DRUG FACTS AND COMPARISONS®

2007

DRUG FACTS AND COMPARISONS®

2007

Wolters Kluwer Health | Facts & Comparisons™

Drug Facts and Comparisons,® 2007 Edition

Adapted from *Facts and Comparisons 4.0* online drug reference.

Manuscript indexed by Graves Editorial Service, Colorado Springs, Colorado.

ISBN 1-57439-256-5
978-1-57439-256-2

Printed in the United States of America.

The information contained in *Drug Facts and Comparisons®* is available for licensing as source data. For more information on data licensing, please call 1-800-223-0554.

Wolters Kluwer Health
77 Westport Plaza, Suite 450
St. Louis, Missouri 63146-3125
Phone 314-216-2100 • 800-223-0554
Fax 314-878-5563
factsandcomparisons.com

DRUG FACTS AND COMPARISONS®

2007

Wolters Kluwer Health | Facts & Comparisons™

Facts & Comparisons™ Editorial Advisory Panel

Contributing Review Panel

Jonathan Abrams, MD
Professor of Medicine
Cardiology Division
University of New Mexico
Albuquerque, New Mexico

Danial E. Baker, PharmD, FASHP, FASCP
Associate Dean for Clinical Programs
Professor of Pharmacotherapy
Director, Drug Information Center
Washington State University
Spokane, Washington

Jimmy D. Bartlett, OD, DOS, ScD
Professor of Optometry, School of Optometry
Professor of Pharmacology, School of Medicine
University of Alabama at Birmingham
Birmingham, Alabama

Edward S. Bennett, OD, MSEd
Associate Professor
Co-Chief, Contact Lens Service
Director of Student Services
College of Optometry
University of Missouri – St. Louis
St. Louis, Missouri

Daniel L. Brown, PharmD
Director of Early Practice Education
Wingate University
School of Pharmacy
Wingate, North Carolina

R. Keith Campbell, RPh, FAPhA, FASHP, MBA, CDE
Associate Dean/Professor of Pharmacotherapy
Washington State University
College of Pharmacy
Pullman, Washington

Melvin D. Cheitlin, MD
Emeritus Professor of Medicine
University of California, San Francisco, Cardiology Division
Former Chief, Cardiology Division
San Francisco General Hospital
San Francisco, California

Richard J. Duma, MD, PhD
Director, Department of Infectious Diseases
Infectious Disease Division
Halifax Medical Center
Daytona Beach, Florida

Kathryn M. Edwards, MD
Vice Chair for Clinical Research
Department of Pediatrics
Professor of Pediatrics
Vanderbilt University
School of Medicine
Nashville, Tennessee

Michael S. Edwards, PharmD, MBA
Assistant Director, Pharmacy Operations
The Sidney Kimmel Comprehensive Cancer Center at Johns Hopkins
Bethesda, Maryland

Mary J. Ferrill, PharmD, FASHP
Assistant Dean for Professionalization
Professor
Wingate University
School of Pharmacy
Wingate, North Carolina

Thomas A. Golper, MD
Professor of Medicine
Medical Director – Nephrology, Hypertension, and Diabetes Patient Care Center
Division of Nephrology
Vanderbilt University
Nashville, Tennessee

COL. John D. Grabenstein, RPh, PhD, FAPhA, FASHP, FRSH
Medical Service Corp.
Deputy Director for Clinical Operations
Military Vaccine Agency
U.S. Army Medical Command

Edward A. Hartshorn, PhD
Professor, Physician Assistant Studies
University of Texas Medical Branch
School of Allied Health Sciences
Galveston, Texas
Instructor
University of Texas Health Science Center
School of Nursing in Houston
Houston, Texas

Siret D. Jaanus, PhD
Professor of Pharmacology
Southern California College of Optometry
Fullerton, California

Robert E. Kates, PharmD, PhD
President
Analytical Solutions, Inc.
Sunnyvale, California

Julio R. Lopez, PharmD
Chief, Pharmacy Service
VA Northern California Health Care System
Martinez, California

Richard M. Oksas, PharmD, MPh
Family Practice Pharmacist
Natividad Medical Center
Salinas, California

J. James Rowsey, MD
St. Luke's Cataract and Laser Institute
Tarpon Springs, Florida

Mary Beth Shirk, PharmD
Specialty Practice Pharmacist, Critical Care Medicine
Clinical Assistant Professor
The Ohio State University Medical Center
Columbus, Ohio

Udho Thadani, MD, MRCP, FRCP(C), FACC, FAHA
Professor Emeritus of Medicine
Cardiovascular Section
University of Oklahoma Health Sciences Center
Consultant Cardiologist, Oklahoma University Medical Center and VA Medical Center
Oklahoma City, Oklahoma

Thom J. Zimmerman, MD, PhD
Emeritus Professor and Chairman
Department of Ophthalmology and Visual Sciences
Emeritus Professor of Pharmacology & Toxicology
University of Louisville
School of Madicine
Global Ophthalmic Medical Director
Global Medical Affairs
Pharmacia Corporation
Louisville, Kentucky

Table of Contents

Foreword

Facts & Comparisons™, a part of Wolters Kluwer Health, has served the drug information needs of pharmacists and other health care professionals since its inception in 1946 by providing timely, accurate, comprehensive, unbiased, comparative information on prescription and nonprescription medications. *Drug Facts and Comparisons® (DFC),* our flagship product, is the primary source of drug information and the reference of choice for more than 100,000 loyal subscribers because of its uncompromising editorial quality, reliability, and ease of use. *DFC* has remained unique among other drug information resources because of its organization by therapeutic use, providing single drug monographs with complete prescribing information as well as in-depth comparisons of closely related agents. Over the years, *DFC* has changed in size and scope, but the concept has never changed. That is why health care professionals continue to look to Facts & Comparisons™ to keep them abreast of important information in their practice.

In addition to the annual bound edition, *DFC* is also available as the popular monthly updated loose-leaf publication and as an annual pocket-size softbound abridged version. These versions allow customers to choose the format that is best suited to their practice site and workflow.

Customers who prefer the speed and efficiency of electronic products can access *DFC* through *Facts & Comparisons 4.0,* our electronic library of reference information, which is available on-line or CD ROM. *Facts & Comparisons 4.0* is the latest enhanced version of *eFacts*. In addition to *DFC,* other content sets include *Drug Interaction Facts, Med Facts* (patient drug information handouts), *Review of Natural Products, Cancer Chemotherapy,* and *Medi-Span Image and Imprint Database.* Information about *Facts & Comparisons 4.0,* can be accessed through www.factsandcomparisons.com. Facts & Comparisons™ also offers drug information for handheld personal data assistants, available for downloading at www.factsandcomparisons.com.

Drug Facts and Comparisons® monographs are now integrated into Medi-Span's Drug Information Bridge, a pre-programmed application programming interface (API) that includes Medi-Span's drug files and clinical databases. The integration of the *DFC* referential content with Medi-Span's premier databases provides superior point-of-care solutions for our professional customers.

Facts & Comparisons™ takes our mission of providing drug information to health care professionals very seriously, which is why we continue to invest in technology, improve our current publications, and stay in contact with our customers to make sure we maintain the high standards we set many years ago when Erwin Kastrup, RPh, first developed this concept. We have many people to thank for helping us achieve these goals, including our Editorial Advisory Panel, reviewers, contributors, and our excellent, dedicated employees, but more than anything we want to thank our loyal subscribers who have helped us develop and improve our drug information publications that are so widely used today.

We are dedicated to maintaining the traditions that are important to both Facts & Comparisons™ and our customers, but we are also dedicated to evolving our products to meet the changing technologies and the changing needs of health care professionals. These goals only can be accomplished by responding to the comments and suggestions from our subscribers, which we encourage and appreciate. As always, let us know how we can better serve you and your drug information needs.

Cathy H. Reilly
Publisher

Preface

As the premier publisher of drug information, Facts & Comparisons™ provides a broad range of print, electronic, and on-line resources to fulfill the day-to-day needs of practicing health care professionals. *Drug Facts and Comparisons® (DFC)*, our flagship publication developed in 1945 by pharmacist Erwin K. Kastrup, was initially designed to provide objective information in a format that facilitated unbiased comparisons of drug products in a timely manner. After more than 60 years, the basic concepts remain the same. However, the content and presentation of material in *DFC* continues to evolve to reflect the changing needs of the health care environment.

The biggest change to this latest edition is that we have created route-specific monographs for the majority of drugs that are available in different routes of administration. This should enable you to locate the appropriate information for a given drug more quickly.

In order to maintain the valued comparative aspect, product tables continue to list all products for a drug regardless of the route of administration. The product table is followed by separate monographs for each route of administration for that drug.

The annual bound edition is one of several formats in which *DFC* is available. The original loose-leaf version is kept up to date through monthly print updates. An electronic version, now updated continously, is available as part of *Facts & Comparisons 4.0* and can be accessed via www.factsandcomparisons.com.

Facts & Comparisons 4.0 now also provides full monographs with complete prescribing information for nearly every single agent drug product, while the print versions continue to present abbreviated drug monographs in instances where a class monograph exists.

The new 61st edition of *DFC* incorporates 27 new drugs: Abatacept (*Orencia*), alglucosidase alfa (*Myozyme*), anidulafungin (*Eraxis*), conivaptan hydrochloride (*Vaprisol*), deferasirox (*Exjade*), decitabine (*Dacogen*), galsulfase (*Naglazyme*), human papillomavirus (*Gardasil*), insulin detemir (*Levemir*), lenalidomide (*Revlimid*), lubiprostone (*Amitiza*), mecasermin (*Increlex*), mecasermin rinfabate (*Iplex*), nabilone (*Cesamet*), napafenac (*Nevanac*), nelarabine (*Arranon*), nitisinone (*Orfadin*), pregabalin (*Lyrica*), prussian blue (*Radiogardase*), ramelteon (*Rozerem*), ranolazine (*Ranexa*), rasagiline (*Azilect*), sorafenib (*Nexavir*), sunitinib malate (*Sutent*), tigecycline (*Tygacil*), tipranavir (*Aptivus*), and zoster vaccine live (*Zostavax*).

Significant new indications added include the following: Adalimumab for psoriatic arthritis; bivalirudin for use as an anticoagulant in patients undergoing PCI and for heparin-induced thrombocytopenia and thrombosis syndrome; candesartan cilexetil for heart failure; docetaxel for prostate cancer; doxorubicin liposomal for ovarian cancer; erlotinib for pancreatic cancer; fondaparinux sodium for prophylaxis of deep vein thrombosis in patients undergoing abdominal surgery; infliximab for psoriatic arthritis and ulcerative colitis; letrozole for treatment of early breast cancer; meloxicam for rheumatoid arthritis and pauciarticular/polyarticular course juvenile arthritis; moxifloxacin hydrochloride for complicated intra-abdominal infections and uncomplicated skin and skin structure infections; meropenem for skin and skin structure infections; mometasone furoate monohydrate for nasal polyps in patients 18 years of age and older; peginterferon alfa-2a for treatment of hepatitis B; ropinirole hydrochloride for restless legs syndrome; rosiglitazone maleate for monotherapy and for use with a sulfonylurea plus metformin when diet, exercise, and both agents do not result in adequate glycemic control; temozolomide for newly diagnosed glioblastoma multiforme; valsartan for reduction of cardiovascular mortality following myocardial infarction; and voriconazole for candidemia.

Sections that have undergone major revisions include the following: Bile acid sequestrants, childhood immunization schedule, nitrates, phosphodiesterase type 5 inhibitors, and histamine H_2 antagonists.

As this edition goes to press, we continue to update our database daily for use in future editions and formats of *DFC*. We also continue to expand our extensive library of drug information resources to remain the full service drug information provider that our customers have come to expect. However, this can only be accomplished with feedback from the loyal health care professionals who use our information on a daily basis. Comments, criticisms, and suggestions are always welcome and encouraged. Please call or visit us at www.factsandcomparisons.com.

Renee M. Wickersham
Senior Managing Editor

Kirsten K. Novak
Managing Editor

Introduction

Drug Facts and Comparisons® is a comprehensive drug information compendium. Organized by therapeutic drug class, the format is designed to provide a wide scope of drug information in a manner that facilitates evaluations and comparisons. A comprehensive index, a detailed table of contents for each chapter, and numerous cross references within monographs enable the reader to quickly locate needed information.

Editorial Policy

The principal editorial policy remains unchanged from the inception of *Drug Facts and Comparisons®* in 1945: Accurate, unbiased information; concise, standardized presentation; comparative, objective format; timely delivery. Review of FDA-approved product labeling, thousands of biomedical journal articles and textbooks, and policies and recommendations from many authoritative and official groups (eg, Centers for Disease Control; National Academy of Sciences; Joint National Committee on Detection, Evaluation, and Treatment of High Blood Pressure; National Heart, Lung and Blood Institute; American Thoracic Society; National Cancer Institute; FDA Office of Orphan Products Development; Food and Drug Administration) form the base of evaluation of information for *Drug Facts and Comparisons®*.

Editorial policy is guided by the distinguished Facts & Comparisons™ Editorial Advisory Panel. This is an authoritative group of nationally and internationally recognized clinicians, scholars, scientists, physicians, pharmacists, and pharmacologists. In addition, many other prominent health care professionals serve on various expert panels and provide review in their specific areas of expertise for *Drug Facts and Comparisons®*. Indications and dosage recommendations are FDA-approved unless otherwise specified. Legitimate "unlabeled" uses and dosages are included when appropriate and given special emphasis. Input from an expert panel on drug interactions is also a feature.

This collection of wisdom and the world drug information literature is then molded and refined into the *Drug Facts and Comparisons®* database, monographs, and product listings. Many sources of drug information are constantly monitored so that *Drug Facts and Comparisons®* contains the most comprehensive, current drug information database available. There is not a more complete drug information compendium available presenting such clinical prescribing and drug product information.

Most of the products listed in *Drug Facts and Comparisons®* are protected by letters of patent, and their names are trademarked and registered by the firm whose name appears with the product. Identification of the product distributor is given in parentheses next to the brand name. The distributor may or may not be the actual manufacturer or fabricator of the final dosage form. When more than one company distributes a generic product, the generic product name is listed, followed by "Various, eg," in parentheses with a selected list of distributors. Listing of specific products is an indication only of market availability and is not an endorsement or recommendation. Most products listed have national or significant regional distribution.

Products that contain the same active ingredients are listed together for comparison and as an aid in product selection. However, drug product interchange is regulated by state laws; listing of products together does not imply that products are therapeutically equivalent or legally interchangeable. Caution is particularly advised when attempting to compare extended-release or delayed-release dosage forms.

How To Use *Drug Facts And Comparisons*®

Efficient use of *Drug Facts and Comparisons® (DFC)* requires an understanding of its organization and format.

Organization:

Information in *DFC* is organized by therapeutic use. Each of the 14 chapters is divided into groups and subgroups to facilitate comparisons of drugs and drug products with similar uses. The first page of each chapter provides a detailed outline, including page references of the information presented in that chapter.

Products most similar in content or use are listed together. This format of presenting the FACTS makes it easy to make COMPARISONS of identical, similar, or related products. Drugs with multiple uses may be listed in more than one section of the book.

Drug Monographs:

Prescribing information is presented in comprehensive drug monographs. General information on a group of closely related drugs (eg, ACE inhibitors) may be presented in a group monograph. Specific information for each drug follows the product listing; often there are separate monographs for each route of administration. All monographs are divided into sections identified with bold titles for ease in locating the desired information.

Indications: All indications or uses listed are FDA-approved unless specifically designated as "Unlabeled uses."

Administration and Dosage: Dosage ranges and methods of administration are presented.

Actions: This section gives a brief summary of the known pharmacologic and pharmacokinetic properties.

Contraindications: This section specifies those conditions in which the drug should NOT be used.

Warnings and Precautions: These sections list conditions in which use of the drug may be hazardous, precautions to observe, and parameters to monitor during therapy.

Drug Interactions: A brief summary of documented, clinically significant drug-drug, drug-lab test and drug-food interactions is provided.

Adverse Reactions: Reported adverse reactions are presented. Incidence data on adverse effects are included when available.

Overdosage: The clinical manifestations of toxicity and treatment of overdosage are given for most agents.

Patient Information: Essential information required by the patient for safe and effective self-administration of the medication is included.

Keeping Up:

The Keeping Up section enables the health care professional to stay up-to-date with the latest developments in drug therapy.

Orphan Drugs: Profiles the generic name and trade name of a drug, its sponsor, and the proposed use of an agent approved for marketing under the terms of the Orphan Drug Act.

Investigational Drugs: Provides brief reports on significant developments in drug therapy, including drugs currently under investigation.

Index:

The alphabetical index includes page references for all drugs by their generic name, brand name, synonyms, common abbreviations and therapeutic group names. Generic names are listed in bold type face for easy identification. A separate index of drug trade names unique to Canada is also a feature.

Product Listings:

Individual products are listed at the beginning of each monograph. The format and components of the product listings are discussed below and illustrated on the opposite page.

NOTE: Products that contain the same active ingredients are listed together for comparison and as an aid in product selection. However, drug product interchange is regulated by state laws; listing of products together does not imply that products are therapeutically equivalent or legally interchangeable. Caution is particularly advised when attempting to compare extended-release or delayed-release dosage forms.

1. Products are grouped by dosage form and strength.
2. Brand name products with the same amount of active ingredient and in the same doseform are listed in alphabetical order.
3. The name of the distributor is given in parentheses next to the product name.
4. Products available by their generic name from multiple sources are indicated as available from (Various) distributors and in selected cases, examples of generic manufacturers are listed.
5. Package sizes are given for all dosage forms and strengths of each product.
6. Product identification imprint codes are listed in parentheses.
7. Cross references to the appropriate drug monograph(s) for complete prescribing information appear at the beginning of the monograph.
8. Controlled substances are designated by their schedule (*c-II, c-III, c-IV,* or *c-V*).
9. Distribution status of products is indicated as *Rx* or *otc* (products listed as *otc* may include nutritional or dietary supplements).
10. Sugar-free liquid preparations are designated by *sf.*
11. Combination products are listed in tables to facilitate comparisons. Products most similar in formulation are listed next to each other.
12. Products with identical active ingredients are listed together.

		PENICILLINS		1231
		Aminopenicillins		

AMOXICILLIN

Callout	Status	Product & Distributor	Dosage form	Description
	Rx	**Amoxil** (SK-Beecham)	**Tablets:** 500 mg (as trihydrate)	(Amoxil 500). Film-coated. Capsule shape. Pink. In 20s, 100s, 500s
			875 mg (as trihydrate)	(Amoxil 875). Film coated, scored. Capsule shape. Pink. In 20s, 100s, 500s.
2	*Rx*	**Amoxicillin** (Various, eg, Biocraft, Major, Rugby, Teva, URL)	**Capsules:** 250 mg (as trihydrate) (1)	In 21s, 30s, 100s, 250s, 500s, 1000s and UD 45s and 100s.
2	*Rx*	**Amoxil** (SK-Beecham)		(Amoxil 250). Blue and pink. In 100s, 500s and UD 100s.
2	*Rx*	**Trimox** (Apothecon)		In 30s, 100s, 500s and UD 100s.
2, 3	*Rx*	**Wymox** (Wyeth-Ayerst)		(Wyeth 559). Gray and green. In 100s and 500s.
4, 5	*Rx*	**Amoxicillin** (Various, eg, Biocraft, Major, Rugby, Teva, URL)	**Capsules:** 500 mg (as trihydrate)	In 21s, 30s, 50s, 100s, 250s, 500s and UD 45s and 100s.
6	*Rx*	**Amoxil** (SK-Beecham)		(Amoxil 500). Blue and pink. In 100s, 500s and UD 100s.
	Rx	**Trimox** (Apothecon)		In 30s, 100s, 500s and UD 100s.
	Rx	**Wymox** (Wyeth-Ayerst)		(Wyeth 560). Gray and green. In 50s and 500s.
	Rx	**Amoxil Pediatric Drops** (SK-Beecham)	**Powder for Oral Suspension:** 50 mg/ml (as trihydrate) when reconstituted	Sucrose. Bubble gum flavor. In 15 and 30 ml.
	Rx	**Trimox Pediatric Drops** (Apothecon)		Sucrose. In 15 ml.
	Rx	**Amoxicillin** (Various, eg, Biocraft, Major, Teva, URL)	**Powder for Oral Suspension:** 125 mg/5 ml (as trihydrate) when reconstituted	In 80, 100, 150 and 200 ml.
	Rx	**Amoxil** (SK-Beecham)		Sucrose. Strawberry flavor. In 80, 100 and 150 ml and UD 5 ml.
	Rx	**Trimox** (Apothecon)		Sucrose. In 80, 100 and 150 ml.
	Rx	**Wymox** (Wyeth-Ayerst)		Sucrose. In 100 and 150 ml.
	Rx	**Amoxicillin** (Various, eg, Biocraft, Major, Teva, URL)	**Powder for Oral Suspension:** 250 mg/5 ml (as trihydrate) when reconstituted	In 80, 100, 150 and 200 ml.
	Rx	**Amoxil** (SK-Beecham)		Sucrose. Bubble gum flavor. In 80, 100 and 150 ml and UD 5 ml.
	Rx	**Trimox** (Apothecon)		Sucrose. In 80, 100 and 150 ml.
	Rx	**Wymox** (Wyeth-Ayerst)		Sucrose. In 100 and 150 ml.

(7) For complete prescribing information, refer to the Penicillins group monograph.

the advantage of more complete absorption than ampicillin, a 3-times a day regimen for most infections and less diarrhea than ampicillin.

COUGH PREPARATIONS

ANTITUSSIVE AND EXPECTORANT COMBINATIONS

Content given per tablet, 5 mL, or packet.

Callout	Status	Product & Distributor	Antitussive	Expectorant	Decongestant
11	*Rx*	**Levall Liquid**[1] (Athlon Pharmaceuticals[2])	20 mg carbetapentane citrate	100 mg guaifenesin	15 mg phenylephrine HCl
11, 12	*c-v*	**Dihistine Expectorant Liquid** (Alpharma)	10 mg codeine phosphate	100 mg guaifenesin	30 mg pseudoephedrine HCl
11, 12	*c-v*	**Guiatuss DAC Liquid**[1] (Various, eg, Alpharma, Ivax)			
11, 12	*c-v sf*	**Halotussin DAC Syrup**[1] (Watson Laboratories)			
11, 12	*c-v sf*	**Mytussin DAC Liquid**[1] (Morton Grove Pharmaceuticals)			
11, 12	*c-v*	**Novagest Expectorant with Codeine Liquid**[1] (Major)			
11	*c-iii*	**Nucofed Expectorant Syrup**[1] (Monarch)			
11, 8	*c-iii*	**Nucotuss Expectorant Syrup**[1] (Alpharma)	12.5% alcohol. In 473 mL.		
11	*c-v*	**Tussirex Syrup** (Scot-Tussin)	10 mg codeine phosphate	83.3 mg sodium citrate	4.17 mg phenylephrine HCl
11, 10	*c-v sf*	**Tussirex Sugar Free Liquid** (Scot-Tussin)			
11	*Rx*	**Donatussin Syrup**[1] (Laser)	7.5 mg dextromethorphan HBr	100 mg guaifenesin	10 mg phenylephrine HCl
11, 9	*otc sf*	**Tussex Cough Syrup**[1] (Alpharma)	10 mg dextromethorphan HBr	100 mg guaifenesin	5 mg phenylephrine HCl
11, 9	*Rx*	**Tussafed Ex Syrup**[1] (Everett Laboratories)	30 mg dextromethorphan HBr	200 mg guaifenesin	10 mg phenylephrine HCl
11	*otc*	**Guiatuss CF Syrup**[1] (Alpharma)	10 mg dextromethorphan HBr	100 mg guafenesin	30 mg pseudoephedrine HCl
11	*otc*	**Robafen CF Syrup**[1] (Major)			
11	*otc*	**Robitussin CF Syrup**[1] (Whitehall-Robins)			

Recommended Dietary Allowances (RDA) are published by the Food and Nutrition Board, National Research Council-National Academy of Sciences, as a guide for nutritional problems and to provide standards of good nutrition for different age groups. They are revised periodically.

The RDA values are *not requirements;* they are *recommended* daily intakes of certain essential nutrients. Based on available scientific knowledge, they are believed to be adequate for known nutritional needs for most *healthy* people under usual environmental stresses. The recommended allowances vary for age and sex, with extra allowances for women during pregnancy and lactation. The most commonly used RDA values (the "reference male" and "reference female") are those of adults 23 to 50 years of age. With the exception of energy (kilocalories), the RDA provide for individual requirement variations and prevent symptoms of clinical deficiency of 97% of the population.

RDA have been established for many essential nutrients; however, present knowledge of human nutritional needs of pantothenic acid and biotin is incomplete. Therefore, to ensure adequate nutrient intake, obtain the recommended allowances from as varied a selection of foods as possible. Nutritionists suggest that dietary planning include regular intake of each of the four basic food groups:

1.) Milk, cheese, dairy products – Minimum 2 servings/day.
2.) Meat, poultry, fish, beans – Minimum 2 servings/day.
3.) Vegetables, fruit – Minimum 4 servings/day.
4.) Bread, cereal (whole-grain and enriched or fortified) – Minimum 4 servings/day.

Such a balance, in sufficient quantities will provide about 1200 kcal, enough protein, and most of the vitamins and minerals required daily. A person may increase nutrient and energy intake by consuming larger quantities (or more servings/day) of the 4 basic food groups. Nutrient and energy intake may also be increased by selecting food from the fifth group, fats-sweets-alcohol, which provides mainly energy.

RDA quantities apply only to healthy people and are not intended to cover therapeutic nutritional requirements in disease or other abnormal states (ie, metabolic disorders, weight reduction, chronic disease, drug therapy). Although certain single nutrients in larger quantities may have pharmacologic actions, these are unrelated to nutritional functions. There is no convincing evidence that consuming excessive quantities of single nutrients will cure or prevent nonnutritional diseases.

The "official" listings of United States Recommended Daily Allowances (US-RDAs) should not be confused with the RDA values. US-RDA are derived from the 1968 RDA and serve as legal standards for nutritional labeling of food and dietary food and dietary supplement products controlled by the FDA. Generally, they represent the higher value of the male or female RDA and are grouped into only 3 age brackets plus 1 category for pregnant or lactating women. Prior to 1972, these allowances were erroneously listed as minimum daily requirements (MDR). A second fallacy perpetuated by US-RDA labeling of foods is the implication that a food is defective if it does not contain all the officially established nutrients in their full US-RDA quantities. No individual food is nutritionally complete, but several foods together should complement each other to provide maximal nutrient balance and to minimize naturally occurring toxic principles consumed from any individual foodstuff.

The RDA for adult males and adult females are included in each individual vitamin monograph. The table on the following page presents the listing of vitamin and mineral RDA values for all age groups as published in *Recommended Dietary Allowances*, 10th Edition, National Academy of Sciences, Washington, DC, 1989.

RECOMMENDED DIETARY ALLOWANCES[1]

Patient parameters						Fat-soluble vitamins				Water-soluble vitamins							Minerals						
Age (years) or Condition	Weight[2]		Height[2]		Protein	Vitamin A	Vitamin D	Vitamin E	Vitamin K	Ascorbic acid (C)	Thiamine (B_1)	Riboflavin (B_2)	Niacin (B_3)	Pyridoxine (B_6)	Folate	Cyanocobalamin (B_{12})	Calcium	Phosphorus	Magnesium	Iron	Zinc	Iodine	Selenium
	(kg)	(lb)	(cm)	(in)	g	IU[3]	IU[4]	IU[5]	μmg	mg	mg	mg	mg	mg	μmg	μmg	mg	mg	mg	mg	mg	μmg	μmg
Infants																							
0.0-0.5	6	13	60	24	13	1249	300	4	5	30	0.3	0.4	5	0.3	25	0.3	400	300	40	6	5	40	10
0.5-1	9	20	71	28	14	1249	400	6	10	35	0.4	0.5	6	0.6	35	0.5	600	500	60	10	5	50	15
Children																							
1-3	13	29	90	35	16	1332	400	9	15	40	0.7	0.8	9	1	50	0.7	800	800	80	10	10	70	20
4-6	20	44	112	44	24	1665	400	10	20	45	0.9	1.1	12	1.1	75	1	800	800	120	10	10	90	20
7-10	28	62	132	52	28	2331	400	10	30	45	1	1.2	13	1.4	100	1.4	800	800	170	10	10	120	30
Males																							
11-14	45	99	157	62	45	3330	400	15	45	50	1.3	1.5	17	1.7	150	2	1200	1200	270	12	15	150	40
15-18	66	145	176	69	59	3330	400	15	65	60	1.5	1.8	20	2	200	2	1200	1200	400	12	15	150	50
19-24	72	160	177	70	58	3330	400	15	70	60	1.5	1.7	19	2	200	2	1200	1200	350	10	15	150	70
25-50	79	174	176	70	63	3330	200	15	80	60	1.5	1.7	19	2	200	2	800	800	350	10	15	150	70
51+	77	170	173	68	63	3330	200	15	80	60	1.2	1.4	15	2	200	2	800	800	350	10	15	150	70
Females																							
11-14	46	101	157	62	46	2664	400	12	45	50	1.1	1.3	15	1.4	150	2	1200	1200	280	15	12	150	45
15-18	55	120	163	64	44	2664	400	12	55	60	1.1	1.3	15	1.5	180	2	1200	1200	300	15	12	150	50
19-24	58	128	164	65	46	2664	400	12	60	60	1.1	1.3	15	1.6	180	2	1200	1200	280	15	12	150	55
25-50	63	138	163	64	50	2664	200	12	65	60	1.1	1.3	15	1.6	180	2	800	800	280	15	12	150	55
51+	65	143	160	63	50	2664	200	12	65	60	1	1.2	13	1.6	180	2	800	800	280	10	12	150	55
Pregnant					60	2664	400	15	65	70	1.5	1.6	17	2.2	400	2.2	1200	1200	320	30	15	175	65
Lactating – 1st 6 mo.					65	4329	400	18	65	95	1.6	1.8	20	2.1	280	2.6	1200	1200	355	15	19	200	75
2nd 6 mo.					62	3996	400	16	65	90	1.6	1.7	20	2.1	260	2.6	1200	1200	340	15	16	200	75

Reproduced from: *Recommended Dietary Allowances*, 10th edition, 1989, National Academy of Sciences, National Academy Press, Washington, DC.

[1] The allowances, expressed as average daily intakes over time, are intended to provide for individual variations among most normal people as they live in the US under usual environmental stresses. Diets should be based on a variety of common foods in order to provide other nutrients for which human requirements have been less well defined.

[2] Weights and heights of Reference Adults are actual medians for the US population of the designated age, as reported by NHANES II. The median weights and heights of those < 19 years of age were taken from Hamill PV, et al. *Am J Clin Nutr.* 1979;32:607-629. The use of these figures does not imply that the height-to-weight ratios are ideal.

[3] Conversion of IU to retinol equivalents (RE): 3.33 IU = 1 mcg of retinol = 1 RE or 6 mcg, β-carotene.

[4] As cholecalciferol. 10 mcg cholecalciferol = 400 IU of vitamin D.

[5] α-Tocopherol equivalents. 1 mg d-α-tocopherol = α-TE = 1.49 IU.

Dietary Reference Intakes (DRIs) refer to nutrient intake values estimated to be adequate for 50% of age- and gender-specific groups. As seen in the table below, DRIs are comprised of RDAs in bold type and Adequate Intakes (AIs) in ordinary type followed by asterisk (*). These values may be used as goals for individual intake. RDAs are estimated to meet the needs of most individuals (97% to 98%). For healthy breastfed infants, the AI represents mean intake. For all other life-stage groups, the AI is believed to cover the needs of all individuals, but a lack of data or uncertainty in the data prevent specifying with confidence with percentage of individuals covered by this intake.

Food and Nutrition Board, Institute of Medicine – National Academy of Science Dietary Reference Intakes: Recommended Intakes for Individuals

Life-stage group		Calcium (mg/d)	Phosphorus (mg/d)	Magnesium (mg/d)	Vitamin A (mcg/d)	Vitamin C (mg/d)	Vitamin D (mcg/d)[a,b]	Vitamin E (mg/d)	Vitamin K (mcg/d)	Fluoride (mg/d)	Thiamine (mg/d)	Riboflavin (mg/d)	Niacin (mg/d)[c]	Vitamin B_6 (mg/d)	Folate (mcg/d)[d]	Vitamin B_{12} (mcg/d)	Pantothenic acid (mg/d)	Biotin (mcg/d)	Choline[e] (mg/d)
Infants	0-6 mo.	210*	100*	30*	400*	40*	5*	4*	2*	0.01*	0.2*	0.3*	2*	0.1*	65*	0.4*	1.7*	5*	125*
	7-12 mo	270*	275*	75*	500*	50*	5*	5*	2.5*	0.5*	0.3*	0.4*	4*	0.3*	80*	0.5*	1.8*	6*	150*
Children	1-3 yr	500*	**460**	**80**	300	15	5*	6	30*	0.7*	**0.5**	**0.5**	**6**	**0.5**	**150**	**0.9**	2*	8*	200*
	4-8 yr	800*	**500**	**130**	400	25	5*	7	55*	1*	**0.6**	**0.6**	**8**	**0.6**	**200**	**1.2**	3*	12*	250*
Males	9-13 yr	1300*	**1250**	**240**	600	45	5*	11	60*	2*	**0.9**	**0.9**	**12**	**1.0**	**300**	**1.8**	4*	20*	375*
	14-18 yr	1300*	**1250**	**410**	900	75	5*	15	75*	3*	**1.2**	**1.3**	**16**	**1.3**	**400**	**2.4**	5*	25*	550*
	19-30 yr	1000*	**700**	**400**	900	90	5*	15	120*	4*	**1.2**	**1.3**	**16**	**1.3**	**400**	**2.4**	5*	30*	550*
	31-50 yr	1000*	**700**	**420**	900	90	5*	15	120*	4*	**1.2**	**1.3**	**16**	**1.3**	**400**	**2.4**	5*	30*	550*
	51-70 yr	1200*	**700**	**420**	900	90	10*	15	120*	4*	**1.2**	**1.3**	**16**	**1.7**	**400**	**2.4**[f]	5*	30*	550*
	> 70 yr	1200*	**700**	**420**	900	90	15*	15	120*	4*	**1.2**	**1.3**	**16**	**1.7**	**400**	**2.4**[f]	5*	30*	550*
Females	9-13 yr	1300*	**1250**	**240**	600	45	5*	11	60*	2*	**0.9**	**0.9**	**12**	**1.0**	**300**	**1.8**	4*	20*	375*
	14-18 yr	1300*	**1250**	**360**	700	65	5*	15	75*	3*	**1**	**1**	**14**	**1.2**	**400**[g]	**2.4**	5*	25*	400*
	19-30 yr	1000*	**700**	**310**	700	75	5*	15	90*	3*	**1.1**	**1.1**	**14**	**1.3**	**400**[g]	**2.4**	5*	30*	425*
	31-50 yr	1000*	**700**	**320**	700	75	5*	15	90*	3*	**1.1**	**1.1**	**14**	**1.3**	**400**[g]	**2.4**	5*	30*	425*
	51-70 yr	1200*	**700**	**320**	700	75	10*	15	90*	3*	**1.1**	**1.1**	**14**	**1.5**	**400**	**2.4**[f]	5*	30*	425*
	> 70 yr	1200*	**700**	**320**	700	75	15*	15	90*	3*	**1.1**	**1.1**	**14**	**1.5**	**400**	**2.4**[f]	5*	30*	425*
Pregnancy	≤ 18 yr	1300*	**1250**	**400**	750	80	5*	15	75*	3*	**1.4**	**1.4**	**18**	**1.9**	**600**[h]	**2.6**	6*	30*	450*
	19-30 yr	1000*	**700**	**350**	770	85	5*	15	90*	3*	**1.4**	**1.4**	**18**	**1.9**	**600**[h]	**2.6**	6*	30*	450*
	31-50 yr	1000*	**700**	**360**	770	85	5*	15	90*	3*	**1.4**	**1.4**	**18**	**1.9**	**600**[f]	**2.6**	6*	30*	450*
Lactation	≤ 18 yr	1300*	**1250**	**360**	1200	115	5*	19	75*	3*	**1.4**	**1.6**	**17**	**2**	**500**	**2.8**	7*	35*	550*
	19-30 yr	1000*	**700**	**310**	1300	120	5*	19	90*	3*	**1.4**	**1.6**	**17**	**2**	**500**	**2.8**	7*	35*	550*
	31-50 yr	1000*	**700**	**320**	1300	120	5*	19	90*	3*	**1.4**	**1.6**	**17**	**2**	**500**	**2.8**	7*	35*	550*

[a] As cholecalciferol. 1 mcg cholecalciferol = 40 IU vitamin D.
[b] In the absence of adequate exposure to sunlight.
[c] As niacin equivalents (NE). 1 mg of niacin = 60 mg of tryptophan; 0 to 6 months = preformed niacin (not NE).
[d] As dietary folate equivalents (DFE). 1 DFE = 1 mcg food folate = 0.6 mcg of folic acid (from fortified food or supplement) consumed with food = 0.5 mcg of synthetic (supplemental) folic acid taken on an empty stomach.
[e] Although AIs have been set for choline, there are few data to assess whether a dietary supply of choline is needed at all stages of the life-cycle, and it may be that the choline requirement can be met by endogenous synthesis at some of these stages.
[f] Because 10% to 30% of older people may malabsorb food-bound B_{12}, it is advisable for those > 50 years to meet their RDA mainly by consuming foods fortified with B_{12} or a supplement containing B_{12}.
[g] In view of evidence linking folate intake with neural tube defects in the fetus, it is recommended that all women capable of becoming pregnant consume 400 mcg of synthetic folic acid from fortified foods and/or supplements in addition to intake of food folate from a varied diet.
[h] It is assumed that women will continue consuming 400 mcg of folic acid until their pregnancy is confirmed and they enter prenatal care, which ordinarily occurs after the end of the periconceptional period – the critical time for formation of the neural tube.

VITAMINS

Fat Soluble Vitamins

VITAMIN A

otc	**Palmitate-A 5000** (Akorn[a])	**Tablets:** 5000 IU vitamin A	In 100s.
otc	**Vitamin A** (Various, eg, Freeda,[b] Naturally Vitamins[c])	**Capsules:** 10,000 IU	In 100s, 250s, and 500s.
otc	**Vitamin A** (Various, eg, Freeda)	**Capsules:** 15,000 IU[a]	In 100s and 250s.
Rx[4]	**Vitamin A** (Various, eg, Naturally Vitamins[c])	**Capsules:** 25,000 IU	In 100s.
Rx	**Aquasol A** (Astra USA)	**Injection:** 50,000 IU/mL[a]	In 2 mL vials.[d]

[a] As vitamin A palmitate.
[b] As vitamin A palmitate or beta carotene.
[c] As retinol.
[d] With 0.5% chlorobutanol, polysorbate 80, butylated hydroxyanisole, and butylated hydroxytoluene.
[e] Some products may be available *otc* according to distributor discretion.

VITAMIN A — ORAL

Indications

➤*Dietary supplement:* As a dietary supplement when vitamin A intake may be inadequate.

➤*Unlabeled uses:* Reduction in falciparum malaria episodes in children older than 12 months.

Administration and Dosage

➤*Recommended daily allowance (RDA):* In the past, the recommended daily allowance (RDA) for vitamin A has been expressed in units. This term units has been replaced by retinol equivalents (RE) or micrograms (mcg) of retinol, with 1 RE equal to 1 mcg of retinol. One RE of vitamin A is equal to 3.33 units of retinol and 10 units of beta-carotene. One tablet contains 5000 IU of vitamin A, 1 capsule contains 10,000 IU, 15,000 IU, or 25,000 IU of vitamin A.

Dosage – The US RDA for males greater than 14 years of age is 900 mcg/day of retinol equivalents and 700 mcg/day of retinol equivalents for females greater than 14 years of age. The US RDA for children 1 to 3 years is 300 mcg/day of retinol equivalents, 400 mcg/day of retinol equivalents in children 4 to 8 years, and 600 mcg/day retinol equivalents in children 9 to 13 years.

Pregnancy and lactation – Avoid use of vitamin A in excess of the RDA during normal pregnancy. The RDA of vitamin A is 1300 mcg retinol equivalents for nursing mothers in the first 6 months and 1200 mg retinol equivalents for the second 6 months. Human breast milk supplies sufficient vitamin A for infants unless maternal diet is grossly inadequate.

Vitamin A absorption is enhanced if taken with food.

Multivitamin preparations contain vitamin A in 1 of these forms: A combination of vitamin A and beta-carotene or beta-carotene alone. Rarely are doses higher than 5000 IU of vitamin A exceeded in these formulas. Supplemental doses of vitamin A greater than 10,000 IU daily are not recommended.

➤*Storage/Stability:* Store away from heat and direct light.

Actions

➤*Pharmacology:* Vitamin A comes in 2 different forms: Retinols and provitamins. Retinols are found in foods that come from animals (eg, meat, milk, eggs) and include retinol, retinal, and retinoic acid. Provitamins come from plants (which are then converted to vitamin A in the body) and include alpha-, beta- and gamma-carotene. Food processing may destroy some vitamins (eg, freezing may reduce the amount of vitamin A in foods). Remind patients the total amount of vitamin A includes what is received from foods that are eaten and from what is taken as a supplement.

Sources of vitamin A include 3 natural compounds from animal sources (retinol, retinal, and retinoic acid) and 3 provitamins from plants (alpha-, beta- and gamma-carotene). Sources rich in vitamin A include liver, butter, cheese, whole milk, egg yolk, meat, and fish. Plants that are good sources of beta-carotene include dark green leafy vegetables, carrots, sweet potatoes, squash, and cantaloupes.

Vitamin A activity is expressed in multiple ways (eg, units, retinol equivalents, retinol activity equivalents). Traditionally, food composition tables used "units" to express vitamin A, and used the following conversion factors: 1 mcg of retinol = 3.33 units of vitamin A activity from retinol. However, the use of "units" is no longer preferred when calculating and reporting the amount of dietary and supplemental vitamin A consumed.

VITAMIN A — ORAL

Vitamin A derivatives are essential for vision, dental development, growth, hydrocortisone synthesis, epithelial tissue differentiation, embryonic development, and reproduction. Vitamin A is also required for maintenance of the mucous membranes of the eyes, skin, mouth, gastrointestinal tract, and genitourinary tract.

Physiological roles of vitamin A derivatives	
Vitamin A derivatives	Physiological role
Retinol	Supports the reproductive cycle
Retinal	Functions in the visual cycle
Retinoic acid	Promotes growth, differentiation, and maintenance of epithelial tissue
Beta-carotene	Visual adaptation to darkness

Deficiency – Vitamin A deficiency leads to suppressed mucus production resulting in irritation and infection. Common symptoms of vitamin A deficiency include nyctalopia (night blindness), keratomalacia (corneal necrosis), keratinization of the skin including secondary xerophthalmia, impaired resistance to infection, retardation of growth, thickening of bone, decreased production of cortical steroids, and fetal malformations. Vitamin A deficiency may also be associated with an increased susceptibility to bacterial, parasitic, and viral infections.

Conditions which may cause vitamin A deficiency: Biliary tract or pancreatic disease, sprue, hepatic cirrhosis, extreme dietary inadequacy, partial gastrectomy, and cystic fibrosis.

➤*Pharmacokinetics:*

Absorption/Distribution – Vitamin A is fat soluble; absorption from the proximal small intestine requires bile salts, pancreatic lipase and dietary fat. Retinol reaches a peak plasma concentration 4 hours after ingestion. Absorption for retinol preparations is greatest for aqueous preparations, intermediate for emulsions, and slowest for oil solutions. Water-miscible preparations should be used in patients where retinol absorption is reduced, such as in pancreatic/hepatic disease, intestinal disease/infections, and cystic fibrosis. Half of absorbed vitamin A is oxidized (or conjugated) and excreted in the feces and urine, while the other half is stored in the Kupffer cells of the liver, mainly as retinyl esters (eg, retinyl palmitate). Retinol is absorbed by intestinal cells through the presence of cellular retinol-binding protein (CRBPs), incorporated into chylomicrons, and transported to the liver.

In contrast to retinol, only 33% of beta-carotene is absorbed due to a high dependence on the presence of bile and absorbable fat in the intestinal tract. Only 50% of ingested beta-carotene is converted to retinol.

Normal serum vitamin A concentrations are 360 to 1200 mcg/L (retinol plasma range is 30 to 70 mcg/dL) and 270 to 753 Units/100 mL for carotenoids. The normal adult liver contains approximately 100 to 300 mcg/g (mostly as retinol palmitate), providing vitamin A requirements for 2 years. A plasma concentration less than 10 to 20 mcg/g or a retinoid hepatic concentration less than 5 to 20 mcg/g is associated with vitamin A deficiency. Plasma retinol concentrations are reduced in cystic fibrosis, alcohol-related cirrhosis, hepatic diseases, proteinuria, and febrile infections. Plasma retinol concentrations are elevated in patients with chronic renal disease.

Vitamin A absorption is enhanced if taken with food.

Metabolism/Excretion – Vitamin A is mobilized from liver stores and transported in the plasma as retinol bound to retinol-binding protein (RBP). RBP protects retinol from oxidation during transport. 11-cis-retinol is converted to 11-cis-retinal and combines with opsin (the rod pigment in the retina) to form rhodopsin, which is necessary for visual adaptation to darkness. Approximately 10% of vitamin A is not absorbed in the intestine and excreted in the feces.

Contraindications

Hypervitaminosis A; oral use in malabsorption syndrome; hypersensitivity; IV use.

Warnings

➤*Renal function impairment:* Vitamin A toxicity has been reported in chronic renal failure patients.

➤*Pregnancy: Category A.* (*Category C* in doses exceeding the RDA). The US RDA of vitamin A is 800 mcg retinol equivalents. Safety of amounts exceeding 5000 IU oral or 6000 IU parenteral daily during pregnancy has not been established. Avoid use of vitamin A in excess of the RDA during normal pregnancy. In pregnant women, vitamin A is necessary for the growth of a healthy fetus.

Animal reproduction studies have shown fetal abnormalities associated with overdosage in several species. One case of an infant with congenital renal anomalies has been reported. High doses and deficiency of vitamin A are considered to be *Category X*. Prolonged high doses of vitamin A (greater than 25,000 IU/day) have been associated with microtia, craniofacial and CNS anomalies, facial palsy, micro/anophthalmia, facial clefts, cardiac defects, limb reductions, GI atresia, and urinary tract defects.

➤*Lactation:* The US RDA of vitamin A is 1300 mcg retinol equivalents for nursing mothers in the first 6 months and 1200 mg retinol equivalents for the second 6 months. Human milk supplies sufficient vitamin A for infants unless maternal diet is grossly inadequate.

Precautions

➤*Prolonged administration:* Closely supervise prolonged administration over 25,000 IU/day. Evaluate vitamin A intake from fortified foods, dietary supplements, self-administered drugs, and prescription drug sources.

➤*Blood level assays:* Blood level assays are not a direct measure of liver storage. Liver storage should be adequate before discontinuing therapy.

➤*Multiple vitamin deficiency:* Single vitamin A deficiency is rare. Multiple vitamin deficiency is expected in any dietary deficiency.

➤*Acne:* Efficacy of large systemic doses of vitamin A (100,000 to 300,000 IU/day) in the treatment of acne has not been established. However, see topical retinoic acid (tretinoin) and isotretinoin monographs.

➤*Special risk:* Use vitamin A cautiously in patients who abuse alcohol or have kidney and liver disease or in patients being treated with etretinate or isotretinoin.

Drug Interactions

➤*Mineral oil:* Mineral oil may decrease the GI absorption of vitamin A.

Adverse Reactions

➤*Dermatologic:* Side effects involve the skin and mucous membranes and include cheilitis, facial dermatitis, dry mucous membranes, stratum corneum fragility, sticky skin, conjunctivitis, palmoplantar peeling, alopecia, pyogenic granuloma-like lesions in acne, paronychia, and corneal opacities.

Overdosage

➤*Symptoms:* Toxicity manifestations depend on patient's age, dosage, and duration of administration.

Acute toxicity – Nausea, vomiting, drowsiness, headache, vertigo, and blurred vision in adults, or bulging fontanelles in infants.

Infants (less than 1 year old) – 100,000 IU/dose.

Children (1 to 6 years old) – 100,000 IU/dose.

Adults – Greater than 1,000,000 IU/dose.

Chronic toxicity – Hypercalcemia; dry scaly skin; bone pain; changes in texture of hair and nails, increased cerebrospinal pressure; pruritus; headache; nausea; irreversible bone changes (eg, demineralization); thinning of long bones; cortical hyperostosis, periostosis; premature closing of epiphyses.

Infants (3 to 6 months old) – 18,500 IU (water dispersed) daily for 1 to 3 months.

Adults – 1 million IU daily for 3 days, 50,000 IU daily for longer than 18 months, or 500,000 IU daily for 2 months.

Hypervitaminosis A syndrome (plasma retinol concentration greater than 100 mcg/dL) – Hypervitaminosis A syndrome generally manifests as a cirrhotic-like liver syndrome. The following have been reported as manifestations of chronic overuse:

CNS: Irritability; headache; vertigo; increased intracranial pressure as manifested by bulging fontanelles, papilledema and exophthalmos.

Dermatologic: Lip fissures; drying and cracking skin; alopecia; scaling; massive desquamation; increased pigmentation; generalized pruritus; erythema.

Musculoskeletal: Slow growth; hard tender cortical thickening over radius and tibia; migratory arthralgia; premature closure of epiphyses; bone pain.

Miscellaneous: Hypomenorrhea; hepatosplenomegaly; edema; leukopenia; vitamin A plasma levels greater than 1200 IU/dL; hypercalcemia; fatigue; malaise; lethargy; abdominal discomfort; jaundice; anorexia; vomiting.

➤*Treatment:* Treatment includes discontinuation of the retinoid. Desquamation and hyperostoses are evident for months. Bone malformations and liver damage may be irreversible.

Patient Information

Avoid prolonged use of mineral oil while taking this drug. Do not exceed recommended dosage, especially during pregnancy. Notify physician if signs of overdosage (eg, nausea, vomiting, drowsiness, headache, dizziness/feeling of whirling motion, blurred vision) or bulging fontanelles in infants occur.

VITAMIN A PALMITATE — INJECTION

Indications

➤*Vitamin A deficiency:* For the treatment of vitamin A deficiency.

The parenteral administration is indicated when the oral administration is not feasible as in anorexia, nausea, vomiting, pre- and postoperative conditions, or it is not available as in the "malabsorption syndrome" with accompanying steatorrhea.

➤*Unlabeled uses:* Reduction in falciparum malaria episodes in children older than 12 months of age.

Promyelocytic leukemia (retinoic acid); acne; diminishing malignant cell growth; enhancing the immune system; lower incidence of lung cancer and cardiovascular disease; reduction in mortality of HIV-infected children.

Administration and Dosage

➤*For intramuscular use:*

Adults – 100,000 IU daily for 3 days followed by 50,000 daily for 2 weeks.

Children 1 to 8 years of age – 17,500 to 35,000 IU daily for 10 days.

Infants – 7500 to 15,000 IU daily for 10 days.

VITAMIN A PALMITATE — INJECTION

Follow-up therapy with an oral therapeutic multi-vitamin preparation, containing 10,000 to 20,000 IU vitamin A for persons over 8 years old and 5000 to 10,000 IU for infants and children, is recommended daily for 2 months. In malabsorption, the parenteral route must be used for an equivalent preparation.

Poor dietary habits should be corrected and an abundant and well-balanced dietary intake should be prescribed.

➤*Storage / Stability:* Store at 2° to 8°C (36° to 46°F). Do not freeze. Protect from light.

Actions

➤*Pharmacology:* Beta-carotene, retinol, and retinal have effective and reliable vitamin A activity. Retinal and retinol are in chemical equilibrium in the body and have equivalent antixerophthalmic activity. Retinal combines with the rod pigment, opsin, in the retina to form rhodopsin, necessary for visual dark adaptation. Vitamin A prevents retardation of growth and preserves the epithelial cells' integrity. Normal adult liver storage is sufficient to satisfy 2 years' requirements of vitamin A.

Vitamin A is readily absorbed from the gastrointestinal tract, where the biosynthesis of vitamin A from beta-carotene takes place. Vitamin A absorption requires bile salts, pancreatic lipase, and dietary fat. It is transported in the blood to the liver by the chylomicron fraction of the lymph. Vitamin A is stored in Kupffer cells of the liver mainly as the palmitate. Normal serum vitamin A is 80 to 300 IU/per 100 mL (plasma range is 30 to 70 mcgdL) and for carotenoids 270 to 753 IU/per 100 mL. The normal adult liver contains approximately 100 to 300 mcg/g, mostly as retinol palmitate.

Contraindications

Intravenous administration; hypervitaminosis A; sensitivity to any of the ingredients in this preparation.

Warnings

➤*Pregnancy: Category X.* Safety of amounts exceeding 6000 IU of vitamin A daily during pregnancy has not been established at this time. The use of vitamin A in excess of the recommended dietary allowance may cause fetal harm when administered to a pregnant woman. Animal reproduction studies have shown fetal abnormalities associated with overdosage in several species. Malformations of the central nervous system, the eye, the palate, and the urogenital tract are recorded. Vitamin A in excess of the recommended dietary allowance is contraindicated in women who are or may become pregnant. If vitamin A is used during pregnancy, or if the patient becomes pregnant while taking vitamin A, the patient should be apprised of the potential hazard to the fetus.

➤*Lactation:* The US Recommended Daily Allowance (RDA) of vitamin A (5000 IU) is recommended for nursing mothers.

Precautions

➤*Prolonged administration:* Avoid overdosage. Prolonged daily dose administration over 25,000 IU vitamin A should be under close supervision.

➤*Blood level assays:* Blood level assays are not a direct measure of liver storage. Liver storage should be adequate before discontinuing therapy.

➤*Multiple vitamin deficiency:* Single vitamin A deficiency is rare. Multiple vitamin deficiency is expected in any dietary deficiency.

Drug Interactions

➤*Oral contraceptives:* Women on oral contraceptives have shown a significant increase in plasma vitamin A levels.

Adverse Reactions

See Overdosage. Anaphylactic shock and death have been reported using the intravenous route. Allergic reactions have been reported rarely with administration of vitamin A palmitate including 1 case of an anaphylactoid type reaction.

Overdosage

The following amounts have been found to be toxic orally. Toxicity manifestations depend on the age, dosage, size, and duration of administration.

➤*Acute toxicity:* Single dose (25,000 IU/kg body weight).

Infant – 350,000 IU.

Adult – Over 2 million IU.

➤*Chronic toxicity (4000 units / kg body weight for 6 to 15 months):*

Infants 3 to 6 months old – 18,500 IU (water dispersed)/day for 1 to 3 months.

Adult – 1 million IU daily for 3 days; 50,000 Units daily for longer than 18 months; 500,000 IU daily for 2 months.

➤*Hypervitaminosis a syndrome:*

General manifestations – Fatigue, malaise, lethargy, abdominal discomfort, anorexia, and vomiting.

Specific manifestations –

Skeletal: Slow growth, hard tender cortical thickening over the radius and tibia, migratory arthralgia and premature closure of the epiphysis.

Central nervous system: Irritability, headache, and increased intracranial pressure as manifested by bulging fontanels, papilledema, and exophthalmos.

Dermatologic: Fissures of the lips, drying and cracking of the skin, alopecia, scaling, massive desquamation, and increased pigmentation.

Systemic: Hypomenorrhea, hepatosplenomegaly, jaundice, leukopenia, vitamin A plasma level over 1200 IU/100 mL.

➤*Treatment:* The treatment of hypervitaminosis A consists of immediate withdrawal of the vitamin along with symptomatic and supportive treatment.

BETA-CAROTENE

otc *sf*	**Beta-carotene** (Various, eg, Pharmavite, Rugby, Tyson Nutraceuticals)	**Softgel capsule:** 15 mg (25,000 IU vitamin A)	In 60s and 100s.

BETA-CAROTENE — ORAL

Indications

➤*Dietary supplement:* As a dietary supplement when vitamin A intake may be inadequate.

➤*Unlabeled uses:* Beta-carotene may also be used to treat or prevent a reaction to sun in patients with erythropoietic protoporphyria or polymorphous light eruption. Beta-carotene has a controversial role in lowering the incidence of cardiovascular disease and cancer, particularly lung cancer.

Administration and Dosage

➤*Vitamin A activity:* 1 mg of beta-carotene contains approximately 1667 IU of vitamin A activity. 1 capsule contains either 6 mg of beta-carotene (10,000 IU of vitamin A) or 15 mg of beta-carotene (25,000 IU of vitamin A); 1 tablet contains 25 mg of beta-carotene (41,666 IU of vitamin A). In terms of vitamin activity, 0.6 mcg of dietary beta-carotene is equivalent to 0.3 mcg of vitamin A (retinol). One retinol activity equivalent (RAE) is equivalent to 1 mcg retinol which is equivalent to 12 mcg of beta-carotene.

➤*Recommended daily allowance (RDA):* The US recommended daily allowance (RDA) for males greater than 14 years of age is 10.8 mg of beta-carotene and 8.4 mg of beta-carotene for females greater than 14 years of age.

The US RDA is 3.6 mg of beta-carotene for children 1 to 3 years of age, 4.8 mg of beta-carotene in children 4 to 8 years of age, and 7.2 mg beta-carotene in children 9 to 13 years of age.

➤*Adults:* As a dietary supplement, take 1 tablet or capsule (generally 6 to 25 mg/day) daily or as recommended by a healthcare provider.

➤*Children:* As a dietary supplement, the recommended daily dose varies. Consult a healthcare provider.

➤*Storage / Stability:* Store away from heat and direct light. Store in a cool, dry place.

Do not freeze or refrigerate. Do not keep outdated dietary supplements or those no longer needed.

Actions

➤*Pharmacology:* Beta-carotene is a provitamin A carotenoid converted in the body to vitamin A (retinol), and is required for normal vision, gene expression, reproduction, embryonic development, immune function, and skin. A lack of vitamin A may cause a rare condition called night blindness, dry eyes, eye infections, skin problems, and slowed growth. Beta-carotene is also an immune system enhancer and antioxidant.

Beta-carotene is converted to retinol primarily in the intestinal mucosa.

Beta-carotene's antioxidant properties protect cell membranes from lipid preoxidation, alter the metabolism of carcinogens, and enhance immune function. By stimulating the release of natural killer cells, lymphocytes, and monocytes, beta-carotene helps the body resist precancerous changes. In contrast to vitamin A, beta-carotene exerts the greatest activity in the early, initiation phase of cancer.

➤*Pharmacokinetics:*

Absorption / Distribution – Bioavailability of beta-carotene depends on fat in the diet to act as a carrier and on bile in the intestinal tract for its absorption. Bioavailability is greatly decreased by steatorrhea, chronic diarrhea, and very low-fat diets. Approximately 50% of beta-carotene is converted to 2 molecules of retinol in the wall of the small intestine. Some retinal is further oxidized to retinoic acid. Once absorbed, carotenoids such as beta-carotene are transported via lymphatics to the liver where further conversion to vitamin A may occur.

Beta-carotene absorption is enhanced if taken with food.

Contraindications

Hypersensitivity to beta-carotene.

Warnings

➤*Pregnancy: Category C.* Beta-carotene has not been studied in pregnant women.

Use only when clearly needed and when potential benefits outweigh potential hazards to the fetus. Beta-carotene use during pregnancy should not exceed 5000 IU of vitamin A.

BETA-CAROTENE — ORAL

➤*Lactation:* Avoid taking large amounts of a dietary supplement while breastfeeding. Beta-carotene has not been reported to cause problems in nursing babies.

It is not known whether this drug is excreted in breast milk. Exercise caution when administering to a nursing mother.

Precautions

➤*Special risk:* Use beta-carotene cautiously in patients with eating disorders, kidney, or liver disease. These conditions may cause high blood levels of beta-carotene, which may increase the chance of side effects.

Adverse Reactions

➤*More common:* Yellowing of palms, hands, or soles of feet, and to a lesser extent the face (this may be a sign that the dose of beta-carotene as a nutritional supplement is too high).

➤*Rare:* Diarrhea; dizziness; joint pain; unusual bleeding or bruising.

Overdosage

➤*Symptoms:* Beta-carotene has been used at dosages of 180 mg/day or more without any adverse effects other than hypercarotenemia. Hypercarotenemia occurs when there is excessive unconverted carotene in the blood causing a yellow discoloration of the skin. Unrelated to jaundice because of the absence of scleral pigmentation, hypercarotenemia usually reverses upon discontinuation of the vitamin A source.

Patient Information

The presence of other medical problems may affect the use of beta-carotene. Tell your healthcare provider if you have any other medical problems, especially eating disorders, kidney disease, or liver disease. These conditions may cause high blood levels of beta-carotene, which may increase the chance for side effects.

Do not take with dairy products.

Skin may appear slightly yellow-orange while receiving beta-carotene therapy.

VITAMIN D

Indications

Refer to individual product listings.

Administration and Dosage

Individualize dosage. The effectiveness of therapy is predicated on adequate daily intake of calcium either by calcium supplementation or proper dietary measures. Refer to the Recommended Dietary Allowances table for a complete listing.

Actions

➤*Pharmacology:* Vitamin D is a fat-soluble vitamin derived from natural sources (fish liver oils) or from conversion of provitamins (7-dehydrocholesterol and ergosterol). In humans, natural supplies of vitamin D depend on ultraviolet light for conversion of 7-dehydrocholesterol to vitamin D_3 or ergosterol to vitamin D_2. Following exposure to UV light, vitamin D_3 must then be converted to the active form of vitamin D (calcitriol) by the liver and kidneys. Vitamin D is hydroxylated by the hepatic microsomal enzymes to 25-hydroxy-vitamin D_3 (25-]-D_3 or calcifediol). Calcifediol is hydroxylated primarily in the kidney to 1, 25-dihydroxy-vitamin D (1, 25-]$_2$-D_3 or calcitriol) and 24,25-dihydroxycholecalciferol (24,25-$(OH)_2D_3$). Doxercalciferol does not require activation by the kidneys. Calcitriol is believed to be the most active form of vitamin D_3 in stimulating intestinal calcium and phosphate transport.

One USP unit or one IU vitamin D activity is equal to 0.025 mcg vitamin D (1 mg = 40,000 units). "Vitamin D" refers to both ergocalciferol (D_2) and cholecalciferol (D_3). Vitamin D_2, essentially a plant vitamin, is used to fortify milk and cereals.

Dihydrotachysterol is a synthetic reduction product of tachysterol, a close isomer of vitamin D. Dihydrotachysterol is hydroxylated in liver to 25-hydroxydihydrotachy-sterol, the major circulating active form of the drug. It does not undergo further hydroxylation by kidney, and is the analog of 1,25-dihydroxy-vitamin D.

Paricalcitol is a synthetic vitamin D analog that reduces parathyroid hormone (PTH) levels. Paricalcitol suppresses PTH levels in patients with chronic renal failure (CRF) with no significant changes in the incidence of hypercalcemia or hyperphosphatemia when compared with placebo. However, the serum phosphorus, calcium, and calcium times phosphorus product (Ca x P) may increase when paricalcitol is administered.

Doxercalciferol is a synthetic vitamin D analog that undergoes metabolic activation in vivo to form 1α,25-dihydroxyvitamin D_2 (1α,25-$(OH)_2D_2$), a naturally occurring, biologically active form of vitamin D_2. Activation of doxercalciferol does not require involvement of the kidneys.

The Metabolic Pathway of Vitamin D Activation

Ergosterol (Provitamin D_2) —UV light→ Ergocalciferol (Vitamin D_2) —Liver→ 25-hydroxyergocalciferol[1] (25 [OH]-D_2) —Kidney→ 1,25-dihydroxyergocalciferol[2] (1,25 $[OH]_2$-D_2)

7-dehydrocholesterol (Provitamin D_3) —Skin via UV light→ Cholecalciferol[1] (Vitamin D_3) —Liver→ Calcifediol[2] (25 [OH]-D_3) —Kidney→ Calcitriol[3] (1,25 $[OH]_2$-D_3)

Dihydrotachysterol —Liver→ 25-hydroxy-dihydrotachysterol[2]

[1] The kidney, in the absence of PTH, converts vitamin D_3 to 24,25$(OH)_2$-D_3, which is much less active than 1,25$(OH)_2$-D_3.
[2] Major transport form of vitamin D; minor intrinsic activity.
[3] Physiologically active forms.

Physiological function – Vitamin D is considered a hormone. Although not a natural human hormone, vitamin D_2 can substitute for D_3 in every metabolic step. Biologically active vitamin D metabolites control the intestinal absorption of dietary calcium, the tubular reabsorption of calcium by the kidney, and, in conjunction with parathyroid hormone (PTH), the mobilization of calcium from the skeleton. They act directly on bone cells (osteoblasts) to stimulate skeletal growth and on the parathyroid glands to suppress PTH synthesis and secretion. Vitamin D is also involved in magnesium metabolism.

Deficiency – Vitamin D deficiency leads to rickets in children and osteomalacia in adults. Vitamin D reverses symptoms of nutritional rickets.

➤*Pharmacokinetics:*

Absorption – Vitamin D is readily absorbed from the small intestine. Vitamin D_3 may be absorbed more rapidly and more completely than vitamin D_2. Bile is essential for adequate absorption. Absorption is reduced in liver or biliary disease. **Calcifediol's** maximum concentration (C_{max}) is 4 hours following oral administration.

Distribution – Stored chiefly in the liver, vitamin D is also found in fat, muscle, skin, and bones. In plasma, it is bound to α globulins and albumin.

Metabolism – There is a 10- to 24-hour lag between administration of **ergocalciferol** and its onset of action. Maximal hypercalcemic effects occur ≈ 4 weeks after using a daily fixed dose; duration of action can be ≥ 2 months. Serum half-life of **calcifediol** is ≈ 16 days. Elimination half-life of **calcitriol**is 5 to 8 hours; pharmacologic activity persists for 3 to 5 days. **Dihydrotachysterol** has a rapid onset of effect and is less persistent after treatment cessation. **Paracalcitol** has a mean half-life of ≈ 15 hours. In healthy volunteers, peak blood levels of the major metabolite of **doxercalciferol**, 1α,25-$(OH)_2D_2$, has a mean half-life of ≈ 32 to 37 hours, with a range of up to 96 hours. Half-life in patients with end-stage renal disease on dialysis appear to be similar. The elimination half-life of **calcitriol** increased by at least twofold in chronic renal failure and hemodialysis patients compared with healthy subjects. Peak serum levels in patients with nephrotic syndrome were reached in 4 hours. For patients requiring hemodialysis, peak serum levels were reached in 8 to 12 hours; half-lives were estimated to be 16.2 and 21.9 hours, respectively.

Excretion – The primary route of vitamin D excretion is in the bile; only a small percentage is found in the urine.

Contraindications

Hypercalcemia; evidence of vitamin D toxicity; malabsorption syndrome; hypervitaminosis D; abnormal sensitivity to the effects of vitamin D; decreased renal function.

Warnings

➤*Concomitant calcium administration:* Adequate dietary calcium is necessary for a clinical response to vitamin D therapy.

➤*Hypercalcemia:* Calcium phosphate may precipitate if the product of serum calcium multiplied by phosphate (Ca x P) exceeds 70. Progressive hypercalcemia due to overdosage of vitamin D and its metabolites may require emergency attention. Chronic hypercalcemia can lead to generalized vascular calcification, nephrocalcinosis and other soft tissue calcification.

VITAMIN D

Radiographic or slit lamp evaluation of suspect anatomical regions may be useful for early detection.

In patients with normal renal function, chronic hypercalcemia may be associated with an increase in serum creatinine. While this is usually reversible, it is important to pay careful attention to factors that may lead to hypercalcemia.

A fall in serum alkaline phosphatase levels usually precedes hypercalcemia. Should hypercalcemia develop, discontinue the drug immediately. After achieving normocalcemia, readminister at a lower dosage.

➤*Bone lesions:* Adynamic bone lesions may develop if PTH levels are suppressed to abnormal levels (**calcitriol**, **paricalcitol**).

➤*Hypersensitivity reactions:* Hypersensitivity to vitamin D may be one etiological factor in infants with idiopathic hypercalcemia. In these cases, severely restrict vitamin D intake.

➤*Renal function impairment:* The kidneys of uremic patients cannot adequately synthesize calcitriol, the active hormone formed from precursor vitamin D. Resultant hypocalcemia and secondary hyperparathyroidism are a major cause of the metabolic bone disease of renal failure.

The beneficial effect of calcitriol in renal osteodystrophy appears to result from correction of hypocalcemia and secondary hyperparathyroidism. It is uncertain whether calcitriol produces other independent beneficial effects. In patients with renal osteodystrophy accompanied by hyperphosphatemia, maintain a normal serum phosphorus level by dietary phosphate restriction or administration of aluminum gels to prevent metastatic calcification.

Because of the effect on serum calcium, administer to patients with renal stones only when potential benefits outweigh possible hazards.

➤*Pregnancy: Category A.* (*Category C* when used in doses that exceed the RDA). Safety of vitamin D in amounts more than 400 IU/day is not established. Avoid doses greater than the RDA during a normal pregnancy. Animal studies have shown fetal abnormalities associated with hypervitaminosis D. Calcifediol and calcitriol are teratogenic in animals when given in doses several times the human dose. The offspring of a woman administered 17 to 36 mcg/day of calcitriol (17 to 36 times the recommended dose) during pregnancy manifested mild hypercalcemia in the first 2 days of life, which returned to normal at day 3. There are no adequate and well controlled studies in pregnant women; use during pregnancy only if the potential benefits outweigh the potential hazards to the fetus.

➤*Lactation:* Vitamin D is excreted in breast milk in limited amounts. In a mother given large doses of vitamin D, 25-hydroxycholecalciferol appeared in the milk and caused hypercalcemia in the child. Monitoring of the infant's serum calcium concentration was required. Do not nurse while taking **calcitriol**; otherwise, exercise caution when administering to a nursing mother.

➤*Children:* Safety and efficacy of vitamin D and its metabolites in children in doses exceeding the RDA and in children undergoing dialysis have not been established. Long-term *Rocaltrol* therapy is well-tolerated by pediatric patients not undergoing dialysis. Individualize pediatric doses and monitor under close medical supervision.

Precautions

➤*Monitoring:* Dosage adjustment is required as soon as there is clinical improvement. Start therapy at the lowest possible dose, and do not increase without careful monitoring of the serum calcium. Estimate daily dietary calcium intake and adjust the intake when indicated. Patients with normal renal function taking calcitriol should avoid dehydration. Maintain adequate fluid intake. In vitamin D-resistant rickets, the range between therapeutic and toxic doses is narrow. When high therapeutic doses are used, follow progress with frequent serum and urinary calcium, phosphate, and blood urea nitrogen determinations.

Periodically monitor serum calcium, phosphate, magnesium, and alkaline phosphatase; monitor 24-hour urinary calcium and phosphate, especially in hypoparathyroid and dialysis patients. During the initial phase, determine serum calcium once or twice weekly. Maintain serum calcium levels between 9 and 10 mg/dL.

Paricalcitol – During the initial phase of therapy, frequently determine serum calcium and phosphate (eg, twice weekly). Once dosage has been established, measure serum calcium and phosphate at least monthly. Measurements of serum or plasma PTH are recommended every 3 months. An intact PTH (iPTH) assay is recommended for reliable detection of biologically active PTH. During dose adjustment of paricalcitol, laboratory tests may be required more frequently.

➤*Concomitant vitamin D intake:* Evaluate vitamin D ingested in fortified foods, dietary supplements, and other concomitantly administered drugs. It may be necessary to limit dietary vitamin D and its derivatives during treatment.

➤*Hypoparathyroidism:* May need calcium, parathyroid hormone, dihydrotachysterol.

➤*Special risk:* Use caution in patients, especially in the elderly with coronary disease, renal function impairment, and arteriosclerosis.

➤*Tartrazine sensitivity:* Some of these products contain tartrazine, which may cause allergic-type reactions (including bronchial asthma) in susceptible individuals. Although the incidence of sensitivity is low, it is frequently seen in patients with aspirin hypersensitivity. Products containing tartrazine are identified in product listings.

Drug Interactions

Vitamin D Drug Interactions

Precipitant drug	Object drug[a]		Description
Vitamin D	Antacids, magnesium-containing	⬆	Hypermagnesemia may develop in patients on chronic renal dialysis.
Vitamin D	Digitalis glycosides	⬆	Hypercalcemia in patients on digitalis may precipitate cardiac arrhythmias.
Vitamin D	Verapamil	⬆	Atrial fibrillation has occurred when supplemental calcium and calciferol have induced hypercalcemia.
Cholestyramine	Vitamin D	⬇	Intestinal absorption of vitamin D may be reduced.
Ketoconazole	Vitamin D	⬇	Ketoconazole may inhibit both synthetic and catabolic enzymes of calcitriol. Reductions in serum endogenous calcitriol concentrations have been observed following the administration of 300 to 1200 mg/day ketoconazole for a week to healthy men.
Mineral oil	Vitamin D	⬇	Absorption of vitamin D is reduced with prolonged use of mineral oil.
Phenytoin Phenobarbital	Vitamin D	⬇	Endogenous synthesis of calcitriol will be inhibited. Higher doses of calcitriol may be necessary if these drugs are administered simultaneously.
Thiazide diuretics	Vitamin D	⬆	Hypoparathyroid patients on vitamin D may develop hypercalcemia due to thiazide diuretics.

[a] ⬆ = Object drug increased. ⬇ = Object drug decreased.

Adverse Reactions

Early – Weakness; headache; somnolence; nausea; vomiting; dry mouth; constipation; muscle pain; bone pain; metallic taste.

Late – Polyuria; polydipsia; anorexia; irritability; weight loss; nocturia; mild acidosis; hypercalciuria; anemia; reversible azotemia, generalized vascular calcification, nephrocalcinosis; conjunctivitis (calcific); pancreatitis; photophobia; rhinorrhea; pruritus; hyperthermia; decreased libido; elevated BUN; albuminuria; hypercholesterolemia; elevated AST and ALT; ectopic calcification; hypertension; cardiac arrhythmias; overt psychosis (rare).

In clinical studies on hypoparathyroidism and pseudohypoparathyroidism, hypercalcemia was noted on at least one occasion in ≈ 1 in 3 patients and hypercalciuria in ≈ 1 in 7. Elevated serum creatinine levels were observed in ≈ 1 in 6 patients (approximately one half of whom had normal levels at baseline).

Occasional mild pain on injection has been observed (*Calcijex*).

Ergocalciferol – Hypercalciuria and mental retardation have been associated with ergocalciferol.

➤*Paricalcitol:*

Lab test abnormalities – **Paricalcitol** may reduce serum total alkaline phosphatase levels.

Miscellaneous – Discontinuation of therapy caused by any adverse event occurred in 6.5% of 62 patients treated with paricalcitol and 2% of 51 patients treated with placebo for 1 to 3 months.

Nausea (13%); vomiting (13%); edema (7%); chills, fever, flu, GI bleeding, lightheadedness, pneumonia, sepsis (5%); dry mouth, feeling unwell, palpitation (3%).

Overdosage

➤*Symptoms:* Administration of vitamin D to patients in excess of their daily requirements may cause hypercalcemia, hypercalciuria, and hyperphosphatemia. Concomitant high intake of calcium and phosphate may lead to similar abnormalities. **Dihydrotachysterol** may be toxic in doses as low as 25 mg/day, and is manifested by symptoms of hypercalcemia.

Hypercalcemia leads to anorexia, nausea, weakness, headache, somnolence, vomiting, dry mouth, metallic taste, weight loss, vague aches and stiffness, constipation, diarrhea, mental retardation, tinnitus, ataxia, hypotonia, depression, amnesia, disorientation, hallucinations, syncope, coma, anemia, and mild acidosis. Impairment of renal function may cause polyuria, nocturia, hypercalciuria, polydipsia, reversible azotemia, hypertension, nephrocalcinosis, generalized vascular calcification, irreversible renal insufficiency, or proteinuria. Widespread calcification of soft tissues, including heart, blood vessels, renal tubules, skin, and lungs may occur. Bone demineralization (osteoporosis) may occur in adults; decline in average linear growth rate and increased bone mineralization may occur in infants and children (dwarfism). Effects can persist ≥ 2 months after ergocalciferol treatment, 1 month after cessation of dihydrotachysterol therapy, 2 to 4 weeks for calcifediol and

VITAMIN D

2 to 7 days for calcitriol. Death may result from cardiovascular or renal failure. Obtain serum calcium levels at least weekly after all dosage changes and subsequent dosage titration. In patients receiving digitalis, obtain serial serum calcium determination, rate of urinary calcium excretion, and an assessment of ECG abnormalities due to hypercalcemia.

➤*Treatment:* Treatment of accidental overdose consists of general supportive measures. Refer to General Management of Acute Overdosage. If ingestion is discovered within a short time, emesis or gastric lavage may be beneficial. Mineral oil may promote fecal elimination.

Treatment of hypervitaminosis D with hypercalcemia consists of immediate withdrawal of vitamin D and calcium supplements, administration of a low-calcium diet, bed rest, administration of a laxative (mineral oil), attention to electrolyte imbalances, assessment of ECG abnormalities (critical in patients receiving digitalis), hemodialysis or peritoneal dialysis against a calcium-free dialysate, generous fluid intake, and urine acidification along with symptomatic and supportive treatment.

Hypercalcemic crisis with dehydration, stupor, coma, and azotemia requires more vigorous treatment. The first step is hydration; saline IV may quickly and significantly increase urinary calcium excretion. A loop diuretic (eg, furosemide) may be given with the saline infusion to further increase calcium excretion. Other measures include administration of citrates, sulfates, phosphates (do not administer with **paricalcitol**), corticosteroids, EDTA, possibly mithramycin and plicamycin. Persistent or markedly elevated serum calcium levels may be corrected by dialysis against a calcium-free dialysate. With appropriate therapy and when no permanent damage has occurred, recovery is probable.

Patient Information

Compliance with dosage instructions, diet, phosphate-binder use, and calcium supplementation is essential. Avoid use of nonprescription drugs, including magnesium-containing antacids, and natural products, unless such use has been discussed with a physician.

➤*Paricalcitol:* Instruct the patient that, to ensure effectiveness of paricalcitol therapy, it is important to adhere to a dietary regimen of calcium supplementation and phosphorus restriction. Appropriate types of phosphate-binding compounds may be needed; avoid excessive use of aluminum-containing compounds. Inform patients about the symptoms of elevated calcium.

Swallow whole; do not crush or chew.

Eating a balanced diet and periodic exposure to sunlight usually satisfies normal vitamin D requirements. Do not use vitamin supplements as a substitute for a balanced diet.

Notify physician if any of the following occurs: Weakness, lethargy, headache, anorexia, weight loss, nausea, vomiting, abdominal cramps, diarrhea, constipation, vertigo, excessive thirst, excessive urine output, dry mouth, or muscle or bone pain.

Avoid concurrent, prolonged use of mineral oil. If on chronic renal dialysis, avoid magnesium-containing antacids while taking these drugs. See Drug Interactions.

DIHYDROTACHYSTEROL (DHT)

Dihydrotachysterol is a synthetic reduction product of tachysterol, a close isomer of vitamin D; 1 mg is approximately equivalent to 3 mg (120,000 IU) vitamin D_2.

Rx	**DHT** (Roxane)	**Tablets**: 0.125 mg	Lactose, sucrose. (54 280). White. In 50s and UD 100s.
		0.2 mg	Lactose, sucrose. (54 903). Pink. In 100s and UD 100s.
		0.4 mg	Lactose, sucrose. (54 772). White. In 50s.
		Intensol Solution: 0.2 mg/mL	20% alcohol. In 30 mL w/dropper.

DIHYDROTACHYSTEROL — ORAL

For complete and comparative prescribing information, see the Vitamin D group monograph.

Indications

➤*Tetany:* For the treatment of acute, chronic, and latent forms of postoperative tetany and idiopathic tetany.

➤*Hypoparathyroidism:* For the treatment of hypoparathyroidism.

Administration and Dosage

The dosage depends on the nature and seriousness of the disorder and should be adapted to each individual patient. Serum calcium levels should be maintained between 9 to 10 mg per 100 mL.

➤*Initial dose:* Take 0.8 mg to 2.4 mg daily for several days.

➤*Maintenance dose:* Take 0.2 mg to 1 mg daily as required for normal serum calcium levels. The average maintenance dose is 0.6 mg daily. This dose may be supplemented with 10 to 15 g of calcium lactate or gluconate by mouth daily.

➤*Storage/Stability:* Store at 25°C (77°F); excursions permitted to 15° to 30°C (59° to 86°F).

CALCITRIOL (1α,25 dihydroxycholecalciferol; 1,25 $[OH]_2D_3$)

Rx	**Calcitriol** (Teva)	**Capsules**: 0.25 mcg	Mannitol, sorbitol. (93 and 657). Opaque red-brown and yellow-brown, oval. In 100s.
Rx	**Rocaltrol** (Roche)		Sorbitol, parabens. (Rocaltrol 0.25 Roche). Light orange. Oval. In 30s and 100s.
Rx	**Calcitriol** (Teva)	0.5 mcg	Mannitol, sorbitol. (93 and 658). Opaque brown and pink. In 100s.
Rx	**Rocaltrol** (Roche)		Sorbitol, parabens. (Rocaltrol 0.5 Roche). Dark orange. Oblong. In 100s.
Rx	**Calcitriol** (Roxane)	**Oral solution**: 1 mcg/mL	In 15 mL with single-use graduated oral dispensers.
Rx	**Rocaltrol** (Roche)		In 15 mL bottle w/dispensers.
Rx	**Calcitriol Injection** (aaiPharma)	**Injection**: 1 mcg/mL	Sodium chloride, EDTA. In 1 mL vials.
Rx	**Calcijex** (Abbott)		In 1 mL amps.[a]
Rx	**Calcitriol Injection** (aaiPharma)	**Injection**: 2 mcg/mL	Sodium chloride, EDTA. In 1 mL vials.

[a] With 4 mg polysorbate 20, 1.5 mg sodium chloride, 10 mg sodium ascorbate, 7.6 mg dibasic sodium phosphate, anhydrous, and EDTA.

CALCITRIOL — ORAL

For complete and comparative prescribing information, see the Vitamin D group monograph.

Indications

➤*Predialysis patients:* Management of secondary hyperparathyroidism and resultant metabolic bone disease in patients with moderate to severe chronic renal failure (Ccr 15 to 55 mL/min) not yet on dialysis.

➤*Dialysis patients:* Management of hypocalcemia and the resultant metabolic bone disease in patients undergoing chronic renal dialysis.

➤*Hypoparathyroidism patients:* Management of hypocalcemia and its clinical manifestations in patients with postsurgical hypoparathyroidism, idiopathic hypoparathyroidism, and pseudohypoparathyroidism.

➤*Unlabeled uses:* Calcitriol, orally (initial dose of 0.25 mcg twice daily) and topically (0.1 to 0.5 mcg/g petrolatum), decreased the severity of psoriatic lesions.

Administration and Dosage

The optimal daily dose of calcitriol must be carefully determined for each patient. Calcitriol can be administered orally either as a capsule (0.25 mcg or 0.5 mcg) or as an oral solution (1 mcg/mL). Calcitriol therapy should always be started at the lowest possible dose and should not be increased without careful monitoring of serum calcium.

➤*Adjunct calcium therapy:* The effectiveness of calcitriol therapy is predicated on the assumption that each patient is receiving an adequate but

CALCITRIOL — ORAL

not excessive daily intake of calcium. Patients are advised to have a dietary intake of calcium at a minimum of 600 mg daily. The US RDA for calcium in adults is 800 mg to 1200 mg. To ensure that each patient receives an adequate daily intake of calcium, the physician should either prescribe a calcium supplement or instruct the patient in proper dietary measures.

Because of improved calcium absorption from the gastrointestinal tract, some patients on calcitriol may be maintained on a lower calcium intake. Patients who tend to develop hypercalcemia may require only low doses of calcium or no supplementation at all.

During the titration period of treatment with calcitriol, serum calcium levels should be checked at least twice weekly. When the optimal dosage of calcitriol has been determined, serum calcium levels should be checked every month (or as given below for individual indications). Samples for serum calcium estimation should be taken without a tourniquet.

➤*Dialysis patients:* The recommended initial dose of calcitriol is 0.25 mcg/day. If a satisfactory response in the biochemical parameters and clinical manifestations of the disease state is not observed, dosage may be increased by 0.25 mcg/day at 4- to 8-week intervals. During this titration period, serum calcium levels should be obtained at least twice weekly, and if hypercalcemia is noted, the drug should be immediately discontinued until normocalcemia ensues. Phosphorus, magnesium, and alkaline phosphatase should be determined periodically.

Patients with normal or only slightly reduced serum calcium levels may respond to calcitriol doses of 0.25 mcg every other day. Most patients undergoing hemodialysis respond to doses between 0.5 and 1 mcg/day.

Oral calcitriol may normalize plasma ionized calcium in some uremic patients, yet fail to suppress parathyroid hyperfunction. In these individuals with autonomous parathyroid hyperfunction, oral calcitriol may be useful to maintain normocalcemia, but has not been shown to be adequate treatment for hyperparathyroidism.

➤*Hypoparathyroidism:* The recommended initial dosage of calcitriol is 0.25 mcg/day given in the morning. If a satisfactory response in the biochemical parameters and clinical manifestations of the disease is not observed, the dose may be increased at 2- to 4-week intervals. During the dosage titration period, serum calcium levels should be obtained at least twice weekly and, if hypercalcemia is noted, calcitriol should be immediately discontinued until normocalcemia ensues. Careful consideration should also be given to lowering the dietary calcium intake. Serum calcium, phosphorus, and 24-hour urinary calcium should be determined periodically.

Most adult patients and pediatric patients greater than or equal to 6 years of age have responded to dosages in the range of 0.5 mcg to 2 mcg daily. Pediatric patients in the 1- to 5-year age group with hypoparathyroidism have usually been given 0.25 mcg to 0.75 mcg daily. The number of treated patients with pseudohypoparathyroidism less than 6 years of age is too small to make dosage recommendations.

Malabsorption is occasionally noted in patients with hypoparathyroidism; hence, larger doses of calcitriol may be needed.

➤*Predialysis patients:* The recommended initial dosage of calcitriol is 0.25 mcg/day in adults and pediatric patients greater than or equal to 3 years of age. This dosage may be increased if necessary to 0.5 mcg/day.

➤*Children:* For pediatric patients younger than 3 years of age, the recommended initial dosage of calcitriol is 10 to 15 ng/kg/day.

➤*Storage/Stability:* Protect from light. Store at 25°C (77°F); excursions permitted to 15° to 30°C (59° to 86°F).

CALCITRIOL — INJECTION

For complete and comparative prescribing information, see the Vitamin D group monograph.

Indications

➤*Hypocalcemia:* Management of hypocalcemia in patients undergoing chronic renal dialysis. It has been shown to significantly reduce elevated parathyroid hormone (PTH) levels. Reduction of PTH has been shown to result in an improvement in renal osteodystrophy.

Administration and Dosage

➤*Approved by the FDA:* September 25, 1986.

➤*Adjunct calcium therapy:* The effectiveness of calcitriol injection therapy is predicated on the assumption that each patient is receiving an adequate and appropriate daily intake of calcium. The RDA for calcium in adults is 800 mg. To ensure that each patient receives an adequate daily intake of calcium, the physician should either prescribe a calcium supplement or instruct the patient in proper dietary measures.

➤*Dosage:* The recommended initial dose of calcitriol injection, depending on the severity of the hypocalcemia and/or secondary hyperparathyroidism, is 1 mcg (0.02 mcg/kg) to 2 mcg administered 3 times weekly, approximately every other day. Doses as small as 0.5 mcg and as large as 4 mcg 3 times weekly have been used as an initial dose.

➤*Unsatisfactory response:* If a satisfactory response is not observed, the dose may be increased by 0.5 to 1 mcg at 2- to 4-week intervals. During this titration period, serum calcium and phosphorus levels should be obtained at least twice weekly.

If hypercalcemia or a serum calcium times phosphate product greater than 70 is noted, the drug should be immediately discontinued until these parameters are appropriate. Then, the calcitriol injection dose should be reinitiated at a lower dose. Doses may need to be reduced as the PTH levels decrease in response to the therapy. Thus, incremental dosing must be individualized and commensurate with PTH, serum calcium and phosphorus levels. The following is a suggested approach in dose titration:

PTH levels	Calcitriol injection
The same or increasing	Increase
Decreasing by less than 30%	Increase
Decreasing by more than 30%, less than 60%	Maintain
Decreasing by more than 60%	Decrease
1.5 to 3 times the upper limit of normal	Maintain

➤*Storage/Stability:* Store at controlled room temperature 15° to 30°C (59° to 86°F). Discard unused portion.

ERGOCALCIFEROL (D_2)

Ergocalciferol 1 mg provides 40,000 units of vitamin D activity.

otc	**Calciferol Drops** (Schwarz Pharma)	**Liquid**: 8,000 units/mL	In 60 mL.[a]
otc	**Drisdol Drops** (Sanofi Pharm.)		In 60 mL.[a]
Rx	**Vitamin D** (Pliva)	**Capsules**: 50,000 units	Soybean oil. (PA140). Green, oval. In 100s or 1,000s.
Rx	**Drisdol** (Sanofi Pharm.)		Tartrazine. (D92 W). In 50s.

[a] In propylene glycol. [b] In sesame oil.

ERGOCALCIFEROL — ORAL

For complete and comparative prescribing information, see the Vitamin D group monograph.

Indications

➤*Hypoparathyroidism:* For the treatment of hypoparathyroidism.

➤*Rickets:* For the treatment of refractory rickets, also known as vitamin D-resistant rickets.

➤*Familial hypophosphatemia:* For the treatment of familial hypophosphatemia.

Administration and Dosage

The range between therapeutic and toxic doses is narrow.

➤*Vitamin D-resistant rickets:* 12,000 to 500,000 units daily.

➤*Hypoparathyroidism:* 50,000 to 200,000 units daily concomitantly with calcium lactate 4 g 6 times per day.

Dosage must be individualized under close medical supervision.

Calcium intake should be adequate. Blood calcium and phosphorus determinations must be made every 2 weeks or more frequently if necessary.

X-rays of the bones should be taken every month until condition is corrected and stabilized.

➤*Storage/Stability:* Store at controlled room temperature between 15° and 30°C (59° to 86°F). Protect from light.

CHOLECALCIFEROL (D_3)

Cholecalciferol 1 mg provides 40,000 IU vitamin D activity.

otc sf	**Delta-D** (Freeda)	**Tablets:** 400 IU	In 250s and 500s.
otc sf	**Vitamin D_3** (Freeda)	**Tablets:** 1000 IU_3	In 100s and 500s.

CHOLECALCIFEROL (VITAMIN D3) — ORAL

For complete and comparative prescribing information, see the Vitamin D group monograph.

Indications

➤*Dietary supplement:* As a dietary supplement when vitamin D intake may be inadequate.

Administration and Dosage

➤*Recommended daily allowance (RDA):* The US recommended daily allowance (RDA) for vitamin D is based on 1 mcg calciferol equaling 40 IU vitamin D; cholecalciferol 1 mg provides 40,000 IU of vitamin D activity. The RDA for infants and children (birth to 3 years of age) is 7.5 to 10 mcg. The RDA for children 4 to 10 years of age is 10 mcg. The RDA for adolescents and adults is 5 to 10 mcg. The RDA for pregnant and breastfeeding females is 10 mcg.

One tablet contains between 400 IU and 1000 IU of vitamin D.

➤*Adults:* As a dietary supplement, take 1 tablet or capsule daily or as recommended by a healthcare provider.

➤*Children:* As a dietary supplement, the recommended daily dose varies. Consult a healthcare provider.

➤*Storage/Stability:* Store away from heat and direct light in a cool, dry place. Heat or moisture may cause the dietary supplement to break down.

PARICALCITOL

Rx	**Zemplar** (Abbott)	**Capsules:** 1 mcg	Alcohol, medium chain triglycerides. (ZA). Gray, oval. In 30s.
		2 mcg	Alcohol, medium chain triglycerides. (ZF). Orange-brown, oval. In 30s.
		4 mcg	Alcohol, medium chain triglycerides. (ZK). Gold, oval. In 30s.
		Injection: 2 mcg/mL	In 1 mL single-dose. *Fliptop* vials.
		5 mcg/mL	In 1 and 2 mL single-dose *Fliptop* vials.

PARICALCITOL — ORAL

For complete and comparative prescribing information, see the Vitamin D group monograph.

Indications

➤*Hyperparathyroidism:* For the prevention and treatment of secondary hyperparathyroidism associated with chronic kidney disease (CKD) stage 3 and 4.

Administration and Dosage

➤*Approved by the FDA:* May 26, 2005.

➤*Administration:* Paricalcitol may be administered daily or 3 times a week. When dosing 3 times weekly, the dose should be administered no more frequently than every other day. The average weekly doses for daily and 3-times-a-week dosage regimens are similar.

Paricalcitol may be taken without regard to food.

➤*Initial dose:* The initial dose of paricalcitol is based on baseline intact parathyroid hormone (iPTH) levels.

Paricalcitol Initial Dosage Recommendations

Baseline iPTH level	Daily dose	3 times weekly dosage[a]
≤ 500 pg/mL	1 mcg	2 mcg
more than 500 pg/mL	2 mcg	4 mcg

[a] To be administered not more often than every other day.

➤*Dose titration:* Dosing must be individualized and based on serum or plasma iPTH levels, with monitoring of serum calcium and serum phosphorus. The following is a suggested titration approach.

Paricalcitol Dosage Titration Recommendations

iPTH level relative to baseline	Paricalcitol dose	Dosage adjustment at 2- to 4-week intervals	
		Daily dosage	3 times weekly dosage[a]
The same or increased	Increase	1 mcg	2 mcg
Decreased less than 30%			
Decreased 30% to 60%	Maintain		
Decreased more than 60%	Decrease	1 mcg	2 mcg
iPTH less than 60 pg/mL			

[a] To be administered not more often than every other day.

➤*Dose reduction:* If a patient is taking the lowest dose on the daily regimen and a dosage reduction is needed, the dosage can be decreased to 1 mcg 3 times a week. If a further dosage reduction is required, the drug should be withheld as needed and can be restarted at a lower dose.

➤*Calcium-based phosphate binder:* If a patient is on a calcium-based phosphate binder, the binder dose may be decreased or withheld, or the patient may be switched to a non-calcium-based phosphate binder.

➤*Hypercalcemia:* If hypercalcemia or an elevated calcium-phosphorus product (Ca× P) is observed, the dose of paricalcitol should be reduced or interrupted until these parameters are normalized.

➤*Storage/Stability:* Store paricalcitol capsules at 25°C (77°F). Excursions permitted between 15° and 30°C (59° and 86°F).

PARICALCITOL — INJECTION

For complete and comparative prescribing information, see the Vitamin D group monograph.

Indications

➤*Hyperparathyroidism:* For the prevention and treatment of secondary hyperparathyroidism associated with chronic kidney disease (CKD) stage 5.

Administration and Dosage

➤*Approved by the FDA:* April 17, 1998.

➤*Dosage:* The currently accepted target range for intact parathyroid hormone (iPTH) levels in CKD stage 5 patients is no more than 1.5 to 3 times the nonuremic upper limit of normal (ULN).

The recommended initial dose of paricalcitol is 0.04 to 0.1 mcg/kg (2.8 to 7 mcg) administered as a bolus dose no more frequently than every other day at any time during dialysis.

➤*Dosage adjustments:* If a satisfactory response is not observed, the dose may be increased by 2 to 4 mcg at 2- to 4-week intervals. During any dose adjustment period, serum calcium and phosphorus levels should be monitored more frequently, and if an elevated calcium level or a Ca × P product greater than 75 is noted, the drug dosage should be immediately reduced or interrupted until these parameters are normalized. Then, paricalcitol should be reinitiated at a lower dose. If a patient is on a calcium-based phaosphate binder, the dose may be decreased or withheld, or the patient may be switched to a noncalcium-based phosphate binder.Doses may need to be decreased as the PTH levels decrease in response to therapy. Thus, incremental dosing must be individualized.

➤*Dose titration:*

Paricalcitol Dosage Titration Recommendations

PTH level	Paricalcitol injection dose
The same or increasing	Increase
Decreasing by less than 30%	Increase
Decreasing by more than 30%, less than 60%	Maintain
Decreasing by more than 60%	Decrease
1.5 to 3 times ULN	Maintain

➤*Storage/Stability:* Store at 25°C (77°F). Excursions permitted to 15° to 30°C (59° to 86°F). Discard unused portion.

DOXERCALCIFEROL

Rx	**Hectorol** (Bone Care International)	**Capsules:** 2.5 mcg	Butylated hydroxyanisole, ethanol. (BCI). Yellow. Oval. In 50s.
		Injection: 2 mcg/mL	In 2 mL amps.[a]

[a] Each milliliter contains polysorbate 20, 4 mg; sodium chloride 1.5 mg; sodium ascorbate 10 mg; sodium phosphate dibasic 7.6 mg; sodium phosphate monobasic 1.8 mg; EDTA 1.1 mg.

DOXERCALCIFEROL — ORAL

For complete and comparative prescribing information, see the Vitamin D group monograph.

Indications

For the reduction of elevated intact parathyroid hormone iPTH levels in the management of secondary hyperparathyroidism in patients undergoing chronic renal dialysis.

Administration and Dosage

➤*Approved by the FDA:* June 9, 1999.

The optimal dose of doxercalciferol must be carefully determined for each patient.

The recommended initial dose of doxercalciferol is 10 mcg administered 3 times weekly at dialysis (approximately every other day) (for iPTH levels > 400 pg/mL). The initial dose should be adjusted, as needed, in order to lower blood iPTH into the range of 150 to 300 pg/mL. The dose may be increased at 8-week intervals by 2.5 mcg if iPTH is not lowered by 50% and fails to reach the target range. The maximum recommended dose of doxercalciferol is 20 mcg administered 3 times a week at dialysis for a total of 60 mcg/week. Drug administration should be suspended if iPTH falls below 100 pg/mL and restarted 1 week later at a dose that is at least 2.5 mcg lower than the last administered dose. During titration, iPTH, serum calcium, and serum phosphorus levels should be obtained weekly. If hypercalcemia, hyperphosphatemia, or a serum calcium times serum phosphorus product > 70 is noted, the drug should be immediately suspended until these parameters are appropriately lowered. Then, the drug should be restarted at a dose that is at least 2.5 mcg lower.

Dosing must be individualized and based on iPTH levels with monitoring of serum calcium and serum phosphorus levels. The following is a suggested approach in dose titration:

Initial Doxercalciferol Dosing	
iPTH level	Doxercalciferol capsule dose
> 400 pg/mL	10 mcg 3 times per week at dialysis
Dose titration	
iPTH level	Doxercalciferol capsule dose
Decreased by < 50% and above 300 pg/mL	Increase by 2.5 mcg at 8-week intervals as necessary
150 to 300 pg/mL	Maintain
< 100 pg/mL	Suspend for 1 week, then resume at a dose that is at least 2.5 mcg lower

➤*Storage/Stability:* Store at controlled room temperature 20° to 25°C (68° to 77°F) [see USP].

DOXERCALCIFEROL — INJECTION

For complete and comparative prescribing information, see the Vitamin D group monograph.

Indications

➤*Secondary hyperparathyroidism:* For the treatment of secondary hyperparathyroidism in adult patients with chronic kidney disease on dialysis.

Administration and Dosage

➤*Approved by the FDA:* June 9, 1999 (oral doseform).

The optimal dose must be carefully determined for each patient.

➤*Initial dosage:* 4 mcg administered as a bolus dose 3 times weekly at the end of dialysis (approximately every other day).

➤*Dosage adjustments:* The initial dose should be adjusted, as needed, in order to lower blood intact parathyroid hormone (iPTH) into the range of 150 to 300 pg/mL. The dose may be increased at 8-week intervals by 1 to 2 mcg if iPTH is not lowered by 50% and fails to reach the target range. Dosages higher than 18 mcg weekly have not been studied. Drug administration should be suspended if iPTH falls below 100 pg/mL and restarted 1 week later at a dose that is at least 1 mcg lower than the last administered dose. During titration, iPTH, serum calcium, and serum phosphorus levels should be obtained weekly. If hypercalcemia, hyperphosphatemia, or a serum calcium times phosphorus product of greater than 55 mg^2/dL^2 is noted, doxercalciferol should be decreased or suspended and/or the dose of phosphate binders should be appropriately adjusted. If suspended, the drug should be restarted at a dose that is 1 mcg lower.

Dosing must be individualized and based on iPTH levels with monitoring of serum calcium and serum phosphorus levels. The following is a suggested approach for dose titration:

Initial Doxercalciferol Dosing	
iPTH level	Doxercalciferol dosage
> 400 pg/mL	4 mcg 3 times/week at the end of dialysis, or approximately every other day
Dose titration	
iPTH level	Doxercalciferol dose
Decreased by < 50% and > 300 pg/mL	Increase by 1 to 2 mcg at 8-week intervals as necessary
150 to 300 pg/mL	Maintain
< 100 pg/mL	Suspend for 1 week, then resume at a dose that is at least 1 mcg lower

➤*Storage/Stability:* Store at 15° to 25°C (59° to 77°F). Protect from light. Discard unused portion.

VITAMIN E

otc	**Vitamin E** (Various, eg, Freeda)	**Tablets:** 100 IU[a]	In 100s and 250s.
		200 IU[a]	In 100s, 250s, and 500s.
		400 IU[a]	In 100s, 250s, and 500s.
		500 IU[a]	In 100s and 250s.
		800 IU[a]	In 100s.
otc	**Vitamin E with Mixed Tocopherols** (Freeda)	**Tablets:** 100 IU[b]	In 100s and 250s.
		200 IU[b]	In 100s and 250s.
		400 IU[b]	In 100s, 250s, and 500s.
otc	**Vitamin E** (Various, eg, Apothecary, Goldline, Nature's Bounty)	**Capsules:** 100 IU[b]	In 100s.
		200 IU[b]	In 100s.
		400 IU[b]	In 100s and 250s.
		1000 IU[b]	In 50s and 100s.
otc	**Mixed E 400 Softgels** (Naturally)	**Capsules:** 400 IU[b]	In 60s, 90s, and 180s.
otc sf	**Vita-Plus E** (Scot-Tussin)	**Capsules:** 400 IU[c]	In 50s.
otc	**d' ALPHA E 1000 Softgels** (Naturally)	**Capsules:** 1000 IU[a]	In 30s and 60s.
otc	**Mixed E 1000 Softgels** (Naturally)	**Capsules:** 1000 IU[b]	In 30s and 60s.
otc	**Aquavit-E** (Cypress)	**Drops:** 15 IU[d] per 0.3 mL	In 30 mL.
otc	**Vitamin E** (Freeda)	**Liquid:** 15 IU[b] per 30 mL	In 30, 60, and 120 mL.

VITAMIN E

otc sf	**Nutr-E-Sol** (Advanced Nutritional Technology)	**Liquid:** 798 IU[b] per 30 mL	Dye free. In 473 mL.

[a] As d-alpha tocopherol.
[b] Form of vitamin E unknown; content given in IU.
[c] As d-alpha tocopheryl acetate.
[d] As dL-alpha tocopheryl acetate.

VITAMIN E — ORAL

Indications

➤*Dietary supplement:* As a dietary supplement when vitamin E intake may be inadequate.

➤*Unlabeled uses:* Vitamin E has been used in certain premature infants to reduce the toxic effects of oxygen therapy on the lung parenchyma (bronchopulmonary dysplasia) and the retina (retrolental fibroplasia). It has been investigated for the prevention of periventricular hemorrhage in premature infants.

It has also been used in cancer, skin conditions, sexual dysfunction, to reduce the incidence of non-fatal MI, to lower the incidence of coronary artery disease, aging, fibrocystic breast disease (cystic mastitis), to treat dapsone-associated hemolysis, arthritis, and tardive dyskinesia. Use of vitamin E in combination with vitamin A has been reported in the treatment of keratosis follicularis (Darier's disease), pityriasis rubra pilaris, ichthyosis, and acne. Use of vitamin E (400 IU) in combination with vitamin C (1 g/day) has resulted in significant risk reduction for preeclampsia during the second half of pregnancy.

Administration and Dosage

➤*Recommended daily allowance (RDA):* In the past, the recommended daily allowance (RDA) for vitamin E has been expressed in units. The term units has been replaced by alpha tocopherol equivalents (alpha-TE) or milligrams (mg) of d-alpha tocopherol. One unit is equivalent to 1 mg of dl-alpha tocopherol acetate or 0.6 mg d-alpha tocopherol. Most products available in stores continue to be labeled in units. 1 mg alpha-tocopherol equivalents equals 1.5 IU.

The US RDA for males and females greater than 14 years of age is 15 mg/day of alpha-tocopherol equivalents (or 22 IU). The US RDA for children 1 to 3 years is 6 mg/day of alpha-tocopherol equivalents (or 9 IU), 7 mg/day of alpha-tocopherol equivalents (or 10.5 IU) in children 4 to 8 years, and 11 mg/day of alpha-tocopherol equivalents (or 16.5 IU) in children 9 to 13 years of age.

Pregnancy and lactation – Avoid the use of vitamin E in excess of the RDA during normal pregnancy and breastfeeding. The RDA of vitamin E is 15 mg/day alpha-tocopherol equivalents (or 22 IU) during pregnancy and 19 mg/day alpha-tocopherol equivalents (or 28 IU) for nursing mothers.

➤*Storage/Stability:* Store away from heat and direct light.

Keep the oral liquid form of this supplement from freezing.

Actions

➤*Pharmacology:* Vitamin E is a fat-soluble vitamin with actions related to its antioxidant properties. Vitamin E protects cellular constituents from oxidation and prevents the formation of toxic oxidation products; it preserves red blood cell (RBC) wall integrity and protects RBCs against hemolysis; it stimulates a cofactor in steroid metabolism; inhibits prostaglandin production; and suppresses platelet aggregation. In combination with selenium, vitamin E protects cell membranes from oxidative damage.

There are 8 naturally occurring compounds with vitamin E activity; 4 are tocopherols and 4 are tocotrienols. Free d-alpha tocopherol is the most biologically active form of vitamin E. One IU of vitamin E activity is equivalent to 1 mg all- rac-alpha-tocopheryl acetate. Normal plasma levels of vitamin E are between 1 and 3 mg/dL in low-birth-weight infants. Infants receiving either oral or parenteral vitamin E should maintain serum vitamin levels less than 3.5 mg/dL. Sources of vitamin E include vegetables, oils, seeds, corn, soy, whole wheat flour, margarine, nuts, leafy vegetables, milk, eggs, and meats.

Deficiency – Clinical deficiency of vitamin E is rare because adequate amounts are supplied in the normal diet. Symptoms of deficiency include ataxia, muscle weakness, nystagmus, and losses in touch and pain sensations. Low tocopherol levels have been noted in the following: Premature infants; malnourished infants with macrocyticanemia; prolonged fat malabsorption (ie, cystic fibrosis, hepatic cirrhosis, sprue); malabsorption syndromes (ie, celiac disease, GI resections); patients with abetalipoproteinemia. Vitamin E deficiency in premature infants may result in hemolytic anemia, thrombocytosis, and increased platelet aggregation. Vitamin E levels less than 0.5 mg/dL are suggestive of a deficiency.

Vitamin E requirements – The daily vitamin E requirement is related to the dietary intake of polyunsaturated fatty acids (PUFA), primarily linoleic acid. Vitamin E requirements may be increased in patients taking large doses of iron. Commercial infant formulas currently available provide an adequate ratio of vitamin E to PUFA; formulas for premature infants have a lower level of iron to preclude interference with vitamin E use. Thus, there is no longer a need to routinely administer vitamin E supplementation to prevent anemia.

➤*Pharmacokinetics:*

Absorption/Distribution – Vitamin E is 20% to 50% absorbed by intestinal epithelial cells in the small intestine. Bile and pancreatic juice are needed for tocopherol absorption. Absorption is increased when administered with medium-chain triglycerides. Distribution to tissues via the lymphatic system occurs as a lipoprotein complex. High concentrations of vitamin E are found in the adrenals, pituitary, testes, and thrombocytes.

Metabolism/Excretion – Vitamin E is stored unmodified in tissues (principally the liver and adipose tissue) and excreted via the feces. Excess vitamin E is converted to a lactone, esterified to glucuronic acid, and subsequently excreted in the urine.

Warnings

➤*Pregnancy:* See Administration and Dosage for more information.

➤*Lactation:* See Administration and Dosage for more information.

➤*Children:* Vitamin E supplements may be recommended for premature infants with low levels of vitamin E.

See Overdosage for more information.

Drug Interactions

Vitamin E Drug Interactions

Precipitant drug	Object drug[a]		Description
Vitamin E	Anticoagulants, oral warfarin	⬆	Vitamin E in high doses (greater than 4000 IU) may increase the hypoprothrombinemic effects of oral anticoagulants.
Vitamin E	Iron	⬇	Vitamin E may impair the hematologic response to iron therapy in children with iron-deficiency anemia.

[a] ⬆ = Object drug increased; ⬇ = Object drug decreased.

Adverse Reactions

➤*Hypervitaminosis:* See Overdosage for more information.

Overdosage

➤*Symptoms:* Doses less than 2,000 IU are not likely to cause side effects. However, large doses (greater than 3,000 IU) have been noted to produce symptoms of hypervitaminosis E, which include nausea, weakness, intestinal cramps, headache, flatulence, diarrhea, thrombophlebitis, pulmonary embolism, severe fatigue syndrome, gynecomastia, breast tumors, increased cholesterol and triglycerides, decrease in serum thyroid hormone, and altered immunity.

Infants – Sepsis and necrotizing enterocolitis have been reported when vitamin E levels are maintained at 5 mg/dL in low-birth-weight infants.

Patient Information

Swallow capsules whole; do not crush or chew.

VITAMIN K (PHYTONADIONE)

Rx	**Mephyton** (Merck)	**Tablets:** 5 mg	Lactose. (MSD 43 Mephyton). Yellow, scored. In 100s.
Rx	**Phytonadione** (Hospira)	**Injection, emulsion:** 2 mg per mL	Dextrose, 9 mg benzyl alcohol. In 0.5 mL ampul.
		10 mg/mL	Dextrose, 9 mg benzyl alcohol. In 1 mL ampul.

PHYTONADIONE — ORAL

Indications

➤*Coagulation disorders:* Phytonadione is indicated in the following coagulation disorders which are due to faulty formation of factors II, VII, IX and X when caused by vitamin K deficiency or interference with vitamin K activity.

Phytonadione tablets are indicated in the following: Anticoagulant-induced prothrombin deficiency caused by coumarin or indanedione derivatives; hypoprothrombinemia secondary to antibacterial therapy; hypoprothrombinemia secondary to administration of salicylates; hypoprothrombinemia secondary to obstructive jaundice or biliary fistulas but only if bile salts are administered concurrently, since otherwise the oral vitamin K will not be absorbed.

PHYTONADIONE — ORAL

Administration and Dosage

➤*Approved by the FDA:* July 25, 1983.

Oral Phytonadione (Summary of Dosage Guidelines)	
Adults	Initial dosage
Anticoagulant-induced prothrombin deficiency (caused by coumarin or indanedione derivatives)	2.5 to 10 mg or up to 25 mg (rarely 50 mg)
Hypoprothrombinemia due to other causes (Antibiotics; salicylates or other drugs; factors limiting absorption or synthesis)	2.5 to 25 mg or more (rarely up to 50 mg)

➤*Anticoagulant-induced prothrombin deficiency in adults:* Frequency and amount of subsequent doses should be determined by prothrombin time response or clinical condition (see Warnings). If, in 12 to 48 hours after oral administration, the prothrombin time has not been shortened satisfactorily, the dose should be repeated.

➤*Hypoprothrombinemia due to other causes in adults:* If possible, discontinuation or reduction of the dosage of drugs interfering with coagulation mechanisms (such as salicylates, antibiotics) is suggested as an alternative to administering concurrent phytonadione. The severity of the coagulation disorder should determine whether the immediate administration of phytonadione is required in addition to discontinuation or reduction of interfering drugs.

The oral route should be avoided when the clinical disorder would prevent proper absorption. Bile salts must be given with the tablets when the endogenous supply of bile to the gastrointestinal tract is deficient.

➤*Storage/Stability:* Store in a tightly closed container at 25°C (77°F); excursions permitted to 15° to 30°C (59° to 86°F). Protect from light. Store container in carton until contents have been used.

Actions

➤*Pharmacology:* Phytonadione tablets possess the same type and degree of activity as does naturally-occurring vitamin K, which is necessary for the production via the liver of active prothrombin (factor II), proconvertin (factor VII), plasma thromboplastin component (factor IX), and Stuart factor (factor X). The prothrombin test is sensitive to the levels of three of these four factors (factors II, VII, and X). Vitamin K is an essential cofactor for a microsomal enzyme that catalyzes the post-translational carboxylation of multiple, specific, peptide-bound glutamic acid residues in inactive hepatic precursors of factors II, VII, IX, and X. The resulting gamma-carboxyglutamic acid residues convert the precursors into active coagulation factors that are subsequently secreted by liver cells into the blood.

In healthy animals and humans, phytonadione is virtually devoid of pharmacodynamic activity. However, in animals and humans deficient in vitamin K, the pharmacological action of vitamin K is related to its normal physiological function; that is, to promote the hepatic biosynthesis of vitamin K-dependent clotting factors.

➤*Pharmacokinetics:* Phytonadione is only absorbed from the GI tract via intestinal lymphatics in the presence of bile salts. Although initially concentrated in the liver, vitamin K is rapidly metabolized and very little tissue accumulation occurs. Little is known about the metabolic fate of vitamin K. Almost no free unmetabolized vitamin K appears in bile or urine.

Phytonadione tablets generally exert their effect within 6 to 10 hours.

Contraindications

Hypersensitivity to any component of this medication.

Warnings

➤*Oral anticoagulant — induced hypoprothrombinemia:* An immediate coagulant effect should not be expected after administration of phytonadione. Phytonadione will not counteract the anticoagulant action of heparin.

When vitamin K_1 is used to correct excessive anticoagulant-induced hypoprothrombinemia, anticoagulant therapy still being indicated, the patient is again faced with the clotting hazards existing prior to starting the anticoagulant therapy. Phytonadione is not a clotting agent, but overzealous therapy with vitamin K_1 may restore conditions which originally permitted thromboembolic phenomena. Dosage should be kept as low as possible, and prothrombin time should be checked regularly as clinical conditions indicate.

➤*Hepatic function impairment:* Repeated large doses of vitamin K are not warranted in liver disease if the response to initial use of the vitamin is unsatisfactory. Failure to respond to vitamin K may indicate a congenital coagulation defect or that the condition being treated is unresponsive to vitamin K.

➤*Pregnancy: Category C.* Animal reproduction studies have not been conducted with phytonadione. It is also not known whether phytonadione can cause fetal harm when administered to a pregnant woman or can affect reproduction capacity. Phytonadione should be given to a pregnant woman only if clearly needed.

➤*Lactation:* It is not known whether this drug is excreted in human milk. Because many drugs are excreted in human milk, caution should be exercised when phytonadione is administered to a nursing woman.

➤*Children:* Safety and effectiveness in pediatric patients have not been established with phytonadione. Hemolysis, jaundice, and hyperbilirubinemia in newborns, particularly in premature infants, have been reported with vitamin K.

Precautions

➤*Monitoring:* Prothrombin time should be checked regularly as clinical conditions indicate.

Drug Interactions

Vitamin K Drug Interactions			
Precipitant drug	Object drug*		Description
Vitamin K	Anticoagulants	⬇	Anticoagulant effects are antagonized by vitamin K. Temporary resistance to oral anticoagulants may result. It may be necessary to increase the anticoagulant dose.
Mineral oil	Vitamin K	⬇	Mineral oil may decrease GI absorption of vitamin K with concurrent oral administration.

* ⬇ = Object drug decreased.

Adverse Reactions

➤*Hyperbilirubinemia:* Hyperbilirubinemia has been observed in the newborn following administration of parenteral phytonadione. This has occurred rarely and primarily with doses above those recommended.

Overdosage

The intravenous and oral LD_{50}s in the mouse are ≈ 1.17 g/kg and greater than 24.18 g/kg, respectively.

PHYTONADIONE — INJECTION

WARNING

IV or IM use – Severe reactions, including fatalities, have occurred during and immediately after intravenous (IV) injection of phytonadione, even when precautions have been taken to dilute the phytonadione and to avoid rapid infusion. Severe reactions, including fatalities, also have been reported following intramuscular (IM) administration. Typically, these severe reactions have resembled hypersensitivity or anaphylaxis, including shock and cardiac or respiratory arrest. Some patients have exhibited these severe reactions on receiving phytonadione for the first time. Therefore, restrict the IV and IM routes to those situations where the subcutaneous route is not feasible and the serious risk involved is considered justified.

Indications

➤*Coagulation disorders:* Phytonadione is indicated in the following coagulation disorders which are due to faulty formation of factors II, VII, IX and X when caused by vitamin K deficiency or interference with vitamin K activity.

Phytonadione injection is indicated in anticoagulant-induced prothrombin deficiency caused by coumarin or indanedione derivatives, prophylaxis and therapy of hemorrhagic disease of the newborn, hypoprothrombinemia secondary to factors limiting absorption or synthesis of vitamin K (eg, obstructive jaundice, biliary fistula, sprue, ulcerative colitis, celiac disease, intestinal resection, cystic fibrosis of the pancreas, regional enteritis), and other drug-induced hypoprothrombinemia where it is definitely shown that the result is due to interference with vitamin K metabolism (eg, salicylates, antibacterial therapy).

Administration and Dosage

➤*Approved by the FDA:* September 30, 1955.

➤*Treatment of hemorrhagic disease of the newborn:* Empiric administration of vitamin K_1 should not replace proper laboratory evaluation of the coagulation mechanism. A prompt response (shortening of the prothrombin time in 2 to 4 hours) following administration of vitamin K_1 is usually diagnostic of hemorrhagic disease of the newborn, and failure to respond indicates another diagnosis or coagulation disorder.

Whole blood or component therapy may be indicated if bleeding is excessive. This therapy, however, does not correct the underlying disorder; give phytonadione concurrently.

➤*Anticoagulant-induced prothrombin deficiency in adults:* Determine frequency and amount of subsequent doses by prothrombin time response or clinical condition. If in 6 to 8 hours after parenteral administration the prothrombin time has not been shortened satisfactorily, repeat the dose.

PHYTONADIONE — INJECTION

Phytonadione Injection Summary of Dosage Guidelines	
Newborns	Dosage
Hemorrhagic disease of the newborn	
Prophylaxis	0.5 to 1 mg IM within 1 hour of birth
Treatment	1 mg subcutaneously or IM (higher doses may be necessary if the mother has been receiving oral anticoagulants)
Adults	Initial dosage
Anticoagulant-induced prothrombin deficiency (caused by coumarin or indanedione derivatives)	2.5 mg to 10 mg or up to 25 mg (rarely 50 mg)
Hypoprothrombinemia due to other causes (antibiotics; salicylates or other drugs; factors limiting absorption or synthesis)	2.5 mg to 25 mg or more (rarely up to 50 mg)

In the event of shock or excessive blood loss, the use of whole blood or component therapy is indicated.

➤*Hypoprothrombinemia due to other causes in adults:* If possible, discontinuation or reduction of the dosage of drugs interfering with coagulation mechanisms (eg, salicylates, antibiotics) is suggested as an alternative to administering concurrent vitamin K_1 injection. The severity of the coagulation disorder should determine whether the immediate administration of vitamin K_1 injection is required in addition to discontinuation or reduction of interfering drugs.

➤*Preparation:* Phytonadione may be diluted with 0.9% sodium chloride injection, 5% dextrose injection, or 5% dextrose and sodium chloride injection. Benzyl alcohol as a preservative has been associated with toxicity in newborns. Therefore, all of the above diluents should be preservative-free. Do not use other diluents. When dilutions are indicated, start administration immediately after mixture with the diluent, and discard unused portions of the dilution, as well as unused contents of the ampul.

➤*Administration of injection:* Whenever possible, give phytonadione by the subcutaneous route. When IV administration is considered unavoidable, inject the drug very slowly, not exceeding 1 mg per minute.

➤*Storage / Stability:* Store at controlled room temperature 15° to 30°C (59° to 86°F). Protect from light. Store ampules in tray until time of use.

Actions

➤*Pharmacology:* Phytonadione aqueous colloidal solution of vitamin K_1 for parenteral injection, possesses the same type and degree of activity as does naturally occurring vitamin K, which is necessary for the production via the liver of active prothrombin (factor II), proconvertin (factor VII), plasma thromboplastin component (factor IX), and Stuart factor (factor X). The prothrombin test is sensitive to the levels of 3 of these 4 factors: II, VII, and X. Vitamin K is an essential cofactor for a microsomal enzyme that catalyzes the post-translational carboxylation of multiple, specific, peptide-bound glutamic acid residues in inactive hepatic precursors of factors II, VII, IX, and X. The resulting gamma-carboxy-glutamic acid residues convert the precursors into active coagulation factors that are subsequently secreted by liver cells into the blood.

In healthy animals and humans, phytonadione is virtually devoid of pharmacodynamic activity. However, in animals and humans deficient in vitamin K, the pharmacological action of vitamin K is related to its normal physiological function, that is, to promote the hepatic biosynthesis of vitamin K-dependent clotting factors.

Contraindications

Hypersensitivity to any component of this medication.

Warnings

➤*Benzyl alcohol:* Benzyl alcohol as a preservative in bacteriostatic sodium chloride injection has been associated with toxicity in newborns. Data are unavailable on the toxicity of other preservatives in this age group. There is no evidence to suggest that the small amount of benzyl alcohol contained in phytonadione, when used as recommended, is associated with toxicity.

➤*Aluminum:* This product may contain aluminum that may be toxic. Aluminum may reach toxic levels with prolonged parenteral administration if kidney function is impaired. Premature neonates are particularly at risk because their kidneys are immature, and they require large amounts of calcium and phosphate solutions, which contain aluminum.

➤*Oral anticoagulant — induced hypoprothrombinemia:* Do not expect an immediate coagulant effect after administration of phytonadione. It takes a minimum of 1 to 2 hours for measurable improvement in the prothrombin time. Whole blood or component therapy may also be necessary if bleeding is severe.

Phytonadione will not counteract the anticoagulant action of heparin.

When vitamin K_1 is used to correct excessive anticoagulant-induced hypoprothrombinemia, anticoagulant therapy still being indicated, the patient is again faced with the clotting hazards existing prior to starting the anticoagulant therapy. Phytonadione is not a clotting agent, but overzealous therapy with vitamin K_1 may restore conditions which originally permitted thromboembolic phenomena. Keep the dosage as low as possible, and check prothrombin time regularly as clinical conditions indicate.

➤*Renal function impairment:* Research indicates that patients with impaired kidney function, including premature neonates, who receive parenteral levels of aluminum at greater than 4 to 5 mcg/kg/day accumulate aluminum at levels associated with CNS and bone toxicity. Tissue loading may occur at even lower rates of administration.

➤*Hepatic function impairment:* Repeated large doses of vitamin K are not warranted in liver disease if the response to initial use of the vitamin is unsatisfactory. Failure to respond to vitamin K may indicate that the condition being treated is inherently unresponsive to vitamin K.

➤*Pregnancy: Category C.* Animal reproduction studies have not been conducted with phytonadione. It is also not known whether phytonadione can cause fetal harm when administered to a pregnant woman or can affect reproduction capacity. Give phytonadione to a pregnant woman only if clearly needed.

➤*Lactation:* It is not known whether this drug is excreted in human milk. Because many drugs are excreted in human milk, exercise caution when phytonadione is administered to a nursing woman.

➤*Children:* Benzyl alcohol has been reported to be associated with a fatal "gasping syndrome" in premature infants.

Hemolysis, jaundice, and hyperbilirubinemia in newborns, particularly in premature infants, may be related to the dose of phytonadione. Therefore, do not exceed the recommended dose.

Precautions

➤*Monitoring:* Check prothrombin time regularly as clinical conditions indicate.

Drug Interactions

Vitamin K Drug Interactions			
Precipitant drug	Object drug*		Description
Vitamin K	Anticoagulants	⬇	Anticoagulant effects are antagonized by vitamin K. Temporary resistance to oral anticoagulants may result. It may be necessary to increase the anticoagulant dose.
Mineral oil	Vitamin K	⬇	Mineral oil may decrease GI absorption of vitamin K with concurrent oral administration.

* ⬇ = Object drug decreased.

Adverse Reactions

➤*Parenteral administration:* Severe reactions, including fatalities, have occurred during and immediately after IV injection of phytonadione, even when precautions have been taken to dilute the phytonadione and to avoid rapid infusion. Severe reactions, including fatalities, also have been reported following IM administration. Typically, these severe reactions have resembled hypersensitivity or anaphylaxis, including shock and cardiac or respiratory arrest. Some patients have exhibited these severe reactions on receiving phytonadione for the first time. Therefore, restrict the IV and IM routes to those situations where the subcutaneous route is not feasible and the serious risk involved is considered justified.

➤*Allergic:* Keep in mind the possibility of allergic sensitivity, including an anaphylactoid reaction.

➤*Miscellaneous:* Transient "flushing sensations" and "peculiar" sensations of taste have been observed, as well as rare instances of dizziness, rapid and weak pulse, profuse sweating, brief hypotension, dyspnea, and cyanosis.

Pain, swelling, and tenderness at the injection site may occur. Infrequently, usually after repeated injection, erythematous, indurated, pruritic plaques have occurred; rarely, these have progressed to scleroderma-like lesions that have persisted for long periods. In other cases, these lesions have resembled erythema perstans.

Hyperbilirubinemia – Hyperbilirubinemia has been observed in the newborn following administration of phytonadione. This has occurred rarely and primarily with doses above those recommended.

Overdosage

The intravenous LD_{50} of phytonadione injection in the mouse is 41.5 and 52 mL/kg for the 0.2% and 1% concentrations, respectively.

Water-Soluble Vitamins

THIAMIN (B_1)

otc	**Thiamine HCl** (Various, eg, Goldline, Rugby)	**Tablets:** 50 mg	In 100s and 250s.
		100 mg	In 100s, 250s, 1000s, and UD 100s.
		250 mg	In 100s, 250s.
otc	**Thiamilate** (Tyson)	**Tablets, enteric-coated:** 20 mg	In 100s.
Rx	**Thiamine HCl** (Various, eg, American Pharmaceutical Partners, ESI)	**Injection:** 100 mg/mL	≤ 9 mg benzyl alcohol. In 1 mL in 2 mL *Tubex* and 2 mL multiple-dose vials.

THIAMIN (B_1) — ORAL

Indications

➤*Thiamin deficiency:* Treatment of thiamin deficiency.

➤*Unlabeled uses:* Oral thiamin has been studied as a mosquito repellant; further verification is needed.

Administration and Dosage

➤*Recommended dietary allowances (RDAs):* Adult males, 1.2 to 1.5 mg/day; adult females, 1 to 1.1 mg/day. Thiamin is recommended at 0.5 mg/1000 Kcal intake. The need for thiamin is greater when the carbohydrate content of the diet is high. For a complete listing of RDAs by age, sex, and condition, refer to the RDA table.

Actions

➤*Pharmacology:* Thiamin is a water-soluble vitamin. Sources include brewer's yeast, legumes, beef, pork, milk, liver, nuts, whole grains, enriched flour, and cereals. The primary functions of thiamin include metabolism of carbohydrates, maintenance of normal growth, transmission of nerve impulses, and acetylcholine synthesis.

Thiamin is essential for normal aerobic metabolism. Thiamin combines with adenosine triphosphate (ATP) and the enzyme thiamin diphosphokinase to form thiamin pyrophosphate, a coenzyme also known as cocarboxylase. Thiamin pyrophosphate is the active form of thiamin. It serves as a coenzyme in the carbohydrate metabolism for the decarboxylation of α keto acids (such as pyruvate) and α-ketoglutarate, as well as serving for the activity of transketolase in the pentose phosphate pathway.

➤*Pharmacokinetics:*

Absorption/Distribution – Thiamin is absorbed by a Na+ dependent active, carrier-mediated process at low concentrations in the jejunum and by passive diffusion in the jejunum and ileum at high concentrations. Maximum oral absorption is 8 to 15 mg/day. Oral absorption may be increased by administering in divided doses with food. Thiamin is mainly stored in the liver but is also found in the brain, kidney, heart, intestine, lung, spleen, and muscle. Tissue stores are saturated when intake exceeds the minimal requirement. For a complete listing of RDAs by age, sex, and condition, refer to the RDA table.

Metabolism/Excretion – Excess thiamin is excreted in the urine both as thiamin acetic acid and metabolites. Approximately 100 mcg/day of thiamin are excreted in the urine with a daily intake of 0.5 mg/1000 kcal. With normal renal function, 80% to 96% of an IV dose is excreted in the urine.

Contraindications

Hypersensitivity to thiamin.

Warnings

➤*Multiple vitamin deficiency:* Simple vitamin B_1 deficiency is rare. Suspect multiple vitamin deficiencies.

➤*Hypersensitivity reactions:* Serious hypersensitivity/anaphylactic reactions can occur.

➤*Pregnancy: Category A* (parenteral). (*Category C* if used in doses greater than the RDA). Studies have not shown an increased risk of fetal abnormalities if administered during pregnancy. The possibility of fetal harm appears remote; however, use during pregnancy only if clearly needed.

➤*Lactation:* It is not known whether this drug is excreted in breast milk. Use with caution in nursing women.

Adverse Reactions

Feeling of warmth; pruritus; urticaria; weakness; sweating; nausea; restlessness; tightness of the throat; angioneurotic edema; cyanosis; pulmonary edema; hemorrhage into the GI tract; cardiovascular collapse; hypersensitivity; anaphylactic shock; death.

Overdosage

Hypersensitivity; anaphylactic shock. Doses of 500 mg/day for a month were administered without toxic effects.

THIAMINE — INJECTION

Indications

➤*Thiamine deficiency:* For the treatment of thiamin deficiency.

➤*Beriberi:* For the treatment of beriberi whether of the dry (major symptoms related to the nervous system) or wet (major symptoms related to the cardiovascular system) variety.

Thiamine HCl injection should be used where rapid restoration of thiamin is necessary, as in Wernicke's encephalopathy, infantile beriberi with acute collapse, cardiovascular disease due to thiamin deficiency, or neuritis of pregnancy if vomiting is severe. It is also indicated when giving IV dextrose to individuals with marginal thiamin status to avoid precipitation of heart failure. Thiamine HCl injection is also indicated in patients with established thiamin deficiency who cannot take thiamine orally due to coexisting severe anorexia, nausea, vomiting, or malabsorption. Thiamine HCl injection is not usually indicated for conditions of decreased oral intake or decreased GI absorption, because multiple vitamins should usually be given.

Administration and Dosage

➤*Beriberi:* "Wet" beriberi with myocardial failure must be treated as an emergency cardiac condition, and thiamin must be administered slowly by the IV route in this situation (see Warnings). In the treatment of beriberi, 10 to 20 mg of thiamine hydrochloride are given IM 3 times daily for as long as 2 weeks (see Warnings). An oral therapeutic multivitamin preparation containing 5 to 10 mg thiamin, administered daily for 1 month, is recommended to achieve body tissue saturation.

➤*Infantile beriberi:* Infantile beriberi that is mild may respond to oral therapy, but if collapse occurs, doses of 25 mg may cautiously be given IV.

Poor dietary habits should be corrected, and an abundant and well-balanced dietary intake should be prescribed.

➤*Neuritis of pregnancy:* Patients with neuritis of pregnancy in whom vomiting is severe enough to preclude adequate oral therapy should receive 5 to 10 mg/day of thiamine hydrochloride IM.

➤*Thiamin deficiency:* IV doses as large as 100 mg/L to correct the deficiency as rapidly as possible. Continue parenteral doses at daily requirements only when GI disturbances prevent adequate oral absorption.

➤*Wernicke-Korsakoff syndrome:* In the treatment of Wernicke-Korsakoff syndrome, thiamine hydrochloride has been administered IV in an initial dose of 100 mg, followed by IM doses of 50 to 100 mg daily until the patient is consuming a regular, balanced diet (see Warnings).

➤*Dextrose and patients with marginal thiamin status:* Patients with marginal thiamin status to whom dextrose is being administered should receive 100 mg thiamine hydrochloride in each of the first few liters of IV fluid to avoid precipitating heart failure.

➤*Incompatibility:* Vitamin B_1 is unstable in neutral or alkaline solutions; do not use in combination with alkaline solutions (eg, carbonates, citrates, barbiturates, acetates, copper ions). Solutions containing sulfites are incompatible with thiamin as are other oxidizing and reducing agents. In vitro testing of thiamin 0.1% reduced activity of erythromycin estolate, kanamycin sulfate, and streptomycin sulfate.

➤*Storage/Stability:* Store at controlled room temperature 15° to 30°C (59° to 86°F). Protect from light.

Use only if solution is clear and seal intact.

Actions

➤*Pharmacokinetics:*

Absorption/Distribution – The water-soluble vitamins are widely distributed in both plants and animals. They are absorbed in man by both diffusion and active transport mechanisms. These vitamins are structurally diverse (derivatives of sugar, pyridine, purines, pyrimidine, organic acid complexes and nucleotide complex) and act as coenzymes, as oxidation-reduction agents, possibly as mitochondrial agents. Thiamin is distributed in all tissues. The highest concentrations occur in the liver, brain, kidney and heart. When thiamin intake is greatly in excess of need, tissue stores increase 2 to 3 times. If intake is insufficient, tissues become depleted of their vitamin content. Absorption of thiamin following IM administration is rapid and complete.

Metabolism/Excretion – Metabolism is rapid, and the excess is excreted in the urine. Thiamin combines with adenosine triphosphate (ATP) to form thiamin pyrophosphate, also known as cocarboxylase, a coenzyme. Its role in carbohydrate metabolism is the decarboxylation of pyruvic acid in the blood and α-ketoacids to acetaldehyde and carbon dioxide. Increased levels of pyruvic acid in the blood indicate vitamin B_1 deficiency. The requirement for thiamin is greater when the carbohydrate content of the diet is raised. Body depletion of vitamin B_1 can occur after ≈ 3 weeks of total absence of thiamin in the diet.

Contraindications

A history of sensitivity to thiamin or to any of the ingredients in this drug is a contraindication (see Warnings).

Warnings

➤*Wernicke's-Korsakoff syndrome:* Thiamin-deficient patients may experience a sudden onset or worsening of Wernicke's encephalopathy following glucose administration; in suspected thiamin deficiency, administer thiamin

THIAMINE — INJECTION

before or along with dextrose-containing fluids.

➤*Hypersensitivity reactions:* Serious hypersensitivity/anaphylactic reactions can occur, especially after repeated administration. Deaths have resulted from IV or IM administration of thiamin (see Adverse Reactions). Routine testing for hypersensitivity, in many cases, may not detect hypersensitivity. Nevertheless, a skin test should be performed on patients who are suspected of drug allergies or previous reactions to thiamin, and any positive responders should not receive thiamin by injection.

If hypersensitivity to thiamin is suspected (based on history of drug allergy or occurrence of adverse reactions after thiamin administration), administer one-hundredth of the dose intradermally and observe for 30 minutes. If no reaction occurs, full dose can be given; the patient should be observed for at least 30 minutes after injection. Be prepared to treat anaphylactic reactions regardless of the precautions taken.

Treatment of anaphylactic reactions includes maintaining a patent airway and the use of epinephrine, oxygen, vasopressors, steroids and antihistamines.

➤*Pregnancy: Category A.* Studies in pregnant women have not shown that thiamine hydrochloride increases the risk of fetal abnormalities if administered during pregnancy. If the drug is used during pregnancy, the possibility of fetal harm appears remote. Because studies cannot rule out the possibility of harm however, thiamine hydrochloride should be used during pregnancy only if clearly needed.

➤*Lactation:* It is not known whether this drug is excreted in human milk. Because many drugs are excreted in human milk, caution should be exercised when thiamine hydrochloride is administered to a nursing mother.

Precautions

➤*Multiple vitamin deficiency:* Simple vitamin B_1 deficiency is rare. Multiple vitamin deficiencies should be suspected in any case of dietary inadequacy.

Adverse Reactions

➤*Hypersensitivity:* An occasional individual may develop a hypersensitivity or life-threatening anaphylactic reaction to thiamin, especially after repeated injection. Collapse and death have been reported.

➤*Local:* Some tenderness and induration may follow IM use (see Warnings).

➤*Miscellaneous:* A feeling of warmth, pruritus, urticaria, weakness, sweating, nausea, restlessness, tightness of the throat, angioneurotic edema, cyanosis, pulmonary edema, and hemorrhage into the GI tract have also been reported.

Overdosage

Parenteral doses of 100 to 500 mg singly have been administered without toxic effects. However, dosages exceeding 30 mg 3 times a day are not utilized effectively. When the body tissues are saturated with thiamin, it is excreted in the urine as pyrimidine. As the intake of thiamin is further increased, it appears unchanged in the urine.

Patient Information

The patient should be advised as to proper dietary habits during treatment so that relapses will be less likely to occur with reduction in dosage or cessation of injection therapy.

RIBOFLAVIN (B_2)

otc	**Riboflavin** (Various, eg, Freeda)	**Tablets:** 50 mg	In 100s and 250s.
		100 mg	In 100s and 250s.

RIBOFLAVIN — ORAL

Indications

Riboflavin is used as a dietary supplement to treat and prevent riboflavin deficiency.

➤*Unlabeled uses:* Lactic acidosis (with hepatic steatosis) in AIDS patients taking nucleoside reverse-transcriptase inhibitors (NRTI) has been successfully treated with riboflavin 50 mg.

Riboflavin is used for the treatment of infants with hyperbilirubinemia.

Riboflavin (400 mg) has been found to be an effective migraine prophylaxis in some patients.

Administration and Dosage

➤*Recommended daily allowances:* The US recommended daily allowance (RDA) of riboflavin for males 14 to 50 years of age is 1.3 mg/day, 1 mg/day in females 14 to 18 years of age, and 1.1 in females 19 years of age and older.

Children (younger than 14 years of age) – The US RDA of riboflavin for children 1 to 3 years is 0.5 mg/day, 0.6 mg/day in children 4 to 8 years, and 0.9 mg/day in children 9 to 13 years of age.

Pregnancy and lactation – Avoid riboflavin use in excess of the RDA during normal pregnancy and breastfeeding. The US RDA of riboflavin is 1.4 mg/day during pregnancy and 1.6 mg/day for nursing mothers.

Dosage ranges are 5 mg to 10 mg/day.

➤*Storage/Stability:* Store away from heat and direct light.

Actions

➤*Pharmacology:* Riboflavin is a water-soluble vitamin that functions as 2 coenzymes. Flavin adenine dinucleotide (FAD) and flavin mononucleotide (FMN) catalyze many oxidation-reduction reactions including glucose oxidation, amino acid deamination, and fatty acid breakdown. Sources of riboflavin include meats, poultry, fish, dairy products, broccoli, turnips, asparagus, spinach, and enriched and fortified grains, cereals, and bakery products.

➤*Pharmacokinetics:* Riboflavin is absorbed from the duodenum and is excreted with its metabolites in the urine. Small amounts of riboflavin are also excreted in the bile, feces, and sweat.

Warnings

➤*Pregnancy: Category A.* (*Category C* in doses that exceed the RDA.)

See Administration and Dosage for more information.

➤*Lactation:* Riboflavin is excreted in breast milk.

See Administration and Dosage for more information.

Precautions

➤*Multiple vitamin deficiency:* Riboflavin deficiency seldom occurs alone and is often associated with deficiency of other vitamin deficiencies.

Adverse Reactions

➤*GU:* Riboflavin may cause urine to have a more yellow color than normal, especially if large doses are taken. This is to be expected and is no cause for alarm. Usually, however, riboflavin does not cause any side effects.

Overdosage

Riboflavin is not toxic in humans because of the limited absorption from the GI tract.

Patient Information

Riboflavin may cause a yellow discoloration of the urine when taken in large doses.

PANTOTHENIC ACID (B_5)

otc	**Calcium Pantothenate** (Various, eg, Freeda)	**Tablets:** 100 mg (equiv. to 92 mg pantothenic acid)	In 100s and 250s.
		218 mg (equiv. to 200 mg pantothenic acid)	In 100s and 250s.
		545 mg (equiv. to 500 mg pantothenic acid)	In 100s and 250s.

CALCIUM PANTOTHENATE — ORAL

Indications

➤*Pantothenic acid deficiency:* As a dietary supplement to treat pantothenic acid deficiency.

Administration and Dosage

An approximate daily dietary intake of 4 to 7 mg/day has been recommended for adults; 2 to 3 mg/day for infants less than or equal to 3 years of age; 3 to 4 mg/day for children 4 to 6 years of age; and 4 to 5 mg/day for children 7 to 10 years of age.

➤*Storage/Stability:* Store in a cool, dry place, away from direct heat and light.

Actions

➤*Pharmacology:* Pantothenic acid is a water-soluble vitamin. Pantothenic acid is a precursor of coenzyme A, which is a cofactor for a variety of enzyme-catalyzed reactions involving transfer of acetyl groups. Functions of pantothenic acid include oxidative metabolism of carbohydrates, gluconeogensis, synthesis and degradation of fatty acids, and synthesis of steroids (cholesterol), steroid hormones, sphingosine, citrate, acetoacetate, and porphyrins. Sources of pantothenic acid include meat, poultry, fish, cereals, fruits, vegetables, milk, and egg yolks.

Deficiency – Deficiency includes neuromuscular degeneration and adrenocortical insufficiency. Pantothenic acid deficiency has not been recognized in humans with a normal diet because of the ubiquitous occurrence of this vitamin in ordinary foods. Deficiency typically is seen only with severe multiple B-complex deficiencies. However, a deficiency syndrome was experimentally

CALCIUM PANTOTHENATE — ORAL

induced in volunteers with the following symptoms: Fatigue, headache, sleep disturbances, abdominal cramps, vomiting, and flatulence. Numbness or tingling in the extremities, muscle cramps, and impaired coordination also occurred.

➤*Pharmacokinetics:*

Absorption/Distribution – Pantothenic acid is absorbed from the GI tract and is distributed to all tissues.

Excretion – Approximately 70% of absorbed pantothenic acid is excreted from the urine.

Warnings

➤*Pregnancy:* Category A (Category C in doses that exceed the RDA). The RDA for pantothenic acid in pregnancy is 10 mg.

➤*Lactation:* Pantothenic acid is excreted in breast milk.

Overdosage

Nontoxic in humans. Diarrhea has been reported with 10 to 20 g/day of calcium pantothenate.

NIACIN (B_3; Nicotinic Acid)

otc[1]	**Nicotinic Acid (Niacin)** (Various, eg, Freeda, Goldline)	**Tablets:** 50 mg	In 100s and 250s.
otc[1]	**Nicotinic Acid (Niacin)** (Various, eg, Freeda, Goldline)	**Tablets:** 100 mg	In 100s and 250s.
otc[1]	**Nicotinic Acid (Niacin)** (Various, eg, Goldline)	**Tablets:** 250 mg	In 100s.
otc[1]	**Nicotinic Acid (Niacin)** (Various, eg, Freeda, Goldline)	**Tablets:** 500 mg	In 100s and 1,000s.
otc[1]	**Nicotinic Acid (Niacin)** (Various, eg, Freeda)	**Tablets, timed-release:** 250 mg	In 100s and 250s.
otc[1]	**Nicotinic Acid (Niacin)** (Various, eg, Goldline)	**Tablets, timed-release:** 500 mg	In 100s and 1,000s.
otc[1]	**Nicotinic Acid (Niacin)** (Various, eg, Naturally)	**Tablets, sustained-release:** 500 mg	In 100s.
otc[1] sf	**Slo-Niacin** (Upsher-Smith)	**Tablets, controlled-release:** 250 mg	(250). Pink. In 100s.
		Tablets, controlled-release: 500 mg	(500). Pink. In 100s.
		Tablets, controlled-release: 750 mg	Pink. In 100s.
otc[1]	**Nicotinic Acid (Niacin)** (Various, eg, Rugby)	**Capsules, extended-release:** 250 mg	In 100s and 1,000s.
otc[1]	**Nicotinic Acid (Niacin)** (Various, eg, Rugby)	**Capsules, extended-release:** 400 mg	In 100s.
otc[1]	**Nicotinic Acid (Niacin)** (Various, eg, Rugby)	**Capsules, sustained-release:** 125 mg	In 100s.
otc[1]	**Nicotinic Acid (Niacin)** (Various, eg, Rugby)	**Capsules, sustained-release:** 500 mg	In 100s.
otc[1]	**Nicotinic Acid (Niacin)** (Various, eg, Goldline, Rugby)	**Capsules, timed-release:** 250 mg	In 100s.
otc[1]	**Nicotinic Acid (Niacin)** (Various, eg, Goldline, Rugby)	**Capsules, timed-release:** 500 mg	In 100s and 1,000s.
Rx	**Niacor** (Upsher-Smith)	**Tablets:** 500 mg	Lactose. (W 901). White, scored. In 100s.
Rx	**Niaspan** (Kos Pharmaceuticals)	**Tablets, extended-release:** 500 mg	(KOS/500). Off-white, capsule shape. In 100s.
		750 mg	(KOS/750). Off-white, capsule shape. In 100s.
		1000 mg	(KOS/1000). Off-white, capsule shape. In 100s.

[1] Some products may be available *Rx*, according to distributor discretion. Most of these products are marketed as nutritional supplements.

NIACIN — ORAL

Also refer to the general discussion of these products in the Antihyperlipidemic Agents Introduction.

Indications

➤*Niacin deficiency:* Treatment of niacin deficiency.

➤*Pellagra:* Prevention and treatment of pellagra.

➤*Hypercholesterolemia:* Adjunct to diet for the reduction of elevated total and LDL levels in patients with primary hypercholesterolemia when the response to diet and other nonpharmacologic measures alone has been inadequate.

➤*Hypertriglyceridemia (Types IV and V):* Adjunctive therapy for treatment in adult patients with very high serum triglyceride levels (Type IV and V hyperlipidemia) who present a risk of pancreatitis and who do not respond adequately to dietary control.

➤*Niacor:*

Hypercholesterolemia – Niacin, alone or in combination with a bile-acid binding resin, is indicated as an adjunct to diet for the reduction of elevated total and LDL cholesterol levels in patients with primary hypercholesterolemia (Types IIa and IIb), (see classification of hyperlipoproteinemias) when the response to a diet restricted in saturated fat and cholesterol and other nonpharmacologic measures alone has been inadequate (see NCEP treatment guidelines).

Hypertriglyceridemia – Niacin is also indicated as adjunctive therapy for treatment of adult patients with very high serum triglyceride levels (Type IV and V hyperlipidemia; see table below) who present a risk of pancreatitis and who do not respond adequately to a determined dietary effort to control them.

➤*Niaspan:*

Hypercholesterolemia – Niacin extended-release tablets are indicated as an adjunct to diet for reduction of elevated TC, LDL-C, Apo B and TG levels, and to increase HDL-C in patients with primary hypercholesterolemia (heterozygous familial and nonfamilial) and mixed dyslipidemia (Frederickson Types IIa and IIb; see table), when the response to an appropriate diet has been inadequate.

Niacin extended-release tablets in combination with a bile acid binding resin is indicated as an adjunct to diet for reduction of elevated TC and LDL-C levels in adult patients with primary hypercholesterolemia (Type IIa, see table), when the response to an appropriate diet, or diet plus monotherapy, has been inadequate.

Combination therapy is not indicated as initial therapy.

Prevention of recurring MI – In patients with a history of MI and hypercholesterolemia, niacin is indicated to reduce the risk of recurrent nonfatal MI.

Atherosclerotic disease – In patients with a history of coronary artery disease (CAD) and hypercholesterolemia, niacin, in combination with a bile acid binding resin, is indicated to slow progression or promote regression of atherosclerotic disease.

Administration and Dosage

➤*Recommended dietary allowances (RDAs):* Adult males, 15 to 20 mg; adult females, 13 to 15 mg. Niacin is recommended at 6.6 mg/1,000 Kcal intake.

To reduce flushing associated with niacin therapy, begin therapy by slowly increasing the dose (100 mg 3 times a day each week).

➤*OTC sustained-release formulations:* Do not substitute sustained-release (modified-release, timed-release) nicotinic acid preparations for equivalent doses of immediate-release (crystalline) nicotinic acid.

➤*Pellagra:* Up to 500 mg/day.

➤*Hyperlipidemia:* 1 to 2 g 2 or 3 times daily. Do not exceed 6 g/day.

➤*OTC:*

Slo-Niacin controlled-release tablets –

Adults:

- *250 or 500 mg* – 1 niacin tablet morning or evening, or as directed by a physician.
- *750 mg* – One-half niacin tablet morning or evening, or as directed by a physician. Before using more than 500 mg daily, consult a physician.

Niacin tablets may be broken on the score line, but should not be crushed or chewed. The inactive matrix of the tablet is not absorbed and may be excreted intact in the stool.

Niacin timed-release capsules – For adults, take 1 capsule daily, or as directed by a physician.

Niacin 500 mg flush-free capsules, *Niacin* 100 mg tablets – For adults, take 1 capsule or tablet daily, preferably with a meal.

➤*Niaspan:* *Niaspan* extended-release tablets should be taken at bedtime, after a low-fat snack, and doses should be individualized according to patient response. Therapy with *Niaspan* extended-release tablets must be initiated at 500 mg every bedtime in order to reduce the incidence and sever-

NIACIN — ORAL

ity of side effects which may occur during early therapy. The recommended dose escalation is shown in the table below.

Recommended Dosing			
	Weeks	Daily dose	*Niaspan* dosing
Initial titration schedule	1 to 4	500 mg	1 *Niaspan* 500 mg tablet at bedtime
	5 to 8	1000 mg	2 *Niaspan* 500 mg tablets at bedtime
	[a]	1500 mg	2 *Niaspan* 750 mg tablets or 3 *Niaspan* 500 mg tablets at bedtime
	[a]	2000 mg	2 *Niaspan* 1000 mg tablets or 4 *Niaspan* 500 mg tablets at bedtime

[a] After week 8, titrate to patient response and tolerance. If response to 1000 mg daily is inadequate, increase dose to 1500 mg daily; may subsequently increase dose to 2000 mg daily. Daily dose should not be increased more than 500 mg in a 4-week period, and doses above 2000 mg daily are not recommended. Women may respond at lower doses than men.

If *Niaspan* extended-release tablet therapy is discontinued for an extended period, reinstitution of therapy should include a titration phase.

Maintenance dose – The daily dosage of *Niaspan* should not be increased by more than 500 mg in any 4-week period.

The recommended maintenance dose is 1000 mg (two 500 mg tablets) to 2000 mg (two 1000 mg tablets or four 500 mg tablets) once daily at bedtime. Doses greater than 2000 mg daily are not recommended. Women may respond at lower *Niaspan* extended-release tablets doses than men.

To reduce flushing: Flushing of the skin may be reduced in frequency or severity by pretreatment with aspirin (taken 30 minutes prior to *Niaspan* extended-release tablet dose) or nonsteroidal anti-inflammatory drugs. Tolerance to this flushing develops rapidly over the course of several weeks. Flushing, pruritus, and gastrointestinal distress are also greatly reduced by slowly increasing the dose of niacin and avoiding administration on an empty stomach.

Tablet interchangeability: Equivalent doses of *Niaspan* extended-release tablets should not be substituted for sustained-release (modified-release, timed-release) niacin preparations or immediate-release (crystalline) niacin. Patients previously receiving other niacin products should be started with the recommended *Niaspan* extended-release tablet titration schedule, and the dose should subsequently be individualized based on patient response. Single-dose bioavailability studies have demonstrated that *Niaspan* extended-release tablet strengths are not interchangeable.

Niaspan extended-release tablets should be taken whole and should not be broken, crushed or chewed before swallowing.

Combination therapy: If lipid response to *Niaspan* extended-release tablets alone is insufficient, or if higher doses of *Niaspan* extended-release tablets are not well tolerated, some patients may benefit from combination therapy with a bile-acid binding resin or an HMG-CoA reductase inhibitor.

Concomitant therapy with lovastatin – Patients already receiving a stable dose of lovastatin who require further TG-lowering or HDL-raising (eg, to achieve NCEP non-HDL-C goals), may receive concomitant dosage titration with *Niaspan* per *Niaspan* recommended initial titration schedule (see table above). For patients already receiving a stable dose of *Niaspan* who require further LDL-lowering (eg, to achieve NCEP LDL-C goals, see table above), the usual recommended starting dose of lovastatin is 20 mg once a day. Dose adjustments should be made at intervals of 4 weeks or more. Combination therapy with *Niaspan* and lovastatin should not exceed doses of 2000 mg and 40 mg daily, respectively.

Renal / hepatic function impairment – Use of *Niaspan* extended-release tablets in patients with renal or hepatic insufficiency has not been studied. *Niaspan* extended-release tablets are contraindicated in patients with significant or unexplained hepatic dysfunction. *Niaspan* extended-release tablets should be used with caution in patients with renal insufficiency.

➤*Niacor*: The usual adult dosage of nicotinic acid is 1 to 2 g 2 or 3 times a day. Doses should be individualized according to the patient's response. Start with one-half tablet (250 mg) as a single daily dose following the evening meal. The frequency of dosing and total daily dose can be increased every 4 to 7 days until the desired LDL cholesterol or triglyceride level is achieved or the first-level therapeutic dose of 1.5 to 2 g/day is reached. If the patient's hyperlipidemia is not adequately controlled after 2 months at this level, the dosage can then be increased at 2- to 4-week intervals to 3 g/day (1 g 3 times per day). In patients with marked lipid abnormalities, a higher dose is occasionally required, but generally should not exceed 6 g/day.

To reduce flushing – Flushing of the skin appears frequently and can be minimized by pretreatment with aspirin or nonsteroidal anti-inflammatory drugs. Tolerance to this flushing develops rapidly over the course of several weeks. Flushing, pruritus, and gastrointestinal distress are also greatly reduced by slowly increasing the dose of nicotinic acid and avoiding administration on an empty stomach.

Tablet interchangeability – Sustained-release (modified-release, timed-release) nicotinic acid preparations should not be substituted for equivalent doses of immediate-release (crystalline) nicotinic acid.

➤*Storage / Stability:* Store at room temperature, 20° to 25°C (68° to 77°F).

Slo-Niacin and *Niacor* – Store at room temperature, 15° to 30°C (59° to 86°F).

Actions

➤*Pharmacology:* Niacin, vitamin B_3, is the common name for nicotinic acid and niacinamide (nicotinamide). Nicotinic acid is present in the body as its active form, nicotinamide (niacinamide). Nicotinamide functions in the body as a component of 2 coenzymes: NAD (nicotinamide adenine dinucleotide, coenzyme I) and NADP (nicotinamide adenine dinucleotide phosphate, coenzyme II), which serve a role in oxidation-reduction reactions. Sources of niacin include niacinamide and tryptophan as well as liver, meat, fish, poultry, whole-grain and enriched breads and cereals, nuts, legumes, green vegetables, yeast, and potatoes. Approximately 60 mg of tryptophan is equivalent to 1 mg of niacin.

The mechanism by which niacin alters lipid profiles has not been well defined. It may involve several actions including partial inhibition of release of free fatty acids from adipose tissue, and increased lipoprotein lipase activity, which may increase the rate of chylomicron triglyceride removal from plasma. Niacin decreases the rate of hepatic synthesis of VLDL and LDL, and does not appear to affect fecal excretion of fats, sterols, or bile acids.

Nicotinic acid (but not nicotinamide) in gram doses produces an average 10% to 20% reduction in total and LDL cholesterol, a 30% to 70% reduction in triglycerides, and an average 20% to 35% increase in HDL cholesterol. The magnitude of individual lipid and lipoprotein responses may be influenced by the severity and type of underlying lipid abnormality. The increase in total HDL is associated with a shift in the distribution of HDL subfractions (as defined by ultra-centrifugation) with an increase in the HDL_2:HDL_3 ratio and an increase in apolipoprotein A-I content.

➤*Pharmacokinetics:*

Absorption –

Niaspan extended-release tablets: Niacin is rapidly and extensively absorbed (at least 60% to 76% of dose) when administered orally. To maximize bioavailability and reduce the risk of gastrointestinal (GI) upset, administration of *Niaspan* extended-release tablets with a low-fat meal or snack is recommended.

Single-dose bioavailability studies have demonstrated that *Niaspan* extended-release tablet strengths are not interchangeable.

Niacor tablets: Following an oral dose, the pharmacokinetic profile of nicotinic acid is characterized by rapid absorption from the gastrointestinal tract and a short plasma elimination half-life. At a 1 g dose, peak plasma concentrations of 15 to 30 mcg/mL are reached within 30 to 60 minutes.

Distribution –

Niaspan extended-release tablets: Studies using radiolabeled niacin in mice show that niacin and its metabolites concentrate in the liver, kidney and adipose tissue.

Metabolism –

Niaspan extended-release tablets: The pharmacokinetic profile of niacin is complicated due to rapid and extensive first-pass metabolism, which is species and dose-rate specific. In humans, 1 pathway is through a simple conjugation step with glycine to form nicotinuric acid (NUA). NUA is then excreted in the urine, although there may be a small amount of reversible metabolism back to niacin. The other pathway results in the formation of nicotinamide adenine dinucleotide (NAD). It is unclear whether nicotinamide is formed as a precursor to, or following the synthesis of, NAD. Nicotinamide is further metabolized to at least N-methylnicotinamide (MNA) and nicotinamide-N-oxide (NNO). MNA is further metabolized to 2 other compounds, N-methyl-2-pyridone-5-carboxamide (2PY) and N-methyl-4-pyridone-5-carboxamide (4PY). The formation of 2PY appears to predominate over 4PY in humans. At the doses used to treat hyperlipidemia, these metabolic pathways are saturable, which explains the nonlinear relationship between niacin dose and plasma concentrations following multiple-dose *Niaspan* extended-release tablet administration.

Nicotinamide does not have hypolipidemic activity; the activity of the other metabolites is unknown.

Excretion – Niacin and its metabolites are rapidly eliminated in the urine. Following single and multiple doses, approximately 60% to 76% of the niacin dose administered as *Niaspan* extended-release tablets were recovered in urine as niacin and metabolites; up to 12% was recovered as unchanged niacin after multiple dosing. The ratio of metabolites recovered in the urine was dependent on the dose administered.

Niacor tablets: Approximately 88% of an oral pharmacologic dose is eliminated by the kidneys as unchanged drug and nicotinuric acid, its primary metabolite.

The plasma elimination half-life of nicotinic acid ranges from 20 to 45 minutes.

Special populations –

Renal function impairment: There are no data in this population. *Niaspan* extended-release tablets should be used with caution in patients with renal disease.

Hepatic function impairment: No studies have been performed. *Niaspan* extended-release tablets should be used with caution in patients with a history of liver disease, who consume substantial quantities of alcohol, or have unexplained transaminase elevations. *Niaspan* extended-release tablets are contraindicated in patients with active liver disease.

Gender: Steady-state plasma concentrations of niacin and metabolites after administration of *Niaspan* are generally higher in women than in men, with the magnitude of the difference varying with dose and metabolite. Recovery of niacin and metabolites in urine, however, is generally similar for men and women, indicating that absorption is similar for both genders. The gender differences observed in plasma levels of niacin and its metabolites may be due to gender-specific differences in metabolic rate or volume of distribution. Data from the clinical trials suggest that women have a greater hypolipidemic response than men at equivalent doses of *Niaspan* extended-release tablets.

NIACIN — ORAL

Contraindications

Niacin should not be administered unless recommended by and taken under the supervision of a physician if any of the following conditions exist: Gallbladder disease, gout, arterial bleeding, glaucoma, diabetes, impaired liver function, peptic ulcer, pregnancy, or lactation.

Known hypersensitivity to niacin or any component of this medication; significant or unexplained hepatic dysfunction; active peptic ulcer disease; arterial bleeding.

Warnings

➤*Schizophrenia:* There is no evidence to support the use of nicotinic acid in the treatment of schizophrenia as part of what is referred to as "orthomolecular psychiatry".

➤*Heart disease:* Persons with heart disease, particularly those who have recurrent chest pain (angina) or who recently suffered a heart attack, should take niacin only under the supervision of a physician. Persons taking high blood pressure or cholesterol-lowering drugs should contact a physician before taking niacin because of possible interactions. Increased uric acid and glucose levels and abnormal liver function tests have been reported in persons taking daily doses of 500 mg or more of niacin.

Discontinue use if adverse reactions occur.

➤*Skeletal muscle effects:* Rare cases of rhabdomyolysis have been associated with concomitant administration of lipid-altering doses (greater than or equal to 1 g/day) of niacin and HMG-CoA reductase inhibitors. In clinical studies with a combination tablet of *Niaspan* and lovastatin, no cases of rhabdomyolysis and 1 suspected case of myopathy have been reported in 1079 patients who were treated with doses of up to 2000 mg of *Niaspan* and 40 mg of lovastatin daily for periods of up to 2 years. Physicians contemplating combined therapy with HMG-CoA reductase inhibitors and nicotinic acid should carefully weigh the potential benefits and risks and should carefully monitor patients for any signs and symptoms of muscle pain, tenderness, or weakness, particularly during the initial months of therapy and during any periods of upward dosage titration of either drug. Periodic serum creatine phosphokinase (CPK) and potassium determinations should be considered in such situations, but there is no assurance that such monitoring will prevent the occurrence of severe myopathy.

➤*Extended-release preparations:* Niacin extended-release tablet preparations should not be substituted for equivalent doses of immediate-release (crystalline) niacin. For patients switching from immediate-release niacin to niacin extended-release tablets, therapy with niacin extended-release tablets should be initiated with low doses (ie, 500 mg every night) and the niacin extended-release tablet dose should then be titrated to the desired therapeutic response.

➤*Hepatic effects:* Cases of severe hepatic toxicity, including fulminant hepatic necrosis, have occurred in patients who have substituted sustained-release (modified-release, timed-release) niacin products for immediate-release (crystalline) niacin at equivalent doses.

Niacin preparations, like some other lipid-lowering therapies, have been associated with abnormal liver tests. In 3 placebo-controlled clinical trials involving titration to final daily nicotinic acid doses ranging from 500 to 3000 mg, 245 patients received nicotinic acid for a mean duration of 17 weeks. No patient with normal serum transaminase levels (AST, ALT) at baseline experienced elevations to more than 3 times the upper limit of normal (ULN) during treatment with nicotinic acid. In these studies, fewer than 1% (2/245) of nicotinic acid patients discontinued due to transaminase elevations greater than 2 times the ULN.

In 3 safety and efficacy studies with a combination tablet of *Niaspan* and lovastatin involving titration to final daily doses (expressed as mg of *Niaspan*/mg of lovastatin) 500 mg/10 mg to 2500 mg/40 mg, 10 of 1028 patients (1%) experienced reversible elevations in AST/ALT to more than 3 times the ULN. Three of 10 elevations occurred at doses outside the recommended dosing limit of 2000 mg/40 mg; no patients receiving 1000 mg/20 mg had 3-fold elevations in AST/ALT.

In the placebo-controlled clinical trials and the long-term extension study, elevations in transaminases did not appear to be related to treatment duration; elevations in AST levels did appear to be dose related. Transaminase elevations were reversible upon discontinuation of nicotinic acid.

➤*Renal/Hepatic function impairment:* Nicotinic acid should be used with caution in patients who have a history of liver disease. Active liver diseases or unexplained transaminase elevations are contraindications to the use of nicotinic acid.

Niaspan – Niacin is rapidly metabolized by the liver, and excreted through the kidneys. *Niaspan* extended-release tablets are contraindicated in patients with significant or unexplained hepatic dysfunction and should be used with caution in patients with renal dysfunction.

➤*Pregnancy: Category A* (*Category C* if used in doses above the RDA). Animal reproduction studies have not been conducted with niacin. It is not known whether nicotinic acid at doses typically used for lipid disorders can cause fetal harm when administered to pregnant women. If a woman receiving niacin or nicotinic acid for primary hypercholesterolemia (Types IIa or IIb) becomes pregnant, discontinue the drug. If a woman being treated with niacin or nicotinic acid for hypertriglyceridemia (Types IV or V) conceives, assess the benefits and risks of continued drug therapy on an individual basis.

➤*Lactation:* Niacin has been reported to be excreted in human milk. Because of the potential for serious adverse reactions in nursing infants from lipid-altering doses of nicotinic acid, a decision should be made whether to discontinue nursing or to discontinue the drug, taking into account the importance of the drug to the mother.

➤*Children:* Safety and effectiveness of niacin therapy in pediatric patients (less than or equal to 16 years for niacin extended-release tablets) have not been established. No studies in patients under 21 years of age have been conducted with niacin extended-release tablets.

Precautions

➤*Monitoring:* Patients with a history of jaundice, hepatobiliary disease, or peptic ulcer should be observed closely during niacin therapy. Frequent monitoring of liver function tests and blood glucose should be performed to ascertain that the drug is producing no adverse effects on these organ systems.

Liver tests should be performed on all patients during therapy with niacin. Serum transaminase levels, including AST and ALT, should be monitored before treatment begins, every 6 to 12 weeks for the first year, and periodically thereafter (eg, at approximately 6-month intervals). Special attention should be paid to patients who develop elevated serum transaminase levels, and in these patients, measurements should be repeated promptly and then performed more frequently. If the transaminase levels show evidence of progression, particularly if they rise to 3 times the upper limit of normal and are persistent, or if they are associated with symptoms of nausea, fever, or malaise, the drug should be discontinued.

➤*Diabetes:* Diabetic patients may experience a dose-related rise in glucose intolerance, the clinical significance of which is unclear. Diabetic or potentially diabetic patients should be observed closely. Adjustment of diet or hypoglycemic therapy may be necessary.

➤*Flushing:* Flushing appears frequently with oral therapy and generally begins 20 minutes after ingestion and lasts 30 to 60 minutes. Flushing is transient and will usually subside after 3 to 6 weeks of continued therapy. The flush response can be attenuated by slowly increasing the niacin dose (100 mg 3 times daily each week), administering with food or milk, or by administering either a prostaglandin inhibitor, such as aspirin 325 mg 60 minutes prior to niacin administration, or sustained-release niacin preparations.

➤*Hyperlipidemia:* Before instituting therapy with niacin, an attempt should be made to control hyperlipidemia with appropriate diet, exercise, and weight reduction in obese patients, and to treat other underlying medical problems.

➤*Alcohol:* Use with caution in patients who consume substantial quantities of alcohol or have a history of liver disease.

➤*Heart disease:* Caution should also be used when niacin is used in patients with unstable angina or in the acute phase of MI, particularly when such patients are also receiving vasoactive drugs such as nitrates, calcium channel blockers, or adrenergic blocking agents.

➤*Gout:* Elevated uric acid levels have occurred with niacin therapy; therefore, use with caution in patients predisposed to gout.

➤*Lab test abnormalities:* In placebo-controlled trials, *Niaspan* extended-release tablets have been associated with small but statistically significant, dose-related reductions in phosphorus levels (mean of −13% with 2000 mg). Although these reductions were transient, phosphorus levels should be monitored periodically in patients at risk for hypophosphatemia.

Drug Interactions

➤*HMG-CoA reductase inhibitors:* Rare cases of rhabdomyolysis have been associated with concomitant administration of lipid-altering doses (greater than or equal to 1 g/day) of niacin and HMG-CoA reductase inhibitors. In clinical studies with a combination tablet of *Niaspan* and lovastatin, no cases of rhabdomyolysis and 1 suspected case of myopathy have been reported in 1079 patients who were treated with doses of up to 2000 mg of *Niaspan* and 40 mg of lovastatin daily for periods of up to 2 years. Physicians contemplating combined therapy with HMG-CoA reductase inhibitors and nicotinic acid should carefully weigh the potential benefits and risks and should carefully monitor patients for any signs and symptoms of muscle pain, tenderness, or weakness, particularly during the initial months of therapy and during any periods of upward dosage titration of either drug. Periodic serum creatine phosphokinase (CPK) and potassium determinations should be considered in such situations, but there is no assurance that such monitoring will prevent the occurrence of severe myopathy.

➤*Anticoagulants: Niaspan* extended-release tablets have been associated with small but statistically significant dose-related reductions in platelet count (mean of −11% with 2000 mg). In addition, *Niaspan* extended-release tablets have been associated with small but statistically significant increases in prothrombin time (mean of approximately +4%); accordingly, patients undergoing surgery should be carefully evaluated. Caution should be observed when *Niaspan* extended-release tablets are administered concomitantly with anticoagulants; prothrombin time and platelet counts should be monitored closely in such patients.

➤*Antihypertensive therapy:* Niacin may potentiate the effects of ganglionic blocking agents and vasoactive drugs resulting in postural hypotension.

➤*Aspirin:* Concomitant aspirin may decrease the metabolic clearance of nicotinic acid. The clinical relevance of this finding is unclear.

➤*Alcohol or hot drinks:* Concomitant alcohol or hot drinks may increase the side effects of flushing and pruritus and should be avoided around the time of nicotinic acid ingestion.

➤*Bile-acid sequestrants:* An in vitro study was carried out investigating the niacin-binding capacity of colestipol and cholestyramine. About 98% of available niacin was bound to colestipol, with 10% to 30% binding to cholestyramine. These results suggest that 4 to 6 hours, or as great an interval as

NIACIN — ORAL

possible, should elapse between the ingestion of bile acid-binding resins and the administration of niacin extended-release tablets or other niacin products.

➤*Other sources of niacin:* Vitamins or other nutritional supplements containing large doses of niacin or related compounds such as nicotinamide may potentiate the adverse effects of niacin extended-release tablets or other niacin products.

➤*Drug/Lab test interactions:* Niacin may produce false elevations in some fluorometric determinations of plasma or urinary catecholamines. Niacin may also give false-positive reactions with cupric sulfate solution (Benedict's reagent) in urine glucose tests.

Adverse Reactions

➤*Miscellaneous:* Niacin may cause temporary flushing, itching and tingling, feelings of warmth and headache, particularly when beginning, increasing amount or changing brands of niacin. These effects seldom require discontinuing niacin use. Skin rash, upset stomach, and low blood pressure when standing are less common symptoms; if they persist, contact a physician.

➤*Niaspan* extended-release tablets: *Niaspan* extended-release tablets are generally well tolerated; adverse reactions have been mild and transient. In the placebo-controlled clinical trials, flushing episodes (ie, warmth, redness, itching or tingling) were the most common treatment-emergent adverse events (reported by as many as 88% of patients) for *Niaspan* extended-release tablets. Spontaneous reports suggest that flushing may also be accompanied by symptoms of dizziness, tachycardia, palpitations, shortness of breath, sweating, chills, or edema, which in rare cases may lead to syncope. In pivotal studies, fewer than 6% (14/245) of *Niaspan* extended-release tablet patients discontinued due to flushing. In comparisons of immediate-release niacin and *Niaspan* extended-release tablets, although the proportion of patients who flushed was similar, fewer flushing episodes were reported by patients who received *Niaspan* extended-release tablets. Following 4 weeks of maintenance therapy at daily doses of 1500 mg, the incidence of flushing over the 4-week period averaged 8.56 events per patient for IR niacin versus 1.88 following *Niaspan* extended-release tablets.

Other adverse reactions occurring in 5% or greater of patients treated with *Niaspan* extended-release tablets, at least remotely related to *Niaspan* extended-release tablets, are shown in the table below.

Treatment-Emergent Adverse Reactions by Dose Level in ≥ 5% of Patients; Reactions Considered at Least Remotely Related to Study Medication

Placebo-controlled studies *Niaspan* extended-release tablets treatment[1]							
			Recommended daily maintenance doses			Greater than recommended daily doses	
Adverse reaction	Placebo (n = 157) %	500 mg[2] (n = 87) %	1,000 mg (n = 110) %	1,500 mg (n = 136) %	2,000 mg (n = 95) %	2,500 mg[2] (n = 49) %	3,000 mg[2] (n = 46) %
Headache	15%	5%[3]	9%	11%	8%	4%[3]	4%
Pain	3%	1%	2%	5%	3%	0%	2%
Pain, abdominal	3%	3%	2%	3%	5%	0%	0%
Diarrhea	8%	6%	7%	6%	8%	10%	11%
Dyspepsia	8%	2%	4%	5%	5%	6%	0%
Nausea	4%	2%	5%	3%	8%	10%	4%
Vomiting	2%	0%	2%	3%	8%[3]	8%	2%
Rhinitis	7%	2%	5%	4%	3%	0%	0%
Pruritus	1%	6%	less than 1%	3%	1%	0%	0%
Rash	less than 1%	5%	5%	4%	0%	0%	0%

[1] Pooled results from placebo-controlled studies; for *Niaspan* extended-release tablets, (n = 245) and mean treatment duration = 17 weeks. Number of *Niaspan* extended-release tablet patients (n) are not additive across doses.
[2] The 500 mg, 2500 mg and 3000 mg/day doses are outside the recommended daily maintenance dosing range.
[3] Significantly different from placebo at P ≤ 0.05; Chi-square test (cell sizes greater than 5), Fisher's Exact test (cell sizes less than or equal to 5). In general, the incidence of adverse events was higher in women compared to men.

➤*Niaspan* extended-release tablets: The following adverse reactions have also been reported with niacin products, either during clinical trials or in routine patient management.

Cardiovascular – Atrial fibrillation, and other cardiac arrhythmias; tachycardia; palpitations; orthostasis; syncope; hypotension.

CNS – Dizziness, insomnia.

Dermatologic – Hyperpigmentation; acanthosis nigricans; maculopapular rash; urticaria; dry skin; sweating.

Hematologic – Slight reductions in platelet counts and prolongation in prothrombin time.

GI – Activation of peptic ulcers and peptic ulceration; jaundice.

Lab test abnormalities – Elevations in serum transaminases, LDH, fasting glucose, uric acid, total bilirubin, and amylase; reductions in phosphorus.

Metabolic – Decreased glucose tolerance; gout.

Musculoskeletal – Myalgia.

Ophthalmic – Toxic amblyopia, cystoid macular edema.

Miscellaneous – Edema, asthenia, chills, migraine.

➤*Niacor* tablets:

Cardiovascular – Atrial fibrillation and other cardiac arrhythmias; orthostasis; hypotension.

CNS – Headache.

Dermatologic – Mild to severe cutaneous flushing; pruritus; hyperpigmentation; acanthosis nigricans; dry skin.

GI – Dyspepsia; vomiting; diarrhea; peptic ulceration; jaundice; abnormal liver function tests.

Metabolic – Decreased glucose-tolerance; hyperuricemia; gout.

Ophthalmic – Toxic amblyopia; cystoid macular edema.

Overdosage

➤*Treatment:* Supportive measures should be undertaken in the event of an overdosage.

Patient Information

➤*OTC:* Use of niacin may cause skin flushing, burning, itching, or rash.

May cause GI upset; take with meals.

Do not take more than 500 mg of niacin per day or switch to more than 250 mg of timed-release niacin per day, except under the supervision of a doctor.

Discontinue use and consult a physician immediately if any of the following symptoms occur: Persistent flu-like symptoms (nausea, vomiting, a general "not well" feeling); loss of appetite; a decrease in urine output associated with dark-colored urine; muscle discomfort such as tender, swollen muscles or muscle weakness; irregular heartbeat; or cloudy or blurry vision.

If you are pregnant or breastfeeding, consult with your doctor prior to use.

If dizziness (postural hypotension) occurs, avoid sudden changes in posture.

Extended-release products – Swallow whole; do not break, crush, or chew.

➤*Rx:* Cutaneous flushing and a sensation of warmth, especially of the face and upper body, may occur. Itching or tingling and headache also may occur. These effects are transient and usually subside with continued therapy.

Niaspan extended-release tablets – Take *Niaspan* extended-release tablets at bedtime after a low-fat snack. Administration on an empty stomach is not recommended.

Carefully follow the prescribed dosing regimen, including the recommended titration schedule, in order to minimize side effects.

Flushing is a common side effect of niacin therapy. Flushing may vary in severity, may last for several hours after dosing, and will, by taking *Niaspan* extended-release tablets at bedtime, most likely occur during sleep; however, if awakened by flushing at night, get up slowly, especially if feeling dizzy, feeling faint, or taking blood pressure medications.

Taking aspirin (approximately 30 minutes before taking *Niaspan* extended-release tablets) or a nonsteroidal anti-inflammatory drug (eg, ibuprofen) may minimize flushing.

Avoid ingestion of alcohol or hot drinks around the time of *Niaspan* extended-release tablets administration, to minimize flushing.

If *Niaspan* extended-release tablet therapy is discontinued for an extended length of time, the physician should be contacted prior to re-starting therapy; retitration is recommended.

Notify physician if they are taking vitamins or other nutritional supplements containing niacin or related compounds such as nicotinamide.

Notify physician if symptoms of dizziness occur. Avoid sudden changes in posture.

If diabetic, notify physician of changes in blood glucose.

Niaspan extended-release tablets should not be broken, crushed or chewed, but should be swallowed whole.

NIACINAMIDE (NICOTINAMIDE)

otc[1]	**Niacinamide (Nicotinamide)** (Various, eg, Freeda, Rugby)	**Tablets:** 100 mg	In 100s and 250s.
		500 mg	In 100s and 250s.

[1] Some products may be available *Rx*, according to distributor discretion.

NIACINAMIDE — ORAL

For complete and comparative prescribing information, refer to the Niacin monograph.

Indications

➤*Dietary supplement:* Niacinamide, 1 of 2 principle forms of niacin, is used as a dietary supplement when niacin intake may be inadequate.

➤*Pellagra:* Niacinamide is used in the prophylaxis and treatment of pellagra, a niacin deficiency condition. Symptoms of pellagra include stomach problems, sores in the mouth, anemia, and a triad of symptoms including dermatitis, diarrhea, and dementia.

➤*Unlabeled uses:* Treatment of several dermatologic conditions, including necrobiosis lipoidica, erythema multiforme, dermatitis herpetiformis, erythema elevatum diutinum, polymorphic light eruption, erythema induration, granuloma annulare, and psoriasis (500 mg 3 times daily).

Administration and Dosage

➤*Recommended daily allowance (RDA):* The US recommended daily allowance (RDA) of niacin equivalents for males 14 years of age and older is 16 mg/day and 14 mg/day in females 14 years of age and older.

The US RDA for children 1 to 3 years is 6 mg/day, 8 mg/day in children 4 to 8 years, and 12 mg/day niacin equivalents in children 9 to 13 years of age.

Pregnancy and lactation – The RDA of niacin equivalents is 18 mg/day during pregnancy and 17 mg/day for breastfeeding women.

Niacinamide is available as a single ingredient product and in multivitamin and multivitamin/multimineral products. Typical supplemental dosage ranges from 20 to 100 mg daily.

Pre- and postnatal vitamin/mineral supplements typically deliver a dose of 20 mg daily.

To treat deficiency, the dose is determined by the prescriber for each individual based on the severity of deficiency.

➤*Storage/Stability:* Store away from heat and direct light.

Actions

➤*Pharmacology:* Niacinamide is synonymous with nicotinamide, 3-pyridine carboxamide, and nicotinic acid amide. Nicotinic acid is present in the body as its active form, nicotinamide (niacinamide). Nicotinamide and nicotinic acid have identical vitamin activities, but they have very different pharmacological activities. Nicotinamide functions in the body as a component of 2 coenzymes: NAD (nicotinamide adenine dinucleotide, coenzyme I) and NADP (nicotinamide adenine dinucleotide phosphate, coenzyme II). These coenzymes participate in glycogenolysis, fatty metabolism, and tissue respiration. Although nicotinic acid and nicotinamide function identically as vitamins, their pharmacologic effects differ. Nicotinamide does not have the hypolipidemic or vasodilating effects characteristic of niacin (nicotinic acid). Nicotinamide has been shown to inhibit activated macrophage killing of beta cells in vitro and reduce induction of class II MHC protein on mouse beta cells.

Contraindications

Hepatic dysfunction; active peptic ulcer; hypersensitivity to nicotinamide or any ingredient.

Warnings

➤*Pregnancy:* Avoid niacinamide use in excess of the RDA during normal pregnancy.

➤*Lactation:* Avoid niacinamide use in excess of the RDA during normal breastfeeding.

Precautions

➤*Special risk:* Use niacinamide cautiously in patients with diabetes mellitus, gout, liver disease, or stomach ulcers.

Adverse Reactions

➤*GI:* Nausea, vomiting, diarrhea, abdominal pain, dyspepsia.

➤*Hepatic:* Liver dysfunction at high doses.

Patient Information

Cutaneous flushing and a sensation of warmth, especially in the face, may occur. Itching or tingling and headache may also occur. These effects are transient and will usually subside with continued therapy.

May cause GI upset; take with meals.

Discontinue use and consult a physician immediately if any of the following symptoms occur: Persistent flu-like symptoms (nausea, vomiting, a general "not well" feeling; loss of appetite; a decrease in urine output associated with dark-colored urine; muscle discomfort such as tender, swollen muscles or muscle weakness; irregular heartbeat; or cloudy or blurry vision.

If dizziness (postural hypotension) occurs, avoid sudden changes in posture.

PYRIDOXINE HCl (B_6)

otc	**Vitelle Nestrex** (Fielding)	**Tablets:** 25 mg	Dextrose. In 100s.
otc	**Vitamin B_6** (Various, eg, Freeda, Goldline, Nutro Labs)	**Tablets:** 50 mg	In 100s, 250s, and 1000s.
otc	**Vitamin B_6** (Various, eg, Freeda, Goldline, Naturally)	**Tablets:** 100 mg	In 100s and 250s.
otc	**Vitamin B_6** (Various, eg, Freeda)	**Tablets:** 250 mg	In 100s.
otc	**Vitamin B_6** (Various, eg, Naturally)	**Tablets:** 500 mg	In 100s.
otc	**Aminoxin** (Tyson & Assoc.)	**Tablets, enteric-coated:** 20 mg[1]	In 100s.
Rx	**Pyridoxine HCl** (Various, eg, American Pharm. Assoc.)	**Injection:** 100 mg/mL[2]	In 1 mL vials.[3]

[1] As pyridoxal-5′-phosphate.
[2] As pyridoxine HCl.
[3] Also contains 5 mg chorobutanol anhydrous.

PYRIDOXINE HYDROCHLORIDE — ORAL

Indications

➤*Pyridoxine deficiency:* Pyridoxine is used as a dietary supplement to treat pyridoxine deficiency, including drug-induced deficiency (eg, isoniazid, hydralazine, oral contraceptives).

➤*Unlabeled uses:* Treatment of palmar-plantar erythrodysesthesia syndrome (hand-foot syndrome).

Hydrazine poisoning – Although experience is limited, reversal of neurologic symptoms and CNS depression have been reported.

Premenstrual syndrome (PMS) – PMS has been treated with pyridoxine 40 to 500 mg/day, but with conflicting results.

Hyperoxaluria type I – Hyperoxaluria type I (and oxalate kidney stones) has been treated with pyridoxine in low doses (25 to 300 mg/day).

Nausea and vomiting in pregnancy – Pyridoxine may treat nausea and vomiting during pregnancy.

Carpal tunnel syndrome – 100 to 200 mg/day for greater than or equal to 12 weeks.

Tardive dyskinesia induced by antipsychotic treatment – 100 mg/day for 4 weeks.

Administration and Dosage

➤*Recommended daily allowance (RDAs):* The US recommended daily allowance (RDA) for males and females 14 to 50 years of age is 1.2 to 1.3 mg/day and 1.5 to 1.7 mg/day in males and females greater than 50 years of age.

The US RDA for children 1 to 3 years is 0.5 mg/day, 0.6 mg/day in children 4 to 8 years, and 1 mg/day in children 9 to 13 years of age.

Pregnancy and lactation – Avoid pyridoxine use in excess of the RDA during normal pregnancy and breastfeeding. The RDA of pyridoxine is 1.9 mg/day during pregnancy and 2 mg/day for nursing mothers.

Pyridoxine is available in multivitamin and multivitamin/multimineral products, as well as products that, in addition to vitamins and minerals, contain other nutritional substances. Single ingredient products are also available. Typical doses of pyridoxine used for nutritional supplementation range from 100 to 200 mg daily.

To treat deficiency, the dose is determined by the prescriber for each individual based on the severity of disease.

➤*Storage/Stability:* Store away from heat and direct light.

Actions

➤*Pharmacology:* Pyridoxine, pyridoxal, or pyridoxamine (in animals) are converted to the physiologically active forms of vitamin B6, pyridoxal phosphate and pyridoxamine phosphate.

Pyridoxine is a coenzyme in the metabolism of amino acids, glycogen, and sphingoid bases and necessary for normal breakdown of proteins, carbohydrates, and fats. Vitamin B_6 is essential to make hemoglobin and helps increase the amount of oxygen carried by hemoglobin. Vitamin B_6 is also involved in maintaining the health of the immune system including maintaining the health of lymphoid organs (thymus, spleen, and lymph nodes) that make white blood cells. Vitamin B_6 maintains normal levels of blood

PYRIDOXINE HYDROCHLORIDE — ORAL

glucose by helping convert stored carbohydrates or other nutrients to glucose. Vitamin B_6 also is needed for the conversion of tryptophan to niacin.

Vitamin E deficiency is extremely rare in humans; symptoms include ataxia, muscle weakness, nystagmus, and losses in touch and pain sensations.

➤*Pharmacokinetics:*

Absorption/Distribution – Vitamin B_6 is absorbed by passive diffusion in the jejunum and to a lesser extent in the ileum.

Metabolism/Excretion – Vitamin B_6 is converted to pyridoxal-5-phosphate in the liver and excreted mostly as 4-pyridoxic acid in the urine.

Contraindications

Sensitivity to pyridoxine.

Warnings

➤*Pregnancy: Category A* (*Category C* in doses that exceed the RDA). Avoid pyridoxine use in excess of the RDA during normal pregnancy. The RDA of pyridoxine is 1.9 mg/day during pregnancy.

➤*Lactation:* Vitamin B_6 is excreted in breast milk and is directly proportional to maternal intake. Convulsions have been reported in infants fed a pyridoxine-deficient diet. Neonatal seizures have been noted following birth in a mother consuming pyridoxine 80 mg/day or in infants whose mothers' breast milk contained 67 mcg/day (less than 20 ng/mL in a separate report). These seizures responded to pyridoxine therapy. Pyridoxine has been reported to inhibit lactation at oral doses of 600 mg/day.

Avoid pyridoxine use in excess of the RDA during normal breastfeeding. The RDA of pyridoxine is 2 mg/day for nursing mothers.

➤*Children:* Safety and efficacy have not been established for use in children in doses that exceed the RDA.

Precautions

➤*Pyridoxine deficiency:* Pyridoxine deficiency alone is rare; multiple vitamin deficiencies can be expected in any inadequate diet. Some drugs may result in increased pyridoxine requirements, including the following: Cycloserine, hydralazine, isoniazid, oral contraceptives, and penicillamine.

➤*Special risk:* Use pyridoxine cautiously in patients being treated with levodopa and phenytoin.

➤*Drug abuse and dependence:* Noted in adults withdrawn from 200 mg/day.

Drug Interactions

Pyridoxine drug interactions			
Precipitant drug	Object drug[a]		Description
Pyridoxine	Levodopa	⬇	Pyridoxine reduces levodopa's effectiveness by increasing its peripheral metabolism; therefore, lower levels are available for CNS penetration.
Pyridoxine	Phenytoin	⬇	Phenytoin serum levels may be decreased.

[a] ⬇ = Object drug decreased.

Adverse Reactions

Sensory neuropathic syndromes; unstable gait; numb feet; awkwardness of hands; perioral numbness; decreased sensation to touch, temperature, and vibration; paresthesia; photoallergic reaction; ataxia.

Overdosage

➤*Symptoms:* Patients receiving 2 to 7 g/day (or greater than 0.2 g/day for longer than 2 months) have developed sensory neuropathy with associated ataxia and numbness of the hands and feet. When pyridoxine is discontinued, symptoms will lessen. It may take 6 months for sensation to normalize.

PYRIDOXINE HYDROCHLORIDE — INJECTION

Indications

➤*Pyridoxine deficiency:* For the treatment of pyridoxine deficiency as seen in the following: Inadequate dietary intake, drug-induced deficiency, as from isoniazid (INH) or oral contraceptives, and inborn errors of metabolism, eg, vitamin B_6-dependent convulsions or vitamin B_6-responsive anemia.

The parenteral route is indicated when oral administration is not feasible as in anorexia, nausea and vomiting, and preoperative and postoperative conditions. It is also indicated when GI absorption is impaired.

➤*Unlabeled uses:*

Hydrazine poisoning – Although experience is limited, reversal of neurologic symptoms and CNS depression have been reported.

Premenstrual syndrome (PMS) – PMS has been treated with pyridoxine 40 to 500 mg/day, but with conflicting results.

Hyperoxaluria type I – Hyperoxaluria type I (and oxalate kidney stones) has been treated with pyridoxine in low doses (25 to 300 mg/day).

Administration and Dosage

➤*Dietary deficiency:* Pyridoxine HCl may be administered IM or IV. In cases of dietary deficiency, the dosage is 10 to 20 mg daily for 3 weeks. Follow-up treatment is recommended daily for several weeks with an oral therapeutic multivitamin preparation containing 2 to 5 mg pyridoxine. Poor dietary habits should be corrected, and an adequate, well-balanced diet should be prescribed.

➤*Vitamin B_6-dependency syndrome:* The vitamin B_6-dependency syndrome may require a therapeutic dosage of as much as 600 mg a day and a daily intake of 30 mg for life.

➤*INH deficiencies:* In deficiencies due to INH, the dosage is 100 mg daily for 3 weeks followed by a 30 mg maintenance dose daily.

In poisoning caused by ingestion of more than 10 g of INH, an equal amount of pyridoxine should be given: 4 g IV followed by 1 g IM every 30 minutes.

➤*Storage/Stability:* Protect from light. Use only if solution is clear and seal intact.

Store at controlled room temperature 15° to 30°C (59° to 86°F).

Actions

➤*Pharmacology:* Natural substances that have vitamin B_6 activity are pyridoxine in plants and pyridoxal or pyridoxamine in animals. All 3 are converted to pyridoxal phosphate by the enzyme pyridoxal kinase. The physiologically active forms of vitamin B_6 are pyridoxal phosphate (codecarboxylase) and pyridoxamine phosphate. Riboflavin is required for the conversion of pyridoxine phosphate to pyridoxal phosphate.

Vitamin B_6 acts as a coenzyme in the metabolism of protein, carbohydrate, and fat. In protein metabolism, it participates in the decarboxylation of amino acids, conversion of tryptophan to niacin or to serotonin (5-hydroxytryptamine), deamination, and transamination and transulfuration of amino acids. In carbohydrate metabolism, it is responsible for the breakdown of glycogen to glucose-1-phosphate.

➤*Pharmacokinetics:*

Metabolism/Excretion – The total adult body pool consists of 16 to 25 mg of pyridoxine. Its half-life appears to be 15 to 20 days. Vitamin B_6 is degraded to 4-pyridoxic acid in the liver. This metabolite is excreted in the urine. The need for pyridoxine increases with the amount of protein in the diet. The tryptophan load test appears to uncover early vitamin B_6 deficiency by detecting xanthinurea. The average adult minimum daily requirement is about 1.25 mg. The dietary reference intake (DRI) is as much as 1.7 mg for adult males, 1.5 mg for adult females, 1.9 mg for pregnant women, and 2 mg for lactating women. The requirements are more in persons having certain genetic defects or those being treated with isonicotinic acid hydrazide (INHJ) or oral contraceptives.

Contraindications

Sensitivity to pyridoxine or to any ingredient in this preparation.

Warnings

➤*Pregnancy: Category A.* The requirement for pyridoxine appears to be increased during pregnancy. Pyridoxine is sometimes of value in the treatment of nausea and vomiting of pregnancy.

➤*Lactation:* The need for pyridoxine is increased during lactation. It is not known whether this drug is excreted in human milk. Because many drugs are excreted in human milk, caution should be exercised when pyridoxine HCl is administered to a nursing woman.

➤*Children:* Safety and efficacy in children have not been established.

Precautions

➤*Multiple vitamin deficiency:* Single deficiency, as of pyridoxine alone, is rare. Multiple vitamin deficiency is to be expected in any inadequate diet.

Women taking oral contraceptives may exhibit increased pyridoxine requirements.

➤*Drug abuse and dependence:* Symptoms of dependence have been noted in adults given only 200 mg daily, followed by withdrawal.

Drug Interactions

Pyridoxine drug interactions			
Precipitant drug	Object drug[a]		Description
Pyridoxine	Levodopa	⬇	Pyridoxine reduces levodopa's effectiveness by increasing its peripheral metabolism; therefore, lower levels are available for CNS penetration.
Pyridoxine	Phenytoin	⬇	Phenytoin serum levels may be decreased.

[a] ⬇ = Object drug decreased.

➤*Levodopa:* Pyridoxine supplements (greater than 5 mg/day) should not be given to patients receiving levodopa, because the action of the latter drug is antagonized by pyridoxine. However, this vitamin may be used concur-

PYRIDOXINE HYDROCHLORIDE — INJECTION

rently in patients receiving a preparation containing both carbidopa and levodopa.

Adverse Reactions

Paresthesia, somnolence, and low serum folic acid levels have been reported.

Overdosage

➤*Symptoms:* Pyridoxine given to animals in amounts of 3 to 4 g/kg of body weight produces convulsions and death. In man, a dose of 25 mg/kg of body weight is well tolerated.

CYANOCOBALAMIN (B_{12})

otc	**Vitamin B_{12}** (Various, eg, Apothecary, Goldline, Rugby)	**Tablets:** 100 mcg	In 100s.
otc	**Vitamin B_{12}** (Various, eg, Goldline, Rugby)	**Tablets:** 500 mcg	In 100s.
		1000 mcg	In 100s.
otc	**Twelve Resin-K** (Key Company)	**Tablets:** 1000 mcg on resin.	In 60s, 250s, and 1000s.
otc	**Big Shot B-12** (Naturally)	**Tablets:** 5000 mcg	In 30s and 60s.
otc	**Big Shot B-12** (Naturally)	**Tablets:** 5000 mcg	In 30s and 60s.
otc	**Big Shot B-12** (Naturally)	**Tablets:** 5000 mcg	In 30s and 60s.
otc	**Vitamin B_{12}** (Freeda)	**Lozenges:** 50 mcg	Sorbitol, mannitol. In 100s.
		100 mcg	In 100s.
		250 mcg	In 100s and 250s.
		500 mcg	In 100s and 250s.

CYANOCOBALAMIN — ORAL

For complete and comparative prescribing information, refer to the vitamin B_{12} monograph.

Indications

➤*B_{12} deficiency:* Nutritional vitamin B $_{12}$ deficiency.

These products are NOT indicated for treatment of pernicious anemia.

Administration and Dosage

➤*Recommended Dietary Allowances (RDAs):* Adults, 2 mcg/day. For a complete listing of RDAs by age, sex, or condition, refer to the RDA table.

➤*Nutritional supplement:* Dosage varies. See individual product literature.

Actions

➤*Pharmacology:* Vitamin B_{12} is essential to growth, cell reproduction, hematopoiesis, nucleic acid, and myelin synthesis. Sources of vitamin B_{12} include liver, meat, fish, and dairy products (eg, milk and cheese). Vitamin B_{12} is not present in foods of plant origin. Deficiency may result in megaloblastic anemia or pernicious anemia. Ten percent to 30% of Americans older than 60 years of age experience atrophic gastritis, resulting in an inability to absorb vitamin B_{12} bound to food protein. Because of enterohepatic recycling, patients who do not absorb, or have a diet deficient in, vitamin B_{12} may not see signs of deficiency for 3 to 5 years.

➤*Pharmacokinetics:* The parietal cells of the stomach secrete intrinsic factor, which regulates the amount of vitamin B_{12} absorbed in the terminal ileum. Simple diffusion is responsible for absorption when more than 30 mcg of vitamin B_{12} is ingested. Bioavailability of oral preparations is ≈ 25%. Vitamin B_{12} is primarily stored in the liver. Enterohepatic circulation plays a key role in recycling vitamin B_{12} from bile and other intestinal secretions. If plasma-binding proteins are saturated, excess free vitamin B_{12} will be excreted in the kidney.

Contraindications

Hypersensitivity to cyanocobalamin.

Warnings

➤*Pregnancy: Category A.* (*Category C* in doses that exceed the RDA).

➤*Lactation:* Vitamin B_{12} is excreted into breast milk.

Overdosage

➤*Symptoms:* Vitamin B_{12} is essentially nontoxic in humans. Allergic reactions and hypersensitivity have been reported.

CYANOCOBALAMIN (B_{12})

Rx	**Nascobal** (Questcor)	**Gel, intranasal:** 500 mcg per 0.1 mL (500 mcg/actuation)	Benzalkonium chloride. In 5 mL bottles (approximately 8 doses/bottle).
		Spray, intranasal: 500 mcg per 0.1 mL (500 mcg/actuation)	Benzalkonium chloride. In 2.3 mL (approximately 8 doses/bottle).

CYANOCOBALAMIN — INTRANASAL

For complete and comparative prescribing information, refer to the vitamin B_{12} monograph.

Indications

➤*Maintenance of hematologic status:* For maintenance of the hematologic status of patients who are in remission following IM vitamin B_{12} therapy for the following conditions:

- Pernicious anemia in hematologic remission with no nervous system involvement.
- Dietary deficiency of vitamin B_{12} occurring in strict vegetarians (isolated vitamin B_{12} deficiency is very rare).
- Malabsorption of vitamin B_{12} resulting from structural or functional damage to the stomach where intrinsic factor is secreted, or to the ileum where intrinsic factor facilitates B_{12} absorption. These conditions include HIV infection, AIDS, Crohn's disease, tropical sprue, and nontropical sprue (idiopathic steatorrhea, gluten-induced enteropathy). Folate deficiency in these patients is usually more severe than vitamin B_{12} deficiency.
- Inadequate secretion of intrinsic factor resulting from lesions that destroy the gastric mucosa (ingestion of corrosives, extensive neoplasia) and conditions associated with a variable degree of gastric atrophy (eg, multiple sclerosis, HIV infection, AIDS, certain endocrine disorders, iron deficiency, subtotal gastrectomy). Total gastrectomy always produces vitamin B_{12} deficiency. Structural lesions leading to vitamin B_{12} deficiency include regional ileitis, ileal resections, and malignancies.
- Competition for vitamin B_{12} by intestinal parasites or bacteria. The fish tapeworm (*Diphyllobothrium latum*) absorbs huge quantities of vitamin B_{12} and infested patients often have associated gastric atrophy. The blind loop syndrome may produce deficiency of vitamin B_{12} or folate.
- Inadequate utilization of vitamin B_{12}. This may occur if antimetabolites for the vitamin are employed in the treatment of neoplasia.

Administration and Dosage

Prime the spray pump prior to initial use. Repriming between doses is not necessary if the unit is upright. Administer at least 1 hour before or 1 hour after ingestion of hot foods or liquids.

➤*Vitamin B_{12} malabsorption in remission following injectable vitamin B_{12} therapy:* 500 mcg intranasally (one nostril) once weekly.

➤*Storage/Stability:* Protect from light. Keep covered in prescription vial until ready to use. Store upright at controlled room temperature (15° to 30°C; 59° to 86°F). Protect from freezing.

Actions

➤*Pharmacokinetics:* Peak concentration of B_{12} after intranasal administration is 1 to 2 hours. Bioavailability is 8.9%.

Contraindications

Sensitivity to cobalt and/or vitamin B_{12} or to any component of this preparation.

Warnings

➤*Optic atrophy:* Patients with early Leber's disease treated with vitamin B_{12} suffered severe and swift optic atrophy.

➤*Megaloblastic anemia:* Patients with severe megaloblastic anemia intensely treated with vitamin B_{12} may develop hypokalemia and sudden death. Folic acid is not a substitute for vitamin B_{12}, although it may improve vitamin B_{12}-deficient megaloblastic anemia. Exclusive use of folic acid in treating vitamin B_{12}-deficient megaloblastic anemia could result in progressive and irreversible neurologic damage.

Precautions

➤*Monitoring:* Obtain hematocrit, reticulocyte count, vitamin B_{12}, folate, and iron levels prior to treatment. All parameters should be normal when beginning treatment.

CYANOCOBALAMIN — INTRANASAL

Monitor vitamin B_{12} blood levels and peripheral blood counts 1 month after the start of treatment and then at 3- to 6-month intervals.

Patients with pernicious anemia have about 3 times the incidence of stomach carcinoma when compared with the general population. Perform appropriate tests.

➤*Test dose:* An intradermal test dose of parenteral vitamin B_{12} is recommended before intranasal administration to patients suspected of cyanocobalamin sensitivity.

➤*Nasal symptoms:* The effectiveness of intranasal cyanocobalamin in patients with nasal congestion, allergic rhinitis, and upper respiratory tract infections has not been determined. Defer treatment until symptoms have subsided.

Drug Interactions

Colchicine, para-aminosalicylic acid, and heavy alcohol intake for longer than 2 weeks may result in vitamin B_{12} malabsorption.

➤*Drug/Lab test interactions:* Most antibiotics, methotrexate, or pyrimethamine invalidate folic acid and vitamin B_{12} diagnostic blood assays.

Adverse Reactions

Asthenia; headache; infection; glossitis; nausea; paresthesia; rhinitis.

Overdosage

No overdose has been reported.

Patient Information

Administer at least 1 hour before or 1 hour after ingestion of hot foods or liquids.

Patients with pernicious anemia will require weekly vitamin B_{12} for the remainder of their lives.

Blood tests are recommended every 3 to 6 months to ensure therapy is appropriate.

AMINOBENZOATE POTASSIUM

Rx	**Potaba** (Glenwood)	**Tablets**: 500 mg	In 100s and 1000s.
Rx	**Aminobenzoate Potassium** (Hope Pharm)	**Capsules**: 500 mg	In 250s.
Rx	**Potaba** (Glenwood)		In 250s and 1000s.
Rx	**Potaba** (Glenwood)	**Envules (Powder)**: 2 g	In 50s.

AMINOBENZOATE POTASSIUM — ORAL

Indications

"Possibly effective" in the treatment of scleroderma, dermatomyositis, morphea, linear scleroderma, pemphigus, and Peyronie's disease.

Administration and Dosage

➤*Adults:* The average adult daily dose of aminobenzoate potassium for scleroderma, morphea, linear scleroderma, and Peyronie's disease is 12 g, usually given in 4 to 6 divided doses. Higher doses (15 to 20 g daily) are initially used in dermatomyositis. Tablets and capsules 500 mg are given at the rate of 4 tablets or capsules 6 times daily, or 6 tablets or capsules given 4 times daily usually with meals and at bedtime with a snack. Tablets must be dissolved in an adequate amount of liquid to prevent GI upset. Aminobenzoate potassium envules contain 2 g pure drug powder and constitute the individual average dose. Six envules are given for a total of 12 g aminobenzoate potassium daily.

Therapy usually requires the maintenance of adequate dosage for 2 to 3 months.

➤*Children:* 1 g daily in divided doses for each 10 lbs of body weight.

Actions

➤*Pharmacology:* Small amounts of para-aminobenzoate are present in cereal, eggs, milk, and meats. Detectable amounts are found in human blood, spinal fluid, urine, and sweat. It is suggested that aminobenzoate potassium has an antifibrosis action caused by mediation of increased oxygen uptake at the tissue level. Fibrosis is believed to occur from either too much serotonin or too little monoamine oxidase (MAO) activity over a period of time. MAO requires an adequate supply of oxygen to function properly. By increasing oxygen supply at the tissue level, aminobenzoate potassium may enhance MAO activity and prevent or cause regression of fibrosis.

Contraindications

Concurrent sulfonamide use.

Warnings

➤*Renal function impairment:* Use cautiously.

➤*Pregnancy:* Safety has not been established.

➤*Lactation:* Safety for use during lactation has not been established.

Precautions

➤*Anorexia or nausea:* If anorexia or nausea occurs, interrupt therapy until the patient is eating normally again to avoid hypoglycemia.

➤*Hypersensitivity:* If a hypersensitivity reaction occurs, discontinue the drug. Refer to Management of Acute Hypersensitivity Reactions.

Adverse Reactions

Anorexia, nausea, fever, and rash have occurred infrequently and subside with omission of the drug. Desensitization can be accomplished and treatment resumed. Hepatotoxicity also has occurred.

Overdosage

➤*Symptoms:* Nausea and vomiting are the most common events associated with overdose. Drug fever, dermatitis, depression of the leukocyte count, and an alleged fatal case of toxic hepatitis have been reported.

VITAMIN C

Indications

➤*Scurvy:* Prevention and treatment of scurvy. Parenteral administration is desirable in an acute deficiency or when absorption of oral ascorbic acid is uncertain.

➤*Unlabeled uses:* Vitamin C in high doses has been advocated for prevention of the common cold, for treatment of asthma, atherosclerosis, wounds, schizophrenia, and cancer; however, clinical data do not justify these uses.

Vitamin C (≥ 2 g/day) may be used as a urinary acidifier either alone or in combination with methenamine therapy. Data regarding the efficacy of ascorbic acid for this purpose are conflicting. Failure to significantly lower urine pH may be attributed to inadequate dosage (less than 2 g/day).

Vitamin C in doses of ≥ 150 mg have been used to control idiopathic methemoglobinemia (less effective than methylene blue).

Doses greater than the recommended RDA for vitamin C have been associated with a low incidence of senile cataract, cancer, coronary artery disease, and increase in HDL.

Risk reduction for pre-eclampsia in combination with vitamin E during the second half of pregnancy (1 g/day).

Topical – Topical vitamin C may photoprotect against UVR because of its antioxidant and anti-inflammatory properties.

Administration and Dosage

Chronic illness, infection, febrile states, hemovascular disorders, and wound healing require an increase in daily intake.

➤*Recommended Dietary Allowances (RDAs):* Adults, 60 mg. For a complete listing of RDAs by age, sex, or condition, refer to the RDA table.

➤*Nicotine use:* The RDA for smokers is 100 mg/day because of an increased utilization of vitamin C.

IM route is preferred; may administer IV or SC. Avoid rapid IV injection. IM injections may cause pain, local swelling, tenderness, and tissue necrosis.

➤*Adults:* The average protective dose is 70 to 150 mg/day. For scurvy, 300 mg to 1 g/day is recommended. However, up to 6 g/day has been administered parenterally to healthy adults without evidence of toxicity.

High-dose therapy – Taper vitamin C prior to discontinuing supplementation. Adults who abruptly stopped high-dose therapy have experienced loosened teeth and bleeding gums.

Enhanced wound healing – Doses of 300 to 500 mg/day for 7 to 10 days both preoperatively and postoperatively are adequate, although considerably larger amounts have been recommended.

Burns – Individualize dosage. For severe burns, daily doses of 1 to 2 g are recommended.

In other conditions in which the need for vitamin C is increased, 3 to 5 times the daily optimum allowance appears adequate.

Actions

➤*Pharmacology:* Vitamin C is a water-soluble vitamin with antioxidant properties. Sources of vitamin C include citrus fruits (eg, lemons, limes), strawberries, tomatoes, cabbage greens, leafy vegetables, and melons.

Physiological Roles of Vitamin C	
Catecholamine biosynthesis	Stimulates peptide synthesis and hydroxylation of proline and lysine in collagen formation
Carnitine synthesis	Epinephrine synthesis
Conversion of folic acid to folinic acid	Facilitates GI iron absorption
Tyrosine metabolism	Dopamine hydroxylation to form norepinephrine

VITAMIN C

Deficiency – Symptoms include impaired wound healing, impaired collagen synthesis, joint pain, anemia, and increased susceptibility to infections. A serum level less than 0.3 mg/dL is considered to be associated with a decreased intake of vitamin C.

Scurvy: Scurvy is characterized by degenerative changes in capillaries, bone, and connective tissues manifested as perifollicular hyperkeratotic papules, dry skin, ecchymosis, muscle weakness, loose teeth caused by gum inflammation, joint pain, easy bruising, and fatigue.

➤*Pharmacokinetics:*

Absorption / Distribution – Absorption of dietary ascorbate from the distal small intestine is nearly complete. Ascorbic acid is distributed throughout water-soluble compartments of the body. The adrenal cortex, leukocytes, platelets, and the pituitary contain high ascorbic acid concentrations. Ascorbic acid body pools are more than 1400 mg; ≈ 4% of this pool is used daily.

Metabolism / Excretion – Ascorbic acid is excreted in the urine.

Warnings

➤*Excessive vitamin C doses:* Diabetic patients, patients prone to recurrent renal calculi, those undergoing stool occult blood tests, and those on sodium-restricted diets or anticoagulant therapy should not take excessive doses of vitamin C over an extended period of time.

➤*Pregnancy: Category A.* (*Category C* in doses greater than the RDA.) It is not known whether ascorbic acid can cause fetal harm or can affect reproduction capacity. Give to pregnant women only if clearly needed.

Do not administer ascorbic acid to pregnant women in excess of the amount needed for treatment. The fetus may adapt to high levels of vitamin C resulting in a scorbutic condition after birth when intake drops to normal levels. Clinical significance is unknown.

➤*Lactation:* Administer with caution to a nursing mother. Ascorbic acid is excreted in breast milk.

Precautions

➤*Tartrazine sensitivity:* Some of these products contain tartrazine, which may cause allergic-type reactions (including bronchial asthma) in susceptible individuals. Although the incidence of sensitivity is low, it is frequently seen in patients who also have aspirin hypersensitivity. Specific products containing tartrazine are identified in the product listings.

➤*Sulfite sensitivity:* Some of these products contain sulfites, which may cause allergic-type reactions in certain susceptible people. The overall prevalence of sulfite sensitivity in the general population is unknown and probably low. Sulfite sensitivity is seen more frequently in asthmatic than in nonasthmatic people.

Drug Interactions

➤*Drug / Lab test interactions:* Large doses (greater than 500 mg) of vitamin C may cause false-negative urine **glucose determinations**.

No exogenous vitamin C should be ingested for 48 to 72 hours before conducting amine-dependent stool **occult blood tests** because false-negative results may occur.

Adverse Reactions

Transient mild soreness may occur at the site of IM or SC injection. Rapid IV administration may cause temporary faintness or dizziness.

Overdosage

Nausea, vomiting, gout precipitation, rebound scurvy, increased iron absorption, impaired bacterial activity, and diarrhea (≥ 1 g). Monitor risk for developing renal calcium oxalate stones (1 to 3 g) due to excessive oxalate excretion produced by ascorbic acid metabolism.

ASCORBIC ACID

otc	**Ascorbic Acid** (Various, eg, Goldline, Nutro Labs)	**Tablets:** 250 mg	In 100s and UD 100s.
otc	**Ascorbic Acid** (Various, eg, Goldline, Naturally, Nutro Labs, Rugby[1])	**Tablets:** 500 mg	In 100s, 250s, 1000s, and UD 100s.
otc	**Cevi-Bid** (Lee)		In 100s, 500s, and UD 12s and 96s.
otc	**Ascorbic Acid** (Various, eg, Goldline, Naturally, Rugby[1])	**Tablets:** 1000 mg	In 100s and 250s.
otc	**Ascorbic Acid** (Various, eg, Naturally)	**Tablets:** 1500 mg	In 100s.
otc	**Ascorbic Acid** (Various, eg, Freeda)	**Tablets, timed-release:** 500 mg	In 100s, 250s, and 500s.
otc	**Ascorbic Acid** (Freeda)	**Tablets, timed-release:** 1000 mg	In 100s, 250s, and 500s.
otc	**Ascorbic Acid** (Various, eg, Goldine)	**Capsules:** 500 mg	In 100s.
otc	**Asco-Caps** (Key Company)		In 100s and 500s.
otc sf	**Vita-C** (Freeda)	**Crystals:** 1000 mg/¼ tsp	In 120 g and 1 lb.
otc sf	**Dull-C** (Freeda)	**Powder:** 1060 mg/¼ tsp	In 120 g and 1 lb.
otc	**Ascorbic Acid** (Humco)	**Powder:** 60 mg/¼ tsp	In 454 g.
otc	**Cecon** (Abbott)	**Solution:** 100 mg/mL	In 50 mL w/dropper.
otc	**Ascorbic Acid** (Various, eg, Rugby)	**Liquid:** 500 mg/5 mL	In 120 and 480 mL.
Rx	**Ascorbic Acid** (Various, eg, American Regent)	**Injection:** 500 mg/mL	In 50 mL vials.
Rx	**Ascor L 500** (McGuff)		0.025% EDTA. Preservative-free. In 50 mL.

[1] With or without rose hips.

For complete and comparative prescribing information, see the Vitamin C group monograph.

SODIUM ASCORBATE

Rx	**Cenolate** (Abbott)	**Injection:** 562.5 mg/mL (equiv. to 500 mg/mL ascorbic acid)	In 1 and 2 mL amps.[1]

[1] With 0.5% sodium hydrosulfite.

For complete prescribing information, refer to the Vitamin C group monograph.

CALCIUM ASCORBATE

otc sf	**Calcium Ascorbate** (Freeda)	**Tablets:** 500 mg	75 mg calcium. Buffered. In 100s, 250s, and 500s.
otc sf	**Calcium Ascorbate** (Freeda)	**Powder:** 814 mg/¼ tsp	100 mg calcium/¼ tsp. Buffered. In 120 g and 1 lb.
otc	**Ascocid** (Key)	**Granules:** 4,000 mg/tsp (as vitamin C)	In 8 oz.

For complete and comparative prescribing information, see the Vitamin C group monograph.

ASCORBIC ACID COMBINATIONS

otc	**SunKist Vitamin C** (Novartis)	**Tablets, chewable:** 60 mg vitamin C as sodium ascorbate and ascorbic acid	Sorbitol, sucrose, lactose. Orange flavor. In 11s.
otc sf	**Fruit C 100** (Freeda)	**Tablets, chewable:** 100 mg vitamin C as calcium ascorbate and ascorbic acid	In 250s.
otc sf	**Fruit C 200** (Freeda)	**Tablets, chewable:** 200 mg vitamin C as calcium ascorbate and ascorbic acid	Rose hips. In 100s and 250s.

ASCORBIC ACID COMBINATIONS

otc	**Chewable Vitamin C** (Various, eg, Goldline)	**Tablets, chewable:** 250 mg vitamin C as sodium ascorbate and ascorbic acid	In 100s.
otc	**SunKist Vitamin C** (Novartis)		Fructose, sorbitol, sucrose, lactose. Orange flavor. In 60s.
otc	**Chewable Vitamin C** (Various, eg, Goldline)	**Tablets, chewable:** 500 mg vitamin C as sodium ascorbate and ascorbic acid	In 100s.
otc	**SunKist Vitamin C** (Novartis)		Fructose, sorbitol, sucrose, lactose. Orange flavor. In 75s.
otc	**Chew-C** (Key Company)		Sugar. Orange flavor. In 100s.
otc *sf*	**Fruit C 500** (Freeda)	**Tablets, chewable:** 500 mg vitamin C as calcium ascorbate and ascorbic acid	Rose hips. In 100s and 250s.
otc	**Vicks Vitamin C Drops** (Proctor and Gamble)	**Lozenges:** 25 mg vitamin C as sodium ascorbate and ascorbic acid	Sucrose, corn syrup. Orange flavor. In 20s.

For complete and comparative prescribing information, refer to the Vitamin C group monograph.

BIOFLAVONOIDS (Vitamin P)

otc *sf*	**Pan C-500** (Freeda)	**Tablets:** 100 mg hesperidin, 100 mg citrus bioflavonoids, and 500 mg vitamin C	Sodium free. In 100s, 250s, and 500s.
otc *sf*	**C Factors "1000" Plus** (Solgar)	**Tablets:** 1000 mg vitamin C, 25 mg rose hips, 250 mg citrus bioflavonoids complex, 50 mg rutin, 25 mg hesperidin	Sodium free. In 50s.
otc *sf*	**Flavons** (Freeda)	**Tablets:** 500 mg bioflavonoids[1]	In 100s and 250s.
otc	**Tri-Super Flavons 1000** (Freeda)	**Tablets:** 1000 mg bioflavonoids	In 100s, 250s, and 500s.
otc	**Peridin-C** (Beutlich)	**Tablets:** 150 mg hesperidin complex, 50 mg hesperidin methyl cholcone (bioflavonoids), 200 mg ascorbic acid	In 100s and 500s.
otc *sf*	**Span C** (Freeda)	**Tablets:** 300 mg citrus bioflavonoids, 200 mg vitamin C (ascorbic acid and rose hips)[1]	In 100s, 250s, and 500s.
otc *sf*	**Flavons-500** (Freeda)	**Tablets:** 500 mg citrus bioflavonoids	In 100s and 250s.
otc *sf*	**Ester-C Plus 1000 mg Vitamin C** (Solgar)	**Tablets:** 1000 mg vitamin C, 200 mg citrus bioflavonoid complex, 25 mg acerola, 25 mg rutin, 25 mg rose hips, 125 mg calcium	Sodium free. In 90s.
otc *sf*	**Quercetin** (Freeda)	**Tablets:** 50 mg quercetin (from eucalyptus)	Sodium free. In 100s and 250s.
		Tablets: 250 mg quercetin (from eucalyptus)	Sodium free. In 100s and 250s.
otc	**Amino-Opti-C** (Tyson)	**Tablets, sustained-release:** 1000 mg vitamin C, 250 mg lemon bioflavonoids. Rose hips powder, rutin, hesperidin[2]	In 100s.
otc *sf*	**Ester-C Plus Multi-Mineral** (Solgar)	**Capsules:** 425 mg vitamin C, 50 mg citrus bioflavonoid complex, 12.5 mg acerola, 12.5 mg rose hips, 5 mg rutin, 25 mg calcium, 13 mg magnesium, 12.5 mg potassium, 2.5 mg zinc	Sodium free. In 60s and 90s.
otc *sf*	**Ester-C Plus 500 mg Vitamin C** (Solgar)	**Capsules:** 500 mg vitamin C, 62 mg calcium, 25 mg citrus bioflavonoids, 10 mg acerola, 10 mg rose hips, 5 mg rutin	Sodium free. In 250s.

[1] Also contains calcium carbonate, calcium stearate.

[2] Also contains dicalcium phosphate, hydrogenated soybean oil.

BIOFLAVONOIDS (VITAMIN P) — ORAL

Indications

➤*Dietary supplement:* Bioflavonoids may be used as a dietary supplement. Bioflavonoids help strengthen the capillaries, as well as increase the absorption of vitamin C.

➤*Unlabeled uses:* Bioflavonoids possess widespread activity. Some biological activities include the following: Anthelmintic, antimicrobial, antimalarial, antineoplastic, cytotoxic, mutagenic, carcinogenic, anticarcinogenic, antioxidant (free radical scavengers), inhibition of prostaglandin synthesis (anti-inflammatory), antiallergic, antiviral, antithrombotic, spasmolitic, and estrogenic. Certain flavonoids have been noted to increase lymphatic drainage and improve venous tone. Bioflavonoids are considered investigational in the treatment of HIV via HIV-1 reverse transcriptase, protease, and integrase inhibition. Unfortunately, many of these uses have not been tested in controlled clinical trials; therefore, there is little evidence that they are effective for any indication.

Administration and Dosage

➤*Recommended daily allowance (RDA):* A recommended daily allowance (RDA) for bioflavonoids has not been established. However, it has been estimated that daily intake ranges from 20 mg to 1 g.

Use to increase the absorption of vitamin C is typically in a ratio of 500 mg vitamin C to 200 mg bioflavonoids taken once or twice daily with food.

➤*Adults:* As a dietary supplement, take as recommended by a healthcare provider.

➤*Children:* As a dietary supplement, take as recommended by a healthcare provider.

➤*Storage/Stability:* Store in a cool, dry place. Do not refrigerate.

Actions

➤*Pharmacology:* Flavonoids are naturally occurring, low-molecular-weight polyphenols of plant origin, historically named "vitamin P." More than 4000 naturally occurring flavonoids have been described. Groups of flavonoids include flavones, flavonols, flavanones, and flavanols, which differ by the number and positions of hydroxyl substituents in 2 aromatic rings. Flavonoids generally occur as aglycones, glycosides, and methylated derivatives. Flavonoids are present in fruits, vegetables, nuts, seeds, grains, tea, wine, stems, and flowers. Bioflavonoid refers to extracts of citrus including lemon, orange, mandarin, or grapefruit varieties. Bioflavonoids extracted from citrus contain a variety of flavonoids. The majority of citrus flavonoids are flavanones bound as glycosides.

Flavonoid	Source
Naringin[a]	Grapefruit, pummelo
Narirutin[a]	Grapefruit
Hesperidin	Oranges, tangerines, lemons, limes
Ericotirin	Lemon, limes
Tangeretin	Tangerines, lemons, limes
Nobiletin	Tangerines, lemons, limes
Genistein	Soybeans
Quercetin	Onions, tomatoes, french beans, apples, berries, red wine

[a] Naringenin glycosides.

BIOFLAVONOIDS (VITAMIN P) — ORAL

➤*Pharmacokinetics:*

Absorption / Distribution –

Quercetin: Quercetin peak levels are attained in less than 0.7 and 2.5 hours following onion and apple ingestion, respectively. Quercetin crosses the intestinal mucosa and is transported to the liver primarily bound to albumin.

Metabolism / Excretion –

Quercetin: Frequent intake of quercetin-rich food resulted in elimination half-lives of 23 hours for apples and 28 hours for onion sources. Quercetin undergoes methylation, sulphation, and glucuronidation to form various conjugates of quercetin. Multiple dosing of grapefruit and orange juice (containing 323 mg naringenin and 44 mg hesperidin) resulted in less than 25% urinary recovery.

Contraindications

None known.

Warnings

➤*Pregnancy:* Consult a healthcare provider.

➤*Lactation:* Consult a healthcare provider.

Drug Interactions

➤*Warfarin:* Use bioflavonoids cautiously in patients being treated with warfarin.

Patient Information

Notify your doctor if you go in for surgery because the presence of bioflavonoids can interfere with some medical tests.

FOLIC ACID AND DERIVATIVES (Folacin; Pteroylglutamic Acid; Folate)

otc[1]	**Folic Acid** (Various, eg, Fibertone, Major, Rugby)	**Tablets:** 0.4 mg	In 100s.
otc[1]	**Folic Acid** (Various, eg, Fibertone, Rugby)	**Tablets:** 0.8 mg	In 100s.
Rx	**Folic Acid** (Various, eg, Genetco, Goldline, Moore, Parmed, Qualitest, Rugby)	**Tablets:** 1 mg	In 30s, 100s, 1000s and UD 100s.
Rx sf	**Deplin** (Pamlab)	**Tablets:** 7.5 mg (as L-methylfolate)	(PAL 7.5). Lt. blue. In 30s, 90s, and 500s.
Rx	**Folic Acid** (American Pharmaceutical Partners)	**Injection:** 5 mg/mL	In 10 mL vials.[2]
Rx	**Folvite** (Lederle)		In 10 mL vials.[3]

[1] Although most folic acid products carry the *Rx* legend, products which provide 0.4 mg or less (or 0.8 mg for pregnant or lactating women) may be *otc* items.

[2] With 1.5% benzyl alcohol and EDTA.

[3] With 1.5% benzyl alcohol.

FOLIC ACID — ORAL

Indications

➤*Megaloblastic anemia:* For the treatment of megaloblastic anemias due to deficiency of folic acid (as may be seen in tropical or nontropical sprue) and in anemias of nutritional origin, pregnancy, infancy, or childhood.

Administration and Dosage

Oral administration is preferred. Although most patients with malabsorption cannot absorb food folates, they are able to absorb folic acid given orally. Doses greater than 0.1 mg should not be used unless anemia due to vitamin B_{12} deficiency has been ruled out or is being adequately treated with cobalamin. Daily doses greater than 1 mg do not enhance the hematologic effect, and most of the excess is excreted unchanged in the urine.

➤*Usual therapeutic dosage:* The usual therapeutic dosage in adults and children (regardless of age) is up to 1 mg daily. Resistant cases may require larger doses.

➤*Maintenance:* When clinical symptoms have subsided and the blood picture has become normal, a daily maintenance level should be used (eg, 0.1 mg for infants and up to 0.3 mg for children less than 4 years of age, 0.4 mg for adults and children greater than or equal to 4 years of age, 0.8 mg for pregnant and lactating women) but never less than 0.1 mg/day. Patients should be kept under close supervision and adjustment of maintenance level made if relapse appears imminent.

In the presence of alcoholism, hemolytic anemia, anticonvulsant therapy, or chronic infection, the maintenance level may need to be increased.

➤*Storage / Stability:* Store at controlled room temperature 15° to 30°C (59° to 86°F). Protect from light and moisture.

Actions

➤*Pharmacology:* Folic acid acts on megaloblastic bone marrow to produce a normoblastic marrow. In man, an exogenous source of folate is required for nucleoprotein synthesis and the maintenance of normal erythropoiesis. Folic acid is the precursor of tetrahydrofolic acid, which is involved as a cofactor for transformylation reactions in the biosynthesis of purines and thymidylates of nucleic acids. Impairment of thymidylate synthesis in patients with folic acid deficiency is thought to account for the defective deoxyribonucleic acid (DNA) synthesis that leads to megaloblast formation and megaloblastic and macrocytic anemias.

➤*Pharmacokinetics:*

Absorption / Distribution – Folic acid is absorbed rapidly from the small intestine, primarily from the proximal portion. Naturally occurring conjugated folates are reduced enzymatically to folic acid in the gastrointestinal tract prior to absorption. Folic acid appears in the plasma approximately 5 to 30 minutes after an oral dose; peak levels are generally reached within 1 hour. After intravenous administration, the drug is rapidly cleared from the plasma. Cerebrospinal fluid levels are several times greater than serum levels of the drug. Folic acid is metabolized in the liver to 7,8-dihydrofolic acid and eventually to 5,6,7,8-tetrahydrofolic acid with the aid of reduced diphosphopyridine nucleotide (DPNH) and folate reductases. Tetrahydrofolic acid is linked in the N^5 or N^{10} positions with formyl, hydroxymethyl, methyl, or formimino groups. N^5 formyltetrahydrofolic acid is leucovorin. Tetrahydrofolic acid derivatives are distributed to all body tissues but are stored primarily in the liver. Normal serum levels of total folate have been reported to be 5 to 15 ng/mL; normal cerebrospinal fluid levels are approximately 16 to 21 ng/mL. Normal erythrocyte folate levels have been reported to range from 175 to 316 ng/mL. In general, folate serum levels below 5 ng/mL indicate folate deficiency, and levels below 2 ng/mL usually result in megaloblastic anemia.

Metabolism / Excretion – After a single oral dose of 100 mcg of folic acid in a limited number of healthy adults, only a trace amount of the drug appeared in the urine. An oral dose of 5 mg in 1 study and a dose of 40 mcg/kg of body weight in another study resulted in approximately 50% of the dose appearing in the urine. After a single oral dose of 15 mg, up to 90% of the dose was recovered in the urine. A majority of the metabolic products appeared in the urine after 6 hours; excretion was generally complete within 24 hours. Small amounts of orally administered folic acid have also been recovered in the feces. Folic acid is also excreted in the milk of lactating mothers.

Contraindications

Previous intolerance to the drug.

Warnings

➤*Pernicious anemia:* Folic acid in doses greater than 0.1 mg daily may obscure pernicious anemia in that hematologic remission can occur while neurologic manifestations remain progressive.

Administration of folic acid alone is improper therapy for pernicious anemia and other megaloblastic anemias in which vitamin B_{12} is deficient.

Except during pregnancy and lactation, folic acid should not be given in therapeutic doses greater than 0.4 mg daily until pernicious anemia has been ruled out. Patients with pernicious anemia receiving greater than 0.4 mg of folic acid daily who are inadequately treated with vitamin B_{12} may show reversion of the hematologic parameters to normal, but neurologic manifestations due to vitamin B_{12} deficiency will progress. Doses of folic acid exceeding the Recommended Dietary Allowance (RDA) should not be included in multivitamin preparations; if therapeutic amounts are necessary, folic acid should be given separately.

There is a potential danger in administering folic acid to patients with undiagnosed anemia, since folic acid may obscure the diagnosis of pernicious anemia by alleviating the hematologic manifestations of the disease while allowing the neurologic complications to progress. This may result in severe nervous system damage before the correct diagnosis is made. Adequate doses of vitamin B_{12} may prevent, halt, or improve the neurologic changes caused by pernicious anemia.

➤*Pregnancy: Category A.*

Folic acid is usually indicated in the treatment of megaloblastic anemias of pregnancy. Folic acid requirements are markedly increased during pregnancy, and deficiency will result in fetal damage.

Studies in pregnant women have not shown that folic acid increases the risk of abnormalities if administered during pregnancy. If the drug is used during pregnancy, the possibility of fetal harm appears remote. Because studies cannot rule out the possibility of harm, however, folic acid should be used during pregnancy only if clearly needed.

➤*Lactation:* Folic acid is excreted in the milk of lactating mothers. During lactation, folic acid requirements are markedly increased; however, amounts present in human milk are adequate to fulfill infant requirements, although supplementation may be needed in low-birth-weight infants, in those who are breastfed by mothers with folic acid deficiency (50 mcg daily), or in those with infections or prolonged diarrhea.

FOLIC ACID — ORAL

Drug Interactions

Folic Acid Drug Interactions			
Precipitant drug	Object drug*		Description
Aminosalicylic acid	Folic acid	⬇	Decreased serum folate levels may occur during concurrent use.
Contraceptives, oral	Folic acid	⬇	Oral contraceptives may impair folate metabolism and produce folate depletion, but the effect is mild and unlikely to cause anemia or megaloblastic changes.
Dihydrofolate reductase inhibitors (eg, methotrexate, trimethoprim)	Folic acid	⬇	A dihydrofolate reductase deficiency caused by administration of folic acid antagonists may interfere with folic acid utilization.
Sulfasalazine	Folic acid	⬇	Signs of folate deficiency have occurred.
Folic acid	Hydantoins	⬇	An increase in seizure frequency and a decrease in serum concentration to subtherapeutic levels have been reported in patients receiving folic acid (particularly 5 to 30 mg/day) with phenytoin. **Phenytoin** may cause a decrease in serum folate levels, and may produce symptoms of folic acid deficiency in 27% to 91% (but clinically important megaloblastic anemia in < 1%) of patients on long-term therapy. If folic acid is required, a higher dose of phenytoin may be needed.

* ⬇ = Object drug decreased.

➤*Phenytoin and other anticonvulsant drugs:* There is evidence that the anticonvulsant action of phenytoin is antagonized by folic acid. A patient whose epilepsy is completely controlled by phenytoin may require increased doses to prevent convulsions if folic acid is given.

In an uncontrolled study, orally administered folic acid was reported to increase the incidence of seizures in some epileptic patients receiving phenobarbital, primidone, or phenytoin. Another investigator reported decreased phenytoin serum levels in folate-deficient patients receiving phenytoin who were treated with 5 mg or 15 mg of folic acid daily.

➤*Drugs causing folate deficiency:* Folate deficiency may result from increased loss of folate, as in renal dialysis or interference with metabolism (eg, folic acid antagonists such as methotrexate); the administration of anticonvulsants, such as phenytoin, primidone, and barbiturates, alcohol consumption and, especially, alcoholic cirrhosis; and the administration of pyrimethamine and nitrofurantoin.

➤*Drug/Lab test interactions:* False low serum and red cell folate levels may occur if the patient has been taking antibiotics, such as tetracycline, which suppress the growth of *Lactobacillus casei*.

Adverse Reactions

➤*CNS:* Other side effects reported in patients receiving 15 mg daily include altered sleep patterns, difficulty in concentrating, irritability, overactivity, excitement, mental depression, confusion, and impaired judgement.

➤*GI:* One patient experienced symptoms suggesting anaphylaxis following injection of the drug. GI side effects, including anorexia, nausea, abdominal distention, flatulence, and a bitter or bad taste, have been reported in patients receiving 15 mg of folic acid daily for 1 month.

➤*Hypersensitivity:* Allergic sensitization has been reported following oral administration of folic acid.

Folic acid is relatively nontoxic in man. Rare instances of allergic responses to folic acid preparations have been reported and have included erythema, skin rash, itching, general malaise, and respiratory difficulty due to bronchospasm.

➤*Miscellaneous:* Decreased vitamin B_{12} serum levels may occur in patients receiving prolonged folic acid therapy.

FOLIC ACID — INJECTION

Indications

➤*Megaloblastic anemia:* For the treatment of megaloblastic anemias due to a deficiency of folic acid as may be seen in tropical or nontropical sprue, in anemias of nutritional origin, pregnancy, infancy or childhood.

Administration and Dosage

➤*Approved by the FDA:* February 18, 1986.

➤*Parenteral administration:* Parenteral administration is not advocated but may be necessary in some individuals (eg, patients receiving parenteral or enteral alimentation). IM, IV and SC routes may be used if the disease is exceptionally severe or if gastrointestinal absorption may be, or is known to be, impaired.

➤*Usual therapeutic dosage in adults and children (regardless of age):* Up to 1 mg daily. Resistant cases may require larger doses.

➤*Maintenance level:* When clinical symptoms have subsided and the blood picture has become normal, a maintenance level should be used, ie, 0.1 mg for infants and up to 0.3 mg for children under four years of age, 0.4 mg for adults and children 4 or more years of age and 0.8 mg for pregnant and lactating women, per day, but never less than 0.1 mg per day. Patients should be kept under close supervision and adjustment of the maintenance level made if relapse appears imminent.

In the presence of alcoholism, hemolytic anemia, anticonvulsant therapy or chronic infection, the maintenance level may need to be increased.

➤*Storage/Stability:* Store at controlled room temperature 15° to 30°C (59° to 86°F).

Protect from light. Retain vial in carton until contents are used.

Actions

➤*Pharmacology:* In man, an exogenous source of folate is required for nucleoprotein synthesis and maintenance of normal erythropoiesis. Folic acid, whether given by mouth or parenterally, stimulates specifically the production of red blood cells, white blood cells and platelets in persons suffering from certain megaloblastic anemias.

Warnings

➤*Pernicious anemia:* Folic acid in doses above 0.1 mg daily may obscure pernicious anemia in that hematologic remission can occur while neurological manifestations remain progressive.

Folic acid alone is improper therapy in the treatment of pernicious anemia and other megaloblastic anemias where vitamin B_{12} is deficient.

Adverse Reactions

➤*Hypersensitivity:* Allergic sensitization has been reported following parenteral administration of folic acid.

LEUCOVORIN CALCIUM (Folinic Acid; Citrovorum Factor)

Rx	**Leucovorin Calcium** (Various, eg, Barr, Lederle)	**Tablets**: 5 mg (as calcium)	In 30s, 100s and UD 50s.
Rx	**Leucovorin Calcium** (Lederle)	**Tablets**: 15 mg (as calcium)	Lactose. (LL 15 C 35). Yellowish white, scored. Oval, convex. In 12s, 24s and UD 50s.
Rx	**Leucovorin Calcium** (Barr)	**Tablets**: 25 mg (as calcium)	(485). Light green. In 25s.
Rx	**Leucovorin Calcium** (Lederle)	**Injection**: 3 mg/mL (as calcium)	In 1 mL amps.[1]
Rx	**Leucovorin Calcium** (American Regent)	**Injection**: 10 mg/mL (as calcium)	In 5 mg single-dose vials (25s).
Rx	**Leucovorin Calcium** (Lederle)	**Powder for Injection**: 50 mg/vial (as calcium)[2]	In vials.
Rx	**Leucovorin Calcium** (Lederle)	**Powder for Injection**: 100 mg/vial (as calcium)[2]	In vials.
Rx	**Leucovorin Calcium** (Mayne)	**Powder for Injection**: 350 mg/vial (as calcium)[2]	In vials.

[1] With 0.9% benzyl alcohol.
[2] Preservative free.

LEUCOVORIN CALCIUM — ORAL

Indications

➤*Methotrexate toxicity:* After high-dose methotrexate therapy in osteosarcoma. Leucovorin is also indicated to diminish the toxicity and counteract the effects of impaired methotrexate elimination and of inadvertent overdosages of folic acid antagonists.

➤*Unlabeled uses:* Treatment of non-Hodgkin lymphoma.

Administration and Dosage

Leucovorin calcium tablets are intended for oral administration. Because absorption is saturable, oral administration of doses more than 25 mg is not recommended.

➤*Leucovorin rescue after high-dose methotrexate therapy:* The recommendations for leucovorin rescue are based on a methotrexate dose of 12 to 15 g/m² administered by IV infusion over 4 hours (see methotrexate

LEUCOVORIN CALCIUM — ORAL

monograph for full prescribing information). Leucovorin rescue at a dose of 15 mg (≈ 10 mg/m²) every 6 hours for 10 doses starts 24 hours after the beginning of the methotrexate infusion. In the presence of GI toxicity, nausea or vomiting, leucovorin should be administered parenterally.

Serum creatinine and methotrexate levels should be determined at least once daily. Leucovorin administration, hydration, and urinary alkalinization (pH of ≥ 7) should be continued until the methotrexate level is less than 5×10^{-8} M (0.05 micromolar). The leucovorin dose should be adjusted or leucovorin rescue extended based on the following guidelines:

Normal methotrexate elimination – Patients with normal methotrexate elimination with serum methotrexate levels ≈ 10 micromolar at 24 hours after administration, 1 micromolar at 48 hours, and less than 0.2 micromolar at 72 hours should receive leucovorin 15 mg orally, IM, or IV every 6 hours for 60 hours (10 doses starting at 24 hours after the start of the methotrexate infusion).

Delayed late methotrexate elimination – Patients with delayed late methotrexate elimination with serum methotrexate levels remaining above 0.2 micromolar at 72 hours, and more than 0.05 micromolar at 96 hours after administration should continue to receive leucovorin 15 mg orally, IM, or IV every 6 hours, until the methotrexate level is less than 0.05 micromolar.

Delayed early methotrexate elimination – Patients with delayed early methotrexate elimination or evidence of acute renal injury with serum methotrexate levels of ≥ 50 micromolar at 24 hours, or ≥ 5 micromolar at 48 hours after administration, or a ≥ 100% increase in serum creatinine level at 24 hours after methotrexate administration (eg, an increase from 0.5 mg/dL to a level of ≥ 1 mg/dL) should receive leucovorin 150 mg IV every 3 hours, until methotrexate level is less than 1 micromolar; then 15 mg IV every 3 hours until the methotrexate level is less than 0.05 micromolar.

Patients who experience delayed early methotrexate elimination are likely to develop reversible renal failure. In addition to appropriate leucovorin therapy, these patients require continuing hydration and urinary alkalinization, and close monitoring of fluid and electrolyte status, until the serum methotrexate level has fallen to less than 0.05 micromolar and the renal failure has resolved.

Some patients will have abnormalities in methotrexate elimination or renal function following methotrexate administration, which are significant but less severe than the abnormalities described above. These abnormalities may or may not be associated with significant clinical toxicity. If significant clinical toxicity is observed, leucovorin rescue should be extended for an additional 24 hours (total of 14 doses over 84 hours) in subsequent courses of therapy. The possibility that the patient is taking other medications which interact with methotrexate (eg, medications which may interfere with methotrexate elimination or binding to serum [albumin]) should always be reconsidered when laboratory abnormalities or clinical toxicities are observed.

➤*Impaired methotrexate elimination or inadvertent overdosage:* The same dosage and administration guidelines may be used. However, leucovorin administration should begin as soon as possible after an inadvertent overdosage is recognized.

➤*Storage/Stability:* Store between 15° to 30°C (59° to 86°F). Protect from light.

Actions

➤*Pharmacology:* Leucovorin is a mixture of the diastereoisomers of the 5-formyl derivative of tetrahydrofolic acid. The biologically active component of the mixture is the (−)-L-isomer, known as Citrovorum factor, or (−)-folinic acid. Leucovorin does not require reduction by the enzyme dihydrofolate reductase in order to participate in reactions utilizing folates as a source of "1-carbon" moieties. Following oral administration, leucovorin is rapidly absorbed and enters the general body pool of reduced folates.

The increase in plasma and serum reduced folate activity (determined microbiologically with *Lactobacillus casei*) seen after oral administration of leucovorin is predominantly due to 5-methyltetrahydrofolate.

Following a 20 mg dose of leucovorin calcium, the mean maximum serum total reduced folate concentrations were the following:

Tablet – Three hundred sixty-four ± 12.1 ng/mL at 2 ± 0.07 hours.

➤*Pharmacokinetics:*

Absorption – Oral tablets produced equivalent bioavailability (8% difference) when compared to the parenteral administration. The parenteral solution also provided equal bioavailability to the tablets when administered orally (2% difference). Oral absorption of leucovorin is saturable at doses above 25 mg. The apparent bioavailability of leucovorin was 97% for 25 mg, 75% for 50 mg and 37% for 100 mg.

Following oral administration, leucovorin is rapidly absorbed and expands the serum pool of reduced folates. After oral administration of leucovorin reconstituted with aromatic elixir, the mean peak concentration of serum total reduced folates was 393 ng/mL (range 160 to 550). At a dose of 25 mg, almost 100% of the l-isomer but only 20% of the d-isomer is absorbed. Oral absorption of leucovorin is saturable at doses above 25 mg. The apparent bioavailability of leucovorin was 97% for 25 mg, 75% for 50 mg, and 37% for 100 mg.

The mean time to peak was 2.3 hours and the terminal half-life was 5.7 hours. The mean peak of 5-methyl-THF was 367 ng/mL at 2.4 hours.

Metabolism – The major component was the metabolite 5-methyltetrahydrofolate to which leucovorin is primarily converted in the intestinal mucosa. The peak level of the parent compound was 51 ng/mL at 1.2 hours. The AUC of total reduced folates after oral administration of the 25 mg dose was 92% of the AUC after IV administration.

Excretion – The half-life of plasma 5-formyltetrahydrofolate was 1.5 ± 0.08 hours and that of the 5-methyltetrahydrofolate was 3 ± 0.09 hours. The terminal half-life was 5.7 hours.

Contraindications

Pernicious anemia and other megaloblastic anemias secondary to the lack of vitamin B_{12}.

Warnings

➤*Folic acid antagonists overdosage:* In the treatment of accidental overdosages of folic acid antagonists, leucovorin should be administered as promptly as possible. As the time interval between antifolate administration (eg, methotrexate) and leucovorin rescue increases, leucovorin's effectiveness in counteracting toxicity diminishes.

➤*Methotrexate concentrations:* Monitoring of serum methotrexate concentration is essential in determining the optimal dose and duration of treatment with leucovorin.

Delayed methotrexate excretion may be caused by a third-space fluid accumulation (ie, ascites, pleural effusion), renal insufficiency, or inadequate hydration. Under such circumstances, higher doses of leucovorin or prolonged administration may be indicated. Doses higher than those recommended for oral use must be given IV.

➤*5-fluorouracil toxicity:* Leucovorin may enhance the toxicity of fluorouracil. Deaths from severe enterocolitis, diarrhea, and dehydration have been reported in elderly patients receiving weekly leucovorin and fluorouracil. Concomitant granulocytopenia and fever were present in some but not all of the patients.

➤*Seizures:* Seizures or syncope have been reported rarely in cancer patients receiving leucovorin, usually in association with fluoropyrimidine administration, and most commonly in those with CNS metastases or other predisposing factors; however, a causal relationship has not been established.

➤*Anemias:* Leucovorin is improper therapy for pernicious anemia and other megaloblastic anemias secondary to the lack of vitamin B_{12}. A hematologic remission may occur while neurologic manifestations remain progressive.

➤*Methotrexate toxicities:* Leucovorin has no effect on other established toxicities of methotrexate such as the nephrotoxicity resulting from drug or metabolite precipitation in the kidney.

➤*Pregnancy: Category C.* Animal reproduction studies have not been conducted with leucovorin. It is also not known whether leucovorin can cause fetal harm when administered to a pregnant woman or can affect reproduction capacity. Leucovorin should be given to a pregnant woman only if clearly needed.

➤*Lactation:* It is not known whether this drug is excreted in human milk. Because many drugs are excreted in human milk, caution should be exercised when leucovorin is administered to a nursing mother.

➤*Children:* Folic acid in large amounts may counteract the antiepileptic effect of phenobarbital, phenytoin and primidone, and increase the frequency of seizures in susceptible children.

Precautions

➤*Parenteral administration:* Parenteral administration is preferable to oral dosing if there is a possibility that the patient may vomit or not absorb the leucovorin.

Drug Interactions

Leucovorin Drug Interactions

Precipitant drug	Object drug*		Description
Leucovorin	Anticonvulsants	⬇	Folic acid in large amounts may counteract the antiepileptic effect of phenobarbital, phenytoin and primidone, and increase the frequency of seizures in susceptible children. Although this interaction has not been reported with leucovorin, consider the possibility when using these drugs concomitantly.
Leucovorin	5-Fluorouracil	⬆	Leucovorin may enhance the toxicity of 5-FU (see Warnings).
Leucovorin	Methotrexate	⬇	Small quantities of systemically administered leucovorin enter the CSF primarily as 5-methyltetrahydrofolate and remain 1 to 3 orders of magnitude lower than the usual MTX concentrations following intrathecal administration. However, high doses of leucovorin may reduce the efficacy of intrathecally administered MTX.

* ⬆ = Object drug increased. ⬇ = Object drug decreased.

LEUCOVORIN CALCIUM — ORAL

Adverse Reactions

Allergic sensitization, including anaphylactoid reactions and urticaria, has been reported following the administration of both oral and parenteral leucovorin.

Overdosage

Excessive amounts of leucovorin may nullify the chemotherapeutic effect of folic acid antagonists.

LEUCOVORIN CALCIUM — INJECTION

Indications

➤*Methotrexate toxicity:* After high-dose methotrexate therapy in osteosarcoma. Leucovorin calcium is also indicated to diminish the toxicity and counteract the effects of impaired methotrexate elimination and of inadvertent overdosage of folic acid antagonists.

➤*Megaloblastic anemia:* Treatment of megaloblastic anemias due to folic acid deficiency when oral therapy is not feasible.

➤*Advanced colorectal cancer:* For use in combination with 5-fluorouracil to prolong survival in the palliative treatment of patients with advanced colorectal cancer.

➤*Unlabeled uses:* Treatment of non-Hodgkin lymphoma.

Administration and Dosage

➤*Advanced colorectal cancer:* Either of the following 2 regimens is recommended:

200 mg/m^2 by slow IV injection over a minimum of 3 minutes, followed by 5-fluorouracil at 370 mg/m^2 by IV injection.

20 mg/m^2 by IV injection followed by 5-fluorouracil at 425 mg/m^2 by IV injection.

5-flurouracil and leucovorin should be administered separately to avoid the formation of a precipitate.

Treatment is repeated daily for 5 days. This 5-day treatment course may be repeated at 4-week (28-day) intervals for 2 courses, and then repeated at 4- to 5-week (28- to 35-day) intervals, provided that the patient has completely recovered from the toxic effects of the prior treatment course.

In subsequent treatment courses, the dosage of 5-fluorouracil should be adjusted based on patient tolerance of the prior treatment course. The daily dosage of 5-fluorouracil should be reduced by 20% for patients who experienced moderate hematologic or GI toxicity in the prior treatment course, and by 30% for patients who experienced severe toxicity. For patients who experienced no toxicity in the prior treatment course, 5-fluorouracil dosage may be increased by 10%. Leucovorin dosages are not adjusted for toxicity.

Several other doses and schedules of leucovorin/5-fluorouracil therapy have also been evaluated in patients with advanced colorectal cancer; some of these alternative regimens may also have efficacy in the treatment of this disease. However, further clinical research will be required to confirm the safety and effectiveness of these alternative leucovorin/5-fluorouracil treatment regimens.

Leucovorin should not be administered intrathecally.

➤*Guidelines for methotrexate toxicity (leucovorin rescue):* The following are guidelines for leucovorin dosage and administration.

In patients with healthy methotrexate elimination, serum methotrexate levels are approximately 10 micromolar at 24 hours after administration, 1 micromolar at 48 hours, and less than 0.2 micromolar at 72 hours; administer 15 mg orally, IM, or IV every 6 hours for 60 hours (10 doses starting at 24 hours after start of methotrexate infusion).

In patients with delayed late methotrexate elimination, serum methotrexate levels remain above 0.2 micromolar at 72 hours, and greater than 0.05 micromolar at 96 hours after administration; continue 15 mg orally, IM, or IV every 6 hours until methotrexate level is less than 0.05 micromolar.

In patients with delayed early methotrexate elimination or evidence of acute renal injury, serum methotrexate levels are greater than or equal to 50 micromolar at 24 hours, or greater than or equal to 5 micromolar at 48 hours after administration; or a greater than or equal to 100% increase in serum creatinine level occurs at 24 hours after methotrexate administration; administer 150 mg IV every 3 hours until methotrexate level is less than 1 micromolar, then 15 mg IV every 3 hours until methotrexate level is less than 0.05 micromolar.

➤*Leucovorin rescue after high-dose methotrexate therapy:* The recommendations for leucovorin rescue are based on a methotrexate dose of 12 to 15 g/m^2 administered by IV infusion over 4 hours.

Leucovorin rescue at a dose of 15 mg (approximately 10 mg/m^2) every 6 hours for 10 doses starts 24 hours after the beginning of the methotrexate infusion. In the presence of GI toxicity, nausea, or vomiting, leucovorin should be administered parenterally.

Serum creatinine and methotrexate levels should be determined at least once daily. Leucovorin administration, hydration, and urinary alkalinization (pH of greater than or equal to 7) should be continued until the methotrexate level is below 5 times 10^{-8} M (0.05 micromolar). The leucovorin dose should be adjusted or leucovorin rescue extended based on the above guidelines.

Patients who experience delayed early methotrexate elimination are likely to develop reversible renal failure. In addition to appropriate leucovorin therapy, these patients require continuing hydration and urinary alkalinization, and close monitoring of fluid and electrolyte status, until the serum methotrexate level has fallen to below 0.05 micromolar and the renal failure has resolved.

Some patients will have abnormalities in methotrexate elimination or renal function following methotrexate administration, which are significant but less severe than the abnormalities described in the data above. Those abnormalities may or may not be associated with significant clinical toxicity. If significant clinical toxicity is observed, leucovorin rescue should be extended for an additional 24 hours (total of 14 doses over 84 hours) in subsequent courses of therapy. The possibility that the patient is taking other medications which interact with methotrexate (eg, medications which may interfere with methotrexate elimination or binding to serum albumin) should always be reconsidered when laboratory abnormalities or clinical toxicities are observed.

➤*Impaired methotrexate elimination or inadvertent overdosage:* Leucovorin rescue should begin as soon as possible after an inadvertent overdosage and within 24 hours of methotrexate administration when there is delayed excretion. Delayed methotrexate excretion may be caused by a third-space fluid accumulation (ie, ascites, pleural effusion), renal insufficiency, or inadequate hydration. Under such circumstances, higher doses of leucovorin or prolonged administration may be indicated. Doses higher than those recommended for oral use must be given IV. Leucovorin 10 mg/m^2 should be administered IV, IM, or orally every 6 hours until the serum methotrexate level is less than 10^{-8} M. In the presence of GI toxicity, nausea, or vomiting, leucovorin should be administered parenterally.

Serum creatinine and methotrexate levels should be determined at 24-hour intervals. If the 24-hour serum creatinine has increased 50% over baseline or if the 24 hour methotrexate level is greater than 5×10^{-8} M or the 48-hour level is greater than 9×10^{-7} M the dose of leucovorin should be increased to 100 mg/m^2 IV every 3 hours until the methotrexate level is less than 10^{-8} M.

Hydration (3 L/day) and urinary alkalinization with sodium bicarbonate solution should be employed concomitantly. The bicarbonate dose should be adjusted to maintain the urine pH at greater than or equal to 7.

➤*Megaloblastic anemia due to folic acid deficiency:* Up to 1 mg daily. There is no evidence that doses greater than 1 mg/day have greater efficacy than those of 1 mg; additionally, loss of folate in urine becomes roughly logarithmic as the amount administered exceeds 1 mg.

➤*Administration:* Because of the calcium content of the leucovorin solution, no more than 160 mg of leucovorin should be injected IV per minute (16 mL of a 10 mg/mL, or 8 mL of a 20 mg/mL solution per minute).

➤*Admixture incompatibility:* Leucovorin should not be mixed in the same infusion as 5-fluorouracil, since this may lead to the formation of a precipitate.

➤*Storage/Stability:* Store at 25°C (77°F): Excursions permitted to 15° to 30°C (59° to 86°F). Protect from light.

Each 350 mg vial of leucovorin calcium for injection when reconstituted with 17 mL of sterile diluent yields a leucovorin concentration of 20 mg leucovorin/mL. Leucovorin calcium for injection contains no preservative. Reconstitute with Bacteriostatic Water for Injection, USP, which contains benzyl alcohol, or with Sterile Water for Injection, USP. When reconstituted with Bacteriostatic Water for Injection, USP, the resulting solution must be used within 7 days. If the product is reconstituted with Sterile Water for Injection, USP, it must be used immediately.

Because of the benzyl alcohol contained in Bacteriostatic Water for Injection, USP, when doses greater than 10 mg/m^2 are administered leucovorin calcium for injection should be reconstituted with Sterile Water for Injection, USP, and used immediately.

Actions

➤*Pharmacology:* Leucovorin is a mixture of the diastereoisomers of the 5-formyl derivative of tetrahydrofolic acid (THF). The biologically active compound of the mixture is the (−)-l-isomer, known as citrovorum factor or (−)-folinic acid. Leucovorin does not require reduction by the enzyme dihydrofolate reductase in order to participate in reactions utilizing folates as a source of "1-carbon" moieties. l-Leucovorin (l-5-formyltetrahydrofolate) is rapidly metabolized (via, 5,10-methenyltetrahydrofolate then 5,10-methylenetetrahydrofolate) to l-5-methyltetrahydrofolate. l – 5-Methyltetrahydrofolate can in turn be metabolized via other pathways back to 5,10-methylenetetrahydrofolate, which is converted to 5-methyltetrahydrofolate by an irreversible, enzyme catalyzed reduction using the cofactors $FADH_2$ and NADPH.

Administration of leucovorin can counteract the therapeutic and toxic effects of folic acid antagonists such as methotrexate, which act by inhibiting dihydrofolate reductase.

In contrast, leucovorin can enhance the therapeutic and toxic effects of fluoropyrimidines used in cancer therapy, such as 5-fluorouracil. Concurrent administration of leucovorin does not appear to alter the plasma pharmacokinetics of 5-fluorouracil. 5-fluorouracil is metabolized to fluorodeoxyuridylic acid, which binds to and inhibits the enzyme thymidylate synthase (an enzyme important in DNA repair and replication).

LEUCOVORIN CALCIUM — INJECTION

Leucovorin is readily converted to another reduced folate, 5, 10-methylenetetrahydrofolate, which acts to stabilize the binding of fluorodeoxyuridylic acid to thymidylate synthase and thereby enhances the inhibition of this enzyme.

➤*Pharmacokinetics:*

Absorption –

IV: The pharmacokinetics after IV, IM, and oral administration of a 25 mg dose of leucovorin were studied in male volunteers. After IV administration, serum total reduced folates (as measured by *Lactobacillus casei* assay) reached a mean peak of 1259 ng/mL (range 897 to 1625). The mean time to peak was 10 minutes. This initial rise in total reduced folates was primarily due to the parent compound 5-formyl-THF (measured by *Streptococcus faecalis* assay) which rose to 1206 ng/mL at 10 minutes. A sharp drop in parent compound followed and coincided with the appearance of the active metabolite 5-methyl-THF which became the predominant circulating form of the drug.

The mean peak of 5-methyl-THF was 258 ng/mL and occurred at 1.3 hours.

IM: After IM injection, the mean peak of serum total reduced folates was 436 mg/mL (range 240 to 725) and occurred at 52 minutes. Similar to IV administration, the initial sharp rise was due to the parent compound.

The mean peak of 5-formyl-THF was 360 ng/mL and occurred at 28 minutes. The level of the metabolite 5-methyl-THF increased subsequently over time until at 1.5 hours it represented 50% of the circulating total folates. The mean peak of 5-methyl-THF was 226 ng/mL at 2.8 hours.

Metabolism / Excretion –

IV: The terminal half-life for total reduced folates was 6.2 hours. The area under the concentration versus time curves (AUCs) for l-leucovorin, d-leucovorin and 5-methyltetrahydrofolate were 28.4 ± 3.5, 956 ± 97 and 129 ± 12 (mg.min/L ± S.E.). When a higher dose of d,l-leucovorin (200 mg/m^2) was used, similar results were obtained. The d-isomer persisted in plasma at concentrations greatly exceeding those of the l-isomer.

IM: The terminal half-life of total reduced folates was 6.2 hours. There was no difference of statistical significance between IM and IV administration in the AUC for total reduced folates. 5-formyl-THF, or 5-methyl-THF.

Contraindications

Pernicious anemia and other megaloblastic anemias secondary to the lack of vitamin B_{12}.

Warnings

➤*Folic acid antagonists overdosage:* In the treatment of accidental overdosage of folic acid antagonists, IV leucovorin should be administered as promptly as possible. As the time interval between antifolate administration (eg, methotrexate) and leucovorin rescue increases, leucovorin's effectiveness in counteracting toxicity decreases. In the treatment of accidental overdosages of intrathecally administered folic acid antagonists, do not administer leucovorin intrathecally. Leucovorin may be harmful or fatal if given intrathecally.

➤*Methotrexate concentrations:* Monitoring of the serum methotrexate concentration is essential in determining the optimal dose and duration of treatment with leucovorin.

Delayed methotrexate excretion may be caused by a third-space fluid accumulation (ie, ascites, pleural effusion), renal insufficiency, or inadequate hydration. Under such circumstances, higher doses of leucovorin or prolonged administration may be indicated. Doses higher than those recommended for oral use must be given IV.

➤*Benzyl alcohol:* Because of the benzyl alcohol contained in certain diluents used for leucovorin calcium for injection, when doses greater than 10 mg/m^2 are administered, leucovorin calcium for injection should be reconstituted with Sterile Water for Injection, USP, and used immediately.

➤*Calcium content:* See Administration and Dosage for more information.

➤*5-fluorouracil dosage / toxicity:* Leucovorin enhances the toxicity of 5-fluorouracil. When those drugs are administered concurrently in the palliative therapy of advanced colorectal cancer, the dosage of 5-fluorouracil must be lower than usually administered. Although the toxicities observed in patients treated with the combination of leucovorin plus 5-fluorouracil are qualitatively similar to those observed in patients treated with 5-fluorouracil alone, GI toxicities (particularly stomatitis and diarrhea) are observed more commonly and may be more severe and of prolonged duration in patients treated with the combination.

In the first Mayo/NCCTG controlled trial, toxicity, primarily gastrointestinal, resulted in 7% of patients requiring hospitalization when treated with 5-fluorouracil alone or 5-fluorouracil in combination with 200 mg/m^2 of leucovorin and 20% when treated with 5-fluorouracil in combination with 20 mg/m^2 of leucovorin. In the second Mayo/NCCTG trial, hospitalizations related to treatment toxicity also appeared to occur more often in patients treated with the low-dose leucovorin/5-fluorouracil combination than in patients treated with the high-dose combination: 11% vs 3%. Therapy with leucovorin/5-fluorouracil must not be initiated or continued in patients who have symptoms of GI toxicity of any severity, until those symptoms have completely resolved. Patients with diarrhea must be monitored with particular care until the diarrhea has resolved, as rapid clinical deterioration leading to death can occur. In an additional study utilizing higher weekly doses of 5-FU and leucovorin, elderly or debilitated patients were found to be at greater risk for severe GI toxicity.

Since leucovorin enhances the toxicity of fluorouracil, leucovorin/5-fluorouracil combination therapy for advanced colorectal cancer should be administered under the supervision of a physician experienced in the use of antimetabolite cancer chemotherapy. Particular care should be taken in the treatment of elderly or debilitated colorectal cancer patients, as these patients may be at increased risk of severe toxicity.

➤*Seizures:* Seizures or syncope have been reported rarely in cancer patients receiving leucovorin, usually in association with fluoropyrimidine administration, and most commonly in those with CNS metastases or other predisposing factors; however, a causal relationship has not been established.

➤*Pneumocystis carinii pneumonia patients:* The concomitant use of leucovorin with trimethoprim-sulfamethoxazole for the acute treatment of *Pneumocystis carinii* pneumonia in patients with HIV infection was associated with increased rates of treatment failure and morbidity in a placebo-controlled study.

➤*Anemias:* Leucovorin is improper therapy for pernicious anemia and other megaloblastic anemias secondary to the lack of vitamin B_{12}. A hematologic remission may occur while neurologic manifestations continue to progress.

➤*Renal function impairment:* This drug is known to be excreted by the kidney, and the risk of toxic reactions to the drug may be greater in patients with impaired renal function.

➤*Elderly:* Clinical studies of leucovorin calcium did not show differences in safety or efficacy between subjects over age 65 and younger subjects. Other clinical experience has not identified differences in responses between the elderly and younger patients, but greater sensitivity of some older patients cannot be ruled out. This drug is known to be excreted by the kidney, and the risk of toxic reactions to the drug may be greater in patients with impaired renal function. Because elderly patients are more likely to have decreased renal function, care should be taken in dose selection in this patient population.

➤*Pregnancy: Category C.*

Adequate animal reproduction studies have not been conducted with leucovorin. It is also not known whether leucovorin can cause fetal harm when administered to a pregnant woman or can affect reproduction capacity. Leucovorin should be given to a pregnant woman only if clearly needed.

➤*Lactation:* It is not known whether this drug is excreted in human milk. Because many drugs are excreted in human milk, caution should be exercised when leucovorin is administered to a nursing mother.

➤*Children:* See Drug Interactions for more information.

Precautions

➤*Monitoring:* Patients being treated with the leucovorin/5-fluorouracil combination should have a CBC with differential and platelets prior to each treatment. During the first 2 courses, a CBC with differential and platelets has to be repeated weekly and thereafter once each cycle at the time of anticipated WBC nadir. Electrolytes and liver function tests should be performed prior to each treatment for the first 3 cycles then prior to every other cycle. Dosage modifications of fluorouracil should be instituted as follows, based on the most severe toxicities:

For moderate diarrhea or stomatitis, WBC nadir 1000 to 1900 mm^3, or platelet nadir 25 to 75,000 mm^3, decrease 5-FU dosage by 20%. For severe diarrhea or stomatitis, WBC nadir less than 1000 mm^3, or platelet nadir less than 25,000 mm^3, decrease 5-FU dosage by 30%.

If no toxicity occurs, the 5-fluorouracil dose may increase 10%. Treatment should be deferred until WBCs are 4000/mm^3 and platelets 130,000/mm^3. If blood counts do not reach these levels within 2 weeks, treatment should be discontinued. Patients should be followed up with physical examination prior to each treatment course and appropriate radiological examination as needed. Treatment should be discontinued when there is clear evidence of tumor progression.

➤*Parenteral administration:* Parenteral administration is preferable to oral dosing if there is a possibility that the patient may vomit or not absorb the leucovorin. Leucovorin has no effect on nonhematologic toxicities of methotrexate such as the nephrotoxicity resulting from drug or metabolite precipitation in the kidney.

Drug Interactions

Leucovorin Drug Interactions

Precipitant drug	Object drug*		Description
Leucovorin	Anticonvulsants	⬇	Folic acid in large amounts may counteract the antiepileptic effect of phenobarbital, phenytoin and primidone, and increase the frequency of seizures in susceptible children. Although this interaction has not been reported with leucovorin, consider the possibility when using these drugs concomitantly.
Leucovorin	5-Fluorouracil	⬆	Leucovorin may enhance the toxicity of 5-FU (see Warnings).

LEUCOVORIN CALCIUM — INJECTION

Leucovorin Drug Interactions			
Precipitant drug	Object drug*		Description
Leucovorin	Methotrexate	⬇	Small quantities of systemically administered leucovorin enter the CSF primarily as 5-methyltetrahydrofolate and remain 1 to 3 orders of magnitude lower than the usual MTX concentrations following intrathecal administration. However, high doses of leucovorin may reduce the efficacy of intrathecally administered MTX.

* ⬆ = Object drug increased. ⬇ = Object drug decreased.

Adverse Reactions

Allergic sensitization, including anaphylactoid reactions and urticaria, has been reported following administration of both oral and parenteral leucovorin. No other adverse reactions have been attributed to the use of leucovorin per se.

Percentage of Patients Treated With Leucovorin/Fluorouracil for Advanced Colorectal Carcinoma Reporting Adverse Reactions or Hospitalized for Toxicity						
Adverse reaction	(High LV) [a]/5-FU (n = 155)		(Low LV)[b]/5-FU (n = 161)		5-FU alone (n = 70)	
	Any [c](%)	Grade 3+ [d](%)	Any [c] (%)	Grade 3+ [d](%)	Any [c] (%)	Grade 3+ [d](%)
Leukopenia	69%	14%	83%	23%	93%	48%
Thrombocytopenia	8%	2%	8%	1%	18%	3%
Infection	8%	1%	3%	1%	7%	2%
Nausea	74%	10%	80%	9%	60%	6%
Vomiting	46%	8%	44%	9%	40%	7%
Diarrhea	66%	18%	67%	14%	43%	11%
Stomatitis	75%	27%	84%	29%	59%	16%
Constipation	3%	0%	4%	0%	1%	
Lethargy/malaise/fatigue	13%	3%	12%	2%	6%	3%
Alopecia	42%	5%	43%	6%	37%	7%
Dermatitis	21%	2%	25%	1%	13%	
Anorexia	14%	1%	22%	4%	14%	
Hospitalization for toxicity	5%		15%		7%	

[a] High LV = leucovorin 200 mg/m^2.
[b] Low LV = leucovorin 20 mg/m^2.
[c] Any = percentage of patients reporting toxicity of any severity.
[d] Grade 3+ = percentage of patients reporting toxicity of grade 3 or higher.

Overdosage

Excessive amounts of leucovorin may nullify the chemotherapeutic effect of folic acid antagonists.

VITAMIN B_{12}

Indications

➤*Vitamin B_{12} deficiency:* Vitamin B_{12} deficiency due to malabsorption syndrome as seen in pernicious anemia; GI pathology, dysfunction or surgery; fish tapeworm infestation; malignancy of pancreas or bowel; gluten enteropathy; sprue; small bowel bacterial overgrowth; total or partial gastrectomy; accompanying folic acid deficiency.

➤*Increased vitamin B_{12} requirements:* Increased vitamin B_{12} requirements associated with pregnancy, thyrotoxicosis, hemolytic anemia, hemorrhage, malignancy and hepatic and renal disease.

➤*Vitamin B_{12} absorption test:* (Schilling test).

Cyanocobalamin (oral) is used for nutritional vitamin B_{12} deficiency (see monograph).

➤*Unlabeled uses:* Hydroxocobalamin has been used to prevent and to treat cyanide toxicity associated with sodium nitroprusside. It lowers red blood cell and plasma cyanide concentrations by combining with cyanide to form cyanocobalamin, which is nontoxic and excreted in the urine.

Actions

➤*Pharmacology:* Vitamin B_{12} (cyanocobalamin and hydroxocobalamin) is essential to growth, cell reproduction, hematopoiesis and nucleoprotein and myelin synthesis. Its physiologic role is associated with methylation, participating in nucleic acid and protein synthesis. Cyanocobalamin participates in red blood cell formation through activation of folic acid coenzymes. Cyanocobalamin has hematopoietic activity apparently identical to that of the anti-anemia factor in purified liver extract. Hydroxocobalamin (vitamin B_{12a}), an analog of cyanocobalamin in which a hydroxyl radical replaces the cyano radical, functions the same as cyanocobalamin.

The normal range of plasma B_{12} is 200 to 750 pg/mL, which represents ≈ 0.1% of the total body content. The total daily loss ranges from 2 to 5 mcg. Because of its slow rate of utilization and considerable body stores, vitamin B_{12} deficiency may take many months to appear.

The average diet supplies ≈ 5 to 15 mcg/day of vitamin B_{12}. Vitamin B_{12} is bound to intrinsic factor during transit through the stomach; separation occurs in the terminal ileum in the presence of calcium, and vitamin B_{12} enters the mucosal cell for absorption. It is then transported by specific B_{12} binding proteins, transcobalamin I and II. Transcobalamin II is the delivery protein for vitamin B_{12}. In addition, ≈ 1% of the total amount ingested is absorbed by simple diffusion, but this mechanism is significant only with large doses.

For use of oral vitamin B_{12} in the treatment of nutritional deficiency, see the individual monograph.

➤*Pharmacokinetics:* Absorption of vitamin B_{12} depends on the presence of sufficient intrinsic factor and calcium. In general, absorption of oral B_{12} is inadequate in malabsorptive states and in pernicious anemia (unless intrinsic factor is simultaneously administered).

Cyanocobalamin – Cyanocobalamin is rapidly absorbed from IM and SC injection sites; the plasma level peaks within 1 hour. Once absorbed, it is bound to plasma proteins, stored mainly in the liver and is slowly released when needed to carry out normal cellular metabolic functions. Within 48 hours after injection of 100 to 1000 mcg of vitamin B_{12}, 50% to 98% of the dose appears in the urine. The major portion is excreted within the first 8 hours. More rapid excretion occurs with IV administration; there is little opportunity for liver storage.

Hydroxocobalamin – Hydroxocobalamin (vitamin B_{12a}) is more highly protein bound and is retained in the body longer than cyanocobalamin. However, it has no advantage over cyanocobalamin. Administration of hydroxocobalamin has resulted in antibody formation to the hydroxocobalamin-transcobalamin II complex and thus cyanocobalamin may be preferred.

Contraindications

Hypersensitivity to cobalt, vitamin B_{12} or any component of these products.

Warnings

➤*Inadequate response:* Parenteral administration is preferred for pernicious anemia. Avoid the IV route.

A blunted or impeded therapeutic response may be due to infection, uremia, bone marrow suppressant drugs (ie, chloramphenicol), concurrent iron or folic acid deficiency or misdiagnosis.

➤*Vitamin B_{12} deficiency:* Vitamin B_{12} deficiency allowed to progress for more than 3 months may produce permanent degenerative lesions of the spinal cord.

➤*Optic nerve atrophy:* Patients with early Leber's disease (hereditary optic nerve atrophy) treated with cyanocobalamin suffer severe and swift optic atrophy.

➤*Hypokalemia:* Hypokalemia and sudden death may occur in severe megaloblastic anemia which is treated intensely.

➤*Benzyl alcohol:* Some of these products contain benzyl alcohol, which has been associated with a fatal "gasping syndrome" in premature infants.

VITAMIN B_{12}

➤*Pregnancy: Category C* (parenteral). Adequate and well-controlled studies have not been performed in pregnant women. However, B_{12} is an essential vitamin and needs are increased during pregnancy. The National Academy of Sciences has recommended that 2.2 mcg/day should be consumed during pregnancy.

➤*Lactation:* Vitamin B_{12} is excreted in breast milk in concentrations that approximate the mother's vitamin B_{12}blood level. Amounts of B_{12} recommended by the Food and Nutrition Board, National Academy of Sciences-National Research Council (2.6 mcg daily) should be consumed during lactation.

➤*Children:* The Food and Nutrition Board, National Academy of Sciences-National Research Council recommends a daily intake of 0.3 to 0.5 mcg/day for infants younger than 1 year of age and 0.7 to 1.4 mcg/day for children 1 to 10 years of age.

Precautions

➤*Monitoring:* During treatment of severe megaloblastic anemia, monitor serum potassium levels closely for the first 48 hours and replace potassium if necessary. Obtain reticulocyte counts, hematocrit and vitamin B_{12}, iron and folic acid plasma levels prior to treatment and between the fifth and seventh days of therapy, and then frequently until the hematocrit is normal. If folate levels are low, also administer folic acid. Continue periodic hematologic evaluations throughout the patient's lifetime.

➤*Test dose:* Anaphylactic shock and death have occurred after parenteral vitamin B_{12} administration. Give an intradermal test dose in patients sensitive to the cobalamins.

➤*Folate:* Doses more than 10 mcg daily may produce hematologic response in patients with folate deficiency. Indiscriminate use may mask the true diagnosis of pernicious anemia.

Doses of folic acid more than 0.1 mg/day may result in hematologic remission in patients with vitamin B_{12} deficiency. Neurologic manifestations will not be prevented with folic acid, and if not treated with vitamin B_{12}, irreversible damage will result.

Single deficiency – Single deficiency (vitamin B_{12} alone) is rare. Expect multiple vitamin deficiency in any dietary deficiency.

➤*Polycythemia vera:* Vitamin B_{12} deficiency may suppress the signs of polycythemia vera. Treatment with vitamin B_{12} may unmask this condition.

➤*Vegetarian diets:* Vegetarian diets containing no animal products (including milk products or eggs) do not supply any vitamin B_{12}. Vegetarians should take oral vitamin B_{12} regularly.

➤*Stomach carcinoma:* Pernicious anemia patients have about 3 times the incidence of stomach carcinoma as the general population; perform appropriate tests for this condition when indicated.

➤*Immunodeficient patients:* Vitamin B_{12} malabsorption may occur in patients with AIDS or HIV infection. Consider monitoring vitamin B_{12} levels in these patients.

Drug Interactions

Vitamin B_{12} Drug Interactions			
Precipitant drug	Object drug[a]		Description
Aminosalicylic acid	Vitamin B_{12}	⬇	Biologic and therapeutic action of vitamin B_{12} may be reduced. An abnormal Schilling test and symptoms of vitamin B_{12} deficiency may also occur.
Chloramphenicol	Vitamin B_{12}	⬇	The hematologic effects of vitamin B_{12} may be decreased in patients with pernicious anemia.
Colchicine Alcohol	Vitamin B_{12}	⬇	Colchicine or excessive alcohol intake (more than 2 weeks) may cause malabsorption of vitamin B_{12}.

[a] ⬇ = Object drug decreased.

➤*Drug/Lab test interactions:* Methotrexate, pyrimethamine and most antibiotics invalidate folic acid and vitamin B_{12} diagnostic microbiological blood assays.

Adverse Reactions

The following reactions are associated with parenteral vitamin B_{12}:

➤*Cardiovascular:* Pulmonary edema; congestive heart failure early in treatment; peripheral vascular thrombosis.

➤*Dermatologic:* Itching; transitory exanthema.

➤*Hypersensitivity:* Anaphylactic shock and death.

➤*Miscellaneous:* Feeling of swelling of the entire body; mild transient diarrhea; polycythemia vera; pain at injection site; severe and swift optic nerve atrophy (see Warnings).

Patient Information

Patients with pernicious anemia will require monthly injections of vitamin B_{12} for the rest of their lives. Failure to do so will result in return of the anemia and in development of incapacitating and irreversible damage to the nerves of the spinal cord.

A well balanced dietary intake is necessary; correct poor dietary habits.

Do not take folic acid instead of vitamin B_{12} because folic acid may prevent anemia, but allow progression of subacute combined degeneration.

HYDROXOCOBALAMIN CRYSTALLINE (Vitamin B_{12})

Rx	**Hydro-Crysti-12** (Roberts Hauck)	**Injection:** 1000 mcg/mL	In 30 mL.
Rx	**LA-12** (Hyrex)		In 30 mL.

HYDROXOCOBALAMIN — INJECTION

For complete and comparative prescribing information, refer to the Vitamin B_{12} monograph.

Indications

➤*Pernicious anemia:* Pernicious anemia both uncomplicated and accompanied by nervous system involvement.

➤*Dietary deficiency of vitamin B_{12}:* Dietary deficiency of vitamin B_{12}, occurring in strict vegetarians and in their breastfed infants. (Isolated vitamin B_{12} deficiency is very rare).

➤*Malabsorption of vitamin B_{12}:* Malabsorption of vitamin B_{12} resulting from structural or functional damage to the stomach, where intrinsic factor is secreted or to the ileum, where intrinsic factor facilitates vitamin B_{12} absorption. These conditions include tropical sprue, and nontropical sprue (idiopathic steatorrhea, gluten-induced enteropathy). Folate deficiency in these patients is usually more severe than vitamin B_{12} deficiency.

➤*Inadequate secretion of intrinsic factor:* Inadequate secretion of intrinsic factor, resulting from lesions that destroy the gastric mucosa (ingestion of corrosives, extensive neoplasia), and a number of conditions associated with a variable degree of gastric atrophy (such as multiple sclerosis, certain endocrine disorders, iron deficiency, and subtotal gastrectomy). Total gastrectomy always produces vitamin B_{12} deficiency.

Structural lesions leading to vitamin B_{12} deficiency include regional ileitis, ileal resections, malignancies, etc.

➤*Competition for vitamin B_{12}:* Competition for vitamin B_{12} by intestinal parasites or bacteria.

➤*Inadequate utilization of vitamin B_{12}:* Inadequate utilization of vitamin B_{12}. This may occur if antimetabolites for the vitamin are employed in the treatment of neoplasia.

➤*Schilling test:* For the Schilling test.

➤*Unlabeled uses:* Hydroxocobalamin has been used to prevent and to treat cyanide toxicity associated with sodium nitroprusside. It lowers red blood cell and plasma cyanide concentrations by combining with cyanide to form cyanocobalamin, which is nontoxic and excreted in the urine.

Administration and Dosage

Hydroxocobalamin injection should be given only IM.

➤*Pernicious anemia:* In patients with Addisonian pernicious anemia, parenteral therapy with vitamin B_{12} is the recommended method of treatment and will be required for the remainder of the patient's life. Oral therapy is not dependable. In other patients with vitamin B_{12} deficiency, the duration of therapy and route of administration will depend upon the cause and whether or not it is reversible.

Confirmatory diagnostic studies should be performed prior to initiating therapy, if possible, and the patient should be followed with appropriate studies to demonstrate hematologic improvement (Hgb, hematocrit, RBC, reticulocyte count). A diagnostic trial utilizing physiologic doses of vitamin B_{12} (1 mcg daily) and observing daily reticulocyte counts after establishing a baseline may also be performed. The observation of reticulocytosis which usually occurs between the third and tenth day of therapy confirms the diagnosis of vitamin B_{12} deficiency.

In seriously ill patients it may be advisable to administer both vitamin B_{12} and folic acid while awaiting the results of distinguishing laboratory studies. It is not necessary to withhold vitamin B_{12} therapy until the precise cause of B_{12} deficiency is established since absorption studies can be performed at any time.

➤*Concomitant potassium therapy:* Serum potassium should be closely observed the first 48 hours and potassium should be administered if necessary.

➤*Vitamin B_{12} deficiency:* 30 mcg daily for 5 to 10 days followed by 100 to 200 mcg monthly injected IM. If the patient is critically ill, or has neurologic disease, an infectious disease or hyperthyroidism, considerably higher doses may be indicated. However, current data indicate that the optimum obtainable neurologic response may be expected with a dosage of vitamin B_{12} sufficient to produce good hematologic response. Children may be given a total of 1 to 5 mg over a period of 2 or more weeks in doses of 100 mcg, then 30 to 50 mcg every 4 weeks for maintenance.

Water-Soluble Vitamins

HYDROXOCOBALAMIN — INJECTION

Patients who have normal intestinal absorption may be treated with an oral therapeutic multivitamin preparation, containing 15 mcg vitamin B_{12} daily.

➤*Schilling test:* The flushing dose is 1000 mcg.

➤*Storage / Stability:* Store at controlled room temperature 15° to 30°C (59° to 86°F). Protect from light.

CYANOCOBALAMIN CRYSTALLINE

otc	**Vitamin B_{12}** (Goldline)	**Tablets:** 500 mcg	Pink. In 100s.
		1000 mcg	Pink. In 100s.
Rx	**Vitamin B_{12}** (Various, eg, Goldline, Rugby)	**Injection:** 100 mcg per mL	In 30 mL vials.
Rx	**Vitamin B_{12}** (Various, eg, American Regent, Geneva, Goldline, Major, Pasadena, Rugby, Schein, Warner Chilcott)	**Injection:** 1000 mcg per mL	In 10 and 30 mL multi-dose vials.
Rx	**Crystamine** (Dunhall)		In 10 and 30 mL multi-dose vials.[1]
Rx	**Crysti 1000** (Roberts Hauck)		In 10 mL vials.
Rx	**Cyanoject** (Mayrand)		In 10 and 30 mL.[1]
Rx	**Cyomin** (Forest)		In 30 mL multi-dose vials.[1]
Rx	**Rubesol-1000** (Central)		In 10 and 30 mL vials[1].

[1] With benzyl alcohol.

CYANOCOBALAMIN CRYSTALLINE

For complete prescribing information, refer to the Vitamin B_{12} monograph.

Administration and Dosage

➤*Addisonian pernicious anemia:* Parenteral therapy is required for life; oral therapy is not dependable. Administer 100 mcg daily for 6 or 7 days by IM or deep SC injection. If there is clinical improvement and a reticulocyte response, give the same amount on alternate days for 7 doses, then every 3 to 4 days for another 2 to 3 weeks. By this time, hematologic values should have become normal. Follow this regimen with 100 mcg monthly for life. Administer folic acid concomitantly if needed.

➤*Other patients with vitamin B_{12} deficiency:* In seriously ill patients, administer both vitamin B_{12} and folic acid. It is not necessary to withhold therapy until the precise cause of B_{12} deficiency is established. For hematologic signs, children may be given 10 to 50 mcg/day for 5 to 10 days followed by 100 to 250 mcg/dose every 2 to 4 weeks; for neurologic signs, 100 mcg/day for 10 to 15 days, then once or twice weekly for several months, possibly tapering to 250 to 1000 mcg monthly by 1 year.

Oral – Up to 1000 mcg/day. Oral vitamin B_{12} therapy is not usually recommended for vitamin B_{12} deficiency. The maximum amount of vitamin B_{12} that can be absorbed from a single oral dose is 1 to 5 mcg. The percent absorbed decreases with increasing doses.

IM or SC – 30 mcg daily for 5 to 10 days followed by 100 to 200 mcg monthly. Larger doses (eg, 1000 mcg) have been recommended, even though a larger amount is lost through excretion. However, it is possible that a greater amount is retained, allowing for fewer injections.

➤*Schilling test:* The flushing dose is 1000 mcg IM.

➤*Storage / Stability:* Protect parenterals from light. Avoid freezing.

MINERALS

Calcium

For information on parenteral calcium products, refer to Intravenous Nutritional Therapy, Minerals section.

Indications

As a dietary supplement when calcium intake may be inadequate. Conditions that may be associated with calcium deficiency include the following: Vitamin D deficiency, sprue, pregnancy and lactation, achlorhydria, chronic diarrhea, hypoparathyroidism, steatorrhea, menopause, renal failure, pancreatitis, hyperphosphatemia, and alkalosis. Some diuretics and anticonvulsants may precipitate hypocalcemia, which may validate calcium replacement therapy. Calcium salt therapy should not preclude the use of other corrective measures intended to treat the underlying cause of calcium depletion.

Oral calcium may also be used in the treatment of osteoporosis, osteomalacia, rickets, and latent tetany.

Calcium taken daily may help reduce typical premenstrual syndrome (PMS) symptoms such as bloating, cramps, fatigue, and moodiness.

➤*Calcium acetate (PhosLo):* Control of hyperphosphatemia in end-stage renal failure; does not promote aluminum absorption.

Administration and Dosage

➤*Recommended dietary allowances (RDAs):*

Men and women (19 to 24 years of age) – 1200 mg/day

Men and women (25 to 50 years of age) – 800 mg/day

Men and women (≥ 51 years of age) – 800 mg/day

➤*Dietary reference intakes (DRIs):*

Men and women (19 to 50 years of age) – 1000 mg/day

Men and women (older than 51 years of age) – 1200 mg/day

Pregnant and breastfeeding women – 1000 mg/day

➤*Dietary supplement:* The usual daily dose is 500 mg to 2 g, 2 to 4 times/day.

Calcium is recommended in doses of 1500 mg/day for men older than 65 years of age and for postmenopausal women not taking estrogen replacement therapy.

➤*PhosLo:* For adult dialysis patients, the initial dose is 2 tablets/capsules/gelcaps with each meal. The dosage may be increased gradually to bring the serum phosphate value less than 6 mg/dL, as long as hypercalcemia does not develop. Most patients require 3 to 4 tablets with each meal.

The recommended initial dose of the half-size (333.5 mg) *PhosLo* for the adult dialysis patient is 4 capsules with each meal. The dosage may be increased gradually to bring the serum phosphate value below 6 mg/dL, as long as hypercalcemia does not develop. Most patients require 6 to 8 capsules with each meal.

➤*Florical:* 1 capsule or tablet daily.

Actions

➤*Pharmacology:* Calcium is the fifth most abundant element in the body; the major fraction is in bone. It is essential for the functional integrity of the nervous and muscular systems, for normal cardiac function, for cell permeability, and for blood coagulation. It also functions as an enzyme cofactor and affects the secretory activity of endocrine and exocrine glands.

Adequate calcium intake is particularly important during periods of bone growth in childhood and adolescence and during pregnancy and lactation. An adequate supply of calcium is necessary in adults, especially those older than 40 years of age, to prevent a negative calcium balance, which may contribute to the development of osteoporosis.

Patients with advanced renal insufficiency (Ccr less than 30 mL/min) exhibit phosphate retention and some degree of hyperphosphatemia. The retention of phosphate plays a pivotal role in causing secondary hyperparathyroidism associated with osteodystrophy and soft-tissue calcification. Calcium acetate, when taken with meals, combines with dietary phosphate to form insoluble calcium phosphate, which is excreted in the feces.

Elemental Calcium Content of Calcium Salts[a]

Calcium salt	% Calcium	mEq Ca^{++}/g
Calcium glubionate	6.5	3.3
Calcium gluconate	9	4.5
Calcium lactate	13	6.5
Calcium citrate	21	10.6
Calcium acetate	25	12.6
Tricalcium phosphate	39	19.3
Calcium carbonate	40	20

[a] 1 mEq of elemental calcium = 20 mg

➤*Pharmacokinetics:*

Absorption – Calcium is absorbed from the GI tract by passive diffusion and active transport. Calcium must be in a soluble, ionized form for absorption to occur. Vitamin D is required for calcium absorption and increases the capability of the absorptive mechanisms. Calcium absorption is increased in the presence of food. Oral bioavailability in adults ranges from 25% to 35% when a 250 mg dose is given with a standardized breakfast. Absorption from milk was ≈ 29% under the same conditions. Calcium absorption varies with age, being highest during infancy (≈ 60%), decreasing to ≈ 28% in prepubertal children, and increasing again during puberty (≈ 34%). Fractional absorption remains at ≈ 25% in young adults, and increases during the last 2 trimesters of pregnancy. Calcium absorption decreases ≈ 0.21% annually in postmenopausal women and similarly in aging men.

Distribution – Calcium enters the extracellular fluid and is rapidly incorporated into skeletal tissue. Normal total serum calcium concentrations range from 9 to 10.4 mg/dL (4.5 to 5.2 mEq/L), but only ionized calcium is active. Calcium crosses the placenta and reaches higher concentrations in fetal blood than maternal blood. Calcium also is distributed in milk.

Excretion – Calcium is mainly excreted in the feces. Only small amounts are excreted in the urine. Urinary excretion of calcium may be as high as 250 to 300 mg/day in healthy adults who eat a regular diet. However, urinary excretion does not exceed 150 mg/day in patients on low calcium diets. Urinary excretion decreases with age, in the early stages of renal failure, and during pregnancy. Calcium also is excreted by the sweat glands.

Contraindications

Hypercalcemia, ventricular fibrillation.

Warnings

➤*PhosLo:* End-stage renal failure patients may develop hypercalcemia when given calcium with meals. Do not give other calcium supplements concurrently with *PhosLo*. Chronic hypercalcemia may lead to vascular and other soft tissue calcification. Monitor serum calcium levels twice weekly during the early dose adjustment period. Do not allow serum calcium times phosphate product to exceed 66.

➤*GI effects:* Calcium salts may be irritating to the GI tract when administered orally and also may cause constipation.

➤*Hypercalcemia:* Hypercalcemia may occur when large doses of calcium are administered to patients with chronic renal failure. Mild hypercalcemia may exhibit as nausea, vomiting, anorexia, or constipation, with mental changes such as stupor, delirium, coma, or confusion. By reducing calcium intake, mild hypercalcemia is usually readily controlled.

➤*Renal calculi:* Recent evidence from studies in men 40 to 75 years of age with no history of kidney stones and women 34 to 59 years of age show that high dietary intake of calcium decreases the risk of symptomatic renal calculi, while intake of supplemental calcium may increase the risk of symptomatic stones. This conflicts with the previous theory that high calcium intake contributes to the risk of renal calculi.

➤*Pregnancy: Category C* (*PhosLo*). It is not known whether *PhosLo* can cause fetal harm when administered to a pregnant woman or can affect reproduction capacity. Give to a pregnant woman only if clearly needed.

➤*Children:* Safety and efficacy in children have not been established (*PhosLo*).

Precautions

➤*Monitoring:* Perform frequent determinations of serum calcium concentrations. Maintain serum calcium concentrations at 9 to 10.4 mg/dL (4.5 to 5.2 mEq/L). Do not allow levels to exceed 12 mg/dL.

➤*Calcium citrate:*

Renal function impairment – Avoid concurrent aluminum-containing antacids.

➤*Phenylketonurics:* Inform phenylketonuric patients that some of these products contain phenylalanine.

➤*Special risk:* Use calcium salts cautiously in patients with sarcoidosis, cardiac or renal disease, and in patients receiving cardiac glycosides.

➤*Tartrazine sensitivity:* Some of these products contain tartrazine (FD&C yellow #5), which may cause allergic-type reactions (including bronchial asthma) in susceptible individuals. Although the incidence of sensitivity is low, it is frequently seen in patients who also have aspirin hypersensitivity. Specific products containing tartrazine are identified in the product listings.

Drug Interactions

Calcium Drug Interactions

Precipitant	Object drug[a]		Description
Calcium salts	Iron salts	⬇	GI absorption of iron may be reduced. In order to avoid a possible interaction, separate administration times whenever possible.
Calcium carbonate	Quinolones	⬇	GI absorption of quinolones may be decreased. The bioavailability of norfloxacin may be reduced; lomefloxacin and ofloxacin do not appear to be affected. Give antacids ≥ 6 hours before or 2 hours after the quinolone.
Calcium salts	Sodium polystyrene sulfonate	⬇	Coadministration in patients with renal impairment may result in an unanticipated metabolic alkalosis and a reduction of the resin's binding of potassium. Separate drugs by several hours.
Calcium salts	Tetracyclines	⬇	The absorption and serum levels of tetracyclines are decreased; a decreased anti-infective response may occur. Avoid simultaneous administration. Separate administration by 3 to 4 hours.
Calcium salts	Verapamil	⬇	Clinical effects and toxicities of verapamil may be reversed.

[a] ⬆ = Object drug increased. ⬇ = Object drug decreased.

Adverse Reactions

May cause constipation and headache. Mild hypercalcemia (Ca^{++} greater than 10.5 mg/dL) may be asymptomatic or manifest itself as anorexia, nausea, and vomiting. More severe hypercalcemia (Ca^{++} greater than 12 mg/dL) is associated with confusion, delirium, stupor, and coma.

Overdosage

Administration of *PhosLo* in excess of the appropriate daily dosage can cause severe hypercalcemia (see Adverse Reactions). Severe hypercalcemia can be treated by acute hemodialysis and discontinuing therapy.

Patient Information

Notify physician if any of the following occur: Anorexia, nausea, vomiting, constipation, abdominal pain, dry mouth, thirst, polyuria.

Inform phenylketonuric patients that some of these products contain phenylalanine.

Take with or following meals to enhance absorption.

Take with a large glass of water.

CALCIUM GLUCONATE

otc	**Calcium Gluconate** (Various, eg, Dixon-Shane, Freeda, Roxane, Rugby)	**Tablets:** 500 mg (45 mg elemental calcium)	In 100s.
		Tablets: 50 mg elemental calcium	In 100s and 500s.
		648 to 650 mg (58.5 to 60 mg elemental calcium)	In 1,000s.
		972 to 975 mg (87.75 to 90 mg elemental calcium)	In 1,000s.
otc	**Cal-G** (Key)	**Capsules:** 700 mg (50 mg elemental calcium)	In 100s.
otc	**Calcium Gluconate** (Freeda)	**Powder for oral suspension:** 346.7 mg elemental calcium/15 mL	In 454 g.

Complete and comparative prescribing information for these products begins in the Calcium group monograph.

CALCIUM GLUBIONATE

otc	**Calcionate** (Various, eg, Rugby, Watson)	**Syrup:** 1.8 g/5 mL	In 473 mL.
otc	**Calciquid** (Breckenridge)		In 473 mL.

Complete and comparative prescribing information for these products begins in the Calcium group monograph.

CALCIUM LACTATE

otc	**Calcium Lactate** (Various, eg, Dixon-Shane, Rugby)	**Tablets**: 648 to 650 mg (84.5 mg elemental calcium)	In 100s and 1000s.
otc	**Calcium Lactate** (Various, eg, Freeda)	**Tablets**: 100 mg elemental calcium	In 100s and 250s.
otc sf	**Cal-Lac** (Bio-Tech)	**Capsules**: 500 mg (96 mg elemental calcium)	In 100s.

Complete and comparative prescribing information for these products begins in the Calcium group monograph.

CALCIUM CITRATE

otc	**Citracal** (Mission)	**Tablets**: 200 mg elemental calcium	(CITRACAL MPC). In 100s.
otc	**Citrus Calcium** (Rugby)	**Tablets**: 200 mg as calcium citrate	Lactose free. Coated. In 100s.
otc	**Calcium Citrate** (Various, eg, Freeda, Vitaline)	**Tablets**: 250 mg elemental calcium	In 100s, 120s, 250s, 500s, and 1,000s.
otc	**Cal-Citrate-250** (Bio-Tech)		In 250s.
otc	**Calcium Citrate** (Various, eg, Major)	**Tablets**: 950 mg	In 100s.
otc sf	**Cal-Cee** (Key)	**Tablets**: 1,150 mg (250 mg elemental calcium)	In 100s.
otc	**Citracal Liquitab** (Mission)	**Tablets, effervescent**: 500 mg elemental calcium	Aspartame, 12 mg phenylalanine, saccharin. Orange flavor. In 30s.
otc	**Cal-C-Caps** (Key)	**Capsules**: 180 mg elemental calcium	In 100s.
otc	**Cal-Citrate-225** (Bio-Tech)	**Capsules**: 225 mg elemental calcium	In 100s and 250s.
otc	**Calcium Citrate** (Various, eg, Freeda)	**Powder for oral suspension**: 760 mg elemental calcium/5 mL	In 454 g.

Complete prescribing information for these products begins in the Calcium group monograph.

CALCIUM ACETATE

Rx	**PhosLo** (Nabi)	**Tablets**: 667 mg (169 mg elemental calcium)	Polyethylene glycol 8000. (BRA 200). White. In 200s.
		Capsules: 333.5 mg (half-size) (84.5 mg elemental calcium)	Polyethylene glycol 8000. (PhosLo 333.5 mg). White. In 400s.
		667 mg (169 mg elemental calcium)	Polyethylene glycol 8000. (PhosLo 667 mg). Blue/white. In 200s.
		Gelcaps: 667 mg (169 mg elemental calcium)	Polyethylene glycol 8000. (PhosLo 667 mg). Blue/white. In 200s.

Complete and comparative prescribing information for these products begins in the Calcium group monograph.

TRICALCIUM PHOSPHATE (Calcium Phosphate, Tribasic)

otc sf	**Posture** (Iverness Medical)	**Tablets**: 600 mg elemental calcium	Preservative-free. In 90s.

Complete and comparative prescribing information for these products begins in the Calcium group monograph.

CALCIUM CARBONATE

otc	**Calcium Carbonate** (Various, eg, Medirex, Vangard)	**Tablets**: 500 mg (200 mg elemental calcium)	In 100s, 120s, and UD 100s.
otc	**Calcium Carbonate** (Various, eg, Major, Moore)	**Tablets**: 600 mg (240 mg elemental calcium)	In 60s, 72s, 150s and UD 100s.
otc	**Calcium Carbonate** (Various, eg, Freeda, Lilly, Major, Roxane, Rugby)	**Tablets**: 648 to 650 mg (260 mg elemental calcium)	In 100s, 250s, 500s, and 1,000s.
otc	**Calcium Carbonate** (Various, eg, Roxane)	**Tablets**: 1,250 mg (500 mg elemental calcium)	In 100s.
otc	**Cal-Carb Forte** (Vitaline)		Capsule shape, scored. In 100s.
otc	**Oyster Shell Calcium** (Various, eg, Major)		In 60s, 150s, 300s, 1,000s, and UD 100s.
otc	**Oysco 500** (Rugby)		As oyster shell calcium. In 60s and 250s.
otc sf	**Oyst-Cal 500** (Goldline)		As oyster shell calcium. Preservative free. Tartrazine. In 60s and 120s.
otc sf	**Os-Cal 500** (GlaxoSmithKline Consumer)		Oyster shell powder, corn syrup, parabens. In 75s.
otc	**Calcium Carbonate** (Various, eg, Major)	**Tablets**: 1,500 mg (600 mg elemental calcium)	In 60s and 150s.
otc	**Calcium 600** (Various, eg, Key, Rugby)		In 60s and 100s.
otc sf	**Caltrate 600** (Whitehall Robins)		Preservative free. (CALTRATE). In 60s.
otc	**Nephro-Calci** (Watson)		(RD26). White, oval, scored. In 100s.
otc	**Calci-Mix** (Watson)	**Capsules**: 1,250 mg (500 mg elemental calcium)	In 100s.
otc	**Florical** (Mericon)	**Capsules and tablets**: 364 mg calcium carbonate (145.6 mg elemental calcium) and 8.3 mg sodium fluoride	In 100s and 500s.
otc	**Mylanta Children's** (J&J/Merck)	**Tablets, chewable**: 400 mg (160 mg elemental calcium)	Sorbitol. Bubble gum flavor. In 24s.
otc	**Trial Antacid** (Zee Medical)	**Tablets, chewable**: 420 mg (168 mg elemental calcium)	Sorbitol. Spearmint flavor. In 24s.

CALCIUM CARBONATE

	Antacid Tablets (Goldline)	**Tablets, chewable:** 500 mg (200 mg elemental calcium)	Sucrose, ≤ 2 mg sodium.[a] Assorted flavors. In 150s.
otc	**Cal•Gest** (Rugby)		Dextrose. Assorted flavors. In 150s.
otc	**Dicarbosil** (BIRA)		Less than 2 mg sodium, 10 mEq ANC.[a] Peppermint flavor. White. In rolls of 12.
otc	**Equilet** (Mission)		≤ 0.35 mg sodium.[a] In 150s.
otc	**Maalox Antacid Barrier Maximum Strength** (Novartis)		Aspartame, sugar, mannitol, sucrose, 1.45 mg phenylalanine (mint flavor), 1.1 mg phenylalanine (cherry flavor), 23 mg sodium. In 65s.
otc	**Tums** (GlaxoSmithKline Consumer)		Sucrose, ≤ 2 mg sodium.[a] Assorted fruit and peppermint flavors. In 75s and 150s.
otc	**Calcium Antacid Extra Strength** (Various, eg, Major)	**Tablets, chewable:** 750 mg (300 mg elemental calcium)	In 96s.
otc	**Tums E-X** (GlaxoSmithKline Consumer)		Sucrose, talc. Mixed berry, assorted fruit, and sugar free orange (aspartame, less than 1 mg phenylalanine, sorbitol) flavors. In 96s.
otc	**Tums Calcium for Life PMS** (GlaxoSmithKline Consumer)		Sucrose. Strawberry flavor. In 120s.
otc	**Tums Smooth Dissolve** (GlaxoSmithKline)		Sorbitol, dextrose, sucrose (2 g sugar). In peppermint and assorted fruit flavors. In 45s.
otc	**Alka-Mints** (Bayer)	**Tablets, chewable:** 850 mg (340 mg elemental calcium)	Sorbitol, sugar, less than 5 mg sodium.[a] (Alka-Mints). Assorted flavors and spearmint. In 75s.
otc	**Tums Ultra** (GlaxoSmithKline Consumer)	**Tablets, chewable:** 1,000 mg (400 mg elemental calcium)	Sucrose, talc. Mint flavor. In 86s.
otc	**Rolaids Extra Strength Softchews** (Pfizer Consumer Health)	**Tablets, chewable:** 1177 mg (470.8 mg elemental calcium)	Sucrose, corn syrup, corn syrup solids, nonfat dry milk. Vanilla creme and wild cherry flavors. In 18s.
otc	**Calcium Carbonate** (Various, eg, Major, Roxane)	**Tablets, chewable:** 1,250 mg (500 mg elemental calcium)	In 60s.
otc	**Cal-Carb Forte** (Vitaline)		Mint flavor. In 100s.
otc	**Calci-Chew** (Watson)		(RD05). Sugar. White. Cherry and assorted flavors. In 100s.
otc	**Os-Cal 500** (GlaxoSmithKline Consumer)		Dextrose. In 60s.
otc	**Tums Calcium for Life Bone Health** (GlaxoSmithKline Consumer)		In 90s.
otc	**Chooz** (Schering-Plough)	**Gum tablets:** 500 mg (200 mg elemental calcium)	Sucrose, glucose. Mint flavor. In 16s.
otc	**Surpass** (Wrigley)	**Gum:** 300 mg (120 mg elemental calcium)	Aspartame, sorbitol. 3.9 mg phenylalanine. Wintergreen flavor. In 10s.
otc	**Surpass Extra Strength** (Wrigley)	**Gum:** 450 mg (180 mg elemental calcium)	Aspartame, sorbitol, 3.9 mg phenylalanine. Fruit flavor. In 10s.
otc	**Calcium Carbonate** (Various, eg, Roxane)	**Oral suspension:** 1,250 mg (500 mg elemental calcium)/5 mL	In 500 mL and UD 5 mL.
otc	**Calcium Carbonate** (Various, eg, Freeda, Humco)	**Powder**	In 454 g.

[a] Acid-neutralizing capacity and sodium content per tablet or 5 mL.

Complete and comparative prescribing information for these products begins in the Calcium group monograph. Also see the Antacids monograph in the Gastrointestinal Agents chapter.

PHOSPHORUS REPLACEMENT PRODUCTS

Contents given per tablet or 75 mL reconstituted liquid.

	Product and distributor	Phosphorus		Potassium		Sodium		Recommended adult dose	How supplied
		mg	mEq	mg	mEq	mg	mEq		
Rx	**Uro-KP-Neutral Tablets** (Star)	250	14.25	49.4	1.27	250.5	10.9	1 or 2 tablets 4 times/day with full glass of water	Lt. peach, capsule shape. Film-coated. In 100s.
Rx	**K-Phos Neutral Tablets** (Beach)	250	14.25	45	1.1	298	13		(Beach 1125). White, capsule shape. Film-coated. In 100s and 500s.
otc sf	**Neutra-Phos Powder**[a] (Ortho-McNeil)	250	14.25	278	7.125	164	7.125	1 powder packet reconstituted in 75 mL water 4 times/day after meals and at bedtime. Provides 250 mg phosphorus por dose (1 g/day)	Fruit flavor. In 64 g bottle and UD 1.25 g packets.
otc sf	**PHOS-NaK** (Cypress)	250	unknown	280	unknown	160	unknown	Mix 1 packet with 75 mL water or juice. Take 1 packet qid.	Fruit flavor. In 1.5 g packets (100s)
otc sf	**Neutra-Phos-K Powder**[b] (Ortho-McNeil)	250	14.25	556	14.25	0	0	1 powder packet reconstituted in 75 mL water 4 times/day after meals and at bedtime. Provides 250 mg phosphorus per dose (1 g/day)	In 71 g bottle and UD 1.45 g packets.

[a] From monobasic and dibasic sodium and potassium phosphates.

[b] From dibasic and monobasic potassium phosphates.

PHOSPHORUS REPLACEMENT PRODUCTS — ORAL

For information on parenteral phosphate, refer to the monograph in the IV Nutritional Therapy section.

Indications

➤*Dietary supplement:* Dietary supplements of phosphorus, particularly if the diet is restricted or needs are increased.

Neutra-Phos and *Neutra-Phos-K* are useful in the treatment of children and adults with conditions associated with excessive renal phosphate loss or inadequate GI absorption of phosphate. They are also useful as adjunct supplementation in the management of phosphate diabetes.

Administration and Dosage

➤*Recommended dietary allowances (RDAs):*

Adults (older than 10 years of age) – 800 to 1200 mg.

Children (1 to 10 years of age) – 800 mg.

Infants (0.5 to 1 year of age) – 500 mg.

Infants (0 to 0.5 years of age) – 300 mg. For a complete listing of RDAs by age, sex, and condition, refer to the RDA table.

➤*Neutra-Phos* and *Neutra-Phos-K* powder:

Dosage		
Age	Dose	Equivalent phosphorus dose
Younger than 4 years of age	60 mL of oral solution 4 times/day	60 mL supplies 200 mg
Adult	75 to 600 mL (or 1 to 8 packets) taken after meals and at bedtime	75 mL (1 packet) supplies 250 mg

Powder concentrate – Patient should dissolve entire contents of 1 bottle in 3.8 L (1 gallon) of water or other desirable liquid. This solution should not be further diluted, but can be chilled to increase palatability, and can be stored for up to 60 days.

Unit-dose packets – Empty contents of 1 packet into ⅓ glassful of water (≈ 75 mL) or other liquid, such as juice, and stir well before taking.

Solubility – *Neutra-Phos* and *Neutra-Phos-K* form an oral solution by reconstitution with water or other liquids, such as juice, per label directions. The solution is neutral (pH 7.3) and isotonic active components will dissolve rapidly, while the excipients will remain in suspension.

➤*Uro-KP-Neutral:*

Adults – 1 or 2 caplets 4 times/day with a full glass of water, providing 1 g of elemental phosphorus. Dosage may be increased or decreased. Optimum daily dosage should provide 1 to 1.5 g phosphorus daily.

➤*K-Phos Neutral*: Take with a full glass of water with meals and at bedtime.

Adults – 1 or 2 tablets 4 times/day.

Children older than 4 years of age – 1 tablet 4 times/day. For patients younger than 4 years of age, use only as directed by a physician.

➤*Storage/Stability:*

Powder – Store the powder concentrate and unit-dose packets in a dry place. When reconstituted to solution, chill if desired. Can be stored up to 60 days.

Tablets – Keep tightly closed. Store at controlled room temperature (20° to 25°C; 68° to 77°F).

Actions

➤*Pharmacology:* Phosphorus has a number of important functions in the biochemistry of the body. The bulk of the body's phosphorus is located in the bones, where it plays a key role in osteoblastic and osteoclastic activities. Enzymatically catalyzed phosphate-transfer reactions are numerous and vital in the metabolism of carbohydrate, lipid, and protein, and a proper concentration of the anion is of primary importance in assuring an orderly biochemical sequence. In addition, phosphorus plays an important role in modifying steady-state tissue concentrations of calcium. Phosphate ions are important buffers of the intracellular fluid, and also play a primary role in the renal excretion of hydrogen ion.

➤*Pharmacokinetics:*

Absorption – Approximately ⅔ of phosphate consumed by adults is absorbed from the bowel, primarily through sodium-dependent active transport, although passive diffusion does play a role mainly within the jejunum and ileum.

When reconstituted to an oral solution, phosphorus shows rapid absorption and utilization from the alimentary tract. Oral phosphate may allow serum levels to rise by as much as 1.5 mg/dL within 60 to 120 minutes after ingestion of 1000 mg phosphorus. The liquid products have an advantage over coated or uncoated tablets, as slow-dissolving tablets may cause local GI irritation or inflammation in sensitive individuals.

Metabolism – Phosphate metabolism is closely associated with calcium metabolism through vitamin D_1 parathyroid hormone, calcitonin, and the mineralization of osteoid. Reduction of plasma phosphate concentrations cause higher serum calcium levels and inhibit deposition of bone salt. An elevated plasma concentration of the phosphate anion promotes the effect of calcitonin on calcium deposition in bone.

Excretion – Over 90% of phosphate absorbed from the GI tract is excreted in the urine through filtration. The majority is then actively reabsorbed by the initial segment of the proximal tubule. A lesser amount is absorbed in the pars recta and/or loop of Henle, distal convulated tubule, and collecting duct. Phosphate excreted into the urine represents a difference between the amount filtered and amount reabsorbed. Tubule secretion is not known to occur in the mammalian kidney. Phosphate reduces levels of urinary calcium and elevates levels of urinary pyrophosphate inhibitor. Orthophosphates have been shown to decrease the crystallization of oxalate in the urine of calculous patients.

Contraindications

Addison's disease; hyperkalemia; acidification of urine in urinary stone disease; patients with infected urolithiasis or struvite stone formation; severely impaired renal function (less than 30% of normal); presence of hyperphosphatemia; hypersensitivity to active or inactive ingredients.

Warnings

➤*Pregnancy: Category C.* It is not known whether this product can cause fetal harm or affect reproduction capacity when administered to a pregnant woman. Use only when clearly needed.

➤*Lactation:* It is not known whether this drug is excreted in breast milk. Exercise caution when administering to a nursing woman.

➤*Children:* For pediatric patients younger than 4 years of age, use only as directed by a physician.

Precautions

➤*Monitoring:* The following determinations are important in patient monitoring (other tests may be warranted in some patients): Renal function; serum calcium; serum phosphorus; serum potassium; serum sodium. Monitor at periodic intervals during therapy.

➤*Potential GI problems:* There have been reports in the literature of small bowel lesions with some long-acting and coated potassium tablets. Orthophosphates may cause dyspepsia in patients with a history of peptic ulcer; other modes of therapy may be necessary in such patients.

➤*Sodium/Potassium restriction:* Use with caution if patient is on a sodium- or potassium-restricted diet. These products provide significant amounts of sodium or potassium.

PHOSPHORUS REPLACEMENT PRODUCTS — ORAL

➤*Kidney stones:* Warn patients with kidney stones of the possibility of passing stones when phosphate therapy is started.

➤*Special risk:* Use with caution when the following medical problems exist: Cardiac disease (particularly in digitalized patients); acute dehydration; renal function impairment or chronic renal disease; extensive tissue breakdown; myotonia congenita; cardiac failure; cirrhosis of the liver or severe hepatic disease; peripheral and pulmonary edema; hypernatremia; hypertension; pre-eclampsia; hypoparathyroidism; osteomalacia; acute pancreatitis; rickets (rickets may benefit from phosphate therapy; however, use caution); severe adrenal insufficiency.

Drug Interactions

Phosphate Drug Interactions

Precipitant drug	Object drug[a]		Description
Androgens	Potassium and phosphate	↑	Androgens may cause retention of potassium and phosphate. Therefore, concurrent use with potassium phosphate may cause hyperkalemia or hyperphosphatemia.
Antacids	Phosphates	↓	Antacids containing magnesium, aluminum, or calcium may bind to phosphate and prevent its absorption.
Calcium Vitamin D	Phosphates	↓	The effects of phosphates may be antagonized in the treatment of hypercalcemia.
Iron supplements	Phosphate	↓	Iron-containing medications have the ability to bind phosphate and form an insoluble complex, thus preventing absorption.
Phosphate	Anorexiants	↓	Acidification of urine may increase elimination and decrease therapeutic effect of anorexiants.
Phosphate	Chlorpropamide (sulfonylurea)	↑	Acidification of urine may increase bioavailability of chlorpropamide and enhance the hypoglycemic actions.
Phosphate	Methadone	↓	Acidification of the urine increases renal clearance of methadone because of increased ionization.
Phosphate	Sympathomimetics	↓	Acidification of urine may increase elimination and decrease therapeutic effect of sympathomimetics.

[a] ↑ = Object drug increased. ↓ = Object drug decreased.

Adverse Reactions

Individuals may experience a mild laxative effect for the first few days. If this persists, reduce the daily intake until this effect subsides, or, if necessary, discontinue use.

GI upset (eg, diarrhea, nausea, stomach pain, vomiting) may occur with phosphate therapy. The following side effects have been reported less frequently: Headaches; dizziness; mental confusion; seizures; weakness or heaviness of legs; unusual tiredness or weakness; muscle cramps; numbness, tingling, pain, or weakness of hands or feet; numbness or tingling around lips; fast or irregular heartbeat; shortness of breath or troubled breathing; swelling of feet or lower legs; unusual weight gain; low urine output; unusual thirst; bone and joint pain. High serum phosphate levels may increase the incidence of extraskeletal calcification.

MAGNESIUM

For more information on parenteral magnesium, refer to the IV Nutritional Therapy monograph in this chapter and the Anticonvulsant monograph in the CNS chapter.

Indications

As a dietary supplement.

Administration and Dosage

1 g Mg = 83.3 mEq (41.7 mmol).

➤*Dietary supplement:* 40 to 400 mg/day in divided doses. Refer to product labeling.

➤*Recommended dietary allowances (RDAs):*

Adult – Males, 270 to 400 mg; females, 280 to 300 mg. For a complete listing of RDAs by age, sex, and condition, refer to the RDA table.

Magnesium-containing antacids also may be used; refer to the Antacids monograph in the GI Agents chapter.

Actions

➤*Pharmacology:* Magnesium is the fourth most abundant mineral in the body and the second most abundant in muscles and other organs. Only potassium levels are higher than magnesium in soft tissues (non-bone tissues). Potassium cannot be retained in soft tissues and leaks out if magnesium is deficient. An adequate amount of magnesium also is required for the absorption and utilization of calcium, favoring the deposition of calcium in bone where it belongs and preventing deposition of calcium in the soft tissues and kidneys where it does not belong. Magnesium is required in adequate amount for the normal activity of 300 enzymes, including those involved in the transfer of energy from foods to physical and mental activities. It is a very important stabilizer of polynucleic acids, substances where genetic information is stored. Unstable nucleic acids predispose to cancer.

Warnings

➤*Pregnancy:* It is unknown whether magnesium supplementation will harm an unborn child or a breastfeeding child. Do not take this mineral without speaking to a physician if pregnant, planning a pregnancy, or breastfeeding.

Precautions

➤*Renal disease:* Do not use without physician supervision because of potential accumulation.

➤*Excessive dosage:* Excessive dosage may cause diarrhea and GI irritation.

➤*Heart disease:* Magnesium supplements may make this condition worse.

Drug Interactions

Magnesium Drug Interactions

Precipitant drug	Object drug[a]		Description
Magnesium salts	Aminoquinolines (eg, chloroquine)	↓	The absorption and therapeutic effect of the aminoquinolines may be decreased.
Magnesium salts	Nitrofurantoin	↓	Adsorption of nitrofurantoin onto magnesium salts may occur, decreasing the bioavailability and possibly the anti-infective effect of nitrofurantoin.
Magnesium salts	Penicillamine	↓	The GI absorption of penicillamine may be decreased, possibly decreasing its pharmacologic effects; however, this only has been reported for magnesium-containing antacids.
Magnesium salts	Tetracyclines	↓	The GI absorption and serum levels of tetracyclines may be decreased; a decreased antimicrobial response may occur.

[a] ↓ = Object drug decreased.

Overdosage

➤*Symptoms:* It is possible to overdose on any electrolyte if large quantities are given; magnesium is no exception. Administer magnesium cautiously, especially to patients with decreased renal function. The most common symptom of overdose is diarrhea. At serum levels between 3 to 5 mEq/L, there is a propensity for hypotension because of peripheral dilation. Severe hypotension may be seen at higher levels. Facial flushing may be seen, associated with a feeling of warmth or thirst. Nausea and vomiting may occur but are not always present. Lethargy, dysarthria, and drowsiness can appear when levels reach 5 to 7 mEq/L. Deep tendon reflexes are lost when levels reach 7 mEq/L. Shallow respirations, irregular brief periods of apnea, and, finally, prolonged apnea are expected when levels exceed 10 mEq/L. Coma occurs when serum levels are between 12 and 15 mEq/L. Finally, when levels exceed 15 to 20 mEq/L, cardiac arrest may be expected.

➤*Treatment:* Terminate exposure. Calcium administration improves many toxic symptoms. Forced diuresis intensifies the elimination of magnesium; hemodialysis is extremely effective at magnesium removal but is infrequently necessary in the absence of renal failure.

MAGNESIUM

otc	**Magnesium Gluconate** (Various, eg, Freeda, Rugby)	**Tablets:** ≈ 27 mg elemental magnesium	In 100s and 500s.
otc	**Magnesium** (Various, eg, Ivax)	**Tablets:** 30 mg elemental magnesium	In 100s.
otc	**Magnesium Citrate** (Various, eg, Freeda)	**Tablets:** 100 mg elemental magnesium	In 100s and 250s.
otc	**Mag-200** (Optimox)	**Tablets:** 200 mg elemental magnesium (as oxide)	300 mg PABA. In 120s.

MAGNESIUM

otc sf	**Mag-Ox 400** (Blaine)	**Tablets**: 400 mg magnesium oxide (241.3 mg elemental magnesium)	(BLAINE). In 120s, 1000s, and UD 100s.
otc	**Magnesium Oxide** (Various, eg, Breckenridge, Cypress, Plus Pharma)		In 120s and 400s.
otc	**Maox 420** (Manne Co.)	**Tablets**: 420 mg magnesium oxide (253 mg elemental magnesium)	Tartrazine. 21 mEq acid neutralizing capacity per tablet. In 250s and 1000s.
otc	**Mag-G** (Cypress)	**Tablets**: 500 mg magnesium gluconate dihydrate (27 mg elemental magnesium)	In 100s.
otc	**Magonate** (Fleming)		87.5 mg Ca, 66 mg P (376 mg dibasic calcium phosphate dihydrate). In 1000s.
otc	**Magtrate** (Mission)	**Tablets**: 500 mg magnesium gluconate (29 mg elemental magnesium)	In 100s.
otc	**Magnesium Oxide** (Various, eg, Major)	**Tablets**: 500 mg magnesium oxide (302 mg elemental magnesium)	In 100s.
otc sf	**Maginex** (Geist)	**Tablets, enteric coated**: 615 magnesium-L-aspartate HCl (61 mg elemental magnesium)	In blister pack 100s, UD 100s, and robot ready 100s.
otc	**Slow-Mag** (Purdue)	**Tablets, enteric-coated**: 64 mg elemental magnesium (as chloride hexahydrate)	Calcium carbonate. In 60s.
otc	**Mag-Tab SR** (Niche)	**Tablets, sustained-release**: 84 mg elemental magnesium (as L-lactate dihydrate)	Lt. yellow, capsule shape, scored. In 60s, 100s, and 1000s.
otc sf	**Uro-Mag** (Blaine)	**Capsules**: 140 mg magnesium oxide (84.5 mg elemental magnesium)	In 100s, 1000s, and UD 100s.
otc	**Mag-Caps** (Genesis)	**Capsules**: ≈ 140 mg magnesium oxide (85 mg elemental magnesium)	In 100s.
otc sf	**Magonate Natal** (Fleming)	**Liquid**: 3.52 mg elemental magnesium (as gluconate)/mL	In 480 mL.
otc	**Magonate** (Fleming)	**Liquid**: 1000 mg magnesium gluconate dihydrate/5 mL (54 mg elemental magnesium/5 mL)	Sorbitol, magnesium carbonate. Melon flavor. In 473 mL.
otc	**Maginex DS** (Geist)	**Powder**: 1230 mg magnesium-L-aspartate HCl (122 mg elemental magnesium)/packet	Preservative-free. Sucrose. Lemon flavor. In 30s and robot ready 30s.

For prescribing information for oral magnesium, refer to the Magnesium introduction. For more information on parenteral magnesium, refer to the IV Nutritional Therapy monograph in this chapter and the Anticonvulsant monograph in the CNS chapter.

TRACE ELEMENTS

Iron

IRON-CONTAINING PRODUCTS

WARNING

Accidental overdose of iron-containing products is a leading cause of fatal poisoning in children younger than 6 years of age. Keep products out of the reach of children. In case of accidental overdose, call a doctor or a poison control center immediately.

Indications

➤*Iron deficiency:* For the prevention and treatment of iron deficiency and iron deficiency anemias.

➤*Iron supplement:* As a dietary supplement for iron.

➤*Unlabeled uses:* Iron supplementation may be required by most patients receiving epoetin therapy. Failure to administer iron supplements (oral or intravenous [IV]) during epoetin therapy can impair the hematologic response to epoetin.

Administration and Dosage

Due to the availability of multiple salt forms, close attention is warranted when administering iron. Substitution of 1 salt for another without proper adjustment may result in serious over or under dosing.

Carbonyl iron and polysaccharide-iron complex are reported to be associated with fewer GI effects and are less toxic than other forms of iron.

The length of iron therapy depends upon the cause and severity of the iron deficiency. In general, approximately 4 to 6 months of oral iron therapy is required to reverse uncomplicated iron deficiency anemias. Iron therapy should increase hemoglobin levels by 1 g/week.

➤*Iron replacement therapy in deficiency states:* Iron doses are given as elemental iron.

Premature infants – 2 to 4 mg/kg/day given in 1 to 2 divided doses. Maximum dosage is 15 mg/day.

Children – 3 to 6 mg/kg/day given in 1 to 3 divided doses.

Adults – 150 to 300 mg/day given in 3 divided doses. Alternatively, 60 mg given 2 to 4 times/day may help lessen GI effects.

➤*Prevention of iron deficiency:*

Premature infants – 2 mg/kg/day given in 1 to 3 divided doses. Maximum dosage is 15 mg/day.

Children – 1 to 2 mg/kg/day given in 1 to 3 divided doses. Maximum dosage is 15 mg/day.

Adults – 60 mg/day given in 1 to 2 divided doses.

➤*Recommended dietary allowances (RDAs):* For a complete listing of RDAs, refer to the RDAs section of the Nutrients and Nutritionals chapter.

RDAs for Iron

Patients	RDA for iron (mg/day)
Children	
7 to 12 months of age	11
1 to 3 years of age	7
4 to 8 years of age	10
Males	
9 to 13 years of age	8
14 to 18 years of age	11
≥ 19 years of age	8
Females	
9 to 13 years of age	8
14 to 18 years of age	15
19 to 50 years of age	18
older than 50 years of age	8
Pregnancy	27
Lactation	
≤ 18 years of age	10
≥ 19 years of age	9

➤*Iron supplementation:*

Pregnancy – Elemental iron 15 to 30 mg/day should be adequate to meet the daily requirement of the last 2 trimesters.

Actions

➤*Pharmacology:* Iron, an essential mineral, is a component of hemoglobin, myoglobin, and a number of enzymes (eg, cytochromes, catalase, peroxidase). The total body content of iron is approximately 50 mg/kg in men (3.5 g in the average 70 kg man), and 37 mg/kg in women. Iron is primarily stored as hemosiderin or aggregated ferritin, found in the reticuloendothelial system and hepatocytes. Approximately two thirds of total body iron is in the circulating red blood cell mass in hemoglobin, the major factor in oxygen transport.

Iron deficiency can affect muscle metabolism, heat production, and catecholamine metabolism and has been associated with behavioral or learning problems in children.

➤*Pharmacokinetics:*

Absorption/Distribution – The average dietary intake of iron is 12 to 20 mg/day for males and 8 to 15 mg/day for females; however, only approximately 10% of this iron is absorbed (1 to 2 mg/day) in individuals with adequate iron stores. Absorption is enhanced when storage iron is depleted or when erythropoiesis occurs at an increased rate.

IRON-CONTAINING PRODUCTS

Iron is primarily absorbed from the duodenum and jejunum. The ferrous salt form is absorbed 3 times more readily than the ferric form. The common ferrous salts (ie, sulfate, gluconate, fumarate) are absorbed almost on a milligram-for-milligram basis but differ in the content of elemental iron. Polysaccharide-complex is a product of ferric iron complexed to a low molecular weight polysaccharide. A radioisotope tracer study in humans demonstrated that absorption of polysaccharide-iron complex is comparable with that of ferrous sulfate. Sustained-release or enteric-coated preparations reduce the amount of available iron; absorption from these doseforms is reduced because iron is transported beyond the duodenum. Dose also influences the amount of iron absorbed. The amount of iron absorbed increases progressively with larger doses; however, the percentage absorbed decreases. Food can decrease the absorption of iron at least 50%; however, gastric intolerance may often necessitate administering the drug with food.

Excretion – Iron is transported via the blood and bound to transferrin. The daily loss of iron from urine, sweat, and sloughing of intestinal mucosal cells amounts to approximately 0.5 to 1 mg in healthy men. In menstruating women, approximately 1 to 2 mg is the normal daily loss.

Elemental Iron Content of Iron Salts

Iron salt	% Iron
Ferrous fumarate	≈ 33
Ferrous gluconate	≈ 12
Ferrous sulfate	≈ 20
Ferrous sulfate, exsiccated (dried)	≈ 32

Contraindications

Hemochromatosis; hemosiderosis; hemolytic anemias; known hypersensitivity to any ingredient.

Warnings

➤*Chronic iron intake:* Individuals with normal iron balance should not take iron chronically.

➤*Accidental overdose:* Accidental overdose of iron-containing products is a leading cause of fatal poisoning in children younger than 6 years of age. Keep this product out of reach of children.

➤*Pregnancy:* *Category A.*

Precautions

➤*Intolerance:* Discontinue use if symptoms of intolerance appear.

➤*GI effects:* Occasional GI discomfort, such as nausea, may be minimized by taking with meals and by slowly increasing to the recommended dosage.

➤*Tartrazine sensitivity:* Some of these products contain tartrazine, which may cause allergic-type reactions (including bronchial asthma) in susceptible individuals. Although the incidence of tartrazine sensitivity in the general population is low, it is frequently seen in patients who also have aspirin hypersensitivity. Specific products containing tartrazine are identified in the product listings.

➤*Sulfite sensitivity:* Some of the products contain sulfites, which may cause allergic-type reactions (eg, hives, itching, wheezing, anaphylaxis) in certain susceptible people. Although the overall prevalence of sulfite sensitivity in the general population is probably low, it is seen more frequently in asthmatic or in atopic nonasthmatic people. Specific products containing sulfites are identified in the product listings.

Drug Interactions

Iron Salts Drug Interactions

Precipitant drug	Object drug[a]		Description
Acetohydroxamic acid (AHA)	Iron salts	⬇	AHA chelates heavy metals, notably iron. The absorption of iron may be decreased. When iron is indicated, administer intramuscularly (IM).
Antacids	Iron salts	⬇	GI absorption of iron may be reduced.
Ascorbic acid	Iron salts	⬆	Ascorbic acid at doses ≥ 200 mg have been shown to enhance the absorption of iron ≥ 30%.
Calcium salts	Iron salts	⬇	GI absorption of iron may be reduced. When possible, separate administration times.
Chloramphenicol	Iron salts	⬆	Serum iron levels may be increased.
Digestive enzymes	Iron salts	⬇	The serum iron response to oral iron may be decreased by concomitant pancreatic extracts.
H_2 antagonists	Iron salts	⬇	GI absorption of iron may be reduced.
Proton pump inhibitors	Iron salts	⬇	GI absorption of iron may be reduced.
Trientine	Iron salts	⬇	The 2 agents inhibit the absorption of each other. If iron is needed, administer the agents at least 2 hours apart.
Iron salts	Trientine		
Iron salts	Captopril	⬇	Concomitant use within 2 hours may promote formation of inactive captopril disulfide dimer.
Iron salts	Cephalosporins (eg, cefdinir)	⬇	Iron supplements and foods fortified with iron may reduce the absorption of cefdinir 80% and 30%, respectively. If iron supplements are needed during cefdinir therapy, cefdinir should be taken 2 hours before or after the supplement. Iron-fortified infant formula (elemental iron 2.2 mg per 6 oz) has no effect on cefdinir absorption.
Iron salts	Fluoroquinolones (eg, ciprofloxacin)	⬇	GI absorption of fluoroquinolones may be decreased because of formation of iron-quinolone complex. Avoid coadministration of these drugs. (See individual fluoroquinolone monographs for administration recommendations.)
Iron salts	Levodopa	⬇	Levodopa appears to form chelates with iron salts, decreasing levodopa absorption and serum levels.
Iron salts	Levothyroxine	⬇	The efficacy of levothyroxine may be decreased, resulting in hypothyroidism. Avoid coadministration.
Iron salts	Methyldopa	⬇	Extent of methyldopa absorption may be decreased, possibly resulting in decreased efficacy.
Iron salts	Mycophenolate mofetil	⬇	Absorption of mycophenolate mofetil may be decreased. Avoid simultaneous administration.
Iron salts	Penicillamine	⬇	Marked reduction in GI absorption of penicillamine may occur, possibly because of chelation.
Iron salts	Tetracyclines	⬇	Concomitant use within 2 hours may decrease absorption and serum levels of tetracyclines. Absorption of iron salts also may be decreased.
Tetracyclines	Iron salts		
Iron salts	Thyroid hormones	⬇	Absorption of thyroid hormones may be decreased. Avoid coadministration.

[a] ⬆ = Object drug increased. ⬇ = Object drug decreased.

➤*Drug/Food interactions:* Administration of iron with food decreases the iron absorption by at least 50%.

Adverse Reactions

Iron-containing liquids may temporarily stain the teeth (enamel is not affected). Dilute the liquid and/or drink through a straw to reduce this possibility. When iron-containing drops are given to infants, the membrane covering the teeth may darken.

➤*GI:* Abdominal pain, constipation, diarrhea, GI irritation, nausea, vomiting. Stools may appear darker in color.

Overdosage

➤*Symptoms:* Symptoms may present when at least 20 mg/kg is ingested. Acute poisoning will produce symptoms in the following 4 stages:

1.) Within 6 hours: abdominal pain, coma, diminished tissue perfusion, dyspnea, fever, hyperglycemia, hypotension, lethargy, leukocytosis, metabolic acidosis, nausea, tarry stools, vomiting, weak-rapid pulse.
2.) If not immediately fatal, symptoms may subside within 12 to 24 hours.
3.) Symptoms return 12 to 48 hours after ingestion and may include the following: anuria, convulsions, death, diffuse vascular congestion, hyperthermia, metabolic acidosis, pulmonary edema, shock.
4.) If patient survives, in 2 to 6 weeks after ingestion pyloric or antral stenosis, hepatic cirrhosis, and CNS damage may be seen.

➤*Treatment:* Maintain proper airway, respiration, and circulation. Perform gastric lavage in patients who are candidates for GI decontamination. Systemic chelation therapy with deferoxamine is generally recommended for patients with serum iron levels greater than 350 to 500 mcg/dL or in patients with symptoms of iron toxicity. IM therapy may suffice, but severe poisoning (eg, shock, coma) may require IV administration (see defero-

IRON-CONTAINING PRODUCTS

amine mesylate in the Detoxification Agents section). Specific treatment for shock, convulsions, acidosis, and renal failure may be necessary. Treatment includes usual supportive measures. Refer to General Management of Acute Overdosage.

Patient Information

Inform patients to take on an empty stomach; if GI upset occurs, advise to take after meals or with food.

Advise patients not to take within 2 hours of antacids, tetracyclines, or fluoroquinolones.

Inform patients to drink liquid iron preparations in water or juice and through a straw to prevent tooth staining.

Inform patients that medication may cause black stools, constipation, or diarrhea.

Advise patients not to crush or chew sustained-release preparations.

FERROUS SULFATE

20% elemental iron.

otc	**Ferrous Sulfate** (Various, eg, Goldline, Upsher-Smith)	**Tablets**: 325 mg (65 mg iron)	In 100s, 1,000s, and UD 100s.
otc	**Feosol** (GlaxoSmithKline)		Capsule shape. In 100s.
otc	**FeroSul** (Major)		Green or red. In 100s and 1,000s.
otc	**Ferrous Sulfate** (Various, eg, Goldline, Major, URL)	**Elixir**: 220 mg per 5 mL (44 mg iron per 5 mL)	May contain alcohol. In 473 mL.
otc	**Ferrous Sulfate** (Various, eg, Alpharma)	**Drops**: 75 mg per 0.6 mL (15 mg iron per 0.6 mL)	May contain alcohol. In 50 mL.
otc	**Fer-In-Sol** (Mead Johnson Nutritionals)		0.2% alcohol. Sodium bisulfite, sorbitol, sugar. In 50 mL with dropper.
otc	**Fer-Gen-Sol** (Goldline)		0.2% alcohol. Sorbitol, sugar, potassium sorbate, sodium bisulfite. Lemon flavor. In 50 mL.
otc	**Ferrous Sulfate** (Pharmaceutical Associates)	**Liquid**: 300 mg per 5 mL (60 mg iron per 5 mL)	Sucrose. Cinnamon flavor. In UD 100s of 5 mL each.

For complete and comparative prescribing information, refer to the Iron-Containing Products group monograph.

FERROUS SULFATE EXSICCATED (DRIED)

Approximately 30% elemental iron.

otc	**Feosol** (GlaxoSmithKline)	**Tablets**: 200 mg (65 mg iron)	Glucose. (Fe). In 100s.
otc	**Feratab** (Upsher-Smith)	**Tablets**: 300 mg (60 mg iron)	Red. In UD 100s.
otc	**Ferrous Sulfate** (Rugby)	**Tablets, slow release**: 160 mg (50 mg iron)	In blister pack 60s.
otc	**Slow Release Iron** (Cardinal Health)		Maltodextrin, mineral oil. In 30s.
otc	**Slow FE** (Ciba)		Cetostearyl alcohol, lactose. (NR CIBA). In 30s.

For complete and comparative prescribing information, refer to the Iron-Containing Products group monograph.

FERROUS GLUCONATE

Approximately 12% elemental iron.

otc	**Ferrous Gluconate** (Various, eg, Goldline)	**Tablets**: 225 mg (27 mg iron)	In 100s.
otc	**Fergon** (Bayer)		In 100s.
otc	**Ferrous Gluconate** (Various, eg, Upsher-Smith)	**Tablets**: 300 mg (35 mg iron)	In 100s.
otc	**Ferrous Gluconate** (Various, eg, Paddock Laboratories)	**Tablets**: 324 mg (38 mg iron)	In 100s.
otc	**Ferrous Gluconate** (Various, eg, Akyma Pharmaceuticals)	**Tablets**: 325 mg (36 mg iron)	In 1,000s.

For complete and comparative prescribing information, refer to the Iron-Containing Products group monograph.

FERROUS FUMARATE

33% elemental iron.

otc	**Ferrous Fumarate** (Mission)	**Tablets**: 90 mg (29.5 mg iron)	Sugar. In 100s.
otc	**Ferrous Fumarate** (Various, eg, Cypress)	**Tablets**: 324 mg (106 mg iron)	In 100s.
otc	**Hemocyte** (U.S. Pharmaceutical Corp.)		In 30s and 100s.
otc	**Ferretts** (Pharmics)	**Tablets**: 325 mg (106 mg iron)	Polydextrose. (P-Fe). Red, oblong, scored. Film-coated. In 60s.
otc sf	**Nephro-Fer** (Watson)	**Tablets**: 350 mg (115 mg iron)	Lactose, tartrazine. In 30s.
otc	**Ferro Sequels** (Inverness)	**Tablets, timed release**: 150 mg (50 mg iron)	Lactose, sodium docusate 100 mg. In 30s and 90s.

For complete and comparative prescribing information, refer to the Iron-Containing Products group monograph.

CARBONYL IRON

Pure iron micro particles.

otc	**Feosol** (GlaxoSmithKline)	**Tablets**: 45 mg iron	In 30s and 60s.
otc	**Ircon** (Kenwood)	**Tablets**: 66 mg iron	In blister pack 100s.
otc	**Icar** (Hawthorn)	**Tablets, chewable**: 15 mg carbonyl iron	Sorbitol. Grape flavor. In 60s.
		Suspension: 15 mg carbonyl iron per 1.25 mL	Fructose, parabens. Grape and lemon flavors. In 118 mL.
otc	**Iron Chews** (Midlothian)	**Tablets, chewable**: 15 mg carbonyl iron	Sorbitol. Grape flavor. In 60s.

For complete and comparative prescribing information, refer to the Iron-Containing Products group monograph.

POLYSACCHARIDE IRON COMPLEX

otc	**Niferex** (Ther-Rx)	**Capsules:** 60 mg iron	Lactose. (THX 0134). Brown/Clear. In UD 100s.
otc	**Polysaccharide Iron Complex** (Various, eg, Contract Pharmacol Corp.)	**Capsules:** 150 mg iron	In 100s.
Rx	**Fe-Tinic 150** (Ethex Corp.)		(ETHEX 024). Opaque orange. In 1,000s and UD 100s.
otc	**Ferrex 150** (Breckenridge)		(B-203). Orange/brown. In UD 100s.
otc	**Hytinic** (Hyrex)		Parabens, EDTA, castor oil. In 50s.
otc	**Nu-Iron 150** (Merz)		Parabens, EDTA, castor oil, sucrose. In 100s.
otc	**EZFE 200** (McNeil)	**Capsules:** 200 mg iron	In 100s.
otc sf	**Niferex** (Ther-Rx)	**Elixir:** 100 mg iron per 5 mL	Sorbitol, 10% alcohol. Dye free. In 237 mL.

For complete and comparative prescribing information, refer to the Iron-Containing Products group monograph.

MISCELLANEOUS IRON COMBINATIONS

Rx	**Tandem** (US Pharmaceutical)	**Capsules:** 106 mg elemental Fe (as 162 mg ferrous fumarate, 115.2 mg polysaccharide iron complex)	(Tandem US). Lt. brown, opaque. In blister pack 90s.

MISCELLANEOUS IRON COMBINATIONS — ORAL

For complete prescribing information, refer to the Iron-Containing Products group monograph.

IRON WITH VITAMIN C

Content given per capsule or tablet.

				Vitamin C			
	Product and Distributor	Dose form	Fe (mg)	Ascorbic Acid	Sodium Ascorbate (mg)	Calcium Ascorbate and Calcium Threonate (mg)	Other Content & How Supplied (mg)
otc	**Ferrex 150 Plus** (Breckenridge)	**Capsules**	150[a]	50			(B 303). Clear/yellow. In UD 100s.
otc	**Fero-Grad-500** (Abbott)	**Tablets, controlled release**	105[b]		500		Castor oil. In blister pack 30s.
otc	**Niferex-150** (Ther-Rx)	**Capsules**	150[c]			50	(THX 0135). Brown/clear. In UD 100s.
otc	**Vitelle Irospan** (Fielding)		65[d]	150			Sugar. In 60s.
otc	**Vitron-C** (Heritage Consumer Products)	**Tablets**	66[e]	125			In 60s.

[a] From polysaccharide iron and ferrous bisglycinate.
[b] From ferrous sulfate.
[c] From polysaccharide-iron complex.
[d] From ferrous sulfate exsiccated.
[e] From ferrous fumarate.

For complete prescribing information, refer to the Iron-Containing Products group monograph.

IRON DEXTRAN

Rx	**InFeD** (Schein)	**Injection:** 50 mg iron/mL (as dextran)	Approximately 0.9% sodium chloride. In 2 mL single-dose vials.
Rx	**DexFerrum** (American Regent)		In 1 and 2 mL single-dose vials.

IRON DEXTRAN — INJECTION

WARNING

The parenteral use of complexes of iron and carbohydrates has resulted in anaphylactic-type reactions. Deaths associated with such administration have been reported. Therefore, use iron dextran for injection only in those patients in whom the indications have been clearly established and laboratory investigations confirm an iron-deficient state not amenable to oral iron therapy. Because fatal anaphylactic reactions have been reported after administration of iron dextran injection, only give the drug when resuscitation techniques and treatment of anaphylactic and anaphylactoid shock are readily available.

Indications

➤*Iron deficiency:* For treatment of patients with documented iron deficiency in whom oral administration is unsatisfactory or impossible.

➤*Unlabeled uses:* Iron supplementation may be required by most patients receiving epoetin therapy. Failure to administer iron supplements (oral or IV) during epoetin therapy can impair the hematologic response to epoetin.

Administration and Dosage

➤*Approved by the FDA:* February 23, 1996.

Discontinue oral iron prior to administration of iron dextran.

➤*Iron-deficiency anemia:* Periodic hematologic determination (hemoglobin and hematocrit) is a simple and accurate technique for monitoring hematological response, and should be used as a guide in therapy. It should be recognized that iron storage may lag behind the appearance of healthy blood morphology. Serum iron, total iron-binding capacity (TIBC), and percent saturation of transferrin are other important tests for detecting and monitoring the iron-deficient state.

Although there are significant variations in body build and weight distribution among males and females, the information below and formula represent a convenient means for estimating the total iron required. This total iron requirement reflects the amount of iron needed to restore hemoglobin concentration to normal or near-normal levels plus an additional allowance to provide adequate replenishment of iron stores in most individuals with moderately or severely reduced levels of hemoglobin. It should be remembered that iron-deficiency anemia will not appear until essentially all iron stores have been depleted. Therapy, thus, should aim at not only replenishment of hemoglobin iron but iron stores as well.

The following table and accompanying formula are applicable for dosage determinations only in patients with iron-deficiency anemia; they are not to be used for dosage determinations in patients requiring iron replacement for blood loss.

Total Iron Dextran Requirement for Hemoglobin Restoration and Iron Stores Replacement[a]

Patient lean body weight		Milliliter requirement of iron dextran injection based on observed hemoglobin of							
kg	lb	3 (g/dL)	4 (g/dL)	5 (g/dL)	6 (g/dL)	7 (g/dL)	8 (g/dL)	9 (g/dL)	10 (g/dL)
5	11	3	3	3	3	2	2	2	2
10	22	7	6	6	5	5	4	4	3
15	33	10	9	9	8	7	7	6	5
20	44	16	15	14	13	12	11	10	9
25	55	20	18	17	16	15	14	13	12
30	66	23	22	21	19	18	17	15	14
35	77	27	26	24	23	21	20	18	17

IRON DEXTRAN — INJECTION

Total Iron Dextran Requirement for Hemoglobin Restoration and Iron Stores Replacement[a]

Patient lean body weight		Milliliter requirement of iron dextran injection based on observed hemoglobin of							
kg	lb	3 (g/dL)	4 (g/dL)	5 (g/dL)	6 (g/dL)	7 (g/dL)	8 (g/dL)	9 (g/dL)	10 (g/dL)
40	88	31	29	28	26	24	22	21	19
45	99	35	33	31	29	27	25	23	21
50	110	39	37	35	32	30	28	26	24
55	121	43	41	38	36	33	31	28	26
60	132	47	44	42	39	36	34	31	28
65	143	51	48	45	42	39	36	34	31
70	154	55	52	49	45	42	39	36	33
75	165	59	55	52	49	45	42	39	35
80	176	63	59	55	52	48	45	41	38
85	187	66	63	59	55	51	48	44	40
90	198	70	66	62	58	54	50	46	42
95	209	74	70	66	62	57	53	49	45
100	220	78	74	69	65	60	56	52	47
105	231	82	77	73	68	63	59	54	50
110	242	86	81	76	71	67	62	57	52
115	253	90	85	80	75	70	64	59	54
120	264	94	88	83	78	73	67	62	57

[a] Table values were calculated based on a normal adult hemoglobin of 14.8 g/dL for weights greater than 15 kg (33 lbs) and a hemoglobin of 12 g/dL for weights less than or equal to 15 kg (33 lbs).

The total amount of iron dextran in mL required to treat the anemia and replenish iron stores may be approximated as follows:

Adults and children over 15 kg (33 lbs) – See dosage table. Alternatively, the total dose may be calculated:

Dose (mL) = 0.0442 (desired Hb - observed Hb) × LBW + (0.26 × LBW).

Based on: Desired Hb = the target Hb in g/dL.
Observed Hb = the patient's current hemoglobin in g/dL.
LBW = Lean body weight in kg. Utilize a patient's lean body weight (or actual body weight if less than lean body weight) when determining dosage.

Children 5 to 15 kg (11 to 33 lbs) – See dosage table. Iron dextran should not normally be given in the first 4 months of life (see Warnings).

➤*Iron replacement for blood loss:* Some individuals sustain blood losses on an intermittent or repetitive basis. Such blood losses may occur periodically in patients with hemorrhagic diatheses (familial telangiectasia; hemophilia; GI bleeding) and on a repetitive basis from procedures such as renal hemodialysis.

Direct iron therapy in these patients toward replacement of the equivalent amount of iron represented in the blood loss. The previously described dosage information and formulas for iron-deficiency anemia are not applicable for simple iron replacement values.

Quantitative estimates of the individual's periodic blood loss and hematocrit during the bleeding episode provide a convenient method for the calculation of the required iron dose.

The formula shown below is based on the approximation that 1 mL of normocytic, normochromic red cells contains 1 mg of elemental iron:

Replacement iron (in mg) = blood loss (in mL) × hematocrit.

Example: Blood loss of 500 mL with 20% hematocrit.

Replacement iron = 500 × 0.2 = 100 mg.

Iron dextran dose = 100 mg/50 = 2 mL.

➤*Administration:* The total amount of iron dextran required for the treatment of iron-deficiency anemia or iron replacement for blood loss is determined from the dosage information or appropriate formula (see above for dosage information).

IV injection – Prior to receiving their first iron dextran therapeutic dose, give all patients an IV test dose of 0.5 mL. Administer the test dose at a gradual rate over at least 5 minutes. Although anaphylactic reactions known to occur following iron dextran administration are usually evident within a few minutes, or sooner, it is recommended that a period of an hour or longer elapse before the remainder of the initial therapeutic dose is given.

Individual doses of less than or equal to 2 mL may be given on a daily basis until the calculated total amount required has been reached. Iron dextran is given undiluted at a slow gradual rate not to exceed 50 mg (1 mL) per minute.

IM injection – Prior to receiving their first iron dextran injection therapeutic dose, give all patients an IM test dose of 0.5 mL. Administer the test dose in the same recommended test site and by the same technique as described above. Although anaphylactic reactions known to occur following iron dextran injection administration are usually evident within a few minutes or sooner, it is recommended that at least an hour or longer elapse before the remainder of the initial therapeutic dose is given.

Iron dextran injection should be injected only into the muscle mass of the upper outer quadrant of the buttock - never into the arm or other exposed areas - and should be injected deeply, with a 2-inch or 3-inch 19 or 20 gauge needle. If the patient is standing, he/she should be bearing his/her weight on the leg opposite the injection site, or if in bed, he/she should be in the lateral position with injection site uppermost. To avoid injection or leakage into the subcutaneous tissue, a Z-track technique (displacement of the skin laterally prior to injection) is recommended.

If no adverse reactions are observed, iron dextran can be given according to the following schedule until the calculated total amount required has been reached. Each day's dose should ordinarily not exceed 0.5 mL (25 mg of iron) for infants less than 5 kg (11 lbs); 1 mL (50 mg of iron) for children less than 10 kg (22 lbs); 2 mL (100 mg of iron) for other patients.

Do not mix iron dextran with other medications or add to parenteral nutrition solutions for IV infusion.

➤*Storage / Stability:* Store at controlled room temperature 15° to 30°C (59° to 86°F).

Actions

➤*Pharmacokinetics:*

Absorption / Distribution – After IM injection, iron dextran is absorbed from the injection site into the capillaries and the lymphatic system. Circulating iron dextran is removed from the plasma by cells of the reticuloendothelial system, which split the complex into its components of iron and dextran. The iron is immediately bound to the available protein moieties to form hemosiderin or ferritin, the physiological forms of iron, or to a lesser extent to transferrin. This iron which is subject to physiological control replenishes hemoglobin and depleted iron stores.

The major portion of IM injections of iron dextran is absorbed within 72 hours; most of the remaining iron is absorbed over the ensuing 3 to 4 weeks.

Metabolism / Excretion – Dextran, a polyglucose, is either metabolized or excreted. Negligible amounts of iron are lost via the urinary or alimentary pathways after administration of iron dextran.

Various studies involving IV administered ^{59}Fe iron dextran to iron deficient subjects, some of whom had coexisting diseases, have yielded half-life values ranging from 5 hours to more than 20 hours. The 5-hour value was determined for ^{59}Fe iron dextran from a study that used laboratory methods to separate the circulating ^{59}Fe iron dextran from the transferrin-bound ^{59}Fe. The 20-hour value reflects a half-life determined by measuring total ^{59}Fe, both circulating and bound. It should be understood that these half-life values do not represent clearance of iron from the body. Iron is not easily eliminated from the body and the accumulation of iron can be toxic.

In vitro studies have shown that removal of iron dextran by dialysis is negligible. Six different dialyzer membranes were investigated (polysulphone, cuprophane, cellulose acetate, cellulose triacetate, polymethylmethacrilate and polyacrylonitrile), including those considered high efficiency and high flux.

Contraindications

Hypersensitivity to the product. All anemias not associated with iron deficiency.

Warnings

➤*Total dose infections:* Large IV doses, such as those used with total dose infusions (TDI), have been associated with an increased incidence of adverse effects. The adverse effects frequently are delayed (1 to 2 days) reactions typified by one or more of the following symptoms: Arthralgia, backache, chills, dizziness, moderate-to-high fever, headache, malaise, myalgia, nausea, and vomiting. The onset is usually 24 to 48 hours after administration, and symptoms generally subside within 3 to 4 days. These symptoms have also been reported following IM injection and generally subside within 3 to 7 days. The etiology of these reactions is not known. The potential for a delayed reaction must be considered when estimating the risk/benefit of treatment.

➤*Maximum dose:* The maximum daily dose should not exceed 2 mL undiluted iron dextran.

➤*Cardiovascular disease:* Adverse reactions experienced following administration of iron dextran may exacerbate cardiovascular complications in patients with preexisting cardiovascular disease.

➤*Infectious kidney disease:* Do not use this medication during the acute phase of infectious kidney disease.

➤*Hypersensitivity reactions:* Anaphylaxis and other hypersensitivity reactions have been reported after uneventful test doses as well as therapeutic doses of iron dextran injection. Therefore, consider administration of subsequent test doses during therapy.

Epinephrine should be immediately available in the event of acute hypersensitivity reactions (usual adult dose: 0.5 mL of a 1:1,000 solution, by subcutaneous or IM injection).

IRON DEXTRAN — INJECTION

Patients using beta-blocking agents may not respond adequately to epinephrine. Isoproterenol or similar beta agonist agents may be required in these patients.

➤*Hepatic function impairment:* Use this preparation with extreme care in patients with serious impairment of liver function.

➤*Carcinogenesis:* A risk of carcinogenesis may attend the IM injection of iron-carbohydrate complexes. Such complexes have been found under experimental conditions to produce sarcoma when large doses or small doses injected repeatedly at the same site were given to rats, mice, and rabbits, and possibly in hamsters.

The long latent period between the injection of a potential carcinogen and the appearance of a tumor makes it impossible to measure accurately the risk in man. There have, however, been several reports in the literature describing tumors at the injection site in humans who had previously received IM injections of iron-carbohydrate complexes.

➤*Pregnancy: Category C.*

Various animal studies and studies in pregnant humans have demonstrated inconclusive results with respect to the placental transfer of iron dextran as iron dextran. It appears that some iron does reach the fetus, but the form in which it crosses the placenta is not clear.

Teratogenic – Iron dextran has been shown to be teratogenic and embryocidal in mice, rats, rabbits, dogs, and monkeys when given in doses of about 3 times the maximum human dose.

No consistent adverse fetal effects were observed in mice, rats, rabbits, dogs, and monkeys at doses of less than or equal to 50 mg iron/kg. Fetal and maternal toxicity has been reported in monkeys at a total IV dose of 90 mg iron/kg over a 14-day period. Similar effects were observed in mice and rats on administration of a single dose of 125 mg iron/kg. Fetal abnormalities in rats and dogs were observed at doses of greater than or equal to 250 mg iron/kg. The animals used in these tests were not iron deficient. There are no adequate and well-controlled studies in pregnant women. Use during pregnancy only if the potential benefit justifies the potential risk to the fetus.

➤*Lactation:* Exercise caution when iron dextran is administered to a nursing woman. Traces of unmetabolized iron dextran are excreted in human milk.

➤*Children:* Not recommended for use in infants younger than 4 months of age (see Administration and Dosage).

Reports in the literature from countries outside the United States (in particular, New Zealand) have suggested that the use of IM iron dextran in neonates has been associated with an increased incidence of gram-negative sepsis, primarily due to *E. coli*.

Precautions

➤*Monitoring:* Serum iron determinations (especially by colorimetric assays) may not be meaningful for 3 weeks following the administration of iron dextran. Serum ferritin peaks approximately 7 to 9 days after an IV dose of iron dextran and slowly returns to baseline after about 3 weeks.

Examination of the bone marrow for iron stores may not be meaningful for prolonged periods following iron dextran therapy because residual iron dextran may remain in the reticuloendothelial cells.

➤*Iron overload:* Unwarranted therapy with parenteral iron will cause excess storage of iron with the consequent possibility of exogenous hemosiderosis. Such iron overload is particularly apt to occur in patients with hemoglobinopathies and other refractory anemias that might be erroneously diagnosed as iron-deficiency anemias.

➤*Rheumatoid arthritis:* Patients with rheumatoid arthritis may have an acute exacerbation of joint pain and swelling following the administration of iron dextran.

➤*Allergies/Asthma:* Use with caution in individuals with histories of significant allergies or asthma.

Drug Interactions

➤*Chloramphenicol:* Serum iron levels may be increased because of decreased iron clearance and erythropoiesis due to direct bone marrow toxicity from chloramphenicol.

➤*Drug/Lab test interactions:* Large doses of iron dextran (greater than or equal to 5 mL) have been reported to give a brown color to serum from a blood sample drawn 4 hours after administration.

The drug may cause falsely elevated values of serum bilirubin and falsely decreased values of serum calcium.

Bone scans involving 99m Tc-diphosphonate have been reported to show a dense, crescentic area of activity in the buttocks, following the contour of the iliac crest, 1 to 6 days after IM injections of iron dextran.

Bone scans with 99 m Tc-labeled bone seeking agents, in the presence of high serum ferritin levels or following iron dextran infusions, have been reported to show reduction of bony uptake, marked renal activity, and excessive blood pool and soft tissue accumulation.

Adverse Reactions

➤*Cardiovascular:* Arrhythmias, bradycardia, cardiac arrest, chest pain, chest tightness, flushing, hypertension, hypotension, shock, tachycardia. Flushing and hypotension may occur from too rapid injections by the IV route.

➤*CNS:* Chills, convulsions, disorientation, dizziness, febrile episodes, headache, numbness, paresthesia, seizures, syncope, unconsciousness, unresponsiveness, weakness.

➤*Dermatologic:* Cyanosis, pruritus, purpura, rash, urticaria.

➤*GI:* Abdominal pain, diarrhea, nausea, vomiting.

➤*GU:* Hematuria.

➤*Hematologic/Lymphatic:* Leucocytosis, lymphadenopathy.

➤*Severe/fatal reactions:* Anaphylactic reactions have been reported with the use of iron dextran injection; on occasions these reactions have been fatal. Such reactions, which occur most often within the first several minutes of administration, have been generally characterized by sudden onset of respiratory difficulty or cardiovascular collapse. Because fatal anaphylactic reactions have been reported after administration of iron dextran injection, give the drug only when resuscitation techniques and treatment of anaphylactic and anaphylactoid shock are readily available.

➤*Musculoskeletal:* Arthralgia, arthritis (may represent reactivation in patients with quiescent rheumatoid arthritis); backache; brown skin or underlying tissue discoloration (staining); cellulitis; inflammation; local phlebitis at or near IV injection site; myalgia; sterile abscess, atrophy/fibrosis (IM injection site); swelling.

➤*Respiratory:* Bronchospasm, dyspnea, respiratory arrest, wheezing.

➤*Miscellaneous:* Altered taste, chills, febrile episodes, malaise, shivering, sweating.

Delayed reactions – Arthralgia, backache, chills, dizziness, fever, headache, malaise, myalgia, nausea, vomiting.

Overdosage

➤*Symptoms:* Overdosage with iron dextran is unlikely to be associated with any acute manifestations. Dosages of iron dextran in excess of the requirements for restoration of hemoglobin and replenishment of iron stores may lead to hemosiderosis.

➤*Treatment:* Periodic monitoring of serum ferritin levels may be helpful in recognizing a deleterious progressive accumulation of iron resulting from impaired uptake of iron from the reticuloendothelial system in concurrent medical conditions such as chronic renal failure, Hodgkin's disease, and rheumatoid arthritis. The LD_{50} of iron dextran is not less than 500 mg/kg in the mouse.

Patient Information

Advise patients of the potential adverse reactions associated with the use of iron dextran.

SODIUM FERRIC GLUCONATE COMPLEX

Rx	**Ferrlecit** (Watson Pharma)	**Injection:** 62.5 mg per 5 mL (12.5 mg/mL) elemental iron	9 mg/mL of benzyl alcohol, 20% sucrose. In 5 mL amps.

SODIUM FERRIC GLUCONATE COMPLEX — INJECTION

Indications

➤*Iron deficiency:* For the treatment of iron deficiency anemia in patients 6 years of age and older undergoing chronic hemodialysis who are receiving supplemental epoetin therapy.

Administration and Dosage

➤*Approved by the FDA:* February 18, 1999.

The dosage of sodium ferric gluconate complex is expressed in milligrams of elemental iron. Each 5 mL ampule contains elemental iron 62.5 mg (12.5 mg/mL).

➤*Iron deficiency:*

Adults – 10 mL (elemental iron 125 mg), may be diluted in 100 mL of 0.9% sodium chloride administered by intravenous (IV) infusion over 1 hour. It may also be administered undiluted as a slow IV injection (at a rate of up to 12.5 mg/min). Most patients will require a minimum cumulative dose of 1 g elemental iron administered over 8 sessions at sequential dialysis treatments to achieve a favorable hemoglobin or hematocrit response. Patients may continue to require therapy with IV iron at the lowest dose necessary to maintain the target levels of hemoglobin, hematocrit, and laboratory parameters of iron storage within acceptable limits.

Sodium ferric gluconate complex has been administered at sequential dialysis sessions by infusion or by slow IV injection during the dialysis session itself.

Children – 0.12 mL/kg (1.5 mg/kg of elemental iron) diluted in 25 mL 0.9% sodium chloride and administered by IV infusion over 1 hour at 8 sequential dialysis sessions. The maximum dosage should not exceed 125 mg/dose.

➤*Admixture incompatibility:* Do not mix with other medications or add to parenteral nutrition solutions for IV infusion. The compatibility of sodium ferric gluconate complex with IV infusion vehicles other than 0.9% sodium chloride has not been evaluated.

SODIUM FERRIC GLUCONATE COMPLEX — INJECTION

➤*Storage/Stability:* Store at 20° to 25°C (68° to 77°F); excursions permitted to 15° to 30°C (59° to 86°F). Do not freeze. Use immediately after dilution in saline.

Actions

➤*Pharmacology:* Sodium ferric gluconate complex in sucrose injection is a stable macromolecular complex used to replete the total body content of iron. Iron is critical for normal hemoglobin synthesis to maintain oxygen transport. Additionally, iron is necessary for metabolism and various enzymatic processes.

The total body iron content of an adult ranges from 2 to 4 g (approximately two thirds in hemoglobin and one third in reticuloendothelial storage [bone marrow, spleen, liver] bound to intracellular ferritin). The body highly conserves iron (daily loss of 0.03%), requiring supplementation of approximately 1 mg/day to replenish losses in healthy, nonmenstruating adults. The etiology of iron deficiency in hemodialysis patients is varied and can include increased iron use (eg, from epoetin therapy) and blood loss. The administration of exogenous epoetin increases red blood cell production and iron use. The increased iron use and blood losses in the hemodialysis patient may lead to absolute or functional iron deficiency. Iron deficiency is absolute when hematologic indicators of iron stores are low. Patients with functional iron deficiency do not meet laboratory criteria for absolute iron deficiency but demonstrate an increase in hemoglobin/hematocrit or a decrease in epoetin dosage with stable hemoglobin/hematocrit when parenteral iron is administered.

➤*Pharmacokinetics:*

Absorption/Distribution – In multiple, sequential, adult, single-dose IV studies, peak drug levels (C_{max}) varied significantly by dosage and by rate of administration with the highest C_{max} observed in the regimen in which 125 mg was administered in 7 minutes (19 mg/L). In single dose IV studies, pediatric patients receiving a dose of 1.5 mg/kg had a C_{max} and area under the curve (AUC) of 12.9 mg/L and 95 mg•h/L, respectively. Pediatric patients who received a dose of 3 mg/kg (maximum dose, 125 mg) had a C_{max} and AUC of 22.8 mg/L and 170.9 mg•h/L, respectively. The initial volume of distribution of 6 L corresponds well to calculated blood volume. The AUC for bound iron varied by dose from 17.5 mg•h/L (62.5 mg) to 35.6 mg•h/L (125 mg). Approximately 80% of drug bound iron was delivered to transferrin as a mononuclear ionic iron species within 24 hours of administration in each dosage regimen. Mean peak transferrin saturation did not exceed 100% and returned to near baseline by 40 hours after administration of each dosage regimen.

Metabolism/Excretion – The terminal elimination half-life for drug bound iron was approximately 1 hour for adults and 2 to 2.5 hours for pediatrics, varying by dose but not by rate of administration. Total clearance was 3.02 to 5.35 L/h. In vitro, less than 1% of the iron species within sodium ferric gluconate complex can be dialyzed through membranes with pore sizes corresponding to 12,000 to 14,000 daltons over a period of up to 270 minutes.

Contraindications

All anemias not associated with iron deficiency; hypersensitivity to sodium ferric gluconate complex or any of its inactive components; evidence of iron overload.

Warnings

➤*Hypotension:* Hypotension associated with light-headedness, malaise, fatigue, weakness, or severe pain in the chest, back, flanks, or groin has been associated with administration of IV iron. These hypotensive reactions are not associated with signs of hypersensitivity and have usually resolved within 1 or 2 hours. Successful treatment may consist of observation or, if the hypotension causes symptoms, volume expansion.

➤*Hypersensitivity reactions:* Serious hypersensitivity reactions have been rarely reported. One case of a life-threatening hypersensitivity reaction has been observed in a patient who received a single dose of sodium ferric gluconate complex in a postmarketing study. Three serious hypersensitivity reactions have been reported from the spontaneous reporting system (see Adverse Reactions).

➤*Mutagenesis:* A clastogenic effect was produced in an in vitro chromosomal aberration assay in Chinese hamster ovary cells.

➤*Elderly:* Cautiously select dose for an elderly patient, usually starting at the low end of the dosing range, reflecting the greater frequency of decreased hepatic, renal, or cardiac function and of concomitant disease or other drug therapy.

➤*Pregnancy: Category B.* There are no adequate and well-controlled studies in pregnant women. Use during pregnancy only if the potential benefit justifies the potential risk to the fetus.

➤*Lactation:* It is not known whether this drug is excreted in breast milk. Because many drugs are excreted in human milk, exercise caution when administering to a breastfeeding woman.

➤*Children:* Safety and efficacy have not been established in pediatric patients younger than 6 years of age. Sodium ferric gluconate complex contains benzyl alcohol; therefore, do not use in neonates.

Precautions

➤*Benzyl alcohol:* This product contains benzyl alcohol, which has been associated with a fatal "gasping syndrome" in premature infants.

➤*Iron overload:* Iron is not easily eliminated from the body and accumulation can be toxic. Unnecessary therapy with parenteral iron will cause excess storage of iron with consequent possibility of iatrogenic hemosiderosis. Iron overload is particularly apt to occur in patients with hemoglobinopathies and other refractory anemias. Do not administer to patients with iron overload.

Drug Interactions

➤*Oral iron preparations:* Coadministration of parenteral iron preparations may reduce absorption of oral iron preparations.

Adverse Reactions

➤*Hypotension:* (See Warnings). Of 226 renal dialysis patients exposed to sodium ferric gluconate complex, 3 (1.3%) patients experienced hypotensive events, which were accompanied by flushing in 2 patients. All completely reversed after 1 hour without sequelae.

Sodium ferric gluconate complex administered to patients during dialysis may cause transient hypotension. Administration may augment hypotension caused by dialysis.

Among the 126 patients evaluated in clinical studies, 1 patient experienced a transient decreased level of consciousness without hypotension. Another patient discontinued treatment prematurely because of dizziness, lightheadedness, diplopia, malaise, and weakness without hypotension that resulted in a 3- to 4-hour hospitalization for observation following drug administration. The syndrome resolved spontaneously.

➤*Hypersensitivity:* (See Warnings). In the single-dose, postmarketing safety study, 1 patient experienced a life-threatening hypersensitivity reaction (diaphoresis, nausea, vomiting, severe lower back pain, dyspnea, and wheezing for 20 minutes) following administration. There were 9 patients (0.8%) who had an adverse reaction that precluded further sodium ferric gluconate complex administration (drug intolerance). These included 1 life-threatening reaction, 6 allergic reactions (2 pruritus reactions and facial flushing, chills, dyspnea/chest pain, and rash), and 2 other reactions (hypotension and nausea). Another 2 patients (0.2%) experienced allergic reactions not deemed to represent drug intolerance (nausea/malaise and nausea/dizziness) following administration.

In multiple-dose studies, hypersensitivity events associated with sodium ferric gluconate complex resulting in premature study discontinuation occurred in 3 out of a total 88 (3.4%) treated patients. The first patient withdrew after the development of pruritus and chest pain following the test dose. The second patient, in the high-dose group, experienced nausea, abdominal and flank pain, fatigue, and rash following the first dose. The third patient, in the low-dose group, experienced a "red, blotchy rash" following the first dose. Of the 38 patients exposed, none reported hypersensitivity reactions.

Many chronic renal failure patients experience cramps, pain, nausea, rash, flushing, and pruritus.

➤*Other adverse reactions (adults):*

Cardiovascular – Hypotension (29%); hypertension (13%); syncope (6%); tachycardia (5%); angina pectoris; bradycardia; myocardial infarction; pulmonary edema; vasodilation.

CNS – Cramps (25%); dizziness (13%); fatigue, paresthesias (6%); agitation; somnolence.

Dermatologic – Pruritus (6%); increased sweating; rash.

GI – Diarrhea, nausea, vomiting (35%); abdominal pain (6%); anorexia; dyspepsia; eructation; flatulence; GI disorder; melena; rectal disorder.

Hematologic – Abnormal erythrocytes (11%); anemia; leukocytosis; lymphadenopathy.

Metabolic – Hyperkalemia (6%); generalized edema (5%); edema; hypervolemia; hypoglycemia; hypokalemia; leg edema; peripheral edema.

Musculoskeletal – Leg cramps (10%); arthralgia; myalgia.

Respiratory – Dyspnea (11%); coughing, upper respiratory tract infections (6%); pneumonia; rhinitis.

Special senses – Abnormal vision; conjunctivitis; ear disorder.

Miscellaneous – Injection-site reaction (33%); chest pain, pain (10%); asthenia, headache (7%); fever (5%); abscess; arm pain; back pain; carcinoma; chills; flu-like syndrome; infection; malaise; rigors; sepsis; urinary tract infection.

➤*Other adverse reactions (children):*

Cardiovascular – Hypertension (23%); hypotension (28% to 41%); tachycardia (13% to 21%); thrombosis (6%).

GI – Abdominal pain (3% to 15%); diarrhea (8%); nausea (6% to 12%); vomiting (9% to 12%).

Respiratory – Pharyngitis (6% to 12%); rhinitis (3% to 9%).

Miscellaneous – Fever (3% to 15%); headache (19% to 29%); infection (8%).

➤*Postmarketing:* Dry mouth, hemorrhage, hypertonia, nervousness.

Overdosage

➤*Symptoms:* Serum iron levels greater than 300 mcg/dL may indicate iron poisoning, which is characterized by abdominal pain, diarrhea, or vomiting that progresses to pallor or cyanosis, lassitude, drowsiness, hyperventilation due to acidosis, and cardiovascular collapse.

➤*Treatment:* Dosages in excess of iron needs may lead to accumulation of iron in iron storage sites and hemosiderosis. Periodic monitoring of laboratory parameters of iron storage may assist in recognition of iron accumulation. Do not administer sodium ferric gluconate complex in patients with iron overload. Sodium ferric gluconate complex is not dialyzable.

IRON SUCROSE

Rx	**Venofer** (American Regent Labs)	**Injection:** 20 mg elemental iron/mL	Preservative free. 300 mg/mL sucrose w/v. In 5 mL single-dose vials.

IRON SUCROSE — INJECTION

Indications

➤*Iron-deficiency anemia:* For the treatment of iron-deficiency anemia in the following patients:
- non-dialysis-dependent chronic kidney disease (NDD-CKD) patients receiving an erythropoietin
- NDD-CKD patients not receiving an erythropoietin
- hemodialysis-dependent chronic kidney disease (HDD-CKD) patients receiving an erythropoietin
- peritoneal dialysis-dependent chronic kidney disease (PDD-CKD) patients receiving an erythropoietin

Administration and Dosage

➤*Approved by the FDA:* November 6, 2000.

The dosage of iron sucrose is expressed in terms of mg of elemental iron. Each mL contains elemental iron 20 mg.

Most CKD patients will require a minimum cumulative repletion dose of elemental iron 1,000 mg administered over sequential sessions to achieve a favorable hemoglobin response and to replenish iron stores (ferritin, transferrin saturation [TSAT]). Hemodialysis patients may continue to require therapy with iron sucrose or other intravenous (IV) iron preparations at the lowest dose necessary to maintain target levels of hemoglobin and laboratory parameters of iron storage within acceptable limits.

➤*Administration:* Iron sucrose must only be administered IV either by slow injection or by infusion.

➤*Adult dosage:*

HDD-CKD patients – Iron sucrose may be administered undiluted as a 100 mg slow IV injection over 2 to 5 minutes or as an infusion of 100 mg, diluted in a maximum of 100 mL of sodium chloride (NaCl) 0.9% over a period of at least 15 minutes per consecutive hemodialysis session for a total cumulative dose of 1,000 mg.

NDD-CKD patients – Iron sucrose is administered as a total cumulative dose of 1,000 mg over a 14-day period as a 200 mg slow IV injection undiluted over 2 to 5 minutes on 5 different occasions within the 14-day period. There is limited experience with administration of an infusion of iron sucrose 500 mg, diluted in a maximum of 250 mL of NaCl 0.9% over a period of 3.5 to 4 hours on day 1 and day 14; hypotension occurred in 2 of 30 patients treated.

PDD-CKD patients – Iron sucrose is administered as a total cumulative dose of 1,000 mg in 3 divided doses, given by slow IV infusion, within a 28-day period: 2 infusions of 300 mg over 1.5 hours 14 days apart, followed by one 400 mg infusion over 2.5 hours 14 days later. The iron sucrose dose should be diluted in a maximum of 250 mL of NaCl 0.9%.

➤*Storage/Stability:* Store in original carton at 25°C (77°F). Excursions permitted to 15° to 30°C (59° to 86°F). Do not freeze. Contains no preservatives.

Actions

➤*Pharmacology:* Iron sucrose is used to replenish body iron stores in NDD-CKD patients receiving erythropoietin and in NDD-CKD patients not receiving erythropoietin, and in HDD-CKD and PDD-CKD patients receiving erythropoietin. Iron deficiency may be caused by blood loss during dialysis, increased erythropoiesis secondary to erythropoietin use, and insufficient absorption of iron from the GI tract. Iron is essential to the synthesis of hemoglobin to maintain oxygen transport and to the function and formation of other physiologically important heme and nonheme compounds. Most dialysis patients require IV iron to maintain sufficient iron stores.

➤*Pharmacokinetics:*

Absorption/Distribution – In healthy adults treated with IV doses of iron sucrose, its iron component exhibits first order kinetics. In healthy adults receiving IV doses of iron sucrose, its iron component appears to distribute mainly in blood and, to some extent, in extravascular fluid. Iron sucrose has a nonsteady state apparent volume of distribution of 10 L, and steady state apparent volume of distribution of 7.9 L. A study evaluating iron sucrose containing iron 100 mg labeled with $^{52}Fe/^{59}Fe$ in patients with iron deficiency shows that a significant amount of the administered iron distributes in the liver, spleen, and bone marrow and that the bone marrow is an iron-trapping compartment and not a reversible volume of distribution.

Metabolism/Excretion – Because iron disappearance from serum depends on the need for iron in the iron stores and iron-utilizing tissues of the body, serum clearance of iron is expected to be more rapid in iron-deficient patients treated with iron sucrose as compared with healthy individuals.

Following IV administration, iron sucrose is dissociated into iron and sucrose by the reticuloendothelial system. The sucrose component is eliminated mainly by urinary excretion with an elimination half-life of 6 hours and total clearance of 1.2 L/h. In a study evaluating a single IV dose of iron sucrose containing sucrose 1,510 mg and iron 100 mg in 12 healthy adults (9 women, 3 men; age range, 32 to 52 years), 68.3% of the sucrose was eliminated in urine in 4 hours and 75.4% in 24 hours. Some iron is also eliminated in the urine. Neither transferrin nor transferrin receptor levels changed immediately after the dose administration. In this study and another study evaluating a single IV dose of iron sucrose containing iron 500 to 700 mg in 26 anemic patients on erythropoietin therapy (23 women, 3 men; age range, 16 to 60 years), approximately 5% of the iron was eliminated in urine in 24 hours at each dose level.

Contraindications

Evidence of iron overload; known hypersensitivity to iron sucrose or any of its inactive components; anemia not caused by iron deficiency.

Warnings

➤*Hypersensitivity reactions:* See Adverse Reactions for more information.

➤*Elderly:* No overall differences in safety were observed between these subjects and younger subjects, and other reported clinical experience has not identified differences in responses between the elderly and younger patients, but greater sensitivity of some older individuals cannot be ruled out.

➤*Pregnancy:* *Category B.*

There are no adequate and well controlled studies in pregnant women. Because animal reproduction studies are not always predictive of human response, administer this drug during pregnancy only if clearly needed.

➤*Lactation:* Iron sucrose is excreted in milk of rats. It is not known whether this drug is excreted in human milk. Because many drugs are excreted in human milk, exercise caution when iron sucrose is administered to a breast-feeding woman.

➤*Children:* Safety and efficacy of iron sucrose in children have not been established.

Precautions

➤*Monitoring:* Patients receiving iron sucrose require periodic monitoring of hematologic and hematinic parameters (hemoglobin, hematocrit, serum ferritin, and transferrin saturation). Withhold iron therapy in patients with evidence of iron overload and discontinue use when serum ferritin levels equal or exceed established guidelines. Transferrin saturation values increase rapidly after IV administration of iron sucrose; thus, serum iron values may be reliably obtained 48 hours after IV dosing.

➤*Iron overload:* Because body iron excretion is limited and excess tissue iron can be hazardous, exercise caution to withhold iron administration in the presence of evidence of tissue iron overload. Dosages of iron sucrose in excess of iron needs may lead to accumulation of iron in storage sites, leading to hemosiderosis. Exercise particular caution to avoid overload where anemia unresponsive to treatment has been incorrectly diagnosed as iron deficiency anemia. Do not administer iron sucrose to patients with iron overload.

➤*Hypotension:* Hypotension has been reported frequently in HDD-CKD patients receiving IV iron. Hypotension also has been reported in NND- and PDD-CKD patients receiving IV iron. Hypotension following administration of iron sucrose may be related to rate of administration and total dose administered. Cautiously administer iron sucrose according to recommended guidelines.

Drug Interactions

➤*Oral iron preparations:* Drug-drug interactions involving iron sucrose have not been studied. However, like other parenteral iron preparations, iron sucrose may be expected to reduce the absorption of concomitantly administered oral iron preparations.

Adverse Reactions

Iron Sucrose Adverse Reactions (≥ 2%) by Indication

	HDD-CKD	NDD-CKD		PDD-CKD	
Adverse reaction	Iron sucrose (n = 231)	Iron sucrose (n = 139)	Oral iron (n = 139)	Iron sucrose (n = 75)	Erythropoietin only (n = 46)
Any adverse reaction	78.8%	76.3%	73.4%	72%	65.2%
CNS					
Asthenia	2.2%	0.7%	2.2%	2.7%	0
Dizziness	6.5%	6.5%	1.4%	1.3%	4.3%
Fatigue	1.7%	3.6%	5.8%	0	4.3%
Headache	12.6%	2.9%	0.7%	4%	0
Hyposthesia	0	0.7%	0.7%	0	4.3%
Cardiovascular					
Cardiac murmur	0.4%	2.2%	2.2%	0	0
Chest pain	6.1%	1.4%	0	2.7%	0
Hypertension	6.5%	6.5%	4.3%	8%	6.5%
Hypotension	39.4%	2.2%	0.7%	2.7%	2.2%

IRON SUCROSE — INJECTION

Iron Sucrose Adverse Reactions (≥ 2%) by Indication					
	HDD-CKD	NDD-CKD		PDD-CKD	
Adverse reaction	Iron sucrose (n = 231)	Iron sucrose (n = 139)	Oral iron (n = 139)	Iron sucrose (n = 75)	Erythropoietin only (n = 46)
Dermatologic					
Pruritus	3.9%	2.2%	4.3%	2.7%	0
Rash	0.4%	1.4%	2.2%	0	2.2%
GI					
Abdominal pain	3.5%	1.4%	2.9%	4%	6.5%
Constipation	1.3%	4.3%	12.9%	4%	6.5%
Diarrhea	5.2%	7.2%	10.1%	8%	4.3%
Nausea	14.7%	8.6%	12.2%	5.3%	4.3%
Vomiting	9.1%	5%	8.6%	8%	2.2%
Local					
Catheter site infection	0	0	0	4%	8.7%
Infusion site burning	0	3.6%	0	0	0
Injection site extravasation	0	2.2%	0	0	0
Injection site pain	0	2.2%	0	0	0
Metabolic/Nutritional					
Fluid overload	3%	1.4%	0.7%	1.3%	0
Gout	0	2.9%	1.4%	0	0
Hyperglycemia	0	2.9%	0	0	2.2%
Hypoglycemia	0.4%	0.7%	0.7%	4%	0
Musculoskeletal					
Arthralgia	3.5%	1.4%	2.2%	4%	4.3%
Arthritis	0	0	0	0	4.3%
Back pain	2.2%	2.2%	3.6%	1.3%	4.3%
Muscle cramp	29.4%	0.7%	0.7%	2.7%	0
Myalgia	0	3.6%	0	1.3%	0
Pain in extremity	5.6%	4.3%	0	2.7%	6.5%
Respiratory					
Cough	3%	2.2%	0.7%	1.3%	0
Dyspnea	3.5%	3.6%	0.7%	1.3%	2.2%
Dyspnea exacerbated	0	2.2%	0.7%	0	0
Nasal congestion	0	1.4%	2.2%	1.3%	0
Nasopharyngitis	0.9%	0.7%	2.2%	2.7%	2.2%
Pharyngitis	0.4%	0	0	6.7%	0
Rhinitis allergic	0	0.7%	2.2%	0	0
Sinusitis	0	0.7%	0.7%	4%	0
Upper respiratory tract infection	1.3%	0.7%	1.4%	2.7%	2.2%
Special senses					
Conjunctivitis	0.4%	0	0	2.7%	0
Dysgeusia	0.9%	7.9%	0	0	0
Ear pain	0	2.2%	0.7%	0	0
Miscellaneous					
Edema	0.4%	6.5%	6.5%	0	2.2%
Fecal occult blood positive	0	1.4%	3.6%	2.7%	4.3%
Feeling abnormal	3%	0	0	0	0
Graft complications	9.5%	1.4%	0	0	0
Peripheral edema	2.6%	7.2%	5%	5.3%	10.9%
Peritoneal infection	0	0	0	8%	10.9%
Pyrexia	3%	0.7%	0.7%	1.3%	0
Urinary tract infection NOS	0.4%	0.7%	5%	1.3%	2.2%

Drug-related adverse reactions reported by at least 2% of iron sucrose-treated patients are shown by dose group in the following table.

Iron Sucrose Adverse Reactions (≥ 2%) by Dose				
	HDD-CKD	NDD-CKD		PDD-CKD
Adverse reaction	100 mg (n = 231)	200 mg (n = 109)	500 mg (n = 30)	300 mg for 2 doses followed by 400 mg for 1 dose (n = 75)
Any adverse reaction	14.7%	23.9%	20%	10.7%
CNS				
Dizziness	0	2.8%	6.7%	0
Headache	0	2.8%	0	0
GI				
Diarrhea	0.9%	0	0	2.7%
Nausea	1.7%	2.8%	0	1.3%
Local				
Infusion site burning	0	3.7%	0	0
Injection site pain	0	2.8%	0	0
Miscellaneous				
Dysgeusia	0.9%	7.3%	3.3%	0
Hypotension	5.2%	0	6.7%	0
Peripheral edema	0	1.8%	6.7%	0

➤*HDD-CKD patients:* Adverse reactions, whether or not related to iron sucrose administration, reported more than 5% of treated patients from a total of 231 patients in HDD-CKD studies A, B, and C were as follows: hypotension (39.4%); muscle cramps (29.4%); nausea (14.7%); headache (12.6%); graft complications (9.5%); vomiting (9.1%); dizziness, hypertension (6.5%); chest pain (6.1%); diarrhea (5.2%).

Postmarketing –

Adverse reactions reported by more than 1% of 1,051 treated patients were congestive cardiac failure, sepsis, and dysgeusia.

NDD-CKD patients – In study D of 182 treated NDD-CKD patients, 91 were exposed to iron sucrose. Adverse reactions, whether or not related to iron sucrose, reported by at least 5% of the iron sucrose exposed patients were as follows: dysgeusia, peripheral edema (7.7%); constipation, diarrhea, dizziness, hypertension, nausea (5.5%).

One serious related adverse reaction was reported (hypotension and shortness of breath not requiring hospitalization in an iron sucrose patient). Two patients experienced possible hypersensitivity/allergic reactions (local edema/hypotension) during the study. Of the 5 patients who prematurely discontinued the treatment phase of the study because of adverse reactions (2 oral iron group and 3 iron sucrose group), 3 iron sucrose patients had reactions that were considered drug-related (hypotension, dyspnea, and nausea).

In an additional study of iron sucrose with varying erythropoietin doses in 96 treated NDD-CKD patients, adverse reactions, whether or not related to iron sucrose, reported by at least 5% of iron sucrose exposed patients are as follows: diarrhea, edema (16.5%); nausea (13.2%); vomiting (12.1%); arthralgia, back pain, dysgeusia, headache, hypertension (7.7%); dizziness (6.6%); extremity pain, injection site burning (5.5%).

No patient experienced a hypersensitivity/allergic reaction during the study. Of the patients who prematurely discontinued the treatment phase of the study because of adverse reactions (2.1% oral iron group and 12.5% iron sucrose group), only 1 patient (iron sucrose group) had reactions that were considered drug-related (anxiety, headache, and nausea). Ninety-one patients in this study were exposed to iron sucrose during the treatment or extending follow-up phase.

PDD-CKD patients – In study E of 121 treated PDD-CKD patients, 75 patients were exposed to iron sucrose. Adverse reactions, whether or not related to iron sucrose, reported by at least 5% of these patients are as follows: diarrhea, hypertension, nausea, peripheral edema, peritoneal infection, pharyngitis, and vomiting.

Of these 75 patients exposed to iron sucrose, 9 patients experienced serious adverse reactions as follows: peritoneal infection (2 patients) and 1 patient each with cardiopulmonary arrest, myocardial infarction, upper respiratory tract infection not otherwise specified (NOS), anemia, gangrene, hypovolemia, tuberculosis. None of these reactions were considered drug related. Two iron sucrose patients experienced a moderate hypersensitivity/allergic reaction (rash or swelling/itching) during the study.

The only drug-related adverse reaction to iron sucrose administration reported by at least 2% of patients was diarrhea.

Three patients in the iron sucrose study group discontinued study treatment because of adverse reactions (cardiopulmonary arrest, peritonitis and myocardial infarction, hypertension), which were considered to be not drug-related.

IRON SUCROSE — INJECTION

➤*Hypersensitivity:* In clinical studies, several patients experienced hypersensitivity reactions presenting with wheezing, dyspnea, hypotension, rashes, or pruritus. Serious episodes of hypotension occurred in 2 patients treated with iron sucrose 500 mg.

From the postmarketing spontaneous reporting system, there were 104 reports of anaphylactoid reactions, including patients who experienced serious or life-threatening reactions (anaphylactic shock, loss of consciousness or collapse, bronchospasm with dyspnea, or convulsion) associated with iron sucrose administration.

One hundred thirty (11%) of the 1,151 patients evaluated in the 4 US trials in HDD-CKD patients (studies A, B, and the 2 postmarketing studies) had prior other IV iron therapy and were reported to be intolerant (defined as precluding further use of the iron product). When these patients were treated with iron sucrose, there were no occurrences of adverse reactions that precluded further use of iron sucrose.

Overdosage

➤*Symptoms:* Symptoms associated with overdosage or infusing iron sucrose too rapidly included hypotension, dyspnea, headache, vomiting, nausea, dizziness, joint aches, paresthesia, abdominal and muscle pain, edema, and cardiovascular collapse.

➤*Treatment:* Most symptoms have been successfully treated with IV fluids, hydrocortisone, and/or antihistamines. Infusing the solution as recommended or at a slower rate may also alleviate symptoms.

IRON WITH VITAMINS

Content given per capsule or tablet.

	Product & Distributor	Fe mg	A IU	D IU	E IU	B_1 mg	B_2 mg	B_3 mg	B_5 mg	B_6 mg	B_{12} mcg	C mg	FA mg	Other Content	How Supplied
Rx	**Chromagen Forte Capsules** (Ther-Rx)	151									10	60	1	Parabens	(THX 0131). In UD 100s.
Rx	**FeoGen Forte Capsules** (Rising Pharmaceuticals)[b]	151									10	60	1		(109). Brown. In UD 100s.
Rx	**Repliva 21/7 Tablets** (Ther-Rx)	151									10	200	1	150 mg succinic acid	Lactose. Red = (Ther-Rx 155). Purple = (Ther-Rx). Oval. Film coated. In 28s. With 7 inert tablets.
Rx	**Hemocyte-F Tablets** (US Pharm)	106[a]											1		Maroon. In 100s
Rx	**Cenogen-OB Capsules** (US Pharm)	106[a]				10	6	30	10	5	15	200	1	18.2 mg Zn, Cu, Mg, Mn	In 100s.
otc	**Ircon-FA Tablets** (Kenwood)	82[n]											0.8		In blister pack 100s.
Rx	**Chromagen FA Capsules** (Ther-Rx)	70									10	150	1	Parabens	(THX 0130). Green/Brown. In UD 100s.
Rx	**FeoGen FA Capsules** (Ther-Rx)	66									10	250	1		(116). Maroon. In UD 100s.
Rx	**Hematinic Tablets** (Cypress)	106[a]											1		In 100s.
otc	**Slow FE Slow Release Iron with Folic Acid Tablets** (Ciba)	50[d]											0.4		Lactose. In 20s.
Rx	**Nestabs CBF** (Fielding)	50	4,000	400	30	3	3	20[5]		3	8	120	1	200 mg Ca, 150 mcg I, 15 mg Zn	(CBF). In 100s
otc	**Tolfrinic Tablets** (B.F. Ascher)	200[a]									25	100			Lactose. Dk. brown. Film coated. In 100s.
Rx	**Niferex-150 Forte Capsules** (Ther-Rx)	150[f]									25		1		(SP 4330). Red, brown, and white. In 100s and 1,000s.
Rx	**Ferrex 150 Forte Plus Capsules** (Breckenridge)	150[m]									25	60	1		(B 398). Orange In UD 100s.
Rx	**Fumatinic Capsules** (Laser)	66[a]									5	60			Extended release. (Laser 0181). Natural/maroon with brown, white, and off-white pellets. In 100s.
otc	**Ferralet Plus Tablets** (Mission)	46[g]									25	400	0.8		Sugar. In 60s.
otc	**Generet-500 Tablets** (Goldline)	105[h]													Timed release. In 60s.
otc	**Iberet Filmtabs** (Abbott)					6	6	30	10	5	25	150[g]			Controlled release. Film coated. In 60s.
otc	**Iron-Folic 500 Tablets** (Major)	105[d]				6	6	30	10	5	25	500[h]	0.8		(AK A101). Timed release. In 100s and 500s.
Rx	**Hematinic Plus Tablets** (Cypress)	106[a]				10	6	30	10	5	15	200	1	Cu, Mg, Mn, 18.2 mg Zn	In 100s.
otc	**Vita-Feron** (Vitaline)	150									6		0.8		In 90s.
Rx	**Ferrex 150 Forte** (Breckenridge)	150[f]									25		1		(B-198). Opaque maroon. In UD 100s.
Rx	**Ferrex PC Tablets** (Breckenridge)	60[e]	4,000	400		3	3		2		3	50[i]	1	10 mg niacinamide, 125 mg Ca, 18 mg Zn	(B-200). Blue, oval. Scored. Film coated. In UD 100s.
Rx	**Ferrex PC Forte** (Breckenridge)	60[f]	5,000	400	30[j]	3	3.4			4	12	80[i]	1	250 mg Ca, 20 mg niacinamide, 0.2 mg I, 10 mg Mg, 25 mg Zn, 2 mg Cu	(B-202). White, oval. Scored. Film coated. In UD 100s.
Rx	**Hemocyte Plus Tablets** (US Pharm)	106[a]				10	6	30	10	5	15	200[h]	1	Cu, Mg, Mn, 18.2 mg Zn	In 100s.
otc sf	**Parvlex Tablets** (Freeda)	100[a]				20	20	20	1	10	50	50[i]	0.1	Cu, Mn	In 100s and 250s.
otc	**Prenatal H.P.** (Mission)	30	4,000	400		4	2	10	1	20	2	100	0.8	50 mg Ca. Sugar.	In 100s.
Rx	**Prenatal Rx** (Mission)	29.5[a]	3,000	400		4	2	20	10	20	8	240[i]	1	175 mg Ca, 2 mg Cu, 0.3 mg I, 15 mg Zn	In 100s.
Rx	**Advanced Formula Zenate Tablets** (Solvay)	65[a]	3000	400	10[j]	1.5	1.6	17		2.2	2.2	70	1	Ca, I, Mg, Zn	In UD 30s.
otc	**Gentle Iron Capsules** (Nature's Bounty)	28[o]									8	60	0.4		In 90s.
otc	**Allbee C-800 Plus Iron Tablets** (Robins)	27[a]			45[l]	15	17	100	25	25	12	800	0.4	Lactose	Red. Film coated. Elliptical. In 60s.
otc	**Theragran Stress Formula Tablets** (Mead Johnson)	27[a]			30[j]	15	15	100	20	25	12	600	0.4	45 mcg biotin	In 75s.
otc sf	**StressForm "605" with Iron Tablets** (NTBY)	27[j]			30[l]	15	15	100	20	5	12	605	0.4	45 mcg biotin	In 60s.
otc	**Stress Formula w/Iron Tablets** (Goldline)	27[a]			30[j]	10	10	100	20	5	12	500[h]	0.4	45 mcg biotin	In 60s.

IRON WITH VITAMINS

	Product & Distributor	Fe mg	A IU	D IU	E IU	B_1 mg	B_2 mg	B_3 mg	B_5 mg	B_6 mg	B_{12} mcg	C mg	FA mg	Other Content	How Supplied
otc	**Stress Formula with Iron Tablets** (NTBY)	27[k]			30[l]	10	10	100	20	5	12	500	0.4	45 mcg biotin	In 60s.
otc	**Stresstabs + Iron Tablets** (Lederle)	18[a]			30[j]	10	10	100	20	5	12	500	0.4	45 mcg biotin	(LL S2). Orange-red. Capsule shape. Film coated. In 60s.
Rx	**Niferex-PN Tablets** (Ther-Rx)	60[f]	4,000	400		3	3	10		2	3	50[h]	1	Ca, 18 mg Zn.	(SP 2209 131/05). Blue. Film coated. Oval. In 30s, 100s, and 1,000s.
Rx	**Nu-Iron V Tablets** (Mayrand)													Ca.	Maroon. Film coated. In 100s.
Rx	**B C w/Folic Acid Plus Tablets** (Geneva)	27[a]	5,000		30[j]	20	20	100	25	25	50	500	0.8	0.15 mg biotin, Cr, Cu, Mg, Mn, 22.5 mg Zn	In 100s.
Rx	**Berocca Plus Tablets** (Roche)													0.15 mg biotin, Cr, Cu, Mg, Mn, 22.5 mg Zn	(Berocca Plus/Roche). Yellow. Capsule shape. In 100s.
Rx	**Formula B Plus Tablets** (Major)													0.15 mg biotin, Cr, Cu, Mg, Mn, Zn	In 100s and 500s.
otc	**Mission Prenatal H.P. Tablets** (Mission)	30[g]	4,000	400		5	2	10	1	25	2	100	0.8	Ca, sugar	In 100s.
otc	**Mission Prenatal F.A. Tablets** (Mission)	30[g]	4,000	400		5	2	10	1	10	2	100	0.8	Ca, 15 mg Zn, sugar	In 100s.
otc	**Mission Prenatal Tablets** (Mission)	30[g]	4,000	400		5	2	10	1	3	2	100	0.4	Ca, sugar	In 100s.
otc	**Iromin-G Tablets** (Mission)	30[g]	4,000	400		5	2	10	1	20.6	2	100	0.8	Ca, sugar	In 100s.
Rx *sf*	**Vitafol Caplets** (Everett)	65[a]	6,000	400	30[c]	1.1	1.8	15		2.5	5	60	1	Ca	(EV0072). Film coated. In 100s and 1,000s.
otc	**Compete Tablets** (Mission)	27[g]	5,000	400	45[j]	2	2.6	30		20.6	9	90	0.4	22.5 mg Zn, sugar	In 100s.
otc *sf*	**Freedavite Tablets** (Freeda)	10[a]	5,000	400	3[j]	5	3	25	5	2	2	60		Choline, inositol, potassium iodide, Ca, Cu, K, Mg, Mn, Se, 0.2 mg Zn	In 100s and 250s.
otc	**Mission Surgical Supplement Tablets** (Mission)	27[g]	5,000	400	45[j]	2.5	2.6	30	16.3	3.6	9	500		22.5 mg Zn, sugar	In 100s.
otc	**Therapeutic-H Tablets** (Goldline)	66.7[a]	8,333	133	5[j]	3.3	3.3	33.3	11.7	3.3	50	100[g]	0.33	Cu, Mg	In 100s.
otc	**Thera Hematinic Tablets** (Major)													Cu, Mg	In 250s and 1,000s.
otc *sf*	**Yelets Tablets** (Freeda)	20[a]	10,000	400	10[l]	10	10	25	10	10	10	100	0.1	PABA, lysine, glutamic acid, Ca, I, Mg, Mn, Se, 4 mg Zn	In 100s and 250s.
Rx	**Zodeac-100 Tablets** (Econo Med)	60[a]	8,000	400	30[i]	1.7	2	20	11	4	8	120	1	300 mcg biotin, Ca, Cu, I, Mg, 15 mg Zn	Orange. Film coated. In 100s.
otc *sf*	**Geritol Complete Tablets** (SK-Beecham)	18[k]	6,000	400	30[j]	1.5	1.7	20	10	2	6	60	0.4	45 mcg biotin, Ca, Cl, Cr, Cu, I, K, Mg, Mn, Mo, Ni, P, Se, Si, Sn, V, Zn, vitamin K	In 14s, 40s, 100s, and 180s.
otc	**Thera-M Tablets** (Various, eg, Major)	27[k]	5,000	400	30[l]	3	3.4	20	10	3	9	90	0.4	30 mcg biotin, 15 mg Zn, P, Ca, Cu, Cr, Se, Mo, K, Cl, I, Mg, Mn	In 130s and 1,000s.
otc	**Multi-Vitamin Mineral w/Beta-Carotene Tablets** (Mission)	27[a]	5,000	400	30[l]	2.25	2.6	20	10	3	9	90	0.4	0.45 mg biotin, Ca, Cl, Cr, Cu, I, K, Mg, Mn, Mo, P, Se, 15 mg Zn, vitamin K_1	In 130s.

IRON WITH VITAMINS

	Product & Distributor	Fe mg	A IU	D IU	E IU	B_1 mg	B_2 mg	B_3 mg	B_5 mg	B_6 mg	B_{12} mcg	C mg	FA mg	Other Content	How Supplied
otc	**CertaVite Tablets** (Major)	13[a]	5,000	400	30[i]	1.5	1.7	20	10	2	6	60	0.4	30 mcg biotin, Ca, P, I, Mg, Cu, Mn, K, Cl, Cr, Mo, Se, Ni, Si, Sn, V, B, vitamin K_1, 15 mg Zn	In 130s and 300s.
otc *sf*	**ABC to Z Tablets** (NTBY)													30 mcg biotin, Ca, Cl, Cr, Cu, I, K, Mg, Mn, Mo, Ni, P, Se, Si, Sn, V, Zn, vitamin K_1	In 100s.
otc	**Advanced Formula Centrum Tablets** (Lederle)													30 mcg biotin, B, Ca, Cl, Cr, Cu, I, K, Mg, Mn, Mo, Ni, P, Se, Si, Sn, V, 15 mg Zn, vitamin K_1	In 60s, 130s, and 200s.
otc	**Cerovite Advanced Formula Tablets** (Rugby)	18[a]	3,500	400	30[j]	1.5	1.7	20	10	2	6	60	0.4	30 mcg biotin, B, Ca, Cl, Cr, Cu, I, K, Mg, Mn, Mo, N , P, Se, Si, Sn, V, 15 mg Zn, vitamin K_1, lutein, lycopene	In 130s.
Rx	**Nephron FA** (Nephro-Tech)	200[a]				1.5	1.7	20		10	6	40	1	300 mcg biotin, 75 mg docusate sodium	(FA). In 100s.

[a] From ferrous fumarate.
[b] Rising Pharmaceuticals, 411 Sette Drive, Paramus, NJ 07652; 201-262-4200, fax 201-262-4284.
[c] As d-alpha tocopherol succinate.
[d] From ferrous sulfate.
[e] As niacinamide.
[f] From polysaccharide-iron complex.
[g] From ferrous gluconate.
[h] As sodium ascorbate.
[i] From ascorbic acid.
[j] As dL-alpha tocopheryl acetate.
[k] Form of iron content unknown.
[l] Form of vitamin E content unknown.
[m] From polysaccharide iron and ferrous bisglycinate.
[n] As carbonyl iron.
[o] From iron glycinate.

IRON WITH VITAMINS — ORAL

For complete and comparative prescribing information, refer to the Iron-Containing Products monograph.

Indications

➤*Iron:* Iron in combination with folic acid is used to treat iron deficiency anemia in conjunction with certain nutritional deficiencies.

➤*B complex vitamins:* B complex vitamins function as coenzymes in carbohydrate, protein or amino acid metabolism, synthesis of DNA and other molecules, maturation of red blood cells, nerve cell function or oxidation-reducation reactions.

➤*Ascorbic acid (vitamin C):* Ascorbic acid may enhance the absorption of iron.

Warnings

➤*Pernicious anemia:* Folic acid alone is improper therapy in the treatment of pernicious anemia and other megaloblastic anemias where vitamin B_{12} is deficient. Where anemia exists, establish its nature and determine underlying causes.

Folic acid, especially in doses greater than 0.1 mg daily, may obscure pernicious anemia, in that hematologic remission may occur while neurological manifestations remain progressive. Concomitant parenteral therapy with vitamin B_{12} may be necessary in patients with deficiency of vitamin B_{12}.

Precautions

➤*Sulfite sensitivity:* Some of these products contain sulfites that may cause allergic-type reactions (including anaphylactic symptoms and life-threatening or less severe asthmatic episodes) in certain susceptible persons. The overall prevalence of sulfite sensitivity in the general population is unknown and probably low. It is seen more frequently in asthmatic or atopic nonasthmatic persons.

IRON WITH VITAMINS, LIQUIDS

Content given per 15 mL.

	Product & Distributor	Fe mg	B_1 mg	B_2 mg	B_3 mg	B_5 mg	B_6 mg	B_{12} mcg	C mg	FA mg	Other Content	How Supplied
Rx *sf*	**Nu-Iron Plus Elixir** (Mayrand)	300[a]						75		3	10% alcohol	Dye-free. In 237 mL.
Rx	**Hemocyte-F Elixir** (US Pharm)	300[a]						75		3	10% alcohol, parabens, saccharin, sorbitol	Sherry wine flavor. In 473 mL.
otc	**Trophite + Iron Liquid** (Menley & James)	60[b]	30					75			Saccharin, glucose, parabens	In 120 mL.
Rx	**Vitafol Syrup** (Everett)	90[b]			39.9		6	25.02		0.75		Raspberry-mint flavor. In 473 mL.

IRON WITH VITAMINS, LIQUIDS

	Product & Distributor	Fe mg	B_1 mg	B_2 mg	B_3 mg	B_5 mg	B_6 mg	B_{12} mcg	C mg	FA mg	Other Content	How Supplied
otc sf	**Vitalize SF Liquid** (Scot-Tussin)	66[b]	30				15	75			300 mg L-lysine, sorbitol, alcohol	Dye-free. In 120 mL.
otc	**Geritol Tonic Liquid** (SmithKline Beecham)	18[b]	2.5	2.5	50	2	0.5				25 mg methionine, 50 mg choline bitartrate, 12% alcohol	In 120 and 360 mL.

[a] From polysaccharide-iron complex.
[b] From ferric pyrophosphate.

IRON WITH VITAMINS — LIQUIDS

For complete and comparative prescribing information, refer to the Iron-Containing Products group monograph.

IRON AND LIVER COMBINATIONS

For complete prescribing information refer to the Iron-Containing Products, Oral group monograph.

Indications

➤*Iron deficiency:* Iron and liver combinations are recommended for iron deficiency anemia in conjunction with certain nutritional deficiencies.

Precautions

➤*Pernicious anemia:* The ingredients in these products are not sufficient, nor are they intended, for the treatment of pernicious anemia. The use of folic acid without adequate vitamin B_{12} therapy in patients with pernicious anemia may result in hematologic remission, but neurological progression.

➤*Benzyl alcohol:* Some parenteral products contain benzyl alcohol, which has been associated with a fatal "gasping syndrome" in premature infants.

➤*Liver:* Liver (concentrate, fraction or desiccated) is used as a source of vitamin B complex.

➤*B complex vitamins:* B complex vitamins function as coenzymes in nutrient metabolism and maturation of red blood cells.

➤*Ascorbic acid (vitamin C):* Ascorbic acid (vitamin C) may enhance the absorption of iron.

IRON AND LIVER COMBINATIONS, TABLETS

Content given per capsule or tablet.

	Product & Distributor	Fe mg	Liver	B_1 mg	B_2 mg	B_3 mg	B_5 mg	B_6 mg	B_{12} mcg	C mg	Other Content	How Supplied
otc sf	**I-L-X B_{12} High Potency Hematinic Caplets** (Kenwood)	37.5[a]	130 mg (desiccated)	2	2	20			12	120		In 100s.

[a] From *Ferronyl* carbonyl iron.

For complete and comparative prescribing information, refer to the Iron-Containing Products group monograph.

IRON AND LIVER COMBINATIONS, LIQUIDS

Content given per 15 mL.

	Product & Distributor	Fe mg	Liver	B_1 mg	B_2 mg	B_3 mg	B_5 mg	B_6 mg	B_{12} mcg	Other Content	How Supplied
otc	**I-L-X B_{12} Elixir** (Kenwood/Bradley)	102[a]	98 mg liver fraction 1	5	2	10			10	8% alcohol	In 240 mL.
otc	**I-L-X Elixir** (Kenwood/Bradley)	70[b]	98 mg liver concentrate 1:20	5	2	10				8% alcohol	In 240 mL.

[a] From iron ammonium citrate, brown.
[b] From ferrous gluconate.

Refer to the general discussion of these products in the Iron-Containing Products group monograph.

IRON AND LIVER COMBINATIONS, PARENTERAL

	Product & Distributor	Fe mg	Liver[a] mcg	B_1 mg	B_2 mg	B_3 mg	B_5 mg	B_6 mg	B_{12} mcg	Other Content	How Supplied
Rx	**Hytinic** (Hyrex)	3[b]	1		0.75	50	1.25		15	2% procaine HCl, 2% benzyl alcohol	In 30 mL vials.

[a] B_{12} equivalent.
[b] From ferrous gluconate.

IRON AND LIVER COMBINATIONS, — PARENTERAL

Refer to the general discussion of this product in the Iron-Containing Products group monograph.

Administration and Dosage

1 to 2 mL IM 1 to 3 times weekly.

IRON WITH VITAMIN B_{12} AND INTRINSIC FACTOR

Content given per capsule or tablet.

	Product & Distributor	Fe mg	B_{12}[a] mcg	IFC[b]	B_1 mg	B_2 mg	B_3 mg	C mg	FA mg	Other Content	How Supplied
Rx	**Foltrin Capsules** (Vitarine)	110[c]	15	240 mg				75	0.5		(E 5380). Maroon/red. In 100s and 1000s.
Rx	**Livitrinsic-f Capsules** (Goldline)										In 100s and 1000s.
Rx	**Trinsicon Capsules** (UCB Pharmaceuticals)										(364). Pink and red. In 60s, 500s and UD 100s.
Rx	**Chromagen Capsules** (Ther-Rx)	70	10 mcg B_{12}	100 mg desiccated stomach substance				150			(THX 0129). Red. In UD 100s.
Rx	**FeoGen Capsules** (Rising)	66	10 mcg B_{12}	100 mg desiccated stomach substance				250			(115). Maroon. IN UD 100S.

[a] B_{12} activity derived from cobalamin or liver.
[b] Intrinsic factor as concentrate or from stomach preparations.
[c] From ferrous fumarate.

IRON WITH VITAMIN B_{12} AND INTRINSIC FACTOR — ORAL

Indications

➤*Absorption of vitamin B_{12}:* These products contain Intrinsic Factor derived from stomach extract to promote the absorption of vitamin B_{12}.

➤*Anemias:* For treatment of anemias that respond to hematinics, including pernicious anemia and other megaloblastic anemias and also iron deficiency anemia.

MANGANESE

otc *sf*	**Chelated Manganese** (Freeda)	**Tablets:** 20 mg	In 100s, 250s and 500s.
		50 mg	In 100s, 250s and 500s.

MANGANESE — ORAL

For information on parenteral manganese, refer to the monograph in the IV Nutritional Therapy section.

Indications

➤*Manganese deficiency:* As a dietary supplement to prevent or treat manganese deficiency.

Administration and Dosage

The need for manganese in human nutrition has been established, but because a lack of manganese is rare, there is no recommended daily allowance (RDA) for it. For adults and adolescents, 2 to 5 mg/day via the diet is recommended.

➤*Adequate intake amounts:* The adequate intake for manganese is 2.3 mg/day in males 19 years of age and older, 2.2 mg/day in males 14 to 18 years of age, and 1.9 mg/day in males 9 to 13 years of age.

The adequate intake for females 9 to 18 years of age is 1.6 mg/day and 1.8 mg/day in females 19 years of age and older.

The adequate intake for manganese for children 1 to 3 years is 1.2 mg/day and 1.5 mg/day in children 4 to 8 years.

The adequate intake during pregnancy is 2 mg/day and 2.6 mg/day for lactating women.

➤*Storage/Stability:* Store at room temperature away from heat and direct light. Do not freeze or refrigerate. Discard outdated supplements.

Actions

➤*Pharmacology:* Manganese is a cofactor in many enzyme systems; it stimulates synthesis of cholesterol and fatty acids in the liver and influences mucopolysaccharide synthesis. It is concentrated in mitochondria, primarily of the pituitary gland, pancreas, liver, kidney and bone.

Warnings

➤*Pregnancy:* Pregnant women should avoid manganese use in excess of the adequate intake.

➤*Lactation:* Breastfeeding women should avoid manganese use in excess of the adequate intake.

Precautions

➤*Special risk:* Use manganese cautiously in patients with biliary disease and liver disease.

Patient Information

The presence of other medical problems may affect the use of manganese. Make sure to tell your healthcare provider if you have any other medical problems, especially biliary disease or liver disease.

Do not keep outdated dietary supplements or those no longer needed. Be sure that any discarded dietary supplement is out of the reach of children.

Zinc Supplements

For information on parenteral zinc, refer to the monograph in the IV Nutritional Therapy section.

Indications

As a dietary supplement; use to treat or prevent zinc deficiencies.

➤*Unlabeled uses:* For acrodermatitis enteropathica and delayed wound healing associated with zinc deficiency, doses of 220 mg zinc sulfate 3 times daily are used. Zinc sulfate has also been used to treat acne, rheumatoid arthritis and Wilson's disease. However, data conflict and are insufficient to recommend these uses.

In one study, zinc gluconate appeared to significantly shorten the duration of the common cold. Patients (n = 65) dissolved one tablet containing 23 mg zinc (one-half tablet for children) in the mouth every 2 hours until all symptoms were absent for 6 hours; 11% were asymptomatic within 12 hours, 22% within 24 hours. Zinc sulfate should not be used. Further study is needed.

Administration and Dosage

➤*Recommended dietary allowances (RDAs):* Adults, 12 to 15 mg. For a complete listing of RDAs by age, sex and condition, refer to the RDA table.

➤*Dietary supplement:* Average adult dose is 25 to 50 mg zinc daily. Take zinc with food to avoid gastric distress; however, some studies indicate that ingestion with some foods (eg, those that contain bran, phytates, protein, some minerals) may inhibit zinc absorption.

Actions

➤*Pharmacology:* Normal growth and tissue repair depend upon adequate zinc. Zinc acts as an integral part of several enzymes important to protein and carbohydrate metabolism.

Zinc deficiency – Zinc deficiency manifestations include: Anorexia; growth retardation; impaired taste and olfactory sensation; hypogonadism; alopecia; hepatosplenomegaly; dwarfism; rashes; cutaneous lesions; glossitis; stomatitis; blepharitis; paronychia; impaired healing.

➤*Pharmacokinetics:* Zinc salts are poorly absorbed from the GI tract; 20% to 30% of dietary zinc is absorbed. The major stores of zinc are in skeletal muscle and bone; zinc is also found in hair, nails, prostate, spermatazoa and choroid of the eye. The main excretion route is through the intestine. Only minor amounts are lost in urine (≈ 2%).

Contraindications

Pregnancy (see Warnings); lactation.

Warnings

➤*Excessive intake:* Excessive intake in healthy persons may be deleterious. Eleven healthy men who ingested 150 mg zinc twice daily for 6 weeks showed significant impairment of lymphocyte and polymorphonuclear leukocyte functions and a significant decrease in high-density lipoproteins (HDL). No clinical side effects were seen during the study.

➤*Pregnancy:* Although zinc deficiency during pregnancy has been associated with adverse perinatal outcomes, other studies report no such occurrences. Therefore, since zinc deficiency is very rare, the routine use of zinc supplementation during pregnancy is not recommended. However, a dietary zinc intake of 15 mg/day is recommended.

➤*Lactation:* Breast milk concentrations of zinc decrease over time following delivery; extra dietary intake of zinc of 7 mg/day for the first 6 months of lactation and 4 mg/day during the second 6 months are recommended.

Precautions

➤*Do not exceed:* Do not exceed prescribed dosage; will cause emesis if administered in single 2 g doses.

Drug Interactions

Zinc Drug Interactions

Precipitant drug	Object drug [a]		Description
Zinc salts	Fluoroquinolones	⬇	The GI absorption and serum levels of some fluoroquinolones may be decreased, possibly resulting in a decreased anti-infective response.
Zinc salts	Tetracyclines	⬇	The GI absorption and serum levels of tetracyclines may be decreased, possibly resulting in a decreased anti-infective response. Doxycycline does not appear to be affected.

[a] ⬇ = Object drug decreased.

➤*Drug/Food interactions:* Bran products (including brown bread) and some foods (eg, protein, phytates, some minerals) may decrease zinc absorption.

Adverse Reactions

Nausea; vomiting.

Overdosage

➤*Symptoms:* Nausea; severe vomiting; dehydration; restlessness; sideroblastic anemia (secondary to zinc-induced copper deficiency).

➤*Treatment:* Reduce dosage or discontinue to control symptoms.

Patient Information

If GI upset occurs, take with food, but avoid foods high in calcium, phosphorus or phytate.

Zinc Supplements

ZINC SULFATE

otc	**Zinc 15** (Mericon)	**Tablets:** 66 mg (15 mg zinc)	In 100s.
otc	**Orazinc** (Mericon)	**Tablets:** 110 mg (25 mg zinc)	In 100s.
otc	**Zinc Sulfate** (Various, eg, Rugby)	**Tablets:** 200 mg (45 mg zinc)	In 1000s.
Rx	**Zinc Sulfate** (Various)	**Capsules:** 220 mg (50 mg zinc)	In 100s, 1000s and UD 100s.
otc	**Orazinc** (Mericon)		In 100s and 1000s.
otc	**Verazinc** (Forest)		In 100s.
otc	**Zinc-220** (Alto)		(401).Pink and blue. In 100s, 1000s and UD 100s.
Rx	**Zincate** (Paddock)		In 100s and 1000s.

Complete and comparative prescribing information for these products begins in the Zinc Supplements group monograph.

ZINC GLUCONATE (14.3% zinc)

otc	**Zinc Gluconate** (Various)	**Tablets:** 10 mg (1.4 mg zinc)	In 250s.
otc	**Zinc Gluconate** (Various, eg, Freeda)	**Tablets:** 15 mg (2 mg zinc)	In 250s.
otc	**Zinc Gluconate** (Various, eg, Major, Mission)	**Tablets:** 50 mg (7 mg zinc)	In 100s and 250s.

Complete and comparative prescribing information for these products begins in the Zinc Supplements group monograph.

ZINC ACETATE

otc	**Halls Zinc Defense** (Warner Lambert)	**Lozenges:** 5 mg	Sugar. Cherry or peppermint flavor. In 24s.

Complete and comparative prescribing information for these products begins in the Zinc Supplements group monograph.

COMPLEX ZINC CARBONATES

otc	**Zinc** (Sublingual Products)	**Liquid:** 15 mg/mL	Fructose, corn syrup solids, sorbitol, parabens. Fruit flavor. In 30 mL with dropper.

Complete and comparative prescribing information for these products begins in the Zinc Supplements group monograph.

ZINC COMBINATIONS

otc	**Zinc** (Zenith-Goldline)	**Lozenges:** 23 mg (zinc citrate/zinc gluconate)	Fructose. In 30s.

Complete and comparative prescribing information for these products begins in the Zinc Supplements group monograph.

Fluoride

Indications

➤*Prevention of dental caries:* Both neutral and acidulated phosphate fluoride effectively control dental decay. Use where water supplies are low in fluoride (less than 0.7 ppm). Fluoride also controls rampant dental decay which frequently follows xerostomia-producing radiotherapy of head and neck tumors.

In communities without fluoridated water, the American Dental Association's Council on Dental Therapeutics recommends continuing fluoride supplements until the age of 13; the American Academy of Pediatrics recommends supplementation until 16 years of age.

➤*Unlabeled uses:* Sodium fluoride may be effective in treating osteoporosis. Doses (as fluoride) up to 60 mg daily or more are used in conjunction with calcium supplements, vitamin D or estrogen. However, large doses may result in a higher frequency of side effects. Some data suggest that doses less than 50 mg/day are efficacious with fewer adverse reactions. No commercially available products contain high sodium fluoride doses for this use; therefore a large number of tablets would be required to obtain this dosage. Fluoride supplementation is not recommended for the prophylaxis of osteoporosis due to the potential for increased incidence of fractures (see Precautions).

Administration and Dosage

Use according to directions accompanying the product.

Fluoride Dosage

Route/Age	Daily dose
Oral:	
Fluoride ion level in drinking water[a] (less than 0.3 ppm):	
Birth to 6 months	None
6 months to 3 years	0.25 mg/day[b]
3 to 6 years	0.5 mg/day
6 to 16 years	1 mg/day
Fluoride content of drinking water (0.3 - 0.6 ppm):	
Birth to 6 months	None
6 months to 3 years	None
3 to 6 years	0.25 mg/day
6 to 16 years	0.5 mg/day
Fluoride content of drinking water (greater than 0.6 ppm):	
Birth to 6 months	None
6 months to 3 years	None
3 to 6 years	None
6 to 16 years	None

Fluoride Dosage

Route/Age	Daily dose
Topical (rinse):	
Children (6 to 12 years)	5 to 10 mL[c]
Adults and children (older than 12 years of age)	10 mL[c]

[a] 1 ppm = 1 mg/L.
[b] 2.2 mg sodium fluoride contains 1 mg fluoride ion.
[c] Use once daily (*Point-Two*, once weekly) after thoroughly brushing teeth and rinsing mouth. Rinse around and between teeth for 1 minute, then spit out.

Actions

➤*Pharmacology:* Sodium fluoride acts systemically before tooth eruption, and topically posteruption, by increasing tooth resistance to acid dissolution, by promoting remineralization and by inhibiting the cariogenic microbial process. Acidulation provides greater topical fluoride uptake by dental enamel than neutral solutions. Phosphate protects enamel from demineralization by the acidulated formulation. Topical application of fluoride works superficially on enamel and plaque, and can reduce dental caries by 30% to 40%. Fluoride supplements may reduce the incidence of caries by up to 60%.

➤*Pharmacokinetics:* Fluoride is absorbed in the GI tract, lungs and skin. About 90% of oral fluoride is absorbed in the stomach. Absorption is related to solubility; sodium fluoride is almost completely absorbed. Calcium, iron or magnesium ions may delay absorption. Following ingestion, 50% of fluoride is deposited in bone and teeth. The major route of excretion is the kidneys; it is also excreted by sweat glands, the GI tract and in breast milk.

Contraindications

When the fluoride content of drinking water exceeds 0.7 ppm; low sodium or sodium free diets; hypersensitivity to fluoride. Do not use 1 mg tablets in children younger than 3 years old or when the drinking water fluoride content is ≥ 0.3 ppm. Do not use 1 mg/5 mL rinse (as a supplement) in children younger than 6 years old.

Warnings

➤*Pregnancy:* Consult physician before using.

➤*Lactation:* Consult physician before using.

➤*Children:* See Contraindications.

Precautions

➤*Fractures:* Some epidemiological studies suggest that the incidence of certain types of bone fractures (crippling skeletal fluorosis) may be higher in some communities with naturally high or adjusted fluoride levels. However, other studies have not detected increased incidence of bone fractures. Crippling skeletal fluorosis is more common in parts of the world with high natural fluoride (greater than 10 ppm), but is extremely rare in the US.

➤*Mucositis:* Gingival tissues may be hypersensitive to some flavors or alcohol.

➤*Tartrazine sensitivity:* Some of these products contain tartrazine, which may cause allergic-type reactions (including bronchial asthma) in susceptible individuals. Although the incidence of tartrazine sensitivity in the general population is low, it is frequently seen in patients who also have aspirin hypersensitivity. Specific products containing tartrazine are identified in the product listings.

Drug Interactions

➤*Drug/Food interactions:* Incompatibility of dairy foods with systemic fluoride has occurred due to formation of calcium fluoride, which is poorly absorbed.

Adverse Reactions

➤*Dermatologic:* Eczema; atopic dermatitis; urticaria; allergic rash and other idiosyncrasies (rare).

➤*Miscellaneous:* Gastric distress; headache; weakness. Rinses and gels containing stannous fluoride may produce surface staining of the teeth; this does not occur with nonstannous fluoride topical preparations. Acidulated fluoride may dull porcelain and composite restorations.

Overdosage

➤*Chronic overdosage:* Chronic overdosage of fluorides may result in dental fluorosis (a mottling of tooth enamel) and osseous changes.

➤*Acute overdosage:*

Symptoms – In children, acute ingestion of 10 to 20 mg sodium fluoride may cause excessive salivation and GI disturbances; 500 mg may be fatal. The oral lethal dose is 70 to 140 mg/kg (5 to 10 g in adults).

GI – Salivation, nausea, abdominal pain, vomiting and diarrhea are frequent due to conversion of sodium fluoride to corrosive hydrofluoric acid in the stomach.

CNS – Because of the calcium-binding effect of fluoride, CNS irritability, paresthesias, tetany, convulsions and respiratory and cardiac failure may occur. Fluoride has a direct toxic action on muscle and nerve tissue, and it interferes with many enzyme systems. Hypocalcemia, hypoglycemia and delayed hyperkalemia are frequent laboratory findings.

➤*Treatment:* Usual supportive measures. Refer to General Management of Acute Overdosage. Precipitate the fluoride by using gastric lavage with 0.15% calcium hydroxide. Administer IV glucose in saline for a forced diuresis; IV calcium may be indicated for tetany. Administer calcium IM (10 mL of 10% calcium gluconate, 5 mL in children) every 4 to 6 hours until recovery is complete. Maintain electrolytes, normal blood pH and adequate urine output. Removing fluoride with dialysis and hemoperfusion may also be beneficial.

Patient Information

➤*Tablets and drops:* Milk and other dairy products may decrease absorption of sodium fluoride; avoid simultaneous ingestion.

➤*Tablets:* Dissolve in the mouth, chew, swallow whole, add to drinking water or fruit juice or add to water for use in infant formulas or other food.

➤*Drops:* Take orally, undiluted, or mix with fluids or food.

➤*Rinses and gels:* Rinses and gels are most effective immediately after brushing or flossing and just prior to sleep. Expectorate any excess. Do not swallow. Do not eat, drink or rinse mouth for 30 minutes after application. Notify dentist if tooth enamel becomes discolored.

FLUORIDE, ORAL

Rx	**EtheDent** (Ethex)	**Tablets, chewable:** 0.25 mg	In 120s.
Rx *sf*	**Luride Lozi-Tabs** (Colgate-Hoyt)		(COP 186). Vanilla flavor. In 120s.
Rx	**Sodium Fluoride**[a] (Various, eg, Rugby)	**Tablets, chewable:** 0.5 mg (from 1.1 mg sodium fluoride)	In 1000s.
Rx	**EtheDent** (Ethex)		In 120s and 1000s.
Rx	**Fluoritab** (Fluoritab)		Dye free. Pineapple flavor. In 1000s and 5000s.
Rx *sf*	**Luride Lozi-Tabs** (Colgate-Hoyt)		(COP 014). Grape and assorted fruit flavors. In 120s. Grape also in 1200s.
Rx *sf*	**Pharmaflur 1.1** (Pharmics)		Grape flavor. In 120s.
Rx	**Sodium Fluoride**[a] (Various, eg, Major, Rugby)	**Tablets, chewable:** 1 mg (from 2.2 mg sodium fluoride)	In 100s, 1000s and UD 1000s.
Rx	**EtheDent** (Ethex)		In 120s and 1000s.
Rx	**Karidium** (Lorvic)		White. In 180s and 1000s.
Rx *sf*	**Luride Lozi-Tabs** (Colgate-Hoyt)		(COP 006). Cherry and assorted fruit flavors. In 120s and 1000s. Cherry also in 5000s.
Rx *sf*	**Luride-SF Lozi-Tabs** (Colgate-Hoyt)		In 120s.
Rx *sf*	**Pharmaflur** (Pharmics)		Cherry flavor. In 1000s.
Rx *sf*	**Pharmaflur df** (Pharmics)		Dye free. Cherry flavor. In 120s.
Rx	**Fluoride** (Kirkman)	**Tablets:** 1 mg (from 2.2 mg sodium fluoride)	In 1000s.
Rx *sf*	**Flura** (Kirkman)		In 100s and 1000s.
Rx	**Sodium Fluoride** (Rugby)	**Drops:** 0.125 mg per drop (from ≈ 0.275 mg sodium fluoride)	In 30 mL.
Rx *sf*	**Fluoritab** (Fluoritab)	**Drops:** 0.25 mg per drop (from 0.55 mg sodium fluoride)	In 22.8 mL.
Rx *sf*	**Sodium Fluoride** (Hi-Tech)	**Drops:** 0.5 mg per mL (from 1.1 mg sodium fluoride)	In 50 mL.
Rx *sf*	**Pediaflor** (Ross)		Less than 0.5% alcohol, sorbitol. Cherry flavor. In 50 mL w/dropper.
Rx *sf*	**Luride** (Colgate)		Peach flavor. In 50 mL.
Rx *sf*	**Fluoride Loz** (Kirkman)	**Lozenges:** 1 mg (from 2.2 mg sodium fluoride)	In 1000s.
Rx	**Flura-Loz** (Kirkman)		Raspberry flavor. In 100s and 1000s.
Rx *sf*	**Phos-Flur** (Colgate-Hoyt)	**Solution:**[b] 0.2 mg per mL (from 0.44 mg sodium fluoride)	Cherry flavor. In 250, 500 mL & gal. Cinnamon (w/saccharin), grape, wintergreen flavors. In 500 mL.

[a] May be regular or chewable.

[b] May be used as a rinse or supplement.

Complete and comparative prescribing information begins in the Fluoride group monograph.

FLUORIDE, TOPICAL

otc	**ACT** (Johnson & Johnson)	**Rinse:** 0.02% (from 0.05% sodium fluoride)	7% alcohol. In 90, 360 and 480 mL.
otc	**Fluorigard** (Colgate-Palmolive)	**Rinse:** 0.02% (from 0.05% sodium fluoride)	6% alcohol. Tartrazine. In 180, 300 & 480 mL.
otc	**Gel-Kam** (Colgate-Palmolive)	**Rinse:** 0.04% sodium fluoride	Mint, fruit and berry, bubblegum, and cinnamon flavors. In 4.3 and 7 oz.
otc sf	**MouthKote F/R** (Parnell)	**Rinse:** 0.04% sodium fluoride	Benzyl alcohol, sorbitol, menthol, EDTA. In 237 mL.
Rx	**Fluorinse** (Oral-B)	**Rinse:** 0.09% (from 0.2% sodium fluoride)	Alcohol free. Mint and cinnamon flavors. In 480 mL.
Rx	**Point-Two** (Colgate-Hoyt)	**Rinse:** 0.09% (from 0.2% sodium fluoride)	6% alcohol. Mint flavor. In 240 mL and gal.
Rx	**PreviDent Rinse** (Colgate Oral)	**Rinse:** 0.2% neutral sodium fluoride	6% alcohol. Mint flavor. In 250 mL and gal (with pump dispenser).
Rx	**Stannous Fluoride** (Cypress)	**Rinse concentrate:** 0.63% stannous fluoride	Mint flavor. In 122 g.
Rx	**Gel-Kam** (Colgate Oral)	**Rinse concentrate:** 0.63% stannous fluoride	Glycerin. Cinnamon and mint flavors. In 283 g.
otc	**Gel-Kam** (Colgate Oral)	**Gel:** 0.1% (from 0.4% stannous fluoride)	Bubble gum, cinnamon, fruit and berry, and mint flavor. In 122 g and 105 g Dental Therapy-Pak.
otc	**Gel-Tin** (Young Dental)	**Gel:** 0.1% (from 0.4% stannous fluoride)	Lime, grape, cinnamon, raspberry, mint and orange flavors. In 60 g.
otc	**Stop** (Oral-B)	**Gel:** 0.1% (from 0.4% stannous fluoride)	Grape, cinnamon, bubblegum, piña colada and mint flavors. In 120 g.
otc	**Stannous Fluoride** (Cypress)	**Gel:** 0.4% stannous fluoride	Parabens. Mint flavor. In 122 g.
Rx	**Karigel** (Lorvic)	**Gel:** 0.5% (from 1.1% sodium fluoride)	pH 5.6. Orange flavor. In 30, 130 and 250 g.
Rx	**Karigel-N** (Lorvic)	**Gel:** 0.5% (from 1.1% sodium fluoride)	Neutral pH. In 24 and 120 g.
Rx	**Prevident** (Colgate-Hoyt)	**Gel:** 0.5% (from 1.1% sodium fluoride)	Mint, berry, cherry and fruit sherbet flavors. In 24 and 60 g. Lime flavor in 60 g.
Rx	**Thera-Flur** (Colgate-Hoyt)	**Gel-Drops:** 0.5% (from 1.1% sodium fluoride)	pH 4.5. Lime flavor. In 24 mL.
Rx	**Thera-Flur-N** (Colgate-Hoyt)	**Gel-Drops:** 0.5% (from 1.1% sodium fluoride)	Neutral pH. In 24 mL.
Rx	**DentaGel 1.1%** (Rising Pharmaceuticals)	**Gel:** 1.1% sodium fluoride	Saccharin, parabens, sorbitol. Fresh mint flavor. In 56 g.
Rx	**NeutraGard Advanced** (Pascal)	**Gel:** 1.1% sodium fluoride	Wintermint flavor. In 60 g.
Rx	**Luride** (Colgate Oral)	**Gel:** 1.2% (from sodium fluoride and hydrogen fluoride)	Mint flavor. In 7 g.
Rx	**Prevident Plus** (Colgate-Hoyt)	**Gel:** 1.2% (from sodium fluoride and hydrogen fluoride)	Mint, berry, cherry and fruit sherbet flavors. In 24 and 60 g. Lime flavor in 60 g.
Rx	**Denta 5000 Plus** (Rising Pharmaceuticals)	**Cream:** 1.1%	Spearmint flavor. In 51 g (2s).
Rx	**EtheDent** (Ethex)	**Cream:** 1.1%	Sorbitol, saccharin. In 51 g.
Rx	**PreviDent 5000 Plus** (Colgate)	**Cream:** 1.1%	Sorbitol, saccharin. In spearmint and fruit flavors. In 51 g (1s and 2s).

Complete and comparative prescribing information for these products begins in the Fluoride group monograph.

SODIUM CHLORIDE

otc	**Sustain** (Zee Medical)	**Tablets:** 220 mg sodium chloride, 18 mg calcium carbonate, 15 mg potassium chloride	In 24s.
otc	**Sodium Chloride** (Purepac)	**Tablets:** 650 mg	In 100s.
otc	**Sodium Chloride** (Various)	**Tablets:** 1 g	In 100s and 1000s.
otc	**Sodium Chloride** (Lilly)	**Tablets:** 2.25 g	In 100s and 500s.
otc	**Slo-Salt** (Mission)	**Tablets, slow release:** 600 mg	In 100s.
otc	**Slo-Salt-K** (Mission)	**Tablets, slow release:** 410 mg sodium chloride and 150 mg potassium chloride in wax matrix	In 1000s.

SODIUM CHLORIDE — ORAL

Indications

➤*Volume depletion:* Prevention or treatment of extracellular volume depletion, dehydration or sodium depletion.

➤*Heat prostration:* Aid in the prevention of heat prostration.

Administration and Dosage

Refer to specific product labeling for dosage guidelines.

Warnings

➤*Acclimatization:* Inappropriate salt administration in an effort to acclimatize to a hot environment can be dangerous. Balanced electrolytes and adequate hydration are essential.

➤*Salt tablets:* Salt tablets may pass through the GI tract undigested. Avoid their use in treating heat cramps since they may cause vomiting, pooling of oral fluids and potassium depletion. Use oral salt solutions instead.

➤*Pregnancy:* Seek professional advice before using these products while pregnant.

➤*Lactation:* Seek professional advice before using these products while breastfeeding.

Precautions

➤*Supplementation:* Individuals with adequate dietary sodium intake and normal renal function should not require sodium chloride supplementation. Balanced electrolyte supplements may be preferred to prevent hypokalemia.

➤*Special risk:* Caution should be used in the presence of CHF, kidney dysfunction, peripheral or pulmonary edema or preeclampsia.

Overdosage

➤*Symptoms:* Overdosage may cause serious electrolyte disturbances. Ingestion of large amounts of sodium chloride irritates the GI mucosa and may result in nausea, vomiting, diarrhea and abdominal cramps. Edema is a sign of excess total body sodium.

Manifestations of hypernatremia may include:

Neurologic – Irritability; restlessness; weakness; obtundation progressing to convulsions and coma.

Cardiovascular – Hypertension, tachycardia, fluid accumulation.

Respiratory – Pulmonary edema; respiratory arrest.

➤*Treatment:* Treatment includes usual supportive measures. Refer to General Management of Acute Overdosage. Use appropriate measures to empty the stomach. Magnesium sulfate may be given as a cathartic. Provide an adequate airway and ventilation. Maintain vascular volume and tissue perfusion.

POTASSIUM

Rx	**Potassium Chloride** (Various, eg, Abbott, Goldline, Rugby, Warner Chilcott)	**Tablets, controlled release:** 8 mEq (600 mg) potassium chloride in a wax matrix	In 100s and 1,000s.
Rx	**Klor-Con 8** (Upsher-Smith)		(KLOR–CON 8). Blue. Film coated. In 100s, 500s and UD 100s.
Rx	**K⁺8** (Alra)	**Tablets, extended release:** 8 mEq potassium chloride	In 100s and 500s.
Rx	**K + 10** (Alra)	**Tablets, controlled release:** 10 mEq (750 mg) potassium chloride in a wax matrix	Film coated. In 100s, 500s, 1000s and UD 100s.
Rx	**Kaon Cl-10** (Savage)		Sucrose. (10). Green. Sugar coated. Capsule shape. In 1000s and Stat-Pak 100s.
Rx	**Klor-Con 10** (Upsher-Smith)		(KLOR–CON 10).Yellow. Film coated. In 100s, 500s and UD 100s.
Rx	**Klotrix** (Bristol)		(KLOTRIX BL 10 meq 770). Orange. Film coated. In 100s, 1000s and UD 100s.
Rx	**K-Tab** (Abbott)		(NM A 101)Yellow. Film coated. Oval. In 100s, 1000s, 5000s and Abbo-Pac 100s.
Rx	**Klor-Con M10** (Upsher-Smith)	**Tablets, extended-release:** 10 mEq potassium (from 750 mg potassium chloride	(KC M10). Oblong. In 90s, 100s, 1000s, and UD 100s.
Rx	**Klor-Con M15** (Upsher-Smith)	**Tablets, extended-release:** 15 mEq potassium (from 1125 mg potassium chloride	(M 15). Oblong, scored. In 100s, 1000s, and UD 100s.
Rx	**Klor-Con M20** (Upsher-Smith)	**Tablets, extended-release:** 20 mEq potassium (from 1500 mg potassium chloride	(KC M20). Oblong, scored. In 90s, 100s, 500s, 1000s, and UD 100s.
Rx	**Potassium Chloride** (Various, eg, Major, Rugby)	**Tablets, extended release:** 750 mg potassium chloride equivalent to 10 mEq potassium in a wax matrix	In 100s and 1000s.
Rx	**K-Dur 10** (Key)	**Tablets, controlled release:** 750 mg microencapsulated potassium chloride equivalent to 10 mEq potassium	(K-Dur 10). White. Oblong. In 100s and UD 100s.
Rx	**Potassium Chloride** (Ethex)	**Tablets, controlled release:** 1,500 mg microencapsulated potassium chloride equivalent to 20 mEq potassium	(ETH 2 0). White to off-white, capsule shape. In 100s, 500s, 1,000s, and UD 100s.
Rx	**K-Dur 20** (Key)		(20). White, scored. Oblong. In 100s, 500s, 1,000s and UD 100s.
otc	**Potassium** (Cardinal Health)	**Tablets:** 99 mg potassium (as potassium gluconate)	Film coated. In 100s.
otc	**Potassium Gluconate** (Various)	**Tablets:** 500 mg potassium gluconate (83.45 mg potassium)	In 100s and 1000s.
otc	**Potassium Gluconate** (Mission)	**Tablets:** 595 mg potassium gluconate (99 mg potassium)	In 100s.
Rx	**K + Care ET** (Alra)	**Tablets, effervescent:** 20 mEq potassium (from potassium bicarbonate)	Saccharin. In 30s and 100s.
Rx sf	**Klorvess** (Sandoz)	**Tablets, effervescent:** 20 mEq potassium (from potassium chloride and bicarbonate and lysine hydrochloride)	Sodium free. Saccharin. White. In 60s and 1000s.
Rx	**K•Lyte/Cl** (Bristol)	**Tablets, effervescent:** 25 mEq potassium (from potassium Cl and bicarbonate, l-lysine monohydrochloride and citric acid)	Saccharin, docusate sodium. Fruit punch or citrus flavors. In 30s, 100s and 250s.
Rx	**K•Lyte/Cl 50** (Bristol)	**Tablets, effervescent:** 50 mEq potassium (from potassium Cl and bicarbonate, l-lysine monohydrochloride and citric acid)	Saccharin, docusate sodium. Fruit punch or citrus flavors. In 30s & 100s.

POTASSIUM

Rx	**K + Care ET** (Alra)	**Tablets, effervescent**: 25 mEq potassium (from potassium bicarbonate)	Saccharin. Orange or lime flavors. In 30s and 100s.
Rx	**Effer-K** (Nomax)	**Tablets, effervescent**: 25 mEq potassium (as bicarbonate and citrate)	Saccharin. Orange or lime flavors. In 30s, 100s & 250s.
Rx	**Effervescent Potassium** (Rugby)		Saccharin. Lime, orange or fruit punch flavors. In 30s.
Rx sf	**Klor-Con/EF** (Upsher-Smith)		Saccharin. Orange flavor. In 30s and 100s.
Rx	**K•Lyte** (Bristol)		Saccharin, docusate sodium, dextrose. Orange or lime flavor. In 30s, 100s and 250s.
Rx	**Effervescent Potassium/ Chloride** (Qualitest)	**Tablets, effervescent**: 25 mEq potassium and chloride (from 1.5 g potassium chloride, 0.5 g potassium bicarbonate, 0.91 g l-lysine monohydrochloride, 0.55 g citric acid)	Saccharin. Fruit-punch flavor. In 30s, 100s, and 250s.
Rx	**K•Lyte DS** (Bristol)	**Tablets, effervescent**: 50 mEq potassium (from potassium bicarbonate and citrate and citric acid)	Saccharin, docusate sodium, lactose. Orange or lime flavor. In 30s and 100s.
Rx	**Micro-K Extencaps** (Robins)	**Capsules, controlled release**: 600 mg potassium chloride equivalent to 8 mEq potassium. Microencapsulated particles	(Micro-K THER-RX 010). Orange. In 100s, 500s and UD 100s.
Rx	**Potassium Chloride** (Various, eg, EtheX, Goldline, Moore, Parmed, Rugby, Warner-Chilcott)	**Capsules, controlled release**: 10 mEq (750 mg) potassium chloride. Microencapsulated particles	In 100s and 500s.
Rx	**Micro-K 10 Extencaps** (Thera-Rx)		(Micro-K 10 AHR/ 5730). Orange/white. In 100s, 500s and UD 100s.
Rx	**Potassium Chloride** (Various, eg, Barre-National, Geneva, Major, Parmed, PBI, Rugby, Schein)	**Liquid**: 20 mEq/15 mL potassium and chloride (10% KCl)	In pt and gal.
Rx sf	**Cena-K** (Century)		In pt and gal.
Rx sf	**Potasalan** (Lannett)		4% alcohol. Orange flavor. In pt and gal.
Rx	**Rum-K** (Fleming)	**Liquid**: 30 mEq/15 mL potassium and chloride (15% KCl)	Butter-rum flavor. In pt and gal.
Rx	**Potassium Chloride** (Various, eg, Barre-National, Major, PBI, Rugby)	**Liquid**: 40 mEq/15 mL potassium and chloride (20% KCl)	In pt and gal.
Rx sf	**Kaon-Cl 20%** (Adria)		5% alcohol, saccharin. Cherry flavor. In 480 mL.
Rx	**Potassium Gluconate** (Various, eg, PBI)	**Liquid**: 20 mEq/15 mL potassium (as potassium gluconate)	In 118 mL, pt, gal and UD 5 and 15 mL (100s).
Rx sf	**Kaon** (Adria)		5% alcohol. Saccharin. Grape flavor. In 480 mL.
Rx	**Kaylixir** (Lannett)		5% alcohol. Saccharin. In pt and gal.
Rx	**Twin-K** (Boots)	**Liquid**: 20 mEq/15 mL potassium (as potassium gluconate & potassium citrate)	Sorbitol, saccharin. In 480 mL.
Rx sf	**Kolyum** (Fisons)	**Liquid**: 20 mEq potassium and 3.4 mEq chloride/15 mL (from potassium gluconate and potassium chloride)	Sorbitol, saccharin. Cherry flavor. In pt and gal.
Rx	**K + Care** (Alra)	**Powder**: 15 mEq potassium chloride per packet	Saccharin. Fruit or orange flavors. In 30s and 100s.
Rx	**Potassium Chloride** (Various, eg, Schein)	**Powder**: 20 mEq potassium chloride per packet	In 30s and 100s.
Rx sf	**Gen-K** (Goldline)		Orange/fruit flavor. In 30s.
Rx sf	**Kay Ciel** (Forest)		Saccharin. In 30s and 100s.
Rx	**K + Care** (Alta)		Saccharin. Fruit or orange flavor. In 30s and 100s.
Rx	**K-Lor** (Abbott)		Saccharin. Fruit flavor. In 30s and 100s.
Rx sf	**Klor-Con** (Upsher-Smith)		Saccharin. Fruit flavor. In 30s and 100s.
Rx	**Micro-K LS** (Robins)		Extended-release. Sucrose. In 30s and 100s.
Rx	**K + Care** (Alra)	**Powder**: 25 mEq potassium chloride per packet	Saccharin. Orange flavor. In 30s and 100s.
Rx sf	**Klor-Con/25** (Upsher-Smith)		Saccharin. Fruit flavor. In 30s, 100s and 250s.
Rx	**K•Lyte/Cl** (Mead Johnson Nutritionals)	**Powder**: 25 mEq potassium chloride per dose	Fruit punch flavor. In 225 g (30 doses).
Rx	**K-vescent Potassium Chloride** (Major)	**Powder**: 20 mEq potassium and chloride from 1.5 g potassium chloride	Saccharin. In 30 and 100 packets.

POTASSIUM — ORAL

For information on parenteral potassium, refer to the IV Nutritional Therapy section.

Indications

➤*Hypokalemia:*

Treatment – Treatment of hypokalemia in the following conditions: With or without metabolic alkalosis; digitalis intoxication; familial periodic paralysis; diabetic acidosis; diarrhea and vomiting; surgical conditions accompanied by nitrogen loss, vomiting, suction drainage, diarrhea and increased urinary excretion of potassium; certain cases of uremia; hyperadrenalism; starvation and debilitation; corticosteroid or diuretic therapy.

Prevention – Prevention of potassium depletion when dietary intake is inadequate in the following conditions: Patients receiving digitalis and diuretics for congestive heart failure; significant cardiac arrhythmias; hepa-

POTASSIUM — ORAL

tic cirrhosis with ascites; states of aldosterone excess with normal renal function; potassium-losing nephropathy; certain diarrheal states.

When hypokalemia is associated with alkalosis, use potassium chloride. When acidosis is present, use the bicarbonate, citrate, acetate or gluconate potassium salts.

➤*Unlabeled uses:* In patients with mild hypertension, the use of potassium supplements (24 to 60 mmol/day) appears to result in a long-term reduction of blood pressure.

Administration and Dosage

The usual dietary intake of potassium ranges between 40 to 150 mEq/day.

Individualize dosage.

➤*Prevention:* Usual range is 16 to 24 mEq/day for the prevention of hypokalemia.

➤*Treatment:* Usual range is 40 to 100 mEq/day or more for the treatment of potassium depletion.

Potassium intoxication may result from any therapeutic dosage.

Actions

➤*Pharmacology:* Potassium, the principal intracellular cation of most body tissues, participates in a number of essential physiological processes, such as maintenance of intracellular tonicity and a proper relationship with sodium across cell membranes, cellular metabolism, transmission of nerve impulses, contraction of cardiac, skeletal and smooth muscle, acid-base balance and maintenance of normal renal function. Normal potassium serum levels range from 3.5 to 5 mEq/L. The active ion transport system maintains this gradient across the plasma membrane.

mEq/g of Various Potassium Salts

Potassium salt	mEq/g
Potassium gluconate	4.3
Potassium citrate	9.8
Potassium bicarbonate	10
Potassium acetate	10.2
Potassium chloride	13.4

Potassium homeostasis – The potassium concentration in extracellular fluid is normally 4 to 5 mEq/L; the concentration in intracellular fluid is approximately 150 to 160 mEq/L. Plasma concentration provides a useful clinical guide to disturbances in potassium balance. By producing large differences in the ratio of intracellular to extracellular potassium, relatively small absolute changes in extracellular concentration may have important effects on neuromuscular activity.

Despite wide variations in dietary intake of potassium (eg, 40 to 120 mEq/day), plasma potassium concentration is normally stabilized within the narrow range of 4 to 5 mEq/L by virtue of close renal regulation of potassium balance. Renal potassium excretion is accomplished largely by potassium secretion in the distal portion of the nephron; essentially all filtered potassium is reabsorbed in the proximal tubule. The potassium that appears in the urine is added to the filtrate by a distal process of sodium-cation exchange. Fecal excretion of potassium is normally only a few mEq per day and does not play a significant role in potassium homeostasis.

Natural potassium sources – Foods rich in potassium include: Beef; veal; ham; chicken; turkey; fish; milk; bananas; dates; prunes; raisins; avocado; watermelon; cantaloupes; apricots; molasses; beans; yams; broccoli; brussels sprouts; lentils; potatoes; spinach.

Hypokalemia – Gradual potassium depletion may occur whenever the rate of potassium loss through renal excretion or GI loss exceeds the rate of potassium intake. Potassium depletion is usually a consequence of prolonged therapy with oral diuretics, primary or secondary hyperaldosteronism, diabetic ketoacidosis, severe diarrhea (especially if associated with vomiting) or inadequate replacement during prolonged parenteral nutrition. Potassium depletion due to these causes is usually accompanied by a concomitant deficiency of chloride and is manifested by hypokalemia and metabolic alkalosis.

The use of potassium salts in patients receiving diuretics for uncomplicated essential hypertension is often unnecessary when such patients have a normal diet. However, if hypokalemia occurs, dietary supplementation with potassium-containing foods may be adequate. In more severe cases, potassium salt supplementation may be indicated.

Potassium depletion sufficient to cause 1 mEq/L drop in serum potassium requires a loss of about 100 to 200 mEq potassium from the total body store.
Symptoms: Weakness; fatigue; ileus; tetany; polydipsia; flaccid paralysis or impaired ability to concentrate urine (in advanced cases). ECG may reveal atrial and ventricular ectopy, prolongation of QT interval, ST segment depression, conduction defects, broad or flat T waves or appearance of U waves.

Contraindications

Severe renal impairment with oliguria or azotemia; untreated Addison's disease; hyperkalemia from any cause (eg, systemic acidosis, acute dehydration, extensive tissue breakdown); adynamia episodica hereditaria; acute dehydration; heat cramps; patients receiving potassium-sparing diuretics (spironolactone, triamterene or amiloride) or aldosterone-inhibiting agents. Solid dosage forms of potassium supplements are contraindicated in any patient in whom there is cause for arrest or delay in tablet passage through the GI tract. Wax matrix potassium chloride preparations have produced esophageal ulceration in cardiac patients with esophageal compression due to an enlarged left atrium; give potassium supplementation as a liquid preparation to these patients.

Warnings

➤*Hyperkalemia:* In patients with impaired potassium excretion, potassium salts can produce hyperkalemia or cardiac arrest. This occurs most commonly in patients given IV potassium, but may also occur in patients given oral potassium. Potentially fatal hyperkalemia can develop rapidly and may be asymptomatic.

Hyperkalemia may be manifested only by an increased serum potassium concentration and characteristic ECG changes (eg, peaking of T waves, loss of P wave, depression of ST segment, prolongation of the QT interval, lengthened P-R interval, widened QRS complex). However, the following may also occur: Parasthesias; heaviness; muscle weakness and flaccid paralysis of the extremities; listlessness; mental confusion; decreased blood pressure; shock; cardiac arrhythmias; heart block.

In response to a rise in the concentration of body potassium, renal excretion of the ion is increased. With normal kidney function, it is difficult to produce potassium intoxication by oral administration. However, administer potassium supplements with caution, since the amount of deficiency and corresponding daily dose is unknown. Frequently monitor the clinical status, periodic ECG and serum potassium levels. This is particularly important in patients receiving digitalis and in patients with cardiac disease. There is a hazard in prescribing potassium in digitalis intoxication manifested by atrioventricular (AV) conduction disturbance.

➤*GI lesions:* Potassium chloride tablets have produced stenotic or ulcerative lesions of the small bowel and death. These lesions are caused by a concentration of potassium ion in the region of a rapidly dissolving tablet, which injures the bowel wall and produces obstruction, hemorrhage or perforation. The reported frequency of small bowel lesions is much less with wax matrix tablets (less than 1 per 100,000 patient-years) and microencapsulated tablets than with enteric coated tablets (40 to 50 per 100,000 patient-years). Upper GI bleeding, esophageal ulceration and stricture, gastric ulceration and lower GI ulceration have occurred with wax matrix preparations. The total number of GI lesions is less than 1 per 47,000 patient-years. Discontinue either type of tablet immediately and consider the possibility of bowel obstruction or perforation if severe vomiting, abdominal pain or distention or GI bleeding occurs.

Patients at greatest risk for developing potassium chloride-induced GI lesions include: The elderly, the immobile and those with scleroderma, diabetes mellitus, mitral valve replacement, cardiomegaly or esophageal stricture/compression.

Reserve slow release potassium chloride preparations for patients who cannot tolerate liquids or effervescent potassium preparations, or for patients in whom there is a problem of compliance with these preparations.

Some studies suggest the "microencapsulated" preparations are less likely to cause GI damage; however, evidence conflicts and a specific recommendation of one solid oral product over another (wax matrix or microencapsulated) cannot be made. Avoid enteric coated products.

➤*Metabolic acidosis and hyperchloremia:* In some patients (eg, those with renal tubular acidosis), potassium depletion is rarely associated with metabolic acidosis and hyperchloremia. Replace with potassium bicarbonate, citrate, acetate or gluconate.

➤*Renal function impairment:* Renal function impairment requires careful monitoring of the serum potassium concentration and appropriate dosage adjustment.

➤*Pregnancy:* *Category C.* It is not known whether potassium salts can cause fetal harm when administered to a pregnant woman or can affect reproduction capacity. Give to a pregnant woman only if clearly needed.

➤*Lactation:* It is not known whether this drug is excreted in breast milk. Exercise caution when administering to a nursing woman. The normal potassium content of breast milk is ≈ 13 mEq/L. As long as body potassium is not excessive, the contribution of potassium salts should have little or no effect on the level of breast milk.

➤*Children:* Safety and efficacy for use in children have not been established.

Precautions

➤*Monitoring:* When blood is drawn for analysis of plasma potassium, it is important to recognize that artificial elevations can occur after improper venipuncture technique or as a result of in vitro hemolysis of the sample.

➤*Hypokalemia:* Hypokalemia is ordinarily diagnosed by demonstrating potassium depletion in a patient and by a careful clinical history. In interpreting the serum potassium level, consider that acute alkalosis can produce hypokalemia in the absence of a deficit in total body potassium, while acute acidosis can increase the serum potassium concentration to the normal range, even in the presence of a reduced total body potassium. Treatment, particularly in the presence of cardiac disease, renal disease or acidosis, requires careful attention to acid-base balance and monitoring of serum electrolytes, ECG and clinical status of the patient.

The administration of concentrated dextrose or sodium bicarbonate may cause an intracellular potassium shift. This may cause hypokalemia which, in turn, may lead to serious cardiac arrhythmias.

Giving potassium to hypokalemic hypertensives may lower blood pressure.

POTASSIUM — ORAL

Drug Interactions

Potassium Preparation Drug Interactions			
Precipitant drug	Object drug[a]		Description
ACE inhibitors	Potassium preparations	↑	Concurrent use may result in elevated serum potassium concentrations in certain patients.
Potassium-sparing diuretics	Potassium preparations	↑	Potassium-sparing diuretics will increase potassium retention and can produce severe hyperkalemia.
Potassium preparations	Digitalis	↑	In patients receiving digoxin, hypokalemia may result in digoxin toxicity. Therefore, use caution if discontinuing a potassium preparation in patients maintained on digoxin.

[a] ↑ = Object drug increased

In addition, potassium citrate, a urinary alkalinizer, may affect the renal excretion and pharmacologic effects of various agents (refer to the Citrate and Citric Acid Solutions monograph).

Adverse Reactions

Most common – Nausea, vomiting, diarrhea, flatulence and abdominal discomfort due to GI irritation are best managed by diluting the preparation further, by taking with meals or by dose reduction.

Rare – Skin rash.

Most severe – Hyperkalemia; GI obstruction, bleeding, ulceration or perforation.

Overdosage

For symptoms and treatment of potassium overdosage and hyperkalemia, refer to the monograph in the IV Nutritional Therapy section.

Patient Information

May cause GI upset; take after meals or with food and with a full glass of water.

Do not chew or crush tablets; swallow whole.

➤*Oral liquids, soluble powders and effervescent tablets:* Mix or dissolve completely in 3 to 8 ounces of cold water, juice or other suitable beverage and drink slowly.

Following release of potassium chloride, the expended wax matrix, which is not absorbable, can be found in the stool. This is no cause for concern.

Do not use salt substitutes concurrently, except on the advice of a physician.

Notify physician if tingling of the hands and feet, unusual tiredness or weakness, a feeling of heaviness in the legs, severe nausea, vomiting, abdominal pain or black stools (GI bleeding) occurs.

ORAL ELECTROLYTE MIXTURES

	Product	Electrolyte content							Other Content	Calories per fl. oz.	How Supplied
		Na+	K+	Cl–	Citrate	Ca++	Mg++	Phosphate			
otc	**Rehydralyte Solution** (Ross)	75[a]	20[a]	65[a]	30[a]				25 g/L dex-trose	3	In 240 mL ready-to-use.
otc	**Infalyte Oral Solution** (Mead Johnson)	50[a]	25[a]	45[a]	34[a]				30 g/L rice syrup solids	4.2	Fruit flavor. In ≈ 1 L ready-to-use.
otc	**Resol Solution** (Wyeth-Ayerst)	50[a]	20[a]	50[a]	34[a]	4[a]	4[a]	5[a]	20 g/L glu-cose	2.5	In 240 mL ready-to-use.
otc	**Naturalyte Solution** (UBI)	45[a]	20[a]	35[a]	48[a]				25 g/L dextrose		Unflavored, fruit or bubble gum flavors. In 240 mL and 1 L.
otc	**Pedialyte Solution** (Ross)	45[a]	20[a]	35[a]	30[a]				25 g/L dex-trose	3	Regular or fruit flavor. In 240 & 960 mL ready-to-use.
otc	**Pedialyte Freezer Pops** (Ross)	45[a]	20[a]	35[a]	30[a]				25 g/L dextrose, phenylalanine, aspartame	3	Grape, cherry, orange and blue raspberry flavors. In 2.1 fl oz ready-to-freeze pops (16s).
otc	**Temp Tab** (National Vitamin)	180[b]	15[b]	287[b]							Preservative- and sugar-free. In 100s.

[a] mEq/L [b] Mg/tablet.

ORAL ELECTROLYTE MIXTURES — ORAL

Indications

➤*Fluid/Electrolyte depletion:* For maintenance of water and electrolytes following corrective parenteral therapy for severe diarrhea; for maintenance to replace mild to moderate fluid losses when food and liquid intake are discontinued; to restore fluid and minerals lost in diarrhea and vomiting in infants and children.

➤*Temp Tab:* For minimizing chronic fatigue, muscle cramps, or heat prostration because of excessive perspiration.

For use by people that are exposed to high temperatures which can cause heat fatigue.

Administration and Dosage

Individualize dosage. Follow the guidelines listed on the product labeling.

➤*Resol:* Individualize dosage based on extent of weight loss and dehydration as assessed by the physician.

➤*Pedialyte/Rehydralyte:* Offer frequently in amounts tolerated. Adjust total daily intake to meet individual needs, based on thirst and response to therapy. In the following table, suggested intakes for replacement are based on fluid losses of 5% or 10% of body weight, including maintenance requirement.

Pedialyte/Rehydralyte Dosage for Infants/Young Children					
	Weight (approx.)			*Rehydralyte*	
Age	kg	lb	Pedialyte oz/day	Replacement for 5% dehydration (oz/day)	Replacement for 10% dehydration (oz/day)
2 wks	3.2	7	13-16	18-21	23-26
3 mos	6	13	28-32	38-42	48-52
6 mos	7.8	17	34-40	47-53	60-66
9 mos	9.2	20	38-44	53-59	68-74
1 yr	10.2	23	41-46	58-63	75-80
1.5 yr	11.4	25	45-50	64-69	83-88
2 yr	12.6	28	48-53	69-74	90-95
2.5 yr	13.6	30	51-56	74-79	97-102
3 yr	14.6	32	54-58	78-82	102-106
3.5 yr	16	35	56-60	83-87	110-114
4 yr	17	38	57-62	85-90	113-118

Extemporaneous oral rehydration solution[a] (Developed by the World Health Organization)				
	Na+/Cl–	K+	Citrate	Glucose
Source	NaCl or table salt	KCl or potassium salt[b]	sodium bicarbonate (baking soda)	Glucose or sucrose (cane sugar)
Weight (g)	3.5	1.5	2.5	20[c]
Household measure	0.5 tsp	0.25 tsp	0.5 tsp	2 tbsp[d]
mmol/L	90/80	20	30	111

[a] To be added to 1 L water. Follow physician's administration instructions.
[b] See potassium salt substitutes.
[c] If sucrose is used, 40 g.
[d] If sucrose is used, 4 tbsp.

➤*Temp Tab:* Take one tablet with 8 ounces of water up to 5 to 7 times/day, depending on working conditions.

Actions

➤*Pharmacology:* Used properly, mixtures with electrolytes, water and glucose prevent dehydration or achieve rehydration, and maintain strength and feeling of well being. They contain sodium, chloride, potassium and bicarbonate to replace depleted electrolytes and restore acid-base balance. Glucose facilitates sodium transport, which aids in sodium and water absorption.

Contraindications

Severe, continuing diarrhea or other critical fluid losses; intractable vomiting; prolonged shock, renal dysfunction (anuria, oliguria). These require parenteral therapy.

PERITONEAL DIALYSIS SOLUTIONS

	Product and Distributor	Icodextrin (g/liter)	Dextrose (g/liter)	Na+	Ca++	Mg++	Cl-	Lactate	Osmolarity (mOsm/liter)	How Supplied
Rx	**Dialyte Pattern LM w/1.5% Dextrose** (Gambro)	0	15	131	3.5	0.5	94	40	345	In 1000, 2000 and 4000 mL.
Rx	**Dialyte Pattern LM w/2.5% Dextrose** (Gambro)	0	25	131.5	3.5	0.5	94	40	395	In 1000, 2000 and 4000 mL.
Rx	**Dialyte Pattern LM w/4.25% Dextrose** (Gambro)	0	42.5	131.5	3.5	0.5	94	40	485	In 1000, 2000 and 4000 mL.
Rx	**Extraneal** (Baxter)	75	0	132	3.5	0.5	96	40	282-286	In 1.5, 2, and 2.5 L *Ultrabag* and 1.5, 2, and 2.5 L *Ambu-Flex*.

PERITONEAL DIALYSIS SOLUTIONS

Indications

Acute or chronic renal failure; acute poisoning by dialyzable toxins; intractable edema; hyperkalemia, hypercalcemia, azotemia and uremia; hepatic coma. Refer to manufacturer's package literature for specific prescribing information.

Electrolyte content given in mEq/liter.

SYSTEMIC ALKALINIZERS

CITRATE AND CITRIC ACID SOLUTIONS

	Product	Content	How Supplied
Rx	**Cytra-3** (Cypress)	**Syrup:** 550 mg potassium citrate monohydrate, 500 mg sodium citrate dihydrate, 334 mg citric acid monohydrate per 5 mL (1 mEq potassium and 1 mEq sodium per mL and is equivalent to 2 mEq bicarbonate)	Sugar free. In 16 oz. bottles.
Rx	**Cytra-LC** (Cypress)	**Solution:** 550 mg potassium citrate monohydrate, 500 mg sodium citrate dihydrate, 334 mg citric acid monohydrate per 5 mL (1 mEq potassium and 1 mEq sodium per mL and is equivalent to 2 mEq bicarbonate)	In 16 oz. bottles.
Rx	**Cytra-K** (Cypress)	**Solution:** 1100 mg potassium citrate monohydrate and 334 mg citric acid monohydrate per 5 mL (2 mEq potassium per mL and is equivalent to 2 mEq bicarbonate)	Alcohol free. In 473 mL.
Rx	**Oracit** (Carolina Medical Products)	**Solution:** 490 mg sodium citrate and 640 mg citric acid per 5 mL (1 mEq sodium per mL and is equivalent to 1 mEq bicarbonate)	Parabens. In 500 mL and UD 15 and 30 mL.
Rx *sf*	**Sodium Citrate/Citric Acid** (Pharmaceutical Associates)	**Solution:** 500 mg sodium citrate dihydrate and 334 mg citric acid monohydrate per 5 mL (1 mEq sodium per mL and is equivalent to 1 mEq bicarbonate)	In 473 mL.
Rx *sf*	**Bicitra** (Alza Corp.)		Alcohol free. In 120 and 473 mL, gal and UD 15 and 30 mL.
Rx	**Cytra-2** (Cypress)		Grape flavored. In 16 oz. bottles.
otc	**Naturalyte Oral Electrolyte Solution** (Unico)	**Solution:** 20 mEq potassium, 30 mEq citrate (20 g dextrose, 5 g fructose, 35 mEq chloride, 45 mEq sodium)/L	In unflavored, artificial fruit, bubble gum, and grape flavors. In 1 liter.

CITRATE AND CITRIC ACID SOLUTIONS — ORAL

Indications

➤*Chronic metabolic acidosis:* Treatment of chronic metabolic acidosis, particularly when caused by renal tubular acidosis.

➤*Urinary alkalizer:* Conditions where long-term maintenance of an alkaline urine is desirable, in treatment of patients with uric acid and cystine calculi of the urinary tract and in conjunction with uricosurics in gout therapy to prevent uric acid nephropathy.

➤*Neutralizing buffer:* Nonparticulate neutralizing buffers.

Administration and Dosage

Dilute in water before taking; follow with additional water, if desired. Monitor urinary pH with *Hydrion* paper (pH 6 to 8) or *Nitrazine* paper (pH 4.5 to 7.5).

➤*Dosage:*

Adults – 15 to 30 mL diluted with water, after meals and before bedtime.

Children – 5 to 10 mL diluted with water, after meals and before bedtime. The solution, not the crystals, is recommended for pediatric administration since dosage can be more easily regulated.

➤*Neutralizing buffer:* A single dose of 15 mL diluted with 15 mL water.

Actions

➤*Pharmacology:* Citrate and citric acid solutions are systemic and urinary alkalinizers. Preparations containing potassium citrate are preferred in patients requiring potassium or those who require sodium restriction. Conversely, sodium citrate may be administered when potassium is undesirable or contraindicated. Potassium citrate and sodium citrate are capable of buffering gastric acidity (pH greater than 2.5). The effects are essentially those of chlorides before absorption, and subsequently, those of bicarbonates.

➤*Pharmacokinetics:* Potassium citrate and sodium citrate are absorbed and metabolized to potassium bicarbonate and sodium bicarbonate, thus acting as systemic alkalinizers. The citric acid is metabolized to carbon dioxide and water; therefore, it has only a transient effect on systemic acid-base status. It functions as a temporary buffer component.

Oxidation is virtually complete; less than 5% of the citrates are excreted in the urine unchanged.

Contraindications

Severe renal impairment with oliguria, azotemia or anuria; untreated Addison's disease; adynamia episodica hereditaria; acute dehydration; heat cramps; severe myocardial damage; hyperkalemia; sodium restricted patients.

Warnings

➤*Lactation:* Exercise caution when administered to a nursing woman.

Precautions

➤*Urolithiasis:* Citrate mobilizes calcium from bones and increases its renal excretion; this, along with the elevated urine pH, may predispose to urolithiasis.

➤*Hyperkalemia / Alkalosis:* Patients with low urinary output and abnormal renal mechanisms may develop hyperkalemia or alkalosis, especially in the presence of hypocalcemia.

➤*Sodium salts:* Use cautiously in patients with cardiac failure, hypertension, impaired renal function, peripheral and pulmonary edema and preeclampsia. Monitor serum electrolytes, particularly the serum bicarbonate level, in patients with renal disease.

➤*GI effects:* Dilute with water to minimize GI injury associated with the oral ingestion of concentrated potassium salts. Take after meals to avoid saline laxative effect.

CITRATE AND CITRIC ACID SOLUTIONS — ORAL

Drug Interactions

Urinary Alkalinizer Drug Interactions

Precipitant drug	Object drug [a]		Description
Urinary alkalinizers (eg, potassium citrate, sodium citrate)	Chlorpropamide Lithium Methenamine Methotrexate Salicylates Tetracyclines	⬇	Urinary alkalinizers may increase the excretion and decrease the serum levels of these agents, possibly decreasing their pharmacologic effects.
Urinary alkalinizers (eg, potassium citrate, sodium citrate)	Anorexiants Flecainide Mecamylamine Quinidine Sympathomimetics	⬆	Urinary alkalinizers may decrease the excretion and increase the serum levels of these agents, possibly increasing their pharmacologic effects.

[a] ⬆ = Object drug increased. ⬇ = Object drug decreased.

Adverse Reactions

Hyperkalemia – Listlessness, weakness, mental confusion, tingling of extremities and other symptoms associated with high serum potassium. Hyperkalemia may exhibit the following ECG abnormalities: Disappearance of the P wave; widening or slurring of the QRS complex; changes of the ST segment; tall peaked T waves.

Overdosage

➤*Symptoms:* Overdosage with sodium salts may cause diarrhea, nausea, vomiting, hypernoia (excessive mental activity) and convulsions. Overdosage with potassium salts may cause hyperkalemia and alkalosis, especially in the presence of renal disease. Treat hyperkalemia immediately, because lethal levels can be reached in a few hours.

➤*Treatment:* For treatment of hyperkalemia, refer to the Potassium monograph in the IV Nutritional Therapy section; for treatment of sodium overdosage, refer to the Sodium Chloride monograph in the Salt Replacement Products section.

Patient Information

Dilute with water; follow with additional water, if desired.

Take after meals.

Notify physician if diarrhea, nausea, stomach pain, vomiting or convulsions occur.

SODIUM BICARBONATE

One g of sodium bicarbonate provides 11.9 mmol sodium and 11.9 mmol bicarbonate.

otc	**Sodium Bicarbonate** (Various, eg, Rugby)	**Tablets:** 325 mg	In 1000s.
		650 mg	In 1000s.
		Powder	In 120 and 300 g and 1 lb.

SODIUM BICARBONATE — ORAL

For information on parenteral sodium bicarbonate products, refer to the monograph in the IV Nutritional Therapy section.

Also see the Antacids group monograph in the Gastrointestinal Agents chapter.

Indications

➤*Antacid:* Sodium bicarbonate relieves acid indigestion, heartburn, sour stomach, and upset stomach associated with these symptoms.

➤*Alkalinizer:* Sodium bicarbonate may also be used for systemic or for urinary alkalinization.

Sodium bicarbonate oral powder is not for injections.

Administration and Dosage

➤*Antacid:*

Tablets – Do not use the maximum dosage for more than 2 weeks.

Adults 60 years of age and over: 1 to 2 tablets every 4 hours, but do not take more than 12 tablets in 24 hours.

Adults younger than 60 years of age: 1 to 4 tablets every 4 hours, but do not take more than 24 tablets in 24 hours.

Oral powder – Take a level ½ teaspoonful in ½ glass (120 mL) of water every 2 hours up to maximum dosage or as directed by a physician. Accurately measure ½ teaspoonful. Each ½ teaspoonful contains 30 mg (0.7 g) sodium.

Except under the advice and supervision of a physician:

- Do not administer to children under 6 years of age.
- Do not take more than six ½ teaspoonfuls per person up to 60 years old, or three ½ teaspoonfuls per person 60 years or older in a 24-hour period.

➤*Systemic alkalinizer:* In severe metabolic acidosis, the initial dose should be 12 to 24 sodium bicarbonate 650 mg tablets (7,800 mg to 15,600 mg). Dissolve in 1 to 2 L of water and consume in 1 hour. A physician should decide the follow-up dose.

➤*Urinary alkalinizer:* The initial dose should be six 650 mg tablets (3,900 mg) of sodium bicarbonate, and then 2 to 4 tablets (1,300 mg to 2,600 mg) every 4 hours. A physician should decide the duration of treatment.

➤*Storage / Stability:* Keep out of the reach of children.

Tablets – Store at room temperature 15° to 30°C (59° to 86°F).

Warnings

➤*Duration of treatment:* Do not use the maximum dose for more than 2 weeks.

➤*Sodium-restricted diet:* Do not use this product if you are on a sodium-restricted diet.

➤*Pregnancy:* Pregnant women should ask a health professional before use.

➤*Lactation:* Nursing women should ask a health professional before use.

Overdosage

➤*Treatment:* In case of accidental ingestion, patients should seek professional assistance or should contact a poison control center immediately.

Patient Information

Ask a doctor or pharmacist before use if you are on a sodium-restricted diet or taking a prescription drug. Sodium bicarbonate may interact with certain prescription drugs.

Stop use and ask a doctor if your symptoms last more than 2 weeks.

If pregnant, ask a health professional before use.

If breast-feeding, ask a health professional before use.

AMINO ACIDS

GLUTAMIC ACID

otc	**Glutamic Acid** (Various, eg, Freeda)	**Tablets:** 500 mg	In 100s and 500s.
otc	**Glutamic Acid** (J.R. Carlson)	**Powder**	In 100 g bottles.

GLUTAMIC ACID — ORAL

Indications

Dietary supplement.

Administration and Dosage

500 to 1000 mg daily or as directed. Take with liquids.

L-LYSINE

otc	**L-Lysine** (Various, eg, Rugby)	**Tablets**: 312 mg	In 100s.
otc	**Enisyl** (Person & Covey)	**Tablets**: 334 mg	In 100s.
otc	**L-Lysine** (Various, eg, Goldline, Moore, Mission, Pasadena, Rugby, URL)	**Tablets**: 500 mg	In 100s.
otc	**Enisyl** (Person & Covey)		In 100s and 250s.
otc	**L-Lysine** (Approved Pharm.)	**Tablets**: 1000 mg	In 60s.
otc	**L-Lysine** (Various, eg, Miller, Tyson & Assoc.)	**Capsules**: 500 mg	In 100s and 250s.

L-LYSINE — ORAL

Indications

Dietary supplement.

➤*Unlabeled uses:* Oral L-lysine has been promoted as treatment and as a prophylactic agent in herpes simplex infections; however, controlled studies do not support these claims.

Administration and Dosage

312 to 1500 mg daily.

Actions

➤*Pharmacology:* An essential amino acid which improves utilization of vegetable proteins.

METHIONINE

Rx	**Methionine** (Tyson & Assoc.)	**Capsules**: 500 mg	In 30s.

METHIONINE — ORAL

Refer to the Dermatologicals chapter for additional prescribing information.

Indications

Dietary supplement.

Administration and Dosage

500 mg daily. The recommended daily allowance has not been established.

THREONINE

otc	**Threonine** (Freeda)	**Tablets**: 500 mg	In 100s and 250s.
otc	**Threonine** (Various, eg, Solgar, Tyson & Assoc.)	**Capsules**: 500 mg	In 60s.

THREONINE — ORAL

Indications

➤*Dietary supplement:* As a dietary supplement.

Administration and Dosage

500 mg daily, preferably on an empty stomach, or as directed.

➤*Pregnancy and lactation:* Avoid threonine use in excess of the adequate intake during pregnancy and breastfeeding.

➤*Storage / Stability:* Store away from heat and direct light.

Actions

➤*Pharmacology:* Threonine is an essential amino acid important for the formation of many proteins and tooth enamel, collagen, and elastin. It aids liver and lipotropic function when combined with aspartic acid and methionine. It metabolizes fat and prevents the build-up of fat in the liver, and is useful with intestinal disorders and indigestion.

Threonine is a precursor of glycine and serine. Threonine is an alcohol-containing amino acid that cannot be produced by metabolism and must be consumed in the diet. There are good levels of threonine in most meats, dairy foods, and eggs, and moderate levels in wheat germ, many nuts, beans, and seeds, as well as some vegetables.

AMINO ACIDS WITH VITAMINS AND MINERALS

otc	**Dequasine** (Miller)	**Tablets**: 20 mg L-lysine, 50 mg L-cysteine, 150 mg dL-methionine, 50 mg N-acetyl cysteine, 200 mg vitamin C, 40 mg Ca, 1 mg Cu, 5 mg Fe, 0.015 mg I, 20 mg K, 40 mg Mg, 5 mg Mn, 150 mcg Mo, 5 mg Zn. *Dose:* 1 tablet/day, or as recommended.	In 100s.
otc sf	**NeuroSlim** (NeuroGenesis)	**Capsules**: 500 mg dL-phenylalanine, 15 mg L-glutamine, 25 mg L-tyrosine, 10 mg L-carnitine, 10 mg L-arginine pyroglutamate, 10 mg ornithine aspartate, 0.033 mg Cr, 0.012 mg Se, 0.33 mg vitamin B_1, 0.5 mg B_2, 3.3 mg B_3, 0.012 mg B_5, 0.333 mg B_6, 1 mcg B_{12}, 5 IU E, 0.05 mg biotin, 0.066 mg FA, 1 mg Fe, 2.5 mg Zn, 35 mg Ca, 0.025 mg I, 0.33 mg Cu, 25 mg Mg. *Dose:* 2 capsules 3 times/day, 1 hour before or 2 hours after meals.	In 180s.
otc sf	**NeuRecovery-DA** (NeuroGenesis)	**Capsules**: 460 mg dL-phenylalanine, 25 mg L-glutamine, 333.3 IU vitamin A, 1.65 mg B_1, 0.85 mg B_2, 33 mg B_3, 15 mg B_5, 3 mg B_6, 5 mcg B_{12}, 0.065 mg FA, 100 mg C, 5 IU E, 0.05 mg biotin, 25 mg Ca, 0.01 mg Cr, 1.5 mg Fe, 25 mg Mg, 2.5 mg Zn. *Dose:* 2 capsules 3 times/day.	In 180s.
otc sf	**NeuRecovery-SA** (NeuroGenesis)	**Capsules**: 250 mg dL-phenylalanine, 150 mg L-tyrosine, 50 mg L-glutamine, 1.65 mg vitamin B_1, 2.5 mg B_2, 16.6 mg B_3, 15 mg B_5, 3.36 mg B_6, 5 mcg B_{12}, 0.067 mg FA, 100 mg C, 25 mg Ca, 1.5 mg Fe, 25 mg Mg, 5 mg Zn. *Dose:* ≤ 6 capsules/day.	In 180s.
otc	**A/G-Pro** (Miller)	**Tablets**: 542 mg protein hydrolysate, 50 mg L-lysine, 12.5 mg L-methionine, 0.33 mg vitamin B_6, 16.7 mg C, 1.66 mg iron. Cu, I, K, Mg, Mn, Zn. *Dose:* 2 tablets 3 times/day.	In 180s.
otc sf	**Jets** (Freeda)	**Tablets, chewable**: 300 mg L-lysine, 10 mg vitamin B_1, 5 mg B_6, 25 mcg B_{12}, 25 mg C.	In 100s.
otc sf	**Body Fortress Natural Amino** (Nature's Bounty)	**Tablets**: 1.67 g protein, 1500 mg lactalbumin hydrolysate *Dose:* 2 to 3 tablets with each meal and directly after each workout, or as directed.	Yeast and preservative free. In 150s.
otc sf	**Amina-21** (Miller)	**Capsules**: 556 mg free-form amino acids *Dose:* 1 or 2 capsules 3 times/day or as recommended.	In 100s and 300s.
otc	**PowerSleep** (Green Turtle Bay Vitamin Co.)	**Tablets**: 250 mg L-glutamine, 25 mg 5-HTP, 0.25 mg melatonin, 25 mg vitamin B_3, 5 mg B_6, 100 mg inositol, 25 mg Ca, 100 mg passion flower extract, 75 mg valerian powder *Dose:* 2 tablets 1 hour before bedtime.	In 60s.
otc sf	**PowerMate** (Green Turtle Bay Vitamin Co.)	**Tablets**: 25 mg N-acetyl-L-cysteine, 5 mg glutathione, 5000 IU vitamin A, 12.5 mg B_3, 250 mg C, 100 IU E, 2.5 mg Zn, 7.5 mcg Se, 5 mg ginkgo biloba, 100 mg green tea extract, 5 mg pine bark extract, 50 mg echinacea, 20 mg golden seal root, 2 mg coenzyme Q10 *Dose:* 2 tablets daily for 2 weeks/month.	Yeast free. In 50s.

AMINO ACIDS WITH VITAMINS AND MINERALS

otc	**EMF** (Wesley Pharmacal)	**Liquid:** Alanine, arginine, aspartic acid, cysteine, glutamic acid, glycine, histidine, hydroxylysine, hydroxyproline, isoleucineline, leucine, lysine, methionine, phenylalanine, proline, serine, threonine, tyrosine, valine, 15 g protein. *Dose:* 30 mL/day.	Sorbitol, saccharin. Cherry flavor. In qt.

Amino Acid Derivatives

LEVOCARNITINE (L-Carnitine)

Rx	**Levocarnitine** (Rising)	**Tablets:** 330 mg	(cor 160). White. In blisters of 90.
Rx	**Carnitor** (Sigma-Tau)		(CARNITOR ST). In 90s.
otc	**L-Carnitine** (Freeda Vitamins)	**Tablets:** 500 mg	In 50s and 100s.
otc	**L-Carnitine** (Various, eg, Miller Pharmacal Group, Nature's Bounty, Tyson, Watson)	**Capsules:** 250 mg	In 30s, 60s, and 100s.
Rx	**Levocarnitine** (Rising)	**Solution:** 100 mg/mL	Sucrose, parabens. Cherry flavor. In 118 mL.
Rx	**Carnitor** (Sigma-Tau)		Sucrose, parabens. Cherry flavor. In 118 mL.
Rx	**Levocarnitine** (Various, eg, American Regent, Bedford)	**Injection:** 200 mg/mL	In single-dose vials.
Rx	**Carnitor** (Sigma-Tau)		Preservative-free. In single-dose vials and amps.

LEVOCARNITINE — ORAL

Indications

➤*Primary systemic carnitine deficiency:* Treatment of primary systemic carnitine deficiency.

➤*Secondary carnitine deficiency:* For acute and chronic treatment of patients with an inborn error of metabolism which results in a secondary carnitine deficiency.

➤*Unlabeled uses:* Carnitine has been used to improve athletic performance and may be of use in valproate toxicity.

Administration and Dosage

➤*Approved by the FDA:* December 27, 1985.

➤*Tablets:*

Adults – 990 mg 2 or 3 times a day using the 330 mg tablets, depending on clinical response.

Infants and children – Between 50 and 100 mg/kg/day in divided doses, with a maximum of 3 g/day. Dosage should begin at 50 mg/kg/day. The exact dosage will depend on clinical response. Monitoring should include periodic blood chemistries, vital signs, plasma carnitine concentrations and overall clinical condition.

➤*Capsules:*

Adults 18 and over – Take 1 capsule daily with meals.

➤*Oral solution:*

Adults – 1 to 3 g/day for a 50 kg subject, which is equivalent to 10 to 30 mL/day of levocarnitine oral solution. Higher doses should be administered only with caution and only where clinical and biochemical considerations make it seem likely that higher doses will be of benefit. Dosage should start at 1 g/day, (10 mL/day), and be increased slowly while assessing tolerance and therapeutic response. Monitoring should include periodic blood chemistries, vital signs, plasma carnitine concentrations, and overall clinical condition.

Infants and children – 50 to 100 mg/kg/day which is equivalent to 0.5 mL/kg/day levocarnitine oral solution. Higher doses should be administered only with caution and only where clinical and biochemical considerations make it seem likely that higher doses will be of benefit. Dosage should start at 50 mg/kg/day, and be increased slowly to a maximum of 3 g/day (30 mL/day) while assessing tolerance and therapeutic response. Monitoring should include periodic blood chemistries, vital signs, plasma carnitine concentrations, and overall clinical condition. Levocarnitine oral solution may be consumed alone or dissolved in drink or other liquid food. Doses should be spaced evenly throughout the day (every 3 or 4 hours) preferably during or following meals and should be consumed slowly in order to maximize tolerance.

➤*Storage/Stability:* Store products at controlled room temperature (25°C; 77°F) (see USP).

Actions

➤*Pharmacology:* Levocarnitine is a naturally occurring substance required in mammalian energy metabolism. It has been shown to facilitate long-chain, fatty-acid entry into cellular mitochondria, thereby delivering substrate for oxidation and subsequent energy production. Fatty acids are utilized as an energy substrate in all tissues except the brain. In skeletal and cardiac muscle, fatty acids are the main substrate for energy production.

Primary systemic carnitine deficiency – Primary systemic carnitine deficiency is characterized by low concentrations of levocarnitine in plasma, red blood cells, or tissues. It has not been possible to determine which symptoms are due to carnitine deficiency and which are due to an underlying organic acidemia, as symptoms of both abnormalities may be expected to improve with levocarnitine. The literature reports that carnitine can promote the excretion of excess organic or fatty acids in patients with defects in fatty acid metabolism or specific organic acidopathies that bioaccumulate acylCoA esters.

Secondary carnitine deficiency – Secondary carnitine deficiency can be a consequence of inborn errors of metabolism. Levocarnitine may alleviate the metabolic abnormalities of patients with inborn errors that result in accumulation of toxic organic acids. Conditions for which this effect has been demonstrated are the following: Glutaric aciduria II, methyl malonic aciduria, propionic acidemia, and medium chain fatty acylCoA dehydrogenase deficiency. Autointoxication occurs in these patients due to the accumulation of acylCoA compounds that disrupt intermediary metabolism. The subsequent hydrolysis of the acylCoA compound to its free acid results in acidosis which can be life-threatening. Levocarnitine clears the acylCoA compound by formation of acylcarnitine, which is quickly excreted. Carnitine deficiency is defined biochemically as abnormally low plasma concentrations of free carnitine, less than 20 mcmol/L at 1 week postterm and may be associated with low tissue or urine concentrations. Further, this condition may be associated with a plasma concentration ratio of acylcarnitine/levocarnitine greater than 0.4 or abnormally elevated concentrations of acylcarnitine in the urine. In premature infants and newborns, secondary deficiency is defined as plasma levocarnitine concentrations below age-related normal concentrations.

➤*Pharmacokinetics:*

Absorption/Distribution – The absolute bioavailability of levocarnitine from the 2 oral formulations of levocarnitine, calculated after correction for circulating endogenous plasma concentrations of levocarnitine, was 15.1 ± 5.3% for levocarnitine tablets and 15.9 ± 4.9% for levocarnitine oral solution.

In a relative bioavailability study in 15 healthy, adult, male volunteers, levocarnitine tablets were found to be bioequivalent to levocarnitine oral solution. Following 4 days of dosing with 6 tablets of levocarnitine 330 mg twice daily or 2 g of levocarnitine oral solution twice daily, the maximum plasma concentration (C_{max}) was about 80 mcmol/L, and the time to maximum plasma concentration (t_{max}) occurred at 3.3 hours.

Levocarnitine was not bound to plasma protein or albumin when tested at any concentration or with any species, including the human.

Metabolism/Excretion – In a pharmacokinetic study where 5 healthy, adult, male volunteers received an oral dose of [^{3}H-methyl]-L-carnitine following 15 days of a high-carnitine diet, and additional carnitine supplement, 58% to 65% of the administered radioactive dose was recovered in the urine and feces in 5 to 11 days. Maximum concentration of [^{3}H-methyl]-L-carnitine in serum occurred from 2 to 4.5 hours after drug administration. Major metabolites found were trimethylamine N-oxide, primarily in urine (8% to 49% of the administered dose) and [^{3}H]-γ-butyrobetaine, primarily in feces (0.44% to 45% of the administered dose). Urinary excretion of levocarnitine was about 4% to 8% of the dose. Fecal excretion of total carnitine was less than 1% of the administered dose.

After attainment of steady state following 4 days of oral administration of levocarnitine tablets (1980 mg every 12 hours) or oral solution (2000 mg every 12 hours) to 15 healthy male volunteers, the mean urinary excretion of levocarnitine during a single dosing interval (12 hours) was about 9% of the orally administered dose (uncorrected for endogenous urinary excretion).

Total body clearance of levocarnitine (Dose/AUC including endogenous baseline concentrations) was a mean of 4 L/hr.

Contraindications

None known.

Warnings

➤*Renal function impairment:* The safety and efficacy of oral levocarnitine has not been evaluated in patients with renal insufficiency. Chronic administration of high doses of oral levocarnitine in patients with severely compromised renal function or in ESRD patients on dialysis may result in accumulation of the potentially toxic metabolites, trimethylamine (TMA) and trimethylamine-N-oxide (TMAO), since these metabolites are normally excreted in the urine.

LEVOCARNITINE — ORAL

➤*Pregnancy: Category B.*

There are no adequate and well-controlled studies in pregnant women. Because animal reproduction studies are not always predictive of human response, this drug should be used during pregnancy only if clearly needed.

➤*Lactation:* Levocarnitine supplementation in breast-feeding mothers has not been specifically studied.

Studies in dairy cows indicate that the concentration of levocarnitine in milk is increased following exogenous administration of levocarnitine. In breast-feeding mothers receiving levocarnitine, any risks to the child of excess carnitine intake need to be weighed against the benefits of levocarnitine supplementation to the mother. Consideration may be given to discontinuation of breast-feeding or of levocarnitine treatment.

➤*Children:* Levocarnitine may be used in infants and children.

Precautions

➤*Monitoring:* Monitoring should include periodic blood chemistries, vital signs, plasma carnitine concentrations and overall clinical condition.

➤*Oral solution:* Not for parenteral use. GI reactions may result from a too-rapid consumption of carnitine.

See Administration and Dosage for more information.

Adverse Reactions

➤*CNS:* Seizures have been reported to occur in patients with or without preexisting seizure activity receiving either oral or IV levocarnitine. In patients with preexisting seizure activity, an increase in seizure frequency or severity has been reported.

➤*GI:* Various mild GI complaints have been reported during the long-term administration of oral L- or D,L-carnitine; these include transient nausea and vomiting, abdominal cramps, and diarrhea. Mild myasthenia has been described only in uremic patients receiving D,L-carnitine. GI adverse reactions with levocarnitine oral solution dissolved in liquids might be avoided by a slow consumption of the solution or by a greater dilution. Decreasing the dosage often diminishes or eliminates drug-related patient body odor or GI symptoms when present. Tolerance should be monitored very closely during the first week of administration, and after any dosage increases.

Overdosage

➤*Symptoms:* There have been no reports of toxicity from levocarnitine overdosage. Large doses of levocarnitine may cause diarrhea.

➤*Treatment:* Levocarnitine is easily removed from plasma by dialysis.

LEVOCARNITINE — INJECTION

Indications

➤*Secondary carnitine deficiency:* For the acute and chronic treatment of patients with an inborn error of metabolism which results in secondary carnitine deficiency.

➤*End-stage renal disease (ESRD):* For the prevention and treatment of carnitine deficiency in patients with end-stage renal disease who are undergoing dialysis.

➤*Primary systemic carnitine deficiency:* For treatment of primary systemic carnitine deficiency.

➤*Unlabeled uses:* Carnitine has been used to improve athletic performance and may be of use in valproate toxicity.

Administration and Dosage

➤*Approved by the FDA:* December 16, 1992.

Levocarnitine injection is administered IV.

➤*Metabolic disorders:* 50 mg/kg given as a slow, 2- to 3-minute bolus injection or by infusion. Often a loading dose is given in patients with severe metabolic crisis followed by an equivalent dose over the following 24 hours. It should be administered every 3 hours or every 4 hours, and never less than every 6 hours, either by infusion or by IV injection. All subsequent daily doses are recommended to be in the range of 50 mg/kg or as therapy may require. The highest dose administered has been 300 mg/kg.

It is recommended that a plasma carnitine level be obtained prior to beginning this parenteral therapy. Weekly and monthly monitoring is recommended as well. This monitoring should include blood chemistries, vital signs, plasma carnitine concentrations (the plasma-free carnitine concentration should be between 35 and 60 mcmol/L) and overall clinical condition.

➤*ESRD patients on hemodialysis:* The recommended starting dose is 10 to 20 mg/kg dry body weight as a slow 2- to 3-minute bolus injection into the venous return line after each dialysis session. Initiation of therapy may be prompted by trough (predialysis) plasma levocarnitine concentrations that are below normal (40 to 50 mcmol/L). Dose adjustments should be guided by trough (predialysis) levocarnitine concentrations, and downward dose adjustments (eg, to 5 mg/kg after dialysis) may be made as early as the third or fourth week of therapy.

➤*Storage/Stability:* Levocarnitine injection USP is compatible and stable when mixed in parenteral solutions of Sodium Chloride 0.9% or Lactated Ringer's in concentrations ranging from 250 mg/500 mL (0.5 mg/mL) to 4,200 mg/500 mL (8 mg/mL) and stored at room temperature (25°C; 77°F) for up to 24 hours in PVC plastic bags.

Store vials at controlled room temperature 25°C (77°F). Retain vial in carton until time of use. Protect from light. Discard unused portion of an opened vial, as they contain no preservative.

Actions

➤*Pharmacology:* Levocarnitine is a naturally occurring substance required in mammalian energy metabolism. It has been shown to facilitate long-chain, fatty-acid entry into cellular mitochondria, thereby delivering substrate for oxidation and subsequent energy production. Fatty acids are utilized as an energy substrate in all tissues except the brain. In skeletal and cardiac muscle, fatty acids are the main substrate for energy production.

Primary systemic carnitine deficiency – Primary systemic carnitine deficiency is characterized by low concentrations of levocarnitine in plasma, red blood cells (RBC), or tissues. It has not been possible to determine which symptoms are due to carnitine deficiency and which are due to the underlying organic acidemia, as symptoms of both abnormalities may be expected to improve with carnitine. The literature reports that levocarnitine can promote the excretion of excess organic or fatty acids in patients with defects in fatty acid metabolism or specific organic acidopathies that bioaccumulate acylCoA esters.

Secondary carnitine deficiency – Secondary carnitine deficiency can be a consequence of inborn errors of metabolism or iatrogenic factors such as hemodialysis. Levocarnitine may alleviate the metabolic abnormalities of patients with inborn errors that result in accumulation of toxic organic acids. Conditions for which this effect was demonstrated are as follows: Glutaric aciduria 2, methyl malonic aciduria, propionic acidemia, and medium chain fatty acylCoA dehydrogenase deficiency. Autointoxication occurs in these patients due to the accumulations of acylCoA compounds that disrupt intermediary metabolism. The subsequent hydrolysis of the acylCoA compound to its free acid results in acidosis that can be life-threatening. Levocarnitine clears the acylCoA compound by formation of acyl carnitine which is quickly excreted. Levocarnitine deficiency is defined biochemically as abnormally low plasma levels of free carnitine, less than 20 mcmol/L at 1 week postterm and may be associated with low tissue or urine concentrations. Further, this condition may be associated with a plasma-concentration ratio of acylcarnitine/levocarnitine greater than 0.4 or abnormally elevated concentrations of acylcarnitine in the urine. In premature infants and newborns, secondary deficiency is defined as plasma-free levocarnitine levels below age-related normal concentrations.

ESRD – ESRD patients on maintenance hemodialysis may have low plasma carnitine concentrations and an increased ratio of acylcarnitine/levocarnitine because of reduced intake of meat and dairy products, reduced renal synthesis and dialytic losses. Certain clinical conditions common in hemodialysis patients such as malaise, muscle weakness, cardiomyopathy and cardiac arrhythmias may be related to abnormal carnitine metabolism.

Pharmacokinetic and clinical studies with levocarnitine have shown that administration of levocarnitine to ESRD patients on hemodialysis results in increased plasma levocarnitine concentrations.

➤*Pharmacokinetics:*

Absorption – The plasma-concentration profiles of levocarnitine after a slow, 3-minute IV bolus dose of 20 mg/kg of levocarnitine were described by a 2-compartment model.

Distribution – Levocarnitine was not bound to plasma protein or albumin when tested at any concentration or with any species, including human.

Metabolism/Excretion – Following a single IV administration, approximately 76% of the levocarnitine dose was excreted in urine during the 0- to 24-hour interval. Using plasma concentrations uncorrected for endogenous levocarnitine, the mean distribution half-life was 0.585 hours and the mean apparent terminal elimination half-life was 17.4 hours.

Total body clearance of levocarnitine (dose/AUC including endogenous baseline concentrations) was a mean of 4 L/hr.

Contraindications

None known.

Warnings

➤*Renal function impairment:* The safety and efficacy of oral levocarnitine have not been evaluated in patients with renal insufficiency. Chronic administration of high doses of oral levocarnitine in patients with severely compromised renal function or in ESRD patients on dialysis may result in accumulation of the potentially toxic metabolites, trimethylamine (TMA) and trimethylamine-N-oxide (TMAO), since these metabolites are normally excreted in the urine.

➤*Pregnancy: Category B.*

There are no adequate and well-controlled studies in pregnant women. Because animal reproduction studies are not always predictive of human response, this drug should be used during pregnancy only if clearly needed.

➤*Lactation:* Levocarnitine supplementation in nursing mothers has not been specifically studied.

Studies in dairy cows indicate that the concentration of levocarnitine in milk is increased following exogenous administration of levocarnitine. In nursing mothers receiving levocarnitine, any risks to the child of excess carnitine intake need to be weighed against the benefits of levocarnitine supplementation to the mother. Consideration may be given to discontinuation of nursing or of levocarnitine treatment.

Precautions

➤*Monitoring:* See Administration and Dosage for more information.

LEVOCARNITINE — INJECTION

Adverse Reactions

Transient nausea and vomiting have been observed. Less frequent adverse reactions are body odor, nausea, and gastritis. An incidence for these reactions is difficult to estimate due to the confounding effects of the underlying pathology.

➤*Seizures:* Seizures have been reported to occur in patients with or without preexisting seizure activity receiving either oral or IV levocarnitine. In patients with preexisting seizure activity, an increase in seizure frequency or severity has been reported.

➤*Adverse reactions (≥ 5%):*

Adverse Reactions with a Frequency ≥ 5% Regardless of Causality by Body System					
Adverse reaction	Placebo (n = 63)	Levocarnitine 10 mg (n = 34)	Levocarnitine 20 mg (n = 62)	Levocarnitine 40 mg (n = 34)	Levocarnitine 10, 20 and 40 mg (n = 130)
Cardiovascular					
Arrhythmia	5	3	—	3	2
Atrial fibrillation	—	—	2	6	2
Cardiovascular disorder	6	3	5	6	5
Electrocardiogram abnormal	—	3	—	6	2
Hemorrhage	6	9	2	3	4
Hypertension	14	18	21	21	20
Hypotension	19	15	19	3	14
Palpitations	—	3	8	—	5
Tachycardia	5	6	5	9	6
Vascular disorder	2	—	2	6	2
CNS					
Anxiety	5	—	2	—	1
Depression	3	6	5	6	5
Dizziness	11	18	10	15	13
Drug dependence	2	6	—	—	2
Hypertonia	5	3	—	—	1
Insomnia	6	3	6	—	4
Paresthesia	3	3	3	12	5
Vertigo	—	6	—	—	2
Dermatologic					
Pruritus	13	—	8	3	5
Rash	3	—	5	3	3
Endocrine					
Parathyroid disorder	2	6	2	6	4
GI					
Anorexia	3	3	5	6	5
Constipation	6	3	3	3	3
Diarrhea	19	9	10	35	16
Dyspepsia	10	9	6	—	5
GI disorder	2	3	—	6	2
Melena	3	6	—	—	2
Nausea	10	9	5	12	8
Stomach atony	5	—	—	—	—
Vomiting	16	9	16	21	15
GU					
Urinary tract infection	6	3	3	—	2
Kidney failure	5	6	6	6	6
Hematologic/lymphatic					
Anemia	3	3	5	12	6
Metabolic/nutritional					
Hypercalcemia	3	15	8	6	9
Hyperkalemia	6	6	6	6	6
Hypervolemia	17	3	3	12	5
Peripheral edema	3	6	5	3	5
Weight decrease	3	3	8	3	5
Weight increase	2	3	—	6	2
Musculoskeletal					
Leg cramps	13	—	8	—	4
Myalgia	6	—	—	—	—
Respiratory					
Bronchitis	—	—	5	3	3
Cough increase	16	—	10	18	9
Dyspnea	19	3	11	3	7
Pharyngitis	33	24	27	15	23
Respiratory disorder	5	—	—	—	—
Rhinitis	10	6	11	6	9
Sinusitis	5	—	2	3	2
Special senses					
Amblyopia	2	—	6	—	3
Eye disorder	3	6	3	—	3
Taste perversion	—	—	2	9	3
Miscellaneous					
Abdominal pain	17	21	5	6	9
Accidental injury	10	12	8	12	10
Allergic reaction	5	6	—	—	2
Asthenia	8	9	8	12	9
Back pain	10	9	8	6	8
Chest pain	14	6	15	12	12
Fever	5	6	5	12	7
Flu syndrome	40	15	27	29	25
Headache	16	12	37	3	22
Injection	17	15	10	24	15
Injection site reaction	59	38	27	38	33
Pain	49	21	32	35	30

Overdosage

➤*Symptoms:* Large doses of levocarnitine may cause diarrhea. There have been no reports of toxicity from levocarnitine overdosage.

➤*Treatment:* Levocarnitine is easily removed from plasma by dialysis.

Actions

➤*Pharmacology:* The need for lipotropics in human nutrition is not established. The lipotropic factors choline, inositol and betaine, not proven therapeutically valuable, have been used for treatment of liver disorders and disturbed fat metabolism.

Choline (trimethylethanolamine), a component of the major phospholipid, lecithin, demonstrates lipotropic action, functions as a methyl group donor and is a precursor of the neurochemical transmitter acetylcholine. Choline and lecithin (because of its choline content) have been advocated for tardive dyskinesia, Huntington's chorea, Tourette's syndrome, Friedreich's ataxia, presenile dementia, fatty liver and cirrhosis. Intestinal bacteria metabolize choline to trimethylamine, which imparts an unpleasant odor to the breath and body. Lecithin does not produce this odor. Choline also causes clinical depression in some patients.

Inositol, an isomer of glucose, is present in cell membrane phospholipids and plasma lipoproteins. No specific role in human nutrition has been established.

Linoleic and linolenic acid are polyunsaturated fatty acids that serve as precursors of important biochemical compounds, such as arachidonic acid, which gives rise to a wide variety of prostaglandins. Linoleic acid is regarded as an essential fatty acid because it cannot be synthesized in vivo and because it has a defined metabolic significance; it helps support normal growth and development and prevent essential fatty acid deficiency (EFAD). The metabolic significance of linolenic acid is unclear. Use of these precursors to alter disease states requires more research.

CHOLINE

otc	**Choline** (Various, eg, Approved Pharm, Rugby)	**Tablets:** 250 mg, 300 and 500 mg	In 100s.
		650 mg	In 90s and 100s.
otc	**Choline** (Freeda)	**Powder:** ¼ tsp equals 375 mg choline	In 16 oz.
otc	**Choline Bitartrate** (Various, eg, City Chem, Fibertone, Spectrum)	**Tablets:** 250 mg	In 100s, 250s, 500s, 1000s.
		Powder	In 120 g and 1 lb.
Rx	**Choline Chloride** (Various, eg, Baker, Biochemical, City Chem, Spectrum)	**Powder**	In 120 and 500 g and 1 and 5 lb.
otc	**Choline Dihydrogen** Citrate (Freeda)	**Tablets:** 650 mg	In 250s.
		Powder	In 120 g and 1 lb.

CHOLINE — ORAL

Refer to additional information in the Lipotropic Products monograph.

Administration and Dosage

650 mg to 2 g daily or as directed.

INOSITOL

otc	**Inositol** (Various, eg, Biochemical, Freeda, Nature's Bounty, Rugby)	**Tablets:** 250 mg	In 100s.
		500 mg	In 100s.
		650 mg	In 90s and 100s.
		Powder: ¼ tsp equals 375 mg	In 25, 60, 100, 120, 500 g & lb.
otc *sf*	**Inositech** (Bio-tech)	**Capsules:** 324 mg	In 100s.

INOSITOL — ORAL

Refer to additional information in the Lipotropic Products monograph.

Indications

➤*Dietary supplement:* Inositol is an essential component of cell walls, and plays an important role in cell growth and function.

Administration and Dosage

➤*Directions:* Take 1 tablet 1 to 3 times daily, preferably with a meal.

This supplement is coated for ease of swallowing.

➤*Storage/Stability:* Keep out of the reach of children. Inositol should be stored in a cool, dry place.

Actions

➤*Pharmacology:* The need for lipotropics in human nutrition is not established. The lipotropic factors choline, inositol, and betaine, not proven therapeutically valuable, have been used for treatment of liver disorders and disturbed fat metabolism.

Choline (trimethylethanolamine), a component of the major phospholipid, lecithin, demonstrates lipotropic actions, functions as a methyl group donor and is a precursor of the neurochemical transmitter acetylcholine. Choline and lecithin (because of its choline content) have been advocated for tardive dyskinesia, Huntington's chorea, Tourette's syndrome, Friedreich's ataxia, presentile dementia, fatty liver, and cirrhosis. Intestinal bacteria metabolize choline to trimethylamine, which imparts an unpleasant odor to the breath and body. Lecithin does not produce this odor. Choline also causes clinical depression in some patients.

Inositol, an isomer of glucose, is present in cell membrane phospholipids and plasma lipoproteins. No specific role in human nutrition has been established.

Linoleic and linolenic acid are polyunsaturated fatty acids that serve as precursors of important biochemical compounds, such as arachidonic acid, which gives rise to a wide variety of prostaglandins. Linoleic acid is regarded as an essential fatty acid because it cannot be synthesized in vivo and because it has a defined metabolic significance; it helps support normal growth and development and prevent essential fatty acid deficiency (EFAD). The metabolic significance of linolenic acid is unclear. Use of these precursors to alter disease states requires more research.

LIPOTROPIC COMBINATIONS

otc	**Lecithin** (Various, eg, Approved Pharm, Dixon-Shane, Goldline, Moore, Nature's Bounty, Rugby, West-Ward)	A source of choline, inositol, phosphorus, linoleic & linolenic acids	
		Capsules: 420 mg	In 60s.
		1.2 g	In 100s, 250s, 1000s.
		Tablets: 1.2 g	In 50s.
		Granules	In 210, 240, 420 g & lb.
		Liquid	In 480 mL.
otc	**PhosChol** (American Lecithin)	Phosphatidylcholine (highly purified lecithin)	
		Softgels: 565 mg	In 100s and 300s
		Softgels: 900 mg	In 100s and 300s.
		Liquid concentrate: 3000 mg/5 mL	In 240 and 480 mL.
otc	**Pertropin** (Lannett)	**Capsules:** 7 mins. linolenic acid, other essential unsaturated free fatty acids, 5 IU vitamin E	In 100s.

LIPOTROPIC COMBINATIONS — ORAL

Refer to additional information in the Lipotropic Products monograph.

Administration and Dosage

➤*Lecithin:* One to 2 capsules daily.

➤*Pertropin:* One or 2 capsules 3 or 4 times daily.

FISH OILS

OMEGA-3 (N-3) POLYUNSATURATED FATTY ACIDS

	Product/Distributor	mg/ capsule	N-3 fat content (mg) EPA	DHA	Other Content	How Supplied
Rx	**Animi 3 Capsules** (PBM Pharm[a])	500	35	350	12.5 mg vitamin B_6, 500 mcg B_{12}, 1 mg folic acid	(PBM 540). Opaque red, oblong. In 60s.
otc sf	**Promega Pearls Softgels** (Parke-Davis)	600	168	72	< 2 mg cholesterol, 1 IU vitamin E,[b] < 2% RDA of vitamins A, B_1, B_2, B_3, Fe and Ca	In 60s and 90s.
Rx	**Omacor Capsules** (Ross)	≥ 900	≈ 465	≈ 375	4 mg α-tocopherol	(OMACOR). Lt. yellow. In 120s.
otc	**Cardi-Omega 3 Capsules** (Thompson Medical)	1000	180	120	< 2% RDA of vitamins A, B_1, B_2, B_3, C, D, Fe and Ca	Sodium free. Peppermint flavor. In 60s.
otc sf	**EPA Capsules** (Nature's Bounty)				1 IU vitamin E[b]	In 50s and 100s.
otc	**Max EPA Capsules** (Various, eg, Jones Medical, Moore, Rexall, Schein)				5 mg cholesterol, < 2% RDA of vitamins A, B_1, B_2, B_3, C, Ca, Fe	In 60s, 90s & 100s.
otc sf	**Promega Softgels** (Parke-Davis)	1000	280	120	< 1 mg cholesterol, 1 IU vitamin E[b] (6% RDA), vitamins A, B_1, B_2, B_3, Ca & Fe (< 2% RDA)	Sodium free. In 30s and 60s.
otc sf	**Sea-Omega 50 Softgels** (Rugby)	1000	300	200	1 IU vitamin E[b]	Sodium free. In 50s.
otc	**Sea-Omega 30 Softgels** (Rugby)	1200	180	140	2 IU vitamin E[b]	In 100s.
otc	**Marine Lipid Concentrate Softgels** (Vitaline)	1200	360	240	5 IU vitamin E[b]	Sodium free. In 90s.
otc	**SuperEPA 1200 Softgels** (Advanced Nutritional)	1200	360	240	5 IU vitamin E[b]	In 60s, 90s and 180s.
otc	**SuperEPA 2000 Capsules** (Advanced Nutritional)	1000	563	312	20 IU vitamin E[b]	In 30s, 60s and 90s.

[a] PBM Pharmaceuticals, Linney House, 204 North Main Street, Gordonsville, VA 22942; (800)485-9828.

[b] As d-alpha tocopherol.

OMEGA-3 (N-3) POLYUNSATURATED FATTY ACIDS — ORAL

Indications

➤*Dietary supplement:* As dietary supplements for patients at early risk of coronary artery disease primarily because of effects on platelets and lipids.

The American Heart Association recommends consumption of fish; however, it does not find justification for fish oil capsule supplementation.

➤*Unlabeled uses:* Omega-3 fatty acids have been studied as adjunctive treatment of rheumatoid arthritis (20 g/day have been used). These agents may also be of benefit in the treatment of psoriasis (10 to 15 g/day); however, data is conflicting. Omega-3 fatty acids (18 g/day) may be beneficial in preventing early restenosis after coronary angioplasty in combination with dipyridamole and aspirin in high risk male patients.

Administration and Dosage

➤*Nutritional supplement:* 1 to 2 capsules 3 times daily with meals.

Actions

➤*Pharmacology:* Cold water fish oils contain large amounts of omega-3 (N-3) polyunsaturated fatty acids, eicosapentaenoic acid (EPA) and docosahexaenoic acid (DHA). Diets high in omega-3 fatty acids may lower very low-density lipoproteins (VLDL), triglyceride and total cholesterol concentrations; increase concentrations of high-density lipoproteins (HDL); prolong bleeding times; decrease platelet aggregation; reduce plasma fibrinogen (data conflict); inhibit leukocyte function.

Studies on the effects of omega-3 fatty acids on the lipoproteins closely associated with atherosclerosis (LDL and HDL) show variable results and require further investigation.

Some studies have actually shown an increase in LDL-cholesterol levels in patients and healthy subjects receiving omega-3 fatty acids at doses currently recommended by the manufacturers (4.6 to 13.3 g/day). Although the optimal dose has not been established, significant effects of the omega-3 fatty acids may only be observed with 20 g or more per day. Some of the available products contain cholesterol and saturated fat, which may play a role in the increased LDL-cholesterol levels.

Patients on diets with high levels of fish oils have increased EPA levels and decreased arachidonic acid levels in plasma lipids and platelet membranes. Also, increased synthesis of prostaglandin I_3 and decreased platelet synthesis of thromboxane A_2 have been noted. Prostaglandin I_3, an antiaggregation substance, and thromboxane A_2, a potent stimulator of platelet aggregation and secretion, are usually in balance. It is believed EPA is utilized by vessel walls to synthesize prostaglandin I_3, and arachidonic acid is utilized by platelets to synthesize thromboxane A_2. Therefore, the higher EPA levels and lower arachidonic acid levels produced by a diet high in fish oils could cause decreased platelet aggregation. Vitamin E in the product could also contribute to decreased platelet aggregation.

Warnings

➤*Diarrhea:* Diarrhea has occurred in patients taking 4 to 6 capsules per day.

➤*Bleeding:* Increased bleeding time and inhibition of platelet aggregation have occurred. Use caution in patients receiving **anticoagulants** or **aspirin**.

➤*Diabetes mellitus:* In one study the fasting and mean glucose levels increased and insulin secretion was impaired in six patients with type 2 diabetes mellitus following 1 month of omega-3 fatty acid administration (5.4 g/day). However, increased insulin sensitivity in type 2 diabetes mellitus patients has occurred. Use with caution in type 2 diabetes mellitus patients.

➤*Pregnancy:* Until further information is available, do not use omega-3 fatty acids in these patients.

➤*Children:* Until further information is available, do not use omega-3 fatty acids in these patients.

LACTASE ENZYME

otc	**Lactrase** (Schwarz Pharma)	**Capsules:** 250 mg standardized enzyme lactase	(Kremers Urban 505). Orange/white. In 100s and blisterpack 10s and 30s.
otc	**Dairy Ease** (Blistex)	**Tablets, chewable:** 3000 FCC lactase units	Mannitol, sucrose. In 60 and 100s.

LACTASE ENZYME — ORAL

Indications

➤*Lactose intolerance:* Lactase enzyme may be used in persons who are lactose intolerant and experience gas, cramps, bloating or diarrhea from eating dairy foods, such as milk, ice cream or cheese. Lactase enzyme dietary supplements aid in dairy food digestion in lactose-intolerant individuals without gas, cramping, bloating or diarrhea.

Administration and Dosage

Lactase enzyme is natural and may be used every day with every meal.

➤*Maximum strength tablets and chewable tablets:* The recommended serving size is 1 maximum strength tablet to be swallowed with the first bite of dairy food or 1 maximum strength chewable tablet to be chewed and swallowed with the first bite of dairy food. Patients who suffer from severe lactose intolerance may require more than 1 tablet or chewable tablet, but should not exceed 2 maximum strength tablets or chewable tablets at one time.

➤*Extra strength tablets:* The recommended serving size is 2 extra strength tablets to be swallowed or chewed with the first bite of dairy food. For best results, patients may increase or decrease the number of tablets taken.

➤*Original strength tablets:* The recommended serving size is 3 original strength tablets to be swallowed or chewed with the first bite of dairy food. For best results, patients may increase or decrease the number of tablets taken.

➤*Storage/Stability:* Store at room temperature (below 25°C; 77°F); do not refrigerate. Keep away from heat.

ALPHA-D-GALACTOSIDASE ENZYME

otc	**Beano** (AK Pharma)	**Liquid:** Alpha-D-galactosidase-derived from *Aspergillus niger* (≥ 175 galactose units per 5 drop dosage)	Glycerol. In 75 serving size at 5 drops per dose.
		Tablets: Alpha-galactosidase enzyme derived from *Aspergillus niger*	Cornstarch, sucrose, hydrogenated cottonseed oil, sorbitol. In 12s, 30s and 100s.

ALPHA-D-GALACTOSIDASE — ORAL

Indications

➤*Intestinal gas/bloating:* Treatment of gassiness or bloating as a result of eating a variety of grains, cereals, nuts, seeds, or vegetables containing the sugars raffinose, stachyose, or verbascose. This includes all or most legumes and all or most cruciferous vegetables (eg, oats, wheats, beans, peas, lentils, peanuts, soy-content foods, pistachios, broccoli, brussels sprouts, cabbage, carrots, corn, onions, squash, cauliflower).

Administration and Dosage

The patient should take 1 tablet or 5 drops of alpha-D-galactosidase liquid per ½ cup serving of gassy food. A typical meal consists of 2 or 3 servings of food, so the patient should take 3 tablets or 15 drops with each meal. The patient can take as many drops or tablets as needed. For best results, the patient should adjust the number of tablets or drops according to the number of servings. The patient should use a higher or lower amount depending on the quantity of food eaten, levels of alpha-linked sugars in the food, and the gas-producing propensity and tolerance of the person.

Actions

➤*Pharmacology:* Alpha-D-galactosidase enzyme hydrolyzes raffinose, verbascose and stachyose into the digestible sugars sucrose, fructose, glucose, and galactose.

Precautions

➤*Galactosemics:* Galactosemics should not use this supplement without physician advice since one of the breakdown sugars is galactose.

SACROSIDASE

Rx	**Sucraid** (Orphan Medical)	**Solution:** 8500 IU/mL	In 118 mL bottles (2) with 1 mL measuring scoop.

SACROSIDASE — ORAL

Indications

➤*Sucrase deficiency:* As oral replacement therapy of the genetically determined sucrase deficiency, which is part of congenital sucrase-isomaltase deficiency (CSID).

Administration and Dosage

The recommended dosage is 1 or 2 mL (8500 to 17,000 IU), or 1 to 2 full measuring scoops (each full measuring scoop equals 1 mL; 22 drops from the sacrosidase container tip equals 1 mL) taken orally with each meal or snack diluted with 2 to 4 ounces of water, milk, or infant formula. The beverage or infant formula should be served cold or at room temperature. The beverage or infant formula should not be warmed or heated before or after addition of sacrosidase because heating is likely to decrease potency. Sacrosidase should not be reconstituted or consumed with fruit juice, since its acidity may reduce the enzyme activity.

It is recommended that approximately half of the dosage be taken at the beginning of each meal or snack, and the remainder be taken at the end of each meal or snack.

➤*Patients less than or equal to 15 kg (33 pounds):* 1 mL/8500 IU (1 full measuring scoop or 22 drops) per meal or snack.

➤*Patients greater than 15 kg (33 pounds):* 2 mL/17,000 IU (2 full measuring scoops or 44 drops) per meal or snack.

Dosage may be measured with the 1 mL measuring scoop (provided) or by drop count method (1 mL equals 22 drops from the sacrosidase container tip).

➤*Storage/Stability:* Store in a refrigerator at 2° to 8°C (36° to 46°F). Discard 4 weeks after first opening due to the potential for bacterial growth. Protect from heat and light.

Actions

➤*Pharmacology:* Congenital sucrase-isomaltase deficiency (CSID) is a chronic, autosomal recessive, inherited, phenotypically heterogenous disease with very variable enzyme activity. CSID is usually characterized by a complete or almost complete lack of endogenous sucrase activity, a very marked reduction in isomaltase activity, a moderate decrease in maltase activity and normal lactase levels.

Sucrase is naturally produced in the brush border of the small intestine, primarily the distal duodenum and jejunum. Sucrase hydrolyzes the disaccharide sucrose into its component monosaccharides, glucose and fructose. Isomaltase breaks down disaccharides from starch into simple sugars. Sacrosidase does not contain isomaltase.

In the absence of endogenous human sucrase, as in CSID, sucrose is not metabolized. Unhydrolyzed sucrose and starch are not absorbed from the intestine and their presence in the intestinal lumen may lead to osmotic retention of water. This may result in loose stools. Unabsorbed sucrose in the colon is fermented by bacterial flora to produce increased amounts of hydrogen, methane and water. As a consequence, excessive gas, bloating, abdominal cramps, nausea and vomiting may occur.

Chronic malabsorption of disaccharides may result in malnutrition. Undiagnosed/untreated CSID patients often fail to thrive and fall behind in their expected growth and development curves. Previously, the treatment of CSID has required the continual use of a strict sucrose-free diet.

CSID is often difficult to diagnose. Approximately 4 to 10% of pediatric patients with chronic diarrhea of unknown origin have CSID. Measurement of expired breath hydrogen under controlled conditions following a sucrose challenge (a measurement of excess hydrogen excreted in exhalation) in CSID patients has shown levels as great as 6 times that in healthy subjects.

A generally accepted clinical definition of CSID is that of a condition characterized by the following: Stool pH of less than 6, an increase in breath hydrogen of greater than 10 ppm when challenged with sucrose after fasting and a negative lactose breath test. However, because of the difficulties in diagnosing CSID, it may be warranted to conduct a short therapeutic trial (eg, one week) to assess response in patients suspected of having CSID.

Contraindications

Hypersensitivity to yeast, yeast products, or glycerin (glycerol).

Warnings

➤*Severe wheezing:* Severe wheezing, 90 minutes after a second dose of sacrosidase, necessitated admission into the ICU for a 4-year old boy. The wheezing was probably caused by sacrosidase. He had asthma and was being treated with steroids. A skin test for sacrosidase was positive.

➤*Hypersensitivity reactions:* Care should be taken to administer initial doses of sacrosidase near (within a few minutes' travel) a facility where acute hypersensitivity reactions can be adequately treated. Alternatively, the patient may be tested for hypersensitivity to sacrosidase through skin

SACROSIDASE — ORAL

abrasion testing. Should symptoms of hypersensitivity appear, discontinue medication and initiate symptomatic and supportive therapy.

Skin testing as a rechallenge has been used to verify hypersensitivity in one asthmatic child who displayed wheezing after oral sacrosidase.

➤*Pregnancy: Category C.* Animal reproduction studies have not been conducted with sacrosidase. Sacrosidase is not expected to cause fetal harm when administered to a pregnant woman or to affect reproductive capacity. Sacrosidase should be given to a pregnant woman only if clearly needed.

➤*Lactation:* The sacrosidase enzyme is broken down in the stomach and intestines and the component amino acids and peptides are then absorbed as nutrients.

➤*Children:* Sacrosidase has been used in patients as young as 5 months of age. Evidence from one controlled trial in primarily pediatric patients shows that sacrosidase is safe and effective for the treatment of the genetically acquired sucrase deficiency, which is part of CSID.

Precautions

➤*Starch restriction:* Although sacrosidase provides replacement therapy for the deficient sucrase, it does not provide specific replacement therapy for the deficient isomaltase. Therefore, restricting starch in the diet may still be necessary to reduce symptoms as much as possible. The need for dietary starch restriction for patients using sacrosidase should be evaluated in each patient.

➤*CSID diagnosis:* The definitive test for diagnosis of CSID is the measurement of intestinal disaccharidases following small bowel biopsy.

Other tests used alone may be inaccurate: For example, the breath hydrogen test (high incidence of false-negatives) or oral sucrose tolerance test (high incidence of false positives). Differential urinary disaccharide testing has been reported to show good agreement with small intestinal biopsy for diagnosis of CSID.

It may sometimes be clinically inappropriate, difficult, or inconvenient to perform a small bowel biopsy or breath hydrogen test to make a definitive diagnosis of CSID. If the diagnosis of CSID is in doubt, it may be warranted to conduct a short therapeutic trial (eg, one week) with sacrosidase to assess response in a patient suspected of sucrase deficiency.

The effects of sacrosidase have not been evaluated in patients with secondary (acquired) disaccharidase deficiencies.

➤*Diabetics:* The use of sacrosidase will enable the products of sucrose hydrolysis (eg, glucose and fructose) to be absorbed. This fact must be carefully considered in planning the diet of diabetic CSID patients using sacrosidase.

Drug Interactions

➤*Drug/Food interactions:* Sacrosidase should not be reconstituted or consumed with fruit juice, since its acidity may reduce the enzyme activity.

Adverse Reactions

In clinical studies of up to 54 months duration, physicians treated a total of 52 patients with sacrosidase. The adverse experiences and respective number of patients reporting each event (in parenthesis) were as follows: abdominal pain (4), vomiting (3), nausea (2), diarrhea (2), constipation (2), insomnia (1), headache (1), nervousness (1), and dehydration (1).

Diarrhea and abdominal pain can be a part of the clinical presentation of the genetically determined sucrase deficiency, which is part of congenital sucrase-isomaltase deficiency (CSID).

➤*Hypersensitivity:* One asthmatic child experienced a serious hypersensitivity reaction (wheezing) probably related to sacrosidase (see Warnings). The event resulted in withdrawal of the patient from the trial but resolved with no sequelae.

➤*Most frequent adverse reactions:* The most frequent adverse reactions reported while taking sacrosidase were abdominal pain (8%) and vomiting (6%). One patient experienced a serious reaction; hypersensitivity (wheezing). This event resolved with no sequelae.

Overdosage

Overdosage with sacrosidase has not been reported.

Patient Information

Patients should be instructed to discard bottles of sacrosidase 4 weeks after first opening due to the potential for bacterial growth.

Sacrosidase is fully soluble with water, milk, and infant formula, but it is important to note that this product is sensitive to heat. Sacrosidase should not be reconstituted or consumed with fruit juice, since its acidity may reduce the enzyme activity.

ORAL NUTRITIONAL SUPPLEMENTS

LACTOBACILLUS

otc	**Intestinex** (A.G. Marin)	**Capsules**: 100 million units *Lactobacillus acidophilus*	In 24s.
otc	**Acidophilus** (Nature's Bounty)	**Capsules**: greater than 100 million units *Lactobacillus acidophilus*	Soybean oil, beeswax/ soybean oil mixture. In 100s.
otc	**Bacid** (Ciba)	**Capsules**: Cultured strain ≥ 500 million viable *Lactobacillus acidophilus*	Mineral oil. In 50s and 100s.
otc	**Lacto-Key-100** (Key)	**Capsules**: ≥ 1 billion CFU *Lactobacillus acidophilus*	In 60s, 120s, and 500s.
otc	**SynBiotics-3** (NutraCea)	**Capsules**: 4.5 billion CFU *Bifidobacterium longum, Lactobacillus rhamnosus* A, *Lactobacillus plantarum, Saccharomyces boulardii*	Maltodextrin. In 60s and UD 200s.
otc	**Lacto-Key-600** (Key)	**Capsules**: ≥ 6 billion CFU *Lactobacillus acidophilus*	In 60s and 120s.
otc sf	**Kala** (Freeda)	**Tablets**: 200 million units soy-based *Lactobacillus acidophilus*	In 100s, 250s, and 500s.
otc	**Floranex** (Rising)	**Tablets, chewable**: 1 million CFU *Lactobacillus acidophilus* and *Lactobacillus bulgaricus*	Sucrose, lactose. In 50s.
otc	**Lactinex** (Becton Dickinson)	**Tablets, chewable**: Mixed culture of *Lactobacillus acidophilus* and *Lactobacillus bulgaricus*	Lactose, sucrose, and mineral oil. In 50s.
		Granules: Mixed culture of *Lactobacillus acidophilus* and *Lactobacillus bulgaricus*	In 1 g packets (12s).
otc	**Acidophilus** (Mason)	**Wafers**: 20 million units *Lactobacillus acidophilus*	Preservative free. 1 g sugar. Vanilla-banana flavor. In 100s.
otc	**Acidophilus with Bifidus** (Various, eg, Mason, Nature's Bounty)	**Wafers**: 1 billion units *Lactobacillus acidophilus* and *Lactobacillus bifidus*	1 g sugar. Strawberry flavor. In 100s.
otc sf	**MoreDophilus** (Freeda)	**Powder**: 4 billion units of acidophilus-carrot derivative per g	In 120 g.
otc	**Superdophilus** (Natren)	**Powder**: 2 billion *Lactobacillus acidophilus* strain DDS-1 per g	In 37.5, 75, and 135 g.

LACTOBACILLUS ACIDOPHILUS — ORAL

Indications

➤*Restoration of intestinal flora:* *Lactobacillus acidophilus* has been found to be useful in the restoration and stabilization of normal intestinal flora.

➤*Unlabeled uses:* The FDA has determined that *Lactobacillus acidophilus* ingredients are not generally recognized to be as safe and effective as antidiarrheal drug products.

Treatment of acute fever blisters (cold sores).

Administration and Dosage

The suggested use is 1 or 2 capsules daily or as directed by a physician.

➤*Storage/Stability:* *Lactobacillus acidophilus* products contain a specially prepared cultured strain on viable *Lactobacillus acidophilus* microorganisms which has been grown on rice and not milk. These microorganisms are encapsulated for stability and are viable for a year from the shipping date.

Actions

➤*Pharmacology:* This supplement is a viable culture of the naturally occurring metabolic products produced by *Lactobacillus acidophilus* and *Lactobacillus bulgaricus.*

LACTOBACILLUS ACIDOPHILUS — ORAL

Warnings

➤*Children:* Unless directed by a physician, do not use in children younger than 3 years of age.

Precautions

➤*Duration:* Do not use for longer than 2 days unless directed by your physician.

➤*Fever:* Unless directed by a physician, do not use in the presence of high fever.

Patient Information

This supplement is recommended for diarrhea, fever, constipation, flatulence (excess gas pressure), anorexia (loss of appetite), emesis (vomiting), obesity. Many of these symptoms occur after antibiotic use, and many physicians recommend the use of yogurt or other sources of acidophilus subsequent to antibiotic treatment.

These *Lactobacillus acidophilus* microorganisms are encapsulated for stability and are viable for a year from the shipping date.

Lactobacillus acidophilus products contain no milk, soy, yeast or other allergens.

FLAVOCOXID

Rx	**Limbrel** (Primus)	**Capsule:** 250 mg	Dextrose, maltodextrin. (LIMBREL 52001). Turquoise green. In 60s.

FLAVOCOXID — ORAL

Indications

➤*Osteoarthritis (OA):* For the clinical dietary management of OA, including associated inflammation.

Administration and Dosage

Take one 250 mg capsule every 12 hours for a total of 500 mg/day. Consume more than 500 mg/day only under direction of a physician. Do not consume food 1 hour before or after taking flavocoxid.

➤*Storage/Stability:* Store at room temperature of 15° to 30°C (59° to 86°F). Protect from light and moisture. Dispense in a light-resistant container with a child-resistant closure.

Actions

➤*Pharmacology:* Flavocoxid consists of a proprietary blend of free B-ring flavonoids and flavans from phytochemical food source materials, which are Generally Recognized as Safe.

Flavocoxid exhibits anti-inflammatory and analgesic properties in animal and human models. The mechanism of action is believed to exist because of inhibition of prostaglandin synthesis, via the inhibition of cyclo-oxygenase (COX). In addition to COX, flavocoxid has been observed to inhibit another important inflammatory pathway of arachidonic acid metabolism known as the 5-lipoxygenase (5-LO or 5-LOX) pathway. In cell-based assays, inhibition of 5-LOX has been shown to reduce the production of leukotriene-B4 (LTB4), an agent that fosters white blood cell chemotaxis and the subsequent release of reactive oxygen species and pro-inflammatory cytokines. Direct inhibition of the 5-LOX enzyme also has been observed. Reactive oxygen species (ROS) have been shown to play a key role in the degradation of cartilage in OA.

Flavocoxid also is believed to act through an antioxidant mechanism by reduction of ROS including hydroxyl radical, superoxide anion radical, and hydrogen peroxide.

Flavocoxid also has been found to reduce the pro-inflammatory cytokines interleukin-1-beta (IL-1 β) and tumor necrosis factor alpha (TNF-α) in in vitro models. This mechanism may account for the anti-inflammatory action of flavocoxid beyond that of traditional COX and 5-LOX inhibition.

Through these mechanisms, flavocoxid is beneficial for the specific dietary management of OA.

➤*Pharmacokinetics:*

Absorption – Do not consume food 1 hour before or after taking flavocoxid. Absorption under conditions of co-ingestion of flavocoxid with food is believed to be safe, but may present modest absorption limitations. This observation is based upon limited clinical experience, and testing has not been performed to confirm this observation.

Metabolism – Flavocoxid is primarily metabolized via glucuronidation and sulfation, with little hepatic metabolism involving cytochrome P450 isoenzymes (CYP). A primary ingredient constituent, baicalin, undergoes hydrolysis of the glucuronide moiety at the gut mucosal border and is absorbed as the aglycone, baicalein. Glucuronidation and sulfation of baicalein occurs intrahepatically. In vitro CYP assays using a microsomal enzyme system show CYP inhibition is nominal, ranging from 11% to 23% inhibition of selected isozymes when studied at a 10 micromolar concentration.

Contraindications

Hypersensitivity to flavocoxid or any component of flavocoxid.

Warnings

➤*General:* Flavocoxid has not been investigated for use in the clinical dietary management of rheumatoid arthritis, acute pain, or primary dysmenorrhea.

➤*Pregnancy:* There are no formal studies among pregnant patients; as a precaution, flavocoxid is not recommended for pregnant patients.

➤*Lactation:* There are no formal studies among lactating patients; as a precaution, flavocoxid is not recommended for lactating patients.

➤*Children:* Because there are no formal studies among patients younger than 18 years of age, as a precaution, flavocoxid is not recommended for patients younger than 18 years of age.

Precautions

➤*Corticosteroids:* Flavocoxid cannot be expected to substitute for the use of corticosteroids or to treat corticosteroid insufficiency.

➤*GI effects:* Because there are no formal studies among patients with a history of GI disorders, as a precaution, flavocoxid is not recommended for patients with a history of stomach ulcers. As with many products, GI side effects such as bleeding, ulceration, and stomach perforation can occur at any time, with or without symptoms, in patients concomitantly or previously treated with NSAIDs or COX-2 inhibitors.

Adverse Reactions

In a 90 day, well-controlled, clinical trial, the incidence of side effects for flavocoxid was comparable with placebo. Some of the adverse events reported appear to have been because of preexisting conditions.

➤*GI:* In 1 study, an isolated number of patients using flavocoxid and placebo products were found to test positive for fecal occult blood. However, the limited incidence of these adverse events was statistically the same between the flavocoxid and placebo legs of this trial. Patients experiencing these events were found to have a history of GI illness. To confirm the isolated nature of these findings, 2 fecal occult blood studies were performed, and all patients tested negative.

➤*Adverse events (at least 2% incidence):*

125 mg twice/day – Fluid accumulation in the knee; hypertension (elevation); varicose veins (increase).

250 mg twice/day – Psoriasis.

Overdosage

There are no known human cases of flavocoxid being overused. Animal studies have shown that consuming the equivalent of up to 20 times the recommended human use (500 mg/day) did not produce adverse events. However, as in most overusage situations, symptoms following an overuse of flavocoxid could vary according to the patient.

➤*Treatment:* If an overusage occurs, manage patients by systematic and supportive care as soon as possible following product consumption. There are no known specific antidotes for an overuse of flavocoxid.

NUTRITIONAL COMBINATION PRODUCTS

VITAMIN A & D COMBINATIONS

	Product & Distributor	A IU	D IU	C mg	Content Given Per	Other Content and How Supplied
otc	**Vitamin A & D Tablets** (Nature's Bounty)	10,000	400		tablet	In 100s.
otc	**White Cod Liver Oil Concentrate w/ Vitamin C Tablets** (Schering-Plough)	4000	200	50	chewable tablet	Tartrazine, sugar. In 100s.
otc sf	**Tri-Vi-Sol Drops** (Mead Johnson Nutritional)	1500	400	35	1 mL	In 30 and 50 mL w/dropper.
otc	**Tri-Vitamin Infants' Drops** (Schein)					Pineapple flavor. In 50 mL w/dropper.
otc sf	**Vi-Daylin ADC Drops** (Ross)					< 0.5% alcohol, parabens. Pineapple flavor. In 50 mL.
otc	**Cod Liver Oil Capsules** (Various, eg, Apothecon, Goldline, IDE, Moore, Nature's Bounty, Rugby, Bristol-Myers Squibb)	1250	≈ 135		capsule	In 100s, 250s and 1000s.
otc	**Scott's Emulsion** (SK-Beecham)	1250	100		5 mL	Benzyl alcohol, parabens. In 187.5 and 375 mL.

VITAMIN A & D COMBINATIONS

	Product & Distributor	A IU	D IU	C mg	Content Given Per	Other Content and How Supplied
otc	**Cod Liver Oil USP** (Humco)	1000	100		g	In 120 mL, pt and gal.
otc	**Cod Liver Oil Liquid USP** (Various, eg, Apothecon, Humco, Bristol-Myers Squibb)	850	85		g	In 120 and 360 mL and pt.

For additional information, refer to the Recommended Dietary Allowances monograph.

CALCIUM AND VITAMIN D

Content given per tablet or softgel.

	Product & Distributor	Ca[1] mg	D IU	P mg	Other Content and How Supplied
otc sf	**Caltrate 600 + D Tablets** (Whitehall Robins)	600	200		(C 40). (CALTRATE). In 60s.
otc sf	**Caltrate Plus Tablets** (Whitehall Robins)				7.5 mg Zn, Mg, Cu, Mn, B. (CALTRATE). In 60s.
otc	**Os-Cal Ultra** (GlaxoSmithKline Consumer)				60 mg vitamin C, 20 mg Mg, 7.5 mg Zn, 15 Units vitamin E, 1 mg Cu, 1 mg Mn, 250 mcg B, sucrose, lactose. In 120s.
otc sf	**Super Calcium '1200' Softgels** (Schiff)				In 60s and 120s.
otc	**Calcium Carbonate 600 mg + Vitamin D Tablets** (Major)	600	125		In 72s.
otc sf	**Calcium 600 + D Tablets** (Nature's Bounty)				In 60s.
otc sf	**Calcarb with Vitamin D** (Zenith Goldline)				In 60s.
otc sf	**Caltrate 600 + Iron/Vitamin D Tablets** (Lederle)				18 mg Fe.[2] (LL). Film coated. Capsule shape. In 60s.
otc sf	**Posture-D Tablets** (Whitehall)				Scored. Film coated. In 60s.
otc	**Calcium 600 with Vitamin D Tablets** (Mission)	600	100		In 60s.
otc sf	**Calel D Tablets** (Rhone-Poulenc Rorer)	500	200		In 75s.
otc sf	**Os-Cal 500 + D Tablets** (GlaxoSmithKline Consumer)				Parabens, corn syrup solids. Green, oblong. In 75s and 160s.
otc sf	**Oyster Calcium 500 mg + D Tablets** (Nion)				In 120s.
otc sf	**Desert Pure Calcium** (Cal•White Mineral Co.)	500	125		Film coated. Oval. In 200s.
otc sf	**Oyster Calcium Tablets** (Nature's Bounty)	375	200		800 IU vitamin A. In 100s.
otc	**Citracal Caplets + D** (Mission)	315	200		(CITRACAL +D MISSION). In 60s.
otc	**Citracal Plus with Magnesium Tablets** (Mission)	250	125		5 mg B_6, B, Cu, Mg, Mn, Zn. In 150s.
otc	**Os-Cal 250 + D Tablets** (GlaxoSmithKline Consumer)				Parabens, EDTA, corn syrup solids. (OS-CAL 250 + D). In 100s and 240s.
otc	**Oysco D Tablets** (Rugby)				In 100s, 250s and 1000s.
otc	**Oyst-Cal-D Tablets** (Goldline)				Tartrazine. Green. Film coated. In 100s, 240s and 1000s.
otc sf	**Oyster Calcium with Vitamin D Tablets** (Nion)				In 100s.
otc	**Oyster Shell Calcium with Vitamin D Tablets** (Major)				In 100s, 1000s and UD 100s.
otc	**Amino-Min-D Capsules** (Tyson)	250	100		7.5 mg Fe, 5.6 mg Zn, Mg, I, Mn, Cu, K, Cr, Se, betaine HCl, glutamic acid HCl. In 100s.
otc	**Calcet Tablets** (Mission)	150	100		Tartrazine. In 100s.
otc sf	**Bone Meal Tablets** (Nion)	236		118	In 250s.
otc sf	**Super CalciCaps Tablets** (Nion)	400	133	42	In 90s and 180s.
otc	**CalciCaps Tablets** (Nion)	125[3]	67	60	In 100s and 500s.
otc	**CalciCaps with Iron Tablets** (Nion)				7 mg Fe.[4] Tartrazine. In 100s and 500s.
otc	**Dical-D Tablets** (Abbott)	105	120	81	In 100s.

[1] Expressed in mg elemental calcium.
[2] As ferrous fumarate.
[3] Dibasic calcium phosphate, calcium gluconate and calcium carbonate.
[4] As ferrous gluconate.

For additional information, refer to the Recommended Dietary Allowances monograph.

VITAMIN COMBINATIONS, MISCELLANEOUS

Content given per capsule, tablet or mL.

	Product and Distributor	Ca[1] mg	E IU	B_6 mg	C mg	Other Content	How Supplied
otc sf	**Ze Caps Capsules** (Everett)		200[2]			9.6 mg Zn (as gluconate), sorbitol	In 60s.
otc sf	**Dolomite Tablets**(Nature's Bounty)	130				78 mg Mg	In 100s and 250s.
otc	**Beelith Tablets** (Beach)			20		362 mg Mg	In 100s.
otc sf	**Calcium Magnesium Zinc Tablets** (Nature's Bounty)	333				133 mg Mg, 8.3 mg Zn	In 100s.
otc sf	**KLB6 Softgels** (Nature's Bounty)			3.5		100 mg soya lecithin, 25 mg kelp, 40 mg cider vinegar	In 100s.
otc	**Ultra KLB6 Tablets** (Nature's Bounty)			16.7		400 mg lecithin, 33.3 mg kelp, 80 mg cider vinegar	In 100s.
otc sf	**Mag-Cal Tablets** (Fibertone)	416.7[3] 166.7[1]				66.7 IU D_3, 83.3 mg Mg, Cu, Mn, K, Zn	In 180s.
otc sf	**Bo-Cal Tablets** (Fibertone)	250				125 mg Mg, 100 IU D_3, B	In 120s.
otc sf	**Oesto-Mins Powder**[4] (Tyson)	250			500	250 mg Mg, 45 mg K, 100 IU vitamin D	In 200 g.
otc sf	**Mag-Cal Mega Tablets** (Freeda)	400				800 mg Mg	Kosher. In 100s and 250s.
otc sf	**Super CalciCaps M-Z Tablets** (Nion)	400				133 mg Mg, 5 mg Zn, 1667 mg vitamin A, 133 IU vitamin D, Se	In 90s.
otc	**MagneBind 200** (Nephro-Tech)	400[3] 160[1]				200 mg Mg[3]	In 150s.
otc	**MagneBind 300** (Nephro-Tech)	250[3] 101[1]				300 mg Mg[3]	In 150s.
Rx	**MagneBind 400 Rx** (Nephro-Tech)	200[3]				400 mg Mg,[3] 1 mg folic acid	In 150s.
otc	**ProSight Lutein** (Major)	22	30		60	15 mg Zn, 2 mg Cu.	In 36s.

[1] Calcium content expressed in mg elemental calcium.
[2] As dL-alpha tocopheryl acetate.
[3] Carbonate.
[4] Content given per 4.5 g.

For additional information, refer to the Recommended Dietary Allowances monograph.

VITAMIN COMBINATIONS, MISCELLANEOUS, WITH C

Content given per capsule, tablet or mL.

	Product and Distributor	A IU	E mg	B_3 mg	C mg	Other Content	How Supplied
otc	**Antiox** (Mayrand)	42,000[1]	100[2]		120		In 60s.
otc	**Ocuvite Extra Tablets** (Bausch & Lomb)	1000	100[2]	40	300	40 mg Zn, 3 mg B_2, Cu, Se, Mn, L-glutathione, 2 mg lutein	In 50s.
otc	**Pro Skin Capsules** (Marlyn)	6250[3]	100[4]		100	10 mg B_5, 10 mg Zn, Se	In 60s.
otc	**Protegra Softgels** (Lederle)	5000[1]	200[2]		250	7.5 mg Zn, Cu, Se, Mn	In 50s.
otc	**OcuCaps Tablets** (Akorn)	5000[1]	182[5]		400	40 mg Zn, 5 mg L-glutathione, sodium pyruvate, Cu, Se	Capsule shape. In 60s.
otc	**Ocuvite Tablets** (Bausch & Lomb)	5000[1]	30[4]		60	40 mg Zn, Cu, 40 mcg Se	In 120s.
otc	**Ocuvite Lutein Capsules** (Bausch & Lomb)		30		60	15 mg Zn, Cu, 6 mg lutein, lactose	In 36s.
otc sf	**C & E Softgels** (Nature's Bounty)		400[5]		500		In 50s.
otc sf	**Vitamin C + E Tablets** (Triage)		400[4]		500		Protein coated. Capsule shape. In 50s.
otc	**Ecee Plus Tablets** (Edwards)		165[6]		100	70 mg Mg sulfate, 80 mg Zn sulfate	In 100s.
otc	**Occuvite PreserVision Tablets** (Bausch & Lomb)	7160	100		113	17.4 mg Zn, Cu, lactose	In 120s.

[1] As beta-carotene.
[2] Form of vitamin E unknown; content given in mg.
[3] As beta, alpha and gamma carotene and lycopenes.
[4] As dL-alpha tocopheryl acetate.
[5] In IU; as mixed tocopherols complex.
[6] As d-alpha tocopheryl acid succinate.

For additional information, refer to the Recommended Dietary Allowances monograph.

B VITAMIN COMBINATIONS, ORAL

Content given per capsule, tablet or 5 mL.

	Product & Distributor	B_1 mg	B_2 mg	B_3 mg	B_5 mg	B_6 mg	B_{12} mcg	FA mg	Other Content	How Supplied
otc	**B 100 Tablets** (Fibertone)	100	100	100	100	100	100	0.4	50 mcg biotin, 100 mg PABA, 100 mg choline bitartrate, 100 mg inositol	Sustained-release. In 100s.
otc sf	**B-100 Tablets** (NBTY)	100	100	100	100	100	100	0.1	100 mcg d-biotin, 100 mg base of PABA, choline, inositol and lecithin	In 50s and 100s.
otc	**Mega-B Tablets** (Arco)								100 mg PABA, 100 mg inositol, 100 mcg d-biotin, 100 mg choline bitartrate and lecithin	In 100s.
otc sf	**Super Quints-50 Tablets** (Freeda)	50	50	50	50	50	50	0.4	30 mg PABA, 50 mcg d-biotin, 50 mg inositol	Kosher. In 100s, 250s and 500s.
otc sf	**B Complex-50 Tablets** (Nion)								50 mcg biotin, 50 mg PABA, 50 mg choline bitartrate, 50 mg inositol	Sustained-release. In 100s.
otc sf	**B-50 Tablets** (NBTY)	50	50	50	50	50	50	0.1	50 mcg d-biotin, PABA, choline bitartrate, inositol	In 50s and 100s.
otc	**Iso-B Capsules** (Tyson)	25	25	75	125	50	100	0.2	2.5 mg pyridoxal 5 phosphate, 50 mg PABA, 50 mg inositol, 125 mg choline bitartrate, 100 mcg biotin	In 120s.
otc	**Neurodep-Caps Capsules** (Medical Products)	125				125	1000			In 50s.
otc	**Apatate Liquid** (Kenwood/Bradley)	15				0.5	25			Cherry flavor. In 120 and 240 mL.
otc	**Apatate Tablets** (Kenwood/Bradley)	15				0.5	25			Chewable. Cherry flavor. In 50s.
otc	**B-Complex and B-12 Tablets** (NBTY)	7	14	4.5			25		10 mg protease	In 90s.
Rx sf	**Cerefolin Tablets** (Pan American Labs)		5			50	1000		5.635 mg L-methylfolate	(PAL M5). Blue. In 90s.
otc	**Apetil Liquid** (Kenwood/Bradley)	1.7	0.3	6.7		2.5	5		14.6 mg Zn, Mg, Mn, l-lysine, sucrose, parabens, sorbitol	Alcohol free. In 237 mL.
otc	**B-Complex with B-12 Tablets** (Major)	3	2	20	0.1	1	5			In 100s.
otc sf	**B-Complex with B-12 Tablets** (Goldline)	1.5	1.7	20	10	2	6	0.4		In 100s.
otc	**Almebex Plus B_{12} Liquid** (Dayton)	1	2	5		0.4	5		33 mg choline, parabens, sucrose	In 473 mL with vitamin B_{12} in separate glass container.
otc	**Gevrabon Liquid** (Lederle)	0.83	0.42	8.3	1.67	0.17	0.17		2.5 mg Fe, choline, I, Mg, Mn, 0.3 mg Zn, 18% alcohol, sucrose	In 480 mL.
otc	**Vitamin-Mineral-Supplement Liquid** (Pennex)								I, 2.5 mg Fe, Mg, 0.3 mg Zn, Mn, choline, 18% alcohol, sorbitol, methylparaben, corn syrup	Sherry wine flavor. In 473 mL.
Rx	**Senilezol Liquid** (Edwards)	0.42	0.42	1.67	0.83	0.17	0.83		3.3 mg ferric pyrophosphate, 15% alcohol, sucrose, methylparaben	In 473 mL.
otc	**Eldertonic Liquid** (Mayrand)	0.17	0.19	2.22	1.11	0.22	0.67		1.7 mg Zn, Mg, Mn, 13.5% alcohol	In 240 mL, pt and gal.
otc sf	**Brewers Yeast Tablets** (NBTY)	0.06	0.02	0.2						In 250s.
otc	**Folgard Tablets** (Upsher-Smith)		0.5			10	115	0.8		In 60s.
Rx	**Megaton Elixir** (Hyrex)			4.4	1.1	0.44	1.33	0.1	4 mg Fe, Mn, 1.7 mg Zn, 13% alcohol, parabens, sucrose	Sherry wine flavor. In 473 mL.
Rx	**PremesisRx** (Ther-Rx Corp.)					75	12	1	200 mg Ca	(Ther-Rx 019). Blue, oval. In 100s.
Rx sf	**Cardiotek Rx Tablets** (Stewart-Jackson)					50	500	2	L-arginine hydrochloride	(CAR/RX) Orange, football shape. Coated. In 30s.
Rx sf	**FOLTX Tablets** (PAMLAB)					25	2000	2.5		Dye free. (PAL). Peach. In 90s.
Rx	**ComBgen Tablets** (Ethex)					25	500	2.2		(ETH 440). Beige, oval. In 100s.
Rx	**Folgard RX 2.2** (Upsher-Smith)					25	500	2.2		(US 016). Yellow, oval. Film-coated. In 100s.
Rx sf	**Folpace Tablets** (Alaven)					25	425	2.05	100 units E, 100 mg Mg	(AP 18). In 90s.

B VITAMIN COMBINATIONS, ORAL

	Product & Distributor	B1 mg	B2 mg	B3 mg	B5 mg	B6 mg	B12 mcg	FA mg	Other Content	How Supplied
Rx *sf*	**Calafol Tablets** (Alaven)					25	425	1.6	400 mg Ca, 400 units D_3	(AP 90). In 90s.
Rx	**Folgard** (Upsher-Smith)					10	115	0.8		In 60s.

For additional information, refer to the Recommended Dietary Allowances monograph.

B VITAMINS WITH VITAMIN C, ORAL

Content given per capsule, tablet or 5 mL.

	Product & Distributor	B1 mg	B2 mg	B3 mg	B5 mg	B6 mg	B12 mcg	C mg	Other Content	How Supplied
otc *sf*	**Enviro-Stress Tablets** (Vitaline)	50	50	100	50	50	25	600	0.4 mg FA, 30 mg Zn, 30 IU vitamin E, Mg, Se, PABA	Slow release. In 90s and 1000s.
otc *sf*	**T-Vites Tablets** (Freeda)	25	25	150	25	25		100	30 mcg biotin, PABA, K, Mg carbonate, 2 mg Mn and 20 mg Zn gluconate	Kosher. In 100s.
otc *sf*	**Beminal 500 Tablets** (Whitehall)	25	12.5	100	20	10	5	500	Lactose	In 100s.
otc	**ThexForte Tablets** (Lee)	25	15	100	10	5		500		Capsule shape. In 75s.
otc	**Vicon-C Capsules** (UCB Pharma)	17.9	10	95	22	4		300	6.4 mg Mg, 15.9 mg Zn	In 60s.
otc *sf*	**Viogen-C Capsules** (Goldline)	20	10	100	20	5		300	Mg, 50 mg dried Zn sulfate, tartrazine	In 100s.
Rx	**Berocca Tablets** (Roche)	15	15	100	18	4	5	500	0.5 mg folic acid, sugar	(Berocca Roche). Light green. Capsule shaped. In 100s and 500s.
Rx	**B-Plex Tablets** (Goldline)								0.5 mg folic acid	In 100s.
Rx	**Formula B Tablets** (Major)									In 250s.
Rx	**Strovite Tablets** (Everett)								0.5 mg folic acid, lactose	In 100s.
otc	**Allbee with C Tablets** (Robins)	15	10.2	50	10	5		300	Saccharin, lactose	Capsule shape. In 130s.
otc	**Therapeutic B Complex with C Capsules** (Upsher-Smith)									Yellow/green. In UD 100s.
otc	**B-Complex/Vitamin C Tablets** (Geneva)									Capsule shape. Yellow. In 100s.
otc	**Econo B & C Tablets** (Vangard)									Capsule shape. In 100s and UD 100s.
otc	**Arcobee with C Tablets** (NBTY)								Tartrazine	Capsule shape. In 100s.
otc *sf*	**Farbee with Vitamin C Tablets** (Major)									Capsule shape. In 100s, 130s and 1000s.
otc *sf*	**Gen-bee with C Tablets** (Goldline)									Capsule shape. In 130s and 1000s.
otc *sf*	**Superplex T Tablets** (Major)	15	10	100	20	5	10	500		In 100s.
otc	**Surbex-T Filmtabs** (Abbott)									Orange. In 100s.
otc	**High Potency N-Vites Tablets** (Nion)									In 100s.
otc	**Probec-T Tablets** (Roberts)	12.2	10	100	18.4	4.1	5	600	Sucrose	In 60s.
otc	**3 mg Biotin Forte Tablets** (Vitaline)	10	10	40	10	25	10	200	3 mg biotin, 800 mcg FA, 30 mg Zn	In 60s and 1000s.
otc	**Extra Strength 5 mg Biotin Forte Tablets** (Vitaline)	10	10	40	10	25	10	100	5 mg biotin, 800 mcg FA	In 60s and 1000s.
otc	**B Complex + C Tablets** (Various, eg, Nion)	15	10	100	20	5	10	500		Timed release. In 100s.
otc	**Surbex with C Filmtabs** (Abbott)	6	6	30	10	2.5	5	250	Lactose	Film coated. In 100s.
otc	**Sublingual B Total Liquid** (Pharmaceutical Lab)		1.7	20	30	2	1000	60	Sorbitol	Alcohol free. In 30 mL with dropper.

B VITAMINS WITH VITAMIN C, ORAL

	Product & Distributor	B_1 mg	B_2 mg	B_3 mg	B_5 mg	B_6 mg	B_{12} mcg	C mg	Other Content	How Supplied
Rx	**Nephplex Rx Tablets** (Nephro-Tech)	1.5	1.7	20	10	10	6	60	1 mg FA, 300 mcg d–biotin, 12.5 mg Zn	In 100s.
Rx	**Nephro-Vite Rx Tablets** (R & D)									(RD 12). Yellow. Film coated. In 100s.
Rx *sf*	**Hemovit Tablets** (Dayton)								1 mg FA, 300 mcg d–biotin	Dye-free. (HT). Yellow. Film-coated. In blister 100s.
otc	**Nephro-Vite Vitamin B Complex and C Supplement Tablets** (R & D)								800 mcg FA, 300 mcg d-biotin	(RD 02). Yellow. Film coated. In 100s.
Rx	**Nephrocaps Capsules** (Fleming)	1.5	1.7	20	5	10	6	100	1 mg FA, 150 mcg biotin	(F). Black. Oval. In 100s.
otc	**Full Spectrum B** (National Vitamin)	1.5	1.7	20	10	10	6	60	800 mcg FA, 3 mg biotin	Preservative- and sugar-free. In 100s.
otc	**Dialyvite 3000** (Hillestad)	1.5	1.7	20	10	25	1000	100	3 mg FA, 300 mcg biotin, 30 units E, 70 mcg Zn.	In 90s.
Rx *sf*	**DexFol Tablets** (Rising)	1.5	1.5	20	10	50	1	60	5 mg FA, 300 mcg biotin	(R128). White. In 90s.
Rx	**Diatx Tablets** (Pan American)	1.5	1.5	20	10	50	1	60	5 mg FA, 300 mcg D-biotin.	Dye free. (PAL 5). Yellow. In 90s.
otc	**Stress B Complex with Vitamin C Tablets** (Mission)	13.8	10	50		4.1		300	15 mg Zn	Timed- release. In 60s.

For additional information, refer to the Recommended Dietary Allowances monograph.

LIPOTROPICS WITH VITAMINS

Content given per capsule or tablet.

	Product & Distributor	Choline (mg)	Inositol (mg)	Methionine (mg)	B_1 mg	B_2 mg	B_3 mg	B_5 mg	B_6 mg	B_{12} mcg	C mg	Other Content	How Supplied
otc	**Lipogen Capsules** (Various, eg, Rugby)	111[1]	†		0.33	0.33	3.33	1.7	0.33	1.7	100	Bioflavonoids, sorbitol, lecithin	In 60s.
otc	**Lipotriad Tablets** (Numark)	†	†		1.5	1.7	20	10	2	6	60	5000 IU vitamin A (as beta carotene), 30 IU E,[2] 30 mg Zn, Cu, Se	In 60s.
otc	**Lipoflavonoid Tablets** (Numark)	111	111		0.33	0.33	3.33	1.66	0.33	1.66	100	100 mg lemon bioflavonoid complex	In 100s and 500s.
otc *sf*	**Cholinoid Capsules** (Goldline)	111[1]	111		0.33	0.33	3.33	1.7	0.33	1.7	100	100 mg lemon bioflavonoid complex	In 100s.

* † – Amount not supplied by manufacturer.
[1] From choline bitartrate.
[2] Form of vitamin E unknown.

For additional information, refer to the Recommended Dietary Allowances monograph.

MULTIVITAMINS, CAPSULES, TABLETS, AND WAFERS

Content given per capsule, tablet, or wafer.

	Product & Distributor	A IU	D IU	E IU	B_1 mg	B_2 mg	B_3 mg	B_5 mg	B_6 mg	B_{12} mcg	C mg	FA mg	Other Content and How Supplied
otc	**Oncovite** (Mission)	10,000	400	200	0.37	0.5	5	2.5	25	1.5	500	0.4	Sugar. 7.5 mg Zn. In 100s.
otc *sf*	**Quintabs Tablets** (Freeda)	10,000	400	29[1]	25	25	100	25	25	25	300	0.1	Inositol, PABA. Kosher. In 100s and 250s.
otc	**Nutrox Capsules** (Tyson)	10,000		150[2]	25	25	50	22			80		L-cysteine, taurine, glutathione, 15 mg zinc oxide, Se. In 90s.
otc	**Optilets-500 Filmtabs** (Abbott)	50,000	400	30[3]	15	10	100	20	5	12	500[4]		Film-coated. In 120s.
otc	**Adavite Tablets** (Hudson)	5000	400	30[1]	3	3.4	30	10	3	9	90	0.4	35 mcg biotin, 1250 IU beta carotene. In 130s.
otc	**Theravee Tablets** (Vangard)	5500	400	30[1]	3	3.4	30	10	3	9	120	0.4	15 mcg biotin. In 100s and UD 100s.
otc	**One-A-Day Men's Vitamin Tablets** (Bayer)	5000	400	45[1]	2.25	2.55	20	10	3	9	200	0.4	(One-A-Day). In 60s and 100s.
otc	**Therapeutic Tablets** (Goldline)	5000	400	30[3]	3	3.4	20	10	3	9	90	0.4	30 mcg d-biotin. In 100s and 130s.

MULTIVITAMINS, CAPSULES, TABLETS, AND WAFERS

	Product & Distributor	A IU	D IU	E IU	B_1 mg	B_2 mg	B_3 mg	B_5 mg	B_6 mg	B_{12} mcg	C mg	FA mg	Other Content and How Supplied
otc	**Therems Tablets** (Rugby)	5000	400	30[3]	3	3.4	30	10	3	9	120	0.4	15 mcg biotin, 1250 IU beta carotene. In 130s and 1000s.
otc sf	**One-A-Day Essential Tablets** (Bayer)	5000	400	30[1]	1.5	1.7	20	10	2	6	60	0.4	In 75s and 130s.
otc	**One-Tablet-Daily Tablets** (Various, eg, Goldline)												In 365s and 1000s.
otc	**Tab-A-Vite Tablets** (Major)			30[3]									In 30s, 100s, 250s, 1000s and UD 100s.
otc	**Sigtab Tablets** (Roberts)	5000	400	15[1]	10.3	10	100	20	6	18	333	0.4	Sucrose. In 90s and 500s.
otc	**Multi-Day Tablets** (NBTY)	5000	400	30[1]	1.5	1.7	20	10	2	6	60	0.4	In 100s.
otc sf	**Unicap Tablets** (Upjohn)	5000	400	15[1]	1.5	1.7	20		2	6	60	0.4	Tartrazine. In 120s.
otc	**Multivitamins Capsules** (Solvay)	5000	400	10[3]	2.5	2.5	20	5	0.5	2	50		(0032–1204). Oval. Brown. In 100s and UD 100s.
otc sf	**Oxi-Freeda Tablets** (Freeda)			150[1]	20	20	40	20	20	10	100		5000 IU beta carotene, glutathione, L-cysteine, Se, 15 mg Zn. Kosher. In 100s and 250s.
otc	**Sesame Street Plus Extra C Tablets** (McNeil-CPC)	2750	200	10[1]	0.75	0.85	10	5	0.7	3	80	0.2	Sucrose, lactose. Chewable. Character shapes. In 50s.
otc sf	**Bugs Bunny with Extra C Children's Tablets** (Bayer)	2500	400	15[1]	1.05	1.2	13.5		1.05	4.5	250	0.3	Chewable. Fruit flavors. In 60s.
otc	**Flintstones Plus Extra C Children's Tablets** (Bayer)												Chewable. Character shapes. In 60s and 100s.
otc sf	**Sunkist Multi-Vitamins + Extra C Tablets** (Ciba)												5 mcg vitamin K, sorbitol, aspartame, phenylalanine. Citrus flavor. In 60s.
otc	**Animal Shapes Tablets** (Major)	2500	400		1.05	1.2	13.5		1.05	4.5	60	0.3	In 100s and 250s.
otc	**Garfield Chewable Tablets** (Menley & James)												Sucrose, lactose. Character shapes. In 60s.
otc	**Bounty Bears Tablets** (NBTY)												In 100s.
otc	**Mediplex Plus Tablets** (US Pharm)			50[3]	25	10	100	25	10	25	300	0.4	18 mg Zn, Cu, Mg, Mn. In 100s.
otc	**Allbee C-800 Tablets** (Robins)			45[1]	15	17	100	25	25	12	800		Lactose. (AHR). Elliptical. In 60s.
otc	**Stress Formula Vitamins Capsules and Tablets** (Various, eg, Goldline)			30[1]	10	10	100	20	5	12	500	0.4	**Capsules**: 45 mcg biotin. In 100s. **Tablets**: 45 mcg biotin. In 60s.
otc	**Stress Formula w/Zinc Tablets** (Various)												45 mcg biotin, 23.9 mg Zn, Cu. In 60s.
otc	**Stress Formula 600 Tablets** (Vangard)			30[3]	15	10	100	20	5	12	500	0.4	45 mcg biotin. In UD 100s.
otc	**Stresstabs Tablets** (Lederle)			30[3]	10	10	100	20	5	12	500	0.4	45 mcg biotin. In 60s.
Rx	**Cefol Filmtab Tablets** (Abbott)			30[3]	15	10	100	20	5	6	750	0.5	(NJ). Green. Film coated. In 100s.

[1] Form of vitamin E unknown.
[2] As d-alpha tocopheryl acid succinate.
[3] As dL-alpha tocopheryl acetate.
[4] As d-alpha tocopheryl succinate.

For a comparison of the potencies of the various forms of vitamin E, see the vitamin E monograph.

MULTIVITAMINS, DROPS AND LIQUIDS

	Product & Distributor	Content Given Per	A IU	D IU	E IU	B_1 mg	B_2 mg	B_3 mg	B_5 mg	B_6 mg	B_{12} mcg	C mg	Other Content	How Supplied
otc	**Certagen Liquid** (Goldline)	15 mL	2500	400	30[1]	1.5	1.7	20	10	2	6	60	6.6% alcohol. 300 mcg biotin, 9 mg Fe, 3 mg Zn, Cr, I, Mn, Mo	In 237 mL.
otc	**Syrvite Liquid**[1] (Various, eg, Major)	5 mL	2500	400	15[2]	1.05	1.2	13.5		1.05	4.5	60		In 480 mL.
otc	**Daily Vitamins Liquid** (Rugby)												Sugar, parabens, corn syrup,	In 237 and 473 mL.
otc	**Vi-Daylin Multivitamin Liquid** (Ross)				15[3]								≤ 0.5% alcohol, glucose, sucrose, methylparaben	Lemon/orange flavor. In 240 and 480 mL.
otc sf	**LKV Infant Drops** (Freeda)	0.6 mL	2500	400	5[2]	1	1	10	3	1	4	50	75 mcg biotin	In 60 mL after mixing powder and liquid.

MULTIVITAMINS, DROPS AND LIQUIDS

	Product & Distributor	Content Given Per	A IU	D IU	E IU	B_1 mg	B_2 mg	B_3 mg	B_5 mg	B_6 mg	B_{12} mcg	C mg	Other Content	How Supplied
otc	**ADEKs Pediatric Drops** (Scandipharm)	1 mL	1500	400	40[4]	0.5	0.6	6	3	0.6	4	45	0.1 mg vitamin K, 15 mcg biotin, 5 mg zinc, 1 mg beta carotene	In 60 mL.
otc	**Poly-Vi-Sol Drops** (Mead Johnson)	1 mL	1500	400	5[2]	0.5	0.6	8		0.4	2	35		In 30 and 50 mL.
otc sf	**Baby Vitamin Drops** (Goldline)													Alcohol free. In 50 mL.
otc sf	**Poly-Vitamin Drops** (Schein)				5[3]									Alcohol free. In 50 mL.
otc sf	**Vi-Daylin Multivitamin Drops** (Ross)	1 mL	1500	400	5[5]	0.5	0.6	8		0.4	1.5	35	< 0.5% alcohol, methylparaben, EDTA	Fruit flavor. In 50 mL.
otc	**Thera Multi-Vitamin Liquid** (Major)	5 mL	10,000	400		10	10	100	21.4	4.1	5	200	Sucrose, methylparaben	In 118 mL.
otc	**Theravite Liquid** (Barre-National)												Sugar, methylparaben	In 118 mL.

[1] May contain alcohol.
[2] Form of vitamin E unknown.
[3] As d-alpha tocopheryl acetate.
[4] As d-alpha tocopheryl polyethylene glycol-1000 succinate.
[5] As d-alpha tocopheryl acid succinate.

For a comparison of the potencies of various forms of vitamin E, see the Vitamin E monograph.

MULTIVITAMINS WITH IRON

Content given per capsule, tablet or liquid dose.

	Product & Distributor	Fe[1] mg	A IU	D IU	E IU	B_1 mg	B_2 mg	B_3 mg	B_5 mg	B_6 mg	B_{12} mcg	C mg	FA mg	Other Content and How Supplied
otc	**CenogenUltra** (US Pharmaceutical)	106				10	6	30	10	5	15	200	1	Cu, Mn. (US CENOGEN ULTRA/140). Blue/Pink. In UD 100s.
otc	**Dayalets + Iron Filmtabs** (Abbott)	18	5000	400	30[3]	1.5	1.7	20		2	6	60	0.4	Film coated. In 100s.
otc sf	**One-Tablet-Daily with Iron** (Goldline)	18	5000	400	30[3]	1.5	1.7	20	10	2	6	60	0.4	In 100s.
otc	**Tab-A-Vite + Iron Tablets** (Major)													Tartrazine. In 100s.
otc sf	**Multi-Day Plus Iron Tablets** (NBTY)	18	5000	400	15[2]	1.5	1.7	20		2	6	60	0.4	In 100s.
otc	**Sesame Street Plus Iron Tablets** (McNeil-CPC)	10	2750	200	10[2]	0.75	0.85	10	5	0.7	3	40	0.2	Chewable. Character shapes. In 50s.
otc	**Animal Shapes + Iron Tablets** (Major)	15	2500	400	15[3]	1.05	1.2	13.5		1.05	4.5	60	0.3	In 100s and 250s.
otc	**Bounty Bears Plus Iron Tablets** (NBTY)				15[2]									Chewable. In 100s.
otc sf	**Bugs Bunny Plus Iron Tablets** (Bayer)													Chewable. In 60s.
otc	**Flintstones Plus Iron Tablets** (Bayer)													Chewable. Character shapes. In 60s and 100s.
otc	**Vi-Daylin Multivitamin + Iron Liquid** (Ross)	10	2500	400	15[4]	1.05	1.2	13.5		1.05	4.5	60		Per 5 mL. ≤ 0.5% alcohol, glucose, sucrose, parabens. Lemon/lime flavor. In 237 and 473 mL.
otc sf	**Baby Vitamin Drops with Iron** (Goldline)	10	1500	400	5[2]	0.5	0.6	8		0.4		35		Per 1 mL. In 50 mL.
otc	**Poly-Vi-Sol with Iron Drops** (Mead Johnson)													Per 1 mL. In 50 mL.
otc	**Polyvitamin Drops with Iron** (Various, eg, Rugby)													Per 1 mL. In 50 mL.
otc sf	**Multi-Vit Drops w/Iron** (Barre-National)													Per 1 mL. Methylparaben. In 50 mL.
otc sf	**Vi-Daylin Multivitamin + Iron Drops** (Ross)													Per 1 mL. Methylparaben, flavor. In 50 mL.
Rx sf	**Diatx Fe Tablets** (Pan American)	100				1.5	1.5	20	10	50	1	60	5	300 mcg D-biotin. Dye free. (PAL 5FE). Red. In 90s.

MULTIVITAMINS WITH IRON

	Product & Distributor	Fe[1] mg	A IU	D IU	E IU	B_1 mg	B_2 mg	B_3 mg	B_5 mg	B_6 mg	B_{12} mcg	C mg	FA mg	Other Content and How Supplied
otc sf	**Vi-Daylin ADC Vitamins + Iron Drops** (Ross)	10	1500	400								35		Per 1 mL. Methylparaben. Fruit flavor. In 50 mL.
otc	**Tri-Vi-Sol with Iron Drops** (Mead Johnson)													Per 1 mL. Fruit-like flavor. In 50 mL.
otc	**Simron Plus Capsules** (SmithKline Beecham)	10								1	3.3	50	0.1	Parabens. In 100s.
Rx	**NataChew** (Warner Chilcott)	29[5]	1000	400	11[3]	2	3			10	12	120	1	20 mg niacinamide. Chewable. (WC 227). Tan, speckled, bisected. Wildberry flavor. In 90s.
Rx	**NataFort** (Warner Chilcott)	60[6]	1000	400	11	2	3			10	12	120	1	20 mg niacinamide. (NataFort). Lactose. White. Film-coated. In UDs 90s.

[1] Iron content expressed in mg elemental iron.
[2] Form of vitamin E unknown.
[3] As dL-alpha tocopheryl acetate.
[4] As d-alpha tocopheryl acid succinate.
[5] As ferrous fumarate.
[6] As carbonyl iron and ferrous sulfate.

These products contain supplemental iron; products containing therapeutic amounts of iron (> 25 mg) with vitamins are listed in the blood modifiers section. For a comparison of the potencies of various forms of vitamin E, see the Vitamin E monograph.

MULTIVITAMINS WITH FLUORIDE, CAPSULES AND TABLETS

Content given per capsule or tablet.

	Product & Distributor	F[1] mg	A IU	D IU	E IU	B_1 mg	B_2 mg	B_3 mg	B_5 mg	B_6 mg	B_{12} mcg	C mg	FA mg	Other Content and How Supplied
otc	**Monocal Tablets** (Mericon)	3												250 mg Ca. In 100s.
Rx	**Adeflor M Tablets** (Kenwood/Bradley)	1	6000	400		1.5	2.5	20	10	10	2	100		250 mg Ca, 30 mg Fe, sorbitol, sucrose. Pink. Elliptical. In 100s.
Rx	**Mulvidren-F Softab Tablets** (Wyeth-Ayerst)	1	4000	400		1.6	2	10	2.8	1	3	75		Saccharin. (Stuart 710). Chewable. Orange, scored. In 100s.
Rx	**Poly Vitamins Fluoride Tablets**[2] (Various, eg, Schein)	1	2,500	400	15[3]	1.05	1.2	13.5		1.05	4.5	60	0.3	In 100s.
Rx	**Chewable Multivitamins w/Fluoride Tablets** (Moore)				15[4]									Sucrose. Fruit flavor. In 100s.
Rx	**Florvite Tablets** (Everett)													Sucrose. Chewable. Fruit flavors. In 100s.
Rx	**Poly-Vi-Flor Tablets 1.0 mg** (Mead Johnson Nutritionals)													Sucrose. (MJ 474). Chewable. In 100s and 1000s.
Rx	**Poly-Vi-Flor with Iron 1.0 mg Tablets** (Mead Johnson Nutritionals)													Cu, 12 mg Fe, 10 mg Zn, sucrose. Chewable. In 100s and 1000s.
Rx	**Polyvitamin Fluoride Tablets w/Iron** (Various, eg, Rugby, Schein)													Cu, 12 mg Fe, 10 mg Zn. Chewable. In 100s.
Rx	**Vi-Daylin/F Chewable Multivitamin Tablets** (Ross)													Chewable. In 100s.
Rx	**Vi-Daylin/F Multivitamins + Iron Chewable Tablets** (Ross)													12 mg Fe, sucrose. Cherry flavor. In 100s.
Rx	**Tri-Vi-Flor 1.0 mg Tablets** (Mead Johnson Nutritionals)	1	2500	400								60		Sucrose. Chewable. Fruit flavor. In 100s.
Rx	**Chewable Triple Vitamins with Fluoride Tablets** (Major)													Dextrose, sucrose. Fruit flavor. In 100s.
Rx	**Trivitamin Fluoride Tablets** (Schein)													Sucrose. Chewable. Fruit flavor. In 100s.

MULTIVITAMINS WITH FLUORIDE, CAPSULES AND TABLETS

	Product & Distributor	F[1] mg	A IU	D IU	E IU	B_1 mg	B_2 mg	B_3 mg	B_5 mg	B_6 mg	B_{12} mcg	C mg	FA mg	Other Content and How Supplied
Rx	**Poly Vitamins w/Fluoride 0.5 Tablets**[2] (Various, eg, Goldline, Rugby, Schein)	0.5	2500	400	15[4]	1.05	1.2	13.5		1.05	4.5	60	0.3	In 100s and 1000s.
Rx	**Poly-Vi-Flor 0.5 mg Tablets** (Mead Johnson Nutritionals)													Lactose, sucrose. (MJ 468). Chewable. Fruit flavor. In 100s.
Rx	**Poly-Vi-Flor 0.5 mg w/Iron Tablets** (Mead Johnson Nutritionals)													Cu, 12 mg Fe, 10 mg Zn, lactose, sucrose. (482 MJ). Chewable. Fruit flavor. In 100s.
Rx	**Polyvitamins w/Fluoride 0.5 mg and Iron Tablets** (Rugby)													Cu, 12 mg Fe, 10 mg Zn, sucrose. Chewable. Cherry flavor. In 100s.
Rx	**Poly-Vi-Flor Tablets 0.25 mg** (Mead Johnson Nutritionals)	0.25	2500	400	15[4]	1.05	1.2	13.5		1.05	4.5	60	0.3	Lactose, sucrose. (MJ 487)Chewable. Fruit flavor. In 100s.
Rx	**Poly-Vi-Flor 0.25 mg Tablets w/Iron** (Mead Johnson Nutritionals)													Cu, 12 mg Fe, 10 mg Zn, lactose, sucrose. (MJ 488). Chewable. Fruit flavor. In 100s.

[1] Fluoride content expressed in mg elemental fluoride.
[2] May be chewable.
[3] Form of vitamin E unknown.
[4] As dL–alpha tocopheryl acetate.

MULTIVITAMINS WITH FLUORIDE CAPSULES AND TABLETS

For a comparison of the potencies of various forms of vitamin E, see the Vitamin E monograph.

Indications

Used for prophylaxis of vitamin deficiencies and as an aid in the prevention of dental caries in infants and children where the fluoride content of the drinking water does not exceed 0.7 ppm. For complete prescribing information on fluoride-containing products, refer to the Fluoride group mongraph.

MULTIVITAMINS WITH FLUORIDE, DROPS

	Product & Distributor	Content Given Per	F[1] mg	A IU	D IU	E IU	B_1 mg	B_2 mg	B_3 mg	B_5 mg	B_6 mg	B_{12} mcg	C mg	Other Content and How Supplied
Rx	**Polyvitamin w/Fluoride Drops** (Various, eg, Rugby	1 mL	0.5	1,500	400	5[2]	0.5	0.6	8		0.4	2	35	In 50 mL.
Rx	**Poly-Vi-Flor 0.5 mg Drops** (Mead Johnson Nutritionals)					5[3]								Fruit flavor. In 50 mL.
Rx	**Poly-Vi-Flor with Iron 0.5 mg Drops** (Mead Johnson Nutritionals)	1 mL	0.5	1,500	400	5[3]	0.5	0.6			0.4		35	10 mg Fe.[4] Fruit flavor. In 50 mL.
Rx	**ADC with Fluoride Drops** (Various, eg, Hi-Tech, Major)	1 mL	0.5	1,500	400								35	Methylparaben. In 50 mL.
Rx	**Tri-A-Vite F Drops** (Major)													In 50 mL.
Rx	**Tri-Vi-Flor 0.5 mg Drops** (Mead-Johnson)													Fruit flavor. In 50 mL.
Rx	**Tri-Vitamin w/Fluoride Drops** (Rugby)													In 50 mL.
Rx	**Tri Vit w/Fluoride 0.5 mg Drops** (Barre-National)													In 50 mL.
Rx *sf*	**Polyvitamin Fluoride Drops** (Various, eg, Goldline, Hi-Tech, Major, Rugby)	1 mL	0.25	1,500	400	5[5]	0.5	0.6	8		0.4	2	35	Alcohol free. In 50 mL.
Rx	**Poly-Vi-Flor 0.25 mg Drops** (Mead Johnson Nutritionals)					5[3]								Fruit flavor. In 50 mL.
Rx	**Florvite Drops** (Everett)					5[2]								Fruit flavor. In 50 mL.
Rx	**Multivitamin and Fluoride Drops** (Major)													In 50 mL.
Rx	**Polyvitamin Drops w/Iron and Fluoride** (Various, eg, Goldline, Hi-Tech, Rugby, Schein)	1 mL	0.25	1,500	400	5[3]	0.5	0.6	8		0.4		35	10 mg Fe.[4] In 50 mL.
Rx	**Poly-Vi-Flor with Iron 0.25 mg Drops** (Mead Johnson Nutritionals)													10 mg Fe.[4] In 50 mL.
Rx *sf*	**Vi-Daylin/F Multivitamin Drops** (Ross)													Methylparaben, < 0.1% alcohol. Fruit flavor. In 50 mL.
Rx *sf*	**Vi-Daylin/F Multivitamin + Iron Drops** (Ross)													10 mg Fe,[5] < 0.1% alcohol, methylparaben. Fruit flavor. In 50 mL.

MULTIVITAMINS WITH FLUORIDE, DROPS

	Product & Distributor	Content Given Per	F[1] mg	A IU	D IU	E IU	B_1 mg	B_2 mg	B_3 mg	B_5 mg	B_6 mg	B_{12} mcg	C mg	Other Content and How Supplied
Rx	**Tri-Vi-Flor 0.25 mg Drops** (Mead Johnson Nutritionals)	1 mL	0.25	1500	400								35	Fruit flavor. In 50 mL.
Rx sf	**Trivitamin Fluoride Drops** (Various, eg, Schein)													Alcohol free. In 50 mL.
Rx sf	**Vi-Daylin/F ADC Vitamins Drops** (Ross)													≈ 0.3% alcohol, parabens. Fruit flavor. In 50 mL.
Rx	**Tri-Vi-Flor 0.25 mg with Iron Drops** (Mead Johnson Nutritionals)	1 mL												10 mg Fe.[4] In 50 mL.
Rx sf	**Vi-Daylin/F ADC + Iron Drops** (Ross)													10 mg Fe,[4] methylparaben. Fruit flavor. In 50 mL.
Rx	**Tri Vit w/Fluoride 0.25 mg Drops** (Barre-National)													In 50 mL.
Rx	**Apatate w/Fluoride Liquid** (Kenwood/Bradley)	5 mL	0.5				15				0.5	25		Cherry flavor. In 120 mL.

[1] Fluoride content expressed in mg elemental fluoride.
[2] As dL–alpha tocopheryl acetate.
[3] As d-alpha tocopheryl acid succinate.
[4] Iron content expressed in mg elemental iron.
[5] Form of vitamin E unknown.

For complete prescribing information on fluoride-containing products, refer to the Fluoride group monograph. For a comparison of the potencies of the various forms of vitamin E, see the vitamin E monograph.

MULTIVITAMINS WITH CALCIUM AND IRON

Content given per tablet or capsule.

	Product & Distributor	Ca[a] mg	Fe[s] mg	A IU	D IU	E IU	B_1 mg	B_2 mg	B_3 mg	B_5 mg	B_6 mg	B_{12} mcg	C mg	FA mg	Other Content	How Supplied
otc sf	**One-A-Day Women's Formula Tablets** (Bayer)	450	27	5,000	400	30[b]	1.5	1.7	20	10	2	6	60	0.4	15 mg Zn, tartrazine	In 60s and 100s.
otc sf	**K.P.N. Tablets** (Freeda)	333[c]	11	2,667	133	10[b]	2	2	10	3.3	0.83	2	33	0.27	Cu, I, K, Mg, Mn, 6.7 mg Zn, bioflavonoids	Kosher. In 100s and 250s.
Rx	**Mynatal Capsules** (ME Pharm)	300	65	5,000	400	30[d]	3	3.4	20	10	10	12	120	1	30 mcg biotin, Cr, Cu, I, Mg, Mn, Mo, 25 mg Zn	In 100s and 500s.
otc	**One-A-Day WeightSmart Tablets** (Bayer)	300	18[f]	2,500	400	30[b]	1.9	2.125	25	12.5	2.5	7.5		400[e]	Vitamin K, Mg, Zn, Se, Cu, Mn, Cr, EGCG, dextrose, glucose.	In 50s and 100s.
Rx	**Obstetrix-100** (Seyer[g])	250	100	2,700	400	30[b]	3	3.4	20		20	12	250	1	25 mg Zn, 50 mg sodium docusate	(SEYER OBX-100). Pink, oval, scored. In UD 30s.
Rx	**Prenate 90 Tablets** (Bock)	250	90	4,000	400	30[b]	3	3.4	20		20	12	120	1	DSS, Cu, I, 25 mg Zn	Dye free. Delayed-release. (Bock PN90). Film-coated. In 100s.
Rx	**Mynate 90 Plus Caplets** (ME Pharm)															Delayed-release. In 100s.
Rx	**Prenatal MR 90 Tablets** (Ethex)															Delayed-release. (Ethex 212). Oval. Film coated. In 100s.
Rx	**Par-F Tablets** (Pharmics)	250	60	5,000	400	30[b]	3	3.4	20	10	12	12	120	1	Cu, I, Mg, 15 mg Zn	In 100s.
Rx	**Mynatal FC Caplets** (ME Pharm)	250	60	5,000	400	30[b]	3	3.4	20	10	10	12	100	1	30 mcg biotin, 25 mg Zn, I, Mg, Cr, Cu, Mo, Mn	In 100s.
Rx	**Mynatal P.N. Forte Caplets** (ME Pharm)	250	60	5,000	400	30[b]	3	3.4	20		4	12	80	1	25 mg Zn, I, Mg, Cu	In 100s.
Rx	**Niferex-PN Forte Tablets** (Ther-Rx)					30[d]									Cu, I, Mg, 25 mg Zn	Dye free. (SP 2309 1 0). White. Capsule shape. Film-coated. In 100s.
Rx	**Prenatal Maternal Tablets** (Ethex)	250	60	5,000	400	30[b]	2.9	3.4	20	10	12.2	12	100	1	Cr, Cu, I, Mg, Mn, Mo, 25 mg Zn, 30 mcg biotin	In 100s.
Rx	**Marnatal-F Tablets** (Marnel)	250	60	4,000	400	30[d]	3	3.4	20		5	12	100	1	Mg, 25 mg Zn, Cu, I	(Marnatal-F). Lt. pink. Film-coated. In 30s and 100s.
Rx	**NovaCare Tablets** (Fielding)	250	40		240	3.5[d]	3	3.4	20		20	12	50	1	15 mg Zn, Cu, Mg.	(SU 01). Peach. Film-coated. In blister card 100s.
Rx	**Prenatal PC 40** (Integrity)														15 mg Zn, Cu, Mg	Polydextrose. Capsule shape. Film coated. In UD 100s.
Rx	**PreCare** (Ther-Rx Corp.)	250	40			3.5					2		50	1	6 mcg vit. D_3, 50 mg Mg, 15 mg Zn, 2 mg Cu, mannitol, sucrose	(THER-RX 025). Orange. Vanilla flavor. In UD 100s.
otc sf	**Os-Cal Fortified** (GlaxoSmithKline)	250	5		125	0.8	1.7	1.7	15		2		50		3 mg Mg, 0.5 mg Zn, 0.5 mg Mn, corn syrup solids, parabens, EDTA	In 100s.

MULTIVITAMINS WITH CALCIUM AND IRON

	Product & Distributor	Ca[a] mg	Fe[s] mg	A IU	D IU	E IU	B_1 mg	B_2 mg	B_3 mg	B_5 mg	B_6 mg	B_{12} mcg	C mg	FA mg	Other Content	How Supplied
Rx	**Embrex 600 Chewable Tablets** (Andrx)	240	90	3500	400	30[h]	2	3			3	12	60	1	20 mg Zn, Cu, Mg, 50 mg dioctylsulfosuccinate sodium.	(CTEX P N). Blue, oval, scored. Orange flavor. In blister pack 35s and 91s.
Rx	**Advanced-RF Natal Care Tablets** (Ethex)	200	90		400	30[b]	3	3.4			20	12	120	1	2 mg Cu, 50 mg docusate sodium, 20 mg niacinamide, 30 mg Mg, 25 mg Zn.	Dye-free. (ETHEX/458). White, oval. In 90s.
Rx	**Ultra-NatalCare** (Ethex)	200[i]	90[j]	2,700	400	30[d]	3	3.4			20	12	120	1	200 mg I, 2 mg Cu, 25 mg Zn, 20 mg niacinamide, 50 mg docusate sodium.	Dye free. (PEC 123). White, oval, bisected. In UD 100s.
Rx	**Vinate GT Tablets** (Breckenridge)	200	90	2,700	400	10[b]	3	3.4	20	6	20	12	120	1	30 mcg biotin, 50 mg docusate sodium, 15 mg Zn, Cu, Mg.	Purple, oval. In UD 90s.
Rx	**Prenatal AD Tablets** (Cypress)	200	90	2700	400	30[d]	3	3.4	20		20	12	120	1	25 mg Zn, Cu, Mg, 50 mg docusate sodium.	(CYP 194). White, oval. In 90s.
Rx	**Nu-Natal Advanced Tablets** (Rising)	200	90		400	30[d]	3	3.4	20		20	12	120	1	50 mg dioctyl sodium sulfosuccinate, 30 mg Mg, 25 mg Zn, 2 mg Cu	(RIS 125). White, oval, film coated. In UD 90s.
Rx sf	**O-Cal f.a. Tablets** (Pharmics)	200	66	5,000	400	30[b]	3	3	20		4	12	90	1	1.1 mg F, Mg, I, Cu, 15 mg Zn	In 100s.
Rx	**Prenatal Plus** (Goldline)	200	65	4,000	400	22[b]	1.84	3	20		10	12	120	1	2 mg Cu, 25 mg Zn	In 100s.
Rx	**Prenatal Plus w/ Betacarotene Tablets** (Rugby)	200	65	4,000	400	11	1.84	3	20		10	12	120	1	25 mg Zn, Cu	In 100s and 500s.
Rx	**Prenatal Plus-Improved Tablets** (Rugby)	200	65	4,000	400	11[b]	1.5	3	20		10	12	120	1	Cu, 25 mg Zn	In 100s.
Rx	**Prenatal-1 + Iron Tablets** (Various, eg, ESI, Goldline, Qualitest, Schein)															In 100s and 500s.
Rx	**Par-Natal Plus 1 Improved Tablets** (Parmed)															In 500s.
Rx	**Lactocal-F Tablets** (Laser)	200	65	4,000	400	30[d]	3	3.4	20		5	12	100	1	Cu, I, Mg, 15 mg Zn	(Laser 173). White. Oval. Film-coated. In 100s and 1000s.
Rx	**Prenatal Z Advanced Formula** (Ethex)	200	65	3,000	400	10	1.5	1.6	17		2.2	2.2	70	1	175 mcg potassium iodide, 100 mg magnesium oxide, 15 mg zinc oxide	In 100s.
Rx	**NataTab Rx Tablets** (Ethex)	200	29	4,000	400	30	3	3	20	7	3	8	120	1	30 mcg biotin, 15 mg Zn, Cu, I, Mg	(ETHEX 376). Yellow, oval, scored. Film-coated. In 90s.
Rx	**Prenatabs RX Tablets** (Cypress)														30 mcg biotin, 15 mg Zn, Cu, I, Mg	(CYP 193). White, oval. Film-coated. In 90s.
Rx	**Duet Tablets** (Integrity)	200	29	3,000	400	30	1.8	4	20		25	12	120	1	Cu, Zn, Mg	Sucrose. (82). Yellow, oval. In 100s.
Rx	**Prenatal 19 Tablets** (Cypress)	200	29	1000	400	30[d]	3	3	15	7	20	12	100	1	20 mg Zn, 25 mg docusate sodium.	(CYP196). White, oval, scored. In 100s.
Rx	**Prenatal 19 Chewable Tablets** (Cypress)														20 mg Zn, 25 mg docusate sodium.	(CYP 197). Orange. Orange flavor. In 100s.
Rx	**Vinate Good Start Chewable Prenatal Formula Tablets** (Breckenridge)														20 mg Zn.	(B 151). Off-white, mottled. In 100s.
otc	**Stuart Prenatal Tablets** (Integrity)	200	28	4000	400	30	1.8	1.7	20		2.6	8	120	0.8	25 mg Zn	In 100s.
Rx	**StuartNatal Plus 3 Tablets** (Integrity)	200	28	3000	400	22[d]	1.8	4	20		25	12	120	1	25 mg Zn, Cu, Mg	(Plus 3). Yellow, oval. In 100s.
Rx	**Trinate Tablets** (Cypress)														25 mg Zn, Cu, Mg.	(CYP 192). White, oval. In 100s.
Rx	**Anemagen OB Capsules** (Ethex)	200	28		400	30	1.6	1.8			20	12	60	1	Docusate calsium	Parabens. (ETH 052). Green. In 100s.
Rx	**NatalCare Three Tablets** (Ethex)	200	27	3000	400	22	1.8	4	20		25	12	120	1	25 mg Zn, Cu, Mg	(ETHEX 375). Beige, oval. In 100s.
Rx	**Enfamil Natalins Rx Tablets** (Mead-Johnson)	100	27	2000	200	7.5[e]	0.75	0.8	8.5	3.5	2	1.25	40	0.5	15 mcg biotin, 1.5 mg Cu, 50 mg Mg	(MJ 702). White. Oval. In 200s.
Rx	**Mynatal Rx Caplets** (ME Pharm)	200	60	4,000	400	15[b]	1.5	1.6	17	7	4	2.5	80	1	30 mcg biot n, 25 mg Zn, Cu, Mg	In 100s.
Rx	**Prenatal Rx Tablets** (Various, eg, Ethex, Goldline, Moore, Qualitest, Schein)														30 mcg biot n, Cu, Mg, 25 mg Zn	In 100s and 500s.
Rx	**Prenatal Rx 1** (Ethex)														30 mcg biot n, 25 mg Zn, 3 mg Cu, 100 mg Mg	(ETHEX 216). White, oval. Film coated. In 100s.
Rx	**Natarex Prenatal Tablets** (Major)	200	60	4,000	400	15[d]	1.5	1.6	17	7	4	2.5	80	1	Cu, Mg, 25 mg Zn, 30 mcg biotin	In 100s.

MULTIVITAMINS WITH CALCIUM AND IRON

	Product & Distributor	Ca[a] mg	Fe[s] mg	A IU	D IU	E IU	B_1 mg	B_2 mg	B_3 mg	B_5 mg	B_6 mg	B_{12} mcg	C mg	FA mg	Other Content	How Supplied
Rx	**NataTab FA** (Ethex)	200	29	4,000	400	30	3	3	20		3	8	120	1	150 mcg iodine, 15 mg Zn, lactose	(ETHEX 329). Purple, oval. Film-coated. In 100s.
Rx	**NataTab CFe** (Ethex)	200	50	4,000	400	30	3	3	20		3	8	120	1	150 mcg iodine, 15 mg Zn, lactose	(ETHEX 328). White, oval. Film-coated. In UD 10s (100s).
Rx	**Prenatal Plus Iron Tablets** (Major)	200	27	4000	400	22	1.84	3			10	12	120	1	20 mg niacinamide, 2 mg Cu, and 25 mg Zn.	In 100s.
otc	**Prenatal w/Folic Acid Tablets** (Geneva)	200	60	4000	400	11[b]	1.5	1.7	18		2.6	4	100	0.8	25 mg Zn	Salmon. Oval. In 100s.
Rx	**Nestabs FA Tablets** (Fielding)	200	29	4,000	400	30[b]	3	3	20[k]		3	8	120	1	150 mcg I, 15 mg Zn	In 100s. Sugar coated.
Rx	**NatalCare Plus** (Ethex)	200	27	4,000	400	22	1.84	3	20		10	12	120	1	25 mg Zn,2 mg Cu,	(Ethex/225). Pink. Film coated. In 100s.
otc	**Vitelle Nestabs OTC** (Fielding)	200	29	5,000	400	30[b]	3	3	20[k]		3	8	120	0.8	150 mcg I, 15 mg Zn	In 100s.
Rx	**Nestabs CBF** (Fielding)	200	50	4,000	400	30	3	3	20[k]		3	8	120	1	150 mcg I, 15 mg Zn	In 100s.
otc	**Nutricon Tablets** (Pasadena)	200	20	2,500	200	15[j]	1.5	1.5	10	5	2	5	50	0.4	Cu, I, Mg, 3.75 mg Zn, 150 mcg biotin	In 120s.
Rx	**StrongStart Caplets** (Savage)	200	29	1000	400	30[e]	3	3	15	7	20	12	100	1	25 mg docusate sodium, 20 mg Zn	(0343). In 30s and 100s.
Rx	**StrongStart Chewable Tablets** (Savage)														20 mg Zn	(0344). In 30s and 100s.
Rx	**O-Cal Prenatal Tablets** (Mission)	200	15	2,500	400	30	1.5	1.6	17		12	12	70	1	Cu, I, Mg, 15 mg Zn	(Pharmics). White, oblong. In 100s.
otc	**Centrum, Jr. + Extra Calcium Tablets** (Lederle)	160	18	5,000	400	30[b]	1.5	1.7	20	10	2	6	60	0.4	Cr, Cu, I, Mg, Mn, Mo, P, 15 mg Zn, vitamin K, 45 mcg biotin, sugar	Chewable. Fruit flavor. In 60s.
otc	**Calcet Plus Tablets** (Mission)	152.8	18	5,000	400	30[b]	2.25	2.55	30	15	3	9	500	0.8	15 mg Zn, sugar	In 60s.
otc	**My-Vitalife Capsules** (ME Pharm)	130	27	6,500	400	30[b]	1.5	1.7	20	10	2	6	60	0.4	Cr, Cu, K, I, Mg, Mn, Mo, P, Se, 15 mg Zn, 30 mcg biotin	In 60s.
Rx	**Vitafol-PN** (Everett Laboratories	125	65	1,700	400	30	1.6	1.8	15		2.5	5	60	1	25 mg Mg, 15 mg Zn.	Capsule shape. In UD 100s.
Rx	**Multifol** (Breckenridge)	125	65[f]	6000	400	30	1.1	1.8	15		2.5	5	60	1		(B126). Purple, capsule shape. In UD 100s.
Rx	**Cal-Nate Tablets** (Ethex)	125	27	2700	400	30[b]	3	3.4	20		20		120	1	25 mg Zn, 150 mcg iodine, 2 mg Cu, 50 mg docusate sodium.	(ETHEX/439). White, oval. In 100s.
otc	**Centrum, Jr. + Extra C Tablets** (Lederle)	108	18	5,000	400	30[b]	1.5	1.7	20	10	2	6	300	0.4	Cr, Cu, I, Mg, Mn, Mo, P, 15 mg Zn, vitamin K, 45 mcg biotin, sugar, lactose	Chewable. Fruit flavor. In 60s.
otc	**Centrum Performance** (Wyeth)	100	18	5,000	400	60	4.5	5.1	40	10	6	18	120	0.4	25 mcg vitamin K, 40 mcg biotin, chloride, 60 mg *Ginkgo biloba* leaf, 50 mg ginseng root, B, Cr, Cu, I, K, Mg, Mn, Mo, Ni, P, Se, Si, Sn, V, 15 mg Zn. Glucose, lactose, malto-dextrin, sucrose	In 120s.
otc sf	**Bugs Bunny Complete Tablets** (Bayer)	100	18	5,000	400	30[d]	1.5	1.7	20	10	2	6	60	0.4	40 mcg biotin, Cu, I, Mg, P, aspartame, phenylalanine, 15 mg Zn	Chewable. Fruit flavor. In 60s.
Rx	**Natelle-EZ** (Pharmelle)	100	25	2700	400	20	3	3.5	20	8	30	12	120	1	30 mcg biotin, Cu, Mg, Se, 15 mg Zn, choline bitartrate.	(P 004). Lt. Pink, sugar-coated. Capsule shape. In 90s.
otc	**4 Nails Softgel Capsules** (Marlyn)	167	3	833	67	10[b]	3.3	1.7	8.3	8.3	8.3	8.3	10	33.3	8.3 mcg biotin, P, I, Mg, Cu, 3.3 mg Zn, Cr, Mn, methionine, inositol, choline bitartrate, Se, PABA, protein isolate, gelatin, lecithin, unsaturated fatty acid, predigested protein, L-cysteine, B mucopolysaccharides, silicon amino acid chelate, S	In 60s.
otc	**Optimox Prenatal Tablets** (Optimox)	100	5	833	67	2[k]	0.5	0.6	6.7	3.3	0.73	0.87	30	0.13	Cr, Cu, I, Mg, Mn, Se, 3.17 mg Zn	In 360s.
otc	**Gynovite Plus Tablets** (Optimox)	83	3	833	67	67[k]	1.7	1.7	3.3	1.7	3.3	21	30	0.07	B, betaine, biotin, Cr, Cu, hesperi-din, I, inositol, Mg, Mn, PABA, pancreatin, rutin, Se, 2.5 mg Zn	In 100s.

MULTIVITAMINS WITH CALCIUM AND IRON

	Product & Distributor	Ca[a] mg	Fe[a] mg	A IU	D IU	E IU	B_1 mg	B_2 mg	B_3 mg	B_5 mg	B_6 mg	B_{12} mcg	C mg	FA mg	Other Content	How Supplied
otc	**Alkavite** (Vitality)	68.5	60	5000	400	30	100	3			3	12	250	1	20 mg niacin, 0.03 mg biotin, 150 mg Mg, 4 mg Zn, 0.01 mg Se.	Brown, oblong. Film-coated. In UD 100s.
otc sf	**Hipotest Tablets** (Marlop Pharm)	53.5	50	10,000	400	12.5[l]	25	25	50	13	15	50	150		Choline, betaine, PABA, rutin, bio-flavonoids, 1 mg biotin, desiccated liver, bone meal, Cu, Mg, Mn, 2.2 mg Zn, I, P, lecithin	In 100s
otc	**One-A-Day Kids Scooby-Doo! Fizzy Vites Chewable Tablets** (Bayer)	50	9[f]	1500	200	15	0.75	0.85	7.5	5	1	3	170	200[e]	20 mcg biotin, P, I, Mg, Zn, Cu, Na, aspartame, phenylalanine, sucrose, vegetable oil.	In 60s.
Rx	**Mynatal PN Captabs** (ME Pharm)	125	60	4,000	400		3	3	10		2	3	50	1	18 mg Zn	Blue. Film-coated. In 100s.
Rx	**PreCare Prenatal Caplets** (Ther-Rx)	250	40		≈240	3.5[d]	3	3.4	20		50	12	50	1	Cu, Mg, 15 mg Zn	(Ther-Rx/118). Peach, scored. Film-coated. In UD 100s.
Rx	**PreCare Conceive Tablets** (Ther-Rx)	200	30			30[d]	3	3.4	20		50	12	60	1	2 mg Cu, 100 mg Mg, 15 mg Zn	Lactose. (Ther-Rx 014). Yellow, diamond-shape. Film-coated. In UD 100s.
Rx	**S.S.S. High Potency Vitamin Tablets** (S.S.S. Company)	100	27			50	7.5	7.5	50	10	12.5	12.5	300	200[i]	50 mg magnesium, 12 mg zinc, 1.5 mg copper, 22.5 mcg biotin.	In 20s, 40s, and 80s.

[a] Calcium and iron content expressed in mg elemental calcium and iron.
[b] Form of vitamin E unknown.
[c] As calcium carbonate and gluconate.
[d] As dL-alpha tocopheryl acetate.
[e] Content listed as mcg.
[f] As ferrous fumarate.
[g] Seyer Pharmatec, Inc., 413 St. George Street, San Juan, PR 00936; (787) 728-7044, (787) 728-7055.
[h] As dL-alpha tocopherol acetate.
[i] As calcium citrate.
[j] As carbonyl iron.
[k] As niacinamide.
[l] As d-alpha tocopheryl acid succinate.

For a comparison of the potencies of the various forms of vitamin E, see the vitamin E monograph.

MULTIVITAMINS WITH MINERALS

Content given per capsule, tablet, or 5 mL.

	Product & Distributor	A IU	D IU	E IU	B_1 mg	B_2 mg	B_3 mg	B_5 mg	B_6 mg	B_{12} mcg	C mg	FA mg	Zn[a] mg	Other Content	How Supplied
otc	**Vademin-Z Capsules** (Roberts/Hauck)	12,500	50	50[b]	10	5	25	10	2		150		2.6	Mg, Mn	In 60s.
otc sf	**Total Formula-3 without Iron Tablets** (Vitaline)	10,000	400	30[c]	15	15	25	25	25	25	100	0.4	30	Ca, Cr, Cu, I, K, Mg, Mn, Mo, V, B, Se, Si, vitamin K, 300 mcg biotin, hesperidin[d]	In 60s and 1,000s.
Rx	**Vicon Forte Capsules** (Whitby)	8,000		50[e]	10	5	25	10	2	10	150	1	18	Mg, Mn, lactose	(ucb 316). Orange/black. In 60s, 500s, and UD 100s.
otc sf	**ICAPS Time ReleaseTablets** (Ciba Vision)	7,000		100[e]		20					200		14.25	Cu, Se	In 60s and 120s.
otc	**Ondrox Tablets** (LSI)	6,000	300	50	0.75	0.75	10	5	1	3	125	200	7.5	50 mg Ca, 15 mcg biotin, I, Mg, Cu, P, vitamin K, K, Cr, Mn, Mo, Se, V, B, Si, citrus bioflavonoid, inositol, N-acetylcysteine, N-methionine, L-glutamine, taurine	In 60s.
otc sf	**ICAPS Plus Tablets** (Ciba Vision)	6,000		60[e]		20					200		14.25	Cu, Se, Mn	In 60s, 120s, and 180s.
Rx	**Nutrifac ZX Tablets** (Rising Pharmaceuticals)[f]	5,000	400	50	20	20	100	25	25	50	500	1	20	Ca, Cr, Cu, Mg, Mn, Se, 200 mcg biotin	Tartrazine, mineral oil. Capsule shape. In 60s.
Rx	**Glutofac-ZX Tablets** (Kenwood)														Parabens, sorbitol. (GLUTOFAC-ZX). Aqua green, capsule shape. In 60s.
otc	**Garfield Complete with Minerals Tablets** (Menley & James)	5,000	400	30[e]	1.5	1.7	20	10	2	6	60	0.4	15	Fe, Ca, Cu, P, I, Mg, 40 mcg biotin, aspartame, phenylalanine	Chewable. Character shapes. In 60s.
otc	**PowerMate Tablets** (Green Turtle Bay)[g]	5,000		100[e]			12.5				250		2.5	Se, n-acetyl-L-cysteine	In 50s.
otc	**One-A-Day Extras Antioxidant Softgel Capsules** (Bayer)	5,000		200[e]							250		7.5	Cu, Se, Mn, tartrazine	(One-A-Day). In 50s.
otc	**Vi-Zac Capsules** (Whitby)	5,000		50[e]							500		18	Lactose	Orange/banded. In 60s.
otc sf	**Glutofac Caplets** (Kenwood/Bradley)	5,000		30[e]	15	10	50	20	50		300		5	Ca, Cr, Cu, Fe, K, Mg, Mn, P, Se	In 90s.

MULTIVITAMINS WITH MINERALS

	Product & Distributor	A IU	D IU	E IU	B_1 mg	B_2 mg	B_3 mg	B_5 mg	B_6 mg	B_{12} mcg	C mg	FA mg	Zn[a] mg	Other Content	How Supplied
otc	**OCuSoft VMS Tablets** (OCuSoft)	5,000		30[e]							60			Cu, Se, 40 mg Zn	Film coated. In 60s.
Rx	**Zincvit Capsules** (Kenwood/Bradley)	5,000	50	50[e]	10	5	25		2		300	1	9.2	Mg, Mn	(Ram/Ram). Aqua green. In 60s.
otc	**Vitelle Nesentials** (Fielding)	5,000	400	30	3	3	25		2	6	120			Ca, P, Zn	In 60s.
otc	**ADEKs Tablets** (Scandipharm)	4,000	400	150[e]	1.2	1.3	10	10	1.5	12	60	0.2	1.1	Vitamin K, 50 mcg biotin, 3 mg beta carotene, fructose	Chewable. Tan. Capsule shape. In 60s.
Rx	**Eldercaps Capsules** (Mayrand)	4,000	400	25[e]	10	5	25	10	2		200	1	15.8	Mg, Mn	In 100s.
otc	**Vicon Plus Capsules** (Whitby)	4,000		50[e]	10	5	25	10	2		150		18	Mg, Mn, lactose	In 60s.
otc	**DermaVite** (Stiefel)	3,500		60		8.5			10		120	0.4	45	600 mcg biotin, 5 mg lycopene, Ca, Cr, Cu, Mn, Se, Si, sucrose	In 60s.
otc sf	**Kenwood Therapeutic Liquid** (Kenwood/Bradley)	3,333	133	1.5[h]	2	1	20	2	0.33		50			Ca, K, Mg, Mn, P	Alcohol free. In 240 mL.
otc	**Obtrex Tablets** (Pronova)	2,700	400	18	3	3.4	20		40	2	120	1	25	Se, Mg, 50 mg sodium docusate	In 60s.
otc	**Flintstones Plus Calcium Tablets** (Bayer)	2,500	400	15[e]	1.05	1.2	13.5		1.05	4.5	60	0.3		200 mg Ca, sorbitol	Chewable. Character shapes. In 60s.
otc sf	**Maximum Green Label Tablets** (Vitaline)	2,500	16.7	66.7[c]	16.7	8.3	31.7	66.7	16.7	16.7	200	0.13	5	Ca, Cr, I, K, Mg, Mn, Mo, Se, Si, V, 50 mcg biotin, SOD, L-lysine[d]	In 180s.
otc sf	**Maximum BlueLabel Tablets** (Vitaline)													Ca, Cr, Cu, I, K, Mg, Mn, Mo, Se, Si, V, 50 mcg biotin, SOD, L-lysine[d]	In 180s.
otc sf	**PowerVites Tablets** (Green Turtle Bay)[g]	2,500	150	12.5[i]	6.3	6.3	25	25	12.5	6.3	125	0.15	2.5	B, Ca, Mg, Cu, Cr, Mn, K, Se, betaine, hesperidin, biotin[d]	In 40s, 100s, and 200s.
otc sf	**Vita-PMS Tablets** (Bajamar)	2,083	16.7	16.7[i]	4.2	4.2	4.2	4.2	50	10.4	250	0.33	4.2	Mg, Ca, Cu, Mn, K, Se, Cr, I, Fe, biotin, betaine[d]	In 100s.
otc	**Po-Pon-S Tablets** (Shionogi)	2,000	100	5[e]	5	3	35	15	4	6	100			Ca, P	Sugar coated. In 60s and 240s.
otc	**Maxovite Tablets** (Tyson)	2,083	16.7	16.7[i]	5	4.2	4.2	4.2	54.2	10.8	250	0.33	5	Ca, Cr, Cu, Fe, I, K, Mg, Mn, Se, 11.7 mcg biotin[d]	Sustained release. In 120s and 240s.
otc sf	**Vita-PMS Plus Tablets** (Bajamar)	667	16.7	16.7[i]	4.2	4.2	4.2	4.2	16.7	10.4	250	0.33	4.2	Mg, Ca, Cu, Mn, K, Se, Cr, I, Fe, biotin, betaine[d]	In 100s.
otc sf	**Stress 600 w/Zinc Tablets** (Nion)			45[h]	20	10	100	25	10	25	600	0.4	5.5	Cu, 45 mcg biotin	In 60s.
otc	**Mediplex Tabules (Tablets)** (JS Pharm)			60[h]	25	10	100	25	10	25	300		4	Cu, Mg, Mn	In 100s.
otc	**Bee-Zee Tablets** (Rugby)			45[h]	15	10.2	100	25	10	6	600		5.2		In 60s.
otc sf	**Z-gen Tablets** (Goldline)														In 60s.
otc	**Z-Bec Tablets** (Robins)			45[e]									22.5	Parabens	In 60s, 500s and *Dis-Co* pack 100s.
Rx	**Renax Caplets** (Everett)			35[i]	3	2	20	10	15	12	50	2.5	20	300 mcg biotin, Cr, Se	*For azotemic patients with low levels of essential vitamins/minerals.* White, oblong. Film coated. In 90s.
otc sf	**Stress B-Complex Tablets** (Moore)			30[h]	15	10	100	20	5	12	500	0.4	23.9	Cu, 45 mcg biotin	In 60s.
otc	**Stresstabs + Zinc Tablets** (Lederle)			30[e]	10	10	100	20	5	12	500	0.4	23.9	Cu, 45 mcg biotin	(S 3). In 60s.
otc sf	**OstiGen Melts** (US Food & Pharmaceuticals)		150											Vitamin K, 350 mg Ca, P, Mg, Cu, Na, K	In chocolate, chocolate mint, and caramel flavors. In 90s.
Rx	**Nicomide Tablets** (Sirius)											0.5		750 mg nicotinamide, 25 mg zinc oxide	In 60s.

[a] Zinc content expressed in mg elemental zinc.
[b] As dL-alpha tocopheryl succinate.
[c] As d-alpha tocopheryl succinate.
[d] Also contains bioflavonoids, choline, inositol, PABA and rutin.
[e] Form of vitamin E unknown.
[f] Rising Pharmaceuticals, Inc., 411 Sette Drive, Paramus, NJ 07652; 201-262-4200, fax 201-262-4284.
[g] The Green Turtle Bay Vitamin Co., P.O. Box 642, Summit, NJ 07902; (908) 277-2240.
[h] As dL-alpha tocopheryl acetate.
[i] As d-alpha tocopherol.

For a comparison of the potencies of various forms of vitamin E, see the Vitamin E monograph.

GERIATRIC SUPPLEMENTS WITH MULTIVITAMINS AND MINERALS

Content given per capsule, tablet or 5 mL.

	Product & Distributor	A IU	D IU	E U	B_1 mg	B_2 mg	B_3 mg	B_5 mg	B_6 mg	B_{12} mcg	C mg	Fe[1] mg	FA mg	Ca[1] mg	Zn mg	Other Content	How Supplied
otc *sf*	**Mega VM-80 Tablets** (NBTY)	10,000	1000	100[2]	80	80	80	80	80	80	250	1.2	0.4	4.5	3.58	Choline, inositol, 80 mcg biotin, PABA, bioflavonoids, betaine, hesperidin, Cu, I, K, Mg, Mn, Se	In 60s and 100s.
otc	**Vita-Plus G Softgel Capsules** (Scot-Tussin)	10,000	400	2[2]	5	2.5	40	4	1	2	75	30		75	0.5	Mg, Mn, P, K	In 100s.
otc	**One-A-Day 55 Plus Tablets** (Bayer)	6000	400	60[2]	4.5	3.4	20	20	6	25	120		0.4	220	15	30 mcg biotin, vitamin K, I, Mg, Cu, Cr, Se, Mo, Mn, K, Cl	(One-A-Day). In 50s and 80s.
otc	**Cerovite Senior Tablets** (Rugby)	6000	400	45[3]	1.5	1.7	20	10	3	25	60	9	0.2	200	15	30 mcg biotin, Cu, I, Mg, P, Cl, Cr, Mn, Mo, Ni, Se, Si, V, K, vitamin K	In 60s.
otc	**Centrum Silver Tablets** (Wyeth)	3500	400	45	1.5	1.7	20	10	3	25	60		0.4	200	15	30 mcg biotin, chloride, 250 mcg lutein, B, Cr, Cu, I, K, Mg, Mn, Mo, Ni, P, Se, Si, V, vitamin K	Sucrose, glucose. In 220s.
otc	**Certagen Senior Tablets** (Goldline)	6000	400	45[3]	1.5	1.7	20	10	3	25	60	3	0.2	80	15	30 mcg biotin, Cl, Cr, Cu, I, Mg, Mn, Mo, Ni, P, K, Se, Si, V, vitamin K	In 60s.
otc	**Gerimed Tablets** (Fielding)	5000	400	30[2]	3	3	25		2	6	120			370	15	P	In 60s.
Rx	**Strovite Plus Caplets** (Everett)	5000		30[3]	20	20	100	25	25	50	500	9	0.8		22.5	150 mcg biotin, Cr, Cu, Mg, Mn	(EV201). Dark red. In 100s.
otc *sf*	**Ultra-Freeda Tablets** (Freeda)	4166	133	66.7[2]	16.7	16.7	33	33	16.7	33	333	2	0.27	27	1.1	Choline, inositol, bioflavonoids, PABA, 100 mcg biotin, Cr, I, K, Mg, Mn, Mo, Se	In 90s, 180s and 270s.
otc *sf*	**Iron Free Ultra-Freeda Tablets** (Freeda)	4166	133	66.7[2]	16.7	16.7	33	33	16.7	33	333		0.27	27	1.1		In 90s, 180s and 270s.
otc	**Optivite P.M.T. Tablets** (Optimox)	2083	†	16.6[4]	4.2	4.2	4.2	4.2	50	10.4	250	2.5	0.03	†	4.2	Choline, Cr, Cu, I, K, Mg, Mn, Se, bioflavonoids, betaine, PABA, pancreatin, rutin, inositol, biotin	In 180s.
otc	**Hep-Forte Capsules** (Marlyn)	1200		10[2]	1	1	10	2	0.5	1	10		0.06		0.5	Choline, inositol, biotin, dL-methionine, desiccated liver, liver concentrate, liver fraction number 2	In 100s, 300s and 500s.
otc	**Vigortol Liquid** (Rugby)				0.8	0.4	8.3	1.7	0.2	0.2		0.3			0.3	Choline, I, Mg, Mn, 18% alcohol, sugar, methylparaben	Sherry wine flavor. In 473 mL.
otc	**Gerivite Liquid** (Goldline)															Choline, I, Mg, Mn, 18% alcohol, methylparaben, sorbitol	Rum and sherry wine flavors. In 473 mL.
otc	**Viminate Liquid** (Various)				2.5	1.25	25	5	0.5	0.5		7.5			1	Choline, I, Mg, Mn	In 480 mL.
otc	**Geravite Elixir** (Roberts-Hauck)				0.3	0.4	33.3			3.3						L-lysine, 15% alcohol, parabens, sorbitol, sucrose	Wine flavor. In 480 mL.
Rx	**Strovite Advance** (Everett)		400	100	20	5	25	15	25	50	300		1		Zn	Carotenoids, 100 mcg biotin, alpha lipoic acid, lutein, Cr, Cu, Mg, Mn, Se, mineral oil	(EV 0208). White, oblong. In 100s.

* † – Amount not supplied by manufacturer.
[1] Calcium and iron content expressed in mg elemental calcium and iron.
[2] Form of vitamin E unknown.
[3] As dL-alpha tocopheryl acetate.
[4] As d-alpha tocopheryl acid succinate.

For a comparison of the potencies of various forms of vitamin E, see the Vitamin E monograph.

MULTIVITAMINS WITH IRON AND OTHER MINERALS

Content given per capsule, tablet or 5 mL.

	Product & Distributor	Fe[1] mg	A IU	D IU	E IU	B_1 mg	B_2 mg	B_3 mg	B_5 mg	B_6 mg	B_{12} mcg	C mg	FA mg	Other Content	How Supplied
Rx	**Prenatal-H Capsules** (Cypress)	106.5				10	6	30	10	5	15	200	1	Cu, Mg, Mn, 18.2 mg Zn	(CYP187). White. In 100s.
otc	**One-Tablet-Daily with Minerals** (Goldline)	18	5,000	400	30[2]	1.5	1.7	20	10	2	6	60	0.4	Ca, Cl, Cr, Cu, I, K, Mg, Mn, Mo, P, Se, 30 mcg biotin, 15 mg Zn	In 100s and 1000s.
otc	**Theravee-M Tablets** (Vangard)	27	5,000	400	30[2]	3	3.4	30	10	3	9	120	0.4	Ca, Cl, Cr, Cu, K, I, Mg, Mn, Mo, Se, 15 mg Zn, P, 15 mcg biotin, 2,500 IU beta carotene	In 100s, 1000s and UD 100s.
otc	**Therems-M Tablets** (Rugby)	27	5,000[3]	400	30[2]	3	3.4	20	10	3	9	90	0.4	Ca, Cl, Cr, Cu, I, K, Mg, Mn, Mo, P, Se, 15 mg Zn, 30 mcg biotin	In 130s and 1000s.
otc	**Adavite-M Tablets** (Hudson)				30[3]									Ca, Cl, Cr, Cu, I, K, Mg, Mn, Mo, P, Se, 15 mg Zn, 30 mcg biotin	In 130s.
otc *sf*	**Therapeutic-M Tablets** (Goldline)				30[2]									Ca, Cl, Cr, Cu, I, K, Mg, Mn, Mo, P, Se, 15 mg Zn, 30 mcg biotin	In 1000s.
otc	**Theravim-M Tablets** (NBTY)				30[3]									Ca, Cl, Cr, Cu, I, K, Mg, Mn, Mo, P, Se, 15 mg Zn, 30 mcg biotin	In 130s.
Rx	**Bacmin Tablets** (Marnel)	27	5,000		30[2]	20	20	100	25	25	50	500	0.8	Cr, Cu, Mg, Mn, 22.5 mg Zn, 0.15 mg biotin	(EV201). Dark red. In 100s.
otc	**Multi-Day with Calcium and Extra Iron Tablets** (NBTY)	27	5,000	400	30[3]	1.5	1.7	20	10	2	6	60	0.4	Ca, 15 mg Zn, tartrazine	In 100s.
otc *sf*	**Total Formula Tablets** (Vitaline)	20	10,000	400	30[3]	15	15	25	25	25	25	100	0.4	Ca, Cr, Cu, I, K, Mg, Mn, Mo, P, Se, Si, V, vitamin K, 300 mcg biotin, 30 mg Zn, choline, bioflavonoids, hesperidin, inositol, PABA, rutin	In 90s and 100s.
otc *sf*	**Total Formula-2 Tablets** (Vitaline)														With boron. In 60s.
otc	**Optilets-M-500 Filmtabs** (Abbott)	20	5,000	400	30[2]	15	10	100	20	5	12	500		Cu, I, Mg, Mn, 1.5 mg Zn	Film coated. In 120s.
otc *sf*	**Unicap T Tablets** (Upjohn)	18	5,000	400	30[3]	10	10	100	25	6	18	500	0.4	Cu, I, K, Mn, Se, 15 mg Zn, tartrazine	In 60s.
otc *sf*	**Avail Tablets** (Menley & James)	18	5,000	400	30[3]	2.25	2.55	20		3	9	90	0.4	Ca, Cr, I, Mg, Se, 22.5 mg Zn	In 60s.
otc	**Myadec Tablets** (Parke-Davis)	18	5,000	400	30[2]	1.7	2	20	10	3	6	60	0.4	30 mcg biotin, vitamin K, Ca, P, I, Mg, Cu, 15 mg Zn, Mn, K, Cl, Cr, Mo, Se, Ni, Si, V, B, Sn	In 130s.
otc	**One-A-Day Kids Tablets** (Bayer)	18	5,000	400	30	1.5	1.7	20	10	2	6	60	0.4	40 mcg biotin, Ca, Cu, P, I, Mg, 15 mg Zn	Chewable. Sorbitol, aspartame, phenylalanine. In 50s.
otc	**Centrum Jr. with Iron Tablets** (Lederle)	18	5,000	400	30[3]	1.5	1.7	20	10	2	6	60	0.4	Ca, Cr, Cu, I, Mg, Mn, Mo, P, 15 mg Zn, 45 mcg biotin, vitamin K	Chewable. In 60s.
otc	**Cerovite Tablets** (Rugby)													Ca, Cl, Cr, Cu, I, K, Mg, Mn, Mo, Ni, P, Se, Si, Sn, V, 30 mcg biotin, vitamin K, 15 mg Zn	In 130s.
otc *sf*	**Children's SunKist Multivitamins Complete Tablets** (Ciba)													Ca, 10 mg Zn, 40 mcg biotin, vitamin K_1, Cu, I, K, Mg, Mn, P, sorbitol, aspartame, phenylalanine, tartrazine.	Chewable. Citrus flavor. In 60s.
otc	**Flintstones Complete Tablets** (Bayer)													Ca, Cu, I, Mg, P, 15 mg Zn, 40 mcg biotin	Chewable. In 60s and 120s.
otc *sf*	**Unicap M Tablets** (Upjohn)													Ca, Cu, I, K, Mn, P, 15 mg Zn, tartrazine	In 120s.
otc	**One-A-Day Maximum Formula Tablets** (Bayer)													Ca, Cl, Cr, Cu, I, K, Mg, Mn, Mo, P, Se, 15 mg Zn, 30 mcg biotin	(One-A-Day). In 60s and 100s.
otc	**Stuart Formula Tablets** (J & J-Merck)	5	5,000	400	10[2]	1.5	1.7	20		1	3	50	0.1	Ca, Cu, I	In 100s.
otc	**Cerovite Jr. Tablets** (Rugby)	18	5,000	400	15[3]	1.5	1.7	20	10	2	6	60	0.4	Cu, I, Mg, Zn, Mn, Mo, 45 mcg biotin, Cr, sugar	In 60s.
otc	**Multi-Day Plus Minerals Tablets** (NBTY)	18	6,500	400	30[2]	1.5	1.7	20	10	2	6	60	0.4	Ca, Cl, Cr, Cu, I, K, Mg, Mn, Mo, P, Se, 15 mg Zn, 30 mcg biotin	In 100s.
otc *sf*	**Hair Booster Vitamin Tablets** (NBTY)	18						35	100		6		0.4	Cu, I, Mn, 15 mg Zn, inositol, PABA, protein, choline bitartrate	In 60s.
otc *sf*	**Quintabs-M Tablets** (Freeda)	15	10,000	400	50[3]	30	30	150	30	30	30	300	0.4	Ca, Cu, Mg, Mn, Se, 30 mg Zn, PABA, K	Kosher. In 100s, 250s and 500s.
otc	**Generix-T Tablets** (Goldline)	15	10,000	400	5.5[3]	15	10	100	10	2	7.5	150		Cu, I, Mg, Mn, 1.5 mg Zn	In 100s.
otc	**Multilex T & M Tablets** (Rugby)														Sugar. In 100s and 1000s.
otc *sf*	**Multilex Tabs** (Rugby)	15	10,000	400	5.5[2]	10	5	30	10	1.7	3	100		Cu, I, Mg, Mn, 1.5 mg Zn	In 100s.
otc	**Vitarex Tablets** (Pasadena)	15	10,000	200	15[3]	15	10	100	20	5	5	250		Ca, Cu, I, K, Mg, Mn, P, 10 mg Zn	In 100s.

MULTIVITAMINS WITH IRON AND OTHER MINERALS

	Product & Distributor	Fe[1] mg	A IU	D IU	E IU	B_1 mg	B_2 mg	B_3 mg	B_5 mg	B_6 mg	B_{12} mcg	C mg	FA mg	Other Content	How Supplied
otc	**Fosfree Tablets** (Mission)	29	3,000	300		9	4	21	2	5	4	100		351 mg Ca	Sugar. In 120s.
otc	**Fosfree** (Mission)	14.5	1500	150		4.5	2	10.5	1	2.5	2	50		175.5 mg Ca	Sugar. In 120s.
otc sf	**Monocaps Tablets** (Freeda)	14	10,000	400	15[4]	15	15	41	15	15	15	125	0.1	Ca, Cu, I, K, Mg, Mn, Se, 12 mg Zn, 15 mcg biotin, L-lysine, PABA, lecithin	Kosher. In 100s, 250s and 500s.
otc	**Vigomar Forte Tablets** (Marlop Pharm)	12	10,000	400	15[3]	10	10	100	20	5	5	200		I, Mg, Cu, Mn, 1.5 mg Zn	In 100s.
otc	**Poly-Vi-Sol w/Iron Tablets** (Mead-Johnson)	12	2,500	400	15[3]	1.05	1.2	13.5		1.05	4.5	60	0.3	Cu, 8 mg Zn, sugar	Chewable. Peter Rabbit shapes. Fruit flavors. In 100s.
otc sf	**Unicap Sr. Tablets** (Upjohn)	10	5,000	200	15[3]	1.2	1.4	16	10	2.2	3	60	0.4	Ca, Cu, I, K, Mg, Mn, P, 15 mg Zn	In 120s.
Rx	**Strovite Forte** (Everett Laboratories)	10	4000[3]	400	60	20	20	100	25	25	50	500	1.0	0.15 biotin, 50 mcg Se, 50 mg MG, 15 mg Zn, 20 mcg Mo, 3 mg Cu, 0.05 mg Cr	(EV 0204). Dark green, oblong, bisect. Capsule shape. In 100s.
otc sf	**Geritol Extend Caplets** (SmithKline-Beecham)	10	3,333	200	15[3]	1.2	1.4	15		2	2	60	0.2	Vitamin K, Ca, I, Mg, Se, 15 mg Zn	In 40s and 100s.
otc	**Advanced Formula Centrum Liquid** (Lederle)	3	833	133	10[2]	0.5	0.57	6.7	3.3	0.67	2	20		100 mcg biotin, Cr, I, Mn, Mo, 1 mg Zn, 5.4% alcohol, sucrose	In 236 mL.
otc sf	**Ultra Vita Time Tablets** (NBTY)	6	10,000	400	13[4]	25	25	50	12.5	15	50	150	0.4	B, Ca, Cr, Cu, I, K, Mg, Mn, Mo, P, Se, 5 mg Zn, 1 mg biotin, bioflavonoids, bone meal, PABA, choline bitartrate, betaine, inositol, lecithin, desiccated liver, rutin	In 100s.
otc sf	**Formula VM-2000 Tablets** (Solgar)	5	12,500	200	100[3]	50	50	50	50	50	50	150	0.2	B, Ca, Cr, Cu, I, K, Mg, Mn, Mo, Se, 7.5 mg Zn, betaine, 50 mcg biotin, choline, bioflavonoids, amino acids, hesperidin, inositol, l-glutathione, PABA, rutin	In 30s, 60s, 90s and 180s.
otc	**M.V.M. Capsules** (Tyson & Associates)	3.6	400		60[2]	20	10	10	100	31	160	50	0.08	Ca, Cr, Cu, I, K, Mg, Mo, 6 mg Zn, 160 mcg biotin, PABA, Mn, Se, tryptophan	In 150s.
otc sf	**Maximum Red Label Tablets** (Vitaline)	3.3	2,500	67	66.7[3]	16.7	8.3	31.7	66.7	16.7	16.7	200	0.13	Ca, Cr, Cu, I, K, Mg, Mn, Mo, Se, Si, V, 5 mg Zn, 50 mcg biotin, choline, inositol, bioflavonoids, l-lysine, PABA	In 180s.
otc	**Androvite Tablets** (Optimox)	3	4,167	67	67[4]	8.3	8.3	8.3	16.7	16.7	20.8	167	0.06	PABA, inositol, biotin, betaine, B, Cr, Cu, I, Mg, Mn, Se, 8.3 mg Zn, pancreatin, hesperidin, rutin	In 180s.
otc sf	**ProCycle Gold Tablets** (Cyclin Pharm)	3	833.3	67	67	1.7	1.7	3.3	1.7	3.3	21	30	0.07	167 mg Ca, 2.5 mg Zn, B, Cu, Cr, I, Mg, Mn, Se, PABA, inositol, rutin, biotin, hesperidin, pancreatin, betaine	In 100s.
otc	**4 Hair Softgel Capsules** (Marlyn)	2.5	1,250		10[4]			5	25	1.5	44	25	33.3	250 mcg biotin, I, Mg, Cu, 7.5 mg Zn, choline bitartrate, inositol, Mn, methionine, PABA, B, L-cysteine, tyrosine, Si	In 60s.
otc	**S.S.S. Vitamin and Mineral Complex Liquid** (S.S.S. Company)	3	833	133[5]	10	1.7	0.57	6.7[6]	3	0.67	2	20		100 mcg biotin, 50 mcg iodine, 1 mg zinc, 0.8 mg manganese, 8 mcg chromium, 8 mcg molybdenum/5 mL	With 6.6% alcohol, sugar. In 236 mL.

[1] Iron content expressed in mg elemental iron.
[2] As dL-alpha tocopheryl acetate.
[3] Form of vitamin E unknown.
[4] As d-alpha tocopheryl acid succinate.
[5] As cholecalciferol.
[6] As niacinamide.

For a comparison of the potencies of various forms of vitamin E, see the Vitamin E monograph.

Enteral nutrition products may be administered orally, via nasogastric tube, via feeding gastrostomy or via needle-catheter jejunostomy. The defined formula diets may be monomeric or oligomeric (amino acids or short peptides and simple carbohydrates) or polymeric (more complex protein and carbohydrate sources) in composition. Modular supplements are used for individual supplementation of protein, carbohydrate or fat when formulas do not offer sufficient flexibility.

There are different criteria for evaluating and categorizing these products; no single system is ideal. Caloric density, generally in the range of 1, 1.5 or 2 Cal/mL, influences the density of other nutrients. Protein content is also a major determinant. Osmolality may be important in patients who experience diarrhea and cramping with high osmolality formulas. Consider products with low fat content in patients with significant malabsorption, hyperlipidemia or severe exocrine pancreatic insufficiency. Medium chain triglycerides are a useful energy source in patients with malabsorption, but do not provide essential fatty acids. Lactose, poorly tolerated by patients lacking lactase activity, has been eliminated from many of the nutritionally complete enteral formulas. In general, with the exception of lactose or specific allergies (eg, corn, gluten), the source of the protein or carbohydrate is not critical. Various amounts of vitamins, electrolytes and minerals are included in the formulations. Consider sodium and potassium content in patients with renal or hepatic disease. Also, consider vitamin K content in patients receiving warfarin, since the hypoprothrombinemic effect may be decreased. Although many of the products have been formulated to contain lesser amounts of vitamin K, caution is still warranted.

Some enteral preparations list the osmolality or osmolarity of the formula at standard dilution. However, when the term osmolarity is used, it cannot be determined whether the osmolarity was calculated from osmolality or if the term osmolarity is being used erroneously. Also, when samples of a specific product from the same lot or different lots were reconstituted, or if the powder was reconstituted by using the provided scoop vs reconstitution by weight, there was a wide variation in osmolality. Be aware of these potential discrepancies when utilizing osmolality information.

Cost of products is influenced by composition (oligomeric or polymeric) and form (ready-to-use or powder). In general, polymeric products cost less than oligomeric products. The form of the product indirectly affects its cost due to the amount of labor involved in preparation.

Specialized formulas are indicated for specific disease states and may be nutritionally incomplete.

Hepatic failure/encephalopathy formulas contain high concentrations of branched chain amino acids (BCAA) and low concentrations of aromatic amino acids (AAA) in an attempt to correct the abnormal plasma amino acid profiles.

Renal failure formulas contain only essential amino acids as the source of protein.

Trauma or high stress formulas contain high concentrations of BCAA, but unlike the hepatic products, are not restricted in the amounts of AAA.

Monitoring of patients receiving enteral nutritional therapy includes the following: Weight, fluid balance, serum electrolytes, glucose tolerance, liver and renal function, albumin and general condition. Watch for GI overload or obstruction and abdominal distention; check tube placement for proper position. Initiate therapy with a slow but gradual advancement in administration rate.

Several case reports and single-dose studies suggest that phenytoin administration during enteral nutritional therapy may result in decreased phenytoin concentrations; however, this has not been substantiated. Monitor phenytoin concentrations in these patients. Consider giving phenytoin 2 hours before and after the enteral feeding, or stopping the enteral therapy for 2 hours before and after phenytoin administration.

Enteral Nutritional Product Categories	
Modular Supplements Protein Carbohydrate Fat	*Defined Formulas* Milk-based formulas Specialized formulas Hepatic failure/encephalopathy Renal failure Trauma/stress Pulmonary Nutritionally complete, lactose free formulas

Content listed is based on standard dilutions. Refer to manufacturer's literature for mixing directions, other dilutions and storage conditions.

Modular Supplements

PROTEIN PRODUCTS

otc	**Gevral Protein** (Lederle)	**Powder:** Ca caseinate and sucrose. Each cup (≈ 26 g) contains: 15.6 g protein, 7.05 g carbohydrate, 0.52 g fat, < 50 mg Na, ≥ 13 mg K and 95.3 Calories *Dose:* 26 g in 8 oz liquid.	< 1% alcohol. In 8 oz and 5 lb.
otc	**ProMod** (Ross)	**Powder:** D-whey protein concentrate and soy lecithin. Each 26.4 g provides 20 g protein, 2.4 g fat, 2.68 g carbohydrate, 176 mg Ca, 60 mg Na, 260 mg K, 132 mg P and 112 Calories *Dose:* Add 1 scoop (6.6 g) to liquid, food or enteral formula.	In 275 g cans.
otc	**Propac** (Sherwood)	**Powder:** Each tablespoon (4 g) contains 3 g protein (from whey protein), 0.24 g carbohydrate from lactose, 0.32 g fat, 2 mg Cl, 20 mg K, 9 mg Na, 14 mg Ca, 12 mg P, 2 mg Mg and 16 Calories *Dose:* Add 1 tablespoon to liquid.	In 20 g packets and 350 g cans.
otc	**Essential ProPlus** (NutriSOY International, Inc.[1])	**Powder:** 16.3 g protein, 0.2 g fat, 6.4 g carbohydrates, 242.5 mg Na, 112.5 mg K, 70 mg Ca, 31.3 mg Mg, 3 mg Fe, 187.5 mg P, 0.4 mg Cu, 0.5 mg Zn, 12.9 mcg I, 0.1 mg B_1, 0.2 mg B_3, 0.1 mg folic acid/25 g. *Dose:* Add 2 tablespoons to liquid or food.	In 2 lb. containers.
otc	**Immunocal** (Immunotech Research)	**Powder:** ≈ 18 to 28 g whey protein/100g, ≥ 1.5 mg vitamin B_1/100 g. *Dose:* Mix 1 packet with liquid or food.	In 10 g packets.

[1] (888) 769-0769.

Refer to additional information in the Enteral Nutritional Therapy introduction.

GLUCOSE POLYMERS

These glucose polymers are derived from cornstarch by hydrolysis. Content given per 100 mL liquid or 100 g powder.

	Product & Distributor	CHO (g)	Calories	Sodium (mg)	Chloride (mg)	Potassium (mg)	Calcium (mg)	Phosphorus (mg)	How Supplied
otc	**Polycose Liquid** (Ross)	50	200	70	140	6	20	3	In 126 mL.
otc	**Polycose Powder** (Ross)	94	380	110	223	10	30	5	In 350 g.
otc	**Moducal Powder** (Mead Johnson Nutritional)	95[1]	380	70	150	< 10	—	—	In 368 g.[2]
otc	**Sumacal Powder** (Sherwood)	95[1]	380	100	210	< 39	< 20	< 31	In 400 g.[2]

[1] Maltodextrin.

[2] Contains 0.4 g/100 g minerals (ash).

GLUCOSE POLYMERS — ORAL

Refer to additional information in the Enteral Nutritional Therapy introduction.

Indications

➤*Nutritional supplements:* Supplies calories in persons with increased caloric needs or persons unable to meet their caloric needs with usual food intake. Supplies carbohydrate calories in protein, electrolyte and fat restricted diets. Also used to increase the caloric density of traditional foods, liquid and tube feedings.

Administration and Dosage

Add to foods or beverages or mix in water. Small, frequent feedings are more desirable than large amounts given infrequently. May be used for extended periods with diets containing all other essential nutrients, or as an oral adjunct to IV administration of nutrients. Not a balanced diet; do not use as a sole source of nutrition.

Modular Supplements

CORN OIL

otc	**Lipomul** (Roberts)	**Liquid**: 10 g corn oil per 15 mL in a vehicle containing polysorbate 80, glyceride phosphates and 6.3 mg saccharin (from sodium saccharin) with 0.05% sodium benzoate, 0.05% benzoic acid, 0.07% sorbic acid, BHA and vitamin E. Each serving (45 mL) contains 270 Calories and 30 g fat.	Citrus-vanilla flavor. In 473 mL.

CORN OIL — ORAL

Refer to additional information in the Enteral Nutritional Therapy introduction.

Indications

➤*Caloric supplementation:* Increasing caloric intake.

Administration and Dosage

➤*Adults:* 45 mL 2 to 4 times daily, after or between meals.

➤*Children:* 30 mL 1 to 4 times daily, after or between meals.

SAFFLOWER OIL

otc	**Microlipid** (Sherwood)	**Emulsion**: 50% fat emulsion. Safflower oil, polyglycerol esters of fatty acids, soy lecithin, xanthan gum and ascorbic acid. Contains 4500 Calories and 500 g fat per L. *Osmolality* - 60 mOsm/kg water	In 120 mL.

SAFFLOWER OIL — ORAL

Refer to additional information in the Enteral Nutritional Therapy introduction.

Indications

➤*Caloric supplementation:* Dietary management of patients requiring caloric supplementation (ie, fatty acid deficiencies). Supplies essential fatty acids.

Administration and Dosage

➤*Oral:* May give by tablespoon. Flavor additives may improve patient acceptance.

➤*Tube feeding:* Can be added to a patient's formula depending upon the degree of caloric supplementation needed.

Shake well before using.

MEDIUM CHAIN TRIGLYCERIDES (MCT)

otc	**MCT** (Mead Johnson Nutritionals)	**Oil**: Lipid fraction of coconut oil consisting primarily of the triglycerides of C_8 (≈ 67%) and C_{10} (≈ 23%) saturated fatty acids. Contains 115 Calories/15 mL	In qt.

MEDIUM CHAIN TRIGLYCERIDES (MCT) — ORAL

Refer to additional information in the Enteral Nutritional Therapy introduction.

Indications

➤*Dietary supplement:* A special dietary supplement for use in the nutritional management of patients who cannot efficiently digest and absorb conventional long chain food fats.

Administration and Dosage

15 mL, 3 to 4 times per day. Mix with fruit juices, use on salads and vegetables, incorporate into sauces or use in cooking or baking. Do not use plastic containers or utensils.

Actions

➤*Pharmacology:* Medium chain triglycerides are more rapidly hydrolyzed than conventional food fat, require less bile acid for digestion, are carried by the portal circulation and are not dependent on chylomicron formation or lymphatic transport. Does not provide essential fatty acids.

Precautions

➤*Hepatic cirrhosis:* In persons with advanced cirrhosis, large amounts of MCT may elevate blood and spinal fluid levels of medium chain fatty acids (MCFA) due to impaired hepatic clearance of MCFA which are rapidly absorbed via the portal vein. These elevated levels have caused reversible coma and precoma in subjects with advanced cirrhosis, particularly with portacaval shunts. Use with caution in persons with hepatic cirrhosis and complications such as portacaval shunts or tendency to encephalopathy.

MILK-BASED FORMULAS

	Product & Distributor	Protein g	Protein Source	Carbohydrate g	Carbohydrate Source	Fat g	Fat Source	Na (mg)	K (mg)	mOsm/ kg H_2O	Cal/ mL	Other Content	How Supplied
		Content per Liter											
otc	**Epulor** (VistaPharm)	89	milk protein, isoleucine, leucine, lysine, methionine/cystine, phenylalanine/tyrosine, threonine, tryptophan, valine			755	soybean oil				7.1	Vit. A, B_1, B_2, B_3, B_5, B_6, B_{12}, C, D, E, K, B, Ca, Cl, Cr, Cu, Fe, I, Mg, Mn, Mo, Ni, P, Se, Si, Sn, V, Zn, biotin, folate	Lemon flavor. In 1.5 oz pouches.
otc	**NovaSource Renal** (Novartis Nutrition)	74	sodium and calcium caseinates, arginine, taurine, carnitine	200	corn syrup, fructose, hydrolyzed corn starch	100	high oleic sunflower oil, corn oil, medium chain triglycerides, soy lecithin	1000 (43.5 mEq) (complete feeding *Brik Paks*; 1600 (70 mEq) (closed system)	810 (20.8 mEq) (complete feeding *Brik Paks*); 1100 (28.2 mEq) (closed system)	700 (complete feeding *Brik Paks*); 960 (closed system)	2	Vit. A, B_1, B_2, B_3, B_5, B_6, B_{12}, C, D, E, K, Ca, Cl, Cu, Fe, I, Mg, Mn, P, Se, Zn, folic acid, biotin, choline	Vanilla flavor. In 237 mL *Tetra Brik Paks* (27s) and 1000 mL closed system containers (6s).
otc	**Meritene Powder**[1] (Sandoz Nutrition)	69.2	nonfat milk, whole milk, Ca caseinate, amino acids	119	sugar, hydrolyzed corn starch, fructose	34	soy lecithin	1077 (47 mEq)	2808 (72 mEq)	690	1.06	Vit A, B_1, B_2, B_3, B_5, B_6, B_{12}, C, D, E, K, Ca, Cl, Cu, Fe, I, Mg, Mn, P, Zn^2	Plain (sugar free), chocolate, eggnog, vanilla and milk chocolate flavors. In 1 and 4.5 lb.
otc	**Forta Shake Powder**[3] (Ross)	9	nonfat milk	26	sucrose	< 1	unknown	115 (5 mEq)	440 (11.3 mEq)	NA	140	Vit A, B_1, B_2, B_3, B_5, B_6, B_{12}, C, D, E, Ca, Cu, Fe, I, Mg, Mn, P, Zn^4	Vanilla, strawberry and eggnog flavors. In 470 g cans. Dutch chocolate flavor. In 530 g cans.
otc	**Ensure Pudding**[5] (Ross)	6.8	nonfat milk	34	sucrose, modified food starch	9.7	partially hydrogenated soybean oil	240	330	unknown	250	Vitamin A, D, E, K, C, folic acid, B_1, B_2, B_6, B_{12}, B_3, choline, biotin, B_5, Cl, Ca, Zn, Fe, P, Mg, I, Mn, Cu, tartrazine	Vanilla, chocolate, and butterscotch flavors. In 150 g cans.
otc	**Sustacal Pudding**[5] (Mead Johnson Nutritionals)	6.8	nonfat milk, amino acids	32	sugar, lactose, modified food starch	9.5	partially hydrogenated soy oil	120 (5.2 mEq)	320 (8.2 mEq)	NA	240	Vit A, B_1, B_2, B_3, B_5, B_6, B_{12}, C, D, E, Ca, Cl, Cu, Fe, I, Mg, Mn, P, Zn^4, tartrazine (vanilla flavor)	Vanilla, chocolate and butterscotch flavors. In 150 g.
otc	**Nepro Liquid** (Ross)	6.6	Ca, Mg and Na caseinates	51.1	sucrose, hydrolyzed cornstarch	22.7	high-oleic safflower oil, soy oil	197	251	NA	2	Vit A, D, E, C, B_1, B_3, B_5, B_6, B_{12}, I, biotin, FA, Na, K, Cl, Ca, P, Mg, Mn, Cu, Zn, Fe, Se^6	Lactose free. Vanilla flavor. In 240 mL ready-to-use cans.
otc	**Nutraloric Powder**[1] (Nutraloric)	91.5	Na and Ca caseinates	175	corn syrup solids, fructose	125	soybean oil, soy lecithin, mono- and diglycerides	874 (38 mEq)	3166.2 (81 mEq)	unknown	2.2	Vit A, B_1, B_2, B_3, B_5, B_6, B_{12}, C, D, E, K, Ca, Cl, Cu, Fe, I, Mg, Mn, P, Zn^2	Chocolate, strawberry, banana nut and vanilla flavors. In 1 lb.
otc	**Immunocal**[6] (Immunotec)	37.5	milk protein isolate	0.42		0		25	30	unknown	0.15	Ca, Mg, P	In 10 g packets (30s).

[1] Content given for powder mixed with whole milk.
[2] Also contains folic acid, biotin and choline.
[3] Content given per serving (42 g mix).
[4] Also contains folic acid and biotin.
[5] Content given per serving (150 g).
[6] Mixed with 8 oz. of fluid per directions.

MILK-BASED FORMULAS — ORAL

See individual product listings for specific labeled indications.

SPECIALIZED FORMULAS

	Product & Distributor	Content per Liter: Protein g	Protein Source	Carbohydrate g	Carbohydrate Source	Fat g	Fat Source	Na (mg)	K (mg)	mOsm/ kg H_2O	Cal/ mL	Other Content	How Supplied
otc	**Amin-Aid Instant Drink Powder**[1] (McGaw)	6.6	amino acids (including phenylalanine)	124.3	maltodextrins, sucrose	15.7	partially hydrogenated soybean oil, lecithin, mono- and diglycerides	< 115 (5 mEq)	NA	700	2	Tartrazine (lemon-lime flavor)	*For acute or chronic renal failure.* Lemon-lime flavor. In 156 g packets (12s).
otc	**Boost Nutritional Pudding** (Mead Johnson Nutritionals)	7	unknown	32	unknown	9	unknown	120	320	unknown	240	Vit A, C, D, E, K, B_6, B_{12}, B_1, B_2, B_3, B_5, Ca, Fe, folic acid, biotin, P, I, Mg, Zn, Se, Cu, Mn, Cr, Mo	Sugar. Vanilla, chocolate, and butterscotch flavors. In 142 g.
otc	**Boost Pudding**[2] (Mead Johnson)	10	unknown	35	unknown	7	unknown	130	400	unknown	240	Vit A, C, D, E, B_1, B_2, B_3, B_5, B_6, B_9, B_{12}, biotin, Ca, P, , Mg, Zn, Cu, sugar, corn syrup	Vanilla, chocolate, strawberry and mocha flavors. In 237 mL.
otc	**Optimental Liquid** (Ross)	12.2	unknown	32.9	unknown	6.7	unknown	250	420	unknown	unknown	Vit. A, D, E, K, C, folic acid, B_1, B_2, B_{12}, B_3, choline, biotin, B_5, chloride, Ca, P, Mg, I, Mn, Cu, Zn, Fe, Se, Cr, Mo	Sucrose, canola oil, soy oil. Vanilla and chocolate flavors. In 237 mL.
otc	**Hepatic-Aid II Instant Drink Powder**[3] (McGaw)	15	amino acids (high BCAA, low AAA)	57.3	maltodextrins, sucrose	12.3	partially hydrogenated soybean oil, lecithin, mono- and diglycerides	< 115 (5 mEq)	unknown	560	1.2	May contain tartrazine	*For chronic liver disease.* Chocolate, eggnog and custard flavors. In 93 g packets (12s).
otc	**Cyclinex-2 Powder**[4] (Ross)	15	amino acids (including carnitine, phenylalanine, tryptophan)	40	hydrolyzed cornstarch	20.7	palm oil, hydrogenated coconut oil, soy oil, mono-and diglycerides	1175 (51.1 mEq)	1830 (47 mEq)	NA	480	Vit A, B_1, B_2, B_3, B_5, B_6, B_{12}, C, D, E, K, inositol, Cl, Cu, I, Mg, Mn, P, Se, Zn, Ca, Fe[5]	*For urea cycle disorder or gyrate atrophy.* Nonessential amino acid free. In 325 g.
otc	**Immun-Aid Powder**[6] (McGaw)	18.5	lactalbumin, amino acids (including carnitine, phenylalanine, taurine)	60	maltodextrins	11	medium chain triglycerides, canola oil	290 (12.6 mEq)	530 (13.6 mEq)	460	1	Vit A, B_1, B_2, B_3, B_5, B_6, B_{12}, C, D, E, K, Ca, Fe, Cl, Cu, Cr, I, Mg, Mn, Mo, P, Se, Zn[5]	*For immunocompromised patients.* Custard flavor. In 123 g packets (24s).
otc	**BCAD 2 Powder**[4] (Mead Johnson Nutritionals)	24	L-glutamine, potassium aspartate, L-lysine HCl, L-tyrosine, L-proline, L-alanine, L-arginine, L-phenylalanine, L-threonine, L-serine, glycine, L-histidine, L-methionine, L-tryptophan, L-cystine, L-carnitine, taurine	57	corn syrup solids, sugar, modified corn starch	8.5	soy oil	610	1220	unknown	410	Vit A, B_1, B_2, B_3, B_5, B_6, B_{12}, C, D, E, K, inositol, Ca, Cl, Cr, Cu, Fe, I, Mg, Mn, Mo, F, Se, Zn[5]	*For Maple Syrup Urine Disease or other inborn errors of branched chain amino acid metabolism.* In 1 lb cans.
otc	**Arginaid Extra Liquid** (Novartis Nutrition)	25.3	Whey protein isolate, L-arginine, L-cysteine	219.4	Sugar, hydrolyzed corn starch	0		< 295	< 93	unknown	1.05	Vitamins A, B_1, B_2, B_3, B_5, B_6, B_{12}, C, D, E, K, biotin, folic acid, Cu, Fe, I, Mn, P, Zn	For promotion of wound healing. Orange and wild berry flavors. In 8 oz *Tetra Brik* Paks.
otc	**Suplena Liquid** (Ross)	29.6	Ca and Na caseinates, carnitine, taurine	252.5	hydrolyzed corn starch, sucrose	95	high-oleic safflower oil, soy oil, soy lecithin	775 (34 mEq)	1104 (28.3 mEq)	unknown	2	Vit A, B_1, B_2, B_3, B_5, B_6, B_{12}, C, D, E, K, Ca, Cl, Cu, Fe, I, Mg, Mn, P, Se, Zn[5]	*For renal conditions.* Vanilla flavor. In 240 mL ready-to-use cans.
otc	**Glutarex-2 Powder**[4] (Ross)	30	amino acids (including carnitine and phenylalanine)	30	hydrolyzed cornstarch	15.5	palm oil, hydrogenated coconut oil, soy oil, mono-and diglycerides	880 (38.3 mEq)	1370 (35 mEq)	NA	410	Vit A, B_1, B_2, B_3, B_5, B_6, B_{12}, C, D, E, inositol, K, Cl, Cu, I, Mg, Mn, P, Se, Zn, Ca, Fe[5]	*For glutaric aciduria type I.* Lysine- and tryptophan-free. In 325 g.

Defined Formula Diets

SPECIALIZED FORMULAS

	Product & Distributor	Protein g	Protein Source	Carbohydrate g	Carbohydrate Source	Fat g	Fat Source	Na (mg)	K (mg)	mOsm/ kg H_2O	Cal/ mL	Other Content	How Supplied
otc	**Hominex-2 Powder**[4] (Ross)	30	amino acids (including carnitine, phenylalanine, tryptophan)	30	hydrolyzed cornstarch	15.5	palm oil, hydrogenated coconut oil, soy oil, mono-and diglycerides	880 (38.3 mEq)	1370 (35.1 mEq)	NA	410	Vit A, B_1, B_2, B_3, B_5, B_6, B_{12}, C, D, E, K, inositol, Cl, Cu, I, Mg, Mn, P, Se, Zn[5]	*For vitamin B_6-nonresponsive homocystinuria or hypermethioninemia.* Methionine free. In 325 g.
otc	**I-Valex-2 Powder**[4] (Ross)	30	carnitine, phenylalanine, tryptophan, amino acids	30	hydrolyzed cornstarch	15.5	palm oil, hydrogenated coconut oil, soy oil, mono-and diglycerides	880 (38.3 mEq)	1370 (35.1 mEq)	NA	410	Vit A, B_1, B_2, B_3, B_5, B_6, B_{12}, C, D, E, K, inositol, Ca, Cl, Cu, I, Mg, Mn, P, Se, Zn[5]	*For disorder of leucine catabolism.* Leucine free. In 325 g.
otc	**Ketonex-2 Powder**[4] (Ross)	30	carnitine, phenylalanine, tryptophan, amino acids	30	hydrolyzed cornstarch	15.5	palm oil, hydrogenated coconut oil, soy oil, mono-and diglycerides	880 (38.3 mEq)	1370 (35.1 mEq)	NA	410	Vit A, B_1, B_2, B_3, B_5, B_6, B_{12}, C, D, E, K, inositol, Ca, Cl, Cu, I, Mg, Mn, P, Se, Zn[5]	*For maple syrup urine disease (MSUD).* Isoleucine, leucine and valine free. In 325 g.
otc	**Phenex-2 Powder**[2] (Ross)	30	amino acids (including carnitine, tryptophan)	30	hydrolyzed cornstarch	15.5	palm oil, hydrogenated coconut oil, soy oil, mono-and diglycerides	880 (38.3 mEq)	1370 (35.1 mEq)	NA	410	Vit A, B_1, B_2, B_3, B_5, B_6, B_{12}, C, D, E, K, inositol, Ca, Cl, Cu, I, Mg, Mn, P, Se, Zn[5]	*For phenylketonuria (PKU).* Phenylalanine free. In 325 g.
otc	**Propimex-2 Powder**[4] (Ross)	30	amino acids (including carnitine, phenylalanine, tryptophan)	30	hydrolyzed cornstarch	15.5	palm oil hydrogenated coconut oil, soy oil, mono-and diglycerides	880 (38.3 mEq)	1370 (35.1 mEq)	NA	410	Vit A, B_1, B_2, B_3, B_5, B_6, B_{12}, C, D, E, K, inositol, Ca, Cl, Cu, I, Mg, Mn, P, Se, Zn[5]	*For propionic or methylmalonic acidemia.* Methionine and valine free. In 325 g.
otc	**Tyrex-2 Powder**[4] (Ross)	30	amino acids (including carnitine, tryptophan)	30	hydrolyzed cornstarch	15.5	palm oil, hydrogenated coconut oil, soy oil	880 (38.3 mEq)	1370 (35.1 mEq)	NA	410	Vit A, B_1, B_2, B_3, B_5, B_6, B_{12}, C, D, E, K, inositol, Ca, Cl, Cu, I, Mg, Mn, P, Se, Zn[5]	*For tyrosinemia type* II. Phenylalanine and tyrosine free. In 325 g.
otc	**Epulor Liquid**[7] (VistaPharm)	31	unknown	4	unknown	5	unknown	7	35	NA	315	Biotin, Ca, chloride, Cr, Cu, folic acid, I, Fe, Mg, Mn, Mo, B_3, Ni, B_5, P, Se, Si, Sn,V, Vit. A, B_1, B_{12}, B_2, B_5, C, D, E, K, Zn	Caramel flavor. In 24s.
otc	**Peptamen Liquid** (Nestle Clinical Nutrition)	40	enzymatically hydrolyzed whey proteins, amino acids (including carnitine, taurine)	127.2	maltodextrin, starch	39.2	MCT (fractionated coconut oil), sunflower oil, soy lecithin					Vit. A, B_1, B_2, B_3, B_5, B_6, B_{12}, C, D, E, K, Cl, Ca, P, Mg, I, Mn, Cu, Zn, Fe, Se, Cr, Mo[2]	*For GI impairment.* Unflavored. In ready-to-use 250 mL cans and 500 mL, 1 L, and 1.5 L *UltraPak* bags.
otc	**Glucerna Liquid** (Ross)	41	amino acids (including carnitine, taurine), Ca and Na caseinate	93	hydrolyzed cornstarch, fructose, soy fiber	55	high-oleic safflower oil, soy oil, soy lecithin	917 (40 mEq)	1542 (40 mEq)	375	1	Vit A, B_1, B_2, B_3, B_5, B_6, B_{12}, C, D, E, K, Cl, Ca, P, Mg, I, Mn, Cu, Zn, Fe, Se, Cr, Mo[5]	*For abnormal glucose tolerance.* Vanilla flavor. In 240 mL ready-to-use cans and 1 liter ready-to-hang feeding containers.
otc	**Nutrament Liquid** (Mead Johnson Nutritionals)	44.5	Ca and Na caseinates, skim milk, soy protein isolates (in all flavors except chocolate	144.6	Sugar, corn syrup	27.8	canola oil, high oleic sunflower oil, corn oil, soy lecithin	695	1390	unknown	1	Vit A, B_1, B_2, B_3, B_5, B_6, B_{12}, C, D, E, K, biotin, folate, Ca, Cr, Cu, Fe, I, Mg, Mn, Mo, P, Se, Zn.	In vanilla, strawberry, chocolate, banana, coconut, and eggnog flavors. In 12 oz cans.
otc	**Peptinex Liquid** (Novartis Nutrition)	50	Whey protein hydrolysate, taurine, L-carnitine	160	Hydrolyzed corn starch	17	Soybean oil, medium chain triglycerides, soy lecithin	1010 (44 mEq)	1490 (38 mEq)	320	1	Vitamins A, B_1, B_2, B_3, B_5, B_6, B_{12}, C, D, E, K, biotin, choline, folic acid, Ca, Cl, Cr, Cu, Fe, I, Mg, Mn, Mo, P, Se, Zn	*For GI impaired patients.* Vanilla flavor. In 8 oz *Tetra Brik Paks.*

SPECIALIZED FORMULAS

		Content per Liter											
		Protein		Carbohydrate		Fat							
	Product & Distributor	g	Source	g	Source	g	Source	Na (mg)	K (mg)	mOsm/ kg H_2O	Cal/ mL	Other Content	How Supplied
otc	**Pulmocare Liquid**[8] (Ross)	62	Ca and Na caseinate, amino acids (including carnitine, taurine)	104	hydrolyzed cornstarch, sucrose	92	corn oil, soy lecithin, canola oil, MCT (fractionated coconut oil), high-oleic safflower oil	1292 (56 mEq)	1708 (44 mEq)	475	1.5	Vit A, B_1, B_2, B_3, B_5, B_6, B_{12}, C, D, E, K, Cl, Ca, P, Mg, I, Mn, Cu, Zn, Fe, Se, Cr, Mo[5]	*For pulmonary patients.* Lactose free. Vanilla and strawberry flavors. In 240 mL ready-to-use cans and 1 liter ready-to-hang containers.
otc	**NutriHeal** (Nestle)	62.4	ca-K caseinate (from cow's milk), taurine	112.8	corn syrup solids, fructooligosaccharides, sugar (sucrose)	33.2	canola oil, corn oil, soy lecithin	876	1248		1	Vit A, B_1, B_2, B_3, B_5, B_6, B_{12}, C, D, E, K, beta carotene, biotin, chloride, choline, folic acid, Ca, Cr, Cu, Fe, I, Mg, Mn, Mo, P, Se, Zn	Vanilla flavor. In 250 mL cans.
otc	**Jevity 1.5 Cal** (Ross)	63.4	Ca and Na caseinates, soy protein isolate, taurine, L-carnitine	214.2	corn syrup solids, corn maltodextrin, fructooligosaccharides, oat fiber, soy fiber	49.6	high oleic safflower oil, canola oil	1386	1848		1.5	Vit A, B_1, B_2, B_3, B_5, B_6, B_{12}, C, D, E, K, Cr, Ca, Cu, Fe, I, Mg, Mn, Mo, P, Se, Zn, biotin, chloride, choline, folic acid	In 237 mL cans and 1 and 1.5 L ready-to-hang containers.
otc	**Respalor Liquid** (Mead Johnson Nutritionals)	75	Ca and Na caseinate	146	corn syrup, sugar	70	MCT (fractionated coconut oil), soy lecithin, canola oil	1250 (54 mEq)	1458 (37 mEq)	580	1.5	Vit A, B_1, B_2, B_3, B_5, B_6, B_{12}, C, D, E, K, Cl, Ca, P, Mg, I, Mn, Cu, Zn, Fe, Se, Cr, Mo[5]	*For pulmonary patients.* Lactose free. Vanilla flavor. In ready-to-use 240 mL.
otc	**TraumaCal Liquid** (Mead Johnson Nutritionals)	83	Ca and Na caseinate, amino acids (including phenylalanine, tryptophan)	195	corn syrup, sugar	69	soybean oil, MCT (fractionated coconut oil), lecithin	1200 (52 mEq)	1400 (36 mEq)	490	1.5	Vit A, B_1, B_2, B_3, B_5, B_6, B_{12}, C, D, E, K, Ca, P, I, Fe, Mg, Mn, Cu, Zn, Cl[5]	*For moderately and severely stressed patients.* Lactose free. Vanilla flavor. In 237 mL ready-to-use cans.
otc	**Pro-Stat 64 Liquid**[9] (Medical Nutrition)	500	collagen hydrolysate, amino acids (including histidine, isoleucine, leucine, lysine, methionine, phenylalanine, threonine, tryptophan, valine, alanine, aspartic acid, cystine, glutamic acid, glycine, proline, serine, tyrosine, hydroxylysine, hydroxyproline)	33	sorbitol, sucralose	0	N/A	2438	390	unknown	2.1	Cl, Mg, P, Cu	Butter pecan and cherry flavors. In 946 mL

SPECIALIZED FORMULAS

	Product & Distributor	Protein g	Protein Source	Carbohydrate g	Carbohydrate Source	Fat g	Fat Source	Na (mg)	K (mg)	mOsm/ kg H_2O	Cal/ mL	Other Content	How Supplied
otc	**Pro-Stat 101 Liquid**[9] (Medical Nutrition)	500	collagen hydrolysate, amino acids (including histidine, isoleucine, leucine, lysine, methionine, phenylalanine, threonine, tryptophan, valine, alanine, arginine, aspartic acid, cystine, glutamic acid, glycine, proline, serine, tyrosine, hydroxylysine, hydroxyproline)	340	fructose, sucralose	0	N/A	2438	390	unknown	3.4	Cl, Mg, P, Cu	Butter pecan and cherry flavors. In 946 mL

(Columns Protein through K are grouped under "Content per Liter".)

[1] Content given per 156 g package.
[2] Content given per 237 mL.
[3] Content given per ≈ 93 g packets.
[4] Content given per 100 g.
[5] Also contains folic acid, biotin and choline.
[6] Content given per 123 g.
[7] Content given per 240 mL.
[8] Content given for vanilla flavor.
[9] Content given per 946 mL.

SPECIALIZED FORMULAS — ORAL

See individual product listings for specific labeled indications.

LACTOSE-FREE PRODUCTS

	Product & Distributor	Protein g	Protein Source	Carbohydrate g	Carbohydrate Source	Fat g	Fat Source	Na (mg)	K (mg)	mOsm/ kg H_2O	Cal/ mL	Other Content	How Supplied
otc	**Nestle VHC 2.25 Liquid** (Nestle Clinical Nutrition)	90	Calcium potassium caseinate, taurine, isolated soy protein	196	Corn syrup solids, sugar (sucrose)	120	Canola oil, corn oil, soy lecithin	1,200	1,732	950	2.25	Vit A, B_1, B_2, B_3, B_5, B_6, B_{12}, C, D, E, K, biotin, chloride, choline, FA, Ca, Cr, Cu, Fe, I, Mg, Mn, Mo, P, Se, Zn	Gluten free. Vanilla flavor. In 250 mL cans.
otc	**Nepro Liquid** (Clintec)	69.7	Ca, Mg and Na caseinates	214.6	sucrose, hydrolyzed cornstarch	95.3	90% high-oleic safflower oil, 10% soy oil	215	1,054	NA	2	Vit A, B_1, B_3, B_5, B_6, B_{12}, biotin, FA, Na, K, Cl, Ca, P, Mg, Mn, I, Cu, Zn, Fe, Se	Vanilla flavor. In 240 mL ready-to-use-cans.
otc	**NutriFocus** (Abbott)	62.16	arginine, sodium caseinates, soy and milk protein isolate	213.78	corn syrup, fiber blend, fructooligosaccharides, sucrose	49.14	canola oil, corn oil, high oleic safflower oil, lecithin	924 (40.32 mEq)	1,680 (42.84 mEq)	NA	1.5	Vit A, B_1, B_2, B_3, B_5, B_6, B_{12}, C, D, E, K, Ca, Cl, Cu, Cr, Fe, I, Mg, Mn, Mo, P, Se, Zn[a]	Gluten free. Chocolate and vanilla flavors. In 237 mL.
otc	**Entrition 0.5 Liquid** (Clintec)	17.5	Na and Ca caseinate	68	maltodextrin	17.5	corn oil, soy lecithin, mono- and diglycerides	350 (15.2 mEq)	600 (15.4 mEq)	120	0.5	Vit A, B_1, B_2, B_3, B_5, B_6, B_{12}, C, D, E, K, Ca, P, Mg, I, Fe, Zn, Mn, Cu, Cl[a]	Unflavored. In 1 L closed system pouches.
otc	**Pre-Attain Liquid** (Sherwood)	20	Na caseinate	60	maltodextrin	20	corn oil, soy lecithin	340 (15 mEq)	575 (15 mEq)	150	0.5	Vit A, B_1, B_2, B_3, B_5, B_6, B_{12}, C, D, E, K, Ca, Cl, Cu, I, Fe, Mg, Mn, P, Zn[a]	In 1 L prefilled closed system containers.
otc	**Citrotein Powder and Liquid**[b] (Novartis)	41	egg white solids, amino acids (including phenylalanine, tryptophan)	122	sugar, hydrolyzed cornstarch	1.6	mono- and diglycerides, partially hydrogenated soybean oil	669 (29 mEq)	551 (14 mEq)	500	0.67	Vit A, B_1, B_2, B_3, B_5, B_6, B_{12}, C, D, E, Ca, P, I, Fe, Mg, Cu, Zn, Cl, Mn[a]	Cholesterol and gluten free. Orange and grape flavors. In 47.1 g packets (72s) and 424 mL cans (12s).
otc	**Choice DM** (Bristol-Myers Squibb)	38.1	unknown	101.5	unknown	42.3	unknown	846	1,818.9	unknown	0.93	Vit A, D, E, K, C, B_1, B_2, B_3, B_5, B_6, B_{12}, FA, biotin, Ca, P, I, Fe, Mg, Cu, Zn, Mn, Cl, K, Na, Se, Cr, Mo, sucrose	Vanilla and chocolate flavors. In 237 mL ready-to-use cans.

(Columns Protein through K are grouped under "Content per Liter".)

Defined Formula Diets

LACTOSE-FREE PRODUCTS

	Product & Distributor	Content per Liter: Protein g	Protein Source	Carbohydrate g	Carbohydrate Source	Fat g	Fat Source	Na (mg)	K (mg)	mOsm/kg H_2O	Cal/mL	Other Content	How Supplied
otc *sf*	**Choice DM Sugar Free Shakes** (Bristol-Myers Squibb)	30.7	unknown	33.8	unknown	7.7	unknown	460.5	1,043.8	un-known	0.38	Vit A, D, E, K, B_1, B_2, B_3, B_5, B_6, B_{12}, Ca, Fe, FA, biotin, P, I, Mg, Zn, Se, Cu, Cr, Mc	Mocha cappuccino flavor. In 325 mL.
		30.7	unknown	36.8	unknown	6.1	unknown	460.5	1,043.8	un-known	0.38		Chocolate fudge flavor. In 325 mL.
		30.7	unknown	24.6	unknown	6.1	unknown	399.1	337.7	un-known	0.31		French vanilla flavor. In 325 mL.
		30.7	unknown	21.5	unknown	7.7	unknown	399.1	337.7	un-known	0.31		Strawberries 'n cream flavor. In 325 mL.
otc	**Vitaneed Liquid** (Sherwood)	40	pureed beef. Ca and Na caseinate, dietary fiber from soy	128	maltodextrin, pureed fruits and vegetables	40	corn oil, soy lecithin	630 (27.4 mEq)	1,250 (32 mEq)	300	1	Vit A, B_1, B_2, B_3, B_5, B_6, B_{12}, C, D, E, K, Ca, Cl, Cu, Fe, I, Mg, Mn, P, Zn[a]	In 250 mL cans and 1 L prefilled closed system containers.
otc	**Lipisorb Powder** (Mead Johnson Nutritionals)	35	Na caseinate, carnitine	117	corn syrup solids, sucrose	48	MCT, corn oil, soy lecithin	733 (32 mEq)	1,250 (32 mEq)	320	1	Vit A, B_1, B_2, B_3, B_5, B_6, B_{12}, C, D, E, K, Ca, Cl, Cu, Fe, I, Mg, Mn, P, Zn[a]	Vanilla flavor. In 1 lb.
otc	**Introlan Half-Strength Liquid** (Elan Pharma)	22.5	Na and Ca caseinate	70	maltodextrin	18	corn oil, MCT, soy lecithin	345 (15 mEq)	585 (15 mEq)	150	0.5	Vit A, B_1, B_2, B_3, B_5, B_6, B_{12}, C, D, E, K, Ca, Cl, Cu, Cr, Fe, I, Mg, Mn, Mo, P, Se, Zn[a]	Gluten free. Unflavored. In 1 L closed system containers. Also available with color check.
otc	**Kindercal** (Mead Johnson Nutritionals)	34	Na and Ca caseinate	135	maltodextrin, sucrose	44	(oils) canola, high oleic sunflower, corn, MCT	370 (16 mEq)	1,310 (34 mEq)	310	1	Vit A, B_1, B_2, B_3, B_5, B_6, B_{12}, C, D, E, K, Ca, Cr, Cu, Fe I, Mg, Mn, Mo, P, Se, Zn, biotin, folic acid, chlorides, L-carnitine, taurine	Vanilla flavor. In 240 mL cans.
otc	**Profiber Liquid** (Sherwood)	40	Na and Ca caseinate, dietary fiber from soy	132	hydrolyzed cornstarch	40	corn oil, soy lecithin	730 (32 mEq)	1,250 (32 mEq)	300	1	Vit A, B_1, B_2, B_3, B_5, B_6, B_{12}, C, D, E, K, Ca, Cl, Cr, Cu, Fe, I, Mg, Mn, Mo, P, Se, Zn[a]	In 1 L prefilled closed system containers.
otc	**Peptinex DT Liquid** (Novartis Nutrition)	50	Casein hydrolysate, amino acids	164	Maltodextrin, modified corn starch	17.4	Medium chain triglycerides, soybean oil	1,700 (74 mEq)	800 (2[illegible] mEq)	460	1	Vit A, B_1, B_2, B_3, B_5, B_6, B_{12}, C, D, E, K, biotin, choline, folic acid, Ca, Cl, Cr, Cu, Fe, I, Mg, Mn, Mo, P, Se, Zn	*For GI impaired patients.* Lactose and gluten free. In 250 mL cans and 1 and 1.5 L closed system containers.
otc	**Impact Liquid** (Sandoz Nutrition)	56	Na and Ca caseinate, L-arginine	130	hydrolyzed cornstarch	28	structured lipids from palm kernel oil and sunflower oil, refined menhaden oil, hydroxylated soy lecithin	1,100 (48 mEq)	1,300 (33 mEq)	375	1	Vit A, B_1, B_2, B_3, B_5, B_6, B_{12}, C, E, D, K, Ca, Fe, P, I, Mg, Zn, Cu, Cl, Mn, Se, Cr, Mo[a]	In 250 mL ready-to-use cans.
otc	**Glucerna Weight Loss Shake** (Abbott)	40.3	sodium and calcium caseinates, soy protein isolate	120.9	fructose, fructooligosaccharides, maltodextrin, soy fiber, sugar alcohols	34.1	canola oil, high oleic safflower oil, soy lecithin	868 (37.82 mEq)	1,550 (39.68 mEq)	NA	0.89	Vit A, B_1, B_2, B_3, B_5, B_6, B_7, B_9, B_{12}, C, D, E, K, choline, Ca, Cl, Cu, Cr, Fe, I, Mg, Mn, Mo, P, Se, Zn	Gluten free. Vanilla, chocolate, banana, peach, and dulce de leche flavors. In 325 mL.
otc	**Glucerna Select** (Abbott)	50	sodium and calcium caseinates, soy protein isolate	95.7	fructose, fructooligosaccharides, maltodextrin, soy fiber, sugar alcohols	54.4	canola oil, high oleic safflower oil, soy lecithin	940 (40.9 mEq)	1,810 (46.3 mEq)	470	1	Vit A, B_1, B_2, B_3, B_5, B_6, B_7, B_9, B_{12}, C, D, E, K, choline, Ca, Cl, Cu, Cr, Fe, I, Mg, Mn, Mo, P, Se, Zn	Gluten free. Vanilla flavor. In 240, 1,000, and 1,500 mL.
otc	**Enlive!** (Abbott)	41.2	whey protein isolate	273	maltodextrin, sucrose	0	NA	273	168	840	1.25	Vit A, B_1, B_2, B_3, B_5, B_3, B_{12}, C, D, E, K, biotin, choline, Ca, Cl, Cu, Cr, Fe, I, Mg, Mn, Mo, P, Se, Zn	Gluten free. Apple and peach flavors. In 240 mL.

LACTOSE-FREE PRODUCTS

		Content per Liter											
		Protein		Carbohydrate		Fat		Na	K	mOsm/	Cal/	Other	
	Product & Distributor	g	Source	g	Source	g	Source	(mg)	(mg)	kg H_2O	mL	Content	How Supplied
otc	**Nutren 1.0 Liquid** (Clintec Nutrition)	40	K and Ca caseinates, taurine, carnitine	127	maltodextrin, corn syrup solids	38	MCT (fractionated coconut oil), corn oil, soy lecithin, canola oil	500 (21.7 mEq)	1,252 (32 mEq)	300 to 390	1	Vit A, B_1, B_2, B_3, B_5, B_6, B_{12}, C, D, E, K, Ca, Cl, Cr, Cu, Fe, I, Mg, Mn, Mo, P, Se, Zn[a]	Gluten free. Unflavored and vanilla, chocolate, and strawberry flavors. In 250 mL and *UltraPak* prefilled bags in 1 and 1.5 L.
otc	**Sustacal Liquid** (Mead Johnson Nutritionals)	60.4	Ca and Na caseinate, soy protein isolate	138	sugar, corn syrup	23	partially hydrogenated soy oil, soy lecithin	1,000 (40 mEq)	2,042 (52.4 mEq)	NA	1	Vit A, B_1, B_2, B_3, B_5, B_6, B_{12}, C, D, E, K, Ca, P, I, Fe, Mg, Cu, Zn, Mn, Cl[a]	Vanilla, chocolate, strawberry, and eggnog flavors. In 240 and 360 mL and qt ready-to-use cans.
otc	**Vivonex T.E.N. Powder** (Sandoz Nutrition)	38.2	free amino acids (phenylalanine and tryptophan)	205	unknown	2.77	linoleic acid	460 (20 mEq)	782 (20 mEq)	630	1	Vit A, B_1, B_2, B_3, B_5, B_6, B_{12}, C, D, E, K, Ca, P, I, Fe, Mg, Cu, Zn, Mn, Se, Mo, Cr, Cl[a]	In 80.4 g packets.
otc	**Portagen Powder** (Mead Johnson Nutritionals)	23.3	Na caseinate, amino acids (including taurine, carnitine)	77	corn syrup solids, sucrose	32	MCT (fractionated coconut oil), corn oil, soy lecithin	367 (16 mEq)	833 (21 mEq)	NA	unknown	Vit A, B_1, B_2, B_3, B_5, B_6, B_{12}, C, D, E, K, inositol, Ca, P, I, Fe, Mg, Cu, Zn, Mn, Cl[a]	In 1 lb cans.
otc	**Vital High Nitrogen Powder** (Ross)	41.7	essential amino acids (including phenylalanine, tryptophan), partially hydrolyzed whey, meat and soy	184.7	hydrolyzed cornstarch, sucrose	10.8	safflower oil, MCT (fractionated coconut oil), mono- and diglycerides, soy lecithin	566.7 (24.6 mEq)	1,400 (36 mEq)	500	1	Vit A, B_1, B_2, B_3, B_5, B_6, B_{12}, C, D, E, K_1, Ca, P, Mg, Fe, Cu, Zn, Mn, I, Cl, folic acid, biotin, choline[a]	Vanilla flavor. In 79 g packets.
otc	**TwoCal HN Liquid** (Ross)	83	Na and Ca caseinates	214.2	hydrolyzed cornstarch, sucrose	90	MCT (fractionated coconut oil), corn oil, soy lecithin	1,292 (56 mEq)	2,417 (62 mEq)	unknown	2	Vit A, B_1, B_2, B_3, B_5, B_6, B_{12}, C, D, E, K, Ca, P, Mg, Fe, Cr, Cu, Se, Zn, Mn, Mo, I, Cl[a]	Vanilla flavor. In ready-to-use 240 mL cans.
otc	**Criticare HN Liquid** (Mead Johnson Nutritionals)	38	enzymatically hydrolyzed casein, amino acids (including phenylalanine, tryptophan)	220	maltodextrin, modified cornstarch	5.3	safflower oil, mono- and diglycerides	630 (27 mEq)	1,320 (34 mEq)	650	1.06	Vit A, B_1, B_2, B_3, B_5, B_6, B_{12}, C, D, E, K, Ca, P, I, Fe, Mg, Cu, Zn, Mn, Cl[a]	Unflavored. In 240 mL ready-to-use bottles.
otc	**Isocal HN Liquid** (Mead Johnson Nutritionals)	44	Ca and Na caseinate, soy protein isolate, amino acids (including taurine, carnitine)	123	maltodextrin	45	soy oil, MCT (fractionated coconut oil)	930 (40 mEq)	1,610 (41 mEq)	270	1.06	Vit A, B_1, B_2, B_3, B_5, B_6, B_{12}, C, D, E, K, Ca, P, I, Fe, Mg, Cu, Zn, Mn, Cl, Se, Cr, Mo[a]	Vanilla flavor. In 240 mL and qt ready-to-use cans. Unflavored in 1 L ready-to-hang bottles.
otc	**Isolan Liquid** (Elan)	40	caseinates	144	maltodextrin	36	MCT, corn oil	690 (30 mEq)	1,170 (30 mEq)	300	1.06	Vit A, B_1, B_2, B_3, B_5, B_6, B_{12}, C, D, E, K, Ca, P, I, Fe, Mg, Cu, Zn, Mn, Cl, Se, Cr, Mo[a]	Gluten free. Unflavored. In 237 mL ready-to-use open system containers and 1 L closed system containers.
otc	**Isotein HN Powder**[c] (Sandoz Nutrition)	20	Na and Ca caseinate, lactalbumin, amino acids (including tryptophan, phenylalanine)	46.7	maltodextrin, fructose	10	MCT, hydrogenated soybean oil, mono- and diglycerides	183 (8 mEq)	317 (8.1 mEq)	300	1.19	Vit A, B_1, B_2, B_3, B_5, B_6, B_{12}, C, D, E, K, Ca, P, I, Fe, Mg, Cu, Zn, Mn, Cl, Se, Cr, Mo[a]	Gluten free. Vanilla flavor. In 87 g packets (36s).
otc	**Jevity Liquid** (Ross)	44	Ca and Na caseinate, soy fiber, carnitine, taurine	150.8	hydrolyzed cornstarch	35	MCT (fractionated coconut oil) canola oil, high-oleic safflower oil, soy lecithin	917 (40 mEq)	1,542 (40 mEq)	300	1.06	Vit A, B_1, B_2, B_3, B_5, B_6, B_{12}, C, D, E, K, Ca, P, Mg, Fe, Mn, Cu, Zn, I, Cl, Se, Cr, Mo[a]	In 240 mL and qt ready-to-use cans and 1 L ready-to-hang bottles.

LACTOSE-FREE PRODUCTS

		Content per Liter											
		Protein		Carbohydrate		Fat		Na (mg)	K (mg)	mOsm/ kg H_2O	Cal/ mL	Other Content	How Supplied
	Product & Distributor	g	Source	g	Source	g	Source						
otc	**Resource Liquid** (Sandoz Nutrition)	37	Ca and Na caseinate, soy protein isolate, amino acids (including phenylalanine and tryptophan)	145	sugar, hydrolyzed cornstarch	37	corn oil, soy lecithin	886 (39 mEq)	1,603 (41 mEq)	430	1.06	Vit A, B_1, B_2, B_3, B_5, B_6, B_{12}, C, D, E, K, Ca, P, I, Fe, Mg, Cu, Zn, Mn, Cl[a]	Gluten free. Vanilla, chocolate, and strawberry flavors. In 240 mL ready-to-use *TetraBrik paks.*
otc	**Osmolite Liquid** (Ross)	37	Ca and Na caseinate, soy protein isolate, carnitine, taurine	143	hydrolyzed cornstarch	37	MCT (fractionated coconut oil), canola oil, high-oleic safflower oil, soy lecithin	625 (27 mEq)	1,000 (26 mEq)	300	1.06	Vit A, B_1, B_2, B_3, B_5, B_6, B_{12}, C, D, E, K, Cl, Ca, Cr, P, Se, Mg, I, Mn, Mo, Cu, Zn, Fe[a]	Unflavored. In 240 mL and qt ready-to-use cans and 1 L ready-to-hang containers.
otc	**Introlite Liquid** (Ross)	22.2	Na and Ca caseinates	70.5	hydrolyzed cornstarch	18.4	MCT (fractionated coconut oil), corn oil, soy oil, soy lecithin	930 (40 mEq)	1,570 (40 mEq)	200	0.53	Vit A, B_1, B_2, B_3, B_5, B_6, B_{12}, C, D, E, K, Cl, Ca, P, Mg, I, Mn, Cu, Zn, Fe, Se, Cr, Mo[a]	In 1 L ready-to-use ready-to-hang containers.
otc	**Osmolite HN Liquid** (Ross)	44	Ca and Na caseinate, soy protein isolate, carnitine, taurine	140	hydrolyzed cornstarch	35	MCT (fractionated coconut oil), high-oleic safflower oil, soy lecithin, canola oil	917 (40 mEq)	1,541 (40 mEq)	300	1.06	Vit A, B_1, B_2, B_3, B_5, B_6, B_{12}, C, D, E, K, Cl, Ca, Cr, P, Se, Mg, I, Mn, Mo, Cu, Zn, Fe[a]	In 240 mL and qt ready-to-use cans and 1 L ready-to-hang containers.
otc	**Nutrilan Liquid** (Elan)	38	caseinates	143	maltodextrin	37	MCT, corn oil	632.5 (27.5 mEq)	1,057 (27.1 mEq)	320	1.06	Vit A, B_1, B_2, B_3, B_5, B_6, B_{12}, C, D, E, K, Cl, Ca, P, Mg, I, Mn, Cu, Zn, Fe, Se, Cr, Mo[a]	Chocolate, vanilla, and strawberry flavors. In ready-to-use 240 mL *TetraPak* open system containers.
otc	**Ensure Liquid and Powder**[d] (Ross)	37	Ca and Na caseinate, soy protein isolate	143	corn syrup, sucrose	37	corn oil, soy lecithin	833 (36.2 mEq)	1,542 (40 mEq)	470	1.06	Vit A, B_1, B_2, B_3, B_5, B_6, B_{12}, C, D, E, K, Cl, Ca, Cr, P, Se, Mn, Mo, I, Mg, Cu, Zn, Fe[a]	Vanilla, chocolate, coffee, black walnut, strawberry, and eggnog flavors. In 240 mL and qt ready-to-use cans and 400 g powder.
otc	**Ensure HN Liquid** (Ross)	44	Ca and Na caseinate, soy protein isolate	140	corn syrup, sucrose	35	corn oil, soy lecithin	792 (34 mEq)	1,042 (40 mEq)	470	1.06	Vit A, B_1, B_2, B_3, B_5, B_6, B_{12}, C, D, E, K, Cl, Ca, P, Mg, Fe, Mn, Cu, Zn, I[a]	Vanilla flavor. In 240 mL and qt ready-to-use cans. Chocolate flavor. In 240 mL ready-to-use cans.
otc	**Ensure High Protein Liquid** (Ross)	50.4	Ca and Na caseinates, soy protein isolate	129.4	sucrose, maltodextrin	25.2	safflower oil, canola oil, soy oil	1,218	2,100	unknown	1	Vit A, B_1, B_2, B_3, B_5, B_6, B_{12}, C, D, E, K_1, Ca, Cl, Cr, Cu, Fe, I, Mg Mn, Mo, P, Se, Zr, folic acid	Banana, chocolate, wild berry, and vanilla flavors. In 237 mL.
otc	**Ultracal Liquid** (Mead Johnson Nutritional)	44	Ca and Na caseinate, soy fiber, oat fiber, taurine, carnitine	123	maltodextrin	45	MCT (fractionated coconut oil), canola oil, mono- and diglycerides, soy lecithin	930 (40 mEq)	1,610 (41 mEq)	310	1.06	Vit A, B_1, B_2, B_3, B_5, B_6, B_{12}, C, D, E, K, Ca, P, I, Fe, Mg, Cu, Zn, Mn, Cl, Se, Cr, Mo[a]	Vanilla flavor. In 240 mL and qt ready-to-use cans and 1 L ready-to-hang containers.
otc	**Compleat Modified Formula Liquid** (Sandoz Nutrition)	43	beef, Ca caseinate, amino acids (including phenylalanine, tryptophan)	140	maltodextrin, pureed fruits & vegetables	37	canola oil, mono- and diglycerides	1,000 (43.5 mEq)	1,400 (36 mEq)	300	1.07	Vit A, B_1, B_2, B_3, B_5, B_6, B_{12}, C, D, E, K, Ca, P, I, Fe, Mg, Cu, Zn, Cl, Mn, Se, Cr, Mo[a]	In ready-to-use 250 mL cans and 1,000 and 1,500 mL closed system containers.
otc	**Ensure with Fiber Liquid** (Ross)	39	Ca and Na caseinate, soy protein isolate, soy fiber	160	hydrolyzed cornstarch, sucrose	37	corn oil, soy lecithin	833 (36 mEq)	1,667 (43 mEq)	480	1.1	Vit A, B_1, B_2, B_3, B_5, B_6, B_{12}, C, D, E, K, Cl, Ca, P, Mg, Fe, Mn, Cu, Zn, I, Se, Cr, Mo[a]	Vanilla and chocolate flavors. In 240 mL and qt (vanilla only) ready-to-use cans.
otc	**Fiberlan Liquid** (Elan)	50	Na and Ca caseinates	160	maltodextrin	40	MCT, corn oil, soy lecithin	920 (40 mEq)	1,560 (40 mEq)	310	1.2	Vit A, B_1, B_2, B_3, B_5, B_6, B_{12}, C, D, E, K, Cl, Ca, P, Mg, Fe, Mn, Cu, Zn, I, Se, Cr, Mo[a]	Gluten free. Unflavored. In ready-to-use 237 mL open system containers and 1 L unflavored closed system containers.

Defined Formula Diets

LACTOSE-FREE PRODUCTS

		Content per Liter											
		Protein		Carbohydrate		Fat		Na	K	mOsm/	Cal/	Other	
	Product & Distributor	g	Source	g	Source	g	Source	(mg)	(mg)	kg H_2O	mL	Content	How Supplied
otc	**Isosource Liquid** (Sandoz Nutrition)	43	Ca and Na caseinate, soy protein isolate	170	hydrolyzed cornstarch	41	MCT, canola oil, soy lecithin	1,200 (52.2 mEq)	1,700 (44 mEq)	360	1.2	Vit A, B_1, B_2, B_3, B_5, B_6, B_{12}, C, D, E, K, Ca, Cl, Cu, Fe, I, Mg, Mn, P, Zn, Se, Cr, Mo[a]	Fiber and gluten free. Vanilla flavor. In ready-to-use 250 mL cans, 240 mL *TetraBrik* packs and 1 and 1.5 L closed system containers.
otc	**Nitrolan Liquid** (Elan)	60	caseinates	160	maltodextrin	40	MCT, corn oil, soy lecithin	690 (30 mEq)	1,170 (30 mEq)	310	1.24	Vit A, B_1, B_2, B_3, B_5, B_6, B_{12}, C, D, E, K, Ca, P, I, Fe, Mg, Cu, Zn, Cl, Mn, Se, Cr, Mo[a]	Gluten free. Unflavored. In ready-to-use 240 mL open system containers and 1 L closed system containers with or without color check.
otc	**Isosource HN Liquid** (Sandoz Nutrition)	53	Ca and Na caseinate, soy protein isolate, amino acids (including phenylalanine, tryptophan)	160	hydrolyzed cornstarch	41	MCT, canola oil, soy lecithin	1,100 (48 mEq)	1,700 (44 mEq)	330	1.2	Vit A, B_1, B_2, B_3, B_5, B_6, B_{12}, C, D, E, K, Ca, P, I, Fe, Mg, Cu, Zn, Cl, Mn, Se, Cr, Mo[a]	Vanilla flavor. In ready-to-use 250 mL cans, 240 mL *TetraBrik* packs, and 1 and 1.5 L closed system containers.
otc	**Comply Liquid** (Sherwood)	60	Ca and Na caseinate	180	maltodextrin, sucrose[e]	60	corn oil, soy lecithin	1,100 (48 mEq)	1,850 (47 mEq)	410	1.5	Vit A, B_1, B_2, B_3, B_5, B_6, B_{12}, C, D, E, K, Ca, Cl, Cu, Fe, I, Mg, Mn, P, Zn[a]	Unflavored. In 250 mL cans. Vanilla, orange, and banana flavors. In 250 mL cans and 1,000 mL prefilled systems.
otc	**Nutren 1.5 Liquid** (Clintec Nutrition)	60	Ca K and Na caseinate	169.2	maltodextrin	67.6	MCT (fractionated coconut oil), corn oil, canola oil, soy lecithin	752 (33 mEq)	1,872 (48 mEq)	410 to 590	1.5	Vit A, B_1, B_2, B_3, B_5, B_6, B_{12}, C, D, E, K, Ca, Cl, Cu, Fe, I, Mg, Mn, P, Zn, Cr, Mo, Se[a]	Gluten free. Unflavored and vanilla and chocolate flavors. In 250 mL ready-to-use cans. Unflavored in 1 L prefilled closed system containers.
otc	**Ensure Plus Liquid**[f] (Ross)	54.2	Ca and Na caseinate, soy protein isolate	197.1	corn syrup, sucrose	53	corn oil, soy lecithin	1,042 (45.3 mEq)	1,917 (49 mEq)	690	1.5	Vit A, B_1, B_2, B_3, B_5, B_6, B_{12}, C, D, E, K, Cl, Ca, P, Mg, Mn, I, Fe, Cu, Zn, Cr, Se, Mo[a]	Chocolate, vanilla, eggnog, strawberry, and coffee flavors. In ready-to-use 240 mL and qt cans and 1 L ready-to-hang containers.
otc	**Resource Plus Liquid**[f] (Sandoz Nutrition)	55	Ca and Na caseinate, soy protein isolate	200	hydrolyzed cornstarch, sugar	53	corn oil, soy lecithin	1,266 (55 mEq)	2,068 (53 mEq)	600	1.5	Vit A, B_1, B_2, B_3, B_5, B_6, B_{12}, C, D, E, K, Ca, P, I, Fe, Mg, Cu, Zn, Cl, Mn[a]	Gluten free. Vanilla, chocolate, and strawberry flavors. In 240 mL ready-to-use *BrikPaks*.
otc	**Ensure Plus HN Liquid** (Ross)	62	Ca and Na caseinate, soy protein isolate, amino acid (including carnitine, taurine)	197	hydrolyzed cornstarch, sucrose	49	corn oil, soy lecithin	1,167 (51 mEq)	1,792 (46 mEq)	unknown	1.5	Vit A, B_1, B_2, B_3, B_5, B_6, B_{12}, C, D, E, K, choline, Cl, Ca, P, Mg, I, Mn, Cu, Zn, Fe, Se, Cr, Mo[a]	Vanilla and chocolate flavors. In 240 mL ready-to-use cans and 1 L ready-to-hang containers.
otc	**NutriFocus** (Ross)	61.7	Na caseinate, milk protein isolate, soy protein isolate, arginine	212.3	corn syrup, sugar, fructooligosaccharides	48.8	canola oil, high oleic safflower oil, corn oil, lecithin	917	1,668	unknown	1.5	Vit A, B_1, B_2, B_3, B_5, B_6, B_{12}, C, D, E, K, Ca, Cl, Cr, Cu, Fe, P, Mg, I, Mn, Zn, Fe, Se, Mo, beta carotene, biotin, choline, 417 mcg folic acid/L	20.85 g fiber/L. Lactose and gluten free. In chocolate and vanilla flavors. In 240 mL cans.
otc	**Ultralan Liquid** (Elan)	60	caseinates	202	maltodextrin	50	MCT, corn oil	1,035 (45 mEq)	1,755 (45 mEq)	610	1.5	Vit A, B_1, B_2, B_3, B_5, B_6, B_{12}, C, D, E, K, Cl, Ca, P, Mg, I, Mn, Cu, Zn, Fe, Se, Cr, Mo[a]	Gluten free. Unflavored. In ready-to-use 1,000 mL *NewPak* closed system containers with and without color check.
otc	**Advera** (Ross)	60	soy protein hydrolysate, sodium caseinate, 127 mg/L carnitine, 212 mg/L taurine	215.8	hydrolyzed cornstarch, sucrose	22.8	canola oil, medium-chain triglycerides (fractionated coconut oil), refined deodorized sardine oil	1,046	2,827	unknown	1.3	8.9 g dietary fiber (from soy fiber), Vit A, D, E, K, C, folic acid, B_1, B_2, B_3, biotin, B_5, B_6, B_{12}, Cl, Ca, Zn, Fe, P, Mg, I, Mn, Cu, Se, Cr, Mo, choline	*For dietary management in HIV infection or AIDS.* Gluten free. Chocolate flavor. In 240 mL cans.

Defined Formula Diets

LACTOSE-FREE PRODUCTS

	Product & Distributor	Protein g	Protein Source	Carbohydrate g	Carbohydrate Source	Fat g	Fat Source	Na (mg)	K (mg)	mOsm/ kg H_2O	Cal/ mL	Other Content	How Supplied
otc	**Magnacal Liquid** (Sherwood)	70	Ca and Na caseinate	250	maltodextrin, sucrose	80	partially hydrogenated soy oil, soy lecithin, mono- and diglycerides	1,000 (43.5 mEq)	1,250 (32 mEq)	590	2	Vit A, B_1, B_2, B_3, B_5, B_6, B_{12}, C, D, E, K, choline, Ca, Cl, Cu, Fe, I, Mg, Mn, P, Zn	Vanilla flavor. In ready-to-use 120 and 240 mL bottles and 250 mL cans.
otc	**Isocal HCN Liquid** (Mead Johnson Nutritionals)	75	Ca and Na caseinate, amino acids (including phenylalanine, tryptophan)	200	corn syrup	102	soy oil, MCT (fractionated coconut oil), soy lecithin	800 (35 mEq)	1,700 (43 mEq)	640	2	Vit A, B_1, B_2, B_3, B_5, B_6, B_{12}, C, D, E, K, Ca, P, I, Fe, Mg, Cu, Zn, Mn, Cl, Se, Cr, Mo[a]	Vanilla flavor. In 240 mL ready-to-use cans.
otc	**Nutren 2.0 Liquid** (Clintec Nutrition)	80	Ca and K caseinate, amino acids	196	maltodextrin, corn syrup solids, sucrose	106	MCT (fractionated coconut oil), corn oil, soy lecithin, canola oil	1,000 (44 mEq)	2,500 (64 mEq)	710	2	Vit A, B_1, B_2, B_3, B_5, B_6, B_{12}, C, D, E, K, Ca, Cl, Cu, Fe, I, Mg, Mn, P, Zn, Cr, Se, Mo[a]	Gluten free. Vanilla flavor. In 250 mL ready-to-use cans.
otc	**Forta Drink Powder**[g] (Ross)	5	whey protein concentrate	15	sucrose, pineapple juice solids	< 1	unknown	50 (2.2 mEq)	70 (1.8 mEq)	NA	85	Vit A, B_1, B_2, B_3, B_5, B_6, B_{12}, C, D, E, Ca, Cu, Fe, I, Mg, Mn, P, Zn[a]	Orange and fruit punch flavors. In 482 g cans.
otc	**Neocate One + Liquid** (SHS)	≈ 2.5	amino acids	14.6	sucrose, maltodextrin	3.5	fractionated coconut oil, canola oil, high oleic sunflower oil	20 (0.9 mEq)	93 (2.4 mEq)	835	100	Vit A, B_1, B_2, B_3, B_5, B_6, B_{12}, C, D, E, K, Ca, Cl, Cr, Cu, Fe, I, Mg, Mn, Mo, Se, Zn, FA, biotin, choline, inositol	Gluten free. Orange and pineapple flavors. In 237 mL with straw.
otc	**ReSource Just for Kids** (Novartis Nutrition)	30	sodium and calcium caseinates, whey protein concentrate, carnitine, taurine	110	hydrolyzed cornstarch, sucrose	50	high oleic sunflower oil, soybean oil, medium chain triglycerides oil	380 (17 mEq)	1,300 (33 mEq)	390	1	Vit A, B_1, B_2, B_3, B_5, B_6, B_{12}, C, D, E, K, biotin, choline, folic acid, m-inositol, Ca, Cl, Cr, Cu, Fe, I, Mo, Mg, Mn, P, Se, Zn	French vanilla, chocolate, and strawberry flavors. In 237 mL *Tetra Brik Paks* (27s).
otc	**ReSource Fruit Beverage** (Novartis Nutrition)	38	whey protein concentrates	150	sugar, hydrolyzed cornstarch	0	NA	< 295 (< 13 mEq)	< 93 (< 2.4 mEq)	700	0.76	Vit A, B_1, B_2, B_3, B_5, B_6, B_{12}, C, D, E, K, biotin, choline, folic acid, Ca, Cl, Cu, Fe, I Mg, Mn, P, Zn	Orange, peach, and wild berry flavors. In 237 mL *Tetra Brik Paks* (27s).
otc	**ReSource Diabetic** (Novartis Nutrition)	63	sodium and calcium caseinates, soy protein isolates, carnitine, taurine	99	hydrolyzed cornstarch, fructose	47	high oleic sunflower oil, soybean oil	970 (42 mEq)	1,100 (29 mEq)	450	1.06	Vit A, B_1, B_2, B_3, B_5, B_6, B_{12}, C, D, E, K, biotin, choline, folic acid, m-inositol, Ca, Cl, Cu, Fe, I, Mg, Mn, Mo, P, Se, Zn	French vanilla, chocolate, and strawberry flavors. In 237 mL *Tetra Brik Paks* (27s) and 1,000 and 1,500 mL closed system containers (6s).
otc	**Pediasure with Fiber** (Ross)	30	sodium caseinate, low-lactose whey, carnitine, taurine	113.5	maltodextrin, sucrose, soy fiber (5 g total dietary fiber)	49.7	high-oleic safflower oil, soy oil, medium chain triglyceride oil, lecithin	380 (16.5 mEq)	1,310 (33.5 mEq)	unknown	1	Vit A, B_1, B_2, B_3, B_6, B_{12}, C, D, E, K, folic acid, Ca, Fe, I Mg, P, Se, Zn	Gluten free. Vanilla flavor. In 8 oz.

[a] Also contains folic acid, biotin, and choline.
[b] Content given per orange flavor.
[c] Content given per 87 g packet.
[d] Content given per ready-to-use liquid.
[e] Unflavored does not contain sucrose.
[f] Content given per vanilla flavor.
[g] Content given per 100 mL.

LACTOSE-FREE PRODUCTS — ORAL

See individual product listings for specific labeled indications.

INFANT FOODS

	Product & Distributor	Dilution	Protein g	Protein Source	Carbohydrate g	Carbohydrate Source	Fat g	Fat Source	Na (mg)	K (mg)	Cal	Other Content	How Supplied
otc	**Enfamil Human Milk Fortifier Powder** (Mead Johnson Nutritionals)	4 packets (3.8 g) added to breast milk	0.7	whey protein, Na caseinate	2.7	corn syrup solids, lactose	< 0.1	unknown	7 (0.3 mEq)	15.6 (0.4 mEq)	14	Vit A, B_1, B_2, B_3, B_5, B_6, B_{12}, C, D, E, K, Ca, P, Zn, Mg, Mn, Cu, Cl[1]	In 0.96 g packets (100s).
otc	**Enfamil Premature Formula Liquid** (Mead Johnson Nutritionals)	150 mL	3	nonfat milk, whey protein concentrate, amino acids	11.1	corn syrup solids, lactose	5.1	soy oil, MCT (fractionated coconut oil), mono- and diglycerides, linoleic acid	39 (1.7 mEq)	103 (2.6 mEq)	80	Vit A, B_1, B_2, B_3, B_5, B_6, B_{12}, C, D, E, K, inositol, Ca, P, Mg, Zn, Fe, Mn, Cu, I, Cl[1]	In 90 mL nursettes.
otc	**Enfamil Liquid and Powder** (Mead Johnson Nutritionals)	1 liter	15	nonfat milk, reduced minerals whey	69	lactose	37.3	soy and coconut oils, soy lecithin, mono- and diglycerides, high-oleic sunflower oil, palm olein, linoleic acid	180 (7.8 mEq)	720 (18.4 mEq)	667	Vit A, B_1, B_2, B_3, B_5, B_6, B_{12}, C, D, E, K, inositol, Ca, P, Mg, Zn, Fe, Mn, Cu, I, Cl[1]	In 390 mL concentrate, 240 mL and 1 qt ready-to-use cans 90, 180 and 240 mL nursettes and 1 and 2 lb powder.
otc	**Carnation Good-Start Liquid and Powder** (Carnation)	1 liter	16	reduced minerals whey, taurine	74.4	lactose, maltodextrin	34.5	palm olein, soy oil, coconut oil, high-oleic safflower oil	162 (7 mEq)	663 (17 mEq)	0.68	Vit A, B_1, B_2, B_3, B_5, B_6, B_{12}, C, D, E, K, inositol, Ca, Mg, P, Zn, Fe, Mn, Cu, I, Cl[1]	In 390 mL concentrated liquid, 1 qt ready-to-feed containers and 360 g powder.
otc	**PediaSure Liquid** (Ross)	1 liter	30	Na caseinate, whey protein concentrate, taurine, carnitine	108	hydrolyzed cornstarch, sucrose	49	high-oleic safflower oil , soy oil, MCT (fractionated coconut oil, mono- and diglycerides, soy lecithin	375 (16.3 mEq)	1292 (33 mEq)	1000	Vit A, B_1, B_2, B_3, B_5, B_6, B_{12}, C, D, E, K, inositol, Ca, Mg, P, Zn, Fe, Mn, Cu, I, Cl, Cr, Mo, Se[1]	Gluten free. Vanilla flavor. In ready-to-use 240 mL cans.
otc	**Enfamil Next Step Liquid and Powder** (Mead Johnson Nutritionals)	1 liter	17.3	nonfat milk	74	corn syrup solids, lactose	33.3	palm olein, soy oil, coconut oil, high- oleic sunflower oil, linoleic acid	273 (11.9 mEq)	867 (22.2 mEq)	100	Vit A, B_1, B_2, B_3, B_5, B_6, B_{12}, C, D, E, K, inositol, Ca, Mg, P, Zn, Fe, Mn, Cu, I, Cl, Se[1]	In 390 mL concentrate, 1 qt ready-to-use liquid and 360 and 720 g powder.
otc	**Carnation Follow-Up Formula Liquid and Powder** (Carnation)	1 liter	17.3	nonfat milk	88	corn syrup	27.3	palm olein, coconut oil, high oleic safflower oil, soy lecithin, soy oil	260 (11.5 mEq)	900 (23 mEq)	676	Vit A, B_1, B_2, B_3, B_5, B_6, B_{12}, C, D, E, K, inositol, Ca, Mg, P, Zn, Fe, Mn, Cu, I, Cl[1]	In 390 mL concentrate, 1 qt ready-to-feed containers and 360 g powder.
otc	**Similac Human Milk Fortifier** (Ross)	4 packets (3.6 g)	1	nonfat milk, whey protein concentrate	1.8	corn syrup solids	0.36	fractionated coconut oil (medium chain triglycerides), soy lecithin	15	63	14	Vit. A, B1, B2, B3, B5, B6, B12, C, D, E, K, folic acid, (folacin), biotin, Ca, Cl, Cu, Fe, Mg, Mn, P, Zn	In 0.9 g packets (50s).

[1] Also contains folic acid, biotin and choline.

INFANT FOODS — ORAL

See individual product listings for specific labeled indications.

Indications

➤*Formula:* Formula for bottle-fed infants; as a supplement to breast-feeding.

Precautions

In conditions where the infant is losing abnormal quantities of one or more electrolytes, it may be necessary to supply electrolytes from sources other than the formula. With premature infants weighing less than 1500 g at birth, it may be necessary to supply an additional source of sodium, calcium and phosphorus during the period of very rapid growth.

INFANT FOODS WITH IRON

	Product & Distributor	Dilution	Protein g	Protein Source	Carbohydrate g	Carbohydrate Source	Fat g	Fat Source	Iron (mg)	Na (mg)	K (mg)	Cal	Other Content	How Supplied
otc	**Phenyl-Free 1** (Mead Johnson Nutritionals)	1 liter	22	casein hydrolysate, amino acids (including tryptophan, taurine, carnitine	54.2	corn syrup solids, modified tapioca starch	16.3	corn oil	12.5	313 (14 mEq)	680 (17.4 mEq)	667	Vit A, B_1, B_2, B_3, B_5, B_6, B_{12}, C, D, E, K, inositol, Ca, P, Mg, Zn, Mn, Cu, I, Cl[1]	Low phenylalanine. In 1 lb powder.

INFANT FOODS WITH IRON

	Product & Distributor	Dilution	Protein g	Protein Source	Carbohydrate g	Carbohydrate Source	Fat g	Fat Source	Iron (mg)	Na (mg)	K (mg)	Cal	Other Content	How Supplied
otc	**Similac w/Iron Liquid and Powder** (Ross)	1 liter	15	nonfat milk, taurine	72.3	lactose	37	Coconut oil, corn oil, soy oil, mono- and diglycerides, soy lecithin, linoleic acid	12	180 (8 mEq)	700 (18 mEq)	676	Vit A, B_1, B_2, B_3, B_5, B_6, B_{12}, C, D, E, K, inositol, Ca, P, Mg, Zn, Mn, Cu, I, Cl[1]	In 390 mL concentrate, 240 mL and 1 qt ready-to-use cans, 120 and 240 mL nursettes and 1 lb powder.
otc	**SMA Iron Fortified Liquid and Powder** (Wyeth-Ayerst)	1 liter	15	nonfat milk, reduced minerals whey, taurine	71	lactose	35.3	oleo, coconut, safflower, sunflower and soybean oils, soy lecithin, linoleic acid	12	147 (6.4 mEq)	553 (14.2 mEq)	667	Vit A, B_1, B_2, B_3, B_5, B_6, B_{12}, C, D, E, K, Ca, P, Mg, Cl, Cu, Zn, Mn, I[1]	In 384 mL concentrate, ready-to-use 240 mL and 1 qt and 1 and 2 lb powder.
otc	**Enfamil w/Iron Liquid and Powder** (Mead Johnson Nutritionals)	1 liter	15	nonfat milk, reduced minerals whey	69	lactose	37	soy and coconut oils, soy lecithin, mono- and diglycerides, palm olein, high-oleic sunflower oil, linoleic acid	12.5	180 (8 mEq)	720 (18.4 mEq)	666	Vit A, B_1, B_2, B_3, B_5, B_6, B_{12}, C, D, E, K, inositol, Ca, P, Mg, Zn, Mn, Cu, I, Cl[1]	In 390 mL concentrate, ready-to-use 240 mL and 1qt , 180 mL nursettes and 1 and 2 lb powder.
otc	**Bonamil Infant Formula w/Iron Powder or Liquid** (Wyeth-Ayerst)	150 mL	2.3	nonfat milk, taurine	10.7	lactose	5.4	soybean oil, coconut oil, soy lecithin, linoleic acid	1.8	27	93	100	Vit A, B_1, B_2, B_3, B_5, B_6, B_{12}, C, D, E, K, biotin, choline, Ca, P, Mg, Zn, Mn, Cu, I, Cl, folic acid	In 453 g powder or 946 mL ready-to-feed liquid.
otc	**EnfaCare Powder or Liquid** (Mead Johnson Nutritionals)	≈ 130 mL	2.8	nonfat milk, whey protein concentrate, taurine, L-carnitine	10.7	maltodextrin, lactose	5.3	high oleic sunflower oil, soy oil, medium chain triglycerides, coconut oil, mono- and diglycerides, soy lecithin	1.8	35	105	100	Vit A, B_1, B_2, B_3, B_5, B_6, B_{12}, C, D, E, K, 26 mcg folic acid, biotin, choline, inositol, linoleic acid, Ca, Cl, Cu, I, Mg, Mn, P, Se, Zn.	In 3 oz *Nursette* bottles (liquid) and 14 oz cans (powder).
otc	**Enfamil LIPIL with Iron** (Mead Johnson Nutritionals)	per 100 calories	2.1	reduced minerals whey, nonfat milk, taurine	10.9	lactose	5.3	vegetable oil (palm olein, soy, coconut, and high oleic sunflower oils), < 1% mortierella alpina oil, crypthecodinium cohnii oil, mono- and diglycerides, soy lecithin	1.8	27	108	20 cal/oz	Vit A, B_1, B_2, B_3, B_5, B_6, B_{12}, C, D, E, K, 16 mcg folic acid/100 cal, biotin, chloride, choline, inositol, linoleic acid, Ca, Cu, I, Mg, Mn, P, Se, Zn.	In 32 oz cans and 3 and 6 oz *Nursette* bottles (ready-to-use liquid), 13 oz cans (liquid concentrate), and 12.9 and 25.7 oz cans (powder).

[1] Also contains folic acid, biotin and choline.

INFANT FOODS WITH IRON — ORAL

See individual product listings for specific labeled indications.

SPECIALIZED INFANT FOODS

	Product & Distributor	Dilution	Protein g	Protein Source	Carbohydrate g	Carbohydrate Source	Fat g	Fat Source	Iron (mg)	Na (mg)	K (mg)	Cal	Other Content	How Supplied
otc	**RCF Liquid** (Ross)	1 liter	39.3	soy protein isolate, amino acids (including carnitine and taurine)	0.08	unknown	71	soy oil, coconut oil, mono- and diglycerides, soy lecithin	3	579 (25.2 mEq)	1429 (37 mEq)	818	Vit A, B_1, B_2, B_3, B_5, B_6, B_{12}, C, D, E, K, inositol, Ca, P, Cu, Mg, Zn, Mn, I, Cl[1]	Carbohydrate free. In 390 mL concentrate.
otc	**Nursoy Liquid and Powder** (Wyeth-Ayerst)	1 liter	21	soy protein isolate, methionine	69	sucrose	36	oleo, coconut, safflower and soybean oils, soy lecithin	11.5	200 (9 mEq)	700 (18 mEq)	667	Vit A, B_1, B_2, B_3, B_5, B_6, B_{12}, C, D, E, K, inositol, Ca, P, Cl, Mg, Mn, Cu, Zn, I[1]	In 390 mL concentrate, 1 qt ready-to-use and 1 lb powder.
otc	**Gerber Soy Formula Liquid** (Gerber)	1 liter	20	soy protein isolate, amino acids (including taurine, carnitine)	67	corn syrup solids, sugar	35.3	palm olein, soy, coconut and high oleic sunflower oils, soy lecithin, mono- and diglycerides, linoleic acid	12	313 (14 mEq)	767 (20 mEq)	667	Vit A, B_1, B_2, B_3, B_5, B_6, B_{12}, C, D, E, K, inositol, Ca, P, Cu, Mg, Zn, Mn, I, Cl[1]	In 1 qt ready-to-use.

SPECIALIZED INFANT FOODS

	Product & Distributor	Dilution	Protein g	Protein Source	Carbohydrate g	Carbohydrate Source	Fat g	Fat Source	Iron (mg)	Na (mg)	K (mg)	Cal	Other Content	How Supplied
otc	**ProSobee Liquid and Powder** (Mead Johnson Nutritionals)	1 liter	20	soy protein isolate, amino acids (including taurine, carnitine)	67	corn syrup solids	35.3	linoleic acid, coconut, corn and soy oil, palm olein, high oleic sunflower oils[2]	12.5	240 (10.5 mEq)	813 (21 mEq)	667	Vit A, B_1, B_2, B_3, B_5, B_6, B_{12}, C, D, E, K, inositol, Ca, P, Cu, Mg, Zn, Mn, I, Cl[1]	*For infants with a family history of allergies.* Sucrose, milk and lactose free. In 390 mL concentrate, 240 mL and 1 qt ready-to-use and 420 g powder.
otc	**Alimentum Liquid** (Ross)	1 liter	19	casein hydrolysate, amino acids (including tryptophan, taurine, carnitine)	69	sucrose, modified tapioca starch	36	MCT (fractionated coconut oil), safflower oil, soy oil	12	297 (13 mEq)	798 (21 mEq)	676	Vit A, B_1, B_2, B_3, B_5, B_6, B_{12}, C, D, E, K, inositol, Ca, Cl, Cu, I, Mg, Mn, P, Zn[1]	*For infants and children with severe food allergies, sensitivity to intact protein, protein maldigestion or fat malabsorption.* Corn and lactose free. In ready-to-use 240 and 360 mL.
otc	**Nutramigen Liquid and Powder** (Mead Johnson Nutritionals)	1 liter	19	enzymatically hydrolyzed casein, amino acids (including tryptophan, taurine, carnitine)	89.3	corn syrup solids, modified cornstarch	26	corn oil, soy oil, linoleic acid	12.5	313 (14 mEq)	727 (19 mEq)	667	Vit A, B_1, B_2, B_3, B_5, B_6, B_{12}, C, D, E, K, inositol, Ca, P, Cu, Mg, Zn, Mn, I, Cl[1]	*For infants and children sensitive to intact proteins of milk and other foods.* Lactose and sucrose free. In 1 lb powder, 390 mL concentrate and 1 qt ready-to-use.
otc	**Pregestimil Powder** (Mead Johnson Nutritionals)	1 liter	18.7	enzymatically hydrolyzed casein, amino acids (including tryptophan, taurine, carnitine)	69	corn syrup solids, modified corn starch, dextrose	37.3	corn oil, MCT (fractionated coconut oil), high-oleic safflower oil, linoleic acid	12.5	260 (11.3 mEq)	726 (19 mEq)	667	Vit A, B_1, B_2, B_3, B_5, B_6, B_{12}, C, D, E, K, inositol, Ca, P, Cu, Mg, Zn, Mn, I, Cl[1]	*For infants with severe malabsorption disorders.* In 1 lb powder.
otc	**Isomil SF Liquid** (Ross)	1 liter	18	soy protein isolate, amino acids (including carnitine)	68.3	hydrolyzed cornstarch	37	soy oil, coconut oil, mono- and diglycerides, soy lecithin, linoleic acid	12	297 (13 mEq)	730 (19 mEq)	676	Vit A, B_1, B_2, B_3, B_5, B_6, B_{12}, C, D, E, K, inositol, Ca, P, Cu, Mg, Zn, Mn, I, Cl[1]	*For infants and children with an allergy sensitivity to cow's milk protein or intolerance to sucrose.* Sucrose and lactose free. In 390 mL concentrate.
otc	**Isomil Liquid and Powder** (Ross)	1 liter	17	soy protein isolate, amino acids (including carnitine)	70	corn syrup, sucrose, cornstarch[2]	37	corn, soy and coconut oils, mono- and diglycerides, soy lecithin	12	297 (13 mEq)	730 (18.4 mEq)	676	Vit A, B_1, B_2, B_3, B_5, B_6, B_{12}, C, D, E, K, inositol, Ca, P, Mg, Zn, Mn, Cu, I, Cl[1]	*For infants and children who are allergic or sensitive to cow's milk, lactose intolerant or deficient or are galactosemic.* Lactose free. In 390 mL concentrate, 120 mL nursing bottles, 240 mL and 1 qt ready-to-use and 420 g powder.
otc	**Similac PM 60/40 Low-Iron Liquid** (Ross)	1 liter	15.6	whey protein concentrate, Na caseinate, carnitine, taurine	68	lactose	37	coconut oil, mono- and diglycerides, soy oil, linoleic acid	1.5	160 (7 mEq)	573 (15 mEq)	100	Vit A, B_1, B_2, B_3, B_5, B_6, B_{12}, C, D, E, K, inositol, Ca, P, Cu, Mg, Zn, Mn, I, Cl	*For infants who are predisposed to hypocalcemia or those who would benefit from lowered mineral levels.* In 120 mL bottles.
otc	**Glutarex-1 Powder** (Ross)	100 g powder[3]	15	amino acids (including carnitine, phenylalanine, taurine)	47	hydrolyzed cornstarch	24	palm oil, hydrogenated coconut oil, soy oil, mono- and diglycerides, linoleic acid	9	190 (8.3 mEq)	675 (17.3 mEq)	480	Vit A, B_1, B_2, B_3, B_5, B_6, B_{12}, C, D, E, K, inositol, Ca, P, Cu, Mg, Zn, Mn, I, Cl, Se[1]	*Nutritional support of infants and toddlers with glutaric aciduria type I.* Lysine and tryptophan free. In 350 g powder.

SPECIALIZED INFANT FOODS

			Content per Dilution										Other Content	How Supplied
			Protein		Carbohydrate		Fat							
	Product & Distributor	Dilution	g	Source	g	Source	g	Source	Iron (mg)	Na (mg)	K (mg)	Cal		
otc	**Hominex-1 Powder** (Ross)	100 g powder[3]	15	amino acids (including phenylalanine, tryptophan, taurine, carnitine)	46.3	hydrolyzed cornstarch	24	palm oil, hydrogenated coconut oil, soy oil, mono- and diglycerides, linoleic acid	9	190 (8.3 mEq)	675 (17.3 mEq)	480	Vit A, B_1, B_2, B_3, B_5, B_6, B_{12}, C, D, E, K, inositol, Ca, P, Cu, Mg, Zn, Mn, I, Cl, Se[1]	*Nutritional support of infants and toddlers with vitamin B_6-nonresponsive homocystinuria or hypermethioninemia.* Methionine free. In 350 g powder.
otc	**I-Valex-1 Powder** (Ross)	100 g powder[3]	15	amino acids (including carnitine, phenylalanine, tryptophan, taurine)	46.3	hydrolyzed cornstarch	24	palm oil, hydrogenated coconut oil, soy oil, mono- and diglycerides, linoleic acid	9	190 (8.3 mEq)	675 (17.3 mEq)	480	Vit A, B_1, B_2, B_3, B_5, B_6, B_{12}, C, D, E, K, inositol, Ca, P, Cu, Mg, Zn, Mn, I, Cl, Se[1]	*Nutritional support of infants and toddlers with a disorder of leucine catabolism.* Leucine free. In 350 g.
otc	**Ketonex-1 Powder** (Ross)	100 g powder[3]	15	amino acids (including phenylalanine, tryptophan, carnitine, taurine)	46.3	hydrolyzed cornstarch	24	palm oil, hydrogenated coconut oil, soy oil, mono-and diglycerides, linoleic acid	9	190 (8.3 mEq)	675 (17.3 mEq)	480	Vit A, B_1, B_2, B_3, B_5, B_6, B_{12}, C, D, E, K, inositol, Ca, P, Cu, Mg, Zn, Mn, I, Cl, Se[1]	*For nutritional support of infants and toddlers with maple syrup urine disease (MSUD).* Isoleucine, leucine and valine free. In 350 g powder.
otc	**Phenex-1 Powder** (Ross)	100 g powder[3]	15	amino acids (including tryptophan, taurine, carnitine)	46.3	hydrolyzed cornstarch	24	palm oil, hydrogenated coconut oil, soy oil, mono- and diglycerides	9	190 (8.3 mEq)	675 (17.2 mEq)	480	Vit A, B_1, B_2, B_3, B_5, B_6, B_{12}, C, D, E, K, inositol, Ca, P, Cu, Mg, Zn, Mn, I, Cl, Se[1]	*Nutritional support of infants and toddlers with phenylketonuria (PKU).* Phenylalanine free. In 350 g.
otc	**Propimex-1 Powder** (Ross)	100 g powder[3]	15	amino acids (including carnitine, phenylalanine, tryptophan, taurine)	46.3	hydrolyzed cornstarch	24	palm oil, hydrogenated coconut oil, soy oil, mono- and diglycerides, linoleic acid	9	190 (8.3 mEq)	675 (18 mEq)	480	Vit A, B_1, B_2, B_3, B_5, B_6, B_{12}, C, D, E, K, inositol, Ca, P, Cu, Mg, Zn, Mn, I, Cl, Se[1]	*For nutritional support of infants and toddlers with propionic or methylmalonic acidemia.* Methionine- and valine-free. In 350 g powder.
otc	**SMA Lo-Iron Infant Formula** (Wyeth Ayerst)	1 liter	15	nonfat milk, reduced minerals whey, taurine	71	lactose	353	oleo oil, coconut oil, high oleic safflower or sunflower oil, soybean oil, soy lecithin, linoleic acid	1.3	147 (6.4 mEq)	553 (14.2 mEq)	667	Vit A, B_1, B_2, B_3, B_5, B_6, B_{12}, C, D, E, K, inositol, Ca, P, Cu, Mg, Zn, Mn, I, Cl[1]	In 390 mL concentrate, 1 qt ready-to-use liquid and 1 lb powder.
otc	**Tyromex-1 Powder** (Ross)	100 g powder[3]	15	amino acids (including tryptophan, taurine, carnitine)	46.3	hydrolyzed cornstarch	29	palm oil, hydrogenated coconut oil, soy oil, mono- and diglycerides, linoleic acid	9	190 (8.3 mEq)	675 (17.3 mEq)	480	Vit A, B_1, B_2, B_3, B_5, B_6, B_{12}, C, D, E, K, inositol, Ca, P, Cu, Mg, Zn, Mn, I, Cl, Se[1]	*For nutritional support of infants and toddlers with tyrosinemia type I.* Phenylalanine, tyrosine and methionine free. In 350 g powder.
otc	**Lactofree Liquid and Powder** (Mead Johnson Nutritionals)	1 liter	14.7	milk protein isolate, taurine, carnitine	69.3	corn syrup solids	37	palm olein, soy, coconut and high -oleic sunflower oils, linoleic acid	12	200 (9 mEq)	733 (19 mEq)	676	Vit A, B_1, B_2, B_3, B_5, B_6, B_{12}, C, D, E, K, inositol, Ca, P, Cu, Mg, Zn, Mn, I, Cl, Se[1]	Lactose free. In 1 qt ready-to-use liquid, 390 mL concentrate and 400 g powder.
otc	**Similac Low-Iron Liquid and Powder** (Ross)	1 liter	14.3	nonfat milk, taurine	72	lactose	36	Corn, coconut and soy oils, mono- and diglycerides, soy lecithin, linoleic acid	1.5	180 (7.8 mEq)	700 (17.9 mEq)	676	Vit A, B_1, B_2, B_3, B_5, B_6, B_{12}, C, D, E, K, inositol, Ca, P, Cu, Mg, Zn, Mn, I, Cl[1]	In 390 mL concentrate, 240 mL and 1 qt ready-to-use, 120 and 240 mL nursettes and 1 lb powder.
otc	**Cyclinex-1 Powder** (Ross)	100 g powder[3]	7.5	amino acids (including phenylalanine, tryptophan, carnitine, taurine)	52	hydrolyzed cornstarch	27	palm oil, hydrogenated coconut oil, soy oil, mono- and diglycerides, linoleic acid	10	215 (9.3 mEq)	760 (19.4 mEq)	515	Vit A, B_1, B_2, B_3, B_5, B_6, B_{12}, C, D, E, K, inositol, Ca, P, Cu, Mg, Zn, Mn, I, Cl, Se[1]	*For nutritional support of infants and toddlers with a urea cycle disorder or gyrate atrophy.* Nonessential amino acid free. In 350 g.

SPECIALIZED INFANT FOODS

	Product & Distributor	Dilution	Protein g	Protein Source	Carbohydrate g	Carbohydrate Source	Fat g	Fat Source	Iron (mg)	Na (mg)	K (mg)	Cal	Other Content	How Supplied
otc	**Soyalac Liquid and Powder** (Nutricia-Loma Linda)	per 100 calories	3.1	soybean extract	10	corn syrup, sucrose	5.5	soy oil, linoleic acid	1.5	‡	‡	667	unknown	Lactose free. In 390 mL concentrate, 1 qt ready-to-use and 420 g powder.
otc	**I-Soyalac Liquid and Powder** (Nutricia-Loma Linda)	per 100 calories	3.1	soy protein isolate, amino acids	10	sucrose, tapioca dextrin, potato maltodextrin	5.5	soy oil, linoleic acid	1.9	‡	‡	100	unknown	Corn syrup solids and lactose free. In 390 mL concentrate and 1 qt ready-to-use and 420 g powder.
otc	**Isomil DF** (Ross)	per 100 calories	2.7	soybean solids, amino acids	10.1	corn syrup, sucrose	5.5	soy oil, coconut oil	1.8	44 (1.9 mEq)	108 (2.8 mEq)	676	Vit A, B_1, B_2, B_3, B_5, B_6, B_{12}, C, D, E, K, inositol, Ca, P, Cu, Mg, Zn, Mn, I, Cl, Se[1]	*For management of diarrhea in infants and toddlers.* Lactose free. In 960 mL, pre-diluted, ready-to-use cans.
otc	**Enfamil LactoFree Liquid, Liquid Concentrate, and Powder** (Mead Johnson Nutritionals)	—	2.1	‡	10.9	‡	5.3	‡	1.8	30	8 mcg	100 per serving	860 mg linoleic acid, 300 IU vit. A, 60 IU vit. D, 2 IU vit. E, 80 mcg vit. B_1, 140 mcg vit. B_2, 60 mcg vit. B_6, 0.3 mcg vit. B_{12}, 1000 mcg vit. B_3, 16 mcg folic acid, 600 mcg vit. B_5, 3 mcg biotin, 12 mg vit. C, 12 mg choline, 17 mg inositol (liquid only), 6 mg inositol (powder only), 82 mg Ca, 55 mg P, 8 mg Mg, 1 mg Zn, 15 mcg Mn, 75 mcg Xu, 15 mcg I, 2.8 mcg Se, 110 mg K, 67 mg chloride	In 397 g (powder), 384 mL (liquid concentrate, or 946 mL liquid)
otc	**Pro-Phree Powder** (Ross)	100 g powder[3]	‡	‡	60	hydrolyzed cornstarch	31	palm oil, hydrogenated coconut oil, soy oil, mono- and diglycerides, linoleic acid	11.9	250 (11 mEq)	875 (22.4 mEq)	520	Vit A, B_1, B_2, B_3, B_5, B_6, B_{12}, C, D, E, K, inositol, Ca, P, Cu, Mg, Zn, Mn, I, Cl, Se[1,4]	*For nutritional support of infants and toddlers who require extra calories, minerals, vitamins and/or protein restriction.* Protein free. In 350 g powder.

* ‡ Amount Unknown.
[1] Also contains folic acid, biotin and choline
[2] Ready-to-use contains soy lecithin and mono- and diglycerides.
[3] Content given from unreconstituted powder.
[4] Contains trace amounts of taurine and carnitine.

SPECIALIZED INFANT FOODS — ORAL

See individual product listings for specific labeled indications.

Food Modifiers

LACTOSE

otc	**Lactose** (Various, eg, Humco, Paddock)	**Powder**	In 1 lb.

LACTOSE — ORAL

Refer to additional information in the Enteral Nutritional Therapy introduction.

CALCIUM CASEINATE

otc	**Casec** (Mead Johnson Nutritionals)	**Powder**: Contains 88 g protein, 1.6 g calcium, 120 mg sodium, 2 g fat and 370 calories per 100 g	In 75 g.

CALCIUM CASEINATE — ORAL

Refer to additional information in the Enteral Nutritional Therapy introduction.

Intravenous nutritional therapy is required when normal enteral feeding is not possible or is inadequate for nutritional requirements. Specific nutritional requirements and administration mode depend on the nutritional status of the patient and the duration of parenteral therapy. To meet IV nutritional requirements, one or more of the following nutrients may be required:

Protein Substrates
- Amino Acids - General Formulations
- Amino Acids - Renal Failure Formulations
- Amino Acids - Hepatic Failure/Encephalopathy Formulations
- Amino Acids - Metabolic Stress Formulations

Energy Substrates
- Dextrose
- IV Fat Emulsion

Electrolytes

Vitamins

Trace Metals

The following general discussion reviews peripheral and central administration routes, and provides basic guidelines for use of various components of IV nutritional therapy.

➤*PERIPHERAL PARENTERAL NUTRITION:*

Peripheral protein sparing – Amino acids with maintenance electrolytes (with or without dextrose) prevent protein catabolism, for short periods of time, in patients with adequate body fat and no clinically significant protein malnutrition. Lipolysis provides energy from oxidation of free fatty acids and ketone bodies; minimal nitrogen is lost since proteolysis does not occur. For peripheral IV infusion, 1 to 1.5 g/kg/day of amino acids achieves optimal fat mobilization and spares protein catabolism.

ProcalAmine: ProcalAmine is a unique product that provides a physiological ratio of biologically useable essential and nonessential amino acids, glycerin (glycerol) and maintenance electrolytes. Glycerin preserves body protein and participates as an active energy substrate through its phosphorylation to α-glycerophosphate.

Peripheral total parenteral nutrition (TPN) – TPN is for patients requiring parenteral nutrition when the central venous route is not indicated. Amino acids with electrolytes, combined with 5% or 10% dextrose and used with IV fat emulsions (and usually vitamins and trace metals), reduce protein catabolism in patients moderately catabolic or depleted and minimize liver glycogen depletion. Peripheral infusions may provide inadequate maintenance requirements for those with greatly increased metabolic demands or severe nutritional deficiencies requiring repletion. May add oral calories as tolerated.

➤*CENTRAL TOTAL PARENTERAL NUTRITION:* Amino acids combined with hypertonic dextrose and IV fat emulsions infused via a central venous catheter promote protein synthesis in hypercatabolic or severely depleted patients or those requiring long-term parenteral nutrition. Appropriate electrolytes, vitamins and trace minerals are added to provide total parenteral nutrition.

➤*Indications:* Parenteral nutrition is indicated to prevent nitrogen and weight loss or to treat negative nitrogen balance when: (1) The alimentary tract, by the oral, gastrostomy or jejunostomy route, cannot or should not be used; (2) GI absorption of protein is impaired by obstruction, inflammatory disease or its complications or antineoplastic therapy; (3) bowel rest is needed because of GI surgery or its complications such as ileus, fistulae or anastomotic leaks; (4) metabolic requirements for protein are substantially increased, as with extensive burns, infections, trauma or other hypermetabolic states; (5) morbidity and mortality may be reduced by replacing amino acids lost from tissue breakdown, thereby preserving tissue reserves, as in acute renal failure; (6) tube feeding methods alone cannot provide adequate nutrition.

After the patient's nutritional deficits, reserves and current status are assessed, set rational and precise nutritional goals. Dosage, route of administration and concomitant infusion of nonprotein calories depend on nutritional and metabolic status, anticipated duration of parenteral nutritional support and vein tolerance.

Peripheral parenteral nutrition – Administration of nutritional solutions through peripheral veins is appropriate if caloric needs are minimal, if they can be partially met by enteral alimentation, if nutritional therapy will only be required for 5 to 14 days, or if central venous access is not feasible.

Central parenteral nutrition – Amino acids, with hypertonic dextrose and IV fat emulsions infused via central venous catheter, promote protein synthesis in the hypercatabolic or severely depleted or in those requiring long-term parenteral nutrition.

Total nutrient admixtures (TNA) – A combination of amino acids, dextrose and lipids in one container has been used. Also known as multicomponent admixtures, all-in-one, 3-in-1 or triple mix, TNA offers the advantage of substituting some dextrose calories with lipids, reducing carbohydrate-related complications (eg, impaired glucose control). It also appears to be used better by the liver due to continuous lipid administration, and is less likely to interfere with immune functions. See also admixture incompatibilities/compatibilities under Administration and Dosage.

Specific disease states – Specific disease states in which TPN requires special considerations are: Renal failure, acute metabolic stress, hepatic failure/hepatic encephalopathy. See individual sections for specific discussions.

➤*Administration and Dosage:*

Total daily dose – Total daily dose depends on daily protein requirements and on the patient's metabolic and clinical responses. The determination of nitrogen balance and accurate daily body weights, corrected for fluid balance, are probably the best means of assessing protein requirements. In addition, guide dosage by the patient's fluid intake limits, glucose and nitrogen tolerances and metabolic and clinical response.

Protein – Recommended dietary allowances of protein are approximately 0.9 g/kg for a healthy adult and 1.4 to 2.2 g/kg for healthy growing infants and children. Protein and caloric requirements in traumatized or malnourished patients may be substantially increased. Daily doses of approximately 1 to 1.5 g/kg for adults and 2 to 3 g/kg for infants are generally sufficient to promote positive nitrogen balance, although higher doses may be required in severely catabolic states. Such higher doses require frequent laboratory evaluation.

Energy requirements – To ensure proper caloric intake, estimate required calorie and energy needs using basal metabolic rate; also consider energy expenditure and disease states. The energy required for proper amino acid utilization is derived from glycogenolysis, lipolysis or infusion of dextrose or fat emulsions. After glycogen is depleted, in the absence of exogenous calories, fat becomes the major energy source. Parenteral amino acids will not be retained and utilized for anabolic purposes unless adequate nonprotein calories are provided simultaneously.

IV fat emulsion: IV fat emulsion should comprise no more than 60% of the total caloric intake, with carbohydrates and amino acids comprising the remaining 40% or more.

Electrolyte requirements – In adults, ≈ 60 to 180 mEq of potassium, 10 to 30 mEq of magnesium and 10 to 40 mM of phosphate per day appear necessary to achieve optimum metabolic response; individualize each requirement. Give sufficient quantities of the major extracellular electrolytes, sodium, calcium and chloride. (Calcium prevents hypocalcemia that may accompany phosphate administration.) Consider content of amino acid infusion when calculating daily electrolyte intake.

HepatAmine: HepatAmine contains less than 3 mEq chloride/L and ≤ 10 mM/L of phosphate. Some patients, especially hypophosphatemics, may require additional phosphate.

Fluid balance – Provide sufficient water to compensate for insensible, urinary and other (eg, nasogastric suction, fistula drainage, diarrhea) fluid losses. Average daily adult fluid requirements are between 2500 and 3000 mL, but may be much higher with losses such as fistula drainage or in burn patients.

Vitamin therapy – If a patient's nutritional intake is primarily parenteral, provide vitamins (especially the water soluble vitamins). Iron is added to the solution or given IM in depot form as indicated. Folic acid and vitamin K are required additives.

Pediatric – Pediatric requirements are constrained by the greater relative fluid and caloric requirements per kg of the infant. Amino acids are best administered in a 2.5% concentration. For most pediatric patients, 2.5 g amino acids/kg/day with dextrose alone or with IV fat calories of 100 to 130 kcal/kg/day are recommended for maintenance. Start with nutritional solution of half strength at a rate of about 60 to 70 mL/kg/day. Within 24 to 48 hours, the volume and concentration of the solution can be increased until full strength pediatric solution is given at a rate of 125 to 150 mL/kg/day.

A basic central line solution for pediatric use should contain 25 g of amino acids and 200 to 250 g of glucose per 1000 mL. Such a solution given at a rate of 145 mL/kg/day provides 100 to 130 kcal/kg/day.

Give supplemental electrolytes and vitamins (including agents such as carnitine) as needed. Iron is more critical in infants because of increasing red cell mass needed for growth. Monitor serum lipids for EFAD in patients maintained on fat-free TPN.

To ensure the precise delivery of the small volumes of fluid necessary, use accurately calibrated and reliable infusion systems.

Preparation/stability of solutions – Aseptically prepare solutions under a laminar flow hood. Use promptly after mixing. Store under refrigeration for a brief period of time only (less than 24 hours). Do not exceed 24 hours for administration time of a single bottle.

Admixture incompatibilities/compatibilities – Because of the potential for incompatibility in the complex formulations, keep additives to a minimum. Do not administer simultaneously with **blood** through the same infusion site because of possible pseudoagglutination. **Antibiotics, steroids** and **pressor agents** should not be added to these solutions. **Bleomycin** is incompatible with amino acids.

Vitamins, electrolytes, trace minerals, heparin and **insulin** are compatible with these solutions.

Total nutrient admixture: Total nutrient admixture (TNA; all-in-one; 3-in-1; triple mix): The combination of amino acids, dextrose and lipids (also known as total nutrient admixture) in one container is generally compatible. When utilizing this type of admixture, consider the following: (1) The order of mixing is important – add amino acids to the fat emulsion or the dextrose; (2) do not add the electrolytes directly to the fat emulsion – add them to the dextrose or amino acids first; (3) TNAs with electrolytes will eventually aggregate; (4) if not used immediately, refrigerate.

Administration sets – Replace all IV sets every 24 hours. Follow appropriate guidelines for care and maintenance of long-term indwelling catheters (eg, Broviac or Hickman).

➤*Actions:*

Pharmacology –

Amino acids: Amino acids promote the production of proteins (anabolism) needed for synthesis of structural components, reduce the rate of protein breakdown (catabolism), promote wound healing and act as buffers in the extracellular and intracellular fluids.

Dextrose: Dextrose is a source of calories; nonprotein calories are required for efficient use of amino acids. It decreases protein and nitrogen losses, promotes glycogen deposition and prevents ketosis (see individual monograph).

IV fat emulsions: IV fat emulsions provide a mixture of fatty acids to be used as a source of energy and to prevent essential fatty acid deficiency (EFAD) (see individual monograph).

Fluid/Electrolytes/Trace metals: Fluid, electrolytes, and trace metals are provided to compensate for normal sensible and insensible losses, as well as the additional losses often present in patients requiring parenteral nutrition (see individual section).

➤*Contraindications:*

Protein substrates – Hypersensitivity to any component; decreased (subcritical) circulating blood volume; inborn errors of amino acid metabolism (eg, maple syrup urine disease, isovaleric acidemia); anuria.

General amino acid formulations – Severe renal failure or liver disease; hepatic coma or encephalopathy; metabolic disorders involving impaired nitrogen utilization.

Renal failure formulations – Severe electrolyte and acid-base imbalance; hyperammonemia.

Hepatic failure/Hepatic encephalopathy formulations – Anuria.

High metabolic stress formulations – Anuria; hyperammonemia; hepatic coma; severe electrolyte or acid-base imbalance.

➤*Warnings:*

Prevention of complications – IV nutritional therapy may be associated with complications that can be prevented or minimized by careful attention to solution preparation, administration and patient monitoring. It is essential to follow a carefully prepared protocol based on current medical practices, preferably administered by an experienced team.

Amino acid metabolism – Hyperchloremic metabolic acidosis may result from amino acids provided as hydrochloride salts that release hydrochloride when utilized. To prevent or control this, supply a portion of the cations as acetate or lactate salts. Sodium and potassium phosphates are also available.

Hepatic function impairment – Hepatic function impairment may result in serum amino acid imbalances, metabolic alkalosis, prerenal azotemia, hyperammonemia, stupor and coma. Instances of asymptomatic hyperammonemia have occurred in patients without overt liver dysfunction. Amino acid products specifically formulated for patients with hepatic failure are discussed separately in this section. Give conservative doses of amino acids to patients with known or suspected hepatic dysfunction.

Hyperammonemia: Hyperammonemia occurs most often in children and adults with renal or hepatic disease and results from a diminished ability to handle a protein load. It is of special significance in infants as it can result in mental retardation. This reaction is dose-related and more likely to develop during prolonged therapy; treatment involves adjusting the dosage or decreasing amino acids.

Ketosis: Administration of amino acids without carbohydrates may result in the accumulation of ketones; correct ketonemia by administering carbohydrates.

Infection control – Parenteral nutrition is associated with a constant risk of sepsis. Careful, aseptic technique in the preparation of solutions and insertion and maintenance of central venous catheters is imperative. A 0.22 micron filter is often recommended to block particulate matter and bacteria. Presence of *Staphylococcus* or *Candida* suggests catheter sepsis. Early symptoms of infection include fever, chills, glucose intolerance and a change in the level of consciousness.

If other sources are not apparent and if fever persists, change solution, delivery system and catheter site. Culture catheter tip and draw blood cultures.

Pregnancy – *Category C.* It is not known whether IV nutritional therapy can cause fetal harm when given to a pregnant woman or can affect reproduction capacity. Use only when clearly needed and potential benefits outweigh hazards to the fetus.

Lactation – Exercise caution when administering to a nursing woman.

Children – The effect of amino acid infusions without dextrose on carbohydrate metabolism of children is not known. Use special caution in pediatric patients with acute renal failure, especially low birth weight infants. Laboratory and clinical monitoring must be extensive and frequent.

➤*Precautions:*

Monitoring – Laboratory monitoring and clinical evaluation are necessary before and during use. Do not withdraw venous blood for blood chemistries through the same peripheral infusion site; interference with estimations of nitrogen-containing substances may occur. The following general protocol is suggested:

General Patient Monitoring During IV Nutritional Therapy
Baseline studies: CBC, platelet count, prothrombin time, weight, body length and head circumference (in infants), electrolytes, CO_2, BUN, glucose, creatinine, total protein, cholesterol, triglycerides (if on fat emulsion), uric acid, bilirubin, alkaline phosphatase, LDH, AST, albumin and other appropriate parameters.
Daily studies during stabilization (average 3 to 5 days): Urine glucose, acetone and ketones each shift, intake/output, weight, plasma and urine osmolarity, electrolytes, trace elements, CO_2, BUN, creatinine.
Routine studies after stabilization: *Daily* - Intake/output, weight, urine glucose and osmolarity and ketones.
Two to three times weekly: Electrolytes, BUN, blood glucose, plasma transaminases, bilirubin, blood acid-base status, ammonia, creatinine.
Weekly: CBC, prothrombin time, plasma total protein and fractions, hemoglobin, body length and head circumference (in infants), cholesterol, triglycerides, uric acid, albumin, LDH, AST, alkaline phosphatase.
Periodic: Nitrogen balance, trace elements, total lymphocyte count, iron status.

BUN – IV amino acid infusion may induce a rise in BUN, especially in GI bleeding or impaired hepatic or renal function. Perform appropriate laboratory tests periodically; discontinue if BUN exceeds normal postprandial limits and continues to rise. A modest rise in BUN normally results from increased protein intake. Azotemic patients should not receive amino acids without regard to total nitrogen intake.

Protein sparing: If daily increases in BUN (range, 10 to 15 mg/dL) for longer than 3 days occur, discontinue protein sparing therapy and institute a regimen with full nonprotein caloric substrates.

Cardiac effects – Avoid circulatory overload, particularly in patients with cardiac insufficiency. In patients with myocardial infarction, infusion of amino acids should always be accompanied by dextrose; in anoxia, free fatty acids cannot be used by the myocardium, and energy must be produced anaerobically from glycogen or glucose.

Hypertonic solutions – Hypertonic solutions containing dextrose should not be administered by peripheral vein infusions. Do not use hypertonic solutions in the presence of intracranial or intraspinal hemorrhage or if the patient is already dehydrated.

Glucose imbalances –

Hyperglycemia: Glucose intolerance is the most common metabolic complication; metabolic adaptation to large glucose loads requires up to 72 hours, although severely septic or hypermetabolic patients may not be able to handle the glucose load. A too rapid infusion of amino acid-carbohydrate mixtures may result in hyperglycemia, glycosuria and a hyperosmolar syndrome, characterized by mental confusion and loss of consciousness. Reducing the administration rate, decreasing the dextrose concentration or administering insulin will minimize these reactions.

Hyperglycemia may not be reflected by glycosuria in renal failure. Therefore, determine blood glucose frequently, often every 6 hours, to guide dosage of dextrose and insulin if required. Infusion of hypertonic dextrose carries a greater risk of hyperglycemia in low birth weight or septic infants.

Excess carbohydrate calories may result in fatty infiltration of the liver. Excess carbon dioxide from too much glucose can compromise weaning hypermetabolic patients from mechanical ventilation or can precipitate acute respiratory failure.

Rebound hypoglycemia: Rebound hypoglycemia may result from sudden cessation of a concentrated dextrose solution due to continued endogenous insulin production. Withdraw parenteral nutrition mixtures slowly. Administer a solution containing 5% or 10% dextrose when hypertonic dextrose infusions are abruptly discontinued.

Essential fatty acid deficiency (EFAD) – Essential fatty acid deficiency (EFAD) results from long-term fat-free IV feeding; symptoms include dry, scaly skin, eczematous rash, hair loss, poor wound healing and fatty degeneration of the liver. In adults, administer at least 500 mL fat emulsion per week to prevent EFAD (see individual monograph).

Electrolyte abnormalities – Intracellular ion deficits may arise due to two mechanisms. As protein is used for increased energy demands in a catabolic patient, intracellular ions are lost. In addition, as anabolism occurs, ions are employed in building new cells. Focus attention on supplying adequate potassium, phosphate, magnesium and calcium. Observe patients for clinical signs of paresthesias, neuromuscular weakness and changes in level of consciousness; monitor laboratory results.

The presence of impaired renal function, pulmonary disease, or cardiac insufficiency presents danger of retention of fluids.

Sodium: Use solutions containing sodium ions cautiously in patients with CHF, severe renal insufficiency, and edema with sodium retention.

Potassium: Use solutions containing potassium ions cautiously in patients with hyperkalemia or severe renal failure, and in conditions in which potassium retention is present.

Acetate: Use solutions containing acetate ions cautiously in patients with metabolic or respiratory alkalosis and in those conditions in which there is an increased level or impaired utilization of this ion, such as severe hepatic insufficiency.

Cancer chemotherapy patients – The American College of Physicians discourages the routine use of parenteral nutrition in patients undergoing cancer chemotherapy since no benefit has been determined (ie, there was no improvement in overall or short-term survival and no greater improvement in chemotherapy response).

Sulfite sensitivity – Some of these products contain sulfites which may cause allergic-type reactions including anaphylactic symptoms and life-threatening or less severe asthmatic episodes in certain susceptible persons. The overall prevalence of sulfite sensitivity in the general population is unknown and probably low. Sulfite sensitivity is seen more frequently in asthmatic or atopic persons.

➤*Drug Interactions:*

Tetracycline – Tetracycline may reduce the protein sparing effects of infused amino acids because of its antianabolic activity.

➤*Adverse Reactions:*

Catheter complications – Phlebitis and venous thrombosis may occur at the site of venipuncture or along the vein. If this occurs, discontinue use or choose another administration site. Use of large peripheral veins, inline filters and slower infusion rates may reduce the incidence of local venous irritation. Infection at the injection site and extravasation may occur.

Nausea, fever and flushing of the skin have occurred.

Metabolic complications include – Metabolic acidosis and alkalosis; hypophosphatemia; hypocalcemia; osteoporosis; glycosuria; hyperglycemia; hypo- or hypermagnesemia; osmotic diuresis; dehydration; hypervolemia; rebound hypoglycemia; hypo- or hypervitaminosis; electrolyte imbalances; hyperammonemia; elevated hepatic enzymes.

Phosphorus deficiency may lead to impaired tissue oxygenation and acute hemolytic anemia. Relative to calcium, excessive phosphorus intake can precipitate hypocalcemia with cramps, tetany and muscular hyperexcitability.

Complications known to occur from the placement of central venous catheters are pneumothorax, hemothorax, hydrothorax, artery puncture and transection, injury to the brachial plexus, malposition of the catheter, formation of arteriovenous fistula, phlebitis, thrombosis and air and catheter embolus.

Reactions reported in clinical studies as a result of infusion of the parenteral fluid were water weight gain, edema, increase in BUN and mild acidosis.

Protein Substrates

AMINO ACID INJECTION (General formulations)

For a complete discussion of the use of protein substrates as a compound of intravenous nutritional therapy, refer to the IV Nutritional Therapy general monograph.

Indications

➤*Nutritional supplement:* Six percent and 10% sulfite-free amino acid injections are indicated for the nutritional support of infants (including those of low birth weight) and young children requiring total parenteral nutrition (TPN) via either central or peripheral infusion routes. Parenteral nutrition with sulfite-free amino acid injections is indicated to prevent nitrogen and weight loss or treat negative nitrogen balance in infants and young children where the alimentary tract, by the oral, gastrostomy, or jejunostomy route, cannot or should not be used, or adequate protein intake is not feasible by these routes; gastrointestinal absorption of protein is impaired; or protein requirements are substantially increased, as with extensive burns. Dosage, route of administration, and concomitant infusion of nonprotein calories are dependent on various factors, such as nutritional and metabolic status of the patient, anticipated duration of parenteral nutritional support, and vein tolerance.

➤*Central venous nutrition:* Central venous infusion should be considered when amino acid solutions are to be admixed with hypertonic dextrose to promote protein synthesis in hypercatabolic or severely depleted infants, or those requiring long-term parenteral nutrition.

➤*Peripheral parenteral nutrition:* For moderately catabolic or depleted patients in whom the central venous route is not indicated, diluted amino acid solutions mixed with 5% to 10% dextrose solutions may be infused by peripheral vein, supplemented, if desired, with fat emulsion.

Administration and Dosage

➤*Nutritional support for children:* The objective of nutritional management of infants and young children is the provision of sufficient amino acid and caloric support for protein synthesis and growth.

The total daily dose of 6% and 10% sulfite-free amino acid injections depends on daily protein requirements and on the patient's metabolic and clinical response. The determination of nitrogen balance and accurate daily body weights, corrected for fluid balance, are probably the best means of assessing individual protein requirements. Dosage should also be guided by the patient's fluid intake limits and glucose and nitrogen tolerances, as well as by metabolic and clinical response.

➤*Protein allowances:* Recommendations for allowances of protein in infant nutrition have ranged from 2 to 4 g of protein per kilogram of body weight per day (2 to 4 g/kg/day). The recommended dosage of sulfite-free amino acid injections is 2 to 2.5 g of amino acids per kilogram of body weight per day (2 to 2.5 g/kg/day) for infants up to 10 kg. For infants and young children larger than 10 kg, the total dosage of amino acids should include the 20 to 25 g/day for the first 10 kg of body weight plus 1 to 1.25 g/day for each kg of body weight over 10 kg.

Typically, sulfite-free amino acid injections are admixed with 50% or 70% Dextrose Injection, supplemented with electrolytes and vitamins and administered continuously over a 24-hour period.

Total daily fluid intake should be appropriate for the patient's age and size. A fluid dose of 125 mL per kg body weight per day is appropriate for most infants on TPN. Although nitrogen requirements may be higher in severely hypercatabolic or depleted patients, provision of additional nitrogen may not be possible due to fluid intake limits, nitrogen, or glucose intolerance.

➤*Cysteine supplement:* Cysteine is considered to be an essential amino acid in infants and young children. An admixture of cysteine HCl to the TPN solution is therefore recommended. Based on clinical studies, the recommended dosage is 1 mmol of L-cysteine hydrochloride monohydrate per kilogram of body weight per day.

In many patients, provision of adequate calories in the form of hypertonic dextrose may require the administration of exogenous insulin to prevent hyperglycemia and glycosuria. To prevent rebound hypoglycemia, a solution containing 5% dextrose should be administered when hypertonic dextrose solutions are abruptly discontinued.

➤*Fat emulsion therapy:* Fat emulsion coadministration should be considered when prolonged (more than 5 days) parenteral nutrition is required in order to prevent essential fatty acid deficiency (EFAD). Serum lipids should be monitored for evidence of EFAD in patients maintained on fat-free TPN.

➤*Other electrolytes:* The provision of sufficient intracellular electrolytes, principally potassium, magnesium, and phosphate, is required for optimum utilization of amino acids. In addition, sufficient quantities of the major extracellular electrolytes sodium, calcium, and chloride, must be given. In patients with hyperchloremic or other metabolic acidoses, sodium and potassium may be added as the acetate salts to provide bicarbonate precursor. The electrolyte content of 6% and 10% sulfite-free amino acid injections must be considered when calculating daily electrolyte intake. Serum electrolytes, including magnesium and phosphorus, should be monitored frequently.

Appropriate vitamins, minerals and trace elements should also be provided.

➤*Central venous nutrition:* Hypertonic mixtures of amino acids and dextrose may be safely administered by continuous infusion through a central venous catheter with the tip located in the superior vena cava. Initial infusion rates should be slow, and gradually increased to the recommended 60 to 125 mL per kilogram of body weight per day. If administration rate should fall behind schedule, no attempt to "catch up" to planned intake should be made. In addition to meeting protein needs, the rate of administration, particularly during the first few days of therapy, is governed by the patient's glucose tolerance. Daily intake of amino acids and dextrose should be increased gradually to the maximum required dose as indicated by frequent determinations of glucose levels in blood and urine.

➤*Peripheral parenteral nutrition:* For patients in whom the central venous route is not indicated and who can consume adequate calories enterally, sulfite-free amino acid injections may be administered by peripheral vein with or without parenteral carbohydrate calories. Such infusates can be prepared by dilution with Sterile Water for Injection or 5% to 10% Dextrose Injection to prepare isotonic or slightly hypertonic solutions for peripheral infusion. It is essential that peripheral infusion be accompanied by adequate caloric intake.

Admixture incompatibility/compatibility – Sulfite-free amino acid injections may be admixed with solutions which contain phosphate or which have been supplemented with phosphate. The presence of calcium and magnesium ions in an additive solution should be considered when phosphate is also present, in order to avoid precipitation.

Care must be taken to avoid incompatible admixtures. Consult with pharmacist.

➤*Storage/Stability:* Protect from light until immediately prior to use. Do not remove container from overpouch until ready to use. Do not use if overpouch has been previously opened or damaged.

Exposure of pharmaceutical products to heat should be minimized. Avoid excessive heat. Protect from freezing. It is recommended that the product be stored at room temperature (25°C/77°F). Brief exposure up to 40°C (104°F) does not adversely affect the product.

Parenteral nutrition solutions should be used promptly after mixing. Any storage should be under refrigeration and limited to a brief period of time, preferably less than 24 hours.

Do not use unless solution is clear and seal is intact.

Actions

➤*Pharmacology:* Six percent and 10% sulfite-free amino acid injections provide a mixture of essential and nonessential amino acids as well as taurine and a soluble form of tyrosine, N-acetyl-L-tyrosine (NAT). This amino acid composition has been specifically formulated to provide a well-tolerated nitrogen source for nutritional support and therapy for infants and young children. When administered in conjunction with cysteine HCl, 6% and 10% amino acid injections result in the normalization of the plasma amino acid concentrations to a profile consistent with that of a breastfed infant.

The rationale for 6% and 10% amino acid injections is based on the observation of inadequate levels of essential amino acids in the plasma of infants receiving TPN using conventional amino acid solutions. These formulas were developed through the application of specific pharmacokinetic multiple regression analysis relating amino acid intake to the resulting plasma amino acid concentrations.

Clinical studies in infants and young children who required TPN therapy showed that infusion of 6% and 10% amino acid injections with a cysteine hydrochloride admixture resulted in a normalization of the plasma amino acid concentrations. In addition, weight gains, nitrogen balance, and serum protein concentrations were consistent with an improving nutritional status.

When infused with hypertonic dextrose as a calorie source, supplemented with cysteine hydrochloride, electrolytes, vitamins, and minerals, sulfite-free amino acid injections provide total parenteral nutrition in infants and young children, with the exception of essential fatty acids.

It is thought that the acetate from lysine acetate and acetic acid, under the conditions of parenteral nutrition, does not impact net acid-base balance when renal and respiratory functions are normal. Clinical evidence seems to support this thinking; however, confirmatory experimental evidence is not available.

The amount of chloride present in sulfite-free amino acid injections is not of clinical significance. The addition of cysteine hydrochloride will contribute to the chloride load.

The electrolyte content of any additives that are introduced should be carefully considered and included in total input computations.

Contraindications

Sulfite-free amino acid injections are contraindicated in patients with untreated anuria, hepatic coma, inborn errors of amino acid metabolism, including those involving branched chain amino acid metabolism such as maple syrup urine disease and isovaleric acidemia, or hypersensitivity to 1 or more amino acids present in the solution.

AMINO ACID INJECTION (General formulations)

Warnings

This injection is for compounding only, not for direct infusion.

➤*Azotemia:* Administration of amino acids in the presence of gastrointestinal bleeding may augment an already elevated blood urea nitrogen. Patients with azotemia from any cause should not be infused with amino acids without regard to total nitrogen intake.

➤*Fluid/solute overload:* Administration of IV fluids can cause fluid or solute overload, resulting in dilution of serum electrolyte concentrations, overhydration, congested states, or pulmonary edema. The risk of dilutional states is inversely proportional to the electrolyte concentrations of the solutions. The risk of solute overload causing congested states with peripheral and pulmonary edema is directly proportional to the electrolyte concentrations of the solution.

➤*Hyperammonemia:* Hyperammonemia is of special significance in infants, as its occurrence in the syndrome caused by genetic metabolic defects is sometimes associated, although not necessarily in a causal relationship, with mental retardation. This reaction appears to be dose related and is more likely to develop during prolonged therapy. It is essential that blood ammonia be measured frequently in infants. The mechanisms of this reaction are not clearly defined but may involve genetic defects and immature or subclinically impaired liver function.

Conservative doses of amino acids should be given, dictated by the nutritional status of the patient. Should symptoms of hyperammonemia develop, amino acid administration should be discontinued and patient's clinical status reevaluated.

➤*Renal function impairment:* Administration of amino acids in the presence of impaired renal function may augment an already elevated blood urea nitrogen.

➤*Hepatic function impairment:* Administration of amino acid solutions to a patient with hepatic insufficiency may result in plasma amino acid imbalances, hyperammonemia, prerenal azotemia, stupor and coma.

➤*Pregnancy: Category C.*

Animal reproduction studies have not been conducted with 6% and 10% sulfite-free amino acid injections. It is also not known whether sulfite-free amino acid injections can cause fetal harm when administered to a pregnant woman or can affect reproduction capacity.

Precautions

➤*Monitoring:* Clinical evaluation and periodic laboratory determinations are necessary to monitor changes in fluid balance, electrolyte concentrations, and acid-base balance during prolonged parenteral therapy or whenever the condition of the patient warrants such evaluation. Significant deviations from normal concentrations may require the use of additional electrolyte supplements.

Safe, effective use of parenteral nutrition requires a knowledge of nutrition as well as clinical expertise in recognition and treatment of the complications which can occur. Frequent evaluation and laboratory determinations are necessary for proper monitoring of parenteral nutrition. Studies should include blood sugar, serum proteins, kidney and liver function tests, electrolytes, hemogram, carbon dioxide content, serum osmolalities, blood cultures, and blood ammonia levels.

➤*Hypertonic solutions:* Strongly hypertonic nutrient solutions should be administered via an IV catheter placed in a central vein, preferably the superior vena cava.

➤*Ketone bodies:* Administration of amino acids without carbohydrates may result in the accumulation of ketone bodies in the blood. Correction of this ketonemia may be achieved by the administration of carbohydrates.

➤*Peripheral administration:* Peripheral administration of 6% and 10% sulfite-free amino acid injections requires appropriate dilution and provision of adequate calories. Care should be taken to ensure proper placement of the needle within the lumen of the vein. The venipuncture site should be inspected frequently for signs of infiltration. If venous thrombosis or phlebitis occurs, discontinue infusions or change infusion site and initiate appropriate treatment.

➤*Electrolyte supplementation:* Extraordinary electrolyte losses such as may occur during protracted nasogastric suction, vomiting, diarrhea, or gastrointestinal fistula drainage may necessitate additional electrolyte supplementation.

Metabolic acidosis can be prevented or readily controlled by adding a portion of the cations in the electrolyte mixture as acetate salts and, in the case of hyperchloremic acidosis, by keeping the total chloride content of the infusate to a minimum. Sulfite-free amino acid injections contain less than 3 mEq chloride per liter.

Sulfite-free amino acid injections contain no added phosphorus. Patients, especially those with hypophosphatemia, may require the addition of phosphate. To prevent hypocalcemia, calcium supplementation should always accompany phosphate administration. To ensure adequate intake, serum levels should be monitored frequently.

➤*Admixture incompatibilities:* To minimize the risk of possible incompatibilities arising from mixing this solution with other additives that may be prescribed, the final infusate should be inspected for cloudiness or precipitation immediately after mixing, prior to administration, and periodically during administration.

➤*Central venous nutrition:* Administration by central venous catheter should be used only by those familiar with this technique and its complications.

Central venous nutrition may be associated with complications which can be prevented or minimized by careful attention to all aspects of the procedure, including solution preparation, administration, and patient monitoring. It is essential that a carefully prepared protocol, based on current medical practices, be followed, preferably by an experienced team.

➤*Diabetes patients:* Special care must be taken when giving hypertonic dextrose to a diabetic or prediabetic patient. To prevent severe hyperglycemia in such patients, insulin may be required.

Administration of glucose at a rate exceeding the patient's utilization rate may lead to hyperglycemia, coma, and death.

➤*Special risk:* Care should be taken to avoid circulatory overload, particularly in patients with cardiac insufficiency.

Adverse Reactions

If an adverse reaction does occur, discontinue the infusion, evaluate the patient, institute appropriate therapeutic countermeasures and save the remainder of the fluid for examination if deemed necessary.

➤*Infusion-related reactions:* Reactions reported in clinical studies as a result of infusion of the parenteral fluid were water weight gain, edema, increase in blood urea nitrogen (BUN), and mild acidosis.

➤*Reactions due to solution or administration technique:* Reactions which may occur because of the solution or the technique of administration include febrile response, infection at the site of injection, venous thrombosis or phlebitis extending from the site of injection, extravasation and hypervolemia.

➤*Local:* Local reaction at the infusion site, consisting of a warm sensation, erythema, phlebitis and thrombosis, have been reported with peripheral amino acid infusions, especially if other substances are also administered through the same site.

If electrolyte supplementation is required during peripheral infusion, it is recommended that additives be administered throughout the day in order to avoid possible venous irritation. Irritating additive medications may require injection at another site and should not be added directly to the amino acid infusate.

Symptoms may result from an excess or deficit of 1 or more of the ions present in the solution; therefore, frequent monitoring of electrolyte levels is essential.

➤*Phosphorus deficiency:* Phosphorus deficiency may lead to impaired tissue oxygenation and acute hemolytic anemia. Relative to calcium, excessive phosphorus intake can precipitate hypocalcemia with cramps, tetany and muscular hyperexcitability.

Overdosage

➤*Treatment:* In the event of a fluid or solute overload during parenteral therapy, reevaluate the patient's condition, and institute appropriate corrective treatment.

Protein Substrates

CRYSTALLINE AMINO ACID INFUSIONS

	Aminosyn 3.5% (Abbott)	Aminosyn II 3.5% (Abbott)	Aminosyn 5% (Abbott)	Aminosyn II 5% (Abbott)	Travasol 5.5% (Clintec)	TrophAmine 6% (McGaw)
Amino Acid Concentration	3.5%	3.5%	5%	5%	5.5%	6%
Nitrogen (g/100 mL)	0.55	0.54	0.79	0.77	0.925	0.93
Amino Acids (Essential) (mg/100 mL)						
Isoleucine	252	231	360	330	263	490
Leucine	329	350	470	500	340	840
Lysine	252	368	360	525	318	490
Methionine	140	60	200	86	318	200
Phenylalanine	154	104	220	149	340	290
Threonine	182	140	260	200	230	250
Tryptophan	56	70	80	100	99	120
Valine	280	175	400	250	252	470
Amino Acids (Nonessential) (mg/100 mL)						
Alanine	448	348	640	497	1140	320
Arginine	343	356	490	509	570	730
Histidine[a]	105	105	150	150	241	290
Proline	300	253	430	361	230	410
Serine	147	186	210	265		230
Taurine						15
Tyrosine	31	95	44	135	22	140
Aminoacetic Acid (Glycine)	448	175	640	250	1140	220
Glutamic Acid		258		369		300
Aspartic Acid		245		350		190
Cysteine						< 14
Electrolytes (mEq/L)						
Sodium	7	16.3		19.3		5
Potassium			5.4			
Chloride					22	< 3
Acetate	46	25.2	86	35.9	48	56
Phosphate (mM/L)						
Osmolarity (mOsm/L)	357	308	500	438	575	525
Supplied in (mL)	1000[b]	1000[c]	500[d] 1000[d]	500[c] 1000[c]	500[e] 1000[e] 2000[e]	500[f]
Labeled Indications						
Peripheral Parenteral Nutrition	Yes	Yes	Yes	Yes	Yes	Yes
Central TPN	No	No	Yes	Yes	Yes	Yes
Protein Sparing	Yes	Yes	Yes	Yes	Yes	No

	Aminosyn 7% (Abbott)	Aminosyn-PF 7% (Abbott)	Aminosyn II 7% (Abbott)	Aminosyn 8.5% (Abbott)
Amino Acid Concentration	7%	7%	7%	8.5%
Nitrogen (g/100 mL)	1.1	1.07	1.07	1.34
Amino Acids (Essential) (mg/100 mL)				
Isoleucine	510	534	462	620
Leucine	660	831	700	810
Lysine	510	475	735	624
Methionine	280	125	120	340
Phenylalanine	310	300	209	380
Threonine	370	360	280	460
Tryptophan	120	125	140	150
Valine	560	452	350	680
Amino Acids (Nonessential) (mg/100 mL)				
Alanine	900	490	695	1100
Arginine	690	861	713	850
Histidine[a]	210	220	210	260
Proline	610	570	505	750
Serine	300	347	371	370
Taurine		50		
Tyrosine	44	44	189	44
Aminoacetic Acid (Glycine)	900	270	350	1100
Glutamic Acid		576	517	
Aspartic Acid		370	490	
Cysteine				
Electrolytes (mEq/L)				
Sodium		3.4	31.3	
Potassium	5.4			5.4
Chloride				35
Acetate	105	32.5	50.3	90
Phosphate (mM/L)				
Osmolarity (mOsm/L)	700	586	612	850
Supplied in (mL)	500[d]	250[g] 500[g]	500[c]	500[d] 1000[d]
Labeled Indications				
Peripheral Parenteral Nutrition	Yes	Yes	Yes	Yes
Central TPN	Yes	Yes	Yes	Yes
Protein Sparing	Yes	No	Yes	Yes

	Aminosyn II 8.5% (Abbott)	Travasol 8.5% without electrolytes (Clintec)	FreAmine III 8.5% (B. Braun)
Amino Acid Concentration	8.5%	8.5%	8.5%
Nitrogen (g/100 mL)	1.3	1.43	
Amino Acids (Essential) (mg/100 mL)			
Isoleucine	561	406	590
Leucine	850	526	770
Lysine	893	492	620
Methionine	146	492	450
Phenylalanine	253	526	480
Threonine	340	356	340
Tryptophan	170	152	130
Valine	425	390	560
Amino Acids (Nonessential) (mg/100 mL)			
Alanine	844	1760	600
Arginine	865	880	810
Histidine[a]	255	372	240
Proline	614	356	950
Serine	450		500
Taurine			
Tyrosine	230	34	
Aminoacetic Acid (Glycine)	425	1760	1190
Glutamic Acid	627		
Aspartic Acid	595		
Cysteine			< 20
Electrolytes (mEq/L)			
Sodium	33.3		10
Potassium			
Chloride		34	< 3
Acetate	61.1	73	72
Phosphate (mM/L)			10
Osmolarity (mOsm/L)	742	890	810
Supplied in (mL)	500[c] 1000[c]	500[h] 1000[h] 2000[h]	500[i] 1000[i]
Labeled Indications			
Peripheral Parenteral Nutrition	Yes	Yes	Yes
Central TPN	Yes	Yes	Yes
Protein Sparing	Yes	Yes	Yes

CRYSTALLINE AMINO ACID INFUSIONS

	TrophAmine 10% (McGaw)	Aminosyn 10% (Abbott)	Aminosyn-PF 10% (Abbott)	Aminosyn II 10% (Abbott)
Amino Acid Concentration	10%	10%	10%	10%
Nitrogen (g/100 mL)	1.55	1.57	1.52	1.53
Amino Acids (Essential) (mg/100 mL)				
Isoleucine	820	720	760	660
Leucine	1400	940	1200	1000
Lysine	820	720	677	1050
Methionine	340	400	180	172
Phenylalanine	480	440	427	298
Threonine	420	520	512	400
Tryptophan	200	160	180	200
Valine	780	800	673	500
Amino Acids (Nonessential) (mg/100 mL)				
Alanine	540	1280	698	993
Arginine	1200	980	1227	1018
Histidine[a]	480	300	312	300
Proline	680	860	812	722
Serine	380	420	495	530
Taurine	25		70	
Tyrosine	240	44	40	270
Aminoacetic Acid (Glycine)	360	1280	385	500
Glutamic Acid	500		620	738
Aspartic Acid	320		527	700
Cysteine	< 16			
Electrolytes (mEq/L)				
Sodium	5		3.4	45.3
Potassium		5.4		
Chloride	< 3			
Acetate	97	148	46.3	71.8
Phosphate (mM/L)10				
Osmolarity (mOsm/L)	875	1000	829	873
Supplied in (mL)	500[f]	500[d] 1000[d]	1000[j]	500[c] 1000[c]
Labeled Indications				
Peripheral Parenteral Nutrition	Yes	Yes	Yes	Yes
Central TPN	Yes	Yes	Yes	Yes
Protein Sparing	No	Yes	No	Yes

	Travasol 10% (Clintec)	FreAmine III 10% (McGaw)	Novamine (Clintec)	Novamine 15% (Clintec)	Aminosyn II 15% (Abbott)
Amino Acid Concentration	10%	10%	11.4%	15%	15%
Nitrogen (g/100 mL)	1.65	1.53	1.8	2.37	2.3
Amino Acids (Essential) (mg/100 mL)					
Isoleucine	600	690	570	749	990
Leucine	730	910	790	1040	1500
Lysine	580	730	900	1180	1575
Methionine	400	530	570	749	258
Phenylalanine	560	560	790	1040	447
Threonine	420	400	570	749	600
Tryptophan	180	150	190	250	300
Valine	580	660	730	960	750
Amino Acids (Nonessential) (mg/100 mL)					
Alanine	2070	710	1650	2170	1490
Arginine	1150	950	1120	1470	1527
Histidine[a]	480	280	680	894	450
Proline	680	1120	680	894	1083
Serine	500	590	450	592	795
Taurine					
Tyrosine	40		30	39	405
Aminoacetic Acid (Glycine)	1030	1400	790	1040	750
Glutamic Acid			570	749	1107
Aspartic Acid			330	434	1050
Cysteine		< 24			
Electrolytes (mEq/L)					
Sodium		10			62.7
Potassium					
Chloride	40	< 3			
Acetate	87	≈89	114	151	107.6
Phosphate (mM/L)		10			
Osmolarity (mOsm/L)	1000	≈ 950	1057	1388	1300
Supplied in (mL)	250[l,m] 500[l,m] 1000[l,m] 2000[l]	500[i] 1000[i]	500[n] 1000[n]	500[n] 1000[n]	2000[o]
Labeled Indications					
Peripheral Parenteral Nutrition	Yes	Yes	Yes	Yes	Yes
Central TPN	Yes	Yes	Yes	Yes	Yes
Protein Sparing	Yes	Yes	Yes	No	No

[a] Histidine is considered an essential amino acid in infants and in renal failure.
[b] With 7 mEq/L sodium from the antioxidant sodium hydrosulfite.
[c] Includes 20 mg/dL sodium hydrosulfite.
[d] Includes 5.4 mEq/L potassium from the antioxidant potassium metabisulfite.
[e] With ≈ 3 mEq/L sodium bisulfite.
[f] With less than 50 mg sodium metabisulfite per 100 mL.
[g] From the antioxidant sodium hydrosulfite.
[h] With 3 mEq/L sodium bisulfite.
[i] With less than 0.1 g sodium bisulfite per 100 mL.
[j] With 230 mg sodium hydrosulfite per 100 mL.
[k] Potassium derived from the antioxidant potassium metabisulfite.
[l] Acetate in Viaflex container = 60 mEq/L; osmolarity is 970 mOsm/L.
[m] Sizes also come in Viaflex containers.
[n] With 30 mg sodium metabisulfite.
[o] With 60 mg sodium hydrosulfite per 100 mL.

CRYSTALLINE AMINO ACID INFUSIONS WITH ELECTROLYTES

	ProcalAmine (McGaw)	FreAmine III 3% w/Electrolytes (McGaw)	Aminosyn 3.5% M (Abbott)	Aminosyn II 3.5% M (Abbott)	3.5% Travasol w/Electrolytes (Clintec)	5.5% Travasol w/Electrolytes (Clintec)
Amino Acid Concentration	3%	3%	3.5%	3.5%	3.5%	5.5%
Nitrogen (g/100 mL)	0.46	0.46	0.55	0.54	0.591	0.925
Amino Acids (Essential) (mg/100 mL)						
Isoleucine	210	210	252	231	168	263
Leucine	270	270	329	350	217	340
Lysine	220	220	252	368	203	318
Methionine	160	160	140	60	203	318
Phenylalanine	170	170	154	104	217	340
Threonine	120	120	182	140	147	230
Tryptophan	46	46	56	70	63	99
Valine	200	200	280	175	161	252
Amino Acids (Nonessential) (mg/100 mL)						
Alanine	210	210	448	348	728	1140
Arginine	290	290	343	356	364	570
Histidine[a]	85	85	105	105	154	241
Proline	340	340	300	253	147	230
Serine	180	180	147	186		
Tyrosine			31	95	14	22
Glycine	420	420	448	175	728	1140
Glutamic Acid				258		
Aspartic Acid				245		
Cysteine	< 20	< 20				
Electrolytes (mEq/L)						
Sodium	35	35	47	36	25	70
Potassium	24	24.5	13	13	15	60
Magnesium	5	5	3	3	5	10
Chloride	41	41	40	37	25	70
Acetate	47	44	58	25	52	102
Phosphate (mM/L)	3.5	3.5	3.5	3.5	7.5	30
Osmolarity (mOsm/L)	735	≈ 405	477	425	450	850
Nonprotein Calories (g/100 mL) (glycerin)	3					
Supplied in (mL)	1000[b]	1000[c]	1000[d]	1000[e]	500[f] 1000[f]	500[f] 1000[f] 2000[f]
Labeled Indications						
Peripheral Parenteral Nutrition	Yes	Yes	Yes	Yes	Yes	Yes
Central TPN	No	No	No	No	No	Yes
Protein Sparing	Yes	Yes	Yes	Yes	Yes	Yes

	Aminosyn 7% w/Electrolytes (Abbott)	Aminosyn II 7% with Electrolytes (Abbott)	Aminosyn 8.5% w/Electrolytes (Abbott)	Aminosyn II 8.5% with Electrolytes (Abbott)	FreAmine III 8.5% w/ Electrolytes (McGaw)	Travasol 8.5% w/Electrolytes (Clintec)
Amino Acid Concentration	7%	7%	8.5%	8.5%	8.5%	8.5%
Nitrogen g/100 mL	1.1	1.07	1.34	1.3	1.3	1.43
Amino Acids (Essential) (mg/100 mL)						
Isoleucine	510	462	620	561	590	406
Leucine	660	700	810	850	770	526
Lysine	510	735	624	893	620	492
Methionine	280	120	340	146	450	492
Phenylalanine	310	209	380	253	480	526
Threonine	370	280	460	340	340	356
Tryptophan	120	140	150	170	130	152
Valine	560	350	680	425	560	390
Amino Acids (Nonessential) (mg/100 mL)						
Alanine	900	695	1100	844	600	1760
Arginine	690	713	850	865	810	880
Histidine[a]	210	210	260	255	240	372
Proline	610	505	750	614	950	356
Serine	300	371	370	450	500	
Tyrosine	44	189	44	230		34
Glycine	900	350	1100	425	1190	1760
Glutamic Acid		517		627		
Aspartic Acid		490		595		
Cysteine					< 20	
Electrolytes (mEq/L)						
Sodium	70	76	70	80	60	70
Potassium	66	66	66	66	60	60
Magnesium	10	10	10	10	10	10
Chloride	96	86	98	86	60	70
Acetate	124	50	142	61	125	141
Phosphate (mM/L)	30	30	30	30	20	30
Osmolarity (mOsm/L)	1013	869	1160	999	1045	1160
Supplied in (mL)	500[g]	500[h]	500[g]	500[h]	500[i] 1000[i]	500[f] 1000[f] 2000[f]
Labeled Indications						
Peripheral Parenteral Nutrition	Yes	Yes	Yes	Yes	Yes	Yes
Central TPN	Yes	Yes	Yes	Yes	Yes	Yes
Protein Sparing	Yes	Yes	Yes	Yes	Yes	Yes

[a] Histidine is considered an essential amino acid in infants and in renal failure.
[b] With less than 50 mg K+ metabisulfite and 3 mEq Ca/L.
[c] With less than 0.05 g of the antioxidant potassium metabisulfite.
[d] Includes 7 mEq/L sodium from the antioxidant sodium hydrosulfite.
[e] With 20 mg sodium hydrosulfite per 100 mL.
[f] With 3 mEq/L sodium bisulfite.
[g] Includes 5.4 mEq/L potassium from the antioxidant potassium metabisulfite.
[h] Includes sodium from the antioxidant sodium hydrosulfite.
[i] With less than 0.1 g sodium bisulfite per 100 mL.

CRYSTALLINE AMINO ACID INFUSIONS WITH DEXTROSE

	Travasol 2.75% in 5% Dextrose[a] (Clintec)	Travasol 2.75% in 10% Dextrose[a] (Clintec)	Travasol 2.75% in 25% Dextrose[a] (Clintec)	Aminosyn II 3.5% in 5% Dextrose[a] (Hospira)	Aminosyn II 3.5% in 25% Dextrose[a] (Hospira)
Amino Acid Concentration	2.75%	2.75%	2.75%	3.5%	3.5%
Dextrose Concentration	5%	10%	25%	5%	25%
Nitrogen (g/100 mL)	0.46	0.46	0.46	0.54	0.54
Amino Acids (Essential) (mg/100 mL)					
Isoleucine	132	132	132	231	231
Leucine	170	170	170	350	350
Lysine	159	159	159	368	368
Methionine	159	159	159	60	60
Phenylalanine	170	170	170	104	104
Threonine	115	115	115	140	140
Tryptophan	50	50	50	70	70
Valine	126	126	126	175	175
Amino Acids (Nonessential) (mg/100 mL)					
Alanine	570	570	570	348	348
Arginine	285	285	285	356	356
Histidine[b]	120	120	120	105	105
Proline	115	115	115	252	252
Serine				186	186
Tyrosine	11	11	11	94	94
Aminoacetic Acid (Glycine)	570	570	570	175	175
Glutamic Acid				258	258
Aspartic Acid				245	245
Cysteine					
Electrolytes (mEq/L)					
Sodium				18	18
Potassium					
Magnesium					
Chloride	11	11	11		
Acetate	16	16	16	25.2	25.2
Phosphate (mM/L)					
Osmolarity (mOsm/L)	530	785	1540	585	1515
Supplied in (mL)	500 mL with 500 mL dextrose	500 mL with 500 mL dextrose	500 mL with 500 mL dextrose	1000 mL with 1000 mL dextrose[c]	500 mL with 500 mL dextrose[c]
Labeled Indications					
Peripheral Parenteral Nutrition	Yes	Yes	Yes	Yes	No
Central TPN	Yes	Yes	Yes	No	Yes

	Travasol 4.25% in 5% Dextrose[a] (Clintec)	Aminosyn II 4.25% in 10% Dextrose[a] (Abbott)	Travasol 4.25% in 10% Dextrose[a] (Clintec)	Aminosyn II 4.25% in 20% Dextrose[a] (Abbott)
Amino Acid Concentration	4.25%	4.25%	4.25%	4.25%
Dextrose Concentration	5%	10%	10%	20%
Nitrogen (g/100 mL)	0.7	0.65	0.7	0.65
Amino Acids (Essential) (mg/100 mL)				
Isoleucine	203	280	203	280
Leucine	263	425	263	425
Lysine	246	446	246	446
Methionine	246	73	246	73
Phenylalanine	263	126	263	126
Threonine	178	170	178	170
Tryptophan	76	85	76	85
Valine	195	212	195	212
Amino Acids (Nonessential) (mg/100 mL)				
Alanine	880	422	880	422
Arginine	440	432	440	432
Histidine[b]	186	128	186	128
Proline	178	307	178	307
Serine		225		225
Tyrosine	17	115	17	115
Aminoacetic Acid (Glycine)	880	212	880	212
Glutamic Acid		314		314
Aspartic Acid		298		298
Cysteine				
Electrolytes (mEq/L)				
Sodium		19		19
Potassium				
Magnesium				
Chloride	17		17	
Acetate	22	30.6	22	30.6
Phosphate (mM/L)				
Osmolarity (mOsm/L)	680	894	935	1295
Supplied in (mL)	500 mL with 500 mL dextrose	1000 mL w/ 1000 mL dextrose[c]	500 mL with 500 mL dextrose	1000 mL with 1000 mL dextrose[c]
Labeled Indications				
Peripheral Parenteral Nutrition	Yes	Yes	Yes	No
Central TPN	Yes	No	Yes	Yes

Protein Substrates

CRYSTALLINE AMINO ACID INFUSIONS WITH DEXTROSE

	Aminosyn II 4.25% in 25% Dextrose[a] (Abbott)	Travasol 4.25% in 25% Dextrose[a] (Clintec)	Aminosyn II 5% in 25% Dextrose[a] (Abbott)
Amino Acid Concentration	4.25%	4.25%	5%
Dextrose Concentration	25%	25%	25%
Nitrogen (g/100 mL)	0.65	0.65	0.77
Amino Acids (Essential) (mg/100 mL)			
Isoleucine	280	203	330
Leucine	425	263	500
Lysine	446	246	525
Methionine	73	246	86
Phenylalanine	126	263	149
Threonine	170	178	200
Tryptophan	85	76	100
Valine	212	195	250
Amino Acids (Nonessential) (mg/100 mL)			
Alanine	422	880	496
Arginine	432	440	509
Histidine[b]	128	186	150
Proline	307	178	361
Serine	225		265
Tyrosine	115	17	135
Aminoacetic Acid (Glycine)	212	880	250
Glutamic Acid	314		369
Aspartic Acid	298		350
Cysteine			
Electrolytes (mEq/L)			
Sodium	19		22.2
Potassium			
Magnesium			
Chloride		17	
Acetate	30.6	22	35.9
Phosphate (mM/L)			
Osmolarity (mOsm/L)	1536	1690	1539
Supplied in (mL)	750 and 1000 mL and 750 and 1000 mL dextrose[c]	500 mL with 500 mL dex- trose[c]	500, 750 and 1000 mL and 500, 750 and 1000 mL dextrose[c]
Labeled Indications			
Peripheral Parenteral Nutrition	No	Yes	No
Central TPN	Yes	Yes	Yes

[a] Solution composition represents admixture of dual-chamber *Quick Mix* or *Nutrimix* container.
[b] Histidine is considered an essential amino acid in infants and in renal failure.
[c] With 30 mg sodium hydrosulfite per 100 mL.

CRYSTALLINE AMINO ACID INFUSIONS WITH ELECTROLYTES IN DEXTROSE

	Aminosyn II 3.5% M[a] in 5% Dextrose[b] (Abbott)	Aminosyn II 4.25% M[a] in 10% Dextrose[b] (Abbott)
Amino Acid Concentration	3.5%	4.25%
Dextrose Concentration	5%	10%
Nitrogen (g/100 mL)	0.535	0.65
Amino Acids (Essential) (mg/100 mL)		
Isoleucine	231	280
Leucine	350	425
Lysine	368	446
Methionine	60	73
Phenylalanine	104	126
Threonine	140	170
Tryptophan	70	85
Valine	175	212
Amino Acids (Nonessential) (mg/100 mL)		
Alanine	348	422
Arginine	356	432
Histidine[c]	105	128
Proline	252	307
Serine	186	225
Tyrosine	94	115
Aminoacetic Acid (Glycine)	175	212
Glutamic Acid	258	314
Aspartic Acid	245	298
Cysteine		
Electrolytes (mEq/L)		
Sodium	41	43.7
Potassium	13	13
Magnesium	3	3
Chloride	36.5	36.5
Acetate	25.1	30.5
Phosphorus (mM/L)	3.5	3.5
Osmolarity (mOsm/L)	616	919
Supplied in (mL)	500 and 1000 mL and 500 and 1000 mL dextrose[d]	500 mL and 500 mL dex- trose[d]
Labeled Indications		
Peripheral Parenteral Nutri- tion	Yes	Yes
Central TPN	No	Yes
Protein Sparing	No	No

[a] With maintenance electrolytes.
[b] Solution composition represents admixture of *Nutrimix* dual-chamber container.
[c] Histidine is considered an essential amino acid in infants and in renal failure.
[d] With 30 mg sodium hydrosulfite per 100 mL.

AMINO ACID FORMULATIONS FOR RENAL FAILURE

	Aminosyn-RF 5.2% (Abbott)	Aminess 5.2% (Clintec)	5.4% NephrAmine (McGaw)	RenAmin (Clintec)
Amino Acid Concentration	5.2%	5.2%	5.4%	6.5%
Nitrogen (g/100 mL)	0.79	0.66	0.65	1
Amino Acids (Essential) (mg/100 mL)				
Isoleucine	462	525	560	500
Leucine	726	825	880	600
Lysine	535	600	640	450
Methionine	726	825	880	500
Phenylalanine	726	825	880	490
Threonine	330	375	400	380

AMINO ACID FORMULATIONS FOR RENAL FAILURE

	Aminosyn-RF 5.2% (Abbott)	Aminess 5.2% (Clintec)	5.4% NephrAmine (McGaw)	RenAmin (Clintec)
Tryptophan	165	188	200	160
Valine	528	600	640	820
Histidine	429	412	250	420
Amino Acids (Nonessential) (mg/100 mL)				
Cysteine			< 20	
Arginine	600			630
Alanine				560
Proline				350
Glycine				300
Serine				300
Tyrosine				40
Electrolytes (mEq/L)				
Sodium			5	
Acetate	≈ 105	50	≈ 44	60
Potassium	5.4			
Chloride			< 3	31
Osmolarity (mOsm/L)	475	416	435	600
Supplied in (mL)	300[a]	400[b]	250[c]	250[d] 500[d]

[a] With 60 mg potassium metabisulfite per 100 mL.
[b] In 500 mL bottle.
[c] With less than 0.05 g sodium bisulfite per 100 mL.
[d] With ≈ 3 mEq sodium bisulfite.

AMINO ACID FORMULATIONS FOR RENAL FAILURE — INTRAVENOUS

For a complete discussion of the use of protein substrates for intravenous nutritional therapy, refer to the IV Nutritionals monograph.

Indications

➤*Nutritional support:* For nutritional support of uremic patients, particularly when oral nutrition is impractical, not feasible or insufficient.

Essential amino acid injection does not replace dialysis and conventional supportive therapy in patients with renal failure. To promote urea reutilization, provide adequate calories with minimal amounts of essential amino acids and restrict the intake of nonessential nitrogen.

➤*Children:* Use with caution in pediatric patients, especially low birth weight infants, due to limited clinical experience. Laboratory and clinical monitoring must be extensive and frequent. Use a low initial dose and increase slowly.

The absence of arginine in *NephrAmine* and *Aminess* may accentuate the risk of hyperammonemia in infants. *Aminosyn-RF* and *RenAmin* contain arginine.

Administration and Dosage

Provide adequate calories simultaneously. Administer essential amino acid/dextrose mixtures by continuous infusion through a central venous catheter. Use slow initial infusion rates, generally 20 to 30 mL/hour for the first 6 to 8 hours. Increase by 10 mL/hour each 24 hours, up to a maximum of 60 to 100 mL/hour.

Administration rate is governed by the patient's nitrogen, fluid and glucose tolerance. Uremic patients are frequently glucose intolerant, especially in association with peritoneal dialysis, and may require exogenous insulin to prevent hyperglycemia. To prevent rebound hypoglycemia when hypertonic dextrose infusions are abruptly discontinued, administer a 5% dextrose solution.

➤*Adults:*

Aminosyn-RF – 300 to 600 mL. Mix 300 mL with 500 mL of 70% dextrose to provide a solution of 1.96% essential amino acids in 44% dextrose (calorie:nitrogen ratio = 504:1).

Aminess – 400 mL. Mix 400 mL with 500 mL of 70% dextrose to yield a solution of 2.3% essential amino acids in 39% dextrose (calorie:nitrogen ratio = 450:1).

NephrAmine – 250 to 500 mL. Mix 250 mL w/500 mL of 70% dextrose to yield solution of 1.8% essential amino acids in 47% dextrose (calorie: nitrogen ratio = 744:1).

RenAmin – 250 to 500 mL.

➤*Children:* Individualize dosage. A dosage of 0.5 to 1 g/kg/day will meet the requirements of the majority of pediatric patients. Use a low initial daily dosage and increase slowly; more than 1 g/kg/day is not recommended.

Actions

➤*Pharmacology:* Patients with renal decompensation have different amino acid requirements than those with normal renal function. Use in uremic patients is based on the minimal requirements for each of the 8 essential amino acids. These products contain histidine, an amino acid considered essential for infant growth and for uremic patients.

In renal failure, nonspecific nitrogen-containing compounds are broken down in the intestine. The ammonia formed is absorbed and incorporated by the liver into nonessential amino acids, provided essential amino acid requirements are being met. Exogenously supplying only essential amino acids allows urea nitrogen to be recycled which can serve as a precursor for nonessential amino acid synthesis. Therefore, administration to uremic patients, particularly those who are protein deficient, results in the utilization of retained urea, and may be followed by a drop in BUN and resolution of many azotemic symptoms.

Infusion of essential amino acids and hypertonic dextrose promotes protein synthesis, improves cellular metabolic balance, decreases the rate of rise of BUN and minimizes deterioration of serum potassium, magnesium and phosphorus balance in patients with impaired renal function. This therapy may decrease morbidity associated with acute renal failure and promote earlier return of renal function. Although controversial, these formulations may have no clinically significant advantage over the general formulations containing both essential and nonessential amino acids in most uremic patients.

AMINO ACID FORMULATIONS FOR HIGH METABOLIC STRESS — INTRAVENOUS

For a complete discussion of the use of protein substrates as a compound of intravenous nutritional therapy, refer to the IV Nutritionals monograph.

Indications

➤*Nitrogen imbalance:* To prevent nitrogen loss or treat negative nitrogen balance in adults if: (1) The alimentary tract, by oral, gastrostomy or jejunostomy route, cannot or should not be used, or adequate protein intake is not feasible by these routes; (2) GI protein absorption is impaired; or (3) nitrogen homeostasis is substantially impaired as with severe trauma or sepsis.

Administration and Dosage

➤*Adults:* Daily amino acid doses of ≈ 1.5 g/kg for adults with adequate calories generally satisfy protein needs and promote positive nitrogen balance. May need higher doses in severely catabolic states. Fat emulsion may help meet energy requirements.

➤*Severely catabolic patients:* For severely catabolic, depleted patients or those requiring long-term TPN, consider central venous nutrition. Start with infusates containing lower dextrose concentrations; gradually increase dextrose to estimated caloric needs as glucose tolerance increases. *FreAmine HBC* 750 mL and 250 mL 70% dextrose or 500 mL *Aminosyn-HBC* 7% and 500 mL concentrated dextrose, with added electrolytes, trace metals and vitamins, may be given over 8 hours. *BranchAmin* 4% must be admixed with a complete amino acid injection, with or without a concentrated caloric source.

➤*Moderately catabolic patients:* For moderately catabolic, depleted patients in whom central venous route is not indicated, may infuse diluted *FreAmine HBC* or *Aminosyn-HBC* 7% with minimal caloric supplementation by peripheral vein; supplement, if desired, with fat emulsion.

Usual administration of 4% BCAA Injection is used as a supplement to parenteral nutrition solutions to achieve an amino acid solution that is ≈ 50% w/w BCAA. One method for achieving this ratio is the admixture of two volumes of 4% BCAA Injection at 4 g/dL concentration with one volume of an amino acid solution of 8 to 10 g/dL concentration. The supplemental amino acid mixture is given with energy substrates to provide at least 35 kcal/kg ideal body weight as nonprotein calories.

Protein Substrates

AMINO ACID FORMULATIONS FOR HIGH METABOLIC STRESS — INTRAVENOUS

Actions

➤*Pharmacology:* These are mixtures of essential and nonessential amino acids with high concentrations of branched chain amino acids (BCAA): Isoleucine, leucine, valine.

Acute metabolic stress – Acute metabolic stress is characterized by increased urinary nitrogen excretion and hyperglycemia; glucose utilization and fat store mobilization are impaired. The primary substrates used to meet energy requirements of muscle are BCAAs.

AMINO ACID FORMULATION IN HEPATIC FAILURE/HEPATIC ENCEPHALOPATHY — INTRAVENOUS

Indications

➤*Hepatic encephalopathy:* For the treatment of hepatic encephalopathy in patients with cirrhosis or hepatitis. Provides nutritional support for patients with these diseases of the liver who require parenteral nutrition and are intolerant of general purpose amino acid injections, which are contraindicated in patients with hepatic coma.

Administration and Dosage

Give 80 to 120 g amino acids (12 to 18 g nitrogen)/day. Typically, 500 mL *HepatAmine* with ≈ 500 mL 50% dextrose and electrolytes and vitamins is given over 8 to 12 hours. This results in total daily fluid intake of ≈ 2 to 3 L. Patients with fluid restrictions may only tolerate 1 to 2 L. Although nitrogen requirements may be higher in severely hypercatabolic or depleted patients, provision of additional nitrogen may not be possible due to fluid intake limits, nitrogen or glucose intolerance.

Use slow initial infusion rates; gradually increase to 60 to 125 mL/hr.

➤*Peripheral vein:* Peripheral vein administration is indicated with or without parenteral carbohydrate calories for patients in whom the central venous route is not indicated and who can consume adequate calories enterally. Prepare infusates by dilution of *HepatAmine* with Sterile Water for Injection or 5% to 10% Dextrose to prepare isotonic or slightly hypertonic solutions; accompany with adequate caloric supplementation.

Actions

➤*Pharmacology:* This formulation is a mixture of essential and nonessential amino acids with high concentrations of the BCAAs, isoleucine, leucine and valine.

Hepatic failure/Hepatic encephalopathy – Etiopathology of hepatic encephalopathy is unknown and multifactorial. Rationale for BCAA therapy is based on studies in which BCAA infusions reversed abnormal plasma amino acid pattern characterized by lower BCAA levels and elevated aromatic amino acids and methionine. Normalization of these amino acids improved mental status and EEG patterns. Nitrogen balance was significantly improved and mortality reduced in these typically protein-intolerant patients who received substantial amounts of protein equivalents.

AMINO ACID FORMULATION FOR HIGH METABOLIC STRESS AND IN HEPATIC FAILURE/HEPATIC ENCEPHALOPATHY

	STRESS FORMULATION			HEPATIC FORMULATION
	4% BranchAmin (Clintec)	FreAmine HBC 6.9% (McGaw)	Aminosyn-HBC 7% (Abbott)	HepatAmine (McGaw)
Amino Acid Concentration	4%	6.9%	7%	8%
Nitrogen (g/100 mL)	0.443	0.97	1.12	1.2
Amino Acids (Essential) (mg/100 mL)				
Isoleucine	1380	760	789	900
Leucine	1380	1370	1576	1100
Lysine		410	265	610
Methionine		250	206	100
Phenylalanine		320	228	100
Threonine		200	272	450
Tryptophan		90	88	66
Valine	1240	880	789	840
Amino Acids (Nonessential) (mg/100 mL)				
Alanine		400	660	770
Arginine		580	507	600
Histidine[a]		160	154	240
Proline		630	448	800
Serine		330	221	500
Tyrosine			33	
Glycine		330	660	900
Cysteine		< 20		< 20
Electrolytes (mEq/L)				
Sodium		10	7[b]	10
Chloride		< 3		< 3
Acetate		≈ 57	72	≈ 62
Phosphate (mM/L)				10
Osmolarity (mOsm/L)	316	620	665	785
Supplied in (mL)	500	750[c,d]	500[b] 1000[b]	500[c]
Labeled Indications				
Peripheral Parenteral Nutrition	Yes[e]	Yes	Yes	Yes
Central TPN	Yes[e]	Yes	Yes	Yes

[a] Histidine is considered an essential amino acid in infants and in renal failure.
[b] With 60 mg sodium hydrosulfite.
[c] With less than 100 mg sodium bisulfite/100 mL.
[d] In 1000 mL bottles.
[e] Must be admixed with a complete amino acid injection.

CYSTEINE HYDROCHLORIDE

Rx	**Cysteine HCl** (Various, eg, Abbott, Gensia)	**Injection:** 50 mg per mL	In 10 mL additive syringe and single dose vials.

CYSTEINE HYDROCHLORIDE — INJECTION

For a complete discussion of the use of protein substrates as a component of intravenous nutritional therapy, refer to the IV Nutritionals monograph.

Indications

➤*Cysteine supplement:* For use only after dilution as an additive to *Aminosyn* (a crystalline amino acid solution) to meet the IV amino acid nutritional requirements of infants receiving total parenteral nutrition.

Administration and Dosage

Use only after dilution in *Aminosyn*. Each 10 mL of cysteine HCl injection should be combined aseptically with 12.5 g of amino acids, such as that present in 250 mL of *Aminosyn* 5%. The admixture is then diluted with 250 mL of dextrose 50% or such lesser volume as indicated. Equal volumes of *Aminosyn* 5% and dextrose 50% produce a final solution which contains *Aminosyn* 2.5% in dextrose 25%, which is suitable for administration by central venous infusion. Administration of the final admixture should begin within 1 hour of mixing. Otherwise, the admixture should be refrigerated immediately and used within 24 hours of the time of mixing.

➤*Storage/Stability:* Store at controlled room temperature 15° to 30°C (59° to 86°F).

Actions

➤*Pharmacology:* Cysteine is synthesized from methionine via the transsulfuration pathway in the adult, but newborn infants lack the enzyme, cystathionase, necessary to effect this conversion. Therefore, cysteine HCl injection is generally considered to be an essential amino acid in infants.

Metabolism of cysteine produces pyruvate and inorganic sulfate as end products. Cysteine is introduced directly into the pathway of carbohydrate metabolism at the pyruvate stage with all 3 carbons convertible to glucose. The sulfur is primarily transformed to inorganic sulfate, which is introduced into complex polysaccharides among other structural components.

Contraindications

The contraindications, warnings, precautions, and adverse reactions associated with cysteine HCl injection additive are the same as those cited for *Aminosyn* 5%, given as part of a total parenteral nutrition program. This preparation should not be used in patients with hepatic coma or metabolic disorders involving impaired nitrogen utilization.

Warnings

➤*Hyperammonemia:* Hyperammonemia is of special significance in infants, as it can result in mental retardation. Therefore, it is essential that blood ammonia levels be measured frequently in infants.

Instances of asymptomatic hyperammonemia have been reported in patients without overt liver dysfunction. The mechanisms of this reaction are not clearly defined but may involve genetic defects and immature or subclinically impaired liver function.

➤*Aluminum toxicity:* This product contains aluminum that may be toxic. Aluminum may reach toxic levels with prolonged parenteral administration if kidney function is impaired. Premature neonates are particularly at risk because their kidneys are immature, and they require large amounts of calcium and phosphate solutions, which contain aluminum.

Research indicates that patients with impaired kidney function, including premature neonates, who receive parenteral levels of aluminum at greater than 4 to 5 mcg/kg/day accumulate aluminum at levels associated with central nervous system and bone toxicity. Tissue loading may occur at even lower rates of administration.

➤*Renal/Hepatic function impairment:* Peripheral IV infusion of amino acids may induce a rise in blood urea nitrogen (BUN) especially in patients with impaired hepatic or renal function. Appropriate laboratory tests should be performed periodically and infusion discontinued if BUN levels exceed normal postprandial limits and continue to rise. It should be noted that a modest rise in BUN normally occurs as a result of increased protein intake.

Administration of amino acid solutions in the presence of impaired renal function may augment an increasing BUN, as does any protein dietary component.

Administration of amino acid solutions to a patient with hepatic insufficiency may result in serum amino acid imbalances, metabolic alkalosis, prerenal azotemia, hyperammonemia, stupor, and coma.

➤*Pregnancy: Category C.*

Animal reproduction studies have not been conducted with cysteine HCl injection. It is also not known whether this additive can cause fetal harm when administered to pregnant women or can affect reproductive capacity. Safe use during pregnancy has not been established, therefore, infusion of amino acids should be undertaken during pregnancy only when this is deemed essential to the patient's welfare, as judged by the physician.

➤*Children:* The effect of infusion of amino acids, without dextrose, upon carbohydrate metabolism of children is not known at this time. Hyperammonemia is of special significance in infants, as it can result in mental retardation.

Precautions

➤*Monitoring:* Frequent clinical evaluations and laboratory determinations are necessary for proper monitoring during administration. Blood studies should include glucose, urea nitrogen, serum electrolytes, ammonia, cholesterol, acid-base balance, serum proteins, kidney and liver function tests, osmolarity and hemogram. White blood count and blood cultures are to be determined if indicated. Urinary osmolarity and glucose should be determined frequently.

Nitrogen intake should be carefully monitored in patients with impaired renal function. For long-term total nutrition, or if a patient has inadequate fat stores, it is essential to provide adequate exogenous calories concurrently with the amino acids. Concentrated dextrose solutions are an effective source of such calories. Such strong hypertonic nutrient solutions should be administered through an indwelling IV catheter with the tip located in the superior vena cava.

➤*Solutions with sodium:* Solutions containing sodium ion should be used with great care, if at all, in patients with congestive heart failure, severe renal insufficiency, and in clinical states in which there exists edema with sodium retention.

➤*Solutions with potassium:* Solutions which contain potassium ion should be used with great care, if at all, in patients with hyperkalemia, severe renal failure, and in conditions in which potassium retention is present.

➤*Solutions with acetate:* Solutions containing acetate ion should be used with great care in patients with metabolic or respiratory alkalosis. Acetate should be administered with great care in those conditions in which there is an increased level or an impaired utilization of this ion such as severe hepatic insufficiency.

➤*Special risk:* Special care must be taken when administering hypertonic glucose to provide calories in diabetic or prediabetic patients.

IV feeding regimens which include amino acids should be used with caution in patients with a history of renal disease, pulmonary disease, or with cardiac insufficiency so as to avoid excessive fluid accumulation.

Drug Interactions

➤*Tetracycline:* Because of its antianabolic activity, coadministration of tetracycline may reduce the nitrogen sparing effects of infused amino acids.

➤*Drug/Lab test interactions:* Do not withdraw venous blood for blood chemistries through the peripheral infusion site, as interference with estimations of nitrogen containing substances may occur.

Adverse Reactions

Local reactions consisting of a warm sensation, erythema, phlebitis, and thrombosis at the infusion site have occurred with peripheral intravenous infusion of amino acids, particularly if other substances, such as antibiotics, are also administered through the same site. In such cases, the infusion site should be changed promptly to another vein. Use of large peripheral veins, in-line filters, and slowing the rate of infusion may reduce the incidence of local venous irritation.

Electrolyte additives should be spread throughout the day. Irritating additive medications may need to be injected at another venous site.

Generalized flushing, fever, and nausea also have been reported during peripheral infusions of amino acid solutions.

Overdosage

Feeding regimens which include amino acids should be used with caution in patients with a history of renal disease, pulmonary disease, or with cardiac insufficiency to avoid excess fluid accumulation. In the event of overhydration or solute overload, reevaluate the patient and institute appropriate corrective measures.

Protein Substrates

TROMETHAMINE

Rx	**Tham** (Abbott)	**Injection:** 18 g (150 mEq) per 500 mL (0.3 M)	In 500 mL single dose container.[a]

[a] With acetic acid.

TROMETHAMINE — INJECTION

Indications

➤*Metabolic acidosis:* For the prevention and correction of metabolic acidosis.

Administration and Dosage

Tromethamine solution is administered by slow intravenous infusion, by addition to pump-oxygenator ACD blood or other priming fluid or by injection into the ventricular cavity during cardiac arrest. For infusion by peripheral vein, a large needle should be used in the largest antecubital vein or an indwelling catheter placed in a large vein of an elevated limb to minimize chemical irritation of the alkaline solution during infusion. Catheters are recommended.

Dosage and rate of administration should be carefully supervised to avoid overtreatment (alkalosis). Pretreatment and subsequent determinations of blood values (eg, pH, PCO_2, PO_2, glucose and electrolytes) and urinary output should be made as necessary to monitor dosage and progress of treatment. In general, dosage should be limited to an amount sufficient to increase blood pH to normal limits (7.35 to 7.45) and to correct acid-base derangements. The total quantity to be administered during the period of illness will depend upon the severity and progression of the acidosis. The possibility of some retention of tromethamine, especially in patients with impaired renal function, should be kept in mind.

The intravenous dosage of tromethamine solution (tromethamine injection) may be estimated from the buffer base deficit of the extracellular fluid in mEq/L determined by means of the Siggaard-Andersen nomogram. The following formula is intended as a general guide:

Tromethamine solution (mL of 0.3 M) Required =
Body Weight (kg) × Base Deficit (mEq/L) × 1.1.

Factor of 1.1 accounts for an approximate reduction of 10% in buffering capacity due to the presence of sufficient acetic acid to lower pH of the 0.3 M solution to approximately 8.6).

The need for administration of additional tromethamine solution is determined by serial determinations of the existing base deficit.

➤*Acidosis associated with cardiac bypass surgery:* An adverse dose of approximately 9 mL/kg (324 mg/kg) has been used in clinical studies with tromethamine solution (tromethamine injection). This is equivalent to a total dose of 630 mL (189 mEq) for 70 kg patient. A total single dose of 500 mL (150 mEq) is considered adequate for most adults. Larger single doses (up to 1000 mL) may be required in unusually severe cases.

It is recommended that individual doses should not exceed 500 mg/kg (227 mg/lb) over a period of not less than 1 hour. Thus, for a 70 kg (154 pound) patient the dose should not exceed a maximum of 35 g per hour (1078 mL of a 0.3 M solution). Repeated determinations of pH and other clinical observations should be used as a guide to the need for repeat doses.

➤*Acidity of ACD blood in cardiac bypass surgery:* The pH of stored blood ranges from 6.80 to 6.22 depending upon the duration of storage. The amount of tromethamine solution used to correct this acidity ranges from 0.5 to 2.5 g (15 to 77 mL of a 0.3 M solution) added to each 500 mL of ACD blood used for priming the pump-oxygenator. Clinical experience indicates that 2 g (62 mL of a 0.3 M solution) added to 500 mL of ACD blood is usually adequate.

➤*Acidosis associated with cardiac arrest:* In the treatment of cardiac arrest, tromethamine solution should be given at the same time that other standard resuscitative measures, including manual systole, are being applied. If the chest is open, tromethamine solution is injected directly into the ventricular cavity. From 2 to 6 g (62 to 185 mL of a 0.3 M solution) should be injected immediately. **Do not inject into the cardiac muscle.**

If the chest is not open, from 3.6 to 10.8 g (111 to 333 mL of a 0.3 M solution) should be injected immediately into a larger peripheral vein. Additional amounts may be required to control acidosis persisting after cardiac arrest is reversed.

➤*Admixture incompatibility:* Additives may be incompatible. Consult with pharmacist, if available. When introducing additives, use aseptic technique, mix thoroughly and do not store.

➤*Storage / Stability:* Protect from freezing and extreme heat.

Do not administer unless solution is clear and seal is intact. Discard unused portion.

Actions

➤*Pharmacology:* When administered intravenously as a 0.3 M solution, tromethamine act as a proton acceptor and prevents or corrects acidosis by actively binding hydrogen ions (H^+). It binds not only cations of fixed or metabolic acids, but also hydrogen ions of carbonic acid, thus increasing bicarbonate anion (HCO_3^-). Tromethamine also acts as an osmotic diuretic, increasing urine flow, urinary pH, and excretion of fixed acids, carbon dioxide and electrolytes. A significant fraction of tromethamine (30% at pH 7.4) is not ionized and therefore is capable of reaching equilibrium in total body water. This portion may penetrate cells and may neutralize acidic ions of the intracellular fluid.

➤*Pharmacokinetics:* The drug is rapidly eliminated by the kidney; 75% or more appears in the urine after 8 hours. Urinary excretion continues over a period of 3 days.

Contraindications

Anuria; uremia.

Warnings

➤*Respiratory depression:* Large doses of tromethamine solution may depress ventilation, as a result of increased blood pH and reduced CO_2 concentration. Thus, dosage should be adjusted so that blood pH is not allowed to increase above normal. In situations in which respiratory acidosis may be present concomitantly with metabolic acidosis, the drug may be used with mechanical assistance to ventilation.

➤*Perivascular infiltration:* Care must be exercised to prevent perivascular infiltration since this can cause inflammation, necrosis and sloughing of tissue. Venospasm and intravenous thrombosis, which may occur during infusion, can be minimized by insuring that the injection needle is well within the largest available vein and that solutions are slowly infused. Intravenous catheters are recommended. If perivascular infiltration occurs, institute appropriate countermeasures. See Adverse Reactions.

➤*Administration:* Tromethamine solution for injection should be administered slowly and in amounts sufficient only to correct the existing acidosis, and to avoid overdosage and alkalosis.

➤*Hypoglycemia:* Overdosage in terms of total drug or too rapid administration, may cause hypoglycemia of a prolonged duration (several hours). Therefore, frequent blood glucose determinations should be made during and after therapy.

➤*Duration of therapy:* Because clinical experience has been limited generally to short-term use, the drug should not be administered for more than a period of 1 day except in a life-threatening situation.

➤*Fluid / solute overload:* The intravenous administration of tromethamine solution can cause fluid or solute overloading resulting in dilution of serum electrolyte concentrations, overhydration, congested states or pulmonary edema.

➤*Renal function impairment:* Extreme care should be exercised in patients with renal disease or reduced urinary output because of potential hyperkalemia and the possibility of a decreased excretion of tromethamine. In such patients, the drug should be used cautiously with electrocardiographic monitoring and frequent serum potassium determinations.

➤*Elderly:* Clinical studies of tromethamine solution did not include sufficient numbers of subjects aged 65 and over to determine whether they respond differently from younger subjects. Other reported clinical experience has not identified differences in response between the elderly and younger patients. In general, dose selection for an elderly patient should be cautious, usually starting at the low end of the dosing range, reflecting the greater frequency of decreased hepatic, renal, or cardiac function, and of concomitant disease or other drug therapy.

This drug is known to be substantially excreted by the kidney, and the risk of toxic reactions to this drug may be greater in patients with impaired renal function. Because elderly patients are more likely to have decreased renal function, care should be taken in dose selection, and it may be useful to monitor renal function.

➤*Pregnancy: Category C.* Animal reproduction studies have not been conducted with tromethamine. It is also not known whether tromethamine can cause fetal harm when administered to a pregnant woman or can affect reproduction capacity. Tromethamine should be given to a pregnant woman only if clearly needed.

➤*Children:* Hypoglycemia may occur when this product is used in premature and even full-term neonates. See Adverse Reactions.

Precautions

➤*Monitoring:* Blood pH, PCO_2 bicarbonate, glucose and electrolyte determinations should be performed before, during and after administration of tromethamine solution.

➤*Coagulation abnormalities:* While it has not been shown that the drug increases coagulation time in humans, this possibility should be kept in mind since this has been noted experimentally in dogs.

Adverse Reactions

Generally, side effects have been infrequent.

➤*Hematologic:* Transient depression of blood glucose may occur.

➤*Local:* Extreme care should be taken to avoid perivascular infiltration. Local tissue damage and subsequent sloughing may occur if extravasation occurs. Chemical phlebitis and venospasm also have been reported.

➤*Respiratory:* Although the incidence of ventilatory depression is low, it is important to keep in mind that such depression may occur. Respiratory depression may be more likely to occur in patients who have chronic hypoventilation or those who have been treated with drugs which depress respiration. In patients with associated respiratory acidosis, tromethamine should be administered with mechanical assistance to ventilation.

Protein Substrates

TROMETHAMINE — INJECTION

➤*Miscellaneous:* Reactions which may occur because of the solution or the technique of administration include febrile response, infection at the site of injection, venous thrombosis or phlebitis extending from the site of injection extravasation and hypervolemia.

If an adverse reaction does occur, discontinue the infusion, evaluate the patient, institute appropriate therapeutic countermeasures and save the remainder of the fluid for examination if deemed necessary.

Overdosage

➤*Symptoms:* Too rapid administration or excessive amounts of tromethamine may cause alkalosis, hypoglycemia, overhydration or solute overload.

➤*Treatment:* In the event of overdosage, discontinue the infusion, evaluate the patient and institute appropriate countermeasures.

Caloric Intake

DEXTROSE (d-GLUCOSE)

Rx	**D-2.5-W** (Various, eg, Abbott, Clintec)	2.5%	In 1000 mL.
Rx	**D-5-W** (Various, eg, Abbott, Clintec, IMS, McGaw)	5%	In 25, 50, 100, 150, 250, 500 and 1000 mL vials and 10 mL syringes, 25 mL fill in 150 mL, 50 mL fill in 250 mL and 100 mL fill in 250 mL vials.
Rx	**D-10-W** (Various, eg, Clintec, Elkins-Sinn, Hospira, Solopak, Winthrop)	10%	In 3 mL amps, 250, 500 and 1000 mL vials, 17 mL fill in 20 mL, 500 mL fill in 1000 mL, and 1000 mL fill in 2000 mL vials.
Rx	**D-20-W** (Various, eg, Abbott, Clintec)	20%	In 500 mL vials, 500 mL fill in 1000 mL and 1000 mL fill in 2000 mL.
Rx	**D-25-W** (Various, eg, Abbott, IMS)	25%	In 10 mL syringes.
Rx	**D-30-W** (Various, eg, Abbott, Clintec, McGaw)	30%	In 500 and 1000 mL, 500 mL fill in 1000 mL and 1000 mL fill in 2000 mL.
Rx	**D-40-W** (Various, eg, Abbott, Clintec, McGaw)	40%	In 500 and 1000 mL, 500 mL fill in 1000 mL and 1000 mL fill in 2000 mL.
Rx	**D-50-W** (Various, eg, Abbott, Astra, Clintec, IMS, McGaw, Pasadena)	50%	In 500, 1000 and 2000 mL and 50 mL amps, vials and syringes and 500 mL fill in 1000 mL and 1000 mL fill in 2000 mL.
Rx	**D-60-W** (Various, eg, Abbott, Clintec, McGaw)	60%	In 500 and 1000 mL, 500 mL fill in 1000 mL and 1000 mL fill in 2000 mL.
Rx	**D-70-W** (Various, eg, Abbott, Clintec, McGaw)	70%	In 70, 1000 and 2000 mL, 500 mL fill in 1000 mL and 1000 mL fill in 2000 mL.

DEXTROSE — INJECTION

Indications

➤*2.5%, 5%, and 10% solutions:* Used for peripheral infusion to provide calories whenever fluid and caloric replacement are required.

➤*25% (hypertonic) solutions):* Acute symptomatic episodes of hypoglycemia in the neonate or older infant to restore depressed blood glucose levels and control symptoms.

➤*50% solution:* Used in the treatment of insulin hypoglycemia (hyperinsulinemia or insulin shock) to restore blood glucose levels.

➤*10%, 20%, 30%, 40%, 50%, 60%, and 70% (hypertonic) solutions:* For infusion after admixture with amino acids or dilution with other compatible IV fluids to provide variable final dextrose concentrations for intravenous infusion in patients whose condition requires parenteral nutrition.

➤*Unlabeled uses:* Hypertonic solutions of 25% to 50% have been used as a sclerosing agent for the treatment of varicose veins, as an irritant to produce adhesive pleuritis and to reduce cerebrospinal pressure and cerebral edema caused by delirium tremens or acute alcohol intoxication.

Administration and Dosage

➤*20%, 30%, 40%, 50%, 60%, and 70% solutions:*

Glycosuria – The maximum rate at which dextrose can be infused without producing glycosuria is 0.5 g/kg of body weight/hr. About 95% of the dextrose is retained when infused at a rate of 0.8 g/kg/hr.

Dosage is to be directed by a physician and is dependent upon age, weight, clinical condition of the patient and laboratory determinations. Frequent laboratory determinations and clinical evaluation are essential to monitor changes in blood glucose and electrolyte concentrations, and fluid and electrolyte balance during prolonged parenteral therapy.

Fluid administration should be based on calculated maintenance or replacement fluid requirements for each patient.

Admixture incompatibilities – Some additives may be incompatible. Consult with pharmacist. When introducing additives, use aseptic techniques. Mix thoroughly. Do not store.

Do not administer dextrose simultaneously with blood through the same infusion set because pseudoagglutination of red cells may occur.

Do not administer concentrated solutions subcutaneously or IM.

➤*Insulin-induced hypoglycemia:* Determine blood glucose before injecting dextrose. In emergencies, promptly administer without waiting for pretreatment test results.

Adults – 10 to 25 g. Repeated doses may be required in severe cases.

Children – There is no specific pediatric dose. The dose is dependent on weight, clinical condition, and laboratory results. Follow recommendations of appropriate pediatric reference text.

Neonates – 250 to 500 mg/kg/dose (5 to 10 mL of 25% dextrose in a 5 kg infant) to control acute symptomatic hypoglycemia.

Severe cases or older infants – Larger or repeated single doses up to 10 or 12 mL of 25% dextrose may be required. Subsequent continuous IV infusion of 10% dextrose may be needed to stabilize blood glucose levels.

➤*Storage/Stability:* Do not use unless solution is clear. Discard unused portion. Protect from freezing and extreme heat.

Actions

➤*Pharmacology:* Dextrose injection provides calories and is a source of water for hydration. It is capable of inducing diuresis depending on the clinical condition of the patient.

When administered intravenously, solutions containing carbohydrate in the form of dextrose restore blood glucose levels and provide calories. Carbohydrate in the form of dextrose may aid in minimizing liver glycogen depletion and exerts a protein sparing action. Dextrose injection undergoes oxidation to carbon dioxide and water.

Dextrose is readily metabolized, may decrease losses of body protein and nitrogen, promotes glycogen deposition, and decreases or prevents ketosis if sufficient doses are provided.

Caloric content and osmolarity of the various concentrations of dextrose

Dextrose concentration			
%	g/L	Caloric content (Cal/L)	Osmolarity (mOsm/L)
2.5	25	85	126
5	50	170	253
10	100	340	505
20	200	680	1,010
25	250	850	1,330
30	300	1,020	1,515
40	400	1,360	2,020
50	500	1,700	2,525
60	600	2,040	3,030
70	700	2,380	3,535

Contraindications

In diabetic coma while blood sugar is excessively high and in patients with hypersensitivity to corn products. When intracranial or intraspinal hemorrhage is present; in the presence of delirium tremens in dehydrated patients; in patients with severe hydration, anuria, hepatic coma, or glucose-galactose malabsorption syndrome.

Warnings

➤*Fluid/solute overload:* The administration of intravenous solutions can cause fluid and/or solute overload resulting in dilution of serum electrolyte concentrations, overhydration, congested states or pulmonary edema. The risk of dilutional states is inversely proportional to the electrolyte concentration.

➤*Prolonged infusion:* Prolonged infusion of isotonic or hypotonic dextrose in water may increase the volume of extracellular fluid and cause water intoxication.

➤*Admixture incompatibility:* See Administration and Dosage for more information.

DEXTROSE — INJECTION

➤*Hypokalemia:* Excessive administration of potassium-free dextrose solutions may result in significant hypokalemia. Serum potassium levels should be maintained and potassium supplemented as required.

Hypokalemia may develop during parenteral administration of hypertonic dextrose solutions. Sufficient amounts of potassium should be added to dextrose solutions administered to fasting patients with good renal function, especially those on digitalis therapy.

➤*Hypertonic dextrose solutions:* Hypertonic dextrose solutions (above 5% concentration) should be given slowly, preferably through a small bore needle into a large vein, to minimize venous irritation. If infused via peripheral veins, thrombosis may result; therefore, administration via a central venous catheter is recommended.

➤*Rapid administration:* Concentrated dextrose in water should be administered only after suitable dilution. Hypertonic dextrose solutions should be given slowly. Significant hyperglycemia and possible hyperosmolar syndrome may result from too rapid administration. The physician should be aware of the symptoms of hyperosmolar syndrome, such as mental confusion and loss of consciousness, especially in patients with chronic uremia and those with known carbohydrate intolerance.

➤*Aluminum toxicity:* Dextrose injection contains aluminum that may be toxic. Aluminum may reach toxic levels with prolonged parenteral administration if kidney function is impaired. Premature neonates are particularly at risk because their kidneys are immature, and they require large amounts of calcium and phosphate solutions, which contain aluminum.

Dextrose injection contains no more than 25 mcg/L of aluminum.

Research indicates that patients with impaired kidney function, including premature neonates, who receive parenteral levels of aluminum at greater than 4 to 5 mcg/kg/day accumulate aluminum at levels associated with central nervous system and bone toxicity. Tissue loading may occur at even lower rates of administration.

➤*Elderly:* An evaluation of current literature revealed no clinical experience identifying differences in responses between the elderly and younger patients. In general, dose selection for an elderly patient should be cautious, usually starting at the low end of the dosing range, reflecting the greater frequency of decreased hepatic, renal, or cardiac function, and of concomitant disease or other drug therapy.

These drugs are known to be substantially excreted by the kidney, and the risk of toxic reactions to these drugs may be greater in patients with impaired renal function. Because elderly patients are more likely to have decreased renal function, care should be taken in dose selection, and it may be useful to monitor renal function.

➤*Pregnancy: Category C.* Animal reproduction studies have not been conducted with dextrose. It is also not known whether dextrose can cause fetal harm when administered to a pregnant woman or can affect reproduction capacity. Dextrose should be given to a pregnant woman only if clearly needed.

Dextrose crosses the placenta; however, insulin does not cross the placenta and the fetus is responsible for its own insulin production in response to the dextrose. Therefore, administer dextrose to a pregnant woman with caution. One report recommends an infusion rate of 3.5 to 7 g/hr since doses greater than 10 g/hr cause increases in fetal insulin.

Labor and delivery – As reported in the literature, dextrose solutions have been administered during labor and delivery. Caution should be exercised, and the fluid balance, glucose and electrolyte concentrations and acid-base balance, of both mother and fetus should be evaluated periodically or whenever warranted by the condition of the patient or fetus.

➤*Lactation:* Because many drugs are excreted in human milk, caution should be exercised when dextrose injections are administered to a nursing woman.

➤*Children:* The safety and effectiveness in the pediatric population are based on the similarity of the clinical conditions of the pediatric and adult populations. In neonates or very small infants the volume of fluid may affect fluid and electrolyte balance.

Serum glucose concentrations should be frequently monitored when dextrose is prescribed to pediatric patients, particularly infants, neonates, and low birth weight infants.

In very low birth weight infants, excessive or rapid administration of dextrose injection may result in increased serum osmolality and possible intracerebral hemorrhage.

Precautions

➤*Monitoring:* Clinical evaluation and periodic laboratory determinations are necessary to monitor changes in fluid balance, electrolyte concentrations, and acid-base balance during prolonged parenteral therapy or whenever the condition of the patient warrants such evaluation. Significant deviations from normal concentrations may require tailoring of the electrolyte pattern, in these or alternative solutions.

Blood electrolyte monitoring is essential, and fluid and electrolyte imbalances should be corrected. Essential vitamins and minerals also should be provided as needed.

Hyperglycemia and glycosuria – To minimize hyperglycemia and consequent glycosuria, it is desirable to monitor blood and urine glucose and if necessary, add insulin. When concentrated dextrose infusion is abruptly withdrawn, it is advisable to follow with the administration of 5% or 10% dextrose to avoid rebound hypoglycemia.

➤*Concentrated solutions:* Some opacity of the plastic due to moisture absorption during sterilization process may be observed. This is normal and does not affect the solution quality or safety. The opacity will diminish gradually.

➤*Pumping device:* If administration is controlled by a pumping device, care must be taken to discontinue pumping action before the container runs dry or air embolism may result.

➤*Precipitation:* To minimize the risk of possible incompatibilities arising from mixing this solution with other additives that may be prescribed, the final infusate should be inspected for cloudiness or precipitation immediately after mixing, prior to administration, and periodically during administration.

➤*Extravasation:* Care should be exercised to ensure that the needle (or catheter) is well within the lumen of the vein and that extravasation does not occur.

➤*Diabetes mellitus:* Solutions containing dextrose should be used with caution in patients with overt or known subclinical diabetes mellitus or carbohydrate intolerance for any reason.

➤*Special risk:* These solutions should be used with care in patients with hypervolemia, renal insufficiency, urinary tract obstruction, or impending or frank cardiac decompensation.

Drug Interactions

➤*Corticosteroids:* Cautiously administer parenteral fluids, especially those containing sodium ions, to patients receiving corticosteroids or corticotropin.

Adverse Reactions

Reactions which may occur because of the solution or the technique of administration include febrile response, infection at the site of injection, venous thrombosis or phlebitis extending from the site of injection, extravasation and hypervolemia.

Too rapid infusion of hypertonic solutions may cause local pain and venous irritation. Rate of administration should be adjusted according to tolerance. Use of the largest peripheral vein and a small bore needle is recommended.

➤*Concentrated solutions:* Hyperosmolar syndrome, resulting from excessively rapid administration of concentrated dextrose may cause hypovolemia, dehydration, mental confusion, or loss of consciousness.

Reactions which may occur because of the solution or the technique of administration include febrile response, infection at the site of injection, venous thrombosis or phlebitis extending from the site of injection, extravasation and hypervolemia.

Overdosage

➤*Treatment:* In the event of a fluid or solute overload during parenteral therapy, reevaluate the patient's condition and institute appropriate corrective treatment.

ALCOHOL (ETHANOL) IN DEXTROSE INFUSIONS

	Product/Distributor	Cal/L	mOsm/L	How Supplied
Rx	**5% Alcohol and 5% Dextrose in Water** (Various, eg, Abbott, Clintec)	450	1114	In 1000 mL.
Rx	**5% Alcohol and 5% Dextrose in Water** (McGaw)		1125	In 1000 mL.
Rx	**10% Alcohol and 5% Dextrose in Water** (McGaw)	720	1995	In 1000 mL.

ALCOHOL (ETHANOL) IN DEXTROSE INFUSIONS — INTRAVENOUS

For specific information on dextrose, refer to the individual monograph.

Indications

➤*Caloric/fluid supplement:* Increasing caloric intake and replenishing fluids.

➤*Unlabeled uses:*

Premature labor – Infusion of a 10% solution of ethyl alcohol IV causes a decrease in uterine activity during labor, presumably by inhibiting the release of oxytocin from the posterior pituitary, and has been used to prevent premature delivery. However, this use has largely been replaced by other therapies (eg, β-adrenergic therapy).

Administration and Dosage

Administer by slow IV infusion only; do not give SC. Individualize dosage. The average adult can metabolize approximately 10 mL/hour (200 mL of 5% solution or 100 mL of 10% solution). The usual adult dosage is 1 to 2 L and rarely exceeds 3 L of a 5% solution in a 24 hour period. Children may be given 40 mL/kg/24 hours or from 350 to 1000 mL, depending on size and clinical response.

ALCOHOL (ETHANOL) IN DEXTROSE INFUSIONS — INTRAVENOUS

➤*Storage / Stability:* Do not use unless solution is clear and seal is intact. Discard unused portion. Protect from freezing and extreme heat.

Actions

➤*Pharmacology:* Alcohol in dextrose solutions are an intravenous source of carbohydrate calories that restore blood glucose levels. Each mL of alcohol provides 5.6 calories; each gram of d–glucose monohydrate provides 3.4 calories. Dextrose may aid in minimizing liver glycogen depletion and exerts a protein-sparing action.

➤*Pharmacokinetics:* Ethyl alcohol is metabolized at a rate of ≈ 10 to 20 mL/hour. Sedative effects of alcohol occur if infusion rate exceeds metabolism rate. Dextrose (d-glucose) can be infused at a maximum of ≈ 0.5 to 0.85 g/kg/hour without producing significant glycosuria. Thus, the maximum rate that alcohol can be infused without producing sedative effects is well below maximum rate of dextrose utilization. Alcohol is metabolized (mostly in liver) to acetaldehyde or acetate; oxidation rate is linear with time. Starvation lowers metabolism rate and insulin increases it.

Contraindications

Epilepsy; urinary tract infection; alcoholism; diabetic coma.

Warnings

➤*Special risk patients:* Use alcohol cautiously in shock, following cranial surgery and in actual or anticipated postpartum hemorrhage.

➤*Diabetic patients:* Alcohol decreases blood sugar in these patients. In the untreated diabetic, the rate of alcohol metabolism is slowed.

➤*Vitamin deficiencies:* As a nutrient, alcohol supplies only calories; given alone it may cause or potentiate vitamin deficiencies and liver function disturbances.

➤*IV administration:* IV administration can cause fluid or solute overload resulting in dilution of serum electrolyte concentrations, overhydration, congested states or pulmonary edema.

➤*Extravasation:* Avoid extravasation during IV administration; do not give SC.

➤*Pseudoagglutination / Hemolysis:* Do not administer simultaneously with blood because of possibility of pseudoagglutination or hemolysis.

➤*Renal / Hepatic function impairment:* Use alcohol cautiously.

➤*Pregnancy: Category C.* It is not known whether alcohol can cause fetal harm when administered to a pregnant woman or can affect reproduction capacity. Use only when clearly needed. It crosses the placenta rapidly and enters fetal circulation.

Fetal Alcohol Syndrome (FAS) – Fetal alcohol syndrome (FAS), a pattern of fetal anomalies, is associated with chronic maternal alcohol consumption of 60 to 75 mL absolute alcohol (4 to 5 drinks) per day; mild FAS is associated with ingestion of as little as 30 mL per day. Features of FAS involve craniofacial, limb, growth, and CNS anomalies. Other reported problems involve cardiac and urogenital defects, liver abnormalities and hemangiomas. Behavioral problems may be long-term. Moderate drinking (more than 1 ounce absolute alcohol twice/week) is associated with second trimester spontaneous abortions.

Administration of alcohol prior to delivery may cause intoxication and depression of the newborn.

➤*Lactation:* Alcohol passes freely into breast milk approximately equivalent to maternal serum levels; however, effects on the infant are generally insignificant until maternal blood levels reach 300 mg/dL. The American Academy of Pediatrics considers alcohol use in the mother compatible with breastfeeding, although adverse effects may occur.

Alcohol may cause potentiation of severe hypoprothrombic bleeding, a pseudo-Cushing syndrome and a reduction in the milk-ejecting response.

➤*Children:* Safety and efficacy are not established. See Administration and Dosage.

Precautions

➤*Monitoring:* Clinical evaluation and periodic laboratory determinations are necessary to monitor changes in electrolyte concentrations and fluid and acid-base balance.

➤*Administer slowly:* Administer slowly and observe patient for restlessness or narcosis.

➤*Gout:* Alcohol increases serum uric acid and can precipitate acute gout.

Drug Interactions

The following interactions may occur with alcohol administration. Those interactions that may only occur with long-term oral alcohol ingestion have not been included.

Alcohol Drug Interactions

Precipitant drug	Object drug[a]		Description
Barbiturates Benzodiazepines Chloral hydrate Glutethimide Meprobamate Metoclopramide Phenothiazines	Alcohol	↑	Increased CNS depressant effects may occur.
Cephalosporins[b] Chlorpropamide Disulfiram Furazolidone Metronidazole Procarbazine	Alcohol	↑	A disulfiram-like reaction consisting of facial flushing, lightheadedness, weakness, sweating, tachycardia, nausea or vomiting may occur.
Alcohol	Antidiabetic agents (insulin, phenformin, sulfonylureas)	↑	Because of altered glucose metabolism, the pharmacologic effects of these agents may be increased by alcohol resulting in hypoglycemia. In addition, alcohol may contribute to the lactic acidosis that is sometimes observed following phenformin administration. Both hypo- and hyperglycemia have occurred with sulfonylureas and alcohol.
Alcohol	Bromocriptine	↑	Intolerance of bromocriptine due to the severity of side effects has occurred with concurrent alcohol.
Alcohol	Salicylates	↑	Alcohol may potentiate aspirin-induced GI blood loss and bleeding time prolongation.

[a] ↑ = Object drug increased.
[b] Those agents with a methyltetrazolethiol moiety.

Adverse Reactions

Fever; injection site infection; venous thrombosis or phlebitis; extravasation; hypervolemia. These may occur because of the solution or administration technique.

Alcoholic intoxication may occur with too rapid infusion. Vertigo, flushing, disorientation (especially in elderly patients), or sedation may also occur. An alcoholic odor may be noted on the breath. Generally, these effects can be avoided by slowing the rate of infusion. Too rapid infusion of hypertonic solutions may cause local pain and, rarely, excessive vein irritation. Use the largest available peripheral vein and a well placed small bore needle.

Overdosage

In the event of alcoholic intoxication or sedation, slow the infusion or discontinue temporarily. If overhydration or solute overload occurs, reevaluate the patient and institute appropriate corrective measures.

INTRAVENOUS FAT EMULSION

Product & Distributor	Oil (%)		Fatty acid content (%)					Egg yolk phospholipids (%)	Glycerin (%)	Calories/mL	Osmolarity (mOsm/L)	How Supplied
	Safflower	Soybean	Linoleic	Oleic	Palmitic	Linolenic	Stearic					
Intralipid[a] 10% (Clintec)		10	50	26	10	9	3.5	1.2	2.25	1.1	260	In 50, 100, 250 and 500 mL.
Intralipid[a] 20% (Clintec)		20	50	26	10	9	3.5	1.2	2.25	2	260	In 50, 100, 250 and 500 mL.
Liposyn II[b] 10% (Hospira)	5	5	65.8	17.7	8.8	4.2	3.4	1.2	2.5	1.1	276	In 100, 200 and 500 mL.
Liposyn II[b] 20% (Hospira)	10	10	65.8	17.7	8.8	4.2	3.4	1.2	2.5	2	258	In 200 and 500 mL.
Liposyn III[b] 10% (Hospira)		10	54.5	22.4	10.5	8.3	4.2	1.2	2.5	1.1	284	In 100, 200 and 500 mL.
Liposyn III[b] 20% (Hospira)		20	54.5	22.4	10.5	8.3	4.2	1.2	2.5	2	292	In 200 and 500 mL.

[a] Store at 25°C (77°F) or below; do not freeze.
[b] Store at 30°C (86°F) or below; do not freeze.

FAT EMULSION — INTRAVENOUS

Refer to the general discussion beginning in the IV Nutritional Therapy monograph.

WARNING

Deaths in preterm infants – Death in preterm infants after infusion of IV fat emulsions have occurred. Autopsy findings included intravascular fat accumulation in the lungs. Treatment of premature and low birth weight infants with IV fat emulsion must be based on careful benefit-risk assessment. Strict adherence to the recommended total daily dose is mandatory; hourly infusion rate should be as slow as possible and should not exceed 1 g/kg in 4 hours. Premature and small for gestational age infants have poor clearance of IV fat emulsion and increased free fatty acid plasma levels following fat emulsion infusion; therefore, administer less than the maximum recommended doses in these patients to decrease the likelihood of IV fat overload. Monitor the infant's ability to eliminate the infused fat from the circulation (such as triglycerides or plasma free fatty acid levels). The lipemia must clear between daily infusions.

Indications

➤*Caloric/fatty acid source:* Source of calories and essential fatty acids for patients requiring parenteral nutrition for extended periods of time (usually for longer than 5 days).

Source of essential fatty acids when a deficiency occurs.

Administration and Dosage

➤*Total parenteral nutrition:* As part of TPN, administer IV via a peripheral vein or by central venous catheter. Fat emulsion should comprise no more than 60% of the patient's total caloric intake, with carbohydrates and amino acids comprising the remaining 40% or more of caloric intake.

Adults –

10%: Initial infusion rate is 1ml/min for the first 15 to 30 minutes. If no adverse reactions occur, the infusion rate can be increased to 2 mL/min. Infuse only 500 mL the first day and increase dose the following day. Do not exceed a daily dosage of 2.5 g/kg.

20%: Initial infusion rate is 0.5 mL/min for the first 15 to 30 minutes. Infuse only 250 mL (Liposyn II;) or 500 mL *(Intralipid)* the first day and increase dose the following day. Do not exceed a daily dosage of 3 g/kg.

➤*Children:*

10% – Initial infusion rate is 0.1 mL/min for the first 10 to 15 minutes.

20% – Initial infusion rate is 0.05 mL/min for the first 10 to 15 minutes.

If no untoward reactions occur, increase rate to 1 g/kg in 4 hours. Do not exceed daily dosage of 3 g/kg. The dosage for premature infants starts at 0.5 g fat/kg/24 hours (5 mL *Intralipid* 10%; 2.5 mL *Intralipid* 20%) and may be increased in relation to the infant's ability to eliminate fat. The maximum dosage recommended by the American Academy of Pediatrics is 3 g fat/kg/24 hours.

➤*Fatty acid deficiency:* To correct EFAD, supply 8% to 10% of the caloric intake by IV fat emulsion to provide an adequate amount of linoleic acid (4% of caloric intake as linoleate).

Fat emulsion is supplied in single dose containers; do not store partially used bottles or resterilize for later use. Do not use filters. Do not use any bottle in which there appears to be separation of the emulsion.

Fat emulsions may be simultaneously infused with amino acid-dextrose mixtures by means of a Y–connector located near the infusion site using separate flow rate controls for each solution. Keep the lipid infusion line higher than the amino acid-dextrose line. Since the lipid emulsion has a lower specific gravity, it may be taken up into the amino acid-dextrose line.

Fat emulsions may also be infused through a separate peripheral site.

➤*Total nutrient admixture (TNA):* IV fat emulsions are compatible with dextrose and amino acids, when properly mixed, for use in TPN therapy. This is also referred to as all-in-one, 3-in-1 and triple-mix. The following proper mixing sequence must be followed to minimize pH-related problems by ensuring that typically acidic dextrose injections are not mixed with lipid emulsions alone: (1) Transfer dextrose injection to the TPN admixture container; (2) transfer amino acid injection; (3) transfer the IV fat emulsion.

Amino acid injection, dextrose injection and the IV fat emulsion may be simultaneously transferred to the admixture container. Use gentle agitation to avoid localized concentration effects. Additives must not be added directly to the fat emulsion and in no case should the fat emulsion be added to the TPN container first. Shake bags gently after each addition to minimize localized concentration. If evacuated glass containers are used, add the dextrose and amino acid injections first, followed by the fat emulsion and then additives. Shake bottles gently after each addition.

The prime destabilizers of emulsions are excessive acidity (low pH) and inappropriate electrolyte content. Give careful consideration to additions of divalent cations (calcium and magnesium) which cause emulsion instability. Amino acid solutions exert a buffering effect protecting the emulsion.

Inspect the admixture carefully for "breaking or oiling out" of the emulsion, which is described as the separation of the emulsion and can be visibly identified by a yellowish streaking or the accumulation of yellowish droplets in the admixed emulsion. Also examine the admixture for particulates. The admixture must be discarded if any of the above is observed.

Heparin may be added to activate lipoprotein lipase at a concentration of 1 or 2 units/mL prior to administration.

Lipid-containing fluids have a propensity to extract phthalates from phthalate-plasticized polyvinyl chloride (PVC). Although the amount is very small and no adverse clinical effects have been reported from administration of such amounts of phthalate, consider administration through a nonphthalate infusion set. Commercially available products may be accompanied by nonphthalate infusion sets.

➤*Storage/Stability:* Use these admixtures promptly; store under refrigeration (2° to 8°C; 36° to 46°F) for 24 hours or less and use completely within 24 hours after removal from refrigeration.

Actions

➤*Pharmacology:* Intravenous fat emulsions are prepared from either soybean or safflower oil and provide a mixture of neutral triglycerides, predominantly unsaturated fatty acids. The major component of fatty acids are linoleic, oleic, palmitic, stearic and linolenic acids; see product listings for content. In addition, these products contain 1.2% egg yolk phospholipids as an emulsifier and glycerol to adjust tonicity. The emulsified fat particles are approximately 0.4 to 0.5 microns in diameter, similar to naturally occurring chylomicrons. IV fat emulsions are isotonic and may be given by central or peripheral venous routes.

These products are metabolized and utilized as a source of energy, causing an increase in heat production, decrease in respiratory quotient and an increase in oxygen consumption following use. The infused fat particles are cleared from the blood stream in a manner thought to be comparable to the clearing of chylomicrons.

Essential Fatty Acid Deficiency (EFAD) – Linoleic, linolenic and arachidonic acids are essential in humans. Linoleic acid, the metabolic precursor to both linolenic and arachidonic acid, cannot be synthesized in vivo. When there is a deficiency of linoleic acid, the enzyme system that converts linoleic acid to arachidonic acid (a tetraene) acts on oleic acid to synthesize eicosatrienoic acid (a triene) which lacks the physiologic functions of arachidonic acid. Biochemically, EFAD is defined as a triene to tetraene ratio greater than 0.4. Clinical manifestations of EFAD include scaly dermatitis, alopecia, growth retardation, poor wound healing, thrombocytopenia and fatty liver. IV fat emulsion prevents or reverses biochemical and clinical manifestations of EFAD.

Contraindications

Disturbance of normal fat metabolism such as pathologic hyperlipemia, lipoid nephrosis or acute pancreatitis, if accompanied by hyperlipemia. Egg yolk phospholipids are present; do not give to patients with severe egg allergies.

Warnings

➤*Special risk patients:* Exercise caution in severe liver damage, pulmonary disease, anemia, blood coagulation disorders, or when there is danger of fat embolism.

➤*Pregnancy: Category C.* It is not known whether IV fat emulsions can cause fetal harm when administered to a pregnant woman or can affect reproduction capacity. Use only when clearly needed.

Precautions

➤*Monitoring:* When IV fat emulsion is administered, monitor the patient's capacity to eliminate the infused fat from the circulation. The lipemia must clear between daily infusions. Closely monitor the hemogram, blood coagulation, liver function tests, plasma lipid profile and platelet count (especially in neonates). Discontinue use if a significant abnormality in any of these parameters is attributed to therapy.

➤*Jaundiced or premature infants:* Use with caution because free fatty acids displace bilirubin bound to albumin.

➤*Too rapid administration:* Too rapid administration can cause fluid or fat overloading. This can result in dilution of serum electrolyte concentrations, overhydration, pulmonary edema, impaired pulmonary diffusion capacity or metabolic acidosis.

Adverse Reactions

Most frequent – Sepsis due to administration equipment and thrombophlebitis due to vein irritation from concurrently administered hypertonic solutions. These adverse reactions are inseparable from the TPN procedure with or without IV fat emulsion.

Less frequent (more directly related to IV fat emulsion) –

Immediate (acute): (Less than 1%) – Dyspnea; cyanosis; hyperlipemia; hypercoagulability; nausea; vomiting; headache; flushing; increase in temperature; sweating; sleepiness; chest and back pain; slight pressure over the eyes; dizziness; irritation at the infusion site; thrombocytopenia in neonates (rare).

Long-term (chronic): Hepatomegaly; jaundice due to central lobular cholestasis; splenomegaly; thrombocytopenia; leukopenia; transient increases in liver function tests; overloading syndrome (focal seizures, fever, leukocytosis, splenomegaly and shock).

The deposition of brown pigmentation in the reticuloendothelial system (the so-called "IV fat pigment") has occurred. Cause and significance of this phenomenon are unknown.

Overdosage

➤*Treatment:* Stop the infusion until visual inspection of the plasma, determination of triglyceride concentrations or measurement of plasma light-scattering activity by nephelometry indicates the lipid has cleared. Reevaluate the patient and institute appropriate corrective measures.

B VITAMINS, PARENTERAL

Content given per mL.

	Product & Distributor	B_1 mg	B_2 mg	B_3 mg	B_5 mg	B_6 mg	How Supplied
Rx	**B-Ject-100 Injection** (Hyrex)	100	2	100	2	2	In 30 mL vials.[a]
Rx	**Vitamin B Complex 100 Injection** (McGuff)						In 10 and 30 mL vials.[a]

[a] May contain benzyl alcohol.

B VITAMINS WITH VITAMIN C, PARENTERAL

Content given per mL.

	Product & Distributor	B_1 mg	B_2 mg	B_3 mg	B_5 mg	B_6 mg	B_{12} mcg	C mg	Other Content	How Supplied
Rx	**Key-Plex Injection** (Hyrex)	50	5	125	6	5	1000	50		In 10 mL multiple dose vials.
Rx	**Lypholized Vitamin B Complex & Vitamin C with B_{12} Injection** (McGuff)									In 10 mL vials.
Rx	**Vicam Injection** (Keene)								Benzyl alcohol	In 10 mL vials.

MULTIVITAMINS, PARENTERAL

	Product & Distributor	Content[a] given per	A IU	D IU	E IU	B_1 mg	B_2 mg	B_3 mg	B_5 mg	B_6 mg	B_{12} mcg	C mg	biotin mcg	FA mg	Other Content and How Supplied
Rx	**Berocca Parenteral Nutrition** (Roche)	1 mL	3300	200	10[b]	3	3.6	40	15	4	5	100	60	0.4	In 2 vial or ampule sets: Soln 1[c] (1 or 2 mL) and soln 2[c] (1 or 2 mL).
Rx	**M.V.I.-12 Injection** (Astra)	5 mL													In 2 vial sets: Vial 1[d] (5 mL single dose or 50 mL multiple dose) and vial 2[e] (5 mL single dose or 50 mL multiple dose).
Rx	**M.V.I.-12 Unit Vial** (Astra)	10 mL													In 10 mL two chambered vials.[d]
Rx	**M.V.I. Pediatric** (Astra)	5 mL	2300	400	7[b]	1.2	1.4	17	5	1	1	80	20	0.14	200 mcg vitamin K_1 and 375 mg mannitol. In single and multiple dose vials.[f]
Rx	**Cernevit-12** (Baxter Healthcare)	5 mL	3500	200	11.2[2]	3.51	4.14	46	17.25	4.53	5.5	125	60	414	In 5 mL single-dose vials.
Rx	**Infuvite Adult** (Baxter)	10 mL (after combining vials)	3300	200 IU D_3	10	6	3.6	40	15	6	5	200	60	600	150 mcg vitamin K. Polysorbate 80. In two 5 mL vials to be combined together.
Rx	**Infuvite Pediatric** (Baxter)	5 mL (after combining vials)	2300	400 IU D_3	7	1.2	1.4	17	5	1	1	80	20	140	0.2 mg vitamin K. Polysorbate 80. In two vials (4 mL and 1 mL to be combined together).
Rx	**B Complex with C and B-12 Injection** (Goldline)	1 mL				50	5	125	6	5	1,000	50			1% benzyl alcohol. In 10 mL multiple dose vials.

[a] After combining vials, if necessary.
[b] As dL-alpha tocopheryl acetate.
[c] With propylene glycol, EDTA and 1% benzyl alcohol.
[d] With propylene glycol, polysorbate 80 and polysorbate 20.
[e] With propylene glycol.
[f] With polysorbate 20 and polysorbate 80.

Minerals

CALCIUM

For information on oral calcium, refer to the Minerals, Oral section.

Indications

➤*Hypocalcemia:* For a prompt increase in plasma calcium levels (eg, neonatal tetany and tetany due to parathyroid deficiency, vitamin D deficiency, alkalosis); prevention of hypocalcemia during exchange transfusions; conditions associated with intestinal malabsorption.

➤*Calcium chloride and gluconate:* Adjunctive therapy in the treatment of insect bites or stings, such as Black Widow spider bites to relieve muscle cramping; sensitivity reactions, particularly when characterized by urticaria; depression due to overdosage of magnesium sulfate; acute symptoms of lead colic; rickets; osteomalacia.

➤*Calcium chloride:* To combat the deleterious effects of severe hyperkalemia as measured by ECG, pending correction of increased potassium in the extracellular fluid.

Cardiac resuscitation – Particularly after open heart surgery, when epinephrine fails to improve weak or ineffective myocardial contractions.

➤*Calcium gluconate:* To decrease capillary permeability in allergic conditions, nonthrombocytopenic purpura and exudative dermatoses such as dermatitis herpetiformis; for pruritus of eruptions caused by certain drugs; in hyperkalemia, calcium gluconate may aid in antagonizing the cardiac toxicity, provided the patient is not receiving digitalis therapy.

➤*Unlabeled uses:* Calcium salts have been used to treat verapamil overdose, treat acute hypotension from verapamil and prevent initial hypotension in patients requiring verapamil for whom decreases in blood pressure could be detrimental.

Administration and Dosage

Elemental Calcium Content of Calcium Salts		
Salt	% Calcium	mEq/g
Calcium chloride	27.3	13.6
Calcium gluconate	9.3	4.65

Calcium gluconate is generally preferred over calcium chloride as it is less irritating.

➤*IV:* Warm solutions to body temperature and give slowly (0.5 to 2 mL/min); stop if patient complains of discomfort. Resume when symptoms disappear. Following injection, patient should remain recumbent for a short time. Repeated injections may be needed because of the rapid calcium excretion. Inject **calcium chloride** and **gluconate** through a small needle into a large vein to minimize venous irritation.

➤*IM administration:* IM administration of **calcium gluconate** may be tolerated; however, reserve this route for emergencies when technical diffi-

CALCIUM

culty makes IV injection impossible. Administer **calcium gluconate** only by the IV route and **calcium chloride** by the IV or intraventricular route.

➤*Admixture incompatibilities:* Calcium salts should not generally be mixed with carbonates, phosphates, sulfates or tartrates in parenteral admixtures; they are conditionally compatible with potassium phosphates, depending on concentration. Calcium ions will chelate tetracycline.

Actions

➤*Pharmacology:* Calcium is the fifth most abundant element in the body with greater than 99.5% of total body stores in skeletal bone. It is essential for the functional integrity of the nervous and muscular systems, for normal cardiac contractility and the coagulation of blood. It also functions as an enzyme cofactor and affects the secretory activity of endocrine and exocrine glands. Normal levels are 8.5 to 10.5 mg/dL.

Hypocalcemia –
Symptoms: Tetany; paresthesias; laryngospasm; muscle spasms; seizures (usually grand mal); irritability; depression; psychosis; prolonged QT interval; intestinal cramps and malabsorption; respiratory arrest. Prolonged hypocalcemia may be associated with ectodermal defects including the nails, skin and teeth.

➤*Pharmacokinetics:* Approximately 80% of body calcium is excreted in the feces as insoluble salts; urinary excretion accounts for the remaining 20%.

Contraindications

Hypercalcemia; ventricular fibrillation; digitalized patients.

Warnings

➤*Extravasation:* **Calcium chloride** and **gluconate** can cause severe necrosis, sloughing and abscess formation with IM or SC administration. Take great care to avoid extravasation or accidental injection into perivascular tissues.

➤*Hypocalcemia of renal insufficiency:* **Calcium chloride** is an acidifying salt and is therefore usually undesirable for treating this condition.

➤*Pregnancy:* *Category C.* It is not known whether this drug can cause fetal harm when given to a pregnant woman or can affect reproduction capacity. Use only when clearly needed.

➤*Lactation:* It is not known whether **calcium gluconate** is excreted in breast milk. Exercise caution when administering to a pregnant woman.

Precautions

➤*Cardiovascular effects:* It is particularly important to prevent a high concentration of calcium from reaching the heart because of the danger of cardiac syncope.

Drug Interactions

Calcium Drug Interactions

Precipitant	Object drug[a]		Description
Thiazide diuretics	Calcium salts	⬆	Hypercalcemia resulting from renal tubular reabsorption, or bone release of calcium by thiazides may be amplified by exogenous calcium.

Calcium Drug Interactions

Precipitant	Object drug[a]		Description
Calcium salts	Atenolol	⬇	Mean peak plasma levels and bioavailability of atenolol may be decreased, possibly resulting in decreased beta blockade.
Calcium salts	Digitalis glycosides	⬆	Inotropic and toxic effects are synergistic; arrhythmias may occur, especially if calcium is given IV. Avoid IV calcium in patients on digitalis glycosides; if necessary, give slowly in small amounts.
Calcium salts	Sodium polystyrene sulfonate	⬇	Coadministration in patients with renal impairment may result in an unanticipated metabolic alkalosis and a reduction of the resin's binding of potassium.
Calcium salts	Verapamil	⬇	Clinical effects and toxicities of verapamil may be reversed.

[a] ⬆ = Object drug increased. ⬇ = Object drug decreased.

➤*Drug/Lab test interactions:* Transient elevations of plasma 11-hydroxy-corticosteroid levels (Glenn-Nelson technique) may occur when IV calcium is administered, but levels return to control values after 1 hour. In addition, IV calcium gluconate can produce false-negative values for serum and urinary magnesium.

Adverse Reactions

IM administration – Local necrosis and abscess formation may occur with **calcium gluconate**, and severe necrosis and sloughing may occur with IM or SC administration of **calcium chloride**.

IV administration – Rapid IV administration may cause bradycardia, sense of oppression, tingling, metallic, calcium or chalky taste or "heat waves". Rapid IV **calcium gluconate** may cause vasodilation, decreased blood pressure, cardiac arrhythmias, syncope and cardiac arrest. **Calcium chloride** injections cause peripheral vasodilation and a local burning sensation; blood pressure may fall moderately.

Overdosage

➤*Symptoms:* Inadvertent systemic overloading with calcium ions can produce an acute hypercalcemic syndrome characterized by a markedly elevated plasma calcium level, weakness, lethargy, intractable nausea and vomiting, coma and sudden death.

➤*Treatment:* It may be life-saving to rapidly lower blood calcium to safe levels. It is now agreed the most effective therapy is IV sodium chloride infusion plus potent natriuretic agents, (eg, furosemide). Sodium competes with calcium for reabsorption in the distal renal tubule and furosemide potentiates this effect. Together they markedly increase renal calcium clearance and reduce hypercalcemia.

CALCIUM GLUCONATE

1 g (10 mL) contains 93 mg (4.65 mEq) calcium.

Rx	**Calcium Gluconate** (Various, eg, American Regent, Astra, Elkins-Sinn, IDE, IMS, McGuff, Rugby)	**Injection:** 10%	In 10 mL amps and syringes, 10 and 50 mL single dose vials and 100 and 200 mL pharmacy bulk vials.[a]

[a] Not for direct infusion; dilute prior to use.

CALCIUM GLUCONATE — INJECTION

For complete and comparative prescribing information, refer to the Calcium group monograph in the Intravenous Nutritional Therapy, Electrolytes section.

CALCIUM CHLORIDE

1 g (10 mL) contains 273 mg (13.6 mEq) calcium.

Rx	**Calcium Chloride** (Various, eg, Abbott, American Regent, Astra, IMS, Moore, VHA)	**Injection:** 10%	In 10 mL amps, vials and syringes.

CALCIUM CHLORIDE — INJECTION

For complete and comparative prescribing information, refer to the Calcium group monograph in the Intravenous Nutritional Therapy, Electrolytes section.

CALCIUM PRODUCTS COMBINED, PARENTERAL

Rx	**Calphosan** (Glenwood)	**Injection:** 50 mg calcium glycerophosphate and 50 mg calcium lactate per 10 mL in sodium chloride solution (0.08 mEq Ca/mL)	In 60 mL vials.[a]

[a] With 0.25% phenol.

CALCIUM PRODUCTS COMBINED — PARENTERAL

For complete and comparative prescribing information, refer to the Calcium group monograph in the Intravenous Nutritional Therapy, Electrolytes group monograph.

Minerals

MAGNESIUM

Rx	**Magnesium Chloride** (Various, eg, American Regent)	**Injection**: 20% (1.97 mEq/mL)	In 50 mL multiple dose vials.
Rx	**Magnesium Sulfate** (Various, eg, Astra, Pasadena)	**Injection**: 10% (0.8 mEq/mL)	In 20 and 50 mL vials and 20 mL amps.
Rx	**Magnesium Sulfate** (Various, eg, Abbott)	**Injection**: 12.5% (1 mEq/mL)	In 20 mL vials.
Rx	**Magnesium Sulfate** (Various, eg, Abbott, American Regent, Astra, IMS,Pasadena, Smith & Nephew Solopak)	**Injection**: 50% (4 mEq/mL)	In 2, 5, 10, 20 and 50 mL vials, 5 and 10 mL syringes, 2 and 10 mL amps.

MAGNESIUM CHLORIDE — INJECTION

For information on oral magnesium, refer to the Minerals and Electrolytes, Oral section.

Indications

➤*Magnesium deficiency:* As an electrolyte replenisher in magnesium deficiencies.

Administration and Dosage

➤*For IV infusion:* Use 4 g in 250 mL of 5% dextrose injection, at a rate not exceeding 3 mL per minute. Serum magnesium levels should serve as a guide to continued dosage.

➤*Usual dosage:* Ranges from 1 to 40 g daily.

➤*Storage / Stability:* Store at controlled room temperature 15° to 30°C (59° to 86°F).

Do not use if a precipitate is present.

Actions

➤*Pharmacology:* Magnesium is the second most plentiful cation within cellular fluids. It is an important activator of many enzyme systems, and deficits are accompanied by a variety of functional disturbances.

Contraindications

Renal impairment; marked myocardial disease; coma.

Warnings

➤*Aluminum toxicity:* This product contains aluminum that may be toxic. Aluminum may reach toxic levels with prolonged parenteral administration if kidney function is impaired. Premature neonates are particularly at risk because their kidneys are immature, and they require large amounts of calcium and phosphate solutions, which contain aluminum.

Research indicates that patients with impaired kidney function, including premature neonates, who receive parenteral levels of aluminum at greater than 4 to 5 mcg/kg/day accumulate aluminum at levels associated with central nervous system and bone toxicity. Tissue loading may occur at even lower rates of administration.

➤*Elderly:* Geriatric patients often require reduced dosage because of impaired renal function. In patients with severe impairment, dosage should not exceed 20 g in 48 hours. Monitor serum magnesium in such patients.

➤*Pregnancy: Category C.* Animal reproduction studies have not been conducted with magnesium chloride. It is also not known whether magnesium chloride can cause fetal harm when administered to a pregnant woman or can affect reproduction capacity. Magnesium chloride should be given to a pregnant woman only if clearly needed.

Precautions

➤*Monitoring:* Respiration and blood pressure should be carefully observed during and after administration of magnesium chloride injection.

➤*Parenteral administration:* The usual precautions for parenteral administration should be observed. A preparation of a calcium salt should be readily available for intravenous injection to counteract potential serious signs of magnesium intoxication. As long as deep tendon reflexes are active, it is probable that the patient will not develop respiratory paralysis.

➤*Flushing / sweating:* Administer with caution if flushing and sweating occurs.

Adverse Reactions

➤*Cardiovascular:* Sharply lowered blood pressure, circulatory collapse.

➤*Respiratory:* Respiratory depression (the most life-threatening effect).

➤*Miscellaneous:* Flushing, sweating, hypothermia, stupor, depressed reflexes, flaccid paralysis.

Overdosage

➤*Symptoms:* Sharp drop in blood pressure and respiratory paralysis. ECG changes may include increased PR interval, increased QRS complex and prolonged QT interval. Disappearance of the patellar reflex is a useful clinical sign to detect the onset of magnesium intoxication.

Although patients usually tolerate high concentrations of magnesium in plasma, there are occasional instances when cardiac consequences may be seen in the form of complete heart block at concentrations well below 10 mEq/L.

Other signs include muscle weakness, hypotension, sedation and confusion. As plasma concentrations of magnesium begin to exceed 4 mEq/L, deep-tendon reflexes are decreased and may be absent at levels approaching 10 mEq/L.

Approximate correlation of magnesium toxicity vs serum level

Serum level (mEq/L)	Effect
1.5 to 2.5	Normal serum concentration
4 to 7	"Therapeutic" level for preeclampsia/eclampsia/convulsions
7 to 10	Loss of deep tendon reflexes, hypotension, narcosis
12 to 15	Respiratory paralysis
> 15	Cardiac conduction affected. PR interval lengthening, QRS widening, dysrhythmias
> 25	Cardiac arrest

➤*Treatment:* Provide artificial ventilation until a calcium salt (10 to 20 mL of a 5% solution, diluted with isotonic sodium chloride for injection if desired) can be injected IV to antagonize the effects of magnesium. A dose of 5 to 10 mEq calcium will usually reverse the respiratory depression and heart block. Physostigmine 0.5 to 1 mg administered subcutaneously may be helpful. Peritoneal dialysis or hemodialysis are also effective.

Hypermagnesemia in the newborn may require resuscitation and assisted ventilation via endotracheal intubation or intermittent positive pressure ventilation as well as IV calcium.

MAGNESIUM SULFATE — INJECTION

For information on oral magnesium, refer to the Minerals and Electrolytes, Oral section. For information on the use of magnesium sulfate as an anticonvulsant, refer to the Anticonvulsants monograph in the CNS chapter.

Indications

➤*Magnesium deficiency:* For replacement therapy in magnesium deficiency, especially in acute hypomagnesemia accompanied by signs of tetany similar to those observed in hypocalcemia. In such cases, the serum magnesium level is usually below the lower limit of normal (1.5 to 2.5 mEq/L) and the serum calcium level is normal (4.3 to 5.3 mEq/L) or elevated.

In total parenteral nutrition (TPN), magnesium sulfate may be added to the nutrient admixture to correct or prevent hypomagnesemia which can arise during the course of therapy.

➤*Seizures in toxemia of pregnancy:* For the prevention and control of seizures (convulsions) in severe toxemia of pregnancy. It effectively prevents and controls the convulsions of eclampsia without producing deleterious depression of the CNS of the mother or infant. However, other effective drugs are available for this purpose.

➤*Acute nephritis:* For acute nephritis in children to control hypertension, encephalopathy, and convulsions.

➤*Unlabeled uses:* Magnesium has demonstrated some effectiveness as an agent to inhibit premature labor (tocolytic); however, it is not a first-line agent. It also appears to be beneficial when added to ritodrine therapy, although efficacy has been questioned and an increase in adverse reactions has been observed.

In asthmatic patients who respond poorly to beta-agonists, IV magnesium sulfate (1.2 g) may be a beneficial adjunct for treatment of acute exacerbations of moderate to severe asthma.

The use of IV magnesium sulfate appears to be effective in reducing early mortality in patients with acute myocardial infarction when given as soon as possible after the MI and continued for 24 to 48 hours.

Administration and Dosage

➤*Approved by the FDA:* September 8, 1986.

Dosage of magnesium sulfate must be carefully adjusted according to individual requirements and response, and administration of the drug should be discontinued as soon as the desired effect is obtained.

➤*Administration:* Both IV and IM administration are appropriate. IM administration of the undiluted 50% solution results in therapeutic plasma levels in 60 minutes, whereas IV doses will provide a therapeutic level almost immediately. The rate of IV injection should generally not exceed 150 mg/min (1.5 mL of a 10% concentration or its equivalent), except in severe eclampsia with seizures (see below).

Solutions for IV infusion must be diluted to a concentration of 20% or less prior to administration. The diluents commonly used are 5% Dextrose Injection and 0.9% Sodium Chloride Injection. Deep IM injection of the undiluted (50%) solution is appropriate for adults, but the solution should be diluted to a 20% or less concentration prior to such injection in children.

➤*Magnesium deficiency:* In the treatment of mild magnesium deficiency, the usual adult dose is 1 g, equivalent to 8.12 mEq of magnesium (2 mL of the 50% solution) injected IM every 6 hours for 4 doses (equivalent to a total

MAGNESIUM SULFATE — INJECTION

of 32.5 mEq of magnesium per 24 hours). For severe hypomagnesemia, as much as 250 mg (approximately 2 mEq) per kg of body weight (0.5 mL of the 50% solution) may be given IM within a period of 4 hours if necessary. Alternatively, 5 g (approximately 40 mEq) can be added to 1 L of 5% Dextrose Injection or 0.9% Sodium Chloride Injection for slow IV infusion over a 3-hour period. In the treatment of deficiency states, caution must be observed to prevent exceeding the renal excretory capacity.

➤*Hyperalimentation:* In TPN, maintenance requirements for magnesium are not precisely known. The maintenance dose used in adults ranges from 8 to 24 mEq (1 to 3 g) daily; for infants, the range is 2 to 10 mEq (0.25 to 1.25 g) daily.

➤*Eclampsia:* In severe pre-eclampsia or eclampsia, the total initial dose is 10 to 14 g of magnesium sulfate. Intravenously, a dose of 4 to 5 g in 250 mL of 5% Dextrose Injection or 0.9% Sodium Chloride Injection may be infused. Simultaneously, IM doses of up to 10 g (5 g or 10 mL of the undiluted 50% solution in each buttock) are given. Alternatively, the initial IV dose of 4 g may be given by diluting the 50% solution to a 10 or 20% concentration; the diluted fluid (40 mL of a 10% solution or 20 mL of a 20% solution) may then be injected IV over a period of 3 to 4 minutes. Subsequently, 4 to 5 g (8 to 10 mL of the 50% solution) are injected IM into alternate buttocks every 4 hours as needed, depending on the continuing presence of the patellar reflex and adequate respiratory function. Alternatively, after the initial IV dose, some clinicians administer 1 to 2 g/hr by constant IV infusion. Therapy should continue until paroxysms cease. A serum magnesium level of 6 mg/100 mL is considered optimal for control of seizures. A total daily (24 hr) dose of 30 to 40 g should not be exceeded. In the presence of severe renal insufficiency, the maximum dosage of magnesium sulfate is 20 g/48 hr and frequent serum magnesium concentrations must be obtained.

➤*Barium poisoning:* In counteracting the muscle-stimulating effects of barium poisoning, the usual dose of magnesium sulfate is 1 to 2 g given IV.

➤*Seizures:* For controlling seizures associated with epilepsy, glomerulonephritis or hypothyroidism, the usual adult dose is 1 g administered IM or IV.

➤*Paroxysmal atrial tachycardia:* In paroxysmal atrial tachycardia, magnesium should be used only if simpler measures have failed and there is no evidence of myocardial damage. The usual dose is 3 to 4 g (30 to 40 mL of a 10% solution) administered IV over 30 seconds with extreme caution.

➤*Cerebral edema:* For reduction of cerebral edema, 2.5 g (25 mL of a 10% solution) is given IV.

➤*Admixture incompatibilities:* Magnesium sulfate in solution may result in a precipitate formation when mixed with solutions containing: alcohol (in high concentrations); alkali carbonates and bicarbonates; alkali hydroxides; arsenates; barium; clindamycin phosphate; calcium; heavy metals; hydrocortisone sodium succinate; phosphates; polymyxin B sulfate; procaine hydrochloride; strontium; salicylates; tartrates.

The potential incompatibility will often be influenced by the changes in the concentration of reactants and the pH of the solutions.

It has been reported that magnesium may reduce the antibiotic activity of streptomycin, tetracycline, and tobramycin when given together.

➤*Storage/Stability:* Store at controlled room temperature 15° to 30°C (59° to 86°F).

Actions

➤*Pharmacology:* Magnesium is an important cofactor for enzymatic reactions and plays an important role in neurochemical transmission and muscular excitability.

As a nutritional adjunct in hyperalimentation, the precise mechanism of action for magnesium is uncertain. Early symptoms of hypomagnesemia (less than 1.5 mEq/L) may develop as early as 3 to 4 days or within weeks.

Magnesium deficiency – Predominant deficiency effects are neurological (eg, muscle irritability, clonic twitching, tremors). Hypocalcemia and hypokalemia often follow low serum levels of magnesium. While there are large stores of magnesium present intracellularly and in the bones of adults, these stores often are not mobilized sufficiently to maintain plasma levels. Parenteral magnesium therapy repairs the plasma deficit and causes deficiency symptoms and signs to cease.

Magnesium prevents or controls convulsions by blocking neuromuscular transmission and decreasing the amount of acetylcholine liberated at the end-plate by the motor nerve impulse. Magnesium is said to have a depressant effect on the CNS, but it does not adversely affect the mother, fetus, or neonate when used as directed in eclampsia or pre-eclampsia. Normal plasma magnesium levels range from 1.5 to 2.5 mEq/L.

One gram of magnesium sulfate provides 8.12 mEq of magnesium.

As plasma magnesium rises above 4 mEq/L, the deep tendon reflexes are first decreased and then disappear as the plasma level approaches 10 mEq/L. At this level, respiratory paralysis may occur. Heart block also may occur at this or lower plasma levels of magnesium. Serum magnesium concentrations in excess of 12 mEq/L may be fatal.

Magnesium acts peripherally to produce vasodilation. With low doses only flushing and sweating occur, but larger doses cause lowering of blood pressure. The central and peripheral effects of magnesium poisoning are antagonized to some extent by IV administration of calcium.

➤*Pharmacokinetics:* With IV administration the onset of anticonvulsant action is immediate and lasts about 30 minutes. Following IM administration, the onset of action occurs in about 1 hour and persists for 3 to 4 hours. Effective anticonvulsant serum levels range from 2.5 to 7.5 mEq/L. Magnesium is excreted solely by the kidney at a rate proportional to the plasma concentration and glomerular filtration.

Contraindications

Heart block or myocardial damage. Do not give in toxemia of pregnancy during the 2 hours preceding delivery.

Warnings

➤*Life-threatening convulsions:* IV use in eclampsia should be reserved for immediate control of life-threatening convulsions.

➤*Renal function impairment:* Because magnesium is removed from the body solely by the kidneys, parenteral use in the presence of renal insufficiency may lead to magnesium intoxication. Use caution in patients with renal impairment.

➤*Elderly:* Geriatric patients often require reduced dosage because of impaired renal function. In patients with severe impairment, dosage should not exceed 20 g in 48 hours. Serum magnesium should be monitored in such patients.

➤*Pregnancy: Category A.* Studies in pregnant women have not shown that magnesium sulfate injection increases the risk of fetal abnormalities if administered during all trimesters of pregnancy. If this drug is used during pregnancy, the possibility of fetal harm appears remote. However, because studies cannot rule out the possibility of harm, magnesium sulfate injection should be used during pregnancy only if clearly needed.

When administered by continuous IV infusion (especially for more than 24 hours preceding delivery) to control convulsions in toxemic mothers, the newborn may show signs of magnesium toxicity, including neuromuscular or respiratory depression. In the event of overdosage, artificial ventilation must be provided until a calcium salt can be injected IV to antagonize the effects of magnesium.

➤*Lactation:* Because magnesium is distributed into milk during parenteral magnesium sulfate administration, the drug should be used with caution in nursing women.

➤*Children:* The 50% magnesium sulfate solution should be diluted to 20% or less for IM injection in infants and children.

Precautions

➤*Monitoring:* Monitor the serum concentration of magnesium. The normal serum level is 1.5 to 2.5 mEq/L.

Urine output should be maintained at a level of 100 mL or more during the 4 hours preceding each dose. Monitoring serum magnesium levels and the patient's clinical status is essential to avoid the consequences of overdosage in toxemia. Clinical indications of a safe dosage regimen include the presence of the patellar reflex (knee jerk) and absence of respiratory depression (approximately 16 breaths or more/min). When repeated doses of the drug are given parenterally, knee jerk reflexes should be tested before each dose and if they are absent, no additional magnesium should be given until they return. Serum magnesium levels usually sufficient to control convulsions range from 3 to 6 mg/100 mL (2.5 to 5 mEq/L). The strength of the deep tendon reflexes begins to diminish when magnesium levels exceed 4 mEq/L. Reflexes may be absent at 10 mEq magnesium/L, where respiratory paralysis is a potential hazard. An injectable calcium salt should be immediately available to counteract the potential hazards of magnesium intoxication in eclampsia.

➤*Hypomagnesemia:* Magnesium sulfate injection should not be given unless hypomagnesemia has been confirmed.

➤*Parenteral administration:* Magnesium sulfate injection (50%) must be diluted to a concentration of 20% or less prior to IV infusion. Rate of administration should be slow and cautious, to avoid producing hypermagnesemia. The 50% solution also should be diluted to 20% or less for IM injection in infants and children.

➤*Flushing/sweating:* Administer with caution if flushing and sweating occurs.

Drug Interactions

➤*CNS depressants:* When barbiturates, narcotics or other hypnotics (or systemic anesthetics), or other CNS depressants are to be given in conjunction with magnesium, their dosage should be adjusted with caution because of additive CNS depressant effects of magnesium. CNS depression and peripheral transmission defects produced by magnesium may be antagonized by calcium.

➤*Neuromuscular-blocking agents:* Excessive neuromuscular block has occurred in patients receiving parenteral magnesium sulfate and a neuromuscular blocking agent; these drugs should be administered concomitantly with caution.

➤*Cardiac glycosides:* Magnesium sulfate should be administered with extreme caution in digitalized patients, because serious changes in cardiac conduction which can result in heart block may occur if administration of calcium is required to treat magnesium toxicity.

Adverse Reactions

The adverse reactions of parenterally administered magnesium usually are the result of magnesium intoxication. These include flushing, sweating, hypotension, depressed reflexes, flaccid paralysis, hypothermia, circulatory collapse, cardiac and CNS depression proceeding to respiratory paralysis. Hypocalcemia with signs of tetany secondary to magnesium sulfate therapy for eclampsia has been reported.

MAGNESIUM SULFATE — INJECTION

Overdosage

➤*Symptoms:* Magnesium intoxication is manifested by a sharp drop in blood pressure and respiratory paralysis. Disappearance of the patellar reflex is a useful clinical sign to detect the onset of magnesium intoxication. In the event of overdosage, artificial ventilation must be provided until a calcium salt can be injected IV to antagonize the effects of magnesium.

➤*Treatment:* Artificial respiration is often required. Intravenous calcium, 10 to 20 mL of a 5% solution (diluted if desirable with isotonic sodium chloride for injection), is used to counteract effects of hypermagnesemia. Subcutaneous physostigmine, 0.5 to 1 mg may be helpful. Peritoneal dialysis or hemodialysis is also effective.

Hypermagnesemia in the newborn may require resuscitation and assisted ventilation via endotracheal intubation or intermittent positive pressure ventilation as well as IV calcium.

PHOSPHATE

Rx	**Potassium Phosphate** (Various, eg, Abbott, American Regent)	**Injection**: Provides 3 mM phosphate and 4.4 mEq potassium per mL	In 5, 10, 15, 30, and 50 mL vials.
Rx	**Sodium Phosphate** (Various, eg, Abbott, American Regent)	**Injection**: Provides 3 mM phosphate and 4 mEq sodium per mL	In 10, 15, 30 and 50 mL vials.

PHOSPHATES — INJECTION

Indications

➤*Hypophosphatemia:* As a source of phosphate, for addition to large volume IV fluids, to prevent or correct hypophosphatemia in patients with restricted or no oral intake. It is also useful as an additive for preparing specific parenteral fluid formulas when the needs of the patient cannot be met by standard electrolyte or nutrient solutions.

Administration and Dosage

Sodium phosphates injection is administered intravenously only after dilution and thorough mixing in a larger volume of fluid. The dose and rate of administration are dependent upon the individual needs of the patient. Using aseptic technique, all or part of the contents of 1 or more vials may be added to other IV fluids to provide any desired number of millimoles (mM) of phosphate and milliequivalents of sodium.

The concomitant amount of sodium (4 mEq/mL) must be calculated into total electrolyte dose of such prepared solutions.

➤*Total parenteral nutrition (TPN):* In patients on TPN, approximately 10 to 15 mM of phosphorus (equivalent to 310 to 465 mg elemental phosphorus) per liter bottle of TPN solution containing 250 g dextrose is usually adequate to maintain normal serum phosphorus, though larger amounts may be required in hypermetabolic states. The amount of sodium and phosphorus that accompanies the addition of sodium phosphate also should be kept in mind, and if necessary, serum sodium levels should be monitored.

Children – The suggested dose of phosphorus for infants receiving TPN is 1.5 to 2 mmol/kg/day.

➤*Storage/Stability:* Store at controlled room temperature 15° to 30°C (59° to 86°F).

Do not administer unless the solution is clear and the seal is intact. Discard any unused portion.

Actions

➤*Pharmacology:* Phosphorus in the form of organic and inorganic phosphate has a variety of important biochemical functions in the body and is involved in many significant metabolic and enzyme reactions in almost all organs and tissues. It exerts a modifying influence on the steady state of calcium levels, a buffering effect on acid-base equilibrium and a primary role in the renal excretion of hydrogen ion.

Phosphorus, present in large amounts in erythrocytes and other tissue cells, plays a significant intracellular role in the synthesis of high energy organic phosphates. It has been shown to be essential to maintain red cell glucose utilization, lactate production, and the concentration of both erythrocyte adenosine triphosphate (ATP) and 2, 3 diphosphoglycerate (DPG), and must be deemed as important to other tissue cells. Hypophosphatemia should be avoided during periods of TPN, or other lengthy periods of IV infusions. It has been suggested that patients receiving TPN receive 20 mEq phosphate (13 mmol phosphate)/1000 kcal from dextrose. Serum phosphorus levels should be regularly monitored and appropriate amounts of phosphorus should be added to the infusions to maintain normal serum phosphorus levels. IV infusion of inorganic phosphorus may be accompanied by a decrease in the serum level and urinary excretion of calcium. The normal level of serum phosphorus is 3 to 4.5 mg/100 mL in adults; 4 to 7 mg/100 mL in children.

➤*Pharmacokinetics:* Intravenously infused phosphorus not taken up by the tissues is excreted almost entirely in the urine. Plasma phosphorus is believed to be filterable by the renal glomeruli, and the major portion of filtered phosphorus (greater than 80%) is actively reabsorbed by the tubules. Many modifying influences tend to alter the amount excreted in the urine.

Contraindications

High phosphorus or low calcium levels; hypernatremia.

Warnings

➤*Parenteral administration:* Sodium phosphates injection must be diluted and thoroughly mixed before use.

To avoid phosphorus intoxication, infuse solutions containing sodium phosphate slowly. Infusing high concentrations of phosphorus may result in a reduction of serum calcium and symptoms of hypocalcemic tetany. Calcium levels should be monitored.

➤*Sodium retention:* Solutions containing sodium ion should be used with great care, if at all, in patients with congestive heart failure, severe renal insufficiency, and in clinical states in which edema with sodium retention exists.

➤*Renal function impairment:* In patients with diminished renal function, administration of solutions containing sodium ions may result in sodium retention.

➤*Elderly:* An evaluation of current literature revealed no clinical experience identifying differences in response between elderly and younger patients. In general, dose selection for an elderly patient should be cautious, usually starting at the low end of the dosing range, reflecting the greater frequency of decreased hepatic, renal, or cardiac function, and of concomitant disease or other drug therapy.

Sodium ions and phosphorus ions are known to be substantially excreted by the kidney, and the risk of toxic reactions may be greater in patients with impaired renal function. Because elderly patients are more likely to have decreased renal function, care should be taken in dose selection, and it may be useful to monitor renal function.

➤*Pregnancy: Category C.* Animal reproduction studies have not been conducted with sodium phosphate. It is also not known whether sodium phosphate can cause fetal harm when administered to a pregnant woman or can affect reproduction capacity. Sodium phosphate should be given to a pregnant woman only if clearly needed.

➤*Lactation:* It is not known whether this drug is excreted in human milk. Because many drugs are excreted in human milk, caution should be exercised when sodium phosphate is administered to a nursing woman.

➤*Children:* The safety and efficacy of sodium phosphate have been established in children (neonates, infants, children, and adolescents).

Precautions

➤*Monitoring:* Phosphate replacement therapy with sodium phosphate should be guided primarily by serum inorganic phosphate levels and the limits imposed by the accompanying sodium (Na+) ion. Frequent monitoring of serum sodium, phosphorus, and calcium levels as well as renal function is recommended.

➤*Special risk:* Use with caution in patients with renal impairment, cirrhosis, cardiac failure, or in conjunction with other edematous medications. It should not be used with sodium-retaining medications.

Drug Interactions

➤*Thiazides:* Concurrent use with thiazides may cause renal damage.

➤*Corticosteroids and corticotropin:* Caution must be exercised in the administration of parenteral fluids, especially those containing sodium ion, to patients receiving corticosteroids or corticotropin.

Adverse Reactions

Adverse reactions involve the possibility of combined sodium and phosphorus intoxication from overdosage.

Phosphorus intoxication results in hypocalcemic tetany.

Overdosage

➤*Symptoms:* Phosphorus intoxication results in a reduction of serum calcium and the symptoms are those of hypocalcemic tetany.

➤*Treatment:* In the event of overdosage, discontinue infusions containing sodium phosphate immediately and institute corrective therapy to restore depressed serum calcium and to reduce elevated serum sodium levels.

SODIUM CHLORIDE

For information on oral sodium chloride, refer to Minerals and Electrolytes, Oral section.

Indications

➤*0.45% and 0.9% flexible plastic containers:* IV solutions containing sodium chloride are indicated for parenteral replenishment of fluid and sodium chloride as required by the clinical condition of the patient.

➤*0.9% syringe:* Sodium chloride injection, 0.9% is intended for use in flushing the indwelling venipuncture device where the medication to be administered is incompatible with heparin.

➤*0.9% vial:* Sodium chloride injection, 0.9% preparations are indicated for diluting or dissolving drugs for intramuscular, intravenous or subcutaneous injection according to instructions of the manufacturer of the drug to be administered.

Sodium chloride injection, 0.9% is also indicated for use in flushing of intravenous catheters.

➤*3% and 5% concentrates:* These intravenous solutions are indicated for use in adults and children as sources of electrolytes and water for hydration.

Sodium chloride injections, 3% and 5% are of particular value in severe salt depletion when rapid electrolyte restoration is of paramount importance. The low salt syndrome may occur in the presence of heart failure, renal impairment, during surgery, and postoperatively. In these conditions, chloride loss frequently exceeds sodium loss.

These hypertonic sodium chloride solutions are also indicated for the following clinical conditions: hyponatremia and hypochloremia due to electrolyte and fluid loss replaced with sodium-free fluids; drastic dilution of extracellular body fluid following excessive water intake sometimes resulting from multiple enemas or perfusion of irrigating fluids into open venous sinuses during transurethral prostatic resections; emergency treatment of severe salt depletion due to excess sweating, vomiting, diarrhea, and other conditions.

➤*14.6% concentrate:* For use as an electrolyte replenisher in parenteral fluid therapy. It serves as an intravenous sodium supplement in hyponatremia or low salt syndrome, as an additive for total parenteral nutrition (TPN), and as an additive for carbohydrate-containing IV fluids.

Toxicity secondary to intestinal obstruction is usually accompanied by a marked reduction in serum chloride, and sodium chloride supplements can have a lifesaving effect. Symptoms of sodium chloride deficiency are very similar to those of Addison's disease, and large doses of sodium chloride will produce temporary alleviation of symptoms. Other disorders where sodium chloride is of clinical benefit include extensive burns, failure of gastric secretion, and postoperative intestinal paralysis.

➤*23.4% concentrate:* As an additive in parenteral fluid therapy for use in patients who have special problems of sodium electrolyte intake or excretion. It is intended to meet the specific requirement of the patient with unusual fluid and electrolyte needs. After available clinical and laboratory information is considered and correlated, determine the appropriate number of milliequivalents of concentrated sodium chloride injection and dilute for use.

Administration and Dosage

➤*Dosage:* Dosage is to be directed by a physician and is dependent on age, weight, clinical condition of the patient, and laboratory determinations. Frequent laboratory determinations and clinical evaluation are essential to monitor changes in blood glucose and electrolyte concentrations, and fluid and electrolyte balance during prolonged parenteral therapy.

Fluid administration should be based on calculated maintenance or replacement fluid requirements for each patient.

Consult the manufacturer's instructions for choice of vehicle, appropriate dilution or volume for dissolving the drugs to be injected, including the route and rate of injection. Inspect reconstituted (diluted or dissolved) drugs for clarity (if soluble) and freedom from unexpected precipitation or discoloration prior to administration.

➤*Admixture incompatibilities:* Before sodium chloride injection, 0.9% is used as a vehicle for the administration of a drug, specific references should be checked for any possible incompatibility with sodium chloride.

To minimize the risk of possible incompatibilities arising from mixing this solution with other additives that may be prescribed, the final infusate should be inspected for cloudiness or precipitation immediately after mixing, prior to administration, and periodically during administration.

Some additives may be incompatible. Consult with pharmacist. When introducing additives, use aseptic techniques. Mix thoroughly. Do not store.

➤*IV catheters:* Sodium chloride injection, 0.9% is also indicated for use in flushing intravenous catheters. Prior to and after administration of the medication, the intravenous catheter should be flushed in its entirety with sodium chloride injection, 0.9%. Use in accord with any warnings or precautions appropriate to the medication being administered.

➤*3% and 5% concentrates:* Do not use plastic container in series connection.

If administration is controlled by a pumping device, care must be taken to discontinue pumping action before the container runs dry or air embolism may result.

When a hypertonic solution is to be administered peripherally, it should be slowly infused through a small bore needle, placed well within the lumen of a large vein to minimize venous irritation. Carefully avoid infiltration.

Maximum IV dosage should be 100 mL given over a period of 1 hour. Before additional amount are given, the serum electrolyte concentrations, including chloride and bicarbonate, should be determined to evaluate the need for more sodium chloride.

IV administration of these solutions should not exceed 100 mL/hour or 400 mL/24 hours.

➤*14.6% concentrate:* Sodium chloride injection, 14.6% is administered intravenously, but only after dilution in a larger volume of fluid. Maintenance electrolyte solutions usually contain sodium at a concentration of 33 to 40 mEq/L, on the assumption the patient will receive 2 to 3 L of fluid/day. A typical oral salt intake of 10 g/day is equivalent to 171 mEq/day. But intake can range from 5 to 15 g of sodium chloride/day, and patients on a sodium-restricted diet may receive 1 to 2 g of sodium/day. The actual dose of sodium chloride administered depends upon specific patient requirements, which are usually determined by review of serial blood samples and clinical evaluation. In solutions for total parenteral nutrition (TPN), adults typically receive 120 mEq of sodium/day (range: 75 to 180 mEq/day), whereas preterm infants receive 3 to 4 mEq/kg/day.

➤*23.4% concentrate:* Concentrated sodium chloride injection is strongly hypertonic and must be diluted prior to administration. The dosage of concentrated sodium chloride injection as an additive in parenteral fluid therapy is predicted on the specific requirement of the patient after necessary clinical and laboratory information is considered and correlated. The appropriate volume is then withdrawn for proper dilution. Having determined the milliequivalents of sodium chloride to be added, divide by 4 to calculate the number of mL of concentrated solution to be used. Withdraw this volume aseptically and transfer this additive solution into appropriate intravenous solutions such as 5% dextrose injection. The properly diluted solutions may be given IV or SC.

➤*Storage/Stability:* Exposure of pharmaceutical products to heat should be minimized. Avoid excessive heat. Protect from freezing. Store at controlled room temperature 15° to 30°C (59° to 86°F).

3% and 5% concentrates – It is recommended that the product be stored at room temperature, 25°C (77°F); however, brief exposure up to 40°C (104°F) does not adversely affect the product.

Some products may not contain preservatives.

Do not administer unless solution is clear and the container or seal is intact. Discard unused portion.

Actions

➤*Pharmacology:* Solutions which provide combinations of hypotonic or isotonic concentrations of sodium chloride are suitable for parenteral maintenance or replacement of water and electrolyte requirements.

Sodium, the major cation of the extracellular fluid, functions primarily in the control of water distribution, fluid balance, and osmotic pressure of body fluids. Sodium is also associated with chloride and bicarbonate in the regulation of the acid-base equilibrium of body fluid.

Chloride, the major extracellular anion, closely follows the metabolism of sodium, and changes in the acid-base balance of the body are reflected by changes in the chloride concentration.

Water balance is maintained by various regulatory mechanisms. Water distribution depends primarily on the concentration of electrolytes in the body compartments and sodium (Na^+) plays a major role in maintaining physiologic equilibrium. Sodium chloride is an electrolyte replenisher. Sodium is the principal cation of extracellular fluid. With a normal plasma concentration of 142 mEq/L, sodium comprises more than 90% of the total plasma cations. While sodium can diffuse across membranes, the intracellular sodium concentration is maintained at a much lower level than extracellular concentrations, the so-called "sodium pump." Compensation for loss of intracellular potassium occurs through an increase in intracellular sodium. Sodium is the principal ion that determines osmotic pressure of interstitial fluids and the degree of tissue hydration.

Adult serum chloride values typically range from 100 to 106 mEq/L. Serum chloride levels decrease in metabolic alkalosis, as serum bicarbonate levels generally increase. In parenteral nutrition when acidosis occurs, it is common practice to reduce chloride intake by substituting acetate salts in place of chloride salts.

Contraindications

Hypernatremic and fluid retention syndromes. Elevated, normal, or only slightly decreased plasma electrolyte concentrations, or when additives of sodium and chloride could be clinically detrimental.

Warnings

➤*Fluid/solute overload:* The risk of dilutional states is inversely proportional to the electrolyte concentrations of administered parenteral solutions. The risk of solute overload causing congested states with peripheral and pulmonary edema is directly proportional to the electrolyte concentrations of such solutions.

Excessive amounts of sodium chloride by any route may cause hypokalemia and acidosis. Excessive amounts by the parenteral route may precipitate congestive heart failure and acute pulmonary edema, especially in patients with cardiovascular disease and in patients receiving corticosteroids or corticotropin or drugs that may give rise to sodium retention.

Excessive infusion of hypertonic sodium chloride solutions may supply more sodium and chloride than normally found in serum and can exceed normal tolerance, resulting in hypernatremia. Infusion of excess chloride ions may cause a loss of bicarbonate, resulting in an acidifying effect.

SODIUM CHLORIDE

➤*Sodium retention:* Solutions containing sodium ions should be used with great care, if at all, in patients with congestive heart failure, severe renal insufficiency, and in clinical states in which there exists edema with sodium retention.

➤*Hypokalemia:* Excessive administration of potassium-free solutions may result in significant hypokalemia.

➤*Surgical patients:* Surgical patients should seldom receive salt-containing solutions immediately following surgery unless factors producing salt depletion are present. Because renal retention of salt occurs during surgery, additional electrolytes given intravenously may result in fluid retention, edema and circulatory overload.

➤*3% and 5% concentrates:* These are very concentrated hypertonic sodium chloride solutions. Infuse very slowly with constant observation of the patient to avoid pulmonary edema.

➤*14.6% and 23.4% concentrates:* Sodium chloride injection is hypertonic and must be diluted prior to administration. Inadvertent direct injection or absorption of concentrated sodium chloride solution may give rise to sudden hypernatremia and such complications as cardiovascular shock, central nervous system disorders, extensive hemolysis and cortical necrosis of the kidneys and severe local tissue necrosis (if administered extravascularly).

➤*Aluminum toxicity (23.4% concentrate):* This product contains aluminum that may be toxic. Aluminum may reach toxic levels with prolonged parenteral administration if kidney function is impaired. Premature neonates are particularly at risk because their kidneys are immature, and they require large amounts of calcium and phosphate solutions, which contain aluminum.

Research indicates that patients with impaired kidney function, including premature neonates, who receive parenteral levels of aluminum at greater than 4 to 5 mcg/kg/day accumulate aluminum at levels associated with central nervous system and bone toxicity. Tissue loading may occur at even lower rates of administration.

➤*Renal function impairment:* In patients with diminished renal function, administration of solutions containing sodium may result in sodium retention. The intravenous administration of this solution (after appropriate dilution) can cause fluid or solute overloading resulting in dilution of other serum electrolyte concentrations, overhydration, congested states or pulmonary edema.

➤*Pregnancy: Category C.* Animal reproduction studies have not been conducted with sodium chloride injection. It is also not known whether sodium chloride can cause fetal harm when administered to a pregnant woman or can affect reproduction capacity. Sodium chloride should be given to a pregnant woman only if clearly needed.

➤*Lactation:* It is not known whether sodium chloride injection is excreted in human milk. Because many drugs are excreted in human milk, caution should be exercised when sodium chloride is administered to a nursing woman.

➤*Children:* Safety and efficacy of sodium chloride injection have not been established in pediatric patients. Its limited use in pediatric patients has been inadequate to fully define proper dosage and limitations for use.

0.45% and 0.9% flexible plastic containers – The safety and efficacy in the pediatric population are based on the similarity of the clinical conditions of the pediatric and adult populations. In neonates or very small infants, the volume of fluid may affect fluid and electrolyte balance.

Precautions

➤*Monitoring:* Clinical evaluation and periodic laboratory determinations are necessary to monitor changes in fluid balance, electrolyte concentrations and acid-base balance during prolonged parenteral therapy or whenever the condition of the patient warrants such evaluation.

➤*Electrolyte losses:* Extraordinary electrolyte losses may occur during protracted nasogastric suction, vomiting, diarrhea, or gastrointestinal fistula drainage and may necessitate additional electrolyte supplementation.

Additional essential electrolytes, minerals, and vitamins should be supplied as needed.

➤*0.9%:*

Children – For use in newborns, when a sodium chloride solution is required for preparation or diluting medications or in flushing intravenous catheters, only preservative free sodium chloride injection, 0.9% should be used.

➤*Special risk:*

3% and 5% concentrates – These solutions should be used with care in patients with hypervolemia, renal insufficiency, urinary tract obstruction, or impending or frank cardiac decompensation.

Care should be exercised in administering solutions containing sodium to patients with renal or cardiovascular insufficiency, with or without congestive heart failure, particularly if they are postoperative or elderly. Special caution should be used in administering sodium-containing solutions to patients with severe renal impairment, cirrhosis of the liver or other edematous or sodium-retaining states.

Drug Interactions

➤*Corticosteroids and corticotropin:* Caution must be exercised in the administration of parenteral fluids, especially those containing sodium ions to patients receiving corticosteroids or corticotropin.

Adverse Reactions

➤*Reactions due to solution or technique of administration:* Reactions which may occur because of the solution or the technique of administration include febrile response, infection at the site of injection, venous thrombosis or phlebitis extending from the site of injection, extravasation and hypervolemia.

➤*Too rapid infusion:* Too rapid infusion of hypertonic solutions may cause local pain and venous irritation. Rate of administration should be adjusted according to tolerance. Use the largest peripheral vein and a well-placed small bore needle is recommended.

Ion excess/deficit – Symptoms may result from an excess or deficit of 1 or more of the ions present in the solution; therefore, frequent monitoring of electrolyte levels is essential.

If infused in large amounts, chloride ions may cause a loss of bicarbonate ions, resulting in an acidifying effect.

Hypernatremia – Hypernatremia may be associated with edema and exacerbation of congestive heart failure due to the retention of water, resulting in an expanded extracellular fluid volume.

➤*14.6% concentrate:* Sodium overload can occur with intravenous infusion of excessive amounts of sodium-containing solutions.

Under rapid infusion – Overzealous administration can result in edema and symptoms resembling congestive heart failure.

Postoperative salt intolerance – Signs of postoperative salt intolerance include cellular dehydration, weakness, disorientation, anorexia, nausea, distention, deep respiration, oliguria, and increased BUN. If an adverse reaction does occur, discontinue the infusion, evaluate the patient, institute appropriate therapeutic countermeasures, and save the remainder of the fluid for examination if deemed necessary.

Overdosage

➤*Symptoms:* Excessive administration of sodium chloride injection may result in electrolyte imbalance with water retention, edema, loss of potassium, and aggravation of an existing acidosis.

Excessive sodium chloride intake is accompanied by excretion of crystalloids, in an attempt to maintain normal osmotic pressure. Increased excretion of potassium and bicarbonate can result in acidosis. There is also a rapid elimination of any foreign salt, such as iodide and bromide, being used therapeutically.

When used as a diluent, solvent or intravascular flushing solution, this parenteral preparation is unlikely to pose a threat of sodium chloride or fluid overload except possibly in very small infants.

➤*Treatment:* In the event of a fluid or solute overload during parenteral therapy, reevaluate the patient's condition and institute appropriate corrective treatment.

SODIUM CHLORIDE INTRAVENOUS INFUSIONS FOR ADMIXTURES

		Sodium (mEq/L)	Chloride (mEq/L)	Osmolarity (mOsm/L)	How Supplied
Rx	**0.45% Sodium Chloride (½ Normal Saline)** (Various, eg, Abbott, Astra, Clintec, McGaw)	77	77	≈ 155	In 25, 50, 150, 250, 500 and 1000 mL.
Rx	**0.9% Sodium Chloride (Normal Saline)** (Various, eg, Abbott, Astra, Clintec, Gensia, McGaw, Rugby, Smith & Nephew SoloPak)	154	154	≈ 310	In 2, 3, 5, 10, 20, 25, 30, 50, 100, 150, 250, 500, 1000ml and 2 mL fill in 3 mL.
Rx	**3% Sodium Chloride**(Various, eg, Clintec, McGaw)	513	513	1030	In 500 mL.
Rx	**5% Sodium Chloride** (Various, eg, Abbott, Clintec, McGaw)	855	855	1710	In 500 mL.

For complete and comparative prescribing information, refer to Sodium Chloride group monograph.

SODIUM CHLORIDE DILUENTS

otc	**Sodium Chloride 0.45%** (Dey)	**Solution**: 0.45% sodium chloride	Preservative free. In single-use 3 and 5 mL vials.
otc	**Sodium Chloride 0.9%** (Dey)	**Solution**: 0.9% sodium chloride	Preservative free. In 3, 5, and 15 mL.
Rx	**Sodium Chloride** (Various, eg, American Regent, ESI Lederle, Hospira)	**Injection**: 0.9% sodium chloride	In 1, 2, 2.5, 3, 5, 10, and 30 mL.[a]

[a] May contain 9 mg benzyl alcohol.

For complete and comparative prescribing information, refer to Sodium Chloride group monograph.

CONCENTRATED SODIUM CHLORIDE INJECTION

Rx	**Sodium Chloride Injection** (Various, eg, IMS)	14.6% sodium chloride	In 20, 40 and 200 mL.
Rx	**Sodium Chloride Injection** (Various, eg, American Regent, Gensia, IMS, Pasadena)	23.4% sodium chloride	In 30, 50, 100 and 200 mL.

CONCENTRATED SODIUM CHLORIDE — INJECTION

For complete and comparative prescribing information, refer to Sodium Chloride group monograph.

Administration and Dosage

Not for direct infusion. *Must* be diluted before use.

POTASSIUM SALTS

For information on oral potassium, refer to Mineral and Electrolytes, Oral section. For information on potassium phosphate, refer to specific monograph in this section.

Indications

➤*Hypokalemia:* Prevention and treatment of moderate or severe potassium deficit when oral replacement therapy is not feasible.

➤*Potassium acetate:* Potassium acetate is useful as an additive for preparing specific IV fluid formulas when patient needs cannot be met by standard electrolyte or nutrient solutions.

Also indicated for marked loss of GI secretions by vomiting, diarrhea, GI intubation or fistulas; prolonged diuresis; prolonged parenteral use of potassium-free fluids (eg, normal saline, dextrose solutions); diabetic acidosis, especially during vigorous insulin and dextrose treatment; metabolic alkalosis; attacks of hereditary or familial periodic paralysis; hyperadrenocorticism; primary aldosteronism; overmedication with adrenocortical steroids, testosterone or corticotropin; healing phase of scalds or burns; cardiac arrhythmias, especially due to digitalis glycosides.

Administration and Dosage

mEq/g of Various Potassium Salts	
Potassium salt	mEq/g
Potassium acetate	10.2
Potassium chloride	13.4
Dibasic potassium phosphate[a]	11.5
Monobasic potassium phosphate[a]	7.3

[a] Commercial preparations of potassium phosphate injection contain a mixture of both mono- and dibasic salts (see Potassium Phosphate monograph).

➤*Do not administer undiluted potassium:* Potassium preparations must be diluted with suitable large volume parenteral solutions, mixed well and given by slow IV infusion.

Too rapid infusion of hypertonic solutions may cause local pain and, rarely, vein irritation. Adjust rate of administration according to tolerance. Use of the largest peripheral vein and a small bore needle is recommended.

The usual additive dilution of potassium chloride is 40 mEq/L of IV fluid. The maximum desirable concentration is 80 mEq/L, although extreme emergencies may dictate greater concentrations.

In critical states, potassium chloride may be administered in saline (unless saline is contraindicated) since dextrose may lower serum potassium levels by producing an intracellular shift.

Avoid "layering" of potassium by proper agitation of the prepared IV solution. Do not add potassium to an IV bottle in the hanging position.

Individualize dosage. Guide dosage and rate of infusion by ECG and serum electrolyte determinations. The following may be used as a guide:

Potassium Dosage/Rate of Infusion Guidelines			
Serum K+	Maximum infusion rate	Maximum concentration	Maximum 24 hour dose
> 2.5 mEq/L	10 mEq/hr	40 mEq/L	200 mEq
< 2 mEq/L	40 mEq/hr	80 mEq/L	400 mEq

Add electrolytes to the mixed solutions only after considering electrolytes already present and potential incompatibilities such as calcium and phosphate or sulfate.

➤*Children:* IV infusion up to 3 mEq/kg or 40 mEq/m²/day. Adjust volume of administered fluids to body size.

Actions

➤*Pharmacology:* The principal intracellular cation, potassium is essential for maintenance of intracellular tonicity; transmission of nerve impulses; contraction of cardiac, skeletal and smooth muscle; and maintenance of normal renal function. Potassium participates in carbohydrate utilization and protein synthesis and is critical in regulating nerve conduction and muscle contraction, particularly in the heart.

Hypokalemia – Gradual potassium depletion occurs via renal excretion, through GI loss or because of inadequate intake (excretion greater than intake). Depletion usually results from diuretic therapy, primary or secondary hyperaldosteronism, diabetic ketoacidosis, severe diarrhea (especially if associated with vomiting) or inadequate replacement during prolonged parenteral nutrition.

Potassium depletion sufficient to cause 1 mEq/L drop in serum potassium requires a loss of about 100 to 200 mEq of potassium from the total body store.

Symptoms: Weakness; fatigue; ileus; polydipsia; flaccid paralysis or impaired ability to concentrate urine (in advanced cases).

ECG may reveal premature atrial and ventricular contractions, prolongation of QT interval, ST segment depression, broad and flat T waves or appearance of U waves. Severe cases may lead to muscular weakness, paralysis, respiratory failure.

➤*Pharmacokinetics:* Normally about 80% to 90% of potassium intake is excreted in urine with the remainder voided in stool and, to a small extent, in perspiration. Kidneys do not conserve potassium well; during fasting or in patients on a potassium-free diet, potassium loss from the body continues, resulting in potassium depletion. A deficiency of either potassium or chloride will lead to a deficit of the other.

Contraindications

Diseases where high potassium levels may be encountered; hyperkalemia; renal failure and conditions in which potassium retention is present; oliguria or azotemia; anuria; crush syndrome; severe hemolytic reactions; adrenocortical insufficiency (untreated Addison's disease); adynamica episodica hereditaria; acute dehydration; heat cramps; hyperkalemia from any cause; early postoperative oliguria except during GI drainage.

Warnings

➤*Potassium intoxication:* Do not infuse rapidly. High plasma concentrations of potassium may cause death through cardiac depression, arrhythmias or arrest. Monitor potassium replacement therapy whenever possible by continuous or serial ECG. In addition to ECG effects, local pain and phlebitis may result when a greater than 40 mEq/L concentration is infused.

Renal impairment or adrenal insufficiency – Renal impairments or adrenal insufficiency may cause potassium intoxication. Potassium salts can produce hyperkalemia and cardiac arrest. Potentially fatal hyperkalemia can develop rapidly and be asymptomatic. Use with great caution, if at all.

➤*Concentrated potassium:* Concentrated potassium solutions are for IV admixtures only; do not use undiluted. Direct injection may be instantaneously fatal.

➤*Metabolic alkalosis:* Potassium depletion is usually accompanied by an obligatory loss of chloride resulting in hypochloremic metabolic alkalosis. Treat the underlying cause of potassium depletion and administer IV potassium chloride.

Use solutions containing acetate ion carefully in metabolic or respiratory alkalosis, and when there is an increased level or impairment of utilization of this ion.

➤*Metabolic acidosis:* Treat associated hypokalemia with an alkalinizing potassium salt (eg, bicarbonate, citrate, gluconate, acetate).

➤*Musculoskeletal/Cardiac effects:* When serum sodium or calcium concentration is reduced, moderate elevation of serum potassium may cause toxic effects on the heart and skeletal muscle. Weakness and later paralysis of voluntary muscles, with consequent respiratory distress and dysphagia, are generally late signs, sometimes significantly preceding dangerous or fatal cardiac toxicity.

POTASSIUM SALTS

➤*Renal function impairment:* Normal kidney function permits safe potassium therapy. Although temporary elevation of serum potassium level due to renal insufficiency secondary to dehydration or shock may mask an intracellular potassium deficit, do not replenish potassium until renal function is reestablished by overcoming dehydration and shock. Discontinue potassium-containing solutions if signs of renal insufficiency develop during infusions.

➤*Pregnancy: Category C.* It is not known whether potassium salts can cause fetal harm when administered to a pregnant woman or can affect reproduction capacity. Give to a pregnant woman only if clearly needed.

➤*Lactation:* Exercise caution when administering to a nursing woman.

Precautions

➤*Monitoring:* Close medical supervision with frequent ECGs and serum potassium determinations. Plasma levels are not necessarily indicative of tissue levels.

➤*Fluid/Solute overload:* IV administration can cause fluid or solute overloading resulting in dilution of serum electrolyte concentrations, overhydration, congested states or pulmonary edema.

The risk of dilutional states is inversely proportional to the electrolyte concentration of administered parenteral solutions. The risk of solute overload causing congested states with peripheral and pulmonary edema is directly proportional to the electrolyte concentrations of such solutions.

➤*Special risk:* Use with caution in the presence of cardiac disease, particularly in digitalized patients or in the presence of renal disease, metabolic acidosis, Addison's disease, acute dehydration, prolonged or severe diarrhea, familial periodic paralysis, hypoadrenalism, hyperkalemia, hyponatremia and myotonia congenita.

Drug Interactions

Potassium Preparation Drug Interactions

Precipitant drug	Object drug[a]		Description
ACE inhibitors	Potassium preparations	↑	Concurrent use may result in elevated serum potassium concentrations in certain patients.
Potassium-sparing diuretics/potassium-containing salt substitutes	Potassium preparations	↑	Potassium-sparing diuretics and potassium-containing salt substitutes will increase potassium retention and can produce severe hyperkalemia.
Potassium preparations	Digitalis	↑	In patients on digoxin, hypokalemia may result in digoxin toxicity. Use caution if discontinuing a potassium preparation in patients maintained on digoxin.

[a] ↑ = Object drug increased.

Adverse Reactions

Hyperkalemia – Adverse reactions involve the possibility of potassium intoxication. Signs and symptoms include: Paresthesias of extremities; flaccid paralysis; muscle or respiratory paralysis; areflexia; weakness; listlessness; mental confusion; weakness and heaviness of legs; hypotension; cardiac arrhythmias; heart block; ECG abnormalities such as disappearance of P waves, spreading and slurring of the QRS complex with development of a biphasic curve and cardiac arrest. See Overdosage.

➤*GI:* Nausea; vomiting; abdominal pain; diarrhea.

Reactions due to solution or technique of administration – Febrile response; infection at injection site; venous thrombosis; phlebitis extending from injection site; extravasation; hypervolemia; hyperkalemia; venospasm.

Overdosage

If excretory mechanisms are impaired or if potassium is administered too rapidly IV, potentially fatal hyperkalemia can result (see Contraindications and Warnings). It is important to consider the entire clinical picture and not rely solely on potassium levels since only extracellular potassium can be measured, yet intracellular potassium accounts for 98% of the total body amount.

➤*Symptoms:* Mild (greater than 5.5 to 6.5 mEq/L) to moderate (greater than 6.5 to 8 mEq/L) hyperkalemia may be asymptomatic and manifested only by increased serum potassium concentration and characteristic ECG changes. Other symptoms include muscular weakness, progressing to flaccid quadriplegia and respiratory paralysis; however, these generally do not develop unless potassium concentrations exceed 8 mEq/L. Dangerous cardiac arrhythmias often occur before onset of complete paralysis. Note that hyperkalemia produces symptoms paradoxically similar to those of hypokalemia.

ECG – Progressive increase in height and peaking of T waves; lowering of the R wave; decreased amplitude and ultimate disappearance of P waves; prolongation of PR interval and QRS complex; shortening of the QT interval; and finally, ventricular fibrillation and death.

➤*Treatment:* Terminate potassium administration. Monitor ECG. Infusion of combined dextrose and insulin in a ratio of 3 g dextrose to 1 unit regular insulin may be administered to shift potassium into cells. Administer sodium bicarbonate 50 to 100 mEq IV to reverse acidosis and also produce an intracellular shift. Give 10 to 100 mL calcium gluconate or calcium chloride 10% to reverse ECG changes. To remove potassium from the body use sodium polystyrene sulfonate resin or hemodialysis or peritoneal dialysis.

In digitalized patients, too rapid lowering of serum potassium can cause digitalis toxicity (see Drug Interactions).

POTASSIUM ACETATE

Rx	**Potassium Acetate** (Various, eg, Abbott, American Regent, IMS)	**Injection:** 2 mEq/mL	In 20, 50 and 100 mL vials.
Rx	**Potassium Acetate** (Various)	**Injection:** 4 mEq/mL	In 50 mL vials.

POTASSIUM ACETATE — INJECTION

Indications

➤*Hypokalemia:* Treatment of potassium deficiency states when oral replacement therapy is not feasible.

The solution is intended as an alternative to potassium chloride to provide potassium (K^+) for addition to large volume infusion fluids for IV use.

Administration and Dosage

➤*Approved by the FDA:* July 20, 1984.

Potassium acetate injection (2 mEq/mL) must be diluted before administration.

The dose and rate of administration are dependent upon the individual condition of each patient. ECG and serum potassium should be monitored as a guide to dosage. Withdraw the calculated volume aseptically and transfer to appropriate intravenous fluids to provide the desired number of milliequivalents of potassium (K^+) with an equal number of milliequivalents of acetate (CH_3COO^-).

➤*Storage/Stability:* Store at controlled room temperature between 15° to 30°C (59° to 86°F).

Discard vial within 4 hours of initial entry.

POTASSIUM CHLORIDE FOR INJECTION CONCENTRATE

Rx	**Potassium Chloride** (McGaw)	**Injection:** 2 mEq/mL	In 250 and 500 mL.
Rx	**Potassium Chloride** (Various, eg, Abbott, Baxter)	**Injection:** 10 mEq	In 5, 10, 50 and 100 mL vials and 5 mL additive syringes.
Rx	**Potassium Chloride** (Various, eg, Abbott, American Regent, Baxter)	**Injection:** 20 mEq	In 10 and 20 mL vials, 10 mL additive syringes, 10 mL amps.
Rx	**Potassium Chloride** (Various, eg, Abbott, Baxter)	**Injection:** 30 mEq	In 15, 20, 30 and 100 mL vials and 20 mL additive syringes.
Rx	**Potassium Chloride** (Various, eg, Abbott, American Regent, Baxter, McGuff)	**Injection:** 40 mEq	In 20, 30, 50 and 100 mL vials, 20 mL amps, 20 mL additive syringes.
Rx	**Potassium Chloride** (Various, eg, American Regent, McGuff)	**Injection:** 60 mEq	In 30 mL vials.
Rx	**Potassium Chloride** (Various)	**Injection:** 90 mEq	In 30 mL vials.

POTASSIUM CHLORIDE — INJECTION

Indications

➤*Hypokalemia:* Treatment of potassium deficiency states when oral replacement is not feasible.

Administration and Dosage

Potassium chloride for injection concentrate must be diluted before administration. Care must be taken to ensure there is complete mixing of the potassium chloride with the large volume fluid, particularly if soft or bag-type containers are used.

➤*Hypokalemia:* The dose and rate of administration are dependent upon the specific condition of each patient.

If the serum potassium level is greater than 2.5 mEq/L, potassium can be given at a rate not to exceed 10 mEq/hour and in a concentration of up to 40 mEq/L. The 24 hour total dose should not exceed 200 mEq.

If urgent treatment is indicated (serum potassium level less than 2 mEq/L and electrocardiographic changes or muscle paralysis), potassium chloride may be infused very cautiously at a rate of up to 40 mEq/hour. In such cases, continuous cardiac monitoring is essential. As much as 400 mEq may be administered in a 24 hour period. In critical conditions, potassium chloride may be administered in saline (unless contraindicated) rather than in dextrose containing fluids, as dextrose may lower serum potassium levels.

➤*Storage/Stability:* Store at controlled room temperature 15° to 30°C (59° to 86°F). Use only if solution is clear and the seal is intact and undamaged.

SODIUM BICARBONATE

Rx	**Sodium Bicarbonate** (Hospira)	**Injection:** 4.2% (0.5 mEq/mL)	In 10 mL (5 mEq) syringes.
Rx	**Sodium Bicarbonate** (American Pharmaceutical Partners)		In 10 mL (5 mEq) *Bristoject* syringes.
Rx	**Sodium Bicarbonate** (Hospira)	**Injection:** 5% (0.6 mEq/mL)	In 500 mL[a] (297.5 mEq).
Rx	**Sodium Bicarbonate** (Baxter)		In 500 mL (297.5 mEq).
Rx	**Sodium Bicarbonate** (McGaw)		In 500 mL[a] (297.5 mEq).
Rx	**Sodium Bicarbonate** (Hospira)	**Injection:** 7.5% (0.9 mEq/mL)	In 50 mL (44.6 mEq) amps and 50 mL (44.6 mEq) syringes.
Rx	**Sodium Bicarbonate** (American Regent)		In 50 mL (44.6 mEq) vials.
Rx	**Sodium Bicarbonate** (American Pharmaceutical Partners)		In 50 mL (44.6 mEq) single-dose vials, 50 mL (44.6 mEq) *Bristoject* syringes and 200 mL (179 mEq) *MaxiVials.*
Rx	**Sodium Bicarbonate** (Hospira)	**Injection:** 8.4% (1 mEq/mL)	In 50 mL (50 mEq) fliptop vials and 10 mL (10 mEq) and 50 mL (50 mEq) syringes.
Rx	**Sodium Bicarbonate** (American Regent)		In 50 mL (50 mEq) vials.
Rx	**Sodium Bicarbonate** (American Pharmaceutical Partners)		In 50 mL (50 mEq) vials and 10 and 50 mEq *Bristoject* syringes.
Rx	**Neut** (Abbott)	**Neutralizing Additive Solution**[2]: 4% (0.48 mEq/mL)	In 5 mL (2.4 mEq) fliptop and pintop vials.[a]
Rx	**Sodium Bicarbonate** (American Pharmaceutical Partners)	**Neutralizing Additive Solution**[b]: 4.2% (0.5 mEq/mL)	In 5 mL fill in 6 mL vials (2.5 mEq).

[a] With EDTA.
[b] For use as a neutralizing additive solution to acidic large volume parenterals.

SODIUM BICARBONATE — INJECTION

For information on oral sodium bicarbonate, refer to Systemic Alkalinizers.

Indications

➤*Metabolic acidosis:* In severe renal disease, uncontrolled diabetes, circulatory insufficiency due to shock, anoxia or severe dehydration, extracorporeal circulation of blood, cardiac arrest and severe primary lactic acidosis where a rapid increase in plasma total CO_2 content is crucial. Treat metabolic acidosis in addition to measures designed to control the cause of the acidosis (eg, insulin in uncomplicated diabetes, blood volume restoration in shock). Since an appreciable time interval may elapse before all ancillary effects occur, bicarbonate therapy is indicated to minimize risks inherent to acidosis itself.

At one time it was suggested to administer bicarbonate during cardiopulmonary resuscitation following cardiac arrest; however, recent evidence suggests that little benefit is provided and its use may be detrimental. For treatment of acidosis in this clinical situation, concentrate efforts on restoring ventilation and blood flow. According to the American Heart Association guidelines, use as a last resort after other standard measures have been utilized.

➤*Urinary alkalinization:* In the treatment of certain drug intoxications (eg, salicylates, lithium) and in hemolytic reactions requiring alkalinization of urine to diminish nephrotoxicity of blood pigments.

➤*Severe diarrhea:* Severe diarrhea, which is often accompanied by a significant loss of bicarbonate.

➤*Neutralizing additive solution:* To reduce the incidence of chemical phlebitis and patient discomfort due to vein irritation at or near the infusion site by raising the pH of IV acid solutions.

➤*Unlabeled uses:* Prevention of contrast media nephrotoxicity.

Administration and Dosage

Administer IV or SC following dilution to isotonicity (1.5%). For IV administration, suitable concentrations range from 1.5% (isotonic) to 8.4% (undiluted), depending on the clinical condition and requirements of the patient. Suitable dilution can be calculated from the following formula:

$$conc_1 \times volume_1 = conc_2 \times volume_2$$

Thus, 8.4% × 50 mL = 1.5% × 280 mL; or 7.5% × 50 mL = 1.5% × 250 mL; or 4.2% × 10 mL = 1.5% × 28 mL.

The diluent may be Sterile Water for Injection, Sodium Chloride Injection, 5% Dextrose or other standard electrolyte solutions. For SC administration, an isotonic solution (1.5%) of sodium bicarbonate can be prepared by diluting 1 mL (84 mg) of 8.4% solution with 4.6 mL Sterile Water for Injection. For 7.5% solution, dilute 1 mL (75 mg) with 4 mL Sterile Water for Injection. For 4.2% solution, dilute 1 mL (42 mg) with 1.8 mL Sterile Water for Injection.

➤*Cardiac arrest:* Bicarbonate administration in this situation may be detrimental. See Indications. Administer according to results of arterial blood pH and $PaCO_2$ and calculation of base deficit. Flush IV lines before and after use.

Adults – A rapid IV dose of 200 to 300 mEq of bicarbonate, given as a 7.5% or 8.4% solution. Observe caution where rapid infusion of large quantities of bicarbonate is indicated. Bicarbonate solutions are hypertonic and may produce an undesirable rise in plasma sodium concentration. In cardiac arrest, however, the risks from acidosis exceed those of hypernatremia.

In emergencies, administer 300 to 500 mL of 5% sodium bicarbonate injection as rapidly as possible without overalkalinizing the patient. To avoid overalkalinizing a patient whose own body mechanisms for correcting metabolic acidosis may be maximally stimulated, only one-third to one-half of the calculated dose is administered as rapidly as indicated by the patient's cardiovascular and fluid balance status. Then, redetermine serum pH and bicarbonate concentration.

Infants (≤ 2 years of age) – 4.2% solution for IV administration at a rate not to exceed 8 mEq/kg/day to guard against the possibility of producing hypernatremia, decreasing CSF pressure and inducing intracranial hemorrhage.

Initial dose – 1 to 2 mEq/kg/min given over 1 to 2 minutes followed by 1 mEq/kg every 10 minutes of arrest. If base deficit is known, give calculated dose of 0.3 × kg × base deficit. If only 7.5% or 8.4% sodium bicarbonate is available, dilute 1:1 with 5% Dextrose in Water before administration.

➤*Severe metabolic acidosis:* Administer 90 to 180 mEq/L (≈ 7.5 to 15 g) at a rate of 1 to 1.5 L during the first hour. Adjust to patient's needs for further management.

➤*Less urgent forms of metabolic acidosis:* Sodium Bicarbonate Injection may be added to other IV fluids. The amount of bicarbonate to be given to older children and adults over a 4 to 8 hour period is approximately 2 to 5 mEq/kg, depending on the severity of the acidosis as judged by the lowering of total CO_2 content, blood pH and clinical condition. Initially, an infusion of 2 to 5 mEq/kg over 4 to 8 hours will produce improvement in the acid-base status of the blood.

Alternatively, estimates of the initial dose of sodium bicarbonate may be based on the following equation:

$$0.5\ (L/kg) \times \text{body weight (kg)} \times \text{desired increase in serum } HCO_3^-\ (mEq/L) = \text{bicarbonate dose (mEq) or } 0.5\ (L/kg) \times \text{body weight (kg)} \times \text{base deficit (mEq/L)} = \text{bicarbonate dose (mEq)}.$$

SODIUM BICARBONATE — INJECTION

The next step of therapy is dependent on the clinical response of the patient. If severe symptoms have abated, reduce frequency of administration and dose.

If the CO_2 plasma content is unknown, a safe average dose of sodium bicarbonate is 5 mEq (420 mg)/kg.

It is unwise to attempt full correction of a low total CO_2 content during the first 24 hours, since this may accompany an unrecognized alkalosis due to delayed readjustment of ventilation to normal. Thus, achieving total CO_2 content of about 20 mEq/L at the end of the first day will usually be associated with a normal blood pH. Further modification of the acidosis to completely normal values usually occurs in the presence of normal kidney function when and if the cause of the acidosis can be controlled. Total CO_2 brought to normal or above normal within the first day may be associated with grossly alkaline blood pH.

If administration is controlled by a pumping device, discontinue pumping action before the container runs dry or air embolism may result.

➤*Neutralizing additive solution:* One vial of neutralizing additive solution added to 1 L of any of the commonly used parenteral solutions including Dextrose, Sodium Chloride, Ringer's, etc, will increase the pH to a more physiologic range (specific pH may vary slightly).

Note – Some products such as amino acid solutions and multiple electrolyte solutions containing dextrose will not be brought to near physiologic pH by the addition of sodium bicarbonate neutralizing additive solution. This is due to the relatively high buffer capacity of these fluids.

➤*Admixture incompatibilities:* Avoid adding sodium bicarbonate to parenteral solutions containing **calcium**, except where compatibility is established; precipitation or haze may result. **Norepinephrine** and **dobutamine** are incompatible.

➤*Storage/Stability:* Store at 15° to 30°C (59° to 86°F). Avoid excessive heat. Protect from freezing. Brief exposure up to 40°C does not adversely affect the product. Replace administration apparatus at least once every 24 hours.

Actions

➤*Pharmacology:* Increases plasma bicarbonate; buffers excess hydrogen ion concentration; raises blood pH; reverses the clinical manifestations of acidosis.

One g sodium bicarbonate provides 11.9 mEq each of sodium and bicarbonate.

➤*Pharmacokinetics:* Sodium bicarbonate in water dissociates to provide sodium (Na^+) and bicarbonate (HCO_3^-) ions. Sodium is the principal cation of extracellular fluid. Bicarbonate is a normal constituent of body fluids and normal plasma level ranges from 24 to 31 mEq/L. Plasma concentration is regulated by the kidney. Bicarbonate anion is considered "labile" since, at a proper concentration of hydrogen ion (H^+), it may be converted to carbonic acid (H_2CO_3), then to its volatile form, carbon dioxide (CO_2), excreted by lungs. Normally, a ratio of 1:20 (carbonic acid: bicarbonate) is present in extracellular fluid. In a healthy adult with normal kidney function, almost all the glomerular filtered bicarbonate ion is reabsorbed; less than 1% is excreted in urine.

Contraindications

Losing chloride by vomiting or from continuous GI suction; receiving diuretics known to produce a hypochloremic alkalosis; metabolic and respiratory alkalosis; hypocalcemia in which alkalosis may produce tetany, hypertension, convulsions or congestive heart failure (CHF); when sodium use could be clinically detrimental.

➤*Neutralizing additive solution:* Do not use as a systemic alkalinizer.

Warnings

➤*Cardiac effects:*

Cardiac arrest – The risk of rapid infusion must be weighed against the potential for fatality due to acidosis.

CHF – Since sodium accompanies bicarbonate, use cautiously in patients with CHF or other edematous or sodium-retaining states.

➤*Fluid/Solute overload:* IV administration can cause fluid or solute overloading resulting in dilution of serum electrolyte concentrations, overhydration, congested states or pulmonary edema. The risk of dilutional states is inversely proportional to the electrolyte concentrations of administered parenteral solutions. The risk of solute overload causing congested states with peripheral and acute pulmonary edema is directly proportional to the electrolyte concentrations of such solutions. Rapid or excessive administration of Sodium Bicarbonate Injection may produce tetany due to a decrease in ionized calcium and hypokalemia as potassium reenters the cells. Hypertonic solutions may cause vein damage. Avoid extravasation.

➤*Neonates and children (younger than 2 years old):* Rapid injection (10 mL/min) of hypertonic sodium bicarbonate solutions may produce hypernatremia, a decrease in cerebrospinal fluid pressure and possible intracranial hemorrhage. Do not administer more than 8 mEq/kg/day. A 4.2% solution is preferred for such slow administration.

➤*Renal function impairment:* Administration of solutions containing sodium ions may result in sodium retention. Use with caution. Also use cautiously in oliguria or anuria.

➤*Elderly:* Exercise particular care when administering sodium-containing solutions to elderly or postoperative patients with renal or cardiovascular insuffiency, with or without CHF.

➤*Pregnancy: Category C.* It is not known whether sodium bicarbonate can cause fetal harm when administered to a pregnant woman. Use only if clearly needed.

➤*Lactation:* It is not known whether this drug is excreted in breast milk. Exercise caution when administering to a nursing woman.

Precautions

➤*Monitoring:* Adverse reactions may result from an excess or deficit of one or more of the ions in the solution; frequent monitoring of electrolyte levels is essential.

➤*Avoid overdosage and alkalosis:* Avoid overdosage and alkalosis by giving repeated small doses and periodic monitoring by appropriate laboratory tests.

➤*Potassium depletion:* Potassium depletion may predispose to metabolic alkalosis, and coexistent hypocalcemia may be associated with carpopedal spasm as the plasma pH rises. Minimize by treating electrolyte imbalances prior to or concomitantly with bicarbonate.

➤*Chloride loss:* Patients losing chloride by vomiting or GI intubation are more susceptible to developing severe alkalosis if given alkalinizing agents.

➤*Neutralizing additive solution:* Administer this solution promptly. When introducing additives, mix thoroughly and do not store. Raising pH of IV fluids with neutralizing additive solution will only reduce incidence of chemical irritation caused by infusate; it will not diminish any foreign body effects caused by needle or catheter.

Extraordinary electrolyte losses such as may occur during protracted nasogastric suction, vomiting, diarrhea or GI fistula drainage may necessitate additional electrolyte supplementation.

Drug Interactions

Sodium Bicarbonate Drug Interactions

Precipitant drug	Object drug[a]		Description
Sodium bicarbonate	Chlorpropamide Lithium Methotrexate Salicylates Tetracyclines	⬇	The renal clearance of these agents may be increased due to alkalinization of the urine, possibly resulting in a decreased pharmacologic effect.
Sodium bicarbonate	Anorexiants Flecainide Mecamylamine Quinidine Sympathomimetics	⬆	The renal clearance of these agents may be decreased due to alkalinizaton of the urine, possibly resulting in increased pharmacologic or toxic effects.

[a] ⬆ = Object drug increased. ⬇ = Object drug decreased.

Adverse Reactions

If an adverse reaction does occur, discontinue the infusion, evaluate the patient, institute appropriate therapeutic countermeasures and save the remainder of the fluid for examination if deemed necessary.

➤*Clinical cellulitis:* Extravasation of IV hypertonic solutions of sodium bicarbonate may cause chemical cellulitis (because of their alkalinity), with tissue necrosis, ulceration or sloughing at the site of infiltration. Prompt elevation of the part, warmth and local injection of lidocaine or hyaluronidase are recommended to prevent sloughing.

Rapid infusion – Too rapid infusion of hypertonic solutions may cause local pain and venous irritation. Adjust the rate of administration according to tolerance. Use of the largest peripheral vein and a well placed small bore needle is recommended.

Too rapid or excessive administration may result in hypernatremia and alkalosis accompanied by hyperirritability or tetany. Hypernatremia may be associated with edema and exacerbation of CHF due to the retention of water, resulting in an expanded extracellular fluid volume.

Reactions due to solution or administration technique – Reactions that may occur because of the solution or the technique of administration include febrile response, infection at the site of injection, venous thrombosis or phlebitis extending from the injection site, extravasation and hypervolemia.

Overdosage

➤*Symptoms:* Excessive or too rapid administration may produce alkalosis. Severe alkalosis may be accompanied by hyperirritability or tetany.

➤*Treatment:* Discontinue sodium bicarbonate. Control symptoms of alkalosis by rebreathing expired air from a paper bag or rebreathing mask or, if more severe, by parenteral injections of calcium gluconate (to control tetany and hyperexcitability). Correct severe alkalosis by IV infusion of 2.14% ammonium chloride solution, except in patients with hepatic disease, in whom ammonia use is contraindicated. Sodium chloride (0.9%) IV or potassium chloride may be indicated if there is hypokalemia.

SODIUM LACTATE

Rx	**1/6 Molar Sodium Lactate** (Various, eg, Abbott, Baxter)	**Injection:** 167 mEq/L each of sodium and lactate ions	In 500 and 1000 mL.

SODIUM LACTATE — INJECTION

Complete and comparative prescribing information for these products begins in the Sodium Bicarbonate monograph.

Indications

➤*Metabolic acidosis:* As a source of bicarbonate for prevention or control of mild to moderate metabolic acidosis in patients with restricted oral intake whose oxidative processes are not seriously impaired.

Administration and Dosage

Sodium lactate injection, 50 mEq (5 mEq/mL), is administered intravenously only after addition to a larger volume of fluid. The amount of sodium ion and lactate ion to be added to larger volume intravenous fluids should be determined in accordance with the electrolyte requirements of each individual patient.

All or part of the contents of 1 (50 mEq in 10 mL) or more vial containers may be added to other intravenous solutions to provide any desired number of milliequivalents of lactate anion (with the same number of milliequivalents of Na^+). The contents of 1 container (50 mEq in 10 mL) added to 290 mL of a nonelectrolyte solution or of Sterile Water for Injection will provide 300 mL of an approximately isotonic (⅙ molar) concentration of sodium lactate (1.9%), containing 167 mEq/L each of Na^+ and lactate anion.

➤*Storage/Stability:* Store at controlled room temperature 15° to 30°C (59° to 86°F).

Do not administer unless solution is clear and seal is intact. Discard unused portion.

Actions

➤*Pharmacology:* Lactate anion ($CH_3CH(OH)COO^-$) serves the important purpose of providing "raw material" for subsequent regeneration of bicarbonate (HCO_3^- and thus acts as a source (alternate) of bicarbonate when normal production and utilization of lactic acid is not impaired as a result of disordered lactate metabolism. Lactate anion is usually present in extracellular fluid at a level of less than 1 mEq/L, but may attain a level of 10 mEq/L during exercise. It is seldom measured as such and thus is one of the "unmeasured anions" ("anion gap") in determinations of the ionic composition of plasma.

Since metabolic conversion of lactate to bicarbonate is dependent on the integrity of cellular oxidative processes, lactate may be inadequate or ineffective as a source of bicarbonate in patients suffering from acidosis associated with shock or other disorders involving reduced perfusion of body tissues. When oxidative activity is intact, 1 to 2 hours time is required for conversion of lactate to bicarbonate.

The sodium (Na^+) ion combines with bicarbonate ion produced from carbon dioxide of the body and thus retains bicarbonate to combat metabolic acidosis (bicarbonate deficiency). The normal plasma level of lactate ranges from 0.9 to 1.9 mEq/L.

Contraindications

Hypernatremia or fluid retention. It should not be used in conditions in which lactate levels are increased (eg, shock, congestive heart failure, respiratory alkalosis) or in which utilization of lactate is diminished (eg, anoxia, beriberi). Not for use in the treatment of lactic acidosis.

Warnings

➤*Sodium solutions:* Solutions containing sodium ions should be used with great care, if at all, in patients with congestive heart failure, severe renal insufficiency, and in clinical states in which there exists edema with sodium retention.

➤*Fluid/solute overload:* The IV administration of this solution (after appropriate dilution) can cause fluid or solute overloading resulting in dilution of other serum electrolyte concentrations, overhydration, congested states, or pulmonary edema.

➤*Hypokalemia:* Excessive administration of potassium-free solutions may result in significant hypokalemia.

➤*Severe acidosis:* It is not intended nor effective for correcting severe acidotic states which require immediate restoration of plasma bicarbonate levels. Sodium lactate has no advantage over sodium bicarbonate and may be detrimental in the management of lactic acidosis.

➤*Renal function impairment:* In patients with diminished renal function, administration of solutions containing sodium ions may result in sodium retention.

➤*Pregnancy: Category C.* Animal reproduction studies have not been conducted with sodium lactate. It is also not known whether sodium lactate can cause fetal harm when administered to a pregnant woman or can affect reproduction capacity. Sodium lactate should be given to a pregnant woman only if clearly needed.

Precautions

➤*Administration:* Sodium lactate injection must be suitably diluted before infusion to avoid a sudden increase in the level of sodium or lactate. Too rapid administration and overdosage should be avoided.

➤*Sodium-retaining states:* The potentially large loads of sodium given with lactate require that caution be exercised in patients with congestive heart failure or other edematous or sodium-retaining states, as well as in patients with oliguria or anuria.

➤*Lactase solution:* Solutions containing lactate ions should be used with caution as excess administration may result in metabolic alkalosis.

Drug Interactions

➤*Corticosteroids or corticotropin:* Caution must be exercised in the administration of parenteral fluids especially those containing sodium ions, to patients receiving corticosteroids or corticotropin.

Adverse Reactions

Adverse reactions to sodium lactate are essentially limited to overdosage of either sodium or lactate ions.

Overdosage

➤*Treatment:* In the event of overdosage, discontinue infusion containing sodium lactate immediately and institute corrective therapy as indicated to reduce elevated serum sodium levels and restore acid-base balance if necessary.

SODIUM ACETATE

Rx	**Sodium Acetate** (Various, eg, Abbott, American Regent)	**Injection:** 2 mEq each of sodium and acetate per mL (16.4%)	In 20, 50 and 100 mL vials.
Rx	**Sodium Acetate** (Various, eg, American Regent)	**Injection:** 4 mEq each of sodium and acetate per mL (32.8%)	In 50 and 100 mL vials.

SODIUM ACETATE — INJECTION

Complete and comparative prescribing information for these products begins in the Sodium Bicarbonate monograph.

Indications

➤*Hyponatremia:* As a source of sodium for addition to large volume IV fluids to prevent or correct hyponatremia in patients with restricted or no oral intake. It is also useful as an additive for preparing specific IV fluid formulas when the needs of the patient cannot be met by standard electrolyte or nutrient solutions.

Administration and Dosage

➤*Approved by the FDA:* May 4, 1983.

Sodium acetate is administered intravenously only after dilution in a larger volume of fluid. The dose and rate of administration are dependent upon the individual needs of the patient. Serum sodium should be monitored as a guide to dosage. Using aseptic technique, all or part of the contents of 1 or more vials may be added to other IV fluids to provide any desired number of milliequivalents (mEq) of sodium with an equal number of acetate.

Once the sterile dispensing set has been inserted into the container, withdrawal of the contents should be accomplished without delay. However, if this is not possible, a maximum time of 4 hours from the initial entry may be allowed to complete fluid aliquoting/transferring operations.

➤*Storage/Stability:* Store at controlled room temperature 15° to 30°C (59° to 86°F).

Discard the container no later than 4 hours after initial closure puncture. Do not administer unless solution is clear and seal is intact.

Actions

➤*Pharmacology:* Sodium (NA^+) is the principal cation of extracellular fluid. It comprises more than 90% of total cations at its normal plasma concentration of approximately 140 mEq/L. The sodium ion exerts a primary role in controlling total body water and its distribution.

Acetate (CH_3COO^-), a source of hydrogen ion acceptors, is an alternate source of bicarbonate (HCO_3^-) by metabolic conversion in the liver. This has been shown to proceed readily, even in the presence of severe liver disease.

Contraindications

Hypernatremia or fluid retention.

Warnings

➤*Administration:* Sodium acetate must be diluted before use.

To avoid sodium overload and water retention, infuse sodium-containing solutions slowly.

Electrolytes

SODIUM ACETATE — INJECTION

➤*Sodium solutions:* Solutions containing sodium ions should be used with great care, if at all, in patients with congestive heart failure, severe renal insufficiency and in clinical states in which there exists edema with sodium retention.

➤*Acetate solutions:* Solutions containing acetate ions should be used with great care in patients with metabolic or respiratory alkalosis. Acetate should be administered with great care in those conditions in which there is an increased level or an impaired utilization of this ion, such as severe hepatic insufficiency.

Solutions containing acetate ions should be used with caution as excess administration may result in metabolic alkalosis.

➤*Fluid/solute overload:* The IV administration of this solution (after appropriate dilution) can cause fluid or solute overloading resulting in dilution of other serum electrolyte concentrations, overhydration, congested states, or pulmonary edema. Excessive administration of potassium free solutions may result in significant hypokalemia.

➤*Renal function impairment:* In patients with diminished renal function, administration of solutions containing sodium ions may result in sodium retention.

➤*Pregnancy:* *Category C.* Animal reproduction studies have not been conducted with sodium acetate. It is also not known whether sodium acetate can cause fetal harm when administered to a pregnant woman or can affect reproduction capacity. Sodium acetate should be given to a pregnant woman only if clearly needed.

➤*Children:* Sodium acetate is not intended for pediatric use.

Precautions

➤*Monitoring:* Sodium replacement therapy should be guided primarily by the serum sodium level.

➤*Sodium retaining states:* Caution should be exercised in administering sodium-containing solutions to patients with severe renal function impairment, cirrhosis, cardiac failure or other edematous or sodium-retaining states, as well as in patients with oliguria or anuria.

Drug Interactions

➤*Corticosteroids or corticotropin:* Caution must be exercised in the administration of parenteral fluids, especially those containing sodium ions, to patients receiving corticosteroids or corticotropin.

Overdosage

➤*Treatment:* In the event of overdosage, discontinue infusion-containing sodium acetate immediately and institute corrective therapy as indicated to reduce elevated serum sodium levels and restore acid-base balance, if necessary.

AMMONIUM CHLORIDE

Rx	**Ammonium Chloride** (Hospira)	**Injection**: 26.75% (5 mEq/mL) To be diluted before infusion	In 20 mL (100 mEq) vials.[a]

[a] With 2 mg EDTA.

AMMONIUM CHLORIDE — INJECTION

Indications

➤*Hypochloremia/metabolic alkalosis:* Treatment of patients with hypochloremic states and metabolic alkalosis.

Administration and Dosage

Ammonium chloride injection, USP is administered intravenously and must be diluted before use. Solutions for intravenous infusion should not exceed a concentration of 1% to 2% of ammonium chloride.

Dosage is dependent upon the condition and tolerance of the patient. It is recommended that the contents of 1 to 2 vials (100 to 200 mEq) be added to 500 or 1000 mL of isotonic (0.9%) sodium chloride injection. The rate of intravenous infusion should not exceed 5 mL/min in adults (approximately 3 hours for infusion of 1000 mL). Dosage should be monitored by repeated serum bicarbonate determinations.

➤*Storage/Stability:* Store at controlled room temperature 15° to 30°C (59° to 86°F).

When exposed to low temperatures, concentrated solutions of ammonium chloride may crystallize. If crystals are observed, the vial should be warmed to room temperature in a water bath prior to use. Do not administer unless the solution is clear and seal is intact. Discard unused portion.

Actions

➤*Pharmacology:* The ammonium ion (NH_4^+) in the body plays an important role in the maintenance of acid-base balance. The kidney uses ammonium (NH_4^+) in place of sodium (Na^+) to combine with fixed anions in maintaining acid-base balance, especially as a homeostatic compensatory mechanism in metabolic acidosis.

When a loss of hydrogen ions (H^+) occurs and serum chloride (Cl^-) decreases, sodium is made available for combination with bicarbonate (HCO_3^-). This creates an excess of sodium bicarbonate ($NaHCO_3$) which leads to a rise in blood pH and a state of metabolic alkalosis.

The therapeutic effects of ammonium chloride depend upon the ability of the kidney to utilize ammonia in the excretion of an excess of fixed anions and the conversion of ammonia to urea by the liver, thereby liberating hydrogen (H^+) and chloride (Cl^-) ions into the extracellular fluid.

One g of ammonium chloride provides 18.7 mEq of chloride.

Contraindications

Severe impairment of renal or hepatic function; metabolic alkalosis due to vomiting of hydrochloric acid is accompanied by loss of sodium (excretion of sodium bicarbonate in the urine).

Warnings

➤*Pregnancy:* *Category C.* Animal reproduction studies have not been conducted with ammonium chloride. It is also not known whether ammonium chloride can cause fetal harm when administered to a pregnant woman or can affect reproduction capacity. Ammonium chloride should be given to a pregnant woman only if clearly needed.

Precautions

➤*Ammonium toxicity:* Patients receiving ammonium chloride should be constantly observed for symptoms of ammonia toxicity (pallor, sweating, retching, irregular breathing, bradycardia, cardiac arrhythmias, local and general twitching, tonic convulsions and coma).

➤*Respiratory acidosis:* It should be used with caution in patients with high total CO_2 and buffer base secondary to primary respiratory acidosis.

➤*Administration:* IV administration should be slow to avoid local irritation and toxic effects.

Adverse Reactions

Rapid intravenous administration of ammonium chloride may be accompanied by pain or irritation at the site of injection or along the venous route.

If an adverse reaction does occur, discontinue the infusion, evaluate the patient, institute appropriate therapeutic countermeasures and save the remainder of the fluid for examination if deemed necessary.

➤*Reactions due to solution or administration technique:* Reactions which may occur because of the solution or the technique of administration include febrile response, infection at the site of injection, venous thrombosis or phlebitis extending from the site of injection, extravasation and hypervolemia (from large volume diluent).

Overdosage

➤*Symptoms:* Overdosage of ammonium chloride has resulted in a serious degree of metabolic acidosis, disorientation, confusion and coma.

➤*Treatment:* Should metabolic acidosis occur following overdosage, the administration of an alkalinizing solution such as sodium bicarbonate or sodium lactate will serve to correct the acidosis.

Trace Metals

Refer to the Trace Elements section for information on oral iodine, manganese, and zinc. Iodine is used as a thyroid agent (see monograph in Thyroid Drugs section) and as an expectorant (see monograph in Respiratory Drugs chapter).

Indications

Supplement to IV solutions given for TPN.

Administration and Dosage

Administer IV after dilution. Frequently monitor plasma levels and clinical status.

➤*Preparation:* Trace metals are usually physically compatible together, and with the electrolytes usually present in amino acid/dextrose solution used for TPN.

Actions

➤*Pharmacology:*

Chromium – Trivalent chromium is part of glucose tolerance factor, an essential activator of insulin-mediated reactions. Chromium helps maintain normal glucose metabolism and peripheral nerve function.

Serum chromium is bound to transferrin (siderophilin). Administration of chromium supplements to chromium deficient patients can result in normalization of the glucose tolerance curve from the diabetic-like curve typical of chromium deficiency. This response is viewed as a more meaningful indicator than serum chromium levels.

Copper – Copper serves as a cofactor for serum ceruloplasmin, an oxidase necessary for proper formation of the iron carrier protein, transferrin. Copper also helps maintain normal rates of red and white blood cell formation. The daily turnover of copper through ceruloplasmin is approximately 0.5 mg.

Iodine – Absorption from the GI tract is rapid and complete. Skin and lungs can also absorb iodine. On administration, iodide equilibrates in extracellular fluids and although all body cells contain iodide, it is specifically concentrated by the thyroid gland, which is estimated to contain 7 to 8 mg total iodine.

Other important organs to take up iodide are salivary glands, gastric mucosa, choroid plexus, skin, hair, mammary glands and placenta. Iodine in saliva and gastric mucosal secretions is reabsorbed and recycled. The circulating iodine is hormonal thyroxine of which 30 to 70 mcg is protein bound and 0.5 mcg is free thyroxine.

Manganese – Manganese serves as an activator for several enzymes. During minimal intake, 20 mcg/day is retained. Manganese is bound to a specific transport protein, transmanganin, and is widely distributed, but it concentrates in mitochondria-rich tissues such as brain, kidney, pancreas and liver.

Molybdenum – Molybdenum is a constituent of the enzymes xanthine oxidase, sulfite oxidase and aldehyde oxidase. Tissue storage of molybdenum varies with the intake levels and is affected by the amount of copper and sulfate in the diet. Consistent levels are observed in liver, kidney and adrenal cortex.

Selenium – Selenium is part of glutathione peroxidase which protects cell components from oxidative damage due to peroxides produced in cellular metabolism.

Pediatric conditions, Keshan disease and Kwashiorkor have been associated with low dietary intake of selenium. The conditions are endemic to geographic areas with low selenium soil content. Dietary supplementation with selenium salts reduces the incidence of the conditions among affected children.

Zinc – Zinc serves as a cofactor for more than 70 different enzymes. Zinc facilitates wound healing, helps maintain normal growth rates, normal skin hydration and the senses of taste and smell. Zinc resides in muscle, bone, skin, kidney, liver, pancreas, retina, prostate and particularly in the red and white blood cells. Zinc binds to plasma albumin, α_2–macroglobulin and some plasma amino acids including histidine, cysteine, threonine, glycine and asparagine.

At plasma levels less than 20 mcg/dL, dermatitis followed by alopecia has been reported for TPN patients. The following table summarizes deficiency symptoms, excretion routes and normal plasma levels for various trace metals. The serum level at which deficiency symptoms appear for many of these elements is not well defined.

Trace Metals: Deficiency/Excretion/Plasma Levels

Trace metal	Symptoms of deficiency	Excretion	Normal plasma levels
Copper	Leukopenia, neutropenia, anemia, decreased ceruloplasmin levels, impaired transferrin formation of secondary iron deficiency, skeletal abnormalities, defective tissue formation.	Bile (80%), intestinal wall (16%), urine (4%)	80-163 mcg/dL
Chromium	Impaired glucose tolerance, peripheral neuropathy, ataxia, confusion.	Kidneys (3-50 mcg/day), bile	1-5 mcg/L[a]
Iodine	Impaired thyroid function, goiter, cretinism.	Kidneys, bile	0.5-1.5 mcg/dL
Manganese	Nausea, vomiting, weight loss, dermatitis, changes in growth and hair color.	Bile; if obstruction present, then pancreatic juice or return to intestinal lumen. Urine (negligible)	6-12 mcg/L (whole blood)
Molybdenum	Tachycardia, tachypnea, headache, night blindness, nausea, vomiting, central scotomas, edema, lethargy, disorientation, coma, hypermethioninemia, hypouricemia, hypouricuria, low urinary excretion of inorganic sulfate and elevated urinary excretion of thiosulfate.	Primarily renal, some biliary	nd
Selenium	Muscle pain & tenderness, cardiomyopathy, Kwashiorkor, Keshan disease.	Urine, feces, lungs, skin	nd[b]
Zinc	Diarrhea, apathy, depression, parakeratosis, hypogeusia, anorexia, dysosmia, geophagia, hypogonadism, growth retardation, anemia, hepatosplenomegaly, impaired wound healing.	90% in stools; urine, perspiration	100 ± 12 mcg/dL

[a] Not considered a meaningful index of tissue stores.

[b] nd = No data

Contraindications

Do not give undiluted by direct injection into a peripheral vein because of the potential for infusion phlebitis, tissue irritation and potential to increase renal loss of minerals from a bolus injection. Copper-deficient patients. See Warnings.

Warnings

➤*Renal failure or biliary tract obstruction:* Metals may accumulate. Serial determinations of serum trace metal concentrations may be a valuable guideline.

Consider the possibility of **copper** and **manganese** retention in patients with biliary tract obstruction. Ancillary routes of manganese excretion include pancreatic secretions or reabsorption into the lumen of the duodenum, jejunum or ileum.

Adjust, reduce or omit use in renal dysfunction or GI malfunction. Consider contributions from blood transfusions. Frequently determine plasma levels.

➤*Wilson's disease:* Avoid administering **copper** supplements to patients with this genetic disorder of copper metabolism.

➤*Decreased serum levels:* Administration of **copper** in the absence of **zinc** and of zinc in the absence of copper may cause decreases in plasma levels. Perform periodic determinations of plasma zinc and copper for subsequent administrations.

➤*Copper deficiency:* **Molybdenum** promotes tissue **copper** mobilization and increases urinary copper excretion; excessive amounts produce a copper deficiency. Frequently check the metabolism of copper in patients receiving molybdenum.

➤*Multiple trace element solutions:* Multiple trace element solutions present a risk of overdosage when the need for one trace element is appreciably higher than that for the other trace elements in the formulation. Administration of trace metals as separate entities may be required.

➤*Hypersensitivity reactions:* Sensitization to **iodides** and deaths due to anaphylactic shock after use have occurred (see Adverse Reactions). Evaluate patient for hypersensitivity before initiating TPN. If patient develops a reaction, withdraw TPN immediately and institute appropriate measures. Refer to Management of Acute Hypersensitivity.

➤*Pregnancy: Category C.* It is not known whether trace metals can cause fetal harm or can affect reproductive capacity. Give to a pregnant woman only if clearly needed.

Molybdenum crosses the placenta. Presence of **selenium** in placenta and umbilical cord blood has been reported.

Precautions

➤*Replacement trace metal therapy:* Replacement trace metal therapy beyond maintenance requirements may be necessary in protracted vomiting or diarrhea, in patients with fistula drainage or nasogastric suction or in acute catabolic states.

➤*Diabetes mellitus:* In assessing the contribution of chromium supplements to maintenance of glucose homeostasis, consider that the patient may be diabetic.

➤*Iodine:* Iodine is readily absorbed through skin, lungs and mucous membranes. Give consideration to the environment, topical skin disinfection and wound treatment practices with surgical swabs and solutions containing iodine and povidone iodine. Air in the coastal areas is known to contain more iodine than inland areas.

➤*Benzyl alcohol:* Some of these products contain benzyl alcohol, which has been associated with a fatal gasping syndrome in premature infants.

Adverse Reactions

Symptoms of toxicity are unlikely to occur at recommended doses.

Hypersensitivity to **iodides** may result in angioneurotic edema, cutaneous and mucosal hemorrhages, fever, arthralgia, lymph node enlargement and eosinophilia. (See Warnings.)

Overdosage

➤*Chromium:* Nausea, vomiting, GI ulcers, renal/hepatic damage, convulsions, coma.

➤*Copper:* Prostration, behavior change, diarrhea, progressive marasmus, hypotonia, photophobia, hepatic damage and peripheral edema have occurred with a serum copper level of 286 mcg/dL. Penicillamine is an effective antidote.

➤*Iodine:* Symptoms of chronic poisoning include metallic taste, sore mouth, increased salivation, coryza, sneezing, swelling of the eyelids, severe headache, pulmonary edema, tenderness of salivary glands, acneiform skin lesions and skin eruptions. Abundant fluid and salt intake helps in elimination of iodides.

➤*Manganese:* "Manganese madness," irritability, speech disturbances, abnormal gait, headache, anorexia, apathy and impotence.

➤*Molybdenum:* Gout-like syndrome with increased blood levels of molybdenum, uric acid and xanthine oxidase.

No data on treatment of molybdenosis in humans is available. Among animals, treatment with copper, sulfate ions and tungsten enhances excretion of molybdenum. The sulfur-containing amino acids, methionine and cysteine, may afford limited protection.

➤*Selenium:* Toxicity symptoms include hair loss, weak nails, dermatitis, dental defects, GI disorders, nervousness, mental depression, metallic taste, vomiting and garlic odor of breath and sweat. Acute poisoning due to ingestion has resulted in death with histopathological changes including fulminating peripheral vascular collapse, internal vascular congestion, diffusely hemorrhagic, congested and edematous lungs and brick-red color gastric mucosa. Death was preceded by coma. No effective antidote is known.

➤*Zinc:* Single IV doses of 1 to 2 mg/kg have been given to adult leukemic patients without toxic manifestations. However, acute toxicity was reported in an adult when 10 mg zinc was infused over 1 hour on each of 4 consecutive days. Profuse sweating, decreased consciousness, blurred vision, tachycardia (140/min) and marked hypothermia (94.2°F) on the fourth day were accompanied by a serum zinc concentration of 207 mcg/dL. Symptoms abated within 3 hours.

Patients receiving an inadvertent overdose (50 to 70 mg zinc/day) developed hyperamylasemia (557 to 1850 Klein units; normal, 130 to 310).

Death resulted from 1683 mg zinc IV over 60 hours to a 72-year-old patient. Symptoms included hypotension (80/40 mm Hg), pulmonary edema, diarrhea, vomiting, jaundice and oliguria with a serum zinc level of 4184 mcg/dL.

Calcium supplements may confer a protective effect against zinc toxicity.

ZINC

Rx	**Zinc Sulfate** (Various, eg, American Regent, Loch)	**Injection**: 1 mg/mL (as sulfate [as 4.39 mg heptahydrate or 2.46 mg anhydrous])	In 10 and 30 mL vials.
Rx	**Zinca-Pak** (Smith & Nephew SoloPak)		In 10 and 30[a] mL vials.
Rx	**Zinc Sulfate** (Various, eg, Loch)	**Injection**: 5 mg/mL (as 21.95 mg sulfate)	In 5 and 10 mL vials.
Rx	**Zinca-Pak** (Smith & Nephew SoloPak)		In 5 mL vials.
Rx	**Zinc** (Various, eg, Abbott)	**Injection**: 1 mg/mL (as 2.09 mg chloride)	In 10 mL vials.

[a] With 0.9% benzyl alcohol.

ZINC SULFATE — INJECTION

Complete and comparative prescribing information for these products begins in the Zinc Supplements group monograph.

Indications

➤*Zinc supplement:* As a supplement to intravenous solutions given for TPN. Administration helps to maintain plasma levels and to prevent depletion of endogenous stores.

Administration and Dosage

➤*Adults:* Zinc sulfate injection, USP provides 1 mg/mL. For metabolically stable adults receiving total parenteral nutrition (TPN), the suggested intravenous dosage level is 2.5 mg to 4 mg/day. An additional 2 mg/day is suggested for acute catabolic states. For the stable adult with fluid loss from the small bowel, an additional 12.2 mg/L of TPN solution, or an additional 17.1 mg/kg of stool or ileostomy output is recommended. Frequent monitoring of zinc blood levels is suggested for patients receiving more than the usual maintenance dosage level of zinc.

➤*Children:* For full-term infants and children up to 5 years of age, 100 mcg/kg/day is recommended. For premature infants (birth weight less than 1500 g) up to 3 kg in body weight, 300 mcg/kg/day is suggested.

➤*Admixture compatibility:* Zinc is physically compatible with the electrolytes and vitamins usually present in the amino acid/dextrose solution used for TPN.

➤*Storage / Stability:* Store at controlled room temperature 15° to 30°C (59° to 86°F) (See USP).

Actions

➤*Pharmacology:* Zinc has been identified as a cofactor for over 70 different enzymes, including alkaline phosphatase, lactic dehydrogenase, and both RNA and DNA polymerase. Zinc facilitates wound healing, helps maintain normal growth rates, normal skin hydration and the senses of taste and smell.

Providing zinc during TPN prevents development of the following deficiency symptoms: Parakeratosis, hypogeusia, anorexia, dysosmia, geophagia, hypogonadism, growth retardation and hepatosplenomegaly. At plasma levels less than 20 mcg/100 mL, dermatitis followed by alopecia has been reported by TPN patients.

Contraindications

Should not be given undiluted by direct injection into a peripheral vein because of the likelihood of infusion phlebitis and the potential to increase renal loss of zinc from a bolus injection.

Warnings

➤*Aluminum toxicity:* This product contains aluminum that may be toxic. Aluminum may reach toxic levels with prolonged parenteral administration if kidney function is impaired. Premature neonates are particularly at risk because their kidneys are immature, and they require large amounts of calcium and phosphate solutions, which contain aluminum.

Research indicates that patients with impaired kidney function, including premature neonates, who receive parenteral levels of aluminum at greater than 4 to 5 mcg/kg/day accumulate aluminum at levels associated with central nervous system and bone toxicity. Tissue loading may occur at even lower rates of administration.

➤*Renal function impairment:* As zinc is eliminated via the kidneys, zinc supplements may be reduced or omitted in renal dysfunction, unless assays of plasma zinc levels are performed.

➤*Pregnancy:* Safety for use in pregnancy has not been established. Use of zinc in women of childbearing potential requires that anticipated benefits be weighed against possible hazards.

Precautions

➤*Concomitant copper therapy:* Administration of zinc in the absence of copper may cause a decrease in serum copper levels. Periodic determination of serum copper as well as zinc are suggested as a guideline for subsequent zinc administration.

Overdosage

➤*Symptoms:* Symptoms of zinc overdosage resulting from oral ingestion of zinc sulfate in large amounts (30 and 44 g, respectively) have resulted in death. Symptoms include nausea, vomiting, dehydration, electrolyte imbalances, dizziness, abdominal pain, lethargy and incoordination. Single intravenous doses of 1 to 2 mg zinc/kg body weight have been given to adult leukemic patients without toxic manifestations. Normal plasma levels for zinc vary from approximately 88 to 112 mcg/100 mL. Plasma levels sufficient to produce symptoms of toxic manifestations in humans are not known. Calcium supplements may confer a protective effect against zinc toxicity.

COPPER

Rx	**Copper** (Abbott)	**Injection**: 0.4 mg/mL (as 1.07 mg cupric Cl)	In 10 mL vials.
Rx	**Cupric Sulfate** (Various, eg, American Regent, Loch)	**Injection**: 0.4 mg/mL (as 1.57 mg sulfate)	In 10 and 30 mL vials.
Rx	**Cupric Sulfate** (Various, eg, Loch)	**Injection**: 2 mg/mL (as 7.85 mg sulfate)	In 10 mL vials.

COPPER — INJECTION

Complete and comparative prescribing information begins in the Trace Metals group monograph.

Indications

➤*Copper supplement:* Copper is indicated for use as a supplement to IV solutions given for total parenteral nutrition (TPN).

Administration and Dosage

Copper contains 0.4 mg copper/mL and is administered IV only after dilution. The additive should be diluted in a volume of fluid not less than 100 mL.

➤*Adults:* The suggested additive dosage is 0.5 to 1.5 mg copper/day (1.25 to 3.75 mL/day).

➤*Children:* The suggested additive dosage is 20 mcg copper/kg/day (0.05 mL/kg/day).

➤*Storage / Stability:* Store at controlled room temperature 15° to 30°C (59° to 86°F).

Do not use unless the solution is clear and the seal is intact. Solution contains no preservatives; discard unused portion immediately after admixture procedure is completed.

Trace Metals

MANGANESE

Rx	**Manganese Chloride** (Various, eg, Abbott)	**Injection:** 0.1 mg/mL (as 0.36 mg manganese chloride)	In 10 mL vials.
Rx	**Manganese Sulfate** (Various, eg, American Regent)	**Injection:** 0.1 mg/mL (as 0.31 mg sulfate)	In 10 and 30 mL vials.

MANGANESE SULFATE — INJECTION

Complete and comparative prescribing information begins in the Trace Metals group monograph.

Indications

➤*Manganese supplement:* As a supplement to IV solutions given for total parenteral nutrition (TPN).

Administration and Dosage

Manganese sulfate injection provides 0.1 mg manganese/mL.

➤*Adults:* For the metabolically stable adult receiving TPN, the suggested additive dosage level for manganese is 0.15 to 0.8 mg/day.

➤*Children:* A dosage level of 2 to 10 mcg manganese/kg/day is recommended.

Manganese is physically compatible with the electrolytes and vitamins usually present in the amino acid/dextrose solution used for TPN. Periodic monitoring of manganese plasma levels is suggested as a guideline for subsequent administration.

➤*Storage/Stability:* Store at controlled room temperature 15° to 30°C (59° to 86°F).

MOLYBDENUM

Rx	**Ammonium Molybdate** (Various, eg, American Regent)	**Injection:** 25 mcg/mL (as 46 mcg/mL ammonium molybdate tetrahydrate)	In 10 mL vials.
Rx	**Molypen** (American Pharmaceutical Partners)		In 10 mL vials.

MOLYBDENUM — INJECTION

Complete and comparative prescribing information for these products begins in the Trace Metals group monograph.

Administration and Dosage

➤*Metabolically stable adults:* 20 to 120 mcg/day. For pediatric patients, calculate the additive dosage level by extrapolation.

➤*Deficiency state resulting from prolonged TPN support:* 163 mcg/day for 21 days reverses deficiency symptoms without toxicity.

CHROMIUM

Rx	**Chromium** (Various, eg, Abbott, McGuff)	**Injection:** 4 mcg/mL (as 20.5 mcg chromic chloride hexahydrate)	In 10 and 30 mL vials.
Rx	**Chromic Chloride** (Various)		In 10 and 30[a] mL vials.
Rx	**Chromium Chloride** (Various, eg, American Regent, Raway)		In 10 and 30 mL vials.
Rx	**Chroma-Pak** (Smith & Nephew SoloPak)		In 10 and 30[a] mL vials.
Rx	**Chromic Chloride** (Various)	**Injection:** 20 mcg/mL (as 102.5 mcg chromic chloride hexahydrate)	In 10 mL vials.
Rx	**Chroma-Pak** (Smith & Nephew SoloPak)		In 5 mL vials.

[a] With 0.9% benzyl alcohol.

CHROMIC CHLORIDE — INJECTION

Complete and comparative prescribing information for these products begins in the Trace Metals group monograph.

Indications

➤*Chromium supplement:* As a supplement to IV solutions given for total parenteral nutrition (TPN).

Administration and Dosage

➤*Approved by the FDA:* June 26, 1986

Chromic chloride contains 4 mcg chromium/mL and is administered IV only after dilution. The additive should be administered in a volume of fluid not less than 100 mL.

➤*Adults:* The suggested additive dosage is 10 to 15 mcg chromium/day (2.5 to 3.75 mL/day). The metabolically stable adult with intestinal fluid loss may require 20 mcg chromium/day (5 mL/day), with frequent monitoring of blood levels as a guideline for subsequent administration.

➤*Children:* The suggested additive dosage is 0.14 to 0.2 mcg/kg/day (0.035 to 0.05 mL/kg/day).

➤*Storage/Stability:* Store at controlled room temperature 15° to 30°C (59° to 86°F).

Do not use unless solution is clear and seal is intact. Solution contains no preservatives; discard unused portion immediately after admixture procedure is completed.

SELENIUM

Rx	**Selenium** (Various, eg, American Regent)	**Injection:** 40 mcg/mL (as 65.4 mcg selenious acid)	In 10 mL vials.
Rx	**Sele-Pak** (Smith & Nephew SoloPak)		In 10 and 30[a] mL vials.
Rx	**Selepen** (American Pharmaceutical Partners)		In 10 and 30[a] mL vials.

[a] With 0.9% benzyl alcohol.

SELENIUM — INJECTION

Complete and comparative prescribing information for these products begins in the Trace Metals group monograph.

Indications

➤*Selenium supplement:* As a supplement to IV solutions given for total parenteral nutrition (TPN).

Administration and Dosage

Selenium injection provides 40 mcg selenium/mL.

➤*Adults:* For metabolically stable adults receiving TPN, the suggested additive dosage level is 20 to 40 mcg selenium/day.

In adults with selenium deficiency states resulting from long-term TPN support, selenium as selenomethionine or selenious acid, administered IV at 100 mcg/day for a period of 24 and 31 days, respectively, has been reported to reverse deficiency symptoms without toxicity.

➤*Children:* The suggested additive dosage level is 3 mcg/kg/day.

Selenium is physically compatible with the electrolytes and other trace elements usually present in amino-acid/dextrose solution used for TPN. The normal whole blood range for selenium is ≈ 10 to 37 mcg/100 mL.

➤*Storage/Stability:* Store at controlled room temperature 15° to 30°C (59° to 86°F).

IODINE

Rx	**Iodopen** (American Pharmaceutical Partners)	**Injection:** 100 mcg/mL (as 118 mcg sodium iodide)	In 10 mL vials.

IODINE — INJECTION

Complete and comparative prescribing information for these products begins in the Trace Metals group monograph.

Administration and Dosage

➤*Metabolically stable adults:* 1 to 2 mcg/kg/day (normal adults, 75 to 150 mcg/day).

➤*Pregnant and lactating women, growing children:* 2 to 3 mcg/kg/day.

TRACE METAL COMBINATIONS

Content given per mL solution.

	Product and Distributor	Chromium (as chloride) mcg	Copper (as sulfate) mg	Iodine (as sodium iodine) mcg	Manganese (as sulfate) mg	Selenium (as selenious acid) mcg	Zinc (as sulfate) mg	How Supplied
Rx	**Pedtrace-4** (Fujisawa)	0.85	0.1		0.025		0.5	In 3 and 10 mL vials.
Rx	**Multiple Trace Element Neonatal** (American Regent)	0.85	0.1		0.025		1.5	In 2 mL vials.
Rx	**Neotrace-4** (American Pharmaceutical Partners)							In 2 mL single-dose vials.
Rx	**PedTE-PAK-4** (SoloPak)	1	0.1		0.025		1	In 3 mL vials.
Rx	**PTE-4** (American Pharmaceutical Partners)							In 3 mL vials.
Rx	**4 Trace Elements** (Hospira)	6	0.42[1]		0.37[a]		1.67[a]	In 5 mL vial.
Rx	**M.T.E.-4** (Fujisawa)	4	0.4		0.1		1	In 3, 10 and 30[b] mL vials.
Rx	**MulTE-PAK-4** (SoloPak)							In 3, 10 and 30 mL vials.
Rx	**M.T.E.-4 Concentrated** (Fujisawa)	10	1		0.5		5	In 1 and 10[b] mL vials.
Rx	**PTE-5** (Fujisawa)	1	0.1		0.025	15	1	In 3 and 10 mL vials.
Rx	**M.T.E.-5** (Fujisawa)	4	0.4		0.1	20	1	In 10 mL vials.
Rx	**MulTE-PAK-5** (SoloPak)							In 3 and 10 mL vials.
Rx	**Multiple Trace Element with Selenium** (American Regent)							In 3, 10 and 30[b] mL vials.
Rx	**M.T.E.-5 Concentrated** (Fujisawa)	10	1		0.5	60	5	In 1 and 10[b] mL vials.
Rx	**Multiple Trace Element with Selenium Concentrated** (American Regent)							In 1 mL fill in 2 mL vials and 10[b] mL vials.
Rx	**Multitrace-5 Concentrate** (American Regent)							In 1 mL single-dose and 10 mL multiple-dose vials.[b]
Rx	**M.T.E.-6** (Fujisawa)	4	0.4	25	0.1	20	1	In 10 mL vials.
Rx	**M.T.E.-7[c]** (Fujisawa)							In 10 mL vials.
Rx	**M.T.E.-6 Concentrated** (Fujisawa)	10	1	75	0.5	60	5	In 1 and 10[b] mL vials.

[a] As chloride.
[b] With 0.9% benzyl alcohol.
[c] With 25 mcg molybdenum.

TRACE METAL COMBINATIONS — INJECTION

Complete and comparative prescribing information begins in the Trace Metals group monograph.

Administration and Dosage

See manufacturers' product labeling for individual dosing information.

Therapeutic supplements to provide replacement for extraordinary losses of individual trace metals may be added.

COMBINED ELECTROLYTE SOLUTIONS

Electrolyte content given in mEq/L.

	Product and distributor	Na^+	K^+	Ca^{++}	Mg^{++}	Cl^-	Lactate	Acetate	Gluconate	Phosphate	Osmolarity (mOsm/L)	How supplied
Rx	**Normosol-M[a]** (Abbott)	40	13		3	40		16			109	In 1000 mL single-dose container.
Rx	**Ringer's Injection** (Various, eg, Abbott, Baxter, B. Braun)	≈ 147	4	≈ 4		≈ 156					≈ 310	In 500 and 1000 mL.
Rx	**Lactated Ringer's Injection** (Various, eg, Abbott, Baxter, B. Braun)	130	4	≈ 3		≈ 109	28				≈ 274	In 250, 500, and 1000 mL.
Rx	**Plasma-Lyte R[b]** (Baxter)	140	10	5	3	103	8	47			312	In 1000 mL.
Rx	**Isolyte S pH 7.4** (B. Braun)	141	5		3	98		27	23	1	295	Preservative free. In 500 and 1000 mL.
Rx	**Normosol-R[c]** (Abbott)	140	5		3	98		27	23		294	Preservative free. In 500 and 1000 mL single-dose containers.
Rx	**Normosol-R pH 7.4** (Abbott)										295	Preservative free. In 500 and 1000 mL single-dose containers.
Rx	**Plasma-Lyte 148[b]** (Baxter)										294	In 500 and 1000 mL.
Rx	**Plasma-Lyte A pH 7.4** (Baxter)										294	In 500 and 1000 mL.

COMBINED ELECTROLYTE SOLUTIONS

	Product and distributor	Na^+	K^+	Ca^{++}	Mg^{++}	Cl^-	Lactate	Acetate	Gluconate	Phosphate	Osmolarity (mOsm/L)	How supplied
Rx	**Potassium Chloride in 0.9% Sodium Chloride Injection** (Various, eg, Baxter, B. Braun)	154	20			174					≈ 350	In 1000 mL.
		154	40			194					≈ 390	In 1000 mL.

[a] pH ≈ 6.
[b] pH ≈ 5.5.
[c] pH ≈ 6.6.

COMBINED ELECTROLYTE SOLUTIONS — INTRAVENOUS

Indications

For use in adults and children as a source of electrolytes and water for hydration. Additives to the solutions may help prevent certain electrolyte deficiencies in patients receiving prolonged parenteral fluid therapy (eg, magnesium) or act as alkalinizing agents.

Normosol-R and *Normosol R pH 7.4* are indicated for replacement of acute extracellular fluid volume losses in surgery, trauma, burns, or shock. Both can be used as adjunctive therapy to restore decreased circulatory volume in patients with moderate blood loss. *Normosol-R pH 7.4* also is indicated for use in starting blood (eg, as a priming solution for infusion sets) or as a diluent in packed red blood cell transfusions.

COMBINED ELECTROLYTE CONCENTRATES

Electrolyte content given in mEq/20 mL or mEq/25 mL after dilution.

	Product and distributor	Na^+	K^+	Ca^{++}	Mg^{++}	Cl^-	Acetate	Gluconate	Osmolarity (mOsm/L)	How supplied
Rx	**Lypholyte**[a] (American Pharmaceutical Partners)	25	≈ 40	5	8	≈ 33	≈ 41	5	≈ 7562	In 20 and 40 mL single-dose vials, and 100 and 200 mL *Maxivials*.[b]
Rx	**Multilyte-40**[c] (American Pharmaceutical Partners)								≈ 6015	In 25 mL single-dose vials.
Rx	**Nutrilyte**[a] (American Regent)								≈ 7562	In 20 mL single-dose vials and 100 mL.[b]
Rx	**Lypholyte-II**[a] (American Pharmaceutical Partners)	35	20	4.5	5	35	29.5		≈ 6200	In 20 and 40 mL single-dose vials and 100 and 200 mL *Maxivials*[b].
Rx	**TPN Electrolytes**[a] (Hospira)	35	20	4.5	5	35	29.5		6220	In 100 mL vials.[b]
Rx	**Nutrilyte II**[a] (American Regent)	35	20	4.5	5	35	29.5		≈ 6212	In 20 mL single-dose vials and 100 mL vials.[b]
Rx	**TPN Electrolytes II**[a] (Hospira)	18	18	4.5	5	35	10.5		4320	In 20 mL single-dose and additive syringes.
Rx	**TPN Electrolytes III**[a] (Hospira)	25	40.6	5	8	33.5	40.6	5	7520	In 100 mL vials.[b]
Rx	**Hyperlyte CR**[a] (B. Braun)	25	20	5	5	30	30		5500	In 250 mL *Super-Vials*.[b]
Rx	**Multilyte-20**[c] (American Pharmaceutical Partners)	25	20	5	5	30	25		≈ 4205	In 25 mL single-dose vials.

[a] In mEq/20 mL.
[b] Pharmacy bulk packaging.
[c] In mEq/25 mL.

COMBINED ELECTROLYTE CONCENTRATES — INTRAVENOUS

Indications

To facilitate amino acid utilization and maintain electrolyte balance in adults receiving parenteral nutritional solutions containing amino acids, dextrose, and other sources of calories administered by central or peripheral venous infusion. Also indicated for electrolyte replacement in adult parenteral therapy patients.

Administration and Dosage

These concentrated solutions are not for direct infusion. They are for prescription compounding of IV admixtures only. Dilute to appropriate strength with suitable IV fluid prior to administration. Recommended dosage is 20 mL (*Multilyte-40* and *Multilyte-20* is 25 mL) added to 1 L of amino acid/dextrose solution (TPN). Osmolarity is based on the concentrate.

DEXTROSE-ELECTROLYTE SOLUTIONS

Electrolyte content given in mEq/L.

	Product and distributor	Dextrose (g/L)	Calories (Cal/L)	Na^+	K^+	Ca^{++}	Mg^{++}	Cl^-	Phosphate	Lactate	Acetate	Gluconate	Osmolarity (mOsm/L)	How supplied
Rx	**Ionosol B and 5% Dextrose Injection** (Hospira)	50		57	25		5	49	7[a]	25			426	In 500 and 1,000 mL single-dose containers.
Rx	**Dextrose 2.5% with 0.45% Sodium Chloride** (Various, eg, Abbott, Baxter, B. Braun)	25	85	77				77					280	In 500 and 1000 mL.
Rx	**Dextrose 3.3% and 0.3% Sodium Chloride** (B. Braun)	33	110	51				51					270	In 250, 500, and 1000 mL.
Rx	**Dextrose 5% with 0.2% Sodium Chloride** (Various, eg, Baxter, B. Braun)	50	170	34				34					≈ 320	In 250, 500, and 1000 mL.
Rx	**Dextrose 5% and 0.225% Sodium Chloride** (Hospira)	50	170	38.5				38.5					329	In 250, 500, and 1000 mL.
Rx	**Dextrose 5% with 0.3% Sodium Chloride** (Hospira)	50	170	51				51					355	In 250, 500, and 1000 mL.
Rx	**Dextrose 5% with 0.33% Sodium Chloride** (Various, eg, Baxter, B. Braun)	50	170	56				56					365	In 250, 500, and 1000 mL.
Rx	**Dextrose 5% with 0.45% Sodium Chloride** (Various, eg, Hospira, Baxter, B. Braun)	50	170	77				77					≈ 405	In 250, 500, and 1000 mL.
Rx	**Dextrose 5% with 0.9% Sodium Chloride** (Various, eg, Hospira, Baxter, B. Braun)	50	170	154				154					≈ 560	In 250, 500, and 1000 mL.
Rx	**Dextrose 10% with 0.2% Sodium Chloride** (Various, eg, B. Braun)	100	340	34				34					575	In 250 mL.
Rx	**Dextrose 10% with 0.225% Sodium Chloride** (Abbott)	100	340	38.5				38.5					582	In 250 and 500 mL.

DEXTROSE-ELECTROLYTE SOLUTIONS

	Product and distributor	Dextrose (g/L)	Calories (Cal/L)	Na^+	K^+	Ca^{++}	Mg^{++}	Cl^-	Phosphate	Lactate	Acetate	Gluconate	Osmolarity (mOsm/L)	How supplied
Rx	**Dextrose 10% with 0.45% Sodium Chloride** (B. Braun)	100	340	77				77					660	In 1000 mL.
Rx	**Dextrose 10% and 0.9% Sodium Chloride** (Various, eg, Baxter, B. Braun)	100	340	154				154					813-815	In 500 and 1000 mL.
Rx	**Potassium Chloride in 5% Dextrose and Lactated Ringer's** (Baxter)	50	170	130	24	3		129		28			565	In 1000 mL.
		50	170	130	44	3		149		28			605	In 1000 mL.
Rx	**Potassium Chloride in 5% Dextrose and Lactated Ringer's** (Hospira)	50	179	130	24	2.7		129		28			563	In 1000 mL.
		50	179	130	44	2.7		149		28			604	In 1000 mL.
Rx	**Potassium Chloride in 5% Dextrose** (Various, eg, Baxter, B. Braun, Hospira)	50	170		10			10					≈ 272	In 1000 mL.
		50	170		20			20					292-295	In 1000 mL.
		50	170		30			30					310-312	In 1000 mL.
		50	170		40			40					330-333	In 500 and 1000 mL.
Rx	**Potassium Chloride in 3.3% Dextrose and 0.3% Sodium Chloride** (B. Braun)	33	110	51	20			71					310	In 1000 mL.
Rx	**Potassium Chloride in 5% Dextrose and 0.2% Sodium Chloride** (Various, eg, Baxter, B. Braun)	50	170	34	10			44					≈ 340	In 1000 mL.
		50	170	34	20			54					≈ 360	In 250, 500, and 1000 mL.
		50	170	34	30			64					≈ 380	In 1000 mL.
		50	170	34	40			74					≈ 400	In 1000 mL.
Rx	**Potassium Chloride in 5% Dextrose and 0.33% Sodium Chloride** (Various, eg, Baxter, B. Braun)	50	170	56	20			76					405	In 500 and 1000 mL.
		50	170	56	30			86					425	In 1000 mL.
		50	170	56	40			96					446	In 1000 mL.
Rx	**Potassium Chloride in 5% Dextrose and 0.45% Sodium Chloride** (Various, eg, Baxter, B. Braun)	50	170	77	10			87					≈ 425	In 1000 mL.
		50	170	77	20			97					445-447	In 500 and 1000 mL.
		50	170	77	30			107					≈ 465	In 1000 mL.
		50	170	77	40			117					487-490	In 1000 mL.
Rx	**Potassium Chloride in 5% Dextrose and 0.9% Sodium Chloride** (Various, eg, Baxter, B. Braun)	50	170	154	20			174					≈ 600	In 1000 mL.
		50	170	154	40			194					≈ 640	In 1000 mL.
Rx	**Potassium Chloride in 10% Dextrose and 0.2% Sodium Chloride** (B. Braun)	100	340	34	20			54					615	In 250 mL.
Rx	**Dextrose 5% and Electrolyte No. 75** (Baxter)	50	180	40	35			48	15	20			402	In 250, 500, and 1000 mL.
Rx	**Isolyte M in 5% Dextrose** (B. Braun)	50	170	36	35			49	15		20		390	In 500 and 1000 mL
Rx	**Ringer's in 5% Dextrose** (Various, eg, Abbott, Baxter, B. Braun)	50	170	≈147	4	≈4.5		≈156					≈560	In 500 and 1000 mL.
Rx	**Half-Strength Lactated Ringer's in 2.5% Dextrose** (Various, eg, Abbott, Baxter, B. Braun)	25	85-89	≈65.5	2	≈1.5		≈55		14			≈264	In 250, 500, and 1000 mL.
Rx	**Lactated Ringer's in 5% Dextrose** (Various, eg, Abbott, Baxter, B. Braun)	50	170	130	4	≈ 3		109-112		28			525-530	In 250, 500, and 1000 mL.
Rx	**Dextrose 5% and Electrolyte No. 48** (Baxter)	50	180	25	20		3	24	3	23			348	In 250 mL.
Rx	**Isolyte H in 5% Dextrose** (B. Braun)	50	170	39	13		3	44			16		360	In 1000 mL.
Rx	**Normosol-M and 5% Dextrose** (Hospira)	50	170	40	13		3	40			16		363	In 500 and 1000 mL.
Rx	**Plasma-Lyte 56 and 5% Dextrose** (Baxter)													In 500 and 1000 mL.
Rx	**Isolyte P in 5% Dextrose** (B. Braun)	50	170	23	20		3	29	3		23		340	In 250, 500, and 1000 mL.
Rx	**Isolyte S with 5% Dextrose** (B. Braun)	50	170	140	5		3	106			27	23	550	In 1000 mL.
Rx	**Normosol-R and 5% Dextrose** (Abbott)	50	185	140	5		3	98			27	23	547	In 500 and 1000 mL.
Rx	**Plasma-Lyte 148 and 5% Dextrose** (Baxter)	50	190	140	5		3	98			27	23	547	In 500 and 1000 mL.
Rx	**Dextrose 10% and Electrolyte No. 48** (Baxter)	100	350	25	20		3	24	3	23			600	In 250 mL.[b]
Rx	**Isolyte R in 5% Dextrose** (B. Braun)	50	170	39	16	5	3	46			24		375	In 1000 mL.
Rx	**Plasma-Lyte M and 5% Dextrose** (Baxter)	50	180	40	16	5	3	40		12	12		377	In 500 and 1000 mL.
Rx	**Plasma-Lyte R and 5% Dextrose** (Baxter)	50	180	140	10	5	3	103		8	47		564	In 1000 mL.[b]

[a] Millimoles per liter.

[b] With sodium bisulfite.

DEXTROSE-ELECTROLYTE SOLUTIONS

Indications

For use as a parenteral source of electrolytes, calories, or water for hydration, or as an alkalinizing agent.

INVERT SUGAR-ELECTROLYTE SOLUTIONS

Electrolyte content given in mEq/L.

	Product and distributor	Invert Sugar (g/L)	Calories (Cal/L)	Na+	K+	Mg++	Cl-	Phosphate	Lactate	Osmolarity (mOsm/L)	How supplied
Rx	**Multiple Electrolytes and 5% Travert** (Baxter)	50	196	56	25	6	56	12.5	25	449	In 1000 mL.[a]
Rx	**Multiple Electrolytes and 10% Travert** (Baxter)	100	384	56	25	6	56	12.5	25	726	In 1000 mL.[a]

[a] With sodium 5 mEq/L sodium bisulfite.

INVERT SUGAR-ELECTROLYTE SOLUTIONS — INTRAVENOUS

Refer to dextrose monograph for further information.

Indications

Used as a source of calories and hydration. Invert sugar is composed of equal parts of dextrose and fructose and shares the same actions and caloric value.

Any supposed advantage of using invert sugar solutions would be from the fructose component.

EPOETIN ALFA, RECOMBINANT (Erythropoietin; EPO)

Rx	**Epogen** (Amgen)	**Injection**: 2,000 units/mL	In 1 mL single-dose vials.[a]
Rx	**Procrit** (Ortho Biotech)		In 1 mL single-dose vials.[a]
Rx	**Epogen** (Amgen)	**Injection**: 3,000 units/mL	In 1 mL single-dose vials.[a]
Rx	**Procrit** (Ortho Biotech)		In 1 mL single-dose vials.[a]
Rx	**Epogen** (Amgen)	**Injection**: 4,000 units/mL	In 1 mL single-dose vials.[a]
Rx	**Procrit** (Ortho Biotech)		In 1 mL single-dose vials.[a]
Rx	**Epogen** (Amgen)	**Injection**:10,000 units/mL	In 1 mL single-dose vials[a] and 2 mL multidose vials.[b]
Rx	**Procrit** (Ortho Biotech)		In 1 mL single-dose vials[a] and 2 mL multidose vials.[b]
Rx	**Epogen** (Amgen)	**Injection**: 20,000 units/mL	In 1 mL multidose vials.[b]
Rx	**Procrit** (Ortho Biotech)		In 1 mL multidose vials.[b]
Rx	**Epogen** (Amgen)	**Injection**: 40,000 units/mL	In 1 mL single-dose vials.[a]
Rx	**Procrit** (Ortho Biotech)		In 1 mL single-dose vials.[a]

[a] Preservative free with 2.5 mg albumin (human) per mL.

[b] Preserved with 1% benzyl alcohol. With 2.5 mg albumin (human) per mL.

EPOETIN ALFA — INJECTION

Indications

➤*Treatment of anemia of chronic renal failure patients (CRF):* For the treatment of anemia associated with chronic renal failure, including patients on dialysis (end-stage renal disease [ESRD]) and patients not on dialysis. Epoetin alfa is indicated to elevate or maintain the RBC level (as manifested by the hematocrit or hemoglobin determinations) and to decrease the need for transfusions in these patients.

Nondialysis patients with symptomatic anemia considered for therapy should have a hemoglobin less than 10 g/dL.

Epoetin alfa is not intended for patients who require immediate correction of severe anemia. Epoetin alfa may obviate the need for maintenance transfusions but is not a substitute for emergency transfusion.

Prior to initiation of therapy, evaluate the patient's iron stores. Transferrin saturation should be at least 20% and ferritin at least 100 ng/mL. Adequately control blood pressure prior to initiation of epoetin alfa therapy, and closely monitor and control during therapy.

➤*Treatment of anemia in zidovudine-treated HIV-infected patients:* For the treatment of anemia related to therapy with zidovudine (AZT) in HIV-infected patients. Epoetin alfa is indicated to elevate or maintain the red blood cell (RBC) level (as manifested by the hematocrit or hemoglobin determinations) and to decrease the need for transfusions in these patients. Epoetin alfa is not indicated for the treatment of anemia in HIV-infected patients because of other factors such as iron or folate deficiencies, hemolysis, or GI bleeding; manage these conditions appropriately.

Epoetin alfa, at a dose of 100 units/kg 3 times/week, is effective in decreasing the transfusion requirement and increasing the RBC level of anemic, HIV-infected patients treated with zidovudine, when the endogenous serum erythropoietin level is less than or equal to 500 milliunits/mL and when patients are receiving a dose of zidovudine less than or equal to 4,200 mg/week.

➤*Treatment of anemia in cancer patients on chemotherapy:* For the treatment of anemia in patients with nonmyeloid malignancies where anemia is due to the effect of concomitantly administered chemotherapy. Epoetin alfa is indicated to decrease the need for transfusions in patients who will be receiving concomitant chemotherapy for a minimum of 2 months. Epoetin alfa is not indicated for the treatment of anemia in cancer patients due to other factors such as iron or folate deficiencies, hemolysis, or GI bleeding; manage these conditions appropriately.

➤*Reduction of allogeneic blood transfusion in surgery patients:* For the treatment of anemic patients (hemoglobin greater than 10 to less than or equal to 13 g/dL) scheduled to undergo elective, noncardiac, nonvascular surgery to reduce the need for allogeneic blood transfusions. Epoetin alfa is indicated for patients at high risk for perioperative transfusions with significant, anticipated blood loss. Epoetin alfa is not indicated for anemic patients who are willing to donate autologous blood. The safety of the perioperative use of epoetin alfa has been studied only in patients who are receiving anticoagulant prophylaxis.

➤*Unlabeled uses:* Use in critically ill patients to reduce the number of RBC transfusions; anemia of prematurity in preterm infants (25 to 100 units/kg/dose subcutaneously 3 times/week; alternatively, 200 to 300 units/kg/dose IV/subcutaneously 3 to 5 times/week for 2 to 6 weeks [total dose per week is 600 to 1,400 units/kg]); anemia associated with myelodysplastic syndrome; anemia associated with chronic inflammatory disorders (eg, rheumatoid arthritis); prophylaxis of anemia associated with frequent blood donation; treatment of anemia associated with ribavirin combination therapy in hepatitis C-infected patients; treatment of anemia in cancer patients not receiving chemotherapy; once-weekly dosing regimen of cancer patients on chemotherapy: 40,000 to 60,000 units/week subcutaneously; treatment of anemia associated with CRF in children not requiring dialysis (3 months to 20 years of age: 50 to 250 units/kg subcutaneously or IV, weekly to 3 times/week); treatment of anemia related to zidovudine therapy in HIV-infected children (8 months to 17 years of age: 50 to 400 units/kg subcutaneously or IV, 2 to 3 times/week); treatment of anemia in children with cancer on chemotherapy (6 months to 18 years of age: 25 to 300 units/kg subcutaneously or IV, 3 to 7 times/week).

Administration and Dosage

➤*Approved by the FDA:* June 1, 1989.

➤*Chronic renal failure (CRF) patients:* The recommended range for the starting dose of epoetin alfa is 50 to 100 units/kg 3 times/week for adult patients. The recommended starting dose for pediatric CRF patients on dialysis is 50 units/kg 3 times/week. Reduce the dose of epoetin alfa as the hemoglobin approaches 12 g/dL or increases by more than 1 g/dL in any 2-week period. The dosage of epoetin alfa must be individualized to maintain the hemoglobin within the suggested target range. At the physician's discretion, the suggested target hemoglobin range may be expanded to achieve maximal patient benefit.

Administration – Epoetin alfa may be given either as an IV or subcutaneous injection. In patients on hemodialysis, epoetin alfa usually has been administered as an IV bolus 3 times/week. While the administration of epoetin alfa is independent of the dialysis procedure, epoetin alfa may be administered into the venous line at the end of the dialysis procedure to obviate the need for additional venous access. In patients with CRF not on dialysis, epoetin alfa may be given either as an IV or subcutaneous injection.

Patients who have been judged competent by their physicians to self-administer epoetin alfa without medical or other supervision may give themselves either an IV or subcutaneous injection. The information below provides general therapeutic guidelines for patients with CRF:

Starting dose –
Adults: 50 to 100 units/kg 3 times/week IV or subcutaneously.
Pediatric patients: 50 units/kg 3 times/week IV or subcutaneously.

Dose reduction – Reduce dose when hemoglobin approaches 12 g/dL or when hemoglobin increases more than 1 g/dL in any 2-week period.

Dose increase – Increase dose if hemoglobin does not increase by 2 g/dL after 8 weeks of therapy, and hemoglobin is below suggested target range.

Maintenance dose – Individually titrate.

Suggested target hemoglobin range – Range, 10 to 12 g/dL.

Monitoring – See Precautions for more information.

Pretherapy iron evaluation – See Precautions for more information.

Dose adjustment – Adjust the dose for each patient to achieve and maintain a target hemoglobin not to exceed 12 g/dL.

Do not increase dose more frequently than once a month. If the hemoglobin is increasing and approaching 12 g/dL, reduce the dose by approximately 25%. If the hemoglobin continues to increase, temporarily withhold the dose until the hemoglobin begins to decrease, resume therapy at that point at a dose approximately 25% below the previous dose. If the hemoglobin increases by more than 1 g/dL in a 2-week period, decrease the dose by approximately 25%.

If the increase in the hemoglobin is less than 1 g/dL over 4 weeks and iron stores are adequate, the dose of epoetin alfa may be increased by approximately 25% of the previous dose. Further increases may be made at 4-week intervals until the specified hemoglobin is obtained.

Maintenance dose – The maintenance dose must be individualized for each patient on dialysis. In the US phase 3 multicenter trial in patients on hemodialysis, the median maintenance dose was 75 units/kg 3 times/week, with a range from 12.5 to 525 units/kg 3 times/week. Almost 10% of the patients required a dose of 25 units/kg, or less, and approximately 10% of the patients required more than 200 units/kg 3 times/week to maintain their hemoglobin in the suggested target range. In pediatric hemodialysis and peritoneal dialysis patients, the median maintenance dose was 167 units/kg/week (49 to 447 units/kg per week) and 76 units/kg per week (24 to 323 units/kg/week) administered in divided doses (2 or 3 times a week), respectively, to achieve the target range of 30% to 36%.

If the hemoglobin remains below, or falls below, the suggested target range, reevaluate the iron stores. If the transferrin saturation is less than 20%, administer supplemental iron. If the transferrin saturation is greater than 20%, the dose of epoetin alfa may be increased. Do not make such dose increases more frequently than once a month unless clinically indicated, as the response time of the hemoglobin to a dose increase can be 2 to 6 weeks. Measure hemoglobin twice weekly for 2 to 6 weeks following dose increases. In patients with CRF not on dialysis, the maintenance dose must also be individualized. Epoetin alfa doses of 75 to 150 units/kg/week have been shown to maintain hematocrits of 36% to 38% for up to 6 months.

EPOETIN ALFA — INJECTION

Lack or loss of response – Over 95% of patients with CRF responded with clinically significant increases in hematocrit, and virtually all patients were transfusion-independent within approximately 2 months of initiation of epoetin alfa therapy.

See Precautions for more information.

➤*Zidovudine-treated HIV-infected patients:* Prior to beginning epoetin alfa, it is recommended that the endogenous serum erythropoietin level be determined (prior to transfusion). Available evidence suggests that patients receiving zidovudine with endogenous serum erythropoietin levels greater than 500 milliunits/mL are unlikely to respond to therapy with epoetin alfa.

Starting dose – For adult patients with serum erythropoietin levels less than or equal to 500 milliunits/mL who are receiving a dose of zidovudine of less than or equal to 4,200 mg/week, the recommended starting dose of epoetin alfa is 100 units/kg as an IV or subcutaneous injection 3 times/week for 8 weeks. Published literature has reported the use of epoetin alfa in 20 zidovudine-treated anemic HIV-infected pediatric patients ages 8 months to 17 years, treated with 50 to 400 units/kg subcutaneously or IV, 2 to 3 times per week. Increases in hemoglobin levels and in reticulocyte counts, and decreases in or elimination of blood transfusions were observed.

Dose adjustment – During the dose adjustment phase of therapy, monitor the hemoglobin weekly. If the response is not satisfactory in terms of reducing transfusion requirements or increasing hemoglobin after 8 weeks of therapy, the dose of epoetin alfa can be increased by 50 to 100 units/kg 3 times/week. Evaluate response every 4 to 8 weeks thereafter and adjust the dose accordingly by 50 to 100 units/kg increments 3 times/week. If patients have not responded satisfactorily to an epoetin alfa dose of 300 units/kg 3 times/week, it is unlikely that they will respond to higher doses of epoetin alfa.

Maintenance dose – After attainment of the desired response (ie, reduced transfusion requirements or increased hemoglobin), titrate the dose of epoetin alfa to maintain the response based on factors such as variations in zidovudine dose and the presence of intercurrent infectious or inflammatory episodes. If the hemoglobin exceeds 13 g/dL, discontinue the dose until the hemoglobin drops to 12 g/dL. Reduce the dose by 25% when treatment is resumed and then titrate to maintain the desired hemoglobin.

➤*Cancer patients on chemotherapy:* Although no specific serum erythropoietin level can be stipulated above which patients would be unlikely to respond to epoetin alfa therapy, treatment of patients with grossly elevated serum erythropoietin levels (eg, more than 200 milliunits/mL) is not recommended. Monitor the hemoglobin on a weekly basis in patients receiving epoetin alfa therapy until hemoglobin becomes stable. Titrate the dose of epoetin alfa to maintain the desired hemoglobin.

Two epoetin alfa dosing regimens may be used in adults; 150 units/kg subcutaneously 3 times/week or 40,000 units subcutaneously weekly.

3 times/week dosing –

Starting dose:

- *Adults* – 150 units/kg subcutaneously 3 times/week.
- *Pediatric patients* – Published literature has reported the use of epoetin alfa in approximately 64 anemic pediatric cancer patients 6 months to 18 years of age, treated with 25 to 300 units/kg subcutaneously or IV, 3 to 7 times per week. Increases in hemoglobin and decreases in transfusion requirements were noted.

Reduce dose by 25% when: Hemoglobin approaches 12 g/dL.

Hemoglobin increases more than 1 g/dL in any 2-week period.

Withhold dose if: Hemoglobin exceeds 13 g/dL, until the hemoglobin falls to 12 g/dL, and restart dose at 25% below the previous dose.

Increase dose to 300 units/kg 3 times/week if: Response is not satisfactory (no reduction in transfusion requirements or rise in hemoglobin) after 8 weeks.

Suggested target hemoglobin range: 10 to 12 g/dL

Weekly dosing – The starting dose in adults is 40,000 units subcutaneously weekly. If after 4 weeks of therapy, the hemoglobin has not increased by at least 1 g/dL, in the absence of RBC transfusion, increase the epoetin alfa dose to 60,000 units weekly.

If patients have not responded satisfactorily to an epoetin alfa dose of 60,000 units weekly after 4 weeks, it is unlikely that they will respond to higher doses of epoetin alfa.

Withhold epoetin alfa if the hemoglobin exceeds 13 g/dL and reinitiate with a 25% dose reduction when the hemoglobin is less than 12 g/dL.

If epoetin alfa treatment produces a very rapid hemoglobin response (eg, an increase of more than 1 g/dL in any 2-week period), reduce the dose of epoetin alfa by 25%.

➤*Surgery patients:* Prior to initiating treatment with epoetin alfa, obtain a hemoglobin to establish that it is greater than 10 to less than or equal to 13 g/dL. The recommended dose of epoetin alfa is 300 units/kg/day subcutaneously for 10 days before surgery, on the day of surgery, and for 4 days after surgery.

An alternate dose schedule is 600 units/kg epoetin alfa subcutaneously in once weekly doses (21, 14, and 7 days before surgery) plus a fourth dose on the day of surgery.

All patients should receive adequate iron supplementation. Initiate iron supplementation no later than the beginning of treatment with epoetin alfa and continue throughout the course of therapy.

➤*Preparation and administration:*

1.) Do not shake. It is not necessary to shake epoetin alfa. Prolonged vigorous shaking may denature any glycoprotein, rendering it biologically inactive.
2.) Visually inspect parenteral drug products for particulate matter and discoloration prior to administration. Do not use any vials exhibiting particulate matter or discoloration.
3.) Using aseptic techniques, attach a sterile needle to a sterile syringe. Remove the flip top from the vial containing epoetin alfa, and wipe the septum with a disinfectant. Insert the needle into the vial, and withdraw into the syringe an appropriate volume of solution.
4.) Single-dose 1 mL vial contains no preservative. Use 1 dose per vial; do not reenter the vial. Discard unused portions. Multidose 1 mL and 2 mL vials contain preservative. Store at 2° to 8°C (35.6° to 46.4°F) after initial entry and between doses. Discard 21 days after initial entry.
5.) Do not dilute or administer in conjunction with other drug solutions. However, at the time of subcutaneous administration, preservative-free epoetin alfa from single-use vials may be admixed in a syringe with bacteriostatic 0.9% sodium chloride injection with benzyl alcohol 0.9% (bacteriostatic saline) at a 1:1 ratio using aseptic technique. The benzyl alcohol in the bacteriostatic saline acts as a local anesthetic which may ameliorate the subcutaneous injection site discomfort. Admixing is not necessary when using the multidose vials of epoetin alfa containing benzyl alcohol.

➤*Storage/Stability:* Store at 2° to 8°C (35.6° to 46°F). Do not freeze or shake.

Actions

➤*Pharmacology:*

Chronic renal failure patients – Endogenous production of erythropoietin is normally regulated by the level of tissue oxygenation. Hypoxia and anemia generally increase the production of erythropoietin, which in turn stimulates erythropoiesis. In healthy subjects, plasma erythropoietin levels range from 0.01 to 0.03 units/mL and increase up to 100- to 1,000-fold during hypoxia or anemia. In contrast, in patients with CRF, production of erythropoietin is impaired, and this erythropoietin deficiency is the primary cause of their anemia.

Chronic renal failure is the clinical situation in which there is a progressive and usually irreversible decline in kidney function. Such patients may manifest the sequelae of renal dysfunction, including anemia, but do not necessarily require regular dialysis. Patients with ESRD are those patients with CRF who require regular dialysis or kidney transplantation for survival.

Epoetin alfa has been shown to stimulate erythropoiesis in anemic patients with CRF, including both patients on dialysis and those who do not require regular dialysis. The first evidence of a response to the 3 times/week administration of epoetin alfa is an increase in the reticulocyte count within 10 days, followed by increases in the red cell count, hemoglobin, and hemoglobin, usually within 2 to 6 weeks. Because of the length of time required for erythropoiesis (several days for erythroid progenitors to mature and be released into the circulation) a clinically significant increase in hematocrit is usually not observed in less than 2 weeks and may require up to 6 weeks in some patients. Once the hematocrit reaches the suggested target range (30% to 36%), that level can be sustained by epoetin alfa therapy in the absence of iron deficiency and concurrent illnesses.

The rate of hematocrit increase varies between patients and is dependent upon the dose of epoetin alfa, within a therapeutic range of approximately 50 to 300 units/kg 3 times/week. A greater biologic response is not observed at doses exceeding 300 units/kg 3 times/week. Other factors affecting the rate and extent of response include availability of iron stores, the baseline hemoglobin, and the presence of concurrent medical problems.

Zidovudine-treated HIV-infected patients – Responsiveness to epoetin alfa in HIV-infected patients is dependent upon the endogenous serum erythropoietin level prior to treatment. Patients with endogenous serum erythropoietin levels less than or equal to 500 milliunits/mL, and who are receiving a dose of zidovudine of less than or equal to 4,200 mg/week, may respond to epoetin alfa therapy. Patients with endogenous serum erythropoietin levels greater than 500 milliunits/mL do not appear to respond to epoetin alfa therapy. In a series of 4 clinical trials involving 255 patients, 60% to 80% of HIV-infected patients treated with zidovudine had endogenous serum erythropoietin levels less than or equal to 500 milliunits/mL.

Response to epoetin alfa in zidovudine-treated HIV-infected patients is manifested by reduced transfusion requirements and increased hemoglobin.

Cancer patients on chemotherapy – A series of clinical trials enrolled 131 anemic cancer patients who received epoetin alfa 3 times/week and who were receiving cyclic cisplatin- or noncisplatin-containing chemotherapy. Endogenous baseline serum erythropoietin levels varied among patients in these trials with approximately 75% (n = 83/110) having endogenous serum erythropoietin levels less than or equal to 132 milliunits/mL, and approximately 4% (n = 4/110) of patients having endogenous serum erythropoietin levels greater than 500 milliunits/mL. In general, patients with lower baseline serum erythropoietin levels responded more vigorously to epoetin alfa than patients with higher baseline erythropoietin levels. Although no specific serum erythropoietin level can be stipulated above which patients would be unlikely to respond to epoetin alfa therapy, treatment of patients with grossly elevated serum erythropoietin levels (eg, greater than 200 milliunits/mL) is not recommended.

➤*Pharmacokinetics:* In adult and pediatric patients with CRF, the elimination half-life of plasma erythropoietin after IV administered epoetin alfa ranges from 4 to 13 hours. The half-life is approximately 20% longer in CRF patients than that in healthy subjects. After subcutaneous administration, peak plasma levels are achieved within 5 to 24 hours. The half-life is similar between adult patients with serum creatinine level greater than 3 and not

EPOETIN ALFA — INJECTION

on dialysis and those maintained on dialysis.

A pharmacokinetic study comparing 150 units/kg subcutaneously 3 times/week to 40,000 units subcutaneous weekly dosing regimen was conducted for 4 weeks in healthy subjects (n = 12) and for 6 weeks in anemic cancer patients (n = 32) receiving cyclic chemotherapy. There was no accumulation of serum erythropoietin after the 2 dosing regimens during the study period. The 40,000 units weekly regimen had a higher C_{max} (3- to 7-fold), longer T_{max} (2- to 3-fold), higher AUC_{0-168h} (2- to 3-fold) of erythropoietin and lower clearance (50%) than the 150 units/kg 3 times/week regimen. In anemic cancer patients, the average $t_{1/2}$ was similar (40 hours with range of 16 to 67 hours) after both dosing regimens. After the 150 units/kg 3-times-weekly dosing, the values of T_{max} and clearance are similar (13.3 ± 12.4 vs 14.2 ± 6.7 hours, and 20.2 ± 15.9 vs 23.6 ± 9.5 mL/hr/kg) between week 1 when patients were receiving chemotherapy (n = 14) and week 3 when patients were not receiving chemotherapy (n = 4). Differences were observed after the 40,000 units weekly dosing with longer T_{max} (38 ± 18 hours) and lower clearance (9.2 ± 4.7 mL/hr/kg) during week 1 when patients were receiving chemotherapy (n = 18) compared with those (22 ± 4.5 hours, 13.9 ± 7.6 mL/hr/kg) during week 3 when patients were not receiving chemotherapy (n = 7).

The bioequivalence between the 10,000 units/mL citrate-buffered epoetin alfa formulation and the 40,000 units/mL phosphate-buffered epoetin alfa formulation has been demonstrated after subcutaneous administration of single 750 units/kg doses to healthy subjects.

Contraindications

Uncontrolled hypertension; known hypersensitivity to mammalian cell-derived products; known hypersensitivity to albumin (human).

Warnings

➤*Thrombotic events and increased mortality:* A randomized, prospective trial of 1,265 hemodialysis patients with clinically evident cardiac disease (ischemic heart disease or congestive heart failure) was conducted in which patients were assigned to epoetin alfa treatment targeted to a maintenance hematocrit of either 42 ± 3% or 30 ± 3%. Increased mortality was observed in 634 patients randomized to a target hemoglobin of 42% (221 deaths [35% mortality]) compared with 631 patients targeted to remain at a hematocrit of 30% (185 deaths [29% mortality]). The reason for the increased mortality observed in these studies is unknown; however, the incidence of nonfatal myocardial infarctions (3.1% vs 2.3%), vascular access thromboses (39% vs 29%), and all other thrombotic events (22% vs 18%) also were higher in the group randomized to achieve a hematocrit of 42%.

Increased mortality also was observed in a randomized placebo-controlled study of epoetin alfa in patients who did not have CRF who were undergoing coronary artery bypass surgery (7 deaths in 126 patients randomized to epoetin alfa versus no deaths among 56 patients receiving placebo). Four of these deaths occurred during the period of study drug administration and all 4 deaths were associated with thrombotic events. While the extent of the population affected is unknown, in patients at risk for thrombosis, weigh the anticipated benefits of epoetin alfa treatment against the potential for increased risks associated with therapy.

In a randomized, prospective trial conducted with another epoetin alfa product, in 939 women with metastatic carcinoma of the breast who were receiving chemotherapy, patients were assigned to receive either epoetin alfa or placebo for up to a year, in a weekly schedule, with the primary goal of showing improved survival and improved quality of life in the epoetin alfa treatment arm. This study utilized a treatment strategy designed to maintain hemoglobin levels of 12 to 14 g/dL (hematocrit 36% to 42%). Increased mortality in the first 4 months after randomization was observed among 469 patients who received the erythropoietin product (41 deaths [8.7% mortality]) compared with 470 patients who received placebo (16 deaths [3.4% mortality]). In the first 4 months of the study, the incidence of fatal thrombotic vascular events (1.1% vs 0.2%) and death attributed to disease progression (6% vs 2.8%) were higher in the group randomized to receive epoetin alfa as compared with placebo. Based on Kaplan-Meier estimates, the proportion of subjects surviving at 12 months after randomization was lower in the epoetin alfa group than in the placebo group (70% vs 76%), $P = 0.012$, log rank. However, due to insufficient monitoring and data collection, reliable comparisons cannot be made concerning the effect of epoetin alfa on overall time to disease progression, progression-free survival, and overall survival.

Cancer patients on chemotherapy – In double-blind, placebo-controlled trials, 3.2% (n = 2/63) of patients treated with epoetin alfa 3 times/week and 11.8% (n = 8/68) of placebo-treated patients had thrombotic events (eg, pulmonary embolism, cerebrovascular accident).

In a placebo-controlled, double-blind trial utilizing weekly dosing with epoetin alfa , 6% (n = 10/168) of safety-evaluable patients treated with epoetin alfa and 3.6% (n = 6/165) ($P = 0.444$) of placebo-treated patients had clinically significant thrombotic events (deep vein thrombosis requiring anticoagulant therapy, embolic event including pulmonary embolism, myocardial infarction, cerebral ischemia, left ventricular failure and thrombotic microangiopathy). A definitive relationship between the rate of hemoglobin increase and the occurrence of clinically significant thrombotic events could not be evaluated because of the limited schedule of hemoglobin measurements in this study.

Surgery patients – In perioperative clinical trials with orthopedic patients, the overall incidence of thrombotic/vascular events was similar in epoetin alfa and placebo treated patients who had a pretreatment hemoglobin of greater than 10 to less than or equal to 13 g/dL. In patients with a hemoglobin of greater than 13 g/dL treated with 300 units/kg of epoetin alfa, the possibility that epoetin alfa treatment may be associated with an increased risk of postoperative thrombotic/vascular events cannot be excluded.

In 1 study in which epoetin alfa was administered in the perioperative period to patients undergoing coronary artery bypass graft surgery, there were 7 deaths in the group treated with epoetin alfa (n = 126) and no deaths in the placebo-treated group (n = 56). Among the 7 deaths in the patients treated with epoetin alfa, 4 were at the time of therapy (between study day 2 and 8). The 4 deaths at the time of therapy (3%) were associated with thrombotic/vascular events. A causative role of epoetin alfa cannot be excluded. While the extent of the population affected is unknown, in patients at risk for thrombosis, weigh the anticipated benefits of epoetin alfa treatment against the potential for increased risks associated with therapy.

➤*Pure red cell aplasia:* Pure red cell aplasia (PRCA), in association with neutralizing antibodies to native erythropoietin, has been observed in patients treated with recombinant erythropoietins. PRCA has been reported in a limited number of patients exposed to epoetin alfa. This has been reported predominantly in patients with CRF. Evaluate any patient with loss of response to epoetin alfa for the etiology of loss of effect. Discontinue epoetin alfa in any patient with evidence of PRCA and evaluate the patient for the presence of binding and neutralizing antibodies to epoetin alfa, native erythropoietin, and any other recombinant erythropoietin administered to the patient. Contact the manufacturer to assist in this evaluation. In patients with PRCA secondary to neutralizing antibodies to erythropoietin, do not administer epoetin alfa and do not switch such patients to another product as antierythropoietin antibodies cross-react with other erythropoietins.

➤*Albumin (human):* Epoetin alfa contains albumin, a derivative of human blood. Based on effective donor screening and product manufacturing processes, it carries an extremely remote risk for transmission of viral diseases. A theoretical risk for transmission of Creutzfeldt-Jakob disease (CJD) also is considered extremely remote. No cases of transmission of viral diseases or CJD have ever been identified for albumin.

➤*Renal function impairment:*

Hypertension –

Chronic renal failure patients: Do not treat patients with uncontrolled hypertension with epoetin alfa; control blood pressure adequately before initiation of therapy. Up to 80% of patients with CRF have a history of hypertension. Although there does not appear to be any direct pressor effects of epoetin alfa, blood pressure may rise during epoetin alfa therapy. During the early phase of treatment when the hematocrit is increasing, approximately 25% of patients on dialysis may require initiation of, or increases in, antihypertensive therapy. Hypertensive encephalopathy and seizures have been observed in patients with CRF treated with epoetin alfa.

In contrast to CRF patients, epoetin alfa therapy has not been linked to exacerbation of hypertension, seizures, and thrombotic events in HIV-infected patients.

Take special care to closely monitor and aggressively control blood pressure in patients treated with epoetin alfa. Advise patients as to the importance of compliance with antihypertensive therapy and dietary restrictions. If blood pressure is difficult to control by initiation of appropriate measures, the hemoglobin may be reduced by decreasing or withholding the dose of epoetin alfa. A clinically significant decrease in hemoglobin may not be observed for several weeks.

It is recommended that the dose of epoetin alfa be decreased if the hemoglobin increase exceeds 4 points in any 2-week period, because of the possible association of excessive rate of rise of hemoglobin with an exacerbation of hypertension. In CRF patients on hemodialysis with clinically evident ischemic heart disease or congestive heart failure, manage the hemoglobin carefully, not to exceed 12 g/dL.

Zidovudine-treated HIV-infected patients: Exacerbation of hypertension has not been observed in zidovudine-treated HIV-infected patients treated with epoetin alfa. However, withhold epoetin alfa in these patients if preexisting hypertension is uncontrolled, and do not start until blood pressure is controlled. In double-blind studies, a single seizure has been experienced by a patient treated with epoetin alfa.

Cancer patients on chemotherapy: Hypertension, associated with a significant increase in hemoglobin, has been noted rarely in patients treated with epoetin alfa. Nevertheless, carefully monitor blood pressure in patients treated with epoetin alfa, particularly in patients with an underlying history of hypertension or cardiovascular disease.

Surgery patients: Blood pressure may rise in the perioperative period in patients being treated with epoetin alfa. Therefore, carefully monitor blood pressure.

Seizures –

Chronic renal failure patients: Seizures have occurred in patients with CRF participating in epoetin alfa clinical trials.

In adult patients on dialysis, there was a higher incidence of seizures during the first 90 days of therapy (occurring in approximately 2.5% of patients) as compared with later timepoints.

Given the potential for an increased risk of seizures during the first 90 days of therapy, closely monitor blood pressure and the presence of premonitory neurologic symptoms. Caution patients to avoid potentially hazardous activities such as driving or operating heavy machinery during this period.

While the relationship between seizures and the rate of rise of hemoglobin is uncertain, it is recommended that the dose of epoetin alfa be decreased if the hemoglobin increase exceeds 1 g/dL in any 2-week period.

Cancer patients on chemotherapy: In double-blind, placebo-controlled trials, 3.2% (n = 2/63) of patients treated with epoetin alfa and 2.9% (n = 2/68) of placebo-treated patients had seizures. Seizures in 1.6% (n = 1/63) of patients treated with epoetin alfa 3 times/week occurred in the context of a significant increase in blood pressure and hematocrit from baseline values. However, both patients treated with epoetin alfa also had underlying CNS pathology which may have been related to seizure activity.

EPOETIN ALFA — INJECTION

In a placebo-controlled, double-blind trial utilizing weekly dosing with epoetin alfa, 1.2% (n = 2/168) of safety-evaluable patients treated with epoetin alfa and 1% (n = 1/165) of placebo-treated patients had seizures. Seizures in the patients treated with weekly epoetin alfa occurred in the context of a significant increase in hemoglobin from baseline values; however, significant increases in blood pressure were not seen. These patients may have had other CNS pathology.

Thrombotic events – During hemodialysis, patients treated with epoetin alfa may require increased anticoagulation with heparin to prevent clotting of the artificial kidney.

Other thrombotic events (eg, myocardial infarction, cerebrovascular accident, transient ischemic attack) have occurred in clinical trials at an annualized rate of less than 0.04 events per patient-year of epoetin alfa therapy. These trials were conducted in patients with CRF (whether on dialysis or not) in whom the target hematocrit was 32% to 40%. However, the risk of thrombotic events, including vascular access thrombosis, was significantly increased in patients with ischemic heart disease or congestive heart failure receiving epoetin alfa therapy with the goal of reaching a normal hematocrit (42%) as compared with a target hematocrit of 30%. Closely monitor patients with preexisting cardiovascular disease.

➤*Fertility impairment:* In female rats treated with epoetin alfa IV, there was a trend for slightly increased fetal wastage at doses of 100 and 500 units/kg.

➤*Pregnancy: Category C.* Epoetin alfa has been shown to have adverse effects in rats when given in doses 5 times the human dose. There are no adequate and well-controlled studies in pregnant women. Only use epoetin alfa during pregnancy if potential benefit justifies the potential risk to the fetus. In studies in female rats, there were decreases in body weight gain, delays in appearance of abdominal hair, delayed eyelid opening, delayed ossification, and decreases in the number of caudal vertebrae in the F1 fetuses of the 500 units/kg group. In female rats treated IV, there was a trend for slightly increased fetal wastage at doses of 100 and 500 units/kg.

In some female patients, menses have resumed following epoetin alfa therapy; discuss the possibility of pregnancy and the need for contraception evaluation.

➤*Lactation:* Postnatal observations of the live offspring (F1 generation) of female rats treated with epoetin alfa during gestation and lactation revealed no effect of epoetin alfa at doses of up to 500 units/kg. There were, however, decreases in body weight gain, delays in appearance of abdominal hair, eyelid opening, and decreases in the number of caudal vertebrae in the F1 fetuses of the 500 units/kg group. There were no epoetin alfa-related effects on the F2 generation fetuses. It is not known whether epoetin alfa is excreted in human milk. Because many drugs are excreted in human milk, exercise caution when epoetin alfa is administered to a nursing woman.

➤*Children:*

Pediatric patients on dialysis – Epoetin alfa is indicated in infants (1 month to 2 years), children (2 years to 12 years), and adolescents (12 years to 16 years) for the treatment of anemia associated with CRF requiring dialysis. Safety and effectiveness in pediatric patients less than 1 month old have not been established. The safety data from these studies show that there is no increased risk to pediatric CRF patients on dialysis when compared with the safety profile of epoetin alfa in adult CRF patients. Published literature provides supportive evidence of the safety and effectiveness of epoetin alfa in pediatric CRF patients on dialysis.

Pediatric patients not requiring dialysis – Published literature has reported the use of epoetin alfa in 133 pediatric patients with anemia associated with CRF not requiring dialysis, ages 3 months to 20 years, treated with 50 to 250 units/kg subcutaneously or IV, weekly to 3 times a week. Dose-dependent increases in hemoglobin and hematocrit were observed with reductions in transfusion requirements.

Pediatric HIV-infected patients – Published literature has reported the use of epoetin alfa in 20 zidovudine-treated anemic HIV-infected pediatric patients ages 8 months to 17 years, treated with 50 to 400 units/kg subcutaneously or IV, 2 to 3 times per week. Increases in hemoglobin levels and in reticulocyte counts, and decreases in or elimination of blood transfusions were observed.

Pediatric cancer patients on chemotherapy – Published literature has reported the use of epoetin alfa in approximately 64 anemic pediatric cancer patients ages 6 months to 18 years, treated with 25 to 300 units/kg subcutaneously or IV, 3 to 7 times per week. Increases in hemoglobin and decreases in transfusion requirements were noted.

Precautions

➤*Monitoring:* Determine the hemoglobin twice a week until it has stabilized in the suggested target range and the maintenance dose has been established. After any dose adjustment, also determine the hemoglobin twice weekly for at least 2 to 6 weeks until it has been determined that the hemoglobin has stabilized in response to the dose change. Then monitor the hemoglobin at regular intervals.

Regularly perform a complete blood count with differential and platelet count. During clinical trials, modest increases were seen in platelets and white blood cell counts. While these changes were statistically significant, they were not clinically significant and the values remained within normal ranges.

In patients with CRF, regularly monitor serum chemistry values (including blood urea nitrogen [BUN], uric acid, creatinine, phosphorus, and potassium). During clinical trials in patients on dialysis, modest increases were seen in BUN, creatinine, phosphorus, and potassium. In some patients with CRF not on dialysis treated with epoetin alfa, modest increases in serum uric acid and phosphorus were observed. While changes were statistically significant, the values remained within the ranges normally seen in patients with CRF.

Patients with CRF not requiring dialysis – Monitor blood pressure and hemoglobin no less frequently than for patients maintained on dialysis. Closely monitor renal function and fluid and electrolyte balance, as an improved sense of well-being may obscure the need to initiate dialysis in some patients.

Renal function – In adult patients with CRF not on dialysis, closely monitor renal function and fluid and electrolyte balance, as an improved sense of well-being may obscure the need to initiate dialysis in some patients. In patients with CRF not on dialysis, placebo-controlled studies of progression of renal dysfunction over periods of greater than 1 year have not been completed. In shorter term trials in patients with CRF not on dialysis, changes in creatinine and creatinine clearance were not significantly different in patients treated with epoetin alfa, compared with placebo-treated patients. Analysis of the slope of 1/serum creatinine versus time plots in these patients indicates no significant change in the slope after the initiation of epoetin alfa therapy.

➤*Hypersensitivity reaction:* Attend the parenteral administration of any biologic product by appropriate precautions in case allergic or other untoward reactions occur. In clinical trials, while transient rashes were occasionally observed concurrently with epoetin alfa therapy, no serious allergic or anaphylactic reactions were reported.

➤*Seizure disorder/underlying hematologic disease:* The safety and efficacy of epoetin alfa therapy have not been established in patients with a known history of a seizure disorder or underlying hematologic disease (eg, sickle cell anemia, myelodysplastic syndromes, or hypercoagulable disorders).

➤*Hematology:* Exacerbation of porphyria has been observed rarely in patients with CRF treated with epoetin alfa. However, epoetin alfa has not caused increased urinary excretion of porphyrin metabolites in healthy volunteers, even in the presence of a rapid erythropoietic response. Nevertheless, use epoetin alfa with caution in patients with known porphyria.

In preclinical studies in dogs and rats, but not in monkeys, epoetin alfa therapy was associated with subclinical bone marrow fibrosis. Bone marrow fibrosis is a known complication of CRF in humans and may be related to secondary hyperparathyroidism or unknown factors. The incidence of bone marrow fibrosis was not increased in a study of patients on dialysis who were treated with epoetin alfa for 12 to 19 months, compared with the incidence of bone marrow fibrosis in a matched group of patients who had not been treated with epoetin alfa.

Measure hemoglobin in CRF patients twice a week; measure hemoglobin in zidovudine-treated HIV-infected and cancer patients once a week until hemoglobin has been stabilized, and measure periodically thereafter.

➤*Lack or loss of response:* If the patient fails to respond or to maintain a response to doses within the recommended dosing range, evaluate and consider the following etiologies:

1.) Iron deficiency: Virtually all patients will eventually require supplemental iron therapy.
2.) Underlying infectious, inflammatory or malignant processes.
3.) Occult blood loss.
4.) Underlying hematologic diseases (ie, thalassemia, refractory anemia or other myelodysplastic disorders).
5.) Vitamin deficiencies: Folic acid or vitamin B12.
6.) Hemolysis.
7.) Aluminum intoxication.
8.) Osteitis fibrosa cystica.
9.) Pure red cell aplasia (PRCA): In the absence of another etiology, evaluate the patient for evidence of PRCA and test sera for the presence of antibodies to recombinant erythropoietins.

➤*Iron evaluation:* During epoetin alfa therapy, absolute or functional iron deficiency may develop. Functional iron deficiency, with normal ferritin levels but low transferrin saturation, is presumably due to the inability to mobilize iron stores rapidly enough to support increased erythropoiesis. Transferrin saturation should be at least 20% and ferritin should be at least 100 ng/mL.

Prior to and during epoetin alfa therapy, evaluate the patient's iron status, including transferrin saturation (serum iron divided by iron-binding capacity) and serum ferritin. Virtually all patients will eventually require supplemental iron to increase or maintain transferrin saturation to levels which will adequately support erythropoiesis stimulated by epoetin alfa. All surgery patients being treated with epoetin alfa should receive adequate iron supplementation throughout the course of therapy in order to support erythropoiesis and avoid depletion of iron stores.

➤*Lipid profile:* In 1 study, total cholesterol, apoprotein B and serum triglycerides fell significantly after initiation of epoetin therapy.

➤*Chronic renal failure patients:*

Hematology – Allow sufficient time to determine a patient's responsiveness to a dosage of epoetin alfa before adjusting the dose. Because of the time required for erythropoiesis and the red cell half-life, an interval of 2 to 6 weeks may occur between the time of a dose adjustment (initiation, increase, decrease, or discontinuation), and a significant change in hemoglobin.

In order to avoid reaching the suggested target hemoglobin too rapidly, or exceeding the suggested target range (hemoglobin of 10 to 12 g/dL), follow the guidelines for dose and frequency of dose adjustments.

For patients who respond to epoetin alfa with a rapid increase in hemoglobin (eg, more than 1 g/dL in any 2-week period), reduce the dose of epoetin

EPOETIN ALFA — INJECTION

alfa because of the possible association of excessive rate of rise of hemoglobin with an exacerbation of hypertension.

The elevated bleeding time characteristic of CRF decreases toward normal after correction of anemia in patients treated with epoetin alfa. Reduction of bleeding time also occurs after correction of anemia by transfusion.

Diet – As the hemoglobin increases and patients experience an improved sense of well-being and quality of life, reinforce the importance of compliance with dietary and dialysis prescriptions. In particular, hyperkalemia is not uncommon in patients with CRF. In US studies in patients on dialysis, hyperkalemia has occurred at an annualized rate of approximately 0.11 episodes per patient-year of epoetin alfa therapy, often in association with poor compliance to medication, diet, or frequency of dialysis.

Dialysis management – Therapy with epoetin alfa results in an increase in hematocrit and a decrease in plasma volume which could affect dialysis efficiency. In studies to date, the resulting increase in hematocrit did not appear to adversely affect dialyzer function or the efficiency of high flux hemodialysis. During hemodialysis, patients treated with epoetin alfa may require increased anticoagulation with heparin to prevent clotting of the artificial kidney.

Patients who are marginally dialyzed may require adjustments in their dialysis prescription. As with all patients on dialysis, regularly monitor the serum chemistry values (including BUN, creatinine, phosphorus, and potassium) in patients treated with epoetin alfa to ensure the adequacy of the dialysis prescription.

➤*Cancer patients on chemotherapy:*

Tumor growth factor potential – Epoetin alfa is a growth factor that primarily stimulates red cell production. Erythropoietin receptors also are found to be present on the surface of some malignant cell lines and tumor biopsy specimens. However, it is not known if these receptors are functional. A randomized, placebo-controlled trial was conducted in 224 chemotherapy-naïve, nonanemic patients with small cell lung cancer receiving cisplatin-based combination chemotherapy, to investigate whether the concurrent use of epoetin alfa stimulated tumor growth as assessed by impact on overall response rate. Patients were randomized to receive epoetin alfa 150 units/kg or placebo subcutaneously 3 times/week during chemotherapy. The overall response rates, after 3 cycles of treatment, were 72% and 67%, in the epoetin alfa and placebo arms, respectively. Complete response rates (17% vs 14%) and median overall survival (10.5 mos vs 10.4 mos) were similar in the epoetin alfa and placebo arms.

Two additional studies explored effect on survival and/or progression of administrations of other exogenous erythropoietin with higher hemoglobin targets.

In a randomized, placebo-controlled study using another epoetin alfa product, conducted in 939 women with metastatic breast cancer, study drug dosing was titrated to attempt to maintain hemoglobin levels between 12 and 14 g/dL. At 4 months, death attributed to disease progression was higher (6% vs 3%) in women receiving epoetin alfa. Overall mortality was significantly higher at 12 months in the epoetin alfa arm.

In a randomized, placebo-controlled study using epoetin beta, conducted in 351 patients with head and neck cancer, study drug was administered with the aim of achieving a hemoglobin level of 14 g/dL in women and 15 g/dL in men. Locoregional progression-free survival was significantly shorter (median PFS: 406 days epoetin beta vs 745 days placebo, P = 0.04) in patients receiving epoetin beta.

There is insufficient information to establish whether use of epoetin products have an adverse effect on time to tumor progression or progression-free survival.

These trials permitted or required dosing to achieve hemoglobin of greater than 12 g/dL. Until further information is available, the recommended target hemoglobin should not exceed 12 g/dL in men or women.

➤*Benzyl alcohol:* The multidose preserved formulation contains benzyl alcohol. Benzyl alcohol has been reported to be associated with an increased incidence of neurological and other complications in premature infants which are sometimes fatal.

➤*Hazardous tasks:* Given the potential for an increased risk of seizures during the first 90 days of therapy, closely monitor blood pressure and the presence of premonitory neurologic symptoms. Caution patients to avoid potentially hazardous activities such as driving or operating heavy machinery during this period.

Drug Interactions

No evidence of interaction of epoetin alfa with other drugs was observed in the course of clinical trials.

Adverse Reactions

➤*Immunogenicity:* As with all therapeutic proteins, there is the potential for immunogenicity. The observed incidence of antibody positivity in an assay may be influenced by several factors including assay methodology, sample handling, timing of sample collection, concomitant medications, and underlying disease. For these reasons, comparison of the incidence of antibodies to epoetin alfa with the incidence of antibodies to other products may be misleading.

A few cases of PRCA associated with antibodies with neutralizing activity have been reported in patients receiving epoetin alfa. These cases were observed in patients treated by either subcutaneous or IV routes of administration and occurred predominantly in CRF patients.

➤*Chronic renal failure patients:* Epoetin alfa is generally well-tolerated. The adverse events reported are frequent sequelae of CRF and are not necessarily attributable to epoetin alfa therapy. In double-blind, placebo-controlled studies involving over 300 patients with CRF, the events reported in greater than 5% of patients treated with epoetin alfa during the blinded phase were:

Epoetin Alfa Adverse Reactions in CRF Patients		
Adverse reaction	Patients treated with epoetin alfa (n = 200)	Placebo-treated patients (n = 135)
Arthralgias	11%	6%
Asthenia	7%	12%
Chest pain	7%	9%
Clotted access	7%	2%
Diarrhea	9%	6%
Dizziness	7%	13%
Edema	9%	10%
Fatigue	9%	14%
Headache	16%	12%
Hypertension	24%	19%
Nausea	11%	9%
Skin reaction (administration site)	7%	12%
Vomiting	8%	5%

➤*Significant adverse events:* Significant adverse events of concern in patients with CRF treated in double-blind, placebo-controlled trials occurred in the following percent of patients during the blinded phase of the studies:

Epoetin Alfa Adverse Reactions in CRF Patients		
Seizure	1.1%	1.1%
CVA/TIA	0.4%	0.6%
Death	0	1.7%
MI	0.4%	1.1%

➤*Adverse events in patients on dialysis:* In the US epoetin alfa studies in patients on dialysis (over 567 patients), the incidence (number of events per patient-year) of the most frequently reported adverse events were the following: Clotted vascular access (0.25), diarrhea (0.11), headache (0.4), hyperkalemia (0.11), hypertension (0.75), nausea/vomiting (0.26), shortness of breath (0.14), and tachycardia (0.31). Other reported events occurred at a rate of less than 0.1 events per patient per year.

➤*Events that occurred within several hours of administration:* Events reported to have occurred within several hours of administration of epoetin alfa were rare, mild, and transient, and included injection site stinging in dialysis patients and flu-like symptoms such as arthralgias and myalgias.

➤*Adverse events in all studies analyzed:* In all studies analyzed to date, epoetin alfa administration was generally well-tolerated, irrespective of the route of administration.

Pediatric CRF patients – In pediatric patients with CRF on dialysis, the pattern of most adverse events was similar to that found in adults. Additional adverse events reported during the double-blind phase in greater than 10% of pediatric patients in either treatment group were the following: Abdominal pain, constipation, cough, dialysis access complications including access infections and peritonitis in those receiving peritoneal dialysis, fever, pharyngitis, and upper respiratory tract infection. The rates are similar between the treatment groups for each event.

Hypertension – Increases in blood pressure have been reported in clinical trials, often during the first 90 days of therapy. On occasion, hypertensive encephalopathy and seizures have been observed in patients with CRF treated with epoetin alfa. When data from all patients in the US phase 3 multicenter trial were analyzed, there was an apparent trend of more reports of hypertensive adverse events in patients on dialysis with a faster rate of rise of hematocrit (greater than 4 hematocrit points in any 2-week period). However, in a double-blind, placebo-controlled trial, hypertensive adverse events were not reported at an increased rate in the group treated with epoetin alfa (150 units/kg 3 times/week) relative to the placebo group.

Seizures – There have been 47 seizures in 1010 patients on dialysis treated with epoetin alfa in clinical trials, with an exposure of 986 patient-years for a rate of approximately 0.048 events per patient-year. However, there appeared to be a higher rate of seizures during the first 90 days of therapy (occurring in approximately 2.5% of patients) when compared with subsequent 90-day periods. The baseline incidence of seizures in the untreated dialysis population is difficult to determine; it appears to be in the range of 5% to 10% per patient-year.

Thrombotic events – In clinical trials where the maintenance hematocrit was 35 ± 3% on epoetin alfa, clotting of the vascular access (A-V shunt) has occurred at an annualized rate of about 0.25 events per patient-year, and other thrombotic events (eg, myocardial infarction, cerebral vascular accident, transient ischemic attack, and pulmonary embolism) occurred at a rate of 0.04 events per patient-year. In a separate study of 1111 untreated dialysis patients, clotting of the vascular access occurred at a rate of 0.5 events per patient-year. However, in CRF patients on hemodialysis who also had clinically evident ischemic heart disease or congestive heart failure, the risk of A-V shunt thrombosis was higher (39% vs 29%, $P < 0.001$), and myocardial infarctions, vascular ischemic events, and venous thrombosis were increased, in patients targeted to a hematocrit of 42 ± 3% compared with those maintained at 30 ± 3%. Increased mortality was observed in 634 patients randomized to a target hematocrit of 42% (221 deaths [35%

EPOETIN ALFA — INJECTION

mortality]) compared with 631 patients targeted to remain at a hematocrit of 30% (185 deaths [29% mortality]). The reason for the increased mortality observed in these studies is unknown; however, the incidence of nonfatal myocardial infarctions (3.1% vs 2.3%), vascular access thromboses (39% vs 29%), and all other thrombotic events (22% vs 18%) also were higher in the group randomized to achieve a hematocrit of 42%.

In patients treated with commercial epoetin alfa, there have been rare reports of serious or unusual thromboembolic events including migratory thrombophlebitis, microvascular thrombosis, pulmonary embolus, and thrombosis of the retinal artery, and temporal and renal veins. A causal relationship has not been established.

Allergic reactions – There have been no reports of serious allergic reactions or anaphylaxis associated with epoetin alfa administration during clinical trials. Skin rashes and urticaria have been observed rarely and when reported have generally been mild and transient in nature.

There have been rare reports of potentially serious allergic reactions including urticaria with associated respiratory symptoms or circumoral edema, or urticaria alone. Most reactions occurred in situations where a causal relationship could not be established. Symptoms recurred with rechallenge in a few instances, suggesting that allergic reactivity may occasionally be associated with epoetin alfa therapy. If an anaphylactoid reaction occurs, immediately discontinue epoetin alfa and initiate appropriate therapy.

➤*Zidovudine-treated HIV-infected patients:* Adverse events reported in clinical trials with epoetin alfa in zidovudine-treated HIV-infected patients were consistent with the progression of HIV infection. In double-blind, placebo-controlled studies of 3 months duration involving approximately 300 zidovudine-treated HIV-infected patients, adverse events with an incidence of greater than or equal to 10% in either patients treated with epoetin alfa or placebo-treated patients were:

Epoetin Alfa Adverse Reactions in Zidovudine-Treated Patients

Adverse reaction	Patients treated with epoetin alfa (n = 144)	Placebo-treated patients (n = 153)
Asthenia	11%	14%
Cough	18%	14%
Diarrhea	16%	18%
Dizziness	9%	10%
Fatigue	25%	31%
Headache	19%	14%
Nausea	15%	12%
Pyrexia	38%	29%
Rash	16%	8%
Respiratory congestion	15%	10%
Shortness of breath	14%	13%
Skin reaction, medication site	10%	7%

In the 297 patients studied, epoetin alfa was not associated with significant increases in opportunistic infections or mortality. In 71 patients from this group treated with epoetin alfa at 150 units/kg 3 times/week, serum p24 antigen levels did not appear to increase. Preliminary data showed no enhancement of HIV replication in infected cell lines in vitro.

Peripheral white blood cell and platelet counts are unchanged following epoetin alfa therapy.

Allergic reactions – Two zidovudine-treated HIV-infected patients had urticarial reactions within 48 hours of their first exposure to study medication. One patient was treated with epoetin alfa and 1 was treated with placebo (epoetin alfa vehicle alone). Both patients had positive immediate skin tests against their study medication with a negative saline control. The basis for this apparent preexisting hypersensitivity to components of the epoetin alfa formulation is unknown, but may be related to HIV-induced immunosuppression or prior exposure to blood products.

Seizures – In double-blind and open-label trials of epoetin alfa in zidovudine-treated HIV-infected patients, 10 patients have experienced seizures. In general, these seizures appear to be related to underlying pathology such as meningitis or cerebral neoplasms, not epoetin alfa therapy.

➤*Cancer patients on chemotherapy:* Adverse experiences reported in clinical trials with epoetin alfa administered 3 times/week in cancer patients were consistent with the underlying disease state. In double-blind, placebo-controlled studies of up to 3 months duration involving 131 cancer patients, adverse events with an incidence greater than 10% in either patients treated with epoetin alfa vs placebo-treated patients were as indicated:

Epoetin Alfa Adverse Reactions in Cancer Patients

Adverse reaction	Patients treated with epoetin alfa (n = 63)	Placebo-treated patients (n = 68)
Asthenia	13%	16%
Diarrhea	21%[a]	7%
Dizziness	5%	12%
Edema	17%[a]	1%
Fatigue	13%	15%
Nausea	17%[a]	32%
Paresthesia	11%	6%
Pyrexia	29%	19%
Shortness of breath	13%	9%
Trunk pain	3%[a]	16%
Upper respiratory tract infection	11%	4%
Vomiting	17%	15%

[a] Statistically significant

Although some statistically significant differences between patients being treated with epoetin alfa and placebo-treated patients were noted, the overall safety profile of epoetin alfa appeared to be consistent with the disease process of advanced cancer. During double-blind and subsequent open-label therapy in which patients (n = 72 for total exposure to epoetin alfa) were treated for up to 32 weeks with doses as high as 927 units/kg, the adverse experience profile of epoetin alfa was consistent with the progression of advanced cancer.

Three hundred thirty-three cancer patients enrolled in a placebo-controlled double-blind trial utilizing weekly dosing with epoetin alfa for up to 4 months were evaluable for adverse events. The incidence of adverse events was similar in the treatment and placebo arms.

➤*Surgery patients:* Adverse events with an incidence of greater than or equal to 10% are shown in the table below:

Epoetin Alfa Adverse Reactions in Surgery Patients

Adverse reaction	Patients treated with epoetin alfa 300 units/kg (n = 112)[a]	Patients treated with epoetin alfa 100 units/kg (n = 101)[a]	Placebo-treated patients (n = 103)[a]	Patients treated with epoetin alfa 600 units/kg (n = 73)[b]	Patients treated with epoetin alfa 300 units/kg (n = 72)[b]
Anxiety	7%	2%	11%	11%	4%
Constipation	43%	42%	43%	51%	53%
Diarrhea	10%	7%	12%	10%	6%
Dizziness	12%	9%	12%	11%	21%
Deep venous thrombosis	10%	3%	5%	0%[c]	0%[c]
Dyspepsia	9%	11%	6%	7%	8%
Edema	6%	11%	8%	11%	7%
Headache	13%	11%	9%	10%	19%
Hypertension	10%	11%	10%	5%	10%
Insomnia	13%	16%	13%	21%	18%
Nausea	48%	43%	45%	45%	58%
Pruritus	16%	16%	14%	14%	22%
Pyrexia	51%	50%	60%	47%	42%
Skin pain	18%	18%	17%	5%	4%
Skin reaction, medication site	25%	19%	22%	26%	29%
Urinary tract infection	12%	3%	11%	11%	8%
Vomiting	22%	12%	14%	21%	29%

[a] Study including patients undergoing orthopedic surgery treated with epoetin alfa or placebo for 15 days.
[b] Study including patients undergoing orthopedic surgery treated with epoetin alfa 600 units/kg/week × 4 or 300 units/kg daily × 15.
[c] Determined by clinical symptoms.

Thrombotic / vascular events – In 3 double-blind, placebo-controlled orthopedic surgery studies, the rate of deep venous thrombosis (DVT) was similar among epoetin alfa and placebo-treated patients in the recommended population of patients with a pretreatment hemoglobin of greater than 10 to less than or equal to 13 g/dL. However, in 2 of 3 orthopedic surgery studies the overall rate (all pretreatment hemoglobin groups combined) of DVTs detected by postoperative ultrasonography and/or surveillance venography was higher in the group treated with epoetin alfa than in the placebo-treated group (11% vs 6%). This finding was attributable to the difference in DVT rates observed in the subgroup of patients with pretreatment hemoglobin greater than 13 g/dL. However, the incidence of DVTs was within the range of that reported in the literature for orthopedic surgery patients.

In the orthopedic surgery study of patients with pretreatment hemoglobin of more than 10 to up to 13 g/dL which compared 2 dosing regimens (600 units/kg/week × 4 and 300 units/kg daily × 15); 4 subjects in the 600 units/kg/week epoetin alfa group (5%) and no subjects in the 300 units/kg daily group had a thrombotic vascular event during the study period.

In a study examining the use of epoetin alfa in 182 patients scheduled for coronary artery bypass graft surgery, 23% of patients treated with epoetin alfa and 29% treated with placebo experienced thrombotic/vascular events. There were 4 deaths among the epoetin alfa-treated patients that were associated with a thrombotic/vascular event. A causative role of epoetin alfa cannot be excluded.

EPOETIN ALFA — INJECTION

Overdosage

The maximum amount of epoetin alfa that can be safely administered in single or multiple doses has not been determined. Doses of up to 1,500 units/kg 3 times a week for 3 to 4 weeks have been administered without any direct toxic effects of epoetin alfa itself. Therapy with epoetin alfa can result in polycythemia if the hemoglobin is not carefully monitored and the dose appropriately adjusted. If the suggested target range is exceeded, epoetin alfa may be temporarily withheld until the hemoglobin returns to the suggested target range; epoetin alfa therapy may then be resumed using a lower dose. If polycythemia is of concern, phlebotomy may be indicated to decrease the hemoglobin.

Patient Information

In those situations in which the physician determines that a home dialysis patient can safely and effectively self-administer epoetin alfa, instruct the patient as to the proper dosage and administration. Inform patients of the signs and symptoms of allergic drug reaction and advise of appropriate actions. If home use is prescribed for a home dialysis patient, thoroughly instruct the patient in the importance of proper disposal and caution against the reuse of needles, syringes, or drug product. A puncture-resistant container for the disposal of used syringes and needles should be available to the patient. Dispose of the full container according to the directions provided by the physician.

DARBEPOETIN ALFA

Rx	**Aranesp** (Amgen)	**Solution for injection**: 25 mcg per 0.42 mL	Preservative-free. In polysorbate or albumin solutions.[a] In single-dose, prefilled, *SingleJect* syringes.
		25 mcg per 1 mL	Preservative-free. In polysorbate or albumin solutions.[a] In 1 mL single-dose vials.
		40 mcg per 0.4 mL	Preservative-free. In polysorbate or albumin solutions.[a] In single-dose, prefilled, *SingleJect* syringes.
		40 mcg per 1 mL	Preservative-free. In polysorbate or albumin solutions.[a] In 1 mL single-dose vials.
		60 mcg per 0.3 mL	Preservative-free. In polysorbate or albumin solutions.[a] In single-dose, prefilled, *SingleJect* syringes.
		60 mcg per 1 mL	Preservative-free. In polysorbate or albumin solutions.[a] In 1 mL single-dose vials.
		100 mcg per 0.5 mL	Preservative-free. In polysorbate or albumin solutions.[a] In single-dose, prefilled, *SingleJect* syringes.
		100 mcg per 1 mL	Preservative-free. In polysorbate or albumin solutions.[a] In 1 mL single-dose vials.
		150 mcg per 0.3 mL	Preservative-free. In polysorbate or albumin solutions.[a] In single-dose, prefilled, *SingleJect* syringes.
		150 mcg per 1 mL	Preservative-free. In polysorbate or albumin solutions.[a] In single-dose vials.
		200 mcg per 0.4 mL	Preservative-free. In polysorbate or albumin solutions.[a] In single-dose, prefilled, *SingleJect* syringes.
		200 mcg per 1 mL	Preservative-free. In polysorbate or albumin solutions.[a] In 1 mL single-dose vials.
		300 mcg per 0.6 mL	Preservative-free. In polysorbate or albumin solutions.[a] In single-dose, prefilled, *SingleJect* syringes.
		300 mcg per 1 mL	Preservative-free. In polysorbate or albumin solutions.[a] In 1 mL single-dose vials.
		500 mcg per 1 mL	Preservative-free. In polysorbate or albumin solutions.[a] In 1 mL single-dose vials and single-dose, prefilled, *SingleJect* syringes.

[a] Each mL of the polysorbate solution contains 0.05 mg polysorbate 80, sodium phosphate monobasic monohydrate 2.12 mg, sodium phosphate dibasic anhydrous 0.66 mg, and sodium chloride 8.18 mg. Each mL of the albumin solution contains albumin (human) 2.5 mg, sodium phosphate monobasic monohydrate 2.23 mg, sodium phosphate dibasic anhydrous 0.53 mg, and sodium chloride 8.18 mg.

DARBEPOETIN ALFA — INJECTION

Indications

➤*Anemia:* For the treatment of anemia associated with chronic renal failure (CRF), including patients on dialysis and patients not on dialysis, and for the treatment of anemia in patients with nonmyeloid malignancies in which anemia is caused by the effect of coadministered chemotherapy.

Administration and Dosage

➤*Approved by the FDA:* September 17, 2001.

Darbepoetin alfa dosing regimens are different for each of the indications described. Darbepoetin alfa should be administered under the supervision of a health care provider.

Darbepoetin alfa is supplied in vials or prefilled syringes with *UltraSafe* needle guards. Following administration of darbepoetin alfa from the prefilled syringe, the *UltraSafe* needle guard should be activated to prevent accidental needle sticks.

➤*CRF patients:* Administered either intravenously (IV) or subcutaneously as a single weekly injection. In patients on hemodialysis, the IV route is recommended. The dose should be started and slowly adjusted as described in the following sections based on hemoglobin levels. If a patient fails to respond or maintain a response, this should be evaluated. When darbepoetin alfa therapy is initiated or adjusted, the hemoglobin should be followed weekly until stabilized and should be monitored at least monthly thereafter.

For patients who respond to darbepoetin alfa with a rapid increase in hemoglobin (eg, greater than 1 g/dL in any 2-week period), the dose of darbepoetin alfa should be reduced because of the association of excessive rate of rise of hemoglobin with adverse reactions.

The dose should be adjusted for each patient to achieve and maintain a target hemoglobin level not to exceed 12 g/dL.

Starting dose –

Correction of anemia: 0.45 mcg/kg body weight, administered as a single IV or subcutaneous injection once weekly. Because of individual variability, doses should be titrated not to exceed a target hemoglobin concentration of 12 g/dL. For many patients, the appropriate maintenance dose will be lower than this starting dose. Predialysis patients, in particular, may require lower maintenance doses. Also, some patients have been treated successfully with a subcutaneous dose of darbepoetin alfa administered once every 2 weeks.

Conversion from epoetin alfa to darbepoetin alfa: The starting weekly dose of darbepoetin alfa should be estimated on the basis of the weekly epoetin alfa dose at the time of substitution (see the following table). Because of individual variability, doses should then be titrated to maintain the target hemoglobin. Because of the longer serum half-life, darbepoetin alfa should be administered less frequently than epoetin alfa. Darbepoetin alfa should be administered once a week if a patient was receiving epoetin alfa 2 to 3 times weekly. Darbepoetin alfa should be administered once every 2 weeks if a patient was receiving epoetin alfa once per week. The route of administration (IV or subcutaneous) should be maintained.

Estimated Darbepoetin Starting Doses (mcg/wk) Based on Previous Epoetin Alfa Dose (units/wk)	
Previous weekly epoetin alfa dose (units/wk)	Weekly starting darbepoetin alfa dose (mcg/wk)
< 2,500	6.25
2,500 to 4,999	12.5
5,000 to 10,999	25
11,000 to 17,999	40
18,000 to 33,999	60
34,000 to 89,999	100
≥ 90,000	200

Dose adjustment – The dose should be adjusted for each patient to achieve and maintain a target hemoglobin not to exceed 12 g/dL.

Increases in dose should not be made more frequently than once a month. If the hemoglobin is increasing and approaching 12 g/dL, the dose should be reduced approximately 25%. If the hemoglobin continues to increase, doses should be temporarily withheld until the hemoglobin begins to decrease, at which point therapy should be reinitiated at a dose approximately 25% below the previous dose. If the hemoglobin increases by greater than 1 g/dL in a 2-week period, the dose should be decreased approximately 25%.

If the increase in hemoglobin is less than 1 g/dL over 4 weeks and iron stores are adequate, the dose of darbepoetin alfa may be increased approximately 25% of the previous dose. Further increases may be made at 4-week intervals until the specified hemoglobin is obtained.

Maintenance dose – Darbepoetin alfa dosage should be adjusted to maintain a target hemoglobin not to exceed 12 g/dL. If the hemoglobin exceeds 12 g/dL, the dose may be adjusted as previously described. Doses must be individualized to ensure that hemoglobin is maintained at an appropriate level for each patient.

DARBEPOETIN ALFA — INJECTION

➤*Cancer patients receiving chemotherapy:* 2.25 mcg/kg administered as a weekly subcutaneous injection.

The dose should be adjusted for each patient to achieve and maintain a target hemoglobin. If there is less than a 1 g/dL increase in hemoglobin after 6 weeks of therapy, the dose of darbepoetin alfa should be increased up to 4.5 mcg/kg. If hemoglobin increases by more than 1 g/dL in a 2-week period or if the hemoglobin exceeds 12 g/dL, the dose should be reduced approximately 25%. If the hemoglobin exceeds 13 g/dL, doses should be temporarily withheld until the hemoglobin falls to 12 g/dL. At this point, therapy should be reinitiated at a dose approximately 25% below the previous dose.

➤*Preparation and administration:*

1.) Do not shake darbepoetin alfa or leave vials or syringes exposed to bright light. After removing the vials or prefilled syringes from the cartons, keep them covered to protect from room light until administration. Vigorous shaking or exposure to light may denature darbepoetin alfa, causing it to become biologically inactive. Always store vials or prefilled syringes of darbepoetin alfa in their cartons until use.
2.) Parenteral drug products should be inspected visually for particulate matter and discoloration prior to administration. Do not use any vials exhibiting particulate matter or discoloration.
3.) Do not dilute darbepoetin alfa.
4.) Do not administer darbepoetin alfa in conjunction with other drug solutions.
5.) Darbepoetin alfa is packaged in single-use vials and prefilled syringes and contains no preservative. Discard any unused portion. Do not pool unused portions from the vials or prefilled syringes. Do not use the vial or prefilled syringe more than 1 time.
6.) Following administration of darbepoetin alfa from the prefilled syringe, activate the *UltraSafe* needle guard. Place hands behind the needle, grasp the guard with one hand, and slide the guard forward until the needle is completely covered and the guard clicks into place. If an audible click is not heard, the needle guard may not be completely activated. The prefilled syringe should be disposed of by placing the entire prefilled syringe with guard activated into an approved puncture-proof container.

➤*Storage/Stability:* Store at 2° to 8°C (36° to 46°F). Do not freeze or shake. Protect from light.

Actions

➤*Pharmacology:* Darbepoetin alfa stimulates erythropoiesis by the same mechanism as endogenous erythropoietin. A primary growth factor for erythroid development, erythropoietin is produced in the kidney and released into the bloodstream in response to hypoxia. In responding to hypoxia, erythropoietin interacts with progenitor stem cells to increase red blood cell (RBC) production. Production of endogenous erythropoietin is impaired in patients with CRF, and erythropoietin deficiency is the primary cause of their anemia. Increased hemoglobin levels are not generally observed until 2 to 6 weeks after initiating treatment with darbepoetin alfa. In patients with cancer receiving concomitant chemotherapy, the etiology of anemia is multifactorial.

➤*Pharmacokinetics:*

Absorption/Distribution – The pharmacokinetics of darbepoetin alfa were studied in patients with CRF and in cancer patients receiving chemotherapy. Over the therapeutic range of 0.45 to 4.5 mcg/kg, pharmacokinetic measures (maximum effective plasma concentration [C_{max}], half-life, area under the plasma concentration-time curve [AUC]) were linear with respect to dose, and no evidence of accumulation was observed beyond an expected less than 2-fold increase in blood levels when compared with the initial dose.

Following subcutaneous administration, absorption is slow and rate-limiting. Postsubcutaneous administration, CRF patients' peak concentrations occur at 34 hours (range, 24 to 72 hours) whereas cancer patients' peak concentrations are at 90 hours (range, 71 to 123 hours).

The bioavailability of darbepoetin alfa as measured in CRF patients after subcutaneous administration is 37% (range, 30% to 50%).

Metabolism/Excretion – The observed half-life in CRF patients, which reflected the rate of absorption, was 49 hours (range, 27 to 89 hours). Following IV administration to these patients, darbepoetin alfa serum concentration-time profiles are biphasic, with a distribution half-life of approximately 1.4 hours and a mean terminal half-life of 21 hours.

When administered IV, the terminal half-life of darbepoetin alfa is approximately 3-fold longer than epoetin alfa.

Contraindications

Uncontrolled hypertension; hypersensitivity to the active substance or any of the excipients.

Warnings

➤*Cardiovascular events, hemoglobin, and rate of rise of hemoglobin:* Darbepoetin alfa and other erythropoietic therapies may increase the risk of cardiovascular events, including death. The higher risk of cardiovascular events may be associated with higher hemoglobin and/or higher rates of rise of hemoglobin. Manage the hemoglobin level carefully to avoid exceeding a target level of 12 g/dL.

In a clinical trial of epoetin alfa treatment in hemodialysis patients with clinically evident cardiac disease, patients were randomized to a target hemoglobin of 14 ± 1 g/dL or 10 ± 1 g/dL. Higher mortality (35% vs 29%) was observed in the 634 patients randomized to a target hemoglobin of 14 g/dL than in the 631 patients assigned a target hemoglobin of 10 g/dL. The reason for the increased mortality observed in this study is unknown; however, the incidence of nonfatal myocardial infarction, vascular access thrombosis, and other thrombotic events was also higher in the group randomized to a target hemoglobin of 14 g/dL.

In patients treated with darbepoetin alfa or other recombinant erythropoietins in darbepoetin alfa clinical trials, increases in hemoglobin greater than approximately 1 g/dL during any 2-week period were associated with increased incidence of cardiac arrest, neurologic events (eg, seizures, stroke), exacerbations of hypertension, congestive heart failure, vascular thrombosis/ischemia/infarction, acute myocardial infarction, and fluid overload/edema. It is recommended that the dose of darbepoetin alfa be decreased if the hemoglobin increase exceeds 1 g/dL in any 2-week period because of the association of excessive rate of rise of hemoglobin with these events.

➤*Hypertension:* Do not treat patients with uncontrolled hypertension with darbepoetin alfa; adequately control blood pressure before initiation of therapy. Blood pressure may rise during treatment of anemia with darbepoetin alfa or epoetin alfa. In darbepoetin alfa clinical trials, approximately 40% of patients with CRF required initiation or intensification of antihypertensive therapy during the early phase of treatment when the hemoglobin was increasing. Hypertensive encephalopathy and seizures have been observed in patients with CRF who were treated with darbepoetin alfa or epoetin alfa.

Take special care to closely monitor and control blood pressure in patients treated with darbepoetin alfa. During darbepoetin alfa therapy, advise patients of the importance of compliance with antihypertensive therapy and dietary restrictions. If blood pressure is difficult to control by pharmacologic or dietary measures, reduce or withhold the dose of darbepoetin alfa. A clinically significant decrease in hemoglobin may not be observed for several weeks.

➤*Seizures:* Seizures have occurred in patients with CRF participating in clinical trials of darbepoetin alfa and epoetin alfa. During the first several months of therapy, closely monitor blood pressure and the presence of premonitory neurologic symptoms. While the relationship between seizures and the rate of rise of hemoglobin is uncertain, it is recommended that the dose of darbepoetin alfa be decreased if the hemoglobin increase exceeds 1 g/dL in any 2-week period.

➤*Thrombotic events and increased mortality:* An increased incidence of thrombotic events has been observed in patients treated with erythropoietic agents. In patients with cancer who received darbepoetin alfa, pulmonary emboli, thrombophlebitis, and thrombosis occurred more frequently than in placebo controls.

In a randomized controlled study with another erythropoietic product in 939 women with metastatic breast cancer receiving chemotherapy, patients received weekly epoetin alfa or placebo for up to a year. This study was designed to prevent anemia (maintain hemoglobin levels between 12 and 14 g/dL or hematocrit 36% to 42%). Treatment with epoetin alfa was associated with a higher rate of fatal thrombotic events (1.1% epoetin alfa vs 0.2% placebo) in the first 4 months of the study. Based on Kaplan-Meier estimates, the proportion of subjects surviving at 12 months after randomization was lower in the epoetin alfa group than in the placebo group (70% vs 76%), $P = 0.012$, log rank. However, because of insufficient monitoring and data collection, reliable comparisons cannot be made concerning the effect of epoetin alfa on overall time with disease progression, progression-free survival, and overall survival. Until further information is available, the recommended target hemoglobin should not exceed 12 g/dL in men or women.

➤*Pure red cell aplasia (PRCA):* Cases of PRCA and severe anemia, with or without other cytopenias, associated with neutralizing antibodies to erythropoietin, have been reported in patients treated with darbepoetin alfa. This has been reported predominantly in patients with CRF receiving darbepoetin alfa by subcutaneous administration. Evaluate any patient who develops a sudden loss of response to darbepoetin alfa, accompanied by severe anemia and low reticulocyte count, for the etiology of loss of effect, including the presence of neutralizing antibodies to erythropoietin. If anti-erythropoietin antibody–associated anemia is suspected, withhold darbepoetin alfa and other erythropoietic proteins. Contact the manufacturer (1-800-772-6436) to perform assays for binding and neutralizing antibodies. Permanently discontinue darbepoetin alfa in patients with antibody-mediated anemia. Do not switch patients to other erythropoietic proteins as antibodies may crossreact.

➤*Albumin (human):* Darbepoetin alfa is supplied in 2 formulations with different excipients, one containing polysorbate 80 and another containing albumin (human), a derivative of human blood. Based on effective donor screening and product manufacturing processes, darbepoetin alfa formulated with albumin carries an extremely remote risk for transmission of viral diseases. A theoretical risk for transmission of Creutzfeldt-Jakob disease (CJD) also is considered extremely remote. No cases of transmission of viral diseases or CJD have ever been identified for albumin.

➤*Hypersensitivity reactions:* There have been rare reports of potentially serious allergic reactions, including skin rash and urticaria, associated with darbepoetin alfa. Symptoms have recurred with rechallenge, suggesting a causal relationship exists in some instances. If a serious allergic or anaphylactic reaction occurs, immediately and permanently discontinue darbepoetin alfa and administer appropriate therapy.

➤*Fertility impairment:* When administered IV to male and female rats prior to and during mating, reproductive performance, fertility, and sperm assessment parameters were not affected at any doses evaluated (up to 10 mcg/kg/dose, administered 3 times weekly). An increase in postimplantation fetal loss was seen at doses greater than or equal to 0.5 mcg/kg/dose, administered 3 times weekly.

DARBEPOETIN ALFA — INJECTION

➤*Elderly:* Of the 1,598 CRF patients in clinical studies of darbepoetin alfa, 42% were 65 years of age and older, while 15% were 75 years of age and older. Of the 873 cancer patients in clinical studies receiving darbepoetin alfa and concomitant chemotherapy, 45% were 65 years of age and older, while 14% were 75 years of age and older. No overall differences in safety or efficacy were observed between older and younger patients.

➤*Pregnancy: Category C.* When darbepoetin alfa was administered IV to rats and rabbits during gestation, no evidence of a direct embryotoxic, fetotoxic, or teratogenic outcome was observed at doses up to 20 mcg/kg/day. The only adverse reaction observed was a slight reduction in fetal weight, which occurred at doses causing exaggerated pharmacological effects in the dams (1 mcg/kg/day and higher). No deleterious effects on uterine implantation were seen in either species. No significant placental transfer of darbepoetin alfa was observed in rats. An increase in postimplantation fetal loss was observed in studies assessing fertility.

IV injection of darbepoetin alfa to female rats every other day from day 6 of gestation through day 23 of lactation at doses of 2.5 mcg/kg/dose and higher resulted in offspring (F1 generation) with decreased body weights, which correlated with a low incidence of deaths, as well as delayed eye opening and delayed preputial separation. No adverse reactions were seen in the F2 offspring.

There are no adequate and well-controlled studies in pregnant women. Use darbepoetin alfa during pregnancy only if the potential benefit justifies the potential risk to the fetus.

➤*Lactation:* It is not known whether darbepoetin alfa is excreted in human milk. Because many drugs are excreted in human milk, exercise caution when darbepoetin alfa is administered to a breast-feeding woman.

➤*Children:* The safety and efficacy of darbepoetin alfa in children have not been established. Pharmacokinetic data obtained in 14 subjects suggest that the pharmacokinetics in children between 5 and 18 years of age with nonhematologic malignancies were similar to those seen in adults with nonhematologic malignancies.

Precautions

➤*Monitoring:* After initiation of darbepoetin alfa therapy, determine the hemoglobin weekly until it has stabilized and the maintenance dose has been established. After a dose adjustment, determine the hemoglobin weekly for at least 4 weeks until it has been determined that the hemoglobin has stabilized in response to the dose change. Then monitor the hemoglobin at regular intervals.

In order to ensure effective erythropoiesis, evaluate iron status for all patients before and during treatment because the majority of patients will eventually require supplemental iron therapy. Supplemental iron therapy is recommended for all patients whose serum ferritin is less than 100 mcg/L or whose serum transferrin saturation is less than 20%.

During the first several months of therapy, closely monitor blood pressure and the presence of premonitory neurologic symptoms. In patients with CRF not requiring dialysis, closely monitor renal function and electrolyte balance.

➤*Lack or loss of response:* A lack of response or failure to maintain a hemoglobin response with darbepoetin alfa doses within the recommended dosing range should prompt a search for causative factors. Exclude or correct deficiencies of folic acid, iron, or vitamin B_{12}. Depending on the clinical setting, intercurrent infections, inflammatory or malignant processes, osteofibrosis cystica, occult blood loss, hemolysis, severe aluminum toxicity, and bone marrow fibrosis may compromise an erythropoietic response. In the absence of another etiology, evaluate the patient for evidence of PRCA and test sera for the presence of antibodies to erythropoietin.

➤*Hematology:* Allow sufficient time to determine a patient's responsiveness to a dosage of darbepoetin alfa before adjusting the dose. Because of the time required for erythropoiesis and the RBC half-life, an interval of 2 to 6 weeks may occur between the time of a dose adjustment (eg, initiation, increase, decrease, discontinuation) and a significant change in hemoglobin.

See Administration and Dosage for more information.

➤*Patients with CRF not requiring dialysis:* Patients with CRF not yet requiring dialysis may require lower maintenance doses of darbepoetin alfa than patients receiving dialysis. Though predialysis patients generally receive less frequent monitoring of blood pressure and laboratory parameters than dialysis patients, predialysis patients may be more responsive to the effects of darbepoetin alfa and require judicious monitoring of blood pressure and hemoglobin. Closely monitor renal function and fluid and electrolyte balance.

➤*Dialysis management:* Therapy with darbepoetin alfa results in an increase in RBCs and a decrease in plasma volume, which could reduce dialysis efficiency; patients who are marginally dialyzed may require adjustments in their dialysis prescription.

➤*Tumor growth factor potential:* Darbepoetin alfa is a growth factor that primarily stimulates RBC production. Erythropoietin receptors are also found on the surfaces of normal nonhematopoietic tissues and some malignant cell lines and tumor biopsy specimens. However, it is not known if these receptors are functional. The possibility that darbepoetin alfa can act as a growth factor for any tumor type, particularly myeloid malignancies, has not been evaluated.

In a randomized placebo-controlled study in 314 anemic patients with advanced lung cancer randomized to darbepoetin alfa or placebo, there were no statistically significant differences in time-to-progression or overall survival observed; however, the study was not designed to detect or exclude clinically meaningful differences in time-to-progression or overall survival.

In a randomized controlled study in 351 head and neck cancer patients, epoetin beta or placebo was administered to achieve target hemoglobins of 14 and 15 g/dL for women and men, respectively. Locoregional progression-free survival was significantly shorter (median, 406 days with epoetin beta vs 745 days with placebo; $P = 0.04$) in patients receiving epoetin beta.

There is insufficient information to establish whether use of epoetin products, including darbepoetin alfa, has an adverse effect on time to tumor progression or progression-free survival.

These studies permitted or required dosing to achieve a hemoglobin level greater than 12 g/dL. Until further information is available, do not exceed the recommended target hemoglobin of 12 g/dL in men or women.

See Warnings for more information.

➤*Special risk:* The safety and efficacy of darbepoetin alfa therapy have not been established in patients with underlying hematologic diseases (eg, hemolytic anemia, sickle cell anemia, thalassemia, porphyria).

Drug Interactions

No formal drug interaction studies of darbepoetin alfa with other medications commonly used in CRF patients have been performed.

Adverse Reactions

Because clinical trials are conducted under widely varying conditions, adverse reaction rates observed in the clinical trials of darbepoetin alfa cannot be directly compared with rates in the clinical trials of other drugs and may not reflect the rates observed in practice.

➤*Immunogenicity:* As with all therapeutic proteins, there is a potential for immunogenicity. Neutralizing antibodies to erythropoietin, in association with PRCA or severe anemia (with or without other cytopenias), have been reported in patients receiving darbepoetin alfa during postmarketing experience.

In clinical studies, the percentage of patients with antibodies to darbepoetin alfa was examined using the BIAcore assay. Sera from 1,501 CRF patients and 1,159 cancer patients were tested. At baseline, prior to darbepoetin alfa treatment, binding antibodies were detected in 59 (4%) of CRF patients and 36 (3%) of cancer patients. While receiving darbepoetin alfa therapy (range, 22 to 177 weeks), a follow-up sample was taken. One additional CRF patient and 8 additional cancer patients developed antibodies capable of binding darbepoetin alfa. None of the patients had antibodies capable of neutralizing the activity of darbepoetin alfa or endogenous erythropoietin at baseline or at end of study. No clinical sequelae consistent with PRCA were associated with the presence of these antibodies.

The incidence of antibody formation is highly dependent on the sensitivity and specificity of the assay. Additionally, the observed incidence of antibody (including neutralizing antibody) positivity in an assay may be influenced by several factors, including assay methodology, sample handling, timing of sample collection, concomitant medications, and underlying disease. For these reasons, comparison of the incidence of antibodies across products within this class (erythropoietic proteins) may be misleading.

CRF patients – In all studies, the most frequently reported serious adverse reactions with darbepoetin alfa were cardiac arrhythmia, congestive heart failure, sepsis, and vascular access thrombosis. The most commonly reported adverse reactions were diarrhea, headache, hypertension, hypotension, infection, and myalgia. The most frequently reported adverse reactions resulting in clinical intervention (eg, discontinuation of darbepoetin alfa, adjustment in dosage, the need for concomitant medication to treat an adverse reaction symptom) were chest pain, fever, hypertension, hypotension, myalgia, and nausea.

The following data reflect exposure to darbepoetin alfa in 1,598 CRF patients, including 675 exposed for at least 6 months, of whom 185 were exposed for greater than 1 year. Darbepoetin alfa was evaluated in active-controlled (n = 823) and uncontrolled studies (n = 775).

The rates of adverse reactions and association with darbepoetin alfa are best assessed in the results from studies in which darbepoetin alfa was used to stimulate erythropoiesis in patients anemic at study baseline (n = 348), and, in particular, the subset of these patients in randomized controlled trials (n = 276). Because there were no substantive differences in the rates of adverse reactions between these subpopulations, or between these subpopulations and the entire population of patients treated with darbepoetin alfa, data from all 1,598 patients were pooled.

The population encompassed an age range from 18 to 91 years. Fifty-seven percent of the patients were men. The percentages of white, black, Asian, and Hispanic patients were 83%, 11%, 3%, and 1%, respectively. The median weekly dose of darbepoetin alfa was 0.45 mcg/kg (25th, 75th percentiles: 0.29, 0.66 mcg/kg).

Some of the adverse reactions reported are typically associated with CRF or recognized complications of dialysis, and may not necessarily be attributable to darbepoetin alfa therapy. No important differences in adverse reaction rates between treatment groups were observed in controlled studies in which patients received darbepoetin alfa or other recombinant erythropoietins. The data in the following table reflect those adverse reactions occurring in at least 5% of patients treated with darbepoetin alfa.

DARBEPOETIN ALFA — INJECTION

Darbepoetin Alfa Adverse Reactions in CRF Patients (≥ 5%)	
Adverse reaction	Patients treated with darbepoetin alfa (n = 1,598)
Cardiovascular	
Angina pectoris/cardiac chest pain	8%
Cardiac arrhythmias/cardiac arrest	10%
Chest pain, unspecified	6%
Congestive heart failure	6%
Hypertension	23%
Hypotension	22%
Thrombosis vascular access	8%
CNS	
Dizziness	8%
Fatigue	9%
Headache	16%
Dermatologic	
Pruritus	8%
GI	
Abdominal pain	12%
Constipation	5%
Diarrhea	16%
Nausea	14%
Vomiting	15%
Musculoskeletal	
Arthralgia	11%
Back pain	8%
Limb pain	10%
Myalgia	21%
Respiratory	
Bronchitis	6%
Cough	10%
Dyspnea	12%
Upper respiratory tract infection	14%
Miscellaneous	
Access hemorrhage	6%
Access infection	6%
Asthenia	5%
Death	7%
Fever	9%
Fluid overload	6%
Infection[a]	27%
Influenza-like symptoms	6%
Injection site pain	7%
Peripheral edema	11%

[a] Infection includes abscess, bacteremia, peritonitis, pneumonia, and sepsis. The incidence rates for other clinically significant reactions are shown in the following table.

Darbepoetin Alfa (Other Adverse Reactions in CRF Patients)	
Adverse reaction	Patients treated with darbepoetin alfa (n = 1,598)
Acute myocardial infarction	2%
Seizure	1%
Stroke	1%
Transient ischemic attack	1%

➤*Thrombotic events:* Vascular access thrombosis in hemodialysis patients occurred in clinical trials at an annualized rate of 0.22 reactions per patient year of darbepoetin alfa therapy. Rates of thrombotic reactions (eg, pulmonary emboli, vascular access thrombosis, venous thrombosis) with darbepoetin alfa therapy were similar to those observed with other recombinant erythropoietins in these trials; the median duration of exposure was 12 weeks.

Cancer patients receiving chemotherapy – The following data reflect the exposure to darbepoetin alfa in 873 cancer patients. Darbepoetin alfa was evaluated in 7 studies that were active- or placebo-controlled studies of up to 6 months' duration. The darbepoetin alfa–treated patient demographics were as follows: median age of 63 years (range, 20 to 91 years); 40% men; 88% white, 5% Hispanic, 4% black, and 3% Asian. Over 90% of patients had locally advanced or metastatic cancer, with the remainder having early stage disease. Patients with solid tumors (eg, lung, breast, colon, ovarian cancers) and lymphoproliferative malignancies (eg, lymphoma, multiple myeloma) were enrolled in the clinical studies. All of the 873 darbepoetin alfa–treated subjects also received concomitant cyclic chemotherapy.

The most frequently reported serious adverse reactions included death (10%), dehydration (3%), dyspnea (2%), fever (4%), pneumonia (3%), and vomiting (2%). The most commonly reported adverse reactions were diarrhea, dyspnea, edema, fatigue, fever, nausea, and vomiting (see the following table). Except for those reactions listed in the following tables, the incidence of adverse reactions in clinical studies occurred at a similar rate compared with patients who received placebo and were generally consistent with the underlying disease and its treatment with chemotherapy. The most frequently reported reasons for discontinuation of darbepoetin alfa were asthenia, death, discontinuation of the chemotherapy, dyspnea, GI hemorrhage, pneumonia, and progressive disease. No important differences in adverse reaction rates between treatment groups were observed in controlled studies in which patients received darbepoetin alfa or other recombinant erythropoietins.

Darbepoetin Alfa Adverse Reactions in Chemotherapy Patients (≥ 5%)		
Adverse reaction	Darbepoetin alfa (n = 873)	Placebo (n = 221)
CNS		
Dizziness	14%	8%
Fatigue	33%	30%
Headache	12%	9%
Dermatologic		
Rash	7%	3%
GI		
Constipation	18%	17%
Diarrhea	22%	12%
Metabolic/Nutritional		
Dehydration	5%	3%
Musculoskeletal		
Arthralgia	13%	6%
Myalgia	8%	5%
Miscellaneous		
Edema	21%	10%
Fever	19%	16%

Darbepoetin Alfa (Other Adverse Reactions in Chemotherapy Patients)		
Adverse reaction	All darbepoetin alfa (n = 873)	Placebo (n = 221)
Hypertension	3.7%	3.2%
Pulmonary embolism	1.3%	0%
Seizures[a]	0.6%	0.5%
Thrombosis[b]	5.6%	4.1%
Thrombotic events	6.2%	4.1%

[a] Seizures include the following preferred terms: seizures, seizures local, and tonic-clonic seizures.
[b] Thrombosis includes the following: thromboembolism, thrombophlebitis deep, thrombosis, thrombosis venous, and thrombosis venous deep.

➤*Thrombotic and cardiovascular events:* Overall, the incidence of thrombotic events was 6.2% for darbepoetin alfa and 4.1% for placebo. However, the following reactions were reported more frequently in darbepoetin alfa–treated patients than in placebo controls: pulmonary embolism, thromboembolism, thrombophlebitis (deep and/or superficial), and thrombosis. In addition, edema of any type was more frequently reported in darbepoetin alfa–treated patients (21%) than in patients who received placebo (10%).

Overdosage

➤*Symptoms:* The maximum amount of darbepoetin alfa that can be safely administered in single or multiple doses has not been determined. Doses over 3 mcg/kg/week for up to 28 weeks have been administered to CRF patients. Doses up to 8 mcg/kg every week and 15 mcg/kg every 3 weeks have been administered to cancer patients for up to 12 to 16 weeks. Excessive rise and rate of rise in hemoglobin, however, have been associated with adverse reactions. In patients treated with darbepoetin alfa or other recombinant erythropoietins in darbepoetin alfa clinical trials, increases in hemoglobin greater than approximately 1 g/dL during any 2-week period were associated with increased incidence of cardiac arrest, neurologic events (eg, seizures, stroke), exacerbations of hypertension, congestive heart failure, vascular thrombosis/ischemia/infarction, acute myocardial infarction, and fluid overload/edema. It is recommended that the dose of darbepoetin alfa be decreased if the hemoglobin increase exceeds 1 g/dL in any 2-week period because of the association of excessive rate of rise of hemoglobin with these events.

DARBEPOETIN ALFA — INJECTION

➤*Treatment:* In the event of polycythemia, temporarily withhold darbepoetin alfa. If clinically indicated, phlebotomy may be performed.

Patient Information

Inform patients of the possible adverse reactions of darbepoetin alfa and instruct them to report these reactions to the prescribing health care provider. Inform patients of the signs and symptoms of allergic drug reactions and advise them of appropriate actions. Counsel patients on the importance of compliance with their darbepoetin alfa treatment and dietary and dialysis prescriptions, and stress the importance of judicious monitoring of blood pressure and hemoglobin concentration.

It is recommended that darbepoetin alfa be administered by a health care provider. In those rare cases in which it is determined that a patient can safely and effectively administer darbepoetin alfa at home, provide appropriate instruction on the proper use of darbepoetin alfa for patients and their health care providers. Caution patients and their health care providers against the reuse of needles, syringes, or drug product, and thoroughly instruct them in proper disposal. Give a puncture-resistant container for the disposal of used syringes and needles to the patient.

FILGRASTIM (Granulocyte Colony Stimulating Factor; G-CSF)

Rx	**Neupogen** (Amgen)	**Injection**: 300 mcg/mL[1]	Preservative free. In 1 and 1.6 mL single-dose vials.
		Injection: 300 mcg per 0.5 mL[2]	Preservative free. In 0.5 mL and 0.8 mL prefilled syringes.

[1] With 0.59 mg acetate, 50 mg sorbitol, 0.004% *Tween* 80 and 0.035 mg Na/mL in water for injection.

[2] With 0.295 mg acetate, 25 mg sorbitol, 0.004% *Tween* 80, and 0.0175 mg Na/mL in water for injection.

FILGRASTIM — INJECTION

Indications

➤*Cancer patients:*

Myelosuppressive chemotherapy – To decrease the incidence of infection, as manifested by febrile neutropenia, in patients with nonmyeloid malignancies receiving myelosuppressive anticancer drugs associated with a significant incidence of severe neutropenia with fever. A complete blood count (CBC) and platelet count should be obtained prior to chemotherapy, and twice a week (see Precautions, Monitoring) during filgrastim therapy to avoid leukocytosis and to monitor the neutrophil count. In phase 3 clinical studies, filgrastim therapy was discontinued when the ANC was greater than or equal to 10,000/mm^3 after the expected chemotherapy-induced nadir.

Acute myeloid leukemia (AML) receiving induction or consolidation chemotherapy – For reducing the time to neutrophil recovery and the duration of fever, following induction or consolidation chemotherapy treatment of adults with AML.

Bone marrow transplant – To reduce the duration of neutropenia and neutropenia-related clinical sequelae (eg, febrile neutropenia) in patients with nonmyeloid malignancies undergoing myeloablative chemotherapy followed by marrow transplantation. It is recommended that CBCs and platelet counts be obtained at a minimum of 3 times a week (see Precautions, Monitoring) following marrow infusion to monitor the recovery of marrow reconstitution.

Peripheral blood progenitor cell (PBPC) collection and therapy – for the mobilization of hematopoietic progenitor cells into the peripheral blood for collection by leukapheresis. Mobilization allows for the collection of increased numbers of progenitor cells capable of engraftment compared with collection by leukapheresis without mobilization or bone marrow harvest. After myeloablative chemotherapy, the transplantation of an increased number of progenitor cells can lead to more rapid engraftment, which may result in a decreased need for supportive care.

➤*Severe chronic neutropenia (SCN):* For chronic administration to reduce the incidence and duration of sequelae of neutropenia (eg, fever, infections, oropharyngeal ulcers) in symptomatic patients with congenital neutropenia, cyclic neutropenia, or idiopathic neutropenia. It is essential that serial CBCs with differential and platelet counts and an evaluation of bone marrow morphology and karyotype be performed prior to initiation of filgrastim therapy (see Warnings). The use of filgrastim prior to confirmation of SCN may impair diagnostic efforts and may thus impair or delay evaluation and treatment of an underlying condition, other than SCN, causing the neutropenia.

➤*Unlabeled uses:* Treatment of graft failure after bone marrow transplantation; neutropenia associated with myelodysplastic syndrome; hairy cell leukemia; aplastic anemia; AIDS; zidovudine- and other drug-induced neutropenias.

Administration and Dosage

➤*Approved by the FDA:* February 1991.

➤*Myelosuppressive chemotherapy:* The recommended starting dose of filgrastim is 5 mcg/kg/day, administered as a single daily injection by SC bolus injection, by short IV infusion (15 to 30 minutes), or by continuous SC or continuous IV infusion. A CBC and platelet count should be obtained before instituting filgrastim therapy, and monitored twice weekly during therapy. Doses may be increased in increments of 5 mcg/kg for each chemotherapy cycle, according to the duration and severity of the ANC nadir.

Filgrastim should be administered no earlier than 24 hours after the administration of cytotoxic chemotherapy. Filgrastim should not be administered in the period 24 hours before the administration of chemotherapy (see Precautions). Filgrastim should be administered daily for up to 2 weeks, until the ANC has reached 10,000/mm^3 following the expected chemotherapy-induced neutrophil nadir. The duration of filgrastim therapy needed to attenuate chemotherapy-induced neutropenia may be dependent on the myelosuppressive potential of the chemotherapy regimen employed. Filgrastim therapy should be discontinued if the ANC surpasses 10,000/mm^3 after the expected chemotherapy-induced neutrophil nadir (see Precautions). In phase 3 trials, efficacy was observed at doses of 4 to 8 mcg/kg/day.

➤*Bone marrow transplant (BMT):* The recommended dose of filgrastim following BMT is 10 mcg/kg/day given as an IV infusion of 4 or 24 hours, or as a continuous 24-hour SC infusion. For patients receiving BMT, the first dose of filgrastim should be administered at least 24 hours after cytotoxic chemotherapy and at least 24 hours after bone marrow infusion.

During the period of neutrophil recovery, the daily dose of filgrastim should be titrated against the neutrophil response as follows:

When the ANC is greater than 1000/mm^3 for 3 consecutive days, reduce the dose to 5 mcg/kg/day. (If, at any time during dosing with 5 mcg/kg/day, the ANC decreases to less than 1000/mm^3, the filgrastim dose should be increased to 10 mcg/kg/day, and the above steps repeated.)

If the ANC remains greater than 1000 mm^3 for 3 more consecutive days, filgrastim should be discontinued.

If the ANC decreases to less than 1000/mm^3, filgrastim should be resumed at 5 mcg/kg/day.

➤*Peripheral blood progenitor cell collection (PBPC) and therapy in cancer patients:* The recommended dose of filgrastim for the mobilization of PBPC is 10 mcg/kg/day SC, either as a bolus or a continuous infusion. It is recommended that filgrastim be given for at least 4 days before the first leukapheresis procedure and continued until the last leukapheresis. Although the optimal duration of filgrastim administration and leukapheresis schedule have not been established, administration of filgrastim for 6 to 7 days with leukaphereses on days 5, 6, and 7 was found to be safe and effective. Neutrophil counts should be monitored after 4 days of filgrastim, and filgrastim dose modification should be considered for those patients who develop a WBC count greater than 100,000/mm^3.

In all clinical trials of filgrastim for the mobilization of PBPC, filgrastim was also administered after reinfusion of the collected cells.

➤*SCN:* Filgrastim should be administered to those patients in whom a diagnosis of congenital, cyclic, or idiopathic neutropenia has been definitively confirmed. Other diseases associated with neutropenia should be ruled out.

Starting dose –

Congenital neutropenia: The recommended daily starting dose is 6 mcg/kg twice daily SC every day.

Idiopathic or cyclic neutropenia: The recommended daily starting dose is 5 mcg/kg as a single injection SC every day.

Dose adjustments – Chronic daily administration is required to maintain clinical benefit. Absolute neutrophil count should not be used as the sole indication of efficacy. The dose should be individually adjusted based on the patients' clinical course as well as ANC. In the severe chronic neutropenia (SCN) postmarketing surveillance study, the reported median daily doses of filgrastim were 6 mcg/kg (congenital neutropenia), 2.1 mcg/kg (cyclic neutropenia), and 1.2 mcg/kg (idiopathic neutropenia). In rare instances, patients with congenital neutropenia have required doses of filgrastim greater than or equal to 100 mcg/kg/day.

➤*Dilution of solution:* If required, filgrastim may be diluted in 5% dextrose. Filgrastim diluted to concentrations between 5 and 15 mcg/mL should be protected from adsorption to plastic materials by the addition of albumin (human) to a final concentration of 2 mg/mL. When diluted in 5% dextrose or 5% dextrose plus albumin (human), filgrastim is compatible with glass bottles, PVC and polyolefin IV bags, and polypropylene syringes.

Dilution of filgrastim to a final concentration of less than 5 mcg/mL is not recommended at any time. Do not dilute with saline at any time; product may precipitate.

➤*Storage / Stability:* Filgrastim should be stored in the refrigerator at 2° to 8°C (36° to 46°F). Avoid shaking. Prior to injection, filgrastim may be allowed to reach room temperature for a maximum of 24 hours. Any vial or prefilled syringe left at room temperature for greater than 24 hours should be discarded. Parenteral drug products should be inspected visually for particulate matter and discoloration prior to administration, whenever solution and container permit; if particulates or discoloration are observed, the container should not be used.

Actions

➤*Pharmacology:* Colony-stimulating factors are glycoproteins which act on hematopoietic cells by binding to specific cell-surface receptors and stimulating proliferation, differentiation commitment, and some end-cell functional activation.

FILGRASTIM — INJECTION

Endogenous G-CSF is a lineage-specific, colony-stimulating factor which is produced by monocytes, fibroblasts, and endothelial cells. G-CSF regulates the production of neutrophils within the bone marrow and affects neutrophil-progenitor proliferation, differentiation, and selected end-cell functional activation (including enhanced phagocytic ability, priming of the cellular metabolism associated with respiratory burst, antibody-dependent killing, and the increased expression of some functions associated with cell surface antigens). G-CSF is not species-specific and has been shown to have minimal direct in vivo or in vitro effects on the production of hematopoietic cell types other than the neutrophil lineage.

➤*Pharmacokinetics:*

Absorption/Distribution – Absorption and clearance of filgrastim follows first-order pharmacokinetic modeling without apparent concentration dependence. A positive linear correlation occurred between the parenteral dose and both the serum concentration and area under the concentration-time curves (AUCs). Continuous IV infusion of 20 mcg/kg of filgrastim over 24 hours resulted in mean and median serum concentrations of approximately 48 and 56 ng/mL, respectively. SC administration of 3.45 mcg/kg and 11.5 mcg/kg resulted in maximum serum concentrations of 4 and 49 ng/mL, respectively, within 2 to 8 hours. The volume of distribution averaged 150 mL/kg in both healthy subjects and cancer patients.

Excretion – The elimination half-life, in both healthy subjects and cancer patients, was approximately 3.5 hours. Clearance rates of filgrastim were approximately 0.5 to 0.7 mL/minute/kg. Single parenteral doses or daily IV doses, over a 14-day period, resulted in comparable half-lives. The half-lives were similar for IV administration (231 minutes, following doses of 34.5 mcg/kg) and for SC administration (210 minutes, following filgrastim doses of 3.45 mcg/kg). Continuous 24-hour IV infusions of 20 mcg/kg over an 11- to 20-day period produced steady-state serum concentrations of filgrastim with no evidence of drug accumulation over the time period investigated.

Contraindications

Hypersensitivity to *E. coli*-derived proteins, filgrastim, or any component of the product.

Warnings

➤*Patients with SCN:* The safety and efficacy of filgrastim in the treatment of neutropenia due to other hematopoietic disorders (eg, myelodysplastic syndrome [MDS]) have not been established. Care should be taken to confirm the diagnosis of SCN before initiating filgrastim therapy.

MDS and AML have been reported to occur in the natural history of congenital neutropenia without cytokine therapy. Cytogenetic abnormalities, transformation to MDS, and AML have also been observed in patients treated with filgrastim for SCN. Based on available data, including a postmarketing surveillance study, the risk of developing MDS and AML appears to be confined to the subset of patients with congenital neutropenia (see Adverse Reactions). Abnormal cytogenetics and MDS have been associated with the eventual development of myeloid leukemia. The effect of filgrastim on the development of abnormal cytogenetics, and the effect of continued filgrastim administration in patients with abnormal cytogenetics or MDS are unknown. If a patient with SCN develops abnormal cytogenetics or myelodysplasia, the risks and benefits of continuing filgrastim should be carefully considered.

➤*Hypersensitivity reactions:* Allergic-type reactions occurring on initial or subsequent treatment have been reported in less than 1 in 4000 patients treated with filgrastim. These have generally been characterized by systemic symptoms involving at least 2 body systems, most often skin (rash, urticaria, facial edema), respiratory (wheezing, dyspnea), and cardiovascular (hypotension, tachycardia). Some reactions occurred on initial exposure. Reactions tended to occur within the first 30 minutes after administration and appeared to occur more frequently in patients receiving filgrastim IV. Rapid resolution of symptoms occurred in most cases after administration of antihistamines, steroids, bronchodilators, or epinephrine. Symptoms recurred in more than half the patients who were rechallenged.

➤*Pregnancy: Category C.* Filgrastim has been shown to have adverse effects in pregnant rabbits when given in doses 2 to 10 times the human dose. Since there are no adequate and well-controlled studies in pregnant women, the effect, if any, of filgrastim on the developing fetus or the reproductive capacity of the mother is unknown. However, the scientific literature describes transplacental passage of filgrastim when administered to pregnant rats during the latter part of gestation and apparent transplacental passage of filgrastim when administered to pregnant humans by less than or equal to 30 hours prior to preterm delivery (less than or equal to 30 weeks gestation). Filgrastim should be used during pregnancy only if the potential benefit justifies the potential risk to the fetus.

In rabbits, increased abortion and embryolethality were observed in animals treated with filgrastim at 80 mcg/kg/day. Filgrastim administered to pregnant rabbits at doses of 80 mcg/kg/day during the period of organogenesis was associated with increased fetal resorption, genitourinary bleeding, developmental abnormalities, decreased body weight, live births, and food consumption. External abnormalities were not observed in the fetuses of dams treated at 80 mcg/kg/day. Reproductive studies in pregnant rats have shown that filgrastim was not associated with lethal, teratogenic, or behavioral effects on fetuses when administered by daily IV injection during the period of organogenesis at dose levels up to 575 mcg/kg/day.

In segment III studies in rats, offspring of dams treated at greater than 20 mcg/kg/day exhibited a delay in external differentiation (detachment of auricles and descent of testes) and slight growth retardation, possibly due to lower body weight of females during rearing and nursing. Offspring of dams treated at 100 mcg/kg/day exhibited decreased body weights at birth, and a slightly reduced 4-day survival rate.

➤*Lactation:* It is not known whether filgrastim is excreted in human milk. Because many drugs are excreted in human milk, caution should be exercised if filgrastim is administered to a nursing woman.

➤*Children:* In a phase 3 study to assess the safety and efficacy of filgrastim in the treatment of SCN, 120 patients with a median age of 12 years were studied. Of the 120 patients, 12 were infants (1 month to 2 years of age), 47 were children (2 to 12 years of age), and 9 were adolescents (12 to 16 years of age). Additional information is available from a SCN postmarketing surveillance study, which includes long-term follow-up of patients in the clinical studies and information from additional patients who entered directly into the postmarketing surveillance study. Of the 531 patients in the surveillance study as of December 31, 1997, 32 were infants, 200 were children, and 68 were adolescents (see Indications, Precautions, Administration and Dosage).

Pediatric patients with congenital types of neutropenia (Kostmann's syndrome, congenital agranulocytosis, or Schwachman-Diamond syndrome) have developed cytogenetic abnormalities and have undergone transformation to MDS and AML while receiving chronic filgrastim treatment. The relationship of these events to filgrastim administration is unknown (see Warnings and Adverse Reactions).

Long-term follow-up data from the postmarketing surveillance study suggest that height and weight are not adversely affected in patients who received up to 5 years of filgrastim treatment. Limited data from patients who were followed in the phase 3 study for 1.5 years did not suggest alterations in sexual maturation or endocrine function.

The safety and efficacy in neonates and patients with autoimmune neutropenia of infancy have not been established.

In the cancer setting, 12 pediatric patients with neuroblastoma have received up to 6 cycles of cyclophosphamide, cisplatin, doxorubicin, and etoposide chemotherapy concurrently with filgrastim; in this population, filgrastim was well-tolerated. There was 1 report of palpable splenomegaly associated with filgrastim therapy; however, the only consistently reported adverse event was musculoskeletal pain, which is no different from the experience in the adult population.

Precautions

➤*Monitoring:* Left upper abdominal pain or shoulder tip pain accompanied by rapid increase in spleen size should be carefully monitored due to the rare but serious risk of splenic rupture.

Cancer patients receiving myelosuppressive chemotherapy – A CBC and platelet count should be obtained prior to chemotherapy, and at regular intervals (twice a week) during filgrastim therapy. Following cytotoxic chemotherapy, the neutrophil nadir occurred earlier during cycles when filgrastim was administered, and WBC differentials demonstrated a left shift, including the appearance of promyelocytes and myeloblasts. In addition, the duration of severe neutropenia was reduced, and was followed by an accelerated recovery in the neutrophil counts. Therefore, regular monitoring of WBC counts, particularly at the time of the recovery from the postchemotherapy nadir, is recommended in order to avoid excessive leukocytosis.

Cancer patients receiving bone marrow transplant – Frequent CBCs and platelet counts are recommended (at least 3 times a week) following marrow transplantation.

Patients with SCN – During the initial 4 weeks of filgrastim therapy and during the 2 weeks following any dose adjustment, a CBC with differential and platelet count should be performed twice weekly. Once a patient is clinically stable, a CBC with differential and platelet count should be performed monthly during the first year of treatment. Thereafter, if clinically stable, routine monitoring with regular CBCs (ie, as clinically indicated but at least quarterly) is recommended. Additionally, for those patients with congenital neutropenia, annual bone marrow and cytogenetic evaluations should be performed throughout the duration of treatment (see Warnings and Adverse Reactions).

Hematologic effects – In studies of filgrastim administration following chemotherapy, most reported side effects were consistent with those usually seen as a result of cytotoxic chemotherapy (see Adverse Reactions). Because of the potential of receiving higher doses of chemotherapy (ie, full doses on the prescribed schedule), the patient may be at greater risk of thrombocytopenia, anemia, and nonhematologic consequences of increased chemotherapy doses (please refer to the monograph information for the specific chemotherapy agents used). Regular monitoring of the hematocrit and platelet count is recommended. Furthermore, care should be exercised in the administration of filgrastim in conjunction with other drugs known to lower the platelet count. In septic patients receiving filgrastim, the physician should be alert to the possibility of adult respiratory distress syndrome, due to the possible influx of neutrophils at the site of inflammation.

There have been rare reports (less than 1 in 7000 patients) of cutaneous vasculitis in patients treated with filgrastim. In most cases, the severity of cutaneous vasculitis was moderate or severe. Most of the reports involved patients with SCN receiving long-term filgrastim therapy. Symptoms of vasculitis generally developed simultaneously with an increase in the ANC and abated when the ANC decreased. Many patients were able to continue filgrastim at a reduced dose.

➤*Simultaneous use with chemotherapy and radiation therapy:* The safety and efficacy of filgrastim given simultaneously with cytotoxic chemotherapy have not been established. Because of the potential sensitivity of rapidly dividing myeloid cells to cytotoxic chemotherapy, do not use filgrastim in the period 24 hours before through 24 hours after the administration of cytotoxic chemotherapy (see Administration and Dosage).

FILGRASTIM — INJECTION

The efficacy of filgrastim has not been evaluated in patients receiving chemotherapy associated with delayed myelosuppression (eg, nitrosoureas) or with mitomycin C or with myelosuppressive doses of antimetabolites such as 5-fluorouracil.

The safety and efficacy of filgrastim have not been evaluated in patients receiving concurrent radiation therapy. Simultaneous use of filgrastim with chemotherapy and radiation therapy should be avoided.

➤*Potential effect on malignant cells:* Filgrastim is a growth factor that primarily stimulates neutrophils. However, the possibility that filgrastim can act as a growth factor for any tumor type cannot be excluded. In a randomized study evaluating the effects of filgrastim vs placebo in patients undergoing remission induction for AML, there was no significant difference in remission rate, disease-free or overall survival.

The safety of filgrastim in chronic myeloid leukemia (CML) and myelodysplasia has not been established.

When filgrastim is used to mobilize PBPC, tumor cells may be released from the marrow and subsequently collected in the leukapheresis product. The effect of reinfusion of tumor cells has not been well studied, and the limited data available are inconclusive.

➤*Leukocytosis:*

Cancer patients receiving myelosuppressive chemotherapy – White blood cell counts of greater than or equal to 100,000/mm^3 were observed in approximately 2% of patients receiving filgrastim at doses above 5 mcg/kg/day. There were no reports of adverse events associated with this degree of leukocytosis. In order to avoid the potential complications of excessive leukocytosis, a CBC is recommended twice a week during filgrastim therapy (see Monitoring).

➤*Premature discontinuation of filgrastim therapy:*

Cancer patients receiving myelosuppressive chemotherapy – A transient increase in neutrophil counts is typically seen 1 to 2 days after initiation of filgrastim therapy. However, for a sustained therapeutic response, filgrastim therapy should be continued following chemotherapy until the post nadir ANC reaches 10,000/mm^3. Therefore, the premature discontinuation of filgrastim therapy, prior to the time of recovery from the expected neutrophil nadir, is generally not recommended (see Administration and Dosage).

➤*Lab test abnormalities:* In clinical trials, the following laboratory results were observed:

- Cyclic fluctuations in the neutrophil counts were frequently observed in patients with congenital or idiopathic neutropenia after initiation of filgrastim therapy.
- Platelet counts were generally at the upper limits of normal prior to filgrastim therapy. With filgrastim therapy, platelet counts decreased but usually remained within normal limits (see Adverse Reactions).
- Early myeloid forms were noted in peripheral blood in most patients, including the appearance of metamyelocytes and myelocytes. Promyelocytes and myeloblasts were noted in some patients.
- Relative increases were occasionally noted in the number of circulating eosinophils and basophils. No consistent increases were observed with filgrastim therapy.
- As in other trials, increases were observed in serum uric acid, lactic dehydrogenase, and serum alkaline phosphatase.

Drug Interactions

Drug interactions between filgrastim and other drugs have not been fully evaluated. Drugs which may potentiate the release of neutrophils, such as lithium, should be used with caution.

Adverse Reactions

➤*Cancer patients receiving myelosuppressive chemotherapy:* In clinical trials involving greater than 350 patients receiving filgrastim following nonmyeloablative cytotoxic chemotherapy, most adverse reactions were the sequelae of the underlying malignancy or cytotoxic chemotherapy. In all phase 2 and 3 trials, medullary bone pain, reported in 24% of patients, was the only consistently observed adverse reaction attributed to filgrastim therapy. This bone pain was generally reported to be of mild-to-moderate severity, and could be controlled in most patients with nonnarcotic analgesics; infrequently, bone pain was severe enough to require narcotic analgesics. Bone pain was reported more frequently in patients treated with higher doses (20 to 100 mcg/kg/day) administered IV, and less frequently in patients treated with lower SC doses of filgrastim (3 to 10 mcg/kg/day).

In the randomized double-blind, placebo-controlled trial of filgrastim therapy following combination chemotherapy in patients (n = 207) with small cell lung cancer, the following adverse events were reported during blinded cycles of study medication (placebo or filgrastim at 4 to 8 mcg/kg/day). Events are reported as exposure-adjusted since patients remained on double-blind filgrastim a median of 3 cycles vs 1 cycle for placebo.

Filgrastim Adverse Reactions in Patients Receiving Myelosuppressive Chemotherapy

Adverse reaction	Filgrastim (n = 384) Patient cycles	Placebo (n = 257) Patient cycles
Nausea/vomiting	57%	64%
Skeletal pain	22%	11%
Alopecia	18%	27%
Diarrhea	14%	23%
Neutropenic fever	13%	35%
Mucositis	12%	20%
Fever	12%	11%
Fatigue	11%	16%
Anorexia	9%	11%
Dyspnea	9%	11%
Headache	7%	9%
Cough	6%	8%
Skin rash	6%	9%
Chest pain	5%	6%
Generalized weakness	4%	7%
Sore throat	4%	9%
Stomatitis	5%	10%
Constipation	5%	10%
Pain (unspecified)	2%	7%

In this study, there were no serious, life-threatening, or fatal adverse reactions attributed to filgrastim therapy. Specifically, there were no reports of flu-like symptoms, pleuritis, pericarditis, or other major systemic reactions to filgrastim.

Spontaneously reversible elevations in uric acid, lactate dehydrogenase, and alkaline phosphatase occurred in 27% to 58% of 98 patients receiving blinded filgrastim therapy following cytotoxic chemotherapy; increases were generally mild to moderate. Transient decreases in blood pressure (less than 90/60 mmHg), which did not require clinical treatment, were reported in 7 of 176 patients in phase 3 clinical studies following administration of filgrastim. Cardiac events (myocardial infarctions [MIs], arrhythmias) have been reported in 11 of 375 cancer patients receiving filgrastim in clinical trials; the relationship to filgrastim therapy is unknown. No evidence of interaction of filgrastim with other drugs was observed in the course of clinical trials (see Drug Interactions).

There has been no evidence for the development of antibodies or of a blunted or diminished response to filgrastim in treated patients, including those receiving filgrastim daily for almost 2 years.

➤*Patients with acute myeloid leukemia:* In a randomized phase 3 clinical trial, 259 patients received filgrastim, and 262 patients received placebo postchemotherapy. Overall, the frequency of all reported adverse events was similar in both the filgrastim and placebo groups (83% vs 82% in induction 1; 61% vs 64% in consolidation 1). Adverse events reported more frequently in the filgrastim-treated group included the following: Petechiae (17% vs 14%); epistaxis (9% vs 5%); transfusion reactions (10% vs 5%). There were no significant differences in the frequency of these reactions.

There were a similar number of deaths in each treatment group during induction (25 filgrastim vs 27 placebo). The primary causes of death included infection (9 vs 18), persistent leukemia (7 vs 5), and hemorrhage (6 vs 3). Of the hemorrhagic deaths, 5 cerebral hemorrhages were reported in the filgrastim group and 1 in the placebo group. Other serious nonfatal hemorrhagic events were reported in the respiratory tract (4 vs 1), skin (4 vs 4), GI tract (2 vs 2), urinary tract (1 vs 1), ocular (1 vs 0), and other nonspecific sites (2 vs 1). While nineteen (7%) patients in the filgrastim group and five (2%) patients in the placebo group experienced severe or fatal hemorrhagic events, overall, hemorrhagic adverse events were reported at a similar frequency in both groups (40% vs 38%). The time to transfusion-independent platelet recovery and the number of days of platelet transfusions were similar in both groups.

➤*Cancer patients receiving bone marrow transplant (BMT):* In clinical trials, the reported adverse effects were those typically seen in patients receiving intensive chemotherapy followed by BMT. The most common events reported in both control and treatment groups included stomatitis, nausea, and vomiting, generally of mild-to-moderate severity and were considered unrelated to filgrastim. In the randomized studies of BMT involving 167 patients who received study drug, the following events occurred more frequently in patients treated with filgrastim than in controls: Nausea (10% vs 4%); vomiting (7% vs 3%); hypertension (4% vs 0%); rash (12% vs 10%); peritonitis (2% vs 0%). None of these events were reported by the investigator to be related to filgrastim. One event of erythema nodosum was reported moderate in severity and possibly related to filgrastim.

Generally, adverse reactions observed in nonrandomized studies were similar to those seen in randomized studies, occurred in a minority of patients, and were of mild-to-moderate severity. In 1 study (n = 45), 3 serious adverse events reported by the investigator were considered possibly related to filgrastim. These included 2 events of renal insufficiency and 1 event of capillary leak syndrome. The relationship of these events to filgrastim remains unclear since they occurred in patients with culture-proven infection with clinical sepsis who were receiving potentially nephrotoxic antibacterial and antifungal therapy.

➤*Cancer patients undergoing PBPC collection and therapy:* In clinical trials, 126 patients received filgrastim for PBPC mobilization. In this set-

FILGRASTIM — INJECTION

ting, filgrastim was generally well tolerated. Adverse events related to filgrastim consisted primarily of mild-to-moderate musculoskeletal symptoms, reported in 44% of patients. These symptoms were predominantly events of medullary bone pain (33%). Headache was reported related to filgrastim in 7% of patients. Transient increases in alkaline phosphatase related to filgrastim were reported in 21% of the patients who had serum chemistries measured; most were mild to moderate.

All patients had increases in neutrophil counts during mobilization, consistent with the biological effects of filgrastim. Two patients had a WBC count greater than 100,000/mm^3. No sequelae were associated with any grade of leukocytosis.

Sixty-five percent (65%) of patients had mild-to-moderate anemia, and 97% of patients had decreases in platelet counts; 5 patients (out of 126) had decreased platelet counts to less than 50,000/mm^3. Anemia and thrombocytopenia have been reported to be related to leukapheresis; however, the possibility that filgrastim mobilization may contribute to anemia or thrombocytopenia has not been ruled out.

➤*Patients with SCN:* Mild-to-moderate bone pain was reported in approximately 33% of patients in clinical trials. This symptom was readily controlled with nonnarcotic analgesics. Generalized musculoskeletal pain was also noted in higher frequency in patients treated with filgrastim. Palpable splenomegaly was observed in approximately 30% of patients. Abdominal or flank pain was seen infrequently, and thrombocytopenia (less than 50,000/mm^3) was noted in 12% of patients with palpable spleens. Fewer than 3% of all patients underwent splenectomy, and most of these had a history of splenomegaly. Fewer than 6% of patients had thrombocytopenia (less than 50,000/mm^3) during filgrastim therapy, most of whom had a history of thrombocytopenia. In most cases, thrombocytopenia was managed by filgrastim dose reduction or interruption. An additional 5% of patients had platelet counts between 50,000 to 100,000/mm^3. There were no associated serious hemorrhagic sequelae in these patients. Epistaxis was noted in 15% of patients treated with filgrastim, but was associated with thrombocytopenia in 2% of patients. Anemia was reported in approximately 10% of patients, but in most cases appeared to be related to frequent diagnostic phlebotomy, chronic illness, or concomitant medications. Other adverse reactions infrequently observed and possibly related to filgrastim therapy were the following: Injection site reaction, rash, hepatomegaly, arthralgia, osteoporosis, cutaneous vasculitis, hematuria/proteinuria, alopecia, and the exacerbation of some preexisting skin disorders (eg, psoriasis).

Cytogenetic abnormalities, transformation to MDS, and AML have been observed in patients treated with filgrastim for SCN (see Warnings). As of December 31, 1997, data were available from a postmarketing surveillance study of 531 SCN patients with an average follow-up of 4 years. Based on analysis of these data, the risk of developing MDS and AML appears to be confined to the subset of patients with congenital neutropenia. A life-table analysis of these data revealed that the cumulative risk of developing leukemia or MDS by the end of the eighth year of filgrastim treatment in a patient with congenital neutropenia was 16.5% (95% confidence interval [CI] = 9.8%, 23.3%); this represents an annual rate of approximately 2%. Cytogenetic abnormalities, most commonly involving chromosome 7, have been reported in patients treated with filgrastim who had previously documented normal cytogenetics. It is unknown whether the development of cytogenetic abnormalities, MDS, or AML is related to chronic daily filgrastim administration, or to the natural history of congenital neutropenia. It is also unknown if the rate of conversion in patients who have not received filgrastim is different from that of patients who have received filgrastim. Routine monitoring through regular CBCs is recommended for all SCN patients. Additionally, annual bone marrow and cytogenetic evaluations are recommended in all patients with congenital neutropenia (see Precautions).

Overdosage

➤*Symptoms:* In cancer patients receiving filgrastim as an adjunct to myelosuppressive chemotherapy, it is recommended, to avoid the potential risks of excessive leukocytosis, that filgrastim therapy be discontinued if the ANC surpasses 10,000/mm^3 after the chemotherapy-induced ANC nadir has occurred. Doses of filgrastim that increase the ANC beyond 10,000/mm^3 may not result in any additional clinical benefit.

The maximum tolerated dose of filgrastim has not been determined. Efficacy was demonstrated at doses of 4 to 8 mcg/kg/day in the phase 3 study of nonmyeloablative chemotherapy. Patients in the BMT studies received up to 138 mcg/kg/day without toxic effects, although there was a flattening of the dose-response curve above daily doses of greater than 10 mcg/kg/day.

In filgrastim clinical trials of cancer patients receiving myelosuppressive chemotherapy, WBC counts greater than 100,000/mm^3 have been reported in less than 5% of patients, but were not associated with any reported adverse clinical effects.

➤*Treatment:* In cancer patients receiving myelosuppressive chemotherapy, discontinuation of filgrastim therapy usually results in a 50% decrease in circulating neutrophils within 1 to 2 days, with a return to pretreatment levels in 1 to 7 days.

Patient Information

In those situations in which the physician determines that the patient can safely and effectively self-administer filgrastim, the patient should be instructed as to the proper dosage and administration. Patients should be referred to the "Information for Patients" labeling included with each dispensing carton of filgrastim. This patient information, however, is not intended to be a disclosure of all known or possible effects. If home use is prescribed, patients should be thoroughly instructed in the importance of proper disposal and cautioned against the reuse of needles, syringes, or drug product. A puncture-resistant container for the disposal of used syringes and needles should be available to the patient. The full container should be disposed of according to the directions provided by the physician.

PEGFILGRASTIM

Rx	**Neulasta** (Amgen)	**Solution for injection:** 10 mg/mL	Preservative free. In dispensing pack containing single-dose syringe with needle.

PEGFILGRASTIM — INJECTION

Indications

➤*Myelosuppressive chemotherapy:* To decrease the incidence of infection, as manifested by febrile neutropenia, in patients with nonmyeloid malignancies receiving myelosuppressive anticancer drugs associated with a clinically significant incidence of febrile neutropenia.

Administration and Dosage

➤*Approved by the FDA:* January 31, 2002.

➤*Dosage:* The recommended dosage of pegfilgrastim is a single subcutaneous (SC) injection of 6 mg administered once per chemotherapy cycle. Pegfilgrastim should not be administered in the period between 14 days before and 24 hours after administration of cytotoxic chemotherapy because of the potential for an increase in sensitivity of rapidly dividing myeloid cells to cytotoxic chemotherapy.

The 6 mg fixed dose formulation should not be used in infants, children and smaller adolescents weighing less than 45 kg.

➤*Administration:* Pegfilgrastim is supplied in prefilled syringes with *UltraSafe Needle Guards.* Following administration of pegfilgrastim from the prefilled syringe, the *UltraSafe Needle Guard* should be activated to prevent accidental needle sticks. To activate the *UltraSafe Needle Guard,* place your hands behind the needle, grasp the guard with one hand, and slide the guard forward until the needle is completely covered and the guard clicks into place. Note: If an audible click is not heard, the needle guard may not be completely activated. The prefilled syringe should be disposed of by placing the entire prefilled syringe with guard activated into an approved puncture-proof container.

Pegfilgrastim should be visually inspected for discoloration and particulate matter before administration. Pegfilgrastim should not be administered if discoloration or particulates are observed.

➤*Storage/Stability:* Pegfilgrastim should be stored refrigerated at 2° to 8°C (36° to 46°F); syringes should be kept in their carton to protect from light until time of use. Shaking should be avoided. Before injection, pegfilgrastim may be allowed to reach room temperature for a maximum of 48 hours but should be protected from light. Pegfilgrastim left at room temperature for more than 48 hours should be discarded. Freezing should be avoided; however, if accidentally frozen, pegfilgrastim should be allowed to thaw in the refrigerator before administration. If frozen a second time, pegfilgrastim should be discarded.

Actions

➤*Pharmacology:* Both filgrastim and pegfilgrastim are colony stimulating factors that act on hematopoietic cells by binding to specific cell surface receptors thereby stimulating proliferation, differentiation, commitment, and end cell functional activation. Studies on cellular proliferation, receptor binding, and neutrophil function demonstrate that filgrastim and pegfilgrastim have the same mechanism of action. Pegfilgrastim has reduced renal clearance and prolonged persistence in vivo as compared to filgrastim.

➤*Pharmacokinetics:*

Special populations – No gender-related differences were observed in the pharmacokinetics of pegfilgrastim, and no differences were observed in the pharmacokinetics of geriatric patients (greater than or equal to 65 years old) compared to younger patients (less than 65 years old). However, due to the small number of elderly subjects studied, small but clinically relevant differences cannot be excluded. The pharmacokinetic profile in pediatric populations or in patients with hepatic or renal insufficiency has not been assessed. The pharmacokinetics and pharmacodynamics of pegfilgrastim were studied in 379 patients with cancer. The pharmacokinetics of pegfilgrastim were nonlinear in cancer patients and clearance decreased with increases in dose. Neutrophil receptor binding is an important component of the clearance of pegfilgrastim, and serum clearance is directly related to the number of neutrophils. For example, the concentration of pegfilgrastim declined rapidly at the onset of neutrophil recovery that followed myelosuppressive chemotherapy. In addition to numbers of neutrophils, body weight appeared to be a factor. Patients with higher body weights experienced higher systemic exposure to pegfilgrastim after receiving a dose normalized for body weight. A large variability in the pharmacokinetics of pegfilgrastim was observed in cancer patients. The half-life of pegfilgrastim ranged from 15 to 80 hours after SC injection.

Contraindications

Hypersensitivity to *E coli*-derived proteins, pegfilgrastim, filgrastim, or any other component of the product.

PEGFILGRASTIM — INJECTION

Warnings

➤*Splenic rupture:* Rare cases of splenic rupture have been reported following the administration of the parent compound of pegfilgrastim, filgrastim, for peripheral blood progenitor cell (PBPC) mobilization in both healthy donors and patients with cancer. Some of these cases were fatal. Pegfilgrastim has not been evaluated in this setting, therefore, pegfilgrastim should not be used for PBPC mobilization. Patients receiving pegfilgrastim who report left upper abdominal or shoulder tip pain should be evaluated for an enlarged spleen or splenic rupture.

➤*Adult respiratory distress syndrome (ARDS):* Adult respiratory distress syndrome (ARDS) has been reported in neutropenic patients with sepsis receiving filgrastim, the parent compound of pegfilgrastim, and is postulated to be secondary to an influx of neutrophils to sites of inflammation in the lungs. Neutropenic patients receiving pegfilgrastim who develop fever, lung infiltrates, or respiratory distress should be evaluated for the possibility of ARDS. In the event that ARDS occurs, pegfilgrastim should be discontinued or withheld until resolution of ARDS and patients should receive appropriate medical management for this condition.

➤*Sickle cell disease:* Severe sickle cell crises have been reported in patients with sickle cell disease (specifically homozygous sickle cell anemia, sickle/hemoglobin C disease, and sickle/β+ thalassemia) who received filgrastim, the parent compound of pegfilgrastim, for PBPC mobilization or following chemotherapy. One of these cases was fatal. Pegfilgrastim should be used with caution in patients with sickle cell disease, and only after careful consideration of the potential risks and benefits. Patients with sickle cell disease who receive pegfilgrastim should be kept well hydrated and monitored for the occurrence of sickle cell crises. In the event of severe sickle cell crisis, supportive care should be administered, and interventions to ameliorate the underlying event, such as therapeutic red blood cell exchange transfusion, should be considered.

➤*Hypersensitivity reactions:* Allergic-type reactions, including anaphylaxis, skin rash and urticaria, occurring on initial or subsequent treatment have been reported with the parent compound of pegfilgrastim, filgrastim. In some cases, symptoms have recurred with rechallenge, suggesting a causal relationship. Allergic-type reactions to pegfilgrastim have not been observed in clinical trials. If a serious allergic reaction or an anaphylactic reaction occurs, appropriate therapy should be administered and further use of pegfilgrastim should be discontinued.

➤*Elderly:* Of the 465 subjects with cancer who received pegfilgrastim in clinical studies, 85 (18%) were age 65 and over, and 14 (3%) were age 75 and over. No overall differences in safety or effectiveness were observed between these patients and younger patients; however, due to the small number of elderly subjects, small but clinically relevant differences cannot be excluded.

➤*Pregnancy: Category C.* Pegfilgrastim has been shown to have adverse effects in pregnant rabbits when administered SC every other day during gestation at doses as low as 50 mcg/kg/dose (approximately 4-fold higher than the recommended human dose). Decreased maternal food consumption, accompanied by a decreased maternal body weight gain and decreased fetal body weights were observed at 50 to 1000 mcg/kg/dose. Pegfilgrastim doses of 200 and 250 mcg/kg/dose resulted in an increased incidence of abortions. Increased postimplantation loss due to early resorptions, was observed at doses of 200 to 1000 mcg/kg/dose and decreased numbers of live rabbit fetuses were observed at pegfilgrastim doses of 200 to 1000 mcg/kg/dose, given every other day.

Subcutaneous injections of pegfilgrastim of up to 1000 mcg/kg/dose every other day during the period of organogenesis in rats were not associated with an embryotoxic or fetotoxic outcome. However, an increased incidence (compared to historical controls) of wavy ribs was observed in rat fetuses at 1000 mcg/kg/dose every other day. Very low levels (less than 0.5%) of pegfilgrastim crossed the placenta when administered subcutaneously to pregnant rats every other day during gestation.

There are no adequate and well-controlled studies in pregnant women. Pegfilgrastim should be used during pregnancy only if the potential benefit to the mother justifies the potential risk to the fetus.

➤*Lactation:* It is not known whether pegfilgrastim is excreted in human milk. Because many drugs are excreted in human milk, caution should be exercised when pegfilgrastim is administered to a nursing woman.

➤*Children:* The safety and effectiveness of pegfilgrastim in pediatric patients have not been established. The 6 mg fixed dose single-use syringe formulation should not be used in infants, children and smaller adolescents weighing less than 45 kg.

Precautions

➤*Use with chemotherapy or radiation therapy:* Pegfilgrastim should not be administered in the period between 14 days before and 24 hours after administration of cytotoxic chemotherapy because of the potential for an increase in sensitivity of rapidly dividing myeloid cells to cytotoxic chemotherapy.

The use of pegfilgrastim has not been studied in patients receiving chemotherapy associated with delayed myelosuppression (eg, nitrosoureas, mitomycin C).

The administration of pegfilgrastim concomitantly with 5-fluorouracil or other antimetabolites has not been evaluated in patients. Administration of pegfilgrastim at 0, 1 and 3 days before 5-fluorouracil resulted in increased mortality in mice; administration of pegfilgrastim 24 hours after 5-fluorouracil did not adversely affect survival.

The use of pegfilgrastim has not been studied in patients receiving radiation therapy.

➤*Potential effect on malignant cells:* Pegfilgrastim is a growth factor that primarily stimulates neutrophils and neutrophil precursors; however, the granulocyte colony-stimulating factor (G-CSF) receptor through which pegfilgrastim and filgrastim act has been found on tumor cell lines, including some myeloid, T-lymphoid, lung, head and neck, and bladder tumor cell lines. The possibility that pegfilgrastim can act as a growth factor for any tumor type cannot be excluded. Use of pegfilgrastim in myeloid malignancies and myelodysplasia (MDS) has not been studied. In a randomized study comparing the effects of the parent compound of pegfilgrastim, filgrastim, to placebo in patients undergoing remission induction and consolidation chemotherapy for acute myeloid leukemia, important differences in remission rate between the 2 arms were excluded. Disease-free survival and overall survival were comparable; however, the study was not designed to detect important differences in these endpoints.

Drug Interactions

No formal drug interaction studies between pegfilgrastim and other drugs have been performed. Drugs such as lithium may potentiate the release of neutrophils; patients receiving lithium and pegfilgrastim should have more frequent monitoring of neutrophil counts.

Adverse Reactions

➤*Splenic rupture:* See Warnings for more information.

➤*Adult respiratory distress syndrome (ARDS):* See Warnings for more information.

➤*Hypersensitivity:* See Warnings for more information.

➤*Sickle cell disease:* See Warnings for more information. Safety data are based upon 465 subjects with lymphoma and solid tumors (breast, lung, and thoracic tumors) enrolled in 6 randomized clinical studies. Subjects received pegfilgrastim after nonmyeloablative cytotoxic chemotherapy. Most adverse experiences were attributed by the investigators to the underlying malignancy or cytotoxic chemotherapy and occurred at similar rates in subjects who received pegfilgrastim (n = 465) or filgrastim (n = 331). These adverse experiences occurred at rates between 72% and 15% and included: Nausea, fatigue, alopecia, diarrhea, vomiting, constipation, fever, anorexia, skeletal pain, headache, taste perversion, dyspepsia, myalgia, insomnia, abdominal pain, arthralgia, generalized weakness, peripheral edema, dizziness, granulocytopenia, stomatitis, mucositis, and neutropenic fever.

The most common adverse event attributed to pegfilgrastim in clinical trials was medullary bone pain, reported in 26% of subjects, which was comparable to the incidence in filgrastim-treated patients. This bone pain was generally reported to be of mild-to-moderate severity. Approximately 12% of all subjects utilized nonnarcotic analgesics and less than 6% utilized narcotic analgesics in association with bone pain. No patient withdrew from study due to bone pain.

In clinical studies, leukocytosis (WBC counts greater than 100×10^9/L) was observed in less than 1% of 465 subjects with non-myeloid malignancies receiving pegfilgrastim. Leukocytosis was not associated with any adverse effects.

In subjects receiving pegfilgrastim in clinical trials, the only serious event that was not deemed attributable to underlying or concurrent disease, or to concurrent therapy was a case of hypoxia.

Reversible elevations in lactic dehydrogenase (LDH), alkaline phosphatase, and uric acid, which did not require treatment intervention, were observed. The incidences of these changes, presented for pegfilgrastim relative to filgrastim, were: LDH (19% vs 29%), alkaline phosphatase (9% vs 16%), and uric acid (8% vs 9% [1% of reported cases for both treatment groups were classified as severe]).

➤*Immunogenicity:* As with all therapeutic proteins, there is a potential for immunogenicity. The incidence of antibody development in patients receiving pegfilgrastim has not been adequately determined. While available data suggest that a small proportion of patients developed binding antibodies to filgrastim or pegfilgrastim, the nature and specificity of these antibodies has not been adequately studied. No neutralizing antibodies have been detected using a cell-based bioassay in 46 patients who apparently developed binding antibodies. The detection of antibody formation is highly dependent on the sensitivity and specificity of the assay, and the observed incidence of antibody positivity in an assay may be influenced by several factors including sample handling, concomitant medications, and underlying disease. Therefore, comparison of the incidence of antibodies to pegfilgrastim with the incidence of antibodies to other products may be misleading.

Cytopenias resulting from an antibody response to exogenous growth factors have been reported on rare occasions in patients treated with other recombinant growth factors. There is a theoretical possibility that an antibody directed against pegfilgrastim may cross-react with endogenous G-CSF, resulting in immune-mediated neutropenia, but this has not been observed in clinical studies.

Overdosage

The maximum amount of pegfilgrastim that can be safely administered in single or multiple doses has not been determined. Single doses of 300 mcg/kg have been administered SC to 8 healthy volunteers and 3 patients with non-small cell lung cancer without serious adverse effects. These subjects experienced a mean maximum ANC of 55×10^9/L, with a corresponding mean maximum WBC of 67×10^9/L. The absolute maximum ANC observed was 96×10^9/L with a corresponding absolute maximum WBC observed of 120×10^9/L. The duration of leukocytosis ranged from 6 to 13 days. Leukapheresis should be considered in the management of symptomatic individuals.

SARGRAMOSTIM (Granulocyte Macrophage Colony Stimulating Factor; GM-CSF)

Rx	**Leukine** (Berlex)	**Powder for injection, lyophilized:** 250 mcg	Preservative-free. In vials.[a]
		Liquid: 500 mcg/mL	1.1% benzyl alcohol. In multiple-dose vials.[a]

[a] With 40 mg mannitol, 10 mg sucrose, 1.2 mg tromethamine per mL.

SARGRAMOSTIM — INJECTION

Indications

➤*Following induction chemotherapy in acute myelogenous leukemia:* For use following induction chemotherapy in older adult patients with acute myelogenous leukemia (AML) to shorten time to neutrophil recovery and to reduce the incidence of severe and life-threatening infections and infections resulting in death. The safety and efficacy of sargramostim have not been assessed in patients with AML under 55 years of age.

➤*Mobilization and following transplantation of autologous peripheral blood progenitor cells:* For the mobilization of hematopoietic progenitor cells into peripheral blood for collection by leukapheresis. Mobilization allows for the collection of increased numbers of progenitor cells capable of engraftment as compared with collection without mobilization. After myeloablative chemotherapy, the transplantation of an increased number of progenitor cells lead to more rapid engraftment, which result in a decreased need for supportive care. Myeloid reconstitution is further accelerated by administration of sargramostim following peripheral blood progenitor cell transplantation.

➤*Myeloid reconstitution after autologous bone marrow transplantation (BMT):* For acceleration of myeloid recovery in patients with non-Hodgkin lymphoma (NHL), acute lymphoblastic leukemia (ALL), and Hodgkin disease undergoing autologous BMT. After autologous BMT in patients with NHL, ALL, or Hodgkin disease, sargramostim has been found to be safe and effective in accelerating myeloid engraftment, decreasing median duration of antibiotic administration, reducing the median duration of infectious episodes, and shortening the median duration of hospitalization. Hematologic response to sargramostim can be detected by complete blood count (CBC) with differential performed twice per week.

➤*Myeloid reconstitution after allogeneic bone marrow transplantation:* For acceleration of myeloid recovery in patients undergoing allogeneic BMT from HLA-matched related donors. Sargramostim has been found to be safe and effective in accelerating myeloid engraftment, reducing the incidence of bacteremia and other culture positive infections, and shortening the median duration of hospitalization.

➤*Bone marrow transplantation failure or engraftment delay:* In patients who have undergone allogeneic or autologous BMT in whom engraftment is delayed or has failed. Sargramostim has been found to be safe and effective in prolonging survival of patients who are experiencing graft failure or engraftment delay, in the presence or absence of infection, following autologous or allogeneic BMT. Survival benefit may be relatively greater in those patients who demonstrate one or more of the following characteristics: Autologous BMT failure or engraftment delay, no previous total body irradiation, malignancy other than leukemia or a multiple organ failure (MOF) score of 2 or less. Hematologic response to sargramostim can be detected by CBC with differential performed twice weekly.

➤*Unlabeled uses:* Crohn's disease, melanoma, wound healing, mucositis, stomatitis, vaccine adjuvancy; adjunct to high-dose chemotherapy; neutropenia associated with myelodysplastic syndrome or aplastic anemia; zidovudine and other drug-induced neutropenia.

Administration and Dosage

➤*Approved by the FDA:* March 1991.

➤*Neutrophil recovery following chemotherapy in acute myelogenous leukemia:* 250 mcg/m^2/day administered intravenously over a 4-hour period starting approximately on day 11 or 4 days following the completion of induction chemotherapy, if the day 10 bone marrow is hypoplastic with less than 5% blasts. If a second cycle of induction chemotherapy is necessary, sargramostim should be administered approximately 4 days after the completion of chemotherapy if the bone marrow is hypoplastic with less than 5% blasts. Sargramostim should be continued until an ANC more than 1,500/mm^3 for 3 consecutive days or a maximum of 42 days. Sargramostim should be discontinued immediately if leukemic regrowth occurs. If a severe adverse reaction occurs, the dose can be reduced 50% or temporarily discontinued until the reaction abates.

In order to avoid potential complications of excessive leukocytosis (WBC more than 50,000 cells/mm^3 or ANC more than 20,000 cells/mm^3) a CBC with differential is recommended twice a week during sargramostim therapy. Sargramostim treatment should be interrupted or the dose reduced 50% if the ANC exceeds 20,000 cells/mm^3.

➤*Mobilization of peripheral blood progenitor cells:* 250 mcg/m^2/day administered IV over 24 hours or subcutaneously once daily. Dosing should continue at the same dose through the period of peripheral blood progenitor cells (PBPC) collection. The optimal schedule for PBPC collection has not been established. In clinical studies, collection of PBPC was usually begun by day 5 and performed daily until protocol specified targets were achieved. If WBC more than 50,000 cells/mm^3, the sargramostim dose should be reduced 50%. If adequate numbers of progenitor cells are not collected, other mobilization therapy should be considered.

➤*Post-PBPC transplantation:* 250 mcg/m^2/day administered IV over 24 hours or subcutaneously once daily beginning immediately following infusion of progenitor cells and continuing until an ANC greater than 1,500/mm^3 for 3 consecutive days is attained.

➤*Myeloid reconstitution after autologous or allogeneic bone marrow transplantation:* 250 mcg/m^2/day administered IV over a 2-hour period beginning 2 to 4 hours after bone marrow infusion, and not less than 24 hours after the last dose of chemotherapy or radiotherapy. Patients should not receive sargramostim until the post-marrow infusion ANC is less than 500 cells/mm^3. Sargramostim should be continued until an ANC greater than 1,500/mm^3 for 3 consecutive days is attained. If a severe adverse reaction occurs, the dose can be reduced 50% or temporarily discontinued until the reaction abates. Sargramostim should be discontinued immediately if blast cells appear or disease progression occurs.

In order to avoid potential complications of excessive leukocytosis (WBC more than 50,000 cells/mm^3, ANC greater than 20,000 cells/mm^3) a CBC with differential is recommended twice weekly during sargramostim therapy. Sargramostim treatment should be interrupted or the dose reduced 50% if the ANC exceeds 20,000 cells/mm^3.

➤*Bone marrow transplantation failure or engraftment delay:* 250 mcg/m^2/day for 14 days as a 2-hour IV infusion. The dose can be repeated after 7 days off therapy if engraftment has not occurred. If engraftment still has not occurred, a third course of 500 mcg/m^2/day for 14 days may be tried after another 7 days off therapy. If there is still no improvement, it is unlikely that further dose escalation will be beneficial. If a severe adverse reaction occurs, the dose can be reduced 50% or temporarily discontinued until the reaction abates. Sargramostim should be discontinued immediately if blast cells appear or disease progression occurs.

In order to avoid potential complications of excessive leukocytosis (WBC more than 50,000 cells/mm^3, ANC greater than 20,000 cells/mm^3) a CBC with differential is recommended twice weekly during sargramostim therapy. Sargramostim treatment should be interrupted or the dose reduced by half if the ANC exceeds 20,000 cells/mm^3.

➤*Preparation:*

1.) Sargramostim liquid is formulated as a sterile, preserved (1.1% benzyl alcohol), injectable solution (500 mcg/mL) in a vial. Lyophilized sargramostim is a sterile, white, preservative-free powder (250 mcg) that requires reconstitution with 1 mL sterile water for injection, or 1 mL bacteriostatic water for injection.
2.) Lyophilized sargramostim (250 mcg) should be reconstituted aseptically with 1 mL of diluent (see below). The contents of vials reconstituted with different diluents should not be mixed together. Previously reconstituted solutions mixed with freshly reconstituted solutions must be administered within 6 hours following mixing. Preparations containing benzyl alcohol (including sargramostim liquid and lyophilized sargramostim reconstituted with bacteriostatic water for injection) should not be used in neonates (see Storage and Warnings).
3.) During reconstitution the diluent should be directed at the side of the vial and the contents gently swirled to avoid foaming during dissolution. Avoid excessive or vigorous agitation; do not shake.
4.) Sargramostim should be used for subcutaneous injection without further dilution. Dilution for IV infusion should be performed in 0.9% sodium chloride injection. If the final concentration of sargramostim is below 10 mcg/mL, albumin (human) at a final concentration of 0.1% should be added to the saline prior to addition of sargramostim to prevent adsorption to the components of the drug delivery system. To obtain a final concentration of 0.1% albumin (human), add 1 mg albumin (human) per 1 mL 0.9% sodium chloride injection (eg, use 1 mL 5% albumin [human] in 50 mL 0.9% sodium chloride injection).
5.) An in-line membrane filter should not be used for intravenous infusion of sargramostim.
6.) In the absence of compatibility and stability information, no other medication should be added to infusion solutions containing sargramostim. Use only 0.9% sodium chloride injection to prepare IV infusion solutions.
7.) Aseptic technique should be employed in the preparation of all sargramostim solutions. To ensure correct concentration following reconstitution, care should be exercised to eliminate any air bubbles from the needle hub of the syringe used to prepare the diluent. Parenteral drug products should be inspected visually for particulate matter and discoloration prior to administration whenever solution and container permit.

➤*Storage/Stability:* The sterile, preserved, injectable solution; the sterile powder; the reconstituted solution; and the diluted solution for injection should be refrigerated at 2° to 8°C (36° to 46°F). Do not freeze or shake. Do not use beyond the expiration date printed on the vial.

Sargramostim liquid may be stored for up to 20 days at 2° to 8°C (36° to 46°F) once the vial has been entered. Discard any remaining solution after 20 days.

Sterile water for injection (without preservative) – Sargramostim vials contain no antibacterial preservative, and therefore solutions prepared with sterile water for injection should be administered as soon as possible, and within 6 hours following reconstitution or dilution for IV infusion. The vial should not be re-entered or reused. Do not save any unused portion for administration more than 6 hours following reconstitution.

SARGRAMOSTIM — INJECTION

Bacteriostatic water for injection (0.9% benzyl alcohol) – Reconstituted solutions prepared with bacteriostatic water for injection (0.9% benzyl alcohol) may be stored for up to 20 days at 2° to 8°C (36° to 46°F) prior to use. Discard reconstituted solution after 20 days.

Actions

➤*Pharmacology:* Granulocyte-macrophage colony stimulating factor (GM-CSF) belongs to a group of growth factors termed colony stimulating factors that support survival, clonal expansion, and differentiation of hematopoietic progenitor cells. GM-CSF induces partially committed progenitor cells to divide and differentiate in the granulocyte-macrophage pathways.

GM-CSF is also capable of activating mature granulocytes and macrophages. GM-CSF is a multilineage factor and, in addition to dose-dependent effects on the myelomonocytic lineage, can promote the proliferation of megakaryocytic and erythroid progenitors. However, other factors are required to induce complete maturation in these 2 lineages. The various cellular responses (division, maturation, activation) are induced through GM-CSF binding to specific receptors expressed on the cell surface of target cells.

In vitro studies of sargramostim in human cells – The biological activity of GM-CSF is species-specific. Consequently, in vitro studies have been performed on human cells to characterize the pharmacological activity of sargramostim. In vitro exposure of human bone marrow cells to sargramostim at concentrations ranging from 1 to 100 ng/mL results in the proliferation of hematopoietic progenitors and in the formation of pure granulocyte, pure macrophage, and mixed granulocyte-macrophage colonies. Chemotactic, anti-fungal and anti-parasitic activities of granulocytes and monocytes are increased by exposure to sargramostim in vitro. Sargramostim increases the cytotoxicity of monocytes toward certain neoplastic cell lines and activates polymorphonuclear neutrophils to inhibit the growth of tumor cells.

Antibody formation – Serum samples collected before and after sargramostim treatment from 214 patients with a variety of underlying diseases have been examined for the presence of antibodies. Neutralizing antibodies were detected in 5 of 214 patients (2.3%) after receiving sargramostim by continuous IV infusion (3 patients) or subcutaneous injection (2 patients) for 28 to 84 days in multiple courses. All 5 patients had impaired hematopoiesis before the administration of sargramostim and consequently the effect of the development of anti-GM-CSF antibodies on normal hematopoiesis could not be assessed. Drug-induced neutropenia, neutralization of endogenous GM-CSF activity and diminution of the therapeutic effect of sargramostim secondary to formation of neutralizing antibody remain a theoretical possibility.

➤*Pharmacokinetics:* Pharmacokinetic profiles have been analyzed in controlled studies of 24 healthy men. Liquid and lyophilized sargramostim, at the recommended dose of 250 mcg/m^2, have been determined to be bioequivalent based on the statistical evaluation of AUC. When sargramostim (either liquid or lyophilized) was administered IV over 2 hours to healthy volunteers, the mean beta half-life was approximately 60 minutes. Peak concentrations of GM-CSF were observed in blood samples obtained during or immediately after completion of sargramostim infusion. For sargramostim liquid, the mean maximum concentration (C_{max}) was 5 ng/mL, the mean clearance rate was approximately 420 mL/min/m^2 and the mean $AUC_{0-\infty}$ was 640 ng/mL•min. Corresponding results for lyophilized sargramostim in the same subjects were mean C_{max} of 5.4 ng/mL, mean clearance rate of 431 mL/min/m^2, and mean $AUC_{0-\infty}$ of 677 ng/mL•min. GM-CSF was last detected in blood samples obtained at 3 or 6 hours. When sargramostim (either liquid or lyophilized) was administered subcutaneously to healthy volunteers, GM-CSF was detected in the serum at 15 minutes, the first sample point. The mean beta half-life was approximately 162 minutes. Peak levels occurred at 1 to 3 hours postinjection, and sargramostim remained detectable for up to 6 hours after injection. The mean C_{max} was 1.5 ng/mL. For sargramostim liquid, the mean clearance was 549 mL/min/m^2 and the mean $AUC_{0-\infty}$ was 549 ng/mL•min. For lyophilized sargramostim, the mean clearance was 529 mL/min/m^2 and the mean $AUC_{0-\infty}$ was 501 ng/mL•min.

Contraindications

In patients with excessive leukemic myeloid blasts in the bone marrow or peripheral blood (≥ 10%); hypersensitivity to GM-CSF, yeast-derived products or any component of the product; concomitant use with chemotherapy and radiotherapy.

Because of the potential sensitivity of rapidly dividing hematopoietic progenitor cells, sargramostim should not be administered simultaneously with cytotoxic chemotherapy or radiotherapy or within 24 hours preceding or following chemotherapy or radiotherapy. In 1 controlled study, patients with small cell lung cancer received sargramostim and concurrent thoracic radiotherapy and chemotherapy or the identical radiotherapy and chemotherapy without sargramostim. The patients randomized to sargramostim had significantly higher incidence of adverse events, including higher mortality and a higher incidence of grade 3 and 4 infections and grade 3 and 4 thrombocytopenia.

Warnings

➤*Benzyl alcohol:* Benzyl alcohol is a constituent of sargramostim liquid and bacteriostatic water for injection diluent. Benzyl alcohol has been reported to be associated with a fatal gasping syndrome in premature infants. Liquid solutions containing benzyl alcohol (including sargramostim liquid) or lyophilized sargramostim reconstituted with bacteriostatic water for injection (0.9% benzyl alcohol) should not be administered to neonates (see Children and Administration and Dosage).

➤*Fluid retention:* Edema, capillary leak syndrome, pleural or pericardial effusion have been reported in patients after sargramostim administration. In 156 patients enrolled in placebo-controlled studies using sargramostim at a dose of 250 mcg/m^2/day by 2-hour IV infusion, the reported incidences of fluid retention (sargramostim versus placebo) were as follows: Peripheral edema, 11% versus 7%; pleural effusion, 1% versus 0%; and pericardial effusion, 4% versus 1%. Capillary leak syndrome was not observed in this limited number of studies; based on other uncontrolled studies and reports from users of marketed sargramostim, the incidence is estimated to be less than 1%. In patients with preexisting pleural and pericardial effusions, administration of sargramostim may aggravate fluid retention; however, fluid retention associated with or worsened by sargramostim has been reversible after interruption or dose reduction of sargramostim with or without diuretic therapy. Sargramostim should be used with caution in patients with preexisting fluid retention, pulmonary infiltrates, or congestive heart failure.

➤*Respiratory symptoms:* Sequestration of granulocytes in the pulmonary circulation has been documented following sargramostim infusion, and dyspnea has been reported occasionally in patients treated with sargramostim. Special attention should be given to respiratory symptoms during or immediately following sargramostim infusion, especially in patients with preexisting lung disease. In patients displaying dyspnea during sargramostim administration, the rate of infusion should be reduced by half. If respiratory symptoms worsen despite infusion rate reduction, the infusion should be discontinued. Subsequent IV infusions may be administered following the standard dose schedule with careful monitoring. Use caution when administering sargramostim to patients with hypoxia.

➤*Cardiovascular symptoms:* Occasional transient supraventricular arrhythmia has been reported in uncontrolled studies during sargramostim administration, particularly in patients with a previous history of cardiac arrhythmia. However, these arrhythmias have been reversible after discontinuation of sargramostim. Use caution when administering sargramostim to patients with preexisting cardiac disease.

➤*Renal/Hepatic function impairment:* In some patients with preexisting renal or hepatic dysfunction enrolled in uncontrolled clinical trials, administration of sargramostim has induced elevation of serum creatinine or bilirubin and hepatic enzymes. Dose reduction or interruption of sargramostim administration has resulted in a decrease to pretreatment values. However, in controlled clinical trials the incidences of renal and hepatic dysfunction were comparable between sargramostim (250 mcg/m^2/day by 2-hour IV infusion) and placebo-treated patients. Monitoring of renal and hepatic function in patients displaying renal or hepatic dysfunction prior to initiation of treatment is recommended at least every other week during sargramostim administration.

➤*Pregnancy:* *Category C.* Animal reproduction studies have not been conducted with sargramostim. It is not known whether sargramostim can cause fetal harm when administered to a pregnant woman or can affect reproductive capability. Give sargramostim to a pregnant woman only if clearly needed.

➤*Lactation:* It is not known whether sargramostim is excreted in human milk. Because many drugs are excreted in human milk, administer sargramostim to a nursing woman only if clearly needed.

➤*Children:* Safety and effectiveness in children have not been established; however, available safety data indicate that sargramostim does not exhibit any greater toxicity in children than adults. A total of 124 pediatric subjects between the ages of 4 months and 18 years of age have been treated with sargramostim in clinical trials at doses ranging from 60 to 1,000 mcg/m^2/day intravenously and 4 to 1,500 mcg/m^2/day subcutaneously. In 53 pediatric patients enrolled in controlled studies at a dose of 250 mcg/m^2/day by 2-hour IV infusion, the type and frequency of adverse events were comparable with those reported for the adult population. Do not administer liquid solutions containing benzyl alcohol (including sargramostim liquid) or lyophilized sargramostim reconstituted with bacteriostatic water for injection (0.9% benzyl alcohol) to neonates.

Precautions

➤*Monitoring:* Monitoring of renal and hepatic function in patients displaying renal or hepatic dysfunction prior to initiation of treatment is recommended at least biweekly during sargramostim administration. Body weight and hydration status should be carefully monitored during sargramostim administration.

➤*Hypersensitivity reactions:* Parenteral administration of recombinant proteins should be attended by appropriate precautions in case an allergic or untoward reaction occurs. Serious allergic or anaphylactic reactions have been reported. If any serious allergic or anaphylactic reaction occurs, immediately discontinue sargramostim therapy and initiate appropriate therapy.

➤*First dose effect:* A syndrome characterized by respiratory distress, hypoxia, flushing, hypotension, syncope, or tachycardia has been reported following the first administration of sargramostim in a particular cycle. These signs have resolved with symptomatic treatment and usually do not recur with subsequent doses in the same cycle of treatment.

➤*Hematologic effects:* Stimulation of marrow precursors with sargramostim may result in a rapid rise in white blood cell (WBC) count. If the ANC exceeds 20,000 cells/mm^3 or if the platelet count exceeds 500,000/mm^3, interrupt sargramostim administration or reduce the dose by half. Base the decision to reduce the dose or interrupt treatment on the clinical condition of the patient. Excessive blood counts have returned to normal or baseline levels within 3 to 7 days following cessation of sargramostim therapy. Perform twice weekly monitoring of CBC with differential (including examination for the presence of blast cells) to preclude development of excessive counts.

➤*Growth factor potential:* Sargramostim is a growth factor that primarily stimulates normal myeloid precursors. However, the possibility that sar-

SARGRAMOSTIM — INJECTION

gramostim can act as a growth factor for any tumor type, particularly myeloid malignancies, cannot be excluded. Because of the possibility of tumor growth potentiation, exercise precaution when using this drug in any malignancy with myeloid characteristics.

Should disease progression be detected during sargramostim treatment, discontinue sargramostim therapy.

Sargramostim has been administered to patients with myelodysplastic syndromes (MDS) in uncontrolled studies without evidence of increased relapse rates. Controlled studies have not been performed in patients with MDS.

➤*Use in patients receiving purged bone marrow:* Sargramostim is effective in accelerating myeloid recovery in patients receiving bone marrow purged by anti-B lymphocyte monoclonal antibodies. Data obtained from uncontrolled studies suggest that if in vitro marrow purging with chemical agents causes a significant decrease in the number of responsive hematopoietic progenitors, the patient may not respond to sargramostim. When the bone marrow purging process preserves a sufficient number of progenitors (more than 1.2×10^4/kg), a beneficial effect of sargramostim on myeloid engraftment has been reported.

➤*Use in patients previously exposed to intensive chemotherapy/radiotherapy:* In patients who before autologous BMT, have received extensive radiotherapy to hematopoietic sites for the treatment of primary disease in the abdomen or chest, or have been exposed to multiple myelotoxic agents (alkylating agents, anthracycline antibiotics, antimetabolites), the effect of sargramostim on myeloid reconstitution may be limited.

➤*Use in patients with malignancy undergoing sargramostim-mobilized PBPC collection:* When using sargramostim to mobilize PBPC, the limited in vitro data suggest that tumor cells may be released and reinfused into the patient in the leukapheresis product. The effect of reinfusion of tumor cells has not been well studied and the data are inconclusive.

➤*Lab test abnormalities:* Sargramostim can induce variable increases in WBC or platelet counts. In order to avoid potential complications of excessive leukocytosis (WBC greater than 50,000 cells/mm^3; ANC greater than 20,000 cells/mm^3), a CBC is recommended twice weekly during sargramostim therapy.

Drug Interactions

Interactions between sargramostim and other drugs have not been fully evaluated. Use caution when administering drugs that may potentiate the myeloproliferative effects of sargramostim (eg, lithium, corticosteroids).

Adverse Reactions

➤*Autologous and allogeneic BMT:* Sargramostim is generally well tolerated. In 3 placebo-controlled studies enrolling a total of 156 patients after autologous BMT or PBPC transplantation, reactions reported in at least 10% of patients who received IV sargramostim or placebo were as follows:

Sargramostim AuBMT Adverse Reactions

Reactions by body system	Sargramostim (n = 79)	Placebo (n = 77)
Cardiovascular		
Hemorrhage	23%	30%
CNS		
CNS disorder	11%	16%
Dermatologic		
Alopecia	73%	74%
Rash	44%	38%
GI		
Nausea	90%	96%
Diarrhea	89%	82%
Vomiting	85%	90%
Anorexia	54%	58%
GI disorder	37%	47%
GI hemorrhage	27%	33%
Stomatitis	24%	29%
Liver damage	13%	14%
GU		
Urinary tract disorder	14%	13%
Kidney function abnormal	8%	10%
Hematologic/lymphatic		
Blood dyscrasia	25%	27%
Metabolic/nutritional		
Edema	34%	35%
Peripheral edema	11%	7%
Respiratory		
Dyspnea	28%	31%
Lung disorder	20%	23%
Miscellaneous		
Fever	95%	96%
Mucous membrane disorder	75%	78%
Asthenia	66%	51%
Malaise	57%	51%
Sepsis	11%	14%

No significant differences were observed between sargramostim and placebo-treated patients in the type or frequency of laboratory abnormalities, including renal and hepatic parameters. In some patients with preexisting renal or hepatic dysfunction enrolled in uncontrolled clinical trials, administration of sargramostim has induced elevation of serum creatinine or bilirubin and hepatic enzymes (see Warnings). In addition, there was no significant difference in relapse rate and 24 month survival between the sargramostim and placebo-treated patients. In the placebo-controlled trial of 109 patients after allogeneic BMT, reactions reported in at least 10% of patients who received IV sargramostim or placebo were the following:

Sargramostim Allogeneic BMT Adverse Reactions

Reactions by body system	Sargramostim (n = 53)	Placebo (n = 56)
Miscellaneous		
Fever	77%	80%
Abdominal pain	38%	23%
Headache	36%	36%
Chills	25%	20%
Pain	17%	36%
Asthenia	17%	20%
Chest pain	15%	9%
Back pain	9%	18%
GI		
Diarrhea	81%	66%
Nausea	70%	66%
Vomiting	70%	57%
Stomatitis	62%	63%
Anorexia	51%	57%
Dyspepsia	17%	20%
Hematemesis	13%	7%
Dysphagia	11%	7%
GI hemorrhage	11%	5%
Constipation	8%	11%
Dermatologic		
Rash	70%	73%
Alopecia	45%	45%
Pruritus	23%	13%
Musculoskeletal		
Bone pain	21%	5%
Arthralgia	11%	4%
Ophthalmic		
Eye hemorrhage	11%	0%
Cardiovascular		
Hypertension	34%	32%
Tachycardia	11%	9%
Metabolic/nutritional		
Bilirubinemia	30%	27%
Hyperglycemia	25%	23%
Peripheral edema	15%	21%
Increased creatinine	15%	14%
Hypomagnesemia	15%	9%
Increased ALT	13%	16%
Edema	13%	11%
Increased alkaline phosphatase	8%	14%
Respiratory		
Pharyngitis	23%	13%
Epistaxis	17%	16%

SARGRAMOSTIM — INJECTION

Sargramostim Allogeneic BMT Adverse Reactions		
Reactions by body system	Sargramostim (n = 53)	Placebo (n = 56)
Dyspnea	15%	14%
Rhinitis	11%	14%
Hematologic/lymphatic		
Thrombocytopenia	19%	34%
Leukopenia	17%	29%
Petechia	6%	11%
Agranulocytosis	6%	11%
GU		
Hematuria	9%	21%
CNS		
Paresthesia	11%	13%
Insomnia	11%	9%
Anxiety	11%	2%
Laboratory abnormalities*		
High glucose	41%	49%
Low albumin	27%	36%
High BUN	23%	17%
Low calcium	2%	7%
High cholesterol	17%	8%

* Grade 3 and 4 laboratory abnormalities only. Denominators may vary due to missing laboratory measurements.

There were no significant differences in the incidence or severity of GVHD, relapse rates and survival between the sargramostim and placebo-treated patients.

Adverse reactions observed for the patients treated with sargramostim in the historically controlled BMT failure study were similar to those reported in the placebo-controlled studies. In addition, headache (26%), pericardial effusion (25%), arthralgia (21%) and myalgia (18%) were also reported in patients treated with sargramostim in the graft failure study.

In uncontrolled Phase I/II studies with sargramostim in 215 patients, the most frequent adverse events were fever, asthenia, headache, bone pain, chills and myalgia. These systemic events were generally mild or moderate and were usually prevented or reversed by the administration of analgesics and antipyretics such as acetaminophen. In these uncontrolled trials, other infrequent events reported were dyspnea, peripheral edema, and rash.

Reports of reactions occurring with marketed sargramostim include arrhythmia, fainting, eosinophilia, dizziness, hypotension, injection site reactions, pain (including abdominal, back, chest, and joint pain), tachycardia, thrombosis, and transient liver function abnormalities.

In patients with preexisting edema, capillary leak syndrome, pleural or pericardial effusion, administration of sargramostim may aggravate fluid retention (see Warnings). Body weight and hydration status should be carefully monitored during sargramostim administration.

Adverse reactions observed in pediatric patients in controlled studies were comparable to those observed in adult patients.

➤*Acute myelogenous leukemia:* Adverse reactions reported in at least 10% of patients who received sargramostim or placebo were the following:

Sargramostim AML Adverse Reactions		
Reactions by body system	Sargramostim (n = 52)	Placebo (n = 47)
Miscellaneous		
Fever (no infection)	81%	74%
Infection	65%	68%
Weight loss	37%	28%
Weight gain	8%	21%
Chills	19%	26%
Allergy	12%	15%
Sweats	6%	13%
GI		
Nausea	58%	55%
Liver	77%	83%
Diarrhea	52%	53%
Vomiting	46%	34%
Stomatitis	42%	43%
Anorexia	13%	11%
Abdominal distention	4%	13%
Dermatologic		
Skin	77%	45%
Alopecia	37%	51%
Metabolic/nutritional		
Metabolic	58%	49%
Edema	25%	23%
Respiratory		
Pulmonary	48%	64%
Hematologic/lymphatic		
Coagulation	19%	21%
Cardiovascular		
Hemorrhage	29%	43%
Hypertension	25%	32%
Cardiac	23%	32%
Hypotension	13%	26%
GU		
Genitourinary	50%	57%
CNS		
Neuro-clinical	42%	53%
Neuromotor	25%	26%
Neuropsychiatric	15%	26%
Neurosensory	6%	11%

Nearly all patients reported leukopenia, thrombocytopenia and anemia. The frequency and type of adverse reactions observed following induction were similar between sargramostim and placebo groups. The only significant difference in the rates of these adverse reactions was an increase in skin associated reactions in the sargramostim group ($p = 0.002$). No significant differences were observed in laboratory results, renal or hepatic toxicity. No significant differences were observed between the sargramostim and placebo-treated patients for adverse reactions following consolidation. There was no significant difference in response rate or relapse rate.

In a historically controlled study of 86 patients with acute myelogenous leukemia (AML), the sargramostim treated group exhibited an increased incidence of weight gain ($p = 0.007$), low serum proteins and prolonged prothrombin time ($p = 0.02$) when compared to the control group. Two sargramostim treated patients had progressive increase in circulating monocytes and promonocytes and blasts in the marrow which reversed when sargramostim was discontinued. The historical control group exhibited an increased incidence of cardiac events ($p = 0.018$), liver function abnormalities ($p = 0.008$), and neurocortical hemorrhagic events ($p = 0.025$).

Overdosage

➤*Symptoms:* The maximum amount of sargramostim that can be safely administered in single or multiple doses has not been determined. Doses up to 100 mcg/kg/day (4000 mcg/m^2/day or 16 times the recommended dose) were administered to 4 patients in a Phase I uncontrolled clinical study by continuous IV infusion for 7 to 18 days. Increases in WBC up to 200,000 cells/mm^3 were observed. Adverse reactions reported were dyspnea, malaise, nausea, fever, rash, sinus tachycardia, headache and chills. All these reactions were reversible after discontinuation of sargramostim.

➤*Treatment:* In case of overdosage, sargramostim therapy should be discontinued and the patient carefully monitored for WBC increase and respiratory symptoms.

OPRELVEKIN (Interleukin 11; IL-11)

Rx	**Neumega** (Wyeth)	**Powder for injection, lyophilized:** 5 mg	1.6 mg dibasic sodium phosphate heptahydrate, 0.55 mg monobasic sodium phosphate monohydrate. Preservative free. In single-dose vials with diluent.

OPRELVEKIN — INJECTION

WARNING

Allergic reactions including anaphylaxis – Oprelvekin has caused allergic or hypersensitivity reactions, including anaphylaxis. Permanently discontinue administration of oprelvekin in any patient who develops an allergic or hypersensitivity reaction.

Indications

➤*Thrombocytopenia, prevention:* For the prevention of severe thrombocytopenia and the reduction of the need for platelet transfusions following myelosuppressive chemotherapy in adult patients with nonmyeloid malignancies who are at high risk of severe thrombocytopenia. Efficacy was demonstrated in patients who had experienced severe thrombocytopenia following the previous chemotherapy cycle. Oprelvekin is not indicated following myeloablative chemotherapy. The safety and efficacy of oprelvekin have not been established in pediatric patients.

➤*Unlabeled uses:* Treatment of Crohn disease.

Administration and Dosage

➤*Approved by the FDA:* November 25, 1997.

➤*Dosage:* The recommended dosage of oprelvekin in adults without severe renal impairment is 50 mcg/kg given once daily. Administer oprelvekin subcutaneously as a single injection in either the abdomen, thigh, or hip (or upper arm if not self-injecting). A safe and effective dose has not been established in children.

Initiate dosing 6 to 24 hours after the completion of chemotherapy. Monitor platelet counts periodically to assess the optimal duration of therapy. Continue dosing until the postnadir platelet count is greater than or equal to 50,000/mcL. In controlled clinical studies, doses were administered in courses of 10 to 21 days. Dosing beyond 21 days per treatment course is not recommended.

Discontinue treatment with oprelvekin at least 2 days before starting the next planned cycle of chemotherapy.

➤*Renal function impairment:* The recommended dose of oprelvekin in adults with severe renal impairment (creatinine clearance [Ccr] less than 30 mL/min) is 25 mcg/kg. An estimate of the patient's Ccr in mL/min is required. Ccr in mL/min may be estimated from a spot serum creatinine (mg/dL) determination using the following formula:

$$\text{Males: } \frac{\text{Weight (kg)} \times (140 - \text{age})}{72 \times \text{serum creatinine (mg/dL)}} = \text{Ccr}$$

Females: 0.85 × above value

➤*Preparation for administration:* Oprelvekin is a sterile, white, preservative-free, lyophilized powder for subcutaneous injection upon reconstitution. Reconstitute oprelvekin (5 mg vials) aseptically with 1 mL of sterile water for injection (without preservative). The reconstituted oprelvekin solution is clear, colorless, and isotonic, with a pH of 7, and contains oprelvekin 5 mg/mL. Do not reenter or reuse the single-use vial. Discard any unused portion of either reconstituted oprelvekin solution or sterile water for injection.

During reconstitution, direct the sterile water for injection at the side of the vial and gently swirl the contents. Avoid excessive or vigorous agitation.

Inspect parenteral drug products visually for particulate matter and discoloration prior to administration, whenever solution and container permit. If particulate matter is present or the solution is discolored, do not use the vial.

Because neither oprelvekin powder for injection nor its accompanying diluent, sterile water for injection, contains a preservative, use oprelvekin within 3 hours of reconstitution. Reconstituted oprelvekin may be refrigerated at 2° to 8°C (36° to 46°F) or stored at room temperature up to 25°C (77°F). Do not freeze or shake the reconstituted solution.

➤*Storage / Stability:* Store lyophilized oprelvekin and diluent in a refrigerator at 2° to 8°C (36° to 46°F). Protect from light. Do not freeze. Reconstituted oprelvekin must be used within 3 hours of reconstitution and can be stored in the vial either at 2° to 8°C (36° to 46°F) or at room temperature up to 25°C (77°F).

Actions

➤*Pharmacology:* The primary hematopoietic activity of oprelvekin is stimulation of megakaryocytopoiesis and thrombopoiesis. Oprelvekin has shown potent thrombopoietic activity in animal models of compromised hematopoiesis, including moderately to severely myelosuppressed mice and nonhuman primates. In these models, oprelvekin improved platelet nadirs and accelerated platelet recoveries compared with controls.

Preclinical trials have shown that mature megakaryocytes that develop during in vivo treatment with oprelvekin are ultrastructurally normal. Platelets produced in response to oprelvekin were morphologically and functionally normal and possessed a normal lifespan.

IL-11 also has been shown to have nonhematopoietic activities in animals, including the following: the regulation of intestinal epithelium growth (enhanced healing of GI lesions), inhibition of adipogenesis, induction of acute phase protein synthesis, inhibition of proinflammatory cytokine production by macrophages, and stimulation of osteoclastogenesis and neurogenesis. Nonhematopoietic pathologic changes observed in animals include fibrosis of tendons and joint capsules, periosteal thickening, papilledema, and embryotoxicity.

IL-11 is produced by bone marrow stromal cells and is part of the cytokine family that shares the gp130 signal transducer. Primary osteoblasts and mature osteoclasts express mRNAs for both IL-11 receptor (IL-11R alpha) and gp130. Both bone-forming and bone-resorbing cells are potential targets of IL-11.

Pharmacodynamics – In a study in which oprelvekin was administered to nonmyelosuppressed cancer patients, daily subcutaneous dosing for 14 days with oprelvekin increased the platelet count in a dose-dependent manner. Platelet counts began to increase relative to baseline between 5 and 9 days after the start of dosing with oprelvekin. After cessation of treatment, platelet counts continued to increase for up to 7 days then returned toward baseline within 14 days. No change in platelet reactivity as measured by platelet activation in response to adenosine diphosphate, and platelet aggregation in response to adenosine diphosphate, epinephrine, collagen, ristocetin, and arachidonic acid has been observed in association with oprelvekin treatment.

In a randomized, double-blind, placebo-controlled study in healthy volunteers, subjects receiving oprelvekin had a mean increase in plasma volume of greater than 20% and all subjects receiving oprelvekin had at least a 10% increase in plasma volume. Red blood cell volume decreased similarly (because of repeated phlebotomy) in the oprelvekin and placebo groups. As a result, whole blood volume increased approximately 10% and hemoglobin concentration decreased approximately 10% in subjects receiving oprelvekin compared with subjects receiving placebo. Mean 24 hour sodium excretion decreased, and potassium excretion did not increase, in subjects receiving oprelvekin compared with subjects receiving placebo.

➤*Pharmacokinetics:*

Special populations –

Renal function impairment: In a clinical study, a single dose of oprelvekin was administered to subjects with severely impaired renal function (Ccr less than 30 mL/min). The mean ± SD values for C_{max} and AUC were 30.8 ± 8.6 ng/mL and 373 ± 106 ng•h/mL, respectively. When compared with control subjects in this study with normal renal function, the mean C_{max} was 2.2-fold higher and the mean AUC was 2.6-fold (95% confidence interval 1.7% to 3.8%) higher in the subjects with severe renal impairment. In the subjects with severe renal impairment, clearance was approximately 40% of the value seen in subjects with normal renal function. The average terminal half-life was similar in subjects with severe renal impairment and those with normal renal function.

A second clinical study of 24 subjects with varying degrees of renal function also was performed and confirmed the results observed in the first study. Single 50 mcg/kg subcutaneous and IV doses were administered in a randomized fashion. As the degree of renal impairment increased, the oprelvekin AUC increased, although half-life remained unchanged. In the 6 patients with severe impairment, the mean ± SD C_{max} and AUC were 23.6 ± 6.7 ng/mL and 373 ± 55.2 ng•h/mL, respectively, compared with 13.1 ± 3.8 ng/mL and 195 ± 49.3 ng•hr/mL, respectively, in the 6 subjects with normal renal function. A comparable increase in exposure was observed after IV administration of oprelvekin.

The pharmacokinetic studies suggest that overall exposure to oprelvekin increases as renal function decreases, indicating that a 50% dose reduction of oprelvekin is warranted for patients with severe renal impairment. No dosage reduction is required for smaller changes in renal function.

Children: In a dose-escalation phase 1 study, oprelvekin also was administered to 43 pediatric patients (age, 8 months to 18 years) and 1 adult patient receiving ICE (ifosfamide, carboplatin, etoposide) chemotherapy. Administered doses ranged from 25 to 125 mcg/kg. Analysis of data from 40 pediatric patients showed that C_{max}, T_{max}, and terminal half-life were comparable with that in adults. The mean area under the concentration-time curve (AUC) for pediatric patients, receiving 50 mcg/kg was approximately half that achieved in healthy adults receiving 50 mcg/kg. Available data suggest that clearance of oprelvekin decreases with increasing age. The pharmacokinetics of oprelvekin have been evaluated in healthy, adults and cancer patients receiving chemotherapy. In a study in which a single 50 mcg/kg subcutaneous dose was administered to 18 healthy men, the peak serum concentration (C_{max}) of 17.4 ± 5.4 ng/mL (mean ± standard deviation [SD]) was reached at 3.2 ± 2.4 hours (T_{max}) following dosing. The terminal half life was 6.9 ± 1.7 hours. In a second study in which single 75 mcg/kg subcutaneous and intravenous (IV) doses were administered to 24 healthy subjects, the pharmacokinetic profiles were similar between men and women. The absolute bioavailability of oprelvekin was greater than 80%. In a study in which multiple subcutaneous doses of 25 and 50 mcg/kg were administered to cancer patients receiving chemotherapy, oprelvekin did not accumulate and clearance of oprelvekin was not impaired following multiple doses.

In preclinical studies in rats, radiolabeled oprelvekin was rapidly cleared from the serum and distributed to highly perfused organs. The kidney was the primary route of elimination. The amount of intact oprelvekin in urine was low, indicating that the molecule was metabolized before excretion.

OPRELVEKIN — INJECTION

Contraindications

Hypersensitivity to oprelvekin or any component of the product.

Warnings

➤*Myeloablative chemotherapy:* Oprelvekin is not indicated following myeloablative chemotherapy. In a randomized, placebo-controlled phase 2 study, the efficacy of oprelvekin was not demonstrated. In this study, a statistically significant increased incidence in edema, conjunctival bleeding, hypotension, and tachycardia was observed in patients receiving oprelvekin as compared with placebo.

The following severe or fatal adverse reactions have been reported in postmarketing use in patients who received oprelvekin following bone marrow transplantation: fluid retention or overload (eg, facial edema, pulmonary edema), capillary leak syndrome, pleural and pericardial effusion, papilledema, and renal failure.

➤*Fluid retention:* Oprelvekin is known to cause serious fluid retention that can result in peripheral edema, dyspnea on exertion, pulmonary edema, capillary leak syndrome, atrial arrhythmias, and exacerbation of preexisting pleural effusions. Severe fluid retention, some cases resulting in death, was reported following recent bone marrow transplantation in patients who have received oprelvekin. Oprelvekin is not indicated following myeloablative chemotherapy. Use with caution in patients with clinically evident congestive heart failure, patients receiving aggressive hydration, patients who may be susceptible to developing congestive heart failure, patients with a history of heart failure who are well compensated and receiving appropriate medical therapy, and patients who may develop fluid retention as a result of associated medical conditions or whose medical condition may be exacerbated by fluid retention.

Fluid retention is reversible within several days following discontinuation of oprelvekin. During dosing with oprelvekin, monitor fluid balance; appropriate medical management is advised.

Perform close monitoring of fluid and electrolyte status in patients receiving chronic diuretic therapy. Sudden deaths have occurred in oprelvekin-treated patients receiving chronic diuretic therapy and ifosfamide who developed severe hypokalemia.

Monitor preexisting fluid collections, including pericardial effusions or ascites. Consider drainage if medically indicated.

➤*Dilutional anemia:* Moderate decreases in hemoglobin concentration, hematocrit, and red blood cell count (approximately 10% to 15%) without a decrease in red blood cell mass have been observed. These changes are predominantly because of an increase in plasma volume (dilutional anemia) that is primarily related to renal sodium and water retention. The decrease in hemoglobin concentration typically begins within 3 to 5 days of the initiation of oprelvekin and is reversible over approximately a week following discontinuation of oprelvekin.

➤*Cardiovascular effects:* Oprelvekin use is associated with cardiovascular reactions, including arrhythmias and pulmonary edema. Cardiac arrest has been reported, but the causal relationship to oprelvekin is uncertain. Use with caution in patients with a history of atrial arrhythmias, and only after consideration of the potential risks in relation to anticipated benefit. In clinical trials, cardiac reactions, including atrial arrhythmias (atrial fibrillation or atrial flutter), occurred in 15% (23/157) of patients treated with oprelvekin at doses of 50 mcg/kg. Arrhythmias were usually brief in duration; conversion to sinus rhythm typically occurred spontaneously or after rate-control drug therapy. Approximately one half (11/24) of the patients who were rechallenged had recurrent atrial arrhythmias. Clinical sequelae, including stroke, have been reported in patients who experienced atrial arrhythmias while receiving oprelvekin.

The mechanism for induction of arrhythmias is not known. Oprelvekin was not directly arrhythmogenic in animal models. In some patients, development of atrial arrhythmias may be because of increased plasma volume associated with fluid retention.

➤*CNS effects:* Stroke has been reported in the setting of patients who develop atrial fibrillation/flutter while receiving oprelvekin. Patients with a history of stroke or transient ischemic attack also may be at increased risk for these reactions.

➤*Papilledema:* Papilledema has been reported in 2% (10/405) of patients receiving oprelvekin in clinical trials following repeated cycles of exposure. Nonhuman primates treated with oprelvekin at a dose of 1,000 mcg/kg subcutaneously once daily for 4 to 13 weeks developed papilledema that was not associated with inflammation or any other histologic abnormality and was reversible after dosing was discontinued. Use oprelvekin with caution in patients with preexisting papilledema, or with tumors involving the CNS because it is possible that papilledema could worsen or develop during treatment.

➤*Hypersensitivity reactions:* In the postmarketing setting, oprelvekin has caused allergic or hypersensitivity reactions, including anaphylaxis. The administration of oprelvekin should be attended by appropriate precautions in case allergic reactions occur. In addition, counsel patients about the symptoms for which they should seek medical attention. Signs and symptoms reported included edema of the face, tongue, or larynx; shortness of breath; wheezing; chest pain; hypotension (including shock); dysarthria; loss of consciousness; mental status changes; rash; urticaria; flushing; and fever. Reactions occurred after the first dose or subsequent doses of oprelvekin. Permanently discontinue administration of oprelvekin in any patient who develops an allergic or hypersensitivity reaction.

➤*Renal function impairment:* Oprelvekin is eliminated primarily by the kidneys. The pharmacokinetics of oprelvekin were studied in subjects with varying degrees of renal dysfunction. $AUC_{0-\infty}$, C_{max}, and absolute bioavailability were significantly increased in subjects with severe renal impairment (Ccr less than 30 mL/min). There were no significant changes in the pharmacokinetic parameters in subjects with mild or moderate impairment. A significant decrease in the hemoglobin concentration was noted on day 2 after a single dose of oprelvekin in subjects with all degrees of renal impairment. By day 14, the hemoglobin was decreased only in patients with severe renal impairment. Fluid retention associated with oprelvekin treatment has not been studied in patients with renal impairment, but carefully monitor fluid balance in these patients.

➤*Pregnancy: Category C.* Oprelvekin has been shown to have embryocidal effects in pregnant rats and rabbits when given in doses of 0.2 to 20 times the human dose. There are no adequate and well-controlled studies of oprelvekin in pregnant women. Use oprelvekin during pregnancy only if the potential benefit justifies the potential risk to the fetus.

Oprelvekin has been tested in studies of fertility, early embryonic development, and pre- and postnatal development in rats, and in studies of organogenesis (teratogenicity) in rats and rabbits. Parental toxicity has been observed when oprelvekin is given at doses of 2 to 20 times the human dose (greater than or equal to 100 mcg/kg/day) in the rat and 0.02 to 2 times the human dose (greater than or equal to 1 mcg/kg/day) in the rabbit. Findings in pregnant rats consisted of transient hypoactivity and dyspnea after administration (maternal toxicity), as well as prolonged estrus cycle, increased early embryonic deaths, and decreased numbers of live fetuses. In addition, low fetal body weights and a reduced number of ossified sacral and caudal vertebrae (ie, retarded fetal development) occurred in rats at 20 times the human dose. Findings in pregnant rabbits consisted of decreased (fecal/urine) eliminations (the only toxicity noted at 1 mcg/kg/day in dams) as well as decreased food consumption, body weight loss, abortion, increased embryonic and fetal deaths, and decreased numbers of live fetuses. No teratogenic effects of oprelvekin were observed in rabbits at doses up to 0.6 times the human dose (30 mcg/kg/day).

Adverse reactions in the first-generation offspring of rats given oprelvekin at maternally toxic doses greater than or equal to 2 times the human dose (greater than or equal to 100 mcg/kg/day) during gestation and lactation included increased newborn mortality, decreased viability index on day 4 of lactation, and decreased body weights during lactation. In rats given 20 times the human dose (1,000 mcg/kg/day) during both gestation and lactation, maternal toxicity and growth retardation of the first-generation offspring resulted in an increased rate of fetal death of the second-generation offspring.

➤*Lactation:* It is not known if oprelvekin is excreted in human milk. Because many drugs are excreted in human milk and because of the potential for serious adverse reactions in breast-feeding infants from oprelvekin, decide whether to discontinue breast-feeding or to discontinue oprelvekin, taking into account the importance of the drug to the mother.

➤*Children:* A safe and effective dose of oprelvekin has not been established in children. In a phase 1, single-arm, dose-escalation study, 43 pediatric patients were treated with oprelvekin at dosages ranging from 25 to 125 mcg/kg/day following ICE chemotherapy. All patients required platelet transfusions and the lack of a comparator arm made the study design inadequate to assess efficacy. The projected effective dose (based on comparable AUC observed for the effective dose in healthy adults) in children appears to exceed the maximum tolerated pediatric dosage of 50 mcg/kg/day. Papilledema was dose limiting and occurred in 16% of children.

The most common adverse reactions seen in pediatric studies included tachycardia (84%), conjunctival injection (57%), radiographic and echocardiographic evidence of cardiomegaly (21%), and periosteal changes (11%). These reactions occurred at a higher frequency in children than adults. The incidence of other adverse reactions was generally similar to those observed using oprelvekin at a dose of 50 mcg/kg in the randomized studies in adults receiving chemotherapy.

Studies in animals were predictive of the effect of oprelvekin on developing bone in children. In growing rodents treated with 100, 300, or 1,000 mcg/kg/day for a minimum of 28 days, thickening of femoral and tibial growth plates, that did not completely resolve after a 28-day nontreatment period was noted. A nonhuman primate toxicology study of oprelvekin animals treated for 2 to 13 weeks at doses of 10 to 1,000 mcg/kg showed partially reversible joint capsule and tendon fibrosis and periosteal hyperostosis. An asymptomatic, laminated periosteal reaction in the diaphyses of the femur, tibia, and fibula has been observed in 1 patient during pediatric studies involving multiple courses of oprelvekin treatment. The relationship of these findings to treatment with oprelvekin is unclear. No studies have been performed to assess the long-term effects of oprelvekin on growth and development.

Precautions

➤*Monitoring:* Obtain a complete blood cell count prior to chemotherapy and at regular intervals during oprelvekin therapy. Monitor platelet counts during the time of the expected nadir and until adequate recovery has occurred (postnadir counts at least 50,000/mcL).

Begin dosing with oprelvekin 6 to 24 hours following the completion of chemotherapy dosing. The safety and efficacy of oprelvekin given immediately prior to or concurrently with cytotoxic chemotherapy or initiated at the time of expected nadir have not been established.

The efficacy of oprelvekin has not been evaluated in patients receiving chemotherapy regimens of more than 5 days duration or regimens associated with delayed myelosuppression (eg, nitrosoureas, mitomycin-C).

Attend the parenteral administration of oprelvekin by appropriate precautions in case allergic reactions occur.

OPRELVEKIN — INJECTION

During dosing with oprelvekin, monitor fluid balance and appropriate medical management is advised.

Perform close monitoring of fluid and electrolyte status in patients receiving chronic diuretic therapy. Sudden deaths have occurred in oprelvekin-treated patients receiving chronic diuretic therapy and ifosfamide who developed severe hypokalemia.

Monitor preexisting fluid collections, including pericardial effusions or ascites. Consider drainage if medically indicated.

➤*Chronic administration:* Oprelvekin has been administered safely using the recommended dosing schedule for up to 6 cycles following chemotherapy. The safety and efficacy of chronic administration of oprelvekin have not been established. Continuous dosage (2 to 13 weeks) in nonhuman primates produced joint capsule and tendon fibrosis and periosteal hyperostosis. The relevance of these findings to humans is unclear.

➤*Timing of therapy:* Begin dosing with oprelvekin 6 to 24 hours following the completion of chemotherapy dosing. The safety and efficacy of oprelvekin given immediately prior to or concurrently with cytotoxic chemotherapy or initiated at the time of expected nadir have not been established.

➤*Duration:* The effectiveness of oprelvekin has not been evaluated in patients receiving chemotherapy regimens of more than 5 days duration or regimens associated with delayed myelosuppression (eg, nitrosoureas, mitomycin-C).

Drug Interactions

No drug interactions known.

Adverse Reactions

Because clinical trials are conducted under widely varying conditions, adverse reaction rates observed in the clinical studies of a drug cannot be directly compared with rates in the clinical studies of another drug and may not reflect the rates observed in practice. The adverse reaction information from clinical trials does, however, provide a basis for identifying the adverse reactions that appear to be related to drug use and for approximating rates.

Three hundred twenty-four subjects, with ages ranging from 8 months to 75 years, have been exposed to oprelvekin treatment. Subjects have received up to 6 (8 in pediatric patients) sequential courses of oprelvekin treatment in clinical studies, with each course lasting from 1 to 28 days. Apart from the sequelae of the underlying malignancy or cytotoxic chemotherapy, most adverse reactions were mild or moderate in severity and reversible after discontinuation of oprelvekin dosing.

In general, the incidence and type of adverse reactions were similar between oprelvekin 50 mcg/kg and placebo groups. The most frequently reported serious adverse reactions were neutropenic fever, syncope, atrial fibrillation, fever, and pneumonia. The most commonly reported adverse reactions were edema, dyspnea, tachycardia, conjunctival injection, palpitations, atrial arrhythmias, and pleural effusions. The most frequently reported adverse reactions resulting in clinical intervention (eg, discontinuation of oprelvekin, adjustment in dosage, need for concomitant medication to treat an adverse reaction symptom) were atrial arrhythmias, syncope, dyspnea, congestive heart failure, and pulmonary edema. Selected adverse reactions that occurred in greater than or equal to 10% of oprelvekin-treated patients are listed in the following table.

Oprelvekin Adverse Reactions (%)

Adverse reaction	Placebo (n = 67)	50 mcg/kg (n = 69)
Cardiovascular		
Atrial fibrillation/flutter[a]	1 (1%)	8 (12%)
Palpitations[a]	2 (3%)	10 (14%)
Syncope	4 (6%)	9 (13%)
Tachycardia[a]	2 (3%)	14 (20%)
Vasodilatation	6 (9%)	13 (19%)
CNS		
Dizziness	19 (28%)	26 (38%)
Headache	24 (36%)	28 (41%)
Insomnia	18 (27%)	23 (33%)
Dermatologic		
Rash	11 (16%)	17 (25%)
GI		
Diarrhea	22 (33%)	30 (43%)
Mucositis	25 (37%)	30 (43%)
Nausea/Vomiting	47 (70%)	53 (77%)
Oral moniliasis[a]	1 (1%)	10 (14%)
Respiratory		
Cough increased	15 (22%)	20 (29%)
Dyspnea[a]	15 (22%)	33 (48%)
Pharyngitis	11 (16%)	17 (25%)
Pleural effusion[a]	0 (0%)	7 (10%)
Rhinitis	21 (31%)	29 (42%)
Special senses		
Conjunctival injection[a]	2(3%)	13 (19%)
Miscellaneous		
Edema[a]	10 (15%)	41 (59%)
Fever	19 (28%)	25 (36%)
Neutropenic fever	28 (42%)	33 (48%)

[a] Occurred in significantly more oprelvekin-treated than placebo-treated patients.

➤*Other adverse reactions:* The following adverse reactions also occurred more frequently in cancer patients receiving oprelvekin than in those receiving placebo: amblyopia, paresthesia, dehydration, skin discoloration, exfoliative dermatitis, and eye hemorrhage. A statistically significant association of oprelvekin to these reactions has not been established. Other than a higher incidence of severe asthenia in oprelvekin-treated patients (10 [14%] in oprelvekin patients vs 2 [3%] in placebo patients), the incidence of severe or life-threatening adverse reactions was comparable in the oprelvekin and placebo treatment groups.

Two patients with cancer treated with oprelvekin experienced sudden death, which the investigator considered possibly or probably related to oprelvekin. Both deaths occurred in patients with severe hypokalemia (less than 3 mEq/L) who had received high doses of ifosfamide and were receiving daily doses of a diuretic.

Other serious reactions associated with oprelvekin were papilledema and cardiovascular reactions, including atrial arrhythmias and stroke. In addition, cardiomegaly was reported in children.

The following adverse reactions, occurring in greater than or equal to 10% of patients, were observed at equal or greater frequency in placebo-treated patients: asthenia, pain, chills, abdominal pain, infection, anorexia, constipation, dyspepsia, ecchymosis, myalgia, bone pain, nervousness, and alopecia. The incidence of fever, neutropenic fever, flu-like symptoms, thrombocytosis, and thrombotic reactions; the average number of units of red blood cells transfused per patient; and the duration of neutropenia is less than 500/mcL were similar in the oprelvekin 50 mcg/kg and placebo groups.

➤*Immunogenicity:* In clinical studies that evaluated the immunogenicity of oprelvekin, 2 of 181 patients (1%) developed antibodies to oprelvekin. In 1 of these 2 patients, neutralizing antibodies to oprelvekin were detected in an unvalidated assay. The clinical relevance of the presence of these antibodies is unknown. In the postmarketing setting, cases of allergic reactions, including anaphylaxis, have been reported. The presence of antibodies to oprelvekin was not assessed in these patients.

The data reflect the percentage of patients whose test results were considered positive for antibodies to oprelvekin and are highly dependent on the sensitivity and specificity of the assay. Additionally, the observed incidence of antibody positivity in an assay may be influenced by several factors, including sample handling, concomitant medications, and underlying disease. For these reasons, comparisons of the incidence of antibodies to oprelvekin with incidence of antibodies to other products may be misleading.

➤*Lab test abnormalities:* The most common laboratory abnormality reported in patients in clinical trials was a decrease in hemoglobin concentration predominantly as a result of expansion of the plasma volume. The increase in plasma volume also is associated with a decrease in the serum concentration of albumin and several other proteins (eg, transferrin and gamma globulins). A parallel decrease in calcium without clinical effects has been documented.

After daily subcutaneous injections, treatment with oprelvekin resulted in a 2-fold increase in plasma fibrinogen. Other acute-phase proteins also increased. These protein levels returned to normal after dosing with oprelvekin was discontinued. Von Willebrand factor concentrations increased with a normal multimer pattern in healthy subjects receiving oprelvekin.

➤*Postmarketing:* The following adverse reactions have been reported during the postmarketing use of oprelvekin: allergic reactions; anaphylaxis/anaphylactoid reactions; capillary leak syndrome; injection site reactions described as dermatitis, pain, and discoloration; papilledema; and renal failure.

Because these reactions are reported voluntarily from a population of uncertain size, it is not always possible to reliably estimate their frequency or establish a causal relationship to drug exposure. Decisions to include these reactions in labeling are typically based on 1 or more of the following factors: (1) seriousness of the reactions, (2) frequency of reporting, or (3) strength of causal connection to oprelvekin.

Overdosage

Doses of oprelvekin greater than 125 mcg/kg have not been administered to humans. While clinical experience is limited, doses of oprelvekin greater than 50 mcg/kg may be associated with an increased incidence of cardiovascular reactions in adult patients. If an overdose of oprelvekin is administered, discontinue oprelvekin and closely observe the patient for signs of toxicity. Base reinstitution of oprelvekin therapy upon individual patient factors (eg, evidence of toxicity, continued need for therapy).

Patient Information

Use oprelvekin under the guidance and supervision of a health care provider. However, when the health care provider determines that oprelvekin may be used outside of the hospital or office setting, instruct persons who will be administering oprelvekin as to the proper dose and the method for reconstituting and administering oprelvekin. If home use is prescribed, instruct patients in the importance of proper disposal and caution against the reuse of needles, syringes, drug product, and diluent. Instruct patients to use a puncture resistant container for the disposal of used needles.

Inform patients of the most serious and common adverse reactions associated with oprelvekin administration, including those symptoms related to allergic or hypersensitivity reactions. Advise patients to immediately seek medical attention if any of the following signs or symptoms develop: swelling of the face, tongue, or throat; difficulty breathing, swallowing, or talking; shortness of breath; wheezing; chest pain; throat tightness; light-headedness; loss of consciousness; confusion; drowsiness; rash; itching; hives; flushing; and/or fever. Mild to moderate peripheral edema and shortness of breath on exertion can occur within the first week of treatment and may con-

OPRELVEKIN — INJECTION

tinue for the duration of administration of oprelvekin. Advise patients who have preexisting pleural or other effusions or a history of congestive heart failure to contact their health care provider for worsening of dyspnea. Most patients who receive oprelvekin develop anemia. Advise patients to contact their health care provider if symptoms attributable to atrial arrhythmia develop. Caution patients who are older or who have other risk factors for the development of atrial arrhythmias to contact their health care provider if symptoms attributable to atrial arrhythmia develop and are not transient. Advise women of childbearing potential of the possible risks to the fetus on oprelvekin.

Oprelvekin is intended for use under the guidance and supervision of a health care provider. If, however, self-injection is recommended, instruct patients in the preparation of oprelvekin, the proper method for self-injection, and the correct dose to use. Instruct patients not to try self-administration until the health care provider's instructions are understood. Give each dose at about the same time each day. If a dose is missed, instruct patients to continue with the next scheduled dose.

Venous thrombi consist mainly of fibrin and red blood cells. Arterial thrombi are composed mainly of platelet aggregates. Theoretically, anticoagulant drugs should be effective for reducing risks involved with venous thrombi formation and antiplatelet drugs should be more effective for reducing risks of arterial thrombi formation. The drugs most commonly used for their antiplatelet effects are aspirin, sulfinpyrazone, dipyridamole and ticlopidine.

Aggregation Inhibitors

CILOSTAZOL

Rx	**Cilostazol** (Various, eg, Andrx, Teva)	**Tablets:** 50 mg	In 60s.
Rx	**Pletal** (Otsuka America Pharmaceuticals)		(PLETAL 50). White, triangular. In 60s
Rx	**Cilostazol** (Various, eg, Andrx, Eon, Teva)	**Tablets:** 100 mg	In 60s and 500s.
Rx	**Pletal** (Otsuka America Pharmaceuticals)		(PLETAL 100). White. In 60s

CILOSTAZOL - ORAL

WARNING

Cilostazol and several of its metabolites are inhibitors of phosphodiesterase (PDE) 3. Several drugs with this pharmacologic effect have caused decreased survival compared with placebo in patients with class III to IV congestive heart failure. Cilostazol is contraindicated in patients with congestive heart failure of any severity.

Indications

➤*Intermittent claudication:* For the reduction of symptoms of intermittent claudication, as indicated by an increased walking distance.

Administration and Dosage

➤*Approved by the FDA:* January 15, 1999.

➤*Recommended dosage:* 100 mg twice daily taken at least 30 minutes before or 2 hours after breakfast and dinner.

➤*Concomitant medications:* A dosage of 50 mg twice daily should be considered during coadministration of inhibitors of CYP3A4 such as diltiazem, erythromycin, itraconazole, and ketoconazole, and during coadministration of inhibitors of CYP2C19 such as omeprazole.

➤*Treatment response:* Patients may respond as early as 2 to 4 weeks after the initiation of therapy, but treatment for up to 12 weeks may be needed before a beneficial effect is experienced.

➤*Discontinuation:* The available data suggest that the dosage of cilostazol can be reduced or discontinued without rebound (ie, platelet hyperaggregability).

➤*Storage/Stability:* Store cilostazol tablets at 25°C (77°F); excursions are permitted to 15° to 30°C (59° to 86°F).

Actions

➤*Pharmacology:* The mechanism of the effects of cilostazol on the symptoms of intermittent claudication is not fully understood. Cilostazol and several of its metabolites are cyclic adenosine monophosphate (cAMP) PDE 3 inhibitors, inhibiting PDE activity and suppressing cAMP degradation with a resultant increase in cAMP in platelets and blood vessels, leading to inhibition of platelet aggregation and vasodilation, respectively.

Cilostazol reversibly inhibits platelet aggregation induced by a variety of stimuli, including thrombin, adenosine diphosphate (ADP), collagen, arachidonic acid, epinephrine, and shear stress. Effects on circulating plasma lipids have been examined in patients taking cilostazol. After 12 weeks, as compared with placebo, cilostazol 100 mg twice daily produced a reduction in triglycerides of 29.3 mg/dL (15%) and an increase in high-density lipoprotein cholesterol of 4 mg/dL (approximately 10%).

Cilostazol affects both vascular beds and cardiovascular function. It produces nonhomogeneous dilation of vascular beds, with greater dilation in femoral beds than in vertebral, carotid, or superior mesenteric arteries. Renal arteries were not responsive to the effects of cilostazol.

In dogs or cynomolgous monkeys, cilostazol increased heart rate, myocardial contractile force, and coronary blood flow as well as ventricular automaticity, as would be expected for a PDE 3 inhibitor. Left ventricular contractility was increased at doses required to inhibit platelet aggregation. Atrio ventricular conduction was accelerated. In humans, heart rate increased in a dose-proportional manner by a mean of 5.1 and 7.4 beats per minute in patients treated with 50 and 100 mg twice daily, respectively. In 264 patients evaluated with Holter monitors, numerically more cilostazol-treated patients had increases in ventricular premature beats and nonsustained ventricular tachycardia events than did placebo-treated patients; the increases were not dose-related.

➤*Pharmacokinetics:*

Absorption – Cilostazol is absorbed after oral administration. A high-fat meal increases absorption, with an approximately 90% increase in a maximum plasma cocentration(C_{max}) and a 25% increase in the area under the plasma concentration-time curve (AUC). Absolute bioavailability is not known.

Distribution – Cilostazol is 95% to 98% protein bound, predominantly to albumin. The mean percent binding for 3,4-dehydro–cilostazol is 97.4% and for 4'-trans-hydroxy–cilostazol is 66%.

Metabolism/Excretion – Cilostazol is extensively metabolized by hepatic cytochrome P-450 enzymes, mainly 3A4, and, to a lesser extent, 2C19, with metabolites largely excreted in urine. Two metabolites are active, with 1 metabolite (3,4-dehydro–cilostazol) appearing to account for at least 50% of the pharmacologic (PDE 3 inhibition) activity after administration of cilostazol. Pharmacokinetics are approximately dose proportional. Cilostazol and its active metabolites have apparent elimination half-lives of about 11 to 13 hours. Cilostazol and its active metabolites accumulate about 2-fold with chronic administration and reach steady-state blood levels within a few days.

Following oral administration of radio-labeled cilostazol 100 mg, 56% of the total analytes in plasma was cilostazol, 15% was 3,4-dehydro–cilostazol (4 to 7 times as active as cilostazol), and 4% was 4'–trans-hydroxy-cilostazol (one fifth as active as cilostazol). The primary route of elimination was via the urine (74%), with the remainder excreted in the feces (20%). No measurable amount of unchanged cilostazol was excreted in the urine, and less than 2% of the dose was excreted as 3,4-dehydro–cilostazol. About 30% of the dose was excreted in the urine as 4'-trans-hydroxy–cilostazol. The remainder was excreted as other metabolites, none of which exceeded 5%. There was no evidence of induction of hepatic microenzymes.

Special populations –

Renal function impairment: The free fraction of cilostazol was 27% higher in subjects with renal function impairment than in healthy volunteers. The total pharmacologic activity of cilostazol and its metabolites was similar in subjects with mild to moderate renal impairment and in healthy subjects. Severe renal function impairment increases metabolite levels and alters protein binding of the parent and metabolites. The expected pharmacologic activity, based on plasma concentrations and relative to PDE 3 inhibiting potency of parent drug and metabolites, appeared little changed.

Patients on dialysis have not been studied, but it is unlikely that cilostazol can be removed efficiently by dialysis because of its high protein binding (95% to 98%).

Special caution is advised when cilostazol is used in patients with severe renal function impairment: (estimated creatine clearance less than 25 mL/min).

Smokers: Population pharmacokinetic analysis suggests that smoking decreased cilostazol exposure by about 20%.

Patients with intermittent claudication due to peripheral arterial disease (PAD): The pharmacokinetics of cilostazol and its 2 major active metabolites were similar in healthy subjects and patients with intermittent claudication due to PAD.

Contraindications

➤*Congestive heart failure:* Cilostazol and several of its metabolites are inhibitors of PDE 3. Several drugs with this pharmacologic effect have caused decreased survival compared with placebo in patients with class III to IV congestive heart failure. Cilostazol is contraindicated with patients with congestive heart failure of any severity.

➤*Other contraindications:* In patients with hemostatic disorders or active pathologic bleeding, such as bleeding peptic ulcer and intracranial bleeding. Cilostazol inhibits platelet aggregation in a reversible manner, and in patients with known or suspected hypersensitivity to any of its components.

Warnings

➤*Mutagenesis:* Cilostazol tested negative in bacterial gene mutation, bacterial deoxyribonucleic acid (DNA) repair, mammalian cell gene mutation, and mouse in vivo bone marrow chromosomal aberration assays. It was, however, associated with a significant increase in chromosomal aberrations in the in vitro Chinese hamster ovary cell assay.

➤*Fertility impairment:* Cilostazol did not affect fertility or mating performance of male and female rats at dosages as high as 1,000 mg/kg/day. At this dose, systemic exposures (AUCs) to unbound cilostazol were less than 1.5 times (in males) and about 5 times (in females) the exposure in humans at the MRHD.

➤*Elderly:* Of the total number of subjects (N = 2,274) in clinical studies of cilostazol, 56% were 65 years of age and older, while 16% were 75 years of age and older.

➤*Pregnancy:* *Category C.* In a rat developmental toxicity study, oral administration of cilostazol 1,000 mg/kg/day was associated with decreased fetal weights and increased incidences of cardiovascular, renal, and skeletal anomalies (eg, ventricular septal, aortic arch, and subclavian artery abnormalities; renal pelvic dilation; 14th rib; retarded ossification). At this dose, systemic exposure to unbound cilostazol in nonpregnant rats was about 5 times the exposure in humans given the MRHD. Increased incidences of ventricular septal defect and retarded ossification were also noted at 150 mg/kg/day (5 times the MRHD on a systemic exposure basis). In a rabbit developmental toxicity study, an increased incidence of retardation of ossification of the sternum was seen at dosages as low as 150 mg/kg/day. In nonpregnant rabbits given 150 mg/kg/day, exposure to unbound cilostazol was

CILOSTAZOL - ORAL

considerably lower than that seen in humans given the MRHD, and exposure to 3,4-dehydro–cilostazol was barely detectable.

When cilostazol was administered to rats during late pregnancy and lactation, an increased incidence of stillbirth and decreased birth weights of offspring was seen at dosages of 150 mg/kg/day (5 times the MRHD on a systemic exposure basis).

There are no adequate and well-controlled studies in pregnant women.

➤*Lactation:* Transfer of cilostazol into milk has been reported in experimental animals (rats). Because of the potential risk to breast-feeding infants, decide whether to discontinue breast-feeding or cilostazol.

➤*Children:* The safety and efficacy of cilostazol in children have not been established.

Precautions

➤*Congestive heart failure:* Cilostazol is contraindicated in patients with congestive heart failure. In patients without congestive heart failure, the long-term effects of PDE 3 inhibitors (including cilostazol) are unknown. Patients in the 3- to 6-month placebo-controlled trials of cilostazol were relatively stable (no recent myocardial infarction or strokes, no rest pain or other signs of rapidly progressing disease), and only 19 patients died (0.7% in the placebo group and 0.8% in the cilostazol group). The calculated relative risk of death of 1.2 has a wide 95% confidence limit (0.5 to 3.1). There are no data as to longer-term risk or risk in patients with more severe underlying heart disease.

➤*Hematologic effects:* Rare cases of thrombocytopenia or leukopenia progressing to agranulocytosis have been reported when cilostazol was not immediately discontinued. The agranulocytosis, however, was reversible on discontinuation of cilostazol.

Drug Interactions

Cilostazol Drug Interactions

Precipitant drug	Object drug[a]		Description
Clopidogrel	Cilostazol	↑	Additive effects on bleeding times not determined. Monitor bleeding times during coadministration.
CYP3A4 inhibitors (eg, erythromycin, ketoconazole)	Cilostazol	↑	Concurrent use may increase the systemic exposure of cilostazol and/or its major metabolites. Consider a reduced dose of cilostazol.
CYP2C19 (eg, omeprazole)	Cilostazol	↑	Concurrent use may increase the systemic exposure of cilostazol and/or its major metabolites. Consider a reduced dose of cilostazol.
Diltiazem	Cilostazol	↑	Diltiazem 180 mg decreased the clearance of cilostazol by approximately 30% and increased the C_{max} and AUC approximately 30% and 40%, respectively.
Aspirin	Cilostazol	↑	Coadministration of aspirin with cilostazol increased the inhibition of platelet aggregation compared to either product alone. Coadministration had no clinically significant impact on PT, aPTT, or bleeding time.
Cilostazol	Aspirin		
Lovastatin	Cilostazol	↓↑	The coadministration of lovastatin with cilostazol decreased cilostazol $C_{ss,\ max}$ and AUC by 15%. There is also a decrease, although nonsignificant, in cilostazol metabolite concentrations. Coadministration increases lovastatin AUC by approximately 70%.
Cilostazol	Lovastatin		

[a] ↑ = Object drug increased; ↓ = Object drug decreased.

➤*Drug/Food interactions:* Grapefruit juice increased the C_{max} of cilostazol by approximately 50%, but had no effect on AUC. A high-fat meal increases absorption with an approximately 90% increase in C_{max} and a 25% increase in the AUC.

Adverse Reactions

Adverse reactions were assessed in 8 placebo-controlled clinical trials involving 2,274 patients exposed to either 50 or 100 mg of cilostazol twice daily (n = 1,301) or placebo (n = 973), with a median treatment duration of 127 days for patients on cilostazol and 134 days for patients on placebo.

The only adverse reaction resulting in discontinuation of therapy in greater than or equal to 3% of patients treated with cilostazol 50 or 100 mg twice daily was headache, which occurred with an incidence of 1.3%, 3.5%, and 0.3% in patients treated with cilostazol 50 mg twice daily, 100 mg twice daily, or placebo, respectively. Other frequent causes of discontinuation included palpitation and diarrhea, both 1.1% for cilostazol (all doses) versus 0.1% for placebo.

Cilostazol Adverse Reactions (≥2%)

Adverse reaction	Cilostazol 50 mg twice daily (n = 303)	Cilostazol 100 mg twice daily (n = 998)	Placebo (n = 973)
Cardiovascular			
Palpitation	5%	10%	1%
Tachycardia	4%	4%	1%
CNS			
Dizziness	9%	10%	6%
Headache	27%	34%	14%
Vertigo	3%	1%	1%
GI			
Abdominal pain	4%	5%	3%
Abnormal stools	12%	15%	4%
Diarrhea	12%	19%	7%
Dyspepsia	6%	6%	4%
Flatulence	2%	3%	2%
Nausea	6%	7%	6%
Metabolic/Nutritional			
Peripheral edema	9%	7%	4%
Musculoskeletal			
Back pain	6%	7%	6%
Myalgia	2%	3%	2%
Respiratory			
Cough increased	3%	4%	3%
Pharyngitis	7%	10%	7%
Rhinitis	12%	7%	5%
Miscellaneous			
Infection	14%	10%	8%

➤*Other Adverse Reactions:* Other adverse reactions seen with an incidence of greater than or equal to 2%, but occurring in the placebo group at least as frequently as in the 100 mg twice-daily group, were as follows:

Cardiovascular – Angina pectoris, hypertension.

CNS – Hypesthesia, paresthesia.

Dermatologic – Rash.

GI – Vomiting.

GU – Hematuria, urinary tract infection.

Respiratory – Bronchitis, dyspnea.

Miscellaneous – Arthritis, asthenia, flu syndrome, leg cramps.

Less frequent adverse reactions (less than 2%) that were experienced by patients exposed to cilostazol 50 or 100 mg twice daily in the 8 controlled clinical trials, and that occurred at a greater frequency in the 100 mg twice-daily group than in the placebo group, regardless of suspected drug relationship, were as follows:

➤*Cardiovascular:* Atrial fibrillation, atrial flutter, cerebral infarct, cerebral ischemia, congestive heart failure, heart arrest, hemorrhage, hypotension, myocardial infarction, myocardial ischemia, nodal arrhythmia, postural hypotension, supraventricular tachycardia, syncope, varicose vein, vasodilation, ventricular extrasystoles, ventricular tachycardia.

➤*CNS:* Anxiety, insomnia, malaise, neuralgia.

➤*Dermatologic:* Dry skin, furunculosis, skin hypertrophy, urticaria.

➤*Endocrine:* Diabetes mellitus.

➤*GI:* Anorexia, cholelithiasis, colitis, duodenal ulcer, duodenitis, esophageal hemorrhage, esophagitis, gastritis, gastroenteritis, gum hemorrhage, hematemesis, increased gamma-glutamyltransferase, melena, peptic ulcer, periodontal abscess, rectal hemorrhage, stomach ulcer, tongue edema.

➤*GU:* Albuminuria, cystitis, urinary frequency, vaginal hemorrhage, vaginitis.

➤*Hematologic/Lymphatic:* Anemia, ecchymosis, iron deficiency anemia, polycythemia, purpura.

➤*Metabolic/Nutritional:* Gout, hyperlipemia, hyperuricemia, increased creatinine.

➤*Musculoskeletal:* Arthralgia, bone pain, bursitis, neck rigidity.

➤*Respiratory:* Asthma, epistaxis, hemoptysis, pneumonia, sinusitis.

➤*Special senses:* Amblyopia, blindness, conjunctivitis, diplopia, ear pain, eye hemorrhage, retinal hemorrhage, tinnitus.

➤*Miscellaneous:* Chills, face edema, fever, generalized edema, pelvic pain, retroperitoneal hemorrhage.

➤*Postmarketing:* The following events have been reported spontaneously from worldwide postmarketing experience since the launch of cilostazol in the United States.

CILOSTAZOL - ORAL

Cardiovascular – Subacute thrombosis. (These cases of subacute thrombosis occurred in patients treated with aspirin and "off-label" use of cilostazol for prevention of thrombotic complication after coronary stenting.)

Torsades de pointes, QTc prolongation. (Torsades de pointes and QTc prolongation occurred in patients with cardiac disorders [eg, complete atrioventricular block, cardiac failure, bradycardia] when treated with cilostazol. Cilostazol was used "off label" because of its positive chronotropic action.)

CNS – Cerebral hemorrhage, cerebrovascular accident, intracranial hemorrhage.

Dermatologic – Hemorrhage subcutaneous; pruritus; skin eruptions including, skin drug eruption (dermatitis medicamentosa), Stevens-Johnson syndrome.

GI – GI hemorrhage.

Hematologic/Lymphatic – Agranulocytosis, bleeding tendency, granulocytopenia, leukopenia, platelet count decreased, thrombocytopenia, white blood cell count decreased.

Hepatic – Hepatic dysfunction/abnormal liver function tests, jaundice.

Lab test abnormalities – Blood glucose increased, blood uric acid increased, increase in serum urea nitrogen (BUN) abnormalities (serum urea increased)

Respiratory – Interstitial pneumonia, pulmonary hemorrhage.

Miscellaneous – Chest pain, extradural hematoma, hot flashes, subdural hematoma pain.

Overdosage

➤*Symptoms:* Information on acute overdosage with cilostazol in humans is limited. The signs and symptoms of an acute overdose can be anticipated to be those of excessive pharmacologic effect, including the following: severe headache, diarrhea, hypotension, tachycardia, and possibly cardiac arrhythmias.

The oral median lethal dose of cilostazol is greater than 5 g/kg in mice and rats and greater than 2 g/kg in dogs.

Animal toxicity – Repeated oral administration of cilostazol to dogs (greater than or equal to 30 mg/kg/day for 52 weeks, greater than or equal to 150 mg/kg/day for 13 weeks, and 450 mg/kg/day for 2 weeks) produced cardiovascular lesions that included endocardial hemorrhage, hemosiderin deposition and fibrosis in the left ventricle, hemorrhage in the right atrial wall, hemorrhage and necrosis of the smooth muscle in the wall of the coronary artery, intimal thickening of the coronary artery, and coronary arteritis and periarteritis. At the lowest dose associated with cardiovascular lesions in the 52-week study, systemic exposure (AUC) to unbound cilostazol was less than that seen in humans at the MRHD of 100 mg twice daily. Similar lesions have been reported in dogs following the administration of other positive inotropic agents (including PDE 3 inhibitors) or vasodilation agents. No cardiovascular lesions were seen in rats following 5 or 13 weeks of administration of cilostazol at dosages up to 1,500 mg/kg/day. At this dose, systemic exposures (AUCs) to unbound cilostazol were only about 1.5 and 5 times (male and female rats, respectively) the exposure seen in humans at the MRHD. Cardiovascular lesions were also not seen in rats following 52 weeks of administration of cilostazol at dosages up to 150 mg/kg/day. At this dose, systemic exposures (AUCs) to unbound cilostazol were about 0.5 and 5 times (male and female rats, respectively) the exposure in humans at the MRHD. In female rats, cilostazol AUCs were similar at 150 and 1,500 mg/kg/day. Cardiovascular lesions were also not observed in monkeys after oral administration of cilostazol for 13 weeks at dosages up to 1,800 mg/kg/day. While this dose of cilostazol produced pharmacologic effects in monkeys, plasma cilostazol levels were less than those seen in humans given the MRHD and those seen in dogs given doses associated with cardiovascular lesions.

➤*Treatment:* Carefully observe the patient and provide supportive treatment. Since cilostazol is highly protein bound, it is unlikely that it can be efficiently removed by hemodialysis or peritoneal dialysis.

Patient Information

Advise patients to read the package information for cilostazol carefully before starting therapy and to reread it each time therapy is renewed in case the information has changed.

Advise patients to take cilostazol at least 30 minutes before or 2 hours after food.

Inform patients that the beneficial effects of cilostazol on the symptoms of intermittent claudication may not be immediate. Although the patient may experience benefits in 2 to 4 weeks after initiation of therapy; however, treatment for up to 12 weeks may be required before a beneficial effect is experienced.

Inform patients about the uncertainty concerning cardiovascular risk in long-term use or in patients with severe underlying heart disease.

CLOPIDOGREL

Rx	**Plavix** (Bristol-Myers Squibb)	**Tablets:** 75 mg (as base)	Lactose, castor oil, mannitol. (75 1171). Pink. Film-coated. In 30s, 90s, 500s, and UD 100s.

CLOPIDOGREL — ORAL

Indications

Clopidogrel bisulfate is indicated for the reduction of atherosclerotic events as follows:

➤*Recent MI, recent stroke or established peripheral arterial disease:* For patients with a history of recent MI, recent stroke, or established peripheral arterial disease, clopidogrel bisulfate has been shown to reduce the rate of a combined endpoint of new ischemic stroke (fatal or not), new MI (fatal or not), and other vascular death.

➤*Acute coronary syndrome:* For patients with acute coronary syndrome (unstable angina/non-Q-wave MI), including patients who are to be managed medically and those who are to be managed with percutaneous coronary intervention (PCI) (with or without stent) or coronary artery bypass graft (CABG), clopidogrel bisulfate has been shown to decrease the rate of a combined endpoint of cardiovascular death, MI, or stroke as well as the rate of a combined endpoint of cardiovascular death, MI, stroke, or refractory ischemia.

➤*Unlabeled uses:* As a loading dose regimen of clopidogrel with aspirin to prevent cardiac adverse events in patients receiving coronary stent implantation.

Administration and Dosage

➤*Approved by the FDA:* November 18, 1997.

➤*Recent MI, recent stroke or established peripheral arterial disease:* The recommended daily dose of clopidogrel bisulfate is 75 mg once daily.

➤*Acute coronary syndrome:* For patients with acute coronary syndrome (unstable angina/non-Q-wave MI), clopidogrel bisulfate should be initiated with a single 300 mg loading dose and then continued at 75 mg once daily. Aspirin (75 mg to 325 mg once daily) should be initiated and continued in combination with clopidogrel bisulfate. In CURE, most patients with acute coronary syndrome also received heparin acutely.

Clopidogrel bisulfate can be administered with or without food.

➤*Elderly:* Plasma concentrations of the main circulating metabolite are significantly higher in elderly (greater than or equal to 75 years) compared to young healthy volunteers but these higher plasma levels were not associated with differences in platelet aggregation and bleeding time. No dosage adjustment is needed for the elderly.

➤*Renal function impairment:* After repeated doses of 75 mg clopidogrel bisulfate per day, plasma levels of the main circulating metabolite were lower in patients with severe renal impairment (creatinine clearance from 5 to 15 mL/min) compared to subjects with moderate renal impairment (creatinine clearance 30 to 60 mL/min) or healthy subjects. Although inhibition of ADP-induced platelet aggregation was lower (25%) than that observed in healthy volunteers, the prolongation of bleeding time was similar to healthy volunteers receiving 75 mg of clopidogrel bisulfate per day.

➤*Storage/Stability:* Store at 25°C (77°F); excursions permitted to 15° to 30°C (59° to 86°F).

Actions

➤*Pharmacology:* It is an inhibitor of platelet aggregation. A variety of drugs that inhibit platelet function have been shown to decrease morbid events in people with established atherosclerotic cardiovascular disease as evidenced by stroke or transient ischemic attacks, MI, or need for vascular bypass or angioplasty. This indicates that platelets participate in the initiation and/or evolution of these events and that inhibiting them can reduce the event rate.

Pharmacodynamic properties – Clopidogrel selectively inhibits the binding of adenosine diphosphate (ADP) to its platelet receptor and the subsequent ADP-mediated activation of the GPIIb/IIIa complex, thereby inhibiting platelet aggregation. Biotransformation of clopidogrel is necessary to produce inhibition of platelet aggregation, but an active metabolite responsible for the activity of the drug has not been isolated. Clopidogrel also inhibits platelet aggregation induced by agonists other than ADP by blocking the amplification of platelet activation by released ADP. Clopidogrel does not inhibit phosphodiesterase activity.

Clopidogrel acts by irreversibly modifying the platelet ADP receptor. Consequently, platelets exposed to clopidogrel are affected for the remainder of their lifespan. Dose-dependent inhibition of platelet aggregation can be seen 2 hours after single oral doses of clopidogrel. Repeated doses of 75 mg clopidogrel per day inhibit ADP-induced platelet aggregation on the first day, and inhibition reaches steady state between day 3 and day 7. At steady state, the average inhibition level observed with a dose of 75 mg clopidogrel bisulfate per day was between 40% and 60%. Platelet aggregation and bleeding time gradually return to baseline values after treatment is discontinued, generally in approximately 5 days.

➤*Pharmacokinetics:*

Absorption/Distribution – Clopidogrel is rapidly absorbed after oral administration of repeated doses of 75 mg clopidogrel (base), with peak plasma levels (approximately equal to 3 mg/L) of the main circulating metabolite occurring approximately 1 hour after dosing. The pharmacokinetics of the main circulating metabolite are linear (plasma concentrations increased in proportion to dose) in the dose range of 50 to 150 mg of clopidogrel. Absorption is greater than or equal to 50% based on urinary excretion of clopidogrel-related metabolites.

CLOPIDOGREL — ORAL

Administration of clopidogrel bisulfate with meals did not significantly modify the bioavailability of clopidogrel as assessed by the pharmacokinetics of the main circulating metabolite.

Clopidogrel and the main circulating metabolite bind reversibly in vitro to human plasma proteins (98% and 94%, respectively). The binding is nonsaturable in vitro up to a concentration of 100 mcg/mL.

Metabolism/Excretion – In vitro and in vivo, clopidogrel undergoes rapid hydrolysis into its carboxylic acid derivative. In plasma and urine, the glucuronide of the carboxylic acid derivative is also observed.

After repeated 75 mg oral doses of clopidogrel (base), plasma concentrations of the parent compound, which has no platelet inhibiting effect, are very low and are generally below the quantification limit (0.00025 mg/L) beyond 2 hours after dosing. Clopidogrel is extensively metabolized by the liver. The main circulating metabolite is the carboxylic acid derivative, and it too has no effect on platelet aggregation. It represents approximately 85% of the circulating drug-related compounds in plasma.

Following an oral dose of ^{14}C-labeled clopidogrel in humans, approximately 50% was excreted in the urine and approximately 46% in the feces in the 5 days after dosing. The elimination half-life of the main circulating metabolite was 8 hours after single and repeated administration. Covalent binding to platelets accounted for 2% of radiolabel with a half-life of 11 days.

Special populations –

Renal function impairment: After repeated doses of 75 mg clopidogrel bisulfate per day, plasma levels of the main circulating metabolite were lower in patients with severe renal impairment (creatinine clearance from 5 to 15 mL/min) compared to subjects with moderate renal impairment (creatinine clearance 30 to 60 mL/min) or healthy subjects. Although inhibition of ADP-induced platelet aggregation was lower (25%) than that observed in healthy volunteers, the prolongation of bleeding time was similar to healthy volunteers receiving 75 mg of clopidogrel bisulfate per day. No dosage adjustment is needed in renally impaired patients.

Elderly: Plasma concentrations of the main circulating metabolite are significantly higher in elderly (greater than or equal to 75 years) compared to young healthy volunteers but these higher plasma levels were not associated with differences in platelet aggregation and bleeding time. No dosage adjustment is needed for the elderly.

Gender: No significant difference was observed in the plasma levels of the main circulating metabolite between males and females. In a small study comparing men and women, less inhibition of ADP-induced platelet aggregation was observed in women, but there was no difference in prolongation of bleeding time. In the large, controlled clinical study (Clopidogrel vs Aspirin in Patients at Risk of Ischemic Events; CAPRIE), the incidence of clinical outcome events, other adverse clinical events, and abnormal clinical laboratory parameters was similar in men and women.

Contraindications

Hypersensitivity to the drug substance or any component of the product; active pathological bleeding such as peptic ulcer or intracranial hemorrhage.

Warnings

➤*Thrombotic thrombocytopenic purpura (TTP):* TTP has been reported rarely following use of clopidogrel bisulfate, sometimes after a short exposure (less than 2 weeks). TTP is a serious condition requiring prompt treatment. It is characterized by thrombocytopenia, microangiopathic hemolytic anemia (schistocytes [fragmented RBCs] seen on peripheral smear), neurological findings, renal dysfunction, and fever. TTP was not seen during clopidogrel's clinical trials, which included over 17,500 clopidogrel-treated patients. In worldwide postmarketing experience, however, TTP has been reported at a rate of about 4 cases per million patients exposed, or about 11 cases per million patient-years. The background rate is thought to be about 4 cases per million person-years.

➤*Renal function impairment:* Experience is limited in patients with severe renal impairment. Clopidogrel bisulfate should be used with caution in this population.

➤*Hepatic function impairment:* Experience is limited in patients with severe hepatic disease, who may have bleeding diatheses. Clopidogrel bisulfate should be used with caution in this population.

➤*Pregnancy:* *Category B.* Reproduction studies performed in rats and rabbits at doses up to 500 and 300 mg/kg/day (respectively, 65 and 78 times the recommended daily human dose on a mg/m^2 basis), revealed no evidence of impaired fertility or fetotoxicity due to clopidogrel. There are, however, no adequate and well-controlled studies in pregnant women. Because animal reproduction studies are not always predictive of a human response, clopidogrel bisulfate should be used during pregnancy only if clearly needed.

➤*Lactation:* Studies in rats have shown that clopidogrel and/or its metabolites are excreted in the milk. It is not known whether this drug is excreted in human milk. Because many drugs are excreted in human milk and because of the potential for serious adverse reactions in nursing infants, a decision should be made whether to discontinue nursing or to discontinue the drug, taking into account the importance of the drug to the mother.

➤*Children:* Safety and efficacy in children have not been established.

Precautions

➤*Monitoring:* Due to the risk of bleeding and undesirable hematological effects, blood cell count determination and/or other appropriate testing should be promptly considered, whenever such suspected clinical symptoms arise during the course of treatment.

➤*Bleeding risk:* As with other antiplatelet agents, clopidogrel bisulfate should be used with caution in patients who may be at risk of increased bleeding from trauma, surgery, or other pathological conditions. If a patient is to undergo elective surgery and an antiplatelet effect is not desired, clopidogrel bisulfate should be discontinued 5 days prior to surgery.

➤*GI bleeding:* Clopidogrel bisulfate prolongs the bleeding time. In CAPRIE, clopidogrel bisulfate was associated with a rate of GI bleeding of 2%, vs 2.7% on aspirin. In CURE, the incidence of major GI bleeding was 1.3% vs 0.7% (clopidogrel bisulfate + aspirin vs placebo + aspirin, respectively.) Clopidogrel bisulfate should be used with caution in patients who have lesions with a propensity to bleed (such as ulcers). Drugs that might induce such lesions should be used with caution in patients taking clopidogrel bisulfate.

Drug Interactions

At high concentrations in vitro, clopidogrel inhibits P450 2C9. Accordingly, clopidogrel may interfere with the metabolism of phenytoin, tamoxifen, tolbutamide, warfarin, torsemide, fluvastatin, and many nonsteroidal anti-inflammatory agents, but there are no data with which to predict the magnitude of these interactions. Use caution when any of these drugs is coadministered with clopidogrel.

Clopidogrel Drug Interactions

Precipitant drug	Object drug*		Description
NSAIDs	Clopidogrel	↑	Coadministration of clopidogrel with naproxen was associated with increased occult GI blood loss. Administer NSAIDs and clopidogrel with caution.
Warfarin	Clopidogrel	↔	Clopidogrel prolongs bleeding time. The safety of coadministration with warfarin has not been established. Administer these 2 agents with caution.
Clopidogrel	Warfarin		

* ↑ = Object drug increased. ↔ = Undetermined clinical effect.

Study of specific drug interactions yielded the following results:

➤*Aspirin:* Aspirin did not modify the clopidogrel-mediated inhibition of ADP-induced platelet aggregation. Concomitant administration of 500 mg of aspirin twice a day for 1 day did not significantly increase the prolongation of bleeding time induced by clopidogrel bisulfate. Clopidogrel bisulfate potentiated the effect of aspirin on collagen-induced platelet aggregation. Clopidogrel bisulfate and aspirin have been administered together for up to 1 year.

➤*Heparin:* In a study in healthy volunteers clopidogrel bisulfate did not necessitate modification of the heparin dose or alter the effects of heparin on coagulation. Coadministration of heparin had no effect on inhibition of platelet aggregation induced by clopidogrel bisulfate.

➤*Other concomitant therapy:* No clinically significant pharmacodynamic interactions were observed when clopidogrel bisulfate was coadministered with atenolol, nifedipine, or both atenolol and nifedipine. The pharmacodynamic activity of clopidogrel bisulfate was also not significantly influenced by the coadministration of phenobarbital, cimetidine, or estrogen.

The pharmacokinetics of digoxin or theophylline were not modified by the coadministration of clopidogrel bisulfate.

At high concentrations in vitro, clopidogrel inhibits P450 (2C9). Accordingly, clopidogrel bisulfate may interfere with the metabolism of phenytoin, tamoxifen, tolbutamide, warfarin, torsemide, fluvastatin, and many nonsteroidal anti-inflammatory agents, but there are no data with which to predict the magnitude of these interactions. Caution should be used when any of these drugs are coadministered with clopidogrel bisulfate.

In addition to the above specific interaction studies, patients entered into clinical trials with clopidogrel bisulfate received a variety of concomitant medications including diuretics, beta-blocking agents, angiotensin-converting enzyme inhibitors, calcium antagonists, cholesterol-lowering agents, coronary vasodilators, antidiabetic agents (including insulin), antiepileptic agents, hormone replacement therapy, heparins (unfractionated and LMWH) and GPIIb/IIIa antagonists without evidence of clinically significant adverse interactions. The use of oral anticoagulants, nonstudy antiplatelet drug and chronic NSAIDs was not allowed in CURE and there are no data on their concomitant use with clopidogrel.

Adverse Reactions

Clopidogrel bisulfate has been evaluated for safety in greater than 17,500 patients, including greater than 9000 patients treated for 1 year or more. The overall tolerability of clopidogrel bisulfate in CAPRIE was similar to that of aspirin regardless of age, gender and race, with an approximately equal incidence (13%) of patients withdrawing from treatment because of adverse reactions. The clinically important adverse events observed in CAPRIE and CURE are discussed below.

Hemorrhagic – In patients receiving clopidogrel bisulfate in CAPRIE, GI hemorrhage occurred at a rate of 2%, and required hospitalization in 0.7%. In patients receiving aspirin, the corresponding rates were 2.7% and 1.1%, respectively. The incidence of intracranial hemorrhage was 0.4% for clopidogrel bisulfate compared to 0.5% for aspirin.

In CURE, clopidogrel bisulfate use with aspirin was associated with an increase in bleeding compared to placebo with aspirin (see CURE incidence of bleeding complications). There was an excess in major bleeding in patients receiving clopidogrel bisulfate plus aspirin compared with placebo plus aspirin, primarily gastrointestinal and at puncture sites. The incidence of intracranial hemorrhage (0.1%), and fatal bleeding (0.2%), was the same in both groups.

In patients receiving both clopidogrel bisulfate and aspirin in CURE, the incidence of bleeding is described in the table below.

CLOPIDOGREL — ORAL

CURE incidence of bleeding complications (% patients)			
Event	Clopidogrel bisulfate (+ aspirin)[1] (n = 6259)	Placebo (+ aspirin)[1] (n = 6303)	P-value
Major bleeding[2]	3.7[3]	2.7[4]	0.001
Life-threatening bleeding	2.2	1.8	0.13
Fatal	0.2	0.2	
5 g/dL hemoglobin drop	0.9	0.9	
Requiring surgical intervention	0.7	0.7	
Hemorrhagic strokes	0.1	0.1	
Requiring inotropes	0.5	0.5	
Requiring transfusion (≥ 4 units)	1.2	1	
Other major bleeding	1.6	1	0.005
Significantly disabling	0.4	0.3	
Intraocular bleeding with significant loss of vision	0.05	0.03	
Requiring 2 to 3 units of blood	1.3	0.9	
Minor bleeding[5]	5.1	2.4	< 0.001

[1] Other standard therapies were used as appropriate.
[2] Life threatening and other major bleeding.
[3] Major bleeding event rate for clopidogrel bisulfate + aspirin was dose-dependent on aspirin: Less than 100 mg = 2.6%; 100 to 200 mg = 3.5%; greater than 200 mg = 4.9%.
[4] Major bleeding event rate for placebo + aspirin was dose-dependent on aspirin: Less than 100 mg = 2%; 100 to 200 mg = 2.3%; greater than 200 mg = 4%.
[5] Led to interruption of study medication.

Ninety-two percent (92%) of the patients in the CURE study received heparin/LMWH, and the rate of bleeding in these patients was similar to the overall results.

There was no excess in major bleeds within 7 days after coronary bypass graft surgery in patients who stopped therapy more than 5 days prior to surgery (event rate 4.4% clopidogrel bisulfate + aspirin; 5.3% placebo + aspirin). In patients who remained on therapy within 5 days of bypass graft surgery, the event rate was 9.6% for clopidogrel bisulfate + aspirin, and 6.3% for placebo + aspirin.

Neutropenia / agranulocytosis – Ticlopidine, a drug chemically similar to clopidogrel bisulfate, is associated with a 0.8% rate of severe neutropenia (less than 450 neutrophils/mcL). In CAPRIE severe neutropenia was observed in 6 patients, 4 on clopidogrel bisulfate and 2 on aspirin. Two (2) of the 9599 patients who received clopidogrel bisulfate and none of the 9586 patients who received aspirin had neutrophil counts of zero. One (1) of the 4 clopidogrel bisulfate patients in CAPRIE was receiving cytotoxic chemotherapy, and another recovered and returned to the trial after only temporarily interrupting treatment with clopidogrel bisulfate. In CURE, the numbers of patients with thrombocytopenia (19 clopidogrel bisulfate + aspirin vs 24 placebo + aspirin) or neutropenia (3 vs 3) were similar.

Although the risk of myelotoxicity with clopidogrel bisulfate thus appears to be quite low, this possibility should be considered when a patient receiving clopidogrel bisulfate demonstrates fever or other sign of infection.

Gastrointestinal – Overall, the incidence of GI events (eg, abdominal pain, dyspepsia, gastritis and constipation) in patients receiving clopidogrel bisulfate was 27.1%, compared to 29.8% in those receiving aspirin in the CAPRIE trial. In the CURE trial the incidence of these GI events for patients receiving clopidogrel bisulfate + aspirin was 11.7% compared to 12.5% for those receiving placebo + aspirin.

In the CAPRIE trial, the incidence of peptic, gastric or duodenal ulcers was 0.7% for clopidogrel bisulfate and 1.2% for aspirin. In the CURE trial, the incidence of peptic, gastric or duodenal ulcers was 0.4% for clopidogrel bisulfate + aspirin and 0.3% for placebo + aspirin.

Cases of diarrhea were reported in the CAPRIE trial in 4.5% of patients in the clopidogrel bisulfate group compared to 3.4% in the aspirin group. However, these were rarely severe (clopidogrel bisulfate = 0.2% and aspirin = 0.1%). In the CURE trial, the incidence of diarrhea for patients receiving clopidogrel bisulfate + aspirin was 2.1% compared to 2.2% for those receiving placebo + aspirin.

In the CAPRIE trial, the incidence of patients withdrawing from treatment because of GI adverse reactions was 3.2% for clopidogrel bisulfate and 4% for aspirin. In the CURE trial, the incidence of patients withdrawing from treatment because of GI adverse reactions was 0.9% for clopidogrel bisulfate + aspirin compared with 0.8% for placebo + aspirin.

Rash and other skin disorders – In the CAPRIE trial, the incidence of skin and appendage disorders in patients receiving clopidogrel bisulfate was 15.8% (0.7% serious); the corresponding rate in aspirin patients was 13.1% (0.5% serious). In the CURE trial, the incidence of rash or other skin disorders in patients receiving clopidogrel bisulfate + aspirin was 4% compared to 3.5% for those receiving placebo + aspirin.

In the CAPRIE trial, the overall incidence of patients withdrawing from treatment because of adverse reactions due to skin and appendage disorders was 1.5% for clopidogrel bisulfate and 0.8% for aspirin. In the CURE trial, the incidence of patients withdrawing because of adverse reactions due to skin and appendage disorders was 0.7% for clopidogrel bisulfate + aspirin compared with 0.3% for placebo + aspirin. Adverse events occurring in greater than or equal to 2.5% of patients on clopidogrel bisulfate in the CAPRIE controlled clinical trial are shown below regardless of relationship to clopidogrel bisulfate. The median duration of therapy was 20 months, with a maximum of 3 years. Incidence of discontinuation, regardless of relationship to therapy, is shown in parentheses.

Adverse events occurring in ≥ 2.5% of clopidogrel bisulfate patients in CAPRIE		
	% Incidence (% discontinuation)	
Body system event	Clopidogrel bisulfate (n = 9599)	Aspirin (n = 9586)
Miscellaneous		
Chest pain	8.3% (0.2%)	8.3% (0.3%)
Accidental/inflicted injury	7.9% (0.1%)	7.3% (0.1%)
Influenza-like symptoms	7.5% (< 0.1%)	7% (< 0.1%)
Pain	6.4% (0.1%)	6.3% (0.1%)
Fatigue	3.3% (0.1%)	3.4% (0.1%)
Cardiovascular		
Edema	4.1% (< 0.1%)	4.5% (< 0.1%)
Hypertension	4.3% (< 0.1%)	5.1% (< 0.1%)
Central and peripheral nervous		
Headache	7.6% (0.3%)	7.2% (0.2%)
Dizziness	6.2% (0.2%)	6.7% (0.3%)
GI		
Abdominal pain	5.6% (0.7%)	7.1% (1%)
Dyspepsia	5.2% (0.6%)	6.1% (0.7%)
Diarrhea	4.5% (0.4%)	3.4% (0.3%)
Nausea	3.4% (0.5%)	3.8% (0.4%)
Metabolic/nutritional		
Hypercholesterolemia	4% (0%)	4.4% (< 0.1%)
Musculoskeletal		
Arthralgia	6.3% (0.1%)	6.2% (0.1%)
Back pain	5.8% (0.1%)	5.3% (< 0.1%)
Hematologic		
Purpura/bruise	5.3% (0.3%)	3.7% (0.1%)
Epistaxis	2.9% (0.2%)	2.5% (0.1%)
Psychiatric		
Depression	3.6% (0.1%)	3.9% (0.2%)
Respiratory		
Upper respiratory tract infection	8.7% (< 0.1%)	8.3% (< 0.1%)
Dyspnea	4.5% (0.1%)	4.7% (0.1%)
Rhinitis	4.2% (0.1%)	4.2% (< 0.1%)
Bronchitis	3.7% (0.1%)	3.7% (0%)
Coughing	3.1% (< 0.1%)	2.7% (< 0.1%)
Dermatologic		
Rash	4.2% (0.5%)	3.5% (0.2%)
Pruritus	3.3% (0.3%)	1.6% (0.1%)
GU		
Urinary tract infection	3.1% (0%)	3.5% (0.1%)

Adverse events occurring in greater than or equal to 2% of patients on clopidogrel bisulfate in the CURE controlled clinical trial are shown below regardless of relationship to clopidogrel bisulfate.

Adverse events occurring in ≥ 2% of clopidogrel patients in CURE		
	% Incidence (% Discontinuation)	
Body system/event	Clopidogrel bisulfate (+ aspirin)* [n = 6259]	Placebo (+ aspirin)* [n = 6303]
Miscellaneous		
Chest pain	2.7% (< 0.1%)	2.8% (0%)
CNS		
Headache	3.1% (0.1%)	3.2% (0.1%)
Dizziness	2.4% (0.1%)	2% (< 0.1%)
GI		
Abdominal pain	2.3% (0.3%)	2.8% (0.3%)
Dyspepsia	2% (0.1%)	1.9% (< 0.1%)
Diarrhea	2.1% (0.1%)	2.2% (0.1%)

* Other standard therapies were used as appropriate.

CLOPIDOGREL — ORAL

Other adverse experiences of potential importance occurring in 1% to 2.5% of patients receiving clopidogrel bisulfate in the CAPRIE or CURE controlled clinical trial are listed below regardless of relationship to clopidogrel bisulfate. In general, the incidence of these events was similar to that in patients receiving aspirin (in CAPRIE) or placebo + aspirin (in CURE).

Other potentially serious adverse events which may be of clinical interest but were rarely reported (less than 1%) in patients who received clopidogrel bisulfate in the CAPRIE or CURE controlled clinical trials are listed below regardless of relationship to clopidogrel bisulfate. In general, the incidence of these events was similar to that in patients receiving aspirin (in CAPRIE) or placebo + aspirin (in CURE).

➤*Allergic:* Allergic reaction (less than 1%).

➤*Cardiovascular:* Edema generalized (less than 1%); cardiac failure, fibrillation atrial (1% to 2.5%).

➤*CNS:* Syncope, palpitation, leg cramps, hypoaesthesia, neuralgia, paresthesia, vertigo (1% to 2.5%).

➤*Dermatologic:* Eczema, skin ulceration (1% to 2.5%); bullous eruption, rash erythematous, rash maculopapular, urticaria (less than 1%).

➤*GI:* Gastric ulcer perforated, gastritis hemorrhagic, upper GI ulcer hemorrhagic (less than 1%); constipation, vomiting (1% to 2.5%).

➤*GU:* Cystitis (1% to 2.5%).

➤*Hematologic:* GI hemorrhage, hematoma, platelets decreased, anemia (1% to 2.5%); menorrhagia in females, anemia aplastic, anemia hypochromic, agranulocytosis, granulocytopenia, leukemia, leukopenia, neutrophils decreased, hemarthrosis, hematuria, hemoptysis, hemorrhage intracranial, hemorrhage retroperitoneal, hemorrhage of operative wound, ocular hemorrhage, pulmonary hemorrhage, purpura allergic, thrombocytopenia (less than 1%).

➤*Hepatic:* Bilirubinemia, hepatitis infectious, liver fatty (less than 1%); hepatic enzymes increased (1% to 2.5%).

➤*Metabolic/Nutritional:* Gout, hyperuricemia, nonprotein nitrogen (NPN) increased (1% to 2.5%).

➤*Musculoskeletal:* Arthritis, arthrosis (1% to 2.5%).

➤*Psychiatric:* Anxiety, insomnia (1% to 2.5%).

➤*Renal:* Abnormal renal function, acute renal failure (less than 1%).

➤*Respiratory:* Pneumonia, sinusitis (1% to 2.5%); hemothorax (less than 1%).

➤*Special senses:* Cataract, conjunctivitis (1% to 2.5%).

➤*Miscellaneous:* Asthenia, fever, hernia (1% to 2.5%); necrosis ischemic (less than 1%).

➤*Postmarketing Experience:* The following events have been reported spontaneously from worldwide postmarketing experience:

CNS – Confusion, hallucinations, taste disorders.

Dermatologic – Angioedema, erythema multiforme.

Endocrine – Vasculitis.

GI – Colitis (including ulcerative or lymphocytic colitis).

GU – Glomerulopathy, abnormal creatinine levels.

Hematologic – Cases of bleeding with fatal outcome (especially intracranial, gastrointestinal and retroperitoneal hemorrhage). Agranulocytosis, aplastic anemia/pancytopenia, thrombotic thrombocytopenic purpura (TTP). TTP is a serious condition requiring prompt treatment. It is characterized by thrombocytopenia, microangiopathic hemolytic anemia (schistocytes [fragmented RBCs] seen on peripheral smear), neurological findings, renal dysfunction, and fever. TTP was not seen during clopidogrel's clinical trials, which included over 17,500 clopidogrel-treated patients. In worldwide postmarketing experience, however, TTP has been reported at a rate of about 4 cases per million patients exposed, or about 11 cases per million patient-years. The background rate is thought to be about 4 cases per million person-years.

Conjunctival, ocular and retinal bleeding.

Hepatic – Abnormal liver function test, hepatitis (noninfectious).

Respiratory – Bronchospasm.

Miscellaneous – Hypersensitivity reactions, anaphylactoid reactions.

Overdosage

➤*Symptoms:* One case of deliberate overdosage with clopidogrel bisulfate was reported in the large, controlled clinical study, CAPRIE. A 34-year-old woman took a single 1050 mg dose of clopidogrel bisulfate (equivalent to 14 standard 75 mg tablets). There were no associated adverse events. No special therapy was instituted, and she recovered without sequelae.

No adverse events were reported after single oral administration of 600 mg (equivalent to 8 standard 75 mg tablets) of clopidogrel bisulfate in healthy volunteers. The bleeding time was prolonged by a factor of 1.7, which is similar to that typically observed with the therapeutic dose of 75 mg of clopidogrel bisulfate per day.

A single oral dose of clopidogrel at 1500 or 2000 mg/kg was lethal to mice and to rats and at 3000 mg/kg to baboons. Symptoms of acute toxicity were vomiting (in baboons), prostration, difficult breathing, and GI hemorrhage in all species.

➤*Treatment:* Based on biological plausibility, platelet transfusion may be appropriate to reverse the pharmacological effects of clopidogrel bisulfate if quick reversal is required.

Patient Information

Patients should be told that it may take them longer than usual to stop bleeding when they take clopidogrel bisulfate, and that they should report any unusual bleeding to their physician. Patients should inform physicians and dentists that they are taking clopidogrel bisulfate before any surgery is scheduled and before any new drug is taken.

TICLOPIDINE HYDROCHLORIDE

Rx	**Ticlopidine HCl** (Various, eg, Apotex Corp., Teva)	**Tablets:** 250 mg	In 30s, 60s, 100s, 500s, and 1000s.
Rx	**Ticlid** (Syntex)		(Ticlid 250). White. Oval. Film coated. In 30s, 60s, and 500s.

TICLOPIDINE HYDROCHLORIDE — ORAL

WARNING

Ticlopidine HCl can cause life-threatening hematological adverse reactions, including neutropenia/agranulocytosis and thrombotic thrombocytopenic purpura (TTP) and aplastic anemia.

Neutropenia/agranulocytosis – Among 2048 patients in clinical trials, there were 50 cases (2.4%) of neutropenia (less than 1200 neutrophils/mm^3), and the neutrophil count was below 450/mm^3 in 17 of these patients (0.8% of the total population).

TTP – One case of TTP was reported during clinical trials. Based on postmarketing data, US physicians reported about 100 cases between 1992 and 1997. Based on an estimated patient exposure of 2 million to 4 million, and assuming an event reporting rate of 10% (the true rate is not known), the incidence of ticlopidine-associated TTP may be as high as 1 case in every 2000 to 4000 patients exposed.

Aplastic anemia – Aplastic anemia was not seen during clinical trials in stroke patients, but US physicians reported about 50 cases between 1992 and 1998. Based on an estimated patient exposure of 2 million to 4 million, and assuming an event reporting rate of 10% (the true rate is not known), the incidence of ticlopidine-associated aplastic anemia may be as high as 1 case in every 4000 to 8000 patients exposed.

WARNING (cont.)

Monitoring of clinical and hematologic status – Severe hematologic adverse reactions may occur within a few days of the start of therapy. The incidence of TTP peaks after about 3 to 4 weeks of therapy and neutropenia peaks at approximately 4 to 6 weeks. The incidence of aplastic anemia peaks after about 4 to 8 weeks of therapy. The incidence of the hematologic adverse reactions declines thereafter. Only a few cases of neutropenia, TTP, or aplastic anemia have arisen after more than 3 months of treatment.

Hematological adverse reactions cannot be reliably predicted by any identified demographic or clinical characteristics. During the first 3 months of treatment, patients receiving ticlopidine HCl must, therefore, be hematologically and clinically monitored for evidence of neutropenia or TTP. If any such evidence is seen, ticlopidine HCl should be immediately discontinued.

Indications

➤*Stroke:* To reduce the risk of thrombotic stroke (fatal or nonfatal) in patients who have experienced stroke precursors, and in patients who have had a completed thrombotic stroke. Because ticlopidine is associated with a risk of life-threatening blood dyscrasias, including thrombotic thrombocytopenic purpura (TTP), neutropenia/agranulocytosis and aplastic anemia, ticlopidine should be reserved for patients who are intolerant or allergic to aspirin therapy or who have failed aspirin therapy.

TICLOPIDINE HYDROCHLORIDE — ORAL

➤*Stent thrombosis, adjunctive therapy:* As adjunctive therapy with aspirin to reduce the incidence of subacute stent thrombosis in patients undergoing successful coronary stent implantation.

Administration and Dosage

➤*Approved by the FDA:* October 1991.

➤*Administration:* Administration of ticlopidine HCl with food is recommended to maximize GI tolerance. In controlled trials, ticlopidine HCl was taken with meals.

➤*Stroke:* 250 mg twice daily taken with food.

➤*Coronary artery stenting:* 250 mg twice daily taken with food together with antiplatelet doses of aspirin for up to 30 days of therapy following successful stent implantation.

➤*Storage/Stability:* Store at 15° to 30°C (59° to 86°F).

Actions

➤*Pharmacology:* When taken orally, ticlopidine HCl causes a time- and dose-dependent inhibition of both platelet aggregation and release of platelet granule constituents, as well as a prolongation of bleeding time. The intact drug has no significant in vitro activity at the concentrations attained in vivo; and, although analysis of urine and plasma indicates at least 20 metabolites, no metabolite which accounts for the activity of ticlopidine has been isolated.

Ticlopidine HCl, after oral ingestion, interferes with platelet membrane function by inhibiting ADP-induced platelet-fibrinogen binding and subsequent platelet-platelet interactions. The effect on platelet function is irreversible for the life of the platelet, as shown both by persistent inhibition of fibrinogen binding after washing platelets ex vivo and by inhibition of platelet aggregation after resuspension of platelets in buffered medium.

Pharmacodynamics – In healthy volunteers over the age of 50, substantial inhibition (greater than 50%) of ADP-induced platelet aggregation is detected within 4 days after administration of ticlopidine HCl 250 mg twice daily, and maximum platelet aggregation inhibition (60% to 70%) is achieved after 8 to 11 days. Lower doses cause less, and more delayed, platelet aggregation inhibition, while doses above 250 mg twice daily give little additional effect on platelet aggregation but an increased rate of adverse effects. The dose of 250 mg twice daily is the only dose that has been evaluated in controlled clinical trials.

After discontinuation of ticlopidine HCl, bleeding time and other platelet function tests return to normal within 2 weeks, in the majority of patients.

At the recommended therapeutic dose (250 mg twice daily), ticlopidine HCl has no known significant pharmacological actions in man other than inhibition of platelet function and prolongation of the bleeding time.

➤*Pharmacokinetics:*

Absorption – After oral administration of a single 250 mg dose, ticlopidine HCl is rapidly absorbed, with peak plasma levels occurring at approximately 2 hours after dosing and is extensively metabolized. Absorption is greater than 80%.

The oral bioavailability of ticlopidine is increased by 20% when taken after a meal. Administration of ticlopidine HCl with food is recommended to maximize GI tolerance. In controlled trials, ticlopidine HCl was taken with meals.

Distribution – Ticlopidine HCl binds reversibly (98%) to plasma proteins, mainly to serum albumin and lipoproteins. The binding to albumin and lipoproteins is nonsaturable over a wide concentration range. Ticlopidine also binds to alpha-1 acid glycoprotein. At concentrations attained with the recommended dose, only 15% or less ticlopidine in plasma is bound to this protein.

Excretion – Ticlopidine HCl is metabolized extensively by the liver; only trace amounts of intact drug are detected in the urine. Following an oral dose of radioactive ticlopidine HCl administered in solution, 60% of the radioactivity is recovered in the urine and 23% in the feces. Approximately ⅓ of the dose excreted in the feces is intact ticlopidine HCl, possibly excreted in the bile. Ticlopidine HCl is a minor component in plasma (5%) after a single dose, but at steady-state is the major component (15%). Approximately 40% to 50% of the radioactive metabolites circulating in plasma are covalently bound to plasma proteins, probably by acylation.

Clearance of ticlopidine decreases with age. Steady-state trough values in elderly patients (mean age 70 years) are about twice those in younger volunteer populations.

Ticlopidine HCl displays nonlinear pharmacokinetics and clearance decreases markedly on repeated dosing. In older volunteers the apparent half-life of ticlopidine after a single 250 mg dose is about 12.6 hours; with repeat dosing at 250 mg twice daily, the terminal elimination half-life rises to 4 to 5 days and steady-state levels of ticlopidine HCl in plasma are obtained after approximately 14 to 21 days.

Special populations –

Renal function impairment: Patients with mildly (Ccr 50 to 80 mL/min) or moderately (Ccr 20 to 50 mL/min) impaired renal function were compared to healthy subjects (Ccr 80 to 150 mL/min) in a study of the pharmacokinetic and platelet pharmacodynamic effects of ticlopidine HCl (250 mg twice daily) for 11 days. Concentrations of unchanged ticlopidine HCl were measured after a single 250 mg dose and after the final 250 mg dose on Day 11.

AUC values of ticlopidine increased by 28% and 60% in mild and moderately impaired patients, respectively, and plasma clearance decreased by 37% and 52%, respectively, but there were no statistically significant differences in ADP-induced platelet aggregation. In this small study (26 patients), bleeding times showed significant prolongation only in the moderately impaired patients.

Hepatic function impairment: The effect of decreased hepatic function on the pharmacokinetics of ticlopidine HCl was studied in 17 patients with advanced cirrhosis. The average plasma concentration of ticlopidine in these subjects was slightly higher than that seen in older subjects in a separate trial. In patients with severe liver impairment, ticlopidine HCl is contraindicated.

Contraindications

Hypersensitivity to the drug; presence of hematopoietic disorders such as neutropenia and thrombocytopenia or a history of TTP or aplastic anemia; presence of a hemostatic disorder or active pathological bleeding (such as bleeding peptic ulcer or intracranial bleeding); patients with severe liver impairment.

Warnings

➤*Hematological effects:*

Neutropenia – Neutropenia may occur suddenly. Bone marrow examination typically shows a reduction in myeloid precursors. After withdrawal of ticlopidine, the neutrophil count usually rises to greater than $1200/mm^3$ within 1 to 3 weeks.

Thrombocytopenia – Rarely, thrombocytopenia may occur in isolation or together with neutropenia.

Thrombotic thrombocytopenic purpura (TTP) – TTP is characterized by thrombocytopenia, microangiopathic hemolytic anemia (schistocytes [fragmented RBCs] seen on peripheral smear), neurological findings, renal dysfunction, and fever. The signs and symptoms can occur in any order, in particular, clinical symptoms may precede laboratory findings by hours or days. With prompt treatment (often including plasmapheresis), 70% to 80% of patients will survive with minimal or no sequelae. Because platelet transfusions may accelerate thrombosis in patients with TTP on ticlopidine, they should, if possible, be avoided.

Aplastic anemia – Aplastic anemia is characterized by anemia, thrombocytopenia and neutropenia together with a bone marrow examination that shows decreases in the precursor cells for red blood cells, white blood cells, and platelets. Patients may present with signs or symptoms suggestive of infection, in association with low white blood cell and platelet counts. Prompt treatment, which may include the use of drugs to stimulate the bone marrow, can minimize the mortality associated with aplastic anemia.

Monitoring for hematologic adverse reactions – See Precautions for more information.

➤*Other hematological effects:* Rare cases of agranulocytosis, pancytopenia or aplastic anemia have been reported in postmarketing experience, some of which have been fatal. All forms of hematological adverse reactions are potentially fatal.

➤*Cholesterol elevation:* Ticlopidine HCl therapy causes increased serum cholesterol and triglycerides. Serum total cholesterol levels are increased 8% to 10% within 1 month of therapy and persist at that level. The ratios of the lipoprotein subfractions are unchanged.

➤*Renal function impairment:* There is limited experience in patients with renal impairment. Decreased plasma clearance, increased AUC values and prolonged bleeding times can occur in renally impaired patients. In controlled clinical trials, no unexpected problems have been encountered in patients having mild renal impairment, and there is no experience with dosage adjustment in patients with greater degrees of renal impairment. Nevertheless, for renally impaired patients, it may be necessary to reduce the dosage of ticlopidine or discontinue it altogether if hemorrhagic or hematopoietic problems are encountered.

See Actions for more information.

➤*Hepatic function impairment:* Since ticlopidine is metabolized by the liver, dosing of ticlopidine HCl or other drugs metabolized in the liver may require adjustment upon starting or stopping concomitant therapy. Because of limited experience in patients with severe hepatic disease, who may have bleeding diatheses, the use of ticlopidine HCl is not recommended in this population.

See Actions for more information.

➤*Elderly:* Clearance of ticlopidine is somewhat lower in elderly patients and trough levels are increased. The major clinical trials with ticlopidine HCl were conducted in an elderly population with an average age of 64 years. Of the total number of patients in the therapeutic trials, 45% of patients were over 65 years old and 12% were over 75 years old. No overall differences in efficacy or safety were observed between these patients and younger patients, and other reported clinical experience has not identified differences in responses between the elderly and younger patients, but greater sensitivity of some older individuals cannot be ruled out.

➤*Pregnancy:* *Category B.* There are no adequate and well-controlled studies in pregnant women. Because animal reproduction studies are not always predictive of a human response, this drug should be used during pregnancy only if clearly needed.

➤*Lactation:* Studies in rats have shown ticlopidine is excreted in the milk. It is not known whether this drug is excreted in human milk. Because many drugs are excreted in human milk and because of the potential for serious adverse reactions in nursing infants from ticlopidine, a decision should be made whether to discontinue nursing or to discontinue the drug, taking into account the importance of the drug to the mother.

TICLOPIDINE HYDROCHLORIDE — ORAL

➤*Children:* Safety and efficacy in pediatric patients have not been established.

Precautions

➤*Monitoring:* Starting just before initiating treatment and continuing through the third month of therapy, patients receiving ticlopidine HCl must be monitored every 2 weeks. Because of ticlopidine's long plasma half-life, patients who discontinue ticlopidine during this 3-month period should continue to be monitored for 2 weeks after discontinuation. More frequent monitoring, and monitoring after the first 3 months of therapy, is necessary only in patients with clinical signs (eg, signs or symptoms suggestive of infection) or laboratory signs (eg, neutrophil count less than 70% of the baseline count, decrease in hematocrit or platelet count) that suggest incipient hematological adverse reactions.

Clinically, fever might suggest either neutropenia, TTP or aplastic anemia; TTP might also be suggested by weakness, pallor, petechiae or purpura, dark urine (due to blood, bile pigments, or hemoglobin) or jaundice, or neurological changes. Patients should be told to discontinue ticlopidine HCl and to contact the physician immediately upon the occurrence of any of these findings.

Laboratory monitoring should include a complete blood count, with special attention to the absolute neutrophil count (WBC × percent neutrophils), platelet count, and the appearance of the peripheral smear. Ticlopidine is occasionally associated with thrombocytopenia unrelated to TTP or aplastic anemia. Any acute, unexplained reduction in hemoglobin or platelet count should prompt further investigation for a diagnosis of TTP, and the appearance of schistocytes (fragmented RBCs) on the smear should be treated as presumptive evidence of TTP. A simultaneous decrease in platelet count and WBC count should prompt further investigation for a diagnosis of aplastic anemia. If there are laboratory signs of TTP, or aplastic anemia, or if the neutrophil count is confirmed to be less than 1200/mm^3, then the drug should be discontinued.

➤*GI bleeding:* Ticlopidine HCl prolongs template bleeding time. The drug should be used with caution in patients who have lesions with a propensity to bleed (such as ulcers). Drugs that might induce such lesions should be used with caution in patients on ticlopidine HCl.

➤*Special risk:* Ticlopidine HCl should be used with caution in patients who may be at risk of increased bleeding from trauma, surgery or pathological conditions. If it is desired to eliminate the antiplatelet effects of ticlopidine HCl prior to elective surgery, the drug should be discontinued 10 to 14 days prior to surgery. Several controlled clinical studies have found increased surgical blood loss in patients undergoing surgery during treatment with ticlopidine. In TASS and CATS it was recommended that patients have ticlopidine discontinued prior to elective surgery. Several hundred patients underwent surgery during the trials, and no excessive surgical bleeding was reported.

Prolonged bleeding time is normalized within 2 hours after administration of 20 mg IV methylprednisolone. Platelet transfusions may also be used to reverse the effect of ticlopidine HCl on bleeding. Because platelet transfusions may accelerate thrombosis in patients with TTP on ticlopidine, they should, if possible, be avoided.

➤*Lab test abnormalities:*

Liver function – Ticlopidine HCl therapy has been associated with elevations of alkaline phosphatase, bilirubin, and transaminases, which generally occurred within 1 to 4 months of therapy initiation. In controlled clinical trials in stroke patients, the incidence of elevated alkaline phosphatase (greater than 2 times upper limit of normal [ULN]) was 7.6% in ticlopidine patients, 6% in placebo patients and 2.5% in aspirin patients. The incidence of elevated AST (greater than 2 times ULN) was 3.1% in ticlopidine patients, 4% in placebo patients and 2.1% in aspirin patients. No progressive increases were observed in closely monitored clinical trials (eg, no transaminase greater than 10 times the ULN was seen), but most patients with these abnormalities had therapy discontinued. Occasionally, patients had developed minor elevations in bilirubin.

Postmarketing experience includes rare individuals with elevations in their transaminases and bilirubin to greater than 10 × above upper limits of normal. Based on postmarketing and clinical trial experience, liver function testing, including ALT, AST, and GGT, should be considered whenever liver dysfunction is suspected, particularly during the first 4 months of treatment.

Drug Interactions

The dose of drugs with low therapeutic ratios metabolized by hepatic microsomal enzymes may require adjustment to maintain optimal therapeutic blood levels when starting or stopping concomitant therapy with ticlopidine.

Ticlopidine Drug Interactions

Precipitant drug	Object drug*		Description
Antacids	Ticlopidine	↓	Giving ticlopidine after antacids has resulted in an 18% decrease in ticlopidine plasma levels.
Cimetidine	Ticlopidine	↑	Chronic cimetidine administration has reduced the clearance of a single ticlopidine dose by 50%.
Ticlopidine	Aspirin	↑	Ticlopidine potentiated the effect of aspirin on collagen-induced platelet aggregation. Ticlopidine-mediated inhibition of ADP-induced platelet aggregation is not affected. Coadministration is not recommended.
Ticlopidine	Digoxin	↓	Digoxin plasma levels may decrease slightly (≈ 15%).
Ticlopidine	Phenytoin	↑	Elevated phenytoin plasma levels with associated somnolence and lethargy have been reported. Exercise caution when administering with ticlopidine. Remeasuring phenytoin levels may be useful.
Ticlopidine	Theophylline	↑	Theophylline elimination half-life was significantly increased (from 8.6 to 12.2 hr) with a comparable reduction in total plasma clearance.

* ↑ = Object drug increased. ↓ = Object drug decreased.

Therapeutic doses of ticlopidine HCl caused a 30% increase in the plasma half-life of antipyrine and may cause analogous effects on similarly metabolized drugs. Therefore, the dose of drugs metabolized by hepatic microsomal enzymes with low therapeutic ratios or being given to patients with hepatic impairment may require adjustment to maintain optimal therapeutic blood levels when starting or stopping concomitant therapy with ticlopidine. Studies of specific drug interactions yielded the following results:

➤*Anticoagulant drugs:* The tolerance and safety of coadministration of ticlopidine HCl with heparin, oral anticoagulants or fibrinolytic agents have not been established. In trials for cardiac stenting, patients received heparin and ticlopidine tablets concomitantly for approximately 12 hours. If a patient is switched from an anticoagulant or fibrinolytic drug to ticlopidine HCl, the former drug should be discontinued prior to ticlopidine HCl administration.

➤*Aspirin and other NSAIDs:* Ticlopidine potentiates the effect of aspirin or other NSAIDs on platelet aggregation. The safety of concomitant use of ticlopidine with aspirin or other NSAIDs has not been established. The safety of concomitant use of ticlopidine and aspirin beyond 30 days has not been established. Aspirin did not modify the ticlopidine-mediated inhibition of ADP-induced platelet aggregation, but ticlopidine potentiated the effect of aspirin on collagen-induced platelet aggregation. Caution should be exercised in patients who have lesions with a propensity to bleed, such as ulcers. Long-term concomitant use of aspirin and ticlopidine is not recommended.

➤*Propranolol:* In vitro studies demonstrated that ticlopidine does not alter the plasma protein binding of propranolol. However, the protein binding interactions of ticlopidine and its metabolites have not been studied in vivo. Caution should be exercised in coadministering this drug with ticlopidine HCl.

➤*Drug/Food interactions:* See Administration and Dosage for more information.

Adverse Reactions

Adverse reactions were relatively frequent, with greater than 50% of patients reporting at least one. Most (30% to 40%) involved the GI tract. Most adverse effects are mild, but 21% of patients discontinued therapy because of an adverse reaction, principally diarrhea, rash, nausea, vomiting, GI pain and neutropenia. Most adverse effects occur early in the course of treatment, but a new onset of adverse effects can occur after several months.

The incidence rates of adverse reactions listed in the following table were derived from multicenter, controlled clinical trials described above comparing ticlopidine HCl, placebo and aspirin over study periods of up to 5.8 years. Adverse events considered by the investigator to be probably drug related that occurred in at least 1% of patients treated with ticlopidine HCl are shown in the following table:

Percent of Patients With Adverse Reactions in Controlled Studies

	Ticlopidine HCl (n =2048)	Aspirin (acetylsalicylic acid) (n = 1527)	Placebo (n = 536)
Adverse reaction	Incidence	Incidence	Incidence
Any reactions	60% (20.9%)*	53.2% (14.5%)	34.3% (6.1%)
Diarrhea	12.5% (6.3%)	5.2% (1.8%)	4.5% (1.7%)
Nausea	7% (2.6%)	6.2% (1.9%)	1.7% (0.9%)
Dyspepsia	7% (1.1%)	9% (2%)	0.9% (0.2%)
Rash	5.1% (3.4%)	1.5% (0.8%)	0.6% (0.9%)
GI pain	3.7% (1.9%)	5.6% (2.7%)	1.3% (0.4%)
Neutropenia	2.4% (1.3%)	0.8 (0.1%)	1.1% (0.4%)
Purpura	2.2% (0.2%)	1.6% (0.1%)	0% (0%)

TICLOPIDINE HYDROCHLORIDE — ORAL

Percent of Patients With Adverse Reactions in Controlled Studies			
	Ticlopidine HCl (n =2048)	Aspirin (acetylsalicylic acid) (n = 1527)	Placebo (n = 536)
Adverse reaction	Incidence	Incidence	Incidence
Vomiting	1.9% (1.4%)	1.4% (0.9%)	0.9% (0.4%)
Flatulence	1.5% (0.1%)	1.4% (0.3%)	0% (0%)
Pruritus	1.3% (0.8%)	0.3% (0.1%)	0% (0%)
Dizziness	1.1% (0.4%)	0.5% (0.4%)	0% (0%)
Anorexia	1% (0.4%)	0.5% (0.3%)	0% (0%)
Abnormal liver function test	1% (0.7%)	0.3% (0.3%)	0% (0%)

* Incidence of discontinuation, regardless of relationship to therapy, is shown in parentheses.

➤*Dermatologic:* Ticlopidine has been associated with a maculopapular or urticarial rash (often with pruritus). Rash usually occurs within 3 months of initiation of therapy with a mean onset time of 11 days. If drug is discontinued, recovery occurs within several days. Many rashes do not recur on drug rechallenge. There have been rare reports of severe rashes, including Stevens-Johnson syndrome, erythema multiforme and exfoliative dermatitis.

➤*GI:* Ticlopidine HCl therapy has been associated with a variety of GI complaints including diarrhea and nausea. The majority of cases are mild, but about 13% of patients discontinued therapy because of these. They usually occur within 3 months of initiation of therapy and typically are resolved within 1 to 2 weeks without discontinuation of therapy. If the effect is severe or persistent, therapy should be discontinued. In some cases of severe or bloody diarrhea, colitis was later diagnosed.

➤*Hematologic:* Neutropenia/thrombocytopenia, TTP, aplastic anemia, leukemia, agranulocytosis, eosinophilia, pancytopenia, thrombocytosis and bone marrow depression have been reported.

Hemorrhagic – Ticlopidine HCl has been associated with increased bleeding, spontaneous posttraumatic bleeding and perioperative bleeding including, but not limited to, GI bleeding. It has also been associated with a number of bleeding complications such as ecchymosis, epistaxis, hematuria and conjunctival hemorrhage.

Intracerebral bleeding was rare in clinical trials with ticlopidine HCl, with an incidence no greater than that seen with comparator agents (ticlopidine 0.5%, aspirin 0.6%, placebo 0.75%). It has also been reported postmarketing.

➤*Less frequent adverse reactions (probably related):* Clinical adverse experiences occurring in 0.5% to 1% of patients in the controlled trials include the following:

CNS – Headache.

Dermatologic – Urticaria.

GI – GI fullness.

Hematologic – Epistaxis.

Special senses – Tinnitus.

Miscellaneous – Asthenia, pain.

➤*Postmarketing experience:*

Miscellaneous – In addition, the following rarer, relatively serious events have also been reported from postmarketing experience: Hemolytic anemia with reticulocytosis, immune thrombocytopenia, hepatitis, hepatocellular jaundice, cholestatic jaundice, hepatic necrosis, hepatic failure, peptic ulcer, renal failure, nephrotic syndrome, hyponatremia, vasculitis, sepsis, angioedema, allergic pneumonitis and anaphylaxis, systemic lupus (positive ANA), peripheral neuropathy, serum sickness, arthropathy and myositis.

Overdosage

➤*Symptoms:* One case of deliberate overdosage with ticlopidine HCl has been reported by a foreign postmarketing surveillance program. A 38-year-old male took a single 6000 mg dose of ticlopidine HCl (equivalent to 24 standard 250 mg tablets). The only abnormalities reported were increased bleeding time and increased ALT. No special therapy was instituted and the patient recovered without sequelae.

Patient Information

Patients should be told that a decrease in the number of white blood cells (neutropenia) or platelets (thrombocytopenia) can occur with ticlopidine HCl, especially during the first 3 months of treatment and that neutropenia, if it is severe, can result in an increased risk of infection. They should be told it is critically important to obtain the scheduled blood tests to detect neutropenia or thrombocytopenia. Patients should also be reminded to contact their physicians if they experience any indication of infection such as fever, chills, or sore throat, any of which might be a consequence of neutropenia. Thrombocytopenia may be part of a syndrome called TTP. Symptoms and signs of TTP, such as fever, weakness, difficulty speaking, seizures, yellowing of skin or eyes, dark or bloody urine, pallor or petechiae (pinpoint hemorrhagic spots on the skin), should be reported immediately.

All patients should be told that it may take them longer than usual to stop bleeding when they take ticlopidine HCl and that they should report any unusual bleeding to their physician. Patients should tell physicians and dentists that they are taking ticlopidine HCl before any surgery is scheduled and before any new drug is prescribed.

Patients should be told to promptly report side effects of ticlopidine HCl such as severe or persistent diarrhea, skin rashes or subcutaneous bleeding or any signs of cholestasis, such as yellow skin or sclera, dark urine, or light-colored stools.

Patients should be told to take ticlopidine HCl with food or just after eating in order to minimize GI discomfort.

Glycoprotein IIb/IIIa Inhibitors

Indications

➤*Acute coronary syndrome:* For the treatment of acute coronary syndrome, including patients who are to be managed medically and those undergoing percutaneous coronary intervention (PCI). See individual monographs for specific indications.

Actions

➤*Pharmacology:* Tirofiban and eptifibatide are antagonists of the platelet glycoprotein (GP) IIb/IIIa receptor, the major platelet surface receptor involved in platelet aggregation. GP IIb/IIIa is found only on platelets and their progenitors. Activation of its receptor function leads to the binding of fibrinogen and von Willebrand's factor to platelets and thus, platelet aggregation. These agents reversibly prevent fibrinogen, von Willebrand's factor, and other adhesion ligands from binding to the GP IIb/IIIa receptor, thereby inhibiting platelet aggregation. They inhibit ex vivo platelet aggregation in a dose- and concentration-dependent manner. Inhibition persists over the duration of the maintenance infusion and is reversible following infusion cessation.

➤*Pharmacokinetics:*

Absorption/Distribution – The recommended regimen of a loading infusion followed by a maintenance infusion produces an early peak plasma concentration that is similar to the steady-state concentration during the infusion. Steady state is reportedly achieved within 4 to 6 hours with eptifibatide. In patients with coronary artery disease, the plasma clearance of tirofiban ranges from 152 to 267 mL/min; renal clearance accounts for 39% of plasma clearance. The steady-state volume of distribution ranges from 22 to 42 L. Unbound fraction of tirofiban in human plasma is 35%, whereas eptifibatide is 75% unbound (25% bound).

Metabolism/Excretion – The half-life is ≈ 2 hours for tirofiban and ≈ 2.5 hours for eptifibatide. Metabolism appears to be limited. Clearance of eptifibatide in patients with coronary artery disease is 55 to 58 mL/kg/hr. These agents are cleared from the plasma largely by renal excretion, ≈ 65% for tirofiban and ≈ 50% for eptifibatide.

Special populations –

Renal function impairment: Plasma clearance of **tirofiban** is significantly decreased (more than 50%) in patients with creatinine clearance < 30 mL/min, including patients requiring hemodialysis (see Administration and Dosage). Tirofiban is removed by hemodialysis.

Elderly: Plasma clearance of **tirofiban** is ≈ 19% to 26% lower in elderly (older than 65 years of age) patients with coronary artery disease than in younger (≤ 65 years of age) patients.

Contraindications

Hypersensitivity to any component of the product; active internal bleeding or a history of bleeding diathesis within the previous 30 days; a history of thrombocytopenia following prior exposure to tirofiban; history of stroke within 30 days or any history of hemorrhagic stroke; major surgical procedure or severe physical trauma within the previous month; severe hypertension (systolic blood pressure over 180 mmHg [tirofiban], over 200 mmHg [eptifibatide] or diastolic blood pressure over 110 mmHg); concomitant use of another parenteral GP IIb/IIIa inhibitor, a history of intracranial hemorrhage, intracranial neoplasm, arteriovenous malformation or aneurysm, history, symptoms, or findings suggestive of aortic dissection, acute pericarditis (tirofiban). A platelet count < 100,000/mm^3, serum creatinine ≥ 2 mg/dL (for the 180 mcg/kg bolus and the 2 mcg/kg/min infusion) or ≥ 4 mg/dL (for the 135 mcg/kg bolus and the 0.5 mcg/kg/min infusion), dependency on renal dialysis (eptifibatide).

Warnings

➤*Bleeding:* Major and minor bleeding events are the most common complications encountered during therapy with tirofiban and eptifibatide. Most major bleeding occurs at the arterial access site for cardiac catheterization.

Use with caution in patients with a platelet count < 150,000/mm^3 and in patients with hemorrhagic retinopathy.

Because these agents inhibit platelet aggregation, use caution when employed with other drugs that affect hemostasis (eg, warfarin, thrombolytics, NSAIDs, dipyridamole, ticlopidine, clopidogrel). The safety of tirofiban when used in combination with thrombolytic agents has not been established. Study regimens (n = 180) of eptifibatide administered concomitantly with the approved "accelerated" regimen of alteplase did not increase the incidence of major bleeding or transfusion compared with the incidence seen when alteplase was given alone. At high study infusion rates (1.3 mcg/kg/min and 2 mcg/kg/min), eptifibatide was associated with an increase in the incidence of bleeding and transfusions compared with the incidence seen when streptokinase was given alone.

During therapy, monitor patients for potential bleeding. When bleeding cannot be controlled with pressure, discontinue infusion of the GP IIb/IIIa inhibitor and heparin.

➤*Percutaneous coronary intervention:*

Care of the femoral artery access site – Therapy with tirofiban and eptifibatide is associated with increases in bleeding rates particularly at the site of arterial access for femoral sheath placement. Take care when attempting vascular access that only the anterior wall of the femoral artery is punctured. Prior to pulling the sheath, discontinue heparin for 3 to 4 hours and document activated clotting time (ACT) < 180 seconds or APTT < 45 seconds. Obtain proper hemostasis after removal of the sheaths using standard compressive techniques followed by close observation. While the vascular sheath is in place, maintain patients on complete bed rest with the head of the bed elevated 30° and the affected limb restrained in a straight position. Achieve sheath hemostasis ≥ 4 hours before hospital discharge.

Minimize vascular and other trauma – Minimize other arterial and venous punctures, IM injections, and the use of urinary catheters, nasotracheal intubation, and nasogastric tubes. When obtaining IV access, avoid noncompressible sites (eg, subclavian or jugular veins).

➤*Renal function impairment:* Patients with severe renal insufficiency (creatinine clearance < 30 mL/min) showed decreased plasma clearance of **tirofiban**. Reduce the dosage of tirofiban in these patients (see Administration and Dosage).

Dose adjustment is unnecessary for **eptifibatide** in mild to moderate renal impairment; no data are available for severe impairment or dialysis.

➤*Elderly:* Elderly patients receiving **tirofiban** with heparin or heparin alone had a higher incidence of bleeding complications than younger patients. The incremental risk of bleeding in patients treated with tirofiban in combination with heparin compared with heparin alone was similar regardless of age; however, the incremental risk of **eptifibatide**-associated bleeding was greater in the older patients. The overall incidence of nonbleeding adverse events was higher in older patients both for tirofiban with heparin and heparin alone. No dose adjustment is recommended.

➤*Pregnancy: Category B.* Tirofiban crosses the placenta in pregnant rats and rabbits. There are no adequate and well-controlled studies in pregnant women. Use during pregnancy only if clearly needed.

➤*Lactation:* It is not known whether GP IIb/IIIa inhibitors are excreted in breast milk. However, significant levels of tirofiban were shown to be present in rat milk. Because of the potential for adverse effects on the nursing infant, decide whether to discontinue nursing or discontinue the drug, taking into account the importance of the drug to the mother.

➤*Children:* Safety and efficacy in pediatric patients have not been established.

Precautions

➤*Monitoring:* Monitor platelet counts, hemoglobin, hematocrit, serum creatinine, and PT/APTT prior to treatment, within 6 hours following the loading infusion, and at least daily thereafter during therapy with tirofiban (or more frequently if there is evidence of significant decline). In eptifibatide patients undergoing PCI, also measure the ACT. Maintain the APTT between 50 and 70 seconds unless PCI is to be performed; during PCI, maintain the ACT between 300 and 350 seconds. If the patient experiences a platelet decrease to < 100,000/mm^3, perform additional platelet counts to exclude pseudothrombocytopenia. If thrombocytopenia is confirmed, discontinue GP IIb/IIIa inhibitors and heparin, and appropriately monitor and treat the condition.

To monitor unfractionated heparin, monitor APTT 6 hours after the start of the heparin infusion; adjust heparin to maintain APTT at ≈ 2 times control.

Drug Interactions

Glycoprotein IIb/IIIa Inhibitor Drug Interactions

Precipitant drug	Object drug*		Description
Aspirin	GP IIb/IIIa inhibitors	↑	Concurrent use with heparin and aspirin has been associated with an increase in bleeding compared with heparin and aspirin alone. Use caution when using with other drugs that affect hemostasis (eg, warfarin) (see Warnings).
Heparin			
Levothyroxine	Tirofiban	↔	Concomitant administration increased tirofiban clearance. Clinical significance is unknown.
Omeprazole			

* ↑ = Object drug increased. ↔ = Undetermined clinical effect.

Adverse Reactions

➤*Bleeding:* The most common drug-related adverse event reported during therapy was bleeding (see Warnings).

In clinical trials, incidence of major bleeding ranged from 1.4% to 2.2% (vs 0.8% to 1.6% with heparin alone) for **tirofiban** and 4.4% to 10.8% for **eptifibatide**. Incidence of minor bleeding was 10.5% to 12% (vs 6.3% to 8% with heparin alone) for tirofiban and 10.5% to 14.2% for eptifibatide.

Intracranial bleeding in 1 study was 0.1% for **tirofiban** with heparin and 0.3% for heparin alone. The overall incidence of stroke was 0.5% to 0.7% in patients receiving **eptifibatide** and 0.7% to 0.8% in placebo patients. The incidences of retroperitoneal bleeding for tirofiban with heparin and heparin alone were 0% to 0.6% and 0.1% to 0.3%, respectively. The incidences of major GI and GU bleeding for tirofiban with heparin were 0.1% to 0.2% and 0% to 0.1%, respectively.

Female and elderly patients receiving **tirofiban** with heparin or heparin alone had a higher incidence of bleeding complications than male patients or younger patients. The incremental risk of bleeding in patients treated with tirofiban in combination with heparin over the risk in patients treated with heparin alone was comparable regardless of age or gender. No dose adjustment is recommended.

Tirofiban Nonbleeding Adverse Reactions (> 1%)

Adverse reaction	Tirofiban + Heparin (n = 1953)	Heparin (n = 1887)
Bradycardia	4	3
Dissection, coronary artery	5	4
Dizziness	3	2
Edema/Swelling	2	1
Pain, leg	3	2
Pain, pelvic	6	5
Reaction, vasovagal	2	1
Sweating	2	1

Other nonbleeding side effects reported at more than a 1% rate with **tirofiban** administered concomitantly with heparin were nausea, fever, and headache; these side effects were reported at a similar rate in the heparin group.

The only serious nonbleeding adverse event that occurred at a rate of ≥ 1% and was more common with **eptifibatide** than placebo (7% vs 6%) was hypotension.

➤*Lab test abnormalities:* Decreases in hemoglobin (2.1%) and hematocrit (2.2%) were observed in the group receiving **tirofiban** compared with 3.1% and 2.6%, respectively, in the heparin group. Increases in the presence of urine and fecal occult blood also were observed (10.7% and 18.3%, respectively) in the group receiving tirofiban compared with 7.8% and 12.2%, respectively, in the heparin group.

Patients treated with **tirofiban** with heparin were more likely to experience decreases in platelet counts than the control group. These decreases were reversible upon discontinuation of tirofiban. The incidence of thrombocytopenia and platelet transfusions were similar between patients treated with **eptifibatide** and placebo.

Overdosage

➤*Symptoms:* In clinical trials, inadvertent overdosage with tirofiban occurred at doses ≤ 5 times and 2 times the recommended dose for bolus administration and loading infusion, respectively. Inadvertent overdosage occurred in doses ≤ 9.8 times the 0.15 mcg/kg/min maintenance infusion rate.

The most frequently reported manifestation of overdosage was bleeding, primarily minor mucocutaneous bleeding events and minor bleeding at the sites of cardiac catheterization (see Warnings).

➤*Treatment:* Treat tirofiban overdosage by assessment of the patient's clinical condition and cessation or adjustment of the drug infusion as appropriate. Tirofiban can be removed by hemodialysis.

TIROFIBAN HYDROCHLORIDE

Rx	**Aggrastat** (Merck)	**Injection:** 50 mcg/mL	Preservative-free. In 250[1] and 500 mL[2] single-dose *IntraVia* containers.
		Injection, concentrate: 250 mcg/mL	Preservative-free. In 25 and 50 mL vials.[3]

[1] With 2.25 g sodium chloride and 135 mg sodium citrate dihydrate.
[2] With 4.5 g sodium chloride and 270 mg sodium citrate dihydrate.
[3] With 8 mg sodium chloride and 2.7 mg sodium citrate dihydrate.

TIROFIBAN HYDROCHLORIDE — INJECTION

For complete and comparative prescribing information, refer to the Glycoprotein IIb/IIIa Inhibitors group monograph.

Indications

Tirofiban HCl, in combination with heparin, is indicated for the treatment of acute coronary syndrome, including patients who are to be managed medically and those undergoing percutaneous transluminal coronary angioplasty (PTCA) or atherectomy. In this setting, tirofiban HCl has been shown to decrease the rate of a combined endpoint of death, new myocardial infarction (MI) or refractory ischemia/repeat cardiac procedure.

Tirofiban HCl has been studied in a setting that included aspirin and heparin.

Administration and Dosage

➤*Approved by the FDA:* May 14, 1998.

Tirofiban concentrated injection must first be diluted to the same strength as tirofiban injection premixed, as noted under Directions for use.

➤*Use with aspirin and heparin:* In the clinical studies, patients received aspirin, unless it was contraindicated, and heparin. Tirofiban HCl and heparin can be administered through the same IV catheter.

➤*Precautions:* Tirofiban HCl is intended for IV delivery using sterile equipment and technique. Do not add other drugs or remove solution directly from the bag with a syringe. Do not use plastic containers in series connections; such use can result in air embolism by drawing air from the first container if it is empty of solution. Any unused solution should be discarded.

➤*Directions for use:* Tirofiban concentrated injection is first diluted to the same strength as tirofiban injection premixed as follows: Withdraw and discard 100 mL from a 500 mL bag of sterile 0.9% sodium chloride or 5% dextrose in water and replace this volume with 100 mL of tirofiban HCl injection (from two 50 mL vials), or withdraw and discard 50 mL from a 250 mL bag of sterile 0.9% sodium chloride or 5% dextrose in water and replace this volume with 50 mL of tirofiban HCl injection (from one 50 mL vial), to achieve a final concentration of 50 mcg/mL. Mix well prior to administration.

Tirofiban HCl injection premixed is supplied as 500 mL of 0.9% sodium chloride containing 50 mcg/mL tirofiban. It is supplied in plastic containers (PL 2408 plastic). To open the container, first tear off its dust cover. The plastic may be somewhat opaque because of moisture absorption during sterilization; the opacity will diminish gradually. Check for leaks by squeezing the inner bag firmly; if any leaks are found, the sterility is suspect and the solution should be discarded. Do not use unless the solution is clear and the seal is intact. Suspend the container from its eyelet support, remove the plastic protector from the outlet port, and attach a conventional administration set.

➤*Admixture compatibility/incompatibility:* Tirofiban HCl may be administered in the same IV line as dopamine, lidocaine, potassium chloride, and famotidine injection. Tirofiban HCl should not be administered in the same IV line as diazepam.

➤*Recommended dosage:* In most patients, tirofiban HCl should be administered IV, at an initial rate of 0.4 mcg/kg/min for 30 minutes and then continued at 0.1 mcg/kg/min. Patients with severe renal insufficiency (creatinine clearance < 30 mL/min) should receive half the usual rate of infusion (see Warnings and Pharmacokinetics). The information below is provided as a guide to dosage adjustment by weight.

	Most patients		Severe renal impairment	
Patient weight (kg)	30-minute loading infusion rate (mL/hr)	Maintenance infusion rate (mL/hr)	30-minute loading infusion rate (mL/hr)	Maintenance infusion rate (mL/hr)
30 to 37	16	4	8	2
38 to 45	20	5	10	3
46 to 54	24	6	12	3
55 to 62	28	7	14	4
63 to 70	32	8	16	4
71 to 79	36	9	18	5
80 to 87	40	10	20	5
88 to 95	44	11	22	6
96 to 104	48	12	24	6
105 to 112	52	13	26	7
113 to 120	56	14	28	7
121 to 128	60	15	30	8
129 to 137	64	16	32	8
138 to 145	68	17	34	9
146 to 153	72	18	36	9

No dosage adjustment is recommended for elderly or female patients (see Warnings). In PRISM-PLUS, tirofiban HCl was administered in combination with heparin for 48 to 108 hours. The infusion should be continued through angiography and for 12 to 24 hours after angioplasty or atherectomy.

➤*Storage/Stability:*

Tirofiban concentrated injection – Store at 25°C (77°F) with excursions permitted between 15° to 30°C (59° to 86°F) (see USP controlled room temperature). Do not freeze. Protect from light during storage.

Tirofiban injection (premixed) – Store at 25°C (77°F) with excursions permitted between 15° to 30°C (59° to 86°F) (see USP controlled room temperature). Do not freeze. Protect from light during storage.

EPTIFIBATIDE

Rx	**Integrilin** (Schering)	**Injection for solution:** 0.75 mg/mL	In 100 mL vials.
		2 mg/mL	In 10 and 100 mL vials.

EPTIFIBATIDE — INJECTION

For complete and comparative prescribing information, refer to the Glycoprotein IIb/IIIa Inhibitors group monograph.

Indications

➤*Acute coronary syndrome:* For the treatment of patients with acute coronary syndrome (unstable angina [UA]/non-ST-segment elevation myocardial infarction [NSTEMI]), including patients who are to be managed medically and those undergoing percutaneous coronary intervention (PCI). In this setting, eptifibatide has been shown to decrease the rate of a combined endpoint of death or new myocardial infarction.

➤*Patients undergoing PCI:* For the treatment of patients undergoing PCI, including those undergoing intracoronary stenting. In this setting, eptifibatide has been shown to decrease the rate of a combined endpoint of death, new myocardial infarction, or need for urgent intervention.

In the IMPACT II, PURSUIT, and ESPRIT studies of eptifibatide, most patients received heparin and aspirin.

Administration and Dosage

➤*Approved by the FDA:* May 18, 1998.

➤*Acute coronary syndrome:* The recommended adult dosage of eptifibatide in patients with acute coronary syndrome and normal renal function is an IV bolus of 180 mcg/kg as soon as possible following diagnosis, followed by a continuous infusion of 2 mcg/kg/min until hospital discharge or initiation of coronary artery bypass graft (CABG) surgery, up to 72 hours. If a patient is to undergo a PCI while receiving eptifibatide, the infusion should be continued up to hospital discharge, or for up to 18 to 24 hours after the procedure, whichever comes first, allowing for up to 96 hours of therapy.

The recommended adult dosage of eptifibatide in patients with acute coronary syndrome with an estimated creatinine clearance (using the Cockroft-Gault equation) less than 50 mL/min or, if creatinine clearance is not available, a serum creatinine greater than 2 mg/dL, is an intravenous bolus of 180 mcg/kg as soon as possible following diagnosis, immediately followed by a continuous infusion of 1 mcg/kg/min.

➤*Percutaneous coronary intervention (PCI):* The recommended adult dosage of eptifibatide in patients with normal renal function is an IV bolus of 180 mcg/kg administered immediately before the initiation of PCI followed by a continuous infusion of 2 mcg/kg/min and a second 180 mcg/kg bolus 10 minutes after the first bolus. Infusion should be continued until hospital discharge, or for up to 18 to 24 hours, whichever comes first. A minimum of 12 hours of infusion is recommended.

The recommended adult dose of eptifibatide in patients with an estimated creatinine clearance (using the Cockroft-Gault equation) less than 50 mL/min or, if creatinine clearance is not available, a serum creatinine greater than 2 mg/dL, is an IV bolus of 180 mcg/kg administered immediately before the initiation of the procedure, immediately followed by a continuous infusion of 1 mcg/kg/min and a second 180 mcg/kg bolus administered 10 minutes after the first.

In patients who undergo coronary artery bypass graft surgery, eptifibatide infusion should be discontinued prior to surgery.

➤*Aspirin and heparin dosing recommendations:* The safety and efficacy of eptifibatide has been established in clinical studies that employed concomitant use of heparin and aspirin. Different dose regimens of eptifibatide were used in the major clinical studies. In the clinical trials that showed eptifibatide to be effective, most patients received concomitant aspi-

EPTIFIBATIDE — INJECTION

rin and heparin. The recommended aspirin and heparin doses to be used are as follows:

Acute coronary syndrome –

Aspirin: 160 to 325 mg orally (by mouth) initially and daily thereafter.

Heparin: Target activated partial thromboplastin time (aPTT) 50 to 70 seconds during medical management for the following:

- If weight is greater than or equal to 70 kg, 5000 U bolus followed by infusion of 1000 U/hr.
- If weight is less than 70 kg, 60 U/kg bolus followed by infusion of 12 U/kg/hr. Target activated clotting time (ACT) 200 to 300 seconds during PCI for the following:
- If heparin is initiated prior to PCI, additional boluses during PCI to maintain an ACT target of 200 to 300 seconds.
- Heparin infusion after the PCI is discouraged.

PCI –

Aspirin: 160 to 325 mg orally (by mouth) 1 to 24 hours prior to PCI and daily thereafter.

Heparin: Target ACT 200 to 300 seconds for the following:

- 60 U/kg bolus initially in patients not treated with heparin within 6 hours prior to PCI.
- Additional boluses during PCI to maintain ACT within target.
- Heparin infusion after the PCI is strongly discouraged. Patients requiring thrombolytic therapy should have eptifibatide infusions stopped.

➤*Administration:*

1.) Like other parenteral drug products, eptifibatide solutions should be inspected visually for particulate matter and discoloration prior to administration, whenever solution and container permit.
2.) Eptifibatide may be administered in the same IV line as alteplase, atropine, dobutamine, heparin, lidocaine, meperidine, metoprolol, midazolam, morphine, nitroglycerin, or verapamil. Eptifibatide should not be administered through the same IV line as furosemide.
3.) Eptifibatide may be administered in the same IV line with 0.9% NaCl or 0.9% NaCl/5% dextrose. With either vehicle, the infusion may also contain up to 60 mEq/L of potassium chloride. No incompatibilities have been observed with IV administration sets. No compatibility studies have been performed with PVC bags.
4.) The bolus dose(s) of eptifibatide should be withdrawn from the 10 mL vial into a syringe. The bolus dose(s) should be administered by IV push.
5.) Immediately following the bolus dose administration, a continuous infusion of eptifibatide should be initiated. When using an IV infusion pump, eptifibatide should be administered undiluted directly from the 100 mL vial. The 100 mL vial should be spiked with a vented infusion set. Care should be taken to center the spike within the circle on the stopper top.

Eptifibatide is to be administered by volume according to patient weight. Patients should receive eptifibatide according to the following table:

Eptifibatide Dosing Charts by Weight

Patient weight		180 mcg/kg bolus volume	2 mcg/kg/min infusion volume		1 mcg/kg/min infusion volume	
kg	lb	(from 2 mg/mL vial)	(from 2 mg/mL 100 mL vial)	(from 0.75 mg/mL 100 mL vial)	(from 2 mg/mL 100 mL vial)	from 0.75 mg/mL 100 mL vial)
37 to 41 kg	81 to 91 lb	3.4 mL	2 mL/hr	6 mL/hr	1 mL/hr	3 mL/hr
42 to 46 kg	92 to 102 lb	4 mL	2.5 mL/hr	7 mL/hr	1.3 mL/hr	3.5 mL/hr
47 to 53 kg	103 to 117 lb	4.5 mL	3 mL/hr	8 mL/hr	1.5 mL/hr	4 mL/hr
54 to 59 kg	118 to 130 lb	5 mL	3.5 mL/hr	9 mL/hr	1.8 mL/hr	4.5 mL/hr
60 to 65 kg	131 to 143 lb	5.6 mL	3.8 mL/hr	10 mL/hr	1.9 mL/hr	5 mL/hr
66 to 71 kg	144 to 157 lb	6.2 mL	4 mL/hr	11 mL/hr	2 mL/hr	5.5 mL/hr
72 to 78 kg	158 to 172 lb	6.8 mL	4.5 mL/hr	12 mL/hr	2.3 mL/hr	6 mL/hr
79 to 84 kg	173 to 185 lb	7.3 mL	5 mL/hr	13 mL/hr	2.5 mL/hr	6.5 mL/hr
85 to 90 kg	186 to 198 lb	7.9 mL	5.3 mL/hr	14 mL/hr	2.7 mL/hr	7 mL/hr
91 to 96 kg	199 to 212 lb	8.5 mL	5.6 mL/hr	15 mL/hr	2.8 mL/hr	7.5 mL/hr
97 to 103 kg	213 to 227 lb	9 mL	6 mL/hr	16 mL/hr	3 mL/hr	8 mL/hr
104 to 109 kg	228 to 240 lb	9.5 mL	6.4 mL/hr	17 mL/hr	3.2 mL/hr	8.5 mL/hr
110 to 115 kg	241 to 253 lb	10.2 mL	6.8 mL/hr	18 mL/hr	3.4 mL/hr	9 mL/hr
116 to 121 kg	254 to 267 lb	10.7 mL	7 mL/hr	19 mL/hr	3.5 mL/hr	9.5 mL/hr
> 121 kg	> 267 lb	11.3 mL	7.5 mL/hr	20 mL/hr	3.7 mL/hr	10 mL/hr

➤*Storage / Stability:* Vials should be stored refrigerated at 2° to 8°C (36° to 46°F). Vials may be transferred to room temperature storage for a period not to exceed 2 months. Upon transfer, vial cartons must be marked by the dispensing pharmacist with a "discard by" date (2 months from the transfer date or the labeled expiration date, whichever comes first).

Protect from light until administration. Discard any unused portion left in the vial.

Store at controlled room temperature 25°C (77°F); excursions permitted between 15° and 30°C (59° and 86°F).

ABCIXIMAB

Rx	**ReoPro** (Lilly)	**Injection:** 2 mg/mL	In buffered solution of 0.01 M sodium phosphate, 0.15 M NaCl, and 0.001% polysorbate 80. Preservative-free. In 5 mL vials.

ABCIXIMAB — INJECTION

Indications

➤*Adjunct to percutaneous coronary intervention (PCI):* Adjunct to percutaneous coronary intervention for the prevention of cardiac ischemic complications:

- In patients undergoing PCI.
- In patients with unstable angina not responding to conventional medical therapy when PCI is planned within 24 hours.

Abciximab use in patients not undergoing PCI has not been studied.

Abciximab is intended for use with aspirin and heparin and has been studied only in that setting.

➤*Unlabeled uses:* For the early treatment of acute MI, abciximab has been shown to facilitate the rate and extent of thrombolysis when combined with low-dose alteplase or low-dose reteplase. Abciximab also has been shown to be safe and effective in a small study evaluating its use in the treatment of acute ischemic stroke.

Administration and Dosage

➤*Approved by the FDA:* December 22, 1994.

➤*Failed PCIs:* In patients with failed percutaneous coronary interventions, the continuous infusion of abciximab should be stopped because there is no evidence for abciximab efficacy in that setting.

➤*Serious bleeding:* In the event of serious bleeding that cannot be controlled by compression, abciximab and heparin should be discontinued immediately.

➤*Recommended dosage:* The recommended dosage of abciximab in adults is a 0.25 mg/kg IV bolus administered 10 to 60 minutes before the start of percutaneous coronary intervention, followed by a continuous IV infusion of 0.125 mcg/kg/min (to a maximum of 10 mcg/min) for 12 hours.

Patients with unstable angina not responding to conventional medical therapy and who are planned to undergo percutaneous coronary intervention within 24 hours may be treated with an abciximab 0.25 mg/kg IV bolus followed by an 18- to 24-hour IV infusion of 10 mcg/min, concluding 1 hour after the percutaneous coronary intervention.

➤*Administration instructions:*

1.) Parenteral drug products should be inspected visually for particulate matter prior to administration. Preparations of abciximab containing visibly opaque particles should not be used.
2.) Hypersensitivity reactions should be anticipated whenever protein solutions such as abciximab are administered. Epinephrine, dopamine, theophylline, antihistamines, and corticosteroids should be available for immediate use. If symptoms of an allergic reaction or anaphylaxis appear, the infusion should be stopped and appropriate treatment given.
3.) As with all parenteral drug products, aseptic procedures should be used during the administration of abciximab.
4.) Withdraw the necessary amount of abciximab for bolus injection into a syringe. Filter the bolus injection using a sterile, nonpyrogenic, low-protein-binding 0.2 or 0.22 mcm filter.
5.) Withdraw the necessary amount of abciximab for the continuous infusion into a syringe. Inject into an appropriate container of sterile 0.9% saline or 5% dextrose and infuse at the calculated rate via a continuous infusion pump. The continuous infusion should be filtered either upon admixture using a sterile, nonpyrogenic, low-protein-binding 0.2 or 0.22 mcm syringe filter or upon administration using an inline, sterile, nonpyrogenic, low-protein-binding 0.2 or 0.22 mcm filter. Discard the unused portion at the end of the infusion.

➤*Admixture incompatibilities:* No incompatibilities have been shown with IV infusion fluids or commonly used cardiovascular drugs. Nevertheless, abciximab should be administered in a separate IV line whenever possible and not mixed with other medications.

No incompatibilities have been observed with glass bottles or polyvinyl chloride bags and administration sets.

➤*Storage / Stability:* Vials should be stored at 2° to 8°C (36° to 46°F). Do not freeze. Do not shake. Discard any unused portion left in the vial.

Actions

➤*Pharmacology:* Abciximab binds to the intact platelet GPIIb/IIIa receptor, which is a member of the integrin family of adhesion receptors and the major platelet surface receptor involved in platelet aggregation. Abciximab inhibits platelet aggregation by preventing the binding of fibrinogen, von Willebrand factor, and other adhesive molecules to GPIIb/IIIa receptor sites

ABCIXIMAB — INJECTION

on activated platelets. The mechanism of action is thought to involve steric hindrance or conformational effects to block access of large molecules to the receptor rather than direct interaction with the RGD (arginine-glycine-aspartic acid) binding site of GPIIb/IIIa.

Abciximab binds with similar affinity to the vitronectin receptor, also known as the $\alpha_v\beta_3$ integrin. The vitronectin receptor mediates the procoagulant properties of platelets and the proliferative properties of vascular endothelial and smooth muscle cells. In in vitro studies using a model cell line derived from melanoma cells, abciximab blocked $\alpha_v\beta_3$-mediated effects including cell adhesion (IC_{50} = 0.34 mcg/mL). At concentrations which, in vitro, provide greater than 80% GPIIb/IIIa receptor blockade, but above the in vivo therapeutic range, abciximab more effectively blocked the burst of thrombin generation that followed platelet activation than select comparator antibodies which inhibit GPIIb/IIIa alone. The relationship of these in vitro data to clinical efficacy is unknown.

Abciximab also binds to the activated Mac-1 receptor on monocytes and neutrophils. In in vitro studies, abciximab and 7E3 IgG blocked Mac-1 receptor function as evidenced by inhibition of monocyte adhesion. In addition, the degree of activated Mac-1 expression on circulating leukocytes and the numbers of circulating leukocyte-platelet complexes has been shown to be reduced in patients treated with abciximab compared to control patients. The relationship of these in vitro data to clinical efficacy is uncertain.

Pharmacodynamics – IV administration in humans of single bolus doses of abciximab from 0.15 mg/kg to 0.3 mg/kg produced rapid dose-dependent inhibition of platelet function as measured by ex vivo platelet aggregation in response to adenosine diphosphate (ADP) or by prolongation of bleeding time. At the 2 highest doses (0.25 and 0.3 mg/kg) at 2 hours post injection (the first time point evaluated), over 80% of the GPIIb/IIIa receptors were blocked and platelet aggregation in response to 20 mcM ADP was almost abolished. The median bleeding time increased to over 30 minutes at both doses compared with a baseline value of approximately 5 minutes.

IV administration in humans of a single bolus dose of 0.25 mg/kg followed by a continuous infusion of 10 mcg/min for periods of 12 to 96 hours produced sustained high-grade GPIIb/IIIa receptor blockade (greater than or equal to 80%) and inhibition of platelet function (ex vivo platelet aggregation in response to 5 mcM or 20 mcM ADP less than 20% of baseline and bleeding time greater than 30 minutes) for the duration of the infusion in most patients. Similar results were obtained when a weight-adjusted infusion dose (0.125 mcg/kg/min to a maximum of 10 mcg/min) was used in patients weighing up to 80 kg. Results in patients who received the 0.25 mg/kg bolus followed by a 5 mcg/min infusion for 24 hours showed a similar initial receptor blockade and inhibition of platelet aggregation, but the response was not maintained throughout the infusion period. The onset of abciximab-mediated platelet inhibition following a 0.25 mg/kg bolus and 0.125 mcg/kg/min infusion was rapid, and platelet aggregation was reduced to less than 20% of baseline in 8 of 10 patients at 10 minutes after treatment initiation.

Low levels of GPIIb/IIIa receptor blockade are present for more than 10 days following cessation of the infusion. After discontinuation of abciximab infusion, platelet function returns gradually to normal. Bleeding time returned to less than or equal to 12 minutes within 12 hours following the end of infusion in 15 of 20 patients (75%) and within 24 hours in 18 of 20 patients (90%). Ex vivo platelet aggregation in response to 5 mcM ADP returned to greater than or equal to 50% of baseline within 24 hours following the end of infusion in 11 of 32 patients (34%) and within 48 hours in 23 of 32 patients (72%). In response to 20 mcM ADP, ex vivo platelet aggregation returned to greater than or equal to 50% of baseline within 24 hours in 20 of 32 patients (62%) and within 48 hours in 28 of 32 patients (88%).

➤*Pharmacokinetics:* Following IV bolus administration, free plasma concentrations of abciximab decrease rapidly with an initial half-life of less than 10 minutes and a second phase half-life of about 30 minutes, probably related to rapid binding to the platelet GPIIb/IIIa receptors. Platelet function generally recovers over the course of 48 hours, although abciximab remains in the circulation for 15 days or more in a platelet-bound state. IV administration of a 0.25 mg/kg bolus dose of abciximab followed by continuous infusion of 10 mcg/min (or a weight-adjusted infusion of 0.125 mcg/kg/min to a maximum of 10 mcg/min) produces approximately constant free plasma concentrations throughout the infusion. At the termination of the infusion period, free plasma concentrations fall rapidly for approximately 6 hours then decline at a slower rate.

Contraindications

Because abciximab may increase the risk of bleeding, abciximab is contraindicated in the following clinical situations:

- Active internal bleeding.
- Recent (within 6 weeks) gastrointestinal or genitourinary bleeding of clinical significance.
- History of cerebrovascular accident (CVA) within 2 years, or CVA with a significant residual neurological deficit.
- Bleeding diathesis.
- Administration of oral anticoagulants within 7 days unless prothrombin time less than or equal to 1.2 times control.
- Thrombocytopenia (less than 100,000 cells/mcL).
- Recent (within 6 weeks) major surgery or trauma.
- Intracranial neoplasm, arteriovenous malformation, or aneurysm.
- Severe uncontrolled hypertension.
- Presumed or documented history of vasculitis.
- Use of IV dextran before percutaneous coronary intervention, or intent to use it during an intervention.

Abciximab is also contraindicated in patients with known hypersensitivities to any component of this product or to murine proteins.

Warnings

➤*Bleeding:* Abciximab has the potential to increase the risk of bleeding, particularly in the presence of anticoagulation (eg, from heparin, other anticoagulants, or thrombolytics).

The risk of major bleeds due to abciximab therapy may be increased in patients receiving thrombolytics and should be weighed against the anticipated benefits.

Should serious bleeding occur that is not controllable with pressure, the infusion of abciximab and any concomitant heparin should be stopped.

➤*Hypersensitivity reactions:* Anaphylaxis has not been reported for abciximab-treated patients in any of the phase 3 clinical trials. However, anaphylaxis may occur. If it does, administration of abciximab should be immediately stopped and standard appropriate resuscitative measures should be initiated.

➤*Elderly:* Of the total number of 7,860 patients in the 4 phase 3 trials, 2,933 (37%) were 65 and over, while 653 (8%) were 75 and over. No overall differences in safety or efficacy were observed between patients of age 65 to less than 75 as compared to younger patients. The clinical experience is not adequate to determine whether patients of age 75 or greater respond differently than younger patients.

➤*Pregnancy: Category C.* Animal reproduction studies have not been conducted with abciximab. It is also not known whether abciximab can cause fetal harm when administered to a pregnant woman or can affect reproduction capacity. Abciximab should be given to a pregnant woman only if clearly needed.

➤*Lactation:* It is not known whether this drug is excreted in human milk or absorbed systemically after ingestion. Because many drugs are excreted in human milk, caution should be exercised when abciximab is administered to a nursing woman.

➤*Children:* Safety and effectiveness in pediatric patients have not been studied.

Precautions

➤*Monitoring:* Before infusion of abciximab, platelet count, prothrombin time, ACT, and APTT should be measured to identify preexisting hemostatic abnormalities.

Based on an integrated analysis of data from all studies, the following guidelines may be utilized to minimize the risk for bleeding:

- When abciximab is initiated 18 to 24 hours before PCI, the APTT should be maintained between 60 and 85 seconds during the abciximab and heparin infusion period.
- During PCI, the ACT should be maintained between 200 and 300 seconds.
- If anticoagulation is continued in these patients following PCI, the APTT should be maintained between 55 and 75 seconds.
- The APTT or ACT should be checked prior to arterial sheath removal. The sheath should not be removed unless APTT less than or equal to 50 seconds or ACT less than or equal to 175 seconds.

➤*Bleeding precautions:* To minimize the risk of bleeding with abciximab, it is important to use a low-dose, weight-adjusted heparin regimen, a weight-adjusted abciximab bolus and infusion, strict anticoagulation guidelines, careful vascular access site management, discontinuation of heparin after the procedure and early femoral arterial sheath removal.

Therapy with abciximab requires careful attention to all potential bleeding sites (including catheter insertion sites, arterial and venous puncture sites, cutdown sites, needle puncture sites, and gastrointestinal, genitourinary, and retroperitoneal sites).

Arterial and venous punctures, intramuscular injections, and use of urinary catheters, nasotracheal intubation, nasogastric tubes, and automatic blood pressure cuffs should be minimized. When obtaining IV access, noncompressible sites (eg, subclavian or jugular veins) should be avoided. Saline or heparin locks should be considered for blood drawing. Vascular puncture sites should be documented and monitored. Gentle care should be provided when removing dressings.

Femoral artery access site – Arterial access site care is important to prevent bleeding. Care should be taken when attempting vascular access that only the anterior wall of the femoral artery is punctured, avoiding a Seldinger (through and through) technique for obtaining sheath access. Femoral vein sheath placement should be avoided unless needed. While the vascular sheath is in place, patients should be maintained on complete bed rest with the head of the bed less than or equal to 30° and the affected limb restrained in a straight position. Patients may be medicated for back/groin pain as necessary.

Discontinuation of heparin immediately upon completion of the procedure and removal of the arterial sheath within 6 hours is strongly recommended if APTT less than or equal to 50 sec or ACT less than or equal to 175 sec. In all circumstances, heparin should be discontinued at least 2 hours prior to arterial sheath removal.

Following sheath removal, pressure should be applied to the femoral artery for at least 30 minutes using either manual compression or a mechanical device for hemostasis. A pressure dressing should be applied following hemostasis. The patient should be maintained on bed rest for 6 to 8 hours following sheath removal or discontinuation of abciximab, or 4 hours following discontinuation of heparin, whichever is later. The pressure dressing should be removed prior to ambulation. The sheath insertion site and distal pulses of affected leg(s) should be frequently checked while the femoral artery

ABCIXIMAB — INJECTION

sheath is in place and for 6 hours after femoral artery sheath removal. Any hematoma should be measured and monitored for enlargement.

The following conditions have been associated with an increased risk of bleeding and may be additive with the effect of abciximab in the angioplasty setting: PCI within 12 hours of the onset of symptoms for acute myocardial infarction, prolonged PCI (lasting more than 70 minutes), and failed PCI.

➤*Thrombocytopenia:* Platelet counts should be monitored prior to treatment, 2 to 4 hours following the bolus dose of abciximab and at 24 hours or prior to discharge, whichever is first. If a patient experiences an acute platelet decrease (eg, a platelet decrease to less than 100,000 cells/mcL and a decrease of at least 25% from pretreatment value), additional platelet counts should be determined. These platelet counts should be drawn in 3 separate tubes containing ethylenediaminetetraacetic acid (EDTA), citrate, and heparin, respectively, to exclude pseudothrombocytopenia due to in vitro anticoagulant interaction. If true thrombocytopenia is verified, abciximab should be immediately discontinued and the condition appropriately monitored and treated. For patients with thrombocytopenia in the clinical trials, a daily platelet count was obtained until it returned to normal. If a patient's platelet count dropped to 60,000 cells/mcL, heparin and aspirin were discontinued. If a patient's platelet count dropped below 50,000 cells/mcL, platelets were transfused. Most cases of severe thrombocytopenia (less than 50,000 cells/mcL) occurred within the first 24 hours of abciximab administration.

➤*Restoration of platelet function:* In the event of serious uncontrolled bleeding or the need for emergency surgery, abciximab should be discontinued. If platelet function does not return to normal, it may be restored, at least in part, with platelet transfusions.

➤*Readministration:* Administration of abciximab may result in human antichimeric antibody (HACA) formation that could potentially cause allergic or hypersensitivity reactions (including anaphylaxis), thrombocytopenia, or diminished benefit upon readministration of abciximab. In the EPIC, EPILOG, and CAPTURE trials, positive HACA responses occurred in approximately 5.8% of the abciximab-treated patients. There was no excess of hypersensitivity or allergic reactions related to abciximab treatment.

Readministration of abciximab to 29 healthy volunteers who had not developed HACA responses after first administration has not led to any change in abciximab pharmacokinetics or to any reduction in antiplatelet potency. However, results in this small group of patients suggest that the incidence of HACA response may be increased after readministration. Readministration to patients who have developed positive HACA responses after initial administration has not been evaluated in clinical trials.

Drug Interactions

Patients with HACA titers may have allergic or hypersensitivity reactions when treated with other diagnostic or therapeutic monoclonal antibodies.

➤*Use of thrombolytics, anticoagulants and other antiplatelet agents:* In the EPIC, EPILOG, CAPTURE, and EPISTENT trials, abciximab was used concomitantly with heparin and aspirin. Because abciximab inhibits platelet aggregation, caution should be employed when it is used with other drugs that affect hemostasis, including thrombolytics, oral anticoagulants, nonsteroidal anti-inflammatory drugs, dipyridamole, and ticlopidine.

In the EPIC trial, there was limited experience with the administration of abciximab with low molecular weight dextran. Low molecular weight dextran was usually given for the deployment of a coronary stent, for which oral anticoagulants were also given. In the 11 patients who received low molecular weight dextran with abciximab, 5 had major bleeding events and 4 had minor bleeding events. None of the 5 placebo patients treated with low molecular weight dextran had a major or minor bleeding event.

There are limited data on the use of abciximab in patients receiving thrombolytic agents. Because of concern about synergistic effects on bleeding, systemic thrombolytic therapy should be used judiciously.

Adverse Reactions

➤*Bleeding:* Abciximab has the potential to increase the risk of bleeding, particularly in the presence of anticoagulation (eg, from heparin, other anticoagulants, or thrombolytics). Bleeding in the phase 3 trials was classified as major, minor, or insignificant by the criteria of the Thrombolysis in Myocardial Infarction study group. Major bleeding events were defined as either an intracranial hemorrhage or a decrease in hemoglobin greater than 5 g/dL. Minor bleeding events included spontaneous gross hematuria, spontaneous hematemesis, observed blood loss with a hemoglobin decrease of more than 3 g/dL, or a decrease in hemoglobin of at least 4 g/dL without an identified bleeding site. Insignificant bleeding events were defined as a decrease in hemoglobin of less than 3 g/dL or a decrease in hemoglobin between 3 to 4 g/dL without observed bleeding. In patients who received transfusions, the number of units of blood lost was estimated through an adaptation of the method of Landefeld, et al.

In the EPIC trial, in which a non-weight-adjusted, longer-duration heparin dose regimen was used, the most common complication during abciximab therapy was bleeding during the first 36 hours. The incidences of major bleeding, minor bleeding, and transfusion of blood products were significantly increased. Major bleeding occurred in 10.6% of patients in the abciximab bolus plus infusion arm compared with 3.3% of patients in the placebo arm. Minor bleeding was seen in 16.8% of abciximab bolus plus infusion patients and 9.2% of placebo patients. Approximately 70% of abciximab-treated patients with major bleeding had bleeding at the arterial access site in the groin. Abciximab-treated patients also had higher incidences of major bleeding events from gastrointestinal, genitourinary, retroperitoneal, and other sites.

Bleeding rates were reduced in the CAPTURE trial, and further reduced in the EPILOG and EPISTENT trials by use of modified dosing regimens and specific patient management techniques. In EPILOG and EPISTENT, using the heparin and abciximab dosing, sheath removal, and arterial access site guidelines, the incidence of major bleeding in patients treated with abciximab and low-dose, weight-adjusted heparin was not significantly different from that in patients receiving placebo.

Subgroup analyses in the EPIC and CAPTURE trials showed that non-CABG major bleeding was more common in abciximab patients weighing less than or equal to 75 kg. In the EPILOG and EPISTENT trials which used weight-adjusted heparin dosing, the non-CABG major bleeding rates for abciximab-treated patients did not differ substantially by weight subgroup.

Although data are limited, abciximab treatment was not associated with excess major bleeding in patients who underwent CABG surgery. (The range among all treatment arms was 3% to 5% in EPIC and 1% to 2% in the CAPTURE, EPILOG, and EPISTENT trials.) Some patients with prolonged bleeding times received platelet transfusions to correct the bleeding time prior to surgery.

The rates of major bleeding, minor bleeding, and bleeding events requiring transfusions in the CAPTURE, EPILOG, and EPISTENT trials are shown in the following table. The rates of insignificant bleeding events are not included in the following table.

Non-CABG bleeding in trials of percutaneous coronary intervention (EPILOG, EPISTENT, and CAPTURE)

Number of patients with bleeds (%)			
EPILOG and EPISTENT			
	Placebo[c] (n = 1748)	Abciximab + low-dose heparin[d] (n = 2525)	Abciximab + standard-dose heparin[e] (n = 918)
Major[a]	18 (1)	21 (0.8)	17 (1.9)
Minor	46 (2.6)	82 (3.2)	70 (7.6)
Requiring transfusion[b]	15 (0.9)	13 (0.5)	7 (0.8)
CAPTURE			
	Placebo[f] (n = 635)		Abciximab[f] (n = 630)
Major[a]	12 (1.9)		24 (3.8)
Minor	13 (2)		30 (4.8)
Requiring transfusion[b]	9 (1.4)		15 (2.4)

[a] Patients who had bleeding in more than 1 classification are counted only once according to the most severe classification. Patients with multiple bleeding events of the same classification are also counted once within that classification.
[b] Patients with major non-CABG bleeding who received packed red blood cells or whole blood.
[c] Standard-dose heparin with or without stent (EPILOG and EPISTENT).
[d] Low-dose heparin with or without stent (EPILOG and EPISTENT).
[e] Standard-dose heparin (EPILOG).
[f] Standard-dose heparin (CAPTURE).

Intracranial hemorrhage and stroke – The total incidence of intracranial hemorrhage and nonhemorrhagic stroke across all 4 trials was not significantly different, $\frac{9}{3,023}$ for placebo patients and $\frac{15}{4,680}$ for abciximab-treated patients. The incidence of intracranial hemorrhage was $\frac{3}{3,023}$ for placebo patients and $\frac{7}{4,680}$ for abciximab patients.

Thrombocytopenia – In the clinical trials, patients treated with abciximab were more likely than patients treated with placebo to experience decreases in platelet counts.

Among patients in the EPILOG and EPISTENT trials who were treated with abciximab plus low-dose heparin, the proportion of patients with any thrombocytopenia (platelets less than 100,000 cells/µL) ranged from 2.5% to 3%. The incidence of severe thrombocytopenia (platelets less than 50,000 cells/µL) ranged from 0.4% to 1%, and platelet transfusions were required in 0.9% to 1.1%, respectively. Modestly lower rates were observed among patients treated with placebo plus standard-dose heparin. Overall higher rates were observed among patients in the EPIC and CAPTURE trials treated with Abciximab plus longer duration heparin: 2.6% to 5.2% were found to have any thrombocytopenia, 0.9% to 1.7% had severe thrombocytopenia, and 2.1% to 5.5% required platelet transfusion, respectively.

Other adverse reactions – The table below shows adverse events other than bleeding and thrombocytopenia from the combined EPIC, EPILOG, and CAPTURE trials which occurred in patients in the bolus plus infusion arm at an incidence of more than 0.5% higher than in those treated with placebo.

ABCIXIMAB — INJECTION

Adverse events among treated patients in the EPIC, EPILOG, and CAPTURE trials		
Event	Placebo (n = 2226)	Bolus + infusion (n = 3111)
	Number of patients (%)	
Cardiovascular		
Hypotension	230 (10.3)	447 (14.4)
Bradycardia	79 (3.5)	140 (4.5)
Gastrointestinal		
Nausea	255 (11.5)	423 (13.6)
Vomiting	152 (6.8)	226 (7.3)
Abdominal pain	49 (2.2)	97 (3.1)
Miscellaneous		
Back pain	304 (13.7)	546 (17.6)
Chest pain	208 (9.3)	356 (11.4)
Headache	122 (5.5)	200 (6.4)
Puncture site pain	58 (2.6)	113 (3.6)
Peripheral edema	25 (1.1)	49 (1.6)

➤*Additional adverse reactions:* The following additional adverse events from the EPIC, EPILOG, and CAPTURE trials were reported by investigators for patients treated with a bolus plus infusion of abciximab at incidences which were less than 0.5% higher than for patients in the placebo arm.

Cardiovascular – Ventricular tachycardia (1.4%), pseudoaneurysm (0.8%), palpitation (0.5%), arteriovenous fistula (0.4%), incomplete AV block (0.3%), nodal arrhythmia (0.2%), complete AV block (0.1%), embolism (limb) (0.1%), thrombophlebitis (0.1%).

CNS – Dizziness (2.9%), anxiety (1.7%), abnormal thinking (1.3%), agitation (0.7%), hypesthesia (0.6%), confusion (0.5%), muscle contractions (0.4%), coma (0.2%), hypertonia (0.2%), diplopia (0.1%).

GI – Dyspepsia (2.1%), diarrhea (1.1%), ileus (0.1%), gastroesophageal reflux (0.1%).

GU – Urinary retention (0.7%), dysuria (0.4%), abnormal renal function (0.4%), frequent micturition (0.1%), cystalgia (0.1%), urinary incontinence (0.1%), prostatitis (0.1%).

Hematologic / Lymphatic – Anemia (1.3%), leukocytosis (0.5%), petechiae (0.2%).

Musculoskeletal – Myalgia (0.2%).

Respiratory – Pneumonia (0.4%), rales (0.4%), pleural effusion (0.3%), bronchitis (0.3%), bronchospasm (0.3%), pleurisy (0.2%), pulmonary embolism (0.2%), rhonchi (0.1%).

Miscellaneous – Pain (5.4%), sweating increased (1%), asthenia (0.7%), incisional pain (0.6%), pruritus (0.5%), abnormal vision (0.3%), edema (0.3%), wound (0.2%), abscess (0.2%), cellulitis (0.2%), peripheral coldness (0.2%), injection site pain (0.1%), dry mouth (0.1%), pallor (0.1%), diabetes mellitus (0.1%), hyperkalemia (0.1%), enlarged abdomen (0.1%), bullous eruption (0.1%), inflammation (0.1%), drug toxicity (0.1%).

Overdosage

There has been no experience of overdosage in human clinical trials.

ANAGRELIDE HYDROCHLORIDE

Rx	**Anagrelide Hydrochloride** (Various, eg, IVAX, Roxane)	**Capsules:** 0.5 mg	In 100s and 500s.
Rx	**Agrylin** (Shire)		Lactose. (S 063). White, opaque. In 100s.
Rx	**Anagrelide Hydrochloride** (Various, eg, IVAX, Roxane)	**Capsules:** 1 mg	In 100s and 500s.
Rx	**Agrylin** (Shire)		Lactose. (S 064). Gray, opaque. In 100s.

ANAGRELIDE HYDROCHLORIDE — ORAL

Indications

➤*Thrombocythemia:* For the treatment of patients with thrombocythemia, secondary to myeloproliferative disorders, to reduce the elevated platelet count and the risk of thrombosis and to ameliorate associated symptoms including thrombohemorrhagic events.

Administration and Dosage

➤*Approved by the FDA:* March 17, 1997.

➤*Dosage:* Treatment with anagrelide should be initiated under close medical supervision. The recommended starting dosage of anagrelide for adult patients is 0.5 mg 4 times daily or 1 mg 2 times daily, which should be maintained for at least 1 week. Starting dosages in pediatric patients have ranged from 0.5 mg/day to 0.5 mg 4 times daily. Because there are limited data on the appropriate starting dosage for pediatric patients, an initial dosage of 0.5 mg/day is recommended. In both adult and pediatric patients, dosage should then be adjusted to the lowest effective dosage required to reduce and maintain platelet count below 600,000/mcL, and ideally to the normal range. The dosage should be increased by not more than 0.5 mg/day in any 1 week. Maintenance dosing is not expected to be different between adult and pediatric patients. Dosage should not exceed 10 mg/day or 2.5 mg in a single dose.

➤*Hepatic function impairment:* It is recommended that patients with moderate hepatic impairment start anagrelide therapy at a dosage of 0.5 mg/day and be maintained for a minimum of 1 week with careful monitoring of cardiovascular effects. The dosage increment must not exceed more than 0.5 mg/day in any 1 week. The potential risks and benefits of anagrelide therapy in a patient with mild and moderate impairment of hepatic function should be assessed before treatment is commenced. Use of anagrelide in patients with severe hepatic impairment has not been studied. Use of anagrelide in patients with severe hepatic impairment is contraindicated.

➤*Response to therapy:* Typically, platelet count begins to respond within 7 to 14 days at the proper dosage. The time to complete response, defined as platelet count less than or equal to 600,000/mcL, ranged from 4 to 12 weeks. Most patients will experience an adequate response at a dosage of 1.5 to 3 mg/day. Patients with known or suspected heart disease, renal insufficiency, or hepatic dysfunction should be monitored closely.

➤*Storage/Stability:* Store at 25°C (77°F) in a light-resistant container. Excursions permitted to 15° to 30°C (59° to 86°F).

Actions

➤*Pharmacology:* The mechanism by which anagrelide reduces blood platelet count is still under investigation. Studies in patients support a hypothesis of dose-related reduction in platelet production resulting from a decrease in megakaryocyte hypermaturation. In blood withdrawn from healthy volunteers treated with anagrelide, a disruption was found in the postmitotic phase of megakaryocyte development and a reduction in megakaryocyte size and ploidy. At therapeutic doses, anagrelide does not produce significant changes in white cell counts or coagulation parameters, and may have a small, but clinically insignificant effect on red cell parameters. Anagrelide inhibits cyclic AMP phosphodiesterase III (PDE III). PDE III inhibitors can also inhibit platelet aggregation. However, significant inhibition of platelet aggregation is observed only at doses of anagrelide higher than those required to reduce platelet count.

➤*Pharmacokinetics:*

Absorption/Distribution – The available plasma concentration time data at steady state in patients showed that anagrelide does not accumulate in plasma after repeated administration.

There were no apparent differences between patient groups (pediatric vs adult patients) for T_{max} and $t_{1/2}$ for anagrelide, 3-hydroxy anagrelide, or RL603.

Pharmacokinetic data obtained from healthy volunteers comparing the pharmacokinetics of anagrelide in the fed and fasted states showed that administration of an anagrelide 1 mg dose with food decreased the C_{max} 14% and increased the area under the curve (AUC) 20%.

Metabolism/Excretion – Following oral administration of ^{14}C-anagrelide in people, more than 70% of radioactivity was recovered in urine. Based on limited data, there appears to be a trend toward dose linearity between doses of 0.5 and 2 mg. At fasting and at a dose of anagrelide 0.5 mg, the plasma half-life is 1.3 hours. Two major metabolites have been identified (RL603 and 3-hydroxy anagrelide).

Special populations –

Hepatic function impairment: A pharmacokinetic study at a single dose of anagrelide 1 mg in subjects with moderate hepatic impairment showed an 8-fold increase in total exposure (AUC) to anagrelide.

Children: Pharmacokinetic data from pediatric (range, 7 to 14 years of age) and adult (range, 16 to 86 years of age) patients with thrombocythemia secondary to a myeloproliferative disorder indicate that dose and body weight-normalized exposure, C_{max}, and AUC of anagrelide were lower in the pediatric patients compared with the adult patients (C_{max} 48%, AUC_t 55%).

Contraindications

Severe hepatic impairment. Exposure to anagrelide is increased 8-fold in patients with moderate hepatic impairment. Use of anagrelide in patients with severe hepatic impairment has not been studied.

Warnings

➤*Cardiovascular:* Use anagrelide with caution in patients with known or suspected heart disease, and only if the potential benefits of therapy outweigh the potential risks. Because of the positive inotropic effects and side effects of anagrelide, a pretreatment cardiovascular examination is recommended along with careful monitoring during treatment. In humans, therapeutic doses of anagrelide may cause cardiovascular effects, including vasodilation, tachycardia, palpitations, and congestive heart failure.

➤*Hepatic function impairment:* Exposure to anagrelide is increased 8-fold in patients with moderate hepatic impairment. Use of anagrelide in patients with severe hepatic impairment has not been studied. Assess the potential risks and benefits of anagrelide therapy in a patient with mild and moderate hepatic impairment before treatment begins. In patients with moderate hepatic impairment, dose reduction is required; carefully monitor patients for cardiovascular effects.

➤*Fertility impairment:* Anagrelide at oral dosages up to 240 mg/kg/day (1,440 mg/m²/day, 195 times the maximum recommended human dose [MRHD] based on body surface area) was found to have no effect on fertility and reproductive performance of male rats. However, in female rats, at oral doses of 60 mg/kg/day (360 mg/m²/day, 49 times the MRHD based on body surface area) or higher, it disrupted implantation when administered in early pregnancy and retarded or blocked parturition when administered in late pregnancy.

➤*Pregnancy: Category C.*

Nonteratogenic – A fertility and reproductive performance study performed in female rats revealed that anagrelide at oral dosages of 60 mg/kg/day (360 mg/m²/day, 49 times the MRHD based on body surface area) or higher disrupted implantation and exerted adverse effect on embryo/fetal survival.

A perinatal and postnatal study performed in female rats revealed that anagrelide at oral dosages of 60 mg/kg/day (360 mg/m²/day, 49 times the MRHD based on body surface area) or higher produced delay or blockage of parturition, deaths of nondelivering pregnant dams and their fully developed fetuses, and increased mortality in the pups born.

Five women became pregnant while on anagrelide treatment at dosages of 1 to 4 mg/day. Treatment was stopped as soon as they realized that they were pregnant. All delivered healthy babies. There are no adequate and well-controlled studies in pregnant women. Use anagrelide during pregnancy only if the potential benefit justifies the potential risk to the fetus.

Anagrelide is not recommended in women who are or may become pregnant. If this drug is used during pregnancy, or if the patient becomes pregnant while taking this drug, apprise the patient of the potential harm to the fetus. Instruct women of childbearing potential that they must not be pregnant and that they should use contraception while taking anagrelide. Anagrelide may cause fetal harm when administered to a pregnant woman.

➤*Lactation:* It is not known whether this drug is excreted in human milk. Because many drugs are excreted in human milk and because of the potential for serious adverse reactions in breast-feeding infants from anagrelide, decide whether to discontinue breast-feeding or discontinue the drug, taking into account the importance of the drug to the mother.

➤*Children:* The frequency of adverse reactions observed in pediatric patients was similar to adult patients. The most common adverse reactions observed in pediatric patients were fever, epistaxis, headache, and fatigue during 3 months of anagrelide treatment in the study. Adverse reactions that had been reported in these pediatric patients prior to the study and were considered to be related to anagrelide treatment based on retrospective review were palpitation, headache, nausea, vomiting, abdominal pain, back pain, anorexia, fatigue, and muscle cramps. Episodes of increased pulse rate and decreased systolic or diastolic blood pressure beyond the normal ranges in the absence of clinical symptoms were observed in some patients. Reported adverse reactions were consistent with the known pharmacological profile of anagrelide and the underlying disease. There were no apparent trends or differences in the types of adverse reactions observed between the pediatric patients compared with those of the adult patients. No overall difference in dosing and safety were observed between pediatric and adult patients.

In another open-label study, anagrelide had been used successfully in 12 pediatric patients (range, 6.8 to 17.4 years of age; 6 men and 6 women), including 8 patients with ET, 2 patients with CML, 1 patient with PV, and 1 patient with OMPD. Patients were started on therapy with 0.5 mg 4 times daily up to a maximum daily dose of 10 mg. The median duration of treatment was 18.1 months with a range of 3.1 to 92 months. Three patients received treatment for more than 3 years. Other adverse reactions reported

ANAGRELIDE HYDROCHLORIDE — ORAL

in spontaneous reports and literature reviews include anemia, cutaneous photosensitivity, and elevated leukocyte count.

Precautions

➤*Monitoring:* Anagrelide therapy requires close clinical supervision of the patient. While the platelet count is being lowered (usually during the first 2 weeks of treatment), monitor blood counts (hemoglobin, white blood cells), liver function (AST, ALT), and renal function (serum creatinine, serum urea nitrogen [BUN]).

Closely monitor patients with known or suspected heart disease, renal insufficiency, or hepatic dysfunction.

To monitor the effect of anagrelide and prevent the occurrence of thrombocytopenia, platelet counts should be performed every 2 days during the first week of treatment and at least weekly thereafter until the maintenance dosage is reached.

➤*Cessation of treatment:* In general, interruption of anagrelide treatment is followed by an increase in platelet count. After sudden stoppage of anagrelide therapy, the increase in platelet count can be observed within 4 days.

➤*Blood pressure:* In 9 subjects receiving a single 5 mg dose of anagrelide, standing blood pressure fell an average of 22/15 mm Hg, usually accompanied by dizziness. Only minimal changes in blood pressure were observed following a dose of 2 mg.

Drug Interactions

Anagrelide Drug Interactions

Precipitant drug	Object drug[a]		Description
CYP1A2 inhibitors (eg, theophylline)	Anagrelide	↑	Anagrelide demonstrates some limited inhibitory activity towards CYP1A2, which may present a theoretical potential for interaction with other coadministered medicinal products sharing that clearance mechanism.
Sucralfate	Anagrelide	↓	There is a single case report that suggests that sucralfate may interfere with anagrelide absorption.
Anagrelide	Aspirin	↑	Anagrelide slightly enhanced the inhibition of platelet aggregation by aspirin.
Anagrelide	Cyclic AMP PDE III (eg, milrinone, enoximone, amrinone, olprinone, cilostazol)	↑	Anagrelide is an inhibitor of cyclic AMP PDE III. The effects of medicinal products with similar properties may be exacerbated by anagrelide.

[a] ↑ = Object drug increased. ↓ = Object drug decreased.

Adverse Reactions

Analysis of the adverse reactions in a population consisting of 942 patients in 3 clinical trials diagnosed with myeloproliferative diseases of varying etiology (ET: 551; PV: 117; OMPD: 274) has shown that all disease groups have the same adverse reaction profile. While most reported adverse reactions during anagrelide therapy have been mild in intensity and have decreased in frequency with continued therapy, serious adverse reactions were reported in these patients. These included the following: atrial fibrillation, cardiomegaly, cardiomyopathy, cerebrovascular accident, complete heart block, congestive heart failure, gastric/duodenal ulceration, myocardial infarction, pancreatitis, pericardial effusion, pericarditis, pleural effusion, pulmonary fibrosis, pulmonary hypertension, pulmonary infiltrates, and seizure.

Of the 942 patients treated with anagrelide for a mean duration of approximately 65 weeks, 161 (17%) were discontinued from the study because of adverse reactions or abnormal laboratory test results. The most common adverse reactions for treatment discontinuation were abdominal pain, diarrhea, edema, headache, and palpitation. Overall, the occurrence rate of all adverse reactions was 17.9 per 1,000 treatment days. The occurrence rate of adverse reactions increased at higher dosages of anagrelide.

➤*Adverse reactions with an incidence of 5% or more:*

Cardiovascular – Palpitations (26.1%); tachycardia (7.5%).

CNS – Headache (43.5%); asthenia (23.1%); dizziness (15.4%); paresthesia (5.9%).

Dermatologic – Rash, including urticaria (8.3%); pruritus (5.5%).

GI – Diarrhea (25.7%); nausea (17.1%); abdominal pain (16.4%); flatulence (10.2%); vomiting (9.7%); anorexia (7.7%); dyspepsia (5.2%).

Respiratory – Dyspnea (11.9%).

Miscellaneous – Edema (20.6%); pain, other (15%); fever (8.9%); peripheral edema (8.5%); chest pain (7.8%); pharyngitis (6.8%); malaise (6.4%); cough (6.3%); back pain (5.9%).

➤*Events with an incidence of 1% to less than 5%:*

Cardiovascular – Angina pectoris, arrhythmia, cardiovascular disease, heart failure, hypertension, postural hypotension, syncope, thrombosis, vasodilation.

CNS – Amnesia, confusion, depression, insomnia, migraine, nervousness, somnolence.

Dermatologic – Alopecia, skin disease.

GI – Aphthous stomatitis, constipation, eructation, gastritis, GI distress, GI hemorrhage, melena.

GU – Dysuria, hematuria.

Hematologic/Lymphatic – Anemia, ecchymosis, lymphadenopathy, thrombocytopenia.

Platelet counts below 100,000/mcL occurred in 84 patients (ET: 35; PV: 9; OMPD: 40), reduction below 50,000/mcL occurred in 44 patients (ET: 7; PV: 6; OMPD: 31) while on anagrelide therapy. Thrombocytopenia promptly recovered upon discontinuation of anagrelide.

Hepatic – Elevated liver enzymes were observed in 3 patients (ET: 2; OMPD: 1) during anagrelide therapy.

Musculoskeletal – Arthralgia, leg cramps, myalgia.

Renal – Renal abnormalities occurred in 15 patients (ET: 10; PV: 4; OMPD: 1). Six ET patients, 4 PV patients, and 1 with OMPD experienced renal failure (approximately 1%) while on anagrelide treatment; in 4 cases, the renal failure was considered to be possibly related to anagrelide treatment. The remaining 11 were found to have preexisting renal impairment. Doses ranged from 1.5 to 6 mg/day, with exposure periods of 2 to 12 months. No dose adjustment was required because of renal insufficiency.

Respiratory – Asthma, bronchitis, epistaxis, pneumonia, respiratory disease, rhinitis, sinusitis.

Special senses – Abnormal vision, amblyopia, diplopia, tinnitus, visual field abnormality.

Miscellaneous – Chills, dehydration, flu symptoms, hemorrhage, photosensitivity.

Overdosage

➤*Symptoms:* There are no reports of overdosage with anagrelide. Platelet reduction from anagrelide therapy is dose-related; therefore, thrombocytopenia, which can potentially cause bleeding, is expected from overdosage. If overdosage occurs, cardiac and CNS toxicity also can be expected.

➤*Treatment:* In case of overdosage, close clinical supervision of the patient is required; this especially includes monitoring of the platelet count for thrombocytopenia. Decrease or stop dosage, as appropriate, until the platelet count returns to within the normal range.

DIPYRIDAMOLE

Rx	**Dipyridamole** (Various, eg, Barr, Genetco, Moore)	**Tablets:** 25 mg	In 90s, 100s, 500s, 1000s, 5000s and UD 100s,
Rx	**Persantine** (Boehringer Ingelheim)		(BI/17). Orange, sugar coated. In 100s, 1000s and UD 100s.
Rx	**Dipyridamole** (Various, eg, Barr, Genetco, Moore)	**Tablets:** 50 mg	In 100s, 500s, 1000s and UD 100s,
Rx	**Persantine** (Boehringer Ingelheim)		(BI/18). Orange, sugar coated. In 100s, 1000s and UD 100s.
Rx	**Dipyridamole** (Various, eg, Barr, Genetco, Moore)	**Tablets:** 75 mg	In 100s, 500s, 1000s and UD 100s.
Rx	**Persantine** (Boehringer Ingelheim)		(BI/19). Orange, sugar coated. In 100s, 500s and UD 100s.

DIPYRIDAMOLE — ORAL

Indications

➤*Thromboembolic complications:* As an adjunct to coumarin anticoagulants in the prevention of postoperative thromboembolic complications of cardiac valve replacement.

➤*Unlabeled uses:* At one time, dipyridamole was indicated as a "possibly effective" long-term therapy for chronic angina pectoris. The FDA, however, has withdrawn approval for this indication.

Dipyridamole in combination with aspirin has been commonly used in the prevention of myocardial reinfarction and reduction of mortality post MI. However, combination therapy appears to be no more beneficial than the use of aspirin alone.

Administration and Dosage

➤*Adjunctive use in prophylaxis of thromboembolism after cardiac valve replacement:* 75 to 100 mg 4 times daily as an adjunct to the usual warfarin therapy. Please note that aspirin is not to be administered concomitantly with coumarin anticoagulants.

DIPYRIDAMOLE — ORAL

➤*Storage/Stability:* Store at 25°C (77°F); excursions permitted to 15° to 30°C (59° to 86°F). Keep out of the reach of children.

Actions

➤*Pharmacology:* It is believed that platelet reactivity and interaction with prosthetic cardiac valve surfaces, resulting in abnormally shortened platelet survival time, is a significant factor in thromboembolic complications occurring in connection with prosthetic heart valve replacement.

Dipyridamole tablets have been found to lengthen abnormally shortened platelet survival time in a dose-dependent manner.

Dipyridamole inhibits the uptake of adenosine into platelets, endothelial cells, and erythrocytes in vitro and in vivo; the inhibition occurs in a dose-dependent manner at therapeutic concentrations (0.5 to 1.9 mcg/mL). This inhibition results in an increase in local concentrations of adenosine which acts on the platelet A_2-receptor, thereby stimulating platelet adenylate cyclase and increasing platelet cyclic-3',5'-adenosine monophosphate (cAMP) levels. Via this mechanism, platelet aggregation is inhibited in response to various stimuli such as platelet activating factor (PAF), collagen, and adenosine diphosphate (ADP).

Dipyridamole inhibits phosphodiesterase (PDE) in various tissues. While the inhibition of cAMP-PDE is weak, therapeutic levels of dipyridamole inhibit cyclic-3',5'-guanosine monophosphate-PDE (cGMP-PDE), thereby augmenting the increase in cGMP produced by endothelium-derived relaxing factor (EDRF), now identified as nitric oxide.

Hemodynamics – In dogs, intraduodenal doses of dipyridamole of 0.5 to 4 mg/kg produced dose-related decreases in systemic and coronary vascular resistance leading to decreases in systemic blood pressure and increases in coronary blood flow. Onset of action was in about 24 minutes and effects persisted for about 3 hours.

Similar effects were observed following IV dipyridamole in doses ranging from 0.025 to 2 mg/kg.

In man, the same qualitative hemodynamic effects have been observed. However, acute intravenous administration of dipyridamole may worsen regional myocardial perfusion distal to partial occlusion of coronary arteries.

➤*Pharmacokinetics:*

Absorption/Distribution – Following an oral dose of dipyridamole tablets, the average time to peak concentration is about 75 minutes. The decline in plasma concentration following a dose of dipyridamole tablets fits a 2-compartment model. The alpha half-life (the initial decline following peak concentration) is approximately 40 minutes. The beta half-life (the terminal decline in plasma concentration) is approximately 10 hours. Dipyridamole is highly bound to plasma proteins.

Metabolism/Excretion – It is metabolized in the liver where it is conjugated as a glucuronide and excreted with the bile.

Contraindications

Hypersensitivity to dipyridamole or any of the other components.

Warnings

➤*Hepatic effects:* Elevations of hepatic enzymes and hepatic failure have been reported in association with dipyridamole administration.

➤*Fertility impairment:* A significant reduction in number of corpora lutea with consequent reduction in implantations and live fetuses was, however, observed at 1250 mg/kg (25 times the maximum recommended human dose on a mg/m^2 basis).

➤*Pregnancy: Category B.*

Teratogenic – There are no adequate and well-controlled studies in pregnant women. Because animal reproduction studies are not always predictive of human response, this drug should be used during pregnancy only if clearly needed.

➤*Lactation:* As dipyridamole is excreted in human milk, caution should be exercised when dipyridamole tablets are administered to a nursing woman.

➤*Children:* Safety and effectiveness in the pediatric population below the age of 12 years have not been established.

Precautions

➤*Special risk:*

Coronary artery disease – Dipyridamole has a vasodilatory effect and should be used with caution in patients with severe coronary artery disease (eg, unstable angina, recently sustained MI). Chest pain may be aggravated in patients with underlying coronary artery disease who are receiving dipyridamole.

Hypotension – Dipyridamole tablets should be used with caution in patients with hypotension since it can produce peripheral vasodilation.

➤*Lab test abnormalities:* Dipyridamole has been associated with elevated hepatic enzymes.

Drug Interactions

➤*Adenosine:* Dipyridamole has been reported to increase the plasma levels and cardiovascular effects of adenosine. Adjustment of adenosine dosage may be necessary.

➤*Cholinesterase inhibitors:* Dipyridamole may counteract the anticholinesterase effect of cholinesterase inhibitors, thereby potentially aggravating myasthenia gravis.

Adverse Reactions

Adverse reactions at therapeutic doses are usually minimal and transient. On long-term use of dipyridamole tablets initial side effects usually disappear.

Adverse reactions reported in 2 heart valve replacement trials		
Adverse reaction	Dipyridamole tablets/warfarin (n = 147)	Placebo/warfarin (n = 170)
Dizziness	13.6%	8.2%
Abdominal distress	6.1%	3.5%
Headache	2.3%	0%
Rash	2.3%	1.1%

When dipyridamole tablets were administered concomitantly with warfarin, bleeding was no greater in frequency or severity than that observed when warfarin was administered alone.

➤*Other reactions from uncontrolled studies:*

Miscellaneous – Other reactions from uncontrolled studies include diarrhea, vomiting, flushing and pruritus. In addition, angina pectoris has been reported rarely, and there have been rare reports of liver dysfunction. On those uncommon occasions when adverse reactions have been persistent or intolerable, they have ceased on withdrawal of the medication.

➤*Postmarketing experience:*

Miscellaneous – In postmarketing reporting experience, there have been rare reports of hypersensitivity reactions (eg, rash, urticaria, severe bronchospasm, angioedema), laryngeal edema, fatigue, malaise, myalgia, arthritis, nausea, dyspepsia, paresthesia, hepatitis, thrombocytopenia, alopecia, cholelithiasis, hypotension, palpitation, and tachycardia.

Overdosage

➤*Symptoms:* Hypotension, if it occurs, is likely to be of short duration, but a vasopressor drug may be used if necessary. Symptoms of acute toxicity included ataxia, decreased locomotion and diarrhea in rodents and emesis, ataxia and depression in dogs.

In case of real or suspected overdose, seek medical attention or contact a poison control center immediately. Careful medical management is essential. Based upon the known hemodynamic effects of dipyridamole, symptoms such as warm feeling, flushes, sweating, restlessness, feeling of weakness, and dizziness may occur. A drop in blood pressure and tachycardia might also be observed.

➤*Treatment:* Symptomatic treatment is recommended, possibly including vasopressor drug. Gastric lavage should be considered. Administration of xanthine derivatives (eg, aminophylline) may reverse the hemodynamic effects of dipyridamole overdose. Since dipyridamole tablets are highly protein bound, dialysis is not likely to be of benefit.

Antiplatelet Combination Agents

DIPYRIDAMOLE AND ASPIRIN

Rx	**Aggrenox** (Boehringer Ingelheim)	**Capsules:** 200 mg extended-release dipyridamole/25 mg aspirin	Lactose, sucrose. (01A). Red/Ivory. In 60s.

DIPYRIDAMOLE AND ASPIRIN — ORAL

For more information, refer to the individual monographs for dipyridamole and aspirin.

Indications

➤*Stroke:* To reduce the risk of stroke in patients who have had transient ischemia of the brain or complete ischemic stroke due to thrombosis.

Administration and Dosage

➤*Dosage:* 1 capsule given orally twice daily, 1 in the morning and 1 in the evening. Swallow whole; do not crush or chew.

Do not interchange with individual components of aspirin and dipyridamole tablets.

➤*Storage/Stability:* Store at 25°C (77°F). Protect from excessive moisture.

Actions

➤*Pharmacology:* Antithrombotic action is the result of the additive antiplatelet effects of dipyridamole and aspirin.

Dipyridamole inhibits the uptake of adenosine into platelets, endothelial cells, and erythrocytes in vitro and in vivo; the inhibition occurs in a dose-dependent manner at therapeutic concentrations (0.5 to 1.9 mcg/mL). This inhibition results in an increase in local concentrations of adenosine that acts on the platelet A_2-receptor thereby stimulating platelet adenylate cyclase and increasing platelet cyclic-3′,5′-adenosine monophosphate (cAMP) levels. Platelet aggregation is inhibited in response to various stimuli such as platelet activation factor, collagen, and adenosine diphosphate (ADP). Dipyridamole inhibits phosphodiesterase (PDE) in various tissues. While the inhibition of cAMP-PDE is weak, therapeutic levels of dipyridamole inhibit cyclic-3′,5′-guanosine monophosphate-PDE (cGMP-

DIPYRIDAMOLE AND ASPIRIN — ORAL

PDE), thereby augmenting the increase in cGMP produced by endothelium-derived relaxing factor (now identified as nitric oxide).

Aspirin inhibits platelet aggregation by irreversible inhibition of platelet cyclooxygenase and thus inhibits the generation of thromboxane A_2, a powerful inducer of platelet aggregation and vasoconstriction.

➤*Pharmacokinetics:*

Absorption –

Dipyridamole: Peak plasma levels of dipyridamole are achieved ≈ 2 hours after administration of a daily dose of 400 mg dipyridamole and aspirin combination (given as 200 mg twice daily). The peak plasma concentration at steady-state is ≈ 1.98 mcg/mL and the steady state trough concentration is ≈ 0.53 mcg/mL.

Aspirin: Peak plasma levels of aspirin are achieved ≈ 0.63 hours after administration of a 50 mg aspirin daily dose from dipyridamole and aspirin combination (given as 25 mg twice daily). The peak plasma concentration at steady-state is ≈ 319 ng/mL. Aspirin undergoes moderate hydrolysis to salicylic acid in the liver and the GI wall, with 50% to 75% of an administered dose reaching the systemic circulation as intact aspirin.

Distribution –

Dipyridamole: Dipyridamole is highly lipophilic; however, it has been shown that the drug does not cross the blood-brain barrier to any significant extent in animals. The steady-state volume of distribution of dipyridamole is ≈ 92 L. Approximately 99% of dipyridamole is bound to plasma proteins, predominantly to α1-acid glycoprotein and albumin.

Aspirin: Aspirin is poorly bound to plasma proteins and its apparent volume of distribution is low (10 L). Its metabolite, salicylic acid, is highly bound to plasma proteins, but its binding is concentration-dependent (nonlinear). At low concentrations (< 100 mcg/mL), ≈ 90% of salicylic acid is bound to albumin. Salicylic acid is widely distributed to all tissues and fluids in the body, including the CNS, breast milk, and fetal tissues.

Metabolism / Excretion –

Dipyridamole: Dipyridamole is metabolized in the liver, primarily by conjugation with glucuronic acid, of which monoglucuronide, which has low pharmacodynamic activity, is the primary metabolite. In plasma, ≈ 80% of the total amount is present as parent compound and 20% as monoglucuronide. Most of the glucuronide metabolite (≈ 95%) is excreted via bile into the feces, with some evidence of enterohepatic circulation. Renal excretion of parent compound is negligible and urinary excretion of the glucuronide metabolite is low (≈ 5%). With IV treatment of dipyridamole, a triphasic profile is obtained: A rapid alpha phase with a half-life of ≈ 3.4 minutes, a beta phase with a half-life of ≈ 39 minutes, (which, together with the alpha phase accounts for ≈ 70% of the total area under the curve, AUC), and a prolonged elimination phase λ_Z with a half-life of ≈ 15.5 hours.

Aspirin: Aspirin is rapidly hydrolized in plasma to salicylic acid with a half-life of 20 minutes. Plasma levels of aspirin are essentially undetectable 2 to 2.5 hours after dosing, and peak salicylic acid concentration occurs 1 hour (range, 0.5 to 2 hours) after aspirin administration. Salicylic acid is primarily conjugated in the liver to form salicyluric acid, a phenolic glucuronide, an acyl glucuronide, and a number of minor metabolites. Salicylate metabolism is saturable and the total body clearance decreases at higher serum concentrations because of the limited ability of the liver to form both salicyluric acid and phenolic glucuronide. Following toxic doses (10 to 20 g), the plasma half-life may increase to > 20 hours.

The elimination of acetylsalicylic acid follows first-order kinetics with the dipyridamole and aspirin combination and has a half-life of 0.33 hours. The half-life of salicylic acid is 1.71 hours. Both values correspond well with data from the literature at a lower dose which state a resultant half-life of ≈ 2 to 3 hours. At higher doses, the elimination of salicylic acid follows zero-order kinetics (ie, the rate of elimination is constant in relation to plasma concentration) with an apparent half-life of ≥ 6 hours. Renal excretion of unchanged drug depends upon urinary pH. As urinary pH rises above 6.5, the renal clearance of free salicylate increases from < 5% to > 80%. Following therapeutic doses, ≈ 10% is excreted as salicylic acid and 75% as salicyluric acid, as the phenolic and acyl glucuronides, in urine.

Special risk –

Elderly: Plasma concentrations (determined as AUC) of dipyridamole in healthy elderly subjects > 65 years of age were ≈ 40% higher than in subjects < 55 years of age receiving treatment with the dipyridamole and aspirin combination.

Hepatic function impairment: In a study conducted with an IV formulation of **dipyridamole**, patients with mild-to-severe hepatic insufficiency showed no change in plasma concentrations of dipyridamole but showed an increase in the pharmacologically inactive monoglucuronide metabolite. Dipyridamole can be dosed without restriction as long as there is no evidence of hepatic failure. Avoid **aspirin** in patients with severe hepatic insufficiency.

Renal function impairment: No changes were observed in the pharmacokinetics of **dipyridamole** or its glucuronide metabolite with creatinine clearances ranging from ≈ 15 mL/min to > 100 mL/min if data were corrected for differences in age. Avoid **aspirin** in patients with severe renal failure (glomerular filtration rate < 10 mL/min).

Contraindications

Hypersensitivity to dipyridamole, aspirin, or any of the other product components.

➤*Allergy:* Aspirin is contraindicated in patients with a known allergy to NSAIDs and in patients with asthma, rhinitis, and nasal polyps. Aspirin may cause severe urticaria, angioedema, or bronchospasms (asthma).

➤*Reye's syndrome:* Do not use in children or teenagers with viral infections with or without fever. There is a risk of Reye's syndrome with concomitant use of aspirin in certain viral illnesses.

Warnings

➤*Alcohol:* Counsel patients who consume ≥ 3 alcoholic drinks every day about the bleeding risks involved with chronic, heavy alcohol use while taking **aspirin**.

➤*Coagulation abnormalities:* Even low doses of **aspirin** can inhibit platelet function leading to an increase in bleeding time. This can adversely affect patients with inherited or acquired bleeding disorders (eg, liver disease, vitamin K deficiency).

➤*GI side effects:* GI side effects include stomach pain, heartburn, nausea, vomiting, and gross GI bleeding. Minor upper GI symptoms, such as dyspepsia, are common and can occur anytime during therapy. Watch for signs of ulceration and bleeding, even in the absence of previous GI symptoms. Inform patients about the signs and symptoms of GI side effects and what steps to take if they occur.

➤*Peptic ulcer disease:* Avoid using **aspirin**, which can cause gastric mucosal irritation and bleeding in patients with a history of active peptic ulcer disease.

➤*Hepatic effects:* Elevations of hepatic enzymes and hepatic failure have been reported in association with **dipyridamole** administration.

➤*Renal function impairment:* Avoid aspirin in patients with severe renal failure (glomerular filtration rate < 10 mL/min).

➤*Mutagenesis:* **Aspirin** induced chromosome aberrations in cultured human fibroblasts.

➤*Fertility impairment:*

Dipyridamole: A significant reduction in number of corpora lutea with consequent reduction in implantations and live fetuses was observed at dose of dipyridamole 1250 mg/kg/day or 7500 mg/m²/day in rats (≈ 25 times the recommended human dose on a body surface area basis).

Aspirin: Aspirin inhibits ovulation in rats.

➤*Pregnancy: Category B* (dipyridamole); *Category D* (aspirin).

Reproduction studies have been performed with the dipyridamole and aspirin combination in a ratio of 1:4.4 in rats and rabbits and have revealed no teratogenic evidence at doses of up to 405 mg/kg/day in rats and 135 mg/kg/day in rabbits. However, treatment with the dipyridamole and aspirin combination at 405 mg/kg/day induced abortion in rats. The doses of dipyridamole at 75 mg/kg/day represent 1.5 times the recommended human dose on a body surface area (BSA) basis. In these studies, aspirin itself was teratogenic at doses of 330 mg/kg/day (1980 mg/m²/day) in rats (eg, spina bifida, exencephaly, microphthalmia, coelosomia) and 110 mg/kg/day (1320 mg/m²/day) in rabbits (eg, congested fetuses, agenesis of skull and upper jaw, generalized edema with malformation of the head, diaphanous skin). The doses of aspirin at 330 mg/kg/day in rats and at 110 mg/kg/day in rabbits were ≈ 54 and 36 times the recommended human dose, respectively, on a BSA basis.

There are no adequate and well-controlled studies in pregnant women. Use this combination during pregnancy only if the potential benefit justifies the risk to the fetus. Because of the aspirin component, avoid the combination in the third trimester of pregnancy.

➤*Lactation:* Dipyridamole and aspirin are excreted in human breast milk in low concentrations. Exercise caution when dipyridamole and aspirin combination capsules are administered to a nursing woman.

➤*Children:* Safety and efficacy of dipyridamole and aspirin combination capsules in pediatric patients have not been studied. Because of the aspirin component, use of this product in the pediatric population is not recommended.

Precautions

➤*Individual component interchangeability:* Dipyridamole and aspirin combination is not interchangeable with the individual components of aspirin and dipyridamole tablets.

➤*Coronary artery disease:* Due to the vasodilatory effect of **dipyridamole**, use with caution in patients with severe coronary artery disease (eg, unstable angina, recently sustained MI). Chest pain may be aggravated in patients with underlying coronary artery disease who are receiving dipyridamole. For stroke or transient ischemic attack patients for whom **aspirin** is indicated to prevent recurrent MI or angina pectoris, the aspirin in this product may not provide adequate treatment for the cardiac indications.

➤*Hypotension:* **Dipyridamole** can produce peripheral vasodilation; use with caution in patients with hypotension.

➤*Risk of bleeding:* In 1 study, the incidence of GI bleeding was 68 patients (4.1%) in the dipyridamole and aspirin combination group, 36 patients (2.2%) in the dipyridamole group, 52 patients (3.2%) in the aspirin group, and 34 patients (2.1%) in the placebo groups. The incidence of intracranial hemorrhage was 9 patients (0.6%) in the dipyridamole and aspirin combination group, 6 patients (0.5%) in the dipyridamole group, 6 patients (0.4%) in the aspirin group, and 7 patients (0.4%) in the placebo groups.

➤*Lab test abnormalities:* **Aspirin** has been associated with elevated hepatic enzymes, blood urea nitrogen and serum creatinine, hyperkalemia, proteinuria, and prolonged bleeding time. **Dipyridamole** has been associated with elevated hepatic enzymes.

DIPYRIDAMOLE AND ASPIRIN — ORAL

Over the course of 24 months, patients treated with dipyridamole and aspirin combination therapy showed a decline (mean change from baseline) in hemoglobin of 0.25 g/dL, hematocrit of 0.75%, and erythrocyte count of $0.13 \times 10^6/mm^3$.

Drug Interactions

No drug-drug interaction studies were conducted with the combination of dipyridamole and aspirin. The following drug interactions are representative of the literature for each agent (dipyridamole or aspirin).

Dipyridamole and Aspirin Combination Drug Interactions

Precipitant drug	Object drug*		Description
Dipyridamole	Adenosine	↑	Dipyridamole increases the plasma levels and cardiovascular effects of adenosine. Adjust adenosine dose as necessary.
Aspirin	ACE inhibitors	↓	Due to the indirect effect of aspirin on the renin-angiotensin conversion pathway, the hyponatremic and hypotensive effects of ACE inhibitors may be diminished by concomitant administration of aspirin.
Aspirin	Acetazolamide	↑	Concurrent use can lead to high serum concentrations of acetazolamide (and toxicity) due to competition at the renal tubule for secretion.
Aspirin	Anticoagulants	↑	Patients on anticoagulation therapy are at increased risk for bleeding because of effects on platelets. Aspirin can displace warfarin from protein binding sites, leading to prolongation of the prothrombin time and the bleeding time. Aspirin can also increase the anticoagulant activity of heparin, increasing bleeding risk.
Aspirin	Anticonvulsants (hydantoins, valproic acid)	↑	Increased free fraction of valproic acid, possibly leading to toxic effects of valproic acid, has occurred. The pharmacologic and toxic effects of hydantoins may be increased by coadministration of high doses of salicylates.
Aspirin	Beta blockers	↓	The hypotensive effects of beta blockers may be diminished by concomitant aspirin because of inhibition of renal prostaglandins, leading to decreased renal blood flow and salt and fluid retention.
Dipyridamole	Cholinesterase inhibitors	↓	Dipyridamole may counteract the anticholinesterase effect of cholinesterase inhibitors, thereby potentially aggravating myasthenia gravis.
Aspirin	Diuretics	↓	The effectiveness of diuretics in patients with underlying renal or cardiovascular disease may be diminished by concomitant aspirin because of inhibition of renal prostaglandins, leading to decreased renal blood flow and salt and fluid retention.
Aspirin	Methotrexate	↑	Salicylates can inhibit renal clearance of methotrexate, leading to bone marrow toxicity, especially in the elderly or renally impaired.
Aspirin	NSAIDs	↑	The concurrent use of aspirin with other NSAIDs may increase bleeding or lead to decreased renal function.
Aspirin	Oral hypoglycemics	↑	Moderate doses of aspirin may increase the effectiveness of oral hypoglycemic drugs, leading to hypoglycemia.
Aspirin	Uricosuric agents (eg, probenecid, sulfinpyrazone)	↓	Salicylates antagonize the uricosuric action of uricosuric agents.

* ↑ = Object drug increased. ↓ = Object drug decreased.

Adverse Reactions

Dipyridamole and Aspirin Combination Therapy Adverse Events (%)

	Individual treatment group (n = 6602)			
Adverse reaction	Dipyridamole/ Aspirin combination (n = 1650)	ER[1]-DP alone (n = 1654)	ASA alone (n = 1649)	Placebo (n = 1649)
% of patients with ≥ 1 on-treatment adverse event	79.9	78.9	80.2	70.1
CNS				
Headache	39.2	38.3	33.8	32.9
Amnesia	2.4	2.4	3.5	2.1
Convulsions	1.7	0.9	1.7	1.6
Anorexia	1.2	1	0.6	0.9
Somnolence	1.2	0.8	1.1	0.5
Confusion	1.1	0.5	1.3	0.9
GI				
Abdominal pain	17.5	15.4	15.9	14.5
Dyspepsia	18.4	17.4	18.1	16.7
Nausea	16	15.4	12.7	14.1
Vomiting	8.4	7.8	6.1	7.2
Diarrhea	12.7	15.5	6.8	9.8
Melena	1.9	0.6	1.2	0.8
Rectal hemorrhage	1.6	1.3	1	0.8
GI hemorrhage	1.2	0.3	0.9	0.4
Hemorrhoids	1	0.8	0.6	0.6
Hematologic				
Hemorrhage NOS[2]	3.2	1.5	2.8	1.5
Epistaxis	2.4	1	2.7	1.5
Anemia	1.6	1	1.2	0.5
Purpura	1.4	0.5	0.5	0.4
Musculoskeletal				
Arthralgia	5.5	4.5	5.5	4.6
Arthritis	2.1	1.5	1	1.2
Myalgia	1.2	1	0.7	0.7
Arthrosis	1.1	1.3	0.8	0.8
Respiratory				
Coughing	1.5	1.1	1.9	1.3
Upper respiratory tract infection	1	0.5	1	0.8
Miscellaneous				
Pain	6.4	5.3	6.2	6
Fatigue	5.8	5.6	5.9	5.5
Back pain	4.6	4.7	4.5	3.9
Accidental injury	2.5	1.5	3.1	2.2
Asthenia	1.8	1.1	1	1.1
Neoplasm NOS[2]	1.7	1	1.4	1.2
Cardiac failure	1.6	1	1.0	1.5
Malaise	1.6	1.4	1.6	1.3
Syncope	1	0.8	1	0.5

[1] Extended release.
[2] NOS = Not otherwise specified.

Adverse reactions that occurred in < 1% or patients treated with dipyridamole and aspirin combination therapy and that were medically judged to be possibly related to either dipyridamole or aspirin are listed below.

➤*Cardiovascular:* Hypotension; tachycardia; palpitation; arrhythmia; supraventricular tachycardia.

➤*CNS:* Coma; dizziness; paresthesia; cerebral hemorrhage; intracranial hemorrhage; subarachnoid hemorrhage; agitation.

➤*Dermatologic:* Pruritus; urticaria.

➤*GI:* Gastritis; ulceration; perforation.

➤*Hematologic:* Hematoma; gingival bleeding.

➤*Hepatic:* Cholelithiasis; jaundice; abnormal hepatic function.

➤*Metabolic/Nutritional:* Hyperglycemia; thirst.

DIPYRIDAMOLE AND ASPIRIN — ORAL

➤*Respiratory:* Hyperpnea; asthma; bronchospasm; hemoptysis; pulmonary edema.

➤*Special senses:* Tinnitus; deafness; taste loss. Patients with high frequency hearing loss may have difficulty perceiving tinnitus. In these patients, tinnitus cannot be used as a clinical indication of salicylism.

➤*Miscellaneous:* Allergic reaction; fever; flushing; uterine hemorrhage; renal insufficiency and failure; hematuria.

➤*Postmarketing reports:* The following is a list of additional adverse reactions that have been reported either in the literature or are from postmarketing spontaneous reports for either dipyridamole or aspirin.

Dermatologic – Rash; alopecia; angioedema; Stevens-Johnson syndrome.

GI – Pancreatitis; Reye's syndrome; hematemesis.

GU – Prolonged pregnancy and labor; stillbirths; lower birth weight infants; antipartum and postpartum bleeding; interstitial nephritis; papillary necrosis; proteinuria.

Hematologic – Prolongation of the prothrombin time; disseminated intravascular coagulation; coagulopathy; thrombocytopenia.

Hepatic – Hepatitis; hepatic failure.

Hypersensitivity – Acute anaphylaxis; laryngeal edema.

Lab test abnormalities – Hyperkalemia; metabolic acidosis; respiratory alkalosis; hypokalemia.

Metabolic/Nutritional – Hypoglycemia; dehydration.

Respiratory – Tachypnea; dyspnea.

Miscellaneous – Hypothermia; chest pain; angina pectoris; cerebral edema; hearing loss; rhabdomyolysis; allergic vasculitis.

Overdosage

Because of the dose ratio of dipyridamole to aspirin, overdosage of the dipyridamole and aspirin combination is likely to be dominated by signs and symptoms of dipyridamole overdose. In case of real or suspected overdose, seek medical attention or contact a Poison Control Center immediately.

➤*Symptoms:*

Dipyridamole – Based upon the known hemodynamic effects of dipyridamole, symptoms such as warm feeling, flushes, sweating, restlessness, feeling of weakness, and dizziness may occur. A drop in blood pressure and tachycardia might also be observed.

Aspirin – Salicylate toxicity may result from acute ingestion (overdose) or chronic intoxication. The early signs of salicylic overdose (salicylism), including tinnitus (ringing in the ears), occur at plasma concentrations approaching 200 mcg/mL. Plasma concentrations of aspirin > 300 mcg/mL are clearly toxic. Severe toxic effects are associated with levels > 400 mcg/mL. A single lethal dose of aspirin in adults is not known with certainty but death may be expected at 30 g.

➤*Treatment:*

Dipyridamole – Symptomatic treatment is recommended, possibly including a vasopressor drug. Consider gastric lavage. Because dipyridamole is highly protein bound, dialysis is not likely to be of benefit.

Aspirin – Treatment consists primarily of supporting vital functions, increasing salicylate elimination, and correcting the acid-base disturbance. Gastric emptying or lavage are recommended as soon as possible after ingestion, even if the patient has vomited spontaneously. After lavage or emesis, administration of activated charcoal (as a slurry) is beneficial, if < 3 hours have passed since ingestion. Do not employ charcoal absorption prior to emesis and lavage.

Severity of aspirin intoxication is determined by measuring the blood salicylate level. Closely follow acid-base status with serial blood gas and serum pH measurements. Maintain fluid and electrolyte balance.

In severe cases, hyperthermia and hypervolemia are the major immediate threats to life. Sponge children with tepid water. Administer replacement fluid IV and augment with correction of acidosis. Monitor plasma electrolytes and pH to promote alkaline diuresis of salicylate if renal function is normal. Infusion of glucose may be required to control hypoglycemia.

Hemodialysis and peritoneal dialysis can be performed to reduce the body drug content. In patients with renal insufficiency or in cases of life-threatening intoxication, dialysis is usually required. Exchange transfusion may be indicated in infants and young children.

Patient Information

Counsel patients who consume ≥ 3 alcoholic drinks every day about the bleeding risks involved with chronic, heavy alcohol use while taking **aspirin**.

Inform patients about the signs and symptoms of GI side effects and what steps to take if they occur.

Avoid using **aspirin**, which can cause gastric mucosal irritation and bleeding in patients with a history of active peptic ulcer disease.

Aspirin is contraindicated in patients with known allergy to NSAIDs and in patients with asthma, rhinitis, and nasal polyps. Aspirin may cause severe urticaria, angioedema, or bronchospasms (asthma).

Do not use in children or teenagers with viral infections with or without fever. There is a risk of Reye's syndrome with concomitant use of **aspirin** in certain viral illnesses.

Blood coagulation resulting in the formation of a stable fibrin clot involves a cascade of proteolytic reactions involving the interaction of clotting factors, platelets, and tissue materials. Clotting factors (see table) exist in the blood in inactive form and must be converted to an enzymatic or activated (a) form before the next step in the clotting mechanism can be stimulated. Each factor is stimulated in turn until an insoluble fibrin clot is formed.

Two separate pathways, intrinsic and extrinsic, lead to the formation of a fibrin clot. Both pathways must function for hemostasis.

➤*Intrinsic pathway:* All the protein factors necessary for coagulation are present in circulating blood. Clot formation may take several minutes and is initiated by activation of factor XII.

➤*Extrinsic pathway:* Coagulation is activated by release of tissue thromboplastin, a factor not found in circulating blood. Clotting occurs in seconds because factor III bypasses the early reactions.

Refer to the complete coagulation pathway.

Anticoagulants used therapeutically include fractionated and unfractionated heparin, warfarin (a coumarin derivative), and anisindione (an indandione derivative).

Blood Clotting Factors

Factor	Synonym	Vitamin K-dependent
I	Fibrinogen	no
II	Prothrombin	yes
III	Tissue thromboplastin, tissue factor	no
IV	Calcium	no
V	Labile factor, proaccelerin	no
VII	Proconvertin	yes
VIII	Antihemophilic factor, AHF	no
IX	Christmas factor, plasma thromboplastin component, PTC	yes
X	Stuart factor, Stuart-Prower factor	yes
XI	Plasma thromboplastin antecedent, PTA	no
XII	Hageman factor	no
XIII	Fibrin stabilizing factor, FSF	no
HMW-K	High molecular weight kininogen, Fitzgerald factor	no
PL	Platelets or phospholipids	no
PK	Prekallikrein, Fletcher factor	no
Protein C[1]		yes
Protein S[2]		yes

[1] Partially responsible for inhibition of the extrinsic pathway. Inactivates factors V and VIII and promotes fibrinolysis. Activity declines following warfarin administration.
[2] A cofactor to accelerate the anticoagulant activity of protein C. Decreased levels occur following warfarin administration.

COAGULATION PATHWAY

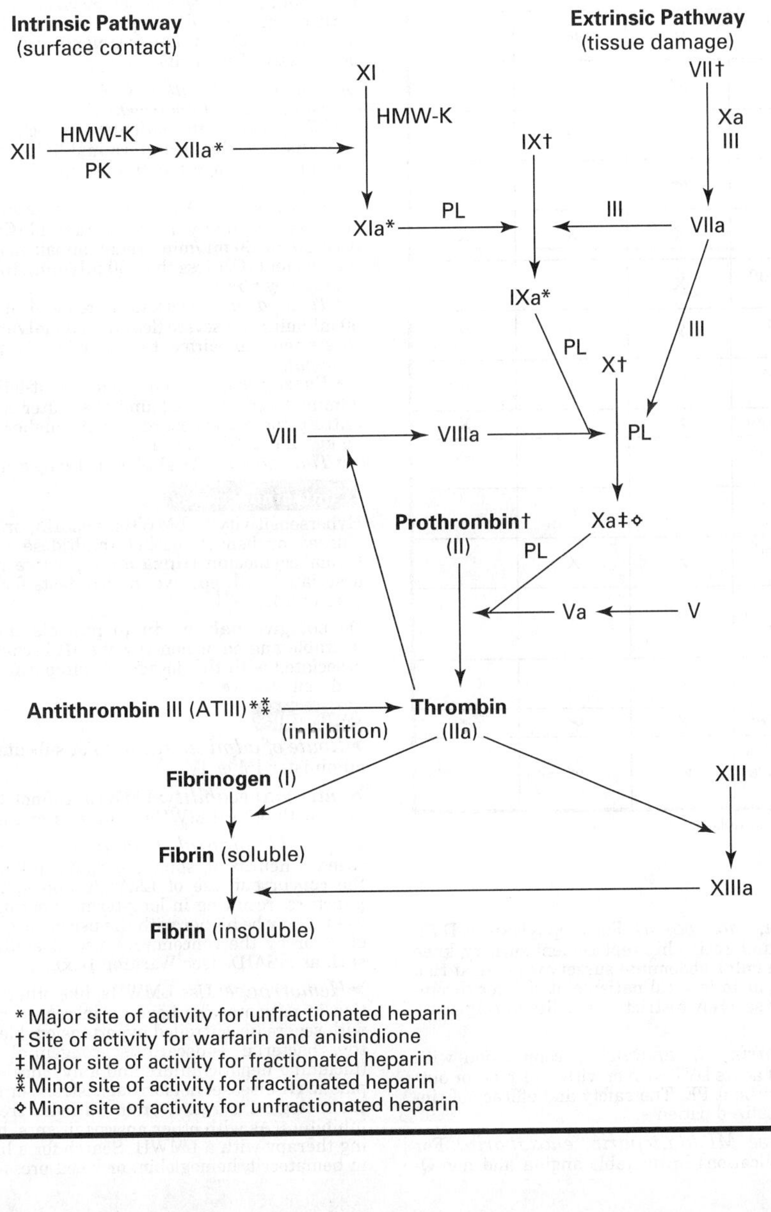

* Major site of activity for unfractionated heparin
† Site of activity for warfarin and anisindione
‡ Major site of activity for fractionated heparin
⁑ Minor site of activity for fractionated heparin
◇ Minor site of activity for unfractionated heparin

WARNING

Spinal/Epidural hematomas – When neuraxial anesthesia (epidural/spinal anesthesia) or spinal puncture is employed, patients who are anticoagulated or scheduled to be anticoagulated with low molecular weight heparins (LMWHs) or heparinoids for prevention of thromboembolic complications are at risk of developing an epidural or spinal hematoma, which can result in long-term or permanent paralysis.

The risk of these events is increased by the use of indwelling epidural catheters for administration of analgesia or by the concomitant use of drugs affecting hemostasis, such as nonsteroidal anti-inflammatory drugs (NSAIDs), platelet inhibitors, or other anticoagulants. The risk also appears to be increased by traumatic or repeated epidural or spinal puncture.

Frequently monitor patients for signs and symptoms of neurological impairment. If neurological compromise is noted, urgent treatment is necessary.

The physician should consider the potential benefit versus risk before neuraxial intervention in patients anticoagulated or scheduled to be anticoagulated for thromboprophylaxis (see Warnings, Precautions, Drug Interactions).

Indications

LMWHs - Summary of Indications

Indications ✓ = labeled X = unlabeled	Dalteparin	Enoxaparin	Tinzaparin
Prophylaxis of DVT that may lead to PE[a]			
In patients undergoing abdominal surgery	✓	✓	
In patients undergoing hip replacement surgery	✓	✓	
In patients undergoing knee replacement surgery		✓	
In patients with severely restricted mobility during acute illness	✓	✓	
In patients undergoing surgery, moderate risk	X	X	X
In patients undergoing surgery, high risk	X	X	
In patients undergoing orthopedic surgery	X	X	X
In patients undergoing hip fracture surgery	X	X	X
In patients undergoing neurosurgery	X	X	X
In patients having undergone major trauma		X	
In patients with acute spinal cord injury		X	
In patients with ischemic stroke and impaired mobility	X	X	
In general medical patients (ie, cancer, bed rest, heart failure, severe lung disease)	X	X	
In pregnancy-related thromboembolism	X	X	
Treatment of DVT with or without PE[b]	X	✓	✓
Prophylaxis of ischemic complications in unstable angina and non-Q-wave MI[c]	✓	✓	

[a] In patients at risk for thromboembolic complications.
[b] In conjunction with warfarin therapy.
[c] In conjunction with aspirin therapy.
DVT = Deep vein thrombosis
PE = Pulmonary embolism

➤*DVT prophylaxis (dalteparin, enoxaparin):* For prophylaxis of DVT, which may lead to PE in patients undergoing hip replacement surgery, knee replacement surgery (**enoxaparin** only), abdominal surgery who are at risk for thromboembolic complications, or in medical patients at risk for thromboembolic complications caused by severely restricted mobility during acute illness.

➤*DVT/PE treatment (enoxaparin, tinzaparin):* In conjunction with warfarin for inpatient treatment of acute DVT with or without PE or for outpatient treatment of acute DVT without PE. The safety and efficacy of tinzaparin were established in hospitalized patients.

➤*Unstable angina/Non-Q-wave MI (dalteparin, enoxaparin):* For the prophylaxis of ischemic complications in unstable angina and non-Q-wave MI when concurrently administered with aspirin therapy.

Actions

➤*Pharmacology:* **Enoxaparin** (average molecular weight is approximately 2,000 to 8,000 daltons), **tinzaparin** (average molecular weight between 5,500 to 7,500 daltons), and **dalteparin** (average molecular weight between 2,000 to 9,000 daltons) are LMWHs obtained by depolymerization of unfractioned porcine heparin. They have antithrombotic properties. These agents enhance the inhibition of Factor Xa and thrombin by binding to and accelerating antithrombin activity. They preferentially potentiate the inhibition of Factor Xa, while only slightly affecting thrombin and clotting time (eg, thrombin time [TT] or activated partial thromboplastin time [aPTT]).

➤*Pharmacokinetics:*

LMWHs Pharmacokinetics Based on Anti-Xa Activity[a]

LMWH	Max activity (h)	Duration (h)	Bio-availability	T_{max} (h)	Vd	Terminal t½ (h)
Dalteparin	-	-	≈ 87%	4	40 to 60 mL/kg	3 to 5
Enoxaparin	3 to 5[b]	12 (40 mg daily dose)	≈ 100%	3 to 4.5	4.3 L	4.5 (single dose) 7 (repeated doses)
Tinzaparin	-	-	86.7%	3.7 (single dose)	3.1 to 5 L	3 to 4

[a] Information listed without regard to dosage or indication.
[b] Maximum anti-Factor Xa and antithrombin activities.

Metabolism/Excretion – LMWHs are primarily metabolized in the liver by desulfation and/or depolymerization to lower molecular weight species with much reduced biological potency. Total renal clearance of active and nonactive **enoxaparin** fragments represents 40% of the dose, with 10% being active fragments.

Special populations –

Renal function impairment:

• *Dalteparin* – In patients with chronic renal insufficiency requiring hemodialysis, the mean terminal half-life of anti-Factor Xa activity may be considerably longer; therefore, greater accumulation can be expected in these patients.

• *Enoxaparin* – Anti-Factor Xa exposure represented by AUC, at steady-state, is marginally increased in mild (Ccr 50 to 80 mL/min) and moderate (Ccr 30 to 50 mL/min) renal impairment. In patients with severe renal impairment (Ccr less than 30 mL/min), the AUC is significantly increased on average by 65%.

• *Tinzaparin* – Clearance is reduced in patients with moderate (Ccr 30 to 50 mL/min) and severe (less than 30 mL/min) renal impairment. Patients with severe renal impairment exhibited a 24% reduction in tinzaparin clearance.

Weight:

• *Enoxaparin* – When non-weight-adjusted enoxaparin dosing was administered, it was found that after a single subcutaneous 40 mg dose, anti-Factor Xa exposure is 52% higher in low-weight women (less than 45 kg) and 27% higher in low-weight men (less than 57 kg).

• *Tinzaparin* – Weight-based dosing is appropriate for heavy/obese patients.

Contraindications

Hypersensitivity to LMWHs, heparin, or pork products; hypersensitivity to sulfites or benzyl alcohol (multidose vials); history of heparin-induced thrombocytopenia (**tinzaparin**); active major bleeding; thrombocytopenia associated with positive in vitro tests for antiplatelet antibody in the presence of a LMWH.

Do not give **dalteparin** to patients undergoing regional anesthesia for unstable angina or non-Q-wave MI because of an increased risk of bleeding associated with the dosage of dalteparin recommended for unstable angina and non-Q-wave MI.

Warnings

➤*Route of administration:* For subcutaneous administration only; do not administer IM or IV.

➤*Interchangeability:* LMWHs cannot be used interchangeably (unit for unit) with other LMWHs or unfractionated heparin.

➤*Spinal/Epidural hematomas:* As with other anticoagulants, rare cases of neuraxial, spinal, or epidural hematomas have been reported with the concurrent use of LMWHs and spinal/epidural anesthesia or spinal puncture, resulting in long-term or permanent paralysis. The risk of these events may be higher with the use of postoperative indwelling epidural catheters or by the concomitant use of additional drugs affecting hemostasis such as NSAIDs (see Warning Box).

➤*Hemorrhage:* Use LMWHs, like other anticoagulants, with extreme caution in patients who have an increased risk of hemorrhage, such as those with severe uncontrolled hypertension; bleeding diathesis; diabetic retinopathy; bacterial endocarditis; congenital or acquired bleeding disorders (including hepatic failure and amyloidosis); active ulceration and angiodysplastic GI disease; hemorrhagic stroke or shortly after brain, spinal, or ophthalmological surgery; or in patients treated concomitantly with platelet inhibitors. As with other anticoagulants, bleeding can occur at any site during therapy with a LMWH. Search for a bleeding site if an unexpected drop in hematocrit, hemoglobin, or blood pressure occurs.

Hemorrhage in some cases has been reported to result in death or permanent disability. If severe hemorrhage occurs, discontinue LMWH.

Major hemorrhages, including retroperitoneal and intracranial bleeding, have been reported. Some of these cases have been fatal.

Discontinue agents that might affect hemostasis (eg, oral anticoagulants, platelet inhibitors) prior to therapy with LMWHs. Concomitant use may increase the risk of hemorrhage. Monitor patient closely if coadministration cannot be avoided (see Drug Interactions).

➤*Thrombocytopenia:* The incidence of thrombocytopenia with platelet counts between 50,000/mm^3 and 100,000/mm^3 was 1.3% in patients treated with **enoxaparin**, 1% with **tinzaparin**, and less than 1% with **dalteparin**. Severe thrombocytopenia (platelet count less than 50,000/mm^3) occurred in 0.13% of tinzaparin-treated patients and 0.1% of enoxaparin-treated patients.

Use extreme caution in patients with a history of heparin-induced thrombocytopenia. Do not use tinzaparin in these patients. Closely monitor thrombocytopenia of any degree. If the platelet count falls to less than 100,000/mm^3, discontinue the LMWH.

Cases of thrombocytopenia with disseminated thrombosis also have been observed in clinical practice with LMWHs, including tinzaparin. Some of these cases were complicated by organ infarction with secondary organ dysfunction or limb ischemia, and have resulted in death.

➤*Priapism:* Priapism has been reported from postmarketing surveillance of **tinzaparin** as a rare occurrence. In some cases, surgical intervention was required.

➤*Renal / Hepatic function impairment:* Delayed elimination of LMWHs may occur with severe liver or kidney insufficiency. Use with caution.

In patients with renal impairment, there is an increase in exposure of **enoxaparin**. Observe all such patients carefully for signs and symptoms of bleeding. Because exposure of enoxaparin is significantly increased in patients with severe renal impairment (Ccr less than 30 mL/min), a dosage adjustment is recommended for therapeutic and prophylactic dosage ranges.

➤*Elderly:* Delayed elimination of **enoxaparin** and **tinzaparin** may occur. Use with caution.

The incidence of bleeding complications was higher in elderly patients as compared with younger patients when enoxaparin injection was administered at doses of 1.5 mg/kg once a day or 1 mg/kg every 12 hours. The risk of enoxaparin injection-associated bleeding increased with age. Serious adverse events increased with age for patients receiving enoxaparin injection. Careful attention to dosing intervals and concomitant medications (especially antiplatelet medications) is advised. Consider monitoring of elderly patients with low body weight (less than 45 kg) and those predisposed to decreased renal function.

➤*Pregnancy: Category B.* There are no adequate and well-controlled studies in pregnant women. There were 72 hemorrhagic events (11 serious) in 63 women. There were 14 cases of neonatal hemorrhage. A few spontaneous postmarketing fetal deaths have been reported in **enoxaparin**-treated patients. Use during pregnancy only if clearly needed. See Precautions for pregnant women with mechanical prosthetic heart valves.

There have been cases reported of cleft palate, optic nerve hypoplasia, trisomy 21 (Down's) syndrome, and cutis aplasia of the scalp in infants of women who received **tinzaparin** during pregnancy. A cause-and-effect relationship has not been established.

There have been reports of fetal death/miscarriage in pregnant women receiving tinzaparin who had high-risk pregnancies or a history of spontaneous abortion. Approximately 6% of pregnancies were complicated by fetal distress. There have been spontaneous reports of 1 case each of pulmonary hypoplasia or muscular hypotonia in infants of women receiving tinzaparin during pregnancy. A cause-and-effect relationship to the above observations has not been established.

Approximately 10% of pregnant women receiving tinzaparin experienced significant vaginal bleeding. A cause-and-effect relationship has not been established.

If tinzaparin is used during pregnancy, or if the patient becomes pregnant while taking this drug, apprise the patient of potential hazards to the fetus.

➤*Lactation:* It is not known whether these drugs are excreted in breast milk. In studies where **tinzaparin** was administered subcutaneously to lactating rats, very low levels of tinzaparin were found in breast milk. Exercise caution when administering to a nursing woman.

➤*Children:* Safety and efficacy in children have not been established.

Precautions

➤*Monitoring:* Perform periodic complete blood counts, including platelet counts and hematocrit or hemoglobin and stool occult blood tests, during the course of treatment. Closely monitor thrombocytopenia of any degree. If the platelet count falls below 100,000/mm^3, discontinue the LMWH (see Warnings). No special monitoring of blood clotting times (eg, aPTT) is needed. At recommended prophylaxis doses, routine coagulation tests such as PT and aPTT are relatively insensitive measures of activity and are, therefore, unsuitable for monitoring. Anti-Factor Xa may be used to monitor the anticoagulant effect in patients with significant renal impairment or if abnormal coagulation parameters or bleeding should occur. Consider monitoring of elderly patients with low body weight (less than 45 kg) and those predisposed to decreased renal function.

➤*Special risk patients:* Use with care in patients with bleeding diathesis, uncontrolled arterial hypertension, or a history of recent GI ulceration or bleeding, diabetic retinopathy, hemorrhage, and severe liver or kidney insufficiency.

➤*Thromboembolic event:* If a thromboembolic event occurs despite LMWH prophylaxis, discontinue the drug and initiate appropriate therapy.

➤*Mechanical prosthetic heart valves:* The use of **enoxaparin** injection has not been adequately studied for thromboprophylaxis or long-term use in patients with mechanical prosthetic heart valves. Isolated cases of prosthetic heart valve thrombosis have been reported in patients with mechanical prosthetic heart valves who have received enoxaparin for thromboprophylaxis. Some of these cases were pregnant women in whom thrombosis led to maternal and fetal deaths. Insufficient data, the underlying disease, and the possibility of inadequate anticoagulation complicate the evaluation of these cases. Women with mechanical prosthetic heart valves may be at higher risk for thromboembolism during pregnancy, and, when pregnant, have a higher rate of fetal loss from stillbirth, spontaneous abortion, and premature delivery. Therefore, frequent monitoring of peak and trough anti-Factor Xa levels and dose adjustment may be needed.

➤*Low-weight patients:* An increase in exposure of **enoxaparin** with prophylactic dosages (less than 45 kg) and low-weight men (less than 57 kg) has been observed. Observe all such patients carefully for signs and symptoms of bleeding.

➤*Benzyl alcohol:* The multidose vials of **dalteparin**, **enoxaparin**, and **tinzaparin** contain benzyl alcohol as a preservative. Benzyl alcohol has been associated with a fatal "gasping syndrome" in premature infants (when large amounts have been administered [99 to 405 mg/kg/day]). Because benzyl alcohol may cross the placenta; do not use LMWHs preserved with benzyl alcohol in pregnant women.

➤*Lab test abnormalities:* Asymptomatic reversible increases in aspartate (AST) and alanine (ALT) aminotransferase levels have occurred in patients treated with LMWHs and heparin (see Adverse Reactions). Because ALT determinations are important in the differential diagnosis of MI, liver disease, and pulmonary emboli, interpret elevations that might be caused by LMWHs with caution.

➤*Sulfite sensitivity:* **Tinzaparin** contains metabisulfite, a sulfite that may cause allergic-type reactions, including anaphylactic symptoms and life-threatening asthmatic episodes, in certain susceptible people. The overall prevalence of sulfite sensitivity in the general population is unknown and probably low. Sulfite sensitivity is seen more frequently in asthmatic than in nonasthmatic people.

Drug Interactions

➤*Anticoagulants / Platelet inhibitors:* Use LMWHs with care in patients receiving oral anticoagulants or platelet inhibitors (eg, aspirin, salicylates, NSAIDs including ketorolac tromethamine, dipyridamole, sulfinpyrazone, dextran, ticlopidine, clopidogrel) and thrombolytics because of increased risk of bleeding. Unless needed, discontinue agents that may enhance the risk of hemorrhage prior to initiation of **enoxaparin** therapy. If coadministration is essential, use close clinical and laboratory monitoring of these patients. Aspirin, unless contraindicated, is recommended in patients treated for unstable angina or non-Q-wave MI.

Adverse Reactions

LMWH Adverse Reactions (%)[a]			
Adverse reaction	Dalteparin	Enoxaparin	Tinzaparin
Hemorrhagic events			
Clinically significant bleeding[b]	0% to 3.6%	0% to 4%	0.8%
Hemorrhage	-	4% to 13%	1.5%
Injection- site hematoma	0.2% to 7.1%	✓	16%
Wound hematoma	0.1% to 3.4%	-	✓
Nonhemorrhagic events			
Cardiovascular			
Angina pectoris	-	-	≥ 1%
Hypertension	-	-	≥ 1%
Hypotension	-	-	≥ 1%
Pulmonary embolism	-	-	2.3%
Tachycardia	-	-	≥ 1
CNS			
Confusion	-	2.2%	≥ 1%
Dizziness	-	-	≥ 1%
Insomnia	-	-	≥ 1%
Headache	-	-	1.7%
Dermatologic			
Bullous eruption	-	-	≥ 1%
Erythematous rash	-	-	≥ 1%
Pruritus/Rash	✓	✓	≥ 1%
Skin disorder	-	-	≥ 1%
GI			
Abdominal pain	-	-	0.8%
Constipation	-	-	1.3%
Diarrhea	-	2.2%	0.6%
Dyspepsia	-	-	≥ 1%
Flatulence	-	-	≥ 1%
GI disorder (NOS)	-	-	≥ 1%
Nausea	-	3%	1.7%
Vomiting	-	-	1%

Low Molecular Weight Heparins (LMWHs)

LMWH Adverse Reactions (%)[a]			
Adverse reaction	Dalteparin	Enoxaparin	Tinzaparin
GU			
Dysuria	-	-	≥ 1%
Hematuria	2.9%	< 1 to 2%	1%
Urinary retention	-	-	≥ 1%
Urinary tract infection	-	-	3.7%
Hematologic			
Anemia	-	< 2% to 16%	≥ 1%
Hematoma	-	✓	≥ 1%
Thrombocythemia	-	✓	-
Thrombocytopenia	< 1%	2.8%	≥ 1%
Respiratory			
Dyspnea	-	3.3%	1.2%
Epistaxis	-	-	1.9%
Pneumonia	-	-	≥ 1%
Respiratory disorder	-	-	≥ 1%
Miscellaneous			
Allergic reactions[c]	✓	✓	✓
Back pain, pain	-	-	1.5%
Cerebrovascular accident	-	-	-
Chest pain	-	-	2.3%
Edema	-	2%	-
Fever	✓	0% to 8%	1.5%
Healing impaired	-	-	≥ 1%
Infection	-	-	≥ 1%
Injection site reactions	✓	✓	✓
Peripheral edema	-	0% to 6%	-
Thrombophlebitis, deep	-	-	≥ 1%
Thrombophlebitis, leg deep	-	-	≥ 1%

[a] Data pooled from several studies and are not necessarily comparable. Percentages listed without regard to specific dosage or indication.
[b] Defined as overt bleeding resulting in a decrease in hemoglobin ≥ 2 g/dL, transfusion of ≥ 2 units of blood, intracranial, intraocular, retroperitoneal, or intra-articular bleeding or moderate to severe bleeding that required discontinuation from the study or required an invasive diagnostic or therapeutic procedure.
[c] Includes maculopapular rash, vesiculobullous rash, urticaria, and bullous eruption.
✓ = Occurs; incidence unknown.

➤*Hemorrhagic complications:* Fatal or nonfatal hemorrhage from any tissue or organ can occur. The signs, symptoms, and severity will vary according to the location and degree or extent of the bleeding. Hemorrhagic complications may present as, but are not limited to, paralysis; paresthesia; headache, chest, abdomen, joint, muscle, or other pain; dizziness; shortness of breath, difficult breathing or swallowing; swelling; weakness; hypotension; shock; or coma. Therefore, consider the possibility of hemorrhage when evaluating the condition of any anticoagulated patient that complaints that do not indicate an obvious diagnosis.

➤*Lab test abnormalities:* Asymptomatic increases in transaminase levels (AST and ALT) greater than 3 times the upper limit of normal of the laboratory reference range have been reported in 1.7% to 8.8% and 4.3% to 13% of patients, respectively, during treatment with LMWHs. Similar significant increases in transaminase levels have been observed in patients treated with heparin. Such elevations are fully reversible and are rarely associated with increases in bilirubin. Because transaminase determinations are important in the differential diagnosis of MI, liver disease, and pulmonary emboli, interpret elevations that might be caused by LMWHs with caution.

➤*Dalteparin:*

Hematologic – Since 1985, there have been 9 reports of epidural or spinal hematoma formation with concurrent use of dalteparin and spinal/epidural anesthesia or spinal puncture (see Warnings). Five of the 9 patients had postoperative indwelling epidural catheters placed for analgesia or received additional drugs affecting hemostasis. The hematomas caused long-term or permanent paralysis (partial or complete) in 7 of these cases.

Miscellaneous – Pain at the injection site (4.5% to 12%); few cases of anaphylactoid reactions.

➤*Enoxaparin:*

Cardiovascular – Atrial fibrillation (0.7%); heart failure (0.95%).

Hematologic – Since 1993, there have been 80 reports of epidural or spinal hematoma formation with concurrent use of enoxaparin and spinal/epidural anesthesia or spinal puncture (see Warnings). Rare cases of hypersensitivity, cutaneous vasculitis, purpura, thrombocytosis, and thrombocytopenia with thrombosis have occurred.

Local – Injection-site hemorrhage (3% to 5%); injection-site pain (2%); injection-site reactions (eg, inflammation, nodules, skin necrosis, oozing).

Respiratory – Lung edema (0.7%); pneumonia (0.82%).

Miscellaneous – Very rare cases of hyperlipidemia have been reported, with 1 case of hyperlipidemia with marked hypertriglyceridemia reported in a diabetic patient; anaphylactoid reactions.

➤*Tinzaparin:*

Cardiovascular – Cardiac arrhythmia, dependent edema, MI/coronary thrombosis, thromboembolism.

Dermatologic – Bullous eruption, erythematous rash, maculopapular rash, skin disorder, skin necrosis.

Hematologic – Anorectal bleeding, cerebral/intracranial bleeding, ecchymosis, GI hemorrhage, granulocytopenia, hemarthrosis, hematemesis, hemopericardium, injection-site bleeding, melena, purpura, retroperitoneal/intra-abdominal bleeding, vaginal hemorrhage.

Approximately 10% of pregnant women receiving tinzaparin experienced significant vaginal bleeding. A cause-and-effect relationship has not been established.

Local – Ecchymosis; hematoma; mild, local irritation; pain.

Miscellaneous – Allergic reaction; anaphylactic/anaphylactoid reactions; cellulitis (local); congenital anomaly; fetal death; fetal distress; neoplasm.

Postmarketing – Abscess; acute febrile reaction; agranulocytosis; allergic purpura; angioedema; cholestatic hepatitis; cutis aplasia of the scalp (fetal/neonatal); epidermal necrolysis; hemoptysis; increase in hepatic enzymes; ischemic necrosis; necrosis; neonatal hypotonia; ocular hemorrhage; pancytopenia; peripheral ischemia; priapism; rectal bleeding; Stevens-Johnson syndrome; thrombocythemia; urticaria.

There has been at least 1 case of spinal epidural hematoma with tinzaparin at a therapeutic dose in a patient who had not received neuraxial anesthesia or spinal puncture.

Overdosage

➤*Symptoms:* An excessive amount of a LMWH may lead to dose-related hemorrhagic complications.

➤*Treatment:* Effects of LMWHs may generally be stopped by the slow IV injection of protamine sulfate (1% solution) at a dose of 1 mg for every 100 anti-Xa units of **dalteparin** and **tinzaparin** or 1 mg for every 1 mg of **enoxaparin** if enoxaparin was administered in the previous 8 hours. An infusion of 0.5 mg protamine/mg of enoxaparin may be administered if enoxaparin was administered more than 8 hours previous to the protamine administration. A second infusion of 0.5 mg protamine per 100 anti-Xa units of dalteparin and tinzaparin or per 1 mg enoxaparin may be administered if the aPTT measured 2 to 4 hours after the first infusion remains prolonged. After 12 hours of the enoxaparin injection, protamine administration may not be required. Even with these additional doses of protamine, the aPTT may remain more prolonged than would usually be found following administration of conventional heparin. In all cases, the anti-Factor Xa activity is never completely neutralized (maximum, approximately 60% to 75%). Take particular care to avoid overdosage with protamine.

Administration of protamine sulfate can cause severe hypotensive and anaphylactoid reactions. Because fatal reactions, often resembling anaphylaxis, have been reported, give protamine only when resuscitation techniques and treatment of anaphylactic shock are readily available.

Patient Information

Instruct patients to contact the physician if they experience bleeding, bruising, dizziness, lightheadedness, itching, rash, fever, swelling, or difficulty breathing.

Instruct patients to notify physician if pregnant, planning to become pregnant, or if breastfeeding.

Instruct patients to change the injection site daily.

Instruct patients to use proper injection technique; inject under the skin, not into muscle.

To minimize bruising, advise patients not to rub the injection site after completion of injection.

Low Molecular Weight Heparins (LMWHs)

DALTEPARIN SODIUM

Rx	**Fragmin** (Pfizer)	**Injection**: 2,500 units/0.2 mL[a] (16 mg/0.2 mL)	Preservative-free. In 0.2 mL single-dose prefilled syringes with 27-gauge × ½-inch needle.
		5,000 units/0.2 mL[a] (32 mg/0.2 mL)	Preservative-free. In 0.2 mL single-dose prefilled syringes with 27-gauge × ½-inch needle.
		7,500 units/0.3 mL[a] (48 mg/0.3 mL)	Preservative-free. In 0.3 mL single-dose prefilled syringes with 27-gauge × ½-inch needle.
		10,000 units/mL[a] (64 mg/mL)	Preservative-free. In 1 mL single-dose, graduated syringes with 27-gauge × ½-inch needle. In 9.5 mL multidose vials with 14 mg/mL benzyl alcohol.
		25,000 units/mL[a] (160 mg/mL)	Contains 14 mg/mL benzyl alcohol. In 3.8 mL multidose vials.

[a] Anti-Factor Xa International Units.

DALTEPARIN SODIUM — INJECTION

For complete and comparative prescribing information, refer to the LMWH group monograph.

WARNING

Spinal/Epidural hematomas – When neuraxial anesthesia (epidural/spinal anesthesia) or spinal puncture is employed, patients who are anticoagulated or scheduled to be anticoagulated with low molecular weight heparins or heparinoids for prevention of thromboembolic complications are at risk of developing an epidural or spinal hematoma, which can result in long-term or permanent paralysis.

The risk of these events is increased by the use of indwelling epidural catheters for administration of analgesia or by concomitant use of drugs affecting hemostasis, such as nonsteroidal anti-inflammatory drugs (NSAIDs), platelet inhibitors, or other anticoagulants. The risk also appears to be increased by traumatic or repeated epidural or spinal puncture.

Frequently monitor patients for signs and symptoms of neurological impairment. If neurological compromise is noted, urgent treatment is necessary.

The physician should consider the potential benefit vs risk before neuraxial intervention in patients anticoagulated or scheduled to be anticoagulated for thromboprophylaxis.

Indications

➤*Unstable angina/non-Q-wave myocardial infarction:* For the prophylaxis of ischemic complications in unstable angina and non-Q-wave myocardial infarction, when concurrently administered with aspirin therapy.

➤*Deep vein thrombosis (DVT) prophylaxis:* For the prophylaxis of DVT, which may lead to pulmonary embolism (PE) in patients undergoing hip replacement surgery, in patients undergoing abdominal surgery who are at risk for thromboembolic complications, and in medical patients who are at risk for thromboembolic complications due to severely restricted mobility during acute illness.

Administration and Dosage

➤*Approved by the FDA:* December 22, 1994 (1S classification).

➤*Unstable angina and non-Q-wave MI:* In patients with unstable angina or non-Q-wave MI, the recommended dose of dalteparin injection is 120 Units/kg of body weight, but not more than 10,000 Units, Subcutaneously every 12 hours with concurrent oral aspirin (75 to 165 mg/day) therapy. Treatment should be continued until the patient is clinically stabilized. In clinical trials, the usual duration of treatment was 5 to 8 days. Concurrent aspirin therapy is recommended except when contraindicated.

Volume of dalteparin sodium to be administered by patient weight, based on 9.5 mL vial (10,000 Units/mL)

Patient weight (lb)	< 110	110 to 131	132 to 153	154 to 175	176 to 197	≥ 198
Patient weight (kg)	< 50	50 to 59	60 to 69	70 to 79	80 to 89	≥ 90
Volume of dalteparin sodium (mL)	0.55	0.65	0.75	0.9	1	1

➤*Hip-replacement surgery:* The table below presents the dosing options for patients undergoing hip replacement surgery. The usual duration of administration is 5 to 10 days after surgery; up to 14 days of treatment with dalteparin sodium have been well tolerated in clinical trials.

Dosing options for patients undergoing hip replacement surgery

Timing of first dose of dalteparin sodium	Dose of dalteparin sodium to be given subcutaneously			
	10 to 14 hours before surgery	Within 2 hours before surgery	4 to 8 hours after surgery[1]	Postoperative period[2]
Postoperative start	-	-	2,500 Units[3]	5,000 Units every day
Preoperative start-day of surgery	-	2,500 Units	2,500 Units[3]	5,000 Units every day

Dosing options for patients undergoing hip replacement surgery

Timing of first dose of dalteparin sodium	Dose of dalteparin sodium to be given subcutaneously			
	10 to 14 hours before surgery	Within 2 hours before surgery	4 to 8 hours after surgery[1]	Postoperative period[2]
Preoperative start-evening before surgery[4]	5,000 Units	-	5,000 Units	5,000 Units every day

[1] Or later, if hemostasis has not been achieved.
[2] Up to 14 days of treatment was well tolerated in controlled clinical trials, where the usual duration of treatment was 5 to 10 days postoperatively.
[3] Allow a minimum of 6 hours between this dose and the dose to be given on postoperative day 1. Adjust the timing of the dose on postoperative day 1 accordingly.
[4] Allow approximately 24 hours between doses.

➤*Abdominal surgery:* In patients undergoing abdominal surgery with a risk of thromboembolic complications, the recommended dose of dalteparin is 2,500 Units administered by Subcutaneous injection once daily, starting 1 to 2 hours prior to surgery and repeated once daily for 5 to 10 days postoperatively.

In patients undergoing abdominal surgery associated with a high risk of thromboembolic complications, such as malignant disorder, the recommended dose of dalteparin is 5,000 Units Subcutaneously the evening before surgery, then once daily for 5 to 10 days postoperatively. Alternatively, in patients with malignancy, 2,500 Units of dalteparin can be administered Subcutaneously 1 to 2 hours before surgery followed by 2,500 Units Subcutaneously 12 hours later, and then 5,000 Units once daily for 5 to 10 days postoperatively.

Dosage adjustment and routine monitoring of coagulation parameters are not required if the dosage and administration recommendations specified above are followed.

➤*Patients with severely restricted mobility during acute illness:* In medical patients with severely restricted mobility during acute illness, the recommended dose of dalteparin sodium is 5,000 Units administered by Subcutaneous injection once daily. In clinical trials, the usual duration of administration was 12 to 14 days.

➤*Administration:* Dalteparin is administered by Subcutaneous injection. It must not be administered by IM injection.

Subcutaneous injection technique – Patients should be sitting or lying down and dalteparin administered by deep Subcutaneous injection. Dalteparin may be injected in a U-shape area around the navel, the upper outer side of the thigh, or the upper outer quadrangle of the buttock. The injection site should be varied daily. When the area around the navel or the thigh is used, using the thumb and forefinger, you must lift up a fold of skin while giving the injection. The entire length of the needle should be inserted at a 45 to 90 degree angle.

Parenteral drug products should be inspected visually for particulate matter and discoloration prior to administration, whenever solution and container permit.

After first penetration of the rubber stopper, store the multiple-dose vials at room temperature for up to 2 weeks. Discard any unused solution after 2 weeks.

Fixed dose syringes – To ensure delivery of the full dose, do not expel the air bubble from the prefilled syringe before injection. Hold the syringe assembly by the open sides of the device. Remove the needle shield. Insert the needle into the injection area as instructed above. Depress the plunger of the syringe while holding the finger flange until the entire dose has been given. The needle guard will not be activated unless the entire dose has been given. Remove needle from the patient. Let go of the plunger and allow the syringe to move up inside the device until the entire needle is guarded. Discard the syringe assembly in approved containers.

Graduated syringes – Hold the syringe assembly by the open sides of the device. Remove the needle shield. With the needle pointing up, prepare the syringe by expelling the air bubble and then continuing to push the plunger down to the desired dose or volume, discarding the extra solution in an appropriate manner. Insert the needle into the injection area as instructed above. Depress the plunger of the syringe while holding the finger flange until the entire dose remaining in the syringe has been given. The needle guard will not be activated unless the entire dose has been given. Remove the needle from the patient. Let go of the plunger and allow syringe to move up inside the device until the entire needle is guarded. Discard the syringe assembly in approved containers.

➤*Storage/Stability:* Store at controlled room temperature 20° to 25°C (68° to 77°F).

Low Molecular Weight Heparins (LMWHs)

ENOXAPARIN SODIUM

Rx	**Lovenox** (Aventis)	**Injection**: 30 mg/0.3 mL[a]	Preservative-free. In amps and single-dose prefilled syringes with a 27-gauge × ½-inch needle.
		40 mg/0.4 mL[a]	Preservative-free. In single-dose prefilled syringes with a 27-gauge × ½-inch needle.
		60 mg/0.6 mL[a]	Preservative-free. In graduated, single-dose prefilled syringes with a 27-gauge × ½-inch needle.
		80 mg/0.8 mL[a]	Preservative-free. In graduated, single-dose prefilled syringes with a 27-gauge × ½-inch needle.
		100 mg/1 mL[a]	Preservative-free. In graduated, single-dose prefilled syringes with a 27-gauge × ½-inch needle.
		120 mg/0.8 mL[a]	Preservative-free. In graduated, single-dose prefilled syringes with a 27-gauge × ½-inch needle.
		150 mg/1 mL[a]	Preservative-free. In graduated, single-dose prefilled syringes with a 27-gauge × ½-inch needle.
		300 mg/3 mL[a]	Contains 15 mg/mL benzyl alcohol. In 3 mL multidose vials.

[a] Approximate anti-Factor Xa activity of 100 units/1 mg enoxaparin sodium (with reference to the WHO First International Low Molecular Weight Heparin Reference Standard).

ENOXAPARIN SODIUM — INJECTION

For complete and comparative prescribing information, refer to the LMWH group monograph.

WARNING

Spinal/Epidural hematomas – When neuraxial anesthesia (epidural/spinal anesthesia) or spinal puncture is employed, patients anticoagulated or scheduled to be anticoagulated with low molecular weight heparins or heparinoids for prevention of thromboembolic complications are at risk of developing an epidural or spinal hematoma that can result in long-term or permanent paralysis.

The risk of these events is increased by the use of indwelling epidural catheters for administration of analgesia or by the concomitant use of drugs affecting hemostasis such as nonsteroidal anti-inflammatory drugs (NSAIDs), platelet inhibitors, or other anticoagulants. The risk also appears to be increased by traumatic or repeated epidural or spinal puncture.

Patients should be frequently monitored for signs and symptoms of neurological impairment. If neurologic compromise is noted, urgent treatment is necessary.

The physician should consider the potential benefit vs risk before neuraxial intervention in patients anticoagulated or to be anticoagulated for thromboprophylaxis.

Indications

➤*Deep vein thrombosis (DVT) prophylaxis:* For the prophylaxis of DVT, which may lead to pulmonary embolism in the following patients: In patients undergoing abdominal surgery who are at risk for thromboembolic complications; in patients undergoing hip replacement surgery, during and following hospitalization; in patients undergoing knee replacement surgery; in medical patients who are at risk for thromboembolic complications due to severely restricted mobility during acute illness.

➤*Unstable angina/non-Q-wave myocardial infarction (MI):* For the prophylaxis of ischemic complications of unstable angina and non-Q-wave MI, when concurrently administered with aspirin.

➤*DVT/Pulmonary embolism:* For the inpatient treatment of acute DVT with or without pulmonary embolism, when administered in conjunction with warfarin sodium; the outpatient treatment of acute DVT without pulmonary embolism when administered in conjunction with warfarin sodium.

Administration and Dosage

➤*Approved by the FDA:* March 29, 1993.

All patients should be evaluated for a bleeding disorder before administration of enoxaparin injection, unless the medication is needed urgently. Since coagulation parameters are unsuitable for monitoring enoxaparin sodium injection activity, routine monitoring of coagulation parameters is not required.

➤*DVT prophylaxis:*

Abdominal surgery – In patients undergoing abdominal surgery who are at risk for thromboembolic complications, the recommended dose of enoxaparin injection is 40 mg once a day administered by SC injection with the initial dose given 2 hours prior to surgery. The usual duration of administration is 7 to 10 days; up to 12 days administration has been well tolerated in clinical trials.

Hip or knee replacement surgery – In patients undergoing hip or knee replacement surgery, the recommended dose of enoxaparin injection is 30 mg every 12 hours administered by SC injection. Provided that hemostasis has been established, the initial dose should be given 12 to 24 hours after surgery. For hip replacement surgery, a dose of 40 mg once a day SC, given initially 12 (± 3) hours prior to surgery, may be considered. Following the initial phase of thromboprophylaxis in hip replacement surgery patients, continued prophylaxis with enoxaparin injection 40 mg once a day administered by SC injection for 3 weeks is recommended. The usual duration of administration is 7 to 10 days; up to 14 days administration has been well tolerated in clinical trials.

Medical patients during acute illness – In medical patients at risk for thromboembolic complications due to severely restricted mobility during acute illness, the recommended dose of enoxaparin injection in 40 mg once a day administered by SC injection. The usual duration of administration is 6 to 11 days; up to 14 days of enoxaparin injection has been well tolerated in the controlled clinical trial.

➤*Unstable angina and non-Q-wave MI:* In patients with unstable angina or non-Q-wave MI, the recommended dose of enoxaparin sodium injection is 1 mg/kg administered SC every 12 hours in conjunction with oral aspirin therapy (100 to 325 mg once daily). Treatment with enoxaparin injection should be prescribed for a minimum of 2 days and continued until clinical stabilization. To minimize the risk of bleeding following vascular instrumentation during the treatment of unstable angina, adhere precisely to the intervals recommended between enoxaparin sodium injection doses. The vascular access sheath for instrumentation should remain in place for 6 to 8 hours following a dose of enoxaparin sodium injection. The next scheduled dose should be given no sooner than 6 to 8 hours after sheath removal. The site of the procedure should be observed for signs of bleeding or hematoma formation. The usual duration of treatment is 2 to 8 days; up to 12.5 days of enoxaparin sodium injections have been well tolerated in clinical trials.

➤*Treatment of DVT with or without pulmonary embolism:* In outpatient treatment, patients with acute DVT without pulmonary embolism who can be treated at home, the recommended dose of enoxaparin injection is 1 mg/kg every 12 hours administered SC. In inpatient (hospital) treatment, patients with acute DVT with pulmonary embolism or patients with acute DVT without pulmonary embolism (who are not candidates for outpatient treatment), the recommended dose of enoxaparin injection is 1 mg/kg every 12 hours administered SC or 1.5 mg/kg once a day administered SC at the same time every day. In both outpatient and inpatient (hospital) treatments, warfarin sodium therapy should be initiated when appropriate (usually within 72 hours of enoxaparin injection). Enoxaparin injection should be continued for a minimum of 5 days and until a therapeutic oral anticoagulant effect has been achieved (International Normalization Ratio 2 to 3). The average duration of administration is 7 days; up to 17 days enoxaparin sodium injection administration has been well tolerated in controlled clinical trials.

➤*Renal function impairment:* Although no dose adjustment is recommended in patients with moderate (Ccr 30 to 50 mL/min) and mild (Ccr 50 to 80 mL/min) renal impairment, all such patients should be observed carefully for signs and symptoms of bleeding.

Dosage Regimens For Patients With Severe Renal Function Impairment (Ccr less than 30 mL/min)

Indication	Dosage regimen
Prophylaxis in abdominal surgery	30 mg administered SC once daily
Prophylaxis in hip or knee replacement surgery	30 mg administered SC once daily
Prophylaxis in medical patients during acute illness	30 mg administered SC once daily
Prophylaxis of ischemic complications of unstable angina and non-Q-wave MI, when concurrently administered with aspirin	1 mg/kg administered SC once daily
Inpatient treatment of acute deep vein thrombosis with or without pulmonary embolism, when administered in conjunction with warfarin sodium	1 mg/kg administered SC once daily

ENOXAPARIN SODIUM — INJECTION

Dosage Regimens For Patients With Severe Renal Function Impairment (Ccr less than 30 mL/min)	
Indication	Dosage regimen
Outpatient treatment of acute deep vein thrombosis without pulmonary embolism, when administered in conjunction with warfarin sodium	1 mg/kg administered SC once daily

➤*Administration:* Enoxaparin injection is a clear, colorless to pale yellow sterile solution, and as with other parenteral drug products, should be inspected visually for particulate matter and discoloration prior to administration.

The use of a tuberculin syringe or equivalent is recommended when using enoxaparin sodium multiple-dose vials to ensure withdrawal of the appropriate volume of drug.

Enoxaparin injection is administered by SC injection. It must not be administered by IM injection. Enoxaparin sodium injection is intended for use under the guidance of a physician. Patients may self-inject only if their physicians determine that it is appropriate, and with medical follow-up as necessary. Proper training in SC injection technique (with or without the assistance of an injection device) should be provided.

SC injection technique – Patients should be lying down and enoxaparin injection administered by deep SC injection. To avoid the loss of drug when using the 30 and 40 mg prefilled syringes, do not expel the air bubble from the syringe before the injection. Administration should be alternated between the left and right anterolateral and left and right posterolateral abdominal wall. The whole length of the needle should be introduced into a skin fold held between the thumb and forefinger; the skin fold should be held throughout the injection. To minimize bruising, do not rub the injection site after completion of the injection. enoxaparin injection prefilled syringes and graduated prefilled syringes are available with a system that shields the needle after injection.

Remove the needle shield by pulling it straight off the syringe. If adjusting the dose is required, the dose adjustment must be done prior to injecting the prescribed dose to the patient.

Note:

- The safety system can only be activated once the syringe has been emptied.
- Activation of the safety system must be done only after removing the needle from the patient's skin.
- Do not replace the needle shield after injection.
- The safety system should not be sterilized.
- Activation of the safety system may cause minimal splatter of fluid. For optimal safety, activate the system while orienting it downwards away from yourself and others.

➤*Incompatibility:* Enoxaparin injection should not be mixed with other injections or infusions.

➤*Storage / Stability:* Store at 25°C (77°F); excursions permitted to 15° to 30°C (59° to 86°F). Keep out of the reach of children.

TINZAPARIN SODIUM

Rx	**Innohep** (Pharmion Corp)	**Injection:** 20,000 units/mL[a]	Each vial contains 3.1 mg/mL sodium metabisulfite, 10 mg/mL benzyl alcohol. In 2 mL multidose vials.

[a] Anti-Factor Xa International Units.

TINZAPARIN SODIUM — INJECTION

For complete and comparative prescribing information, refer to the LMWH group monograph.

WARNING

Spinal/Epidural hematomas – When neuraxial anesthesia (epidural/spinal anesthesia) or spinal puncture is employed, patients anticoagulated or scheduled to be anticoagulated with LMWHs or heparinoids for prevention of thromboembolic complications are at risk of developing an epidural or spinal hematoma, that can result in long-term or permanent paralysis.

The risk of these events is increased by the use of indwelling epidural catheters for administration of analgesia or by the concomitant use of drugs affecting hemostasis, such as nonsteroidal anti-inflammatory drugs (NSAIDs), platelet inhibitors, or other anticoagulants. The risk also appears to be increased by traumatic or repeated epidural or spinal puncture.

Frequently monitor patients for signs and symptoms of neurological impairment. If neurological compromise is noted, urgent treatment is necessary.

The physician should consider the potential benefit versus risk before neuraxial intervention in patients anticoagulated or to be anticoagulated for thromboprophylaxis.

Indications

➤*Deep vein thrombosis (DVT):* Treatment of acute symptomatic DVT, with or without pulmonary embolism (PE), when administered in conjunction with warfarin. The safety and effectiveness of tinzaparin were established in hospitalized patients.

➤*Unlabeled uses:* Prophylaxis of DVT, which may lead to PE, in patients undergoing surgery (moderate risk), orthopedic surgery, hip fracture surgery, or neurosurgery at risk for thromboembolic complications.

Administration and Dosage

➤*Approved by the FDA:* July 18, 2000.

Evaluate all patients for bleeding disorders before administration of tinzaparin. Because coagulation parameters are unsuitable for monitoring tinzaparin activity, routine monitoring of coagulation parameters is not required.

➤*Adults:* The recommended dose of tinzaparin for the treatment of DVT with or without PE is 175 anti-Xa units/kg of body weight, administered subcutaneously once daily for at least 6 days and until the patient is adequately anticoagulated with warfarin (international normalized ratio [INR] of at least 2 for 2 consecutive days). Initiate warfarin therapy when appropriate (usually within 1 to 3 days of tinzaparin initiation).

Because tinzaparin may theoretically affect the prothrombin time (PT)/INR, draw blood for PT/INR determination just prior to the next scheduled dose of tinzaparin for patients receiving tinzaparin and warfarin.

The following table provides doses for the treatment of DVT with or without PE. It is necessary to calculate the appropriate tinzaparin dose for patient weights not displayed in the table.

Use an appropriately calibrated syringe to assure withdrawal of the correct volume of drug from vials.

Tinzaparin Weight-Based Dosing for Treatment of DVT With or Without Symptomatic PE

		DVT treatment 175 units/kg subcutaneously once daily 20,000 units/mL	
Body weight (lbs)	Body weight (kg)	Dose (units)	Amount (mL)
68 to 80	31 to 36	6,000	0.3
81 to 94	37 to 42	7,000	0.35
95 to 107	43 to 48	8,000	0.4
108 to 118	49 to 53	9,000	0.45
119 to 131	54 to 59	10,000	0.5
132 to 144	60 to 65	11,000	0.55
145 to 155	66 to 70	12,000	0.6
156 to 168	71 to 76	13,000	0.65
169 to 182	77 to 82	14,000	0.7
183 to 195	83 to 88	15,000	0.75
196 to 206	89 to 93	16,000	0.8
207 to 219	94 to 99	17,000	0.85
220 to 232	100 to 105	18,000	0.9
233 to 243	106 to 110	19,000	0.95
244 to 256	111 to 116	20,000	1
257 to 270	117 to 122	21,000	1.05
271 to 283	123 to 128	22,000	1.1
284 to 294	129 to 133	23,000	1.15
295 to 307	134 to 139	24,000	1.2
308 to 320	140 to 145	25,000	1.25
321 to 331	146 to 150	26,000	1.3
332 to 344	151 to 156	27,000	1.35
345 to 358	157 to 162	28,000	1.4

Use the following equation to calculate the volume (mL) of tinzaparin 175 anti-Xa units/kg subcutaneous dose for treatment of DVT:

Patient weight (kg) × 0.00875 mL/kg = volume to be given (mL) subcutaneously.

➤*Administration:* Administer tinzaparin by subcutaneous injection. Do not administer by IM or IV injection.

➤*Admixture incompatibilities:* Do not mix with other injections or infusions.

➤*Subcutaneous injection technique:* Position patients either lying down (supine) or sitting, and administer tinzaparin by deep subcutaneous injection. Alternate administration between left and right anterolateral and left and right posterolateral abdominal wall. Vary the injection site daily. Introduce the whole length of the needle into a skin fold held between the thumb

TINZAPARIN SODIUM — INJECTION

and forefinger; hold the skin fold throughout the injection. To minimize bruising, do not rub the injection site after completion of the injection.

➤*Storage/Stability:* Store at 25°C (77°F); excursions permitted to 15° to 30°C (59° to 86°F).

Heparin

Indications

➤*Thrombosis/Embolism:* Prophylaxis and treatment of venous thrombosis and its extension; pulmonary embolism; peripheral arterial embolism; atrial fibrillation with embolization.

➤*Coagulopathies:* Diagnosis and treatment of acute and chronic consumption coagulopathies (disseminated intravascular coagulation [DIC]).

➤*Prophylaxis:* Low-dose regimen for prevention of postoperative deep venous thrombosis (DVT) and pulmonary embolism in patients undergoing major abdominothoracic surgery or who are at risk of developing thromboembolic disease.

According to the National Institutes of Health Consensus Development Conference, low-dose heparin is the treatment of choice as prophylaxis for DVT and pulmonary embolism in urology patients > 40 years of age; pregnant patients with prior thromboembolism; stroke patients; those with heart failure, acute MI or pulmonary infection; also recommended as suggested prophylaxis in high-risk surgery patients, moderate and high-risk gynecologic patients without malignancy, neurology patients with extracranial problems and patients with severe musculoskeletal trauma.

➤*Clotting prevention:* Prevention of clotting in arterial and heart surgery, blood transfusions, extracorporeal circulation, dialysis procedures and blood samples.

➤*Unlabeled uses:* Prophylaxis of left ventricular thrombi and cerebrovascular accidents post-MI.

Continuous infusion for treatment of myocardial ischemia in unstable angina refractory to conventional treatment. Heparin decreases the number of anginal attacks and silent ischemic episodes and reduces the daily duration of ischemia. Intermittent heparin is not as effective.

Prevention of cerebral thrombosis in the evolving stroke.

As an adjunct in treatment of coronary occlusion with acute MI. Although there is some controversy regarding the efficacy of heparin therapy with concurrent antiplatelet therapy (eg, aspirin) in the prevention of rethrombosis/reocclusion after primary thrombolysis with thrombolytics (eg, alteplase, anistreplase, streptokinase) during acute MI, it is recommended by the American College of Cardiology and the American Heart Association. Generally, administer heparin IV immediately after thrombolytic therapy, usually within 2 to 8 hours (depending on the thrombolytic used), and maintain the infusion for ≥ 24 hours. Begin aspirin therapy immediately as soon as the patient is admitted, and continue its administration.

Administration and Dosage

➤*Administration:* Give by intermittent IV injection, continuous IV infusion or deep SC (ie, above the iliac crest of abdominal fat layer) injection. Avoid IM injection.

Continuous IV infusion is generally preferable due to the higher incidence of bleeding complications with other routes.

Adjust dosage according to coagulation test results prior to each injection. Dosage is adequate when whole blood clotting time (WBCT) is ≈ 2.5 to 3 times control value, or when aPTT is 1.5 to 2 times normal.

When given by continuous IV infusion, perform coagulation tests every 4 hours in the early stages. When administered by intermittent IV infusion, perform coagulation tests before each dose during early stages and at appropriate intervals thereafter. After deep SC injection, perform tests 4 to 6 hours after the injections.

➤*General heparin dosage guidelines:* Although dosage must be individualized, the following guidelines may be used:

Heparin Dosage Guidelines

Method of administration	Frequency	Recommended dose[a]
Subcutaneous[b]	Initial dose	10,000 – 20,000 units[c]
	Every 8 hours	8000 – 10,000 units
	Every 12 hours	15,000 – 20,000 units
Intermittent IV	Initial dose	10,000 units[d]
	Every 4 to 6 hours	5000 – 10,000 units[d]
IV Infusion	Initial dose	In 1000 mL 0.9% sodium chloride
	Continuous	20,000 – 40,000 units/day[c]

[a] Based on a 68 kg (150 lb) patient.
[b] Use a concentrated solution.
[c] Immediately preceded by IV loading dose of 5000 units.
[d] Administer undiluted or in 50 to 100 mL 0.9% NaCl.

Heparin Dosage for DVT Treatment

PTT (secs)	Action	Rate change
< 45	5000 units bolus	increase by 250 units/hr
45 to 54	—	increase by 150 units/hr
55 to 85	—	no change
86 to 110	stop infusion × 1 hr	decrease by 150 units/hr
> 110	stop infusion × 1 hr	decrease by 250 units/hr

➤*Children:* In general, the following dosage schedule may be used as a guideline:

Initial dose – 50 units/kg IV bolus.

Maintenance dose – 100 units/kg/dose IV drip every 4 hours, or 20,000 units/m²/24 hours continuous IV infusion.

➤*Low-dose prophylaxis of postoperative thromboembolism:* Low-dose heparin prophylaxis, prior to and after surgery, will reduce the incidence of postoperative DVT in the legs and clinical pulmonary embolism. Give 5000 units SC 2 hours before surgery and 5000 units every 8 to 12 hours thereafter for 7 days or until the patient is fully ambulatory, whichever is longer. Administer by deep SC injection above the iliac crest or abdominal fat layer, arm, or thigh using a concentrated solution. Use a fine-gauge needle (25 to 26 gauge) to minimize tissue trauma. Reserve such prophylaxis for patients > 40 years of age undergoing major surgery. Exclude patients on oral anticoagulants or drugs that affect platelet function (see Drug Interactions) or in patients with bleeding disorders, brain or spinal cord injuries, spinal anesthesia, eye surgery, or potentially sanguineous operations.

If bleeding occurs during or after surgery, discontinue heparin and neutralize with protamine sulfate. If clinical evidence of thromboembolism develops despite low-dose prophylaxis, give full therapeutic doses of anticoagulants until contraindicated. Prior to heparinization, rule out bleeding disorders; perform appropriate coagulation tests just prior to surgery. Coagulation test values should be normal or only slightly elevated at these times.

➤*Surgery of the heart and blood vessels:* Give an initial dose of not less than 150 units/kg to patients undergoing total body perfusion for open heart surgery. Often, 300 units/kg is used for procedures < 60 minutes and 400 units/kg is used for procedures > 60 minutes.

➤*Extracorporeal dialysis:* Follow equipment manufacturers' operating directions.

➤*Blood transfusion:* Add 400 to 600 units per 100 mL whole blood to prevent coagulation. Add 7500 units to 100 mL 0.9% Sodium Chloride Injection (or 75,000 units/L of 0.9% Sodium Chloride Injection); from this sterile solution, add 6 to 8 mL per 100 mL whole blood. Perform leukocyte counts on heparinized blood within 2 hours of addition of heparin. Do not use heparinized blood for isoagglutinin, complement, erythrocyte fragility tests, or platelet counts.

➤*Laboratory samples:* Add 70 to 150 units per 10 to 20 mL sample of whole blood to prevent coagulation of sample (see Blood transfusion).

➤*Clearing intermittent infusion (heparin lock) sets:* To prevent clot formation in a heparin lock set, inject diluted heparin solution (Heparin Lock Flush Solution, USP; or a 10 to 100 units/mL heparin solution) via the injection hub to fill the entire set to the needle tip. Replace this solution each time the heparin lock is used. Aspirate before administering any solution via the lock to confirm patency and location of needle or catheter tip. If the administered drug is incompatible with heparin, flush the entire heparin lock set with sterile water or normal saline before and after the medication is administered; following the second flush, the dilute heparin solution may be reinstilled into the set. Consult the set manufacturer's instructions.

Because repeated injections of small doses of heparin can alter aPTT, obtain a baseline aPTT prior to insertion of a heparin lock set.

➤*Preparation of solution:* Slight discoloration does not alter potency.

When heparin is added to infusion solution for continuous IV administration, invert container ≥ 6 times to ensure adequate mixing and to prevent pooling of heparin.

➤*Converting to oral anticoagulant therapy:* Perform baseline coagulation tests to determine prothrombin activity when heparin activity is too low to affect prothrombin time (PT) or the International Normalized Ratio (INR). For immediate anticoagulant effect, give heparin in usual therapeutic doses. When results of initial prothrombin determinations are known, initiate the oral anticoagulant in the usual amount. Perform coagulation tests and prothrombin activity at appropriate intervals. To ensure continuous anticoagulation, continue full heparin therapy for several days after PT or INR has reached therapeutic range. Heparin therapy may then be discontinued. Measure PT or INR ≥ 6 hours after last IV bolus dose and 24 hours after last SC dose of heparin. If continuous IV heparin infusion is used, PT or INR can usually be measured at any time. When prothrombin activity reaches the desired therapeutic range, discontinue heparin and continue oral anticoagulants.

Actions

➤*Pharmacology:* Commercial preparations of heparin are derived from bovine lung or porcine intestinal mucosa; although chemical and biological differences exist, there are no clinical differences in the antithrombotic effects. The anticoagulant potency of heparin is standardized by bioassay and is expressed in "units" of activity. Because the number of units per milligram varies, express dosage only in "units." (Heparin sodium should contain not less than 140 heparin units/mg.)

The major rate-limiting step in the coagulation cascade is the activation of factor X, which is involved in both intrinsic and extrinsic pathways (refer to the Anticoagulant introduction). Small amounts of heparin in combination with antithrombin III (ATIII) inhibit thrombosis by inactivating factor Xa and inhibiting the conversion of prothrombin to thrombin. Once active thrombosis has developed, larger amounts of heparin in combination with heparin cofactor (HC-II) can inhibit further coagulation by inactivating thrombin and preventing the conversion of fibrinogen to fibrin. In combination with ATIII, heparin inactivates activated coagulation factors IX, X, XI, XII, plasmin, kallikrein and thrombin, inhibiting conversion of fibrinogen to fibrin. The heparin-antithrombin III complex is 100 to 1000 times more potent as an anticoagulant than antithrombin III alone. Heparin also prevents the formation of a stable fibrin clot by inhibiting the activation of factor XIII (the fibrin stabilizing factor). Other effects include the inhibition of thrombin-induced activation of factors V and VIII and variable inhibitions of platelet aggregates.

Commercial products contain both low and high molecular weight heparin fractions. Low molecular weight heparin has a greater inhibitory effect on factor Xa and less antithrombin activity than the high molecular weight fraction.

Heparin inhibits reactions that lead to clotting but does not significantly alter the concentration of the normal clotting factors of blood. Although clotting time is prolonged by full therapeutic doses, in most cases it is not measurably affected by low doses of heparin. Bleeding time is usually unaffected. The drug has no fibrinolytic activity; it will not lyse existing clots, but it can prevent extension of existing clots.

Heparin also enhances lipoprotein lipase release, (which clears plasma of circulating lipids), increases circulating free fatty acids and reduces lipoprotein levels.

➤*Pharmacokinetics:*

Absorption/Distribution – Heparin is not adsorbed from the GI tract and must be given IV or SC. An IV bolus results in immediate anticoagulant effects, the anticoagulant response to heparin at therapeutic doses is not linear but increases disproportionately both in its intensity and duration with increasing dose. Peak plasma levels of heparin are achieved 2 to 4 hours following SC use, although there are considerable individual variations. Once absorbed, heparin is distributed in plasma and is extensively and nonspecifically protein bound.

Metabolism/Excretion – Heparin is rapidly cleared from plasma with an average half-life of 30 to 180 minutes. Half-life is dose-dependent and nonlinear and may be disproportionately prolonged at higher doses (30 min at 25 u/kg vs 150 minutes at 400 u/kg). Heparin is partially metabolized by liver heparinase and the reticuloendothelial system. There may be a secondary site of metabolism in the kidneys. Apparent volume of distribution is 40 to 60 mL/kg. In patients with deep venous thrombosis, plasma clearance is more rapid and half-life is shorter than in patients with pulmonary embolism. Heparin half-life may be prolonged in liver disease. Heparin is excreted in urine as unchanged drug (up to 50%), particularly after large doses. Some urinary degradation products have anticoagulant activity.

Contraindications

Hypersensitivity to heparin; severe thrombocytopenia; uncontrolled bleeding (except when it is due to DIC); any patient for whom suitable blood coagulation tests cannot be performed at the appropriate intervals (there is usually no need to monitor coagulation parameters in patients receiving low-dose heparin).

Warnings

➤*IM administration:* Avoid because of the danger of hematoma formation.

➤*Hemorrhage:* Hemorrhage can occur at virtually any site in patients receiving heparin. An unexplained fall in hematocrit, fall in blood pressure or any other unexplained symptom should lead to serious consideration of a hemorrhagic event. An overly prolonged coagulation test or bleeding can usually be controlled by withdrawing the drug. Signs and symptoms will vary according to the location and extent of bleeding and may be present as paralysis, headache, chest, abdomen, joint or other pain, shortness of breath, difficulty breathing or swallowing, unexplained swelling or unexplained shock. GI or urinary tract bleeding may indicate an underlying occult lesion. Certain hemorrhagic complications may be difficult to detect.

Adrenal hemorrhage – Adrenal hemorrhage resulting in acute adrenal insufficiency has occurred. Discontinue therapy in patients who develop signs and symptoms of acute adrenal hemorrhage or insufficiency. Initiation of therapy should not depend on laboratory confirmation of diagnosis, since any delay in an acute situation may result in death.

Ovarian (corpus luteum) hemorrhage – This type of hemorrhage has developed in a number of reproductive age women receiving anticoagulants. If unrecognized, this may be fatal.

Retroperitoneal hemorrhage – Retroperitoneal hemorrhage may occur.

Germinal matrix-intraventricular hemorrhage – Occurs fourfold higher in low-birth-weight infants receiving heparin therapy.

Use heparin with extreme caution in disease states in which there is increased danger of hemorrhage. These include:

Cardiovascular: Subacute bacterial endocarditis; severe hypertension.

CNS: During and immediately following spinal tap, spinal anesthesia or major surgery, especially of the brain, spinal cord or eye.

Hematologic: Hemophilia; some vascular purpuras; thrombocytopenia.

GI: Ulcerative lesions, diverticulitis or ulcerative colitis; continuous tube drainage of the stomach or small intestine.

Obstetric: Menstruation.

Other: Liver disease with impaired hemostasis; severe renal disease.

➤*Hyperlipidemia:* Heparin may increase free fatty acid serum levels by induction of lipoprotein lipase. The catabolism of serum lipoproteins by this enzyme produces lipid fragments rapidly processed by the liver. Patients with dysbetalipoproteinemia (type III) cannot catabolize the lipid fragments, resulting in hyperlipidemia.

➤*Benzyl alcohol:* Benzyl alcohol, which is contained in some of these products as a preservative, has been associated with a fatal "gasping syndrome" in premature infants.

➤*Resistance:* Increased resistance to the drug is frequently encountered in fever, thrombosis, thrombophlebitis, infections with thrombosing tendencies, MI, cancer and postoperative states.

➤*Thrombocytopenia:* Thrombocytopenia has occurred in patients receiving heparin with a reported incidence of up to 30%. The development of thrombocytopenia does not necessarily imply a causal relationship. Often patients have other potential causes for thrombocytopenia; they can be ill, receiving several medications or in a postoperative phase. Exclude these potential causes for thrombocytopenia before implicating heparin. The incidence of heparin-associated thrombocytopenia is higher with bovine than with porcine heparin (15.6% vs 5.8%). The severity also appears to be related to heparin dosage, with low-dose therapy resulting in fewer complications.

Early thrombocytopenia – (Type I) develops 2 to 3 days after starting heparin, tends to be mild and is due to a direct action of heparin on platelets.

Delayed thrombocytopenia – (Type II) develops 7 to 12 days after either low-dose or full-dose heparin, can have serious consequences and may reflect the presence of an immunoglobulin that induces platelet aggregation.

Mild thrombocytopenia – Mild thrombocytopenia (platelet count > 100,000/mm^3) may remain stable or reverse even if heparin is continued. However, closely monitor thrombocytopenia of any degree. If a count falls < 100,000/mm^3 or if recurrent thrombosis develops, discontinue heparin. If continued heparin therapy is essential, administration of heparin from a different organ source can be reinstituted with caution.

White clot syndrome – Patients may develop new thrombus formation in association with thrombocytopenia resulting from irreversible aggregation of platelets induced by heparin, the so-called "white clot syndrome." The process may lead to severe thromboembolic complications (eg, skin necrosis, gangrene of the extremities possibly leading to amputation, MI, pulmonary embolism, stroke, possibly death). Monitor platelet counts before and during therapy. If significant thrombocytopenia occurs, immediately terminate heparin and institute other therapeutic measures.

➤*Hypersensitivity reactions:* Give heparin to patients with documented hypersensitivity only in life-threatening situations. Before a therapeutic dose is given, a trial dose may be advisable. Have epinephrine 1:1000 immediately available. Refer to Management of Acute Hypersensitivity Reactions.

Vasospastic reactions – Vasospastic reactions may develop 6 to 10 days after starting therapy and last 4 to 6 hours. The affected limb is painful, ischemic and cyanotic. An artery to this limb may have been recently catheterized. After repeated injections, the reaction may gradually increase to generalized vasospasm with cyanosis, tachypnea, feeling of oppression and headache. Protamine sulfate has no marked effect. Itching and burning, especially on the plantar side of the feet, is possibly based on a similar allergic vasospastic reaction. Chest pain, elevated blood pressure, arthralgias or headache have also been reported in the absence of definite peripheral vasospasm.

➤*Elderly:* A higher incidence of bleeding has occurred in women > 60 years of age.

➤*Pregnancy: Category C.* Safety for use during pregnancy has not been established. Heparin does not cross the placenta. However, its use during pregnancy has been associated with 13% to 22% unfavorable outcomes, including stillbirths and prematurity. This contrasts with a 31% incidence with coumarin derivatives. Heparin is probably the preferred anticoagulant during pregnancy, but it is not risk free. Heparin-induced osteoporosis has occurred, including collapse of vertebrae. Use with caution during pregnancy, especially during the last trimester and during the immediate postpartum period, because of the risk of maternal hemorrhage.

➤*Lactation:* Heparin is not excreted in breast milk.

➤*Children:* See Administration and Dosage. Safety and efficacy have not been determined in newborns; germinal matrix intraventricular hemorrhage occurs more often in low-birth-weight infants receiving heparin.

Use heparin lock flush solution with caution in infants with disease states in which there is an increased danger of hemorrhage. The use of the 100 unit/mL concentration is not advised because of bleeding risk, especially in low-birth-weight infants.

Precautions

➤*Monitoring:* The most common test used to monitor heparin's effect is Activated Partial Thromboplastin Time (APTT). The APTT is widely used, quick, easily done and reproducible. Other tests used include Activated Coagulation Time (ACT) and Lee White-Whole Blood Clotting Time (WBCT). The ACT is also rapid and readily available. The WBCT is time consuming and unreliable; it is used as a standard with which to compare newer tests. If the coagulation test is unduly prolonged or if hemorrhage occurs, discontinue the drug promptly (see Overdosage). Perform periodic platelet counts, hematocrit and tests for occult blood in stool during the entire course of therapy, regardless of route of administration.

➤*Hyperkalemia:* May develop, probably due to induced hypoaldosteronism. Use with caution in patients with diabetes or renal insufficiency. Monitor patient closely.

Drug Interactions

Heparin Drug Interactions

Precipitant drug	Object drug[a]		Description
Cephalosporins	Heparin	↑	Several parenteral cephalosporins have caused coagulopathies; this might be additive with heparin, possibly increasing the risk of bleeding.
Nitroglycerin	Heparin	↓	The pharmacologic effects of heparin may be decreased, although information on the interaction is conflicting.
Penicillins	Heparin	↑	Parenteral penicillins can produce alterations in platelet aggregation and coagulation tests. These effects might be additive with heparin, possibly increasing the risk of bleeding.
Platelet inhibitors (eg, ibuprofen, indomethacin, dipyridamole, hydroxychloroquine, NSAIDs, ticlopidine phenylbutazone, aspirin, dextran)	Heparin	↑	An increased risk of bleeding is possible during concurrent administration due to interference with platelet aggregation.
Digitalis, tetracyclines, nicotine, antihistamines	Heparin	↓	May partially counteract the anticoagulant action of heparin sodium.
Streptokinase	Heparin	↓	Relative resistance to heparin anticoagulation following administration of streptokinase as a systemic thrombolytic agent may occur.

[a] ↑ = Object drug increased. ↓ = Object drug decreased.

➤*Drug/Lab test interactions:* Significant elevations of **aminotransferase** (AST and ALT) levels have occurred in a high percentage of patients. Cautiously interpret aminotransferase increases that might be caused by heparin.

Adverse Reactions

Hemorrhage – Hemorrhage is the chief complication (≤ 10%). See Warnings.

➤*Local: Avoid IM use.* Local irritation, erythema, mild pain, hematoma or ulceration may follow deep SC use, but are more common after IM use. Histamine-like reactions and subcutaneous and cutaneous necrosis have been observed.

➤*Hypersensitivity:*

Most common – Chills; fever; urticaria.

Rare – Asthma; rhinitis; lacrimation; headache; nausea; vomiting; shock; anaphylactoid reactions. Allergic vasospastic reactions with painful, ischemic, cyanotic limbs may develop 6 to 10 days after starting therapy and last 4 to 6 hours. Whether these are identical to thrombocytopenia-associated complications is undetermined. See Warnings.

➤*Miscellaneous:* Thrombocytopenia (see Warnings); osteoporosis (after long-term, high doses); cutaneous necrosis, suppressed aldosterone synthesis, delayed transient alopecia, priapism, rebound hyperlipidemia (after discontinuation).

Overdosage

➤*Symptoms:* Bleeding is the chief sign of heparin overdosage. Nosebleeds, hematuria or tarry stools may be the first sign of bleeding. Easy bruising or petechial formations may precede frank bleeding.

➤*Treatment:* Protamine sulfate (1% solution) will neutralize heparin (see individual monograph). Each mg of protamine neutralizes ≈ 100 USP heparin units.

HEPARIN SODIUM INJECTION

A sterile solution of heparin sodium in water for injection.

	Multiple Dose Vials		
Rx	**Heparin Sodium** (Various, eg, Elkins-Sinn, Fujisawa, Pasadena, Solopak, Pharmacia & Upjohn)	**Injection:** 1,000 units per mL	In 1, 10 and 30 mL vials.
Rx	**Heparin Sodium** (Hospira)	**Injection:** 2,000 units per mL	In 5 and 10 mL vials.
Rx	**Heparin Sodium** (Hospira)	**Injection:** 2,500 units per mL	In 5 and 10 mL vials.
Rx	**Heparin Sodium** (Various, eg, Elkins-Sinn, Fujisawa, Pasadena,Pharmacia & Upjohn, URL)	**Injection:** 5,000 units per mL	In 1 and 10 mL vials.
Rx	**Heparin Sodium** (Various, eg, Elkins-Sinn, Lilly, Fujisawa, Pasadena, Phamacia & Upjohn)	**Injection:** 10,000 units per mL	In 0.5, 1, 4, 5 and 10 mL vials.
Rx	**Heparin Sodium** (Various, eg, Pasadena, Schein)	**Injection:** 20,000 units per mL	In 1, 2 and 5 mL vials.
Rx	**Heparin Sodium** (Various, eg, Pasadena, Schein)	**Injection:** 40,000 units per mL	In 1, 2 and 5 mL vials.
	Single-Dose Ampules and Vials		
Rx	**Heparin Sodium** (Various, eg, Fujisawa)	**Injection:**1000 units per mL	In 1 mL vials.
Rx	**Heparin Sodium** (Various, eg, Fujisawa, Sanofi Winthrop)	**Injection:** 5000 units per mL	In 1 mL vials.
Rx	**Heparin Sodium** (Various, eg, Fujisawa, Pasadena, Pharmacia & Upjohn, Sanofi Winthrop)	**Injection:** 10,000 units per mL	In 1 mL vials.
Rx	**Heparin Sodium** (Various, eg, Fujisawa, Pasadena, Schein)	**Injection:** 20,000 units per mL	In 1 mL vials.
Rx	**Heparin Sodium** (Various, eg, Pasadena)	**Injection:** 40,000 units per mL	In 1 mL vials.
	Unit-Dose		
Rx	**Heparin Sodium**[a] (Elkins-Sinn)	**Injection:** 1,000 units per dose	In 1, 10 and 30 mL *Dosette* vials.[b]
Rx	**Heparin Sodium**[a] (Wyeth-Ayerst)		In 1 mL *Tubex*.[b]
Rx	**Heparin Sodium**[a] (Wyeth-Ayerst)	**Injection:** 2,500 units per dose	In 1 mL *Tubex*.[2]
Rx	**Heparin Sodium**[1] (Elkins-Sinn)	**Injection:** 5,000 units per dose	In 1 and 10 mL vial.[b]
Rx	**Heparin Sodium**[a] (Wyeth-Ayerst)		In 0.5 and 1 mL *Tubex*.[b]
Rx	**Heparin Sodium**[a] (Sanofi Winthrop)		In 1 mL fill in 2 mL *Carpuject*.[b]
Rx	**Heparin Sodium**[a] (Wyeth-Ayerst)	**Injection:** 7,500 units per dose	In 1 mL *Tubex*.[b]
Rx	**Heparin Sodium**[a] (Elkins-Sinn)	**Injection:** 10,000 units per dose	In 0.5, 1 and 4 mL vials.[b]
Rx	**Heparin Sodium**[a] (Wyeth-Ayerst)		In 1 mL *Tubex*.[b]
Rx	**Heparin Sodium**[a] (Wyeth-Ayerst)	**Injection:** 20,000 units per dose	In 1 mL *Tubex*.[b]

[a] From porcine intestinal mucosa.
[b] With benzyl alcohol.

Heparin

HEPARIN SODIUM — INJECTION

For complete and comparative prescribing information, refer to the Heparin Group Monograph.

HEPARIN SODIUM AND SODIUM CHLORIDE

Rx	**Heparin Sodium**[a] **and 0.9% Sodium Chloride** (Baxter Healthcare)	**Injection:** 1000 units	In 500 mL *Viaflex*.
		2000 units	In 1000 mL *Viaflex*.
Rx	**Heparin Sodium**[a] **and 0.45% Sodium Chloride** (Abbott)	**Injection:** 12,500 units	In 250 mL.[b]
		25,000 units	In 250 and 500 mL.[b]

[a] From porcine intestinal mucosa. [b] With EDTA.

For complete and comparative prescribing information, refer to the Heparin Group Monograph.

HEPARIN SODIUM LOCK FLUSH — SOLUTION

Used as an IV flush to maintain patency of indwelling IV catheters in intermittent IV therapy or blood sampling; not intended for therapeutic use.

Rx	**Heparin I.V. Flush** (Medefil)	**Injection:** 1 unit per mL	In 1, 2, 2.5, 5, and 10 mL syringes.
Rx	**Heparin Lock Flush** (Various, eg, Abbott, Fujisawa)	**Injection:** 10 units per mL	In 1, 2, 5, 10, 30 and 50 mL vials; 1, 2, 2.5, 3, 5 mL disposable syringes.
Rx	**Hep-Lock**[a] (Elkins-Sinn)		In 1, 2 mL *Dosette* vials; 1, 2.5 mL *Dosette* cartridge needle units; 10, 30 mL vials.[b]
Rx	**Hep-Lock U/P**[a] (Elkins-Sinn)		Preservative free. In 1 mL *Dosette* vials.
Rx	**Hepflush-10** (American Pharmaceutical Partners)		Preservative-free. In 10 mL single-dose vials.
Rx	**Heparin Lock Flush** (Various, eg, Abbott, Fujisawa)	**Injection:** 100 units per mL	In 1, 2, 5, 10, 30 and 50 mL vials; 1 mL amps; 1, 2, 2.5, 3, 5 mL disposable syringes.
Rx	**Hep-Lock U/P**[a] (Elkins-Sinn)		Preservative free. In 1 mL *Dosette* vials.

[a] From porcine intestinal mucosa. [b] With benzyl alcohol.

HEPARIN LOCK FLUSH — IRRIGATION SOLUTION

For complete and comparative prescribing information, refer to the Heparin Group Monograph.

Antithrombin Agents

ANTITHROMBIN III (HUMAN)

Rx	**Thrombate** III (Bayer)	**Powder for injection, lyophilized:** 500 IU	Preservative-free. In single-use vials with 10 mL Sterile Water for Injection.
		1000 IU	Preservative-free. In single-use vials with 20 mL Sterile Water for Injection.

ANTITHROMBIN III (HUMAN) — INJECTION

Indications

➤*Antithrombin III deficiency:* Antithrombin III (human) is indicated for the treatment of patients with hereditary antithrombin III (AT-III) deficiency in connection with surgical or obstetrical procedures or when they suffer from thromboembolism.

Administration and Dosage

Each bottle of antithrombin III (human) has the functional activity, in international units (Units), stated on the label of the bottle. The potency assignment has been determined with a standard calibrated against a World Health Organization (WHO) AT-III reference preparation.

Determine dosage on an individual basis based on the pretherapy plasma AT-III level, in order to increase plasma AT-III levels to the level found in normal human plasma (100%). Dosage of antithrombin III (human) can be calculated from the following formula: The international units required equals the difference between the desired and baseline AT-III level (expressed as % normal level based on functional AT-III assay) times the patient's weight in kg divided by 1.4.

The formula is based on an expected incremental in vivo recovery above baseline levels for antithrombin III (human), of 1.4% per Unit per kg administered. Thus, if a 70 kg individual has a baseline AT-III level of 57%, in order to increase plasma AT-III to 120%, the initial antithrombin III (human) dose would be

$$[(120 - 57) \times 70]/1.4 = 3{,}150 \text{ Units total.}$$

However, recovery may vary, and levels should be initially drawn at baseline and 20 minutes postinfusion. Subsequent doses can be calculated based on the recovery of the first dose. These recommendations are intended only as a guide for therapy. Individualize the exact loading dose and maintenance intervals for each patient.

It is recommended that following an initial dose of antithrombin III (human), plasma levels of AT-III be initially monitored at least every 12 hours and before the next infusion of antithrombin III (human) to maintain plasma AT-III levels greater than 80%. In some situations (eg, following surgery, hemorrhage or acute thrombosis, during IV heparin administration), the half-life of antithrombin III (human) has been reported to be shortened. In such conditions, monitor plasma AT-III levels more frequently, and administer antithrombin III (human) as necessary.

When an infusion of antithrombin III (human) is indicated for a patient with hereditary deficiency to control an acute thrombotic episode or prevent thrombosis following surgical or obstetrical procedures, it is desirable to raise the AT-III level to normal and maintain this level for 2 to 8 days, depending on the indication for treatment, type and extent of surgery, patient's medical condition and history, and doctor's judgment. Concomitant administration of heparin in each of these situations should be based on the medical judgment of the doctor.

➤*Dosing recommendations:* As a general recommendation, the following therapeutic program may be utilized as a starting program for treatment, modifying the program based on the actual plasma AT-III levels achieved:

1.) An initial loading dose of antithrombin III (human) calculated to elevate the plasma AT-III level to 120%, assuming an expected rise over the baseline plasma AT-III level of 1.4% (functional activity) per Unit per kg of antithrombin III (human) administered. Thus, if an individual has a baseline AT-III level of 57%, the initial antithrombin III (human) dose would be (120−57)/1.4 = 45 Units/kg.

2.) Measure preinfusion and 20 minutes postinfusion (peak) plasma antithrombin III levels following the initial loading dose, plasma antithrombin III level after 12 hours, then preceding the next infusion (trough level). Subsequently measure antithrombin III levels preceding and 20 minutes after each infusion until predictable peak and trough levels have been achieved, generally between 80% to 120%. Plasma levels between 80% to 120% may be maintained by administration of maintenance doses of 60% of the initial loading dose, administered every 24 hours. Make adjustments in the maintenance dose or interval between doses based on actual plasma AT-III levels achieved.

The above recommendations for dosing are provided as only a general guideline for therapy. Individualize the exact loading and maintenance dosages and dosing intervals for each subject, based on the individual clinical conditions, response to therapy, and actual plasma AT-III levels achieved. In some situations (eg, following surgery, with hemorrhage or acute thrombosis, during IV heparin administration), in vivo survival of infused antithrombin III has been reported to be shortened, resulting in the need to administer antithrombin III more frequently.

➤*Reconstitution:* Reconstitute antithrombin III (human) with sterile water for injection and bring it to room temperature prior to administration. Filter antithrombin III (human) through a sterile filter needle as supplied in the package prior to use, and administer within 3 hours following reconstitution. Antithrombin III (human) may be infused over 10 to 20 minutes. Antithrombin III (human) must be administered IV.

Visually inspect parenteral drug products for particulate matter and discoloration prior to administration, whenever solution and container permit.

➤*Rate of administration:* Adapt the rate of administration to the response of the individual patient; administration of the entire dose in 10 to 20 minutes is generally well tolerated.

➤*Storage/Stability:* Store under refrigeration (2° to 8°C [36° to 46°F]). Avoid freezing because breakage of the diluent bottle might occur.

Actions

➤*Pharmacology:* AT-III, an alpha$_2$-glycoprotein of molecular weight 58,000, is normally present in human plasma at a concentration of approxi-

ANTITHROMBIN III (HUMAN) — INJECTION

mately 12.5 mg/dL and is the major plasma inhibitor of thrombin. Inactivation of thrombin by AT-III occurs by formation of a covalent bond resulting in an inactive 1:1 stoichiometric complex between the two, involving an interaction of the active serine of thrombin and an arginine reactive site on AT-III. AT-III is also capable of inactivating other components of the coagulation cascade including factors IXa, Xa, XIa, and XIIa, as well as plasmin.

The neutralization rate of serine proteases by AT-III proceeds slowly in the absence of heparin, but is greatly accelerated in the presence of heparin. As the therapeutic antithrombotic effect in vivo of heparin is mediated by AT-III, heparin is ineffective in the absence or near absence of AT-III.

The prevalence of the hereditary deficiency of AT-III is estimated to be 1 per 2,000 to 5,000 in the general population. The pattern of inheritance is autosomal dominant. In affected individuals, spontaneous episodes of thrombosis and pulmonary embolism may be associated with AT-III levels of 40% to 60% of normal. These episodes usually appear after the age of 20, the risk increasing with age and in association with surgery, pregnancy, and delivery. The frequency of thromboembolic events in hereditary AT-III deficiency during pregnancy has been reported to be 70%, and several studies of the beneficial use of antithrombin III (human) concentrates during pregnancy in women with hereditary deficiency have been reported. In many cases, however, no precipitating factor can be identified for venous thrombosis or pulmonary embolism. Greater than 85% of individuals with hereditary AT-III deficiency have had at least 1 thrombotic episode by 50 years of age. In about 60% of patients thrombosis is recurrent. Clinical signs of pulmonary embolism occur in 40% of affected individuals. In some individuals, treatment with oral anticoagulants leads to an increase of the endogenous levels of AT-III, and treatment with oral anticoagulants may be effective in the prevention of thrombosis in such individuals.

Contraindications

None known.

Warnings

➤*Viral infections:* Antithrombin III (human) is made from human plasma. Products made from human plasma may contain infectious agents, such as viruses, that can cause disease. The risk that such products will transmit an infectious agent has been reduced by screening plasma donors for prior exposure to certain viruses, testing for the presence of certain current virus infections, and inactivating or removing certain viruses. Despite these measures, such products can still potentially transmit disease. There is also the possibility that unknown infectious agents may be present in such products. Individuals who receive infusions of blood or plasma products may develop signs or symptoms of some viral infections, particularly hepatitis C.

Report all infections possibly transmitted by this product to the manufacturer at (888) 765-3203.

Discuss the risks and benefits of this product with the patient, before prescribing or administering it to a patient.

➤*Pregnancy: Category B.* Reproduction studies have been performed in rats and rabbits at doses up to 4 times the human dose and have revealed no evidence of impaired fertility or harm to the fetus due to antithrombin III (human). It is not known whether antithrombin III (human) can cause fetal harm when administered to a pregnant woman or can affect reproduction capacity. Because animal reproduction studies are not always predictive of human response, use this drug during pregnancy only if clearly needed.

➤*Children:* Safety and efficacy in the pediatric population have not been established. The AT-III level in neonates of parents with hereditary AT-III deficiency should be measured immediately after birth. (Fatal neonatal thromboembolism, such as aortic thrombi in children of women with hereditary antithrombin III deficiency, has been reported.)

Plasma levels of AT-III are lower in neonates than adults, averaging approximately 60% in healthy term infants. AT-III levels in premature infants may be much lower. Low plasma AT-III levels, especially in a premature infant, therefore, do not necessarily indicate hereditary deficiency. It is recommended that testing and treatment with antithrombin III of neonates be discussed with an expert on coagulation.

Precautions

➤*Monitoring:* It is recommended that AT-III plasma levels be monitored during the treatment period. Functional levels of AT-III in plasma may be measured by amidolytic assays using chromogenic substrates or by clotting assays.

➤*Administration general information:*

1.) Administer within 3 hours after reconstitution. Do not refrigerate after reconstitution.
2.) Administer only by the IV route.
3.) Once reconstituted, give antithrombin III (human) alone, without mixing with other agents or diluting solutions.
4.) Product administration and handling of needles must be done with caution. Percutaneous puncture with a needle contaminated with blood can transmit infectious virus including HIV (the virus that causes AIDS) and hepatitis. Obtain immediate medical attention if injury occurs.

Place needles in sharps container after single use. Discard all equipment, including any reconstituted antithrombin III (human) product in accordance with biohazard procedures.

➤*Antithrombin III deficiency diagnosis:* Base the diagnosis of hereditary AT-III deficiency on a clear family history of venous thrombosis as well as decreased plasma AT-III levels, and the exclusion of acquired deficiency.

Drug Interactions

➤*Heparin:* The anticoagulant effect of heparin is enhanced by concurrent treatment with antithrombin III (human) in patients with hereditary AT-III deficiency. Thus, in order to avoid bleeding, reduced dosage of heparin is recommended during treatment with antithrombin III (human).

Adverse Reactions

In clinical studies involving antithrombin III (human), adverse reactions were reported in association with 17 of the 340 infusions during the clinical studies. Included were dizziness (7), chest tightness (3), nausea (3), foul taste in mouth (3), chills (2), cramps (2), shortness of breath (1), chest pain (1), film over eye (1), light-headedness (1), bowel fullness (1), hives (1), fever (1), and oozing and hematoma formation (1). If adverse reactions are experienced, decrease the infusion rate, or, if indicated, interrupt the infusion until symptoms abate.

Thrombin Inhibitor

DESIRUDIN

Rx	**Iprivask** (Aventis)	**Powder for injection, lyophilized:** 15 mg	Preservative free. In single-use vials with diluent.[1]

[1] Diluent includes 0.6 mL mannitol (3%) in water for injection.

DESIRUDIN — INJECTION

WARNING

Spinal/Epidural hematomas – When neuraxial anesthesia (epidural/spinal anesthesia) or spinal puncture is employed, patients anticoagulated or scheduled to be anticoagulated with selective inhibitors of thrombin such as desirudin may be at risk of developing an epidural or spinal hematoma which can result in long-term or permanent paralysis.

The risk of these events may be increased by the use of indwelling spinal catheters for administration of analgesia or by the concomitant use of drugs affecting hemostasis such as nonsteroidal anti-inflammatory drugs (NSAIDs), platelet inhibitors, or other anticoagulants. Likewise with such agents, the risk appears to be increased by traumatic or repeated epidural or spinal puncture.

Patients should be frequently monitored for signs and symptoms of neurological impairment. If neurological compromise is noted, urgent treatment is necessary.

The physician should consider the potential benefit versus risk before neuraxial intervention, in patients anticoagulated or to be anticoagulated for thromboprophylaxis.

Indications

➤*Deep vein thrombosis, prophylaxis:* Desirudin is indicated for the prophylaxis of deep vein thrombosis, which may lead to pulmonary embolism, in patients undergoing elective hip-replacement surgery.

Administration and Dosage

➤*Approved by the FDA:* April 4, 2003.

All patients should be evaluated for bleeding disorder risk before prophylactic administration of desirudin. Any agent which may enhance the risk of hemorrhage should be discontinued prior to initiation of desirudin therapy. These agents include medications such as dextran 40, systemic glucocorticoids, thrombolytics, and anticoagulants.

➤*Initial dosage:* In patients undergoing hip-replacement surgery, the recommended dose of desirudin is 15 mg every 12 hours administered by SC injection, with the initial dose given up to 5 to 15 minutes prior to surgery, but after induction of regional block anesthesia, if used. Up to 12 days administration (average duration 9 to 12 days) of desirudin has been well tolerated in controlled clinical trials.

DESIRUDIN — INJECTION

➤*Renal function impairment:*

Desirudin Use in Renal Function Impairment		
Degree of renal insufficiency	Creatinine clearance (mL/min/1.73 m² body surface area)	aPTT monitoring and dosing instructions
Moderate	≥ 31 to 60	Initiate therapy at 5 mg every 12 hours by SC injection. Monitor aPTT and serum creatinine at least daily. If aPTT exceeds 2 times control: 1) Interrupt therapy until the value returns to less than 2 times control. 2) Resume therapy at a reduced dose guided by the initial degree of aPTT abnormality.
Severe	< 31	Initiate therapy at 1.7 mg every 12 hours. Monitor aPTT and serum creatinine at least daily. If aPTT exceeds 2 times control: 1) Interrupt therapy until the value returns to less than 2 times control. 2) Consider further dose reductions guided by the initial degree of aPTT abnormality.

➤*Hepatic function impairment:* In the absence of clinical studies in this population, dosing recommendations cannot be made at this time. Although desirudin is not significantly metabolized by the liver, hepatic impairment or serious liver injury (eg, liver cirrhosis) may alter the anticoagulant effect of desirudin due to coagulation defects secondary to reduced generation of vitamin K-dependent coagulation factors. Desirudin should be used with caution in these patients.

➤*Preparation for administration:*

1.) Reconstitution should be carried out under sterile conditions.
2.) Reconstitute each vial with 0.5 mL of provided diluent [mannitol USP (3%) in Water for Injection]. Once reconstituted, each 0.5 mL contains 15.75 mg of desirudin.
3.) Shake the vial gently until the drug is fully reconstituted.
4.) Reconstituted desirudin is a clear colorless solution. Inspect desirudin visually for particulate matter and discoloration prior to administration. Do not use solutions that are cloudy or contain particles.
5.) Use a syringe with a 26- or 27-gauge needle which is approximately ½ inch in length to withdraw all of the reconstituted solution (15.75 mg desirudin/0.5 mL) and inject the entire contents of the syringe SC, which will deliver 15 mg.
6.) The reconstituted solution should be used immediately; however, it is stable for up to 24 hours when stored at room temperature and protected from light. Discard any unused solution appropriately.

Desirudin should not be mixed with other injections, solvents, or infusions. Desirudin is administered by SC injection. It must not be administered by IM injection.

➤*SC injection technique:* Select a syringe with a 26- or 27-gauge needle which is approximately ½ inch in length for administration of desirudin. Withdraw the entire reconstituted solution (15.75 mg desirudin/0.5 mL) into the syringe and inject the total volume SC.

Patients should be sitting or lying down, and desirudin injection should be administered by deep SC injection. Administration should be alternated between the left and right anterolateral and left and right posterolateral thigh or abdominal wall. The whole length of the needle should be introduced into a skin fold held between the thumb and forefinger; the skin fold should be held throughout the injection. To minimize bruising, do not rub the injection site after completion of the injection.

➤*Storage/Stability:* Protect from light.

Unopened vials or ampules – Store at 25°C (77°F); excursions permitted to 15° to 30°C (59° to 86°F).

Actions

➤*Pharmacology:* Desirudin is a selective inhibitor of free circulating and clot-bound thrombin. The anticoagulant properties of desirudin are demonstrated by its ability to prolong the clotting time of human plasma. One molecule of desirudin binds to 1 molecule of thrombin and thereby blocks the thrombogenic activity of thrombin. As a result, all thrombin-dependent coagulation assays are affected. Activated partial thromboplastin time (aPTT) is a measure of the anticoagulant activity of desirudin and increases in a dose-dependent fashion. The pharmacodynamic effect of desirudin on proteolytic activity of thrombin was assessed as an increase in aPTT. A mean peak aPTT prolongation of about 1.38 times baseline value (range 0.58 to 3.41) was observed following SC twice-daily injections of 15 mg desirudin. Thrombin time (TT) frequently exceeds 200 seconds even at low plasma concentrations of desirudin, which renders this test unsuitable for routine monitoring of desirudin therapy. At therapeutic serum concentrations, desirudin has no effect on other enzymes of the hemostatic system such as factors IXa, Xa, kallikrein, plasmin, tissue plasminogen activator, or activated protein C. In addition, it does not display any effect on other serine proteases, such as the digestive enzymes trypsin, chymotrypsin, or on complement activation by the classical or alternative pathways.

➤*Pharmacokinetics:*

Absorption – Pharmacokinetic parameters were calculated based on plasma concentration data obtained by a nonspecific enzyme-linked immunosorbent assay (ELISA) method that does not discriminate between native desirudin and its metabolites. It is not known if the metabolites are pharmacologically active.

The absorption of desirudin is complete when administered SC at doses of 0.3 mg/kg or 0.5 mg/kg. Following SC administration of single doses of 0.1 to 0.75 mg/kg, plasma concentrations of desirudin increased to a maximum level (C_{max}) between 1 and 3 hours. Both C_{max} and area-under-the-curve (AUC) values are dose proportional.

Distribution – The pharmacokinetic properties of desirudin following IV administration are well described by a 2- or 3- compartment disposition model. Desirudin is distributed in the extracellular space with a volume of distribution at steady state of 0.25 L/kg, independent of the dose. Desirudin binds specifically and directly to thrombin, forming an extremely tight, noncovalent complex with an inhibition constant of approximately 2.6×10^{-13} M. Thus, free or protein bound desirudin immediately binds circulating thrombin. The pharmacological effect of desirudin is not modified when coadministered with highly protein-bound drugs (greater than 99%).

Metabolism – Human and animal data suggest that desirudin is primarily eliminated and metabolized by the kidney. The total urinary excretion of unchanged desirudin amounts to 40% to 50% of the administered dose. Metabolites lacking 1 or 2 C-terminal amino acids constitute a minor proportion of the material recovered from urine (less than 7%). There is no evidence for the presence of other metabolites. This indicates that desirudin is metabolized by stepwise degradation from the C-terminus probably catalyzed by carboxypeptidase(s) such as carboxypeptidase A, originating from the pancreas. Total clearance of desirudin is approximately 1.5 to 2.7 mL/min/kg following either SC or IV administration and is independent of dose. This clearance value is close to the glomerular filtration rate.

Excretion – The elimination of desirudin from plasma is rapid after IV administration, with approximately 90% of the dose disappearing from the plasma within 2 hours of the injection. Plasma concentrations of desirudin then decline with a mean terminal elimination half-life of 2 to 3 hours. After SC administration, the mean terminal elimination half-life is also approximately 2 hours.

Special populations –

Renal function impairment: In a pharmacokinetic study of renally impaired subjects, subjects with mild (creatinine clearance [Ccr] between 61 and 90 mL/min/1.73 m² body surface area), moderate (Ccr between 31 and 60 mL/min/1.73 m² body surface area), and severe (Ccr below 31 mL/min/1.73 m² body surface area) renal insufficiency, were administered a single IV dose of 0.5, 0.25, or 0.125 mg/kg desirudin, respectively. This resulted in mean dose-normalized AUC_{effect} ($AUC_{0\text{-}60th}$ for aPTT prolongation) increases of approximately 3-, and 9-fold for the moderate and severe renally impaired subjects, respectively, compared with healthy individuals. In subjects with mild renal impairment, there was no increase in AUC_{effect} compared with healthy individuals. In subjects with severe renal insufficiency, terminal elimination half-lives were prolonged up to 12 hours compared with 2 to 4 hours in healthy volunteers or subjects with mild-to-moderate renal insufficiency. Dose adjustments are recommended in certain circumstances in relation to the degree of impairment or degree of aPTT abnormality.

Age/Gender: The mean plasma clearance of desirudin in patients greater than or equal to 65 years of age (n = 12; 110 mL/min) is approximately 28% lower than in patients younger than 65 years of age (n = 8; 153 mL/min). Population pharmacokinetics conducted in 301 patients undergoing elective total hip replacement indicate that age or gender do not affect the systemic clearance of desirudin when renal creatinine clearance is considered. This drug is substantially excreted by the kidney, and the risk of adverse events due to it may be greater in patients with impaired renal function. Because elderly patients are more likely to have decreased renal function, care should be taken in dose selection, and it may be useful to monitor renal function. Dosage adjustment in the case of moderate and severe renal impairment is necessary.

Contraindications

Hypersensitivity to natural or recombinant hirudins; active bleeding or irreversible coagulation disorders.

Warnings

➤*Hemorrhagic events:* Desirudin is not intended for IM injection, as local hematoma formation may result.

Desirudin, like other anticoagulants, should be used with caution in patients with increased risks of hemorrhage such as those with recent major surgery, organ biopsy or puncture of a noncompressible vessel within the last month; a history of hemorrhagic stroke, intracranial or intraocular bleeding including diabetic (hemorrhagic) retinopathy; recent ischemic stroke, severe uncontrolled hypertension, bacterial endocarditis, a known hemostatic disorder (congenital or acquired [eg, hemophilia, liver disease]) or a history of GI or pulmonary bleeding within the past 3 months.

Bleeding can occur at any site during therapy with desirudin. An unexplained fall in hematocrit or blood pressure should lead to a search for a bleeding site.

➤*Spinal/epidural anesthesia:* As with other anticoagulants, there is a risk of neuraxial hematoma formation with the concurrent use of desirudin and spinal/epidural anesthesia, which has the potential to result in long term or permanent paralysis. The risk may be greater with the use of postoperative indwelling catheters or the concomitant use of additional drugs affecting hemostasis such as nonsteroidal anti-inflammatory drugs

DESIRUDIN — INJECTION

(NSAIDs), platelet inhibitors or other anticoagulants. The risk may also be increased by traumatic or repeated neuraxial puncture.

To reduce the potential risk of bleeding associated with the concurrent use of desirudin and epidural or spinal anesthesia/analgesia, the pharmacokinetic profile of the drug should be considered when scheduling or using epidural or spinal anesthesia in proximity to desirudin administration. The physician should consider placement of the catheter prior to initiating desirudin and removal of the catheter when the anticoagulant effect of desirudin is low.

Should the physician decide to administer anticoagulation in the context of epidural/spinal anesthesia, extreme vigilance and frequent monitoring must be exercised to detect any signs and symptoms of neurological impairment such as midline back pain, sensory and motor deficits (numbness or weakness in lower limbs), bowel or bladder dysfunction. Patients should be instructed to inform their physicians immediately if they experience any of the above signs or symptoms. If signs or symptoms of spinal hematoma are suspected, urgent diagnosis and treatment including spinal cord decompression should be initiated.

The physician should consider the potential benefit versus risk before neuraxial intervention in patients anticoagulated or to be anticoagulated for thromboprophylaxis.

Interchangeability – Desirudin cannot be used interchangeably with other hirudins as they differ in manufacturing process and specific biological activity (ATUs). Each of these medicines has its own instructions for use.

➤*Hypersensitivity reactions:*

Antibodies/reexposure – Antibodies have been reported in patients treated with hirudins. Potential for cross-sensitivity to hirudin products cannot be excluded. Irritative skin reactions were observed in 9/322 volunteers exposed to desirudin by SC injection or IV bolus or infusion in single or multiple administrations of the drug. Allergic events were reported in less than 2% of patients who were administered desirudin in phase III clinical trials. Allergic events were reported in 1% of patients receiving unfractionated heparin and 1% of patients receiving enoxaparin. Hirudin-specific IgE evaluations may not be indicative of sensitivity to desirudin as this test was not always positive in the presence of symptoms. Very rarely, antihirudin antibodies have been detected upon reexposure to desirudin. Fatal anaphylactoid reactions have been reported during hirudin therapy.

➤*Renal function impairment:* Desirudin must be used with caution in patients with renal impairment, particularly in those with moderate and severe renal impairment (creatinine clearance less than or equal to 60 mL/min/1.73 m^2 body surface area). Dose reductions by factors of 3 and 9 are recommended for patients with moderate and severe renal impairment respectively. In addition, daily aPTT and serum creatinine monitoring are recommended for patients with moderate or severe renal impairment.

➤*Hepatic function impairment:* No information is available about the use of desirudin in patients with hepatic insufficiency/liver injury. Although desirudin is not significantly metabolized by the liver, hepatic impairment or serious liver injury (eg, liver cirrhosis) may alter the anticoagulant effect of desirudin due to coagulation defects secondary to reduced generation of vitamin K-dependent coagulation factors. Desirudin should be used with caution in these patients.

➤*Elderly:* In 3 clinical studies of desirudin, the percentage of patients greater than 65 years of age treated with 15 mg of desirudin SC every 12 hours was 58.5%, while 20.8% were 75 years of age or older. Elderly patients treated with desirudin had a reduction in the incidence of VTE similar to that observed in the younger patients, and a slightly lower incidence of VTE compared to those patients treated with heparin or enoxaparin.

Regarding safety, in the clinical studies the incidence of hemorrhage (major or otherwise) in patients 65 years of age or older was similar to that in patients less than 65 years of age. In addition, the elderly had a similar incidence of total, treatment-related, or serious adverse events compared to those patients less than 65 years of age. Serious adverse events occurred more frequently in patients 75 years of age or older as compared to those less than 65 years of age. In general, 15 mg desirudin every 12 hours can be used safely in the geriatric population as in the population of patients younger than 65 years of age so long as renal function is adequate.

➤*Pregnancy: Category C.* Teratology studies have been performed in rats at SC doses in a range of 1 to 15 mg/kg/day (about 0.3 to 4 times the recommended human dose based on body surface area) and in rabbits at IV doses in a range of 0.6 to 6 mg/kg/day (about 0.3 to 3 times the recommended human dose based on body surface area) and have revealed desirudin to be teratogenic. Observed teratogenic findings were omphalocele, asymmetric and fused sternebrae, edema, shortened hind limbs in rats; and spina bifida, malrotated hind limb, hydrocephaly, gastroschisis in rabbits. There are no adequate and well-controlled studies in pregnant women. Desirudin should be used during pregnancy only if the potential benefit justifies the potential risk to the fetus.

➤*Lactation:* It is not known whether desirudin is excreted in human milk. Because many drugs are excreted in human milk, caution should be exercised when desirudin is administered to a nursing woman.

➤*Children:* Safety and efficacy in pediatric patients have not been established.

Precautions

➤*Monitoring:* Activated partial thromboplastin time (aPTT) should be monitored daily in patients with increased risk of bleeding or renal impairment. Serum creatinine should be monitored daily in patients with renal impairment. Peak aPTT should not exceed 2 times control. Should peak aPTT exceed this level, dose reduction is advised, based on the degree of aPTT abnormality. If necessary, therapy with desirudin should be interrupted until aPTT falls to less than 2 times control, at which time treatment with desirudin can be resumed at a reduced dose). Thrombin time (TT) is not a suitable test for routine monitoring of desirudin therapy. Dose adjustments based on serum creatinine may be necessary.

Drug Interactions

Desirudin Drug Interactions			
Precipitant drug	Object drug*		Description
Thrombolytics (eg,alteplase, streptokinase), Glucocorticoids Dextran	Desirudin	↑	Concomitant treatment with thrombolytics may increase the risk of bleeding. Discontinue before initiations of desirudin therapy.
Anticoagulants (eg, heparin [unfractionated and LMWH])	Desirudin	↑	During prophylaxis of venous thromboembolism, concomitant treatment is not recommended. The effects include prolongation of aPTT. As with other anticoagulants, desirudin should be used with caution.
Antiplatelets and glycoprotein IIb/IIIa antagonists (eg, salicylates, NSAIDs, ketorolac, acetylsalicylic acid, triclopidine, dipyridamole, sulfinpyrazone, clopidogrel, abciximab)	Desirudin	↑	Use with caution in conjunction with desirudin

* ↑ = Object drug increased.

Adverse Reactions

In the phase II and III clinical studies, desirudin was administered to 2159 patients undergoing elective hip-replacement surgery to determine the safety and efficacy of desirudin in preventing VTE in this population. Below is the safety profile of the desirudin 15 mg (every 12 hours) regimen from these 5 multicenter clinical trials.

Hemorrhagic events –

Hemorrhage in Patients Undergoing Hip-replacement Surgery			
	Dosing regimen		
	Desirudin 15 mg every 12 hours SC (n = 1561) n (%)	Heparin 5000 IU every 8 hours SC (n = 501) n (%)	Enoxaparin 40 mg every day SC (n = 1036) n (%)
Patients with any hemorrhage [a]	464 (30%)	111 (22%)	341 (33%)
Patients with serious hemorrhage [b]	41 (3%)	15 (3%)	21 (2%)
Patients with major hemorrhage [c]	13 (< 1%)	0 (0%)	2 (< 1%)

[a] Includes hematomas which occurred at an incidence of 6% in the desirudin and enoxaparin treatment groups and 5% in the heparin treatment group.
[b] Bleeding complications were considered serious if perioperative transfusion requirements exceeded 5 units of whole blood or packed red cells, or if total transfusion requirements up to postoperative day 6 inclusive exceeded 7 units of whole blood or packed red cells, or total blood loss up to postoperative day 6 inclusive exceeded 3500 mL.
[c] Bleeding complications were considered major if the hemorrhage was overt and it produced a fall in hemoglobin of greater than or equal to 2 g/dL or if it lead to a transfusion of 2 or more units of whole or packed cells outside the perioperative period (the time from start of surgery until up to 12 hours after) and retroperitoneal, intracranial, intraocular, intraspinal, or occurred in a major prosthetic joint.

Nonhemorrhagic reactions –

Adverse Reactions Occurring at ≥ 2% in Desirudin-treated Patients Undergoing Hip-replacement Surgery[a,b]			
Body system (Preferred term)	Desirudin 15 mg every 12 hours SC (n = 1561) n (%)	Heparin 5000 IU every 8 hours SC (n = 501) n (%)	Enoxaparin 40 mg every day SC (n = 1036) n (%)
Injection site mass	56 (4%)	32 (6%)	7 (< 1%)
Wound secretion	59 (4%)	23 (5%)	34 (3%)
Anemia	51 (3%)	11 (2%)	37 (4%)

DESIRUDIN — INJECTION

Adverse Reactions Occurring at ≥ 2% in Desirudin-treated Patients Undergoing Hip-replacement Surgery[a,b]			
Body system (Preferred term)	Desirudin 15 mg every 12 hours SC (n = 1561) n (%)	Heparin 5000 IU every 8 hours SC (n = 501) n (%)	Enoxaparin 40 mg every day SC (n = 1036) n (%)
Deep thrombophlebitis	24 (2%)	41 (8%)	22 (2%)
Nausea	24 (2%)	6 (< 1%)	10 (< 1%)

[a] Represents reactions reported while on treatment, excluding unrelated adverse reactions.

[b] All hemorrhages that occurred are included in Adverse Reactions.

Related adverse reactions with a frequency of less than 2% and greater than 0.2% (in decreasing order of frequency) – Thrombosis, hypotension, leg edema, fever, decreased hemoglobin, hematuria, dizziness, epistaxis, vomiting, impaired healing, cerebrovascular disorder, leg pain, hematemesis.

Hypersensitivity reactions – In clinical studies, allergic events were reported less than 2% overall and in 2% of patients who were administered 15 mg desirudin.

Postmarketing – In addition to adverse reactions reported from clinical trials the following adverse reactions have been identified during postapproval use of desirudin. These events were reported voluntarily from a population of unknown size and the frequency of occurrence cannot be determined precisely: Rare reports of major hemorrhages, some of which were fatal, and anaphylactic/anaphylactoid reactions.

Overdosage

➤*Animal pharmacology and toxicology:*

General toxicity – Desirudin produced bleeding, local inflammation, and granulation at injection sites in rat and dog toxicity studies. In a 28-day study in rhesus monkeys, there was also evidence of SC bleeding and local inflammation at the injection sites. In addition, desirudin was immunogenic in dogs and formed antibody complexes resulting in prolonged half-life and accumulation. Desirudin showed sensitization potential in guinea pig immediate and delayed hypersensitivity models.

➤*Treatment:* In case of overdose, most likely reflected in hemorrhagic complications or suggested by excessively high aPTT values, desirudin therapy should be discontinued. Emergency procedures should be instituted as appropriate (for example, determination of aPTT and other coagulation levels, hemoglobin, the use of blood transfusion or plasma expanders).

No specific antidote for desirudin is available; however, the anticoagulant effect of desirudin is partially reversible using thrombin-rich plasma concentrates while aPTT levels can be reduced by the IV administration of 0.3 mcg/kg DDAVP (desmopressin). The clinical effectiveness of DDAVP in treating bleeding due to desirudin overdose has not been studied. In an open, pilot, dose-ascending study to assess safety, the highest dose of desirudin (40 mg every 12 hours) caused excessive hemorrhage.

LEPIRUDIN

Rx	**Refludan** (Hoechst-Marion Roussel)	**Powder for injection:** 50 mg	Mannitol. Freeze-dried. In boxes of 10.

LEPIRUDIN — INJECTION

Indications

➤*Thrombocytopenia, heparin-induced:* Lepirudin is indicated for anticoagulation in patients with heparin-induced thrombocytopenia (HIT) and associated thromboembolic disease in order to prevent further thromboembolic complications.

Administration and Dosage

➤*Approved by the FDA:* March 6, 1998.

➤*Initial dosage:*

Anticoagulation in adult patients with HIT and associated thromboembolic disease – 0.4 mg/kg body weight (up to 110 kg) slowly IV (eg, over 15 to 20 seconds) as a bolus dose, followed by 0.15 mg/kg body weight (up to 110 kg)/hour as a continuous IV infusion for 2 to 10 days or longer if clinically needed. Normally the initial dosage depends on the patient's body weight. This is valid up to a body weight of 110 kg. In patients with a body weight exceeding 110 kg, the initial dosage should not be increased beyond the 110 kg body weight dose (maximal initial bolus dose of 44 mg, maximal initial infusion dose of 16.5 mg/hr.

In general, therapy with lepirudin is monitored using the aPTT ratio (patient aPTT at a given time over an aPTT reference value, usually median of the laboratory normal range for aPTT) (see Monitoring and adjusting therapy). A patient baseline aPTT should be determined prior to initiation of therapy with lepirudin, since lepirudin should not be started in patients presenting with a baseline aPTT ratio of 2.5 or more, in order to avoid initial overdosing.

➤*Dose modifications:* Any aPTT ratio out of the target range is to be confirmed at once before drawing conclusions with respect to dose modifications, unless there is a clinical need to react immediately.

If the confirmed aPTT ratio is above the target range, the infusion should be stopped for 2 hours. At restart, the infusion rate should be decreased by 50% (no additional IV bolus should be administered). The aPTT ratio should be determined again 4 hours later.

If the confirmed aPTT ratio is below the target range, the infusion rate should be increased in steps of 20%. The aPTT ratio should be determined again 4 hours later.

In general, an infusion rate of 0.21 mg/kg/hr should not be exceeded without checking for coagulation abnormalities which might be preventive of an appropriate aPTT response.

➤*Monitoring therapy:* In general, the dosage (infusion rate) should be adjusted according to the aPTT ratio (patient aPTT at a given time over an aPTT reference value, usually median of the laboratory normal range for aPTT).

The target range for the aPTT ratio during treatment (therapeutic window) should be 1.5 to 2.5. Data from clinical trials in HIT patients suggest that with aPTT ratios higher than this target range, the risk of bleeding increases, while there is no incremental increase in clinical efficacy.

Lepirudin should not be started in patients presenting with a baseline aPTT ratio of 2.5 or more, in order to avoid initial overdosing.

The first aPTT determination for monitoring treatment should be done 4 hours after start of the lepirudin infusion.

Follow-up aPTT determinations are recommended at least once daily, as long as treatment with lepirudin is ongoing.

More frequent aPTT monitoring is highly recommended in patients with renal impairment or serious liver injury (see Use in renal impairment) or with an increased risk of bleeding.

➤*Renal function impairment:* As lepirudin is almost exclusively excreted in the kidneys, individual renal function should be considered prior to administration. In case of renal impairment, relative overdose might occur even with the standard dosage regimen. Therefore, the bolus dose and the infusion rate must be reduced in case of known or suspected renal insufficiency (creatinine clearance below 60 mL/min or serum creatinine above 1.5 mg/dL).

There is only limited information on the therapeutic use of lepirudin in HIT patients with significant renal impairment. The following dosage recommendations are mainly based on single-dose studies in a small number of patients with renal impairment. Therefore, these recommendations are only tentative and aPTT monitoring should be used along with monitoring of renal status.

Dose adjustments should be based on creatinine clearance values, whenever available, as obtained from a reliable method (24-hour urine sampling). If creatinine clearance is not available, the dose adjustments should be based on the serum creatinine.

In all patients with renal insufficiency, the bolus dose is to be reduced to 0.2 mg/kg body weight. The standard initial infusion rate given in initial dosage and IV infusion must be reduced according to the recommendations given in the following data. Additional aPTT monitoring is highly recommended.

Reduction of Infusion Rate in Patients With Renal Impairment			
		Adjusted infusion rate	
Creatinine clearance (mL/min)	Serum creatinine (mg/dL)	% of standard initial infusion rate	(mg/kg/hr)
45 to 60 mL/min	1.6 to 2 mg/dL	50%	0.075 mg/kg/hr
30 to 44 mL/min	2.1 to 3 mg/dL	30%	0.045 mg/kg/hr
15 to 29 mL/min	3.1 to 6 mg/dL	15%	0.0225 mg/kg/hr
below 15*	above 6*	avoid or stop infusion*	

* In hemodialysis patients or in case of acute renal failure (creatinine clearance below 15 mL/min or serum creatinine above 6 mg/dL), infusion of lepirudin is to be avoided or stopped. Additional IV bolus doses of 0.1 mg/kg body weight should be considered every other day only if the aPTT ratio falls below the lower therapeutic limit of 1.5.

➤*Concomitant use with thrombolytic therapy:* Clinical trials in HIT patients have provided only limited information on the combined use of lepirudin and thrombolytic agents. The following dosage regimen of lepirudin was used in a total of 9 HIT patients in the historically controlled clinical trials (HAT-1 and HAT-2) studies who presented with thromboembolic complications (TECs) at baseline and were started on both lepirudin and thrombolytic therapy (rt-PA, urokinase or streptokinase): Initial IV bolus, 0.2 mg/kg body weight; continuous IV infusion, 0.1 mg/kg body weight/hr.

The number of patients receiving combined therapy was too small to identify differences in clinical outcome of patients who were started on both lepirudin and thrombolytic therapy as compared to those who were started on lepirudin alone. The combined incidences of death, limb amputation, or new TEC were 22.2% and 20.7%, respectively. While there was a 47% relative increase in the overall bleeding rate in patients who were started on both lepirudin and thrombolytic therapy (55.6% vs 37.9%), there were no differences in the rates of serious bleeding events (fatal or life-threatening bleeds,

LEPIRUDIN — INJECTION

bleeds that were permanently or significantly disabling, overt bleeds requiring transfusion of 2 or more units of packed red blood cells, bleeds necessitating surgical intervention, intracranial bleeds) between the groups (11.1% vs 11.2%). Although no intracranial bleeding has been observed in any of these patients, there have been reports of intracranial bleeding in the presence or absence of concomitant thrombolytic therapy.

Special attention should be paid to the fact that thrombolytic agents per se may increase the aPTT ratio. Therefore, aPTT ratios with a given plasma level of lepirudin are usually higher in patients who receive concomitant thrombolysis than in those who do not.

➤*Patients scheduled for a switch to oral anticoagulation:* If a patient is scheduled to receive coumarin derivatives (vitamin K antagonists) for oral anticoagulation after lepirudin therapy, the dose of lepirudin should first be gradually reduced in order to reach an aPTT ratio just above 1.5 before initiating oral anticoagulation. Coumarin derivatives should be initiated only when platelet counts are normalizing. The intended maintenance dose should be started with no loading dose. To avoid prothrombotic effects when initiating coumarin, continue parenteral anticoagulation for 4 to 5 days (see oral anticoagulant monograph for information). The parenteral agent can be discontinued when the INR stabilizes within the desired target range.

➤*Administration:*

Directions on preparation and dilution – Lepirudin should not be mixed with other drugs except for Sterile Water for Injection, 0.9% Sodium Chloride Injection or 5% Dextrose Injection.

Reconstitution and further dilution are to be carried out under sterile conditions:

- For reconstitution, Sterile Water for Injection or 0.9% Sodium Chloride Injection are to be used.
- For further dilution, Sodium Chloride Injection or 5% Dextrose Injection are suitable.
- For rapid, complete reconstitution, inject 1 mL of diluent into the vial and shake it gently. After reconstitution a clear, colorless solution is usually obtained in a few seconds, but definitely in less than 3 minutes.
- Parenteral drug products should be inspected visually for particulate matter and discoloration prior to administration whenever solution and container permit. Do not use solutions that are cloudy or contain particles.
- The reconstituted solution is to be used immediately. It remains stable for up to 24 hours at room temperature (eg, during infusion).
- The preparation should be warmed to room temperature before administration.
- Discard any unused solution appropriately.

➤*Initial IV bolus:* For IV bolus injection, use a solution with a concentration of 5 mg/mL.

Preparation of a lepirudin solution with a concentration of 5 mg/mL:

- Reconstitute 1 vial (50 mg of lepirudin) with 1 mL of Sterile Water for Injection or 0.9% Sodium Chloride Injection.
- The final concentration of 5 mg/mL is obtained by transferring the contents of the vial into a sterile, single-use syringe (of at least 10 mL capacity) and diluting the solution to a total volume of 10 mL, using Sterile Water for Injection, 0.9% Sodium Chloride Injection or 5% Dextrose Injection.
- The final solution is to be administered according to body weight (see table below and Initial dose).

IV injection of the bolus is to be carried out slowly (eg, over 15 to 20 seconds).

Standard Bolus Injection Volumes According to Body Weight for a 5 mg/mL Concentrate		
	Injection volume	
Body weight (kg)	Dosage 0.4 mg/kg	Dosage 0.2 mg/kg*
50 kg	4 mL	2 mL
60 kg	4.8 mL	2.4 mL
70 kg	5.6 mL	2.8 mL
80 kg	6.4 mL	3.2 mL
90 kg	7.2 mL	3.6 mL
100 kg	8 mL	4 mL
≥ 110 kg	8.8 mL	4.4 mL

* Dosage recommended for all patients with renal insufficiency.

➤*IV infusion:* For continuous IV infusion, solutions with concentration of 0.2 mg/mL or 0.4 mg/mL may be used.

Preparation of a lepirudin solution with a concentration of 0.2 or 0.4 mg/mL:

- Reconstitute 2 vials (each containing 50 mg of lepirudin) with 1 mL each using either Sterile Water for Injection or 0.9% Sodium Chloride Injection.
- The final concentrations of 0.2 mg/mL or 0.4 mg/mL are obtained by transferring the contents of both vials into an infusion bag containing 500 mL or 250 mL of 0.9% Sodium Chloride Injection or 5% Dextrose Injection.

The infusion rate (mL/hr) is to be set according to body weight (see Initial dosage).

Standard Infusion Rates According to Body Weight		
	Infusion rate at 0.15 mg/kg/hr	
Body weight (kg)	500 mL infusion bag 0.2 mg/mL	250 mL infusion bag 0.4 mg/mL
50 kg	38 mL/hr	19 mL/hr
60 kg	45 mL/hr	23 mL/hr
70 kg	53 mL/hr	26 mL/hr
80 kg	60 mL/hr	30 mL/hr
90 kg	68 mL/hr	34 mL/hr
100 kg	75 mL/hr	38 mL/hr
≥ 110 kg	83 mL/hr	41 mL/hr

➤*Storage/Stability:* Store unopened vials at 2° to 25°C (36° to 77°F). Once reconstituted, use lepirudin immediately.

Actions

➤*Pharmacology:* The pharmacodynamic effect of lepirudin on the proteolytic activity of thrombin was routinely assessed as an increase in aPTT. This was observed with increasing plasma concentrations of lepirudin, with no saturable effect up to the highest tested dose (0.5 mg/kg body weight IV bolus). Thrombin time (TT) frequently exceeded 200 seconds even at low plasma concentrations of lepirudin, which renders this test unsuitable for routine monitoring of lepirudin therapy.

The pharmacodynamic response defined by the aPTT ratio (aPTT at a time after lepirudin administration over an aPTT reference value, usually median of the laboratory normal range for aPTT) depends on plasma drug levels which in turn depend on the individual patient's renal function. For patients undergoing additional thrombolysis, elevated aPTT ratios were already observed at low lepirudin plasma concentrations, and further response to increasing plasma concentrations was relatively flat. In other populations, the response was steeper. At plasma concentrations of 1500 ng/mL, aPTT ratios were nearly 3 for healthy volunteers, 2.3 for patients with heparin-induced thrombocytopenia, and 2.1 for patients with deep venous thrombosis.

➤*Pharmacokinetics:*

Absorption/Distribution – The pharmacokinetic properties of lepirudin following IV administration are well described by a 2-compartment model. Distribution is essentially confined to extracellular fluids and is characterized by an initial half-life of approximately 10 minutes. Elimination follows a first-order process and is characterized by a terminal half-life of about 1.3 hours in young healthy volunteers. As the IV dose is increased over the range of 0.1 to 0.4 mg/kg, the maximum plasma concentration and the area-under-the-curve increase proportionally.

Metabolism/Excretion – Lepirudin is thought to be metabolized by release of amino acids via catabolic hydrolysis of the parent drug. However, conclusive data are not available. About 48% of the administered dose is excreted in the urine, which consists of unchanged drug (35%) and other fragments of the parent drug.

The systemic clearance of lepirudin is proportional to the glomerular filtration rate or creatinine clearance. Dose adjustment based on creatinine clearance is recommended. In patients with marked renal insufficiency (creatinine clearance below 15 mL/min) and on hemodialysis, elimination half-lives are prolonged up to 2 days.

The systemic clearance of lepirudin in women is about 25% lower than in men. In elderly patients, the systemic clearance of lepirudin is 20% lower than in younger patients. This may be explained by the lower creatinine clearance in elderly patients compared to younger patients.

The table below summarizes systemic clearance (Cl) and volume of distribution at steady state (Vss) of lepirudin for various study populations.

Cl and Vss of Lepirudin		
	Cl (mL/min) mean (% CV*)	Vss (L) mean (% CV*)
Healthy young subjects (n = 18, age 18 to 60 years)	164 (19.3%)	12.2 (16.4%)
Healthy elderly subjects (n = 10, age 65 to 80 years)	139 (22.5%)	18.7 (20.6%)
Renally impaired patients (n = 16, creatinine clearance below 80 mL/min)	61 (89.4%)	18 (41.1%)
HIT** patients (n = 73)	114 (46.8%)	32.1 (98.9%)

* CV is coefficient of variation.
** HIT is heparin-induced thrombocytopenia.

Contraindications

Known hypersensitivity to hirudins or to any of the components in lepirudin (rDNA) for injection.

LEPIRUDIN — INJECTION

Warnings

➤*Hemorrhagic events:* As with other anticoagulants, hemorrhage can occur at any site in patients receiving lepirudin. An unexpected fall in hemoglobin, fall in blood pressure or any unexplained symptom should lead to consideration of a hemorrhagic event. While patients are being anticoagulated with lepirudin, the anticoagulation status should be monitored closely using an appropriate measure such as the aPTT.

Intracranial bleeding following concomitant thrombolytic therapy with rt-PA or streptokinase may be life-threatening. There have been reports of intracranial bleeding with lepirudin in the absence of concomitant thrombolytic therapy.

For patients with increased risk of bleeding, a careful assessment weighing the risk of lepirudin administration vs its anticipated benefit has to be made by the treating physician.

In particular, this includes the following conditions: recent puncture of large vessels or organ biopsy; anomaly of vessels or organs; recent cerebrovascular accident, stroke, intracerebral surgery, or other neuraxial procedures; severe uncontrolled hypertension; bacterial endocarditis; advanced renal impairment (see Renal impairment); hemorrhagic diathesis; recent major surgery; recent major bleeding (eg, intracranial, gastrointestinal, intraocular, or pulmonary bleeding); recent active peptic ulcer.

➤*Hypersensitivity reactions:* There have been reports of allergic and hypersensitivity reactions, including anaphylactic reactions. Serious anaphylactic reactions that have resulted in shock or death have been reported. These reactions have been reported during initial administration or upon second or subsequent reexposure(s).

➤*Renal function impairment:* With renal impairment, relative overdose might occur even with standard dosage regimen. Therefore, the bolus dose and the rate of infusion must be reduced in patients with known or suspected renal insufficiency.

➤*Hepatic function impairment:* Serious liver injury (eg, liver cirrhosis) may enhance the anticoagulant effect of lepirudin due to coagulation defects secondary to reduced generation of vitamin K-dependent coagulation factors.

➤*Pregnancy: Category B.* There are no adequate and well-controlled studies in pregnant women. Because animal reproduction studies are not always predictive of human response, this drug should be used during pregnancy only if clearly needed.

Lepirudin (1 mg/kg) by IV administration crosses the placental barrier in pregnant rats. It is not known whether the drug crosses the placental barrier in humans.

Following IV administration of lepirudin at 30 mg/kg/day (180 mg/m^2/day, 1.2 times the recommended maximum human total daily dose based on body surface area) during organogenesis and perinatal-postnatal periods, pregnant rats showed an increased maternal mortality due to undetermined causes.

➤*Lactation:* It is not known whether lepirudin is excreted in human milk. Because many drugs are excreted in human milk and because of the potential for serious adverse reactions in nursing infants from lepirudin, a decision should be made whether to discontinue nursing or to discontinue the drug, taking into account the importance of the drug to the mother.

➤*Children:* Safety and effectiveness in pediatric patients have not been established. In the HAT-2 study, two children, an 11-year-old girl and a 12-year-old boy, were treated with lepirudin. Both children presented with TECs at baseline. Lepirudin doses given ranged from 0.15 mg/kg/hr to 0.22 mg/kg/hr for the girl, and from 0.1 mg/kg/hr (in conjunction with urokinase) to 0.7 mg/kg/hr for the boy. Treatment with lepirudin was completed after 8 and 58 days, respectively, without serious adverse events.

Precautions

➤*Antibodies:* Formation of antihirudin antibodies was observed in about 40% of HIT patients treated with lepirudin. This may increase the anticoagulant effect of lepirudin possibly due to delayed renal elimination of active lepirudin-antihirudin complexes. Therefore, strict monitoring of aPTT is necessary also during prolonged therapy. No evidence of neutralization of lepirudin or of allergic reactions associated with positive antibody test results was found.

➤*Reexposure:* During the HAT-1 and HAT-2 studies, a total of 13 patients were reexposed to lepirudin. One of these patients experienced a mild allergic skin reaction during the second treatment cycle. In postmarketing experience, anaphylaxis after reexposure has been reported.

➤*Lab test abnormalities:* In general, the dosage (infusion rate) should be adjusted according to the aPTT ratio (patient aPTT at a given time over an aPTT reference value, usually median of the laboratory normal range for aPTT). Other thrombin-dependent coagulation assays are changed by lepirudin.

Drug Interactions

Lepirudin Drug Interactions

Precipitant drug	Object drug*		Description
Thrombolytics (eg, alteplase, streptokinase)	Lepirudin	↑	Concomitant treatment with thrombolytics may increase the risk of bleeding complications and considerably enhance the effect of lepirudin on aPTT prolongation.

Lepirudin Drug Interactions

Precipitant drug	Object drug*		Description
Coumarin derivatives (vitamin K antagonists)	Lepirudin	↑	Concomitant treatment with coumarin derivatives and drugs that affect platelet function may increase the risk of bleeding.

* ↑ = Object drug increased.

Adverse Reactions

➤*Adverse events reported in HIT patients:* The following safety information is based on all 198 patients treated with lepirudin in the HAT-1 and HAT-2 studies. The safety profile of 113 lepirudin patients from these studies who presented with TECs at baseline is compared to 91 such patients in the historical control.

Hematologic –

Hemorrhagic events: Bleeding was the most frequent adverse event observed in patients treated with lepirudin. The following table gives an overview of all hemorrhagic events which occurred in at least 2 patients. Patients may have suffered more than one event.

Overview of Hemorrhagic Events

	HAT-1 HAT-2 (all patients) (n = 198)	Patients with TECs	
		Lepirudin (n = 113)	Historical control (n = 91)
Bleeding from puncture sites and wounds	14.1%	10.6%	4.4%
Anemia or isolated drop in hemoglobin	13.1%	12.4%	1.1%
Other hematoma and unclassified bleeding	11.1%	10.6%	4.4%
Hematuria	6.6%	4.4%	0%
GI and rectal bleeding	5.1%	5.3%	6.6%
Epistaxis	3%	4.4%	1.1%
Hemothorax	3%	0%	1.1%
Vaginal bleeding	1.5%	1.8%	0%
Intracranial bleeding	0%	0%	2.2%

Other hemorrhagic events (hemoperitoneum, hemoptysis, liver bleeding, lung bleeding, mouth bleeding, retroperitoneal bleeding) each occurred in one individual among all 198 patients treated with lepirudin.

Miscellaneous –

Nonhemorrhagic events: The following table gives an overview of the most frequently observed nonhemorrhagic events. Patients may have suffered more than 1 event.

Overview of the Most Frequently Observed Nonhemorrhagic Events

	HAT-1 HAT-2 (all patients) (n = 198)	Patients with TECs	
		Lepirudin (n = 113)	Historical control (n = 91)
Fever	6.1%	4.4%	8.8%
Abnormal liver function	6.1%	5.3%	0%
Pneumonia	4%	4.4%	5.5%
Sepsis	4%	3.5%	5.5%
Allergic skin reactions	3%	3.5%	1.1%
Heart failure	3%	1.8%	2.2%
Abnormal kidney function	2.5%	1.8%	4.4%
Unspecified infections	2.5%	1.8%	1.1%
Multiorgan failure	2%	3.5%	0%
Pericardial effusion	1%	0%	1.1%
Ventricular fibrillation	1%	0%	0%

➤*Adverse events reported in other populations:* The following safety information is based on a total of 2302 individuals who were treated with lepirudin in clinical pharmacology studies (n = 323) or for clinical indications other than HIT (n = 1979).

Intracranial bleeding – Intracranial bleeding was the most serious adverse reaction found in populations other than HIT patients. It occurred in patients with acute myocardial infarction who were started on both lepirudin and thrombolytic therapy with rt-PA or streptokinase. The overall frequency of this potentially life-threatening complication among patients receiving both lepirudin and thrombolytic therapy was 0.6% (7 out of 1134 patients). Although no intracranial bleeding was observed in 1168 subjects or patients who did not receive concomitant thrombolysis, there have been

LEPIRUDIN — INJECTION

postmarketing reports of intracranial bleeding with lepirudin (rDNA) for injection in the absence of concomitant thrombolytic therapy.

Allergic –

Allergic or Suspected Allergic Reactions in non-HIT Patients	
Airway reactions (cough, bronchospasm, stridor, dyspnea)	common
Unspecified allergic reactions	uncommon
Skin reactions (pruritus, urticaria, rash, flushes, chills)	uncommon
General reactions (anaphylactoid or anaphylactic reactions)	uncommon
Edema (facial edema, tongue edema, larynx edema, angioedema)	rare

The Council for International Organization of Medical Sciences (CIOMS) III standard categories are used for classification frequencies:

CIOMS III Standard Categories	
Very common	10% or more
Common (frequent)	1% to < 10%
Uncommon (infrequent)	0.1% to < 1%
Rare	0.01% to < 0.1%
Very rare	0.01% or less

About 53% (n = 46) of all allergic reactions or suspected allergic reactions occurred in patients who concomitantly received thrombolytic therapy (eg, streptokinase) for acute myocardial infarction and/or contrast media for coronary angiography.

➤*Adverse events from postmarketing reports:* Serious anaphylactic reactions that have resulted in shock or death have been reported.

Intracranial bleeding has been reported in patients treated with lepirudin, with or without concomitant thrombolytic therapy. Although no intracranial bleeding was observed in clinical trials in those patients who did not receive concomitant thrombolytic therapy, there have been postmarketing reports of intracranial bleeding in patients who received lepirudin without concomitant thrombolytic therapy.

Overdosage

➤*General toxicity:* Lepirudin caused bleeding in animal toxicity studies.

➤*Symptoms:* In case of overdose (eg, suggested by excessively high aPTT values) the risk of bleeding is increased.

➤*Treatment:* No specific antidote for lepirudin is available. If life-threatening bleeding occurs and excessive plasma levels of lepirudin are suspected, the following steps should be followed:

1.) Immediately STOP lepirudin administration.
2.) Determine aPTT and other coagulation levels as appropriate.
3.) Determine hemoglobin and prepare for blood transfusion.
4.) Follow the current guidelines for treating patients with shock.

Individual clinical case reports and in vitro data suggest that either hemofiltration or hemodialysis (using high-flux dialysis membranes with a cutoff point of 50,000 daltons, eg, AN/69) may be useful in this situation. In studies in pigs, the application of von Willebrand Factor (vWF, 66 IU/kg body weight) markedly reduced the bleeding time. The clinical significance of this data is unknown.

ARGATROBAN

Rx	**Argatroban** (GlaxoSmithKline)	**Injection:** 100 mg/mL	750 mg D-sorbitol, 1000 mg dehydrated alcohol. In 2.5 mL single-use vials.

ARGATROBAN — INJECTION

Indications

➤*Heparin-induced thrombocytopenia (prophylaxis and treatment):* As an anticoagulant for prophylaxis or treatment of thrombosis in patients with heparin-induced thrombocytopenia.

➤*Thrombosis, percutaneous coronary intervention:* As an anticoagulant in patients with or at risk for heparin-induced thrombocytopenia undergoing percutaneous coronary interventions (PCI).

Administration and Dosage

➤*Approved by the FDA:* June 30, 2000.

Each 2.5 mL vial contains 250 mg of argatroban; and, as supplied, is a concentrated drug (100 mg/mL), which must be diluted 100-fold prior to infusion. Argatroban should not be mixed with other drugs prior to dilution in a suitable intravenous fluid.

➤*Preparation for IV administration:* Argatroban should be diluted in 0.9% Sodium Chloride Injection, 5% Dextrose Injection, or Lactated Ringer's Injection to a final concentration of 1 mg/mL. The contents of each 2.5 mL vial should be diluted 100-fold by mixing with 250 mL of diluent. Use 250 mg (2.5 mL) per 250 mL of diluent or 500 mg (5 mL) per 500 mL of diluent. The constituted solution must be mixed by repeated inversion of the diluent bag for 1 minute. Upon preparation, the solution may show slight but brief haziness due to the formation of microprecipitates that rapidly dissolve upon mixing. The pH of the IV solution prepared as recommended is 3.2 to 7.5.

➤*Heparin-induced thrombocytopenia (HIT/HITTS):* Before administering argatroban, discontinue heparin therapy and obtain a baseline activated partial thromboplastin time (aPTT). The recommended initial dose of argatroban for adult patients without hepatic impairment is 2 mcg/kg/min, administered as a continuous infusion.

Recommended Doses And Infusion Rates for 2 mcg/kg/min Dose of Argatroban for Patients with HIT/HITTS (without Hepatic Impairment) (1 mg/mL Final Concentration)

Body weight (kg)	Dose (mcg/min)	Infusion rate (mL/hr)
50	100	6
60	120	7
70	140	8
80	160	10
90	180	11
100	200	12
110	220	13
120	240	14
130	260	16
140	280	17

Monitoring therapy – In general, therapy with argatroban is monitored using the aPTT. Tests of anticoagulant effects (including the aPTT) typically attain steady-state levels within 1 to 3 hours following initiation of argatroban. Dose adjustment may be required to attain the target aPTT. Check the aPTT 2 hours after initiation of therapy to confirm that the aPTT is within the desired therapeutic range.

Dosage adjustment – After the initial dose of argatroban, the dose can be adjusted as clinically indicated (not to exceed 10 mcg/kg/min), until the steady-state aPTT is 1.5 to 3 times the initial baseline value (not to exceed 100 seconds). Argatroban therapy should be continued until platelet counts have recovered substantially (ie, greater than 100×10^9/L or to pre-HIT/-HITTS.

➤*Percutaneous coronary interventions (PCI) in HIT/HITTS patients:*

Initial dosage – An infusion of argatroban should be started at 25 mcg/kg/min and a bolus of 350 mcg/kg administered via a large bore IV line over 3 to 5 minutes. Activated clotting time (ACT) should be checked 5 to 10 minutes after the bolus dose is completed. The procedure may proceed if the ACT is greater than 300 seconds.

Dosage adjustment – If the ACT is less than 300 seconds, an additional IV bolus dose of 150 mcg/kg should be administered, the infusion dose increased to 30 mcg/kg/min, and the ACT checked 5 to 10 minutes later. If the ACT is greater than 450 seconds, the infusion rate should be decreased to 15 mcg/kg/min, and the ACT checked 5 to 10 minutes later (see table below). Once a therapeutic ACT (between 300 and 450 seconds) has been achieved, this infusion dose should be continued for the duration of the procedure.

Recommended Doses and Infusion Rates of Argatroban for Patients Undergoing PCI (without Hepatic Impairment) (1 mg/mL Final Concentration)**

	For ACT 300 to 450 seconds initial dosage*; 25 mcg/kg/min			If ACT < 300 seconds dosage adjustment[1]; 30 mcg/kg/min			If ACT > 450 seconds dosage adjustment; 15 mcg/kg/min	
Body weight (kg)	Bolus dose (mcg)	Infusion dose (mcg/min)	Infusion rate (mL/hr)	Bolus dose (mcg)	Infusion dose (mcg/min)	Infusion rate (mL/hr)	Infusion dose (mcg/min)	Infusion rate (mL/hr)
50	17500	1250	75	7500	1500	90	750	45
60	21000	1500	90	9000	1800	108	900	54
70	24500	1750	105	10500	2100	126	1050	63
80	28000	2000	120	12000	2400	144	1200	72
90	31500	2250	135	13500	2700	162	1350	81
100	35000	2500	150	15000	3000	180	1500	90
110	38500	2750	165	16500	3300	198	1650	99
120	42000	3000	180	18000	3600	216	1800	108
130	45500	3250	195	19500	3900	234	1950	117
140	49000	3500	210	21000	4200	252	2100	126

* Initial IV bolus dose of 350 mcg/kg should be administered.
** Note: 1 mg = 1000 mcg; 1 kg = 2.2 lbs.
[1] Additional IV bolus dose of 150 mcg/kg should be administered if ACT is less than 300 seconds.

ARGATROBAN — INJECTION

In case of dissection, impending abrupt closure, thrombus formation during the procedure, or inability to achieve or maintain an ACT over 300 seconds, additional bolus doses of 150 mcg/kg may be administered and the infusion dose increased to 40 mcg/kg/min. The ACT should be checked after each additional bolus or change in the rate of infusion.

Monitoring therapy – Therapy with argatroban is monitored using ACT. ACTs should be obtained before dosing, 5 to 10 minutes after bolus dosing and after change in the infusion rate, and at the end of the PCI procedure. Additional ACTs should be drawn about every 20 to 30 minutes during a prolonged procedure.

Continued anticoagulation after PCI – If a patient requires anticoagulation after the procedure, argatroban may be continued, but at a lower infusion dose (see Heparin-induced Thrombocytopenia [HIT/HITTS] above). If the patient has HIT or HITTS, argatroban therapy should be continued until the platelet counts have recovered substantially (ie, greater than 100 × 10^9/L or to pre-HIT/-HITTS baseline value).

➤*Hepatic function impairment:* For patients with heparin-induced thrombocytopenia with hepatic impairment, the initial dose of argatroban should be reduced. For patients with moderate hepatic impairment, an initial dose of 0.5 mcg/kg/min is recommended, based on the approximate 4-fold decrease in argatroban clearance relative to those with healthy hepatic function. The aPTT should be monitored closely, and the dosage should be adjusted as clinically indicated.

Hepatic impairment in HIT/HITTS patients undergoing PCI – Use of high doses of argatroban in PCI patients with clinically significant hepatic disease or AST/ALT levels greater than or equal to 3 times the upper limit of normal should be avoided. Such patients were not studied in PCI trials.

➤*Conversion to oral anticoagulant therapy:*

Initiating oral anticoagulant therapy – Once the decision is made to initiate oral anticoagulant therapy, recognize the potential for combined effects on INR with coadministration of argatroban and warfarin. Continue to monitor argatroban using aPTT. Oral anticoagulation therapy (warfarin) should be initiated only after substantial recovery of platelet counts (eg, greater than 100 × 10^9/L or to pre-HIT/-HITTS baseline value). A loading dose of warfarin should not be used. Initiate therapy using the expected daily dose of warfarin. To avoid prothrombotic effects and to ensure continuous anticoagulation when initiating warfarin, it is recommended to overlap argatroban and warfarin therapy for 4 or 5 days (see warfarin monograph).

Coadministration of warfarin and argatroban at doses up to 2 mcg/kg/min – Use of argatroban with warfarin results in prolongation of INR beyond that produced by warfarin alone. To avoid prothrombotic effects and to ensure continuous anticoagulation when initiating warfarin, it is recommended to continue coadministration for at least 4 or 5 days before discontinuing argatroban. The previously established relationship between INR and bleeding risk is altered. The combination of argatroban and warfarin does not cause further reduction in the vitamin K-dependent factor Xa activity than that which is seen with warfarin alone. The relationship between INR obtained on combined therapy and INR obtained on warfarin alone is dependent on both the dose of argatroban and the thromboplastin reagent used. The INR value on warfarin alone (INR_W) can be calculated from the INR value on combination argatroban and warfarin therapy.

INR should be measured daily while argatroban and warfarin are coadministered. In general, with doses of argatroban up to 2 mcg/kg/min, argatroban can be discontinued when the INR is greater than 4 on combined therapy. After argatroban is discontinued, repeat the INR measurement in 4 to 6 hours. If the repeat INR is below the desired therapeutic range, resume the infusion of argatroban and repeat the procedure daily until the desired therapeutic range on warfarin alone is reached.

Coadministration of warfarin and argatroban at doses greater than 2 mcg/kg/min – For doses greater than 2 mcg/kg/min, the relationship of INR between warfarin alone to the INR on warfarin plus argatroban is less predictable. In this case, in order to predict the INR on warfarin alone, temporarily reduce the dose of argatroban to a dose of 2 mcg/kg/min. Repeat the INR on argatroban and warfarin 4 to 6 hours after reduction of the argatroban dose and follow the process outlined above for administering argatroban at doses up to 2 mcg/kg/min.

➤*Storage/Stability:* Argatroban is a clear, colorless to pale yellow, slightly viscous solution. If the solution is cloudy, or if an insoluble precipitate is noted, the vial should be discarded.

Solutions prepared as recommended are stable at 25°C (77°F) with excursions permitted to 15° to 30°C (59° to 86°F) in ambient indoor light for 24 hours; therefore, light-resistant measures such as foil protection for IV lines are unnecessary. Solutions are physically and chemically stable for up to 48 hours when stored at 2° to 8°C (36° to 46°F) in the dark. Prepared solutions should not be exposed to direct sunlight. No significant potency losses have been noted following simulated delivery of the solution through IV tubing.

Store the vials in original cartons at room temperature 25°C (77°F); excursions permitted to 15° to 30°C (59° to 86°F). Do not freeze. Retain in the original carton to protect from light.

Actions

➤*Pharmacology:* Argatroban is a direct thrombin inhibitor that reversibly binds to the thrombin active site. Argatroban does not require the co-factor antithrombin III for antithrombotic activity. Argatroban exerts its anticoagulant effects by inhibiting thrombin-catalyzed or induced reactions, including fibrin formation; activation of coagulation factors V, VIII, and XIII; protein C; and platelet aggregation.

Argatroban is highly selective for thrombin with an inhibitory constant (K_1) of 0.04 mcM. At therapeutic concentrations, argatroban has little or no effect on related serine proteases (trypsin, factor Xa, plasmin, and kallikrein).

Argatroban is capable of inhibiting the action of both free and clot-associated thrombin.

Argatroban does not interact with heparin-induced antibodies. Evaluation of sera from 12 healthy subjects and 8 patients who received multiple doses of argatroban did not reveal antibody formation to argatroban.

➤*Pharmacokinetics:*

Distribution – Argatroban distributes mainly in the extracellular fluid as evidenced by an apparent steady state volume of distribution of 174 mL/kg (12.18 L in a 70 kg adult). Argatroban is 54% bound to human serum proteins, with binding to albumin and α_1-acid glycoprotein being 20% and 34%, respectively.

Metabolism – The main route of argatroban metabolism is hydroxylation and aromatization of the 3-methyltetrahydroquinoline ring in the liver. The formation of each of the 4 known metabolites is catalyzed in vitro by the human liver microsomal cytochrome P450 enzymes CYP3A4/5. The primary metabolite (M1) exerts 3- to 5-fold weaker anticoagulant effects than argatroban. Unchanged argatroban is the major component in plasma. The plasma concentrations of M1 range between 0% to 20% of that of the parent drug. The other metabolites (M2 to M4) are found only in very low quantities in the urine and have not been detected in plasma or feces. These data, together with the lack of effect of erythromycin (a potent CYP3A4/5 inhibitor) on argatroban pharmacokinetics suggest that CYP3A4/5 mediated metabolism is not an important elimination pathway in vivo.

There is no interconversion of the 21-(R): 21-(S) diastereoisomers. The plasma ratio of these diastereoisomers is unchanged by metabolism or hepatic impairment, remaining constant at 65:35 (± 2%).

Excretion – Total body clearance is approximately 5.1 mL/min/kg (0.31 L/hr/kg) for infusion doses up to 40 mcg/kg/min. The terminal elimination half-life of argatroban ranges between 39 and 51 minutes.

Argatroban is excreted primarily in the feces, presumably through biliary secretion. In a study in which ^{14}C-argatroban (5 mcg/kg/min) was infused for 4 hours into healthy subjects, approximately 65% of the radioactivity was recovered in the feces within 6 days of the start of infusion with little or no radioactivity subsequently detected. Approximately 22% of the radioactivity appeared in the urine within 12 hours of the start of infusion. Little or no additional urinary radioactivity was subsequently detected. Average percent recovery of unchanged drug, relative to total dose, was 16% in urine and at least 14% in feces.

Special populations –

Hepatic function impairment: The dosage of argatroban should be decreased in patients with hepatic impairment. Patients with hepatic impairment were not studied in percutaneous coronary intervention (PCI) trials. At a dose of 2.5 mcg/kg/min, hepatic impairment is associated with decreased clearance and increased elimination half-life of argatroban (to 1.9 mL/kg/min and 181 minutes, respectively, for patients with a Child-Pugh score greater than 6).

Pharmacokinetic/pharmacodynamic relationship – When argatroban is administered by continuous infusion, anticoagulant effects and plasma concentrations of argatroban follow similar, predictable temporal response profiles, with low intersubject variability. Immediately upon initiation of argatroban infusion, anticoagulant effects are produced as plasma argatroban concentrations begin to rise. Steady-state levels of both drug and anticoagulant effect are typically attained within 1 to 3 hours and are maintained until the infusion is discontinued or the dosage adjusted. Steady-state plasma argatroban concentrations increase proportionally with dose (for infusion doses up to 40 mcg/kg/min in healthy subjects) and are well correlated with steady-state anticoagulant effects. For infusion doses up to 40 mcg/kg/min, argatroban increases in a dose-dependent fashion, the activated partial thromboplastin time (aPTT), the activated clotting time (ACT), the prothrombin time (PT) and International Normalized Ratio (INR), and the thrombin time (TT) in healthy volunteers and cardiac patients. Representative steady-state plasma argatroban concentrations and anticoagulant effects are shown below for argatroban infusion doses up to 10 mcg/kg/min.

Effect on International Normalized Ratio (INR) – Because argatroban is a direct thrombin inhibitor, coadministration of argatroban and warfarin produces a combined effect on the laboratory measurement of the INR. However, concurrent therapy, compared to warfarin monotherapy, exerts no additional effect on vitamin K dependent factor Xa activity.

The relationship between INR on co-therapy and warfarin alone is dependent on both the dose of argatroban and the thromboplastin reagent used. This relationship is influenced by the international sensitivity index (ISI) of the thromboplastin.Thromboplastins with higher ISI values than shown result in higher INRs on combined therapy of warfarin and argatroban. These data are based on results obtained in healthy individuals.

Contraindications

Overt major bleeding; hypersensitivity to this product or any of its components.

Warnings

➤*Route of administration:* Argatroban is intended for IV administration. All parenteral anticoagulants should be discontinued before administration of argatroban.

➤*Hemorrhage:* Hemorrhage can occur at any site in the body in patients receiving argatroban. An unexplained fall in hematocrit, fall in blood pressure, or any other unexplained symptom should lead to consideration of a

ARGATROBAN — INJECTION

hemorrhagic event. Argatroban should be used with extreme caution in disease states and other circumstances in which there is an increased danger of hemorrhage. These include the following: Severe hypertension; immediately following lumbar puncture; spinal anesthesia; major surgery, especially involving the brain, spinal cord, or eye; hematologic conditions associated with increased bleeding tendencies such as congenital or acquired bleeding disorders and gastrointestinal lesions such as ulcerations.

➤*Hepatic function impairment:* Caution should be exercised when administering argatroban to patients with hepatic disease by starting with a lower dose and carefully titrating until the desired level of anticoagulation is achieved. Also, upon cessation of argatroban infusion in the hepatically impaired patient, full reversal of anticoagulant effects may require longer than 4 hours due to decreased clearance and increased elimination half-life of argatroban. For patients with moderate hepatic impairment, an initial dose of 0.5 mcg/kg/min is recommended, based on the approximate 4-fold decrease in argatroban clearance relative to those with healthy hepatic function. The aPTT should be monitored closely and the dosage should be adjusted as clinically indicated.

Use of high doses of argatroban in PCI patients with clinically significant hepatic disease or AST/ALT levels greater than or equal to 3 times the upper limit of normal should be avoided. Such patients were not studied in PCI trials.

➤*Elderly:* In the clinical studies of adult patients with HIT or HITTS, the effectiveness of argatroban was not affected by age.

➤*Pregnancy: Category B.* There are no adequate and well-controlled studies in pregnant women. Because animal reproduction studies are not always predictive of human response, this drug should be used during pregnancy only if clearly needed.

➤*Lactation:* Experiments in rats show that argatroban is detected in milk. It is not known whether this drug is excreted in human milk. Because many drugs are excreted in human milk and because of the potential for serious adverse reactions in nursing infants from argatroban, a decision should be made whether to discontinue nursing or to discontinue the drug, taking into account the importance of the drug to the mother.

➤*Children:* The safety and effectiveness of argatroban in patients below the age of 18 years have not been established.

Precautions

➤*Lab test abnormalities:* Anticoagulation effects associated with argatroban infusion at doses up to 40 mcg/kg/min are well correlated with the activated partial thromboplastin time (aPTT). Although other global clot-based tests including prothrombin time (PT), the International Normalized Ratio (INR), the activated clotting time (ACT) and thrombin time (TT) are affected by argatroban; the therapeutic ranges for these tests have not been identified for argatroban therapy. Plasma argatroban concentrations also correlate well with anticoagulant effects.

In clinical trials in PCI, the activated clotting time (ACT) was used for monitoring argatroban activity during the procedure.

The concomitant use of argatroban and warfarin results in prolongation of the PT and INR beyond that produced by warfarin alone. INR should be measured daily while argatroban and warfarin are coadministered. In general, with doses of argatroban up to 2 mcg/kg/min, argatroban can be discontinued when the INR is greater than 4 on combined therapy. After argatroban is discontinued, repeat the INR measurement in 4 to 6 hours. If the repeat INR is below the desired therapeutic range, resume the infusion of argatroban and repeat the procedure daily until the desired therapeutic range on warfarin alone is reached. The relationship between INR obtained on combined therapy and INR obtained on warfarin alone is dependent on both the dose of argatroban and the thromboplastin reagent used.

For doses greater than 2 mcg/kg/min, the relationship of INR on warfarin alone to the INR on warfarin plus argatroban is less predictable. In this case, in order to predict the INR on warfarin alone, temporarily reduce the dose of argatroban to a dose of 2 mcg/kg/min. Repeat the INR on argatroban and warfarin 4 to 6 hours after reduction of the argatroban dose and follow the process outlined above for administering argatroban at doses up to 2 mcg/kg/min.

Drug Interactions

➤*Heparin:* Since heparin is contraindicated in patients with heparin-induced thrombocytopenia, the coadministration of argatroban and heparin is unlikely for this indication. However, if argatroban is to be initiated after cessation of heparin therapy, allow sufficient time for heparin's effect on the aPTT to decrease prior to initiation of argatroban therapy.

➤*Oral anticoagulant agents:* Pharmacokinetic drug-drug interactions between argatroban and warfarin (7.5 mg single oral dose) have not been demonstrated. However, the concomitant use of argatroban and warfarin (5 to 7.5 mg initial oral dose followed by 2.5 to 6 mg/day orally for 6 to 10 days) results in prolongation of the prothrombin time (PT) and International Normalized Ratio (INR).

➤*Other drugs affecting coagulation:* Concomitant use of argatroban with antiplatelet agents, thrombolytics, and other anticoagulants may increase the risk of bleeding. Drug-drug interactions have not been observed between argatroban and digoxin or erythromycin.

Adverse Reactions

➤*Adverse events reported in HIT/HITTS patients:* The following safety information is based on all 568 patients treated with argatroban in Study 1 and Study 2. The safety profile of the patients from these studies is compared with that of 193 historical controls in which the adverse events were collected retrospectively. The adverse events reported in this section include all events regardless of relationship to treatment. Adverse events are separated into hemorrhagic and non-hemorrhagic events.

Major bleeding was defined as bleeding that was overt and associated with a hemoglobin decrease greater than or equal to 2 g/dL, that led to a transfusion of greater than or equal to 2 units, or that was intracranial, retroperitoneal, or into a major prosthetic joint. Minor bleeding was overt bleeding that did not meet the criteria for major bleeding.

The table below gives an overview of the most frequently observed hemorrhagic events, presented separately by major and minor bleeding, sorted by decreasing occurrence among argatroban-treated patients.

Major and minor hemorrhagic adverse events in HIT/HITTS patients

	Argatroban-treated patients (Study 1 and Study 2) (n = 568)%	Historical control (n = 193)%
Major hemorrhagic events*		
Overall bleeding	5.3%	6.7%
Gastrointestinal	2.3%	1.6%
Genitourinary and hematuria	0.9%	0.5%
Decrease hemoglobin/hematocrit	0.7%	0%
Multisystem hemorrhage and DIC	0.5%	1%
Limb and BKA stump	0.5%	0%
Intracranial hemorrhage	0%[1]	0.5%
Minor hemorrhagic events*		
Gastrointestinal	14.4%	18.1%
Genitourinary and hematuria	11.6%	0.8%
Decrease in hemoglobin and hematocrit	10.4%	0%
Groin	5.4%	3.1%
Hemoptysis	2.9%	0.8%
Brachial	2.4%	0.8%

* Patients may have experienced more than 1 adverse event.
[1] One patient experienced intracranial hemorrhage 4 days after discontinuation of argatroban and following therapy with urokinase and oral anticoagulation.DIC = disseminated intravascular coagulation.BKA = below the knee amputation.

The table below gives an overview of the most frequently observed nonhemorrhagic events sorted by decreasing frequency of occurrence (greater than or equal to 2%) among argatroban-treated patients.

Nonhemorrhagic adverse events in HIT/HITTS patients*

	Argatroban-treated patients (Study 1 and Study 2) (n = 568)%	Historical control (n = 193)%
Dyspnea	8.1%	8.8%
Hypotension	7.2%	2.6%
Fever	6.9%	2.1%
Diarrhea	6.2%	1.6%
Sepsis	6%	12.4%
Cardiac arrest	5.8%	3.1%
Nausea	4.8%	0.5%
Ventricular tachycardia	4.8%	3.1%
Pain	4.6%	3.1%
Urinary tract infection	4.6%	5.2%
Vomiting	4.2%	0%
Infection	3.7%	3.6%
Pneumonia	3.3%	9.3%
Atrial fibrillation	3%	11.4%
Coughing	2.8%	1.6%
Abnormal renal function	2.8%	4.7%
Abdominal pain	2.6%	1.6%
Cerebrovascular disorder	2.3%	4.1%

* Patients may have experienced more than 1 adverse event.

➤*Adverse events reported in HIT/HITTS patients undergoing PCI:* The following safety information is based on 91 patients initially treated with argatroban and 21 patients subsequently reexposed to argatroban for a total of 112 PCIs with argatroban anticoagulation. The adverse events reported in this section include all events regardless of relationship to treatment. Adverse events are separated into hemorrhagic (see below) and nonhemorrhagic (see below) events.

Major bleeding was defined as bleeding that was overt and associated with a hemoglobin decrease greater than or equal to 5 g/dL, that led to a transfusion of greater than or equal to 2 units, or that was intracranial, retroperitoneal, or into a major prosthetic joint.

ARGATROBAN — INJECTION

The rate of major bleeding events and intracranial hemorrhage in the PCI trials was 1.8% and in the placebo arm of the EPILOG trial (placebo plus standard dose, weight-adjusted heparin) was 3.1%.

Major and minor hemorrhagic adverse events in HIT/HITTS patients undergoing PCI	
Major hemorrhagic events*	
	Argatroban-treated patients (n = 112)+%
Retroperitoneal	0.9%
Gastrointestinal	0.9%
Intracranial hemorrhage	0%
Minor hemorrhagic events*	
	Argatroban-treated patients (n = 112)+%
Groin (bleeding or hematoma)	3.6%
Gastrointestinal (includes hematemesis)	2.6%
Genitourinary (includes hematuria)	1.8%
Decrease in hemoglobin or hematocrit	1.8%
CABG (coronary arteries)	1.8%
Access site	0.9%
Hemoptysis	0.9%
Other	0.9%

* Patients may have experienced more than 1 adverse event.
+ 91 patients who underwent 112 interventions.CABG = coronary artery bypass graft.

The table below gives an overview of the most frequently observed nonhemorrhagic events (greater than 2%), sorted by decreasing frequency of occurrence among argatroban-treated PCI patients.

Non-hemorrhagic adverse events * in HIT/HITTS patients undergoing PCI		
	Argatroban procedures* (n = 112)+%	Controls (n = 2226)++%
Chest pain	15.2%	9.3%
Hypotension	10.7%	10.3%
Back pain	8%	13.7%
Nausea	7.1%	11.5%
Vomiting	6.3%	6.8%
Headache	5.4%	5.5%
Bradycardia	4.5%	3.5%
Abdominal pain	3.6%	2.2%
Fever	3.6%	< 0.5%
Myocardial infarction	3.6%	NR+++

* Patients may have experienced more than 1 adverse event.
+ 91 patients who underwent 112 interventions.
++ Controls from EPIC (Evaluation of c7E3 Fab in the Prevention of Ischemic Complications), EPILOG (Evaluation in PTCA to Improve Long-Term Outcome with abciximab GP IIb/IIIa Blockade Study) and CAPTURE (Chimeric 7E3 Antiplatelet Therapy in Unstable angina Refractory to standard treatment) trials.
+++ NR = not reported.

There were 22 serious adverse events in 17 PCI patients (19.6% in 112 interventions). The types of events, which are listed regardless of relationship to treatment, are shown in the table below. The table below lists the serious adverse events occurring in argatroban-treated HIT/HITTS patients undergoing PCI.

Serious adverse events in HIT/HITTS patients undergoing PCI*	
Coded term	Argatroban procedures+ (n = 112)
Chest pain	1 (0.9%)
Fever	1 (0.9%)
Retroperitoneal hemorrhage	1 (0.9%)
Angina pectoris	2 (1.8%)
Aortic stenosis	1 (0.9%)
Coronary thrombosis	2 (1.8%)
Arterial thrombosis	1 (0.9%)
Myocardial infarction	4 (3.5%)
Myocardial ischemia	2 (1.8%)
Coronary occlusion	2 (1.8%)
Gastrointestinal hemorrhage	1 (0.9%)
Gastrointestinal disorder (GERD)	1 (0.9%)
Cerebrovascular disorder	1 (0.9%)
Lung edema	1 (0.9%)
Vascular disorder	1 (0.9%)

* Individual events may also have been reported elsewhere (see previous tables).
+ 91 patients underwent 112 procedures. Some patients may have experienced more than 1 event.

➤*Adverse events reported in other populations:* The following safety information is based on a total of 1127 individuals who were treated with argatroban in clinical pharmacology studies (n = 211) or for other clinical indications (n = 916).

Allergic – One hundred and fifty-six (156) allergic reactions or suspected allergic reactions were observed in 1127 individuals who were treated with argatroban in clinical pharmacology studies or for other clinical indications. About 95% (148/156) of these reactions occurred in patients who concomitantly received thrombolytic therapy (eg, streptokinase) for acute myocardial infarction or contrast media for coronary angiography.

Allergic reactions or suspected allergic reactions in populations other than HIT/HITTS patients include (in descending order of frequency [The Council for International Organization of Medical Sciences III standard categories are used for classification of frequencies.]):

- Airway reactions (coughing, dyspnea): 10% or more.
- Skin reactions (rash, bullous eruption): 1% to less than 10%.
- General reactions (vasodilation): 1% to 10%.

Intracranial bleeding – In the HIT/HITTS population, intracranial bleeding was not observed. Intracranial bleeding only occurred in patients with acute myocardial infarction who were started on both argatroban and thrombolytic therapy with streptokinase. The overall frequency of this potentially life-threatening complication among patients receiving both argatroban and thrombolytic therapy (streptokinase or tissue plasminogen activator) was 1% (8 out of 810 patients). Intracranial bleeding was not observed in 317 subjects or patients who did not receive concomitant thrombolysis.

Overdosage

➤*Symptoms:* Single IV doses of argatroban at 200, 124, 150, and 200 mg/kg were lethal to mice, rats, rabbits, and dogs, respectively. The symptoms of acute toxicity were loss of righting reflex, tremors, clonic convulsions, paralysis of hind limbs, and coma.

➤*Treatment:* Excessive anticoagulation, with or without bleeding, may be controlled by discontinuing argatroban or by decreasing the argatroban infusion dosage. In clinical studies at therapeutic levels, anticoagulation parameters generally return to baseline within 2 to 4 hours after discontinuation of the drug. Reversal of anticoagulant effect may take longer in patients with hepatic impairment.

No specific antidote to argatroban is available; if life-threatening bleeding occurs and excessive plasma levels of argatroban are suspected, argatroban should be discontinued immediately, aPTT and other coagulation tests should be determined. Symptomatic and supportive therapy should be provided to the patient.

BIVALIRUDIN

Rx	**Angiomax** (Medicines Company)	**Powder for injection, lyophilized:** 250 mg	In single-use vials.

BIVALIRUDIN — INJECTION

Indications

➤*Concomitant aspirin therapy:* Bivalirudin is intended for use with aspirin and has been studied only in patients receiving concomitant aspirin.

The safety and efficacy of bivalirudin have not been established in patients with acute coronary syndromes who are not undergoing percutaneous transluminal coronary angioplasty (PTCA) or percutaneous coronary intervention (PCI).

➤*PCI:* Bivalirudin with provisional use of glycoprotein IIb/IIIa inhibitor (GPIIb/IIIa inhibitor) is indicated for use as an anticoagulant in patients undergoing PCI.

➤*PTCA:* Bivalirudin is indicated for use as an anticoagulant in patients with unstable angina undergoing PTCA.

➤*Heparin-induced thrombocytopenia / heparin-induced thrombocytopenia and thrombosis syndrome (HIT / HITTS):* Bivalirudin is indicated for patients with, or at risk of, HIT/HITTS undergoing PCI.

Administration and Dosage

➤*Approved by the FDA:* December 15, 2000.

➤*Dosage:* The recommended dosage of bivalirudin is an intravenous (IV) bolus dose of 0.75 mg/kg. This should be followed by an infusion of 1.75 mg/kg/h for the duration of the PCI procedure. Five minutes after the bolus dose has been administered, an activated clotting time (ACT) should be per-

BIVALIRUDIN — INJECTION

formed and an additional bolus of 0.3 mg/kg should be given if needed.

GPIIb/IIIa inhibitor administration should be considered in the event that any of the following conditions are present: decreased thrombosis in myocardial infarction (TIMI) flow (0 to 2) or slow reflow; dissection with decreased flow; new or suspected thrombus; persistent residual stenosis; distal embolization; unplanned stent; suboptimal stenting; side branch closure; abrupt closure; clinical instability; prolonged ischemia.

HIT/HITTS – The recommended dose of bivalirudin in patients with HIT/HITTS undergoing PCI is an IV bolus dose of 0.75 mg/kg. This should be followed by a continuous infusion at a rate of 1.75 mg/kg/h for the duration of the procedure.

Continuation of the infusion following PCI for up to 4 hours postprocedure is optional, at the discretion of the treating health care provider. After 4 hours, an additional IV infusion of bivalirudin may be initiated at a rate of 0.2 mg/kg/h for up to 20 hours, if needed. Bivalirudin is intended for use with aspirin (300 to 325 mg daily) and has been studied only in patients receiving concomitant aspirin.

The dose to be administered is adjusted according to the patient's weight (see the following table).

Bivalirudin Dosing			
	Using 5 mg/mL concentration		Using 0.5 mg/mL concentration
Weight (kg)	Bolus 0.75 mg/kg (mL)	Infusion 1.75 mg/kg/h (mL/h)	Subsequent low-rate infusion 0.2 mg/kg/h (mL/h)
43 to 47	7	16	18
48 to 52	7.5	17.5	20
53 to 57	8	19	22
58 to 62	9	21	24
63 to 67	10	23	26
68 to 72	10.5	24.5	28
73 to 77	11	26	30
78 to 82	12	28	32
83 to 87	13	30	34
88 to 92	13.5	31.5	36
93 to 97	14	33	38
98 to 102	15	35	40
103 to 107	16	37	42
108 to 112	16.5	38.5	44
113 to 117	17	40	46
118 to 122	18	42	48
123 to 127	19	44	50
128 to 132	19.5	45.5	52
133 to 137	20	47	54
138 to 142	21	49	56
143 to 147	22	51	58
148 to 152	22.5	52.5	60

➤*Preparation for administration:* Bivalirudin is intended for IV injection and infusion after dilution. To each 250 mg vial, add 5 mL of sterile water for injection. Gently swirl until all material is dissolved. Each reconstituted vial should be further diluted in 50 mL of 5% dextrose in water or 0.9% sodium chloride for injection to yield a final concentration of 5 mg/mL (eg, 1 vial in 50 mL; 2 vials in 100 mL; 5 vials in 250 mL). The dose to be administered is adjusted according to the patient's weight, see the Bivalirudin Dosing table.

If the low-rate infusion is used after the initial infusion, a lower concentration bag should be prepared. In order to prepare this bag, reconstitute the 250 mg vial with 5 mL of sterile water for injection. Gently swirl until all material is dissolved. Each reconstituted vial should be further diluted in 500 mL of 5% dextrose in water or 0.9% sodium chloride for injection to yield a final concentration of 0.5 mg/mL. The infusion rate to be administered should be selected from the subsequent low-rate infusion column in the previous table.

➤*IV compatibilities/incompatibilities:* Bivalirudin should be administered via an IV line. No incompatibilities have been observed with glass bottles or polyvinyl chloride bags and administration sets. The following drugs should not be administered in the same IV line with bivalirudin because they resulted in haze formation, microparticulate formation, or gross precipitation when mixed with bivalirudin: alteplase, amiodarone, amphotericin B, chlorpromazine, diazepam, prochlorperazine edisylate, reteplase, streptokinase, and vancomycin. Dobutamine was compatible at concentrations up to 4 mg/mL but incompatible at a concentration of 12.5 mg/mL.

Parenteral drug products should be inspected visually for particulate matter and discoloration prior to administration. Preparations of bivalirudin containing particulate matter should not be used. Reconstituted material will be a clear to slightly opalescent, colorless to slightly yellow solution.

➤*Renal function impairment:* The infusion dose of bivalirudin may need to be reduced and anticoagulant status monitored in patients with renal function impairment. Patients with moderate renal function impairment (creatinine clearance [Ccr], 30 to 59 mL/min) should receive 1.75 mg/kg/h. If the Ccr is less than 30 mL/min, reduction of the infusion rate to 1 mg/kg/h should be considered. If a patient is on hemodialysis, the infusion should be reduced to 0.25 mg/kg/h. No reduction in the bolus dose is needed.

➤*Storage/Stability:* Store bivalirudin dosage units at 20° to 25°C (68° to 77°F); excursions to 15° to 30°C (59° to 86°F) permitted.

Do not freeze reconstituted or diluted bivalirudin. Reconstituted material may be stored at 2° to 8°C (36° to 46°F) for up to 24 hours. Diluted bivalirudin with a concentration between 0.5 and 5 mg/mL is stable at room temperature for up to 24 hours. Discard any unused portion of reconstituted solution remaining in the vial.

Actions

➤*Pharmacology:* Bivalirudin directly inhibits thrombin by specifically binding both to the catalytic site and to the anion-binding exosite of circulating and clot-bound thrombin. Thrombin is a serine proteinase that plays a central role in the thrombotic process, acting to cleave fibrinogen into fibrin monomers and to activate factor XIII to factor XIIIa, allowing fibrin to develop a covalently cross-linked framework that stabilizes the thrombus; thrombin also activates factors V and VIII, promoting further thrombin generation, and activates platelets, stimulating aggregation and granule release. The binding of bivalirudin to thrombin is reversible as thrombin slowly cleaves the bivalirudin-Arg_3-Pro_4 bond, resulting in recovery of thrombin active site functions.

In in vitro studies, bivalirudin inhibited both soluble (free) and clot-bound thrombin, was not neutralized by products of the platelet-release reaction, and prolonged the activated partial thromboplastin time (aPTT), thrombin time (TT), and prothrombin time (PT) of normal human plasma in a concentration-dependent manner. The clinical relevance of these findings is unknown.

Pharmacodynamics – In healthy volunteers and patients (with 70% or more vessel occlusion undergoing routine angioplasty), bivalirudin exhibits linear dose- and concentration-dependent anticoagulant activity as evidenced by prolongation of the ACT, aPTT, PT, and TT. IV administration of bivalirudin produces an immediate anticoagulant effect. Coagulation times return to baseline approximately 1 hour following cessation of bivalirudin administration.

In 291 patients with 70% or more vessel occlusion undergoing routine angioplasty, a positive correlation was observed between the dose of bivalirudin and the proportion of patients achieving ACT values of 300 or 350 seconds. At a bivalirudin dose of 1 mg/kg IV bolus plus 2.5 mg/kg/h IV infusion for 4 hours, followed by 0.2 mg/kg/h, all patients reached maximal ACT values greater than 300 seconds.

➤*Pharmacokinetics:*

Special populations –
Renal function impairment:

Pharmacokinetic Parameters in Patients with Renal Function Impairment[a]		
Renal function (GFR, mL/min)	Clearance (mL/min/kg)	Half-life (min)
Normal renal function (≥ 90 mL/min)	3.4	25
Mild renal impairment (60 to 89 mL/min)	3.4	22
Moderate renal impairment (30 to 59 mL/min)	2.7	34
Severe renal impairment (10 to 29 mL/min)	2.8	57
Dialysis-dependent patients (off dialysis)	1	3.5 h

[a] Monitor the ACT in renally impaired patients.

Bivalirudin exhibits linear pharmacokinetics following IV administration to patients undergoing PTCA. In these patients, a mean steady-state bivalirudin concentration of 12.3 ± 1.7 mcg/mL is achieved following an IV bolus of 1 mg/kg and a 4-hour 2.5 mg/kg/h IV infusion. Bivalirudin is cleared from plasma by a combination of renal mechanisms and proteolytic cleavage, with a half-life in patients with healthy renal function of 25 minutes. The disposition of bivalirudin was studied in PTCA patients with mild and moderate renal function impairment and in patients with severe renal function impairment. Drug elimination was related to glomerular filtration rate (GFR). Total body clearance was similar for patients with healthy renal function and with mild renal impairment (60 to 89 mL/min). Clearance was reduced approximately 20% in patients with moderate and severe renal impairment and was reduced approximately 80% in dialysis-dependent patients. See the following table for pharmacokinetic parameters. For patients with renal function impairment, monitor the ACT. Bivalirudin is hemodialyzable. Approximately 25% is cleared by hemodialysis.

Bivalirudin does not bind to plasma proteins (other than thrombin) or to red blood cells.

Contraindications

Active major bleeding; hypersensitivity to bivalirudin or its components.

BIVALIRUDIN — INJECTION

Warnings

➤*Hematologic effects:* Bivalirudin is not intended for intramuscular administration. Although most bleeding associated with the use of bivalirudin in PCI occurs at the site of arterial puncture, hemorrhage can occur at any site. An unexplained fall in blood pressure or hematocrit, or any unexplained symptom, should lead to serious consideration of a hemorrhagic event and cessation of bivalirudin administration.

➤*Brachytherapy:* An increased risk of thrombus formation has been associated with the use of bivalirudin in gamma brachytherapy, including fatal outcomes.

Use caution when bivalirudin is used as the antithrombin during brachytherapy procedures. Operators are advised to maintain meticulous catheter technique, with frequent aspiration and flushing, paying special attention to minimizing conditions of stasis within the catheter or vessels.

➤*Antidote:* There is no known antidote to bivalirudin. Bivalirudin is hemodialyzable.

➤*Renal function impairment:* The disposition of bivalirudin was studied in PTCA patients with mild and moderate renal function impairment and in patients with severe renal function impairment. Drug elimination was related to GFR. Total body clearance was similar for patients with healthy renal function and with mild renal impairment (60 to 89 mL/min). Clearance was reduced approximately 20% in patients with moderate and severe renal impairment and was reduced approximately 80% in dialysis-dependent patients.

➤*Mutagenesis:* Bivalirudin displayed no genotoxic potential in the in vitro bacterial cell reverse mutation assay (Ames test), the in vitro Chinese hamster ovary cell forward gene mutation test (CHO/HGPRT), the in vitro human lymphocyte chromosomal aberration assay, the in vitro rat hepatocyte unscheduled deoxyribonucleic acid (DNA) synthesis (UDS) assay, and the in vivo rat micronucleus assay.

➤*Elderly:* In studies of patients undergoing PCI, 44% were 65 years of age and older, and 12% were older than 75 years of age. Elderly patients experienced more bleeding events than younger patients. Patients treated with bivalirudin experienced fewer bleeding events in each age stratum, compared with heparin.

➤*Pregnancy: Category B.* Bivalirudin is intended for use with aspirin. Because of the possible adverse reactions on the neonate and the potential for increased maternal bleeding, particularly during the third trimester, use bivalirudin and aspirin together during pregnancy only if clearly needed.

There are no adequate and well-controlled studies in pregnant women. Because animal reproduction studies are not always predictive of human response, use this drug during pregnancy only if clearly needed.

➤*Lactation:* It is not known whether bivalirudin is excreted in human milk. Because many drugs are excreted in human milk, exercise caution when bivalirudin is administered to a breast-feeding woman.

➤*Children:* The safety and efficacy of bivalirudin in pediatric patients have not been established.

Precautions

➤*Immunogenicity/Reexposure:* Among 494 subjects who received bivalirudin in clinical trials and were tested for antibodies, 2 subjects had treatment-emergent positive bivalirudin antibody tests. Neither subject demonstrated clinical evidence of allergic or anaphylactic reactions, and repeat testing was not performed. Nine additional patients who had initial positive tests were negative on repeat testing.

➤*Special risk:* Use bivalirudin with caution in patients with disease states associated with an increased risk of bleeding.

Drug Interactions

Bivalirudin does not exhibit binding to plasma proteins (other than thrombin) or red blood cells.

➤*Hematological agents:* In clinical trials in patients undergoing PTCA/PCI, coadministration of bivalirudin with heparin, warfarin, thrombolytics, or GPIIb/IIIa inhibitors was associated with increased risks of major bleeding events compared with patients not receiving these concomitant medications. There is no experience with coadministration of bivalirudin and plasma expanders such as dextran.

Adverse Reactions

➤*Bleeding:*

Major Hematologic Outcomes in the REPLACE-2 Study (Safety Population)			
	Bivalirudin plus "provisional" GPIIb/IIIa inhibitor[a] (n = 2,914)	Heparin plus GPIIb/IIIa inhibitor (n = 2,987)	*P* value
Protocol-defined major hemorrhage[b] (%)	2.3%	4%	< 0.001
Protocol-defined minor hemorrhage[c] (%)	13.6%	25.8%	< 0.001
TIMI-defined bleeding[d]			
Major	0.6%	0.9%	0.259
Minor	1.3%	2.9%	< 0.001
Non-access site bleeding			
Retroperitoneal bleeding	0.2%	0.5%	0.069
Intracranial bleeding	< 0.1%	0.1%	1
Access site bleeding			
Sheath site bleeding	0.9%	2.4%	< 0.001
Thrombocytopenia[e]			
< 100,000/mm^3	0.7%	1.7%	< 0.001
< 50,000/mm^3	0.3%	0.6%	0.039
Transfusions			
Red blood cells (RBC)	1.3%	1.9%	0.08
Platelets	0.3%	0.6%	0.095

[a] GPIIb/IIIa inhibitors were administered to 7.2% of patients in the bivalirudin plus "provisional" GPIIb/IIIa inhibitor group.
[b] Defined as the occurrence of any of the following: intracranial bleeding, retroperitoneal bleeding, a transfusion of 2 units or more of blood/blood products, a fall in hemoglobin greater than 4 g/dL, whether or not bleeding site is identified, spontaneous or nonspontaneous blood loss with a decrease in hemoglobin greater than 3 g/dL.
[c] Defined as observed bleeding that does not meet the criteria for major hemorrhage.
[d] TIMI major bleeding is defined as: intracranial, or a fall in adjusted hemoglobin (Hgb) greater than 5 g/dL or hematocrit of greater than 15%; TIMI minor bleeding is defined as a fall in adjusted hemoglobin of 3 to less than 5 g/dL or a fall in adjusted hematocrit of 9% to less than 15%, with a bleeding site such as hematuria, hematemesis, hematomas, retroperitoneal bleeding, or a decrease in hemoglobin of greater than 4 g/dL with no bleeding site.
[e] If less than 100,000/mm^3 and greater than 25% reduction from baseline, or less than 50,000/mm^3.

Bivalirudin Major Bleeding and Transfusions: All Patients[a]		
	Bivalirudin (n = 2,161)	Heparin (n = 2,151)
Number (%) patients with major hemorrhage[b]	79 (3.7%)	199 (9.3%)
with ≥ 3 g/dL fall in hemoglobin	41 (1.9%)	124 (5.8%)
with ≥ 5 g/dL fall in hemoglobin	14 (0.6%	47 (2.2%)
Retroperitoneal bleeding	5 (0.2%)	15 (0.7%)
Intracranial bleeding	1 (< 0.1%)	2 (< 0.1%)
Required transfusion	43 (2%)	123 (5.7%)

[a] No monitoring of ACT (or PTT) was done after a target ACT was achieved.
[b] Major hemorrhage was defined as the occurrence of any of the following: intracranial bleeding, retroperitoneal bleeding, clinically overt bleeding with a decrease in hemoglobin greater than or equal to 3 g/dL or leading to a transfusion of greater than or equal to 2 units of blood. This table includes data from the entire hospitalization period.

➤*Other adverse reactions:* Adverse reactions observed in clinical trials are similar between the bivalirudin-treated patients and the control groups. Adverse reactions seen are those typical of PCI trials.

Bivalirudin Adverse Reactions (> 5%)		
Adverse reaction	Bivalirudin (n = 2,161)	Heparin (n = 2,151)
Cardiovascular		
Bradycardia	118 (5%)	164 (8%)
Hypertension	135 (6%)	115 (5%)
Hypotension	262 (12%)	371 (17%)
CNS		
Headache	264 (12%)	225 (10%)
Insomnia	142 (7%)	139 (6%)
Nervousness	102 (5%)	87 (4%)

Thrombin Inhibitor

BIVALIRUDIN — INJECTION

Bivalirudin Adverse Reactions (> 5%)

Adverse reaction	Bivalirudin (n = 2,161)	Heparin (n = 2,151)
GI		
Abdominal pain	103 (5%)	104 (5%)
Dyspepsia	100 (5%)	111 (5%)
Nausea	318 (15%)	347 (16%)
Vomiting	138 (6%)	169 (8%)
GU		
Urinary retention	89 (4%)	98 (5%)
Miscellaneous		
Anxiety	127 (6%)	140 (7%)
Back pain	916 (42%)	944 (44%)
Fever	103 (5%)	108 (5%)
Injection-site pain	174 (8%)	274 (13%)
Pain	330 (15%)	358 (17%)
Pelvic pain	130 (6%)	169 (8%)

➤*Other adverse reactions:* Serious, nonbleeding adverse reactions were experienced in 2% of 2,161 bivalirudin-treated patients and 2% of 2,151 heparin-treated patients. The following individual serious, nonbleeding adverse reactions were rare (greater than 0.1% to less than 1%) and similar in incidence between bivalirudin- and heparin-treated patients.

Cardiovascular – Hypotension, syncope, vascular anomaly, ventricular fibrillation.

CNS – Cerebral ischemia, confusion, facial paralysis.

GU – Kidney failure, oliguria.

Respiratory – Lung edema.

Miscellaneous – Fever, infection, sepsis. In the double-blind, randomized REPLACE-2 trial described above that compared bivalirudin plus "provisional" GPIIb/IIIa inhibitor with heparin plus GPIIb/IIIa inhibitor, similar adverse reactions were reported in both treatment groups:

Bivalirudin Adverse Reactions (≥ 2%)

Adverse reaction	Bivalirudin plus "provisional" GPIIb/IIIa inhibitor (n = 2,914)	Heparin plus GPIIb/IIIa inhibitor (n = 2,987)
Cardiovascular		
Angina pectoris	155 (5.3%)	156 (5.2%)
Hypotension	91 (3.1%)	120 (4%)
CNS		
Headache	75 (2.6%)	83 (2.8%)
GI		
Nausea	86 (3%)	96 (3.2%)
Miscellaneous		
Back pain	268 (9.2%)	263 (8.8%)
Chest pain	68 (2.3%)	69 (2.3%)
Injection-site pain	80 (2.7%)	80 (2.7%)
Pain	98 (3.4%)	72 (2.4%)

Postmarketing – The following reactions have been reported: fatal bleeding; hypersensitivity and allergic reactions, including very rare reports of anaphylaxis; thrombus formation during PCI with and without intracoronary brachytherapy, including reports of fatal outcomes.

Overdosage

➤*Symptoms:* Single bolus doses of bivalirudin up to 7.5 mg/kg have been reported without associated bleeding or other adverse reactions. Discontinuation of bivalirudin leads to a gradual reduction in anticoagulant effects caused by metabolism of the drug.

➤*Treatment:* In case of overdosage, discontinue bivalirudin immediately and closely monitor the patient for signs of bleeding. Bivalirudin is hemodialyzable. There is no known antidote to bivalirudin.

Selective Factor Xa Inhibitor

FONDAPARINUX SODIUM

Rx	**Arixtra** (GlaxoSmithKline)	**Injection**: 2.5 mg per 0.5 mL	Preservative free. In single-dose, prefilled syringes with 27-gauge needle. In 10s.
		5 mg per 0.4 mL	Preservative free. In single-dose, prefilled syringes with 27-gauge needle. In 10s.
		7.5 mg per 0.6 mL	Preservative free. In single-dose, prefilled syringes with 27-gauge needle. In 10s.
		10 mg per 0.8 mL	Preservative free. In single-dose, prefilled syringes with 27-gauge needle. In 10s.

FONDAPARINUX SODIUM — INJECTION

WARNING

Spinal/Epidural hematomas – When neuraxial anesthesia (epidural/spinal anesthesia) or spinal puncture is employed, patients anticoagulated or scheduled to be anticoagulated with low molecular weight heparins (LMWHs), heparinoids, or fondaparinux for prevention of thromboembolic complications are at risk of developing an epidural or spinal hematoma that can result in long-term or permanent paralysis.

The risk of these events is increased by the use of indwelling epidural catheters for administration of analgesia or by the concomitant use of drugs affecting hemostasis, such as nonsteroidal anti-inflammatory drugs (NSAIDs), platelet inhibitors, or other anticoagulants. The risk also appears to be increased by traumatic or repeated epidural or spinal puncture.

Frequently monitor patients for signs and symptoms of neurological impairment. If neurologic compromise is noted, urgent treatment is necessary.

Consider the potential benefit versus risk before neuraxial intervention in patients anticoagulated or scheduled to be anticoagulated for thromboprophylaxis. Use fondaparinux injection, like other anticoagulants, with extreme caution in conditions with increased risk of hemorrhage, such as congenital or acquired bleeding disorders; active ulcerative and angiodysplastic GI disease; hemorrhagic stroke; or shortly after brain, spinal, or ophthalmological surgery; or in patients treated concomitantly with platelet inhibitors.

Indications

➤*Prophylaxis of deep vein thrombosis (DVT):* For the prophylaxis of DVT, which may lead to pulmonary embolism (PE):

- in patients undergoing hip fracture surgery, including extended prophylaxis;
- in patients undergoing hip replacement surgery;
- in patients undergoing knee replacement surgery;
- in patients undergoing abdominal surgery who are at risk for thromboembolic complications.

➤*Treatment of acute DVT:* For the treatment of acute DVT when administered in conjunction with warfarin.

➤*Treatment of acute PE:* For the treatment of acute PE when administered in conjunction with warfarin when initial therapy is administered in the hospital.

Administration and Dosage

➤*Approved by the FDA:* December 7, 2001.

➤*DVT prophylaxis following hip fracture or hip or knee replacement surgeries:* In patients undergoing hip fracture, hip replacement, or knee replacement surgery, the recommended dose of fondaparinux is 2.5 mg administered by subcutaneous injection once daily. After hemostasis has been established, give the initial dose 6 to 8 hours after surgery. Administration before 6 hours after surgery has been associated with an increased risk of major bleeding. The usual duration of administration is 5 to 9 days; up to 11 days administration has been tolerated. In patients undergoing hip fracture surgery, an extended prophylaxis course of up to 24 additional days is recommended. In patients undergoing hip fracture surgery, a total of 32 days (perioperative and extended prophylaxis) has been tolerated. If thrombotic events occur despite fondaparinux prophylaxis, initiate appropriate therapy.

➤*DVT prophylaxis following abdominal surgery:* In patients undergoing abdominal surgery, the recommended dose of fondaparinux is 2.5 mg administered by subcutaneous injection once daily after hemostasis has been established. The initial dose should be given 6 to 8 hours after surgery. Administration before 6 hours after surgery has been associated with an increased risk of major bleeding. The usual duration of administration is 5 to 9 days; up to 10 days of fondaparinux injection has been administered. If thrombotic events occur despite fondaparinux prophylaxis, initiate appropriate therapy.

FONDAPARINUX SODIUM — INJECTION

➤*DVT and PE treatment:* In patients with acute symptomatic DVT and in patients with acute symptomatic PE, the recommended dose of fondaparinux is 5 mg (body weight less than 50 kg), 7.5 mg (body weight 50 to 100 kg), or 10 mg (body weight greater than 100 kg) by subcutaneous injection once daily (fondaparinux treatment regimen). Continue fondaparinux injection treatment for at least 5 days and until a therapeutic oral anticoagulant effect is established (International Normalized Ratio [INR] 2 to 3). Initiate concomitant treatment with warfarin as soon as possible, usually within 72 hours. The usual duration of administration of fondaparinux is 5 to 9 days; up to 26 days of fondaparinux injection has been administered.

➤*Administration:* Administer fondaparinux injection according to the recommended regimen, especially with respect to the timing of the first dose after surgery. In the hip fracture, hip replacement, knee replacement, or abdominal surgery clinical studies, the administration of fondaparinux before 6 hours after surgery has been associated with an increased risk of major bleeding.

Fondaparinux injection is provided in a single-dose, prefilled syringe affixed with an automatic needle protection system. Fondaparinux is administered by subcutaneous injection. It must not be administered by intramuscular injections. Fondaparinux is intended for use under a health care provider's guidance. Patients may self-inject only if their health care providers determine that it is appropriate and with medical follow-up as necessary. Provide proper training in subcutaneous injection technique.

To avoid the loss of drug when using the prefilled syringe, do not expel the air bubble from the syringe before the injection. Administer in the fatty tissue, alternating injection sites (eg, between the left and right anterolateral or the left and right posterolateral abdominal wall).

➤*Admixture incompatibilities:* Do not mix fondaparinux with other injections or infusions.

➤*Storage/Stability:* Store at 25°C (77°F); excursions permitted to 15° to 30°C (59° to 86°F). Keep out of the reach of children.

Actions

➤*Pharmacology:* The antithrombotic activity of fondaparinux is the result of antithrombin III (ATIII)-mediated selective inhibition of factor Xa. By selectively binding to ATIII, fondaparinux potentiates (about 300 times) the innate neutralization of factor Xa by ATIII. Neutralization of factor Xa interrupts the blood coagulation cascade and inhibits thrombin formation and thrombus development.

Fondaparinux does not inactivate thrombin (activated factor II) and has no known effect on platelet function. At the recommended dose, fondaparinux does not affect fibrinolytic activity or bleeding time.

Anti-Xa activity – The pharmacodynamics/pharmacokinetics of fondaparinux are derived from fondaparinux plasma concentrations quantified via anti-factor Xa activity. Only fondaparinux can be used to calibrate the anti-Xa assay. (The international standards of heparin or LMWH are not appropriate for this use.) As a result, the activity of fondaparinux is expressed as milligrams (mg) of the fondaparinux calibrator. The anti-Xa activity of the drug increases with increasing drug concentration, reaching maximum values in approximately 3 hours.

➤*Pharmacokinetics:*

Absorption – Fondaparinux administered by subcutaneous injection is rapidly and completely absorbed (absolute bioavailability is 100%). Following a single subcutaneous dose of fondaparinux 2.5 mg in young male subjects, C_{max} of 0.34 mg/L is reached in approximately 2 hours. In patients undergoing treatment with fondaparinux injection 2.5 mg once daily, the peak steady-state plasma concentration is, on average, 0.39 to 0.5 mg/L and is reached approximately 3 hours postdose. In these patients, the minimum steady-state plasma concentration is 0.14 to 0.19 mg/L. In patients with symptomatic DVT and PE undergoing treatment with fondaparinux injection 5 mg (body weight less than 50 kg), 7.5 mg (body weight 50 to 100 kg), and 10 mg (body weight greater than 100 kg) once daily, the body-weight-adjusted doses provide similar mean steady-state peaks and minimum plasma concentrations across all body weight categories. The mean peak steady-state plasma concentration is in the range of 1.2 to 1.26 mg/L. In these patients, the mean minimum steady-state plasma concentration is in the range of 0.46 to 0.62 mg/L.

Distribution – In healthy adults, intravenously (IV) or subcutaneously administered fondaparinux distributes mainly in blood and only to a minor extent in extravascular fluid as evidenced by steady state and nonsteady state apparent volume of distribution of 7 to 11 L. Similar fondaparinux distribution occurs in patients undergoing elective hip surgery or hip fracture surgery. In vitro, fondaparinux is highly (at least 94%) and specifically bound to ATIII and does not bind significantly to other plasma proteins (including platelet factor 4 [PF4]) or red blood cells.

Metabolism – In vivo metabolism of fondaparinux has not been investigated since the majority of the administered dose is eliminated unchanged in urine in individuals with normal kidney function.

Excretion – In individuals with normal kidney function, fondaparinux is eliminated in urine mainly as unchanged drug. In healthy individuals up to 75 years of age, up to 77% of a single subcutaneous or IV fondaparinux dose is eliminated in urine as unchanged drug in 72 hours. The elimination half-life is 17 to 21 hours.

Special populations –

Renal function impairment: Fondaparinux elimination is prolonged in patients with renal impairment because the major route of elimination is urinary excretion of unchanged drug. In patients undergoing prophylaxis following elective hip surgery or hip fracture surgery, the total clearance of fondaparinux is approximately 25% lower in patients with mild renal impairment (creatinine clearance [Ccr] 50 to 80 mL/min), approximately 40% lower in patients with moderate renal impairment (Ccr 30 to 50 mL/min) and approximately 55% lower in patients with severe renal impairment (less than 30 mL/min) compared with patients with normal renal function. A similar relationship between fondaparinux clearance and extent of renal impairment was observed in DVT treatment patients.

Elderly: Fondaparinux elimination is prolonged in patients older than 75 years of age. In studies evaluating 2.5 mg fondaparinux prophylaxis in hip fracture surgery or elective hip surgery, the total clearance of fondaparinux was approximately 25% lower in patients older than 75 years of age as compared with patients younger than 65 years of age. A similar relationship between fondaparinux clearance and age was observed in DVT treatment patients.

Patients weighing less than 50 kg: Total clearance of fondaparinux is decreased by approximately 30% in patients weighing less than 50 kg. Fondaparinux prophylactic therapy is contraindicated in patients with body weight less than 50 kg undergoing hip fracture, hip replacement, knee replacement surgery, and abdominal surgery. During the randomized clinical trials of prophylaxis in the perioperative period following hip fracture, hip replacement, or knee replacement surgery, occurrence of major bleeding was doubled in patients with body weight less than 50 kg compared with those with body weight greater than or equal to 50 kg (5.4% vs 2.1%). In the clinical trial in patients undergoing abdominal surgery, the major bleeding rate was also higher in patients with a body weight less than 50 kg as compared with those with a body weight of at least 50 kg (5.3% vs 3.3%), respectively.

Contraindications

Fondaparinux injection is contraindicated in patients with severe renal impairment (Ccr less than 30 mL/min). Fondaparinux is eliminated primarily by the kidneys, and such patients are at increased risk for major bleeding episodes.

Fondaparinux prophylactic therapy is contraindicated in patients with body weight less than 50 kg undergoing hip fracture, hip replacement, knee replacement surgery, or abdominal surgery. During the randomized clinical trials of prophylaxis in the perioperative period following hip fracture, hip replacement, or knee replacement surgery, occurrence of major bleeding was doubled in patients with a body weight less than 50 kg compared with those with a body weight greater than or equal to 50 kg (5.4% vs 2.1%). In the clinical trial in patients undergoing abdominal surgery, the major bleeding rate was also higher in patients with a body weight less than 50 kg as compared with those with a body weight of 50 kg or greater (5.3% vs 3.3%), respectively.

The use of fondaparinux is contraindicated in patients with active major bleeding, bacterial endocarditis, in patients with thrombocytopenia associated with a positive in vitro test for antiplatelet antibody in the presence of fondaparinux, or in patients with known hypersensitivity to fondaparinux.

Warnings

➤*Interchangeability:* Fondaparinux injection cannot be used interchangeably (unit for unit) with heparin, LMWHs, or heparinoids, as they differ in manufacturing process, anti-Xa and anti-IIa activity, units, and dosage. Each of these medicines has its own instructions for use.

➤*Hemorrhage:* See the Warning box for more information.

➤*Neuraxial anesthesia and postoperative indwelling epidural catheter use:* See the Warning box for more information.

➤*Thrombocytopenia:* Thrombocytopenia can occur with the administration of fondaparinux. Moderate thrombocytopenia (platelet counts between 100,000/mm^3 and 50,000/mm^3) occurred at a rate of 3% in patients given fondaparinux 2.5 mg in the perioperative hip fracture, hip replacement, or knee replacement surgery, and abdominal surgery clinical trials. Severe thrombocytopenia (platelet counts less than 50,000/mm^3) occurred at a rate of 0.2% in patients given fondaparinux 2.5 mg in these clinical trials. During extended prophylaxis, no cases of moderate or severe thrombocytopenia were reported.

Moderate thrombocytopenia occurred at a rate of 0.5% in patients given the fondaparinux treatment regimen in the DVT and PE treatment clinical trials. Severe thrombocytopenia occurred at a rate of 0.04% in patients given the fondaparinux treatment regimen in the DVT and PE treatment clinical trials.

Closely monitor thrombocytopenia of any degree. If the platelet count falls below 100,000/mm^3, discontinue fondaparinux.

➤*Renal function impairment:*

Hip fracture, hip replacement, and knee replacement surgeries – Major bleeding in patients receiving prophylactic therapy in hip fracture, hip replacement, or knee replacement surgery occurred in 1.6% (25/1,565) of patients with normal renal function, in 2.4% (31/1,288) with mild renal impairment, in 3.8% (19/504) with moderate renal impairment, and in 4.8% (4/83) with severe renal impairment. When fondaparinux was used according to the recommended timing of the first injection (6 to 8 hours after surgery), major bleeding occurred in 1.8% (16/905) of patients with normal renal function, in 2.2% (15/675) with mild renal impairment, in 2.3% (6/265) with moderate renal impairment, and in 0% (0/40) with severe renal impairment.

Abdominal surgery – Major bleeding in patients receiving prophylactic therapy in abdominal surgery occurred in 2.1% (13/606) of patients with normal renal function, in 3.6% (22/613) with mild renal impairment, in 6.7% (12/179) with moderate renal impairment, and in 7.1% (1/14) with severe renal impairment. When fondaparinux was used according to the recom-

FONDAPARINUX SODIUM — INJECTION

mended timing of the first injection (6 to 8 hours after surgery), major bleeding occurred in 2.1% (10/467) of patients with normal renal function, in 3.3% (16/481) with mild renal impairment, in 5.8% (8/137) with moderate renal impairment, and in 7.7% (1/13) with severe renal impairment.

Treatment of DVT and PE – Major bleeding in patients receiving treatment for DVT and PE occurred in 0.4% (4/1,132) of patients with normal renal function, in 1.6% (12/733) with mild renal impairment, in 2.2% (7/318) with moderate renal impairment, and in 7.3% (4/55) with severe renal impairment.

Use fondaparinux with caution in patients with moderate renal impairment (Ccr 30 to 50 mL/min). Periodically assess renal function in patients receiving fondaparinux. Immediately discontinue the drug in patients who develop severe renal impairment while on therapy. After discontinuation of fondaparinux, its anticoagulant effects may persist for 2 to 4 days in patients with normal renal function (ie, at least 3 to 5 half-lives). The anticoagulant effects of fondaparinux may persist even longer in patients with renal impairment.

➤*Elderly:* Use fondaparinux injection with caution in elderly patients. Over 3,000 patients, 65 years of age and older, have received 2.5 mg fondaparinux in randomized clinical trials. Over 1,200 patients, 65 years of age and older, have received the fondaparinux treatment regimen in the DVT and PE treatment clinical trials. The efficacy of fondaparinux in the elderly (65 years of age and older) was similar to that seen in younger patients (younger than 65 years). In the perioperative hip fracture, hip replacement, or knee replacement surgery clinical trials with patients receiving fondaparinux 2.5 mg the risk of fondaparinux-associated major bleeding increased with age: 1.8% (23/1,253) in patients younger than 65 years, 2.2% (24/1,111) in those 65 to 74 years, and 2.7% (33/1,227) in those 75 years or older. Serious adverse reactions increased with age for patients receiving fondaparinux. In patients undergoing 3 weeks of extended prophylaxis following 1 week of perioperative prophylaxis after hip fracture surgery, the incidence of major bleeding was 1.9% (1/52) in patients younger than 65 years of age, 1.4% (1/71) in those 65 to 74 years, and 2.9% (6/204) in those 75 years of age or older. In the abdominal surgery clinical trial, the risk of fondaparinux-associated major bleeding increased with age: 3% (19/644) in patients younger than 65 years of age, 3.2% (16/507) in those 65 to 74 years of age, and 5% (14/282) in those 75 years of age and older. In the DVT and PE treatment clinical trials with patients receiving the fondaparinux treatment regimen, the risk of fondaparinux-associated major bleeding increased with age: 0.6% (7/1151) in patients younger than 65 years of age, 1.6% (9/560) in those 65 to 74 years of age, and 2.1% (12/583) in those 75 years of age or older. Careful attention to dosing directions and concomitant medications (especially antiplatelet medication) is advised.

Fondaparinux is substantially excreted by the kidney, and the risk of toxic reactions to fondaparinux may be greater in patients with impaired renal function. Because elderly patients are more likely to have decreased renal function, it may be useful to monitor renal function.

➤*Pregnancy: Category B.* There are no adequate and well-controlled studies in pregnant women. Because animal reproduction studies are not always predictive of human response, use this drug during pregnancy only if clearly needed.

➤*Lactation:* Fondaparinux was found to be excreted in the milk of lactating rats. However, it is not known whether this drug is excreted in human milk. Because many drugs are excreted in human milk, exercise caution when fondaparinux is administered to a nursing mother.

➤*Children:* Safety and effectiveness of fondaparinux in pediatric patients have not been established.

Precautions

➤*Monitoring:* Frequently monitor patients for signs and symptoms of neurological impairment.

Periodic routine complete blood counts (including platelet count), serum creatinine level, and stool occult blood tests are recommended during the course of treatment with fondaparinux injection.

When administered at the recommended doses, routine coagulation tests such as prothrombin time (PT) and activated partial thromboplastin time (aPTT) are relatively insensitive measures of fondaparinux activity, and are therefore, unsuitable for monitoring.

The anti-factor Xa activity of fondaparinux can be measured by anti-Xa assay using the appropriate calibrator (fondaparinux). Since the international standards of heparin or LMWH are not appropriate calibrators, the activity of fondaparinux is expressed in milligrams (mg) of the fondaparinux and cannot be compared with activities of heparin or LMWHs.

Because routine coagulation tests such as PT and aPTT are relatively insensitive measures of fondaparinux activity and international standards of heparin or LMWH are not calibrators to measure anti-factor Xa activity of fondaparinux, if during fondaparinux therapy unexpected changes in coagulation parameters or major bleeding occurs, discontinue fondaparinux.

➤*Special risk:* Use fondaparinux injection with care in patients with a bleeding diathesis, uncontrolled arterial hypertension, or a history of recent GI ulceration, diabetic retinopathy, and hemorrhage.

Drug Interactions

Discontinue agents that may enhance the risk of hemorrhage prior to initiation of fondaparinux therapy. If coadministration is essential, close monitoring may be appropriate.

➤*Coumarin:* In an in vitro study in human liver microsomes, inhibition of CYP2A6 hydroxylation of coumarin by fondaparinux (200 mcM [ie, 350 mg/L]) was 17% to 28%. Inhibition of the other isozymes evaluated (CYPs 2A1, 2C9, 2C19, 2D6, 3A4, and 3E1) was 0% to 16%. Since fondaparinux does not markedly inhibit CYP450s (CYP1A2, CYP2A6, CYP2C9, CYP2C19, CYP2D6, CYP2E1, or CYP3A4) in vitro, fondaparinux is not expected to significantly interact with other drugs in vivo by inhibition of metabolism mediated by these isozymes.

Adverse Reactions

➤*Hemorrhage:* During fondaparinux administration, the most common adverse reactions were bleeding complications.

Hip fracture, hip replacement, and knee replacement surgery –

Fondaparinux Major Bleeding Episodes[a] in Randomized, Controlled, Hip Fracture, Hip Replacement, and Knee Replacement Surgery Studies

	Perioperative prophylaxis (day 1 to day 7 ± 1 postsurgery)		Extended prophylaxis (day 8 to day 28 ± 2 postsurgery)	
Indications	2.5 mg Fondaparinux subcutaneously once daily	Enoxaparin[b,c]	2.5 mg Fondaparinux subcutaneously once daily	Placebo subcutaneously once daily
Hip fracture	18/831 (2.2%)	19/842 (2.3%)	8/327 (2.4%)[d]	2/329 (0.6%)
Hip replacement	67/2,268 (3%)	55/2,597 (2.1%)		
Knee replacement	11/517 (2.1%)[e]	1/517 (0.2%)		

[a] Major bleeding was defined as clinically overt bleeding that was (1) fatal, (2) bleeding at critical site (eg, intracranial, retroperitoneal, intra-ocular, pericardial, spinal, into adrenal gland), (3) associated with reoperation at operative site, or (4) with a bleeding index (BI) greater than or equal to 2 calculated as [number of whole blood or packed red blood cell units transfused ± [(prebleeding) − (post-bleeding)] hemoglobin (g/dL) values].
[b] Enoxaparin dosing regimen: 30 mg every 12 hours or 40 mg once daily.
[c] Not approved for use in patients undergoing hip fracture surgery.
[d] During noncomparative, unblinded, perioperative prophylaxis, major bleeding was reported in 22/737 (3%) patients. Fifteen of these 22 patients continued to receive fondaparinux in extended prophylaxis. After randomization, 4/327 (1.2%) patients experienced major bleeding for the first time.
[e] *P*-value vs enoxaparin: less than 0.01, 95% CI, [1.1% to 3.3%] in fondaparinux group versus [0% to 1.1%] in enoxaparin group.

Fondaparinux Bleeding Across Randomized, Controlled Hip Fracture, Hip Replacement and Knee Replacement Surgery Studies

	Perioperative prophylaxis (day 1 to day 7 ± 1 postsurgery)		Extended prophylaxis (day 8 to day 28 ± 2 postsurgery)	
	2.5 mg Fondaparinux subcutaneously once daily	Enoxaparin[a,b]	2.5 mg Fondaparinux subcutaneously once daily	Placebo subcutaneously once daily
	(n = 3,616)	(n = 3,956)	(n = 327)	(n = 329)
Major bleeding[c]	96 (2.7%)	75 (1.9%)	8 (2.4%)[d]	2 (0.6%)
Fatal bleeding	0 (0%)	1 (< 0.1%)	0 (0%)	0 (0%)
Non-fatal bleeding at critical site	0 (0%)	1 (< 0.1%)	0 (0%)	0 (0%)
Re-operation due to bleeding	12 (0.3%)	10 (0.3%)	2 (0.6%)	2 (0.6%)
BI ≥ 2[e]	84 (2.3%)	63 (1.6%)	6 (1.8%)	0 (0%)
Minor bleeding[f]	109 (3%)	116 (2.9%)	5 (1.5%)	2 (0.6%)

[a] Enoxaparin dosing regimen: 30 mg every 12 hours or 40 mg once daily.
[b] Not approved for use in patients undergoing hip fracture surgery.
[c] Major bleeding was defined as clinically overt bleeding that was (1) fatal, (2) bleeding at critical site (eg, intracranial, retroperitoneal, intra-ocular, pericardial, spinal, into adrenal gland), (3) associated with reoperation at operative site, or (4) with a BI greater than or equal to 2.
[d] During noncomparative, unblinded, perioperative prophylaxis, 2 fatal bleeds were reported (1 in a 50 kg patient, 1 in a severe renal failure patient).
[e] BI greater than or equal to 2: overt bleeding associated only with a BI greater than or equal to 2 calculated as [number of whole blood or packed red blood cell units transfused + [(prebleeding) − (postbleeding)] hemoglobin (g/dL) values].
[f] Minor bleeding was defined as clinically overt bleeding that was not major.

A separate analysis of major bleeding across all randomized, controlled, perioperative, prophylaxis, clinical studies of hip fracture, hip replacement, or knee replacement surgery according to the time of the first injection of fondaparinux after surgical closure was performed in patients who received fondaparinux only postoperatively. In this analysis the incidences of major bleeding were as follows: less than 4 hours was 4.8% (5/104), 4 to 6 hours was 2.3% (28/1,196), 6 to 8 hours was 1.9% (38/1,965). In all studies, the majority (greater than or equal to 75%) of the major bleeding events occurred during the first 4 days after surgery.

FONDAPARINUX SODIUM — INJECTION

Abdominal surgery:

Major Bleeding Episodes[a] in Randomized, Controlled, Abdominal Surgery Study

	Fondaparinux 2.5 mg subcutaneously once daily	Dalteparin 5,000 units subcutaneously once daily
	n = 1,433	n = 1, 425
Major bleeding	49 (3.4%)	34 (2.4%)
Fatal bleeding	2 (0.1%)	2 (0.1%)
Nonfatal bleeding at critical site	0 (0%)	0 (0%)
Other nonfatal major bleeding		
Surgical site	38 (2.7%)	26 (1.8%)
Nonsurgical site	9 (0.6%)	6 (0.4%)
Minor bleeding[b]	31 (2.2%)	23 (1.6%)

[a] Major bleeding was defined as bleeding that was (1) fatal, (2) bleeding at the surgical site leading to intervention, (3) nonsurgical bleeding at a critical site (eg, intracranial, retroperitoneal, intraocular, pericardial, spinal, into adrenal gland) or leading to an intervention, and/or with a bleeding index (BI) ≥ 2. (BI ≥ 2 calculated as [number of whole blood or packed red blood cell units transfused + [(prebleeding) − (postbleeding)] hemoglobin (g/dL) values].)
[b] Minor bleeding was defined as clinically overt bleeding that was not major.

A separate analysis of major bleeding according to the time of the first injection of fondaparinux after surgical closure was performed. In this analysis, the incidences of major bleeding were as follows: less than 6 hours was 3.4% (9/263) and 6 to 8 hours was 2.9% (32/1,112).

Treatment of DVT and PE –

Bleeding[a] in DVT and PE Treatment Studies

	Fondaparinux treatment regimen	1 mg/kg enoxaparin subcutaneously every 12 hours	Heparin aPTT adjusted IV
	(n = 2,294)	(n = 1,101)	(n = 1,092)
Major bleeding[b]	28 (1.2%)	13 (1.2%)	12 (1.1%)
Fatal bleeding	3 (0.1%)	0 (0%)	1 (0.1%)
Nonfatal bleeding at a critical site	3 (0.1%)	0 (0%)	2 (0.2%)
Intracranial bleeding	3 (0.1%)	0 (0%)	1 (0.1%)
Retroperitoneal bleeding	0 (0%)	0 (0%)	1 (0.1%)
Clinically overt bleeding with a 2 g/dL fall in hemoglobin and/or leading to transfusion of PRBC or whole blood ≥ 2 units	22 (1%)	13 (1.2%)	10 (0.9%)
Minor bleeding[c]	70 (3.1%)	33 (3%)	57 (5.2%)

[a] Bleeding rates are during the study drug treatment period (approximately 7 days). Patients were also treated with vitamin K antagonists initiated within 72 hours after the first study drug administration.
[b] Major bleeding was defined as clinically overt: and/or contributing to death - and/or in a critical organ including intracranial, retroperitoneal, intraocular, spinal, pericardial, or adrenal gland - and/or associated with a fall in hemoglobin level greater than or equal to 2 g/dL - and/or leading to a transfusion greater than or equal to 2 units of packed red blood cells or whole blood.
[c] Minor bleeding was defined as clinically overt bleeding that was not major.

Thrombocytopenia – Thrombocytopenia can occur with the administration of fondaparinux. Moderate thrombocytopenia (platelet counts between 100,000/mm^3 and 50,000/mm^3) occurred at a rate of 2.9% in patients given fondaparinux 2.5 mg in the perioperative hip fracture, hip replacement, or knee replacement surgery clinical trials. Severe thrombocytopenia (platelet counts less than 50,000/mm^3) occurred at a rate of 0.2% in patients given fondaparinux 2.5 mg in these clinical trials. During extended prophylaxis, no cases of moderate or severe thrombocytopenia were reported.

Moderate thrombocytopenia occurred at a rate of 0.5% in patients given the fondaparinux treatment regimen in the DVT and PE treatment clinical trials. Severe thrombocytopenia occurred at a rate of 0.04% in patients given the fondaparinux treatment regimen in the DVT and PE treatment clinical trials.

Closely monitor thrombocytopenia of any degree. If the platelet count falls below 100,000/mm^3, discontinue fondaparinux.

➤*Local:* Mild local irritation (injection site bleeding, rash and pruritus) may occur following subcutaneous injection of fondaparinux.

➤*Elevations of serum aminotransferases:* In the perioperative prophylaxis randomized clinical trials of 7 ± 2 days asymptomatic increases in AST and ALT aminotransferase levels greater than 3 times the upper limit of normal of the laboratory reference range have been reported in 1.7% and 2.6% of patients, respectively, during treatment with fondaparinux 2.5 mg injection versus 3.2% and 3.9%, of patients, respectively, during treatment with enoxaparin 30 mg every 12 hours or enoxaparin 40 mg once daily. Such elevations are fully reversible and are rarely associated with increases in bilirubin. In the extended prophylaxis clinical trial no significant differences in AST and ALT between fondaparinux 2.5 mg injection and placebo-treated patients were observed.

In the DVT and PE treatment clinical trials asymptomatic increases in AST and ALT aminotransferase levels greater than 3 times the upper limit of normal of the laboratory reference range have been reported in 0.7% and 1.3% of patients, respectively, during treatment with the fondaparinux injection treatment regimen. In comparison, these increases have been reported in 4.8% and 12.3%, of patients, respectively, in the DVT treatment trial during treatment with enoxaparin 1 mg/kg every 12 hours, and in 2.9% and 8.7% of patients, respectively, in the PE treatment trial during treatment with aPTT adjusted heparin.

Since aminotransferase determinations are important in the differential diagnosis of myocardial infarction, liver disease, and pulmonary emboli, interpret elevations that might be caused by drugs like fondaparinux with caution.

➤*Other adverse reactions:*

Adverse Reactions Occurring in ≥ 2% of Fondaparinux Sodium, Enoxaparin, or Placebo-Treated Patients in Randomized, Controlled, Surgery Studies

	Perioperative prophylaxis (day 1 to day 7 ± 1 postsurgery)		Extended prophylaxis (day 8 to day 28 ± 2 postsurgery)	
Adverse reactions	2.5 mg fondaparinux subcutaneously once daily (n = 3,616)	Enoxaparin[a,b] (n = 3,956)	2.5 mg fondaparinux subcutaneously once daily (n = 327)	Placebo subcutaneously once daily (n = 329)
Cardiovascular				
Hypotension	126 (3.5%)	125 (3.2%)	1 (0.3%)	0 (0%)
CNS				
Confusion	113 (3.1%)	132 (3.3%)	4 (1.2%)	1 (0.3%)
Dizziness	131 (3.6%)	165 (4.2%)	2 (0.6%)	0 (0%)
Headache	72 (2%)	97 (2.5%)	0 (0%)	2 (0.6%)
Insomnia	179 (5%)	214 (5.4%)	3 (0.9%)	1 (0.3%)
Dermatologic				
Bullous eruption[c]	112 (3.1%)	102 (2.6%)	0 (0%)	1 (0.3%)
Purpura	128 (3.5%)	137 (3.5%)	0 (0%)	0 (0%)
Rash	273 (7.5%)	329 (8.3%)	2 (0.6%)	4 (1.2%)
Surgical site reaction	29 (0.8%)	41 (1%)	5 (1.5%)	8 (2.4%)
GI				
Constipation	309 (8.5%)	416 (10.5%)	6 (1.8%)	7 (2.1%)
Diarrhea	90 (2.5%)	102 (2.6%)	6 (1.8%)	8 (2.4%)
Dyspepsia	87 (2.4%)	102 (2.6%)	1 (0.3%)	2 (0.6%)
Nausea	409 (11.3%)	484 (12.2%)	1 (0.3%)	4 (1.2%)
Vomiting	212 (5.9%)	236 (6%)	2 (0.6%)	4 (1.2%)
GU				
Urinary retention	106 (2.9%)	117 (3%)	0 (0%)	1 (0.3%)
Urinary tract infection	136 (3.8%)	135 (3.4%)	13 (4%)	13 (4%)
Hematologic				
Anemia	707 (19.6%)	670 (16.9%)	5 (1.5%)	4 (1.2%)
Hematoma	103 (2.8%)	109 (2.8%)	7 (2.1%)	1 (0.3%)
Hypokalemia	152 (4.2%)	164 (4.1%)	0 (0%)	0 (0%)
Postoperative hemorrhage	85 (2.4%)	69 (1.7%)	2 (0.6%)	2 (0.6%)
Miscellaneous				
Edema	313 (8.7%)	348 (8.8%)	3 (0.9%)	2 (0.6%)
Fever	491 (13.6%)	610 (15.4%)	1 (0.3%)	4 (1.2%)
Pain	62 (1.7%)	101 (2.6%)	0 (0%)	0 (0%)
Wound drainage increased	161 (4.5%)	184 (4.7%)	2 (0.6%)	0 (0%)

[a] Enoxaparin dosing regimen: 30 mg every 12 hours or 40 mg once daily.
[b] Not approved for use in patients undergoing hip fracture surgery.
[c] Localized blister coded as bullous eruption.

Selective Factor Xa Inhibitor

FONDAPARINUX SODIUM — INJECTION

Adverse Reactions Occurring in ≥ 2% of Fondaparinux- or Dalteparin-Treated Patients Undergoing Abdominal Surgery

Adverse reaction	Fondaparinux 2.5 mg subcutaneously once daily	Dalteparin 5,000 units subcutaneously once daily
	n = 1,433	n = 1,425
Cardiovascular		
Hypertension	35 (2.4%)	41 (2.9%)
Dermatologic		
Postoperative wound infection	70 (4.9%)	69 (4.8%)
Surgical site reaction	46 (3.2%)	40 (2.8%)
GI		
Vomiting	31 (2.2%)	26 (1.8%)
Hematologic		
Anemia	35 (2.4%)	26 (1.8%)
Postoperative hemorrhage	61 (4.3%)	42 (2.9%)
Respiratory		
Pneumonia	33 (2.3%)	23 (1.6%)
Miscellaneous		
Fever	53 (3.7%)	54 (3.8%)

Adverse Reactions Occurring in ≥ 2% of Fondaparinux Sodium, Enoxaparin, or Heparin-treated Patients Across VTE Treatment Studies

Adverse reactions	Fondaparinux (n = 2,294)	Enoxaparin (n = 1,101)	Heparin (n = 1,092)
Cardiovascular			
Chest pain	33 (1.4%)	8 (0.7%)	26 (2.4%)
CNS			
Anxiety	18 (0.8%)	8 (0.7%)	22 (2%)
Headache	104 (4.5%)	37 (3.4%)	65 (6%)
Insomnia	86 (3.7%)	19 (1.7%)	75 (6.9%)
GI			
Abdominal pain	33 (1.4%)	14 (1.3%)	28 (2.6%)
Constipation	106 (4.6%)	32 (2.9%)	93 (8.5%)
Diarrhea	43 (1.9%)	22 (2%)	27 (2.5%)
Nausea	76 (3.3%)	29 (2.6%)	53 (4.9%)
Vomiting	26 (1.1%)	14 (1.3%)	27 (2.5%)

Adverse Reactions Occurring in ≥ 2% of Fondaparinux Sodium, Enoxaparin, or Heparin-treated Patients Across VTE Treatment Studies

Adverse reactions	Fondaparinux (n = 2,294)	Enoxaparin (n = 1,101)	Heparin (n = 1,092)
GU			
Urinary tract infection	53 (2.3%)	20 (1.8%)	24 (2.2%)
Hematologic			
Anemia	28 (1.2%)	3 (0.3%)	23 (2.1%)
Epistaxis	30 (1.3%)	12 (1.1%)	41 (3.8%)
Prothrombin decreased	30 (1.3%)	3 (0.3%)	34 (3.1%)
Hepatic			
ALT increased	4 (0.2%)	31 (2.8%)	3 (0.3%)
AST increased	7 (0.3%)	47 (4.3%)	8 (0.7%)
Hepatic enzymes increased	7 (0.3%)	52 (4.7%)	30 (2.7%)
Hepatic function abnormal	10 (0.4%)	14 (1.3%)	24 (2.2%)
Metabolic/Nutritional			
Hypokalemia	25 (1.1%)	2 (0.2%)	23 (2.1%)
Respiratory			
Coughing	48 (2.1%)	7 (0.6%)	26 (2.4%)
Miscellaneous			
Back pain	30 (1.3%)	11 (1%)	34 (3.1%)
Bruise	24 (1%)	24 (2.2%)	14 (1.3%)
Fever	81 (3.5%)	32 (2.9%)	47 (4.3%)
Leg pain	31 (1.4%)	10 (0.9%)	22 (2%)

Overdosage

➤*Symptoms:* There is no known antidote for fondaparinux injection. Overdose of fondaparinux may lead to hemorrhagic complications.

➤*Treatment:* Overdosage associated with bleeding complications should lead to treatment discontinuation and initiation of appropriate therapy. Data obtained in patients undergoing chronic intermittent hemodialysis suggest that fondaparinux clearance can increase by 20% during hemodialysis.

Patient Information

Advise patients not to take any aspirin or NSAIDs without consulting a doctor. The risk of bleeding is increased when taken with fondaparinux.

Administer as a subcutaneous injection. Instruct patient on proper injection technique.

Advise patients to notify a doctor immediately if any unusual bleeding or symptoms occur (eg, bruising, petechiae, hematuria, nosebleeds, black, tarry stools).

Inform patients that regular visits to a doctor or clinic are needed to monitor therapy.

Warfarin

WARFARIN SODIUM

Rx	**Warfarin Sodium** (Various, eg, Barr, Geneva, Taro)	Tablets: 1 mg	In 100s and 1000s.
Rx	**Coumadin** (Bristol-Myers Squibb)		Lactose. (COUMADIN 1). Pink, scored. In 100s, 1000s, and UD 100s.
Rx	**Jantoven** (Upsher-Smith)		Lactose, povidone. (WRF 1 832). Pink, scored. In 100s and 1000s.
Rx	**Warfarin Sodium** (Various, eg, Barr, Geneva, Taro)	2 mg	In 100s and 1000s.
Rx	**Coumadin** (Bristol-Myers Squibb)		Lactose. (COUMADIN 2). Lavender, scored. In 100s, 1000s, and UD 100s.
Rx	**Jantoven** (Upsher-Smith)		Lactose, povidone. (WRF 2 832). Lavender, scored. In 100s and 1000s.
Rx	**Warfarin Sodium** (Various, eg, Barr, Geneva, Taro)	2.5 mg	In 100s and 1000s.
Rx	**Coumadin** (Bristol-Myers Squibb)		Lactose. (COUMADIN 2½). Green, scored. In 100s, 1000s, and UD 100s.
Rx	**Jantoven** (Upsher-Smith)		Lactose, povidone. (WRF 2½ 832). Green, scored. In 100s and 1000s.
Rx	**Warfarin Sodium** (Various, eg, Barr, Geneva, Taro)	3 mg	In 100s and 1000s.
Rx	**Coumadin** (Bristol-Myers Squibb)		Lactose. (COUMADIN 3). Tan, scored. In 100s, 1000s, and UD 100s.
Rx	**Jantoven** (Upsher-Smith)		Lactose, povidone. (WRF 3 832). Tan, scored. In 100s and 1000s.
Rx	**Warfarin Sodium** (Various, eg, Barr, Geneva, Taro)	4 mg	In 100s and 1000s.
Rx	**Coumadin** (Bristol-Myers Squibb)		Lactose. (COUMADIN 4). Blue, scored. In 100s, 1000s, and UD 100s.
Rx	**Jantoven** (Upsher-Smith)		Lactose, povidone. (WRF 4 832). Blue, scored. In 100s and 1000s.

WARFARIN SODIUM

Rx	**Warfarin Sodium** (Various, eg, Barr, Geneva, Taro)	5 mg	In 100s and 1000s.
Rx	**Coumadin** (Bristol-Myers Squibb)		Lactose. (COUMADIN 5). Peach, scored. In 100s, 1000s, and UD 100s.
Rx	**Jantoven** (Upsher-Smith)		Lactose, povidone. (WRF 5 832). Peach, scored. In 100s and 1000s.
Rx	**Warfarin Sodium** (Various, eg, Barr, Geneva, Taro)	6 mg	In 100s and 1000s.
Rx	**Coumadin** (Bristol-Myers Squibb)		Lactose. (COUMADIN 6). Teal, scored. In 100s, 1000s, and UD 100s.
Rx	**Jantoven** (Upsher-Smith)		Lactose, povidone. (WRF 6 832). Teal, scored. In 100s and 1000s.
Rx	**Warfarin Sodium** (Various, eg, Barr, Geneva, Taro)	7.5 mg	In 100s and 1000s.
Rx	**Coumadin** (Bristol-Myers Squibb)		Lactose. (COUMADIN 7½). Yellow, scored. In 100s and UD 100s.
Rx	**Jantoven** (Upsher-Smith)		Lactose, povidone. (WRF 7½ 832). Yellow, scored. In 100s and 500s.
Rx	**Warfarin Sodium** (Various, eg, Barr, Geneva, Taro)	10 mg	In 100s.
Rx	**Coumadin** (Bristol-Myers Squibb)		Dye free. Lactose. (COUMADIN 10). White, scored. In 100s and UD 100s.
Rx	**Jantoven** (Upsher-Smith)		Dye free. Lactose, povidone. (WRF 10 832). White, scored. In 100s and 500s.
Rx	**Coumadin** (Bristol-Myers Squibb)	**Powder for injection, lyophilized**: 5.4 mg (2 mg/mL when reconstituted)	Mannitol. Preservative-free. In 5 mg vials.

WARFARIN SODIUM — ORAL

Indications

For the prophylaxis or treatment of venous thrombosis and its extension, and pulmonary embolism.

For the prophylaxis or treatment of the thromboembolic complications associated with atrial fibrillation or cardiac valve replacement.

To reduce the risk of death, recurrent myocardial infarction, and thromboembolic events such as stroke or systemic embolization after myocardial infarction.

Administration and Dosage

➤*Approved by the FDA:* June 8, 1954.

The dosage and administration of warfarin sodium must be individualized for each patient according to the particular patients prothrombin time (PT)/ International Normalized Ratio (INR) response to the drug. The dosage should be adjusted based upon the patient's PT/INR (see Laboratory control below for full discussion on INR).

➤*Venous thromboembolism (including pulmonary embolism):* Available clinical evidence indicates that an INR of 2 to 3 is sufficient for prophylaxis and treatment of venous thromboembolism and minimizes the risk of hemorrhage associated with higher INRs. In patients with risk factors for recurrent venous thromboembolism including venous insufficiency, inherited thrombophilia, idiopathic venous thromboembolism, and a history of thrombotic events, consideration should be given to longer term therapy.

➤*Atrial fibrillation:* Five recent clinical trials evaluated the effects of warfarin in patients with non-valvular atrial fibrillation (AF). Meta-analysis findings of these studies revealed that the effects of warfarin in reducing thromboembolic events including stroke were similar at either moderately high INR (2 to 4.5) or low INR (1.4 to 3). There was a significant reduction in minor bleeds at the low INR. Similar data from clinical studies in valvular atrial fibrillation patients are not available. The trials in non-valvular atrial fibrillation support the American College of Chest Physicians' (ACCP) recommendation that an INR of 2 to 3 be used for long-term warfarin therapy in appropriate AF patients.

➤*Post-myocardial infarction:* In post-myocardial infarction patients, warfarin sodium therapy should be initiated early (2 to 4 weeks post-infarction) and dosage should be adjusted to maintain an INR of 2.5 to 3.5 long-term. The recommendation is based on the results of the Warfarin Re-Infarction Study (WARIS) in which treatment was initiated 2 to 4 weeks after the infarction. In patients thought to be at an increased risk of bleeding complications or on aspirin therapy, maintenance of warfarin sodium therapy at the lower end of this INR range is recommended.

➤*Mechanical and bioprosthetic heart valves:* In patients with mechanical heart valve(s), long-term prophylaxis with warfarin to an INR of 2.5 to 3.5 is recommended. In patients with bioprosthetic heart valve(s), based on limited data, the ACCP recommends warfarin therapy to an INR of 2 to 3 for 12 weeks after valve insertion. In patients with additional risk factors such as atrial fibrillation or prior thromboembolism, consideration should be given for longer term therapy.

➤*Recurrent systemic embolism:* In cases where the risk of thromboembolism is great, such as in patients with recurrent systemic embolism, a higher INR may be required.

An INR of greater than 4 appears to provide no additional therapeutic benefit in most patients and is associated with a higher risk of bleeding.

➤*Initial dosage:* The dosing of warfarin sodium must be individualized according to patient's sensitivity to the drug as indicated by the PT/INR. Use of a large loading dose may increase the incidence of hemorrhagic and other complications, does not offer more rapid protection against thrombi formation, and is not recommended. Low initiation doses are recommended for elderly or debilitated patients and patients with potential to exhibit greater than expected PT/INR response to warfarin sodium. Based on limited data, Asian patients may also require lower initiation and maintenance doses of warfarin sodium. It is recommended that warfarin sodium therapy be initiated with a dose of 2 to 5 mg per day with dosage adjustments based on the results of PT/INR determinations.

➤*Maintenance:* Most patients are satisfactorily maintained at a dose of 2 to 10 mg daily. Flexibility of dosage is provided by breaking scored tablets in half. The individual dose and interval should be gauged by the patient's prothrombin response.

➤*Duration of therapy:* The duration of therapy in each patient should be individualized. In general, anticoagulant therapy should be continued until the danger of thrombosis and embolism has passed.

➤*Missed dose:* The anticoagulant effect of warfarin sodium persists beyond 24 hours. If the patient forgets to take the prescribed dose of warfarin sodium at the scheduled time, the dose should be taken as soon as possible on the same day. The patient should not take the missed dose by doubling the daily dose to make up for missed doses, but should refer back to his or her physician.

➤*Treatment during dentistry and surgery:* The management of patients who undergo dental and surgical procedures requires close liaison between attending physicians, surgeons and dentists. PT/INR determination is recommended just prior to any dental or surgical procedure. In patients undergoing minimal invasive procedures who must be anticoagulated prior to, during, or immediately following these procedures, adjusting the dosage of warfarin sodium to maintain the PT/INR at the low end of the therapeutic range may safely allow for continued anticoagulation. The operative site should be sufficiently limited and accessible to permit the effective use of local procedures for hemostasis. Under these conditions, dental and minor surgical procedures may be performed without undue risk of hemorrhage. Some dental or surgical procedures may necessitate the interruption of warfarin sodium therapy. When discontinuing warfarin sodium even for a short period of time, the benefits and risks should be strongly considered.

➤*Conversion from heparin therapy:* Since the anticoagulant effect of warfarin sodium is delayed, heparin is preferred initially for rapid anticoagulation. Conversion to warfarin sodium may begin concomitantly with heparin therapy or may be delayed 3 to 6 days. To ensure continuous anticoagulation, it is advisable to continue full dose heparin therapy and that warfarin sodium therapy be overlapped with heparin for 4 to 5 days, until the warfarin sodium has produced the desired therapeutic response as determined by PT/INR. When warfarin sodium has produced the desired PT/INR or prothrombin activity, heparin may be discontinued. Warfarin sodium may increase the aPTT test, even in the absence of heparin. During initial therapy with warfarin sodium, the interference with heparin anticoagulation is of minimal clinical significance. As heparin may affect the PT/INR, patients receiving both heparin and warfarin sodium should have blood for PT/INR determination drawn at least:

- 5 hours after the last IV bolus dose of heparin.
- 4 hours after cessation of a continuous IV infusion of heparin.
- 24 hours after the last subcutaneous heparin injection.

➤*Storage / Stability:* Protect from light. Store at controlled room temperature (15° to 30°C; 59° to 86°F). Dispense in a tight, light-resistant container.

Hospital unit-dose blister packages are to be stored in carton until contents have been used.

Actions

➤*Pharmacology:* Warfarin sodium and other coumarin anticoagulants act by inhibiting the synthesis of vitamin K dependent clotting factors, which include Factors II, VII, IX, and X, and the anticoagulant proteins C and S. Half-lives of these clotting factors are as follows: Factor II, 60 hours; VII, 4 to 6 hours; IX, 24 hours; and X, 48 to 72 hours. The half-lives of proteins C and S are approximately 8 hours and 30 hours, respectively. The resultant in vivo effect is a sequential depression of Factors VII, IX, X, and II activi-

WARFARIN SODIUM — ORAL

ties. Vitamin K is an essential cofactor for the post ribosomal synthesis of the vitamin K dependent clotting factors. The vitamin promotes the biosynthesis of α-carboxyglutamic acid residues in the proteins which are essential for biological activity. Warfarin is thought to interfere with clotting factor synthesis by inhibition of the regeneration of vitamin K_1 epoxide. The degree of depression is dependent upon the dosage administered. Therapeutic doses of warfarin decrease the total amount of the active form of each vitamin K dependent clotting factor made by the liver by approximately 30% to 50%.

An anticoagulation effect generally occurs within 24 hours after drug administration. However, peak anticoagulant effect may be delayed 72 to 96 hours. The duration of action of a single dose of racemic warfarin is 2 to 5 days. The effects of warfarin sodium may become more pronounced as effects of daily maintenance doses overlap. Anticoagulants have no direct effect on an established thrombus, nor do they reverse ischemic tissue damage. However, once a thrombus has occurred, the goal of anticoagulant treatment is to prevent further extension of the formed clot and prevent secondary thromboembolic complications, which may result in serious and possibly fatal sequelae.

➤*Pharmacokinetics:*

Absorption – Warfarin sodium is a racemic mixture of the R- and S-enantiomers. The S-enantiomer exhibits 2 to 5 times more anticoagulant activity than the R-enantiomer in humans, but generally has a more rapid clearance.

Warfarin sodium is essentially completely absorbed after oral administration with peak concentration generally attained within the first 4 hours.

Distribution – There are no differences in the apparent volumes of distribution after intravenous and oral administration of single doses of warfarin solution. Warfarin distributes into a relatively small apparent volume of distribution of about 0.14 L/kg. A distribution phase lasting 6 to 12 hours is distinguishable after rapid intravenous or oral administration of an aqueous solution. Using a one compartment model, and assuming complete bioavailability, estimates of the volumes of distribution of R- and S-warfarin are similar to each other and to that of the racemate. Concentrations in fetal plasma approach the maternal values, but warfarin has not been found in human milk. The same limited published data report that some breastfed infants, whose mothers were treated with warfarin, had prolonged prothrombin times, although not as prolonged as those of the mothers. The decision to breastfeed should be undertaken only after careful consideration of the available alternatives. Women who are breastfeeding and anticoagulated with warfarin should be very carefully monitored so that recommended PT/INR values are not exceeded. It is prudent to perform coagulation tests and to evaluate vitamin K status in infants at risk for bleeding tendencies before advising women taking warfarin to breastfeed. Effects in premature infants have not been evaluated. Approximately 99% of the drug is bound to plasma proteins.

Metabolism – The elimination of warfarin is almost entirely by metabolism. Warfarin sodium is stereoselectively metabolized by hepatic microsomal enzymes (cytochrome P450) to inactive hydroxylated metabolites (predominant route) and by reductases to reduced metabolites (warfarin alcohols). The warfarin alcohols have minimal anticoagulant activity. The metabolites are principally excreted into the urine; and to a lesser extent into the bile. The metabolites of warfarin that have been identified include dehydrowarfarin, 2 diastereoisomer alcohols, 4-, 6-, 7-, 8- and 10-hydroxywarfarin. The cytochrome P450 isozymes involved in the metabolism of warfarin include 2C9, 2C19, 2C8, 2C18, 1A2, and 3A4. 2C9 is likely to be the principal form of human liver P450, which modulates the in vivo anticoagulant activity of warfarin.

Excretion – The terminal half-life of warfarin after a single dose is approximately 1 week; however, the effective half-life ranges from 20 to 60 hours, with a mean of about 40 hours. The clearance of R-warfarin is generally half that of S-warfarin, thus as the volumes of distribution are similar, the half-life of R-warfarin is longer than that of S-warfarin. The half-life of R-warfarin ranges from 37 to 89 hours, while that of S-warfarin ranges from 21 to 43 hours. Studies with radiolabeled drug have demonstrated that up to 92% of the orally administered dose is recovered in urine. Very little warfarin is excreted unchanged in urine. Urinary excretion is in the form of metabolites.

Special populations –

Hepatic function impairment: Hepatic dysfunction can potentiate the response to warfarin through impaired synthesis of clotting factors and decreased metabolism of warfarin. The administration of warfarin sodium via the IV route should provide the patient with the same concentration of an equal oral dose, but maximum plasma concentration will be reached earlier. However, the full anticoagulant effect of a dose of warfarin may not be achieved until 72 to 96 hours after dosing, indicating that the administration of IV warfarin sodium should not provide any increased biological effect or earlier onset of action.

Elderly: Patients 60 years or older appear to exhibit greater than expected PT/INR response to the anticoagulant effects of warfarin. The cause of the increased sensitivity to the anticoagulant effects of warfarin in this age group is unknown. This increased anticoagulant effect from warfarin may be due to a combination of pharmacokinetic and pharmacodynamic factors. Racemic warfarin clearance may be unchanged or reduced with increasing age. Limited information suggests there is no difference in the clearance of S-warfarin in the elderly versus young subjects. However, there may be a slight decrease in the clearance of R-warfarin in the elderly as compared to the young. Therefore, as patient age increases, a lower dose of warfarin is usually required to produce a therapeutic level of anticoagulation.

Race: Asian patients may require lower initiation and maintenance doses of warfarin. One noncontrolled study conducted in 151 Chinese outpatients reported a mean daily warfarin requirement of 3.3 ± 1.4 mg to achieve an INR of 2 to 2.5. These patients were stabilized on warfarin for various indications. Patient age was the most important determinant of warfarin requirement in Chinese patients with a progressively lower warfarin requirement with increasing age.

Contraindications

Any localized or general physical condition or personal circumstance in which the hazard of hemorrhage might be greater than the potential clinical benefits of anticoagulation; pregnancy (see warnings).

Hemorrhagic tendencies or blood dyscrasias; recent or contemplated surgery of (1) central nervous system, (2) eye, or (3) traumatic surgery resulting in large open surfaces; bleeding tendencies associated with active ulceration or overt bleeding of (1) gastrointestinal, genitourinary or respiratory tracts, (2) cerebrovascular hemorrhage, (3) aneurysms-cerebral, dissecting aorta, (4) pericarditis and pericardial effusions, or (5) bacterial endocarditis; threatened abortion, eclampsia and preeclampsia; inadequate laboratory facilities; unsupervised patients with senility, alcoholism, or psychosis or other lack of patient cooperation; spinal puncture and other diagnostic or therapeutic procedures with potential for uncontrollable bleeding; major regional, lumbar block anesthesia, malignant hypertension and known hypersensitivity to warfarin or to any other components of this product.

Warnings

➤*Hemorrhage/Necrosis:* The most serious risks associated with anticoagulant therapy with warfarin sodium are hemorrhage in any tissue or organ and, less frequently (less than 0.1%), necrosis or gangrene of skin and other tissues. The risk of hemorrhage is related to the level of intensity and the duration of anticoagulant therapy. Hemorrhage and necrosis have in some cases been reported to result in death or permanent disability. Necrosis appears to be associated with local thrombosis and usually appears within a few days of the start of anticoagulant therapy. In severe cases of necrosis, treatment through debridement or amputation of the affected tissue, limb, breast or penis has been reported. Careful diagnosis is required to determine whether necrosis is caused by an underlying disease. Warfarin therapy should be discontinued when warfarin is suspected to be the cause of developing necrosis and heparin therapy may be considered for anticoagulation. Although various treatments have been attempted, no treatment for necrosis has been considered uniformly effective. See below for information on predisposing conditions. These and other risks associated with anticoagulant therapy must be weighed against the risk of thrombosis or embolization in untreated cases.

➤*Conversion from heparin therapy:* See Administration and Dosage for more information.

➤*Atheroemboli/Microemboli:* Anticoagulation therapy with warfarin sodium may enhance the release of atheromatous plaque emboli, thereby increasing the risk of complications from systemic cholesterol microembolization, including the "purple toes syndrome." Discontinuation of warfarin sodium therapy is recommended when such phenomena are observed.

Systemic atheroemboli and cholesterol microemboli can present with a variety of signs and symptoms including purple toes syndrome, livedo reticularis, rash, gangrene, abrupt and intense pain in the leg, foot, or toes, foot ulcers, myalgia, penile gangrene, abdominal pain, flank or back pain, hematuria, renal insufficiency, hypertension, cerebral ischemia, spinal cord infarction, pancreatitis, symptoms simulating polyarteritis, or any other sequelae of vascular compromise due to embolic occlusion. The most commonly involved visceral organs are the kidneys followed by the pancreas, spleen, and liver. Some cases have progressed to necrosis or death.

➤*Purple toes syndrome:* Purple toes syndrome is a complication of oral anticoagulation characterized by a dark, purplish or mottled color of the toes, usually occurring between 3 to 10 weeks, or later, after the initiation of therapy with warfarin or related compounds. Major features of this syndrome include purple color of plantar surfaces and sides of the toes that blanches on moderate pressure and fades with elevation of the legs; pain and tenderness of the toes; waxing and waning of the color over time. While the purple toes syndrome is reported to be reversible, some cases progress to gangrene or necrosis, which may require debridement of the affected area, or may lead to amputation.

➤*Heparin-induced thrombocytopenia:* Warfarin sodium should be used with caution in patients with heparin-induced thrombocytopenia and deep venous thrombosis. Cases of venous limb ischemia, necrosis, and gangrene have occurred in patients with heparin-induced thrombocytopenia and deep venous thrombosis when heparin treatment was discontinued and warfarin therapy was started or continued. In some patients sequelae have included amputation of the involved area or death.

A severe elevation (greater than 50 seconds) in activated partial thromboplastin time (aPTT) with a PT/INR in the desired range has been identified as an indication of increased risk of postoperative hemorrhage.

➤*Special risk patients:* Warfarin sodium is a narrow therapeutic range (index) drug, and caution should be observed when warfarin sodium is administered to certain patients such as the elderly or debilitated or when administered in any situation or physical condition where added risk of hemorrhage is present.

The decision to administer anticoagulants in the following conditions must be based upon clinical judgment in which the risks of anticoagulant therapy are weighed against the benefits:

- Severe to moderate hepatic or renal insufficiency.
- Infectious diseases or disturbances of intestinal flora: Sprue, antibiotic therapy.
- Trauma which may result in internal bleeding.
- Surgery or trauma resulting in large exposed raw surfaces.

WARFARIN SODIUM — ORAL

- Indwelling catheters.
- Severe to moderate hypertension.
- Known or suspected deficiency in protein C mediated anticoagulant response: Hereditary or acquired deficiencies of protein C or its cofactor, protein S, have been associated with tissue necrosis following warfarin administration. Not all patients with these conditions develop necrosis, and tissue necrosis occurs in patients without these deficiencies. Inherited resistance to activated protein C has been described in many patients with venous thromboembolic disorders but has not yet been evaluated as a risk factor for tissue necrosis. The risk associated with these conditions, both for recurrent thrombosis and for adverse reactions, is difficult to evaluate since it does not appear to be the same for everyone. Decisions about testing and therapy must be made on an individual basis. It has been reported that concomitant anticoagulation therapy with heparin for 5 to 7 days during initiation of therapy with warfarin sodium may minimize the incidence of tissue necrosis. Warfarin therapy should be discontinued when warfarin is suspected to be the cause of developing necrosis and heparin therapy may be considered for anticoagulation.
- Miscellaneous: Polycythemia vera, vasculitis, and severe diabetes.

➤*Acquired / Inherited warfarin resistance:* In patients with acquired or inherited warfarin resistance, decreased therapeutic responses to warfarin sodium have been reported. Exaggerated therapeutic responses have been reported in other patients.

➤*Hypersensitivity reactions:* Minor and severe allergic/hypersensitivity reactions and anaphylactic reactions have been reported.

➤*Elderly:* Patients 60 years or older appear to exhibit greater than expected PT/INR response to the anticoagulant effects of warfarin. Warfarin sodium is contraindicated in any unsupervised patient with senility. Caution should be observed with administration of warfarin sodium to elderly patients in any situation or physical condition where added risk of hemorrhage is present. It is recommended that warfarin sodium therapy be initiated with a dose of 2 to 5 mg per day with dosage adjustments based on the results of PT/INR determinations.

Warfarin sodium is a narrow therapeutic range (index) drug, and caution should be observed when warfarin sodium is administered to certain patients such as the elderly.

➤*Pregnancy: Category X.* Warfarin sodium is contraindicated in women who are or may become pregnant because the drug passes through the placental barrier and may cause fatal hemorrhage to the fetus in utero. Furthermore, there have been reports of birth malformations in children born to mothers who have been treated with warfarin during pregnancy.

Embryopathy characterized by nasal hypoplasia with or without stippled epiphyses (chondrodysplasia punctata) has been reported in pregnant women exposed to warfarin during the first trimester. Central nervous system abnormalities also have been reported, including dorsal midline dysplasia characterized by agenesis of the corpus callosum, Dandy-Walker malformation, and midline cerebellar atrophy. Ventral midline dysplasia, characterized by optic atrophy, and eye abnormalities have been observed. Mental retardation, blindness, and other central nervous system abnormalities have been reported in association with second and third trimester exposure. Although rare, teratogenic reports following in utero exposure to warfarin include urinary tract anomalies such as single kidney, asplenia, anencephaly, spina bifida, cranial nerve palsy, hydrocephalus, cardiac defects and congenital heart disease, polydactyly, deformities of toes, diaphragmatic hernia, corneal leukoma, cleft palate, cleft lip, schizencephaly, and microcephaly.

Spontaneous abortion and still birth are known to occur and a higher risk of fetal mortality is associated with the use of warfarin. Low birth weight and growth retardation have also been reported.

Women of childbearing potential who are candidates for anticoagulant therapy should be carefully evaluated and the indications critically reviewed with the patient. If the patient becomes pregnant while taking this drug, she should be apprised of the potential risks to the fetus, and the possibility of termination of the pregnancy should be discussed in light of those risks.

➤*Lactation:* Based on very limited published data, warfarin has not been detected in the breast milk of mothers treated with warfarin. The same limited published data report that some breastfed infants, whose mothers were treated with warfarin, had prolonged prothrombin times, although not as prolonged as those of the mothers. The decision to breastfeed should be undertaken only after careful consideration of the available alternatives. Women who are breastfeeding and anticoagulated with warfarin should be very carefully monitored so that recommended PT/INR values are not exceeded. It is prudent to perform coagulation tests and to evaluate vitamin K status in infants at risk for bleeding tendencies before advising women taking warfarin to breastfeed. Effects in premature infants have not been evaluated.

➤*Children:* Safety and effectiveness in pediatric patients below the age of 18 years have not been established in randomized, controlled clinical trials. However, the use of warfarin sodium in pediatric patients is well-documented for the prevention and treatment of thromboembolic events. Difficulty achieving and maintaining therapeutic PT/INR ranges in the pediatric patient has been reported. More frequent PT/INR determinations are recommended because of possible changing warfarin requirements.

Precautions

➤*Monitoring:* It cannot be emphasized too strongly that treatment of each patient is a highly individualized matter. Warfarin sodium, a narrow therapeutic range (index) drug, may be affected by factors such as other drugs and dietary vitamin K. Dosage should be controlled by periodic determinations of PT/INR or other suitable coagulation tests. Determinations of whole blood clotting and bleeding times are not effective measures for control of therapy. Heparin prolongs the one-stage PT.

Patients with congestive heart failure may exhibit greater than expected PT/INR response to warfarin sodium, thereby requiring more frequent laboratory monitoring, and reduced doses of warfarin sodium. Concomitant use of anticoagulants with streptokinase or urokinase is not recommended and may be hazardous. (Please note recommendations accompanying these preparations.)

Periodic determination of PT/INR or other suitable coagulation test is essential.

Numerous factors, alone or in combination, including travel, changes in diet, environment, physical state and medication may influence response of the patient to anticoagulants. It is generally good practice to monitor the patient's response with additional PT/INR determinations in the period immediately after discharge from the hospital, and whenever other medications, including botanicals, are initiated, discontinued or taken irregularly.

IM injections of concomitant medications should be confined to the upper extremities which permits easy access for manual compression, inspections for bleeding and use of pressure bandages.

Acquired or inherited warfarin resistance should be suspected if large daily doses of warfarin sodium are required to maintain a patient's PT/INR within a normal therapeutic range.

➤*Concomitant NSAIDs and aspirin:* Caution should be observed when warfarin is administered concomitantly with nonsteroidal anti-inflammatory drugs (NSAIDs), including aspirin, to be certain that no change in anticoagulation dosage is required. In addition to specific drug interactions that might affect PT/INR, NSAIDs, including aspirin, can inhibit platelet aggregation, and can cause gastrointestinal bleeding, peptic ulceration or perforation.

Drug Interactions

Careful monitoring and appropriate dosage adjustments usually will permit combination therapy. Critical times during therapy occur when an interacting drug is added to or discontinued from a patient stabilized on anticoagulants.

Oral Anticoagulant Drug Interactions

Precipitant drug	Object drug*		Description
Acetaminophen Androgens Beta blockers (propranolol) Capecitabine Cephalosporins, parenteral Chenodiol Chlorpropamide Cisapride Dextran Dextrothyroxine Diazoxide Disulfiram Fibric acids Flutamide Glucagon Halothane Heparin Influenza virus vaccine Isoniazid Levamisole Methyldopa Methylphenidate NSAIDs, COX-2 selective Pentoxifylline Propoxyphene Quinolones (eg, ciprofloxacin, levofloxacin, norfloxacin, ofloxacin) SSRIs[1] (ie, fluoxetine, fluvoxamine, paroxetine, sertraline)	Anticoagulants	⬆	These agents may increase the anticoagulant effect. The risk of bleeding may be increased. The mechanism of the interaction is unknown or complicated.

WARFARIN SODIUM — ORAL

Oral Anticoagulant Drug Interactions

Precipitant drug	Object drug*		Description
Streptokinase Sulfonamides Tamoxifen Thrombolytics (ie, tissue plasminogen activator [t-PA]) Thyroid hormones Tolbutamide Tramadol Urokinase Zafirlukast Zileuton	Anticoagulants	⬆	These agents may increase the anticoagulant effect. The risk of bleeding may be increased. The mechanism of the interaction is unknown or complicated.
Allopurinol Amiodarone Azole antifungals[2] Chloramphenicol Cimetidine HMG-CoA reductase inhibitors (ie, fluvastatin, lovastatin, simvastatin) Ifosfamide[3] Metronidazole Omeprazole Phenylbutazone[3] Propafenone Quinidine Quinine SMZ-TMP Sulfinpyrazone	Anticoagulants	⬆	These agents may increase the anticoagulant effect of warfarin by inhibition of the anticoagulant's hepatic metabolism. The risk of bleeding may be increased.
Macrolide antibiotics	Anticoagulants	⬆	These agents may increase the anticoagulant effect by reducing body clearance of warfarin. The risk of bleeding may be increased.
Loop diuretics (ie, ethacrynic acid, furosemide) Nalidixic acid Valproate	Anticoagulants	⬆	These agents may increase the anticoagulant effect of warfarin caused by displacement from binding sites. The risk of bleeding may be increased.
Aminoglycosides (oral) Tetracyclines Vitamin E	Anticoagulants	⬆	These agents may increase the anticoagulant effect of warfarin through an interference with vitamin K. The risk of bleeding may be increased.
Aminosalicylic acid Diflunisal NSAIDs Penicillins, high-dose IV Salicylates Methylsalicylate ointment, topical Ticlopidine	Anticoagulants	⬆	These agents may increase the anticoagulant effect of warfarin and increase the risk of bleeding caused by effects on platelet function, and, in the case of NSAIDs, GI irritant effects.
Alcohol[4] Atorvastatin Chloral hydrate Cholestyramine[5] Corticosteroids Cyclophosphamide Methimazole Moricizine Hydantoins (eg, phenytoin) Pravastatin Prednisone Propylthiouracil Ranitidine	Anticoagulants	⬆⬇	Increased and decreased PT/INR responses have been reported. May increase or decrease anticoagulant effect of warfarin; mechanism unknown.
Ascorbic acid, high doses Chlordiazepoxide Clozapine Contraceptives, oral[6] Cyclosporine[7] Estrogens Ethchlorvynol Griseofulvin Haloperidol Meprobamate Paraldehyde Trazodone	Anticoagulants	⬇	These agents may decrease the anticoagulant effect of warfarin. The mechanism of the interaction is unknown.
Aminoglutethimide Barbiturates Carbamazepine Dicloxacillin[8] Glutethimide Nafcillin[8] Rifamycins Terbinafine	Anticoagulants	⬇	These agents may decrease the anticoagulant effect of warfarin caused by induction of the anticoagulant's hepatic microsomal enzymes.
Spironolactone[9] Sucralfate Thiazide diuretics[9] Thiopurines[10] Vitamin K[11]	Anticoagulants	⬇	These agents may decrease the anticoagulant effect of warfarin by various mechanisms (eg, possible decreased absorption or increased elimination).

* ⬆ = Object drug increased. ⬇ = Object drug decreased.
[1] Bleeding has been reported with fluoxetine alone.
[2] Miconazole includes both intravaginal and systemic formulations.
[3] May also displace the anticoagulant from protein binding sites.
[4] Chronic consumption may increase the clearance of the anticoagulant; moderate to small doses do not alter the anticoagulant effect.
[5] Reduced anticoagulant absorption and possibly increased elimination.
[6] Rarely, increased risk of thromboembolism; this is in contrast to intended effect.
[7] Cyclosporine levels also may be decreased.
[8] Associated with warfarin resistance.
[9] Diuretic-induced hemoconcentration of clotting factors.
[10] Thiopurine-induced increase in synthesis or activation of prothrombin.
[11] Vitamin K overcomes interference of vitamin K-dependent clotting factors by anticoagulants.

➤*Herbal medicines:* Exercise caution when herbal medicines are taken concomitantly with warfarin. Specific herbals reported to affect warfarin therapy include the following:

- Bromelains, danshen, dong quai (*Angelica sinensis*), garlic, boldo, *Lycium barbarum* L. , and *Ginkgo biloba* are associated most often with an increase in the effects of warfarin.
- Coenzyme Q_{10} (ubidecarenone), St. John's wort, green tea, and ginseng are associated most often with a decrease in the effects of warfarin.

Some herbals may cause bleeding events when taken alone (eg, garlic, *Ginkgo biloba*) and may have anticoagulant, antiplatelet, and/or fibrinolytic properties. These effects would be expected to be additive to the anticoagulant effects of warfarin.

Some herbals that may affect coagulation are listed in the following table; however, this list should not be considered all-inclusive.

Herbals That Contain Coumarins With Potential Anticoagulant Effects

Alfalfa	Celery	Parsley
Angelica (dong quai)	Chamomile (German and Roman)	Passion flower
Aniseed	Dandelion[3]	Prickly ash (Northern)
Arnica	Fenugreek	Quassia
Asa foetida	Horse chestnut	Red clover
Bogbean[1]	Horseradish	Sweet clover
Boldo	Licorice[3]	Sweet woodruff
Buchu	Meadowsweet[1]	Tonka beans
Capsicum[2]	Nettle	Wild carrot
Cassia[3]		Wild lettuce

[1] Contains coumarins and salicylates.
[2] Contains coumarins and has fibrinolytic properties.
[3] Contains coumarins and has antiplatelet properties.

Miscellaneous Herbals With Anticoagulant Properties

Bladder wrack (*Fucus*)	Pau d'arco

WARFARIN SODIUM — ORAL

Herbals That Contain Salicylate and/or Have Antiplatelet Properties		
Agrimony[1]	Dandelion[3]	Meadowsweet[2]
Aloe gel	Feverfew	Onion[4]
Aspen	Garlic[4]	Policosanol
Black cohosh	German sarsaparilla	Poplar
Black haw	Ginger	Senega
Bogbean[2]	*Ginkgo biloba*	Tamarind
Cassia[3]	Ginseng (*Panax*)[4]	Willow
Clove	Licorice[3]	Wintergreen

[1] Contains salicylate and has coagulant properties.
[2] Contains coumarins and salicylates.
[3] Contains coumarins and has antiplatelet properties.
[4] Has antiplatelet and fibrinolytic properties.

Herbals With Fibrinolytic Properties		
Bromelains	Garlic[2]	Inositol nicotinate
Capsicum[1]	Ginseng (*Panax*)[2]	Onion[2]

[1] Contains coumarins and has fibrinolytic properties.
[2] Has antiplatelet and fibrinolytic properties.

Herbals with Coagulant Properties		
Agrimony[1]	Mistletoe	Yarrow
Goldenseal		

[1] Contains salicylate and has coagulant properties.

➤*Drug/Food interactions:* Vitamin K-rich vegetables may decrease the anticoagulant effects of warfarin by interfering with absorption. Minimize consumption of vitamin K-rich foods (eg, spinach, seaweed, broccoli, turnip greens) or nutritional supplements. Mango has been shown to increase warfarin's effect.

Adverse Reactions

➤*Dermatologic:* Necrosis of skin and other tissues. Necrosis appears to be associated with local thrombosis and usually appears within a few days of the start of anticoagulant therapy. In severe cases of necrosis, treatment through debridement or amputation of the affected tissue, limb, breast or penis has been reported. Careful diagnosis is required to determine whether necrosis is caused by an underlying disease. Warfarin therapy should be discontinued when warfarin is suspected to be the cause of developing necrosis and heparin therapy may be considered for anticoagulation. Although various treatments have been attempted, no treatment for necrosis has been considered uniformly effective. Priapism has been associated with anticoagulant administration, however, a causal relationship has not been established. Rash and dermatitis, including bullous eruptions, pruritus, alopecia.

➤*GI:* Abdominal pain including cramping, flatulence/bloating, nausea, vomiting, diarrhea.

➤*Hematologic:* Fatal or nonfatal hemorrhage from any tissue or organ. This is a consequence of the anticoagulant effect. The signs, symptoms, and severity will vary according to the location and degree or extent of the bleeding. Hemorrhagic complications may present as paralysis; paresthesia; headache, chest, abdomen, joint, muscle or other pain; dizziness; shortness of breath, difficult breathing or swallowing; unexplained swelling; weakness; hypotension; or unexplained shock. Therefore, the possibility of hemorrhage should be considered in evaluating the condition of any anticoagulated patient with complaints that do not indicate an obvious diagnosis. Bleeding during anticoagulant therapy does not always correlate with PT/INR. Bleeding that occurs when the PT/INR is within the therapeutic range warrants diagnostic investigation since it may unmask a previously unsuspected lesion, eg, tumor, ulcer.

➤*Hepatic:* Hepatitis, cholestatic hepatic injury, jaundice, elevated liver enzymes.

➤*Respiratory:* Rare events of tracheal or tracheobronchial calcification have been reported in association with long-term warfarin therapy. The clinical significance of this event is unknown.

➤*Miscellaneous:* Hypersensitivity/allergic reactions, systemic cholesterol microembolization, purple toes syndrome, vasculitis, edema, fever, urticaria, fatigue, lethargy, malaise, asthenia, pain, headache, dizziness, taste perversion, cold intolerance, and paresthesia including feeling cold and chills.

Overdosage

➤*Symptoms:* Suspected or overt abnormal bleeding (eg, appearance of blood in stools or urine, hematuria, excessive menstrual bleeding, melena, petechiae, excessive bruising or persistent oozing from superficial injuries) are early manifestations of anticoagulation beyond a safe and satisfactory level.

➤*Treatment:* Excessive anticoagulation with or without bleeding may be controlled by discontinuing warfarin sodium therapy and if necessary, by administration of oral or parenteral vitamin K_1. (Please see recommendations accompanying vitamin K_1 preparations prior to use.)

Such use of vitamin K_1 reduces response to subsequent warfarin sodium therapy. Patients may return to a pretreatment thrombotic status following the rapid reversal of a prolonged PT/INR. Resumption of warfarin sodium administration reverses the effect of vitamin K, and a therapeutic PT/INR can again be obtained by careful dosage adjustment. If rapid anticoagulation is indicated, heparin may be preferable for initial therapy.

If minor bleeding progresses to major bleeding, give 5 to 25 mg (rarely up to 50 mg) parenteral vitamin K_1. In emergency situations of severe hemorrhage, clotting factors can be returned to normal by administering 200 to 500 mL of fresh whole blood or fresh frozen plasma, or by giving commercial Factor IX complex.

A risk of hepatitis and other viral diseases is associated with the use of these blood products Factor IX complex is also associated with an increased risk of thrombosis. Therefore, these preparations should be used only in exceptional or life-threatening bleeding episodes secondary to warfarin sodium overdosage.

Purified Factor IX preparations should not be used because they cannot increase the levels of prothrombin, Factor VII and Factor X which are also depressed along with the levels of Factor IX as a result of warfarin sodium treatment. Packed red blood cells may also be given if significant blood loss has occurred. Infusions of blood or plasma should be monitored carefully to avoid precipitating pulmonary edema in elderly patients or patients with heart disease.

Patient Information

The objective of anticoagulant therapy is to decrease the clotting ability of the blood so that thrombosis is prevented, while avoiding spontaneous bleeding. Effective therapeutic levels with minimal complications are in part dependent upon cooperative and well-instructed patients who communicate effectively with their physicians.

Strict adherence to prescribed dosage schedule is necessary.

Do not take or discontinue any other medication, including salicylates (eg, aspirin and topical analgesics) and other over-the-counter medications except on advice of the physician.

Avoid alcohol consumption.

Do not take warfarin sodium during pregnancy and do not become pregnant while taking it.

Avoid any activity or sport that may result in traumatic injury.

Prothrombin time tests and regular visits to physician or clinic are needed to monitor therapy. Carry identification stating that warfarin sodium is being taken.

If the prescribed dose of warfarin sodium is forgotten, notify the physician immediately. Take the dose as soon as possible on the same day, but do not take a double dose of warfarin sodium the next day to make up for missed doses.

The amount of vitamin K in food may affect therapy with warfarin sodium. Eat a healthy, balanced diet maintaining a consistent amount of vitamin K. Avoid drastic changes in dietary habits, such as eating large amounts of green leafy vegetables. Contact physician to report any illness, such as diarrhea, infection or fever.

Notify a physician immediately if any unusual bleeding or symptoms occur. Signs and symptoms of bleeding include pain, swelling or discomfort, prolonged bleeding from cuts, increased menstrual flow or vaginal bleeding, nosebleeds, bleeding of gums from brushing, unusual bleeding or bruising, red or dark brown urine, red or tar black stools, headache, dizziness, or weakness. If therapy with warfarin sodium is discontinued, patients should be cautioned that the anticoagulant effects of warfarin sodium may persist for about 2 to 5 days.

Patients should be informed that all warfarin sodium products represent the same medication, and should not be taken concomitantly, as overdosage may result.

WARFARIN SODIUM — INJECTION

Indications

For the prophylaxis and/or treatment of venous thrombosis and its extension, and pulmonary embolism.

For the prophylaxis and/or treatment of the thromboembolic complications associated with atrial fibrillation and/or cardiac valve replacement.

To reduce the risk of death, recurrent myocardial infarction, and thromboembolic events such as stroke or systemic embolization after myocardial infarction.

Administration and Dosage

➤*Approved by the FDA:* June 8, 1954.

The dosage and administration of warfarin sodium must be individualized for each patient according to the particular patients prothrombin time (PT)/International Normalized Ratio (INR) response to the drug. The dosage should be adjusted based upon the patient's PT/INR.

➤*Venous thromboembolism (including pulmonary embolism):* Available clinical evidence indicates that an INR of 2 to 3 is sufficient for prophylaxis and treatment of venous thromboembolism and minimizes the risk of hemorrhage associated with higher INRs. In patients with risk factors for recurrent venous thromboembolism including venous insufficiency, inherited thrombophilia, idiopathic venous thromboembolism, and a history of thrombotic events, consideration should be given to longer term therapy.

➤*Atrial fibrillation:* Five recent clinical trials evaluated the effects of warfarin in patients with non-valvular atrial fibrillation (AF). Meta-analysis findings of these studies revealed that the effects of warfarin in reducing thromboembolic events including stroke were similar at either moderately high INR (2 to 4.5) or low INR (1.4 to 3). There was a significant reduction in minor bleeds at the low INR. Similar data from clinical studies in valvular

WARFARIN SODIUM — INJECTION

atrial fibrillation patients are not available. The trials in non-valvular atrial fibrillation support the American College of Chest Physicians' (ACCP) recommendation that an INR of 2 to 3 be used for long-term warfarin therapy in appropriate AF patients.

➤*Post-myocardial infarction:* In post-myocardial infarction patients, warfarin sodium therapy should be initiated early (2 to 4 weeks post-infarction) and dosage should be adjusted to maintain an INR of 2.5 to 3.5 long-term. The recommendation is based on the results of the Warfarin Re-Infarction Study (WARIS) in which treatment was initiated 2 to 4 weeks after the infarction. In patients thought to be at an increased risk of bleeding complications or on aspirin therapy, maintenance of warfarin sodium therapy at the lower end of this INR range is recommended.

➤*Mechanical and bioprosthetic heart valves:* In patients with mechanical heart valve(s), long-term prophylaxis with warfarin to an INR of 2.5 to 3.5 is recommended. In patients with bioprosthetic heart valve(s), based on limited data, the ACCP recommends warfarin therapy to an INR of 2 to 3 for 12 weeks after valve insertion. In patients with additional risk factors such as atrial fibrillation or prior thromboembolism, consideration should be given for longer term therapy.

➤*Recurrent systemic embolism:* In cases where the risk of thromboembolism is great, such as in patients with recurrent systemic embolism, a higher INR may be required.

An INR of greater than 4 appears to provide no additional therapeutic benefit in most patients and is associated with a higher risk of bleeding.

➤*Initial dosage:* The dosing of warfarin sodium must be individualized according to patient's sensitivity to the drug as indicated by the PT/INR. Use of a large loading dose may increase the incidence of hemorrhagic and other complications, does not offer more rapid protection against thrombi formation, and is not recommended. Low initiation and maintenance doses are recommended for elderly and/or debilitated patients and patients with potential to exhibit greater than expected PT/INR response to warfarin sodium. Based on limited data, Asian patients may also require lower initiation and maintenance doses of warfarin. It is recommended that warfarin sodium therapy be initiated with a dose of 2 to 5 mg per day with dosage adjustments based on the results of PT/INR determinations.

➤*Maintenance:* Most patients are satisfactorily maintained at a dose of 2 to 10 mg daily. Flexibility of dosage is provided by breaking scored tablets in half. The individual dose and interval should be gauged by the patient's prothrombin response.

➤*Duration of therapy:* The duration of therapy in each patient should be individualized. In general, anticoagulant therapy should be continued until the danger of thrombosis and embolism has passed.

➤*Missed dose:* The anticoagulant effect of warfarin sodium persists beyond 24 hours. If the patient forgets to take the prescribed dose of warfarin sodium at the scheduled time, the dose should be taken as soon as possible on the same day. The patient should not take the missed dose by doubling the daily dose to make up for missed doses, but should refer back to his or her physician.

➤*IV route of administration:* Warfarin sodium for injection provides an alternate administration route for patients who cannot receive oral drugs. The IV dosages would be the same as those that would be used orally if the patient could take the drug by the oral route. Warfarin sodium injection should be administered as a slow bolus injection over 1 to 2 minutes into a peripheral vein. It is not recommended for IM administration. The vial should be reconstituted with 2.7 mL of Sterile Water for Injection and inspected for particulate matter and discoloration immediately prior to use. Do not use if either particulate matter or discoloration is noted. After reconstitution, warfarin sodium injection is chemically and physically stable for 4 hours at room temperature. It does not contain any antimicrobial preservative and, thus, care must be taken to assure the sterility of the prepared solution. The vial is not recommended for multiple use and unused solution should be discarded.

➤*Treatment during dentistry and surgery:* The management of patients who undergo dental and surgical procedures requires close liaison between attending physicians, surgeons, and dentists. PT/INR determination is recommended just prior to any dental or surgical procedure. In patients undergoing minimal invasive procedures who must be anticoagulated prior to, during, or immediately following these procedures, adjusting the dosage of warfarin sodium to maintain the PT/INR at the low end of the therapeutic range may safely allow for continued anticoagulation. The operative site should be sufficiently limited and accessible to permit the effective use of local procedures for hemostasis. Under these conditions, dental and minor surgical procedures may be performed without undue risk of hemorrhage. Some dental or surgical procedures may necessitate the interruption of warfarin sodium therapy. When discontinuing warfarin sodium even for a short period of time, the benefits and risks should be strongly considered.

➤*Conversion from heparin therapy:* Since the anticoagulant effect of warfarin sodium is delayed, heparin is preferred initially for rapid anticoagulation. Conversion to warfarin sodium may begin concomitantly with heparin therapy or may be delayed 3 to 6 days. To ensure continuous anticoagulation, it is advisable to continue full dose heparin therapy and that warfarin sodium therapy be overlapped with heparin for 4 to 5 days, until the warfarin sodium has produced the desired therapeutic response as determined by PT/INR. When warfarin sodium has produced the desired PT/INR or prothrombin activity, heparin may be discontinued. Warfarin sodium may increase the aPTT test, even in the absence of heparin. During initial therapy with warfarin sodium, the interference with heparin anticoagulation is of minimal clinical significance. As heparin may affect the PT/INR, patients receiving both heparin and warfarin sodium should have blood for PT/INR determination drawn at least:

- 5 hours after the last IV bolus dose of heparin.
- 4 hours after cessation of a continuous IV infusion of heparin.
- 24 hours after the last subcutaneous heparin injection.

➤*Storage/Stability:* Warfarin for injection is available for intravenous use only. Not recommended for intramuscular administration. Reconstitute with 2.7 mL of Sterile Water for Injection to yield 2 mg/mL. Net contents 5.4 mg lyophilized powder. Maximum yield 2.5 mL.

Protect from light. Keep vial in box until used. Store at controlled room temperature (15° to 30°C; 59° to 86°F). After reconstitution, store at controlled room temperature (15° to 30°C; 59° to 86°F) and use within 4 hours. Do not refrigerate. Discard any unused solution.

Actions

➤*Pharmacology:* Warfarin sodium and other coumarin anticoagulants act by inhibiting the synthesis of vitamin K dependent clotting factors, which include Factors II, VII, IX, and X, and the anticoagulant proteins C and S. Half-lives of these clotting factors are as follows: Factor II, 60 hours; VII, 4 to 6 hours; IX, 24 hours; and X, 48 to 72 hours. The half-lives of proteins C and S are approximately 8 hours and 30 hours, respectively. The resultant in vivo effect is a sequential depression of Factors VII, IX, X, and II activities. Vitamin K is an essential cofactor for the post ribosomal synthesis of the vitamin K dependent clotting factors. The vitamin promotes the biosynthesis of α-carboxyglutamic acid residues in the proteins which are essential for biological activity. Warfarin is thought to interfere with clotting factor synthesis by inhibition of the regeneration of vitamin K_1 epoxide. The degree of depression is dependent upon the dosage administered. Therapeutic doses of warfarin decrease the total amount of the active form of each vitamin K dependent clotting factor made by the liver by approximately 30% to 50%.

An anticoagulation effect generally occurs within 24 hours after drug administration. However, peak anticoagulant effect may be delayed 72 to 96 hours. The duration of action of a single dose of racemic warfarin is 2 to 5 days. The effects of warfarin sodium may become more pronounced as effects of daily maintenance doses overlap. Anticoagulants have no direct effect on an established thrombus, nor do they reverse ischemic tissue damage. However, once a thrombus has occurred, the goal of anticoagulant treatment is to prevent further extension of the formed clot and prevent secondary thromboembolic complications which may result in serious and possibly fatal sequelae.

➤*Pharmacokinetics:*

Absorption – Warfarin sodium is a racemic mixture of the R- and S-enantiomers. The S-enantiomer exhibits 2 to 5 times more anticoagulant activity than the R-enantiomer in humans, but generally has a more rapid clearance.

Warfarin sodium is essentially completely absorbed after oral administration with peak concentration generally attained within the first 4 hours.

Distribution – There are no differences in the apparent volumes of distribution after IV and oral administration of single doses of warfarin solution. Warfarin distributes into a relatively small apparent volume of distribution of about 0.14 L/kg. A distribution phase lasting 6 to 12 hours is distinguishable after rapid IV or oral administration of an aqueous solution. Using a one compartment model, and assuming complete bioavailability, estimates of the volumes of distribution of R- and S-warfarin are similar to each other and to that of the racemate. Concentrations in fetal plasma approach the maternal values, but warfarin has not been found in human milk. Based on very limited published data, warfarin has not been detected in the breast milk of mothers treated with warfarin. The same limited published data report that some breastfed infants, whose mothers were treated with warfarin, had prolonged prothrombin times, although not as prolonged as those of the mothers. The decision to breastfeed should be undertaken only after careful consideration of the available alternatives. Women who are breastfeeding and anticoagulated with warfarin should be very carefully monitored so that recommended PT/INR values are not exceeded. Approximately 99% of the drug is bound to plasma proteins.

Metabolism – The elimination of warfarin is almost entirely by metabolism. Warfarin sodium is stereoselectively metabolized by hepatic microsomal enzymes (cytochrome P-450) to inactive hydroxylated metabolites (predominant route) and by reductases to reduced metabolites (warfarin alcohols). The warfarin alcohols have minimal anticoagulant activity. The metabolites are principally excreted into the urine; and to a lesser extent into the bile. The metabolites of warfarin that have been identified include dehydrowarfarin, 2 diastereoisomer alcohols, 4-, 6-, 7-, 8- and 10-hydroxywarfarin. The cytochrome P-450 isozymes involved in the metabolism of warfarin include 2C9, 2C19, 2C8, 2C18, 1A2, and 3A4. 2C9 is likely to be the principal form of human liver P-450 which modulates the in vivo anticoagulant activity of warfarin.

Excretion – The terminal half-life of warfarin after a single dose is approximately 1 week; however, the effective half-life ranges from 20 to 60 hours, with a mean of about 40 hours. The clearance of R-warfarin is generally half that of S-warfarin, thus as the volumes of distribution are similar, the half-life of R-warfarin is longer than that of S-warfarin. The half-life of R-warfarin ranges from 37 to 89 hours, while that of S-warfarin ranges from 21 to 43 hours. Studies with radiolabeled drug have demonstrated that up to 92% of the orally administered dose is recovered in urine. Very little warfarin is excreted unchanged in urine. Urinary excretion is in the form of metabolites.

Special populations –

Hepatic function impairment: Hepatic dysfunction can potentiate the response to warfarin through impaired synthesis of clotting factors and decreased metabolism of warfarin. The administration of warfarin sodium

WARFARIN SODIUM — INJECTION

via the IV route should provide the patient with the same concentration of an equal oral dose, but maximum plasma concentration will be reached earlier. However, the full anticoagulant effect of a dose of warfarin may not be achieved until 72 to 96 hours after dosing, indicating that the administration of IV warfarin sodium should not provide any increased biological effect or earlier onset of action.

Elderly: Patients 60 years or older appear to exhibit greater than expected PT/INR response to the anticoagulant effects of warfarin. The cause of the increased sensitivity to the anticoagulant effects of warfarin in this age group is unknown. This increased anticoagulant effect from warfarin may be due to a combination of pharmacokinetic and pharmacodynamic factors. Racemic warfarin clearance may be unchanged or reduced with increasing age. Limited information suggests there is no difference in the clearance of S-warfarin in the elderly versus young subjects. However, there may be a slight decrease in the clearance of R-warfarin in the elderly as compared to the young. Therefore, as patient age increases, a lower dose of warfarin is usually required to produce a therapeutic level of anticoagulation.

Race: Asian patients may require lower initiation and maintenance doses of warfarin. One non-controlled study conducted in 151 Chinese outpatients reported a mean daily warfarin requirement of 3.3 ± 1.4 mg to achieve an INR of 2 to 2.5. These patients were stabilized on warfarin for various indications. Patient age was the most important determinant of warfarin requirement in Chinese patients with a progressively lower warfarin requirement with increasing age.

Contraindications

Any localized or general physical condition or personal circumstance in which the hazard of hemorrhage might be greater than the potential clinical benefits of anticoagulation; pregnancy (see Warnings).

Hemorrhagic tendencies or blood dyscrasias; recent or contemplated surgery of: Central nervous system, eye, or traumatic surgery resulting in large open surfaces; bleeding tendencies associated with active ulceration or overt bleeding of: Gastrointestinal, genitourinary or respiratory tracts, cerebrovascular hemorrhage, aneurysms-cerebral, dissecting aorta, pericarditis and pericardial effusions, or bacterial endocarditis; threatened abortion, eclampsia and preeclampsia; inadequate laboratory facilities; unsupervised patients with senility, alcoholism, or psychosis or other lack of patient cooperation; spinal puncture and other diagnostic or therapeutic procedures with potential for uncontrollable bleeding; major regional, lumbar block anesthesia, malignant hypertension and known hypersensitivity to warfarin or to any other components of this product.

Warnings

➤*Hemorrhage/Necrosis:* The most serious risks associated with anticoagulant therapy with warfarin sodium are hemorrhage in any tissue or organ and, less frequently (less than 0.1%), necrosis or gangrene of skin and other tissues. The risk of hemorrhage is related to the level of intensity and the duration of anticoagulant therapy. Hemorrhage and necrosis have in some cases been reported to result in death or permanent disability. Necrosis appears to be associated with local thrombosis and usually appears within a few days of the start of anticoagulant therapy. In severe cases of necrosis, treatment through debridement or amputation of the affected tissue, limb, breast or penis has been reported. Careful diagnosis is required to determine whether necrosis is caused by an underlying disease. Warfarin therapy should be discontinued when warfarin is suspected to be the cause of developing necrosis and heparin therapy may be considered for anticoagulation. Although various treatments have been attempted, no treatment for necrosis has been considered uniformly effective. See below for information on predisposing conditions. These and other risks associated with anticoagulant therapy must be weighed against the risk of thrombosis or embolization in untreated cases.

➤*Atheroemboli/Microemboli:* Anticoagulation therapy with warfarin sodium may enhance the release of atheromatous plaque emboli, thereby increasing the risk of complications from systemic cholesterol microembolization, including the "purple toes syndrome." Discontinuation of warfarin sodium therapy is recommended when such phenomena are observed.

Systemic atheroemboli and cholesterol microemboli can present with a variety of signs and symptoms including purple toes syndrome, livedo reticularis, rash, gangrene, abrupt and intense pain in the leg, foot, or toes, foot ulcers, myalgia, penile gangrene, abdominal pain, flank or back pain, hematuria, renal insufficiency, hypertension, cerebral ischemia, spinal cord infarction, pancreatitis, symptoms simulating polyarteritis, or any other sequelae of vascular compromise due to embolic occlusion. The most commonly involved visceral organs are the kidneys followed by the pancreas, spleen, and liver. Some cases have progressed to necrosis or death.

➤*Purple toes syndrome:* Purple toes syndrome is a complication of oral anticoagulation characterized by a dark, purplish or mottled color of the toes, usually occurring between 3 to 10 weeks, or later, after the initiation of therapy with warfarin or related compounds. Major features of this syndrome include purple color of plantar surfaces and sides of the toes that blanches on moderate pressure and fades with elevation of the legs; pain and tenderness of the toes; waxing and waning of the color over time. While the purple toes syndrome is reported to be reversible, some cases progress to gangrene or necrosis, which may require debridement of the affected area, or may lead to amputation.

➤*Heparin-induced thrombocytopenia:* Warfarin sodium should be used with caution in patients with heparin-induced thrombocytopenia and deep venous thrombosis. Cases of venous limb ischemia, necrosis, and gangrene have occurred in patients with heparin-induced thrombocytopenia and deep venous thrombosis when heparin treatment was discontinued and warfarin therapy was started or continued. In some patients sequelae have included amputation of the involved area or death.

A severe elevation (greater than 50 seconds) in activated partial thromboplastin time (aPTT) with a PT/INR in the desired range has been identified as an indication of increased risk of postoperative hemorrhage.

➤*Special risks patients:* Warfarin sodium is a narrow therapeutic range (index) drug, and caution should be observed when warfarin sodium is administered to certain patients such as the elderly or debilitated or when administered in any situation or physical condition where added risk of hemorrhage, necrosis, or gangrene is present.

Acquired or inherited warfarin resistance should be suspected if large daily doses of warfarin sodium are required to maintain a patient's PT/INR within a normal therapeutic range.

The decision to administer anticoagulants in the following conditions must be based upon clinical judgment in which the risks of anticoagulant therapy are weighed against the benefits.

- Severe to moderate hepatic or renal insufficiency.
- Infectious diseases or disturbances of intestinal flora: Sprue, antibiotic therapy.
- Trauma which may result in internal bleeding.
- Surgery or trauma resulting in large exposed raw surfaces.
- Indwelling catheters.
- Severe to moderate hypertension.
- Known or suspected deficiency in protein C mediated anticoagulant response: Hereditary or acquired deficiencies of protein C or its cofactor, protein S, have been associated with tissue necrosis following warfarin administration. Not all patients with these conditions develop necrosis, and tissue necrosis occurs in patients without these deficiencies. Inherited resistance to activated protein C has been described in many patients with venous thromboembolic disorders but has not yet been evaluated as a risk factor for tissue necrosis. The risk associated with these conditions, both for recurrent thrombosis and for adverse reactions, is difficult to evaluate since it does not appear to be the same for everyone. Decisions about testing and therapy must be made on an individual basis. It has been reported that concomitant anticoagulation therapy with heparin for 5 to 7 days during initiation of therapy with warfarin sodium may minimize the incidence of tissue necrosis. Warfarin therapy should be discontinued when warfarin is suspected to be the cause of developing necrosis and heparin therapy may be considered for anticoagulation.
- Miscellaneous: Polycythemia vera, vasculitis, and severe diabetes.

➤*Acquired/Inherited warfarin resistance:* In patients with acquired or inherited warfarin resistance, decreased therapeutic responses to warfarin sodium have been reported. Exaggerated therapeutic responses have been reported in other patients.

➤*Enhanced anticoagulant effect:* Patients with congestive heart failure may exhibit greater than expected PT/INR response to warfarin sodium, thereby requiring more frequent laboratory monitoring, and reduced doses of warfarin sodium. Concomitant use of anticoagulants with streptokinase or urokinase is not recommended and may be hazardous. (Please note recommendations accompanying these preparations.)

➤*Hypersensitivity reactions:* Minor and severe allergic/hypersensitivity reactions and anaphylactic reactions have been reported.

➤*Elderly:* Patients 60 years or older appear to exhibit greater than expected PT/INR response to the anticoagulant effects of warfarin. The cause of the increased sensitivity to the anticoagulant effects of warfarin in this age group is unknown. This increased anticoagulant effect from warfarin may be due to a combination of pharmacokinetic and pharmacodynamic factors. Racemic warfarin clearance may be unchanged or reduced with increasing age. Limited information suggests there is no difference in the clearance of S-warfarin in the elderly versus young subjects. However, there may be a slight decrease in the clearance of R-warfarin in the elderly as compared to the young. Therefore, as patient age increases, a lower dose of warfarin is usually required to produce a therapeutic level of anticoagulation. Warfarin sodium is contraindicated in any unsupervised patient with senility. Caution should be observed with administration of warfarin sodium to elderly patients in any situation or physical condition where added risk of hemorrhage is present.

➤*Pregnancy: Category X.* Warfarin sodium is contraindicated in women who are or may become pregnant because the drug passes through the placental barrier and may cause fatal hemorrhage to the fetus in utero. Furthermore, there have been reports of birth malformations in children born to mothers who have been treated with warfarin during pregnancy.

WARFARIN SODIUM — INJECTION

Embryopathy characterized by nasal hypoplasia with or without stippled epiphyses (chondrodysplasia punctata) has been reported in pregnant women exposed to warfarin during the first trimester. Central nervous system abnormalities also have been reported, including dorsal midline dysplasia characterized by agenesis of the corpus callosum, Dandy-Walker malformation, and midline cerebellar atrophy. Ventral midline dysplasia, characterized by optic atrophy, and eye abnormalities have been observed. Mental retardation, blindness, and other central nervous system abnormalities have been reported in association with second and third trimester exposure. Although rare, teratogenic reports following in utero exposure to warfarin include urinary tract anomalies such as single kidney, asplenia, anencephaly, spina bifida, cranial nerve palsy, hydrocephalus, cardiac defects and congenital heart disease, polydactyly, deformities of toes, diaphragmatic hernia, corneal leukoma, cleft palate, cleft lip, schizencephaly, and microcephaly.

Spontaneous abortion and still birth are known to occur and a higher risk of fetal mortality is associated with the use of warfarin. Low birth weight and growth retardation have also been reported.

Women of childbearing potential who are candidates for anticoagulant therapy should be carefully evaluated and the indications critically reviewed with the patient. If the patient becomes pregnant while taking this drug, she should be apprised of the potential risks to the fetus, and the possibility of termination of the pregnancy should be discussed in light of those risks.

➤*Lactation:* Based on very limited published data, warfarin has not been detected in the breast milk of mothers treated with warfarin. The same limited published data report that some breastfed infants, whose mothers were treated with warfarin, had prolonged prothrombin times, although not as prolonged as those of the mothers. The decision to breastfeed should be undertaken only after careful consideration of the available alternatives. Women who are breastfeeding and anticoagulated with warfarin should be very carefully monitored so that recommended PT/INR values are not exceeded. It is prudent to perform coagulation tests and to evaluate vitamin K status in infants at risk for bleeding tendencies before advising women taking warfarin to breastfeed. Effects in premature infants have not been evaluated.

➤*Children:* Safety and effectiveness in pediatric patients below the age of 18 have not been established in randomized, controlled clinical trials. However, the use of warfarin sodium in pediatric patients is well-documented for the prevention and treatment of thromboembolic events. Difficulty achieving and maintaining therapeutic PT/INR ranges in the pediatric patient has been reported. More frequent PT/INR determinations are recommended because of possible changing warfarin requirements.

Precautions

➤*Monitoring:* It cannot be emphasized too strongly that treatment of each patient is a highly individualized matter. Warfarin sodium, a narrow therapeutic range (index) drug, may be affected by factors such as other drugs and dietary vitamin K. Dosage should be controlled by periodic determinations of PT/INR or other suitable coagulation tests. Determinations of whole blood clotting and bleeding times are not effective measures for control of therapy. Heparin prolongs the one-stage PT. When heparin and warfarin sodium are administered concomitantly, refer to Conversion from Heparin Therapy above, under Administration and Dosage, for recommendations.

Periodic determination of PT/INR or other suitable coagulation test is essential.

Patients with congestive heart failure may exhibit greater than expected PT/INR response to warfarin sodium, thereby requiring more frequent laboratory monitoring, and reduced doses of warfarin sodium. Concomitant use of anticoagulants with streptokinase or urokinase is not recommended and may be hazardous. (Please note recommendations accompanying these preparations.)

Numerous factors, alone or in combination, including travel, changes in diet, environment, physical state and medication may influence response of the patient to anticoagulants. It is generally good practice to monitor the patient's response with additional PT/INR determinations in the period immediately after discharge from the hospital, and whenever other medications are initiated, discontinued or taken irregularly.

➤*Concomitant NSAIDs / aspirin:* Caution should be observed when warfarin is administered concomitantly with nonsteroidal anti-inflammatory drugs (NSAIDs), including aspirin, to be certain that no change in anticoagulation dosage is required. In addition to specific drug interactions that might affect PT/INR, NSAIDs, including aspirin, can inhibit platelet aggregation, and can cause gastrointestinal bleeding, peptic ulceration or perforation.

Drug Interactions

Careful monitoring and appropriate dosage adjustments usually will permit combination therapy. Critical times during therapy occur when an interacting drug is added to or discontinued from a patient stabilized on anticoagulants.

Oral Anticoagulant Drug Interactions

Precipitant drug	Object drug*		Description
Acetaminophen Androgens Beta blockers (propranolol) Capecitabine Cephalosporins, parenteral Chenodiol Chlorpropamide Cisapride Dextran Dextrothyroxine Diazoxide Disulfiram Fibric acids Flutamide Glucagon Halothane Heparin Influenza virus vaccine Isoniazid Levamisole Methyldopa Methylphenidate NSAIDs, COX-2 selective Pentoxifylline Propoxyphene Quinolones (eg, ciprofloxacin, levofloxacin, norfloxacin, ofloxacin) SSRIs[1] (ie, fluoxetine, fluvoxamine, paroxetine, sertraline) Streptokinase Sulfonamides Tamoxifen Thrombolytics (ie, tissue plasminogen activator [t-PA]) Thyroid hormones Tolbutamide Tramadol Urokinase Zafirlukast Zileuton	Anticoagulants	↑	These agents may increase the anticoagulant effect. The risk of bleeding may be increased. The mechanism of the interaction is unknown or complicated.
Allopurinol Amiodarone Azole antifungals[2] Chloramphenicol Cimetidine HMG-CoA reductase inhibitors (ie, fluvastatin, lovastatin, simvastatin) Ifosfamide[3] Metronidazole Omeprazole Phenylbutazone[3] Propafenone Quinidine Quinine SMZ-TMP Sulfinpyrazone	Anticoagulants	↑	These agents may increase the anticoagulant effect of warfarin by inhibition of the anticoagulant's hepatic metabolism. The risk of bleeding may be increased.
Macrolide antibiotics	Anticoagulants	↑	These agents may increase the anticoagulant effect by reducing body clearance of warfarin. The risk of bleeding may be increased.

WARFARIN SODIUM — INJECTION

Oral Anticoagulant Drug Interactions

Precipitant drug	Object drug*		Description
Loop diuretics (ie, ethacrynic acid, furosemide) Nalidixic acid Valproate	Anticoagulants	↑	These agents may increase the anticoagulant effect of warfarin caused by displacement from binding sites. The risk of bleeding may be increased.
Aminoglycosides (oral) Tetracyclines Vitamin E	Anticoagulants	↑	These agents may increase the anticoagulant effect of warfarin through an interference with vitamin K. The risk of bleeding may be increased.
Aminosalicylic acid Diflunisal NSAIDs Penicillins, high-dose IV Salicylates Methylsalicylate ointment, topical Ticlopidine	Anticoagulants	↑	These agents may increase the anticoagulant effect of warfarin and increase the risk of bleeding caused by effects on platelet function, and, in the case of NSAIDs, GI irritant effects.
Alcohol[4] Atorvastatin Chloral hydrate Cholestyramine[5] Corticosteroids Cyclophosphamide Methimazole Moricizine Hydantoins (eg, phenytoin) Pravastatin Prednisone Propylthiouracil Ranitidine	Anticoagulants	↑↓	Increased and decreased PT/INR responses have been reported. May increase or decrease anticoagulant effect of warfarin; mechanism unknown.
Ascorbic acid, high doses Chlordiazepoxide Clozapine Contraceptives, oral[6] Cyclosporine[7] Estrogens Ethchlorvynol Griseofulvin Haloperidol Meprobamate Paraldehyde Trazodone	Anticoagulants	↓	These agents may decrease the anticoagulant effect of warfarin. The mechanism of the interaction is unknown.
Aminoglutethimide Barbiturates Carbamazepine Dicloxacillin[8] Glutethimide Nafcillin[8] Rifamycins Terbinafine	Anticoagulants	↓	These agents may decrease the anticoagulant effect of warfarin caused by induction of the anticoagulant's hepatic microsomal enzymes.
Spironolactone[9] Sucralfate Thiazide diuretics[9] Thiopurines[10] Vitamin K[11]	Anticoagulants	↓	These agents may decrease the anticoagulant effect of warfarin by various mechanisms (eg, possible decreased absorption or increased elimination).

* ↑ = Object drug increased. ↓ = Object drug decreased.
[1] Bleeding has been reported with fluoxetine alone.
[2] Miconazole includes both intravaginal and systemic formulations.
[3] May also displace the anticoagulant from protein binding sites.
[4] Chronic consumption may increase the clearance of the anticoagulant; moderate to small doses do not alter the anticoagulant effect.
[5] Reduced anticoagulant absorption and possibly increased elimination.
[6] Rarely, increased risk of thromboembolism; this is in contrast to intended effect.
[7] Cyclosporine levels also may be decreased.
[8] Associated with warfarin resistance.
[9] Diuretic-induced hemoconcentration of clotting factors.
[10] Thiopurine-induced increase in synthesis or activation of prothrombin.
[11] Vitamin K overcomes interference of vitamin K-dependent clotting factors by anticoagulants.

➤*Herbal medicines:* Exercise caution when herbal medicines are taken concomitantly with warfarin. Specific herbals reported to affect warfarin therapy include the following:

- Bromelains, danshen, dong quai (*Angelica sinensis*), garlic, boldo, *Lycium barbarum* L. , and *Ginkgo biloba* are associated most often with an increase in the effects of warfarin.
- Coenzyme Q_{10} (ubidecarenone), St. John's wort, green tea, and ginseng are associated most often with a decrease in the effects of warfarin.

Some herbals may cause bleeding events when taken alone (eg, garlic, *Ginkgo biloba*) and may have anticoagulant, antiplatelet, and/or fibrinolytic properties. These effects would be expected to be additive to the anticoagulant effects of warfarin.

Some herbals that may affect coagulation are listed in the following table; however, this list should not be considered all-inclusive.

Herbals That Contain Coumarins With Potential Anticoagulant Effects

Alfalfa	Celery	Parsley
Angelica (dong quai)	Chamomile (German and Roman)	Passion flower
Aniseed	Dandelion[3]	Prickly ash (Northern)
Arnica	Fenugreek	Quassia
Asa foetida	Horse chestnut	Red clover
Bogbean[1]	Horseradish	Sweet clover
Boldo	Licorice[3]	Sweet woodruff
Buchu	Meadowsweet[1]	Tonka beans
Capsicum[2]	Nettle	Wild carrot
Cassia[3]		Wild lettuce

[1] Contains coumarins and salicylates.
[2] Contains coumarins and has fibrinolytic properties.
[3] Contains coumarins and has antiplatelet properties.

Miscellaneous Herbals With Anticoagulant Properties

Bladder wrack (*Fucus*)	Pau d'arco

Herbals That Contain Salicylate and/or Have Antiplatelet Properties

Agrimony[1]	Dandelion[3]	Meadowsweet[2]
Aloe gel	Feverfew	Onion[4]
Aspen	Garlic[4]	Policosanol
Black cohosh	German sarsaparilla	Poplar
Black haw	Ginger	Senega
Bogbean[2]	*Ginkgo biloba*	Tamarind
Cassia[3]	Ginseng (*Panax*)[4]	Willow
Clove	Licorice[3]	Wintergreen

[1] Contains salicylate and has coagulant properties.
[2] Contains coumarins and salicylates.
[3] Contains coumarins and has antiplatelet properties.
[4] Has antiplatelet and fibrinolytic properties.

Herbals With Fibrinolytic Properties

Bromelains	Garlic[2]	Inositol nicotinate
Capsicum[1]	Ginseng (*Panax*)[2]	Onion[2]

[1] Contains coumarins and has fibrinolytic properties.
[2] Has antiplatelet and fibrinolytic properties.

Herbals with Coagulant Properties

Agrimony[1]	Mistletoe	Yarrow
Goldenseal		

[1] Contains salicylate and has coagulant properties.

➤*Drug/Food interactions:* Vitamin K-rich vegetables may decrease the anticoagulant effects of warfarin by interfering with absorption. Minimize consumption of vitamin K-rich foods (eg, spinach, seaweed, broccoli, turnip greens) or nutritional supplements. Mango has been shown to increase warfarin's effect.

Adverse Reactions

➤*Dermatologic:* Necrosis of skin and other tissues. Necrosis appears to be associated with local thrombosis and usually appears within a few days of the start of anticoagulant therapy. In severe cases of necrosis, treatment through debridement or amputation of the affected tissue, limb, breast or penis has been reported. Careful diagnosis is required to determine whether necrosis is caused by an underlying disease. Warfarin therapy should be discontinued when warfarin is suspected to be the cause of developing necrosis and heparin therapy may be considered for anticoagulation. Priapism has been associated with anticoagulant administration, however, a causal relationship has not been established. Rash and dermatitis, including bullous eruptions, pruritus, alopecia.

➤*GI:* Abdominal pain including cramping, flatulence/bloating, nausea, vomiting, diarrhea.

➤*Hematologic:* Fatal or nonfatal hemorrhage from any tissue or organ. This is a consequence of the anticoagulant effect. The signs, symptoms, and severity will vary according to the location and degree or extent of the bleeding. Hemorrhagic complications may present as paralysis; paresthesia; headache, chest, abdomen, joint, muscle or other pain; dizziness; shortness of breath, difficult breathing or swallowing; unexplained swelling; weakness; hypotension; or unexplained shock. Therefore, the possibility of hem-

WARFARIN SODIUM — INJECTION

orrhage should be considered in evaluating the condition of any anticoagulated patient with complaints that do not indicate an obvious diagnosis. Bleeding during anticoagulant therapy does not always correlate with PT/INR. Bleeding that occurs when the PT/INR is within the therapeutic range warrants diagnostic investigation since it may unmask a previously unsuspected lesion, eg, tumor, ulcer.

➤*Hepatic:* Hepatitis, cholestatic hepatic injury, jaundice, elevated liver enzymes.

➤*Respiratory:* Rare events of tracheal or tracheobronchial calcification have been reported in association with long-term warfarin therapy. The clinical significance of this event is unknown.

➤*Miscellaneous:* Hypersensitivity/allergic reactions, systemic cholesterol microembolization, purple toes syndrome, vasculitis, edema, fever, urticaria, fatigue, lethargy, malaise, asthenia, pain, headache, dizziness, taste perversion, cold intolerance, and paresthesia including feeling cold and chills.

Overdosage

➤*Symptoms:* Suspected or overt abnormal bleeding (eg, appearance of blood in stools or urine, hematuria, excessive menstrual bleeding, melena, petechiae, excessive bruising or persistent oozing from superficial injuries) are early manifestations of anticoagulation beyond a safe and satisfactory level.

➤*Treatment:* Excessive anticoagulation with or without bleeding may be controlled by discontinuing warfarin sodium therapy and if necessary, by administration of oral or parenteral vitamin K_1. (Please see recommendations accompanying vitamin K_1 preparations prior to use.)

Such use of vitamin K_1 reduces response to subsequent warfarin sodium therapy. Patients may return to a pretreatment thrombotic status following the rapid reversal of a prolonged PT/INR. Resumption of warfarin sodium administration reverses the effect of vitamin K, and a therapeutic PT/INR can again be obtained by careful dosage adjustment. If rapid anticoagulation is indicated, heparin may be preferable for initial therapy.

If minor bleeding progresses to major bleeding, give 5 to 25 mg (rarely up to 50 mg) parenteral vitamin K_1. In emergency situations of severe hemorrhage, clotting factors can be returned to normal by administering 200 to 500 mL of fresh whole blood or fresh frozen plasma, or by giving commercial Factor IX complex.

A risk of hepatitis and other viral diseases is associated with the use of these blood products. Factor IX complex is also associated with an increased risk of thrombosis. Therefore, these preparations should be used only in exceptional or life-threatening bleeding episodes secondary to warfarin sodium overdosage.

Purified Factor IX preparations should not be used because they cannot increase the levels of prothrombin, Factor VII and Factor X which are also depressed along with the levels of Factor IX as a result of warfarin sodium treatment. Packed red blood cells may also be given if significant blood loss has occurred. Infusions of blood or plasma should be monitored carefully to avoid precipitating pulmonary edema in elderly patients or patients with heart disease.

Patient Information

The objective of anticoagulant therapy is to decrease the clotting ability of the blood so that thrombosis is prevented, while avoiding spontaneous bleeding. Effective therapeutic levels with minimal complications are in part dependent upon cooperative and well-instructed patients who communicate effectively with their physician.

Strict adherence to prescribed dosage schedule is necessary.

Do not take or discontinue any other medication, including salicylates (eg, aspirin and topical analgesics) and other over-the-counter medications, and botanical (herbal) products (eg, bromelains, coenzyme Q_{10}, danshen, dong quai, garlic, ginkgo biloba, ginseng, and St. John's wort) except on advice of the physician.

Avoid alcohol consumption.

Do not take warfarin sodium during pregnancy and do not become pregnant while taking it. Warfarin sodium is contraindicated in women who are or may become pregnant because the drug passes through the placental barrier and may cause fatal hemorrhage to the fetus in utero. Furthermore, there have been reports of birth malformations in children born to mothers who have been treated with warfarin during pregnancy.

Avoid any activity or sport that may result in traumatic injury.

Prothrombin time tests and regular visits to physician or clinic are needed to monitor therapy.

Carry identification stating that warfarin sodium is being taken.

If the prescribed dose of warfarin sodium is forgotten, notify the physician immediately. Take the dose as soon as possible on the same day, but do not take a double dose of warfarin sodium the next day to make up for missed doses.

The amount of vitamin K in food may affect therapy with warfarin sodium. Eat a normal, balanced diet maintaining a consistent amount of vitamin K. Avoid drastic changes in dietary habits, such as eating large amounts of green leafy vegetables.

Contact physician to report any illness, such as diarrhea, infection, or fever.

Notify physician immediately if any unusual bleeding or symptoms occur. Signs and symptoms of bleeding include: Pain, swelling or discomfort, prolonged bleeding from cuts, increased menstrual flow or vaginal bleeding, nosebleeds, bleeding of gums from brushing, unusual bleeding or bruising, red or dark brown urine, red or tar black stools, headache, dizziness, or weakness.

If therapy with warfarin sodium is discontinued, patients should be cautioned that the anticoagulant effects of warfarin sodium may persist for about 2 to 5 days.

Patients should be informed that all warfarin sodium products represent the same medication, and should not be taken concomitantly, as overdosage may result.

COAGULANTS

Heparin Antagonist

PROTAMINE SULFATE

Rx	**Protamine Sulfate** (Various, eg, American Pharmaceutical Partners "APP], Lilly)	**Injection:** 10 mg/mL	Preservative-free. In 5 and 25 mL vials.

PROTAMINE SULFATE — INJECTION

Indications

➤*Heparin overdose:* Treatment of heparin overdosage.

Administration and Dosage

➤*Approved by the FDA:* April 7, 1987.

Each mg of protamine sulfate, calculated on the dried basis, neutralizes not less than 100 heparin units.

Protamine sulfate injection should be given by very slow IV injection over a 10-minute period in doses not to exceed 50 mg (see Warnings).

Because heparin disappears rapidly from the circulation, the dose of protamine sulfate required also decreases rapidly with the time elapsed following IV injection of heparin. For example, if the protamine sulfate is administered 30 minutes after the heparin, one-half the usual dose may be sufficient.

The dosage of protamine sulfate should be guided by blood coagulation studies (see Warnings).

➤*Dilution (if desired):* Protamine sulfate is intended for injection without further dilution; however, if further dilution is desired, D5-W or normal saline may be used. Diluted solutions should not be stored since they contain no preservative.

➤*Incompatibilities:* Protamine sulfate should not be mixed with other drugs without knowledge of their compatibility, because protamine sulfate has been shown to be incompatible with certain antibiotics, including several of the cephalosporins and penicillins.

➤*Storage/Stability:* Store at controlled room temperature 15° to 30°C (59° to 86°F). Do not permit to freeze.

Parenteral drug products should be visually inspected for particulate matter and discoloration prior to administration, whenever solution and container permit.

Actions

➤*Pharmacology:* When administered alone, protamine has an anticoagulant effect. However, when it is given in the presence of heparin (which is strongly acidic), a stable salt is formed and the anticoagulant activity of both drugs is lost.

➤*Pharmacokinetics:*

Absorption/Distribution – Protamine sulfate has a rapid onset of action. Neutralization of heparin occurs within 5 minutes after IV administration of an appropriate dose of protamine sulfate.

Metabolism – Although the metabolic fate of the heparin-protamine complex has not been elucidated, it has been postulated that protamine sulfate in the heparin-protamine complex may be partially metabolized or may be attacked by fibrinolysin, thus freeing heparin.

Contraindications

Previous intolerance to the drug.

Warnings

➤*Hyperheparinemia or bleeding:* Hyperheparinemia or bleeding has been reported in experimental animals and in some patients 30 minutes to 18 hours after cardiac surgery (under cardiopulmonary bypass) in spite of complete neutralization of heparin by adequate doses of protamine sulfate at the end of the operation. It is important to keep the patient under close observation after cardiac surgery. Additional doses of protamine sulfate should be administered if indicated by coagulation studies, such as the hepa-

Heparin Antagonist

PROTAMINE SULFATE — INJECTION

rin titration test with protamine and the determination of plasma thrombin time.

➤*Hypersensitivity reactions:* Too-rapid administration of protamine sulfate can cause severe hypotensive and anaphylactoid reactions (see Administration and Dosage and Warnings). Facilities to treat shock should be available.

Patients with a history of allergy to fish may develop hypersensitivity reactions to protamine, although to date no relationship has been established between allergic reactions to protamine and fish allergy.

Fatal anaphylaxis has been reported in one patient with no history of allergies.

➤*Pregnancy: Category C.* Animal reproduction studies have not been conducted with protamine sulfate. It is also not known whether protamine sulfate can cause fetal harm when administered to a pregnant woman or can affect reproduction capacity. Protamine sulfate should be given to a pregnant woman only if clearly needed.

➤*Lactation:* It is not known whether this drug is excreted in human milk. Because many drugs are excreted in human milk, caution should be exercised when protamine sulfate is administered to a nursing woman.

➤*Children:* Safety and effectiveness in children have not been established.

Precautions

➤*Anticoagulant effect:* Because of the anticoagulant effect of protamine, it is unwise to give more than 100 mg over a short period unless a larger dose is clearly needed.

➤*Previous exposure to protamine:* Previous exposure to protamine through use of protamine-containing insulins or during heparin neutralization may predispose susceptible individuals to the development of untoward reactions from the subsequent use of this drug. Reports of the presence of antiprotamine antibodies in the sera of infertile or vasectomized men suggest that some of these individuals may react to the use of protamine sulfate.

Drug Interactions

➤*Antibiotics:* Protamine sulfate has been shown to be incompatible with certain antibiotics, including several of the cephalosporins and penicillins (see Administration and Dosage).

Adverse Reactions

➤*Cardiovascular:* The IV administration of protamine sulfate may cause a sudden fall in blood pressure and bradycardia.

Back pain has been reported in conscious patients undergoing such procedures as cardiac catheterization.

Severe and potentially irreversible circulatory collapse associated with MI and reduced cardiac output can also occur. The mechanism(s) of this reaction and the role played by concurrent factors are unclear.

High-protein, noncardiogenic pulmonary edema associated with the use of protamine has been reported in patients on cardiopulmonary bypass who are undergoing cardiovascular surgery. The etiologic role of protamine in the pathogenesis of this condition is uncertain, and multiple factors have been present in most cases. The condition has been reported in association with administration of certain blood products, other drugs, cardiopulmonary bypass alone, and other etiologic factors. It is difficult to treat, and it can be life-threatening. Because fatal anaphylactic and anaphylactoid reactions have been reported after the administration of protamine sulfate, the drug should be given only when resuscitation techniques and treatment of anaphylactic and anaphylactoid shock are readily available.

➤*Hypersensitivity:* Severe adverse reactions have been reported including: Anaphylaxis that resulted in severe respiratory distress, circulation collapse and capillary leak (see Warnings). Fatal anaphylaxis has been reported in one patient with no prior history of allergies; anaphylactoid reactions with circulatory collapse, capillary leak, and noncardiogenic pulmonary edema; acute pulmonary hypertension.

Complement activation by the heparin-protamine complexes, release of lysosomal enzymes from neutrophils, and prostaglandin and thomboxane generation have been associated with the development of anaphylactoid reactions.

➤*Miscellaneous:* Other reactions include transitory flushing and feeling of warmth, dyspnea, nausea, vomiting and lassitude.

Overdosage

The median lethal dose of protamine sulfate is 100 mg/kg in mice. Serum concentrations of protamine sulfate are not clinically useful. Information is not available on the amount of drug in a single dose that is associated with overdosage or is likely to be life-threatening.

➤*Symptoms:* Overdose of protamine sulfate may cause bleeding. Protamine has a weak anticoagulant effect due to an interaction with platelets and with many proteins including fibrinogen. This effect should be distinguished from the rebound anticoagulation that may occur 30 minutes to 18 hours following the reversal of heparin with protamine.

Rapid administration of protamine is more likely to result in bradycardia, dyspnea, a sensation of warmth, flushing, and severe hypotension. Hypertension has also occurred.

➤*Treatment:* To obtain up-to-date information about the treatment of overdose, a good resource is your certified regional poison control center. In managing overdosage, consider the possibility of multiple drug overdoses, interaction among drugs and unusual drug kinetics in your patient.

Replace blood loss with blood transfusions of fresh frozen plasma.

If the patient is hypotensive, consider fluids, epinephrine, dobutamine, or dopamine.

THROMBOLYTIC AGENTS

Tissue Plasminogen Activators

ALTEPLASE, RECOMBINANT

Rx	Activase (Genentech)	**Lyophilized powder for injection**[a]: 50 mg (29 million units)	In vials with diluent (50 mL sterile water for injection) and vacuum.
		100 mg (58 million units)	In vials with diluent (100 mL sterile water for injection) and 1 transfer device.
Rx	Cathflo Activase (Genentech)	**Lyophilized powder for injection**[a]: 2 mg	In vials.

[a] With L-arginine, phosphoric acid, and polysorbate 80.

ALTEPLASE, RECOMBINANT — INJECTION

Indications

➤*Acute myocardial infarction (AMI) (Activase* only): For the management of AMI in adults for the improvement of ventricular function following AMI, the reduction of the incidence of congestive heart failure, and the reduction of mortality associated with AMI. Initiate treatment as soon as possible after the onset of AMI symptoms.

➤*Acute ischemic stroke (AIS) (Activase* only): For the management of AIS in adults for improving neurological recovery and reducing the incidence of disability. Initiate treatment only within 3 hours after the onset of stroke symptoms and after exclusion of intracranial hemorrhage (ICH) by a cranial computerized tomography (CT) scan or other diagnostic imaging method sensitive for the presence of hemorrhage (see Contraindications).

➤*Pulmonary embolism (PE) (Activase* only): For the management of acute massive PE in adults for the lysis of acute PE, defined as obstruction of blood flow to a lobe or multiple segments of the lungs, and for the lysis of PE accompanied by unstable hemodynamics (eg, failure to maintain blood pressure without supportive measures).

Confirm the diagnosis by objective means such as pulmonary angiography or noninvasive procedures such as lung scanning.

➤*Restoration of function to central venous access device (Cathflo Activase* only): For the restoration of function to central venous access devices as assessed by the ability to withdraw blood.

➤*Unlabeled uses:* Administered as a bolus for the reversal of occluded catheters.

Administration and Dosage

➤*Approved by the FDA:* February 23, 1989 (*Activase*); September 4, 2001 (*Cathflo Activase*).

For IV administration only

➤*Restoration of function to central venous catheter (Cathflo Activase* only): Instill into dysfunctional catheter at a concentration of 1 mg/mL. For patients weighing 30 kg or more, use 2 mg in 2 mL. For patients weighing 10 kg or more to less than 30 kg, use 110% of the internal lumen volume of the catheter, not to exceed 2 mg in 2 mL. If catheter function is not restored in 120 minutes after 1 dose, a second dose may be instilled.

➤*AMI:* Administer as soon as possible after the onset of symptoms. Do not use a dose of 150 mg because it has been associated with an increase in intracranial bleeding.

Accelerated infusion – The recommended total dose is based upon patient weight, not to exceed 100 mg. For patients weighing more than 67 kg, the recommended dose administered is 100 mg as a 15 mg IV bolus, followed by 50 mg infused over the next 30 minutes, and then 35 mg infused over the next 60 minutes.

For patients weighing 67 kg or less, the recommended dose is administered as a 15 mg IV bolus, followed by 0.75 mg/kg infused over the next 30 minutes not to exceed 50 mg, and then 0.50 mg/kg over the next 60 minutes not to exceed 35 mg.

The safety and efficacy of this accelerated infusion of alteplase regimen has only been investigated with coadministration of heparin and aspirin.

ALTEPLASE, RECOMBINANT — INJECTION

3-hour infusion – The recommended dose is 100 mg administered as 60 mg (34.8 million units) in the first hour (with 6 to 10 mg administered as a bolus), 20 mg (11.6 million units) over the second hour, and 20 mg (11.6 million units) over the third hour. For smaller patients (less than 65 kg), a dose of 1.25 mg/kg administered over 3 hours, as described above, may be used.

Coadministration – Although the use of anticoagulants during and following alteplase administration has not been fully studied, heparin has been administered concomitantly for 24 hours or longer in more than 90% of patients. Aspirin and/or dipyridamole has been given either during or following heparin treatment (see Drug Interactions).

➤*AIS:* The recommended dose is 0.9 mg/kg (not to exceed 90 mg total dose) infused over 60 minutes with 10% of the total dose administered as an initial IV bolus over 1 minute. The safety and efficacy of this regimen with coadministration of heparin and aspirin during the first 24 hours after symptom onset has not been investigated. Doses greater than 0.9 mg/kg may be associated with an increased incidence of ICH. Do not use doses greater than 0.9 mg/kg (maximum 90 mg) in the management of acute ischemic stroke.

➤*PE:* The recommended dose is 100 mg administered by IV infusion over 2 hours. Institute or reinstitute heparin therapy near the end of or immediately following the alteplase infusion when the partial thromboplastin time or thrombin time returns to twice normal or less.

➤*Reconstitution:* Reconstitute only with sterile water for injection without preservatives. Do not use bacteriostatic water for injection. The reconstituted preparation results in a colorless to pale yellow, transparent solution. Slight foaming upon reconstitution is usual; standing undisturbed for several minutes is usually sufficient to allow dissipation of any large bubbles.

50 mg vial – Do not use if vacuum is not present. Reconstitute with a large bore needle (eg, 18-gauge), directing the stream of sterile water for injection into the lyophilized cake.

100 mg vial – Use transfer device provided for reconstitution. 100 mg vials do not contain vacuum.

➤*Admixture compatibility:* May be administered as reconstituted at 1 mg/mL. As an alternative, the reconstituted solution may be further diluted immediately before administration with an equal volume of 0.9% sodium chloride injection or 5% dextrose injection to yield a concentration of 0.5 mg/mL.

➤*Admixture incompatibilities:* Do not add other medications to infusion solution.

➤*Storage/Stability:* Store lyophilized alteplase at controlled room temperature not to exceed 30°C (86°F) or under refrigeration (2° to 8°C; 36° to 46°F). During extended storage, protect from excessive exposure to light. Discard any unused solution.

The solution may be used for direct IV administration within 8 hours following reconstitution when stored between 2° and 30°C (36° and 86°F). Avoid excessive agitation during dilution; mix by gentle swirling or slow inversion. Do not use other infusion solutions.

Actions

➤*Pharmacology:* Alteplase, a tissue plasminogen activator (tPA) produced by recombinant DNA, is synthesized using the complementary DNA for natural human tissue-type plasminogen activator obtained from a human melanoma cell line. Biological potency, determined by an in vitro clot lysis assay, is expressed in international units. The specific activity is 580,000 units/mg.

Alteplase is an enzyme (serine protease) that has the property of fibrin-enhanced conversion of plasminogen to plasmin. It produces limited conversion of plasminogen in the absence of fibrin. When introduced into the systemic circulation at pharmacologic concentration, alteplase binds to fibrin in a thrombus and converts the entrapped plasminogen to plasmin. This initiates local fibrinolysis with limited systemic proteolysis. Following administration of 100 mg, there is a decrease (16% to 36%) in circulating fibrinogen. In a controlled trial, 8 of 73 patients (11%) receiving alteplase (1.25 mg/kg over 3 hours) experienced a decrease in fibrinogen to below 100 mg/dL.

➤*Pharmacokinetics:*

Absorption/Distribution – Because of its large molecular size, alteplase cannot easily diffuse across biological membranes and must be given parenterally, usually IV. Maximal plasma concentrations of 3 to 4 mg/L are achieved after standard administration of 90 to 100 mg doses. Steady-state concentrations for the initial infusion period were 45% higher when administered in an accelerated regimen.

Metabolism/Excretion – Alteplase is cleared rapidly from plasma at a rate of 380 to 570 mL/min, primarily by the liver. More than 50% of the drug present in plasma is cleared within 5 minutes after the infusion has been terminated, and approximately 80% is cleared within 10 minutes. Initial volume of distribution is 2.8 to 4.6 L, and it approximately doubles at steady state. Total body clearance is 34.3 to 38.4 L/h.

Contraindications

Hypersensitivity to alteplase or any of the components.

➤*AMI or PE (Activase only):* Active internal bleeding; history of cerebrovascular accident; recent intracranial or intraspinal surgery or trauma; intracranial neoplasm, arteriovenous malformation, or aneurysm; bleeding diathesis; severe uncontrolled hypertension.

➤*AIS (Activase only):* Evidence of ICH on pretreatment evaluation; suspicion of subarachnoid hemorrhage; recent (within 3 months) intracranial or intraspinal surgery, serious head trauma, or previous stroke; history of ICH; uncontrolled hypertension at time of treatment (eg, greater than 185 mm Hg systolic or greater than 110 mm Hg diastolic); seizure at the onset of stroke; active internal bleeding; intracranial neoplasm, arteriovenous malformation, or aneurysm; bleeding diathesis.

➤*Bleeding diathesis:* Bleeding diathesis includes, but is not limited to: Current use of oral anticoagulants (eg, warfarin sodium) with prothrombin time (PT) longer than 15 seconds; administration of heparin within 48 hours preceding stroke onset with an elevated activated partial thromboplastin time (aPTT) at presentation; platelet count below 100,000/mm^3.

Warnings

➤*Bleeding:* Bleeding is the most common complication. The bleeding associated with thrombolytic therapy can be divided into 2 broad categories:

1.) Internal bleeding involving intracranial or retroperitoneal sites or the GI, GU, or respiratory tracts.
2.) Superficial or surface bleeding, observed mainly at invaded or disturbed sites (eg, venous cutdowns, arterial punctures, sites of recent surgical intervention).

The concomitant use of heparin anticoagulation may contribute to the bleeding. Some of the hemorrhagic episodes occurred 1 or more days after alteplase effects had dissipated but while heparin therapy was continuing.

As fibrin is lysed during alteplase therapy, bleeding from recent puncture sites may occur. Therefore, thrombolytic therapy requires careful attention to all potential bleeding sites (including catheter insertion sites, arterial and venous puncture sites, cutdown sites, and needle puncture sites). Avoid IM injections and nonessential handling of the patient during treatment with alteplase. Perform venipunctures carefully and only as required. Minimize arterial and venous punctures.

Should an arterial puncture be necessary during an infusion, it is preferable to use an upper extremity vessel accessible to manual compression. Apply pressure for at least 30 minutes, apply a pressure dressing, and check the puncture site frequently for bleeding evidence. Avoid noncompressible arterial puncture (ie, avoid internal jugular and subclavian venous punctures to minimize noncompressible site bleeding).

If serious bleeding (not controllable by local pressure) occurs, immediately terminate alteplase infusion and any concomitant heparin. Protamine can be given to reverse heparin effects.

In the following conditions, the risks of alteplase therapy may be increased and should be weighed against the anticipated benefits: recent major surgery (eg, coronary artery bypass graft, obstetrical delivery, organ biopsy, previous puncture of noncompressible vessels); cerebrovascular disease; recent GI or GU bleeding; recent trauma; hypertension: systolic BP 175 mm Hg or more or diastolic BP 110 mm Hg or more; likelihood of left heart thrombus (eg, mitral stenosis with atrial fibrillation); acute pericarditis; subacute bacterial endocarditis; hemostatic defects including those secondary to severe hepatic or renal disease; significant hepatic dysfunction; pregnancy; diabetic hemorrhagic retinopathy or other hemorrhagic ophthalmic conditions; septic thrombophlebitis or occluded AV cannula at seriously infected site; advanced age (eg, older than 75 years of age); patients currently receiving oral anticoagulants (eg, warfarin sodium); any other condition in which bleeding constitutes a significant hazard or would be particularly difficult to manage because of its location.

➤*Cholesterol embolism:* Cholesterol embolism has been reported rarely in patients treated with all thrombolytic agents; the incidence is unknown. This serious condition, which can be lethal, is associated with invasive vascular procedures (eg, cardiac catheterization, angiography, vascular surgery) or anticoagulant therapy. Clinical features of cholesterol embolism may include livedo reticularis, "purple toe" syndrome, acute renal failure, gangrenous digits, hypertension, pancreatitis, MI, cerebral infarction, spinal cord infarction, retinal artery occlusion, bowel infarction, and rhabdomyolysis.

➤*Arrhythmias:* Coronary thrombolysis may result in arrythmias associated with reperfusion. These arrhythmias (such as sinus bradycardia, accelerated idioventricular rhythm, ventricular premature depolarizations, ventricular tachycardia) are not different from those often seen in the ordinary course of AMI and may be managed with standard antiarrhythmic measures. Have antiarrhythmic therapy for bradycardia or ventricular irritability available when alteplase infusions are administered.

➤*PE:* The treatment of PE with alteplase has not been shown to constitute treatment of underlying deep vein thrombosis. Consider the possible risk of re-embolization caused by lysis of underlying deep venous thrombi.

➤*AMI:* In AMI patients who are at low risk of death from cardiac causes (ie, no previous myocardial infarction, Killip class I) and who have high blood pressure at the time of presentation, the risk for stroke may offset the survival benefit produced by thrombolytic therapy.

➤*AIS:* The risks of alteplase therapy to treat AIS may be increased in the following conditions and should be weighed against the anticipated benefits: Severe neurological deficit (eg, NIHSS greater than 22) at presentation (increases risk of ICH) and major early infarct signs on a CT scan (eg, substantial edema, mass effect, or midline shift).

In patients without recent use of oral anticoagulants or heparin, initiate alteplase treatment prior to the availability of coagulation study results. However, discontinue infusion if either a pretreatment PT longer than 15 seconds or an elevated aPTT is identified.

In AIS, neither the incidence of ICH nor the benefits of therapy are known in patients treated with alteplase more than 3 hours after the onset of symp-

ALTEPLASE, RECOMBINANT — INJECTION

toms. Therefore, do not treat patients with AIS more than 3 hours after symptom onset. Because of the increased risk for misdiagnosis of AIS, special diligence is required in making this diagnosis in patients whose blood glucose values are less than 50 mg/dL or greater than 400 mg/dL.

➤*Neurological deficit:* The safety and efficacy of treatment with alteplase in patients with minor neurological deficit or with rapidly improving symptoms prior to the start of alteplase administration has not been evaluated; therefore, treatment with alteplase is not recommended.

➤*Carcinogenesis:* Cytotoxicity, as reflected by a decrease in mitotic index, was evidenced only after prolonged exposure at high concentrations.

➤*Pregnancy: Category C.* Alteplase has been shown to have an embryocidal effect because of an increased postimplantation loss rate in rabbits when administered by IV at doses approximately 100 times (3 mg/kg) the human dose. There are no adequate and well-controlled studies in pregnant women. Use during pregnancy only if the potential benefit justifies the potential risk to the fetus.

➤*Lactation:* It is not known whether alteplase is excreted in human milk. Exercise caution when administering to nursing women.

➤*Children:* Safety and efficacy of alteplase in pediatric patients have not been established (*Activase*); safety and efficacy in patients younger than 2 years of age or who weigh less than 10 kg have not been established (*Cathflo Activase*).

Precautions

➤*Monitoring:* With coadministration of heparin or aspirin, monitor for bleeding especially at arterial puncture sites. Control and monitor blood pressure frequently during and following alteplase administration to manage AIS.

Heparin has been given with and after alteplase infusions to reduce risk of rethrombosis. Either heparin or alteplase may cause bleeding complications; carefully monitor for bleeding, especially at arterial puncture sites.

➤*Infection (Cathflo Activase* only): Use with caution in the presence of suspected infection in a catheter. Use during infection may release a localized infection into the systemic circulation.

➤*Hypersensitivity reaction:* There is no experience with readministration of alteplase. If an anaphylactoid reaction occurs, discontinue the infusion immediately and initiate appropriate therapy. Refer to Management of Acute Hypersensitivity Reactions.

Readministration – Sustained antibody formation in patients receiving 1 dose of alteplase has not been documented, but readminister with caution. Detectable antibody levels (single point measurement) were reported in 1 patient but subsequent antibody test results were negative.

➤*Lab test abnormalities:* During therapy, if coagulation tests or measures of fibrinolytic activity are performed, the results may be unreliable unless specific precautions are taken to prevent in vitro artifacts. Alteplase present in blood in pharmacologic concentrations remains active in vitro. This can lead to degradation of fibrinogen in blood samples removed for analysis. Collection of blood samples in the presence of aprotinin (150 to 200 units/mL) can, to some extent, mitigate this phenomenon.

Drug Interactions

➤*Anticoagulants:* A potential increased risk exists when alteplase is used concomitantly with heparin and vitamin K antagonists.

➤*Drugs affecting platelet function:* Drugs that alter platelet function (ie, aspirin, dipyridamole, and abciximab) may increase the risk of bleeding if administered prior to or after alteplase therapy.

➤*Nitroglycerin:* Concomitant use decreases alteplase concentrations, therefore decreasing thrombolytic effect. Avoid use of nitroglycerin with alteplase.

Adverse Reactions

Bleeding (most frequent) – Should serious bleeding in a critical location (intracranial, GI, retroperitoneal, pericardial) occur, immediately discontinue alteplase therapy along with any concomitant therapy with heparin.

Incidence of Significant Bleeding with Alteplase for 3-Hour Infusion Regimen

Site of bleeding	Total dose ≤ 100 mg/3 h
GI	5%
GU	4%
Ecchymosis	1%
Retroperitoneal	< 1%
Epistaxis	< 1%
Gingival	< 1%

The incidence of ICH in AMI patients treated with alteplase is as follows:

Incidence of Intracranial Bleeding in AMI Patients with Alteplase

Dose	Patients	%
100 mg, 3 hours	3,272	0.4
≤ 100 mg, accelerated	10,396	0.7
150 mg	1,779	1.3
1 to 1.4 mg/kg	237	0.4

Accelerated infusion – All strokes (1.6%); nonfatal stroke (0.9%); hemorrhagic stroke (0.7%). The incidence of all strokes, as well as that for hemorrhagic stroke, increased with increasing age.

Hypersensitivity – Allergic-type reactions (eg, anaphylactoid reaction, laryngeal edema, orolingual angioedema, rash, and urticaria) have been reported. Most reports were of patients treated for AIS and some from treatment for AMI. Many of these patients received concomitant angiotensin-converting enzyme inhibitors (ACEIs). Most cases resolved with prompt treatment.

Other adverse reactions (Activase only) –
AMI: Arrhythmia; AV block; cardiogenic shock; heart failure; cardiac arrest; recurrent ischemia; myocardial reinfarction; myocardial rupture; electromechanical dissociation; pericardial effusion; pericarditis; mitral regurgitation; cardiac tamponade; thromboembolism; pulmonary edema; nausea and/or vomiting; hypotension; fever.
PE: Pulmonary re-embolization; pulmonary edema; pleural effusion; thromboembolism; hypotension; fever.
AIS: Cerebral edema; cerebral herniation; seizure; new ischemic stroke.

Other adverse reactions (Cathflo Activase only) – GI bleeding; sepsis; venous thrombosis; death; major hemorrhage; ICH; pulmonary emboli; arterial emboli; injection-site hemorrhage; upper extremity deep venous thrombosis.

RETEPLASE, RECOMBINANT

Rx	**Retavase** (Centocor)	**Powder for injection, lyophilized:** 10.4 units (18.1 mg)	Preservative-free. In kits[a] and half-kits.[b]

[a] Each kit includes a package insert, 2 single-use reteplase vials of 10.4 units (18.1 mg), 2 single-use diluent vials for reconstitution (10 mL sterile water for injection), 2 sterile 10 mL syringes, 2 sterile dispensing pins, 4 sterile needles, and 2 alcohol swabs.

[b] Each half-kit includes a package insert, 1 single-use reteplase vial 10.4 units (18.1 mg), 1 single-use diluent vial for reconstitution (10 mL sterile water for injection), and a sterile dispensing pin.

RETEPLASE RECOMBINANT — INJECTION

Indications

➤*Acute myocardial infarction (AMI):* For use in the management of AMI in adults for the improvement of ventricular function following AMI, the reduction of the incidence of congestive heart failure and the reduction of mortality associated with AMI. Initiate treatment as soon as possible after the onset of AMI symptoms.

➤*Unlabeled uses:* For clearance of occluded venous catheters; thrombolytic treatment of acute and chronic deep venous thrombosis (DVT); treatment of massive pulmonary embolism with a double bolus; use in conjunction with heparin and percutaneous transluminal angioplasty (PTA) in the treatment of thrombosed polytetrafluoroethylene hemodialysis arteriovenous grafts (AVGs).

Administration and Dosage

➤*Approved by the FDA:* October 30, 1996.

➤*Dosage:* Reteplase is for IV administration only. Reteplase is administered as a 10 + 10 unit double-bolus injection. Two 10 unit bolus injections are required for a complete treatment. Administer each bolus as an IV injection over 2 minutes. Give the second bolus 30 minutes after initiation of the first bolus injection. Give each bolus injection via an IV line in which no other medication is being simultaneously injected or infused. No other medication should be added to the injection solution containing reteplase. There is no experience with patients receiving repeat courses of therapy with reteplase.

➤*Admixture incompatibility:* Heparin and reteplase are incompatible when combined in solution. Do not administer heparin and reteplase simultaneously in the same IV line. If reteplase is to be injected through an IV line containing heparin, flush a normal saline or 5% dextrose (D5W) solution through the line prior to and following the reteplase injection.

➤*Adjunctive therapy:* Although the value of anticoagulants and antiplatelet drugs during and following administration of reteplase has not been studied, heparin has been administered concomitantly in greater than 99% of patients. Aspirin has been given either during and/or following heparin treatment. Studies assessing the safety and efficacy of reteplase without adjunctive therapy with heparin and aspirin have not been performed.

➤*Reconstitution:* Reconstitute using the diluent and dispensing pin provided with reteplase. It is important that reteplase be reconstituted only with the supplied Sterile Water for Injection (without preservatives). The reconstituted preparation results in a colorless solution containing reteplase 1 unit/mL. Slight foaming upon reconstitution is not unusual; allowing the vial to stand undisturbed for several minutes is usually sufficient to allow dissipation of any large bubbles.

➤*Reconstitution instructions: Reteplase kit and reteplase half-kit:* Use aseptic technique throughout.

1.) Withdraw 10 mL of Sterile Water for Injection (SWFI) from the supplied vial into a sterile 10 mL syringe.
2.) Open the package containing the dispensing pin. Remove the protective cap from the luer lock port of the dispensing pin and connect the sterile 10 mL syringe to the dispensing pin. Remove the protective flip-cap from 1 vial of reteplase.

RETEPLASE RECOMBINANT — INJECTION

3.) Remove the protective cap from the spike end of the dispensing pin, and insert the spike into the vial of reteplase until the security clips lock onto the vial. Transfer the 10 mL of SWFI through the dispensing pin into the vial of reteplase.
4.) With the dispensing pin and syringe still attached to the vial, swirl the vial gently to dissolve the reteplase. Do not shake.
5.) Withdraw 10 mL of reteplase reconstituted solution back into the syringe. A small amount of solution will remain in the vial due to overfill.
6.) Detach the syringe from the dispensing pin, and attach a sterile needle.
7.) The 10 mL bolus dose is now ready for administration.

Safely discard all used reconstitution components and the empty reteplase vial according to institutional procedures.

➤*Storage/Stability:* Because reteplase contains no antibacterial preservatives, reconstitute it immediately before use. When reconstituted as directed, the solution may be used within 4 hours when stored at 2° to 30°C (36° to 86°F). Prior to administration, visually inspect the product for particulate matter and discoloration.

Store reteplase at 2° to 25°C (36° to 77°F). The box should remain sealed until use to protect the lyophilisate from exposure to light.

Actions

➤*Pharmacology:* Reteplase is a recombinant plasminogen activator which catalyzes the cleavage of endogenous plasminogen to generate plasmin. Plasmin in turn degrades the fibrin matrix of the thrombus, thereby exerting its thrombolytic action. In a controlled trial, 36 of 56 patients treated for an acute myocardial infarction (AMI) had a decrease in fibrinogen levels to below 100 mg/dL by 2 hours following the administration of reteplase as a double-bolus IV injection (10 + 10 unit) in which 10 unit (17.4 mg) was followed 30 minutes later by a second bolus of 10 unit (17.4 mg). The mean fibrinogen level returned to the baseline value by 48 hours.

➤*Pharmacokinetics:*

Metabolism/Excretion – Based on the measurement of thrombolytic activity, reteplase is cleared from plasma at a rate of 250 to 450 mL/min, with an effective half-life of 13 to 16 minutes. Reteplase is cleared primarily by the liver and kidney.

Contraindications

Active internal bleeding; history of cerebrovascular accident; recent intracranial or intraspinal surgery or trauma; intracranial neoplasm, arteriovenous malformation, or aneurysm; known bleeding diathesis; severe uncontrolled hypertension

Warnings

➤*Bleeding:* The most common complication encountered during reteplase therapy is bleeding. The sites of bleeding include both internal bleeding sites (intracranial, retroperitoneal, GI, GU, or respiratory) and superficial bleeding sites (venous cutdowns, arterial punctures, sites of recent surgical intervention). The concomitant use of heparin anticoagulation may contribute to bleeding. In clinical trials, some of the hemorrhage episodes occurred 1 or more days after the effects of reteplase had dissipated, but while heparin therapy was continuing.

Injection sites – As fibrin is lysed during reteplase therapy, bleeding from recent puncture sites may occur. Therefore, thrombolytic therapy requires careful attention to all potential bleeding sites (including catheter insertion sites, arterial and venous puncture sites, cutdown sites, and needle puncture sites). Noncompressible arterial puncture must be avoided and internal jugular and subclavian venous punctures should be avoided to minimize bleeding from noncompressible sites.

IM injections – Avoid IM injections and nonessential handling of the patient during treatment with reteplase. Perform venipunctures carefully and only as required.

High-risk conditions – Carefully evaluate each patient being considered for therapy with reteplase and weigh anticipated benefits against the potential risks associated with therapy. In the following conditions, the risks of reteplase therapy may be increased and should be weighed against the anticipated benefits: recent major surgery (eg, coronary artery bypass graft, obstetrical delivery, organ biopsy); previous puncture of noncompressible vessels; cerebrovascular disease; recent GI or GU bleeding; recent trauma; hypertension: systolic BP greater than or equal to 180 mm Hg and/or diastolic BP greater than or equal to 110 mm Hg; high likelihood of left heart thrombus (eg, mitral stenosis with atrial fibrillation); acute pericarditis; subacute bacterial endocarditis; hemostatic defects including those secondary to severe hepatic or renal disease; severe hepatic or renal dysfunction; pregnancy; diabetic hemorrhagic retinopathy or other hemorrhagic ophthalmic conditions; septic thrombophlebitis or occluded AV cannula at a seriously infected site; advanced age; patients currently receiving oral anticoagulants (eg, warfarin sodium); any other condition in which bleeding constitutes a significant hazard or would be particularly difficult to manage because of its location.

Should an arterial puncture be necessary during the administration of reteplase, it is preferable to use an upper extremity vessel that is accessible to manual compression. Apply pressure for at least 30 minutes, apply a pressure dressing, and frequently check the puncture site for evidence of bleeding.

Should serious bleeding (not controllable by local pressure) occur, immediately terminate concomitant anticoagulant therapy. In addition, do not give the second bolus of reteplase if serious bleeding occurs before it is administered.

➤*Cholesterol embolization:* Cholesterol embolism has been reported rarely in patients treated with thrombolytic agents; the true incidence is unknown. This serious condition, which can be lethal, is also associated with invasive vascular procedures (eg, cardiac catheterization, angiography, vascular surgery) and/or anticoagulant therapy. Clinical features of cholesterol embolism may include livedo reticularis, "purple toe" syndrome, acute renal failure, gangrenous digits, hypertension, pancreatitis, myocardial infarction, cerebral infarction, spinal cord infarction, retinal artery occlusion, bowel infarction, and rhabdomyolysis.

➤*Arrhythmias:* Coronary thrombolysis may result in arrhythmias associated with reperfusion. These arrhythmias (such as sinus bradycardia, accelerated idioventricular rhythm, ventricular premature depolarizations, ventricular tachycardia) are not different from those often seen in the ordinary course of AMI and should be managed with standard antiarrhythmic measures. Antiarrhythmic therapy for bradycardia and/or ventricular irritability should be available when reteplase is administered.

➤*Pregnancy: Category C.* Reteplase has been shown to have an abortifacient effect in rabbits when given in doses 3 times the human dose (0.86 unit/kg). Reproduction studies performed in rats at doses less than or equal to 15 times the human dose (4.31 unit/kg) revealed no evidence of fetal anomalies; however, reteplase administered to pregnant rabbits resulted in hemorrhaging in the genital tract, leading to abortions in mid-gestation. There are no adequate and well-controlled studies in pregnant women. The most common complication of thrombolytic therapy is bleeding, and certain conditions, including pregnancy, can increase this risk. Use reteplase during pregnancy only if the potential benefit justifies the potential risk to the fetus.

➤*Lactation:* It is not known whether reteplase is excreted in human milk. Because many drugs are excreted in human milk, exercise caution when reteplase is administered to a nursing woman.

➤*Children:* Safety and efficacy of reteplase in children have not been established.

Precautions

➤*Monitoring:* Because heparin, aspirin, or reteplase may cause bleeding complications, careful monitoring for bleeding is advised, especially at arterial puncture sites.

➤*General:* Implement standard management of MI concomitantly with reteplase treatment. Minimized arterial and venous punctures. In addition, do not give the second bolus of reteplase if the serious bleeding occurs before it is administered. In the event of serious bleeding, terminate any concomitant heparin immediately. Heparin effects can be reversed by protamine.

➤*Readministration:* There is no experience with patients receiving repeat courses of therapy with reteplase. Reteplase did not induce the formation of reteplase specific antibodies in any of the approximately 2,400 patients who were tested for antibody formation in clinical trials. If an anaphylactoid reaction occurs, do not give the second bolus of reteplase, and initiate appropriate therapy.

Drug Interactions

The interaction of reteplase with other cardioactive drugs has not been studied. In addition to bleeding associated with heparin and vitamin K antagonists, drugs that alter platelet function (such as aspirin, dipyridamole, and abciximab) may increase the risk of bleeding if administered prior to or after reteplase therapy.

➤*Use of antithrombotics:* Heparin and aspirin have been administered concomitantly with and following the administration of reteplase in the management of AMI. Because heparin, aspirin, or reteplase may cause bleeding complications, careful monitoring for bleeding is advised, especially at arterial puncture sites.

➤*Drug/Lab test interactions:* Administration of reteplase may cause decreases in plasminogen and fibrinogen. During reteplase therapy, if coagulation tests and/or measurements of fibrinolytic activity are performed, the results may be unreliable unless specific precautions are taken to prevent in vitro artifacts. Reteplase is an enzyme that when present in blood in pharmacologic concentrations remains active under in vitro conditions. This can lead to degradation of fibrinogen in blood samples removed for analysis. Collection of blood samples in the presence of PPACK (chloromethylketone) at 2 mm concentrations was used in clinical trials to prevent in vitro fibrinolytic artifacts.

Adverse Reactions

➤*Bleeding:* The most frequent adverse reaction associated with reteplase is bleeding. The types of bleeding events associated with thrombolytic therapy may be broadly categorized as either intracranial hemorrhage or other types of hemorrhage.

- Intracranial hemorrhage. In the INJECT clinical trial the rate of in-hospital, intracranial hemorrhage among all patients treated with reteplase was 0.8% (23 of 2,965 patients). As seen with reteplase and other thrombolytic agents, the risk for intracranial hemorrhage is increased in patients with advanced age or with elevated blood pressure.
- Other types of hemorrhage. The incidence of other types of bleeding events in clinical studies of reteplase varied depending upon the use of arterial catheterization or other invasive procedures and whether the study was performed in Europe or the USA. The overall incidence of any bleeding event in patients treated with reteplase in clinical studies (n = 3,805) was 21.1%. The rates for bleeding events, regardless of severity, for the 10 + 10 unit reteplase regimen from controlled clinical studies are summarized in the following table.

RETEPLASE RECOMBINANT — INJECTION

➤*Reteplase hemorrhage rates:*

Reteplase, Recombinant Hemorrhage Rates			
	INJECT	RAPID 1 and RAPID 2	
Bleeding site	Europe (n = 2,965)	US (n = 210)	Europe (n = 113)
Anemia, site unknown	2.6%	1.4%	0.9%
GI	2.5%	9%	1.8%
GU	1.6%	9.5%	0.9%
Injection site[a]	4.6%	48.6%	19.5%

[a] Includes the arterial catheterization site (all patients in the RAPID studies underwent arterial catheterization). In these studies the severity and sites of bleeding events were comparable for reteplase and the comparison thrombolytic agents.

Should serious bleeding in a critical location (intracranial, GI, retroperitoneal, pericardial) occur, immediately terminate any concomitant heparin. In addition, do not give the second bolus of reteplase if the serious bleeding occurs before it is administered. Death and permanent disability are not uncommonly reported in patients who have experienced stroke (including intracranial bleeding) and other serious bleeding episodes.

Fibrin which is part of the hemostatic plug formed at needle puncture sites will be lysed during reteplase therapy. Therefore, reteplase therapy requires careful attention to potential bleeding sites (eg, catheter insertion sites, arterial puncture sites).

➤*Allergic:* Among the 2,965 patients receiving reteplase in the INJECT trial, serious allergic reactions were noted in 3 patients, with 1 patient experiencing dyspnea and hypotension. No anaphylactoid reactions were observed among the 3,856 patients treated with reteplase in initial clinical trials. In an ongoing clinical trial 2 anaphylactoid reactions have been reported among approximately 2,500 patients receiving reteplase.

➤*Miscellaneous:* Patients administered reteplase as treatment for MI have experienced many events which are frequent sequelae of myocardial infarction and may or may not be attributable to reteplase therapy. These events include cardiogenic shock, arrhythmias (eg, sinus bradycardia, accelerated idioventricular rhythm, ventricular premature depolarizations, supraventricular tachycardia, ventricular tachycardia, ventricular fibrillation), AV block, pulmonary edema, heart failure, cardiac arrest, recurrent ischemia, reinfarction, myocardial rupture, mitral regurgitation, pericardial effusion, pericarditis, cardiac tamponade, venous thrombosis and embolism, and electromechanical dissociation. These events can be life-threatening and may lead to death. Other adverse events have been reported, including nausea and/or vomiting, hypotension, and fever.

TENECTEPLASE

Rx	**TNKase** (Genentech)	**Powder for Injection, lyophilized:** 50 mg	In vials[a] with one 10 mL vial of sterile water for injection and syringe.

[a] With 0.55 g L-arginine, 0.17 g phosphoric acid, 4.3 mg polysorbate 20.

TENECTEPLASE — INJECTION

Indications

➤*Acute myocardial infarction (AMI):* For use in the reduction of mortality associated with AMI. Treatment should be initiated as soon as possible after the onset of AMI symptoms.

Administration and Dosage

➤*Approved by the FDA:* June 2, 2000.

➤*Dosage:* Tenecteplase is for intravenous administration only. The recommended total dose should not exceed 50 mg and is based upon patient weight.

A single bolus dose should be administered over 5 seconds based on patient weight. Treatment should be initiated as soon as possible after the onset of AMI symptoms.

Tenecteplase Dose Information		
Patient weight (kg)	Tenecteplase (mg)	Volume tenecteplase[a] to be administered (mL)
< 60	30	6
≥ 60 to < 70	35	7
≥ 70 to < 80	40	8
≥ 80 to < 90	45	9
≥ 90	50	10

[a] From 1 vial of tenecteplase reconstituted with 10 mL of sterile water for injection.

The safety and efficacy of tenecteplase has only been investigated with concomitant administration of heparin and aspirin.

➤*Reconstitution:* Because tenecteplase contains no antibacterial preservatives, it should be reconstituted immediately before use. If the reconstituted tenecteplase is not used immediately, refrigerate the tenecteplase vial at 2° to 8°C (36° to 46°F) and use within 8 hours.

Read all instructions completely before beginning reconstitution and administration.

1.) Remove the shield assembly from the supplied *B-D* 10 cc syringe with *TwinPak* Dual Cannula Device (see figure) and aseptically withdraw 10 mL of Sterile Water for Injection (SWFI), USP, from the supplied diluent vial using the red hub cannula syringe filling device. Do not use Bacteriostatic Water for Injection, USP. Note: Do not discard the shield assembly.
2.) Inject the entire contents of the syringe (10 mL) into the tenecteplase vial directing the diluent stream into the powder. Slight foaming upon reconstitution is not unusual; any large bubbles will dissipate if the product is allowed to stand undisturbed for several minutes.
3.) Gently swirl until contents are completely dissolved. Do not shake. The reconstituted preparation results in a colorless to pale yellow transparent solution containing tenecteplase at 5 mg/mL at a pH of approximately 7.3. The osmolality of this solution is approximately 290 mOsm/kg.
4.) Determine the appropriate dose of tenecteplase (see Dosage) and withdraw this volume (in milliliters) from the reconstituted vial with the syringe. Any unused solution should be discarded.
5.) Once the appropriate dose of tenecteplase is drawn into the syringe, stand the shield vertically on a flat surface (with green side down) and passively recap the red hub cannula.
6.) Remove the entire shield assembly, including the red hub cannula, by twisting counter clockwise. Note: The shield assembly also contains the clear-ended blunt plastic cannula; retain for split septum IV access.

➤*Administration:* The product should be visually inspected prior to administration for particulate matter and discoloration. Tenecteplase may be administered as reconstituted at 5 mg/mL.

Reconstituted tenecteplase should be administered as a single IV bolus over 5 seconds.

Although the supplied syringe is compatible with a conventional needle, this syringe is designed to be used with needleless IV systems. From the information below, follow the instructions applicable to the IV system in use.

- Split septum IV system: Remove the green cap. Attach the clear-ended blunt plastic cannula to the syringe. Remove the shield and use the blunt plastic cannula to access the split septum injection port. Because the blunt plastic cannula has two side ports, air or fluid expelled through the cannula will exit in two sideways directions; direct away from face or mucous membranes.
- *Luer-Lok* system: Connect syringe directly to IV port.
- Conventional needle (not supplied in this kit): Attach a large bore needle, eg, 18 gauge, to the syringe's universal *Luer-Lok*.

Dispose of the syringe, cannula, and shield per established procedures.

➤*Compatibility:* Precipitation may occur when tenecteplase is administered in an IV line containing dextrose. Dextrose-containing lines should be flushed with a saline-containing solution prior to and following single bolus administration of tenecteplase.

➤*Storage/Stability:* Store lyophilized tenecteplase at controlled room temperature not to exceed 30°C (86°F) or under refrigeration 2° to 8°C (36° to 46°F). Do not use beyond the expiration date stamped on the vial.

Actions

➤*Pharmacology:* Tenecteplase is a modified form of human tissue plasminogen activator (tPA) that binds to fibrin and converts plasminogen to plasmin. In the presence of fibrin, in vitro studies demonstrate that tenecteplase conversion of plasminogen to plasmin is increased relative to its conversion in the absence of fibrin. This fibrin specificity decreases systemic activation of plasminogen and the resulting degradation of circulating fibrinogen as compared to a molecule lacking this property. Following administration of 30, 40, or 50 mg of tenecteplase, there are decreases in circulating fibrinogen (4% to 15%) and plasminogen (11% to 24%). The clinical significance of fibrin-specificity on safety (eg, bleeding) or efficacy has not been established. Biological potency is determined by an in vitro clot lysis assay and is expressed in tenecteplase-specific units. The specific activity of tenecteplase has been defined as 200 units/mg.

➤*Pharmacokinetics:* In patients with acute myocardial infarction (AMI), tenecteplase administered as a single bolus exhibits a biphasic disposition from the plasma. Tenecteplase was cleared from the plasma with an initial half-life of 20 to 24 minutes. The terminal phase half-life of tenecteplase was 90 to 130 minutes. In 99 of 104 patients treated with tenecteplase, mean plasma clearance ranged from 99 to 119 mL/min.

The initial volume of distribution is weight related and approximates plasma volume. Liver metabolism is the major clearance mechanism for tenecteplase.

TENECTEPLASE — INJECTION

Contraindications

Tenecteplase therapy in patients with acute myocardial infarction is contraindicated in the following situations because of an increased risk of bleeding (see Warnings): active internal bleeding; history of cerebrovascular accident; intracranial or intraspinal surgery or trauma within 2 months; intracranial neoplasm, arteriovenous malformation, or aneurysm; known bleeding diathesis; severe uncontrolled hypertension.

Warnings

➤*Bleeding:* The most common complication encountered during tenecteplase therapy is bleeding. The type of bleeding associated with thrombolytic therapy can be divided into two broad categories:

- Internal bleeding, involving intracranial and retroperitoneal sites, or the gastrointestinal, genitourinary, or respiratory tracts.
- Superficial or surface bleeding, observed mainly at vascular puncture and access sites (eg, venous cutdowns, arterial punctures) or sites of recent surgical intervention.

Should serious bleeding (not controlled by local pressure) occur, any concomitant heparin or antiplatelet agents should be discontinued immediately.

In clinical studies of tenecteplase, patients were treated with both aspirin and heparin. Heparin may contribute to the bleeding risks associated with tenecteplase. The safety of the use of tenecteplase with other antiplatelet agents has not been adequately studied (see Drug Interactions). Intramuscular injections and nonessential handling of the patient should be avoided for the first few hours following treatment with tenecteplase. Venipunctures should be performed and monitored carefully.

Should an arterial puncture be necessary during the first few hours following tenecteplase therapy, it is preferable to use an upper extremity vessel that is accessible to manual compression. Pressure should be applied for at least 30 minutes, a pressure dressing applied, and the puncture site checked frequently for evidence of bleeding.

High-risk patients – Each patient being considered for therapy with tenecteplase should be carefully evaluated and anticipated benefits weighed against potential risks associated with therapy. In the following conditions, the risk of tenecteplase therapy may be increased and should be weighed against the anticipated benefits:

- Recent major surgery, eg, coronary artery bypass graft, obstetrical delivery, organ biopsy, previous puncture of noncompressible vessels
- Cerebrovascular disease
- Recent gastrointestinal or genitourinary bleeding
- Recent trauma
- Hypertension: Systolic BP at least 180 mmHg and/or diastolic BP at least 110 mmHg
- High likelihood of left heart thrombus (eg, mitral stenosis with atrial fibrillation)
- Acute pericarditis
- Subacute bacterial endocarditis
- Hemostatic defects, including those secondary to severe hepatic or renal disease
- Severe hepatic dysfunction
- Pregnancy
- Diabetic hemorrhagic retinopathy or other hemorrhagic ophthalmic conditions
- Septic thrombophlebitis or occluded AV cannula at seriously infected site
- Advanced age (see Warnings, Elderly)
- Patients currently receiving oral anticoagulants (eg, warfarin sodium)
- Recent administration of GP IIb/IIIa inhibitors
- Any other condition in which bleeding constitutes a significant hazard or would be particularly difficult to manage because of its location

➤*Cholesterol embolization:* Cholesterol embolism has been reported rarely in patients treated with all types of thrombolytic agents; the true incidence is unknown. This serious condition, which can be lethal, is also associated with invasive vascular procedures (eg, cardiac catheterization, angiography, vascular surgery) and/or anticoagulant therapy. Clinical features of cholesterol embolism may include livedo reticularis, "purple toe" syndrome, acute renal failure, gangrenous digits, hypertension, pancreatitis, myocardial infarction, cerebral infarction, spinal cord infarction, retinal artery occlusion, bowel infarction, and rhabdomyolysis.

➤*Arrhythmias:* Coronary thrombolysis may result in arrhythmias associated with reperfusion. These arrhythmias (such as sinus bradycardia, accelerated idioventricular rhythm, ventricular premature depolarizations, ventricular tachycardia) are not different from those often seen in the ordinary course of acute myocardial infarction and may be managed with standard antiarrhythmic measures. It is recommended that antiarrhythmic therapy for bradycardia and/or ventricular irritability be available when tenecteplase is administered.

➤*Elderly:* Of the patients in ASSENT-2 who received tenecteplase, 4,958 (59%) were under the age of 65; 2256 (27%) were between the ages of 65 and 74; and 1244 (15%) were 75 and over. The 30-day mortality rates by age were 2.5% in patients under the age of 65, 8.5% in patients between the ages of 65 and 74, and 16.2% in patients age 75 and over. The ICH rates were 0.4% in patients under the age of 65, 1.6% in patients between the ages of 65 and 74, and 1.7% in patients age 75 and over. The rates of any stroke were 1% in patients under the age of 65, 2.9% in patients between the ages of 65 and 74, and 3% in patients age 75 and over. Major bleeding rates, defined as bleeding requiring blood transfusion or leading to hemodynamic compromise, were 3.1% in patients under the age of 65, 6.4% in patients between the ages of 65 and 74, and 7.7% in patients age 75 and over. In elderly patients, the benefits of tenecteplase on mortality should be carefully weighed against the risk of increased adverse events, including bleeding.

➤*Pregnancy: Category C.* Tenecteplase has been shown to elicit maternal and embryo toxicity in rabbits given multiple IV administrations. In rabbits administered 0.5, 1.5, and 5 mg/kg/day, vaginal hemorrhage resulted in maternal deaths. Subsequent embryonic deaths were secondary to maternal hemorrhage and no fetal anomalies were observed. Tenecteplase does not elicit maternal and embryo toxicity in rabbits following a single IV administration. Thus, in developmental toxicity studies conducted in rabbits, the no observable effect level (NOEL) of a single IV administration of tenecteplase on maternal or developmental toxicity was 5 mg/kg (approximately 8 to 10 times the human dose). There are no adequate and well-controlled studies in pregnant women. Tenecteplase should be given to pregnant women only if the potential benefits justify the potential risk to the fetus.

➤*Lactation:* It is not known if tenecteplase is excreted in human milk. Because many drugs are excreted in human milk, caution should be exercised when tenecteplase is administered to a breast-feeding woman.

➤*Children:* The safety and efficacy of tenecteplase in pediatric patients have not been established.

Precautions

➤*General information:* Standard management of myocardial infarction should be implemented concomitantly with tenecteplase treatment. Arterial and venous punctures should be minimized. Noncompressible arterial puncture must be avoided and internal jugular and subclavian venous punctures should be avoided to minimize bleeding from the noncompressible sites. In the event of serious bleeding, heparin and antiplatelet agents should be discontinued immediately. Heparin effects can be reversed by protamine.

➤*Readministration:* Readministration of plasminogen activators, including tenecteplase, to patients who have received prior plasminogen activator therapy has not been systematically studied. Three of 487 patients tested for antibody formation to tenecteplase had a positive antibody titer at 30 days. The data reflect the percentage of patients whose test results were considered positive for antibodies to tenecteplase in a radioimmunoprecipitation assay, and are highly dependent on the sensitivity and specificity of the assay. Additionally, the observed incidence of antibody positivity in an assay may be influenced by several factors including sample handling, concomitant medications, and underlying disease. For these reasons, comparison of the incidence of antibodies to tenecteplase with the incidence of antibodies to other products may be misleading. Although sustained antibody formation in patients receiving one dose of tenecteplase has not been documented, readministration should be undertaken with caution. If an anaphylactic reaction occurs, appropriate therapy should be administered.

Drug Interactions

Formal interaction studies of tenecteplase with other drugs have not been performed. Patients studied in clinical trials of tenecteplase were routinely treated with heparin and aspirin. Anticoagulants (such as heparin and vitamin K antagonists) and drugs that alter platelet function (such as acetylsalicylic acid, dipyridamole, and GP IIb/IIIa inhibitors) may increase the risk of bleeding if administered prior to, during, or after tenecteplase therapy.

➤*Drug/Lab test interactions:* During tenecteplase therapy, results of coagulation tests and/or measures of fibrinolytic activity may be unreliable unless specific precautions are taken to prevent in vitro artifacts. Tenecteplase is an enzyme that, when present in blood in pharmacologic concentrations, remains active under in vitro conditions. This can lead to degradation of fibrinogen in blood samples removed for analysis.

Adverse Reactions

➤*Allergic:* Allergic-type reactions (eg, anaphylaxis, angioedema, laryngeal edema, rash, urticaria) have rarely (less than 1%) been reported in patients treated with tenecteplase. Anaphylaxis was reported in less than 0.1% of patients treated with tenecteplase; however, causality was not established. When such reactions occur, they usually respond to conventional therapy.

➤*Hematologic:* The most frequent adverse reaction associated with tenecteplase is bleeding (see Warnings).

Should serious bleeding occur, concomitant heparin and antiplatelet therapy should be discontinued. Death or permanent disability can occur in patients who experience stroke or serious bleeding episodes.

For tenecteplase-treated patients in ASSENT-2, the incidence of intracranial hemorrhage was 0.9% and any stroke was 1.8%. The incidence of all strokes, including intracranial bleeding, increases with increasing age (see Warnings).

ASSENT-2 Non-ICH Bleeding Events

	Tenecteplase (n = 8,461)	Accelerated activase (n = 8,488)	Relative risk tenecteplase/activase (95% CI)
Major bleeding[a]	4.7%	5.9%	0.78 (0.69, 0.89)
Minor bleeding	21.8%	23%	0.94 (0.89, 1)

Tissue Plasminogen Activators

TENECTEPLASE — INJECTION

ASSENT-2 Non-ICH Bleeding Events			
	Tenecteplase (n = 8,461)	Accelerated activase (n = 8,488)	Relative risk tenecteplase/activase (95% CI)
Units of transfused blood			
Any	4.3%	5.5%	0.77 (0.67, 0.89)
1 to 2	2.6%	3.2%	
> 2	1.7%	2.2%	

[a] Major bleeding is defined as bleeding requiring blood transfusion or leading to hemodynamic compromise.

Nonintracranial major bleeding and the need for blood transfusions were lower in patients treated with tenecteplase.

Types of major bleeding reported in 1% or more of the patients were hematoma (1.7%) and gastrointestinal tract (1%). Types of major bleeding reported in less than 1% of the patients were urinary tract, puncture site (including cardiac catheterization site), retroperitoneal, respiratory tract, and unspecified. Types of minor bleeding reported in 1% or more of the patients were hematoma (12.3%), urinary tract (3.7%), puncture site (including cardiac catheterization site) (3.6%), pharyngeal (3.1%), GI tract (1.9%), epistaxis (1.5%), and unspecified (1.3%).

➤*Miscellaneous:* The following adverse reactions have been reported among patients receiving tenecteplase in clinical trials. These reactions are frequent sequelae of the underlying disease, and the effect of tenecteplase on the incidence of these events is unknown.

These events include cardiogenic shock, arrhythmias, atrioventricular block, pulmonary edema, heart failure, cardiac arrest, recurrent myocardial ischemia, myocardial reinfarction, myocardial rupture, cardiac tamponade, pericarditis, pericardial effusion, mitral regurgitation, thrombosis, embolism, and electromechanical dissociation. These events can be life-threatening and may lead to death. Nausea and/or vomiting, hypotension, and fever have also been reported.

Recombinant Human Activated Protein C

DROTRECOGIN ALFA (ACTIVATED)

Rx	**Xigris** (Eli Lilly)	**Powder for injection, lyophilized:** 5 mg	Preservative-free. Sodium chloride 40.3 mg, sucrose. In single-use vials.
		20 mg	Preservative-free. Sodium chloride 158.1 mg, sucrose. In single-use vials.

DROTRECOGIN ALFA (ACTIVATED) — INJECTION

Indications

➤*Sepsis:* For the reduction of mortality in adult patients with severe sepsis (sepsis associated with acute organ dysfunction) who have a high risk of death (eg, as determined by the APACHE II score).

Safety and efficacy have not been established in adult patients with severe sepsis and lower risk of death. Safety and efficacy have not been established in pediatric patients with severe sepsis.

Administration and Dosage

➤*Approved by the FDA:* November 21, 2001.

Administer drotrecogin alfa intravenously (IV) at an infusion rate of 24 mcg/kg/h (based on actual body weight) for a total duration of infusion of 96 hours. Dose adjustment based on clinical or laboratory parameters is not recommended.

If the infusion is interrupted, restart drotrecogin alfa at the 24 mcg/kg/h infusion rate. Dose escalation or bolus doses of drotrecogin alfa are not recommended.

In the event of clinically important bleeding, immediately stop the infusion.

➤*Preparation and administration:*

1.) Use appropriate aseptic technique during the preparation of drotrecogin alfa for IV administration.
2.) Calculate the approximate amount of drotrecogin alfa needed based upon the patient's actual body weight and duration of this infusion period. The maximum duration of infusion from one preparation step is 12 hours. Multiple infusion periods will be needed to cover the entire 96-hour duration of administration.

mg of drotrecogin alfa = (patient weight, kg) × 24 mcg/kg/h × (hours of infusion) ÷ 1,000 Round the actual drotrecogin alfa to be prepared to the nearest 5 mg increment to avoid discarding reconstituted drotrecogin alfa.

3.) Determine the number of vials of drotrecogin alfa needed to make up this amount.
4.) Reconstitute each vial of drotrecogin alfa with sterile water for injection. The 5 mg vials must be reconstituted with 2.5 mL; the 20 mg vials with 10 mL. Slowly add the sterile water for injection to the vial and avoid inverting or shaking the vial. Gently swirl each vial until the powder is completely dissolved. The resulting drotrecogin alfa concentration of the solution is 2 mg/mL.
5.) Drotrecogin alfa contains no antibacterial preservatives; immediately prepare the IV solution after reconstitution of the drotrecogin alfa in the vial(s). If the reconstituted vial is not used immediately, it may be stored at controlled room temperature 20° to 25°C (68° to 77°F), but must be used within 3 hours.
6.) Inspect the reconstituted drotrecogin alfa for particulate matter and discoloration before further dilution. Do not use vials if particulate matter is visible or solution is discolored.
7.) Administer drotrecogin alfa via a dedicated IV line or a dedicated lumen of a multilumen central venous catheter. The only other solutions that can be administered through the same line are 0.9% sodium chloride injection, Ringer's lactate injection, dextrose injection, and dextrose and sodium chloride injection.
8.) Avoid exposing drotrecogin alfa solutions to heat and/or direct sunlight. Studies conducted at the recommended concentrations indicate the drotrecogin alfa IV solution to be compatible with glass infusion bottles, and infusion bags and syringes made of polyvinylchloride, polyethylene, polypropylene, or polyolefin.

➤*Dilution and administration for an IV infusion pump:*

1.) Complete preparation and administration steps 1 through 8, then complete the next 6 steps.
2.) The solution of reconstituted drotrecogin alfa must be further diluted into an infusion bag containing 0.9% sodium chloride injection to a final concentration between 0.1 and 0.2 mg/mL. Bag volumes between 50 and 250 mL are typical.
3.) Confirm that the intended bag volume will result in an acceptable final concentration.

Final concentration, mg/mL = (actual drotrecogin alfa amount, mg) ÷ (bag volume, mL) If the calculated final concentration is not between 0.1 and 0.2 mg/mL, select a different bag volume and recalculate the final concentration.

4.) Slowly withdraw the reconstituted drotrecogin alfa solution from the vial(s) and add the reconstituted drotrecogin alfa into the infusion bag of 0.9% sodium chloride injection. When injecting the drotrecogin alfa into the infusion bag, direct the stream to the side of the bag to minimize the agitation of the solution. Gently invert the infusion bag to obtain a homogeneous solution. Do not transport the infusion bag using mechanical transport systems, such as pneumatic-tube systems, that may cause vigorous agitation of the solution.
5.) Calculate the actual duration of the infusion period for the diluted drotrecogin alfa.

Infusion period, hours = (actual drotrecogin alfa amount, mg) × 1,000 ÷ (patient weight, kg) ÷ 24 mcg/kg/h

6.) Account for the added volume of reconstituted drotrecogin alfa (0.5 mL per mg drotrecogin alfa used) and the volume of bag solution removed (if saline solution is removed prior to adding the reconstitute drotrecogin alfa).

Final bag volume, mL = starting bag volume, mL + reconstituted drotrecogin alfa volume, mL − saline volume removed (if any), mL Calculate the actual infusion rate of the diluted drotrecogin alfa.

Infusion rate, mL/h = final bag volume, mL ÷ infusion period, hours

7.) After preparation for an IV infusion pump, use the IV solution at controlled room temperature 20° to 25°C (68° to 77°F) within 14 hours. If the IV solution is not administered immediately, the solution may be stored refrigerated 2° to 8°C (36° to 46°F) for up to 12 hours. If the prepared solution is refrigerated prior to administration, the maximum time limit for use of the IV solution, including preparation, refrigeration, and administration, is 24 hours.

➤*Dilution and administration for a syringe pump:*

1.) Complete preparation and administration steps 1 through 8, then complete the next 7 steps.
2.) The solution of reconstituted drotrecogin alfa must be further diluted with 0.9% sodium chloride injection to a final concentration between 0.1 and 1 mg/mL.
3.) Confirm that the intended volume will result in an acceptable final concentration.

Final concentration, mg/mL = (actual drotrecogin alfa amount, mg) ÷ (solution volume, mL) If the calculated final concentration is not between 0.1 and 1 mg/mL select a different bag volume and recalculate the final concentration.

DROTRECOGIN ALFA (ACTIVATED) — INJECTION

4.) Slowly withdraw the reconstituted drotrecogin alfa solution from the vial(s) into a syringe that will be used in the syringe pump. Into the same syringe, slowly withdraw 0.9% sodium chloride injection to obtain the desired final volume of diluted drotrecogin alfa. Gently invert or rotate the syringe to obtain a homogenous solution.
5.) Calculate the actual duration of the infusion period for the diluted drotrecogin alfa.

Infusion period, hours = (actual drotrecogin alfa amount, mg) × 1,000 ÷ (patient weight, kg) ÷ 24 mcg/kg/h

6.) Calculate the actual infusion rate of the diluted drotrecogin alfa.

Infusion rate, mL/h = solution volume, mL ÷ infusion period, hours

7.) When administering drotrecogin alfa using a syringe pump at low concentrations (less than approximately 0.2 mg/mL) at low flow rates (less than approximately 5 mL/h), the infusion set must be primed for approximately 15 minutes at a flow rate of approximately 5 mL/h.
8.) After preparation for a syringe pump, the IV solution should be used at controlled room temperature 20° to 25°C (68° to 77°F) within 12 hours. The maximum time limit for use of the IV solution, including preparation and administration, is 12 hours.

➤*Storage/Stability:* Store drotrecogin alfa in a refrigerator 2° to 8°C (36° to 46°F). Do not freeze. Protect unreconstituted vials of drotrecogin alfa from light. Retain in carton until time of use.

If the reconstituted vial is not used immediately, it may be stored at controlled room temperature 20° to 25°C (68° to 77°F), but must be used within 3 hours.

After preparation for an IV infusion pump, use the IV solution at controlled room temperature 20° to 25°C (68° to 77°F) within 14 hours. If the IV solution is not administered immediately, the solution may be stored refrigerated 2° to 8°C (36° to 46°F) for up to 12 hours. If the prepared solution is refrigerated prior to administration, the maximum time limit for use of the IV solution, including preparation, refrigeration, and administration, is 24 hours.

After preparation for a syringe pump, the IV solution should be used at controlled room temperature 20° to 25°C (68° to 77°F) within 12 hours. The maximum time limit for use of the IV solution, including preparation and administration, is 12 hours.

Actions

➤*Pharmacology:* Activated protein C exerts an antithrombotic effect by inhibiting Factors VA and VIIIa. In vitro data indicate that activated protein C has indirect profibrinolysic activity through its ability to inhibit plasminogen activator inhibitor-1 (PAI-1) and limiting generation of activated thrombin-activatable-fibrinolysis-inhibitor. Additionally, in vitro data indicate that activated protein C may exert an anti-inflammatory effect by inhibiting human tumor necrosis factor production by monocytes, blocking leukocyte adhesion to selectins, and by limiting the thrombin-induced inflammatory responses within the microvascular endothelium.

Pharmacodynamics – The specific mechanisms by which drotrecogin alfa exerts its effect on survival in patients with severe sepsis are not completely understood. In patients with severe sepsis, drotrecogin alfa infusions of 48 or 96 hours produced dose-dependent declines in D-dimer and IL-6. Compared with placebo, drotrecogin alfa-treated patients experienced more rapid declines in D-dimer, PAI-1 levels, thrombin-antithrombin levels, prothrombin F1.2, IL-6, more rapid increases in protein C and antithrombin levels, and normalization of plasminogen. As assessed by infusion duration, the maximum observed pharmacodynamic effect of drotrecogin alfa on D-dimer levels occurred at the end of 96 hours of infusion for the 24 mcg/kg/h treatment group.

➤*Pharmacokinetics:*

Absorption/Distribution – Drotrecogin alfa and endogenous activated protein C are inactivated by endogenous plasma protease inhibitors. Plasma concentrations of endogenous activated protein C in healthy subjects and patients with severe sepsis are usually below detection limits. The median C_{ss} of 45 ng/mL (interquartile range, 35 to 62 ng/mL) was attained within 2 hours after starting infusion. In the majority of patients, plasma concentrations of drotrecogin alfa fell below the assay's quantitation limit of 10 ng/mL within 2 hours after stopping infusion.

In patients with severe sepsis, drotrecogin alfa infusions of 12 to 30 mcg/kg/h rapidly produce steady-state concentrations (C_{ss}) that are proportional to infusion rates.

Metabolism/Excretion – In a phase 3 trial, median clearance of drotrecogin alfa was 40 L/h (interquartile range, 27 to 52 L/h). Plasma clearance of drotrecogin alfa in patients with severe sepsis is approximately 50% higher than that in healthy subjects.

Special populations –

Severe sepsis: In adult patients with severe sepsis, small differences were detected in the plasma clearance of drotrecogin alfa with regard to age, gender, hepatic dysfunction, or renal dysfunction. Dose adjustment is not required based on these factors alone or in combination.

End-stage renal disease: Patients with end-stage renal disease requiring chronic renal replacement therapy were excluded from the phase 3 study. In patients without sepsis undergoing hemodialysis (n = 6), plasma clearance (mean ± SD) of drotrecogin alfa administered on nondialysis days was 30 ± 8 L/h. Plasma clearance of drotrecogin alfa was 23 ± 4 L/h in patients without sepsis undergoing peritoneal dialysis (n = 5). These clearance rates did not meaningfully differ from those in healthy subjects (28 ± 9 L/h) (n = 190).

Contraindications

Hypersensitivity to drotrecogin alfa or any component of this product. Drotrecogin alfa increases the risk of bleeding. Drotrecogin alfa is contraindicated in patients with the following clinical situations in which bleeding could be associated with a high risk of death or significant morbidity: active internal bleeding; recent (within 3 months) hemorrhagic stroke; recent (within 2 months) intracranial or intraspinal surgery, or severe head trauma; trauma with an increased risk of life-threatening bleeding; presence of an epidural catheter; intracranial neoplasm or mass lesion or evidence of cerebral herniation.

Warnings

➤*Single organ dysfunction and recent surgery:* Among the small number of patients enrolled in PROWESS with single organ dysfunction and recent surgery (surgery within 30 days prior to study treatment), all-cause mortality was numerically higher in the drotrecogin alfa group (28-day: 10/49; in-hospital: 14/48) compared with the placebo group (28-day: 8/49; in-hospital: 8/47).

In a preliminary analysis of the subset of patients with single organ dysfunction and recent surgery from a separate, randomized, placebo-controlled study (ADDRESS) of septic patients at lower risk of death (APACHE II score less than 25 or single sepsis-induced organ failure at any APACHE II score), all-cause mortality was also higher in the drotrecogin alfa group (28-day: 67/323; in-hospital: 76/325) compared with the placebo group (28-day: 44/313; in-hospital: 62/314).

Patients with single organ dysfunction and recent surgery may not be at high risk of death irrespective of APACHE II score and, therefore, may not be among the indicated population. Use drotrecogin alfa in these patients only after careful consideration of the risks and benefits.

➤*Bleeding:* Bleeding is the most common serious adverse reaction associated with drotrecogin alfa therapy. Carefully evaluate each patient being considered for therapy with drotrecogin alfa and weigh the anticipated benefits against potential risks associated with therapy.

Certain conditions, many of which led to exclusion from the phase 3 trial, are likely to increase the risk of bleeding with drotrecogin alfa therapy. For individuals with 1 or more of the following conditions, carefully consider the increased risk of bleeding when deciding whether to use drotrecogin alfa therapy:

- Concurrent therapeutic dosing of heparin to treat an active thrombotic or embolic event.
- Platelet count less than 30,000 × 10^6/L, even if the platelet count is increased after transfusions.
- Prothrombin time - international normalized ratio (INR) greater than 3.
- Recent (within 6 weeks) GI bleeding.
- Recent administration (within 3 days) of thrombolytic therapy.
- Recent administration (within 7 days) of oral anticoagulants or glycoprotein IIb/IIIa inhibitors.
- Recent administration (within 7 days) of aspirin greater than 650 mg/day or other platelet inhibitors.
- Recent (within 3 months) ischemic stroke.
- Intracranial arteriovenous malformation or aneurysm.
- Known bleeding diathesis.
- Chronic severe hepatic disease.
- Any other condition in which bleeding constitutes a significant hazard or would be particularly difficult to manage because of its location.

Should clinically important bleeding occur, immediately stop the infusion of drotrecogin alfa. Carefully assess continued use of other agents affecting the coagulation system. Once adequate hemostasis has been achieved, continued use of drotrecogin alfa may be reconsidered.

Discontinue drotrecogin alfa 2 hours prior to undergoing an invasive surgical procedure or procedures with an inherent risk of bleeding. Once adequate hemostasis has been achieved, initiation of drotrecogin alfa may be reconsidered 12 hours after major invasive procedures or surgery, or restarted immediately after uncomplicated less invasive procedures.

➤*Pregnancy: Category C.* Animal reproductive studies have not been conducted with drotrecogin alfa. It is not known whether drotrecogin alfa can cause fetal harm when administered to a pregnant woman or can affect reproduction capacity. Administer drotrecogin alfa to pregnant women only if clearly needed.

➤*Lactation:* It is not known whether drotrecogin alfa is excreted in human milk or absorbed systemically after ingestion. Because many drugs are excreted in human milk, and because of the potential for adverse reactions of the breast-feeding infant, decide whether to discontinue breast-feeding or discontinue the drug, taking into account the importance of the drug to the mother.

➤*Children:* The safety and efficacy of drotrecogin alfa have not been established in the age group newborn (38 weeks gestation age) to 18 years of age. The efficacy of drotrecogin alfa in adult patients with severe sepsis and high risk of death cannot be extrapolated to pediatric patients with severe sepsis.

Recombinant Human Activated Protein C

DROTRECOGIN ALFA (ACTIVATED) — INJECTION

Precautions

➤*Readministration:* Drotrecogin alfa has not been readministered to patients with severe sepsis.

➤*Immunogenicity:* As with all therapeutic proteins, there is a potential for immunogenicity. The incidence of antibody development in patients receiving drotrecogin alfa has not been adequately determined, as the assay sensitivity is inadequate to reliably detect all potential antibody responses. One patient in the phase 2 trial developed antibodies to drotrecogin alfa without clinical sequelae. One patient in the phase 3 trial who developed antibodies to drotrecogin alfa developed superficial and deep vein thrombi during the study, and died of multiorgan failure on day 36 posttreatment but the relationship of this event to antibody is not clear.

➤*Lab test abnormalities:* Most patients with severe sepsis have a coagulopathy that is commonly associated with prolongation of the activated partial thromboplastin time (APTT) and the prothrombin time (PT). Drotrecogin alfa may variably prolong the APTT. Therefore, the APTT cannot be reliably used to assess the status of the coagulopathy during drotrecogin alfa infusion. Drotrecogin alfa has minimal effect on the PT and the PT can be used to monitor the status of the coagulopathy in these patients.

Drug Interactions

Drug interactions with drotrecogin alfa have not been performed in patients with severe sepsis. However, because there is an increased risk of bleeding with drotrecogin alfa, employ caution when drotrecogin alfa is used with other drugs that affect hemostasis. Approximately two thirds of the patients in the phase 3 study received either prophylactic low-dose heparin (unfractionated heparin up to 15,000 units/day) or prophylactic doses of low molecular weight heparins as indicated in the prescribing information for the specific products. Concomitant use of prophylactic low-dose heparin did not appear to affect safety; however, its effects on the efficacy of drotrecogin alfa has not been evaluated in an adequate and well-controlled clinical trial.

➤*Drug/Lab test interactions:* Because drotrecogin alfa may affect the APTT assay, drotrecogin alfa present in plasma samples may interfere with one-stage coagulation assays based on the APTT (eg, factor VIII, IX, XI assays). This interference may result in an apparent factor concentration that is lower than the true concentration. Drotrecogin alfa present in plasma samples does not interfere with one-stage factor assays based on the PT (eg, factor II, V, VII, X assays).

Adverse Reactions

➤*Bleeding:* Bleeding is the most common adverse reaction associated with drotrecogin alfa.

In the phase 3 study, serious bleeding events were observed during the 28-day study period in 3.5% of drotrecogin alfa-treated and 2% of placebo-treated patients, respectively. The difference in serious bleeding between drotrecogin alfa and placebo occurred primarily during the infusion period and is shown in the following table. Serious bleeding events were defined as any intracranial hemorrhage, life-threatening bleed, bleeding event requiring the administration of 3 units or more of packed red blood cells per day for 2 consecutive days, or bleeding event assessed as a serious adverse reaction.

Number of Patients Experiencing a Serious Bleeding Event by Site of Hemorrhage During the Study Drug Infusion Period[a] in PROWESS

Adverse reaction	Drotrecogin alfa (n = 850)	Placebo (n = 840)
Total	20 (2.4%)	8 (1%)
Site of hemorrhage		
GI	5	4
GU	2	0
Intra-abdominal	2	3
Intracranial	2	0
Intrathoracic	4	0
Retroperitoneal	3	0
Skin/soft tissue	1	0
Miscellaneous[b]	1	1

[a] Study drug infusion period is defined as the date of initiation of study drug to the date of study drug discontinuation plus the next calendar day.
[b] Patients requiring the administration of greater than or equal to 3 units of packed red blood cells per day for 2 consecutive days without an identified site of bleeding.

In PROWESS, 2 cases of intracranial hemorrhage (ICH) occurred during the infusion period for drotrecogin alfa-treated patients and no cases were reported in the placebo patients. The incidence of ICH during the 28-day study period was 0.2% for drotrecogin alfa-treated patients and 0.1% for placebo-treated patients. ICH has been reported in patients receiving drotrecogin alfa in non-placebo-controlled trials with an incidence of approximately 1% during the infusion period. The risk of ICH may be increased in patients with risk factors for bleeding, such as severe coagulopathy and severe thrombocytopenia.

In PROWESS, 25% of the drotrecogin alfa-treated patients and 18% of the placebo-treated patients experienced at least 1 bleeding event during the 28-day study period. In both treatment groups, the majority of bleeding events were ecchymoses or GI tract bleeding.

➤*Miscellaneous:* Patients administered drotrecogin alfa as treatment for severe sepsis experienced many events that are potential sequelae of severe sepsis and may or may not be attributable to drotrecogin alfa therapy. In clinical trials, there were no types of nonbleeding adverse reactions, suggesting a causal association with drotrecogin alfa.

Overdosage

➤*Treatment:* There is no known antidote for drotrecogin alfa. In case of overdose, immediately stop the infusion and monitor closely for hemorrhagic complications.

In postmarketing experience, there have been a limited number of medication error reports of excessive rate of drotrecogin alfa infusion for short periods of time (median, 2 hours). No unexpected adverse reactions were observed during the overdose period. However, this information is insufficient to assess whether drotrecogin alfa overdose is associated with an increased hemorrhage risk beyond that observed with drotrecogin alfa administered at the recommended dose.

Thrombolytic Enzymes

STREPTOKINASE — INJECTION

Rx	**Streptase** (Aventis Behring)	**Powder for injection, lyophilized**[a]: 250,000 units	Preservative-free. In 6 mL vials.
		750,000 units	Preservative-free. In 6 mL vials.
		1,500,000 units	Preservative-free. In 6 mL vials and 50 mL infusion bottle.

[a] With 25 mg cross-linked gelatin polypeptides, 25 mg sodium l-glutamate, and 100 mg albumin (human).

STREPTOKINASE — INJECTION

Indications

➤*Acute evolving transmural myocardial infarction:* Streptokinase is indicated for use in the management of acute myocardial infarction (AMI) in adults, for the lysis of intracoronary thrombi, the improvement of ventricular function and the reduction of mortality associated with AMI, when administered by either the IV or the intracoronary route, as well as for the reduction of infarct size and congestive heart failure associated with AMI when administered by the IV route. Earlier administration of streptokinase is correlated with greater clinical benefit.

➤*Pulmonary embolism:* Streptokinase is indicated for the lysis of objectively diagnosed (angiography or lung scan) pulmonary emboli, involving obstruction of blood flow to a lobe or multiple segments, with or without unstable hemodynamics.

➤*Deep vein thrombosis:* Streptokinase is indicated for the lysis of objectively diagnosed (preferably ascending venography), acute, extensive thrombi of the deep veins such as those involving the popliteal and more proximal vessels.

➤*Arterial thrombosis and embolism:* Streptokinase is indicated for the lysis of acute arterial thrombi and emboli. Streptokinase is not indicated for arterial emboli originating from the left side of the heart due to the risk of new embolic phenomena such as cerebral embolism.

➤*Unlabeled uses:* Appears to be an effective local thrombolytic for occluded catheters; however, its use may be limited by adverse effects. Also used to treat chronic arterial occlusions; retinal vessel thrombosis; hemolytic-uremic syndrome; renal artery thrombosis; renal cortical necrosis.

Administration and Dosage

➤*Acute evolving transmural MI:* Administer as soon as possible after symptom onset. The greatest benefit in mortality reduction was observed when streptokinase was administered within 4 hours, but statistically significant benefit has been reported up to 24 hours.

IV infusion – Administer a total dose of 1,500,000 units within 60 minutes.

Intracoronary infusion – Administer 20,000 units by bolus followed by 2,000 units/min for 60 minutes for a total dose of 140,000 units.

➤*PE, DVT, arterial thrombosis, or embolism:* Institute treatment as soon as possible after thrombotic event onset, preferably within 7 days. Any delay in instituting lytic therapy to evaluate the effect of heparin therapy decreases the potential for optimal efficacy. Because human exposure to streptococci is common, antibodies to streptokinase are prevalent. Thus, a loading dose of streptokinase sufficient to neutralize these antibodies is required. A dose of 250,000 units streptokinase infused into a peripheral vein over 30 minutes was appropriate in over 90% of patients. If the thrombin time, or any other parameter of lysis after 4 hours of therapy is not significantly different from the normal control level, discontinue streptokinase because excessive resistance is present.

STREPTOKINASE — INJECTION

Streptokinase Dosages		
Indication	Loading dose	IV infusion dosage/duration
PE	250,000 units over 30 min	100,000 units/h for 24 h (72 h if concurrent DVT is suspected)
DVT	250,000 units over 30 min	100,000 units/h for 72 h
Arterial thrombosis or embolism	250,000 units over 30 min	100,000 units/h for 24 to 72 h

➤*AV cannulae occlusion:* Before using, try to clear the cannula by syringe technique, using heparinized saline solution. If adequate flow is not re-established, use streptokinase. Allow the effect of any pretreatment anticoagulants to diminish. Slowly instill 250,000 units in 2 mL solution into each occluded limb of the cannula. Clamp off cannula limb(s) for 2 hours. Observe closely for adverse effects. After treatment, aspirate contents of infused cannula limb(s), flush with saline, and reconnect cannula.

➤*Pediatric use:* Controlled clinical studies have not been conducted in children to determine safety and efficacy. The evidence of clinical benefits and risks is solely based on anecdotal reports in patients ranging in age from less than 1 month to 16 years. The largest number of patient reports have pertained to the use of streptokinase in arterial occlusions. For arterial occlusions, the most frequently used loading dose was 1,000 units/kg; fewer numbers of patients received 3,000 units/kg. Loading dose durations typically have ranged from 5 to 30 minutes. Continuous infusion doses were frequently 1,000 units/kg/h; fewer were at 1,500 units/kg/h. Infusions were maintained for 12 hours or less in approximately half of the published cases; a smaller proportion were between 12 and 24 hours. Reported adverse events associated with the use of streptokinase in the pediatric population are similar in nature to those associated with its use in adults. Rates of all bleeding complications have been variable and as high as 50% at catheter sites in some studies. Occasionally, bleeding has required transfusion. Careful monitoring of patient status is necessary.

➤*Reconstitution (vials and infusion bottles):*
1.) Slowly add 5 mL NaCl injection or 5% dextrose injection to the streptokinase vial, directing the diluent at the side of the vacuum-packed vial rather than into the drug powder.
2.) Roll and tilt the vial gently to reconstitute. Avoid shaking (shaking may cause foaming). If necessary, total volume may be increased to a maximum of 500 mL in glass or 50 mL in plastic containers; adjust the infusion pump rate accordingly. To facilitate setting the infusion pump rate, a total volume of 45 mL, or a multiple thereof, is recommended.
3.) Withdraw the entire reconstituted contents of the vial; slowly and carefully dilute further to a total volume as recommended. Avoid shaking and agitation on dilution.
4.) When diluting the 1,500,000 units infusion bottle (50 mL), slowly add 5 mL NaCl injection or 5% dextrose injection, directing it at the side of the bottle rather than into the drug powder. Roll and tilt the bottle gently to reconstitute. Avoid shaking as it may cause foaming. Add an additional 40 mL of diluent to the bottle, avoiding shaking and agitation (total volume = 45 mL). Administer by infusion pump at the rate indicated.
5.) Inspect parenteral drug products visually for particulate matter and discoloration prior to administration (the human albumin may impart a slightly yellow color to the solution).
6.) The reconstituted solution can be filtered through a 0.8 mcm or larger pore size filter.
7.) Because streptokinase contains no preservatives, reconstitute immediately before use. The solution may be used for direct IV administration within 8 hours following reconstitution if stored at 2° to 8°C (36° to 46°F).
8.) Do not add other medication to the container.
9.) Discard unused reconstituted drug.

Streptokinase Suggested Dilutions and Infusion Rates				
Indication	Infusion type	Vial size (units)	Total solution volume	Dosage and infusion rate
AMI	Intravenous infusion	1,500,000	45 mL	Infuse 45 mL over 60 min
AMI	Intracoronary infusion	250,000	125 mL	Loading dose of 10 mL (20,000 IU); then 60 mL/h (2000 IU/min)
PE, DVT, arterial thrombosis, embolism	IV infusion 1. Loading dose	1,500,000	90 mL	1. Infuse 30 mL/h for 30 min (250,000 IU)
	2. Maintenance dose			2. Then infuse at 6 mL/h (100,000 units/h)
	IV infusion 1. Loading dose	1,500,000 infusion bottle	45 mL	1. 15 mL/h for 30 min (250,000 units)
	2. Maintenance dose			2. Then infuse 3 mL/h (100,000 IU/h)

AV cannula – Slowly reconstitute contents of the 250,000 units, vacuum-packed vial with 2 mL sodium chloride injection or 5% dextrose injection.

➤*IV incompatibilities:* Do not add other medication to streptokinase.

➤*Storage/Stability:* Store unopened vials at room temperature (15° to 30°C or 59° to 86°F). The solution may be used for direct IV administration within 8 hours following reconstitution if stored at 2° to 8°C (36° to 46°F). Discard unused reconstituted drug.

Actions

➤*Pharmacology:* Streptokinase acts with plasminogen to produce an "activator complex" that converts plasminogen to the proteolytic enzyme plasmin. The $t_{½}$ of the activator complex is about 23 minutes; the complex is inactivated, in part, by antistreptococcal antibodies. The mechanism by which dissociated streptokinase is eliminated is clearance by sites in the liver; however no metabolites have yet been identified. Plasmin degrades fibrin clots as well as fibrinogen and other plasma proteins. Plasmin is inactivated by circulating inhibitors such as alpha-2-plasmin inhibitor or alpha-2-macroglobulin. These inhibitors are rapidly consumed at high doses of streptokinase.

IV infusion of streptokinase is followed by increased fibrinolytic activity, which decreases plasma fibrinogen levels for 24 to 36 hours. The decrease in plasma fibrinogen is associated with decreases in plasma and blood viscosity and red blood cell aggregation. The hyperfibrinolytic effect disappears within a few hours after discontinuation, but a prolonged thrombin time may persist up to 24 hours due to a decrease in plasma levels of fibrinogen and an increase in the amount of circulating fibrin(ogen) degradation products (FDP). Depending on the dosage and duration of infusion of streptokinase, the thrombin time will decrease to < 2 times the normal control value within 4 hours, and return to normal by 24 hours.

IV administration has been shown to reduce blood pressure and total peripheral resistance with corresponding reduction in cardiac afterload. However, these expected responses were not studied with the intracoronary administration of streptokinase. The quantitative benefit has not been evaluated.

Variable amounts of circulating antistreptokinase antibody are present in individuals as a result of recent streptococcal infections. The recommended dosage schedule usually obviates the need for antibody titration.

Contraindications

Because thrombolytic therapy increases the risk of bleeding, streptokinase is contraindicated in the following situations: Active internal bleeding; recent (within 2 months) cerebrovascular accident, or intracranial or intraspinal surgery (see Warnings); intracranial neoplasm; severe uncontrolled hypertension.

Streptokinase should not be administered to patients having experienced a severe allergic reaction to the product.

Warnings

➤*Bleeding:* Following IV high-dose brief-duration streptokinase therapy in acute MI, severe bleeding complications requiring transfusion are extremely rare (0.3% to 0.5%) and combined therapy with low-dose aspirin does not appear to increase the risk of major bleeding. The addition of aspirin to streptokinase may cause a slight increase in the risk of minor bleeding (3.1% without aspirin vs 3.9% with aspirin). Streptokinase will cause lysis of hemostatic fibrin deposits such as those occurring at sites of needle punctures, particularly when infused over several hours, and bleeding may occur from such sites. In order to minimize the risk of bleeding during treatment with streptokinase, venipunctures and physical handling of the patient should be performed carefully and as infrequently as possible, and IM injections must be avoided.

Should an arterial puncture be necessary during IV therapy, it is preferable to use an upper extremity vessel. Pressure should be applied for at least 30 minutes, a pressure dressing applied, and the puncture site checked frequently for evidence of bleeding.

Increased risks of therapy – In the following conditions, the risks of therapy may be increased and should be weighed against the anticipated benefits:

Recent (within 10 days) major surgery, obstetrical delivery, organ biopsy, previous puncture of noncompressible vessels.
Recent (within 10 days) serious GI bleeding.
Recent (within 10 days) trauma including cardiopulmonary resuscitation.
Hypertension: systolic BP ≥ 180 mm Hg or diastolic BP ≥ 110 mm Hg.
High likelihood of left heart thrombus, eg, mitral stenosis with atrial fibrillation.
Subacute bacterial endocarditis.
Hemostatic defects including those secondary to severe hepatic or renal disease.
Age > 75 years.
Pregnancy.
Cerebrovascular disease.
Diabetic hemorrhagic retinopathy.
Septic thrombophlebitis or occluded AV cannula at seriously infected site.
Any other condition in which bleeding constitutes a significant hazard or would be particularly difficult to manage because of its location.

Should serious spontaneous bleeding (not controllable by local pressure) occur, the infusion of streptokinase should be terminated immediately and treatment instituted as described under Adverse Reactions.

Bleeding into the pericardium, sometimes associated with myocardial rupture, has been seen in individual cases and has resulted in fatalities.

➤*Arrhythmias:* Rapid lysis of coronary thrombi has been shown to cause atrial reperfusion or ventricular dysrhythmias requiring immediate treatment. Careful monitoring for arrhythmia is recommended during and

STREPTOKINASE — INJECTION

immediately following administration of streptokinase for acute MI. Occasionally, tachycardia and bradycardia have been observed.

➤*Hypotension:* Hypotension, sometimes severe, not secondary to bleeding or anaphylaxis has been observed during IV streptokinase infusion in 1% to 10% of patients. Patients should be monitored closely and, if symptomatic or alarming hypotension occurs, appropriate treatment administered, which may include a decrease in the IV streptokinase infusion rate. Smaller hypotensive effects are common and have not required treatment.

➤*Cholesterol embolism:* Cholesterol embolism has been reported rarely in patients treated with all types of thrombolytic agents; the true incidence is unknown. This serious condition, which can be lethal, is also associated with invasive vascular procedures (eg, cardiac catheterization, angiography, vascular surgery) or anticoagulant therapy. Clinical features of cholesterol embolism include livedo reticularis, "purple toe" syndrome, acute renal failure, gangrenous digits, hypertension, pancreatitis, MI, cerebral infarction, spinal cord infarction, retinal artery occlusion, bowel infarction, and rhabdomyolysis.

Non-cardiogenic pulmonary edema has been reported rarely in patients treated with streptokinase. The risk of this appears greatest in patients who have large MIs and are undergoing thrombolytic therapy by the intracoronary route.

Rarely, polyneuropathy has been temporally related to the use of streptokinase, with some cases described as Guillain Barré syndrome.

Should pulmonary embolism or recurrent pulmonary embolism occur during streptokinase therapy, the originally planned course of treatment should be completed in an attempt to lyse these emboli. While pulmonary embolism may occasionally occur during streptokinase treatment, the incidence is no greater than when patients are treated with heparin alone. In addition to pulmonary embolization, embolization to other sites during streptokinase treatment has been observed.

➤*Fertility impairment:* It is not known whether streptokinase can affect reproduction capacity.

➤*Pregnancy: Category C.* Animal reproduction studies have not been conducted with streptokinase. It is also not known whether streptokinase can cause fetal harm when administered to a pregnant woman or can affect reproduction capacity. Streptokinase should be given to a pregnant woman only if clearly needed.

➤*Children:* Controlled clinical studies have not been conducted in children to determine safety and efficacy in children. The evidence of clinical benefits and risks is solely based on anecdotal reports in patients ranging in age from younger than 1 month to 16 years of age. The largest number of patient reports have pertained to the use of streptokinase in arterial occlusions. For arterial occlusions, the most frequently used loading dose was 1000 IU/kg; fewer numbers of patients received 3000 IU/kg. Loading dose durations have typically ranged from 5 to 30 minutes. Continuous infusion doses were frequently 1000 IU/kg/hour; fewer were at 1500 IU/kg/hour. Infusions were maintained for 12 hours or less in approximately half of the published cases; a smaller proportion were between 12 and 24 hours. Reported adverse events associated with the use of streptokinase in children are similar in nature to those associated with its use in adults. Rates of all bleeding complications have been variable, and as high as 50% at catheter sites in some studies. Occasionally bleeding has required transfusion. Careful monitoring of patient status is necessary.

Precautions

There have been rare cases where streptokinase has been administered for suspected AMI subsequently diagnosed as pancreatitis. Fatalities have occurred under these circumstances.

➤*Repeated administration:* Because of the increased likelihood of resistance due to antistreptokinase antibodies, streptokinase may not be effective if administered between 5 days and 12 months of prior streptokinase or anistreplase administration or streptococcal infections, such as streptococcal pharyngitis, acute rheumatic fever, or acute glomerulonephritis secondary to a streptococcal infection.

➤*IV infusion for other indications:* Before commencing thrombolytic therapy, it is desirable to obtain an APTT, a PT, a TT, or fibrinogen levels, and a hematocrit and platelet count. If heparin has been given, it should be discontinued and the TT or APTT should be less than twice the normal control value before thrombolytic therapy is started.

During the infusion, decreases in the plasminogen and fibrinogen level and an increase in the level of FDP (the latter 2 causing a prolongation in the clotting times of coagulation tests) will generally confirm the existence of a lytic state. Therefore, lytic therapy can be confirmed by performing the TT, APTT, PT or fibrinogen levels ≈ 4 hours after initiation of therapy.

➤*Special risk:* If heparin is to be reinstituted following the streptokinase infusion, the TT or APTT should be less than twice the normal control value.

➤*Lab test abnormalities:*

IV or intracoronary infusion for MI – IV administration of streptokinase will cause marked decreases in plasminogen and fibrinogen and increase in thrombin time (TT), activated partial thromboplastin time (APTT) and prothrombin time (PT); these should normalize within 12 to 24 hours. These changes may occur in some patients with intracoronary administration of streptokinase.

Drug Interactions

The interaction of streptokinase with other drugs has not been well studied.

➤*Use of anticoagulants and antiplatelet agents:* Streptokinase, alone or in combination with antiplatelet agents, and anticoagulants, may cause bleeding complications. Therefore, careful monitoring is advised. In the treatment of acute MI, aspirin when not otherwise contraindicated, should be administered with streptokinase (see below).

➤*Anticoagulation after treatment for MI:* In the treatment of acute MI, the use of aspirin has been shown to reduce the incidence of reinfarction and stroke. The addition of aspirin to streptokinase causes a minimal increase in the risk of minor bleeding (3.9% vs 3.1%), but does not appear to increase the incidence of major bleeding (see Adverse Reactions). The use of anticoagulants following administration of streptokinase increases the risk of bleeding, but has not yet been shown to be of unequivocal clinical benefit. Therefore, whereas the use of aspirin is recommended unless otherwise contraindicated, the use of anticoagulants should be individualized.

➤*Anticoagulation after IV treatment for other indications:* Continuous IV infusion of heparin, without a loading dose, has been recommended following termination of streptokinase infusion for treatment of pulmonary embolism or deep vein thrombosis to prevent rethrombosis. The effect of streptokinase on thrombin time (TT) and activated partial thromboplastin time (APTT) will usually diminish within 3 to 4 hours after streptokinase therapy, and heparin therapy without a loading dose can be initiated when the TT or the APTT is less than twice the normal control value.

Adverse Reactions

The following adverse reactions have been associated with IV therapy and may also occur with intracoronary artery infusion:

➤*Allergic:* Fever and shivering, occurring in 1% to 4% of patients, are the most commonly reported allergic reactions with IV use of streptokinase in acute MI. Anaphylactic and anaphylactoid reactions ranging in severity from minor breathing difficulty to bronchospasm, periorbital swelling or angineurotic edema have been observed rarely. Other milder allergic effects such as urticaria, itching, flushing, nausea, headache and musculoskeletal pain have also been observed, as have pulmonary edema and delayed hypersensitivity reactions such as vasculitis and interstitial nephritis. Anaphylactic shock is very rare, having been reported in 0% to 0.1% of patients.

Mild or moderate allergic reactions may be managed with concomitant antihistamine or corticosteroid therapy. Severe allergic reactions require immediate discontinuation of streptokinase with adrenergics, antihistamines, or corticosteroids administered IV as required.

➤*Hematologic:* The reported incidence of bleeding (major or minor) has varied widely depending on the indication, dose, route and duration of administration and concomitant therapy.

Minor bleeding can be anticipated mainly from sites of invasive procedures. If such bleeding occurs, local measures should be taken to control the bleeding.

Severe internal bleeding involving GI (including hepatic bleeding), GU, retroperitoneal, or intracerebral sites has occurred and has resulted in fatalities. In the treatment of acute MI with IV streptokinase, the GISSI and ISIS-2 studies reported a rate of major bleeding (requiring transfusion) of 0.3% to 0.5%. However, rates as high as 16% have been reported in studies that required administration of anticoagulants and invasive procedures.

Major bleed rates are difficult to determine for other dosages and patient populations because of the different dosing and intervals of infusions. The rates reported appear to be within the ranges reported for IV administration in acute MI.

Should uncontrollable bleeding occur, streptokinase infusion should be terminated immediately rather than slowing the rate of administration or reducing the dose of streptokinase. If necessary, bleeding can be reversed and blood loss effectively managed with appropriate replacement therapy. Although the use of aminocaproic acid in humans as an antidote for streptokinase has not been documented, it may be considered in an emergency situation.

➤*Respiratory:* There have been reports of respiratory depression in patients receiving streptokinase. In some cases, it was not possible to determine whether the respiratory depression was associated with streptokinase or was a symptom of the underlying process. If respiratory depression is associated with streptokinase, the occurrence is believed to be rare.

➤*Miscellaneous:* Transient elevations of serum transaminases have been observed. There have been reports in the literature of cases of back pain associated with the use of streptokinase. In most cases the pain developed during streptokinase IV infusion and ceased within minutes of discontinuation of the infusion.

HYDROXYUREA

For complete and comparative prescribing and other indications information, refer to the Hydroxyurea monograph in the Antineoplastics chapter.

HEMORRHEOLOGIC AGENTS

PENTOXIFYLLINE

Rx	**Pentoxifylline** (Copley)	**Tablets, controlled-release:** 400 mg	Film-coated. In 100s, 500s, and bulk pack 5000s.
Rx	**Trental** (Hoechst Marion Roussel)		(Trental). Pink. Film coated. Oblong. In 100s and bulk pack 5000s.
Rx	**Pentoxifylline Extended-Release** (Purepac)	**Tablets, extended-release:** 400 mg	In 100s, 500s and 1000s.

PENTOXIFYLLINE — ORAL

Indications

➤*Intermittent claudication:* For the treatment of intermittent claudication on the basis of chronic occlusive arterial disease of the limbs. Pentoxifylline can improve function and symptoms but is not intended to replace more definitive therapy, such as surgical bypass, or removal of arterial obstructions when treating peripheral vascular disease.

➤*Unlabeled uses:* Pentoxifylline was found superior to placebo in improving psychopathological symptoms in patients with cerebrovascular insufficiency. The drug has also been studied in diabetic angiopathies and neuropathies, transient ischemic attacks, leg ulcers, sickle cell thalassemias, strokes, high-altitude sickness, asthenozoospermia, acute and chronic hearing disorders, severe idiopathic recurrent aphthous stomatitis (400 mg 3 times a day for 1 month), eye circulation disorders, and Raynaud's phenomenon.

Administration and Dosage

➤*Approved by the FDA:* August 30, 1984.

The usual dosage is 1 tablet (400 mg) 3 times a day with meals.

While the effect of pentoxifylline may be seen within 2 to 4 weeks, it is recommended that treatment be continued for at least 8 weeks. Efficacy has been demonstrated in double-blind clinical studies of 6 month's duration.

Digestive and central nervous system side effects are dose related. If patients develop these effects, it is recommended that the dosage be lowered to 1 tablet twice a day (800 mg/day). If side effects persist at this lower dosage, discontinue the administration of pentoxifylline.

➤*Storage/Stability:* Store between 15° and 30°C (59° and 86°F). Dispense in well-closed, light-resistant containers. Protect blisters from light.

Actions

➤*Pharmacology:* Pentoxifylline and its metabolites improve the flow properties of blood by decreasing its viscosity. In patients with chronic peripheral arterial disease, this increases blood flow to the affected microcirculation and enhances tissue oxygenation. The precise mode of action of pentoxifylline and the sequence of events leading to clinical improvement are still to be defined. Pentoxifylline administration has been shown to produce dose-related hemorrheologic effects, lowering blood viscosity, and improving erythrocyte flexibility. Leukocyte properties of hemorrheologic importance have been modified in animal and in vitro human studies. Pentoxifylline has been shown to increase leukocyte deformability and to inhibit neutrophil adhesion and activation. Tissue oxygen levels have been shown to be significantly increased by therapeutic doses of pentoxifylline in patients with peripheral arterial disease.

➤*Pharmacokinetics:*

Absorption/Distribution – After oral administration in aqueous solution pentoxifylline is almost completely absorbed. It undergoes a first-pass effect and the various metabolites appear in plasma very soon after dosing. Peak plasma levels of the parent compound and its metabolites are reached within 1 hour. The major metabolites are Metabolite I (1-[5-hydroxyhexyl]-3,7-dimethylxanthine) and Metabolite V (1-[3-carboxypropyl]-3,7-dimethylxanthine), and plasma levels of these metabolites are 5 and 8 times greater, respectively, than pentoxifylline.

After administration of the 400 mg controlled-release pentoxifylline tablet, plasma levels of the parent compound and its metabolites reach their maximum within 2 to 4 hours and remain constant over an extended period of time. Coadministration of pentoxifylline tablets with meals resulted in an increase in mean C_{max} and AUC by about 28% and 13% for pentoxifylline, respectively. C_{max} for Metabolite I also increased by about 20%. The controlled release of pentoxifylline from the tablet eliminates peaks and troughs in plasma levels for improved gastrointestinal tolerance.

Metabolism/Excretion – Following oral administration of aqueous solutions containing 100 to 400 mg of pentoxifylline, the pharmacokinetics of the parent compound and Metabolite I are dose-related and not proportional (nonlinear), with half-life and area under the blood-level time curve (AUC) increasing with dose. The elimination kinetics of Metabolite V are not dose-dependent. The apparent plasma half-life of pentoxifylline varies from 0.4 to 0.8 hours and the apparent plasma half-lives of its metabolites vary from 1 to 1.6 hours. There is no evidence of accumulation or enzyme induction (cytochrome P450) following multiple oral doses.

Excretion is almost totally urinary; the main biotransformation product is Metabolite V. Essentially no parent drug is found in the urine. Despite large variations in plasma levels of parent compound and its metabolites, the urinary recovery of Metabolite V is consistent and shows dose proportionality. Less than 4% of the administered dose is recovered in feces. Food intake shortly before dosing delays absorption of an immediate-release dosage form but does not affect total absorption. The pharmacokinetics and metabolism of pentoxifylline have not been studied in patients with renal and/or hepatic dysfunction, but AUC was increased and elimination rate decreased in an older population (60 to 68 years) compared to younger individuals (22 to 30 years).

Contraindications

Recent cerebral and/or retinal hemorrhage; previous intolerance to this product or methylxanthines such as caffeine, theophylline, and theobromine.

Warnings

➤*Carcinogenesis:* Long-term studies of the carcinogenic potential of pentoxifylline were conducted in mice and rats by dietary administration of the drug at doses up to 450 mg/kg (approximately 19 times the maximum recommended human daily dose [MRHD] in both species when based on body weight; 1.5 times the MRHD in the mouse and 3.3 times the MRHD in the rat when based on body surface area). In mice, the drug was administered for 18 months, whereas in rats, the drug was administered for 18 months followed by an additional 6 months without drug exposure. In the rat study, there was a statistically significant increase in benign mammary fibroadenomas in females of the 450 mg/kg group. The relevance of this finding to human use is uncertain.

➤*Pregnancy: Category C.* Teratogenicity studies have been performed in rats and rabbits using oral doses up to 576 and 264 mg/kg, respectively. On a weight basis, these doses are 24 and 11 times the MRHD; on a body-surface-area basis, they are 4.2 and 3.5 times the MRHD. No evidence of fetal malformation was observed. Increased resorption was seen in rats of the 576 mg/kg group. There are no adequate and well controlled studies in pregnant women. Use pentoxifylline during pregnancy only if the potential benefit justifies the potential risk to the fetus.

➤*Lactation:* Pentoxifylline and its metabolites are excreted in human milk. Because of the potential for tumorigenicity shown for pentoxifylline in rats, a decision should be made whether to discontinue nursing or discontinue the drug, taking into account the importance of the drug to the mother.

➤*Children:* Safety and effectiveness in pediatric patients have not been established.

Precautions

➤*Monitoring:* Patients on warfarin should have more frequent monitoring of prothrombin times, while patients with other risk factors complicated by hemorrhage (eg, recent surgery, peptic ulceration, cerebral and/or retinal bleeding) should have periodic examinations for bleeding including, hematocrit and/or hemoglobin.

➤*Arterial disease of the limbs:* Patients with chronic occlusive arterial disease of the limbs frequently show other manifestations of arteriosclerotic disease. Pentoxifylline has been used safely for treatment of peripheral arterial disease in patients with concurrent coronary artery and cerebrovascular diseases, but there have been occasional reports of angina, hypotension, and arrhythmia. Controlled trials do not show that pentoxifylline causes such adverse effects more often than placebo, but, as it is a methylxanthine derivative, it is possible some individuals will experience such responses.

Drug Interactions

➤*Anticoagulants:* Although a causal relationship has not been established, there have been reports of bleeding and/or prolonged prothrombin time in patients treated with pentoxifylline with and without anticoagulants or platelet aggregation inhibitors. Patients on warfarin should have more frequent monitoring of prothrombin times, while patients with other risk factors complicated by hemorrhage (eg, recent surgery, peptic ulceration) should have periodic examinations for bleeding including, hematocrit and/or hemoglobin.

➤*Theophylline:* Concomitant administration of pentoxifylline and theophylline-containing drugs leads to increased theophylline levels and theophylline toxicity in some individuals. Closely monitor such patients for signs of toxicity and have their theophylline dosage adjusted as necessary.

➤*Antihypertensives:* Pentoxifylline has been used concurrently with antihypertensive drugs, beta blockers, digitalis, diuretics, antidiabetic agents, and antiarrhythmics, without observed problems. Small decreases in blood pressure have been observed in some patients treated with pentoxifylline; periodic systemic blood pressure monitoring is recommended for patients receiving concomitant antihypertensive therapy. If indicated, reduce the dosage of the antihypertensive agents.

Adverse Reactions

Clinical trials were conducted using either controlled-release pentoxifylline tablets for up to 60 weeks or immediate-release pentoxifylline capsules for up to 24 weeks. Dosage ranges in the tablet studies were 400 mg twice daily

PENTOXIFYLLINE — ORAL

to 3 times daily and in the capsule studies, 200 to 400 mg 3 times daily. The data below summarize the incidence (in percent) of adverse reactions considered drug related, as well as the numbers of patients who received controlled-release pentoxifylline tablets, immediate-release pentoxifylline capsules, or the corresponding placebos. The incidence of adverse reactions was higher in the capsule studies (where dose related increases were seen in digestive and nervous system side effects) than in the tablet studies. Studies with the capsule include domestic experience, whereas studies with the controlled-release tablets were conducted outside the US.

Incidence (%) of Adverse Reactions				
	Controlled-release tablets (commercially available)		Immediate-release capsules (used only for controlled clinical trials)	
	Pentoxifylline	Placebo	Pentoxifylline	Placebo
(Number of patients at risk)	(321)	(128)	(177)	(138)
Discontinued for side effect	3.1%	0	9.6%	7.2%
Cardiovascular				
Angina/chest pain	0.3%	-	1.1%	2.2%
Arrhythmia/palpitation	-	-	1.7%	0.7%
Flushing	-	-	2.3%	0.7%
CNS				
Agitation/nervousness	-	-	1.7%	0.7%
Blurred vision	-	-	2.3%	1.4%
Dizziness	1.9%	3.1%	11.9%	4.3%
Drowsiness	-	-	1.1%	5.8%
Headache	1.2%	1.6%	6.2%	5.8%
Insomnia	-	-	2.3%	2.2%
Tremor	0.3%	0.8%	-	-
GI				
Abdominal discomfort	-	-	4%	1.4%
Belching/flatus/bloating	0.6%	-	9%	3.6%
Diarrhea	-	-	3.4%	2.9%
Dyspepsia	2.8%	4.7%	9.6%	2.9%
Nausea	2.2%	0.8%	28.8%	8.7%
Vomiting	1.2%	-	4.5%	0.7%

➤*Other reactions less than 1%:* Pentoxifylline has been marketed in Europe and elsewhere since 1972. In addition to the above symptoms, the following have been reported spontaneously since marketing or occurred in other clinical trials with an incidence of less than 1%; the causal relationship was uncertain:

Cardiovascular – Dyspnea, edema, hypotension.

CNS – Anxiety, aseptic meningitis, confusion, depression, seizures.

Dermatologic – Angioedema, brittle fingernails, pruritus, rash, urticaria.

GI – Anorexia, cholecystitis, constipation, dry mouth/thirst.

Respiratory – Epistaxis, flu-like symptoms, laryngitis, nasal congestion.

Special senses – Blurred vision, conjunctivitis, earache, scotoma.

Miscellaneous – Bad taste, excessive salivation, leukopenia, malaise, sore throat/swollen neck glands, weight change.

➤*Rare events:* A few rare events have been reported spontaneously worldwide since marketing in 1972. Although they occurred under circumstances in which a causal relationship with pentoxifylline could not be established, they are listed to serve as information for physicians:

Cardiovascular – Anaphylactoid reactions, angina, arrhythmia, tachycardia.

GI – Hepatitis, jaundice, increased liver enzymes.

Hematologic/Lymphatic – Aplastic anemia, decreased serum fibrinogen, leukemia, pancytopenia, purpura, thrombocytopenia.

Overdosage

➤*Symptoms:* Overdosage with pentoxifylline has been reported in pediatric patients and adults. Symptoms appear to be dose related. A report from a poison control center on 44 patients taking overdoses of enteric-coated pentoxifylline tablets noted that symptoms usually occurred 4 to 5 hours after ingestion and lasted about 12 hours. The highest amount ingested was 80 mg/kg; flushing, hypotension, convulsions, somnolence, loss of consciousness, fever, and agitation occurred. All patients recovered.

➤*Treatment:* In addition to symptomatic treatment and gastric lavage, special attention must be given to supporting respiration, maintaining systemic blood pressure, and controlling convulsions. Activated charcoal has been used to absorb pentoxifylline in patients who have overdosed.

ANTIHEMOPHILIC AGENTS

COAGULATION FACTOR VIIa (RECOMBINANT)

Rx	**NovoSeven** (Novo Nordisk)	**Powder for injection, lyophilized**: 1.2 mg/vial (1,200 mcg/vial) recombinant human coagulation Factor VIIa (rFVIIa)	In single-use vials.
		2.4 mg/vial (2,400 mcg/vial) recombinant human coagulation Factor VIIa (rFVIIa)	In single-use vials.
		4.8 mg/vial (4,800 mcg/vial) recombinant human coagulation Factor VIIa (rFVIIa)	In single-use vials.

COAGULATION FACTOR VIIA — INJECTION

Indications

➤*Bleeding episodes in hemophilia patients:* For the treatment of bleeding episodes in hemophilia A or B patients with inhibitors to Factor VIII or Factor IX. Coagulation factor VIIa should be administered to patients only under the direct supervision of a physician experienced in the treatment of hemophilia.

Administration and Dosage

➤*Approved by the FDA:* March 25, 1999.

➤*Dosage:* Coagulation factor VIIa is intended for IV bolus administration only. Evaluation of hemostasis should be used to determine the effectiveness of coagulation factor VIIa and to provide a basis for modification of the coagulation factor VIIa treatment schedule; coagulation parameters do not necessarily correlate with or predict the effectiveness of coagulation factor VIIa.

The recommended dose of coagulation factor VIIa for hemophilia A or B patients with inhibitors is 90 mcg/kg given every 2 hours until hemostasis is achieved, or until the treatment has been judged to be inadequate. Doses between 35 and 120 mcg/kg have been used successfully in clinical trials, and both the dose and administration interval may be adjusted based on the severity of the bleeding and degree of hemostasis achieved. The minimal effective dose has not been established. For patients treated for joint or muscle bleeds, a decision on outcome was reached for a majority of patients within 8 doses although more doses were required for severe bleeds. A majority of patients who reported adverse experiences received more than 12 doses.

Posthemostatic dosing – The appropriate duration of posthemostatic dosing has not been studied. For severe bleeds, dosing should continue at 3- to 6-hour intervals after hemostasis is achieved, to maintain the hemostatic plug. The biological and clinical effects of prolonged elevated levels of factor VIIa have not been studied; therefore, the duration of post-hemostatic dosing should be minimized, and patients should be appropriately monitored by a physician experienced in the treatment of hemophilia during this time period.

➤*Reconstitution:* Reconstitution should be performed using the following procedures.

1.) Always use aseptic technique.
2.) Bring coagulation factor VIIa (white, lyophilized powder) and the specified volume of sterile water for injection (diluent) to room temperature, but not above 37°C (98.6°F). The specified volume of diluent corresponding to the amount of coagulation factor VIIa is as follows. 1.2 mg (1,200 mcg) vial + 2.2 mL Sterile Water for Injection, 4.8 mg (4,800 µg) vial + 8.5 mL Sterile Water for Injection. After reconstitution with the specified volume of diluent, each vial contains ≈ 0.6 mg/mL coagulation factor VIIa (600 mcg/mL).
3.) Remove caps from the coagulation factor VIIa vials to expose the central portion of the rubber stopper. Cleanse the rubber stoppers with an alcohol swab and allow to dry prior to use.
4.) Draw back the plunger of a sterile syringe (attached to sterile needle) and admit air into the syringe.
5.) Insert the needle of the syringe into the Sterile Water for Injection vial. Inject air into the vial and withdraw the quantity required for reconstitution.
6.) Insert the syringe needle containing the diluent into the coagulation factor VIIa vial through the center of the rubber stopper, aiming the needle against the side so that the stream of liquid runs down the vial wall (the coagulation factor VIIa vial does not contain a vacuum). Do not inject the diluent directly on the coagulation factor VIIa powder.
7.) Gently swirl the vial until all the material is dissolved. The reconstituted solution is a clear, colorless solution which may be used up to 3 hours after reconstitution.

COAGULATION FACTOR VIIA — INJECTION

➤*Administration:* Administration should take place within 3 hours after reconstitution. Any unused solution should be discarded. Do not store reconstituted coagulation factor VIIa in syringes. Coagulation factor VIIa is intended for IV bolus injection only and should not be mixed with infusion solutions. As with all parenteral drug products, reconstituted coagulation factor VIIa should be inspected visually for particulate matter and discoloration prior to administration. Do not use if particulate matter or discoloration is observed. Administration should be performed using the following procedures.

1.) Always use aseptic technique.
2.) Draw back the plunger of a sterile syringe (attached to sterile needle) and admit air into the syringe.
3.) Insert needle into the vial of reconstituted coagulation factor VIIa. Inject air into the vial and then withdraw the appropriate amount of reconstituted coagulation factor VIIa into the syringe.
4.) Remove and discard the needle from the syringe; attach a suitable intravenous injection needle and administer as a slow bolus injection over 2 to 5 minutes, depending on the dose administered.
5.) Discard any unused reconstituted coagulation factor VIIa after 3 hours.

➤*Admixture incompatibility:* Coagulation factor VIIa should not be mixed with infusion solutions until clinical data are available to direct this use.

➤*Storage / Stability:* Prior to reconstitution, keep refrigerated (2° to 8°C; 36° to 46°F). Avoid exposure to direct sunlight. Do not use past the expiration date.

After reconstitution, coagulation factor VIIa may be stored either at room temperature or refrigerated for up to 3 hours. Do not freeze reconstituted coagulation factor VIIa or store it in syringes.

Actions

➤*Pharmacology:* Coagulation factor VIIa is recombinant factor VIIa and, when complexed with tissue factor can activate coagulation factor X to factor Xa, as well as coagulation factor IX to factor IXa. Factor Xa, in complex with other factors, then converts prothrombin to thrombin, which leads to the formation of a hemostatic plug by converting fibrinogen to fibrin and thereby inducing local hemostasis.

➤*Pharmacokinetics:* Single-dose pharmacokinetics of coagulation factor VIIa (17.5, 35, and 70 mcg/kg) exhibited dose-proportional behavior in 15 subjects with hemophilia A or B. Factor VII clotting activities were measured in plasma drawn prior to and during a 24-hour period after coagulation factor VIIa administration. The median apparent volume of distribution at steady state was 103 mL/kg (range, 78 to 139). Median clearance was 33 mL/kg/hr (range, 27 to 49). The median residence time was 3 hours (range, 2.4 to 3.3), and the $t_{1/2}$ was 2.3 hours (range, 1.7 to 2.7). The median in vivo plasma recovery was 44% (30% to 71%).

Contraindications

Hypersensitivity to mouse, hamster, or bovine proteins. Coagulation factor VIIa (recombinant) should not be administered to patients with known hypersensitivity to coagulation factor VIIa or any of the components of coagulation factor VIIa.

Warnings

➤*Thrombotic events:* The extent of the risk of thrombotic adverse reactions after treatment with coagulation factor VIIa is not known, but is considered to be low. Patients with disseminated intravascular coagulation (DIC), advanced atherosclerotic disease, crush injury, or septicemia may have an increased risk of developing thrombotic events due to circulating TF or predisposing coagulopathy (see Adverse Reactions).

Additional data on the adverse reaction profile in general and regarding the frequency of thrombotic events in particular is being collected through a postmarket surveillance program. The coagulation factor VIIa cooperative registry surveillance program is designed to collect data on all uses of coagulation factor VIIa to expand the base of experience regarding the use of coagulation factor VIIa. All prescribers can obtain information regarding contribution of patient data to this program by calling 1-877-362-7355.

➤*Pregnancy: Category C.*

Treatment of rats and rabbits with coagulation factor VIIa in reproduction studies has been associated with mortality at doses up to 6 mg/kg and 5 mg/kg. At 6 mg/kg in rats, the abortion rate was 0 out of 25 litters; in rabbits at 5 mg/kg, the abortion rate was 2 out of 25 litters. Twenty-three out of 25 female rats given 6 mg/kg of coagulation factor VIIa gave birth successfully; however, 2 of the 23 litters died during the early period of lactation. No evidence of teratogenicity was observed after dosing with coagulation factor VIIa. There are no adequate and well controlled studies in pregnant women. Coagulation factor VIIa should be used during pregnancy only if the potential benefit justifies the potential risk to the fetus. The patients in whom coagulation factor VIIa is indicated are male.

➤*Lactation:* It is not known whether coagulation factor VIIa is excreted in human milk. Because many drugs are excreted in human milk, and because of the potential for serious adverse reactions in nursing infants, a decision should be made whether to discontinue nursing or to discontinue the drug, taking into account the importance of the drug to the mother.

➤*Children:* The safety and efficacy of coagulation factor VIIa were not determined to be different in various age groups, from infants to adolescents (0 to 16 years of age). Clinical trials were conducted with dosing determined according to body weight and not according to age.

Precautions

➤*Monitoring:* Patients who receive coagulation factor VIIa should be monitored if they develop signs or symptoms of activation of the coagulation system or thrombosis. When there is laboratory confirmation of intravascular coagulation or presence of clinical thrombosis, the rFVIIa dosage should be reduced or the treatment stopped, depending on the patient's symptoms.

Due to limited clinical studies which clearly address the effect of post-hemostatic dosing, precautions should be exercised when coagulation factor VIIa is used for prolonged dosing (see Administration and Dosage).

➤*Lab test abnormalities:* Laboratory coagulation parameters may be used as an adjunct to the clinical evaluation of hemostasis in monitoring the effectiveness and treatment schedule of coagulation factor VIIa although these parameters have shown no direct correlation to achieving hemostasis. Assays of prothrombin time (PT), activated partial thromboplastin time (aPTT), and plasma FVII clotting activity (FVII:C), may give different results with different reagents. Treatment with coagulation factor VIIa has been shown to produce the following characteristics:

PT – In patients with hemophilia A/B with inhibitors, the PT shortened to about a 7-second plateau at a FVII:C level of approximately 5 units/mL. For FVII:C levels more than 5 units/mL, there is no further change in PT.

aPTT – While administration of coagulation factor VIIa shortens the prolonged aPTT in hemophilia A/B patients with inhibitors, normalization has usually not been observed in doses shown to induce clinical improvement. Data indicate that clinical improvement was associated with a shortening of aPTT of 15 to 20 seconds.

FVIIa:C – FVIIa:C levels were measured 2 hours after coagulation factor VIIa administration of 35 mcg/kg and 90 mcg/kg following 2 days of dosing at 2 hour intervals. Average steady state levels were 11 and 28 units/mL for the 2 dose levels, respectively.

Drug Interactions

➤*Coagulation factor concentrates:* The risk of a potential interaction between coagulation factor VIIa and coagulation factor concentrates has not been adequately evaluated in preclinical or clinical studies. Simultaneous use of activated prothrombin complex concentrates or prothrombin complex concentrates should be avoided.

Adverse Reactions

Coagulation factor VIIa has been generally well tolerated in clinical studies in 298 patients with hemophilia A or B with inhibitors treated for 1,939 bleeding episodes. The paragraph below lists adverse events that were reported in at least 2% of coagulation factor VIIa patients and were considered to be at least possibly related or of unknown relationship to coagulation factor VIIa administration.

Body system	Number of episodes reported	Number of unique patients
Event	(n = 1,939 treatments)	(n = 298 patients)
Miscellaneous		
Fever	16	13
Platelets, bleeding, and clotting		
Hemorrhage NOS	15	8
Fibrinogen plasma decreased	10	5
Dermatologic and musculoskeletal		
Hemarthrosis	14	8
Cardiovascular		
Hypertension	9	6

Events which were reported in 1% of patients and were considered to be at least possibly or of unknown relationship to coagulation factor VIIa administration were allergic reaction, arthrosis, bradycardia, coagulation disorder, DIC, edema, fibrinolysis increased, headache, hypotension, injection site reaction, pain, pneumonia, prothrombin decreased, pruritus, purpura, rash, renal function abnormal, therapeutic response decreased, and vomiting.

In the 298 hemophilia patients, thrombosis was reported in 2 patients.

Serious adverse events that were probably or possibly related, or where the relationship to coagulation factor VIIa was not specified occurred in 14 of the 298 patients (4.7%). Six of these 14 patients died of the following conditions: worsening of chronic renal failure, anesthesia complications during proctoscopy, renal failure complicating a retroperitoneal bleed, ruptured abscess leading to sepsis and DIC, pneumonia, and splenic hematoma and GI bleeding.

Overdosage

Dose-limiting toxicities of coagulation factor VIIa (recombinant) have not been investigated in clinical trials. Two cases of accidental overdose by bolus administration have occurred in the clinical program. One hemophilia B patient (16 years of age, 68 kg) received a single dose of 352 mcg/kg and one hemophilia A patient (2 years of age, 14.6 kg) received doses ranging from 246 mcg/kg to 986 mcg/kg on 5 consecutive days. There were no reported complications in either case. The recommended dose schedule should not be intentionally increased, even in the case of lack of effect, due to the absence of information on the additional risk that may be incurred.

Patient Information

Patients receiving coagulation factor VIIa should be informed of the benefits and risks associated with treatment. Patients should be warned about the early signs of hypersensitivity reactions, including hives, urticaria, tightness of the chest, wheezing, hypotension, and anaphylaxis.

ANTIHEMOPHILIC FACTOR (Factor VIII; AHF)

Indications

➤*Classical hemophilia:* Classical hemophilia (hemophilia A) in which there is a deficiency of the plasma clotting factor, Factor VIII. Provides a means of temporarily replacing the missing clotting factor to correct, and/or prevent bleeding episodes. Also indicated for perioperative management of hemophilic patients.

➤*Short-term prophylaxis (ReFacto only):* For short-term routine prophylaxis to reduce the frequency of spontaneous bleeding episodes. The effect of regular routine prophylaxis on long-term morbidity and mortality is unknown.

➤*Hyate:C:* For the treatment and prevention of bleeding in congenital hemophilia A patients with antibodies (inhibitors) to human Factor VIII and also for previously nonhemophilic patients with spontaneously acquired inhibitors to human Factor VIII (acquired hemophilia). In patients with acquired hemophilia, consider porcine Factor VIII infusion as first-line therapy regardless of the initial anti-human inhibitor titer. Because of the wide individual variation in the interaction of antihuman Factor VIII antibodies with porcine Factor VIII, directly measure the patient's antibody titer against porcine Factor VIII.

Circulating antibodies (inhibitors) generally show a weaker neutralizing activity against porcine Factor VIII than against human Factor VIII. Therefore, antihemophilic factor can be used to produce a hemostatic level of Factor VIII in patients whose antibody level and kinetics preclude treatment with human Factor VIII concentrates. Determine the activity of a patient's antibody in the laboratory using porcine Factor VIII as a substrate in a modified Bethesda assay.

Administration and Dosage

Administer IV only. Use a plastic syringe; solutions may stick to the surface of glass.

Individualize dosage. The dose depends on patient weight, severity of the deficiency, severity of hemorrhage, presence of inhibitors, and the Factor VIII level desired. Clinical effect on the patient is the most important factor of therapy. When inhibitors are present, dosage requirements are extremely variable; determine by clinical response. It may be necessary to administer more AHF to obtain the desired result.

There is a linear dose-response relation with an approximate yield of 2% to 2.5% rise in Factor VIII activity for each unit of Factor VIII/kg transfused, from which an approximate factor of 0.5 IU/kg can be calculated. The following formulas provide a guide for dosage calculations:

$$\text{Expected Factor VIII increase (in \% of normal)} = \frac{\text{AHF/IU administered} \times 2}{\text{body weight (in kg)}}$$

$$\text{AHF/IU required} = \text{body weight (kg)} \times \text{desired Factor VIII increase (\% normal)} \times 0.5$$

Physician supervision of the dosage is required. The following dosage schedule may be used as a guide.

Antihemophilic Factor Recommended Dosage Schedule		
Hemorrhage: Degree of hemorrhage	Required peak postinfusion AHF activity in the blood (as % of normal or IU/dL plasma)	Frequency of infusion
Early hemarthrosis, muscle bleed, or oral bleed	20 to 40	Begin infusion every 12 to 24 hours for 1 to 3 days until the bleeding episode as indicated by pain is resolved or healing is achieved.
More extensive hemarthrosis, muscle bleed, or hematoma	30 to 60	Repeat infusion every 12 to 24 hours for usually ≥ 3 days until pain and disability are resolved.
Life threatening bleeds such as head injury, throat bleed, severe abdominal pain	60 to 100	Repeat infusion every 8 to 24 hours until threat is resolved.
Surgery: Minor surgery, including tooth extraction	60 to 80 60 to 100 (*Advate* only)[a]	A single infusion plus oral antifibrinolytic therapy within 1 hour is sufficient in ≈ 70% of cases.
Major surgery	80 to 100 (pre- and postoperative) 80 to 120 (pre and postoperative, *Advate* only)[b]	Repeat infusion every 8 to 24 hours depending on state of healing.

[a] Give a single bolus infusion beginning within 1 hour of the operation, with optional additional dosing every 12 to 24 hours as needed to control bleeding. For dental procedures, adjunctive therapy may be considered.
[b] For bolus infusion replacement, repeat infusions every 8 to 24 hours, depending on the desired level of Factor VIII and state of wound healing.

The careful control of the substitution therapy is especially important in cases of major surgery or life-threatening hemorrhages.

Although dosage can be estimated by the calculations above, it is strongly recommended that whenever possible, appropriate laboratory tests including serial AHF assays be performed on the patient's plasma at suitable intervals to assure that adequate AHF levels have been reached and are maintained.

➤*Mild hemorrhage:* Do not repeat therapy unless further bleeding occurs. Minor episodes generally subside with a single infusion of 10 IU/kg if level ≥ 20% to 30% of normal is attained.

➤*Moderate hemorrhage and minor surgery:* These instances require plasma Factor VIII level to be raised to 30% to 50% of normal for optimum hemostasis. This usually requires an initial dose of 15 to 25 AHF/IU/kg; if further therapy is required, administer a maintenance dose of 10 to 15 AHF/IU/kg every 8 to 12 hours.

➤*Severe hemorrhage:* For life-threatening bleeding, or hemorrhage involving vital structures (CNS, retropharyngeal and retroperitoneal spaces, iliopsoas sheath), raise the Factor VIII level to 80% to 100% of normal. Administer an initial AHF dose of 40 to 50 AHF/IU/kg and a maintenance dose of 20 to 25 AHF/IU/kg every 8 to 12 hours.

➤*Major surgery:* Major surgery procedures require a dose of AHF sufficient to achieve a level of 80% to 100% of normal; give 1 hour before the procedure. Check the Factor VIII level prior to surgery to assure the level is achieved. Repeat infusions may be necessary every 6 to 12 hours initially. Maintain the Factor VIII level at a daily minimum of ≥ 30% of normal for a healing period of 10 to 14 days.

➤*Dental extraction:* Dental extraction procedures require a peak postinfusion AHF activity in the blood of 60% to 80%. A single infusion plus oral antifibrinolytic therapy within 1 hour is sufficient in ≈ 70% of cases.

➤*Prophylaxis:* Factor VIII concentrates may be administered on a regular schedule for prophylaxis of bleeding.

Incorrect diagnosis, inappropriate dosage, method of administration, and biological differences in individual patients could reduce the efficacy of these products or even result in an ill effect following its use. It is important that these products be stored properly, the directions for use be followed carefully during use, the risk of transmitting viruses be carefully weighed before a product is prescribed, and that plasma Factor VIII levels be measured in initial treatment situations or if clinical response appears inadequate.

➤*ReFacto:* For short-term routine prophylaxis to prevent or reduce the frequency of spontaneous musculoskeletal hemorrhage in patients with hemophilia A, give ≥ 2 times/week. In pediatric patients, shorter dosage intervals or higher doses may be necessary. Pharmacokinetic/pharmacodynamic modeling predicts that routine prophylactic dosing 3 times/week may be associated with a lower bleeding risk than with dosing twice weekly. No randomized comparison of different doses or frequency regimens for routine prophylaxis has been performed.

➤*Rate of administration:* Administer preparations IV at a rate of ≈ 2 mL/min. Can be given at up to 10 mL/min. Administration of the entire dose in 5 to 10 minutes is generally well tolerated. As a precaution, determine the pulse rate before and during administration of the AHF concentrate. Should a significant increase of pulse rate occur, reduce the rate of administration or discontinue.

➤*Storage/Stability:* Store between 2° and 8°C (35° to 46°F) (except *Hyate:C*). Do not freeze. See additional storage information below. Use before the expiration date.

AHF Room Temperature Storage Recommendations	
Product	Recommendation
Advate	22° to 28°C (72° to 82°F) for ≤ 6 months[a]
Alphanate	< 30°C (80°F) for < 2 months
Bioclate	< 30°C (80°F) until expiration date
Helixate FS	< 25°C (77°F) for ≤ 2 months
Hemofil M	< 30°C (80°F) until expiration date
Koate-DVI	< 25°C (77°F) for ≤ 6 months
Kogenate	< 25°C (77°F) for ≤ 3 months
Kogenate FS	< 25°C (77°F) for ≤ 2 months
Monoclate P	< 30°C (80°F) for < 6 months
Recombinate	< 30°C (80°F) until expiration date
ReFacto	< 25°C (77°F) for ≤ 3 months

[a] Should be refrigerated but may be stored at room temperature.

Advate – Refrigerate at 2° to 8°C (36° to 46°F). Avoid freezing to prevent damage to the diluent vial. Use before expiration date.

Hyate:C – Store at -15° to -20°C (5° to -4°F). Use before expiration date.

Actions

➤*Pharmacology:* AHF is a protein found in normal plasma necessary for clot formation. Administration of AHF can temporarily correct the coagulation defect of patients with classical hemophilia (hemophilia A). Activated Factor VIII acts as a cofactor for activated Factor IX accelerating the conversion of Factor X to activated Factor X. Activated Factor X converts prothrombin into thrombin. Thrombin then converts fibrinogen into fibrin and a clot is formed. Factor VIII activity is greatly reduced in patients with hemophilia A and, therefore, replacement therapy is necessary. The biological half-life is ≈ 10 to 18 hours.

Contraindications

Hypersensitivity to mouse, hamster, or bovine protein (see Precautions), or to porcine or murine factor.

Warnings

➤*von Willebrand's disease:* Not effective in controlling the bleeding of patients with von Willebrand's disease.

➤*Hepatitis and AIDS:* Because antihemophilic factor is made from pooled human plasma, it may carry a risk of transmitting infectious agents (eg, viruses, and theoretically, the Creutzfeldt-Jakob disease [CJD] agent). Stringent procedures designed to reduce the risk of adventitious agent transmission have been employed in the manufacture of these products, from the screening of plasma donors and the collection and testing of plasma, through the application of viral elimination/reduction steps such as solvent detergent and heat treatment in the manufacturing process. Despite these measures, such products can still potentially transmit disease; therefore, the risk of infectious agents cannot be totally eliminated. All infections thought by a physician possibly to have been transmitted by antihemophilic factor should be reported to the manufacturer. The physician should weigh the risks and benefits of use of the product and discuss these with the patient.

Individuals who receive infusions of blood or plasma products may develop signs or symptoms of some viral infections, particularly hepatitis C. Incubation in a solvent detergent mixture during the manufacturing process is designed to reduce the risk of transmitting viral infection. However, scientific opinion encourages hepatitis A and B vaccinations for patients with hemophilia at birth or time of diagnosis.

➤*Pregnancy: Category C.* Safety for use during pregnancy has not been established. Use only if clearly needed.

➤*Children:*

Bioclate, Helixate FS, Kogenate, Kogenate FS, Recombinate, ReFacto – Appropriate for use in all ages, including newborns.

Alphanate – Clinical trials in patients < 16 years of age have not been conducted. In a small, well-controlled clinical trial with patients previously treated with AHF FVII, a pediatric patient treated with *Alphanate* responded similarly to adults. No adverse events were reported.

Koate DVI – *Koate DVI* has not been studied in pediatric patients.

Advate – A total of 54 subjects 16 years of age and younger have been treated across all studies to date. Interim pharmacokinetic data for 34 subjects (per protocol analysis population) 16 years of age and younger were obtained from a combined dataset comprising subjects 10 to 16 years of age treated on the phase 2/3 pivotal study and subjects enrolled and treated on the ongoing study of pediatric previously treated subjects younger than 6 years of age. Among these, 0 were neonates (birth to younger than 1 month of age), 2 were infants (1 month to younger than 2 years of age), 15 were children (2 to 12 years of age), and 17 were adolescents (12 to 16 years of age or younger). Pharmacokinetic parameters were not significantly different for the different age categories. The mean plasma half-life was 11.21 hours (range, 8.31 to 24.7 hours). The mean $AUC_{0\text{-}48h}$ was 1363 IU•h/dL. The mean values for C_{max} and adjusted recovery were 109 IU/dL and 2.17 IU/dL/IU/kg, respectively.

Precautions

Identification of the clotting defect as a Factor VIII deficiency is essential before the administration of AHF FVIII:C is initiated.

➤*Factor VIII inhibitor:* The formation of inhibitors to Factor VIII is a known complication in the management of individuals with hemophilia A. The reported prevalence of these antibodies in patients receiving plasma derived AHF is 10% to 20%. These inhibitors are invariably IgG immunoglobulins, the Factor VIII procoagulant inhibitory activity of which is expressed as Bethesda Units (BU) per mL of plasma or serum. Carefully monitor patients treated with rAHF for the development of antibodies to rAHF by appropriate clinical observations and laboratory tests. Inhibitor formation is especially common in young children with severe hemophilia during their first years of treatment, or in patients of any age who have received little previous treatment with FVIII. Nonetheless, inhibitor formation may occur at any time in the treatment of a patient with hemophilia A. Anti-inhibitor complex is available (see the Anti-Inhibitor Coagulant Complex monograph).

➤*Hemolysis:* AHF contains naturally occurring blood group-specific antibodies (Anti-A and Anti-B isoagglutinins). When large or frequently repeated doses are needed in patients of blood group A, B, or AB, intravascular hemolysis may occur; monitor the hematocrit and Direct Coombs' test. Correct hemolytic anemia with compatible group O red blood cells or AHF from group-specific plasma.

➤*Monoclonal antibody-derived Factor VIII:*

Formation of antibodies to mouse protein – Although no hypersensitivity reactions have been observed, they may possibly occur because of trace amounts of mouse protein.

➤*Laboratory tests:* Ensure that adequate AHF levels have been reached and are maintained. If the AHF level fails to reach expected levels or if bleeding is not controlled after apparently adequate dosage, inhibitors may be present. The presence of inhibitors can be demonstrated and quantitated in terms of AHF units neutralized by each mL of plasma or by the total estimated plasma volume. After sufficient dosage to neutralize inhibitor, additional dosage produces predicted clinical response.

➤*Porcine parvovirus (PPV) (Hyate:C only):* PPV is endemic in pigs throughout the world and can frequently be identified in pooled collections of porcine plasmas. The virus is highly resistant to chemical and physical methods of sterilization. The available evidence is that PPV does not cause clinical or subclinical infection in humans. The porcine plasma used in the manufacture of *Hyate:C* is screened for the presence of PPV DNA using a sensitive polymerase chain reaction test. Only plasma that is nonreactive in the test is used for the manufacture of *Hyate:C*. It is possible that extremely low levels of PPV or of other viruses, present at levels below the limit of detection of the cell screens, or small quantities of noninfective viral subunits including DNA may be present in the final product. There is no evidence that these materials are a health hazard. However, the effects, if any, of long-term exposure have not been studied systematically and are therefore unknown.

Adverse Reactions

➤*Cardiovascular:* Mild hypotension; chest discomfort; vasodilation; angina pectoris; tachycardia.

➤*CNS:* Headache; somnolence; lethargy; dizziness; tingling in arm, ear, and face; jittery feeling; asthenia.

➤*Dermatologic:* Rash; facial flushing; increased perspiration; acne; pruritus.

➤*GI:* Nausea; vomiting; taste changes; constipation; stomachache; diarrhea; anorexia; gastroenteritis; abdominal pain; dysgeusia.

➤*Hematologic:* Forearm bleeding following venapuncture; anemia; permanent venous access catheter complications; infected hematoma; forehead bruises.

➤*Musculoskeletal:* Myalgia; muscle weakness; joint swelling.

➤*Respiratory:* Nose bleeds; rhinitis; dyspnea; coughing.

➤*Special senses:* Serous otitis media; blurred vision; sore throat; eye disorder/vision abnormal.

➤*Miscellaneous:* Fever; chills; urticaria; fatigue; depersonalization; adenopathy; pallor in an inhibitor patient with gastroenteritis; cold feet; increased amino transferase; increased bilirubin; CPK increase; cold sensation; finger pain; rigors; hot flushes; hematocrit decreased; coagulation factor VIII decreased; chest pain.

Allergic reactions – Hives, fever, urticaria, mild chills, nausea, stinging at the infusion site, tightness of the chest, hypotension, and anaphylaxis may occur.

Thrombocytopenia (Hyate:C) – Acute thrombocytopenia has been reported to occur on rare occasions following infusion of *Hyate:C*. Consider monitoring of the platelet count during treatment.

Patient Information

Inform patients of the early symptoms and signs of hypersensitivity reaction, including hives, generalized urticaria, chest tightness, dyspnea, wheezing, faintness, hypotension, and anaphylaxis. Advise patients to discontinue use of the product and contact their physician or seek emergency care, depending on the severity of the reaction, if these symptoms occur.

Some viruses, such as parvovirus B19 or hepatitis A, are particularly difficult to remove or inactivate at this time. Parvovirus B19 most seriously affects seronegative pregnant women or immune-compromised individuals. The majority of parvovirus B19 and hepatitis A infections are acquired by environmental (natural) sources. Symptoms of parvovirus B19 infection include fever, drowsiness, chills, and runny nose followed ≈ 2 weeks later by a rash and joint pain. Evidence of hepatitis A may include several days to weeks of poor appetite, tiredness, and low-grade fever followed by nausea, vomiting, and pain in the belly. Dark urine and a yellowed complexion are also common symptoms. Encourage patients to consult their physician if such symptoms appear.

Factor VIII inhibitors are circulating antibodies that neutralize the procoagulant activity of Factor VIII. Patients with these inhibitors may not respond to treatment with AHF or the response may be much less than would otherwise be expected. Therefore, larger doses of AHF are often required. The management of bleeding in patients with inhibitors requires careful monitoring, especially if surgical procedures are indicated.

ANTIHEMOPHILIC FACTOR (Factor VIII; AHF)

Rx **Advate** (Baxter)	**Powder for Injection**: Concentrated recombinant AHF-PFM (plasma/albumin-free method). When reconstituted, contains 38 mg/mL mannitol, 10 mg/mL trehalose, 12mM histidine, 12mM Tris, 1.9 mM calcium, 0.17 mg/mL polysorbate-80, 0.1 mg/mL glutathione, and no more than 2 ng vWF/units rAHF. Monoclonal purified and solvent-detergent treated.	108 mEq/L sodium. Preservative free. In 250, 500, 1,000, and 1,500 units/single-dose vials with 5 mL of sterile water for injection, double-ended needle, filter needle, infusion set/blood collection set, and 10 mL sterile syringe.
Rx **Alphanate** (Grifols)	**Injection, lyophilized**: Concentrate of human Factor VIII. When reconstituted, contains ≥ 5 units FVIII:C/mg total protein, 0.3 to 0.9 g/100 mL albumin (human), ≤ 5 mmol Ca/L, ≤ 750 mcg glycine/units FVIII:C, ≤ 1 units heparin/mL, ≤ 10 to 40 mmol histidine/L, ≤ 0.1 mg imidazole/mL, ≤ 50 to 200 mmol arginine/L, ≤ 1 mcg PEG and polysorbate 80. Solvent/detergent- and heat-treated.	≤ 0.1 mcg TNBP[a]/units FVIII:C. In single-dose vials with diluent.[b]
Rx **Bioclate** (Aventis)	**Powder for Injection, lyophilized**: Concentrated recombinant AHF. When reconstituted, contains 12.5 mg/mL albumin (human), 1.5 mg/mL PEG 3350, 55 mM histidine, 0.2 mg/mL Ca^{++}. Monoclonal purified.	180 mEq Na/L. Preservative free. In 250, 500, and 1,000 units/ single-dose bottle with diluent, double-ended needle, and filter needle.
Rx **Helixate FS** (Aventis)	**Injection, lyophilized**: Concentrate of AHF (recombinant). When reconstituted, contains 21 to 25 mg/mL glycine, ≤ 20 mcg/ 1,000 units imidazole, 2 to 3 mM CaCl, 32 to 40 mEq/L chloride, 18 to 23 mM histidine, < 0.6 mcg/1,000 units Cu. Solvent/detergent-treated.	27 to 36 mEq Na/L, < 5 mcg/1,000 units TNBP,[a] 28 mg sucrose. Preservative and albumin free. In 250, 500, and 1,000 units with diluent[b], double-ended needle, filter needle, and administration set.
Rx **Hemofil M** (Baxter Healthcare)	**Injection**: A preparation of human AHF in concentrated form. When reconstituted, contains ≤ 12.5 mg/mL albumin (human), 0.07 mg/mL PEG 3,350, 0.39 mg histidine, 0.1 mg glycine, and ≤ 1 ng of mouse protein. Solvent/detergent-treated. Monoclonal purified.	18 ng TNBP. In single-dose bottles with diluent,[b] double-ended needle, and filter needle.
Rx **Hyate:C (Porcine)** (IPSEN[c])	**Powder for Injection, lyophilized**: Concentrate of AHF (VIII):C. Each vial contains 400 to 700 porcine units and 10 to 30 mmol/L citrate ions.	110 to 135 mmol/L sodium ions. Preservative free. In vials[b] with filter needle.
Rx **Koate-DVI** (Bayer)	**Injection, lyophilized**: Concentrate of AHF (human). When reconstituted, contains ≤ 1,500 mcg/mL PEG, ≤ 0.05 M glycine, ≤ 25 mcg/mL polysorbate 80, ≤ 3 mM Ca, ≤ 1 mcg/mL Al, ≤ 0.06 M histidine, ≤ 10 mg/mL albumin (human). Solvent/detergent- and heat-treated.	≤ 5 mcg/g TNBP.[a] In ≈ 250 or 500 units Factor VIII activity and ≈ 1000 units Factor VIII activity with diluent,[b] double-ended needle, filter needle, and administration set.
Rx **Kogenate FS** (Bayer)	**Injection, lyophilized**: Recombinant AHF. 21 to 25 mg/mL glycine, 18 to 23 mM histidine; 2 to 3 mM CaCl, 32 to 40 mEq/L Cl, ≤ 35 mcg/mL polysorbate 80, ≤ 20 mcg/1,000 units imidazole, ≤ 0.6 mcg/1,000 units Cu. Solvent/detergent-treated. Monoclonal purified.	≤ 5 mcg/1,000 units TNBP,[a] 27 to 36 mEq Na/L, 28 mg sucrose/ vial. Preservative and albumin free. In 250, 500, and 1000 units with diluent, double-ended transfer needle, filter needle, and administration set.
Rx **Monarc-M** (American Red Cross)	**Powder for injection**: A concentrated preparation of AHF. 2 to 15 AHF units/mg total protein, and a maximum of 12.5 mg/mL albumin (human) and 0.07 mg PEG 3350, 0.39 mg histidine, and 0.1 mg glycine/AHF IU. ≤ 0.1 ng/AHF units mouse protein, 18 ng organic solvent (tri-n-butyl phosphate), and 50 ng detergent (octoxynol 9). Monoclonal purified.	In single-dose bottles with 10 mL Sterile Water for Injection, double-ended needle, and filter needle.
Rx **Monoclate-P** (Aventis)	**Powder for injection, lyophilized**: Concentrate of human Factor VIII: C. When reconstituted, contains ≈ 2 to 5 mM CaCl per L, ≈ 1% to 2% albumin (human), 0.8% mannitol, 1.2 mM histidine, and < 50 ng/100 units trace murine monoclonal antibody. Heat-treated. Monoclonal purified.	≈ 300 to 450 mM/L Na ions. With diluent, double-ended needle, vented filter spike, winged infusion set, and alcohol swabs.[b]
Rx **Recombinate** (Baxter)	**Powder for injection, lyophilized**: Concentrated recombinant AHF. When reconstituted, contains 12.5 mg/mL albumin (human), 1.5 mg/mL PEG, 55 mM histidine, 0.2 mg/mL Ca. Monoclonal purified.	180 mEq Na/L. In single-dose 250, 500, and 1,000 units bottles[b] with diluent, double-ended needle, and filter needle.
Rx **ReFacto** (Genetics Institute)	**Powder for injection, lyophilized**: Recombinant AHF. When reconstituted, contains L-histidine, CaCl, and polysorbate 80.	NaCl, sucrose. Preservative free. In single-use vials with 250, 500, or 1,000 units/vial, with diluent, double-ended needle, filter needle for withdrawal, infusion set, and alcohol swabs.

[a] Tri-n-butyl-phosphate.
[b] Actual number of AHF units are indicated on the vials.
[c] IPSEN Inc., 27 Maple Street, Milford, MA 01757; (800) 456-7322.

For prescribing information on all products, refer to the Antihemophilic Factor (Factor VIII) group monograph.

ANTI-INHIBITOR COAGULANT COMPLEX

Rx	**Autoplex T** (Nabi)	Dried anti-inhibitor coagulant complex. Maximum of 2 units heparin and 2 mg polyethylene glycol/mL reconstituted material. Heat-treated.	≈ 177 mEq/L Na. In vials with diluent and needles. Each bottle is labeled with the units of Factor VIII correctional activity it contains.
Rx	**Feiba VH Immuno** (Immuno-US)	Freeze-dried anti-inhibitor coagulant complex. Heparin free. Vapor-heated.	≈ 8 mg/mL Na. In vials with diluent and needles. Each bottle is labeled with the units of Factor VIII inhibitor bypassing activity it contains.

ANTI-INHIBITOR COAGULANT COMPLEX, HEAT TREATED, *AUTOPLEX T*

WARNING

This is a potent drug with potential hazards. For maximal safety and efficacy, carefully read and follow directions below.

Indications

➤*Factor VIII inhibitors:* Anti-inhibitor coagulant complex, heat treated, is indicated for use in patients with Factor VIII inhibitors who are bleeding or are to undergo surgery. The intravenous administration of this preparation is intended to control bleeding episodes in such patients.

Approximately 10% of individuals with hemophilia A (classical hemophilia) have laboratory-measurable inhibitors to Factor VIII. For these patients, the treatment of choice depends upon the following factors: The severity of the bleeding episode, the existing level of inhibitor and whether the patient responds to infusion of Factor VIII with increasing antibody titers (anamnestic rise of Factor VIII antibody).

Patients whose present Factor VIII inhibitor levels are greater than 10 BU, as well as patients whose inhibitor levels are historically known to rise to greater than 10 BU following treatment with antihemophilic factor (human), should be treated with anti-inhibitor coagulant complex.

Patients whose present Factor VIII inhibitor levels are between 2 and 10 BU and whose inhibitor levels are historically known to remain in this range following treatment with antihemophilic factor (human) may be treated with either antihemophilic factor (human) or anti-inhibitor coagulant complex, depending on the patient's clinical history and the severity of the bleeding episode.

Patients with Factor VIII inhibitor levels of less than 2 BU whose inhibitor levels are historically known to remain at 2 BU or less following treatment with antihemophilic factor (human) may be treated with appropriate doses of antihemophilic factor (human).

For patients who have low levels of Factor VIII inhibitor and whose history does not include adequate laboratory indications of an anamnestic response to antihemophilic factor (human), the treatment of choice should be based on clinical judgement. In such patients who are having non-critical or minor bleeding episodes, the use of anti-inhibitor coagulant complex, heat treated, will maintain the inhibitor at a low level and allow the use of other coagulant therapeutic agents in subsequent major emergencies.

Administration and Dosage

Each bottle of anti-inhibitor coagulant complex, heat treated, is labeled with the number of Hyland Factor VIII Correctional Units that it contains. One Hyland Factor VIII Correctional Unit is that quantity of activated prothrombin complex which, upon addition to an equal volume of Factor VIII deficient or inhibitor plasma, will correct the clotting time (ellagic acid-activated partial thromboplastin time) to 35 seconds (normal).

➤*Dosage:* The recommended dosage range is 25 to 100 Hyland Factor VIII Correctional Units per kg of body weight, depending upon the severity of hemorrhage. If no hemostatic improvement is observed approximately 6 hours following the initial administration, the dosage should be repeated.

Subsequent dosage and administration intervals should be adjusted according to the patient's clinical response.

➤*Reconstitution (use aseptic technique):*

1.) Bring anti-inhibitor coagulant complex, heat treated (dry concentrate) and Sterile Water for Injection, USP, (diluent) to room temperature.
2.) Remove caps from concentrate and diluent bottles to expose central portions of rubber stoppers.
3.) Cleanse stoppers with germicidal solution.
4.) Remove protective covering from one end of the double-ended needle and insert exposed needle through diluent stopper.
5.) Remove protective covering from the other end of the double-ended needle. Invert diluent bottle over the upright concentrate bottle, then rapidly insert free end of the needle through the concentrate bottle stopper at its center. Vacuum in the concentrate bottle will draw in diluent.
6.) Disconnect the 2 bottles by removing needle from the diluent bottle, then remove needle from concentrate bottle stopper. Swirl or rotate the concentrate bottle until all material is dissolved. Do not shake vigorously.

Parenteral drug products should be inspected visually for particulate matter and discoloration prior to administration, whenever solution and container permit.

Do not refrigerate after reconstitution.

➤*Rate of administration:* It is recommended that anti-inhibitor coagulant complex, heat treated, be infused initially at a rate of 2 mL/min. If infusion at this rate is well tolerated the administration rate may be gradually increased to 10 mL/min.

➤*Administration (use aseptic technique):* When reconstitution of anti-inhibitor coagulant complex, heat treated, is complete, its infusion should commence as soon as practical; however, it must be completed within 1 hour. The reconstituted solution should be at room temperature during infusion.

➤*Intravenous drip infusion:* Follow directions for use printed on the administration set container. The use of a Hyland administration set is recommended as it contains a suitable filter.

➤*Intravenous syringe injection:*

1.) Attach filter needle to syringe and draw back plunger to admit air into the syringe.
2.) Insert needle into the reconstituted anti-inhibitor coagulant complex, heat treated.
3.) Inject air into bottle and then withdraw the reconstituted material into the syringe.
4.) Remove and discard the filter needle from the syringe; attach a suitable needle and inject intravenously as instructed under Rate of administration.
5.) If patient is to receive more than 1 bottle of concentrate, the contents of 2 bottles may be drawn into the same syringe by drawing up each bottle through a separate unused filter needle. This practice lessens the loss of concentrate. Please note: Filter needles are intended to filter the contents of a single bottle of anti-inhibitor coagulant complex, heat treated, only.

➤*Storage/Stability:* Anti-inhibitor coagulant complex, heat treated, should be stored under ordinary refrigeration 2° to 8°C (36° to 46°F). Avoid freezing to prevent damage to the diluent bottle.

Actions

➤*Pharmacology:* In work with human immunodeficiency virus (HIV), substantial reduction in viral content has been reported in a recent study of the effects of ethanol fractionation, the process by which anti-inhibitor coagulant complex, heat treated, is manufactured. The study reports 1 to 4 log reduction in each fractionation step they examined.

The effectiveness of the 6-day heating step in reducing viral infectivity was assessed by in vitro viral inactivation studies, using as markers, viruses not commonly found in plasma. When known quantities of these viruses were added to the product, the heat treatment employed inactivated the following quantities of virus:

Sindbis	$10\ Log_{10}$
Vesicular stomatitis	$5\ Log_{10}$
Herpes simplex	$1.6\ Log_{10}$
HIV	$4.5\ Log_{10}$

In separate experiments, HIV was also studied and these data are reported in the table above.

A retrospective study conducted with patients receiving unheated anti-inhibitor coagulant complex, supports the effectiveness of the purification process in reducing viral burden in the product. In the study, none of the patients who received that product exclusively seroconverted for HIV antibodies, while 56% of those patients who received other treatment modalities seroconverted during the 3-year study.

Contraindications

The use of anti-inhibitor coagulant complex, heat treated, is contraindicated in patients with signs of fibrinolysis and in patients with disseminated intravascular coagulation (DIC).

Warnings

➤*Infectious disease transmission:* Anti-inhibitor coagulant complex, heat treated, is made from human plasma. Products made from human plasma may contain infectious agents, such as viruses, that can cause disease. The risk that such products will transmit an infectious agent has been reduced by screening plasma donors for prior exposure to certain viruses, by testing for the presence of certain current virus infections, and by inactivating or removing certain viruses (see Pharmacology). Despite these measures, such products can still potentially transmit disease. There is also the possibility that unknown infectious agents may be present in such products. All infections thought by a physician possibly to have been transmitted by this product should be reported by the physician or other healthcare provider to the US distributor. The physician should discuss the risks and benefits of this product with the patient. Physicians should also report adverse reactions or any disease condition which may occur concomitantly with the administration of this product to the US distributor.

➤*Reconstitution/Infusion time:* If the infusion of the concentrate occurs more than 1 hour following reconstitution, there may be increased prekallikrein activator (PKA) with consequent hypotension.

➤*Pregnancy: Category C.* Animal reproduction studies have not been conducted with anti-inhibitor coagulant complex, heat treated. It is also not known whether anti-inhibitor coagulant complex, heat treated, can cause fetal harm when administered to a pregnant woman or can affect reproduction capacity. Anti-inhibitor coagulant complex, heat treated, should be given to a pregnant woman only if clearly needed.

ANTI-INHIBITOR COAGULANT COMPLEX, HEAT TREATED, *AUTOPLEX T*

➤*Children:* Special caution should be taken in the use of this concentrate in newborns, where a high morbidity and mortality may be associated with hepatitis, and in individuals with preexisting liver disease.

Precautions

➤*Monitoring:* In children, fibrinogen levels should be determined prior to the initial infusion and monitored during the course of the treatment.

➤*Parvovirus B19 / Hepatitis A:* Some viruses, such as parvovirus B19 or hepatitis A, are particularly difficult to remove or inactivate at this time. Parvovirus B19 most seriously affects pregnant women, or immune-compromised individuals.

Symptoms of parvovirus B19 infection include fever, drowsiness, chills, and runny nose followed about 2 weeks later by a rash, and joint pain. Evidence of hepatitis A may include several days to weeks of poor appetite, tiredness, and low-grade fever followed by nausea, vomiting, and pain in the belly. Dark urine and a yellowed complexion are also common symptoms. Patients should be encouraged to consult their physician if such symptoms appear.

➤*Latex sensitivity:* Certain components used in the packaging of this product contain natural rubber latex.

➤*Identification of clotting deficiency:* Identification of the clotting deficiency as that caused by the presence of Factor VIII inhibitors is essential before the administration of anti-inhibitor coagulant complex, heat treated, is initiated.

➤*Hypotension:* Signs or symptoms of hypotension may occur with this product. In these cases, stopping the infusion allows the symptoms to disappear. With all but the most reactive individuals, the infusion may be resumed at a slower rate.

➤*DIC:* If clinical signs of intravascular coagulation occur, the infusion should be stopped promptly and the patient monitored for DIC by the appropriate laboratory tests. Symptoms of DIC include changes in blood pressure and pulse rate, respiratory distress, chest pain and cough. Laboratory indications of DIC include prolonged thrombin time, prothrombin time and partial thromboplastin time tests. Other indications of DIC are decreased fibrinogen concentration, decreased platelet count or the presence of fibrinogen/fibrin degradation products.

➤*Factor VIII inhibitors:* This product is to be used only in patients with inhibitors to Factor VIII.

➤*Lab test abnormalities:* In some cases, laboratory tests such as the activated partial thromboplastin time test may not correlate with clinical response, in that the appearance of hemostatic improvement may occur without a reduction of partial thromboplastin time. However, the prothrombin time would be expected to be shortened.

Drug Interactions

➤*Epsilon-aminocaproic acid (EACA) or tranexamic acid:* Because only limited data are available on the administration of highly activated prothrombin complex products together with antifibrinolytic agents such as EACA or tranexamic acid, the concomitant use of anti-inhibitor coagulant complex, heat treated, with such agents is not recommended.

Adverse Reactions

As with other plasma preparations, reactions manifested by fever, chills or indications of protein sensitivity may be observed with the administration of anti-inhibitor coagulant complex, heat treated. Signs or symptoms of high prekallikrein activity, such as changes in blood pressure or pulse rate may also be observed. It is advisable that appropriate medications be available for the treatment of acute allergic reactions or acute vasoactive reactions, should they occur.

A rate of infusion that is too rapid may cause headache, flushing, and changes in pulse rate and blood pressure. In such instances, stopping the infusion allows the symptoms to disappear promptly. With all but the most reactive individuals, infusion may be resumed at a slower rate.

ANTI-INHIBITOR COAGULANT COMPLEX (*FEIBA VH IMMUNO*)

Indications

Anti-inhibitor coagulant complex, vapor heated, is indicated for the control of spontaneous bleeding episodes or to cover surgical interventions in hemophilia A and B patients with inhibitors.

In addition, the use of anti-inhibitor coagulant complex, has been described in a few non-hemophiliacs with acquired inhibitors to Factors VIII, XI, and XII. One case has been reported where anti-inhibitor coagulant complex, was effective in a patient with von Willebrand's disease with an inhibitor.

Clinical experience suggests that patients with a Factor VIII inhibitor titer of less than 5 Bethesda units (BU) may be successfully treated with antihemophilic factor. Patients with titers ranging between 5 and 10 BU may either be treated with antihemophilic factor or anti inhibitor coagulant complex, vapor heated. Cases with Factor VIII inhibitor titers more than 10 BU have generally been refractory to treatment with antihemophilic factor.

➤*Guidelines to first and second choice treatment:*

Patient's inhibitor	Clinical situation		
Titer	Minor bleeding	Major bleeding	Surgery (emergency)
Less than 5 BU	AHF[a]	AHF	AHF
5 to 10 BU	AHF	AHF	AHF
	AICC[b]	AICC	AICC
More than 10 BU	AICC	AICC	AICC

[b] AICC = Anti-inhibitor coagulant complex, vapor heated, *Feiba VH Immuno*.
[a] AHF = Antihemophilic factor. Inadequate response to treatment may result from an abnormal platelet count or impaired platelet function, which were present before treatment with anti-inhibitor coagulant complex.

Administration and Dosage

Clinical trials have demonstrated that the response to treatment with anti-inhibitor coagulant complex, may differ from patient to patient with no correlation to the patient's inhibitor titer. Response may also vary between different types of hemorrhage (eg, joint hemorrhage vs CNS hemorrhage).

➤*General dosage guideline:* As a general guideline a dosage range of 50 to 100 Immuno Units of anti-inhibitor coagulant complex per kg of body weight is recommended. However, care should be taken to distinguish between the following 4 indications, all of which have undergone careful clinical evaluation.

Single doses of 100 units per kg of body weight of anti-inhibitor coagulant complex and daily doses of 200 units/kg of body weight of anti-inhibitor coagulant complex should not be exceeded. Patients receiving more than 100 units/kg of body weight of anti-inhibitor coagulant complex must be monitored for the development of DIC or symptoms of acute coronary ischemia.

➤*Joint hemorrhage:* In joint hemorrhage, a dose of 50 units/kg of body weight is recommended at 12-hour intervals, which may be increased to doses of 100 unit0/kg of body weight at 12-hour intervals.

Treatment should be continued until clear signs of clinical improvement appear, such as relief of pain, reduction of swelling or mobilization of the joint.

➤*Mucous membrane bleeding:* A dose of 50 units/kg of body weight is recommended to be given at 6-hour intervals under careful monitoring (visible bleeding site, repeated measurements of the patient's hematocrit). Again, if hemorrhage does not stop, the dose may be increased to 100 units/kg of body weight at 6-hour intervals. However, 2 such administrations or 200 units/kg of body weight a day should not be exceeded.

➤*Soft tissue hemorrhage:* For serious soft tissue bleeding, such as retroperitoneal bleeding, doses of 100 units/kg of body weight at 12-hour intervals are recommended. A daily dosage of 200 units/kg of body weight should not be exceeded.

➤*Other severe hemorrhages:* Severe hemorrhages, such as CNS bleedings have been effectively treated with doses of 100 units/kg of body weight at 12-hour intervals. Sometimes, anti-inhibitor coagulant complex, may be indicated at 6-hour intervals until clear clinical improvement is achieved.

➤*Reconstitution:*
1.) Warm the unopened bottle containing Sterile Water for Injection (diluent) to room temperature (not above 37°C; 98°F).
2.) Remove caps from the concentrate and diluent bottles to expose central portions of the rubber stoppers.
3.) Cleanse exposed surface of the rubber stoppers with germicidal solution and allow to dry.
4.) Using aseptic technique, remove protective covering from one end of the double-ended needle, and completely insert the exposed end through the diluent bottle stopper.
5.) Remove protective covering from the other end of the double-ended needle, taking care not to touch the exposed end. Invert diluent bottle over the concentrate bottle, then rapidly insert free end of the needle to its full length through the concentrate bottle stopper. Diluent will be drawn into the concentrate bottle by vacuum.
6.) Disconnect the 2 bottles by removing needle from the concentrate bottle stopper. Gently agitate or rotate the concentrate bottle until all material is dissolved.

Parenteral drug products should be inspected visually for particulate matter and discoloration prior to administration, whenever solution and container permit.

Do not refrigerate after reconstitution.

After complete reconstitution of anti-inhibitor coagulant complex, its injection or infusion should be commenced as promptly as practicable, but must be completed within 3 hours following reconstitution.

The solution must be given by intravenous injection or intravenous drip infusion and the maximum injection or infusion rate must not exceed 2 units/kg of body weight per minute. In a patient with a body weight of 75 kg, this corresponds to an infusion rate of 2.5 to 7.5 mL/minute depending on the number of units per vial (see label on vial).

➤*For intravenous injection:*
1.) After reconstituting the concentrate as described under Reconstitution, attach the enclosed filter needle to a sterile disposable syringe. Insert filter needle through the concentrate bottle stopper.
2.) Inject air and withdraw solution into the syringe.
3.) Remove and discard the filter needle. Attach a suitable intravenous needle or infusion set with winged adapter, and inject solution intravenously.

➤*For Intravenous Infusion:* Prepare a solution of anti-inhibitor coagulant complex, as described under Reconstitution.

Follow manufacturer's instructions for the administration set used. Make sure that the set contains an adequate filter.

➤*Storage / Stability:* Store at refrigerator temperature 2° to 8°C (36° to 46°F).

Avoid freezing, which may damage the diluent bottle.

ANTI-INHIBITOR COAGULANT COMPLEX (*FEIBA VH IMMUNO*)

Actions

➤*Pharmacology:* In a preclinical study to determine the virus inactivating efficacy of vapor heating, samples of bulk anti-inhibitor coagulant complex were spiked with 2×10^6/mL infectious units of HIV and subjected to vapor heat treatment. The residual virus titer was found to be less than 1 infectious unit/0.5 mL. A clinical study testing antihemophilic factor treated by a similar vapor heating procedure has shown none of 4 lots used in the study to produce non-A, non-B hepatitis in intensively followed patients naive to blood product administration.

Contraindications

The use of anti-inhibitor coagulant complex is contraindicated in patients who are known to have a normal coagulation mechanism.

Warnings

➤*Identification of clotting deficiency:* Anti-inhibitor coagulant complex must be used only in patients with circulating inhibitors to one or more coagulation factors and should not be used for the treatment of bleeding episodes resulting from coagulation factor deficiencies. It should not be given to patients with significant signs of disseminated intravascular coagulation (DIC) or fibrinolysis.

➤*Thromboembolic events:* In the course of treatment with preparations containing the prothrombin complex thromboembolic events may occur, particularly following the administration of high doses or in patients with thrombotic risk factors.

➤*High doses:* High doses of anti-inhibitor coagulant complex should be given only as long as absolutely necessary to stop bleeding.

➤*Concomitant antifibrinolytics:* It has been reported that anti-inhibitor coagulant complex and antifibrinolytics have been given simultaneously without complications. It is, however, recommended not to use antifibrinolytics until 12 hours after the administration of anti-inhibitor coagulant complex.

➤*Anamnestic responses:* Anamnestic responses with rise in Factor VIII inhibitor titer have been observed in 20% of the cases.

➤*Infectious disease transmission:* This product is prepared from pooled human plasma which may contain the causative agents of hepatitis and other viral diseases. Prescribed manufacturing procedures utilized at the plasma collection centers, plasma testing laboratories, and the fractionation facilities are designed to reduce the risk of transmitting viral infection. However, the risk of viral infectivity from this product cannot be totally eliminated.

➤*Viral infections:* Individuals who receive infusions of blood or plasma products may develop signs or symptoms of some viral infections, particularly non-A, non-B hepatitis.

➤*Pregnancy: Category C.* Animal reproduction studies have not been conducted with anti-inhibitor coagulant complex. It is also not known whether anti-inhibitor coagulant complex can cause fetal harm when administered to a pregnant woman or can affect reproduction capacity. Anti-inhibitor coagulant complex should be given to a pregnant woman only if clearly needed.

➤*Children:* No data are available regarding the use of anti-inhibitor coagulant complex in newborns.

Precautions

➤*Monitoring:* If clinical signs of intravascular coagulation occur, which include changes in blood pressure, pulse rate, respiratory distress, chest pain and cough, the infusion should be stopped promptly and appropriate diagnostic and therapeutic measures are to be initiated.

Laboratory indications of DIC are decreased fibrinogen, decreased platelet count, or presence of fibrin-fibrinogen degradation products (FDP). Other indications of DIC include significantly prolonged thrombin time, prothrombin time, or partial thromboplastin time.

➤*Non hemophilic patients:* Non-hemophilic patients with acquired inhibitors against Factors VIII, IX or XII may have both a bleeding tendency and an increased risk of thrombosis at the same time.

➤*Lab test abnormalities:* Tests used to control efficacy such as APTT, WBCT, and TEG do not correlate with clinical improvement. For this reason, attempts at normalizing these values by increasing the dose of anti-inhibitor coagulant complex may not be successful and are strongly discouraged because of the potential hazard of producing DIC by overdosage.

Adverse Reactions

In the course of treatment with preparations containing the prothrombin complex thromboembolic events may occur, particularly after high doses or in patients with thrombotic risk factors.

After application of high doses (single infusion of beyond 100 units/kg of body weight, and daily doses of 200 units/kg of body weight) of anti-inhibitor coagulant complex laboratory or clinical signs of DIC have occasionally been observed.

In individual instances myocardial infarction was found to occur after high doses or prolonged administration or in the presence of risk factors predisposing to myocardial infarction.

As with all human plasma products, any kind of allergic reaction may be seen, ranging from mild, short-term urticarial rashes to severe anaphylactoid reactions.

Administration of anti-inhibitor coagulant complex should be discontinued immediately, if such signs appear. Allergic reactions should be treated with antihistamines and glucocorticoids. Shock should be treated in the usual way.

FACTOR IX CONCENTRATES

Rx	**AlphaNine SD** (Grifols)	**Powder for injection**: Dried plasma fraction of Factor IX.[a] Solvent/detergent-treated. Virus-filtered.	In single-dose vials with diluent, needle, and filter.[b]
Rx	**BeneFix** (Genetics Institute)	**Powder for injection**: Nonpyrogenic lyophilized. Purified protein produced by recombinant DNA for use in Factor IX deficiency.[a]	Preservative free. In 250, 500 or 1,000 international units/single-dose vial with diluent, needle, filter, infusion set, and alcohol swabs.
Rx	**Mononine** (Aventis)	**Powder for injection**: Sterile, lyophilized concentrate of Factor IX, plasma-derived.	In 250, 500, and 1,000 units single-dose vials with diluent, double-ended needle, vented filter spike, winged infusion set, and alcohol swabs.[c]
Rx	**Profilnine SD** (Grifols)	**Powder for injection**: Sterile, lyophilized concentrate of Factor IX, plasma-derived. Solvent/detergent-treated.	Heparin free. Preservative free. In 250, 500, and 1,000 units single-dose vials with diluent.
Rx	**Proplex T** (Baxter)	**Powder for injection**: Plasma derived concentrate of clotting Factors II, VII, IX and X.[a] Heat-treated.	In 30 mL vials with diluent and needles.[c]
Rx	**Bebulin VH** (Baxter)	**Powder for injection**: Purified freeze-dried concentrate of coagulation Factor IX, II, and X. Heat-treated.[a]	In single-dose vials with Sterile Water for Injection, double-ended needle, and filter needle.

[a] Actual number of units shown on each bottle.
[b] Contains heparin and dextrose.
[c] Contains heparin.

FACTOR IX CONCENTRATES — INJECTION

Indications

➤*Factor IX deficiency (hemophilia B [Christmas disease]):* To prevent or control bleeding episodes. Do not use in mild Factor IX deficiency if fresh frozen plasma is effective. (See individual package inserts for product specifications.)

➤*Factor VII deficiency (Proplex T only):* Factor IX complex has been used in hemarthroses occurring in hemophiliacs with inhibitors to Factor VIII.

The Factor VII content present in *Proplex T* has been shown to be effective in prevention or control of bleeding episodes in patients with Factor VII deficiency.

Administration and Dosage

➤*Factor IX Deficiency (hemophilia B [Christmas disease]):* For IV use only. One international unit is defined as the activity present in 1 mL of pooled normal fresh plasma. The potency is standardized in terms of Factor IX content.

When reconstitution of Factor IX concentrate is complete, its infusion should commence within 3 hours. However, begin the infusion as promptly as is practical.

The amount of Factor IX concentrate required to restore normal hemostasis varies with circumstances and patient. Dosage depends on the degree of deficiency and desired hemostatic level of the deficient factor. Use the following formula as a guide to calculate dosage.

Units required to raise blood level percentages:

Recombinant Factor IX –

1.2 international units/kg × body weight (kg) × desired increase (% of normal)

Human-derived Factor IX –

1 international unit/kg × body weight (kg) × desired increase (% of normal).

If a 70 kg (154 lb) patient needs a 25% increase in Factor IX, give 1 unit/kg × 70 kg × 25 = 1,750 units.

FACTOR IX CONCENTRATES — INJECTION

Factor IX Dosing Guidelines in Bleeding Episodes and Surgery[a]			
Type of hemorrhage	Circulating Factor IX activity required (% or [international units/dL])	Dosing interval (hours)	Duration of therapy (days)
Minor Uncomplicated hemarthroses, superficial muscle, or soft tissue	20 to 30	12 to 24	1 to 2
Moderate Intramuscle or soft tissue with disconnection, mucous membranes, dental extractions, or hematuria	25 to 50	12 to 24	Treat until bleeding stops and healing begins; about 2 to 7 days.
Major Pharynx, retropharynx, retroperitoneum, CNS, surgery	50 to 100	12 to 24	7 to 10

[a] Adapted from: Roberts HR, Eberst ME. Current management of hemophilia B. *Hematol Oncol Clin North Am*. 1993;7:1269-1280.

As a general rule, 1 unit of human-derived Factor IX activity per kg will increase the circulating level of Factor IX by 1% of normal, and 1 international unit of recombinant Factor IX per kg of body weight will increase the circulatory activity of Factor IX by 0.8 international units/dL. Determine exact dosage based on the physician's judgment of circumstances, patient condition, degree of deficiency, and the desired level of Factor IX to be achieved. If inhibitors to Factor IX appear, use sufficient additional dosage to overcome the inhibitors.

To maintain an elevated level of the deficient factor, repeat dosage as needed. Clinical studies suggest relatively high levels may be maintained by daily or twice daily doses, while the lower effective levels may require injections only once every 2 or 3 days. A single dose may stop a minor bleeding episode.

➤*Factor VII deficiency (Proplex T only):* Units required to raise blood level percentages:

0.5 unit/kg × body weight (in kg) × desired increase (% of normal).

Repeat dose every 4 to 6 hours as needed.

If a 70 kg (154 lb) patient with a Factor VII level of 0% needs to be elevated to 25%, give 0.5 unit/kg × 70 kg × 25 = 875 units.

In preparation for and following surgery, maintain levels more than 25% for ≥ 1 week. Use laboratory control to assure such levels. To maintain levels more than 25% for a reasonable time, calculate each dose to raise levels to 40% to 60% of normal.

➤*Factor VIII inhibitor (Proplex T only):* Employ dosage levels approximating 75 international units/kg.

Proplex T is recommended when hemarthroses occurring in hemophiliacs with inhibitors to Factor VII cannot be resolved by administration of Factor IX complex and in other types of bleeding episodes in Factor VII-inhibitor patients.

➤*Rate of administration:* This varies with the individual product; adapt to response of the patient. Infuse slowly; 2 to 3 mL/min is suggested. If headache, flushing, or changes in pulse rate or blood pressure appear, stop the infusion until symptoms subside, then resume at a slower rate.

➤*Storage/Stability:* Refrigerate between 2° to 8°C (35° to 46°F). Do not freeze diluent.

➤*Pharmacology:* Factor IX is activated by factor VII in the extrinsic coagulation pathway as well as by Factor XIa in the intrinsic coagulation pathway. Activated Factor IX, in combination with activated Factor VIII, activates Factor X. This results in the conversion of prothrombin to thrombin. Thrombin then converts fibrinogen to fibrin, and a clot can be formed.

Factor IX is the specific clotting factor deficient in patients with hemophilia B and in patients with acquired factor IX deficiencies.

The administration of Factor IX concentrate raises Factor IX plasma levels, thus minimizing the hazards of hemorrhage in patients with Factor IX deficiency .

Proplex T, Bebulin VH – Plasma levels of factors II, VII, and X may be increased following administration of these preparations.

➤*Pharmacokinetics:* The mean half-life of Factor IX administered to Factor IX-deficient patients is ≈ 22 hours (range, 11 to 36 hours). The mean increase in circulating factor IX activity after IV infusion is 0.67 to 1.15 international units/dL rise per international units/kg body weight.

Known hypersensitivity to mouse protein (*Mononine*) or hamster protein (*BeneFix*).

➤*Hepatitis and AIDS:* Human-derived Factor IX products are prepared from pooled units of human plasma that may contain the causative agents of hepatitis and other viral and infectious diseases. Prescribed manufacturing procedures used at the plasma collection centers, plasma testing facilities, and the fractionation facility are designed to reduce the risk of transmitting viral infection. However, the risk of viral infectivity from these products cannot be totally eliminated.

Individuals receiving human-derived plasma product infusions may develop signs or symptoms of a viral infection, especially non-A, non-B hepatitis. Scientific opinion encourages hepatitis B and hepatitis A vaccination at birth or diagnosis for patients with hemophilia.

➤*Thromboembolic complications:* The administration of human Factor IX concentrates containing factors II, VII, IX, and X has been associated with the development of thromboembolic complications, MI, disseminated intravascular coagulation (DIC), venous thrombosis, and pulmonary embolism. Signs include change in pulse rate, blood pressure, respiratory distress, chest pain, and cough. Because of the potential risk of thromboembolic complications, exercise caution when administering these products to patients with liver disease, postoperative patients, neonates, or patients at risk for thromboembolic phenomena or DIC. In each of these situations, weigh the benefit of treatment against the risk of these complications.

If signs of DIC occur, stop the infusion promptly. To reduce the risk of enhancing intravascular coagulation, do not attempt to raise Factor IX or Factor VII levels to more than 50% of normal. If it is necessary to raise the patient's Factor IX or Factor VII level higher than 50% of normal, monitor infusion to detect signs and symptoms of DIC.

➤*Nephrotic syndrome:* Nephrotic syndrome has been reported following attempted immune tolerance induction with Factor IX products in hemophilia B patients with Factor IX inhibitors and a history of severe allergic reactions to Factor IX. The safety and efficacy of using Factor IX in attempted immune tolerance induction has not been established.

➤*Hypersensitivity reactions:* Activity-neutralizing antibodies (inhibitors) have been detected in patients receiving Factor IX-containing products. Monitor patients for the development of Factor IX inhibitors. Patients with these inhibitors may be at increased risk of anaphylaxis upon subsequent challenge with Factor IX. Evaluate patients experiencing allergic reactions for the presence of inhibitor.

Allergic-type hypersensitivity reactions, including anaphylaxis, have been reported for all Factor IX products. Frequently, these events have occurred in close temporal association with the development of Factor IX inhibitors. Inform patients of the early symptoms and signs of hypersensitivity reactions, including hives, generalized urticaria, angioedema, chest tightness, dyspnea, wheezing, faintness, hypotension, tachycardia, and anaphylaxis. Advise patients to discontinue use of the product, contact physician, and seek immediate emergency care, depending on the severity of the reactions, if any of these symptoms occur.

➤*Pregnancy: Category C.* It is not known whether Factor IX can cause fetal harm when administered to a pregnant woman. Give to a pregnant woman only if clearly needed.

➤*Children:* Safety and efficacy trials in pediatric patients 6 years of age or younger have not been conducted. Studies have been small or ongoing.

Mononine – A small trial evaluation of safety and effectiveness of *Mononine* in patients from 1 day of age to 20 years of age showed excellent hemostasis without thrombotic complications. Dosing in children is based on body weight and is based on the same adult guidelines.

➤*Monitoring:* Monitoring the Factor IX activity using the Factor IX activity assay is advised.

During clinical studies conducted in previously treated patients, 60 mild adverse reactions definitely, probably, or possibly related to therapy were reported. These were nausea (16), discomfort at the IV site (13), altered taste (10), burning sensation in the jaw and skull (6), allergic rhinitis (3), lightheadedness (2), headache (2), dizziness (1), chest tightness (1), fever (1), phlebitis/cellulitis at IV site (1), drowsiness (1), dry cough/sneeze (1), rash (1), and a single hive (1). Twelve days after a dose of Factor IX, 1 hepatitis C antibody-positive patient developed a renal infarct. The relationship of the infarct to Factor IX administration is uncertain.

➤*High doses:* The use of high doses of Factor IX concentrates may be associated with MI, DIC, venous thrombosis, and pulmonary embolism (see Warnings).

Postmarketing adverse reactions – Postmarketing adverse reactions included the following: Inadequate Factor IX recovery, inadequate therapeutic response, inhibitor development, anaphylaxis, laryngeal edema, angioedema, cyanosis, dyspnea, hypotension, thrombosis.

Rapid infusion rate – Headache, flushing, changes in blood pressure or pulse rate, transient fever, chills, tingling, urticaria, nausea, and vomiting may occur. Symptoms disappear promptly upon discontinuation. Except in the most reactive individuals, the infusion may be resumed at a slower rate.

Pyrogenic reactions – Chills and fever (particularly when large doses are used).

Profilnine SD – Adverse reactions may include the following: Urticaria, fever, chills, nausea, vomiting, headache, somnolence, lethargy, flushing, or tingling.

Patient Information

Advise patients of the early signs of hypersensitivity reactions including hives, generalized urticaria, tightness of the chest, wheezing, hypotension, anaphylaxis, dyspnea, faintness, angioedema, tachycardia, fever, nausea, rashes, and retching. Advise patients to discontinue use of the product and contact their physician if these symptoms occur.

ANTIHEMOPHILIC FACTOR/von WILLEBRAND FACTOR COMPLEX (Factor VIII/VWF; AHF/VWF)

Rx	Humate-P (Aventis Behring)	**Powder for injection, lyophilized:** 250 units AHF and 500 units VWF:RCo/vial[a]	In single-dose vials with 10 mL diluent, sterile transfer set for reconstitution, and a sterile filter spike for withdrawal.
		500 units AHF and 1000 units VWF:RCo/vial[a]	In single-dose vials with 20 mL diluent, sterile transfer set for reconstitution, and a sterile filter spike for withdrawal.
		1000 units AHF and 2000 units VWF:RCo/vial[a]	In single-dose vials with 30 mL diluent, sterile transfer set for reconstitution, and a sterile filter spike for withdrawal.

[a] Heat-treated. Upon reconstitution with the volume of diluent provided, each milliliter contains 20 to 40 units Factor VIII activity, 50 to 100 units von Willebrand factor:Ristocetin cofactor (VWF:RCo) activity, 15 to 33 mg of glycine, 3.5 to 9.3 mg of sodium citrate, 2 to 5.3 mg of sodium chloride, 4 to 8 mg of albumin (human), 1 to 7 mg of other proteins and 5 to 15 mg of total proteins. Contains anti-A and anti-B blood group isoagglutinins.

ANTIHEMOPHILIC FACTOR/von WILLEBRAND FACTOR COMPLEX (Factor VIII/VWF; AHF/VWF) — INJECTION

Indications

➤*Classical hemophilia:* In adult patients for treatment and prevention of bleeding in hemophilia A (classical hemophilia).

➤*von Willebrand disease:* In adult and pediatric patients for treatment of spontaneous and trauma-induced bleeding episodes in severe von Willebrand disease, and in mild and moderate von Willebrand disease where use of desmopressin is known or suspected to be inadequate.

Controlled clinical trials to evaluate the safety and efficacy of prophylactic dosing with *Humate-P* to prevent spontaneous bleeding and to prevent excessive bleeding related to surgery have not been evaluated in von Willebrand disease patients. Adequate data are not presently available on which to evaluate or to base dosing recommendations in either of these settings.

Administration and Dosage

➤*Approved by the FDA:* April 1, 1999.

Strongly consider administration of hepatitis A and hepatitis B vaccines to individuals receiving plasma derivatives. Potential risks and benefits of vaccination should be carefully weighed by the physician and discussed with the patient.

For IV administration only.

➤*Hemophilia A:* As a general rule, 1 unit of Factor VIII activity per kilogram body weight will increase the circulating Factor VIII level by approximately 2 units/dL. Adequacy of treatment must be judged by the clinical effects; thus, the dosage may vary with individual cases. Although dosage must be individualized according to the needs of the patient (weight, severity of hemorrhage, presence of inhibitors), the following general dosages are recommended for adult patients

Adult Dosage Recommendations for the Treatment of Hemophilia A

Hemorrhagic event	Dosage
Minor hemorrhage: •Early joint or muscle bleed •Severe epistaxis	Loading dose 15 units/kg to achieve FVIII:C plasma level of approximately 30% of normal; 1 infusion may be sufficient. If needed, half of the loading dose may be given once or twice daily for 1 to 2 days.
Moderate hemorrhage: •Advanced joint or muscle bleed •Neck, tongue or pharyngeal hematoma (without airway compromise) •Tooth extraction •Severe abdominal pain	Loading dose 25 units/kg to achieve FVIII:C plasma level of approximately 50% of normal, followed by 15 units/kg every 8 to 12 hours for first 1 to 2 days to maintain FVIII:C plasma level at 30% of normal, and then the same dose once or twice a day for a total of up to 7 days, or until adequate wound healing.
Life-threatening hemorrhage: •Major operations •GI bleeding •Neck, tongue, or pharyngeal hematoma with potential for airway compromise •Intracranial, intra-abdominal or intrathoracic bleeding •Fractures	Initially 40 to 50 units/kg, followed by 20 to 25 units/kg every 8 hours to maintain FVIII:C plasma level at 80% to 100% of normal for 7 days, then continue the same dose once or twice a day for another 7 days in order to maintain the FVIII:C level at 30% to 50% of normal.

Individualize dosage by clinical judgement of the potential for compromise of a vital structure, and by frequent monitoring of factor VIII activity in the patient's plasma.

➤*von Willebrand disease:* The dosage should be adjusted according to the extent and location of bleeding. As a rule, 40 to 80 units VWF:RCo (corresponding to 16 to 32 units factor VIII in *Humate-P*) per kilogram body weight are given every 8 to 12 hours. Repeat doses are administered for as long as needed based on repeat monitoring of appropriate clinical and laboratory measures. Expected levels of VWF:RCo are based on an expected in vivo recovery of 1.5 units/dL rise per units/kg VWF:RCo administered. The administration of 1 units of Factor VIII per kilogram body weight can be expected to lead to a rise in circulating VWF:RCo of approximately 3.5 to 4 units/dL. The following table provides dosing guidelines for pediatric and adult patients.

Dosing Recommendations for the Treatment of von Willebrand Disease

Classification of VWD	Hemorrhage	Dosage (units VWF:RCo/kg body weight)
Type 1 •Mild, if desmopressin is inappropriate (baseline VWF:RCo activity typically > 30%)	Major (eg, severe or refractory epistaxis, GI bleeding, CNS trauma, or traumatic hemorrhage)	Loading dose 40 to 60 units/kg, then 40 to 50 units/kg every 8 to 12 hours for 3 days to keep the nadir level of VWF:RCo > 50%; then 40 to 50 units/kg daily for a total of up to 7 days of treatment.
Type 1 •Moderate or severe (baseline VWF:RCo activity typically < 30%)	Minor (eg, epistaxis, oral bleeding, menorrhagia) Major (eg, severe or refractory epistaxis, GI bleeding, CNS trauma, hemarthrosis or traumatic hemorrhage	40 to 50 units/kg (1 or 2 doses). Loading dose 50 to 75 units/kg, then 40 to 60 units/kg every 8 to 12 hours for 3 days to keep the nadir level of VWF:RCo > 50%; then 40 to 60 units/kg/day for a total of up to 7 days of treatment. Monitor and maintain FVIII:C levels according to the guidelines for hemophilia A therapy. See above table.
Types 2 (all variants) and 3	Minor (clinical indications above) Major (clinical indications above)	40 to 50 units/kg (1 or 2 doses). Loading dose of 60 to 80 units/kg, then 40 to 60 units/kg every 8 to 12 hours for 3 days to keep the nadir level of VWF:RCo > 50% then 40 to 60 units/kg/day for a total of up to 7 days of treatment. Monitor and maintain FVIII:C levels according to the guidelines for hemophilia A therapy. See above table.

➤*Reconstitution:*

1.) Warm both diluent and *Humate-P* in unopened vials to room temperature (not above 37°C [98°F]).
2.) Pierce the double needle of the transfer set into the diluent vial. Remove the protective cap and insert the exposed (longer) needle into the upright *Humate-P* vial. The diluent will be transferred into the *Humate-P* by vacuum.
3.) Remove the diluent vial and the transfer set and discard.
4.) Gently rotate the vial. DO NOT SHAKE VIAL. Vigorous shaking will prolong the reconstitution time. Continue swirling until the powder is dissolved and the solution is ready for administration. To assure product sterility, administer within 3 hours after reconstitution.
5.) When the reconstitution procedure is precisely followed, it is not uncommon for a few small flakes or particles to remain. The filter spike provided with *Humate-P* should remove those particles and this should not influence dosage calculations.

➤*Administration:* Plastic disposable syringes are recommended for administration of *Humate-P* solution. The ground glass surface of all-glass syringes tend to adhere protein solutions of this type.

1.) Attach the filter spike to a sterile disposable syringe and take the filter spike out of the package.
2.) Remove the protective cap and - without touching the tip of the filter spike - insert the disposable filter spike into the stopper of the *Humate-P* vial; inject air.
3.) Draw up the solution slowly (when using several syringes leave the filter spike in the vial). Separate the syringe from the filter spike and attach the syringe to an infusion kit or a suitable injection needle. Discard the filter spike.
4.) Slowly inject the solution (maximally 4 mL/minute) intravenously with an infusion kit or with a suitable injection needle.

➤*Storage/Stability:* When stored at refrigerator temperature, 2° to 8°C (36° to 46°F), *Humate-P* is stable for the period indicated by the expiration date on its label. Within this period, *Humate-P* may be stored at room temperature not to exceed 30°C (86°F), for up to six months. Avoid freezing, which may damage the diluent container.

Actions

➤*Pharmacology:* The Antihemophilic Factor/VWF complex consists of two different noncovalently bound proteins (Factor VIII and von Willebrand factor). Factor VIII is an essential cofactor in activation of Factor X leading

ANTIHEMOPHILIC FACTOR/von WILLEBRAND FACTOR COMPLEX (Factor VIII/VWF; AHF/VWF) — INJECTION

ultimately to formation of thrombin and fibrin. The VWF promotes platelet aggregation and platelet adhesion on damaged vascular endothelium; it also serves as a stabilizing carrier protein for the procoagulant protein Factor VIII. The activity of VWF is measured as VWF:RCo.

➤*Pharmacokinetics:* After intravenous injection of *Humate-P* in humans, there is a rapid increase of plasma Factor VIII activity (FVIII:C) followed by a rapid decrease in activity and a subsequent slower rate of decrease in activity. Studies with *Humate-P* in hemophilic patients have demonstrated a mean half-life of 12.2 hours (range, 8.4 to 17.4 hours).

The pharmacokinetics of *Humate-P* have been evaluated in 8 VWD patients (type 1, n = 1; type 2, n = 1; type 2A, n = 4; type 3, n = 2) in the non-bleeding state. The median half-life of VWF:RCo was 10.3 hours (range, 6.4 to 13.3 hours). The median in vivo recovery for VWF:RCo activity was 1.89 (units/dL)/(units/kg) (range, 1.1 to 2.74 [units/dL]/]). In all patients, the administration of *Humate-P* resulted in a transient shortening of the bleeding time. *Humate-P* was effective in improving the VWF multimer pattern in VWD patients and in most cases this improvement was sustained through 22 to 26 hours postinfusion.

Contraindications

None known.

Warnings

➤*Thromboembolism:* Thromboembolic events have been reported in VWD patients receiving Antihemophilic Factor/von Willebrand Factor Complex replacement therapy, especially in the setting of known risk factors for thrombosis. Early reports might indicate a higher incidence in females. In addition, endogenous high levels of FVIII have also been associated with thrombosis but no causal relationship has been established. In all VWD patients in situations of high thrombotic risk receiving coagulation factor replacement therapy, caution should be exercised and antithrombotic measures should be considered (see Administration and Dosage).

➤*Transmission of infectious agents:* Antihemophilic Factor/von Willebrand Factor Complex is made from human plasma. Products made from human plasma may contain infectious agents, such as viruses, that can cause disease. The risk that such products will transmit an infectious agent has been reduced by screening plasma donors for prior exposure to certain viruses, by testing for the presence of certain current viral infections and by inactivating and/or removing certain viruses during manufacture. Despite these measures, such products can still potentially transmit disease. There is also the theoretical possibility that infectious agents not yet known or identified may be present in such products. Any infections thought by a physician possibly to have been transmitted by this product should be reported by the physician or other healthcare provider to Aventis Behring at (800) 504-5434 (in the U.S. and Canada). The physician should discuss the risks and benefits of this product with the patient.

➤*Hypersensitivity reactions:* Rare cases of allergic reaction and rise in temperature have been observed. Anaphylactic reactions can occur in rare instances. If allergic/anaphylactic reactions occur, the infusion should be discontinued and appropriate treatment given as required. In some cases, inhibitors of Factor VIII may occur. Allergic symptoms, including allergic reaction, urticaria, chest tightness, rash, pruritus, and edema, were reported in 6% of patients in a Canadian retrospective study; 2% experienced other adverse events that were considered to have a possible or probable relationship to the product. These included chills, phlebitis, vasodilation, and paresthesia. All adverse events were mild or moderate in intensity.

➤*Pregnancy: Category C.* It is not known whether *Humate-P* can cause fetal harm when administered to a pregnant woman or can affect reproduction capacity. *Humate-P* should be given to a pregnant woman only if clearly needed.

➤*Children:* Adequate and well-controlled studies with long term evaluation of joint damage have not been done in pediatric patients. Joint damage may result from suboptimal treatment of hemarthroses. For immediate control of bleeding for Hemophilia A, the general recommendations for dosing and administration for adults may be referenced (see Administration and Dosage).

The safety and effectiveness of *Humate-P* for the treatment of von Willebrand disease was demonstrated in 26 pediatric patients, including infants, children and adolescents but has not yet been evaluated in neonates. As in adults, pediatric patients should be dosed based upon weight (kg) (see Administration and Dosage).

Precautions

➤*Identification of clotting deficiency:* It is important to determine that the coagulation disorder is caused by factor VIII or VWF deficiency, since no benefit in treating other deficiencies can be expected.

➤*Isoagglutinin:* This Antihemophilic Factor/von Willebrand Factor preparation contains blood group isoagglutinins (anti-A and anti-B). When very large or frequently repeated doses are needed, as when inhibitors are present or when pre- and postsurgical care is involved, patients of blood groups A, B and AB should be monitored for signs of intravascular hemolysis and decreasing hematocrit values and be treated appropriately as required.

The replacement therapy should be monitored with the aid of coagulation tests, especially in cases of major surgery.

Adverse Reactions

Antihemophilic Factor/von Willebrand Factor (Human), Dried, Pasteurized, *Humate-P* is usually tolerated without reaction.

➤*Hypersensitivity:* See Warnings.

➤*Thromboembolism:* Reports of thromboembolic events in VWD patients with other thrombotic risk factors receiving coagulation factor replacement therapy have been obtained from spontaneous reports, published literature, and a European clinical study. Early reports might indicate a higher incidence in females. Caution should be exercised and antithrombotic measures should be considered in all VWD patients in situations of high thrombotic risk (see Warnings).

Patient Information

Some viruses, such as parvovirus B19 or hepatitis A, are particularly difficult to remove or inactivate at this time. Parvovirus B19 may most seriously affect pregnant women, or immune-compromised individuals.

Although the overwhelming number of hepatitis A and parvovirus B19 cases are community acquired, there have been reports of these infections associated with the use of some plasma-derived products. Therefore, physicians should be alert to the potential symptoms of parvovirus B19 and hepatitis A infections and inform patients under their supervision receiving plasma-derived products to report potential symptoms promptly.

Symptoms of parvovirus B19 may include low-grade fever, rash, arthralgias and transient symmetric, nondestructive arthritis. Diagnosis is often established by measuring B19 specific IgM and IgG antibodies. Symptoms of hepatitis A include low grade fever, anorexia, nausea, vomiting, fatigue and jaundice. A diagnosis may be established by determination of specific IgM antibodies.

HEMOSTATICS

Systemic

AMINOCAPROIC ACID

Rx	**Aminocaproic Acid** (VersaPharm)	**Tablets:** 500 mg	(VP 045). White, scored. In 100s.
Rx	**Amicar** (Xanodyne)		(LL A10). White, scored. In 100s.
Rx	**Amicar** (Xanodyne)	**Tablets:** 1,000 mg	(XP A 20). White, oblong, scored. In 100s.
Rx	**Amicar** (Xanodyne)	**Syrup:** 250 mg/mL	Parabens, EDTA, saccharin, sorbitol. Raspberry flavor. In 473 mL.
Rx	**Aminocaproic Acid** (VersaPharm)	**Oral solution:** 250 mg/mL	Saccharin, sorbitol, parabens. Raspberry flavor. In 237 and 473 mL.
Rx	**Aminocaproic Acid** (Various, eg, Abbott, American Regent)	**Injection:** 250 mg/mL	In 20 mL vials.

AMINOCAPROIC ACID — ORAL

Indications

➤*Excessive bleeding:* Aminocaproic acid is useful in enhancing hemostasis when fibrinolysis contributes to bleeding. In life-threatening situations, fresh whole blood transfusions, fibrinogen infusions, and other emergency measures may be required.

➤*Unlabeled uses:* Oral or IV aminocaproic acid, 36 g/day in six divided doses, has been used to prevent recurrence of subarachnoid hemorrhage (SAH).

In the management of amegakaryocytic thrombocytopenia, the need for platelet transfusion may be decreased by use of aminocaproic acid 8 to 24 g/day for 3 days to 13 months.

To abort and prevent attacks of hereditary angioneurotic edema.

In patients with acute promyelocytic leukemia who develop coagulopathy associated with low levels of alpha-2 – plasmin inhibitor.

To reduce postsurgical bleeding complications in patients undergoing cardiopulmonary bypass procedures (eg, 5 g IV followed by 1 g/hr infusions for 6 to 8 hours).

Administration and Dosage

➤*Plasma levels:* An initial dose of 5 g, followed by 1 to 1.25 g hourly, should achieve and sustain drug plasma levels at 0.13 mg/mL. This is the concentration apparently necessary for inhibition of fibrinolysis. Administration of more than 30 g/24 hours is not recommended.

➤*Tablets and Syrup:* If the patient is able to take medication by mouth, an identical dosage regimen may be followed by administering aminocaproic acid tablets or aminocaproic acid syrup, 25% as follows: For the treatment of acute bleeding syndromes due to elevated fibrinolytic activity, it is suggested that 10 tablets (5 g) or 4 teaspoonfuls of syrup (5 g) of aminocaproic acid be administered during the first hour of treatment, followed by a continuing rate of 2 tablets (1 g) or 1 teaspoonful of syrup (1.25 g) per hour. This method

AMINOCAPROIC ACID — ORAL

of treatment would ordinarily be continued for about 8 hours or until the bleeding situation has been controlled.

➤*Storage/Stability:* Store between 15° to 30°C (59° to 86°F). Dispense in tight containers. Do not freeze.

Actions

➤*Pharmacology:* The fibrinolysis-inhibitory effects of aminocaproic acid appear to be exerted principally via inhibition of plasminogen activators and to a lesser degree through antiplasmin activity.

➤*Pharmacokinetics:*

Absorption – In adults, oral absorption appears to be a zero-order process with an absorption rate of 5.2 g/hr. The mean lag time in absorption is 10 minutes. After a single oral dose of 5 g, absorption was complete (F = 1). Mean ± SD peak plasma concentrations (164 ± 28 mcg/mL) were reached within 1.2 ± 0.45 hours. A single IV dose has a duration of action of < 3 hours.

Distribution – After oral administration, the apparent volume of distribution was estimated to be 23.1 ± 6.6 L (mean ± SD). Correspondingly, the volume of distribution after intravenous administration has been reported to be 30 ± 8.2 L. After prolonged administration, aminocaproic acid has been found to distribute throughout extravascular and intravascular compartments of the body, penetrating human red blood cells as well as other tissue cells.

Excretion – Renal excretion is the primary route of elimination, whether aminocaproic acid is administered orally or intravenously. Sixty-five percent of the dose is recovered in the urine as unchanged drug and 11% of the dose appears as the metabolite adipic acid. Renal clearance (116 mL/min) approximates endogenous creatinine clearance. The total body clearance is 169 mL/min. The terminal elimination half-life for aminocaproic acid is approximately 2 hours.

Contraindications

Evidence of an active intravascular clotting process.

When there is uncertainty as to whether the cause of bleeding is primary fibrinolysis or disseminated intravascular coagulation (DIC), this distinction must be made before administering aminocaproic acid because aminocaproic acid administered to a patient with DIC may produce potentially fatal thrombus formation.

Aminocaproic acid must not be used in the presence of DIC without concomitant heparin.

Warnings

➤*Upper urinary tract bleeding:* In patients with upper urinary tract bleeding, aminocaproic acid administration has been known to cause intrarenal obstruction in the form of glomerular capillary thrombosis or clots in the renal pelvis and ureters. For this reason, aminocaproic acid should not be used in hematuria of upper urinary tract origin, unless the possible benefits outweigh the risk.

➤*Skeletal muscle weakness:* Rarely, skeletal muscle weakness with necrosis of muscle fibers has been reported following prolonged administration. Clinical presentation may range from mild myalgias with weakness and fatigue to a severe proximal myopathy with rhabdomyolysis, myoglobinuria, and acute renal failure. Muscle enzymes, especially creatine phosphokinase (CPK) are elevated. CPK levels should be monitored in patients on long-term therapy. Aminocaproic acid administration should be stopped if a rise in CPK is noted. Resolution follows discontinuation of aminocaproic acid; however, the syndrome may recur if aminocaproic acid is restarted.

➤*Cardiac/Hepatic lesions:* The possibility of cardiac muscle damage should also be considered when skeletal myopathy occurs. One case of cardiac and hepatic lesions observed in man has been reported. The patient received 2 g of aminocaproic acid every 6 hours for a total dose of 26 g. Death was due to continued cerebrovascular hemorrhage. Necrotic changes in the heart and liver were noted at autopsy.

➤*Fertility impairment:* Impairment of fertility consistent with the antifibrinolytic activity of aminocaproic acid has been suggested in some rodent studies. Dietary administration of an equivalent of the maximum human therapeutic dose of aminocaproic acid to rats of both sexes impaired fertility as evidenced by decreased implantations, litter sizes and number of pups born.

➤*Pregnancy: Category C.* Animal teratological studies have not been conducted with aminocaproic acid. It is also not known whether aminocaproic acid can cause fetal harm when administered to a pregnant woman or can affect reproduction capacity. Aminocaproic acid should be given to a pregnant woman only if clearly needed.

➤*Lactation:* It is not known whether this drug is excreted in human milk. Because many drugs are excreted in human milk, caution should be exercised when aminocaproic acid is administered to a nursing woman.

➤*Children:* Safety and effectiveness in pediatric patients have not been established.

Precautions

➤*Hyperfibrinolysis:* Aminocaproic acid inhibits both the action of plasminogen activators and to a lesser degree, plasmin activity. The drug should not be administered without a definite diagnosis and/or laboratory finding indicative of hyperfibrinolysis (hyperplasminemia).

Fibrinolysis is a normal process, presumably active at all times to ensure the fluidity of blood. Inhibition of fibrinolysis by aminocaproic acid may theoretically result in clotting or thrombosis. However, there is no definite evidence that administration of aminocaproic acid has been responsible for the few reported cases of intravascular clotting which followed this treatment. Rather, it appears that such intravascular clotting was most likely due to the patient's preexisting clinical condition, eg, the presence of DIC. It has been postulated that extravascular clots formed in vivo may not undergo spontaneous lysis as do normal clots.

➤*Neurological events:* Reports have appeared in the literature of an increased incidence of certain neurological deficits such as hydrocephalus, cerebral ischemia, or cerebral vasospasm associated with the use of antifibrinolytic agents in the treatment of subarachnoid hemorrhage (SAH). All of these events have also been described as part of the natural course of SAH, or as a consequence of diagnostic procedures such as angiography. Drug relatedness remains unclear.

➤*Thrombophlebitis:* Thrombophlebitis, a possibility with all intravenous therapy, should be guarded against by strict attention to the proper insertion of the needle and the fixing of its position.

➤*Thrombosis:* Epsilon-aminocaproic acid should not be administered with Factor IX Complex concentrates or Anti-Inhibitor Coagulant concentrates, as the risk of thrombosis may be increased.

➤*Special risk:*

Cardiac, hepatic or renal disease – Administer with caution to these patients. Animal pathology has shown endocardial hemorrhages, myocardial fat degeneration, and kidney concretions.

Subendocardial hemorrhages have been observed in dogs given intravenous infusions of 0.2 times the maximum human therapeutic dose of aminocaproic acid and in monkeys given 8 times the maximum human therapeutic dose of aminocaproic acid.

Fatty degeneration of the myocardium has been reported in dogs given intravenous doses of aminocaproic acid at 0.8 to 3.3 times the maximum human therapeutic dose and in monkeys given intravenous doses of aminocaproic acid at 6 times the maximum human therapeutic dose.

➤*Lab test abnormalities:* The use of aminocaproic acid should be accompanied by tests designed to determine the amount of fibrinolysis present. There are presently available: general tests such as those for the determination of the lysis of a clot of blood or plasma; and more specific tests for the study of various phases of fibrinolytic mechanisms.

These latter tests include both semiquantitative and quantitative techniques for the determination of profibrinolysin, fibrinolysin, and antifibrinolysin.

Drug Interactions

➤*Oral contraceptives or estrogens:* An increase in clotting factors leading to a hypercoagulable state may be produced by coadministration.

➤*Drug/Lab test interactions:* Prolongation of the template bleeding time has been reported during continuous intravenous infusion of aminocaproic acid at dosages exceeding 24 g/day. Platelet function studies in these patients have not demonstrated any significant platelet dysfunction. However, in vitro studies have shown that at high concentrations (7.4 mmol/L or 0.97 mg/mL and greater) EACA inhibits ADP and collagen-induced platelet aggregation, the release of ATP and serotonin, and the binding of fibrinogen to the platelets in a concentration-response manner. Following a 10 g bolus of aminocaproic acid, transient peak plasma concentrations of 4.6 mmol/L or 0.6 mg/mL have been obtained. The concentration of aminocaproic acid necessary to maintain inhibition of fibrinolysis is 0.99 mmol/L or 0.13 mg/mL. Administration of a 5 g bolus followed by 1 to 1.25 g/hr should achieve and sustain plasma levels of 0.13 mg/mL. Thus, concentrations which have been obtained in vivo clinically in patients with normal renal function are considerably lower than the in vitro concentrations found to induce abnormalities in platelet function tests. However, higher plasma concentrations of aminocaproic acid may occur in patients with severe renal failure.

Serum potassium may be elevated by aminocaproic acid, especially in patients with impaired renal function.

Adverse Reactions

Aminocaproic acid is generally well tolerated. The following adverse experiences have been reported:

➤*Cardiovascular:* Bradycardia; hypotension; peripheral ischemia; thrombosis.

➤*CNS:* Confusion; convulsions; delirium; dizziness; hallucinations; intracranial hypertension; stroke; syncope. Two cases of convulsions following IV administration have been reported.

➤*Dermatologic:* Pruritus; rash.

➤*GI:* Abdominal pain; diarrhea; nausea; vomiting.

➤*GU:* BUN increased; renal failure.

➤*Hematologic:* Agranulocytosis; coagulation disorder; leukopenia; thrombocytopenia.

➤*Hypersensitivity:* Allergic and anaphylactoid reactions; anaphylaxis.

➤*Local:* Injection site reactions; pain and necrosis.

➤*Musculoskeletal:* CPK increased; muscle weakness; myalgia; myopathy (see Warnings); myositis; rhabdomyolysis.

➤*Respiratory:* Dyspnea; nasal congestion; pulmonary embolism.

➤*Special senses:* Tinnitus; vision decreased; watery eyes.

➤*Miscellaneous:* Edema; headache; malaise.

AMINOCAPROIC ACID — ORAL

There have been some reports of dry ejaculation during the period of aminocaproic acid treatment. These have been reported to date only in hemophilia patients who received the drug after undergoing dental surgical procedures. However, this symptom resolved in all patients within 24 to 48 hours of completion of therapy.

There have been reports of an increased incidence of certain neurological deficits (eg, hydrocephalus, cerebral ischemia, cerebral vasospasm) associated with use of fibrinolytic agents in the treatment of SAH. All of these events have also been described as part of the natural course of SAH, or as a consequence of diagnostic procedures such as angiography. Drug relatedness remains unclear.

Overdosage

A few cases of acute overdosage with aminocaproic acid have been reported with the injection formulation. See the aminocaproic acid injection monograph for specific details.

The intravenous and oral LD_{50} of aminocaproic acid were 3 and 12 g/kg, respectively, in the mouse and 3.2 and 16.4 g/kg, respectively, in the rat. An intravenous infusion dose of 2.3 g/kg was lethal in the dog. On intravenous administration, tonic-clonic convulsions were observed in dogs and mice. No treatment for overdosage is known, although evidence exists that aminocaproic acid is removed by hemodialysis and may be removed by peritoneal dialysis. Pharmacokinetic studies have shown that total body clearance of aminocaproic acid is markedly decreased in patients with severe renal failure.

AMINOCAPROIC ACID — INJECTION

Indications

➤*Excessive bleeding:* Aminocaproic acid is useful in enhancing hemostasis when fibrinolysis contributes to bleeding. In life-threatening situations, fresh whole blood transfusions, fibrinogen infusions, and other emergency measures may be required.

➤*Unlabeled uses:* Oral or IV aminocaproic acid, 36 g/day in 6 divided doses, has been used to prevent recurrence of subarachnoid hemorrhage (SAH).

In the management of amegakaryocytic thrombocytopenia, the need for platelet transfusion may be decreased by use of aminocaproic acid 8 to 24 g/day for 3 days to 13 months.

To abort and prevent attacks of hereditary angioneurotic edema.

In patients with acute promyelocytic leukemia who develop coagulopathy associated with low levels of alpha-2–plasmin inhibitor.

To reduce postsurgical bleeding complications in patients undergoing cardiopulmonary bypass procedures (eg, 5 g IV followed by 1 g/hr infusions for 6 to 8 hours).

Administration and Dosage

➤*Plasma levels:* An initial dose of 5 g, followed by 1 to 1.25 g hourly, should achieve and sustain drug plasma levels at 0.13 mg/mL. This is the concentration apparently necessary for inhibition of fibrinolysis. Administration of more than 30 g/24 hours is not recommended.

➤*Intravenous:* Aminocaproic acid injection is administered by infusion, utilizing the usual compatible intravenous vehicles (eg, Sterile Water for Injection, Sodium Chloride for Injection, 5% Dextrose or Ringer's Injection). Although Sterile Water for Injection is compatible for intravenous injection the resultant solution is hypo-osmolar. Rapid injection of aminocaproic acid injection undiluted into a vein is not recommended. Hypotension, bradycardia, or arrhythmia may result.

For the treatment of acute bleeding syndromes due to elevated fibrinolytic activity, it is suggested that 16 to 20 mL (4 to 5 g) of aminocaproic acid injection in 250 mL of diluent be administered by infusion during the first hour of treatment, followed by a continuing infusion at the rate of 4 mL (1 g) per hour in 50 mL of diluent. This method of treatment would ordinarily be continued for about 8 hours or until the bleeding situation has been controlled.

➤*Storage / Stability:* Store between 15° to 30°C (59° to 86°F). Do not freeze.

Parenteral drug products should be inspected visually for particulate matter and discoloration prior to administration, whenever solution and container permit.

Actions

➤*Pharmacology:* The fibrinolysis-inhibitory effects of aminocaproic acid appear to be exerted principally via inhibition of plasminogen activators and to a lesser degree through antiplasmin activity.

➤*Pharmacokinetics:*

Distribution – After oral administration, the apparent volume of distribution was estimated to be 23.1 ± 6.6 L (mean ± SD). Correspondingly, the volume of distribution after intravenous administration has been reported to be 30 ± 8.2 L. After prolonged administration, aminocaproic acid has been found to distribute throughout extravascular and intravascular compartments of the body, penetrating human red blood cells as well as other tissue cells.

Metabolism – A single IV dose has a duration of action less than 3 hours.

Excretion – Renal excretion is the primary route of elimination, whether aminocaproic acid is administered orally or intravenously. Sixty-five percent of the dose is recovered in the urine as unchanged drug and 11% of the dose appears as the metabolite adipic acid. Renal clearance (116 mL/min) approximates endogenous creatinine clearance. The total body clearance is 169 mL/min. The terminal elimination half-life for aminocaproic acid is approximately 2 hours.

Contraindications

Evidence of an active intravascular clotting process.

When there is uncertainty as to whether the cause of bleeding is primary fibrinolysis or disseminated intravascular coagulation (DIC), this distinction must be made before administering aminocaproic acid because aminocaproic acid administered to a patient with DIC may produce potentially fatal thrombus formation.

Aminocaproic acid must not be used in the presence of DIC without concomitant heparin.

Warnings

➤*Upper urinary tract bleeding:* In patients with upper urinary tract bleeding, aminocaproic acid administration has been known to cause intrarenal obstruction in the form of glomerular capillary thrombosis or clots in the renal pelvis and ureters. For this reason, aminocaproic acid should not be used in hematuria of upper urinary tract origin, unless the possible benefits outweigh the risk.

Subendocardial hemorrhages have been observed in dogs given intravenous infusions of 0.2 times the maximum human therapeutic dose of aminocaproic acid and in monkeys given 8 times the maximum human therapeutic dose of aminocaproic acid.

Fatty degeneration of the myocardium has been reported in dogs given intravenous doses of aminocaproic acid at 0.8 to 3.3 times the maximum human therapeutic dose and in monkeys given intravenous doses of aminocaproic acid at 6 times the maximum human therapeutic dose.

➤*Skeletal muscle weakness:* Rarely, skeletal muscle weakness with necrosis of muscle fibers has been reported following prolonged administration. Clinical presentation may range from mild myalgias with weakness and fatigue to a severe proximal myopathy with rhabdomyolysis, myoglobinuria, and acute renal failure. Muscle enzymes, especially creatine phosphokinase (CPK) are elevated. CPK levels should be monitored in patients on long-term therapy. Aminocaproic acid administration should be stopped if a rise in CPK is noted. Resolution follows discontinuation of aminocaproic acid; however, the syndrome may recur if aminocaproic acid is restarted.

➤*Cardiac and hepatic lesions:* The possibility of cardiac muscle damage should also be considered when skeletal myopathy occurs. One case of cardiac and hepatic lesions observed in man has been reported. The patient received 2 g of aminocaproic acid every 6 hours for a total dose of 26 g. Death was due to continued cerebrovascular hemorrhage. Necrotic changes in the heart and liver were noted at autopsy.

➤*Fertility impairment:* Impairment of fertility consistent with the antifibrinolytic activity of aminocaproic acid has been suggested in some rodent studies. Dietary administration of an equivalent of the maximum human therapeutic dose of aminocaproic acid to rats of both sexes impaired fertility as evidenced by decreased implantations, litter sizes, and number of pups born.

➤*Pregnancy: Category C.* Animal teratological studies have not been conducted with aminocaproic acid. It is also not known whether aminocaproic acid can cause fetal harm when administered to a pregnant woman or can affect reproduction capacity. Aminocaproic acid should be given to a pregnant woman only if clearly needed.

➤*Lactation:* It is not known whether this drug is excreted in human milk. Because many drugs are excreted in human milk, caution should be exercised when aminocaproic acid is administered to a nursing woman.

➤*Children:* Safety and effectiveness in pediatric patients have not been established.

Precautions

➤*Benzyl alcohol:* Aminocaproic acid injection contains benzyl alcohol as a preservative and is not recommended for use in newborns.

➤*Hyperfibrinolysis:* Aminocaproic acid inhibits both the action of plasminogen activators and to a lesser degree, plasmin activity. The drug should not be administered without a definite diagnosis or laboratory finding indicative of hyperfibrinolysis (hyperplasminemia).

Fibrinolysis is a normal process, presumably active at all times to ensure the fluidity of blood. Inhibition of fibrinolysis by aminocaproic acid may theoretically result in clotting or thrombosis. However, there is no definite evidence that administration of aminocaproic acid has been responsible for the few reported cases of intravascular clotting which followed this treatment. Rather, it appears that such intravascular clotting was most likely due to the patient's preexisting clinical condition, eg, the presence of DIC. It has been postulated that extravascular clots formed in vivo may not undergo spontaneous lysis as do normal clots.

➤*Neurologic events:* Reports have appeared in the literature of an increased incidence of certain neurological deficits such as hydrocephalus, cerebral ischemia, or cerebral vasospasm associated with the use of antifibrinolytic agents in the treatment of subarachnoid hemorrhage (SAH). All of these events have also been described as part of the natural course of SAH, or as a consequence of diagnostic procedures such as angiography. Drug relatedness remains unclear.

➤*Thrombophlebitis:* Thrombophlebitis, a possibility with all intravenous therapy, should be guarded against by strict attention to the proper insertion of the needle and the fixing of its position.

AMINOCAPROIC ACID — INJECTION

➤*Thrombosis:* Thrombosis with severe sequelae (acute myocardial infarction, gangreno) has been rarely reported in patients with hemophilia receiving combined treatment with Factor IX concentrate and aminocaproic acid. Aminocaproic acid should not be administered concomitantly with prothrombin complex concentrates or with activated prothrombin concentrates unless the increased risk of thrombosis is outweighed by the anticipated clinical benefit.

Epsilon-aminocaproic acid should not be administered with Factor IX complex concentrates or anti-inhibitor coagulant concentrates, as the risk of thrombosis may be increased.

➤*Special risk:*

Cardiac, hepatic, or renal disease – Administer with caution to these patients. Animal pathology has shown endocardial hemorrhages, myocardial fat degeneration, and kidney concretions.

➤*Lab test abnormalities:* The use of aminocaproic acid should be accompanied by tests designed to determine the amount of fibrinolysis present. There are presently available: General tests such as those for the determination of the lysis of a clot of blood or plasma; and more specific tests for the study of various phases of fibrinolytic mechanisms.

These latter tests include both semiquantitative and quantitative techniques for the determination of profibrinolysin, fibrinolysin, and antifibrinolysin.

Drug Interactions

➤*Drug/Lab test interactions:* Prolongation of the template bleeding time has been reported during continuous IV infusion of aminocaproic acid at dosages exceeding 24 g/day. Platelet function studies in these patients have not demonstrated any significant platelet dysfunction. However, in vitro studies have shown that at high concentrations (7.4 mMol/L or 0.97 mg/mL or greater) EACA inhibits ADP and collagen-induced platelet aggregation, the release of ATP and serotonin, and the binding of fibrinogen to the platelets in a concentration-response manner. Following a 10 g bolus of aminocaproic acid, transient peak plasma concentrations of 4.6 mMol/L or 0.6 mg/mL have been obtained. The concentration of aminocaproic acid necessary to maintain inhibition of fibrinolysis is 0.99 mMol/L or 0.13 mg/mL. Administration of a 5 g bolus followed by 1 to 1.25 g/hr should achieve and sustain plasma levels of 0.13 mg/mL. Thus, concentrations which have been obtained in vivo clinically in patients with normal renal function are considerably lower than the in vitro concentrations found to induce abnormalities in platelet function tests. However, higher plasma concentrations of aminocaproic acid may occur in patients with severe renal failure.

Adverse Reactions

Aminocaproic acid is generally well tolerated. The following adverse reactions have been reported:

➤*Cardiovascular:* Bradycardia; hypotension; peripheral ischemia; thrombosis.

➤*CNS:* Confusion; convulsions; delirium; dizziness; hallucinations; intracranial hypertension; stroke; syncope.

➤*Dermatologic:* Pruritus; rash.

➤*GI:* Abdominal pain; diarrhea; nausea; vomiting.

➤*GU:* BUN increased; renal failure.

➤*Hematologic:* Agranulocytosis; coagulation disorder; leukopenia; thrombocytopenia.

➤*Hypersensitivity:* Allergic and anaphylactoid reactions; anaphylaxis.

➤*Local:* Injection site reactions; pain and necrosis.

➤*Musculoskeletal:* CPK increased; muscle weakness; myalgia; myopathy; myositis; rhabdomyolysis.

➤*Respiratory:* Dyspnea; nasal congestion; pulmonary embolism.

➤*Special senses:* Tinnitus; vision decreased; watery eyes.

➤*Miscellaneous:* Edema; headache; malaise.

There have been some reports of dry ejaculation during the period of aminocaproic acid treatment. These have been reported to date only in hemophilia patients who received the drug after undergoing dental surgical procedures. However, this symptom resolved in all patients within 24 to 48 hours of completion of therapy.

There have been reports of an increased incidence of certain neurological deficits (eg, hydrocephalus, cerebral ischemia, cerebral vasospasm) associated with use of fibrinolytic agents in the treatment of SAH. All of these events have also been described as part of the natural course of SAH, or as a consequence of diagnostic procedures such as angiography. Drug relatedness remains unclear.

Overdosage

➤*Symptoms:* A few cases of acute overdosage with aminocaproic acid administered intravenously have been reported. The effects have ranged from no reaction to transient hypotension to severe acute renal failure leading to death. One patient with a history of brain tumor and seizures experienced seizures after receiving an 8 g bolus injection of aminocaproic acid. The single dose of aminocaproic acid causing symptoms of overdosage or considered to be life-threatening is unknown. Patients have tolerated doses as high as 100 grams while acute renal failure has been reported following a dose of 12 g.

➤*Treatment:* The intravenous and oral LD_{50} of aminocaproic acid were 3 and 12 g/kg, respectively, in the mouse and 3.2 and 16.4 g/kg, respectively, in the rat. An intravenous infusion dose of 2.3 g/kg was lethal in the dog. On intravenous administration, tonic-clonic convulsions were observed in dogs and mice. No treatment for overdosage is known, although evidence exists that aminocaproic acid is removed by hemodialysis and may be removed by peritoneal dialysis. Pharmacokinetic studies have shown that total body clearance of aminocaproic acid is markedly decreased in patients with severe renal failure.

TRANEXAMIC ACID

Rx	**Cyklokapron** (Kabi Pharmacia)	**Tablets:** 500 mg	(CY). White. In 100s.
		Injection: 100 mg/mL	In 10 mL amps.

TRANEXAMIC ACID — ORAL

Indications

➤*Hemorrhage:* In patients with hemophilia for short-term use (2 to 8 days) to reduce or prevent hemorrhage and reduce the need for replacement therapy during and following tooth extraction.

➤*Unlabeled uses:* Tranexamic acid has been used for many hemostatic purposes including prevention of bleeding after surgery or trauma (eg, tonsillectomy and adenoidectomy, prostatic surgery, and cervical conization), and to prevent rebleeding of subarachnoid hemorrhage. It has also been used to treat primary or IUD-induced menorrhagia, gastric and intestinal hemorrhage, recurrent epistaxis, and hereditary angioneurotic edema. Tranexamic acid has been used with systemic therapy topically as a mouthwash to reduce bleeding after oral surgery in patients on anticoagulant therapy. The drug also inhibits induced hyperfibrinolysis during thrombolytic treatment with plasminogen activators.

Administration and Dosage

Following surgery, a dose of 25 mg per kg body weight may be given orally 3 or 4 times daily for 2 to 8 days.

Alternatively, tranexamic acid can be administered entirely orally, 25 mg per kg body weight 3 to 4 times a day beginning 1 day prior to surgery.

➤*Renal function impairment:*

Tranexamic Acid Dosage for Moderate to Severe Renal Function Impairment

Serum creatinine (mcmol/L)	Tablets
120 to 250 (1.36 to 2.83 mg/dL)	15 mg/kg twice daily
250 to 500 (2.83 to 5.66 mg/dL)	15 mg/kg daily
> 500 (> 5.66 mg/dL)	15 mg/kg every 48 hours or 7.5 mg/kg every 24 hours

➤*Storage/Stability:* Store tranexamic acid tablets at room temperature, 15° to 30°C (59° to 86°F).

Actions

➤*Pharmacology:* Tranexamic acid is a competitive inhibitor of plasminogen activation, and at much higher concentrations, a noncompetitive inhibitor of plasmin, ie, actions similar to aminocaproic acid. Tranexamic acid is about 10 times more potent in vitro than aminocaproic acid.

Tranexamic acid binds more strongly than aminocaproic acid to both the strong and weak receptor sites of the plasminogen molecule in a ratio corresponding to the difference in potency between the compounds. Tranexamic acid in a concentration of 1 mg/mL does not aggregate platelets in vitro.

Tranexamic acid in concentrations up to 10 mg/mL blood has no influence on the platelet count, the coagulation time or various coagulation factors in whole blood or citrated blood from healthy subjects. On the other hand, tranexamic acid in concentrations of 10 mg and 1 mg per mL blood prolongs the thrombin time.

The plasma protein binding of tranexamic acid is about 3% at therapeutic plasma levels and seems to be fully accounted for by its binding to plasminogen. Tranexamic acid does not bind to serum albumin.

➤*Pharmacokinetics:*

Absorption – Absorption of tranexamic acid after oral administration in humans represents approximately 30% to 50% of the ingested dose and bioavailability is not affected by food intake.

Distribution – The plasma peak level after 1 g orally is 8 mg/L and after 2 g, 15 mg/L, both obtained 3 hours after dosing.

Tranexamic acid passes through the placenta. The concentration in cord blood after an IV injection of 10 mg/kg to pregnant women is about 30 mg/L, as high as in the maternal blood. Tranexamic acid diffuses rapidly into joint fluid and the synovial membrane. In the joint fluid the same concentration is obtained as in the serum. The biological half-life of tranexamic acid in the joint fluid is about 3 hours.

TRANEXAMIC ACID — ORAL

The concentration of tranexamic acid in a number of other tissues is lower than in blood. In breast milk the concentration is about one-hundredth of the serum peak concentration. Tranexamic acid concentration in cerebrospinal fluid is about one-tenth of that of the plasma. The drug passes into the aqueous humor, the concentration being about one-tenth of the plasma concentration.

Tranexamic acid has been detected in semen where it inhibits fibrinolytic activity but does not influence sperm migration.

Metabolism – Only a small fraction of the drug is metabolized.

Excretion – Urinary excretion is the main route of elimination via glomerular filtration. Overall renal clearance is equal to overall plasma clearance (110 to 116 mL/min) and more than 95% of the dose is excreted in the urine as the unchanged drug. After oral administration of 10 to 15 mg per kg body weight, the cumulative urinary excretion at 24 hours is 39% and at 48 hours, 41% of the ingested dose or 78% and 82% of the absorbed material.

After oral administration, 1% of the dicarboxylic acid and 0.5% of the acetylated compound are excreted.

An antifibrinolytic concentration of tranexamic acid remains in different tissues for about 17 hours, and in the serum, up to 7 or 8 hours.

Contraindications

Acquired defective color vision, since this prohibits measuring one endpoint that should be followed as a measure of toxicity (see Warnings); subarachnoid hemorrhage (anecdotal experience indicates that cerebral edema and cerebral infarction may be caused by tranexamic acid in such patients); active intravascular clotting.

Warnings

➤*Visual abnormalities and retinal degeneration:* Focal areas of retinal degeneration have developed in cats, dogs and rats following tranexamic acid at doses between 250 to 1600 mg/kg/day (6 to 40 times the recommended usual human dose) from 6 days to 1 year. The incidence of such lesions has varied from 25% to 100% of animals treated and was dose-related. At lower doses some lesions have appeared to be reversible.

Limited data in cats and rabbits showed retinal changes in some animals with doses as low as 126 mg/kg/day (only about 3 times the recommended human dose) administered for several days to 2 weeks.

No retinal changes have been reported or noted in eye examinations in patients treated with tranexamic acid for weeks to months in clinical trials.

However, visual abnormalities, often poorly characterized, represent the most frequently reported postmarketing adverse reaction in Sweden. For patients who are to be treated continually for longer than several days, an ophthalmological examination, including visual acuity, color vision, eye-ground and visual fields, is advised, before commencing and at regular intervals during the course of treatment. Tranexamic acid should be discontinued if changes in examination results are found.

➤*Renal function impairment:* The dose of tranexamic acid tablets should be reduced in patients with renal insufficiency because of the risk of accumulation (see Administration and Dosage).

➤*Carcinogenesis:* An increased incidence of leukemia in male mice receiving tranexamic acid in food at a concentration of 4.8% (equivalent to doses as high as 5 g/kg/day) may have been related to treatment. Female mice were not included in this experiment. Hyperplasia of the biliary tract and cholangioma and adenocarcinoma of the intrahepatic biliary system have been reported in one strain of rats after dietary administration of doses exceeding the maximum tolerated dose for 22 months. Hyperplastic, but not neoplastic, lesions were reported at lower doses. Subsequent long term dietary administration studies in a different strain of rat, each with an exposure level equal to the maximum level employed in the earlier experiment, have failed to show such hyperplastic/neoplastic changes in the liver.

➤*Pregnancy: Category B.* There are no adequate and well-controlled studies in pregnant women. However, tranexamic acid is known to pass the placenta and appears in cord blood at concentrations approximately equal to maternal concentration. Because animal reproduction studies are not always predictive of human response, this drug should be used during pregnancy only if clearly needed.

➤*Lactation:* Tranexamic acid is present in the mother's milk at a concentration of about a hundredth of the corresponding serum levels. Caution should be exercised when tranexamic acid is administered to a nursing woman.

➤*Children:* The drug has had limited use in pediatric patients, principally in connection with tooth extraction. The limited data suggest that dosing instructions for adults can be used for pediatric patients needing tranexamic acid therapy.

Precautions

➤*Ureteral obstruction:* Ureteral obstruction due to clot formation in patients with upper urinary tract bleeding has been reported in patients treated with tranexamic acid.

➤*Thrombosis/Thromboembolism:* Venous and arterial thrombosis or thromboembolism has been reported in patients treated with tranexamic acid. In addition, cases of central retinal artery and central retinal vein obstruction have been reported.

Patients with a history of thromboembolic disease may be at increased risk for venous or arterial thrombosis.

Tranexamic acid should not be administered concomitantly with factor IX complex concentrates or anti-inhibitor coagulant concentrates, as the risk of thrombosis may be increased.

➤*Disseminated intravascular coagulation (DIC):* Patients with DIC, who require treatment with tranexamic acid, must be under strict supervision of a physician experienced in treating this disorder.

Adverse Reactions

➤*Cardiovascular:* Hypotension has been observed when intravenous injection is too rapid. To avoid this response, the solution should not be injected more rapidly than 1 mL/min. This adverse reaction has not been reported with oral administration.

Hypotension has been reported occasionally.

➤*GI:* GI disturbances (nausea, vomiting, diarrhea) may occur but disappear when the dosage is reduced.

➤*Miscellaneous:* Giddiness.

➤*Worldwide postmarketing reports:* Thromboembolic events (eg, deep vein thrombosis, pulmonary embolism, cerebral thrombosis, and central retinal artery and vein obstruction) have been rarely reported in patients receiving tranexamic acid for indications other than hemorrhage prevention in patients with hemophilia. However, due to the spontaneous nature of the reporting of medical events and the lack of controls, the actual incidence and causal relationship of drug and event cannot be determined.

Overdosage

There is no known case of overdosage of tranexamic acid tablets.

➤*Symptoms:* Symptoms of overdosage may be nausea, vomiting, orthostatic symptoms or hypotension.

TRANEXAMIC ACID — INJECTION

Indications

➤*Hemorrhage:* In patients with hemophilia for short-term use (2 to 8 days) to reduce or prevent hemorrhage and reduce the need for replacement therapy during and following tooth extraction.

➤*Unlabeled uses:* Tranexamic acid has been used for many hemostatic purposes including prevention of bleeding after surgery or trauma (eg, tonsillectomy and adenoidectomy, prostatic surgery, and cervical conization), and to prevent rebleeding of subarachnoid hemorrhage. It has also been used to treat primary or IUD-induced menorrhagia, gastric and intestinal hemorrhage, recurrent epistaxis, and hereditary angioneurotic edema. Tranexamic acid has been used with systemic therapy topically as a mouthwash to reduce bleeding after oral surgery in patients on anticoagulant therapy. The drug also inhibits hyperfibrinolysis during thrombolytic treatment with plasminogen activators.

Administration and Dosage

Parenteral therapy, 10 mg per kg body weight 3 to 4 times daily can be used for patients unable to take oral medication.

➤*Dental extraction in patients with hemophilia:* Immediately before dental extraction in patients with hemophilia, administer 10 mg per kg body weight of tranexamic acid intravenously together with replacement therapy.

➤*Renal function impairment:*

Moderate to Severe Renal Function Impairment Dosage	
Serum creatinine (mcmol/L)	IV dosage
120 to 250 (1.36 to 2.83 mg/dL)	10 mg/kg twice daily
250 to 500 (2.83 to 5.66 mg/dL)	10 mg/kg daily
> 500 (> 5.66 mg/dL)	10 mg/kg every 48 hours or 5 mg/kg every 24 hours

➤*Admixture compatibility/incompatibilities:* For IV infusion, tranexamic acid injection may be mixed with most solutions for infusion such as electrolyte solutions, carbohydrate solutions, amino acid solutions and Dextran solutions. The mixture should be prepared the same day the solution is to be used. Heparin may be added to tranexamic acid injection. Tranexamic acid injection should not be mixed with blood. The drug is a synthetic amino acid, and should not be mixed with solutions containing penicillin.

➤*Storage/Stability:* Store tranexamic injection at room temperature, 15° to 30°C (59° to 86°F).

TRANEXAMIC ACID — INJECTION

Actions

➤*Pharmacology:*

Electrophysiology – Tranexamic acid is a competitive inhibitor of plasminogen activation, and at much higher concentrations, a noncompetitive inhibitor of plasmin, ie, actions similar to aminocaproic acid. Tranexamic acid is about 10 times more potent in vitro than aminocaproic acid.

Tranexamic acid binds more strongly than aminocaproic acid to both the strong and weak receptor sites of the plasminogen molecule in a ratio corresponding to the difference in potency between the compounds. Tranexamic acid in a concentration of 1 mg/mL does not aggregate platelets in vitro.

Tranexamic acid in concentrations up to 10 mg/mL blood has no influence on the platelet count, the coagulation time or various coagulation factors in whole blood or citrated blood from healthy subjects. On the other hand, tranexamic acid in concentrations of 10 mg and 1 mg/mL blood prolongs the thrombin time.

The plasma protein binding of tranexamic acid is about 3% at therapeutic plasma levels and seems to be fully accounted for by its binding to plasminogen. Tranexamic acid does not bind to serum albumin.

➤*Pharmacokinetics:*

Distribution – After an intravenous dose of 1 g, the plasma concentration time curve shows a triexponential decay with a half-life of about 2 hours for the terminal elimination phase. The initial volume of distribution is about 9 to 12 L.

Tranexamic acid passes through the placenta. The concentration in cord blood after an intravenous injection of 10 mg/kg to pregnant women is about 30 mg/L, as high as in the maternal blood. Tranexamic acid diffuses rapidly into joint fluid and the synovial membrane. In the joint fluid the same concentration is obtained as in the serum. The biological half-life of tranexamic acid in the joint fluid is about 3 hours.

The concentration of tranexamic acid in a number of other tissues is lower than in blood. In breast milk the concentration is about one-hundredth of the serum peak concentration. Tranexamic acid concentration in cerebrospinal fluid is about one-tenth of that of the plasma. The drug passes into the aqueous humor, the concentration being about one-tenth of the plasma concentration.

Tranexamic acid has been detected in semen where it inhibits fibrinolytic activity but does not influence sperm migration.

Metabolism – Only a small fraction of the drug is metabolized.

Excretion – Urinary excretion is the main route of elimination via glomerular filtration. Overall renal clearance is equal to overall plasma clearance (110 to 116 mL/min) and more than 95% of the dose is excreted in the urine as the unchanged drug. Excretion of tranexamic acid is about 90% at 24 hours after intravenous administration of 10 mg per kg body weight. After oral administration of 10 to 15 mg per kg body weight, the cumulative urinary excretion at 24 hours is 39% and at 48 hours, 41% of the ingested dose or 78% and 82% of the absorbed material.

An antifibrinolyic concentration of tranexamic acid remains in different tissues for about 17 hours, and in the serum up to 7 to 8 hours.

Contraindications

Acquired defective color vision, since this prohibits measuring one endpoint that should be followed as a measure of toxicity (see Warnings); subarachnoid hemorrhage (anecdotal experience indicates that cerebral edema and cerebral infarction may be caused by tranexamic acid in such patients); active intravascular clotting.

Warnings

➤*Visual abnormalities and retinal degeneration:* Focal areas of retinal degeneration have developed in cats, dogs and rats following intravenous tranexamic acid at doses between 250 to 1600 mg/kg/day (6 to 40 times the recommended usual human dose) from 6 days to 1 year. The incidence of such lesions has varied from 25% to 100% of animals treated and was dose-related. At lower doses some lesions have appeared to be reversible.

Limited data in cats and rabbits showed retinal changes in some animals with doses as low as 126 mg/kg/day (only about 3 times the recommended human dose) administered for several days to 2 weeks.

No retinal changes have been reported or noted in eye examinations in patients treated with tranexamic acid for weeks to months in clinical trials.

However, visual abnormalities, often poorly characterized, represent the most frequently reported postmarketing adverse reaction in Sweden. For patients who are to be treated continually for longer than several days, an ophthalmological examination, including visual acuity, color vision, eyeground and visual fields, is advised, before commencing and at regular intervals during the course of treatment. Tranexamic acid should be discontinued if changes in examination results are found.

➤*Renal function impairment:* The dose of tranexamic acid should be reduced in patients with renal insufficiency because of the risk of accumulation (see Administration and Dosage).

➤*Carcinogenesis:* An increased incidence of leukemia in male mice receiving tranexamic acid in food at a concentration of 4.8% (equivalent to doses as high as 5 g/kg/day) may have been related to treatment. Female mice were not included in this experiment.

Hyperplasia of the biliary tract and cholangioma and adenocarcinoma of the intrahepatic biliary system have been reported in one strain of rats after dietary administration of doses exceeding the maximum tolerated dose for 22 months. Hyperplastic, but not neoplastic, lesions were reported at lower doses. Subsequent long-term dietary administration studies in a different strain of rat, each with an exposure level equal to the maximum level employed in the earlier experiment, have failed to show such hyperplastic/neoplastic changes in the liver.

➤*Pregnancy: Category B.* There are no adequate and well-controlled studies in pregnant women. However, tranexamic acid is known to pass the placenta and appears in cord blood at concentrations approximately equal to maternal concentration. Because animal reproduction studies are not always predictive of human response, this drug should be used during pregnancy only if clearly needed.

➤*Lactation:* Tranexamic acid is present in the mother's milk at a concentration of about a hundredth of the corresponding serum levels. Caution should be exercised when tranexamic acid is administered to a nursing woman.

➤*Children:* The drug has had limited use in pediatric patients, principally in connection with tooth extraction. The limited data suggest that dosing instructions for adults can be used for pediatric patients needing tranexamic acid therapy.

Precautions

➤*Ureteral obstruction:* Ureteral obstruction due to clot formation in patients with upper urinary tract bleeding has been reported in patients treated with tranexamic acid.

➤*Thrombosis/Thromboembolism:* Venous and arterial thrombosis or thromboembolism has been reported in patients treated with tranexamic acid. In addition, cases of central retinal artery and central retinal vein obstruction have been reported.

Patients with a previous history of thromboembolic disease may be at increased risk for venous or arterial thrombosis.

Tranexamic acid should not be administered concomitantly with factor IX complex concentrates or anti-inhibitor coagulant concentrates, as the risk of thrombosis may be increased.

➤*Disseminated intravascular coagulation (DIC):* Patients with DIC who require treatment with tranexamic acid, must be under strict supervision of a physician experienced in treating this disorder.

Adverse Reactions

➤*Cardiovascular:* Hypotension has been reported occasionally. Hypotension has been observed when intravenous injection is too rapid. To avoid this response, the solution should not be injected more rapidly than 1 mL/min.

➤*GI:* GI disturbances (nausea, vomiting, diarrhea) may occur but disappear when the dosage is reduced.

➤*Miscellaneous:* Giddiness.

➤*Worldwide postmarketing reports:* Thromboembolic events (eg, deep vein thrombosis, pulmonary embolism, cerebral thrombosis, and central retinal artery and vein obstruction) have been rarely reported in patients receiving tranexamic acid for indications other than hemorrhage prevention in patients with hemophilia. However, due to the spontaneous nature of the reporting of medical events and the lack of controls, the actual incidence and causal relationship of drug and event cannot be determined.

Overdosage

There is no known case of overdosage of tranexamic acid injection.

➤*Symptoms:* Symptoms of overdosage may be nausea, vomiting, orthostatic symptoms or hypotension.

APROTININ

Rx	**Trasylol** (Bayer)	**Injection:** 10,000 KIU[1]/mL	In 100 and 200 mL vials.[2]

[1] KIU = Kallikrein Inhibitor Units.
[2] With 9 mg sodium chloride/mL.

APROTININ — INJECTION

WARNING

Anaphylactic or anaphylactoid reactions are possible when aprotinin is administered. Hypersensitivity reactions are rare in patients with no prior exposure to aprotinin. The risk of anaphylaxis is increased in patients who are re-exposed to aprotinin-containing products. The benefit of aprotinin to patients undergoing primary coronary artery bypass graft (CABG) surgery should be weighed against the risk of anaphylaxis should a second exposure to aprotinin be required (see Warnings and Precautions).

Indications

➤*Hemorrhage, coronary artery bypass graft surgery:* Aprotinin is indicated for prophylactic use to reduce perioperative blood loss and the need for blood transfusion in patients undergoing cardiopulmonary bypass in the course of coronary artery bypass graft surgery.

Administration and Dosage

➤*Approved by the FDA:* December 29, 1993.

➤*Dosage regimens:* Aprotinin given prophylactically in both Regimen A and Regimen B (half Regimen A) to patients undergoing CABG surgery significantly reduced the donor blood transfusion requirement relative to placebo treatment. In low risk patients there is no difference in efficacy between regimens A and B. Therefore, the dosage used (A vs B) is at the discretion of the practitioner.

Aprotinin is supplied as a solution containing 10,000 (kallikrein inhibitor units) KIU/mL, which is equal to 1.4 mg/mL. All intravenous doses of aprotinin should be administered through a central line. Do not administer any other drug using the same line. Both regimens include a 1 mL test dose, a loading dose, a dose to be added while recirculating the priming fluid of the cardiopulmonary bypass circuit ("pump prime" dose), and a constant infusion dose. To avoid physical incompatibility of aprotinin and heparin when adding to the pump prime solution, each agent must be added during recirculation of the pump prime to assure adequate dilution prior to admixture with the other component. Regimens A and B (both incorporating a 1 mL test dose) are described below:

Aprotinin Dosage

	Test dose	Loading dose	"Pump prime" dose	Constant infusion dose
Aprotinin Regimen A	1 mL (1.4 mg or 10,000 KIU)	200 mL (280 mg or 2 million KIU)	200 mL (280 mg or 2 million KIU)	50 mL/hr (70 mg/hr or 500,000 KIU/hr)
Aprotinin Regimen B	1 mL (1.4 mg or 10,000 KIU)	100 mL (140 mg or 1 million KIU)	100 mL (140 mg or 1 million KIU)	25 mL/hr (35 mg/hr or 250,000 KIU/hr)

➤*Administration:* The 1 mL test dose should be administered intravenously at least 10 minutes before the loading dose. With the patient in a supine position, the loading dose is given slowly over 20 to 30 minutes, after induction of anesthesia but prior to sternotomy. In patients with known previous exposure to aprotinin, the loading dose should be given just prior to cannulation. When the loading dose is complete, it is followed by the constant infusion dose, which is continued until surgery is complete and the patient leaves the operating room. The "pump prime" dose is added to the recirculating priming fluid of the cardiopulmonary bypass circuit, by replacement of an aliquot of the priming fluid, prior to the institution of cardiopulmonary bypass. Total doses of more than 7 million KIU have not been studied in controlled trials.

➤*Storage/Stability:* Aprotinin should be stored between 2° and 25°C (36° to 77°F). Protect from freezing.

Parenteral drug products should be inspected visually for particulate matter and discoloration prior to administration whenever solution and container permit. Discard any unused portion.

Actions

➤*Pharmacology:* Aprotinin is a broad-spectrum protease inhibitor which modulates the systemic inflammatory response (SIR) associated with cardiopulmonary bypass (CPB) surgery. SIR results in the interrelated activation of the hemostatic, fibrinolytic, cellular and humoral inflammatory systems. Aprotinin, through its inhibition of multiple mediators (eg, kallikrein, plasmin) results in the attenuation of inflammatory responses, fibrinolysis, and thrombin generation.

Aprotinin inhibits pro-inflammatory cytokine release and maintains glycoprotein homeostasis. In platelets, aprotinin reduces glycoprotein loss (eg, GpIb, GpIIb/IIIa), while in granulocytes it prevents the expression of pro-inflammatory adhesive glycoproteins (eg, CD11b).

The effects of aprotinin use in CPB involves a reduction in inflammatory response which translates into a decreased need for allogeneic blood transfusions, reduced bleeding, and decreased mediastinal re-exploration for bleeding.

➤*Pharmacokinetics:* The studies comparing the pharmacokinetics of aprotinin in healthy volunteers, cardiac patients undergoing surgery with cardiopulmonary bypass, and women undergoing hysterectomy suggest linear pharmacokinetics over the dose range of 50,000 KIU to 2 million KIU. After IV injection, rapid distribution of aprotinin occurs into the total extracellular space, leading to a rapid initial decrease in plasma aprotinin concentration. Following this distribution phase, a plasma half-life of about 150 minutes is observed. At later time points, (ie, beyond 5 hours after dosing) there is a terminal elimination phase with a half-life of about 10 hours.

Average steady state intraoperative plasma concentrations were 137 KIU/mL (n = 10) after administration of the following dosage regimen: 1 million KIU IV loading dose, 1 million KIU into the pump prime volume, 250,000 KIU per hour of operation as continuous intravenous infusion (Regimen B). Average steady state intraoperative plasma concentrations were 250 KIU/mL in patients (n = 20) treated with aprotinin during cardiac surgery by administration of Regimen A (exactly double Regimen B): 2 million KIU IV loading dose, 2 million KIU into the pump prime volume, 500,000 KIU per hour of operation as continuous intravenous infusion.

Following a single IV dose of radiolabeled aprotinin, approximately 25% to 40% of the radioactivity is excreted in the urine over 48 hours. After a 30 minute infusion of 1 million KIU, about 2% is excreted as unchanged drug. After a larger dose of 2 million KIU infused over 30 minutes, urinary excretion of unchanged aprotinin accounts for approximately 9% of the dose.

Animal studies have shown that aprotinin is accumulated primarily in the kidney. Aprotinin, after being filtered by the glomeruli, is actively reabsorbed by the proximal tubules in which it is stored in phagolysosomes. Aprotinin is slowly degraded by lysosomal enzymes. The physiological renal handling of aprotinin is similar to that of other small proteins (eg, insulin).

Contraindications

Hypersensitivity to aprotinin.

Warnings

➤*Reexposure to aprotinin:* In a retrospective review of 387 European patient records with documented reexposure to aprotinin, the incidence of hypersensitivity/anaphylactic reactions was 2.7%. Two patients who experienced hypersensitivity/anaphylactic reactions subsequently died, 24 hours and 5 days after surgery, respectively. The relationship of these 2 deaths to aprotinin is unclear. This retrospective review also showed that the incidence of a hypersensitivity or anaphylactic reaction following reexposure is increased when the reexposure occurs within 6 months of the initial administration (5% for reexposure within 6 months and 0.9% for reexposure > 6 months). Other smaller studies have shown that in case of reexposure, the incidence of hypersensitivity/anaphylactic reactions may reach the 5% level.

Before initiating treatment with aprotinin in a patient with a history of exposure to aprotinin or products containing aprotinin, the recommendations below should be followed to manage a potential hypersensitivity or anaphylactic reaction:

1.) Have standard emergency treatments for hypersensitivity or anaphylactic reactions readily available in the operating room (eg, epinephrine, corticosteroids).
2.) Administration of the test dose and loading dose should be done only when the conditions for rapid cannulation (if necessary) are present.
3.) Delay the addition of aprotinin into the pump prime solution until after the loading dose has been safely administered. Additionally, administration of H_1 and H_2 blockers 15 minutes before the test dose may be considered.

➤*Hypersensitivity reactions:* Anaphylactic or anaphylactoid reactions are possible when aprotinin is administered. Hypersensitivity reactions are rare in patients with no prior exposure to aprotinin. Hypersensitivity reactions can range from skin eruptions, itching, dyspnea, nausea, and tachycardia to fatal anaphylactic shock with circulatory failure. If a hypersensitivity reaction occurs during injection or infusion of aprotinin, administration should be stopped immediately and emergency treatment should be initiated. It should be noted that severe (fatal) hypersensitivity/anaphylactic reactions can also occur in connection with application of the 1 mL test dose. Even when a second exposure to aprotinin has been tolerated without symptoms, a subsequent administration may result in severe hypersensitivity/anaphylactic reactions.

➤*Elderly:* Of the total of 3083 subjects in clinical studies of aprotinin, 1100 (35.7%) were 65 and over, while 297 (9.6%) were 75 and over. Of patients 65 years and older, 479 (43.5%) received Regimen A and 237 (21.5%) received Regimen B. No overall differences in safety or effectiveness were observed between these subjects and younger subjects for either dose regimen, and other reported clinical experience has not identified differences in responses between the elderly and younger patients.

➤*Pregnancy: Category B.* There are no adequate and well-controlled studies in pregnant women. Because animal reproduction studies are not always predictive of human response, this drug should be used during pregnancy only if clearly needed.

APROTININ — INJECTION

➤*Lactation:* Not applicable.

➤*Children:* Safety and effectiveness in pediatric patient(s) have not been established.

Precautions

➤*Test dose:* All patients treated with aprotinin should first receive a test dose to assess the potential for allergic reactions. The test dose of 1 mL aprotinin should be administered intravenously at least 10 minutes prior to the loading dose. However, even after the uneventful administration of the initial 1 mL test-dose, the therapeutic dose may cause an anaphylactic reaction. If this happens the infusion of aprotinin should immediately be stopped, and standard emergency treatment for anaphylaxis be applied. It should be noted that hypersensitivity/anaphylactic reactions can also occur in connection with application of the test dose (see Warnings). In reexposure cases, IV administration of an antihistamine is recommended shortly before the loading dose of aprotinin.

➤*Loading dose:* The loading dose of aprotinin should be given intravenously to patients in the supine position over a 20 to 30 minute period. Rapid intravenous administration of aprotinin can cause a transient fall in blood pressure (see Administration and Dosage).

➤*Special risk:*

Allergic reactions – Patients with a history of allergic reactions to drugs or other agents may be at greater risk of developing a hypersensitivity or anaphylactic reaction upon exposure to aprotinin (see Warnings).

Use in patients undergoing deep hypothermic circulatory arrest – Two US case control studies have reported contradictory results in patients receiving aprotinin while undergoing deep hypothermic circulatory arrest in connection with surgery of the aortic arch.

Renal failure/mortality: The first study showed an increase in both renal failure and mortality compared to age-matched historical controls. Similar results were not observed, however, in a second case control study. The strength of this association is uncertain because there are no data from randomized studies to confirm or refute these findings.

Drug Interactions

Aprotinin Drug Interactions			
Precipitant drug	Object drug*		Description
Aprotinin	Captopril	⬇	In a study of nine patients with untreated hypertension, aprotinin IV infused in a dose of 2 million KIU over 2 hours blocked the acute hypotensive effect of 100 mg captopril.
Aprotinin	Fibrinolytic agents	⬇	Aprotinin is known to have antifibrinolytic activity and, therefore, may inhibit the effects of fibrinolytic agents.
Aprotinin	Heparin	⬆	Aprotinin, in the presence of heparin, has been found to prolong the activated clotting time. However, aprotinin should not be viewed as a heparin-sparing agent.

* ⬆ = Object drug increased. ⬇ = Object drug decreased.

➤*Laboratory monitoring of anticoagulation during cardiopulmonary bypass:* Aprotinin prolongs whole blood clotting times by a different mechanism than heparin. In the presence of aprotinin, prolongation is dependent on the type of whole blood clotting test employed. If an ACT is used to determine the effectiveness of heparin anticoagulation, the prolongation of the ACT by aprotinin may lead to an overestimation of the degree of anticoagulation, thereby leading to inadequate anticoagulation. During extended extracorporeal circulation, patients may require additional heparin, even in the presence of ACT levels that appear adequate.

Methods to maintain adequate anticoagulation – In patients undergoing CPB with aprotinin therapy, 1 of the following methods may be employed to maintain adequate anticoagulation:

ACT: An activated clotting time (ACT) is not a standardized coagulation test, and different formulations of the assay are affected differently by the presence of aprotinin. The test is further influenced by variable dilution effects and the temperature experienced during cardiopulmonary bypass. It has been observed that kaolin-based ACTs are not increased to the same degree by aprotinin as are diatomaceous earth-based (celite) ACTs. Although protocols vary, a minimal celite ACT of 750 seconds or kaolin ACT of 480 seconds, independent of the effects of hemodilution and hypothermia, is recommended in the presence of aprotinin. Consult the manufacturer of the ACT test regarding the interpretation of the assay in the presence of aprotinin.

Fixed heparin dosing: A standard loading dose of heparin, administered prior to cannulation of the heart, plus the quantity of heparin added to the prime volume of the cardiopulmonary bypass (CPB) circuit, should total at least 350 IU/kg. Additional heparin should be administered in a fixed-dose regimen based on patient weight and duration of CPB.

Heparin titration: Protamine titration, a method that is not affected by aprotinin, can be used to measure heparin levels. A heparin dose response, assessed by protamine titration, should be performed prior to administration of aprotinin to determine the heparin loading dose. Additional heparin should be administered on the basis of heparin levels measured by protamine titration. Heparin levels during bypass should not be allowed to drop below 2.7 U/mL (2 mg/kg) or below the level indicated by heparin dose response testing performed prior to administration of aprotinin. In patients treated with aprotinin, the amount of protamine administered to reverse heparin activity should be based on the actual amount of heparin administered, and not on the ACT values.

Adverse Reactions

Studies of patients undergoing CABG surgery, either primary or repeat, indicate that aprotinin is generally well tolerated. The adverse events reported are frequent sequelae of cardiac surgery and are not necessarily attributable to aprotinin therapy. Adverse events reported, up to the time of hospital discharge, from patients in US placebo-controlled trials are listed in the following table. The table lists only those events that were reported in 2% or more of the aprotinin treated patients without regard to causal relationship.

Aprotinin Adverse Reactions (≥ 2%)		
Adverse reaction	Aprotinin (n = 2002) values in %	Placebo (n = 1084) values in %
Any event	76	77
Miscellaneous		
Fever	15	14
Infection	6	7
Chest pain	2	2
Asthenia	2	2
Cardiovascular		
Atrial fibrillation	21	23
Hypotension	8	10
Myocardial infarct	6	6
Atrial flutter	6	5
Ventricular extrasystoles	6	4
Tachycardia	6	7
Ventricular tachycardia	5	4
Heart failure	5	4
Pericarditis	5	5
Peripheral edema	5	5
Hypertension	4	5
Arrhythmia	4	3
Supraventricular tachycardia	4	3
Atrial arrhythmia	3	3
GI		
Nausea	11	9
Constipation	4	5
Vomiting	3	4
Diarrhea	3	2
Liver function tests abnormal	3	2
Hematologic and lymphatic		
Anemia	2	8
Metabolic and nutritional		
Creatine phosphokinase increased	2	1
Musculoskeletal		
Any event	2	3
CNS		
Confusion	4	4
Insomnia	3	4
Respiratory		
Lung disorder	8	8
Pleural effusion	7	9
Atelectasis	5	6
Dyspnea	4	4
Pneumothorax	4	4
Asthma	2	3
Hypoxia	2	1
Dermatologic		
Rash	2	2

APROTININ — INJECTION

Aprotinin Adverse Reactions (≥ 2%)		
Adverse reaction	Aprotinin (n = 2002) values in %	Placebo (n = 1084) values in %
GU		
Kidney function abnormal	3	2
Urinary retention	3	3
Urinary tract infection	2	2

In comparison to the placebo group, no increase in mortality in patients treated with aprotinin was observed. Additional events of particular interest from controlled US trials with an incidence of < 2%, are listed below:

Aprotinin Adverse Reactions (< 2%)		
Adverse reaction	% of patients treated with aprotinin (n = 2002)	% of patients treated with placebo (n = 1084)
Thrombosis	1	0.6
Shock	0.7	0.4
Cerebrovascular accident	0.7	2.1
Thrombophlebitis	0.2	0.5
Deep thrombophlebitis	0.7	1
Lung edema	1.3	1.5
Pulmonary embolus	0.3	0.6
Kidney failure	1	0.6
Acute kidney failure	0.5	0.6
Kidney tubular necrosis	0.8	0.4

➤*Additional events, incidence between 1% and 2%:* Listed below are additional events, from controlled US trials with an incidence between 1% and 2%, and also from uncontrolled, compassionate use trials and spontaneous postmarketing reports. Estimates of frequency cannot be made for spontaneous postmarketing reports.

Cardiovascular – Ventricular fibrillation, heart arrest, bradycardia, congestive heart failure, hemorrhage, bundle branch block, myocardial ischemia, ventricular tachycardia, heart block, pericardial effusion, ventricular arrhythmia, shock, pulmonary hypertension (1% to 2%).

CNS – Agitation, dizziness, anxiety, convulsion (1% to 2%).

Dermatologic – Skin discoloration (spontaneous postmarketing reports).

GI – Dyspepsia, gastrointestinal hemorrhage, jaundice, hepatic failure (1% to 2%).

GU – Oliguria, kidney failure, acute kidney failure, kidney tubular necrosis (1% to 2%).

Hematologic/Lymphatic – Although thrombosis was not reported more frequently in aprotinin versus placebo-treated patients in controlled trials, it has been reported in uncontrolled trials, compassionate use trials, and spontaneous postmarketing reporting. These reports of thrombosis encompass the following terms: Thrombosis, occlusion, arterial thrombosis, coronary occlusion, embolus, pulmonary embolus, thrombophlebitis, deep thrombophlebitis, cerebrovascular accident, cerebral embolism (1% to 2%); pulmonary thrombosis (spontaneous postmarketing reports). Other hematologic events reported include leukocytosis, thrombocytopenia, coagulation disorder (which includes disseminated intravascular coagulation), decreased prothrombin (1% to 2%).

Metabolic/Nutritional – Hyperglycemia, hypokalemia, hypervolemia, acidosis (1% to 2%).

Musculoskeletal – Arthralgia (1% to 2%).

Respiratory – Pneumonia, apnea, increased cough, lung edema (1% to 2%).

Miscellaneous – Sepsis, death, multisystem organ failure, immune system disorder (1% to 2%); hemoperitoneum (spontaneous postmarketing reports).

➤*Myocardial infarction:* In the pooled analysis of all patients undergoing CABG surgery, there was no significant difference in the incidence of investigator-reported myocardial infarction (MI) in aprotinin-treated patients as compared to placebo-treated patients. However, because no uniform criteria for the diagnosis of myocardial infarction were utilized by investigators, this issue was addressed prospectively in 3 later studies (2 studies evaluated Regimen A, Regimen B, and Pump Prime Regimen; 1 study evaluated only Regimen A), in which data were analyzed by a blinded consultant employing an algorithm for possible, probable or definite MI. Utilizing this method, the incidence of definite myocardial infarction was 5.9% in the aprotinin-treated patients versus 4.7% in the placebo-treated patients. This difference in the incidence rates was not statistically significant. Data from these 3 studies are summarized below.

Incidence of Myocardial Infarctions with Aprotinin			
Treatment	Definite MI %	Definite or probable MI %	Definite, probable, or possible MI
Pooled data from 3 studies that evaluated Regimen A			
Aprotinin regimen A (n = 646)	4.6	10.7	14.1
Placebo (n = 661)	4.7	11.3	13.4
Pooled data from 2 studies that evaluated Regimen B and Pump Prime Regimen			
Aprotinin Regimen B (n = 241)	8.7	15.9	18.7
Aprotinin Pump Prime Regimen (n = 239)	6.3	15.7	18.1
Placebo (n = 240)	6.3	15.1	15.8

➤*Graft patency:* In a recently completed multicenter, multinational study to determine the effects of aprotinin Regimen A vs placebo on saphenous vein graft patency in patients undergoing primary CABG surgery, patients were subjected to routine postoperative angiography. Of the 13 study sites, 10 were in the United States and 3 were non-US centers (Denmark 1, Israel 2). The results of this study are summarized below.

Incidence of Graft Closure, Myocardial Infarction and Death with Aprotinin				
	Overall closure rates[1]		Incidence of MI[2]	Incidence of death[3]
	All centers (n = 703), %	US centers (n = 381), %	All centers (n = 831), %	All centers (n = 870), %
Aprotinin	15.4	9.4	2.9	1.4
Placebo	10.9	9.5	3.8	1.6
CI for the difference (%) (drug-placebo)	(1.3, 9.6)[4]	(−3.8, 5.9)[4]	(−3.3, 1.5)[5]	(−1.9, 1.4)[5]

[1] Population: All patients with assessable saphenous vein grafts.
[2] Population: All patients assessable by blinded consultant.
[3] All patients.
[4] 90%; per protocol.
[5] 95%; not specified in protocol.

Although there was a statistically significantly increased risk of graft closure for aprotinin-treated patients compared to patients who received placebo (p = 0.035), further analysis showed a significant treatment by site interaction for 1 of the non-US sites vs the US centers. When the analysis of graft closures was repeated for US centers only, there was no statistically significant difference in graft closure rates in patients who received aprotinin vs placebo. These results are the same whether analyzed as the proportion of patients who experienced at least 1 graft closure postoperatively or as the proportion of grafts closed. There were no differences between treatment groups in the incidence of myocardial infarction as evaluated by the blinded consultant (2.9% aprotinin vs 3.8% placebo) or of death (1.4% aprotinin vs 1.6% placebo) in this study.

➤*Hypersensitivity:* See Warnings. Hypersensitivity and anaphylactic reactions during surgery were rarely reported in US controlled clinical studies in patients with no prior exposure to aprotinin (1/1424 patients or < 0.1% on aprotinin vs 1/861 patients or 0.1% on placebo). In case of reexposure the incidence of hypersensitivity/anaphylactic reactions has been reported to reach the 5% level. A review of 387 European patient records involving reexposure to aprotinin showed that the incidence of hypersensitivity or anaphylactic reactions was 5% for reexposure within 6 months and 0.9% for reexposure > 6 months.

➤*Lab test abnormalities:*

Serum creatinine – Data pooled from all patients undergoing CABG surgery in US placebo-controlled trials showed no statistically or clinically significant increase in the incidence of postoperative renal dysfunction in patients treated with aprotinin. The incidence of serum creatinine elevations > 0.5 mg/dL above pretreatment levels was 9% in the aprotinin group vs 8% in the placebo group (p = 0.248), while the incidence of elevations > 2 mg/dL above baseline was only 1% in each group (p = 0.883). In the majority of instances, postoperative renal dysfunction was not severe and was reversible. Patients with baseline elevations in serum creatinine were not at increased risk of developing postoperative renal dysfunction following aprotinin treatment.

Serum transaminases – Data pooled from all patients undergoing CABG surgery in US placebo-controlled trials showed no evidence of an increase in the incidence of postoperative hepatic dysfunction in patients treated with aprotinin. The incidence of treatment-emergent increases in ALT (formerly SGPT) > 1.8 times the upper limit of normal was 14% in both the aprotinin and placebo-treated patients (p = 0.687), while the incidence of increases > 3 times the upper limit of normal was 5% in both groups (p = 0.847).

Other laboratory findings – The incidence of treatment-emergent elevations in plasma glucose, AST (formerly SGOT), LDH, alkaline phosphatase,

Systemic

APROTININ — INJECTION

and CPK-MB was not notably different between aprotinin - and placebo-treated patients undergoing CABG surgery. Significant elevations in the partial thromboplastin time (PTT) and celite activated clotting time (celite ACT) are expected in aprotinin-treated patients in the hours after surgery due to circulating concentrations of aprotinin, which are known to inhibit activation of the intrinsic clotting system by contact with a foreign material (eg, celite), a method used in these tests (see Laboratory monitoring of anti-coagulation during cardiopulmonary bypass.)

Overdosage

The maximum amount of aprotinin that can be safely administered in single or multiple doses has not been determined. Doses up to 17.5 million KIU have been administered within a 24 hour period without any apparent toxicity. There is 1 poorly documented case, however, of a patient who received a large, but not well determined, amount of aprotinin (in excess of 15 million KIU) in 24 hours. The patient, who had preexisting liver dysfunction, developed hepatic and renal failure postoperatively and died. Autopsy showed hepatic necrosis and extensive renal tubular and glomerular necrosis. The relationship of these findings to aprotinin therapy is unclear.

Topical

THROMBIN, TOPICAL

Rx	**Thrombin-JMI** (Jones Medical)	**Powder**	In 10,000 and 20,000 unit vials.
Rx	**Thrombogen** (Johnson & Johnson)	**Powder**	In 5,000[3], 10,000[4] or 20,000[4] unit vials.
Rx	**Thrombostat** (Parke-Davis)	**Powder**	In 5,000[5], 10,000[6] or 20,000[6] unit vials.

[1] With 50% mannitol and 45% sodium chloride.
[2] With 50% mannitol, 45% sodium chloride and Sterile Water for Injection diluent.
[3] With Isotonic Saline diluent and transfer needle.
[4] With Isotonic Saline diluent. benzethonium chloride and transfer needle. Also in spray kit.
[5] With Isotonic Saline diluent containing 0.02 mg benzethonium chloride/mL.
[6] With Isotonic Saline diluent containing 0.02 mg benzethonium chloride/mL. Also in spray kit.

THROMBIN — TOPICAL

WARNING

Topical thrombin (bovine) must not be injected! Apply on the surface of bleeding tissue.

The use of topical bovine thrombin preparations has occasionally been associated with abnormalities in hemostasis ranging from asymptomatic alterations in laboratory determinations, such as prothrombin time (PT) and partial thromboplastin time (PTT), to severe bleeding or thrombosis which rarely have been fatal. These hemostatic effects appear to be related to the formation of antibodies against bovine thrombin or factor V which in some cases may cross react with human factor V, potentially resulting in factor V deficiency. Repeated clinical applications of topical bovine thrombin increase the likelihood that antibodies against thrombin or factor V may be formed. Consultation with an expert in coagulation disorders is recommended if a patient exhibits abnormal coagulation laboratory values, abnormal bleeding, or abnormal thrombosis following the use of topical thrombin. Any interventions should consider the immunologic basis of this condition. Patients with antibodies to bovine thrombin preparations should not be re-exposed to these products.

Indications

➤*Hemostasis:* As an aid to hemostasis whenever oozing blood and minor bleeding from capillaries and small venules is accessible.

In various types of surgery, solutions of thrombin topical may be used in conjunction with an absorbable gelatin sponge for hemostasis.

Administration and Dosage

➤*Reconstitution:* Solutions of thrombin topical (bovine origin), USP, may be reconstituted with sterile isotonic saline at a recommended concentration of 1000 to 2000 US U/mL. Where bleeding is profuse, as from abraded surfaces of liver or spleen, concentrations of 1000 US U/mL may be required. For general use in plastic surgery, dental extractions, skin grafting, etc, solutions containing ≈ 100 US U/mL are frequently used. Intermediate strengths to suit the needs of the case may be prepared by diluting the contents of the thrombin topical container with an appropriate volume of sterile isotonic saline. In many situations, it may be advantageous to use thrombin topical in a dry form on oozing surfaces.

In instances where a concentration of ≈ 1000 U/mL is desired, the contents of the vial of sterile isotonic saline diluent may be transferred into the thrombin topical container with a sterile syringe or sterile transfer needle. If the transfer needle is used for reconstitution, transfer the diluent in the following manner:

1.) Remove the plastic cap off of the diluent vial.
2.) Twist the clear plastic cover on the transfer needle and remove.
3.) Insert the exposed needle into the diaphragm of the diluent vial.
4.) Flip the plastic cover up on the thrombin topical container. Do not remove the cover and aluminum seal.
5.) Remove the pink plastic cap from the transfer needle exposing the needle.
6.) Invert the vial of diluent and insert the exposed needle into the diaphragm of the thrombin topical container.

➤*Thrombin topical spray kit:* Each spray kit contains one vial of thrombin topical and one spray pump and actuator.

1.) Remove the outer lid by pulling up at the indicated edge. The inner tray is sterile and suitable for introduction into any operating field.
2.) Remove the cover on inner tray to expose sterile contents.
3.) Reconstitute the thrombin topical to desired potency by introducing sterile isotonic saline with a sterile syringe or a sterile transfer needle. If the transfer needle is used, follow the previously described procedure.
4.) When the thrombin topical is completely dissolved, open vial by flipping up metal and tearing counterclockwise.
5.) Remove the rubber diaphragm from vial. Remove pump with protective cap from tray and snap onto vial. Remove protective cap and attach actuator.
6.) To spray, hold vial upright or at a slight angle. Several strokes of the pump will be required to expel the solution.
7.) Discard unused contents and pump. Do not transfer spray pump to another vial.

➤*Thrombin topical syringe spray kit:* Each syringe kit contains one vial of thrombin topical and one spray tip and syringe.

1.) Remove the outer lid by pulling up at the indicated edge. The inner tray is sterile and suitable for introduction into any operating field.
2.) Remove the cover on the inner tray to expose sterile contents.
3.) Using the sterile syringe equipped with a needle, draw the desired amount of saline diluent from the vial into the syringe.
4.) Inject the saline diluent into the thrombin topical vial from the syringe to reconstitute the thrombin topical powder.
5.) When the thrombin topical powder is completely dissolved, draw the thrombin topical solution into the syringe.
6.) Replace the needle guard.
7.) Turn needle guard counterclockwise and remove and discard the needle.
8.) Affix spray tip by pushing down and turning clockwise until the spray tip locks in place.
9.) To spray, depress the syringe plunger in a normal fashion to dispense the thrombin topical solution through the tip in a fine spray.
10.) Discard unused contents and syringe.

➤*Application techniques:* The following techniques are suggested for the topical application of thrombin topical.

1.) The recipient surface should be sponged (not wiped) free of blood before thrombin topical is applied.
2.) A spray may be used or the surface may be flooded using a sterile syringe and small gauge needle. The most effective hemostasis results occur when the thrombin topical mixes freely with the blood as soon as it reaches the surface.
3.) Sponging of the treated surfaces should be avoided to assure that the clot remains securely in place.

➤*Thrombin topical with absorbable gelatin sponge:* Thrombin topical may be used in conjunction with absorbable gelatin sponge as follows:

1.) Prepare thrombin topical solution to desired strength.
2.) Immerse sponge strips of the desired size in thrombin topical solution. Knead the sponge strips vigorously with moistened, gloved fingers to remove trapped air, thereby facilitating saturation of the sponge.
3.) Apply saturated sponge to bleeding area. Hold in place with a pledget of cotton or a small gauze sponge until hemostasis occurs.

➤*Storage/Stability:* Store 1000 unit vial thrombin topical (bovine) at 2° to 8°C (36° to 46°F). Store 5000, 10,000, 20,000 and 50,000 U/vial sizes of thrombin topical at 2° to 25°C (36° to 77°F).

Solutions should be used promptly upon removal from the container. However, the solution may be refrigerated at 2° to 8°C (36° to 46°F) for up to 3 hours.

Actions

➤*Pharmacology:* Thrombin topical requires no intermediate physiological agent for its action. It clots the fibrinogen of the blood directly. Failure to clot blood occurs in the rare case where the primary clotting defect is the absence of fibrinogen itself. The speed with which thrombin clots blood is dependent upon the concentration of both thrombin and fibrinogen.

Contraindications

Sensitivity to any of its components or to material of bovine origin.

Topical

THROMBIN — TOPICAL

Warnings

➤*Do not inject:* Because of its action in the clotting mechanism, thrombin topical must not be injected or otherwise allowed to enter large blood vessels. Extensive intravascular clotting and even death may result.

➤*Pregnancy: Category C.* Animal reproduction studies have not been conducted with thrombin topical. It is also not known whether thrombin topical can cause fetal harm when administered to a pregnant woman or can affect reproduction capacity. Thrombin topical should be given to a pregnant woman only if clearly indicated.

➤*Children:* Safety and effectiveness in children have not been established.

Precautions

Consult the absorbable gelatin sponge labeling for complete information for use prior to utilizing the thrombin saturated sponge procedure.

Adverse Reactions

➤*Allergic:* Allergic reactions may be encountered in persons known to be sensitive to bovine materials. Inhibitory antibodies which interfere with hemostasis may develop in a small percentage of patients (see Warnings).

MICROFIBRILLAR COLLAGEN HEMOSTAT

Rx	**Hemopad** (Astra)	**Fibrous absorbable collagen hemostat:** 2.5 cm x 5 cm, 5 cm x 8 cm and 8 cm x 10 cm	In 10s.
Rx	**Hemotene** (Astra)	**Fibrous absorbable collagen hemostat:** 1 g	In dispenser packs of 5.

MICROFIBRILLAR COLLAGEN HEMOSTAT — TOPICAL

Indications

➤*Hemostasis:* Used in surgical procedures as an adjunct to hemostasis when control of bleeding by ligature or conventional procedures is ineffective or impractical.

Administration and Dosage

This product should not be resterilized. It is not for injection or intraocular use. Moistening or wetting with saline or thrombin impairs its hemostatic efficacy. It should be used dry. Discard any unused portion.

➤*Fibrous form:* Must be applied directly to the source of bleeding. Because of its adhesiveness, it may seal over the exit site of deeper hemorrhage and conceal an underlying hematoma as in penetrating liver wounds.

Surface preparation – Compress with dry sponges immediately prior to application of the dry product, then apply pressure over the hemostat with a dry sponge; the length of time varies with the force and severity of bleeding. A minute may suffice for capillary bleeding (eg, skin graft donor sites, dermatologic curettage), but ≥ 3 to 5 minutes may be required for brisk bleeding (eg, splenic tears) or high pressure leaks in major artery suture holes.

Control of oozing from cancellous bone – Pack firmly into the spongy bone surface. After 5 to 10 minutes, tease excess away; this can usually be accomplished with blunt forceps and is facilitated by wetting with sterile 0.9% saline solution and irrigation. If breakthrough bleeding occurs in areas of thin application, apply additional hemostat. The amount required depends on the severity of bleeding.

Capillary bleeding – 1 g is usually sufficient for a 50 cm^2 area. Thicker coverage is required for more brisk bleeding.

Application – Adheres to wet gloves, instruments or tissue surfaces. To facilitate handling, use dry smooth forceps. Do not use gloved fingers to apply pressure.

➤*Nonwoven web form:* In neurosurgical and other procedures, apply small squares to bleeding areas; then cover the sites with moist cottonoid "patties." To prevent wetting of the MCH, and to apply needed pressure, hold a suction tip against the cottonoid for one to several minutes, depending on the briskness of bleeding. After 5 to 10 minutes, remove excess MCH by teasing and irrigation.

Actions

➤*Pharmacology:* Microfibrillar collagen hemostat (MCH) is an absorbable topical hemostatic agent prepared as a dry, sterile, fibrous, water insoluble, partial hydrochloric acid salt of purified bovine corium collagen.

In contact with a bleeding surface, MCH attracts platelets that adhere to the fibrils and undergo the release phenomenon to trigger aggregation of platelets into thrombi in the interstices of the fibrous mass. The effect on platelet adhesion and aggregation is not inhibited by heparin in vitro. Platelets of patients with clinical thrombasthenia do not adhere to the hemostat in vitro. However, in clinical trials, it was effective in 50 of 68 patients receiving aspirin. It cannot control bleeding due to systemic coagulation disorders. Institute appropriate therapy to correct the underlying coagulopathy prior to use of the drug. It is tenaciously adherent to surfaces wet with blood, but excess material not involved in the hemostatic clot may be removed by teasing or irrigation, usually without restarting bleeding.

MCH stimulates a mild, chronic cellular inflammatory response. When implanted in animal tissues, it is absorbed in less than 84 days and does not predispose to stenosis at vascular anastomotic sites. These findings have not been confirmed in humans. In human studies of hemostasis in osteotomy cuts, it does not interfere with bone regeneration or healing.

Contraindications

Closure of skin incisions; it may interfere with the healing of the skin edges due to simple mechanical interposition of dry collagen.

Bone surfaces to which prosthetic materials are to be attached with methylmethacrylate adhesives. By filling porosities of cancellous bone, MCH may significantly reduce the bond strength of methylmethacrylate adhesives.

Warnings

➤*Sterilization:* MCH is inactivated by autoclaving. Ethylene oxide reacts with bound hydrochloric acid to form ethylene chlorohydrin.

➤*Infection:* The presence of the hemostat does not enhance or initiate experimental staphylococcus wound infections to a greater or lesser extent than control agents. The effects on experimental wounds contaminated with a gram-negative aerobic rod and an anaerobic non-spore-forming bacteria are currently under investigation. Use in contaminated wounds may enhance infection.

➤*Pregnancy:* There are no well controlled studies in pregnant women. Safety for use during pregnancy has not been established. Use only when clearly needed and when the potential benefits outweigh the potential hazards to the fetus.

Precautions

➤*Excess material:* After several minutes, remove excess material; this is usually possible without the reinitiation of active bleeding. Failure to remove excess material may result in bowel adhesion or mechanical pressure sufficient to compromise the ureter. In otolaryngological surgery, precautions against aspiration should include removal of all excess dry material and thorough irrigation of the pharynx.

➤*Antibodies:* Contains a low level of intercalated bovine serum protein that reacts immunologically as does beef serum albumin (BSA). Increases in anti-BSA titer have been observed following treatment. About two-thirds of individuals exhibit antibody titers because of ingestion of food products of bovine origin. Intradermal skin tests have occasionally shown weak positive reactions to BSA or MCH, but these have not been correlated with IgG titers to BSA. Tests have failed to demonstrate clinically significant elicitation of antibodies of the IgE class against BSA following therapy.

➤*Blood from operative sites:* Fragments of MCH may pass through filters of blood scavenging systems. Therefore, avoid reintroduction of blood from operative sites treated with MCH.

➤*Autologous blood salvage circuits:* MCH should not be used in conjunction with autologous blood salvage circuits.

➤*Handling:* Avoid spillage on nonbleeding surfaces, particularly in abdominal or thoracic viscera.

Adverse Reactions

Most serious – Potentiation of infection (including abscess formation, hematoma, wound dehiscence and mediastinitis). Adhesion formation; allergic reaction; foreign body reaction; subgaleal seroma (single case).

The use of MCH in dental extraction sockets increases the incidence of alveolalgia. Transient laryngospasm due to aspiration of dry materials has been reported following use in tonsillectomy.

Topical

ABSORBABLE GELATIN SPONGE

Rx	**Gelfoam** (Upjohn)	**Sponges:** Size 12: 2 x 6 cm x 3 or 7 mm	In 4s and 12s (7 mm only).
		Size 50: 8 x 6.25 cm	In 4s.
		Size 100: 8 x 12.5 cm	In regular and compressed. In 6s.
		Size 200: 8 x 25 cm	In 6s.
		Packs: Size 2: 40 x 2 cm	In single jars.
		Size 6: 40 x 6 cm	In 6s.
		Dental pk: Size 4: 2 x 2 cm	In 15s.
		Prostatectomy cones: Size 13: 5″ diameter	In 6s.
		Size 18: 7″ diameter	In 6s.

ABSORBABLE GELATIN — SPONGE

Indications

➤*Hemostasis:* For use in surgical procedures as an adjunct to hemostasis when control of bleeding by ligature or conventional procedures is ineffective or impractical.

Also used in oral and dental surgery as an aid in providing hemostasis.

In open prostatic surgery, insertion into the prostatic cavity provides hemostasis.

Administration and Dosage

➤*Hemostasis:* Apply dry or saturated with NaCl injection. When bleeding is controlled, leave pieces in place. Since sponge causes little more cellular infiltration than the blood clot, the wound may be closed over it. When applied, the sponge will stay in place until it liquefies. When applied dry, compress pieces before application to bleeding surface, then hold in place with moderate pressure for 10 to 15 seconds. When used with saline solutions, immerse in solution, withdraw, squeeze to remove the air bubbles present and replace in solution where it will swell to original size. If it does not, remove and knead vigorously until all air is expelled. Leave piece wet, or blot to dampness on gauze, and apply to bleeding point. Hold in place with moderate pressure with a cotton pledget or small gauze sponge until hemostasis results.

➤*Dentistry:* When used dry, roll between fingers and lightly compress to diameter of cavity or socket. After insertion, apply light finger pressure for 1 or 2 min. When used moist, immerse in NaCl solution, then remove, squeeze thoroughly to remove air bubbles and replace in solution where it will swell to original size. Take from solution, blot on sterile gauze to remove excess fluid and place in cavity or wound.

➤*Prostatectomy cones:* These are designed for use with the Foley bag catheter.

➤*Storage/Stability:* Once package is opened, contents are subject to contamination.

Actions

➤*Pharmacology:* A sterile, pliable surgical sponge prepared from purified gelatin solution and capable of absorbing and holding many times its weight of whole blood.

When implanted into tissues, it is absorbed completely within 4 to 6 weeks without inducing excessive scar tissue formation. When applied to bleeding areas of nasal, rectal or vaginal mucosa, it completely liquefies within 2 to 5 days.

Contraindications

Closure of skin incisions (may interfere with the healing of skin edges); control of postpartum bleeding or menorrhagia.

Warnings

➤*Sterilization:* Do not resterilize by heat, since heating may change absorption time. Ethylene oxide is not recommended for resterilization; it may be trapped in the interstices of the foam and trace amounts may cause burns or irritation to tissue.

Precautions

➤*Infection:* Not recommended in the presence of infection. If signs of infection or abscess develop in the area where the sponge has been placed, reoperation may be necessary to remove the infected material and allow drainage.

➤*Compression:* Sponge may expand and impinge on nearby structures. When placing into cavities or closed tissue spaces, use minimal preliminary compression; avoid overpacking.

Adverse Reactions

Sponge may form infection and abscess (see Precautions). Giant cell granuloma in the brain has occurred at implantation site, as well as brain and spinal cord compression due to sterile fluid accumulation. Excessive fibrosis and prolonged fixation of the tendon were seen when the sponge was used at a tendon juncture.

ABSORBABLE GELATIN FILM, STERILE

Rx	**Gelfilm** (Upjohn)	**Film:** 100 mm x 125 mm	In 1s.
Rx	**Gelfilm Ophthalmic** (Upjohn)	**Film:** 25 mm x 50 mm	In 6s.

GELATIN ABSORBABLE — FILM

Indications

➤*Neurosurgery:* As a dural substitute; absorbable gelatin film is nonconducive to undue inflammatory reaction and absorbable at a rate slow enough to permit dural regeneration and healing of the arachnoid layer. Its use in patients undergoing craniotomies reportedly prevented the development of meningocerebral adhesions, thereby reducing the risk of postoperative sequelae.

➤*Thoracic surgery:* In the repair of pleural defects in connection with thoracotomies, thoracoplasties and extrapleural procedures, implantation has been followed by minimal tissue reaction and subsequent closure of the defect by ingrowth of regenerating pleural and fibrous tissue across the gradually resorbed implant.

➤*Ocular surgery:* In glaucoma filtration operations (ie, iridencleisis and trephination), extraocular muscle surgery and diathermy or scleral "buckling" operations for retinal detachment. There is a remarkable lack of cellular reaction to the film implanted subconjunctivally or used as a seton into the anterior chamber. Evidence shows that implants help prevent formation of adhesions between contiguous ocular structures.

Administration and Dosage

➤*Preparation:* Immerse in sterile saline solution; soak until quite pliable; cut to the desired size and shape; apply as follows:

➤*Covering dural defects:* Place over the surface of the brain. Tuck the edges of the implant beneath the dura and the wound; close the wound in the usual manner. If desired, the film can be sutured loosely to the dura. The moist film tears easily.

➤*Covering pleural defects:* Place over the defect and anchor in place by means of small interrupted sutures.

➤*As a seton in iridencleisis:* Place a small piece (≈ 4 mm x 10 mm) over the prolapsed iris pillar parallel to the limbus; Tenon's capsule and the conjunctiva are then closed with continuous absorbable sutures closely spaced to ensure tight wound closure.

➤*Diathermy or scleral "buckling" operations:* Place film over the sclera, then suture the muscle and the conjunctiva over the underlying film.

➤*Extraocular muscle surgery:* Place film over and beneath the muscle before Tenon's capsule and the conjunctiva are closed in layers.

➤*Storage/Stability:* Once the envelopes have been opened, contents are subject to contamination. To ensure sterility, use immediately after withdrawal from the envelope. Store at room temperature 15° to 30°C (59° to 86°F).

Actions

➤*Pharmacology:* A sterile, absorbable gelatin film for use in neurosurgery, thoracic and ocular surgery.

In the dry state, absorbable gelatin film has the appearance and texture of cellophane of equivalent thickness; when moistened, it assumes a rubbery consistency and can then be cut to the desired size and fitted to rounded or irregular surfaces. The rate of absorption after implantation ranges from 1 to 6 months, depending on the size of the implant and the site of implantation. Pleural and muscle implants are completely absorbed in 8 to 14 days; dural and ocular implants usually require at least 2 to 5 months for complete absorption. The absence of undue tissue reactions, with the consequent decreased likelihood of developing adhesions, has been of particular value in the case of dural and ocular implants.

Contraindications

Because the rate of absorption is likely to be increased in the presence of purulent exudation, do not implant in grossly contaminated or infected surgical wounds.

OXIDIZED CELLULOSE

Rx	**Oxycel** (Becton-Dickinson)	**Pads:** 3″ x 3″, 8 ply **Pledgets:** 2″ x 1″ x 1″ **Strips:** 18″ x 2″, 4 ply	In 10s.
Rx	**Surgicel** (Johnson & Johnson)	**Strips:** 2″ x 14″ 4″ x 8″ 2″ x 3″ ½″ x 2″	In 1s.
		Surgical Nu-knit: 1″ x 1″ 3″ x 4″ 6″ x 9″	In 1s.

OXIDIZED CELLULOSE — TOPICAL

Indications

➤*Hemorrhage:* Used adjunctively in surgical procedures to assist in the control of capillary, venous and small arterial hemorrhage when ligation or other conventional methods of control are impractical or ineffective. Also indicated for use in oral surgery and exodontia.

Administration and Dosage

Withdraw hemostat from the container with dry sterile forceps. Minimal amounts of an appropriate size are laid on the bleeding site or held firmly against the tissues until hemostasis is obtained.

➤*Storage / Stability:* Discard opened, unused oxidized cellulose. It cannot be resterilized.

Actions

➤*Pharmacology:* An absorbable hemostatic agent prepared from cellulose by a special process that converts it into polyanhydroglucuronic acid (cellulosic acid). Oxidation of cellulose yields an absorbable product of known acidity, soluble in alkali.

Provides hemostatic action when applied to sites of bleeding. The mechanism of action is not completely understood, but it appears to be a physical effect rather than any alteration of the normal physiologic clotting mechanism. Upon contact with blood, oxidized cellulose becomes a dark reddish-brown or almost black, tenacious, adhesive mass. It conforms and adheres readily to the bleeding surface. After 24 to 48 hours, it becomes gelatinous and can be removed, usually without causing additional bleeding. If left in situ, absorption depends on several factors, including the amount used, degree of saturation with blood and the tissue bed.

Oxidized cellulose swells upon contact with blood; the resultant pressure adds to its hemostatic action. It does not enter the normal clotting mechanism; however, within a few minutes of contact with blood, it forms an artificially produced clot in the bleeding area.

Bactericidal effects – The hemostat is bactericidal in vitro against many gram-positive and gram-negative organisms including aerobes and anaerobes: *Staphylococcus aureus, S. epidermidis, Micrococcus luteus, Streptococcus pyogenes* Groups A and B, *S. salivarius, Bacillus subtilis, Proteus vulgaris, Corynebacterium xerosis, Mycobacterium phlei, Clostridium tetani, Branhamella catarrhalis, Escherichia coli, Klebsiella aerogenes, Lactobacillus* sp, *Salmonella enteritidis, Shigella dysenteriae, Serratia marcescens, C. perfringens, Bacteroides fragilis, Enterococcus, Enterobacter cloacae, Pseudomonas aeruginosa, P. stutzeri* and *Proteus mirabilis.* In contrast to other hemostatic agents, it does not tend to enhance experimental infection.

Contraindications

Packing or wadding as a hemostatic agent; packing or implantation in fractures or laminectomies (it interferes with bone regeneration and can cause cyst formation); control of hemorrhage from large arteries or on nonhemorrhagic serous oozing surfaces since body fluids other than whole blood (eg, serum) do not react with oxidized cellulose to produce satisfactory hemostatic effects; do not use around the optic nerve and chiasm; as a wrap in vascular surgery because it has a stenotic effect.

Warnings

➤*Sterilization:* Do not autoclave; autoclaving causes physical breakdown.

➤*Surgery:* Not intended as a substitute for careful surgery and proper use of sutures and ligatures.

➤*Contaminated wound:* Closing oxidized cellulose in a contaminated wound without drainage may lead to complications and should be avoided.

➤*Application / Removal:* The hemostatic effect is greater when applied dry; therefore, do not moisten with water or saline. Do not impregnate with materials such as buffering or hemostatic substances. Its hemostatic effect is not enhanced by the addition of thrombin; the activity of thrombin is destroyed by the low pH of the product. If used temporarily to line the cavity of large open wounds, place so as not to overlap the skin edges.

May be left in situ when necessary, but remove it once hemostasis is achieved. It must always be removed if used in, around or in proximity to foramina in bone, areas of bony confine, the spinal cord or the optic nerve and chiasm; by swelling, it may cause nerve damage by pressure in a bony confine. Paralysis has been reported when used around the spinal cord, particularly in surgery for herniated intervertebral disc. Remove from open wounds by forceps or by irrigation with sterile water or saline solution after bleeding has stopped.

➤*Infections:* Although it is bactericidal against a wide range of pathogenic microorganisms, it is not a substitute for systemic antimicrobial agents to control or prevent postoperative infections. Do not impregnate with anti-infective agents.

Precautions

➤*Packing:* Apply by loosely packing against the bleeding surface. Avoid wadding or packing tightly, especially within the bony enclosure of the CNS and within other relatively rigid cavities where swelling may interfere with normal function or possibly cause necrosis.

➤*Use sparingly:* To control bleeding in open reduction of fractures and in cancellous bone, use sparingly. To minimize the possibility of interference with callus formation and the theoretical chance of cyst formation, remove any excess after bleeding is controlled.

➤*Urological procedures:* Use minimal amounts and exercise care to prevent plugging of the urethra, ureter or catheter.

Since absorption is prevented in chemically cauterized areas, its use should not be preceded by application of silver nitrate or any other escharotic chemicals.

➤*Otorhinolaryngologic surgery:* Exercise care so that none of the material is aspirated by the patient (eg, when controlling hemorrhage after tonsillectomy; controlling epistaxis).

Adverse Reactions

Encapsulation of fluid and foreign body reactions, with or without infection, have been reported.

Possible prolongation of drainage in cholecystectomies and difficulty passing urine per urethra after prostatectomy have been reported. There has been one report of a blocked ureter after kidney resection.

Burning has been reported when applied after nasal polyp removal and after hemorrhoidectomy. Headache, burning, stinging and sneezing in epistaxis and other rhinological procedures and stinging when applied on surface wounds (varicose ulcerations, dermabrasions and donor sites) have also been reported. These are believed to be due to the low pH of the product.

Intestinal obstruction has occurred, due to transmigration of a bolus of oxidized cellulose from gallbladder bed to terminal ileum or to adhesions in a loop of denuded intestine to which oxidized cellulose had been applied.

➤*Miscellaneous:* Necrosis of nasal mucous membrane or perforation of nasal septum due to tight packing; urethral obstruction following retropubic prostatectomy and introduction of oxidized cellulose within enucleated prostatic capsule.

Indications

Unless the condition responsible for the hypoproteinemia can be corrected, albumin in any form can provide only symptomatic relief or supportive treatment.

➤*Shock:* For shock due to burns, trauma, surgery and infections; in the treatment of injuries of such severity that shock, although not immediately present, is likely to ensue; in other similar conditions where the restoration of blood volume is urgent.

In cases in which there has been a considerable loss of red blood cells, transfusion with whole blood or red blood cells is indicated.

For the earliest emergency treatment of shock, it may be more convenient to have 25% normal serum albumin available because it is so highly concentrated. However, the concentrated solution depends (for its maximum osmotic effect) on holding additional fluids in the circulation, which are drawn from the tissues or administered separately; if patient is dehydrated, maximum effect cannot be obtained without additional fluids. Therefore, for routine hospital use, normal serum albumin 5% may be preferred, as maximum osmotic effect is obtained with no additional fluids.

Albumin 25% with appropriate crystalloids may offer therapeutic advantages in oncotic deficits or in long-standing shock where treatment has been delayed. Removal of ascitic fluid from the patient with cirrhosis may cause changes in cardiovascular function and even result in hypovolemic shock.

➤*Burns:* Albumin 5% or plasma protein 5% may be used in conjunction with adequate infusions of crystalloid to prevent hemoconcentration and to combat the water, protein and electrolyte losses which usually follow serious burns. After 24 hours, albumin 25% can be used to maintain plasma colloid osmotic pressure.

➤*Hypoproteinemia:* In clinical situations usually associated with a low concentration of plasma protein and, consequently, a reduced volume of circulating blood.

Normal serum albumin 5% or plasma protein fraction 5% may be used in hypoproteinemic patients, providing sodium restriction is not a problem. If sodium restriction is imperative, use 25% normal serum albumin.

For acute complications of chronic hypoproteinemia, use albumin 25% possibly in conjunction with a diuretic.

➤*Adult respiratory distress syndrome (ARDS):* This syndrome is characterized by deficient oxygenation caused by pulmonary interstitial edema complicating shock and postsurgical conditions. When clinical signs are those of hypoproteinemia with a fluid volume overload, albumin 25%, together with a diuretic, may play a role in therapy.

➤*Cardiopulmonary bypass:* Preoperative dilution of the blood using albumin and crystalloid is safe and well tolerated. Although the limit to which the hematocrit and plasma protein concentration can be safely lowered has not been defined, it is common to achieve a hematocrit of 20% and a plasma albumin concentration of 2.5 g/100 mL.

➤*Acute liver failure with or without coma:* Administration of albumin may serve the double purpose of supporting the colloid osmotic pressure of the plasma as well as binding excess plasma bilirubin. Albumin 25% may be considered.

➤*Sequestration of protein rich fluids:* This occurs in such conditions as acute peritonitis, pancreatitis, mediastinitis and extensive cellulitis. The magnitude of loss into the third space may require treatment of reduced volume or oncotic activity with albumin.

➤*Erythrocyte resuspension:* Albumin may be required to avoid excessive hypoproteinemia during certain types of exchange transfusion or with the use of very large volumes of previously frozen or washed red cells.

➤*Acute nephrosis:* Certain patients may not respond to cyclophosphamide or steroid therapy. A loop diuretic and albumin 25% may help control the edema and the patient may then respond to steroid treatment.

➤*Renal dialysis:* Albumin 25% may be of value in treating shock or hypotension.

➤*Hyperbilirubinemia and erythroblastosis fetalis:* Albumin can be a useful adjunct in exchange transfusions; it reduces the necessity for re-exchange and increases the amount of bilirubin removed with each transfusion, lessening the risk of kernicterus.

Actions

➤*Pharmacology:* The plasma protein fractions include plasma protein fraction 5% (83% albumin with alpha and beta globulins), normal serum albumin 5% and normal serum albumin 25%.

The albumin fraction of human blood has two known functions: Maintenance of plasma colloid osmotic pressure and carrier of intermediate metabolites in the transport and exchange of tissue products. It comprises about 50% to 60% of the plasma proteins and provides approximately 70% to 80% of their colloid osmotic pressure. Thus, it is important in regulating the volume of circulating blood; its loss is critical, particularly in shock with hemorrhage or reduced plasma volume. When plasma volume is reduced, an adequate amount of albumin quickly restores the volume in most instances. Twenty-five grams of albumin is the osmotic equivalent of approximately 2 units (500 mL) of fresh frozen plasma; or 100 mL of normal serum albumin 25% provides about as much plasma protein as does 500 mL plasma or 2 pints whole blood. Normal serum albumin 5% is osmotically equivalent to an approximately equal volume of citrated plasma. The 25% albumin solution is osmotically equivalent to 5 times the volume of citrated plasma.

Plasma protein fraction is effective in the maintenance of a normal blood volume, but it has not been proven effective to maintain oncotic pressure. When the circulating blood volume has been depleted, the hemodilution following albumin administration persists for many hours. In individuals with normal blood volume, it usually lasts only a few hours. The half-life of albumin is 15 to 20 days with a turnover of ≈ 15 g per day.

Albumin 5% increases the circulating plasma volume by approximately equal to the amount infused. Albumin 25% draws about 3.5 times its volume of additional fluid into the circulation within 15 minutes except when the patient is dehydrated. Both 5% and 25% decrease blood viscosity.

There is no evidence that normal serum albumin (human) interferes with normal coagulation mechanisms. Antibodies, especially isoagglutinins, have been removed, enabling the product to be used without regard to the patient's blood group or blood factors.

Unlike whole blood or plasma, plasma protein fractions are free of the danger of homologous serum hepatitis, because these solutions are heat treated at 60°C (140°F) for 10 hours; thus, the possibility of transmitting serum hepatitis is reduced to a minimum. No crossmatching is required and the absence of cellular elements removes the risk of sensitization with repeated infusions.

Contraindications

A history of allergic reactions to albumin; severe anemia; cardiac failure; the presence of normal or increased intravascular volume; patients on cardiopulmonary bypass.

In chronic nephrosis, infused albumin is promptly excreted by the kidneys with no relief of the chronic edema or effect on the underlying renal lesion. It is of occasional use in the rapid "priming" diuresis of nephrosis. Similarly, in hypoproteinemic states associated with chronic cirrhosis, malabsorption, protein losing enteropathies, pancreatic insufficiency and undernutrition, the infusion of albumin as a source of protein nutrition is not justified.

Warnings

➤*Pregnancy: Category C.* Safety for use has not been established. Use only when clearly needed and when the potential benefits outweigh the hazards to the fetus.

Precautions

➤*Concomitant blood administration:* When large quantities of albumin are given, supplement with or replace by whole blood to combat relative anemia.

Not a substitute for whole blood in situations where the oxygen carrying capacity of whole blood is required in addition to plasma volume expansion. Contains no recognized blood coagulating factors and should not be used for control of hemorrhage due to deficiencies or defects in the clotting mechanism.

➤*Hypotension:* Rapid infusion (> 10 mL/min) may produce hypotension. Monitor blood pressure during use and slow or discontinue infusion if hypotension occurs. Vasopressors may also help correct the hypotension.

➤*Hemorrhage:* Supplement albumin with hemodilution. When circulating blood volume has been reduced, hemodilution following the administration of albumin persists for many hours. In patients with a normal blood volume, hemodilution lasts for a much shorter period.

➤*Shock:* Monitor blood pressure frequently. Widening of the pulse pressure is correlated with an increase in stroke volume or cardiac output.

➤*Dehydration:* Patients with marked dehydration require additional fluids.

➤*Special risk patients:* Use with caution in patients with hepatic or renal failure because of the added protein load.

Certain patients (eg, those with congestive cardiac failure, renal insufficiency or with stabilized chronic anemia) are at risk of developing circulatory overload. Rapid infusion may cause vascular overload with resultant pulmonary edema. Monitor for signs of increased venous pressure.

Use caution in patients with low cardiac reserve or with no albumin deficiency. A rapid increase in plasma volume may cause circulatory embarrassment or pulmonary edema.

The quick rise in blood pressure that may follow administration of albumin after injuries or surgery necessitates observation to detect bleeding points that may have failed to bleed at the lower blood pressure; otherwise, new hemorrhage and shock may occur.

Adverse Reactions

Allergic or pyrogenic reactions – Such reactions are characterized primarily by fever and chills. Flushing, urticaria, back pain, headache, rash, nausea, vomiting, increased salivation and febrile reactions, tachycardia, hypotension, and changes in respiration, pulse and blood pressure have also been reported. If such reactions occur, discontinue the infusion and institute appropriate therapy.

➤*Cardiovascular:* Hypotension (see Precautions). In addition, rapid administration may result in vascular overload, dyspnea and pulmonary edema.

PLASMA PROTEIN FRACTION

Rx	**Plasmanate** (Bayer)	**Injection:** 5%	In 50, 250, and 500 mL vials.
Rx	**Plasma-Plex** (Centeon)		In 50, 250, and 500 mL vials with injection set.
Rx	**Protenate** (Baxter Healthcare)		In 250 and 500 mL vials.

PLASMA PROTEIN FRACTION (HUMAN) — INJECTION

For complete and comparative prescribing information, refer to the Plasma Protein Fractions group monograph.

Indications

➤*Treatment of shock:* Treatment of shock due to burns, crushing injuries, abdominal emergencies, and any other cause where there is a predominant loss of plasma fluids and not red blood cells. It is also effective in the emergency treatment of shock due to hemorrhage. Following the emergency phase of therapy, blood transfusions may be indicated depending on the severity of the blood loss.

Infants and small children – Found to be very useful in the initial therapy of shock due to dehydration and infection.

Administration and Dosage

➤*Dosage:* Dosage is based almost entirely on the nature of the individual case and response to therapy. The usual minimum effective dose in adults is 250 to 500 mL. As with any plasma expander, the rate should be adjusted or slowed according to the clinical response and rising blood pressure.

➤*Administration:* Administration should be by vein and preferably through an area of skin at some distance from any site of infection or trauma.

First swab the stopper with iodine tincture, followed by a sterile antiseptic swab.

Parenteral drug products should be inspected visually for particulate matter and discoloration prior to administration, whenever solution and container permit.

Only 16 gauge needles or dispensing pins should be used with 20 mL vial sizes and larger. Needles or dispensing pins should only be inserted within the stopper area delineated by the raised ring. The stopper should be penetrated perpendicular to the plane of the stopper within the ring.

➤*Admixture compatibility:* Plasma protein fraction (human) is compatible with the usual carbohydrate and electrolyte solutions.

➤*Storage/Stability:* Store at room temperature not exceeding 30°C (86°F). Solution that has been frozen should not be used.

ALBUMIN HUMAN (Normal Serum Albumin)

Rx	**Albuminar-5** (Centeon)	**Injection:** 5%	In 50 and 1,000 mL vials.
Rx	**Albutein 5%** (Alpha Therapeutic)		In 250 and 500 mL vials.
Rx	**Normal Serum Albumin (Human) 5% Solution** (Immuno-US)		In 50, 250, and 500 mL vials with IV set.
Rx	**Plasbumin-5** (Bayer)		In 50, 250, and 500 mL vials.
Rx	**Plasbumin-20** (Talecris)	**Injection:** 20%	In 50 and 100 mL vials.
Rx	**Albuminar-25** (Centeon)	**Injection:** 25%	In 20 mL vials.
Rx	**Albutein 25%** (Alpha Therapeutic)		In 20, 50, and 100 mL vials.
Rx	**Human Albumin Grifols** (Grifols)		In 50 and 100 mL vials.
Rx	**Normal Serum Albumin (Human) 25% Solution** (Immuno-US)		In 20, 50, and 100 mL vials with IV set.
Rx	**Plasbumin-25** (Bayer)		In 20, 50, and 100 mL vials.

ALBUMIN (HUMAN) — INJECTION

For complete and comparative prescribing information, refer to the Plasma Protein Fractions group monograph.

Indications

➤*Hypovolemic shock:*

25% and 20% solutions – For emergency treatment of hypovolemic shock.

Albumin (human) 25% and 20% solutions are hyperoncotic and on IV infusion will expand the plasma volume by an additional amount, 3 to 4 times the volume actually administered, by withdrawing fluid from the interstitial spaces, provided the patient is normally hydrated interstitially or there is interstitial edema. If the patient is dehydrated, additional crystalloids must be given, or, alternatively, albumin (human) 5% solution, should be used. The patient's hemodynamic response should be monitored and the usual precautions against circulatory overload observed. The total dose should not exceed the level of albumin found in the healthy individual (ie, about 2 g/kg body weight) in the absence of active bleeding). Although albumin (human) 5% solution is to be preferred for the usual volume deficits, albumin (human) 25% or 20% solution with appropriate crystalloids may offer therapeutic advantages in oncotic deficits or in long-standing shock where treatment has been delayed.

Removal of ascitic fluid from a patient with cirrhosis may cause changes in cardiovascular function and even result in hypovolemic shock. In such circumstances, the use of an albumin infusion may be required to support the blood volume.

5% solution – For the treatment of hypovolemic shock.

➤*Hypoproteinemia (with or without edema):*

25% and 20% solutions – During major surgery, patients can lose over half of their circulating albumin, with the attendant complications of oncotic deficit. A similar situation can occur in sepsis or intensive-care patients. Treatment with albumin (human) 25% or 20% solutions may be of value in such cases.

5% solution – For treatment in conditions in which there is severe hypoalbuminemia. However, unless the pathologic condition responsible for the hypoalbuminemia can be corrected, administration of albumin can afford only symptomatic or supportive relief.

➤*Cardiopulmonary bypass:*

25% and 20% solutions – With the relatively small priming volume required with modern pumps, preoperative dilution of the blood using albumin and crystalloid has been shown to be safe and well tolerated. Although the limit to which the hematocrit and plasma protein concentration can be safely lowered has not been defined, it is common practice to adjust the albumin and crystalloid pump prime to achieve a hematocrit of 20% and a plasma albumin concentration of 2.5 g/100 mL in the patient.

5% solution – May be used as an adjunct in cardiopulmonary bypass procedures.

➤*Renal dialysis:*

25% and 20% solutions – Although not part of the regular regimen of renal dialysis, albumin (human) 25% or 20% solutions may be of value in the treatment of shock or hypotension in these patients. The usual volume administered is about 100 mL, taking particular care to avoid fluid overload, as these patients are often fluid overloaded and cannot tolerate substantial volumes of salt solution.

5% solution – May be used as an adjunct in hemodialysis.

Note – In those conditions in which the colloid requirement is high, and there is less need for fluid, albumin should be administered as a 25% solution.

➤*Burn therapy:*

25% and 20% solutions – An optimal therapeutic regimen with respect to the administration of colloids, crystalloids, and water following extensive burns has not been established. During the first 24 hours after sustaining thermal injury, large volumes of crystalloids are infused to restore the depleted extracellular fluid volume. Beyond 24 hours, albumin (human) 25% or 20% solutions can be used to maintain plasma colloid osmotic pressure.

➤*Adult respiratory distress syndrome (ARDS):*

25% and 20% solutions – ARDS is characterized by deficient oxygenation caused by pulmonary interstitial edema complicating shock and postsurgical conditions. When clinical signs are those of hypoproteinemia with a fluid volume overload, albumin (human) 25% or 20% solution together with a diuretic may play a role in therapy.

➤*Acute liver failure:*

25% and 20% solutions – In the uncommon situation of rapid loss of liver function with or without coma, administration of albumin may serve the double purpose of supporting the colloid osmotic pressure of the plasma as well as binding excess plasma bilirubin.

➤*Sequestration of protein-rich fluids:*

25% and 20% solutions – Sequestration of protein-rich fluids occurs in such conditions as acute peritonitis, pancreatitis, mediastinitis, and extensive cellulitis. The magnitude of loss into the third space may require treatment of reduced volume or oncotic activity with an infusion of albumin.

➤*Erythrocyte resuspension:*

25% and 20% solutions – Albumin may be required to avoid excessive hypoproteinemia during certain types of exchange transfusion or with the use of very large volumes of previously frozen or washed red cells. About 25 g of albumin per liter of erythrocytes is commonly used, although the requirements in preexistent hypoproteinemia or hepatic impairment can be greater. Albumin human 25% or 20% solutions are added to the isotonic sus-

ALBUMIN (HUMAN) — INJECTION

pension of washed red cells immediately prior to transfusion.

➤*Acute nephrosis:*

25% and 20% solutions – Certain patients with acute nephrosis may not respond to cyclophosphamide or steroid therapy. The steroids may even aggravate the underlying edema. In this situation, a loop diuretic and 100 mL of albumin (human) 25% or 20% solutions repeated daily for 7 to 10 days may be helpful in controlling the edema, and the patient may then respond to steroid treatment.

➤*Pediatric use:*

25% and 20% solutions –

Neonatal hemolytic disease: The administration of albumin (human) 25% or 20% solutions may be indicated prior to exchange transfusion in order to bind free bilirubin, thus lessening the risk of kernicterus. A dosage of 1 g/kg body weight is given about 1 hour prior to exchange transfusion. Caution must be observed in hypervolemic infants.

5% solution – The pediatric use of albumin (human) 5% solution has not been clinically evaluated. Therefore, physicians should weigh the risks and benefits of the use of albumin (human) 5% solution in the pediatric population.

➤*Situations in which albumin administration is not warranted:* In chronic nephrosis, infused albumin is promptly excreted by the kidneys, with no relief of the chronic edema or effect on the underlying renal lesion. It is of occasional use in the rapid "priming" diuresis of nephrosis. Similarly, in hypoproteinemic states associated with chronic cirrhosis, malabsorption, protein losing enteropathies, pancreatic insufficiency, and undernutrition, the infusion of albumin as a source of protein nutrition is not justified.

Administration and Dosage

Albumin (human) 25%, 20% and 5% solutions are administered IV.

➤*Dosage:*

5% solution – The total dosage will vary with the individual. In adults, an initial infusion of 500 mL is suggested. Additional amounts may be administered as clinically indicated.

Hypovolemic shock –

25% and 20% solutions: For treatment of hypovolemic shock, the volume administered and the speed of infusion should be adapted to the response of the individual patient.

5% solution: In the treatment of the patient in shock with greatly reduced blood volume, albumin (human) 5% solution may be administered as rapidly as necessary in order to improve the clinical condition and restore normal blood volume. This may be repeated in 15 to 30 minutes if the initial dose fails to prove adequate. In the patient with a slightly low or normal blood volume, the rate of administration should be 1 to 2 mL/min.

Burns –

25% and 20% solutions: After a burn injury (usually beyond 24 hours), there is a close correlation between the amount of albumin infused and the resultant increase in plasma colloid osmotic pressure. The aim should be to maintain the plasma albumin concentration in the region of 2.5 ± 0.5 g/100 mL, with a plasma oncotic pressure of 20 mm Hg (equivalent to a total plasma protein concentration of 5.2 g/100 mL). This is best achieved by the IV administration of albumin (human) 25% or 20% solutions. The duration of therapy is decided by the loss of protein from the burned areas and in the urine. In addition, oral or parenteral feeding with amino acids should be initiated, as the long-term administration of albumin should not be considered as a source of nutrition.

Hypoproteinemia, with or without edema –

25% and 20% solutions: Unless the underlying pathology responsible for the hypoproteinemia can be corrected, the IV administration of albumin (human) 25% or 20% solutions must be considered purely symptomatic or supportive. The usual daily dose of albumin for adults is 50 to 75 g and, for children, 25 g. Patients with severe hypoproteinemia who continue to lose albumin may require larger quantities. Since hypoproteinemic patients usually have approximately normal blood volumes, the rate of administration of albumin (human) 25% or 20% solutions should not exceed 2 mL/min, as more rapid injection may precipitate circulatory embarrassment and pulmonary edema. Other dosage recommendations are given under the specific indications referred to above.

Pediatric use –

5% solution: The pediatric use of albumin (human) 5% solution has not been clinically evaluated. The dosage will vary with the clinical state and body weight of the individual. Typically, a dose one-quarter to one-half the adult dose may be administered, or dosage may be calculated on the basis of 0.6 to 1 g/kg of body weight (12 to 20 mL of human albumin 5% solution). The usual rate of administration in children should be one-quarter the adult rate.

➤*Administration:* Parenteral drug products should be inspected visually for particulate matter and discoloration prior to administration, whenever solution and container permit.

Albumin (human) must be administered IV. It may be administered either in conjunction with or combined with other parenterals such as whole blood, plasma, saline, glucose or sodium lactate. The volume of the total dose and the rate of infusion depends on the patient's condition and response.

25% and 20% solutions – Albumin (human) 25% and 20% solutions may be administered either undiluted or diluted in 0.9% sodium chloride or 5% dextrose in water. If sodium restriction is required, albumin (human) 25% or 20% solutions should only be administered either undiluted or diluted in a sodium-free carbohydrate solution such as 5% dextrose in water.

Preparation for administration – Remove seal to expose stopper. Always swab stopper top immediately with a suitable antiseptic prior to entering vial.

Only 16-gauge needles or dispensing pins should be used with 20 mL vial sizes and larger. Needles or dispensing pins should only be inserted within the stopper area delineated by the raised ring. The stopper should be penetrated perpendicular to the plane of the stopper within the ring.

➤*5% solution:*

Directions for use (250 mL and 500 mL with administration set) – Flip off plastic cap on the top of the vial and expose rubber stopper. Cleanse exposed rubber stopper with a suitable germicidal solution, being sure to remove any excess. Observe aseptic technique and prepare sterile IV equipment as follows:

1.) Close clamp on administration set (delivers approximately 15 drops/mL).
2.) With bottle upright, thrust piercing pin straight through stopper center. Do not twist or angle.
3.) Immediately invert bottle to automatically establish proper fluid level in drip chamber (half full).
4.) Attach infusion set to administration set, open clamp and allow solution to expel air from tubing and needle, then close clamp.
5.) Make venipuncture and adjust flow.
6.) Discard all administration equipment after use. Discard any unused contents.

➤*Storage/Stability:* Solutions of albumin (human) should not be used if they appear turbid or if there is sediment in the bottle. Do not begin administration more than 4 hours after the container has been entered. Discard unused portion.

Solutions which have been frozen should not be used. Vials which are cracked or which have been previously entered or damaged should not be used, as this may have allowed the entry of microorganisms. Albumin (human) 25%, 20% and 5% solutions contain no preservative.

5% solution – Albumin (human) 5% solution is stable for 3 years, providing storage temperature does not exceed 30°C (89°F). Protect from freezing.

25% and 20% solutions – Store at room temperature not exceeding 30°C (86°F). Do not freeze. Do not use after expiration date.

HETASTARCH (Hydroxyethyl Starch; HES)

Rx	**Hetastarch** (Gensia Sicor Pharm)	**Injection:** 6 g/100 mL in 0.9% sodium chloride	In 500 mL IV infusion containers.

HETASTARCH (Hydroxyethyl Starch; HES) — INJECTION

Indications

➤*Shock:* Adjunct for plasma volume expansion in shock due to hemorrhage, burns, surgery, sepsis or other trauma.

➤*Leukapheresis:* Adjunct to improve harvesting and increase yield of granulocytes.

Administration and Dosage

➤*Administration:* Administer by IV infusion only. Total dosage and rate of infusion depend upon the amount of blood lost and the resultant hemoconcentration.

➤*Plasma volume expansion:* The usual amount is 500 to 1000 mL. Total dosage does not usually exceed 1500 mL/day (20 mL/kg). In acute hemorrhagic shock, rates approaching 20 mL/kg/hour may be used.

➤*Leukapheresis:* In continuous flow centrifugation (CFC) procedures, 250 to 700 mL is typically infused at a constant fixed ratio of 1:8 to 1:13 to venous whole blood.

➤*Storage/Stability:* Store at room temperature not exceeding 40°C (104°F). Do not freeze. Do not use if solution is turbid deep brown or if crystalline precipitate forms.

Actions

➤*Pharmacology:* Hetastarch (HES) is a complex mixture of ethoxylated amylopectin molecules of various sizes; average molecular weight (MW) is 450,000 (range, 10,000 to > 1 million). Colloidal properties of 6% HES approximate those of human albumin. After IV infusion, plasma volume expands slightly in excess of volume infused and decreases over 24 to 36 hours. Hemodynamic status will decrease after 24 hours. Adding HES to whole blood increases the erythrocyte sedimentation rate and improves the efficiency of granulocyte collection by centrifugal means.

➤*Pharmacokinetics:* Molecules < 50,000 MW are rapidly eliminated renally; ≈ 33% appear in urine in 24 hours. Larger molecules are broken down; ≈ 90% of the dose is eliminated (avg. half-life, 17 days; the remainder has a half-life of 48 days). The hydroxyethyl group remains intact and attached to glucose units when excreted.

Contraindications

Severe bleeding disorders; severe cardiac failure; renal failure with oliguria or anuria.

Warnings

➤*Blood/Plasma substitute:* Not a substitute for blood or plasma, as it does not have oxygen-carrying capacity or contain plasma proteins (eg, coagulation factors).

➤*Coagulation effects:* Large volumes may alter coagulation and result in transient prolongation of prothrombin time (PT), partial thromboplastin time (PTT), bleeding and clotting times, decreased hematocrit and excessive dilution of plasma proteins.

➤*Leukapheresis:* Slight declines in platelet count and hemoglobin levels have been observed in donors undergoing repeated leukapheresis procedures due to the volume expanding effects of hetastarch. Hemoglobin levels usually return to normal within 24 hours. Hemodilution by hetastarch and saline may also result in 24 hour declines of total protein, albumin, calcium, and fibrinogen values.

➤*Hypersensitivity reactions:* Anaphylactoid reactions (periorbital edema, urticaria, wheezing) have been reported. If these occur, discontinue the drug. If necessary, give antihistamines. See Management of Acute Hypersensitivity Reactions. Also, use caution when administering HES to a person allergic to corn.

➤*Pregnancy: Category C.* Safety for use has not been established. Use only when clearly needed and when potential benefits outweigh potential hazards to the fetus.

➤*Lactation:* It is not known whether hetastarch is excreted in breast milk. Exercise caution when administering to a nursing woman.

➤*Children:* Safety and efficacy have not been established.

Precautions

➤*Monitoring:* During leukapheresis, monitor CBC, total leukocyte and platelet counts, leukocyte differential count, hemoglobin, hematocrit, PT and PTT.

➤*Special risk:* The possibility of circulatory overload exists. Take special care in patients with impaired renal clearance and when the risk of pulmonary edema or congestive heart failure is increased. Indirect bilirubin levels increased in two subjects receiving multiple infusions; levels returned to normal by 96 hours after infusion. Total bilirubin remained normal. Use caution in liver disease.

Adverse Reactions

Vomiting; mild temperature elevation; chills; itching; submaxillary and parotid glandular enlargement; mild influenza-like symptoms; headache; muscle pain; peripheral edema of the lower extremities; allergic reactions (see Warnings).

DEXTRAN, LOW MOLECULAR WEIGHT (Dextran 40)

Rx	**Dextran 40** (McGaw)	**Injection:** 10% dextran 40 in 0.9% sodium chloride	In 500 mL.
Rx	**Gentran 40** (Baxter)		In 500 mL.
Rx	**10% LMD** (Abbott)		In 500 mL.
Rx	**Rheomacrodex** (Medisan)		In 500 mL.
Rx	**Dextran 40** (McGaw)	**Injection:** 10% dextran 40 in 5% dextrose	In 500 mL.
Rx	**Gentran 40** (Baxter)		In 500 mL.
Rx	**10% LMD** (Abbott)		In 500 mL.
Rx	**Rheomacrodex** (Medisan)		In 500 mL.

DEXTRAN, LOW MOLECULAR WEIGHT (Dextran 40) — INJECTION

Indications

➤*Shock:* Adjunctive treatment of shock or impending shock due to hemorrhage, burns, surgery or other trauma. The solution is for emergency treatment when whole blood products are not available; it is not a substitute for whole blood or plasma proteins.

➤*Priming fluid:* As a priming fluid, either as the sole primer or as an additive, in pump oxygenators during extracorporeal circulation.

➤*Deep venous thrombosis (DVT)/Pulmonary embolism (PE) prophylaxis:* Prophylaxis against DVT and PE in patients undergoing procedures associated with a high incidence of thromboembolic complications, such as hip surgery.

Administration and Dosage

For IV use only.

➤*Adjunctive therapy in shock:* Total dosage during the first 24 hours should not exceed 20 mL/kg. The first 10 mL/kg should be infused rapidly, with the remaining dose being administered more slowly. Monitor the central venous pressure frequently during the initial infusion. Should therapy continue beyond 24 hours, total daily dosage should not exceed 10 mL/kg, and therapy should not continue beyond 5 days.

➤*Hemodiluent in extracorporeal circulation:* The dosage employed in the priming fluid will vary with the volume of pump oxygenator employed. It may be added as sole primer or as an additive. Generally, 10 to 20 mL/kg are added to the perfusion circuit. Do not exceed total dosage of 20 mL/kg; this can be limited and controlled by adding other priming fluids.

➤*Prophylactic therapy of venous thrombosis and thromboembolism:* Select dosage according to the risk of thromboembolic complications (eg, type of surgery and duration of immobilization). In general, initiate treatment during surgery. Administer 500 to 1000 mL (approximately 10 mL/kg) on the day of the operation. Continue treatment at a dose of 500 mL/day for an additional 2 to 3 days. Thereafter, and according to the risk of complications, 500 mL may be administered every second or third day during the period of risk for up to 2 weeks.

➤*Children:* The best guide is the body weight or surface area, and the total dosage should not exceed 20 mL/kg.

➤*Storage/Stability:* Store at a constant temperature between 15° to 30°C (59° to 86°F). Protect from freezing.

Actions

➤*Pharmacology:* Dextran 40 is a branched polysaccharide plasma-volume expander with an average molecular weight of 40,000 (range 10,000 to 90,000). A 2.5% solution of dextran 40 is equivalent in colloid osmotic pressure to normal plasma. Generally, plasma volume is increased onefold to twofold over the volume of dextran 40 infused. The extent and duration of volume expansion produced will depend on the preexisting blood volume, rate of infusion and rate of dextran clearance by the kidneys.

➤*Pharmacokinetics:* Dextran 40 is evenly distributed in the vascular system. Its distribution according to molecular weight shifts toward higher molecular weights as the smaller molecules are excreted by the kidney. Approximately 50% administered to a normovolemic subject is excreted in the urine within 3 hours, 60% within 6 hours and 75% within 24 hours. The remaining 25% is partially hydrolyzed and excreted in the urine, partially excreted in the feces and partially oxidized. Unexcreted dextran molecules diffuse into the extravascular compartment and are temporarily taken up by

DEXTRAN, LOW MOLECULAR WEIGHT (Dextran 40) — INJECTION

the reticuloendothelial system. Some of these molecules are returned to the intravascular compartment via the lymphatics. Dextran is slowly degraded to glucose by the enzyme dextranase.

Adjunctive therapy in shock – Enhances blood flow, particularly in the microcirculation, by a combination of the following mechanisms: Increases blood volume, venous return and cardiac output; decreases blood viscosity and peripheral vascular resistance; reduces aggregation of erythrocytes and other cellular elements of blood by coating them and maintaining their electronegative charges.

Administration to a patient in shock usually increases blood volume, central venous pressure, cardiac output, stroke volume, arterial blood pressure, pulse pressure, capillary perfusion, venous return and urinary output; it also decreases blood viscosity, heart rate, peripheral resistance and mean transit time and prevents or reverses cellular aggregation. Hematocrit is lowered in proportion to the infusion volume.

The intense but relatively short-lived plasma expansion volume produced by dextran 40 is advantageous in the treatment of early shock because it acts rapidly to correct hypovolemia while allowing control of the plasma volume. If overexpansion occurs, the discontinuation of the infusion will result in a decline in plasma volume due to loss of dextran from the intravascular space.

Priming solution for extracorporeal circulation – Dextran 40's advantages over homologous blood and other priming fluids include: Decreased destruction of erythrocytes and platelets; reduced intravascular hemagglutination; maintenance of electronegativity of erythrocytes and platelets.

Prophylaxis against venous thrombosis, thromboembolism – The infusion of dextran 40 during and after surgical trauma reduces the incidence of DVT and PE in surgical patients subject to procedures with a high incidence of thromboembolic complications. Dextran 40 simultaneously inhibits mechanisms essential to thrombus formation such as vascular stasis and platelet adhesiveness, and alters the structure and lysability of fibrin clots.

Dextran 40 increases cardiac output, arterial, venous and microcirculatory flow and reduces mean transit time, chiefly by expanding plasma volume, by reducing blood viscosity through hemodilution and by reducing red cell aggregation.

Contraindications

Hypersensitivity to dextran; marked hemostatic defects of all types (eg, thrombocytopenia, hypofibrinogenemia), including those caused by drugs (eg, heparin, warfarin); marked cardiac decompensation; renal disease with severe oliguria or anuria.

Decreased urinary output, secondary to shock, is not a contraindication unless there is no improvement in urine output after the initial dose.

If administration of sodium or chloride could be clinically detrimental, 10% Dextran in 0.9% Sodium Chloride Injection is contraindicated.

Warnings

➤*Fluid imbalance:* These products are colloid hypertonic solutions and will attract water from the extravascular space. Poorly hydrated patients will need additional fluid therapy. If given in excess, vascular overload could occur. This can be avoided by monitoring central venous pressure.

Administration of dextran IV can cause fluid or solute overloading, resulting in dilution of serum electrolyte concentrations, overhydration, congested states or pulmonary edema. The risk of dilutional states is inversely proportional to electrolyte concentrations of administered parenteral solutions.

➤*Hemorrhage:* Use with caution in patients with active hemorrhage; the increase in perfusion pressure and improved microcirculatory flow may result in additional blood loss.

Avoid administering infusions that exceed the recommended dose, as a dose-related increase in the incidence of wound hematoma, wound seroma, wound bleeding, distant bleeding (hematuria and melena) and pulmonary edema has been observed.

➤*Hematologic effects:* Use with caution in patients with thrombocytopenia. Hematocrit should not be depressed below 30% by volume. When large volumes of dextran are administered, plasma protein levels will be decreased. Do not give dextran 40 to patients with marked thrombocytopenia or hypofibrinogenemia.

In individuals with normal hemostasis, dosages of up to 15 mL/kg or > 1000 mL may prolong bleeding time and decrease coagulation due to depressed platelet function. Dosages in this range also markedly decrease factor VIII; they also decrease factors V and IX to a slightly greater degree than would be expected from hemodilution alone. Because these changes tend to be more pronounced following trauma or major surgery, observe all patients for early signs of bleeding complications.

➤*Special risk patients:* Use solutions containing sodium ions with great care, if at all, in patients with congestive heart failure, severe renal insufficiency, in clinical states in which edema exists with sodium retention (particularly in postoperative or elderly patients) and in patients receiving corticosteroids.

Use dextrose-containing solutions with caution in overt or known subclinical diabetes mellitus.

➤*Hypersensitivity reactions:* Antigenicity of dextrans is directly related to their degree of branching. Because dextran 40 has a low degree of branching, it is relatively free of antigenic effect. Hypersensitivity reactions have, however, been reported (see Adverse Reactions). Infrequently, severe and fatal anaphylactoid reactions (eg, marked hypotension, cardiac and respiratory arrest) have been reported. Most of these reactions occurred early in the infusion period in patients not previously exposed to IV dextran and have appeared after administration of as little as 10 mL. Stop infusion immediately if an anaphylactoid reaction is imminent. Refer to Management of Acute Hypersensitivity Reactions. In circulatory collapse due to anaphylaxis, institute rapid volume substitution with an agent other than dextran. Dextran 1 is indicated for prophylaxis of serious anaphylactic reactions to dextran infusions.

➤*Renal function impairment:* Renal excretion causes elevation of the specific gravity of the urine. In the presence of adequate urine flow, only minor elevations occur, but in patients with diminished urine flow, urine viscosity and specific gravity can be increased markedly. As osmolarity is only slightly affected by the presence of dextran molecules, assess a patient's state of hydration by determination of urine or serum osmolarity. If signs of dehydration are noted, administer additional fluids. An osmotic diuretic such as mannitol is useful in maintaining adequate urine flow.

Renal failure, sometimes irreversible, has been reported. While the preexisting clinical condition of these patients could account for the oliguria or anuria, it is possible that dextran use may have contributed to its development. Evidence of tubular vacuolization (osmotic nephrosis) has been found following administration. The exact clinical significance is unknown.

In patients with diminished renal function, use of solutions containing sodium ions may result in sodium retention. Excessive doses may precipitate renal failure.

➤*Pregnancy: Category C.* Safety for use during pregnancy has not been established. Use only when clearly needed and when the potential benefits outweigh the potential hazards to the fetus.

➤*Lactation:* It is not known whether this drug is excreted in breast milk. Exercise caution when dextran 40 is administered to a nursing woman.

Precautions

➤*Monitoring:* Urine output should be carefully monitored. Usually, an increase in urine output occurs in oliguric patients after administration. If no increase is observed after the infusion of 500 mL, discontinue the drug until adequate diuresis develops spontaneously or can be induced by other means.

Exercise care to prevent a depression of the hematocrit below 30%.

Infusion of dextran may lead to excessive dilution of red blood cells and plasma proteins, dilution of other blood constituents (platelets, fibrinogen) or dilutional acidosis caused by dilution of the bicarbonate ion.

➤*Bleeding complications:* Observe patients for early signs of bleeding complications, particularly following surgery, major trauma or if anticoagulant drugs are being administered.

Drug Interactions

➤*Drug/Lab test interactions:* Blood sugar determinations that employ high concentrations of acid (acetic or sulfuric) may cause hydrolysis of dextran; falsely elevated glucose assays may be reported in patients receiving dextran. In other laboratory tests, the presence of dextran may result in the development of turbidity, which can interfere with bilirubin assays in which alcohol has been employed, in total protein assays employing biuret reagent and in blood sugar determinations with the ortho-toluidine method. Consider withdrawal of blood for chemical laboratory tests prior to initiating therapy.

Blood typing and crossmatching procedures employing enzyme techniques may give unreliable readings if the samples are taken after infusion. Other blood typing and crossmatching procedures are not affected. Draw blood samples for the above determinations prior to initiating infusion or, alternatively, inform the laboratory that the patient has received dextran so that suitable assay methods can be applied.

Occasional abnormal renal and hepatic function values have been reported following IV use. The specific effect on renal and hepatic function could not be determined, as most of these patients had also undergone surgery or cardiac catheterization.

Adverse Reactions

➤*Hypersensitivity:* Mild cutaneous eruptions, generalized urticaria, hypotension, nausea, vomiting, headache, dyspnea, fever, tightness of the chest, bronchospasm, wheezing and, rarely, anaphylactoid (allergic) shock (see Warnings).

➤*Miscellaneous:* Reactions which may occur because of the solution or the technique of administration include febrile response, infection at the injection site, venous thrombosis or phlebitis extending from the injection site, extravasation and hypervolemia.

Hypernatremia may be associated with edema and exacerbation of congestive heart failure due to the retention of water, resulting in expanded extracellular fluid volume.

If solutions containing sodium chloride are infused in large volumes, chloride ions may cause a loss of bicarbonate ions, resulting in an acidifying effect.

DEXTRAN, HIGH MOLECULAR WEIGHT (Dextran 70 and 75)

Rx	**Dextran 75** (Abbott)	**Injection:** 6% dextran 75 in 0.9% sodium chloride	In 500 mL.
Rx	**Dextran 70** (McGaw)	**Injection:** 6% dextran 70 in 0.9% sodium chloride	In 500 mL.
Rx	**Gentran 70** (Baxter)		In 500 mL.
Rx	**Macrodex** (Medisan)		In 500 mL.
Rx	**Dextran 75** (Abbott)	**Injection:** 6% dextran 75 in 5% dextrose	In 500 mL.
Rx	**Macrodex** (Medisan)	**Injection:** 6% dextran 70 in 5% dextrose	In 500 mL.

DEXTRAN, HIGH MOLECULAR WEIGHT (Dextran 70 and 75) — INJECTION

Indications

➤*Shock:* Treatment of shock or impending shock due to surgery or other trauma, hemorrhage or burns. Intended for emergency treatment only when whole blood or blood products are not available; do not regard as a substitute for whole blood or plasma proteins. It should not replace other forms of therapy known to be of value in the treatment of shock.

Administration and Dosage

Administer by IV infusion only. Total dose and rate of infusion depend upon the magnitude of fluid loss and the resultant hemoconcentration. It is suggested that the total dosage not exceed 20 mL/kg during the first 24 hours.

➤*Adults:* The amount usually administered is 500 to 1000 mL, which may be given at a rate of from 20 to 40 mL/minute in an emergency.

➤*Children:* The best guide to dosage is the body weight or surface area of the patient; total dosage should not exceed 20 mL/kg.

No additives should be delivered via plasma volume expanders.

➤*Storage / Stability:* The solution has no bacteriostat; discard partially used containers. The solution must be clear. Store at a constant temperature not > 25°C (77°F).

Actions

➤*Pharmacology:* Dextrans are synthetic polysaccharides used to approximate the colloidal properties of albumin. Dextran 70 has an average molecular weight (MW) of 70,000 (range 20,000 to 200,000), and dextran 75 has an average MW of 75,000 . Dextran 70 improves blood pressure, pulse rate, respiratory exchange and renal function in patients with hypovolemia or hypotensive shock. IV infusion results in an expansion of plasma volume slightly in excess of volume infused and decreases from this maximum over the next 24 hours. This plasma volume expansion improves hemodynamic status for ≥ 24 hours.

➤*Pharmacokinetics:* Dextran molecules below 50,000 molecular weight are eliminated by renal excretion, with approximately 50% appearing in the urine in 24 hours in the normovolemic patient. The remaining dextran is enzymatically degraded to glucose at a rate of about 70 to 90 mg/kg/day. This is a variable process.

Contraindications

Hypersensitivity to dextran; marked hemostatic defects of all types (thrombocytopenia, hypofibrinogenemia, etc), including those induced by drugs; marked cardiac decompensation; renal disease with severe oliguria or anuria; severe congestive heart failure, pulmonary edema and severe bleeding disorders; where use of sodium or chloride could be clinically detrimental.

Warnings

➤*Fluid imbalance:* Fluid or solute overloading may occur, resulting in dilution of serum electrolyte concentrations, overhydration, congested states (CHF) and peripheral or pulmonary edema. The risk of dilutional states is inversely proportional to the electrolyte concentration of administered parenteral solutions.

The risk of solute overload causing congested states with peripheral and pulmonary edema is directly proportional to electrolyte concentrations of such solutions.

➤*Hematologic effects:* In individuals with normal hemostasis, dosages approximating 15 mL/kg or > 1000 mL prolong bleeding time and decrease coagulation due to depressed platelet function; use with caution in patients with thrombocytopenia. Such dosages also markedly decrease factor VIII and decrease factor V and factor IX more than would be expected from hemodilution alone. These changes tend to be more pronounced following trauma or major surgery; observe patients for early signs of bleeding complications. Transient prolongation of bleeding time may occur following doses > 1000 mL, particularly if the patient is on concomitant anticoagulation therapy. Take care to prevent depression of hematocrit below 30% by volume. When large volumes of dextran are given, plasma protein level will be decreased.

➤*Special risk patients:* Use solutions containing sodium ions with great care, if at all, in patients with congestive heart failure, pulmonary edema, severe renal insufficiency, patients receiving corticosteroids or corticotropin and in clinical states in which edema exists with sodium retention. Circulatory overload may occur. Exercise special care in patients with impaired renal clearance.

Exercise care in patients with pathological abdominal conditions and in those undergoing bowel surgery.

➤*Hypersensitivity reactions:* Severe and fatal anaphylactoid reactions (eg, marked hypotension, cardiac and respiratory arrest) have occurred early in the infusion period in patients not previously exposed to IV dextran. Stop infusion immediately if an anaphylactoid reaction is imminent, provided that other means of sustaining the circulation are available. Refer to Management of Acute Hypersensitivity Reactions. In circulatory collapse due to anaphylaxis, institute rapid volume substitution with an agent other than dextran. Antihistamines may be effective in relieving some symptoms. Dextran 1 is indicated for prophylaxis of serious anaphylactic reactions associated with dextran infusions.

➤*Pregnancy: Category C.* Safety for use during pregnancy has not been established. There are no adequate and well controlled studies in pregnant women. Use only when clearly needed and when potential benefits outweigh potential hazards.

➤*Lactation:* It is not known whether this drug is excreted in breast milk. Exercise caution when administering to a nursing woman.

Precautions

➤*Monitoring:* Urine output should be carefully observed. An increase in urine output usually occurs in oliguric patients after the administration of dextran. If no increase is observed after the infusion of 500 mL of dextran, discontinue the drug until adequate diuresis develops spontaneously or can be provoked by other means.

Monitoring central venous blood pressure is recommended to detect overexpansion of blood volume. When signs of overexpansion appear, discontinuing IV infusion allows blood volume to readjust and decline, primarily by loss of fluid to urine.

➤*Bleeding complications:* Observe patients for early signs of bleeding complications, particularly following surgery or major trauma, or if anticoagulant drugs are being administered.

Drug Interactions

➤*Drug / Lab test interactions:* Blood sugar determinations that employ high concentrations of acid (acetic or sulfuric) may cause hydrolysis of dextran; falsely elevated glucose assays may be reported in patients receiving dextran. In other laboratory tests, the presence of dextran may result in the development of turbidity, which can interfere with bilirubin assays in which alcohol has been employed, in total protein assays employing biuret reagent and in blood sugar determinations with the ortho-toluidine method.

Blood typing and crossmatching procedures employing enzyme techniques may give unreliable readings if the samples are taken after infusion. If blood is drawn after the infusion, the saline-agglutination and indirect antiglobulin methods may be used for typing and crossmatching. Draw blood samples for the above determinations prior to initiating infusion or, alternatively, inform the laboratory that the patient has received dextran so that suitable assay methods can be applied.

Adverse Reactions

➤*Infusion technique:* Reactions which may occur because of the solution or the technique of administration include febrile response, infection at the injection site, venous thrombosis or phlebitis extending from the injection site, extravasation and hypervolemia. If a reaction develops, discontinue use and treat accordingly.

➤*Hypersensitivity:* Allergic reactions include urticaria, nasal congestion, wheezing, tightness of the chest, dyspnea, mild hypotension and, rarely, anaphylactoid (allergic) shock (see Warnings).

➤*Miscellaneous:* Sudden marked hypotension; nausea; vomiting; fever; joint pains.

Hypernatremia may be associated with edema and exacerbation of congestive heart failure due to water retention, resulting in expanded extracellular fluid volume.

If solutions containing sodium chloride are infused in large volumes, chloride ions may cause a loss of bicarbonate ions, resulting in an acidifying effect.

Dextran Adjunct

DEXTRAN 1

Rx	**Promit** (Medisan)	**Injection:** 150 mg/mL	In 20 mL vials.

DEXTRAN 1 — INJECTION

Indications

➤*Serious anaphylactic reactions to dextran:* Prophylaxis of serious anaphylactic reactions to IV infusion of clinical dextran. Mild dextran-induced anaphylactic (allergic) reactions are not prevented by dextran 1.

Administration and Dosage

For IV use only. Do not dilute or admix with clinical dextran.

➤*Adults:* 20 mL (150 mg/mL) IV rapidly, 1 to 2 minutes before IV infusion of clinical dextran.

➤*Children:* 0.3 mL/kg in a corresponding manner.

➤*Administration:* The time interval between administration of dextran 1 and clinical dextran solutions should not exceed 15 minutes; if a longer period elapses, repeat dextran 1 dose. Repeat dextran 1 injection if 48 hours have elapsed since the last infusion of clinical dextran. Administer 1 to 2 minutes before every IV clinical dextran infusion.

May give IV through Y injection site if minimally diluted with primary solution. Do not give through an IV set used to infuse clinical dextran. May give through heparin lock.

➤*Storage / Stability:* Do not exceed 25°C (77°F). Protect from freezing.

Actions

➤*Pharmacology:* Clinical dextran is not antigenic, but its structure is similar to other antigenic polysaccharides. Some polysaccharide-reacting antibodies may crossreact with clinical dextran, forming antibody-antigen complexes that can trigger an anaphylactic reaction. This may occur in patients who have never received clinical dextran, but have enough dextran-reacting antibodies (DRA) to form large immune complexes. Dextran 1, a monovalent hapten, reacts with dextran-reactive immunoglobulin (IgG) without bridge formation and with no tendency for the formation of large immune complexes. A molar excess of monovalent hapten, given just before a clinical IV dextran solution, competitively prevents the formation of immune complexes with polyvalent clinical dextrans and impedes anaphylaxis. During the initial phase of a clinical dextran infusion, protection is affected by hapten inhibition. During the later phase and the following day, protection is exerted by dextran molecules in clinical dextran solutions because an antigen excess develops in the circulation and only small nonanaphylactogenic immune complexes can be formed. An additional injection of dextran 1 is recommended if 48 hours or more have elapsed since the previous infusion of clinical dextran.

Dextran-induced anaphylactic reactions have an incidence range of 0.002% to 0.025% per unit used (0.002% to 0.013% for dextran 40 and 0.017% to 0.025% for dextran 60/75). By means of hapten inhibition, the incidence is 15 to 20 times lower.

➤*Pharmacokinetics:* Because of its low molecular weight of 1000, dextran 1 is rapidly and completely excreted by glomerular filtration. After IV injection of a single 20 mL dose, ≈ 50% is cleared from the blood within 30 minutes. Mean urinary elimination half-life was 41 ± 11 minutes in 12 healthy individuals.

Contraindications

Do not give dextran 1 if IV use of clinical dextran solutions is contraindicated. This includes marked hemostatic defects of all types or hemorrhagic tendencies, marked cardiac decompensation and renal disease with severe oliguria or anuria.

Warnings

➤*Cardiac effects:* Severe hypotension and bradycardia have been reported.

➤*Pregnancy: Category B.* In rabbits, doses 35 to 70 times the human dose increased the incidence of fetal resorption, postimplantation fetal loss, retardation of fetal long-bone ossification and marginal fetal growth retardation. There are no adequate and well-controlled studies in pregnant women. Use only if clearly needed.

➤*Lactation:* It is not known whether dextran 1 is excreted in breast milk. Exercise caution when administering to nursing women.

Precautions

➤*Reactions:* If any reaction occurs, do not administer clinical dextran solutions.

Adverse Reactions

Cutaneous (0.016%); moderate hypotension (systolic BP > 60 mmHg; 0.014%); bradycardia (< 60 bpm) with moderate hypotension (0.013%); nausea, pallor, shivering (0.011%); bradycardia (0.004%); bradycardia with severe hypotension (systolic BP < 60 mmHg; 0.001%). Do not give subsequent infusion if adverse reactions occur.

Overdosage

The drug is rapidly cleared by renal excretion. Therefore, any overdosage should be of short duration and of minimal consequence.

HEMIN

Rx	**Panhematin** (Ovation)	**Powder for injection, lyophilized:** 313 mg hemin (301 mg hematin/vial [equivalent to 7 mg hematin/mL] after reconstitution with 43 mL sterile water for injection)	Preservative free. With 300 mg sorbitol. In single-dose vials.

HEMIN — INJECTION

WARNING

Hemin for injection should only be used by physicians experienced in the management of porphyrias in hospitals where the recommended clinical and laboratory diagnostic and monitoring techniques are available.

Consider hemin therapy after an appropriate period of alternate therapy (ie, 400 g glucose/day for 1 to 2 days).

Indications

➤*Porphyria:* For the amelioration of recurrent attacks of acute intermittent porphyria temporally related to the menstrual cycle in susceptible women. Manifestations such as pain, hypertension, tachycardia, abnormal mental status, and mild to progressive neurologic signs may be controlled in selected patients.

Similar findings have been reported in other patients with acute intermittent porphyria, porphyria variegata, and hereditary coproporphyria.

Administration and Dosage

For IV use only. Use a large arm vein or a central venous catheter to avoid phlebitis.

Before administering hemin for injection, consider alternate therapy (ie, 400 g glucose/day for 1 to 2 days). If improvement is unsatisfactory for the treatment of acute attacks of porphyria, administer an IV infusion containing a dose of 1 to 4 mg/kg/day of hematin over a period of 10 to 15 minutes for 3 to 14 days, based on clinical signs. In more severe cases, this dose may be repeated no earlier than every 12 hours. Give no more than 6 mg/kg in any 24-hour period.

➤*Preparation of solution:* Reconstitute by adding 43 mL of Sterile Water for Injection to the dispensing vial. Shake well for a period of 2 to 3 minutes to aid dissolution.

After reconstitution, each mL contains the equivalent of approximately 7 mg hematin (301 mg hemin/43 mL), 5 mg sodium carbonate (215 mg/43 mL), and 7 mg sorbitol (301 mg/43 mL). The drug may be administered directly from the vial.

Hemin Solution Preparation
Dosage Calculation Table
1 mg hematin equivalent = 0.14 mL
2 mg hematin equivalent = 0.28 mL
3 mg hematin equivalent = 0.42 mL
4 mg hematin equivalent = 0.56 mL

Because reconstituted hemin is not transparent, any undissolved particulate matter is difficult to see; therefore, terminal filtration through a sterile 0.45 micron or smaller filter is recommended.

➤*Admixture incompatibility:* Do not add any drug or chemical agent fluid admixture unless its effect on the chemical and physical stability has first been determined.

➤*Storage / Stability:* Because this product contains no preservative and undergoes rapid chemical decomposition in solution, do not reconstitute until immediately before use. Refrigerate lyophilized powder at 2° to 8°C (36° to 46°F) until time of use. Discard any unused portion.

Actions

➤*Pharmacology:* Hemin for injection is an enzyme inhibitor derived from processed red blood cells. It was known previously as hematin. The term hematin has been used to describe the chemical reaction product of hemin and sodium carbonate solution. Hemin is an iron-containing metalloporphyrin.

Porphyrias are rare metabolic disorders that, as a group, represent disturbances of heme synthesis and are differentiated on the basis of specific enzymatic defects. Porphyrias are characterized clinically by neurologic (psychoses, seizures, paresis) or cutaneous (photosensitivity) manifestations, and chemically by overproduction of porphyrins or their precursors. Porphyrins are byproducts of heme synthesis; heme is the iron-containing constituent of hemoglobin and respiratory pigments and is produced and required by nearly every body tissue. Heme limits the hepatic or marrow synthesis of porphyrin, which is likely due to inhibition of delta-aminolevulinic acid synthetase, the enzyme that limits the rate of porphyrin/heme biosynthetic pathway. However, the exact mechanism by which hematin produces symptomatic improvement in patients with acute episodes of the hepatic porphyrias is not known.

➤*Pharmacokinetics:* Following IV administration of hematin in non-jaundiced patients, an increase in fecal urobilinogen can be observed, which is roughly proportional to the amount of hematin administered. This suggests an enterohepatic pathway as at least 1 route of elimination. Bilirubin metabolites also are excreted in the urine following hematin injections.

Contraindications

Hypersensitivity to hemin; porphyria cutanea tarda.

Warnings

➤*Pregnancy: Category C.* Safety for use during pregnancy has not been established. Use only when clearly needed and when the potential benefits outweigh the potential hazards to the fetus.

➤*Lactation:* It is not known whether hemin for injection is excreted in breast milk. Safety for use in the nursing mother has not been established.

➤*Children:* Safety and efficacy for use in children have not been established.

Precautions

➤*Monitoring:* Drug effect will be demonstrated by a decrease in urinary concentration of 1 or more of the following compounds: ALA (delta-aminolevulinic acid); UPG (uroporphyrinogen); PBG (porphobilinogen coproporphyrin).

➤*Neuronal damage:* Clinical benefit depends on prompt administration. Attacks of porphyria may progress to irreversible neuronal damage. Hemin therapy is intended to prevent an attack from reaching the critical stage of neuronal degeneration. This agent is not effective in repairing neuronal damage.

➤*Renal effects:* Reversible renal shutdown has been observed where an excessive hematin dose (12.2 mg/kg) was administered in a single infusion. Oliguria and increased nitrogen retention occurred, although the patient remained asymptomatic. No worsening of renal function has been seen with use of recommended dosages.

➤*Diagnostic tests:* Before beginning therapy, diagnose the presence of acute porphyria using the following criteria: Presence of clinical symptoms and positive Watson-Schwartz or Hoesch test.

Drug Interactions

Hemin Drug Interactions			
Precipitant drug	Object drug*		Description
Hemin	Anticoagulants	⬆	Hemin has exhibited transient, mild anticoagulant effects during clinical studies; therefore, avoid concurrent anticoagulant therapy. The extent and duration of the hypocoagulable state have not been established.
Barbiturates Estrogens Steroid metabolites	Hemin	⬌	These agents increase the activity of delta-amino-levulinic acid synthetase. Because hemin therapy limits the rate of porphyria/heme biosynthesis, possibly by inhibiting the enzyme delta-aminolevulinic acid synthetase, avoid concurrent use of these agents.

* ⬆ = Object drug increased. ⬌ = Undetermined effect.

Adverse Reactions

Phlebitis with or without leukocytosis and with or without mild pyrexia has occurred after administration of hematin through small arm veins.

There has been 1 report of coagulopathy. This patient exhibited prolonged prothrombin time, partial thromboplastin time, thrombocytopenia, mild hypofibrinogenemia, mild elevation of fibrin split products, and a 10% fall in hematocrit.

Overdosage

Reversible renal shutdown has been observed in a case where an excessive hematin dose (12.2 mg/kg) was administered in a single infusion (see Precautions). Treatment of this case consisted of ethacrynic acid and mannitol.

WARNING

Estrogens have been reported to increase the risk of endometrial carcinoma in postmenopausal women – Studies have shown an increased risk of endometrial cancer in postmenopausal women exposed to exogenous estrogens for more than 1 year. The risk of endometrial cancer in estrogen users was 4.5 to 13.9 times higher than in nonusers and appears to depend on duration of treatment and dose. Therefore, when estrogens are used for the treatment of menopausal symptoms, use the lowest dose and discontinue medication as soon as possible. When prolonged treatment is indicated, reassess the patient at least semiannually by endometrial sampling to determine the need for continued therapy.

Close clinical surveillance of women taking estrogens is important. Adequate diagnostic measures, including endometrial sampling when indicated, should be undertaken to rule out malignancy in all cases of undiagnosed persistent or recurring abnormal vaginal bleeding.

There is no evidence that natural estrogens are more or less hazardous than synthetic estrogens at equiestrogenic doses.

Do not use estrogens during pregnancy – Estrogen therapy during pregnancy is associated with an increased risk of congenital defects in the reproductive organs of the fetus and possibly other birth defects. Studies of women who received diethylstilbestrol (DES) during pregnancy have shown that female offspring have an increased risk of vaginal adenosis, squamous cell dysplasia of the uterine cervix, and clear cell vaginal cancer later in life; male offspring have an increased risk of urogenital abnormalities and possibly testicular cancer later in life.

There is no indication for estrogen therapy during pregnancy or during the immediate postpartum period. Estrogens are ineffective for the prevention or treatment of threatened or habitual abortion. Estrogens are not indicated for the prevention of postpartum breast engorgement.

If estrogens are used during pregnancy, or if the patient becomes pregnant while taking estrogens, inform her of the potential risks to the fetus.

Cardiovascular and other risks – Do not use estrogens with or without progestins for the prevention of cardiovascular disease.

The Women's Health Initiative (WHI) reported increased risks of MI, stroke, invasive breast cancer, pulmonary emboli, and deep vein thrombosis in postmenopausal women during 5 years of treatment with conjugated equine estrogens 0.625 mg combined with medroxyprogesterone acetate 2.5 mg relative to placebo. Other doses of conjugated estrogens and medroxyprogesterone acetate and other combinations of estrogens and progestins were not studied in the WHI and, in the absence of comparable data, these risks should be assumed to be similar. Because of these risks, prescribe estrogens with or without progestins at the lowest effective doses and for the shortest duration consistent with treatment goals and risks for the individual woman.

Dementia – The Women's Health Initiative Memory Study (WHIMS), a substudy of WHI, reported increased risk of developing probable dementia in postmenopausal women 65 years of age or older during 4 years of treatment with conjugated estrogens plus medroxyprogesterone acetate relative to placebo. It is unknown whether this finding applies to younger postmenopausal women or to women taking estrogen alone therapy.

Indications

Estrogens are most commonly used as a component of combination contraceptives or as hormone replacement therapy in postmenopausal women. Benefits in postmenopausal women include relief of moderate to severe vasomotor symptoms and decreased risk of osteoporosis. Hormone replacement therapy also may be used in vaginal and vulvar atrophy and in hypoestrogenism caused by hypogonadism, castration, or primary ovarian failure. Less commonly, select breast or prostate cancer patients with advanced disease may receive estrogens as palliative therapy. Refer to individual agents for specific indications.

➤*Unlabeled uses:* In the treatment of Turner syndrome (ovarian dysgenesis), estrogen therapy replicates the events of puberty.

Administration and Dosage

Refer to individual agents for specific administration and dosage recommendations.

➤*Moderate to severe vasomotor symptoms and/or moderate to severe symptoms of vulvar and vaginal atrophy associated with menopause:* Start at the lowest dose and discontinue as promptly as possible. Attempts to discontinue or taper medication should be made at 3- to 6-month intervals. Therapy may be given continuously with no interruption in therapy or in cyclical regimens (such as 25 days on followed by 5 days off drug) as is medically appropriate on an individualized basis.

➤*Hypoestrogenism caused by hypogonadism, castration, or primary ovarian failure:* Therapy usually is given cyclically (such as 3 weeks on and 1 week off). Adjust dose depending on severity of symptoms and patient responsiveness.

➤*Osteoporosis prevention:* Therapy may be given continuously with no interruption in therapy or in cyclical regimens (such as 25 days on followed by 5 days off drug) as is medically appropriate on an individualized basis. Discontinuation of therapy may re-establish the natural rate of bone loss.

➤*Prostate cancer (advanced androgen-dependent):* For palliation only. The effectiveness of therapy can be judged by phosphatase determinations as well as by symptomatic improvement of the patient.

➤*Breast cancer (metastatic):* For palliation only. Therapy usually is given for at least 3 months.

➤*Concomitant progestin therapy when a woman has not had a hysterectomy:* Addition of a progestin for 10 or more days of a cycle of estrogen has lowered the incidence of endometrial hyperplasia. Morphological and biochemical studies of endometrium suggest that 10 to 14 days of progestin are needed to provide maximal maturation of the endometrium and to reduce the likelihood of any hyperplastic changes. It is not established whether this will provide protection from endometrial carcinoma. There may be additional risks with the inclusion of progestin in estrogen replacement regimens, including possible increased risk of breast cancer; adverse effects on carbohydrate and lipid metabolism (lowering HDL and raising LDL); impairment of glucose tolerance; possible enhancement of mitotic activity in breast epithelial tissue, although few epidemiological data are available to address this point. Choice of progestin, regimen, and dosage may be important in minimizing risks.

Actions

➤*Pharmacology:* Estrogens occur naturally in several forms. The primary source of estrogen in normally cycling adult women is the ovarian follicle, which secretes 70 to 500 mcg of estradiol daily, depending on the phase of the menstrual cycle. This is converted primarily to estrone, which circulates in roughly equal proportion to estradiol, and to small amounts of estriol. After menopause, most endogenous estrogen is produced by conversion of androstenedione, secreted by the adrenal cortex, to estrone by peripheral tissues. Thus, estrone—especially in its sulfate ester form—is the most abundant circulating estrogen in postmenopausal women. Although circulating estrogens exist in a dynamic equilibrium of metabolic interconversions, estradiol is the principal intracellular human estrogen and is substantially more potent than estrone or estriol at the receptor.

Estrogens, important in developing and maintaining the female reproductive system and secondary sex characteristics, promote growth and development of the vagina, uterus, and fallopian tubes. With other hormones, such as pituitary hormones and progesterone, they cause enlargement of the breasts through promotion of ductal growth, stromal development, and the accretion of fat. Estrogens are intricately involved with other hormones, especially progesterone, in the processes of the ovulatory menstrual cycle and pregnancy and affect release of pituitary gonadotropins. Indirectly, they contribute to the following: Shaping of the skeleton; maintenance of tone and elasticity of urogenital structures; changes in epiphyses of long bones that allow for pubertal growth spurt and its termination; growth of axillary and pubic hair; pigmentation of nipples and genitals.

Menstruation – Decline of estrogenic activity at the end of the menstrual cycle can induce menstruation, although cessation of progesterone secretion is the most important factor in the mature ovulatory cycle. However, in the preovulatory or nonovulatory cycle, estrogen is the primary determinant of the onset of menstruation.

Menopause – After menopause, estradiol secretion from the ovaries ceases and the primary circulating estrogen is estrone. Estrone has approximately one-third the estrogenic potency of estradiol, but the estrone concentrations are about 4-fold that of estradiol after menopause.

Osteoporosis – Immobilization and prolonged bed rest produce rapid bone loss, while weight-bearing exercise has been shown to reduce bone loss and to increase bone mass. The optimal type and amount of physical activity that would prevent osteoporosis have not been established.

Estrogen reduces bone resorption and retards or halts postmenopausal bone loss. Studies have shown an approximately 60% reduction in hip and wrist fractures in women whose estrogen replacement began within a few years of menopause. Studies also suggest that estrogen reduces the rate of vertebral fractures. Even when started as late as 6 years after menopause, estrogen prevents further loss of bone mass but does not restore it to premenopausal levels.

➤*Pharmacokinetics:*

Absorption/Distribution – Estrogens used in therapy are well absorbed through the skin, mucous membranes, and GI tract. When applied for a local action, absorption is usually sufficient to cause systemic effects. When conjugated with aryl and alkyl groups for parenteral administration, the rate of absorption of oily preparations is slowed with a prolonged duration of action, such that a single IM injection of estradiol valerate or estradiol cypionate is absorbed over several weeks. Conjugated estrogens are well absorbed from the GI tract after release from the drug formulation. The tablet releases conjugated estrogens slowly over several hours. The distribution of exogenous estrogens is similar to that of endogenous estrogens. Estrogens are widely distributed in the body and are generally found in higher concentration in the sex hormone target organs. Estrogens circulate in the blood largely bound to sex hormone-binding globulin (SHBG) and albumin.

Transdermal system: In contrast to oral estradiol, the skin metabolizes estradiol via the transdermal system only to a small extent. Therefore, transdermal use produces therapeutic serum levels of estradiol with lower circulating levels of estrone and estrone conjugates and requires smaller total doses.

Metabolism/Excretion – When given orally, naturally occurring estrogens and their esters are extensively metabolized (first-pass effect) and circulate primarily as estrone sulfate, with smaller amounts of other conjugated and unconjugated estrogenic species. This results in limited oral potency. By contrast, synthetic estrogens, such as ethinyl estradiol and the nonsteroidal estrogens, are degraded very slowly in the liver and other tissues, which results in their high intrinsic potency. Estrogen drug products administered by non-oral routes are not subject to first-pass metabolism but also undergo significant hepatic uptake, metabolism, and enterohepatic recycling.

Metabolic conversion of estrogens occurs primarily in the liver (first-pass effect) but also at local target tissue sites. Complex metabolic processes result in a dynamic equilibrium of circulating conjugated and unconjugated estrogenic forms that are continually interconverted, especially between estrone and estradiol and between esterified and nonesterified forms. A certain proportion of the estrogen is excreted into the bile and then reabsorbed from the intestine. During this enterohepatic recirculation, estrogens are desulfated and resulfated and undergo degradation through conversion to less active estrogens (estriol and other estrogens), oxidation to nonestrogenic substances (catecholestrogens, which interact with catecholamine metabolism, especially in the CNS), and conjugation with glucuronic acids (which are then rapidly excreted in the urine).

Contraindications

Known or suspected breast cancer, except in appropriately selected patients being treated for metastatic disease; known or suspected estrogen-dependent neoplasia; undiagnosed abnormal genital bleeding; active deep vein thrombosis, PE, or a history of these conditions; active or recent (eg, within past year) arterial thromboembolic disease (eg, stroke, MI); active thrombophlebitis or thromboembolic disorders; history of thrombophlebitis, thrombosis or thromboembolic disorders associated with previous estrogen use (except when used in treatment of breast or prostatic malignancy); known or suspected pregnancy (see Warning Box); porphyria (estradiol vaginal tablets only); hypersensitivity to any product component.

Warnings

➤*Induction of malignant neoplasms:*

Endometrial cancer – The use of unopposed estrogens in women with intact uteri has been associated with an increased risk of endometrial cancer. The reported endometrial cancer risk among unopposed estrogen users is about 2- to 12-fold greater than in nonusers and appears dependent on duration of treatment and on estrogen dose. Most studies show no significant increased risk associated with use of estrogens for less than 1 year. The greatest risk appears associated with prolonged use, with increased risks of 15- to 24-fold for 5 to 10 years or more and this risk has been shown to persist for at least 8 to 15 years after estrogen therapy is discontinued.

Clinical surveillance of all women taking estrogen/progestin combinations is important. Adequate diagnostic measures, including endometrial sampling when indicated, should be undertaken to rule out malignancy in all cases of undiagnosed persistent or recurring abnormal vaginal bleeding. There is no evidence that the use of natural estrogens results in a different endometrial risk profile than synthetic estrogens of equivalent estrogen dose. Adding a progestin to postmenopausal estrogen therapy has been shown to reduce the risk of endometrial hyperplasia, which may be a precursor to endometrial cancer.

Breast cancer – Estrogen and estrogen/progestin therapy in postmenopausal women have been associated with an increased risk of breast cancer. In the 0.625 mg conjugated equine estrogens plus 2.5 mg medroxyprogesterone acetate per day substudy of the WHI, 26% of the women reported prior use of estrogen alone and/or estrogen/progestin combination hormone therapy. After a mean follow-up of 5.6 years during the clinical trial, the overall relative risk of invasive breast cancer was 1.24 (95% confidence interval 1.01 to 1.54), and the overall absolute risk was 41 vs 33 cases per 10,000 women-years, for estrogen plus progestin compared with placebo. among women who reported prior use of hormone therapy, the relative risk of invasive breast cancer was 1.86, and absolute risk was 46 vs 25 cases per 10,000 women-years, for estrogen plus progestin compared with placebo. Among women who reported no prior use of hormone therapy, the relative risk of invasive breast cancer was 1.09, and the absolute risk was 40 vs 36 cases per 10,000 women-years for estrogen plus progestin compared with placebo. In the WHI trial invasive breast cancers were larger and diagnosed at a more advanced stage in the estrogen plus progestin group compared with the placebo group. Metastatic disease was rare with no apparent difference between the 2 groups. Other prognostic factors such as histologic subtype, grade, and hormone receptor status did not differ between the groups.

A postmenopausal woman without a uterus who requires estrogen should receive estrogen-alone therapy and should not be exposed unnecessarily to progestins. All postmenopausal women should receive yearly breast exams by a health care provider and perform monthly breast self-examinations. In addition, mammography examinations should be scheduled based on patient age and risk factors.

Ovarian cancer – Use of estrogen-only products, in particular for 10 years or more, has been associated with an increased risk of ovarian cancer in some epidemiological studies. Other studies did not show a significant association. Data are insufficient to determine whether there is an increased risk with combined estrogen/progestin therapy in postmenopausal women.

➤*Gallbladder disease:* There is a 2-fold to 4-fold increase in risk of gallbladder disease requiring surgery in women receiving postmenopausal estrogens.

➤*Cardiovascular disorders:* Estrogen and estrogen/progestin therapy have been associated with an increased risk of cardiovascular events (eg, MI and stroke, venous thrombosis, PE [venous thromboembolism (VTE)]). Should any of these occur or be suspected, discontinue estrogens immediately.

Risk factors for cardiovascular disease (eg, hypertension, diabetes mellitus, tobacco use, hypercholesterolemia, obesity) should be managed appropriately.

CHD – In the 0.625 mg conjugated equine estrogens per day substudy of the WHI, an increase in the number of MIs and strokes has been observed compared with placebo. These observations are preliminary and the study is continuing.

In the 0.625 mg conjugated equine estrogens plus 2.5 mg medroxyprogesterone acetate per day substudy of the WHI, an increased risk of CHD events (defined as nonfatal MI and CHD death) was observed compared with placebo (37 vs 30 per 10,000 person-years). The increase in risk was observed in year 1 and persisted.

In the same substudy of the WHI, an increased risk of stroke also was observed compared with placebo (29 vs 21 per 10,000 person-years). The increase in risk was observed after the first year and persisted.

In postmenopausal women with documented heart disease (n = 2763; average age, 66.7 years) a controlled clinical trial of secondary prevention of cardiovascular disease (Heart and Estrogen/progestin Replacement Study; HERS) treatment with 0.625 mg conjugated equine estrogens plus 2.5 mg medroxyprogesterone acetate per day demonstrated no cardiovascular benefit. During an average follow-up of 4.1 years, treatment with 0.625 mg conjugated equine estrogens plus 2.5 mg medroxyprogesterone acetate per day did not reduce the overall rate of CHD events in postmenopausal women with established CHD. There were more CHD events in the 0.625 mg conjugated equine estrogens plus 2.5 mg medroxyprogesterone acetate per day-treated group than in the placebo group in year 1, but not during subsequent years.

Large doses of estrogen (5 mg conjugated estrogens per day), comparable with those used to treat cancer of the prostate and breast, have been shown in a large prospective clinical trial in men to increase the risks of nonfatal MI, PE, and thrombophlebitis.

VTE – In the 0.625 mg conjugated equine estrogens per day substudy of the WHI, an increase in VTE has been observed compared with placebo. These observations are preliminary, and the study is continuing.

In the 0.625 mg conjugated equine estrogens plus 2.5 mg medroxyprogesterone acetate per day substudy of the WHI, a 2-fold greater rate of VTE, including deep venous thrombosis and PE, was observed compared with placebo. The rate of VTE was 34 per 10,000 woman-years in the 0.625 mg conjugated equine estrogens plus 2.5 mg medroxyprogesterone acetate per day group compared with 16 per 10,000 woman-years in the placebo group. The increase in VTE risk was observed during the first year and persisted.

If feasible, discontinue estrogens at least 4 to 6 weeks before surgery of the type associated with an increased risk of thromboembolism or during periods of prolonged immobilization.

➤*Dementia:* In the WHIMS, 4,532 generally healthy postmenopausal women 65 years of age and older were studied, of whom 35% were 70 to 74 years of age and 18% were 75 years of age or older. After an average follow-up of 4 years, 40 women being treated with 0.625 mg conjugated estrogens plus 2.5 mg medroxyprogesterone acetate (1.8%, n = 2,229) and 21 women in the placebo group (0.9%, n = 2,303) received diagnoses of probable dementia. The relative risk for estrogen/progestin vs placebo was 2.05 (95% confidence interval 1.21 to 3.48), and was similar for women with and without histories of menopausal hormone use before WHIMS. The absolute risk of probable dementia for estrogen/progestin vs placebo was 45 vs 22 cases per 10,000 women-years, and the absolute excess risk for estrogen/progestin was 23 cases per 10,000 women-years. It is unknown whether these findings apply to younger postmenopausal women.

The results of the estrogen alone substudy of the WHIMS have not been reported. It is unknown whether these findings apply to estrogen alone therapy.

➤*Hepatic adenoma:* Benign hepatic adenomas appear to be associated with the use of oral contraceptives (OCs). Although benign and rare, they may rupture and may cause death through intra-abdominal hemorrhage. Such lesions have not been reported in association with other estrogen or progestogen preparations but should be considered in estrogen users having abdominal pain and tenderness, abdominal mass, or hypovolemic shock. Hepatocellular carcinoma also has been reported in women taking estrogen-containing OCs. The relationship of this malignancy to these drugs is not known.

➤*Familial hyperlipoproteinemia:* Estrogen therapy may be associated with elevations of plasma triglycerides leading to pancreatitis and other complications in patients with familial defects of lipoprotein metabolism.

➤*Hypercalcemia:* Estrogens may lead to severe hypercalcemia in patients with breast cancer and bone metastases. If this occurs, discontinue the drug and take appropriate measures to reduce the serum calcium level.

➤*Glucose tolerance:* A worsening of glucose tolerance has been observed in a significant percentage of patients on estrogen-containing OCs. Carefully observe diabetic patients receiving estrogen.

➤*Visual abnormalities:* Retinal vascular thrombosis has been reported in patients receiving estrogens. Discontinue medication pending examination if there is sudden partial or complete loss of vision or a sudden onset of proptosis, diplopia, or migraine. If examination reveals papilledema or retinal vascular lesions, discontinue estrogens.

➤*Hypothyroidism:* Estrogen administration leads to increased thyroid-binding globulin (TBG) levels. Patients with normal thyroid function can compensate for the increased TBG by making more thyroid hormone, thus maintaining free T_4 and T_3 serum concentrations in the normal range. Patients dependent on thyroid hormone replacement therapy who are also receiving estrogens may require increased doses of their thyroid replacement therapy. Monitor thyroid function in these patients in order to maintain their free thyroid hormone levels in an acceptable range.

➤*Depression:* OCs appear to be associated with an increased incidence of mental depression. Although it is not clear whether this is caused by the estrogenic or progestogenic component of the contraceptive, carefully observe patients with a history of depression.

➤*Uterine leiomyomata:* Pre-existing uterine leiomyomata may increase in size during estrogen use.

➤*Hepatic function impairment:* Exercise caution in patients with a history of cholestatic jaundice associated with past estrogen use or with pregnancy and, in the case of recurrence, discontinue medication. Estrogens may be poorly metabolized in impaired liver function; use with caution.

➤*Pregnancy: Category X.* Do not use estrogens during pregnancy. See Warning Box.

➤*Lactation:* Estrogens have been shown to decrease the quantity and quality of breast milk and detectable amounts are excreted in breast milk. Administer only when clearly needed.

➤*Children:* Estrogen therapy has been used for the induction of puberty in adolescents with some forms of pubertal delay. Safety and efficacy in pediatric patients have not otherwise been established.

Large and repeated doses of estrogen over an extended period of time have been shown to accelerate epiphyseal closure, which could result in short adult stature if treatment is initiated before the completion of physiologic puberty in normally developing children. If estrogen is administered to patients whose bone growth is not complete, periodic monitoring of bone maturation and effects on epiphyseal centers is recommended during estrogen administration.

Estrogen treatment of prepubertal girls also induces premature breast development and vaginal cornification and may induce vaginal bleeding. In boys, estrogen treatment may modify the normal pubertal process and induce gynecomastia.

Precautions

➤*Elevated blood pressure:* In a small number of case reports, substantial increases in blood pressure have been attributed to idiosyncratic reactions to estrogens. In a large, randomized, placebo-controlled clinical trial, a generalized effect of estrogen therapy on blood pressure was not seen. Monitor blood pressure at regular intervals with estrogen use.

➤*Hypercoagulability:* Some studies have shown that women taking estrogen replacement therapy have hypercoagulability, primarily related to decreased antithrombin activity. This effect appears dose- and duration-dependent and is less pronounced than that associated with oral contraceptive use. Also, postmenopausal women tend to have increased coagulation parameters at baseline compared with premenopausal women. There is some suggestion that low-dose postmenopausal mestranol may increase the risk of thromboembolism, although the majority of studies (of primarily conjugated estrogens users) report no such increase. There is insufficient information on hypercoagulability in women who have had previous thromboembolic disease. Therefore, do not use in people with active thrombophlebitis or thromboembolic disorders or in people with a history of such disorders associated with estrogen use (except in treatment of malignancy).

➤*History/Physical exam:* Before initiating estrogens, take complete medical and family history. Pretreatment and periodic history and physical exams every 12 months should include blood pressure, breasts, abdomen, pelvic organs, and a Papanicolaou smear. Generally, do not prescribe for longer than 1 year between physical examinations.

➤*Vaginal products:* Estradiol vaginal ring may not be suitable for women with narrow, short, or stenosed vaginas. Narrow vagina, vaginal stenosis, prolapse, and vaginal infections are conditions that make the vagina more susceptible to estradiol vaginal ring-caused irritation or ulceration. Women with signs or symptoms of vaginal irritation should alert their physician.

Vaginal infection is generally more common in postmenopausal women because of the lack of the normal flora of fertile women, especially lactobacillus, and the subsequent higher pH. Treat vaginal infections with appropriate antimicrobial therapy before initiation of therapy. If a vaginal infection develops during use of the estradiol vaginal ring, remove the ring and reinsert only after the infection has been appropriately treated.

Conjugated estrogens vaginal cream exposure has been reported to weaken latex condoms. Consider its potential to weaken and contribute to the failure of condoms, diaphragms, or cervical caps made of latex or rubber.

➤*Excessive estrogenic stimulation:* Certain patients may develop undesirable manifestations of excessive estrogenic stimulation (eg, abnormal or excessive uterine bleeding, mastodynia). Advise the pathologist of estrogen therapy when relevant specimens are submitted.

➤*Fluid retention:* Estrogens may cause some degree of fluid retention; conditions that might be influenced by this factor (eg, asthma, epilepsy, migraine, cardiac or renal dysfunction) require careful observation.

➤*Calcium and phosphorus metabolism:* Calcium and phosphorus metabolism is influenced by estrogens; use caution in metabolic bone diseases associated with hypercalcemia or in renal insufficiency. Use estrogens with caution in individuals with severe hypocalcemia.

➤*Endometrial hyperplasia:* Prolonged unopposed estrogen therapy may increase risk of endometrial hyperplasia.

➤*Exacerbations of other conditions:* Endometriosis may be exacerbated with administration of estrogen therapy. Estrogen therapy also may cause an exacerbation of asthma, diabetes mellitus, epilepsy, migraine, or porphyria; use with caution in patients with these conditions.

➤*Benzyl alcohol:* Benzyl alcohol, contained in some of these products as a preservative, has been associated with a fatal "gasping syndrome" in premature infants.

➤*Lab test abnormalities:* Certain endocrine and liver function tests may be affected by estrogen-containing OCs. Expect the following similar changes with larger doses:

Increased sulfobromophthalein retention.

Increased prothrombin time, partial thromboplastin time, platelet aggregation time, platelet count, and factors II, VII, VIII, IX, X, XII, VII-X complex, II-VII-X complex, and β-thromboglobulin; decreased antithrombin III, anti-factor Xa; increased fibrinogen, plasminogen, and norepinephrine-induced platelet aggregability.

Increased thyroid binding globulin (TBG) leading to increased circulating total thyroid hormone, as measured by protein bound iodine (PBI), T_4 by column or T_4 or T_3 by radioimmunoassay. Free T_3 resin uptake is decreased, reflecting the elevated TBG; free T_4 and free T_3 concentration is unaltered.

Impaired glucose tolerance; decreased pregnanediol excretion; reduced response to metyrapone test; reduced serum folate concentration; increased serum triglyceride and phospholipid concentration.

Other binding proteins may be elevated in serum (ie, corticosteroid binding globulin [CBG], SHBG), leading to increased circulating corticosteroids and sex steroids, respectively. Free or biologically active hormone concentrations are unchanged. Other plasma proteins may be increased (angiotensinogen/renin substrate, α-1-antitrypsin, ceruloplasmin).

Increased plasma HDL and HDL-2 subfraction concentrations, reduced LDL cholesterol concentration levels, increased triglyceride levels.

➤*Tartrazine sensitivity:* Some of these products contain tartrazine (FD&C yellow #5), which may cause allergic-type reactions (including bronchial asthma) in susceptible individuals. Although the incidence of sensitivity is low, it is frequently seen in patients who also have aspirin hypersensitivity. Specific products containing tartrazine are identified in the product listings.

Drug Interactions

Refer to the drug interaction section in the Oral Contraceptives group monograph for more information.

Estrogen Drug Interactions

Precipitant drug	Object drug[a]		Description
Estrogens	Anticoagulants, oral	↓	Estrogens may theoretically reduce the effect of anticoagulants.
Estrogens	Antidepressants, tricyclic	↔	Pharmacologic effects of these agents may be altered by estrogens; the effects of this interaction may depend on the dose of the estrogen. An increased incidence of toxic reactions also may occur.
Estrogens	Corticosteroids	↑	An increase in the pharmacologic and toxicologic effects of corticosteroids may occur via inactivation of hepatic P-450 enzyme.
Estrogens	Thyroid hormones	↓	In hypothyroid women, estrogens may increase serum thyroxine-binding globulin concentrations, therefore changing serum thyroxine and thyrotropin concentrations. Thyroid hormone requirements may be increased.
CYP 3A4 inducers Barbiturates Carbamazepine Rifampin St. John's wort	Estrogens	↓	Coadministration may reduce plasma concentrations of estrogens, possibly resulting in a decrease in therapeutic effects and/or changes in the uterine bleeding profile.
CYP 3A4 inhibitors Itraconazole Ketoconazole Macrolide antibiotics Ritonavir	Estrogens	↑	Coadministration may increase plasma concentrations of estrogens and may result in side effects.
Hydantoins	Estrogens	↓	Breakthrough bleeding, spotting, and pregnancy have resulted when these medications were used concurrently. A loss of seizure control also has been suggested and may be caused by fluid retention.
Estrogens	Hydantoins		
Topiramate	Estrogens	↓	Topiramate may increase the metabolism of estrogens, decreasing their efficacy.

[a] ↑ = Object drug increased. ↓ = Object drug decreased. ↔ = Undetermined clinical effect.

➤*Drug/Food interactions:* Grapefruit juice may inhibit CYP3A4-mediated estrogen metabolism, increasing plasma concentrations of estrogens and possibly resulting in side effects.

Adverse Reactions

See Warnings regarding induction of neoplasia, adverse effects on the fetus, increased incidence of gallbladder disease, hypercalcemia, cardiovascular disease, elevated blood pressure, and adverse effects similar to those of OCs.

➤*Cardiovascular:* Venous thromboembolism; pulmonary embolism; syncope; deep and superficial venous thrombosis; thrombophlebitis; MI; stroke; increased blood pressure.

➤*CNS:* Headache; migraine; dizziness; mental depression; chorea; insomnia; anxiety; emotional lability; nervousness; mood disturbances; irritability; exacerbation of epilepsy; fatigue; sinus headache; tension headaches.

➤*Dermatologic:* Chloasma or melasma (may persist when drug is discontinued); erythema nodosum/multiforme; hemorrhagic eruption; dermatitis; skin hypertrophy; loss of scalp hair; hirsutism; pruritus; rash; pruritus ani; acne.

➤*GI:* Nausea; vomiting; abdominal cramps/pain; bloating; cholestatic jaundice; pancreatitis; diarrhea; dyspepsia; flatulence; gastritis; gastroenteritis; enlarged abdomen; hemorrhoids; increased incidence of gallbladder disease; constipation.

➤*GU:* Breakthrough bleeding; abnormal withdrawal bleeding; spotting; change in menstrual flow; dysmenorrhea; premenstrual-like syndrome; amenorrhea during and after treatment; vaginal candidiasis; change in cervical ectropion and degree of cervical secretion; cystitis-like syndrome; urinary tract infection; leukorrhea; vaginitis; vaginal discomfort/pain; vaginal hemorrhage; asymptomatic genital bacterial growth; genital moniliasis; cystitis; dysuria; genital pruritus; genital eruption; urinary incontinence; endometrial hyperplasia; increase in size of uterine leiomyomata/fibromyomata; ovarian cancer; endometrial cancer; micturition frequency; urethral disorder; vaginosis fungal; vaginal discharge.

➤*Local:* Redness/erythema and irritation at application site with the estradiol transdermal system; rash (rare).

➤*Ophthalmic:* Steepening of corneal curvature; intolerance to contact lenses; retinal vascular thrombosis.

➤*Respiratory:* Upper respiratory tract infection; sinusitis; rhinitis; bronchitis; pharyngitis; nasopharyngitis; cough; nasal congestion; pharyngolaryngeal pain.

➤*Miscellaneous:* Aggravation of porphyria; edema; changes in libido; breast pain, tenderness, enlargement, or secretion; galactorrhea; fibrocystic breast changes; breast cancer; reduced carbohydrate tolerance; pain; hypersensitivity reactions; increase or decrease in weight; back pain; arthritis; arthralgia; skeletal pain; flu-like symptoms; hot flushes; allergy; chest pain; leg edema; otitis media; toothache; tooth disorder; infection; accidental injury; asthenia; anemia; paresthesia; leg cramps; anaphylactoid/anaphylactic reactions (including urticaria and angioedema); hypocalcemia; exacerbation of asthma; increased triglycerides; neck pain; neck rigidity; candidal infection; fungal infection; herpes simplex; fluid retention.

Overdosage

Serious ill effects have not been reported following ingestion of large doses of estrogen-containing OCs by young children. Overdosage of estrogen may cause nausea and vomiting; withdrawal bleeding may occur in females.

Patient Information

Patient package insert is available with products.

Estrogens increase the chances of getting cancer of the uterus. Report any unusual vaginal bleeding right away. Vaginal bleeding after menopause may be a warning sign of cancer of the uterus.

Do not use estrogens with or without progestins to prevent heart disease, heart attacks, or strokes. Using estrogens with or without progestins may increase the chances of heart attacks, strokes, breast cancer, and blood clots.

Notify physician if any of the following occur: Pain in the calves; sharp chest pain or sudden shortness of breath; coughing blood; abnormal vaginal bleeding; missed menstrual period or suspected pregnancy; lumps in the breast; severe headache or vomiting; dizziness or fainting; vision or speech disturbance; weakness or numbness in an arm or leg; abdominal pain, swelling, or tenderness; yellowing of the skin or eyes; depression.

ESTRADIOL TOPICAL EMULSION

For topical estradiol prescribing information, see the Topical Estrogens, Miscellaneous monograph.

ESTRADIOL TRANSDERMAL SYSTEM

	Product/ Distributor	Release rate (mg/24 h)	Surface area (cm^2)	Total estradiol content (mg)	How Supplied
Rx	**Menostar** (Berlex)	0.014	3.25	1	In 4s.
Rx	**Estradiol Transdermal System** (Mylan)	0.025	7.75	0.97	In 4s.
Rx	**Alora** (Watson)		9	0.77	In calendar packs (8 systems).
Rx	**Climara** (Berlex)		6.5	2	In 4s.
Rx	**Esclim** (Women First Healthcare)		11	5	In patient packs (8s).
Rx	**Vivelle-Dot** (Novartis)		2.5	0.39	In calendar packs (8s and 24s).
Rx	**Esclim** (Women First Healthcare)	0.0375	16.5	7.5	In patient packs (8s).
Rx	**Climara** (Berlex)		9.375	2.85	In 4s.
Rx	**Vivelle** (Novartis)		11	3.28	In calendar packs (8 and 24 systems).
Rx	**Vivelle-Dot** (Novartis)		3.75	0.585	In calendar packs (8 systems).
Rx	**Estradiol Transdermal System** (Mylan)	0.05	15.5	1.94	In 4s.
Rx	**Alora** (Watson)		18	1.5	In calendar packs (8s).
Rx	**Climara** (Berlex)		12.5	3.8	In 4s.
Rx	**Estraderm** (Novartis)		10	4	In calendar packs (8 and 24 systems).
Rx	**Vivelle** (Novartis)		14.5	4.33	In calendar packs (8 and 24 systems).
Rx	**Vivelle-Dot** (Novartis)		5	0.78	In calendar packs (8 systems).
Rx	**Climara** (Berlex)	0.06 mg	15	4.55	In 4s.
Rx	**Estradiol Transdermal System** (Mylan)	0.075	23.25	2.91	In 4s.
Rx	**Alora** (Watson)		27	2.3	In calendar packs (8 systems).
Rx	**Climara** (Berlex)		18.75	5.7	In 4s.
Rx	**Vivelle** (Novartis)		22	6.57	In calendar packs (8 and 24 systems).
Rx	**Vivelle–Dot** (Novartis)		7.5	1.17	In calendar packs (8 systems).
Rx	**Estradiol Transdermal System** (Mylan)	0.1	31	3.88	In 4s.
Rx	**Alora** (Watson)		36	3.1	In calendar packs (8 systems).
Rx	**Climara** (Berlex)		25	7.6	In 4s.
Rx	**Estraderm** (Novartis)		20	8	In calendar packs (8 and 24 systems).
Rx	**Vivelle** (Novartis)		29	8.66	In calendar packs (8 and 24 systems).
Rx	**Vivelle-Dot** (Novartis)		10	1.56	In calendar packs (8 systems).

ESTRADIOL — TRANSDERMAL

For complete and comparative prescribing information, refer to the Estrogens group monograph.

WARNING

Estrogens increase the risk of endometrial cancer – Close clinical surveillance of all women taking estrogens is important. Use adequate diagnostic measures, including endometrial sampling when indicated, to rule out malignancy in all cases of undiagnosed persistent or recurring abnormal vaginal bleeding. There is currently no evidence that "natural" estrogens results in a different endometrial risk profile than synthetic estrogens at equivalent estrogen dose(s).

Cardiovascular and other risks – Do not use estrogens with or without progestins for the prevention of cardiovascular disease or dementia.

The Women's Health Initiative (WHI) study reported increased risks of myocardial infarction (MI), stroke, invasive breast cancer, pulmonary emboli (PE), and deep vein thrombosis in postmenopausal women during 5 years of treatment with conjugated equine estrogens 0.625 mg combined with medroxyprogesterone acetate 2.5 mg relative to placebo.

The Women's Health Initiative Memory Study (WHIMS), a substudy of WHI, reported increased risk of developing probable dementia in postmenopausal women 65 years of age or older during 4 years of treatment with oral conjugated estrogens plus medroxyprogesterone acetate relative to placebo. It is unknown whether this finding applies to younger postmenopausal women or to women taking estrogen alone therapy.

Other doses of conjugated estrogens with medroxyprogesterone, and other combinations of estrogens and progestins were not studied in the WHI and, in the absence of comparable data, these risks should be assumed to be similar. Because of these risks, prescribe estrogens with or without progestins at the lowest effective doses and for the shortest duration consistent with treatment goals and risks for the individual woman.

Indications

Estradiol transdermal system is indicated for use in the following:

➤*Vasomotor symptoms (except Menostar)*: Treatment of moderate to severe vasomotor symptoms associated with menopause.

➤*Vulvular / Vaginal atrophy (except Menostar)*: Treatment of moderate to severe symptoms of vulvar and vaginal atrophy associated with menopause. When prescribing solely for the treatment of symptoms of vulvar and vaginal atrophy, consider topical vaginal products.

➤*Hypoestrogenism (except Menostar)*: Treatment of hypoestrogenism because of hypogonadism, castration, or primary ovarian failure.

➤*Prevention of postmenopausal osteoporosis:* When prescribing solely for the prevention of postmenopausal osteoporosis, consider therapy only for women at significant risk of osteoporosis. Carefully consider nonestrogen medications. The mainstays for decreasing the risk of postmenopausal osteoporosis are weight-bearing exercise, adequate calcium and vitamin D intake, and when indicated, pharmacologic therapy. Postmenopausal women require an average of 1,500 mg/day of elemental calcium. Therefore, when not contraindicated, calcium supplementation may be helpful for women with suboptimal dietary intake. Vitamin D supplementation of 400 to 800 units/day may also be required to ensure adequate daily intake in postmenopausal women.

Administration and Dosage

➤*Application of system:* Place the adhesive side of the estradiol transdermal system on a clean, dry area of the lower abdomen, femoral triangle (upper inner thigh), upper arm, upper quadrant of the buttock, or outer aspect of the hip. The site selected should be one that is not exposed to sunlight. Do not apply transdermal estradiol to or near the breasts or other parts of the body. Replace the estradiol transdermal system once or twice weekly, depending on the product specification. The sites of application must be rotated, with an interval of at least 1 week allowed between applications to a particular site. The area selected should not be oily, damaged, or irritated. Avoid the waistline because tight clothing may rub the patch off. Also avoid application to areas where sitting would dislodge the patch. Apply the patch immediately after opening the pouch and removing the protective liner. Press the patch firmly in place with the palm of the hand for about 10 seconds, making sure there is good contact, especially around the edges. In the unlikely event that a patch should fall off, the same patch may be reapplied (except *Climara* or *Menostar*). If necessary, a new patch may be applied. In the event that a *Climara* or *Menostar* system falls off, apply a new system for the remainder of the 7-day dosing interval. In either case, continue the original treatment schedule.

If a patient has forgotten to apply a patch, she should apply a new patch as soon as possible. Apply the new patch on the original treatment schedule. The interruption of treatment in women taking estradiol transdermal might increase the likelihood of breakthrough bleeding, spotting, and recurrence of symptoms. Wear only 1 patch at any given time. Swimming, bathing, or using a sauna while using the estradiol transdermal system may decrease the adhesion of the patch and the delivery of estradiol.

➤*Removal of the transdermal system:* Carefully and slowly remove the system to avoid irritation of the skin. Should any adhesive remain on the skin after removal of the system, allow the area to dry for 15 minutes. Then gently rub the area with an oil-based cream or lotion to remove the adhesive residue. Used patches still contain some active hormones. Carefully fold each patch in half so that it sticks to itself before throwing it away.

➤*Initiation of therapy:* When estrogen is prescribed for a postmenopausal woman with a uterus, initiate progestin also to reduce the risk of endometrial cancer. A woman without a uterus does not need progestin. Limit use of estrogen alone or in combination with a progestin to the shortest duration consistent with treatment goals and risks for the individual woman. Reevaluate patients periodically as clinically appropriate (eg, 3- to 6-month intervals) to determine whether treatment is still necessary. For women who have a uterus, undertake adequate diagnostic measures, such as endometrial sampling, when indicated, to rule out malignancy in cases of undiagnosed persistent or recurring abnormal vaginal bleeding.

Estradiol transdermal systems are available in a variety of sizes as once-weekly dosing formulations that provide estradiol 0.014, 0.025, 0.0375, 0.05, 0.06, 0.075, or 0.1 mg/day and as twice-weekly dosing formulations that provide estradiol 0.025, 0.0375, 0.05, 0.075, and 0.1 mg/day. *Alora*, *Estraderm*, *Vivelle*, and *Vivelle-Dot* are applied twice a week. *Climara* and *Menostar* last for 7 days and are applied once a week.

Treatment of menopausal symptoms – For the treatment of vasomotor symptoms, initiate treatment with an estradiol transdermal system that provides estradiol 0.025 mg/day. For the treatment of moderate to severe vasomotor symptoms, vulvar and vaginal atrophy associated with menopause, hypoestrogenism caused by hypogonadism, castration, or primary ovarian failure, treatment is usually initiated with an estradiol transdermal system that delivers estradiol 0.025 to 0.05 mg/day.

Depending on the specific product chosen, apply the transdermal system to the skin once or twice weekly. Adjust the dosage as necessary to control symptoms. Choose the lowest dose and regimen that will control symptoms. In order to use the lowest dosage necessary for the control of symptoms, do not make decisions to increase dosage until after the first month of therapy. Discontinue the medication as promptly as possible. Make attempts to taper or discontinue the medication at 3- to 6-month intervals.

Prophylaxis of postmenopausal osteoporosis – For the prevention of postmenopausal osteoporosis, the minimum dosage that has been shown to be effective is the estradiol 0.025 mg/day transdermal system. Initiate prophylactic therapy with transdermal estradiol to prevent postmenopausal bone loss with the lowest available dosage as soon as possible after menopause. The dosage may be adjusted if necessary. Response to therapy can be predicted by pretreatment serum estradiol, and can be assessed during treatment by measuring biochemical markers of bone formation/resorptions and/or bone mineral density. Discontinuation of estrogen therapy may reestablish bone loss at a rate comparable with the immediate postmenopausal period. Reproductive-system-associated adverse reactions were encountered more frequently in the highest dosage group (0.1 mg/day) than in other active treatment groups or in placebo-treated patients.

In women not currently taking oral estrogens, treatment with transdermal estradiol may be initiated at once. In women who are currently taking oral estrogen, initiate treatment with transdermal estradiol 1 week after withdrawal of oral hormone therapy, or sooner if menopausal symptoms reappear in less than 1 week.

➤*Therapeutic regimen:* Estradiol transdermal therapy may be given continuously in patients who do not have an intact uterus. In those patients with an intact uterus, transdermal estradiol may be given on a cyclic schedule (eg, 3 weeks on drug followed by 1 week off drug); *Vivelle* may be given continuously or on a cyclic schedule (eg, 3 weeks on drug followed by 1 week off drug) with a progestin.

Concomitant progestin therapy – When estrogen is prescribed for a postmenopausal woman with a uterus, also initiate progestin to reduce the risk of endometrial cancer. A women without a uterus does not need progestin.

➤*Menostar* (estradiol 1 mg): *Menostar* should only be prescribed to postmenopausal women who are at significant risk of osteoporosis. Carefully consider nonestrogen medications. Risk factors for osteoporosis include low bone mineral density, low estrogen levels, family history of osteoporosis, previous fracture, small frame (low BMI), light skin color, smoking, and alcohol intake. Response to therapy can be predicted by pretreatment serum estradiol, and can be assessed during treatment by measuring biochemical markers of bone formation/resorption and/or bone mineral density.

It is recommended that women who have a uterus and be treated with *Menostar* receive a progestin for 14 days every 6 to 12 months and undergo an endometrial biopsy at yearly intervals or as clinically indicated.

Application of the system – Place the adhesive side of the *Menostar* transdermal system on a clean, dry area of the lower abdomen. Do not apply *Menostar* to or near the breasts. The sites of application must be rotated, with an interval of at least 1-week allowed between applications to a particular site. The area selected should not be oily, damaged, or irritated. Avoid the waistline because tight clothing may rub and remove the transdermal system. Avoid application to areas where sitting would dislodge the transdermal system. Apply the transdermal system immediately after opening the pouch and removing the protective liner. Press the transdermal system firmly in place with the fingers for about 10 seconds, making sure there is good contact, especially around the edges. If the transdermal system lifts, apply pressure to maintain adhesion. In the event that a transdermal system should fall off, apply a new transdermal system for the remainder of the 7-day dosing interval. Wear only 1 system at any one time during the 7-day dosing interval. Swimming, bathing, or using a sauna while using *Menostar* has not been studied, and these activities may decrease the adhesion of the transdermal system and the delivery of estradiol.

➤*Storage / Stability:* Store at controlled room temperature at 25°C (77°F). Do not store above 30°C (86°F). Do not store unpouched. Apply immediately upon removal from the protective pouch.

Discard used estradiol transdermal systems in household trash in a manner that prevents accidental application or ingestion by children, pets, or others.

ESTRADIOL

Rx	**Femtrace** (Warner Chilcott)	**Tablets:** 0.45 mg estradiol acetate	Lactose. (WC 389). Cream. In 100s.
Rx	**Estradiol** (Various, eg, Geneva, Mylan)	**Tablets:** 0.5 mg micronized estradiol	May contain lactose. In 100s.
Rx	**Estrace** (Warner Chilcott)		Lactose. (021 MJ). White, scored. In 100s.
Rx	**Gynodiol** (Fielding)		Lactose. (0768). Lavender, scored. In 30s and 100s.
Rx	**Femtrace** (Warner Chilcott)	**Tablets:** 0.9 mg estradiol acetate	Lactose. (WC 390). White. In 100s.
Rx	**Estradiol** (Various, eg, Geneva, Mylan)	**Tablets:** 1 mg micronized estradiol	May contain lactose. In 100s and 500s.
Rx	**Estrace** (Warner Chilcott)		Lactose. (755 MJ). Lavender, scored. In 100s, 500s.
Rx	**Gynodiol** (Fielding)		Lactose. (1259). Rose, scored. In 30s and 100s.
Rx	**Gynodiol** (Fielding)	**Tablets:** 1.5 mg micronized estradiol	Lactose. (0158). Aqua, scored. In 30s and 100s.
Rx	**Femtrace** (Warner Chilcott)	**Tablets:** 1.8 mg estradiol acetate	Lactose. (WC 391). Yellow. In 100s.
Rx	**Estradiol** (Various, eg, Geneva, Mylan)	**Tablets:** 2 mg micronized estradiol	May contain lactose. In 100s and 500s.
Rx	**Estrace** (Warner Chilcott)		Lactose, tartrazine. (756 MJ). Turquoise, scored. In 100s and 500s.
Rx	**Gynodiol** (Fielding)		Lactose. (0748). Blue, scored. In 30s and 100s.

ESTRADIOL — ORAL

For complete and comparative prescribing information, refer to the Estrogens group monograph.

WARNING

Endometrial cancer – Estrogens increase the risk of endometrial cancer. Close clinical surveillance of all women taking estrogens is important. Undertake adequate diagnostic measures, including endometrial sampling when indicated, to rule out malignancy in all cases of undiagnosed persistent or recurring abnormal vaginal bleeding.

Cardiovascular and other risks – Do not use estrogens with or without progestins for the prevention of cardiovascular disease.

The Women's Health Initiative (WHI) study reported increased risks of myocardial infarction (MI), stroke, invasive breast cancer, pulmonary emboli, and deep vein thrombosis (DVT) in postmenopausal women (50 to 79 years of age) during 5 years of treatment with oral conjugated estrogens 0.625 mg combined with medroxyprogesterone acetate 2.5 mg relative to placebo.

The Women's Health Initiative Memory Study (WHIMS), a substudy of WHI, reported increased risk of developing probable dementia in postmenopausal women 65 years of age or older during 4 years of treatment with oral conjugated estrogens combined with medroxyprogesterone acetate relative to placebo.

Because of these risks, prescribe estrogens with or without progestins at the lowest effective doses and for the shortest duration consistent with treatment goals and risks for the individual woman.

Indications

➤*Breast cancer (except Femtrace)*: For palliation only in appropriately selected women and men with metastatic disease.

➤*Hypoestrogenism caused by hypogonadism, castration, or primary ovarian failure (except Femtrace)*: Treatment of hypoestrogenism caused by hypogonadism, castration, or primary ovarian failure.

➤*Moderate to severe vasomotor symptoms:* Treatment of moderate to severe vasomotor symptoms associated with menopause.

➤*Osteoporosis prevention (except Femtrace)*: For the prevention of osteoporosis.

➤*Prostate cancer (except Femtrace)*: For palliation only in advanced androgen-dependent prostate carcinoma.

➤*Vulval and vaginal atrophy (except Femtrace)*: Treatment of vulval and vaginal atrophy associated with menopause.

Administration and Dosage

➤*Breast cancer:* For palliation only. The usual dosage is 10 mg 3 times daily for at least 3 months.

➤*Hypoestrogenism caused by hypogonadism, castration, or primary ovarian failure:* Treatment usually is initiated with a dosage of 1 to 2 mg daily and adjusted as necessary to control presenting symptoms; determine the minimal effective dose for maintenance therapy by titration.

➤*Moderate to severe vasomotor symptoms, vulval and vaginal atrophy:* Use the lowest dose and for the shortest duration consistent with treatment goals and risks for the individual woman. Periodically reevaluate patients as clinically appropriate (eg, 3- to 6-month intervals) to determine if treatment is still necessary. Attempt to discontinue or taper medication at 3- to 6-month intervals.

Initiate treatment at the lowest dose. Titrate to determine the minimal effective dose for maintenance therapy. Administer micronized estradiol cyclically (eg, 3 weeks on and 1 week off). Administer estradiol acetate once daily.

➤*Osteoporosis prevention:* Administer 0.5 mg/day cyclically (eg, 23 days on and 5 days off) as soon as possible after menopause. Adjust dosage if necessary to control concurrent menopausal symptoms. Discontinuation may re-establish natural rate of bone loss. The mainstays of prevention and management of osteoporosis are estrogen and calcium; exercise and nutrition may be important adjuncts.

➤*Prostate cancer:* For palliation only. Administer 1 to 2 mg 3 times daily. Judge the efficacy of therapy by phosphatase determinations and symptomatic improvement of the patient.

➤*Concomitant progestin therapy:* When estrogen is prescribed for a postmenopausal woman with a uterus, also initiate progestin to reduce the risk of endometrial cancer. A woman without a uterus does not need progestin.

➤*Storage/Stability:* Store at controlled room temperature, 15° to 30°C (59° to 86°F). Dispense in a tight, light-resistant container.

ESTRADIOL VALERATE IN OIL

Rx	**Delestrogen** (Monarch)	**Injection:** 10 mg/mL	In 5 mL multidose vials.[a]
		20 mg/mL	In 5 mL multidose vials.[b]
		40 mg/mL	In 5 mL multidose vials.[b]

[a] In sesame oil with chlorobutanol.

[b] In castor oil with benzyl benzoate and benzyl alcohol.

ESTRADIOL VALERATE — INJECTION

For complete and comparative prescribing information, refer to the Estrogens group monograph.

WARNING

Estrogens increase the risk of endometrial cancer – Close clinical surveillance of all women taking estrogens is important. Adequate diagnostic measures, including endometrial sampling when indicated, should be undertaken to rule out malignancy in all cases of undiagnosed persistent or recurring abnormal vaginal bleeding. There is no evidence that "natural" estrogens results in a different endometrial risk profile than synthetic estrogens at equivalent estrogen doses.

Cardiovascular and other risks – Estrogens with and without progestins should not be used for the prevention of cardiovascular disease.

WARNING (cont.)

The Women's Health Initiative (WHI) study reported increased risks of myocardial infarction, stroke, invasive breast cancer, pulmonary emboli, and deep vein thrombosis in postmenopausal women during 5 years of treatment with conjugated equine estrogens (CE 0.625 mg) combined with medroxyprogesterone acetate (MPA 2.5 mg) relative to placebo. Other doses of conjugated estrogens with medroxyprogesterone, and other combinations of estrogens and progestins were not studied in the WHI and, in the absence of comparable data, these risks should be assumed to be similar. Because of these risks, estrogens with or without progestins should be prescribed at the lowest effective doses and for the shortest duration consistent with treatment goals and risks for the individual woman.

Indications

Estradiol valerate injection is indicated for the treatment of the following: moderate-to-severe vasomotor symptoms associated with the menopause; hypoestrogenism caused by hypogonadism, castration or primary ovarian

ESTRADIOL VALERATE — INJECTION

failure; advanced androgen-dependent carcinoma of the prostate (for palliation only); vulval and vaginal atrophy associated with the menopause. When prescribing solely for the treatment of vulvar and vaginal atrophy, topical vaginal products should be considered.

Administration and Dosage

Patients should be started at the lowest effective dose for the indication.

➤*Concomitant progestin therapy:* When estrogen is prescribed for a postmenopausal woman with a uterus, progestin should also be initiated to reduce the risk of endometrial cancer. A woman without a uterus does not need progestin.

Use of estrogen, alone or in combination with a progestin, should be limited to the shortest duration consistent with treatment goals and risks for the individual woman. Patients should be reevaluated periodically as clinically appropriate (eg, 3-month to 6-month intervals) to determine if treatment is still necessary. For women who have a uterus, adequate diagnostic measures, such as endometrial sampling, when indicated, should be undertaken to rule out malignancy in cases of undiagnosed persistent or recurring abnormal vaginal bleeding.

➤*Administration:* Care should be taken to inject deeply into the upper, outer quadrant of the gluteal muscle following the usual precautions for IM administration. By virtue of the low viscosity of the vehicles, the various preparations of estradiol valerate injection may be administered with a small gauge needle. Since the 40 mg potency provides a high concentration in a small volume, particular care should be observed to administer the full dose.

Estradiol valerate for injection should be visually inspected for particulate matter and color prior to administration; the solution is clear, colorless to pale yellow. Storage at low temperatures may result in the separation of some crystalline material which redissolves readily on warming.

A dry needle and syringe should be used. Use of a wet needle or syringe may cause the solution to become cloudy; however, this does not affect the potency of the material.

➤*For treatment of moderate-to-severe vasomotor symptoms, vulval and vaginal atrophy associated with the menopause:* For treatment of moderate-to-severe vasomotor symptoms, vulval and vaginal atrophy associated with the menopause, the lowest dose and regimen that will control symptoms should be chosen, and medication should be discontinued as promptly as possible.

Attempts to discontinue or taper medication should be made at 3- to 6-month intervals.

The usual dosage is 10 to 20 mg estradiol valerate every 4 weeks.

➤*For treatment of female hypoestrogenism caused by hypogonadism, castration, or primary ovarian failure:* The usual dosage is 10 to 20 mg estradiol valerate every 4 weeks.

➤*For treatment of advanced androgen-dependent carcinoma of the prostate, for palliation only:* The usual dosage is 30 mg or more administered every 1 or 2 weeks.

Treated patients with an intact uterus should be monitored closely for signs of endometrial cancer, and appropriate diagnostic measures should be taken to rule out malignancy in the event of persistent or recurrent abnormal vaginal bleeding.

➤*Storage/Stability:* Store at room temperature.

CONJUGATED ESTROGENS

Tablets contain a mixture of conjugated equine estrogens obtained exclusively from natural sources that includes sodium estrone sulfate, sodium equilin sulfate, sodium sulfate conjugates, 17α-dihydroequilin, 17α-estradiol, and 17β dihydroequilin.

Rx	**Premarin** (Wyeth-Ayerst)	**Tablets**: 0.3 mg	Lactose, sucrose. Green, oval. In 100s and 1,000s.
		0.45 mg	Lactose, sucrose. Blue, oval. In 100s and UD 1,00s.
		0.625 mg	Lactose, sucrose. Maroon, oval. In 1,000s and UD 100s.
		0.9 mg	Lactose, sucrose. White, oval. In 100s.
		1.25 mg	Lactose, sucrose. Yellow, oval. In 100s and 1,000s.
Rx	**Premarin Intravenous** (Wyeth-Ayerst)	**Injection**: 25 mg	In *Secules*[a] (vials), each with 5 mL sterile diluent.[b]

[a] With 200 mg lactose, 0.2 mg simethicone, and 12.2 mg sodium citrate.

[b] With 2% benzyl alcohol.

CONJUGATED ESTROGENS — ORAL

For complete prescribing information, refer to the Estrogens group monograph.

WARNING

Estrogens increase the risk of endometrial cancer – Close clinical surveillance of all women taking estrogens is important. Adequate diagnostic measures, including endometrial sampling when indicated, should be undertaken to rule out malignancy in all cases of undiagnosed persistent or recurring abnormal vaginal bleeding. There is no evidence that "natural" estrogens results in a different endometrial risk profile than synthetic estrogens of equivalent estrogen dose.

Cardiovascular and other risks – Estrogens with or without progestins should not be used for the prevention of cardiovascular disease.

The Women's Health Initiative (WHI) study reported increased risks of myocardial infarction, stroke, invasive breast cancer, pulmonary emboli, and deep vein thrombosis in postmenopausal women during 5 years of treatment with conjugated equine estrogens (0.625 mg) combined with medroxyprogesterone acetate (2.5 mg) relative to placebo. Other doses of conjugated estrogens and medroxyprogesterone acetate, and other combinations of estrogens and progestins were not studied in the WHI and, in the absence of comparable data, these risks should be assumed to be similar. Because of these risks, estrogens with or without progestins should be prescribed at the lowest effective doses and for the shortest duration consistent with treatment goals and risks for the individual woman.

Indications

Moderate to severe vasomotor symptoms associated with menopause; moderate to severe symptoms of vulvar and vaginal atrophy associated with menopause; prevention of postmenopausal osteoporosis (loss of bone mass); hypoestrogenism caused by hypogonadism, castration, or primary ovarian failure; breast cancer (for palliation only) in appropriately selected women and men with metastatic disease; advanced androgen-dependent prostatic carcinoma (for palliation only).

Administration and Dosage

➤*Concomitant progestin therapy:* When estrogen is prescribed for a postmenopausal woman with a uterus, also initiate progestin to reduce the risk of endometrial cancer. A woman without a uterus does not need progestin.

➤*Moderate to severe vasomotor symptoms and/or moderate to severe symptoms of vulvar and vaginal atrophy associated with menopause:* Start at the lowest dose. Therapy may be given continuously with no interruption, or in cyclical regimens (regimens such as 25 days on drug followed by 5 days off drug) as is medically appropriate on an individualized basis.

➤*Female hypogonadism:* 0.3 to 0.625 mg daily, administered cyclically (eg, 3 weeks on and 1 week off). Doses are adjusted depending on the severity of symptoms and responsiveness of the endometrium.

The dosage may be gradually titrated upward at 6- to 12-month intervals as needed to achieve appropriate bone age advancement and eventual epiphyseal closure. Chronic dosing with 0.625 mg is sufficient to induce artificial cyclic menses with sequential progestin treatment and to maintain bone mineral density after skeletal maturity is achieved.

➤*Female castration and primary ovarian failure:* 1.25 mg/day cyclically. Adjust according to severity of symptoms and patient response. For maintenance, adjust to lowest effective level.

➤*Osteoporosis prevention:* 0.625 mg/day, continuously or cyclically (such as 25 days on, 5 days off). The mainstays of prevention and management of osteoporosis are estrogen and calcium; exercise and nutrition may be important adjuncts.

➤*Breast cancer, metastatic (for palliation):* 10 mg 3 times daily for at least 3 months.

➤*Prostatic carcinoma (for palliation; advanced androgen-dependent):* 1.25 to 2.5 mg 3 times daily. Effectiveness can be judged by phosphatase determinations as well as by symptomatic improvement.

➤*Duration:* Limit the use of estrogen, alone or in combination with a progestin, to the shortest duration consistent with treatment goals and risks for the individual woman. Periodically re-evaluate patients as clinically appropriate (eg, at 3- to 6-month intervals) to determine if treatment is still necessary.

➤*Storage/Stability:* Store at room temperature (approximately 25°C). Dispense in a well-closed container.

CONJUGATED ESTROGENS – INJECTION

For complete prescribing information, refer to the Estrogens group monograph.

WARNING

Estrogens have been reported to increase the risk of endometrial carcinoma – Three independent, case-controlled studies have reported an increased risk of endometrial cancer in postmenopausal women exposed to exogenous estrogens for more than 1 year. This risk was independent of the other known risk factors for endometrial cancer. These studies are further supported by the finding that incidence rates of endometrial cancer have increased sharply since 1969 in 8 different areas of the United States with population-based cancer-reporting systems, an increase which may be related to the rapidly expanding use of estrogens during the last decade.

The 3 case-controlled studies reported that the risk of endometrial cancer in estrogen users was about 4.5 to 13.9 times greater than in nonusers. The risk appears to depend on both duration of treatment and on estrogen dose. In view of these findings, when estrogens are used for the treatment of menopausal symptoms, the lowest dose that will control symptoms should be utilized and medication should be discontinued as soon as possible. When prolonged treatment is medically indicated, the patient should be reassessed, on at least a semiannual basis, to determine the need for continued therapy. Although the evidence must be considered preliminary, one study suggests that cyclic administration of low doses of estrogen may carry less risk than continuous administration. It therefore appears prudent to utilize such a regimen.

Close clinical surveillance of all women taking estrogens is important. In all cases of undiagnosed persistent or recurring abnormal vaginal bleeding, adequate diagnostic measures should be undertaken to rule out malignancy.

There is no evidence at present that "natural" estrogens are more or less hazardous than "synthetic" estrogens at equiestrogenic doses.

Estrogens should not be used during pregnancy – The use of female sex hormones, both estrogens and progestogens, during early pregnancy may seriously damage the offspring. It has been shown that females exposed in utero to diethylstilbestrol, a nonsteroidal estrogen, have an increased risk of developing, in later life, a form of vaginal or cervical cancer that is ordinarily extremely rare. This risk has been estimated as not more than 4/1,000 exposures. Furthermore, a high percentage of such exposed women (from 30% to 90%) have been found to have vaginal adenosis, epithelial changes of the vagina and cervix. Although these changes are histologically benign, it is not known whether they are precursors of malignancy. Although similar data are not available with the use of other estrogens, it cannot be presumed they would not induce similar changes. Several reports suggest an association between intrauterine exposure to female sex hormones and congenital anomalies, including congenital heart defects and limb-reduction defects. One case-controlled study estimated a 4.7-fold increased risk of limb-reduction defects in infants exposed in utero to sex hormones (oral contraceptives, hormone withdrawal tests for pregnancy, or attempted treatment for threatened abortion). Some of these exposures were very short and involved only a few days of treatment. The data suggest that the risk of limb-reduction defects in exposed fetuses is somewhat less than 1/1,000.

WARNING (cont.)

In the past, female sex hormones have been used during pregnancy in an attempt to treat threatened or habitual abortion. There is considerable evidence that estrogens are ineffective for these indications, and there is no evidence from well-controlled studies that progestogens are effective for these uses.

If conjugated estrogens for injection is used during pregnancy, or if the patient becomes pregnant while taking this drug, she should be apprised of the potential risks to the fetus, and the advisability of pregnancy continuation.

Indications

Conjugated estrogens, USP for injection is indicated in the treatment of abnormal uterine bleeding caused by hormonal imbalance in the absence of organic pathology.

Administration and Dosage

➤*Approved by the FDA:* January 26, 1984.

➤*Abnormal uterine bleeding caused by hormonal imbalance:* One 25 mg injection, intravenously or intramuscularly. Intravenous use is preferred since more rapid response can be expected from this mode of administration. Repeat in 6 to 12 hours if necessary. The use of conjugated estrogens, USP for injection does not preclude the advisability of other appropriate measures.

The usual precautionary measures governing intravenous administration should be adhered to. Injection should be made slowly to obviate the occurrence of flushes.

➤*Compatibility of solutions:* Conjugated estrogens for injection is compatible with normal saline, dextrose, and invert sugar solutions. It is not compatible with protein hydrolysate, ascorbic acid, or any solution with an acid pH.

Infusion of conjugated estrogens, USP for injection with other agents is not generally recommended. In emergencies, however, when an infusion has already been started it may be expedient to make the injection into the tubing just distal to the infusion needle. If so used, compatibility of solutions must be considered.

➤*Storage/Stability:*

Storage before reconstitution – Store package in refrigerator, 2° to 8°C (36° to 46°F).

To reconstitute – First withdraw air from the vial so as to facilitate introduction of sterile diluent. Then, flow the sterile diluent slowly against side of the vial and agitate gently. Do not shake violently.

Storage after reconstitution – It is common practice to utilize the reconstituted solution within a few hours. If it is necessary to keep the reconstituted solution for more than a few hours, store the reconstituted solution under refrigeration (2° to 8°C; 36° to 46°F). Under these conditions, the solution is stable for 60 days, and is suitable for use unless darkening or precipitation occurs.

ESTERIFIED ESTROGENS

These products contain 75% to 85% sodium estrone sulfate and 6% to 15% sodium equilin sulfate, in such proportion that the total of these 2 components is not less than 90% of the total esterified estrogens content.

Rx	**Menest** (Monarch)	**Tablets:** 0.3 mg	Lactose. (M72). Yellow, oblong. Film-coated. In 100s.
		0.625 mg	Lactose. (M73). Orange, oblong. Film-coated. In 100s.
		1.25 mg	Lactose. (M74). Green, oblong. Film-coated. In 100s.
		2.5 mg	Lactose. (M75). Pink, oblong. Film-coated. In 50s.

ESTERIFIED ESTROGENS — ORAL

For complete prescribing information, refer to the Estrogens group monograph.

WARNING

Estrogens have been reported to increase the risk of endometrial carcinoma – Three independent case control studies have shown an increased risk of endometrial cancer in postmenopausal women exposed to exogenous estrogens for prolonged periods. This risk was independent of the other known risk factors for endometrial cancer. These studies are further supported by the finding that incidence rates of endometrial cancer have increased sharply since 1969 in 8 different areas of the United States with population-based cancer reporting systems, an increase which may be related to the rapidly expanding use of estrogens during the last decade.

The 3 case control studies reported that the risk of endometrial cancer in estrogen users was about 4.5 to 13.9 times higher than in nonusers. The risk appears to depend on both duration of treatment and on estrogen dose. In view of these findings, when estrogens are used for the treatment of menopausal symptoms, the lowest dose that will control symptoms should be utilized and medication should be discontinued as soon as possible. When prolonged treatment is medically indicated, the patient should be reassessed on at least a semiannual basis to determine the need for continued therapy. Although the evidence must be considered preliminary, 1 study suggests that cyclic administration of low doses of estrogen may carry less risk than continuous administration; it therefore appears prudent to utilize such a regimen.

Close clinical surveillance of all women taking estrogens is important. In all cases of undiagnosed persistent or recurring abnormal vaginal bleeding, adequate diagnostic measures should be undertaken to rule out malignancy.

There is no evidence at present that "natural" estrogens are more or less hazardous than "synthetic" estrogens at equiestrogenic doses.

Estrogens should not be used during pregnancy – The use of female sex hormones, both estrogens and progestagens, during early pregnancy may seriously damage the offspring. It has been shown that females exposed in utero to diethylstilbestrol, a nonsteroidal estrogen, have an increased risk of developing in later life a form of vaginal or cervical cancer that is ordinarily extremely rare. The risk has been estimated as not more than 4/1,000 exposures. Furthermore, a high percentage of such exposed women (from 30% to 90%) have been found to have vaginal adenosis, epithelial changes of the vagina and cervix. Although these changes are histologically benign, it is not known whether they are precursors of malignancy. Although similar data are not available with the use of other estrogens, it cannot be presumed they would not induce similar changes. Several reports suggest an association between intrauterine exposure to female sex hormones and congenital anomalies, including congenital heart defects and limb reduction defects. One case control study estimated a 4.7-fold increased risk of limb reduction defects in infants exposed in utero to sex hormones (oral contraceptives, hormone withdrawal tests for pregnancy, or attempted treatment for threatened abortion). Some of these exposures were very short and involved only a few days of treatment. The data suggest that the risk of limb reduction defects in exposed fetuses is somewhat less than 1/1,000. In the past, female sex hormones have been used during pregnancy in an attempt to treat threatened or habitual abortion. There is considerable evidence that estrogens are ineffective for these indications, and there is no evidence from well-controlled studies that progestagens are effective for these uses. If esterified estrogens tablets are used during pregnancy, or if the patient becomes pregnant while taking this drug, she should be apprised of the potential risks to the fetus, and the advisability of pregnancy continuation.

Indications

Esterified estrogens is indicated in the treatment of:

1.) Moderate to severe vasomotor symptoms associated with the menopause. (There is no evidence that estrogens are effective for nervous symptoms or depression which might occur during menopause, and they should not be used to treat these conditions.)
2.) Atrophic vaginitis.
3.) Kraurosis vulvae.
4.) Female hypogonadism.
5.) Female castration.
6.) Primary ovarian failure.
7.) Breast cancer (for palliation only) in appropriately selected women and men with metastatic disease.
8.) Prostatic carcinoma. Palliative therapy of advanced disease.

Esterified estrogens tablets have not been shown to be effective for any purpose during pregnancy and its use may cause severe harm to the fetus (see Warning Box).

Administration and Dosage

➤*Given cyclically for short-term use only:* For treatment of moderate to severe vasomotor symptoms, atrophic vaginitis or kraurosis vulvae associated with the menopause.

The lowest dose that will control symptoms should be chosen and medication should be discontinued as promptly as possible.

Administration should be cyclic (eg, 3 weeks on and 1 week off).

Attempts to discontinue or taper medication should be made at 3- to 6-month intervals.

Usual dosage ranges –

Vasomotor symptoms: 1.25 mg daily. If the patient has not menstruated within the last 2 months or more, cyclic administration is started arbitrarily. If the patient is menstruating, cyclic administration is started on day 5 of bleeding.

Atrophic vaginitis and kraurosis vulvae: 0.3 to 1.25 mg or more daily, depending upon the tissue response of the individual patient. Administer cyclically.

➤*Given cyclically:* Female hypogonadism; female castration; primary ovarian failure.

Usual dosage ranges –

Female hypogonadism: 2.5 to 7.5 mg daily, in divided doses for 20 days, followed by a rest period of 10 days' duration. If bleeding does not occur by the end of this period, the same dosage schedule is repeated. The number of courses of estrogen therapy necessary to produce bleeding may vary depending on responsiveness of the endometrium.

If bleeding occurs before the end of the 10-day period, begin a 20-day estrogen-progestin cyclic regimen with esterified estrogens tablets, 2.5 to 7.5 mg daily in divided doses, for 20 days. During the last 5 days of estrogen therapy, give an oral progestin. If bleeding occurs before this regimen is concluded, therapy is discontinued and may be resumed on the fifth day of bleeding.

Female castration and primary ovarian failure: 1.25 mg daily, cyclically. Adjust dosage upward or downward according to severity of symptoms and response of the patient. For maintenance, adjust dosage to lowest level that will provide effective control.

➤*Chronically:*

Inoperable progressing prostatic cancer – 1.25 to 2.5 mg 3 times daily. The effectiveness of therapy can be judged by phosphatase determinations as well as by symptomatic improvement of the patient.

Inoperable progressing breast cancer in appropriately selected men and postmenopausal women (see Indications). Suggested dosage is 10 mg 3 times daily for a period of at least 3 months.

Treated patients with an intact uterus should be monitored closely for signs of endometrial cancer and appropriate diagnostic measures should be taken to rule out malignancy in the event of persistent or recurring abnormal vaginal bleeding.

ESTROPIPATE (Piperazine Estrone Sulfate)

Estropipate is a natural substance prepared from crystalline estrone solubilized as the sulfate and stabilized with piperazine.

Rx	**Estropipate** (Various, eg, Mylan, Watson)	**Tablets:** 0.625 mg sodium estrone sulfate (equiv. to 0.75 mg estropipate)	In 30s, 100s, and 500s.
Rx	**Ogen** (Pharmacia)		Lactose. (U 3772). Yellow, scored. In 100s.
Rx	**Ortho-Est** (Women First Healthcare)		Lactose. (WFHC 101). White, diamond shape, scored. In 100s.
Rx	**Estropipate** (Various, eg, Mylan, Watson)	**Tablets:** 1.25 mg sodium estrone sulfate (equiv. to 1.5 mg estropipate)	In 30s, 100s, and 500s.
Rx	**Ogen** (Pharmacia)		Lactose. (U 3773). Peach, scored. In 100s.
Rx	**Ortho-Est** (Women First Healthcare)		Lactose. (WHFC 102). Lavender, diamond shape, scored. In 100s.
Rx	**Estropipate** (Various, eg, Watson)	**Tablets:** 2.5 mg sodium estrone sulfate (equiv. to 3 mg estropipate)	In 30s, 100s, and 500s.
Rx	**Ogen** (Pharmacia)		Lactose. (U 3774). Blue, scored. In 100s.
Rx	**Estropipate** (Various, eg, Watson)	**Tablets:** 5 mg sodium estrone sulfate (equiv. to 6 mg estropipate)	In 30s, 100s, and 500s.

ESTROPIPATE — ORAL

For complete prescribing information, refer to the Estrogens group monograph.

WARNING

Estrogens have been reported to increase the risk of endometrial carcinoma in postmenopausal women – Close clinical surveillance of all women taking estrogens is important. Adequate diagnostic measures, including endometrial sampling when indicated, should be undertaken to rule out malignancy in all cases of undiagnosed persistent or recurring abnormal vaginal bleeding. There is no evidence that "natural" estrogens are more or less hazardous than "synthetic" estrogens at equiestrogenic doses.

Estrogens should not be use during pregnancy – There is no indication for estrogen therapy during pregnancy or during the immediate postpartum period. Estrogens are ineffective for the prevention or treatment of threatened or habitual abortion. Estrogens are not indicated for the prevention of postpartum breast engorgement.

Estrogen therapy during pregnancy is associated with an increased risk of congenital defects in the reproductive organs of the fetus, and possibly other birth defects. Studies of women who received diethylstilbestrol (DES) during pregnancy have shown that female offspring have an increased risk of vaginal adenosis, squamous cell dysplasia of the uterine cervix, and clear cell vaginal cancer later in life; male offspring have an increased risk of urogenital abnormalities and possibly testicular cancer later in life. The 1985 DES Task Force concluded that use of DES during pregnancy is associated with a subsequent increased risk of breast cancer in the mothers, although a causal relationship remains unproven and the observed level of excess risk is similar to that for a number of other breast cancer risk factors.

Indications

Estropipate tablets are indicated in the following: Treatment of moderate to severe vasomotor symptoms associated with menopause; treatment of vulval and vaginal atrophy; treatment of hypoestrogenism due to hypogonadism, castration or primary ovarian failure; prevention of osteoporosis.

There is no adequate evidence that estrogens are effective for nervous symptoms or depression which might occur during menopause and they should not be used to treat these conditions.

Administration and Dosage

➤*Moderate to severe vasomotor symptoms:* For treatment of moderate to severe vasomotor symptoms, vulval and vaginal atrophy associated with the menopause, the lowest dose and regimen that will control symptoms should be chosen and medication should be discontinued as promptly as possible.

Attempts to discontinue or taper medication should be made at 3- to 6-month intervals.

Usual dosage ranges –

Vasomotor symptoms: Estropipate tablets 0.75 mg to 6 mg per day. The lowest dose that will control symptoms should be chosen. If the patient has not menstruated within the last 2 months or more, cyclic administration is started arbitrarily. If the patient is menstruating, cyclic administration is started on day 5 of bleeding.

➤*Vulval and vaginal atrophy:* Estropipate tablets 0.75 mg to 6 mg daily, depending upon the tissue response of the individual patient. The lowest dose that will control symptoms should be chosen. Administer cyclically.

➤*Female hypoestrogenism:* For treatment of female hypoestrogenism caused by hypogonadism, castration, or primary ovarian failure.

Usual dosage ranges –

Female hypogonadism: A daily dose of 1.5 to 9 mg of estropipate tablets may be given for the first 3 weeks of a theoretical cycle, followed by a rest period of 8 to 10 days. The lowest dose that will control symptoms should be chosen. If bleeding does not occur by the end of this period, the same dosage schedule is repeated. The number of courses of estrogen therapy necessary to produce bleeding may vary depending on the responsiveness of the endometrium. If satisfactory withdrawal bleeding does not occur, an oral progestogen may be given in addition to estrogen during the third week of the cycle.

Female castration or primary ovarian failure: A daily dose of 1.5 to 9 mg of estropipate tablets may be given for the first 3 weeks of a theoretical cycle, followed by a rest period of 8 to 10 days. Adjust dosage upward or downward according to severity of symptoms and response of the patient. For maintenance, adjust dosage to lowest level that will provide effective control. Treated patients with an intact uterus should be monitored closely for signs of endometrial cancer and appropriate diagnostic measures should be taken to rule out malignancy in the event of persistent or recurring abnormal vaginal bleeding.

➤*Osteoporosis:* For prevention of osteoporosis. A daily dose of 0.75 mg of estropipate tablets for 25 days of a 31-day cycle per month.

➤*Storage/Stability:* Store at controlled room temperature 15° to 30°C (59° to 86°F).

Dispense with a child-resistant closure in a tight, light-resistant container.

SYNTHETIC CONJUGATED ESTROGENS, A

Tablets contain a blend of 9 synthetic estrogenic substances: Sodium estrone sulfate, sodium equilin sulfate, sodium 17α-dihydroequilin sulfate, sodium 17α-estradiol sulfate, sodium 17β-dihydroequilin sulfate, sodium 17α-dihydroequilenin sulfate, sodium 17β-dihydroequilenin sulfate, sodium equilenin sulfate, and sodium 17β-estradiol sulfate.

Rx	**Cenestin** (Barr/Duramed)	**Tablets:** 0.3 mg	Lactose. (dp 41). Green. Film-coated. In 30s, 100s, and 1,000s.
		0.45 mg	Lactose. (dp 46). Orange. Film-coated. In 30s, 100s, and 1,000s.
		0.625 mg	Lactose. (dp 42). Red. Film-coated. In 30s, 100s, and 1,000s.
		0.9 mg	Lactose. (dp 43). White. Film-coated. In 30s, 100s, and 1,000s.
		1.25 mg	Lactose. (dp 44). Blue. Film-coated. In 30s, 100s, and 1,000s.

SYNTHETIC CONJUGATED ESTROGENS, A — ORAL

For complete prescribing information, refer to the Estrogens group monograph.

WARNING

Estrogens increase the risk of endometrial cancer – The use of unopposed estrogens in women with intact uteri has been associated with an increased risk of endometrial cancer. The reported endometrial cancer risk among unopposed estrogen users is about 2- to 12-fold higher than in nonusers, and appears dependent on duration of treatment and on estrogen dose. Most studies show no significant increased risk associated with use of estrogens for less than 1 year. The greatest risk appears associated with prolonged use, with increased risks of 15- to 24-fold for 5 to 10 years or more, and this risk has been shown to persist for at least 8 to 15 years after estrogen therapy is discontinued.

Clinical surveillance of all women taking estrogen/progestin combinations is important. Undertake adequate diagnostic measures, including endometrial sampling when indicated to rule out malignancy in all cases of undiagnosed persistent or recurring abnormal vaginal bleeding. There is no evidence that the use of natural estrogens results in a different endometrial risk profile than synthetic estrogens of equivalent estrogen dose. Adding a progestin to estrogen therapy has been shown to reduce the risk of endometrial hyperplasia, which may be a precursor to endometrial cancer.

WARNING (cont.)

Cardiovascular and other risks – Estrogens, with and without progestins, should not be used for the prevention of cardiovascular disease. The Women's Health Initiative (WHI) study reported increased risks of myocardial infarction, stroke, invasive breast cancer, pulmonary emboli, and deep vein thrombosis in postmenopausal women (50 to 79 years of age) during 5 years of treatment with conjugated equine estrogens (CEE 0.625 mg) combined with medroxyprogesterone acetate (MPA 2.5 mg) relative to placebo. Other doses of conjugated estrogens with medroxyprogesterone, and other combinations of estrogens and progestins were not studied in the WHI and, in the absence of comparable data, these risks should be assumed to be similar. Because of these risks, prescribe estrogens, with or without progestins, in the lowest effective doses and for the shortest duration consistent with treatment goals and risks for the individual woman.

Indications

➤*Vasomotor symptoms:* This medication is indicated for the treatment of moderate to severe vasomotor symptoms associated with menopause (ie, 0.45 mg, 0.625 mg, 0.9 mg, 1.25 mg).

➤*Vulvar/Vaginal atrophy:* This medication is indicated for the treatment of moderate to severe symptoms of vulvar and vaginal atrophy associated with the menopause (ie, 0.3 mg). When prescribing solely for the treatment of symptoms of vulvar and vaginal atrophy, consider topical vaginal products.

Administration and Dosage

When estrogen is prescribed for a postmenopausal woman with a uterus, also initiate progestin to reduce the risk of endometrial cancer. A woman without a uterus does not need progestin. Limit use of estrogen, alone or in combination with a progestin, to the shortest duration consistent with treat-

SYNTHETIC CONJUGATED ESTROGENS, A — ORAL

ment goals and risks for the individual woman. Periodically reevaluate patients as clinically appropriate (eg, 3- to 6-month intervals) to determine if treatment is still necessary. The WHI study reported increased risks of myocardial infarction, stroke, invasive breast cancer, pulmonary emboli, and deep vein thrombosis in postmenopausal women during 5 years of treatment with conjugated equine estrogens (CEE 0.625 mg) combined with medroxyprogesterone acetate (MPA 2.5 mg) relative to placebo. Other doses of conjugated estrogens with medroxyprogesterone, and other combinations of estrogens and progestins were not studied in the WHI and, in the absence of comparable data, these risks should be assumed to be similar. For women who have a uterus, undertake adequate diagnostic measures, such as endometrial sampling, when indicated, to rule out malignancy in cases of undiagnosed persistent or recurring abnormal vaginal bleeding.

➤*Storage/Stability:* Store at 20° to 25°C (68° to 77°F); excursions are permitted to 15° to 30°C (59° to 86°F).

Dispense in tight container.

Dispense in child-resistant packaging.

Dispenser – Include one "Information for the patient" leaflet with each package dispensed.

SYNTHETIC CONJUGATED ESTROGENS, B

Rx	**Enjuvia** (Barr/Duramed)	**Tablets**[a]: 0.3 mg	EDTA, lactose. (F1). White, oval. Film-coated. In 100s.
		0.45 mg	EDTA, lactose. (E2). Mauve, oval. Film-coated. In 100s.
		0.625 mg	EDTA, lactose. (E3). Pink, oval. Film-coated. In 100s.
		1.25 mg	EDTA, lactose. (E4). Yellow, oval. Film-coated. In 100s.

[a] Tablets contain a blend of 10 synthetic estrogenic substances: Sodium estrone sulfate, sodium equilin sulfate, sodium 17α-dihydroequilin sulfate, sodium 17α-estradiol sulfate, sodium 17β-dihydroequilin sulfate, sodium 17α-dihydroequilenin sulfate, sodium 17β-dihydroequilenin sulfate, sodium equilenin sulfate, sodium 17β-estradiol sulfate, and sodium Δ8,9-dehydroestrone sulfate.

SYNTHETIC CONJUGATED ESTROGENS, B — ORAL

For complete prescribing information, refer to the Estrogens group monograph.

Indications

➤*Menopause:* For the treatment of moderate to severe vasomotor symptoms associated with menopause.

Administration and Dosage

➤*Approved by the FDA:* May 10, 2004.

➤*Menopause:* Start patients at lowest approved dose of 0.3 mg once daily. Subsequent dosage adjustment may be made based upon the individual patient response. Health care provider should periodically reassess dose.

➤*Concomitant progestin therapy:* When estrogen is prescribed for a postmenopausal woman with a uterus, initiate a progestin to reduce the risk of endometrial cancer. A woman without a uterus does not need a progestin.

Prescribe use of estrogen, alone or in combination with a progestin, with the lowest effective dose and for the shortest duration consistent with treatment goals and risks for the individual woman. Reevaluate patients periodically as clinically appropriate (eg, at 3- to 6-month intervals) to determine if treatment is still necessary (see Boxed Warnings and Warnings). For women who have a uterus, undertake adequate diagnostic measures, such as endometrial sampling, when indicated, to rule out malignancy in cases of undiagnosed persistent or recurring abnormal vaginal bleeding.

➤*Storage/Stability:* Store at controlled room temperature 20° to 25°C (68° to 77°F).

ESTRADIOL CYPIONATE IN OIL

Rx	**Depo-Estradiol** (Pharmacia)	**Injection:** 5 mg/mL	In 5 mL vials.[1]

[1] In cottonseed oil with 5.4 mg chlorobutanol.

ESTRADIOL CYPIONATE — INJECTION

For complete prescribing information, refer to the Estrogens group monograph.

WARNING

Estrogens have been reported to increase the risk of endometrial carcinoma in postmenopausal women – Close clinical surveillance of all women taking estrogens is important. Adequate diagnostic measures including endometrial sampling when indicated, should be undertaken to rule out malignancy in all cases of undiagnosed persistent or recurring abnormal vaginal bleeding. There is currently no evidence that "natural" estrogens are more or less hazardous than "synthetic" estrogens at equi-estrogenic doses.

Estrogens should not be used during pregnancy – There is no indication for estrogen therapy during pregnancy or during the immediate postpartum period. Estrogens are ineffective for the prevention or treatment of threatened or habitual abortion. Estrogens are not indicated for the prevention of postpartum breast engorgement.

Estrogen therapy during pregnancy is associated with an increased risk of congenital defects in the reproductive organs of the fetus, and possibly other birth defects. Studies of women who received diethylstilbestrol (DES) during pregnancy have shown that female offspring have an increased risk of vaginal adenosis, squamous cell dysplasia of the uterine cervix, and clear cell vaginal cancer later in life; male offspring have an increased risk of urogenital abnormalities and possibly testicular cancer later in life. The 1985 DES Task force concluded that use of DES during pregnancy is associated with a subsequent increased risk of breast cancer in the mothers, although a causal relationship remains unproven and the observed level of excess risk is similar to that for a number of other breast cancer risk factors.

Indications

Estradiol cypionate injection is indicated in the treatment of the following: hypoestrogenism caused by hypogonadism; moderate to severe vasomotor symptoms associated with the menopause. (There is no evidence that estrogens are effective for nervous symptoms or depression that might occur during menopause, and they should not be used to treat these conditions.)

Administration and Dosage

Parenteral drug products should be inspected visually for particulate matter and discoloration prior to administration whenever solution and container permit.

Warming and shaking the vial should redissolve any crystals that may have formed during storage at temperatures lower than recommended.

➤*Estradiol cypionate injection is for IM use only:*

1.) Short-term cyclic use for treatment of moderate to severe vasomotor symptoms, vulval and vaginal atrophy associated with the menopause, the lowest dose and regimen that will control symptoms should be chosen and medication should be discontinued as promptly as possible. Attempts to discontinue or taper medication should be made at 3- to 6-month intervals. The usual dosage range is 1 to 5 mg injected every 3 to 4 weeks.

2.) For treatment of female hypoestrogenism caused by hypogonadism 1.5 to 2 mg injected at monthly intervals.

➤*Storage/Stability:* Store at controlled room temperature 20° to 25°C (68° to 77°F).

MISCELLANEOUS ESTROGENS, VAGINAL

Rx	**Vagifem** (Novo Nordisk)	**Tablets, vaginal:** 25 mcg estradiol (equiv. to 25.8 mcg of the hemihydrate)	Lactose. White. Film-coated. In 8s, 15s, and 18s.
Rx	**Estrace Vaginal** (Warner Chilcott)	**Cream:** 0.1 mg estradiol/g in a nonliquefying base	Stearyl alcohol, EDTA, methylparaben. In 42.5 g with calibrated applicator.
Rx	**Premarin Vaginal** (Wyeth-Ayerst)	**Cream:** 0.625 mg conjugated estrogens/g in a nonliquefying base	Benzyl and cetyl alcohols, mineral oil. In 42.5 g with or without calibrated applicator.
Rx	**Ogen Vaginal** (Pharmacia)	**Cream:** 1.5 mg estropipate/g	Cetyl alcohol, parabens, mineral oil. In 42.5 g with calibrated applicator.
Rx	**Estring** (Pharmacia)	**Ring:** 2 mg estradiol[a]	In single packs.

MISCELLANEOUS ESTROGENS, VAGINAL

Rx	Femring (Galen)	Ring: 0.05 mg/day estradiol acetate[b]	In single packs.
		0.1 mg/day estradiol acetate[c]	In single packs.

[a] Releases estradiol, approximately 7.5 mcg/24 hours, in a consistent, stable manner over 90 days. Dimensions: outer diameter, 55 mm; cross-sectional diameter, 9 mm; core diameter, 2 mm.
[b] Central core contains 12.4 mg estradiol acetate that releases 0.05 mg/day for 3 months. Dimensions: outer diameter, 56 mm; cross-sectional diameter, 7.6 mm; core diameter, 2 mm.
[c] Central core contains 24.8 mg estradiol acetate that releases 0.1 mg/day for 3 months. Dimensions: outer diameter, 56 mm; cross-sectional diameter, 7.6 mm; core diameter, 2 mm.

CONJUGATED ESTROGENS — VAGINAL CREAM

WARNING

Estrogens increase the risk of endometrial cancer – Close clinical surveillance of all women taking estrogens is important. Undertake adequate diagnostic measures, including endometrial sampling when indicated, to rule out malignancy in all cases of undiagnosed persistent or recurring abnormal vaginal bleeding. There is no evidence that the use of "natural" estrogens results in a different endometrial risk profile than synthetic estrogens of equivalent estrogen dose.

Cardiovascular and other risks – Do not use estrogens with or without progestins for the prevention of cardiovascular disease or dementia. The Women's Health Initiative (WHI) study reported increased risks of stroke and deep vein thrombosis in postmenopausal women (50 to 79 years of age) during 6.8 years of treatment with conjugated estrogens 0.625 mg relative to placebo. The WHI study reported increased risks of myocardial infarction (MI), stroke, invasive breast cancer, pulmonary emboli, and deep vein thrombosis in postmenopausal women (50 to 79 years of age) during 5 years of treatment with oral conjugated estrogens 0.625 mg combined with medroxyprogesterone 2.5 mg relative to placebo. The Women's Health Initiative Memory Study (WHIMS), a substudy of WHI, reported increased risk of developing probable dementia in postmenopausal women 65 years of age or older during 5.2 years of treatment with oral conjugated estrogens alone and during 4 years of treatment with conjugated estrogens combined with medroxyprogesterone, relative to placebo. It is unknown whether this finding applies to younger postmenopausal women. Other doses of conjugated estrogens and medroxyprogesterone acetate, and other combinations and dosage forms of estrogens and progestins, were not studied in the WHI clinical trials and, in the absence of comparable data, these risks should be assumed to be similar. Because of these risks, prescribe estrogens with or without progestins at the lowest effective doses and for the shortest duration consistent with treatment goals and risks for the individual woman.

Indications

➤*Atrophic vaginitis:* For the treatment of atrophic vaginitis.

➤*Kraurosis vulvae:* For the treatment of kraurosis vulvae.

Administration and Dosage

➤*Approved by the FDA:* May 8, 1942 (oral dosage form).

Estrogen administration should be guided by clinical response at the lowest dose for the treatment of postmenopausal vulvar and vaginal atrophy.

➤*Usual dosage range:* 0.5 to 2 g daily, intravaginally, depending on the severity of the condition. The lowest dose that will control symptoms should be chosen and medication should be discontinued as promptly as possible. Administration should be cyclic (eg, 3 weeks on and 1 week off).

➤*Duration of therapy:* Use of conjugated estrogens vaginal cream, alone or in combination with a progestin, should be limited to the shortest duration consistent with treatment goals and risks for the individual woman. Patients should be reevaluated periodically as clinically appropriate (eg, at 3- to 6-month intervals) to determine if treatment is still necessary. For women who have a uterus, adequate diagnostic measures, such as endometrial sampling, when indicated, should be undertaken to rule out malignancy in cases of undiagnosed persistent or recurring abnormal vaginal bleeding.

➤*Instructions for use:* Remove the cap from the tube and screw the nozzle end of the applicator onto the tube. Gently squeeze the tube from the bottom to force sufficient cream into the barrel to provide the prescribed dose, using the marked stopping points on the applicator as a guideline. Unscrew the applicator from the tube. Lie on back with knees drawn up. To deliver the medication, gently insert the applicator deeply into the vagina and press the plunger downward to its original position. To cleanse the applicator, pull the plunger to remove it from the barrel. Wash the applicator with mild soap and warm water. Do not boil or use hot water.

➤*Storage/Stability:* Store at room temperature (approximately 25°C [77°F]).

ESTRADIOL ACETATE — VAGINAL

For complete prescribing information, refer to the Estrogens group monograph.

WARNING

Estrogens increase the risk of endometrial cancer – Close clinical surveillance of all women taking estrogens is important. Adequate diagnostic measures, including endometrial sampling when indicated, should be undertaken to rule out malignancy in all cases of undiagnosed persistent or recurring abnormal vaginal bleeding. There is no evidence that the use of "natural" estrogens results in a different endometrial risk profile than synthetic estrogens at equivalent estrogen doses.

Cardiovascular and other risks – Estrogens with and without progestins should not be used for the prevention of cardiovascular disease.

The Women's Health Initiative (WHI) study reported increased risks of myocardial infarction, stroke, invasive breast cancer, pulmonary emboli, and deep vein thrombosis in postmenopausal women during 5 years of treatment with conjugated equine estrogens 0.625 mg combined with medroxyprogesterone acetate 2.5 mg relative to placebo. Other doses of conjugated estrogens with medroxyprogesterone acetate, and other combinations of estrogens and progestins were not studied in the WHI and, in the absence of comparable data, these risks should be assumed to be similar. Because of these risks, estrogens with or without progestins should be prescribed at the lowest effective doses and for the shortest duration consistent with treatment goals and risks for the individual woman.

Indications

Estradiol acetate vaginal ring therapy is indicated in thetreatment of the following: moderate to severe vasomotor symptoms associated with the menopause; moderate to severe symptoms of vulvar and vaginal atrophy associated with the menopause. When prescribing solely for the treatment of symptoms of vulvar and vaginal atrophy, other vaginal products should be considered

Administration and Dosage

➤*Approved by the FDA:* March 20, 2003.

➤*Dosage:* Two doses of estradiol acetate vaginal ring are available, 0.05 and 0.1 mg daily, for the treatment of moderate to severe vasomotor symptoms and/or moderate to severe symptoms of vulvar and vaginal atrophy associated with the menopause. Patients should be started at the lowest dose.

➤*Instructions for use:* Hands should be thoroughly washed before and after ring insertion.

Estradiol acetate vaginal ring insertion – Insert upon removal from the protective pouch.

The opposite sides of the vaginal ring should be pressed together and inserted into the vagina. The exact position is not critical to its function. When estradiol acetate vaginal ring is in place, the patient should not feel anything. If the patient feels discomfort, the vaginal ring is probably not far enough inside the vagina. Gently push estradiol acetate vaginal ring further into the vagina.

Estradiol acetate vaginal ring use – Estradiol acetate vaginal ring should remain in place for 3 months and then be replaced by a new estradiol acetate vaginal ring.

The patient should not feel estradiol acetate vaginal ring when it is in place and it should not interfere with sexual intercourse. Straining upon bowel movement may make estradiol acetate vaginal ring move down in the lower part of the vagina. If so, it may be repositioned with a finger.

If estradiol acetate vaginal ring is expelled totally from the vagina, it should be rinsed in lukewarm water and reinserted by the patient (or healthcare provider if necessary).

Estradiol acetate vaginal ring removal – Estradiol acetate vaginal ring may be removed by looping a finger through the ring and pulling it out.

➤*Concomitant progestin therapy:* When estrogen is prescribed for a postmenopausal woman with a uterus, progestin should also be initiated to reduce the risk of endometrial cancer. A woman without a uterus does not need progestin. Use of estrogen, alone or in combination with a progestin, should be limited to the shortest duration consistent with treatment goals and risks for the individual woman. Patients should be reevaluated periodically as clinically appropriate (eg, 3- to 6-month intervals) to determine if treatment is still necessary (see Boxed Warning and Warnings). For women who have a uterus, adequate diagnostic measures, such as endometrial sampling, when indicated, should be undertaken to rule out malignancy in cases of undiagnosed persistent or recurring abnormal vaginal bleeding.

➤*Storage/Stability:* Store at 25°C (77°F); excursions permitted to 15° to 30°C (59° to 86°F).

ESTRADIOL — VAGINAL

For complete prescribing information, refer to the Estrogens group monograph.

WARNING

Estrogens have been reported to increase the risk of endometrial carcinoma in postmenopausal women – Close clinical surveillance of all women taking estrogens is important. Adequate diagnostic measures, including endometrial sampling when indicated, should be undertaken to rule out malignancy in all cases of undiagnosed persistent or recurring abnormal vaginal bleeding. There is no evidence that "natural" estrogens are more or less hazardous than "synthetic" estrogens at equiestrogenic doses.

Three independent, case-controlled studies have reported an increased risk of endometrial cancer in postmenopausal women exposed to exogenous estrogens for more than 1 year. This risk was independent of the other known risk factors for endometrial cancer. These studies are further supported by the finding that incidence rates of endometrial cancer have increased sharply since 1969 in 8 different areas of the United States with population-based, cancer-reporting systems, an increase which may be related to the rapidly expanding use of estrogens during the last decade.

The 3 case-controlled studies reported that the risk of endometrial cancer in estrogen users was about 4.5 to 13.9 times higher than in nonusers. The risk appears to depend on both duration of treatment and on estrogen dose. In view of these findings, when estrogens are used for the treatment of menopausal symptoms, the lowest dose that will control symptoms should be utilized and medication should be discontinued as soon as possible. When prolonged treatment is medically indicated, the patient should be reassessed, on at least a semiannual basis, to determine the need for continued therapy.

Estrogens should not be used during pregnancy – There is no indication for estrogen therapy during pregnancy or during the immediate postpartum period. Estrogens are ineffective for the prevention or treatment of threatened or habitual abortion. Estrogens are not indicated for the prevention of postpartum breast engorgement.

Estrogen therapy during pregnancy is associated with an increased risk of congenital defects in the reproductive organs of the fetus, and possibly other birth defects. Studies of women who received diethylstilbestrol (DES) during pregnancy have shown that female offspring have an increased risk of vaginal adenosis, squamous cell dysplasia of the uterine cervix, and clear cell vaginal cancer later in life; male offspring have an increased risk of urogenital abnormalities and possibly testicular cancer later in life. The 1985 DES Task Force concluded that use of DES during pregnancy is associated with subsequent increased risk of breast cancer in the mothers; although, a causal relationship remains unproven, and the observed level of excess risk is similar to that for a number of other breast cancer risk factors.

Indications

➤*Vaginal cream:* Estradiol vaginal cream is indicated in the treatment of vulval and vaginal atrophy.

➤*Vaginal tablets:* Estradiol vaginal tablets are indicated for the treatment of atrophic vaginitis.

➤*Vaginal ring:* Estradiol vaginal ring is indicated for the treatment of urogenital symptoms associated with postmenopausal atrophy of the vagina (eg, dryness, burning, pruritus, dyspareunia) and/or the lower urinary tract (urinary urgency and dysuria).

Administration and Dosage

➤*Approved by the FDA:* Vaginal cream, January 31, 1984; vaginal ring, April 26, 1996; vaginal tablet, March 26, 1999.

For treatment of vulval and vaginal atrophy and atrophic vaginitis associated with the menopause, the lowest dose and regimen that will control symptoms should be chosen and medication should be discontinued as promptly as possible.

The need to continue therapy should be assessed by the physician with the patient. Attempts to discontinue or taper medication should be made at 3- to 6-month intervals.

➤*Vaginal cream:*

Usual dose – The usual dose range is 2 to 4 g (marked on the applicator or delivered via 1 g tubes) daily for 1 or 2 weeks, then gradually reduced to one-half initial dosage for a similar period. A maintenance dosage of 1 g, 1 to 3 times a week, may be used after restoration of the vaginal mucosa has been achieved. The number of doses per multi-dose tube will vary with dosage requirements and patient handling.

Patients with intact uteri should be monitored closely for signs of endometrial cancer, and appropriate diagnostic measures should be taken to rule out malignancy in the event of persistent or recurring abnormal vaginal bleeding.

➤*Vaginal tablets:* The estradiol vaginal tablet is gently inserted into the vagina as far as it can comfortably go without force, using the supplied applicator.

Initial dose – One estradiol vaginal tablet, inserted vaginally, once daily for 2 weeks. It is advisable to have the patient administer treatment at the same time each day.

Maintenance dose – One estradiol vaginal tablet, inserted vaginally, twice weekly.

➤*Vaginal ring:* One estradiol vaginal ring is to be inserted as deeply as possible into the upper one-third of the vaginal vault. The ring is to remain in place continuously for 3 months, after which it is to be removed and, if appropriate, replaced by a new ring. The need to continue treatment should be assessed at 3- or 6-month intervals.

Should the ring be removed or fall out at any time during the 90-day treatment period, the ring should be rinsed in lukewarm water and re inserted by the patient, or, if necessary, by a physician or nurse.

Retention of the ring for greater than 90 days does not represent overdosage but will result in progressively greater underdosage with the attendant risk of loss of efficacy and increasing risk of vaginal infections and/or erosions.

Estradiol vaginal ring insertion – The ring should be pressed into an oval and inserted into the upper third of the vaginal vault. The exact position is not critical. When estradiol vaginal ring is in place, the patient should not feel anything. If the patient feels discomfort, estradiol vaginal ring is probably not far enough inside. Gently push estradiol vaginal ring further into the vagina.

Estradiol vaginal ring use – The estradiol vaginal ring should be left in place continuously for 90 days and then, if continuation of therapy is deemed appropriate, replaced by a new estradiol vaginal ring.

The patient should not feel estradiol vaginal ring when it is in place and it should not interfere with sexual intercourse. Straining at defecation may make estradiol vaginal ring move down in the lower part of the vagina. If so, it may be pushed up again with a finger.

If estradiol vaginal ring is expelled totally from the vagina, it should be rinsed in lukewarm water and reinserted by the patient (or doctor/nurse if necessary).

Estradiol vaginal ring removal – The estradiol vaginal ring may be removed by hooking a finger through the ring and pulling it out.

➤*Storage / Stability:*

Vaginal cream – Store at room temperature. Protect from temperatures in excess of 40°C (104°F).

Vaginal tablets – Store at 25°C (77°F); excursions permitted to 15° to 30°C (59° to 86°F).

Vaginal ring – Store at controlled room temperature 15° to 30°C (59° to 86°F).

ESTROPIPATE — VAGINAL

For complete prescribing information, refer to the Estrogens group monograph.

WARNING

Estrogens have been reported to increase the risk of endometrial carcinoma in postmenopausal women – Close clinical surveillance of all women taking estrogens is important. Adequate diagnostic measures, including endometrial sampling when indicated, should be undertaken to rule out malignancy in all cases of undiagnosed persistent or recurring abnormal vaginal bleeding. There is no evidence that "natural" estrogens are more or less hazardous than "synthetic" estrogens at equiestrogenic doses.

Estrogens should not be used during pregnancy – There is no indication for estrogen therapy during pregnancy or during the immediate postpartum period. Estrogens are ineffective for the prevention or treatment of threatened, or habitual abortion. Estrogens are not indicated for the prevention of postpartum breast engorgement.

Estrogen therapy during pregnancy is associated with an increased risk of congenital defects in the reproductive organs of the fetus, and possibly other birth defects. Studies of women who received diethylstilbestrol (DES) during pregnancy have shown that female offspring have an increased risk of vaginal adenosis, squamous cell dysplasia of the uterine cervix, and clear cell vaginal cancer later in life; male offspring have an increased risk of urogenital abnormalities and possibly testicular cancer later in life. The 1985 DES Task Force concluded that use of DES during pregnancy is associated with a subsequent increased risk of breast cancer in the mothers, although a causal relationship remains unproven and the observed level of excess risk is similar to that for a number of other breast cancer risk factors.

Indications

Estropipate vaginal cream is indicated for the treatment of vulval and vaginal atrophy.

Administration and Dosage

➤*Approved by the FDA:* November 27, 1996.

➤*Dosage:* Intravaginally, estropipate vaginal cream 2 to 4 g daily, depending upon the severity of the condition.

Attempts to discontinue or taper medication should be made at 3-month to 6-month intervals.

For treatment of vulval and vaginal atrophy associated with the menopause, the lowest dose and regimen that will control symptoms should be chosen and medication should be discontinued as promptly as possible.

Between uses, pull plunger out of barrel and wash applicator in warm, soapy water. Do not put applicator in hot or boiling water.

➤*Storage/Stability:* Store below 30°C (86°F).

MISCELLANEOUS ESTROGENS, TOPICAL

Rx	**Estrogel** (Unimed)	**Gel:** 0.06% estradiol (0.75 mg estradiol/1.25 g unit dose)	Alcohol. In 80 g tubes and 93 g pumps.
Rx	**Estrasorb** (Novavax)	**Topical emulsion:** 2.5 mg estradiol hemihydrage/g	Soybean oil, ethanol. In 1.74 g pouches.

ESTRADIOL — TOPICAL

For complete prescribing information, refer to the Estrogens group monograph.

WARNING

Estrogens increase the risk of endometrial cancer – Close clinical surveillance of all women taking estrogen is important. Adequate diagnostic measures, including endometrial sampling when indicated, should be undertaken to rule out malignancy in all cases of undiagnosed persistent or recurring abnormal vaginal bleeding. There is no evidence that the use of "natural" estrogens results in a different endometrial risk profile than synthetic estrogens at equivalent estrogenic doses.

Cardiovascular and other risks – Estrogens with or without progestins should not be used for the prevention of cardiovascular disease.

The Women's Health Initiative (WHI) study reported increased risks of myocardial infarction, stroke, invasive breast cancer, pulmonary emboli, and deep vein thrombosis in postmenopausal women (50 to 79 years of age) during 5 years of treatment with conjugated equine estrogens 0.625 mg combined with medroxyprogesterone acetate 2.5 mg relative to placebo. Other doses of conjugated estrogens and medroxyprogesterone acetate, and other combinations of estrogens and progestins were not studies in the WHI and, in the absence of comparable data, these risks should be assumed to be similar. Because of these risks, estrogens with or without progestins should be prescribed at the lowest effective doses and for the shortest duration consistent with treatment goals and risks for the individual woman.

Indications

➤*Vasomotor symptoms:* Estradiol topical emulsion and gel are indicated for the treatment of moderate to severe vasomotor symptoms associated with menopause.

➤*Vulvar/Vaginal atrophy (gel only):* Treatment of moderate to severe symptoms of vulvar and vaginal atrophy associated with the menopause. When prescribing solely for the treatment of symptoms of vulvar and vaginal atrophy, topical vaginal products should be considered.

Administration and Dosage

➤*Approved by the FDA:* October 9, 2003.

➤*Estradiol topical emulsion:* For the treatment of moderate to severe vasomotor symptoms associated with the menopause, the single approved dose of estradiol topical emulsion is 3.48 g daily. The lowest effective dose of estradiol topical emulsion for this indication has not been determined.

Instructions for daily application of two 1.74 g foil-laminated pouches –

1.) Estradiol topical emulsion should be applied in a comfortable sitting position to clean, dry skin on both legs each morning. Each foil-laminated pouch of estradiol topical emulsion should be opened individually.
2.) Cut or tear the first foil-laminated pouch at the notches indicated near the top of the pouch.

➤*Estradiol gel:* Estradiol gel 1.25 g is the single approved dose for the treatment of moderate to severe vasomotor symptoms and/or moderate to severe symptoms of vulvar and vaginal atrophy associated with the menopause. The lowest effective dose of estradiol gel for these indications has not been determined. When prescribing solely for the treatment of moderate to severe symptoms of vulvar and vaginal atrophy, topical vaginal products should be considered.

➤*Concomitant progestin therapy:* When estrogen is prescribed for a postmenopausal woman with a uterus, a progestin should also be initiated to reduce the risk of endometrial cancer. A woman without a uterus does not need progestin. Use of estrogen, alone or in combination with a progestin, should be limited to the shortest duration consistent with treatment goals and risks for the individual women. Patients should be re-evaluated periodically as clinically appropriate (eg, at 3- to 6-month intervals) to determine if treatment is still necessary. For women with a uterus, adequate diagnostic measures, such as endometrial sampling, when indicated, should be undertaken to rule out malignancy in cases of undiagnosed persistent or recurring abnormal vaginal bleeding.

➤*Storage/Stability:* Store at 20° to 25°C (68° to 77°F); excursions permitted to 15° to 30°C (59° to 86°F).

Keep out of the reach of children.

Selective Estrogen Receptor Modulator

RALOXIFENE

Rx	**Evista** (Eli Lilly)	**Tablets:** 60 mg	Lactose. (LILLY 4165). White, elliptical. Film coated. In unit-of-use 30s and 100s, and 2000s.

RALOXIFENE HYDROCHLORIDE — ORAL

Indications

➤*Osteoporosis (treatment and prevention):* For the treatment and prevention of osteoporosis in postmenopausal women.

➤*Unlabeled uses:* For the treatment of uterine leiomyomas, prevention of breast cancer, treatment of pubertal gynecomastia, and the prevention of bone loss in men with prostate cancer.

Administration and Dosage

➤*Approved by the FDA:* December 9, 1997.

➤*Dosage:* The recommended dosage is one 60 mg raloxifene tablet daily, which may be administered any time of day without regard to meals.

➤*Calcium / Vitamin D supplements:* For either osteoporosis treatment or prevention, add supplemental calcium or vitamin D to the diet if daily intake is inadequate.

➤*Storage / Stability:* Store at controlled room temperature, 20° to 25°C (68° to 77°F). The USP defines controlled room temperature as a temperature maintained thermostatically that encompasses the usual and customary working environment of 20° to 25°C (68° to 77°F); that results in a mean kinetic temperature calculated to be not more than 25°C (77°F); and that allows for excursions between 15° and 30°C (59° and 86°F) that are experienced in pharmacies, hospitals, and warehouses.

Actions

➤*Pharmacology:* Decreases in estrogen levels after oophorectomy or menopause lead to increases in bone resorption and accelerated bone loss. Bone is initially lost rapidly because the compensatory increase in bone formation is inadequate to offset resorptive losses. In addition to loss of estrogen, this imbalance between resorption and formation may be due to age-related impairment of osteoblasts or their precursors. In some women, these changes will eventually lead to decreased bone mass, osteoporosis, and increased risk for fractures, particularly of the spine, hip, and wrist. Vertebral fractures are the most common type of osteoporotic fracture in postmenopausal women.

The biological actions of raloxifene are largely mediated through binding to estrogen receptors. This binding results in activation of certain estrogenic pathways and blockade of others. Thus, raloxifene is an SERM.

Raloxifene decreases resorption of bone and reduces biochemical markers of bone turnover to the premenopausal range. These effects on bone are manifested as reductions in the serum and urine levels of bone turnover markers, decreases in bone resorption based on radiocalcium kinetics studies, increases in bone mineral density (BMD), and decreases in incidence of fractures. Raloxifene also has effects on lipid metabolism. Raloxifene decreases total and LDL cholesterol levels but does not increase triglyceride levels. It does not change total HDL cholesterol levels. Preclinical data demonstrate that raloxifene is an estrogen antagonist in uterine and breast tissues. Clinical trial data (through a median of 42 months) suggest that raloxifene lacks estrogen-like effects on the uterus and breast tissue.

➤*Pharmacokinetics:*

Absorption – Raloxifene is absorbed rapidly after oral administration. Approximately 60% of an oral dose is absorbed, but presystemic glucuronide conjugation is extensive. Absolute bioavailability of raloxifene is 2%. The time to reach average maximum plasma concentration and bioavailability are functions of systemic interconversion and enterohepatic cycling of raloxifene and its glucuronide metabolites.

Administration of raloxifene with a standardized, high-fat meal increases the absorption of raloxifene (C_{max} 28% and AUC 16%) but does not lead to clinically meaningful changes in systemic exposure. Raloxifene can be administered without regard to meals.

Distribution – Following oral administration of single doses ranging from 30 to 150 mg of raloxifene, the apparent volume of distribution is 2,348 L/kg and is not dose dependent.

Raloxifene and the monoglucuronide conjugates are highly (95%) bound to plasma proteins. Raloxifene binds to both albumin and alpha-1-acid glycoprotein, but not to sex steroid-binding globulin.

Metabolism – Biotransformation and disposition of raloxifene in humans have been determined following oral administration of ^{14}C-labeled raloxifene. Raloxifene undergoes extensive first-pass metabolism to the glucuronide conjugates: raloxifene-4′-glucuronide, raloxifene-6-glucuronide, and raloxifene-6, 4′-diglucuronide. No other metabolites have been detected, providing strong evidence that raloxifene is not metabolized by cytochrome P-450 pathways. Unconjugated raloxifene comprises less than 1% of the total radiolabeled material in plasma. The terminal log-linear portions of the plasma concentration curves for raloxifene and the glucuronides are generally parallel. This is consistent with interconversion of raloxifene and the glucuronide metabolites.

Following IV administration, raloxifene is cleared at a rate approximating hepatic blood flow. Apparent oral clearance is 44.1 L/kg•hr. Raloxifene and its glucuronide conjugates are interconverted by reversible systemic metabolism and enterohepatic cycling, thereby prolonging its plasma elimination half-life to 27.7 hours after oral dosing.

Results from single oral doses of raloxifene predict multiple-dose pharmacokinetics. Following chronic dosing, clearance ranges from 40 to 60 L/kg•hr. Increasing doses of raloxifene (ranging from 30 to 150 mg) result in slightly less than a proportional increase in the area under the plasma time concentration curve (AUC).

Excretion – Raloxifene is primarily excreted in feces, and less than 0.2% is excreted unchanged in urine. Less than 6% of the raloxifene dose is eliminated in urine as glucuronide conjugates. The disposition of raloxifene has been evaluated in more than 3,000 postmenopausal women in selected raloxifene osteoporosis treatment and prevention clinical trials using a population approach. Pharmacokinetic data were also obtained in conventional pharmacology studies in 292 postmenopausal women. Raloxifene exhibits high intra-subject variability (approximately 30% coefficient of variation) of most pharmacokinetic parameters. The following table summarizes the pharmacokinetic parameters of raloxifene.

Summary of Raloxifene Pharmacokinetic Parameters in the Healthy Postmenopausal Women[a]

	C_{max}[b] (ng/mL)/(mg/kg)	$T_{½}$ (hr)	$AUC_{0-\infty}$ (ng•hr/mL)/(mg/kg)	CL/F (L/kg•hr)	V/F (L/kg)
Single dose					
Mean	0.5	27.7	27.2	44.1	2,348
CV (%)	52	10.7 to 273[c]	44	46	52
Multiple dose					
Mean	1.36	32.5	24.2	47.4	2,583
CV (%)	37	15.8 to 86.6[c]	36	41	56

[a] Abbreviations: C_{max} = maximum plasma concentration, $t_{½}$ = half-life, AUC = area under the curve, CL = clearance, V = volume of distribution, F = bioavailability, CV = coefficient of variation.
[b] Data normalized for dose in mg and body weight in kg.
[c] Range of observed half-life.

Contraindications

Lactating women or women who are or may become pregnant (see Pregnancy section); women with active or a history of venous thromboembolic events, including deep vein thrombosis, pulmonary embolism, and retinal vein thrombosis; women known to be hypersensitive to raloxifene or other constituents of the tablets.

Warnings

➤*Venous thromboembolism:* In clinical trials, raloxifene-treated women had an increased risk of venous thromboembolism (deep vein thrombosis and pulmonary embolism). Other venous thromboembolic events could also occur. A less serious event, superficial thrombophlebitis, also has been reported more frequently with raloxifene. The greatest risk for deep vein thrombosis and pulmonary embolism occurs during the first 4 months of treatment, and the magnitude of risk appears to be similar to the reported risk associated with use of hormone replacement therapy. Because immobilization increases the risk for venous thromboembolic events independent of therapy, discontinue raloxifene at least 72 hours prior to and during prolonged immobilization (eg, postsurgical recovery, prolonged bed rest), and resume raloxifene therapy only after the patient is fully ambulatory. In addition, advise women taking raloxifene to move about periodically during prolonged travel. Consider the risk-benefit balance in women at risk of thromboembolic disease for other reasons (eg, congestive heart failure, superficial thrombophlebitis, active malignancy).

➤*Premenopausal use:* There is no indication for premenopausal use of raloxifene. Safety of raloxifene in premenopausal women has not been established and its use is not recommended.

➤*Hepatic function impairment:* Raloxifene was studied, as a single dose, in Child-Pugh class A patients with cirrhosis and serum total bilirubin ranging from 0.6 to 2 mg/dL. Plasma raloxifene concentrations were approximately 2.5 times higher than in controls and correlated with total bilirubin concentrations. Safety and efficacy have not been evaluated further in patients with severe hepatic insufficiency.

➤*Carcinogenesis:* In a 21-month carcinogenicity study in mice, there was an increased incidence of ovarian tumors in female animals given 9 to 242 mg/kg, which included benign and malignant tumors of granulosa/theca cell origin and benign tumors of epithelial cell origin. Systemic exposure (AUC) of raloxifene in this group was 0.3 to 34 times that in postmenopausal women administered a 60 mg dose. There was also an increased incidence of testicular interstitial cell tumors and prostatic adenomas and adenocarcinomas in male mice given 41 or 210 mg/kg (4.7 or 24 times the AUC in humans), and prostatic leiomyoblastoma in male mice given 210 mg/kg.

In a 2-year carcinogenicity study in rats, an increased incidence in ovarian tumors of granulosa/theca cell origin was observed in female rats given 279 mg/kg (approximately 400 times the AUC in humans). The female rodents in these studies were treated during their reproductive lives when their ovaries were functional and responsive to hormonal stimulation.

➤*Fertility impairment:* When male and female rats were given daily doses greater than or equal to 5 mg/kg (greater than or equal to 0.8 times the human dose based on surface area, mg/m^2) prior to and during mating, no pregnancies occurred. In male rats, daily doses less than or equal to 100 mg/kg (16 times the human dose based on surface area, mg/m^2) for greater than or equal to 2 weeks did not affect sperm production or quality, or reproductive performance. In female rats, at doses of 0.1 to 10 mg/kg/day (0.02 to 1.6 times the human dose based on surface area, mg/m^2), raloxifene disrupted estrous cycles and inhibited ovulation. These effects of raloxifene were reversible. In another study in rats in which raloxifene was given during the preimplantation period at doses greater than or equal to 0.1 mg/kg (greater than or equal to 0.02 times the human dose based on surface area, mg/m^2), raloxifene delayed and disrupted embryo implantation resulting in

RALOXIFENE HYDROCHLORIDE — ORAL

prolonged gestation and reduced litter size. The reproductive and developmental effects observed in animals are consistent with the estrogen receptor activity of raloxifene.

➤*Pregnancy: Category X.* Raloxifene should not be used in women who are or may become pregnant.

Raloxifene is contraindicated in women who are or may become pregnant. Raloxifene may cause fetal harm when administered to a pregnant woman. In rabbit studies, abortion and a low rate of fetal heart anomalies (ventricular septal defects) occurred in rabbits at doses greater than or equal to 0.1 mg/kg (greater than or equal to 0.04 times the human dose based on surface area, mg/m^2), and hydrocephaly was observed in fetuses at doses greater than or equal to 10 mg/kg (greater than or equal to 4 times the human dose based on surface area, mg/m^2). In rat studies, retardation of fetal development and developmental abnormalities (wavy ribs, kidney cavitation) occurred at doses greater than or equal to 1 mg/kg (greater than or equal to 0.2 times the human dose based on surface area, mg/m^2). Treatment of rats at doses of 0.1 to 10 mg/kg (0.02 to 1.6 times the human dose based on surface area, mg/m^2) during gestation and lactation produced effects that included delayed and disrupted parturition; decreased neonatal survival and altered physical development; sex- and age-specific reductions in growth and changes in pituitary hormone content; and decreased lymphoid compartment size in offspring. At 10 mg/kg, raloxifene disrupted parturition, which resulted in maternal and progeny death and morbidity. Effects in adult offspring (4 months of age) included uterine hypoplasia and reduced fertility; however, no ovarian or vaginal pathology was observed. Apprise the patient of the potential hazard to the fetus if this drug is used during pregnancy, or if the patient becomes pregnant while taking this drug.

➤*Lactation:* Raloxifene should not be used by lactating women. Treatment of rats at doses of 0.1 to 10 mg/kg (0.02 to 1.6 times the human dose based on surface area, mg/m^2) during gestation and lactation produced effects that included delayed and disrupted parturition; decreased neonatal survival and altered physical development; sex- and age-specific reductions in growth and changes in pituitary hormone content; and decreased lymphoid compartment size in offspring. It is not known whether raloxifene is excreted in human milk.

➤*Children:* Raloxifene should not be used in children.

Precautions

➤*Monitoring:* If raloxifene is given concurrently with warfarin or other coumarin derivatives, monitor prothrombin time more closely when starting or stopping therapy with raloxifene.

➤*Concurrent estrogen therapy:* The concurrent use of raloxifene and systemic estrogen or hormone replacement therapy (ERT or HRT) has not been studied in prospective clinical trials, and, therefore, concomitant use of raloxifene with systemic estrogens is not recommended.

➤*Lipid metabolism:* Raloxifene lowers serum total and LDL cholesterol by 6% to 11%, but does not affect serum concentrations of total HDL cholesterol or triglycerides. Take these effects into account in therapeutic decisions for patients who may require therapy for hyperlipidemia.

Limited clinical data suggest that some women with histories of marked hypertriglyceridemia (more than 5.6 mmol/L or greater than 500 mg/dL) in response to treatment with oral estrogen or estrogen plus progestin may develop increased levels of triglycerides when treated with raloxifene. Women with this medical history should have serum triglycerides monitored when taking raloxifene.

Concurrent use of raloxifene and lipid-lowering agents has not been studied.

➤*Endometrium:* Raloxifene has not been associated with endometrial proliferation. Investigate unexplained uterine bleeding as clinically indicated.

➤*Breast abnormalities:* Raloxifene has not been associated with breast enlargement, breast pain, or an increased risk of breast cancer. Investigate any unexplained breast abnormality occurring during raloxifene therapy.

➤*Use in men:* Safety and efficacy have not been evaluated in men.

➤*Lab test abnormalities:* The following changes in analyte concentrations are commonly observed during raloxifene therapy: Increased apolipoprotein A1; and reduced serum total cholesterol, LDL cholesterol, fibrinogen, apolipoprotein B, and lipoprotein. Raloxifene modestly increases hormone-binding globulin concentrations, including sex steroid-binding globulin, thyroxine-binding globulin, and corticosteroid-binding globulin with corresponding increases in measured total hormone concentrations. There is no evidence that these changes in hormone-binding globulin concentrations affect concentrations of the corresponding free hormones.

There were small decreases in serum total calcium, inorganic phosphate, total protein, and albumin, which were generally of lesser magnitude than decreases observed during ERT/HRT. Platelet count was also decreased slightly and was not different from ERT.

Drug Interactions

➤*Highly protein-bound drugs:* Raloxifene is more than 95% bound to plasma proteins. In vivo, raloxifene did not affect the binding of warfarin, phenytoin, or tamoxifen. However, use caution when raloxifene is coadministered with other highly protein-bound drugs (eg, diazepam, diazoxide, lidocaine).

Raloxifene Drug Interactions

Precipitant drug	Object drug[a]		Description
Ampicillin	Raloxifene	⬇	Peak raloxifene levels and the overall extent of absorption are reduced 28% and 14%, respectively, with coadministration of ampicillin. This is consistent with decreased enterohepatic cycling associated with antibiotic reduction of enteric bacteria. However, the systemic exposure and elimination rate of raloxifene were not affected. Therefore, raloxifene can be coadministered with ampicillin.
Cholestyramine	Raloxifene	⬇	Raloxifene absorption and enterohepatic cycling was reduced 60%; avoid coadministration.
Raloxifene	Warfarin	⬇	In single-dose studies, 10% decreases in prothrombin time (PT) have been observed. Monitor PT closely.

[a] ⬇ = Object drug decreased.

➤*Drug/Food interactions:* Administration of raloxifene with a standardized, high-fat meal increases the absorption of raloxifene (C_{max} 28% and AUC 16%), but does not lead to clinically meaningful changes in systemic exposure. Raloxifene can be administered without regard to meals.

Adverse Reactions

➤*Adverse reactions in the osteoporosis treatment clinical trial:* The safety of raloxifene in the treatment of osteoporosis was assessed in a large (7,705 patients) multinational placebo-controlled trial. Duration of treatment was 36 months and 5,129 postmenopausal women were exposed to raloxifene (2,557 received 60 mg/day and 2,572 received 120 mg/day).

The majority of adverse reactions occurring during the study were mild and generally did not require discontinuation of therapy.

Therapy was discontinued due to an adverse reaction in 10.9% of raloxifene-treated women and 8.8% of placebo-treated women. Common adverse reactions considered to be related to raloxifene therapy were hot flashes and leg cramps. Hot flashes were most commonly reported during the first 6 months of treatment and were not different from placebo thereafter.

➤*Adverse reactions in placebo-controlled clinical trials to support the osteoporosis prevention indication:* The safety of raloxifene has been assessed primarily in 12 phase 2 and 3 studies with placebo, estrogen, and estrogen-progestin replacement therapy (HRT) control groups. The duration of treatment ranged from 2 to 30 months and 2,036 women were exposed to raloxifene (371 patients received 10 to 50 mg/day, 828 received 60 mg/day, and 837 received from 120 to 600 mg/day).

The majority of adverse reactions occurring during clinical trials were mild and generally did not require discontinuation of therapy.

Therapy was discontinued due to an adverse reaction in 11.4% of 581 raloxifene-treated women and 12.2% of 584 placebo-treated women. Common adverse reactions considered to be drug-related were hot flashes and leg cramps (see the following table). The first occurrence of hot flashes was most commonly reported during the first 6 months of treatment.

Discontinuation rates due to hot flashes did not differ significantly between raloxifene and placebo groups (1.7% and 2.2%, respectively).

Adverse reactions occurring in either the osteoporosis treatment or the prevention placebo-controlled clinical trial databases at a frequency greater than or equal to 2% in either group and in more raloxifene-treated women than in placebo-treated women are listed in the table below. Adverse reactions are shown without attribution of causality.

Adverse Reactions Occurring in Placebo-controlled Osteoporosis Clinical Trials at a Frequency ≥ 2% and in More Raloxifene-treated (60 Mg Once Daily) Women than Placebo-treated Women

	Treatment		Prevention	
	Raloxifene (n = 2,557)	Placebo (n = 2,576)	Raloxifene (n = 581)	Placebo (n = 584)
Body system	%	%	%	%
Cardiovascular				
Hot flashes	9.7%	6.4%	24.6%	18.3%
Migraine	[a]	[a]	2.4%	2.1%
Syncope	2.3%	2.1%	[b]	[b]
Varicose vein	2.2%	1.5%	[a]	[a]
CNS				
Depression	[a]	[a]	6.4%	6%
Hypesthesia	2.1%	2%	[b]	[b]
Insomnia	[a]	[a]	5.5%	4.3%
Neuralgia	2.4%	1.9%	[b]	[b]

RALOXIFENE HYDROCHLORIDE — ORAL

Adverse Reactions Occurring in Placebo-controlled Osteoporosis Clinical Trials at a Frequency ≥ 2% and in More Raloxifene-treated (60 Mg Once Daily) Women than Placebo-treated Women

	Treatment		Prevention	
	Raloxifene (n = 2,557)	Placebo (n = 2,576)	Raloxifene (n = 581)	Placebo (n = 584)
Body system	%	%	%	%
Vertigo	4.1%	3.7%	[a]	[a]
Dermatologic				
Rash	[a]	[a]	5.5%	3.8%
Sweating	2.5%	2%	3.1%	1.7%
GI				
Diarrhea	7.2%	6.9%	[a]	[a]
Dyspepsia	[a]	[a]	5.9%	5.8%
Flatulence	[a]	[a]	3.1%	2.4%
Gastroenteritis	[b]	[b]	2.6%	2.1%
GI disorder	[a]	[a]	3.3%	2.1%
Nausea	8.3%	7.8%	8.8%	8.6%
Vomiting	4.8%	4.3%	3.4%	3.3%
GU				
Cystitis	4.6%	4.5%	3.3%	3.1%
Endometrial disorder[c]	[b]	[b]	3.1%	1.9%
Leukorrhea	[a]	[a]	3.3%	1.7%
Urinary tract disorder	2.5%	2.1%	[a]	[a]
Urinary tract infection	[a]	[a]	4%	3.9%
Uterine disorder[c,d]	3.3%	2.3%	[a]	[a]
Vaginal hemorrhage	2.5%	2.4%	[a]	[a]
Vaginitis	[a]	[a]	4.3%	3.6%
Metabolic/nutritional				
Peripheral edema	5.2%	4.4%	3.3%	1.9%
Weight gain	[a]	[a]	8.8%	6.8%
Musculoskeletal				
Arthralgia	15.5%	14%	10.7%	10.1%
Arthritis	[a]	[a]	4%	3.6%
Myalgia	[a]	[a]	7.7%	6.2%
Tendon disorder	3.6%	3.1%	[a]	[a]
Respiratory				
Bronchitis	9.5%	8.6%	[a]	[a]
Increased cough	9.3%	9.2%	6%	5.7%
Laryngitis	[b]	[b]	2.2%	1.4%
Pharyngitis	5.3%	5.1%	7.6%	7.2%
Pneumonia	[a]	[a]	2.6%	1.5%
Rhinitis	10.2%	10.1%	[a]	[a]
Sinusitis	7.9%	7.5%	10.3%	6.5%
Special senses				
Conjunctivitis	2.2%	1.7%	[a]	[a]
Miscellaneous				
Chest pain	[a]	[a]	4%	3.6%
Fever	3.9%	3.8%	3.1%	2.6%
Flu syndrome	13.5%	11.4%	14.6%	13.5%
Headache	9.2%	8.5%	[a]	[a]
Infection	[a]	[a]	15.1%	14.6%
Leg cramps	7%	3.7%	5.9%	1.9%

[a] Placebo incidence greater than or equal to raloxifene incidence.
[b] Less than 2% incidence and more frequent with raloxifene.
[c] Treatment-emergent uterine-related adverse reaction, including only patients with an intact uterus. Prevention trials: raloxifene, n = 354; placebo, n = 364; treatment trial: raloxifene, n = 1,948; placebo, n = 1,999.
[d] Actual terms most frequently referred to endometrial fluid.

➤*Comparison of raloxifene and hormone replacement therapy adverse reactions:* Raloxifene was compared with estrogen-progestin replacement therapy (HRT) in 3 clinical trials for prevention of osteoporosis. Adverse reactions occurring more frequently in 1 treatment group and at an incidence greater than or equal to 2% in any group are shown in the following table. Adverse reactions are shown without attribution of causality.

Adverse Reactions Reported in the Clinical Trials for Osteoporosis Prevention with Raloxifene-treated (60 mg once daily) and Continuous Combined or Cyclic Estrogen Plus Progestin (HRT) at an Incidence ≥ 2% in any Treatment Group[a]

	Raloxifene (n = 317)	HRT-continuous combined (n = 96)	HRT-cyclic (n = 219)
Adverse reaction	%	%	%
Cardiovascular			
Hot flashes	28.7%	3.1%	5.9%
GI			
Flatulence	1.6%	12.5%	6.4%
GU			
Breast pain	4.4%	37.5%	29.7%
Vaginal bleeding[b]	6.2%	64.2%	88.5%
Miscellaneous			
Abdominal pain	6.6%	10.4%	18.7%
Chest pain	2.8%	0%	0.5%
Infection	11%	0%	6.8%

[a] These data are from both blinded and open-label studies.
[b] Treatment-emergent uterine-related adverse reactions, including only patients with an intact uterus: Raloxifene, n = 290; HRT-continuous combined, n = 67; HRT-cyclic, n = 217. Continuous combined HRT = 0.625 mg conjugated estrogens plus 2.5 mg medroxyprogesterone acetate. Cyclic HRT = 0.625 mg conjugated estrogens for 28 days with concomitant 5 mg medroxyprogesterone acetate or 0.15 mg norgestrel on days 1 through 14 or 17 through 28.

➤*Additional safety information:* Incidences of estrogen-dependent carcinoma of the endometrium and breast are being evaluated across all completed and ongoing clinical trials involving 17,151 patients, of which at least 10,850 women have received at least 1 dose of raloxifene. These trials provided over 21,000 person-years of raloxifene exposure, with a maximum exposure of 58 months.

Endometrium – Compared to placebo, raloxifene did not increase the risk of endometrial cancer.

Breast – Compared to placebo, raloxifene did not increase the risk of breast cancer.

Postintroduction reports – Adverse reactions reported since market introduction include retinal vein occlusion (very rarely).

Overdosage

➤*Symptoms:* Incidents of overdose in humans have not been reported. In an 8-week study of 63 postmenopausal women, a dose of raloxifene 600 mg/day was safely tolerated. No mortality was seen after a single oral dose in rats or mice at 5,000 mg/kg (810 times the human dose for rats and 405 times the human dose for mice based on surface area, mg/m^2) or in monkeys at 1,000 mg/kg (80 times the AUC in humans).

➤*Treatment:* There is no specific antidote for raloxifene.

Patient Information

For safe and effective use of raloxifene, physicians should inform patients about the following:

➤*Patient immobilization:* Discontinue raloxifene greater than or equal to 72 hours prior to and during prolonged immobilization (eg, postsurgical recovery, prolonged bed rest). Advise patients to avoid prolonged restrictions of movement during travel because of the increased risk of venous thromboembolic events.

➤*Hot flashes or flushes:* Raloxifene may increase the incidence of hot flashes and is not effective in reducing hot flashes or flushes associated with estrogen deficiency. In some asymptomatic patients, hot flashes may occur upon beginning raloxifene therapy.

Selective Estrogen Receptor Modulator

RALOXIFENE HYDROCHLORIDE — ORAL

➤*Other osteoporosis treatment and prevention measures:* Instruct patients to take supplemental calcium and/or vitamin D, if daily dietary intake is inadequate. Consider weightbearing exercise along with the modification of certain behavioral factors, such as cigarette smoking, or alcohol consumption, if these factors exist.

Instruct patients to read the patient package insert before starting therapy with raloxifene and to reread it each time the prescription is renewed.

Progestins

For progestins recommended only for antineoplastic action in endometrial carcinoma, see megestrol acetate and medroxyprogesterone acetate monographs in the Antineoplastics chapter.

WARNING

Progestins and estrogens should not be used for the prevention of cardiovascular disease.

The Women's Health Initiative (WHI) study reported increased risks of myocardial infarction, stroke, invasive breast cancer, pulmonary emboli, and deep vein thrombosis in postmenopausal women (50 to 79 years of age) during 5 years of treatment with oral conjugated estrogens (CE 0.625 mg) combined with medroxyprogesterone acetate (MPA 2.5 mg) relative to placebo.

The Women's Health Initiative Memory Study (WHIMS), a sub-study of WHI, reported increased risk of developing probable dementia in postmenopausal women 65 years of age or older during 4 years of treatment with oral conjugated estrogens plus medroxyprogesterone acetate relative to placebo. It is unknown whether this finding applies to younger postmenopausal women.

Other doses of oral conjugated estrogens with medroxyprogesterone and other combinations and dosage forms of estrogens and progestins were not studied in the WHI clinical trials. In the absence of comparable data and product-specific studies, the relevance of the WHI findings to other products has not been established. Therefore, the risks should be assumed to be similar for all estrogen and progestin products. Because of these risks, estrogens with or without progestins should be prescribed at the lowest effective doses and for the shortest duration consistent with treatment goals and risks for the individual woman.

Indications

➤*Amenorrhea:* Primary and secondary.

➤*Abnormal uterine bleeding:* Abnormal uterine bleeding caused by hormonal imbalance in the absence of organic pathology, such as fibroids or uterine cancer.

➤*Endometriosis:* Norethindrone only.

➤*AIDS wasting syndrome:* Megestrol acetate suspension only.

➤*Infertility (progesterone gel only):* Progesterone supplementation or replacement as part of an Assisted Reproductive Technology (ART) treatment for infertile women with progesterone deficiency.

➤*Unlabeled uses:* Medroxyprogesterone acetate (10 mg/day) has been used in the treatment of menopausal symptoms.

Adding progestin for at least 7 days of a cycle of estrogen replacement for menopause has lowered incidence of endometrial hyperplasia. Morphological and biochemical endometrium studies suggest 10 to 13 days of progestin provide maximal maturation of endometrium and eliminate any hyperplastic changes. It is not clear whether this provides protection from endometrial carcinoma. There may be additional risks with progestin in estrogen replacement regimens, including adverse effects on carbohydrate and lipid metabolism. Choice of progestin and dosage may be important in minimizing these adverse effects.

Progesterone suppositories (rectal or vaginal, 200 to 400 mg twice daily) have been used in premenstrual syndrome (PMS). Some studies report no improvements in PMS symptoms with progesterone suppositories vs placebo; however, these studies may have had methodologic flaws. One controlled trial suggested oral progesterone (100 mg in the morning, 200 mg at night for 10 days during the luteal phase) improved PMS symptoms. Further controlled studies are needed.

Progesterone has been used successfully in premature labor in late stages of pregnancy. Progesterone suppositories have been used during the luteal phase to the end of the first trimester to decrease spontaneous abortions in previous aborters and in anovulatory women receiving clomiphene citrate or human menopausal gonadotropins, and in luteal phase defects to improve fertility (see Warning Box).

Actions

➤*Pharmacology:* Progesterone, a principle of corpus luteum, is the primary endogenous progestational substance. Progestins (progesterone and derivatives) transform proliferative endometrium into secretory endometrium. Progesterone is necessary to increase endometrial receptivity for implantation of an embryo. Once an embryo is implanted, progesterone acts to maintain the pregnancy. They inhibit (at the usual dose range) or facilitate through positive feedback the secretion of pituitary gonadotropins, which in turn prevents follicular maturation and ovulation or alternatively promotes it for the "primed" follicle. They also inhibit spontaneous uterine contractions as well as other smooth muscles throughout the body. Progestins may demonstrate some anabolic or androgenic activity.

Several investigators have reported on the appetite-enhancing property of megestrol acetate and its possible use in cachexia. The precise mechanism by which megestrol produces effects in anorexia and cachexia is unknown.

➤*Pharmacokinetics:*

Absorption/Distribution –

Oral: Progestins are rapidly absorbed from the GI tract and undergo prompt hepatic degradation. Maximum concentration is achieved in 1 to 2 hours. During the first 6 hours after ingestion, half-life is approximately 2 to 3 hours; half-life is approximately 8 to 9 hours thereafter. Metabolites, present for several days after an oral dose, are excreted in the urine.

IM: Following IM administration, progesterone in oil is rapidly absorbed and undergoes rapid metabolism. Half-life is a few minutes. Effective concentrations of long-acting forms can be maintained for 3 to 6 months. Maximum concentration occurs in approximately 24 hours with a half-life of approximately 10 weeks.

Gel: Because of the gel's sustained release properties, progesterone absorption is prolonged with an absorption half-life of approximately 25 to 50 hours, and an elimination half-life of 5 to 20 minutes. Progesterone is extensively bound to serum proteins (approximately 96% to 99%), primarily to serum albumin and corticosteroid binding globulin.

Metabolism/Excretion –

Oral/IM: The major urinary metabolite of oral progesterone is 5β-pregnan-3α, 20α-diol glucuronide. Progesterone undergoes biliary and renal elimination. Following an injection of labeled progesterone, 50% to 60% of the excretion of progesterone metabolites occurs via the kidney; approximately 10% occurs via the bile and feces, the second major excretory pathway. Overall recovery of labeled material accounts for 70% of an administered dose, with the remainder of the dose not characterized with respect to elimination. Only a small portion of unchanged progesterone is excreted in the bile.

Gel –

Multiple Dose Pharmacokinetics of Progesterone Gel

	Twice daily dosing for 12 days	Once daily dosing for 12 days
C_{max} (ng/ml)	14.57	15.97
C_{avg} (ng/ml)	11.6	8.99
T_{max} (hr)	3.55	5.4
AUC (ng•hr/ml)	138.72	391.98
$t_{1/2}$ (hr)	25.91	45

Mean Single Dose Relative Bioavailability of Progesterone: Gel vs IM

	8% gel	90 mg IM
C_{max} (ng/ml)	14.87	53.76
$C_{avg\ 0\text{-}24}$ (ng/ml)	6.98	28.98
$AUC_{0\text{-}96}$ (ng•hr/ml)	296.78	1378.91
T_{max} (hr)	6.8	9.2
$T_{1/2}$ (hr)	34.8	19.6

Contraindications

Hypersensitivity to progestins; thrombophlebitis, thromboembolic disorders, cerebral hemorrhage, or patients with a history of these conditions; impaired liver function or disease; carcinoma of the breast or genital organs; undiagnosed vaginal bleeding; missed abortion; as a diagnostic test for pregnancy; prophylactic use to avoid weight loss (megestrol acetate suspension).

Warnings

➤*Ophthalmologic effects:* Discontinue medication pending examination if there is a sudden partial or complete loss of vision or if there is sudden onset of proptosis, diplopia, or migraine. If papilledema or retinal vascular lesions occur, discontinue use.

➤*Thrombotic disorders:* Thrombotic disorders (eg, thrombophlebitis, cerebrovascular disorders, retinal thrombosis, pulmonary embolism) occasionally occur in patients taking progestins; be alert to the earliest manifestations of the disease. If these occur or are suspected, discontinue the drug immediately. However, this has not been shown to occur more often than that seen in a control group.

➤*HIV-infected women:* Although **megestrol** has been used extensively in women for endometrial and breast cancers, its use in HIV-infected women has been limited. All the women in

➤*Fertility impairment:* **Medroxyprogesterone acetate** at high doses is an antifertility drug. High doses would be expected to impair fertility until the cessation of treatment.

➤*Pregnancy: Category D* (**progesterone** injection); *Category X* (**norethindrone acetate**). Use is not recommended (see Warning Box). Progesterone gel is used to support embryo implantation and maintain pregnancies as part of ART treatments.

➤*Lactation:* Detectable amounts of progestins enter the milk of mothers receiving these agents. The effect on the nursing infant has not been determined.

Medroxyprogesterone does not adversely affect lactation and may increase milk production and duration of lactation if given in the puerperium.

➤*Children:* Safety and efficacy of **megestrol acetate suspension** in children have not been established.

Precautions

➤*Pretreatment physical examination:* Pretreatment physical examination should include breasts and pelvic organs, as well as Papanicolaou smear. Advise the pathologist of progestin therapy when relevant specimens are submitted. In cases of irregular vaginal bleeding, consider nonfunctional causes. Adequately diagnose all cases of vaginal bleeding.

➤*Fluid retention:* Fluid retention may occur; therefore, conditions influenced by this factor (epilepsy, migraine, asthma, cardiac or renal dysfunction) require careful observation.

➤*Depression:* Observe patients who have a history of psychic depression and discontinue the drug if depression recurs to a serious degree.

➤*Glucose tolerance:* A decrease in glucose tolerance has been observed in a small percentage of patients on estrogen-progestin combination drugs. The mechanism of this decrease is not known. For this reason, carefully observe diabetic patients receiving progestin therapy.

➤*Menopause:* The age of the patient constitutes no absolute limiting factor although treatment with progestins may mask the onset of the climacteric.

➤*Causes of weight loss:* Institute therapy with **megestrol** for weight loss only after treatable causes of weight loss are sought and addressed. These treatable causes include possible malignancies, systemic infections, GI disorders affecting absorption and endocrine, renal or psychiatric diseases.

➤*Benzyl alcohol:* Benzyl alcohol, contained in some of these products as a preservative, has been associated with a fatal "gasping syndrome" in premature infants.

➤*Lab test abnormalities:* Laboratory test results of hepatic function, coagulation tests (increase in prothrombin, Factors VII, VIII, IX and X), thyroid, metyrapone test and endocrine functions, may be affected by progestins.

Drug Interactions

Progestins Drug Interactions

Precipitant drug	Object drug[a]		Description
Aminoglutethimide	Medroxyprogesterone	⬇	Aminoglutethimide may increase the hepatic metabolism of medroxyprogesterone, possibly decreasing its therapeutic effects.
Rifampin	Norethindrone	⬇	Rifampin may reduce the plasma levels of norethindrone via hepatic microsomal enzyme induction, possibly decreasing its pharmacologic effects.

[a] ⬇ = Object drug decreased.

➤*Pregnanediol:* Pregnanediol determination may be altered by the use of progestins.

Adverse Reactions

For information concerning adverse reactions associated with combined estrogen-progestin therapy, refer to the Oral Contraceptives group monograph.

➤*General:*

CNS – Insomnia; somnolence; mental depression.

Dermatologic – Rash (allergic) with and without pruritus; acne; melasma or chloasma. **Progesterone** is irritating at the injection site whether the oil or aqueous vehicle is used; however, the aqueous preparation is particularly painful.

GI – Changes in weight (increase or decrease); nausea.

GU – Breakthrough bleeding; spotting; change in menstrual flow; amenorrhea; changes in cervical eversion, cervical secretions; galactorrhea.

Miscellaneous – Breast changes (tenderness); masculinization of the female fetus; edema; cholestatic jaundice; pyrexia; hirsutism.

➤*Medroxyprogesterone acetate:*

Miscellaneous – Sensitivity reactions ranging from pruritus and urticaria to generalized rash; alopecia; hirsutism.

➤*Progesterone gel:*

Progesterone Gel Adverse Reactions (%)

Adverse reaction	90 mg once daily	90 mg twice daily
CNS		
Somnolence	27	-
Headache	17	13
Nervousness	16	-
Depression	11	-
Libido decreased	10	-
Dizziness	-	5
GI		
Constipation	27	-
Nausea	22	7
Diarrhea	8	-
Vomiting	5	-
GU		
Breast enlargement	40	-
Breast pain	-	13
Moniliasis, genital	-	7
Vaginal discharge	-	7
Dyspareunia	6	-
Miscellaneous		
Nocturia	13	-
Arthralgia	8	-
Pruritus	-	5
Perineal pain	17	-
Cramps	-	15
Abdominal pain	12	-
Pain	-	8
Bloating	-	7

➤*Additional adverse events reported in women at a frequency less than 5% include the following:*

CNS – Emotional lability; insomnia.

Dermatologic – Acne; pruritus.

GI – Dyspepsia; eructation; flatulence.

GU – Dysuria; micturition frequency; UTI.

Miscellaneous – Allergy; fatigue; fever; influenza-like symptoms; water retention; asthma; back pain; leg pain; sinusitis; upper respiratory tract infection.

➤*Megestrol acetate suspension:*

Megestrol Adverse Reactions (%)[a]

Adverse reaction	Megestrol	Placebo
Diarrhea	8 to 15	8 to 15
Impotence	4 to 14	≤ 3
Rash	2 to 12	3 to 9
Flatulence	≤ 10	3 to 9
Hypertension	≤ 8	0
Asthenia	2 to 6	3 to 8
Insomnia	≤ 6	0
Nausea	≤ 5	3 to 9
Anemia	≤ 5	≤ 6
Fever	2 to 6	3
Libido decreased	≤ 5	≤ 3
Dyspepsia	≤ 4	≤ 5
Hyperglycemia	≤ 6	≤ 3
Headache	≤ 10	3 to 6
Pain	≤ 6	5 to 6
Vomiting	≤ 6	3 to 9
Pneumonia	≤ 3	3 to 6
Urinary frequency	≤ 2	≤ 5

[a] Data pooled from several studies. Percentages listed for megestrol without regard to specified dosage.

➤*Other adverse reactions reported in 1% to 3% of patients on megestrol include the following:*

Cardiovascular – Cardiomyopathy; palpitation.

CNS – Paresthesia; confusion; convulsion; depression; neuropathy; hypesthesia; abnormal thinking.

Dermatologic – Alopecia; herpes; pruritus; vesiculobullous rash; sweating; skin disorder.

GI – Constipation; dry mouth; hepatomegaly; increased salivation; oral moniliasis.

GU – Albuminuria; urinary incontinence; urinary tract infection; gynecomastia.

Respiratory – Dyspnea; cough; pharyngitis; lung disorder.

Miscellaneous – Leukopenia; amblyopia; LDH increased; edema; peripheral edema; abdominal pain; chest pain; infection; moniliasis; sarcoma.

Patient Information

Patient package insert is available with product.

If GI upset occurs, take with food.

➤*Diabetic patients:* Glucose tolerance may be decreased; monitor urine sugar closely and report any abnormalities to physician.

Notify physician if pregnancy is suspected or if any of the following occurs: Sudden severe headache; visual disturbance; numbness in an arm or leg.

➤*Vaginal gel:* Do not use concurrently with other local intravaginal therapy. If other local intravaginal therapy is to be used concurrently, administer ≥ 6 hours before or after progesterone gel.

Progestins

PROGESTERONE

Rx	**Prometrium** (Solvay)	**Capsules**: 100 mg (micronized progesterone)	Glycerin, peanut oil. (SV). Peach. In 100s.
		200 mg (micronized progesterone)	Glycerin, peanut oil. (SV2). Oval, pale yellow. In 100s.
Rx	**Progesterone In Oil** (Various, eg, APP, Watson)	**Injection**: 50 mg per mL	In sesame or peanut oil with benzyl alcohol. In 10 mL vials and 10 mL multidose vials.
Rx	**Crinone** (Serono)	**Vaginal gel**: 4% (45 mg)	Glycerin, mineral oil. In single-use, prefilled, disposable applicator delivering 1.125 g gel. In 6s.
Rx	**Prochieve** (Columbia Labs)		Glycerin, mineral oil. In single-use, prefilled, disposable applicator delivering 1.125 g gel. In 6s.
Rx	**Crinone** (Serono)	**Vaginal gel**: 8% (90 mg)	Glycerin, mineral oil. In single-use, prefilled, disposable applicator delivering 1.125 g gel. In 6s and 18s.
Rx	**Prochieve** (Columbia Labs)		Glycerin, mineral oil. In single-use, prefilled, disposable applicator delivering 1.125 g gel. In 6s and 18s.

PROGESTERONE — ORAL

For complete and comparative prescribing information, refer to the Progestins group monograph.

Indications

Progesterone capsules are indicated for use in the prevention of endometrial hyperplasia in non-hysterectomized postmenopausal women who are receiving conjugated estrogens tablets. They are also indicated for use in secondary amenorrhea.

Administration and Dosage

➤*Approved by the FDA:* May 14, 1998.

➤*Prevention of endometrial hyperplasia:* Progesterone capsules should be given as a single daily dose in the evening, 200 mg orally for 12 days sequentially per 28-day cycle, to postmenopausal women with a uterus who are receiving daily conjugated estrogens tablets.

➤*Secondary amenorrhea:* Progesterone capsules may be given as a single daily dose of 400 mg in the evening for 10 days.

➤*Storage/Stability:* Store at 25°C (77°F). Excursions permitted to 15° to 30°C (59° to 86°F).

Dispense in tight, light-resistant container as defined in USP/NF, accompanied by a Patient Insert. Protect from excessive moisture.

PROGESTERONE — VAGINAL

For complete and comparative prescribing information, refer to the Progestins group monograph.

Indications

➤*Assisted Reproductive Technology (ART):* The 8% gel is for progesterone supplementation or replacement as part of an ART treatment for infertile women with progesterone deficiency.

➤*Secondary amenorrhea:* For use in secondary amenorrhea (capsules); the 4% gel is for the treatment of secondary amenorrhea, and the 8% gel is for women who have failed to respond to treatment with the 4% gel.

Administration and Dosage

➤*ART:* Administer 90 mg (8% gel) vaginally once daily in women who require progesterone supplementation. In women with partial or complete ovarian failure who require progesterone replacement, administer 90 mg vaginally twice daily. If pregnancy occurs, continue treatment up to 10 to 12 weeks until placental autonomy is achieved.

➤*Secondary amenorrhea:* Administer 45 mg (4% gel) vaginally every other day up to a total of 6 doses. For women who fail to respond, a trial of 8% gel every other day up to a total of 6 doses may be instituted. It is important to note that a dosage increase from the 4% gel can only be accomplished by using the 8% gel. Increase in the volume of gel administered does not increase the amount of progesterone absorbed.

➤*Storage/Stability:* Store at 25°C (77°F); excursions permitted to 15° to 30°C (59° to 86°F).

PROGESTERONE — INJECTION

For complete and comparative prescribing information, refer to the Progestins group monograph.

Indications

This drug is indicated in amenorrhea and abnormal uterine bleeding caused by hormonal imbalance in the absence of organic pathology, such as submucous fibroids or uterine cancer.

Administration and Dosage

➤*Amenorrhea:* 5 to 10 mg are given for 6 to 8 consecutive days. If there has been sufficient ovarian activity to produce a proliferative endometrium, one can expect withdrawal bleeding 48 to 72 hours after the last injection. This may be followed by spontaneous normal cycles.

➤*Functional uterine bleeding:* 5 to 10 mg are given daily for 6 doses. Bleeding may be expected to cease within 6 days. When estrogen is given as well, the administration of progesterone is begun after 2 weeks of estrogen therapy. If menstrual flow begins during the course of injections of progesterone, they are discontinued.

➤*Administration:* Progesterone is administered by intramuscular injection. It differs from other commonly used steroids in that it is irritating at the place of injection. This is true whether the preparation is an oil or an aqueous vehicle. The latter is particularly painful.

Parenteral drug products should be inspected visually for particulate matter and discoloration prior to administration whenever the solution and container permit.

➤*Storage/Stability:* Store at controlled room temperature 15° to 30°C (59° to 86°F).

MEDROXYPROGESTERONE ACETATE

Rx	**Medroxyprogesterone Acetate** (Various, eg, Barr, Greenstone)	**Tablets**: 2.5 mg	In 30s, 90s, 100s, 500s and 1000s.
Rx	**Provera** (Pharmacia & Upjohn)		(PROVERA 2.5). Lactose, sucrose. Orange, scored. In 30s and 100s.
Rx	**Medroxyprogesterone Acetate** (Various, eg, Barr, Greenstone)	**Tablets**: 5 mg	In 30s, 100s, 500s and 1000s.
Rx	**Provera** (Pharmacia & Upjohn)		(PROVERA 5). Lactose, sucrose. White, scored. Hexagonal. In 30s and 100s.
Rx	**Medroxyprogesterone Acetate** (Various, eg, Barr, Geneva, Greenstone)	**Tablets**: 10 mg	In 30s, 40s, 50s, 100s, 250s and 500s.
Rx	**Provera** (Pharmacia & Upjohn)		(PROVERA 10). Lactose, sucrose. White, scored. In 30s, 100s, 500s and UD 10s.

MEDROXYPROGESTERONE ACETATE — ORAL

For complete and comparative prescribing information, refer to the Progestins group monograph. Parenteral medroxyprogesterone acetate is used as an antineoplastic agent; refer to the monograph in the Antineoplastics section.

Indications

➤*Secondary amenorrhea:* Secondary amenorrhea and abnormal uterine bleeding due to hormonal imbalance in the absence of organic pathology, such as fibroids or uterine cancer.

➤*Endometrial hyperplasia:* To reduce the incidence of endometrial hyperplasia in nonhysterectomized postmenopausal women receiving conjugated estrogen 0.625 mg.

➤*Unlabeled uses:* Treatment of advanced breast cancer.

Administration and Dosage

➤*Abnormal uterine bleeding caused by hormonal imbalance in the absence of organic pathology:* Five or 10 mg daily for 5 to 10 days, beginning day 16 or 21 of the menstrual cycle. To produce an optimum secretory transformation of an endometrium that has been adequately primed with either endogenous or exogenous estrogen, give 10 mg daily for 10 days, beginning on the day 16 of the cycle. Withdrawal bleeding usually occurs 3 to 7 days after discontinuing therapy. Patients with recurrent episodes of abnormal uterine bleeding may benefit from planned menstrual cycling with medroxyprogesterone acetate.

➤*Endometrial hyperplasia:* Five or 10 mg daily for 12 to 14 consecutive days per month, beginning on day 1 or 16 of the cycle.

➤*Secondary amenorrhea:* Five or 10 mg daily for 5 to 10 days. A dose for inducing an optimum secretory transformation of an endometrium that has been adequately primed with endogenous or exogenous estrogen is 10 mg daily for 10 days. Start therapy any time. Withdrawal bleeding usually occurs 3 to 7 days after therapy ends.

➤*Storage/Stability:* Store at controlled room temperature 20° to 25°C (68° to 77°F).

NORETHINDRONE ACETATE

Rx	**Norethindrone Acetate** (Barr)	**Tablets:** 5 mg	(b 211/5). White, oval, scored. In 50s.
Rx	**Aygestin** (Barr)		Lactose. White, scored. In 50s.

NORETHINDRONE ACETATE — ORAL

For complete and comparative prescribing information, refer to the Progestins group monograph.

Indications

For the treatment of secondary amenorrhea, endometriosis, and abnormal uterine bleeding caused by hormonal imbalance in the absence of organic pathology, such as submucous fibroids or uterine cancer.

Administration and Dosage

➤*Approved by the FDA:* April 21, 1982.

Therapy with norethindrone acetate must be adapted to the specific indications and therapeutic response of the individual patient. This dosage schedule assumes the interval between menses to be 28 days.

➤*Secondary amenorrhea, abnormal uterine bleeding due to hormonal imbalance in the absence of organic pathology:* For the treatment of secondary amenorrhea, abnormal uterine bleeding due to hormonal imbalance in the absence of organic pathology, norethindrone acetate 2.5 to 10 mg may be given daily for 5 to 10 days during the second half of the theoretical menstrual cycle to produce an optimum secretory transformation of an endometrium that has been adequately primed with either endogenous or exogenous estrogen.

Progestin withdrawal bleeding usually occurs within 3 to 7 days after discontinuing norethindrone acetate therapy. Patients with a history of recurrent episodes of abnormal uterine bleeding may benefit from planned menstrual cycling with norethindrone acetate.

➤*Endometriosis:* Initial daily dosage should be norethindrone acetate 5 mg for 2 weeks. Dosage should be increased by 2.5 mg/day every 2 weeks until 15 mg/day of norethindrone acetate is reached. Therapy may be held at this level for 6 to 9 months or until annoying breakthrough bleeding demands temporary termination.

➤*Storage/Stability:* Store at controlled room temperature 20° to 25°C (68° to 77°F); excursions permitted to 15° to 30°C (59° to 86°F).

Dispense in a well-closed container.

MEGESTROL ACETATE

Rx	**Megestrol Acetate** (Various, eg, UDL)	**Tablets:** 20 mg	In 100s and UD 100s.
Rx	**Megestrol Acetate** (Various, eg, Major, UDL)	**Tablets:** 40 mg	In 100s, 500s, UD 100s, and blister package 25s.
Rx	**Megace** (Bristol-Myers Oncology)		Lactose. Lt. blue, scored. In 250s and 500s.
Rx	**Megestrol Acetate** (Various, eg, Roxane, Teva)	**Suspension:** 40 mg/mL	Alcohol, sorbitol, sucrose. In 240 mL.
Rx	**Megace** (Bristol-Myers Oncology)		≤ 0.06% alcohol, sucrose. Lemon-lime flavor. In 240 mL.
Rx	**Megace ES** (Par Pharmaceutical, Inc.)	**Suspension:** 125 mg/mL	≤ 0.06% alcohol, sucrose. Lemon-lime flavor. In 150 mL.

MEGESTROL ACETATE — ORAL

For complete and comparative prescribing information, refer to the Progestins group monograph.

Indications

➤*Tablets:* For the palliative treatment of advanced carcinoma of the breast or endometrium (recurrent, inoperable, or metastatic disease). It should not be used in lieu of currently accepted procedures such as surgery, radiation, or chemotherapy.

➤*Oral suspension:* For the treatment of anorexia, cachexia, or an unexplained, significant weight loss in patients with a diagnosis of acquired immunodeficiency syndrome (AIDS).

➤*Unlabeled uses:* Appetite stimulant for cachexia in advanced cancer; treatment of hot flashes.

Administration and Dosage

➤*Tablets:*

Breast cancer – For breast cancer 160 mg/day (40 mg 4 times a day).

Endometrial carcinoma – For endometrial carcinoma 40 to 320 mg/day in divided doses. At least 2 months of continuous treatment is considered an adequate period for determining the efficacy of megestrol acetate.

➤*Oral suspension:* The recommended adult initial dosage of megestrol acetate oral suspension, is 800 mg/day (20 mL/day). Shake container well before using.

In clinical trials evaluating different dose schedules, daily doses of 400 and 800 mg/day were found to be clinically effective.

Extra strength oral suspension – The recommended adult initial dosage of megestrol acetate extra strength oral suspension is 625 mg/day (5 mL/day or one teaspoon daily). Please refer to the table below for correct dosing and administration. Shake container well before using.

Megestrol Oral Suspension Product Differences

	Megestrol extra strength oral suspension	Megestrol oral suspension
mg/mL	125 mg/mL	40 mg/mL
Recommended daily dose	625 mg	800 mg
Daily volume intake	5 mL (teaspoon)	20 mL (dosing cup)
Formulation	Concentrated formula	Regular formula

In clinical trials evaluating the different dose schedules, daily doses of 400 and 800 mg/day of megestrol oral suspension (800 mg/20 mL equivalent to 625 mg/5 mL of megestrol extra strength oral suspension) were found to be clinically effective.

➤*Storage/Stability:*

Tablets – Store at 25°C (77°F); excursions permitted to 15° to 30°C (59° to 86°F). Protect from temperatures above 40°C (104°F).

Oral suspension – Store megestrol acetate oral suspension between 15° to 25°C (59° to 77°F) and dispense in a tight container. Protect from heat.

ESTROGENS AND PROGESTINS COMBINED

Rx	**Prempro** (Wyeth-Ayerst)	**Tablets:** 0.3 mg conjugated estrogens/ 1.5 mg medroxyprogesterone acetate.	Cream, oval. In dial pack 28s.
		0.45 mg conjugated estrogens/1.5 mg medroxyprogesterone acetate	Gold, oval. In *EZ DIAL* 28s.
		0.625 mg conjugated estrogens/2.5 mg medroxyprogesterone acetate	Lactose, sucrose. (PREMPRO). Peach, oval. In dial pack 28s
		0.625 mg conjugated estrogens/5 mg medroxyprogesterone acetate	Lactose, sucrose. (W 0.625/5). Lt. blue, oval. In dial pack 28s.
Rx	**Premphase** (Wyeth-Ayerst)	**Tablets:** 0.625 mg conjugated estrogens; 0.625 mg conjugated estrogens/5 mg medroxyprogesterone acetate	Lactose, sucrose. (PREMARIN or PREMPHASE). **Estrogen only:** Maroon, oval. **Estrogen/Progestin:** Lt. blue, oval. In dial pack 28s (14 of each tablet).
Rx	**Angeliq** (Berlex)	**Tablets:** 0.5 mg drospirenone/ 1 mg estradiol	Lactose. (CK) Round, pink. Film coated. In blister packs 28s.
Rx	**Femhrt** (Warner Chilcott)	**Tablets:** 2.5 mcg ethinyl estradiol/0.5 mg norethindrone acetate	Lactose. White, oval. In 90s and blister card 28s.
		5 mcg ethinyl estradiol/1 mg norethindrone acetate	Lactose. White, D-shaped. In 90s and blister card 28s.
Rx	**Activella** (Novo Nordisk)	**Tablets:** 1 mg estradiol/0.5 mg norethindrone acetate	Lactose. (NOVO 288). White, biconvex. Film-coated. In dial pack 28s.
Rx	**Prefest** (Barr/Duramed)	**Tablets:** 1 mg estradiol; 1 mg estradiol/ 0.09 mg norgestimate	Lactose. **Estradiol only:** (1 J-C E2 O-M). Pink. **Estradiol/Norgestimate:** (1/90 J-C E2/N O-M). White. In blister card 30s (15 of each tablet).
Rx	**ClimaraPro** (Berlex)	**Transdermal patch:** 0.045 mg estradiol/ 0.015 mg levonorgestrel per day	22 cm^2. In 4s.
Rx	**CombiPatch** (Aventis)	**Transdermal patch:** 0.05 mg estradiol/ 0.14 mg norethindrone acetate per day	9 cm^2. In 8s.
		0.05 mg estradiol/0.25 mg norethindrone acetate per day	16 cm^2. In 8s.

ESTROGENS AND PROGESTINS COMBINED

For complete and comparative prescribing information, refer to the Estrogens group monograph and the Progestins group monograph. Consider the information given for Oral Contraceptives (see group monograph) when using these products.

WARNING

Do not use estrogens, with or without progestins, for the prevention of cardiovascular disease or dementia.

The Women's Health Initiative (WHI) study reported increased risks of myocardial infarction, stroke, invasive breast cancer, pulmonary emboli, and deep vein thrombosis in postmenopausal women (50 to 79 years of age) during 5 years of treatment with oral conjugated equine estrogens 0.625 mg combined with medroxyprogesterone acetate 2.5 mg relative to placebo.

The WHI Memory Study (WHIMS), a sub-study of WHI, reported increased risk of developing probable dementia in postmenopausal women 65 years of age and older during 4 years of treatment with oral conjugated estrogens plus medroxyprogesterone acetate relative to placebo. It is unknown whether this finding applies to younger postmenopausal women.

Other doses of oral conjugated estrogens with medroxyprogesterone acetate, and other combinations and dosage forms of estrogens and progestins were not studied in the WHI clinical trials. In the absence of comparable data, these risks should be assumed to be similar. Because of these risks, estrogens with or without progestins should be prescribed at the lowest effective doses and for the shortest duration consistent with treatment goals and risks for the individual woman.

Indications

In women with an intact uterus for:

➤*Hypoestrogenism (CombiPatch* only): Treatment of hypoestrogenism caused by hypogonadism, castration, or primary ovarian failure.

➤*Moderate to severe vasomotor symptoms:* Treatment of moderate to severe vasomotor symptoms associated with menopause.

➤*Moderate to severe vulvar and vaginal atrophy (except Femhrt* and *ClimaraPro*): Treatment of moderate to severe symptoms of vulvar and vaginal atrophy associated with menopause.

When prescribing solely for the treatment of symptoms of vulvar and vaginal atrophy, consider topical vaginal products.

➤*Osteoporosis prevention (except Angeliq* and *CombiPatch*): Prevention of postmenopausal osteoporosis.

When prescribing solely for the prevention of postmenopausal osteoporosis, consider therapy only for women at significant risk of osteoporosis; carefully consider nonestrogen medications.

Administration and Dosage

➤*Approved by the FDA:* November 17, 1995.

Use of estrogen, alone or in combination with a progestin, should be limited to the lowest effective dose available and to the shortest duration consistent with treatment goals and risks for the individual woman.

Patients should be started at the lowest dose.

➤*Prempro:* One 0.625 mg/2.5 mg tablet once daily; can increase to 0.625 mg/5 mg once daily.

➤*Premphase:* One 0.625 mg conjugated estrogens tablet once daily on days 1 through 14 and one 0.625 mg conjugated estrogen/5 mg medroxyprogesterone tablet taken once daily on days 15 through 28.

➤*Femhrt* and *Activella*: One tablet/day.

➤*Angeliq*: One tablet daily. Women who are already using a product containing estrogen should stop taking that product before starting *Angeliq*.

The lowest effective dose of *Angeliq* has not been determined.

➤*Prefest*: One pink tablet/day for 3 days, followed by 1 white tablet/day for 3 days. This regimen is repeated continuously without interruption.

➤*CombiPatch*: Replace the patch system twice weekly. Advise women that monthly withdrawal bleeding often occurs.

Apply to a smooth (fold-free) clean, dry area of the skin on the lower abdomen. Do not apply to or near the breasts and avoid the waistline. The sites of application must be rotated; allow an interval of at least 1 week between applications to the same site.

Continuous combined regimen – Apply twice weekly during a 28-day cycle. Irregular bleeding may occur, particularly in the first 6 months.

Continuous sequential regimen – It can be applied as a sequential regimen in combination with an estradiol-only transdermal delivery system.

➤*ClimaraPro:* Apply a new system weekly during a 28-day cycle. Women often experience withdrawal bleeding at the completion of the cycle. The first day of this bleeding would be an appropriate time to begin therapy.

Place on a smooth (fold-free), clean, dry area of the skin on the lower abdomen. Do not apply to or near the breasts. The area selected should not be oily (which can impair adherence of the system), damaged, or irritated. Avoid the waistline since tight clothing may rub the system off or modify drug delivery. The sites of application must be rotated with an interval of at least 1 week allowed between applications to the same site.

➤*Menopause and vulval / vaginal atrophy:* Reevaluate patients at 3- to 6-month intervals to determine the need for continued treatment.

➤*Osteoporosis:* The mainstays of prevention and management of osteoporosis are estrogen and calcium; exercise and nutrition may be important adjuncts.

➤*Monitoring:* For women who have a uterus, adequate diagnostic measures, such as endometrial sampling, when indicated, should be undertaken to rule out malignancy in cases of undiagnosed persistent or recurring abnormal vaginal bleeding. Patients should be evaluated for breast abnormalities in accordance with good clinical practice.

➤*Storage / Stability:* Store at 20° to 25°C (68° to 77°F); excursions permitted to 15° to 30°C (59° to 86°F).

Activella – Store in a dry place protected from light.

ClimaraPro – Do not store unpouched.

CombiPatch – Prior to dispensing to the patient, store refrigerated 2° to 8°C (36° to 46°F). After dispensing to the patient, *CombiPatch* can be stored

ESTROGENS AND PROGESTINS COMBINED

at room temperature below 25°C (77°F) for up to 6 months, or the expiration date, whichever comes first.

Store the systems in the sealed foil pouch.

Do not store the system in areas where extreme temperatures can occur.

ESTROGEN AND ANDROGEN COMBINATIONS, ORAL

Rx	**Esterified Estrogens and Methyltestosterone H.S.** (Various, eg, Interpharm, Lannett)	**Tablets:** 0.625 mg esterified estrogens and 1.25 mg methyltestosterone	May contain lactose. In 100s and 1,000s.
Rx	**Estratest H.S.** (Solvay)		Lactose, sucrose, parabens. (SOLVAY 1023). Lt. green, capsule shape. Sugar coated. In 100s.
Rx	**Syntest H.S.** (Breckenridge)		Lactose. (Syntho 230). Lt. blue, capsule shape. Film coated. In 100s.
Rx	**Esterified Estrogens and Methyltestosterone** (Various, eg, (Interpharm, Lannett)	**Tablets:** 1.25 mg esterified estrogens and 2.5 mg methyltestosterone	May contain lactose. In 100s and 1,000s.
Rx	**Estratest** (Solvay)		Lactose, sucrose, parabens. (SOLVAY 1026). Dk. green, capsule shape. Sugar-coated. In 100s and 1000s.
Rx	**Syntest D.S.** (Breckenridge)		Lactose. (Syntho 231). Lt. green, capsule shape. Film coated. In 100s.

[a] Syntho Pharmaceuticals, Inc., 230 Sherwood Dr., Farmingdale, NY 11735; 631-755-9898.

ESTROGEN AND ANDROGEN COMBINATIONS — ORAL

For complete and comparative prescribing information, refer to the Estrogens and Androgens group monographs.

WARNING

Estrogens have been reported to increase the risk of endometrial carcinoma.

Close clinical surveillance of all women taking estrogens is important. In all cases of undiagnosed, persistent, or recurring abnormal vaginal bleeding, adequate diagnostic measures should be undertaken to rule out malignancy.

Do not use estrogens during pregnancy.

The use of female sex hormones, estrogens and progestogens, during early pregnancy may seriously damage the offspring.

Refer to the Warning Box in the Estrogens group monograph for more information.

Indications

➤*Moderate to severe vasomotor symptoms:* Moderate to severe vasomotor symptoms associated with menopause in patients not improved with estrogens alone.

Administration and Dosage

Give cyclically for short-term use only.

➤*Usual dosage range:* One 1.25/2.5 mg tablet or one to two 0.625/1.25 mg tablets daily, as recommended by the physician.

Administer cyclically (3 weeks on and 1 week off). Make attempts to discontinue or taper medication at 3- to 6-month intervals.

Use the lowest dose that will control symptoms and discontinue medication as promptly as possible.

➤*Monitoring:* Closely monitor treated patients with an intact uterus for signs of endometrial cancer and take appropriate diagnostic measures to rule out malignancy in the event of persistent or recurring abnormal vaginal bleeding.

➤*Storage/Stability:* Store at controlled room temperature, 15° to 30°C (59° to 86°F).

ORAL CONTRACEPTIVES

WARNING

Smoking – Cigarette smoking increases the risk of serious cardiovascular side effects from oral contraceptives (OCs). This risk increases with age and with heavy smoking (at least 15 cigarettes daily) and is quite marked in women older than 35 years of age. Women who use OCs should not smoke.

Indications

➤*Contraception:* For the prevention of pregnancy.

Because of the positive association between the amount of estrogen and progestin in OCs and the risk of vascular disease and thromboembolism, minimizing exposure to these agents is in keeping with good principles of therapeutics. For any particular combination, prescribe the dosage regimen that contains the least amount of estrogen and progestin compatible with a low failure rate and needs of the individual patient. Start new patients on preparations containing estrogen 35 mcg or less.

➤*Emergency contraception (Plan B and Preven only):* For prevention of pregnancy following unprotected intercourse or a known or suspected contraceptive failure. To obtain efficacy, have the patient take the first dose as soon as possible within 72 hours of intercourse. The second dose must be taken 12 hours later.

➤*Acne vulgaris (Ortho Tri-Cyclen and Estrostep only):* For the treatment of moderate acne vulgaris in females at least 15 years of age who have no known contraindications to oral contraceptive therapy and who desire contraception, have achieved menarche, and are unresponsive to topical antiacne medications.

Administration and Dosage

➤*Acne:* The timing of dosing with *Ortho Tri-Cyclen* or *Estrostep* for acne should follow the guidelines for use of *Ortho Tri-Cyclen* or *Estrostep* as an OC. The dosage regimen for treatment of facial acne uses a 21-day active and a 7-day inert schedule. Have the patient take 1 active tablet daily for 21 days followed by 1 inert for 7 days. After 28 tablets have been taken, the patient should start a new course the next day.

➤*Emergency contraception (Plan B and Preven only):* The *Preven* emergency contraceptive kit contains a pregnancy test. This test can be used to verify an existing pregnancy resulting from intercourse that occurred earlier in the current menstrual cycle or the previous cycle. If a positive pregnancy result is obtained, advise the patient not to take the pills in the kit.

Take the initial 1 (*Plan B*) or 2 (*Preven*) pills as soon as possible but within 72 hours of unprotected intercourse. This is followed by the second dose of 1 (*Plan B*) or 2 (*Preven*) pills 12 hours later. Emergency contraception can be used at any time during the menstrual cycle. If the user vomits within 1 hour of taking either dose of the medication, she should contact her health care professional to discuss whether or not to repeat that dose or take an antinausea medication. Emergency contraceptive pills are not indicated for ongoing pregnancy protection and should not be used as a woman's routine form of contraception.

➤*Contraception:*

Progestin-only – One tablet every day at the same time. Administration is continuous, with no interruption between pill packs. Every time a pill is taken late, especially if a pill is missed, pregnancy is more likely.

Missed dose: If the patient is more than 3 hours late or misses at least 1 tablet, she should take the missed pill as soon as remembered, then go back to taking progestin-only products (POPs) at the regular time, while being sure to use a backup method (eg, condom, spermicide) every time she has sexual intercourse for the next 48 hours.

Combined –

Sunday-start packaging: If the instructions recommend starting the regimen on Sunday, inform the patient to take the first tablet on the first Sunday after menstruation begins. If menstruation begins on Sunday, she should take the first tablet on that day.

21-day regimen: For day-1 start, the first day of menstrual bleeding should be counted as day 1. The cycle is to take 1 tablet per day for 21 days; no tablets are taken for 7 days. Whether bleeding has stopped or not, the patient should start a new course of the 21-day regimen. Withdrawal flow will normally occur approximately 3 days after the last tablet is taken. The patient must follow the schedule whether flow occurs as expected, or whether spotting or breakthrough bleeding (BTB) occurs during the cycle.

28-day regimen: To eliminate the need to count the days between cycles, some products contain 7 inert or iron-containing tablets to permit continu-

ORAL CONTRACEPTIVES

ous daily dosage during the entire 28-day cycle. Inform the patient to take the 7 tablets on the last 7 days of the cycle.

84-day regimen: The dosage of *Seasonale* is 1 pink (active) tablet per day for 84 consecutive days, followed by 7 days of white (inert) tablets. Withdrawal bleeding should occur during the 7 days following discontinuation of pink active tablets. During the first cycle, the patient should not place contraceptive reliance on *Seasonale* until a pink tablet has been taken daily for 7 consecutive days; the patient should use a nonhormonal backup method of birth control (such as condoms or spermicide) during those 7 days. The patient should consider the possibility of ovulation and conception prior to initiation of medication.

The patient begins her next and all subsequent 91-day courses of tablets without interruption on the same day of the week on which she began her first course, following the same schedule. If in any cycle the patient starts tablets later than the proper day, she should protect herself against pregnancy by using a nonhormonal backup method of birth control until she has taken a pink tablet daily for 7 consecutive days.

Biphasic and triphasic OCs: Have the patient follow the instructions on the dispensers or packs; these are clearly marked, usually indicating where to start on the regimen and in what order to take the pills (usually marked with arrows), along with the appropriate week numbers. If there is any question, detailed instructions are provided in the specific package insert. As with the monophasic OCs, 1 tablet is taken each day; however, as the color of the tablet changes, the strength of the tablet also changes (the estrogen/progestin ratio varies).

Missed active dose: While there is little likelihood of ovulation occurring if only 1 tablet is missed, the possibility of spotting or bleeding is increased. The possibility of ovulation occurring increases with each successive day that scheduled tablets are missed. This is particularly likely to occur if at least 2 consecutive tablets are missed. Any time at least 1 active tablets have been missed, the patient should use another method of contraception for the balance of the cycle until tablets have been taken for 7 consecutive days. If a patient forgets to take at least 1 tablet, the following is suggested:

- *One active tablet* – Have the patient take this as soon as remembered or she should take 2 tablets the next day; alternatively, the patient can take 1 tablet, discard the other missed tablet, continue as scheduled, and use another form of contraception until menses.
- *Two consecutive active tablets* – The patient should take 2 tablets as soon as remembered with the next pill at the usual time or she should take 2 tablets daily for the next 2 days, then resume the regular schedule. The patient should use an additional form of contraception for the 7 days after pills are missed , preferably for the remainder of the cycle. If 2 active pills are missed in a row in the third week and the patient is a Sunday starter, 1 pill should be taken every day until Sunday. On Sunday, the rest of the pack should be discarded and a new pack of pills started that same day. If 2 active pills are missed in a row in the third week and the patient is a day-1 starter, the rest of the pill pack should be discarded and a new pack started that same day. Menses may not occur this month but this is expected. However, if menses do not occur 2 months in a row, the health care provider or clinic should be contacted because of the possibility of pregnancy.
- *Three consecutive active tablets* – If the patient is a Sunday starter, she should keep taking 1 pill every day until Sunday. On Sunday, the rest of the pack should be discarded and a new pack of pills started that same day. If she is a day-1 starter, the rest of the pill pack should be discarded and a new pack started that same day. Menses may not occur this month, but this is expected. However, if menses do not occur 2 months in a row, the health care provider or clinic should be contacted because of the possibility of pregnancy. Pregnancy may result from sexual intercourse during the 7 days after the pills are missed. The patient should use another birth control method (eg, condoms, foam) as a backup method for those 7 days.

Switching pills – If switching from the combined pills to POPs, the patient should take the first POP the day after the last active combined pill is finished. She should not take any of the 7 inactive pills from the combined pill pack. Many women have irregular periods after switching to POPs; this is normal and to be expected. If switching from POPs to the combined pills, the patient should take the first active combined pill on the first day of menses, even if the POP pack is not finished. If switching to another brand of POPs, she should start the new brand any time. If the patient is breastfeeding, she can switch to another method of birth control at any time, except she should not switch to the combined pills until breastfeeding is stopped or until at least 6 months after delivery.

Bleeding – Bleeding that resembles menstruation occurs rarely. Persistent bleeding not controlled by this method indicates the need for re-examination of the patient; consider nonhormonal causes. If pathology has been excluded, time or a change to another formulation may solve the problem.

Missed menstrual period – If the patient has not adhered to the prescribed dosage regimen, consider possible pregnancy after the first missed period; withhold OCs until ruling out pregnancy and use a nonhormonal method of contraception. If the patient has adhered to the prescribed regimen and misses 2 consecutive periods, rule out pregnancy before continuing the contraceptive regimen.

After several months of treatment, menstrual flow may reduce to a point of virtual absence. This reduced flow may occur as a result of medication and is not indicative of pregnancy.

Postpartum administration – Postpartum administration in nonnursing mothers may begin at the first postpartum examination (4 to 6 weeks), regardless of whether spontaneous menstruation has occurred. Have the patient consider the possibility of ovulation and conception prior to initiation of medication. Also, the patient should start no earlier than 4 to 6 weeks after a midtrimester pregnancy termination. Immediate postpartum use is associated with increased risk of thromboembolism. If possible, nursing mothers should defer taking OCs until the infant is weaned (see Warnings).

If fully breastfeeding (not giving baby any food or formula), start the patient on POPs 6 weeks after delivery. If partially breastfeeding (giving baby some food or formula), the patient should start taking POPs by 3 weeks after delivery.

In the nonlactating mother, *Seasonale* may be initiated no earlier than day 28 postpartum for contraception because of the increased risk for thromboembolism. When the tablets are administered in the postpartum period, the increased risk of thromboembolic disease associated with the postpartum period must be considered. Advise the patient to use a nonhormonal backup method for the first 7 days of tablet-taking. However, if intercourse has already occurred, consider the possibility of ovulation and conception prior to initiation of medication. *Seasonale* may be initiated immediately after a first-trimester abortion; if the patient starts *Seasonale* immediately, additional contraceptive measures are not needed.

Dosage adjustments – Side effects noted during the initial cycles may be transient; if they continue, dosage adjustments may be indicated. Many side effects are related to the potency of the estrogen or progestin in the products. The following table summarizes these dose-related side effects.

Achieving Proper Hormonal Balance in an Oral Contraceptive

Estrogen		Progestin	
Excess	Deficiency	Excess	Deficiency
Nausea, bloating Cervical mucorrhea, polyposis Melasma Hypertension Migraine headache Breast fullness or tenderness Edema	Early or mid-cycle breakthrough bleeding Increased spotting Hypomenorrhea	Increased appetite Weight gain Tiredness, fatigue Hypomenorrhea Acne, oily scalp[a] Hair loss, hirsutism[a] Depression Monilial vaginitis Breast regression	Late breakthrough bleeding Amenorrhea Hypermenorrhea

[a] Result of androgenic activity of progestins.

Pharmacological Effects of Progestins Used in Oral Contraceptives[a]

	Progestin	Estrogen	Androgen
Desogestrel	++++	0	+++
Levonorgestrel	++++	0	++++
Norgestrel	+++	0	+++
Ethynodiol diacetate	++	+++	+
Norgestimate	++	0	++
Norethindrone acetate	++	++	++
Norethindrone	++	++	++

[a] *Symbol Key: ++++ – pronounced effect; +++ – moderate effect; ++ – low effect; + – slight effect; 0 – no effect*

Minimize the above effects by adjusting the estrogen/progestin balance or dosage. The following table categorizes products by their estrogenic, progestational, and androgenic activity. Because overall activity is influenced by the interaction of components, including androgenic and antiestrogenic activity, it is difficult to precisely classify products; placement in the table is only approximate. Differences between products within a group are probably not clinically significant.

ORAL CONTRACEPTIVES

Estimated Relative Oral Contraceptive Progestin/Estrogen/Androgen Activity

	Ingredients	Brand-name examples	Progestin activity	Estrogen activity	Androgen activity
Monophasic	0.1 mg levonorgestrel/ 20 mcg EE[a]	*Alesse, Aviane, Lessina, Levlite*	Low	Low	Low
	0.25 mg norgestimate/35 mcg EE	*Ortho-Cyclen, Sprintec*		Intermediate	
	0.5 mg norethindrone/35 mcg EE	*Brevicon, Modicon, Necon 0.5/35, Nortrel 0.5/35*		High	
	0.4 mg norethindrone/35 mcg EE	*Ovcon-35*			
	0.15 mg levonorgestrel/30 mcg EE	*Levlen, Levora, Nordette, Portia*	Intermediate	Low	Intermediate
	0.3 mg norgestrel/30 mcg EE	*Cryselle, Lo-Ovral, Low-Ogestrel*			
	1 mg norethindrone/50 mcg mestranol	*Necon 1/50, Norinyl 1+50, Ortho-Novum 1/50*		Intermediate	
	1 mg norethindrone/35 mcg EE	*Necon 1/35, Norinyl 1+35, Nortrel 1/35, Ortho-Novum 1/35*		High	
	1 mg norethindrone/50 mcg EE	*Ovcon-50*			
	1 mg norethindrone acetate/20 mcg EE	*Loestrin 21 1/20, Loestrin Fe 1/20, Microgestin Fe 1/20*	High	Low	
	1.5 mg norethindrone acetate/30 mcg EE	*Loestrin 21 1.5/30, Loestrin Fe 1.5/30, Microgestin Fe 1.5/30*			High
	1 mg ethynodiol diacetate/35 mcg EE	*Demulen 1/35, Zovia 1/35E*			Low
	Desogestrel/EE 0.15 mg-20 mcg and EE 10 mcg	*Kariva, Mircette*			
	0.15 mg desogestrel/30 mcg EE	*Apri, Desogen, Ortho-Cept*	High	Intermediate	
	1 mg ethynodiol diacetate/50 mcg EE	*Demulen 1/50, Zovia 1/50E*			
	0.5 mg norgestrel/50 mcg EE	*Ovral, Ogestrel*		High	High
	3 mg drospirenone/30 mcg EE	*Yasmin*	No data	Intermediate[b]	None[b]
Biphasic	Norethindrone/EE 0.5-35/1-35 mg-mcg	*Necon 10/11, Ortho-Novum 10/11*	Intermediate	High	Low
Triphasic	Norgestimate/EE 0.18-25/0.215-25/0.25-25 mg-mcg	*Ortho Tri-Cyclen Lo*	Low	Low	
	Levonorgestrel/EE 0.05-30/0.075-40/0.125-30 mg-mcg	*Enpresse, Tri-Levlen, Triphasil, Trivora*		Intermediate	
	Norgestimate/EE 0.18-35/0.215-35/0.25-35 mg-mcg	*Ortho Tri-Cyclen*			
	Norethindrone/EE 0.5-35/1-35/0.5-35 mg-mcg	*Tri-Norinyl*		High	
	Norethindrone/EE 0.5-35/0.75-35/1-35 mg-mcg	*Necon 7/7/7, Ortho-Novum 7/7/7*	Intermediate		
	Norethindrone/EE 1-20/1-30/1-35 mg-mcg	*Estrostep 21, Estrostep Fe*	High	Low	Intermediate
	Desogestrel/EE 0.1-25/0.125-25/0.15-25 mg-mcg	*Cyclessa*			Low

[a] EE = ethinyl estradiol.
[b] Preclinical studies have shown that drospirenone has no androgenic, estrogenic, glucocorticoid, antiglucocorticoid, or antiandrogenic activity.

Actions

➤*Pharmacology:* OCs include estrogen-progestin combinations and POPs.

Progestin-only – Progestin-only oral contraceptives prevent conception by suppressing ovulation in approximately 50% of users, thickening the cervical mucus to inhibit sperm penetration, lowering the midcycle luteinizing hormone (LH) and follicle-stimulating hormone (FSH) peaks, slowing the movement of the ovum through the fallopian tubes, and altering the endometrium.

Combination OCs – Combination OCs inhibit ovulation by suppressing the gonadotropins, FSH, and LH. Additionally, alterations in the genital tract, including cervical mucus (which inhibits sperm penetration) and the endometrium (which reduces the likelihood of implantation), may contribute to contraceptive effectiveness.

These products differ in the type and relative potency of the components and in the relative predominance of estrogenic or progestational activity. Their ultimate effects are related to combined estrogenic, progestational, androgenic, and antiestrogenic effects.

Progestins may modify the effects of estrogens; these effects depend on the type or amount of progestin present and the ratio of progestin to estrogen. Dosage, potency, length of administration, and concomitant estrogen administration contribute to total progestational potency, making it difficult to establish equivalent doses of progestins. The total estrogenic potency of an OC is based on the combined effects of the estrogen and the estrogenic/antiestrogenic/androgenic effect of the progestin.

See the table in the Administration and Dosage section for a summary of the effects of the various progestins. Although not in the table, note that drospirenone is a spironolactone analog with antimineralocorticoid activity. Preclinical studies have shown that drospirenone has no androgenic, estrogenic, glucocorticoid, antiglucocorticoid, or antiandrogenic activity.

Contraceptive efficacy – In a study comparing the efficacy and safety of *Plan B* (1 tablet of levonorgestrel 0.75 mg taken within 72 hours of intercourse and 1 tablet taken 12 hours later) with the Yuzpe regimen (2 tablets of levonorgestrel 0.25 mg and ethinyl estradiol 0.05 mg taken within 72 hours of intercourse and 2 tablets taken 12 hours later), *Plan B* was at least as effective as the Yuzpe regimen in preventing pregnancy. After a single act of intercourse, the expected pregnancy rate of 8% (with no contraception) was reduced to approximately 1% with *Plan B*. Thus, *Plan B* reduced the expected number of pregnancies by 89%.

If 100 women used emergency contraceptive pills (ECPs) correctly in 1 month, approximately 2 women would become pregnant after a single act of intercourse. The use of ECPs results in a 75% reduction in the number of pregnancies expected if no ECPs were used after unprotected intercourse. Some clinical trials have shown that efficacy was greatest when ECPs were taken within 24 hours of unprotected intercourse; the efficacy decreases somewhat during each subsequent 24-hour period.

ECPs are not as effective as other forms of contraception. Efficacy in most cases depends greatly upon degree of compliance and user reliability. No other contraceptive drug or device, except levonorgestrel implant and medroxyprogesterone injection, approaches the efficacy of the combined OCs. For effectiveness rates of other contraceptive methods, refer to the following table.

Pregnancy Rates for Various Means of Contraception (%)[a]

Method of contraception	Lowest expected[b]	Typical[c]
Oral contraceptives		3
Combined	0.1	5
Progestin-only	0.5	5
Mechanical/Chemical		
Levonorgestrel implant	0.09	0.09
Medroxyprogesterone injection	0.3	0.3
IUD		
Progesterone	1.5	2
Copper T 380A	0.8	0.6
LNg 20	0.1	0.1
Cervical cap		
Parous	26	40
Nulliparous	9	20
Condom		
Without spermicide	3	14
With spermicide[d]	1.8	4 to 6
Spermicide alone	6	26
Diaphragm (with spermicidal cream or gel)	6	20
Female condom	5	21
Periodic abstinence (ie, rhythm; all methods)	1 to 9	25
Sterility		
Vasectomy	0.1	0.15
Tubal ligation	0.5	0.5

ORAL CONTRACEPTIVES

Pregnancy Rates for Various Means of Contraception (%)[a]		
Method of contraception	Lowest expected[b]	Typical[c]
No contraception	85	85

[a] During first year of continuous use.
[b] Best guess of percentage expected to experience an accidental pregnancy among couples who initiate a method and use it consistently and correctly.
[c] A "typical" couple who initiate a method and experience an accidental pregnancy.
[d] Used as a separate product (not in condom package).

There are 3 types of combination OCs, monophasic, biphasic, and triphasic. The biphasic and triphasic OCs are intended to deliver hormones in a fashion similar to physiologic processes.

Monophasic – There is a fixed dosage of estrogen to progestin throughout the cycle.

Biphasic – The amount of estrogen remains the same for the first 21 days of the cycle. A decreased progestin:estrogen ratio in the first half of the cycle allows endometrial proliferation. An increased ratio in the second half provides adequate secretory development.

Triphasic – The estrogen amount remains the same while the progestin changes, or the dose of both estrogen and progestin change during the cycle.

Noncontraceptive health benefits – The following health benefits related to the use of combination OCs are supported by epidemiological studies that largely utilized OC formulations containing estrogen doses of ethinyl estradiol 35 mcg or more or mestranol 50 mcg.

Effects on menses: Increased menstrual cycle regularity, decreased blood loss and decreased incidence of iron deficiency anemia, decreased incidence of dysmenorrhea.

Effects related to inhibition of ovulation: Decreased incidence of functional ovarian cysts and ectopic pregnancies.

Other effects: Decreased incidence of fibroadenomas and fibrocystic disease of the breast, acute pelvic inflammatory disease, endometrial cancer, ovarian cancer, maintenance of bone density, and decreased symptomatic endometriosis.

➤*Pharmacokinetics:*

Estrogens – Ethinyl estradiol is rapidly absorbed with peak concentrations attained within 2 hours. It undergoes considerable first-pass elimination. Mestranol is demethylated to ethinyl estradiol. Ethinyl estradiol is 97% to 98% bound to plasma albumin. Half-life varies from 6 to 20 hours. It is excreted in bile and urine as conjugates and undergoes some enterohepatic recirculation.

Progestins – Peak concentrations of norethindrone occur 0.5 to 4 hours after oral administration; it undergoes first-pass metabolism with an overall bioavailability of approximately 65%. Levonorgestrel reaches peak concentrations between 0.5 to 2 hours, does not undergo a first-pass effect, and is completely bioavailable. Norethindrone and levonorgestrel are chiefly metabolized by reduction followed by conjugation. Desogestrel is rapidly and completely absorbed and converted into 3-keto-desogestrel, the biologically active metabolite. Relative bioavailability is approximately 84%. Maximum concentrations of the metabolite are reached at approximately 1.4 hours. Norgestimate is well absorbed; peak serum concentrations are observed within 2 hours followed by a rapid decline to levels generally below assay within 5 hours. However, a major metabolite, 17-deacetyl norgestimate, appears rapidly in serum with concentrations greatly exceeding that of the parent. Both norethynodrel and ethynodiol diacetate are converted to norethindrone. Peak serum concentrations of drospirenone are reached 1 to 3 hours after administration. Progestins are bound to albumin (79% to 95%) and to sex hormone binding globulin (except drospirenone). Terminal half-life of the progestins are as follows: Norethindrone, 5 to 14 hours; levonorgestrel, 11 to 45 hours; desogestrel (metabolite), 38 ± 20 hours; norgestimate (metabolite), 12 to 30 hours; drospirenone, 30 hours. Progestin-only administration results in lower steady-state serum progestin levels and a shorter elimination half-life than coadministration with estrogens.

Contraindications

Thrombophlebitis; thromboembolic disorders (eg, valvular heart disease with thrombogenic complications); history of deep-vein thrombophlebitis; cerebral vascular disease; MI; coronary artery disease; known or suspected breast carcinoma or estrogen-dependent neoplasia; carcinoma of endometrium; hepatic adenomas/carcinomas (see Warnings); undiagnosed abnormal genital bleeding; known or suspected pregnancy (see Warnings); cholestatic jaundice of pregnancy/jaundice with prior pill use; hypersensitivity to any component of the product; acute liver disease; uncontrolled hypertension; headaches with focal neurological symptoms; diabetes with vascular complications; major surgery with prolonged immobility.

➤*Yasmin:* Renal insufficiency, hepatic dysfunction, adrenal insufficiency, heavy smoking (at least 15 cigarettes daily) and older than 35 years of age.

Warnings

➤*Smoking:* Cigarette smoking increases the risk of serious cardiovascular side effects from OCs. This risk increases with age and with heavy smoking (at least 15 cigarettes daily) and is quite marked in women older than 35 years of age. Women who use OCs should not smoke.

➤*Hyperkalemia: Yasmin* contains the progestin drospirenone that has antimineralocorticoid activity, including the potential for hyperkalemia in high-risk patients, comparable with spironolactone 25 mg. *Yasmin* should not be used in patients with conditions that predispose to hyperkalemia (eg, renal insufficiency, hepatic dysfunction, adrenal insufficiency). Women receiving daily, long-term treatment for chronic conditions or diseases with medications that may increase serum potassium should have their serum potassium level checked during the first treatment cycle. Drugs that may increase serum potassium include ACE inhibitors, angiotensin-II receptor antagonists, potassium-sparing diuretics, heparin, aldosterone antagonists, and NSAIDs.

➤*Risks of OC use:* The use of OCs is associated with increased risk of thromboembolism, stroke, MI, hypertension, hepatic neoplasia, and gallbladder disease, although risk of serious morbidity or mortality is very small in healthy women without underlying risk factors. Risk of morbidity/mortality increases significantly in the presence of other underlying risk factors such as hypertension, hyperlipidemias, obesity, and diabetes.

➤*Mortality:* Mortality associated with all methods of birth control is low and below that associated with childbirth, with the exception of OC use in women at least 35 years of age who smoke and at least 40 years of age who do not smoke. In 1989, the Fertility and Maternal Health Drugs Advisory Committee concluded that although cardiovascular disease risk may be increased with OC use in healthy nonsmoking women older than 40 years of age (even with the newer low-dose formulations), there also are greater potential health risks associated with pregnancy in older women and with the alternative surgical and medical procedures that may be necessary if such women do not have access to effective and acceptable means of contraception. Therefore, the committee recommended that the benefits of low-dose OC use by healthy nonsmoking women older than 40 years of age may outweigh the possible risks. Of course, like all women, older women who take oral contraceptives should take an oral contraceptive that contains the least amount of estrogen and progestin that is compatible with a low failure rate and individual patient needs.

➤*Thromboembolism:* Be alert to the earliest symptoms of thromboembolic and thrombotic disorders. Should any of these occur or be suspected, discontinue the drug immediately.

In 1998, the American College of Obstetrics and Gynecology Committee on Gynecologic Practice reconfirmed that the risks of nonfatal venous thromboembolism for healthy, nonpregnant nonusers of OCs is 4 cases per 100,000 woman-years versus 10 to 15 cases per 100,000 woman-years and 20 to 30 cases per 100,000 woman-years for users of second- and third-generation OCs, respectively. The risk for pregnant women is 60 cases per 100,000 woman-years. The committee confirms that the risk of nonfatal venous thrombosis with third-generation OCs (desogestrel, gestodene, and norgestimate) is 2 to 3 times the risk of second-generation OCs. The risk of development of deep vein thrombosis was found to be 2 to 5 times higher with low-estrogen, desogestrel-containing OCs than with second-generation monophasic and triphasic preparations. The committee stated that the decision regarding the use of third-generation OCs should be left to the clinician and patient because they might have benefit in some cases (eg, patients requiring suppression of ovarian androgens or those with conditions for which they might be advantageous).

MI – MI risk associated with OC use is increased. This risk is primarily in smokers or women with other underlying risk factors for coronary artery disease such as hypertension, hypercholesterolemia, morbid obesity, and diabetes. The risk is very low in women younger than 30 years of age. It is estimated that the relative risk of heart attack for current OC users is 2 to 6.

Long-term use – Data suggest that the increased risk of MI persists after discontinuation of long-term OC use; the highest risk group includes women 40 to 49 years of age who used OCs for at least 5 years.

Smoking – Smoking in combination with OC use has been shown to contribute substantially to the incidence of MIs in women in their mid-30s or older, with smoking accounting for the majority of excess cases. Mortality rates associated with circulatory disease have been shown to increase substantially in smokers, especially in those at least 35 years of age who use OCs.

Cerebrovascular diseases – OCs increase the risk of cerebrovascular events (thrombotic and hemorrhagic strokes), although, in general, the risk is greatest in hypertensive women older than 35 years of age who also smoke. Relative risk of thrombotic strokes ranges from 3 (normotensive users) to 14 (severe hypertensive users). Relative risk of hemorrhagic stroke for OC users is 1.2 for nonsmokers, 7.6 for smokers, 1.8 for normotensives, and 25.7 for severe hypertensives; for nonuser smokers, risk is 2.6. The attributable risk also is greater in older women.

Vascular disease – A positive association is observed between the amount of estrogen and progestin in OCs and the risk of vascular disease. A decline in serum high-density lipoproteins (HDL) has occurred with progestins and has been associated with an increased incidence of ischemic heart disease. Because estrogens increase HDL cholesterol, the net effect depends on a balance achieved between doses of estrogen and progestin and the activity of the progestin used in the contraceptives.

Age – The risk of cerebrovascular and circulatory disease in OC users is substantially increased in women at least 35 years of age with other risk factors (eg, smoking, uncontrolled hypertension, hypercholesterolemia [LDL 190], obesity, diabetes). Mortality rates associated with circulatory disease have been shown to increase substantially in smokers older than 35 years of age and nonsmokers older than 40 years of age among women who use OCs. Current clinical practice involves use of lower-estrogen dose formulations combined with careful restriction of OC use to women who do not have the various risk factors listed.

Postsurgical thromboembolism – Risk is increased 2- to 4-fold. If possible, discontinue OCs at least 4 weeks before and 2 weeks after surgery and during and following prolonged immobilization because OCs are associated with an increased risk of thromboembolism.

ORAL CONTRACEPTIVES

Subarachnoid hemorrhage – Subarachnoid hemorrhage has been increased by OC use. Smoking alone increases the incidence of these accidents; smoking and OC use appear to work together to produce a combined risk greater than either alone.

Persistence of risk – An increased risk may persist for at least 6 years after discontinuation of OC use for cerebrovascular disease and at least 9 years for MI in users 40 to 49 years of age who had used OCs at least 5 years; this risk was not demonstrated in other age groups. This information is based on studies that used OC formulations containing at least estrogen 50 mcg.

NOTE – The associations between OCs and cardiovascular disease are based on epidemiological studies whose conclusions have been criticized for the following reasons: National trends of cardiovascular mortality are incompatible with these risk estimates; excess deaths may not be attributable entirely to smoking; the clinical diagnosis of thromboembolism is often unreliable.

➤*Ocular lesions:* Ocular lesions such as retinal thrombosis have been associated with the use of OCs. Discontinue medication if there is unexplained loss of vision, onset of proptosis or diplopia, papilledema, or retinal vascular lesions. Immediately undertake appropriate diagnostic therapeutic measures.

➤*Carcinoma:* Numerous epidemiological studies have been performed on the incidence of breast, endometrial, ovarian, and cervical cancer in women using OCs. While there are conflicting reports, the overall evidence in the literature suggests that use of OCs is not associated with an increase in the risk of developing breast cancer, regardless of age and parity of first use. The Cancer and Steroid Hormone study also showed no latent effect on the risk of breast cancer for at least a decade following long-term use. Some studies have shown an increased relative risk of developing breast cancer, particularly at a younger age and apparently related to duration of use. These studies have predominantly involved combined oral contraceptives; there is insufficient data to determine whether the use of POPs similarly increases the risk. Women with breast cancer should not use OCs because the role of female hormones in breast cancer has not been fully determined. Most studies have not shown such a risk; methodologies of earlier studies have been questioned. According to the CDC, there is a small subset of premenopausal-associated breast cancers, but there is no proof of cause and effect; there is no association with the postmenopausal variety.

Some studies suggest that OC use has been associated with an increase in the risk of cervical intraepithelial neoplasia in some populations of women. There is insufficient data to determine whether the use of POPs increases the risk of developing cervical intraepithelial neoplasia. There continues to be controversy about the extent to which such findings may be because of differences in sexual behavior and other factors. Other epidemiologic studies have suggested an increased risk of cervical dysplasia and carcinoma.

In spite of many studies of the relationship between OC use and breast and cervical cancers, a cause and effect relationship has not been established.

Studies have reported an increased risk of endometrial carcinoma associated with the prolonged use of estrogen in postmenopausal women. However, the risk appears to be decreased in OC users because of the progestin component. In fact, there is a protective effect; users appear about half as likely to develop ovarian and endometrial cancer as women who have never used OCs. The protective effect from endometrial cancer lasts up to 15 years after the pills are stopped.

There appears to be no increased risk of breast cancer in OC users or any subgroup of users, although the CDC states that there may be an association with a subset of young, premenopausal users. There is no increased risk of breast cancer in OC users with prior benign breast disease. Another study suggests that use prior to the first full-term pregnancy was associated with a significant relative risk of breast cancer especially when OC use began before 25 years of age.

Close clinical surveillance of all women taking OCs is essential; they should be reexamined at least once a year. In all cases of undiagnosed persistent or recurrent abnormal vaginal bleeding, rule out malignancy. Monitor women with a strong family history of breast cancer or who have breast nodules, fibrocystic disease of the breast, cervical dysplasia, or abnormal mammograms.

➤*Hepatic lesions (eg, adenomas, focal nodular hyperplasia, hepatocellular carcinoma):* Benign and malignant hepatic adenomas have been associated with the use of OCs, but this is a relatively rare disease. Severe abdominal pain, shock, or death may be caused by rupture and hemorrhage of a liver tumor. Fortunately, this is quite rare; there may be some association with higher-dose mestranol preparations or duration (greater after at least 4 years) of OC use. While hepatic adenoma is uncommon, consider it in women presenting with abdominal pain and tenderness, abdominal mass, or shock. A few cases of hepatocellular carcinoma have been reported in women taking OCs long-term; however, an association has not been established.

➤*Gallbladder disease:* Earlier studies have reported an increased risk of gallbladder surgery in OC users. More recent studies, however, have shown that the relative risk of developing gallbladder disease among OC users may be minimal. These recent findings may be related to the use of OC formulations containing lower estrogen and progestin doses.

➤*Carbohydrate metabolism:* Glucose tolerance may decrease, which is directly related to estrogen dose. Progestins increase insulin secretion and create insulin resistance. These effects vary with different agents. However, OCs appear to have no effect on fasting blood glucose in nondiabetic women. Observe prediabetic and diabetic patients receiving OCs. In a recent study, OC users were less likely to develop diabetes than nonusers.

➤*Lipid profile:* A small proportion of women will have persistent hypertriglyceridemia while using OCs. Changes in serum triglycerides and lipoprotein levels have been reported in OC users.

➤*Elevated blood pressure:* Elevated blood pressure and hypertension may occur within a few months of beginning use. The prevalence increases with the duration of use and age. Incidence of hypertension may directly correlate with increasing dosages of progestin.

Encourage women with a history of hypertension, renal disease, or hypertension-related diseases during pregnancy to use another method of contraception. Monitor these patients if they choose to use OCs. Discontinue the OC if elevated blood pressure occurs. High blood pressure returns to normal in most women after OC discontinuation.

➤*Headache:* Onset or exacerbation of migraine or development of headache with focal neurological symptoms of a new pattern that is recurrent, persistent, or severe, requires OC discontinuation and evaluation.

➤*Bleeding irregularities:* BTB and spotting are sometimes encountered in OC patients, especially during the first 3 months of use. BTB, spotting, and amenorrhea are frequent reasons for discontinuing OCs. The type and dose of progestin may be important. In BTB, consider nonhormonal causes. In undiagnosed persistent or recurrent abnormal vaginal bleeding, rule out pregnancy or malignancy. If amenorrhea occurs, rule out pregnancy. If pathology has been excluded, time or formulation change may resolve the problem. Changing to an OC with a higher estrogen content may minimize menstrual irregularity, but consider the increased risk of thromboembolic disease. Consider short-term estrogen supplements.

It was thought that women with a history of oligomenorrhea or secondary amenorrhea or young women without regular cycles may tend to remain anovulatory or become amenorrheic after discontinuation of OCs; however, this is not certain. Other factors may play a role in the development of amenorrhea after OC withdrawal, including stress, previous menstrual irregularity, psychiatric conditions, and marked weight loss. Also, the incidence may have been much higher when higher-dose products were used more regularly. Advise patients of this possibility.

Seasonale – When prescribing *Seasonale*, the convenience of fewer planned menses (4 annually instead of 13 annually) should be weighed against the inconvenience of increased intermenstrual bleeding and/or spotting. More *Seasonale* subjects, compared with subjects on the 28-day cycle regimen enrolled in a clinical trial, discontinued prematurely for unacceptable bleeding (7.7% with *Seasonale* versus 1.8% of 28-day cycle regimen).

Progestin-only products – Episodes of irregular, unpredictable spotting, and BTB within the first year are the most frequently encountered side effects and are the major reasons why women discontinue OC use.

➤*Risks of use immediately preceding pregnancy:* Some extensive epidemiological studies have revealed no increased risk of birth defects in OC users prior to pregnancy.

➤*Menopause:* Treatment with OCs may mask the onset of the climacteric.

➤*Fertility impairment:* Fertility impairment may occur in women discontinuing OCs; however, impairment diminishes with time. In nulliparous women 25 to 29 years of age, the effect is negligible after 48 months. Among nulliparous women 30 to 34 years of age, impairment persists up to 72 months and appears more severe. For parous women, the effect is negligible and short-lived after cessation of contraception.

The limited available data indicated a rapid return of normal ovulation and fertility following discontinuation of progestin-only OCs.

➤*Pregnancy: Category X.* Rule out pregnancy before initiating or continuing OCs and always consider it if withdrawal bleeding does not occur. Rule out pregnancy before continuing OCs for any patient who has missed 2 consecutive periods. If the patient has not adhered to the prescribed schedule, consider the possibility of pregnancy at the time of the first missed period and withhold further use until pregnancy has been ruled out. If pregnancy is confirmed, apprise the patient of the potential risks to the fetus. The majority of recent studies do not indicate a teratogenic effect, particularly cardiac anomalies and limb reduction defects, when OCs are taken inadvertently during early pregnancy.

The use of female sex hormones (eg, estrogens) during early pregnancy may seriously damage the offspring (see the Warning Box in the Estrogens monograph). However, there is no conclusive evidence that OC use is associated with an increase in birth defects when taken inadvertently during early pregnancy. Previously, a few studies reported that OCs might be associated with birth defects, but these findings have not been seen in more recent studies. Nevertheless, do not use during pregnancy unless clearly necessary.

Do not administer OCs to induce withdrawal bleeding as a test for pregnancy.

Do not use OCs during pregnancy to treat threatened or habitual abortion.

Ectopic pregnancy – Ectopic pregnancy, as well as intrauterine pregnancy, may occur in contraceptive failures.

The incidence of ectopic pregnancies for progestin-only OC users is 5 per 1,000 women-years. Up to 10% of pregnancies reported in clinical studies of progestin-only OC users are extrauterine. Although symptoms of ectopic pregnancy should be watched for, a history of ectopic pregnancy need not be considered a contraindication for use of this contraceptive method. Health care providers should be alert to the possibility of an ectopic pregnancy in women who become pregnant or complain of lower abdominal pain while on progestin-only OCs.

➤*Lactation:* Combination OCs given in the postpartum period may interfere with lactation, decreasing the quantity and quality of breast milk. Furthermore, a small amount of OC steroids is excreted in breast milk. A few adverse effects on the breast-feeding infant have been reported, including jaundice and breast enlargement. If possible, defer use until the infant has been weaned; however, in some situations, breast-feeding is the only real alternative (see Administration and Dosage).

Small amounts of progestin pass into the breast milk resulting in steroid levels in infant plasma of 1% to 6% of maternal plasma levels.

➤*Children:* Safety and efficacy has been established in women of reproductive age. Safety and efficacy are expected to be the same for postpubertal adolescents 16 years of age or younger. Use of these products before menarche is not indicated.

Precautions

➤*Monitoring:* It is good medical practice for all women to have annual history and physical examinations, including women using OCs. Physical examination may be deferred until after initiation of OCs if requested by the patient and judged appropriate by the health care provider. The physical exam should evaluate blood pressure, breasts, abdomen, and pelvic organs, including Pap smear. Perform preventative measures (ie, ensure up to date vaccinations) and screening, which should include total and HDL cholesterol within 5-year intervals. Advise the pathologist of OC therapy when relevant specimens are submitted. Do not prescribe for more than 1 year without another physical exam.

➤*Lipid disorders:* Closely follow women taking OCs who are being treated for hyperlipidemias. Some progestins may elevate LDL levels and decrease HDL levels (see Warnings), making hyperlipidemia control more difficult. Consider withholding the OC if the dyslipidemia does not respond (ie, LDL of 190).

HDL and total cholesterol may be increased, LDL may be increased or decreased, while LDL/HDL ratio may be decreased and triglycerides unchanged.

➤*Uterine fibroids:* Pre-existing uterine leiomyomata (uterine fibroids) may increase in size. However, there is no evidence of this with low-dose OCs. In addition, data indicate that the risk of developing uterine fibroids is actually reduced with OC use.

➤*Depression:* The incidence of depression in OC users ranges from less than 5% to 30%. Pyridoxine deficiency may be a factor in the depression. Pyridoxine 25 to 50 mg per day has been recommended. In patients with a history of depression, discontinue if depression recurs to a serious degree. Patients becoming significantly depressed should discontinue medication to determine if the symptom is drug-related.

➤*Fluid retention:* OCs may cause fluid retention; prescribe with caution and monitor patients with conditions that might be aggravated by fluid retention (eg, convulsive disorders; migraine syndrome; asthma; cardiac, hepatic, or renal dysfunction).

➤*Hepatic function:* Patients with a history of jaundice during pregnancy have an increased risk of recurrence of jaundice; if jaundice develops, discontinue use. Steroid hormones may be poorly metabolized in patients with liver dysfunction; administer with caution.

➤*Contact lenses:* Contact lens wearers who develop changes in vision or lens tolerance should be assessed by an ophthalmologist; consider temporary or permanent cessation of wear.

➤*Serum folate levels:* Serum folate levels may be depressed by therapy. Although OCs may impair folate metabolism, the effect is mild and unlikely to cause anemia or megaloblastic changes in women who have a good dietary folate intake. Because the pregnant woman is predisposed to folate deficiency, a woman who becomes pregnant shortly after stopping therapy may have a greater chance of developing folate deficiency and its attendant complications. Folic acid supplements are recommended.

➤*Acute intermittent porphyria:* Estrogens have been reported to precipitate attacks of acute intermittent porphyria; use with caution in susceptible patients.

➤*Vomiting/Diarrhea:* Several cases of OC failure have been reported in association with vomiting or diarrhea. If significant GI disturbance occurs, a backup method of contraception for the remainder of the cycle is recommended.

➤*Sexually transmitted diseases (STDs):* Advise patients that OCs do not protect against HIV infection and other STDs.

➤*Tartrazine sensitivity:* Some of these products contain tartrazine, which may cause allergic-type reactions (including bronchial asthma) in susceptible individuals. Although the incidence of tartrazine sensitivity in the general population is low, it is frequently seen in patients who also have aspirin hypersensitivity. Specific products containing tartrazine are identified in the product listings.

Drug Interactions

Oral Contraceptive Drug Interactions

Precipitant drug	Object drug[a]		Description
Contraceptives, oral	Anticoagulants	↔	Because OCs can increase levels of certain circulating clotting factors and reduce antithrombin III levels, therapeutic efficacy of the anticoagulants may be decreased by OCs. However, both an increased and decreased effect has occurred.
Contraceptives, oral	Antidepressants, tricyclic Beta blockers Caffeine Corticosteroids Theophyllines	↑	The hepatic metabolism of these agents may be decreased by OCs, resulting in increased therapeutic effects or toxicity.
Contraceptives, oral	Benzodiazepines	↑↓	OCs may increase the clearance of the benzodiazepines that undergo glucuronidation (eg, lorazepam, oxazepam, temazepam) because of increased metabolism. Combination OCs with alprazolam, chlordiazepoxide, diazepam, and triazolam may inhibit hepatic mixed-function oxidases leading to a decrease in benzodiazepine oxidation rate (may prolong the half-life of benzodiazepines).
Contraceptives, oral	Cyclosporine	↑	OCs may inhibit the metabolism of cyclosporine, increasing the risk of toxicity. Avoid this combination if possible. If given together, monitor cyclosporine concentrations, as well as renal and hepatic function. Adjust cyclosporine dose as indicated.
Contraceptives, oral	Lamotrigine	↓	OCs may increase lamotrigine metabolism, therefore decreasing the therapeutic effect.
Contraceptives, oral	Selegiline	↑	Coadministration may increase selegiline concentrations because of inhibition of its metabolism.
Antibiotics	Contraceptives, oral	↓	Coadministration of griseofulvin, penicillins, or tetracyclines with OCs may decrease the pharmacologic effects of the OCs, possibly because of altered steroid gut metabolism secondary to changes in the intestinal flora. Menstrual irregularities (eg, spotting, BTB) and pregnancy may occur. An alternate or additional form of birth control may be advisable during concomitant use. OCs and troleandomycin may be associated with an increased risk of intrahepatic cholestasis.
Atorvastatin	Contraceptives, oral	↑	Coadministration increased AUC values for norethindrone and ethinyl estradiol approximately 30% and 20%, respectively.
Barbiturates Carbamazepine Felbamate Griseofulvin Hydantoins[b] Modafinil Oxcarbazepine Phenytoin Protease inhibitors Rifamycins St. John's wort	Contraceptives, oral	↓	These agents may increase the hepatic metabolism of the OCs via hepatic microsomal enzyme induction, possibly resulting in decreased effectiveness of the OC; menstrual irregularities (eg, spotting, BTB) and pregnancy may occur. An alternate or additional form of birth control may be advisable during concomitant use.

[a] ↑ = Object drug increased. ↓ = Object drug decreased. ↔ = Undetermined clinical effect.
[b] Pharmacologic effects of the hydantoins also may be altered.

➤*Drug/Lab test interactions:* Estrogen-containing OCs may cause the following alterations in serum, plasma, or blood, unless specified otherwise.

Increased – Factors I (prothrombin), VII, VIII, IX, X; fibrinogen; norepinephrine-induced platelet aggregation; thyroid-binding globulin (TBG), leading to increased total thyroid hormone (as measured by protein bound iodine, T_4 by column or radioimmunoassay); corticosteroid levels; triglycerides and phospholipids; aldosterone; amylase; gamma-glutamyltranspeptidase; iron-binding capacity; sex-hormone-binding globulins are increased and result in elevated levels of total circulating sex steroids (combination) and corticoids; transferrin; prolactin; renin activity; vitamin A.

Decreased – Antithrombin III; free T_3 resin uptake; response to metyrapone test; folate; glucose tolerance; albumin; cholinesterase; haptoglobin; tissue plasminogen activator; zinc; vitamin B_{12}; sex-hormone-binding globulin, thyroxine caused by decrease in thyroid-binding globulin (progestin-only).

Adverse Reactions

Serious – See Warnings. Arterial thromboembolism; cerebral hemorrhage; cerebral thrombosis; coronary thrombosis; gallbladder disease; hepatic adenomas or benign liver tumors; hypertension; mesenteric thrombosis MI; pulmonary embolism; thrombophlebitis and venous thrombosis with or without embolism.

➤*CNS:* Dizziness; headache; mental depression; migraine.

➤*Dermatologic:* Melasma (may persist); rash (allergic).

➤*Endocrine:* Breast tenderness, enlargement, secretion; diminution in lactation when given immediately postpartum.

ORAL CONTRACEPTIVES

➤*GI:* Abdominal cramps; bloating; cholestatic jaundice; nausea and vomiting (occurring in approximately 10% to 30% of patients during the first cycle, less common with low doses, and the majority resolve in 3 months).

➤*GU:* Amenorrhea during and after treatment; BTB (the majority, more than 80%, resolve in 3 months), spotting, change in menstrual flow; change in cervical erosion and secretions; invasive cervical cancer; temporary infertility after discontinuation; vaginal candidiasis.

➤*Ophthalmic:* Changes in corneal curvature (steepening); contact lens intolerance; neuro-ocular lesions (eg, retinal thrombosis, optic neuritis).

➤*Miscellaneous:* Edema; reduced carbohydrate tolerance; weight change (increase or decrease); prevalence of cervical chlamydia trachomatis may be increased; hirsutism (rare).

The following associations have been neither confirmed nor refuted: acne; acute hepatitis; anemia; Budd-Chiarri syndrome; cataracts; cerebrovascular disease with mitral valve prolapse; changes in appetite; changes in libido; colitis; colonic Crohn disease; cystitis-like syndrome; dizziness; EEG abnormalities; endometrial, cervical, and breast carcinoma (conflicting data; see Warnings); erythema multiforme; erythema nodosum; fatigue; gingivitis; headache; hemolytic uremic syndrome; hemorrhagic eruption; herpes gestationis; hirsutism; itching; loss of scalp hair; lupus erythematosus or lupus-like syndromes; malignant hypertension; malignant melanoma; nervousness; pancreatitis; porphyria; photosensitivity;pituitary tumors; premenstrual syndrome; pulmonary embolism; renal function impairment; rhinitis; sickle cell disease; vaginitis.

➤*Emergency contraceptives:* The most common adverse events in the clinical trial for women receiving emergency contraceptives include the following: abdominal pain/cramps; breast tenderness; diarrhea; dizziness; fatigue; headache; menstrual irregularities; nausea; vomiting.

Overdosage

Serious ill effects have not been reported following acute overdosage of OCs in young children. Overdosage may cause nausea. Withdrawal bleeding may occur in females.

Patient Information

Patient package insert available with product.

To achieve maximum contraceptive effectiveness, inform the patient to take OCs exactly as directed at intervals not exceeding 24 hours, preferably at the same time each day, including throughout all bleeding episodes.Inform the patient to take tablets regularly with a meal or at bedtime. Efficacy depends on strict adherence to the dosage schedule. Missing a pill can cause spotting or light bleeding; the patient may be a little sick to her stomach on the days she takes the missed pill with her regularly scheduled pill. For missed doses, see Administration and Dosage.

Advise the patient to use a backup method (eg, condoms, spermicides) for the following 48 hours whenever a progestin-only OC is taken at least 3 hours late.

If pregnancy is terminated within the first 12 weeks, instruct the patient to start OCs immediately or within 7 days. If pregnancy is terminated after 12 weeks, instruct the patient to start OCs after 2 weeks.

OCs may cause spotting or BTB during the first few months of therapy; if bleeding occurs in more than 1 cycle or lasts more than a few days, advise the patient to notify the health care provider.

Advise the patient to inform the health care provider of prolonged episodes of bleeding, amenorrhea, or severe abdominal pain.

Advise the patient to use an additional method of birth control until after the first week of administration in the initial cycle or for the entire cycle if vomiting or diarrhea occurs.

Inform patients that OCs do not protect against HIV infection and other STDs.

MONOPHASIC ORAL CONTRACEPTIVES

	Product & Distributor	Estrogen (mcg)	Progestin (mg)	How Supplied
Rx	**Necon 1/50** (Watson)	50 mestranol	1 norethindrone	Lactose. (WATSON 510). Lt. blue. In 21s and 28s. With 7 white inert tablets (WATSON P) in the 28s.
Rx	**Norinyl 1 + 50** (Watson)			Lactose. (Watson 265). White. In *Wallette* 28s. With 7 orange inert tablets (Watson P1).
Rx	**Ortho-Novum 1/50** (Ortho-McNeil)			Lactose. (Ortho 150). Yellow. In *Dialpak* 28s. With 7 green inert tablets.
Rx	**Ovcon-50** (Warner Chilcott)	50 ethinyl estradiol	1 norethindrone	Lactose. (MJ 584). Yellow. In 28s. With 7 green, capsule shape inert tablets (MJ 850).
Rx	**Demulen 1/50** (Searle)		1 ethynodiol diacetate	Lactose (inert tablets). (SEARLE 71). White. In *Compack* tablet dispensers of 21s and 28s. With 7 pink inert tablets (SEARLE P) in the 28s.
Rx	**Zovia 1/50E** (Watson)			Lactose. (WATSON 384). Pink. In 21s and 28s. With 7 white inert tablets (WATSON P) in the 28s.
Rx	**Ovral** (Wyeth-Ayerst)		0.5 norgestrel	Lactose. (WYETH 56). White. In *Pilpak* 21s and 28s. With 7 pink inert tablets (WYETH 445) in the 28s.
Rx	**Ogestrel 0.5/50** (Watson)			Lactose. (Watson 848). White. In 28s. With 7 peach inert tablets (Watson P1).
Rx	**Necon 1/35** (Watson)	35 ethinyl estradiol	1 norethindrone	Lactose. (WATSON 508). Dk. yellow. In 21s and 28s. With 7 white inert tablets (WATSON P) in the 28s.
Rx	**Norinyl 1 + 35** (Watson)			Lactose. (WATSON 259). Yellow-green. In *Wallette* 28s. With 7 orange inert tablets (WATSON P1).
Rx	**Nortrel 1/35** (Barr)			Lactose. (b 949). Yellow. In 21s and 28s. With 7 white inert tablets (b 944) in the 28s.
Rx	**Ortho-Novum 1/35** (Ortho-McNeil)			Lactose. (Ortho 135). Peach. In *Dialpak* and *Veridate* 28s. With 7 green inert tablets (Ortho).
Rx	**Brevicon** (Watson)		0.5 norethindrone	Lactose. (Watson 254). Blue. In *Wallette* 28s. With 7 orange inert tablets (Watson P1).
Rx	**Modicon** (Ortho-McNeil)			Lactose. (Ortho 535). White. In *Dialpak* and *Veridate* 28s. With 7 green inert tablets (Ortho).
Rx	**Necon 0.5/35** (Watson)			Lactose. (WATSON 507). Lt. yellow. In 21s and 28s. With 7 white inert tablets (WATSON P) in the 28s.
Rx	**Nortrel 0.5/35** (Barr)			Lactose. (b 941). Lt. yellow. In 21s and 28s. With 7 white inert tablets (b 944) in the 28s.
Rx	**Ovcon-35** (Warner Chilcott)		0.4 norethindrone	Lactose. (MJ 583). Peach. With 7 green capsule shape inert tablets (MJ 850). In 28s.
Rx	**MonoNessa** (Watson)		0.25 norgestimate	(Watson 526). Blue. In 28s.
Rx	**Ortho-Cyclen** (Ortho-McNeil)			Lactose. (Ortho 250). Blue. In *Dialpak* and *Veridate* 28s. With 7 green inert tablets.
Rx	**Sprintec** (Barr)			Lactose. (b 987). Blue. In 28s. With 7 white inert tablets (b 143).
Rx	**Demulen 1/35** (Searle)		1 ethynodiol diacetate	Lactose (inert tablets). (SEARLE 151). White. In *Compack* tablet dispensers of 21s and 28s. With 7 blue inert tablets (SEARLE P) in the 28s.
Rx	**Kelnor 1/35** (Barr)			Lt. yellow. In 28s. With 7 white inert tablets.
Rx	**Zovia 1/35E** (Watson)			Lactose. (WATSON 383). Lt. pink. In 21s and 28s. With 7 white inert tablets (WATSON P) in the 28s.

MONOPHASIC ORAL CONTRACEPTIVES

	Product & Distributor	Estrogen (mcg)	Progestin (mg)	How Supplied
Rx	**Yasmin** (Berlex)	30 ethinyl estradiol	3 drospirenone	Lactose. Yellow. Film-coated. In blister pack 28s. With 7 white inert film-coated tablets.
Rx	**Junel 21 Day 1.5/30** (Barr)		1.5 norethindrone acetate	Lactose, sugar. Pink. In 21s.
Rx	**Junel Fe 1.5/30** (Barr)			Pink. In 28s. With 7 brown tablets (75 mg ferrous fumarate per tablet).
Rx	**Loestrin 21 1.5/30** (Duramed)			Lactose, sugar. Green. In 21s.
Rx	**Loestrin Fe 1.5/30** (Duramed)			Lactose, sugar (active tablets), sucrose (inert tablets). Green. In 28s. With 7 brown tablets (75 mg ferrous fumarate per tablet).
Rx	**Microgestin Fe 1.5/30** (Watson)			Lactose. (WATSON 631). Green. In 28s. With 7 brown tablets (75 mg ferrous fumarate per tablet; WATSON 632).
Rx	**Cryselle** (Barr)		0.3 norgestrel	White. (dp 543). In 21s and 28s. With 7 lt. green inert tablets (dp 331).
Rx	**Lo/Ovral** (Wyeth-Ayerst)			Lactose. (Wyeth 78). White. In *Pilpak* 21s and 28s. With 7 pink inert tablets (Wyeth 486) in the 28s.
Rx	**Low-Ogestrel** (Watson)			Lactose. (WATSON 847). White. In 28s. With 7 peach inert tablets (WATSON P1).
Rx	**Apri** (Barr)		0.15 desogestrel	Lactose. (dp 575). Rose. In blister card 28s. With 7 white inert tablets (dp 570).
Rx	**Desogen** (Organon)			Lactose. (Organon T_5R). White. In 28s. With 7 green inert tablets (Organon K_2H).
Rx	**Ortho-Cept** (Ortho-McNeil)			Lactose. Orange. In *Dialpak* and *Veridate* 28s. With 7 green inert tablets.
Rx	**Reclipsen** (Watson)			Lactose. (WATSON 954). White. In 28s, including 7 green, inert tablets (WATSON P).
Rx	**Levlen** (Berlex)		0.15 levonorgestrel	Lactose . (B 28). Lt. orange. In slidecase dispenser with 7 pink inert tablets.
Rx	**Levora** (Watson)			Lactose. (15/30 WATSON). White. In 28s. With 7 peach inert tablets (WATSON P1).
Rx	**Nordette-28** (Barr/Duramed)			Lactose. (WYETH 75). Lt. orange. In 28s. With 7 pink inert tablets (WYETH 486).
Rx	**Portia** (Barr)			Lactose. (b 992). Pink. Film-coated. In 21s and 28s. With 7 white inert tablets (b 208) in the 28s.
Rx	**Seasonale**[a] (Duramed)			Lactose. (S 62). Pink. Film-coated. In 91s with 7 white inert tablets (S 197).
Rx	**YAZ** (Berlex)	20 ethinyl estradiol	3 mg drospirenone	Lactose. (DS). Lt. pink, hexagon. Film-coated. In 24s. With 4 white, hexagon, inert tablets (DP). In blister pack 3s.
Rx	**Alesse** (Wyeth-Ayerst)		0.1 levonorgestrel	Lactose. (W 912). Pink. In 28s. With 7 lt. green inert tablets (W 650).
Rx	**Aviane** (Barr)			Lactose. (dp 016). Orange. In 28s. With 7 lt. green inert tablets (dp 519).
Rx	**Lessina** (Barr)			Lactose. (b 965). Pink. Film-coated. In 21s and 28s. With 7 white inert tablets (b 208) in the 28s.
Rx	**Levlite** (Berlex)			Lactose, sucrose. (B 22). Pink. In slidecase dispensers of 28s. With 7 white inert tablets (B 29).
Rx	**Lutera** (Watson)			Lactose. (WATSON 949). White. In 28s. With 7 peach inert tablets (WATSON P1).
Rx	**Junel 21 Day 1/20** (Barr)		1 norethindrone acetate	Lactose, sugar. Lt. yellow. In 21s.
Rx	**Junel Fe 1/20** (Barr)			Lt. yellow. In 28s. With 7 brown tablets (75 mg ferrous fumarate per tablet).
Rx	**Loestrin 21 1/20** (Duramed)			Lactose, sugar. White. In 21s.
Rx	**Loestrin Fe 1/20** (Duramed)			Lactose, sugar (active tablets), sucrose (inert tablets). White. In 28s. With 7 brown tablets (75 mg ferrous fumarate per tablet).
Rx	**Microgestin Fe 1/20** (Watson)			Lactose. (WATSON 630). White. In 28s. With 7 brown tablets (75 mg ferrous fumarate per tablet; WATSON 632).
Rx	**Kariva**[b] (Barr)	20 ethinyl estradiol (white tablets)/10 ethinyl estradiol (lt. blue tablets)	0.15 desogestrel (white tablets only)	Lactose. 21 white tablets (021) and 5 lt. blue tablets (022). In blister card 28s. With 2 lt. green inert tablets (331).
Rx	**Mircette**[c] (Organon)	20 ethinyl estradiol (white tablets)/10 ethinyl estradiol (yellow tablets)	0.15 desogestrel (white tablets only)	Lactose. 21 white tablets (T_4R Organon) and 5 yellow tablets (K_2S Organon). In blister card 28s. With 2 green inert tablets (K_2H Organon).
Rx	**Solia** (Prasco)	30 ethinyl estradiol	0.15 desogestrel	Lactose. 21 white tablets (T_5R Prasco). In blister card 28s. With 7 green inert tablets (K_2H Prasco).

[a] Take 1 pink (active) tablet per day for 84 consecutive days, followed by 7 days of white (inert) tablets.
[b] Take 1 white tablet daily for 21 days, followed by 1 light-green (inert) tablet daily for 2 days and 1 light-blue (active) tablet daily for 5 days.
[c] Take 1 white tablet daily for 21 days, followed by 1 green (inert) tablet daily for 2 days and 1 yellow (active) tablet daily for 5 days.

MONOPHASIC ORAL CONTRACEPTIVES

For complete and comparative prescribing information, refer to the Oral Contraceptives group monograph. The combination therapy products are listed in order of decreasing estrogen content.

BIPHASIC ORAL CONTRACEPTIVES

	Product	*Phase 1*	*Phase 2*	How Supplied
Rx	**Necon 10/11** (Watson)	0.5 mg norethindrone, 35 mcg ethinyl estradiol (10 lt. yellow tablets)	1 mg norethindrone, 35 mcg ethinyl estradiol (11 dk. yellow tablets)	Lactose. Lt. yellow = (WATSON 507). Dk. yellow = (WATSON 508). In 28s with 7 white inert tablets (WATSON P).
Rx	**Ortho-Novum 10/11** (Ortho-McNeil)	0.5 mg norethindrone, 35 mcg ethinyl estradiol (10 white tablets)	1 mg norethindrone, 35 mcg ethinyl estradiol (11 peach tablets)	Lactose. White = (Ortho 535). Peach = (Ortho 135). In *Dialpak* 28s. With 7 green inert tablets (Ortho).

BIPHASIC ORAL CONTRACEPTIVES

For complete and comparative prescribing information, refer to the Oral Contraceptives group monograph. The combination therapy products are listed in order of decreasing estrogen content.

TRIPHASIC ORAL CONTRACEPTIVES

	Product	Phase 1	Phase 2	Phase 3	How Supplied
Rx	**Tri-Norinyl** (Watson)	0.5 mg norethindrone, 35 mcg ethinyl estradiol (7 blue tablets)	1 mg norethindrone, 35 mcg ethinyl estradiol (9 yellow-green tablets)	0.5 mg norethindrone, 35 mcg ethinyl estradiol (5 blue tablets)	Lactose. Blue = (Watson 254). Yellow-green = (Watson 259). In *Wallette* 28s. With 7 orange inert tablets (Watson P1).
Rx	**Aranelle** (Barr)	0.5 mg norethindrone, 35 mcg ethinyl estradiol (7 lt. yellow tablets)	1 mg norethindrone, 35 mcg ethinyl estradiol (9 white tablets)	0.5 mg norethindrone, 35 mcg ethinyl estradiol (5 lt. yellow tablets)	Lactose. Lt. yellow = (b 341). White = (b 342). Peach = (b 343). Beveled. In 28s. With 7 peach inert tablets.
Rx	**Leena** (Watson)	0.5 mg norethindrone, 35 mcg ethinyl estradiol (7 lt. blue tablets)	1 mg norethindrone, 35 mcg ethinyl estradiol (9 lt. yellow-green tablets)	0.5 mg norethindrone, 35 mcg ethinyl estradiol (5 lt. blue tablets)	Lactose. Lt. blue = (Watson 243). Lt yellow-green = (Watson 244). Peach = (Watson P1). In 28s. With 7 orange inert tablets.
Rx	**Necon 7/7/7** (Watson)	0.5 mg norethindrone, 35 mcg ethinyl estradiol (7 white tablets)	0.75 mg norethindrone, 35 mcg ethinyl estradiol (7 lt. peach tablets)	1 mg norethindrone, 35 mcg ethinyl estradiol (7 peach tablets)	In 28s. With 7 green inert tablets.
Rx	**Ortho-Novum 7/7/7** (Ortho-McNeil)				Lactose. White = (Ortho 535). Lt. peach = (Ortho 75). Peach = (Ortho 135). In *Dialpak* and *Veridate* 28s. With 7 green inert tablets (Ortho).
Rx	**Enpresse** (Barr)	0.05 mg levonorgestrel, 30 mcg ethinyl estradiol (6 pink tablets)	0.075 mg levonorgestrel, 40 mcg ethinyl estradiol (5 white tablets)	0.125 mg levonorgestrel, 30 mcg ethinyl estradiol (10 orange tablets)	Lactose. Pink = (dp 510). White = (dp 511). Orange = (dp 512). In 28s. With 7 lt. green inert tablets (dp 519).
Rx	**Tri-Levlen** (Berlex)	0.05 mg levonorgestrel, 30 mcg ethinyl estradiol (6 brown tablets)	0.075 mg levonorgestrel, 40 mcg ethinyl estradiol (5 white tablets)	0.125 mg levonorgestrel, 30 mcg ethinyl estradiol (10 lt. yellow tablets)	Lactose. Brown = (B 95). Film-coated. White to off-white = (B 96). Film-coated. Lt. yellow = (B 97). Film-coated. In slidecase dispenser 28s. With 7 lt. green film-coated inert tablets (B 11).
Rx	**Triphasil** (Wyeth Labs)				Lactose. Brown = (W 641). White = (W 642). Lt. yellow = (W 643). In 21s and 28s. With 7 lt. green inert tablets (W 650) in the 28s.
Rx	**Trivora** (Watson)	0.05 mg levonorgestrel, 30 mcg ethinyl estradiol (6 blue tablets)	0.075 mg levonorgestrel, 40 mcg ethinyl estradiol (5 white tablets)	0.125 mg levonorgestrel, 30 mcg ethinyl estradiol (10 pink tablets)	Lactose. Blue, white, and pink tablets. In 28s. With 7 peach inert tablets (WATSON P1).
Rx	**Cyclessa** (Organon)	0.1 mg desogestrel, 25 mcg ethinyl estradiol (7 lt. yellow tablets)	0.125 mg desogestrel, 25 mcg ethinyl estradiol (7 orange tablets)	0.15 mg desogestrel, 25 mcg ethinyl estradiol (7 red tablets)	Lactose, talc. Lt. yellow = (T_0R Organon). Orange = (T_6R Organon). Red = (T_1R Organon). In 28s. With 7 green inert tablets (K_2H Organon).
Rx	**Cesla** (Prasco)				Lactose, talc (lt. yellow, orange, green). Lt. yellow = (T_0R Organon). Orange = (T_6R Organon). Red = (T_1R Organon). Green = (K_2H Organon). With 7 green inert tablets. In 28s.
Rx	**Velivet** (Barr)	0.1 mg desogestrel, 25 mcg ethinyl estradiol (7 beige tablets)	0.125 mg desogestrel, 25 mcg ethinyl estradiol (7 orange tablets)	0.15 mg desogestrel, 25 mcg ethinyl estradiol (7 pink tablets)	With 7 white inert tablets. (b 334). In 28s.
Rx	**Ortho Tri-Cyclen** (Ortho-McNeil)	0.18 mg norgestimate, 35 mcg ethinyl estradiol (7 white tablets)	0.215 mg norgestimate, 35 mcg ethinyl estradiol (7 lt. blue tablets)	0.25 mg norgestimate, 35 mcg ethinyl estradiol (7 blue tablets)	Lactose. White = (Ortho 180). Lt. blue = (Ortho 215). Blue = (Ortho 250). In *Dialpak* and *Veridate* 28s. With 7 green inert tablets.
Rx	**Tri-Previfem** (Teva)				Lactose. White = (746). Lt. blue = (747). Blue = (748). In 28s. With 7 teal inert tablets.
Rx	**TriNessa** (Watson)				With 7 green inert tablets. In 28s.
Rx	**Tri-Sprintec** (Barr)	0.18 mg norgestimate, 35 mcg ethinyl estradiol (7 gray tablets)	0.215 mg norgestimate, 35 mcg ethinyl estradiol (7 lt. blue tablets)	0.25 mg norgestimate, 35 mcg ethinyl estradiol (7 blue tablets)	Lactose. Gray = (b 985). Lt. blue = (b 986). Blue = (b 987). White = (b 143). With 7 white inert tablets. In 28s.
Rx	**Ortho Tri-Cyclen Lo** (Ortho-McNeil)	0.18 mg norgestimate, 25 mcg ethinyl estradiol (7 white tablets)	0.215 mg norgestimate, 25 mcg ethinyl estradiol (7 lt. blue tablets)	0.25 mg norgestimate, 25 mcg ethinyl estradiol (7 dk. blue tablets)	Talc (green inert tablets), lactose. White = (O-M 180). Lt. blue = (O-M 215). Dk. blue = (O-M 250). In *Dialpak* and *Veridate* 28s. With 7 green inert tablets.
Rx	**Estrostep 21** (Pfizer)	1 mg norethindrone acetate, 20 mcg ethinyl estradiol (5 triangular tablets)	1 mg norethindrone acetate, 30 mcg ethinyl estradiol (7 square tablets)	1 mg norethindrone acetate, 35 mcg ethinyl estradiol (9 round tablets)	Lactose. White. In 21s.
Rx	**Estrostep Fe** (Warner Chilcott)	1 mg norethindrone acetate, 20 mcg ethinyl estradiol (5 triangular tablets)	1 mg norethindrone acetate, 30 mcg ethinyl estradiol (7 square tablets)	1 mg norethindrone acetate, 35 mcg ethinyl estradiol (9 round tablets)	Lactose (white), sucrose (brown). White. In 28s. With 7 brown tablets (75 mg ferrous fumarate per tablet).

TRIPHASIC ORAL CONTRACEPTIVES

For complete and comparative prescribing information, refer to the Oral Contraceptives group monograph. The combination therapy products are listed in order of decreasing estrogen content.

PROGESTIN-ONLY PRODUCTS

	Product	Tablets	How Supplied
Rx	**Camila** (Barr)	**Tablets:** 0.35 mg norethindrone	Lactose. (b 715). Lt. pink. In 28s.
Rx	**Errin** (Barr)		Lactose. (b 344). Yellow. In 28s.
Rx	**Jolivette** (Watson)		Lactose. (WATSON 892). Green. In 28s.
Rx	**Nor-QD** (Watson)		Lactose. Yellow. In 28s.
Rx	**Nora-BE** (Watson)		Lactose. (Watson 020). White. In 28s.
Rx	**Ortho Micronor** (Ortho-McNeil)		Lactose. Green. In *Dialpak* 28s.
Rx	**Ovrette** (Wyeth-Ayerst)	**Tablets:** 0.075 mg norgestrel	Tartrazine, lactose. (WYETH 62). Yellow. In *Pilpak* 28s.

NORETHINDRONE — ORAL

For complete and comparative prescribing information, refer to the Oral Contraceptives group monograph.

Indications

➤*Contraception:* Progestin-only oral contraceptives (OCs) are indicated for the prevention of pregnancy.

Administration and Dosage

To achieve maximum contraceptive effectiveness, norethindrone must be taken exactly as directed. One tablet is taken every day, at the same time. Administration is continuous, with no interruption between pill packs.

➤*Storage/Stability:* Store at controlled room temperature 25°C (77°F); excursions permitted to 15° to 30°C (59° to 86°F).

NORGESTREL — ORAL

For complete and comparative prescribing information, refer to the Oral Contraceptives group monograph.

Indications

➤*Contraception:* Oral contraceptives (OCs) are indicated for the prevention of pregnancy in women who elect to use this product as a method of contraception.

Administration and Dosage

➤*Dosage regimen:* To achieve maximum contraceptive effectiveness, norgestrel must be taken exactly as directed and at intervals not exceeding 24 hours.

Norgestrel is administered on a continuous daily-dosage regimen starting on the first day of menstruation (ie, 1 tablet each day, every day of the year).

NORGESTREL — ORAL

Tablets should be taken at the same time each day and continued daily, without interruption, whether bleeding occurs or not. The patient should be advised that, if prolonged bleeding occurs, she should consult her physician. In the nonlactating mother, norgestrel may be initiated postpartum for contraception. When the tablets are administered in the postpartum period, the increased risk of thromboembolic disease associated with the postpartum period must be considered.

➤*Missed dose:* The risk of pregnancy increases with each tablet missed. If the patient misses 1 tablet, she should be instructed to take it as soon as she remembers and to also take her next tablet at the regular time. If she misses 2 tablets, she should take 1 of the missed tablets as soon as she remembers, as well as taking her regular tablet for that day at the proper time. Furthermore, she should use a method of nonhormonal contraception in addition to taking norgestrel until 14 tablets have been taken. If more than 2 tablets have been missed, norgestrel should be discontinued immediately and a method of nonhormonal contraception should be used until menses has appeared or pregnancy has been excluded. If menses does not appear within 45 days from the last period, a method of nonhormonal contraception should be substituted until the start of the next menstrual period or an appropriate diagnostic procedure is performed to rule out pregnancy.

➤*Switching pills:* If switching from the combined pills to progestin-only pills (POPs), take the first POP the day after the last active combined pill is finished. So not take any of the 7 inactive pills from the combined pill pack. Many women have irregular periods after switching to POPs; this is normal and to be expected. If switching from POPs to the combined pills, take the first active combined pill on the first day of menses, even if the POP pack is not finished. If switching to another brand of POPs, start the new brand any time. If breastfeeding, switch to another method of birth control at any time, except do not switch to the combined pills until breastfeeding is stopped or until at least 6 months after delivery.

➤*Missed menstrual period:* If the patient has not adhered to the prescribed dosage regimen, consider possible pregnancy after the first missed period; withhold OCs until ruling out pregnancy. If the patient has adhered to the prescribed regimen and misses 2 consecutive periods, rule out pregnancy before continuing the contraceptive regimen.

➤*Cessation of menstrual flow:* After several months of treatment, menstrual flow may reduce to a point of virtual absence. This reduced flow may occur as a result of medication, and is not indicative of a pregnancy.

➤*Postpartum administration:* Postpartum administration in non-breast-feeding mothers may begin at the first postpartum examination (4 to 6 weeks), regardless of whether spontaneous menstruation has occurred. The possibility of ovulation and conception prior to initiation of medication should be considered. Also, start no earlier than 4 to 6 weeks after a midtrimester pregnancy termination. Immediate postpartum use is associated with increased risk of thromboembolism. If possible, nursing mothers should defer taking OCs until the infant is weaned.

If fully breast-feeding (not giving baby any food or formula), start pills 6 weeks after delivery. If partially breast-feeding (giving baby some food or formula), start taking pills by 3 weeks after delivery.

EMERGENCY CONTRACEPTIVES

Rx	**Plan B** (Duramed)	**Tablets:** 0.75 mg levonorgestrel	Lactose. (INOR). White. In blister packages of 2.
Rx	**Preven** (Gynétics)	**Tablets:** 0.25 mg levonorgestrel, 0.05 mg ethinyl estradiol	Lactose. (G 891). Blue. Film-coated. In blister packages of 4s.[a]

[a] Also available in a kit that contains a pregnancy test.

LEVONORGESTREL/ETHINYL ESTRADIOL EMERGENCY CONTRACEPTIVE — ORAL

Indications

➤*Emergency contraception:* For prevention of pregnancy following unprotected intercourse or a known or suspected contraceptive failure. To obtain optimal efficacy, the first dose should be taken as soon as possible within 72 hours of intercourse. The second dose must be taken 12 hours later.

Administration and Dosage

The emergency contraceptive kit contains a pregnancy test. This test can be used to verify an existing pregnancy resulting from intercourse that occurred earlier in the current menstrual cycle or in the previous cycle. If a positive pregnancy result is obtained, advise the patient not to take the pills in the kit.

The patient should take 2 tablets as soon as possible within 72 hours after unprotected intercourse. She should take the second dose of 2 tablets 12 hours later. Emergency contraception can be used at any time during the menstrual cycle.

Instruct the user that if vomiting occurs within 1 hour of taking either dose of medication, to contact her health care professional to discuss whether or not to repeat that dose or take an antinausea medication.

Emergency contraceptive pills are not indicated for ongoing pregnancy protection and should not be used as a woman's routine form of contraception. Emergency contraceptives are not effective in terminating an existing pregnancy.

➤*Storage/Stability:* Store at 25°C (77°F); excursions permitted to 15° to 30°C (59° to 86°F).

LEVONORGESTREL — ORAL

Indications

➤*Emergency contraception:* Levonorgestrel tablets are intended to prevent pregnancy after known or suspected contraceptive failure or unprotected intercourse. Emergency contraceptive pills (like all oral contraceptives) do not protect against infection with HIV (the virus that causes AIDS) and other sexually transmitted diseases.

Levonorgestrel is an emergency contraceptive that can be used to prevent pregnancy following unprotected intercourse or a known or suspected contraceptive failure. To obtain optimal efficacy, the first tablet should be taken as soon as possible within 72 hours of intercourse. The second tablet must be taken 12 hours later.

Administration and Dosage

➤*Approved by the FDA:* July 28, 1999.

One tablet of levonorgestrel should be taken orally within 72 hours after unprotected intercourse. The second tablet should be taken 12 hours after the first dose. Efficacy is better if levonorgestrel is taken as directed as soon as possible after unprotected intercourse. Levonorgestrel can be used at any time during the menstrual cycle.

The user should be instructed that if she vomits within 1 hour of taking either dose of medication she should contact her healthcare professional to discuss whether to repeat that dose.

➤*Storage/Stability:* Store levonorgestrel tablets at 25°C (77°F); excursions permitted to 15° to 30°C (59° to 86°F). [See USP Controlled Room Temperature.]

NORELGESTROMIN/ETHINYL ESTRADIOL TRANSDERMAL SYSTEM

	Product	Release Rate	Surface Area (cm^2)	Total Content	How Supplied
Rx	**Ortho Evra** (Ortho-McNeil)	0.15 mg norelgestromin, 0.02 mg ethinyl estradiol/24 h	20	6 mg norelgestromin, 0.75 mg ethinyl estradiol/patch	In cycles (3 patches) and single patches.

NORELGESTROMIN/ETHINYL ESTRADIOL — TRANSDERMAL SYSTEM

WARNING

Cigarette smoking increases the risk of serious cardiovascular side effects from hormonal contraceptive use. This risk increases with age and with heavy smoking (at least 15 cigarettes daily) and is quite marked in women older than 35 years of age. Strongly advise women who use hormonal contraceptives, including the norelgestromin/ethinyl estradiol transdermal patch, not to smoke.

Indications

➤*Contraception:* For prevention of pregnancy.

Administration and Dosage

➤*Approved by the FDA:* November 20, 2001.

➤*Use:* This system uses a 28-day (4-week) cycle. A new patch is applied each week for 3 weeks (21 days total). Week 4 is patch-free. Withdrawal bleeding is expected to begin during this time.

Apply every new patch on the same day of the week. This day is known as the "Patch Change Day." For example, if the first patch is applied on a Monday, apply all subsequent patches on a Monday. Wear only 1 patch at a time.

On the day after week 4 ends, a new 4-week cycle is started by applying a new patch. Under no circumstances should there be more than a 7 day patch-free interval between dosing cycles.

The patient must choose 1 option –

First day start: For first day start, the woman should apply her first patch during the first 24 hours of her menstrual period.

If therapy starts after day 1 of the menstrual cycle, a nonhormonal back-up contraceptive (eg, condoms, spermicide, diaphragm) should be used concurrently for the first 7 consecutive days of the first treatment cycle.

NORELGESTROMIN/ETHINYL ESTRADIOL — TRANSDERMAL SYSTEM

Sunday start: For Sunday start, the woman should apply her first patch on the first Sunday after her menstrual period starts. She must use back-up contraception for the first week of her first cycle.

If the menstrual period begins on a Sunday, the first patch should be applied on that day and no back-up contraception is needed.

➤*Application:* Apply the patch to clean, dry, intact, healthy skin on the buttock, abdomen, upper outer arm, or upper torso in a place where it will not be rubbed by tight clothing. The patch should not be placed on skin that is red, irritated, or cut, nor should it be placed on the breasts.

To prevent interference with the adhesive properties of the patch, no makeup, creams, lotions, powders, or other topical products should be applied to the skin area where the patch is or will be placed.

Patch changes may occur at any time on the change day. Apply each new patch to a new spot on the skin to help avoid irritation, although they may be kept within the same anatomic area.

➤*If a patch is partially or completely detached:*

For less than 1 day (up to 24 hours) – The woman should try to reapply it to the same place or replace it with a new patch immediately. No back-up contraception is needed. The woman's "patch change day" will remain the same.

For more than 1 day (≥ 24 hours) or if the woman is not sure how long the patch has been detached – The woman may not be protected from pregnancy. She should stop the current contraceptive cycle and start a new cycle immediately by applying a new patch. There is now a new "day 1" and a new "patch change day." Back-up contraception (eg, condoms, spermicide, diaphragm) must be used for the first week of the new cycle. A patch should not be reapplied if it is no longer sticky, if it has become stuck to itself or another surface, if it has other material stuck to it, or if it has previously become loose or fallen off. If a patch cannot be reapplied, a new patch should be applied immediately. Supplemental adhesives or wraps should not be used to hold the patch in place.

➤*If the woman forgets to change her patch:*

At the start of any patch cycle (week 1/day 1) – She may not be protected from pregnancy. She should apply the first patch of her new cycle as soon as she remembers. There is now a new "patch change day" and a new "day 1." The woman must use back-up contraception (eg, condoms, spermicide, diaphragm) for the first week of the new cycle.

In the middle of the patch cycle (week 2/day 8 or week 3/day 15) –

For 1 or 2 days (up to 48 hours): She should apply a new patch immediately. The next patch should be applied on the usual "patch change day." No back-up contraception is needed.

For more than 2 days (≥ 48 hours): She may not be protected from pregnancy. She should stop the current contraceptive cycle and start a new 4-week cycle immediately by putting on a new patch. There is now a new "patch change day" and a new "day 1." The woman must use back-up contraception for 1 week.

At the end of the patch cycle (week 4/day 22) – If the woman forgets to remove her patch, she should take it off as soon as she remembers. The next cycle should be started on the usual "patch change day," which is the day after day 28. No back-up contraception is needed. Under no circumstances should there be more than a 7-day patch-free interval between cycles. If there are more than 7 patch-free days, the woman may not be protected from pregnancy and back-up contraception (eg, condoms, spermicide, diaphragm) must be used for 7 days. As with combined oral contraceptives, the risk of ovulation increases with each day beyond the recommended drug-free period. If intercourse has occurred during such an extended patch-free interval, the possibility of fertilization should be considered.

➤*Change day adjustment:* If the woman wishes to change her patch change day, she should complete her current cycle, removing the third patch on the correct day. During the patch-free week, she may select an earlier patch change day by applying a new patch on the desired day. In no case should there be more than 7 consecutive patch-free days.

➤*Switching from an oral contraceptive:* Treatment with the norelgestromin/ethinyl estradiol transdermal patch should begin on the first day of withdrawal bleeding. If there is no withdrawal bleeding within 5 days of the last active (hormone-containing) tablet, pregnancy must be ruled out. If therapy starts later than the first day of withdrawal bleeding, a nonhormonal contraceptive should be used concurrently for 7 days. If more than 7 days elapse after taking the last active oral contraceptive tablet, the possibility of ovulation and conception should be considered.

➤*Use after childbirth:* Women who elect not to breastfeed should start contraceptive therapy with the norelgestromin/ethinyl estradiol transdermal patch no sooner than 4 weeks after childbirth. If a woman begins using the patch postpartum and has not yet had a period, the possibility of ovulation and conception occurring prior to use of the patch should be considered, and she should be instructed to use an additional method of contraception (eg, condoms, diaphragm, spermicide) for the first 7 days.

➤*Use after abortion or miscarriage:* After an abortion or miscarriage that occurs in the first trimester, the patch may be started immediately. An additional method of contraception is not needed if the patch is started immediately. If use of the patch is not started within 5 days following a first trimester abortion, the woman should follow the instructions for a woman starting the patch for the first time. In the meantime, she should be advised to use a nonhormonal contraceptive method. Ovulation may occur within 10 days after an abortion or miscarriage.

The patch should be started no earlier than 4 weeks after a second trimester abortion or miscarriage. When the patch is used postpartum or postabortion, the increased risk of thromboembolic disease must be considered.

➤*Breakthrough bleeding or spotting:* In the event of breakthrough bleeding or spotting (bleeding that occurs on the days that the patch is worn), continue treatment. If breakthrough bleeding persists longer than a few cycles, a cause other than the patch should be considered.

In the event of no withdrawal bleeding (bleeding that should occur during the patch-free week), treatment should be resumed on the next scheduled change day. If the patch has been used correctly, the absence of withdrawal bleeding is not necessarily an indication of pregnancy. Nevertheless, the possibility of pregnancy should be considered, especially if absence of withdrawal bleeding occurs in 2 consecutive cycles. Discontinue the patch if pregnancy is confirmed.

➤*Skin irritation:* If patch use results in uncomfortable irritation, the patch may be removed and a new patch may be applied to a different location until the next change day. Only 1 patch should be worn at a time.

➤*Missed menstrual period:* If the woman has not adhered to the prescribed schedule, the possibility of pregnancy should be considered at the time of the first missed period. Discontinue hormonal contraceptive use if pregnancy is confirmed.

If the woman has adhered to the prescribed regimen and misses 1 period, she should continue using her contraceptive patches.

If the woman has adhered to the prescribed regimen and misses 2 consecutive periods, pregnancy should be ruled out. Discontinue use of the patch if pregnancy is confirmed.

➤*Storage/Stability:* Store at 25°C (77°F); excursions permitted to 15° to 30°C (59° to 86°F). Store patches in their protective pouches. Apply immediately upon removal from the protective pouch. Do not store in the refrigerator or freezer. Used patches still contain some active hormones. Each patch should be carefully folded in half so that it sticks to itself before throwing it away.

Actions

➤*Pharmacology:* Norelgestromin is the active progestin largely responsible for the progestational activity that occurs in women following application of norelgestromin/ethinyl estradiol transdermal patch. Norelgestromin also is the primary active metabolite produced following oral administration of norgestimate.

Combination oral contraceptives act by suppression of gonadotropins. Although the primary mechanism of this action is inhibition of ovulation, other alterations include changes in the cervical mucus (which increases the difficulty of sperm entry into the uterus) and the endometrium (which reduces the likelihood of implantation).

Receptor and human sex hormone-binding globulin (SHBG) binding studies, as well as studies in animals and humans, have shown that norgestimate and norelgestromin exhibit high progestational activity with minimal intrinsic androgenicity. Transdermally administered norelgestromin, in combination with ethinyl estradiol, does not counteract the estrogen-induced increases in SHBG, resulting in lower levels of free testosterone in serum compared with baseline.

➤*Pharmacokinetics:*

Absorption – Following application of the product, norelgestromin and ethinyl estradiol rapidly appear in the serum, reach a plateau by approximately 48 hours, and are maintained at an approximate steady state throughout the wear period. C_{ss} for norelgestromin and ethinyl estradiol during 1 week of patch wear are approximately 0.6 to 0.8 ng/mL and 40 to 50 pg/mL, respectively, and are generally consistent from all studies and application sites.

Distribution – Norelgestromin and norgestrel (a serum metabolite of norelgestromin) are highly bound (more than 97%) to serum proteins. Norelgestromin is bound to albumin and not to SHBG, while norgestrel is bound primarily to SHBG, which limits its biological activity. Ethinyl estradiol is extensively bound to serum albumin.

Metabolism – Because the patch is applied transdermally, first-pass metabolism (via the GI tract or liver) of norelgestromin and ethinyl estradiol that would be expected with oral administration is avoided. Hepatic metabolism of norelgestromin occurs and metabolites include norgestrel, which is highly bound to SHBG, and various hydroxylated and conjugated metabolites. Ethinyl estradiol also is metabolized to various hydroxylated products and their glucuronide and sulfate conjugates.

Excretion – Following removal of patches, the elimination kinetics of norelgestromin and ethinyl estradiol were consistent for all studies with half-life values of approximately 28 hours and 17 hours, respectively. The metabolites of norelgestromin and ethinyl estradiol are eliminated by renal and fecal pathways.

Special populations – The effects of age, body weight, and body surface area on the pharmacokinetics of norelgestromin and ethinyl estradiol were evaluated. For norelgestromin and ethinyl estradiol, increasing age, body weight, and body surface area each were associated with slight decreases in C_{ss} and AUC values. However, only a small fraction (10% to 25%) of the overall variability in the pharmacokinetics of norelgestromin and ethinyl estradiol following application of the norelgestromin/ethinyl estradiol transdermal patch may be associated with any or all of the above demographic parameters.

NORELGESTROMIN/ETHINYL ESTRADIOL — TRANSDERMAL SYSTEM

Contraindications

Thrombophlebitis; thromboembolic disorders; history of deep vein thrombophlebitis or thromboembolic disorders; cerebrovascular or coronary artery disease (current or history); valvular heart disease with complications; severe hypertension; diabetes with vascular involvement; headaches with focal neurological symptoms; major surgery with prolonged immobilization; known or suspected carcinoma of the breast or personal history of breast cancer; carcinoma of the endometrium or other known or suspected estrogen-dependent neoplasia; undiagnosed abnormal genital bleeding; cholestatic jaundice of pregnancy or jaundice with prior hormonal contraceptive use; acute or chronic hepatocellular disease with abnormal liver function; hepatic adenomas or carcinomas; known or suspected pregnancy; hypersensitivity to any component of the product.

Warnings

➤*Thromboembolic disorders and other vascular problems:*

Thromboembolism – An increased risk of thromboembolic and thrombotic disease associated with the use of hormonal contraceptives is well established. Case control studies have found the relative risk of users compared with nonusers to be 3 for the first episode of superficial venous thrombosis, 4 to 11 for deep vein thrombosis or pulmonary embolism, and 1.5 to 6 for women with predisposing conditions for venous thromboembolic disease. Cohort studies have shown the relative risk to be somewhat lower, approximately 3 for new cases and approximately 4.5 for new cases requiring hospitalization. The risk of thromboembolic disease associated with hormonal contraceptives is not related to length of use and disappears after hormonal contraceptive use is stopped. A 2- to 4-fold increase in relative risk of postoperative thromboembolic complications has been reported with the use of hormonal contraceptives. The relative risk of venous thrombosis in women who have predisposing conditions is twice that of women without such medical conditions. If feasible, hormonal contraceptives should be discontinued at least 4 weeks prior to and for 2 weeks after elective surgery of a type associated with an increase in risk of thromboembolism and during and following prolonged immobilization. Since the immediate postpartum period is also associated with an increased risk of thromboembolism, hormonal contraceptives should be started no earlier than 4 weeks after delivery in women who elect not to breastfeed.

In large clinical trials (n = 3,330 with 1,704 women-years of exposure), 1 case of nonfatal pulmonary embolism occurred during norelgestromin/ethinyl estradiol transdermal patch use, and 1 case of postoperative nonfatal pulmonary embolism also was reported with use of the patch. It is unknown if the risk of venous thromboembolism with norelgestromin/ethinyl estradiol transdermal patch use is different than with use of combination oral contraceptives.

As with any combination hormonal contraceptives, the clinician should be alert to the earliest manifestations of thrombotic disorders (thrombophlebitis, pulmonary embolism, cerebrovascular disorders, and retinal thrombosis). Should any of these occur or be suspected, discontinue norelgestromin/ethinyl estradiol transdermal patch use immediately.

MI – An increased risk of MI has been attributed to hormonal contraceptive use. This risk is primarily in smokers or women with other underlying risk factors for coronary artery disease (eg, hypertension, hypercholesterolemia, morbid obesity, diabetes). The relative risk of heart attack for current hormonal contraceptive users has been estimated to be 2 to 6, compared with nonusers. The risk is very low under 30 years of age.

Smoking in combination with oral contraceptive use has been shown to contribute substantially to the incidence of MIs in women in their mid-30s or older, with smoking accounting for the majority of excess cases. Mortality rates associated with circulatory disease have been shown to increase substantially in smokers, especially in those at least 35 years of age among women who use oral contraceptives.

Hormonal contraceptives may compound the effects of well-known risk factors (eg, hypertension, diabetes, hyperlipidemias, age, obesity). In particular, some progestins are known to decrease high density lipoprotein (HDL) cholesterol and cause glucose intolerance, while estrogens may create a state of hyperinsulinism. Hormonal contraceptives have been shown to increase blood pressure among some users. Similar effects on risk factors have been associated with an increased risk of heart disease. Hormonal contraceptives, including norelgestromin/ethinyl estradiol transdermal patch, must be used with caution in women with cardiovascular disease risk factors.

Norgestimate and norelgestromin have minimal androgenic activity. There is some evidence that the risk of MI associated with hormonal contraceptives is lower when the progestin has minimal androgenic activity than when the activity is greater.

Cerebrovascular diseases – Hormonal contraceptives have been shown to increase the relative and attributable risks of cerebrovascular events (thrombotic and hemorrhagic strokes), although, in general, the risk is greatest among older (older than 35 years of age), hypertensive women who also smoke. Hypertension was found to be a risk factor for users and nonusers for both types of strokes, and smoking interacted to increase the risk of stroke.

In a large study, the relative risk of thrombotic strokes has been shown to range from 3 for normotensive users to 14 for users with severe hypertension. The relative risk of hemorrhagic stroke is reported to be 1.2 for nonsmokers who used hormonal contraceptives, 2.6 for smokers who did not use hormonal contraceptives, 7.6 for smokers who used hormonal contraceptives, 1.8 for normotensive users, and 25.7 for users with severe hypertension. The attributable risk is also greater in older women.

Dose-related risk – A positive association has been observed between the amount of estrogen and progestin in hormonal contraceptives and the risk of vascular disease. A decline in serum HDL has been reported with many progestational agents. A decline in serum HDL has been associated with an increased incidence of ischemic heart disease. Because estrogens increase HDL cholesterol, the net effect of a hormonal contraceptive depends on a balance achieved between doses of estrogen and progestin and the activity of the progestin used in the contraceptives. The activity and amount of both hormones should be considered in the choice of a hormonal contraceptive.

Persistence of risk – There are 2 studies that have shown persistence of risk of vascular disease for ever-users of combination hormonal contraceptives. In a study in the US, the risk of developing MI after discontinuing combination hormonal contraceptives persists for at least 9 years for women 40 to 49 years of age who had used combination hormonal contraceptives for at least 5 years, but this increased risk was not demonstrated in other age groups. In another study in Great Britain, the risk of developing cerebrovascular disease persisted for at least 6 years after discontinuation of combination hormonal contraceptives, although excess risk was very small. However, both studies were performed with combination hormonal contraceptive formulations containing at least 50 mcg of estrogens.

It is unknown whether norelgestromin/ethinyl estradiol transdermal patch is distinct from other combination hormonal contraceptives with regard to the occurrence of venous and arterial thrombosis.

➤*Mortality:* With the exception of combination oral contraceptive users at least 35 years of age who smoke, and at least 40 years of age who do not smoke, mortality associated with all methods of birth control is low and below that associated with childbirth.

In 1989, the Fertility and Maternal Health Drugs Advisory Committee was asked to review the use of combination hormonal contraceptives in women at least 40 years of age. The Committee concluded that although cardiovascular disease risks may be increased with combination hormonal contraceptive use after 40 years of age in healthy nonsmoking women (even with the newer low-dose formulations), there are also greater potential health risks associated with pregnancy in older women and with the alternative surgical and medical procedures that may be necessary if such women do not have access to effective and acceptable means of contraception. The Committee recommended that the benefits of low-dose combination hormonal contraceptive use by healthy nonsmoking women older than 40 years of age may outweigh the possible risks.

Although the data are mainly obtained with oral contraceptives, this is likely to apply to norelgestromin/ethinyl estradiol transdermal patch as well. Women of all ages who use combination hormonal contraceptives should use the lowest possible dose formulation that is effective and meets their needs.

➤*Carcinoma:* Numerous epidemiological studies give conflicting reports on the relationship between breast cancer and combination oral contraceptive (COC) use. The risk of having breast cancer diagnosed may be slightly increased among current and recent users of COCs. However, this excess risk appears to decrease over time after COC discontinuation and by 10 years after cessation the increased risk disappears. Some studies report an increased risk with duration of use while other studies do not and no consistent relationships have been found with dose or type of steroid. Some studies have found a small increase in risk for women who first use COCs before 20 years of age. Most studies show a similar pattern of risk with COC use regardless of a woman's reproductive history or her family breast cancer history.

In addition, breast cancers diagnosed in current or ever oral contraceptive users may be less clinically advanced than in never-users.

Women who currently have or have had breast cancer should not use hormonal contraceptives because breast cancer is usually a hormonally sensitive tumor.

Some studies suggest that COC use has been associated with an increase in the risk of cervical intraepithelial neoplasia in some populations of women. However, there continues to be controversy about the extent to which such findings may be because of differences in sexual behavior and other factors.

In spite of many studies of the relationship between oral contraceptive use and breast and cervical cancers, a cause-and effect relationship has not been established. It is not known whether norelgestromin/ethinyl estradiol transdermal patch is distinct from oral contraceptives with regard to the above statements.

➤*Hepatic neoplasia:* Benign hepatic adenomas are associated with hormonal contraceptive use, although the incidence of benign tumors is rare in the US. Indirect calculations have estimated the attributable risk to be in the range of 3.3 cases/100,000 for users, a risk that increases after at least 4 more years of use, especially with hormonal contraceptives containing at least 50 mcg of estrogen. Rupture of benign, hepatic adenomas may cause death through intra-abdominal hemorrhage.

Studies from Britain and the US have shown an increased risk of developing hepatocellular carcinoma in long-term (at least 8 years) oral contraceptive users. However, these cancers are extremely rare in the US and the attributable risk (the excess incidence) of liver cancers in oral contraceptive users approaches less than 1 per million users. It is unknown whether the norelgestromin/ethinyl estradiol transdermal patch is distinct from oral contraceptives in this regard.

➤*Ocular lesions:* There have been clinical case reports of retinal thrombosis associated with the use of hormonal contraceptives. Discontinue the norelgestromin/ethinyl estradiol transdermal patch if there is unexplained

NORELGESTROMIN/ETHINYL ESTRADIOL — TRANSDERMAL SYSTEM

partial or complete loss of vision, onset of proptosis or diplopia, papilledema, or retinal vascular lesions. Undertake appropriate diagnostic and therapeutic measures immediately.

➤*Risks of use before or during early pregnancy:* Extensive epidemiological studies have revealed no increased risk of birth defects in women who have used oral contraceptives prior to pregnancy.

➤*Gallbladder disease:* Earlier studies have reported an increased lifetime relative risk of gallbladder surgery in users of hormonal contraceptives and estrogens. More recent studies, however, have shown that the relative risk of developing gallbladder disease among hormonal contraceptive users may be minimal. The recent findings of minimal risk may be related to the use of hormonal contraceptive formulations containing lower hormonal doses of estrogens and progestins.

Combination hormonal contraceptives such as norelgestromin/ethinyl estradiol transdermal patch may worsen existing gallbladder disease and may accelerate the development of this disease in previously asymptomatic women. Women with a history of combination hormonal contraceptive-related cholestasis are more likely to have the condition recur with subsequent combination hormonal contraceptive use.

➤*Carbohydrate and lipid metabolic effects:* Glucose tolerance may decrease in some users. However, in nondiabetic women, combination hormonal contraceptives appear to have no effect on fasting blood glucose. Carefully monitor prediabetic and diabetic women in particular while taking combination hormonal contraceptives such as the norelgestromin/ethinyl estradiol transdermal patch.

A small proportion of women will have persistent hypertriglyceridemia while taking hormonal contraceptives. Changes in serum triglycerides and lipoprotein levels have been reported in hormonal contraceptive users.

➤*Elevated blood pressure:* Do not start women with significant hypertension on hormonal contraception. Encourage women with a history of hypertension or hypertension-related diseases, or renal disease to use another method of contraception. If women elect to use the norelgestromin/ethinyl estradiol transdermal patch, monitor them closely and if a clinically significant elevation of blood pressure occurs, discontinue the patch. For most women, elevated blood pressure will return to normal after stopping hormonal contraceptives, and there is no difference in the occurrence of hypertension between former and never-users.

An increase in blood pressure has been reported in women taking hormonal contraceptives, and this increase is more likely in older hormonal contraceptive users and with extended duration of use. Data from the Royal College of General Practitioners and subsequent randomized trials have shown that the incidence of hypertension increases with increasing progestational activity.

➤*Headaches:* The onset or exacerbation of migraine headache or the development of headache with a new pattern that is recurrent, persistent, or severe requires discontinuation of the norelgestromin/ethinyl estradiol transdermal patch and evaluation of the cause.

➤*Bleeding irregularities and patterns:* Breakthrough bleeding and spotting are sometimes encountered in women using the norelgestromin/ethinyl estradiol transdermal patch. Consider nonhormonal causes and take adequate diagnostic measures to rule out malignancy, other pathology, or pregnancy in the event of breakthrough bleeding, as in the case of any abnormal vaginal bleeding. If pathology has been excluded, time or a change to another contraceptive product may resolve the bleeding. In the event of amenorrhea, rule out pregnancy before initiating use of the norelgestromin/ethinyl estradiol transdermal patch.

Some women may encounter amenorrhea or oligomenorrhea after discontinuation of hormonal contraceptive use, especially when such a condition was pre-existent.

In the clinical trials, most women started their withdrawal bleeding on the fourth day of the drug-free interval, and the median duration of withdrawal bleeding was 5 to 6 days. On average, 26% of women per cycle had 7 or more total days of bleeding or spotting (this includes both withdrawal flow and breakthrough bleeding or spotting).

➤*Pregnancy: Category X.* Norelgestromin was tested for its reproductive toxicity in a rabbit developmental toxicity study by the subcutaneous route of administration. Doses of 0, 1, 2, 4, and 6 mg/kg body weight, which gave systemic exposure of ≈ 25 to 125 times the human exposure with the norelgestromin/ethinyl estradiol transdermal patch, were administered daily on gestation days 7 through 19. Malformations reported were paw hyperflexion at 4 and 6 mg/kg and paw hyperextension and cleft palate at 6 mg/kg.

Ectopic pregnancy – Ectopic as well as intrauterine pregnancy may occur in contraceptive failures.

➤*Lactation:* The effects of the norelgestromin/ethinyl estradiol transdermal patch in breast-feeding mothers have not been evaluated and are unknown. Small amounts of combination hormonal contraceptive steroids have been identified in the milk of breast-feeding mothers and a few adverse effects on the child have been reported, including jaundice and breast enlargement. In addition, combination hormonal contraceptives given in the postpartum period may interfere with lactation by decreasing the quantity and quality of breast milk. Long-term follow-up of infants whose mothers used combination hormonal contraceptives while breast-feeding has shown no deleterious effects. However, advise the breast-feeding mother not to use the norelgestromin/ethinyl estradiol transdermal patch, but to use other forms of contraception until she has completely weaned her child.

➤*Children:* Safety and efficacy are expected to be the same for postpubertal adolescents younger than 16 years of age and for users at least 16 years of age. Use of this product before menarche is not indicated.

Precautions

➤*Sexually transmitted diseases:* Counsel patients that this product does not protect against HIV infection (AIDS) and other sexually transmitted diseases.

➤*Body weight 90 kg (198 lb) or more:* Results of clinical trials suggest that the norelgestromin/ethinyl estradiol transdermal patch may be less effective in women with body weight 90 kg (198 lb) or more than in women with lower body weights.

➤*Hepatic function impairment:* If jaundice develops in any woman using the norelgestromin/ethinyl estradiol transdermal patch, discontinue the medication. The hormones in the patch may be poorly metabolized in women with impaired liver function.

➤*Fluid retention:* Steroid hormones like those in the norelgestromin/ethinyl estradiol transdermal patch may cause some degree of fluid retention. Prescribe this product with caution, and only with careful monitoring, in patients with conditions that might be aggravated by fluid retention.

➤*Depression:* Women who become significantly depressed while using combination hormonal contraceptives such as the norelgestromin/ethinyl estradiol transdermal patch should stop the medication and use another method of contraception in an attempt to determine whether the symptom is drug-related. Carefully observe women with a history of depression and discontinue the product if significant depression occurs.

➤*Contact lenses:* Contact lens wearers who develop visual changes or changes in lens tolerance should be assessed by an ophthalmologist.

Drug Interactions

Most drug interactions are based on oral contraceptives.

Transdermal Contraceptive Patch Drug Interactions

Precipitant drug	Object drug[a]		Description
Acetaminophen	Contraceptives, oral	↑	Ethinyl estradiol plasma levels may increase, whereas acetaminophen plasma concentrations may decrease.
Contraceptives, oral	Acetaminophen	↓	
Antibiotics	Contraceptives, oral	↓	Coadministration of griseofulvin, penicillins, or tetracyclines with OCs may decrease the pharmacologic effects of the OCs, possibly because of altered steroid gut metabolism secondary to changes in the intestinal flora. Menstrual irregularities (spotting, breakthrough bleeding) and pregnancy may occur. An alternate or additional form of birth control may be advisable during concomitant use. OCs and troleandomycin may be associated with an increased risk of intrahepatic cholestasis.
Atorvastatin	Contraceptives, oral	↑	Ethinyl estradiol AUC may increase by approximately 20%.
Ascorbic acid	Contraceptives, oral	↑	Ethinyl estradiol plasma levels may increase.
Barbiturates Carbamazepine Felbamate Griseofulvin Hydantoins[b] Oxcarbazepine Phenylbutazone Phenytoin Primidone Rifampin Topiramate	Contraceptives, oral	↓	These agents may increase the hepatic metabolism of the OCs via hepatic microsomal enzyme induction, possibly resulting in decreased effectiveness of the OC; menstrual irregularities (spotting, breakthrough bleeding) and pregnancy may occur. An alternate or additional form of birth control may be advisable during concomitant use.
CYP3A4 inhibitors (eg, itraconazole, ketoconazole)	Contraceptives, oral	↑	Increase in plasma hormone levels may occur.
Protease inhibitors	Contraceptives, oral	↓	Increased metabolism of the OCs is suspected resulting in a loss of effectiveness of OCs. An alternate or additional form of birth control may be advisable during concomitant use.
St. John's wort	Contraceptives, oral	↓	St. John's wort may induce hepatic enzymes and p-glycoprotein transporter and may reduce the effectiveness of contraceptive steroids.
Contraceptives, oral	Anticoagulants	↔	Because OCs can increase levels of certain circulating clotting factors and reduce antithrombin III levels, therapeutic efficacy of the anticoagulants may be decreased by OCs. However, both an increased and decreased effect has occurred.

NORELGESTROMIN/ETHINYL ESTRADIOL — TRANSDERMAL SYSTEM

Transdermal Contraceptive Patch Drug Interactions

Precipitant drug	Object drug[a]		Description
Contraceptives, oral	Antidepressants, tricyclic Beta blockers Caffeine Corticosteroids Theophyllines	↑	The hepatic metabolism of these agents may be decreased by OCs, resulting in increased therapeutic effects or toxicity.
Contraceptives, oral	Benzodiazepines	↓	OCs may increase the clearance of the benzodiazepines that undergo glucuronidation (lorazepam, oxazepam, temazepam) because of increased metabolism. Combination OCs with alprazolam, chlordiazepoxide, diazepam, and triazolam may inhibit hepatic mixed-function oxidases leading to a decrease in benzodiazepine oxidation rate (may prolong the half-life of benzodiazepines).
Contraceptives, oral	Cyclosporine Prednisolone Theophylline	↑	Increased plasma concentrations of cyclosporine, prednisolone, and theophylline have been reported with coadministration of OCs.
Contraceptives, oral	Clofibric acid Morphine Salicylic acid	↓	Increased clearance of these agents has been noted when administered with OCs.

[a] ↑ = Object drug increased. ↓ = Object drug decreased.
↔ = Undetermined clinical effect.
[b] Pharmacologic effects of the hydantoins also may be altered.

➤*Drug/Lab test interactions:* Certain endocrine and liver function tests and blood components may be affected by hormonal contraceptives:

Increased – Prothrombin and factors VII, VIII, IX, and X; increased norepinephrine-induced platelet aggregability; thyroid-binding globulin (TBG) leading to increased circulating total thyroid hormone as measured by protein-bound iodine (PBI), T4 by column or by radioimmunoassay; other binding proteins may be elevated in serum; sex hormone binding globulins are increased and result in elevated levels of total circulating endogenous sex steroids and corticoids; triglycerides may be increased and levels of various other lipids and lipoproteins may be affected.

Decreased – Antithrombin III; free T3 resin uptake; glucose tolerance may be decreased; serum folate levels may be depressed by hormonal contraceptive therapy. This may be of clinical significance if a woman becomes pregnant shortly after discontinuing the norelgestromin/ethinyl estradiol transdermal patch.

Adverse Reactions

The most common adverse reactions reported by 9% to 22% of women using the norelgestromin/ethinyl estradiol transdermal patch in clinical trials (n = 3,330) were the following, in order of decreasing incidence: breast symptoms, headache, application site reaction, nausea, upper respiratory tract infection, menstrual cramps, and abdominal pain.

The most frequent adverse reactions leading to discontinuation in 1% to 2.4% of women using the norelgestromin/ethinyl estradiol transdermal patch in the trials included the following: nausea or vomiting, application site reaction, breast symptoms, headache, emotional lability.

Listed below are adverse reactions that have been associated with the use of combination hormonal contraceptives. These also are likely to apply to combination transdermal hormonal contraceptives such as the norelgestromin/ethinyl estradiol transdermal patch.

➤*Serious:* Thrombophlebitis and venous thrombosis with or without embolism; arterial thromboembolism; pulmonary embolism; MI; cerebral hemorrhage; cerebral thrombosis; hypertension; gallbladder disease; hepatic adenomas or benign liver tumors; mesenteric thrombosis; retinal thrombosis.

➤*GI:* Cholestatic jaundice; GI symptoms (eg, abdominal cramps, bloating); nausea; vomiting.

➤*GU:* Amenorrhea; breakthrough bleeding; breast changes: tenderness, enlargement, secretion; change in cervical erosion and secretion; change in menstrual flow; diminution in lactation when given immediately postpartum; spotting; temporary infertility after discontinuation of treatment; vaginal candidiasis.

➤*Miscellaneous:* Change in corneal curvature (steepening); change in weight (increase or decrease); edema; intolerance to contact lenses; melasma, which may persist; mental depression; migraine; rash (allergic); reduced tolerance to carbohydrates.

The following adverse reactions have been reported in users of combination hormonal contraceptives and a cause-and-effect association has been neither confirmed nor refuted: Acne; Budd-Chiari syndrome; cataracts; changes in appetite; changes in libido; colitis; cystitis-like syndrome; dizziness; erythema multiforme; erythema nodosum; headache; hemolytic uremic syndrome; hemorrhagic eruption; hirsutism; impaired renal function; loss of scalp hair; nervousness; porphyria; premenstrual syndrome; vaginitis.

Overdosage

Serious ill effects have not been reported following accidental ingestion of large doses of hormonal contraceptives. Overdosage may cause nausea, vomiting, and withdrawal bleeding. Given the nature and design of the norelgestromin/ethinyl estradiol transdermal patch, it is unlikely that overdosage will occur. Serious ill effects have not been reported following acute ingestion of large doses of oral contraceptives by young children. In case of suspected overdose, remove all norelgestromin/ethinyl estradiol transdermal patches and give symptomatic treatment.

Patient Information

Counsel women that the norelgestromin/ethinyl estradiol transdermal patch does not protect against HIV infection (AIDS) and other sexually transmitted diseases.

If any of these adverse effects occur while you are using the patch, call your doctor immediately:

- Sharp chest pain, coughing of blood, sudden shortness of breath (indicating a possible clot in the lung);
- pain in the calf (indicating a possible clot in the leg);
- crushing chest pain or tightness in the chest (indicating a possible heart attack);
- sudden severe headache or vomiting, dizziness or fainting, disturbances of vision or speech, weakness or numbness in an arm or leg (indicating a possible stroke);
- sudden partial or complete loss of vision (indicating a possible clot in the eye);
- breast lumps (indicating possible breast cancer or fibrocystic disease of the breast; ask your doctor or health care professional to show you how to examine your breasts);
- severe pain or tenderness in the stomach area (indicating a possibly ruptured liver tumor);
- severe problems with sleeping, weakness, lack of energy, fatigue, or change in mood (possibly indicating severe depression);
- jaundice or a yellowing of the skin or eyeballs accompanied frequently by fever, fatigue, loss of appetite, dark-colored urine, or light-colored bowel movements (indicating possible liver problems).

➤*Skin irritation:* Skin irritation, redness, or rash may occur at the site of application. If this occurs, the patch may be removed and a new patch may be applied to a new location until the next patch change day. Single replacement patches are available from pharmacies.

➤*Vaginal bleeding:* Irregular bleeding may occur during the first few months of contraceptive patch use, but also may occur after you have been using the contraceptive patch for some time. If the bleeding occurs in more than a few cycles or lasts for more than a few days, talk to your health care professional.

ETONOGESTREL/ETHINYL ESTRADIOL VAGINAL RING

	Product and Distributor	Release Rate	Total Content	How Supplied
Rx	**NuvaRing** (Organon)	0.12 mg etonogestrel, 0.015 mg ethinyl estradiol/day	11.7 mg etonogestrel 2.7 mg ethinyl estradiol/sachet	In single and 3 sachets.

ETONOGESTREL/ETHINYL ESTRADIOL — VAGINAL RING

WARNING

Cigarette smoking increases the risk of serious cardiovascular side effects from combination oral contraceptive use. This risk increases with age and with heavy smoking (at least 15 cigarettes daily) and is quite marked in women older than 35 years of age. Strongly advise women who use combination hormonal contraceptives, including the contraceptive vaginal ring, not to smoke.

Indications

➤*Contraception:* For the prevention of pregnancy.

Administration and Dosage

➤*Approved by the FDA:* October 3, 2001.

➤*Use:* One etonogestrel/ethinyl estradiol vaginal ring is inserted in the vagina by the woman herself. This ring is to remain in place continuously for 3 weeks. It is removed for a 1-week break, during which a withdrawal bleed usually occurs. A new ring is inserted 1 week after the last ring was removed on the same day of the week as it was inserted in the previous cycle. The withdrawal bleed usually starts on day 2 to 3 after removal of the ring and may not have finished before the next ring is inserted. In order to maintain contraceptive effectiveness, insert the new ring 1 week after the previous one was removed even if menstrual bleeding has not finished.

➤*Insertion:* The user can choose the insertion position that is most comfortable to her, for example standing with one leg up, squatting, or lying down. Compress the ring and insert into the vagina. The exact position of the contraceptive vaginal ring inside the vagina is not critical for its function. Insert the contraceptive vaginal ring on the appropriate day and leave in place for 3 consecutive weeks.

ETONOGESTREL/ETHINYL ESTRADIOL — VAGINAL RING

➤*Removal:* The ring is removed 3 weeks later on the same day of the week as it was inserted and at about the same time. Remove the vaginal ring by hooking the index finger under the forward rim or by grasping the rim between the index and middle finger and pulling it out. Place the used ring in the sachet (foil pouch) and discard in a waste receptacle out of the reach of children and pets. Do not flush in the toilet.

➤*Starting the contraceptive vaginal ring:* Consider the possibility of ovulation and conception prior to the first use of the contraceptive vaginal ring.

No preceding hormonal contraceptive use in the past month – Counting the first day of menstruation as day 1, insert the contraceptive vaginal ring on or prior to day 5 of the cycle, even if the patient has not finished bleeding. During the first cycle, an additional method of contraception (eg, male condoms, spermicide) is recommended until after the first 7 days of continuous ring use.

Switching from a combination oral contraceptive – Insert the contraceptive vaginal ring anytime within 7 days after the last combined (estrogen plus progestin) oral contraceptive tablet and no later than the day that a new cycle of pills would have started. No backup method is needed.

Switching from a progestin-only method – There are several types of progestin-only methods. Insert the first contraceptive vaginal ring as follows:

- Any day of the month when switching from a progestin-only pill; do not skip any days between the last pill and the first day of contraceptive vaginal ring use;
- on the same day as contraceptive implant removal;
- on the same day as removal of a progestin-containing IUD; or
- on the day when the next contraceptive injection would be due.

In all of these cases, advise the patient to use an additional method of contraception (eg, male condoms, spermicide) for the first 7 days after insertion of the ring.

➤*Following complete first-trimester abortion:* The patient may start using the contraceptive vaginal ring within the first 5 days following a complete first trimester abortion and does not need to use an additional method of contraception. If use of the contraceptive vaginal ring is not started within 5 days following a first trimester abortion, the patient should follow the instructions for "No preceding hormonal contraceptive use in the past month." In the meantime, advise the patient to use a nonhormonal contraceptive method.

➤*Following delivery or second-trimester abortion:* Initiate the use of the contraceptive vaginal ring 4 weeks postpartum in women who elect not to breastfeed. Advise women who are breastfeeding not to use the contraceptive vaginal ring but to use other forms of contraception until the child is weaned. Initiate use of the contraceptive vaginal ring 4 weeks after a second-trimester abortion. When the contraceptive vaginal ring is used postpartum or postabortion, consider the increased risk of thromboembolic disease (see Contraindications, Warnings, and Precautions). If the patient begins using the contraceptive vaginal ring postpartum and has not yet had a period, consider the possibility of ovulation and conception occurring prior to initiation of the contraceptive vaginal ring, and instruct the patient to use an additional method of contraception (eg, male condoms, spermicide) for the first 7 days.

➤*Inadvertent removal, expulsion, or prolonged ring-free interval:* If the contraceptive vaginal ring has been out during the 3-week use period, rinse with cool to lukewarm (not hot) water and reinsert as soon as possible, at the latest within 3 hours. If the ring has been out of the vagina for more than 3 hours, contraceptive effectiveness may be reduced. Use an additional method of contraception (eg, male condoms, spermicide) until the contraceptive vaginal ring has been used continuously for 7 days.

Consider the possibility of pregnancy if the ring-free interval has been extended beyond 1 week. Use an additional method of contraception (eg, male condoms, spermicide) until the contraceptive vaginal ring has been used continuously for 7 days.

➤*Prolonged use:* If the contraceptive vaginal ring has been left in place for up to 1 extra week (up to 4 weeks total), remove it and insert a new ring after a 1-week ring-free interval. Rule out pregnancy if the contraceptive vaginal ring has been left in place for more than 4 weeks. Use an additional method of contraception (eg, male condoms, spermicide) until the contraceptive vaginal ring has been used continuously for 7 days.

➤*In the event of a missed menstrual period:* If the patient has not adhered to the prescribed regimen (the contraceptive vaginal ring has been out of the vagina for more than 3 hours or the preceding ring-free interval was extended beyond 1 week), consider the possibility of pregnancy at the time of the first missed period and discontinue the use of the contraceptive vaginal ring if pregnancy is confirmed.

Rule out pregnancy if the patient has adhered to the prescribed regimen and misses 2 consecutive periods.

Rule out pregnancy if the patient has retained 1 contraceptive vaginal ring for more than 4 weeks.

➤*Storage / Stability:* Prior to dispensing to the user, store refrigerated 2° to 8°C (36° to 46°F). After dispensing to the user, the contraceptive vaginal ring can be stored for up to 4 months at 15° to 30°C (59° to 86°F). Avoid storing the contraceptive vaginal ring in direct sunlight or at temperatures above 30°C (86°F). When the contraceptive vaginal ring is dispensed to the user, place an expiration date on the label. The date should not be more than 4 months from the date of dispensing or the expiration date, whichever comes first.

Actions

➤*Pharmacology:* The contraceptive vaginal ring is a nonbiodegradable, flexible, transparent, colorless to almost colorless combination contraceptive vaginal ring containing 2 active components: A progestin, etonogestrel, and an estrogen, ethinyl estradiol. When placed in the vagina, each ring releases on average 0.12 mg/day of etonogestrel and 0.015 mg/day of ethinyl estradiol over a 3-week period of use.

Combination hormonal contraceptives act by suppression of gonadotropins. Although the primary effect of this action is inhibition of ovulation, other alterations include changes in the cervical mucus (which increase the difficulty of sperm entry into the uterus) and in the endometrium (which reduce the likelihood of implantation).

Receptor binding studies, as well as studies in animals, have shown that etonogestrel, the biologically active metabolite of desogestrel, combines high progestational activity with low intrinsic androgenicity. The relevance of this latter finding in humans is unknown.

➤*Pharmacokinetics:*

Absorption – Etonogestrel released by the vaginal ring is rapidly absorbed. Bioavailability of etonogestrel after vaginal administration is ≈ 100%.

Ethinyl estradiol released by the vaginal ring is rapidly absorbed. Bioavailability of ethinyl estradiol after vaginal administration is approximately 55.6%, which is comparable to that with oral administration of ethinyl estradiol.

Mean Serum Etonogestrel and Ethinyl Estradiol Concentrations (n = 16)

	1 week	2 weeks	3 weeks
Etonogestrel (pg/mL)	1,578	1,476	1,374
Ethinyl estradiol (pg/mL)	19.1	18.3	17.6

Mean Pharmacokinetic Parameters of Etonogestrel/Ethinyl Estradiol Vaginal Ring (n = 16)

Hormone	C_{max}[a] pg/mL	T_{max}[b] h	$T_{½}$[c] h	CL[d] L/h
Etonogestrel	1,716	200.3	29.3	3.4
Ethinyl estradiol	34.7	59.3	44.7	34.8

[a] C_{max} — maximum serum concentration
[b] T_{max} — time at which maximum serum drug concentration occurs
[c] $t_{½}$ — elimination half-life, calculated by $0.693/K_{elim}$
[d] CL — apparent clearance

Distribution – Etonogestrel is approximately 32% bound to sex hormone binding globulin (SHBG) and approximately 66% bound to albumin in blood.

Ethinyl estradiol is highly but not specifically bound to serum albumin (approximately 98.5%) and induces an increase in the serum concentrations of SHBG.

Metabolism – In vitro data show that both etonogestrel and ethinyl estradiol are metabolized in liver microsomes by the cytochrome P-450 3A4 isoenzyme. Ethinyl estradiol is primarily metabolized by aromatic hydroxylation, but a wide variety of hydroxylated and methylated metabolites are formed. These are present as free metabolites and as sulfate and glucuronide conjugates. The hydroxylated ethinyl estradiol metabolites have weak estrogenic activity. The biological activity of etonogestrel metabolites is unknown.

Excretion – Etonogestrel and ethinyl estradiol are primarily eliminated in urine, bile, and feces.

Contraindications

Thrombophlebitis or thromboembolic disorders; a past history of deep vein thrombophlebitis or thromboembolic disorders; cerebral vascular or coronary artery disease (current or history); valvular heart disease with complications; severe hypertension; diabetes with vascular involvement; headaches with focal neurological symptoms; major surgery with prolonged immobilization; known or suspected carcinoma of the breast or personal history of breast cancer; carcinoma of the endometrium or other known or suspected estrogen-dependent neoplasia; undiagnosed abnormal genital bleeding; cholestatic jaundice of pregnancy or jaundice with prior hormonal contraceptive use; hepatic tumors (benign or malignant); active liver disease; known or suspected pregnancy; heavy smoking (at least 15 cigarettes daily) and older than 35 years of age; hypersensitivity to any of the components of the contraceptive vaginal ring.

Warnings

➤*Thromboembolic disorders and other vascular problems:*

Thromboembolism – An increased risk of thromboembolic and thrombotic disease associated with the use of hormonal contraceptives is well-established. Case control studies have found the relative risk of users compared with nonusers to be 3 for the first episode of superficial venous thrombosis, 4 to 11 for deep vein thrombosis or pulmonary embolism, and 1.5 to 6 for women with predisposing conditions for venous thromboembolic disease. Cohort studies have shown the relative risk to be somewhat lower, approximately 3 for new cases and approximately 4.5 for new cases requiring hos-

ETONOGESTREL/ETHINYL ESTRADIOL — VAGINAL RING

pitalization. The risk of thromboembolic disease associated with hormonal contraceptives is not related to length of use and disappears after pill use is stopped.

Several epidemiology studies indicate that third generation oral contraceptives, including those containing desogestrel (etonogestrel, the progestin in the vaginal ring, is the biologically active metabolite of desogestrel), are associated with a higher risk of venous thromboembolism than certain second generation oral contraceptives. In general, these studies indicate an approximately 2-fold increased risk, which corresponds to an additional 1 to 2 cases of venous thromboembolism per 10,000 women-years of use. However, data from additional studies have not shown this 2-fold increase in risk. It is unknown if the vaginal ring has a different risk of venous thromboembolism than second generation oral contraceptives.

A 2- to 4-fold increase in relative risk of postoperative thromboembolic complications has been reported with the use of oral contraceptives. The relative risk of venous thrombosis in women who have predisposing conditions is twice that of women without such medical conditions. If feasible, discontinue the use of combination hormonal contraceptives, including the vaginal ring, for ≥ 4 weeks prior to and for 2 weeks after elective surgery of a type associated with an increase in risk of thromboembolism and during and following prolonged immobilization. Because the immediate postpartum period is also associated with an increased risk of thromboembolism, start combination hormonal contraceptives (eg, vaginal ring) no earlier than 4 weeks after delivery in women who elect not to breastfeed.

The clinician should be alert to the earliest manifestations of thrombotic disorders (thrombophlebitis, pulmonary embolism, cerebrovascular disorders, and retinal thrombosis). Should any of these occur or be suspected, discontinue the use of the vaginal ring immediately.

MI – An increased risk of MI has been attributed to hormonal contraceptive use. The risk is primarily in smokers or women with other underlying risk factors for coronary artery disease (eg, hypertension, hypercholesterolemia, morbid obesity, and diabetes). The relative risk of heart attack for current combination hormonal contraceptive users has been estimated to be 2 to 6. The risk is very low in women younger than 30 years of age.

Smoking in combination with oral contraceptive use has been shown to contribute substantially to the incidence of MI in women in their mid-30s or older with smoking accounting for the majority of excess cases. Mortality rates associated with circulatory disease have been shown to increase substantially in smokers older than 35 years of age and nonsmokers older than 40 years of age among women who use oral contraceptives.

Hormonal contraceptives may compound the effects of well-known risk factors (eg, hypertension, diabetes, hyperlipidemias, age, obesity). In particular, some progestogens are known to decrease high density lipoprotein (HDL) cholesterol and cause glucose intolerance, while estrogens may create a state of hyperinsulinism. Hormonal contraceptives have been shown to increase blood pressure among users. Similar effects on risk factors have been associated with an increased risk of heart disease. Use the vaginal ring with caution in women with cardiovascular disease risk factors.

Cerebrovascular diseases – Hormonal contraceptives have been shown to increase both the relative and attributable risks of cerebrovascular events (thrombotic and hemorrhagic strokes), although, in general, the risk is highest among older (older than 35 years of age), hypertensive women who also smoke. Hypertension was found to be a risk factor for both users and nonusers, for both types of strokes, while smoking interacted to increase the risk for hemorrhagic strokes.

In a large study, the relative risk of thrombotic strokes has been shown to range from 3 for normotensive users to 14 for users with severe hypertension. The relative risk of hemorrhagic stroke is reported to be 1.2 for nonsmokers who used oral contraceptives, 2.6 for smokers who did not use oral contraceptives, 7.6 for smokers who used oral contraceptives, 1.8 for normotensive users and 25.7 for users with severe hypertension. The attributable risk is also greater in older women.

Dose-related risk – A positive association has been observed between the amount of estrogen and progestogen in hormonal contraceptives and the risk of vascular disease. A decline in serum HDL has been reported with many progestational agents. A decline in serum high-density lipoproteins has been associated with an increased incidence of ischemic heart disease. Because estrogens increase HDL cholesterol, the net effect of a hormonal contraceptive depends on a balance achieved between doses of estrogen and progestogen and the nature and absolute amount of progestogens used in the contraceptives. Consider the activity and amount of both hormones in the choice of a hormonal contraceptive.

Persistence of risk – There are 2 studies that have shown persistence of risk of vascular disease for ever-users of hormonal contraceptives. In a study in the US, the risk of developing MI after discontinuing oral contraceptives persists for at least 9 years for women 40 to 49 years of age who had used oral contraceptives for at least 5 years, but this increased risk was not demonstrated in other age groups. In another study in Great Britain, the risk of developing cerebrovascular disease persisted at least 6 years after discontinuation of oral contraceptives, although excess risk was very small. However, both studies were performed with oral contraceptive formulations containing at least 50 mcg of estrogen.

It is unknown whether the contraceptive vaginal ring is distinct from combination hormonal contraceptives with regard to the occurrence of venous or arterial thrombosis.

➤*Mortality:* With the exception of oral contraceptive users at least 35 years of age who smoke and at least 40 years of age who do not smoke, mortality associated with all methods of birth control is low and below that associated with childbirth.

In 1989, the Fertility and Maternal Health Drugs Advisory Committee was asked to review the use of combination hormonal contraceptives in women at least 40 years of age. The Committee concluded that although cardiovascular disease risks may be increased with oral contraceptive use after 40 years of age in healthy nonsmoking women (even with the newer low-dose formulations), there are also greater potential risks associated with pregnancy in older women and with the alternative surgical and medical procedures that may be necessary if such women do not have access to effective and acceptable means of contraception. Therefore, the Committee recommended that the benefits of low-dose oral contraceptive use by healthy nonsmoking women older than 40 years of age may outweigh the possible risks. Although the data are mainly obtained with oral contraceptives, this is likely to apply to the contraceptive vaginal ring as well. Women of all ages who take hormonal contraceptives should take the lowest possible dose formulation that is effective and meets the needs of the individual patient.

➤*Carcinoma:* Numerous epidemiologic studies have been performed on the incidence of breast, endometrial, ovarian, and cervical cancer in women using combination oral contraceptives.

The risk of having breast cancer diagnosed may be slightly increased among current and recent users of combination oral contraceptives (COCs). However, this excess risk appears to decrease over time after COC discontinuation and by 10 years after cessation the increased risk disappears. Some studies report an increased risk with duration of use while other studies do not and no consistent relationships have been found with dose or type of steroid. Some studies have found a small increase in risk for women who first use COCs before 20 years of age. Most studies show a similar pattern of risk with COC use regardless of a woman's reproductive history or her family breast cancer history.

In addition, breast cancers diagnosed in current or ever oral contraceptive users may be less clinically advanced than in never-users.

Women who currently have or have had breast cancer should not use hormonal contraceptives because breast cancer is usually a hormonal sensitive tumor.

Some studies suggest that combination oral contraceptive use has been associated with an increase in the risk of cervical intraepithelial neoplasia in some populations of women. However, there continues to be controversy about the extent to which such findings may be caused by differences in sexual behavior and other factors.

In spite of many studies of the relationship between oral contraceptive use and breast and cervical cancers, a cause-and-effect relationship has not been established.

It is unknown whether the contraceptive vaginal ring is distinct from oral contraceptives with regard to the previous statements.

➤*Hepatic neoplasia:* Benign hepatic adenomas are associated with oral contraceptive use, although the incidence of benign tumors is rare in the US. Indirect calculations have estimated the attributable risk to be in the range of 3.3 cases per 100,000 for users, a risk that increases after at least 4 years of use. Rupture of rare, benign, hepatic adenomas may cause death through intra-abdominal hemorrhage.

Studies from Great Britain have shown an increased risk of developing hepatocellular carcinoma in long-term (more than 8 years) oral contraceptive users. However, these cancers are extremely rare in the US and the attributable risk (the excess incidence) of liver cancers in oral contraceptive users approaches less than 1 per million users. It is unknown whether the contraceptive vaginal ring is distinct from oral contraceptives in this regard.

➤*Ocular lesions:* There have been clinical case reports of retinal thrombosis associated with the use of oral contraceptives. Discontinue the use of the contraceptive vaginal ring if there is unexplained partial or complete loss of vision, onset of proptosis or diplopia, papilledema, or retinal vascular lesions. Undertake appropriate diagnostic and therapeutic measures immediately.

➤*Risk of use before or during early pregnancy:* Do not use hormonal contraceptives during pregnancy. Extensive epidemiologic studies have revealed no increased risk of birth defects in women who have used oral contraceptives prior to pregnancy. Studies also do not suggest a teratogenic effect, particularly where cardiac anomalies and limb reduction defects are concerned, when oral contraceptives are taken inadvertently during early pregnancy.

➤*Gallbladder disease:* Combination hormonal contraceptives (eg, contraceptive vaginal ring) may worsen existing gallbladder disease and may accelerate the development of this disease in previously asymptomatic women. Women with a history of combination hormonal contraceptive-related cholestasis are more likely to have the condition recur with subsequent combination hormonal contraceptive use.

➤*Carbohydrate and lipid metabolic effects:* Hormonal contraceptives have been shown to cause a decrease in glucose tolerance in some users. However, in the nondiabetic woman, combination hormonal contraceptives appear to have no effect on fasting blood glucose. Carefully observe prediabetic and diabetic women while taking combination hormonal contraceptives (eg, contraceptive vaginal ring). In a clinical study involving 37 contraceptive vaginal ring-treated subjects, glucose tolerance tests showed no clinically significant changes in serum glucose levels from baseline to cycle 6.

A small proportion of women will have persistent hypertriglyceridemia while using hormonal contraceptives. Changes in serum triglycerides and lipoprotein levels have been reported in combination hormonal contraceptive users.

ETONOGESTREL/ETHINYL ESTRADIOL — VAGINAL RING

➤*Elevated blood pressure:* An increase in blood pressure has been reported in women taking hormonal contraceptives; this increase is more likely in older hormonal contraceptive users and with continued use. Data from the Royal College of General Practitioners and subsequent randomized trials have shown that the incidence of hypertension increases with increasing concentrations of progestogens. Encourage women with a history of hypertension or hypertension-related diseases, or renal disease to use another method of contraception. Closely monitor these women if they elect to use the contraceptive vaginal ring. Discontinue use of the contraceptive vaginal ring if significant elevation of blood pressure occurs. For most women, elevated blood pressure will return to normal after stopping hormonal contraceptives.

➤*Headache:* The onset or exacerbation of migraine or development of headache with a new pattern that is recurrent, persistent, or severe requires discontinuation of the contraceptive vaginal ring and evaluation of the cause.

➤*Bleeding irregularities and patterns:* Breakthrough bleeding and spotting are sometimes encountered in women using the contraceptive vaginal ring. If abnormal bleeding while using the contraceptive vaginal ring persists or is severe, investigate to rule out the possibility of organic pathology or pregnancy, and institute appropriate treatment when necessary. Rule out pregnancy in the event of amenorrhea.

Bleeding patterns were evaluated in 2 large clinical studies. During cycles 1 through 13, breakthrough bleeding/spotting occurred in 7.2% to 11.7% of cycles in a study of 1,177 subjects and in 2.6% to 6.4% of cycles in a second study of 1,145 subjects. Absence of withdrawal bleeding occurred in 2.3% to 3.8% of cycles in the first trial subjects and in 0.6% to 2.1% of cycles in the second trial subjects. Bleeding patterns for individual women over multiple cycles were not evaluated. Some women may encounter amenorrhea or oligomenorrhea after discontinuing use of the contraceptive vaginal ring, especially when a condition was preexistent.

➤*Elderly:* This medication has not been studied in women at least 65 years of age and is not indicated in this population.

➤*Pregnancy: Category X.* Teratology studies have been performed in rats and rabbits using the oral route of administration at doses up to 130 and 260 times, respectively, the human contraceptive vaginal ring dose (based on body surface area) and have revealed no evidence of harm to the fetus due to etonogestrel.

Ectopic pregnancy – Ectopic as well as intrauterine pregnancy may occur in contraceptive failures.

➤*Lactation:* The effects of the contraceptive vaginal ring in breast-feeding mothers have not been evaluated and are unknown. Small amounts of contraceptive steroids have been identified in the milk of breast-feeding mothers and a few adverse effects on the child have been reported, including jaundice and breast enlargement. In addition, contraceptive steroids given in the postpartum period may interfere with lactation by decreasing the quantity and quality of breast milk. Long-term follow-up of children whose mothers used combination hormonal contraceptives while breast-feeding has shown no deleterious effects in infants. However, advise women who are breast-feeding not to use the contraceptive vaginal ring but to use other forms of contraception until the child is weaned.

➤*Children:* Safety and efficacy of the contraceptive vaginal ring have been established in women of reproductive age. Safety and efficacy are expected to be the same for postpubertal adolescents younger than 16 years of age and for users at least 16 years of age. Use of this product before menarche is not indicated.

Precautions

➤*Sexually transmitted diseases:* Counsel patients that this product does not protect against HIV infection (AIDS) and other sexually transmitted diseases.

➤*Lipid disorders:* Closely follow women who are being treated for hyperlipidemias if they elect to use the contraceptive vaginal ring. Some progestogens may elevate LDL levels and may render the control of hyperlipidemias more difficult.

➤*Hepatic function impairment:* If jaundice develops in any woman using the contraceptive vaginal ring, discontinue the medication. The hormones in the contraceptive vaginal ring may be poorly metabolized in women with impaired liver function.

➤*Fluid retention:* Steroid hormones like those in the contraceptive vaginal ring may cause some degree of fluid retention. Prescribe this product with caution, and only with careful monitoring, in patients with conditions that might be aggravated by fluid retention.

➤*Depression:* Women who become significantly depressed while using combination hormonal contraceptives such as the contraceptive vaginal ring should stop the medication and use another method of contraception in an attempt to determine whether the symptom is drug-related. Carefully observe women with a history of depression and discontinue the product if significant depression occurs.

➤*Contact lenses:* Contact lens wearers who develop visual changes or changes in lens tolerance should be assessed by an ophthalmologist.

➤*Vaginal use:* The contraceptive vaginal ring may not be suitable for women with conditions that make the vagina more susceptible to vaginal irritation or ulceration. Some women are aware of the ring at random times during the 21 days of use or during intercourse. During intercourse, some sexual partners may feel the contraceptive vaginal ring in the vagina. However, clinical studies revealed that 90% of couples did not find this to be a problem.

If the contraceptive vaginal ring has been removed or expelled during the 3-week use period, it should be rinsed with cool to lukewarm (not hot) water and reinserted as soon as possible, but at the latest within 3 hours of removal or expulsion. If the contraceptive vaginal ring is lost, insert a new vaginal ring and continue the regimen without alteration. If the ring has been out of the vagina for more than 3 hours, contraceptive effectiveness may be reduced and an additional method of contraception (eg, male condom, spermicide) must be used until the ring has been used continuously for 7 days. The contraceptive vaginal ring may interfere with the correct placement and position of a diaphragm. Therefore, a diaphragm is not recommended as a backup method with contraceptive vaginal ring use.

➤*Expulsion:* The contraceptive vaginal ring can be accidentally expelled, for example, when it has not been inserted properly, or while removing a tampon, moving the bowels, straining, or with severe constipation. If this occurs, rinse the vaginal ring with cool to lukewarm (not hot) water and reinsert promptly. If the contraceptive vaginal ring is lost, insert a new vaginal ring and continue the regimen without alteration. If the ring has been out of the vagina for more than 3 hours, contraceptive effectiveness may be reduced and an additional method of contraception (eg, male condom, spermicide) must be used until the ring has been used continuously for 7 days. Vaginal stenosis, cervical prolapse, rectoceles, and cystoceles are conditions that under some circumstances may make expulsion more likely to occur.

Drug Interactions

Most drug interactions are based on oral contraceptives.

Contraceptive Vaginal Ring Drug Interactions

Precipitant drug	Object drug[a]		Description
Acetaminophen	Contraceptives, oral	↑	Ethinyl estradiol plasma levels may increase, whereas acetaminophen plasma concentrations may decrease.
Contraceptives, oral	Acetaminophen	↓	
Antibiotics	Contraceptives, oral	↓	Coadministration of griseofulvin, penicillins, or tetracyclines with OCs may decrease the pharmacologic effects of the OCs, possibly because of altered steroid gut metabolism secondary to changes in the intestinal flora. Menstrual irregularities (spotting, breakthrough bleeding) and pregnancy may occur. An alternate or additional form of birth control may be advisable during concomitant use. OCs and troleandomycin may be associated with an increased risk of intrahepatic cholestasis.
Atorvastatin	Contraceptives, oral	↑	Ethinyl estradiol AUC may increase by approximately 20%.
Ascorbic acid	Contraceptives, oral	↑	Ethinyl estradiol plasma levels may increase.
Barbiturates Carbamazepine Felbamate Griseofulvin Hydantoins[b] Oxcarbazepine Phenylbutazone Phenytoin Primidone Rifampin Topiramate	Contraceptives, oral	↓	These agents may increase the hepatic metabolism of the OCs via hepatic microsomal enzyme induction, possibly resulting in decreased effectiveness of the OC; menstrual irregularities (spotting, breakthrough bleeding) and pregnancy may occur. An alternate or additional form of birth control may be advisable during concomitant use.
CYP3A4 inhibitors (eg, itraconazole, ketoconazole)	Contraceptives, oral	↑	Increase in plasma hormone levels may occur.
Protease inhibitors	Contraceptives, oral	↓	Increased metabolism of the OCs is suspected, resulting in a loss of effectiveness of OCs. An alternate or additional form of birth control may be advisable during concomitant use.
St. John's wort	Contraceptives, oral	↓	St. John's wort may induce hepatic enzymes and p-glycoprotein transporter and may reduce the effectiveness of contraceptive steroids.
Miconazole	Etonogestrel/ ethinyl estradiol vaginal ring	↑	Vaginally administered oil-based miconazole capsule increased serum concentrations of etonogestrel and ethinyl estradiol by approximately 17% and 16%, respectively.
Contraceptives, oral	Anticoagulants	↔	Therapeutic efficacy of the anticoagulants may be decreased by OCs. However, both an increased and decreased effect has occurred.
Contraceptives, oral	Antidepressants, tricyclic Beta blockers Caffeine Corticosteroids Theophyllines	↑	The hepatic metabolism of these agents may be decreased by OCs, resulting in increased therapeutic effects or toxicity.

ETONOGESTREL/ETHINYL ESTRADIOL — VAGINAL RING

Contraceptive Vaginal Ring Drug Interactions			
Precipitant drug	Object drug[a]		Description
Contraceptives, oral	Benzodiazepines	↓	OCs may increase the clearance of the benzodiazepines that undergo glucuronidation (lorazepam, oxazepam, temazepam) because of increased metabolism. Combination OCs with alprazolam, chlordiazepoxide, diazepam, and triazolam may inhibit hepatic mixed-function oxidases, leading to a decrease in benzodiazepine oxidation rate (may prolong the half-life of benzodiazepines).
Contraceptives, oral	Cyclosporine Prednisolone Theophylline	↑	Increased plasma concentrations of cyclosporine, prednisolone, and theophylline have been reported with coadministration of OCs.
Contraceptives, oral	Clofibric acid Morphine Salicylic acid	↓	Increased clearance of these agents has been noted when administered with OCs.

[a] ↑ = Object drug increased. ↓ = Object drug decreased. ↔ = Undetermined clinical effect.
[b] Pharmacologic effects of the hydantoins also may be altered.

➤*Drug/Lab test interactions:* Certain endocrine and liver function tests and blood components may be affected by hormonal contraceptives:

Increased – Prothrombin and factors VII, VIII, IX, and X; increased norepinephrine-induced platelet aggregability; thyroid binding globulin (TBG) leading to increased circulating total thyroid hormone as measured by protein-bound iodine (PBI), T4 by column or by radioimmunoassay; other binding proteins may be elevated in serum; sex hormone binding globulins are increased and result in elevated levels of total circulating endogenous sex steroids and corticoids; triglycerides may be increased and levels of various other lipids and lipoproteins may be affected.

Decreased – Antithrombin III; free T3 resin uptake; glucose tolerance may be decreased; serum folate levels may be depressed by hormonal contraceptive therapy. This may be of clinical significance if a woman becomes pregnant shortly after discontinuing the contraceptive vaginal ring.

Adverse Reactions

The most common adverse reactions reported by 5% to 14% of women using the contraceptive vaginal ring in clinical trials (n = 2501) were the following: vaginitis, headache, upper respiratory tract infection, leukorrhea, sinusitis, weight gain, and nausea.

The most frequent system-organ class adverse reactions leading to discontinuation in 1% to 2.5% of women using the contraceptive vaginal ring in the trials included the following: device-related events (foreign body sensation, coital problems, device expulsion), vaginal symptoms (discomfort/vaginitis/leukorrhea), headache, emotional lability, and weight gain.

Listed below are adverse reactions that have been associated with the use of combination hormonal contraceptives. These are also likely to apply to combination vaginal hormonal contraceptives such as the contraceptive vaginal ring.

➤*Serious:* Thrombophlebitis and venous thrombosis with or without embolism; arterial thromboembolism; pulmonary embolism; MI; cerebral hemorrhage; cerebral thrombosis; hypertension; gallbladder disease; hepatic adenomas or benign liver tumors; mesenteric thrombosis; retinal thrombosis.

➤*GI:* Cholestatic jaundice; GI symptoms (eg, abdominal cramps, bloating); nausea; vomiting.

➤*GU:* Amenorrhea; breakthrough bleeding; breast changes (tenderness, enlargement, secretion); change in cervical erosion and secretion; change in menstrual flow; diminution in lactation when given immediately postpartum; spotting; temporary infertility after discontinuation of treatment; vaginal candidiasis.

➤*Miscellaneous:* Changes in weight (increase or decrease); change in corneal curvature (steepening); edema; intolerance to contact lenses; melasma (which may persist); mental depression; migraine; rash (allergic); reduced tolerance to carbohydrates.

The following additional adverse reactions have been reported in users of combination hormonal contraceptives and a causal association has been neither confirmed nor refuted: Acne; Budd-Chiari syndrome; cataracts; changes in appetite; changes in libido; colitis; cystitis-like syndrome; dizziness; erythema multiforme; erythema nodosum; headache; hemolytic uremic syndrome; hemorrhagic eruption; hirsutism; impaired renal function; loss of scalp hair; nervousness; premenstrual syndrome; porphyria; vaginitis.

Overdosage

Overdosage of combination hormonal contraceptives may cause nausea, vomiting, vaginal bleeding, or other menstrual irregularities. Given the nature and design of the contraceptive vaginal ring, it is unlikely that overdosage will occur. If the contraceptive vaginal ring is broken, it does not release a higher dose of hormones. Serious ill effects have not been reported following acute ingestion of large doses of oral contraceptives by young children. There are no antidotes and further treatment should be symptomatic.

Patient Information

Instruct the patient regarding the proper use of the contraceptive vaginal ring.

Counsel patients that this product does not protect against HIV infection (AIDS) and other sexually transmitted diseases.

Advise patients to call their health care provider right away if they experience any of the following symptoms:

- Sharp chest pain, coughing blood, or sudden shortness of breath (possible clot in the lung);
- pain in the calf (back of lower leg; possible clot in the leg);
- crushing chest pain or heaviness in the chest (possible heart attack);
- sudden severe headache or vomiting, dizziness or fainting, problems with vision or speech, weakness or numbness in an arm or leg (possible stroke);
- sudden partial or complete loss of vision (possible clot in the eye);
- yellowing of the skin or whites of the eyes (jaundice), especially with fever, tiredness, loss of appetite, dark-colored urine, or light-colored bowel movements (possible liver problems);
- severe pain, swelling, or tenderness in the abdomen (gallbladder or liver problems);
- breast lumps (possible breast cancer or benign breast disease);
- irregular vaginal bleeding or spotting that happens in more than 1 menstrual cycle or lasts for more than a few days;
- swelling (edema) of the fingers or ankles;
- difficulty in sleeping, weakness, lack of energy, fatigue, or a change in mood (possible severe depression).

INTRAUTERINE PROGESTERONE CONTRACEPTIVE SYSTEM

Rx	**Progestasert** (Alza)	**Intrauterine System:** T-shaped unit containing a reservoir of 38 mg progesterone with barium sulfate dispersed in medical grade silicone fluid	In 6s w/ inserters.

PROGESTERONE CONTRACEPTIVE SYSTEM — INTRAUTERINE

Indications

➤*Contraception:* Intrauterine contraception in women who have had at least 1 child, are in a stable, mutually monogamous relationship, and have no history of pelvic inflammatory disease (PID).

➤*Unlabeled uses:* This system has been used in the treatment of menorrhagia.

Administration and Dosage

Insert a single system into the uterine cavity. Contraceptive effectiveness is retained for 1 year, and the system must be replaced 1 year after insertion. See manufacturer's literature for insertion and removal instructions.

Actions

➤*Pharmacology:*

Estrogens – Ethinyl estradiol is rapidly absorbed with peak concentrations attained within 2 hours. It undergoes considerable first-pass elimination. Mestranol is demethylated to ethinyl estradiol. Ethinyl estradiol is 97% to 98% bound to plasma albumin. Half-life varies from 6 to 20 hours. It is excreted in bile and urine as conjugates and undergoes some enterohepatic recirculation.

Progestins – Peak concentrations of norethindrone occur 0.5 to 4 hours after oral administration; it undergoes first-pass metabolism with an overall bioavailability of approximately 65%. Levonorgestrel reaches peak concentrations between 0.5 to 2 hours, does not undergo a first-pass effect, and is completely bioavailable. Norethindrone and levonorgestrel are chiefly metabolized by reduction followed by conjugation. Desogestrel is rapidly and completely absorbed and converted into 3-keto-desogestrel, the biologically active metabolite. Relative bioavailability is approximately 84%. Maximum concentrations of the metabolite are reached at approximately 1.4 hours. Norgestimate is well absorbed; peak serum concentrations are observed within 2 hours followed by a rapid decline to levels generally below assay within 5 hours. However, a major metabolite, 17-deacetyl norgestimate, appears rapidly in serum with concentrations greatly exceeding that of the parent. Both norethynodrel and ethynodiol diacetate are converted to norethindrone. Peak serum concentrations of drospirenone are reached 1 to 3 hours after administration. Progestins are bound to albumin (79% to 95%) and to sex hormone binding globulin (except drospirenone). Terminal half-life of the progestins are as follows: Norethindrone, 5 to 14 hours; levonorgestrel, 11 to 45 hours; desogestrel (metabolite), 38 ± 20 hours; norgestimate (metabolite), 12 to 30 hours; drospirenone, 30 hours. Progestin-only administration results in lower steady-state serum progestin levels and a shorter elimination half-life than coadministration with estrogens.

➤*Pharmacokinetics:*

Estrogens – Ethinyl estradiol is rapidly absorbed with peak concentrations attained within 2 hours. It undergoes considerable first-pass elimination. Mestranol is demethylated to ethinyl estradiol. Ethinyl estradiol is 97% to 98% bound to plasma albumin. Half-life varies from 6 to 20 hours. It is excreted in bile and urine as conjugates and undergoes some enterohepatic recirculation.

Progestins – Peak concentrations of norethindrone occur 0.5 to 4 hours after oral administration; it undergoes first-pass metabolism with an overall bioavailability of approximately 65%. Levonorgestrel reaches peak concentrations between 0.5 to 2 hours, does not undergo a first-pass effect, and is

PROGESTERONE CONTRACEPTIVE SYSTEM — INTRAUTERINE

completely bioavailable. Norethindrone and levonorgestrel are chiefly metabolized by reduction followed by conjugation. Desogestrel is rapidly and completely absorbed and converted into 3-keto-desogestrel, the biologically active metabolite. Relative bioavailability is approximately 84%. Maximum concentrations of the metabolite are reached at approximately 1.4 hours. Norgestimate is well absorbed; peak serum concentrations are observed within 2 hours followed by a rapid decline to levels generally below assay within 5 hours. However, a major metabolite, 17-deacetyl norgestimate, appears rapidly in serum with concentrations greatly exceeding that of the parent. Both norethynodrel and ethynodiol diacetate are converted to norethindrone. Peak serum concentrations of drospirenone are reached 1 to 3 hours after administration. Progestins are bound to albumin (79% to 95%) and to sex hormone binding globulin (except drospirenone). Terminal half-life of the progestins are as follows: Norethindrone, 5 to 14 hours; levonorgestrel, 11 to 45 hours; desogestrel (metabolite), 38 ± 20 hours; norgestimate (metabolite), 12 to 30 hours; drospirenone, 30 hours. Progestin-only administration results in lower steady-state serum progestin levels and a shorter elimination half-life than coadministration with estrogens.

Contraindications

Pregnancy or suspected pregnancy; previous ectopic pregnancy; presence or history of PID; patient or partner with multiple sexual partners; sexually transmitted disease; postpartum endometritis or infected abortion; pelvic surgery; abnormalities which result in uterine distortion or uteri that measure less than 6 cm or more than 10 cm by sounding; uterine or cervical malignancy, including an unresolved abnormal Pap smear; genital bleeding of unknown etiology; vaginitis or cervicitis unless infection has been completely controlled and is nongonococcal and nonchlamydial; incomplete involution of the uterus following abortion or childbirth; previously inserted intrauterine device (IUD) still in place; genital actinomycosis; conditions or treatments associated with increased susceptibility to infections with microorganisms (eg, leukemia, diabetes, AIDS); IV drug abuse.

Warnings

➤*Pelvic infection:* An increased risk of PID associated with IUD use has been reported; the highest rate occurs shortly after insertion and up to 4 months thereafter. Teach patients to recognize the symptoms of PID and ectopic pregnancy. Pelvic infection may occur with an IUD in situ, and may result in tubo-ovarian abscesses or general peritonitis. If this occurs, remove the IUD and institute appropriate antibiotic treatment. PID can result in tubal damage and occlusion, threatening future fertility or predisposing to ectopic pregnancy. PID may be asymptomatic but still result in tubal damage and its sequelae.

Following diagnosis of PID, initiate antibiotic therapy promptly and remove the progesterone IUD. Guidelines for treatment are available from the CDC.

Genital actinomycosis has been associated primarily with long-term IUD use.

➤*Embedment:* Partial penetration or lodging of an IUD in the endometrium can result in difficult removal. In some cases, this can result in IUD fragmentation, necessitating surgical removal.

➤*Perforation:* Perforation, partial or total, of the uterine wall or cervix may occur. If perforation occurs, remove the device. Adhesions, foreign body reactions, peritonitis, cystic masses in the pelvis, intestinal penetrations, local inflammatory reaction with abscess formation and erosion of adjacent viscera and intestinal obstruction may result if the IUD is left in the peritoneal cavity.

➤*Mortality risks:* Refer to the Oral Contraceptives group monograph for risk of death associated with various methods of contraception.

➤*Pregnancy:* Long-term effects on the fetus are unknown.

Septic abortion – Septic abortion may be increased, associated in some instances with septicemia, septic shock, and death in patients becoming pregnant with an IUD in place, usually in the second trimester. If pregnancy occurs with a system in situ, remove it if the thread is visible or, if removal is difficult, consider termination of the pregnancy.

Continuation of pregnancy – If pregnancy is maintained and the system remains in situ, warn the patient of the increased risk of spontaneous abortion and sepsis, including death, and premature labor and delivery. Advise her to report immediately all abnormal symptoms, such as flu-like syndrome, fever, chills, abdominal cramping and pain, bleeding or vaginal discharge; generalized symptoms of septicemia may be insidious.

Congenital anomalies – Systemically administered sex steroids, including progestational agents, have been associated with an increased risk of congenital anomalies. It is not known whether there is an increased risk of such anomalies when pregnancy is continued with this system in place.

Ectopic pregnancy – The *Progestasert* system acts in the uterus to prevent uterine pregnancy, but it does not prevent either ovulation or ectopic pregnancy. Therefore, a pregnancy that occurs while a patient is using an IUD is much more likely to be ectopic. Determine whether ectopic pregnancy has occurred in patients with delayed menses or unilateral pelvic pain.

In clinical trials of the progesterone system, 1 of 3.6 pregnancies in parous women and 1 of 6.2 pregnancies in nulliparous women were ectopic. The per-year risk of ectopic pregnancy in progesterone system users is approximately 1 ectopic pregnancy in 200 users per year. This risk is approximately the same as in noncontracepting, sexually active women.

In two clinical studies, for the first year the risk of ectopic pregnancy was approximately 6 times higher among women using progesterone systems than among women using copper systems. Over 2 years, the risk of an ectopic pregnancy with the progesterone-releasing IUD was about 10 times higher than that with copper-releasing IUDs.

Women who have previously had acute PID subsequently have an 8- to 10-fold greater than normal risk of ectopic pregnancy (see Pelvic Infection). Multiple sexual partners or a partner with multiple sexual partners, previous pelvic surgery, endometritis, endometriosis, and retrograde menstruation have also been recognized as risk factors for ectopic pregnancy.

Precautions

➤*Prior to insertion:* Prior to insertion, complete a medical and social history, and determine risk of ectopic pregnancy because of previous PID. Perform pelvic examination, Pap smear, gonorrhea and chlamydia culture and, if indicated, tests for other sexually transmitted diseases. Carefully sound the uterus prior to insertion to determine the degree of patency of the endocervical canal and the internal os, and the direction and depth of the uterine cavity. Occasionally, severe cervical stenosis may be encountered. The uterus should sound to a depth of 6 to 10 cm. Inserting the system into a uterine cavity measuring less than 6.5 cm may increase the incidence of expulsion, bleeding, and pain.

To reduce the possibility of insertion in the presence of an undetermined pregnancy, insert during or shortly following menstruation.

➤*Cervicitis/Vaginitis:* Postpone use in these patients until infection has cleared and until the cervicitis has been shown not to be due to gonorrhea or chlamydia.

➤*Involution of uterus:* Do not insert postpartum or postabortion until involution of the uterus is completed. Incidence of perforation (see Warnings) and expulsion is greater if involution is not completed. Involution may be delayed in nursing mothers.

➤*Anemia:* Use cautiously in those who have anemia or history of menorrhagia or hypermenorrhea. Patients experiencing menorrhagia or metrorrhagia following IUD insertion may be at risk of developing hypochromic microcytic anemia.

➤*Syncope/Bradycardia:* Syncope, bradycardia, or other neurovascular episodes may occur during insertion or removal, especially in patients previously disposed to these conditions or cervical stenosis.

➤*Valvular/Congenital heart disease patients:* Valvular or congenital heart disease patients are more prone to develop subacute bacterial endocarditis. The use of the IUD may represent a potential source of septic emboli.

➤*Reexamine:* Reexamine patient shortly after the first postinsertion menses, since an IUD may be expelled or displaced, but definitely within 3 months after insertion. Thereafter, perform an annual examination.

➤*Replace:* Replace the device every 12 months, since the level of contraceptive efficacy after this time decreases.

➤*Remove:* Remove the device for the following reasons: Menorrhagia/metrorrhagia-producing anemia; pelvic infection; endometritis; genital actinomycosis; intractable pelvic pain; dyspareunia; pregnancy; endometrial or cervical malignancy; uterine or cervical perforation; increase of length of the threads extending from the cervix or any other indication of partial expulsion. If retrieval threads are not visible, they may have retracted into the uterus or have been broken; therefore, consider the system displaced and remove. After menstrual period, determine that the threads still protrude from the cervix. Caution patients not to pull on the threads. If partial expulsion occurs, removal is indicated and a new system may be inserted.

➤*Bleeding and cramps:* Bleeding and cramps may occur during the first few weeks after insertion; if symptoms continue or are severe, consult health care provider.

➤*Prophylactic antibiotics:* Prophylactic antibiotics may be considered prior to IUD insertion to decrease the risk of PID; however, the utility of this treatment is still under evaluation. Regimens include doxycycline 200 mg orally 1 hour before insertion or erythromycin 500 mg orally 1 hour before and 6 hours after insertion.

Drug Interactions

➤*Anticoagulants:* Use IUDs with caution in patients receiving anticoagulants or having a coagulopathy.

Adverse Reactions

Endometritis; spontaneous abortion; septic abortion; septicemia; perforation of uterus and cervix; pelvic infection; cervical erosion; vaginitis; leukorrhea; pregnancy; ectopic pregnancy; uterine embedment; difficult removal; complete or partial expulsion; intermenstrual spotting; prolongation of menstrual flow; anemia; amenorrhea or delayed menses; pain and cramping; dysmenorrhea; backaches; dyspareunia; neurovascular episodes including bradycardia and syncope secondary to insertion; fragmentation of IUD; tubo-ovarian abscess; tubal damage; fetal damage and congenital anomalies. Perforation into the abdomen followed by peritonitis, abdominal adhesions, intestinal penetration, intestinal obstruction, local inflammatory reaction, abscess formation and erosion of adjacent viscera, and cystic masses in the pelvis have occurred. Some of these adverse reactions can lead to loss of fertility, partial or total removal of reproductive organs, hormonal imbalance, or death.

Patient Information

Patient package insert and patient instructions are available with the product. The patient must read and initial each section of the *Patient Information* leaflet, and the Informed Choice Statement must be signed by the patient and by the health care provider.

Notify health care provider if any of the following occurs: Abnormal or excessive bleeding; severe cramping; abnormal or odorous vaginal discharge; fever or flu-like syndrome; pain; genital lesions or sores; missed period.

LEVONORGESTREL-RELEASING INTRAUTERINE SYSTEM

Rx	**Mirena** (Berlex Labs.)	**Intrauterine system:** T-shaped unit containing a reservoir of 52 mg levonorgestrel covered by a silicone membrane	In 1s w/ inserter.

LEVONORGESTREL — INTRAUTERINE SYSTEM

WARNING

Patients should be counseled that this product does not protect against HIV infection (AIDS) and other sexually transmitted diseases.

Indications

➤*Contraception:* The levonorgestrel-releasing intrauterine system is indicated for intrauterine contraception for up to 5 years. Thereafter, if continued contraception is desired, the system should be replaced.

➤*Recommended patient profile:* Levonorgestrel-releasing intrauterine system is recommended for women who have had at least one child, are in a stable, mutually monogamous relationship, have no history of pelvic inflammatory disease, and have no history of ectopic pregnancy or condition that would predispose to ectopic pregnancy.

Administration and Dosage

➤*Approved by the FDA:* December 6, 2000.

➤*Directions for use:*

Note – Healthcare providers are advised to become thoroughly familiar with the insertion instructions before attempting insertion of the levonorgestrel-releasing intrauterine system.

➤*Insertion instructions:* The levonorgestrel-releasing intrauterine system is inserted with the provided inserter into the uterine cavity within 7 days of the onset of menstruation or immediately after first trimester abortion by carefully following the insertion instructions. It can be replaced by a new system at any time during the menstrual cycle.

➤*Important:* If you suspect that the system is not in the correct position, check placement, (eg, with ultrasound). Remove the system if it is not positioned completely within the uterus. Do not reinsert a removed system.

➤*Removal of the levonorgestrel-releasing intrauterine system:* Remove levonorgestrel-releasing intrauterine system by applying gentle traction on the threads with forceps. The arms of the system will fold upward as it is withdrawn from the uterus. The system should not remain in the uterus after 5 years.

➤*Special notes if a patient wants to continue contraception after removal:* You may insert a new levonorgestrel-releasing intrauterine system immediately following removal.

If a patient with regular cycles wants to start a different birth control method, remove the system during the first 7 days of the menstrual cycle and start the new method.

If a patient with irregular cycles or amenorrhea wants to start a different birth control method, or if you remove the system after the seventh day of the menstrual cycle, start the new method at least 7 days before removal.

➤*Storage/Stability:* Store at 25°C (77°F); with excursions permitted between 15° to 30°C (59° to 86°F) [see USP controlled room temperature].

Actions

➤*Pharmacology:* Levonorgestrel is a progestogen used in a variety of contraceptive products. Low doses of levonorgestrel can be administered into the uterine cavity with the levonorgestrel-releasing intrauterine delivery system. Initially, levonorgestrel is released at a rate of ≈ 20 mcg/day. This rate decreases progressively to half that value after 5 years.

The levonorgestrel-releasing intrauterine system has mainly local progestogenic effects in the uterine cavity. Morphological changes of the endometrium are observed, including stromal pseudodecidualization, glandular atrophy, a leucocytic infiltration and a decrease in glandular and stromal mitoses.

Ovulation is inhibited in some women using the levonorgestrel-releasing intrauterine system. In a 1-year study, approximately 45% of menstrual cycles were ovulatory, and in another study, after 4 years, 75% of cycles were ovulatory.

The local mechanism by which continuously released levonorgestrel enhances contraceptive effectiveness of the intrauterine system has not been conclusively demonstrated. Studies of the levonorgestrel-releasing intrauterine system prototypes have suggested several mechanisms that prevent pregnancy: Thickening of cervical mucus preventing passage of sperm into the uterus; inhibition of sperm capacitation or survival; alteration of the endometrium.

➤*Pharmacokinetics:*

Absorption/Distribution – Following insertion of levonorgestrel-releasing intrauterine system, the initial release of levonorgestrel into the uterine cavity is 20 mcg/day. A stable plasma level of levonorgestrel 150 to 200 pg/mL occurs after the first few weeks following insertion of the intrauterine system. Levonorgestrel levels after long-term use of 12, 24, and 60 months were 180 ± 66 pg/mL, 192 ± 140 pg/mL, and 159 ± 59 pg/mL, respectively. The plasma concentrations achieved by the intrauterine system are lower than those seen with levonorgestrel contraceptive implants and with oral contraceptives. Unlike oral contraceptives, plasma levels with the levonorgestrel-releasing intrauterine system do not display peaks and troughs.

The mean ± SD levonorgestrel endometrial tissue concentration in 4 women using levonorgestrel intrauterine systems releasing 30 mcg/day of levonorgestrel for 36 to 49 days was 808 ± 511 ng/g wet tissue weight. The endometrial tissue concentration in 2 women who had been taking a 250 mcg levonorgestrel-containing oral contraceptive for 7 days was 3.5 nanograms/g wet tissue weight. In contrast, fallopian tube and myometrial levonorgestrel tissue concentrations were of the same order of magnitude in the levonorgestrel-releasing intrauterine system group and the oral contraceptive group (between 1 and 5 nanograms/g of wet weight of tissue).

Metabolism/Excretion – The pharmacokinetics of levonorgestrel itself have been extensively studied and reported in the literature. Levonorgestrel in serum is primarily bound to proteins (mainly sex hormone-binding globulin) and is extensively metabolized to a large number of inactive metabolites. Metabolic clearance rates may differ among individuals by several-fold, and this may account in part for wide individual variations in levonorgestrel concentrations seen in individuals using levonorgestrel-containing contraceptive products. The elimination half-life of levonorgestrel after daily oral doses is approximately 17 hours; both the parent drug and its metabolites are primarily excreted in the urine.

Contraindications

Levonorgestrel-releasing intrauterine system insertion is contraindicated when one or more of the following conditions exist: Pregnancy or suspicion of pregnancy; congenital or acquired uterine anomaly including fibroids if they distort the uterine cavity; acute pelvic inflammatory disease or a history of pelvic inflammatory disease, unless there has been a subsequent intrauterine pregnancy; postpartum endometritis or infected abortion in the past 3 months; known or suspected uterine or cervical neoplasia, or unresolved, abnormal Pap smear; genital bleeding of unknown etiology; untreated acute cervicitis or vaginitis, including bacterial vaginosis or other lower genital tract infections until infection is controlled; acute liver disease or liver tumor (benign or malignant); woman or her partner has multiple sexual partners; conditions associated with increased susceptibility to infections with microorganisms (such conditions include, but are not limited to, leukemia, acquired immune deficiency syndrome [AIDS], and IV drug abuse; genital actinomycosis (see Warnings); a previously inserted IUD that has not been removed; hypersensitivity to any component of this product; known or suspected carcinoma of the breast; history of ectopic pregnancy or condition that would predispose to ectopic pregnancy.

Warnings

➤*Ectopic pregnancy:* In large clinical trials of the levonorgestrel-releasing intrauterine system, half of all pregnancies detected during the studies were ectopic. The per-year incidence of ectopic pregnancy in the clinical trials was approximately 1 ectopic pregnancy/1,000 users per year. The rate of ectopic pregnancies associated with the levonorgestrel-releasing intrauterine system use is not significantly different than the rate for sexually active women not using any contraception.

Clinical trials of the levonorgestrel-releasing intrauterine system excluded women with a history of ectopic pregnancy. The intrauterine system is not recommended for use in women with a history of ectopic pregnancy or conditions that increase the risk of ectopic pregnancy. Women who choose the levonorgestrel-releasing intrauterine system must be warned about the risks of ectopic pregnancy. They should be taught to recognize and report to their physician promptly any symptoms of ectopic pregnancy. Women should also be informed that ectopic pregnancy has been associated with complications leading to loss of fertility.

➤*Intrauterine pregnancy:* In the event of an intrauterine pregnancy with the levonorgestrel-releasing intrauterine system, the following should be considered:

Septic abortion – In patients becoming pregnant with an IUD in place, septic abortion, with septicemia, septic shock, and death, may occur. If pregnancy should occur with a levonorgestrel-releasing intrauterine system in place, the system should be removed. Removal or manipulation of the system may result in pregnancy loss.

Continuation of pregnancy – If a woman becomes pregnant with a levonorgestrel-releasing intrauterine system in place, and if the levonorgestrel-releasing intrauterine system cannot be removed or the woman chooses not to have it removed, she should be warned that failure to remove the system increases the risk of miscarriage, sepsis, premature labor and premature delivery. She should be followed closely and advised to report immediately any flu-like symptoms, fever, chills, cramping, pain, bleeding, vaginal discharge or leakage of fluid.

Long-term effects and congenital anomalies – When pregnancy continues with the levonorgestrel-releasing intrauterine system in place, long-term effects on the offspring are unknown. Because of the intrauterine administration of levonorgestrel and local exposure to the hormone, the possibility of teratogenicity following exposure to the intrauterine system cannot be completely excluded. Clinical experience with the outcomes of pregnancies is limited due to the small number of reported pregnancies following exposure to the levonorgestrel-releasing intrauterine system.

Congenital anomalies have occurred infrequently when the levonorgestrel-releasing intrauterine system has been in place during pregnancy. In these cases, the role of the system in the development of the congenital anomalies is unknown. As of September, 1999, 32 live births following exposure to the intrauterine system were reported retrospectively. All but 2 of the infants

LEVONORGESTREL — INTRAUTERINE SYSTEM

were healthy at birth. One infant had pulmonary artery hypoplasia, and another infant had cystic hypoplastic kidneys. (A sibling of this infant had renal agenesis with no levonorgestrel-releasing intrauterine system exposure.)

➤*Sepsis:* As of 1999, four cases of group A streptococcal sepsis (GAS) out of an estimated 1.3 million levonorgestrel-releasing intrauterine system users were reported. All 4 women experienced the symptom of severe pain within hours of insertion, and this was followed by sepsis within a few days (of insertion). All recovered with treatment. Since death from GAS is more likely if treatment is delayed, it is important to be aware of these rare but serious infections. Aseptic technique during the intrauterine system insertion is essential. (GAS sepsis can also occur postpartum, after minor surgery, in wounds and in association with other IUDs.)

➤*Pelvic inflammatory disease (PID):* The levonorgestrel-releasing intrauterine system is contraindicated in the presence of known or suspected PID or in women with a history of PID, unless there has been a subsequent intrauterine pregnancy. Use of IUDs has been associated with an increased risk of PID. The highest risk of PID occurs shortly after insertion (usually within the first 20 days thereafter) (see insertion precautions). A decision to use the intrauterine system must include consideration of the risks of PID.

Women at increased risk for PID – PID is often associated with a sexually transmitted disease, and the levonorgestrel-releasing intrauterine system does not protect against sexually transmitted disease. The risk of PID is greater for women who have multiple sexual partners, and also for women whose sexual partner(s) have multiple sexual partners. Women who have ever had PID are at increased risk for a recurrence or reinfection.

PID warning to levonorgestrel-releasing intrauterine system users – All women who choose the levonorgestrel-releasing intrauterine system must be informed prior to insertion about the possibility of PID, and that PID can cause tubal damage leading to ectopic pregnancy or infertility, or in infrequent cases can necessitate hysterectomy, or can cause death. Patients must be taught to recognize and report to their physician promptly any symptoms of pelvic inflammatory disease. These symptoms include development of menstrual disorders (prolonged or heavy bleeding), unusual vaginal discharge, abdominal or pelvic pain or tenderness, dyspareunia, chills, and fever.

Asymptomatic PID – PID may be asymptomatic but still result in tubal damage and its sequelae.

Treatment of PID – Following a diagnosis of PID, or suspected PID, bacteriologic specimens should be obtained and antibiotic therapy should be initiated promptly. Removal of the levonorgestrel-releasing intrauterine system after initiation of antibiotic therapy is usually appropriate. Guidelines for PID treatment are available from the center for disease control (CDC), Atlanta, Georgia. Adequate PID treatment requires the application of current standards of therapy prevailing at the time of occurrence of the infection with reference to prescription labeling.

Actinomycosis has been associated with IUDs. Symptomatic women with IUDs should have the IUD removed and should receive antibiotics. However, the management of the asymptomatic carrier is controversial because actinomycetes can be found normally in the genital tract cultures in healthy women without IUDs. False-positive findings of actinomycosis on Pap smears can be a problem. When possible, confirm the Pap smear diagnosis with cultures.

➤*Irregular bleeding and amenorrhea:* The levonorgestrel-releasing intrauterine system can alter the bleeding pattern. During the first 3 to 6 months of intrauterine system use, the number of bleeding and spotting days may be increased and bleeding patterns may be irregular. Thereafter the number of bleeding and spotting days usually decreases but bleeding may remain irregular. If bleeding irregularities develop during prolonged treatment, appropriate diagnostic measures should be taken to rule out endometrial pathology.

Amenorrhea develops in approximately 20% of levonorgestrel-releasing intrauterine system users by 1 year. The possibility of pregnancy should be considered if menstruation does not occur within 6 weeks of the onset of previous menstruation. Once pregnancy has been excluded, repeated pregnancy tests are not necessary in amenorrheic subjects unless indicated by other signs of pregnancy or by pelvic pain.

➤*Embedment:* Partial penetration or embedment of the levonorgestrel-releasing intrauterine system in the myometrium may decrease contraceptive effectiveness and can result in difficult removal.

➤*Perforation:* An IUD may perforate the uterus or cervix, most often during insertion, although the perforation may not be detected until some time later. If perforation occurs, the IUD must be removed and surgery may be required. Adhesions, peritonitis, intestinal perforations, intestinal obstruction, abscesses and erosion of adjacent viscera have been reported with IUDs.

It is recommended that postpartum levonorgestrel-releasing intrauterine system insertion be delayed until uterine involution is complete to decrease perforation risk. There is an increased risk of perforation in women who are lactating. Inserting the system immediately after first trimester abortion is not known to increase the risk of perforation, but insertion after second trimester abortion should be delayed until uterine involution is complete.

➤*Ovarian cysts:* Since the contraceptive effect of the levonorgestrel-releasing intrauterine system is mainly due to its local effect, ovulatory cycles with follicular rupture usually occur in women of fertile age using the intrauterine system. Sometimes atresia of the follicle is delayed and the follicle may continue to grow. Enlarged follicles have been diagnosed in about 12% of the subjects using the intrauterine system. Most of these follicles are asymptomatic, although some may be accompanied by pelvic pain or dyspareunia. In most cases the enlarged follicles disappear spontaneously during 2 to 3 months' observation. Surgical intervention is not usually required.

➤*Breast cancer:* Women who currently have or have had breast cancer should not use hormonal contraception because breast cancer is a hormone-sensitive tumor.

➤*Risks of mortality:* The available data from a variety of sources have been analyzed to estimate the risk of death associated with various methods of contraception. The estimates of risk of death include the combined risk of the contraceptive method plus the risk of pregnancy or abortion in the event of method failure.

➤*Pregnancy:* Category X. (See ectopic and intrauterine pregnancy above.)

➤*Lactation:* Levonorgestrel has been identified in small quantities in the breast milk of lactating women using the levonorgestrel-releasing intrauterine system. In a study of 14 breastfeeding women using a levonorgestrel-releasing intrauterine system prototype during lactation, mean infant serum levels of levonorgestrel were approximately 7% of maternal serum levels. Hormonal contraceptives are not recommended as the contraceptive method of first choice during lactation.

➤*Children:* Safety and efficacy of the levonorgestrel-releasing intrauterine system have been established in women of reproductive age. Use of this product before menarche is not indicated (see Indications).

Precautions

➤*Sexually transmitted diseases:* Patients should be counseled that this product does not protect against HIV infection (AIDS) and other sexually transmitted diseases.

➤*Prior to insertion:* Prior to insertion, the physician, nurse, or other trained health professional must provide the patient with the patient package insert. The patient should be given the opportunity to read the information and discuss fully any questions she may have concerning the levonorgestrel-releasing intrauterine system as well as other methods of contraception.

Careful and objective counseling of the user prior to insertion regarding the expected bleeding pattern, the possible interindividual variation in changes in bleeding, and the etiology of the changes may have an effect on the frequency of removal because of bleeding problems and amenorrhea.

The patient should be told that some bleeding such as irregular or prolonged bleeding and spotting, or cramps may occur during the first few weeks after insertion. If her symptoms continue or are severe, she should report them to her healthcare provider. She should also be given instructions on what other symptoms require her to call her healthcare provider. She should be instructed on how to check after her menstrual period to make certain that the thread still protrudes from the cervix and cautioned not to pull on the thread and displace the levonorgestrel-releasing intrauterine system. She should be informed that there is no contraceptive protection if the system is displaced or expelled.

The uterus should be carefully sounded prior to the levonorgestrel-releasing intrauterine system insertion to determine the degree of patency of the endocervical canal and the internal os, and the direction and depth of the uterine cavity. In occasional cases, severe cervical stenosis may be encountered. Do not use excessive force to overcome this resistance.

➤*Patient evaluation and clinical considerations:* A complete medical and social history, including that of the partner, should be obtained to determine conditions that might influence the selection of an IUD for contraception (see Contraindications). A physical examination should include a pelvic examination, a Pap smear, and appropriate tests for any other forms of genital disease, such as gonorrhea and chlamydia laboratory evaluations, if indicated. Special attention must be given to ascertaining whether the woman is at increased risk of ectopic pregnancy or PID. The levonorgestrel-releasing intrauterine system is contraindicated in these women.

The healthcare provider should determine that the patient is not pregnant. The possibility of insertion of a levonorgestrel-releasing intrauterine system in the presence of an existing undetermined pregnancy is reduced if insertion if performed within 7 days of the onset of a menstrual period. The system can be replaced by a new system at any time in the cycle. The system can be inserted immediately after first trimester abortion.

➤*Postpartum:* The levonorgestrel-releasing intrauterine system should not be inserted until 6 weeks postpartum or until involution of the uterus is complete in order to reduce the incidence of perforation and expulsion.

➤*Valvular / Congenital heart disease:* Patients with certain types of valvular or congenital heart disease and surgically constructed systemic-pulmonary shunts are at increased risk of infective endocarditis. Use of a levonorgestrel-releasing intrauterine system in these patients may represent a potential source of septic emboli. Patients with known congenital heart disease who may be at increased risk should be treated with appropriate antibiotics at the time of insertion and removal. Patients requiring chronic corticosteroid therapy or insulin for diabetes should be monitored with special care for infection.

➤*Coagulopathy / Anticoagulant therapy:* Levonorgestrel-releasing intrauterine system should be used with caution in patients who have a coagulopathy or are receiving anticoagulants.

➤*Vaginitis / Cervicitis:* Use of a levonorgestrel-releasing intrauterine system in patients with vaginitis or cervicitis should be postponed until proper treatment has eradicated the infection and until it has been shown that the cervicitis is not due to gonorrhea or chlamydia (see Contraindications).

LEVONORGESTREL — INTRAUTERINE SYSTEM

➤*Prophylactic antibiotics:* Because the presence of organisms capable of establishing PID cannot be determined by appearance, and because IUD insertion may be associated with introduction of vaginal bacteria into the uterus, strict asepsis should be observed at insertion. Administration of antibiotics may be considered, but the utility of this treatment is unknown.

➤*Syncope/Bradycardia:* Syncope, bradycardia, or other neurovascular episodes may occur during insertion or removal of the levonorgestrel-releasing intrauterine system, especially in patients with a predisposition to these conditions or cervical stenosis. If decreased pulse, perspiration, or pallor are observed, the patient should remain supine until these signs have disappeared.

➤*Continuation and removal:* The levonorgestrel-releasing intrauterine system must be replaced every 5 years because contraceptive effectiveness after 5 years has not been established.

User complaints of pain, odorous discharge, bleeding, fever, genital lesions or sores should be promptly responded to and prompt examination recommended (see Warnings).

If examination during visits subsequent to insertion reveals that the length of the threads has changed from the length at time of insertion, and the system is verified as displaced, it should be removed. A new system may be inserted at that time, or during the next menses, if it is certain that conception has not occurred. If the threads are not visible, location of the levonorgestrel-releasing intrauterine system should be verified, for example with x-ray, ultrasound, or gentle probing of the uterine cavity. If the system is in place with no evidence of perforation, no intervention is indicated. If expulsion has occurred, it may be replaced within 7 days of a menstrual period after pregnancy has been ruled out.

Since the levonorgestrel-releasing intrauterine system may be displaced, patients should be reexamined and evaluated shortly after the first postinsertion menses, but definitely within 3 months after insertion. Symptoms of the partial or complete expulsion of any IUD may include bleeding or pain. However, the system can be expelled from the uterine cavity without the woman noticing it. Partial expulsion may decrease the effectiveness of the intrauterine system. As menstrual flow usually decreases after the first 3 to 6 months of the intrauterine system use, increase of menstrual flow may be indicative of an expulsion.

The levonorgestrel-releasing intrauterine system should be removed for the following medical reasons: Menorrhagia or metrorrhagia producing anemia; acquired immune deficiency syndrome (AIDS); sexually transmitted disease; pelvic infection; endometritis; symptomatic genital actinomycosis; intractable pelvic pain; severe dyspareunia; pregnancy; endometrial or cervical malignancy; uterine or cervical perforation.

If the retrieval threads are not visible, they may have retracted into the uterus or have been broken, or the intrauterine system may have been broken, perforated the uterus, or have been expelled. Location of the system may be determined by sonography, x-ray, or by gentle exploration of the uterine cavity with a probe.

Removal of the system should also be considered if any of the following conditions arise for the first time: migraine; focal migraine with asymmetrical visual loss or other symptoms indicating transient cerebral ischemia; exceptionally severe headache; jaundice; marked increase of blood pressure; severe arterial disease such as stroke or myocardial infarction (MI).

➤*Pregnancy during therapy:* In the event a pregnancy is confirmed during levonorgestrel-releasing intrauterine system use, the following steps should be taken:

1.) Determine whether pregnancy is ectopic and take appropriate measures if it is.
2.) Inform patient of the risks of leaving the system in place or removing it during pregnancy, and of the lack of data on long-term effects on the offspring of women who have had the system in place during conception or gestation (see Warnings).
3.) If possible, the levonorgestrel-releasing intrauterine system should be removed after the patient has been warned of the risks of removal. If removal is difficult, the patient should be counseled and offered pregnancy termination.
4.) If the levonorgestrel-releasing intrauterine system is left in place, the patient's course should be followed closely.

➤*Sexually transmitted disease (STDs):* Should the patient's relationship cease to be mutually monogamous, or should her partner become HIV positive, or acquire a sexually transmitted disease, she should be instructed to report this change to her clinician immediately. The use of a barrier method as a partial protection against acquiring sexually transmitted diseases should be strongly recommended. Removal of the system should be considered.

➤*Glucose tolerance:* Levonorgestrel may affect glucose tolerance, and the blood glucose concentration should be monitored in diabetic users of the levonorgestrel-releasing intrauterine system.

Drug Interactions

The effect of hormonal contraceptives may be impaired by drugs which induce liver enzymes. The influence of these drugs on the contraceptive efficacy of the levonorgestrel-releasing intrauterine system has not been studied.

Adverse Reactions

➤*Adverse reactions reported by at least 5%:* The most serious adverse reactions associated with the use of the levonorgestrel-releasing intrauterine system are discussed in Warnings. Others are presented in Precautions. Other adverse reactions reported by at least 5% subjects include the following:

Cardiovascular – Hypertension.

CNS – Headache, depression, nervousness.

Dermatologic – Acne, skin disorder.

GI – Abdominal pain, nausea.

GU – Dysmenorrhea, leukorrhea, vaginitis, abnormal Pap smear.

Respiratory – Upper respiratory tract infection, sinusitis.

Miscellaneous – Back pain, breast pain, weight increase, decreased libido.

➤*Adverse reactions occurring in less than 3%:* Other reported adverse reactions occurring in less than 3% of patients include the following:

CNS – Migraine.

Dermatologic – Hair loss, eczema.

GI – Vomiting.

GU – Cervicitis, dyspareunia, failed insertion.

Hematologic – Anemia.

Patient Information

The levonorgestrel-releasing intrauterine system is used to prevent pregnancy. It does not protect against HIV infection (AIDS) and other sexually transmitted diseases (STDs).

MEDROXYPROGESTERONE CONTRACEPTIVE INJECTION

Rx	**Depo-Sub Q Provera 104** (Pfizer)	**Injection**: 104 mg (160 mg/mL)	In 0.65 mL prefilled single-use syringes.[a]
Rx	**Medroxyprogesterone Acetate** (Various, eg, Greenstone, Sicor)	**Injection**: 150 mg/mL	In 1 mL vials.
Rx	**Depo-Provera** (Pharmacia Corp)		In 1 mL vials.[b]
Rx	**Depo-Provera** (Pharmacia Corp)	**Injection**: 400 mg/mL	In 2.5 and 10 mL vials and 1 mL U-ject.[c]

[a] With methylparaben 1.04 mg, propylparaben 0.098 mg, sodium chloride 5.2 mg, polyethylene glycol 18.688 mg, polysorbate 80 1.95 mg, monobasic sodium phosphate 0.451, dibasic sodium phosphate 0.382 mg, methionine 0.975 mg, povidone 3.25 mg, and possibly sodium hydroxide and/or hydrochloric acid.

[b] With 28.9 mg PEG 3350, 2.41 mg polysorbate 80, 8.68 mg sodium chloride, 1.37 mg methylparaben and 0.15 mg propylparaben.

[c] With polyethylene glycol 3350, sodium sulfate anhydrous, myristyl-gamma-picolinium Cl.

MEDROXYPROGESTERONE ACETATE — INJECTION

WARNING

Contraceptive injection – Patients should be counseled that this product does not protect against HIV infection (AIDS) or other sexually transmitted diseases.

Indications

➤*Endometrial/Renal carcinoma (400 mg/mL):* Adjunctive therapy and palliative treatment of inoperable, recurrent, and metastatic endometrial or renal carcinoma.

➤*Contraception (104 mg subcutaneous and 150 mg/mL IM):* Medroxyprogesterone acetate contraceptive injection is indicated only for the prevention of pregnancy. To ensure that medroxyprogesterone acetate contraceptive injection is not administered inadvertently to a pregnant woman, the first injection must be given only during the first 5 days of a normal menstrual period; only within the first 5 days postpartum if not breastfeeding, and if exclusively breast-feeding; only at the sixth postpartum week. The efficacy of medroxyprogesterone acetate contraceptive injection depends on adherence to the recommended dosage schedule. It is a long-term injectable contraceptive in women when administered at 3-month (13-week) intervals. Dosage does not need to be adjusted for body weight.

Administration and Dosage

➤*Endometrial/Renal carcinoma:*

400 mg/mL – The suspension is intended for intramuscular administration only.

Doses of medroxyprogesterone acetate sterile aqueous suspension 400 to 1,000 mg weekly are recommended initially. If improvement is noted within a few weeks or months and the disease appears stabilized, it may be possible to maintain improvement with as little as 400 mg monthly. Medroxyprogesterone acetate is not recommended as primary therapy, but as adjunctive and palliative treatment in advanced inoperable cases including those with recurrent or metastatic disease.

MEDROXYPROGESTERONE ACETATE — INJECTION

When multi-dose vials are used, special care to prevent contamination of the contents is essential. Although initially sterile, any multi-dose use of vials may lead to contamination unless strict aseptic technique is observed.

➤*Contraception:*

150 mg/mL – Both the 1 mL vial and the 1 mL prefilled syringe of medroxyprogesterone acetate contraceptive injection should be vigorously shaken just before use to ensure that the dose being administered represents a uniform suspension.

The recommended dose is medroxyprogesterone acetate contraceptive injection 150 mg every 3 months (13 weeks) administered by deep, IM injection in the gluteal or deltoid muscle. To ensure the patient is not pregnant at the time of the first injection, the first injection must be given only during the first 5 days of a normal menstrual period; only within the first 5 days postpartum if not breast-feeding; and if exclusively breast-feeding, only at the sixth postpartum week. If the time interval between injections is greater than 13 weeks, the physician should determine that the patient is not pregnant before administering the drug. The efficacy of medroxyprogesterone acetate contraceptive injection depends on adherence to the dosage schedule of administration.

104 mg subcutaneous injection – The recommended dose is 104 mg every 3 months (12 to 14 weeks) administered subcutaneously into the anterior thigh or abdomen.

Switching from other methods of contraception – When switching from other contraceptive methods, give medroxyprogesterone in a manner than ensures continuous contraceptive coverage. For example, patients switching from combined (estrogen plus progestin) contraceptives should have their first injection within 7 days after the last day of using that method (7 days after taking the last active pill, removing the patch or ring). Similarly, contraceptive coverage will be maintained in switching from IM (150 mg) to subcutaneous (104 mg) provided the next injection is given within the prescribed dosing period for the IM (150 mg).

➤*Storage/Stability:* Store at controlled room temperature 20° to 25°C (68° to 77°F).

Actions

➤*Pharmacology:*

400 mg/mL – Medroxyprogesterone acetate, administered parenterally in the recommended doses to women with adequate endogenous estrogen, transforms proliferative endometrium into secretory endometrium.

Medroxyprogesterone acetate inhibits (in the usual dose range) the secretion of pituitary gonadotropin which, in turn, prevents follicular maturation and ovulation.

Because of its prolonged action and the resulting difficulty in predicting the time of withdrawal bleeding following injection, medroxyprogesterone acetate is not recommended in secondary amenorrhea or dysfunctional uterine bleeding. In these conditions, oral therapy is recommended.

150 mg/mL – Medroxyprogesterone acetate contraceptive injection, when administered at the recommended dose to women every 3 months, inhibits the secretion of gonadotropins which, in turn, prevents follicular maturation and ovulation and results in endometrial thinning. These actions produce its contraceptive effect.

➤*Pharmacokinetics:*

Absorption – Following a single IM dose of medroxyprogesterone acetate contraceptive injection 150 mg, medroxyprogesterone acetate concentrations, measured by an extracted radioimmunoassay procedure, increase by approximately 3 weeks to reach peak plasma concentrations of 1 to 7 ng/mL. The levels then decreased exponentially until they become undetectable (less than 100 pg/mL) between 120 to 200 days following injection.

Metabolism – Using an unextracted radioimmunoassay procedure for the assay of medroxyprogesterone acetate in serum, the apparent half-life for medroxyprogesterone acetate following IM administration of medroxyprogesterone acetate contraceptive injection is approximately 50 days.

Women with lower body weights conceive sooner than women with higher body weights after discontinuing medroxyprogesterone acetate contraceptive injection.

Contraindications

Known or suspected pregnancy or as a diagnostic test for pregnancy; undiagnosed vaginal bleeding; known or suspected malignancy of breast; active thrombophlebitis, or current or past history of thromboembolic disorders, or cerebral vascular disease; liver dysfunction or disease; known sensitivity to medroxyprogesterone acetate or any of its other ingredients.

Warnings

➤*Thromboembolic disorders:* The physician should be alert to the earliest manifestations of thrombotic disorder (thrombophlebitis, cerebrovascular disorder, pulmonary embolism, and retinal thrombosis). Should any of these occur or be suspected, the drug should not be readministered.

➤*Ocular disorders:* Medication should be discontinued pending examination if there is a sudden partial or complete loss of vision, or if there is a sudden onset of proptosis, diplopia, or migraine. If examination reveals papilledema or retinal vascular lesions, medication should not be readministered.

➤*400 mg/mL:*

Multi-dose use – Multi-dose use of medroxyprogesterone acetate sterile aqueous suspension from a single vial requires special care to avoid contamination. Although initially sterile, any multi-dose use of vials may lead to contamination unless strict aseptic technique is observed.

➤*150 mg/mL:*

Bleeding irregularities – Most women using medroxyprogesterone acetate contraceptive injection experience disruption of menstrual bleeding patterns. Altered menstrual bleeding patterns include irregular or unpredictable bleeding or spotting, or rarely, heavy or continuous bleeding. If abnormal bleeding persists or is severe, appropriate investigation should be instituted to rule out the possibility of organic pathology, and appropriate treatment should be instituted when necessary.

As women continue using medroxyprogesterone acetate contraceptive injection, fewer experience irregular bleeding and more experience amenorrhea. By month 12, amenorrhea was reported by 55% of women, and by month 24, amenorrhea was reported by 68% of women using medroxyprogesterone acetate contraceptive injection.

Bone mineral density changes – Use of medroxyprogesterone acetate contraceptive injection may be considered among the risk factors for development of osteoporosis. The rate of bone loss is greatest in the early years of use and then subsequently approaches the normal rate of age-related fall.

➤*Hypersensitivity reactions:*

Anaphylaxis and anaphylactoid reaction – Anaphylaxis and anaphylactoid reaction have been reported with the use of medroxyprogesterone acetate contraceptive injection. If an anaphylactic reaction occurs, appropriate therapy should be instituted. Serious anaphylactic reactions require emergency medical treatment.

➤*Carcinogenesis:* Long-term intramuscular administration of medroxyprogesterone acetate (MPA) has been shown to produce mammary tumors in beagle dogs. There is no evidence of a carcinogenic effect associated with the oral administration of MPA to rats and mice.

150 mg/mL:

• *Cancer risks* – Long-term case-controlled surveillance of users of medroxyprogesterone acetate contraceptive injection found slight or no increased overall risk of breast cancer and no overall increased risk of ovarian, liver, or cervical cancer and a prolonged, protective effect of reducing the risk of endometrial cancer in the population of users.

A pooled analysis from 2 case-control studies, the World Health Organization Study and the New Zealand Study, reported the relative risk (RR) of breast cancer for women who had ever used medroxyprogesterone acetate contraceptive injection as 1.1 (95% confidence interval [CI]: 0.97 to 1.4). Overall, there was no increase in risk with increasing duration of use of medroxyprogesterone acetate contraceptive injection. The RR of breast cancer for women of all ages who had initiated use of medroxyprogesterone acetate contraceptive injection within the previous 5 years was estimated to be 2 (95% CI: 1.5 to 2.8). The World Health Organization Study, a component of the pooled analysis described above, showed an increased RR of 2.19 (95% CI: 1.23 to 3.89) of breast cancer associated with use of medroxyprogesterone acetate contraceptive injection in women whose first exposure to drug was within the previous 4 years and who were under 35 years of age. However, the overall RR for ever-users of medroxyprogesterone acetate contraceptive injection was only 1.2 (95% CI: 0.96 to 1.52).

Note: An RR of 1 indicates neither an increased nor a decreased risk of cancer associated with the use of the drug, relative to no use of the drug. In the case of the subpopulation with an RR of 2.19, the 95% CI is fairly wide and does not include the value of 1, thus inferring an increased risk of breast cancer in the defined subgroup relative to nonusers. The value of 2.19 means that women whose first exposure to drug was within the previous 4 years and who are under 35 years of age have a 2.19-fold (95% CI: 1.23- to 3.89-fold) increased risk of breast cancer relative to nonusers. The National Cancer Institute reports an average annual incidence rate for breast cancer for US women, all races, age 30 to 34 years of 26.7 per 100,000. An RR of 2.19, thus, increases the possible risk from 26.7 to 58.5 cases per 100,000 women. The attributable risk, thus, is 31.8 per 100,000 women per year.

A statistically insignificant increase in RR estimates of invasive squamous-cell cervical cancer has been associated with the use of medroxyprogesterone acetate contraceptive injection in women who were first exposed before the age of 35 years (RR: 1.22 to 1.28 and 95% CI: 0.93 to 1.7). The overall, non-significant relative rate of invasive squamous-cell cervical cancer in women who ever used medroxyprogesterone acetate contraceptive injection was estimated to be 1.11 (95% CI: 0.96 to 1.29). No trends in risk with duration of use or times since initial or most recent exposure were observed.

➤*Fertility impairment:* Medroxyprogesterone acetate at high doses is an anti-fertility drug and high doses would be expected to impair fertility until the cessation of treatment.

➤*Pregnancy:* Category X.

The use of progestational drugs during the first 4 months of pregnancy is not recommended. Progestational agents have been used beginning with the first trimester of pregnancy in attempts to prevent abortion, but there is no evidence that such use is effective. Furthermore, the use of progestational agents, with their uterine-relaxant properties, in patients with fertilized defective ova may cause a delay in spontaneous abortion.

Several reports suggest an association between intrauterine exposure to progestational drugs in the first trimester of pregnancy and genital abnormalities in male and female fetuses. The risk of hypospadias (5 to 8 per 1,000 male births in the general population) may be approximately doubled with exposure to these drugs. There are insufficient data to quantify the risk to exposed female fetuses, but insofar as some of these drugs induce mild virilization of the external genitalia of the female fetus, and because of the increased association of hypospadias in the male fetus, it is prudent to avoid the use of these drugs during the first trimester of pregnancy.

MEDROXYPROGESTERONE ACETATE — INJECTION

If the patient is exposed to medroxyprogesterone acetate injection during the first 4 months of pregnancy, or if she becomes pregnant while taking this drug, she should be apprised of the potential risks to the fetus.

150 mg/mL –

Unexpected pregnancies: To ensure that medroxyprogesterone acetate contraceptive injection is not administered inadvertently to a pregnant woman, the first injection must be given only during the first 5 days of a normal menstrual period; only within the first 5 days postpartum if not breast feeding, and if exclusively breastfeeding, only at the sixth postpartum week.

Neonates from unexpected pregnancies that occur 1 to 2 months after injection of medroxyprogesterone acetate contraceptive injection may be at an increased risk of low birth weight, which, in turn, is associated with an increased risk of neonatal death. The attributable risk is low because such pregnancies are uncommon.

A significant increase in incidence of polysyndactyly and chromosomal anomalies was observed among infants of users of medroxyprogesterone acetate contraceptive injection, the former being most pronounced in women younger than 30 years of age. The unrelated nature of these defects, the lack of confirmation from other studies, the distant preconceptual exposure to medroxyprogesterone acetate contraceptive injection, and the chance effects due to multiple statistical comparisons, make a causal association unlikely.

Neonates exposed to medroxyprogesterone acetate in utero and followed to adolescence, showed no evidence of any adverse effects on their health including their physical, intellectual, sexual, or social development.

Ectopic pregnancy: Healthcare providers should be alert to the possibility of an ectopic pregnancy among women using medroxyprogesterone acetate contraceptive injection who become pregnant or complain of severe abdominal pain.

➤*Lactation:* Detectable amounts of drug have been identified in the milk of mothers receiving progestational drugs. The effect of this on the nursing infant has not been determined.

In nursing mothers treated with medroxyprogesterone acetate contraceptive injection, milk composition, quality, and amount are not adversely affected. Neonates and infants exposed to medroxyprogesterone from breast milk have been studied for developmental and behavioral effects through puberty. No adverse effects have been noted.

➤*Children:* Safety and efficacy in children have not been established.

Precautions

➤*History/Physical exam:* It is good medical practice for all women to have annual history and physical examinations, including women using medroxyprogesterone acetate injection. The physical examination, however, may be deferred until after initiation of medroxyprogesterone acetate injection if requested by the woman and judged appropriate by the clinician. The physical examination should include special reference to blood pressure, breasts, abdomen and pelvic organs, including cervical cytology and relevant laboratory tests. In case of undiagnosed, persistent or recurrent abnormal vaginal bleeding, appropriate measures should be conducted to rule out malignancy. Women with strong family histories of breast cancer or who have breast nodules should be monitored with particular care.

➤*Fluid retention:* Because progestational drugs may cause some degree of fluid retention, conditions which might be influenced by this condition, such as epilepsy, migraine, asthma, cardiac or renal dysfunction, require careful observation.

➤*400 mg/mL:*

Vaginal bleeding – In cases of breakthrough bleeding, as in all cases of irregular bleeding per vaginum, nonfunctional causes should be borne in mind and adequate diagnostic measures undertaken.

Masking of climacteric – The age of the patient constitutes no absolute limiting factor although treatment with progestin may mask the onset of the climacteric.

Use with estrogen – Studies of the addition of a progestin product to an estrogen replacement regimen for 7 or more days of a cycle of estrogen administration have reported a lowered incidence of endometrial hyperplasia. Morphological and biochemical studies of endometria suggest that 10 to 13 days of a progestin are needed to provide maximal maturation of the endometrium and to eliminate any hyperplastic changes. Whether this will provide protection from endometrial carcinoma has not been clearly established.

There are possible risks which may be associated with the inclusion of progestin in estrogen replacement regimen, including adverse effects on carbohydrate and lipid metabolism. The dosage used may be important in minimizing these adverse effects.

A decrease in glucose tolerance has been observed in a small percentage of patients on estrogen-progestin combination treatment. The mechanism of this decrease is obscure. For this reason, diabetic patients should be carefully observed while receiving such therapy.

Prolonged use – The effect of prolonged use of medroxyprogesterone acetate injection at the recommended doses on pituitary, ovarian, adrenal, hepatic, and uterine function is not known.

Multi-dose use – When multi-dose vials are used, special care to prevent contamination of the contents is essential. There is some evidence that benzalkonium chloride is not an adequate antiseptic for sterilizing medroxyprogesterone acetate injection multi-dose vials. A povidone-iodine solution or similar product is recommended to cleanse the vial top prior to aspiration of contents.

➤*150 mg/mL:*

Weight changes – There is a tendency for women to gain weight while on therapy with medroxyprogesterone acetate contraceptive injection. From an initial average body weight of 136 lbs, women who completed 1 year of therapy with medroxyprogesterone acetate contraceptive injection gained an average of 5.4 lbs. Women who completed 2 years of therapy gained an average of 8.1 lbs.

Women who completed 4 years gained an average of 13.8 lbs. Women who completed 6 years gained an average of 16.5 lbs. Two percent (2%) of women withdrew from a large-scale clinical trial because of excessive weight gain.

Return of fertility – Medroxyprogesterone acetate contraceptive injection has a prolonged contraceptive effect. In a large US study of women who discontinued use of medroxyprogesterone acetate contraceptive injection to become pregnant, data are available for 61% of them. Based on Life-Table analysis of these data, it is expected that 68% of women who do become pregnant may conceive within 12 months, 83% may conceive within 15 months, and 93% may conceive within 18 months from the last injection. The median time to conception for those who do conceive is 10 months following the last injection with a range of 4 to 31 months, and is unrelated to the duration of use. No data are available for 39% of the patients who discontinued medroxyprogesterone acetate contraceptive injection to become pregnant and who were lost to follow-up or changed their minds.

Convulsions – There have been a few reported cases of convulsions in patients who were treated with medroxyprogesterone acetate contraceptive injection. Association with drug use or preexisting conditions is not clear.

Carbohydrate metabolism – A decrease in glucose tolerance has been observed in some patients on medroxyprogesterone acetate contraceptive injection treatment. The mechanism of this decrease is obscure. For this reason, diabetic patients should be carefully observed while receiving such therapy.

Liver function – If jaundice develops, consideration should be given to not readministering the drug.

Protection against sexually transmitted diseases – Patients should be counseled that this product does not protect against HIV infection (AIDS) and other sexually transmitted diseases.

➤*Depression:* Patients who have a history of psychic depression should be carefully observed and the drug not be readministered if the depression recurs.

Drug Interactions

Aminoglutethimide administered concomitantly with medroxyprogesterone acetate injection may significantly depress the serum concentrations of medroxyprogesterone acetate. Medroxyprogesterone acetate users should be warned of the possibility of decreased efficacy with the use of this or any related drugs.

➤*Drug/Lab test interactions:* The pathologist should be advised of progestin therapy when relevant specimens are submitted. The following laboratory tests may be affected by progestins, including medroxyprogesterone acetate injection:

- Plasma and urinary steroid levels are decreased (eg, progesterone, estradiol, pregnanediol, testosterone, cortisol).
- Gonadotropin levels are decreased.
- Sex-hormone binding globulin concentrations are decreased.
- Protein bound iodine and butanol extractable protein bound iodine may increase. T_3 uptake values may decrease.
- Coagulation test values for prothrombin (Factor II), and Factors VII, VIII, IX, and X may increase.
- Sulfobromophthalein and other liver function test values may be increased.
- The effects of medroxyprogesterone acetate on lipid metabolism are inconsistent. Both increases and decreases in total cholesterol, triglycerides, low-density lipoprotein (LDL) cholesterol, and high-density lipoprotein (HDL) cholesterol have been observed in studies.

Adverse Reactions

➤*400 mg/mL:* Several reports suggest an association between intrauterine exposure to progestational drugs in the first trimester of pregnancy and genital abnormalities in male and female fetuses. The risk of hypospadias (5 to 8 per 1,000 male births in the general population) may be approximately doubled with exposure to these drugs. There are insufficient data to quantify the risk to exposed female fetuses, but insofar as some of these drugs induce mild virilization of the external genitalia of the female fetus, and because of the increased association of hypospadias in the male fetus, it is prudent to avoid the use of these drugs during the first trimester of pregnancy.

CNS – Dizziness, headache, insomnia, mental depression, nervousness.

Dermatologic – Skin sensitivity reactions consisting of urticaria, pruritus, edema, and generalized rash; acne, alopecia, and hirsutism.

Rash (allergic) with and without pruritus.

GU – Breakthrough bleeding, spotting, change in menstrual flow, amenorrhea, changes in cervical erosion and cervical secretions, breast tenderness and galactorrhea.

Hepatic – Cholestatic jaundice, including neonatal jaundice.

Hypersensitivity – Anaphylactoid reactions and anaphylaxis.

Metabolic – Change in weight (increase or decrease).

Miscellaneous – Edema, pyrexia, fatigue, nausea, somnolence.

MEDROXYPROGESTERONE ACETATE — INJECTION

In a few instances there have been undesirable sequelae at the site of injection, such as residual lump, change in skin color, or sterile abscess. A statistically significant association has been demonstrated between use of estrogen-progestin combination drugs and pulmonary embolism and cerebral thrombosis and embolism. For this reason, patients on progestin therapy should be carefully observed. There is also evidence suggestive of an association with neuro-ocular lesions (eg, retinal thrombosis and optic neuritis).

The following adverse reactions have been observed in patients receiving estrogen-progestin combination drugs – Rise in blood pressure in susceptible individuals, premenstrual syndrome, changes in libido, changes in appetite, cystitis-like syndrome, headache, nervousness, fatigue, backache, hirsutism, loss of scalp hair, erythema multiforme, erythema nodosum, hemorrhagic eruption, itching, dizziness.

Lab test abnormalities – The following laboratory results may be altered by the use of estrogen-progestin combination drugs: Increased sulfobromophthalein retention and other hepatic function tests; coagulation tests: Increase in prothrombin factors VII, VIII, IX, and X; metyrapone test; pregnanediol determinations; thyroid function: Increase in PBI, and butanol extractable protein bound iodine and decrease in T_3 uptake values.

➤*150 mg/mL:* In the largest clinical trial with medroxyprogesterone acetate contraceptive injection, with more than 3,900 women, who were treated for up to 7 years, reported the following adverse reactions, which may or may not be related to the use of medroxyprogesterone acetate contraceptive injection.

Adverse reactions reported by more than 5% of subjects using medroxyprogesterone acetate contraceptive injection – Menstrual irregularities (bleeding or amenorrhea, or both), abdominal pain or discomfort, weight changes, dizziness, headache, asthenia (weakness or fatigue), nervousness.

Adverse reactions reported by 1% to 5% of subjects using medroxyprogesterone acetate contraceptive injection – Decreased libido or anorgasmia, pelvic pain, backache, breast pain, leg cramps, no hair growth or alopecia, depression, bloating, nausea, rash, insomnia, edema, leukorrhea, hot flashes, acne, arthralgia, vaginitis.

Events reported by fewer than 1% of subjects using medroxyprogesterone acetate contraceptive injection – Galactorrhea, melasma, chloasma, convulsions, changes in appetite, gastrointestinal disturbances, jaundice, genitourinary infections, vaginal cysts, dyspareunia, paresthesia, chest pain, pulmonary embolus, allergic reactions, anemia, drowsiness, syncope, dyspnea and asthma, tachycardia, fever, excessive sweating and body odor, dry skin, chills, increased libido, excessive thirst, hoarseness, pain at injection site, blood dyscrasia, rectal bleeding, changes in breast size, breast lumps or nipple bleeding, axillary swelling, breast cancer, prevention of lactation, sensation of pregnancy, lack of return to fertility, paralysis, facial palsy, scleroderma, osteoporosis, uterine hyperplasia, cervical cancer, varicose veins, dysmenorrhea, hirsutism, unexpected pregnancy, thrombophlebitis, deep vein thrombosis.

In addition, voluntary reports have been received of anaphylaxis and anaphylactoid reaction with use of medroxyprogesterone acetate contraceptive injection.

Ovulation Stimulants

CLOMIPHENE CITRATE

Rx	**Clomiphene Citrate** (Various, eg, Lemmon)	**Tablets:** 50 mg	In 10s and 30s.
Rx	**Clomid** (Aventis Pharm.)		(Clomid 50). White, scored. In 30s.
Rx	**Milophene** (Milex)		(M50). White, scored. In 30s.
Rx	**Serophene** (Serono)		(S). White, scored. In 10s and 30s.

CLOMIPHENE CITRATE — ORAL

Indications

➤*Treatment of ovulatory failure:* Clomiphene citrate is indicated for the treatment of ovulatory dysfunction in women desiring pregnancy. Impediments to achieving pregnancy must be excluded or adequately treated before beginning clomiphene citrate therapy. Those patients most likely to achieve success with clomiphene therapy include patients with polycystic ovary syndrome, amenorrhea-galactorrhea syndrome, psychogenic amenorrhea, post-oral-contraceptive amenorrhea, and certain cases of secondary amenorrhea of undetermined etiology.

➤*Unlabeled uses:* Clomiphene has been used to treat male infertility (50 to 400 mg/day for 2 to 12 months); however, this use is controversial, and further study is needed.

Administration and Dosage

➤*Approved by the FDA:* March 22, 1982.

➤*General considerations:* The workup and treatment of candidates for clomiphene citrate therapy should be supervised by physicians experienced in management of gynecologic or endocrine disorders. Patients should be chosen for therapy with clomiphene citrate only after careful diagnostic evaluation. The plan of therapy should be outlined in advance. Impediments to achieving the goal of therapy must be excluded or adequately treated before beginning clomiphene citrate. The therapeutic objective should be balanced with potential risks and discussed with the patient and others involved in the achievement of a pregnancy.

Ovulation most often occurs from 5 to 10 days after a course of clomiphene citrate. Coitus should be timed to coincide with the expected time of ovulation. Appropriate tests to determine ovulation may be useful during this time.

➤*Initial therapy:* Treatment of the selected patient should begin with a low dose, 50 mg daily (1 tablet) for 5 days. The dose should be increased only in those patients who do not ovulate in response to cyclic clomiphene citrate 50 mg. A low dosage or duration of treatment course is particularly recommended if unusual sensitivity to pituitary gonadotropin is suspected, such as in patients with polycystic ovary syndrome.

The patient should be evaluated carefully to exclude pregnancy, ovarian enlargement, or ovarian cyst formation between each treatment cycle.

If progestin-induced bleeding is planned, or if spontaneous uterine bleeding occurs prior to therapy, the regimen of 50 mg daily for 5 days should be started on or about the fifth day of the cycle. Therapy may be started at any time in the patient who has had no recent uterine bleeding. When ovulation occurs at this dosage, there is no advantage to increasing the dose in subsequent cycles of treatment.

➤*Second course of therapy:* If ovulation does not appear to occur after the first course of therapy, a second course of 100 mg daily (two 50 mg tablets given as a single daily dose) for 5 days should be given. This course may be started as early as 30 days after the previous one after precautions are taken to exclude the presence of pregnancy. Increasing the dosage or duration of therapy beyond 100 mg/day for 5 days is not recommended.

➤*Third course of therapy:* The majority of patients who are going to ovulate will do so after the first course of therapy. If ovulation does not occur after 3 courses of therapy, further treatment with clomiphene citrate is not recommended and the patient should be reevaluated. If 3 ovulatory responses occur, but pregnancy has not been achieved, further treatment is not recommended. If menses does not occur after an ovulatory response, the patient should be reevaluated. Long-term cyclic therapy is not recommended beyond a total of about 6 cycles.

➤*Storage/Stability:* Store tablets at controlled room temperature (15° to 30°C; 59° to 86°F). Protect from heat, light, and excessive humidity. Store in closed containers.

Actions

➤*Pharmacology:*

Action – Clomiphene citrate is a drug of considerable pharmacologic potency. With careful selection and proper management of the patient, clomiphene citrate has been demonstrated to be a useful therapy for the anovulatory patient desiring pregnancy.

Clomiphene citrate is capable of interacting with estrogen-receptor-containing tissues, including the hypothalamus, pituitary, ovary, endometrium, vagina, and cervix. It may compete with estrogen for estrogen-receptor-binding sites and may delay replenishment of intracellular estrogen receptors. These endocrine events culminate in a preovulatory gonadotropin surge and subsequent follicular rupture.

The first endocrine event in response to a course of clomiphene therapy is an increase in the release of pituitary gonadotropins. This initiates steroidogenesis and folliculogenesis, resulting in growth of the ovarian follicle and an increase in the circulating level of estradiol. Following ovulation, plasma progesterone and estradiol rise and fall as they would in a normal ovulatory cycle.

Available data suggest that both the estrogenic and antiestrogenic properties of clomiphene may participate in the initiation of ovulation. The 2 clomiphene isomers have been found to have mixed estrogenic and antiestrogenic effects, which may vary from one species to another. Some data suggest that zuclomiphene has greater estrogenic activity than enclomiphene.

Although there is no evidence of a "carryover effect" of clomiphene citrate, spontaneous ovulatory menses have been noted in some patients after clomiphene citrate therapy.

➤*Pharmacokinetics:* Based on early studies with ^{14}C-labeled clomiphene citrate, the drug was shown to be readily absorbed orally in humans and excreted principally in the feces. Cumulative urinary and fecal excretion of the ^{14}C averaged about 50% of the oral dose and 37% of an IV dose after 5 days. Mean urinary excretion was approximately 8% with fecal excretion of about 42%.

Some ^{14}C label was still present in the feces 6 weeks after administration. Subsequent single-dose studies in healthy volunteers showed that zuclomiphene (cis) has a longer half-life than enclomiphene (trans). Detectable levels of zuclomiphene persisted for greater than 1 month in these subjects. This may be suggestive of stereo-specific enterohepatic recycling or sequestering of the zuclomiphene. Thus, it is possible that some active drug may remain in the body during early pregnancy in women who conceive in the menstrual cycle during clomiphene citrate therapy.

CLOMIPHENE CITRATE — ORAL

Contraindications

➤*Hypersensitivity:* Clomiphene citrate is contraindicated in patients with a known hypersensitivity or allergy to clomiphene citrate or to any of its ingredients.

➤*Pregnancy:* See Warnings for more information.

➤*Fetal/neonatal anomalies and mortality:* See Warnings for more information.

➤*Animal fetotoxicity:* See Warnings for more information.

➤*Liver disease:* Clomiphene citrate therapy is contraindicated in patients with liver disease or a history of liver dysfunction.

➤*Abnormal uterine bleeding:* Clomiphene citrate is contraindicated in patients with abnormal uterine bleeding of undetermined origin.

➤*Ovarian cysts:* Clomiphene citrate is contraindicated in patients with ovarian cysts or enlargement not due to polycystic ovarian syndrome.

➤*Other:* Clomiphene citrate is contraindicated in patients with uncontrolled thyroid or adrenal dysfunction or in the presence of an organic intracranial lesion such as pituitary tumor.

Warnings

➤*Ophthalmologic effects:* Patients should be advised that blurring or other visual symptoms such as spots or flashes (scintillating scotomata) may occasionally occur during therapy with clomiphene citrate. These visual symptoms increase in incidence with increasing total dose or therapy duration and generally disappear within a few days or weeks after clomiphene citrate is discontinued. Patients should be warned that these visual symptoms may render such activities as driving a car or operating machinery more hazardous than usual, particularly under conditions of variable lighting.

These visual symptoms appear to be due to intensification and prolongation of afterimages. Symptoms often first appear or are accentuated with exposure to a brightly lit environment. While measured visual acuity usually has not been affected, a study patient taking clomiphene citrate 200 mg daily developed visual blurring on the seventh day of treatment, which progressed to severe diminution of visual acuity by the day 10. No other abnormality was found, and the visual acuity returned to normal on the third day after treatment was stopped.

Ophthalmologically definable scotomata and retinal cell function (electroretinographic) changes have also been reported. A patient treated during clinical studies developed phosphenes and scotomata during prolonged clomiphene citrate administration, which disappeared by day 32 after stopping therapy.

Postmarketing surveillance of adverse events has also revealed other visual signs and symptoms during clomiphene citrate therapy (eg, abnormal accommodation, cataract, eye pain, macular edema, optic neuritis, photopsia, posterior vitreous detachment, retinal hemorrhage, retinal thrombosis, retinal vascular spasm, temporary loss of vision). While the etiology of these visual symptoms is not yet understood, patients with any visual symptoms should discontinue treatment and have a complete ophthalmological evaluation carried out promptly.

➤*Ovarian hyperstimulation syndrome:* The ovarian hyperstimulation syndrome (OHSS) has been reported to occur in patients receiving clomiphene citrate therapy for ovulation induction. In some cases, OHSS occurred following cyclic use of clomiphene citrate therapy or when clomiphene citrate was used in combination with gonadotropins. Transient liver function test abnormalities suggestive of hepatic dysfunction, which may be accompanied by morphologic changes on liver biopsy, have been reported in association with OHSS.

OHSS is a medical event distinct from uncomplicated ovarian enlargement. The clinical signs of this syndrome in severe cases can include gross ovarian enlargement, gastrointestinal symptoms, ascites, dyspnea, oliguria, and pleural effusion. In addition, the following symptoms have been reported in association with this syndrome: Pericardial effusion, anasarca, hydrothorax, acute abdomen, hypotension, renal failure, pulmonary edema, intraperitoneal and ovarian hemorrhage, deep venous thrombosis, torsion of the ovary, and acute respiratory distress.

The early warning signs of OHSS are abdominal pain and distention, nausea, vomiting, diarrhea, and weight gain. Elevated urinary steroid levels, varying degrees of electrolyte imbalance, hypovolemia, hemoconcentration, and hypoproteinemia may occur. Death caused by hypovolemic shock, hemoconcentration, or thromboembolism has occurred. Because of fragility of enlarged ovaries in severe cases, abdominal and pelvic examination should be performed very cautiously. If conception results, rapid progression to the severe form of the syndrome may occur.

To minimize the hazard associated with occasional abnormal ovarian enlargement associated with clomiphene citrate therapy, the lowest dose consistent with expected clinical results should be used. Maximal enlargement of the ovary, whether physiologic or abnormal, may not occur until several days after discontinuation of the recommended dose of clomiphene citrate. Some patients with polycystic ovary syndrome who are unusually sensitive to gonadotropin may have an exaggerated response to usual doses of clomiphene citrate. Therefore, patients with polycystic ovary syndrome should be started on the lowest recommended dose and shortest treatment duration for the first course of therapy.

If enlargement of the ovary occurs, additional clomiphene citrate therapy should not be given until the ovaries have returned to pretreatment size, and the dosage or duration of the next course should be reduced. Ovarian enlargement and cyst formation associated with clomiphene citrate therapy usually regress spontaneously within a few days or weeks after discontinuing treatment. The potential benefit of subsequent clomiphene citrate therapy in these cases should exceed the risk. Unless surgical indication for laparotomy exists, such cystic enlargement should always be managed conservatively.

A causal relationship between ovarian hyperstimulation and ovarian cancer has not been determined. However, because a correlation between ovarian cancer and nulliparity, infertility, and age has been suggested, if ovarian cysts do not regress spontaneously, a thorough evaluation should be performed to rule out the presence of ovarian neoplasia.

➤*Carcinogenesis:*

Ovarian cancer: Prolonged use of clomiphene citrate tablets may increase the risk of a borderline or invasive ovarian tumor. Long-term toxicity studies in animals have not been performed to evaluate the carcinogenic potential of clomiphene citrate.

➤*Fertility impairment:* Oral administration of clomiphene citrate to male rats at doses of 0.3 or 1 mg/kg/day caused decreased fertility, while higher doses caused temporary infertility. Oral doses of 0.1 mg/kg/day in female rats temporarily interrupted the normal cyclic vaginal smear pattern and prevented conception. Doses of 0.3 mg/kg/day slightly reduced the number of ovulated ova and corpora lutea, while 3 mg/kg/day inhibited ovulation.

➤*Pregnancy: Category X.*

Clomiphene citrate should not be administered during pregnancy. Clomiphene citrate may cause fetal harm in animals (see Animal Fetotoxicity, below). Although no causative evidence of a deleterious effect of clomiphene citrate therapy on the human fetus has been established, there have been reports of birth anomalies which, during clinical studies, occurred at an incidence within the range reported for the general population.

To avoid inadvertent clomiphene citrate administration during early pregnancy, appropriate tests should be utilized during each treatment cycle to determine whether ovulation occurs. The patient should be evaluated carefully to exclude pregnancy, ovarian enlargement, or ovarian cyst formation between each treatment cycle. The next course of clomiphene citrate therapy should be delayed until these conditions have been excluded.

Fetal/neonatal anomalies and mortality – The following fetal abnormalities have been reported subsequent to pregnancies following ovulation induction therapy with clomiphene citrate during clinical trials. Each of the following fetal abnormalities were reported at a rate of less than 1% (experiences are listed in order of decreasing frequency): Congenital heart lesions, Down's syndrome, club foot, congenital gut lesions, hypospadias, microcephaly, harelip and cleft palate, congenital hip, hemangioma, undescended testicles, polydactyly, conjoined twins and teratomatous malformation, patent ductus arteriosus, amaurosis, arteriovenous fistula, inguinal hernia, umbilical hernia, syndactyly, pectus excavatum, myopathy, dermoid cyst of scalp, omphalocele, spina bifida occulta, ichthyosis, and persistent linqual frenulum. Neonatal death and fetal death/stillbirth in infants with birth defects have also been reported at a rate of less than 1%. The overall incidence of reported birth anomalies from pregnancies associated with maternal clomiphene citrate ingestion during clinical studies was within the range of that reported for the general population.

In addition, reports of birth anomalies have been received during postmarketing surveillance of clomiphene citrate (eg, delayed development; abnormal bone development including skeletal malformations of the skull, face, nasal passages, jaw, hand, limb [ectromelia, including amelia, hemimella, and phocomelia], foot, and joints; tissue malformations including imperforate anus, tracheoesophageal fistula, diaphragmatic hernia, renal agenesis and dysgenesis, and malformations of the eye and lens [cataract], ear, lung, heart [ventricular septal defect and tetralogy of Fallot], and genitalia; as well as dwarfism, deafness, mental retardation, chromosomal disorders, and neural tube defects [including anencephaly]).

Animal fetotoxicity – Oral administration of clomiphene citrate to pregnant rats during organogenesis at doses of 1 to 2 mg/kg/day resulted in hydramnion and weak, edematous fetuses with wavy ribs and other temporary bone changes. Doses of 8 mg/kg/day or more also caused increased resorptions and dead fetuses, dystocia, and delayed parturition, and 40 mg/kg/day resulted in increased maternal mortality. Single doses of 50 mg/kg caused fetal cataracts, while 200 mg/kg caused cleft palate.

Following injection of clomiphene citrate 2 mg/kg to mice and rats during pregnancy, the offspring exhibited metaplastic changes of the reproductive tract. Newborn mice and rats injected during the first few days of life also developed metaplastic changes in uterine and vaginal mucosa, as well as premature vaginal opening and anovulatory ovaries. These findings are similar to the abnormal reproductive behavior and sterility described with other estrogens and antiestrogens.

In rabbits, some temporary bone alterations were seen in fetuses from dams given oral doses of 20 or 40 mg/kg/day during pregnancy, but not following 8 mg/kg/day. No permanent malformations were observed in those studies. Also, rhesus monkeys given oral doses of 1.5 to 4.5 mg/kg/day for various periods during pregnancy did not have any abnormal offspring.

➤*Lactation:* It is not known whether clomiphene citrate is excreted in human milk. Because many drugs are excreted in human milk, caution should be exercised if clomiphene citrate is administered to a breast-feeding woman. In some patients, clomiphene citrate may reduce lactation.

Precautions

➤*Diagnosis prior to therapy:* Careful attention should be given to the selection of candidates for clomiphene citrate therapy. Pelvic examination is necessary prior to clomiphene citrate treatment and before each subsequent course.

CLOMIPHENE CITRATE — ORAL

➤*Drug abuse and dependence:* Tolerance, abuse, or dependence with clomiphene citrate has not been reported.

➤*Hazardous tasks:* Patients should be advised that blurring or other visual symptoms such as spots or flashes (scintillating scotomata) may occasionally occur during therapy with clomiphene citrate. These visual symptoms increase in incidence with increasing total dose or therapy duration and generally disappear within a few days or weeks after clomiphene citrate is discontinued. Patients should be warned that these visual symptoms may render such activities as driving a car or operating machinery more hazardous than usual, particularly under conditions of variable lighting.

Drug Interactions

Drug interactions with clomiphene citrate have not been documented.

Adverse Reactions

➤*Clinical trial adverse reactions:* Clomiphene citrate, at recommended dosages, is generally well tolerated. Adverse reactions usually have been mild and transient, and most have disappeared promptly after treatment has been discontinued. Adverse reactions reported in patients treated with clomiphene citrate during clinical studies are shown in the following table:

Incidence of adverse reactions in clinical studies (reactions greater than 1%) (n = 8,029)[a]

Adverse reaction	%
Ovarian enlargement	13.6%
Vasomotor flushes	10.4%
Abdominal/pelvic discomfort/ distention/bloating	5.5%
Nausea/vomiting	2.2%
Breast discomfort	2.1%
Visual symptoms (blurred vision, lights, floater, waves, unspecified visual complaints, photophobia, diplopia, scotomata, phosphenes	1.5%
Headache	1.3%
Abnormal uterine bleeding (intermenstrual spotting, menorrhagia)	1.3%

[a] Includes 498 patients whose reports may have been duplicated in the event totals and could not be distinguished as such. Also, excludes 47 patients who did not report symptom data.

The following adverse reactions have been reported in less than 1% of patients in clinical trials: Acute abdomen, appetite increase, constipation, dermatitis or rash, depression, diarrhea, dizziness, fatigue, hair loss/dry hair, increased urinary frequency/volume, insomnia, lightheadedness, nervous tension, vaginal dryness, vertigo, weight gain/loss.

Patients on prolonged clomiphene citrate therapy may show elevated serum levels of desmosterol. This is most likely due to a direct interference with cholesterol synthesis. However, the serum sterols in patients receiving the recommended dose of clomiphene citrate are not significantly altered. Ovarian cancer has been infrequently reported in patients who have received fertility drugs. Infertility is a primary risk factor for ovarian cancer; however, epidemiology data suggest that prolonged use of clomiphene may increase the risk of a borderline or invasive ovarian tumor.

➤*Postmarketing adverse reactions:* The following adverse experiences were reported spontaneously with clomiphene citrate. The cause and effect relationship of the listed events to the administration of clomiphene citrate is not known.

Cardiovascular – Arrhythmia, chest pain, edema, hypertension, palpitation, phlebitis, pulmonary embolism, shortness of breath, tachycardia, thrombophlebitis.

CNS – Migraine headache, paresthesia, seizure, stroke, syncope.

Dermatologic – Acne, allergic reaction, erythema, erythema multiforme, erythema nodosum, hypertrichosis, pruritus.

GU – Endometriosis, ovarian cyst (ovarian enlargement or cysts could, as such, be complicated by adnexal torsion), ovarian hemorrhage, tubal pregnancy, uterine hemorrhage.

Hepatic – Transaminases increased, hepatitis.

Musculoskeletal – Arthralgia, back pain, myalgia.

Ophthalmic – Abnormal accommodation, cataract, eye pain, macular edema, optic neuritis, photopsia, posterior vitreous detachment, retinal hemorrhage, retinal thrombosis, retinal vascular spasm, temporary loss of vision.

Psychiatric – Anxiety, irritability, mood changes, psychosis.

Miscellaneous – Fever, tinnitus, weakness, leukocytosis, thyroid disorder.

Neoplasms: Liver (hepatic hemangiosarcoma, liver cell adenoma, hepatocellular carcinoma); breast (fibrocystic disease, breast carcinoma); endometrium (endometrial carcinoma); nervous system (astrocytoma, pituitary tumor, prolactinoma, neurofibromatosis, glioblastoma multiforme, brain abscess); ovary (luteoma of pregnancy, dermoid cyst of the ovary, ovarian carcinoma); trophoblastic (hydatiform mole, choriocarcinoma); miscellaneous (melanoma, myeloma, perianal cysts, renal cell carcinoma, Hodgkin's lymphoma, tongue carcinoma, bladder carcinoma); and neoplasms of offspring (neuroectodermal tumor, thyroid tumor, hepatoblastoma, lymphocytic leukemia).

Fetal/neonatal anomalies: The following fetal neonatal abnormalities have also been reported during postmarketing surveillance: Delayed development; abnormal bone development including skeletal malformations of the skull, face, nasal passages, jaw, hand, limb (ectromelia including amelia, hemimella, and phocomelia), foot, and joints; tissue malformations including imperforate anus, tracheoesophageal fistula, diaphragmatic hernia, renal agenesis and dysgenesis, and malformations of the eye and lens (cataract), ear, lung, heart (ventricular septal defect and tetralogy of Fallot), and genitalia; as well as dwarfism, deafness, mental retardation, chromosomal disorders, and neural tube defects (including anencephaly).

Overdosage

➤*Oral LD_{50}:* The acute oral LD_{50} of clomiphene citrate is 1,700 mg/kg in mice and 5,750 mg/kg in rats. The toxic dose in humans is not known.

➤*Symptoms:* Toxic effects accompanying acute overdosage of clomiphene citrate have not been reported. Signs and symptoms of overdosage as a result of the use of more than the recommended dose during clomiphene citrate therapy include nausea, vomiting, vasomotor flushes, visual blurring, spots or flashes, scotomata, ovarian enlargement with pelvic or abdominal pain. Clomiphene citrate is contraindicated in patients with ovarian cysts or enlargement not caused by polycystic ovarian syndrome.

➤*Treatment:* In the event of overdose, appropriate supportive measures should be employed in addition to gastrointestinal decontamination.

Dialysis – It is not known if clomiphene citrate is dialyzable.

Patient Information

The purpose and risks of clomiphene citrate therapy should be presented to the patient before starting treatment. It should be emphasized that the goal of clomiphene citrate therapy is ovulation for subsequent pregnancy. The physician should counsel the patient with special regard to the following potential risks:

➤*Visual symptoms:* Advise that blurring or other visual symptoms occasionally may occur during or shortly after clomiphene citrate therapy. Warn patients that visual symptoms may render such activities as driving a car or operating machinery more hazardous than usual, particularly under conditions of variable lighting.

The patient should be instructed to inform the physician whenever any unusual visual symptoms occur. If the patient has any visual symptoms, treatment should be discontinued and complete ophthalmologic evaluation performed.

➤*Abdominal/pelvic pain or distention:* Ovarian enlargement may occur during or shortly after therapy with clomiphene citrate. To minimize the risks associated with ovarian enlargement, the patient should be instructed to inform the physician of any abdominal or pelvic pain, weight gain, discomfort, or distention after taking clomiphene citrate.

➤*Multiple pregnancy:* Inform the patient that there is an increased chance of multiple pregnancy, including bilateral tubal pregnancy and coexisting tubal and intrauterine pregnancy, when conception occurs in relation to clomiphene citrate therapy. The potential complications and hazards of multiple pregnancy should be explained.

➤*Pregnancy wastage and birth anomalies:* The physician should explain the assumed risk of any pregnancy, whether ovulation is induced with the aid of clomiphene citrate or occurs naturally. The patient should be informed of the greater risks associated with certain characteristics or conditions of any pregnant woman (eg, age of female and male partner, history of spontaneous abortions, Rh genotype, abnormal menstrual history, infertility history, organic heart disease, diabetes, exposure to infectious agents such as rubella, familial history of birth anomaly, that may be pertinent to the patient for whom clomiphene citrate is being considered). Based upon the evaluation of the patient, genetic counseling may be indicated.

The overall incidence of reported birth anomalies from pregnancies associated with maternal clomiphene citrate ingestion during the investigational studies was within the range of that reported in published references for the general population. Clomiphene citrate should not be administered during pregnancy. During clinical investigation, the experience from patients with known pregnancy outcome shows a spontaneous abortion rate of 20.4% and stillbirth rate of 1%.

FOLLITROPINS

Indications

➤*Ovulation induction:* For the induction of ovulation and pregnancy in anovulatory infertile patients in whom the cause of infertility is functional and not caused by primary ovarian failure.

Refer to individual product monographs for specific indications.

➤*Follicle stimulation:* To stimulate the development of multiple follicles in ovulatory patients undergoing Assisted Reproductive Technologies (ART), eg, in vitro fertilization.

Actions

➤*Pharmacology:* **Urofollitropin** is a preparation of highly purified follicle-stimulating hormone (FSH) extracted from the urine of postmenopausal women. **Follitropin alfa** and **follitropin beta** are human FSH

FOLLITROPINS

preparations of recombinant DNA origin. Follitropins stimulate ovarian follicular growth in women who do not have primary ovarian failure. FSH is required for normal follicular growth, maturation and gonadal steroid production. In the female, the level of FSH is critical for the onset and duration of follicular development, and consequently for the timing and number of follicles reaching maturity. In order to affect ovulation in the absence of endogenous LH surge, human chorionic gonadotropin (hCG) must be given following the administration of urofollitropin, follitropin alfa and beta when clinical and laboratory assessment of the patient indicate that sufficient follicular maturation has occurred.

➤*Pharmacokinetics:*

Absorption / Distribution – Follitropins have absorption-rate limited pharmacokinetics; the absorption rate following IM or subcutaneous administration is slower than the elimination rate. Bioavailability ranges from approximately 66% to 78% depending on the agent. Following a single IM or subcutaneous dose, AUCs are similar for all agents and C_{max} is similar for urofollitropin and follitropin alfa; however, the C_{max} for follitropin beta differs with respect to IM or subcutaneous administration (approximately 6.86 versus approximately 5.41 units/L, respectively).

Following multiple IM or subcutaneous doses, steady-state plasma levels are reached within 4 to 5 days. Peak follitropin alfa plasma levels were 6 to 12 units/L following 150 U/day administered subcutaneous for 7 days; follitropin beta peak levels, following 75, 150 or 225 units either subcutaneous or IM for 7 days, were approximately 4.3 or 4.65, 8.51 or 9.46, and 13.92 or 11.3 units/L, respectively.

Metabolism / Excretion – Total clearance of follitropin alfa following IV administration was 0.6 L/hr; data is lacking regarding clearance for the other two agents. Following multiple dosing, the terminal half-life for follitropin alfa (IM) and beta (subcutaneous) were approximately 30 hours.

Special populations –

Obesity: Body weight, measured as kg or as body mass index (BMI), was shown to influence the absorption rate and thus the AUC of follitropin alfa and beta. Increased body weight or BMI was associated with a decrease in the rate of follitropin absorption and a significantly smaller AUC. Clearance, however was essentially the same on a per kg basis.

Select Pharmacokinetic Parameters of Follitropins Following subcutaneous (IM) Administration

	Mean T_{max} (hrs)	Mean elimination t½ (hrs)[a]	Mean V_d (L)
Follitropin alfa	16 (25)	24 and 32[b]	10
Follitropin beta	(27)	(≈ 30)	8
Urofollitropin	15 (10)	-	

[a] This value increases with body mass index.
[b] In healthy and ART patients, respectively.

Contraindications

High levels of FSH indicating primary ovarian failure; uncontrolled thyroid or adrenal dysfunction; the presence of any cause of infertility other than anovulation; tumor of the ovary, breast, uterus, hypothalamus or pituitary gland; abnormal vaginal bleeding of undetermined origin; ovarian cysts or enlargement not due to polycystic ovary syndrome; hypersensitivity to the product or any of its components; pregnancy (see Warnings).

Warnings

➤*Administration:* These medications should only be used by physicians who are thoroughly familiar with infertility problems and their management. It is a potent gonadotropic substance capable of causing mild to severe adverse reactions. To minimize risks, use only at the lowest effective dose. Monitor ovarian response with serum estradiol and vaginal ultrasound on a regular basis.

➤*Overstimulation of the ovary:*

Ovarian enlargement – Mild to moderate uncomplicated ovarian enlargement, which may be accompanied by abdominal distention or abdominal pain, occurs in approximately 20% of those treated with urofollitropin and hCG, and generally regresses without treatment within 2 or 3 weeks.

Ovarian Hyperstimulation Syndrome (OHSS) – The hyperstimulation syndrome is characterized by severe ovarian enlargement, abdominal pain/distention, nausea, vomiting, diarrhea, dyspnea and oliguria, and may be accompanied by ascites, pleural effusion, hypovolemia, electrolyte imbalance, hemoperitoneum and thromboembolic events. OHSS occurred in 6% of patients in trials.

If hyperstimulation occurs, stop treatment and hospitalize the patient. This syndrome develops rapidly within 24 hours to several days and generally occurs during the 7 to 10 days immediately following treatment. Hemoconcentration associated with fluid loss into the abdominal cavity has occurred and should be assessed in the following manner: 1) Fluid intake and output, 2) weight, 3) hematocrit, 4) serum and urinary electrolytes, 5) urine specific gravity, 6) BUN and creatinine and 7) abdominal girth. Perform these determinations daily or more often if the need arises. Treatment is primarily symptomatic and consists of bed rest, fluid and electrolyte replacement and analgesics. The ascitic, pleural and pericardial fluids should never be removed because of the potential danger of injury.

Hemoperitoneum from ruptured ovarian cysts is usually the result of pelvic examination. If this does occur, and if bleeding becomes such that surgery is required, design the surgical treatment to control bleeding and retain as much ovarian tissue as possible.

Intercourse should be prohibited in patients in whom significant ovarian enlargement occurs after ovulation because of the danger of hemoperitoneum resulting from ruptured ovarian cysts.

➤*Pulmonary and vascular complications:* Serious pulmonary conditions (eg, atelectasis, acute respiratory distress syndrome and exacerbation of asthma) have been reported. In addition, thromboembolic events both in association with, and separate from OHSS have been reported. Intravascular thrombosis and embolism can result in reduced blood flow to critical organs or the extremities. Sequelae of such events have included venous thrombophlebitis, pulmonary embolism, pulmonary infarction, cerebral vascular occlusion (stroke) and arterial occlusion resulting in loss of limb. In rare cases, pulmonary complications and thromboembolic events have resulted in death.

➤*Multiple births:* Reports of multiple pregnancies have been associated with these medications, including triplet and quintuplet gestations. Multiple births have occurred with **urofollitropin** (20.8%), **follitropin alfa** (12.3%) and **follotropin beta** (8%). Advise the patient of the potential risk of multiple births before starting treatment.

➤*Pregnancy: Category X.* Contraindicated in pregnancy.

➤*Lactation:* It is not known if this drug is excreted in breast milk. Exercise caution if administering to a nursing mother.

➤*Children:* Safety and efficacy in pediatric patients have not been established, although this drug is not intended for use in children.

Precautions

➤*Monitoring:* Monitor sufficient follicular maturation. This may be directly estimated by sonographic visualization of the ovaries and endometrial lining or measuring serum estradiol levels. The combination of both ultrasonography and measurement of estradiol levels is useful for monitoring the growth and development of follicles and timing hCG administration, as well as minimizing the risk of OHSS and multiple gestations.

The clinical evaluation of estrogenic activity (changes in vaginal cytology and changes in appearance and volume of cervical mucus) provides an indirect estimate of the estrogenic effect upon the target organs, and therefore it should only be used adjunctively with more direct estimates of follicular development (eg, ultrasonography and serum estradiol determinations).

The clinical confirmation of ovulation is obtained by direct and indirect indices of progesterone production. The indices most generally used are as follows: 1) a rise in basal body temperature, 2) increase in serum progesterone, and 3) menstruation following the shift in basal body temperature.

When used in conjunction with indices of progesterone production, sonographic visualization of the ovaries will assist if ovulation has occurred. Sonographic evidence of ovulation may include the following: 1) fluid in the cul-de-sac, 2) follicle showing marked decrease in size, and 3) collapsed follicle.

➤*Selection of patients:* Give careful attention to diagnosis in candidates for therapy. Before treatment is instituted:

1.) Perform a thorough gynecologic and endocrinologic evaluation including a hysterosalpingogram (to rule out uterine and tubal pathology) and documentation of anovulation by review of patient history, physical examination, determining serum hormonal levels as indicated and optionally performing an endometrial biopsy. Patients with tubal pathology should receive the drug only if enrolled in an in vitro fertilization program.
2.) Exclude primary ovarian failure by the determination of gonadotropin levels.
3.) Make careful examination to rule out early pregnancy.
4.) Patients in late reproductive life have a greater predilection to endometrial carcinoma and a higher incidence of anovulatory disorders. Perform a thorough diagnostic evaluation in patients who demonstrate abnormal uterine bleeding or other signs of endometrial abnormalities before starting therapy.
5.) Evaluate partner's fertility potential.

➤*Ovulation confirmation:* Treatment results in follicular growth and maturation to effect ovulation in the absence of an endogenous LH surge. HCG is given following the administration of urofollitropin and follitropin alfa and beta when clinical assessment indicates sufficient follicular maturation has occurred. This is indirectly estimated by the estrogenic effect upon the target organs. With serum or urinary estrogen determinations and ultrasonography, the estrogenic effect is an acceptable means for monitoring the growth and development of follicles, timing hCG administration and minimizing the risk of hyperstimulation. Clinically confirm ovulation, with the exception of pregnancy, by indirect indices of progesterone production. The indices most generally used are a rise in basal body temperature, increase in serum progesterone and menstruation following the shift in basal body temperature.

Other clinical parameters that may have potential use for monitoring urofollitropin therapy include changes in the vaginal cytology and appearance and volume of the cervical mucus.

Adverse Reactions

The following adverse reactions are listed in decreasing order of potential severity: Pulmonary and vascular complications (see Warnings); OHSS (see Warnings); adnexal torsion (as a complication of ovarian enlargement); mild to moderate ovarian enlargement; abdominal pain; sensitivity to urofollitropin (febrile reactions which may be accompanied by chills, musculoskeletal aches, joint pains, malaise, headache and fatigue have occurred. It is not clear whether or not these were pyrogenic responses or possible allergic

FOLLITROPINS

reactions); ovarian cysts; GI symptoms (nausea, vomiting, diarrhea, abdominal cramps, bloating); pain, rash, swelling or irritation at the site of injection; breast tenderness; headache; dermatological symptoms (dry skin, body rash, hair loss, hives); hemoperitoneum has been reported during menotropins therapy and, therefore, may also occur during follitropin therapy.

The following adverse events have been reported in women treated with gonadotropins: Pulmonary and vascular complications (see Warnings), hemoperitoneum, adnexal torsion (as a complication of ovarian enlargement, abdominal pain), dizziness, tachycardia, dyspnea, tachypnea, febrile reactions, flu-like symptoms including fever, chills, musculoskeletal aches, joint pains, nausea, headache and malaise, ovarian cysts; gastrointestinal symptoms (nausea, vomiting, diarrhea, abdominal cramps, bloating); pain, rash, swelling, or irritation at the site of injection; breast tenderness and dermatological symptoms (dry skin, body rash, hair loss and hives).

Overdosage

Aside from possible ovarian hyperstimulation and multiple gestations (see Warnings), little is known concerning the consequences of acute overdosage.

Patient Information

Prior to therapy, inform patients of the following: Duration of treatment and monitoring required; possible adverse reactions; risk of multiple births.

UROFOLLITROPIN

Rx	**Bravelle** (Ferring)	**Powder for injection, lyophilized:** 75 units FSH activity[a]	In vials[b] with 2 mL vials NaCl as diluent.

[a] Contains up to 2% luteinizing hormone (LH) activity.

[b] With lactose monohydrate 23 mg.

UROFOLLITROPIN — INJECTION

For complete and comparative prescribing information, refer to the Follitropins group monograph.

Indications

➤*Ovulation induction:* In conjunction with human chorionic gonadotropin (hCG) for ovulation induction in patients who previously have received pituitary suppression.

➤*Multifollicular development during ART:* In conjunction with hCG for multiple follicular development (controlled ovarian stimulation) during assisted reproductive technologies (ART) cycles in patients who have previously received pituitary suppression.

Administration and Dosage

➤*Approved by the FDA:* August 26, 1996.

➤*Infertile patients with oligo-anovulation:* The dose to stimulate development of ovarian follicles must be individualized for each patient. Use the lowest dose consistent with achieving good results based on clinical experience and reported clinical data.

The recommended initial dose for patients who have received gonadotropin-releasing hormone (GnRH) agonist or antagonist suppression is 150 units/day subcutaneous or IM for the first 5 days of treatment. Based on clinical monitoring (including serum estradiol levels and vaginal ultrasound results), adjust subsequent dosing according to individual patient response. Do not make adjustments in dose more frequently than once every 2 days and do not exceed more than 75 to 150 units/adjustment. The maximum daily dose should not exceed 450 units and, in most cases, dosing beyond 12 days is not recommended.

If patient response is appropriate, give hCG (5,000 to 10,000 units) 1 day following the last dose of urofollitropin. Withhold the hCG if the serum estradiol is greater than 2,000 pg/mL, if the ovaries are abnormally enlarged, or if abdominal pain occurs, and advise the patient to refrain from intercourse. These precautions may reduce the risk of Ovarian Hyperstimulation Syndrome (OHSS) and multiple gestations. Follow patients closely for at least 2 weeks after hCG administration. If there is inadequate follicle development or ovulation without subsequent pregnancy, the course of treatment may be repeated.

Encourage the couple to have intercourse daily, beginning on the day prior to the administration of hCG until ovulation becomes apparent from indices employed for the determination of progestational activity. In the light of the foregoing indices and parameters mentioned, it should become obvious that unless a physician is willing to devote considerable time to these patients and be familiar with and conduct the necessary laboratory studies, urofollitropin should not be used.

➤*ART:* The recommended initial dose of urofollitropin for patients undergoing in vitro fertilization (IVF) and donor egg patients who have received GnRH agonist or antagonist pituitary suppression is 225 units daily administered subcutaneous for the first 5 days of treatment. Based on clinical monitoring (including serum estradiol levels and vaginal ultrasound results) subsequent dosing should be adjusted according to individual patient response. Adjustments in dose should not be made more frequently than once every 2 days and should not exceed more than 75 to 150 units per adjustment. The maximum daily dose of urofollitropin given should not exceed 450 units and in most cases dosing beyond 12 days is not recommended.

Once adequate follicular development is evident, hCG (5,000 to 10,000 units) should be administered to induce final follicular maturation in preparation for oocyte retrieval. The administration of hCG must be withheld in cases where the ovaries are abnormally enlarged on the last day of therapy. This should reduce the chance of developing OHSS.

➤*Reconstitution:* To prepare the solution, inject 1 mL of sterile saline for injection into the vial of urofollitropin. Do not shake, but gently swirl until the solution is clear. Generally, urofollitropin dissolves immediately. Check the liquid in the container; if it is not clear or contains particles, do not use it.

For patients requiring a single injection from multiple vials of urofollitropin, up to 6 vials can be reconstituted with 1 mL of sterile saline for injection. This can be accomplished by reconstituting a single vial as described above. Then draw the entire contents of the first vial into a syringe and inject the contents into a second vial of lyophilized urofollitropin. Gently swirl the second vial, once again checking to make sure the solution is clear and free of particles. This step can be repeated with 4 additional vials for a total of up to 6 vials of lyophilized urofollitropin into 1 mL of diluent.

➤*Administration:* Immediately administer the reconstituted urofollitropin. The recommended sites for subcutaneous injection are either side of the lower abdomen in alternating fashion. Injection into the thigh is not recommended.

➤*Storage / Stability:* Lyophilized powder may be stored in the refrigerator or at room temperature (3° to 25°C; 37° to 77°F). Protect from light. Use immediately after reconstitution. Discard unused material.

FOLLITROPIN ALFA

Rx	**Gonal-f** (Serono)	**Powder for injection, lyophilized:** 82 units FSH activity (to deliver 75 units)	30 mg sucrose. In 1 and 10 single-dose vials with sterile water for injection as diluent.
		600 units FSH activity (to deliver 450 units)	30 mg sucrose. In 1 multi-dose vial with prefilled syringe of bacteriostatic water[a] for injection as diluent and 6 syringes.
		1,200 units FSH activity (to deliver 1,050 units)	30 mg sucrose. In 1, 5, and 10 multi-dose vials with prefilled syringes of bacteriostatic water[a] for injection as diluent.
Rx	**Gonal-f RFF Pen** (Serono)	**Injection:** 415 units FSH activity (to deliver ≥ 300 units/0.5 mL)	In prefilled pens[b] with needles.
		568 units FSH activity (to deliver ≥ 450 units/0.75 mL)	
		1,026 units FSH activity (to deliver ≥ 900 units/1.5 mL)	

[a] With 0.9% benzyl alcohol.

[b] With 60 mg/mL sucrose, 3.0 mg/mL m-cresol, 1.1 mg/mL disodium hydrogen phosphate, 0.45 mg/mL sodium dihydrogen phosphate monohydrate, 0.1 mg//mL methionine, 0.1 mg/mL poloxamer 188.

FOLLITROPIN ALFA — INJECTION

For complete and comparative prescribing information, refer to the Follitropins group monograph.

Indications

➤*Ovulation induction:* For the induction of ovulation and pregnancy in oligo-anovulatory infertile patients in whom the cause of infertility is functional and not primary ovarian failure.

➤*Multifollicular development during assisted reproductive technology (ART):* To stimulate the development of multiple follicles in ovulatory patients participating in an ART program (eg, in vitro fertilization).

➤*Male infertility (except prefilled pen):* For the induction of spermatogenesis in men with primary and secondary hypogonadotropic hypogonadism in whom the cause of infertility is not primary testicular failure.

FOLLITROPIN ALFA — INJECTION

Administration and Dosage

➤*Approved by the FDA:* September 30, 1997.

For subcutaneous administration only. Individualize dosage.

➤*Ovulation induction:* The initial dose for the first cycle is 75 units/day subcutaneous. An incremental adjustment in dose of up to 37.5 units may be considered after 14 days. Further dose increases of the same magnitude can be made, if necessary, every 7 days. Do not exceed a treatment duration of 35 days unless an estradiol rise indicates imminent follicular development. To complete follicular development and effect ovulation in the absence of an endogenous luteinizing hormone surge, give 5,000 units human chorionic gonadotropin (hCG) 1 day after the last dose of follitropin alfa. Withhold hCG if the serum estradiol is greater than 2,000 pg/mL. If the ovaries are abnormally enlarged or abdominal pain occurs, discontinue follitropin alfa treatment, do not administer hCG, and advise the patient not to have intercourse; this may reduce the chance of developing Ovarian Hyperstimulation Syndrome (OHSS) and, should spontaneous ovulation occur, reduce the chance of multiple gestations. Conduct a follow-up visit in the luteal phase.

Individualize initial dose in subsequent cycles for each patient based on response in the preceding cycle. Doses larger than 300 units/day of follicle stimulating hormone are not routinely recommended. As in the initial cycle, 5,000 units of hCG must be given 1 day after the last dose of follitropin alfa to complete follicular development and induce ovulation. Follow the above precautions to minimize the chances of developing OHSS.

Use the lowest dose consistent with the expectation of good results. Over the course of treatment, doses of follitropin alfa may range up to 300 units/day depending on patient response. Give until adequate follicular development is indicated by serum estradiol and vaginal ultrasonography. A response is generally evident after 5 to 7 days. Base subsequent monitoring intervals on patient response.

Encourage the couple to have intercourse daily, beginning on the day prior to hCG administration until ovulation becomes apparent. Take care to ensure insemination. In light of the indices and parameters mentioned, the drug should not be used unless a physician is willing to devote considerable time to these patients and be familiar with and conduct the necessary lab studies.

➤*Multifollicular development during ART:* Initiate in the early follicular phase (cycle day 2 or 3) at a dose of 150 units/day, until sufficient follicular development is attained. In most cases, therapy should not exceed 10 days.

In patients undergoing ART under 35 years of age, whose endogenous gonadotropin levels are suppressed, initiate follitropin alfa prefilled pens at a dose of 150 units/day. In patients undergoing ART 35 years of age and older, whose endogenous gonadotropin levels are suppressed, initiate follitropin alfa prefilled pens at a dose of 225 units/day. Continue treatment until adequate follicular development is indicated as determined by ultrasound in combination with measurement of serum estradiol levels. Consider dose adjustments after 5 days based on the patient's response; adjust subsequent dosage no more frequently than every 3 to 5 days and by no more than 75 to 150 units additionally at each adjustment. Doses greater than 450 units/day are not recommended. Once adequate follicular development is evident, administer hCG (5,000 to 10,000 units) to induce final follicular maturation in preparation for oocyte retrieval. Withhold hCG in cases where the ovaries are abnormally enlarged on the last day of therapy to reduce the risk of developing OHSS.

➤*Male infertility:* The dose of follitropin alfa to induce spermatogenesis must be individualized for each patient. Give follitropin alfa in conjunction with hCG. Prior to concomitant therapy with follitropin alfa and hCG, pretreatment with hCG alone (1,000 to 2,250 units 2 to 3 times/week) is required. Continue treatment for a period sufficient to achieve serum testosterone levels within the normal range. Such pretreatment may require 3 to 6 months and the dose of hCG may need to be increased to achieve normal testosterone levels.

After normal serum testosterone levels are reached, the recommended dose of follitropin alfa is 150 units administered subcutaneous 3 times/week and the recommended dose of hCG is 1,000 units (or the dose required to maintain serum testosterone levels within the normal range) 3 times/week. Use the lowest dose of follitropin alfa that induces spermatogenesis. If azoospermia persists, the dose may be increased to a maximum of 300 units 3 times/week. Follitropin alfa may need to be administered for up to 18 months to achieve adequate spermatogenesis.

➤*Reconstitution:*

Single-dose amps – Dissolve contents of 1 or more amps in 0.5 to 1 mL of sterile water for injection (concentration should not exceed 225 units/0.5 mL) and immediately give subcutaneous. Discard unused reconstituted material.

Multi-dose vials – Dissolve the contents of 1 multi-dose vial (1,200 units) with the contents of 1 prefilled syringe (2 mL) containing bacteriostatic water for injection (0.9% benzyl alcohol). Resulting concentration will be 600 units/mL. Following reconstitution as directed, product will deliver approximately 1,050 units FSH. Instruct patients to use the accompanying syringes calibrated in FSH units (units FSH) for administration.

➤*Storage/Stability:*

Single-dose vials – Store vials in the refrigerator or at room temperature (2° to 25°C; 36° to 77°F). Protect from light. Use immediately after reconstitution. Discard unused material.

Multi-dose vials – Store multi-dose vials in the refrigerator or at room temperature until reconstituted (25°C; 77°F). Following reconstitution, refrigerate (2° to 8°C; 36° to 46° F) or store at room temperature (2° to 25°C; 36° to 77° F). Protect from light. Discard unused reconstituted solution after 28 days.

Prefilled pens – Store prefilled pens in the refrigerator (2° to 8°C; 36° to 46° F) until dispensed. Upon dispensing, refrigerate pen (2° to 8°C; 36° to 46° F) or store at room temperature (2° to 25°C; 36° to 77° F) for up to 1 month or until the expiration date, whichever occurs first. After the first injection, store pen in the refrigerator (2° to 8°C; 36° to 46° F) or at room temperature (2° to 25°C; 36° to 77° F) for up to 28 days. Protect from light. Do not freeze. Discard unused material after 28 days.

FOLLITROPIN BETA

Rx	**Follistim AQ Cartridge** (Organon)	**Injection:** 175 units per 0.21 mL (delivering 150 units FSH[a] activity)	Benzyl alcohol 10 mg/mL, sucrose 50 mg/mL. In cartridges with *BD micro-fine* pen needles.
		350 units per 0.42 mL (delivering 300 units FSH activity)	Benzyl alcohol 10 mg/mL, sucrose 50 mg/mL. In cartridges with *BD micro-fine* pen needles.
		650 units per 0.78 mL (delivering 600 units FSH activity)	Benzyl alcohol 10 mg/mL, sucrose 50 mg/mL. In cartridges with *BD micro-fine* pen needles.
		975 units per 1.17 mL (delivering 900 units FSH activity)	Benzyl alcohol 10 mg/mL, sucrose 50 mg/mL. In cartridges with *BD micro-fine* pen needles.
	Follistim AQ (Organon)	**Injection:** 75 units per 0.5 mL	Sucrose 25 mg, sodium 7.35 mg. In single-use vials.
		150 units per 0.5 mL	Sucrose 25 mg, sodium 7.35 mg. In single-use vials.

[a] FSH = follicle-stimulating hormone.

FOLLITROPIN BETA — INJECTION

For complete and comparative prescribing information, refer to the Follitropin group monograph.

Indications

➤*Follicle stimulation:* For the development of multiple follicles in ovulatory patients participating in an assisted reproductive technology (ART) program.

➤*OI:* For the induction of ovulation and pregnancy in anovulatory infertile patients in whom the cause of infertility is functional and not due to primary ovarian failure.

Administration and Dosage

➤*Approved by the FDA:* September 29, 1997.

➤*Dose conversion of follitropin beta administered with the Follistim Pen:* Consider a lower starting dose for gonadotropin stimulation and dose adjustments during gonadotropin stimulation for each patient. For that purpose, the following dose conversion table might be a useful reference.

Follitropin Beta Administered with the *Follistim Pen* Dose Conversion Table[a]

Lyophilized recombinant FSH dosing in ampules or vials, using conventional syringe	Follitropin beta dosing with the *Follistim Pen*
75 units	50 units
150 units	125 units
225 units	175 units
300 units	250 units
375 units	300 units
450 units	375 units

[a] Each value represents an 18% difference rounded to the nearest 25 unit increment.

Follitropin beta is delivered by the *Follistim Pen*, which accurately delivers the dose to which it is set. In a clinical bioavailability study that compared administration of the dissolved lyophilized follitropin beta preparation using a conventional syringe with needle and a ready-to-use follitropin beta solution in a cartridge injected with the pen device, it was shown that the pen device delivered, on average, an 18% higher amount of follitropin beta.

FOLLITROPIN BETA — INJECTION

This difference is due to the accurate dosing obtained with the *Follistim Pen* compared with a conventional syringe. This 18% difference corresponds to a similar difference in serum FSH concentrations caused by differences between the anticipated and the actual volume of follitropin beta injected with the conventional syringe.

The net deliverable dose of 150, 300, 600, and 900 units are based upon a maximum of 2 injections of 75 units (for 150 units), 4 injections of 75 units (for 300 units), 6 injections of 100 units (for 600 units), and 9 injections of 100 units (for 900 units).

➤*ART:*

Cartridges – In an open-label, noncontrolled, multicenter study, 60 women who were undergoing controlled ovarian hyperstimulation (COH) for in vitro fertilization (IVF) with and without intracytoplasmic sperm injection (ICSI) were treated with follitropin beta at a starting dose of 150 to 225 units for the first 5 days of treatment. This dose could be adjusted after that time based upon ovarian response. The maximum individualized daily dose of follitropin beta used in this clinical study was 450 units.

A starting dose of 150 to 225 units or lower of follitropin beta is recommended for at least the first 5 days of treatment. If a health care provider generally uses a starting dose of lyophilized gonadotropin 150 to 225 units, then the health care provider should consider using a lower starting dose of follitropin beta (see the preceding table). After this, adjust the dose for the individual patient based upon her ovarian response. For follitropin beta, consider lower maintenance doses for each patient.

During treatment with follitropin beta, when a sufficient number of follicles of adequate size are present, the final maturation of the follicles is induced by administering human chorionic gonadotropin (hCG) at a dose of 5,000 to 10,000 units. Oocyte (egg) retrieval is performed 34 to 36 hours later. The administration of hCG must be withheld in cases where the ovaries are abnormally enlarged on the last day of treatment with follitropin beta. This will reduce the chance of developing ovarian hyperstimulation syndrome (OHSS).

Single-use vial – A starting dose of 150 to 225 units of follitropin beta is recommended for at least the first 4 days of treatment. After this, the dose may be adjusted for the individual patient based upon her ovarian response. In clinical studies with responding patients, it was shown that daily maintenance doses ranging from 75 to 300 units for 6 to 12 days are sufficient, although longer treatment may be necessary. However, in patients that were low or poor responders, maintenance doses of 375 to 600 units were administered according to individual response. This later category comprised approximately 10% of the women evaluated during clinical studies. The maximum individualized daily dose of follitropin beta used in clinical studies is 600 units.

During treatment with follitropin beta, when a sufficient number of follicles of adequate size are present, the final maturation of the follicles is induced by administering hCG at a dose of 5,000 to 10,000 units. Oocyte (egg) retrieval is performed 34 to 36 hours later. The administration of hCG must be withheld in cases where the ovaries are abnormally enlarged on the last day of treatment with follitropin beta. This will reduce the chance of developing OHSS.

➤*OI:* For OI, encourage the couple to have intercourse daily, beginning on the day prior to the administration of hCG and until ovulation becomes apparent from the indices employed for the determination of progestational activity. Take care to ensure insemination.

Cartridges – In an open-label, noncontrolled, multicenter study in 43 clomiphene-resistant women with chronic anovulation (World Health Organization [WHO] group II) who were treated with follitropin beta for induction of ovulation, a stepwise increasing dose regimen was included. The starting dose was follitropin beta 75 units for up to 7 days. The dose was increased by 25 or 50 units at weekly intervals until follicular growth and/or serum estradiol levels indicated an adequate ovarian response. The maximum, individualized daily dose of follitropin beta that had been used for OI patients during this clinical trial is 175 units.

A starting dose of follitropin beta 75 units or lower is recommended for at least the first 7 days of treatment with dose adjustments at weekly intervals based upon patient response. If a health care provider generally uses a starting dose of lyophilized gonadotropin 75 units, then the health care provider should consider using a lower starting dose of follitropin beta (see the preceding table).

Continue treatment until ultrasonic visualizations and/or serum estradiol determinations indicate preovulatory conditions equivalent to or greater than those of the normal individual followed by hCG, 5,000 to 10,000 units. If the ovaries are abnormally enlarged on the last day of treatment with follitropin beta therapy, hCG must be withheld during this course of treatment; this will reduce the chances of developing OHSS.

Single-use vial – In studies using follitropin beta, a stepwise gradually increasing dosing scheme was used. The starting dose was 75 units of follitropin beta for up to 14 days. The dose was then increased by 37.5 units of follitropin at weekly intervals until follicular growth and/or serum estradiol levels indicated an adequate response. The maximum individualized daily dose of follitropin beta that has been safely used for OI in patients during clinical trials is 300 units.

Continue treatment until ultrasonic visualizations and/or serum estradiol determinations indicate preovulatory conditions equivalent to or greater than those of the normal individual followed by hCG, 5,000 to 10,000 units. If the ovaries are abnormally enlarged on the last day of treatment with follitropin beta therapy, hCG must be withheld during this course of treatment; this will reduce the chances of developing OHSS.

➤*Admixture incompatibilities:* Do not add or combine other drugs into the follitropin beta cartridge. Do not mix follitropin beta with any other medicines in the same vial or same syringe. Visually inspect parenteral drug products for particulate matter and clarity prior to administration whenever solution and container permit. Do not use the solution if particulate matter is present.

➤*Storage / Stability:*

Cartridges – Refrigerate at 2° to 8°C (36° to 46°F) until dispensed. Upon dispensing, the product may be stored by the patient at 2° to 8°C (36° to 46°F) until the expiration date or at 25°C (77°F) for 3 months or until expiration date, whichever occurs first. Once the rubber stopper of the follitropin beta cartridge has been pierced by a needle, the product can only be stored for a maximum of 28 days at 2° to 25°C (36° to 77°F). Protect from light. Do not freeze.

Single-use vial – Refrigerate at 2° to 8°C (36° to 46°F) until dispensed. Upon dispensing, the product may be stored by the patient at 2° to 8°C (36° to 46°F) until the expiration date or at or below 25°C (77°F) for 3 months or until expiration date, whichever occurs first. Protect from light; keep container in carton. Do not freeze.

MENOTROPINS

Rx	**Menopur** (Ferring)	**Powder or pellet for injection, lyophilized:** 75 units FSH activity, 75 units LH activity	In vials with diluent.
Rx	**Repronex** (Ferring)		In vials with diluent.
Rx	**Repronex** (Ferring)	**Powder or pellet for injection, lyophilized:** 150 units FSH activity, 150 units LH activity	In vials with diluent.

MENOTROPINS — INJECTION

Indications

➤*Menopur:* Menotropins, administered subcutaneously, are indicated for the development of multiple follicles and pregnancy in the ovulatory patients participating in the assisted reproductive technology (ART) program.

➤*Repronex:* Menotropins, in conjunction with human chorionic gonadotropin (hCG), is indicated for multiple follicular development (controlled ovarian stimulation) and ovulation induction in patients who have previously received pituitary suppression.

➤*Unlabeled uses:* Treatment of male infertility caused by hypogonadotropic hypogonadism when used in conjunction with hCG.

Administration and Dosage

➤*Approved by the FDA:* August 22, 1975.

➤*Dosage:*

Assisted reproductive technologies (Menopur and Repronex) – The recommended initial dose of menotropins for patients who have received gonadotropin-releasing hormone (GnRH) agonist pituitary suppression is 225 units. Based on clinical monitoring (including serum estradiol levels and vaginal ultrasound results), subsequent dosing should be adjusted according to individual patient response. Adjustments in dose should not be made more frequently than once every 2 days and should not exceed more than 75 to 150 units/adjustment for *Repronex* or 150 units/adjustment for *Menopur*.

The maximum daily dose of menotropins given should not exceed 450 units, and dosing beyond 12 days for *Repronex* and 20 days for *Menopur* is not recommended.

Once adequate follicular development is evident, hCG (5,000 to 10,000 units) should be administered to induce final follicular maturation in preparation for oocyte retrieval. The administration of hCG must be withheld in cases in which the ovaries are abnormally enlarged on the last day of therapy. This should reduce the chance of developing Ovarian Hyperstimulation Syndrome (OHSS).

Infertile patients with oligoanovulation (Repronex only) – The dose of menotropins to stimulate development of ovarian follicles must be individualized for each patient. The lowest dose consistent with achieving good results based on clinical experience and reported clinical data should be used.

The recommended initial dosage of menotropins for patients who have received GnRH agonist or antagonist pituitary suppression is 150 units daily for the first 5 days of treatment. Based on clinical monitoring (including serum estradiol levels and vaginal ultrasound results) subsequent dosing should be adjusted according to individual patient response. Adjustments in dose should not be made more frequently than once every 2 days and should not exceed more than 75 to 150 units/adjustment. The maximum daily dose of menotropins should not exceed 450 units and dosing beyond 12 days is not recommended.

If patient response to menotropins is appropriate, hCG (5,000 to 10,000 units) should be given 1 day following the last dose of menotropins.

MENOTROPINS — INJECTION

The hCG should be withheld if the serum estradiol is more than 2,000 pg/mL, the ovaries are abnormally enlarged, or abdominal pain occurs, and the patient should be advised to refrain from intercourse. These precautions may reduce the risk of OHSS and multiple gestation. Patients should be followed closely for at least 2 weeks after hCG administration. If there is inadequate follicle development or ovulation without subsequent pregnancy, the course of treatment with menotropins may be repeated. The couple should be encouraged to have intercourse daily, beginning on the day prior to the administration of hCG until ovulation becomes apparent from the indices employed for the determination of progestational activity. In the light of the foregoing indices and parameters mentioned, it should become obvious that, unless a health care provider is willing to devote considerable time to these patients and be familiar with and conduct the necessary laboratory studies, menotropins should not be used.

➤*Preparation and administration:* Dissolve the contents of 1 to 6 vials of menotropins in 1 mL (*Menopur*) or 1 to 2 mL (*Repronex*) sterile saline and administer subcutaneously or intramuscularly (*Repronex* only) immediately. Any unused reconstituted material should be discarded.

The lower abdomen (alternating sides) should be used for subcutaneous administration.

➤*Storage/Stability:* Lyophilized powder may be stored refrigerated or at room temperature (3° to 25°C; 37° to 77°F). Protect from light. Use immediately after reconstitution. Discard unused material.

Actions

➤*Pharmacology:* Menotropins administered for 7 to 20 days with *Menopur* or 7 to 12 days with *Repronex* produces ovarian follicular growth and maturation in women who do not have primary ovarian failure. In order to produce final follicular maturation and ovulation in the absence of an endogenous LH surge, hCG must be administered following menotropin treatment at a time when patient monitoring indicates sufficient follicular development has occurred.

➤*Pharmacokinetics:*

Absorption –

Menopur: The subcutaneous route of administration trends toward greater bioavailability than the IM route for single and multiple doses of menotropins.

Repronex: The geometric mean of FSH maximum plasma drug concentration (C_{max}) and area under the curve ($AUC_{0-\infty}$) upon single-dose subcutaneous administration of menotropins is 5.62 milliunits/mL and 385.2 milliunits•h/mL, respectively; the corresponding geometric median of FSH time to maximum concentration (T_{max}) is 12 hours. The geometric mean of FSH C_{max} and $AUC_{0-\infty}$ upon single-dose IM administration of menotropins is 4.15 milliunits/mL and 320.1 milliunits•h/mL, respectively; the corresponding geometric median of FSH T_{max} is 18 hours.

Distribution – Human tissue or organ distribution of FSH and LH have not been studied for menotropins.

Metabolism – Metabolism of FSH and LH have not been studied for menotropins in humans.

Excretion –

Menopur: The elimination half-lives for FSH in the multiple-dose phase were similar (11 to 13 hours) for *Menopur* subcutaneous and *Menopur* IM.

Repronex: The mean elimination half-lives of FSH upon single-dose subcutaneous and IM administration of *Repronex* are 53.7 and 59.2 hours, respectively.

Contraindications

Menotropins are contraindicated in women who have: a high FSH level indicating primary ovarian failure; uncontrolled thyroid and adrenal dysfunction; an organic intracranial lesion, such as a pituitary tumor; the presence of any cause of infertility other than anovulation, unless they are candidates for IVF (*Repronex* only); sex hormone-dependent tumors of the reproductive tract and accessory organs (*Menopur* only); abnormal uterine bleeding of undetermined origin; ovarian cysts or enlargement not caused by polycystic ovary syndrome; prior hypersensitivity to menotropins; menotropins is not indicated in women who are pregnant. There are limited human data on the effects of menotropins when administered during pregnancy.

Warnings

➤*Administration:* Menotropins should only be used by health care providers who are thoroughly familiar with infertility problems. It is a potent gonadotropic substance capable of causing OHSS in women with or without pulmonary or vascular complications and mild to severe adverse reactions in women. Gonadotropin therapy requires a certain time commitment by health care providers and supportive health professionals, and its use requires the availability of appropriate monitoring facilities.

➤*Overstimulation of the ovary during menotropins therapy:*

Ovarian enlargement – Mild to moderate uncomplicated ovarian enlargement, which may be accompanied by abdominal distension and/or abdominal pain, occurs in approximately 5% to 10% of women treated with menotropins and hCG and generally regresses without treatment within 2 or 3 weeks. The lowest dose consistent with expectation of good results and careful monitoring of ovarian response can further minimize the risk of overstimulation.

To minimize the hazard associated with the occasional abnormal ovarian enlargement that may occur with menotropins and hCG therapy, use the lowest dose consistent with expectation of good results. Careful monitoring of ovarian response can further minimize the risk of overstimulation.

If the ovaries are abnormally enlarged on the last day of menotropins therapy, do not administer hCG in this course of treatment; this will reduce the chances of development of the OHSS.

OHSS – OHSS is a medical event distinct from uncomplicated ovarian enlargement. OHSS may progress rapidly to become a serious medical event. It is characterized by an apparent dramatic increase in vascular permeability that can result in a rapid accumulation of fluid in the peritoneal cavity, thorax, and, potentially, the pericardium. The early warning signs of development of OHSS are severe pelvic pain, nausea, vomiting, and weight gain. The following symptomatology has been seen with cases of OHSS: abdominal pain; abdominal distension; GI symptoms including nausea, vomiting, and diarrhea; severe ovarian enlargement; weight gain; dyspnea; and oliguria. Clinical evaluation may reveal hypovolemia, hemoconcentration, electrolyte imbalances, ascites, hemoperitoneum, pleural effusions, hydrothorax, acute pulmonary distress, and thromboembolic events. Transient liver function test abnormalities suggestive of hepatic dysfunction, which may be accompanied by morphologic changes on liver biopsy, have been reported in association with the OHSS.

In the IVF clinical study, 0399E, OHSS occurred in 7.2% of 373 menotropin-treated women.

OHSS occurred in 3 of 125 (2.4%) of *Repronex*-treated women during ART clinical studies. None of these cases was classified as severe. In OI clinical studies, 4 of 72 (5.5%) of *Repronex*-treated women developed OHSS and 1 of these cases was classified as severe (1.4%). Cases of OHSS are more common, severe, and protracted if pregnancy occurs. OHSS develops rapidly; therefore, follow patients for at least 2 weeks after hCG administration. Most often, OHSS occurs after treatment has been discontinued and reaches its maximum at about 7 to 10 days following treatment. Usually, OHSS resolves spontaneously with the onset of menses. If there is evidence that OHSS may be developing prior to hCG administration, withhold the hCG.

If severe OHSS occurs, stop treatment and hospitalize the patient.

Consult a health care provider experienced in the management of the syndrome or fluid and electrolyte imbalances.

Repronex: Treatment is primarily symptomatic, consisting of bed rest, fluid and electrolyte management, and analgesics if needed. The phenomenon of hemoconcentration associated with fluid loss into the peritoneal cavity, pleural cavity, and the pericardial cavity has occurred and should be thoroughly assessed in the following manner:

- Fluid intake and output
- Weight
- Hematocrit
- Serum and urinary electrolytes
- Urine specific gravity
- Serum urea nitrogen (BUN) and creatinine
- Abdominal girth

These determinations are to be performed daily or more often if the need arises.

With OHSS there is an increased risk of injury to the ovary. Do not remove the ascitic, pleural, and pericardial fluid unless absolutely necessary to relieve symptoms such as pulmonary distress or cardiac tamponade. Avoid pelvic examination, which may cause rupture of an ovarian cyst and may result in hemoperitoneum. If this does occur, and if bleeding becomes such that surgery is required, design the surgical treatment to control bleeding and to retain as much ovarian tissue as possible. Intercourse is prohibited in patients in whom significant ovarian enlargement occurs after ovulation because of the danger of hemoperitoneum resulting from ruptured ovarian cysts.

• *Management of OHSS* – The management of OHSS may be divided into 3 phases: acute, chronic, and resolution. Because the use of diuretics can accentuate the diminished intravascular volume, avoid diuretics except in the late phase of resolution as described in the following section.

Acute phase: During the acute phase, design management to prevent hemoconcentration due to loss of intravascular volume to the third space and to minimize the risk of thromboembolic phenomena and kidney damage. Treatment is designed to normalize electrolytes while maintaining an acceptable but somewhat reduced intravascular volume. Full correction of the intravascular volume deficit may lead to an unacceptable increase in the amount of third space fluid accumulation. Management includes administration of limited intravenous (IV) fluids, electrolytes, and human serum albumin. Monitoring for the development of hyperkalemia is recommended.

Chronic phase: After stabilizing the patient during the acute phase, limit excessive fluid accumulation in the third space by instituting severe potassium, sodium, and fluid restriction.

Resolution phase: A fall in hematocrit and an increasing urinary output without an increased intake are observed due to the return of third space fluid to the intravascular compartment. Peripheral and/or pulmonary edema may result if the kidneys are unable to excrete third-space fluid as rapidly as it is mobilized. Diuretics may be indicated during the resolution phase if necessary to combat pulmonary edema.

➤*Multiple pregnancies:*

Menopur – In the clinical trial, multiple pregnancy, as diagnosed by ultrasound, occurred in 35.3% (n = 30) of 85 total pregnancies.

Advise the patient and her partner of the potential risk of multiple births before starting treatment.

Repronex – Multiple pregnancies have occurred following treatment with IM and subcutaneous menotropins. In a clinical trial for ovulation induction in which menotropins IM and menotropins subcutaneous were directly compared, the rates of multiple pregnancies were as follows. Of the 4 clinical

MENOTROPINS — INJECTION

pregnancies with menotropins IM, 2 were single and 2 were multiple pregnancies. Both multiple pregnancies were triplet pregnancies. Of the 6 clinical pregnancies with menotropins subcutaneous, 3 were single and 3 were multiple pregnancies. The 3 multiple pregnancies included 1 twin pregnancy and 2 quadruplet pregnancies.

In a clinical trial of IVF patients in which menotropins IM and menotropins subcutaneous were directly compared, the rates of multiple pregnancies were as follows. Of the 24 continuing pregnancies on menotropins IM, 14 were single and 10 were multiple pregnancies. The 10 multiple pregnancies included 3 triplet and 7 twin pregnancies. Of the 29 continuing pregnancies on subcutaneous menotropins, 14 were single and 15 were multiple pregnancies. The 15 multiple pregnancies included 3 quadruplet, 3 triplet, and 9 twin pregnancies. Advise the patient and her partner of the potential risk of multiple births before starting treatment.

➤*Pulmonary and vascular complications:* Serious pulmonary conditions (eg, atelectasis, acute respiratory distress syndrome) have been reported. In addition, thromboembolic events in association with, and separate from, the OHSS have been reported following menotropins therapy. Intravascular thrombosis and embolism, which may originate in venous or arterial vessels, can result in reduced blood flow to critical organs or the extremities. Sequelae of such events have included venous thrombophlebitis, pulmonary embolism, pulmonary infarction, cerebral vascular occlusion (stroke), and arterial occlusion resulting in loss of limb. In rare cases, pulmonary complications and/or thromboembolic events have resulted in death.

➤*Hypersensitivity reactions:* Hypersensitivity/anaphylactic reactions associated with menotropins administration have been reported in some patients. These reactions presented as generalized urticaria, facial edema, angioneurotic edema, or dyspnea suggestive of laryngeal edema. The relationship of these symptoms to uncharacterized urinary proteins is uncertain.

➤*Pregnancy: Category X.* Menotropins are not indicated in women who are pregnant. There are limited human data on the effects of menotropins when administered during pregnancy.

With menotropin therapy, congenital abnormalities have been reported. One infant was shown to have multiple congenital anomalies consisting of aplasia of the sigmoid colon, cecovesicle fistula, bifid scrotum, meningocele, bilateral internal tibial torsion, and right metatarsus adductus. Other reported anomalies include imperforate anus, congenital heart lesions, supernumerary digits, hypospadias, exstrophy of the bladder, Down syndrome, and hydrocephalus. The incidence of congenital abnormalities does not exceed that found in the general population.

➤*Lactation:* It is not known whether this drug is excreted in human milk. Because many drugs are excreted in human milk, exercise caution if administering menotropins to a breast-feeding woman.

➤*Children:* Safety and efficacy in pediatric patients have not been established.

Precautions

➤*Monitoring:*

Treatment for induction of ovulation – The combination of estradiol levels and ultrasonography are useful for monitoring the growth and development of follicles, timing hCG administration, and minimizing the risk of the OHSS and multiple gestation.

The clinical confirmation of ovulation, is determined by the following:
- A rise in basal body temperature.
- Increase in serum progesterone.
- Menstruation following the shift in basal body temperature.

When used in conjunction with indices of progesterone production, sonographic visualization of the ovaries will assist in determining if ovulation has occurred. Sonographic evidence of ovulation may include the following:
- Fluid in the cul-de-sac.
- Ovarian stigmata.
- Collapsed follicle.

Because of the subjectivity of the various tests for the determination of follicular maturation and ovulation, it cannot be overemphasized that the health care provider should choose tests with which he/she is thoroughly familiar.

Give careful attention to a diagnosis of infertility in the selection of candidates for menotropins therapy.

Drug Interactions

No drug/drug interaction studies have been conducted for menotropins in humans.

Adverse Reactions

➤*Menopur:* The safety of menotropins was examined in 3 clinical studies that enrolled a total of 575 patients receiving menotropins in the IVF and OI studies. All adverse reactions (without regard to causality assessment) occurring at an incidence of at least 2% in women treated with menotropins are listed in the following table.

Menopur (IM and Subcutaneous) Adverse Reactions in Women Undergoing IVF and OI (≥ 2%)

Adverse reactions	IVF[a] (n = 499) n (%)	OI[b] (n = 76) n (%)
CNS		
Dizziness	13 (2.6%)	0 (0%)
Headache	170 (34.1%)	12 (15.8%)
Migraine	12 (2.4%)	0 (0%)
GI		
Abdomen enlarged	12 (2.4%)	0 (0%)
Abdominal cramps	30 (6%)	5 (6.6%)
Abdominal fullness	16 (3.2%)	7 (9.2%)
Abdominal pain	88 (17.6%)	7 (9.2%)
Constipation	8 (1.6%)	0 (0%)
Diarrhea	14 (2.8%)	2 (2.6%)
Nausea	60 (12%)	6 (7.9%)
Vomiting	21 (4.2%)	2 (2.6%)
GU		
Breast tenderness	9 (1.8%)	2 (2.6%)
Hot flash	3 (0.6%)	2 (2.6%)
Menstrual disorder	16 (3.2%)	0 (0%)
OHSS	19 (3.8%)	10 (13.2%)
Pelvic cramps	0 (0%)	3 (3.9%)
Pelvic discomfort	2 (0.4%)	2 (2.6%)
Postretrieval pain	32 (6.4%)	0 (0%)
Uterine spasm	8 (1.6%)	3 (3.9%)
Respiratory		
Cough increased	8 (1.6%)	2 (2.6%)
Respiratory disorder	29 (5.8%)	3 (3.9%)
Miscellaneous		
Back pain	16 (3.2%)	0 (0%)
Elevated estradiol	12 (2.4%)	0 (0%)
Flu syndrome	13 (2.6%)	1 (1.3%)
Flushing	12 (2.4%)	0 (0%)
Injection site pain	27 (5.4%)	0 (0%)
Injection site reaction	48 (9.6%)	9 (11.8%)
Malaise	14 (2.8%)	2 (2.6%)
Pain	16 (3.2%)	2 (2.6%)

[a] Includes IM and subcutaneous subjects from protocols MFK/IVF/0399E and *Menopur* 2000-02.
[b] Includes IM and subcutaneous subjects from protocol *Menopur* 2000-01.

➤*Repronex:* The following adverse reactions, reported during menotropins therapy, are listed in decreasing order of potential severity:
- Pulmonary and vascular complications
- OHSS
- Hemoperitoneum
- Adnexal torsion (as a complication of ovarian enlargement)
- Mild-to-moderate ovarian enlargement
- Ovarian cysts
- Abdominal pain
- Sensitivity to menotropins. (Febrile reactions suggestive of allergic response have been reported following the administration of menotropins. Flu-like symptoms including fever, chills, musculoskeletal aches, joint pains, nausea, headaches, and malaise also have been reported.)
- GI symptoms (nausea, vomiting, diarrhea, abdominal cramps, bloating)
- Pain, rash, swelling, or irritation at the site of injection
- Body rashes
- Dizziness, dyspnea, tachycardia, tachypnea

The following medical events have been reported subsequent to pregnancies resulting from menotropins therapy: ectopic pregnancy, congenital abnormalities.

There have been infrequent reports of ovarian neoplasms, both benign and malignant, in women who have undergone multiple-drug regimens for ovulation induction; however, a causal relationship has not been established.

Adverse reactions occurring in at least 1% of patients exposed to menotropins IM or menotropins subcutaneous are described in the following table:

MENOTROPINS — INJECTION

Repronex Adverse Reactions (≥ 1%)		
Adverse reactions	Menotropins IM (n = 101) n (%)	Menotropins subcutaneous (n = 96) n (%)
GI		
Abdominal cramping	7 (6.9%)	5 (5.2%)
Abdominal pain	5 (5%)	7 (7.3%)
Diarrhea	0 (0%)	2 (2.1%)
Enlarged abdomen	6 (6%)	2 (2.1%)
Nausea	4 (4%)	7 (7.3%)
Vomiting	0 (0%)	3 (3.1%)
GU		
Breast tenderness	2 (2%)	2 (2.1%)
Ectopic pregnancy	1 (1%)	1 (1%)
OHSS	2 (2%)	5 (5.2%)
Ovarian disease	3 (3%)	8 (8.3%)
Pelvic pain	3 (3%)	1 (1%)
Vaginal hemorrhage	8 (7.9%)	3 (3.1%)
Local		
Injection site edema	1 (1%)	8 (8.3%)[a]
Injection site reaction	2 (2%)	8 (8.3%)[a]
Miscellaneous		
Dyspnea	1 (1%)	2 (2.1%)
Headache	6 (6%)	5 (5.2%)
Infection	1 (1%)	0 (0%)

[a] Fisher exact/chi-square tests (significant for *Repronex* subcutaneous vs *Repronex* IM).

Overdosage

Aside from possible ovarian hyperstimulation, little is known concerning the consequences of acute overdosage with menotropins.

Patient Information

Prior to therapy, inform patients of the duration of treatment and the monitoring of their condition that will be required. Also discuss possible adverse reactions and the risk of multiple births.

LUTROPIN ALFA

Rx	**Luveris** (Serono)	**Powder for injection, lyophilized:** 82.5 units/vial	48 mg sucrose. In single-dose vials. Delivers 75 units lutropin alfa after reconstitution.

LUTROPIN ALFA — INJECTION

Indications

➤*Follicle stimulation:* Lutropin alfa coadministered with follitropin alfa (Gonal-F®) is indicated for stimulation of follicular development in infertile, hypogonadotropic, hypogonadal women with profound luteinizing hormone (LH) deficiency (LH less than 1.2 units/L). A definitive effect on pregnancy in this population has not been demonstrated. The safety and efficacy of concomitant administration of lutropin alfa with any other preparation of recombinant human follicle stimulating hormone (FSH) or urinary human FSH is unknown.

Administration and Dosage

➤*Approved by the FDA:* October 8, 2004.

For subcutaneous use only.

➤*Dosage:* It is recommended that lutropin alfa 75 units be coadministered subcutaneously with follitropin alfa 75 to 150 units as 2 separate injections in the initial treatment cycle. Coadministration of lutropin alfa with follitropin alfa was studied in clinical trials for lutropin alfa. The safety and efficacy of coadministration of lutropin alfa with any other preparation of recombinant human FSH or urinary human FSH is unknown. Administer Lutropin alfa and follitropin alfa daily until adequate follicular development is indicated by ovary ultrasonography and serum estradiol. Treatment duration should not normally exceed 14 days unless signs of imminent follicular development are present.

To complete follicular development and effect ovulation in the absence of an endogenous LH surge, give human chorionic gonadotropin (hCG) 1 day after the last dose of lutropin alfa and follitropin alfa. Withhold treatment with hCG if the ovaries are abnormally enlarged or if excessive estradiol production has occurred. If the ovaries are abnormally enlarged or abdominal pain occurs, discontinue treatment with lutropin alfa and follitropin alfa and do not administer hCG. Advise the patient not to have intercourse; this may reduce the chances of developing ovarian hyperstimulation syndrome and, should spontaneous ovulation occur, reduce the chances of multiple gestation. Conduct a follow-up visit in the luteal phase.

Individualize doses administered in subsequent cycles for each patient based on her response in the preceding cycle. Doses of follitropin alfa greater than 225 units/day are not routinely recommended. As in the initial cycle, hCG must be given to complete follicular development and induce ovulation. Follow the precautions described above to minimize the chance of developing ovarian hyperstimulation syndrome.

Encourage the couple to have intercourse daily, beginning on the day prior to hCG administration until ovulation becomes apparent in the indices used for the determination of progestational activity.

In light of the indices and parameters mentioned, it should become obvious that, unless a health care provider is willing to devote considerable time to these patients and be familiar with and conduct the necessary laboratory studies, he/she should not prescribe lutropin alfa.

➤*Administration:* Dissolve the contents of 1 vial of lutropin alfa in 1 mL sterile water for injection. Reconstitute and administer follitropin alfa as directed in the prescriber labeling for this product. Administer entire contents of each vial subcutaneously as separate injections. For single use. Use immediately after reconstitution. Discard any unused reconstituted material. Mix gently. Do not shake.

Visually inspect parenteral drug products for particulate matter and discoloration prior to administration.

Lutropin alfa and follitropin alfa may be self-administered by the patient. Follow the directions below for reconstituting and injecting as separate injections of lutropin alfa and follitropin alfa. Reconstitute and administer follitropin alfa as directed in the prescriber labeling for this product. Discard any unused reconstituted material.

Step 1: Prepare the vials – Wash hands thoroughly with soap and water. Begin by opening the cartons of lutropin alfa. Remove the plastic flip-tops from the vial of lutropin alfa powder and the vial of diluent provided with lutropin alfa. After removing the plastic flip-tops, wipe the rubber stoppers with alcohol. Do not touch the rubber stoppers after they are wiped.

Step 2: Withdraw the water into the syringe – Carefully remove the needle cover. Do not touch the needle or allow the needle to touch any surface. After removing the needle cover, draw air into the syringe by slowly pulling back the plunger to the 1 mL mark. Place the vial of diluent on a hard, flat surface. Carefully insert the needle through the rubber stopper into the vial with the sterile water (diluent). Gently inject the air into the vial (the injected air creates pressure, which makes withdrawing the solution easier). Without removing the needle, turn the vial upside down and withdraw all of the water into the syringe, making sure the tip of the needle remains in the water. Remove the needle from the vial.

Step 3: Inject the water into the lutropin alfa vial – Place the vial containing the lutropin alfa powder on a hard, flat surface. Insert the needle through the rubber stopper into the vial. Keep the syringe in a straight, upright position as you insert it through the center of the rubber stopper, or it may be difficult to depress the plunger. After inserting the needle, slowly inject the sterile water (diluent) by depressing the plunger on the syringe into the vial of lutropin alfa powder.

Step 4: Gently dissolve the lutropin alfa powder – Leaving the needle in the vial, gently rotate the vial between your fingers until all of the powder is dissolved. Do not shake. Check that the solution is clear and colorless. Do not use if the solution is cloudy, discolored, or contains particles.

Step 5: Withdraw the lutropin alfa solution from the vial – Without removing the needle, turn the vial upside down and withdraw all of the lutropin alfa solution into the syringe. Make sure the tip of the needle remains in the solution by slowly backing the needle out of the vial to withdraw as much of the solution as possible. Next, remove the needle from the vial.

Step 6: Replace needle and remove air bubbles in the syringe – Recap the syringe needle and twist the cap and needle off of syringe. Twist a new needle onto the end of the syringe and carefully remove the cap of the needle. To remove any air bubbles in the syringe, point the needle up and gently tap the syringe. When all the bubbles float to the top, slightly push the plunger until a small drop or two of solution begins to appear from the tip of the needle.

Step 7: Recap the syringe needle – Recap the syringe needle. Do not touch the needle or allow the needle to touch any surface. Carefully lay the syringe down on a flat, clean surface.

Step 8: Carefully clean the injection site – Suitable injection sites on the stomach (a few inches above or below the navel) will be advised by your fertility specialist. Occasionally your fertility specialist may suggest an alternative site. Make yourself comfortable by sitting or lying down. Carefully clean the injection site with an alcohol wipe and allow it to air-dry.

LUTROPIN ALFA — INJECTION

Step 9: Administer the injection – Remove the needle cap from the syringe needle. Hold the syringe like a pencil. With the other hand, pinch the skin together. Using a dart-like motion, insert the needle at a 45° to 90° angle (just under the skin) into the pad of tissue as shown or as directed by your health care provider.

Do not inject into a vein. Release the hand pinching the skin and depress the plunger in a slow, steady motion until all the medication is injected.

Step 10: Gently withdraw the needle – Withdraw the needle.

Step 11: Storage and clean up – Discard the used needle and syringe into your safety container. Place gauze over the injection site. If any bleeding occurs, apply gentle pressure. If bleeding does not stop within a few minutes, place a clean piece of gauze over the injection site and cover it with an adhesive bandage. Remember that the injection materials must be kept sterile and cannot be reused.

➤*Storage/Stability:* Vials may be refrigerated or stored at room temperature (2° to 25°C; 36° to 77°F). Protect from light. Store in original package. Use immediately after reconstitution. Discard unused material.

Actions

➤*Pharmacology:* The physicochemical, immunological, and biological activities of lutropin alfa are comparable with those of human pituitary LH. In the ovaries during the follicular phase, LH stimulates theca cells to secrete androgens that will be used as the substrate by granulosa cell aromatase enzyme to produce estradiol, supporting FSH-induced follicular development. Lutropin alfa is administered concomitantly with follitropin alfa to stimulate development of a potentially competent follicle and to indirectly prepare the reproductive tract for implantation and pregnancy.

➤*Pharmacokinetics:*

Absorption – Following subcutaneous administration of lutropin alfa, maximum serum concentration is reached after approximately 4 to 16 hours.

The mean absolute bioavailability of lutropin alfa following a single subcutaneous injection (at a much higher dose to allow proper quantification [10,000 units]) to healthy women is 56 ± 23%, supported by an immunoassay method. There were no statistical differences between the intramuscular and subcutaneous routes of administration for C_{max}, T_{max}, or bioavailability.

Distribution – Following an IV dose of 300 units of lutropin alfa, a rapid distribution phase ($t_{½λ1}$ of approximately 1 hour) and a terminal half-life ($t_{½}$) of approximately 11 hours were observed for r-hLH. The steady state volume of distribution (V_{ss}) was approximately 10 L. Mean residence time (MRT) was approximately 6 hours.

Metabolism/Excretion – Following subcutaneous administration of lutropin alfa, r-hLH is eliminated from the body with a mean terminal half-life of about 18 hours. Total body clearance is approximately 2 to 3 L/h with less than 5% of the dose being excreted unchanged renally. When given by IV administration, lutropin alfa demonstrates linear pharmacokinetics over the 300 to 40,000 units dose range. Following a 75 unit dose, the concentration range is too small to allow proper quantification of the pharmacokinetic parameters. The disposition of r-hLH is adequately described by a biexponential model.

Following subcutaneous administration, the terminal half-life is slightly longer than after IV administration. Upon repeated daily administration, a modest accumulation takes place (accumulation ratio of 1.6 ± 0.8). Following administration of lutropin alfa 150 units, r-hLH pharmacokinetics are described in the following table.

Pharmacokinetic Parameters[a] (mean ± SD) of r-hLH After Single-dose Subcutaneous Administration of Lutropin Alfa in Pituitary Desensitized Healthy Female Volunteers

Parameter[a]	Lutropin alfa 150 units subcutaneous
C_{max} (units/L)	1.1 ± 0.3
T_{max} (h)[b]	6 (3-9)
AUC (h•units/L)	44 ± 44
$T_{½}$ (h)	14 ± 8

[a] C_{max}: peak concentration; T_{max}: time of C_{max}; AUC: total area under the curve; $t_{½}$: elimination half-life
[b] Median (range).

Contraindications

Lutropin alfa is contraindicated in women who exhibit the following: prior hypersensitivity to hLH preparations or one of their excipients; primary ovarian failure; uncontrolled thyroid or adrenal dysfunction; uncontrolled organic intracranial lesion such as a pituitary tumor; abnormal uterine bleeding of undetermined origin; ovarian cyst or enlargement of undetermined origin; sex hormone dependent tumors of the reproductive tract and accessory organs; pregnancy.

Warnings

➤*Administration:* Gonadotropins, including lutropin alfa, should only be used by health care providers who are thoroughly familiar with infertility problems and their management. Like other gonadotropin products, lutropin alfa is a potent gonadotropic substance capable of contributing to the development of ovarian hyperstimulation syndrome in women with or without pulmonary or vascular complications. Gonadotropin therapy requires a certain time commitment by health care providers, and requires the availability of appropriate monitoring facilities. Safe and effective use of lutropin alfa requires monitoring of ovarian response with serum estradiol and ovary ultrasound on a regular basis.

➤*Overstimulation of the ovary:*

Ovarian enlargement – Mild to moderate uncomplicated ovarian enlargement, which may be accompanied by abdominal distension and/or abdominal pain, may occur in patients treated with gonadotropins (such as lutropin alfa). These conditions generally regress without treatment within 2 or 3 weeks. Careful monitoring of ovarian response can further minimize the risk of overstimulation.

If the ovaries are abnormally enlarged on the last day of therapy with lutropin alfa and follitropin alfa, do not administer hCG in this course of therapy. This will reduce the risk of development of ovarian hyperstimulation syndrome.

Ovarian hyperstimulation syndrome – Ovarian hyperstimulation syndrome is a medical event distinct from uncomplicated ovarian enlargement. Severe ovarian hyperstimulation syndrome may progress rapidly (within 24 hours to several days) to become a serious medical event. It is characterized by an apparent dramatic increase in vascular permeability which can result in a rapid accumulation of fluid in the peritoneal cavity, thorax, and potentially, the pericardium. The early warning signs of development of ovarian hyperstimulation syndrome are severe pelvic pain, nausea, vomiting, and weight gain. The following symptomatology has been seen with cases of ovarian hyperstimulation syndrome: abdominal pain, abdominal distension, GI symptoms (eg, nausea, vomiting, diarrhea), severe ovarian enlargement, weight gain, dyspnea, and oliguria. Clinical evaluation may reveal hypovolemia, hemoconcentration, electrolyte imbalances, ascites, hemoperitoneum, pleural effusions, hydrothorax, acute pulmonary distress, and thromboembolic events. Transient liver function test abnormalities that are suggestive of hepatic dysfunction have been reported in association with ovarian hyperstimulation syndrome. These liver function test abnormalities may be accompanied by morphological changes on liver biopsy.

In hypogonadotropic hypogonadal women with profound LH and FSH deficiency from 5 clinical trials, 4 cases of ovarian hyperstimulation syndrome were reported in 4 of 70 (5.7%) patients treated with lutropin alfa 75 units and follitropin alfa and 1 case was reported in 1 of 31 (3.2%) patients treated with follitropin alfa alone. Among women treated with any dose of lutropin alfa in these studies, 5 of 96 (5.2%) patients reported 6 cases of ovarian hyperstimulation syndrome after treatment with lutropin alfa and follitropin alfa.

Ovarian hyperstimulation syndrome may be more severe and more protracted if pregnancy occurs. Ovarian hyperstimulation syndrome develops rapidly; therefore, follow patients for at least 2 weeks after hCG administration. Most often, ovarian hyperstimulation syndrome occurs after treatment has been discontinued and reaches its maximum severity at 7 to 10 days following treatment. Usually, ovarian hyperstimulation syndrome resolves spontaneously with the onset of menses. If there is evidence that ovarian hyperstimulation syndrome may be developing prior to hCG administration, hCG must be withheld.

If severe ovarian hyperstimulation syndrome occurs, stop treatment with gonadotropins and hospitalize the patient.

Consult a health care provider experienced in the management of this syndrome or in the management of fluid and electrolyte imbalances.

➤*Multiple births:* Advise patients of the potential risk of multiple births before starting treatment.

➤*Pulmonary and vascular complications:* As with other gonadotropin products, a potential for the occurrence of arterial thromboembolism exists.

➤*Fertility impairment:* Impaired fertility has been reported in animals exposed to high doses of lutropin alfa; increased preimplantation and postimplantation losses were observed in female rats and rabbits given lutropin alfa at dosages of 10 units/kg/day and higher.

➤*Pregnancy: Category X.* When administered to rats during the late period of pregnancy, dosages of 10 units/kg/day and higher were also shown to affect the postnatal survival and growth of the newborns. There was no evidence of teratogenic effect in either rats or rabbits. Lutropin alfa is contraindicated in women who are pregnant and may cause fetal harm when administered to a pregnant woman. Reproductive toxicity studies performed in female rats and rabbits showed that lutropin alfa at doses of 10 units/kg/day and greater caused an increase in preimplantation and postimplantation losses.

➤*Lactation:* It is not known if this drug is excreted in human milk. Because many drugs are excreted in human milk, exercise caution if lutropin alfa is administered to a nursing woman.

➤*Children:* Lutropin alfa is not indicated in pediatric patients. Safety and efficacy in pediatric patients have not been established.

Precautions

➤*Monitoring:* In most instances, treatment of women with LH and FSH results only in follicular recruitment and development. In the absence of an endogenous LH surge, hCG is given when monitoring of the patient indicates that sufficient follicular development has occurred. This may be estimated by ultrasound alone or in combination with measurement of serum estradiol levels. The combination of both ultrasound and serum estradiol measurement are useful for monitoring the development of follicles, for timing of the ovulatory trigger, as well as for detecting ovarian enlargement and minimizing the risk of the ovarian hyperstimulation syndrome and multiple

LUTROPIN ALFA — INJECTION

gestation. It is recommended that the number of growing follicles be confirmed using ultrasonography because serum estrogens do not give an indication of the size or number of follicles.

With the exception of confirmation of pregnancy, the clinical confirmation of ovulation is obtained by direct and indirect indices of progesterone production. The indices most generally used are as follows:

1.) A rise in basal body temperature
2.) Increase in serum progesterone
3.) Menstruation following a shift in basal body temperature

When used in conjunction with the indices of progesterone production, sonographic visualization of the ovaries will assist in determining if ovulation has occurred. Sonographic evidence of ovulation may include the following:

1.) Fluid in the cul-de-sac
2.) Ovarian stigmata
3.) Collapsed follicle
4.) Secretory endometrium

Accurate interpretation of the indices of ovulation require a health care provider who is experienced in the interpretation of these tests.

➤*General:* Give careful attention to the diagnosis of infertility in candidates for lutropin alfa therapy.

Drug Interactions

There are no pharmacokinetic interactions with follitropin alfa when administered simultaneously with lutropin alfa. No drug-drug interaction studies have been conducted with lutropin alfa.

Adverse Reactions

The safety of lutropin alfa was examined in 6 clinical studies that treated 170 infertile women with HH of whom 152 received lutropin alfa and follitropin alfa in 283 treatment cycles. Adverse reactions reported by at least 2% of patients (regardless of causality) treated with any dose of lutropin alfa (25, 75, 150, or 225 units) are listed in the following table.

Adverse Reactions Reported in ≥ 2% Patients in All Cycles in All HH Patients in Studies 6253, 6905,[a] 7798,[b] 8297,[c] 21008, and 21415

	Lutropin alfa 0 units and follitropin alfa patients (n = 43) n (%)	Lutropin alfa 75 units and follitropin alfa patients (n = 118) n (%)	All doses of lutropin alfa and follitropin alfa patients (n = 152) n (%)
Patients with events	20 (46.5%)	50 (42.4%)	72 (47.4%)
CNS			
Headache	2 (4.7%)	12 (10.2%)	15 (9.9%)
GI			
Abdominal pain	5 (11.6%)	6 (5.1%)	13 (8.6%)
Constipation	0	3 (2.5%)	3 (2%)
Diarrhea	1 (2.3%)	3 (2.5%)	3 (2%)
Flatulence	3 (7%)	5 (4.2%)	6 (3.9%)
Nausea	0	8 (6.8%)	11 (7.2%)
GU			
Breast pain (female)	4 (9.3%)	6 (5.1%)	9 (5.9%)
Dysmenorrhea	1 (2.3%)	2 (1.7%)	4 (2.6%)
Ovarian cyst	4 (9.3%)	6 (5.1%)	8 (5.3%)
Ovarian disorder	0	2 (1.7%)	3 (2%)
Ovarian hyperstimulation	1 (2.3%)	7 (5.9%)	9 (5.9%)
Miscellaneous			
Fatigue	0	3 (2.5%)	5 (3.3%)
Injection site reaction	2 (4.7%)	4 (3.4%)	6 (3.9%)
Pain	3 (7%)	3 (2.5%)	6 (3.9)
Upper respiratory tract infection	2 (4.7%)	1 (0.8%)	3 (2%)

[a] Study 6905 was a randomized, open-label, dose-finding study to assess the safety and efficacy of lutropin alfa administered with follitropin alfa 150 units for induction of follicular development in HH women.
[b] Study 7798 was an uncontrolled, multicenter, dose-finding study to assess the safety and efficacy of lutropin alfa administered with follitropin alfa 150 units for induction of follicular development in LH and FSH deficient anovulatory women in Germany.
[c] Study 8297 was an uncontrolled, multicenter, dose-finding study to assess the safety and efficacy of lutropin alfa administered with follitropin alfa 150 units for induction of follicular development in HH women in Spain.

The following medical events have been reported subsequent to pregnancies resulting from administration of gonadotropins for ovulation induction in controlled clinical studies:

- Spontaneous abortion
- Ectopic pregnancy
- Premature labor
- Postpartum fever
- Congenital abnormalities

There is no evidence that use of any gonadotropin drug product for treatment of infertility is associated with an increased risk of congenital malformations.

The following adverse reactions have been previously reported during menotropin therapy:

- Pulmonary and vascular complications
- Adnexal torsion (as a complication of ovarian enlargement)
- Mild to moderate ovarian enlargement
- Hemoperitoneum

There have been infrequent reports of ovarian neoplasms, both benign and malignant, in women who have undergone multiple drug regimens for ovulation induction; however, a causal relationship has not been established.

Overdosage

Aside from possible ovarian hyperstimulation and multiple gestations, there is no information on the consequences of overdosage with lutropin alfa.

Patient Information

Prior to therapy with lutropin alfa, inform patients of the duration of treatment and monitoring of their condition that will be required. Also discuss the risks of ovarian hyperstimulation syndrome and multiple births and other possible adverse reactions.

HUMAN CHORIONIC GONADOTROPIN INJECTION

Rx	**Chorionic Gonadotropin** (Various, eg, Goldline, Rugby, Steris)	**Powder for Injection:** 5,000 units/vial with 10 mL diluent (to make 500 units/mL)	In 10 mL vials.
Rx	**Chorex-5** (Hyrex)		In 10 ml vials.[2]
Rx	**Profasi** (Serono)		In 10 ml vials.[2]
Rx	**Chorionic Gonadotropin** (Various, eg, Goldline, Rugby, Steris)	**Powder for Injection:** 10,000 units/vial with 10 mL diluent (to make 1,000 units/mL)	In 10 mL vials.
Rx	**Choron 10** (Forest)		In 10 mL vials.[2]
Rx	**Gonic** (Hauck)		In 10 mL vials.[2]
Rx	**Novarel** (Ferring)		In 10 mL vials.[2]
Rx	**Pregnyl** (Organon)		In 10 mL vials.[3]
Rx	**Profasi** (Serono)		In 10 mL vials.[2]
Rx	**Chorionic Gonadotropin** (Various, eg, Goldline, Steris)	**Powder for Injection:** 20,000 units/vial with 10 mL diluent (to make 2,000 units/mL)	In 10 mL vials.

[1] With benzyl alcohol, less than 0.2% phenol and lactose.
[2] With mannitol and 0.9% benzyl alcohol.
[3] With 0.9% benzyl alcohol.

HUMAN CHORIONIC GONADOTROPIN — INJECTION

WARNING

Human chorionic gonadotropin (hCG) has no known effect on fat mobilization, appetite, sense of hunger or body-fat distribution. Human chorionic gonadotropin (hCG) has not been demonstrated to be effective adjunctive therapy in the treatment of obesity. There is no substantial evidence that it increases weight loss beyond that resulting from caloric restriction, that it causes a more attractive or "normal" distribution of fat or that it decreases the hunger and discomfort associated with calorie-restricted diets.

Indications

➤*Prepubertal cryptorchidism:* Prepubertal cryptorchidism not caused by anatomic obstruction. In general, chorionic gonadotropin is thought to induce testicular descent in situations when descent would have occurred at puberty. Chorionic gonadotropin thus may help to predict whether or not orchiopexy will be needed in the future. Although, in some cases, descent following chorionic gonadotropin administration is permanent, in most cases the response is temporary. Therapy is usually instituted between the ages of 4 and 9.

➤*Hypogonadism:* Selected cases of hypogonadotropic hypogonadism (hypogonadism secondary to a pituitary deficiency) in males.

➤*Ovulation induction:* Induction of ovulation and pregnancy in the anovulatory, infertile woman in whom the cause of anovulation is secondary and not caused by primary ovarian failure, and who has been appropriately pretreated with human menotropins.

Administration and Dosage

Parenteral drug products should be inspected visually for particulate matter and discoloration prior to administration, whenever solution and container permit.

➤*IM use only:* The dosage regimen to be used will depend upon the indication for use, the age and weight of the patient, and the physician's preference. The following regimens have been advocated by various authorities.

➤*Prepubertal cryptorchidism not caused by anatomical obstruction:* Therapy is usually instituted between the ages of 4 and 9.

1.) 4,000 units 3 times weekly for 3 weeks.
2.) 5,000 units every second day for 4 injections.
3.) 15 injections of 500 to 1,000 units over a period of 6 weeks.
4.) 500 units 3 times weekly for 4 to 6 weeks. If this course of treatment is not successful, another is begun 1 month later, giving 1,000 units/injection.

➤*Selected cases of male hypogonadism secondary to pituitary failure:*

1.) 500 to 1,000 units 3 times a week for 3 weeks, followed by the same dose twice a week for 3 weeks.
2.) 4,000 units 3 times weekly for 6 to 9 months, following which the dosage may be reduced to 2,000 units 3 times weekly for an additional 3 months.

➤*Induction of ovulation and pregnancy:*

1.) Induction of ovulation and pregnancy in the anovulatory, infertile woman in whom the cause of anovulation is secondary and not caused by primary ovarian failure and who has been appropriately pretreated with human menotropins.
2.) 5,000 to 10,000 units 1 day following the last dose of menotropins. A dosage of 10,000 units is recommended in the labeling for menotropins.

➤*Important:* Use completely within 60 days after reconstitution. Refrigerate after reconstitution.

➤*Directions for reconstitution:*

Two-vial package – Withdraw sterile air from lyophilized vial and inject into diluent vial. Remove 10 mL from diluent vial and add to lyophilized vial; agitate gently until solution is complete.

➤*Storage/Stability:* Store dry product at controlled room temperature 15° to 30°C (59° to 86°F). After reconstitution, refrigerate the product at 2° to 8°C (36° to 46°F) and use within 30 days.

Actions

➤*Pharmacology:* The action of hCG is virtually identical to that of pituitary LH, although hCG appears to have a small degree of FSH activity as well. It stimulates production of gonadal steroid hormones by stimulating the interstitial cells (Leydig cells) of the testis to produce androgens and the corpus luteum of the ovary to produce progesterone. Androgen stimulation in the male leads to the development of secondary sex characteristics and may stimulate testicular descent when no anatomical impediment to descent is present. This descent is usually reversible when hCG is discontinued. During the normal menstrual cycle, LH participates with FSH in the development and maturation of the normal ovarian follicle, and the midcycle LH surge triggers ovulation. hCG can substitute for LH in this function.

During a normal pregnancy, hCG secreted by the placenta maintains the corpus luteum after LH secretion decreases, supporting continued secretion of estrogen and progesterone, and preventing menstruation. Human chorionic gonadotropin has no known effect on fat mobilization, appetite or sense of hunger, or body-fat distribution.

➤*Pharmacokinetics:*

Absorption/Distribution – Following IM injection, a detectable rise in serum hCG levels is seen in 2 hours; peak levels are reached in 6 hours and remain at this level for 36 hours. Human chorionic gonadotropin levels begin to decline at 48 hours and approach baseline (undetectable) levels at 72 hours.

Contraindications

Precocious puberty; prostatic carcinoma or other androgen-dependent neoplasia; prior allergic reaction to chorionic gonadotropin.

Warnings

➤*Administration:* Human chorionic gonadotropin should be used in conjunction with human menopausal gonadotropins only by physicians experienced with infertility problems who are familiar with the criteria for patient selection and the contraindications, warnings, precautions, and adverse reactions described in the monograph for menotropins. The principal serious adverse reactions during this use are as follows: Ovarian hyperstimulation, a syndrome of sudden ovarian enlargement; ascites with or without pain, or pleural effusion; enlargement of preexisting ovarian cysts or rupture of ovarian cysts with resultant hemoperitonum; multiple births; and arterial thromboembolism.

➤*Benzyl alcohol:* The diluent used for reconstitution contains benzyl alcohol. Benzyl alcohol has been reported to be associated with a fatal "gasping syndrome" in premature infants.

➤*Carcinogenesis:* There have been sporadic reports of testicular tumors in otherwise healthy young men receiving hCG for secondary infertility. A causative relationship between hCG and tumor development in these men has not been established. There have been rare reports of ovarian malignancy (where information is available, the reports indicate that the malignancies were diagnosed subsequent to multiple-drug regimens utilized for ovulation induction).

➤*Mutagenesis:* Defects of forelimbs and of the CNS, as well as alterations in sex ratio, have been reported in mice on combined gonadotropin and hCG regimens. The dose of gonadotropins used was intended to induce superovulation. No mutagenic effect has been clearly established in humans.

➤*Pregnancy: Category X.* Human chorionic gonadotropin is contraindicated in pregnant women. Combined hCG/PMS therapy has been noted to induce high incidences of external congenital anomalies in the offspring of mice, in a dose-dependent manner. The potential extrapolation to humans has not been determined.

Chorionic gonadotropin may cause fetal harm when administered to a pregnant woman. Defects of forelimbs and central nervous system and alterations in sex ratio have been reported in mice receiving combined gonadotropin and chorionic gonadotropin therapy in dosages to induce superovulation. Multiple ovulations with resulting plural gestations (mostly twins) have been reported to occur in approximately 20% of pregnancies when conception has followed chorionic gonadotropin therapy.

➤*Lactation:* It is not known whether chorionic gonadotropin is excreted in human milk. Because many drugs are excreted in human milk, caution should be exercised when hCG is administered to a nursing woman.

➤*Children:* Safety and efficacy in pediatric patients younger than 4 years of age have not been established.

The diluent used for reconstitution contains benzyl alcohol. Benzyl alcohol has been reported to be associated with a fatal "gasping syndrome" in premature infants.

Precautions

➤*Monitoring:* In adult males and females, the following hormone levels may be monitored depending on the nature of the diagnostic and therapeutic purpose: Testosterone, dihydrotestosterone, 17β-estradiol, 17β-hydroxyprogesterone, progesterone, androstenedione. In prepubertal males, testosterone and dihydrotestosterone should be followed.

Induction of androgen secretion by hCG may induce precocious puberty in patients treated for cryptorchidism. Therapy should be discontinued if signs of precocious puberty occur.

➤*Special risk:* Since androgens may cause fluid retention, chorionic gonadotropin should be used with caution in patients with epilepsy, migraine, asthma, cardiac or renal disease.

Drug Interactions

➤*Drug/Lab test interactions:* Human chorionic gonadotropin can cross-react in the radio-immunoassay of gonadotropins, especially LH. Each individual laboratory should establish the degree of cross-reactivity with their gonadotropin assay. Physicians should make the laboratory aware of patients on hCG if gonadotropin levels are requested.

Adverse Reactions

➤*Cardiovascular:* Arterial thromboembolism.

➤*CNS:* Headache; irritability; restlessness; depression; fatigue; aggressive behavior.

➤*GU:* Precocious puberty; gynecomastia; ovarian hyperstimulation syndrome; enlargement of preexisting ovarian cysts and possible rupture; phallic or testicular enlargement; growth of pubic hair; signs or symptoms of androgen excess. There have been rare reports of ovarian malignancy

➤*Hypersensitivity:* Hypersensitivity reactions both localized and systemic in nature, including erythema, urticaria, rash, angioedema, dyspnea, and shortness of breath, have been reported. The relationship of these allergic-like events to the polypeptide hormone or the diluent containing benzyl alcohol is not clear.

HUMAN CHORIONIC GONADOTROPIN — INJECTION

➤*Local:* Pain at the site of injection.

➤*Miscellaneous:* Edema.

Overdosage

➤*Symptoms:* There is no experience to date with deliberate overdosage of chorionic gonadotropin.

➤*Treatment:* Treatment must be symptomatic and supportive.

CHORIOGONADOTROPIN ALFA

Rx	**Ovidrel** (Serono)	**Injection:** 250 mcg/0.5 mL	28.1 mg mannitol, 505 mcg 85% O-phosphoric acid. In single-dose prefilled syringes.

CHORIOGONADOTROPIN ALFA — INJECTION

Indications

➤*Final follicular maturation:* Choriogonadotropin alfa for injection is indicated for the induction of final follicular maturation and early luteinization in infertile women who have undergone pituitary desensitization and who have been appropriately pretreated with follicle-stimulating hormones (FSH) as part of an assisted reproductive technology (ART) program such as in vitro fertilization and embryo transfer.

➤*Ovulation induction:* Choriogonadotropin alfa is also indicated for the induction of ovulation (OI) and pregnancy in anovulatory infertile patients in whom the cause of infertility is functional and not caused by primary ovarian failure.

Administration and Dosage

➤*Approved by the FDA:* September 22, 2000.

For subcutaneous use only.

➤*Infertile women undergoing ART:* Administer choriogonadotropin alfa 250 mcg 1 day following the last dose of the follicle-stimulating agent. Do not administer choriogonadotropin alfa until adequate follicular development is indicated by serum estradiol and vaginal ultrasonography. Withhold administration in situations where there is an excessive ovarian response, as evidenced by clinically significant ovarian enlargement or excessive estradiol production.

➤*Infertile women undergoing OI:* Do not administer choriogonadotropin alfa until adequate follicular development is indicated by serum estradiol and vaginal ultrasonography.

Administer choriogonadotropin alfa 250 mcg 1 day following the last dose of the follicle-stimulating agent.

Withhold choriogonadotropin alfa administration in situations where there is an excessive ovarian response, as evidenced by multiple follicular development, clinically significant ovarian enlargement, or excessive estradiol production.

➤*Administration of choriogonadotropin alfa:* Choriogonadotropin alfa is intended for a single subcutaneous injection and should be administered following reconstitution with 1 mL of sterile water for injection. Any unused reconstituted material should be discarded.

Choriogonadotropin alfa may be self-administered by the patient. Follow the directions below for reconstituting (mixing) and injecting choriogonadotropin alfa.

➤*Reconstitution and administration directions for choriogonadotropin alfa:*

1.) Wash hands thoroughly with soap and water. Using thumbs, remove the plastic flip-tops from both vials. After removing the plastic flip-tops, wipe the rubber stoppers with alcohol. The rubber stoppers should not be touched after they are wiped.
2.) Store and clean up. The injection materials must be kept sterile and cannot be reused.

➤*Storage/Stability:* Vials may be stored refrigerated or at room temperature 2° to 25°C (36° to 77°F). Protect from light.

Store in original package. Use immediately after reconstitution. Discard unused material.

Prefilled syringe – The choriogonadotropin alfa prefilled syringe must be stored at 2° to 8°C (36° to 46°F) before being dispensed to the patient. Patient may store the prefilled syringe at no more than 25°C (77°F) for up to 30 days prior to administration. Protect from light.

Actions

➤*Pharmacology:* The physicochemical, immunological, and biological activities of r-hCG are comparable with those of placental and human pregnancy u-hCG. Choriogonadotropin alfa stimulates late follicular maturation and resumption of oocyte meiosis, and initiates rupture of the preovulatory ovarian follicle. Choriogonadotropin alfa, the active component of choriogonadotropin alfa, is an analogue of LH and binds to the LH/hCG receptor of the granulosa and theca cells of the ovary to effect these changes in the absence of an endogenous LH surge. In pregnancy, hCG, secreted by the placenta, maintains the viability of the corpus luteum to provide the continued secretion of estrogen and progesterone necessary to support the first trimester of pregnancy. Choriogonadotropin alfa is administered when monitoring of the patient indicates that sufficient follicular development has occurred in response to FSH treatment for ovulation induction.

In women on oral contraception after an initial latency period, choriogonadotropin alfa induced a clear increase in androstenedione serum levels by 24 hours after dosing. Pharmacodynamic studies in females determined that the relationship of choriogonadotropin alfa pharmacokinetics to pharmacologic effect of choriogonadotropin alfa are complex and vary with the pharmacodynamic marker examined. In general, pharmacologic effects are not proportional to exposure and in some cases appear to be near maximal at a 250 mcg dose.

➤*Pharmacokinetics:*

Absorption – When given by intravenous (IV) administration, the pharmacokinetic profile of choriogonadotropin alfa followed a biexponential model and was linear over a range of 25 mcg to 1,000 mcg. Pharmacokinetic parameter estimates following subcutaneous administration of choriogonadotropin alfa 250 mcg to women are presented below:

In the following information, C_{max} is the peak concentration (above baseline), T_{max} is the time of C_{max}, AUC is the total area under the curve, $t_{1/2}$ is the elimination half-life, and F is bioavailability.

Pharmacokinetic Parameters (Mean ± SD) of r-hCG After Single-dose Administration of Choriogonadotropin Alfa in Healthy Women

	Choriogonadotropin alfa 250 mcg subcutaneous
C_{max} (units/L)	121 ± 44
T_{max} (h)[a]	24 (12 to 24)
AUC (h•IU/L)	7,701 ± 2,101
$T_{1/2}$ (h)	29 ± 6
F	0.4 ± 0.1

[a] Median (range).

Following subcutaneous administration of choriogonadotropin alfa 250 mcg, maximum serum concentration (121 ± 44 units/L) is reached after approximately 12 to 24 hours. The mean absolute bioavailability of choriogonadotropin alfa following a single subcutaneous injection to healthy female volunteers is approximately 40%.

Distribution – Following IV administration of choriogonadotropin alfa 250 mcg to healthy down-regulated women, the serum profile of hCG is described by a 2-compartment model with an initial half-life of 4.5 ± 0.5 hours. The volume of the central compartment is 3 ± 0.5 L and the steady state volume of distribution is 5.9 ± 1 L.

Metabolism/Excretion – Following subcutaneous administration of choriogonadotropin alfa, hCG is eliminated from the body with a mean terminal half-life of approximately 29 ± 6 hours. After IV administration of choriogonadotropin alfa 250 mcg to healthy down-regulated women, the mean terminal half-life is 26.5 ± 2.5 hours, and the total body clearance is 0.29 ± 0.04 L/hr. One-tenth of the dose is excreted in the urine.

Prefilled syringe –

Bioequivalence of formulations: Choriogonadotropin alfa prefilled syringe has been determined to be bioequivalent to choriogonadotropin alfa for injection based on the statistical evaluation of AUC and C_{max}. A summary of the choriogonadotropin alfa prefilled syringe pharmacokinetic parameters is presented in the following table.

Summary of Choriogonadotropin Alfa Prefilled Syringe Pharmacokinetic Parameters

Parameter	C_{max} (milliunits/mL)	AUC_{last} (milliunits•h/mL)	AUC (milliunits•h/mL)	$AUC_{extrapolated}$ (%)	T_{max} (h)
Mean (min-max)	125 (68-294)	10,050 (5,646-14,850)	10,350 (5,800-15,100)	2.85 (1.08-6.27)	20 (9-48)

Contraindications

Choriogonadotropin alfa for injection is contraindicated in women who exhibit any of the following: prior hypersensitivity to hCG preparations or one of their excipients, primary ovarian failure, uncontrolled thyroid or adrenal dysfunction, an uncontrolled organic intracranial lesion such as a pituitary tumor, abnormal uterine bleeding of undetermined origin, ovarian cyst or enlargement of undetermined origin, sex hormone-dependent tumors of the reproductive tract and accessory organs, pregnancy.

Warnings

➤*Administration:* Gonadotropins, including choriogonadotropin alfa, should only be used by health care providers who are thoroughly familiar with infertility problems and their management. Like other hCG products, choriogonadotropin alfa is a potent gonadotropic substance capable of causing ovarian hyperstimulation syndrome in women with or without pulmonary or vascular complications. Gonadotropin therapy requires a certain time commitment by health care providers, and requires the availability of appropriate monitoring facilities. Safe and effective induction of ovulation

CHORIOGONADOTROPIN ALFA — INJECTION

and use of choriogonadotropin alfa in women requires monitoring of ovarian response with serum estradiol and transvaginal ultrasound on a regular basis.

➤*Overstimulation of the ovary following hCG therapy:*

Ovarian enlargement – Mild to moderate uncomplicated ovarian enlargement which may be accompanied by abdominal distention or abdominal pain may occur in patients treated with FSH and hCG, and generally regresses without treatment within 2 or 3 weeks. Careful monitoring of ovarian response can further minimize the risk of overstimulation.

If the ovaries are abnormally enlarged on the last day of FSH therapy, do not administer choriogonadotropin alfa in this course of therapy. This will reduce the risk of development of ovarian hyperstimulation syndrome.

Ovarian hyperstimulation syndrome – Ovarian hyperstimulation syndrome is a medical event distinct from uncomplicated ovarian enlargement. Severe ovarian hyperstimulation syndrome may progress rapidly (within 24 hours to several days) to become a serious medical event. It is characterized by an apparent dramatic increase in vascular permeability which can result in a rapid accumulation of fluid in the peritoneal cavity, thorax, and potentially, the pericardium. The early warning signs of development of ovarian hyperstimulation syndrome are severe pelvic pain, nausea, vomiting, and weight gain. The following symptomatology has been seen with cases of ovarian hyperstimulation syndrome: abdominal pain, abdominal distension, GI symptoms including nausea, vomiting and diarrhea, severe ovarian enlargement, weight gain, dyspnea, and oliguria. Clinical evaluation may reveal hypovolemia, hemoconcentration, electrolyte imbalances, ascites, hemoperitoneum, pleural effusions, hydrothorax, acute pulmonary distress, and thromboembolic events. Transient liver function test abnormalities suggestive of hepatic dysfunction, which may be accompanied by morphologic changes on liver biopsy, have been reported in association with ovarian hyperstimulation syndrome.

Ovarian hyperstimulation syndrome occurred in 4 of 236 (1.7%) patients treated with choriogonadotropin alfa 250 mcg during clinical trials for ART and 3 of 99 (3%) patients treated in the OI trial. ovarian hyperstimulation syndrome occurred in 8 of 89 (9%) patients who received choriogonadotropin alfa 500 mcg. Two patients treated with choriogonadotropin alfa 500 mcg developed severe ovarian hyperstimulation syndrome.

Ovarian hyperstimulation syndrome may be more severe and more protracted if pregnancy occurs. Ovarian hyperstimulation syndrome develops rapidly; therefore, patients should be followed for at least 2 weeks after hCG administration. Most often, ovarian hyperstimulation syndrome occurs after treatment has been discontinued and reaches its maximum at about 7 to 10 days following treatment. Usually, ovarian hyperstimulation syndrome resolves spontaneously with the onset of menses. If there is evidence that ovarian hyperstimulation syndrome may be developing prior to hCG administration, the hCG must be withheld.

If severe ovarian hyperstimulation syndrome occurs, stop treatment with gonadotropins and hospitalize the patient.

Consult a health care provider experienced in the management of this syndrome, or who is experienced in the management of fluid and electrolyte imbalances should be consulted.

➤*Multiple births:* As with other hCG products, reports of multiple births have been associated with choriogonadotropin alfa treatment. In ART, the risk of multiple births correlates to the number of embryos transferred. Multiple births occurred in 17 of 55 live deliveries (30.9%) experienced by women receiving choriogonadotropin alfa 250 mcg in the ART studies. In the ovulation induction clinical trial, 2 of 15 live deliveries (13.3%) were associated with multiple births in women receiving choriogonadotropin alfa. Advise the patient of the potential risk of multiple births before starting treatment.

➤*Pulmonary and vascular complications:* As with other hCG products, a potential for the occurrence of arterial thromboembolism exists.

➤*Pregnancy: Category X.* Fetal death and impaired parturition were observed in pregnant rats given a dose of choriogonadotropin alfa (25 mcg/day) equivalent to 6 times the maximum human dose of 250 mcg based on body surface area or for prefilled syringe of choriogonadotropin alfa: u-hCG (500 units) equivalent to 3 times the maximum human dose of 10,000 USP, based on body surface area.

➤*Lactation:* It is not known whether this drug is excreted in human milk. Because many drugs are excreted in human milk, exercise caution if hCG is administered to a breast-feeding woman.

➤*Children:* Safety and efficacy in children have not been established.

Precautions

➤*Monitoring:* Careful attention should be given to the diagnosis of infertility in candidates for hCG therapy.

➤*Lab test abnormalities:* After the exclusion of preexisting conditions, elevations in ALT were found in 10 (3%) of 335 patients receiving choriogonadotropin alfa 250 mcg, 9 (10%) of 89 patients receiving choriogonadotropin alfa 500 mcg, and in 16 (4.8%) of 328 patients receiving u-hCG. The elevations ranged up to 1.2 times the upper limit of normal. The clinical significance of these findings is not known.

In most instances, treatment of women with FSH results only in follicular recruitment and development. In the absence of an endogenous LH surge, hCG is given when monitoring of the patient indicates that sufficient follicular development has occurred. This may be estimated by ultrasound alone or in combination with measurement of serum estradiol levels. The combination of both ultrasound and serum estradiol measurement are useful for monitoring the development of follicles, timing of the ovulatory trigger, as well as detecting ovarian enlargement and minimizing the risk of the ovarian hyperstimulation syndrome and multiple gestation. It is recommended that the number of growing follicles be confirmed using ultrasonography because serum estrogens do not give an indication of the size or number of follicles.

Human chorionic gonadotropins can crossreact in the radioimmunoassay of gonadotropins, especially luteinizing hormone. Each individual laboratory should establish the degree of crossreactivity with their gonadotropin assay. Make the laboratory aware of patients on hCG if gonadotropin levels are requested.

The clinical confirmation of ovulation, with the exception of pregnancy, is obtained by direct and indirect indices of progesterone production. The indices most generally used are as follows: a rise in basal body temperature, increase in serum progesterone, menstruation following a shift in basal body temperature.

When used in conjunction with the indices of progesterone production, sonographic visualization of the ovaries will assist in determining if ovulation has occurred. Sonographic evidence of ovulation may include the following: fluid in the cul-de-sac, ovarian stigmata, collapsed follicle, secretory endometrium.

Accurate interpretation of the indices of ovulation require a health care provider who is experienced in the interpretation of these tests.

Drug Interactions

No drug-drug interaction studies have been conducted.

➤*Drug/Lab test interactions:* Administration of choriogonadotropin alfa may interfere with the interpretation of pregnancy tests.

Adverse Reactions

The safety of choriogonadotropin alfa was examined in 4 clinical studies that treated 752 patients, of whom 335 received choriogonadotropin alfa 250 mcg following follicular recruitment with gonadotropins. When patients enrolled in 4 clinical studies (3 in ART and 1 in OI) were injected subcutaneously with either choriogonadotropin alfa or an approved u-hCG, 14.6 % (49 of 335 patients) in the choriogonadotropin alfa 250 mcg group experienced application site disorders, compared to 28% (92 of 328 patients) in the approved u-hCG group. Adverse reactions reported for choriogonadotropin alfa 250 mcg occurring in at least 2% of patients (regardless of causality) are listed in the following tables. The first table shows the 3 ART studies, and the second table shows the single OI study.

Incidence of Adverse Reactions of r-hCG in ART (Studies 7648, 7927, 9073)

Body system (preferred term)	Choriogonadotropin alfa 250 mcg (n = 236); incidence rate, % (n)
At least 1 adverse reaction	33.1% (78)
Abdominal pain	4.2% (10)
Application site disorders	14% (33)
Injection site bruising	4.7% (11)
Injection site pain	7.6% (18)
GI system disorders	8.5% (20)
Nausea	3.4% (8)
Postoperative pain	4.7% (11)
Secondary terms (postoperative pain)	4.7% (11)
Vomiting	2.5% (6)

Adverse reactions not listed in the above table that occurred in less than 2% of patients treated with choriogonadotropin alfa 250 mcg whether or not considered causally related to choriogonadotropin alfa, included the following: injection site inflammation and reaction; flatulence; diarrhea; hiccup; ectopic pregnancy; breast pain; intermenstrual bleeding; vaginal hemorrhage; cervical lesion; leukorrhea; ovarian hyperstimulation; uterine disorders; vaginitis; vaginal discomfort; body pain; back pain; fever; dizziness; headache; hot flashes; malaise; paresthesias; rash; emotional lability; insomnia; upper respiratory tract infection; cough; dysuria; urinary tract infection; urinary incontinence; albuminuria; cardiac arrhythmia; genital moniliasis; genital herpes; leukocytosis; heart murmur; cervical carcinoma.

Incidence of Adverse Reactions of r-hCG in Ovulation Induction (Study 8209)

Body system (preferred term)	Choriogonadotropin alfa 250 mcg (n = 236); incidence rate, % (n)
At least 1 adverse event	26.2% (26)
Abdominal pain	3% (3)
Application site disorders	16.2% (16)
GI system disorders	4% (4)
Injection site bruising	3% (3)
Injection site inflammation	2% (2)
Injection site pain	8.1% (8)
Injection site reaction	3% (3)
Ovarian cyst	3% (3)
Ovarian hyperstimulation	3% (3)

CHORIOGONADOTROPIN ALFA — INJECTION

Incidence of Adverse Reactions of r-hCG in Ovulation Induction (Study 8209)	
Body system (preferred term)	Choriogonadotropin alfa 250 mcg (n = 236); incidence rate, % (n)
Reproductive disorders, female	7.1% (7)

Additional adverse reactions not listed in the preceding table that occurred in less than 2% of patients treated with choriogonadotropin alfa 250 mcg, whether or not considered causally related to choriogonadotropin alfa, included the following: breast pain; flatulence; abdominal enlargement; pharyngitis; upper respiratory tract infection; hyperglycemia; pruritus.

The following medical events have been reported subsequent to pregnancies resulting from hCG therapy in controlled clinical studies: spontaneous abortion; ectopic pregnancy; premature labor; postpartum fever; congenital abnormalities.

Of 125 clinical pregnancies reported following treatment with FSH and choriogonadotropin alfa 250 or 500 mcg, 3 were associated with a congenital anomaly of the fetus or newborn. Among patients receiving choriogonadotropin alfa 250 mcg, cranial malformation was detected in the fetus of 1 woman and a chromosomal abnormality (47, XXX) in another. These events were judged by the investigators to be of unlikely or unknown relation to treatment. These 3 events represent an incidence of major congenital malformations of 2.4%, which is consistent with the reported rate for pregnancies resulting from natural or assisted conception. In a woman who received choriogonadotropin alfa 500 mcg, 1 birth in a set of triplets was associated with Down syndrome and atrial septal defect. This event was considered to be unrelated to the study drug.

The following adverse reactions have been previously reported during menotropin therapy: pulmonary and vascular complications; adnexal torsion (as a complication of ovarian enlargement); mild to moderate ovarian enlargement; hemoperitoneum.

There have been infrequent reports of ovarian neoplasms, both benign and malignant, in women who have undergone multiple drug regimens for ovulation induction; however, a causal relationship has not been established.

Patient Information

Prior to therapy with hCG, inform patients of the duration of treatment and monitoring of their condition that will be required. Also discuss the risks of ovarian hyperstimulation syndrome and multiple births in women and other possible adverse reactions.

NAFARELIN ACETATE

Rx	**Synarel** (Syntex)	**Nasal Solution:** 2 mg/mL (as nafarelin base)	In 10 mL bottle with metered spray pump (delivers approximately 200 mcg/spray).[a]

[a] With benzalkonium chloride, glacial acetic acid and sorbitol.

NAFARELIN ACETATE — NASAL

Indications

➤*Endometriosis:* Nafarelin acetate is indicated for management of endometriosis, including pain relief and reduction of endometriotic lesions. Experience with nafarelin acetate for the management of endometriosis has been limited to women 18 years of age and older treated for 6 months.

➤*Central precocious puberty:* Nafarelin acetate is indicated for treatment of central precocious puberty (CPP) (gonadotropin-dependent precocious puberty) in children of both sexes.

Administration and Dosage

➤*Approved by the FDA:* 1990.

➤*Endometriosis:* For the management of endometriosis, the recommended daily dose of nafarelin acetate is 400 mcg. This is achieved by one spray (200 mcg) into one nostril in the morning and one spray into the other nostril in the evening. Treatment should be started between days 2 and 4 of the menstrual cycle.

In an occasional patient, the 400 mcg daily dose may not produce amenorrhea. For these patients with persistent regular menstruation after 2 months of treatment, the dose of nafarelin acetate may be increased to 800 µg daily. The 800 mcg dose is administered as one spray into each nostril in the morning (a total of 2 sprays) and again in the evening.

The recommended duration of administration is 6 months. Retreatment cannot be recommended since safety data for retreatment are not available. If the symptoms of endometriosis recur after a course of therapy, and further treatment with nafarelin acetate is contemplated, it is recommended that bone density be assessed before retreatment begins to ensure that values are within normal limits.

There appeared to be no significant effect of rhinitis, ie, nasal congestion, on the systemic bioavailability of nafarelin acetate; however, if the use of a nasal decongestant for rhinitis is necessary during treatment with nafarelin acetate, the decongestant should not be used until at least 2 hours following dosing with nafarelin acetate.

Sneezing during or immediately after dosing with nafarelin acetate should be avoided, if possible, since this may impair drug absorption.

At 400 mcg/day, a bottle of nafarelin acetate provides a 30-day (about 60 sprays) supply. If the daily dose is increased, increase the supply to the patient to ensure uninterrupted treatment for the recommended duration of therapy.

➤*Central Precocious Puberty:* For the treatment of central precocious puberty (CPP), the recommended daily dose of nafarelin acetate is 1,600 mcg. The dose can be increased to 1,800 mcg daily if adequate suppression cannot be achieved at 1,600 mcg/day.

The 1,600 mcg dose is achieved by 2 sprays (400 mcg) into each nostril in the morning (4 sprays) and 2 sprays into each nostril in the evening (4 sprays), a total of 8 sprays daily. The 1,800 mcg dose is achieved by 3 sprays (600 mcg) into alternating nostrils 3 times a day, a total of 9 sprays per day. The patient's head should be tilted back slightly, and 30 seconds should elapse between sprays.

If the prescribed therapy has been well tolerated by the patient, treatment of CPP with nafarelin acetate should continue until resumption of puberty is desired.

There appeared to be no significant effect of rhinitis, ie, nasal congestion, on the systemic bioavailability of nafarelin acetate; however, if the use of a nasal decongestant for rhinitis is necessary during treatment with nafarelin acetate, the decongestant should not be used until at least 2 hours following dosing with nafarelin acetate.

Sneezing during or immediately after dosing with nafarelin acetate should be avoided, if possible, since this may impair drug absorption.

At 1,600 mcg daily, a bottle of nafarelin acetate provides about a 7-day supply (about 56 sprays). If the daily dose is increased, increase the supply to the patient to ensure uninterrupted treatment for the duration of therapy.

➤*Storage/Stability:* Store upright at 25°C (77°F); excursions permitted to 15° to 30°C (59° to 86°F). [See USP Controlled Room Temperature]. Protect from light.

Actions

➤*Pharmacology:* Nafarelin acetate is a potent agonistic analog of gonadotropin-releasing hormone (GnRH). At the onset of administration, nafarelin stimulates the release of the pituitary gonadotropins, LH and FSH, resulting in a temporary increase of ovarian steroidogenesis. Repeated dosing abolishes the stimulatory effect on the pituitary gland. Twice-daily administration leads to decreased secretion of gonadal steroids by about 4 weeks; consequently, tissues and functions that depend on gonadal steroids for their maintenance become quiescent.

Contraindications

Hypersensitivity to GnRH, GnRH agonist analogs or any of the excipients in nafarelin acetate; undiagnosed abnormal vaginal bleeding; use in women who are breast feeding (see Lactation); use in pregnancy or in women who may become pregnant while receiving the drug.

Warnings

➤*Central Precocious Puberty:* The diagnosis of central precocious puberty (CPP) must be established before treatment is initiated. Regular monitoring of CPP patients is needed to assess both patient response as well as compliance. This is particularly important during the first 6 to 8 weeks of treatment to assure that suppression of pituitary-gonadal function is rapid. Testing may include LH response to GnRH stimulation and circulating gonadal sex steroid levels. Assessment of growth velocity and bone age velocity should begin within 3 to 6 months of treatment initiation.

Some patients may not show suppression of the pituitary-gonadal axis by clinical and/or biochemical parameters. This may be due to lack of compliance with the recommended treatment regimen and may be rectified by recommending that the dosing be done by caregivers. If compliance problems are excluded, the possibility of gonadotropin independent sexual precocity should be reconsidered and appropriate examinations should be conducted. If compliance problems are excluded and if gonadotropin independent sexual precocity is not present, the dose of nafarelin acetate may be increased to 1800 mcg/day administered as 600 mcg 3 times daily.

➤*Carcinogenesis:* Carcinogenicity studies of nafarelin were conducted in rats (24 months) at doses up to 100 mcg/kg/day and mice (18 months) at doses up to 500 mcg/kg/day using intramuscular doses (up to 110 times and 560 times the maximum recommended human intranasal dose, respectively). These multiples of the human dose are based on the relative bioavailability of the drug by the two routes of administration. As seen with other GnRH agonists, nafarelin acetate given to laboratory rodents at high doses for prolonged periods induced proliferative responses (hyperplasia and/or neoplasia) of endocrine organs. At 24 months, there was an increase in the incidence of pituitary tumors (adenoma/carcinoma) in high-dose female rats and a dose-related increase in male rats. There was an increase in pancreatic islet cell adenomas in both sexes, and in benign testicular and ovarian tumors in the treated groups. There was a dose-related increase in benign adrenal medullary tumors in treated female rats. In mice, there was a dose-related increase in Harderian gland tumors in males and an increase in pituitary adenomas in high-dose females. No metastases of these tumors

NAFARELIN ACETATE — NASAL

were observed. It is known that tumorigenicity in rodents is particularly sensitive to hormonal stimulation.

➤*Fertility impairment:* Reproduction studies in male and female rats have shown full reversibility of fertility suppression when drug treatment was discontinued after continuous administration for up to 6 months. The effect of treatment of prepubertal rats on the subsequent reproductive performance of mature animals has not been investigated.

➤*Pregnancy: Category X.* Safe use of nafarelin acetate in pregnancy has not been established clinically. Before starting treatment with nafarelin acetate, pregnancy must be excluded.

When used regularly at the recommended dose, nafarelin acetate usually inhibits ovulation and stops menstruation. Contraception is not insured, however, by taking nafarelin acetate, particularly if patients miss successive doses. Therefore, patients should use nonhormonal methods of contraception. Patients should be advised to see their physician if they believe they may be pregnant. If a patient becomes pregnant during treatment, the drug must be discontinued and the patient must be apprised of the potential risk to the fetus.

Teratogenic – (See Contraindications.) Intramuscular nafarelin acetate was administered to rats during the period of organogenesis at 0.4, 1.6, and 6.4 mcg/kg/day (about 0.5, 2, and 7 times the maximum recommended human intranasal dose based on the relative bioavailability by the two routes of administration). An increase in major fetal abnormalities was observed in 4/80 fetuses at the highest dose. A similar, repeat study at the same doses in rats and studies in mice and rabbits at doses up to 600 mcg/kg/day and 0.18 mcg/kg/day, respectively, failed to demonstrate an increase in fetal abnormalities after administration during the period of organogenesis. In rats and rabbits, there was a dose-related increase in fetal mortality and a decrease in fetal weight with the highest dose.

➤*Lactation:* It is not known whether nafarelin acetate is excreted in human milk. Because many drugs are excreted in human milk, and because the effects of nafarelin acetate on lactation and/or the breastfed child have not been determined, nafarelin acetate should not be used by nursing mothers.

➤*Children:* Safety and efficacy of nafarelin acetate for endometriosis in patients younger than 18 years of age have not been established.

Precautions

➤*Ovarian cysts:* As with other drugs that stimulate the release of gonadotropins or that induce ovulation, ovarian cysts have been reported to occur in the first two months of therapy with nafarelin acetate. Many, but not all, of these events occurred in patients with polycystic ovarian disease. These cystic enlargements may resolve spontaneously, generally by about 4 to 6 weeks of therapy, but in some cases may require discontinuation of drug and/or surgical intervention. The relevance, if any, of such events in children is unknown.

Drug Interactions

No pharmacokinetic-based drug-drug interaction studies have been conducted with nafarelin acetate. However, because nafarelin acetate is a peptide that is primarily degraded by peptidase and not by cytochrome P-450 enzymes, and the drug is only about 80% bound to plasma proteins at 4°C (39.2°F), drug interactions would not be expected to occur.

➤*Drug/Lab test interactions:* Administration of nafarelin acetate in therapeutic doses results in suppression of the pituitary-gonadal system. Normal function is usually restored within 4 to 8 weeks after treatment is discontinued. Therefore, diagnostic tests of pituitary gonadotropic and gonadal functions conducted during treatment and up to 4 to 8 weeks after discontinuation of therapy with nafarelin acetate may be misleading.

Adverse Reactions

➤*Endometriosis:* In formal clinical trials of 1,509 healthy adult patients, symptoms suggestive of drug sensitivity, such as shortness of breath, chest pain, urticaria, rash and pruritus occurred in 3 patients (approximately 0.2%).

As would be expected with a drug which lowers serum estradiol levels, the most frequently reported adverse reactions were those related to hypoestrogenism.

In addition, less than 1% of patients experienced paresthesia, palpitations, chloasma, maculopapular rash, eye pain, asthenia, lactation, breast engorgement, and arthralgia.

Lab test abnormalities –

Plasma enzymes: During clinical trials with nafarelin acetate, regular laboratory monitoring revealed that APT and AST levels were more than twice the upper limit of normal in only one patient each. There was no other clinical or laboratory evidence of abnormal liver function and levels returned to normal in both patients after treatment was stopped.

Lipids: At enrollment, 9% of the patients in the group taking nafarelin acetate 400 mcg/day and 2% of the patients in the danazol group had total cholesterol values above 250 mg/dL. These patients also had cholesterol values above 250 mg/dL at the end of treatment.

Of those patients whose pretreatment cholesterol values were below 250 mg/dL, 6% in the group treated with nafarelin acetate and 18% in the danazol group, had post-treatment values above 250 mg/dL.

The mean (± SEM) pretreatment values for total cholesterol from all patients were 191.8 (4.3) mg/dL in the group treated with nafarelin acetate and 193.1 (4.6) mg/dL in the danazol group. At the end of treatment, the mean values for total cholesterol from all patients were 204.5 (4.8) mg/dL in the group treated with nafarelin acetate and 207.7 (5.1) mg/dL in the danazol group. These increases from the pretreatment values were statistically significant (p less than 0.05) in both groups.

Triglycerides were increased above the upper limit of 150 mg/dL in 12% of the patients who received nafarelin acetate and in 7% of the patients who received danazol.

At the end of treatment, no patients receiving nafarelin acetate had abnormally low HDL cholesterol fractions (less than 30 mg/dL) compared with 43% of patients receiving danazol. None of the patients receiving nafarelin acetate had abnormally high LDL cholesterol fractions (greater than 190 mg/dL) compared with 15% of those receiving danazol. There was no increase in the LDL/HDL ratio in patients receiving nafarelin acetate, but there was approximately a 2-fold increase in the LDL/HDL ratio in patients receiving danazol.

Other changes: In comparative studies, the following changes were seen in ≈ 10% to 15% of patients. Treatment with nafarelin acetate was associated with elevations of plasma phosphorus and eosinophil counts, and decreases in serum calcium and WBC counts. Danazol therapy was associated with an increase of hematocrit and WBC.

Musculoskeletal –

Changes in bone density: After 6 months of treatment with nafarelin acetate, vertebral trabecular bone density and total vertebral bone mass, measured by quantitative computed tomography (QCT), decreased by an average of 8.7% and 4.3%, respectively, compared to pretreatment levels. There was partial recovery of bone density in the post-treatment period; the average trabecular bone density and total bone mass were 4.9% and 3.3% less than the pretreatment levels, respectively. Total vertebral bone mass, measured by dual photon absorptiometry (DPA), decreased by a mean of 5.9% at the end of treatment.

After six months treatment with nafarelin acetate, bone mass as measured by dual x-ray bone densitometry (DEXA), decreased 3.2%. Mean total vertebral mass, re-examined by DEXA six months after completion of treatment, was 1.4% below pretreatment. There was little, if any, decrease in the mineral content in compact bone of the distal radius and second metacarpal. Use of nafarelin acetate for longer than the recommended 6 months or in the presence of other known risk factors for decreased bone mineral content may cause additional bone loss.

➤*Central precocious puberty:* In clinical trials of 155 pediatric patients, 2.6% reported symptoms suggestive of drug sensitivity, such as shortness of breath, chest pain, urticaria, rash, and pruritus.

In these 155 patients treated for an average of 41 months and as long as 80 months (6.7 years), adverse events most frequently reported (more than 3% of patients) consisted largely of episodes occurring during the first 6 weeks of treatment as a result of the transient stimulatory action of nafarelin upon the pituitary-gonadal axis:

- acne (10%)
- transient breast enlargement (8%)
- vaginal bleeding (8%)
- emotional lability (6%)
- transient increase in pubic hair (5%)
- body odor (4%)
- seborrhea (3%)

Hot flashes, common in adult women treated for endometriosis, occurred in only 3% of treated children and were transient. Other adverse reactions thought to be drug-related, and occurring in more than 3% of patients were rhinitis (5%) and white or brownish vaginal discharge (3%). Approximately 3% of patients withdrew from clinical trials due to adverse events.

In one male patient with concomitant congenital adrenal hyperplasia, and who had discontinued treatment 8 months previously to resume puberty, adrenal rest tumors were found in the left testis. Relationship to nafarelin acetate is unlikely.

Regular examinations of the pituitary gland by magnetic resonance imaging (MRI) or computer assisted tomography (CT) of children during long-term nafarelin therapy as well as during the post-treatment period has occasionally revealed changes in the shape and size of the pituitary gland. These changes include asymmetry and enlargement of the pituitary gland, and a pituitary microadenoma has been suspected in a few children. The relationship of these findings to nafarelin acetate is not known.

Overdosage

In experimental animals, a single subcutaneous administration of up to 60 times the recommended human dose (on a mcg/kg basis, not adjusted for bioavailability) had no adverse effects. At present, there is no clinical evidence of adverse effects following overdosage of GnRH analogs.

Based on studies in monkeys, nafarelin acetate is not absorbed after oral administration.

Gonadotropin-Releasing Hormone Antagonists

GANIRELIX ACETATE

Rx	Ganirelix Acetate (Organon)	Injection: 250 mcg per 0.5 mL	In 1 mL prefilled, disposable syringes. In 1s.

GANIRELIX ACETATE — INJECTION

Indications

➤*Infertility treatment:* For the inhibition of premature luteinizing hormone (LH) surges in women undergoing controlled ovarian hyperstimulation.

Administration and Dosage

➤*Approved by the FDA:* July 29, 1999.

➤*Infertility treatment:* After initiating follicle-stimulating hormone (FSH) therapy on day 2 or 3 of the cycle, ganirelix 250 mcg may be administered subcutaneously once daily during the early-to-mid follicular phase. By taking advantage of endogenous pituitary FSH secretion, the requirement for exogenously administered FSH may be reduced. Continue treatment with ganirelix daily until the day of chorionic gonadotropin (hCG) administration. When a sufficient number of follicles of adequate size are present, as assessed by ultrasound, final maturation of follicles is induced by administering hCG. Withhold the administration of hCG in cases where the ovaries are abnormally enlarged on the last day of FSH therapy to reduce the chance of developing ovarian hyperstimulation syndrome (OHSS).

➤*Administration:* Ganirelix is intended for subcutaneous administration only. The most convenient sites for subcutaneous injection are in the abdomen around the navel or upper thigh. Swab the injection site with a disinfectant to remove any surface bacteria. Clean approximately 2 inches around the point where the needle will be inserted and let the disinfectant dry for at least 1 minute before proceeding. Pinch up a large area of skin between the finger and thumb. Vary the injection site a little with each injection. Insert the needle at the base of the pinched-up skin at an angle of 45° to 90° to the skin surface. When the needle is correctly positioned, it will be difficult to draw back on the plunger. If any blood is drawn into the syringe, the needle tip has penetrated a vein or artery. If this happens, withdraw the needle slightly and reposition the needle without removing it from the skin. Alternatively, remove the needle and use a new, sterile, prefilled syringe. Cover the injection site with a swab containing disinfectant and apply pressure; the site should stop bleeding within 1 or 2 minutes. Once the needle is correctly placed, depress the plunger slowly and steadily, so the solution is correctly injected and the skin is not damaged. Pull the syringe out quickly and apply pressure to the site with a swab containing disinfectant. Use the sterile, prefilled syringe only once and dispose of it properly.

➤*Storage/Stability:* Store at 25°C (77°F). Protect from light.

Actions

➤*Pharmacology:* Ganirelix is a synthetic decapeptide with high antagonistic activity against naturally occurring gonadotropin-releasing hormone (GnRH). Ganirelix is derived from native GnRH with substitutions of amino acids at positions 1, 2, 3, 6, 8, and 10.

The pulsatile release of GnRH stimulates the synthesis and secretion of LH and FSH. Ganirelix acts by competitively blocking the GnRH receptors on the pituitary gonadotroph and subsequent transduction pathway. It induces a rapid, reversible suppression of gonadotropin secretion. The suppression of pituitary LH secretion by ganirelix is more pronounced than that of FSH. An initial release of endogenous gonadotropins has not been detected with ganirelix, which is consistent with an antagonist effect. Upon discontinuation of ganirelix, pituitary LH and FSH levels are fully recovered within 48 hours.

➤*Pharmacokinetics:* The pharmacokinetic parameters of single and multiple injections of ganirelix in healthy adult females are summarized in the following table. Steady-state serum concentrations are reached after 3 days of treatment. The pharmacokinetics of ganirelix are dose-proportional in the dose range of 125 to 500 mcg.

Mean Pharmacokinetic Parameters of Ganirelix

Absorption	
Mean absolute bioavailability	91.1%[a]
C_{max}	14.8 ng/ml[a], 11.2 ng/ml[b]
T_{max}	1.1[a,b]
Distribution	
Vd	43.7 L[c], 76.5 L[b]
Protein binding	81.9%
Metabolism	
Metabolites	1 to 4 peptide and 1 to 6 peptide
Excretion	
Site	feces (75.1%)[d,e], urine (22.1%)[d,f]
Elimination t½	12.8 h[a], 16.2 h[b]
Clearance	2.4 L/h[c], 3.3[b]

[a] Based on single-dose administration of 250 mcg subcutaneously.
[b] Based on multiple-dose administration of 250 mcg daily subcutaneous × 7 days.
[c] Based on single-dose administration of 250 mcg IV.
[d] Recovered over 288 hours following single-dose administration of 1 mg IV.
[e] Fecal excretion plateaus 192 hours after dosing.
[f] Urinary excretion is complete in 24 hours.

Contraindications

Hypersensitivity to ganirelix, any of its components, GnRH, or any other GnRH analog; known or suspected pregnancy (see Warnings).

Warnings

➤*Latex allergy:* The packaging of this product contains natural rubber latex, which may cause allergic reactions.

➤*Hypersensitivity reactions:* Caution is advised in patients with hypersensitivity to GnRH. Carefully monitor these patients after the first injection. Refer to the Management of Acute Hypersensitivity Reactions. Anaphylactic reactions or ganirelix antibody formation have not been reported in clinical trials.

➤*Pregnancy: Category X.* Ganirelix is contraindicated in pregnant women. When administered from day 7 to near term to pregnant rats and rabbits at doses 10 and 30 mcg/day (approximately 0.4 to 3.2 times the human dose based on body surface area) or more, ganirelix increased the incidence of litter resorption. There was no increase in fetal abnormalities.

The effects on fetal resorption are logical consequences of the alteration in hormonal levels brought about by the antigonadotrophic properties of this drug and could result in fetal loss in humans. Therefore, do not use this drug in pregnant women.

Ganirelix should be prescribed by physicians who are experienced in infertility treatment. Before starting treatment with ganirelix, exclude pregnancy. Safe use of ganirelix during pregnancy has not been established.

Congenital anomalies – Ongoing clinical follow-up studies of 283 newborns of women administered ganirelix were reviewed. There were 3 neonates with major congenital anomalies and 18 neonates with minor congenital anomalies. The major congenital anomalies were the following: Hydrocephalus/Meningocele, omphalocele, and Beckwith-Wiedemann syndrome. The minor congenital anomalies were the following: Nevus, skin tags, sacral sinus, hemangioma, torticollis/asymmetric skull, talipes, supernumerary digit finger, hip subluxation, torticollis/high palate, occiput/abnormal hand crease, hernia unbilicalis, hernia inguinalis, hydrocele, undescended testes, and hydronephrosis. The causal relationship between these congenital anomalies and ganirelix is unknown. Multiple factors, genetic, and others (including, but not limited to intracystoplasmatic sperm injection [ICSI], in vitro fertilization [IVF], gonadotropins, progesterone) may confound assisted reproductive technology (ART) procedures.

➤*Lactation:* It is not known whether this drug is excreted in breast milk. Ganirelix should not be used by breast-feeding women.

Drug Interactions

➤*Gonadotropins:* Because ganirelix can suppress the secretion of pituitary gonadotropins, dose adjustments of exogenous gonadotropins may be necessary when used during controlled ovarian hyperstimulation.

Adverse Reactions

In clinical studies, treatment duration ranged from 1 to 14 days. The following table represents adverse events from the first day of ganirelix administration until confirmation of pregnancy by ultrasound at an incidence of at least 1% in ganirelix-treated subjects without regard to causality.

Ganirelix Adverse Reactions (at least 1%)

Adverse reaction	Ganirelix (n = 794) (%)
Abdominal pain (gynecological)	4.8
Death, fetal	3.7
Headache	3
Ovarian hyperstimulation syndrome	2.4
Vaginal bleeding	1.8
Injection site reaction	1.1
Nausea	1.1
Abdominal pain (GI)	1

➤*Lab test abnormalities:* A neutrophil count at least 8.3 (× 10^9/L) was noted in 11.9% (16.8 × 10^9/L or less) of all subjects in the clinical trials. In addition, downward shifts within the ganirelix group were observed for hematocrit and total bilirubin. The clinical significance of these findings was not determined.

Patient Information

Prior to therapy with ganirelix, inform patients of the duration of treatment and monitoring procedures that will be required. Discuss the risk of possible adverse reactions (see Adverse Reactions). Do not prescribe ganirelix if the patient is pregnant.

Gonadotropin-Releasing Hormone Antagonists

CETRORELIX ACETATE

Rx	**Cetrotide** (ASTA Medica)	**Injection**: 0.25 mg	In trays containing 1 vial of 0.26 to 0.27 mg cetrorelix acetate, 1 mL syringe of sterile water for injection, a 20-gauge needle, a 27-gauge needle, and alcohol swabs. In 1s and 7s.
		3 mg	In trays containing 1 vial of 3.12 to 3.24 mg cetrorelix acetate, a 3 mL syringe of sterile water for injection, a 20-gauge needle, a 27-gauge needle, and alcohol swabs. In 1s.

CETRORELIX ACETATE — INJECTION

Indications

➤*Infertility treatment:* Cetrorelix is indicated for the inhibition of premature luteinizing hormone (LH) surges in women undergoing controlled ovarian stimulation.

Administration and Dosage

➤*Approved by the FDA:* August 11, 2000.

➤*Dosage:* Start ovarian stimulation therapy with gonadotropins (follicle-stimulating hormone [FSH], human menopausal gonadotropin [HMG]) on cycle day 2 or 3. Adjust the dose of gonadotropins according to individual response. Cetrorelix may be administered subcutaneously once daily (0.25 mg dose) or once (3 mg dose) during the early- to midfollicular phase.

When assessment by ultrasound shows a sufficient number of follicles of adequate size, administer hCG to induce ovulation and final maturation of the oocytes. Administer hCG if the ovaries show an excessive response to the treatment with gonadotropins to reduce the chance of developing ovarian hyperstimulation syndrome (OHSS).

Single-dose regimen – In the single-dose regimen, administer cetrorelix 3 mg when the serum estradiol level is indicative of an appropriate stimulation response, usually on stimulation day 7 (range, day 5 to 9). If human chorionic gonadotropin (hCG) has not been administered within 4 days after injection of cetrorelix 3 mg, administer cetrorelix 0.25 mg once daily until the day of hCG administration.

Multiple-dose regimen – In the multiple-dose regimen, administer cetrorelix 0.25 mg on stimulation day 5 (morning or evening) or day 6 (morning) and continue daily until the day of hCG administration.

➤*Administration:* Cetrorelix 0.25 and 3 mg can be administered by the patient herself after appropriate instructions by her health care provider.

Directions for using cetrorelix 0.25 and 3 mg –

1.) Wash hands thoroughly with soap and water.
2.) Flip off the plastic cover of the vial and wipe the aluminum ring and the rubber stopper with an alcohol swab.
3.) Twist the injection needle with the yellow mark (20 gauge) on the prefilled syringe.
4.) Push the needle through the center of the rubber stopper of the vial and slowly inject the solvent into the vial.
5.) Leaving the syringe in the vial, gently swirl the vial until the solution is clear and without residues. Avoid forming bubbles.
6.) Draw the total contents of the vial into the syringe. If necessary, invert the vial and pull back the needle as far as needed to withdraw the entire contents of the vial.
7.) Replace the needle with the yellow mark by the injection needle with the grey mark (27 gauge).
8.) Invert the syringe and push the plunger until all air bubbles have been expelled.
9.) Choose an injection site in the lower abdominal area, preferably around, but staying at least 1 inch away from the navel. If you are on a multiple-dose (0.25 mg) regimen, choose a different injection site each day to minimize local irritation. Use the second alcohol swab to clean the skin at the injection site and allow alcohol to dry. Gently pinch up the skin surrounding the site of injection.
10.) Inject the prescribed dose as directed by your doctor.
11.) Use the syringe and needles only once. Dispose of the syringe and needles properly after use. If available, use a medical waste container for disposal.

➤*Storage/Stability:* Store cetrorelix in a cool, dry place protected from excess moisture and heat. Store 3 mg cetrorelix at 25°C (77°F). Excursions are permitted to 15° to 30°C (59° to 86°F). Store cetrorelix 0.25 mg in the refrigerator at 2° to 8°C (36° to 46°F). Keep the packaged tray in the outer carton in order to protect it from light.

Use immediately after preparation. Discard unused material.

Actions

➤*Pharmacology:* GnRH induces the production and release of LH and follicle-stimulating hormone (FSH) from the gonadotrophic cells of the anterior pituitary. Because of a positive estradiol (E_2) feedback at midcycle, GnRH liberation is enhanced, resulting in an LH surge. This LH surge induces the ovulation of the dominant follicle, resumption of oocyte meiosis and, subsequently, luteinization, as indicated by rising progesterone levels.

Cetrorelix competes with natural GnRH for binding to membrane receptors on pituitary cells and thus controls the release of LH and FSH in a dose-dependent manner. The onset of LH suppression is approximately 1 hour with the 3 mg dose and 2 hours with the 0.25 mg dose. This suppression is maintained by continuous treatment, and there is a more pronounced effect on LH than on FSH. An initial release of endogenous gonadotropins has not been detected with cetrorelix, which is consistent with an antagonist effect.

The effects of cetrorelix on LH and FSH are reversible after discontinuation of treatment. In women, cetrorelix delays the LH surge and, consequently, ovulation in a dose-dependent fashion. FSH levels are not affected at the doses used during controlled ovarian stimulation. Following a single 3 mg dose of cetrorelix, duration of action of at least 4 days has been established. A dose of cetrorelix 0.25 mg every 24 hours has been shown to maintain the effect.

➤*Pharmacokinetics:*

Absorption – Cetrorelix is rapidly absorbed following subcutaneous injection, maximal plasma concentrations being achieved approximately 1 to 2 hours after administration. The mean absolute bioavailability of cetrorelix following subcutaneous administration to healthy women is 85%.

Distribution – The volume of distribution of cetrorelix following a single IV dose of 3 mg is about 1 L/kg. In vitro protein binding to human plasma is 86%.

Cetrorelix concentrations in follicular fluid and plasma were similar on the day of oocyte pick-up in patients undergoing controlled ovarian stimulation. Following subcutaneous administration of cetrorelix 0.25 and 3 mg, plasma concentrations of cetrorelix were below or in the range of the lower limit of quantitation on the day of oocyte pick-up and embryo transfer.

Metabolism – After subcutaneous administration of cetrorelix 10 mg to women and men, cetrorelix and small amounts of (1 to 9), (1 to 7), (1 to 6), and (1 to 4) peptides were found in bile samples over 24 hours.

In in vitro studies, cetrorelix was stable against phase I- and phase II-metabolism. Cetrorelix was transformed by peptidases, and the (1 to 4) peptide was the predominant metabolite.

Excretion – Following subcutaneous administration of cetrorelix 10 mg to men and women, only unchanged cetrorelix was detected in urine. In 24 hours, cetrorelix and small amounts of the (1 to 9), (1 to 7), (1 to 6), and (1 to 4) peptides were found in bile samples. Two percent to 4% of the dose was eliminated in the urine as unchanged cetrorelix, while 5% to 10% was eliminated as cetrorelix and the 4 metabolites in bile. Therefore, only 7% to 14% of the total dose was recovered as unchanged cetrorelix and metabolites in urine and bile up to 24 hours. The remaining portion of the dose may not have been recovered since bile and urine were not collected for a longer period of time. The pharmacokinetic parameters of single and multiple doses of cetrorelix in adult healthy women are summarized in the following table.

Pharmacokinetic Parameters of Cetrorelix Following 3 mg Single or 0.25 mg Single and Multiple (Daily for 14 Days) Subcutaneous Administration

	Single dose 3 mg	Single dose 0.25 mg	Multiple dose 0.25 mg
Number of subjects	12	12	12
T_{max}[a,b] (h)	1.5 (0.5 to 2)	1 (0.5 to 1.5)	1 (0.5 to 2)
$T_{½}$[a,c] (h)	62.8 (38.2 to 108)	5 (2.4 to 48.8)	20.6 (4.1 to 179.3)
C_{max}[d] (ng/mL)	28.5 (22.5 to 36.2)	4.97 (4.17 to 5.92)	6.42 (5.18 to 7.96)
AUC[e] (ng•h/mL)	536 (451 to 636)	31.4 (23.4 to 42)	44.5 (36.7 to 54.2)
CL[f,g] (mL/min•kg)	1.28[h]		
Vz[f,i] (L/kg)	1.16[h]		

[a] Geometric mean (95% CI_{ln}), arithmetic mean.
[b] T_{max} = Time to reach observed maximum plasma concentration.
[c] $T_{½}$ = Elimination half-life.
[d] C_{max} = Maximum plasma concentration; multiple dose $C_{ss,\ max}$.
[e] AUC = Area under the curve; single dose $AUC_{0-\infty}$ multiple dose AUC_{τ}.
[f] Geometric mean (95% CI_{ln}), median (minimum to maximum).
[g] CL = Total plasma clearance.
[h] Based on IV administration (n = 6, separate study 0013).
[i] V_z = Volume of distribution.

Contraindications

Hypersensitivity to cetrorelix acetate, extrinsic peptide hormones, or mannitol; known hypersensitivity to GnRH or any other GnRH analogs; known or suspected pregnancy, and lactation; severe renal impairment.

Warnings

➤*Hypersensitivity reactions:* Caution is advised in patients with hypersensitivity to GnRH. Carefully monitor these patients after the first injection. A severe anaphylactic reaction associated with cough, rash, and hypotension was observed in 1 patient after 7 months of treatment with 10 mg/day cetrorelix in a study for an indication unrelated to infertility.

➤*Mutagenesis:* Cetrorelix was not genotoxic in vitro (Ames test, HPRT test, chromosome aberration test) or in vivo (chromosome aberration test, mouse micronucleus test). Cetrorelix induced polyploidy in CHL Chinese

CETRORELIX ACETATE — INJECTION

hamster lung fibroblasts, but not in V79 Chinese hamster lung fibroblasts, cultured peripheral human lymphocytes, or in an in vitro micronucleus test in the CHL cell line.

➤*Fertility impairment:* Treatment with 0.46 mg/kg cetrorelix for 4 weeks resulted in complete infertility in female rats which was reversed 8 weeks after cessation of treatment.

➤*Elderly:* Cetrorelix is not intended to be used in subjects aged 65 years of age and older.

➤*Pregnancy: Category X.*

Cetrorelix is contraindicated in pregnant women.

Cetrorelix should be prescribed by health care providers who are experienced in fertility treatment. Before starting treatment with cetrorelix acetate, pregnancy must be excluded.

When administered to rats for the first 7 days of pregnancy, cetrorelix did not affect the development of the implanted conceptus at doses up to 38 mcg/kg (approximately 1 times the recommended human therapeutic dose based on body surface area). However, a dose of 139 mcg/kg (approximately 4 times the human dose) resulted in a resorption rate and a postimplantation loss of 100%.

When administered from day 6 to near term to pregnant rats and rabbits, very early resorptions and total implantation losses were seen in rats at doses from 4.6 mcg/kg (0.2 times the human dose) and in rabbits at doses from 6.8 mcg/kg (0.4 times the human dose). In animals that maintained their pregnancies, there was no increase in the incidence of fetal abnormalities.

The fetal resorption observed in animals is a logical consequence of the alteration in hormonal levels effected by the antigonadotrophic properties of cetrorelix acetate, which could result in fetal loss in humans as well. Therefore, do not use this drug in pregnant women.

Congenital anomalies – Clinical follow-up studies of 316 newborns of women administered cetrorelix were reviewed. One infant of a set of twin neonates was found to have anencephaly at birth and died after 4 days. The other twin was healthy. Developmental findings from ongoing baby follow-up included a child with a ventricular septal defect and another child with bilateral congenital glaucoma.

Four pregnancies that resulted in therapeutic abortion in phase 2 and phase 3 controlled ovarian stimulation studies had major anomalies (diaphragmatic hernia, trisomy 21, Klinefelter syndrome, polymalformation, and trisomy 18). In 3 of these 4 cases, intracytoplasmic sperm injection (ICSI) was the fertilization method employed; in the fourth case, in vitro fertilization (IVF) was the method employed.

The minor congenital anomalies reported include supernumerary nipple, bilateral strabismus, imperforate hymen, congenital nevi, hemangiomata, and QT syndrome.

The casual relationship between the reported anomalies and cetrorelix is unknown. Multiple factors, genetic and others (including, but not limited to ICSI, IVF, gonadotropins, and progesterone), make causal attribution difficult to study.

➤*Lactation:* It is not known whether cetrorelix is excreted in human milk. Because many drugs are excreted in human milk, and because the effects of cetrorelix on lactation or the breastfed child have not been determined, do not use cetrorelix acetate in nursing mothers.

Precautions

➤*Monitoring:* Caution is advised in patients with hypersensitivity to GnRH. Carefully monitor these patients after the first injection. A severe anaphylactic reaction associated with cough, rash, and hypotension was observed in 1 patient after 7 months of treatment with cetrorelix 10 mg daily in a study for an indication unrelated to infertility.

➤*Special risk:* Take special care in women with signs and symptoms of active allergic conditions or known history of allergic predisposition. Treatment with cetrorelix is not advised in women with severe allergic conditions.

➤*Lab test abnormalities:* After the exclusion of preexisting conditions, enzyme elevations (ALT, AST, GGT, alkaline phosphatase) were found in 1% to 2% of patients receiving cetrorelix during controlled ovarian stimulation. The elevations ranged up to 3 times the upper limit of normal. The clinical significance of these findings was not determined.

During stimulation with human menopausal gonadotropin, cetrorelix had no notable effects on hormone levels aside from inhibition of LH surges.

Drug Interactions

No formal drug interaction studies have been performed with cetrorelix.

Adverse Reactions

The safety of cetrorelix in 949 patients undergoing controlled ovarian stimulation in clinical studies was evaluated. Women were between 19 and 40 years of age (mean age, 32). Ninety-four percent of them were white patients. Cetrorelix was given in doses ranging from 0.1 to 5 mg as a single or multiple dose.

The following table shows systemic adverse reactions, reported in clinical studies without regard to causality, from the beginning of cetrorelix treatment until confirmation of pregnancy by ultrasound at an incidence greater than or equal to 1% in cetrorelix-treated subjects undergoing COS.

Adverse Reactions in at Least 1% Cetrorelix-Treated Subjects	
(WHO-preferred Term)	Cetrorelix for Injection (n = 949) % (n)
Nausea	1.3% (12)
Headache	1.1% (10)
Ovarian hyperstimulation syndrome[a]	3.5% (33)

[a] Intensity moderate or severe, or WHO grade 2 or 3, respectively.

Local site reactions (eg, redness, erythema, bruising, itching, swelling, pruritus) were reported. Usually they were of a transient nature, mild intensity, and short duration. During postmarketing surveillance, rare cases of hypersensitivity reactions including anaphylactoid reactions have been reported.

Two stillbirths were reported in phase 3 studies of cetrorelix.

Overdosage

There have been no reports of overdosage with 0.25 or 3 mg cetrorelix in humans. Single doses up to 120 mg cetrorelix have been well tolerated in patients treated for other indications without signs of overdosage.

Patient Information

Prior to therapy with cetrorelix, inform patients of the duration of treatment and monitoring procedures that will be required. Discuss the risk of possible adverse reactions. Cetrorelix should not be prescribed if a patient is pregnant.

Gonadotropin-Releasing Hormone Antagonists

ABARELIX

Rx	**Plenaxis** (Praecis[a])	**Powder for injection:** 113 mg	Preservative-free. In kits.[b]

[a] Praecis Pharmaceuticals Incorporated, 830 Winter Street, Waltham, MA 02451-1420; (877) PRAECIS, (877) 772-3247.

[b] Kit contains a single-use 10 mL diluent vial of 0.9% sodium chloride injection, one 3 mL syringe with an 18-gauge 1½ inch needle, and one 22-gauge 1½ inch *Safety Glide* injection needle.

ABARELIX — INJECTION

WARNING

Immediate-onset systemic allergic reactions, some resulting in hypotension and syncope, have occurred after administration of abarelix. These immediate-onset reactions have been reported to occur following any administration of abarelix, including after the initial dose. The cumulative risk of such a reaction increases with the duration of treatment (see Warnings). Following each injection of abarelix, observe patients for at least 30 minutes in the office and in the event of an allergic reaction, manage appropriately.

- Only physicians who have enrolled in the *Plenaxis* PLUS Program (*Plenaxis* User Safety Program), based on their attestation of qualifications and acceptance of prescribing responsibilities, may prescribe abarelix (see Administration and Dosage).
- Abarelix is indicated for the palliative treatment of men with advanced symptomatic prostate cancer, in whom luteinizing hormone release hormone (LHRH) agonist therapy is not appropriate and who refuse surgical castration, and have 1 or more of the following: 1) Risk of neurological compromise because of metastases, 2) ureteral or bladder outlet obstruction because of local encroachment or metastatic disease, or 3) severe bone pain from skeletal metastases persisting on narcotic analgesia.
- The effectiveness of abarelix in suppressing serum testosterone to castrate levels decreases with continued dosing in some patients. Effectiveness beyond 12 months has not been established. Treatment failure can be detected by measuring serum total testosterone concentrations just prior to administration on day 29 and every 8 weeks thereafter (see Warnings).

Indications

➤*Prostate cancer:* For the palliative treatment of men with advanced symptomatic prostate cancer in whom LHRH agonist therapy is not appropriate, who refuse surgical castration, and have 1 or more of the following: 1) Risk of neurological compromise because of metastases, 2) ureteral or bladder outlet obstruction caused by local encroachment or metastatic disease, or 3) severe bone pain from skeletal metastases persisting on narcotic analgesia.

Administration and Dosage

➤*Approved by the FDA:* November 25, 2003.

For safety reasons, abarelix is approved with marketing restrictions. Abarelix will be provided to physicians enrolled in the *Plenaxis* PLUS Program. To enroll in the abarelix prescribing program, call (866) PLENAXIS (866-753-6294) or visit http://www.plenaxisplus.com.

➤*Dose:* The recommended dose of abarelix is 100 mg IM to the buttock on days 1, 15, 29 (week 4), and every 4 weeks thereafter. Treatment failure can be detected by measuring serum testosterone concentrations just prior to abarelix administration, beginning on day 29 and every 8 weeks thereafter.

➤*Preparation for administration:* Reconstitution of 1 vial of abarelix will provide a 100 mg (50 mg/mL) dose as a single IM injection. Abarelix does not contain a preservative; administer within 1 hour following reconstitution.

1.) Prior to reconstitution, gently shake the vial of abarelix for injectable suspension. Hold the vial at a 45 degree angle and tap lightly on the table to break up any caking. Withdraw 2.2 mL of 0.9% sodium chloride injection using the enclosed 18-gauge 1½ inch needle and a 3 mL syringe. Discard the remaining diluent.
2.) Keeping the vial upright, insert the needle all the way into the vial and inject the diluent quickly. Before withdrawing the needle, remove 2.2 mL of air. Shake immediately.
3.) Shake for approximately 15 seconds. Allow the vial to stand for approximately 2 minutes. Tap the vial to reduce foaming and swirl the vial occasionally. Again shake for approximately 15 seconds. Allow the vial to stand for approximately 2 minutes. Tap the vial to reduce foaming and swirl the vial occasionally.
4.) Do not reinject the air into the vial. Locate a second injection spot on the stopper, and then insert the 18-gauge needle. Invert the vial and draw up some of the suspension into the syringe, without removing the needle from the vial, reinject it at any remaining solids in the vial. Repeat the process until all solids are dispersed. Swirl the vial before withdrawal and withdraw the entire contents (at least 2 mL) by positioning the needle at a 45-degree angle.
5.) Pull the plunger back to recover the residual suspension in the 18-gauge 1½ inch needle. Exchange the 18-gauge 1½ inch needle with the enclosed 22-gauge 1½ inch *Safety Glide* injection needle.
6.) Insert the needle at the desired injection site and pull the plunger back to check for backflow of blood. If blood flows into the syringe, do not inject at this site. Select another injection site. Deliver the entire reconstituted suspension IM immediately. Observe the patient after injection for 30 minutes for any sign of an allergic-type response.

➤*Storage/Stability:* Store at 25°C (77°F); excursions permitted to 15° to 30°C (59° to 86°F). Abarelix does not contain a preservative; administer within 1 hour following reconstitution.

Actions

➤*Pharmacology:* Abarelix is a synthetic decapeptide with potent antagonistic activity against naturally occurring gonadotropin releasing-hormone (GnRH). Abarelix inhibits gonadotropin and related androgen production by directly and competitively blocking GnRH receptors in the pituitary. Abarelix exerts its pharmacological action by directly suppressing luteinizing hormone (LH) and follicle stimulating hormone (FSH) secretion and thereby reducing the secretion of testosterone by the testes. Because of the direct inhibition of the secretion of LH by abarelix, there is no initial increase in serum testosterone concentrations.

➤*Pharmacokinetics:*

Absorption – A single 100 mg IM dose of abarelix was given to 14 healthy men 52 to 75 years of age, with body weight of 61.6 to 110.5 kg. The pharmacokinetic information is provided below.

Abarelix Mean Pharmacokinetic Parameters

Single dose (n = 14)	C_{max} (ng/mL)	T_{max} (days)	$AUC_{0-\infty}$ (ng•day/mL)	CL/F (L/day)	$T_{½}$ (days)
100 mg IM	43.4	3	500	208	13.2

Following 100 mg IM administration, abarelix is absorbed slowly with a mean peak concentration of 43.4 ng/mL observed approximately 3 days after the injection.

Distribution – The apparent volume of distribution during the terminal phase determined after IM administration of abarelix was about 4040 L, implying that abarelix probably distributes extensively within the body. Abarelix is highly bound to plasma proteins (96% to 99%).

Metabolism – In vitro hepatocyte (rat, monkey, human) studies and in vivo studies in rats and monkeys showed that the major metabolites of abarelix were formed via hydrolysis of peptide bonds. No significant oxidative or conjugated metabolites of abarelix were found either in vitro or in vivo. There is no evidence of cytochrome P450 involvement in the metabolism of abarelix.

Excretion – In humans, approximately 13% of unchanged abarelix was recovered in urine after a 15 mcg/kg IM injection; there were no detectable metabolites in urine. Renal clearance of abarelix was 14.4 L/day (or 10 mL/min) after administration of 100 mg abarelix.

Contraindications

Known hypersensitivity to any of the components in the abarelix injectable suspension.

Abarelix is not indicated in women or pediatric patients. In addition, abarelix may cause fetal harm if administered to a pregnant woman.

Warnings

➤*QT prolongation:* In a single, active-controlled clinical study comparing abarelix to LHRH agonist plus nonsteroidal antiandrogen, periodic electrocardiograms were performed. Both therapies prolonged the mean Fridericia-corrected QT interval by more than 10 msec from baseline. In approximately 20% of patients in both groups, there were either changes from baseline QTc of more than 30 msec, or end-of-treatment QTc values exceeding 450 msec. Similar results were observed in 2 other phase 3 studies with abarelix and the active-control treatments. It is unclear whether these changes were directly related to study drugs, to androgen deprivation therapy, or to other variables.

Because abarelix may prolong the QT interval, carefully consider whether the risks of abarelix outweigh the benefits in patients with baseline QTc values greater than 450 msec (eg, congenital QT prolongation) and in patients taking Class IA (eg, quinidine, procainamide) or Class III (eg, amiodarone, sotalol) antiarrhythmic medications.

➤*Decrease in effectiveness:* A decrease in overall effectiveness with increased duration of treatment as measured by failure to maintain suppression of serum testosterone below 50 ng/dL, was noted. Treatment failure can be detected by measuring serum total testosterone concentrations just prior to administration on day 29 after the initial dose and every 8 weeks thereafter. The decrease in overall effectiveness of abarelix with increased duration of treatment is greater in patients who weighed more than 102 kg (225 lbs). Strict monitoring of serum testosterone in these patients is warranted.

➤*Hypersensitivity reactions:* Immediate-onset systemic allergic reactions have occurred (see Black Box Warning). In the clinical trial of patients with advanced, symptomatic prostate cancer, 3 of 81 (3.7%) patients experienced an immediate-onset systemic allergic reaction within minutes of receiving abarelix. The allergic reactions were urticaria (day 15), urticaria and pruritus (day 29), and hypotension and syncope (day 141). Monitor patients for at least 30 minutes after each abarelix injection. In the event of an allergic reaction associated with hypotension and/or syncope, use appropriate supportive measures (eg, leg elevation, oxygen, IV fluids, antihistamines, corticosteroids, and epinephrine [alone or in combination]).

Gonadotropin-Releasing Hormone Antagonists

ABARELIX — INJECTION

From all the prostate cancer clinical trials with abarelix (mostly in men without advanced, symptomatic disease), immediate-onset systemic allergic reactions (occurring within 30 minutes of dosing) were observed in 1.1% of patients dosed with abarelix. In 14/15 patients who experienced an allergic reaction, each developed symptoms within 8 minutes of injection. The cumulative risk of such a reaction increased with duration of treatment. The cumulative rates on days 56, 141, 365, and 676 were 0.51%, 0.8%, 1.24%, and 2.91%, respectively. Seven patients experienced hypotension or syncope as part of their allergic reaction, representing 0.5% of all patients. The cumulative rates for these types of reactions on days 56, 141, 365, and 617 after the initial dose were 0.22%, 0.32%, 0.61%, and 1.67%, respectively.

➤*Fertility impairment:* In animals, mating and fertility were significantly decreased at doses of 3 and 10 mg/kg (0.34-fold and 1.135-fold, respectively, the human therapeutic dose of 100 mg based on body surface area [BSA]), but the effects were reversible.

➤*Pregnancy: Category X.* Embryolethality occurred in pregnant rats administered a single subcutaneous dose of abarelix up to 3 mg/kg (0.228-fold the human therapeutic dose of 100 mg based on BSA). In rabbits, a dose-related increase in fetal resorptions and reduced viability was observed at doses up to 30 mg/kg (6.81-fold the human therapeutic dose of 100 mg based on BSA).

➤*Lactation:* It is not known whether abarelix is excreted in human milk. Do not use in nursing mothers.

➤*Children:* The safety and efficacy of abarelix in pediatric patients have not been studied. Abarelix is not indicated for use in pediatric patients.

Precautions

➤*Monitoring:* Monitor the response to abarelix by measuring serum total testosterone concentrations just prior to administration on day 29 and every 8 weeks thereafter. Also consider periodic measurement of serum PSA levels. Clinically meaningful transaminase elevations were observed in some patients who received abarelix or comparator drugs. Obtain serum transaminase levels before starting abarelix treatment and periodically during treatment.

➤*Decrease in bone mineral density:* Extended treatment with GnRH antagonists and LHRH agonists may result in a decrease in bone mineral density.

Adverse Reactions

Abarelix Adverse Reactions (at least 10%)	
Adverse reaction	Abarelix (n = 81)
CNS	
Dizziness	12
Fatigue	10
Headache	12
Sleep disturbance[a]	44
Endocrine	
Breast enlargement[a]	30
Breast pain/nipple tenderness[a]	20
GI	
Constipation	15
Diarrhea	11
Nausea	10
GU	
Dysuria	10
Micturition frequency	10
Urinary retention	10
Urinary tract infection	10
Miscellaneous	
Back pain	17
Hot flushes[a]	79
Pain	31
Peripheral edema	15
Upper respiratory tract infection	12

[a] Pharmacological consequences of androgen deprivation.

➤*Hypersensitivity:* Immediate-onset systemic allergic reactions may occur (see Black Box Warning and Warnings).

➤*Lab test abnormalities:* Clinically meaningful increases in serum transaminases were seen in a small percentage of patients in both treatment groups in each active-controlled abarelix study. In study 1 and 2 combined, the percentage of abarelix patients reporting serum ALT greater than 2.5 times ULN or more than 200 units/L was 8.2% and 1.8%, respectively. The percentage reporting serum AST greater than 2.5 times ULN or more than 200 units/L was 3.1% and 0.8%, respectively. Similar results were reported for active comparators. Slight decreases in hemoglobin, a pharmacological consequence of castration, were observed in patients receiving abarelix and active comparator. Mean increases in serum triglycerides of approximately 10% were seen in abarelix-treated patients.

Overdosage

The maximum tolerated dose of abarelix has not been determined. The maximum dose used in clinical studies was 150 mg. There have been no reports of accidental overdose of abarelix.

Patient Information

Abarelix can cause serious or life-threatening allergic reactions that may need emergency medical treatment right away.

These serious reactions may include the following: Low blood pressure and fainting (shock); swelling of face, eyelids, tongue, or throat; asthma, wheezing, or other breathing problems such as chest tightness or shortness of breath.

Chances of getting a serious or life-threatening allergic reaction may increase with each abarelix injection.

If a serious or life-threatening allergic reaction occurs, it is usually soon after getting an abarelix injection; therefore, instruct patients to wait in the physicians's office or health care facility for 30 minutes after each abarelix injection.

Instruct patients to inform their physician right away if they feel any warmth, redness, lightheadedness, swelling, or thickness in their throat; this could mean they are having a serious allergic reaction.

Inform patients to tell their physician if they or any family member have the rare heart condition known as prolongation of the QTc interval.

Abarelix can cause allergic skin reactions such as rash, hives, itching, tingling, and redness (flushing). A skin reaction may occur immediately after injection or several days later.

The most common side effects are the following: Hot flashes; problems sleeping; pain, including back pain; breast enlargement or breast pain; constipation.

Androgens

Anabolic steroids are classified as a *c-iii* controlled substance under the anabolic steroids act of 1990.

An androgenic agent used in the therapy of carcinoma of the breast is listed under Antineoplastic Agents: Testolactone. (See individual monograph.)

Indications

➤*Males:* For replacement therapy in hypogonadism associated with a deficiency or absence of endogenous testosterone.

Primary hypogonadism (congenital or acquired) – Testicular failure because of cryptorchidism, bilateral torsion, orchitis, vanishing testis syndrome or orchidectomy, Klinefelter syndrome, chemotherapy, or toxic damage from alcohol or heavy metals. These men usually have low serum testosterone levels and gonadotropins (FSH, LH) above the normal range.

Hypogonadotropic hypogonadism (congenital or acquired) – Idiopathic gonadotropin- or luteinizing hormone-releasing hormone (LHRH) deficiency or pituitary-hypothalamic injury from tumors, trauma, or radiation.

If the above conditions occur prior to puberty, androgen replacement therapy is needed for development of secondary sexual characteristics. Prolonged treatment is required to maintain sexual characteristics in these and other males who develop testosterone deficiency after puberty. However, appropriate adrenal cortical and thyroid hormone replacement therapy are still necessary and are of primary importance.

Delayed puberty – To stimulate puberty in carefully selected males with clearly delayed puberty. These patients usually have a familial pattern of delayed puberty that is not secondary to a pathological disorder; puberty is expected to occur spontaneously at a relatively late date. Brief occasional treatment with conservative doses may be justified if these patients do not respond to psychological support. Discuss the potential adverse effect on bone maturation with the patient and parents prior to androgen administration. To assess the effect of treatment on the epiphyseal centers, obtain an x-ray of the hand and wrist to determine bone age every 6 months.

➤*Females:*

Metastatic cancer – May be used secondarily in women with advancing inoperable metastatic (skeletal) mammary cancer who are 1 to 5 years postmenopausal. Primary goals of therapy include ablation of the ovaries. This treatment has been used in premenopausal women with breast cancer who have benefitted from oophorectomy and have a hormone-responsive tumor.

Androgens are not effective (lack of substantial evidence) in treating fractures or managing surgery, convalescence or functional uterine bleeding, or enhancement of athletic performance (see Warnings).

Actions

➤*Pharmacology:* Testosterone, produced by the Leydig cells of the testis, is the primary male androgen.

In many tissues, the activity of testosterone appears to depend on reduction to dihydrotestosterone, which binds to cytosol receptor proteins. The steroid-receptor complex is transported to the nucleus where it initiates transcription events and cellular changes related to androgen action.

Endogenous androgens are responsible for the normal growth and development of the male sex organs and for maintenance of secondary sex characteristics. These effects include the growth and maturation of the prostate, seminal vesicles, penis, and scrotum; the development of male hair distribution, such as facial, pubic, chest, and axillary hair; laryngeal enlargement; vocal cord thickening; alterations in body musculature and fat distribution.

These drugs also cause retention of nitrogen, sodium, potassium, phosphorus, and decreased urinary excretion of calcium. Androgens have been reported to increase protein anabolism and decrease protein catabolism. Nitrogen balance is improved only when there is sufficient intake of calories and protein.

Androgens are responsible for the growth spurt of adolescence and for the termination of linear growth by fusion of the epiphyseal growth centers. In children, exogenous androgens accelerate linear growth rates but may cause a disproportionate advancement in bone maturation. Use over long periods may result in fusion of the epiphyseal growth centers and termination of the growth process. Androgens have been reported to stimulate production of red blood cells by enhancing production of the erythropoietic stimulating factor.

During administration of exogenous androgens, endogenous testosterone release is inhibited through feedback inhibition of pituitary luteinizing hormone (LH). Large doses of exogenous androgens may suppress spermatogenesis through feedback inhibition of pituitary follicle-stimulating hormone (FSH).

➤*Pharmacokinetics:*

Absorption –

Oral: Testosterone is metabolized by the gut and 44% is cleared by the liver in the first pass. Doses as high as 400 mg daily are needed to achieve clinically effective blood levels for full replacement therapy. The synthetic androgen, **methyltestosterone**, is less extensively metabolized by the liver and has a longer half-life. It is more suitable than testosterone for oral administration.

IM: Testosterone esters are less polar than free testosterone. Testosterone esters in oil injected IM are absorbed slowly from the lipid phase; thus, **testosterone cypionate** and **enanthate** can be given at intervals of 2 to 4 weeks. Suspensions of testosterone or its esters in aqueous media may cause local irritation and the rate of absorption is not always uniform.

Topical gel: In a study with the dose of topical testosterone gel 10 g (to deliver testosterone 100 mg), all patients showed an increase in serum testosterone within 30 minutes, and 8 of 9 patients had a serum testosterone concentration within the normal range by 4 hours after the initial application. Absorption of testosterone into the blood continues for the entire 24-hour dosing interval. Serum concentrations approximate the steady-state level by the end of the first 24 hours and are at steady state by the second or third day of dosing.

When the topical gel treatment is discontinued after achieving steady state, serum testosterone levels remain in the normal range for 24 to 48 hours but return to their pretreatment levels by the fifth day after the last application.

Transdermal system:

• *Testoderm* – Following placement of *Testoderm* on scrotal skin, the serum testosterone concentration rises to a maximum at 2 to 4 hours and returns toward baseline within approximately 2 hours after system removal. Serum levels reach a plateau at 3 to 4 weeks. The testosterone levels achieved with *Testoderm* generally are within the range for normal men.

Scrotal skin is at least 5 times more permeable to testosterone than other skin sites. *Testoderm* and *Testoderm with Adhesive* will not produce adequate serum testosterone concentration if applied to nongenital skin.

• *Testoderm TTS* – The 3 recommended skin sites (arm, back, and upper buttocks) are interchangeable based on equivalent testosterone $AUC_{(0-27)}$ values.

• *Androderm* – Following application to nonscrotal skin, testosterone is continuously absorbed during the 24-hour dosing period. Daily application at approximately 10 p.m. results in a serum testosterone concentration profile that mimics the normal circadian variation observed in healthy young men. Maximum concentrations occur in the early morning hours with minimum concentrations in the evening. Normal range morning serum testosterone concentrations are reached during the first day of dosing. There is no accumulation of testosterone during continuous treatment.

Distribution – Testosterone in plasma is approximately 98% bound to a specific testosterone-estradiol-binding globulin. Generally, the amount of binding globulin will determine the percentage of free and bound testosterone; the free testosterone concentration will determine its half-life.

Metabolism/Excretion – There are considerable variations in the reported half-life of testosterone, ranging from 10 to 100 minutes. The half-life of **testosterone cypionate** IM is approximately 8 days; for oral **fluoxymesterone**, it is approximately 9.2 hours; **methyltestosterone** undergoes less extensive first-pass hepatic metabolism than testosterone following oral administration and has a longer half-life. Inactivation of testosterone occurs primarily in the liver. About 90% of a testosterone dose is excreted in the urine as conjugates of testosterone and its metabolites; about 6% of a dose is excreted in the feces.

Contraindications

Patients with serious cardiac, hepatic, or renal diseases; hypersensitivity to the drug or any components of the products; in men with carcinomas of the breast or known or suspected carcinoma of the prostate; women (*Testoderm*); pregnancy.

Pregnant women should avoid skin contact with *AndroGel* application sites in men. Testosterone may cause fetal harm. In the event that unwashed or unclothed skin to which *AndroGel* has been applied does come in direct contact with the skin of a pregnant woman, wash the general area of contact on the woman with soap and water as soon as possible. In vitro studies show that residual testosterone is removed from the skin surface by washing with soap and water.

Warnings

➤*Hepatic effects:* Prolonged use of high doses of androgens has been associated with the development of potentially life-threatening peliosis hepatis, hepatic neoplasms, cholestatic hepatitis, jaundice, and hepatocellular carcinoma. Long-term therapy with **testosterone enanthate**, which elevates blood levels for prolonged periods, has produced multiple hepatic adenomas. Testosterone is not known to produce these adverse effects.

Cholestatic hepatitis and jaundice occur with **fluoxymesterone** and **methyltestosterone** at relatively low doses. If cholestatic hepatitis with jaundice appears with use of any androgen, or if liver function tests become abnormal, discontinue the androgen and determine the etiology. Drug-induced jaundice is reversible when the medication is discontinued.

➤*Athletic performance:* Although the anabolic steroids are generally the agents that are abused for enhancement of athletic performance, these agents also have been used for such purposes. However, these drugs are not safe and effective for this use and have a potential risk of serious side effects.

➤*Sleep apnea:* The treatment of hypogonadal men with testosterone esters may potentiate sleep apnea in some patients, especially those with risk factors such as obesity or chronic lung diseases.

➤*Breast cancer:* In patients with breast cancer, androgen therapy may cause hypercalcemia by stimulating osteolysis. If hypercalcemia occurs, discontinue the drug.

➤*Oligospermia:* Oligospermia and reduced ejaculatory volume may occur after prolonged administration or excessive dosage.

➤*Edema:* Edema, with or without congestive heart failure, may be a serious complication in patients with preexisting cardiac, renal, or hepatic disease. In addition to discontinuation of the drug, diuretic therapy may be required.

➤*Gynecomastia:* Gynecomastia frequently develops and occasionally persists in patients being treated for hypogonadism.

➤*Bone maturation:* Use cautiously in healthy males with delayed puberty. Monitor bone maturation by assessing bone age of the wrist and hand every 6 months.

➤*Product interchange:* Do not use **testosterone cypionate** interchangeably with **testosterone propionate** because of differences in duration of action.

➤*Carcinogenesis:* Testosterone has induced cervical-uterine tumors in mice; these tumors metastasized in some cases. Injection of testosterone into some strains of female mice may increase their susceptibility to hepatoma. Testosterone is also known to increase the number of tumors and decrease the degree of differentiation of chemically-induced carcinomas of the liver in rats. There are rare reports of hepatocellular carcinoma in patients receiving long-term therapy with androgens in high doses. Drug withdrawal did not lead to tumor regression in all cases.

➤*Elderly:* Elderly men, or men in general, treated with androgens may be at an increased risk of developing prostatic hypertrophy, prostatic carcinoma, and prostatic hyperplasia.

➤*Pregnancy: Category X.* Androgens are contraindicated in women who are or who may become pregnant; androgens may cause fetal harm. Androgens cause virilization of the external genitalia of the female fetus (eg, clitoromegaly, abnormal vaginal development, fusion of genital folds to form a scrotal-like structure). The degree of masculinization is related to the amount of drug given and the age of the fetus. Masculinization is most likely to occur in the female fetus when androgens are given in the first trimester. If the patient becomes pregnant while taking these drugs, apprise her of the potential hazards to the fetus.

➤*Lactation:* It is not known whether androgens are excreted in breast milk. Decide whether to discontinue nursing or to discontinue the drug, taking into account the importance of the drug to the mother. Testosterone transdermal systems and testosterone gel are not indicated for women and must not be used in women.

➤*Children:* Use androgens cautiously in children; the drugs should only be given by specialists who are aware of the adverse effects on bone maturation.

Androgens may accelerate bone maturation without producing compensatory gain in linear growth. This adverse effect may result in compromised adult stature. The younger the child, the greater the risk of compromising final mature height.

Safety and efficacy of *Testoderm* and *Androgel* products in children have not been established.

Benzyl alcohol – Benzyl alcohol-containing products have been associated with a fatal "gasping syndrome" in premature infants. Refer to product listings.

Precautions

➤*Monitoring:* Frequently determine urine and serum calcium levels during the course of therapy in women with disseminated breast carcinoma.

Periodically check liver function, prostate specific antigen, cholesterol, and high-density lipoprotein. To ensure proper dosing, measure serum testosterone concentrations.

Make periodic (every 6 months) x-ray examinations of bone age during treatment of prepubertal males to determine the rate of bone maturation and the effects of androgen therapy on the epiphyseal centers.

Check hemoglobin and hematocrit periodically for polycythemia in patients who are receiving high doses of androgens or who are receiving long-term administration.

➤*Virilization:* Observe women for signs of virilization (eg, deepening voice, hirsutism, acne, clitoromegaly, menstrual irregularities). Discontinue therapy at the time of evidence of mild virilism to prevent irreversible virilization. Virilization is usual following high-dose androgens. Some virilization should be tolerated during treatment for breast carcinoma.

Virilization of female partners has been reported with use of topical testosterone. Percutaneous creams leave as much as 90 mg residual testosterone on the skin. The results from one study indicated that, after removal of a *Testoderm* system, the potential for transfer of testosterone to a sexual partner was 6 mg, 1/45th the daily endogenous testosterone production by the female body. *Testoderm TTS* has an occlusive backing that prevents the partner from coming in contact with the active material in the system. If a *Testoderm TTS* system is inadvertently transferred to a female partner, remove it immediately and wash the contacted skin. Changes in body hair distribution or significant increases in acne of the female partner should be brought to the attention of a physician.

➤*Pellets:* Pellet implantation is much less flexible for dosage adjustment than is oral administration or IM injection of oil solutions or aqueous suspensions. Therefore, take great care when estimating the amount of testosterone needed. In the face of complications where the effects of testosterone should be discontinued, the pellets would have to be removed. In addition, there are times when the pellets may slough out. This accident is usually traceable to superficial implantation or to neglect in regard to aseptic precautions.

➤*Hypercholesterolemia:* Serum cholesterol may be altered during therapy.

➤*Special risk:* Patients with benign prostatic hypertrophy may develop acute urethral obstruction. Priapism or excessive sexual stimulation may develop. Oligospermia may occur after prolonged administration or excessive dosage. If any of these effects appear, stop administration. If restarted, use a lower dosage. Avoid stimulation to the point of increasing nervous, mental, and physical activities beyond the patient's cardiovascular capacity.

➤*Tartrazine sensitivity:* Some of these products contain tartrazine, which may cause allergic-type reactions (including bronchial asthma) in susceptible individuals. Although the incidence of tartrazine sensitivity in the general population is low, it is frequently seen in patients who also have aspirin hypersensitivity. Specific products containing tartrazine are identified in the product listings.

Drug Interactions

Androgens Drug Interactions

Precipitant drug	Object drug[a]		Description
Fluoxymesterone, Methyltestosterone	Anticoagulants	⬆	The anticoagulant effect may be potentiated by 17-alkyl testosterone derivatives (eg, fluoxymesterone, methyltestosterone). Although the non-17-alkylated agent (testosterone) appears safer, at least 1 case report described a similar interaction. Avoid the combination with 17-alkyl derivatives if possible.
Androgens	Oxyphenbutazone	⬆	Coadministration of oxyphenbutazone and androgens may result in elevated serum levels of oxyphenbutazone.
Androgens	Insulin	⬇	In diabetic patients, the metabolic effects of androgens may decrease blood glucose and, therefore, insulin requirements.
Testosterone	Propranolol	⬇	In a pharmacokinetic study of an injectable testosterone product, administration of testosterone cypionate led to an increased clearance of propranolol in the majority of men tested.
Testosterone	Corticosteroids, ACTH	⬆	The coadministration of testosterone with ACTH or corticosteroids may enhance edema formation; thus, administer these drugs cautiously, particularly in patients with cardiac or hepatic disease.
Methyltestosterone	Cyclosporine	⬆	Increased cyclosporine blood concentrations with possible toxicity (eg, nephrotoxicity) may occur. Consider monitoring serum bilirubin, serum creatinine, and cyclosporine concentrations in patients receiving cyclosporine and methyltestosterone concurrently. Adjust the doses as needed.

[a] ⬆ = Object drug increased. ⬇ = Object drug decreased.

➤*Drug/Lab test interactions:*

Thyroid function tests – Decreased levels of thyroxine-binding globulin, resulting in decreased total T_4 serum levels and increased resin uptake of T_3 and T_4. Free thyroid hormone levels remain unchanged, and there is no clinical evidence of thyroid dysfunction.

Adverse Reactions

Women –

Most common: Amenorrhea and other menstrual irregularities; inhibition of gonadotropin secretion and virilization, including deepening voice and clitoral enlargement. The latter usually is not reversible after androgens are discontinued. When administered to a pregnant woman, androgens cause virilization of external genitalia of the female fetus.

Androgen Adverse Reactions[a] (%)

Adverse reaction	Oral	Injection	Transdermal	Implant	Topical (5 to 10 g dose)
Cardiovascular					
CHF	—	—	1	—	—
Hypertension	—	—	less than 1	—	less than 3
Tachycardia	—	—	less than 1	—	—
Stroke	—	—	2	—	—
Deep vein phlebitis	—	—	1	—	—
Peripheral edema	—	—	—	—	1.4 to 3.1
Vasodilation	—	—	—	—	less than 1
Peripheral vascular disease	—	—	less than 1	—	—
CNS					
Headache	✓	✓	1 to 6	✓	less than 4
Pain	—	—	2	—	—
Asthenia	—	—	2	—	less than 3
Libido increased	✓	✓	1	✓	—
Memory loss	—	—	1	—	—
Nervousness/Anxiety	✓	✓	less than 1	✓	less than 3
Depression	✓	✓	less than 3	✓	less than 1
Dizziness/Vertigo	—	—	1 to 6	—	less than 1
Dry mouth	—	—	less than 1	—	—
Insomnia	—	—	less than 1	—	—
Libido decreased	✓	✓	less than 1	✓	1 to 3
Personality disorder	—	—	less than 1	—	—
CNS stimulation	—	—	less than 1	—	—
Generalized paresthesia	✓	✓	less than 1	✓	less than 1
Emotional lability	—	—	—	—	less than 3
Amnesia	—	—	—	—	less than 1
Hostility	—	—	—	—	less than 1
Fatigue	—	—	less than 1	—	—
Confusion	—	—	less than 1	—	—
Thinking abnormalities	—	—	less than 1	—	—
Dermatologic					
Application site itching	—	—	7 to 12	—	—
Application site erythema	—	—	3 to 7	—	—
Application site discomfort	—	—	4	—	—
Application site irritation	—	—	2	—	—
Pruritus	—	—	2 to 37	—	—
Burning sensation	—	—	3	—	—
Rash	—	—	1 to 2	—	—
Acne	✓	✓	1 to 4	✓	2.8 to 12.5
Alopecia	—	—	less than 1	—	less than 1
Male pattern baldness	✓	✓	—	✓	—
Hirsutism	✓	✓	less than 1	✓	less than 1
Other application site reactions	—	—	less than 6	—	3.1 to 10
Injection site pain/inflammation	—	✓	—	✓	—
Burn-like blister under system	—	—	12	—	—
Seborrhea	—	✓	—	—	—
Discolored hair	—	—	—	—	less than 1
Dry skin	—	—	—	—	less than 1
GI					
Abdominal pain	—	—	less than 1	—	—
Diarrhea	—	—	less than 1	—	—
Nausea	✓	✓	less than 1	✓	—
Cholestatic jaundice	✓	✓	—	✓	—
Abnormal liver function tests	✓	✓	1	✓	—
Hepatocellular neoplasms	✓	✓	—	✓	—
Peliosis hepatis	✓	✓	—	✓	—
GI bleeding	—	—	2	—	—
Increased appetite	—	—	less than 1	—	—
Stomatitis	—	—	✓	—	—
GU					
Abnormal ejaculation	—	—	less than 1	—	—
Breast pain/tenderness	—	—	1 to 3	—	1 to 3
Dysuria	—	—	less than 1	—	—

Adverse reaction	Oral	Injection	Transdermal	Implant	Topical (5 to 10 g dose)
UTI/Prostatitis	—	—	1 to 4	—	—
Impaired urination	—	—	less than 1	—	less than 2.8
Frequent erections	✓	✓	—	✓	—
Prolonged erection	✓	✓	—	✓	—
Oligospermia	✓	✓	—	✓	—
Scrotal cellulitis	—	—	1	—	—
BPH	—	—	1	—	—
Rectal mucosal lesion over prostate	—	—	1	—	—
Hematuria/Bladder cancer	—	—	1	—	—
Papilloma on scrotum	—	—	1	—	—
Prostate disorder	—	—	less than 5	—	2.8 to 18.8[b]
Testes disorder	—	—	less than 1	—	less than 3
Penis disorder	—	—	less than 1	—	less than 1
Pelvic pain	—	—	less than 1	—	—
Incontinence	—	—	less than 1	—	—
Gynecomastia	✓	✓	1 to 5	✓	less than 3
Hematologic					
Suppression of clotting factors	✓	✓	—	✓	—
Polycythemia	✓	✓	—	✓	—
Motabolic/Nutritional					
Hyperglycemia	—	—	less than 1	—	—
Hyperlipidemia	—	—	less than 1	—	—
Hyponatremia	—	—	less than 1	—	—
Electrolyte imbalance	✓	✓	—	✓	—
Increased serum cholesterol	✓	✓	—	✓	—
Abnormal lab tests[3]	—	—	—	—	4.2 to 6.3

Androgen Adverse Reactions[a] (%)

Adverse reaction	Oral	Injection	Transdermal	Implant	Topical (5 to 10 g dose)
Musculoskeletal					
Myalgia	—	—	2	—	—
Back pain	—	—	less than 1	—	—
Arthralgia	—	—	less than 1	—	—
Miscellaneous					
Accidental injury	—	—	2	—	—
Flu syndrome	—	—	1	—	—
Infection	—	—	less than 1	—	—
Anaphylaxis	✓	✓	—	✓	—
Accelerated growth	—	—	less than 1	—	—
Bronchitis	—	—	less than 1	—	—
Papillary dilation	—	—	1	—	—
Sweating	—	—	—	—	less than 1

– = No data.
✓ = Reported, incidence not listed.
[a] Data pooled from separate studies and are not necessarily comparable.
[b] Including prostate enlargement, BPH, elevated PSA results, new diagnosis of prostate cancer.
[c] Including abnormal hemoglobin, hematocrit, triglycerides, serum lipids, potassium, glucose, creatinine, bilirubin, liver function tests.

Overdosage

There is one report of acute overdosage by injection of testosterone enanthate: Testosterone levels of up to 11,400 ng/dL were implicated in a cerebrovascular accident.

Patient Information

Oral tablets may cause GI upset.

Notify physician if nausea, vomiting, swelling of the ankles (edema), too frequent or persistent erections of the penis, changes in skin color, and breathing disturbances, including those associated with sleep, occur.

➤*Women:* Notify physician if hoarseness, deepening of the voice, increases in facial hair, acne, or menstrual irregularities occur.

Advise male adolescent patients receiving androgens for delayed puberty to have bone development checked every 6 months.

TESTOSTERONE ENANTHATE (IN OIL)

c-iii	**Delatestryl** (Savient[a])	**Injection:** 200 mg/mL	In 5 mL multidose vials and 1 mL single dose syringes with needle.[b]

[a] Savient Pharmaceuticals, Inc., 70 Wood Avenue South, Iselin, NJ, 08830; (732) 632-8800, FAX (732) 632-8844.

[b] In sesame oil with 5 mg chlorobutanol.

TESTOSTERONE ENANTHATE — INJECTION

For complete and comparative prescribing information, refer to the Androgens group monograph.

Indications

➤*Males:* Testosterone enanthate injection is indicated for replacement therapy in conditions associated with a deficiency or absence of endogenous testosterone.

Primary hypogonadism (congenital or acquired) – Testicular failure due to cryptorchidism; bilateral torsion, orchitis, vanishing testis syndrome, or orchidectomy.

Hypogonadotropic hypogonadism (congenital or acquired) – Idiopathic gonadotropin or luteinizing hormone-releasing hormone (LHRH) deficiency, or pituitary-hypothalamic injury from tumors, trauma, or radiation. (Appropriate adrenal cortical and thyroid hormone replacement therapy are still necessary, however, and are actually of primary importance.)

If the above conditions occur prior to puberty, androgen replacement therapy will be needed during the adolescent years for development of secondary sexual characteristics. Prolonged androgen treatment will be required to maintain sexual characteristics in these and other males who develop testosterone deficiency after puberty.

Delayed puberty – Testosterone enanthate injection may be used to stimulate puberty in carefully selected males with clearly delayed puberty. These patients usually have a familial pattern of delayed puberty that is not secondary to a pathological disorder; puberty is expected to occur spontaneously at a relatively late date. Brief treatment with conservative doses may occasionally be justified in these patients if they do not respond to psychological support. The potential adverse effect on bone maturation should be discussed with the patient and parents prior to androgen administration. An x-ray of the hand and wrist to determine bone age should be obtained every 6 months to assess the effect of treatment on the epiphyseal centers.

➤*Females:*

Metastatic mammary cancer – Testosterone enanthate injection may be used secondarily in women with advancing inoperable metastatic (skeletal) mammary cancer who are 1 to 5 years postmenopausal. Primary goals of therapy in these women include ablation of the ovaries. Other methods of counteracting estrogen activity are adrenalectomy, hypophysectomy, or antiestrogen therapy. This treatment has also been used in premenopausal women with breast cancer who have benefited from oophorectomy and are considered to have a hormone-responsive tumor. Judgment concerning androgen therapy should be made by an oncologist with expertise in this field.

Administration and Dosage

Dosage and duration of therapy with testosterone enanthate injection will depend on age, sex, diagnosis, patient's response to treatment, and appearance of adverse effects. When properly given, injections of testosterone enanthate are well tolerated. Care should be taken to inject the preparation deeply into the gluteal muscle following the usual precautions for IM administration. In general, total doses above 400 mg monthly are not required because of the prolonged action of the preparation. Injections more frequently than every 2 weeks are rarely indicated.

Use of a wet needle or wet syringe may cause the solution to become cloudy; however this does not affect the potency of the material. Parenteral drug products should be inspected visually for particulate matter and discoloration prior to administration, whenever solution and container permit. Testosterone enanthate injection is a clear, colorless to pale yellow solution.

➤*Male hypogonadism:* As replacement therapy (ie, for eunuchism) the suggested dosage is 50 to 400 mg every 2 to 4 weeks.

➤*In males with delayed puberty:* Various dosage regimens have been used; some call for lower dosages initially with gradual increases as puberty progresses, with or without a decrease to maintenance levels. Other regimens call for higher dosage to induce pubertal changes and lower dosage for maintenance after puberty. The chronological and skeletal ages must be taken into consideration, both in determining the initial dose and in adjusting the dose. Dosage is within the range of 50 to 200 mg every 2 to 4 weeks for a limited duration, for example, 4 to 6 months. X-rays should be taken at appropriate intervals to determine the amount of bone maturation and skeletal development (see Indications).

➤*Palliation of inoperable mammary cancer in women:* A dosage of 200 to 400 mg every 2 to 4 weeks is recommended. Women with metastatic breast carcinoma must be followed closely because androgen therapy occasionally appears to accelerate the disease.

TESTOSTERONE ENANTHATE — INJECTION

➤*Directions for use:* Directions for use of unimatic single dose syringe:

1.) Screw the threaded tip of the plunger rod clockwise into the cartridge plunger, and push forward a few millimeters to break any friction between the cartridge plunger and syringe barrel.

2.) Remove the needle guard, hold the syringe erect, and push plunger forward until a drop appears at tip of needle and all of the air is evacuated. Following the usual aspiration procedure, complete the injection.

3.) Destroy the needle and syringe immediately after use.

➤*Storage/Stability:* Testosterone enanthate injection should be stored at room temperature. Warming and rotating the syringe unit or vial between the palms of the hands will redissolve any crystals that may have formed during storage at low temperatures.

TESTOSTERONE CYPIONATE (IN OIL)

c-iii	**Depo-Testosterone** (Pharmacia)	**Injection:** 100 mg/mL	In 10 mL vials.[a]
c-iii	**Testosterone Cypionate** (Watson)	**Injection:** 200 mg/mL	Benzyl alcohol, cotton seed oil. In 10 mL multi-dose vials.
c-iii	**Depo-Testosterone** (Pharmacia)		In 1 and 10 mL vials.[b]

[a] In cottonseed oil 736 mg with benzyl benzoate 0.1 mL and benzyl alcohol 9.45 mg.

[b] In cottonseed oil 560 mg with benzyl benzoate 0.2 mL and benzyl alcohol 9.45 mg.

TESTOSTERONE CYPIONATE — INJECTION

For complete and comparative prescribing information, refer to the Androgens group monograph.

Indications

➤*Replacement therapy:* Testosterone cypionate sterile solution is indicated for replacement therapy in the male in conditions associated with symptoms of deficiency or absence of endogenous testosterone.

Primary hypogonadism (congenital or acquired) – Primary hypogonadism (congenital or acquired)-testicular failure caused by cryptorchidism, bilateral torsion, orchitis, vanishing testis syndrome; or orchidectomy.

Hypogonadotropic hypogonadism (congenital or acquired) – Hypogonadotropic hypogonadism (congenital or acquired)-idiopathic gonadotropin or LHRH deficiency, or pituitary-hypothalamic injury from tumors, trauma, or radiation.

Administration and Dosage

Testosterone cypionate sterile solution is for intramuscular use only. IM injections should be given deep in the gluteal muscle.

It should not be given IV.

Testosterone cypionate should not be used interchangeably with testosterone propionate because of differences in duration of action.

The suggested dosage for testosterone cypionate sterile solution varies depending on the age, sex, and diagnosis of the individual patient. Dosage is adjusted according to the patient's response and the appearance of adverse reactions.

Various dosage regimens have been used to induce pubertal changes in hypogonadal males; some experts have advocated lower dosages initially, gradually increasing the dose as puberty progresses, with or without a decrease to maintenance levels. Other experts emphasize that higher dosages are needed to induce pubertal changes and lower dosages can be used for maintenance after puberty. The chronological and skeletal ages must be taken into consideration, both in determining the initial dose and in adjusting the dose.

For replacement in the hypogonadal male, 50 to 400 mg should be administered every 2 to 4 weeks.

➤*Storage/Stability:* Vials should be stored at controlled room temperature 20° to 25°C (68° to 77°F) (see USP). Protect from light.

Parenteral drug products should be inspected visually for particulate matter and discoloration prior to administration, whenever solution and container permit. Warming and shaking the vial should redissolve any crystals that may have formed during storage at temperatures lower than recommended.

TESTOSTERONE PELLETS

c-iii	**Testopel** (Bartor Pharmacal)	**Pellets:** 75 mg	0.2 mg stearic acid, 2 mg polyvinylpyrroidone. 1 pellet/vial. In 3s, 10s, and 100s.

TESTOSTERONE PELLETS

For complete and comparative prescribing information, refer to the Androgens group monograph.

Indications

➤*Replacement therapy:*

Primary hypogonadism (congenital or acquired) – Testicular failure caused by cryptorchidism, bilateral torsion, orchitis, vanishing testis syndrome, or orchidectomy.

Hypogonadotropic hypogonadism (congenital or acquired) – Idiopathic gonadotropin or LHRH deficiency, or pituitary-hypothalamic injury from tumors, trauma, or radiation.

If these conditions occur prior to puberty, androgen replacement therapy will be needed during the adolescent years for development of secondary sexual characteristics. Prolonged androgen treatment will be required to maintain sexual characteristics in these and other males who develop testosterone deficiency after puberty.

Delayed puberty – To stimulate puberty in carefully selected males with clearly delayed puberty. These patients usually have a familial pattern of delayed puberty that is not secondary to a pathological disorder; puberty is expected to occur spontaneously at a relatively late date. Brief treatment with conservative doses may occasionally be justified in these patients if they do not respond to psychological support. Discuss the potential adverse effect on bone maturation with the patient and parents prior to androgen administration. Obtain an x-ray of the hand and wrist every 6 months to determine bone age and assess the effect of treatment on the epiphyseal centers.

Administration and Dosage

The suggested dosage for androgens varies depending on the age and diagnosis of the individual patient. Dosage is adjusted according to the patient's response and the appearance of adverse reactions.

➤*Replacement therapy:* The dosage guideline for testosterone pellets for replacement therapy in androgen-deficient males is 150 to 450 mg SC every 3 to 6 months. Various dosage regimens have been used to induce pubertal changes in hypogonadal males; some experts have advocated lower dosages initially, gradually increasing the dose as puberty progresses, with or without a decrease to maintenance levels. Other experts emphasize that higher dosages are needed to induce pubertal changes and lower dosages can be used for maintenance after puberty. The chronological and skeletal ages must be taken into consideration, both in determining the initial dose and in adjusting the dose.

➤*Delayed puberty:* Dosages used in delayed puberty generally are in the lower range of that listed above, and for a limited time duration, for example 4 to 6 months.

➤*Determination of dose:* The number of pellets to be implanted depends upon the minimal daily requirement of testosterone propionate determined by a gradual reduction of the amount administered parenterally. The usual ratio is as follows: Implant two 75 mg pellets for each 25 mg testosterone propionate required weekly. Thus, when a patient requires injections of 75 mg/week, it is usually necessary to implant 450 mg (6 pellets). With injections of 50 mg/week, implantation of 300 mg (4 pellets) may suffice for ≈ 3 months. With lower requirements by injection, correspondingly lower amounts may be implanted. It has been found that ≈ ⅓ of the material is absorbed in the first month, ¼ in the second month, and ⅙ in the third month. Adequate effect of the pellets ordinarily continues for 3 to 4 months, sometimes as long as 6 months.

➤*Storage/Stability:* Store in a cool place.

TESTOSTERONE TRANSDERMAL SYSTEM

	Product/Distributor	Release rate (mg/24 hr)	Total contact surface area (cm^2)	Total testosterone content (mg)	How supplied
c-iii	**Androderm** (Watson Pharma)	5	44	24.3	In 30s.
c-iii	**Androderm** (Watson Pharma)	2.5	37	12.2	In 60s.

TESTOSTERONE — TRANSDERMAL

For complete and comparative prescribing information, refer to the Androgens group monograph.

Indications

➤*Replacement therapy:* Testosterone transdermal system is indicated for testosterone replacement therapy in adult males for conditions associated with a deficiency or absence of endogenous testosterone:

➤*Primary hypogonadism (congenital or acquired):* Testicular failure due to cryptorchidism, bilateral torsion, orchitis, vanishing testis syndrome, orchidectomy, Klinefelter syndrome, chemotherapy, or toxic damage from alcohol or heavy metals. These men usually have low serum testosterone levels and gonadotropins (follicle-stimulating hormone [FSH], luteinizing hormone [LH]) above the normal range.

➤*Hypogonadotropic hypogonadism (congenital or acquired):* Idiopathic gonadotropin or luteinizing hormone-releasing hormone (LHRH) deficiency or pituitary-hypothalamic injury from tumors, trauma, or radiation. These men have low serum testosterone concentrations without associated elevation in gonadotropins.

Administration and Dosage

➤*Approved by the FDA:* September 29, 1995.

➤*Dosage:* The usual starting dose is 1 testosterone 5 mg transdermal system or 2 testosterone 2.5 mg transdermal systems applied nightly for 24 hours, providing a total dose of 5 mg/day.

To ensure proper dosing, measure the morning serum testosterone concentration following system application the previous evening. If the serum concentration is outside the normal range, repeat sampling with assurance of proper system adhesion as well as appropriate application time. Confirmed serum concentrations outside the normal range may require increasing the daily dose to 7.5 mg (ie, one 5 mg and one 2.5 mg system or three 2.5 mg systems) or decreasing the daily dose to 2.5 mg (one 2.5 mg system), maintaining nightly application. Because of variability in analytical values among diagnostic laboratories, perform this laboratory work and any later analyses for assessing the effect of testosterone transdermal system therapy at the same laboratory so results can be compared.

Application of system – The adhesive side of the testosterone transdermal system should be applied to a clean, dry area of the skin on the back, abdomen, upper arms, or thighs. Avoid application over bony prominences or on a part of the body that may be subject to prolonged pressure during sleep or sitting (eg, deltoid region of the upper arm, greater trochanter of the femur, ischial tuberosity). Do not apply to the scrotum. Rotate the sites of application, with an interval of 7 days between applications to the same site. The area selected should not be oily, damaged, or irritated.

Apply the system immediately after opening the pouch and removing the protective release liner. Press the system firmly in place, making sure there is good contact with the skin, especially around the edges.

➤*Skin irritation:* Mild skin irritation may be ameliorated by treatment of the affected skin with over-the-counter topical hydrocortisone cream applied after system removal.

Applying a small amount of 0.1% triamcinolone acetonide cream (prescription) to the skin under the central drug reservoir of the testosterone transdermal system has been shown to reduce the incidence and severity of skin irritation. The administration of 0.1% triamcinolone acetonide cream (prescription) does not significantly alter transdermal absorption of testosterone from the system. Do not use ointment formulations for pretreatment as they may significantly reduce testosterone absorption.

➤*Nonvirilized patients:* Testosterone transdermal system therapy for nonvirilized patients may be initiated with one 2.5 mg/day system applied nightly.

➤*Storage/Stability:* Store at room temperature, 15° to 30°C (59° to 86°F). Apply to skin immediately upon removal from the protective pouch. Do not store outside the pouch provided. Do not use damaged systems. The drug reservoir may burst from excessive pressure or heat. Discard systems in household trash in a manner that prevents accidental application or ingestion by children, pets, or others.

Disposal – Discard used testosterone products in household trash in a manner that prevents accidental application or ingestion by children or pets. Contents are flammable.

TESTOSTERONE GEL

c-iii	**AndroGel 1%** (Unimed Pharm)	**Gel:** 1% testosterone	67% ethanol. Each packet contains 2.5 or 5 g gel to deliver testosterone 25 or 50 mg. In 30s. In metered-dose pumps to deliver 75 g or 60 metered 1.25 g doses.
c-iii	**Testim** (Auxilium Pharm[a])		74% ethanol, glycerin. In 5 g.

[a] Auxilium Pharmaceuticals, Inc., 160 W. Germantown Pike, Suite D5, Norristown, PA 19401; 610-278-6316.

TESTOSTERONE — TOPICAL

For complete and comparative prescribing information, refer to the Androgens group monograph.

Indications

➤*Replacement therapy:* Testosterone gel is indicated for testosterone replacement therapy in adult males for conditions associated with a deficiency or absence of endogenous testosterone:

Primary hypogonadism (congenital or acquired) – Testicular failure caused by cryptorchidism, bilateral torsion, orchitis, vanishing testis syndrome, orchidectomy, Klinefelter syndrome, chemotherapy, or toxic damage from alcohol or heavy metals. These men usually have low serum testosterone levels and gonadotropins (follicle-stimulating hormone [FSH], luteinizing hormone [LH]) above the normal range.

Hypogonadotropic hypogonadism (congenital or acquired) – Idiopathic gonadotropin or luteinizing hormone-releasing hormone (LHRH) deficiency or pituitary-hypothalamic injury from tumors, trauma, or radiation. These men have low serum testosterone concentrations without associated elevation in gonadotropins.

Administration and Dosage

➤*Approved by the FDA:* October 31, 2002 (*Testim*); February 28, 2000 (*AndroGel*).

The recommended starting dose of 1% testosterone gel is 5 g (to deliver testosterone 50 mg) applied once daily (preferably in the morning) to clean, dry, intact skin of the shoulders and/or upper arms or abdomen (*AndroGel* only). Upon opening the packet(s) or tube, squeeze the entire contents into the palm of the hand and immediately apply it to the application sites. Allow application sites to dry for a few minutes prior to dressing. Wash hands with soap and water after application. Cover the application sites with clothing after gel has dried.

Do not apply the gel to the genitals. Do not apply *Testim* to the abdomen.

It is unknown for how long showering or swimming should be delayed. For optimal absorption of testosterone from *AndroGel*, it appears reasonable to wait at least 5 to 6 hours after application prior to showering or swimming. Nevertheless, showering or swimming after just 1 hour should have a minimal effect on the amount absorbed if done infrequently. Do not wash the sites of application for at least 2 hours after application of *Testim*.

Measure serum testosterone levels 14 days after initiation of therapy to ensure proper dosing. If the serum testosterone concentration is below the normal range, or if the desired clinical response is not achieved, the dose may be increased from 5 to 7.5 g (*AndroGel*) or 10 g (*Testim*) and from 7.5 to 10 g (*AndroGel*), as instructed by the physician.

➤*Transfer of testosterone:*

AndroGel – The potential for dermal testosterone transfer following use was evaluated in vigorous skin-to-skin contact. Under study conditions, all unprotected female partners had a serum testosterone concentration greater than 2 times the baseline value at some time during the study. When a shirt covered the application site(s), the transfer of testosterone from the males to the female partners was completely prevented. Washing the area of contact on the other person as soon as possible with soap and water will remove residual testosterone from the skin surface.

Testim – The potential for dermal testosterone transfer following use was evaluated in 2 clinical trials with males dosed with *Testim* and their untreated female partners.

In couples asked to rub abdomen to abdomen, serum testosterone concentrations in female partners increased from baseline by at least 4 times and potential for transfer was seen at all timepoints.

When a shirt was used to cover the abdomen at 15 minutes postapplication and partners again rubbed abdomens for 15 minutes at the 1-hour timepoint, the potential for transfer was markedly reduced.

In the second trial, 100 mg *Testim* was applied to the male arms and shoulders. In 1 group, 15 minutes of direct skin to skin rubbing began at 4 hours after application. In these 6 women, all of whom showered immediately after the rubbing activity, mean maximum serum testosterone concentrations increased from baseline by approximately 4 times. When males wore a long-sleeved T-shirt and rubbing was started at 1 and at 4 hours after application, the transfer of testosterone from male to female partners was prevented.

In order to prevent transfer to another person, instruct patients to wear clothing to cover the application sites. If direct skin-to-skin contact with another person is anticipated, the application sites must be washed thoroughly with soap and water.

In order to maintain serum testosterone levels in the normal range, instruct patients not to wash the sites of application for at least 2 hours after application.

➤*Storage/Stability:* Store at room temperature 25°C (77°F); excursions permitted to 15° to 30°C (59° to 86°F).

Disposal – Discard used testosterone products in household trash in a manner that prevents accidental application or ingestion by children or pets. Contents are flammable.

TESTOSTERONE, BUCCAL

Rx	**Striant** (Columbia)	**Buccal system:** 30 mg testosterone	Lactose. In blister packs of 10 systems.

TESTOSTERONE — BUCCAL SYSTEM

For complete and comparative prescribing information, refer to the Androgens group monograph.

Indications

➤*Replacement therapy:* Testosterone buccal system is indicated for replacement therapy in men for conditions associated with a deficiency or absence of endogenous testosterone:

Hypogonadotropic hypogonadism (congenital or acquired) – Idiopathic gonadotropin or luteinizing hormone-releasing hormone (LHRH) deficiency, or pituitary hypothalamic injury from tumors, trauma, or radiation. These patients have low serum testosterone levels but have gonadotropins in the normal or low range.

Primary hypogonadism (congenital or acquired) – Testicular failure caused by cryptorchidism, bilateral torsion, orchitis, vanishing testis syndrome, orchidectomy, Klinefelter syndrome, chemotherapy, or toxic damage from alcohol or heavy metals. These men usually have low serum testosterone levels and gonadotropins (follicle-stimulating hormone [FSH], luteinizing hormone [LH]) above the normal range.

Administration and Dosage

➤*Approved by the FDA:* June 19, 2003.

The recommended dosing schedule for testosterone buccal system is the application of 1 buccal system 30 mg to the gum region twice daily; morning and evening (about 12 hours apart). Place testosterone buccal system in a comfortable position just above the incisor tooth (on either side of the mouth). With each application, rotate testosterone buccal system to alternate sides of the mouth.

Upon opening the packet, place the rounded side surface of the buccal system against the gum and hold it firmly in place with a finger over the lip and against the product for 30 seconds to ensure adhesion. Testosterone buccal system is designed to stay in position until removed. If the buccal system fails to properly adhere to the gum or falls off during the 12-hour dosing interval, remove the old buccal system and apply a new one. If the buccal system falls out of position within 4 hours prior to the next dose, apply a new buccal system and leave it in place until the time of next regularly scheduled dosing.

Take care to avoid dislodging the buccal system. Check to see if testosterone buccal system is in place following toothbrushing, use of mouthwash, and consumption of food or alcoholic/nonalcoholic beverages. Do not chew or swallow testosterone buccal system. To remove testosterone buccal system, gently slide it downward from the gum towards the tooth to avoid scratching the gum.

➤*Storage/Stability:* Store at 20° to 25°C (68° to 77°F). Protect from heat and moisture. Damaged blister packages should not be used. Dispose of discarded testosterone buccal systems in household trash in a manner that prevents accidental application or ingestion by children or pets.

METHYLTESTOSTERONE

c-iii	**Methyltestosterone** (Various, eg, Global)	**Tablets:** 10 mg	In 100s.
c-iii	**Methitest** (Global)		Lactose, sugar. (7037). White, scored. In 100s.
c-iii	**Methyltestosterone** (Various, eg, Global)	**Tablets:** 25 mg	In 100s.
c-iii	**Methitest** (Global)		Lactose, sugar. (7038). Yellow, scored. In 100s and 1000s.
c-iii	**Methyltestosterone** (Various, eg, Global)	**Tablets (buccal):** 10 mg	In 100s.
c-iii	**Android** (Valeant)	**Capsules:** 10 mg	(ICN 0901). Red. In 100s.
c-iii	**Testred** (Valeant)		(ICN 0901). Red. In 100s.
c-iii	**Virilon** (Star)		(Virilon 10 mg). Black and clear. In 100s and 1000s.

METHYLTESTOSTERONE — ORAL

For complete and comparative prescribing information, refer to the Androgens group monograph.

Indications

➤*Males:* Methyltestosterone is indicated for replacement therapy in conditions associated with a deficiency or absence of endogenous testosterone.

Primary hypogonadism (congenital or acquired) – Primary hypogonadism (congenital or acquired)—testicular failure caused by cryptorchidism, bilateral torsion, architis, vanishing testis syndrome; or orchidectomy.

Hypogonadotropic hypogonadism (congenital or acquired) – Hypogonadotropic hypogonadism (congenital or acquired) idiopathic gonadotropin or LHRH deficiency, or pituitary hypothalamic injury from tumors, trauma, or radiation. If the above conditions occur prior to puberty, androgen replacement therapy will be needed during the adolescent years to development of secondary sexual characteristics. Prolonged androgen treatment will be required to maintain sexual characteristics in these and other males who develop testosterone deficiency after puberty.

Delayed puberty – Androgens may be used to stimulate puberty in carefully selected males with clearly delayed puberty. These patients usually have a familial pattern of delayed puberty that is not secondary to a pathological disorder; puberty is expected to occur spontaneously at a relatively late date. Brief treatment with conservative doses may occasionally be justified in these patients if they do not respond to psychological support. The potential adverse effect on bone maturation should be discussed with the patient and parents prior to androgen administration. An x-ray of the hand and wrist to determine bone age should be obtained every 6 months to assess the effect of treatment on the epiphyseal centers.

➤*Females:*

Metastatic mammary cancer – Methyltestosterone may be used secondarily in women with advancing inoperable metastatic (skeletal) mammary cancer who are 1 to 5 years postmenopausal. Primary goals of therapy in these women include ablation of the ovaries. Other methods of counteracting estrogen activity are adrenalectomy, hypophysectomy, or antiestrogen therapy. This treatment has also been used in premenopausal women with breast cancer who have benefited from oophorectomy and are considered to have a hormone responsive tumor. Judgment concerning androgen therapy should be made by an oncologist with expertise in this field.

Administration and Dosage

➤*Approved by the FDA:* November 24, 1982.

Dosage must be strictly individualized. The suggested dose for androgens varies depending on the age, sex, and diagnosis of the individual patient. Dosage is adjusted according to the patient's response and the appearance of adverse reactions.

➤*Males:* See below for replacement therapy guidelines in androgen-deficient males. Various dosage recommendations have been used to induce pubertal changes in hypogonadal males. Some experts have advocated lower dosages initially, gradually increasing the dose as puberty progresses, with or without a decrease to maintenance levels. Other experts emphasize that higher dosages are needed to induce pubertal changes, and lower dosages can be used for maintenance after puberty. The chronological and skeletal ages must be taken into consideration, both in determining the initial dose and in adjusting the dose.

Dosages used in delayed puberty generally are in the lower ranges of those given below, and for a limited duration (eg, 4 to 6 months).

Guidelines for androgen replacement therapy in the male – Methyltestosterone (oral) 10 to 50 mg administered daily.

➤*Females:* Women with metastatic breast carcinoma must be followed closely because androgen therapy occasionally appears to accelerate the disease. Thus, many experts prefer to use the shorter-acting androgen preparations rather than those with prolonged activity for treating breast carcinoma, particularly during the early stages of androgen therapy.

Guideline dosages of androgens for use in palliative treatment of women with metastatic breast carcinoma are given below.

Guidelines for androgen replacement therapy in breast carcinoma in females – Methyltestosterone (oral) 50 to 200 mg administered daily.

➤*Storage/Stability:* Keep out of reach of children. Dispense in tight container as defined in the USP, with a child-resistant closure.

Store at controlled room temperature 15° to 30°C (59° to 83°F).

FLUOXYMESTERONE

c-iii	**Fluoxymesterone** (Various, eg, Major, Rosemont, United)	**Tablets:** 10 mg	In 100s.
c-iii	**Androxy** (Upsher-Smith)		Lactose. (832 86). Green, scored. In 100s.

FLUOXYMESTERONE — ORAL

For complete and comparative prescribing information, refer to the Androgens group monograph.

Indications

➤*Men:*

Replacement therapy – Fluoxymesterone is indicated in conditions associated with symptoms of deficiency or absence of endogenous testosterone.

Primary hypogonadism (congenital or acquired): Fluoxymesterone is indicated for testicular failure due to cryptorchidism, bilateral torsion, orchitis, vanishing testis syndrome, or orchidectomy.

Hypogonadotropic hypogonadism (congenital or acquired): Fluoxymesterone is indicated in idiopathic gonadotropin or LHRH deficiency, or pituitary-hypothalamic injury from tumors, trauma, or radiation.

Delayed puberty – Fluoxymesterone is indicated for delayed puberty provided it has been definitely established as such, and is not just a familial trait.

➤*Women:*

Metastatic mammary cancer – Fluoxymesterone tablets may be used secondarily in women with advancing inoperable metastatic (skeletal) mammary cancer who are 1 to 5 years postmenopausal. This treatment has been used in premenopausal women with breast cancer who have benefited from oophorectomy and are considered to have a hormone-responsive tumor. Judgment concerning androgen therapy should be made by an oncologist with expertise in this field.

➤*Unlabeled uses:* Palliative treatment of androgen-responsive, recurrent breast cancer in premenopausal women after oophorectomy.

Administration and Dosage

➤*Approved by the FDA:* October 21, 1983.

May be given as a single daily dose or in divided doses. Dosage and duration of therapy will depend on age, sex, diagnosis, patient's response to treatment, and appearance of adverse effects.

➤*Male delayed puberty:* Dosage is within the range of 2.5 to 20 mg daily, although generally in the lower range of 2.5 to 10 mg daily, and for a limited duration, for example 4 to 6 months. X-rays should be taken at appropriate intervals to determine the amount of bone maturation and skeletal development.

➤*Male hypogonadism:* As replacement therapy (for eunuchism) a daily dose of 5 to 20 mg is suggested. It is usually preferable to start therapy at a higher level within the range (eg, 10 mg) with subsequent adjustment as required.

➤*Metastatic mammary cancer in women:* A daily dose of 10 to 40 mg given in divided doses is recommended. Treatment should be continued for 3 months or more. Patients must be followed closely because androgen therapy occasionally appears to accelerate the disease.

Hormone therapy is adjunctive to and not a replacement for conventional therapy. Duration of therapy will depend on the response of the condition and the appearance of adverse reactions.

➤*Storage/Stability:* Store at controlled room temperature 20° to 25°C (68° to 77°F).

DANAZOL

Rx	Danazol (Various, eg, Barr)	Capsules: 50 mg	In 100s.
		100 mg	In 100s.
		200 mg	In 60s, 100s, and 500s.

DANAZOL — ORAL

WARNING

Use of danazol in pregnancy is contraindicated. A sensitive test (eg, beta subunit test if available) capable of determining early pregnancy is recommended immediately prior to start of therapy. Additionally, a nonhormonal method of contraception should be used during therapy. If a patient becomes pregnant while taking danazol, discontinue administration of the drug and apprise the patient of the potential risk to the fetus.

Thromboembolism, thrombotic and thrombophlebitic events, including sagittal sinus thrombosis and life-threatening or fatal strokes have been reported.

Experience with long-term therapy with danazol is limited. Peliosis hepatis and benign hepatic adenoma have been observed with long-term use. Peliosis hepatis and hepatic adenoma may be silent until complicated by acute, potentially life-threatening intra-abdominal hemorrhage. Therefore, alert the physician to this possibility. Attempts should be made to determine the lowest dose that will provide adequate protection (see Warnings).

Danazol has been associated with several cases of benign intracranial hypertension also known as pseudotumor cerebri. Early signs and symptoms of benign intracranial hypertension include papilledema, headache, nausea and vomiting, and visual disturbances. Screen patients with these symptoms for papilledema and, if present, advise the patients to discontinue danazol immediately and refer them to a neurologist for further diagnosis and care.

Indications

➤*Endometriosis:* For the treatment of endometriosis amenable to hormonal management.

➤*Fibrocystic breast disease:* Most cases of symptomatic fibrocystic breast disease may be treated by simple measures (eg, padded bras, analgesics). Pain and tenderness may be severe enough to warrant suppression of ovarian function. Danazol is usually effective in decreasing modularity, pain, and tenderness, but it considerably alters hormone levels. Recurrence of symptoms is very common after cessation of therapy.

➤*Hereditary angioedema:* For the prevention of attacks of angioedema (eg, cutaneous, abdominal, laryngeal) in men and women.

➤*Unlabeled uses:* Danazol has been used to treat precocious puberty, gynecomastia, and menorrhagia. It has also been studied in the treatment of idiopathic immune thrombocytopenia, lupus-associated thrombocytopenia, and autoimmune hemolytic anemia.

Administration and Dosage

➤*Endometriosis:* Begin therapy during menstruation or make sure the patient is not pregnant. In moderate-to-severe disease, or in patients infertile because of endometriosis, administer 800 mg daily in 2 divided doses to best achieve amenorrhea and rapid response to painful symptoms. Downward titration to a dose sufficient to maintain amenorrhea may be considered depending upon response. Initially, for mild cases, give 200 to 400 mg in 2 divided doses. Individualize dosage. Continue therapy uninterrupted for 3 to 6 months; may extend to 9 months. If symptoms recur after termination, treatment can be reinstituted.

➤*Fibrocystic breast disease:* Begin therapy during menstruation or make sure patient is not pregnant. Dosage ranges from 100 to 400 mg daily in 2 divided doses. A nonhormonal method of contraception is recommended when danazol is administered at this dose because ovulation may not be suppressed.

Breast pain and tenderness are usually relieved by the first month and eliminated in 2 to 3 months; elimination of nodularity requires 4 to 6 months of uninterrupted therapy. Regular or irregular menstrual patterns and amenorrhea each occur in approximately one third of patients treated with at least 100 mg doses. Approximately 50% of patients may have recurring symptoms within 1 year; treatment may be reinstituted.

➤*Hereditary angioedema:* Individualize dosage. Recommended starting dose is 200 mg 2 or 3 times daily. After a favorable initial response, determine continuing dosage by decreasing the dosage by 50% or less at intervals of at least1 to 3 months if frequency of attacks prior to treatment dictates. If an attack occurs, increase dosage by 200 mg daily or less. During the dose-adjusting phase, monitor response closely, particularly if patient has a history of airway involvement.

➤*Storage/Stability:* Store at controlled room temperature, 15° to 30°C (59° to 86°F).

Actions

➤*Pharmacology:* A synthetic androgen derived from ethisterone, danazol suppresses the pituitary-ovarian axis by inhibiting the output of pituitary gonadotropins. It also has weak, androgenic activity. Danazol depresses the output of both follicle-stimulating hormone (FSH) and luteinizing hormone (LH). Evidence suggests direct inhibitory effect at gonadal sites and a binding of danazol to receptors of gonadal steroids at target organs. In addition, danazol has been shown to significantly decrease IgG, IgM, and IgA levels, as well as phospholipid and IgG isotope autoantibodies in patients with endometriosis and associated elevations of autoantibodies. Generally, the pituitary suppressive action is reversible. Ovulation and cyclic bleeding usually return within 60 to 90 days after therapy is discontinued.

Endometriosis – In the treatment of endometriosis, danazol alters the normal and ectopic endometrial tissue so that it becomes inactive and atrophic. Complete resolution of endometrial lesions occurs in the majority of cases. Changes in vaginal cytology and cervical mucus reflect the suppressive effect of danazol on the pituitary-ovarian axis.

Hereditary angioedema – Danazol prevents attacks of the disease characterized by episodic edema of the abdominal viscera, extremities, face, and airway that may be disabling and, if the airway is involved, fatal. In addition, danazol partially or completely corrects the primary biochemical abnormality of hereditary angioedema. It increases the levels of the deficient C1 esterase inhibitor, thereby increasing the serum levels of the C4 component of the complement system.

➤*Pharmacokinetics:* Blood levels of danazol do not increase proportionately with increases in dose. When the dose is doubled, plasma levels increase only approximately 35% to 40%.

Contraindications

Undiagnosed abnormal genital bleeding; markedly impaired hepatic, renal, or cardiac function.

Pregnancy and lactation.

Patients with porphyria. Danazol can induce aminolevulinate acid (ALA) synthetase activity and hence porphyrin metabolism.

Warnings

➤*Thrombotic events:* Thromboembolism, thrombotic and thrombophlebitic events including sagittal sinus thrombosis and life-threatening or fatal strokes have been reported.

➤*Hepatic effects:* Experience with long-term therapy with danazol is limited. Peliosis hepatis and benign hepatic adenoma have been observed with long-term use. Peliosis hepatis and hepatic adenoma may be silent until complicated by acute, potentially life-threatening intra-abdominal hemorrhage. Therefore, alert the physician to this possibility. Make attempts to determine the lowest dose that will provide adequate protection. If the drug was begun at a time of exacerbation of hereditary angioneurotic edema because of trauma, stress, or other cause, consider periodic attempts to decrease or withdraw therapy.

➤*Intracranial hypertension:* Danazol has been associated with several cases of benign intracranial hypertension (also known as pseudotumor cerebri). Early signs and symptoms of benign intracranial hypertension include papilledema, headache, nausea and vomiting, and visual disturbances. Screen patients with these symptoms for papilledema and, if present, advise the patients to discontinue danazol immediately and refer them to a neurologist for further diagnosis and care.

➤*Lipoprotein alterations:* A temporary alteration of lipoproteins in the form of decreased high density lipoproteins (HDL) and possibly increased low density lipoproteins (LDL) has been reported during danazol therapy. These alterations may be marked, and prescribers should consider the potential impact on the risk of atherosclerosis and coronary artery disease in accordance with the potential benefit of the therapy to the patient.

➤*Carcinoma of the breast:* Exclude carcinoma of the breast before initiating therapy for fibrocystic breast disease. Nodularity, pain, and tenderness because of fibrocystic disease may prevent recognition of underlying carcinoma; therefore, if any nodule persists or enlarges during treatment, rule out carcinoma.

➤*Long-term experience:* Long-term experience with danazol is limited. Long-term therapy with other steroids alkylated at the 17 position has been associated with serious toxicity (eg, cholestatic jaundice, peliosis hepatis). Similar toxicity may develop after long-term danazol. Determine the lowest dose that will provide adequate protection. If the drug was begun for exacerbation of angioneurotic edema because of trauma, stress, or another cause, consider decreasing or withdrawing therapy periodically.

➤*Androgenic effects:* Androgenic effects may not be reversible even when the drug is discontinued. Watch patients closely for signs of virilization.

➤*Pregnancy: Category X.* Use of danazol in pregnancy is contraindicated. A sensitive test (eg, beta subunit test if available) capable of determining early pregnancy is recommended immediately prior to start of therapy. Additionally, a nonhormonal method of contraception should be used during therapy. If a patient becomes pregnant while taking danazol, discontinue administration of the drug and apprise the patient of the potential risk to the fetus. Exposure to danazol in utero may result in androgenic effects on the female fetus; reports of clitoral hypertrophy, labial fusion, urogenital sinus defect, vaginal atresia, and ambiguous genitalia have been received.

In rabbits, the administration of danazol on days 6 to 18 of gestation at doses of at least 60 mg/kg daily (2 to 4 times the human dose) resulted in inhibition of fetal development.

➤*Lactation:* Breast-feeding is contraindicated in patients taking danazol.

➤*Children:* Safety and efficacy in children have not been established.

DANAZOL — ORAL

Precautions

➤*Monitoring:*

Fluid retention – Conditions influenced by edema (eg, epilepsy, migraine, cardiac or renal dysfunction) require careful observation.

Hepatic dysfunction – Hepatic dysfunction has been reported manifested by modest increases in serum transaminase levels; perform periodic liver function tests.

Lipoproteins – Monitor HDL and LDL periodically.

Semen – Semen should be checked for volume, viscosity, sperm count, and motility.

➤*Porphyria:* Danazol administration has been reported to cause exacerbation of the manifestations of acute intermittent porphyria.

Drug Interactions

Danazol Drug Interactions			
Precipitant drug	Object drug[a]		Description
Danazol	Carbamazepine	↑	Therapy with danazol may cause an increase in carbamazepine levels in patients taking both drugs.
Danazol	Cyclosporine	↑	Increased cyclosporine blood concentrations with possible toxicity (eg, nephrotoxicity) has occurred. Monitor serum bilirubin, serum creatinine, and cyclosporine concentrations in patients receiving concomitant therapy. Adjust doses of drugs as needed.
Danazol	Warfarin	↑	Prolongation of prothrombin time has been reported with concomitant use.

[a] ↑ = Object drug increased.

➤*Drug/Lab test interactions:* Danazol treatment may interfere with laboratory determinations of testosterone, androstenedione, and dehydroepiandrosterone.

Abnormalities in laboratory tests may occur during therapy with danazol including the following: CPK, glucose tolerance, glucagon, thyroid-binding globulin, sex hormone-binding globulin, other plasma proteins, lipids, and lipoproteins.

Adverse Reactions

Androgenic – Acne; edema; mild hirsutism; changes in the voice (eg, hoarseness, sore throat, instability, deepening of pitch); oily skin or hair; weight gain; seborrhea; hair loss; clitoral hypertrophy (rare).

➤*GU:* Menstrual disturbances including spotting; alteration of the timing of the cycle; amenorrhea. Although cyclical bleeding and ovulation usually return within 60 to 90 days after discontinuation of therapy with danazol, persistent amenorrhea has occasionally been reported. In the male, a modest reduction in spermatogenesis may occur during treatment. Abnormalities in semen volume, viscosity, sperm count, and motility may occur with long-term therapy.

Hypoestrogenic – Flushing; sweating; vaginal dryness/irritation; reduction in breast size; nervousness; emotional lability.

➤*Hepatic:* Dysfunction (elevated serum enzymes or jaundice) has been reported in patients receiving at least 400 mg daily. It is recommended that patients receiving danazol be monitored for hepatic dysfunction by laboratory tests and clinical observation. Serious hepatic toxicity, including cholestatic jaundice, peliosis hepatis, and hepatic adenoma has been reported.

➤*The following have been reported, but the causal relationship is not confirmed:*

CNS – Dizziness; headache; nervousness; emotional lability; fainting; weakness; Guillain-Barré syndrome; sleep disorders; fatigue; tremor; paresthesias; visual disturbances; anxiety; depression and changes in appetite; benign intracranial hypertension, convulsions (rare).

Dermatologic – Rashes (eg, maculopapular, vesicular, papular, purpuric, petechial); sun sensitivity, Stevens-Johnson syndrome (rare).

GI – Gastroenteritis; nausea; vomiting; constipation; pancreatitis (rare).

GU – Hematuria; prolonged posttherapy amenorrhea.

Hematologic – Increase in red cell and platelet count; reversible erythrocytosis, leukocytosis, or polycythemia; eosinophilia; leukopenia; thrombocytopenia.

Hypersensitivity – Urticaria, pruritus; nasal congestion (rare).

Musculoskeletal – Muscle cramps or spasms; pains; joint pain; joint lock-up; joint swelling; pain in back, neck, or extremities; carpal tunnel syndrome (rare, may be secondary to fluid retention).

Miscellaneous – Change in libido; elevated blood pressure; chills; increased insulin requirements in diabetic patients; cataracts, bleeding gums, fever, pelvic pain, nipple discharge, malignant liver tumors (after long-term use) (rare).

Patient Information

Notify physician if masculinizing effects occur (eg, abnormal growth of facial or other fine body hair, deepening of the voice).

Use nonhormonal contraceptive measures during therapy. Discontinue use if pregnancy is suspected.

Androgen Hormone Inhibitor

FINASTERIDE

Rx	**Propecia** (Merck)	**Tablets:** 1 mg	Lactose. (P Propecia). Tan, octagonal. Film-coated. In unit-of-use 30s, and *ProPAK* carton of 3 unit-of-use bottles of 30.
Rx	**Proscar** (Merck)	**Tablets:** 5 mg	Lactose. (MSD 72 Proscar). Blue, apple shape. Film-coated. In 1,000s, unit-of-use 30s and 100s, and UD 100s.

FINASTERIDE — ORAL

Indications

➤*Androgenetic alopecia (Propecia only):* Finasteride is indicated for the treatment of male pattern hair loss (androgenetic alopecia) in men only. Safety and efficacy were demonstrated in men between 18 to 41 years of age with mild to moderate hair loss of the vertex and anterior mid-scalp area.

Efficacy in bitemporal recession has not been established.

➤*Benign prostatic hyperplasia (BPH) (Proscar only):* Finasteride is indicated for the treatment of symptomatic BPH in men with an enlarged prostate to improve symptoms, reduce the risk of acute urinary retention, and reduce the risk of the need for surgery including transurethral resection of the prostate (TURP) and prostatectomy.

Finasteride administered in combination with the alpha-blocker doxazosin is indicated to reduce the risk of symptomatic progression of BPH (a confirmed greater than or equal to 4-point increase in AUA symptom score).

➤*Unlabeled uses:* Possible treatment of prostate cancer; male chronic pelvic pain syndrome (chronic nonbacterial prostatitis).

Administration and Dosage

➤*Approved by the FDA:* June 19, 1992.

Finasteride may be administered with or without meals.

➤*Androgenetic alopecia:* The recommended dosage is 1 mg once a day. In general, daily use for 3 months or more is necessary before benefit is observed. Continued use is recommended to sustain benefit, which should be re-evaluated periodically. Withdrawal of treatment leads to reversal of effect within 12 months.

➤*BPH:* The recommended dose is 5 mg orally once a day. Finasteride can be administered alone or in combination with the alpha blocker doxazosin.

➤*Storage/Stability:* Store at room temperature, 15° to 30°C (59° to 86°F). Keep container tightly closed and protected from moisture and light.

Actions

➤*Pharmacology:*

Propecia – Finasteride is a competitive and specific inhibitor of Type II 5α-reductase, an intracellular enzyme that converts the androgen testosterone into DHT. Two distinct isozymes are found in mice, rats, monkeys, and humans: Type I and II. Each of these isozymes is differentially expressed in tissues and developmental stages. In humans, Type I 5α-reductase is predominant in the sebaceous glands of most regions of skin, including scalp, and liver. Type I 5α-reductase is responsible for approximately one-third of circulating DHT. The Type II 5α-reductase isozyme is primarily found in prostate, seminal vesicles, epididymides, and hair follicles as well as liver, and is responsible for two-thirds of circulating DHT.

In humans, the mechanism of action of finasteride is based on its preferential inhibition of the Type II isozyme. Using native tissues (scalp and prostate), in vitro binding studies examining the potential of finasteride to inhibit either isozyme revealed a 100-fold selectivity for the human Type II 5α-reductase over Type I isozyme (IC_{50} = 500 and 4.2 nM for Type I and II, respectively). For both isozymes, the inhibition by finasteride is accompanied by reduction of the inhibitor to dihydrofinasteride and adduct formation with NADP+. The turnover for the enzyme complex is slow ($t_{½}$ approximately 30 days for the Type II enzyme complex and 14 days for the Type I complex).

Finasteride has no affinity for the androgen receptor and has no androgenic, antiandrogenic, estrogenic, antiestrogenic, or progestational effects. Inhibition of Type II 5α-reductase blocks the peripheral conversion of testosterone to DHT, resulting in significant decreases in serum and tissue DHT concentrations. Finasteride produces a rapid reduction in serum DHT concentration, reaching 65% suppression within 24 hours of oral dosing with a 1 mg tablet.

In men with male pattern hair loss (androgenetic alopecia), the balding scalp contains miniaturized hair follicles and increased amounts of DHT

FINASTERIDE — ORAL

compared with hairy scalp. Administration of finasteride decreases scalp and serum DHT concentrations in these men. The relative contributions of these reductions to the treatment effect of finasteride have not been defined. By this mechanism, finasteride appears to interrupt a key factor in the development of androgenetic alopecia in those patients genetically predisposed.

A 48-week, placebo-controlled study designed to assess by phototrichogram the effect of finasteride 1 mg on total and actively growing (anagen) scalp hairs in vertex baldness enrolled 212 men with androgenetic alopecia. At baseline and 48 weeks, total and anagen hair counts were obtained in a 1 cm^2 target area of the scalp. Men treated with finasteride 1 mg showed increases from baseline in total and anagen hair counts of 7 hairs and 18 hairs, respectively, whereas men treated with placebo had decreases of 10 hairs and 9 hairs, respectively. These changes in hair counts resulted in a between-group difference of 17 hairs in total hair count (P less than 0.001) and 27 hairs in anagen hair count (P less than 0.001), and an improvement in the proportion of anagen hairs from 62% at baseline to 68% for men treated with finasteride.

Finasteride had no effect on circulating levels of cortisol, thyroid-stimulating hormone, or thyroxine, nor did it affect the plasma lipid profile (eg, total cholesterol, low-density lipoproteins, high-density lipoproteins and triglycerides) or bone mineral density. In studies with finasteride, no clinically meaningful changes in luteinizing hormone (LH) or follicle-stimulating hormone (FSH) were detected. In healthy volunteers, treatment with finasteride did not alter the response of LH and FSH to gonadotropin-releasing hormone, indicating that the hypothalamic-pituitary-testicular axis was not affected. Mean circulating levels of testosterone and estradiol were increased by approximately 15% as compared to baseline in the first year of treatment, but these levels were within the physiologic range.

Proscar – The development and enlargement of the prostate gland is dependent on the potent androgen, 5α-dihydrotestosterone (DHT). Type II 5α-reductase metabolizes testosterone to DHT in the prostate gland, liver and skin. DHT induces androgenic effects by binding to androgen receptors in the cell nuclei of these organs.

Finasteride is a competitive and specific inhibitor of Type II 5α-reductase with which it slowly forms a stable enzyme complex. Turnover from this complex is extremely slow ($t_{1/2}$ approximately 30 days). This has been demonstrated both in vivo and in vitro. Finasteride has no affinity for the androgen receptor.

In man, the 5α-reduced steroid metabolites in blood and urine are decreased after administration of finasteride. In man, a single 5 mg oral dose of finasteride produces a rapid reduction in serum DHT concentration, with the maximum effect observed 8 hours after the first dose. The suppression of DHT is maintained throughout the 24-hour dosing interval and with continued treatment. Daily dosing of finasteride at 5 mg/day for up to 4 years has been shown to reduce the serum DHT concentration by approximately 70%. The median circulating level of testosterone increased by approximately 10% to 20% but remained within the physiologic range.

Adult males with genetically inherited Type II 5α-reductase deficiency also have decreased levels of DHT. Except for the associated urogenital defects present at birth, no other clinical abnormalities related to Type II 5α-reductase deficiency have been observed in these individuals. These individuals have a small prostate gland throughout life and do not develop BPH.

In patients with BPH treated with finasteride (1 to 100 mg/day) for 7 to 10 days prior to prostatectomy, an approximate 80% lower DHT content was measured in prostatic tissue removed at surgery, compared to placebo; testosterone tissue concentration was increased up to 10 times over pretreatment levels, relative to placebo. Intraprostatic content of prostate-specific antigen (PSA) also was decreased.

In healthy men treated with finasteride for 14 days, discontinuation of therapy resulted in a return of DHT levels to pretreatment levels in approximately 2 weeks. In patients treated for 3 months, prostate volume, which declined by approximately 20%, returned to close to baseline value after approximately 3 months of discontinuation of therapy.

➤*Pharmacokinetics:*

Absorption –

Propecia: In a study in 15 healthy men, the mean bioavailability of finasteride 1 mg tablets was 65% (range, 26% to 170%), based on the ratio of AUC relative to a 5 mg IV dose infused over 60 minutes. Following IV infusion, mean plasma clearance was 165 mL/min (range, 70 to 279 mL/min) and mean steady-state volume of distribution was 76 L (range, 44 to 96 L). In a separate study, the bioavailability of finasteride was not affected by food.

There is a slow accumulation phase for finasteride after multiple dosing. At steady state following dosing with 1 mg/day, maximum finasteride plasma concentration averaged 9.2 ng/mL (range, 4.9 to 13.7 ng/mL) and was reached 1 to 2 hours postdose; $AUC_{(0-24\ hr)}$ was 53 ng•hr/mL (range, 20 to 154 ng•hr/mL) and mean terminal half-life of elimination was 4.8 hours (range, 3.3 to 13.4 hours).

Semen levels have been measured in 35 men taking finasteride 1 mg daily for 6 weeks. In 60% (21 of 35) of the samples, finasteride levels were undetectable. The mean finasteride level was 0.26 ng/mL and the highest level measured was 1.52 ng/mL. Using this highest semen level measured and assuming 100% absorption from a 5 mL ejaculate daily, human exposure through vaginal absorption would be up to 7.6 ng daily, which is 750 times lower than the exposure from the no-effect dose for developmental abnormalities in rhesus monkeys. The in utero effects of finasteride exposure during the period of embryonic and fetal development were evaluated in the rhesus monkey (gestation days 20 to 100), a species more predictive of human development than rats or rabbits. IV administration of finasteride to pregnant monkeys at doses as high as 800 ng daily (at least 60 to 120 times the highest estimated exposure of pregnant women to finasteride from semen of men taking 5 mg daily) resulted in no abnormalities in male fetuses. In confirmation of the relevance of the rhesus model for human fetal development, oral administration of a very high dose of finasteride (2 mg/kg daily; 20 times the recommended human dose of 5 mg daily or approximately 1 to 2 million times the highest estimated exposure to finasteride from semen of men taking 5 mg daily) to pregnant monkeys resulted in external genital abnormalities in male fetuses. No other abnormalities were observed in male fetuses and no finasteride-related abnormalities were observed in female fetuses at any dose.

Proscar: In a study of 15 healthy young subjects, the mean bioavailability of finasteride 5 mg tablets was 63% (range, 34% to 108%), based on the ratio of area under the curve (AUC) relative to an IV reference dose. Maximum finasteride plasma concentration averaged 37 ng/mL (range, 27 to 49 ng/mL) and was reached 1 to 2 hours postdose. Bioavailability of finasteride was not affected by food.

Distribution – Mean steady-state volume of distribution was 76 L (range, 44 to 96 L). Approximately 90% of circulating finasteride is bound to plasma proteins. There is a slow accumulation phase for finasteride after multiple dosing. After dosing with 5 mg/day of finasteride for 17 days, plasma concentrations of finasteride were 47% and 54% higher than after the first dose in men 45 to 60 years old (n = 12) and greater than or equal to 70 years old (n = 12), respectively. Mean trough concentrations after 17 days of dosing were 6.2 ng/mL (range, 2.4 to 9.8 ng/mL) and 8.1 ng/mL (range, 1.8 to 19.7 ng/mL), respectively, in the 2 age groups. Although steady state was not reached in this study, mean trough plasma concentration in another study in patients with BPH (mean age, 65 years) receiving 5 mg/day was 9.4 ng/mL (range, 7.1 to 13.3 ng/mL; n = 22) after over a year of dosing.

Finasteride has been shown to cross the blood brain barrier but does not appear to distribute preferentially to the CSF.

In 2 studies of healthy subjects (n = 69) receiving finasteride 5 mg/day for 6 to 24 weeks, finasteride concentrations in semen ranged from undetectable (less than 0.1 ng/mL) to 10.54 ng/mL. In an earlier study using a less sensitive assay, finasteride concentrations in the semen of 16 subjects receiving finasteride 5 mg/day ranged from undetectable (less than 1 ng/mL) to 21 ng/mL. Thus, based on a 5 mL ejaculate volume, the amount of finasteride in semen was estimated to be 50- to 100-fold less than the dose of finasteride (5 mcg) that had no effect on circulating DHT levels in men.

Metabolism – Finasteride is extensively metabolized in the liver, primarily via the cytochrome P-450 3A4 enzyme subfamily. Two metabolites, the t-butyl side chain monohydroxylated and monocarboxylic acid metabolites, have been identified that possess no more than 20% of the 5α-reductase inhibitory activity of finasteride.

Excretion –

Propecia: Following an oral dose of ^{14}C-finasteride in man, a mean of 39% (range, 32% to 46%) of the dose was excreted in the urine in the form of metabolites; 57% (range, 51% to 64%) was excreted in the feces. The major compound isolated from urine was the monocarboxylic acid metabolite; virtually no unchanged drug was recovered. The t-butyl side chain monohydroxylated metabolite has been isolated from plasma. These metabolites possessed no more than 20% of the 5 α-reductase inhibitory activity of finasteride.

Proscar: In healthy young subjects (n = 15), mean plasma clearance of finasteride was 165 mL/min (range, 70 to 279 mL/min) and mean elimination half-life in plasma was 6 hours (range, 3 to 16 hours). Following an oral dose of ^{14}C-finasteride in man (n = 6), a mean of 39% (range, 32% to 46%) of the dose was excreted in the urine in the form of metabolites; 57% (range, 51% to 64%) was excreted in the feces.

The mean terminal half-life of finasteride in subjects greater than or equal to 70 years of age was approximately 8 hours (range, 6 to 15 hours; n = 12), compared with 6 hours (range, 4 to 12 hours; n = 12) in subjects 45 to 60 years of age. As a result, mean $AUC_{(0-24\ hr)}$ after 17 days of dosing was 15% higher in subjects greater than or equal to 70 years of age than in subjects 45 to 60 years of age (P = 0.02).

Pharmacokinetic parameters –

Mean (SD) Pharmacokinetic Parameters in Healthy Young Subjects (n = 15)	
	Mean (± SD)
Bioavailability	63% (34% to 108%)[a]
Clearance (mL/min)	165 (55)
Volume of distribution (L)	76 (14)
Half-life (hours)	6.2 (2.1)

[a] Range.

Mean (SD) Noncompartmental Pharmacokinetic Parameters After Multiple Doses of 5 mg/day in Older Men		
	Mean (± SD)	
	45 to 60 years of age (n = 12)	≥ 70 years of age (n = 12)
AUC (ng•hr/mL)	389 (98)	463 (186)
Peak concentration (ng/mL)	46.2 (8.7)	48.4 (14.7)

FINASTERIDE — ORAL

Mean (SD) Noncompartmental Pharmacokinetic Parameters After Multiple Doses of 5 mg/day in Older Men		
	Mean (± SD)	
	45 to 60 years of age (n = 12)	≥ 70 years of age (n = 12)
Time to peak (hours)	1.8 (0.7)	1.8 (0.6)
Half-life (hours)[a]	6 (1.5)	8.2 (2.5)

[a] First-dose values; all other parameters are last-dose values.

Contraindications

Finasteride use is contraindicated in women when they are or may potentially be pregnant. Because of the ability of Type II 5α-reductase inhibitors to inhibit the conversion of testosterone to DHT, finasteride may cause abnormalities of the external genitalia of a male fetus of a pregnant woman who receives finasteride. If this drug is used during pregnancy, or if pregnancy occurs while taking this drug, apprise the pregnant woman of the potential hazard to the male fetus. In female rats, low doses of finasteride administered during pregnancy have produced abnormalities of the external genitalia in male offspring.

Finasteride is contraindicated for hypersensitivity to any component of this medication.

Warnings

➤*Exposure of women / risk to male fetus:* Finasteride is not indicated for use in pediatric patients or women. Women should not handle crushed or broken finasteride tablets when they are pregnant or may potentially be pregnant because of the possibility of absorption of finasteride and the subsequent potential risk to a male fetus. Finasteride tablets are coated and will prevent contact with the active ingredient during normal handling, provided that the tablets have not been broken or crushed.

➤*Carcinogenesis:* In a 19-month carcinogenicity study in CD-1 mice, a statistically significant ($P \leq 0.05$) increase in the incidence of testicular Leydig cell adenomas was observed at a dose of 250 mg/kg/day (228 times the human exposure at 5 mg/day). In mice at a dose of 25 mg/kg/day (23 times the human exposure at 5 mg/day, estimated) and in rats at a dose of greater than or equal to 40 mg/kg/day (39 times the human exposure at 5 mg/day) an increase in the incidence of Leydig cell hyperplasia was observed. A positive correlation between the proliferative changes in the Leydig cells and an increase in serum LH levels (2- to 3-fold above control) has been demonstrated in both rodent species treated with high doses of finasteride. No drug-related Leydig cell changes were seen in either rats or dogs treated with finasteride for 1 year at doses of 20 mg/kg/day and 45 mg/kg/day (30 and 350 times, respectively, the human exposure at 5 mg/day) or in mice treated for 19 months at a dose of 2.5 mg/kg/day (2.3 times the human exposure, estimated).

➤*Fertility impairment:* In sexually mature male rabbits treated with finasteride at 80 mg/kg/day (4,344 times and 543 times the human exposure at 1 mg/day and 5 mg/day, respectively) for up to 12 weeks, no effect on fertility, sperm count, or ejaculate volume was seen. In sexually mature male rats treated with 80 mg/kg/day of finasteride (488 and 61 times the estimated human exposure at 1 mg/day and 5 mg/day, respectively), there were no significant effects on fertility after 6 or 12 weeks of treatment; however, when treatment was continued for up to 24 or 30 weeks, there was an apparent decrease in fertility, fecundity, and an associated significant decrease in the weights of the seminal vesicles and prostate. All these effects were reversible within 6 weeks of discontinuation of treatment. No drug-related effect on testes or on mating performance has been seen in rats or rabbits. This decrease in fertility in finasteride-treated rats is secondary to its effect on accessory sex organs (prostate and seminal vesicles) resulting in failure to form a seminal plug. The seminal plug is essential for normal fertility in rats but is not relevant in man.

➤*Elderly:*

5 mg – Of the total number of subjects included in PLESS, 1,480 and 105 subjects were 65 years of age and older and 75 years of age and older, respectively. No overall differences in safety or effectiveness were observed between these subjects and younger subjects, and other reported clinical experience has not identified differences in responses between the elderly and younger patients. No dosage adjustment is necessary in the elderly.

➤*Pregnancy: Category X.* Finasteride is not indicated for use in women. Administration of finasteride to pregnant rats at doses ranging from 100 mcg/kg/day to 100 mg/kg/day (1 to 1,000 times the maximum recommended human dose of 5 mg/day) resulted in dose-dependent development of hypospadias in 3.6% to 100% of male offspring. Pregnant rats produced male offspring with decreased prostatic and seminal vesicular weights, delayed preputial separation, and transient nipple development when given finasteride at greater than or equal to 30 mcg/kg/day (greater than or equal to 0.3 times the maximum recommended human dose of 5 mg/day) and decreased anogenital distance when given finasteride at greater than or equal to 3 mcg/kg/day (greater than or equal to 0.03 times the maximum recommended human dose of 5 mg/day). The critical period during which these effects can be induced in male rats has been defined to be days 16 to 17 of gestation. The changes described above are expected pharmacological effects of drugs belonging to the class of Type II 5α-reductase inhibitors and are similar to those reported in male infants with a genetic deficiency of Type II 5α-reductase. No abnormalities were observed in female offspring exposed to any dose of finasteride in utero.

The in utero effects of finasteride exposure during the period of embryonic and fetal development were evaluated in the rhesus monkey (gestation days 20 to 100), a species more predictive of human development than rats or rabbits. IV administration of finasteride to pregnant monkeys at doses as high as 800 ng/day (at least 60 to 120 times the highest estimated exposure of pregnant women to finasteride from semen of men taking 5 mg/day) resulted in no abnormalities in male fetuses. In confirmation of the relevance of the rhesus model for human fetal development, oral administration of a very high dose of finasteride (2 mg/kg/day; 20 times the recommended human dose of 5 mg/day or approximately 1 to 2 million times the highest estimated exposure to finasteride from semen of men taking 5 mg/day) to pregnant monkeys resulted in external genital abnormalities in male fetuses. No other abnormalities were observed in male fetuses and no finasteride-related abnormalities were observed in female fetuses at any dose.

➤*Lactation:* Finasteride is not indicated for use in women. It is not known whether finasteride is excreted in human milk.

➤*Children:* Finasteride is not indicated for use in pediatric patients. Safety and efficacy in children have not been established.

Precautions

➤*Monitoring:*

Proscar – Prior to initiating therapy with finasteride for BPH, perform appropriate evaluation to identify other conditions such as infection, prostate cancer, stricture disease, hypotonic bladder or other neurogenic disorders that might mimic BPH.

Carefully monitor patients with large residual urinary volume or severely diminished urinary flow for obstructive uropathy. These patients may not be candidates for finasteride therapy for BPH.

➤*Proscar:*

Effects on PSA and prostate cancer detection – No clinical benefit has been demonstrated in patients with prostate cancer treated with finasteride. Patients with BPH and elevated PSA were monitored in controlled clinical studies with serial PSAs and prostate biopsies. In these studies, finasteride did not appear to alter the rate of prostate cancer detection. The overall incidence of prostate cancer was not significantly different in patients treated with finasteride or placebo.

Finasteride causes a decrease in serum PSA levels by approximately 50% in patients with BPH, even in the presence of prostate cancer. This decrease is predictable over the entire range of PSA values, although it may vary in individual patients. Analysis of PSA data from over 3,000 patients in PLESS confirmed that in typical patients treated with finasteride for 6 months or more, PSA values should be doubled for comparison with normal ranges in untreated men. This adjustment preserves the sensitivity and specificity of the PSA assay and maintains its ability to detect prostate cancer.

Carefully evaluate any sustained increases in PSA levels while on finasteride, including consideration of noncompliance to therapy with finasteride.

Percent free PSA (free to total PSA ratio) is not significantly decreased by finasteride. The ratio of free to total PSA remains constant even under the influence of finasteride. If clinicians elect to use percent free PSA as an aid in the detection of prostate cancer in men undergoing finasteride therapy, no adjustment to its value appears necessary.

➤*Hepatic function impairment:* Use caution in the administration of finasteride in patients with liver function abnormalities, as finasteride is metabolized extensively in the liver.

Drug Interactions

No drug interactions of clinical importance have been identified. Finasteride does not appear to affect the cytochrome P450-linked drug metabolizing enzyme system. Compounds that have been tested in man include antipyrine, digoxin, propranolol, theophylline, and warfarin, and no interactions were found.

➤*Other concomitant therapy:* Although specific interaction studies were not performed, finasteride doses of 1 mg or more were concomitantly used in clinical studies with acetaminophen, α-blockers, analgesics, angiotensin-converting enzyme (ACE) inhibitors, anticonvulsants, benzodiazepines, beta blockers, calcium-channel blockers, cardiac nitrates, diuretics, H_2 antagonists, HMG-CoA reductase inhibitors, prostaglandin synthetase inhibitors (NSAIDs), and quinolone anti-infectives without evidence of clinically significant adverse interactions.

➤*Drug / Lab test interactions:*

Propecia – In clinical studies with finasteride 1 mg in men 18 to 41 years of age, the mean value of serum prostate-specific antigen (PSA) decreased from 0.7 ng/mL at baseline to 0.5 ng/mL at month 12. When finasteride is used in older men who have benign prostatic hyperplasia (BPH), PSA levels are decreased by approximately 50%. Until further information is gathered in men older than 41 years of age without BPH, consider doubling the PSA level in men undergoing this test and taking finasteride.

Proscar – In patients with BPH, finasteride has no effect on circulating levels of cortisol, estradiol, prolactin, thyroid-stimulating hormone, or thyroxine. No clinically meaningful effect was observed on the plasma lipid profile (ie, total cholesterol, low density lipoproteins, high density lipoproteins, and triglycerides) or bone mineral density. Increases of about 10% were observed in luteinizing hormone (LH) and follicle-stimulating hormone (FSH) in patients receiving finasteride, but levels remained within the normal range. In healthy volunteers, treatment with finasteride did not alter the response of LH and FSH to gonadotropin-releasing hormone indicating that the hypothalamic-pituitary-testicular axis was not affected.

FINASTERIDE — ORAL

Treatment with finasteride for 24 weeks to evaluate semen parameters in healthy male volunteers revealed no clinically meaningful effects on sperm concentration, mobility, morphology, or pH. A 0.6 mL (22.1%) median decrease in ejaculate volume with a concomitant reduction in total sperm per ejaculate, was observed. These parameters remained within the normal range and were reversible upon discontinuation of therapy with an average time to return to baseline of 84 weeks.

Adverse Reactions

Finasteride is generally well tolerated; adverse effects usually have been mild and transient.

➤*Propecia*:

Clinical studies for finasteride 1 mg in the treatment of male pattern hair loss – In controlled clinical trials for finasteride of 12-month duration, 1.4% of the patients were discontinued due to adverse experiences that were considered to be possibly, probably or definitely drug-related (1.6% for placebo); 1.2% of patients on finasteride and 0.9% of patients on placebo discontinued therapy because of a drug-related sexual adverse experience. The following clinical adverse reactions were reported as possibly, probably or definitely drug-related in greater than or equal to 1% of patients treated for 12 months with finasteride or placebo, respectively: Decreased libido (1.8%, 1.3%), erectile dysfunction (1.3%, 0.7%) and ejaculation disorder (1.2%, 0.7%; primarily decreased volume of ejaculate [0.8%, 0.4%]). Integrated analysis of clinical adverse experiences showed that during treatment with finasteride, 36 (3.8%) of 945 men had reported 1 or more of these adverse experiences as compared to 20 (2.1%) of 934 men treated with placebo ($P = 0.04$). Resolution occurred in all men who discontinued therapy with finasteride because of these side effects and in most of those who continued therapy. The incidence of each of the above side effects decreased to less than or equal to 0.3% by the fifth year of treatment with finasteride.

In a study of finasteride 1 mg daily in healthy men, a median decrease in ejaculate volume of 0.3 mL (−11%) compared with 0.2 mL (−8%) for placebo was observed after 48 weeks of treatment. Two other studies showed that finasteride at 5 times the dosage of finasteride (5 mg daily) produced significant median decreases of approximately 0.5 mL (−25%) compared with placebo in ejaculate volume but this was reversible after discontinuation of treatment.

In the clinical studies with finasteride, the incidences for breast tenderness and enlargement, hypersensitivity reactions, and testicular pain in finasteride-treated patients were not different from those in patients treated with placebo.

Postmarketing experience for finasteride 1 mg – Breast tenderness and enlargement; hypersensitivity reactions including rash, pruritus, urticaria, and swelling of the lips and face; and testicular pain.

Controlled clinical trials and long-term open extension studies for finasteride 5 mg in the treatment of benign prostatic hyperplasia – In controlled clinical trials for finasteride 5 mg of 12-month duration, 1.3% of the patients were discontinued due to adverse experiences that were considered to be possibly, probably, or definitely drug-related (0.9% for placebo); only 1 patient on finasteride 5 mg (0.2%) and 1 patient on placebo (0.2%) discontinued therapy because of a drug-related sexual adverse experience.

The following clinical adverse reactions were reported as possibly, probably or definitely drug-related in greater than or equal to 1% of patients treated for 12 months with finasteride or placebo, respectively: erectile dysfunction (3.7%, 1.1%), decreased libido (3.3%, 1.6%), and decreased volume of ejaculate (2.8%, 0.9%). The adverse experience profiles for patients treated with finasteride 1 mg/day for 12 months and those maintained on finasteride for 24 to 48 months were similar to that observed in the 12-month controlled studies with finasteride. Sexual adverse experiences resolved with continued treatment in over 60% of patients who reported them.

The relationship between long-term use of finasteride and male breast neoplasia is currently unknown. During a 4- to 6-year placebo- and comparator-controlled study that enrolled 3,047 men, there were 4 cases of breast cancer in men treated with finasteride but no cases in men not treated with finasteride. In another 4-year, placebo-controlled study that enrolled 3,040 men, there were 2 cases of breast cancer in placebo-treated men, but no cases were reported in men treated with finasteride. In a 7-year placebo-controlled trial that enrolled 18,882 healthy men, 9,060 had prostate needle biopsy data available for analysis. In the finasteride group, 280 (6.4%) men had prostate cancer with Gleason scores of 7 to 10 detected on needle biopsy vs 237 (5.1%) men in the placebo group. Of the total cases of prostate cancer diagnosed in this study, approximately 98% were classified as intracapsular (stage T1 or T2). The clinical significance of these findings is unknown.

➤*Proscar*:

Four-year placebo-controlled study – In PLESS, 1,524 patients treated with finasteride and 1,516 patients treated with placebo were evaluated for safety over a period of 4 years. The most frequently reported adverse reactions were related to sexual function. 3.7% (57 patients) treated with finasteride and 2.1% (32 patients) treated with placebo discontinued therapy as a result of adverse reactions related to sexual function, which are the most frequently reported adverse reactions.

The table below presents the only clinical adverse reactions considered possibly, probably or definitely drug related by the investigator, for which the incidence on finasteride was greater than or equal to 1% and greater than placebo over the 4 years of the study. In years 2 to 4 of the study, there was no significant difference between treatment groups in the incidences of impotence, decreased libido and ejaculation disorder, which are the most frequently reported adverse reactions.

Drug-Related Adverse Experiences Which are the Most Frequently Reported Adverse Reactions				
	Year 1 (%)		Years 2, 3, and 4[a] (%)	
	Finasteride	Placebo	Finasteride	Placebo
Breast enlargement	0.5%	0.1%	1.8%	1.1%
Breast tenderness	0.4%	0.1%	0.7%	0.3%
Decreased libido	6.4%	3.4%	2.6%	2.6%
Decreased volume of ejaculate	3.7%	0.8%	1.5%	0.5%
Ejaculation disorder	0.8%	0.1%	0.2%	0.1%
Impotence	8.1%	3.7%	5.1%	5.1%
Rash	0.5%	0.2%	0.5%	0.1%

[a] Combined years 2 to 4.N = 1,524 and 1,516, finasteride vs placebo, respectively.

Phase 3 studies and 5-year open extensions – The adverse experience profile in the 1-year, placebo-controlled, Phase 3 studies, the 5-year open extensions, and PLESS were similar.

Medical Therapy of Prostatic Symptoms (MTOPS) Study: The incidence rates of drug-related adverse experiences reported by greater than or equal to 2% of patients in any treatment group in the MTOPS Study are listed in the following table.

The individual adverse effects which occurred more frequently in the combination group compared to either drug alone were asthenia, postural hypotension, peripheral edema, dizziness, decreased libido, rhinitis, abnormal ejaculation, impotence, and abnormal sexual function (see table below). Of these, the incidence of abnormal ejaculation in patients receiving combination therapy was comparable to the sum of the incidences of this adverse experience reported for the 2 monotherapies.

Combination therapy with finasteride and doxazosin was associated with no new clinical adverse experience.

Four patients in MTOPS reported the adverse experience breast cancer. Three of these patients were on finasteride only and 1 was on combination therapy. (See the following table.)

Incidence ≥ 2% in 1 or More Treatment Groups				
Drug-related clinical adverse experiences in MTOPS				
Adverse experience	Placebo (n = 737) (%)	Doxazosin 4 mg or 8 mg (n = 756) (%)	Finasteride (n = 768) (%)	Combination (n = 786) (%)
Cardiovascular				
Hypotension	0.7%	3.4%	1.2%	1.5%
Postural hypotension	8%	16.7%	9.1%	17.8%
CNS				
Dizziness	8.1%	17.7%	7.4%	23.2%
Libido decreased	5.7%	7%	10%	11.6%
Somnolence	1.5%	3.7%	1.7%	3.1%
GU				
Abnormal ejaculation	2.3%	4.5%	7.2%	14.1%
Gynecomastia	0.7%	1.1%	2.2%	1.5%
Impotence	12.2%	14.4%	18.5%	22.6%
Abnormal sexual function	0.9%	2%	2.5%	3.1%
Metabolic and nutritional				
Peripheral edema	0.9%	2.6%	1.3%	3.3%
Respiratory				
Dyspnea	0.7%	2.1%	0.7%	1.9%
Rhinitis	0.5%	1.3%	1%	2.4%
Miscellaneous				
Asthenia	7.1%	15.7%	5.3%	16.8%
Headache	2.3%	4.1%	2%	2.3%

The MTOPS Study was not specifically designed to make statistical comparisons between groups for reported adverse experiences. In addition, direct comparisons of safety data between the MTOPS study and previous studies of the single agents may not be appropriate based upon differences in patient population, dosage or dose regimen, and other procedural and study design elements.

Long-term data: There is no evidence of increased adverse experiences with increased duration of treatment with finasteride. New reports of drug-related sexual adverse experiences decreased with duration of therapy.

FINASTERIDE — ORAL

During the 4- to 6-year placebo- and comparator-controlled MTOPS study that enrolled 3,047 men, there were 4 cases of breast cancer in men treated with finasteride but no cases in men not treated with finasteride. During the 4-year, placebo-controlled PLESS study that enrolled 3,040 men, there were 2 cases of breast cancer in placebo-treated men, but no cases were reported in men treated with finasteride. The relationship between long-term use of finasteride and male breast neoplasia is currently unknown.

In a 7-year placebo-controlled trial that enrolled 18,882 healthy men, 9,060 had prostate needle biopsy data available for analysis. In the finasteride group, 280 (6.4%) men had prostate cancer with Gleason scores of 7 to 10 detected on needle biopsy vs 237 (5.1%) men in the placebo group. Of the total cases of prostate cancer diagnosed in this study, approximately 98% were classified as intracapsular (stage T1 or T2). The clinical significance of these findings is unknown.

Postmarketing experience – The following additional adverse reactions have been reported in postmarketing experience: Hypersensitivity reactions, including pruritus, urticaria, and swelling of the lips and face, and testicular pain.

Overdosage

In clinical studies, single doses of finasteride up to 400 mg and multiple doses of finasteride up to 80 mg/day for 3 months did not result in adverse reactions. Until further experience is obtained, no specific treatment for an overdose with finasteride can be recommended.

Significant lethality was observed in male and female mice at single oral doses of 1,500 mg/m² (500 mg/kg) and in female and male rats at single oral doses of 2,360 mg/m² (400 mg/kg) and 5,900 mg/m² (1,000 mg/kg), respectively.

Patient Information

Finasteride is for use by men only.

Women should not handle crushed or broken finasteride tablets when they are pregnant or may potentially be pregnant because of the possibility of absorption of finasteride and the subsequent potential risk to a male fetus. Finasteride tablets are coated and will prevent contact with the active ingredient during normal handling, provided that the tablets have not been broken or crushed. Impotence and decreased libido may occur in patients treated with finasteride.

Instruct patients to read the patient package insert before starting therapy with finasteride and to reread it each time the prescription is renewed so that they are aware of current information for patients regarding finasteride.

Instruct patients to promptly report any changes in their breasts such as lumps, pain, or nipple discharge. Breast changes including breast enlargement, tenderness, and neoplasm have been reported.

DUTASTERIDE

Rx	**Avodart** (GlaxoSmithKline)	**Capsules:** 0.5 mg	(GX CE2). Yellow, oblong. In 100s and UD 70s.

DUTASTERIDE — ORAL

Indications

➤*Benign prostatic hyperplasia (BPH):* Dutasteride is indicated for the treatment of symptomatic BPH in men with an enlarged prostate gland to:
- Improve symptoms.
- Reduce the risk of acute urinary retention.
- Reduce the risk of the need for BPH-related surgery.

Administration and Dosage

➤*Approved by the FDA:* November 20, 2001.

➤*Dose:* The recommended dose of dutasteride is 1 capsule (0.5 mg) taken orally once a day. The capsules should be swallowed whole. Dutasteride may be administered with or without food.

➤*Storage / Stability:* Store at 25°C (77°F); excursions permitted to 15° to 30°C (59° to 86°F).

Actions

➤*Pharmacology:* Dutasteride inhibits the conversion of testosterone to 5α-dihydrotestosterone (DHT). DHT is the androgen primarily responsible for the initial development and subsequent enlargement of the prostate gland. Testosterone is converted to DHT by the enzyme 5α-reductase, which exists as 2 isoforms, type 1 and type 2. The type 2 isoenzyme is primarily active in the reproductive tissues while the type 1 isoenzyme is also responsible for testosterone conversion in the skin and liver.

Dutasteride is a competitive and specific inhibitor of both type 1 and type 2 5α-reductase isoenzymes, with which it forms a stable enzyme complex. Dissociation from this complex has been evaluated under in vitro and in vivo conditions and is extremely slow. Dutasteride does not bind to the human androgen receptor.

Effect on DHT and testosterone – The maximum effect of daily doses of dutasteride on the reduction of DHT is dose-dependent and is observed within 1 to 2 weeks. After 1 and 2 weeks of daily dosing with dutasteride 0.5 mg, median serum DHT concentrations were reduced by 85% and 90%, respectively. In patients with BPH treated with dutasteride 0.5 mg/day for 2 years, the median decrease in serum DHT was 94% at 1 year and 93% at 2 years. The median increase in serum testosterone was 19% at both 1 and 2 years but remained within the physiologic range.

In BPH patients treated with 5 mg/day of dutasteride or placebo for up to 12 weeks prior to transurethral resection of the prostate, mean DHT concentrations in prostatic tissue were significantly lower in the dutasteride group compared with placebo (784 and 5,793 pg/g, respectively, *P* less than 0.001). Mean prostatic tissue concentrations of testosterone were significantly higher in the dutasteride group compared with placebo (2,073 and 93 pg/g, respectively, *P* less than 0.001).

Adult males with genetically inherited type 2 5α-reductase deficiency also have decreased DHT levels. These 5α-reductase deficient males have a small prostate gland throughout life and do not develop BPH. Except for the associated urogenital defects present at birth, no other clinical abnormalities related to 5α-reductase deficiency have been observed in these individuals.

Other effects – Plasma lipid panel and bone mineral density were evaluated following 52 weeks of dutasteride 0.5 mg once daily in healthy volunteers. There was no change in bone mineral density as measured by dual energy x-ray absorptiometry (DEXA) compared with either placebo or baseline. In addition, the plasma lipid profile (ie, total cholesterol, low density lipoproteins, high density lipoproteins, and triglycerides) was unaffected by dutasteride. No clinically significant changes in adrenal hormone responses to ACTH stimulation were observed in a subset population (n = 13) of the 1-year healthy volunteer study.

➤*Pharmacokinetics:*

Absorption – Following administration of a single dose of a soft gelatin capsule 0.5 mg, time to peak serum concentrations (t_{max}) of dutasteride occurs within 2 to 3 hours. Absolute bioavailability in 5 healthy subjects is approximately 60% (range, 40% to 94%). When the drug is administered with food, the maximum serum concentrations were reduced by 10% to 15%. This reduction is of no clinical significance.

Distribution – Pharmacokinetic data following single and repeat oral doses show that dutasteride has a large volume of distribution (300 to 500 L). Dutasteride is highly bound to plasma albumin (99%) and alpha-1 acid glycoprotein (96.6%).

In a study of healthy subjects (n = 26) receiving dutasteride 0.5 mg/day for 12 months, semen dutasteride concentrations averaged 3.4 ng/mL (range, 0.4 to 14 ng/mL) at 12 months and, similar to serum, achieved steady-state concentrations at 6 months. On average, at 12 months, 11.5% of serum dutasteride concentrations partitioned into semen.

Metabolism / Excretion – Dutasteride is extensively metabolized in humans. While not all metabolic pathways have been identified, in vitro studies showed that dutasteride is metabolized by the CYP3A4 isoenzyme to 2 minor mono-hydroxylated metabolites. Dutasteride is not metabolized in vitro by human cytochrome P-450 isoenzymes CYP1A2, CYP2C9, CYP2C19, and CYP2D6 at 2,000 ng/mL (50-fold greater than steady-state serum concentrations). In human serum, following dosing to steady state, unchanged dutasteride, 3 major metabolites (4′-hydroxydutasteride, 1,2-dihydrodutasteride, and 6-hydroxydutasteride) and 2 minor metabolites (6,4′-dihydroxydutasteride and 15-hydroxydutasteride), as assessed by mass spectrometric response, have been detected. The absolute stereochemistry of the hydroxyl additions in the 6 and 15 positions is not known. In vitro, 4′-hydroxydutasteride and 1, 2-dihydrodutasteride metabolites are much less potent than dutasteride against both isoforms of human 5AR. The activity of 6β-hydroxydutasteride is comparable to that of dutasteride.

Dutasteride and its metabolites were excreted mainly in feces. As a percent of dose, there was approximately 5% unchanged dutasteride (approximately 1% to approximately 15%) and 40% as dutasteride-related metabolites (approximately 2% to approximately 90%). Only trace amounts of unchanged dutasteride were found in urine (less than 1%). Therefore, on average, the dose unaccounted for approximated 55% (range, 5% to 97%).

The terminal elimination half-life of dutasteride is approximately 5 weeks at steady state. The average steady-state serum dutasteride concentration was 40 ng/mL following 0.5 mg/day for 1 year. Following daily dosing, dutasteride serum concentrations achieve 65% of steady-state concentration after 1 month and approximately 90% after 3 months. Due to the long half-life of dutasteride, serum concentrations remain detectable (more than 0.1 ng/mL) for up to 4 to 6 months after discontinuation of treatment.

Special populations –

Hepatic function impairment: See Warnings for more information.

Gender: Dutasteride is not indicated for use in women. Women who are pregnant or may be pregnant should not handle dutasteride soft gelatin capsules because of the possibility of absorption of dutasteride and the potential risk of a fetal anomaly to a male fetus (see Contraindications). In addition, women should use caution whenever handling dutasteride soft gelatin capsules. If contact is made with leaking capsules, the contact area should be washed immediately with soap and water. The pharmacokinetics of dutasteride in women have not been studied.

Contraindications

Dutasteride is contraindicated for use in women and children. Dutasteride is contraindicated for patients with known hypersensitivity to dutasteride, other 5α-reductase inhibitors, or any component of the preparation.

DUTASTERIDE — ORAL

Warnings

➤*Exposure of women (risk to male fetus):* Dutasteride is absorbed through the skin. Therefore, women who are pregnant or may be pregnant should not handle dutasteride soft gelatin capsules because of the possibility of absorption of dutasteride and the potential risk of a fetal anomaly to a male fetus (see Contraindications). In addition, women should use caution whenever handling dutasteride soft gelatin capsules. If contact is made with leaking capsules, the contact area should be washed immediately with soap and water.

➤*Hepatic function impairment:* The effect of hepatic impairment on dutasteride pharmacokinetics has not been studied. Because dutasteride is extensively metabolized and has a half-life of approximately 5 weeks at steady state, caution should be used in the administration of dutasteride to patients with liver disease.

➤*Carcinogenesis:* In a 2-year carcinogenicity study in B6C3F1 mice, at doses of 3, 35, 250, and 500 mg/kg/day for males and 3, 35, and 250 mg/kg/day for females. An increased incidence of benign hepatocellular adenomas was noted at 250 mg/kg/day (290-fold the expected clinical exposure to a 0.5 mg daily dose) in females only. Two of the 3 major human metabolites have been detected in mice. The exposure to these metabolites in mice is either lower than in humans or is not known.

In a 2-year carcinogenicity study in Han Wistar rats, at doses of 1.5, 7.5, and 53 mg/kg/day for males and 0.8, 6.3, and 15 mg/kg/day for females there was an increase in Leydig cell adenomas in the testes at 53 mg/kg/day (135-fold the expected clinical exposure). An increased incidence of Leydig cell hyperplasia was present at 7.5 mg/kg/day (52-fold the expected clinical exposure) and 53 mg/kg/day in male rats. A positive correlation between proliferative changes in the Leydig cells and an increase in circulating luteinizing hormone levels has been demonstrated with 5α-reductase inhibitors and is consistent with an effect on the hypothalamic-pituitary-testicular axis following 5α-reductase inhibition. At tumorigenic doses in rats, luteinizing hormone levels in rats were increased by 167%. In this study, the major human metabolites were tested for carcinogenicity at approximately 1 to 3 times the expected clinical exposure.

➤*Fertility impairment:* Treatment of sexually mature male rats with dutasteride at doses of 0.05, 10, 50, and 500 mg/kg/day (0.1- to 110-fold the expected clinical exposure of parent drug) for up to 31 weeks resulted in dose- and time-dependent decreases in fertility, reduced cauda epididymal (absolute) sperm counts but not sperm concentration (at 50 and 500 mg/kg/day), reduced weights of the epididymis, prostate, and seminal vesicles, and microscopic changes in the male reproductive organs. The fertility effects were reversed by recovery week 6 at all doses, and sperm counts were normal at the end of a 14-week recovery period. The 5α-reductase-related changes consisted of cytoplasmic vacuolation of tubular epithelium in the epididymides and decreased cytoplasmic content of epithelium, consistent with decreased secretory activity in the prostate and seminal vesicles. The microscopic changes were no longer present at recovery week 14 in the low-dose group and were partly recovered in the remaining treatment groups. Low levels of dutasteride (0.6 to 17 ng/mL) were detected in the serum of untreated female rats mated to males dosed at 10, 50, or 500 mg/kg/day for 29 to 30 weeks.

In a fertility study in female rats, oral administration of dutasteride at doses of 0.05, 2.5, 12.5, and 30 mg/kg/day resulted in reduced litter size, increased embryo resorption and feminization of male fetuses (decreased anogenital distance) at doses of greater than or equal to 2.5 mg/kg/day (2- to 10-fold the clinical exposure of parent drug in men). Fetal body weights were also reduced at greater than or equal to 0.05 mg/kg/day in rats (less than 0.02-fold the human exposure).

➤*Pregnancy: Category X*

Dutasteride is contraindicated for use in women and children.

Dutasteride has not been studied in women because preclinical data suggest that the suppression of circulating levels of dihydrotestosterone may inhibit the development of the external genital organs in a male fetus carried by a woman exposed to dutasteride.

In an intravenous embryo-fetal development study in the rhesus monkey (12/group), administration of dutasteride at 400, 780, 1325, or 2010 ng/day on gestation days 20 to 100 did not adversely affect development of male external genitalia. Reduction of fetal adrenal weights, reduction in fetal prostate weights, and increases in fetal ovarian and testis weights were observed in monkeys treated with the highest dose. Based on the highest measured semen concentration of dutasteride in treated men (14 ng/mL) these doses represent 0.8 to 16 times based on blood levels of parent drug (32 to 186 times based on a ng/kg daily dose) the potential maximum exposure of a 50 kg human female to 5 mL semen daily from a dutasteride-treated man, assuming 100% absorption. Dutasteride is highly bound to proteins in human semen (greater than 96%), potentially reducing the amount of dutasteride available for vaginal absorption.

In an embryo-fetal development study in female rats, oral administration of dutasteride at doses of 0.05, 2.5, 12.5, and 30 mg/kg/day resulted in feminization of male fetuses (decreased anogenital distance) and male offspring (nipple development, hypospadias, and distended preputial glands) at all doses (0.07- to 111-fold the expected male clinical exposure). An increase in stillborn pups was observed at 30 mg/kg/day, and reduced fetal body weight was observed at doses greater than or equal to 2.5 mg/kg/day (15- to 111-fold the expected clinical exposure). Increased incidences of skeletal variations considered to be delays in ossification associated with reduced body weight were observed at doses of 12.5 and 30 mg/kg/day (56- to 111-fold the expected clinical exposure).

In an oral pre- and postnatal development study in rats, dutasteride doses of 0.05, 2.5, 12.5, or 30 mg/kg/day were administered. Unequivocal evidence of feminization of the genitalia (ie, decreased anogenital distance, increased incidence of hypospadias, nipple development) of F1 generation male offspring occurred at doses greater than or equal to 2.5 mg/kg/day (14- to 90-fold the expected clinical exposure in men). At a daily dose of 0.05 mg/kg/day (0.05-fold the expected clinical exposure), evidence of feminization was limited to a small, but statistically significant, decrease in anogenital distance. Doses of 2.5 to 30 mg/kg/day resulted in prolonged gestation in the parental females and a decrease in time to vaginal patency for female offspring and decrease prostate and seminal vesicle weights in male offspring. Effects on newborn startle response were noted at doses greater than or equal to 12.5 mg/kg/day. Increased stillbirths were noted at 30 mg/kg/day.

Feminization of male fetuses is an expected physiological consequence of inhibition of the conversion of testosterone to DHT by 5α-reductase inhibitors. These results are similar to observations in male infants with genetic 5α-reductase deficiency.

In the rabbit, embryo-fetal study doses of 30, 100, and 200 mg/kg (28- to 93-fold the expected clinical exposure in men) were administered orally on days 7 to 29 of pregnancy to encompass the late period of external genitalia development. Histological evaluation of the genital papilla of fetuses revealed evidence of feminization of the male fetus at all doses. A second embryo-fetal study in rabbits at doses of 0.05, 0.4, 3, and 30 mg/kg/day (0.3- to 53-fold the expected clinical exposure) also produced evidence of feminization of the genitalia in male fetuses at all doses. It is not known whether rabbits or rhesus monkeys produce any of the major human metabolites.

➤*Lactation:* Dutasteride is not indicated for use in women. It is not known whether dutasteride is excreted in human milk.

➤*Children:* Dutasteride is not indicated for use in the pediatric population. Safety and effectiveness in the pediatric population have not been established.

Precautions

➤*Monitoring:* Lower urinary tract symptoms of BPH can be indicative of other urological diseases, including prostate cancer. Patients should be assessed to rule out other urological diseases prior to treatment with dutasteride. Patients with a large residual urinary volume or severely diminished urinary flow may not be good candidates for 5α-reductase inhibitor therapy and should be carefully monitored for obstructive uropathy.

➤*Effects on PSA and prostate cancer detection:* Digital rectal examinations, as well as other evaluations for prostate cancer, should be performed on patients with BPH prior to initiating therapy with dutasteride and periodically thereafter.

Dutasteride reduces total serum PSA concentration by approximately 40% following 3 months of treatment and 50% following 6, 12 and 24 months of treatment. This decrease is predictable over the entire range of PSA values, although it may vary in individual patients. Therefore, for interpretation of serial PSAs in a man taking dutasteride, a new baseline PSA concentration should be established after 3 to 6 months of treatment, and this new value should be used to assess potentially cancer-related changes in PSA. To interpret an isolated PSA value in a man treated with dutasteride for 6 months or more, the PSA value should be doubled for comparison with normal values in untreated men.

➤*Special risk:*

Blood donation – Men being treated with dutasteride should not donate blood until at least 6 months have passed following their last dose. The purpose of this deferred period is to prevent administration of dutasteride to a pregnant female transfusion recipient.

Drug Interactions

➤*CYP 450:* Although dutasteride is extensively metabolized, no metabolically based drug interaction studies have been conducted. The effect of potent CYP3A4 inhibitors has not been studied. Because of the potential for drug-drug interactions, care should be taken when administering dutasteride to patients taking potent, chronic CYP3A4 enzyme inhibitors (eg, ritonavir).

Dutasteride does not inhibit the in vitro metabolism of model substrates for the major human cytochrome P-450 isoenzymes (CYP1A2, CYP2C9, CYP2C19, CYP2D6, and CYP3A4) at a concentration of 1000 ng/mL, 25 times greater than steady-state serum concentrations in humans. In vitro studies demonstrate that dutasteride does not displace warfarin, diazepam, or phenytoin from plasma protein binding sites, nor do these model compounds displace dutasteride.

➤*Calcium channel antagonists:* In a population pharmacokinetics analysis, a decrease in clearance of dutasteride was noted when coadministered with the CYP3A4 inhibitors verapamil (−37%, n = 6) and diltiazem (−44%, n = 5). In contrast, no decrease in clearance was seen when amlodipine, another calcium channel antagonist that is not a CYP34A inhibitor, was coadministered with dutasteride (+7%, n = 4).

The decrease in clearance and subsequent increase in exposure to dutasteride in the presence of verapamil and diltiazem is not considered to be clinically significant. No dose adjustment is recommended.

➤*Drug/Lab test interactions:*

Effects on PSA – PSA levels generally decrease in patients treated with dutasteride as the prostate volume decreases. In approximately one-half of the subjects, a 20% decrease in PSA is seen within the first month of therapy. After 6 months of therapy, PSA levels stabilize to a new baseline that is approximately 50% of the pretreatment value. Results of subjects treated with dutasteride for up to 2 years indicate this 50% reduction in

DUTASTERIDE — ORAL

PSA is maintained. Therefore, a new baseline PSA concentration should be established after 3 to 6 months of treatment with dutasteride.

CNS toxicity – In rats and dogs, repeated oral administration of dutasteride resulted in some animals showing signs of nonspecific, reversible, centrally-mediated toxicity, without associated histopathological changes at exposure 425- and 315-fold the expected clinical exposure (of parent drug), respectively.

Adverse Reactions

Most adverse reactions were mild or moderate and generally resolved while on treatment in both the dutasteride and placebo groups. The most common adverse reactions leading to withdrawal in both treatment groups were associated with the reproductive system.

Over 4,300 men with BPH were randomly assigned to receive placebo or 0.5-mg daily doses of dutasteride in 3 identical, placebo-controlled Phase III treatment studies. Of this group, 2167 male subjects were exposed to dutasteride, including 1,772 exposed for 1 year and 1,510 exposed for 2 years. The population was aged 47 to 94 years (mean age, 66 years) and greater than 90% were white.

Over the 2-year treatment period, 376 subjects (9% of each treatment group) were withdrawn from the studies due to adverse experiences, most commonly associated with the reproductive system. Withdrawals due to adverse reactions considered by the investigator to have a reasonable possibility of being caused by the study medication occurred in 4% of the subjects receiving dutasteride and in 3% of the subjects receiving placebo. The table below summarizes clinical adverse reactions that were reported by the investigator as drug-related in at least 1% of subjects receiving dutasteride and at a higher incidence than subjects receiving placebo.

➤*Drug-related adverse reactions:*

Drug-Related Adverse Reactions[a] Reported in ≥ 1% Subjects Over A 24-Month Period and More Frequently in the Dutasteride Group Than the Placebo Group (Pivotal Studies Pooled)

Adverse reaction	Adverse reaction onset Month 0-6	Month 7-12	Month 13-18	Month 19-24
Dutasteride (n)	(n = 2,167)	(n = 1,901)	(n = 1,725)	(n = 1,605)
Placebo (n)	(n = 2,158)	(n = 1,922)	(n = 1,714)	(n =1,555)
Impotence				
Dutasteride	4.7%	1.4%	1%	0.8%
Placebo	1.7%	1.5%	0.5%	0.9%
Decreased libido				
Dutasteride	3%	0.7%	0.3%	0.3%
Placebo	1.4%	0.6%	0.2%	0.1%
Ejaculation disorder				
Dutasteride	1.4%	0.5%	0.5%	0.1%
Placebo	0.5%	0.3%	0.1%	0%
Gynecomastia[b]				
Dutasteride	0.5%	0.8%	1.1%	0.6%
Placebo	0.2%	0.3%	0.3%	0.1%

[a] A drug-related adverse reaction is one considered by the investigator to have a reasonable possibility of being caused by the study medication. In assessing causality, investigators were asked to select from 1 of 2 options: Reasonably related to study medication or unrelated to study medication.

[b] Includes breast tenderness and breast enlargement.

➤*Long-term treatment:* The incidence of most drug-related sexual adverse events (impotence, decreased libido and ejaculation disorder) decreased with duration of treatment. The incidence of drug-related gynecomastia remained constant over the treatment period (see "adverse reactions" table). The relationship between long-term use of dutasteride and male breast neoplasia is currently unknown.

Overdosage

In volunteer studies, single doses of dutasteride up to 40 mg (80 times the therapeutic dose) for 7 days have been administered without significant safety concerns. In a clinical study, daily doses of 5 mg (10 times the therapeutic dose) were administered to 60 subjects for 6 months with no additional adverse effects to those seen at therapeutic doses of 0.5 mg.

There is no specific antidote for dutasteride. Therefore, in cases of suspected overdosage symptomatic and supportive treatment should be given as appropriate, taking the long half-life of dutasteride into consideration.

Patient Information

Dutasteride is for use by men only.

Read this information carefully before you start taking dutasteride. Read the information you get with dutasteride each time you refill your prescription. There may be new information. This information does not take the place of talking with your doctor.

Anabolic Steroids

Effective February 27, 1991, these agents were switched to a ***c-iii*** status by the Drug Enforcement Administration (DEA) because of their abuse potential.

WARNING

Peliosis hepatis – Peliosis hepatis, a condition in which liver and, sometimes, splenic tissue is replaced with blood-filled cysts, has occurred in patients receiving androgenic anabolic steroids. These cysts are sometimes present with minimal hepatic dysfunction and have been associated with liver failure. Often, they are not recognized until life-threatening liver failure or intra-abdominal hemorrhage develops. Withdrawal of drug usually results in complete disappearance of lesions.

Liver cell tumors – Most often these tumors are benign and androgen-dependent, but fatal malignant tumors have occurred. Withdrawal of drug often results in regression or cessation of tumor progression. However, hepatic tumors associated with androgens or anabolic steroids are much more vascular than other hepatic tumors and may be silent until life-threatening, intra-abdominal hemorrhage develops.

Blood lipid changes – Blood lipid changes associated with increased risk of atherosclerosis are seen in patients treated with androgens and anabolic steroids. These changes include decreased high-density lipoprotein (HDL) and, sometimes, increased low-density lipoprotein (LDL). The changes may be very marked and could have a serious impact on the risk of atherosclerosis and coronary artery disease (CAD).

Indications

➤*Anemia (**oxymetholone** only):* For the treatment of anemias caused by deficient red cell production; acquired or congenital aplastic anemias, myelofibrosis, and/or hypoplastic anemias caused by the administration of myelotoxic drugs often respond.

➤*Anemia of renal insufficiency (**nandrolone** only):* For the management of the anemia of renal insufficiency. This drug increases hemoglobin and red cell mass. Surgically induced anephric patients have been reported to be less responsive.

➤*Bone pain (**oxandrolone** only):* For the relief of bone pain frequently accompanying osteoporosis.

➤*Protein catabolism (**oxandrolone** only):* To offset the protein catabolism associated with prolonged administration of corticosteroids.

➤*Weight gain (**oxandrolone** only):* Adjunctive therapy to promote weight gain after weight loss following extensive surgery, chronic infections, or severe trauma, and in some patients who, without definite pathophysiologic reasons, fail to gain or maintain normal weight.

➤*Unlabeled uses:*

Nandrolone and oxymetholone – HIV-associated wasting.

Oxandrolone – Catabolic illnesses, such as alcoholic liver disease and burn injury. The following have been designated orphan drug status: short stature associated with Turner syndrome, HIV-associated wasting, constitutional delay of growth and puberty; moderate/severe acute alcoholic hepatitis in the presence of moderate protein calorie malnutrition, Duchenne and Becker muscular dystrophy.

Actions

➤*Pharmacology:* Anabolic steroids are synthetic derivatives of testosterone. Certain clinical effects and adverse reactions demonstrate the androgenic properties of this class of drugs. Complete dissociation of anabolic and androgenic effects has not been achieved. Therefore, the actions of anabolic steroids are similar to those of male sex hormones, with the possibility of causing serious disturbances of growth and sexual development if given to young children. Anabolic steroids suppress the gonadotropic functions of the pituitary gland and may exert a direct effect upon the testis.

During exogenous administration of anabolic androgens, endogenous testosterone release is inhibited through inhibition of pituitary luteinizing hormone (LH). At large doses, spermatogenesis may be suppressed through feedback inhibition of pituitary follicle-stimulating hormone (FSH).

Anabolic steroids have been reported to increase LDL and decrease HDL. These changes revert to normal on discontinuation of treatment.

Nitrogen balance is improved with anabolic agents but only when there is sufficient intake of calories and protein. Whether this positive nitrogen balance is of primary benefit in the utilization of protein-building dietary substances has not been established. **Oxymetholone** enhances the production and urinary excretion of erythropoietin in patients with anemias caused by bone marrow failure and often stimulates erythropoiesis in anemias caused by deficient red cell production.

➤*Pharmacokinetics:* The pharmacokinetics of **nandrolone** (given as single 50 to 150 mg intramuscular [IM] doses) were studied in healthy young men. The mean T_{max} was found to be 2 to 3 days after injection, and the C_{max} ranged from 2.14 ng/mL (50 mg group) to 5.16 ng/mL (150 mg group). The mean elimination half-life was 7.1 days, 11.7 days, and 11.8 days for the 50 mg, 100 mg, and 150 mg groups, respectively. Nandrolone is metabolized to 2 metabolites that can be detected in the urine.

After oral administration, **oxandrolone** is well absorbed, with T_{max} occurring in approximately 1 hour, and approximately 95% is protein bound. Oxandrolone is relatively resistant to metabolism by the liver, and approximately 28% is excreted unchanged in the urine. Plasma levels decline in a biphasic manner; the distribution half-life is approximately 30 minutes, and the elimination half-life is approximately 9 hours.

Based on the structurally similar testosterone, it is assumed that **oxymetholone** is absorbed completely after oral administration. Oxymetholone undergoes both phase I and phase II metabolism. Along with other various metabolites, approximately 5% of oxymetholone has been recovered in the urine as glucuronic acid conjugates.

Contraindications

Known or suspected carcinoma of the prostate or breast in men; carcinoma of the breast in women with hypercalcemia (androgenic anabolic steroids may stimulate osteolytic resorption of bones); pregnancy (see Warnings); nephrosis or the nephrotic phase of nephritis; hypersensitivity to any component of the product; hypercalcemia (**oxandrolone** only); severe hepatic dysfunction (**oxymetholone** only).

Warnings

➤*Peliosis hepatis:* Peliosis hepatis, a condition in which liver and sometimes splenic tissue is replaced with blood-filled cysts, has occurred in patients receiving androgenic anabolic steroids. These cysts are sometimes present with minimal hepatic dysfunction and have been associated with liver failure. Often, they are not recognized until life-threatening liver failure or intra-abdominal hemorrhage develops. Withdrawal of drug usually results in complete disappearance of lesions.

➤*Hepatitis:* Cholestatic hepatitis and jaundice occur with 17-alpha-alkylated androgens at relatively low doses. Clinical jaundice may be painless, with or without pruritus. It also may be associated with acute hepatic enlargement and right upper quadrant pain, which has been mistaken for acute (surgical) obstruction of the bile duct. If cholestatic hepatitis with jaundice appears or if liver function tests become abnormal, discontinue drug therapy and determine the etiology. Drug-induced jaundice is usually reversible when the medication is discontinued. Continued therapy has been associated with hepatic coma and death. Because of the hepatoxicity associated with drug administration, periodic liver function tests are recommended.

➤*Liver cell tumors:* See the Warning box for more information.

➤*Blood lipid changes:* Blood lipid changes associated with increased risk of atherosclerosis are seen in patients treated with androgens and anabolic steroids. These changes include decreased HDL and, sometimes, increased LDL. The changes may be very marked and could have a serious impact on the risk of atherosclerosis and CAD.

➤*Hypercalcemia:* In patients with breast cancer, anabolic steroids may cause hypercalcemia by stimulating osteolysis. Hypercalcemia may develop spontaneously and as a result of androgen therapy in women with disseminated breast carcinoma. Discontinue therapy if hypercalcemia occurs.

➤*Edema:* Edema, with or without congestive heart failure, may be a serious complication in patients with preexisting cardiac, renal, or hepatic disease. Coadministration with adrenal steroids or corticotropin may increase the edema. This is generally controllable with appropriate diuretics and/or digitalis therapy.

➤*Athletic performance:* Anabolic steroids have not been shown to be safe and effective for the enhancement of athletic ability. Because of the potential risk of serious adverse health effects, do not use this drug for such purpose.

➤*Virilization:* Observe women for signs of virilization (deepening of the voice, hirsutism, acne, and clitoromegaly). To prevent irreversible change, drug therapy must be discontinued when mild virilism is first detected. Virilization is usual following androgenic anabolic steroid use at high doses. Some virilizing changes in women are irreversible, even after prompt discontinuance of therapy, and are not prevented by coadministration of estrogens. Menstrual irregularities, including amenorrhea, also may occur.

➤*Carcinogenesis:*

Liver cell tumors: Liver cell tumors have been reported in patients receiving long-term therapy with androgenic anabolic steroids. Withdrawal of the drugs did not lead to regression of the tumors in all cases. Elderly patients treated with anabolic steroids may be at an increased risk for prostatic hypertrophy and prostate carcinoma.

A 2-year carcinogenicity study in rats given **oxymetholone** orally produced a wide spectrum of neoplastic and non-neoplastic effects. Female rats given 30 mg/kg/day had increased incidences of lung alveolar/bronchiolar adenoma and adenoma or carcinoma combined. At 100 mg/kg/day, female rats had increased incidences of hepatocellular adenoma and adenoma or carcinoma combined; the combined incidence of squamous cell carcinoma and carcinoma of the sweat glands also was increased.

➤*Fertility impairment:* In 2-year chronic oral **oxandrolone** studies in rats, a dose-related reduction of spermatogenesis and decreased organ weights (testes, prostate, seminal vesicles, ovaries, uterus, adrenals, and pituitary) were shown. Oligospermia in men and amenorrhea in women are potential adverse effects of treatment with **oxymetholone**.

➤*Elderly:* Elderly men treated with androgenic anabolic steroids may be at an increased risk for the development of prostate hypertrophy and prostatic carcinoma. In general, exercise caution in dose selection for an elderly patient, usually starting at the low end of the dosing range, reflecting the greater frequency of decreased hepatic, renal, or cardiac function, and concomitant disease or other drug therapy.

➤*Pregnancy: Category X.* Because of possible masculinization of the fetus, the use of anabolic steroids is contraindicated in pregnancy. **Oxandrolone** has been shown to cause embryotoxicity, fetotoxicity, infertility, and masculinization of the female animal offspring when given in doses 9 times the human dose. **Oxymetholone** can cause fetal harm when administered to pregnant women. It is contraindicated in women who are or may become pregnant. If a patient becomes pregnant while taking the drug, apprise her of the potential hazard to the fetus.

➤*Lactation:* It is not known whether anabolic steroids are excreted in human milk. Because of the potential for serious adverse reactions in breast-feeding infants, decide whether to discontinue breast-feeding or to discontinue the drug, taking into account the importance of the drug to the mother. Women who take **oxymetholone** should stop breast-feeding.

➤*Children:* Anabolic steroids may accelerate epiphyseal maturation more rapidly than linear growth in children, and the effect may continue for 6 months after the drug has been stopped. The younger the child the greater the risk of compromising final mature height. Therefore, monitor therapy by x-ray studies (eg, left wrist and hand) at 6-month intervals in order to avoid the risk of compromising the adult height. Use anabolic/androgenic steroids very cautiously in children and only by specialists who are aware of their effects on bone maturation. The safety and efficacy of **nandrolone** in children with metastatic breast cancer (rarely found) has not been established.

Precautions

➤*Monitoring:* Because of the hepatotoxicity associated with the use of 17-alpha-alkylated anabolic steroids, obtain liver function tests periodically.

Periodically determine serum lipids and HDL-cholesterol.

Periodically check hemoglobin and hematocrit for polycythemia in patients who are receiving high doses of anabolic steroids. Because iron deficiency anemia has been observed in some patients treated with **oxymetholone**, periodic determination of the serum iron and iron binding capacity is recommended. If iron deficiency anemia is detected, treat appropriately with supplementary iron.

Women – Women with disseminated breast carcinoma should have frequent determination of urine and serum calcium levels during the course of therapy.

Children – Perform periodic (every 6 months) x-ray examinations of bone age during treatment of prepubertal patients to determine the rate of bone maturation and the effects of androgenic anabolic steroid therapy on the epiphyseal centers.

➤*Leukemia:* Leukemia has been observed in patients with aplastic anemia treated with **oxymetholone**. The role, if any, of oxymetholone is unclear because malignant transformation has been seen in patients with blood dyscrasias, and leukemia has been reported in patients with aplastic anemia who have not been treated with oxymetholone.

➤*Benzyl alcohol:* Benzyl alcohol has been associated with a fatal "gasping syndrome" in premature infants. Refer to product listings.

➤*Special risk:* Because serum cholesterol may increase during therapy, use caution when administering these agents to patients with a history of myocardial infarction or CAD.

The insulin or oral hypoglycemic dosage may need to be adjusted in diabetic patients who receive anabolic steroids. Anabolic steroids have been shown to alter fasting blood sugar and glucose tolerance tests.

➤*Lab test abnormalities:* Anabolic steroids may cause suppression of clotting factors II, V, VII, and X and an increase in prothrombin time.

Oxymetholone has been shown to decrease 17-ketosteroid excretion (see Adverse Reactions).

➤*Drug abuse and dependence:* Anabolic steroids are classified as a schedule III controlled substance under the Anabolic Steroids Control Act of 1990.

Drug Interactions

Anabolic Steroids Drug Interactions

Precipitant drug	Object drug[a]		Description
Anabolic steroids	Anticoagulants, oral	⬆	The anticoagulant effects may be potentiated by anabolic steroids. Unexpected large increases in the international normalized ratio (INR) or the prothrombin time (PT) may occur. Monitor closely and adjust anticoagulant dose as needed.
Anabolic steroids — Oxandrolone	Hypoglycemic agents, oral	⬆	Oxandrolone may inhibit the metabolism of oral hypoglycemic agents.

[a] ⬆ = Object drug increased.

➤*Drug/Lab test interactions:* Anabolic steroids may decrease levels of thyroxine-binding globulin, resulting in decreased total T_4 serum levels and increased resin uptake of T_3 and T_4. Free thyroid hormone levels remain unchanged. Altered tests usually persist for 2 to 3 weeks after stopping anabolic steroid therapy. In addition, a decrease in protein-bound iodine (PBI) and radioactive iodine uptake may occur.

Anabolic steroids have been shown to alter fasting blood sugar and glucose tolerance tests.

Adverse Reactions

Anabolic Steroids Adverse Reactions			
Adverse Reactions	Nandrolone	Oxandrolone	Oxymetholone
CNS			
Depression	X[a]	X	
Excitation	X	X	X
Habituation	X	X	
Insomnia	X	X	X
Dermatologic			
Acne	X	X	X
Hirsutism/male-pattern baldness (women)	X	X	X
Male-pattern hair loss (postpubertal men)			X
GI			
Diarrhea	X		X
Nausea	X		X
Vomiting	X		X
GU			
Gynecomastia	X	X	X
Increased or decreased libido	X	X	X
Men (prepubertal):			
Increased frequency of erections	X	X	X
Phallic enlargement	X	X	X
Men (postpubertal):			
Bladder irritability	X	X	X
Chronic priapism	X	X	X
Decreased seminal volume			X
Epididymitis	X	X	X
Impotence	X	X	X
Inhibition of testicular function	X	X	X
Oligospermia	X	X	X
Testicular atrophy	X	X	X
Women:			
Clitoral enlargement	X	X	X
Menstrual irregularities	X	X	X
Hematologic			
Iron-deficiency anemia			X
Leukemia[b]			X
Hepatic			
Cholestatic jaundice with, rarely, hepatic necrosis and death[b]		X	X
Hepatocellular neoplasms[c]	X	X	X
Peliosis hepatis[c]	X	X	X
Metabolic			
Decreased glucose tolerance	X	X	X
Edema	X	X	X
Retention of serum electrolytes (ie, sodium, chloride, potassium, phosphate, calcium)	X	X	X
Musculoskeletal			
Muscle cramp			X
Premature closure of epiphyses in children[c]	X	X	X
Miscellaneous			
Chills			X
Deepening of the voice (women)	X	X	X
Inhibition of gonadotropin secretion		X	

[a] X = incidence not reported.
[b] See Precautions.
[c] See Warnings.

➤*Lab test abnormalities:* Reversible changes in liver function tests, including increased bromsulfophthalein retention and increases in serum bilirubin, AST, and alkaline phosphatase (see Precautions).

Increased serum levels of LDL and decreased HDL, increased creatine and creatinine excretion, and increased serum levels of creatinine phosphokinase.

Overdosage

➤*Symptoms:* No symptoms or signs associated with overdosage have been reported. It is possible that sodium and water retention may occur. The oral LD_{50} of **oxandrolone** in mice and dogs is greater than 5,000 mg/kg.

➤*Treatment:* No specific antidote is known, but gastric lavage may be used.

Patient Information

Instruct patients to immediately report any use of warfarin and any bleeding.

Instruct patients to also report any of the following side effects: ankle swelling, changes in skin color, nausea, vomiting.

Men: Instruct patients to report appearance or aggravation of acne and too frequent or persistent erections of the penis.

Women: Instruct patients to also report acne, changes in menstrual periods, hoarseness, or more facial hair.

OXYMETHOLONE

c-iii	**Anadrol-50** (Unimed)	**Tablets:** 50 mg	Lactose. (8633 Unimed). White, scored. In 100s.

OXYMETHOLONE — ORAL

For complete prescribing information, refer to the Anabolic Steroids group monograph.

WARNING

Peliosis hepatis – Peliosis hepatis, a condition in which liver and, sometimes, splenic tissue is replaced with blood-filled cysts, has occurred in patients receiving androgenic anabolic steroids. These cysts are sometimes present with minimal hepatic dysfunction and have been associated with liver failure. Often, they are not recognized until life-threatening liver failure or intra-abdominal hemorrhage develops. Withdrawal of drug usually results in complete disappearance of lesions.

Liver cell tumors – Most often these tumors are benign and androgen-dependent, but fatal malignant tumors have occurred. Withdrawal of drug often results in regression or cessation of tumor progression. However, hepatic tumors associated with androgens or anabolic steroids are much more vascular than other hepatic tumors and may be silent until life-threatening, intra-abdominal hemorrhage develops.

Blood lipid changes – Blood lipid changes associated with increased risk of atherosclerosis are seen in patients treated with androgens and anabolic steroids. These changes include decreased high-density lipoprotein (HDL) and, sometimes, increased low-density lipoprotein (LDL). The changes may be very marked and could have a serious impact on the risk of atherosclerosis and coronary artery disease.

Indications

➤*Anemia:* For the treatment of anemias caused by deficient red cell production. Acquired or congenital aplastic anemias, myelofibrosis, and/or hypoplastic anemias caused by the administration of myelotoxic drugs often respond.

Oxymetholone should not replace other supportive measures, such as transfusion; correction of iron, folic acid, vitamin B_{12}, or pyridoxine deficiency; antibacterial therapy; and the appropriate use of corticosteroids.

➤*Unlabeled uses:* HIV-associated wasting.

Administration and Dosage

➤*Approved by the FDA:* January 18, 1972.

➤*Anemias:* 1 to 5 mg/kg daily. The usual effective dosage is 1 to 2 mg/kg daily, but higher dosages may be required. Individualize dosage. Response often is not immediate; give a minimum trial of 3 to 6 months. Following remission, some patients may be maintained without the drug, while others may be maintained on an established lower daily dose. Continuous maintenance is usually necessary in patients with congenital aplastic anemia.

➤*Storage/Stability:* Store at controlled room temperature, 20° to 25°C (68° to 77°F); excursions permitted to 15° to 30°C (59° to 86°F).

OXANDROLONE

c-iii	**Oxandrin** (Savient)	**Tablets:** 2.5 mg	Lactose. (BTG 11). White, oval, scored. In 100s.
		10 mg	Lactose. (BTG 10). White, capsule shape. In 60s.

OXANDROLONE — ORAL

For complete prescribing information, refer to the Anabolic Steroids group monograph.

WARNING

Peliosis hepatis – Peliosis hepatis, a condition in which liver and, sometimes, splenic tissue is replaced with blood-filled cysts, has occurred in patients receiving androgenic anabolic steroids. These cysts are sometimes present with minimal hepatic dysfunction and have been associated with liver failure. Often, they are not recognized until life-threatening liver failure or intra-abdominal hemorrhage develops. Withdrawal of drug usually results in complete disappearance of lesions.

Liver cell tumors – Most often these tumors are benign and androgen-dependent, but fatal malignant tumors have occurred. Withdrawal of drug often results in regression or cessation of tumor progression. However, hepatic tumors associated with androgens or anabolic steroids are much more vascular than other hepatic tumors and may be silent until life-threatening, intra-abdominal hemorrhage develops.

Blood lipid changes – Blood lipid changes associated with increased risk of atherosclerosis are seen in patients treated with androgens and anabolic steroids. These changes include decreased high-density lipoprotein (HDL) and, sometimes, increased low-density lipoprotein (LDL). The changes may be very marked and could have a serious impact on the risk of atherosclerosis and coronary artery disease.

Indications

➤*Bone pain:* For the relief of the bone pain frequently accompanying osteoporosis.

➤*Protein catabolism:* To offset the protein catabolism associated with prolonged administration of corticosteroids.

➤*Weight gain:* Adjunctive therapy to promote weight gain after weight loss following extensive surgery, chronic infections, or severe trauma, and in some patients who, without definite pathophysiologic reasons, fail to gain or maintain normal weight.

➤*Unlabeled uses:* Catabolic illnesses, such as alcoholic liver disease and burn injury.

Orphan drug designation – Short stature associated with Turner syndrome, HIV-associated wasting, constitutional delay of growth and puberty, moderate/severe acute alcoholic hepatitis in the presence of moderate protein calorie malnutrition, Duchenne and Becker muscular dystrophy.

Administration and Dosage

➤*Approved by the FDA:* July 21, 1964.

Individualize dosage. Use intermittent therapy. Therapy with anabolic steroids is adjunctive to and not a replacement for conventional therapy. The duration of therapy with oxandrolone will depend on the response of the patient and the possible appearance of adverse reactions.

➤*Adults:* 2.5 to 20 mg daily in 2 to 4 divided doses. A daily dose of as little as 2.5 mg or as much as 20 mg may be required to achieve the desired response. A course of therapy of 2 to 4 weeks is usually adequate. This may be repeated intermittently as indicated.

➤*Children:* Total daily dose is 0.1 mg/kg or less, or 0.045 mg/lb or less. This may be repeated intermittently as indicated.

➤*Storage/Stability:* Store at room temperature, 15° to 25°C (59° to 77°F).

NANDROLONE DECANOATE

c-iii	**Nandrolone Decanoate** (Watson)	**Injection (in oil):** 100 mg/mL	In 2 mL multiple-dose vials.[a]
c-iii	**Nandrolone Decanoate** (Watson)	**Injection (in oil):** 200 mg/mL	In 1 mL single-dose vials.[a]

[a] In sesame oil with benzyl alcohol.

NANDROLONE DECANOATE — INJECTION

For complete prescribing information, refer to the Anabolic Steroids group monograph.

WARNING

Peliosis hepatis – Peliosis hepatis, a condition in which liver and, sometimes, splenic tissue is replaced with blood-filled cysts, has occurred in patients receiving androgenic anabolic steroids. These cysts are sometimes present with minimal hepatic dysfunction and have been associated with liver failure. Often, they are not recognized until life-threatening liver failure or intra-abdominal hemorrhage develops. Withdrawal of drug usually results in complete disappearance of lesions.

Liver cell tumors – Most often these tumors are benign and androgen-dependent, but fatal malignant tumors have occurred. Withdrawal of drug often results in regression or cessation of tumor progression. However, hepatic tumors associated with androgens or anabolic steroids are much more vascular than other hepatic tumors and may be silent until life-threatening, intra-abdominal hemorrhage develops.

Blood lipid changes – Blood lipid changes associated with increased risk of atherosclerosis are seen in patients treated with androgens and anabolic steroids. These changes include decreased high-density lipoprotein (HDL) and, sometimes, increased low-density lipoprotein (LDL). The changes may be very marked and could have a serious impact on the risk of atherosclerosis and coronary artery disease.

Indications

➤*Anemia:* For the management of the anemia of renal insufficiency. This drug increases hemoglobin and red cell mass. Surgically induced anephric patients have been reported to be less responsive.

➤*Unlabeled uses:* HIV-associated wasting.

Administration and Dosage

➤*Approved by the FDA:* October 30, 1959.

If possible, therapy should be intermittent. Individualize dosage. Duration of therapy depends on response of the condition and appearance of adverse reactions. This drug should be regarded as adjunctive therapy. Instruct patients to consume adequate quantities of nutrients in order to obtain maximal therapeutic effects. For example, when it is used in the treatment of refractory anemia, adequate iron intake is required for a maximal response.

Inject deeply intramuscularly (IM), preferably into the gluteal muscle.

➤*Anemia of renal disease:* Discontinue therapy if no hematologic improvement is seen within the first 6 months.

Women – 50 to 100 mg/week IM.

Men – 100 to 200 mg/week IM.

Children (2 to 13 years of age) – Average dosage is 25 to 50 mg IM every 3 to 4 weeks.

➤*Storage/Stability:* Store at controlled room temperature 15° to 30°C (59° to 86°F). Protect from light. Store in carton until contents are used.

MIFEPRISTONE

Rx[a]	Mifeprex (Danco Labs)	Tablets: 200 mg	(MF). Lt. yellow, cylindrical, biconvex. In single-dose blister packets containing 3 tablets.

[a] Mifepristone will be supplied only to licensed physicians who sign and return a Prescriber's Agreement.

MIFEPRISTONE — ORAL

WARNING

Serious and sometimes fatal infections and bleeding occur very rarely following spontaneous, surgical, and medical abortions, including following mifepristone use. No causal relationship between the use of mifepristone and misoprostol and these reactions has been established. Before prescribing mifepristone, inform the patient about the risk of these serious events and discuss the Medication Guide and the Patient Agreement. Ensure that the patient knows whom to call and what to do, including going to an emergency room, if none of the provided contacts are reachable, if she experiences sustained fever, severe abdominal pain, prolonged heavy bleeding, or syncope, or if she experiences abdominal pain or discomfort or general malaise (including weakness, nausea, vomiting, or diarrhea) more than 24 hours after taking misoprostol.

Atypical infection – Patients with serious bacterial infections (eg, *Clostridium sordelli*) and sepsis can present without fever, bacteremia, or significant findings on pelvic examination following an abortion. Very rarely, deaths have been reported in patients who presented without fever, with or without abdominal pain, but with leukocytosis with a marked left shift, tachycardia, hemoconcentration, and general malaise. A high index of suspicion is needed to rule out serious infection and sepsis.

Bleeding – Prolonged heavy bleeding may be a sign of incomplete abortion or other complications, and prompt medical or surgical intervention may be needed. Advise patients to seek immediate medical attention if they experience prolonged heavy vaginal bleeding.

Advise patients to take their *Medication Guide* with them if they visit an emergency room or another health care provider who did not prescribe mifepristone, so that provider will be aware that the patient is undergoing a medical abortion.

Indications

➤*Termination of intrauterine pregnancy:* Mifepristone is indicated for the medical termination of intrauterine pregnancy through 49 days of pregnancy. For purposes of this treatment, pregnancy is dated from the first day of the last menstrual period in a presumed 28-day cycle with ovulation occurring at mid-cycle. The duration of pregnancy may be determined from menstrual history and by clinical examination. Use ultrasonographic scan if the duration of pregnancy is uncertain, or if ectopic pregnancy is suspected.

Pregnancy termination by surgery is recommended in cases when mifepristone and misoprostol fail to cause termination of intrauterine pregnancy because of the risk of fetal malformation resulting from the treatment.

➤*Unlabeled uses:* Emergency contraception; uterine leiomyomata.

Administration and Dosage

➤*Approved by the FDA:* September 28, 2000.

Treatment with mifepristone and misoprostol for the termination of pregnancy requires 3 office visits by the patient. Mifepristone should be prescribed only by physicians who have read and understood the prescribing information. Mifepristone may be administered only in a clinic, medical office, or hospital, by or under the supervision of a physician able to assess the gestational age of an embryo and to diagnose ectopic pregnancies. Physicians must also be able to provide surgical intervention in cases of incomplete abortion or severe bleeding, or have made plans to provide such care through others, and be able to ensure patient access to medical facilities equipped to provide blood transfusions and resuscitation, if necessary.

Remove any intrauterine device (IUD) before treatment with mifepristone begins.

Patients taking mifepristone must take misoprostol 400 mcg 2 days after taking mifepristone unless a complete abortion has already been confirmed before that time.

➤*Day 1, mifepristone administration:* Patients must read the *Medication Guide* and read and sign the *Patient Agreement* before mifepristone is administered.

Three mifepristone 200 mg tablets (600 mg) are taken in a single oral dose.

➤*Day 3, misoprostol administration:* The patient returns to the health care provider 2 days after ingesting mifepristone. Unless abortion has occurred and has been confirmed by clinical examination or ultrasonographic scan, the patient takes 2 misoprostol 200 mcg tablets (400 mcg) orally.

During the period immediately following the administration of misoprostol, the patient may need medication for cramps or GI symptoms (eg, diarrhea, nausea, vomiting). Give the patient instructions on what to do if significant discomfort, excessive vaginal bleeding, or other adverse reactions occur and a phone number to call if she has questions following the administration of the misoprostol. In addition, provide the name and phone number of the physician who will be handling emergencies for the patient.

➤*Day 14, posttreatment examination:* Patients will return for a follow-up visit approximately 14 days after the administration of mifepristone. This visit is very important to confirm by clinical examination or ultrasonographic scan that a complete termination of pregnancy has occurred.

According to data from the US and French studies, women should expect to experience vaginal bleeding or spotting for an average of 9 to 16 days. Up to 8% of women may experience some type of bleeding for more than 30 days. Persistence of heavy or moderate vaginal bleeding at this visit, however, could indicate an incomplete abortion.

Patients who have an ongoing pregnancy at this visit have a risk of fetal malformation resulting from the treatment. Surgical termination is recommended to manage medical abortion treatment failures.

➤*Reporting of adverse reactions:* Adverse reactions, such as hospitalization, blood transfusion, ongoing pregnancy, or other major complications following the use of mifepristone and misoprostol must be reported to Danco Laboratories. Please provide a brief clinical and administrative synopsis of any such adverse reactions in writing to the following: Medical Director, Danco Laboratories, LLC, P.O. Box 4816, New York, NY 10185 (1-877-4-EARLY OPTION [1-877-432-7596]).

For immediate consultation 24 hours a day, 7 days a week with an expert in mifepristone, call Danco Laboratories at (1-877-4-EARLY OPTION [1-877-432-7596]).

➤*Prescriber's agreement*: Mifepristone will be supplied only to licensed physicians who sign and return a Prescriber's Agreement. Distribution of mifepristone will be subject to specific requirements imposed by the distributor, including procedures for storage, dosage tracking, damaged product returns, and other matters. Mifepristone is a prescription drug, although it will not be available to the public through licensed pharmacies.

➤*Storage / Stability:* Store at 25°C (77°F); excursions permitted to 15° to 30°C (59° to 86°F).

Actions

➤*Pharmacology:* The antiprogestational activity of mifepristone results from competitive interaction with progesterone at progesterone-receptor sites. Based on studies with various oral doses in several animal species (mouse, rat, rabbit, and monkey), the compound inhibits the activity of endogenous or exogenous progesterone. The termination of pregnancy results.

Doses greater than or equal to mifepristone 1 mg/kg have been shown to antagonize the endometrial and myometrial effects of progesterone in women. During pregnancy, the compound sensitizes the myometrium to the contraction-inducing activity of prostaglandins.

Mifepristone also exhibits antiglucocorticoid and weak antiandrogenic activity. The activity of the glucocorticoid dexamethasone in rats was inhibited following doses of mifepristone 10 to 25 mg/kg. Doses of 4.5 mg/kg or greater in humans resulted in a compensatory elevation of adrenocorticotropic hormone (ACTH) and cortisol. Antiandrogenic activity was observed in rats following repeated administration of doses from 10 to 100 mg/kg.

➤*Pharmacokinetics:*

Absorption – Following oral administration of a single dose of 600 mg, mifepristone is rapidly absorbed, with a peak plasma concentration of 1.98 mg/L occurring approximately 90 minutes after ingestion. The absolute bioavailability of a 20 mg oral dose is 69%.

Distribution – Mifepristone is 98% bound to plasma proteins, albumin, and α-1-acid glycoprotein. Binding to the latter protein is saturable, and the drug displays nonlinear kinetics with respect to plasma concentration and clearance.

Metabolism – Metabolism of mifepristone is primarily via pathways involving N-demethylation and terminal hydroxylation of the 17-propynyl chain. In vitro studies have shown that cytochrome P-450 3A4 is primarily responsible for the metabolism. The 3 major metabolites identified in humans are

1.) RU 42 633, the most widely found in plasma, which is the N-monodemethylated metabolite;
2.) RU 42 848, which results from the loss of 2 methyl groups from the 4-dimethylaminophenyl in position 11β; and
3.) RU 42 698, which results from terminal hydroxylation of the 17-propynyl chain.

Excretion – Following a distribution phase, elimination of mifepristone is slow at first (50% eliminated between 12 and 72 hours) and then becomes more rapid with a terminal elimination half-life of 18 hours. By 11 days after a 600 mg dose of tritiated compound, 83% of the drug has been accounted for by the feces and 9% by the urine. Serum levels are undetectable by 11 days.

Contraindications

Administration of mifepristone and misoprostol for the termination of pregnancy (the "treatment procedure") is contraindicated in patients with any one of the following conditions: confirmed or suspected ectopic pregnancy or undiagnosed adnexal mass (the treatment procedure will not be effective to terminate an ectopic pregnancy); IUD in place; chronic adrenal failure; concurrent long-term corticosteroid therapy; history of allergy to mifepristone, misoprostol, or other prostaglandin; hemorrhagic disorders or concurrent anticoagulant therapy; inherited porphyrias.

➤*Access to medical care:* Because it is important to have access to appropriate medical care if an emergency develops, the treatment procedure is contraindicated if a patient does not have adequate access to medical facili-

MIFEPRISTONE — ORAL

ties equipped to provide emergency treatment of incomplete abortion, blood transfusions, and emergency resuscitation during the period from the first visit until discharged by the administering health care provider.

Mifepristone also should not be used by any patient who may be unable to understand the effects of the treatment procedure or to comply with its regimen. Instruct patients to review the *Medication Guide* and the *Patient Agreement* provided with mifepristone carefully and give them a copy of the product label for their review. Patients should discuss their understanding of these materials with their health care providers, and retain the *Medication Guide* for later reference.

Warnings

➤*Vaginal bleeding:* Vaginal bleeding occurs in almost all patients during a medical abortion. Prolonged heavy bleeding (soaking through 2 thick full-size sanitary pads per hour for 2 consecutive hours) may be a sign of incomplete abortion or other complications, and prompt medical or surgical intervention may be needed to prevent the development of hypovolemic shock. Counsel patients to seek immediate medical attention if they experience prolonged heavy vaginal bleeding following a medical abortion.

➤*Infection:* As with other types of abortion, cases of serious bacterial infection, including very rare cases of fatal septic shock, have been reported following the use of mifepristone. No causal relationship between these events and the use of mifepristone and misoprostol has been established. Physicians evaluating a patient who is undergoing a medical abortion should be alert to the possibility of this rare event. In particular, a sustained fever of 38°C (100.4°F) or higher, severe abdominal pain, or pelvic tenderness in the days after a medical abortion may be an indication of infection. Atypical presentations of serious infection and sepsis, without fever, severe abdominal pain, or pelvic tenderness, but with significant leukocytosis, tachycardia, or hemoconcentration can occur.

A high index of suspicion is needed to rule out sepsis (eg, *C. sordelli* if a patients reports abdominal pain or discomfort or general malaise (including weakness, nausea, vomiting, or diarrhea) more than 24 hours after taking misoprostol. Very rarely, deaths have been reported in patients who presented without fever, with or without abdominal pain, but with leukocytosis with a marked left shift, tachycardia, hemoconcentration, and general malaise. These deaths occurred in women who used vaginally administered misoprostol, but no causal relationship between vaginal misoprostol use and an increased risk of infection or death has been established. *C. sordelli* infections also have been reported very rarely following childbirth (vaginal delivery and caesarian section), and in other gynecologic and nongynecologic conditions.

➤*Pregnancy termination confirmation:* Schedule patients to return for a follow-up visit at approximately 14 days after administration of mifepristone to confirm that the pregnancy is completely terminated and to assess the degree of bleeding. Termination can be confirmed by clinical examination or ultrasonographic scan. Lack of bleeding following treatment, however, usually indicates failure; prolonged or heavy bleeding is not proof of a complete abortion. Manage medical abortion failures with surgical termination. Advise the patient whether you will provide such care or will refer her to another provider as part of counseling prior to prescribing mifepristone.

➤*Ectopic pregnancy:* Mifepristone is contraindicated in patients with a confirmed or suspected ectopic pregnancy since mifepristone is not effective for terminating these pregnancies. Remain alert to the possibility that a patient who is undergoing a medical abortion could have an undiagnosed ectopic pregnancy since some of the expected symptoms of a medical abortion may be similar to those of a ruptured ectopic pregnancy. The presence of an ectopic pregnancy may have been missed, even if the patient underwent ultrasonography prior to being prescribed mifepristone.

➤*Fertility impairment:* The pharmacological activity of mifepristone disrupts the estrus cycle of animals, precluding studies designed to assess effects on fertility during drug administration. Three studies have been performed in rats to determine whether there were residual effects on reproductive function after termination of the drug exposure.

In rats, administration of the lowest oral dose of 0.3 mg/kg/day caused severe disruption of the estrus cycles for the 3 weeks of the treatment period. Following resumption of the estrus cycle, animals were mated and no effect on reproductive performance was observed. In a neonatal exposure study in rats, the administration of a subcutaneous dose of mifepristone up to 100 mg/kg on the first day after birth had no adverse effect on future reproductive function in males or females. The onset of puberty was observed to be slightly premature in female rats neonatally exposed to mifepristone. In a separate study in rats, oviduct and ovary malformations in female rats, delayed male puberty, deficient male sexual behavior, reduced testicular size, and lowered ejaculation frequency were noted after exposure to mifepristone 1 mg every other day as neonates.

➤*Pregnancy: Category X.*

Mifepristone is indicated for use in the termination of pregnancy (through 49 days of pregnancy) and has no other approved indication for use during pregnancy.

Human data – As of September 2000, over 620,000 women in Europe have taken mifepristone in combination with a prostaglandin to terminate pregnancy. Among these 620,000 women, about 415,000 have received mifepristone together with misoprostol. As of May 2000, a total of 82 cases have been reported in which women with ongoing pregnancies after using mifepristone alone or mifepristone followed by misoprostol declined to have a surgical procedure at that time. These cases are summarized in the following table.

Pregnancies Not Terminated by Surgical Abortion at the End of Mifepristone Alone or Mifepristone-Misoprostol Treatment[a]

	Mifepristone alone (n = 42)	Mifepristone –Misoprostol (n = 40)	Total (n = 82)
Subsequently had surgical abortion	3	7	10
No abnormalities detected	2	7	9
Abnormalities detected (sirenomelia, cleft palate)	1	0	1
Subsequently resulted in live birth	13	13	26
No abnormalities detected at birth	13	13	26
Abnormalities detected at birth	0	0	0
Other/Unknown	26	20	46

[a] Reported cases as of May 2000.

Prostaglandins: Several reports in the literature indicate that prostaglandins, including misoprostol, may have teratogenic effects in human beings. Skull defects, cranial nerve palsies, delayed growth and psychomotor development, facial malformation, and limb defects have all been reported after first trimester exposure.

Animal data – Teratology studies in mice, rats, and rabbits at doses of 0.25 to 4 mg/kg (less than 1/100 to approximately 1/3 the human exposure level based on body surface area) were carried out. Because of the antiprogestational activity of mifepristone, fetal losses were much higher than in control animals. Skull deformities were detected in rabbit studies at approximately 1/6 the human exposure, although no teratogenic effects of mifepristone have been observed to date in rats or mice. These deformities were most likely due to the mechanical effects of uterine contractions resulting from decreased progesterone levels.

Nonteratogenic – The indication for use of mifepristone in conjunction with misoprostol is for the termination of pregnancy through 49 days' duration of pregnancy (as dated from the first day of the last menstrual period). These drugs together disrupt pregnancy by causing decidual necrosis, myometrial contractions, and cervical softening, leading to the expulsion of the products of conception.

➤*Lactation:* It is not known whether mifepristone is excreted in human milk. Many hormones with a similar chemical structure, however, are excreted in breast milk. Because the effects of mifepristone on infants are unknown, breast-feeding women should consult with their health care provider to decide if they should discard their breast milk for a few days following administration of the medications.

➤*Children:* Safety and efficacy in children have not been established.

Precautions

➤*Monitoring:* Clinical examination is necessary to confirm the complete termination of pregnancy after the treatment procedure. Changes in quantitative human chorionic gonadotropin (hCG) levels will not be decisive until at least 10 days after the administration of mifepristone. A continuing pregnancy can be confirmed by ultrasonographic scan.

The existence of debris in the uterus following the treatment procedure will not necessarily require surgery for its removal.

➤*Administration:* Mifepristone is available only in single-dose packaging. Administration must be under the supervision of a qualified physician. Mifepristone may be administered only in a clinic, medical office, or hospital, by or under the supervision of a physician able to assess the gestational age of an embryo and to diagnose ectopic pregnancies. Physicians must also be able to provide surgical intervention in cases of incomplete abortion or severe bleeding, or have made plans to provide such care through others, and be able to ensure patient access to medical facilities equipped to provide blood transfusions and resuscitation, if necessary.

➤*Rhesus immunization:* The use of mifepristone is assumed to require the same preventive measures as those taken prior to and during surgical abortion to prevent rhesus immunization.

➤*Effectiveness:* Although there is no clinical evidence, the effectiveness of mifepristone may be lower if misoprostol is administered more than 2 days after mifepristone administration.

➤*Special risk:* There are no data on the safety and efficacy of mifepristone in women with chronic medical conditions such as cardiovascular, hypertensive, hepatic, respiratory, or renal disease; type 1 diabetes mellitus; severe anemia; or heavy smoking. Treat women who are older than 35 years of age and who also smoke 10 or more cigarettes per day with caution because such patients were generally excluded from clinical trials of mifepristone.

➤*Lab test abnormalities:* Decreases in hemoglobin concentration, hematocrit, and red blood cell count occur in some women who bleed heavily. Hemoglobin decreases of more than 2 g/dL occurred in 5.5% of subjects during the French clinical trials of mifepristone and misoprostol.

Clinically significant changes in serum enzyme (alanine aminotransferase [ALT], aspartate aminotransferase [AST], alkaline phosphatase, gamma-glutamyltransferase [GT]) activities were rarely reported.

MIFEPRISTONE — ORAL

Drug Interactions

Mifepristone Drug Interactions			
Precipitant Drug	Object Drug[a]		Description
CYP3A4 inducers (eg, rifampin, dexamethasone, St. John's wort, phenytoin, phenobarbital, carbamazepine)	Mifepristone	⬇	Induction of mifepristone metabolism may occur, resulting in lower serum levels.
CYP3A4 inhibitors (eg, ketoconazole, itraconazole, erythromycin, grape fruit juice)	Mifepristone	⬆	Mifepristone's metabolism may be inhibited, resulting in increased serum levels.

[a] ⬆ = Object drug increased. ⬇ = Object drug decreased.

Adverse Reactions

The treatment procedure is designed to induce the vaginal bleeding and uterine cramping necessary to produce an abortion. Nearly all of the women who receive mifepristone and misoprostol will report adverse reactions, and many can be expected to report more than 1 such reaction. About 90% of patients report adverse reactions following administration of misoprostol on day 3 of the treatment procedure. Those adverse reactions that occurred with a frequency greater than 1% in the US and French trials are shown in the following table.

Vaginal bleeding and cramping are expected consequences of the action of mifepristone as used in the treatment procedure. Following administration of mifepristone and misoprostol in the French clinical studies, 80% to 90% of women reported bleeding more heavily than they do during a heavy menstrual period. Women also typically experienced abdominal pain, including uterine cramping. Other commonly reported side effects were nausea, vomiting, and diarrhea. Some adverse reactions reported during the 4 hours following administration of misoprostol were judged by women as being more severe than others. The percentage of women who considered any particular adverse reaction as severe ranged from 2% to 35% in the US and French trials. After the third day of the treatment procedure, the number of reports of adverse reactions declined progressively in the French trials, so that by day 14, reports were rare except for reports of bleeding and spotting.

Mifepristone and Misoprostol Adverse Reactions (> 1%)		
Adverse reaction	US trials	French trials
CNS		
Anxiety	2%	NA[a]
Dizziness	12%	1%
Fainting	NA	2%
Fatigue	10%	NA
Headache	31%	2%
Insomnia	3%	NA
Syncope	1%	NA
GI		
Abdominal pain (cramping)	96%	NA
Diarrhea	20%	12%
Dyspepsia	3%	NA
Nausea	61%	43%
Vomiting	26%	18%
GU		
Endometritis/salpingitis/pelvic inflammatory disease	1%	NA
Leukorrhea	2%	NA
Pelvic pain	NA	2%
Uterine cramping	NA	83%
Uterine hemorrhage	5%	NA
Vaginitis	3%	NA
Hematologic		
Anemia	2%	NA
Decrease in hemoglobin < 2 g/dL	NA	6%
Miscellaneous		
Asthenia	2%	1%
Back pain	9%	NA
Fever	4%	NA
Leg pain	2%	NA
Rigors (chills/shaking)	3%	NA
Sinusitis	2%	NA
Viral infections	4%	NA

[a] NA: Not applicable

➤*Postmarketing:*

Cardiovascular – Hypotension (including orthostatic), shortness of breath, tachycardia (including racing pulse, heart palpitations, heart pounding).

CNS – Light-headedness, loss of consciousness.

Hypersensitivity – Allergic reaction (including rash, hives, itching).

Miscellaneous – Postabortal infection (including endomyometritis, parametritis), ruptured ectopic pregnancy.

Overdosage

No serious adverse reactions were reported in tolerance studies in healthy nonpregnant women and healthy men where mifepristone was administered in single doses greater than 3-fold that recommended for termination of pregnancy. If a patient ingests a massive overdose, observe her closely for signs of adrenal failure.

Patient Information

Fully advise patients of the treatment procedure and its effects. Give patients a copy of the *Medication Guide* and the *Patient Agreement*. (Additional copies of the *Medication Guide* and the *Patient Agreement* are available by contacting Danco Laboratories at 1-877-432-7596.) Advise patients to review both the *Medication Guide* and the *Patient Agreement*, and give them the opportunity to discuss them and obtain answers to any questions they may have prior to receiving mifepristone. Advise patients to take their *Medication Guide* with them if they visit an emergency room or another health care provider who did not prescribe mifepristone, so that provider will be aware that the patient is undergoing a medical abortion.

Each patient must understand:
- the necessity of completing the treatment schedule, including a follow-up visit approximately 14 days after taking mifepristone;
- that vaginal bleeding and uterine cramping probably will occur;
- that prolonged heavy vaginal bleeding is not proof of a complete abortion;
- that if the treatment fails, there is a risk of fetal malformation;
- that medical abortion treatment failures are managed by surgical termination; and
- the steps to take in an emergency situation, including precise instructions and a telephone number that she can call if she has any problems or concerns.

Another pregnancy can occur following termination of pregnancy and before resumption of normal menses. Contraception can be initiated as soon as the termination of the pregnancy has been confirmed, or before the woman resumes sexual intercourse.

Patient information is included with each package of mifepristone.

CARBOPROST TROMETHAMINE

Rx	**Hemabate** (Pharmacia & Upjohn)	**Injection:** carboprost 250 mcg and tromethamine 83 mcg/mL	Sodium chloride 9 mg, benzyl alcohol 9.45 mg. In 1 mL amps.[a]

[a] With 9.45% benzyl alcohol and sodium chloride 9 mg/mL.

CARBOPROST TROMETHAMINE — INJECTION

Indications

➤*Abortion:* For aborting pregnancy between week 13 and 20 of gestation as calculated from the first day of the last normal menstrual period and in the following conditions related to second trimester abortion:

1.) Failure of expulsion of the fetus during the course of treatment by another method;
2.) Premature rupture of membranes in intrauterine methods with loss of drug and insufficient or absent uterine activity;
3.) Requirement of a repeat intrauterine instillation of drug for expulsion of the fetus;
4.) Inadvertent or spontaneous rupture of membranes in the presence of a previable fetus and absence of adequate activity for expulsion.

➤*Postpartum uterine hemorrhage:* For the treatment of postpartum hemorrhage due to uterine atony which has not responded to conventional methods of management. Prior treatment should include the use of intravenously administered oxytocin, manipulative techniques such as uterine massage and, unless contraindicated, intramuscular ergot preparations. Studies have shown that in such cases, the use of carboprost tromethamine has resulted in satisfactory control of hemorrhage, although it is unclear whether or not ongoing or delayed effects of previously administered ecbolic agents have contributed to the outcome. In a high proportion of cases, carboprost tromethamine used in this manner has resulted in the cessation of life threatening bleeding and the avoidance of emergency surgical intervention.

CARBOPROST TROMETHAMINE — INJECTION

Administration and Dosage

➤*Abortion:* An initial dose of 1 mL of carboprost tromethamine sterile solution (containing the equivalent of 250 micrograms of carboprost) is to be administered deep in the muscle with a tuberculin syringe. Subsequent doses of 250 micrograms should be administered at 1.5- to 3.5-hour intervals depending on uterine response.

An optional test dose of 100 micrograms (0.4 mL) may be administered initially. The dose may be increased to 500 micrograms (2 mL) if uterine contractility is judged to be inadequate after several doses of 250 micrograms (1 mL).

The total dose administered of carboprost tromethamine should not exceed 12 milligrams and continuous administration of the drug for more than two days is not recommended.

➤*For Refractory Postpartum Uterine Bleeding:* An initial dose of 250 mcg of carboprost tromethamine sterile solution (1 mL of carboprost tromethamine) is to be given deep, intramuscularly. In clinical trials it was found that the majority of successful cases (73%) responded to single injections. In some selected cases, however, multiple dosing at intervals of 15 to 90 minutes was carried out with successful outcome. The need for additional injections and the interval at which these should be given can be determined only by the attending physicians as dictated by the course of clinical events. The total dose of carboprost tromethamine should not exceed 2 mg (8 doses).

➤*Storage / Stability:* Carboprost tromethamine must be refrigerated at 2° to 8° C (36° to 46° F).

Actions

➤*Pharmacology:* Carboprost tromethamine administered intramuscularly stimulates in the gravid uterus myometrial contractions similar to labor contractions at the end of a full term pregnancy. Whether or not these contractions result from a direct effect of carboprost on the myometrium has not been determined. Nonetheless, they evacuate the products of conception from the uterus in most cases.

Postpartum, the resultant myometrial contractions provide hemostasis at the site of placentation.

Carboprost tromethamine also stimulates the smooth muscle of the human GI tract. This activity may produce the vomiting or diarrhea or both that is common when carboprost tromethamine is used to terminate pregnancy and for use postpartum. In laboratory animals and also in humans carboprost tromethamine can elevate body temperature. With the clinical doses of carboprost tromethamine used for the termination of pregnancy, and for use postpartum, some patients do experience transient temperature increases.

In laboratory animals and in humans large doses of carboprost tromethamine can raise blood pressure, probably by contracting the vascular smooth muscle. With the doses of carboprost tromethamine used for terminating pregnancy, this effect has not been clinically significant. In some patients, carboprost tromethamine may cause transient bronchoconstriction.

➤*Pharmacokinetics:* Drug plasma concentrations were determined by radioimmunoassay in peripheral blood samples collected by different investigators from 10 patients undergoing abortion. The patients had been injected intramuscularly with 250 mcg of carboprost at two hour intervals. Blood levels of drug peaked at an average of 2,060 pg/mL one-half hour after the first injection then declined to an average concentration of 770 pg/mL 2 hours after the first injection just before the second injection. The average plasma concentration one-half hour after the second injection was slightly higher (2,663 pg/mL) than that after the first injection and decreased again to an average of 1,047 pg/mL by 2 hours after the second injection. Plasma samples were collected from 5 of these 10 patients following additional injections of the prostaglandin. The average peak concentrations of drug were slightly higher following each successive injection of the prostaglandin, but always decreased to levels less than the preceding peak values by two hours after each injection.

Five women who had delivery spontaneously at term were treated immediately postpartum with a single injection of 250 mcg of carboprost tromethamine. Peripheral blood samples were collected at several times during the 4 hours following treatment and carboprost tromethamine levels were determined by radioimmunoassay. The highest concentration of carboprost tromethamine was observed at 15 minutes in 2 patients (3,009 and 2,916 pg/mL), at 30 minutes in 2 patients (3,097 and 2,792 pg/mL), and at 60 minutes in 1 patient (2,718 pg/mL).

Six metabolites have been identified. The liver appears to be the primary site for oxidation. Less than 1% of the drug is excreted unchanged in the urine. Urinary excretion of metabolites is rapid and nearly complete within 24 hours following IM administration. About 80% of the dose is excreted in the first 5 to 10 hours and an additional 5% in the next 20 hours.

Contraindications

Hypersensitivity to carboprost tromethamine sterile solution; acute pelvic inflammatory disease; patients with active cardiac, pulmonary, renal or hepatic disease.

Warnings

➤*Viable fetus:* Carboprost tromethamine does not appear to directly affect the fetoplacental unit. Therefore, the possibility does exist that the previable fetus aborted by carboprost tromethamine could exhibit transient life signs. Carboprost tromethamine is not indicated if the fetus in utero has reached the stage of viability. Carboprost tromethamine should not be considered a feticidal agent.

➤*Benzyl alcohol:* This product contains benzyl alcohol. Benzyl alcohol has been reported to be associated with a fatal "Gasping Syndrome" in premature infants.

➤*Pregnancy: Category C.* Animal studies do not indicate that carboprost tromethamine is teratogenic, however, it has been shown to be embryotoxic in rats and rabbits and any dose which produces increased uterine tone could put the embryo or fetus at risk.

Evidence from animal studies has suggested that certain other prostaglandins have some teratogenic potential. Although these studies do not indicate that carboprost tromethamine is teratogenic, any pregnancy termination with carboprost tromethamine that fails should be completed by some other means.

➤*Children:* Safety and effectiveness in pediatric patients have not been established.

Precautions

➤*Bone effects:* Animal studies lasting several weeks at high doses have shown that prostaglandins of the E and F series can induce proliferation of bone. Such effects have also been noted in newborn infants who have received prostaglandin E1 during prolonged treatment. There is no evidence that short term administration of carboprost tromethamine sterile solution can cause similar bone effects.

➤*Concomitant medications:* The pretreatment or coadministration of antiemetic and antidiarrheal drugs decreases considerably the very high incidence of GI effects common with all prostaglandins used for abortion. Their use should be considered an integral part of the management of patients undergoing abortion with carboprost tromethamine. Narcotic analgesics may be given for uterine pain.

➤*Incomplete abortion:* As with spontaneous abortion, a process which is sometimes incomplete, abortion induced by carboprost tromethamine may be expected to be incomplete in about 20% of cases.In such cases, take other measures to ensure complete abortion.

➤*Cervical trauma:* Although the incidence of cervical trauma is extremely small, the cervix should always be carefully examined immediately post-abortion.

➤*Pyrexia:* Use of carboprost tromethamine is associated with transient pyrexia that may be due to its effect on hypothalamic thermoregulation. Temperature elevations exceeding 1.1° C (2° F) were observed in approximately one-eighth of the patients who received the recommended dosage regimen. In all cases, temperature returned to normal when therapy ended. Differentiation of post-abortion endometritis from drug-induced temperature elevations is difficult, but with increasing clinical experience, the distinctions become more obvious and are summarized below:

➤*Endometritis Pyrexia vs Pyrexia Induced By Carboprost Tromethamine:*

Time of onset –

Endometritis Pyrexia: Typically, on third post-abortional day (38° C or higher).

Pyrexia Induced By Carboprost Tromethamine: Within 1 to 16 hours after the first injection.

Duration –

Endometritis Pyrexia: Untreated pyrexia and infection continue and may give rise to other pelvic infections.

Pyrexia Induced By Carboprost Tromethamine: Temperatures revert to pretreatment levels after discontinuation of therapy without any other treatment.

Retention –

Endometritis Pyrexia: Products of conception are often retained in the cervical os or uterine cavity.

Pyrexia Induced By Carboprost Tromethamine: Temperature elevation occurs whether or not tissue is retained.

Histology –

Endometritis Pyrexia: Endometrium is infiltrated with lymphocytes and some areas are necrotic and hemorrhagic.

Pyrexia Induced By Carboprost Tromethamine: Although the endometrial stroma may be edematous and vascular, it is not inflamed.

The uterus –

Endometritis Pyrexia: Often remains boggy and soft with tenderness over the fundus, and pain on moving the cervix on bimanual examination.

Pyrexia Induced By Carboprost Tromethamine: Uterine involution normal and uterus is not tender.

Discharge –

Endometritis Pyrexia: Often associated with foul-smelling lochia and leukorrhea.

Pyrexia Induced By Carboprost Tromethamine: Lochia normal.

Cervical culture – The culture of pathological organisms from the cervix of uterine cavity after abortion alone does not warrant the diagnosis of septic abortion in the absence of clinical evidence of sepsis. Pathogens have been cultured soon after abortion in patients with no infections. Persistent positive culture with clear clinical signs of infections are significant in the differential diagnosis.

Blood count – Leukocytosis and differential white cell counts do not distinguish between endometritis and hyperthermia caused by carboprost tromethamine since total WBC's may increase during infection and transient leukocytosis may also be drug-induced.

Fluids should be forced in patients with drug-induced fever and no clinical or bacteriological evidence of intrauterine infection. Any other simple empirical measures for temperature reduction are unnecessary because all fevers induced by carboprost tromethamine have been transient or self-limiting.

CARBOPROST TROMETHAMINE — INJECTION

➤*Postpartum Hemorrhage:*

Increased Blood Pressure – In the postpartum hemorrhage series, 5/115 (4%) patients had an increase of blood pressure reported as a side effect. The degree of hypertension was moderate and it is not certain as to whether this was in fact due to a direct effect of carboprost tromethamine or a return to a status of pregnancy associated hypertension manifest by the correction of hypovolemic shock. In any event the cases reported did not require specific therapy for the elevated blood pressure.

Use in Patients with Chorioamnionitis – During the clinical trials with carboprost tromethamine, chorioamnionitis was identified as a complication contributing to postpartum uterine atony and hemorrhage in 8/115 (7%) cases, 3 of which failed to respond to carboprost tromethamine. This complication during labor may have an inhibitory effect on the uterine response to carboprost tromethamine similar to what has been reported for other oxytocic agents.

➤*Special risk:* In patients with a history of asthma, hypo- or hypertension, cardiovascular, renal, or hepatic disease, anemia, jaundice, diabetes, or epilepsy, carboprost tromethamine should be used cautiously. As with any oxytocic agent, carboprost tromethamine should be used with caution in patients with compromised (scarred) uteri.

Drug Interactions

➤*Other Oxytocics:* Carboprost tromethamine may augment the activity of other oxytocic agents. Concomitant use with other oxytocic agents is not recommended.

Adverse Reactions

The adverse effects of carboprost tromethamine sterile solution are generally transient and reversible when therapy ends. The most frequent adverse reactions observed are related to its contractile effect on smooth muscle.

In patients studied, approximately two-thirds experienced vomiting and diarrhea, approximately one-third had nausea, one-eighth had a temperature increase greater than 2° F, and one-fourteenth experienced flushing.

The pretreatment or concurrent administration of antiemetic and antidiarrheal drugs decreases considerably the very high incidence of gastrointestinal effects common with all prostaglandins used for abortion. Their use should be considered an integral part of the management of patients undergoing abortion with carboprost tromethamine.

Of those patients experiencing a temperature elevation, approximately one-sixteenth had a clinical diagnosis of endometritis. The remaining temperature elevations returned to normal within several hours after the last injection.

Adverse effects observed during the use of carboprost tromethamine for abortion and for hemorrhage, not all of which are clearly drug related, in decreasing order of frequency include: Vomiting, diarrhea, nausea, flushing or hot flashes, chills or shivering, coughing, headaches, endometritis, hiccough, dysmenorrhea-like pain, paresthesia, backache, muscular pain, breast tenderness, eye pain, drowsiness, dystonia, asthma, injection site pain, tinnitus, vertigo, vaso-vagal syndrome, dryness of mouth, hyperventilation, respiratory distress, hematemesis, taste alterations, urinary tract infection, septic shock, torticollis, lethargy, hypertension, tachycardia, pulmonary edema, endometritis from IUCD, nervousness, nosebleed, sleep disorders, dyspnea, tightness in chest, wheezing, posterior cervical perforation, weakness, diaphoresis, dizziness, blurred vision, epigastric pain, excessive thirst, twitching eyelids, gagging, retching, dry throat, sensation of choking, thyroid storm, syncope, palpitations, rash, upper respiratory infection, leg cramps, perforated uterus, anxiety, chest pain, retained placental fragment, shortness of breath, fullness of throat, uterine sacculation, faintness, lightheadedness, uterine rupture.

The most common complications when carboprost tromethamine was utilized for abortion requiring additional treatment after discharge from the hospital were endometritis, retained placental fragments, and excessive uterine bleeding, occurring in about one in every 50 patients.

DINOPROSTONE (Prostaglandin E_2; PGE_2)

Rx	**Prepidil** (Upjohn)	**Gel:** 0.5 mg	In 3 g (2.5 mL) syringes[a] with 2 shielded catheters (10 and 20 mm tip).
Rx	**Cervidil** (Forest)	**Vaginal insert:** 10 mg	In 1s.
Rx	**Prostin E2** (Pharmacia & Upjohn)	**Vaginal suppositories:** 20 mg	In containers of 1 each.

[a] With colloidal silicon dioxide NF 240 mg and triacetin 2,760 mg, USP.

DINOPROSTONE — VAGINAL

WARNING

Dinoprostone, as with other potent oxytocic agents, should be used only with strict adherence to recommended dosages. Dinoprostone should be used by medically trained personnel in a hospital which can provide immediate intensive care and acute surgical facilities.

Indications

➤*Vaginal suppository:* For the termination of pregnancy from the 12th through the 20th gestational week as calculated from the first day of the last normal menstrual period.

For evacuation of the uterine contents in the management of missed abortion or intrauterine fetal death up to 28 weeks of gestational age as calculated from the first day of the last normal menstrual period.

Management of nonmetastatic gestational trophoblastic disease (benign hydatidiform mole).

➤*Cervical gel and vaginal insert:* For the initiation or continuation of cervical ripening in patients at or near term in whom there is a medical or obstetrical indication for the induction of labor.

Administration and Dosage

➤*Vaginal suppository:* Remove foil before use.

A suppository containing 20 mg of dinoprostone should be inserted high into the vagina. The patient should remain in the supine position for 10 minutes following insertion.

Additional intravaginal administration of each subsequent suppository should be at 3- to 5-hour intervals until abortion occurs. Within the above recommended intervals administration time should be determined by abortifacient progress, uterine contractility response, and by patient tolerance. Continuous administration of the drug for more than 2 days is not recommended.

➤*Cervical gel:*

Note – Use caution in handling this product to prevent contact with skin. Wash hands thoroughly with soap and water after administration. Dinoprostone cervical gel should be brought to room temperature (15° to 30°C; 59° to 86°F) just prior to administration. Do not force the warming process by using a water bath or other source of external heat (eg, microwave oven).

To prepare the product for use, remove the peel-off seal from the end of the syringe. Then remove the protective end cap (to serve as plunger extension) and insert the protective end cap into the plunger stopper assembly in the barrel of syringe. Choose the appropriate length shielded catheter (10 mm or 20 mm) and aseptically remove the sterile shielded catheter from the package. Careful vaginal examination will reveal the degree of effacement which will regulate the size of the shielded endocervical catheter to be used. That is, the 20 mm endocervical catheter should be used if no effacement is present, and the 10 mm catheter should be used if the cervix is 50% effaced.

Firmly attach the catheter hub to the syringe tip as evidenced by a distinct click. Fill the catheter with sterile gel by pushing the plunger assembly to expel air from the catheter prior to administration to the patient.

To properly administer the product, the patient should be in a dorsal position with the cervix visualized using a speculum. Using sterile technique, introduce the gel with the catheter provided into the cervical canal just below the level of the internal os. Administer the contents of the syringe by gentle expulsion and then remove the catheter. The gel is easily extrudable from the syringe. Use the contents of 1 syringe for 1 patient only. No attempt should be made to administer the small amount of gel remaining in the catheter. The syringe, catheter, and any unused package contents should be discarded after use. Following administration of dinoprostone cervical gel, the patient should remain in the supine position for at least 15 to 30 minutes to minimize leakage from the cervical canal. If the desired response is obtained from dinoprostone cervical gel, the recommended interval before giving intravenous oxytocin is 6 to 12 hours. If there is no cervical/uterine response to the initial dose of dinoprostone cervical gel, repeat dosing may be given. The recommended repeat dose is 0.5 mg dinoprostone with a dosing interval of 6 hours. The need for additional dosing and the interval must be determined by the attending physician based on the course of clinical events. The maximum recommended cumulative dose for a 24-hour period is 1.5 mg of dinoprostone (7.5 mL dinoprostone cervical gel).

➤*Vaginal insert:* The dosage in the vaginal insert is 10 mg designed to be released at approximately 0.3 mg/hour over a 12 hour period. Dinoprostone vaginal insert should be removed upon onset of active labor or 12 hours after insertion.

One dinoprostone vaginal insert is placed transversely in the posterior fornix of the vagina immediately after removal from its foil package. The insertion of the vaginal insert does not require sterile conditions. The vaginal insert must not be used without its retrieval system. There is no need for previous warming of the product. A minimal amount of water-miscible lubricant may be used to assist in insertion of dinoprostone vaginal insert. Care should be taken not to permit excess contact or coating with the lubricant and thus prevent optimal swelling and release of dinoprostone from the vaginal insert. Patients should remain in the supine position for 2 hours following insertion, but thereafter may be ambulatory.

➤*Storage / Stability:*

Vaginal suppository – Store in a freezer not above −20°C (−4°F) but bring to room temperature just prior to use.

Cervical gel – Dinoprostone cervical gel has a shelf life of 24 months when stored under continuous refrigeration (2° to 8°C; 36° to 46°F).

Vaginal insert – Store in a freezer between −20° and −10°C (−4° and 14°F). Dinoprostone vaginal insert is packed in foil and is stable when stored in a freezer for a period of 3 years. Vaginal inserts exposed to high humidity will absorb moisture from the air and thereby alter the release characteristics of dinoprostone. Once used, the vaginal insert should be discarded.

DINOPROSTONE — VAGINAL

Actions

➤*Pharmacology:*

Dinoprostone vaginal suppository – Dinoprostone vaginal suppository administered intravaginally stimulates the myometrium of the gravid uterus to contract in a manner that is similar to the contractions seen in the term uterus during labor. Whether or not this action results from a direct effect of dinoprostone on the myometrium has not been determined with certainty at this time. Nonetheless, the myometrial contractions induced by the vaginal administration of dinoprostone are sufficient to produce evacuation of the products of conception from the uterus in the majority of cases.

Dinoprostone is also capable of stimulating the smooth muscle of the gastrointestinal tract of man. This activity may be responsible for the vomiting or diarrhea that is not uncommon when dinoprostone is used to terminate pregnancy.

In laboratory animals, and also in man, large doses of dinoprostone can lower blood pressure, probably as a consequence of its effect on the smooth muscle of the vascular system. With the doses of dinoprostone used for terminating pregnancy this effect has not been clinically significant. In laboratory animals, and also in man, dinoprostone can elevate body temperature. With the clinical doses of dinoprostone used for the termination of pregnancy some patients do exhibit temperature increases.

Dinoprostone cervical gel – Dinoprostone cervical gel administered endocervically may stimulate the myometrium of the gravid uterus to contract in a manner similar to contractions seen in the term uterus during labor. Whether or not this action results from a direct effect of dinoprostone on the myometrium has not been determined. Dinoprostone is also capable of stimulating smooth muscle of the gastrointestinal tract in humans. This activity may be responsible for the vomiting or diarrhea that is occasionally seen when dinoprostone is used for preinduction cervical ripening.

In laboratory animals, and also in humans, large doses of dinoprostone can lower blood pressure, probably as a result of its effect on smooth muscle of the vascular system. With the doses of dinoprostone used for cervical ripening this effect has not been seen. In laboratory animals, and also in humans, dinoprostone can elevate body temperature; however, with the dosing used for cervical ripening this effect has not been seen.

In addition to an oxytocic effect, there is evidence suggesting that this agent has a local cervical effect in initiating softening, effacement, and dilation. These changes, referred to as cervical ripening, occur spontaneously as the normal pregnancy progresses toward term and allow evacuation of uterine contents by decreasing cervical resistance at the same time that myometrial activity increases. While not completely understood, biochemical changes within the cervix during natural cervical ripening are similar to those following PGE_2-induced ripening. Further, it has been shown that these changes can take place independent of myometrial activity; however, it is quite likely that PGE_2 administered endocervically produces effacement and softening by combined contraction-inducing and cervical-ripening properties. There is evidence to suggest that the changes that take place within the cervix are due to collagen degradation resulting from collagenase secretion as a response, at least in part, to PGE_2.

Using an unvalidated assay, the following information was determined. When dinoprostone cervical gel was administered endocervically to women undergoing preinduction ripening, results from measurement of plasma levels of the metabolite 13,14-dihydro-15-keto-PGE_2 (DHK-PGE_2) showed that PGE_2 was relatively rapidly absorbed and the T_{max} was 0.5 to 0.75 hours. Plasma mean C_{max} for gel-treated subjects was 433 ± 51 pg/mL versus 137 ± 24 pg/mL for untreated controls. In those subjects in which a clinical response was observed, mean C_{max} was 484 ± 57 pg/mL versus 213 ± 69 pg/mL in nonresponders and 219 ± 92 pg/mL in control subjects who had positive clinical progression toward normal labor. These elevated levels in gel-treated subjects appear to be largely a result of absorption of PGE_2 from the gel rather than from endogenous sources.

PGE_2 is completely metabolized in humans. PGE_2 is extensively metabolized in the lungs, and the resulting metabolites are further metabolized in the liver and kidney. The major route of elimination of the products of PGE_2 metabolism is the kidneys.

Dinoprostone vaginal insert – Dinoprostone (PGE_2) is a naturally occurring biomolecule. It is found in low concentrations in most tissues of the body and functions as a local hormone. As with any local hormone, it is very rapidly metabolized in the tissues of synthesis (the half-life estimated to be 2.5 to 5 minutes). The rate limiting step for inactivation is regulated by the enzyme 15-hydroxyprostaglandin dehydrogenase (PGDH). Any PGE_2 that escapes local inactivation is rapidly cleared to the extent of 95% on the first pass through the pulmonary circulation.

In pregnancy, PGE_2 is secreted continuously by the fetal membranes and placenta and plays an important role in the final events leading to the initiation of labor. It is known that PGE_2 stimulates the production of PGF_2(alpha) which in turn sensitizes the myometrium to endogenous or exogenously administrated oxytocin. Although PGE_2 is capable of initiating uterine contractions and may interact with oxytocin to increase uterine contractility, the available evidence indicates that, in the concentrations found during the early part of labor, PGE_2 plays an important role in cervical ripening without affecting uterine contractions. This distinction serves as the basis for considering cervical ripening and induction of labor, usually by the use of oxytocin, as two separate processes.

PGE_2 plays an important role in the complex set of biochemical and structural alterations involved in cervical ripening. Cervical ripening involves a marked relaxation of the cervical smooth muscle fibers of the uterine cervix which must be transformed from a rigid structure to a softened, yielding and dilated configuration to allow passage of the fetus through the birth canal. This process involves activation of the enzyme collagenase, which is responsible for digestion of some of the structural collagen network of the cervix. This is associated with a concomitant increase in the amount of hydrophilic glycosaminoglycan, hyaluronic acid, and a decrease in dermatan sulfate. Failure of the cervix to undergo these natural physiologic changes, usually assessed by the method described by Bishop, prior to the onset of effective uterine contractions, results in an unfavorable outcome for successful vaginal delivery and may result in fetal compromise. It is estimated that in approximately 5% of pregnancies the cervix does not ripen normally. In an additional 10% to 11% of pregnancies, labor must be induced for medical or obstetric reasons prior to the time of cervical ripening.

The delivery rate of PGE_2 in vivo is about 0.3 mg/hour over a period of 12 hours. The controlled release of PGE_2 from the hydrogel insert is an attempt to provide sufficient quantities of PGE_2 to the local receptors to satisfy hormonal requirements. In the majority of patients, these local effects are manifested by changes in the consistency, dilatation and effacement of the cervix as measured by the Bishop score. Although some patients experience uterine hyperstimulation as a result of direct PGE_2- or PGF_2(alpha)-mediated sensitization of the myometrium to oxytocin, systemic effects of PGE_2 are rarely encountered. The insert is fitted with a biocompatible retrieval system which facilitates removal at the conclusion of therapy or in the event of an adverse reaction.

No correlation could be established between PGE_2 release and plasma concentrations of PGEm. The relative contributions of endogenously and exogenously released PGE_2 to the plasma levels of the metabolite PGEm could not be determined. Moreover, it is uncertain as to whether the measured concentrations of PGEm reflect the natural progression of PGEm concentrations in blood as birth approaches or to what extent the measured concentrations following PGE_2 administration represent an increase over basal levels that might be measured in control patients.

Contraindications

➤*Dinoprostone vaginal suppository:* Hypersensitivity to dinoprostone; acute pelvic inflammatory disease; patients with active cardiac, pulmonary, renal, or hepatic disease.

➤*Dinoprostone cervical gel:* Endocervically administered dinoprostone cervical gel is not recommended for the following: Patients in whom oxytocic drugs are generally contraindicated or where prolonged contractions of the uterus are considered inappropriate, such as cases with a history of cesarean section or major uterine surgery, cases in which cephalopelvic disproportion is present, cases in which there is a history of difficult labor and/or traumatic delivery, grand multiparae with 6 or more previous term pregnancies cases with non-vertex presentation, cases with hyperactive or hypertonic uterine patterns, cases of fetal distress where delivery is not imminent, and in obstetric emergencies where the benefit-to-risk ratio for either the fetus or the mother favors surgical intervention; patients with hypersensitivity to prostaglandins or constituents of the gel; patients with placenta previa or unexplained vaginal bleeding during this pregnancy; patients for whom vaginal delivery is not indicated, such as vasa previa or active herpes genitalia.

➤*Dinoprostone vaginal insert:* Patients with known hypersensitivity to prostaglandins; patients in whom there is clinical suspicion or definite evidence of fetal distress where delivery is not imminent; patients with unexplained vaginal bleeding during this pregnancy; patients in whom there is evidence or strong suspicion of marked cephalopelvic disproportion; patients already receiving intravenous oxytocic drugs; pultipara with 6 or more previous term pregnancies; patients in whom oxytocic drugs are contraindicated; when prolonged contraction of the uterus may be detrimental to fetal safety or uterine integrity (previous cesarean section or major uterine surgery).

Warnings

Dinoprostone does not appear to directly affect the fetoplacental unit. Therefore, the possibility does exist that the previable fetus aborted by dinoprostone could exhibit transient life signs.

Dinoprostone is not indicated if the fetus in utero has reached the stage of viability. Dinoprostone should not be considered a feticidal agent.

Evidence from animal studies has suggested that certain prostaglandins may have some teratogenic potential. Therefore, any failed pregnancy termination with dinoprostone should be completed by some other means.

➤*Pregnancy: Category C.*

Dinoprostone vaginal suppository – Animal studies do not indicate that dinoprostone is teratogenic, however, it has been shown to be embryotoxic in rats and rabbits and any dose which produces increased uterine tone could put the embryo or fetus at risk.

Dinoprostone cervical gel and vaginal insert – Prostaglandin E_2 produced an increase in skeletal anomalies in rats and rabbits. No effect would be expected clinically, when used as indicated, because dinoprostone cervical gel is administered after the period of organogenesis. Dinoprostone cervical gel has been shown to be embryotoxic in rats and rabbits, and any dose that produces sustained increased uterine tone could put the embryo or fetus at risk (see Precautions).

➤*Children:* Safety and efficacy in children have not been established.

Precautions

➤*Dinoprostone vaginal suppository:* Animal studies lasting several weeks at high doses have shown that prostaglandins of the E and F series can induce proliferation of bone. Such effects have also been noted in newborn infants who have received prostaglandin E_1 during prolonged treatment. There is no evidence that short-term administration of dinoprostone vaginal suppository can cause similar bone effects.

As in spontaneous abortion, where the process is sometimes incomplete, abortion induced by dinoprostone may sometimes be incomplete. In such cases, other measures should be taken to ensure complete abortion.

DINOPROSTONE — VAGINAL

In patients with a history of asthma, hypo- or hypertension, cardiovascular disease, renal disease, hepatic disease, anemia, jaundice, diabetes or history of epilepsy, dinoprostone should be used with caution.

Dinoprostone administered by the vaginal route should be used with caution in the presence of cervicitis, infected endocervical lesions, or acute vaginitis.

As with any oxytocic agent, dinoprostone should be used with caution in patients with compromised (scarred) uteri.

Dinoprostone vaginal therapy is associated with transient pyrexia that may be due to its effect on hypothalamic thermoregulation. In the patients studied, temperature elevations in excess of 1.1°C (2°F) were observed in approximately one-half of the patients on the recommended dosage regimen. In all cases, temperature returned to normal on discontinuation of therapy. Differentiation of post-abortion endometritis from drug-induced temperature elevations is difficult, but with increasing clinical exposure and experience with PGE_2 vaginal therapy the distinctions become more obviously apparent and are summarized below:

Apparent distinctions between endometritis pyrexia and PGE_2-induced pyrexia are compared below.

Time of onset – Endometritis pyrexia (38° C or higher) typically occurs on the third post-abortional day, while PGE_2-induced pyrexia typically occurs within 15 to 45 minutes of suppository administration.

Duration – Untreated endometritis pyrexia and infection continue and may give rise to other infective pelvic pathology. PGE_2-induced pyrexia elevations revert to pretreatment levels within 2 to 6 hours after discontinuation of therapy or removal of the suppository from the vagina without any other treatment.

Retention – In patients experiencing endometritis pyrexia, products of conception are often retained in the cervical os or uterine cavity. In PGE_2-induced pyrexia, elevation occurs irrespective of any retained tissue.

Histology – In patients experiencing endometritis pyrexia, the endometrium may show evidence of inflammatory lymphocytic infiltration with areas of necrotic or hemorrhagic tissue. In PGE_2-induced pyrexia, although the endometrial stroma may be edematous and vascular, there is relative absence of inflammatory reaction.

The uterus – In patients experiencing endometritis pyrexia, the uterus often remains boggy and soft with tenderness over the fundus and pain on moving the cervix on bimanual examination. PGE_2-induced pyrexia is characterized by normal uterine involution without tenderness.

Discharge – Endometritis pyrexia is often associated with foul-smelling lochia and leukorrhea, while lochia are normal in PGE_2-induced pyrexia.

Cervical culture – The culture of pathological organisms from the cervix or uterine cavity after abortion does not, of itself, warrant the diagnosis of septic abortion in the absence of clinical evidence of sepsis. It is not uncommon to culture pathogens from cases of recent abortion not clinically infected. Persistent positive culture with clear clinical signs of infection are significant in the differential diagnosis.

Blood count – Leukocytosis and differential white cell counts are not of major clinical importance in distinguishing between the 2 conditions, since total WBCs may be increased as a result of infection and transient leukocytosis may also be drug induced.

In the absence of clinical or bacteriological evidence of intrauterine infection, supportive therapy for drug induced fevers includes the forcing of fluids. As all PGE_2-induced fevers have been found to be transient or self-limiting, it is doubtful if any simple empirical measures for temperature reduction are indicated.

Laboratory tests – When a pregnancy diagnosed as missed abortion is electively interrupted with intravaginal administration of dinoprostone, confirmation of intrauterine fetal death should be obtained in respect to a negative pregnancy test for chorionic gonadotropic activity (UCG test or equivalent). When a pregnancy with late fetal intrauterine death is interrupted with intravaginal administration of dinoprostone, confirmation of intrauterine fetal death should be obtained prior to treatment.

➤*Dinoprostone cervical gel:* During use, uterine activity, fetal status, and character of the cervix (dilation and effacement) should be carefully monitored either by auscultation or electronic fetal monitoring to detect possible evidence of undesired responses (eg, hypertonus, sustained uterine contractility, or fetal distress). In cases where there is a history of hypertonic uterine contractility or tetanic uterine contractions, it is recommended that uterine activity and the state of the fetus should be continuously monitored. The possibility of uterine rupture should be borne in mind when high-tone myometrial contractions are sustained. Feto-pelvic relationships should be carefully evaluated before use of dinoprostone cervical gel (see Contraindications).

Caution should be exercised in administration of dinoprostone cervical gel in patients with asthma or history of asthma, glaucoma or raised intraocular pressure.

Caution should be taken so as not to administer dinoprostone cervical gel above the level of the internal os. Careful vaginal examination will reveal the degree of effacement which will regulate the size of the shielded endocervical catheter to be used. That is, the 20 mm endocervical catheter should be used if no effacement is present, and the 10 mm catheter should be used if the cervix is 50% effaced. Placement of dinoprostone cervical gel into the extra-amniotic space has been associated with uterine hyperstimulation.

As dinoprostone cervical gel is extensively metabolized in the lung, liver, and kidney, and the major route of elimination is the kidney, dinoprostone cervical gel should be used with caution in patients with renal and hepatic dysfunction.

Patients with ruptured membranes – Caution should be exercised in the administration of dinoprostone cervical gel in patients with ruptured membranes. The safety of use of dinoprostone cervical gel in these patients has not been determined.

➤*Dinoprostone vaginal insert:* Because prostaglandins potentiate the effect of oxytocin, dinoprostone vaginal insert must be removed before oxytocin administration is initiated and the patient's uterine activity carefully monitored for uterine hyperstimulation. If uterine hyperstimulation is encountered or if labor commences, the vaginal insert should be removed. Dinoprostone vaginal insert should also be removed prior to amniotomy.

Caution should be exercised in the administration of dinoprostone vaginal insert for cervical ripening in patients with ruptured membranes, in cases of non-vertex, or non-singleton presentation, and in patients with a history of previous uterine hypertony, glaucoma, or a history of childhood asthma, even though there have been no asthma attacks in adulthood.

Uterine activity, fetal status and the progression of cervical dilatation and effacement should be carefully monitored whenever the dinoprostone vaginal insert is in place. Any evidence of uterine hyperstimulation, sustained uterine contractions, fetal distress, or other fetal or maternal adverse reactions, should be a cause for consideration of removal of the insert.

Drug Interactions

Dinoprostone may augment the activity of other oxytocic drugs. Concomitant use with other oxytocic agents is not recommended.

➤*Dinoprostone cervical gel:* For the sequential use of oxytocin following dinoprostone cervical gel administration, a dosing interval of 6 to 12 hours is recommended.

➤*Dinoprostone vaginal insert:* A dosing interval of at least 30 minutes is recommended for the sequential use of oxytocin following the removal of the dinoprostone vaginal insert. No other drug interactions have been identified.

Adverse Reactions

➤*Dinoprostone vaginal suppository:* The most frequent adverse reactions observed with the use of dinoprostone for abortion are related to its contractile effect on smooth muscle.

In the patients studied, ≈ ⅔ experienced vomiting, ½ temperature elevations, ⅖ diarrhea, ⅓ some nausea, ⅒ headache, and ⅒ shivering and chills.

In addition, ≈ ⅒ of the patients studied exhibited transient diastolic blood pressure decreases of > 20 mmHg.

Two cases of myocardial infarction following the use of dinoprostone have been reported in patients with a history of cardiovascular disease.

It is not known whether these events were related to the administration of dinoprostone.

Adverse effects in decreasing order of their frequency, observed with the use of dinoprostone, not all of which are clearly drug related include: Vomiting; diarrhea; nausea; fever; headache; chills or shivering; backache; joint inflammation or pain, new or exacerbated; flushing or hot flashes; dizziness; arthralgia; vaginal pain; chest pain; dyspnea; endometritis; syncope or fainting sensation; vaginitis or vulvitis; weakness; muscular cramp or pain; tightness in chest; nocturnal leg cramps; uterine rupture; breast tenderness; blurred vision; coughing; rash; myalgia; stiff neck; dehydration; tremor; paresthesia; hearing impairment; urine retention; pharyngitis; laryngitis; diaphoresis; eye pain; wheezing; cardiac arrhythmia; skin discoloration; vaginismus; tension.

➤*Dinoprostone cervical gel:* Dinoprostone cervical gel is generally well-tolerated. In controlled trials, in which 1,731 women were entered, the following events were reported at an occurrence of at least 1%:

Dinoprostone Gel Adverese Reactions

	Dinoprostone cervical gel (n = 884)		Control[a] (n = 847)	
Adverse reaction	n	%	n	%
Maternal				
Uterine contractile abnormality	58	6.6%	34	4%
Any GI effect	50	5.7%	22	2.6%
Back pain	27	3.1%	0	0%
Warm feeling in vagina	13	1.5%	0	0%
Fever	12	1.4%	10	1.2%
Fetal				
Any fetal heart rate abnormality	150	17%	123	14.5%
Bradycardia	36	4.1%	26	3.1%
Deceleration, late	25	2.8%	18	2.1%
Deceleration, variable	38	4.3%	29	3.4%
Deceleration. unspecified	19	2.1%	19	2.2%

[a] Placebo gel or no treatment.

In addition, in other trials amnionitis and intrauterine fetal sepsis have been associated with extra-amniotic intrauterine administration of PGE_2. Uterine rupture has been reported in association with the use of dinoprostone cervical gel intracervically. Additional events reported in the literature, associated by the authors with the use of dinoprostone cervical gel, included premature rupture of membranes, fetal depression (1 min Apgar less than 7), and fetal acidosis (umbilical artery pH less than 7.15).

DINOPROSTONE — VAGINAL

➤*Dinoprostone vaginal insert:* Dinoprostone vaginal insert is well tolerated. In placebo-controlled trials in which 658 women were entered and 320 received active therapy (218 without retrieval system, 102 with retrieval system), the following events were reported.

Total dinoprostone vaginal insert-treated drug related adverse reactions				
	Controlled studies[a]		Study 101-801[b]	
	Active	Placebo	Active	Placebo
Uterine hyperstimulation with fetal distress	2.8%	0.3%	2.9%	0%
Uterine hyperstimulation without fetal distress	4.7%	0%	2%	0%
Fetal distress without uterine hyperstimulation	3.8%	1.2%	2.9%	1%
n	320	338	102	104

[a] Controlled studies (with and without retrieval system).
[b] Controlled study (with retrieval system).

Drug related fever, nausea, vomiting, diarrhea, and abdominal pain were noted in less than 1% of patients who received dinoprostone vaginal insert.

In Study 101-801 (with the retrieval system) cases of hyperstimulation reversed within 2 to 13 minutes of removal of the product. Tocolytics were required in 1 of the 5 cases.

In cases of fetal distress, when product removal was thought advisable there was a return to normal rhythm and no neonatal sequelae.

Five minute Apgar scores were 7 or above in 98.2% (646/658) of studied neonates whose mothers received dinoprostone vaginal insert. In a report of a 3 year pediatric follow-up study in 121 infants, 51 of whose mothers received dinoprostone vaginal insert, there were no deleterious effects on physical examination or psychomotor evaluation.

Overdosage

➤*Dinoprostone cervical gel:* Overdosage with dinoprostone cervical gel may be expressed by uterine hypercontractility and uterine hypertonus. Because of the transient nature of PGE_2 -induced myometrial hyperstimulation, nonspecific, conservative management was found to be effective in the vast majority of the cases; ie, maternal position change and administration of oxygen to the mother. Beta-adrenergic drugs may be used as a treatment of hyperstimulation following the administration of PGE_2 for cervical ripening.

➤*Dinoprostone vaginal insert:* Dinoprostone vaginal insert is used as a single dosage in a single application. Overdosage is usually manifested by uterine hyperstimulation which may be accompanied by fetal distress and is responsive to removal of the insert. Other treatment must be symptomatic since, to date, clinical experience with prostaglandin antagonists is insufficient. The use of beta-adrenergic agents should be considered in the event of undesirable increased uterine activity.

OXYTOCIN

Rx	**Oxytocin** (Various, eg, APP)	**Injection:** 10 units/mL	In 3 and 10 mL vials.
Rx	**Pitocin** (Monarch)		In 1 mL amps[a], 1 mL *Steri-Dose* disposable syringes, and 1 mL *Steri-Vials*.[a]

[a] With 0.5% chlorobutanol.

OXYTOCIN — INJECTION

WARNING

Oxytocin is indicated for the medical, rather than the elective, induction of labor. Available data and information are inadequate to define the benefit-to-risk considerations in the use of oxytocin for elective induction.

Indications

➤*Antepartum:* For the initiation or improvement of uterine contractions, when this is desirable and considered suitable for reasons of fetal or maternal concern, in order to achieve vaginal delivery. It is indicated for patients with a medical indication for the initiation of labor such as Rh problems, maternal diabetes, preeclampsia at or near term, when delivery is in the best interest of mother and fetus, or when membranes are ruptured prematurely and delivery is indicated; stimulation or reinforcement of labor, as in selected cases of uterine inertia; adjunctive therapy for the management of inevitable or incomplete abortion. In the first trimester, curettage generally is considered primary therapy. In second trimester abortion, oxytocin infusion often is successful in emptying the uterus. However, other means of therapy may be required in such cases.

➤*Postpartum:* To produce uterine contractions during the third stage of labor and to control postpartum bleeding or hemorrhage.

Administration and Dosage

The dosage of oxytocin is determined by the uterine response and, therefore, must be individualized and initiated at a very low level. The following dosage information is based upon various regimens and indications in general use.

➤*Induction or stimulation of labor:*

IV infusion (drip method) – IV infusion (drip method) is the only acceptable method of parenteral administration for the induction or stimulation of labor. Accurate control of the rate of infusion flow is essential. An infusion pump or other device and frequent monitoring of strength, frequency, and duration of contractions, resting uterine tone, and fetal heart rate are necessary for the safe administration of oxytocin for the induction or stimulation of labor.

Start an IV infusion of nonoxytocin-containing solution. Use physiologic electrolyte solution, except under unusual circumstances.

Dosage: The initial dose should be no more than 0.5 to 2 milliunits/min. Gradually increase the dose in increments of no more than 1 to 2 milliunits/min at 30- to 60-minute intervals until a contraction pattern has been established that is similar to normal labor.

Infusion rates: Infusion rates up to 6 milliunits/min give the same oxytocin levels that are found in spontaneous labor. At term, give higher infusion rates with great care; rates exceeding 9 to 10 milliunits/min rarely are required. Before term, when the sensitivity of the uterus is lower because of a lower concentration of oxytocin receptors, a higher infusion rate may be required.

Discontinue: Discontinue the oxytocin infusion immediately in the event of uterine hyperactivity or fetal distress. Administer oxygen to the mother, who preferably should be put in a lateral position. Immediately evaluate the condition of the mother and fetus; take appropriate steps. If uterine contractions become too powerful, the infusion can be stopped abruptly; oxytocic stimulation of the uterine musculature will soon wane.

➤*Control of postpartum uterine bleeding:*

IV infusion (drip method) – Add 10 to 40 units (maximum of 40 units) to 1,000 mL of a nonhydrating diluent and run at a rate necessary to control uterine atony.

IM – Administer 10 units after delivery of the placenta.

➤*Treatment of incomplete or inevitable abortion:* IV infusion of 10 units oxytocin with 500 mL physiologic saline solution or 5% dextrose in physiologic saline solution infused at a rate of 10 to 20 milliunits (20 to 40 drops) per minute. Do not exceed 30 units in a 12-hour period because of the risk of water intoxication.

➤*Reconstitution:* Add 1 mL (10 units) to 1,000 mL 0.9% aqueous sodium chloride or Ringer's lactate. The solution contains 10 milliunits/mL (0.01 units/mL). Use a constant infusion pump to accurately control the rate of infusion.

➤*Storage/Stability:*

Pitocin – Store at 2° to 8°C (36° to 46°F); may be held at 15° to 25°C (59° to 77°F) for up to 30 days. Discard after holding at 15° to 25°C (59° to 77°F).

Oxytocin – Store at controlled room temperature 15° to 30°C (59° to 86°F).

Actions

➤*Pharmacology:* Oxytocin acts on the smooth muscle of the uterus to stimulate contractions; response depends on the uterine threshold of excitability. It exerts a selective action on the smooth musculature of the uterus, particularly toward the end of pregnancy, during labor, and immediately following delivery. Oxytocin stimulates rhythmic contractions of the uterus, increases the frequency of existing contractions, and raises the tone of the uterine musculature.

➤*Pharmacokinetics:*

Absorption/Distribution – Oxytocin is distributed throughout the extracellular fluid. Small amounts of the drug probably reach the fetal circulation. Following IV administration, uterine response occurs almost immediately and subsides within 1 hour. Following IM injection, uterine response occurs within 3 to 5 minutes and persists for 2 to 3 hours.

Metabolism/Excretion – The plasma half-life is approximately 1 to 6 minutes, which is decreased in late pregnancy and lactation. Rapid removal from the plasma is accomplished mainly by the kidney and liver. Only small amounts are excreted in urine unchanged.

Contraindications

Significant cephalopelvic disproportion; unfavorable fetal positions or presentations that are undeliverable without conversion prior to delivery (eg, transverse lies); in obstetrical emergencies where the benefit-to-risk ratio for the fetus or the mother favors surgical intervention; cases of fetal distress where delivery is not imminent; prolonged use in uterine inertia or severe toxemia; hypertonic or hyperactive uterine patterns; where adequate uterine activity fails to achieve satisfactory progress; induction or augmentation of labor where vaginal delivery is contraindicated, such as invasive cervical carcinoma, active herpes genitalis, cord presentation or prolapse, total placenta previa, and vasa previa; hypersensitivity to the drug.

Warnings

➤*IV use:* When given for induction or augmentation of uterine activity, administer oxytocin only by the IV route and with adequate medical supervision in hospital. All patients receiving IV oxytocin must be under continuous observation by trained personnel who have a thorough knowledge of the drug and are qualified to identify complications.

OXYTOCIN — INJECTION

➤*Special risk patients:* Except in unusual circumstances, do not administer oxytocin in the following conditions: fetal distress; hydramnios; partial placenta previa; prematurity; borderline cephalopelvic disproportion and any condition in which there is a predisposition for uterine rupture, such as previous major surgery on the cervix or uterus including cesarean section; overdistention of the uterus; grand multiparity; history of uterine sepsis or traumatic delivery; invasive cervical carcinoma. Weigh the potential benefits oxytocin can provide in a given case against rare but definite potential for the drug to produce hypertonicity or tetanic spasm.

➤*Maternal deaths:* Maternal deaths caused by hypertensive episodes, subarachnoid hemorrhage, or rupture of the uterus and fetal deaths caused by various causes have been associated with the use of parenteral oxytocic drugs for induction of labor or for augmentation in the first and second stages of labor.

➤*Pregnancy:* There are no known indications for use in the first and second trimester of pregnancy other than in relation to spontaneous or induced abortion. Oxytocin is not expected to present a risk of fetal abnormalities when used as indicated (see Adverse Reactions in the fetus).

➤*Lactation:* It is not known whether this drug is excreted in human milk. Because many drugs are excreted in human milk, exercise caution when administering to a nursing mother.

➤*Children:* Oxytocin is not intended for use in children.

Precautions

➤*Monitoring:* During the induction or stimulation of labor, monitor fetal heart rate, resting uterine tone, and the frequency, duration, and force of contraction. Keep in mind the possibility of increased blood and afibrinogenemia when administering the drug. Monitor for signs of water intoxication (eg, drowsiness, listlessness, confusion, headache, anuria).

Electronic fetal monitoring provides the best means for early detection of overdosage (see Overdosage). However, keep in mind that only intrauterine pressure recording can accurately measure the intrauterine pressure during contractions. A fetal scalp electrode provides a more dependable recording of the fetal heart rate than any external monitoring system.

➤*Uterine contractions:* When properly administered, oxytocin stimulates uterine contractions comparable with those in normal labor. Overstimulation of the uterus can be hazardous to the mother and fetus. Even with proper administration and adequate supervision, hypertonic contractions can occur in patients whose uteri are hypersensitive to oxytocin. Consider this fact in exercising judgment regarding patient selection.

➤*Water intoxication:* Oxytocin has an intrinsic antidiuretic effect, acting to increase water reabsorption from the glomerular filtrate. Consider the possibility of water intoxication, particularly when oxytocin is administered by continuous infusion and the patient is receiving fluids by mouth. Severe water intoxication with convulsions and coma has occurred and is associated with a slow infusion over a 24-hour period. Maternal death caused by oxytocin-induced water intoxication has been reported.

➤*Existent labor:* When oxytocin is used for induction or reinforcement of already existent labor, carefully select patients. Consider pelvic adequacy and maternal and fetal conditions before use of the drug.

Drug Interactions

➤*Cyclopropane anesthesia:* Cyclopropane anesthesia may modify oxytocin's cardiovascular effects, producing unexpected results such as hypotension. Maternal sinus bradycardia with abnormal atrioventricular rhythms also has been noted when oxytocin was used concomitantly with cyclopropane anesthesia.

➤*Sympathomimetics:* If used concurrently with oxytocic drugs, the pressor effect of the sympathomimetics may be increased, possibly resulting in postpartum hypertension.

➤*Vasoconstrictors/caudal block anesthesia:* Severe hypertension occurred when oxytocin was given 3 to 4 hours following prophylactic administration of a vasoconstrictor in conjunction with caudal block anesthesia.

Adverse Reactions

➤*Maternal:*

Cardiovascular – Cardiac arrhythmia, hypertensive episodes, premature ventricular contractions.

GI – Nausea, vomiting.

GU – Pelvic hematoma, postpartum hemorrhage; rupture of the uterus, spasm, tetanic contraction, or uterine hypertonicity may occur from excessive dosage or hypersensitivity to the drug.

Miscellaneous – Anaphylactic reaction, fatal afibrinogenemia, subarachnoid hemorrhage; severe water intoxication with convulsions, coma, and death have been reported.

➤*Fetal or neonate (caused by induced uterine motility):*

Cardiovascular – Bradycardia, premature ventricular contractions, and other arrhythmias.

CNS – Permanent CNS or brain damage, neonatal seizures.

Miscellaneous – Fetal death, low Apgar scores at 5 minutes, neonatal jaundice, neonatal retinal hemorrhage.

Overdosage

➤*Symptoms:* Overdosage depends essentially on uterine hyperactivity, whether or not caused by hypersensitivity to this agent. Hyperstimulation with strong (hypertonic) or prolonged (tetanic) contractions or a resting tone of at least 15 to 20 mm H_2O between contractions can lead to tumultuous labor, uterine rupture, cervical and vaginal lacerations, postpartum hemorrhage, uteroplacental hypoperfusion, and variable deceleration of fetal heart, fetal hypoxia, hypercapnia, perinatal hepatic necrosis, or death. Water intoxication with convulsions, which is caused by the inherent antidiuretic effect of oxytocin, is a serious complication that may occur if large doses (40 to 50 milliunits/min) are infused for long periods.

➤*Treatment:* To treat, discontinue drug, restrict fluid intake, initiate diuresis, administer IV hypertonic saline solution, correct electrolyte imbalance, control convulsions, and provide supportive therapy.

ERGONOVINE MALEATE

Rx	**Ergotrate** (HPS Rx Enterprises)	**Tablets:** 0.2 mg	Mannitol. (HPS). White. In 100s, 500s, and 1,000s.

ERGONOVINE MALEATE — ORAL

Indications

➤*Postpartum/postabortal hemorrhage:* For the prevention and treatment of postpartum and postabortal hemorrhage caused by uterine atony.

➤*Unlabeled uses:* Oxytocin challenge test.

Administration and Dosage

The immediate postpartum dose of ergonovine is usually 0.2 mg. It is ordinarily administered parenterally. To minimize late postpartum bleeding, 1 or 2 tablets may be given orally 2 to 4 times daily (every 6 to 12 hours) until the danger of uterine atony has passed (usually 48 hours). Severe cramping is evidence of effectiveness but may justify reduction in dosage. Tablets also may be administered sublingually.

➤*Storage/Stability:* Store at controlled room temperature 15° to 30°C (59° to 86°F).

Dispense in a tight, light-resistant container with a child-resistant closure.

Actions

➤*Pharmacology:* Within 6 to 15 minutes, ergonovine produces a firm tetanic contraction of the postpartum uterus that, in the course of about 90 minutes, gradually changes to a series of clonic contractions that persist for another 90 minutes or more.

Contraindications

Induction of labor and in cases of threatened spontaneous abortion; do not administer to those patients who have shown allergic or idiosyncratic reactions to it.

Warnings

➤*Pregnancy:*

Uterine effects – All oxytocic agents are potentially dangerous. Mothers and infants have been injured, and some have died because of their injudicious use. Hyperstimulation of the uterus during labor may lead to uterine tetany and marked impairment of the uteroplacental blood flow, uterine rupture, cervical and perineal lacerations, amniotic fluid embolism, and trauma to the infant (eg, hypoxia, intracranial hemorrhage). Because of hazards that result from overdosage, oxytocic agents must be administered under conditions of meticulous observation.

Labor and delivery – Because of the high uterine tone produced, ergonovine is not recommended for routine use prior to the delivery of the placenta unless the operator is versed in the technique described by Davis and others and has adequate facilities and personnel at his disposal.

Precautions

➤*Monitoring:* Monitor blood pressure, pulse, and uterine response. Note sudden changes in vital signs or frequent periods of uterine relaxation.

➤*Duration:* As is the case with all ergot preparations, avoid prolonged use of ergonovine. Discontinue ergonovine if symptoms of ergotism appear.

➤*Vaginal bleeding:* Observe the character and amount of vaginal bleeding.

➤*Calcium deficiency:* Hypocalcemia may affect patient response to the drug. If the patient is not also taking digitalis, cautious administration of calcium gluconate IV may produce the desired oxytocic action.

➤*Special risk:* Use ergonovine cautiously in patients with hypertension, heart disease, venoatrial shunts, mitral-valve stenosis, obliterative vascular disease, sepsis, or hepatic or renal impairment.

Adverse Reactions

Nausea and vomiting may occur, but they are uncommon. Allergic phenomena, including shock, have been reported. Ergotism has also been reported. Elevation of blood pressure (sometimes extreme) may appear in a small percentage of patients, most frequently in association with regional anesthesia (caudal or spinal), previous administration of a vasoconstrictor, and the IV route of administration of the oxytocic. The mechanism of such hypertension is obscure because it may occur in the absence of anesthesia, vasoconstrictors, and oxytocics. These elevations are no more frequent with ergonovine

ERGONOVINE MALEATE — ORAL

than with other oxytocics. They usually subside promptly following IV administration of 15 mg chlorpromazine.

Overdosage

➤*Symptoms:* The principal manifestations of serious overdosage are convulsions and gangrene. Symptoms of overdosage include the following: vomiting, diarrhea, dizziness, rise or fall in blood pressure, weak pulse, dyspnea, loss of consciousness, numbness and coldness of the extremities, tingling, pain in the chest, gangrene of the fingers and toes, and hypercoagulability.

➤*Treatment:* Treat convulsions. Control hypercoagulability by the administration of heparin, and maintain blood-clotting time at approximately 3 times the normal. Give a vasodilator such as tolazine as an antidote; the rate of administration may be controlled by monitoring pulse rate and blood pressure. For emergency measures, delay absorption of ingested ergonovine by giving tap water, milk, or activated charcoal and then removing by gastric lavage or emesis followed by catharsis. Gangrene will require surgical amputation.

METHYLERGONOVINE MALEATE

Rx	**Methergine** (Sandoz)	**Tablets:** 0.2 mg	Lactose, FD&C Blue No.1, parabens, sucrose. (78-54 SANDOZ). Orchid, round. Coated. In 100s.
		Injection: 0.2 mg/mL	In 1 mL ampuls.

METHYLERGONOVINE MALEATE — ORAL

Indications

➤*Uterine contractions/bleeding:* For routine management after delivery of the placenta; postpartum atony and hemorrhage; subinvolution. Under full obstetric supervision, it may be given in the second stage of labor following delivery of the anterior shoulder.

Administration and Dosage

➤*Approved by the FDA:* November 19, 1946.

➤*Dosage:* 1 tablet (0.2 mg) 3 or 4 times daily in the puerperium for a maximum of 1 week.

➤*Storage/Stability:* Store tablets below 25°C (77°F) in a tight, light-resistant container.

Actions

➤*Pharmacology:* Methylergonovine maleate acts directly on the smooth muscle of the uterus and increases the tone, rate, and amplitude of rhythmic contractions. Thus, it induces a rapid and sustained tetanic uterotonic effect which shortens the third stage of labor and reduces blood loss. The onset of action after oral administration is 5 to 10 minutes.

➤*Pharmacokinetics:*

Absorption/Distribution – The bioavailability after oral administration was reported to be about 60%, with no accumulation after repeated doses.

Bioavailability studies conducted in fasting, healthy female volunteers have shown that oral absorption of a 0.2 mg methylergonovine tablet was fairly rapid, with a mean peak plasma concentration of 3,243 ± 1,308 pg/mL observed at 1.12 ± 0.82 hours. The extent of absorption of the tablet, based upon methylergonovine plasma concentrations, was found to be equivalent to that of the IM solution given orally, and the extent of oral absorption of the IM solution was proportional to the dose following administration of 0.1, 0.2, and 0.4 mg. The volume of distribution (Vd_{ss}/F) of methylergonovine was calculated to be 56.1 ± 17 L, and the plasma clearance (CLp/F) was calculated to be 14.4 ± 4.5 L/hr. A delayed GI absorption (t_{max} about 3 hours) of methylergonovine maleate tablet might be observed in postpartum women during continuous treatment with this oxytocic agent.

Metabolism/Excretion – Ergot alkaloids are mostly eliminated by hepatic metabolism and excretion, and the decrease in bioavailability following oral administration is probably a result of first-pass metabolism in the liver.

The plasma level decline was biphasic with a mean elimination half-life of 3.39 hours (range, 1.5 to 12.7 hours).

Contraindications

Certain ergot alkaloid drugs (eg, dihydroergotamine, ergotamine) are contraindicated for concomitant use with potent CYP3A4 inhibitors (eg, protease inhibitors, macrolide antibiotics, azole antifungals) because of the risk of vasospasm leading to cerebral ischemia and/or ischemia of the extremities. Although there have been no reports of such interactions with methylergonovine alone, potent CYP3A4 inhibitors should not be used concomitantly with methylergonovine.

Hypertension, toxemia, pregnancy, and hypersensitivity.

Warnings

➤*CYP3A4 inhibitors (eg, macrolide antibiotics and protease inhibitors):* There have been rare reports of serious adverse events in connection with the coadministration of certain ergot alkaloid drugs (eg, dihydroergotamine and ergotamine) and potent CYP3A4 inhibitors, resulting in vasospasm leading to cerebral ischemia and/or ischemia of the extremities. Although there have been no reports of such interactions with methylergonovine alone, potent CYP3A4 inhibitors should not be coadministered with methylergonovine.

➤*Pregnancy: Category C.* Animal reproductive studies have not been conducted with methylergonovine maleate. It is also not known whether methylergonovine maleate can cause fetal harm or can affect reproductive capacity. Use of methylergonovine maleate is contraindicated during pregnancy because of its uterotonic effects.

Labor and delivery – The uterotonic effect of methylergonovine maleate is utilized after delivery to assist involution and decrease hemorrhage, shortening the third stage of labor.

➤*Lactation:* Methylergonovine maleate may be administered orally for a maximum of 1 week postpartum to control uterine bleeding. Recommended dosage is 1 tablet (0.2 mg) 3 or 4 times daily. At this dosage level, a small quantity of drug appears in mothers' milk. Caution should be exercised when methylergonovine maleate is administered to a nursing woman.

➤*Children:* Safety and efficacy in children patients have not been established.

Precautions

➤*Special risk:* Exercise caution should be in the presence of sepsis, obliterative vascular disease, hepatic or renal involvement. Also use with caution during the second stage of labor. The necessity for manual removal of a retained placenta should occur only rarely with proper technique and adequate allowance of time for its spontaneous separation.

Drug Interactions

➤*CYP3A4 inhibitors:* Methylergonovine should not be coadministered with potent CYP3A4 inhibitors. Examples of some of the more potent CYP3A4 inhibitors include macrolide antibiotics (eg, clarithromycin, erythromycin, troleandomycin), HIV protease or reverse transcriptase inhibitors (eg, delavirdine, indinavir, nelfinavir, ritonavir) or azole antifungals (eg, ketoconazole, itraconazole, voriconazole). Less potent CYP3A4 inhibitors should be administered with caution. Less potent inhibitors include saquinavir, nefazodone, fluconazole, grapefruit juice, fluoxetine, fluvoxamine, zileuton, and clotrimazole. These lists are not exhaustive, and the prescriber should consider the effects on CYP3A4 of other agents being considered for concomitant use with methylergonovine (see Warnings).

➤*Vasoconstrictors/Ergot alkaloids:* Exercise caution when methylergonovine maleate is used concurrently with other vasoconstrictors or ergot alkaloids.

Adverse Reactions

The most common adverse reaction is hypertension associated in several cases with seizure or headache. Hypotension has also been reported. Nausea and vomiting have occurred occasionally. Rarely observed reactions have included, in order of severity: acute myocardial infarction, transient chest pains, dyspnea, hematuria, thrombophlebitis, water intoxication, hallucinations, leg cramps, dizziness, tinnitus, nasal congestion, diarrhea, diaphoresis, palpitation, and foul taste.

There have been rare isolated reports of anaphylaxis, without a proven causal relationship to the drug product.

Overdosage

Because reports of overdosage with methylergonovine maleate are infrequent, the lethal dose in humans has not been established. The oral LD_{50} (in mg/kg) for the mouse is 187, the rat, 93, and the rabbit, 4.5. Several cases of accidental methylergonovine maleate injection in newborn infants have been reported, and, in such cases, 0.2 mg represents an overdose of great magnitude. However, recovery occurred in all but 1 case following a period of respiratory depression, hypothermia, hypertonicity with jerking movements, and, in 1 case, a single convulsion.

Also, several children 1 to 3 years of age have accidentally ingested up to 10 tablets (2 mg) with no apparent ill effects. A postpartum patient took 4 tablets at 1 time in error and reported paresthesias and clamminess as her only symptoms.

➤*Symptoms:* Symptoms of acute overdose may include the following: abdominal pain, nausea, numbness, tingling of the extremities, vomiting, rise in blood pressure, in severe cases followed by coma, convulsions, hypotension, hypothermia, and respiratory depression.

➤*Treatment:* Treatment of acute overdosage is symptomatic and includes the following usual procedures of: removal of offending drug by inducing emesis, gastric lavage, catharsis, and supportive diuresis; maintenance of adequate pulmonary ventilation, especially if convulsions or coma develop; correction of hypotension with pressor drugs as needed; control of convulsions with standard anticonvulsant agents; control of peripheral vasospasm with warmth to the extremities if needed.

METHYLERGONOVINE MALEATE — INJECTION

Indications

➤*Uterine contractions/bleeding:* For routine management after delivery of the placenta; postpartum atony and hemorrhage; subinvolution. Under full obstetric supervision, it may be given in the second stage of labor following delivery of the anterior shoulder.

Administration and Dosage

➤*Approved by the FDA:* November 19, 1946.

➤*IM:* 1 mL, 0.2 mg, after delivery of the anterior shoulder, after delivery of the placenta, or during the puerperium. May be repeated as required, at intervals of 2 to 4 hours.

➤*IV:* Dosage same as IM. This drug should not be administered IV routinely because of the possibility of inducing sudden hypertensive and cerebrovascular accidents. If IV administration is considered essential as a lifesaving measure, methylergonovine maleate should be given slowly over a period of no less than 60 seconds with careful monitoring of blood pressure. Intra-arterial or periarterial injection should be strictly avoided.

➤*Storage/Stability:*

Ampuls – Store in refrigerator, 2° to 8°C (36° to 46°F). Protect from light. Administer only if solution is clear and colorless.

Actions

➤*Pharmacology:* Methylergonovine maleate injection acts directly on the smooth muscle of the uterus and increases the tone, rate, and amplitude of rhythmic contractions. Thus, it induces a rapid and sustained tetanic uterotonic effect which shortens the third stage of labor and reduces blood loss. The onset of action after IV administration is immediate; after IM administration, it is 2 to 5 minutes.

➤*Pharmacokinetics:*

Absorption/Distribution – Pharmacokinetic studies following an IV injection have shown that methylergonovine is rapidly distributed from plasma to peripheral tissues within 2 to 3 minutes or less. During delivery, with IM injection, bioavailability increased to 78%.

For a 0.2 mg IM injection, a mean peak plasma concentration of 5,918 ± 1,952 pg/mL was observed at 0.41 ± 0.21 hours. When given IM, the extent of absorption of methylergonovine maleate solution was about 25% greater than the tablet. The volume of distribution (Vd_{ss}/F) of methylergonovine was calculated to be 56.1 ± 17 L, and the plasma clearance (CLp/F) was calculated to be 14.4 ± 4.5 L/hr.

Metabolism/Excretion – The plasma level decline was biphasic with a mean elimination half-life of 3.39 hours (range 1.5 to 12.7 hours). Ergot alkaloids are mostly eliminated by hepatic metabolism and excretion, and the decrease in bioavailability following oral administration is probably a result of first-pass metabolism in the liver.

Contraindications

Certain ergot alkaloid drugs (eg, dihydroergotamine and ergotamine) are contraindicated for concomitant use with potent CYP3A4 inhibitors (eg, protease inhibitors, macrolide antibiotics, azole antifungals) because of the risk of vasospasm leading to cerebral ischemia and/or ischemia of the extremities. Although there have been no reports of such interactions with methylergonovine alone, potent CYP3A4 inhibitors should not be used concomitantly with methylergonovine.

Hypertension; toxemia; pregnancy; and hypersensitivity.

Warnings

➤*Administration:* This drug should not be administered IV routinely because of the possibility of inducing sudden hypertensive and cerebrovascular accidents. If IV administration is considered essential as a lifesaving measure, methylergonovine maleate should be given slowly over a period of no less than 60 seconds with careful monitoring of blood pressure. Intra-arterial or periarterial injection should be strictly avoided.

➤*CYP3A4 inhibitors (eg, macrolide antibiotics and protease inhibitors):* There have been rare reports of serious adverse events in connection with the coadministration of certain ergot alkaloid drugs (eg, dihydroergotamine and ergotamine) and potent CYP3A4 inhibitors, resulting in vasospasm leading to cerebral ischemia and/or ischemia of the extremities. Although there have been no reports of such interactions with methylergonovine alone, potent CYP3A4 inhibitors should not be coadministered with methylergonovine.

➤*Pregnancy: Category C.* Animal reproductive studies have not been conducted with methylergonovine maleate. It is also not known whether methylergonovine maleate can cause fetal harm or can affect reproductive capacity. Use of methylergonovine maleate is contraindicated during pregnancy because of its uterotonic effects.

Labor and delivery – The uterotonic effect of methylergonovine maleate is utilized after delivery to assist involution and decrease hemorrhage, shortening the third stage of labor.

➤*Lactation:* Methylergonovine maleate may be administered orally for a maximum of 1 week postpartum to control uterine bleeding. Recommended dosage is 1 tablet (0.2 mg) 3 or 4 times daily. At this dosage level a small quantity of drug appears in mothers' milk. Caution should be exercised when methylergonovine maleate is administered to a nursing woman.

➤*Children:* Safety and efficacy in children have not been established.

Precautions

➤*Special risk:* Exercised caution in the presence of sepsis, obliterative vascular disease, hepatic or renal involvement. Also use with caution during the second stage of labor. The necessity for manual removal of a retained placenta should occur only rarely with proper technique and adequate allowance of time for its spontaneous separation.

Drug Interactions

➤*CYP3A4 inhibitors:* Methylergonovine should not be coadministered with potent CYP3A4 inhibitors. Examples of some of the more potent CYP3A4 inhibitors include macrolide antibiotics (eg, clarithromycin, erythromycin, troleandomycin), HIV protease or reverse transcriptase inhibitors (eg, delavirdine, indinavir, nelfinavir, ritonavir) or azole antifungals (eg, itraconazole, ketoconazole, voriconazole). Less potent CYP3A4 inhibitors should be administered with caution. Less potent inhibitors include saquinavir, nefazodone, fluconazole, grapefruit juice, fluoxetine, fluvoxamine, zileuton, and clotrimazole. These lists are not exhaustive, and the prescriber should consider the effects on CYP3A4 of other agents being considered for concomitant use with methylergonovine (see Warnings).

➤*Vasoconstrictors/Ergo alkaloids:* Exercise caution when methylergonovine maleate injection is used concurrently with other vasoconstrictors or ergot alkaloids.

Adverse Reactions

The most common adverse reaction is hypertension associated in several cases with seizure or headache. Hypotension has also been reported. Nausea and vomiting have occurred occasionally. Rarely observed reactions have included, in order of severity: Acute myocardial infarction, transient chest pains, dyspnea, hematuria, thrombophlebitis, water intoxication, hallucinations, leg cramps, dizziness, tinnitus, nasal congestion, diarrhea, diaphoresis, palpitation, and foul taste.

There have been rare, isolated reports of anaphylaxis, without a proven causal relationship to the drug product.

Overdosage

Because reports of overdosage with methylergonovine maleate are infrequent, the lethal dose in humans has not been established. The oral LD_{50} (in mg/kg) for the mouse is 187, the rat, 93, and the rabbit, 4.5. Several cases of accidental methylergonovine maleate injection in newborn infants have been reported, and, in such cases, 0.2 mg represents an overdose of great magnitude. However, recovery occurred in all but 1 case following a period of respiratory depression, hypothermia, hypertonicity with jerking movements, and, in 1 case, a single convulsion.

Also, several children 1 to 3 years of age have accidentally ingested up to 10 tablets (2 mg) with no apparent ill effects. A postpartum patient took 4 tablets at 1 time in error, and reported paresthesias and clamminess as her only symptoms.

➤*Symptoms:* Symptoms of acute overdose may include the following: nausea, vomiting, abdominal pain, numbness, tingling of the extremities, rise in blood pressure, in severe cases followed by hypotension, respiratory depression, hypothermia, convulsions, and coma.

➤*Treatment:* Treatment of acute overdosage is symptomatic and includes the usual procedures of the following: removal of offending drug by inducing emesis, gastric lavage, catharsis, and supportive diuresis; maintenance of adequate pulmonary ventilation, especially if convulsions or coma develop; correction of hypotension with pressor drugs as needed; control of convulsions with standard anticonvulsant agents; control of peripheral vasospasm with warmth to the extremities if needed.

BISPHOSPHONATES

Indications

➤*Osteoporosis in postmenopausal women (alendronate, risedronate):* For the treatment and prevention of osteoporosis in postmenopausal women.

➤*Osteoporosis in men (alendronate):* To increase bone mass in men with osteoporosis.

➤*Glucocorticoid-induced osteoporosis (alendronate, risedronate):* For the prevention and treatment of glucocorticoid-induced osteoporosis in men and women who are either initiating or continuing systemic glucocorticoid treatment for chronic diseases.

➤*Paget disease (osteitis deformans):* For treatment of patients with Paget disease of bone having alkaline phosphatase at least 2 times the upper limit of normal (ULN), or those who are symptomatic or at risk for future complications from their disease (**alendronate**, **risedronate**, **tiludronate**); treatment of symptomatic Paget disease (oral **etidronate**); treatment of moderate to severe Paget disease (**pamidronate**).

➤*Heterotopic ossification (oral etidronate):* Prevention and treatment of heterotopic ossification following total hip replacement or caused by spinal injury.

➤*Hypercalcemia of malignancy (HCM):* For the treatment of HCM (**zoledronic acid**); in conjunction with adequate hydration (eg, saline hydration, with or without loop diuretics) for the treatment of moderate or severe hypercalcemia associated with malignancy with or without bone metastases (**pamidronate**; patients with epidermoid or nonepidermoid tumors respond to pamidronate); when inadequately managed by dietary modification or oral hydration, concurrent therapy is recommended as soon as there is a restoration of urine output (IV **etidronate**); for HCM that persists after adequate hydration has been restored (IV **etidronate**).

➤*Breast cancer/Multiple myeloma (pamidronate):* In conjunction with standard antineoplastic therapy for the treatment of osteolytic bone metastases of breast cancer and osteolytic lesions of multiple myeloma.

➤*Multiple myeloma and bone metastases of solid tumors (zoledronic acid):* For the treatment of patients with multiple myeloma and patients with documented bone metastases from solid tumors, in conjunction with standard antineoplastic therapy. Prostate cancer should have progressed after treatment with at least 1 hormonal therapy.

➤*Unlabeled uses:*

Etidronate – Treatment and prevention of osteoporosis in postmenopausal women; prevention of corticosteroid-induced osteoporosis.

Pamidronate – Postmenopausal osteoporosis; hyperparathyroidism; prevent glucocorticoid-induced osteoporosis; reduce bone pain in patients with prostatic carcinoma; immobilization-related hypercalcemia.

Actions

➤*Pharmacology:* **Etidronate**, **tiludronate**, **pamidronate**, **risedronate**, and **alendronate** are bisphosphonates that act primarily on the bone. Their major pharmacologic action is the inhibition of normal and abnormal bone resorption. Secondarily, etidronate reduces bone formation because formation is coupled to resorption; pamidronate inhibits bone resorption apparently without inhibiting bone formation and mineralization. Alendronate shows preferential localization to sites of bone resorption, specifically under osteoclasts. The osteoclasts adhere normally to the bone surface but lack the ruffled border that is indicative of active resorption. Alendronate does not interfere with osteoclast recruitment or attachment, but it does inhibit osteoclast activity. Tiludronate disodium appears to inhibit osteoclasts through at least 2 mechanisms: Disruption of the cytoskeletal ring structure, possibly by inhibition of protein-tyrosine-phosphatase, thus leading to detachment of osteoclasts from the bone surface and the inhibition of the osteoclastic proton pump.

Reduction of abnormal bone resorption is responsible for therapeutic benefit in hypercalcemia. The exact mechanism(s) is not fully understood, but may be related to inhibition of hydroxyapatite crystal dissolution or its action on bone-resorbing cells. Pamidronate inhibits accelerated bone resorption resulting from osteoclast hyperactivity induced by various tumors in animals. The number of osteoclasts in active bone turnover sites is substantially reduced after etidronate. Etidronate also can inhibit formation and growth of hydroxyapatite crystals and their amorphous precursors at concentrations in excess of those required to inhibit crystal dissolution.

Alendronate – As a result of bone resorption inhibition, asymptomatic reductions in serum calcium and phosphate concentrations are seen after treatment with alendronate. In long-term studies, reductions from baseline in serum calcium (approximately 2%) and phosphate (approximately 4% to 6%) were seen the first month after initiation of 10 mg alendronate, but no further decreases were seen for the 5-year duration of the studies. The reduction in serum phosphate may reflect not only the positive bone mineral balance caused by alendronate but also a decrease in renal phosphate reabsorption. Alendronate decreases the rate of bone resorption directly, leading to an indirect decrease in bone formation.

In Paget disease, 40 mg alendronate once daily for 6 months produced highly significant decreases in serum alkaline phosphatase as well as in urinary markers of bone collagen degradation. As a result of the inhibition of bone resorption, alendronate induced generally mild, transient, and asymptomatic decreases in serum calcium and phosphate.

Etidronate – Etidronate does not appear to alter renal tubular reabsorption of calcium and does not affect hypercalcemia in patients with hyperparathyroidism where increased calcium reabsorption may be a factor in hypercalcemia. Hyperphosphatemia has been observed with oral etidronate, usually with doses of 10 to 20 mg/kg/day; no adverse effects have been noted, and it is not a contraindication. It is apparently caused by drug-related increased phosphate tubular reabsorption by the kidneys. Serum phosphate levels generally return to normal 2 to 4 weeks post-therapy.

In Paget disease, etidronate slows accelerated bone turnover (resorption and accretion) in pagetic lesions and to a lesser extent, in normal bone. Reduced bone turnover is often accompanied by symptomatic improvement, including reduced bone pain. Incidence of pagetic fractures may decrease, and elevated cardiac output and other vascular disorders improve.

Pamidronate – Pamidronate therapy has decreased serum phosphate levels, presumably caused by decreased release of phosphate from bone and increased renal excretion as parathyroid hormone levels (usually suppressed in HCM) return toward normal. Phosphate therapy was administered in 30% of patients; levels usually returned to normal within 7 to 10 days. Urinary calcium/creatinine and urinary hydroxyproline/creatinine ratios decrease and usually return to normal or below after treatment. The changes occur within the first week after treatment, as do decreases in serum calcium levels.

Risedronate – In pagetic patients treated with 30 mg/day risedronate for 2 months, bone turnover returned to normal in a majority of patients as evidenced by significant reductions in serum alkaline phosphatase (SAP), a marker of bone formation, and in urinary hydroxyproline/creatinine and deoxypyridinoline/creatinine, markers of bone resorption. Radiographic structural changes of bone lesions, especially improvement of a majority of lesions with an osteolytic front in weight-bearing bones, also were observed. In addition, histomorphometric data provide further support that risedronate decreases the extent of osteolysis in the appendicular and axial skeleton. Osteolytic lesions in the lower extremities improved or were unchanged in 15/16 (94%) of assessed patients; 9/16 (56%) patients showed clear improvement in osteolytic lesions. No evidence of new fractures was observed.

Tiludronate – In pagetic patients treated with 400 mg/day tiludronate for 3 months, changes in urinary hydroxyproline, a biochemical marker of bone resorption and in serum alkaline phosphatase, a marker of bone formation, indicate a reduction toward normal in the rate of bone turnover. In addition, reduced numbers of osteoclasts by histomorphometric analysis and radiological improvement of lytic lesions indicate that tiludronate can suppress the pagetic disease process.

Zoledronic acid – In vitro, zoledronic acid inhibits osteoclastic activity and induces osteoclast apoptosis. Zoledronic acid also blocks the osteoclastic resorption of mineralized bone and cartilage through its binding to bone. Zoledronic acid inhibits the increased osteoclastic activity and skeletal calcium release induced by various stimulatory factors released by tumors.

➤*Pharmacokinetics:*

Special populations –

Renal function impairment: The pharmacokinetics of **pamidronate** were studied in cancer patients (n = 19) with normal and varying degrees of renal impairment. Given the recommended dose, 90 mg infused over 4 hours, excessive accumulation of pamidronate in renally impaired patients is not anticipated if pamidronate is administered on a monthly basis.

Alendronate – There is no evidence that alendronate is metabolized. Relative to an IV reference dose, mean oral bioavailability in women was 0.64% for 5 to 70 mg doses after an overnight fast and 2 hours before a standardized breakfast. Oral bioavailability of the 10 mg tablet in men (0.59%) was similar to that in women given after an overnight fast and 2 hours before breakfast. In 49 postmenopausal women, bioavailability was decreased by approximately 40% when 10 mg was given 0.5 or 1 hour before a standardized breakfast when compared with dosing 2 hours before eating. Bioavailability was negligible whether alendronate was given with or up to 2 hours after a standardized breakfast. Concomitant coffee or orange juice reduced bioavailability by approximately 60%. Mean steady-state volume of distribution (exclusive of bone) is at least 28 L. Protein binding in plasma is approximately 78%. After a single IV dose, approximately 50% was excreted in the urine with little or none recovered in the feces. After a single 10 mg IV dose, renal clearance was 71 mL/min; systemic clearance did not exceed 200 mL/min. Plasma levels fell by more than 95% within 6 hours after IV administration. The terminal half-life is estimated to exceed 10 years, probably reflecting alendronate release from the skeleton. Based on the above, it is estimated that after 10 years of 10 mg/day orally, the amount of alendronate released daily from the skeleton is approximately 25% of that absorbed from the GI tract.

Etidronate – Etidronate is not metabolized. The amount of drug absorbed after an oral dose is approximately 3%. In normal subjects, plasma half-life of etidronate, based on noncompartmental pharmacokinetics is 1 to 6 hours. Within 24 hours, about 50% of the absorbed dose is excreted in urine; the remainder is distributed to bone compartments from which it is slowly eliminated. Animal studies have yielded bone clearance estimates up to 165 days. In humans, the residence time on bone may vary due to such factors as specific metabolic condition and bone type. Unabsorbed drug is excreted intact in feces. Preclinical studies indicate etidronate disodium does not cross the blood-brain barrier. The mean residence time for IV etidronate in the exchangeable pool is approximately 8.7 hours. The mean volume of distribution at steady state in healthy subjects is 1370 ± 203 mL/kg while the plasma half-life is approximately 6 hours. In these same subjects, nonrenal clearance from the exchangeable pool amounts to 30% to 50% of the infused dose. This nonrenal clearance is caused by uptake by bone; subsequently, the drug is slowly eliminated through bone turnover. The half-life in bone is in excess of 90 days.

Pamidronate – Cancer patients (n = 24) who had minimal or no bony involvement were given an IV infusion of 30, 60, or 90 mg of pamidronate over 4 hours and 90 mg of pamidronate over 24 hours. The mean ± SD body retention of pamidronate was calculated to be 54% ± 16% of the dose over 120 hours.

Pamidronate is not metabolized and is exclusively eliminated by renal excretion. After administration of 30, 60, and 90 mg of pamidronate over 4 hours, and 90 mg of pamidronate over 24 hours, an overall mean ± SD of 46% ± 16% of the drug was excreted unchanged in the urine within 120 hours. Cumulative urinary excretion was linearly related to dose. The mean ± SD elimination half-life is 28 ± 7 hours. Mean ± SD total and renal clearances of pamidronate were 107 ± 50 mL/min and 49 ± 28 mL/min, respectively. The rate of elimination from bone has not been determined.

After IV administration in rats, approximately 50% to 60% was rapidly adsorbed by bone and slowly eliminated by the kidneys. In rats given 10 mg/kg bolus injections, approximately 30% of the compound was found in the liver shortly after administration and was then redistributed to bone or eliminated by the kidneys over 24 to 48 hours. The drug was rapidly cleared from circulation and taken up mainly by bones, liver, spleen, teeth, and tracheal cartilage. Bone uptake occurred preferentially in areas of high bone turnover. The terminal phase of elimination half-life in bone was approximately 300 days.

Risedronate – Like other bisphosphonates, no evidence supports systemic metabolism of risedronate. Absorption is relatively rapid (T_{max} approximately 1 hour) and is independent of dose. Mean oral bioavailability is 0.63%. Dosing either 0.5 hours prior to breakfast or 2 hours after dinner reduces extent of absorption by 55% as compared with the fasting state. Dosing 1 hour prior to breakfast reduces extent of absorption by 30% as compared with dosing in the fasting state.

Animal studies indicate that approximately 60% of the dose is distributed to bone with the remainder excreted in the urine. The mean steady-state volume of distribution is 6.3 L/kg; plasma protein binding is about 24%.

Approximately 50% of the absorbed dose is excreted in urine within 24 hours, and 85% of an IV dose is recovered in the urine over 28 days. Mean renal clearance is 105 mL/min and mean total clearance is 122 mL/min, with the difference primarily reflecting nonrenal clearance or clearance caused by adsorption to bone. The renal clearance is not concentration-dependent, and there is a linear relationship between renal clearance and creatinine clearance. Unabsorbed drug is eliminated unchanged in feces. Once risedronate is absorbed, the serum concentration-time profile is multiphasic with an initial half-life of about 1.5 hours and a terminal exponential half-life of 480 hours.

Tiludronate – In animals, tiludronic acid undergoes little if any metabolism. In vitro, tiludronic acid is not metabolized in human liver microsomes and hepatocytes.

Relative to IV reference dose, the mean oral bioavailability of tiludronate disodium in healthy men was 6% after an oral dose equivalent to 400 mg tiludronic acid administered after an overnight fast and 4 hours before a standard breakfast. Bioavailability is reduced by food.

After administration of a single dose equivalent to 400 mg tiludronic acid to healthy men, tiludronic acid was rapidly absorbed with peak plasma concentrations of approximately 3 mg/L occurring within 2 hours. In pagetic patients, after repeated administration of doses equivalent to 400 mg/day tiludronic acid (2 hours before or 2 hours after a meal) for durations of 12 days to 12 weeks, average plasma concentrations of tiludronic acid occurring between 1 and 2 hours after dosing ranged between 1 and 4.6 mg/L.

After oral administration of doses equivalent to 400 mg/day tiludronic acid to nonpagetic patients with osteoarthrosis, the steady state in bone was not reached after 30 days of dosing. At plasma concentrations between 1 and 10 mg/L, tiludronic acid was approximately 90% bound to human serum protein (mainly albumin).

The principal route of elimination of tiludronic acid is in the urine. After IV administration to healthy volunteers, approximately 60% of the dose was excreted in the urine as tiludronic acid within 13 days. Renal clearance is dose independent and is approximately 10 mL/min in healthy subjects. In pagetic patients treated with doses equivalent to 400 mg/day tiludronic acid for 12 days, the mean apparent plasma elimination half-life was approximately 150 hours. The elimination rate from human bone is unknown.

Contraindications

Hypersensitivity to bisphosphonates or any component of the products; hypocalcemia (**alendronate**, **risedronate**, see Precautions); abnormalities of the esophagus that delay esophageal emptying such as stricture or achalasia (**alendronate**); inability to stand or sit upright for at least 30 minutes (**alendronate**, **risedronate**); clinically overt osteomalacia (oral **etidronate**); Class Dc and higher renal impairment (serum creatinine more than 5 mg/dL; IV **etidronate** only; see Warnings).

Warnings

➤*GI irritation / disorders:* Bisphosphonates cause local irritation of the upper GI mucosa. Alert physicians to any signs or symptoms signaling a possible esophageal reaction and instruct patients to discontinue bisphosphonates and seek medical attention if they develop dysphagia, odynophagia, retrosternal pain, or new or worsening heartburn.

The risk of severe esophageal adverse experiences appears to be greater in patients who lie down after taking bisphosphonates or who fail to swallow it with a full glass (6 to 8 oz) of water, or who continue to take bisphosphonates after developing symptoms suggestive of esophageal irritation. Therefore, it is very important that the full dosing instructions are provided to and understood by the patient. In patients who cannot comply with dosing instructions because of mental disability, use bisphosphonate therapy under appropriate supervision.

Because of possible irritant effects of bisphosphonates on the upper GI mucosa and a potential for worsening of the underlying disease, use caution when bisphosphonates are given to patients with active upper GI problems (such as dysphagia, esophageal diseases, gastritis, duodenitis, or ulcers). **Etidronate** therapy has been withheld from patients with enterocolitis because diarrhea is seen in some patients, particularly at higher doses.

➤*Osteoporosis (alendronate):* Consider causes of osteoporosis other than estrogen deficiency and aging; consider glucocorticoid use.

➤*Paget disease (oral etidronate):* Response to therapy may be slow and continue for months after treatment discontinuation. Do not increase dosage prematurely. Do not initiate retreatment until after at least a 90-day drug-free interval.

➤*Asthma (zoledronic acid):* While not observed in clinical trials with zoledronic acid, administration of other bisphosphonates has been associated with bronchoconstriction in aspirin-sensitive asthmatic patients. Use zoledronic acid with caution in patients with aspirin-sensitive asthma.

➤*Renal function impairment:*

Alendronate – Although no clinical information is available, it is likely that alendronate elimination via the kidney will be reduced in impaired renal function. Therefore, somewhat greater accumulation of alendronate in bone might be expected in impaired renal function. No dosage adjustment is necessary in mild to moderate renal insufficiency (Ccr 35 to 60 mL/min). Alendronate use is not recommended in more severe renal insufficiency (Ccr less than 35 mL/min).

Etidronate (IV) – Occasional mild to moderate renal function abnormalities (elevated BUN or serum creatinine) have occurred when etidronate IV infusion was given to patients with HCM. These were reversible or remained stable without worsening after therapy completion. In some patients with preexisting renal impairment or who had received potentially nephrotoxic drugs, further renal function depression was sometimes seen. Monitor renal function.

Reduction of the etidronate dose, if used at all, may be advisable in Class Cc (Classification of Renal Function Impairment) renal function impairment (serum creatinine 2.5 to 4.9 mg/dL). Use only if the potential benefit of hypercalcemia correction will substantially exceed the potential for worsening of renal function. In patients with Class Dc and higher renal function impairment (serum creatinine greater than 5 mg/dL), withhold etidronate infusion.

Pamidronate – Bisphosphonates, including pamidronate, have been associated with renal toxicity manifested as deterioration of renal function and potential renal failure.

Because of the risk of clinically significant deterioration in renal function, which may progress to renal failure, single doses of pamidronate should not exceed 90 mg (see Administration and Dosage for appropriate infusion durations).

Pamidronate has not been tested in patients who have Class Dc renal impairment (creatinine greater than 5 mg/dL) and has been tested in few multiple myeloma patients with serum creatinine 3 mg/dL or more. For the treatment of bone metastases, the use of pamidronate in patients with severe renal impairment is not recommended. In other indications, clinical judgement should determine whether the potential benefit outweighs the potential risk in such patients.

Risedronate – Risedronate is not recommended for patients with severe renal impairment (Ccr less than 30 mL/min). No dosage adjustment is needed when Ccr is greater than 30 mL/min.

Tiludronate – Tiludronate is not recommended for patients with severe renal failure (Ccr less than 30 mL/min). The plasma elimination half-life is longer.

Zoledronic acid – Because of the risk of clinically significant deterioration in renal function, which may progress to renal failure, single doses of zoledronic acid should not exceed 4 mg and the duration of infusion should be no less than 15 minutes. Because safety and pharmacokinetic data are limited in patients with severe renal impairment, zoledronic acid treatment is not recommended in patients with bone metastases with severe renal impairment (in the clinical trials, patients with serum creatinine greater than 3 mg/dL were excluded). Consider zoledronic acid treatment in patients with HCM only after evaluating the risks and benefits of treatment (in the clinical trials, patients with serum creatinine greater than 400 mcmol/L or greater than 4.5 mg/dL were excluded).

In clinical trials, the risk for renal function deterioration (defined as an increase in serum creatinine) was significantly increased in patients who received zoledronic acid over 5 minutes compared with patients who received the same dose over 15 minutes. In addition, the risk for renal function deterioration and renal failure was significantly increased in patients who received 8 mg zoledronic acid, even when given over 15 minutes. While this risk is reduced with the 4 mg zoledronic acid dose administered over 15 minutes, deterioration in renal function can still occur. Risk factors for this deterioration include elevated baseline creatinine and multiple cycles of treatment with the bisphosphonate. Patients who receive zoledronic acid should have serum creatinine assessed prior to each treatment.

➤*Carcinogenesis:*

Alendronate: Parafollicular cell (thyroid) adenomas were increased in high-dose male rats ($P = 0.003$) at doses equivalent to 1 and 3.75 mg/kg body weight. These doses are equivalent to 0.26 and 1 times a 40 mg human daily dose based on surface area, mg/m^2.

Pamidronate: In a 104-week carcinogenicity study (daily oral pamidronate administration) in rats, there was a positive dose-response relationship for benign adrenal pheochromocytoma in males ($P < 0.00001$).

Zoledronic acid: Mice were given oral doses of zoledronic acid of 0.1, 0.5, or 2 mg/kg/day. There was an increased incidence of Harderian gland adenomas in males and females in all treatment groups (at doses of 0.002 or more times a human IV dose of 4 mg, based on a comparison of relative body surface areas).

➤*Fertility impairment:*

Pamidronate: In rats, decreased fertility occurred in first-generation offspring of parents who had received 150 mg/kg oral pamidronate; however, this occurred only when animals were mated with members of the same dose group.

Risedronate: In rats, inhibited ovulation at an oral dose of 16 mg/kg/day and decreased implantation with doses of 7 mg/kg/day or more occurred. Testicular and epididymal atrophy and inflammation were noted at 40 mg/kg/day.

Zoledronic acid: Female rats were given SC doses of 0.01, 0.03, or 0.1 mg/kg/day zoledronic acid beginning 15 days before mating and continuing through gestation. Effects observed in the high-dose group (with systemic exposure of 1.2 times the human systemic exposure following an IV dose of 4 mg, based on AUC comparison) included inhibition of ovulation and a decrease in the number of pregnant rats. Effects observed in both the mid-dose group (with systemic exposure of 0.2 times the human systemic exposure following an IV dose of 4 mg, based on AUC comparison) and high-dose group included an increase in preimplantation losses and a decrease in the number of implantations and live fetuses.

➤*Pregnancy:*

Category D. –

Pamidronate: Bolus IV studies conducted in rats and rabbits determined that pamidronate produces maternal toxicity and embryo/fetal effects when given during organogenesis at doses of 0.6 to 8.3 times the highest recommended human dose for a single IV infusion. As it has been shown that pamidronate can cross the placenta in rats and has produced marked maternal and nonteratogenic embryo/fetal effects in rats and rabbits, it should not be given to women during pregnancy.

There are no adequate and well-controlled studies in pregnant women. If the patient becomes pregnant while taking this drug, apprise the patient of the potential harm to the fetus. Advise women of childbearing potential to avoid becoming pregnant.

Zoledronic acid: There are no studies in pregnant women using zoledronic acid. If the patient becomes pregnant while taking this drug, apprise the patient of the potential harm to the fetus. Advise women of childbearing potential to avoid becoming pregnant.

Do not use zoledronic acid during pregnancy. It may cause fetal harm when administered to a pregnant woman. In reproductive studies in the pregnant rat, SC doses equivalent to 2.4 or 4.8 times the human systemic exposure (IV dose of 4 mg based on an AUC comparison) resulted in pre- and postimplantation losses, decreases in viable fetuses and fetal skeletal, visceral, and external malformations.

Category C. –
Alendronate: There are no studies in pregnant women. Use alendronate during pregnancy only if the potential benefit justifies the risk to the mother and fetus.

Reproduction studies in rats showed decreased postimplantation survival at 2 mg/kg/day and decreased body weight gain in normal pups at 1 mg/kg/day. Sites of incomplete fetal ossification were statistically significantly increased in rats beginning at 10 mg/kg/day in vertebral (cervical, thoracic, and lumbar), skull, and sternebral bones. Both total and ionized calcium decreased in pregnant rats at 15 mg/kg/day (3.9 times a 40 mg human daily dose based on surface area, mg/m^2) resulting in delays and failures of delivery. Protracted parturition because of maternal hypocalcemia occurred in rats at doses as low as 0.5 mg/kg/day (0.13 times a 40 mg human daily dose based on surface area, mg/m^2) when rats were treated from before mating through gestation. Maternotoxicity (late pregnancy deaths) occurred in rats treated with 15 mg/kg/day alendronate for varying periods of time; these deaths were lessened but not eliminated by treatment cessation. Calcium could not ameliorate hypocalcemia or prevent maternal and neonatal deaths caused by delay in delivery; IV calcium supplementation prevented maternal but not fetal deaths.

Oral etidronate: There are no adequate and well-controlled studies in pregnant women. Use only when clearly needed and when the potential benefits outweigh potential hazards to the fetus. Etidronate has caused skeletal abnormalities in rats when given at oral dose levels of 300 mg/kg (15 to 60 times the human dose). Other effects on the offspring (including decreased live births) occur at dosages that cause significant toxicity in the parent generation and are 25 to 200 times the human dose. The skeletal effects are thought to be the result of the pharmacological effects of the drug on bone.

IV etidronate: There are no adequate and well-controlled studies.

Risedronate: There are no adequate and well-controlled studies in pregnant women. Use during pregnancy only if the potential benefit justifies the potential risk to the fetus.

Survival of neonates was decreased in rats treated during gestation with oral doses of 16 mg/kg/day or more (approximately 5.2 times the 30 mg/day human dose based on surface area, mg/m^2). Body weight was decreased in neonates from dams treated with 80 mg/kg (approximately 26 times the 30 mg/day human dose based on surface area, mg/m^2). In rats treated during gestation, the number of fetuses exhibiting incomplete ossification of sternebrae or skull was statistically significantly increased at 7.1 mg/kg/day (approximately 2.3 times the 30 mg/day human dose based on surface area, mg/m^2).

Tiludronate: There are no adequate and well-controlled studies in pregnant women. Use tiludronate during pregnancy only if the potential benefit justifies the potential risk to the fetus.

In rabbits at doses of 42 and 130 mg/kg/day (2 and 5 times the 400 mg/day human dose based on body surface area), there was dose-related scoliosis likely attributable to the pharmacologic properties of tiludronate. Mice receiving 375 mg/kg/day (7 times the 400 mg/day human dose based on body surface area mg/m^2) showed slight maternal toxicity. Maternal toxicity also was observed in rats dosed at 375 mg/kg/day (10 times the 400 mg/day human dose).

➤*Lactation:* It is not known whether these drugs are excreted in breast milk. Exercise caution when administering **alendronate**, **etidronate**, **tiludronate**, **risedronate**, **pamidronate**, or **zoledronic acid** to a nursing mother. Because zoledronic acid binds to bone long-term, do not administer to a breast-feeding woman.

➤*Children:* Safety and efficacy for use in children have not been established with most bisphosphonates (in children younger than 18 years of age for **risedronate**).

Children have been treated with oral **etidronate** at doses recommended for adults to prevent heterotopic ossifications or soft tissue calcifications. A rachitic syndrome has been reported infrequently at doses of 10 mg/kg/day or more and for prolonged periods approaching or exceeding 1 year. The epiphyseal radiologic changes associated with retarded mineralization of new osteoid and cartilage, and occasional symptoms reported, have been reversible when medication is discontinued.

Precautions

➤*Monitoring:* Assess serum creatinine in patients who receive **pamidronate** prior to each treatment. Patients treated with pamidronate for bone metastases should have the dose withheld if renal function has deteriorated. Carefully monitor standard hypercalcemia-related metabolic parameters, such as serum levels of calcium, phosphate, magnesium, and potassium following pamidronate and **zoledronic acid** initiation. Asymptomatic hypophosphatemia (16%), hypomagnesemia (11%), hypokalemia (7%), and hypocalcemia (5% to 12%) have occurred. Also, closely monitor electrolytes, creatinine, CBC, differential, and hematocrit/hemoglobin. Carefully monitor patients who have pre-existing anemia, leukopenia, or thrombocytopenia in the first 2 weeks following treatment.

➤*Hypercalcemia:* Carefully monitor standard hypercalcemia-related metabolic parameters, such as serum levels of calcium, phosphate, and magnesium, as well as serum creatinine, following initiation of therapy with **zoledronic acid**. Patients with HCM must be adequately rehydrated prior to administration of zoledronic acid. Do not use loop diuretics until the patient is adequately rehydrated; use with caution in combination with zoledronic acid in order to avoid hypocalcemia. Use zoledronic acid with caution with other nephrotoxic drugs.

➤*Concomitant use with estrogen/hormone replacement therapy (alendronate):* Two clinical studies have shown that the degree of suppression of bone turnover (as assessed by mineralizing surface) was significantly greater with the combination than with either component alone. The safety and tolerability profile of the combination was consistent with those individual treatments.

➤*Nutrition:* Maintain adequate nutrition, particularly an adequate intake of calcium and vitamin D when taking oral **etidronate**, **risedronate**, and **alendronate**.

➤*Osteoid:* Oral **etidronate** suppresses bone turnover and may retard mineralization of osteoid laid down during the bone accretion process. These effects are dose- and time-dependent. Osteoid, which may accumulate noticeably at doses of 10 to 20 mg/kg/day, mineralizes normally post-therapy. In patients with fractures, especially of long bones, it may be advisable to delay or interrupt treatment until callus is evident.

➤*Fracture:* In Paget patients, treatment regimens of oral **etidronate** exceeding the recommended daily maximum dose of 20 mg/kg or continuous administration for periods greater than 6 months may be associated with osteomalacia and an increased risk of fracture.

Long bones predominantly affected by lytic lesions, particularly in those patients unresponsive to therapy, may be especially prone to fracture. Radiographically and biochemically monitor patients with predominantly lytic lesions to permit termination of etidronate in those patients unresponsive to treatment.

➤*Hypocalcemia:* Hypocalcemia (5% to 12%) has occurred with **pamidronate** therapy. Rare cases of symptomatic hypocalcemia (including tetany) occurred during pamidronate treatment. If hypocalcemia occurs, consider short-term calcium therapy.

Hypocalcemia must be corrected before therapy initiation with **alendronate** and **risedronate**. Also effectively treat other disturbances of mineral metabolism (eg, vitamin D deficiency). Presumably because of the effects of alendronate and risedronate on increasing bone mineral, small asymptomatic decreases in serum calcium and phosphate may occur, especially in patients with Paget disease, in whom the pretreatment rate of bone turnover may be greatly elevated and in patients receiving glucocorticoids, in whom calcium absorption may be decreased. Ensure adequate calcium and vitamin D intake to provide for these enhanced needs.

Drug Interactions

Bisphosphonate Drug Interactions

Precipitant drug	Object drug[a]		Description
Aminoglycosides	Bisphosphonates (Zoledronic acid)	↑	Caution is advised when bisphosphonates are administered with aminoglycosides, because these agents may have an additive effect to lower serum calcium levels for prolonged periods.
Aspirin	Tiludronate	↓	Aspirin may decrease the bioavailability of tiludronate by up to 50% when taken 2 hours after tiludronate.
Calcium supplements, antacids	Alendronate, Etidronate, Risedronate, Tiludronate	↓	Products containing calcium and other multivalent cations interfere with alendronate, risedronate, and etidronate absorption. The bioavailability of tiludronate is decreased by 80% by calcium when administered at the same time and 60% by some aluminum- or magnesium-containing antacids when administered 1 hour before tiludronate.
Loop diuretics	Zoledronic acid	↑	Use caution when zoledronic acid is used in combination with loop diuretics because of an increased risk of hypocalcemia.
Indomethacin	Tiludronate	↑	The bioavailability of tiludronate is increased 2- to 4-fold by indomethacin, but is not significantly altered by coadministration of diclofenac.
Ranitidine	Alendronate	↑	IV ranitidine doubled alendronate bioavailability. The clinical significance is unknown.
Alendronate	Aspirin	↑	The risk of upper GI adverse effects associated with aspirin increased with alendronate doses higher than 10 mg/day.

Bisphosphonate Drug Interactions			
Precipitant drug	Object drug[a]		Description
Etidronate	Warfarin	↑	There have been isolated reports of patients experiencing increases in their prothrombin times when etidronate was added to warfarin therapy. Patients on warfarin should have their prothrombin time monitored.

[a] ↑ = Object drug increased. ↓ = Object drug decreased.

➤*Drug/Food interactions:* In 1 study, bioavailability of **alendronate** was decreased by 40% when 10 mg alendronate was given 0.5 or 1 hour before breakfast vs 2 hours before, and bioavailability was negligible when alendronate was given with or 2 hours after breakfast. Concomitant coffee or orange juice reduced bioavailability by 60%. Take alendronate in the morning at least 30 minutes before the first meal, beverage, or medication.

Absorption of **etidronate** may be reduced by foods. Take on an empty stomach 2 hours before a meal.

In single-dose studies, bioavailability of **tiludronate** was reduced by 90% when an oral dose equivalent to 400 mg tiludronic acid was administered with, or 2 hours after, a standard breakfast compared with the same dose administered after an overnight fast and 4 hours before a standard breakfast.

Mean oral bioavailability of **risedronate** is decreased when given with food. Take at least 30 minutes before the first food or drink of the day other than water.

Adverse Reactions

Bisphosphonate Adverse Reactions (%)[a]														
	Pamidronate				Etidronate	Alendronate		Tiludronate	Risedronate				Zoledronic acid	
	Osteolytic bone metastases of breast cancer and osteo- lytic lesions of multiple myeloma (average of 3 trials)	Hypercalcemia of malignancy study comparing these 3 dose regimens			Hyper-calcemia of malignancy	Osteoporosis in post-menopausal women	Fracture intervention trial[b]	Pagetic patients	Pagetic patients	Combined osteoporosis trials	Osteoporosis study in postmeno-pausal women comparing these 2 doseforms		Hyper-calcemia of malignancy	Combined multiple myeloma and bone metastases of solid tumor trials
Adverse reaction	90 mg (n = 572)[c]	60 mg over 4 hr (n = 23)	60 mg over 24 hr (n = 73)	90 mg over 24 hr (n = 17)	7.5 mg/kg x 3 days (n = 35)	10 mg/day[d] (n = 196)	(n = 3236)	400 mg/day (n = 75)	30 mg/day x 2 months (n = 61)[e]	5 mg (n = 1916)	5 mg/day (n = 480)	35 mg/wk (n = 485)	4 mg (n = 86)	4 mg (n = 1099)
Cardiovascular														
Angina pectoris	—	—	—	—	—	—	—	—	—	2.5	—	—	—	—
Atrial fibrillation	—	—	—	6	—	—	—	—	—	—	—	—	—	—
Atrial flutter	—	—	1	—	—	—	—	—	—	—	—	—	—	—
Cardiac failure	—	—	1	—	—	—	—	—	—	—	—	—	—	—
Cardiovascular disorder	—	—	—	—	—	—	—	—	—	2.5	—	—	—	—
Chest pain	—	—	—	—	—	—	—	2.7	6.6	5	2.3	2.7	—	—
Hypertension	—	—	—	6	—	—	—	—	—	10	5.8	4.9	—	—
Hypotension	—	—	—	—	—	—	—	—	—	—	—	—	10.5	—
Syncope	—	—	—	6	—	—	—	—	—	—	0.6	2.1	—	—
Tachycardia	—	—	—	6	—	—	—	—	—	—	—	—	—	—
Vasodilation	—	—	—	—	—	—	—	—	—	—	2.3	1.4	—	—
CNS														
Agitation	—	—	—	—	—	—	—	—	—	—	—	—	12.8	—
Anxiety	14.3	—	—	—	—	—	—	—	—	4.3	0.6	2.7	14	9
Confusion	—	—	—	—	—	—	—	—	—	—	—	—	12.8	—
Convulsions	—	—	—	—	3	—	—	—	—	—	—	—	—	—
Depression	—	—	—	—	—	—	—	—	—	6.8	2.3	2.3	—	12
Dizziness	—	—	—	—	—	—	—	4	6.6	6.4	5.8	4.9	—	14
Headache	26.2	—	—	—	—	2.6	0.2	6.7	18	—	7.3	7.2	—	18
Hypertonia	—	—	—	—	—	—	—	—	—	2.2	—	—	—	—
Hypesthesia	—	—	—	—	—	—	—	—	—	—	—	—	—	10
Insomnia	22.2	—	1	—	—	—	—	—	—	4.7	—	—	15.1	14
Neuralgia	—	—	—	—	—	—	—	—	—	3.8	—	—	—	—
Paresthesia	—	—	—	—	—	—	—	4	—	2.1	—	—	—	12
Psychosis	—	4	—	—	—	—	—	—	—	—	—	—	—	—
Somnolence	—	—	1	6	—	—	—	—	—	—	—	—	—	—
Vertigo	—	—	—	—	—		—	—	—	3.3	2.1	1.6	—	—
Dermatologic														
Alopecia	—	—	—	—	—	—	—	—	—	—	—	—	—	11
Dermatitis		—	—	—	—	—	—	—	—	—	—	—	—	10
Pruritus	—	—	—	—	—	—	—	—	—	3	1.9	2.3	—	—
Rash	—	—	—	—	—	—	—	2.7	11.5	7.7	3.1	4.1	—	—
Skin carcinoma	—	—	—	—	—	—	—	—	—	2	—	—	—	—
Skin disorder	—	—	—	—	—	—	—	2.7	—	—	—	—	—	—
GI														
Abdominal pain	22.6	—	1	—	—	6.6	1.5	—	11.5	11.6	7.3	7.6	16.3	12
Abdominal distension	—	—	—	—	—	1	—	—	—	—	—	—	—	—
Acid regurgitation	—	—	—	—	—	2	1.1	—	—	—	—	—	—	—
Anorexia	26	4	1	12	—	—	—	—	—	—	—	—	9.3	20
Appetite decreased	—	—	—	—	—	—	—	—	—	—	—	—	—	11
Belching	—	—	—	—	—	—	—	—	3.3	—	—	—	—	—
Colitis	—	—	—	—	—	—	—	—	3.3	—	0.8	2.5	—	—
Constipation	33.2	4	—	6	3	3.1	0	—	6.6	—	12.5	12.2	26.7	28
Diarrhea	28.5	—	1	—	—	3.1	0.6	9.3	19.7	10.6	6.3	4.9	17.4	22
Dry mouth	—	—	—	—	—	—	—	—	—	—	2.5	1.4	—	—
Dyspepsia	22.6	4	—	—	—	3.6	1.1	5.3	—	—	6.9	7.6	—	—
Dysphasia	—	—	—	—	—	1	0.1	—	—	—	—	—	—	—
Esophageal ulcer	—	—	—	—	—	1.5	0.1	—	—	—	—	—	—	—
Flatulence	—	—	—	—	—	2.6	0.2	2.7	—	4.6	3.3	3.1	—	—
Gastritis	—	—	—	—	—	0.5	0.6	—	—	2.5	—	—	—	—
Gastroenteritis	—	—	—	—	—	—	—	—	—	—	3.8	3.5	—	—
GI disorder	—	—	—	—	—	—	—	—	—	2.3	1.9	2.5	—	—
GI hemorrhage	—	—	—	6	—	—	—	—	—	—	—	—	—	—

Bisphosphonate Adverse Reactions (%)[a]

Adverse reaction	Pamidronate				Etidronate	Alendronate		Tiludronate	Risedronate				Zoledronic acid	
	Osteolytic bone metastases of breast cancer and osteo- lytic lesions of multiple myeloma (average of 3 trials)	Hypercalcemia of malignancy study comparing these 3 dose regimens			Hyper-calcemia of malignancy	Osteoporosis in post-menopausal women	Fracture intervention trial[b]	Pagetic patients	Pagetic patients	Combined osteoporosis trials	Osteoporosis study in postmeno-pausal women comparing these 2 doseforms		Hyper-calcemia of malignancy	Combined multiple myeloma and bone metastases of solid tumor trials
	90 mg (n = 572)[c]	60 mg over 4 hr (n = 23)	60 mg over 24 hr (n = 73)	90 mg over 24 hr (n = 17)	7.5 mg/kg x 3 days (n = 35)	10 mg/day[d] (n = 196)	(n = 3236)	400 mg/day (n = 75)	30 mg/day x 2 months (n = 61)[e]	5 mg (n = 1916)	5 mg/day (n = 480)	35 mg/wk (n = 485)	4 mg (n = 86)	4 mg (n = 1099)
Nausea	53.5	4	—	18	6	3.6	1.1	9.3	9.8	10.9	8.5	6.2	29.1	43
Rectal disorder	—	—	—	—	—	—	—	—	—	2.2	—	—	—	—
Stomatitis	—	—	1	—	3	—	—	—	—	—	—	—	—	—
Vomiting	35.7	4	—	—	—	1	0.2	4	—	—	1.9	2.5	14	30
Weight decreased	—	—	—	—	—	—	—	—	—	—	—	—	—	13
Hemic/Lymphatic														
Anemia	42.5	—	—	6	—	—	—	—	—	2.4	—	—	22.1	29
Ecchymosis	—	—	—	—	—	—	—	—	—	4.3	—	—	—	—
Granulocytopenia	19.8	—	—	—	—	—	—	—	—	—	—	—	—	—
Leukopenia	—	4	—	—	—	—	—	—	—	—	—	—	—	—
Neutropenia	—	—	1	—	—	—	—	—	—	—	—	—	—	11
Thrombocytopenia	14	—	1	—	—	—	—	—	—	—	—	—	—	—
Lab abnormalities														
Abnormal hepatic function	—	—	—	—	3	—	—	—	—	—	—	—	—	—
Hypocalcemia	3.3	—	1	12	—	—	—	—	—	—	—	—	—	—
Hypokalemia	10.5	4	4	18	—	—	—	—	—	—	—	—	11.6	—
Hypomagnesemia	4.4	4	10	12	3	—	—	—	—	—	—	—	10.5	—
Hypophosphatemia	1.7	—	9	18	3	—	—	—	—	—	—	—	12.8	—
Serum creatinine	18.5	—	—	—	—	—	—	—	—	—	—	—	—	—
Musculoskeletal														
Arthralgia	13.6	—	—	—	—	—	—	2.7	32.8	23.7	11.5	14.2	—	18
Arthritis	—	—	—	—	—	—	—	—	—	—	4.8	4.1	—	—
Arthrosis	—	—	—	—	—	—	—	2.7	—	—	—	—	—	—
Back pain	—	—	—	—	—	—	—	8	—	26.1	9.2	8.7	—	10
Bone disorder	—	—	—	—	—	—	—	—	—	4	—	—	—	—
Bone fracture	—	—	—	—	—	—	—	—	—	—	5	6.4	—	—
Bone/skeletal pain	66.8	—	—	—	—	4.1	0.4	—	4.9	4.6	2.9	1.4	11.6	53
Bursitis	—	—	—	—	—	—	—	—	—	3	1.3	2.5	—	—
Joint disorder	—	—	—	—	—	—	—	—	—	6.8	—	—	—	—
Leg/Muscle cramps	—	—	—	—	—	—	0.2	—	3.3	3.5	—	—	—	—
Myalgia	26	—	1	—	—	—	—	—	—	6.6	4.6	6.2	—	21
Myasthenia	—	—	—	—	—	—	—	—	3.3	—	—	—	—	—
Tendon disorder	—	—	—	—	—	—	—	—	—	3	—	—	—	—
Respiratory														
Bronchitis	—	—	—	—	—	—	—	—	3.3	—	2.3	4.9	—	—
Coughing	25.7	—	—	—	—	—	—	2.7	—	—	3.1	2.5	11.6	19
Dyspnea	30.4	—	—	—	3	—	—	—	—	3.8	—	—	22.1	24
Pharyngitis	—	—	—	—	—	—	—	2.7	—	5.8	4.6	2.9	—	—
Pleural effusion	10.7	—	—	—	—	—	—	—	—	—	—	—	—	—
Pneumonia	—	—	—	—	—	—	—	—	—	3.1	0.8	2.5	—	—
Rales	—	—	—	6	—	—	—	—	—	—	—	—	—	—
Rhinitis	—	—	—	6	—	—	—	5.3	—	5.7	2.3	2.1	—	—
Sinusitis	15.6	—	—	—	—	—	—	5.3	4.9	—	4.6	4.5	—	—
URI	24.1	—	3	—	—	—	—	5.3	—	—	—	—	—	8
Special senses														
Amblyopia	—	—	—	—	—	—	—	—	3.3	—	—	—	—	—
Cataract	—	—	—	—	—	—	—	2.7	—	5.9	2.9	1.9	—	—
Conjunctivitis	—	—	—	—	—	—	—	2.7	—	3.1	—	—	—	—
Dry eye	—	—	—	—	—	—	—	—	3.3	—	—	—	—	—
Glaucoma	—	—	—	—	—	—	—	2.7	—	—	—	—	—	—
Otitis media	—	—	—	—	—	—	—	—	—	2.5	—	—	—	—
Taste perversion	—	—	—	—	3	0.5	0.1	—	—	—	—	—	—	—
Tinnitus	—	—	—	—	—	—	—	—	3.3	—	—	—	—	—
General														
Accidental injury	—	—	—	—	—	—	—	4	—	—	10.6	10.7	—	—
Asthenia	22.2	—	—	—	—	—	—	—	4.9	5.1	3.5	5.4	—	21
Edema/Peripheral edema	—	—	1	—	—	—	—	2.7	8.2	—	4.2	1.6	—	19
Fatigue	37.2	—	—	12	—	—	—	—	—	—	—	—	—	36
Fever	38.5	26	19	18	9	—	—	—	—	—	—	—	44.2	30
Fluid overload	—	—	—	—	6	—	—	—	—	—	—	—	—	—
Influenza-like symptoms	—	—	—	—	—	—	—	4	9.8	—	7.1	8.5	—	—
Infusion-site reaction	—	—	4	18	—	—	—	—	—	—	—	—	—	—
Metastases	20.5	—	—	—	—	—	—	—	—	—	—	—	—	—
Moniliasis	—	—	—	6	—	—	—	—	—	—	—	—	11.6	—
Pain	14.3	—	—	—	—	—	—	21.3	—	13.6	7.7	9.9	—	—
Miscellaneous														
Allergic reaction	—	—	—	—	—	—	—	—	—	—	1.9	2.5	—	—
Cancer progression	—	—	—	—	—	—	—	—	—	—	—	—	16.3	—
Cystitis	—	—	—	—	—	—	—	—	—	4.1	—	—	—	—
Dehydration	—	—	—	—	—	—	—	—	—	—	—	—	—	12

Bisphosphonate Adverse Reactions (%)[a]														
	Pamidronate				Etidronate	Alendronate		Tiludronate	Risedronate				Zoledronic acid	
	Osteolytic bone metastases of breast cancer and osteo- lytic lesions of multiple myeloma (average of 3 trials)	Hypercalcemia of malignancy study comparing these 3 dose regimens			Hyper-calcemia of malignancy	Osteoporosis in post-menopausal women	Fracture intervention trial[b]	Pagetic patients	Pagetic patients	Combined osteoporosis trials	Osteoporosis study in postmeno-pausal women comparing these 2 doseforms		Hyper-calcemia of malignancy	Combined multiple myeloma and bone metastases of solid tumor trials
Adverse reaction	90 mg (n = 572)[c]	60 mg over 4 hr (n = 23)	60 mg over 24 hr (n = 73)	90 mg over 24 hr (n = 17)	7.5 mg/kg x 3 days (n = 35)	10 mg/day[d] (n = 196)	(n = 3236)	400 mg/day (n = 75)	30 mg/day x 2 months (n = 61)[e]	5 mg (n = 1916)	5 mg/day (n = 480)	35 mg/wk (n = 485)	4 mg (n = 86)	4 mg (n = 1099)
Hernia	—	—	—	—	—	—	—	—	—	2.9	—	—	—	—
Hyperparathyroidism	—	—	—	—	—	—	—	2.7	—	—	—	—	—	—
Hypothyroidism	—	—	—	6	—	—	—	—	—	—	—	—	—	—
Infection	—	—	—	—	—	—	—	2.7	—	29.9	19	20.6	—	—
Neck pain	—	—	—	—	—	—	—	—	—	5.3	2.7	1.2	—	—
Neoplasm	—	—	—	—	—	—	—	—	3.3	3.3	0.8	2.1	—	15
Overdose	—	—	—	—	—	—	—	—	—	—	6.9	6.8	—	—
Rigors	—	—	—	—	—	—	—	—	—	—	—	—	—	10
Tooth disorder	—	—	—	—	—	—	—	2.7	—	2.1	—	—	—	—
Vitamin D deficiency	—	—	—	—	—	—	—	2.7	—	—	—	—	—	—
Uremia	—	4	—	—	—	—	—	—	—	—	—	—	—	—
Urinary tract infection	18.5	—	—	—	—	—	—	—	—	10.9	2.9	5.2	14	11

— = No data.

[a] Data are pooled from separate studies and are not necessarily comparable.

[b] 5 mg/day for 2 years and 10 mg/day for either 1 or 2 additional years.

[c] Most of these adverse experiences may have been related to the underlying disease state or cancer therapy.

[d] 10 mg/day for 3 years.

[e] Considered to be possibly or probably causally related in at least 1 patient.

➤*Alendronate:*

Osteoporosis in postmenopausal women: One patient treated with 10 mg/day who had a history of peptic ulcer disease and gastrectomy and was taking concomitant aspirin developed an anastomotic ulcer with mild hemorrhage, which was considered drug-related. Aspirin and alendronate

• *Other* – Rash, erythema (rare).

Adverse Reactions in Osteoporosis Treatment Studies in Postmenopausal Women (≥ 1%)		
Adverse reaction	Alendronate 70 mg once weekly (n = 519)	Alendronate 10 mg/day (n = 370)
GI		
Abdominal distension	1	1.4
Abdominal pain	3.7	3
Acid regurgitation	1.9	2.4
Constipation	0.8	1.6
Dyspepsia	2.7	2.2
Flatulence	0.4	1.6
Gastritis	0.2	1.1
Gastric ulcer	0	1.1
Nausea	1.9	2.4
Musculoskeletal		
Muscle cramp	0.2	1.1
Musculoskeletal (bone, muscle, joint) pain	2.9	3.2

Adverse Reactions in an Osteoporosis Study in Men (≥ 2%)		
Adverse reactions	Alendronate 10 mg/day (n = 146)	Placebo (n = 95)
GI		
Acid regurgitation	4.1	3.2
Flatulence	4.1	1.1
Dyspepsia	3.4	0
Abdominal pain	2.1	1.1
Nausea	2.1	0

Adverse Reactions in Osteoporosis Prevention Studies in Postmenopausal Women (≥ 1%)				
	2- and 3-year studies		1-year study	
Adverse reaction	Alendronate 5 mg/day (n = 642)	Placebo (n = 648)	Alendronate 5 mg/day (n = 361)	Alendronate 35 mg once weekly (n = 362)
GI				
Dyspepsia	1.9	1.4	2.2	1.7
Abdominal pain	1.7	3.4	4.2	2.2
Acid regurgitation	1.4	2.5	4.2	4.7
Nausea	1.4	1.4	2.5	1.4
Diarrhea	1.1	1.7	1.1	0.6
Constipation	0.9	0.5	1.7	0.3
Abdominal distension	0.2	0.3	1.4	1.1
Musculoskeletal				
Musculoskeletal (bone, muscle, or joint) pain	0.8	0.9	1.9	2.2

Adverse Reactions in 1-year Studies in Glucocorticoid-Treated Patients (≥ 1%)			
Adverse reaction	Alendronate 10 mg/day (n = 157)	Alendronate 5 mg/day (n = 161)	Placebo (n = 159)
CNS			
Headache	0.6	0	1.3
GI			
Abdominal pain	3.2	1.9	0
Acid regurgitation	2.5	1.9	1.3
Constipation	1.3	0.6	0
Melena	1.3	0	0
Nausea	0.6	1.2	0.6
Diarrhea	0	0	1.3

Paget disease: In clinical studies in osteoporosis and Paget disease in patients taking 40 mg/day for 3 to 12 months, the adverse experiences were similar to those in the 10 mg/day osteoporosis study. However, there was an increased incidence of upper GI side effects in the 40 mg/day group (17.7% of the patients taking alendronate vs 10.2% placebo). One case of esophagitis and 2 cases of gastritis resulted in treatment discontinuation.

Musculoskeletal pain, which also occurs with other bisphosphonates, occurred in approximately 6% of patients treated with 40 mg/day alendronate vs approximately 1% taking placebo, rarely resulting in discontinuation. Discontinuation caused by any adverse reaction occurred in 6.4% of patients with Paget disease treated with 40 mg/day alendronate vs 2.4% of placebo-treated patients.

Lab test abnormalities – In double-blind, multicenter, controlled studies, asymptomatic, mild, and transient decreases in serum calcium and phosphate occurred in approximately 18% and 10%, respectively, of patients taking alendronate vs approximately 12% and 3% of those taking placebo. However, the incidence of decreases in serum calcium to less than 8 mg/dL (2 mM) and serum phosphate to at least 2 mg/dL (0.65 mM) were similar in both treatment groups.

Postmarketing: Hypersensitivity reactions including urticaria and rarely angioedema; esophagitis; esophageal erosions; esophageal ulcers, rarely esophageal stricture or perforation; oropharyngeal ulceration; gastric or duodenal ulcers, some severe and with complications; rash (occasionally with photosensitivity); uveitis (rare).

➤*Etidronate (oral):* The incidence of GI complaints (diarrhea, nausea) is the same at 5 mg/kg/day as for placebo (approximately 6.7%). At 10 to

20 mg/kg/day, the incidence may increase to 20% or 30%. These complaints are often alleviated by dividing the total daily dose.

Paget disease (oral): Increased or recurrent bone pain at pagetic sites or the onset of pain at previously asymptomatic sites has occurred. At 5 mg/kg/day, about 10% (vs 6.7% with placebo) report these phenomena. At higher doses, the incidence rises to about 20%. When the therapy continues, pain resolves in some patients but persists in others.

Lab test abnormalities (IV): HCM is frequently associated with abnormal elevations of serum creatinine and BUN, which improve in some patients or remain unchanged in most. However, in approximately 10% of patients, occasional mild to moderate abnormalities in renal function (increases of more than 0.5 mg/dL serum creatinine) were observed during or immediately after treatment. The possibility that etidronate IV infusion contributed to these changes cannot be excluded.

IV: Of patients who participated in the controlled hypercalcemia trials, 10 of 221 (5%) in the treatment courses reported a metallic or altered taste, or loss of taste, which usually disappeared within hours during or shortly after etidronate infusion. A few patients with Paget disease of bone have reported allergic skin rashes in association with oral etidronate.

A patient with 1 kidney and slowly rising creatinine prior to therapy received 30 mg/kg/day body weight of etidronate infusion for 18 hours (total dose 60 mg/kg). This patient reported altered taste and further gradual increase in serum creatinine from 2.1 mg/dL to 2.7 mg/dL during the week after therapy was observed.

Postmarketing:

• *Oral* – Other adverse events that have been reported and were thought to be possibly related to etidronate disodium include the following: Alopecia; arthropathies, including arthralgia and arthritis; bone fracture; esophagitis; glossitis; hypersensitivity reactions, including angioedema, follicular eruption, macular rash, maculopapular rash, pruritus, a single case of Stevens-Johnson syndrome, and urticaria; osteomalacia; neuropsychiatric events, including amnesia, confusion, depression, and hallucination; and paresthesias.

In patients receiving etidronate disodium, there have been rare reports of agranulocytosis, pancytopenia, and a report of leukopenia with recurrence on rechallenge. In addition, there have been rare reports of exacerbation of asthma. Exacerbation of existing peptic ulcer disease has been reported in a few patients. In 1 patient, perforation also occurred. In osteoporosis clinical trials, headache, gastritis, leg cramps, and arthralgia occurred at a significantly greater incidence in patients who received etidronate as compared with those who received placebo.

➤*Pamidronate:*

Hypercalcemia of malignancy: Transient mild elevation of temperature by at least 1°C was noted 24 to 48 hours after administration in 34% of patients. In trials, patients treated with pamidronate (60 or 90 mg over 24 hours) developed electrolyte abnormalities more frequently.

Drug-related local soft tissue symptoms (redness, swelling, or induration, and pain on palpation) at the site of catheter insertion were most common in patients treated with 90 mg.

Rare cases of uveitis, iritis, scleritis, and episcleritis have occurred, including 1 case of scleritis and 1 case of uveitis upon separate rechallenges.

Five of 231 patients (2%) had seizures; 2 had preexisting seizure disorders. None of the seizures were considered to be drug-related. However, a possible relationship cannot be ruled out.

Other reactions in at least 15% of patients included the following: Fluid overload; generalized/abdominal/bone pain; hypertension; anorexia; constipation; nausea; vomiting; urinary tract infection.

• *Lab test abnormalities* – Anemia; hypokalemia; hypomagnesemia; hypophosphatemia.

Paget disease: Transient mild elevation of temperature more than 1°C above pretreatment baseline was noted within 48 hours after completion of treatment in 21% of patients treated with 90 mg. Drug-related musculoskeletal pain and CNS symptoms (eg, dizziness, headache, paresthesia, increased sweating) were more common with Paget disease than with HCM treated with the same 90 mg dose.

Adverse experiences considered to be related to trial drug, which occurred in at least 5% of patients with Paget disease treated with 90 mg of pamidronate in 2 US clinical trials, were fever, nausea, back pain, and bone pain.

Other adverse reactions are as follows: Hypertension, arthrosis, bone pain, headache (10%).

Osteolytic bone metastases of breast cancer and osteolytic lesions of multiple myeloma: In multiple myeloma patients, there were 5 pamidronate-related serious and unexpected adverse experiences. Four of these were reported during the 12-month extension of the multiple myeloma trial. Three of the reports were of worsening renal function developing in patients with progressive multiple myeloma or multiple myeloma-associated amyloidosis. The fourth report was the adult respiratory distress syndrome developing in a patient recovering from pneumonia and acute gangrenous cholecystitis. One pamidronate-treated patient experienced an allergic reaction characterized by swollen and itchy eyes, runny nose, and scratchy throat within 24 hours after the sixth infusion.

In the breast cancer trials, there were 4 pamidronate-related adverse experiences, all moderate in severity, that caused a patient to discontinue participation in the trial. One was because of interstitial pneumonitis, another because of malaise and dyspnea. One pamidronate patient discontinued the trial because of asymptomatic hypocalcemia. Another pamidronate patient discontinued therapy because of severe bone pain after each infusion, which the investigator felt was trial drug-related.

Postmarketing: Rare instances of allergic manifestations have been reported, including hypotension, dyspnea, or angioedema, and very rarely, anaphylactic shock.

➤*Tiludronate:* Adverse events associated with tiludronate usually have been mild and generally have not required discontinuation of therapy. Of patients receiving 400 mg tiludronate and placebo, 1.3% and 5.4% respectively, discontinued therapy because of a clinical adverse event.

The most frequently occurring adverse events in patients who received tiludronate 400 mg/day were in the GI system: Nausea (9.3%), diarrhea (9.3%), and dyspepsia (5.3%).

Paget disease: The following reactions occurred in at least 1% of patients.

CNS – Vertigo; involuntary muscle contractions; anxiety; nervousness.

Dermatologic – Pruritus; increased sweating; Stevens-Johnson-type syndrome (rare).

GI – Dry mouth; gastritis; abdominal pain; constipation.

Miscellaneous – Asthenia; pathological fracture; bronchitis; urinary tract infection; flushing; syncope; fatigue; hypertension; anorexia; somnolence; insomnia.

➤*Risedronate:* Duodenitis and glossitis have been reported uncommonly (0.1% to 1%). There have been rare reports of abnormal liver function tests (less than 0.1%). Three patients who received risedronate 30 mg/day experienced acute iritis in 1 supportive study. All 3 patients recovered from their events. All patients were effectively treated with topical steroids.

Lab test abnormalities – Asymptomatic and small decreases were observed in serum calcium and phosphorus levels. Overall, mean decreases of 0.8% in serum calcium and of 2.7% in phosphorus were observed at 6 months in patients receiving risedronate. Throughout the phase 3 studies, serum calcium levels below 8 mg/dL were observed in 18 patients, 9 (0.5%) in each treatment arm (risedronate and placebo). Serum phosphorus levels below 2 mg/dL were observed in 14 patients, 11 (0.6%) treated with risedronate and 3 (0.2%) treated wit

➤*Zoledronic acid:*

Hypercalcemia of malignancy: IV administration has been most commonly associated with fever. Occasionally, patients experience a flu-like syndrome consisting of fever, chills, bone pain or arthralgias, and myalgias. GI reactions such as nausea and vomiting have been reported following IV infusion. Local reactions at the infusion site, such as redness or swelling, were observed infrequently. In most cases, no specific treatment is required and the symptoms subside after 24 to 48 hours. Rare cases of rash, pruritus, chest pain, conjunctivitis, and hypomagnesemia have been reported.

Other adverse reactions greater than or equal to 5% but less than 10% include the following: Asthenia, chest pain, leg edema, mucositis, metastases, dysphagia, granulocytopenia, thrombocytopenia, pancytopenia, nonspecific infection, hypocalcemia, dehydration, arthralgias, headache, somnolence, pleural effusion.

Lab test abnormalities:

Grade 3 to 4 Laboratory Abnormalities in Clinical Trials for Hypercalcemia of Malignancy

	Grade 3				Grade 4			
	Zoledronic acid 4 mg		Pamidronate 90 mg		Zoledronic acid 4 mg		Pamidronate 90 mg	
Laboratory parameter	n/N	%	n/N	%	n/N	%	n/N	%
Serum creatinine[a]	2/86	2.3	3/100	3	0/86	—	1/100	1
Hypocalcemia[b]	1/86	1.2	2/100	2	0/86	—	0/100	—
Hypophosphatemia[c]	36/70	51.4	27/81	33.3	1/70	1.4	4/81	4.9
Hypomagnesemia[d]	0/71	—	0/84	—	0/71	—	1/84	1.2

[a] Grade 3: More than 3 times the ULN; Grade 4: More than 6 times the ULN
[b] Grade 3: Less than 7 mg/dL; Grade 4: Less than 6 mg/dL
[c] Grade 3: Less than 2 mg/dL; Grade 4: Less than 1 mg/dL
[d] Grade 3: Less than 0.8 mEq/L; Grade 4: Less than 0.5 mEq/L

Multiple myeloma and bone metastases of solid tumors:

• *Lab test abnormalities* –

Grade 3 Laboratory Abnormalities in Clinical Trials in Patients with Bone Metastases

	Zoledronic acid 4 mg		Pamidronate 90 mg		Placebo	
Laboratory parameter	n/N	%	n/N	%	n/N	%
Serum creatinine[a]	7/529	1.3	4/268	1.5	2/241	0.8
Hypocalcemia[b]	7/1041	0.7	4/610	0.7	0/415	—
Hypophosphatemia[c]	96/1041	9.2	40/611	6.6	13/415	3.1
Hypermagnesemia[d]	19/1039	1.8	3/609	0.5	8/415	1.9
Hypomagnesemia[e]	0/1039	—	0/609	—	1/415	0.2

[a] Grade 3: More than 3 times the ULN; Grade 4: More than 6 times the ULN. Serum creatinine data for all patients randomized after the 15-minute infusion amendment.
[b] Grade 3: Less than 7 mg/dL; Grade 4: Less than 6 mg/dL
[c] Grade 3: Less than 2 mg/dL; Grade 4: Less than 1 mg/dL
[d] Grade 3: More than 3 mEq/L; Grade 4: More than 8 mEq/L
[e] Grade 3: Less than 0.9 mEq/L; Grade 4: Less than 0.7 mEq/L

Grade 4 Laboratory Abnormalities in Clinical Trials in Patients with Bone Metastases

	Zoledronic acid 4 mg		Pamidronate 90 mg		Placebo	
Laboratory parameter	n/N	%	n/N	%	n/N	%
Serum creatinine[a]	2/529	0.4	1/268	0.4	0/241	—
Hypocalcemia[b]	6/1041	0.6	2/610	0.3	1/415	0.2
Hypophosphatemia[c]	6/1041	0.6	0/611	—	1/415	0.2

Grade 4 Laboratory Abnormalities in Clinical Trials in Patients with Bone Metastases						
	Zoledronic acid 4 mg		Pamidronate 90 mg		Placebo	
Laboratory parameter	n/N	%	n/N	%	n/N	%
Hypermagnesemia[d]	0/1039	—	0/609	—	2/415	0.5
Hypomagnesemia[e]	2/1039	0.2	2/609	0.3	0/415	—

[a] Grade 3: More than 3 times the ULN; Grade 4: More than 6 times the ULN. Serum creatinine data for all patients randomized after the 15-minute infusion amendment.
[b] Grade 3: Less than 7 mg/dL; Grade 4: Less than 6 mg/dL
[c] Grade 3: Less than 2 mg/dL; Grade 4: Less than 1 mg/dL
[d] Grade 3: More than 3 mEq/L; Grade 4: More than 8 mEq/L
[e] Grade 3: Less than 0.9 mEq/L; Grade 4: Less than 0.7 mEq/L

• *Renal* – In the bone metastases trials, renal deterioration was defined as an increase of 0.5 mg/dL for patients with normal baseline creatinine (less than 1.4 mg/dL) or an increase of 1 mg/dL for patients with an abnormal baseline creatinine (greater than 1.4 mg/dL). Percentage of patients with renal function deterioration who were randomized following the 15 minute 4 mg zoledronic acid infusion amendment were as follows:

Multiple myeloma and breast cancer: Normal (9.3%), abnormal (3.8%), total (8.8%)

Solid tumors: Normal (11%), abnormal (9.1%), total (10.9%)

Prostate cancer: Normal (12.2%), abnormal (40%), total (15.2%)

Overdosage

➤*Alendronate:* Hypocalcemia, hypophosphatemia, and upper GI adverse events (eg, upset stomach, heartburn, esophagitis, gastritis, ulcer) may result from overdosage. Consider the administration of milk or antacids to bind alendronate. Dialysis would not be beneficial.

➤*Etidronate:*

Oral – Clinical experience with etidronate overdosage is extremely limited. Decreases in serum calcium following substantial overdosage may be expected in some patients. Signs and symptoms of hypocalcemia also may occur and some patients may develop vomiting. In 1 event, an 18-year-old female who ingested an estimated single dose of 4,000 to 6,000 mg (67 to 100 mg/kg) was mildly hypocalcemic (7.52 mg/dL) and experienced paresthesia of the fingers. Some patients may develop vomiting and expel the drug. Orally administered etidronate disodium may cause hematologic abnormalities in some patients. Etidronate disodium suppresses bone turnover and may retard mineralization of osteoid laid down during the bone accretion process.

Gastric lavage may remove unabsorbed drug. Standard procedures for treating hypocalcemia, including the administration of calcium IV, would be expected to restore physiologic amounts of ionized calcium and relieve signs and symptoms of hypocalcemia. Such treatment has been effective.

IV – Rapid IV administration of etidronate at doses above 27 mg/kg has produced ECG changes and bleeding problems in animals. These abnormalities are probably related to marked or rapid decreases in ionized calcium levels in blood and tissue fluids. They are thought to be caused by chelation of calcium by massive amounts of the diphosphonate. These abnormalities have been reversible in animal studies by use of ionizable calcium salts. Similar problems are not expected to occur in humans if treated with etidronate as recommended. Moreover, signs and symptoms of hypocalcemia such as paresthesias and carpopedal spasms have not been reported with either agent. The chelation effects of the diphosphonate are reversible with IV calcium gluconate.

Administration of IV etidronate at doses and possibly at rates in excess of those recommended has been associated with renal insufficiency.

➤*Pamidronate:* There have been several cases of drug maladministration of IV pamidronate in hypercalcemia patients with total doses of 225 to 300 mg given over 2.5 to 4 days. All survived but experienced hypocalcemia requiring IV or oral calcium.

One obese woman (95 kg) who was treated with pamidronate 285 mg/day for 3 days experienced high fever (39.5°C; 102°F), hypotension, and transient taste perversion noted about 6 hours after the first infusion. Fever and hypotension were rapidly corrected with steroids.

If overdosage occurs, symptomatic hypocalcemia also could result; treat such patients with short-term IV calcium.

➤*Risedronate:* Decreases in serum calcium following substantial overdose may be expected in some patients. Signs and symptoms of hypocalcemia also may occur in some of these patients.

Gastric lavage may remove unabsorbed drug. Administration of milk or antacids to chelate risedronate may be helpful. Standard procedures that are effective for treating hypocalcemia, including IV administration of calcium, would be expected to restore physiologic amounts of ionized calcium and to relieve signs and symptoms of hypocalcemia.

➤*Tiludronate:* Hypocalcemia is a potential consequence of tiludronate overdose. In 1 patient with HCM, IV administration of high doses of tiludronate (800 mg/day total dose, 6 mg/kg/day for 2 days) was associated with acute renal failure and death.

No specific information is available on the treatment of overdose with tiludronate. Dialysis would not be beneficial. Standard medical practices may be used to manage renal insufficiency or hypocalcemia if signs of these develop.

➤*Zoledronic acid:* Overdosage may cause clinically significant hypocalcemia, hypophosphatemia, and hypomagnesemia. Clinically relevant reductions in serum levels of calcium, phosphorus, and magnesium should be corrected by IV administration of calcium gluconate, potassium or sodium phosphate, and magnesium sulfate, respectively.

Patient Information

Bisphosphonates may cause GI upset (eg, nausea, diarrhea).

➤*Alendronate:* Instruct patients that the expected benefits of alendronate only may be obtained when each tablet is taken with plain water first thing in the morning and at least 30 minutes before the first food, beverage, or medication of the day. Also instruct them that waiting more than 30 minutes will improve alendronate absorption. Even dosing with orange juice or coffee markedly reduces the absorption of alendronate.

Instruct patients to take alendronate with a full glass of water (6 to 8 oz; 180 to 240 mL) and not to lie down for at least 30 minutes and until after the first food of the day following administration to facilitate delivery to the stomach and reduce the potential for esophageal irritation.

Patients should not chew or suck on the tablet because of a potential for oropharyngeal ulceration. Specifically instruct patients not to take alendronate at bedtime or before arising for the day. Inform patients that failure to follow these instructions may increase their risk of esophageal problems. Instruct patients that if they develop symptoms of esophageal disease (eg, difficulty or pain upon swallowing, retrosternal pain, new or worsening heartburn) they should stop taking alendronate and consult their physician.

Instruct patients that if they miss a dose of once-weekly alendronate they should take 1 tablet on the morning after they remember. They should not take 2 tablets on the same day but should return to taking 1 tablet once a week as originally scheduled on their chosen day.

Instruct patients to take supplemental calcium and vitamin D if dietary intake is inadequate. Consider weight-bearing exercise along with the modification of certain behavioral factors, such as excessive cigarette smoking or alcohol consumption, if these factors exist.

It is likely that calcium supplements, antacids, and some oral medications will interfere with absorption of alendronate. Therefore, patients must wait at least 30 minutes after taking alendronate before taking any other oral medications.

➤*Etidronate (oral):* Take on an empty stomach 2 hours before or after meals, including vitamin and mineral supplements or antacids, which are high in metals such as calcium, iron, magnesium, or aluminum.

➤*Risedronate:* Inform patients to pay particular attention to the dosing instructions because clinical benefits may be compromised by failure to take the drug according to instructions. Take risedronate at least 30 minutes before the first food or drink of the day other than water.

If a patient forgets to take the 5 or 35 mg risedronate tablet in the morning, inform him/her not to take it later in the day. Take only 1 risedronate 5 or 35 mg tablet the next morning and continue the usual schedule of 5 mg (1 tablet a day) or 35 mg (1 tablet on a chosen day of the week). Do not take 2 tablets on the same day.

In order to facilitate delivery to the stomach and minimize the possibility of esophageal irritation, take risedronate in an upright position, sitting or standing, with a full glass (6 to 8 oz; 180 to 240 mL) of plain water and avoid lying down for 30 minutes after taking this medication. Patients should receive supplemental calcium and vitamin D if dietary intake is inadequate (see Precautions). Calcium, magnesium or aluminum supplements, or antacids may interfere with the absorption of risedronate; take them at a different time of the day as with food. Patients should not chew or suck on tablets because of potential for oropharyngeal irritation.

Instruct patients that if they develop symptoms of esophageal disease (eg, difficulty or pain upon swallowing; retrosternal pain; severe, persistent, or worsening heartburn) they should consult their physician before continuing risedronate.

Weight-bearing exercise should be considered along with the modification of certain behavioral factors, such as excessive cigarette smoking, or alcohol consumption, if these factors exist.

Physicians should instruct their patients to read the patient information before starting therapy with 5 mg risedronate and to reread it each time the prescription is renewed.

➤*Tiludronate:* Take tiludronate with 6 to 8 oz (180 to 240 mL) of plain water. Do not take within 2 hours of food. Maintain adequate vitamin D and calcium intake. Do not take calcium supplements, aspirin, and indomethacin within 2 hours before or after tiludronate. If needed, take aluminum- or magnesium-containing antacids at least 2 hours after tiludronate.

ALENDRONATE SODIUM

Rx	**Fosamax** (Merck)	**Tablets:** 5 mg (as base)	Lactose. (MRK 925). White. In unit-of-use 30s and 100s.
		10 mg (as base)	Lactose. (MRK 936). White, oval. In 1,000s, unit-of-use 30s and 100s, *Uniblister* cards of 31, and UD 100s.
		35 mg (as base)	Lactose. (77). White, oval. In unit-of-use 4s and UD 20s.
		40 mg (as base)	Lactose. (MRK 212/Fosamax). White, triangular. In unit-of-use 30s.
		70 mg (as base)	Lactose. (31). White, oval. In unit-of-use 4s and UD 20s.
		Oral solution: 70 mg (as base)	Saccharin, parabens. Raspberry flavor. In 75 mL.

ALENDRONATE SODIUM — ORAL

For complete and comparative prescribing information, refer to the Bisphosphonates group monograph.

Indications

➤*Glucocorticoid-induced osteoporosis:* For the treatment of glucocorticoid-induced osteoporosis in men and women receiving glucocorticoids in a daily dosage equivalent to prednisone 7.5 mg or greater and who have lowbone mineral density. Patients treated with glucocorticoids should receive adequate amounts of calcium and vitamin D.

➤*Osteoporosis in men:* As a treatment to increase bone mass in men with osteoporosis.

➤*Osteoporosis in postmenopausal women:* For the treatment and prevention of osteoporosis in postmenopausal women.

➤*Paget disease of bone:* For the treatment of Paget disease of bone in men and women. Treatment is indicated in patients with Paget disease of bone having alkaline phosphatase at least 2 times the upper limit of normal, those who are symptomatic, or those at risk for future complications from their disease.

Administration and Dosage

➤*Approved by the FDA:* September 29, 1995.

➤*Administration:* Alendronate must be taken at least 30 minutes before the first food, beverage, or medication of the day with plain water only. Other beverages (including mineral water), food, and some medications are likely to reduce the absorption of alendronate. Waiting less than 30 minutes, or taking alendronate with food, beverages (other than plain water), or other medications, will lessen the effect of alendronate by decreasing its absorption into the body.

Alendronate should only be taken upon arising for the day. To facilitate delivery to the stomach and reduce the potential for esophageal irritation, an alendronate tablet should be swallowed with a full glass of water (180 to 240 mL). To facilitate gastric emptying, alendronate oral solution should be followed by at least 60 mL (one-fourth cup) of water. Patients should not lie down for at least 30 minutes and until after their first food of the day. Alendronate should not be taken at bedtime or before arising for the day. Failure to follow these instructions may increase the risk of esophageal adverse reactions.

➤*Calcium/Vitamin D supplementation:* Patients should receive supplemental calcium and vitamin D if dietary intake is inadequate.

➤*Glucocorticoid-induced osteoporosis:* One 5 mg tablet once daily for men and women, except for postmenopausal women not receiving estrogen, for whom the recommended dosage is one 10 mg tablet once daily.

➤*Osteoporosis in men:* One 70 mg tablet once weekly, 1 bottle of 70 mg oral solution once weekly, or one 10 mg tablet once daily.

➤*Treatment of osteoporosis in postmenopausal women:* One 70 mg tablet once weekly, 1 bottle of 70 mg oral solution once weekly, or one 10 mg tablet once daily.

➤*Prevention of osteoporosis in postmenopausal women:* One 35 mg tablet once weekly or one 5 mg tablet once daily.

The safety of treatment and prevention of osteoporosis with alendronate has been studied for up to 7 years.

➤*Paget disease of bone:* 40 mg once a day for 6 months.

➤*Retreatment of Paget disease:* In clinical studies in which patients were followed every 6 months, relapses during the 12 months following therapy occurred in 9% (3 of 32) of patients who responded to treatment with alendronate. Specific retreatment data are not available; although responses to alendronate were similar in patients who had received prior bisphosphonate therapy and those who had not.

Retreatment with alendronate may be considered following a 6-month post-treatment evaluation period in patients who have relapsed, based on increases in serum alkaline phosphatase, which should be measured periodically. Retreatment may also be considered in those who failed to normalize their serum alkaline phosphatase.

➤*Renal function impairment:* Alendronate is not recommended for patients with more severe renal function impairment (Ccr less than 35 mL/min) because of lack of experience.

➤*Storage/Stability:*

Tablets – Store in a well-closed container at room temperature, 15° to 30°C (59° to 86°F).

Oral solution – Store at 25°C (77°F); excursions are permitted to 15° to 30°C (59° to 86°F). Do not freeze.

ETIDRONATE DISODIUM

Rx	**Etidronate Disodium** (Genpharm)	**Tablets:** 200 mg	(ED 200 G). White, rectangular. In 60s.
Rx	**Didronel** (Procter & Gamble Pharm.)		(P & G 402). White, rectangular. In 60s.
Rx	**Etidronate Disodium** (Genpharm)	**Tablets:** 400 mg	(ED 400 G). White, capsule shape. In 60s.
Rx	**Didronel** (Procter & Gamble Pharm.)		(N E 406). White, scored, capsule shape. In 60s.

ETIDRONATE DISODIUM — ORAL

For complete prescribing information, refer to the Bisphosphonates group monograph.

Indications

➤*Heterotopic ossification:* For the prevention and treatment of heterotopic ossification following total hip replacement or caused by spinal cord injury. Etidronate reduces the incidence of clinically important heterotopic bone by about two-thirds. Among those patients who form heterotopic bone, etidronate retards the progression of immature lesions and reduces the severity by at least 50%. Follow-up data (at least 9 months posttherapy) suggest these benefits persist.

➤*Paget disease:* For the treatment of symptomatic Paget disease of bone. Therapy usually arrests or significantly impedes the disease process as evidenced by symptomatic relief, including decreased pain and/or increased mobility (experienced by 3 of 5 patients), reductions in serum alkaline phosphatase and urinary hydroxyproline levels (30% or more in 4 of 5 patients), histomorphometry showing reduced numbers of osteoclasts and osteoblasts and more lamellar bone formation, and bone scans showing reduced radionuclide uptake at pagetic lesions.

In addition, reductions in pagetically elevated cardiac output and skin temperature have been observed in some patients.

In many patients, the disease process will be suppressed for a period of at least 1 year following cessation of therapy. The upper limit of this period has not been determined.

The effects of etidronate treatment in patients with asymptomatic Paget disease have not been studied. However, etidronate treatment of such patients may be warranted if extensive involvement threatens irreversible neurologic damage, major joints, or major weight-bearing bones.

➤*Unlabeled uses:* For the prevention and treatment of corticosteroid-induced osteoporosis.

Administration and Dosage

➤*Approved by the FDA:* September 1, 1977.

➤*Heterotopic ossification:*

Spinal cord injury – 20 mg/kg/day for 2 weeks, followed by 10 mg/kg/day for 10 weeks; total treatment period is 12 weeks. Institute therapy as soon as medically feasible following the injury, preferably prior to evidence of heterotopic ossification. Retreatment has not been studied.

Total hip replacement – 20 mg/kg/day for 1 month before and 3 months after surgery; total treatment period is 4 months. Retreatment has not been studied.

➤*Paget disease:*

Initial treatment – 5 to 10 mg/kg/day (not to exceed 6 months) or 11 to 20 mg/kg/day (not to exceed 3 months). Reserve doses greater than 10 mg/kg/day for use when lower doses are ineffective or when there is an overriding need to suppress rapid bone turnover (especially when irreversible neurologic damage is possible) or to reduce elevated cardiac output. Doses greater than 20 mg/kg/day are not recommended.

Retreatment – Initiate only after an etidronate-free period of at least 90 days and when there is biochemical, symptomatic, or other evidence of active disease process. Monitor patients every 3 to 6 months, although some patients may go drug-free for extended periods. Retreatment regimens are the same as for initial treatment. For most patients, the original dose will be adequate for retreatment. If not, consider increasing the dose within the recommended guidelines.

ETIDRONATE DISODIUM — ORAL

➤*Administration:* Administer as a single oral dose. However, if GI discomfort occurs, the dose may be divided. To maximize absorption, patients should avoid taking the following within 2 hours of dosing:

1.) Food, especially items high in calcium, such as milk or milk products.

2.) Vitamins with mineral supplements or antacids high in metals (eg, calcium, iron, magnesium, aluminum).

➤*Storage/Stability:* Avoid excessive heat (over 104°F or 40°C).

TILUDRONATE DISODIUM

Rx	**Skelid** (Sanofi-Synthelabo)	**Tablets:** 240 mg (equivalent to 200 mg tiludronic acid)	Lactose. (S.W 200). White. In foil strips in cartons of 56 tablets/carton.

TILUDRONATE DISODIUM — ORAL

For complete and comparative prescribing information, refer to the Bisphosphonates group monograph.

Indications

➤*Paget disease:* Treatment is indicated in patients with Paget disease of bone who have a level of serum alkaline phosphatase (SAP) at least twice the upper limit of normal, who are symptomatic, or who are at risk for future complications of their disease.

Administration and Dosage

➤*Approved by the FDA:* February 7, 1997.

➤*Dosage:* A single daily oral dose of tiludronate disodium 400 mg, taken with 6 to 8 ounces of plain water only, should be administered for a period of 3 months. Beverages other than plain water (including mineral water), food, and some medications are likely to reduce the absorption of tiludronate disodium.

Following therapy, allow an interval of 3 months to assess response. Specific data regarding re-treatment are limited, although results from uncontrolled studies indicate favorable biochemical improvement similar to initial tiludronate disodium treatment.

➤*Administration:* Tiludronate disodium should not be taken within 2 hours of food.

Tiludronate disodium should not be taken within 2 hours of indomethacin.

Calcium or mineral supplements should be taken at least 2 hours before or 2 hours after tiludronate disodium. Aluminum- or magnesium-containing antacids, if needed, should be taken at least 2 hours after taking tiludronate disodium.

➤*Storage/Stability:* Store tiludronate disodium at 25°C (77°F); excursions permitted to 15° to 30°C (59° to 86°F). Do not remove tablets from the foil strips until they are to be used.

RISEDRONATE SODIUM

Rx	**Actonel** (Procter & Gamble)	**Tablets:** 5 mg	Lactose. (RSN 5 mg). Yellow, oval. Film-coated. In 30s and 2000s.
		30 mg	Lactose. (RSN 30 mg). White, oval. Film-coated. In 30s.
		35 mg	Lactose. (RSN 35 mg). Orange, oval. Film-coated. In dose packs of 4

RISEDRONATE SODIUM — ORAL

For complete and comparative prescribing information, refer to the Bisphosphonates group monograph.

Indications

➤*Postmenopausal osteoporosis:* For the treatment and prevention of osteoporosis in postmenopausal women.

Prevention of osteoporosis – Risedronate sodium may be considered in postmenopausal women who are at risk of developing osteoporosis and for whom the desired clinical outcome is to maintain bone mass and to reduce the risk of fracture.

Treatment of osteoporosis – In postmenopausal women with osteoporosis, risedronate sodium increases BMD and reduces the incidence of vertebral fractures and a composite end point of nonvertebral osteoporosis-related fractures. Osteoporosis may be confirmed by the presence or history of osteoporotic fracture, or by the finding of low bone mass (for example, at least 2 SD below the premenopausal mean).

➤*Glucocorticoid-induced osteoporosis:* For the prevention and treatment of glucocorticoid-induced osteoporosis in men and women who are either initiating or continuing systemic glucocorticoid treatment (daily dosage equivalent to 7.5 mg or greater of prednisone) for chronic diseases. Patients treated with glucocorticoids should receive adequate amounts of calcium and vitamin D.

Administration and Dosage

➤*Approved by the FDA:* March 27, 1998.

➤*Administration:* Risedronate sodium should be taken at least 30 minutes before the first food or drink of the day other than water.

To facilitate delivery to the stomach, patients should take risedronate sodium while in an upright position with a full glass of plain water (180 to 240 mL). Patients should not lie down for 30 minutes after taking this medication.

➤*Dietary intake:* Patients should receive supplemental calcium and vitamin D if dietary intake is inadequate.

➤*Concurrent medications:* Calcium supplements and calcium-, aluminum- and magnesium-containing antacids may interfere with the absorption of risedronate sodium and should be taken at a different time of the day.

➤*Renal function impairment:* Risedronate sodium is not recommended for use in patients with severe renal impairment (creatinine clearance less than 30 mL/min).

➤*Treatment of postmenopausal osteoporosis:* The recommended regimen is one 5 mg tablet orally, taken daily, or one 35 mg tablet orally, taken once a week.

➤*Treatment and prevention of glucocorticoid-induced osteoporosis:* The recommended regimen is one 5 mg tablet orally, taken daily.

➤*Paget disease:* The recommended treatment regimen is 30 mg orally once daily for 2 months.

Re-treatment may be considered (following posttreatment observation of at least 2 months) if relapse occurs, or if treatment fails to normalize serum alkaline phosphatase. For retreatment, the dose and duration of therapy are the same as for initial treatment. No data are available on more than 1 course of retreatment.

➤*Storage/Stability:* Store at controlled room temperature 20° to 25°C (68° to 77°F [see USP]).

ZOLEDRONIC ACID

Rx	**Zometa** (Novartis)	**Powder for injection:** 4 mg	Mannitol 220 mg, sodium citrate 24 mg. In 5 mL vials.

ZOLEDRONIC ACID — INJECTION

For complete prescribing information, refer to the Bisphosphonates group monograph.

Indications

➤*Hypercalcemia of malignancy (HCM):* For the treatment of HCM.

➤*Multiple myeloma and bone metastases of solid tumors:* For the treatment of patients with multiple myeloma and patients with documented bone metastases from solid tumors, in conjunction with standard antineoplastic therapy. Prostate cancer should have progressed after treatment with at least 1 hormonal therapy.

➤*Unlabeled uses:* Treatment of postmenopausal osteoporosis. Treatment of Paget disease.

Administration and Dosage

➤*Approved by the FDA:* August 20, 2001.

➤*Hypercalcemia of malignancy:* Consider the severity of, as well as the symptoms of, tumor-induced hypercalcemia when considering use of zoledronic acid for injection. Vigorous saline hydration alone may be sufficient to treat mild, asymptomatic hypercalcemia.

Dose – The maximum recommended dose of zoledronic acid in HCM (albumin-corrected serum calcium† is greater than or equal to 12 mg/dL [3 mmol/L]) is 4 mg. The 4 mg dose must be given as a single-dose intravenous (IV) infusion over no less than 15 minutes.

Hydration – Adequately rehydrate patients prior to administration of zoledronic acid. Promptly initiate vigorous saline hydration, an integral part of hypercalcemia therapy, and make an attempt to restore the urine output to about 2 L/day throughout treatment. Mild or asymptomatic hypercalcemia may be treated with conservative measures (eg, saline hydration, with or without loop diuretics). Adequately hydrate patients throughout the treat-

† Albumin-corrected serum calcium (Cca, mg/dL) = Ca + 0.8 (mid-range albumin-measured albumin in mg/dL).

ZOLEDRONIC ACID — INJECTION

ment, but overhydration, especially in those patients who have cardiac failure, must be avoided. Do not employ diuretic therapy prior to correction of hypovolemia.

Retreatment – Retreatment with zoledronic acid 4 mg, may be considered if serum calcium does not return to normal or remain normal after initial treatment. It is recommended that a minimum of 7 days elapse before retreatment, to allow for full response to the initial dose. Renal function must be carefully monitored in all patients receiving zoledronic acid and possible deterioration in renal function must be assessed prior to retreatment with zoledronic acid.

➤*Multiple myeloma and metastatic bone lesions from solid tumors:* The recommended dose of zoledronic acid in patients with multiple myeloma and metastatic bone lesions from solid tumors for patients with creatinine clearance (Ccr) higher than 60 mL/min is 4 mg infused over no less than 15 minutes every 3 or 4 weeks. The optimal duration of therapy is not known. Also administer patients an oral calcium supplement of 500 mg and a multiple vitamin containing 400 units of vitamin D daily.

Renal function impairment –

Recommended Zoledronic Acid Dose for Patients with Mild to Moderate Renal Function Impairment

Baseline Ccr (mL/min)	Zoledronic acid recommended dose[a]
> 60	4 mg
50 to 60	3.5 mg
40 to 49	3.3 mg
30 to 39	3 mg

[a] Doses calculated assuming target AUC of 0.66 (mg•h/L) (Ccr = 75 mL/min).

During treatment, measure serum creatinine before each zoledronic acid dose and withhold treatment for renal deterioration. In the clinical studies, renal deterioration was defined as follows:

- For patients with normal baseline creatinine, increase of 0.5 mg/dL.
- For patients with abnormal baseline creatinine, increase of 1 mg/dL.

In the clinical studies, zoledronic acid treatment was resumed only when the creatinine returned to within 10% of the baseline value. Reinitiate zoledronic acid at the same dose as that prior to treatment interruption.

➤*Preparation of solution:* Visually inspect parenteral drug products for particulate matter and discoloration prior to administration, whenever solution and container permit.

4 mg dose – Vials of zoledronic acid concentrate for infusion contain overfill allowing for the withdrawal of 5 mL of concentrate (equivalent to zoledronic acid 4 mg). Dilute this concentrate immediately in 100 mL of sterile 0.9% sodium chloride or 5% dextrose injection. Do not store undiluted concentrate in a syringe to avoid inadvertent injection. The dose must be given as a single IV infusion over no less than 15 minutes.

Reduced doses for patients with baseline Ccr less than or equal to 60 mL/min – Withdraw an appropriate volume of the 5 mL zoledronic acid concentrate as needed:

- 4.4 mL for 3.5 mg dose.
- 4.1 mL for 3.3 mg dose.
- 3.8 mL for 3 mg dose.

The withdrawn concentrate must be diluted in 100 mL of sterile 0.9% sodium chloride or 5% dextrose injection. The dose must be given as a single IV infusion over no less than 15 minutes.

Admixture incompatibilities – Zoledronic acid must not be mixed with calcium-containing infusion solutions, such as lactated Ringers solution, and should be administered as a single IV solution in a line separate from all other drugs.

Administration – Because of the risk of clinically significant deterioration in renal function, which may progress to renal failure, single doses of zoledronic acid should not exceed 4 mg and the duration of infusion should be no less than 15 minutes. In the trials and in postmarketing experience, renal deterioration, progression to renal failure and dialysis, have occurred in patients, including those treated with the approved dose of 4 mg infused over 15 minutes. There have been instances of this occurring after the initial zoledronic acid dose.

There must be strict adherence to the IV administration recommendations for zoledronic acid in order to decrease the risk of deterioration in renal function.

➤*Storage/Stability:* Store at 25°C (77°F); excursions permitted to 15° to 30°C (59° to 86°F).

If not used immediately after dilution with infusion media, for microbiological integrity, refrigerate the solution at 2° to 8°C (36° to 46°F). Then equilibrate the refrigerated solution to room temperature prior to administration. The total time between dilution, storage in the refrigerator, and end of administration must not exceed 24 hours.

IBANDRONATE SODIUM

Rx	**Boniva** (Roche)	**Tablets:** 2.5 mg (as base)	Lactose (IT L3). White, oblong. Film-coated. In 30s.
		150 mg (as base)	Lactose (BNVA 150). White, oblong. Film-coated. In unit-dose 1s.
		Injection: 1 mg/mL (as base)	In 5 mL single-use prefilled syringe.

IBANDRONATE SODIUM — ORAL

For complete and comparative prescribing information, refer to the Bisphosphonates group monograph.

Indications

➤*Osteoporosis in postmenopausal women, prevention:* Ibandronate may be considered in postmenopausal women who are at risk of developing osteoporosis and for whom the desired clinical outcome is to maintain bone mass and reduce the risk of fracture.

➤*Osteoporosis in postmenopausal women, treatment:* In postmenopausal women with osteoporosis, ibandronate increases bone mineral density (BMD) and reduces the incidence of vertebral fractures. Osteoporosis may be confirmed by the presence or history of osteoporotic fracture or by a finding of low bone mass (BMD more than 2 SD below the premenopausal mean [T-score]).

➤*Unlabeled uses:* The treatment of metastatic bone disease in breast cancer.

Administration and Dosage

➤*Approved by the FDA:* May 16, 2003.

➤*Prevention or treatment of postmenopausal osteoporosis:* The recommended dose of ibandronate for the prevention or treatment of postmenopausal osteoporosis is one 2.5 mg tablet taken once daily. Alternatively, one 150 mg tablet taken once monthly on the same date each month may be considered.

➤*Administration:* To maximize absorption and clinical benefit, patients should take ibandronate at least 60 minutes before the first food or drink (other than water) of the day or before taking any oral medication or supplementation, including calcium, antacids, or vitamins.

To facilitate delivery to the stomach and reduce the potential for esophageal irritation, ibandronate tablets should be swallowed whole with a full glass of plain water (180 to 240 mL; 6 to 8 oz) while the patient is standing or sitting in an upright position. Patients should not lie down for 60 minutes after taking ibandronate.

Patients should not chew or suck the tablets because of the potential for oropharyngeal ulceration.

A patient should take the ibandronate 150 mg tablet on the same date each month (ie, the patient's ibandronate day).

➤*Missed monthly dose:* If the once-monthly dose is missed, and the patient's next scheduled ibandronate day is more than 7 days away, instruct the patient to take 1 ibandronate 150 mg tablet in the morning following the date that it is remembered. The patient then should return to taking 1 ibandronate 150 mg tablet every month in the morning of his or her chosen day, according to the original schedule.

The patient must not take two 150 mg tablets within the same week. If the patient's next scheduled ibandronate day is only 1 to 7 days away, the patient must wait until his next scheduled ibandronate day to take the tablet. The patient then should return to taking one ibandronate 150 mg tablet every month in the morning of his or her chosen day, according to his original schedule.

➤*Dietary intake:* Patients should receive supplemental calcium or vitamin D if dietary intake is inadequate.

➤*Renal function impairment:* No dose adjustment is necessary for patients with mild or moderate renal impairment where creatinine clearance [Ccr] is greater than or equal to 30 mL/min. Ibandronate is not recommended for use in patients with severe renal function impairment (Ccr less than 30 mL/min).

➤*Storage/Stability:* Store at 25°C (77°F); excursions permitted between 15° and 30°C (59° and 86°F).

IBANDRONATE SODIUM — INJECTION

For complete and comparative prescribing information, refer to the Bisphosphonates group monograph.

Indications

➤*Treatment of postmenopausal osteoporosis:* For the treatment of osteoporosis in postmenopausal women. Ibandronate increases bone mineral density (BMD) and reduces the incidence of vertebral fractures. Osteoporosis may be confirmed by the presence or history of osteoporotic fracture or by a finding of low bone mass (BMD more than 2 SD below the premenopausal mean [T-score]).

Administration and Dosage

➤*Approved by the FDA:* May 16, 2003 (oral).

IBANDRONATE SODIUM — INJECTION

➤*Treatment of postmenopausal osteoporosis:* The recommended dose for the treatment of postmenopausal osteoporosis is 3 mg every 3 months administered over a period of 15 to 30 seconds.

➤*Renal toxicity:* No cases of acute renal failure were observed in controlled clinical trials in which intravenous ibandronate was administered as a 15 to 30 second bolus. The risk of serious renal toxicity with other intravenous bisphosphonates appears to be inversely related to the rate of drug administration.

➤*Administration:* Ibandronate injection must only be administered intravenously. Care must be taken not to administer ibandronate injection intraarterially or paravenously as this could lead to tissue damage.

Do not administer by any other route of administration. The safety and efficacy of ibandronate injection following non-intravenous routes of administration have not been established.

Administer ibandronate injection using the enclosed needle. Prefilled syringes are for single use only.

➤*Missed doses:* If the dose is missed, administer the injection as soon as it can be rescheduled. Thereafter, schedule injections every 3 months from the date of the last injection. Do not administer ibandronate injection (3 mg) more frequently than once every 3 months.

➤*Dietary intake:* Patients must receive supplemental calcium and vitamin D.

➤*Renal function impairment:* Ibandronate is not recommended for use in patients with severe renal impairment, patients with serum creatinine greater than 200 mcmol/L (2.3 mg/dL) or (Ccr [measured or estimated] less than 30 mL/min).

➤*Admixture incompatibilities:* Ibandronate injection must not be mixed with calcium-containing solutions or other intravenously administered drugs.

➤*Storage / Stability:* Store at 25°C (77°F); excursions permitted between 15° and 30°C (59° and 86°F). Discard unused portion.

PAMIDRONATE DISODIUM

Rx	**Pamidronate Disodium** (Sandoz)	**Powder for injection, lyophilized**: 30 mg	470 mg mannitol. In vials.
Rx	**Aredia** (Novartis)		470 mg mannitol. In vials.
Rx	**Pamidronate Disodium** (Sandoz)	**Powder for injection, lyophilized**: 90 mg	375 mg mannitol. In vials.
Rx	**Aredia** (Novartis)		375 mg mannitol. In vials.
Rx	**Pamidronate Disodium** (Various, eg, American Pharm Partners, Faulding)	**Injection**: 3 mg/mL	May contain mannitol. In 10 mL vials.
Rx	**Pamidronate Disodium** (Faulding)	**Injection**: 6 mg/mL	400 mg mannitol. In 10 mL vials.
Rx	**Pamidronate Disodium** (Various, eg, American Pharm Partners, Faulding)	**Injection**: 9 mg/mL	May contain mannitol. In 10 mL vials.

PAMIDRONATE DISODIUM — INJECTION

For complete and comparative prescribing information, refer to the Bisphosphonates group monograph.

Indications

➤*Hypercalcemia of malignancy:* Pamidronate, in conjunction with adequate hydration, is indicated for the treatment of moderate or severe hypercalcemia associated with malignancy, with or without bone metastases. Patients who have either epidermoid or nonepidermoid tumors respond to treatment with pamidronate. Initiate vigorous saline hydration, an integral part of hypercalcemia therapy, promptly and attempt to restore the urine output to about 2 L/day throughout treatment. Mild or asymptomatic hypercalcemia may be treated with conservative measures (ie, saline hydration, with or without loop diuretics). Patients should be hydrated adequately throughout the treatment, but overhydration, especially in those patients who have cardiac failure, must be avoided. Do not employ diuretic therapy prior to correction of hypovolemia. The safety and efficacy of pamidronate in the treatment of hypercalcemia associated with hyperparathyroidism or with other nontumor-related conditions have not been established.

➤*Paget disease:* Pamidronate is indicated for the treatment of patients with moderate to severe Paget disease of bone. The effectiveness of pamidronate was demonstrated primarily in patients with serum alkaline phosphatase greater than or equal to 3 times the upper limit of normal. Pamidronate therapy in patients with Paget disease has been effective in reducing serum alkaline phosphatase and urinary hydroxyproline levels by greater than or equal to 50% in at least 50% of patients, and by greater than or equal to 30% in at least 80% of patients. Pamidronate therapy has also been effective in reducing these biochemical markers in patients with Paget disease who failed to respond, or no longer responded to, other treatments.

➤*Osteolytic bone metastases of breast cancer and osteolytic lesions of multiple myeloma:* Pamidronate is indicated, in conjunction with standard antineoplastic therapy, for the treatment of osteolytic bone metastases of breast cancer and osteolytic lesions of multiple myeloma. The pamidronate treatment effect appeared to be smaller in the study of breast cancer patients receiving hormonal therapy than in the study of those receiving chemotherapy; however, overall evidence of clinical benefit has been demonstrated.

➤*Unlabeled uses:* Postmenopausal osteoporosis; hyperparathyroidism; prevention of glucocorticoid-induced osteoporosis; reduction of bone pain in patients with prostatic carcinoma; immobilization-related hypercalcemia.

Administration and Dosage

➤*Approved by the FDA:* October 31, 1991.

➤*Hypercalcemia of malignancy:* Consider the severity and the symptoms of hypercalcemia. Vigorous saline hydration alone may be sufficient for treating mild, asymptomatic hypercalcemia. Avoid overhydration in patients who have potential for cardiac failure. In hypercalcemia associated with hematologic malignancies, the use of glucocorticoid therapy may be helpful.

➤*Moderate hypercalcemia:* The recommended dose of pamidronate in moderate hypercalcemia (corrected serum calcium [albumin-corrected serum calcium (CCa, mg/dL) = serum calcium, mg/dL + 0.8 (4-serum albumin, g/dL)] of approximately 12 to 13.5 mg/dL) is 60 to 90 mg given as a single dose, intravenous infusion over at least 2 to 24 hours. Longer infusions (ie, greater than 2 hours) may reduce the risk for renal toxicity, particularly in patients with preexisting renal insufficiency.

➤*Severe hypercalcemia:* The recommended dose of pamidronate in severe hypercalcemia (corrected serum calcium [albumin-corrected serum calcium (CCa, mg/dL) = serum calcium, mg/dL + 0.8 (4-serum albumin, g/dL)] greater than 13.5 mg/dL) is 90 mg given as a single dose, intravenous infusion over 2 to 24 hours. Longer infusions (ie, greater than 2 hours) may reduce the risk for renal toxicity, particularly in patients with preexisting renal insufficiency.

➤*Retreatment:* A limited number of patients have received more than 1 treatment with pamidronate for hypercalcemia. Retreatment with pamidronate in patients who show complete or partial response initially may be carried out if serum calcium does not return to normal or remain normal after initial treatment. It is recommended that a minimum of 7 days elapse before retreatment, to allow for full response to the initial dose. The dose and manner of retreatment is identical to that of the initial therapy.

➤*Paget disease:* The recommended dosage of pamidronate in patients with moderate to severe Paget disease of bone is 30 mg/day, administered as a 4-hour infusion on 3 consecutive days for a total dose of 90 mg.

➤*Retreatment:* A limited number of patients with Paget disease have received more than 1 treatment of pamidronate in clinical trials. When clinically indicated, patients should be retreated at the dose of initial therapy.

➤*Osteolytic bone lesions of multiple myeloma:* The recommended dosage of pamidronate in patients with osteolytic bone lesions of multiple myeloma is 90 mg administered as a 4-hour infusion given on a monthly basis.

Give patients with marked Bence-Jones proteinuria and dehydration adequate hydration prior to pamidronate infusion.

Limited information is available on the use of pamidronate in multiple myeloma patients with a serum creatinine greater than or equal to 3 mg/dL.

The optimal duration of therapy is not yet known, however, in a study of patients with myeloma, final analysis after 21 months demonstrated overall benefits.

➤*Osteolytic bone metastases of breast cancer:* The recommended dosage of pamidronate in patients with osteolytic bone metastases is 90 mg administered over a 2-hour infusion given every 3 to 4 weeks.

Pamidronate has been frequently used with doxorubicin, fluorouracil, cyclophosphamide, methotrexate, mitoxantrone, vinblastine, dexamethasone, prednisone, melphalan, vincristine, megesterol, and tamoxifen. It has been given less frequently with etoposide, cisplatin, cytarabine, paclitaxel, and aminoglutethimide. The optimal duration of therapy is not known; however, in 2 breast cancer studies, final analyses performed after 24 months of therapy demonstrated overall benefits.

➤*Preparation of solution:*

Reconstitution – Pamidronate is reconstituted by adding 10 mL of sterile water for injection, to each vial, resulting in a solution of 30 mg per 10 mL or 90 mg per 10 mL. The pH of the reconstituted solution is 6 to 7.4. The drug should be completely dissolved before the solution is withdrawn.

Method of administration – Due to the risk of clinically significant deterioration in renal function, which may progress to renal failure, single doses of pamidronate should not exceed 90 mg.

There must be strict adherence to the IV administration recommendations for pamidronate in order to decrease the risk of deterioration in renal function.

PAMIDRONATE DISODIUM — INJECTION

➤*Hypercalcemia of malignancy:* The daily dose must be administered as an IV infusion over at least 2 to 24 hours for the 60 and 90 mg doses. Dilute the recommended dose in 1,000 mL of sterile 0.45% or 0.9% sodium chloride, or 5% dextrose injection. This infusion solution is stable for up to 24 hours at room temperature.

➤*Paget disease:* The recommended daily dose of 30 mg should be diluted in 500 mL of sterile 0.45% or 0.9% sodium chloride, or 5% dextrose injection, and administered over a 4-hour period for 3 consecutive days.

➤*Osteolytic bone metastases of breast cancer:* The recommended dose of 90 mg should be diluted in 250 mL of sterile 0.45% or 0.9% Sodium Chloride, USP, or 5% Dextrose Injection, USP, and administered over a 2-hour period every 3 to 4 weeks.

➤*Osteolytic bone lesions of multiple myeloma:* The recommended dose of 90 mg should be diluted in 500 mL of sterile 0.45% or 0.9% sodium chloride, or 5% dextrose injection, and administered over a 4-hour period on a monthly basis.

Do not mix pamidronate with calcium-containing infusion solutions, such as Ringer solution. Administer in a single IV solution and line separate from all other drugs.

➤*Note:* Visually inspect parenteral drug products for particulate matter and discoloration prior to administration, whenever solution and container permit.

➤*Storage/Stability:* Pamidronate reconstituted with sterile water for injection may be stored under refrigeration at 2° to 8°C (36° to 46°F) for up to 24 hours.

Do not store vials for reconstitution above 30°C (86°F).

BISPHOSPHONATE COMBINATION

Rx	**Actonel with Calcium** (Procter & Gamble)	**Tablets:** risedronate 35 mg, calcium carbonate 1,250 mg (equiv. to elemental calcium 500 mg)	Lactose. 4 **Actonel** tablets: (RSN 35 mg). Orange, oval. Film coated. 24 calcium carbonate tablets: (NE 2). Lt. blue, oval. Film coated. In 28-day course, blister package.
Rx	**Fosamax Plus D** (Merck)	**Tablets:** alendronate 70 mg sodium/ 2,800 units cholecalciferol	Lactose, sucrose. (710). White to off-white, capsule shape. In unit-of-use blisters of 4, and UD 20s.

BISPHOSPHONATE COMBINATION — ORAL

For complete prescribing information, refer to the Bisphosphonates group monograph and the Vitamin D monograph.

Indications

➤*Osteoporosis in men (Fosamax Plus D* only): For treatment to increase bone mass in men with osteoporosis.

➤*Osteoporosis in postmenopausal women:*

Prevention (Actonel with Calcium only) – Consider in postmenopausal women who are at risk of developing osteoporosis and for whom the desired clinical outcome is to maintain bone mass and to reduce the risk of fracture.

Treatment – For the treatment of osteoporosis in postmenopausal women by increasing bone mass and reducing the incidence of fractures, including those of the hip and spine (vertebral compression fractures).

Administration and Dosage

➤*Approved by the FDA:* April 7, 2005.

➤*Dosage:*

Alendronate/Cholecalciferol – Recommended dosage is 1 alendronate 70 mg/cholecalciferol 2,800 units tablet once weekly.

Risedronate/Calcium – Recommended dosage is 1 risedronate 35 mg tablet taken once a week (day 1 of the 7-day treatment cycle) and 1 calcium 1,250 mg tablet (elemental calcium 500 mg) taken with food daily on each of the remaining 6 days (days 2 through 7 of the 7-day treatment cycle).

➤*Administration:* Must be taken at least 30 minutes before the first food, beverage, or medication of the day with plain water only. Other beverages (including mineral water), food, and some medications (including those containing calcium, aluminum, and magnesium) are likely to reduce the absorption of alendronate or risedronate.

To facilitate delivery to the stomach and thus reduce the potential for esophageal irritation, advise the patient to swallow the tablets with a full glass of water (6 to 8 ounces) upon arising for the day. Patients should not lie down for at least 30 minutes and until after their first food of the day. Instruct the patient not to take alendronate/cholecalciferol at bedtime or before arising for the day. Failure to follow these instructions may increase the risk of esophageal adverse experiences.

➤*Calcium/Vitamin D supplementation:* Patients should receive supplemental calcium if dietary intake is inadequate. The recommended total (diet and otherwise) daily calcium intake in postmenopausal women is elemental calcium 1,200 mg. If patients need calcium in excess of that provided by risedronate with calcium, this should be taken with food at a separate time of day. Patients at increased risk for vitamin D insufficiency (eg, those in nursing homes, chronically ill, older than 70 years of age), should receive vitamin D supplementation in addition to that provided in alendronate/cholecalciferol. Patients with GI malabsorption syndromes may require higher doses of vitamin D supplementation; consider measurement of 25-hydroxyvitamin D.

The recommended intake of vitamin D is 400 to 800 units daily. Alendronate/cholecalciferol is intended to provide 7 days' worth of 400 units daily vitamin D in a single, once-weekly dose.

➤*Renal function impairment:* Not recommended for patients with severe renal insufficiency (creatinine clearance less than 35 mL/minute) for alendronate/cholecalciferol and for patients with creatinine clearance less than 30 mL/minute for risedronate/calcium.

➤*Storage/Stability:* Store at 20° to 25°C (68° to 77°F); excursions between 15° to 30°C (59° to 86°F) are allowed. Protect from moisture and light.

Fosamax Plus D –

Unit-of-use blister and unit dose packages: Store tablets in original blister package until used.

ANTIDIABETIC AGENTS

Insulin

Indications

➤*Type 1 diabetes mellitus (formerly known as insulin-dependent diabetes mellitus [IDDM]):* For the treatment of type 1 diabetes mellitus.

➤*Type 2 diabetes mellitus (formerly known as noninsulin-dependent diabetes mellitus [NIDDM]):* For the treatment of type 2 diabetes mellitus that cannot be controlled properly by diet, exercise, and weight reduction.

➤*Hyperkalemia:* Infusion of glucose and regular insulin produces a shift of potassium into cells and lowers serum potassium levels.

➤*Severe ketoacidosis/diabetic coma:* Insulin injection (regular insulin) may be given IV or IM for rapid effect in severe ketoacidosis or diabetic coma.

➤*Highly purified (single component) and human insulins:* Local insulin allergy, immunologic insulin resistance, injection-site lipodystrophy; temporary insulin use (eg, surgery, acute stress type 2 diabetes, gestational diabetes); newly diagnosed diabetics.

Administration and Dosage

➤*Preparation and administration:* The number and size of daily doses, time of administration, and diet and exercise require continuous medical supervision. Dosage adjustment may be necessary when changing types of insulin, particularly when changing from single-peak to the more purified animal or human insulins.

For insulin suspensions, ensure uniform dispersion by rolling the vial gently between hands. Avoid vigorous shaking that may result in the formation of air bubbles or foam. Regular insulin, insulin glargine, and insulin glulisine should be a clear solution.

Injection site – Administer maintenance doses subcutaneously. Rotate administration sites to prevent lipodystrophy. A general rule is not to administer within 1 inch of the same site for 1 month. The rate of absorption is more rapid when the injection is in the abdomen (possibly greater than 50% faster), followed by the upper arm, thigh, and buttocks. Therefore, it may be best to rotate sites within an area rather than rotating areas. Give regular insulin IV or IM in severe ketoacidosis or diabetic coma.

➤*Dosage guidelines:* Individualize doses and monitor patients with diabetes mellitus closely; the following dosage guidelines may be considered.

Children and adults – 0.5 to 1 unit/kg/day.

Insulin timing: Give insulin lispro within 15 minutes before a meal. Human regular insulin is best given 30 to 60 minutes before a meal. Give insulin glargine once daily subcutaneously at bedtime. Give insulin glulisine within 15 minutes before a meal or within 20 minutes after starting a meal.

Insulin requirements may be altered during intercurrent conditions such as illness, emotional disturbances, or stress.

Adjust doses to achieve premeal and bedtime blood glucose levels of 80 to 140 mg/dL (100 to 200 mg/dL in children younger than 5 years of age).

➤*Insulin mixtures:* When mixing 2 types of insulin, always draw clear regular insulin into the syringe first. Patients stabilized on mixtures should have a consistent response if the mixing is standardized. An unexpected response is most likely to occur when switching from separate injections to the use of mixture or vice versa. To avoid dosage error, do not alter order of mixing insulins or change model or brand of syringe or needle. Each type of insulin used must be of the same concentration (units/mL).

Isophane insulin (NPH)/regular mixtures of insulin are now available from the manufacturer in premixed formulations of 70% NPH and 30% regular. A

50/50 combination also is available. NPH/regular combinations of insulin are stable and are absorbed as if injected separately. In mixtures of regular and lente insulins, binding is detectable 5 minutes to 24 hours after mixing. If the regular/lente mixtures are not administered within the first 5 minutes after mixing, the effect of the regular insulin is diminished. The excess zinc binds with the regular and forms a lente-type insulin. Thus, it is critical that mixtures of regular with the lente insulins be mixed and injected immediately.

These mixtures remain stable for 1 month at room temperature or for 3 months refrigerated. These mixtures also can be stored in prefilled plastic or glass syringes for 1 week to possibly 14 days under refrigeration. Keep filled syringes in a vertical or oblique position with the needle pointing upward to avoid plugging problems. Prior to injection, pull back the plunger and tip the syringe back and forth, slightly agitating to remix the insulins. Check for normal appearance.

Semilente, ultralente, and lente insulins may be mixed in any ratio; they are chemically identical and differ only in size and structure of insulin particles. These mixtures are stable 1 month at room temperature or 3 months under refrigeration.

If insulin glulisine is mixed with NPH human insulin, draw insulin glulisine into the syringe first. Make the injection immediately after mixing. Do not mix insulin glulisine with insulin preparations other than NPH. When it is used in a pump, do not mix insulin glulisine with other insulins or with a diluent.

➤*Insulin adsorption:* Insulin adsorption into plastic IV infusion sets reportedly has removed up to 80% of a dose, but 20% to 30% is more common. The percent adsorbed is inversely proportional to insulin concentration; it takes place within 30 to 60 minutes. Because this phenomenon cannot be predicted accurately, patient monitoring is essential.

➤*Concomitant sulfonylurea therapy:* Insulin and oral sulfonylurea coadministration has been used with some success in type 2 diabetic patients who are difficult to control with diet and sulfonylurea therapy alone.

➤*Storage / Stability:* Proper storage is critical. Insulin preparations are generally stable if stored at room temperature (and not exposed to extreme temperatures or direct sunlight) for 1 month. Always store extra bottles in the refrigerator; do not freeze.

Insulin prefilled in plastic or glass syringes is stable for 28 days under refrigeration. Insulin lispro must be mixed immediately before injection.

Actions

➤*Pharmacology:* Insulin and its analogs lower blood glucose levels by stimulating peripheral glucose uptake, especially by skeletal muscle and fat, and by inhibiting hepatic glucose production. Insulin inhibits lipolysis in the adipocyte, inhibits proteolysis, and enhances protein synthesis. Insulin, secreted by the beta cells of the pancreas, is the principal hormone required for proper glucose use in normal metabolic processes. It is composed of 2 amino acid chains, A (acidic) and B (basic), joined together by disulfide linkages. Human insulin has minor but significant differences from animal insulin with respect to the amino acid sequence on the B-chain (see below). It is derived from a biosynthetic process with strains of *Escherichia coli* (recombinant DNA; rDNA) or yeast (rDNA).

Insulin Amino Acids[a]

	A-Chain Position			B-Chain Position			
Source/Types	A8	A10	A21	B28	B29	B30	B31 and B32
Beef	Ala	Val	Asn	Pro	Lys	Ala	-
Pork	Thr	Ilc	Asn	Pro	Lys	Ala	-
Human	Thr	Ilc	Asn	Pro	Lys	Thr	-
Glargine	Thr	Ilc	Gly	Pro	Lys	Thr	Arg
Aspart	Thr	Ilc	Asn	Aspartic acid	Lys	Thr	-
Lispro	Thr	Ilc	Asn	Lys	Pro	Thr	-
Glulisine	Thr	I1c	Asn	Pro	Glu	Thr	-

[a] Ala = alanine, Arg = arginine, Asn = asparagine, Gly = glycine, Ilc = isoleucine, Lys = lysine, Pro = proline, Thr = threonine, Val = valine, Glu = glutamine.

Human insulin may have a more rapid onset and shorter duration of action than pork insulin in some patients. However, the bioavailability of the insulins is identical when given subcutaneously. The human insulins are slightly less antigenic than pork or beef insulins. Consider the potential for flocculation with NPH insulin. Human insulin is also the insulin of choice for patients with insulin allergy, insulin resistance, all pregnant patients with diabetes, and any patient who uses insulin intermittently.

Insulin preparations are divided into the following 3 categories according to promptness, duration, and intensity of action following subcutaneous administration: rapid-, intermediate-, or long-acting.

Crystalline regular insulin – Crystalline regular insulin is prepared by precipitation in the presence of zinc chloride. Regular insulins available in the United States are prepared at neutral pH; this improves stability. Modified forms have been developed to alter the pattern of activity.

NPH – A modified, crystalline protamine zinc insulin. Its effects are comparable to a mixture of 2 to 3 parts regular insulin and 1 part protamine zinc insulin.

Extended insulin zinc suspension (ultralente) – Large crystals of insulin with high zinc content are collected and resuspended in a sodium acetate/sodium chloride solution. This relatively insoluble insulin is formed without a modifying protein.

Prompt insulin zinc suspension (semilente) – Amorphous (noncrystalline) insulin precipitated at a high pH.

Insulin zinc suspension (lente) – Stable mixture of 70% ultralente and 30% semilente.

Insulin lispro – Consists of zinc-insulin lispro crystals dissolved in clear aqueous fluid. Created when the amino acids at positions 28 and 29 on the insulin B-chain are reversed.

Insulin aspart – Homologous with regular human insulin with the exception of a single substitution of the amino acid proline by aspartic acid in position B28. Produced by recombinant DNA technology utilizing *Saccharomyces cerevisiae* (baker's yeast) as the production organism.

Insulin glargine – Created when the amino acids at position 21 of human insulin are replaced by glycine and 2 arginines are added to the C terminus of the B chain.

Insulin glulisine – Insulin glulisine is produced by recombinant DNA technology utilizing a nonpathogenic laboratory strain of *E. coli* (K12). Insulin glulisine differs from human insulin in that the amino acid asparagine at position B3 is replaced by lysine and the lysine in position B29 is replaced by glutamic acid.

Individual response to insulin varies and is affected by diet, exercise, concomitant drug therapy, and other factors. Characteristics of various insulins given subcutaneously are compared below:

Pharmacokinetics and Compatibility of Various Insulins

	Insulin Preparations	Half-life (hrs)	Onset (hrs)	Peak (hrs)	Duration (hrs)	Compatible mixed with
Rapid-acting	Insulin injection (regular)		0.5 to 1		8 to 12	All
	Prompt insulin zinc suspension (semilente)		1 to 1.5	5 to 10	12 to 16	Lente
	Lispro insulin solution	1	0.25	0.5 to 1.5	2 to 5	Ultralente, NPH
	Insulin aspart solution	1.5	0.25	1 to 3	3 to 5	[a]
	Insulin glulisine	0.7		0.5 to 1.5	1 to 2.5	NPH
Intermediate-acting	Isophane insulin suspension (NPH)		1 to 1.5	4 to 12	24	Regular
	Insulin zinc suspension (lente)		1 to 2.5	7 to 15	24	Regular, semilente
Long-acting	Insulin glargine solution		1.1	5[b]	24[c]	None
	Protamine zinc insulin suspension (PZI)		4 to 8	14 to 24	36	Regular
	Extended insulin zinc suspension (ultralente)		4 to 8	10 to 30	20 to 36	Regular, semilente

[a] See Administration and Dosage in insulin aspart monograph.
[b] No pronounced peak; small amounts of insulin glargine are released slowly, resulting in a relatively constant concentration/time profile over 24 hours.
[c] Studies only conducted up to 24 hours.

Contraindications

During episodes of hypoglycemia and in patients sensitive to any ingredient of the product.

Warnings

➤*Changing insulins:* Change insulins cautiously and under medical supervision. Changes in purity, strength, brand, type, or species source may require dosage adjustment. Teach patients using insulin to self monitor blood glucose levels and keep daily records of results. Concomitant oral antidiabetic treatment may need to be adjusted.

➤*Hypersensitivity reactions:* May require discontinuation of insulin.

Local – Occasionally, redness, swelling, and itching at the injection site may develop. This reaction occurs if the injection is not properly made, if the skin is sensitive to the cleansing solution, or if the patient is allergic to insulin or insulin additives (eg, preservatives). The condition usually resolves in a few days to a few weeks. A change in the type or species source of insulin may be considered.

Systemic – Systemic reactions are less common and may present as a rash, shortness of breath, fast pulse, sweating, a drop in blood pressure, bronchospasm, shock, anaphylaxis, or angioedema and may be life-threatening.

Insulin aspart, insulin glulisine – Localized reactions and generalized myalgias have been reported with the use of cresol as an injectable excipient.

➤*Renal function impairment:* Some studies with human insulin have shown increased circulating levels of insulin in patients with renal failure. Careful glucose monitoring and dose adjustments of insulin may be necessary in patients with renal dysfunction. Insulin requirements may be reduced in patients with renal function impairment.

➤*Hepatic function impairment:* Some studies with human insulin have shown increased circulating levels of insulin in patients with hepatic failure. Careful glucose monitoring and dose adjustments of insulin may be necessary in patients with hepatic dysfunction.

➤*Fertility impairment:*

Insulin glargine – In a combined fertility and prenatal and postnatal study in male and female rats at subcutaneous doses of insulin glargine up to 0.36 mg/kg/day, which is approximately 7 times the recommended human subcutaneous starting dose of 10 units (0.008 mg/kg/day), based on mg/m^2, maternal toxicity caused by dose-dependent hypoglycemia, including some deaths, was observed. Consequently, a reduction of the rearing rate occurred in the high-dose group only. Similar effects were observed with NPH human insulin.

➤*Elderly:* In elderly patients with diabetes, the initial dosing, dosing increments, and maintenance dosing should be conservative to avoid hypoglycemic reactions. Hypoglycemia may be difficult to recognize in the elderly.

➤*Pregnancy: Category B; Category C* (insulin glargine, insulin aspart, insulin glulisine). Pregnancy may make diabetes management more difficult. Human insulin does not cross the placenta, at least when given in the second trimester. Insulin is the drug of choice for diabetes control in pregnancy. Keep patients under close medical supervision. Rigid control of serum glucose and avoidance of ketoacidosis are desired throughout pregnancy. It is essential for patients with diabetes or a history of gestational diabetes to maintain good metabolic control before conception and throughout pregnancy. Insulin requirements usually fall during the first trimester, increase during the second and third trimester, and rapidly decline after delivery.

Insulin glargine – Subcutaneous reproduction and teratology studies have been performed with insulin glargine and regular human insulin in rats and Himalayan rabbits. The drug was given to female rats before mating, during mating, and throughout pregnancy at doses up to 0.36 mg/kg/day, which is approximately 7 times the recommended human subcutaneous starting dose of 10 units (0.008 mg/kg/day), based on mg/m^2. In rabbits, doses of 0.072 mg/kg/day, which is approximately 2 times the recommended human subcutaneous starting dose of 10 units (0.008 mg/kg/day), based on mg/m^2, were administered during organogenesis. The effects of insulin glargine generally did not differ from those observed with regular human insulin in rats or rabbits. However, in rabbits, 5 fetuses from 2 litters of the high-dose group exhibited dilation of the cerebral ventricles. Fertility and early embryonic development appeared normal.

There are no well-controlled clinical studies of the use of insulin glargine in pregnant women. Use this drug during pregnancy only if clearly needed.

Insulin aspart – Subcutaneous reproduction and teratology studies have been performed with insulin aspart and regular human insulin in rats and rabbits. In these studies, insulin aspart was given to female rats before mating, during mating, and throughout pregnancy and to rabbits during organogenesis. The effects of insulin aspart did not differ from those observed with subcutaneous regular human insulin. Insulin aspart, like human insulin, caused pre- and postimplantation losses and visceral/skeletal abnormalities in rats at a dose of 200 units/kg/day (approximately 32 times the human subcutaneous dose of 1 unit/kg/day, based on unit/body surface area) and in rabbits at a dose of 10 units/kg/day (approximately 3 times the human subcutaneous dose of 1 unit/kg/day, based on unit/body surface area). The effects are probably secondary to maternal hypoglycemia at high doses. No significant effects were observed in rats at a dose of 50 units/kg/day and rabbits at a dose of 3 units/kg/day. These doses are approximately 8 times the human subcutaneous dose of 1 unit/kg/day for rats and equal to the human subcutaneous dose of 1 unit/kg/day for rabbits, based on units/body surface area.

There are no well-controlled clinical studies of the use of insulin aspart in pregnant women. Use during pregnancy only if the potential benefit justifies the potential risk to the fetus.

Insulin glulisine – The drug was given to female rabbits throughout pregnancy at subcutaneous doses up to 1.5 units/kg/day (dose resulting in an exposure 0.5 times the average human dose, based on body surface area comparison). Adverse effects on embryo-fetal development were only seen at maternal toxic dose levels inducing hypoglycemia. Increased incidence of postimplantation losses and skeletal defects were observed at a dose level of 1.5 units/kg once daily that also caused mortality in dams. A slight increased incidence of postimplantation losses was seen at the next lower dose level of 0.5 units/kg once daily (dose resulting in an exposure 0.2 times the average human dose, based on body surface area comparison), which also was associated with severe hypoglycemia, but there were no defects at that dose.

There are no well-controlled clinical studies of the use of insulin glulisine in pregnant women. Use this drug during pregnancy only if the potential benefit justifies the potential risk to the fetus.

➤*Lactation:* Insulin is destroyed in the GI tract when administered orally and therefore would not be expected to be absorbed intact by the breastfeeding infant. However, inadequate or excessive insulin treatment of diabetic mothers inhibits milk production. Lactating women may require adjustments in insulin dose and diet.

Insulin glargine, insulin aspart, insulin glulisine – It is unknown whether insulin glargine, insulin aspart, or insulin glulisine are excreted in significant amounts in breast milk. Many drugs, including human insulin, are excreted in breast milk. For this reason, exercise caution when insulin glargine is administered to a nursing woman.

➤*Children:* Safety and efficacy in patients younger than 12 years of age have not been established.

Insulin glargine – Safety and efficacy of insulin glargine have been established in children 6 to 15 years of age with type 1 diabetes.

Humalog – *Humalog* can be used in combination with sulfonylureas in children older than 3 years of age.

Precautions

➤*Insulin resistance:* Insulin resistance occurs rarely. Insulin resistant patients require more than 200 units of insulin/day for more than 2 days in the absence of ketoacidosis or acute infection. Sometimes, the resistance is due to high levels of IgG antibodies to insulin. Insulin resistance also may occur in obese patients, patients with acanthosis nigricans, ketoacidosis, endocrinopathies, and patients with insulin receptor defects; insulin resistance during infection may be caused by a postreceptor defect. Hyperglycemia may be managed by changing the insulin species source (eg, beef or mixed beef-pork to pork or human insulin). Corticosteroids (prednisone 60 to 100 mg/day) may be given if changing the insulin is not effective. Corticosteroids may decrease IgG production or decrease insulin binding to the antibody. Closely monitor for signs of hyperglycemia and for adverse effects of high-dose corticosteroids. Highly concentrated insulin (U-500) also may be given to insulin-resistant patients. Use caution to avoid hypoglycemia. Some type 2 patients with insulin resistance have been treated with a combination of a sulfonylurea plus insulin (see Administration and Dosage).

➤*Hypoglycemia:* Hypoglycemia may result from excessive insulin dose or may be caused by the following: increased work or exercise without eating; food not being absorbed in the usual manner because of postponement or omission of a meal or in illness with vomiting, fever, or diarrhea; when insulin requirements decline (see Overdosage). Early warning symptoms of hypoglycemia may be different or less pronounced under certain conditions, such as long duration of diabetes, diabetic nerve disease, use of medications such as beta blockers, or intensified diabetes control. Such situations may result in severe hypoglycemia (and possibly loss of consciousness) prior to patients' awareness of hypoglycemia. Rapid changes in serum glucose levels may induce symptoms of hypoglycemia in patients with diabetes, regardless of the glucose value.

➤*Diabetic ketoacidosis:* Diabetic ketoacidosis, a potentially life-threatening condition, requires prompt diagnosis and treatment. Hyperglucagonemia, hyperglycemia, and ketoacidosis may result. Diabetic ketoacidosis may result from stress, illness, or insulin omission or may develop slowly after a long period of insulin control. Treat with fluids, correction of acidosis and hypotension, and low-dose regular insulin IM or IV infusion.

Symptoms of Hypoglycemia vs Ketoacidosis

Reaction	Onset	Urine glucose/ acetone	Symptoms				
			CNS	Respiration	Mouth/GI	Skin	Miscellaneous
Hypoglycemic reaction (insulin reaction)	sudden	0/0	fatigue, weakness, nervousness, confusion, headache, diplopia, convulsions, psychoses, dizziness, unconsciousness	rapid, shallow	numbness, tingling, hunger, nausea	pallor, moist, shallow or dry	normal or noncharacteristic pulse, eyeballs normal
Ketoacidosis (diabetic coma)	gradual (hours or days)	+/+	drowsiness, dim vision	air hunger	thirst, acetone breath, nausea, vomiting, abdominal pain, loss of appetite	dry, flushed	rapid pulse, soft eyeballs

➤*Lipodystrophy:*

Lipoatrophy – Lipoatrophy is the breakdown of adipose tissue at the insulin injection site, causing a depression in the skin and possibly delaying insulin absorption. It may be the result of an immune response or when less pure insulins are administered. Injection of human or purified pork insulins into the site over a 2- to 4-week period may result in subcutaneous fat accumulation.

Lipohypertrophy – Lipohypertrophy is the result of repeated insulin injection into the same site. It is the accumulation of subcutaneous fat, and it may interfere with insulin absorption from the site. This condition may be avoided by rotating the injection site.

➤*Diet:* Patients must follow a prescribed diet and exercise regularly. Determine the time, number, and amount of individual doses and distribution of food among the meals of the day. Do not change this regimen unless prescribed otherwise.

➤*Hyperthyroidism / Hypothyroidism:* Hyperthyroidism may cause an increase in the renal clearance of insulin. Therefore, patients may need more insulin to control their diabetes. Hypothyroidism may delay insulin turnover, requiring less insulin to control diabetes.

Drug Interactions

Drugs That Decrease the Hypoglycemic Effect of Insulin

Acetazolamide	Estrogens
AIDS antivirals	Ethacrynic acid
Albuterol	Glucagon
Antipsychotic medications (atypical olanzapine and clozapine])	Isoniazid
	Lithium carbonate
Asparaginase	Morphine sulfate
Calcitonin	Niacin
Contraceptives, oral	Nicotine
Corticosteroids	Phenothiazines
Cyclophosphamide	Phenytoin
Danazol	Progestogens (eg, oral contraceptives)
Dextrothyroxine	

Drugs That Decrease the Hypoglycemic Effect of Insulin	
Diazoxide	Protease inhibitors
Diltiazem	Somatropin
Diuretics	Terbutaline
Dobutamine	Thiazide diuretics
Epinephrine	Thyroid hormones

Drugs That Increase the Hypoglycemic Effect of Insulin	
ACE inhibitors	Lithium carbonate
Alcohol	MAO inhibitors
Anabolic steroids	Mebendazole
Antidiabetic products, oral	Pentamidine[b]
Beta blockers[a]	Pentoxifylline
Calcium	Phenylbutazone
Chloroquine	Propoxyphene
Clofibrate	Pyridoxine
Clonidine	Salicylates
Disopyramide	Somatostatin analog (eg, octreotide)
Fluoxetine	Sulfinpyrazone
Fibrates	Sulfonamides
Guanethidine	Tetracyclines

[a] Nonselective beta blockers may delay recovery from hypoglycemic episodes and mask their signs/symptoms. Cardioselective agents may be alternatives.
[b] May sometimes be followed by hyperglycemia.

Adverse Reactions

➤*Human insulin:* Hypoglycemia and hypokalemia are among the potential clinical adverse events associated with the use of all insulins. Other adverse events commonly associated with human insulin therapy include the following:

Dermatologic – Injection-site reaction, lipodystrophy, pruritus, rash.

Lab test abnormalities – Hypoglycemia; hypokalemia.

Miscellaneous – Allergic reactions. Sodium retention and edema may occur, particularly if previously poor metabolic control is improved by intensified insulin therapy.

➤*Insulin glargine:*

Local – In clinical studies in adult patients, there was a higher incidence of treatment-emergent injection-site pain in insulin glargine-treated patients (2.7%) compared with NPH insulin-treated patients (0.7%). The reports of pain at the injection site were usually mild and did not result in discontinuation of therapy. Other treatment-emergent injection-site reactions occurred at similar incidences with both insulin glargine and NPH human insulin.

Ophthalmic – Retinopathy was evaluated in the clinical studies by means of retinal adverse events reported and fundus photography. The numbers of retinal adverse events reported for insulin glargine and NPH treatment groups were similar for patients with type 1 and 2 diabetes. Progression of retinopathy was investigated by fundus photography using a grading protocol derived from the Early Treatment Diabetic Retinopathy Study (ETDRS). In 1 clinical study involving patients with type 2 diabetes, a difference in the number of subjects with at least a 3-step progression in ETDRS scale over a 6-month period was noted by fundus photography (7.5% in insulin glargine group vs 2.7% in NPH-treated group). The overall relevance of this isolated finding cannot be determined because of the small number of patients involved, the short follow-up period, and the fact that this finding was not observed in other clinical studies.

➤*Insulin aspart:*

Lab test abnormalities – Small but persistent elevations in alkaline phosphatase.

Miscellaneous –

Antibody production: Insulin antibodies may develop during treatment with insulin. In large clinical trials, levels of antibodies that crossreact with human insulin and insulin aspart were higher in patients treated with insulin aspart compared with regular human insulin. The clinical significance of these antibodies is uncertain.

Overdosage

➤*Symptoms:* Hypoglycemia may result from excessive insulin dose or may be caused by the following: Increased work or exercise without eating; food not being absorbed in the usual manner because of postponement or omission of a meal or in illness with vomiting, fever, or diarrhea; when insulin requirements decline.

➤*Treatment:* Mild episodes of hypoglycemia can be treated with oral glucose or carbohydrates. Adjustments in drug dosage, meal patterns, or exercise may be needed. More severe episodes with coma, seizure, or neurologic impairment may be treated with IM/subcutaneous glucagon or concentrated IV glucose. Sustained carbohydrate intake and observation may be necessary because hypoglycemia may recur after apparent clinical recovery.

Patient Information

Patients should use the same type and brand of syringe to avoid dosage errors. Advise patients to rotate sites to prevent lipodystrophy. If using a "pen-filled" device, patients should follow information for proper use.

Advise patients to not change the order of mixing insulins (if applicable) or change the brand, strength, type, species, or dose without your physician's knowledge.

Insulin requirements may change in patients who become ill, especially with vomiting or fever and during stress or emotional disturbances. Consult a physician.

Advise patients to see their dentist twice yearly and to see an ophthalmologist regularly.

Patient information inserts are available; advise patients to read and understand all aspects of insulin use. Patients must receive complete instructions about the nature of diabetes. Strict adherence to prescribed diet, exercise program, and personal hygiene are essential.

Periodic measurement of glycosylated hemoglobin is recommended for the monitoring of long-term glycemic control.

Patients should wear diabetic identification (*Medic-Alert*) so appropriate treatment can be given if complications occur away from home.

Advise patients to monitor blood glucose and urine for glucose and ketones as prescribed and to monitor blood pressure regularly.

Patients should inform their doctor if they are pregnant or are contemplating pregnancy.

Insulin stored at room temperature will be less painful to inject compared with that stored in the refrigerator, so patients should allow refrigerated insulin to come to room temperature prior to injection.

➤*Insulin glargine:* Do not mix or dilute this type of insulin with any other insulin or solution or it will not work as intended (ie, there may be a loss of blood sugar control).

➤*Insulin glulisine:* The syringe must be new and not contain any other medicine.

Advise patient not to mix with any other type of insulin than NPH. If mixing with NPH human insulin, draw insulin glulisine into the syringe first. Inject the mixture right away.

INSULIN REGULAR

otc	**Regular Iletin** II (Lilly)	**Injection**: 100 units/mL purified pork	In 10 mL vials.
otc	**Humulin R** (Lilly)	**Injection**: 100 units/mL human insulin (rDNA)	In 10 mL vials.
otc	**Novolin R** (Novo Nordisk)		In 10 mL vials.
otc	**Novolin R Prefilled** (Novo Nordisk)		In 5 × 1.5 mL prefilled syringes.
otc	**Novolin R PenFill** (Novo Nordisk)	**Cartridges**: 100 units/mL human insulin (rDNA) (Use with *NovoPen* and *Novolin Pen*)	In 5 × 1.5 mL and 5 × 3 mL.

INSULIN REGULAR (PORK) — INJECTION

For complete and comparative prescribing information, refer to the Insulin group monograph.

INSULIN REGULAR (HUMAN) — INJECTION

For complete and comparative prescribing information, refer to the Insulin group monograph.

INSULIN ISOPHANE (NPH)

Insulin combined with protamine and zinc.

otc	**NPH Iletin** II (Lilly)	**Injection (suspension)**: 100 units/mL purified pork	In 10 mL vials.
otc	**Humulin N** (Lilly)	**Injection (suspension)**: 100 units/mL human insulin (rDNA)	In 5 × 3 mL disposable pen insulin delivery devices, and 10 mL vials.
otc	**Novolin N** (Novo Nordisk)		In 10 mL vials.
otc	**Novolin N Prefilled** (Novo Nordisk)		In 5 × 1.5 mL prefilled syringes.

INSULIN ISOPHANE (NPH)

otc	**Novolin N PenFill** (Novo Nordisk)	**Cartridges (suspension)**: 100 units/mL human insulin (rDNA) (Use with *NovoPen* and *Novolin Pen*)	In 5 × 1.5 mL and 5 × 3 mL.

INSULIN ISOPHANE (NPH; HUMAN) — INJECTION

For complete and comparative prescribing information, refer to the Insulin group monograph.

INSULIN ISOPHANE (NPH; PORK) — INJECTION

For complete and comparative prescribing information, refer to the Insulin group monograph.

INSULIN ISOPHANE AND REGULAR — INJECTION

Provides rapid activity (onset 30 minutes) with a duration of up to 24 hours.

otc	**Humulin 70/30** (Lilly)	**Injection (suspension)**: 100 units/mL human insulin (rDNA)	70% isophane insulin (NPH) and 30% insulin injection (regular). In 5 × 3 mL disposable pen insulin delivery devices, and 10 mL vials.
otc	**Novolin 70/30** (Novo Nordisk)		70% isophane insulin (NPH) and 30% insulin injection (regular). In 10 mL vials.
otc	**Novolin 70/30 Prefilled** (Novo Nordisk)		70% isophane insulin (NPH) and 30% insulin injection (regular). In 5 × 1.5 mL prefilled syringes.
otc	**Novolin 70/30 PenFill** (Novo Nordisk)	**Cartridges (suspension)**: 100 units/mL human insulin (rDNA) (Use with *NovoPen* and *Novolin Pen*)	70% isophane insulin (NPH) and 30% insulin injection (regular). In 5 × 1.5 and 5 × 3 mL.
otc	**Humulin 50/50** (Lilly)	**Injection (suspension)**: 100 units/mL human insulin (rDNA)	50% isophane insulin (NPH) and 50% insulin injection (regular). In 10 mL vials.

INSULIN ISOPHANE AND REGULAR (HUMAN) — INJECTION

For complete and comparative prescribing information, refer to the Insulin group monograph.

INSULIN ZINC (LENTE)

70% crystalline and 30% amorphous insulin suspension.

otc	**Lente Iletin II** (Lilly)	**Injection (suspension)**: 100 units/mL purified pork	In 10 mL vials.
otc	**Humulin L** (Lilly)	**Injection (suspension)**: 100 units/mL human insulin (rDNA)	In 10 mL vials.

INSULIN ZINC (LENTE; HUMAN) — INJECTION

For complete and comparative prescribing information, refer to the Insulin group monograph.

INSULIN ZINC (LENTE; PORK) — INJECTION

For complete and comparative prescribing information, refer to the Insulin group monograph.

INSULIN ZINC, EXTENDED (ULTRALENTE)

otc	**Humulin U** (Lilly)	**Injection (suspension)**: 100 units/mL human insulin (rDNA)	In 10 mL vials.

INSULIN ZINC, EXTENDED (ULTRALENTE; HUMAN) — INJECTION

For complete and comparative prescribing information, refer to the Insulin group monograph.

INSULIN ANALOG INJECTION

Rx	**Humalog** (Lilly)	**Injection**: 100 units/mL human insulin lispro (rDNA)	In 10 mL vials, 5 × 1.5 and 5 × 3 mL cartridges, and 5 × 3 mL disposable pen insulin delivery device.
Rx	**Humalog Mix 75/25**[a] (Lilly)		Protamine sulfate 0.28 mg. In 10 mL vials and 5 × 3 mL disposable pen insulin delivery devices.
Rx	**NovoLog** (Novo Nordisk)	**Injection**: 100 units/mL human insulin aspart (rDNA)	In 3 mL *PenFill* cartridges and 10 mL vials.
Rx	**NovoLog Mix 70/30**[b] (Novo Nordisk)	**Injection**: 100 units/mL insulin aspart.	In 3 mL *Penfill* cartridges and 3 mL *FlexPen* prefilled syringes.

[a] Contains 75% insulin lispro protamine suspension and 25% insulin lispro injection (rDNA).

[b] Contains 70% insulin aspart (rDNA) protamine suspension and 30% insulin aspart (rDNA).

INSULIN LISPRO — INJECTION

For complete and comparative prescribing information, refer to the Insulin group monograph.

Indications

➤*Diabetes:* Insulin lispro is an insulin analog that is indicated in the treatment of patients with diabetes mellitus for the control of hyperglycemia. Insulin lispro has a more rapid onset and a shorter duration of action than human regular insulin. Therefore, in patients with type 1 diabetes, insulin lispro should be used in regimens that include a longer-acting insulin. However, in patients with type 2 diabetes, insulin lispro may be used without a longer-acting insulin when used in combination therapy with sulfonylurea agents.

Administration and Dosage

➤*Administration:* Insulin lispro is intended for subcutaneous administration. Dosage regimens of insulin lispro will vary among patients and should be determined by the health care professional familiar with the patient's metabolic needs, eating habits, and other lifestyle variables. Pharmacokinetic and pharmacodynamic studies showed insulin lispro to be equipotent to human regular insulin (ie, one unit of insulin lispro has the same glucose-lowering capability as one unit of human regular insulin), but with more rapid activity.

The quicker glucose-lowering effect of insulin lispro is related to the more rapid absorption rate from subcutaneous tissue. An adjustment of dose or schedule of basal insulin may be needed when a patient changes from other insulins to insulin lispro, particularly to prevent pre-meal hyperglycemia.

When used as a meal-time insulin, insulin lispro should be given within 15 minutes before or immediately after a meal. Human regular insulin is best given 30-60 minutes before a meal. To achieve optimal glucose control, the amount of longer-acting insulin being given may need to be adjusted when using insulin lispro.

Injection site – The rate of insulin absorption and consequently the onset of activity is known to be affected by the site of injection, exercise, and other variables. Insulin lispro was absorbed at a consistently faster rate than human regular insulin in healthy male volunteers given 0.2 units/kg human regular insulin or insulin lispro at abdominal, deltoid, or femoral sites, the 3 sites often used by patients with diabetes. When not mixed in the same syringe with other insulins, insulin lispro maintains its rapid onset of action and has less variability in its onset of action among injection sites compared with human regular insulin. After abdominal administration, insulin lispro concentrations are higher than those following deltoid or thigh injections.

INSULIN LISPRO — INJECTION

Also, the duration of action of insulin lispro is slightly shorter following abdominal injection, compared with deltoid and femoral injections. As with all insulin preparations, the time course of action of insulin lispro may vary considerably in different individuals or within the same individual. Patients must be educated to use proper injection techniques.

➤*Compatibility:* Insulin lispro may be diluted with sterile diluent for insulin lispro, *Humulin N, Humulin 50/50, Humulin 70/30*, and *NPH Iletin* to a concentration of 1:10 (equivalent to U-10) or 1:2 (equivalent to U-50). Diluted insulin lispro may remain in patient use for 28 days when stored at 5°C (41°F) and for 14 days when stored at 30°C (86°F).

➤*Storage/Stability:* Insulin lispro should be stored in a refrigerator (2° to 8°C [36° to 46°F]), but not in the freezer. If refrigeration is impossible, the vial or cartridge of insulin lispro in use can be unrefrigerated for up to 28 days, as long as it is kept as cool as possible (not greater than 30°C [86°F]) and away from direct heat and light. Unrefrigerated vials and cartridges must be used within this time period or be discarded. Do not use insulin lispro if it has been frozen.

Parenteral drug products should be inspected visually prior to administration whenever the solution and the container permit. If the solution is cloudy, contains particulate matter, is thickened, or is discolored, the contents must not be injected. Insulin lispro should not be used after its expiration date.

INSULIN ASPART (rDNA origin) — INJECTION

Indications

Insulin aspart (rDNA origin) injection is indicated for the treatment of adult patients with diabetes mellitus for the control of hyperglycemia. Because insulin aspart has a more rapid onset and a shorter duration of action than regular human insulin, insulin aspart should normally be used in regimens together with an intermediate or long-acting insulin. Insulin aspart may also be infused subcutaneously by external insulin pumps.

Administration and Dosage

➤*Approved by the FDA:* June 7, 2000.

Generally, give immediately before a meal (start of meal within 5 to 10 minutes after injection) because of insulin aspart's fast onset of action. Individualize the dosage of insulin aspart in accordance with the needs of the patient. The total daily individual insulin requirement is usually between 0.5 to 1 units/kg/day. When used in a meal-related subcutaneous injection treatment regimen, 50% to 70% of total insulin requirements may be provided by insulin aspart and the remainder provided by an intermediate-acting or long-acting insulin. When used in external insulin infusion pumps, the initial programming of the pump is based on the total daily insulin dose of the previous regimen. Although there is significant interpatient variability, approximately 50% of the total dose is given as meal-related boluses of insulin aspart and the remainder as basal infusion. Because of insulin aspart's comparatively rapid onset and short duration of glucose lowering activity, some patients may require more basal insulin and more total insulin to prevent premeal hyperglycemia when using insulin aspart than when using human regular insulin. Additional basal insulin injections or higher basal rates in external subcutaneous infusion pumps may be necessary. Infusion sets and the insulin in the infusion sets must be changed every 48 hours or sooner to assure the activity of insulin aspart and proper pump function.

Administer insulin aspart by subcutaneous injection in the abdominal wall, the thigh, or the upper arm or by continuous subcutaneous infusion in the abdominal wall. Injection sites and infusion sites should be rotated within the same region. As with all insulins, the duration of action will vary according to the dose, injection site, blood flow, temperature, and level of physical activity.

Parenteral drug products should be inspected visually for particulate matter and discoloration prior to administration, whenever solution and container permit. Never use any insulin aspart if it has become viscous (thickened) or cloudy; use it only if it is clear and colorless. Insulin aspart should not be used after its expiration date.

➤*Storage/Stability:* Insulin aspart in unopened vials and cartridges, and insulin aspart prefilled syringes should be stored between 2° and 8°C (36° to 46°F). Do not freeze. Do not use insulin aspart if it has been frozen or exposed to temperatures that exceed 37°C (98.6°F). After a vial or cartridge has been punctured, it may be kept at temperatures below 30°C (86°F) for up to 28 days, but do not expose to excessive heat or sunlight. Opened vials may be refrigerated. Do not refrigerate cartridges after insertion into the *NovoPen 3*. Discard infusion sets (reservoirs, tubing, and catheters) and the insulin aspart in the reservoir after no more than 48 hours of use or after exposure to temperatures that exceed 37°C (98.6°F).

INSULIN GLARGINE

Rx	**Lantus** (Aventis)	**Injection:** 100 units/mL insulin glargine (rDNA)	In 10 mL vials and 3 mL cartridge system for use with *OptiClik*.

INSULIN GLARGINE — INJECTION

For complete and comparative prescribing information, refer to the Insulin group monograph.

Indications

➤*Diabetes:* Once-daily subcutaneous administration for the treatment of adults and children with type 1 diabetes mellitus or adults with type 2 diabetes mellitus who require basal (long-acting) insulin for the control of hyperglycemia.

Insulin glargine is not the insulin of choice for the treatment of diabetic ketoacidosis. Short-acting intravenous (IV) insulin is the preferred treatment.

Administration and Dosage

➤*Approved by the FDA:* April 20, 2000.

➤*Administration:* Insulin glargine should be administered subcutaneously once daily at the same time every day. The dose may be administered at any time during the day.

Insulin glargine is not intended for IV administration. The prolonged duration of activity of insulin glargine is dependent on injection into subcutaneous tissue. IV administration of the usual subcutaneous dose could result in severe hypoglycemia.

As with all insulins, injection sites within an injection area (abdomen, deltoid, or thigh) must be rotated from one injection to the next.

In clinical studies, there was no relevant difference in insulin glargine absorption after abdominal, deltoid, or thigh subcutaneous administration. As for all insulins, the rate of absorption and, consequently, the onset and duration of action may be affected by exercise and other variables.

Insulin glargine is a recombinant human insulin analog. Its potency is approximately the same as human insulin. It exhibits a relatively constant blood glucose–lowering profile over 24 hours that permits once-daily dosing. The desired blood glucose levels as well as the doses and timing of antidiabetes medications must be determined individually. Blood glucose monitoring is recommended for all patients with diabetes.

➤*Children:* Insulin glargine can be safely administered to pediatric patients 6 years of age and older. Administration to pediatric patients younger than 6 years of age has not been studied. Based on the results of a study in pediatric patients, the dose recommendation for changeover to insulin glargine is the same as described for adults.

➤*Initial dosing:* In a clinical study with insulin-naïve patients with type 2 diabetes already treated with oral antidiabetic drugs, insulin glargine was started at an average dose of 10 units once daily and subsequently adjusted according to the patient's need to a total daily dose ranging from 2 to 100 units.

➤*Changeover to insulin glargine:* If changing from a treatment regimen with an intermediate- or long-acting insulin to a regimen with insulin glargine, the amount and timing of short-acting insulin, fast-acting insulin analog, or the dose of any oral antidiabetic drug may need to be adjusted. In clinical studies, when patients were transferred from once-daily neutral protamine Hagedorn (NPH) human insulin or ultralente human insulin to once-daily insulin glargine, the initial dose was usually not changed. However, when patients were transferred from twice-daily NPH to insulin glargine once daily to reduce the risk of hypoglycemia, the initial dose was usually reduced by approximately 20% (compared with total daily units of NPH human insulin) and then adjusted based on patient response.

A program of close metabolic monitoring under medical supervision is recommended during transfer and in the initial weeks thereafter. The amount and timing of short- or fast-acting insulin analog may need to be adjusted. This is particularly true for patients with acquired antibodies to human insulin needing high insulin doses and occurs with all insulin analogs. Dose adjustment of insulin glargine and other insulins or oral antidiabetic drugs may be required; for example, if the patient's timing of dosing, weight or lifestyle changes, or other circumstances arise that increase susceptibility to hypoglycemia or hyperglycemia.

The dose also may have to be adjusted during intercurrent illness.

➤*Preparation and handling:* Use only if clear and colorless with no visible particles.

The syringes must not contain any other medicinal product or residue.

If *OptiClik*, the insulin delivery devise for insulin glargine, malfunctions, insulin glargine may be drawn from the cartridge system into a U-100 syringe and injected.

➤*Mixing and diluting:* Insulin glargine must not be diluted or mixed with any other insulin or solution. If insulin glargine is diluted or mixed, the solution may become cloudy and the pharmacokinetic/pharmacodynamic profile (eg, onset of action, time to peak effect) of insulin glargine and/or the mixed insulin may be altered in an unpredictable manner. When insulin glargine and regular human insulin were mixed immediately before injection in dogs, a delayed onset of action and time to maximum effect for regular human insulin was observed. The total bioavailability of the mixture also was slightly decreased compared with separate injections of insulin glargine and regular human insulin. The relevance of these observations in dogs to humans is not known.

INSULIN GLARGINE — INJECTION

➤*Storage/Stability:* Store unopened insulin glargine vials and cartridges in a refrigerator at 2° to 8°C (36° to 46°F). Do not store insulin glargine in the freezer or allow it to freeze. Discard if it has been frozen.

If refrigeration is not possible, the open vial in use can be kept unrefrigerated for up to 28 days away from direct heat and light, as long as the temperature is not above 30°C (86°F). Opened vials, whether or not refrigerated, must be used within a 28-day period or they must be discarded.

Do not refrigerate the opened (in-use) cartridge system in *OptiClik*. Keep the opened cartridge system at room temperature below 30°C (86°F), away from direct heat and light. Discard the opened cartridge system in *OptiClik* that has been kept at room temperature after 28 days. Do not store *OptiClik*, with or without cartridge system, in a refrigerator at any time.

INSULIN GLULISINE

Rx	**Apidra** (Aventis)	**Injection**: 100 units/mL insulin glulisine (rDNA)	In 10 mL vials.

INSULIN GLULISINE (rDNA ORIGIN) — INJECTION

For complete prescribing information, refer to the Insulin group monograph.

Indications

➤*Diabetes:* Insulin glulisine (rDNA origin) injection is indicated for the treatment of adult patients with diabetes mellitus for the control of hyperglycemia.

Insulin glulisine has a more rapid onset of action and a shorter duration of action than regular human insulin. Insulin glulisine should normally be used in regimens that include a longer-acting insulin or basal insulin analog.

Insulin glulisine also may be infused subcutaneously by external insulin infusion pumps.

Administration and Dosage

➤*Approved by the FDA:* April 16, 2004.

➤*Dosage:* Insulin glulisine is a recombinant insulin analog that has been shown to be equipotent to human insulin. One unit of insulin glulisine has the same glucose-lowering effect as 1 unit of regular human insulin. After subcutaneous administration, it has a more rapid onset and shorter duration of action.

Insulin glulisine should be given within 15 minutes before a meal or within 20 minutes after starting a meal.

Insulin glulisine is intended for subcutaneous administration and for use by external infusion pump.

The dosage of insulin glulisine should be individualized and determined based on the physician's advice in accordance with the needs of the patient. Insulin glulisine should normally be used in regimens that include a longer-acting insulin or basal insulin analog.

➤*Administration:* Insulin glulisine should be administered by subcutaneous injection in the abdominal wall, the thigh or the deltoid or by continuous subcutaneous infusion in the abdominal wall. As with all insulins, injection sites and infusion sites within an injection area (abdomen, thigh or deltoid) should be rotated from one injection to the next.

As for all insulins, the rate of absorption, and consequently the onset and duration of action, may be affected by injection site, exercise and other variables. Blood glucose monitoring is recommended for all patients with diabetes.

➤*Preparation and handling:* Parenteral drug products should be inspected visually prior to administration whenever the solution and the container permit. Insulin glulisine must only be used if the solution is clear and colorless with no particles visible.

When it is used in a pump, insulin glulisine should not be mixed with other insulins or with a diluent.

➤*Storage/Stability:*

Unopened vial – Unopened insulin glulisine vials should be stored in a refrigerator, 2° to 8°C (36° to 46°F). Protect from light. Insulin glulisine should not be stored in the freezer and it should not be allowed to freeze. Discard vial if frozen.

Open (in-use) vial – Opened vials, whether or not refrigerated, must be used within 28 days. They must be discarded if not used within 28 days. If refrigeration is not possible, the open vial in use can be kept unrefrigerated for up to 28 days away from direct heat and light, as long as the temperature is not greater than 25°C (77°F).

	Not in-use (unopened) refrigerated	Not in-use (unopened) room temperature, below 25°C (77°F)	In-use (opened) room temperature, below 25°C (77°F)
10 mL vial	Until expiration date	28 days	28 days, refrigerated/room temperature

Infusion sets – Infusion sets (reservoirs, tubing, and catheters) and the insulin glulisine in the reservoir should be discarded after no more than 48 hours of use or after exposure to temperatures that exceed 37°C (98.6°F).

INSULIN DETEMIR

Rx	**Levemir** (Novo Nordisk)	**Injection**: 100 units/mL insulin detemir (rDNA)	In 3 mL *Penfill* cartridges, 3 mL prefilled syringes (use with *FlexPen* and *Innolet*), and 10 mL vials.

INSULIN DETEMIR — INJECTION

Indications

➤*Diabetes:* For once- or twice-daily subcutaneous administration for the treatment of adult and pediatric patients with type 1 diabetes mellitus or adult patients with type 2 diabetes mellitus who require basal (long-acting) insulin for the control of hyperglycemia.

Administration and Dosage

➤*Approved by the FDA:* June 16, 2005.

➤*Dosage:* Insulin detemir can be administered once or twice daily. The dose of insulin detemir should be adjusted according to blood glucose measurements. The dosage of insulin detemir should be individualized in accordance with the needs of the patient.

- For patients treated with insulin detemir once daily, the dose should be administered with the evening meal or at bedtime.
- For patients who require twice-daily dosing for effective blood glucose control, the evening dose can be administered with the evening meal, at bedtime, or 12 hours after the morning dose.

➤*Injection sites:* Insulin detemir should be administered by subcutaneous injection in the thigh, abdominal wall, or upper arm. Injection sites should be rotated within the same region. As with all insulins, the duration of action will vary according to the dose, injection site, blood flow, temperature, and level of physical activity.

➤*Dose determination:* As with all insulins, close glucose monitoring is recommended during the transition and in the initial weeks thereafter. Dose and timing of concurrent short-acting insulins or other concomitant antidiabetic treatment may need to be adjusted.

Basal bolus patients – For patients with type 1 or type 2 diabetes on basal-bolus treatment, changing the basal insulin to insulin detemir can be done on a unit-to-unit basis. The dose of insulin detemir should then be adjusted to achieve glycemic targets. In some patients with type 2 diabetes, more insulin detemir may be required than neutral protamine Hagedorn (NPH) insulin. In a clinical study, the mean dose at end of treatment was 0.77 units/kg for insulin detemir and 0.52 units/kg for NPH human insulin.

Basal insulin only patients – For patients currently receiving only basal insulin, changing the basal insulin to insulin detemir may be done on a unit-to-unit basis.

Insulin-naïve patients – For insulin-naïve patients with type 2 diabetes who are inadequately controlled on oral antidiabetic drugs, insulin detemir should be started at a dose of 0.1 to 0.2 units/kg once daily in the evening or 10 units once or twice daily, and adjust the dose to achieve glycemic targets.

➤*Preparation and handling:*

Mixing and diluting – Do not mix or dilute insulin detemir with any other insulin preparations.

➤*Storage/Stability:* Store unused insulin detemir between 2° and 8°C (36° and 46°F). Do not freeze. Do not use insulin detemir if it has been frozen.

Vials – After initial use, store vials in a refrigerator, never in a freezer. If refrigeration is not possible, the in-use vial can be kept unrefrigerated at room temperature, below 30°C (86°F), for up to 42 days, as long as it is kept as cool as possible and away from direct heat and light.

Unpunctured vials can be used until the expiration date printed on the label if they are stored in a refrigerator. Keep unused vials in the carton so they will stay clean and protected from light.

Cartridges and prefilled syringe cartridges – After initial use, a cartridge or prefilled syringe may be used for up to 42 days if it is kept at room temperature, below 30°C (86°F). In-use cartridges and prefilled syringes must not be stored in a refrigerator or with the needle in place. Keep all cartridges and prefilled syringes away from direct heat and sunlight.

Not in-use (unopened) cartridges and prefilled syringes can be used until the expiration date printed on the label if they are stored in a refrigerator. Keep unused cartridges and prefilled syringes in the carton so they will stay clean and protected from light.

INSULIN HUMAN (INHALATION)

Rx	**Exubera** (Pfizer)	**Powder for inhalation:** 1 mg (rDNA)	In unit dose blister 90s with 2 **Exubera** release units.[a]
		3 mg (rDNA)	In unit dose blister 90s with 2 **Exubera** release units.[a]

[a] Also available in Combination Patient Packs with ninety 1 mg and ninety 3 mg blisters with 2 *Exubera* release units.

INSULIN HUMAN — INHALATION

Indications

➤*Diabetes mellitus:* For the treatment of adult patients with diabetes mellitus for the control of hyperglycemia.

Administration and Dosage

➤*Approved by the FDA:* October 28, 1982 (injection)

➤*Type 1 diabetes:* In patients with type 1 diabetes, inhaled insulin should be used in regimens that include a longer-acting insulin.

➤*Type 2 diabetes:* For patients with type 2 diabetes, inhaled insulin may be used as monotherapy or in combination with oral agents (OAs) or longer-acting insulin.

➤*For inhalation use:* Inhaled insulin is intended for administration by inhalation and must only be administered using the inhaled insulin inhaler. Refer to the Medication Guide for a description of the inhaler and for instructions on how to use the inhaler.

➤*Initial dose:* Inhaled insulin doses should be administered immediately prior to meals (no more than 10 minutes prior to each meal). The initial dosage of inhaled insulin should be individualized and determined based on the physician's advice in accordance with the needs of the patient. Recommended initial premeal doses are based on clinical trials in which patients were requested to eat 3 meals per day. Initial premeal doses may be calculated using the following formula: [Body weight (kg) × 0.05 mg/kg = premeal dose (mg)] rounded down to the nearest whole milligram number (eg, 3.7 mg rounded down to 3 mg).

Approximate guidelines for initial, premeal inhaled insulin doses based on patient body weight are indicated in the following table:

Approximate Guidelines for Initial, Premeal Insulin Inhalation Dose				
Weight (kg)	Weight (lb)	Initial dose per meal	Number of 1 mg blisters/dose	Number of 3 mg blisters/dose
30 to 39.9 kg	66 to 87 lb	1 mg	1	—
40 to 59.9 kg	88 to 132 lb	2 mg	2	—
60 to 79.9 kg	133 to 176 lb	3 mg	—	1
80 to 99.9 kg	177 to 220 lb	4 mg	1	1
100 to 119.9 kg	220 to 264 lb	5 mg	2	1
120 to 139.9 kg	265 to 308 lb	6 mg	—	2

As with all insulins, additional factors that should be taken into consideration when determining the inhaled insulin starting dose include, but are not limited to, the patient's current glycemic control, previous response to insulin, duration of diabetes, and dietary and exercise habits.

Insulin equivalent doses – A 1 mg blister of inhaled insulin is approximately equivalent to 3 units of subcutaneously injected regular human insulin. A 3 mg blister of inhaled insulin is approximately equivalent to 8 units of subcutaneously injected regular human insulin. The following table provides the approximate unit dose of regular subcutaneous human insulin for inhaled insulin doses from 1 to 6 mg.

Approximate Equivalent Unit Dose of Regular Human Subcutaneous Insulin for Inhaled Insulin Doses			
Dose	Approximate regular insulin subcutaneous dose	Number of 1 mg inhaled insulin blisters per dose	Number of 3 mg inhaled insulin blisters per dose
1 mg	3 units	1	—
2 mg	6 units	2	—
3 mg	8 units	—	1

Approximate Equivalent Unit Dose of Regular Human Subcutaneous Insulin for Inhaled Insulin Doses			
Dose	Approximate regular insulin subcutaneous dose	Number of 1 mg inhaled insulin blisters per dose	Number of 3 mg inhaled insulin blisters per dose
4 mg	11 units	1	1
5 mg	14 units	2	1
6 mg	16 units	—	2

Patients should combine 1 and 3 mg blisters so that the least number of blisters per dose are taken (eg, a 4 mg dose should be administered as one 1 mg blister and one 3 mg blister). Consecutive inhalation of three 1 mg unit dose blisters results in significantly greater insulin exposure than inhalation of one 3 mg unit dose blister. Therefore, three 1 mg doses should not be substituted for one 3 mg dose. When a patient is stabilized on a dosing regimen that includes 3 mg blisters, and the 3 mg blisters become temporarily unavailable, the patient can temporarily substitute two 1 mg blisters for one 3 mg blister. Blood glucose should be monitored closely.

➤*Dose adjustments:* Adjustment of dosage of any insulin may be necessary if patients change their physical activity or their usual meal plan. Insulin requirements may be altered during intercurrent conditions, such as illness, emotional disturbances, or stress.

After initiating inhaled insulin therapy, as with other glucose-lowering agents, dose adjustment may be required based on the patient's need (eg, blood glucose concentrations, meal size and nutrient composition, time of day, recent or anticipated exercise). Each patient should be titrated to their optimal dosage based on blood glucose monitoring results. Close monitoring of blood glucose concentrations and dose adjustment may be required on an individual basis.

As for all insulins, the time course of inhaled insulin action may vary in different individuals or at different times in the same individual.

➤*Bronchodilators:* Inhaled medicinal products (eg, bronchodilators) should be administered prior to administration of inhaled insulin.

➤*Renal function impairment:* As with other insulin preparations, the dose requirements for inhaled insulin may be reduced in patients with renal impairment.

➤*Hepatic function impairment:* As with other insulin preparations, the dose requirements for inhaled insulin may be reduced in patients with hepatic impairment.

➤*Respiratory illness:* Inhaled insulin may be used during intercurrent respiratory illness (eg, bronchitis, upper respiratory tract infection, rhinitis).

➤*Storage/Stability:*

Blister storage –

Not in-use (unopened): Store at controlled room temperature, 25°C (77°F); excursions permitted to 15° to 30°C (59° to 86°F). Do not freeze or refrigerate.

In-use: Once the foil overwrap is opened, protect unit dose blisters from moisture, and store at 25°C (77°F); excursions permitted to 15° to 30°C (59° to 86°F). Do not freeze or refrigerate. Use unit dose blisters within 3 months after opening the foil overwrap. Return the blisters to the overwrap to protect from moisture. Take additional care to avoid humid environments (eg, steamy bathroom following a shower). Discard blister if frozen.

Inhaler storage – Store at controlled room temperature, 25°C (77°F); excursions permitted to 15° to 30°C (59° to 86°F). Do not freeze or refrigerate. The inhaled insulin inhaler can be used for up to 1 year from the date of first use.

Exubera release unit: Change the *Exubera* release unit in the *Exubera* inhaler every 2 weeks.

INSULIN REGULAR CONCENTRATE

Rx	**Humulin R Regular U-500 (Concentrated)** (Lilly)	**Injection:** 500 units/mL regular human insulin (rDNA)	In 20 mL vials.[a]

[a] With 2.5 mg m-cresol and 16 mg glycerin per mL.

INSULIN REGULAR CONCENTRATE — INJECTION

For complete prescribing information, refer to the Insulin group monograph.

Indications

➤*Insulin resistance:* Treatment of diabetic patients with marked insulin resistance (requirements greater than 200 units/day), because a large dose may be administered subcutaneously in a reasonable volume.

Administration and Dosage

➤*Administration:* Administer subcutaneously. Do not inject IM or IV. It is inadvisable to inject concentrated insulin IV because of possible inadvertent overdosage.

Use a tuberculin-type or insulin syringe for dosage measurement. Dosage variations are frequent in the insulin-resistant patient because the individual is unresponsive to the pharmacologic effect of the insulin. Nevertheless, encourage accuracy of measurement because of the potential danger of the preparations. Inadvertent overdose may result in irreversible insulin shock. Serious consequences may result if not used under constant medical supervision.

Concentrated insulin injection is not modified by any agent that might prolong its action. It frequently has a duration similar to repository insulin; a single dose demonstrates activity for 24 hours. This has been credited to the high concentration of the preparation.

➤*Dosage adjustments:* Closely observe every patient exhibiting insulin resistance who requires concentrated insulin for diabetic control until appropriate dosing is established. Response will vary among patients. Most patients will show a "tolerance" to insulin, so that minor dosage variations will not cause untoward symptoms of insulin shock. Some may require only 1 dose daily; others may require 2 or 3 injections per day.

Insulin resistance is frequently self-limited; after several weeks or months of high dosage, responsiveness may be regained and dosage reduced.

INSULIN REGULAR CONCENTRATE — INJECTION

➤*Hypoglycemic reactions:* Hypoglycemia when using this concentrated insulin can be prolonged and severe. As with other human insulin preparations, hypoglycemic reactions may be associated with the administration of concentrated insulin. However, deep secondary hypoglycemic reactions may develop 18 to 24 hours after the original injection of concentrated insulin. Consequently, carefully observe patients and promptly initiate treatment with glucagon injections or glucose by IV injection or gavage. A few patients who have experienced hypoglycemic reactions after transfer from animal-source insulin to human insulin have reported that the early warning symptoms of hypoglycemia were less pronounced or different from those experienced with their previous insulin. Refer to Insulin group monograph.

➤*Storage/Stability:* Keep in a cold place, preferably in a refrigerator. Do not freeze. Do not use if it is not water-clear. Discoloration, turbidity, or unusual viscosity indicates deterioration or contamination.

Sulfonylureas

Indications

➤*Type 2 diabetes:* As an adjunct to diet and exercise to lower the blood glucose in patients with type 2 (non-insulin-dependent) diabetes mellitus whose hyperglycemia cannot be controlled by diet and exercise alone.

➤*Unlabeled uses:* **Chlorpropamide** in doses of 200 to 500 mg/day has been used in the treatment of diabetes insipidus.

Sulfonylureas have been used as temporary adjuncts to insulin therapy in selected type 2 diabetes patients to improve diabetes control (see Administration and Dosage).

Administration and Dosage

➤*Institution of therapy:* Individualize therapy. Selection of an individual agent is influenced by the drug's potency, duration of action, metabolism, adverse reactions, patient's lack of response to other oral agents, and the patient's personal preference.

Monitor patient's blood glucose periodically to determine the minimum effective dose for the patient; to detect primary failure (ie, inadequate lowering of blood glucose at the maximum recommended dose of medication); and to detect secondary failure (ie, loss of adequate blood glucose response after an initial period of effectiveness). Glycosylated hemoglobin levels are also valuable in monitoring the patient's response to therapy.

➤*Short-term use:* Short-term administration of sulfonylureas may be sufficient during periods of transient loss of control in patients usually well controlled on diet.

➤*Transfer from other hypoglycemic agents:*

Sulfonylureas – When transferring patients from 1 oral hypoglycemic agent to another, no transitional period and no initial or priming dose is necessary. However, when transferring patients from **chlorpropamide**, exercise particular care during the first 2 weeks because the prolonged retention of chlorpropamide in the body and subsequent overlapping drug effects may provoke hypoglycemia. See specific guidelines for each agent in the individual Administration and Dosage sections.

Insulin – During insulin withdrawal period, test urine for glucose and ketones 3 times daily and report results to physician daily. For specific guidelines for each individual sulfonylurea, refer to the Administration and Dosage section for each agent.

General clinical characteristics which favor successful sulfonylureas monotherapy following insulin withdrawal include the following:

- Onset of diabetes at at least 35 years of age
- Obese or normal body weight
- Duration of diabetes less than 10 years
- Absence of ketoacidosis
- Fasting serum glucose 200 mg/dL or less
- Postprandial blood glucose values less than 250 mg/dL
- Insulin requirement less than 40 units/day
- Absence of renal or hepatic dysfunction

➤*Elderly patients:* Elderly patients may be particularly sensitive to these agents; therefore, start with a lower initial dose before breakfast, and check blood and urine glucoseduring the first 24 hours of therapy. If control is satisfactory, continue or gradually increase dose. If there is a tendency toward hypoglycemia, reduce dose or discontinue the drug.

➤*Acute complications:* During the course of intercurrent complications (eg, ketoacidosis, severe trauma, major surgery, infections, severe diarrhea, nausea, vomiting), supportive therapy with insulin may be necessary. Continue or withdraw sulfonylurea therapy while insulin is used. Insulin is indispensable in managing acute complications; carefully instruct all diabetes patients in its use.

➤*Combination insulin therapy:* Concurrent administration of insulin and an oral sulfonylurea (generally **glipizide** or **glyburide**) has been used with some success in type 2 diabetes patients who are difficult to control with diet and sulfonylurea therapy alone. One proposed method is referred to as the BIDS system: Bedtime Insulin (usually NPH) in combination with a Daytime (morning only or morning and evening) Sulfonylurea, usually glyburide.

Actions

➤*Pharmacology:* The sulfonylurea hypoglycemic agents are sulfonamide derivatives but are devoid of antibacterial activity. These agents are divided into 2 groups: First generation (**acetohexamide**, **chlorpropamide**, **tolazamide**, **tolbutamide**) and second generation (**glipizide**, **glyburide**, **glimepiride**). They are used as adjuncts to diet and exercise in the treatment of type 2 diabetes, previously known as non-insulin-dependent diabetes mellitus (NIDDM). Type 2 diabetes has also been referred to as adult-onset or maturity-onset diabetes and ketosis-resistant diabetes.

Type 2 diabetes not only leads to hyperglycemia but affects several organ systems resulting in dyslipidemia, hypertension, central obesity, and accelerated atherosclerosis. This multisystem disorder, also known as the insulin resistance syndrome, contributes to high rates of morbidity and mortality that are usually manifestations of coronary artery and cerebrovascular disease. Other factors influencing premature death in these patients are the duration of diabetes, lack of glycemic control, and other cardiovascular risk factors such as smoking and physical inactivity.

Type 2 diabetes is characterized by insulin resistance, impaired insulin secretion, and overproduction of hepatic glucose. Evidence suggests that insulin resistance is the predominant factor preceding the onset of hyperglycemia. During the transition from impaired glucose tolerance to frank disease, basal hepatic glucose production rates increase, insulin resistance becomes more severe (which may be partly due to acquired conditions such as age, obesity, and an inactive lifestyle), and beta-cell function decreases affecting insulin secretory ability.

By binding to the plasma membrane of functional beta-cells in the pancreatic islets, sulfonylureas cause a decrease in potassium (K+) permeability and membrane depolarization which, in turn, leads to an increase in intracellular calcium ions and subsequent exocytosis of insulin-containing secretory granules. This process is also stimulated by glucose and other insulin-releasing fuels; however, sulfonylureas increase insulin secretion at stimulatory levels lower than that required for glucose suggesting that they enhance beta-cell response rather than change beta-cell sensitivity to glucose. The role of extrapancreatic effects of sulfonylureas in the treatment of hyperglycemia are of questionable clinical significance with the possible exception of glimepiride, which has demonstrated increased sensitivity of peripheral tissues to insulin.

Other pharmacologic activity includes: Potentiation of the effect of antidiuretic hormone (ADH); tolazamide, acetohexamide, glyburide, and glipizide may produce a mild diuresis; acetohexamide has significant uricosuric activity;chlorpropamide can cause flushing (a disulfiram-like reaction) in some patients who consume alcohol.

➤*Pharmacokinetics:* The sulfonylureas are well absorbed after oral administration. All sulfonylureas except **glipizide** can be taken with food; absorption of glipizide is delayed by food. **Tolbutamide**, **glyburide**, and glipizide are more effective when taken approximately 30 minutes before a meal. **Tolazamide** is absorbed more slowly than the other sulfonylureas. They are metabolized in the liver to active and inactive metabolites and excreted primarily in the urine. The hypoglycemic effects of sulfonylureas may be prolonged in severe liver disease caused by decreased metabolism.

Although the mechanisms of action and maximal hypoglycemic effects are similar, the second and first generation sulfonylureas differ. Second generation compounds possess a more nonpolar or lipophilic side chain. Therapeutically effective doses and serum concentrations of the second generation sulfonylureas are lower, due to their higher intrinsic potency. All sulfonylureas are strongly bound to plasma proteins, primarily albumin. Protein binding of the first generation sulfonylureas is ionic; that of the second generation agents is predominantly nonionic. The clinical therapeutic significance of this difference is unknown; however, because they are bound to albumin by ionic bindings, the first generation agents may be more likely to be displaced by drugs that competitively bind to proteins (eg, warfarin). Displacement of sulfonylurea agents from protein would result in greater hypoglycemic response (see Drug Interactions).

Differences exist among the sulfonylureas in the duration of hypoglycemic effects (see following table). Tolbutamide is short-acting because it is rapidly metabolized to an inactive metabolite; it may be useful in patients with kidney disease. The active metabolite of acetohexamide is 2.5 times as potent as the parent compound. Because the metabolite is excreted in the urine, the duration of action of **acetohexamide** is prolonged in renal disease. Tolazamide has 2 active metabolites which are less potent than the parent compound. The renal elimination of chlorpropamide may be sensitive to changes in urinary pH; urinary alkalinization increases its excretion in the urine. When the urine pH is less than 6, urinary excretion decreases and hepatic metabolism is the primary route of elimination. The half-life of **chlorpropamide** is prolonged in renal disease.

Major Pharmacokinetic Parameters of the Sulfonylureas

Sulfonylureas	Approximate equivalent doses (mg)	Doses/ day	Serum t½ (h)	Onset (h)	Duration (h)	Renal excretion (%)	Active metabolites
First generation							
Acetohexamide	500 to 750	1 to 2	≈ 6 to 8 (parent drug + metabolite)	1	12 to 24	100	Yes
Chlorpropamide	250 to 375	1	36	1	24 to 60	100	Yes
Tolazamide	250 to 375	1 to 2	7	4 to 6	12 to 24	100	Yes
Tolbutamide	1,000 to 1,500	2 to 3	4.5 to 6.5	1	6 to 12	100	No
Second generation							
Glipizide	10	1 to 2	2 to 4	1 to 3	10 to 24	80 to 85	No
Glyburide Nonmicronized	5	1 to 2	10	2 to 4	16 to 24	50	Yes[a]
Micronized	3	1 to 2	≈ 4	1	12 to 24	50	Yes[a]

Major Pharmacokinetic Parameters of the Sulfonylureas							
Sulfonylureas	Approximate equivalent doses (mg)	Doses/ day	Serum t½ (h)	Onset (h)	Duration (h)	Renal excretion (%)	Active metab-olites
Glimepiride	NA[b]	1	≈ 9	2 to 3	24	60	Yes

[a] Weakly active.
[b] Not applicable.

Contraindications

Hypersensitivity to sulfonylureas; diabetes complicated by ketoacidosis, with or without coma; sole therapy of type 1 (insulin-dependent) diabetes mellitus; diabetes when complicated by pregnancy.

Warnings

➤*Cardiovascular risk:* The administration of oral hypoglycemic drugs has been associated with increased cardiovascular mortality as compared with treatment with diet alone or diet plus insulin. Despite controversy regarding its interpretation, this warning is based on the study conducted by the University Group Diabetes Program (UGDP). This long-term prospective clinical trial involving 823 patients evaluated the effectiveness of glucose-lowering drugs in preventing or delaying vascular complications in patients with non-insulin-dependent diabetes. (*Diabetes* 1970;19]:747-830.)

Patients treated for 5 to 8 years with diet plus **tolbutamide** (1.5 g/day) had a rate of cardiovascular mortality approximately 2.5 times that of patients treated with diet alone. A significant increase in total mortality was not observed. Consider this for other sulfonylureas as well.

Sulfonylurea binding to ATP-dependent K+ channels has been shown to inhibit the response to ischemia, potentially delaying the recovery of contractile function and increasing infarct size during a MI. However, prevention of channel opening during ischemia could reduce the occurrence of ventricular fibrillation during ischemia. Inform the patient of potential risks, advantages, and alternative modes of therapy.

➤*Bioavailability:* Micronized **glyburide** 3 mg tablets provide serum concentrations that are *not* bioequivalent to those from the conventional formulation (nonmicronized) 5 mg tablets. Therefore, retitrate patients when transferring patients from any hypoglycemic agent to micronized glyburide.

➤*Renal/Hepatic function impairment:* Oral hypoglycemic agents are metabolized in the liver. The drugs and most of their metabolites are excreted by the kidneys. Hepatic impairment may result in inadequate release of glucose in response to hypoglycemia. Renal impairment may cause decreased elimination of sulfonylureas leading to accumulation producing hypoglycemia. Therefore, use these agents with caution in type 2 diabetes patients with renal or hepatic impairment, and monitor renal and liver function frequently.

➤*Elderly:* In elderly, debilitated, or malnourished patients, and patients with impaired renal or hepatic function, the initial and maintenance dosing should be conservative to avoid hypoglycemic reactions.

➤*Pregnancy:* (*Category C. Category B – Glynase, Micronase*). Sulfonylureas (except **glyburide**) are teratogenic in animals. There are no adequate studies in pregnant women. Use only if clearly needed. In general, avoid sulfonylureas in pregnancy; they will not provide good control in patients who cannot be controlled by diet alone.

Because abnormal blood glucose levels during pregnancy may be associated with a higher incidence of congenital abnormalities, insulin is recommended to maintain blood glucose levels as close to normal as possible. However, fetal mortality and major congenital anomalies generally occur 3 to 4 times more often in offspring of diabetic mothers.

Labor and delivery – Prolonged severe hypoglycemia (4 to 10 days) has occurred in neonates born to mothers on a sulfonylurea at the time of delivery. This has been reported more frequently with agents with prolonged half-lives. If used during pregnancy, discontinue at least 2 days to 4 weeks before expected delivery date.

➤*Lactation:* **Chlorpropamide** and **tolbutamide** are excreted in breast milk. A chlorpropamide breast milk concentration of 5 mcg/ml has been detected following a 500 mg dose (normal peak blood level after 250 mg is 30 mcg/ml). It is not known if other sulfonylureas are excreted in breast milk. Because of the potential for hypoglycemia in nursing infants, decide whether to discontinue nursing or the drug.

➤*Children:* Safety and efficacy in children have not been established.

Precautions

➤*Monitoring:* Keep patients under continuous medical supervision. During the initial test period, the patient should communicate with the physician daily, and report at least weekly for the first month for physical examination and evaluation of diabetes control. After the first month, examine at monthly intervals or as indicated. Uncooperative individuals may be unsuitable for treatment with oral agents.

During the transitional period, test the urine for glucose and acetone at least 3 times daily and have the results reviewed by a physician frequently. Measurement of glycosylated hemoglobin (HbA1c) is also recommended. It is important that patients be taught to correctly and frequently self-monitor blood glucose.

Hyperglycemia is a major risk factor in the development of diabetic complications. Maintaining blood glucose levels helps prevent the progression of nephropathy, neuropathy, and retinopathy. Hyperglycemia is also associated with the risk factors of atherosclerosis.

Treatment Goals for Type 2 Diabetes Mellitus		
Patient population	Average preprandial glucose (mg/dl)	HbA1c[a](%)
ADA general recommendations[b]	80-120	< 7
Healthy, relatively young	80-120	< 8
Elderly and patients with serious medical conditions	100-140	< 9

[a] Glycosylated hemoglobin.
[b] American Diabetes Association 1999 Clinical Practice Recommendations.

➤*Diet and exercise:* Diet and exercise remain the primary considerations of diabetic patient management. Caloric restriction and weight loss are essential in the obese diabetic patient. These drugs are an adjunct to, not a substitute for, dietary regulation. Also, loss of blood glucose control on diet alone may be transient, thus requiring only short-term sulfonylurea therapy. Identify cardiovascular risk factors and take corrective measures where possible.

➤*Hypoglycemia:* All sulfonylureas may produce severe hypoglycemia. Proper patient selection, dosage, and instructions are important to avoid hypoglycemic episodes. Renal or hepatic insufficiency may elevate drug blood levels, and the latter may also diminish gluconeogenic capacity, both of which increase the risk of serious hypoglycemic reactions. Elderly, debilitated, or malnourished patients, and those with adrenal or pituitary insufficiency are particularly susceptible to the hypoglycemic action of glucose-lowering drugs. Hypoglycemia may be difficult to recognize in the elderly and in patients taking β-adrenergic blocking drugs. Hypoglycemia is more likely to occur when caloric intake is deficient, after severe or prolonged exercise, when alcohol is ingested, or when more than 1 glucose-lowering drug is used.

Because of the long half-life of **chlorpropamide**, patients who become hypoglycemic during therapy require careful supervision of the dose and frequent feedings for at least 3 to 5 days. Hospitalization and IV glucose may be necessary.

➤*Asymptomatic patients:* Controlling blood glucose in type 2 diabetes with sulfonylureas has not been definitely established to be effective in preventing the long-term cardiovascular or neural complications of diabetes.

➤*Loss of blood glucose control:* When a patient stabilized on any diabetic regimen is exposed to stress such as fever, trauma, infection, or surgery, a loss of control may occur. At such times, it may be necessary to discontinue the drug and give insulin.

The effectiveness of any oral hypoglycemic in lowering blood glucose to a desired level decreases in many patients over time (secondary failure); this may be due to progression of the severity of the diabetes or to diminished drug responsiveness. Adequately adjust dose and assess adherence to diet before classifying a patient as a secondary failure. Primary failure occurs when the drug is ineffective in a patient when first given. Certain patients who demonstrate an inadequate response or true primary or secondary failure to 1 sulfonylurea may benefit from a transfer to another sulfonylurea.

➤*Disulfiram-like syndrome:* A sulfonylurea-induced facial flushing reaction may occur when some sulfonylureas are administered with alcohol. This syndrome is characterized by facial flushing and occasional breathlessness but without the nausea, vomiting, and hypotension seen with a true alcohol-disulfiram reaction. The facial flushing reaction occurs in approximately 33% of type 2 diabetes patients taking **chlorpropamide** and alcohol. It is uncertain whether **glyburide** and **glipizide** can cause the facial flushing reaction.

➤*Syndrome of inappropriate secretion of antidiuretic hormone (SIADH):* Water retention and dilutional hyponatremia have occurred after administration of sulfonylureas to type 2 diabetes patients, especially those with CHF or hepatic cirrhosis. The drugs stimulate antidiuretic hormone (ADH) release, augmenting hypothalamic-pituitary release of ADH. The result is excessive water retention, hyponatremia, low serum osmolality, and high urine osmolality.

Glipizide, **acetohexamide**, **tolazamide**, and **glyburide** are mildly diuretic.

Drug Interactions

Sulfonylurea Drug Interactions

Precipitant drug	Object drug[a]		Description
Androgens Anticoagulants Azole antifungals Chloramphenicol Clofibrate Fenfluramine Fluconazole Gemfibrozil Histamine H_2 antagonists Magnesium salts Methyldopa MAO inhibitors Probenecid Salicylates Sulfinpyrazone Sulfonamides Tricyclic antidepressants Urinary acidifiers	Sulfonylureas	⬆	The hypoglycemic effect of sulfonylureas may be enhanced because of various mechanisms (eg, decreased hepatic metabolism, inhibition of renal excretion, displacement from protein-binding sites, decreased blood glucose, alteration of carbohydrate metabolism). Monitor blood glucose carefully upon initiation, cessation, or changes in therapy with any of these agents.
Beta blockers Calcium channel blockers Cholestyramine Corticosteroids Diazoxide Estrogens Hydantoins Isoniazid Nicotinic acid Oral contraceptives Phenothiazines Rifampin Sympathomimetics Thiazide diuretics Thyroid agents Urinary alkalinizers	Sulfonylureas	⬇	The hypoglycemic effect of sulfonylureas may be decreased because of various mechanisms (eg, increased hepatic metabolism, decreased insulin release, increased renal excretion).
Charcoal	Sulfonylureas	⬇	Charcoal can reduce the absorption of sulfonylureas; depending on the clinical situation, this will reduce their efficacy or toxicity.
Ciprofloxacin	Glyburide	⬆	A possible interaction between glyburide and ciprofloxacin has been reported, resulting in a potentiation of the hypoglycemic action.
Ethanol	Sulfonylureas	⬌	Ethanol may prolong but not augment glipizide-induced reductions in blood glucose. Chronic ethanol use may decrease the half-life of tolbutamide. Ethanol ingestion by patients taking chlorpropamide may result in a disulfiram-like reaction (see Precautions).
Chlorpropamide	Barbiturates	⬆	Animal studies suggest that the action of barbiturates may be prolonged by therapy with chlorpropamide; coadminister with caution.
Glyburide	Anticoagulants	⬆ ⬇	Possible interactions between glyburide and coumarin derivatives have been reported that may either potentiate or weaken the effects of coumarin derivatives.
Sulfonylureas	Digitalis glycosides	⬆	Concurrent administration may result in increased digitalis serum levels.

[a] ⬆ = Object drug increased. ⬇ = Object drug decreased.
⬌ = Undetermined clinical effect.

➤*Drug/Lab test interactions:* A metabolite of **tolbutamide** in the urine may give a false-positive reaction for albumin if measured by the acidification-after-boiling test, which causes the metabolite to precipitate. There is no interference with the sulfosalicylic acid test.

➤*Drug/Food interactions:* Absorption of **glipizide** is delayed by approximately 40 minutes when taken with food; the drug is more effective when given approximately 30 minutes before a meal. The other sulfonylureas may be taken with food.

Adverse Reactions

Hypoglycemia – See Precautions.

➤*CNS:* Drowsiness; asthenia; nervousness; tremor; pain; insomnia; anxiety; depression; hypesthesia; chills; hypertonia; confusion; somnolence; abnormal gait; decreased libido; migraine; anorexia; arthralgia; myalgia; fatigue; weakness; paresthesia; dizziness; vertigo; malaise; headache (infrequent).

➤*Dermatologic:* Allergic skin reactions; eczema; pruritus; erythema multiforme; urticaria; morbilliform or maculopapular eruptions; lichenoid reactions; rash; sweating; exfoliative dermatitis. These may be transient and may disappear despite continued use of the drug; if skin reactions persist, discontinue the drug. Porphyria cutanea tarda; photosensitivity reactions.

➤*Endocrine:* Reactions identical to the syndrome of inappropriate secretion of antidiuretic hormone (SIADH). (See Precautions.)

➤*GI:* GI disturbances (eg, nausea, epigastric fullness, heartburn) are the most common reactions. They tend to be dose-related and may disappear when dosage is reduced. Diarrhea; taste alteration (tolbutamide); GI pain; constipation; gastralgia; dyspepsia; vomiting; hunger; proctocolitis; flatulence; cholestatic jaundice (rare, discontinue the drug if this occurs).

➤*Hematologic:* Leukopenia; thrombocytopenia (which may present as purpura); aplastic anemia; agranulocytosis; hemolytic anemia; pancytopenia; hepatic porphyria; eosinophilia.

➤*Miscellaneous:* Disulfiram-like reactions (see Precautions); tinnitus; fatigue; rhinitis; hepatic porphyria; hyponatremia; blurred vision; polyuria; trace blood in stool; thirst; edema; arrhythmia; flushing; hypertension; pharyngitis; eye pain; conjunctivitis; retinal hemorrhage; dysuria; hepatitis; dyspnea; leg cramps; syncope; vasculitis.

➤*Lab test abnormalities:* Elevated liver function tests; occasional mild-to-moderate elevations in BUN, creatinine, AST, LDH, alkaline phosphatase.

Overdosage

➤*Symptoms:* Overdosage can produce hypoglycemia. In order of general appearance, the signs and symptoms associated with hypoglycemia include: Tingling of lips and tongue; nausea; vomiting; mild epigastric pain diminished cerebral function (lethargy, yawning, confusion, agitation, nervousness); increased sympathetic activity (tachycardia, sweating, tremor, hunger) and ultimately, convulsions, stupor, coma, and death.

➤*Treatment:* Treat mild hypoglycemia without loss of consciousness or neurologic findings aggressively with oral glucose and adjustments in drug dosage or meal patterns. Continue close monitoring until the patient is stabilized. Severe hypoglycemic reactions occur infrequently, but require immediate hospitalization. If hypoglycemic coma is suspected, rapidly inject concentrated (50%) dextrose IV. Follow by a continuous infusion of more dilute (10%) dextrose at a rate that will maintain the blood glucose at a level more than 100 mg/dl. Closely monitor for a minimum of 24 to 48 hours because hypoglycemia may recur after apparent clinical recovery. Because of the long half-life of **chlorpropamide**, patients who become hypoglycemic from this drug require close supervision for a minimum of 3 to 5 days.

In 1 patient with renal failure on hemodialysis, charcoal hemoperfusion shortened the half-life of chlorpropamide following an overdose. Charcoal administration also reduces the absorption of the sulfonylureas and may reduce their toxicity.

Patient Information

Patients must receive full and complete instructions about the nature of diabetes. Strict adherence to prescribed diet, an exercise program, personal hygiene, and avoidance of infection are essential. It is important to teach patients to self-monitor blood glucose.

Do not discontinue medication except on the advice of a physician.

May cause GI upset; may be taken with food. Take **glipizide** approximately 30 minutes before a meal to increase effectiveness.

Advise patients to avoid alcohol; lack of blood sugar control may occur. Flushing has been reported with **chlorpropamide**.

Monitor urine for glucose and ketones as prescribed; monitor blood glucose as prescribed.

➤*Notify physician:* Notify physician if any of the following occurs:

Hypoglycemia – Fatigue, excessive hunger, profuse sweating, numbness of extremities.

Hyperglycemia – Excessive thirst or urination, urinary glucose, or ketones.

Other – Fever, sore throat, rash, unusual bruising or bleeding.

CHLORPROPAMIDE

Rx	**Chlorpropramide** (Various, eg, Sidmak, UDL)	**Tablets**: 100 mg	In 100s, 500s, 1,000s, and UD 100s and 600s.
Rx	**Diabinese** (Pfizer)		(393). Blue, scored. D-shaped. In 100s, 500s, and UD 100s.
Rx	**Chlorpropamide** (Various, eg, Major, Goldline, Sidmak, UDL)	**Tablets**: 250 mg	In 100s, 250s, 500s, 1,000s, and UD 100s and UD 600s.
Rx	**Diabinese** (Pfizer)		(394). Blue, scored. D-shaped. In 100s, 250s, 1,000s, and UD 100s.

CHLORPROPAMIDE — ORAL

For complete prescribing information, refer to the Sulfonylureas group monograph.

Indications

➤*Type 2 diabetes:* As an adjunct to diet to lower the blood glucose in patients with type 2 diabetes mellitus whose hyperglycemia cannot be controlled by diet alone.

Administration and Dosage

➤*Initial therapy:* The mild to moderately severe, middle-aged, stable, type 2 diabetic patient should be started on 250 mg daily. In elderly patients, debilitated or malnourished patients, and patients with impaired renal or hepatic function, the initial and maintenance dosing should be conservative to avoid hypoglycemic reactions. Older patients should be started on smaller amounts of chlorpropamide, in the range of 100 to 125 mg daily.

Short-term administration of chlorpropamide may be sufficient during periods of transient loss of control in patients usually controlled well on diet.

The total daily dosage is generally taken at a single time each morning with breakfast. Occasionally cases of gastrointestinal intolerance may be relieved by dividing the daily dosage. A loading or priming dose is not necessary and should not be used.

No transition period is necessary when transferring patients from other oral hypoglycemic agents to chlorpropamide. The other agent may be discontinued abruptly and chlorpropamide started at once. In prescribing chlorpropamide, due consideration must be given to its greater potency.

Many mild to moderately severe, middle-aged, stable, type 2 diabetic patients receiving insulin can be placed directly on the oral drug and their insulin abruptly discontinued. For patients requiring more than 40 units of insulin daily, therapy with chlorpropamide may be initiated with a 50% reduction in insulin for the first few days, with subsequent further reductions dependent upon the response.

➤*Transfer from insulin:* During the initial period of therapy with chlorpropamide, hypoglycemic reactions may occasionally occur, particularly during the transition from insulin to the oral drug. Hypoglycemia within 24 hours after withdrawal of the intermediate or long-acting types of insulin will usually prove to be the result of insulin carryover and not primarily due to the effect of chlorpropamide.

During the insulin withdrawal period, the patient should test his urine for sugar and ketone bodies at least 3 times daily and report the results frequently to his physician. If they are abnormal, the physician should be notified immediately. In some cases, it may be advisable to consider hospitalization during the transition period.

General clinical characteristics which favor successful sulfonylureas monotherapy following insulin withdrawal include onset of diabetes at greater than or equal to 35 years of age, obese or normal body weight, duration of diabetes less than 10 years, absence of ketoacidosis, fasting serum glucose less than or equal to 200 mg/dL, postprandial blood glucose values less than 250 mg/dL, insulin requirement less than 40 units/day, absence of renal or hepatic dysfunction.

➤*Dosage adjustment:* Five to 7 days after the initial therapy, the blood level of chlorpropamide reaches a plateau. Dosage may subsequently be adjusted upward or downward by increments of not more than 50 to 125 mg at intervals of 3 to 5 days to obtain optimal control. More frequent adjustments are usually undesirable.

➤*Maintenance therapy:* Most moderately severe, middle-aged, stable, type 2 diabetic patients are controlled by approximately 250 mg daily. Many investigators have found that some milder diabetics do well on daily doses of 100 mg or less. Many of the more severe diabetics may require 500 mg daily for adequate control. Patients who do not respond completely to 500 mg daily will usually not respond to higher doses. Maintenance doses above 750 mg daily should be avoided.

➤*Storage/Stability:* Store below 30°C (86°F).

TOLAZAMIDE

Rx	**Tolazamide** (Various, eg, Zenith Goldline)	**Tablets**: 100 mg	In 100s and 250s.
Rx	**Tolazamide** (Various, eg, Mylan, Zenith Goldline)	**Tablets**: 250 mg	In 100s, 200s, 500s, and 1,000s.
		500 mg	In 100s, 250s, and 500s.

TOLAZAMIDE — ORAL

For complete prescribing information, refer to the Sulfonylureas group monograph.

Indications

➤*Type 2 diabetes:* As an adjunct to diet to lower the blood glucose in patients with type 2 (non-insulin dependent diabetes mellitus) whose hyperglycemia cannot be satisfactorily controlled by diet alone.

In initiating treatment for type 2 diabetes, diet should be emphasized as the primary form of treatment. Caloric restriction and weight loss are essential in the obese diabetic patient. Proper dietary management alone may be effective in controlling the blood glucose and symptoms of hyperglycemia. The importance of regular physical activity should also be stressed and cardiovascular risk factors should be identified and corrective measures taken where possible.

If this treatment program fails to reduce symptoms and/or blood glucose, the use of an oral sulfonylurea or insulin should be considered. Use of tolazamide must be viewed by both the physician and patient as a treatment in addition to diet and not as a substitute for diet or as a convenient mechanism for avoiding dietary restraint. Furthermore, loss of blood glucose control on diet alone may be transient thus requiring only short-term administration of tolazamide.

During maintenance programs, tolazamide should be discontinued if satisfactory lowering of blood glucose is no longer achieved. Judgments should be based on regular clinical and laboratory evaluations.

In considering the use of tolazamide in asymptomatic patients, it should be recognized that controlling the blood glucose in type 2 diabetes has not been definitely established to be effective in preventing the long-term cardiovascular or neural complications of diabetes.

Administration and Dosage

➤*Approved by the FDA:* November 2, 1984.

➤*Usual starting dose:* The usual starting dose of tolazamide tablets for the mild to moderately severe type 2 diabetic patient is 100 to 250 mg daily administered with breakfast or the first main meal. Generally, if the fasting blood glucose is less than 200 mg/dL, the starting dose is 100 mg/day as a single daily dose. If the fasting blood glucose value is greater than 200 mg/dL, the starting dose is 250 mg/day as a single dose. If the patient is malnourished, underweight, elderly, or not eating properly, the initial therapy should be 100 mg once a day. Failure to follow an appropriate dosage regimen may precipitate hypoglycemia. Patients who do not adhere to their prescribed dietary regimen are more prone to exhibit unsatisfactory response to drug therapy.

Short-term administration of tolazamide may be sufficient during periods of transient loss of control in patients usually controlled well on diet.

➤*Transfer from other hypoglycemic therapy:*

Patients receiving other oral antidiabetic therapy – Transfer of patients from other oral antidiabetes regimens to tolazamide should be done conservatively. When transferring patients from oral hypoglycemic agents other than chlorpropamide to tolazamide, no transition period or initial or priming dose is necessary. When transferring from chlorpropamide, particular care should be exercised to avoid hypoglycemia.

Tolbutamide: If receiving less than 1 g/day, begin at tolazamide 100 mg/day. If receiving 1 g or more daily, initiate at tolazamide 250 mg/day as a single dose.

Chlorpropamide: 250 mg of chlorpropamide may be considered to provide approximately the same degree of blood glucose control as 250 mg of tolazamide. The patient should be observed carefully for hypoglycemia during the transition period from chlorpropamide to tolazamide (1 to 2 weeks) due to the prolonged retention of chlorpropamide in the body and the possibility of a subsequent overlapping drug effect.

Acetohexamide: 100 mg of tolazamide may be considered to provide approximately the same degree of blood glucose control as 250 mg of acetohexamide.

Patients receiving insulin – Some type 2 diabetic patients who have been treated only with insulin may respond satisfactorily to therapy with tolazamide. If the patient's previous insulin dosage has been less than 20 units, substitution of 100 mg of tolazamide per day as a single daily dose may be tried. If the previous insulin dosage was less than 40 units, but more than 20 units, the patient should be placed directly on 250 mg of tolazamide per day as a single dose. If the previous insulin dosage was greater than 40 units, the insulin dosage should be decreased by 50% and 250 mg of tolazamide per day started. The dosage of tolazamide should be adjusted weekly (or more often in the group previously requiring more than 40 units of insulin). During this conversion period when both insulin and tolazamide are being used, hypoglycemia may rarely occur. During insulin withdrawal, patients should test their urine for glucose and acetone at least 3 times daily and report results to their physician. The appearance of persistent acetonuria with glycosuria indicates that the patient is a type 1 diabetic patient who requires insulin therapy.

➤*Maximum dose:* Daily doses of greater than 1,000 mg are not recommended. Patients will generally have no further response to doses larger than this.

TOLAZAMIDE — ORAL

➤*Usual maintenance dose:* The usual maintenance dose is in the range of 100 to 1,000 mg/day with the average maintenance dose being 250 to 500 mg/day. Following initiation of therapy, dosage adjustment is made in increments of 100 mg to 250 mg at weekly intervals based on the patient's blood glucose response.

➤*Dosage interval:* Once a day therapy is usually satisfactory. Doses up to 500 mg/day should be given as a single dose in the morning. 500 mg once daily is as effective as 250 mg twice daily. When a dose of more than 500 mg/day is required, the dose may be divided and given twice daily.

➤*Special risk patients:* In elderly patients, debilitated or malnourished patients, and patients with impaired renal or hepatic function, the initial and maintenance dosing should be conservative to avoid hypoglycemic reactions. Renal or hepatic insufficiency may cause elevated blood levels of tolazamide and the latter may also diminish gluconeogenic capacity, both of which increase the risk of serious hypoglycemic reactions. Elderly, debilitated, or malnourished patients and those with adrenal or pituitary insufficiency are particularly susceptible to the hypoglycemic action of glucose-lowering drugs. Hypoglycemia may be difficult to recognize in the elderly and in people who are taking beta-adrenergic blocking drugs. Hypoglycemia is more likely to occur when caloric intake is deficient, after severe or prolonged exercise, when alcohol is ingested, or when more than one glucose-lowering drug is used.

➤*Storage/Stability:* Store at controlled room temperature 20° to 25°C (68° to 77°F) [see USP].

TOLBUTAMIDE

Rx	**Tolbutamide** (Various, eg, Zenith Goldline, Mylan, UDL)	**Tablets:** 500 mg	In 100s and 500s.
Rx	**Orinase** (Upjohn)		Lactose. (ORINASE 500). White, scored. In 200s and unit-of-use 100s.

TOLBUTAMIDE — ORAL

For complete prescribing information, refer to the Sulfonylureas group monograph.

Indications

➤*Type 2 diabetes:* As an adjunct to diet to lower the blood glucose in patients with type 2 diabetes whose hyperglycemia cannot be satisfactorily controlled by diet alone. In initiating treatment for type 2 diabetes, diet should be emphasized as the primary form of treatment. Caloric restriction and weight loss are essential in the obese diabetic patient. Proper dietary management alone may be effective in controlling the blood glucose and symptoms of hyperglycemia. The importance of regular physical activity should also be stressed and cardiovascular risk factors should be identified and corrective measures taken where possible.

Administration and Dosage

➤*Usual starting dose:* The usual starting dose is 1 to 2 g daily. This may be increased or decreased depending on individual patient response. Failure to follow an appropriate dosage regimen may precipitate hypoglycemia. Patients who do not adhere to their prescribed dietary regimens are more prone to exhibit unsatisfactory response to drug therapy.

Short-term administration of tolbutamide may be sufficient during periods of transient loss of control in patients usually controlled well on diet.

➤*Transfer from other hypoglycemic therapy patients receiving other oral antidiabetic therapy:* Transfer of patients from other oral antidiabetes regimens to tolbutamide should be done conservatively. When transferring patients from oral hypoglycemic agents other than chlorpropamide to tolbutamide, no transition period and no initial or priming doses are necessary. When transferring patients from chlorpropamide, however, particular care should be exercised during the first 2 weeks because of the prolonged retention of chlorpropamide in the body and the possibility that subsequent overlapping drug effects might provoke hypoglycemia.

➤*Patients receiving insulin:* Patients requiring 20 units or less of insulin daily may be placed directly on tolbutamide and insulin abruptly discontinued. Patients whose insulin requirement is between 20 and 40 units daily may be started on therapy with tolbutamide with a concurrent 30% to 50% reduction in insulin dose, with further daily reduction of the insulin when response to tolbutamide is observed. In patients requiring more than 40 units of insulin daily, therapy with tolbutamide may be initiated in conjunction with a 20% reduction in insulin dose the first day, with further careful reduction of insulin as response is observed. Occasionally, conversion to tolbutamide in the hospital may be advisable in candidates who require more than 40 units of insulin daily. During this conversion period when both insulin and tolbutamide are being used, hypoglycemia may rarely occur. During insulin withdrawal, patients should test their urine for glucose and acetone at least 3 times daily and report results to their physician. The appearance of persistent acetonuria with glycosuria indicates that the patient is a type 1 diabetic patient who requires insulin therapy.

➤*Maximum dose:* Daily doses of more 3 g are not recommended.

➤*Usual maintenance dose:* The maintenance dose is in the range of 0.25 to 3 g daily. Maintenance doses above 2 g are seldom required.

➤*Dosage interval:* The total daily dose may be taken either in the morning or in divided doses through the day. While either schedule is usually effective, the divided dose system is preferred by some clinicians from the standpoint of digestive tolerance.

➤*Special patient populations:* In elderly, debilitated or malnourished patients, and patients with impaired renal or hepatic function the initial and maintenance dosing should be conservative to avoid hypoglycemic reactions.

➤*Storage/Stability:* Store at controlled room temperature 15° to 30°C (59° to 86°F).

GLIPIZIDE

Rx	**Glipizide** (Various, eg, Endo, Mylan, UDL, Watson, Zenith Goldline)	**Tablets:** 5 mg	In 100s, 500s, 1,000s, and UD 100s.
Rx	**Glucotrol** (Pfizer)		Lactose. (Pfizer 411). Dye free. White, scored. Diamond shape. In 100s, 500s, and UD 100s.
Rx	**Glipizide** (Various, eg, Endo, Mylan, UDL, Watson, Zenith Goldline)	**Tablets:** 10 mg	In 100s, 500s, 1,000s, and UD 100s.
Rx	**Glucotrol** (Pfizer)		Lactose. (Pfizer 412). Dye free. White, scored. Diamond shape. In 100s, 500s, and UD 100s.
Rx	**Glipizide Extended-Release** (Andrx)	**Tablets, extended release:** 2.5 mg	(871). Blue. In 30s.
Rx	**Glucotrol XL** (Pfizer)		(Glucotrol XL 2.5). Blue, biconvex. In 30s.
Rx	**Glipizide Extended-Release** (Various, eg, Andrx, Watson)	5 mg	In 100s and 500s.
Rx	**Glucotrol XL** (Pfizer)		(Glucotrol XL 5). White, biconvex. In 100s and 500s.
Rx	**Glipizide Extended-Release** (Various, eg, Andrx, Watson)	10 mg	In 100s and 500s.
Rx	**Glucotrol XL** (Pfizer)		(GLUCOTROL XL 10). White, biconvex. In 100s and 500s.

GLIPIZIDE — ORAL

For complete prescribing information, refer to the Sulfonylureas group monograph.

Indications

➤*Type 2 diabetes:* As an adjunct to diet for the control of hyperglycemia and its associated symptomatology in patients with type 2 diabetes formerly known as non-insulin-dependent diabetes mellitus (NIDDM) or maturity-onset diabetes, after an adequate trial of dietary therapy has proved unsatisfactory. Glipizide is indicated when diet alone has been unsuccessful in correcting hyperglycemia, but even after the introduction of the drug in the patient's regimen, dietary measures should continue to be considered as important. In 12-week, well-controlled studies, there was a maximal average net reduction in hemoglobin A_{1C} of 1.7% in absolute units between placebo-treated and glipizide-treated patients.

Administration and Dosage

➤*Approved by the FDA:* May 8, 1984.

➤*Extended-release tablets:* There is no fixed dosage regimen for the management of diabetes mellitus with glipizide extended-release tablets or any other hypoglycemic agent. Glycemic control should be monitored with hemoglobin A_{1C} or blood glucose levels to determine the minimum effective dose

GLIPIZIDE — ORAL

for the patient; to detect primary failure (ie, inadequate lowering of blood glucose at the maximum recommended dose of medication); and to detect secondary failure (ie, loss of an adequate blood-glucose-lowering response after an initial period of effectiveness). Home blood glucose monitoring may also provide useful information to the patient and physician. Short-term administration of glipizide extended-release tablets may be sufficient during periods of transient loss of control in patients usually controlled on diet.

In general, glipizide extended-release tablets should be given with breakfast.

Initial dose – The recommended starting dose is 5 mg/day, given with breakfast. The recommended dose for geriatric patients is also 5 mg/day.

Dosage adjustment should be based on laboratory measures of glycemic control. While fasting blood glucose levels generally reach steady state following initiation or change in glipizide dosage, a single fasting glucose determination may not accurately reflect the response to therapy. In most cases, hemoglobin A_{1C} level, measured at 3-month intervals, is the preferred means of monitoring response to therapy.

Hemoglobin A_{1C} should be measured as glipizide therapy is initiated at the 5 mg dose, and repeated approximately 3 months later. If the result of this test suggests that glycemic control over the preceding 3 months was inadequate, the glipizide dose may be increased. Subsequent dosage adjustments should be made on the basis of hemoglobin A_{1C} levels measured at 3-month intervals. If no improvement is seen after 3 months of therapy with a higher dose, the previous dose should be resumed. Decisions which utilize fasting blood glucose to adjust glipizide therapy should be based on at least 2 or more similar, consecutive values obtained 7 days or more after the previous dose adjustment.

Most patients will be controlled with 5 to 10 mg taken once daily. However, some patients may require up to the maximum recommended daily dose of 20 mg. While the glycemic control of selected patients may improve with doses which exceed 10 mg, clinical studies conducted to date have not demonstrated an additional group average reduction of hemoglobin A_{1C} beyond what was achieved with the 10 mg dose.

Based on the results of a randomized crossover study, patients receiving immediate-release glipizide may be switched safely to glipizide extended-release tablets once-a-day at the nearest equivalent total daily dose. Patients receiving immediate-release glipizide also may be titrated to the appropriate dose of glipizide extended-release starting with 5 mg once daily. The decision to switch to the nearest equivalent dose or to titrate should be based on clinical judgment.

Special patient populations: In elderly patients, debilitated or malnourished patients, and patients with impaired renal or hepatic function, the initial and maintenance dosing should be conservative to avoid hypoglycemic reactions. All sulfonylurea drugs are capable of producing severe hypoglycemia. Proper patient selection, dosage, and instructions are important to avoid hypoglycemic episodes. Renal or hepatic insufficiency may affect the disposition of glipizide and the latter may also diminish gluconeogenic capacity, both of which increase the risk of serious hypoglycemic reactions. Elderly, debilitated or malnourished patients, and those with adrenal or pituitary insufficiency are particularly susceptible to the hypoglycemic action of glucose-lowering drugs. Hypoglycemia may be difficult to recognize in the elderly, and in people who are taking beta-adrenergic-blocking drugs. Hypoglycemia is more likely to occur when caloric intake is deficient, after severe or prolonged exercise, when alcohol is ingested, or when more than 1 glucose-lowering drug is used. Therapy with a combination of glucose-lowering agents may increase the potential for hypoglycemia.

When glipizide is used in combination with other oral blood glucose-lowering agents, the second agent should be added at the lowest recommended dose, and patients should be observed carefully. Titration of the added oral agent should be based on clinical judgment.

➤*Immediate-release tablets:* There is no fixed dosage regimen for the management of diabetes mellitus with glipizide or any other hypoglycemic agent. In addition to the usual monitoring of urinary glucose, the patient's blood glucose must also be monitored periodically to determine the minimum effective dose for the patient; to detect primary failure (ie, inadequate lowering of blood glucose at the maximum recommended dose of medication); and to detect secondary failure (ie, loss of an adequate blood glucose-lowering response after an initial period of effectiveness). Glycosylated hemoglobin levels may also be of value in monitoring the patient's response to therapy.

Short-term administration of glipizide may be sufficient during periods of transient loss of control in patients usually controlled well on diet.

In general, glipizide should be given approximately 30 minutes before a meal to achieve the greatest reduction in postprandial hyperglycemia.

Initial dose – The recommended starting dose is 5 mg, given before breakfast. Elderly patients or those with liver disease may be started on 2.5 mg.

Titration – Dosage adjustments should ordinarily be in increments of 2.5 to 5 mg, as determined by blood glucose response. At least several days should elapse between titration steps. If response to a single dose is not satisfactory, dividing that dose may prove effective. The maximum recommended, once-daily dose is 15 mg. Doses above 15 mg should ordinarily be divided and given before meals of adequate caloric content. The maximum recommended total daily dose is 40 mg.

Maintenance – Some patients may be effectively controlled on a once-a-day regimen, while others show better response with divided dosing. Total daily doses above 15 mg should ordinarily be divided. Total daily doses greater than 30 mg have been safely given on a twice-daily basis to long-term patients.

Special patient populations: In elderly patients, debilitated or malnourished patients, and patients with impaired renal or hepatic function, the initial and maintenance dosing should be conservative to avoid hypoglycemic reactions (see Recommended dosing, above).

Combination therapy – When adding other blood glucose-lowering agents to glipizide extended-release tablets for combination therapy, the agent should be initiated at the lowest recommended dose, and patients should be observed carefully for hypoglycemia. Refer to the product information supplied with the oral agent for additional information.

When adding glipizide extended-release tablets to other blood glucose-lowering agents, glipizide can be initiated at 5 mg. Those patients who may be more sensitive to hypoglycemic drugs may be started at a lower dose. Titration should be based on clinical judgment.

➤*Patients receiving insulin:* As with other sulfonylurea-class hypoglycemics, many patients with stable type 2 diabetes receiving insulin may be transferred safely to treatment with glipizide extended- or immediate-release tablets. When transferring patients from insulin to glipizide, the following general guidelines should be considered:

For patients whose daily insulin requirement is less than or equal to 20 units, insulin may be discontinued and glipizide therapy may begin at usual dosages. Several days should elapse between titration steps.

For patients whose daily insulin requirement is greater than 20 units, the insulin dose should be reduced by 50%, and glipizide therapy may begin at usual dosages. Subsequent reductions in insulin dosage should depend on individual patient response. Several days should elapse between titration steps.

During the insulin withdrawal period, the patient should test urine samples for sugar and ketone bodies at least 3 times daily. Patients should be instructed to contact the prescriber immediately if these tests are abnormal. In some cases, especially when the patient has been receiving greater than 40 units of insulin daily, it may be advisable to consider hospitalization during the transition period.

➤*Patients receiving other oral hypoglycemic agents:* As with other sulfonylurea-class hypoglycemics, no transition period is necessary when transferring patients to glipizide extended- or immediate-release tablets. Patients should be observed carefully (1 to 2 weeks) for hypoglycemia when being transferred from longer half-life sulfonylureas (eg, chlorpropamide) to glipizide due to potential overlapping of drug effect.

➤*Storage/Stability:*

Extended-release tablets – The tablets should be protected from moisture and humidity and stored at controlled room temperature, 15° to 30°C (59° to 86°F).

Tablets – Store below 30°C (86°F).

GLIMEPIRIDE

Rx	**Glimepiride** (Various, eg, Dr. Reddy's, Par, Perrigo, Teva)	**Tablets:** 1 mg	May contain lactose. In 30s, 100s, 500s, and 1,000s.
Rx	**Amaryl** (Hoechst-Roussel)		Lactose. (AMA RYL). Pink, flat-faced, double bisect. Oblong. In 100s.
Rx	**Glimepiride** (Various, eg, Dr. Reddy's, Par, Perrigo, Teva)	**Tablets:** 2 mg	May contain lactose. In 30s, 100s, 500s, 1,000s, and UD 100s.
Rx	**Amaryl** (Hoechst-Roussel)		Lactose. (AMA RYL). Green, flat-faced, double bisect. Oblong. In 100s.
Rx	**Glimepiride** (Various, eg, Dr. Reddy's, Par, Perrigo, Teva)	**Tablets:** 4 mg	May contain lactose. In 30s, 100s, 250s, 500s, 1,000s, and UD 100s.
Rx	**Amaryl** (Hoechst-Roussel)		Lactose. (AMA RYL). Blue, flat-faced, double bisect. Oblong. In 100s and UD 100s.

GLIMEPIRIDE — ORAL

For complete prescribing information, refer to the Sulfonylureas group monograph.

Indications

Glimepiride is indicated as an adjunct to diet and exercise to lower the blood glucose in patients with non-insulin-dependent (type 2) diabetes mellitus whose hyperglycemia cannot be controlled by diet and exercise alone. Glimepiride may be used concomitantly with metformin when diet, exercise, and glimepiride or metformin alone do not result in adequate glycemic control.

Glimepiride is also indicated for use in combination with insulin to lower blood glucose in patients whose hyperglycemia cannot be controlled by diet

GLIMEPIRIDE — ORAL

and exercise in conjunction with an oral hypoglycemic agent. Combined use of glimepiride and insulin may increase the potential for hypoglycemia.

In initiating treatment for type 2 diabetes, diet and exercise should be emphasized as the primary form of treatment. Caloric restriction, weight loss, and exercise are essential in the obese diabetic patient. Proper dietary management and exercise alone may be effective in controlling the blood glucose and symptoms of hyperglycemia. In addition to regular physical activity, cardiovascular risk factors should be identified and corrective measures taken where possible.

If this treatment program fails to reduce symptoms and/or blood glucose, the use of an oral sulfonylurea or insulin should be considered. Use of glimepiride must be viewed by both the physician and patient as a treatment in addition to diet and exercise and not as a substitute for diet and exercise or as a convenient mechanism for avoiding dietary restraint. Furthermore, loss of blood glucose control on diet and exercise alone may be transient, thus requiring only short-term administration of glimepiride.

During maintenance programs, glimepiride monotherapy should be discontinued if satisfactory lowering of blood glucose is no longer achieved. Judgments should be based on regular clinical and laboratory evaluations. Secondary failures to glimepiride monotherapy can be treated with glimepiride-insulin combination therapy.

In considering the use of glimepiride in asymptomatic patients, it should be recognized that blood glucose control in type 2 diabetes has not definitely been established to be effective in preventing the long-term cardiovascular and neural complications of diabetes. However, the Diabetes Control and Complications Trial (DCCT) demonstrated that control of HbA1c and glucose was associated with a decrease in retinopathy, neuropathy, and nephropathy for insulin-dependent diabetic (IDDM) patients.

Administration and Dosage

➤*Approved by the FDA:* November 30, 1995.

There is no fixed dosage regimen for the management of diabetes mellitus with glimepiride or any other hypoglycemic agent. The patient's fasting blood glucose and HbA1c must be measured periodically to determine the minimum effective dose for the patient; to detect primary failure, ie, inadequate lowering of blood glucose at the maximum recommended dose of medication; and to detect secondary failure, ie, loss of adequate blood glucose lowering response after an initial period of effectiveness. Glycosylated hemoglobin levels should be performed to monitor the patient's response to therapy.

Short-term administration of glimepiride may be sufficient during periods of transient loss of control in patients usually controlled well on diet and exercise.

➤*Usual starting dose:* The usual starting dose of glimepiride as initial therapy is 1 to 2 mg once daily, administered with breakfast or the first main meal. Those patients who may be more sensitive to hypoglycemic drugs should be started at 1 mg once daily, and should be titrated carefully. No exact dosage relationship exists between glimepiride and the other oral hypoglycemic agents. The maximum starting dose of glimepiride should be no more than 2 mg.

Failure to follow an appropriate dosage regimen may precipitate hypoglycemia. Patients who do not adhere to their prescribed dietary and drug regimen are more prone to exhibit unsatisfactory response to therapy.

➤*Usual maintenance dose:* The usual maintenance dose is 1 to 4 mg once daily. The maximum recommended dose is 8 mg once daily. After reaching a dose of 2 mg, dosage increases should be made in increments of no more than 2 mg at 1 to 2 week intervals based upon the patient's blood glucose response. Long-term efficacy should be monitored by measurement of HbA1c levels, for example, every 3 to 6 months.

➤*Glimepiride-metformin combination therapy:* If patients do not respond adequately to the maximal dose of glimepiride monotherapy, addition of metformin may be considered. Published clinical information exists for the use of other sulfonylureas including glyburide, glipizide, chlorpropamide, and tolbutamide in combination with metformin.

With concomitant glimepiride and metformin therapy, the desired control of blood glucose may be obtained by adjusting the dose of each drug. However, attempts should be made to identify the minimum effective dose of each drug to achieve this goal. With concomitant glimepiride and metformin therapy, the risk of hypoglycemia associated with glimepiride therapy continues and may be increased. Appropriate precautions should be taken.

➤*Glimepiride-insulin combination therapy:* Combination therapy with glimepiride and insulin may also be used in secondary failure patients. The fasting glucose level for instituting combination therapy is in the range of > 150 mg/dL in plasma or serum depending on the patient. The recommended glimepiride dose is 8 mg once daily administered with the first main meal. After starting with low-dose insulin, upward adjustments of insulin can be done approximately weekly as guided by frequent measurements of fasting blood glucose. Once stable, combination-therapy patients should monitor their capillary blood glucose on an ongoing basis, preferably daily. Periodic adjustments of insulin may also be necessary during maintenance as guided by glucose and HbA1c levels.

➤*Specific patient populations:* Glimepiride is not recommended for use in pregnancy, nursing mothers, or children. In elderly, debilitated, or malnourished patients, or in patients with renal or hepatic insufficiency, the initial dosing, dose increments, and maintenance dosage should be conservative to avoid hypoglycemic reactions.

➤*Patients receiving other oral hypoglycemic agents:* As with other sulfonylurea hypoglycemic agents, no transition period is necessary when transferring patients to glimepiride. Patients should be observed carefully (1 to 2 weeks) for hypoglycemia when being transferred from longer half-life sulfonylureas (eg, chlorpropamide) to glimepiride due to potential overlapping of drug effect.

➤*Storage/Stability:* Store between 59° and 86°F (15° and 30°C). Dispense in well-closed containers with safety closures.

GLYBURIDE (Glibenclamide)

Rx	**Glyburide** (Various, eg, Brightstone, Copley, Coventry, Geneva, Greenstone, Novopharm)	**Tablets:** 1.25 mg	In 50s, 100s, and 500s.
Rx	**DiaBeta** (Hoechst Marion Roussel)		(Hoechst Diaβ). Peach, scored. Oblong. In 50s.
Rx	**Micronase** (Pharmacia & Upjohn)		(MICRONASE 1.25). White, scored. In 100s.
Rx	**Glyburide** (Various, eg, Copley, Mova, Novopharm)	**Tablets, micronized:** 1.5 mg	In 100s, 500s, 1,000s, and UD 100s.
Rx	**Glynase PresTab** (Pharmacia & Upjohn)		Lactose. (GLYNASE 1.5/PT PT). White, scored. Oval. In 100s and UD 100s.
Rx	**Glyburide** (Various, eg, Brightstone, Copley, Coventry, Geneva, Greenstone, Novopharm, UDL)	**Tablets:** 2.5 mg	In 90s, 100s, 500s, 1,000s, UD 100s, and blister pack 25s, 100s, and 600s.
Rx	**DiaBeta** (Hoechst Marion Roussel)		(Hoechst Diaβ). Pink, scored. Oblong. In 100s and 500s.
Rx	**Micronase** (Pharmacia & Upjohn)		(MICRONASE 2.5). Pink, scored. In 100s, 1,000s, and UD 100s.
Rx	**Glyburide** (Various, eg, Copley, Mova, Novopharm)	**Tablets, micronized:** 3 mg	In 100s, 500s, 1,000s, and UD 100s.
Rx	**Glynase PresTab** (Pharmacia & Upjohn)		Lactose. (GLYNASE 3/PT PT). Blue, scored. Oval. In 100s, 500s, 1,000s, and UD 100s.
Rx	**Glyburide** (Various, eg, Mova)	**Tablets, micronized:** 4.5 mg	In 100s, 500s, and 1,000s.
Rx	**Glyburide** (Various, eg, Brightstone, Copley, Coventry, Geneva, Greenstone, Novopharm, UDL)	**Tablets:** 5 mg	In 90s, 100s, 500s, 1,000s, UD 100s, and blister pack 25s, 100s, and 600s.
Rx	**DiaBeta** (Hoechst Marion Roussel)		(Hoechst Diaβ). Green, scored. Oblong. In 500s and 1,000s.
Rx	**Micronase** (Pharmacia & Upjohn)		(MICRONASE 5). Blue, scored. In 100s, 500s, 1,000s, and UD 100s.
Rx	**Glyburide** (Various, eg, Mova, Novopharm)	**Tablets, micronized:** 6 mg	In 100s, 500s, and 1,000s.
Rx	**Glynase PresTab** (Pharmacia & Upjohn)		Lactose. (GLYNASE 6/PT PT). Yellow, scored. Oval. In 100s and 500s.

GLYBURIDE — ORAL

For complete prescribing information, refer to the Sulfonylureas group monograph.

Indications

➤*Type 2 diabetes:* Indicated as an adjunct to diet to lower the blood glucose in patients with non-insulin-dependent diabetes mellitus (type 2) whose hyperglycemia cannot be controlled by diet alone.

Administration and Dosage

➤*Approved by the FDA:* May 1, 1984.

Patients should be retitrated when transferred from glyburide or other oral hypoglycemic agents.

There is no fixed dosage regimen for the management of diabetes mellitus with glyburide or any other hypoglycemic agent. The patient's fasting blood glucose must be measured periodically to determine the minimum effective dose for the patient; to detect primary failure (ie, inadequate lowering of blood glucose at the maximum recommended dose of medication) and to detect secondary failure (ie, loss of adequate blood glucose lowering response after an initial period of effectiveness). Periodic glycosylated hemoglobin determinations should be performed.

Short-term administration of glyburide may be sufficient during periods of transient loss of control in patients usually controlled well on diet.

➤*Usual starting dose:* The usual starting dose of glyburide as initial therapy is 2.5 to 5 mg daily, administered with breakfast or the first main meal. Those patients who may be more sensitive to hypoglycemic drugs should be started at 1.25 mg daily (see Precautions section for patients at increased risk). Failure to follow an appropriate dosage regimen may precipitate hypoglycemia. Patients who do not adhere to their prescribed dietary and drug regimen are more prone to exhibit unsatisfactory response to therapy.

The suggested starting dose of micronized glyburide tablets is 1.5 to 3 mg daily, administered with breakfast or the first main meal. Those patients who may be more sensitive to hypoglycemic drugs should be started at 0.75 mg daily.

➤*Transfer from other hypoglycemic therapy for patients receiving other oral antidiabetic therapy:* Transfer of patients from other oral antidiabetic regimens to glyburide should be done conservatively, and the initial daily dose should be 2.5 to 5 mg of glyburide tablets or 1.5 to 3 mg of micronized glyburide tablets. When transferring patients from oral hypoglycemic agents other than chlorpropamide to glyburide, no transition period and no initial or priming dose are necessary. When transferring patients from chlorpropamide, particular care should be exercised during the first 2 weeks because the prolonged retention of chlorpropamide in the body and subsequent overlapping drug effects may provoke hypoglycemia.

➤*Patients receiving insulin:* Some type 2 diabetic patients being treated with insulin may respond satisfactorily to glyburide. If the insulin dose is less than 20 units daily, substitution of glyburide tablets 2.5 to 5 mg or micronized glyburide tablets 1.5 to 3 mg daily as a single dose may be tried. If the insulin dose is between 20 and 40 units daily, the patient may be placed directly on glyburide tablets 5 mg or micronized glyburide tablets 3 mg daily as a single dose. If the insulin dose is more than 40 units daily, a transition period is required for conversion to glyburide. In these patients, insulin dosage is decreased by 50% and glyburide tablets 5 mg or micronized glyburide tablets 3 mg daily is started (see Titration to maintenance dose).

➤*Titration to maintenance dose:* The usual maintenance dose is in the range of 1.25 to 20 mg of glyburide tablets or 0.75 to 12 mg of micronized glyburide tablets daily, which may be given as a single dose or in divided doses (see Dosage interval). Dosage increases should be made in increments of no more than 2.5 mg of glyburide tablets or 1.5 mg of micronized glyburide tablets at weekly intervals based upon the patient's blood glucose response.

No exact dosage relationship exists between glyburide and other oral hypoglycemic agents. Although patients may be transferred from the maximum dose of other sulfonylureas, the maximum starting dose of 5 mg of glyburide tablets or 3 mg of micronized glyburide tablets should be observed. A maintenance dose of 5 mg of glyburide tablets or 3 mg of micronized glyburide tablets provides approximately the same degree of blood glucose control as 250 to 375 mg chlorpropamide, 250 to 375 mg tolazamide, 500 to 750 mg acetohexamide, or 1,000 to 1,500 mg tolbutamide.

When transferring patients receiving more than 40 units of insulin daily, they may be started on a daily dose of glyburide tablets 5 mg or micronized glyburide tablets 3 mg concomitantly with a 50% reduction in insulin dose. Progressive withdrawal of insulin and increase of glyburide in increments of 1.25 to 2.5 mg every 2 to 10 days for glyburide tablets or 0.75 to 1.5 mg every 2 to 10 days for micronized glyburide tablets is then carried out. During this conversion period when both insulin and glyburide are being used, hypoglycemia may rarely occur. During insulin withdrawal, patients should test their urine for glucose and acetone at least 3 times daily and report results to their physician. The appearance of persistent acetonuria with glycosuria indicates that the patient is a type 1 diabetic who requires insulin therapy.

➤*Concomitant glyburide and metformin therapy:* Glyburide tablets should be added gradually to the dosing regimen of patients who have not responded to the maximum dose of metformin monotherapy after 4 weeks (see Usual starting dose and Titration to maintenance dose).

With concomitant glyburide and metformin therapy, the desired control of blood glucose may be obtained by adjusting the dose of each drug. However, attempts should be made to identify the optimal dose of each drug needed to achieve this goal. With concomitant glyburide and metformin therapy, the risk of hypoglycemia associated with sulfonylurea therapy continues and may be increased. Appropriate precautions should be taken.

➤*Maximum dose:* Daily doses of more than 20 mg of glyburide tablets or 12 mg of micronized glyburide tablets are not recommended.

➤*Dosage interval:* Once-a-day therapy is usually satisfactory. Some patients, particularly those receiving more than 10 mg daily of glyburide tablets or 6 mg daily of micronized glyburide tablets, may have a more satisfactory response with twice-a-day dosage.

➤*Special patient populations:* Glyburide is not recommended for use in pregnancy or for use in children.

In elderly patients, debilitated or malnourished patients, and patients with impaired renal or hepatic function, the initial and maintenance dosing should be conservative to avoid hypoglycemic reactions (see Warnings).

➤*Storage / Stability:* Store between 15° and 30°C (59° and 86°F). Dispense in well-closed containers with safety closures.

ACARBOSE

Rx	**Precose** (Bayer)	**Tablets:** 25 mg	(PRECOSE 25). White to yellow. In 100s.
		50 mg	(PRECOSE 50). White to yellow. In 100s and UD 100s.
		100 mg	(PRECOSE 100). White to yellow. In 100s and UD 100s.

ACARBOSE — ORAL

Indications

➤*Type 2 diabetes:* Monotherapy as an adjunct to diet to lower blood glucose in patients with type 2 diabetes mellitus whose hyperglycemia cannot be managed on diet alone. Acarbose may also be used in combination with a sulfonylurea when diet plus either acarbose or a sulfonylurea do not result in adequate glycemic control. Also, acarbose may be used in combination with insulin or metformin. The effect of acarbose to enhance glycemic control is additive to that of sulfonylureas, insulin, or metformin when used in combination, presumably because its mechanism of action is different.

Administration and Dosage

➤*Approved by the FDA:* September 6, 1995

There is no fixed dosage regimen for the management of diabetes mellitus with acarbose or any other pharmacologic agent. Dosage of acarbose must be individualized on the basis of both effectiveness and tolerance while not exceeding the maximum recommended dose of 100 mg 3 times a day. Acarbose should be taken 3 times daily at the start (with the first bite) of each main meal. Acarbose should be started at a low dose, with gradual dose escalation as described below, both to reduce gastrointestinal side effects and to permit identification of the minimum dose required for adequate glycemic control of the patient.

During treatment initiation and dose titration (see below), 1-hour postprandial plasma glucose may be used to determine the therapeutic response to acarbose and identify the minimum effective dose for the patient. Thereafter, glycosylated hemoglobin should be measured at intervals of approximately 3 months. The therapeutic goal should be to decrease both postprandial plasma glucose and glycosylated hemoglobin levels to normal or near normal by using the lowest effective dose of acarbose, either as monotherapy or in combination with sulfonylureas, insulin or metformin.

➤*Initial dosage:* The recommended starting dosage of acarbose is 25 mg given orally 3 times daily at the start (with the first bite) of each main meal. However, some patients may benefit from more gradual dose titration to minimize gastrointestinal side effects. This may be achieved by initiating treatment at 25 mg once per day and subsequently increasing the frequency of administration to achieve 25 mg 3 times daily.

➤*Maintenance dosage:* Once a 25 mg 3 times daily dosage regimen is reached, dosage of acarbose should be adjusted at 4- to 8-week intervals based on 1-hour postprandial glucose or glycosylated hemoglobin levels, and on tolerance. The dosage can be increased from 25 mg 3 times daily to 50 mg 3 times daily. Some patients may benefit from further increasing the dosage to 100 mg 3 times daily. The maintenance dose ranges from 50 mg 3 times daily to 100 mg 3 times daily. However, since patients with low body weight may be at increased risk for elevated serum transaminases, only patients with body weight greater than 60 kg should be considered for dose titration above 50 mg 3 times daily. If no further reduction in postprandial glucose or

ACARBOSE — ORAL

glycosylated hemoglobin levels is observed with titration to 100 mg 3 times daily, consideration should be given to lowering the dose. Once an effective and tolerated dosage is established, it should be maintained.

➤*Maximum dosage:* The maximum recommended dose for patients less than or equal to 60 kg is 50 mg 3 times daily. The maximum recommended dose for patients more than than 60 kg is 100 mg 3 times daily.

➤*Patients receiving sulfonylureas or insulin:* Sulfonylurea agents or insulin may cause hypoglycemia. Acarbose given in combination with a sulfonylurea or insulin will cause a further lowering of blood glucose and may increase the potential for hypoglycemia. If hypoglycemia occurs, appropriate adjustments in the dosage of these agents should be made.

➤*Storage/Stability:* Do not store above 25°C (77°F). Protect from moisture. For bottles, keep container tightly closed.

Actions

➤*Pharmacology:* Acarbose is a complex oligosaccharide that delays the digestion of ingested carbohydrates, thereby resulting in a smaller rise in blood glucose concentration following meals. As a consequence of plasma glucose reduction, acarbose reduces levels of glycosylated hemoglobin in patients with type 2 diabetes mellitus. Systemic nonenzymatic protein glycosylation, as reflected by levels of glycosylated hemoglobin, is a function of average blood glucose concentration over time.

In contrast to sulfonylureas, acarbose does not enhance insulin secretion. The antihyperglycemic action of acarbose results from a competitive, reversible inhibition of pancreatic alpha-amylase and membrane-bound intestinal alpha-glucoside hydrolase enzymes. Pancreatic alpha-amylase hydrolyzes complex starches to oligosaccharides in the lumen of the small intestine, while the membrane-bound intestinal alpha-glucosidases hydrolyze oligosaccharides, trisaccharides, and disaccharides to glucose and other monosaccharides in the brush border of the small intestine. In diabetic patients, this enzyme inhibition results in a delayed glucose absorption and a lowering of postprandial hyperglycemia.

Because its mechanism of action is different, the effect of acarbose to enhance glycemic control is additive to that of sulfonylureas, insulin or metformin when used in combination. In addition, acarbose diminishes the insulinotropic and weight-increasing effects of sulfonylureas.

Acarbose has no inhibitory activity against lactase and consequently would not be expected to induce lactose intolerance.

➤*Pharmacokinetics:*

Absorption – In a study of 6 healthy men, less than 2% of an oral dose of acarbose was absorbed as active drug, while approximately 35% of total radioactivity from a ^{14}C-labeled oral dose was absorbed. An average of 51% of an oral dose was excreted in the feces as unabsorbed drug-related radioactivity within 96 hours of ingestion. Because acarbose acts locally within the gastrointestinal tract, this low systemic bioavailability of parent compound is therapeutically desired. Following oral dosing of healthy volunteers with ^{14}C-labeled acarbose, peak plasma concentrations of radioactivity were attained 14 to 24 hours after dosing, while peak plasma concentrations of active drug were attained at approximately 1 hour. The delayed absorption of acarbose-related radioactivity reflects the absorption of metabolites that may be formed by either intestinal bacteria or intestinal enzymatic hydrolysis.

Metabolism – Acarbose is metabolized exclusively within the GI tract, principally by intestinal bacteria, but also by digestive enzymes. A fraction of these metabolites (approximately 34% of the dose) was absorbed and subsequently excreted in the urine. At least 13 metabolites have been separated chromatographically from urine specimens. The major metabolites have been identified as 4-methylpyrogallol derivatives (ie, sulfate, methyl, glucuronide conjugates). One metabolite (formed by cleavage of a glucose molecule from acarbose) also has alpha-glucosidase inhibitory activity. This metabolite, together with the parent compound, recovered from the urine, accounts for less than 2% of the total administered dose.

Excretion – The fraction of acarbose that is absorbed as intact drug is almost completely excreted by the kidneys. When acarbose was given intravenously, 89% of the dose was recovered in the urine as active drug within 48 hours. In contrast, less than 2% of an oral dose was recovered in the urine as active (ie, parent compound and active metabolite) drug. This is consistent with the low bioavailability of the parent drug. The plasma elimination half-life of acarbose activity is approximately 2 hours in healthy volunteers. Consequently, drug accumulation does not occur with 3 times a day oral dosing.

Contraindications

Hypersensitivity to the drug; diabetic ketoacidosis or cirrhosis; inflammatory bowel disease; colonic ulceration; partial intestinal obstruction; patients predisposed to intestinal obstruction. In addition, acarbose is contraindicated in patients who have chronic intestinal diseases associated with marked disorders of digestion or absorption and in patients who have conditions that may deteriorate as a result of increased gas formation in the intestine.

Warnings

➤*Renal function impairment:* Plasma concentrations of acarbose in renally impaired volunteers were proportionally increased relative to the degree of renal dysfunction. Long-term clinical trials in diabetic patients with significant renal dysfunction (serum creatinine greater than 2 mg/dL) have not been conducted. Therefore, treatment of these patients with acarbose is not recommended.

➤*Carcinogenesis:* Eight carcinogenicity studies were conducted with acarbose. Six studies were performed in rats (2 strains, Sprague-Dawley and Wistar) and 2 studies were performed in hamsters. In the first rat study, Sprague-Dawley rats received acarbose in feed at high doses (up to approximately 500 mg/kg body weight) for 104 weeks. Acarbose treatment resulted in a significant increase in the incidence of renal tumors (adenomas and adenocarcinomas) and benign Leydig cell tumors. This study was repeated with a similar outcome. Further studies were performed to separate direct carcinogenic effects of acarbose from indirect effects resulting from the carbohydrate malnutrition induced by the large doses of acarbose employed in the studies. In 1 study using Sprague-Dawley rats, acarbose was mixed with feed but carbohydrate deprivation was prevented by the addition of glucose to the diet. In a 26-month study of Sprague-Dawley rats, acarbose was administered by daily postprandial gavage so as to avoid the pharmacologic effects of the drug. In both of these studies, the increased incidence of renal tumors found in the original studies did not occur. Acarbose was also given in food and by postprandial gavage in 2 separate studies in Wistar rats. No increased incidence of renal tumors was found in either of these Wistar rat studies. In 2 feeding studies of hamsters, with and without glucose supplementation, there was also no evidence of carcinogenicity.

➤*Elderly:* Of the total number of subjects in clinical studies of acarbose in the United States, 27% were greater than or equal to 65 years of age, while 4% were greater than or equal to 75 years of age. No overall differences in safety and effectiveness were observed between these subjects and younger subjects. The mean steady-state area under the curve (AUC) and maximum concentrations of acarbose were approximately 1.5 times higher in elderly compared to young volunteers; however, these differences were not statistically significant.

➤*Pregnancy: Category B.*

Teratogenic – The safety of acarbose in pregnant women has not been established. In rabbits, reduced maternal body weight gain, probably the result of the pharmacodynamic activity of high doses of acarbose in the intestines, may have been responsible for a slight increase in the number of embryonic losses. However, rabbits given 160 mg/kg acarbose (corresponding to 10 times the dose in man, based on body surface area) showed no evidence of embryotoxicity and there was no evidence of teratogenicity at a dose 32 times the dose in man (based on body surface area). There are, however, no adequate and well-controlled studies of acarbose in pregnant women. Because animal reproduction studies are not always predictive of the human response, this drug should be used during pregnancy only if clearly needed. Because current information strongly suggests that abnormal blood glucose levels during pregnancy are associated with a higher incidence of congenital anomalies as well as increased neonatal morbidity and mortality, most experts recommend that insulin be used during pregnancy to maintain blood glucose levels as close to normal as possible.

➤*Lactation:* A small amount of radioactivity has been found in the milk of lactating rats after administration of radiolabeled acarbose. It is not known whether this drug is excreted in human milk. Because many drugs are excreted in human milk, acarbose should not be administered to a nursing woman.

➤*Children:* Safety and efficacy of acarbose in pediatric patients have not been established.

Precautions

➤*Monitoring:* Therapeutic response to acarbose should be monitored by periodic blood glucose tests. Measurement of glycosylated hemoglobin levels is recommended for the monitoring of long-term glycemic control.

Acarbose, particularly at doses in excess of 50 mg 3 times daily, may give rise to elevations of serum transaminases and, in rare instances, hyperbilirubinemia. It is recommended that serum transaminase levels be checked every 3 months during the first year of treatment with acarbose and periodically thereafter. If elevated transaminases are observed, a reduction in dosage or withdrawal of therapy may be indicated, particularly if the elevations persist.

➤*Calcium/vitamin B_6:* Low serum calcium and low plasma vitamin B_6 levels were associated with acarbose therapy but were thought to be either spurious or of no clinical significance.

➤*Hematocrit:* Small reductions in hematocrit occurred more often in acarbose-treated patients than in placebo-treated patients but were not associated with reductions in hemoglobin.

➤*Hypoglycemia:* Because of its mechanism of action, acarbose when administered alone should not cause hypoglycemia in the fasted or postprandial state. Sulfonylurea agents or insulin may cause hypoglycemia. Because acarbose given in combination with a sulfonylurea or insulin will cause a further lowering of blood glucose, it may increase the potential for hypoglycemia. Hypoglycemia does not occur in patients receiving metformin alone under usual circumstances of use, and no increased incidence of hypoglycemia was observed in patients when acarbose was added to metformin therapy. Oral glucose (dextrose), whose absorption is not inhibited by acarbose, should be used instead of sucrose (cane sugar) in the treatment of mild to moderate hypoglycemia. Sucrose, whose hydrolysis to glucose and fructose is inhibited by acarbose, is unsuitable for the rapid correction of hypoglycemia. Severe hypoglycemia may require the use of either intravenous glucose infusion or glucagon injection.

➤*Loss of control of blood glucose:* When diabetic patients are exposed to stress such as fever, trauma, infection, or surgery, a temporary loss of control of blood glucose may occur. At such times, temporary insulin therapy may be necessary.

➤*Lab test abnormalities:* In long-term studies (up to 12 months, and including acarbose doses up to 300 mg 3 times daily) conducted in the United States, treatment-emergent elevations of serum transaminases (AST and/or ALT) above the upper limit of normal (ULN), greater than 1.8 times the ULN, and greater than 3 times the ULN occurred in 14%, 6%, and 3%,

ACARBOSE — ORAL

respectively, of acarbose-treated patients as compared to 7%, 2%, and 1%, respectively, of placebo-treated patients. Although these differences between treatments were statistically significant, these elevations were asymptomatic, reversible, more common in females, and, in general, were not associated with other evidence of liver dysfunction. In addition, these serum transaminase elevations appeared to be dose related. In US studies including acarbose doses up to the maximum approved dose of 100 mg 3 times daily, treatment-emergent elevations of AST and/or ALT at any level of severity were similar between acarbose-treated patients and placebo-treated patients ($P \geq 0.496$).

In approximately 3 million patient-years of international postmarketing experience with acarbose, 62 cases of serum transaminase elevations greater than 500 units/L (29 of which were associated with jaundice) have been reported. Forty-one of these 62 patients received treatment with 100 mg 3 times daily or greater and 33 of 45 patients for whom weight was reported weighed less than 60 kg. In the 59 cases where follow-up was recorded, hepatic abnormalities improved or resolved upon discontinuation of acarbose in 55 and were unchanged in 2. A few cases of fulminant hepatitis with fatal outcome have been reported; the relationship to acarbose is unclear.

Drug Interactions

Acarbose Drug Interactions

Precipitant drug	Object drug[a]		Description
Acarbose	Digoxin	↓	Serum digoxin concentrations may be reduced, decreasing the therapeutic effects.
Digestive enzymes (eg, amylase, pancreatin)	Acarbose	↓	Effect of acarbose may be reduced. Do not use concomitantly.
Intestinal absorbents (eg, charcoal)	Acarbose	↓	Effect of acarbose may be reduced. Do not use concomitantly.

[a] ↓ = Object drug decreased.

Certain drugs tend to produce hyperglycemia and may lead to loss of blood glucose control. These drugs include the thiazides and other diuretics, corticosteroids, phenothiazines, thyroid products, estrogens, oral contraceptives, phenytoin, nicotinic acid, sympathomimetics, calcium channel-blocking drugs, and isoniazid. When such drugs are administered to a patient receiving acarbose, the patient should be closely observed for loss of blood glucose control. When such drugs are withdrawn from patients receiving acarbose in combination with sulfonylureas or insulin, patients should be observed closely for any evidence of hypoglycemia.

Adverse Reactions

➤*GI:* GI symptoms are the most common reactions to acarbose. In US placebo-controlled trials, the incidences of abdominal pain, diarrhea, and flatulence were 19%, 31%, and 74%, respectively, in 1255 patients treated with acarbose 50 to 300 mg 3 times daily, whereas the corresponding incidences were 9%, 12%, and 29% in 999 placebo-treated patients. In a 1-year safety study, during which patients kept diaries of GI symptoms, abdominal pain and diarrhea tended to return to pretreatment levels over time, and the frequency and intensity of flatulence tended to abate with time. The increased gastrointestinal tract symptoms in patients treated with acarbose are a manifestation of the mechanism of action of acarbose and are related to the presence of undigested carbohydrate in the lower GI tract. Rarely, these GI events may be severe and might be confused with paralytic ileus.

➤*Hypersensitivity:* Rarely, hypersensitive skin reactions such as rash may occur.

➤*Lab test abnormalities:* Elevated serum transaminase levels, small reductions in hematocrit occurred more often in acarbose-treated patients than in placebo-treated patients but were not associated with reductions in hemoglobin. Low serum calcium and low plasma vitamin B_6 levels were associated with acarbose therapy but are thought to be either spurious or of no clinical significance.

➤*Miscellaneous:* Edema in rare instances edema has been reported.

Overdosage

Unlike sulfonylureas or insulin, an overdose of acarbose will not result in hypoglycemia. An overdose may result in transient increases in flatulence, diarrhea, and abdominal discomfort which shortly subside.

Patient Information

Patients should be told to take acarbose orally 3 times a day at the start (with the first bite) of each main meal. It is important that patients continue to adhere to dietary instructions, a regular exercise program, and regular testing of urine or blood glucose.

Acarbose itself does not cause hypoglycemia even when administered to patients in the fasted state. Sulfonylurea drugs and insulin, however, can lower blood sugar levels enough to cause symptoms or sometimes life-threatening hypoglycemia. Because acarbose given in combination with a sulfonylurea or insulin will cause a further lowering of blood sugar, it may increase the hypoglycemic potential of these agents. Hypoglycemia does not occur in patients receiving metformin alone under usual circumstances of use, and no increased incidence of hypoglycemia was observed in patients when acarbose was added to metformin therapy. The risk of hypoglycemia, its symptoms and treatment, and conditions that predispose to its development should be well understood by patients and responsible family members. Because acarbose prevents the breakdown of table sugar, patients should have a readily available source of glucose (dextrose, D-glucose) to treat symptoms of low blood sugar when taking acarbose in combination with a sulfonylurea or insulin.

If side effects occur with acarbose, they usually develop during the first few weeks of therapy. They are most commonly mild-to-moderate gastrointestinal effects, such as flatulence, diarrhea, or abdominal discomfort, and generally diminish in frequency and intensity with time.

MIGLITOL

Rx	**Glyset** (Pfizer)	**Tablets:** 25 mg	(GLYSET 25). White. In 100s.
		50 mg	(GLYSET 50). White. In 100s.
		100 mg	(GLYSET 100). White. In 100s.

MIGLITOL — ORAL

Indications

➤*Type 2 diabetes:* Monotherapy as an adjunct to diet to improve glycemic control in patients with type 2 diabetes whose hyperglycemia cannot be managed with diet alone. Miglitol may also be used in combination with a sulfonylurea when diet plus either miglitol or a sulfonylurea alone do not result in adequate glycemic control. The effect of miglitol to enhance glycemic control is additive to that of sulfonylureas when used in combination, presumably because its mechanism of action is different.

Administration and Dosage

➤*Approved by the FDA:* December 12, 1996.

There is no fixed dosage regimen for the management of diabetes mellitus with miglitol tablets or any other pharmacologic agent. Dosage of miglitol must be individualized on the basis of both effectiveness and tolerance while not exceeding the maximum recommended dosage of 100 mg 3 times daily. Miglitol should be taken 3 times daily at the start (with the first bite) of each main meal. Miglitol should be started at 25 mg, and the dosage gradually increased as described below, both to reduce GI adverse reactions and to permit identification of the minimum dose required for adequate glycemic control of the patient.

During treatment initiation and dose titration (see below), 1-hour postprandial plasma glucose may be used to determine the therapeutic response to miglitol and identify the minimum effective dose for the patient. Thereafter, glycosylated hemoglobin should be measured at intervals of approximately 3 months. The therapeutic goal should be to decrease both postprandial plasma glucose and glycosylated hemoglobin levels to normal or near normal by using the lowest effective dose of miglitol, either as monotherapy or in combination with a sulfonylurea.

➤*Initial dosage:* The recommended starting dosage of miglitol is 25 mg, given orally 3 times daily at the start (with the first bite) of each main meal. However, some patients may benefit by starting at 25 mg once daily to minimize GI adverse reactions, and gradually increasing the frequency of administration to 3 times daily.

➤*Maintenance dosage:* The usual maintenance dose of miglitol is 50 mg 3 times daily, although some patients may benefit from increasing the dose to 100 mg 3 times daily. In order to allow adaptation to potential GI adverse reactions, it is recommended that miglitol therapy be initiated at a dosage of 25 mg 3 times daily, the lowest effective dosage, and then gradually titrated upward to allow adaptation. After 4 to 8 weeks of the 25 mg 3 times daily regimen, the dosage should be increased to 50 mg 3 times daily for approximately 3 months, following which a glycosylated hemoglobin level should be measured to assess therapeutic response. If, at that time, the glycosylated hemoglobin level is not satisfactory, the dosage may be further increased to 100 mg 3 times daily, the maximum recommended dosage. Pooled data from controlled studies suggest a dose response for both HbA1c and 1-hour postprandial plasma glucose throughout the recommended dosage range. However, no single study has examined the effect on glycemic control of titrating patients' doses upwards within the same study. If no further reduction in postprandial glucose or glycosylated hemoglobin levels is observed with titration to 100 mg 3 times daily, consideration should be given to lowering the dose. Once an effective and tolerated dosage is established, it should be maintained.

➤*Maximum dosage:* The maximum recommended dosage of miglitol is 100 mg 3 times daily. In 1 clinical trial, 200 mg 3 times daily gave additional improved glycemic control but increased the incidence of the GI symptoms.

➤*Patients receiving sulfonylureas:* Sulfonylurea agents may cause hypoglycemia. There was no increased incidence of hypoglycemia in patients who took miglitol in combination with sulfonylurea agents compared to the

MIGLITOL — ORAL

incidence of hypoglycemia in patients receiving sulfonylureas alone in any clinical trial. However, miglitol given in combination with a sulfonylurea will cause a further lowering of blood glucose and may increase the risk of hypoglycemia due to the additive effects of the 2 agents. If hypoglycemia occurs, appropriate adjustments in the dosage of these agents should be made.

➤*Storage/Stability:* Store at 25°C (77°F); excursions permitted to 15° to 30°C (59° to 86°F).

Actions

➤*Pharmacology:* Miglitol is a desoxynojirimycin derivative that delays the digestion of ingested carbohydrates, thereby resulting in a smaller rise in blood glucose concentration following meals. As a consequence of plasma glucose reduction, miglitol tablets reduce levels of glycosylated hemoglobin in patients with type 2 diabetes mellitus. Systemic nonenzymatic protein glycosylation, as reflected by levels of glycosylated hemoglobin, is a function of average blood glucose concentration over time.

In contrast to sulfonylureas, miglitol does not enhance insulin secretion. The antihyperglycemic action of miglitol results from a reversible inhibition of membrane-bound intestinal α-glucoside hydrolase enzymes. Membrane-bound intestinal α-glucosidases hydrolyze oligosaccharides and disaccharides to glucose and other monosaccharides in the brush border of the small intestine. In diabetic patients, this enzyme inhibition results in delayed glucose absorption and lowering of postprandial hyperglycemia.

Because its mechanism of action is different, the effect of miglitol to enhance glycemic control is additive to that of sulfonylureas when used in combination. In addition, miglitol diminishes the insulinotropic and weight-increasing effects of sulfonylureas. Miglitol has minor inhibitory activity against lactase and consequently, at the recommended doses, would not be expected to induce lactose intolerance.

➤*Pharmacokinetics:*

Absorption – Absorption of miglitol is saturable at high doses; a dose of 25 mg is completely absorbed, whereas a dose of 100 mg is only 50% to 70% absorbed. For all doses, peak concentrations are reached in 2 to 3 hours. There is no evidence that systemic absorption of miglitol contributes to its therapeutic effect.

Distribution – The protein binding of miglitol is negligible (less than 4%). Miglitol has a volume of distribution of 0.18 L/kg, consistent with distribution primarily into the extracellular fluid.

Metabolism – Miglitol is not metabolized in man or in any animal species studied. No metabolites have been detected in plasma, urine, or feces, indicating a lack of either systemic or presystemic metabolism.

Excretion – Miglitol is eliminated by renal excretion as unchanged drug. Thus, following a 25 mg dose, over 95% of the dose is recovered in the urine within 24 hours. At higher doses, the cumulative recovery of drug from urine is somewhat lower due to the incomplete bioavailability. The elimination half-life of miglitol from plasma is approximately 2 hours.

Special populations –

Renal function impairment: Because miglitol is excreted primarily by the kidneys, accumulation of miglitol is expected in patients with renal impairment. Patients with creatinine clearance less than 25 mL/min taking 25 mg 3 times daily exhibited a more than 2-fold increase in miglitol plasma levels as compared to subjects with creatinine clearance more than 60 mL/min. Dosage adjustment to correct the increased plasma concentrations is not feasible because miglitol acts locally. Little information is available on the safety of miglitol in patients with creatinine clearance less than 25 mL/min.

Contraindications

Diabetic ketoacidosis; inflammatory bowel disease, colonic ulceration, or partial intestinal obstruction, and in patients predisposed to intestinal obstruction; chronic intestinal diseases associated with marked disorders of digestion or absorption, or with conditions that may deteriorate as a result of increased gas formation in the intestine; hypersensitivity to the drug or any of its components.

Warnings

➤*Renal function impairment:* Plasma concentrations of miglitol in renally impaired volunteers were proportionally increased relative to the degree of renal dysfunction. Long-term clinical trials in diabetic patients with significant renal dysfunction (serum creatinine more than 2 mg/dL) have not been conducted. Therefore, treatment of these patients with miglitol is not recommended.

➤*Pregnancy: Category B.*

Teratogenic – The safety of miglitol in pregnant women has not been established. Developmental toxicology studies have been performed in rats at doses of 50, 150 and 450 mg/kg, corresponding to levels of approximately 1.5, 4, and 12 times the maximum recommended human exposure based on body surface area. In rabbits, doses of 10, 45, and 200 mg/kg corresponding to levels of approximately 0.5, 3, and 10 times the human exposure were examined. These studies revealed no evidence of fetal malformations attributable to miglitol. Doses of miglitol up to 4 and 3 times the human dose (based on body surface area), for rats and rabbits, respectively, did not reveal evidence of impaired fertility or harm to the fetus. The highest doses tested in these studies, 450 mg/kg in the rat and 200 mg/kg in the rabbit promoted maternal or fetal toxicity. Fetotoxicity was indicated by a slight but significant reduction in fetal weight in the rat study and slight reduction in fetal weight, delayed ossification of the fetal skeleton and increase in the percentage of non-viable fetuses in the rabbit study. In the peri- and postnatal study in rats, the NOAEL (no observed adverse effect level) was 100 mg/kg (corresponding to approximately 4 times the exposure to humans, based on body surface area). An increase in stillborn progeny was noted at the high dose (300 mg/kg) in the rat peri- and postnatal study, but not at the high dose (450 mg/kg) in the delivery segment of the rat developmental toxicity study. Otherwise, there was no adverse effect on survival, growth, development, behavior, or fertility in either the rat developmental toxicity or peri-postnatal studies. There are, however, no adequate and well-controlled studies in pregnant women. Because animal reproduction studies are not always predictive of human response, this drug should be used during pregnancy only if clearly needed.

➤*Lactation:* Miglitol has been shown to be excreted in human milk to a very small degree. Total excretion into milk accounted for 0.02% of a 100 mg maternal dose. The estimated exposure to a nursing infant is approximately 0.4% of the maternal dose. Although the levels of miglitol reached in human milk are exceedingly low, it is recommended that miglitol not be administered to a nursing woman.

➤*Children:* Safety and efficacy of miglitol in children have not been established.

Precautions

➤*Monitoring:* Therapeutic response to miglitol may be monitored by periodic blood glucose tests. Measurement of glycosylated hemoglobin level is recommended for the monitoring of long-term glycemic control.

➤*Hypoglycemia:* Because of its mechanism of action, miglitol when administered alone should not cause hypoglycemia in the fasted or postprandial state. Sulfonylurea agents may cause hypoglycemia. Because miglitol tablets given in combination with a sulfonylurea will cause a further lowering of blood glucose, it may increase the hypoglycemic potential of the sulfonylurea, although this was not observed in clinical trials. Oral glucose (dextrose), whose absorption is not delayed by miglitol, should be used instead of sucrose (cane sugar) in the treatment of mild-to-moderate hypoglycemia. Sucrose, whose hydrolysis to glucose and fructose is inhibited by miglitol, is unsuitable for the rapid correction of hypoglycemia. Severe hypoglycemia may require the use of either IV glucose infusion or glucagon injection.

➤*Loss of control of blood glucose:* When diabetic patients are exposed to stress such as fever, trauma, infection, or surgery, a temporary loss of control of blood glucose may occur. At such times, temporary insulin therapy may be necessary.

Drug Interactions

Miglitol Drug Interactions

Precipitant	Object drug*		Description
Miglitol	Digoxin	⬇	Coadministration may reduce the average plasma concentrations of digoxin by 19% to 28%. In 1 study in diabetic patients under treatment with digoxin, plasma digoxin concentrations were not altered when coadministered with miglitol 100 mg 3 times/day × 14 days.
Miglitol	Glyburide	⬇	Decreased AUC and C_{max} values for glyburide occurred when coadministered with miglitol. These differences were not statistically significant.
Miglitol	Metformin	⬇	Mean AUC and C_{max} values for metformin were 12% to 13% lower when the volunteers were given miglitol as compared with placebo, but this difference was not statistically significant.
Miglitol	Propranolol	⬇	Miglitol may significantly reduce the bioavailability of propranolol by 40%.
Miglitol	Ranitidine	⬇	Miglitol may significantly reduce the bioavailability of ranitidine by 60%.
Digestive enzymes (eg, amylase, pancreatin)	Miglitol	⬇	Digestive enzyme preparations may reduce the effect of miglitol. Do not take concomitantly.
Intestinal adsorbents (eg, charcoal)	Miglitol	⬇	Intestinal adsorbents may reduce the effect of miglitol. Do not take concomitantly.

* ⬇ = Object drug decreased.

Several studies investigated the possible interaction between miglitol and glyburide. In 6 healthy volunteers given a single dose of 5 mg glyburide on a background of 6 days treatment with miglitol (50 mg 3 times daily for 4 days followed by 100 mg 3 times daily for 2 days) or placebo, the mean C_{max} and AUC values for glyburide were 17% and 25% lower, respectively, when glyburide was given with miglitol. In a study in diabetic patients in which the effects of adding miglitol 100 mg 3 times daily × 7 days or placebo to a background regimen of 3.5 mg glyburide daily were investigated, the mean AUC value for glyburide was 18% lower in the group treated with miglitol,

MIGLITOL — ORAL

although this difference was not statistically significant. Further information on a potential interaction with glyburide was obtained from one of the large US clinical trials (study 7) in which patients were dosed with either miglitol or placebo on a background of glyburide 10 mg twice daily. At the 6-month and 1-year clinic visits, patients taking concomitant miglitol 100 mg 3 times daily exhibited mean C_{max} values for glyburide that were 16% and 8% lower, respectively, compared to patients taking glyburide alone. However, these differences were not statistically significant. Thus, although there was a trend toward lower AUC and C_{max} values for glyburide when coadministered with miglitol, no definitive statement regarding a potential interaction can be made based on the foregoing 3 studies.

In 12 healthy males, concomitantly administered antacid did not influence the pharmacokinetics of miglitol.

Adverse Reactions

➤*Dermatologic:* Skin rash was reported in 4.3% of patients treated with miglitol compared to 2.4% of placebo-treated patients. Rashes were generally transient, and most were assessed as unrelated to miglitol by physician-investigators.

➤*GI:* GI symptoms are the most common reactions to miglitol tablets. In US placebo-controlled trials, the incidences of abdominal pain, diarrhea, and flatulence were 11.7%, 28.7%, and 41.5%, respectively in 962 patients treated with miglitol 25 to 100 mg 3 times daily, whereas the corresponding incidences were 4.7%, 10%, and 12% in 603 placebo-treated patients. The incidence of diarrhea and abdominal pain tended to diminish considerably with continued treatment.

➤*Lab test abnormalities:* Low serum iron occurred more often in patients treated with miglitol (9.2%) than in placebo-treated patients (4.2%) but did not persist in the majority of cases and was not associated with reductions in hemoglobin or changes in other hematologic indices.

Overdosage

➤*Symptoms:* Unlike sulfonylureas or insulin, an overdose of miglitol tablets will not result in hypoglycemia. An overdose may result in transient increases in flatulence, diarrhea, and abdominal discomfort. Because of the lack of extra-intestinal effects seen with miglitol, no serious systemic reactions are expected in the event of an overdose.

Amylin Analog

PRAMLINTIDE ACETATE

Rx	**Symlin** (Amylin Pharmaceuticals, Inc.)	**Solution for injection**: 0.6 mg/mL[a]	In 5 mL vials.

[a] Contains metacresol 2.25 mg/mL as a preservative, D-mannitol as a tonicity modifier, and acetic acid and sodium acetate as pH modifiers.

PRAMLINTIDE ACETATE — INJECTION

WARNING

Pramlintide is used with insulin and has been associated with an increased risk of insulin-induced severe hypoglycemia, particularly in patients with type 1 diabetes. When severe hypoglycemia associated with pramlintide use occurs, it is seen within 3 hours following a pramlintide injection. If severe hypoglycemia occurs while operating a motor vehicle, heavy machinery, or while engaging in other high-risk activities, serious injuries may occur. Appropriate patient selection, careful patient instruction, and insulin dose adjustments are critical elements for reducing this risk.

Indications

➤*Type 1 diabetes mellitus:* As an adjunct treatment in patients who use mealtime insulin therapy and who have failed to achieve desired glucose control despite optimal insulin therapy.

➤*Type 2 diabetes mellitus:* As an adjunct treatment in patients who use mealtime insulin therapy and who have failed to achieve desired glucose control despite optimal insulin therapy, with or without a concurrent sulfonylurea agent and/or metformin.

Administration and Dosage

➤*Approved by the FDA:* March 16, 2005.

➤*Dosage:* Pramlintide dosage differs depending on whether the patient has type 2 or type 1 diabetes (see below). When initiating therapy with pramlintide, initial insulin dose reduction is required in all patients (both type 2 and type 1) to reduce the risk of insulin-induced hypoglycemia. Because this reduction in insulin may lead to glucose elevations, monitor patients at regular intervals to assess pramlintide tolerability and the effect on blood glucose so that individualized insulin adjustments may be initiated. If pramlintide therapy is discontinued for any reason (eg, surgery, illness), follow the same initiation protocol when pramlintide therapy is reinstituted.

➤*Initiation of therapy:*

Patients with insulin-using type 2 diabetes – In patients with insulin-using type 2 diabetes, initiate pramlintide at a dose of 60 mcg and increase to a dose of 120 mcg as tolerated. Instruct patients to:

- Initiate pramlintide at 60 mcg subcutaneously, immediately prior to major meals.
- Reduce preprandial, rapid-acting or short-acting insulin dosages, including fixed-mix insulins (eg, 70/30) by 50%.Dosage adjustments
- Increase the pramlintide dose to 120 mcg when no clinically significant nausea has occurred for 3 to 7 days. Make pramlintide dose adjustments only as directed by the health care provider. If significant nausea persists at the 120 mcg dose, decrease the pramlintide dose to 60 mcg.
- Adjust insulin doses to optimize glycemic control once the target dose of pramlintide is achieved and nausea (if experienced) has subsided. Make insulin dose adjustments only as directed by the health care provider.
- Contact a health care provider skilled in the use of insulin to review pramlintide and insulin dose adjustments at least once weekly until a target dose of pramlintide is achieved, pramlintide is well-tolerated, and blood glucose concentrations are stable.

Patients with type 1 diabetes – In patients with type 1 diabetes, initiate pramlintide at a dose of 15 mcg and titrate at 15 mcg increments to a maintenance dose of 30 or 60 mcg as tolerated. Instruct patients to:

- Initiate pramlintide at a starting dose of 15 mcg subcutaneously, immediately prior to major meals;
- Reduce preprandial, rapid-acting or short-acting insulin dosages, including fixed-mix insulins (eg, 70/30) by 50%;
- Increase the pramlintide dose to the next increment (30, 45, or 60 mcg) when no clinically significant nausea has occurred for at least 3 days. Only make pramlintide dose adjustments as directed by the health care provider. If significant nausea persists at the 45 or 60 mcg dose level, decrease the pramlintide dose to 30 mcg. If the 30 mcg dose is not tolerated, consider discontinuation of pramlintide therapy.
- Adjust insulin doses to optimize glycemic control once the target dose of pramlintide is achieved and nausea (if experienced) has subsided. Only make insulin dose adjustments as directed by the health care provider.
- Contact a health care professional skilled in the use of insulin to review pramlintide and insulin dose adjustments at least once weekly until a target dose of pramlintide is achieved, pramlintide is well-tolerated, and blood glucose concentrations are stable.

➤*Optimizing therapy (type 1 and type 2 diabetic patients):* After a maintenance dose of pramlintide is achieved, instruct both insulin-using patients with type 2 diabetes and patients with type 1 diabetes to:

- Adjust insulin doses to optimize glycemic control once the target dose of pramlintide is achieved and nausea (if experienced) has subsided. Only make insulin dose adjustments as directed by a health care provider.
- Contact a health care provider in the event of recurrent nausea or hypoglycemia. View an increased frequency of mild to moderate hypoglycemia as a warning sign of increased risk for severe hypoglycemia.

➤*Administration:* Administer pramlintide subcutaneously immediately prior to each major meal (250 or more kcal or containing 30 g or more of carbohydrate). If a pramlintide dose is missed, do not give an additional injection.

To administer pramlintide from vials, use a U-100 insulin syringe (preferably a 0.3 mL [0.3 cc] size) for optimal accuracy. If using a syringe calibrated for use with U-100 insulin, use the following chart to measure the microgram dosage in unit increments.

Conversion of Pramlintide Dose to Insulin Unit Equivalents

Pramlintide dosage prescribed (mcg)	Increment using a U-100 syringe (units)	Volume (cc or mL)
15	2.5	0.025
30	5	0.05
45	7.5	0.075
60	10	0.1
120	20	0.2

Administer each pramlintide dose subcutaneously into the abdomen or thigh (administration into the arm is not recommended because of variable absorption). Rotate injection sites so that the same site is not used repeatedly. The injection site selected should also be distinct from the site chosen for any concomitant insulin injection. Always use a new syringe and needle to give pramlintide and insulin injections.

Mixing incompatibilities –

- Always administer pramlintide and insulin as separate injections.
- Do not mix pramlintide with any type of insulin.

➤*Discontinuation of therapy:* Discontinue pramlintide therapy if any of the following occur:

- Recurrent unexplained hypoglycemia that requires medical assistance
- Persistent clinically significant nausea
- Noncompliance with self-monitoring of blood glucose concentrations

PRAMLINTIDE ACETATE — INJECTION

- Noncompliance with insulin dose adjustments
- Noncompliance with scheduled health care professional contacts or recommended clinic visits

➤*Preparation and handling:* Inspect pramlintide visually for particulate matter or discoloration prior to administration whenever the solution and the container permit.

➤*Storage/Stability:*

Unopened (not in-use) vials – Before use, refrigerate pramlintide vials at 36° to 46°F (2° to 8°C), and protect from light. Do not freeze. If a vial has been frozen or overheated, throw it away.

Opened (in-use) vials – Keep opened vials in use (punctured) refrigerated or at room temperature for up to 28 days as long as the temperature is not more than 77°F (25°C). Opened vials, whether or not refrigerated, must be used within 28 days. Discard after 28 days.

Storage Conditions and Stability of Pramlintide (5 mL vials)

	Unopened (not in-use) refrigerated	Open (in-use) refrigerated or room temperature
5 mL vial	Until expiration date	Use within 28 days

Actions

➤*Pharmacology:* Amylin is co-located with insulin in secretory granules and co-secreted with insulin by pancreatic beta cells in response to food intake. Amylin and insulin show similar fasting and postprandial patterns in healthy individuals.

Amylin affects the rate of postprandial glucose appearance through a variety of mechanisms. Amylin slows gastric emptying (ie, the rate at which food is released from the stomach to the small intestine) without altering the overall absorption of nutrients. In addition, amylin suppresses glucagon secretion (not normalized by insulin alone), which leads to suppression of endogenous glucose output from the liver. Amylin also regulates food intake caused by centrally-mediated modulation of appetite.

In patients with insulin-using type 2 or type 1 diabetes, the pancreatic beta cells are dysfunctional or damaged, resulting in reduced secretion of insulin and amylin in response to food.

Pramlintide, by acting as an amylinomimetic agent, has the following effects: 1) modulation of gastric emptying; 2) prevention of the postprandial rise in plasma glucagon; and 3) satiety leading to decreased caloric intake and potential weight loss.

Gastric emptying – The gastric-emptying rate is an important determinant of the postprandial rise in plasma glucose. Pramlintide slows the rate at which food is released from the stomach to the small intestine after a meal, and, thus, it reduces the initial postprandial increase in plasma glucose. This effect lasts for approximately 3 hours after pramlintide administration. Pramlintide does not alter the net absorption of ingested carbohydrate or other nutrients.

Postprandial glucagon secretion – In patients with diabetes, glucagon concentrations are abnormally elevated during the postprandial period, contributing to hyperglycemia. Pramlintide has been shown to decrease postprandial glucagon concentrations in insulin-using patients with diabetes.

Satiety – Pramlintide administered prior to a meal has been shown to reduce total caloric intake. This effect appears to be independent of the nausea that may accompany pramlintide treatment.

➤*Pharmacokinetics:*

Absorption – The absolute bioavailability of a single subcutaneous dose of pramlintide is approximately 30% to 40%. Subcutaneous administration of different doses of pramlintide into the abdominal area or thigh of healthy subjects resulted in dose-proportionate maximum plasma concentrations (C_{max}) and overall exposure (expressed as area under the plasma concentration curve or [AUC]) (see the following table).

Mean Pharmacokinetic Parameters Following Administration of Single Subcutaneous Doses of Pramlintide

Subcutaneous dose (mcg)	$AUC_{(0-\infty)}$ (pmol•min/L)	C_{max} (pmol/L)	T_{max} (min)	Elimination t½ (min)
30	3,750	39	21	55
60	6,778	79	20	49
90	8,507	102	19	51
120	11,970	147	21	48

Injection of pramlintide into the arm showed higher exposure with greater variability compared with exposure after injection of pramlintide into the abdominal area or thigh.

There was no strong correlation between the degree of adiposity as assessed by body mass index (BMI) or skin fold thickness measurements and relative bioavailability. Injections administered with 6 and 12.7 mm needles yielded similar bioavailability.

Distribution – Pramlintide does not bind extensively to blood cells or albumin (approximately 40% of the drug is unbound in plasma), and thus pramlintide's pharmacokinetics should be insensitive to changes in binding sites.

Metabolism/Excretion – In healthy subjects, the half-life of pramlintide is approximately 48 minutes. Pramlintide is metabolized primarily by the kidneys. Des-lys[1] pramlintide (2-37 pramlintide), the primary metabolite, has a similar half-life and is biologically active both in vitro and in vivo in rats. AUC values are relatively constant with repeat dosing, indicating no bioaccumulation.

Pharmacodynamics – In clinical studies in patients with insulin-using type 2 and type 1 diabetes, pramlintide administration resulted in a reduction in mean postprandial glucose concentrations, reduced glucose fluctuations, and reduced food intake. Pramlintide doses differ for insulin-using type 2 and type 1 patients.

Reduction in postprandial glucose concentrations: Pramlintide administered subcutaneously immediately prior to a meal reduced plasma glucose concentrations after the meal when used with regular insulin or rapid-acting insulin analogs. This reduction in postprandial glucose decreased the amount of short-acting insulin required and limited glucose fluctuations based upon 24-hour glucose monitoring. When rapid-acting analog insulins were used, plasma glucose concentrations tended to rise during the interval between 150 minutes following pramlintide injection and the next meal.

Reduced food intake: A single, subcutaneous dose of pramlintide 120 mcg (type 2 diabetes) or 30 mcg (type 1 diabetes) administered 1 hour prior to an unlimited buffet meal was associated with reductions in total caloric intake (placebo-subtracted mean changes of approximately 23% and 21%, respectively), which occurred without decreases in meal duration.

Contraindications

Hypersensitivity to pramlintide or any of its components, including metacresol; a confirmed diagnosis of gastroparesis; hypoglycemia unawareness.

Warnings

➤*Patient selection:* Proper patient selection is critical to safe and effective use of pramlintide.

Before initiation of therapy, review the patient's HbA_{1c}, recent blood glucose monitoring data, history of insulin-induced hypoglycemia, current insulin regimen, and body weight. Only consider pramlintide therapy in patients with insulin-using type 2 or type 1 diabetes who have failed to achieve adequate glycemic control despite individualized insulin management and who are receiving ongoing care under the guidance of a health care professional skilled in the use of insulin and supported by the services of diabetes educator(s).

Do not consider patients meeting any of the following criteria for pramlintide therapy: poor compliance with current insulin regimen; poor compliance with prescribed self-blood glucose monitoring; have an HbA_{1c} greater than 9%; recurrent severe hypoglycemia requiring assistance during the past 6 months; presence of hypoglycemia unawareness; confirmed diagnosis of gastroparesis; require the use of drugs that stimulate GI motility; pediatric patients.

➤*Hypoglycemia:* Pramlintide alone does not cause hypoglycemia. However, pramlintide is indicated to be coadministered with insulin therapy, and, in this setting, pramlintide increases the risk of insulin-induced severe hypoglycemia, particularly in patients with type 1 diabetes. Severe hypoglycemia associated with pramlintide occurs within the first 3 hours following a pramlintide injection. If severe hypoglycemia occurs while operating a motor vehicle, heavy machinery, or while engaging in other high-risk activities, serious injuries may occur. Therefore, when introducing pramlintide therapy, take appropriate precautions to avoid increasing the risk for insulin-induced severe hypoglycemia. These precautions include frequent pre- and post-meal glucose monitoring combined with an initial 50% reduction in pre-meal doses of short-acting insulin.

Symptoms of hypoglycemia may include hunger, headache, sweating, tremor, irritability, or difficulty concentrating. Rapid reductions in blood glucose concentrations may induce such symptoms regardless of glucose values. More severe symptoms of hypoglycemia include loss of consciousness, coma, or seizure.

Early warning symptoms of hypoglycemia may be different or less pronounced under certain conditions, such as long duration of diabetes; diabetic nerve disease; use of medications such as beta-blockers, clonidine, guanethidine, or reserpine; or intensified diabetes control.

Clinical studies employing a controlled hypoglycemic challenge have demonstrated that pramlintide does not alter the counter-regulatory hormonal response to insulin-induced hypoglycemia. Likewise, in pramlintide-treated patients, the perception of hypoglycemic symptoms was not altered with plasma glucose concentrations as low as 45 mg/dL.

Drugs that increase the susceptibility to hypoglycemia – The addition of any antihyperglycemic agent (eg, pramlintide) to an existing regimen of 1 or more antihyperglycemic agents (eg, insulin, sulfonylurea) or to other agents that may increase the risk of hypoglycemia may necessitate further insulin dose adjustments and particularly close monitoring of blood glucose.

The following are examples of substances that may increase the blood glucose-lowering effect and susceptibility to hypoglycemia: oral antidiabetic products, angiotensin-converting enzyme (ACE) inhibitors, disopyramide, fibrates, fluoxetine, monoamine oxidase (MAO) inhibitors, pentoxifylline, propoxyphene, salicylates, and sulfonamide antibiotics.

➤*Hypersensitivity reactions:*

Local – Patients may experience redness, swelling, or itching at the site of injection. These minor reactions usually resolve within a few days to a few weeks. In some instances, these reactions may be related to factors other than pramlintide, such as irritants in a skin-cleansing agent or improper injection technique.

Systemic – In controlled clinical trials up to 12 months, potential systemic allergic reactions were reported in 65 (5%) of type 2 patients and 59 (5%) of type 1 pramlintide-treated patients. Similar reactions were reported by 18 (4%) and 28 (5%) of placebo-treated type 2 and type 1 patients, respectively.

PRAMLINTIDE ACETATE — INJECTION

No patient receiving pramlintide was withdrawn from a trial because of a potential systemic allergic reaction.

➤*Fertility impairment:* Administration of 0.3, 1, or 3 mg/kg/day of pramlintide (8, 17, and 82 times the exposure resulting from the maximum recommended human dose based on body surface area, respectively) had no significant effects on fertility in male or female rats. The highest dose of 3 mg/kg/day resulted in dystocia in 8/12 female rats secondary to significant decreases in serum calcium levels.

➤*Elderly:* Pramlintide has been studied in patients ranging in age from 15 to 84 years of age, including 539 patients 65 years of age or older. The change in HbA_{1c} values and hypoglycemia frequencies did not differ by age, but greater sensitivity in some older individuals cannot be ruled out. Thus, carefully manage pramlintide and insulin regimens to obviate an increased risk of severe hypoglycemia.

➤*Pregnancy: Category C* No adequate and well-controlled studies have been conducted in pregnant women. Studies in perfused human placenta indicate that pramlintide has low potential to cross the maternal/fetal placental barrier. Embryofetal toxicity studies with pramlintide have been performed in rats and rabbits. Increases in congenital abnormalities (neural tube defect, cleft palate, exencephaly) were observed in fetuses of rats treated during organogenesis with 0.3 and 1 mg/kg/day (10 and 47 times the exposure resulting from the maximum recommended human dose based on AUC, respectively). Administration of doses up to 0.3 mg/kg/day pramlintide (9 times maximum recommended dose based on AUC) to pregnant rabbits had no adverse effects in embryofetal development; however, animal reproduction studies are not always predictive of human response. Only use pramlintide during pregnancy if it is determined by the health care provider that the potential benefit justifies the potential risk to the fetus.

➤*Lactation:* It is unknown whether pramlintide is excreted in human milk. Many drugs, including peptide drugs, are excreted in human milk. Therefore, administer pramlintide to nursing women only if it is determined by the health care provider that the potential benefit outweighs the potential risk to the infant.

➤*Children:* Safety and efficacy in children have not been established.

Precautions

➤*Monitoring:* Monitor blood glucose frequently, including pre- and post-meals and at bedtime.

➤*Hazardous tasks:* Severe hypoglycemia associated with pramlintide occurs within the first 3 hours following a pramlintide injection. If severe hypoglycemia occurs while operating a motor vehicle, heavy machinery, or while engaging in other high-risk activities, serious injuries may occur. Therefore, when introducing pramlintide therapy, take appropriate precautions to avoid increasing the risk for insulin-induced severe hypoglycemia. These precautions include frequent pre- and post-meal glucose monitoring combined with an initial 50% reduction in pre-meal doses of short-acting insulin.

Drug Interactions

➤*Drugs that alter GI motility / absorption:* Because of its effects on gastric emptying, do not consider pramlintide therapy for patients taking drugs that alter GI motility (eg, anticholinergic agents such as atropine) and agents that slow the intestinal absorption of nutrients (eg, alpha-glucosidase inhibitors). Patients using these drugs have not been studied in clinical trials.

➤*Pramlintide delays absorption of concomitantly administered drugs:* Pramlintide has the potential to delay the absorption of coadministered oral medications. When the rapid onset of an orally coadministered agent is a critical determinant of effectiveness (eg, analgesics), administer the agent at least 1 hour prior to or 2 hours after pramlintide injection.

Adverse Reactions

Adverse reactions (excluding hypoglycemia) commonly associated with pramlintide when coadministered with a fixed dose of insulin in the long-term, placebo-controlled trials in insulin-using type 2 diabetic patients and type 1 diabetic patients are presented in the table below and the following table, respectively. The same adverse reactions were also shown in the open-label clinical practice study, which employed flexible insulin dosing

Pramlintide Adverse Reactions (≥ 5% and Incidence Greater Than Placebo) in Patients with Insulin-using Type 2 Diabetes

	Long-term, placebo-controlled studies		Open-label, clinical practice study
Adverse reactions	Placebo + Insulin (N = 284)	Pramlintide + Insulin (N = 292)	Pramlintide + Insulin (N = 166)
CNS			
Dizziness	11 (4%)	17 (6%)	3 (2%)
Fatigue	11 (4%)	20 (7%)	5 (3%)
Headache	19 (7%)	39 (13%)	8 (5%)
GI			
Abdominal Pain	19 (7%)	23 (8%)	3 (2%)
Anorexia	5 (2%)	27 (9%)	1 (< 1%)
Nausea	34 (12%)	81 (28%)	53 (30%)
Vomiting	12 (4%)	24 (8%)	13 (7%)

Pramlintide Adverse Reactions (≥ 5% and Incidence Greater Than Placebo) in Patients with Insulin-using Type 2 Diabetes

	Long-term, placebo-controlled studies		Open-label, clinical practice study
Adverse reactions	Placebo + Insulin (N = 284)	Pramlintide + Insulin (N = 292)	Pramlintide + Insulin (N = 166)
Respiratory			
Coughing	12 (4%)	18 (6%)	4 (2%)
Pharyngitis	7 (2%)	15 (5%)	6 (3%)

Pramlintide Adverse Reactions (≥ 5% and Incidence Greater than Placebo) in Patients with Type 1 Diabetes

	Long-term, placebo-controlled studies		Open-label, clinical practice study
Adverse reactions	Placebo + insulin (N = 538)	Pramlintide + insulin (N = 716)	Pramlintide + insulin (N = 265)
CNS			
Dizziness	21 (4%)	34 (5%)	5 (2%)
Fatigue	22 (4%)	51 (7%)	12 (4.5%)
GI			
Anorexia	12 (2%)	122 (17%)	0 (0%)
Nausea	92 (17%)	342 (48%)	98 (37%)
Vomiting	36 (7%)	82 (11%)	18 (7%)
Miscellaneous			
Allergic Reaction	28 (5%)	41 (6%)	1 (< 1%)
Arthralgia	27 (5%)	51 (7%)	6 (2%)
Inflicted Injury	55 (10%)	97 (14%)	20 (8%)

GI – Most adverse events were GI in nature. In patients with type 2 or type 1 diabetes, the incidence of nausea was higher at the beginning of pramlintide treatment and decreased with time in most patients. The incidence and severity of nausea are reduced when pramlintide is gradually titrated to the recommended doses.

➤*Severe hypoglycemia:* Pramlintide alone (without the coadministration of insulin) does not cause hypoglycemia. However, pramlintide is indicated as an adjunct treatment in patients who use mealtime insulin therapy, and coadministration of pramlintide with insulin may increase the risk of insulin-induced hypoglycemia, particularly in patients with type 1 diabetes. The incidence of severe hypoglycemia during the pramlintide clinical development program is summarized in the following tables.

Severe Hypoglycemia in Patients with Insulin-Using Type 2 Diabetes

	Long-term, placebo-controlled studies (no insulin dose-reduction during initiation)				Open-label, clinical practice study (insulin dose-reduction during initiation)	
	Placebo + Insulin		Pramlintide + Insulin		Pramlintide + Insulin	
Severe hypoglycemia	0 to 3 months (n = 284)	More than 3 to 6 months (n = 251)	0 to 3 months (n = 292)	More than 3 to 6 months (n = 255)	0 to 3 months (n = 166)	More than 3 to 6 months (n = 150)
Patient-ascertained[a]						
Reaction rate (reaction rate/ patient year)	0.24	0.13	0.45	0.39	0.05	0.03
Incidence (%)	2.1%	2.4%	8.2%	4.7%	0.6%	0.7%
Medically assisted[b]						
Reaction rate (reaction rate/ patient year)	0.06	0.07	0.09	0.02	0.05	0.03
Incidence (%)	0.7%	1.2%	1.7%	0.4%	0.6%	0.7%

[a] Patient-ascertained severe hypoglycemia: Requiring the assistance of another individual (including aid in ingestion of oral carbohydrate), and/or requiring the administration of glucagon injection, IV glucose, or other medical intervention.

[b] Medically assisted severe hypoglycemia: Requiring glucagon, IV glucose, hospitalization, paramedic assistance, emergency room visit, and/or assessed as a serious adverse event (SAE) by the investigator.

Severe Hypoglycemia in Practice Studies in Patients with Type 1 Diabetes

	Long-term, placebo-controlled studies (no insulin dose-reduction during initiation)				Open-label, clinical practice study (insulin dose-reduction during initiation)	
	Placebo + Insulin		Pramlintide + Insulin		Pramlintide + Insulin	
Severe hypoglycemia	0 to 3 months (n = 538)	More than 3 to 6 months (n = 470)	0 to 3 months (n = 716)	More than 3 to 6 months (n = 576)	0 to 3 months (n = 265)	More than 3 to 6 months (n = 213)
Patient-ascertained[a]						
Reaction rate (reaction rate/ patient year)	1.33	1.06	1.55	0.82	0.29	0.16
Incidence (%)	10.8	8.7	16.8	11.1	5.7	3.8

Amylin Analog

PRAMLINTIDE ACETATE — INJECTION

Severe Hypoglycemia in Practice Studies in Patients with Type 1 Diabetes

	Long-term, placebo-controlled studies (no insulin dose-reduction during initiation)				Open-label, clinical practice study (insulin dose-reduction during initiation)	
	Placebo + Insulin		Pramlintide + Insulin		Pramlintide + Insulin	
Severe hypoglycemia	0 to 3 months (n = 538)	More than 3 to 6 months (n = 470)	0 to 3 months (n = 716)	More than 3 to 6 months (n = 576)	0 to 3 months (n = 265)	More than 3 to 6 months (n = 213)
Medically assisted[b]						
Reaction rate (reaction rate/ patient year)	0.19	0.24	0.50	0.27	0.1	0.04
Incidence (%)	3.3	4.3	7.3	5.2	2.3	0.9

[a] Patient-ascertained severe hypoglycemia: Requiring the assistance of another individual (including aid in ingestion of oral carbohydrate); and/or requiring the administration of glucagon injection, IV glucose, or other medical intervention.

[b] Medically assisted severe hypoglycemia: Requiring glucagon, IV glucose, hospitalization, paramedic assistance, emergency room visit, and/or assessed as an SAE by the investigator.

Overdosage

➤*Symptoms:* Single doses of pramlintide 10 mg (83 times the maximum dose of 120 mcg) were administered to 3 healthy volunteers. Severe nausea was reported in all 3 individuals and was associated with vomiting, diarrhea, vasodilatation, and dizziness. No hypoglycemia was reported.

➤*Treatment:* Pramlintide has a short half-life and, in the case of overdose, supportive measures are indicated.

Patient Information

Inform patients of the potential risks and advantages of pramlintide therapy. Also inform patients about self-management practices including glucose monitoring, proper injection technique, timing of dosing, and proper storage of pramlintide. In addition, advise patients of the importance of adherence to meal planning, physical activity, recognition and management of hypoglycemia and hyperglycemia, and assessment of diabetes complications. Refer patients to the pramlintide Medication Guide for additional information.

Instruct patients on handling of special situations such as intercurrent conditions (illness or stress), an inadequate or omitted insulin dose, inadvertent administration of increased insulin or pramlintide dose, inadequate food intake, or missed meals.

Always administer pramlintide and insulin as separate injections and never mix the injections.

Advise women with diabetes to inform their health care provider if they are pregnant or planning to become pregnant.

Incretin Mimetic Agents

EXENATIDE

Rx	**Byetta** (Amylin Pharmaceuticals, Inc.)	**Subcutaneous injection**: 5 mcg/dose	In 1.2 mL prefilled pens (60 doses).
		10 mcg/dose	In 2.4 mL prefilled pen (60 doses).

EXENATIDE — INJECTION

Indications

➤*Type 2 diabetes mellitus:* As adjunctive therapy to improve glycemic control in patients with type 2 diabetes mellitus who are taking metformin, a sulfonylurea, or a combination of metformin and a sulfonylurea but have not achieved adequate glycemic control.

Administration and Dosage

➤*Approved by the FDA:* April 29, 2005.

➤*Dosage:* Exenatide therapy should be initiated at 5 mcg per dose administered twice daily at any time within the 60-minute period before the morning and evening meals. Exenatide should not be administered exenatide after a meal. Based on clinical response, the dose of exenatide can be increased to 10 mcg twice daily after 1 month of therapy. Each dose should be administered as a subcutaneous injection in the thigh, abdomen, or upper arm.

➤*Concomitant therapy:* Exenatide is recommended for use in patients with type 2 diabetes mellitus who are already receiving metformin, a sulfonylurea, or both and have suboptimal glycemic control. When exenatide is added to metformin therapy, the current dose of metformin can be continued as it is unlikely that the dose of metformin will require adjustment due to hypoglycemia when used with exenatide. When exenatide is added to sulfonylurea therapy, a reduction in the dose of sulfonylurea may be considered to reduce the risk of hypoglycemia.

➤*Storage/Stability:* Refrigerate exenatide at 36° to 46°F (2° to 8°C); protect from light. Discard the pen 30 days after first use, even if some drug remains in the pen. Do not freeze. Do not use exenatide if it has been frozen.

Exenatide is a clear and colorless liquid and should not be used if particles appear or if the solution is cloudy or colored.

Actions

➤*Pharmacology:* Incretins, such as glucagon-like peptide-1 (GLP-1), enhance glucose-dependent insulin secretion and exhibit other antihyperglycemic actions following their release into the circulation from the gut. Exenatide is an incretin mimetic agent that mimics the enhancement of glucose-dependent insulin secretion and several other antihyperglycemic actions of incretins.

The amino acid sequence of exenatide partially overlaps that of human GLP-1. Exenatide has been shown to bind and activate the known human GLP-1 receptor in vitro. This leads to an increase in both glucose-dependent synthesis of insulin, and in vivo secretion of insulin from pancreatic beta cells, by mechanisms involving cyclic adenosine monophosphate (AMP) and/or other intracellular signaling pathways. Exenatide promotes insulin release from beta cells in the presence of elevated glucose concentrations. When administered in vivo, exenatide mimics certain antihyperglycemic actions of GLP-1.

Exenatide improves glycemic control by reducing fasting and postprandial glucose concentrations in patients with type 2 diabetes through the actions described below.

Glucose-dependent insulin secretion – Exenatide has acute effects on pancreatic beta-cell responsiveness to glucose and leads to insulin release only in the presence of elevated glucose concentrations. This insulin secretion subsides as blood glucose concentrations decrease and approach euglycemia.

First-phase insulin response – In healthy individuals, robust insulin secretion occurs during the first 10 minutes following intravenous (IV) glucose administration. This secretion, known as the first-phase insulin response, is characteristically absent in patients with type 2 diabetes. The loss of the first-phase insulin response is an early beta-cell defect in type 2 diabetes. Administration of exenatide at therapeutic plasma concentrations restored first-phase insulin response to an IV bolus of glucose in patients with type 2 diabetes. Both first-phase insulin secretion and second-phase insulin secretion were significantly increased in patients with type 2 diabetes treated with exenatide compared with saline ($P < 0.001$ for both).

Patients received an IV infusion of insulin for 6.5 hours (discontinued at time [t] = -30 minutes) to normalize plasma glucose concentrations and a continuous IV infusion of either exenatide or saline for 5 hours beginning 3 hours prior to an IV bolus of glucose (0.3 g/kg over 30 seconds) at t = 0 minutes.

Glucagon secretion – In patients with type 2 diabetes, exenatide moderates glucagon secretion and lowers serum glucagon concentrations during periods of hyperglycemia. Lower glucagon concentrations lead to decreased hepatic glucose output and decreased insulin demand. However, exenatide does not impair the normal glucagon response to hypoglycemia.

Gastric emptying – Exenatide slows gastric emptying, thereby reducing the rate at which meal-derived glucose appears in the circulation.

Food intake – In both animals and humans, administration of exenatide has been shown to reduce food intake.

Pharmacodynamics –

Postprandial glucose: In patients with type 2 diabetes, exenatide reduces the postprandial plasma glucose concentrations.

Fasting glucose: In a single-dose crossover study in patients with type 2 diabetes and fasting hyperglycemia, an immediate insulin release followed injection of exenatide. Plasma glucose concentrations were significantly reduced with exenatide compared with placebo.

➤*Pharmacokinetics:*

Absorption – After subcutaneous administration to patients with type 2 diabetes, exenatide reaches median peak plasma concentrations in 2.1 hours. Mean peak exenatide concentration (C_{max}) was 211 pg/mL and overall mean area under the curve (AUC_{0-inf}) was 1,036 pg•h/mL following subcutaneous administration of exenatide 10 mcg. Exenatide exposure (AUC) increased proportionally over the therapeutic dose range of 5 to 10 mcg. The C_{max} values increased less than proportionally over the same range. Similar exposure is achieved with subcutaneous administration of exenatide in the abdomen, thigh, or arm.

Distribution – The mean apparent volume of distribution of exenatide after SC administration of a single dose of exenatide is 28.3 L.

Metabolism/Excretion – Nonclinical studies have shown that exenatide is predominantly eliminated by glomerular filtration with subsequent proteolytic degradation. The mean apparent clearance of exenatide in humans is 9.1 L/h and the mean terminal half-life is 2.4 hours. These pharmacokinetic characteristics of exenatide are independent of the dose. In most individuals, exenatide concentrations are measurable for approximately 10 hours post-dose.

Special populations –

Renal function impairment: In patients with mild to moderate renal impairment (Ccr 30 to 80 mL/min), exenatide clearance was only mildly reduced; therefore, no dosage adjustment of exenatide is required in patients with mild to moderate renal impairment. However, in patients with end-stage renal disease receiving dialysis, mean exenatide clearance is reduced to 0.9 L/h compared with 9.1 L/h in healthy subjects.

EXENATIDE — INJECTION

Contraindications

Hypersensitivity to this product or any of its components.

Warnings

➤*Carcinogenesis:* A 104-week carcinogenicity study was conducted in male and female rats at doses of 18, 70, or 250 mcg/kg/day administered by bolus subcutaneous injection. Benign thyroid C-cell adenomas were observed in female rats at all exenatide doses. The incidences in female rats were 8% and 5% in the 2 control groups and 14%, 11%, and 23% in the low-, medium-, and high-dose groups with systemic exposures of 5, 22, and 130 times, respectively, the human exposure resulting from the maximum recommended dose of 20 mcg/day, based on AUC.

➤*Pregnancy: Category C.* Exenatide has been shown to cause reduced fetal and neonatal growth, and skeletal effects in mice at systemic exposures 3 times the human exposure resulting from the maximum recommended dose of 20 mcg/day, based on AUC. Exenatide has been shown to cause skeletal effects in rabbits at systemic exposures 12 times the human exposure resulting from the maximum recommended dose of 20 mcg/day, based on AUC. There are no adequate and well-controlled studies in pregnant women. Use exenatide during pregnancy only if the potential benefit justifies the potential risk to the fetus.

In pregnant mice given subcutaneous doses of 6, 68, 460, or 760 mcg/kg/day from gestation day 6 through 15 (organogenesis), cleft palate (some with holes), and irregular skeletal ossification of rib and skull bones were observed at 6 mcg/kg/day, a systemic exposure 3 times the human exposure resulting from the maximum recommended dose of 20 mcg/kg/day, based on AUC.

In pregnant rabbits given subcutaneous doses of 0.2, 2, 22, 156, or 260 mcg/kg/day from gestation day 6 through 18 (organogenesis), irregular skeletal ossifications were observed at 2 mcg/kg/day, a systemic exposure 12 times the human exposure resulting from the maximum recommended dose of 20 mcg/day, based on AUC.

In pregnant mice given subcutaneous doses of 6, 68, or 760 mcg/kg/day from gestation day 6 through lactation day 20 (weaning), an increased number of neonatal deaths were observed on postpartum days 2-4 in dams given 6 mcg/kg/day, a systemic exposure 3 times the human exposure resulting from the maximum recommended dose of 20 mcg/day, based on AUC.

➤*Lactation:* It is not known whether exenatide is excreted in human milk. Many drugs are excreted in human milk and because of the potential for clinically significant adverse reactions in nursing infants from exenatide, decide whether to discontinue breast-feeding or discontinue the drug, taking into account the importance of the drug to the mother. Studies in lactating mice have demonstrated that exenatide is present at low concentrations in milk (less than or equal to 2.5% of the concentration in maternal plasma following subcutaneous dosing). Exercise caution when exenatide is administered to a breast-feeding woman.

➤*Children:* Safety and efficacy of exenatide have not been established in pediatric patients.

Precautions

➤*Insulin:* Exenatide is not a substitute for insulin in insulin-requiring patients. Do not use exenatide in patients with type 1 diabetes or for the treatment of diabetic ketoacidosis. The concurrent use of exenatide with insulin, thiazolidinediones, D-phenylalanine derivatives, meglitinides, or alpha-glucosidase inhibitors has not been studied.

➤*Renal impairment:* Exenatide is not recommended for use in patients with end-stage renal disease or severe renal impairment (Ccr less than 30 mL/min). In patients with end-stage renal disease receiving dialysis, single doses of exenatide 5 mcg were not well tolerated due to gastrointestinal side effects.

➤*GI disease:* Exenatide has not been studied in patients with severe GI disease, including gastroparesis. Its use is commonly associated with GI adverse effects, including nausea, vomiting, and diarrhea. Therefore, the use of exenatide is not recommended in patients with severe GI disease.

➤*Hypoglycemia:* In the 30-week controlled clinical trials with exenatide, a hypoglycemia episode was recorded as an adverse event if the patient reported symptoms associated with hypoglycemia with an accompanying blood glucose less than 60 mg/dL or if symptoms were reported without an accompanying blood glucose measurement. When exenatide was used in combination with metformin, no increase in the incidence of hypoglycemia was observed over that of placebo in combination with metformin. In contrast, when exenatide was used in combination with a sulfonylurea, the incidence of hypoglycemia was increased over that of placebo in combination with a sulfonylurea. Therefore, patients receiving exenatide in combination with a sulfonylurea may have an increased risk of hypoglycemia. To reduce the risk of hypoglycemia associated with the use of a sulfonylurea, reduction in the dose of sulfonylurea may be considered.

Exenatide did not alter the counter-regulatory hormone responses to insulin-induced hypoglycemia in a randomized, double-blind, controlled study in healthy subjects.

➤*Immunogenicity:* Consistent with the potentially immunogenic properties of protein and peptide pharmaceuticals, patients may develop anti-exenatide antibodies following treatment with exenatide. In most patients who develop antibodies, antibody titers diminish with time. In the 30-week controlled trials, 38% of patients had low titer anti-exenatide antibodies at 30 weeks. For this group, the level of glycemic control (HbA_{1c}) was generally comparable to that observed in those without antibody titers. An additional 6% of patients had higher titer antibodies at 30 weeks. In about half of this 6% (3% of the total patients given exenatide in the controlled studies), the glycemic response to exenatide appeared attenuated; the remainder had a glycemic response consistent with that of patients without antibodies. Patients who developed anti-exenatide antibodies had similar rates and types of adverse events as those with no anti-exenatide antibodies.

Drug Interactions

The effect of exenatide to slow gastric emptying may reduce the extent and rate of absorption of oral drugs. Use exenatide with caution in patients receiving oral medications that require rapid GI absorption. For oral medications that are dependent on threshold concentrations for efficacy, such as contraceptives and antibiotics, advise patients to take those drugs at least 1 hour before exenatide. If such drugs are to be administered with food, advise patients to take them with a meal or snack when exenatide is not administered. The effect of exenatide on the absorption and effectiveness of oral contraceptives has not been characterized.

Exenatide Drug Interactions

Precipitant drug	Object drug[a]		Description
Exenatide	Acetaminophen	⬇	When given concomitantly, acetaminophen AUC and C_{max} decreased and T_{max} increased. Give acetaminophen 1 hour before exenatide injection.
Exenatide	Digoxin	⬇	Coadministration of repeated doses of exenatide decreased digoxin C_{max} 17% and delayed T_{max} approximately 2.5 hours. AUC was not changed.
Exenatide	Lisinopril	⬇	Lisinopril steady-state T_{max} was delayed 2 hours.
Exenatide	Lovastatin	⬇	Lovastatin AUC and C_{max} were decreased ≈ 40% and 28%, respectively, and T_{max} was delayed approximately 4 hours when administered concomitantly with exenatide.
Exenatide	Oral antibiotics	⬇	Advise patients to take oral antibiotics at least 1 hour before exenatide injection.
Exenatide	Oral contraceptives	⬇	Advise patients to take oral contraceptives at least 1 hour before exenatide injection.

[a] ⬇ = drug decrease.

Adverse Reactions

➤*Hypoglycemia:* In the 30-week controlled clinical trials with exenatide, an adverse event of hypoglycemia was recorded if the patient reported symptoms subjectively associated with hypoglycemia with an accompanying blood glucose less than 60 mg/dL or if symptoms were reported without an accompanying blood glucose measurement. In patients treated with exenatide and a sulfonylurea or exenatide with both metformin and a sulfonylurea, hypoglycemia appeared to be dependent on the doses of both exenatide and the sulfonylurea. Most episodes of hypoglycemia were mild to moderate in intensity, and all resolved with oral administration of carbohydrate. Hypoglycemia was rarely observed in patients treated with the combination of exenatide and metformin and was similar in incidence to patients treated with placebo and metformin (see the following table).

Incidence (%) of Hypoglycemia[a] by Concomitant Antidiabetic Therapy

		Exenatide			Exenatide			Exenatide	
	Placebo twice daily	5 mcg twice daily	10 mcg twice daily	Placebo twice daily	5 mcg twice daily	10 mcg twice daily	Placebo twice daily	5 mcg twice daily	10 mcg twice daily
	With metformin			With a sulfonylurea			With metformin/sulfonylurea		
N	113	110	113	123	125	129	247	245	241
Hypoglycemia	5.3%	4.5%	5.3%	3.3%	14.4%	35.7%	12.6%	19.2%	27.8%

[a] In three 30-week placebo-controlled clinical trials, exenatide and placebo were administered before the morning and evening meals.

➤*Other adverse reactions:* Adverse events with an incidence greater than or equal to 5% (excluding hypoglycemia; see previous table) that occurred more frequently in exenatide-treated patients compared with placebo-treated patients are summarized in the following table.

Exenatide Adverse Reactions (≥ 5%) Excluding Hypoglycemia[a]

Adverse Reactions	Placebo twice daily n = 483	All exenatide twice daily n = 963
CNS		
Dizziness	6%	9%
Feeling jittery	4%	9%
Headache	6%	9%
GI		
Diarrhea	6%	13%
Dyspepsia	3%	6%

Incretin Mimetic Agents

EXENATIDE — INJECTION

Exenatide Adverse Reactions (≥ 5%) Excluding Hypoglycemia[a]		
	Placebo twice daily	All exenatide twice daily
Adverse Reactions	n = 483	n = 963
Nausea	18%	44%
Vomiting	4%	13%

[a] In three 30-week, placebo-controlled clinical trials.

In the three, 30-week controlled trials, adverse events associated with exenatide generally were mild to moderate in intensity. The most frequently reported adverse event, mild to moderate nausea, occurred in a dose-dependent fashion. With continued therapy, the frequency and severity decreased over time in most of the patients who initially experienced nausea. Adverse events reported in at least 1% to less than 5% of patients receiving exenatide and reported more frequently than with placebo included asthenia (mostly reported as weakness), decreased appetite, gastroesophageal reflux disease, and hyperhidrosis. Patients in the extension studies at 52 weeks experienced similar types of adverse events observed in the 30-week controlled trials.

In 30-week controlled trials, the incidence of withdrawal due to adverse events was 7% for exenatide-treated patients and 3% for placebo-treated patients. The most common adverse events leading to withdrawal for exenatide-treated patients were nausea (3% of patients) and vomiting (1%). For placebo-treated patients, less than 1% withdrew due to nausea and 0% due to vomiting.

➤*Immunogenicity:* Consistent with the potentially immunogenic properties of protein and peptide pharmaceuticals, patients may develop anti-exenatide antibodies following treatment with exenatide. In most patients who develop antibodies, antibody titers diminish over time. In the 30-week controlled trials, 38% of patients had low titer anti-exenatide antibodies at 30 weeks. For this group, the level of glycemic control (HbA_{1c}) was generally comparable to that observed in those without antibody titers. An additional 6% of patients had higher titer antibodies at 30 weeks. In about half of this 6% (3% of the total patients given exenatide in the controlled studies), the glycemic response to exenatide appeared attenuated; the remainder had a glycemic response consistent with that of patients without antibodies. Patients who developed anti-exenatide antibodies had similar rates and types of adverse events as those with no anti-exenatide antibodies.

Overdosage

➤*Symptoms:* In a clinical study of exenatide, 3 patients with type 2 diabetes each experienced a single overdose of 100 mcg subcutaneously (10 times the maximum recommended dose). Effects of the overdoses included severe nausea, severe vomiting, and rapidly declining blood glucose concentrations. One of the 3 patients experienced severe hypoglycemia requiring parenteral glucose administration. The 3 patients recovered without complication.

➤*Treatment:* In the event of overdose, initiate appropriate supportive treatment according to the patient's clinical signs and symptoms.

Patient Information

Inform patients of the potential risks of exenatide. Also fully inform patients about self-management practices, including the importance of proper storage of exenatide, injection technique, timing of dosage of exenatide as well as concomitant oral drugs, adherence to meal planning, regular physical activity, periodic blood glucose monitoring and HbA_{1c} testing, recognition and management of hypoglycemia and hyperglycemia, and assessment for diabetes complications.

Advise patients to inform their physicians if they are pregnant or intend to become pregnant.

Administer each dose of exenatide as a subcutaneous injection in the thigh, abdomen, or upper arm at any time within the 60-minute period before the morning and evening meals. Do not administer exenatide after a meal. If a dose is missed, resume the treatment regimen as prescribed with the next scheduled dose.

The risk of hypoglycemia is increased when exenatide is used in combination with an agent that induces hypoglycemia, such as a sulfonylurea. Explain to the patient the symptoms, treatment, and conditions that predispose development of hypoglycemia. While the patient's usual instructions for hypoglycemia management do not need to be changed, review these instructions and reinforce them when initiating exenatide therapy, particularly when concomitantly administered with a sulfonylurea. Advise patients that treatment with exenatide may result in a reduction in appetite, food intake, and/or body weight, and that there is no need to modify the dosing regimen due to such effects. Treatment with exenatide may also result in nausea, particularly upon initiation of therapy.

The patient should read the Patient Information insert and the Pen User Manual before starting exenatide therapy and review them each time the prescription is refilled. Instruct the patient on proper use and storage of the pen, emphasizing how and when to set up a new pen and noting that only one setup step is necessary at initial use. Advise the patient not to share the pen and needles.

Inform patients that pen needles are not included with the pen and must be purchased separately. Advise patients which needle length and gauge should be used.

Biguanides

METFORMIN HYDROCHLORIDE

Rx	**Metformin Hydrochloride** (Various, eg, Andrx, Barr, Ivax, Teva)	**Tablets:** 500 mg	In 100s, 500s, 1,000s, 2,000s, and UD 100s.
Rx	**Glucophage** (Bristol-Myers Squibb)		(BMS 6060 500). White to off-white. Film-coated. In 100s and 500s.
Rx	**Metformin Hydrochloride** (Various, eg, Andrx, Barr, Ivax, Teva)	**Tablets:** 850 mg	In 100s, 500s, 1,000s, and UD 100s.
Rx	**Glucophage** (Bristol-Myers Squibb)		(BMS 6070 850). White to off-white. Film-coated. In 100s.
Rx	**Metformin Hydrochloride** (Various, eg, Andrx, Barr, Ivax)	**Tablets:** 1,000 mg	In 100s, 500s, 1,000s, and UD 100s.
Rx	**Glucophage** (Bristol-Myers Squibb)		(BMS 6071 1000). White, oval, bisected. Film-coated. In 100s.
Rx	**Metformin Hydrochloride ER** (PAR)	**Tablets, extended-release:** 500 mg	White to off-white, capsule shape. In 100s.
Rx	**Fortamet** (Andrx)		(574). White, biconvex. Film-coated. In 60s.
Rx	**Glucophage XR** (Bristol-Myers Squibb)		(BMS 6063 500). White to off-white, capsule shape. In 100s and 500s.
Rx	**Metformin Hydrochloride** (Barr Labs)	**Tablets, extended-release:** 750 mg	(b 107). White to off-white, capsule shaped. In 100s.
Rx	**Glucophage XR** (Bristol-Myers Squibb)		(BMS 6064 750). Pale red, capsule shape. In 100s.
Rx	**Fortamet** (Andrx)	**Tablets, extended-release:** 1000 mg	(575). White, biconvex. Film-coated. In 60s.
Rx	**Riomet** (Ranbaxy)	**Oral solution:** 500 mg/5 mL	Saccharin. Cherry flavor. In 120 and 480 mL bottles.

METFORMIN HYDROCHLORIDE — ORAL

WARNING

Lactic acidosis – Lactic acidosis is a rare, but serious, metabolic complication that can occur because of metformin accumulation during treatment with metformin; when it occurs, it is fatal in approximately 50% of cases. Lactic acidosis also may occur in association with a number of pathophysiologic conditions, including diabetes mellitus, and whenever there is significant tissue hypoperfusion and hypoxemia. Lactic acidosis is characterized by elevated blood lactate levels (greater than 5 mmol/L), decreased blood pH, electrolyte disturbances with an increased anion gap, and an increased lactate/pyruvate ratio. When metformin is implicated as the cause of lactic acidosis, metformin plasma levels greater than 5 mcg/mL are generally found.

The reported incidence of lactic acidosis in patients receiving metformin is very low (approximately 0.03 cases/1,000 patient-years, with approximately 0.015 fatal cases/1,000 patient-years). In more than 20,000 patient-years exposure to metformin in clinical trials, there were no reports of lactic acidosis. Reported cases have occurred primarily in diabetic patients with significant renal insufficiency, including both intrinsic renal disease and renal hypoperfusion, often in the setting of multiple concomitant medical/surgical problems and multiple concomitant medications. Patients with congestive heart failure requiring pharmacologic management, in particular those with unstable or acute congestive heart failure who are at risk of hypoperfusion and hypoxemia, are at increased risk of lactic acidosis. The risk of lactic acidosis increases with the degree of renal dysfunction and the patient's age. The risk of lactic acidosis may, therefore, be significantly decreased by regular monitoring of renal function in patients taking metformin and by use of the minimum effective dose of metformin. In particular, treatment of the elderly should be accompanied by careful monitoring of renal function. Do not initiate metformin treatment in patients 80 years of age and older unless measurement of Ccr demonstrates that renal function is not reduced, because these patients are more susceptible to developing lactic acidosis. In addition, promptly withhold metformin in the presence of any condition associated with hypoxemia, dehydration, or sepsis. Because impaired hepatic function may significantly limit the ability to clear lactate, generally avoid using metformin in patients with clinical or laboratory evidence of hepatic disease. Caution patients against excessive alcohol intake, either acute or chronic, when taking metformin because alcohol potentiates the effects of metformin on lactate metabolism. In addition, temporarily discontinue metformin prior to any intravascular radiocontrast study and for any surgical procedure.

The onset of lactic acidosis often is subtle, and accompanied only by nonspecific symptoms such as malaise, myalgias, respiratory distress, increasing somnolence, and nonspecific abdominal distress. There may be associated hypothermia, hypotension, and resistant bradyarrhythmias with more marked acidosis. The patient and the patient's physician must be aware of the possible importance of such symptoms. Instruct the patient to notify the physician immediately if these symptoms occur. Withdraw metformin until the situation is clarified. Serum electrolytes, ketones, blood glucose, and, if indicated, blood pH, lactate levels, and even blood metformin levels may be useful. Once a patient is stabilized on any dose level of metformin, GI symptoms, which are common during initiation of therapy, are unlikely to be drug related. Later occurrence of GI symptoms could be caused by lactic acidosis or other serious disease.

Levels of fasting venous plasma lactate above the upper limit of normal but less than 5 mmol/L in patients taking metformin do not necessarily indicate impending lactic acidosis and may be explained by other mechanisms, such as poorly controlled diabetes or obesity, vigorous physical activity, or technical problems in sample handling.

Suspect lactic acidosis in any diabetic patient with metabolic acidosis lacking evidence of ketoacidosis (ketonuria and ketonemia).

Lactic acidosis is a medical emergency that must be treated in a hospital setting. In a patient with lactic acidosis who is taking metformin, immediately discontinue the drug and promptly institute general supportive measures. Because metformin is dialyzable (with a clearance of up to 170 mL/min under good hemodynamic conditions), prompt hemodialysis is recommended to correct the acidosis and remove the accumulated metformin. Such management often results in prompt reversal of symptoms and recovery.

Indications

➤*Type 2 diabetes:* Monotherapy as an adjunct to diet and exercise to improve glycemic control in patients with type 2 diabetes. Metformin immediate-release (IR) tablets and solution are indicated in patients 10 years of age and older. Metformin extended-release (ER) tablets are indicated in patients 17 years of age and older.

Metformin may be used concomitantly with a sulfonylurea or insulin to improve glycemic control in adults 17 years of age and older.

➤*Unlabeled uses:* Treatment for anovulation in women with polycystic ovary syndrome (PCOS); treatment of antipsychotic-induced weight gain.

Administration and Dosage

➤*Approved by the FDA:* December 29, 1994.

There is no fixed dosage regimen for the management of hyperglycemia in patients with type 2 diabetes with metformin or any other pharmacologic agent. Dosage of metformin must be individualized on the basis of efficacy and tolerance, while not exceeding the maximum recommended daily doses. The maximum recommended daily dose of metformin IR tablets and solution is 2,550 mg in adults and 2,000 mg in children (10 to 16 years of age); the maximum recommended daily dose of metformin ER tablets is 2,000 mg in adults (2,500 mg for *Fortamet*).

Give IR tablets and solution in divided doses with meals, and give ER tablets once daily with the evening meal. Start metformin at a low dose, with gradual dose escalation, both to reduce gastrointestinal (GI) side effects and to permit identification of the minimum dose required for adequate glycemic control of the patient.

During treatment initiation and dose titration, use fasting plasma glucose (FPG) to determine the therapeutic response to metformin and identify the minimum effective dose for the patient. Thereafter, measure glycosylated hemoglobin (HbA_{1c}) at intervals of approximately 3 months. The therapeutic goal should be to decrease both FPG and HbA_{1c} levels to normal or near normal by using the lowest effective dose of metformin, either when used as monotherapy or in combination with a sulfonylurea or insulin.

Monitoring of blood glucose and HbA_{1c} also will permit detection of primary failure (ie, inadequate lowering of blood glucose at the maximum recommended dose of medication) and secondary failure (ie, loss of an adequate blood glucose-lowering response after an initial period of efficacy).

Short-term administration of metformin may be sufficient during periods of transient loss of control in patients usually well controlled on diet alone.

Metformin ER tablets must be swallowed whole and never crushed or chewed. Occasionally, the inactive ingredients will be eliminated in the feces as a soft, hydrated mass.

➤*Recommended dosing schedule:*

Adults – In general, clinically significant responses are not seen at doses below 1,500 mg/day. However, a lower recommended starting dose and gradually increased dosage is advised to minimize GI symptoms.

IR tablets, solution: The usual starting dose is 500 mg twice daily or 850 mg once daily, given with meals. Make dosage increases in increments of 500 mg weekly or 850 mg every 2 weeks, up to a total of 2,000 mg/day, given in divided doses. Patients also can be titrated from 500 mg twice daily to 850 mg twice daily after 2 weeks. For those patients requiring additional glycemic control, metformin may be given to a maximum daily dose of 2,550 mg/day. Doses above 2,000 mg may be better tolerated given 3 times/day with meals.

ER tablets: The usual starting dose is 500 mg once daily with the evening meal. Make dosage increases in increments of 500 mg weekly, up to a maximum of 2,000 mg once daily (2,500 mg for *Fortamet*) with the evening meal. If glycemic control is not achieved on 2,000 mg once daily, consider a trial of 1,000 mg twice daily. If higher doses of metformin are required, use metformin IR tablets at total daily doses up to 2,550 mg administered in divided daily doses.

Conversion from IR to ER tablets: In a randomized trial, patients currently treated with metformin IR tablets were switched to metformin ER tablets. Results of this trial suggest that patients receiving metformin IR treatment may be safely switched to metformin ER treatment once daily at the same total daily dose, up to 2,000 mg once daily. Following a switch from metformin IR to ER tablets, closely monitor glycemic control and make dosage adjustments accordingly.

Children – The usual starting dose of metformin IR tablets and solution is 500 mg twice a day, given with meals. Make dosage increases in increments of 500 mg weekly up to a maximum of 2,000 mg/day, given in divided doses. The safety and efficacy of metformin ER tablets have not been established.

➤*Transfer from other antidiabetic therapy:* When transferring patients from standard oral hypoglycemic agents other than chlorpropamide to metformin, no transition period generally is necessary. When transferring patients from chlorpropamide, exercise care during the first 2 weeks because of the prolonged retention of chlorpropamide in the body, leading to overlapping drug effects and possible hypoglycemia.

➤*Concomitant metformin and oral sulfonylurea therapy in adults:* If a patient has not responded to 4 weeks of the maximum dose of metformin monotherapy, give consideration to gradual addition of an oral sulfonylurea while continuing metformin at the maximum dose, even if prior primary or secondary failure to a sulfonylurea has occurred. Clinical and pharmacokinetic drug-drug interaction data are currently available only for metformin plus glyburide (glibenclamide).

With concomitant metformin and sulfonylurea therapy, the desired control of blood glucose may be obtained by adjusting the dose of each drug. In a clinical trial of patients with type 2 diabetes and prior failure on glyburide, patients started on metformin 500 mg and glyburide 20 mg were titrated to 1,000/20 mg, 1,500/20 mg, 2,000/20 mg, or 2,500/20 mg of metformin and glyburide, respectively, to reach the goal of glycemic control as measured by FPG, HbA_{1c}, and plasma glucose response. However, make attempts to identify the minimum effective dose of each drug to achieve this goal. With concomitant metformin and sulfonylurea therapy, the risk of hypoglycemia associated with sulfonylurea therapy continues and may be increased. Take appropriate precautions (see drug monograph of the respective sulfonylurea).

If a patient has not satisfactorily responded to 1 to 3 months of concomitant therapy with the maximum dose of metformin and the maximum dose of an oral sulfonylurea, consider therapeutic alternatives, including switching to insulin with or without metformin.

➤*Concomitant metformin and insulin therapy in adults:* Continue the current insulin dose upon initiation of metformin therapy. Initiate metformin therapy at 500 mg once daily in patients on insulin therapy. For patients not responding adequately, increase the dose of metformin by 500 mg after approximately 1 week and by 500 mg every week thereafter until adequate glycemic control is achieved. The maximum recommended

METFORMIN HYDROCHLORIDE — ORAL

daily dose is 2,500 mg for metformin IR tablets and solution and 2,000 mg for metformin ER tablets (2,500 mg for *Fortamet*). It is recommended that the insulin dose be decreased 10% to 25% when FPG concentrations decrease to less than 120 mg/dL in patients receiving concomitant insulin and metformin. Individualize further adjustment based on glucose-lowering response.

➤*Special patient populations:* Metformin is not recommended for use in pregnancy. Metformin IR tablets are not recommended in patients younger than 10 years of age. Metformin ER tablets are not recommended in children younger than 17 years of age.

The initial and maintenance dosing of metformin should be conservative in patients with advanced age because of the potential for decreased renal function in this population. Base any dosage adjustment on a careful assessment of renal function. Generally, do not titrate elderly, debilitated, and malnourished patients to the maximum dose of metformin.

Monitoring of renal function is necessary to aid in prevention of lactic acidosis, particularly in the elderly. Metformin is known to be substantially excreted by the kidney, and the risk of metformin accumulation and lactic acidosis increases with the degree of impairment of renal function. Thus, do not give metformin to patients with serum creatinine levels above the upper limit of normal for their age. In patients with advanced age, carefully titrate metformin to establish the minimum dose for adequate glycemic effect, because aging is associated with reduced renal function. In elderly patients, particularly those 80 years of age and older, regularly monitor renal function and, generally, do not titrate metformin to the maximum dose.

➤*Storage/Stability:*

Tablets (IR and ER) – Store at 20° to 25°C (68° to 77°F); excursions permitted to 15° to 30°C (59° to 86°F). Dispense in light-resistant containers.

Solution – Store at controlled room temperature 15° to 30°C (59° to 86°F).

Actions

➤*Pharmacology:* Metformin is an antihyperglycemic agent that improves glucose tolerance in patients with type 2 diabetes, lowering basal and postprandial plasma glucose (PPG). Its pharmacologic mechanisms of action are different from other classes of oral antihyperglycemic agents. Metformin decreases hepatic glucose production, decreases intestinal absorption of glucose, and improves insulin sensitivity by increasing peripheral glucose uptake and utilization. Unlike sulfonylureas, metformin does not produce hypoglycemia in patients with type 2 diabetes or healthy subjects, except in special circumstances (eg, when caloric intake is deficient, when strenuous exercise is not compensated by caloric supplementation, or during concomitant use with other glucose-lowering agents [such as sulfonylureas and insulin] or ethanol), and does not cause hyperinsulinemia. With metformin therapy, insulin secretion remains unchanged, while fasting insulin levels and day-long plasma insulin response may actually decrease.

➤*Pharmacokinetics:*

Absorption –

Tablets (IR and ER): The absolute bioavailability of a metformin 500 mg tablet given under fasting conditions is approximately 50% to 60%. Studies using single oral doses of metformin 500 to 1,500 mg, and 850 to 2,550 mg, indicate that there is a lack of dose proportionality with increasing doses, which is caused by decreased absorption rather than an alteration in elimination. Food decreases the extent and slightly delays the absorption of metformin, as shown by an approximately 40% lower mean peak plasma concentration (C_{max}), a 25% lower area under the plasma concentration versus time curve (AUC), and a 35-minute prolongation of time to peak plasma concentration (T_{max}) following administration of a single 850 mg tablet of metformin with food, compared with the same tablet strength administered fasting. The clinical relevance of these decreases is unknown.

Following a single oral dose of metformin ER, C_{max} is achieved with a median value of 7 hours and a range of 4 to 8 hours. Peak plasma levels are approximately 20% lower compared with the same dose of metformin IR; however, the extent of absorption (as measured by AUC) is similar to metformin IR.

At steady state, the AUC and C_{max} are less than dose proportional for metformin ER within the range of 500 to 2,000 mg administered once daily. Peak plasma levels are approximately 0.6, 1.1, 1.4, and 1.8 mcg/mL for 500, 1,000, 1,500, and 2,000 mg once-daily doses, respectively. The extent of metformin absorption (as measured by AUC) from metformin ER at a 2,000 mg once-daily dose is similar to the same total daily dose administered as metformin IR 1,000 mg twice daily. After repeated administration of metformin ER, metformin did not accumulate in plasma.

Within-subject variability in C_{max} and AUC of metformin from metformin ER is comparable with metformin IR.

Although the extent of metformin absorption (as measured by AUC) from the metformin ER increased approximately 50% when given with food, there was no effect of food on C_{max} and T_{max} of metformin. Both high- and low-fat meals had the same effect on the pharmacokinetics of metformin ER.

Solution: Two pharmacokinetic studies have been performed in healthy volunteers to evaluate the bioavailability of metformin solution in comparison with the commercially available metformin tablets under fasting and fed conditions (study 1 and 2). A third pharmacokinetic study (study 3) assessed effects of food on absorption of metformin solution.

The rate and extent of absorption with metformin solution was found to be comparable with that of metformin tablets under fasting or fed conditions.

The food-effect study (study 3) assessed the effects of a high-fat/high-calorie meal and low-fat/low-calorie meal on the bioavailability of metformin solution in comparison with administration in the fasted state in healthy volunteers. The extent of absorption was increased 21% and 17% with the low-fat/low-calorie meal and the high-fat/high-calorie meal, respectively, compared with the administration in the fasted state. The rate and extent of absorption with high-fat/high-calorie and low-fat/low-calorie meals were similar. The mean T_{max} was 2.5 hours under fasting conditions as compared with 3.9 hours with both low-fat/low-calorie and high-fat/high-calorie meals.

Studies using single oral doses of metformin tablet formulations 500 to 1,500 mg, and 850 to 2,550 mg indicate that there is a lack of dose proportionality with increasing doses, which is caused by decreased absorption rather than an alteration in elimination.

Distribution – The apparent volume of distribution of metformin following single oral doses of metformin 850 mg averaged 654 ± 358 L. Metformin is negligibly bound to plasma proteins, in contrast to sulfonylureas, which are more than 90% protein bound. Metformin partitions into erythrocytes, most likely as a function of time. At usual clinical doses and dosing schedules of metformin, steady-state plasma concentrations of metformin are reached within 24 to 48 hours and are generally less than 1 mcg/mL. During controlled clinical trials of metformin, maximum metformin plasma levels did not exceed 5 mcg/mL, even at maximum doses.

Metabolism/Excretion – IV single-dose studies in healthy subjects demonstrate that metformin is excreted unchanged in the urine and does not undergo hepatic metabolism (no metabolites have been identified in humans) nor biliary excretion. Renal clearance is approximately 3.5 times greater than creatinine clearance (Ccr), which indicates that tubular secretion is the major route of metformin elimination. Following oral administration, approximately 90% of the absorbed drug is eliminated via the renal route within the first 24 hours, with a plasma elimination half-life of approximately 6.2 hours. In blood, the elimination half-life is approximately 17.6 hours, suggesting that the erythrocyte mass may be a compartment of distribution.

Special populations –

Renal function impairment: In patients with decreased renal function (based on measured Ccr), the plasma and blood half-life of metformin are prolonged, and the renal clearance is decreased in proportion to the decrease in Ccr.

Elderly: Limited data from controlled pharmacokinetic studies of metformin in healthy elderly subjects suggest that total plasma clearance of metformin is decreased, the half-life is prolonged, and C_{max} is increased, compared with healthy younger subjects. From these data, it appears that the change in metformin pharmacokinetics with aging is primarily accounted for by a change in renal function. Do not initiate metformin treatment in patients 80 years of age and older unless measurement of Ccr demonstrates that renal function is not reduced.

Base any dosage adjustment on a careful assessment of renal function. Generally, do not titrate elderly, debilitated, and malnourished patients to the maximum dose of metformin.

Monitoring of renal function is necessary to aid in prevention of lactic acidosis, particularly in the elderly.

Contraindications

Renal disease or renal dysfunction (eg, as suggested by serum creatinine levels greater than or equal to 1.5 mg/dL [males], greater than or equal to 1.4 mg/dL [females], or abnormal Ccr) that also may result from conditions such as cardiovascular collapse (shock), acute myocardial infarction, and septicemia; congestive heart failure requiring pharmacologic treatment; known hypersensitivity to metformin; acute or chronic metabolic acidosis, including diabetic ketoacidosis, with or without coma. Treat diabetic ketoacidosis with insulin.

Warnings

➤*Lactic acidosis:* See the Warning box for more information.

➤*Renal function impairment:*

Monitoring of renal function – Metformin is known to be substantially excreted by the kidney, and the risk of metformin accumulation and lactic acidosis increases with the degree of impairment of renal function. Thus, do not give metformin to patients with serum creatinine levels above the upper limit of normal for their age. In patients with advanced age, carefully titrate metformin to establish the minimum dose for adequate glycemic effect, because aging is associated with reduced renal function. In elderly patients, particularly those 80 years of age and older, regularly monitor renal function and, generally, do not titrate metformin to the maximum dose.

Before initiation of metformin therapy and at least annually thereafter, assess renal function and verify as normal. In patients in whom development of renal dysfunction is anticipated, assess renal function more frequently and discontinue metformin if evidence of renal impairment is present.

Use of concomitant medications that may affect renal function or metformin disposition – Concomitant medication(s) that may affect renal function or result in significant hemodynamic change or may interfere with the disposition of metformin, such as cationic drugs that are eliminated by renal tubular secretion, should be used with caution. Cationic drugs (eg, amiloride, digoxin, morphine, procainamide, quinidine, quinine, ranitidine, triamterene, trimethoprim, vancomycin) that are eliminated by renal tubular secretion theoretically have the potential for interaction with metformin by competing for common renal tubular transport systems. Although such interactions remain theoretical (except for cimetidine), careful patient monitoring and dose adjustment of metformin or the interfering drug is recommended in patients who are taking caloric medications that are excreted via the proximal renal tubular secretory systems.

METFORMIN HYDROCHLORIDE — ORAL

➤*Hepatic function impairment:* Because impaired hepatic function has been associated with some cases of lactic acidosis, generally avoid metformin in patients with clinical or laboratory evidence of hepatic disease.

➤*Carcinogenesis:* An increased incidence of benign stromal uterine polyps in female rats treated with 900 mg/kg/day.

➤*Elderly:* Controlled clinical studies of metformin did not include sufficient numbers of elderly patients to determine whether they respond differently than younger patients, although other reported clinical experience has not identified differences in responses between the elderly and younger patients. Metformin is known to be substantially excreted by the kidney; because the risk of serious adverse reactions to the drug is greater in patients with impaired renal function, only use metformin in patients with healthy renal function. Because aging is associated with reduced renal function, use metformin with caution as age increases. Take care in dose selection, and base dose on careful and regular monitoring of renal function. Generally, do not titrate elderly patients to the maximum dose of metformin.

➤*Pregnancy: Category B.*

Teratogenic – Recent information strongly suggests that abnormal blood glucose levels during pregnancy are associated with a higher incidence of congenital abnormalities. Most experts recommend that insulin be used during pregnancy to maintain blood glucose levels as close to normal as possible. Because animal reproduction studies are not always predictive of human response, do not use metformin during pregnancy unless clearly needed.

There are no adequate and well-controlled studies in pregnant women with metformin. Metformin was not teratogenic in rats and rabbits at doses up to 600 mg/kg/day. This represents an exposure of approximately 2 and 6 times the daily MRHD of 2,000 mg based on body surface area comparisons for rats and rabbits, respectively. Determination of fetal concentrations demonstrated a partial placental barrier to metformin.

➤*Lactation:* Studies in lactating rats show that metformin is excreted into milk and reaches levels comparable to those in plasma. It is not known whether this drug is excreted in human milk. Similar studies have not been conducted in nursing mothers. Because the potential for hypoglycemia in nursing infants may exist, decide whether to discontinue nursing or to discontinue the drug, taking into account the importance of the drug to the mother. If metformin is discontinued, and if diet alone is inadequate for controlling blood glucose, consider insulin therapy.

➤*Children:*

IR tablets, solution – The safety and efficacy of metformin for the treatment of type 2 diabetes have been established in children 10 to 16 years of age (studies have not been conducted in children younger than 10 years of age). Use of metformin in this age group is supported by evidence from adequate and well-controlled studies of metformin in adults with additional data from a controlled clinical study in children 10 to 16 years of age with type 2 diabetes, which demonstrated a similar response in glycemic control to that seen in adults. In this study, adverse reactions were similar to those described in adults. A maximum daily dose of 2,000 mg is recommended.

ER tablets – Safety and efficacy of metformin ER tablets in children have not been established.

Precautions

➤*Monitoring:* Monitor response to all diabetic therapies by periodic assessments of FPG and HbA_{1c} levels, with a goal of decreasing these levels toward the normal range. During initial dose titration, fasting glucose can be used to determine the therapeutic response. Thereafter, monitor both glucose and HbA_{1c}. Measurements of HbA_{1c} may be especially useful for evaluating long-term control.

Perform initial and periodic monitoring of hematologic parameters (eg, hemoglobin/hematocrit and red blood cell indices) and renal function (serum creatinine), at least on an annual basis. While megaloblastic anemia has rarely been seen with metformin therapy, if this is suspected, exclude vitamin B_{12} deficiency.

➤*Change in clinical status of patients with previously controlled type 2 diabetes:* Promptly evaluate patients with type 2 diabetes previously well controlled on metformin who develop laboratory abnormalities or clinical illness (especially vague and poorly defined illness) for evidence of ketoacidosis or lactic acidosis. Evaluation should include serum electrolytes and ketones, blood glucose and, if indicated, blood pH, lactate, pyruvate, and metformin levels. If acidosis of either form occurs, stop metformin immediately and initiate other appropriate corrective measures.

➤*Vitamin B_{12} levels:* In controlled clinical trials of metformin of 29 weeks' duration, a decrease to subnormal levels of previously normal serum vitamin B_{12} levels, without clinical manifestations, was observed in approximately 7% of patients. Such decrease, possibly caused by interference with B_{12} absorption from the B_{12}-intrinsic factor complex, is, however, very rarely associated with anemia and appears to be rapidly reversible with discontinuation of metformin or vitamin B_{12} supplementation. Measurement of hematologic parameters on an annual basis is advised in patients on metformin, and any apparent abnormalities should be appropriately investigated and managed.

Certain individuals (those with inadequate vitamin B_{12} or calcium intake or absorption) appear to be predisposed to developing subnormal vitamin B_{12} levels. In these patients, routine serum vitamin B_{12} measurements at 2- to 3-year intervals may be useful.

➤*Hypoxic states:* Cardiovascular collapse (shock) from whatever cause, acute congestive heart failure, acute myocardial infarction and other conditions characterized by hypoxemia have been associated with lactic acidosis and also may cause prerenal azotemia. When such events occur in patients on metformin therapy, promptly discontinue the drug.

➤*Surgical procedures:* Temporarily suspend metformin therapy for any surgical procedure (except minor procedures not associated with restricted intake of food and fluids) and do not restart until the patient's oral intake has resumed and renal function has been evaluated as normal.

➤*Hypoglycemia:* Hypoglycemia does not occur in patients receiving metformin alone under usual circumstances of use, but could occur when caloric intake is deficient, when strenuous exercise is not compensated by caloric supplementation, or during concomitant use with other glucose-lowering agents (eg, sulfonylureas and insulin) or ethanol.

Elderly, debilitated, or malnourished patients, and those with adrenal or pituitary insufficiency or alcohol intoxication are particularly susceptible to hypoglycemic effects. Hypoglycemia may be difficult to recognize in the elderly, and in people who are taking beta-adrenergic-blocking drugs.

➤*Iodinated contrast materials:* Radiologic studies involving the use of intravascular iodinated contrast materials (ie, IV urogram, IV cholangiography, angiography, and computed tomography [CT] scans with intravascular contrast materials) can lead to acute alteration of renal function and have been associated with lactic acidosis in patients receiving metformin. Therefore, in patients in whom any such study is planned, temporarily discontinue metformin at the time of or prior to the procedure, and withhold for 48 hours subsequent to the procedure; reinstitute only after renal function has been reevaluated and found to be normal.

➤*Loss of control of blood glucose:* When a patient stabilized on any diabetic regimen is exposed to stress (eg, fever, trauma, infection, or surgery), a temporary loss of glycemic control may occur. At such times, it may be necessary to withhold metformin and temporarily administer insulin. Metformin may be reinstituted after the acute episode is resolved.

The efficacy of oral antidiabetic drugs in lowering blood glucose to a targeted level decreases in many patients over a period of time. This phenomenon, which may be caused by progression of the underlying disease or to diminished responsiveness to the drug, is known as secondary failure, to distinguish it from primary failure in which the drug is ineffective during initial therapy. Should secondary failure occur with either metformin or sulfonylurea monotherapy, combined therapy with metformin and sulfonylurea may result in a response. Should secondary failure occur with combined metformin/sulfonylurea therapy, it may be necessary to consider therapeutic alternatives including initiation of insulin therapy.

Drug Interactions

Certain drugs tend to produce hyperglycemia and may lead to loss of glycemic control. These drugs include the thiazides and other diuretics, corticosteroids, phenothiazines, thyroid products, estrogens, oral contraceptives, phenytoin, nicotinic acid, sympathomimetics, calcium channel blocking drugs, and isoniazid. When such drugs are administered to a patient receiving metformin, closely observe the patient for loss of blood glucose control. When such drugs are withdrawn from a patient receiving metformin, closely observe the patient for hypoglycemia.

Metformin Drug Interactions

Precipitant drug	Object drug[a]		Description
Alcohol	Metformin	↑	Alcohol potentiates the effect of metformin on lactate metabolism. Warn patients against excessive alcohol intake, acute or chronic, while receiving metformin.
Cationic drugs (eg, amiloride, digoxin, morphine, procainamide, quinidine, quinine, ranitidine, triamterene, trimethoprim, vancomycin)	Metformin	↑	Cationic drugs that are eliminated by renal tubular secretion theoretically have the potential for interaction with metformin by competing for common renal tubular transport systems. Although such interactions remain theoretical, careful patient monitoring and dose adjustment of metformin and/or the interfering drug are recommended in patients who are taking cationic medications excreted via the proximal renal tubular secretory system.
Cimetidine	Metformin	↑	Cimetidine caused a 60% increase in peak metformin plasma concentrations and a 40% increase in AUC.

Biguanides

METFORMIN HYDROCHLORIDE — ORAL

Metformin Drug Interactions

Precipitant drug	Object drug[a]		Description
Furosemide	Metformin	↑	Furosemide increased the metformin plasma and blood C_{max} 22% and blood AUC 15%, without any significant change in metformin renal clearance. When administered with metformin, the C_{max} and AUC of furosemide were 31% and 12% smaller, respectively, than when administered alone, and the terminal half-life was decreased 32%, without any significant change in furosemide renal clearance.
Metformin	Furosemide	↓	
Iodinated contrast material	Metformin	↑	Parenteral contrast studies with iodinated materials can lead to acute renal failure and have been associated with lactic acidosis in patients receiving metformin. Therefore, in patients in whom any such study is planned, withhold metformin for ≥ 48 hours prior to, and 48 hours subsequent to, the procedure, and reinstitute only after renal function has been re-evaluated and found to be normal.
Nifedipine	Metformin	↑	Coadministration increased plasma metformin C_{max} and AUC 20% and 9%, respectively, and increased the amount excreted in the urine. Nifedipine appears to enhance the absorption of metformin.
Metformin	Glyburide	↓	Following coadministration of single doses, decreases in glyburide AUC and C_{max} were observed, but were highly variable. The single-dose nature of this study and the lack of correlation between glyburide blood levels and pharmacodynamic effects makes the clinical significance of this interaction uncertain.

[a] ↑ = Object drug increased. ↓ = Object drug decreased.

Adverse Reactions

➤*IR tablets, solution:*

Most Common Adverse Reactions (> 5%) in a Placebo-Controlled Clinical Study of Metformin Monotherapy[a]

Adverse reaction	Metformin monotherapy (n = 141)	Placebo (n = 145)
Abdominal discomfort	6.4%	4.8%
Asthenia	9.2%	5.5%
Diarrhea	53.2%	11.7%
Flatulence	12.1%	5.5%
Headache	5.7%	4.8%
Indigestion	7.1%	4.1%
Nausea/vomiting	25.5%	8.3%

[a] Reactions that were more common in metformin- than placebo-treated patients.

Diarrhea led to discontinuation of study medication in 6% of patients treated with metformin. Additionally, the following adverse reactions were reported in 1% or more to 5% or less of metformin patients and were more commonly reported with metformin than placebo: abnormal stools, chest discomfort, chills, dyspnea, flushing, flu syndrome, hypoglycemia, lightheadedness, myalgia, nail disorder, palpitation, rash, sweating increased, taste disorder.

➤*ER tablets:*

Most Common Adverse Reactions (> 5%) in Placebo-Controlled Studies of Metformin ER Tablets[a]

Adverse reaction	Metformin ER (n = 781)	Placebo (n = 195)
Diarrhea	9.6%	2.6%
Nausea/Vomiting	6.5%	1.5%

[a] Reactions that were more common in metformin ER tablet than placebo-treated patients.

Diarrhea led to discontinuation of study medication in 0.6% of patients treated with metformin ER tablets. Additionally, the following adverse reactions were reported in 1% or more to 5% or less of metformin ER tablets patients and were more commonly reported with metformin ER tablets than placebo: abdomen distention, abdominal pain, constipation, dizziness, dyspepsia/heartburn, flatulence, headache, taste disturbance, upper respiratory tract infection.

➤*Children:* In clinical trials with metformin in children with type 2 diabetes, the profile of adverse reactions was similar to that observed in adults.

Overdosage

➤*Symptoms:* Overdose of metformin has occurred, including ingestion of amounts greater than 50 g. Hypoglycemia was reported in approximately 10% of cases, but no causal association with metformin has been established. Lactic acidosis has been reported in approximately 32% of metformin overdose cases.

➤*Treatment:* Metformin is dialyzable, with a clearance of up to 170 mL/min under good hemodynamic conditions. Therefore, hemodialysis may be useful for removal of accumulated drug from patients in whom metformin overdosage is suspected.

Patient Information

Inform patients of the potential risks and benefits of metformin and of alternative modes of therapy. Also inform patients about the importance of adherence to dietary instructions, of a regular exercise program, and of regular testing of blood glucose, HbA_{1c}, renal function, and hematologic parameters.

Explain the risks of lactic acidosis, its symptoms, and conditions that predispose to its development to patients. Advise patients to discontinue metformin immediately and to promptly notify their health practitioner if unexplained hyperventilation, myalgia, malaise, unusual somnolence, or other nonspecific symptoms occur. Once a patient is stabilized on any dose level of metformin, GI symptoms, which are common during initiation of metformin therapy, are unlikely to be drug related. Later occurrence of GI symptoms could be caused by lactic acidosis or other serious disease.

Counsel patients against excessive alcohol intake, either acute or chronic, while receiving metformin.

Metformin alone does not usually cause hypoglycemia, although it may occur when metformin is used in conjunction with oral sulfonylureas and insulin. When initiating combination therapy, explain the risks of hypoglycemia, its symptoms and treatment, and conditions that predispose to its development to patients and responsible family members.

Inform patients that metformin ER tablets must be swallowed whole and not crushed or chewed, and that the inactive ingredients may occasionally be eliminated in the feces as a soft mass that may resemble the original tablet.

Meglitinides

REPAGLINIDE

Rx	**Prandin** (Novo Nordisk)	**Tablets:** 0.5 mg	White. In 100s, 500s, and 1,000s.
		1 mg	Yellow. In 100s, 500s, and 1,000s.
		2 mg	Peach. In 100s, 500s, and 1,000s.

REPAGLINIDE — ORAL

Indications

➤*Type 2 diabetes mellitus:* As an adjunct to diet and exercise to lower the blood glucose in patients with type 2 diabetes mellitus (non-insulin-dependent diabetes mellitus [NIDDM]) whose hyperglycemia cannot be controlled satisfactorily by diet and exercise alone.

Repaglinide is also indicated for combination therapy use (with metformin or thiazolidinediones) to lower blood glucose in patients whose hyperglycemia cannot be controlled by diet and exercise plus monotherapy with any of the following agents: Metformin, sulfonylureas, repaglinide, or thiazolidinediones. If glucose control has not been achieved after a suitable trial of combination therapy, give consideration to discontinuing these drugs and using insulin. Base judgments on regular clinical and laboratory evaluations.

Administration and Dosage

➤*Approved by the FDA:* December 23, 1997.

REPAGLINIDE — ORAL

There is no fixed dosage regimen for the management of type 2 diabetes with repaglinide.

The patient's blood glucose should be monitored periodically to determine the minimum effective dose for the patient; to detect primary failure (ie, inadequate lowering of blood glucose at the maximum recommended dose of medication); and to detect secondary failure (ie, loss of an adequate blood glucose-lowering response after an initial period of effectiveness). Glycosylated hemoglobin levels are of value in monitoring the patient's longer-term response to therapy.

Short-term administration of repaglinide may be sufficient during periods of transient loss of control in patients usually well controlled on diet.

➤*Administration:* Repaglinide doses are usually taken within 15 minutes of the meal but time may vary from immediately preceding the meal to as long as 30 minutes before the meal.

➤*Starting dose:* For patients not previously treated or whose HbA_{1c} is less than 8%, the starting dose should be 0.5 mg with each meal. For patients previously treated with blood glucose-lowering drugs and whose HbA_{1c} is greater than or equal to 8%, the initial dose is 1 or 2 mg with each meal preprandially.

➤*Dose adjustment:* Dosing adjustments should be determined by blood glucose response, usually fasting blood glucose. Postprandial glucose levels testing may be clinically helpful in patients whose premeal blood glucose levels are satisfactory but whose overall glycemic control (HbA_{1c}) is inadequate. The preprandial dose should be doubled up to 4 mg with each meal until satisfactory blood glucose response is achieved. At least 1 week should elapse to assess response after each dose adjustment.

➤*Dose range:* The recommended dose range is 0.5 mg to 4 mg taken with meals. Repaglinide may be dosed preprandially 2, 3, or 4 times a day in response to changes in the patient's meal pattern. The maximum recommended daily dose is 16 mg.

➤*Patient management:* Long-term efficacy should be monitored by measurement of HbA_{1c} levels approximately every 3 months. Failure to follow an appropriate dosage regimen may precipitate hypoglycemia or hyperglycemia. Patients who do not adhere to their prescribed dietary and drug regimen are more prone to exhibit unsatisfactory response to therapy, including hypoglycemia. When hypoglycemia occurs in patients taking a combination of repaglinide and a thiazolidinedione or repaglinide and metformin, the dose of repaglinide should be reduced.

➤*Patients receiving other oral hypoglycemic agents:* When repaglinide is used to replace therapy with other oral hypoglycemic agents, repaglinide may be started on the day after the final dose is given. Patients should then be observed carefully for hypoglycemia due to potential overlapping of drug effects. When transferred from longer half-life sulfonylurea agents (eg, chlorpropamide) to repaglinide, close monitoring may be indicated for up to 1 week or longer.

➤*Combination therapy:* If repaglinide monotherapy does not result in adequate glycemic control, metformin or a thiazolidinedione may be added. If metformin or thiazolidinedione monotherapy does not provide adequate control, repaglinide may be added. The starting dose and dose adjustments for repaglinide combination therapy is the same as for repaglinide monotherapy. The dose of each drug should be carefully adjusted to determine the minimal dose required to achieve the desired pharmacologic effect. Failure to do so could result in an increase in the incidence of hypoglycemic episodes. Appropriate monitoring of FPG and HbA_{1c} measurements should be used to ensure that the patient is not subjected to excessive drug exposure or increased probability of secondary drug failure.

➤*Renal function impairment:* Initiate patients with type 2 diabetes who have severe renal function impairment with the repaglinide 0.5 mg dose; subsequently, titrate patients carefully.

➤*Storage/Stability:* Do not store above 25°C (77°F). Protect from moisture. Keep bottles tightly closed. Dispense in tight containers with safety closures.

Actions

➤*Pharmacology:* Repaglinide lowers blood glucose levels by stimulating the release of insulin from the pancreas. This action is dependent upon functioning beta cells in the pancreatic islets. Insulin release is glucose-dependent and diminishes at low glucose concentrations.

Repaglinide closes ATP-dependent potassium channels in the beta-cell membrane by binding at characterizable sites. This potassium channel blockade depolarizes the beta-cell, which leads to an opening of calcium channels. The resulting increased calcium influx induces insulin secretion. The ion channel mechanism is highly tissue-selective, with low affinity for heart and skeletal muscle.

➤*Pharmacokinetics:*

Absorption – After oral administration, repaglinide is rapidly and completely absorbed from the GI tract. After single and multiple oral doses in healthy subjects or in patients, peak plasma drug levels (C_{max}) occur within 1 hour (T_{max}). Repaglinide is rapidly eliminated from the blood stream with a half-life of approximately 1 hour. The mean absolute bioavailability is 56%. When repaglinide was given with food, the mean T_{max} was not changed, but the mean C_{max} and AUC (area under the time/plasma concentration curve) were decreased 20% and 12.4%, respectively.

Distribution – After IV dosing in healthy subjects, the volume of distribution at steady state (V_{ss}) was 31 L, and the total body clearance (CL) was 38L/h. Protein binding and binding to human serum albumin was greater than 98%.

Metabolism – Repaglinide is completely metabolized by oxidative biotransformation and direct conjugation with glucuronic acid after either an IV or oral dose. The major metabolites are an oxidized dicarboxylic acid (M2), the aromatic amine (M1), and the acyl glucuronide (M7). The cytochrome P450 enzyme system, specifically 3A4, has been shown to be involved in the N-dealkylation of repaglinide to M2 and the further oxidation to M1. Metabolites do not contribute to the glucose-lowering effect of repaglinide.

Excretion – Within 96 hours after dosing with ^{14}C-repaglinide as a single, oral dose, approximately 90% of the radiolabel was recovered in the feces and approximately 8% in the urine. Only 0.1% of the dose is cleared in the urine as parent compound. The major metabolite (M2) accounted for 60% of the administered dose. Less than 2% of parent drug was recovered in feces.

Special populations –

Renal function impairment: Single-dose and steady-state pharmacokinetics of repaglinide were compared between patients with type 2 diabetes and healthy renal function (Ccr greater than 80 mL/min), mild-to-moderate renal function impairment (Ccr = 40 to 80 mL/min), and severe renal function impairment (Ccr = 20 to 40 mL/min). Both AUC and C_{max} of repaglinide were similar in patients with normal and mild to moderately impaired renal function (mean values 56.7 ng/mL•h vs 57.2 ng/mL•h and 37.5 ng/mL vs 37.7 ng/mL, respectively.) Patients with severely reduced renal function had elevated mean AUC and C_{max} values (98 ng/mL•h and 50.7 ng/mL, respectively), but this study showed only a weak correlation between repaglinide levels and creatinine clearance. Initial dose adjustment does not appear to be necessary for patients with mild-to-moderate renal dysfunction. However, initiate patients with type 2 diabetes who have severe renal function impairment with the repaglinide 0.5 mg dose; subsequently, titrate patients carefully. Studies were not conducted in patients with creatinine clearances below 20 mL/min or patients with renal failure requiring hemodialysis.

Hepatic function impairment: A single-dose, open-label study was conducted in 12 healthy subjects and 12 patients with chronic liver disease (CLD) classified by Child-Pugh scale and caffeine clearance. Patients with moderate to severe impairment of liver function had higher and more prolonged serum concentrations of both total and unbound repaglinide than healthy subjects (healthy AUC, 91.6 ng/mL•h; CLD patients AUC, 368.9 ng/mL•h; healthy C_{max}, 46.7 ng/mL; CLD patients C_{max}, 105.4 ng/mL). AUC was statistically correlated with caffeine clearance. No difference in glucose profiles was observed across patient groups. Patients with impaired liver function may be exposed to higher concentrations of repaglinide and its associated metabolites than would patients with normal liver function receiving usual doses. Therefore, use repaglinide cautiously in patients with impaired liver function. Utilize longer intervals between dose adjustments to allow full assessment of response.

Gender: A comparison of pharmacokinetics in males and females showed the AUC over the 0.5 to 4 mg dose range to be 15% to 70% higher in females with type 2 diabetes. This difference was not reflected in the frequency of hypoglycemic episodes (male: 16%; female: 17%) or other adverse events. With respect to gender, no change in general dosage recommendation is indicated since dosage for each patient should be individualized to achieve optimal clinical response.

Contraindications

Type 1 diabetes; known hypersensitivity to the drug or its inactive ingredients; diabetic ketoacidosis, with or without coma. Treat this condition with insulin.

Warnings

➤*Hepatic function impairment:* Patients with impaired liver function may be exposed to higher concentrations of repaglinide and its associated metabolites than would patients with normal liver function receiving usual doses. Therefore, use repaglinide cautiously in patients with impaired liver function. Utilize longer intervals between dose adjustments to allow full assessment of response.

➤*Carcinogenesis:* Long-term carcinogenicity studies were performed for 104 weeks at doses up to and including 120 mg/kg body weight/day (rats) and 500 mg/kg body weight/day (mice) or approximately 60 and 125 times clinical exposure, respectively, on a mg/m^2 basis. No evidence of carcinogenicity was found in mice or female rats. In male rats, there was an increased incidence of benign adenomas of the thyroid and liver. The relevance of these findings to humans is unclear. The no-effect doses for these observations in male rats were 30 mg/kg body weight/day for thyroid tumors and 60 mg/kg body weight/day for liver tumors, which are over 15 and 30 times, respectively, clinical exposure on a mg/m^2 basis.

➤*Pregnancy: Category C.*

Teratogenic – Safety in pregnant women has not been established. Because animal reproduction studies are not always predictive of human response, use repaglinide during pregnancy only if it is clearly needed.

Nonteratogenic – Offspring of rat dams exposed to repaglinide at 15 times clinical exposure on a mg/m^2 basis during days 17 to 22 of gestation and during lactation developed nonteratogenic skeletal deformities consisting of shortening, thickening, and bending of the humerus during the postnatal period. This effect was not seen at doses up to 2.5 times clinical exposure (on a mg/m^2 basis) on days 1 to 22 of pregnancy or at higher doses given during days 1 to 16 of pregnancy. Relevant human exposure has not occurred to date and therefore the safety of repaglinide administration throughout pregnancy or lactation cannot be established.

➤*Lactation:* In rat reproduction studies, measurable levels of repaglinide were detected in the breast milk of the dams and lowered blood glucose levels were observed in the pups. Cross fostering studies indicated that skeletal changes could be induced in control pups nursed by treated dams, although this occurred to a lesser degree than those pups treated in utero. Although it is not known whether repaglinide is excreted in human milk

REPAGLINIDE — ORAL

some oral agents are known to be excreted by this route. Because the potential for hypoglycemia in nursing infants may exist, and because of the effects on nursing animals, a decision should be made as to whether repaglinide should be discontinued in nursing mothers, or if mothers should discontinue nursing. If repaglinide is discontinued and if diet alone is inadequate for controlling blood glucose, consider insulin therapy.

➤*Children:* No studies have been performed in children.

Precautions

➤*Monitoring:* Monitor response to all diabetic therapies by periodic measurements of fasting blood glucose and glycosylated hemoglobin levels with a goal of decreasing these levels towards the normal range. During dose adjustment, fasting glucose can be used to determine the therapeutic response. Thereafter, monitor both glucose and glycosylated hemoglobin. Glycosylated hemoglobin may be especially useful for evaluating long-term glycemic control. Postprandial glucose level testing may be clinically helpful in patients whose premeal blood glucose levels are satisfactory but whose overall glycemic control (HbA_{1c}) is inadequate.

➤*Use with insulin:* Repaglinide is not indicated for use in combination with NPH-insulin.

➤*Hypoglycemia:* All oral blood glucose-lowering drugs are capable of producing hypoglycemia. Proper patient selection, dosage, and instructions to the patients are important to avoid hypoglycemic episodes. Hepatic insufficiency may cause elevated repaglinide blood levels and may diminish gluconeogenic capacity, both of which increase the risk of serious hypoglycemia. Elderly, debilitated, or malnourished patients, and those with adrenal, pituitary, hepatic insufficiency or severe renal insufficiency are particularly susceptible to the hypoglycemic action of glucose-lowering drugs.

Hypoglycemia may be difficult to recognize in the elderly and in people taking beta-adrenergic-blocking drugs. Hypoglycemia is more likely to occur when caloric intake is deficient, after severe or prolonged exercise, when alcohol is ingested, or when more than 1 glucose-lowering drug is used.

The frequency of hypoglycemia is greater in patients with type 2 diabetes who have not been previously treated with oral blood glucose-lowering drugs (naive) or whose HbA_{1c} is less than 8%. Administer repaglinide with meals to lessen the risk of hypoglycemia.

➤*Secondary failure:* When a patient stabilized on any diabetic regimen is exposed to stress such as fever, trauma, infection, or surgery, a loss of glycemic control may occur. At such times, it may be necessary to discontinue repaglinide and administer insulin. The effectiveness of any hypoglycemic drug in lowering blood glucose to a desired level decreases in many patients over a period of time, which may be due to progression of the severity of diabetes or to diminished responsiveness to the drug. This phenomenon is known as secondary failure, to distinguish it from primary failure in which the drug is ineffective in an individual patient when the drug is first given. Adequate adjustment of dose and adherence to diet should be assessed before classifying a patient as a secondary failure.

Drug Interactions

➤*CYP-450 inhibitors:* In vitro data indicate that repaglinide metabolism may be inhibited by antifungal agents like ketoconazole and miconazole, and antibacterial agents like erythromycin (cytochrome P-450 enzyme system 3A4 inhibitors).

➤*CYP-450 inducers:* Drugs that induce the cytochrome P-450 enzyme system 3A4 may increase repaglinide metabolism; such drugs include troglitazone, rifampin, barbiturates, and carbamazepine.

Repaglinide Drug Interactions

Precipitant drug	Object drug[a]		Description
Beta blockers Chloramphenicol, Coumarins, MAOIs, NSAIDs, Probenecid, Salicylates, Sulfonamide)	Repaglinide	⬆	The action of repaglinide may be potentiated by certain drugs, including those highly protein bound. Observe for hypoglycemia and loss of glycemic control.
Calcium channel blockers Corticosteroids, Estrogens, Isoniazid, Nicotinic acid, Oral contraceptives, Phenothiazines, Phenytoin, Sympathomimetics, Thiazides and other diuretics, Thyroid products	Repaglinide	⬇	Certain drugs tend to produce hyperglycemia and may lead to loss of glycemic control. Observe closely.
CYP 4503A4 inhibitors (eg, ketoconazole, miconazole, clarithromycin)	Repaglinide	⬆	Coadministration may increase repaglinide plasma levels because of inhibition of its metabolism. Monitor blood glucose and adjust repaglinide dose as needed.
CYP 4503A4 inducers (eg, rifampin, barbiturates, carbamazepine)	Repaglinide	⬇	Coadministration may decrease repaglinide plasma levels because of induction of its metabolism. Monitor blood glucose and adjust repaglinide dose as needed.
Gemfibrozil	Repaglinide	⬆	Concomitant use may result in enhanced and prolonged blood glucose-lowering effects of repaglinide. Use caution in patients already on repaglinide. Monitor blood glucose levels. Repaglinide dose adjustment may be needed.
Gemfibrozil and Itraconazole	Repaglinide	⬆	Gemfibrozil and itraconazole have a synergistic metabolic inhibitory effect on repaglinide. Therefore, patients taking repaglinide and gemfibrozil should not take itraconazole.
Levonorgestrel and ethinyl estradiol	Repaglinide	⬆	Coadministration of a combination tablet of 0.15 mg levonorgestrel and 0.03 mg ethinyl estradiol administered once daily for 21 days with 2 mg repaglinide administered 3 times/day on days 1 to 4 and a single dose on day 5 resulted in 20% increases in repaglinide, levonorgestrel, and ethinyl estradiol C_{max}. Ethinyl estradiol AUC parameters were increased by 20%, while repaglinide and levonorgestrel AUC values remained unchanged.
Repaglinide	Levonorgestrel and ethinyl estradiol		
Simvastatin	Repaglinide	⬆	Coadministration of 20 mg simvastatin and a single dose of 2 mg repaglinide (after 4 days of once-daily 20 mg simvastatin and 2 mg repaglinide 3 times/day) resulted in a 26% increase in repaglinide C_{max}.

[a] ⬆ = Object drug increased. ⬇ = Object drug decreased.

➤*Drug/Food interactions:* When given with food, mean C_{max} and AUC of repaglinide were decreased 20% and 12.4%, respectively. Administer repaglinide before meals.

Adverse Reactions

Repaglinide has been administered to 2,931 individuals during clinical trials. Approximately 1,500 of these individuals with type 2 diabetes have been treated for at least 3 months, 1,000 for at least 6 months and 800 for at least 1 year. The majority of these individuals (1,228) received repaglinide in 1 of five 1-year, active-controlled trials. The comparator drugs in these 1-year trials were oral sulfonylurea drugs including glyburide and glipizide. Over 1 year, 13% of repaglinide patients were discontinued because of adverse reactions vs 14% of sulfonylurea patients. The most common adverse events leading to withdrawal were hyperglycemia, hypoglycemia, and related symptoms. Mild or moderate hypoglycemia occurred in 16% of repaglinide patients, 20% of glyburide patients, and 19% of glipizide patients.

The table below lists common adverse reactions for repaglinide patients compared to both placebo (in trials 12 to 24 weeks duration) and to glyburide and glipizide in 1-year trials. The adverse-event profile of repaglinide was generally comparable to that for sulfonylurea drugs.

Repaglinide Adverse Reactions (%)[a]

Adverse reaction	Repaglinide (n = 352)	Placebo (n = 108)	Repaglinide (n = 1,228)	Sulfonylurea (n = 498)
	Placebo-controlled studies		Active-controlled studies	
CNS				
Headache	11%	10%	9%	8%
Paresthesia	3%	3%	2%	1%
GI				
Constipation	3%	2%	2%	3%
Diarrhea	5%	2%	4%	6%
Dyspepsia	2%	2%	4%	2%
Nausea	5%	5%	3%	2%
Vomiting	3%	3%	2%	1%
Musculoskeletal				
Arthralgia	6%	3%	3%	4%
Back pain	5%	4%	6%	7%
Respiratory				
Bronchitis	2%	1%	6%	7%
Rhinitis	3%	3%	7%	8%

REPAGLINIDE — ORAL

Repaglinide Adverse Reactions (%)[a]				
Adverse reaction	Repaglinide (n = 352)	Placebo (n = 108)	Repaglinide (n = 1,228)	Sulfonylurea (n = 498)
	Placebo-controlled studies		Active-controlled studies	
Sinusitis	6%	2%	3%	4%
Upper respiratory tract infection	16%	8%	10%	10%
Miscellaneous				
Allergy	2%	0%	1%	< 1%
Chest pain	3%	1%	2%	1%
Hypoglycemia	31%[b]	7%	16%	20%
Tooth disorder	2%	0%	< 1%	< 1%
Urinary tract infection	2%	1%	3%	3%

[a] Events greater than or equal to 2% for the repaglinide group in the placebo-controlled studies and events occurring as often or more often than those in the placebo group.
[b] In a double-blind, placebo-controlled, 3 months' dose-titration study, repaglinide or placebo doses for each patient were increased weekly from 0.25 mg through 0.5, 1, and 2 mg, to a maximum of 4 mg, until an FPG level less than 160 mg/dL was achieved or the maximum dose reached. The dose that achieved the targeted control or the maximum dose was continued to end of study. FPG and 2-hour PPG increased in patients receiving placebo and decreased in patients treated with repaglinide. Differences between the repaglinide- and placebo-treated groups were −61 mg/dL (FPG) and −104 mg/dL (PPG). The between-group change in HbA_{1C}, which reflects long-term glycemic control, was 1.7% units.

➤*Hypoglycemia:* All oral blood glucose-lowering drugs are capable of producing hypoglycemia. Proper patient selection, dosage, and instructions to the patients are important to avoid hypoglycemic episodes.

Severe hypoglycemic reactions with coma, seizure, or other neurological impairment occur infrequently, but constitute medical emergencies requiring immediate hospitalization.

➤*Cardiovascular:* Cardiovascular events also occur commonly in patients with type 2 diabetes. In 1-year comparator trials, the incidence of individual events was not greater than 1% except for chest pain (1.8%) and angina (1.8%). The individual incidence of other cardiovascular events (hypertension, abnormal EKG, myocardial infarction, arrhythmias, and palpitations) was less than or equal to 1% and not different for repaglinide and the comparator drugs.

The incidence of total serious cardiovascular adverse events added together, including ischemia, was slightly higher for repaglinide (4%) than for sulfonylurea drugs (3%) in controlled comparator clinical trials. In 1-year controlled trials, repaglinide treatment was not associated with excess mortality rates when compared with rates observed with other oral hypoglycemic agent therapies.

Serious Repaglinide Cardiovascular Reactions (%)		
	Repaglinide (n = 1,228)	Sulfonylurea[a] (n = 498)
Serious CV reactions	4%	3%
Cardiac ischemic reactions	2%	2%
Deaths caused by CV reactions	0.5%	0.4%

[a] Glyburide and glipizide.

Seven controlled clinical trials included repaglinide combination therapy with NPH-insulin (n = 431), insulin formulations alone (n = 388) or other combinations (sulfonylurea plus NPH-insulin or repaglinide plus metformin) (n = 120). There were 6 serious adverse events of myocardial ischemia in patients treated with repaglinide plus NPH-insulin from 2 studies, and 1 event in patients using insulin formulations alone from another study.

Infrequent adverse reactions (less than 1%) – Less common adverse clinical or laboratory events observed in clinical trials included elevated liver enzymes, thrombocytopenia, leukopenia, and anaphylactoid reactions (1 patient).

Combination therapy with thiazolidinediones – During 24-week treatment clinical trials of repaglinide-rosiglitazone or repaglinide-pioglitazone combination therapy (a total of 250 patients in combination therapy), hypoglycemia (blood glucose less than 50 mg/dL) occurred in 7% of combination therapy patients in comparison with 7% for repaglinide monotherapy, and 2% for thiazolidinedione monotherapy.

Peripheral edema was reported in 12 out of 250 repaglinide-thiazolidinedione combination therapy patients and 3 out of 124 thiazolidinedione monotherapy patients, with no cases reported in these trials for repaglinide monotherapy. When corrected for dropout rates of the treatment groups, the percentage of patients having events of peripheral edema per 24 weeks of treatment were 5% for repaglinide-thiazolidinedione combination therapy, and 4% for thiazolidinedione monotherapy. There were reports in 2 of 250 patients (0.8%) treated with repaglinide-thiazolidinedione therapy of episodes of edema with congestive heart failure. Both patients had a history of coronary artery disease and recovered after treatment with diuretic agents. No comparable cases in the monotherapy treatment groups were reported.

Mean change in weight from baseline was +4.9 kg for repaglinide-thiazolidinedione therapy. There were no patients on repaglinide-thiazolidinedione combination therapy who had elevations of liver transaminases (defined as 3 times the upper limit of normal levels).

➤*Postmarketing:* Although no causal relationship has been established, postmarketing experience includes reports of the following rare adverse reactions: Alopecia, hemolytic anemia, pancreatitis, Stevens-Johnson syndrome, and severe hepatic dysfunction.

Overdosage

➤*Symptoms:* In a clinical trial, patients received increasing doses of repaglinide up to 80 mg a day for 14 days. There were few adverse effects other than those associated with the intended effect of lowering blood glucose. Hypoglycemia did not occur when meals were given with these high doses.

➤*Treatment:* Treat hypoglycemic symptoms without loss of consciousness or neurologic findings aggressively with oral glucose and adjustments in drug dosage and/or meal patterns. Close monitoring may continue until the physician is assured that the patient is out of danger. Closely monitor patients for a minimum of 24 to 48 hours, since hypoglycemia may recur after apparent clinical recovery. There is no evidence that repaglinide is dialyzable using hemodialysis.

Severe hypoglycemic reactions with coma, seizure, or other neurological impairment occur infrequently, but constitute medical emergencies requiring immediate hospitalization. If hypoglycemic coma is diagnosed or suspected, the patient should be given a rapid intravenous injection of concentrated (50%) glucose solution. This should be followed by a continuous infusion of more dilute (10%) glucose solution at a rate that will maintain the blood glucose at a level above 100 mg/dL.

Patient Information

Inform patients of the potential risks and advantages of repaglinide and of alternative modes of therapy. Also inform them about the importance of adherence to dietary instructions, of a regular exercise program, and of regular testing of blood glucose and HbA_{1c}. Explain the risks of hypoglycemia, its symptoms and treatment, and its conditions that predispose to its development and concomitant administration of other glucose-lowering drugs to patients and responsible family members. Also explain primary and secondary failure.

Instruct patients to take repaglinide before meals (2, 3, or 4 times a day preprandially). Doses are usually taken within 15 minutes of the meal but time may vary from immediately preceding the meal to as long as 30 minutes before the meal. Instruct patients who skip a meal (or add an extra meal) to skip (or add) a dose for that meal.

NATEGLINIDE

Rx	**Starlix** (Novartis)	**Tablets:** 60 mg	Lactose. (STARLIX 60). Pink. In 100s and 500s.
		120 mg	Lactose. (STARLIX 120). Yellow, oval. In 100s and 500s.

NATEGLINIDE — ORAL

Indications

➤*Type 2 diabetes:* As monotherapy to lower blood glucose in patients with type 2 diabetes whose hyperglycemia cannot be adequately controlled by diet and physical exercise and who have not been chronically treated with other antidiabetic agents.

Nateglinide is also indicated for use in combination with metformin or a thiazolidinedione. In patients whose hyperglycemia is inadequately controlled with metformin or after a therapeutic response to a thiazolidinedione, nateglinide may be added to, but not substituted for, those drugs.

Patients whose hyperglycemia is not adequately controlled with glyburide or other insulin secretagogues should not be switched to nateglinide, nor should nateglinide be added to their treatment regimen.

Administration and Dosage

➤*Approved by the FDA:* December 22, 2000.

➤*Monotherapy and combination with metformin or a thiazolidinedione:* The recommended starting and maintenance dose of nateglinide, alone or in combination with metformin, is 120 mg 3 times daily before meals.

The 60 mg dose of nateglinide, either alone or in combination with metformin or a thiazolidinedione, may be used in patients who are near goal HbA_{1C} when treatment is initiated.

Nateglinide should be taken 1 to 30 minutes prior to meals.

➤*Elderly patients:* See Warnings for more information.

➤*Storage/Stability:* Store at 25°C (77°F); excursions permitted to 15° to 30°C (59° to 86°F). Dispense in a tight container.

Actions

➤*Pharmacology:* Nateglinide is an amino-acid derivative that lowers blood glucose levels by stimulating insulin secretion from the pancreas. This

NATEGLINIDE — ORAL

action is dependent upon functioning beta cells in the pancreatic islets. Nateglinide interacts with the ATP-sensitive potassium ($K+_{ATP}$) channel on pancreatic beta cells. The subsequent depolarization of the beta cell opens the calcium channel, producing calcium influx and insulin secretion. The extent of insulin release is glucose dependent and diminishes at low glucose levels. Nateglinide is highly tissue selective with low affinity for heart and skeletal muscle.

Pharmacodynamics – Nateglinide is rapidly absorbed and stimulates pancreatic insulin secretion within 20 minutes of oral administration. When nateglinide is dosed 3 times daily before meals, there is a rapid rise in plasma insulin, with peak levels approximately 1 hour after dosing and a fall to baseline by 4 hours after dosing.

In a double-blind, controlled clinical trial in which nateglinide was administered before each of 3 meals, plasma glucose levels were determined over a 12-hour daytime period after 7 weeks of treatment. Nateglinide was administered 10 minutes before meals. The meals were based on standard diabetic weight maintenance menus with the total caloric content based on each subject's height. Nateglinide produced statistically significant decreases in fasting and postprandial glycemia compared with placebo.

➤*Pharmacokinetics:*

Absorption – Following oral administration immediately prior to a meal, nateglinide is rapidly absorbed with mean peak plasma drug concentrations (C_{max}) generally occurring within 1 hour (T_{max}) after dosing. When administered to patients with type 2 diabetes over the dosage range 60 to 240 mg 3 times a day for 1 week, nateglinide demonstrated linear pharmacokinetics for both area under the time/plasma concentration curve (AUC) and C_{max}. T_{max} was also found to be independent of dose in this patient population. Absolute bioavailability is estimated to be approximately 73%. When given with or after meals, the extent of nateglinide absorption (AUC) remains unaffected. However, there is a delay in the rate of absorption characterized by a decrease in C_{max} and a delay in time to peak plasma concentration (T_{max}). Plasma profiles are characterized by multiple plasma concentration peaks when nateglinide is administered under fasting conditions. This effect is diminished when nateglinide is taken prior to a meal.

Distribution – Based on data following IV administration of nateglinide, the steady-state volume of distribution of nateglinide is estimated to be approximately 10 L in healthy subjects. Nateglinide is extensively bound (98%) to serum proteins, primarily serum albumin, and to a lesser extent α_1 acid glycoprotein. The extent of serum protein binding is independent of drug concentration over the test range of 0.1 to 10 mcg/mL.

Metabolism – Nateglinide is metabolized by the mixed-function oxidase system prior to elimination. The major routes of metabolism are hydroxylation followed by glucuronide conjugation. The major metabolites are less potent antidiabetic agents than nateglinide. The isoprene minor metabolite possesses potency similar to that of the parent compound nateglinide.

In vitro data demonstrate that nateglinide is predominantly metabolized by cytochrome P450 isoenzymes CYP2C9 (70%) and CYP3A4 (30%).

Excretion – Nateglinide and its metabolites are rapidly and completely eliminated following oral administration. Within 6 hours after dosing, approximately 75% of the administered ^{14}C-nateglinide was recovered in the urine. Eighty-three percent (83%) of the ^{14}C-nateglinide was excreted in the urine with an additional 10% eliminated in the feces. Approximately 16% of the ^{14}C-nateglinide was excreted in the urine as parent compound. In all studies of healthy volunteers and patients with type 2 diabetes, nateglinide plasma concentrations declined rapidly with an average elimination half-life of approximately 1.5 hours. Consistent with this short elimination half-life, there was no apparent accumulation of nateglinide upon multiple dosing of up to 240 mg 3 times daily for 7 days.

Special populations –

Renal function impairment: Compared to healthy matched subjects, patients with type 2 diabetes and moderate to severe renal insufficiency (creatinine clearance [Ccr] 15 to 50 mL/min) not on dialysis displayed similar apparent clearance, AUC, and C_{max}. Patients with type 2 diabetes and renal failure on dialysis exhibited reduced overall drug exposure. However, hemodialysis patients also experienced reductions in plasma protein binding compared with the matched healthy volunteers.

Hepatic function impairment: The peak and total exposure of nateglinide in nondiabetic subjects with mild hepatic insufficiency were increased by 30% compared with matched healthy subjects. Use nateglinide with caution in patients with chronic liver disease.

Contraindications

Known hypersensitivity to the drug or its inactive ingredients; type 1 diabetes; diabetic ketoacidosis. This condition should be treated with insulin.

Warnings

➤*Hepatic function impairment:* Use nateglinide with caution in patients with moderate to severe liver disease because such patients have not been studied.

➤*Elderly:* No differences were observed in safety or efficacy of nateglinide between patients 65 years of age or older, and those younger than 65 years of age. However, greater sensitivity of some older individuals to nateglinide therapy cannot be ruled out.

➤*Pregnancy: Category C.* In the rabbit, embryonic development was adversely affected and the incidence of gallbladder agenesis or small gallbladder was increased at a dose of 500 mg/kg (approximately 40 times the human therapeutic exposure with a recommended nateglinide dose of 120 mg, 3 times daily before meals). There are no adequate and well-controlled studies in pregnant women. Do not use nateglinide during pregnancy.

➤*Lactation:* Studies in lactating rats showed that nateglinide is excreted in the milk; the AUC_{0-48hr} ratio in milk to plasma was approximately 1:4. During the peri- and postnatal period, body weights were lower in offspring of rats administered nateglinide at 1,000 mg/kg (approximately 60 times the human therapeutic exposure with a recommended nateglinide dose of 120 mg, 3 times daily before meals). It is not known whether nateglinide is excreted in human milk. Because many drugs are excreted in human milk, do not administer nateglinide to a nursing woman.

➤*Children:* The safety and efficacy of nateglinide in pediatric patients have not been established.

Precautions

➤*Monitoring:* Periodically assess response to therapies with glucose values and HbA_{1C} levels.

➤*Hypoglycemia:* All oral blood glucose-lowering drugs that are absorbed systemically are capable of producing hypoglycemia. The frequency of hypoglycemia is related to the severity of the diabetes, the level of glycemic control, and other patient characteristics. Geriatric patients, malnourished patients, and those with adrenal or pituitary insufficiency or severe renal impairment are more susceptible to the glucose-lowering effect of these treatments. The risk of hypoglycemia may be increased by strenuous physical exercise, ingestion of alcohol, insufficient caloric intake on an acute or chronic basis, or combinations with other oral antidiabetic agents. Hypoglycemia may be difficult to recognize in patients with autonomic neuropathy or those who use beta blockers. Administer nateglinide prior to meals to reduce the risk of hypoglycemia. Patients who skip meals should also skip their scheduled dose of nateglinide to reduce the risk of hypoglycemia.

➤*Loss of glycemic control:* Transient loss of glycemic control may occur with fever, infection, trauma, or surgery. Insulin therapy may be needed instead of nateglinide therapy at such times. Secondary failure, or reduced effectiveness of nateglinide over a period of time, may occur.

Drug Interactions

➤*Cytochrome P450:* In vitro metabolism studies indicate that nateglinide is predominantly metabolized by the cytochrome P450 isozyme CYP2C9 (70%) and to a lesser extent CYP3A4 (30%). Nateglinide is a potential inhibitor of the CYP2C9 isoenzyme in vivo as indicated by its ability to inhibit the in vitro metabolism of tolbutamide. Inhibition of CYP3A4 metabolic reactions was not detected in in vitro experiments.

Nateglinide Drug Interactions

Precipitant drug	Object drug[a]		Description
Beta-adrenergic blockers, nonselective MAOIs NSAIDS Salicylates	Nateglinide	↑	These drugs may potentiate the hypoglycemic effects of nateglinide and other oral antidiabetic agents. Closely monitor blood glucose when these agents are started or stopped.
Corticosteroids Sympathomimetics Thiazides Thyroid products	Nateglinide	↓	These agents may reduce the hypoglycemic action of nateglinide and other oral antidiabetic agents. Closely monitor blood glucose when these agents are started or stopped.
Rifamycins (eg, rifampin)	Nateglinide	↓	Nateglinide plasma concentrations and pharmacologic effects may be decreased with coadministration. Closely monitor blood glucose levels when starting and stopping rifamycin therapy and adjust nateglinide dose as necessary.

[a] ↑ = Object drug increased. ↓ = Object drug decreased.

➤*Drug/Food interactions:* Peak plasma levels were significantly reduced when nateglinide was administered 10 minutes prior to a liquid meal.

Adverse Reactions

Hypoglycemia was relatively uncommon in all treatment arms of the clinical trials. Only 0.3% of nateglinide patients discontinued due to hypoglycemia. GI symptoms, especially diarrhea and nausea, were no more common in patients using the combination of nateglinide and metformin than in patients receiving metformin alone. Likewise, peripheral edema was no more common in patients using the combination of nateglinide and rosiglitazone than in patients receiving rosiglitazone alone. The following table lists events that occurred more frequently in nateglinide patients than in placebo patients in controlled clinical trials.

NATEGLINIDE — ORAL

Common Adverse Events (≥ 2% in Nateglinide Patients) in Nateglinide Monotherapy Trials (% of Patients)		
Adverse reaction	Placebo (n = 458)	Nateglinide (n = 1,441)
Preferred term		
Accidental trauma	1.7%	2.9%
Arthropathy	2.2%	3.3%
Back pain	3.7%	4%
Bronchitis	2.6%	2.7%
Coughing	2.2%	2.4%
Diarrhea	3.1%	3.2%
Dizziness	2.2%	3.6%
Flu symptoms	2.6%	3.6%
Hypoglycemia	0.4%	2.4%
Upper respiratory tract infection	8.1%	10.5%

During postmarketing experience, rare cases of hypersensitivity reactions such as rash, itching, and urticaria have been reported.

➤*Lab test abnormalities:*

Uric acid – There were increases in mean uric acid levels for patients treated with nateglinide alone, nateglinide in combination with metformin, metformin alone, and glyburide alone. The respective differences from placebo were 0.29 mg/dL, 0.45 mg/dL, 0.28 mg/dL, and 0.19 mg/dL. The clinical significance of these findings is unknown.

Overdosage

➤*Symptoms:* In a clinical study in patients with type 2 diabetes, nateglinide was administered in increasing doses up to 720 mg daily for 7 days and there were no clinically significant adverse events reported. There have been no instances of overdose with nateglinide in clinical trials. However, an overdose may result in an exaggerated glucose-lowering effect with the development of hypoglycemic symptoms.

➤*Treatment:* Treat hypoglycemic symptoms without loss of consciousness or neurological findings with oral glucose and adjustments in dosage or meal patterns. Treat severe hypoglycemic reactions with coma, seizure, or other neurological symptoms with IV glucose. As nateglinide is highly protein bound, dialysis is not an efficient means of removing it from the blood.

Patient Information

Inform patients of the potential risks and benefits of nateglinide and of alternative modes of therapy. Explain the risks and management of hypoglycemia. Instruct patients to take nateglinide 1 to 30 minutes before ingesting a meal, but to skip their scheduled dose if they skip the meal so that the risk of hypoglycemia will be reduced. Discuss drug interactions with patients. Inform patients of potential drug-drug interactions with nateglinide.

Indications

➤*Type 2 diabetes:* Monotherapy as an adjunct to diet and exercise to improve glycemic control.

In combination with metformin, insulin, or a sulfonylurea when diet, exercise, and a single agent do not result in adequate glycemic control.

Actions

➤*Pharmacology:* **Rosiglitazone** and **pioglitazone**, members of the thiazolidinediones class of antidiabetic agents, improve glycemic control by improving insulin sensitivity. They depend on the presence of insulin for their mechanism of action. Studies indicate that they improve sensitivity to insulin in muscle and adipose tissue and inhibit hepatic gluconeogenesis. Thiazolidinediones are highly selective and potent agonists for the peroxisome proliferator-activated receptor-gamma (PPARγ). PPAR receptors are found in adipose tissue, skeletal muscle, and liver. Activation of PPARγ nuclear receptors regulates the transcription of insulin-responsive genes involved in the control of glucose production, transport, and utilization and participates in the regulation of fatty acid metabolism.

➤*Pharmacokinetics:*

Pharmacokinetics of Thiazolidinediones		
Parameters	Pioglitazone	Rosiglitazone
Absorption		
Bioavailability	—	99%
C_{max}[a]	—	1 mg[b]: 76 ng/mL 2 mg[b]: 156 ng/mL 8 mg[b]: 598 ng/mL 8 mg[c]: 432 ng/mL
T_{max}	2 h[b] 3 to 4 h[c]	1 h
Food effect	Delays time to peak concentration; does not alter extent of absorption	28% decrease in C_{max} and delay in T_{max} (1.75 h); no overall change in AUC
Distribution		
Volume of distribution	≈ 0.63 L/kg[a]	17.6 L
Protein binding	> 99%	≈ 99.8%
Metabolism		
Mechanism	Hydroxylation, oxidation, CYP2C8, CYP3A4, CYP1A1	N-demethylation, hydroxylation, conjugation CYP2C8, CYP2C9 (minor)
Active metabolites	MII[d], MIII[e], MIV[d]	—
Excretion		
Site	Urine (15 to 30%), feces	Urine (64%), feces (23%)
Elimination half-life	Pioglitazone: 3 to 7 h Total pioglitazone: 16 to 24 h	3 to 4 h
Oral clearance	5 to 7 L/h	1 mg[b]: 3.03 L/h 2 mg[b]: 2.89 L/h 8 mg[b]: 2.85 L/h 8 mg[c]: 2.97 L/h

[a] Following single oral doses.
[b] In the fasting state.
[c] In the fed state.
[d] Hydroxy derivatives of pioglitazone.
[e] Keto derivative of pioglitazone.

Special populations –

Gender: The mean pioglitazone C_{max} and AUC values were increased 20% to 60% in females.

Hepatic function impairment:

• *Rosiglitazone* – Unbound oral clearance of rosiglitazone was significantly lower in moderate to severe liver disease patients (Child-Pugh class B/C) in comparison with healthy subjects. This resulted in an increased C_{max} by 2-fold and AUC by 3-fold, and a longer elimination half-life by 2 hours. Do not initiate rosiglitazone in patients exhibiting clinical evidence of active liver disease or increased serum transaminase levels (ALT more than 2.5 times the upper limit of normal [ULN]).

• *Pioglitazone* – Compared with healthy controls, subjects with impaired hepatic function (Child-Pugh class B/C) have approximately 45% reduction in pioglitazone and total pioglitazone mean peak concentrations but no change in the mean AUC values. Do not initiate pioglitazone if the patient exhibits clinical evidence of active liver disease or serum transaminase levels (ALT more than 2.5 times the ULN).

Obesity: Both oral clearance (CL/F) and oral steady-state volume of distribution (Vss/F) were shown to increase with increases in body weight. The range of predicted CL/F and Vss/F values varied by less than 1.7-fold and less than 2.3-fold, respectively, over the weight range observed in these analyses (50 to 150 kg).

Contraindications

Hypersensitivity to **pioglitazone** or **rosiglitazone** or any of their components.

Warnings

➤*Hepatotoxicity:* Although available clinical data show no evidence of **pioglitazone**- and **rosiglitazone**-induced hepatotoxicity or ALT elevations, they are related structurally to or very similar to **troglitazone**, a thiazolidinedione no longer marketed in the United States, which was associated with idiosyncratic hepatotoxicity and cases of liver failure, liver transplants, and death during postmarketing clinical use. Do not use in patients who experienced jaundice while taking troglitazone. In preapproval clinical studies of 4,598 patients treated with rosiglitazone, encompassing approximately 3,600 patient-years of exposure, there was no signal of drug-induced hepatotoxicity or elevation of ALT levels. In postmarketing experience with rosiglitazone, reports of hepatitis and hepatic enzyme elevations to 3 or more times the ULN have been received. Very rarely, these reports have involved hepatic failure with and without fatal outcome, although causality has not been established. In preapproval clinical studies worldwide, over 4,500 subjects were treated with pioglitazone. In US clinical studies, over 4,700 patients with type 2 diabetes received pioglitazone. There was no evidence of drug-induced hepatotoxicity or elevation of ALT levels in the clinical studies. In postmarketing experience with pioglitazone, reports of hepatitis and hepatic enzyme elevations to 3 or more times the ULN have been received. Very rarely, these reports have involved hepatic failure with and without fatal outcome, although causality has not been established.

It is recommended that patients treated with pioglitazone and rosiglitazone undergo periodic monitoring of liver enzymes. Check liver enzymes prior to the initiation of therapy in all treated patients. Do not initiate therapy in patients with increased baseline liver enzyme levels (ALT more than 2.5 times the ULN). In patients with normal baseline liver enzymes following initiation of therapy, it is recommended that liver enzymes be monitored every 2 months for the first 12 months and periodically thereafter. Evaluate patients with mildly elevated liver enzymes (ALT levels less than or equal to 2.5 times the ULN) at baseline or during therapy to determine the cause of the liver enzyme elevation. Proceed with caution in the initiation of, or continuation of, therapy in patients with mild liver enzyme elevations and include appropriate close clinical follow-up, including more frequent liver enzyme monitoring, to determine if the liver enzyme elevations resolve or worsen. If, at any time, ALT levels increase to more than 3 times the ULN in patients on therapy, recheck liver enzyme levels as soon as possible. If ALT levels remain more than 3 times the ULN or if the patient is jaundiced, discontinue therapy.

If any patient develops symptoms suggesting hepatic dysfunction (eg, unexplained nausea, vomiting, abdominal pain, fatigue, anorexia, dark urine), check liver enzymes. Guide the decision by clinical judgment whether to continue the patient on therapy with pioglitazone and rosiglitazone pending laboratory evaluations. If jaundice is observed, discontinue therapy.

➤*Cardiac effects:* Thiazolidinediones, alone or in combination with other antidiabetic agents, can cause fluid retention, which may exacerbate or lead to heart failure. Observe patients for signs and symptoms of heart failure. In combination with insulin, thiazolidinediones also may increase the risk of other cardiovascular adverse events. Discontinue if any deterioration in cardiac status occurs. Rosiglitazone and pioglitazone are not recommended in patients with NYHA Class 3 and 4 cardiac status.

In clinical studies, an increased incidence of edema, cardiac failure, and other cardiovascular adverse events was seen in patients on rosiglitazone and insulin combination therapy compared with insulin and placebo. Patients who experienced cardiovascular events were older on average and had a longer duration of diabetes. These cardiovascular events were noted at the 4 and 8 mg daily dose strengths. In this population, however, it was not possible to determine specific risk factors that could be used to identify all patients at risk of heart failure and other cardiovascular events on combination therapy. Three of 10 patients who developed cardiac failure on combination therapy during the double blind part of the studies had no known prior evidence of CHF, or pre-existing cardiac condition.

Monitor patients treated with combination **rosiglitazone** and insulin or combination rosiglitazone/metformin and insulin for cardiovascular adverse events. Discontinue this combination therapy in patients who do not respond as manifested by a reduction in HbA_{1c} or insulin dose after 4 to 5 months of therapy or who develop any significant adverse events.

In a clinical trial involving 566 patients, 2 of 191 patients (1.1%) receiving 15 mg **pioglitazone** plus insulin and 2 of 188 patients (1.1%) receiving 30 mg pioglitazone plus insulin developed CHF compared with none of the 187 patients on insulin therapy alone. All 4 of these patients had previous histories of cardiovascular conditions, including coronary artery disease, previous CABG procedures, and MI. In a 24-week, dose-controlled study in which pioglitazone was coadministered with insulin, 1 of 345 of patients (0.3%) on 30 mg and 3 of 345 of patients (0.9%) on 45 mg reported CHF as a serious adverse event. Analysis of data from these studies did not identify specific factors that predict increased risk of CHF in combination therapy with insulin.

In postmarketing experience with pioglitazone, cases of CHF have been reported in patients with and without previously known heart disease.

➤*Ovulation:* In premenopausal anovulatory patients, thiazolidinedione treatment may result in resumption of ovulation. These patients may be at risk for pregnancy. Recommend adequate contraception in these women.

➤*Carcinogenesis:* There was an increase in incidence of adipose hyperplasia in mice at **rosiglitazone** doses of 1.5 mg/kg/day or more (approximately 2 times human AUC at the maximum recommended human daily dose). In rats, there was a significant increase in the incidence of benign adipose tissue tumors (lipomas) at doses of 0.3 mg/kg/day or more (approximately 2 times human AUC at the maximum recommended human daily dose). These proliferative changes in both species are considered to be caused by the persistent pharmacological overstimulation of adipose tissue.

A 2-year carcinogenicity study was conducted in male and female rats at oral doses up to 63 mg/kg **pioglitazone** (approximately 14 times the maximum recommended human oral dose of 45 mg based on mg/m^2). Drug-induced tumors were not observed in any organ except for the urinary bladder. Benign and/or malignant transitional cell neoplasms were observed in male rats at 4 mg/kg/day and above (approximately equal to the maximum recommended human oral dose based on mg/m^2).

➤*Fertility impairment:* **Rosiglitazone** altered estrous cyclicity (2 mg/kg/day) and reduced fertility (40 mg/kg/day) of female rats in association with lower plasma levels of progesterone and estradiol (approximately 20 to 200 times human AUC at the maximum recommended human daily dose, respectively). In monkeys, rosiglitazone (0.6 and 4.6 mg/kg/day; approximately 3 and 15 times the human AUC at the maximum recommended human daily dose, respectively) diminished the follicular phase rise in serum estradiol with consequential reduction in the luteinizing hormone surge, lower luteal phase progesterone levels, and amenorrhea. The mechanism for these effects appears to be direct inhibition of ovarian steroidogenesis.

➤*Pregnancy: Category C* (**pioglitazone, rosiglitazone**). There are no adequate and well-controlled studies in pregnant women. Do not use pioglitazone or rosiglitazone during pregnancy unless the potential benefit justifies the potential risk to the fetus.

Treatment with rosiglitazone during mid-to-late gestation was associated with fetal death and growth retardation in rats and rabbits. Rosiglitazone caused placental pathology in rats (3 mg/kg/day). Treatment of rats during gestation through lactation reduced litter size, neonatal viability, and postnatal growth, with growth retardation reversible after puberty. For effects on the placenta, embryo/fetus, and offspring, the no-effect dose was 0.2 mg/kg/day in rats and 15 mg/kg/day in rabbits. These no-effect levels are approximately 4 times the human AUC at the maximum recommended human daily dose.

Delayed parturition and embryotoxicty (ie, increased postimplantation losses, delayed development, and reduced fetal weights) were observed in rats at oral doses of 40 mg/kg/day or more (about 10 times the maximum recommended human oral dose based on mg/m^2). No functional or behavioral toxicity was observed in the offspring of rats. In rabbits, embryotoxicity was observed at an oral dose of 160 mg/kg (about 40 times the maximum recommended human oral dose based on mg/m^2). Delayed postnatal development, attributed to decreased body weight, was observed in offspring of rats at oral doses of 10 mg/kg or more during late gestation and lactation periods (about 2 times the maximum recommended human oral dose based on mg/m^2).

Because current information strongly suggests that abnormal blood glucose levels during pregnancy are associated with a higher incidence of congenital anomalies, as well as increased neonatal morbidity and mortality, most experts recommend insulin be used during pregnancy to maintain blood glucose levels as close to normal as possible.

➤*Lactation:* It is not known whether **pioglitazone** or **rosiglitazone** are secreted in human milk. Pioglitazone and rosiglitazone are secreted in the milk of lactating rats. Do not administer to nursing women.

➤*Children:* Safety and efficacy have not been established in patients younger than 18 years of age.

Precautions

➤*Monitoring:* Perform periodic fasting blood glucose and HbA_{1c} measurements to monitor therapeutic response. Liver enzyme monitoring is recommended prior to initiation of therapy in all patients and periodically thereafter (see Warnings).

➤*Type 1 diabetes:* **Pioglitazone** and **rosiglitazone** are active only in the presence of insulin. Therefore, do not use in type 1 diabetes patients or for the treatment of diabetic ketoacidosis.

➤*Hypoglycemia:* Patients receiving **pioglitazone** and **rosiglitazone** in combination with insulin or oral hypoglycemics (eg, sulfonylureas) may be at risk for hypoglycemia; reduction in the dose of the concomitant agent may be necessary.

➤*Hematologic:* Mean decreases in hemoglobin up to 1 g/dL and hematocrit up to 3.3% were observed for **rosiglitazone** alone and in combination with other hypoglycemic agents, primarily occurring during the first 3 months or following an increase in rosiglitazone dose. White blood cell counts also decreased slightly in patients treated with rosiglitazone. **Pioglitazone** also may cause decreases in hemoglobin and hematocrit. Mean hemoglobin values declined by 2% to 4% in pioglitazone-treated patients. These changes primarily occurred within the first 4 to 12 weeks of therapy and remained relatively constant thereafter. The observed changes may be related to the increased plasma volume observed with treatment and have not been associated with any significant hematologic clinical effects.

➤*Edema:* Use **pioglitazone** and **rosiglitazone** with caution in patients with edema. In a clinical study in healthy volunteers who received rosiglitazone 8 mg once daily for 8 weeks, there was a statistically significant increase in median plasma volume compared with placebo. In controlled clinical trials of patients with type 2 diabetes, mild to moderate edema was reported in pioglitazone- and rosiglitazone-treated patients. Patients with ongoing edema are more likely to have adverse events associated with edema if started on combination therapy with insulin and rosiglitazone.

Because thiazolidinediones can cause fluid retention, which can exacerbate or lead to CHF, use with caution in patients at risk for heart failure, and monitor patients at risk for heart failure for signs and symptoms of heart failure.

➤*Weight gain:* Dose-related weight gain was seen with **rosiglitazone** and **pioglitazone** alone and in combination with other hypoglycemic agents. The mechanism of weight gain is unclear but probably involves a combination of fluid retention and fat accumulation.

In postmarketing experience, there have been rare reports of unusually rapid increases in weight and increases in excess of that generally observed in clinical trials. Assess patients who experience such increases for fluid accumulation and volume-related events (eg, excessive edema, CHF).

Drug Interactions

➤*CYP450 system:* In vitro drug metabolism studies suggest that **rosiglitazone** does not inhibit any of the major P450 enzymes at clinically relevant concentrations. In vitro data demonstrate that rosiglitazone is metabolized predominantly by CYP2C8 and, to a lesser extent, 2C9.

In vivo drug interaction studies have suggested that **pioglitazone** may be a weak inducer of CYP450 isoform 3A4 substrate. In vitro, ketoconazole appears to inhibit significantly the metabolism of pioglitazone. Pending the availability of additional data, evaluate patients receiving ketoconazole concomitantly with pioglitazone more frequently with respect to glycemic control.

Thiazolidinediones Drug Interactions

Precipitant drug	Object drug[a]		Description
Atorvastatin	Pioglitazone	⬆	Concurrent use for 7 days resulted in an increase in pioglitazone and atorvastatin serum concentrations.
Pioglitazone	Atorvastatin		
Ketoconazole	Pioglitazone	⬆	Coadministration resulted in an increase in pioglitazone AUC and C_{max}.
Pioglitazone	Midazolam	⬇	Administration of pioglitazone for 15 days followed by a single 7.5 mg dose of midazolam syrup resulted in a 26% reduction in midazolam C_{max} and AUC.
Pioglitazone	Nifedipine	⬆	Concurrent use of pioglitazone and extended-release nifedipine resulted in an increase in nifedipine concentrations. Clinical significance is unknown.

Thiazolidinediones Drug Interactions			
Precipitant drug	Object drug[a]		Description
Pioglitazone	Oral contraceptives	⬇	Coadministration of pioglitazone with an oral contraceptive (eg, ethinyl estradiol/ norethindrone) for 21 days resulted in an 11% decrease in the ethinyl estradiol AUC and an 11% to 14% decrease in the C_{max}. Clinical significance is unknown. Rosiglitazone was not shown to have a clinical effect on these pharmacokinetics.

[a] ⬆ = Object drug increased. ⬇ = Object drug decreased.

Adverse Reactions

Thiazolidinediones Adverse Reactions (%)[a]		
Adverse reaction	Pioglitazone (n = 606)	Rosiglitazone (n = 2,526)
CNS		
Fatigue	—	3.6
Headache	9.1	5.9
GI		
Diarrhea	—	2.3
Tooth disorder	5.3	—
Metabolism		
Aggravated diabetes mellitus	5.1	—
Hyperglycemia	—	3.9
Hypoglycemia	—	0.6
Respiratory		
Pharyngitis	5.1	—
Sinusitis	6.3	3.2
Upper respiratory tract infection	13.2	9.9
Miscellaneous		
Anemia	—	1.9
Back pain	—	4
Edema	4.8	4.8
Injury	—	7.6
Myalgia	5.4	—

[a] Data are pooled from separate studies and are not necessarily comparable.

Pioglitazone – Edema was reported in 7.2% of patients treated with pioglitazone and sulfonylureas compared with 2.1% of patients on sulfonylureas alone. In combination studies with metformin, edema was reported in 6% of patients on combination therapy compared with 2.5% of patients on metformin alone.

In a 16-week, placebo-controlled, pioglitazone plus insulin trial (N = 379), 10 patients treated with pioglitazone plus insulin developed dyspnea and also, at some point during their therapy, developed either weight change or edema. Seven of these 10 patients received diuretics to treat these symptoms. This was not reported in the insulin plus placebo group. In controlled combination therapy studies with either a sulfonylurea or insulin, mild to moderate hypoglycemia, which appears to be dose-related, was reported (see Precautions).

Rosiglitazone – Overall, the types of adverse experiences reported when rosiglitazone was used in combination with metformin or a sulfonylurea were similar to those during monotherapy with rosiglitazone. Reports of anemia (7.1%) were greater in patients treated with a combination of rosiglitazone and metformin compared with rosiglitazone monotherapy or combination therapy with a sulfonylurea. Lower pretreatment hemoglobin/hematocrit levels in patients enrolled in the metformin combination clinical trials may have contributed to the higher reporting rate of anemia in these studies.

Edema was reported with higher frequency in the rosiglitazone plus insulin combination trials (insulin, 5.4%; rosiglitazone in combination with insulin, 14.7%). Reports of new onset or exacerbation of CHF occurred at rates of 1% for insulin alone, and 2% (4 mg) and 3% (8 mg) for insulin in combination with rosiglitazone. In postmarketing experience with rosiglitazone, adverse events potentially related to volume expansion (eg, CHF, pulmonary edema, pleural effusions) have been reported.

➤*Lab test abnormalities:*

Hematologic – Decreases in hemoglobin, hematocrit, and white blood cell counts may be related to increased plasma volume observed with thiazolidinedione treatment. Mean decreases of up to 1 g/dL hemoglobin and up to 3.3% hematocrit occurred in **rosiglitazone**-treated patients. Mean hemoglobin values decreased by 2% to 4% in **pioglitazone**-treated patients (see Precautions).

Lipids – **Rosiglitazone** as monotherapy was associated with increases in total cholesterol, LDL, and HDL and decreases in free fatty acids. Patients treated with **pioglitazone** had mean decreases in triglycerides, mean increases in HDL cholesterol, and no consistent mean changes in LDL and total cholesterol. In placebo-controlled trials, the placebo-corrected mean changes from baseline decreased 5% to 26% for triglycerides and increased 6% to 13% for HDL in patients treated with pioglitazone.

Serum transaminase levels – In controlled trials, 0.2% of patients treated with **rosiglitazone** had reversible elevations in ALT greater than 3 times the ULN compared with 0.2% on placebo and 0.5% on active comparators. Hyperbilirubinemia was found in 0.3% of patients treated with rosiglitazone compared with 0.9% treated with placebo and 1% in patients treated with active comparators. In postmarketing experience with rosiglitazone, reports of hepatic enzyme elevations of 3 or more times the ULN and hepatitis have been received.

During clinical trials in the United States, a total of 0.3% **pioglitazone**-treated patients had ALT values 3 times or more the ULN. All patients with follow-up values had reversible elevations in ALT. In the population of patients treated with pioglitazone, mean values for bilirubin, AST, ALT, alkaline phosphatase, and GGT were decreased at the final visit compared with baseline. Fewer than 0.9% of pioglitazone-treated patients were withdrawn from clinical trials in the United States because of abnormal liver function tests.

CPK levels – During required laboratory testing in clinical trials, sporadic, transient elevations in creatine phosphokinase levels (CPK) were observed. An isolated elevation to more than 10 times the ULN (values of 2150 to 11,400 units/L) was noted in 9 patients. Six of these patients continued to receive **pioglitazone**. Two patients completed receiving study medication at the time of the elevated value and 1 patient discontinued study medication because of the elevation. These elevations resolved without any apparent clinical sequelae. The relationship of these events to pioglitazone therapy is unknown.

Overdosage

Limited data are available with regard to overdosage in humans. In clinical studies in volunteers, **rosiglitazone** has been administered at single oral doses of up to 20 mg and was well tolerated. During controlled clinical trials, 1 case of overdose with **pioglitazone** was reported. A male patient took 120 mg/day for 4 days, then 180 mg/day for 7 days. The patient denied any clinical symptoms during this period. In the event of an overdose, initiate appropriate supportive treatment.

Patient Information

Pioglitazone and **rosiglitazone** may be taken with or without meals. If the dose is missed at the usual meal, it may be taken at the next meal. If the dose is missed on 1 day, the dose should not be doubled the following day.

Management of type 2 diabetes should include diet control. Caloric restriction, weight loss, and exercise are essential for the proper treatment of the diabetic patient because they help improve insulin sensitivity. This is important not only in the primary treatment of type 2 diabetes but in maintaining the efficacy of drug therapy.

It is important for the patient to adhere to dietary instructions and to have blood glucose and glycosylated hemoglobin tested regularly. During periods of stress, such as fever, trauma, infection, or surgery, medication requirements may change, and patients should seek the advice of their physician.

Inform patients that blood will be drawn to check their liver function prior to the start of therapy and every 2 months for the first 12 months and periodically thereafter.

When using combination therapy with insulin or an oral hypoglycemic agent, explain the risks of hypoglycemia, its symptoms, treatment, and predisposing conditions to patients and their family members.

Patients who experience an unusually rapid increase in weight or edema or who develop shortness of breath or other symptoms of heart failure while on therapy should immediately report these symptoms to their physician.

Instruct patients to immediately report any signs or symptoms of hepatic dysfunction (eg, nausea, vomiting, abdominal pain, fatigue, anorexia, dark urine, jaundice) to their physician.

Use of thiazolidinediones can cause resumption of ovulation in women. Therefore, recommend adequate contraception in premenopausal women.

Advise patients that it can take 2 weeks of rosiglitazone therapy to see a reduction in blood glucose and 2 to 3 months to see full effect.

ROSIGLITAZONE MALEATE

Rx	**Avandia** (GlaxoSmithKline)	**Tablets:** 2 mg	Lactose. (SB 2). Pink, pentagonal. Film-coated. In 60s.
		4 mg	Lactose. (SB 4). Orange, pentagonal. Film-coated. In 30s and 100s.
		8 mg	Lactose. (SB 8). Red-brown, pentagonal. Film-coated. In 30s and 100s.

ROSIGLITAZONE MALEATE — ORAL

For complete and comparative prescribing information, refer to the Thiazolidinediones group monograph.

Indications

➤*Type 2 diabetes:* As an adjunct to diet and exercise to improve glycemic control in patients with type 2 diabetes mellitus. Rosiglitazone is indicated as monotherapy.

For use in combination with a sulfonylurea, metformin, or insulin when diet, exercise, and a single agent do not result in adequate glycemic control. For patients inadequately controlled with a maximum dose of a sulfonylurea or metformin, give rosiglitazone as an addition to, rather than as a substitute for, a sulfonylurea or metformin.

For use in combination with a sulfonylurea plus metformin when diet, exercise, and both agents do not result in adequate glycemic control.

➤*Unlabeled uses:* Increased ovulation frequency in women with polycystic ovary syndrome; reduced in-stent restenosis in patients with diabetes.

Administration and Dosage

➤*Approved by the FDA:* May 28, 1999.

Management of type 2 diabetes should include diet control. Caloric restriction, weight loss, and exercise are essential for the proper treatment of the diabetic patient because they help improve insulin sensitivity. This is important not only in the primary treatment of type 2 diabetes but also in maintaining the efficacy of drug therapy. Prior to initiation of therapy with rosiglitazone, secondary causes of poor glycemic control (eg, infection) should be investigated and treated.

The management of antidiabetic therapy should be individualized. All patients should start rosiglitazone at the lowest recommended dose. Further increases in the rosiglitazone dose should be accompanied by careful monitoring for adverse reactions related to fluid retention.

Rosiglitazone may be administered either at a starting dose of 4 mg as a single daily dose or divided and administered in the morning and evening. For patients who respond inadequately following 8 to 12 weeks of treatment, as determined by reduction in fasting plasma glucose (FPG), the dose may be increased to 8 mg daily as monotherapy or in combination with metformin, sulfonylurea, or sulfonylurea plus metformin. Rosiglitazone may be taken with or without food.

➤*Monotherapy:* The usual starting dose of rosiglitazone is 4 mg, administered either as a single dose once daily or in divided doses twice daily. In clinical trials, the 4 mg twice-daily regimen resulted in the highest reduction in FPG and HbA_{1c}.

➤*Combination therapy:* When rosiglitazone is added to existing therapy, the current dose(s) of the agent(s) can be continued upon initiation of rosiglitazone therapy.

➤*Sulfonylurea:* When used in combination with sulfonylurea, the usual starting dose of rosiglitazone is 4 mg administered as either a single dose once daily or in divided doses twice daily. If patients report hypoglycemia, the dose of the sulfonylurea should be decreased.

➤*Metformin:* The usual starting dose of rosiglitazone in combination with metformin is 4 mg administered as either a single dose once daily or in divided doses twice daily. It is unlikely that the dose of metformin will require adjustment because of hypoglycemia during combination therapy with rosiglitazone.

➤*Insulin:* For patients stabilized on insulin, the insulin dose should be continued upon initiation of therapy with rosiglitazone. Rosiglitazone should be dosed at 4 mg daily. Doses of rosiglitazone higher than 4 mg daily in combination with insulin are not currently indicated. It is recommended that the insulin dose be decreased 10% to 25% if the patient reports hypoglycemia or if the FPG concentrations decrease to less than 100 mg/dL. Further adjustments should be individualized based on glucose-lowering response.

➤*Sulfonylurea plus metformin:* The usual starting dose of rosiglitazone in combination with sulfonylurea plus metformin is 4 mg administered as either a single dose once daily or divided doses twice daily. If patients report hypoglycemia, the dose of sulfonylurea should be decreased.

➤*Maximum recommended dose:* The dosage of rosiglitazone should not exceed 8 mg daily, taken as a single dose or divided doses twice daily. The 8 mg daily dose has been shown to be safe and effective in clinical studies as monotherapy and in combination with metformin, sulfonylurea, or sulfonylurea plus metformin. Doses of rosiglitazone higher than 4 mg daily in combination with insulin are not currently indicated.

➤*Renal function impairment:* Because metformin is contraindicated in patients with renal function impairment, coadministration of metformin and rosiglitazone also is contraindicated in such patients.

➤*Hepatic function impairment:* Therapy with rosiglitazone should not be initiated if the patient exhibits clinical evidence of active liver disease or increased serum transaminase levels (ALT more than 2.5 times the upper limit of normal at start of therapy). Liver enzymes should be checked prior to the initiation of therapy with rosiglitazone and periodically thereafter in all patients.

➤*Storage/Stability:* Store at 25°C (77°F); excursions permitted to 15° to 30°C (59° to 86°F). Dispense in a tight, light-resistant container.

PIOGLITAZONE HYDROCHLORIDE

Rx	**Actos** (Takeda Pharmaceuticals North America, Inc.)	**Tablets:** 15 mg	Lactose. (ACTOS 15). White to off-white. In 30s, 90s, and 500s.
		30 mg	Lactose. (ACTOS 30). White to off-white. In 30s, 90s, and 500s.
		45 mg	Lactose. (ACTOS 45). White to off-white. In 30s, 90s, and 500s.

PIOGLITAZONE — ORAL

For complete and comparative prescribing information, refer to the Thiazolidinediones group monograph.

Indications

➤*Type 2 diabetes:* Monotherapy as an adjunct to diet and exercise to improve glycemic control in patients with type 2 diabetes.

Also for use in combination with a sulfonylurea, metformin, or insulin when diet, exercise, and the single agent do not result in adequate glycemic control.

Administration and Dosage

➤*Approved by the FDA:* July 16, 1999.

Management of type 2 diabetes also should include nutritional counseling, weight reduction as needed, and exercise. These efforts are important not only in the primary treatment of type 2 diabetes, but also to maintain the efficacy of drug therapy.

Take once daily without regard to meals. It is recommended that patients be treated with pioglitazone for a period of time adequate to evaluate change in HbA_{1c} (3 months) unless glycemic control deteriorates.

➤*Monotherapy:* Initiate monotherapy in patients not adequately controlled with diet and exercise at 15 or 30 mg once daily. For patients who respond inadequately to the initial dose of pioglitazone, the dose can be increased in increments up to 45 mg once daily. Consider combination therapy for patients not responding adequately to monotherapy.

➤*Combination therapy:*

Sulfonylureas – Initiate pioglitazone in combination with a sulfonylurea at 15 or 30 mg once daily. Continue the current sulfonylurea upon initiation of pioglitazone therapy. Decrease the dose of the sulfonylurea if patient reports hypoglycemia.

Metformin – Initiate pioglitazone in combination with metformin at 15 or 30 mg once daily. Continue the current metformin dose upon initiation of pioglitazone therapy. It is unlikely that the dose of metformin will require adjustment because of hypoglycemia during combination therapy with pioglitazone.

Insulin – Initiate pioglitazone in combination with insulin at 15 or 30 mg once daily. Continue the current insulin dose upon initiation of pioglitazone therapy. Decrease the insulin dose by 10% to 25% if the patient reports hypoglycemia or if plasma glucose concentrations decrease to less than 100 mg/dL. Individualize further adjustments based on glucose-lowering response.

➤*Maximum recommended dose:* Do not exceed 45 mg once daily of pioglitazone because doses more than 45 mg once daily have not been studied in placebo-controlled clinical studies.

➤*Hepatic disease:* Do not initiate pioglitazone therapy if the patient exhibits clinical evidence of active liver disease or increased serum transaminase levels (ALT more than 2.5 times the ULN) at the start of therapy. Liver enzyme monitoring is recommended in all patients prior to initiation of therapy with pioglitazone and periodically thereafter.

➤*Children:* The use of pioglitazone in pediatric patients younger than 18 years of age is not recommended.

➤*Storage/Stability:* Store at 25°C (77°F); excursions permitted to 15° to 30°C (59° to 86°F). Keep container tightly closed, and protect from moisture and humidity.

GLYBURIDE/METFORMIN HYDROCHLORIDE

Rx	**Glyburide/Metformin hydrochloride** (PAR)	**Tablets:** 1.25 mg/250 mg	(6057). Pale yellow, capsule shape. Film-coated. In 100s.
Rx	**Glucovance** (Bristol-Myers Squibb)		(BMS 6072). Pale yellow, capsule shape. Film-coated. In 100s and 500s.
Rx	**Glyburide/Metformin hydrochloride** (PAR)	**Tablets:** 2.5 mg/500 mg	(6058). Pale orange, capsule shape. Film-coated. In 100s.
Rx	**Glucovance** (Bristol-Myers Squibb)		(BMS 6073). Pale orange, capsule shape. Film-coated. In 100s and 500s.
Rx	**Glyburide/Metformin hydrochloride** (PAR)	**Tablets:** 5 mg/500 mg	(6059). Yellow, capsule shape. Film-coated. In 100s.
Rx	**Glucovance** (Bristol-Myers Squibb)		(BMS 6074). Yellow, capsule shape. Film-coated. In 100s.

GLYBURIDE/METFORMIN HYDROCHLORIDE — ORAL

For complete and comparative prescribing information, refer to the Sulfonylureas group monograph and the Metformin and Rosiglitazone individual monographs.

WARNING

Lactic acidosis is a rare, but serious, metabolic complication that can occur because of metformin accumulation during treatment with glyburide/metformin. When it occurs, it is fatal in approximately 50% of cases. See Warnings in the Metformin monograph for more information.

Indications

➤*Type 2 diabetes (initial therapy):* As initial therapy, as an adjunct to diet and exercise, to improve glycemic control in patients with type 2 diabetes whose hyperglycemia cannot be satisfactorily managed with diet and exercise alone.

➤*Type 2 diabetes (second-line therapy):* As second-line therapy when diet, exercise, and initial treatment with a sulfonylurea or metformin do not result in adequate glycemic control in patients with type 2 diabetes. For patients requiring additional therapy, a thiazolidinedione may be added to glyburide/metformin to achieve additional glycemic control.

Administration and Dosage

➤*Approved by the FDA:* July 31, 2000.

Individualize dosage on the basis of effectiveness and tolerance while not exceeding the maximum recommended daily dose of 20 mg glyburide/2000 mg metformin. Give with meals and initiate at a low dose, with gradual dose escalation as described below, in order to avoid hypoglycemia (largely because of glyburide), to reduce GI side effects (largely because of metformin), and to permit determination of the minimum effective dose for adequate control of blood glucose for the individual patient.

With initial treatment and during dose titration, appropriately monitor blood glucose to determine the therapeutic response to glyburide/metformin hydrochloride and to identify the minimum effective dose for the patient. Thereafter, measure HbA_{1c} at intervals of about 3 months to assess the effectiveness of therapy.

No studies have been performed specifically examining the safety and efficacy of switching to glyburide/metformin hydrochloride therapy in patients taking concomitant glyburide (or other sulfonylurea) plus metformin.

➤*Initial therapy:*

Starting dose – 1.25 mg/250 mg once or twice daily with meals. Increase dosage in increments of 1.25 mg/250 mg/day every 2 weeks up to the minimum effective dose necessary to achieve adequate control of blood glucose. Do not use glyburide/metformin 5 mg/500 mg as initial therapy because of an increased risk of hypoglycemia.

➤*Second-line therapy:*

Starting dose – 2.5 mg/500 mg or 5 mg/500 mg twice daily with meals. Titrate the daily dose in increments of no more than 5 mg/500 mg up to the minimum effective dose to achieve adequate control of blood glucose or to a maximum dose of 20 mg/2000 mg/day. If patients previously treated with combination therapy of glyburide (or another sulfonylurea) plus metformin are switching to glyburide/metformin hydrochloride, the starting dose should not exceed the daily dose of glyburide (or equivalent dose of another sulfonylurea) and metformin already being taken. Monitor patients closely for signs and symptoms of hypoglycemia following such a switch and titrate the dose of glyburide/metformin hydrochloride as described above to achieve adequate control of blood glucose.

➤*Addition of thiazolidinediones to glyburide/metformin therapy:* When a thiazolidinedione is added to glyburide/metformin therapy, the current dose of glyburide/metformin can be continued and the thiazolidinedione initiated at its recommended starting dose. For patients needing additional glycemic control, the dose of the thiazolidinedione can be increased based on its recommended titration schedule. The increased glycemic control attainable with glyburide/metformin plus a thiazolidinedione may increase the potential for hypoglycemia at any time of day. In patients who develop hypoglycemia when receiving glyburide/metformin and a thiazolidinedione, consider reducing the dose of the glyburide component of glyburide/metformin. As clinically warranted, also consider adjustment of the dosages of the other components of the antidiabetic regimen.

➤*Lactic acidosis:* See Warnings in metformin monograph.

➤*Specific patient populations:* Glyburide/metformin hydrochloride is not recommended for use during pregnancy or in pediatric patients. Initial and maintenance dosing should be conservative in patients with advanced age because of the potential for decreased renal function in this population. Dosage adjustment requires a careful assessment of renal function. Do not titrate elderly, debilitated, or malnourished patients to the maximum dose to avoid the risk of hypoglycemia. Monitoring of renal function is necessary to aid in prevention of metformin-associated lactic acidosis, particular in the elderly.

➤*Storage/Stability:* Store at temperatures up to 25°C (77°F). Dispense in light-resistant containers.

GLIPIZIDE/METFORMIN HYDROCHLORIDE

Rx	**Glipizide and Metformin Hydrochloride** (Sandoz)	**Tablets:** 2.5 mg/250 mg	(cor 167). Pink. Film-coated. In 100s, 500s, and 1,000s.
Rx	**Metaglip** (Bristol-Myers Squibb)		(BMS 6081). Pink, oval. Film-coated. In 100s.
Rx	**Glipizide and Metformin Hydrochloride** (Sandoz)	**Tablets:** 2.5 mg/500 mg	(cor 168). White. Film-coated. In 100s, 500s, and 1,000s.
Rx	**Metaglip** (Bristol-Myers Squibb)		(BMS 6077). White, oval. Film-coated. In 100s.
Rx	**Glipizide and Metformin Hydrochloride** (Sandoz)	**Tablets:** 5 mg/500 mg	(cor 169). Pink. Film-coated. In 100s, 500s, and 1,000s.
Rx	**Metaglip** (Bristol-Myers Squibb)		(BMS 6078). Pink, oval. Film-coated. In 100s.

GLIPIZIDE/METFORMIN HYDROCHLORIDE — ORAL

For complete and comparative prescribing information, refer to the Sulfonylureas group monograph and the Metformin Hydrochloride monograph.

WARNING

Lactic acidosis is a rare, but serious, metabolic complication that can occur due to metformin accumulation during treatment with glipizide/metformin. When it occurs, it is fatal in approximately 50% of cases. See Warnings in the Metformin Hydrochloride monograph for more information.

Indications

➤*Type 2 diabetes (initial therapy):* As initial therapy as an adjunct to diet and exercise to improve glycemic control in patients with type 2 diabetes whose hyperglycemia cannot be satisfactorily managed with diet and exercise alone.

➤*Type 2 diabetes (second-line therapy):* As second-line therapy when diet, exercise, and initial treatment with a sulfonylurea or metformin do not result in adequate glycemic control in patients with type 2 diabetes.

Administration and Dosage

➤*Approved by the FDA:* October 22, 2002.

Dosage must be individualized on the basis of effectiveness and tolerance while not exceeding the maximum recommended daily dose of 20 mg glipizide/2000 mg metformin. Give glipizide/metformin with meals and initiate at a low dose, with gradual dose escalation as described below in order to avoid hypoglycemia (largely because of glipizide), to reduce GI side effects (largely because of metformin), and to permit determination of the minimum effective dose for adequate control of blood glucose for the individual patient.

With initial treatment and during dose titration, use appropriate blood glucose monitoring to determine the therapeutic response to glipizide/metformin and to identify the minimum effective dose for the patient.

GLIPIZIDE/METFORMIN HYDROCHLORIDE — ORAL

Thereafter, measure HbA_{1c} at intervals of approximately 3 months to assess the effectiveness of therapy.

No studies have been performed specifically examining the safety and efficacy of switching to glipizide/metformin therapy in patients taking concomitant glipizide (or other sulfonylurea) plus metformin.

➤*Initial therapy:* The recommended starting dose of glipizide/metformin is 2.5 mg/250 mg once a day with a meal. For patients whose fasting plasma glucose (FPG) is 280 to 320 mg/dL, consider a starting dose of 2.5 mg/500 mg twice daily. The efficacy of glipizide/metformin tablets in patients whose FPG exceeds 320 mg/dL has not been established. Increase dosage to achieve adequate glycemic control in increments of 1 tablet per day every 2 weeks up to a maximum of 10 mg/1000 mg or 10 mg/2000 mg per day given in divided doses. In clinical trials with glipizide/metformin as initial therapy, there was no experience with total daily doses greater than 10 mg/2000 mg per day.

➤*Second-line therapy:* For patients not adequately controlled on either glipizide (or another sulfonylurea) or metformin alone, the recommended starting dose is 2.5 mg/500 mg or 5 mg/500 mg twice daily with the morning and evening meals. In order to avoid hypoglycemia, the starting dose should not exceed the daily doses of glipizide or metformin already being taken. Titrate the daily dose in increments of no more than 5 mg/500 mg up to the minimum effective dose to achieve adequate control of blood glucose or to a maximum dose of 20 mg/2000 mg per day.

Patients previously treated with combination therapy of glipizide (or another sulfonylurea) plus metformin may be switched to glipizide/metformin 2.5 mg/500 mg or 5 mg/500 mg; the starting dose should not exceed the daily dose of glipizide (or equivalent dose of another sulfonylurea) and metformin already being taken. Base the decision to switch to the nearest equivalent dose or to titrate on clinical judgment. Closely monitor patients for signs and symptoms of hypoglycemia following such a switch and titrate the dose of glipizide/metformin as described above to achieve adequate control of blood glucose.

➤*Lactic acidosis:* See Warnings in the Metformin HCl monograph.

➤*Specific patient populations:* Glipizide/metformin is not recommended for use during pregnancy or for use in pediatric patients. The initial and maintenance dosing should be conservative in patients with advanced age because of the potential for decreased renal function in this population. Any dosage adjustment requires a careful assessment of renal function. Generally, do not titrate elderly, debilitated, and malnourished patients to the maximum dose to avoid the risk of hypoglycemia. Monitoring of renal function is necessary to aid in prevention of metformin-associated lactic acidosis, particularly in the elderly.

➤*Storage/Stability:* Store at 20° to 25°C (68° to 77°F). Excursions permitted to 15° to 30°C (59° to 86°F).

ROSIGLITAZONE MALEATE/METFORMIN HYDROCHLORIDE

Rx	**Avandamet** (GlaxoSmithKline)	**Tablets:** 1 mg/500 mg	Lactose. (gsk 1/500). Yellow, oval. Film-coated. In 60s.
		2 mg/500 mg	Lactose. (gsk 2/500). Pale pink, oval. Film-coated. In 60s.
		2 mg/1,000 mg	Lactose. (gsk 2/1,000). Yellow, oval. Film-coated. In 60s.
		4 mg/500 mg	Lactose. (gsk 4/500). Orange, oval. Film-coated. In 60s.
		4 mg/1,000 mg	Lactose. (gsk 4/1,000). Pink, oval. Film-coated. In 60s.

ROSIGLITAZONE MALEATE/METFORMIN HYDROCHLORIDE — ORAL

For complete and comparative prescribing information, refer to the Thiazolidinediones group monograph and the Metformin monograph.

WARNING

Lactic acidosis is a rare, but serious, metabolic complication that can occur due to metformin accumulation during treatment with rosiglitazone/metformin. When it occurs, it is fatal in approximately 50% of cases. Lactic acidosis may also occur in association with a number of pathophysiologic conditions, including diabetes mellitus (DM), and whenever there is significant tissue hypoperfusion and hypoxemia. Lactic acidosis is characterized by elevated blood lactate levels (greater than 5 mmol/L), decreased blood pH, electrolyte disturbances with an increased anion gap, and an increased lactate/pyruvate ratio. When metformin is implicated as the cause of lactic acidosis, metformin plasma levels greater than 5 mcg/mL are generally found.

The reported incidence of lactic acidosis in patients receiving metformin is very low (approximately 0.03 cases/1,000 patient years of exposure, with approximately 0.015 fatal cases/1,000 patient years of exposure). Reported cases have occurred primarily in diabetic patients with significant renal insufficiency, including both intrinsic renal disease and renal hypoperfusion, often in the setting of multiple concomitant medical/surgical problems and multiple concomitant medications. Patients with congestive heart failure requiring pharmacologic management, in particular those with unstable or acute congestive heart failure who are at risk of hypoperfusion and hypoxemia, are at increased risk of lactic acidosis. The risk of lactic acidosis increases with the degree of renal dysfunction

and the patient's age. The risk of lactic acidosis may, therefore, be significantly decreased by regular monitoring of renal function in patients taking rosiglitazone/metformin and by use of the minimum effective dose of rosiglitazone/metformin. In particular, treatment of the elderly should be accompanied by careful monitoring of renal function. Treatment with rosiglitazone/metformin should not be initiated in patients 80 years of age and older unless measurement of creatinine clearance demonstrates that renal function is not reduced, because these patients are more susceptible to developing lactic acidosis. In addition, rosiglitazone/metformin should be promptly withheld in the presence of any condition associated with hypoxemia, dehydration, or sepsis. Generally, avoid rosiglitazone/metformin therapy in patients with clinical or laboratory evidence of hepatic disease because impaired hepatic function may significantly limit the ability to clear lactate. Caution patients against excessive alcohol intake, either acute or chronic, when taking rosiglitazone/metformin because alcohol potentiates the effects of metformin on lactate metabolism. In addition, temporarily discontinue rosiglitazone/metformin therapy prior to any intravascular radio contrast study and for any surgical procedure.

WARNING (cont.)

The onset of lactic acidosis often is subtle and accompanied only by nonspecific symptoms such as malaise, myalgias, respiratory distress, increasing somnolence, and nonspecific abdominal distress. There may be associated hypothermia, hypotension, and resistant bradyarrhythmias with more marked acidosis. Be aware of the possible importance of such symptoms and instruct the patient to immediately notify their health care provider if they occur. Withdraw rosiglitazone/metformin until the situation is clarified. Serum electrolytes, ketones, blood glucose, blood pH, lactate levels, and blood metformin levels may be useful. Once a patient is stabilized on any dose level of rosiglitazone/metformin, GI symptoms, which are common during initiation of therapy, are unlikely to be drug related. Later occurrence of GI symptoms could be due to lactic acidosis or other serious disease.

Levels of fasting venous plasma lactate above the upper limit of normal but less than 5 mmol/L in patients taking rosiglitazone/metformin do not necessarily indicate impending lactic acidosis and may be explainable by other mechanisms such as poorly controlled diabetes or obesity, vigorous physical activity, or technical problems in sample handling.

Suspect lactic acidosis in any diabetic patient with metabolic acidosis lacking evidence of ketoacidosis (ketonuria and ketonemia).

Lactic acidosis is a medical emergency that must be treated in a hospital setting. Immediately discontinue rosiglitazone/metformin therapy in a patient with lactic acidosis and promptly institute general supportive measures. Because metformin is dialyzable (with a clearance of up to 170 mL/min under good hemodynamic conditions), prompt hemodialysis is recommended to correct the acidosis and remove the accumulated metformin. Such management often results in prompt reversal of symptoms and recovery.

Indications

➤*Type 2 DM:* An adjunct to diet and exercise to improve glycemic control in patients with type 2 DM who are already treated with combination rosiglitazone and metformin or who are not adequately controlled on metformin alone.

Management of type 2 DM should include diet control. Caloric restriction, weight loss, and exercise are essential for the proper treatment of the diabetic patient because they help improve insulin sensitivity. This is important not only in the primary treatment of type 2 DM but also in maintaining the efficacy of drug therapy. Prior to initiation or escalation of oral antidiabetic therapy in patients with type 2 DM, investigation and treat secondary causes of poor glycemic control (eg, infection).

The safety and efficacy of rosiglitazone/metformin as initial pharmacologic therapy for patients with type 2 DM after a trial of caloric restriction, weight loss, and exercise has not been established.

Administration and Dosage

➤*Approved by the FDA:* October 11, 2002.

➤*Dose selection:* Base the dose selection of rosiglitazone/metformin on the patient's current doses of rosiglitazone and/or metformin.

The following recommendations regarding the use of rosiglitazone/metformin in patients inadequately controlled on rosiglitazone and metformin monotherapies are based on clinical practice experience with rosiglitazone and metformin combination therapy

ROSIGLITAZONE MALEATE/METFORMIN HYDROCHLORIDE — ORAL

Individualize the dosage of antidiabetic therapy with rosiglitazone/metformin on the basis of efficacy and tolerability while not exceeding the maximum recommended daily dose of 8 mg/2,000 mg. Give rosiglitazone/metformin in divided doses with meals, with gradual dosage escalation. This reduces GI adverse reactions (largely caused by of metformin) and permits determination of the minimum effective dose for the individual patient. Give sufficient time to assess adequacy of therapeutic response. Use fasting plasma glucose (FPG) to determine the therapeutic response to rosiglitazone/metformin. After an increase in metformin dosage, dosage titration is recommended if patients are not adequately controlled after 1 to 2 weeks. After an increase in rosiglitazone dosage, dose titration is recommended if patients are not adequately controlled after 8 to 12 weeks.

➤*Dosage recommendations:*

Patients inadequately controlled on metformin monotherapy – The usual starting dose is rosiglitazone 4 mg (total daily dose) plus the dose of metformin already being taken (see the following table).

Patients inadequately controlled on rosiglitazone monotherapy –The usual starting dose is metformin 1,000 mg (total daily dose) plus the dose of rosiglitazone already being taken (see the following table).

Rosiglitazone/Metformin Starting Dose

	Usual rosiglitazone/metformin starting dose	
Prior therapy (total daily dose)	Tablet strength	Number of tablets
Metformin[a]		
1,000 mg/day	2 mg/500 mg	1 tablet bid[b]
2,000 mg/day	2 mg/1,000 mg	1 tablet bid
Rosiglitazone		
4 mg/day	2 mg/500 mg	1 tablet bid
8 mg/day	4 mg/500 mg	1 tablet bid

[a] For patients on dosages of metformin between 1,000 and 2,000 mg/day, initiation of rosiglitazone/metformin requires individualization of therapy.
[b] bid = twice a day.

Switching from combination therapy of rosiglitazone plus metformin as separate tablets – The usual starting dose is the dose of rosiglitazone and metformin already being taken.

Dosage adjustments – The daily dose may be increased by increments of rosiglitazone 4 mg and/or metformin 500 mg , up to the maximum recommended total daily dose of 8 mg/2,000 mg.

Other oral hypoglycemic agents – No studies have been performed specifically examining the safety and efficacy of rosiglitazone/metformin in patients previously treated with other oral hypoglycemic agents and switched to rosiglitazone/metformin. Any change in therapy of type 2 DM should be undertaken with care and appropriate monitoring as changes in glycemic control can occur.

➤*Specific risk patients:*

Pregnant patients/children – Rosiglitazone/metformin is not recommended for use in pregnancy or for use in children.

Elderly – The initial and maintenance dosing should be conservative in patients of advanced age because of the potential for decreased renal function in this population. Base any dosage adjustment on a careful assessment of renal function. Generally, elderly, debilitated, and malnourished patients should not be titrated to the maximum dose. Monitoring of renal function is necessary to aid in prevention of metformin-associated lactic acidosis, particularly in elderly patients.

Hepatic function impairment – Therapy with rosiglitazone/metformin should not be initiated if the patient exhibits clinical evidence of active liver disease or increased serum transaminase levels (ALT more than 2.5 times upper limit of normal at start of therapy). Liver enzyme monitoring is recommended in all patients prior to initiation of therapy with rosiglitazone/metformin and periodically thereafter.

➤*Storage/Stability:* Store at 25°C (77°F); excursions are permitted to 15° to 30°C (59° to 86°F). Dispense in a tight, light-resistant container.

PIOGLITAZONE HYDROCHLORIDE AND METFORMIN HYDROCHLORIDE

Rx	**ActoPlus Met** (Takeda)	**Tablets:** 15 mg pioglitazone hydrochloride (as base) and 500 mg metformin hydrochloride	(4833M 15/500). White to off-white, oblong. Film coated. In 60s and 180s.
		15 mg pioglitazone hydrochloride (as base) and 850 mg metformin hydrochloride	(4833M 15/850). White to off-white, oblong. Film coated. In 60s and 180s.

PIOGLITAZONE HYDROCHLORIDE AND METFORMIN HYDROCHLORIDE — ORAL

WARNING

Metformin –

Lactic acidosis: Lactic acidosis is a rare, but serious, metabolic complication that can occur due to metformin accumulation during treatment with pioglitazone/metformin combination tablets; when it occurs, it is fatal in approximately 50% of cases. See Warnings in the Metformin Hydrochloride monograph for more information.

Indications

➤*Type 2 diabetes:* Pioglitazone/metformin is indicated as an adjunct to diet and exercise to improve glycemic control in patients with type 2 diabetes who are already treated with a combination of pioglitazone and metformin or whose diabetes is not adequately controlled with metformin alone, or for those patients who have initially responded to pioglitazone alone and require additional glycemic control.

Management of type 2 diabetes also should include nutritional counseling, weight reduction as needed, and exercise. These efforts are important not only in the primary treatment of type 2 diabetes but also to maintain the efficacy of drug therapy.

Administration and Dosage

➤*Approved by the FDA:* August 29, 2005.

The use of antihyperglycemic therapy in the management of type 2 diabetes should be individualized on the basis of effectiveness and tolerability while not exceeding the maximum recommended daily dose of pioglitazone 45 mg and metformin 2,550 mg.

➤*Dosage recommendations:* Selecting the starting dose of pioglitazone/metformin should be based on the patient's current regimen of pioglitazone and/or metformin. Pioglitazone/metformin should be given in divided daily doses with meals to reduce the GI side effects associated with metformin.

Maximum recommended dose – Pioglitazone/metformin tablets are available as a pioglitazone 15 mg plus metformin 500 mg or a pioglitazone 15 mg plus metformin 850 mg formulation for oral administration. The maximum recommended dose for pioglitazone is 45 mg daily. The maximum recommended daily dose for metformin is 2,550 mg in adults.

Starting dose for patients inadequately controlled on metformin monotherapy – Based on the usual starting dose of pioglitazone (15 to 30 mg daily), pioglitazone/metformin may be initiated at either the 15 mg/500 mg or 15 mg/850 mg tablet strength once or twice daily, and gradually titrated after assessing adequacy of therapeutic response.

Starting dose for patients who initially responded to pioglitazone monotherapy and require additional glycemic control – Based on the usual starting doses of metformin (500 mg twice daily or 850 mg daily), pioglitazone/metformin may be initiated at either the 15 mg/500 mg twice daily or 15 mg/850 mg tablet strength once daily, and gradually titrated after assessing adequacy of therapeutic response.

Starting dose for patients switching from combination therapy of pioglitazone plus metformin as separate tablets – Pioglitazone/metformin may be initiated with either the 15 mg/500 mg or 15 mg/850 mg tablet strengths based on the dose of pioglitazone and metformin already being taken.

No studies have been performed specifically examining the safety and efficacy of pioglitazone/metformin in patients previously treated with other oral hypoglycemic agents and switched to pioglitazone/metformin. Any change in therapy of type 2 diabetes should be undertaken with care and appropriate monitoring because changes in glycemic control can occur.

Sufficient time should be given to assess adequacy of therapeutic response. Ideally, the response to therapy should be evaluated using hemoglobin A_{1C} (HbA_{1C}), which is a better indicator of long-term glycemic control than fasting plasma glucose (FPG) alone. HbA_{1C} reflects glycemia over the previous 2 to 3 months. In clinical use, it is recommended that patients be treated with pioglitazone/metformin for a period of time adequate to evaluate change in HbA_{1C} (8 to 12 weeks) unless glycemic control as measured by FPG deteriorates.

➤*Special patient populations:*

Children – Pioglitazone/metformin is not recommended for use in pediatric patients.

Pregnancy – Pioglitazone/metformin is not recommended for use in pregnancy.

Elderly – The initial and maintenance dosing of pioglitazone/metformin should be conservative in patients with advanced age, due to the potential for decreased renal function in this population. Any dosage adjustment should be based on a careful assessment of renal function. Generally, elderly, debilitated, and malnourished patients should not be titrated to the maximum dose of pioglitazone/metformin. Monitoring of renal function is necessary to aid in prevention of metformin-associated lactic acidosis, particularly in the elderly.

PIOGLITAZONE HYDROCHLORIDE AND METFORMIN HYDROCHLORIDE — ORAL

Liver function impairment – Therapy with pioglitazone/metformin should not be initiated if the patient exhibits clinical evidence of active liver disease or increased serum transaminase levels (ALT greater than 2.5 times the ULN) at start of therapy. Liver enzyme monitoring is recommended in all patients prior to initiation of therapy with pioglitazone/metformin and periodically thereafter.

➤*Storage/Stability:* Store at 25°C (77°F); excursions permitted to 15° to 30°C (59° to 86°F). Keep container tightly closed, and protect from moisture and humidity.

ROSIGLITAZONE/GLIMEPIRIDE

Rx	**Avandaryl** (GlaxoSmithKline)	**Tablets:** 4 mg rosiglitazone/1 mg glimepiride	Lactose. (gsk 4/1). Yellow, rounded triangle. In 30s.
		4 mg rosiglitazone/2 mg glimepiride	Lactose. (gsk 4/2). Orange, rounded triangle. In 30s.
		4 mg rosiglitazone/4 mg glimepiride	Lactose. (gsk 4/4). Pink, rounded triangle. In 30s.

ROSIGLITAZONE/GLIMEPIRIDE — ORAL

Indications

➤*Type 2 diabetes:* Rosiglitazone/Glimepiride is indicated as an adjunct to diet and exercise to improve glycemic control in patients with type 2 diabetes who are already treated with a combination of rosiglitazone and a sulfonylurea or who are not adequately controlled on a sulfonylurea alone or for those patients who have initially responded to rosiglitazone alone and require additional glycemic control.

Administration and Dosage

Rosiglitazone/Glimepiride should be given once daily with the first meal of the day. The dosage of antidiabetic therapy with rosiglitazone/glimepiride should be individualized on the basis of effectiveness and tolerability. No exact dosage relationship exists between rosiglitazone/glimepiride and other antidiabetic agents.

Sufficient time should be given to assess adequacy of therapeutic response. Fasting glucose should be used to determine the therapeutic response to rosiglitazone/glimepiride.

➤*Patients inadequately controlled on sulfonylurea or rosiglitazone monotherapy:* For patients inadequately controlled on sulfonylurea monotherapy or who have initially responded to rosiglitazone alone and require additional glycemic control, the usual starting dose of rosiglitazone/glimepiride is 4 mg/1 mg or 4 mg/2 mg once daily. Patients who may be more sensitive to glimepiride, including the elderly, debilitated, or malnourished, and those with renal, hepatic, or adrenal insufficiency, should be started on rosiglitazone/glimepiride 4 mg/1 mg and carefully titrated. When switching from combination therapy of rosiglitazone plus glimepiride as separate tablets, the usual starting dose of rosiglitazone/glimepiride is the dose of rosiglitazone and glimepiride already being taken. The maximum recommended daily dose of Rosiglitazone/Glimepiride is 8 mg of rosiglitazone and 4 mg of glimepiride.

➤*Switching patients from thiazolidinedione monotherapy:* For patients previously treated with thiazolidinedione monotherapy switched to rosiglitazone/glimepiride, dose titration is recommended if patients are not adequately controlled after 1 to 2 weeks. If additional glycemic control is needed, the daily dose of rosiglitazone/glimepiride may be increased by increasing the glimepiride component in no more than 2 mg increments at 1-to 2-week intervals up to the maximum recommended total daily dose of 8 mg rosiglitazone/4 mg glimepiride.

➤*Switching patients from sulfonylurea monotherapy:* For patients previously treated with sulfonylurea monotherapy switched to rosiglitazone/glimepiride, it may take 2 weeks to see a reduction in blood glucose and 2 to 3 months to see the full effect of the rosiglitazone component. If additional glycemic control is needed, the dose of the glimepiride component may be increased. The dose of the rosiglitazone component should not exceed 8 mg. As with other sulfonylurea-containing antidiabetic agents, no transition period is necessary when transferring patients to rosiglitazone/glimepiride. Patients should be observed carefully (1 to 2 weeks) for hypoglycemia when being transferred from longer half-life sulfonylureas (eg, chlorpropamide) to rosiglitazone/glimepiride due to potential overlapping of drug effect.

➤*Hypoglycemia:* If hypoglycemia occurs during up-titration of the dose or while maintained on therapy, a dosage reduction of the sulfonylurea component of rosiglitazone/glimepiride may be considered.

➤*Pregnancy/Lactation:* Rosiglitazone/Glimepiride should not be used during pregnancy or in nursing mothers.

➤*Children:* There are no data on the use of rosiglitazone/glimepiride in patients younger than 18 years; therefore, use of rosiglitazone/glimepiride in pediatric patients is not recommended.

➤*Elderly, debilitated, or malnourished patients:* In elderly, debilitated, or malnourished patients, the initial dosing, dose increments, and maintenance dosage of rosiglitazone/glimepiride should be conservative to avoid hypoglycemic reactions.

➤*Renal function impairment:* In renal insufficiency, the initial dosing, dose increments, and maintenance dosage of rosiglitazone/glimepiride should be conservative to avoid hypoglycemic reactions.

➤*Hepatic function impairment:* In hepatic insufficiency, the initial dosing, dose increments, and maintenance dosage of rosiglitazone/glimepiride should be conservative to avoid hypoglycemic reactions.

Therapy with rosiglitazone/glimepiride should not be initiated if the patient exhibits clinical evidence of active liver disease or increased serum transaminase levels (ALT greater than 2.5 × upper limit of normal at start of therapy). Liver enzyme monitoring is recommended in all patients prior to initiation of therapy with rosiglitazone/glimepiride and periodically thereafter.

➤*Adrenal insufficiency:* In adrenal insufficiency, the initial dosing, dose increments, and maintenance dosage of rosiglitazone/glimepiride should be conservative to avoid hypoglycemic reactions.

➤*Storage/Stability:* Store at 25°C (77°F); excursions permitted to 15° to 30°C (59° to 86°F). Dispense in a tight, light-resistant container.

GLUCAGON (rDNA Origin)

Rx	**GlucaGen** (Bedford)	**Powder for Injection**: 1 mg (1 unit)	107 mg lactose. In vials with 1 mL diluent.
Rx	**Glucagon Emergency Kit** (Eli Lilly)		49 mg lactose. In vials with 1 ml syringe diluent.[1]
Rx	**Glucagon Diagnostic Kit** (Eli Lilly)		49 mg lactose. In vials with 1 ml syringe diluent.[1]

[1] With 12 mg/ml glycerin.

GLUCAGON — INJECTION

Indications

➤*Hypoglycemia:* Glucagon is indicated as a treatment for severe hypoglycemia. Because patients with type 1 diabetes may have less of an increase in blood glucose levels compared with a stable type 2 diabetes patient, give supplementary carbohydrates as soon as possible, especially to a pediatric patient.

➤*Diagnostic aid:* Glucagon is indicated as a diagnostic aid in the radiologic examination of the stomach, duodenum, small bowel, and colon when diminished intestinal motility would be advantageous.

➤*Unlabeled uses:* Glucagon has been used in the treatment of propranolol overdose and in cardiovascular emergencies.

Administration and Dosage

Patient instructions are provided with the product.

Use the diluent only in preparation of glucagon for parenteral injection. Do not use glucagon at concentrations > 1 mg/ml (1 unit/ml). Use the reconstituted glucagon immediately and only if it is clear and of water-like consistency. Inspect for visual particulate matter and discoloration prior to use. Discard any unused portion.

➤*Severe hypoglycemia:* Treat severe hypoglycemia initially with IV glucose, if possible. If parenteral glucose cannot be used, prepare parenteral glucagon, and use immediately. An unconscious patient will usually awaken within 15 minutes following glucagon injection. If the response is delayed, administer an additional dose of glucagon. However, in view of the deleterious effects of cerebral hypoglycemia, seek emergency aid so that parenteral glucose can be given. After the patient responds, give supplemental carbohydrate to restore liver glycogen and to prevent secondary hypoglycemia.

Adults and children > 20 kg – 1 mg (1 unit) SC, IM, or IV.

Children < 20 kg – 0.5 mg (0.5 unit) or a dose equivalent to 20 to 30 mcg/kg.

➤*Diagnostic aid:* Administer the doses in the following chart for relaxation of the stomach, duodenum, and small bowel, depending on the time of onset of action and the duration of effect required. Because the stomach is less sensitive to the effect of glucagon, 0.5 mg IV or 2 mg IM is recommended.

Glucagon Dosing Parameters as a Diagnostic Aid

Dose	Route	Onset (min)	Duration (min)
0.25 to 0.5 mg (0.25-0.5 unit)	IV	1	9-17
1 mg (1 unit)	IM	8-10	12-27
2 mg (2 units)[1]	IV	1	22-25
2 mg (2 units)[1]	IM	4-7	21-32

[1] 2 mg doses produce a higher incidence of nausea and vomiting.

For examination of the colon, administer 2 mg IM ≈ 10 minutes prior to initiation of the procedure.

➤*Storage/Stability:* Store at room temperature prior to reconstitution (20° to 25°C; 68° to 77°F). After reconstitution, use immediately.

Actions

➤*Pharmacology:* Glucagon, a polypeptide hormone produced by pancreatic alpha cells of the islets of Langerhans, exerts an effect on blood glucose opposite to that of insulin. Elevation in blood glucose by glucagon is due to inhibition of glycogen synthesis, enhanced formation of glucose from noncarbohydrates such as proteins and fats (gluconeogenesis), and increased hydrolysis of glycogen to glucose (glycogenolysis) in the liver. Glucagon accelerates hepatic glycogenolysis by stimulating cyclic AMP synthesis via adenylyl cyclase and enhancing phosphorylase kinase activity. Lipolysis in the adipose tissue is enhanced via adenylyl cyclase stimulation. Glucagon also increases the force of contraction in the heart and has a relaxant effect on the GI tract.

Glucagon for injection (rDNA origin) is identical to human glucagon and is synthesized in a genetically altered *Escherichia coli* strain. Parenteral administration of glucagon converts hepatic glycogen to glucose and produces relaxation of the smooth muscles of the stomach, duodenum, small bowel, and colon.

➤*Pharmacokinetics:*

Absorption/Distribution – A 1 mg dose demonstrated a mean volume of distribution of 0.25 L/kg. Maximum plasma concentrations were 7.9 ng/ml ≈ 20 minutes following SC administration and 6.9 ng/ml ≈ 13 minutes following IM dosing. Peak glucose concentrations in 25 volunteers were 136 mg/dl 30 minutes after a 1 mg SC dose and 138 mg/dl 26 minutes after a 1 mg IM dose.

Metabolism/Excretion – Glucagon is extensively degraded in the liver, kidney, and plasma. Mean clearance of a 1 mg dose was 13.5 ml/min/kg. The half-life ranged from 8 to 18 minutes.

Contraindications

Hypersensitivity to glucagon; patients with pheochromocytoma (see Warnings).

Warnings

➤*Insulinoma/Pheochromocytoma:* Administer cautiously to patients with a history of insulinoma, pheochromocytoma, or both. In patients with insulinoma, IV glucagon will produce an initial increase in blood glucose, but because of its insulin-releasing effect, it may subsequently cause hypoglycemia. Administer glucose orally, intravenously, or by gavage to a patient developing symptoms of hypoglycemia after a dose of glucagon. It also stimulates catecholamine release, causing a sudden marked increase in blood pressure in patients with pheochromocytoma. To control sudden increases in blood pressure, 5 to 10 mg of IV phentolamine mesylate may be administered.

➤*Pregnancy: Category B.* There are no adequate and well-controlled studies in pregnant women. Use during pregnancy only if clearly needed.

➤*Lactation:* It is not known whether this drug is excreted in breast milk. Exercise caution when administering to a nursing mother.

➤*Children:* The use of glucagon in pediatric patients for hypoglycemia is safe and effective. Safety and efficacy have not been established in pediatric patients for use as a diagnostic aid.

Precautions

➤*Monitoring:* Obtain blood glucose determinations in a hypoglycemic patient until the patient is asymptomatic.

➤*Hypoglycemia:* Glucagon is effective in treating hypoglycemia only if sufficient liver glycogen is present. Because glucagon is of little or no help in states of starvation, adrenal insufficiency, or chronic hypoglycemia, treat hypoglycemia in these conditions with glucose. Although glucagon may be used for emergency treatment of hypoglycemia, notify the physician when hypoglycemic reactions occur so that the insulin dose may be adjusted.

Drug Interactions

➤*Anticoagulants:* The anticoagulant effect may be enhanced by coadministration of glucagon, possibly with bleeding. The onset may be delayed. Monitor prothrombin activity and for signs of bleeding, and adjust doses accordingly.

Adverse Reactions

Nausea, vomiting (occasional; this may also occur with hypoglycemia); generalized allergic reactions including urticaria, respiratory distress, and hypotension.

Overdosage

➤*Symptoms:* Expect nausea, vomiting, gastric hypotonicity, and diarrhea without consequential toxicity if overdosage occurs. Decreased serum potassium concentration may occur, and normal limits can be obtained with potassium supplementation. IV administration has demonstrated positive inotropic and chronotropic effects. A transient increase in blood pressure and pulse rate may occur. Patients receiving beta blockers may be expected to have a greater increase in blood pressure and pulse. Increases may be transient because of glucagon's short half-life. Patients with pheochromocytoma and coronary artery disease may require therapy for increased blood pressure and pulse rate.

Because glucagon is a polypeptide, it would be rapidly destroyed by the GI tract if it were to be accidently ingested.

➤*Treatment:* In managing overdosage, consider the possibility of multiple drug overdoses, interaction among drugs, and unusual drug kinetics in the patient.

In view of the extremely short half-life of glucagon and its prompt destruction and excretion, the treatment of overdosage is symptomatic, primarily for nausea, vomiting, and possible hypokalemia.

If the patient develops a dramatic increase in blood pressure, 5 to 10 mg of phentolamine mesylate has been shown to be effective in lowering blood pressure for the short time that control would be needed.

Forced diuresis, peritoneal dialysis, hemodialysis, or charcoal hemoperfusion have not been established as beneficial for an overdose of glucagon; it is extremely unlikely that one of these procedures would ever be indicated.

Patient Information

Refer patients and family members to the patient information supplied with the product for instructions describing the method of preparing and injecting glucagon. Advise the patient and family members to become familiar with the technique of preparing glucagon before an emergency arises. Instruct patients to use 1 mg (1 unit) for adults and half the adult dose (0.5 mg [0.5 unit]) for pediatric patients weighing < 44 lbs (20 kg).

Inform patients and family members of the following measures to prevent hypoglycemic reactions due to insulin:

- Reasonable uniformity from day to day with regard to diet, insulin, and exercise.

GLUCAGON — INJECTION

- Careful adjustment of the insulin program so that the type (or types) of insulin, dose, and time (or times) of administration are suited to the individual patient.
- Frequent testing of the blood or urine for glucose so that a change in insulin requirements can be foreseen.
- Routine carrying of sugar, candy, or other readily absorbable carbohydrate by the patient so that it may be taken at the first warning of an oncoming reaction.

To prevent severe hypoglycemia, inform patients and family members of the symptoms of mild hypoglycemia and how to treat it appropriately.

Inform family members to arouse the patient as quickly as possible because prolonged hypoglycemia may result in damage to the CNS. Glucagon or IV glucose should awaken the patient sufficiently so that oral carbohydrates may be taken.

Advise patients to inform their physician when hypoglycemic reactions occur so that the treatment regimen may be adjusted if necessary.

GLUCOSE

otc	**Glutose** (Paddock)	**Gel:** Liquid glucose (40% dextrose)	Dye free. In 80 g bottle and 25 g tube.
otc	**Insta-Glucose** (ICN)		Cherry flavor. In UD 30.8 g tubes.
otc	**Insulin Reaction** (Sherwood)		Lime flavor. In UD 25 g tubes.
otc	**Dex4 Glucose** (Can-Am Care)	**Tablets:** Glucose	Lemon, orange, raspberry and grape flavors. In 10s and 50s.
otc	**B-D Glucose** (Becton Dickinson)	**Tablets, chewable:** 5 g	In 36s.

GLUCOSE — ORAL

Refer to parenteral dextrose (d-glucose) in Nutrients and Nutritional Agents which is also used in the treatment of acute hypoglycemia.

Indications

Management of hypoglycemia.

Administration and Dosage

Administer 10 to 20 g orally; repeat in 10 minutes if necessary. Response should occur in 10 minutes.

Glucose is not absorbed from the buccal cavity; it must be swallowed to be effective. While swallowing reflexes may be preserved in the unconscious patient, the lack of normal gag reflexes may lead to aspiration. When possible, use other methods of treating hypoglycemia in unconscious patients.

➤*Children:* Do not give to children younger than 2 years of age, unless directed by a physician.

Actions

➤*Pharmacology:* Glucose, a monosaccharide, is absorbed from the intestine after administration and then used, distributed and stored by the tissues. Direct absorption takes place, resulting in a rapid increased blood glucose concentration. Therefore, it is effective in small doses; no evidence of toxicity has been reported. Glucose provides 4 cal/g.

Adverse Reactions

Isolated reports of nausea, which also may occur with hypoglycemia.

ADRENOCORTICAL STEROIDS

Adrenal Steroid Inhibitors

AMINOGLUTETHIMIDE

Rx	**Cytadren** (Ciba)	**Tablets:** 250 mg	(Ciba 24). White, scored. In 100s.

AMINOGLUTETHIMIDE — ORAL

Indications

➤*Cushing syndrome:* For the suppression of adrenal function in selected patients with Cushing syndrome. Morning levels of plasma cortisol in patients with adrenal carcinoma and ectopic ACTH-producing tumors were reduced on the average to about one half of the pretreatment levels, and in patients with adrenal hyperplasia to about two thirds of the pretreatment levels, during 1 to 3 months of therapy with aminoglutethimide. Data available from the few patients with adrenal adenoma suggest similar reductions in plasma cortisol levels. Measurements of plasma cortisol showed reductions to at least 50% of baseline or to normal levels in one third or more of the patients studied, depending on diagnostic groups and time of measurement.

➤*Unlabeled uses:* Aminoglutethimide has been used successfully in postmenopausal patients with advanced breast carcinoma and in patients with metastic prostate carcinoma.

Administration and Dosage

➤*Dosage:* Treatment should be instituted in a hospital until a stable dosage regimen is achieved. Therapy should be initiated with 250 mg orally 4 times daily, preferably at 6-hour intervals. Adrenocortical response should be followed by careful monitoring of plasma cortisol levels until the desired level of suppression is achieved. If the level of cortisol suppression is inadequate, the dosage may be increased in increments of 250 mg daily at intervals of 1 to 2 weeks to a total daily dose of 2 g. Dose reduction or temporary discontinuation of therapy may be required in the event of adverse effects, including extreme drowsiness, severe skin rash, or excessively low cortisol levels. If a skin rash persists for longer than 5 to 8 days or becomes severe, the drug should be discontinued. It may be possible to reinstate therapy at a lower dosage following the disappearance of a mild or moderate rash. Mineralocorticoid replacement (eg, fludrocortisone) may be necessary. If glucocorticoid replacement therapy is needed, 20 to 30 mg of hydrocortisone orally in the morning will replace endogenous secretion.

➤*Storage/Stability:* Protect from light. Do not store above 30°C (86°F).

Actions

➤*Pharmacology:* Aminoglutethimide inhibits the enzymatic conversion of cholesterol to δ^5-pregnenolone, resulting in a decrease in the production of adrenal glucocorticoids, mineralocorticoids, estrogens, and androgens.

Aminoglutethimide blocks several other steps in steroid synthesis, including the C-11, C-18, and C-21 hydroxylations and the hydroxylations required for the aromatization of androgens to estrogens, mediated through the binding of aminoglutethimide to cytochrome P-450 complexes.

A decrease in adrenal secretion of cortisol is followed by an increased secretion of pituitary adrenocorticotropic hormone (ACTH), which will overcome the blockade of adrenocortical steroid synthesis by aminoglutethimide. The compensatory increase in ACTH secretion can be suppressed by the simultaneous administration of hydrocortisone. Since aminoglutethimide increases the rate of metabolism of dexamethasone but not that of hydrocortisone, the latter is preferred as the adrenal glucocorticoid replacement.

Although aminoglutethimide inhibits the synthesis of thyroxine by the thyroid gland, the compensatory increase in thyroid-stimulating hormone (TSH) is frequently of sufficient magnitude to overcome the inhibition of thyroid synthesis due to aminoglutethimide. In spite of an increase in TSH, aminoglutethimide has not been associated with increased prolactin secretion.

Note – Aminoglutethimide was marketed previously as an anticonvulsant but was withdrawn from marketing for that indication in 1966 because of the effects on the adrenal gland.

➤*Pharmacokinetics:* Aminoglutethimide is rapidly and completely absorbed after oral administration. In 6 healthy men, maximum plasma levels of aminoglutethimide averaged 5.9 mc/mL at a median of 1.5 hrs after ingestion of two 250 mg tablets. The bioavailability of tablets is equivalent to equal doses given as a solution. After ingestion of a single oral dose, 34% to 54% is excreted in the urine as unchanged drug during the first 48 hours, and an additional fraction as the N-acetyl derivative.

The half-life of aminoglutethimide in healthy volunteers given single oral doses averaged 12.5 ± 1.6 hours.

Upon withdrawal of therapy with aminoglutethimide, the ability of the adrenal glands to synthesize steroid returns, usually within 72 hours.

Contraindications

Serious forms, or more severe manifestations, of hypersensitivity to glutethimide or aminoglutethimide.

Warnings

➤*Stress:* Aminoglutethimide may cause adrenocortical hypofunction, especially under conditions of stress, such as surgery, trauma, or acute illness. Patients should be carefully monitored and given hydrocortisone and mineralocorticoid supplements as indicated. Dexamethasone should not be used. (See Drug Interactions.)

➤*Hypotension:* Aminoglutethimide also may suppress aldosterone production by the adrenal cortex and may cause orthostatic or persistent hypotension. The blood pressure should be monitored in all patients at appropriate intervals. Patients should be advised of the possible occurrence of weakness and dizziness as symptoms of hypotension, and of measures to be taken should they occur.

The effects of aminoglutethimide may be potentiated if it is taken in combination with alcohol.

➤*Carcinogenesis:* A 2-year carcinogenicity study of aminoglutethimide conducted in rats at doses of 10 to 60 mg/kg/day (approximately 0.04 to 0.2 times the maximum daily therapeutic dose based on surface area, mg/m^2) revealed a highly statistically significant dose-related trend in the incidence of benign and malignant neoplasms of the adrenal cortex and thyroid follicular cells in both sexes. A borderline statistically significant

AMINOGLUTETHIMIDE — ORAL

increase (0.05 level) in ovarian tubular adenomas was observed at 60 mg/kg/day. Urinary bladder papillomas also showed a statistically significant dose-related trend in males.

➤*Fertility impairment:* Aminoglutethimide affects fertility in female rats (see Pregnancy). The relevance of these findings to humans is not known.

➤*Pregnancy: Category D.*

Aminoglutethimide can cause fetal harm when administered to a pregnant woman. In the earlier experience with the drug in about 5,000 patients, 2 cases of pseudohermaphroditism were reported in female infants whose mothers were treated with aminoglutethimide and concomitant anticonvulsants. Normal pregnancies have also occurred in patients treated with aminoglutethimide.

When administered to rats at doses ½ and 1¼ times the maximum daily human dose, aminoglutethimide caused a decrease in fetal implantation, an increase in fetal deaths, and a variety of teratogenic effects. The compound also caused pseudohermaphroditism in rats treated with approximately 3 times the maximum daily human dose. If this drug must be used during pregnancy, or if the patient becomes pregnant while taking the drug, the patient should be apprised of the potential hazard to the fetus.

➤*Lactation:* It is not known whether this drug is excreted in human milk. Because many drugs are excreted in human milk and because of the potential for serious adverse reactions in breast-feeding infants from aminoglutethimide, a decision should be made whether to discontinue breast-feeding or to discontinue the drug, taking into account the importance of the drug to the mother.

➤*Children:* Safety and efficacy in children have not been established.

Precautions

➤*Monitoring:* Hypothyroidism may occur in association with aminoglutethimide; hence, appropriate clinical observations should be made and laboratory studies of thyroid function performed as indicated. Supplementary thyroid hormone may be required.

Hematologic abnormalities in patients receiving aminoglutethimide have been reported (see Adverse Reactions). Therefore, baseline hematologic studies should be performed, followed by periodic hematologic evaluation.

Because elevations in AST, alkaline phosphatase, and bilirubin have been reported, appropriate clinical observations and regular laboratory studies should be performed before and during therapy.

Serum electrolyte levels should be determined periodically.

➤*Administration:* This drug should be administered only by physicians familiar with its use and hazards. Therapy should be initiated in a hospital.

Drug Interactions

Aminoglutethimide Drug Interactions

Precipitant drug	Object drug[a]		Description
Aminoglutethimide	Anticoagulants	⬇	Anticoagulant effects may be decreased.
Aminoglutethimide	Dexamethasone	⬇	Possible loss of dexamethasone-induced adrenal suppression. If a corticosteroid is needed, substitute hydrocortisone.
Aminoglutethimide	Digitoxin	⬇	Digitoxin clearance may be increased.
Aminoglutethimide	Medroxyprogesterone	⬇	Medroxyprogesterone serum levels may be decreased.
Aminoglutethimide	Theophyllines	⬇	The action of theophyllines may be reduced.

[a] ⬇ = Object drug decreased.

Adverse Reactions

Untoward effects have been reported in about 2 out of 3 patients with Cushing syndrome who were treated for 4 or more weeks with aminoglutethimide as the only adrenocortical suppressant.

The most frequent and reversible side effects were drowsiness (approximately 1 in 3 patients), morbilliform skin rash (1 in 6 patients), nausea and anorexia (each approximately 1 in 8 patients), and dizziness (about 1 in 20 patients). The dizziness was possibly caused by lowered vascular resistance or orthostasis. These reactions often disappear spontaneously with continued therapy.

➤*Cardiovascular:* Hypotension, occasionally orthostatic, occurred in 1 in 30 patients receiving aminoglutethimide. Tachycardia occurred in 1 in 40 patients.

➤*CNS:* Headache was reported in about 1 in 20 patients.

➤*Dermatologic:* In addition to rash (1 in 6 patients, and often reversible with continued therapy), pruritus was reported in 1 in 20 patients. These may be allergic or hypersensitive reactions. Urticaria has occurred rarely.

➤*Endocrine:* Adrenal insufficiency occurred in about 1 in 30 patients with Cushing syndrome who were treated with aminoglutethimide for 4 or more weeks. This insufficiency tended to involve glucocorticoids as well as mineralocorticoids. Hypothyroidism is occasionally associated with thyroid enlargement and may be detected or confirmed by measuring plasma levels of the thyroid hormone. Masculinization and hirsutism have occasionally occurred in females, as has precocious sexual development in males.

➤*GI:* Vomiting occurred in 1 in 30 patients.

➤*Hematologic:* Single instances of neutropenia, leukopenia, pancytopenia (patient received concomitant 5-fluorouracil), and agranulocytosis occurred in 4 of 27 patients with Cushing syndrome caused by adrenal carcinoma who were treated for at least 4 weeks. In 1 patient with adrenal hyperplasia, hemoglobin levels and hematocrit decreased during the course of treatment with aminoglutethimide. From the earlier experience with the drug used as an anticonvulsant in 1,214 patients, transient leukopenia was the only hematologic effect and was reported once; Coombs'-negative hemolytic anemia also occurred once. In approximately 300 patients with nonadrenal malignancy, 1 in 25 showed some degree of anemia, and 1 in 150 developed pancytopenia during treatment with aminoglutethimide.

➤*Hepatic:* Isolated instances of abnormal findings on liver function tests were reported. Suspected hepatotoxicity occurred in less than 1 in 1,000 patients.

➤*Miscellaneous:* Fever was reported in several patients who were treated with aminoglutethimide for less than 4 weeks; some of these patients also received other drugs. Myalgia occurred in 1 in 30 patients. Pulmonary hypersensitivity, including allergic alveolitis and interstitial alveolar infiltrates, has occurred rarely.

Overdosage

➤*Acute toxicity:* No deaths caused by overdosage with aminoglutethimide have been reported.

The highest known doses that have been survived are 7 g (33-year-old woman), 7.5 to 10 g (16-year-old girl), and 10 g (10-year-old boy).

Intravenous LD_{50}'s (mg/kg) – Rats, 156; dogs, more than 100.

➤*Symptoms:* An acute overdose with aminoglutethimide may reduce the production of steroids in the adrenal cortex to a degree that is clinically relevant. The following manifestations may be expected:

Cardiovascular – Hypotension, hypovolemic shock due to dehydration.

CNS/muscles – Somnolence, lethargy, coma, ataxia, dizziness, fatigue. (Extreme weakness has been reported with divided doses of 3 g daily.)

GI – Nausea, vomiting.

Laboratory test abnormalities – Hyponatremia, hypochloremia, hyperkalemia, hypoglycemia.

Renal function – Loss of sodium and water.

Respiratory function – Respiratory depression; hypoventilation.

The signs and symptoms of acute overdosage with aminoglutethimide may be aggravated or modified if alcohol, hypnotics, tranquilizers, or tricyclic antidepressants have been taken at the same time.

➤*Treatment:* Symptomatic treatment of overdosage is recommended.

Gastric lavage and unspecified supportive treatment have been employed. Full consciousness following deep coma was regained 40 hours or less after ingestion of 3 or 4 g without lavage. No evidence of hematologic, renal, or hepatic effects was subsequently found.

Close monitoring should be provided, and appropriate measures taken to support vital functions, if necessary.

If deficiency of circulating glucocorticoid develops, an IV infusion of a soluble hydrocortisone preparation (100 mg of hydrocortisone sodium succinate in 500 mL of isotonic sodium chloride solution) and 50 mL of 40% glucose solution should be given within 3 hours. After the initial infusion is completed, an IV administration of hydrocortisone, 10 mg/h, should be continued until the patient is able to take oral cortisone.

If hypovolemia or hypotension occurs, an IV administration of norepinephrine, 10 mg, in 500 mL of isotonic sodium chloride should be administered according to the patient's needs and response. After rehydration, 500 mL of plasma or blood should be given for maintenance of sufficient circulatory volume.

Dialysis may be considered in severe intoxication.

Patient Information

Warn patients that drowsiness may occur and that they should not drive, operate potentially dangerous machinery, or engage in other activities that may become hazardous because of decreased alertness.

Warn patients of the possibility of hypotension and its symptoms (see Warnings).

Indications

➤*ACTH and cosyntropin:* For diagnostic testing of adrenocortical function and in the screening of patients presumed to have adrenocortical insufficiency. Cosyntropin is less allergenic than the exogenous ACTH preparations.

➤*ACTH:* Corticotropin has limited therapeutic value in conditions responsive to corticosteroid therapy; in such cases, corticosteroid therapy is the treatment of choice. Repository corticotropin may be used in the following disorders:

Allergic states – Control of severe or incapacitating allergic conditions intractable to adequate trials of conventional treatment: Seasonal or perennial allergic rhinitis; bronchial asthma; contact dermatitis; atopic dermatitis; serum sickness.

Collagen diseases – During an exacerbation or as maintenance therapy in selected cases of systemic lupus erythematosus; systemic dermatomyositis (polymyositis); acute rheumatic carditis.

Dermatologic diseases – Pemphigus; bullous dermatitis herpetiformis; severe erythema multiforme (Stevens-Johnson syndrome); exfoliative dermatitis; severe psoriasis; severe seborrheic dermatitis; mycosis fungoides.

Edematous state – To induce a diuresis or a remission of proteinuria in the nephrotic syndrome without uremia of the idiopathic type or that due to lupus erythematosus.

Endocrine disorders – Nonsuppurative thyroiditis; hypercalcemia associated with cancer.

GI diseases – To tide the patient over a critical period of the disease in ulcerative colitis and regional enteritis.

Hematologic disorders – Acquired (autoimmune) hemolytic anemia; secondary thrombocytopenia in adults; erythroblastopenia (RBC anemia); congenital (erythroid) hypoplastic anemia.

Neoplastic disease – For palliative management of leukemias and lymphomas in adults and acute leukemia of childhood.

Nervous system diseases – Acute exacerbations of multiple sclerosis.

Ophthalmic diseases – Severe acute and chronic allergic and inflammatory processes involving the eye and its adnexa such as the following: Allergic conjunctivitis; keratitis; herpes zoster ophthalmicus; iritis and iridocyclitis; diffuse posterior uveitis and choroiditis; optic neuritis; sympathetic ophthalmia; chorioretinitis; anterior segment inflammation; allergic corneal marginal ulcers.

Rheumatic disorders – As adjunctive therapy for short-term administration (to tide the patient over an acute episode or exacerbation) in the following: Psoriatic arthritis; rheumatoid arthritis, including juvenile rheumatoid arthritis (selected cases may require low-dose maintenance therapy); ankylosing spondylitis; acute and subacute bursitis; acute nonspecific tenosynovitis; acute gouty arthritis; post-traumatic arthritis; synovitis of osteoarthritis; epicondylitis.

Respiratory diseases – Symptomatic sarcoidosis; Loeffler syndrome not manageable by other means; berylliosis; fulminating or disseminated pulmonary tuberculosis when used concurrently with antituberculous chemotherapy; aspiration pnemonitis.

Miscellaneous – Tuberculous meningitis with subarachnoid block or impending block when accompanied by antituberculous chemotherapy; trichinosis with neurologic or myocardial involvement.

➤*Unlabeled uses:* Treatment of infantile spasms.

Actions

➤*Pharmacology:* ACTH stimulates the adrenal cortex to secrete cortisol, corticosterone, aldosterone, and a number of weakly androgenic substances. Although ACTH does stimulate secretion of aldosterone, the rate is relatively independent. Prolonged administration of large doses of ACTH induces hyperplasia and hypertrophy of the adrenal cortex and continuous high output of cortisol, corticosterone, and weak androgens. The release of ACTH is under the influence of the nervous system via the corticotropin regulatory hormone released from the hypothalamus and by a negative corticosteroid feedback mechanism. Elevated plasma cortisol suppresses ACTH release.

Cosyntropin is a synthetic peptide corresponding to the amino acid residues 1 to 24 of human ACTH, which exhibits the full corticosteroidogenic activity of natural ACTH. A dose of 0.25 mg cosyntropin is pharmacologically equivalent to 25 units of natural ACTH. Cosyntropin is less allergenic than natural ACTH.

➤*Pharmacokinetics:* ACTH rapidly disappears from the circulation following its IV administration; in humans, the plasma half-life is about 15 minutes. The maximal effects of a trophic hormone on a target organ are achieved when optimal amounts of hormone are acting continuously. Thus, a fixed dose of ACTH will demonstrate a linear increase in adrenocortical secretion with increasing duration for the infusion.

Contraindications

➤*Repository corticotropin:* Scleroderma; osteoporosis; systemic fungal infections; ocular herpes simplex; recent surgery; history of or presence of peptic ulcer; congestive heart failure (CHF); hypertension; sensitivity to porcine proteins; IV administration. Treatment of conditions accompanied by primary adrenocortical insufficiency or adrenocortical hyperfunction.

➤*Cosyntropin:* Previous adverse reaction to drug.

Warnings

➤*Do not administer:* Do not administer until adrenal responsiveness has been verified with the route of administration (IM or subcutaneous) that will be used during treatment. A rise in urinary and plasma corticosteroid values provides direct evidence of a stimulatory effect.

➤*Chronic administration:* Chronic administration may lead to irreversible adverse effects. ACTH may suppress signs and symptoms of chronic disease without altering the natural course of the disease. Since complications with corticotropin use are dependent on the dose and duration of treatment, a risk to benefit decision must be made in each case.

➤*Ocular effects:* Prolonged use increases the risk of hypersensitivity reactions and may produce posterior subcapsular cataracts and glaucoma with possible damage to the optic nerve.

➤*Stress:* Although the action of ACTH is similar to that of exogenous adrenocortical steroids, the quantity of adrenocorticoid secreted may be variable. In patients who receive prolonged corticotropin therapy, use additional rapidly acting corticosteroids before, during, and after an unusually stressful situation.

➤*Infection:* ACTH may mask signs of infection including fungal or viral eye infections that may appear during its use. There may be decreased resistance and inability to localize infection. When infection is present, administer appropriate anti-infective therapy.

Tuberculosis – Observe patients with latent tuberculosis. During prolonged ACTH therapy, administer chemoprophylaxis.

➤*Immunosuppression:* Perform immunization procedures with caution, especially when high doses are administered, because of the possible hazards of neurological complications and lack of antibody response. While on corticotropin therapy, patients should not be vaccinated against smallpox.

➤*Blood pressure and electrolytes:* Corticotropin can elevate blood pressure, cause salt and water retention, and increase potassium and calcium excretion. Dietary salt restriction and potassium supplementation may be necessary.

➤*Hypersensitivity:* Cosyntropin exhibits slight immunologic activity, does not contain animal protein, and is less risky to use than natural ACTH. Patients known to be sensitized to natural ACTH with markedly positive skin tests will, with few exceptions, react negatively when tested intradermally with *Cortrosyn*. Most patients with a history of a previous hypersensitivity reaction to natural ACTH or a pre-existing allergic disease will tolerate cosyntropin; however, hypersensitivity reactions are possible. Refer to Management of Acute Hypersensitivity Reactions.

➤*Pregnancy: Category C.* ACTH has embryocidal effects. Use in pregnancy only when clearly needed and when potential benefits outweigh potential hazards to the fetus.

➤*Lactation:* It is not known whether this drug is excreted in breast milk. Because of the potential for serious adverse reactions in breast-feeding infants from ACTH, decide whether to discontinue breast-feeding or to discontinue the drug.

➤*Children:* Prolonged use of corticotropin in children will inhibit skeletal growth. If use is necessary, give intermittently and carefully observe the child.

Precautions

➤*Concomitant therapy:* Because maximal corticotropin stimulation of the adrenals may be limited during the first few days of treatment, administer other drugs when an immediate therapeutic effect is desirable.

Administer for treatment only when disease is intractable to nonsteroid treatment.

➤*Use the lowest possible dose:* Use the lowest possible dose to control the condition, and when reduction in dosage is possible, it should be gradual.

➤*Adrenocortical insufficiency:* Suppression of the pituitary adrenal axis occurs following prolonged therapy, which may be slow in returning to normal. Protect patients from the stress of trauma or surgery by the use of corticosteroids during the period of stress.

➤*Hypothyroidism and cirrhosis:* An enhanced effect of corticotropin may occur.

➤*Multiple sclerosis:* Although ACTH may speed the resolution of acute exacerbations of multiple sclerosis, it does not affect the ultimate outcome or natural course of the disease. Relatively high doses of ACTH are necessary to demonstrate a significant effect.

➤*Acute gouty arthritis:* Limit treatment of acute gouty arthritis to a few days. Since rebound attacks may occur when corticotropin is discontinued, administer conventional concomitant therapy during corticotropin treatment and for several days after it is stopped.

➤*Mental disturbances:* Psychic symptoms may appear, or pre-existing symptoms may be enhanced. These may range from mood alteration to a psychotic state.

➤*Secondary disease:* Patients with a secondary disease may have that disease worsened. Use with caution in patients with diabetes, diverticulitis, renal insufficiency, and myasthenia gravis.

Drug Interactions

Corticotropin (ACTH) Drug Interactions

Precipitant drug	Object drug[a]		Description
Corticotropin, Cosyntropin	Anticholinesterases	⬇	Corticosteroids antagonize the effects of anticholinesterases in myasthenia gravis.
Corticotropin, Cosyntropin	Aspirin	⬇	Corticosteroids will reduce serum salicylate levels and may decrease their effectiveness. Use aspirin cautiously in conjunction with corticotropin in hypoprothrombinemia.
Corticotropin, Cosyntropin	Diuretics	⬆	Corticotropin may accentuate the electrolyte loss associated with diuretic therapy.
Barbiturates	Corticotropin, Cosyntropin	⬇	Decreased pharmacologic effects of the corticosteroid may be observed. Avoid this combination if possible. Monitor closely. Increases in the corticosteroid dosage may be required.
Hydantoins (eg, phenytoin)	Corticotropin, Cosyntropin	⬇	Decreased corticosteroid effects may occur. Phenytoin levels may be reduced. Monitor phenytoin levels and adjust dose of either agent if needed.
Corticotropin, Cosyntropin	Hydantoins (eg, phenytoin)		

[a] ⬆ = Object drug increased. ⬇ = Object drug decreased.

Adverse Reactions

➤*Cardiovascular:* Hypertension; CHF; necrotizing angiitis; bradycardia; tachycardia.

➤*CNS:* Convulsions; vertigo; headache; increased intracranial pressure with papilledema (pseudotumor cerebri), usually after treatment.

➤*Dermatologic:* Impaired wound healing; petechiae and ecchymoses; increased sweating; hyperpigmentation; thin fragile skin; facial erythema; acne; suppression of skin test reactions; rash.

➤*Endocrine:* Menstrual irregularities; suppression of growth in children; hirsutism; development of Cushingoid state; manifestations of latent diabetes mellitus; decreased carbohydrate tolerance; increased requirements for insulin or oral hypoglycemic agents in diabetics; secondary adrenocortical and pituitary unresponsiveness, especially during stress.

➤*GI:* Pancreatitis; ulcerative esophagitis; abdominal distention; peptic ulcer with possible perforation and hemorrhage.

➤*Hypersensitivity:* Allergic reactions may manifest as dizziness, nausea, vomiting, shock, and skin reactions. A rare hypersensitivity reaction usually associated with pre-existing allergic disease and/or a previous reaction to natural ACTH is possible. Symptoms may include slight whealing with splotchy erythema at the injection site. There have been rare reports of anaphylactic reaction.

➤*Metabolic:* Negative nitrogen balance caused by protein catabolism; sodium and fluid retention; potassium and calcium loss; hypokalemic alkalosis; peripheral edema.

➤*Musculoskeletal:* Muscle weakness; steroid myopathy; loss of muscle mass; osteoporosis; vertebral compression fractures; pathologic fracture of long bones; aseptic necrosis of femoral and humeral heads.

➤*Ophthalmic:* Posterior subcapsular cataracts; increased intraocular pressure; glaucoma with possible damage to optic nerve; exophthalmos.

➤*Miscellaneous:* Abscess; prolonged use of ACTH may result in antibody production and subsequent loss of the stimulatory effect.

Overdosage

An acute overdose would present no different adverse reactions.

Patient Information

ACTH may mask signs of infection. There may be decreased resistance and inability to localize infection.

Diabetics may have increased requirements for insulin or oral hypoglycemics.

Notify physician if marked fluid retention, muscle weakness, abdominal pain, seizures, or headache occurs.

REPOSITORY CORTICOTROPIN

Rx	**H.P. Acthar Gel** (Aventis)	**Repository injection:** 80 units/mL	In 5 mL multidose vials.[1]

[1] With 16% gelatin.

REPOSITORY CORTICOTROPIN — INJECTION

For complete and comparative prescribing information, refer to the Corticotropin group monograph.

Indications

For diagnostic testing of adrenocortical function.

Repository corticotropin injection has limited therapeutic value in those conditions responsive to corticosteroid therapy; in such cases, corticosteroid therapy is considered to be the treatment of choice. Repository corticotropin injection may be employed in the following disorders:

➤*Endocrine disorders:* Nonsuppurative thyroiditis; hypercalcemia associated with cancer.

➤*Nervous system diseases:* Acute exacerbations of multiple sclerosis.

➤*Rheumatic disorders:* As adjunctive therapy for short-term administration (to tide the patient over an acute episode or exacerbation) in the following: Psoriatic arthritis; rheumatoid arthritis, including juvenile rheumatoid arthritis (selected cases may require low-dose maintenance therapy); ankylosing spondylitis; acute and subacute bursitis; acute nonspecific tenosynovitis; acute gouty arthritis; posttraumatic arthritis; synovitis of osteoarthritis; epicondylitis.

➤*Collagen diseases:* During an exacerbation or as maintenance therapy in selected cases of the following: Systemic lupus erythematosus; systemic dermatomyositis (polymyositis); acute rheumatic carditis.

➤*Dermatologic diseases:* Pemphigus, bullous dermatitis herpetiformis; severe erythema multiforme (Stevens-Johnson syndrome); exfoliative dermatitis; severe psoriasis; severe seborrheic dermatitis; mycosis fungoides.

➤*Allergic states:* Control of severe or incapacitating allergic conditions intractable to adequate trials of conventional treatment, such as the following: Seasonal or perennial allergic rhinitis; bronchial asthma; contact dermatitis; atopic dermatitis; serum sickness.

➤*Ophthalmic diseases:* Severe acute and chronic allergic and inflammatory processes involving the eye and its adnexa, such as the following: Allergic conjunctivitis; keratitis; herpes zoster ophthalmicus; iritis and iridocyclitis; diffuse posterior uveitis and choroiditis; optic neuritis; sympathetic ophthalmia; chorioretinitis; anterior segment inflammation; allergic corneal marginal ulcers.

➤*Respiratory diseases:* Symptomatic sarcoidosis; Loeffler syndrome not manageable by other means; berylliosis; fulminating or disseminated pulmonary tuberculosis when used concurrently with antituberculous chemotherapy; aspiration pneumonitis.

➤*Hematologic disorders:* Acquired (autoimmune) hemolytic anemia; secondary thrombocytopenia in adults; erythro-blastopenia (RBC anemia); congenital (erythroid) hypoplastic anemia.

➤*Neoplastic diseases:* For palliative management of leukemias and lymphomas in adults or acute leukemia of childhood.

➤*Edematous state:* To induce a diuresis or a remission of proteinuria in the nephrotic syndrome without uremia of the idiopathic type or that due to lupus erythematosus.

➤*GI diseases:* To tide the patient over a critical period of the disease in ulcerative colitis or regional enteritis.

➤*Miscellaneous:* Tuberculous meningitis with subarachnoid block or impending block when used concurrently with appropriate antituberculous chemotherapy; trichinosis with neurologic or myocardial involvement.

➤*Unlabeled uses:* Treatment of infantile spasms.

Administration and Dosage

➤*Verification test:* Standard tests for verification of adrenal responsiveness to corticotropin may utilize as much as 80 units as a single injection or 1 or more injections of a lesser dosage. Verification tests should be performed prior to treatment with corticotropins. The test should utilize the route(s) of administration proposed for treatment. Following verification, dosage should be individualized according to the disease under treatment and the general medical condition of each patient. Frequency and dose of the drug should be determined by considering severity of the disease, plasma and urine corticosteroid levels, and the initial response of the patient. Only gradual change in dosage schedules should be attempted after full drug effects have become apparent.

➤*Dosage reduction:* When reduction in dosage is indicated, this should be done gradually by either reducing the amount of each injection, administering injections at longer intervals or by a combination of both of the above. During reduction of dosage, careful consideration should be given to the disease being treated, the general medical conditions of the patient, and the duration over which corticotropin was administered.

➤*Usual dose:* The usual dose of repository corticotropin injection is 40 to 80 units given IM or subcutaneous every 24 to 72 hours. The chronic administration of greater than 40 units daily may be associated with uncontrollable adverse reactions.

➤*Acute exacerbations of multiple sclerosis:* In the treatment of acute exacerbations of multiple sclerosis, daily IM doses of 80 to 120 units for 2 to 3 weeks may be administered.

➤*Preparation:* Repository corticotropin injection should be warmed to room temperature before using. Do not overpressurize the vial prior to withdrawing the product.

➤*Storage / Stability:* Store repository corticotropin injection under refrigeration between 2° and 8°C (36° and 46°F).

Corticotropin (ACTH)

COSYNTROPIN

Rx	Cortrosyn (Amphastar)	Powder for Injection, lyophilized: 0.25 mg	In vials[a] with diluent.

[a] With 10 mg mannitol.

COSYNTROPIN — INJECTION

For complete and comparative prescribing information, refer to the Corticotropin group monograph.

Indications

➤*Diagnostic agent:* For use as a diagnostic agent in the screening of patients presumed to have adrenocortical insufficiency. Because of its rapid effect on the adrenal cortex it may be utilized to perform a 30-minute test of adrenal function (plasma cortisol response) as an office or outpatient procedure, using only 2 venipunctures.

Administration and Dosage

Cosyntropin may be administered intramuscularly or as a direct intravenous injection when used as a rapid screening test of adrenal function. It may also be given as an intravenous infusion over a 4- to 8-hour period to provide a greater stimulus to the adrenal glands. Doses of cosyntropin 0.25 to 0.75 mg have been used in clinical studies and a maximal response noted with the smallest dose.

Another method for a rapid screening test of adrenal function has also been suggested. A control blood sample of 6 to 7 mL is collected in a heparinized tube. Reconstitute 0.25 mg of cosyntropin in solvent (ampul of 1 mL 0.9% sodium chloride injection) and inject intramuscularly. The reconstituted drug product should be inspected visually for particulate matter and discoloration prior to injection. Reconstituted cosyntropin should not be retained. In the pediatric population, aged 2 years or less, a dose of 0.125 mg will often suffice. A second blood sample is collected exactly 30 minutes later. Both blood samples should be refrigerated until sent to the laboratory for determination of the plasma cortisol response by some appropriate method. If it is not possible to send them to the laboratory or perform the fluorimetric procedure within 12 hours, then the plasma should be separated and refrigerated or frozen according to need.

The usual normal response in most cases is an approximate doubling of the basal level, provided that the basal level does not exceed the normal range. Patients taking inadvertent doses of cortisone or hydrocortisone on the test day and patients taking spironolactone or women taking drugs which contain estrogen may exhibit abnormally high basal plasma cortisol levels. A paradoxical response may be noted in the former group as seen in a decrease in plasma cortisol values following a stimulating dose of cosyntropin. In the latter group only a normal incremental response is to be expected. Many patients with normal adrenal function, however, do not respond to the expected degree so that the following criteria have been established to denote a normal response:

1.) The control plasma cortisol level should exceed 5 mcg/100 mL.
2.) The 30-minute level should show an increment of at least 7 mcg/100 mL above the basal level.
3.) The 30-minute level should exceed 18 mcg/100 mL. Comparable figures have been reported by others. These criteria also apply when the drug is injected intravenously in 2 to 5 mL of saline over a 2-minute period.

Plasma cortisol levels usually peak about 45 to 60 minutes after an injection of cosyntropin for injection and some prefer the 60-minute interval for testing for this reason. While it is true that the 60-minute values are usually higher than the 30-minute values, the difference may not be significant enough in most cases to outweigh the disadvantage of a longer testing period. If the 60-minute test period is used, the criterion for a normal response is an approximate doubling of the basal plasma cortisol value.

Two alternative methods of administration are intravenous injection and infusion. Cosyntropin can be injected IV in 2 to 5 mL of saline over a 2-minute period. When given as an intravenous infusion: Cosyntropin, 0.25 mg may be added to glucose or saline solutions and given at the rate of approximately 40 mcg per hour over a 6-hour period. It should not be added to blood or plasma as it is apt to be inactivated by enzymes. Adrenal response may be measured in the usual manner by determining urinary steroid excretion before and after treatment or by measuring plasma cortisol levels before and at the end of the infusion. The latter is preferable because the urinary steroid excretion does not always accurately reflect the adrenal or plasma cortisol response to ACTH. Patients receiving cortisone, hydrocortisone or spironolactone should omit their pretest doses on the day selected for testing. In patients with a raised plasma bilirubin or in patients where the plasma contains free hemoglobin, falsely high fluorescence measurements will result. The test may be performed at any time during the day but because of the physiological diurnal variation of plasma cortisol the criteria listed by Wood cannot apply. It has been shown that basal plasma cortisol levels and the post cosyntropin increment exhibit diurnal changes. However, the 30-minute plasma cortisol level remains unchanged throughout the day so that only this single criterion should be used.

➤*Storage/Stability:* Store at 15° to 30°C (59° to 86°F).

Parenteral drug products should be inspected visually for particulate matter and discoloration whenever solution and container permit. Reconstituted cosyntropin should not be retained.

Glucocorticoids

Indications

➤*Allergic states:* Control of severe or incapacitating allergic conditions intractable to conventional treatment in serum sickness and drug hypersensitivity reactions.

Parenteral therapy is indicated for urticarial transfusion reactions and acute noninfectious laryngeal edema (epinephrine is the first drug of choice).

➤*Collagen diseases:* For exacerbation or maintenance therapy in selected cases of systemic lupus erythematosus, acute rheumatic carditis or systemic dermatomyositis (polymyositis).

➤*Dermatologic diseases:* Pemphigus; bullous dermatitis herpetiformis; severe erythema multiforme (Stevens-Johnson syndrome); mycosis fungoides; severe psoriasis; angioedema or urticaria; exfoliative, severe seborrheic, contact, or atopic dermatitis.

➤*Edematous states:* To induce diuresis or remission of proteinuria in the nephrotic syndrome (without uremia) of the idiopathic type or that are caused by lupus erythematosus.

➤*Endocrine disorders:* Primary or secondary adrenal cortical insufficiency (hydrocortisone or cortisone is the drug of choice; synthetic analogs may be used in conjunction with mineralocorticoids; in infancy, mineralocorticoid supplementation is important); congenital adrenal hyperplasia; nonsuppurative thyroiditis; hypercalcemia associated with cancer.

Parenteral – Acute adrenal cortical insufficiency (hydrocortisone or cortisone is drug of choice); preoperatively or in serious trauma or illness with known adrenal insufficiency or when adrenal cortical reserve is doubtful; shock unresponsive to conventional therapy if adrenal cortical insufficiency exists or is suspected.

➤*GI diseases:* To tide the patient over a critical period of the disease in ulcerative colitis, regional enteritis (Crohn's disease), and intractable sprue.

➤*Hematologic disorders:* Idiopathic thrombocytopenic purpura and secondary thrombocytopenia in adults (IV only; IM use is contraindicated); acquired (autoimmune) hemolytic anemia; erythroblastopenia (RBC anemia); congenital (erythroid) hypoplastic anemia.

➤*Intra-articular or soft tissue administration:* Short-term adjunctive therapy (to tide the patient over an acute episode) in synovitis of osteoarthritis; rheumatoid arthritis; acute and subacute bursitis; acute gouty arthritis; epicondylitis; acute nonspecific tenosynovitis; post-traumatic osteoarthritis.

➤*Intralesional administration:* Keloids; localized hypertrophic, infiltrated, inflammatory lesions of lichen planus, psoriatic plaques, granuloma annulare, lichen simplex chronicus (neurodermatitis); discoid lupus erythematosus; necrobiosis lipoidica diabeticorum; alopecia areata. May be useful in cystic tumors of an aponeurosis or tendon (ganglia).

➤*Neoplastic diseases:* For palliative management of leukemias and lymphomas in adults and acute leukemia of childhood.

➤*Nervous system:* Acute exacerbations of multiple sclerosis (see Precautions).

➤*Ophthalmic:* Severe acute and chronic allergic and inflammatory processes involving the eye and its adnexa such as in the following: Allergic conjunctivitis; keratitis; allergic corneal marginal ulcers; herpes zoster ophthalmicus; iritis and iridocyclitis; chorioretinitis; diffuse posterior uveitis and choroiditis; optic neuritis; sympathetic ophthalmia and anterior segment inflammation.

➤*Respiratory diseases:* Symptomatic sarcoidosis; bronchial asthma (including status asthmaticus); Loeffler's syndrome not manageable by other means; berylliosis; fulminating or disseminated pulmonary tuberculosis when accompanied by appropriate antituberculous chemotherapy; aspiration pneumonitis; seasonal or perennial allergic rhinitis.

➤*Rheumatic disorders:* Adjunctive therapy for short-term use (acute episode or exacerbation) in the following: Ankylosing spondylitis; acute and subacute bursitis; acute nonspecific tenosynovitis; acute gouty arthritis; psoriatic arthritis; rheumatoid arthritis, including juvenile (selected cases may require low-dose maintenance therapy); post-traumatic osteoarthritis; synovitis of osteoarthritis; epicondylitis.

➤*Miscellaneous:* Tuberculous meningitis with subarachnoid block or impending block when accompanied by appropriate antituberculous chemotherapy; in trichinosis with neurologic or myocardial involvement.

➤*Dexamethasone:* Dexamethasone also is indicated for testing of adrenal cortical hyperfunction; cerebral edema associated with primary or metastatic brain tumor, craniotomy, or head injury.

➤*Triamcinolone:* Triamcinolone also is indicated for the treatment of pulmonary emphysema where bronchospasm or bronchial edema plays a significant role, and diffuse interstitial pulmonary fibrosis (Hamman-Rich syndrome); in conjunction with diuretic agents to induce a diuresis in refractory CHF and in cirrhosis of the liver with refractory ascites; and for postoperative dental inflammatory reactions.

➤*Unlabeled uses:*

Glucocorticoid Unlabeled Uses	
Use	Drug/Comment
Acute mountain sickness	Dexamethasone 4 mg q 6 h; prevention or treatment
Antiemetic	Dexamethasone most common, 16 to 20 mg
Bacterial meningitis	Dexamethasone 0.15 mg/kg q 6 h; to decrease incidence of hearing loss
Bronchopulmonary dysplasia in preterm infants	Dexamethasone 0.5 mg/kg, then taper.
COPD	Prednisone 30 to 60 mg/day for 1 to 2 weeks, then taper
Depression, diagnosis of	Dexamethasone 1 mg
Duchenne's muscular dystrophy	Prednisone 0.75 to 1.5 mg/kg/day; to improve strength and function
Graves ophthalmopathy	Prednisone 60 mg/day, taper to 20 mg/day
Hepatitis, severe alcoholic	Methylprednisolone 32 mg/day; to reduce mortality
Hirsutism	Dexamethasone 0.5 to 1 mg/day
Respiratory distress syndrome	Prevention in premature neonates (betamethasone most common); adults, methylprednisolone 30 mg/kg (controversial)
Septic shock	Methylprednisolone 30 mg/kg IV most common (very controversial)
Spinal cord injury, acute	Methylprednisolone IV within 8 hrs of injury; to improve neurologic function
Tuberculous pleurisy	Prednisolone 0.75 mg/kg/day, then taper; concurrently w/antituberculous therapy

Administration and Dosage

➤*Administration:* The maximal activity of the adrenal cortex is between 2 and 8 am, and it is minimal between 4 pm and midnight. Exogenous corticosteroids suppress adrenocortical activity the least when given at the time of maximal activity (am). Therefore, administer glucocorticoids in the morning prior to 9 am. When large doses are given, administer antacids between meals to help prevent peptic ulcers.

➤*Initiation of therapy:* The initial dosage depends on the specific disease entity being treated. Maintain or adjust the initial dosage until a satisfactory response is noted. If after a reasonable period of time there is a lack of satisfactory clinical response, discontinue the drug and transfer the patient to other appropriate therapy. It should be emphasized that dosage requirements are variable and must be individualized. For infants and children, the recommended dosage should be governed by the same considerations rather than by strict adherence to the ratio indicated by age or body weight.

➤*Maintenance therapy:* After a favorable response is observed, determine the maintenance dosage by decreasing the initial dosage in small amounts at intervals until the lowest dosage that will maintain an adequate clinical response is reached. Constant monitoring of drug dosage is required. Situations that may make dosage adjustments necessary are changes in the disease process, the patient's individual drug responsiveness, and the effect of patient exposure to stress; in this latter situation it may be necessary to increase the dosage for a period of time consistent with the patient's condition.

➤*Withdrawal of therapy:* If, after long-term therapy, the drug is to be stopped, it must be withdrawn gradually. If spontaneous remission occurs in a chronic condition, discontinue treatment gradually. Continued supervision of the patient after discontinuation of corticosteroids is essential, because there may be a sudden reappearance of severe manifestations of the disease.

➤*Alternate-day therapy:* Alternate day therapy is a dosing regimen in which twice the usual daily dose is administered every other morning. The purpose is to provide the patient requiring long-term treatment with the beneficial effects of corticosteroids while minimizing pituitary-adrenal suppression, the cushingoid state, withdrawal symptoms, and growth suppression in children. The benefits of alternate-day therapy are only achieved by using the intermediate-acting agents.

The rationale for this treatment schedule is based on 2 major premises: a) The therapeutic effect of intermediate-acting corticosteroids persists longer than their physical presence and metabolic effects; b) administration of the corticosteroid every other morning allows for reestablishment of a more normal hypothalamic-pituitary-adrenal (HPA) activity on the off-steroid day. Keep the following in mind when considering alternate day therapy:

1.) Benefits of alternate day therapy do not encourage indiscriminate steroid use.
2.) Alternate day therapy is primarily designed for patients in whom long-term corticosteroid therapy is anticipated.
3.) In less severe disease processes, it may be possible to initiate treatment with alternate day therapy. More severe disease states usually require daily divided high-dose therapy for initial control. Continue initial suppressive dose until satisfactory clinical response is obtained, usually 4 to 10 days in the case of many allergic and collagen diseases. Keep the period of initial suppressive dose as brief as possible, particularly when alternate day therapy is intended. Once control is established, 2 courses are available: a) Change to alternate day therapy, then gradually reduce the amount of corticosteroid given every other day, or b) reduce daily corticosteroid dose to the lowest effective level as rapidly as possible, then change over to an alternate day schedule. Theoretically, course a) may be preferable.
4.) Because of the advantages of alternate day therapy, it may be desirable to try patients on this form of therapy who have been on daily corticosteroids for long periods of time (eg, patients with rheumatoid arthritis). Because these patients may already have a suppressed HPA axis, establishing them on alternate day therapy may be difficult and not always successful; however, it is recommended that such regular attempts be made. It may be helpful to triple or even quadruple the daily maintenance dose and administer this every other day rather than just doubling the daily dose if difficulty is encountered. Once the patient is controlled, attempt to reduce this dose to a minimum.
5.) Long-acting corticosteroids (eg, **dexamethasone**, **betamethasone**), because of their prolonged suppressive effect on adrenal activity, are not recommended for alternate day therapy.
6.) It is important to individualize therapy. Complete control of symptoms will not be possible in all patients. An explanation of the benefits of alternate day therapy will help the patient to understand and tolerate the possible flare-up in symptoms that may occur in the latter part of the off-steroid day. Other therapy to relieve symptoms may be added or increased at this time if needed.
7.) In the event of an acute flare-up of the disease process, it may be necessary to return to a full suppressive daily corticosteroid dose for control. Once control is established, alternate day therapy may be reinstituted.

➤*Intra-articular injection:* Dose depends on the joint size and varies with the severity of the condition. In chronic cases, injections may be repeated at intervals of 1 to 5 or more weeks, depending upon the degree of relief obtained from the initial injection. Injection must be made into the synovial space. Do not inject unstable joints. Repeated intra-articular injection may result in joint instability. X-ray follow-up is suggested in selected cases to detect deterioration.

Suitable sites – Suitable sites for injection are the knee, ankle, wrist, elbow, shoulder, hip, and phalangeal joints. Because difficulty is frequently encountered in entering the hip joint, avoid any large blood vessels in the area. Joints not suitable for injection are those that are anatomically inaccessible and devoid of synovial space, such as the spinal joints and the sacroiliac joints. Treatment failures frequently result from failure to enter the joint space; little or no benefit follows injection into surrounding tissue. If failures occur when injections into the synovial spaces are certain, as determined by aspiration of fluid, repeated injections are usually of no benefit. Local therapy does not alter the underlying disease process; whenever possible, employ comprehensive therapy, including physiotherapy and orthopedic correction (see Precautions).

➤*Miscellaneous (tendinitis, epicondylitis, ganglion):* In the treatment of conditions such as tendinitis or tenosynovitis, inject into the tendon sheath rather than into the substance of the tendon. When treating conditions such as epicondylitis, outline the area of greatest tenderness and infiltrate the drug into the area. For ganglia of the tendon sheaths, inject the drug directly into the cyst. In many cases, a single injection markedly decreases size of the cystic tumor and may effect disappearance. The dose varies with the condition being treated. In recurrent or chronic conditions, repeated injections may be needed.

➤*Injections for local effect in dermatologic conditions:* Avoid injection of sufficient material to cause blanching because this may be followed by a small slough. One to four injections are usually employed. Intervals between injections vary with the type of lesion being treated and duration of improvement produced by initial injection.

Actions

➤*Pharmacology:* The naturally occurring adrenocortical steroids have both anti-inflammatory (glucocorticoid) and salt-retaining (mineralocorticoid) properties. Glucocorticoids cause profound and varied metabolic effects. In addition, they modify the body's immune responses to diverse stimuli.

These compounds, including **hydrocortisone** (cortisol) and **cortisone**, are used as replacement therapy in adrenocortical deficiency states and may be used for their anti-inflammatory effects. The synthetic steroid compounds **prednisone**, **prednisolone**, and **fludrocortisone** also have glucocorticoid and mineralocorticoid activity. Prednisone and prednisolone are used primarily for their glucocorticoid effects.

In addition, a group of synthetic compounds with marked glucocorticoid activity are distinguished by the absence of any significant salt-retaining activity. These include **triamcinolone**, **dexamethasone**, **methylprednisolone**, and **betamethasone**. These agents are used for their potent anti-inflammatory effects.

➤*Pharmacokinetics:*

Absorption – **Hydrocortisone** and most of its congeners are readily absorbed from the GI tract; greatly altered onsets and durations are usually achieved with injections of suspensions and esters.

Distribution – **Hydrocortisone** is reversibly bound to corticosteroid-binding globulin (CBG or transcortin) and corticosteroid binding albumin (CBA). Exogenous glucocorticoids are bound to these proteins to a significantly lesser degree. In hypoproteinemic or dysproteinemic states, the total endogenous hydrocortisone levels are decreased. Conversely, with increased CBG (pregnancy, estrogen therapy), the total plasma hydrocortisone levels are elevated. These alterations are not of clinical significance because it is the unbound fraction of the hormone that is metabolically active. However, the administration of exogenous glucocorticoids to patients with altered protein-binding capacities will result in significant differences in glucocorticoid pharmacological effects.

Metabolism/Excretion – Hydrocortisone is metabolized by the liver, which is the rate-limiting step in its clearance. The metabolism and excretion of the synthetic glucocorticoids generally parallel hydrocortisone. Induction of hepatic enzymes will increase the metabolic clearance of hydrocortisone and the synthetic glucocorticoids. About 1% of its usual daily production, or about 200 mcg unchanged hormone is excreted in urine daily. Renal clearance is increased when plasma levels are increased. **Prednisone** is inactive and must be metabolized to **prednisolone**. The following table summarizes the approximate dosage equivalencies (based on glucocorticoid properties) of the various glucocorticoid preparations and several of their pharmacokinetic parameters. The half-life values refer to the intrinsic activity of each agent; insoluble salts of these drugs are used as repository injections and have sustained effects because of delayed absorption from the injection site.

Glucocorticoid Equivalencies, Potencies, and Half-Life

Glucocorticoid	Equivalent potency dose (mg)[a]	Anti-inflammatory potency[a]	Sodium-retaining potency	Half-life plasma (min)
Short-acting				
Cortisone	25	0.8	2	30
Hydrocortisone	20	1	2	80-118
Intermediate-acting				
Prednisone	5	4	1	60
Prednisolone	5	4	1	115-212
Triamcinolone	4	5	0	200+
Methylprednisolone	4	5	0	78-188
Long-acting				
Dexamethasone	0.75	20-30	0	110-210
Betamethasone	0.6-0.75	20-30	0	300+

[a] When converting doses, use only equivalent potency column, not anti-inflammatory potency column.

Contraindications

Systemic fungal infections; hypersensitivity to the drug; IM use in idiopathic thrombocytopenic purpura; administration of live virus vaccines (eg, smallpox) in patients receiving immunosuppressive corticosteroid doses (see Warnings).

Warnings

➤*Infections:* Corticosteroids may mask signs of infection, and new infections may appear during their use. There may be decreased resistance and inability of the host defense mechanisms to prevent dissemination of the infection. If an infection occurs during therapy, it should be promptly controlled by suitable antimicrobial therapy.

Tuberculosis – Restrict use in active tuberculosis to cases of fulminating or disseminated disease in which the corticosteroid is used for disease management with appropriate chemotherapy. If corticosteroids are indicated in latent tuberculosis or tuberculin reactivity, observe closely; disease reactivation may occur. During prolonged corticosteroid use, these patients should receive chemoprophylaxis.

Fungal – Corticosteroids may exacerbate systemic fungal infections; do not use in such infections, except to control drug reactions caused by amphotericin B. Concomitant use of amphotericin B and **hydrocortisone** has been followed by cardiac enlargement and CHF.

Amebiasis – Corticosteroids may activate latent amebiasis. Rule out amebiasis before giving to a patient who has been in the tropics or has unexplained diarrhea.

Cerebral malaria – A double-blind trial has shown corticosteroid use is associated with prolongation of coma and a higher incidence of pneumonia and GI bleeding.

➤*Hepatitis:* Although advocated for use in chronic active hepatitis, corticosteroids may be harmful in chronic active hepatitis positive for hepatitis B surface antigen.

➤*Ocular effects:* Prolonged use may produce posterior subcapsular cataracts, glaucoma with possible damage to the optic nerves, and may enhance the establishment of secondary ocular infections due to fungi or viruses. Use cautiously in ocular herpes simplex because of possible corneal perforation.

➤*Fluid and electrolyte balance:* Average and large doses of **hydrocortisone** or **cortisone** can cause elevation of blood pressure, salt and water retention, and increased excretion of potassium. These effects are less likely to occur with the synthetic derivatives except when used in large doses. Dietary salt restriction and potassium supplementation may be necessary. All corticosteroids increase calcium excretion.

➤*Peptic ulcer:* The relationship between peptic ulceration and glucocorticoid therapy is unclear. Patients who appear to be at risk are those being treated for nephrotic syndrome or liver disease or who are comatose postcraniotomy. Other predisposing factors include a total **prednisone** intake exceeding 1 g, a history of ulcer disease, concomitant use of known gastric irritants (as in arthritic patients), and stress. It may be desirable to use prophylactic antacids pending clarification of the relationship.

➤*Immunosuppression:* During therapy, do not use live virus vaccines (eg, smallpox). Do not immunize patients who are receiving corticosteroids, especially high doses, because of possible hazards of neurological complications and a lack of antibody response. This does not apply to patients receiving corticosteroids as replacement therapy. Corticosteroids may suppress reactions to skin tests.

➤*Adrenal suppression:* Prolonged therapy of pharmacologic doses may lead to hypothalamic-pituitary-adrenal suppression. The degree of adrenal suppression varies with the dosage, relative glucocorticoid activity, biological half-life and duration of glucocorticoid therapy within each individual. Adrenal suppression may be minimized by the use of intermediate-acting glucocorticoids (**prednisone**, **prednisolone**, **methylprednisolone**) on an alternate day schedule (see Administration and Dosage).

Withdrawal of therapy – Following prolonged therapy, abrupt discontinuation may result in a withdrawal syndrome without evidence of adrenal insufficiency. To minimize morbidity associated with adrenal insufficiency, discontinue exogenous corticosteroid therapy gradually. During withdrawal therapy, increased supplementation may be necessary during times of stress. Symptoms of adrenal insufficiency as a result of too rapid withdrawal include the following: Nausea; fatigue; anorexia; dyspnea; hypotension; hypoglycemia; myalgia; fever; malaise; arthralgia; dizziness; desquamation of skin; fainting. Continued supervision after therapy termination is essential; severe disease manifestations may reappear suddenly.

➤*Stress:* In patients receiving or recently withdrawn from corticosteroid therapy subjected to unusual stress, increased dosage of rapidly acting corticosteroids is indicated before, during, and after stressful situations, except in patients on high-dose therapy. Relative adrenocortical insufficiency may persist for months after therapy ends; in any stress situation occurring during that period, reinstitute therapy. Because mineralocorticoid secretion may be impaired, administer salt or a mineralocorticoid concurrently.

➤*Cardiovascular:* Reports suggest an apparent association between corticosteroid use and left ventricular free wall rupture after a recent myocardial infarction. Use with great caution in these patients.

➤*Hypersensitivity reactions:* Anaphylactoid reactions have occurred rarely with corticosteroid therapy; take precautionary measures, especially in patients with a history of allergies. Refer to Management of Acute Hypersensitivity Reactions.

➤*Renal function impairment:* Edema may occur in the presence of renal disease with a fixed or decreased glomerular filtration rate. Use with caution in renal insufficiency, acute glomerulonephritis, and chronic nephritis.

➤*Elderly:* Consider the risk/benefit factors of steroid use. Consider lower doses because of body changes caused by aging (ie, diminution of muscle mass and plasma volume). Monitor blood pressure, blood glucose and electrolytes at least every 6 months.

➤*Pregnancy:* (*Category C* - **Prednisolone sodium phosphate**). Corticosteroids cross the placenta (**prednisone** has the poorest transport). In animal studies, large doses of cortisol administered early in pregnancy produced cleft palate, stillborn fetuses, and decreased fetal size. Chronic maternal ingestion during the first trimester has shown a 1% incidence of cleft palate in humans. If used in pregnancy, or in women of childbearing potential, weigh benefits against the potential hazards to the mother and fetus. Carefully observe infants born of mothers who have received substantial corticosteroid doses during pregnancy for signs of hypoadrenalism.

➤*Lactation:* Corticosteroids appear in breast milk and could suppress growth, interfere with endogenous corticosteroid production or cause other unwanted effects in the nursing infant. Advise mothers taking pharmacologic corticosteroid doses not to nurse. However, several studies suggest that amounts excreted in breast milk are negligible with **prednisone** or **prednisolone** doses ≤ 20 mg/day or **methylprednisolone** doses ≤ 8 mg/day, and large doses for short periods may not harm the infant. Alternatives to consider include waiting 3 to 4 hours after the dose before breastfeeding and using prednisolone rather than prednisone (resulting in a lower corticosteroid dose to the infant).

➤*Children:* Carefully observe growth and development of infants and children on prolonged corticosteroid therapy.

Benzyl alcohol – Some of these products contain benzyl alcohol, which has been associated with a fatal "gasping syndrome" in premature infants.

Precautions

➤*Monitoring:* Observe patients for weight increase, edema, hypertension, and excessive potassium excretion, as well as for less obvious signs of adrenocortical steroid-induced untoward effects. Monitor for a negative nitrogen balance due to protein catabolism. A liberal protein intake is essential during prolonged therapy. Evaluate blood pressure and body weight, and do routine laboratory studies, including 2-hour postprandial blood glucose and serum potassium and a chest x-ray at regular intervals during prolonged therapy. Upper GI x-rays are desirable in patients with known or suspected peptic ulcer disease or significant dyspepsia or in patients complaining of gastric distress. Observe growth and development of infants and children on prolonged therapy.

➤*Use the lowest possible dose:* Make a benefit/risk decision in each individual case as to the size of the dose, duration of treatment, and the use of daily or intermittent therapy because complications of treatment are dependent on these factors.

➤*Use with caution in:*

GI – Nonspecific ulcerative colitis if there is a probability of impending perforation, abscess or other pyogenic infection; diverticulitis; fresh intestinal anastomoses; active or latent peptic ulcer (see Warnings).

Cardiovascular – Hypertension; CHF; thromboembolitic tendencies; thrombophlebitis.

Miscellaneous – Osteoporosis; exanthema; Cushing syndrome; antibiotic-resistant infections; convulsive disorders; metastatic carcinoma; myasthenia gravis; vaccinia; varicella; diabetes mellitus; hypothyroidism, cirrhosis (enhanced effect of corticosteroids).

➤*Steroid psychosis:* Steroid psychosis is characterized by a delirious or toxic psychosis with clouded sensorium. Other symptoms may include euphoria, insomnia, mood swings, personality changes, and severe depression. The onset of symptoms usually occurs within 15 to 30 days. Predisposing factors include doses more than 40 mg **prednisone** equivalent, female predominance, and, possibly, a family history of psychiatric illness. A patient history of psychiatric problems does not correlate well with predisposition to steroid-induced psychosis. Incidence appears to correlate with dose. One study of 718 patients treated with prednisone revealed less than or equal to 40 mg/day = 1.3%; 41 to 80 mg/day = 4.6%; greater than or equal to 80 mg/day = 18.4%. If the steroids cannot be discontinued, psychotropic medication is effective.

➤*Multiple sclerosis:* Although corticosteroids are effective in speeding the resolution of acute exacerbations of multiple sclerosis, they do not affect the ultimate outcome or natural history of the disease. Relatively high doses of corticosteroids are necessary to demonstrate a significant effect.

➤*Repository injections:* To minimize the likelihood and severity of atrophy, do not inject subcutaneous, avoid injection into the deltoid, and avoid repeated IM injections into the same site, if possible. Repository injections are not recommended as initial therapy in acute situations.

➤*Local injections:* Intra-articular injection may produce systemic and local effects. A marked increase in pain accompanied by local swelling, further restriction of joint motion, fever, and malaise is suggestive of septic arthritis. Appropriate examination of any joint fluid present is necessary. If a diagnosis of sepsis is confirmed, institute appropriate antimicrobial therapy. Avoid local injection into an infected site and into unstable joints.

Strongly impress patients with the importance of not overusing joints in which symptomatic benefit has been obtained as long as the inflammatory process remains active. Frequent intra-articular injection may damage joint tissues.

Avoid overdistention of the joint capsule and deposition of steroid along the needle track in intra-articular injection, as it may lead to subcutaneous atrophy. While crystals of adrenal steroids in the dermis suppress inflammatory reactions, their presence may cause disintegration of the cellular elements and physiochemical changes in the ground substance of the connective tissue.

The resultant dermal or subdermal changes may form depressions in the skin at the injection site; the degree will vary with the amount of adrenal steroid injection. Regeneration is usually complete within a few months or after all crystals of the adrenal steroid have been absorbed. In order to minimize the incidence of dermal and subdermal atrophy, exercise care not to exceed recommended doses in injections. Make multiple small injections into the area of the lesion whenever possible.

➤*Tartrazine sensitivity:* Some of these products contain tartrazine, which may cause allergic-type reactions (including bronchial asthma) in susceptible individuals. Although the incidence of tartrazine sensitivity in the general population is low, it is frequently seen in patients who also have aspirin hypersensitivity. Specific products containing tartrazine are identified in the product listings.

➤*Sulfite sensitivity:* Some of these products contain sulfites which may cause severe allergic reactions in certain susceptible individuals, particularly asthmatics. Anaphylactoid and hypersensitivity reactions have occurred. Do not use in patients allergic to sulfites. Products containing sulfites are identified in product listings.

Drug Interactions

Corticosteroid Drug Interactions

Precipitant drug	Object drug[a]		Description
Aminoglutethimide	Dexamethasone	⬇	Possible loss of dexamethasone-induced adrenal suppression.
Barbiturates	Corticosteroids	⬇	Decreased pharmacologic effects of the corticosteroid may be observed.
Cholestyramine	Hydrocortisone	⬇	The hydrocortisone AUC may be decreased.
Contraceptives, oral	Corticosteroids	⬆	Corticosteroid half-life and concentration may be increased and clearance decreased.
Ephedrine	Dexamethasone	⬇	A decreased half-life and increased clearance of dexamethasone may occur.
Estrogens	Corticosteroids	⬆	Corticosteroid clearance may be decreased.
Hydantoins	Corticosteroids	⬇	Corticosteroid clearance may be increased, resulting in reduced therapeutic effects.
Ketoconazole	Corticosteroids	⬆	Corticosteroid clearance may be decreased and the AUC increased.
Macrolide antibiotics	Methylprednisolone	⬆	Significant decrease in methylprednisolone clearance may require a decrease in methylprednisolone dose and the dosing interval.
Rifampin	Corticosteroids	⬇	Corticosteroid clearance may be increased, resulting in decreased therapeutic effects.
Corticosteroids	Anticholinesterases	⬇	Anticholinesterase effects may be antagonized in myasthenia gravis.
Corticosteroids	Anticoagulants, oral	⬌	Anticoagulant dose requirements may be reduced. Conversely, corticosteroids may oppose the anticoagulant action.
Corticosteroids	Cyclosporine	⬆	Although this combination is therapeutically beneficial for organ transplants, toxicity may be enhanced.
Corticosteroids	Digitalis glycosides	⬆	Coadministration may enhance the possibility of digitalis toxicity associated with hypokalemia.
Corticosteroids	Isoniazid	⬇	Isoniazid serum concentrations may be decreased.
Corticosteroids	Nondepolarizing muscle relaxants	⬌	Corticosteroids may potentiate, counteract, or have no effect on the neuromuscular blocking action.
Corticosteroids	Potassium-depleting agents (eg, diuretics)	⬆	Observe patients for hypokalemia.
Corticosteroids	Salicylates	⬇	Corticosteroids will reduce serum salicylate levels and may decrease their effectiveness.
Corticosteroids	Somatrem	⬇	Growth-promoting effect of somatrem may be inhibited.
Corticosteroids	Theophyllines	⬌	Alterations in the pharmacologic activity of either agent may occur.
Theophyllines	Corticosteroids	⬌	Alterations in the pharmacologic activity of either agent may occur.

[a] ⬆ = Object drug increased. ⬇ = Object drug decreased.
⬌ = Undetermined clinical effect.

➤*Drug/Lab test interactions:* Urine glucose and serum cholesterol levels may increase.

Decreased serum levels of potassium, triiodothyronine (T_3), and a minimal decrease of thyroxine (T_4) may occur. Thyroid I^{131} uptake may be decreased. False-negative results with the nitroblue-tetrazolium test for bacterial infection may occur. **Dexamethasone**, given for cerebral edema, may alter the results of a brain scan (decreased uptake of radioactive material).

Adverse Reactions

Parenteral therapy – Rare instances of blindness associated with intralesional therapy around the face and head; hyperpigmentation or hypopigmentation; subcutaneous and cutaneous atrophy; sterile abscess; Charcot-like arthropathy; burning or tingling, especially in the perineal area (after IV injection); scarring, induration, inflammation, paresthesia, occasional irritation at the injection site or occasional brief increase in joint discomfort; transient or delayed pain or soreness; muscle twitching, ataxia, hiccoughs and nystagmus (low incidence following injection); anaphylactic reactions with or without circulatory collapse; cardiac arrest; bronchospasm; arachnoiditis after intrathecal use; foreign body granulomatous reactions involving the synovium with repeated injections.

Intra-articular: Osteonecrosis; tendon rupture; infection; skin atrophy; postinjection flare; hypersensitivity; facial flushing. Systemic reactions may also occur.

Intraspinal: Meningitis (tuberculous, bacterial, cryptococcal, aseptic, chemical); adhesive arachnoiditis; conus medullaris syndrome.

➤*Cardiovascular:* Thromboembolism or fat embolism; thrombophlebitis; necrotizing angiitis; cardiac arrhythmias or ECG changes caused by potassium deficiency; syncopal episodes; aggravation of hypertension; myocardial rupture following recent MI (see Warnings). There are reports of cardiac arrhythmias, fatal arrest, or circulatory collapse following the rapid administration of large IV doses of **methylprednisolone** (0.5 to 1 g in less than 10 to 120 minutes) (see Electrolyte Disturbance).

➤*CNS:* Convulsions; increased intracranial pressure with papilledema (pseudotumor cerebri), usually after stopping treatment; vertigo; headache; neuritis/paresthesias; aggravation of pre-existing psychiatric conditions; steroid psychoses (see Precautions).

➤*Dermatologic:* Impaired wound healing; thin fragile skin; petechiae and ecchymoses; erythema; lupus erythematosus-like lesions; suppression of skin test reactions; subcutaneous fat atrophy; purpura; striae; hirsutism; acneiform eruptions; other cutaneous reactions such as allergic dermatitis; urticaria; angioneurotic edema; perineal irritation.

➤*Endocrine:* Amenorrhea, postmenopausal bleeding and other menstrual irregularities; development of cushingoid state (eg, moonface, buffalo hump, supraclavicular fat pad enlargement, central obesity); suppression of growth in children; secondary adrenocortical and pituitary unresponsiveness, particularly in times of stress (eg, trauma, surgery, illness); increased sweating; decreased carbohydrate tolerance; hyperglycemia; glycosuria; increased insulin or sulfonylurea requirements in diabetics; manifestations of latent diabetes mellitus; negative nitrogen balance caused by protein catabolism; hirsutism.

➤*Electrolyte disturbance:* Sodium and fluid retention; hypokalemia; hypokalemic alkalosis; metabolic alkalosis; hypocalcemia; CHF in susceptible patients; hypotension or shock-like reactions; hypertension (see Warnings).

➤*GI:* Pancreatitis; abdominal distension; ulcerative esophagitis; nausea; vomiting; increased appetite and weight gain; peptic ulcer with perforation and hemorrhage (see Warnings); perforation of the small and large bowel, particularly in inflammatory bowel disease.

➤*Musculoskeletal:* Muscle weakness; steroid myopathy; muscle mass loss; tendon rupture; osteoporosis; aseptic necrosis of femoral and humeral heads (1% to 37%); spontaneous fractures, including vertebral compression fractures and pathologic fracture of long bones.

➤*Ophthalmic:* Posterior subcapsular cataracts; increased IOP; glaucoma; exophthalmos.

➤*Miscellaneous:* Anaphylactoid/hypersensitivity reactions, aggravation/masking of infections (see Warnings); malaise; leukocytosis (including neonates receiving dexamethasone via maternal injection); fatigue; insomnia; increased or decreased motility and number of spermatozoa.

Overdosage

➤*Symptoms:* There are 2 categories of toxic effects from therapeutic use of glucocorticoids:

Acute adrenal insufficiency – Acute adrenal insufficiency caused by too rapid corticosteroid withdrawal after long-term use, resulting in fever, myalgia, arthralgia, malaise, anorexia, nausea, skin desquamation, orthostatic hypotension, dizziness, fainting, dyspnea, and hypoglycemia.

Cushingoid changes – Cushingoid changes from continued use of large doses resulting in moonface, central obesity, striae, hirsutism, acne, ecchymoses, hypertension, osteoporosis, myopathy, sexual dysfunction, diabetes, hyperlipidemia, peptic ulcer, increased susceptibility to infection and electrolyte and fluid imbalance. Reports of acute toxicity or death are rare.

➤*Treatment:* Recovery of normal adrenal and pituitary function may require up to 9 months. Gradually taper the steroid under the supervision of a physician. Frequent lab tests are necessary. Supplementation is required during periods of stress (eg, illness, surgery, injury). Eventually reduce to the lowest dose that will control the symptoms or discontinue the corticosteroid completely. For large, acute overdoses, treatment includes gastric lavage or emesis and usual supportive measures. Refer to General Management of Acute Overdosage.

Patient Information

May cause GI upset; take with meals or snacks. Take single daily or alternate day doses in the morning prior to 9 a.m. Take multiple doses at evenly spaced intervals throughout the day.

Patients on chronic steroid therapy should wear or carry identification to that effect.

Notify physician if unusual weight gain, swelling of the lower extremities, muscle weakness, black tarry stools, vomiting of blood, puffing of the face, menstrual irregularities, prolonged sore throat, fever, cold, or infection occurs.

Signs of adrenal insufficiency include fatigue, anorexia, nausea, vomiting, diarrhea, weight loss, weakness, dizziness, and low blood sugar. Notify physician promptly if these symptoms occur following dosage reduction or withdrawal of therapy.

➤*High-dose or long-term therapy:* Avoid abrupt withdrawal of therapy.

BETAMETHASONE

Rx	**Celestone** (Schering)	**Solution:** 0.6 mg per 5 mL	Alcohol. Sorbitol, sugar. In 118 mL.

BETAMETHASONE — ORAL

For complete and comparative prescribing information, refer to the Glucocorticoids group monograph.

Administration and Dosage

➤*Initial dosage:* 0.6 to 7.2 mg/day; individualize.

➤*Storage/Stability:* Store between 2° and 30°C (36° and 86°F). Protect from excessive moisture.

BETAMETHASONE SODIUM PHOSPHATE AND BETAMETHASONE ACETATE

Rx	**Celestone Soluspan** (Schering)	**Injection:** 3 mg betamethasone acetate and 3 mg betamethasone (as sodium phosphate)/mL suspension	In 5 mL multidose vials.[a]

[a] With EDTA and benzalkonium chloride.

BETAMETHASONE SODIUM PHOSPHATE/BETAMETHASONE ACETATE — INJECTION

For complete and comparative prescribing information, refer to the Glucocorticoids group monograph.

Administration and Dosage

➤*Dosage:* The initial dosage may vary from 0.5 to 9 mg/day, depending on the specific disease entity being treated. In situations of less severity, lower doses will generally suffice, while in selected patients higher initial doses may be required. Usually the parenteral dosage ranges are ⅓ to ½ the oral dose given every 12 hours. However, in certain overwhelming, acute, life-threatening situations, administration in dosages exceeding the usual dosages may be justified and may be in multiples of the oral dosages.

The initial dosage should be maintained or adjusted until a satisfactory response is noted. If, after a reasonable period of time, there is a lack of satisfactory clinical response, betamethasone sodium phosphate/betamethasone acetate should be discontinued and the patient transferred to other appropriate therapy.

It should be emphasized that dosage requirements are variable and must be individualized on the basis of the disease under treatment and the response of the patient.

After a favorable response is noted, the proper maintenance dosage should be determined by decreasing the initial drug dosage in small decrements at appropriate time intervals until the lowest dosage which will maintain an adequate clinical response is reached. It should be kept in mind that constant monitoring is needed in regard to drug dosage. Included in the situations which may make dosage adjustments necessary are changes in clinical status secondary to remissions or exacerbations in the disease process, the patient's individual drug responsiveness, and the effect of patient exposure to stressful situations not directly related to the disease entity under treatment. In this latter situation, it may be necessary to increase the dosage of betamethasone sodium phosphate/betamethasone acetate for a period of time consistent with the patient's condition. If, after long-term therapy, the drug is to be stopped, it is recommended that it be withdrawn gradually rather than abruptly.

If coadministration of a local anesthetic is desired, betamethasone sodium phosphate/betamethasone acetate injectable suspension may be mixed with 1% or 2% lidocaine hydrochloride, using the formulations which do not contain parabens. Similar local anesthetics may also be used. Diluents containing methylparaben, propylparaben, phenol, should be avoided since these compounds may cause flocculation of the steroid. The required dose of betamethasone sodium phosphate/betamethasone acetate is first withdrawn from the vial into the syringe. The local anesthetic is then drawn in, and the syringe shaken briefly. Do not inject local anesthetics into the vial of betamethasone sodium phosphate/betamethasone acetate.

➤*Bursitis, tenosynovitis, peritendinitis:* In acute subdeltoid, subacromial, olecranon, and prepatellar bursitis, 1 intrabursal injection of 1 mL betamethasone sodium phosphate/betamethasone acetate can relieve pain and restore full range of movement. Several intrabursal injections of corticosteroids are usually required in recurrent acute bursitis and in acute exacerbations of chronic bursitis. Partial relief of pain and some increase in mobility can be expected in both conditions after 1 or 2 injections. Chronic bursitis may be treated with reduced dosage once the acute condition is controlled. In tenosynovitis and tendinitis, 3 or 4 local injections at intervals of 1 to 2 weeks between injections are given in most cases. Injections should be made into the affected tendon sheaths, rather than into the tendons themselves. In ganglions of joint capsules and tendon sheaths, injection of 0.5 mL directly into the ganglion cysts has produced marked reduction in the size of the lesions.

➤*Rheumatoid arthritis and osteoarthritis:* Following intra-articular administration of 0.5 to 2 mL, relief of pain, soreness, and stiffness may be experienced. Duration of relief varies widely in both diseases. Intra-articular injection (betamethasone sodium phosphate/betamethasone acetate) is well tolerated in joints and periarticular tissues. There is virtually no pain on injection, and the "secondary flare" that sometimes occurs a few hours after intra-articular injection of corticosteroids has not been reported with betamethasone sodium phosphate/betamethasone acetate. Using sterile technique, a 20- to 24-gauge needle on an empty syringe is inserted into the synovial cavity and a few drops of synovial fluid are withdrawn to confirm that the needle is in the joint. The aspirating syringe is replaced by a syringe containing betamethasone sodium phosphate/betamethasone acetate, and injection is then made into the joint.

The recommended dose is 1 to 2 mL for intra-articular injection into very large joints such as the hip. The recommended dose is 1 mL for large joints such as the knee, ankle or shoulder. The recommended dose is 0.5 to 1 mL for medium joints such as the elbow or wrist. For small joints in the hand (metacarpophalangeal, interphalangeal) or chest (sternoclavicular), the recommended dose is 0.25 to 0.5 mL.

A portion of the administered dose of betamethasone sodium phosphate/betamethasone acetate is absorbed systemically following intra-articular injection. In patients being treated concomitantly with oral or parenteral corticosteroids, especially those receiving large doses, the systemic absorption of the drug should be considered in determining intra-articular dosage.

BETAMETHASONE SODIUM PHOSPHATE/ BETAMETHASONE ACETATE — INJECTION

➤*Dermatologic conditions:* In intralesional treatment, 0.2 mL/cm² is injected intradermally (not subcutaneous) using a tuberculin syringe with a 25-gauge, ½-inch needle. Care should be taken to deposit a uniform depot of medication intradermally. A total of no more than 1 mL at weekly intervals is recommended.

➤*Disorders of the foot:* A tuberculin syringe with a 25-gauge ¾-inch needle is suitable for most injections into the foot. The following doses are recommended at intervals of 3 days to a week.

For the treatment of bursitis, the dose is 0.25 to 0.5 mL when under the heloma durum or the heloma molle, 0.5 mL when under the calcaneal spur, and 0.5 mL when over the hallux rigidus or the digiti quinti varus. For the treatment of tenosynovitis (periostitis of cuboid), the recommended dose is 0.5 mL. For the treatment of acute gouty arthritis, the recommended dose is 0.5 to 1 mL.

➤*Storage/Stability:* Shake well before using. Store between 2° and 25°C (36° and 77°F). Protect from light.

BUDESONIDE

Rx	**Entocort EC** (Prometheus)	**Capsules:** 3 mg budesonide (micronized)	Sugar spheres. (ENTOCORT EC 3 mg). Lt. gray/pink. In 100s.

BUDESONIDE — ORAL

For complete and comparative prescribing information, refer to the Glucocorticoids group monograph.

Indications

➤*Crohn disease:* For the treatment of mild to moderate active Crohn disease involving the ileum or the ascending colon and the maintenance of clinical remission of mild to moderate Crohn disease involving the ileum and/or the ascending colon for up to 3 months.

Administration and Dosage

➤*Dosage:* Budesonide should be swallowed whole and not chewed or broken.

The recommended adult dosage for the treatment of mild to moderate active Crohn disease involving the ileum and/or the ascending colon is 9 mg taken once daily in the morning for up to 8 weeks.

Repeated 8-week courses can be given for recurring episodes of active disease.

➤*Maintenance therapy:* Following an 8-week course(s) of treatment for active disease and once the patient's symptoms are controlled (Crohn Disease Activity Index [CDAI] less than 150), budesonide 6 mg is recommended once daily for maintenance of clinical remission up to 3 months. If symptom control is still maintained at 3 months, an attempt to taper to complete cessation is recommended. Continued treatment with budesonide 6 mg for more than 3 months has not been shown to provide substantial clinical benefit.

➤*Switching from prednisolone:* Patients with mild to moderate active Crohn disease involving the ileum and/or ascending colon have been switched from oral prednisolone to budesonide with no reported episodes of adrenal insufficiency. Because prednisolone should not be stopped abruptly, tapering should begin concomitantly with initiating budesonide treatment.

➤*Hepatic function impairment:* Patients with moderate to severe liver disease should be monitored for increased signs or symptoms of hypercorticism. Reducing the dose of budesonide should be considered in these patients.

➤*Concomitant use with CYP3A4 inhibitors:* If coadministration with ketoconazole or any other CYP3A4 inhibitor is indicated, patients should be closely monitored for increased signs and/or symptoms of hypercorticism. Reduction in the dose of budesonide should be considered.

➤*Storage/Stability:* Store at 25°C (77°F); excursions permitted to 15° to 30°C (59° to 86°F). Keep container tightly closed.

CORTISONE

Rx	**Cortisone Acetate** (Various, eg, Ivax, Major)	**Tablets:** 25 mg	In 8s, 100s, 500s, 1000s, and UD100s.

CORTISONE ACETATE — ORAL

For complete and comparative prescribing information, refer to the Glucocorticoids group monograph.

Indications

➤*Allergic states:* Control of severe or incapacitating allergic conditions intractable to adequate trials of conventional treatment: Seasonal or perennial allergic rhinitis; bronchial asthma; contact dermatitis; atopic dermatitis; serum sickness; drug hypersensitivity reactions.

➤*Collagen diseases:* During an exacerbation or as maintenance therapy in selected cases of: Systemic lupus erythematosus; acute rheumatic carditis; systemic dermatomyositis (polymyositis).

➤*Dermatologic diseases:* Pemphigus; bullous dermatitis herpetiformis; severe erythema multiforme (Stevens-Johnson syndrome); exfoliative dermatitis; mycosis fungoides; severe psoriasis; severe seborrheic dermatitis.

➤*Edematous states:* To induce a diuresis of remission or proteinuria in the nephrotic syndrome, without uremia, of the idiopathic type or that caused by lupus erythematosus.

➤*Endocrine disorders:* Primary or secondary adrenocortical insufficiency (hydrocortisone or cortisone is the first choice; synthetic analogs may be used in conjunction with mineralocorticoids where applicable; in infancy mineralocorticoid supplementation is of particular importance). Congenital adrenal hyperplasia; nonsuppurative thyroiditis; hypercalcemia associated with cancer.

➤*Gastrointestinal diseases:* To tide the patient over a critical period of the disease in: ulcerative colitis; regional enteritis.

➤*Hematologic disorders:* Idiopathic thrombocytopenic purpura in adults; secondary thrombocytopenia in adults; acquired (autoimmune) hemolytic anemia; erythroblastopenia (RBC anemia); congenital (erythroid) hypoplastic anemia.

➤*Neoplastic diseases:* For palliative management of: leukemias and lymphomas in adults; acute leukemia of childhood.

➤*Ophthalmic diseases:* Severe acute and chronic allergic and inflammatory processes involving the eye and its adnexa, such as: allergic conjunctivitis; keratitis; allergic corneal marginal ulcers; herpes zoster ophthalmicus; iritis and iridocyclitis; chorioretinitis; anterior segment inflammation; diffuse posterior uveitis and choroiditis; optic neuritis; sympathetic ophthalmia.

➤*Respiratory diseases:* Symptomatic sarcoidosis; Loeffler syndrome not manageable by other means; berylliosis; fulminating or disseminated pulmonary tuberculosis when used concurrently with appropriate antituberculosis chemotherapy; aspiration pneumonitis.

➤*Rheumatic disorders:* As adjunctive therapy for short-term administration (to tide the patient over an acute episode or exacerbation) in: Psoriatic arthritis; rheumatoid arthritis (RA), including juvenile RA (selected cases may require low-dose maintenance therapy); ankylosing spondylitis; acute and subacute bursitis; acute nonspecific tenosynovitis; acute gouty arthritis; posttraumatic osteoarthritis; synovitis of osteoarthritis; epicondylitis.

➤*Miscellaneous:* Tuberculous meningitis with subarachnoid block or impending block when used concurrently with appropriate antituberculous chemotherapy; trichinosis with neurologic or myocardial involvement.

➤*Unlabeled uses:* For the treatment of acute nonrheumatic carditis; pemphigoid; hemolysis; as an adjunct treatment for brain neoplasm; myasthenia gravis; desquamative gingivitis; recurrent aphthous stomatitis; pericarditis; acute or chronic asthmatic bronchitis; chronic obstructive pulmonary disease; noncardiogenic pulmonary edema; airway obstructing hemangioma in infants; status asthmaticus; rheumatic fever; acute calcium pyrophosphate deposition disease; shock; Reiter disease, prophylaxis and treatment of organ transplant rejection; oral lesions associated with corticosteroid responsive disorders; multiple myeloma; fever caused by malignant neoplasm; malignant neoplasm of the breast and prostate; severe eczema; mixed connective tissue disease; polyarteritis nodosa; relapsing polychondritis; vasculitis.

Administration and Dosage

Dosage requirements are variable and must be individualized based on disease and response of patient.

➤*Initial dosage:* 25 to 300 mg/day (oral). In less severe diseases, lower doses may suffice.

➤*Maintenance dosage:* Decrease initial dosage in small amounts to the lowest dosage that maintains an adequate clinical response. If the drug is to be stopped after more than a few days of treatment, it usually should be withdrawn gradually.

➤*Dosage adjustment:* Changes in clinical status resulting from remissions or exacerbations of the disease, individual drug responsiveness, and the effect of stress (ie, surgery, infection, trauma) may require dosage adjustment. During stress it may be necessary to temporarily increase the dose.

➤*Storage/Stability:* Store at controlled room temperature 15° to 30°C (59° to 86°F). Protect from light and moisture.

Dispense in a tight, light-resistant container using a child-resistant closure.

Glucocorticoids

DEXAMETHASONE

Rx	**Dexamethasone** (Various, eg, Par)	**Tablets:** 0.25 mg	In 100s and 1000s.
Rx	**Dexamethasone** (Various, eg, Ivax, Roxane, Par)	**Tablets:** 0.5 mg	In 100s, 1000s, and UD 100s.
Rx	**Decadron** (Merck)		Lactose. (MSD 41 DECADRON). Yellow, pentagonal, scored. In 100s.
Rx	**Dexamethasone** (Various, eg, Ivax, Roxane, Par)	**Tablets:** 0.75 mg	In 100s, 500s, 1000s, and UD 100s.
Rx	**Decadron** (Merck)		Lactose. (MSD 63 DECADRON). Bluish green, pentagonal, scored. In 12s and 100s.
Rx	**Dexamethasone** (Roxane)	**Tablets:** 1 mg	(54 489). Yellow, scored. In 100s and UD 100s.
Rx	**Dexamethasone** (Various, eg, Ivax, Roxane, Par)	**Tablets:** 1.5 mg	In 50s, 100s, 500s, 1000s, and UD 100s.
Rx	**Dexamethasone** (Roxane)	**Tablets:** 2 mg	(54 662). White, scored. In 100s and UD 100s.
Rx	**Dexamethasone** (Various, eg, Ivax, Roxane, Par)	**Tablets:** 4 mg	In 50s, 100s, 500s, 1000s, and UD 100s.
Rx	**Dexamethasone** (Various, eg, Roxane, Par)	**Tablets:** 6 mg	In 50s, 100s, and UD 100s.
Rx	**Dexamethasone** (Various, eg, Ivax, Alpharma)	**Elixir:** 0.5 mg per 5 mL	May contain alcohol. In 100 and 237 mL.
Rx sf	**Dexamethasone** (Various, eg, Roxane, Morton Groves)	**Oral solution:** 0.5 mg per 5 mL	May contain sorbitol. In 500 mL and UD 5 and 20 mL, and 237 mL.
Rx	**Dexamethasone Intensol** (Roxane)	**Oral solution (concentrate):** 1 mg per mL	30% alcohol. In 30 mL w/dropper.

DEXAMETHASONE — ORAL

For complete and comparative prescribing information, refer to the Glucocorticoids group monograph.

Indications

➤*Allergic states:* Control of severe or incapacitating allergic conditions intractable to adequate trials of conventional treatment: Seasonal or perennial allergic rhinitis; bronchial asthma; contact dermatitis; atopic dermatitis; serum sickness; drug hypersensitivity reactions.

➤*Cerebral edema:* Edema associated with primary or metastatic brain tumor, craniotomy, or head injury. Use in cerebral edema is not a substitute for careful neurosurgical evaluation and definitive management such as neurosurgery or other specific therapy.

➤*Collagen diseases:* During an exacerbation or as maintenance therapy in selected cases of: systemic lupus erythematosus; acute rheumatic carditis.

➤*Dermatologic diseases:* Pemphigus; bullous dermatitis herpetiformis; severe erythema multiforme (Stevens-Johnson syndrome); exfoliative dermatitis; mycosis fungoides; severe psoriasis; severe seborrheic dermatitis.

➤*Diagnostic testing:* Adrenocortical hyperfunction.

➤*Edematous states:* To induce a diuresis or remission of proteinuria in the nephrotic syndrome, without uremia, of the idiopathic type or that because of lupus erythematosus.

➤*Endocrine disorders:* Primary or secondary adrenocortical insufficiency (hydrocortisone or cortisone is the first choice; synthetic analogs may be used in conjunction with mineralocorticoids where applicable; in infancy mineralocorticoid supplementation is of particular importance). Congenital adrenal hyperplasia; nonsuppurative thyroiditis; hypercalcemia associated with cancer.

➤*Gastrointestinal diseases:* To tide the patient over a critical period of the disease in: Ulcerative colitis; regional enteritis.

➤*Hematologic disorders:* Idiopathic thrombocytopenic purpura in adults; secondary thrombocytopenia in adults; acquired (autoimmune) hemolytic anemia; erythroblastopenia (RBC anemia); congenital (erythroid) hypoplastic anemia.

➤*Neoplastic diseases:* For palliative management of: Leukemias and lymphomas in adults; acute leukemia of childhood.

➤*Ophthalmic diseases:* Severe acute and chronic allergic and inflammatory processes involving the eye and its adnexa such as: Allergic conjunctivitis; keratitis; allergic corneal marginal ulcers; herpes zoster ophthalmicus; iritis and iridocyclitis; chorioretinitis; anterior segment inflammation; diffuse posterior uveitis and choroiditis; optic neuritis; sympathetic ophthalmia.

➤*Respiratory diseases:* Symptomatic sarcoidosis; Loeffler syndrome not manageable by other means; berylliosis; fulminating or disseminated pulmonary tuberculosis when used concurrently with appropriate antituberculous chemotherapy; aspiration pneumonitis.

➤*Rheumatic disorders:* As adjunctive therapy for short-term administration (to tide the patient over an acute episode or exacerbation) in: Psoriatic arthritis; rheumatoid arthritis (RA), including juvenile RA (selected cases may require low-dose maintenance therapy); ankylosing spondylitis; acute and subacute bursitis; acute nonspecific tenosynovitis; acute gouty arthritis; posttraumatic osteoarthritis; synovitis of osteoarthritis; epicondylitis.

➤*Miscellaneous:* Tuberculous meningitis with subarachnoid block or impending block when used concurrently with appropriate antituberculous chemotherapy; trichinosis with neurologic or myocardial involvement.

➤*Unlabeled uses:* For the treatment of nonrheumatic carditis; mixed connective tissue disease; polyarteritis nodosa; relapsing polychondritis; vasculitis; diagnosis of endogenous depression; severe eczema; pemphigoid; localized cutaneous sarcoid; sarcoidosis; hemolysis; prevention of nausea and vomiting associated with chemotherapy, especially cisplatin-containing regimens; breast and prostatic carcinoma; adjunct treatment for fever caused by malignant neoplasm; adjunct treatment for brain neoplasm; multiple myeloma; myasthenia gravis; cerebral ischemia; cerebri pseudomotor; desquamative gingivitis; oral lesions associated with corticosteroid responsive disorder; recurrent aphthous stomatitis; pericarditis; nasal polyps; croup; acute and chronic asthmatic bronchitis; noncardiogenic pulmonary edema; airway-obstructing hemangioma in infants; respiratory distress syndrome; acute calcium pyrophosphate deposition disease; Reiter disease; rheumatic fever; organ transplant rejection; prophylaxis for acute mountain sickness; adjunctive treatment for bacterial meningitis.

Administration and Dosage

Dosage requirements are variable and must be individualized based on disease and response of patient.

➤*Initial dosage:* 0.75 to 9 mg/day.

➤*Maintenance dosage:* Decrease initial dosage in small amounts to the lowest dosage that maintains an adequate clinical response. If the drug is to be stopped after more than a few days of treatment, it usually should be withdrawn gradually.

➤*Dosage adjustment:* Changes in clinical status resulting from remissions or exacerbations of the disease, individual drug responsiveness, and the effect of stress (ie, surgery, infection, trauma). During stress it may be necessary to increase the dose temporarily.

➤*Acute, self-limited allergic disorders or acute exacerbations of chronic allergic disorders:* The following dosage schedule combining parenteral and oral therapy (0.75 mg tablets) is suggested: Dexamethasone sodium phosphate injection, 4 mg/mL:

First day – 1 or 2 mL intramuscular.

Second day – Four 0.75 mg tablets in 2 divided doses.

Third day – Four 0.75 mg tablets in 2 divided doses.

Fourth day – Two 0.75 mg tablets in 2 divided doses.

Fifth day – One 0.75 mg tablet.

Sixth day – One 0.75 mg tablet.

Seventh day – No treatment.

Eighth day – Follow-up visit.

➤*Palliative management of recurrent or inoperable brain tumors:* 2 mg 2 or 3 times/day for maintenance therapy.

➤*Administration of Intensol:* Recommend mixing with liquid or semi-solid food such as water, juices, soda or soda-like beverages, applesauce, and puddings. Use the provided calibrated dropper to administer prescribed amount of *Intensol* into a liquid or semi-solid food. Stir gently for a few seconds. Consume the entire amount of the liquid or food immediately; do not store for future use.

➤*Suppression tests:*

For Cushing syndrome – Give 1 mg at 11 pm. Draw blood for plasma cortisol determination the following day at 8 am. For greater accuracy, give 0.5 mg every 6 hours for 48 hours. Collect 24 hour urine to determine 17-hydroxycorticosteroid excretion.

Test to distinguish Cushing syndrome because of pituitary ACTH excess from Cushing syndrome because of other causes – Give 2 mg every 6 hours for 48 hours. Collect 24 hour urine to determine 17-hydroxycorticosteroid excretion.

➤*Storage/Stability:* Keep container of dexamethasone elixir tightly closed.

Tablets – Store at controlled room temperature 15° to 30°C (59° to 86°F).

DEXAMETHASONE ACETATE

Rx	**Dexamethasone Acetate** (Various, eg, Bioline, Dixon-Shane, Goldline, Major, Moore, Rugby, URL)	**Injection:** 8 mg/mL (as acetate) suspension. Not for IV use.	In 5 mL vials.
Rx	**Dexasone L.A.** (Hauck)		In 5 mL vials.[a]
Rx	**Dexone LA** (Keene)		In 5 mL vials.[a]
Rx	**Cortastat LA** (Clint)		In 5 mL vials.[a]
Rx	**Dalalone D.P.** (Forest)	**Injection:** 16 mg/mL (as acetate) suspension. Not for IV or intralesional use.	In 1 and 5 mL vial.[a]

[a] With creatinine, polysorbate 80, carboxymethylcellulose, sodium bisulfite, EDTA, benzyl alcohol.

DEXAMETHASONE ACETATE — INJECTION

For complete and comparative prescribing information, refer to the Glucocorticoids group monograph.

Administration and Dosage

A long-acting repository preparation with prompt onset of action.

Not for IV use.

➤*Systemic:* 8 to 16 mg intramuscular, may repeat in 1 to 3 weeks.

➤*Intralesional:* 0.8 to 1.6 mg.

➤*Intra-articular and soft tissue:* 4 to 16 mg; may repeat at 1 to 3 week intervals.

DEXAMETHASONE SODIUM PHOSPHATE

Rx	**Dexamethasone Sodium Phosphate** (Various, eg, Bioline, Dixon-Shane, Elkins Sinn, Geneva Marsam, Kendall McGaw, Moore, Rugby, URL)	**Injection:** 4 mg/mL dexamethasone phosphate (as sodium phosphate) solution	In 1, 5, 10 and 30 mL vials, 1 mL disp. syringe and 1 mL fill in 2 mL vials.
Rx	**Dalalone** (Forest)		In 5 mL vials.[a]
Rx	**Decadron Phosphate** (MSD)		In 1, 5 and 25 mL vials and 2.5 mL syringes.[b]
Rx	**Dexasone** (Hauck)		In 5, 10 and 30 mL vials.[c]
Rx	**Dexone** (Keene)		In 5 and 10 mL vials.[a]
Rx	**Hexadrol Phosphate** (Organon)		In 1 and 5 mL vials and 1 mL disp. syringe.[a]
Rx	**Cortastat** (Clint)		In 5, 10 and 30 mL multiple-dose vials.[a]
Rx	**Dexamethasone Sodium Phosphate** (Various, eg, Elkins-Sinn)	**Injection:** 10 mg/mL dexamethasone phosphate (as sodium phosphate) solution	In 1 and 10 mL vials and 1 mL disp. syringe.
Rx	**Hexadrol Phosphate** (Organon)		In 10 mL (IV or IM) vials and 1 mL disp. syringe.[a]
Rx	**Hexadrol Phosphate** (Organon)	**Injection:** 20 mg/mL dexamethasone phosphate (as sodium phosphate solution)	In 5 mL vials (IV).[a]
Rx	**Decadron Phosphate** (MSD)	**Injection:** 24 mg/mL dexamethasone phosphate (as sodium phosphate) solution. For IV use only	In 5 and 10 mL vials.[d]

[a] With sodium sulfite and benzyl alcohol.
[b] With methyl and propyl parabens and sodium bisulfite.
[c] With sodium metabisulfite, EDTA and methyl and propyl parabens.
[d] With EDTA, methyl and propyl parabens and sodium bisulfite.

DEXAMETHASONE SODIUM PHOSPHATE — INJECTION

For complete and comparative prescribing information, refer to the Glucocorticoids group monograph.

Administration and Dosage

➤*Preparation and administration:* Dexamethasone sodium phosphate injection, 4 mg/mL is for IV, intramuscular, intra-articular, intralesional, and soft tissue injection.

Dexamethasone sodium phosphate injection, 10 mg/mL is for IV and intramuscular injection only.

Dexamethasone sodium phosphate injection, 24 mg/mL is for IV injection only.

Dexamethasone sodium phosphate injection can be given directly from the vial, or it can be added to sodium chloride injection or dextrose injection and administered by IV drip. Solutions used for IV administration or further dilution of this product should be preservative-free when used in the neonate, especially the premature infant.

When it is mixed with an infusion solution, sterile precautions should be observed. Because infusion solutions generally do not contain preservatives, mixtures should be used within 24 hours.

Parenteral drug products should be inspected visually for particulate matter and discoloration prior to administration, whenever solution and container permit.

Dosage requirements are variable and must be individualized on the basis of the disease and the response of the patient.

This schedule is designed to ensure adequate therapy during acute episodes while minimizing the risk of overdosage in chronic cases.

➤*IV and intramuscular injection:* The initial dosage of dexamethasone sodium phosphate injection varies from 0.5 to 9 mg a day depending on the disease being treated. In less severe diseases, doses lower than 0.5 mg may suffice, while in severe diseases, doses higher than 9 mg may be required.

The initial dosage should be maintained or adjusted until the patient's response is satisfactory. If a satisfactory clinical response does not occur after a reasonable period of time, discontinue dexamethasone sodium phosphate injection and transfer the patient to other therapy.

After a favorable initial response, the proper maintenance dosage should be determined by decreasing the initial dosage in small amounts to the lowest dosage that maintains an adequate clinical response. Patients should be observed closely for signs that might require dosage adjustment, including changes in clinical status resulting from remissions or exacerbations of the disease, individual drug responsiveness, and the effect of stress (eg, surgery, infection, trauma). During stress it may be necessary to increase dosage temporarily.

If the drug is to be stopped after more than a few days of treatment, it usually should be withdrawn gradually.

When the IV route of administration is used, dosage usually should be the same as the oral dosage. In certain overwhelming, acute, life-threatening situations, however, administration in dosages exceeding the usual dosages may be justified and may be in multiples of the oral dosages. The slower rate of absorption by intramuscular administration should be recognized.

➤*Shock:* There is a tendency in current medical practice to use high (pharmacologic) doses of corticosteroids for the treatment of unresponsive shock. The following dosages of dexamethasone sodium phosphate injection have been suggested.

Dexamethasone Sodium Injection Dosage

Author	Dosage
Cavanagh	3 mg/kg of body weight per 24 hours by constant IV infusion after an initial IV injection of 20 mg
Dietzman	2 to 6 mg/kg of body weight as a single IV injection
Frank	40 mg initially followed by repeat IV injection every 4 to 6 hours while shock persists
Oaks	40 mg initially followed by repeat IV injection every 2 to 6 hours while shock persists
Schumer	1 mg/kg of body weight as a single IV injection

Administration of high dose corticosteroid therapy should be continued only until the patient's condition has stabilized and usually not longer than 48 to 72 hours. Although adverse reactions associated with high dose, short-term corticosteroid therapy are uncommon, peptic ulceration may occur.

➤*Cerebral edema:* Dexamethasone sodium phosphate injection is generally administered initially in a dosage of 10 mg IV followed by 4 mg every 6 hours IM until the symptoms of cerebral edema subside. Response is usually noted within 12 to 24 hours and dosage may be reduced after 2 to 4 days and gradually discontinued over a period of 5 to 7 days. For palliative man-

DEXAMETHASONE SODIUM PHOSPHATE — INJECTION

agement of patients with recurrent or inoperable brain tumors, maintenance therapy with 2 mg 2 or 3 times a day may be effective.

➤*Acute allergic disorders:* In acute, self-limited allergic disorders or acute exacerbations of chronic allergic disorders, the following dosage schedule combining parenteral and oral therapy is suggested:

Dexamethasone sodium phosphate injection, 4 mg/mL – First day, 1 or 2 mL (4 or 8 mg), intramuscular.

Dexamethasone tablets, 0.75 mg – Second and third days, 4 tablets in 2 divided doses each day; fourth day, 2 tablets in 2 divided doses; fifth and sixth days, 1 tablet each day; seventh day, no treatment; eighth day, follow-up visit.

This schedule is designed to ensure adequate therapy during acute episodes, while minimizing the risk of overdosage in chronic cases.

➤*Intra-articular, intralesional, and soft tissue injection:* Intra-articular, intralesional, and soft tissue injections are generally employed when the affected joints or areas are limited to 1 or 2 sites. Dosage and frequency of injection varies depending on the condition and the site of injection. The usual dose is from 0.2 to 6 mg. The frequency usually ranges from once every 3 to 5 days to once every 2 to 3 weeks. Frequent intra-articular injection may result in damage to joint tissues.

Some of the usual single doses are:

Dexamethasone Phosphate Dosages

Site of injection	Amount of dexamethasone phosphate (mg)
Large joints (eg, knee)	2 to 4
Small joints (eg, interphalangeal, temporomandibular)	0.8 to 1
Bursae	2 to 3
Tendon sheaths	0.4 to 1
Soft tissue infiltration	2 to 6
Ganglia	1 to 2

Dexamethasone sodium phosphate injection is particularly recommended for use in conjunction with 1 of the less soluble, longer-acting steroids for intra-articular and soft tissue injection.

➤*Storage/Stability:* Store at 25°C (77°F), excursions permitted to 15° to 30°C (59° to 86°F). The product is sensitive to heat. Do not autoclave. Protect from freezing and light. Store container in carton until contents have been used.

DEXAMETHASONE SODIUM PHOSPHATE WITH LIDOCAINE HYDROCHLORIDE

Rx	**Decadron w/Xylocaine** (MSD)	**Injection:** 4 mg dexamethasone sodium phosphate and 10 mg lidocaine hydrochloride/mL solution	In 5 mL vials.[a]

[a] With EDTA, parabens and sodium bisulfite.

DEXAMETHASONE SODIUM PHOSPHATE WITH LIDOCAINE HYDROCHLORIDE — INJECTION

For complete and comparative prescribing information, refer to the Glucocorticoids group monograph.

Administration and Dosage

Dexamethasone sodium phosphate provides prompt activity. Lidocaine hydrochloride is a local anesthetic with a rapid onset and a duration of 45 minutes to 1 hour (see Local Anesthetics). Steroid activity usually begins by the time the anesthesia wears off.

➤*Soft tissue injection: Acute and subacute bursitis:* 0.5 to 0.75 mL.

Acute and subacute nonspecific tenosynovitis – 0.1 to 0.25 mL.

HYDROCORTISONE (Cortisol)

Rx	**Cortef** (Upjohn)	**Tablets:** 5 mg	(Cortef 5). White, scored. In 50s.
Rx	**Hydrocortisone** (Major)	**Tablets:** 10 mg	In 100s.
Rx	**Cortef** (Upjohn)		(Cortef 10). White, scored. In 100s.
Rx	**Hydrocortone** (MSD)		(MSD 619). White, scored. Oval. In 100s.
Rx	**Hydrocortisone** (Various, eg, Major, Moore, Rugby, URL)	**Tablets:** 20 mg	In 100s.
Rx	**Cortef** (Upjohn)		(Cortef 20). White, scored. In 100s.
Rx	**Hydrocortone** (MSD)		(MSD 625). White, scored. Oval. In 100s.

HYDROCORTISONE — ORAL

For complete and comparative prescribing information, refer to the Glucocorticoids group monograph.

Administration and Dosage

For oral administration. Dosage requirements are variable and must be individualized on the basis of the disease and the response of the patient.

➤*Initial dosage:* The initial dosage varies from 20 to 240 mg a day depending on the disease being treated. In less severe diseases doses less than 20 mg may suffice, while in severe diseases doses more than 240 mg may be required. The initial dosage should be maintained or adjusted until the patient's response is satisfactory. If satisfactory clinical response does not occur after a reasonable period of time, discontinue hydrocortisone tablets and transfer the patient to other therapy.

➤*Maintenance dosage:* After a favorable initial response, the proper maintenance dosage should be determined by decreasing the initial dosage in small amounts to the lowest dosage that maintains an adequate clinical response.

➤*Dosage adjustments:* Patients should be observed closely for signs that might require dosage adjustment, including changes in clinical status resulting from remissions or exacerbations of the disease, individual drug responsiveness, and the effect of stress (eg, surgery, infection, trauma). During stress it may be necessary to increase dosage temporarily.

If the drug is to be stopped after more than a few days of treatment, it usually should be withdrawn gradually.

➤*Multiple sclerosis:* In treatment of acute exacerbations of multiple sclerosis, daily doses of 200 mg of prednisolone for a week followed by 80 mg every other day for 1 month have been shown to be effective (20 mg of hydrocortisone is equivalent to 5 mg of prednisolone).

➤*Storage/Stability:* Store at controlled room temperature 20° to 25°C (68° to 77°F).

HYDROCORTISONE ACETATE

Rx	**Hydrocortisone Acetate** (Various, eg, Dixon-Shane, Moore, Rugby, Schein, URL)	**Injection:** 25 mg/mL suspension	In 10 mL vials.
Rx	**Hydrocortone Acetate** (MSD)		In 5 mL vials.[a]
Rx	**Hydrocortisone Acetate** (Various, eg, Moore, Rugby, URL)	**Injection:** 50 mg/mL suspension	In 10 mL vials.

[a] With 4 mg polysorbate 80, 5 mg sodium carboxymethylcellulose and 9 mg benzyl alcohol per mL.

HYDROCORTISONE ACETATE — INJECTION

For complete and comparative prescribing information, refer to the Glucocorticoids group monograph.

Administration and Dosage

Hydrocortisone acetate has a slow onset but long duration of action when compared with more soluble preparations. Because of its insolubility, it is suitable for intra-articular, intralesional and soft tissue injection where its anti-inflammatory effects are confined mainly to the area in which it has been injected, although it is capable of producing systemic hormonal effects.

For intralesional, intra-articular or soft tissue injection only. Not for IV use.

➤*Large joints (eg, knee):* 25 mg; occasionally, 37.5 mg.

➤*Small joints (eg, interphalangeal, temporomandibular):* 10 to 25 mg.

➤*Tendon sheaths:* 5 to 12.5 mg.

➤*Soft tissue infiltration:* 25 to 50 mg; occasionally, 75 mg.

➤*Bursae:* 25 to 37.5 mg.

➤*Ganglia:* 12.5 to 25 mg.

Glucocorticoids

HYDROCORTISONE ACETATE — INJECTION

If desired, a local anesthetic may be injected before hydrocortisone acetate or mixed in a syringe and given simultaneously.

If used prior to intra-articular injection of the steroid, inject most of the anesthetic into the soft tissues of the surrounding area and instill a small amount into the joint.

If given together, mix in the injection syringe by drawing the steroid in first, then the anesthetic. In this way, the anesthetic will not be introduced inadvertently into the vial of the steroid. The mixture must be used immediately and any unused portion discarded.

HYDROCORTISONE CYPIONATE

Rx	**Cortef** (Upjohn)	**Oral Suspension:** 10 mg per 5 mL hydrocortisone (as cypionate)	Sucrose. In 120 mL.

HYDROCORTISONE CYPIONATE — ORAL

For complete and comparative prescribing information, refer to the Glucocorticoids group monograph.

Administration and Dosage

➤*Dosage:* The initial dosage may vary from 2 to 24 teaspoonfuls (10 to 120 mL) per day depending on the specific disease entity being treated. This provides a daily dosage of 26.8 mg to 321.6 mg of hydrocortisone cypionate, equivalent in activity to 20 to 240 mg of hydrocortisone.

➤*Resuspension of product:* Shake well before dispensing and before each use, until all visible sediment in the bottle is resuspended. This may require 5 to 7 minutes of shaking before the first use. Subsequent uses from the same bottle will require shaking for significantly less time to resuspend the sediment.

➤*Storage/Stability:* Store bottle inside carton. Dispense in tight, light-resistant container. Keep container tightly closed.

Store at controlled room temperature 20° to 25°C (68° to 77°F).

HYDROCORTISONE SODIUM PHOSPHATE

Rx	**Hydrocortone Phosphate** (MSD)	**Injection:** 50 mg/mL hydrocortisone (as sodium phosphate) solution	In 2 and 10 mL vials.[a]

[a] With sodium bisulfite 3.2 mg, and methylparaben 1.5 mg and propylparaben 0.2 mg.

HYDROCORTISONE SODIUM PHOSPHATE — INJECTION

For complete and comparative prescribing information, refer to the Glucocorticoids group monograph.

Administration and Dosage

➤*Administration:* For IV, IM, and subcutaneous injection. For single-dose use only. Maintenance of sterility cannot be ensured when used as a multiple-dose vial.

Hydrocortisone sodium phosphate can be given directly from the vial, or it can be added to sodium chloride injection or dextrose injection and administered by IV drip.

When it is mixed with an infusion solution, sterile precautions should be observed. Since infusion solutions generally do not contain preservatives, mixtures should be used within 24 hours.

➤*Dosage:* Dosage requirements are variable and must be individualized on the basis of the disease and the response of the patient.

The initial dosage varies from 15 to 240 mg a day depending on the disease being treated. In less severe diseases, doses less than 15 mg may suffice, while in severe diseases, doses higher than 240 mg may be required. Usually the parenteral dosage ranges are one-third to one-half the oral dose given every 12 hours. However, in certain overwhelming, acute, life-threatening situations, administration in dosages exceeding the usual dosages may be justified and may be in multiples of the oral dosages.

The initial dosage should be maintained or adjusted until the patient's response is satisfactory. If a satisfactory clinical response does not occur after a reasonable period of time, discontinue hydrocortisone sodium phosphate injection and transfer the patient to other therapy.

➤*Maintenance dosage:* After a favorable initial response, the proper maintenance dosage should be determined by decreasing the initial dosage in small amounts to the lowest dosage that maintains an adequate clinical response.

➤*Dosage adjustment:* Patients should be observed closely for signs that might require dosage adjustment, including changes in clinical status resulting from remissions or exacerbations of the disease, individual drug responsiveness, and the effect of stress (eg, surgery, infection, trauma). During stress it may be necessary to increase dosage temporarily.

If the drug is to be stopped after more than a few days of treatment, it usually should be withdrawn gradually.

➤*Storage/Stability:* Sensitive to heat. Do not autoclave.

HYDROCORTISONE SODIUM SUCCINATE

Rx	**A-Hydrocort** (Abbott)	**Injection:** 100 mg hydrocortisone (as sodium succinate) per vial	In 2 mL *Univials*[a] and fliptop vials.
Rx	**Solu-Cortef** (Upjohn)		In vials and 2 mL *Act-O-Vials.*[a]
Rx	**A-Hydrocort** (Abbott)	**Injection:** 250 mg hydrocortisone (as sodium succinate) per vial	In 2 mL *Univials*[a] and fliptop vials.
Rx	**Solu-Cortef** (Upjohn)		In 2 mL *Act-O-Vials.*[a]
Rx	**A-Hydrocort** (Abbott)	**Injection:** 500 mg hydrocortisone (as sodium succinate) per vial	In 4 mL *Univials*[a] and fliptop vials.
Rx	**Solu-Cortef** (Upjohn)		In 4 mL *Act-O-Vials.*[a]
Rx	**A-Hydrocort** (Abbott)	**Injection:** 1,000 mg hydrocortisone (as sodium succinate) per vial	In 8 mL *Univials*[a] and fliptop vials.
Rx	**Solu-Cortef** (Upjohn)		In 8 mL *Act-O-Vials.*[a]

[a] With benzyl alcohol.

HYDROCORTISONE SODIUM SUCCINATE — INJECTION

For complete prescribing information, refer to the Glucocorticoids group monograph

Administration and Dosage

➤*Administration:* This preparation may be administered by IV injection, IV infusion, or IM injection, the preferred method for initial emergency use being IV injection. Following the initial emergency period, consideration should be given to employing a longer-acting injectable preparation or an oral preparation.

➤*Dosage:* Therapy is initiated by administering hydrocortisone sodium succinate injection IV over a period of 30 seconds (eg, 100 mg) to 10 minutes (eg, at least 500 mg). In general, high-dose corticosteroid therapy should be continued only until the patient's condition has stabilized, usually not beyond 48 to 72 hours. Although adverse effects associated with high-dose, short-term corticoid therapy are uncommon, peptic ulceration may occur. Prophylactic antacid therapy may be indicated.

When high-dose hydrocortisone therapy must be continued beyond 48 to 72 hours, hypernatremia may occur. Under such circumstances it may be desirable to replace hydrocortisone sodium succinate with a corticoid such as methylprednisolone sodium succinate which causes little or no sodium retention.

The initial dose of hydrocortisone sodium succinate injection is 100 mg to 500 mg, depending on the severity of the condition. This dose may be repeated at intervals of 2, 4 or 6 hours as indicated by the patient's response and clinical condition. While the dose may be reduced for infants and children, it is governed more by the severity of the condition and response of the patient than by age or body weight but should not be less than 25 mg daily.

Patients subjected to severe stress following corticosteroid therapy should be observed closely for signs and symptoms of adrenocortical insufficiency.

Corticoid therapy is an adjunct to, and not a replacement for, conventional therapy.

➤*Preparation of solutions (100 mg plain):* For IV or IM injection, prepare solution by aseptically adding not more than 2 mL of bacteriostatic water for injection or bacteriostatic sodium chloride injection to the contents of 1 vial. For IV infusion, first prepare solution by adding not more than 2 mL of bacteriostatic water for injection to the vial; this solution may then be added to 100 to 1,000 mL of the following: 5% dextrose in water (or isotonic saline solution or 5% dextrose in isotonic saline solution if patient is not on sodium restriction).

➤*Directions for using the Act-o-Vial* system:

1.) Press down on plastic activator to force diluent into the lower compartment.
2.) Gently agitate to effect solution.
3.) Remove plastic tab covering center of stopper.
4.) Sterilize top of stopper with a suitable germicide.
5.) Insert needle squarely through center of stopper until tip is just visible. Invert vial and withdraw dose.

HYDROCORTISONE SODIUM SUCCINATE — INJECTION

Further dilution is not necessary for IV or IM injection. For IV infusion, first prepare solution as just described. The 100-mg solution may then be added to 100 to 1,000 mL of 5% dextrose in water (or isotonic saline solution or 5% dextrose in isotonic saline solution if patient is not on sodium restriction). The 250-mg solution may be added to 250 to 1,000 mL, the 500-mg solution may be added to 500 to 1,000 mL and the 1,000-mg solution to 1,000 mL of the same diluents. In cases where administration of a small volume of fluid is desirable, 100 mg to 3,000 mg of hydrocortisone sodium succinate injection may be added to 50 mL of the above diluents. The resulting solutions are stable for at least 4 hours and may be administered either directly or by IV piggyback.

When reconstituted as directed, pHs of the solutions range from 7 to 8 and the tonicities are: 100 mg *Act-O-Vial*, 0.36 osmolar; 250 mg *Act-O-Vial*, 500 mg *Act-O-Vial*, and the 1,000 mg *Act-O-Vial*, 0.57 osmolar, (isotonic saline = 0.28 osmolar.)

➤*Storage/Stability:* Store unreconstituted product at controlled room temperature 20° to 25°C (68° to 77°F).

Store solution at controlled room temperature 20° to 25°C (68° to 77°F) and protect from light. Use solution only if it is clear. Unused solution should be discarded after 3 days.

METHYLPREDNISOLONE

Rx	**Medrol** (Upjohn)	**Tablets**: 2 mg	Lactose, sucrose. (MEDROL 2). Pink, scored. Elliptical. In 100s.
Rx	**Methylprednisolone** (Various, eg, Geneva, Major, Moore, Parmed, Prasco, Rugby)	**Tablets**: 4 mg	In 21s, 100s, and unit-of-use 21s.
Rx	**Medrol** (Upjohn)		Lactose, sucrose. White, scored. Elliptical. In 30s, 100s, 500s, UD 100s and Dosepak 21s.
Rx	**Methylprednisolone** (Prasco)	**Tablets**: 8 mg	Lactose. (TL 002). White, oval, scored. In 25s.
Rx	**Medrol** (Upjohn)		Lactose, sucrose. Peach, scored. Elliptical. In 25s.
Rx	**Methylprednisolone** (Various, eg, Rugby, URL)	**Tablets**: 16 mg	In 50s.
Rx	**Medrol** (Upjohn)		Lactose, sucrose. White, scored. Elliptical. In 50s and ADT Pak 14s.
Rx	**Medrol** (Upjohn)	**Tablets**: 24 mg	Lactose, sucrose. Tartrazine. Yellow, scored. Elliptical. In 25s.
		32 mg	Lactose and sucrose. Peach, scored. Elliptical. In 25s.

METHYLPREDNISOLONE — ORAL

For complete and comparative prescribing information, refer to the Glucocorticoids group monograph.

Administration and Dosage

➤*Initial dosage:* The initial dosage of methylprednisolone tablets may vary from methylprednisolone 4 to 48 mg daily depending on the specific disease entity being treated. In situations of less severity lower doses will generally suffice, while in selected patients higher initial doses may be required. The initial dosage should be maintained or adjusted until a satisfactory response is noted. If, after a reasonable period of time, there is a lack of satisfactory clinical response, methylprednisolone should be discontinued and the patient transferred to other appropriate therapy.

It should be emphasized that dosage requirements are variable and must be individualized on the basis of the disease under treatment and the response of the patient. After a favorable response is noted, the proper maintenance dosage should be determined by decreasing the initial drug dosage in small decrements at appropriate time intervals until the lowest dosage that will maintain an adequate clinical response is reached. It should be kept in mind that constant monitoring is needed in regard to drug dosage. Included in the situations which may make dosage adjustments necessary are changes in clinical status secondary to remissions or exacerbations in the disease process, the patient's individual drug responsiveness, and the effect of patient exposure to stressful situations not directly related to the disease entity under treatment; in this latter situation it may be necessary to increase the dosage of methylprednisolone for a period of time consistent with the patient's condition. If, after long-term therapy, the drug is to be stopped, it is recommended that it be withdrawn gradually rather than abruptly.

➤*Multiple sclerosis:* In treatment of acute exacerbations of multiple sclerosis, daily doses of prednisolone 200 mg for a week followed by 80 mg every other day for 1 month have been shown to be effective (methylprednisolone 4 mg is equivalent to prednisolone 5 mg).

➤*ADT (alternate-day therapy):* Alternate-day therapy is a corticosteroid dosing regimen in which twice the usual daily dose of corticoid is administered every other morning. The purpose of this mode of therapy is to provide the patient requiring long-term pharmacologic dose treatment with the beneficial effects of corticoids while minimizing certain undesirable effects, including pituitary-adrenal suppression, the cushingoid state, corticoid withdrawal symptoms, and growth suppression in children.

➤*Storage/Stability:* Store at controlled room temperature 20° to 25°C (68° to 77°F).

METHYLPREDNISOLONE ACETATE

Rx	**Methylprednisolone Acetate** (Various, eg, Rugby)	**Injection**: 20 mg/mL suspension	In 5 and 10 mL vials.
Rx	**Depo-Medrol** (Upjohn)		In 5 mL vials.[a]
Rx	**Methylprednisolone Acetate** (Various, eg, Dixon-Shane, Goldline, Moore, Rugby, URL)	**Injection**: 40 mg/mL suspension	In 5 and 10 ml vials.
Rx	**depMedalone 40** (Forest)		In 5 mL vials.[a]
Rx	**Depo-Medrol** (Upjohn)		In 1, 5 and 10 mL vials.[a]
Rx	**Depopred-40** (Hyrex)		In 5 and 10 mL vials.
Rx	**Duralone-40** (Hauck)		In 10 mL vials.[a]
Rx	**Medralone 40** (Keene)		In 5 mL vials.[a]
Rx	**Methylprednisolone Acetate** (Various, Dixon-Shane, Goldline, Moore, Rugby, URL)	**Injection**: 80 mg/mL suspension	In 5 mL vials.
Rx	**depMedalone 80** (Forest)		In 5 mL vials.[a]
Rx	**Depo-Medrol** (Upjohn)		In 1 and 5 mL vials.[a]
Rx	**Depopred-80** (Hyrex)		In 5 mL vials.
Rx	**Duralone-80** (Hauck)		In 5 mL vials.[a]
Rx	**Medralone 80** (Keene)		In 5 mL vials.[a]

[a] With polyethylene glycol and myristyl-gamma-picolinium chloride.

METHYLPREDNISOLONE ACETATE — INJECTION

For complete and comparative prescribing information, refer to the Glucocorticoids group monograph.

Administration and Dosage

Because of its low solubility, methylprednisolone acetate has a sustained effect.

➤*Systemic:* Not for IV use. As a temporary substitute for oral therapy, administer the total daily dose as a single IM injection. For prolonged effect, give a single weekly dose.

Adrenogenital syndrome – A single 40 mg injection IM every 2 weeks.

METHYLPREDNISOLONE ACETATE — INJECTION

Rheumatoid arthritis – Weekly IM maintenance dose varies from 40 to 120 mg.

Dermatologic lesions – 40 to 120 mg IM weekly for 1 to 4 weeks. In severe dermatitis (eg, poison ivy), relief may result within 8 to 12 hours of a single dose of 80 to 120 mg IM. In chronic contact dermatitis, repeated injections every 5 to 10 days may be necessary. In seborrheic dermatitis, a weekly dose of 80 mg IM may be adequate.

Asthma and allergic rhinitis – 80 to 120 mg IM.

➤*Intra-articular and soft tissue:*

Large joints – 20 to 80 mg.

Medium joints – 10 to 40 mg.

Small joints – 4 to 10 mg.

Ganglion, tendinitis, epicondylitis and bursitis – 4 to 30 mg.

➤*Intralesional:* 20 to 60 mg.

METHYLPREDNISOLONE SODIUM SUCCINATE

Rx	**Methylprednisolone Sodium Succinate** (Various, eg, Elkins Sinn)	**Powder for injection:** 40 mg/vial	In 1 and 3 mL vials.
Rx	**A-Methapred** (Hospira)		In 1 mL *Univial.*[a]
Rx	**Solu-Medrol** (Pfizer)		In 1 mL *Act-O-Vial.*[a]
Rx	**Methylprednisolone Sodium Succinate** (Various, eg, Elkins Sinn)	**Powder for injection:** 125 mg/vial	In 2 and 5 mL vials.
Rx	**A-Methapred** (Hospira)		In 2 mL *Univial.*[b]
Rx	**Solu-Medrol** (Pfizer)		In 2 mL *Act-O-Vial.*[b]
Rx	**Methylprednisolone Sodium Succinate** (Various, eg, Elkins Sinn)	**Powder for injection:** 500 mg/vial	In 1, 4 and 20 mL vials.
Rx	**Solu-Medrol** (Pfizer)		In 8 mL vials and 8 mL vials w/diluent.[c]
Rx	**Methylprednisolone Sodium Succinate** (Various, eg, Elkins Sinn)	**Powder for Injection:** 1 g/vial	In 1, 8 and 50 mL vials.
Rx	**Solu-Medrol** (Pfizer)		In 1 g vials, 1 g vials w/diluent and 8 mL *Act-O-Vial.*[d]
Rx	**Solu-Medrol** (Pfizer)	**Powder for Injection:** 2 g/vial	In 2 g vials w/diluent.

[a] With sodium phosphate anhydrous (1.6 mg monobasic, 17.5 mg dibasic), 25 mg lactose and 9 mg benzyl alcohol.
[b] With sodium phosphate anhydrous (1.6 mg monobasic, 17.4 mg dibasic), approximately 18 mg benzyl alcohol.
[c] With sodium phosphate anhydrous (6.4 mg monobasic, 69.6 mg dibasic). May contain 36 to 70.2 mg benzyl alcohol.
[d] With sodium phosphate anhydrous (12.8 mg monobasic, 139.2 mg dibasic). May contain 66.8 to 141 mg benzyl alcohol.

METHYLPREDNISOLONE SODIUM SUCCINATE — INJECTION

For complete and comparative prescribing information, refer to the Glucocorticoids group monograph.

Administration and Dosage

➤*Approved by the FDA:* February 27, 1985.

➤*Dosage:* When high-dose therapy is desired, the recommended dose of methylprednisolone sodium succinate sterile powder is 30 mg/kg administered IV over at least 30 minutes. This dose may be repeated every 4 to 6 hours for 48 hours.

In general, high-dose corticosteroid therapy should be continued only until the patient's condition has stabilized; usually not beyond 48 to 72 hours.

Although adverse reactions associated with high-dose, short-term corticoid therapy are uncommon, peptic ulceration may occur. Prophylactic antacid therapy may be indicated.

In other indications, initial dosage will vary from 10 to 40 mg of methylprednisolone depending on the clinical problem being treated. The larger doses may be required for short-term management of severe, acute conditions. The initial dose usually should be given IV over a period of several minutes. Subsequent doses may be given IV or IM at intervals dictated by the patient's response and clinical condition. Corticoid therapy is an adjunct to, and not replacement for conventional therapy.

Dosage may be reduced for infants and children but should be governed more by the severity of the condition and response of the patient than by age or size. It should not be less than 0.5 mg/kg every 24 hours.

Dosage must be decreased or discontinued gradually when the drug has been administered for more than a few days. If a period of spontaneous remission occurs in a chronic condition, treatment should be discontinued. Routine laboratory studies, such as urinalysis, 2-hour postprandial blood sugar, determination of blood pressure and body weight, and a chest x-ray should be made at regular intervals during prolonged therapy. Upper GI x-rays are desirable in patients with an ulcer history or significant dyspepsia.

➤*Administration:* Methylprednisolone sodium succinate may be administered by IV or IM injection or by IV infusion, the preferred method for initial emergency use being IV injection. To administer by IV (or IM) injection, prepare solution as directed. The desired dose may be administered IV over a period of several minutes. If desired, the medication may be administered in diluted solutions by adding Water for Injection or other suitable diluent (see below) to the *Act-O-Vial* and withdrawing the indicated dose.

To prepare solutions for IV infusion, first prepare the solution for injection as directed. This solution may then be added to indicated amounts of 5% dextrose in water, isotonic saline solution or 5% dextrose in isotonic saline solution.

➤*Multiple sclerosis:* In treatment of acute exacerbations of multiple sclerosis, daily doses of prednisolone 200 mg for a week followed by 80 mg every other day for 1 month have been shown to be effective (methylprednisolone 4 mg is equivalent to prednisolone 5 mg).

➤*Directions for using the Act-O-Vial* system:

1.) Press down on plastic activator to force diluent into the lower compartment.
2.) Gently agitate to effect the solution.
3.) Remove plastic tab covering center of stopper.
4.) Sterilize top of stopper with a suitable germicide.
5.) Insert needle squarely through center of stopper until tip is just visible. Invert vial and withdraw dose.

Important – Use only the accompanying diluent or bacteriostatic water for injection with benzyl alcohol when reconstituting methylprednisolone sodium succinate. Use within 48 hours after mixing.

➤*Storage / Stability:* Protect from light. Store powder at controlled room temperature, 20° to 25°C (68° to 77°F) [see USP].

Store reconstituted solution at controlled room temperature, 20° to 25°C (68° to 77°F) [see USP]. Use solution within 48 hours after mixing.

PREDNISOLONE

Rx	**Prednisolone** (Various, eg, Geneva, Goldline, Major, Moore, Roxane, Rugby, Schein)	**Tablets:** 5 mg	In 100s, 1,000s, and 5,000s.
Rx	**Prelone** (Aero)	**Syrup:** 15 mg per 5 mL	5% alcohol. Saccharin, sucrose. Cherry flavor. In 240 mL.
Rx	**Prednisolone** (Various, eg, WE Pharmaceuticals)	**Syrup:** 15 mg per 5 mL	Sucrose. In 240 and 480 mL.

PREDNISOLONE — ORAL

For complete and comparative prescribing information, refer to the Glucocorticoids group monograph.

Administration and Dosage

➤*Approved by the FDA:* June 21, 1955.

➤*Dosage:* Dosage of prednisolone should be individualized according to the severity of the disease and the response of the patient. For infants and children, the recommended dosage should be governed by the same considerations rather than strict adherence to the ratio indicated by age or body weight.

Hormone therapy is an adjunct to and not a replacement for conventional therapy.

Dosage should be decreased or discontinued gradually when the drug has been administered for more than a few days.

The severity, prognosis, expected duration of the disease, and the reaction of the patient to medication are primary factors in determining dosage.

If a period of spontaneous remission occurs in a chronic condition, treatment should be discontinued.

PREDNISOLONE — ORAL

The initial dosage of prednisolone may vary from 5 mg to 60 mg per day depending on the specific disease entity being treated. In situations of less severity lower doses will generally suffice, while in selected patients higher initial doses may be required. The initial dosage should be maintained or adjusted until a satisfactory response is noted. If after a reasonable period of time there is a lack of satisfactory clinical response, prednisolone should be discontinued and the patient transferred to other appropriate therapy. It should be emphasized that dosage requirements are variable and must be individualized on the basis of the disease under treatment and the response of the patient.

After a favorable response is noted, the proper maintenance dosage should be determined by decreasing the initial drug dosage in small decrements at appropriate time intervals until the lowest dosage that will maintain an adequate clinical response is reached. It should be kept in mind that constant monitoring is needed in regard to drug dosage. Included in the situations which may make dosage adjustments necessary are changes in clinical status secondary to remissions or exacerbations in the disease process, the patient's individual drug responsiveness, and the effect of patient exposure to stressful situations not directly related to the disease entity under treatment. In this latter situation it may be necessary to increase the dosage of prednisolone for a period of time consistent with the patient's condition. If after long-term therapy the drug is to be stopped, it is recommended that it be withdrawn gradually rather than abruptly.

Dose/volume chart for prednisolone syrup	
prednisolone 15 mg	5 mL (1 teaspoonful)
prednisolone 10 mg	3.33 mL (⅔ teaspoonful)
prednisolone 7.5 mg	2.5 mL (½ teaspoonful)
prednisolone 5 mg	1.66 mL (⅓ teaspoonful)

➤*Alternate-day therapy:* Alternate-day therapy is a corticosteroid dosing regimen in which twice the usual daily dose of corticoid is administered every other morning. The purpose of this mode of therapy is to provide the patient requiring long-term pharmacologic dose treatment with the beneficial effects of corticoids while minimizing certain undesirable effects, including pituitary-adrenal suppression, the cushingoid state, corticoid withdrawal symptoms, and growth suppression in children.

➤*Storage/Stability:* Dispense prednisolone syrup with suitable calibrated measuring device to ensure proper measuring of dose. Dispense in tight, light-resistant and child-resistant container. Store at room temperature 15° to 30°C (59° to 86°F). Do not refrigerate.

PREDNISOLONE ACETATE

Rx	**Prednisolone Acetate** (Various, eg, Rugby, URL)	**Injection:** 25 mg/mL suspension	In 10 and 30 mL vials.
Rx	**Prednisolone Acetate** (Various, eg, Goldline, Moore, Rugby, URL)	**Injection:** 50 mg/mL suspension	In 10 and 30 mL vials.
Rx	**Predcor-50** (Hauck)		In 10 mL vials.[a]

[a] With polysorbate 80, carboxymethylcellulose and benzyl alcohol.

PREDNISOLONE ACETATE — INJECTION

For complete and comparative prescribing information, refer to the Glucocorticoids group monograph.

Administration and Dosage

Relatively insoluble.

➤*Systemic:* Not for IV use.

Initial dosage – 4 to 60 mg/day, IM.

➤*Intralesional, intra-articular or soft tissue injection:* 4 mg, up to 100 mg.

➤*Multiple sclerosis:* 200 mg daily for a week, followed by 80 mg every other day or dexamethasone 4 to 8 mg every other day for 1 month.

PREDNISOLONE SODIUM PHOSPHATE

Rx sf	**Pediapred** (Fisons)	**Oral Liquid:** prednisolone (as sodium phosphate) 5 mg per 5 mL	Alcohol and dye free. Raspberry flavor. In 120 mL.
Rx	**Prednisolone Sodium Phosphate** (Upstate Pharma)	**Oral solution:** prednisolone (6.7 mg prednisolone sodium phosphate) 5 mg per 5 mL	Dye free. Sorbitol, EDTA, methylparaben. Raspberry flavor. In 120 mL.
Rx	**Prednisolone Sodium Phosphate** (Pharmaceutical Associates)	**Oral solution:** prednisolone (20.2 mg prednisolone sodium phosphate) 15 mg per 5 mL	Corn syrup, saccharin. Grape flavor. In 237 mL.
Rx	**Orapred** (BioMarin)		Dye free. 2% alcohol, fructose, sorbitol. Grape flavor. In 237 mL.

[a] With niacinamide, EDTA, phenol and sodium bisulfite.

PREDNISOLONE SODIUM PHOSPHATE — ORAL

For complete and comparative prescribing information, refer to the Glucocorticoids group monograph.

Administration and Dosage

➤*Dosage:* The initial dose of prednisolone sodium phosphate oral solutions may vary from prednisolone base 5 to 60 mg daily, depending on the specific disease entity being treated. In situations of less severity, lower doses will generally suffice, while in selected patients higher initial doses may be required. The initial dosage should be maintained or adjusted until a satisfactory response is noted. If, after a reasonable period of time, there is a lack of satisfactory clinical response, prednisolone sodium phosphate oral solution should be discontinued and the patient placed on other appropriate therapy. It should be emphasized that dosage requirements are variable and must be individualized on the basis of the disease under treatment and the response of the patient. After a favorable response is noted, the proper maintenance dosage should be determined by decreasing the initial drug dosage in small decrements at appropriate time intervals until the lowest dosage which will maintain an adequate clinical response is reached. It should be kept in mind that constant monitoring is needed in regard to drug dosage. Included in the situations which may make dosage adjustments necessary are changes in clinical status secondary to remissions or exacerbations in the disease process, the patient's individual drug responsiveness, and the effect of patient exposure to stressful situations not directly related to the disease entity under treatment; in this latter situation, it may be necessary to increase the dosage of prednisolone sodium phosphate oral solution for a period of time consistent with the patient's condition. If, after long-term therapy, the drug is to be stopped, it is recommended that it be withdrawn gradually rather than abruptly.

➤*Multiple sclerosis:* In the treatment of acute exacerbations of multiple sclerosis, daily doses of prednisolone 200 mg for a week followed by 80 mg every other day or dexamethasone 4 to 8 mg every other day for 1 month have been shown to be effective.

➤*Children:* In children, the initial dose of prednisolone sodium phosphate oral solutions may vary depending on the specific disease entity being treated. The range of initial doses is 0.14 to 2 mg/kg/day in 3 or 4 divided doses (4 to 60 mg/m^2bsa/day).

Nephrotic syndrome – The standard regimen used to treat nephrotic syndrome in children is 60 mg/m^2/day, given in 3 divided doses for 4 weeks, followed by 4 weeks of single dose alternate-day therapy at 40 mg/m^2/day.

Uncontrolled asthma – The National Heart, Lung, and Blood Institute (NHLBI)-recommended dosing for systemic prednisone, prednisolone or methylprednisolone in children whose asthma is uncontrolled by inhaled corticosteroids and long-acting bronchodilators is 1 to 2 mg/kg/day in single or divided doses. It is further recommended that short course, or "burst" therapy, be continued until a child achieves a peak expiratory flow rate of 80% of his or her personal best or symptoms resolve. This usually requires 3 to 10 days of treatment, although it can take longer. There is no evidence that tapering the dose after improvement will prevent a relapse.

➤*Storage/Stability:* Keep tightly closed and out of the reach of children.

15 mg per 5 mL oral solution – Dispense in tight, light-resistant glass or PET plastic containers.

Store refrigerated, 2° to 8°C (36° to 48°F).

5 mg per 5 mL oral solution – Store at 4° to 25°C (39° to 77°F). The solution may be refrigerated.

PREDNISONE

Rx	**Prednisone** (Roxane)	**Tablets:** 1 mg	Lactose. (54 092). White, scored. In 100s, 1,000s, and UD 100s.
Rx	**Meticorten** (Schering)		Lactose. (KEM or 843). White. In 100s.
Rx	**Orasone** (Solvay)		Lactose. (RR 1). Pink, scored. In 100s and 1,000s.
Rx	**Panasol-S** (Seatrace)		Pink, scored. In 100s and 1,000s.
Rx	**Prednisone** (Roxane)	**Tablets:** 2.5 mg	Lactose. (54 339). White, scored. In 100s and UD 100s.
Rx	**Deltasone** (Upjohn)		Lactose, sucrose. (Deltasone 2.5). Scored. In 100s.
Rx	**Prednisone** (Various, eg, Barr, Geneva, Goldline, Lannett, Major, Parmed, Roxane, Rugby)	**Tablets:** 5 mg	In 100s, 500s, 1,000s, 5,000s, and UD 100s.
Rx	**Deltasone** (Upjohn)		Lactose, sucrose. (Deltasone 5). Scored. In 100s, UD 100s, and Dosepak 21s.
Rx	**Orasone** (Solvay)		Lactose. (RR 5). White, scored. In 100s and 1,000s.
Rx	**Prednicen-M** (Central)		(131/07). Red. Film coated. In 100s, 1000s and unit pak 21s.
Rx	**Sterapred** (Merz)		(DAN/5052, mfg. by Danbury). (DELTASONE 5, mfg. by Upjohn). White, scored. In Uni-Pak 21s. **Sterapred 12 day.** In Uni-Pak 48s.
Rx	**Prednisone** (Various, eg, Barr, Geneva, Goldline, Major, Parmed, Roxane, Rugby)	**Tablets:** 10 mg	In 100s, 500s, 1,000s, and UD 100s.
Rx	**Deltasone** (Upjohn)		Lactose, sucrose. (Deltasone 10). Scored. In 100s, 500s and UD 100s.
Rx	**Orasone** (Solvay)		Lactose. (RR 10). Blue, scored. In 100s and 1000s.
Rx	**Sterapred DS** (Merz)		(DAN/5442, mfg. by Danbury). (DELTASONE 10, mfg. by Upjohn). White, scored. In Uni-Pak 21s. **Sterapred DS 12 day.** In Uni-Pak 48s. **Sterapred DS 14 day.** In Uni-Pak 49s.
Rx	**Prednisone** (Various, eg, Barr, Bioline, Geneva, Goldline, Lannett, Major, Parmed, Roxane, Rugby)	**Tablets:** 20 mg	In 100s, 500s, 1,000s, and UD 100s.
Rx	**Deltasone** (Upjohn)		Lactose, sucrose. (Deltasone 20). Scored. In 100s, 500s and UD 100s.
Rx	**Orasone** (Solvay)		Lactose. (RR 20). Yellow, scored. In 100s and 1,000s.
Rx	**Prednisone** (Various, eg, Geneva, Major, Roxane, Rugby)	**Tablets:** 50 mg	In 100s and UD 100s.
Rx	**Orasone** (Solvay)		Lactose. (RR 50). White, scored. Film coated. In 100s.
Rx	**Prednisone** (Roxane)	**Oral Solution:** 5 mg per 5 mL	5% alcohol, EDTA, fructose, saccharin. In 120 and 500 mL and UD 5 mL.
Rx	**Prednisone Intensol Concentrate** (Roxane)	**Oral Solution:** 5 mg/mL	30% alcohol. In 30 mL w/calibrated dropper.
Rx	**Liquid Pred** (Muro)	**Syrup:** 5 mg per 5 mL	5% alcohol. Saccharin, sorbitol and sucrose. In 120 and 240 mL.

PREDNISONE — ORAL

For complete and comparative prescribing information, refer to the Glucocorticoids group monograph.

Administration and Dosage

➤*Dosage:* Dosage of prednisone should be individualized according to the severity of the disease and the response of the patient. For infants and children, the recommended dosage should be governed by the same considerations rather than strict adherence to the ratio indicated by age or body weight.

Hormone therapy is an adjunct to, and not a replacement for, conventional therapy.

Dosage should be decreased or discontinued gradually when the drug has been administered for more than a few days.

The severity, prognosis, expected duration of the disease, and the reaction of the patient to medication are primary factors in determining dosage.

If a period of spontaneous remission occurs in a chronic condition, treatment should be discontinued.

The initial dosage of prednisone tablets may vary from 5 mg to 60 mg of prednisone per day depending on the specific disease entity being treated. In situations of less severity lower doses will generally suffice while in selected patients higher initial doses may be required. The initial dosage should be maintained or adjusted until a satisfactory response is noted. If after a reasonable period of time there is a lack of satisfactory clinical response, prednisone should be discontinued and the patient transferred to other appropriate therapy.

It should be emphasized that dosage requirements are variable and must be individualized on the basis of the disease under treatment and the response of the patient.

After a favorable response is noted, the proper maintenance dosage should be determined by decreasing the initial drug dosage in small decrements at appropriate time intervals until the lowest dosage which will maintain an adequate clinical response is reached. It should be kept in mind that constant monitoring is needed in regard to drug dosage. Included in the situations which may make dosage adjustments necessary are changes in clinical status secondary to remissions or exacerbations in the disease process, the patient's individual drug responsiveness, and the effect of patient exposure to stressful situations not directly related to the disease entity under treatment; in this latter situation it may be necessary to increase the dosage of prednisone for a period of time consistent with the patient's condition. If after long-term therapy the drug is to be stopped, it is recommended that it be withdrawn gradually rather than abruptly.

➤*Multiple sclerosis:* In the treatment of acute exacerbations of multiple sclerosis daily doses of prednisone 200 mg for a week followed by 80 mg every other day for 1 month have been shown to be effective. (Dosage range is the same for prednisone and prednisolone.)

➤*Alternate day therapy (ADT):* ADT is a corticosteroid dosing regimen in which twice the usual daily dose of corticoid is administered every other morning. The purpose of this mode of therapy is to provide the patient requiring long-term pharmacologic dose treatment with the beneficial effects of corticoids while minimizing certain undesirable effects, including pituitary-adrenal suppression, the Cushingoid state, corticoid withdrawal symptoms, and growth suppression in children.

➤*Storage/Stability:* Store at controlled room temperature 15° to 30°C (59° to 86°F).

TRIAMCINOLONE

Rx	**Aristocort** (Astellas[a])	**Tablets:** 4 mg	Lactose. (F A4). White, scored. Oblong, flat. In 30s and 100s.

[a] Astellas Pharma, 3 Parkway North Center, Deerfield, IL 60016; (847) 317-5941, fax (847) 317-5941.

TRIAMCINOLONE — ORAL

For complete and comparative prescribing information, refer to the Glucocorticoids group monograph.

Administration and Dosage

➤*Initial daily dosage in specific disorders is:*

Adrenocortical insufficiency – 4 to 12 mg, in addition to mineralocorticoid therapy.

Rheumatic and dermatological disorders and bronchial asthma – 8 to 16 mg.

Allergic states – 8 to 12 mg.

Ophthalmological diseases – 12 to 40 mg.

Respiratory diseases – 16 to 48 mg.

Hematologic disorders – 16 to 60 mg.

Tuberculous meningitis – 32 to 48 mg.

Acute rheumatic carditis – 20 to 60 mg.

Acute leukemia and lymphoma (adults) – 16 to 40 mg. It may be necessary to give as much as 100 mg/day in leukemia.
Acute leukemia (children): 1 to 2 mg/kg.

Edematous states – 16 to 20 mg (up to 48 mg) until diuresis occurs.

Systemic lupus erythematosus – 20 to 32 mg.

TRIAMCINOLONE ACETONIDE

Rx	**Tac-3** (Herbert)	**Injection:** 3 mg per ml suspension	In 5 ml vials.[1]
Rx	**Kenalog-10** (Westwood-Squibb)	**Injection:** 10 mg per ml suspension	In 5 ml vials.[1]
Rx	**Triamcinolone Acetonide** (Various, eg, Bioline, Dixon-Shane, Geneva Marsam, Goldline)	**Injection:** 40 mg per ml suspension	In 1 and 5 ml vials.
Rx	**Kenalog-40** (Westwood-Squibb)		In 1, 5 and 10 ml vials.[1]
Rx	**Tac-40** (Parnell)		In 5 ml vials.
Rx	**Triamonide 40** (Forest)		In 5 ml vials.[1]
Rx	**Tri-Kort** (Keene)		In 5 ml vials.[1]
Rx	**Trilog** (Hauck)		In 5 ml vials.[1]

[1] With polysorbate 80, carboxymethlcellulose and benzyl alcohol.

TRIAMCINOLONE ACETONIDE — INJECTION

For complete and comparative prescribing information, refer to the Glucocorticoids group monograph.

Administration and Dosage

➤*Approved by the FDA:* October 16, 1987.

➤*Dosage:* The initial dose of triamcinolone acetonide injection for intra-articular or intrabursal administration and for injection into tendon sheaths may vary from 2.5 to 5 mg for smaller joints, and from 5 to 15 mg for larger joints, depending on the specific disease entity being treated. Single injections into several joints for multiple locus involvement, up to a total of 20 mg or more, have been given without incident. For intradermal administration, the initial dose of triamcinolone acetonide will vary depending upon the specific disease entity being treated, but should be limited to 1 mg (0.1 mL) per injection site, since larger volumes are more likely to produce cutaneous atrophy. Multiple sites (separated by 1 centimeter or more) may be so injected, keeping in mind that the greater the total volume employed, the more corticosteroid becomes available for possible systemic absorption and subsequent corticosteroid effects. Such injections may be repeated, if necessary, at weekly or less frequent intervals.

The lower dosages in the initial dosage range of triamcinolone acetonide may produce the desired effect when the corticosteroid is administered to provide a localized concentration. The site of the injection and the volume of the injection should be carefully considered when triamcinolone acetonide is administered for this purpose. The initial dosage should be maintained or adjusted until a satisfactory response is noted. If, after a reasonable period of time, there is a lack of satisfactory clinical response, triamcinolone acetonide injection should be discontinued and the patient transferred to other appropriate therapy. It should be emphasized that dosage requirements are variable and must be individualized on the basis of the disease under treatment and the response of the patient. After a favorable response is noted, the proper maintenance dosage should be determined by decreasing the initial drug dosage in small increments at appropriate time intervals until the lowest dosage which will maintain an adequate clinical response is reached. It should be kept in mind that constant monitoring is needed in regard to drug dosage. Included in the situations which may make dosage adjustments necessary are changes in clinical status secondary to remissions or exacerbations in the disease process, the patient's individual drug responsiveness, and the effect of patient exposure to stressful situations not directly related to the disease entity under treatment; in this latter situation it may be necessary to increase the dosage of triamcinolone acetonide injection for a period of time consistent with the patient's condition. If the drug is to be stopped after long-term therapy, it is recommended that it be withdrawn gradually rather than abruptly.

➤*Administration:* Shake the vial before use to ensure a uniform suspension. Prior to withdrawal, inspect suspension for clumping or granular appearance (agglomeration). An agglomerated product results from exposure to freezing temperatures and should not be used. After withdrawal, inject without delay to prevent settling in the syringe. Careful technique should be employed to avoid the possibility of entering a blood vessel or introducing infection.

Routine laboratory studies, such as urinalysis, 2-hour postprandial blood sugar, determination of blood pressure and body weight, and a chest x-ray should be made at regular intervals during prolonged therapy. Upper GI x-rays are desirable in patients with an ulcer history or significant dyspepsia.

For treatment of joints, the usual intra-articular injection technique, as described in standard textbooks, should be followed. If an excessive amount of synovial fluid is present in the joint, some, but not all, should be aspirated to aid in the relief of pain and to prevent undue dilution of the steroid.

With intra-articular or intrabursal administration, and with injection of triamcinolone acetonide injection into tendon sheaths, the use of a local anesthetic may often be desirable. When a local anesthetic is used, its package insert should be read with care and all the precautions connected with its use should be observed. It should be injected into the surrounding soft tissues prior to the injection of the corticosteroid. A small amount of the anesthetic solution may be instilled into the joint.

In treating acute nonspecific tenosynovitis, care should be taken to ensure that the injection of triamcinolone acetonide injection is made into the tendon sheath rather than the tendon substance. Epicondylitis (tennis elbow) may be treated by infiltrating the preparation into the area of greatest tenderness.

For treatment of dermal lesions, triamcinolone acetonide injection is injected directly into the lesion (ie, intradermally or sometimes SC). For accuracy of dosage measurement and ease of administration, it is preferable to employ a tuberculin syringe and a small-bore needle (23- to 25-gauge). Ethyl chloride spray may be used to alleviate the discomfort of the injection.

➤*Storage/Stability:* Store at room temperature; avoid freezing; protect from light.

Glucocorticoids

TRIAMCINOLONE HEXACETONIDE

Rx	**Aristospan Intralesional** (Fujisawa)	**Injection:** 5 mg/mL suspension	In 5 mL vials.[a]
Rx	**Aristospan Intra-articular** (Fujisawa)	**Injection:** 20 mg/mL suspension	In 1 and 5 mL vials.[a]

[a] With polysorbate 80, sorbitol and benzyl alcohol.

TRIAMCINOLONE HEXACETONIDE — INJECTION

For complete and comparative prescribing information, refer to the Glucocorticoids group monograph.

Administration and Dosage

Relatively insoluble, slowly absorbed and has a prolonged action.

Not for IV use.

➤*Intra-articular:* 2 to 20 mg average.

Large joints (eg, knee, hip, shoulder) – 10 to 20 mg.

Small joints (eg, interphalangeal, metacarpophalangeal) – 2 to 6 mg.

➤*Intralesional or sublesional:* Up to 0.5 mg/square inch of affected area.

Mineralocorticoids

FLUDROCORTISONE ACETATE

Rx	**Fludrocortisone Acetate** (Various, eg, Global)	**Tablets:** 0.1 mg	In 100s.
Rx	**Florinef Acetate** (Monarch)		Lactose. (429). White, scored. In 100s.

FLUDROCORTISONE ACETATE — ORAL

Indications

Partial replacement therapy for primary and secondary adrenocortical insufficiency in Addison disease and for the treatment of salt-losing adrenogenital syndrome.

➤*Unlabeled uses:* Fludrocortisone has been used in the management of symptomatic orthostatic hypotension.

Administration and Dosage

Dosage depends on the severity of the disease and the response of the patient. Continually monitor patients for signs that indicate dosage adjustment is necessary, such as remissions or exacerbations of the disease and stress (surgery, infection, trauma).

➤*Addison disease:* The usual dose is 0.1 mg/day (range, 0.1 mg 3 times weekly to 0.2 mg/day). If transient hypertension develops as a consequence of therapy, reduce the dose to 0.05 mg/day. Administration in conjunction with cortisone (10 to 37.5 mg/day in divided doses) or hydrocortisone (10 to 30 mg/day in divided doses) is preferable. In Addison disease, the combination of fludrocortisone acetate tablets with a glucocorticoid such as hydrocortisone or cortisone provides substitution therapy approximating normal adrenal activity with minimal risks of unwanted effects.

➤*Salt-losing adrenogenital syndrome:* 0.1 to 0.2 mg/day.

➤*Withdrawal:* Use the lowest possible dose of corticosteroid to control the condition being treated. Make a gradual reduction in dosage when possible. Adverse reactions to corticosteroids may be produced by too-rapid withdrawal or by continued use of large doses.

➤*Storage/Stability:* Store at room temperature; avoid excessive heat.

Actions

➤*Pharmacology:* Fludrocortisone is a synthetic, adrenocortical steroid with potent mineralocorticoid properties and high glucocorticoid activity; it is used only for its mineralocorticoid effects.

The physiological action of fludrocortisone is similar to that of hydrocortisone. However, the effects of fludrocortison, particularly on electrolyte balance, but also on carbohydrate metabolism, are considerably heightened and prolonged. Mineralocorticoids act on the renal distal tubules to enhance the reabsorption of sodium. They increase urinary excretion of both potassium and hydrogen ions. The consequence of these 3 primary effects together with similar actions on cation transport in other tissues appears to account for the spectrum of physiological activities characteristic of mineralocorticoids.

In small oral doses, fludrocortisone produces marked sodium retention and increased urinary potassium excretion. It also causes a rise in blood pressure, apparently because of these effects on electrolyte levels. In larger doses, fludrocortisone inhibits endogenous adrenal cortical secretion, thymic activity, and pituitary corticotropin excretion, promotes the deposition of liver glycogen, and, unless protein intake is adequate, induces negative nitrogen balance.

➤*Pharmacokinetics:* Plasma half-life is approximately 3.5 hours; biological half-life ranges from 18 to 36 hours.

Contraindications

Hypersensitivity to fludrocortisone; systemic fungal infections.

Warnings

➤*Sodium retention:* Because of its marked effect on sodium retention, the use of fludrocortisone in the treatment of conditions other than those indicated is not advised.

➤*Infections:* Corticosteroids may mask some signs of infection, and new infections may appear during their use. There may be decreased resistance and inability to localize infection when corticosteroids are used. If an infection occurs during fludrocortisone acetate therapy, it should be controlled promptly by suitable antimicrobial therapy.

Tuberculosis – Restrict the use of fludrocortisone acetate tablets in patients with active tuberculosis to cases of fulminating or disseminated tuberculosis in which the corticosteroid is used for the management of the disease in conjunction with an appropriate antituberculous regimen. If corticosteroids are indicated in patients with latent tuberculosis or tuberculin reactivity, close observation is necessary because reactivation of the disease may occur. During prolonged corticosteroid therapy, these patients should receive chemoprophylaxis.

Children – Children who are on immunosuppressant drugs are more susceptible to infections than healthy children. Chicken pox and measles, for example, can have a more serious or even fatal course in children on immunosuppressant corticosteroids. In such children, or in adults who have not had these diseases, take particular care to avoid exposure. If exposed, therapy with varicella zoster immune globulin or pooled IV immunoglobulin, as appropriate, may be indicated. If chicken pox develops, consider treatment with antiviral agents.

➤*Ocular effects:* Prolonged use of corticosteroids may produce posterior subcapsular cataracts and glaucoma with possible damage to the optic nerves and may enhance the establishment of secondary ocular infections caused by fungi or viruses.

Use corticosteroids cautiously in patients with ocular herpes simplex because of possible corneal perforation.

➤*Adrenal insufficiency:* To avoid drug-induced adrenal insufficiency, supportive dosage may be required in times of stress (eg, trauma, surgery, severe illness), both during treatment with fludrocortisone and for a year afterwards.

➤*Fluid and electrolyte balance:* Average and large doses of hydrocortisone or cortisone can cause elevation of blood pressure, retention of salt and water, and increased excretion of potassium. These effects are less likely to occur with the synthetic derivatives except when they are used in large doses. However, because fludrocortisone is a potent mineralocorticoid, carefully monitor the dosage and salt intake in order to avoid the development of hypertension, edema, or weight gain. Periodic checking of serum electrolyte levels is advisable during prolonged therapy; dietary salt restriction and potassium supplementation may be necessary. All corticosteroids increase calcium excretion.

➤*Vaccinations:* Do not vaccinate patients against smallpox while they are on corticosteroid therapy. Do not undertake other immunization procedures in patients who are on corticosteroids, especially high doses because of possible hazards of neurological complications and a lack of antibody response.

➤*Pregnancy: Category C.* Adequate animal reproduction studies have not been conducted with fludrocortisone acetate. However, many corticosteroids have been shown to be teratogenic in laboratory animals at low doses. Teratogenicity of these agents in humans has not been demonstrated. It is not known whether fludrocortisone acetate can cause fetal harm when administered to a pregnant woman or can affect reproduction capacity. Give fludrocortisone acetate to a pregnant woman only if clearly needed.

Carefully observe infants born of mothers who have received substantial doses of fludrocortisone acetate during pregnancy for signs of hypoadrenalism.

➤*Lactation:* Corticosteroids are found in the breast milk of lactating women. Exercise caution when administering these drugs to nursing women.

➤*Children:* Safety and efficacy in children have not been established. Monitor growth and development of infants and children on prolonged therapy.

Precautions

➤*Monitoring:* Regularly monitor patients for blood pressure and serum electrolyte determinations.

➤*Use with caution:*

GI – Use corticosteroids with caution in patients with nonspecific ulcerative colitis if there is a probability of impending perforation, abscess, or other pyogenic infection and in patients with diverticulitis, fresh intestinal anastomoses, or active or latent peptic ulcer.

Miscellaneous – There is an enhanced corticosteroid effect in patients with hypothyroidism and cirrhosis. Use with caution in patients with renal insufficiency, hypertension, osteoporosis, and myasthenia gravis.

FLUDROCORTISONE ACETATE — ORAL

➤*Psychiatric effects:* Psychic derangements may appear when corticosteroids are used. These may range from euphoria, insomnia, mood swings, personality changes, and severe depression to frank psychotic manifestations. Corticosteroids also may aggravate existing emotional instability or psychotic tendencies.

Drug Interactions

Fludrocortisone Drug Interactions

Precipitant drug	Object drug[a]		Description
Anabolic steroids	Fludrocortisone	↑	Concurrent use may enhance the tendency toward edema. Use with caution, especially in patients with hepatic or cardiac disease.
Barbiturates Hydantoins Rifamycins	Fludrocortisone	↓	Fludrocortisone hepatic metabolism may be increased, resulting in decreased therapeutic effects.
Estrogens	Fludrocortisone	↑	Corticosteroid metabolism may be decreased.
Fludrocortisone	Amphotericin B Potassium-depleting diuretics	↑	Coadministration may enhance hypokalemia. Check serum potassium levels at frequent intervals. Use potassium supplements if necessary.
Fludrocortisone	Anticholinesterases	↓	Although fludrocortisone is not used to treat myasthenia gravis, corticosteroids may antagonize the effects of anticholinesterases in myasthenia gravis.
Fludrocortisone	Anticoagulants, oral	↑↓	Anticoagulant dose requirements may be reduced. Conversely, corticosteroids may oppose the anticoagulant action. Monitor prothrombin time and adjust dose accordingly.
Fludrocortisone	Antidiabetic agents (oral agents and insulin)	↓	Antidiabetic effect may be decreased. Monitor for signs of hyperglycemia; adjust dose of antidiabetic agent if necessary.
Fludrocortisone	Digitalis glycosides	↑	Coadministration may enhance the possibility of arrhythmias or digitalis toxicity associated with hypokalemia. Monitor serum potassium levels and use potassium supplements if necessary.
Fludrocortisone	Nondepolarizing muscle relaxants	↓	Corticosteroids may decrease the actions of the nondepolarizing muscle relaxants.
Fludrocortisone	Salicylates	↑↓	Corticosteroids will reduce serum salicylate levels and may decrease their effectiveness. Coadministration also may increase the ulcerogenic effects of each.
Fludrocortisone	Vaccines	↑↓	Concurrent use may increase neurological complications and decrease antibody response (see Warnings).

[a] ↑ = Object increased. ↓ = Object decreased.

➤*Drug/Lab test interactions:* Corticosteroids may affect the nitroblue-tetrazollum test for bacterial infection and produce false-negative results.

Adverse Reactions

Most adverse reactions are caused by fludrocortisone's mineralocorticoid activity (retention of sodium and water). When fludrocortisone is used in the small dosages recommended, the glucocorticoid side effects often seen with cortisone and its derivatives are not usually a problem; however, keep in mind the following untoward effects, particularly when fludrocortisone is used over a prolonged period of time or in conjunction with cortisone or a similar glucocorticoid.

➤*Cardiovascular:* Hypertension; CHF; cardiac enlargement.

➤*CNS:* Convulsions; increased intracranial pressure with papilledema (pseudotumor cerebri), usually after treatment; vertigo; headache; severe mental disturbances.

➤*Dermatologic:* Allergic skin rash; maculopapular rash; urticaria; impaired wound healing; thin, fragile skin; bruising; petechiae and ecchymoses; facial erythema; increased sweating; SC fat atrophy; purpura; striae; hyperpigmentation of skin and nails; hirsutism; acneiform eruptions; hives. Reactions to skin tests may be suppressed.

➤*Endocrine:* Menstrual irregularities; development of the cushingoid state; suppression of growth in children; secondary adrenocortical and pituitary unresponsiveness, particularly in times of stress (eg, trauma, surgery, illness); decreased carbohydrate tolerance; manifestations of latent diabetes mellitus; increased requirements for insulin or oral hypoglycemic agents in diabetics.

➤*GI:* Peptic ulcer with possible perforation and hemorrhage; pancreatitis; abdominal distention; ulcerative esophagitis.

➤*Metabolic:* Hyperglycemia; glycosuria; negative nitrogen balance caused by protein catabolism; potassium loss; edema; hypokalemic alkalosis.

➤*Musculoskeletal:* Muscle weakness; steroid myopathy; loss of muscle mass; osteoporosis; vertebral compression fractures; aseptic necrosis of femoral and humeral heads; pathologic fracture of long bones; spontaneous fractures.

➤*Ophthalmic:* Posterior subcapsular cataracts; increased intraocular pressure; glaucoma; exophthalmos.

➤*Miscellaneous:* Necrotizing angiitis; thrombophlebitis; aggravation or masking of infections; insomnia; syncopal episodes; anaphylactoid reactions.

Overdosage

➤*Symptoms:* Hypertension; edema; hypokalemia; excessive weight gain; increase in heart size.

➤*Treatment:* Discontinue the drug; symptoms usually subside within several days. Resume subsequent treatment with reduced doses. Muscular weakness may develop because of excessive potassium loss; treat with potassium supplements. Monitor blood pressure and serum electrolytes regularly.

Patient Information

Notify physician if dizziness, severe or continuing headaches, swelling of feet or lower legs, or unusual weight gain occurs.

Warn patients who are on immunosuppressant doses of corticosteroids to avoid exposure to chicken pox or measles and, if exposed, to obtain medical advice.

Advise the patient to use the medicine only as directed, to take a missed dose as soon as possible, unless it is almost time for the next dose, and not to double the next dose.

TERIPARATIDE (rDNA origin)

Rx	**Forteo** (Eli Lilly)	**Injection:** 250 mcg/mL[a]	In 3 mL prefilled pen delivery device.

[a] With mannitol 45.4 mg.

TERIPARATIDE rDNA — INJECTION

WARNING

In male and female rats, teriparatide caused an increase in the incidence of osteosarcoma (a malignant bone tumor) that was dependent on dose and treatment duration. The effect was observed at systemic exposures to teriparatide ranging from 3 to 60 times the exposure in humans given a 20 mcg dose. Because of the uncertain relevance of the rat osteosarcoma finding to humans, teriparatide should be prescribed only to patients for whom the potential benefits are considered to outweigh the potential risk. Teriparatide should not be prescribed for patients who are at increased baseline risk for osteosarcoma (including those with Paget's disease of bone or unexplained elevations of alkaline phosphatase, open epiphyses, or prior radiation therapy involving the skeleton).

Indications

➤*Postmenopausal women:* For the treatment of postmenopausal women with osteoporosis who are at high risk for fracture. These include women with a history of osteoporotic fracture, or who have multiple risk factors for fracture, or who have failed or are intolerant of previous osteoporosis therapy, based upon physician assessment. Teriparatide should not be prescribed for patients who are at increased baseline risk for osteosarcoma (including those with Paget's disease of bone or unexplained elevations of alkaline phosphatase, open epiphyses, or prior radiation therapy involving the skeleton). In postmenopausal women with osteoporosis, teriparatide increases bone mineral density (BMD) and reduces the risk of vertebral and nonvertebral fractures.

➤*Men:* For injection is indicated to increase bone mass in men with primary or hypogonadal osteoporosis who are at high risk for fracture. These include men with a history of osteoporotic fracture, or who have multiple risk factors for fracture, or who have failed or are intolerant to previous osteoporosis therapy, based upon physician assessment (see above). In men with primary or hypogonadal osteoporosis, teriparatide increases BMD. The effects of teriparatide on risk for fracture in men have not been studied.

Administration and Dosage

➤*Approved by the FDA:* November 26, 2002.

➤*Dosage:* Teriparatide injection should be administered as a subcutaneous injection into the thigh or abdominal wall. The recommended dosage is 20 mcg once a day.

Teriparatide injection should be administered initially under circumstances in which the patient can sit or lie down if symptoms of orthostatic hypotension occur. Patients should be instructed that if they feel lightheaded or have palpitations after the injection, they should sit or lie down until the symptoms resolve. If symptoms persist or worsen, patients should be instructed to consult a physician before continuing treatment

The safety and efficacy of teriparatide injection have not been evaluated beyond 2 years of treatment. Consequently, use of the drug for more than 2 years is not recommended.

➤*Instructions for pen use:* Patients and caregivers who administer teriparatide should receive appropriate training and instruction on the proper use of the teriparatide pen from a qualified health professional. It is important to read, understand, and follow the instructions in the teriparatide pen user manual for priming the pen and dosing. Failure to do so may result in inaccurate dosing. Each teriparatide pen can be used for up to 28 days after the first injection. After the 28-day use period, discard the teriparatide pen, even if it still contains some unused solution. Never share a teriparatide pen.

➤*Storage/Stability:* Store at 2° to 8°C (36° to 46°F) at all times. Recap the pen when not in use to protect the cartridge from physical damage and light. During the use period, time out of the refrigerator should be minimized; the dose may be delivered immediately following removal from the refrigerator. Do not freeze. Do not use teriparatide if it has been frozen.

Teriparatide injection is a clear and colorless liquid. Do not use if solid particles appear or if the solution is cloudy or colored.

Actions

➤*Pharmacology:* Endogenous 84-amino-acid parathyroid hormone (PTH) is the primary regulator of calcium and phosphate metabolism in bone and kidney. Physiological actions of PTH include regulation of bone metabolism, renal tubular reabsorption of calcium and phosphate, and intestinal calcium absorption. The biological actions of PTH and teriparatide are mediated through binding to specific high-affinity cell-surface receptors. Teriparatide and the 34 N-terminal amino acids of PTH bind to these receptors with the same affinity and have the same physiological actions on bone and kidney. Teriparatide is not expected to accumulate in bone or other tissues.

The skeletal effects of teriparatide depend upon the pattern of systemic exposure. Once-daily administration of teriparatide stimulates new bone formation on trabecular and cortical (periosteal or endosteal) bone surfaces by preferential stimulation of osteoblastic activity over osteoclastic activity. In monkey studies, teriparatide improved trabecular microarchitecture and increased bone mass and strength by stimulating new bone formation in both cancellous and cortical bone. In humans, the anabolic effects of teriparatide are manifest as an increase in skeletal mass, an increase in markers of bone formation and resorption, and an increase in bone strength. By contrast, continuous excess of endogenous PTH, as occurs in hyperparathyroidism, may be detrimental to the skeleton because bone resorption may be stimulated more than bone formation.

➤*Pharmacokinetics:*

Absorption/Distribution – Teriparatide is extensively absorbed after subcutaneous injection; the absolute bioavailability is approximately 95% based on pooled data from 20, 40, and 80 mcg doses. The rates of absorption and elimination are rapid. The peptide reaches peak serum concentrations about 30 minutes after subcutaneous injection of a 20 mcg dose and declines to non-quantifiable concentrations within 3 hours.

Systemic clearance of teriparatide (approximately 62 L/h in women and 94 L/h in men) exceeds the rate of normal liver plasma flow, consistent with both hepatic and extra-hepatic clearance. Volume of distribution, following intravenous injection, is approximately 0.12 L/kg. Intersubject variability in systemic clearance and volume of distribution is 25% to 50%. The half-life of teriparatide in serum is 5 minutes when administered by intravenous injection and approximately 1 hour when administered by subcutaneous injection. The longer half-life following subcutaneous administration reflects the time required for absorption from the injection site.

Metabolism/Excretion – No metabolism or excretion studies have been performed with teriparatide. However, the mechanisms of metabolism and elimination of PTH(1-34) and intact PTH have been extensively described in published literature. Peripheral metabolism of PTH is believed to occur by non-specific enzymatic mechanisms in the liver followed by excretion via the kidneys.

Special populations –

Renal function impairment: No pharmacokinetic differences were identified in 11 patients with mild or moderate renal insufficiency [creatinine clearance (Ccr) 30 to 72 mL/min] administered a single dose of teriparatide. In 5 patients with severe renal insufficiency (Ccr less than 30 mL/min), the AUC and $t_{½}$ of teriparatide were increased by 73% and 77%, respectively. Maximum serum concentration of teriparatide was not increased. No studies have been performed in patients undergoing dialysis for chronic renal failure.

Gender: Although systemic exposure to teriparatide was approximately 20% to 30% lower in men than women, the recommended dose for both genders is 20 mcg/day.

Contraindications

Hypersensitivity to teriparatide or to any of its excipients.

Warnings

➤*Osteosarcoma:* In male and female rats, teriparatide caused an increase in the incidence of osteosarcoma (a malignant bone tumor) that was dependent on dose and treatment duration. Teriparatide should not be prescribed for patients who are at increased baseline risk for osteosarcoma (including those with Paget's disease of bone or unexplained elevations of alkaline phosphatase, open epiphyses, or prior radiation therapy involving the skeleton). The effect was observed at systemic exposures to teriparatide ranging from 3 to 60 times the exposure in humans given a 20 mcg dose. Because of the uncertain relevance of the rat osteosarcoma finding to humans, teriparatide should be prescribed only to patients for whom the potential benefits are considered to outweigh the potential risk.

The following categories of patients have increased baseline risk of osteosarcoma and therefore should not be treated with teriparatide:

- Paget disease of bone. Teriparatide should not be given to patients with Paget disease of bone. Unexplained elevations of alkaline phosphatase may indicate Paget disease of bone.
- Pediatric populations. Teriparatide has not been studied in pediatric populations. Teriparatide should not be used in pediatric patients or young adults with open epiphyses.
- Prior radiation therapy. Patients with a history of radiation therapy involving the skeleton should be excluded from treatment with teriparatide.

➤*Avoid use in:* Patients with bone metastases or a history of skeletal malignancies should be excluded from treatment with teriparatide.

Patients with metabolic bone diseases other than osteoporosis should be excluded from treatment with teriparatide.

Teriparatide has not been studied in patients with preexisting hypercalcemia. These patients should be excluded from treatment with teriparatide because of the possibility of exacerbating hypercalcemia.

➤*Carcinogenesis:* Two carcinogenicity bioassays were conducted in Fischer 344 rats. In the first study, male and female rats were given daily subcutaneous teriparatide injections of 5, 30, or 75 mcg/kg/day for 24 months from 2 months of age. These doses resulted in systemic exposures that were, respectively, 3, 20, and 60 times higher than the systemic exposure observed in humans following a subcutaneous dose of 20 mcg (based on AUC comparison). Teriparatide treatment resulted in a marked dose-related increase in the incidence of osteosarcoma, a rare malignant bone tumor, in both male and female rats. Osteosarcomas were observed at all doses and the incidence reached 40% to 50% in the high-dose groups. Teriparatide also caused a dose-related increase in osteoblastoma and osteoma in both sexes. No osteosarcomas, osteoblastomas or osteomas were observed in untreated control rats. The bone tumors in rats occurred in association with a large increase in bone mass and focal osteoblast hyperplasia.

TERIPARATIDE rDNA — INJECTION

The second 2-year study was carried out in order to determine the effect of treatment duration and animal age on the development of bone tumors. Female rats were treated for different periods between 2 and 26 months of age with subcutaneous doses of 5 and 30 mcg/kg (equivalent to 3 and 20 times the human exposure at the 20 mcg dose, based on AUC comparison). The study showed that the occurrence of osteosarcoma, osteoblastoma and osteoma was dependent upon dose and duration of exposure. Bone tumors were observed when immature 2-month old rats were treated with 30 mcg/kg/day for 24 months or with 5 or 30 mcg/kg/day for 6 months. Bone tumors were also observed when mature 6-month old rats were treated with 30 mcg/kg/day for 6 or 20 months. Tumors were not detected when mature 6-month old rats were treated with 5 mcg/kg/day for 6 or 20 months. The results did not demonstrate a difference in susceptibility to bone tumor formation, associated with teriparatide treatment, between mature and immature rats.

The relevance of these rat findings to humans is uncertain.

➤*Elderly:* Of the patients receiving teriparatide in the osteoporosis trial of 1637 postmenopausal women, 75% were 65 years of age and over and 23% were 75 years of age and over. Of the patients receiving teriparatide in the osteoporosis trial of 437 men, 39% were 65 years of age and over and 13% were 75 years of age and over. No significant differences in bone response or adverse reactions were seen in geriatric patients receiving teriparatide as compared with younger patients. Nonetheless, as with many medications, elderly patients may have greater sensitivity to the adverse effects of teriparatide.

➤*Pregnancy: Category C.* In pregnant rats given subcutaneous teriparatide doses up to 1,000 mcg/kg/day, there were no findings. In pregnant mice given subcutaneous doses of 225 or 1,000 mcg/kg/day (greater than or equal to 60 times the human dose based on surface area, mcg/m^2) from gestation day 6 through 15, the fetuses showed an increased incidence of skeletal deviations or variations (interrupted rib, extra vertebra or rib).

Developmental effects in a perinatal/postnatal study in pregnant rats given subcutaneous doses of teriparatide from gestation day 6 through postpartum day 20 included mild growth retardation in female offspring at doses greater than or equal to 225 mcg/kg/day (greater than or equal to 120 times the human dose based on surface area, mcg/m^2), and in male offspring at 1,000 mcg/kg/day (540 times the human dose based on surface area, mcg/m^2). There was also reduced motor activity in both male and female offspring at 1,000 mcg/kg/day. There were no developmental or reproductive effects in mice or rats at a dose of 30 mcg/kg (8 or 16 times the human dose based on surface area, mcg/m^2). The effect of teriparatide treatment on human fetal development has not been studied. teriparatide is not indicated for use in pregnancy.

➤*Lactation:* Because teriparatide is indicated for the treatment of osteoporosis in postmenopausal women, it should not be administered to women who are nursing their children. There have been no clinical studies to determine if teriparatide is secreted into breast milk.

➤*Children:* The safety and efficacy of teriparatide have not been established in pediatric populations. Teriparatide is not indicated for use in pediatric patients.

Precautions

➤*Hypotension:* In short-term clinical pharmacology studies with teriparatide, transient episodes of symptomatic orthostatic hypotension were observed infrequently. Typically, an event began within 4 hours of dosing and spontaneously resolved within a few minutes to a few hours. When transient orthostatic hypotension occurred, it happened within the first several doses, it was relieved by placing the person in a reclining position, and it did not preclude continued treatment.

➤*Long-term therapy:* The safety and efficacy of teriparatide have not been evaluated beyond 2 years of treatment. Consequently, use of the drug for more than 2 years is not recommended.

➤*Urolithiasis or preexisting hypercalciuria:* In clinical trials, the frequency of urolithiasis was similar in patients treated with teriparatide and placebo. However, teriparatide has not been studied in patients with active urolithiasis. If active urolithiasis or preexisting hypercalciuria are suspected, measurement of urinary calcium excretion should be considered. Teriparatide should be used with caution in patients with active or recent urolithiasis because of the potential to exacerbate this condition.

➤*Concomitant treatment with digitalis:* In a study of 15 healthy people administered digoxin daily to steady state, a single teriparatide dose did not alter the effect of digoxin on the systolic time interval (from electrocardiographic Q-wave onset to aortic valve closure, a measure of digoxin's calcium-mediated cardiac effect). However, sporadic case reports have suggested that hypercalcemia may predispose patients to digitalis toxicity. Because teriparatide transiently increases serum calcium, teriparatide should be used with caution in patients taking digitalis.

➤*Calcium levels:* Teriparatide transiently increases serum calcium, with the maximal effect observed at approximately 4 to 6 hours post-dose. By 16 hours post-dose, serum calcium generally has returned to or near baseline. These effects should be kept in mind because serum calcium concentrations observed within 16 hours after a dose may reflect the pharmacologic effect of teriparatide. Persistent hypercalcemia was not observed in clinical trials with teriparatide. If persistent hypercalcemia is detected, treatment with teriparatide should be discontinued pending further evaluation of the cause of hypercalcemia.

Patients known to have an underlying hypercalcemia disorder, such as primary hyperparathyroidism, should not be treated with teriparatide.

➤*Urinary calcium:* Teriparatide increases urinary calcium excretion, but the frequency of hypercalciuria in clinical trials was similar for patients treated with teriparatide and placebo.

➤*Uric acid:* Teriparatide increases serum uric acid concentrations. In clinical trials, 2.8% of teriparatide patients had serum uric acid concentrations above the upper limit of normal compared with 0.7% of placebo patients. However, the hyperuricemia did not result in an increase in gout, arthralgia, or urolithiasis.

Drug Interactions

➤*Concomitant treatment with digitalis:* Sporadic case reports have suggested that hypercalcemia may predispose patients to digitalis toxicity. Because teriparatide transiently increases serum calcium, teriparatide should be used with caution in patients taking digitalis.

Adverse Reactions

The safety of teriparatide has been evaluated in 24 clinical trials that enrolled over 2,800 women and men. Four long-term phase 3 clinical trials included 1 large placebo-controlled, double-blind, multinational trial with 1,637 postmenopausal women; 1 placebo-controlled, double-blind, multinational trial with 437 men; and 2 active-controlled trials including 393 postmenopausal women. Teriparatide doses ranged from 5 to 100 mcg/day in short-term trials and 20 to 40 mcg/day in the other trials. A total of 1,943 of the patients studied received teriparatide, including 815 patients at 20 mcg/day and 1,107 patients at 40 mcg/day. In the clinical trials, a total of 1,432 patients were treated with teriparatide for 3 months to 2 years, of whom 1,137 were treated for greater than 1 year (500 at 20 mcg/day and 637 at 40 mcg/day). The maximum duration of treatment was 2 years. Adverse reactions associated with teriparatide usually were mild and generally did not require discontinuation of therapy.

In the two phase 3 placebo-controlled clinical trials in men and postmenopausal women, early discontinuation due to adverse reactions occurred in 5.6% of patients assigned to placebo and 7.1% of patients assigned to teriparatide. Reported adverse reactions that appeared to be increased by teriparatide treatment were dizziness and leg cramps.

The following table lists adverse reactions that occurred in the two phase 3 placebo-controlled clinical trials in men and postmenopausal women at a frequency greater than or equal to 2.0% in the teriparatide groups and in more teriparatide-treated patients than in placebo-treated patients, without attribution of causality.

Adverse reactions are shown without attribution of causality.

Teriparatide Adverse Reactions

Adverse reaction	Teriparatide rDNA (n = 691) (%)	Placebo (n = 691) (%)
Miscellaneous		
Pain	21.3%	20.5%
Headache	7.5%	7.4%
Asthenia	8.7%	6.8%
Neck pain	3%	2.7%
Cardiovascular		
Hypertension	7.1%	6.8%
Angina pectoris	2.5%	1.6%
Syncope	2.6%	1.4%
GI		
Nausea	8.5%	6.7%
Constipation	5.4%	4.5%
Diarrhea	5.1%	4.6%
Dyspepsia	5.2%	4.1%
Vomiting	3%	2.3%
GI disorder	2.3%	2%
Tooth disorder	2%	1.3%
Musculoskeletal		
Arthralgia	10.1%	8.4%
Leg cramps	2.6%	1.3%
CNS		
Dizziness	8%	5.4%
Depression	4.1%	2.7%
Insomnia	4.3%	3.6%
Vertigo	3.8%	2.7%
Respiratory		
Rhinitis	9.6%	8.8%
Increased cough	6.4%	5.5%
Pharyngitis	5.5%	4.8%
Dyspnea	3.6%	2.6%
Pneumonia	3.9%	3.3%
Dermatologic		
Rash	4.9%	4.5%
Sweating	2.2%	1.7%

➤*Serum calcium:* Teriparatide transiently increases serum calcium, with the maximal effect observed at approximately 4 to 6 hours post-dose. Serum calcium measured at least 16 hours post-dose was not different from pretreatment levels. In clinical trials, the frequency of at least 1 episode of transient hypercalcemia in the 4 to 6 hours after teriparatide administration was increased from 1.5% of women and none of the men treated with placebo to 11.1% of women and 6% of men treated with teriparatide. The number of patients treated with teriparatide whose transient hypercalcemia was verified on consecutive measurements was 3% of women and 1.3% of men.

TERIPARATIDE rDNA — INJECTION

➤*Immunogenicity:* In a large clinical trial, antibodies that cross-reacted with teriparatide were detected in 2.8% of women receiving teriparatide. Generally, antibodies were first detected following 12 months of treatment and diminished after withdrawal of therapy. There was no evidence of hypersensitivity reactions, allergic reactions, effects on serum calcium, or effects on BMD response.

Overdosage

➤*Symptoms:* Incidents of overdose in humans have not been reported in clinical trials. Teriparatide has been administered in single doses of up to 100 mcg and in repeated doses of up to 60 mcg/day for 6 weeks. The effects of overdose that might be expected include a delayed hypercalcemic effect and risk of orthostatic hypotension. Nausea, vomiting, dizziness, and headache might also occur.

➤*Treatment:* There is no specific antidote for teriparatide. Treatment of suspected overdose should include discontinuation of teriparatide, monitoring of serum calcium and phosphorus, and implementation of appropriate supportive measures, such as hydration.

Patient Information

Patients should read the Medication Guide and pen user manual before starting therapy with teriparatide and re-read them each time the prescription is renewed.

Patients should be made aware that teriparatide caused osteosarcomas in rats and that the clinical relevance of these findings is unknown.

Teriparatide should be administered initially under circumstances where the patient can immediately sit or lie down if symptoms occur. Patients should be instructed that if they feel lightheaded or have palpitations after the injection, they should sit or lie down until the symptoms resolve. If symptoms persist or worsen, patients should be instructed to consult a physician before continuing treatment.

Although symptomatic hypercalcemia was not observed in clinical trials, physicians should instruct patients to contact a healthcare provider if they develop persistent symptoms of hypercalcemia (ie, nausea, vomiting, constipation, lethargy, muscle weakness).

Patients should be instructed on how to properly use the delivery device (refer to user manual), properly dispose of needles, and be advised not to share their pens with other patients.

Patients should be informed regarding the roles of supplemental calcium or vitamin D, weight-bearing exercise, and modification of certain behavioral factors such as cigarette smoking or alcohol consumption.

THYROID DRUGS

Thyroid Hormones

Synthetic derivatives include levothyroxine (T_4), liothyronine (T_3), and liotrix (a 4 to 1 mixture of T_4 and T_3).

WARNING

Drugs with thyroid hormone activity, alone or with other therapeutic agents, have been used for the treatment of obesity. In euthyroid patients, doses within the range of daily hormonal requirements are ineffective for weight reduction. Larger doses may produce serious or even life-threatening manifestations of toxicity, particularly when given in association with sympathomimetic amines such as those used for their anorectic effects.

Indications

➤*Hypothyroidism:* As replacement or supplemental therapy in hypothyroidism of any etiology, except transient hypothyroidism during the recovery phase of subacute thyroiditis. Specific indications include the following: Cretinism, myxedema, and ordinary hypothyroidism; primary hypothyroidism resulting from functional deficiency, primary atrophy, partial or total absence of thyroid gland, or the effects of surgery, radiation, or drugs, with or without the presence of goiter; secondary (pituitary) or tertiary (hypothalamic) hypothyroidism.

➤*Pituitary TSH suppressants:* In the treatment or prevention of various types of euthyroid goiters, including thyroid nodules, subacute or chronic lymphocytic thyroiditis (Hashimoto), and multinodular goiter and in the management of thyroid cancer (except liothyronine).

➤*Diagnostic use (except levothyroxine):* Diagnostic use in suppression tests to differentiate suspected mild hyperthyroidism or thyroid gland autonomy.

➤*Myxedema coma/precoma (injection only):* For the treatment of myxedema coma/precoma.

➤*Unlabeled uses:* Thyroid hormones have been used to treat obesity; however, they are ineffective and should not be used for this condition (see Warnings).

Administration and Dosage

Individualize dosage. Determine patient response by clinical judgment in conjunction with laboratory findings.

Generally, institute thyroid therapy at relatively low doses and slowly increase in small increments until the desired response is obtained. Administer thyroid as a single daily dose, preferably before breakfast.

➤*Treatment of choice:* Treatment of choice for hypothyroidism is levothyroxine (T_4) under most circumstances because of its predictable potency and prolonged half-life.

➤*Thyroid cancer:* Exogenous thyroid hormone may produce regression of metastases from follicular and papillary carcinoma of the thyroid and is used as ancillary therapy of these conditions with radioactive iodine. Larger doses than those used for replacement therapy are required. Medullary thyroid carcinoma usually is unresponsive.

➤*Laboratory tests:* Laboratory tests useful in the diagnosis and evaluation of thyroid function are listed in the following table, indicating the alterations noted in various thyroid disorders.

Laboratory Tests for Diagnosis and Evaluation of Thyroid Function

↑ = Increased
↓ = Decreased
N = Normal
X = Contraindicated

	Pregnancy	Primary hypothyroidism	Secondary hypothyroidism	Hyperthyroidism	T_3 thyrotoxicosis	Normal values
Free T_4 (unbound)	N	↓	↓	↑	N	12 to 32 pmol/L
Total T_4	↑	↓	↓	↑	N	55 to 160 nmol/L
T_3	↑	↓	↓	↑	↑	0.6 to 3.1 nmol/L
RAIU[a]	X	↓	-	↑	–	5% to 30%
Free thyroxine index (FT_4I)	N	↓	↓	↑	-	6.5 to 12.5[b] 1.3 to 3.9[c]
TSH[a]	N	↑	N/↓	↓	↓	0.4 to 4.2 milliunit/L

[a] RAIU = radioactive iodine uptake; TSH = thyroid-stimulating hormone
[b] T_4 uptake method
[c] $TT_4 \times RT_3U$ method

➤*Dosage equivalents of thyroid products:* In changing from one thyroid product to another, the following dosage equivalents may be used. However, these equivalents are only estimates; each patient still may require fine dosage adjustments.

Approximate Dosage Equivalents of Thyroid Products[a]

Preparation	Composition ratio T_4	Composition ratio T_3	Dosage equivalents
Thyroid desiccated	4	1	≈ 60 to 65 mg (1 grain)
Levothyroxine	1	0	≈ 50 to 60 mcg (range, 50 to 100 mcg)
Liothyronine	0	1	≈ 25 mcg (range, 15 to 37.5 mcg)
Liotrix	4	1	≈ 1 grain (12.5 mcg T_3/50 mcg T_4)

[a] References may vary in dosage equivalent recommendations.

Actions

➤*Pharmacology:* Thyroid hormones include natural and synthetic derivatives. The natural product, desiccated thyroid, is derived from beef or pork. The US Pharmacopeia (USP) has standardized the total iodine content of natural preparations. Thyroid USP contains not less than 0.17% and not more than 0.23% iodine. Iodine content is only an indirect indicator of true hormonal biologic activity.

Physiological effects – The mechanisms by which thyroid hormones exert their physiologic action are not well understood. It is believed that most of their effects are exerted through control of DNA transcription and protein synthesis. These hormones enhance oxygen consumption by most tissues of the body and increase the basal metabolic rate and metabolism of carbohydrates, lipids, and proteins in the body. Thyroid hormones exert a profound influence on every organ system and are particularly important in CNS development. The physiological actions of thyroid hormones are produced predominantly by T_3, the majority of which (approximately 80%) is derived from T_4 by deiodination in peripheral tissues.

Regulation of thyroid secretion: Thyroid hormone synthesis and secretion are controlled by thyrotropin (thyroid-stimulating hormone; TSH) secreted by the anterior pituitary. TSH secretion is, in turn, controlled by a feedback mechanism effected by thyroid hormones and thyrotropin-releasing hormone (TRH), a tripeptide of hypothalamic origin. Endogenous thyroid hormone secretion is suppressed when exogenous thyroid hormones are given to euthyroid individuals in excess of the normal gland's secretion.

The normal thyroid gland contains, per gram of gland, approximately 200 mcg of T_4 and 15 mcg of T_3. The ratio of these 2 hormones in the circulation does not represent the ratio in the thyroid gland because about 80% of peripheral T_3 comes from monodeiodination of T_4. Peripheral monodeiodination of T_4 also results in the formation of reverse triiodothyronine (rT_3), which is calorigenically inactive.

Low triiodothyronine syndrome – The T_3 level is low in the fetus and newborn, in the elderly, and in cases of chronic caloric deprivation, hepatic cirrhosis, renal failure, surgical stress, and chronic illnesses.

➤*Pharmacokinetics:*

Absorption – Absorption of orally administered T_4 varies from 40% to 80% of the administered dose. T_4 absorption is increased by fasting and decreased in malabsorption syndromes and by certain foods, such as soybean infant formula. Dietary fiber decreases bioavailability of T_4. Absorption also may decrease with age. In addition, many drugs and foods affect T_4 absorption. In 4 hours, T_3 is approximately 95% absorbed. The hormones in natural preparations are absorbed in a manner similar to the synthetic hormones.

Distribution – More than 99% of circulating hormones are bound to serum proteins, including thyroxine-binding globulin (TBG) and thyroxine-binding prealbumin (TBPA) and albumin (TBA), whose capacities and affinities vary for the hormones. The higher affinity of T_4 for TBG and TBPA as compared with T_3 partially explains the higher serum levels and longer half-life of T_4. Both protein-bound hormones exist in reverse equilibrium with minute amounts of free hormone, the latter accounting for the metabolic activity.

Metabolism – Approximately 80% of T_3 comes from monodeiodination of T_4. Deiodination of T_4 occurs at a number of sites, including liver, kidney, and other tissues. The conjugated hormone, in the form of glucuronide or sulfate, is found in the bile and gut where it may complete an enterohepatic circulation. Of T_4 metabolized daily, 80% to 85% is deiodinated to yield equal amounts of T_3 and reverse T_3 (rT_3). T_3 and rT_3 are further deiodinated to diiodothyronine.

Excretion – Thyroid hormones are primarily eliminated by the kidneys. A portion of the conjugated hormone reaches the colon unchanged and is eliminated in the feces. Approximately 20% of T_4 is eliminated in the stool. Urinary excretion of T_4 decreases with age.

Various Pharmacokinetic Parameters of Thyroid Hormones

Hormone	Ratio in thyroglobulin	Biologic potency	Half-life (days)	Protein binding (%)[a]
Levothyroxine (T_4)	10 to 20	1	6 to 7[b]	99+
Liothyronine (T_3)	1	4	≤ 2.5	99+

[a] Includes TBG, TBPA, and TBA.
[b] 3 to 4 days in hyperthyroidism, 9 to 10 days in hypothyroidism.

Contraindications

In patients with diagnosed but uncorrected adrenal cortical insufficiency; untreated thyrotoxicosis; hypersensitivity to active or extraneous constituents.

Levothyroxine is contraindicated in patients with untreated subclinical (suppressed serum TSH level with normal T_3 and T_4 levels) and in patients with acute MI.

Concomitant use of *Triostat* and artificial rewarming of patients is contraindicated.

Warnings

➤*Obesity:* Obesity has been treated with thyroid hormones. In euthyroid patients, hormonal replacement doses are ineffective for weight reduction. Larger doses may produce serious or even life-threatening toxicity, particularly when given with sympathomimetic amines such as anorexiants.

➤*Infertility:* Thyroid hormone therapy is unjustified for the treatment of male or female infertility unless the condition is accompanied by hypothyroidism.

➤*Cardiovascular disease:* Use great caution when the integrity of the cardiovascular system, particularly the coronary arteries, is suspected. This includes patients with angina pectoris or the elderly, in whom there is a greater likelihood of occult cardiac disease. In these patients, initiate therapy with low doses. When, in such patients, a euthyroid state only can be reached at the expense of an aggravation of the cardiovascular disease, reduce thyroid hormone dosage.

Overtreatment with levothyroxine sodium may have adverse cardiovascular effects such as an increase in heart rate, cardiac wall thickness, and cardiac contractility and may precipitate angina or arrhythmias. During surgical procedures, closely monitor patients with coronary artery disease who are receiving levothyroxine therapy because the possibility of precipitating cardiac arrhythmias may be greater in those treated with levothyroxine. Concomitant administration of levothyroxine and sympathomimetic agents to patients with coronary artery disease may precipitate coronary insufficiency.

➤*Endocrine disorders:* Thyroid hormone therapy in patients with concomitant diabetes mellitus or insipidus or adrenal cortical insufficiency (Addison disease) exacerbates the intensity of their symptoms. Appropriate adjustments in the therapy of these concomitant endocrine diseases are required.

Autoimmune polyglandular syndrome – Occasionally, chronic autoimmune thyroiditis may occur in association with other autoimmune disorders, such as adrenal insufficiency, pernicious anemia, and insulin-dependent diabetes mellitus. Treat patients with concomitant adrenal insufficiency with replacement glucocorticoids prior to initiation of treatment. Failure to do so may precipitate an acute adrenal crisis when thyroid hormone therapy is initiated because of increased metabolic clearance of glucocorticoids by thyroid hormone. Patients with diabetes mellitus may require upward adjustments of their antidiabetic therapeutic regimens.

In patients with secondary or tertiary hypothyroidism, consider additional hypothalamic/pituitary hormone deficiencies and, if diagnosed, treat.

➤*Nontoxic diffuse goiter or nodular thyroid disease:* Exercise caution when administering levothyroxine to patients with nontoxic diffuse goiter or nodular thyroid disease in order to prevent precipitation of thyrotoxicosis. If the serum TSH is already suppressed, do not administer levothyroxine.

➤*Severe and prolonged hypothyroidism:* Severe and prolonged hypothyroidism can lead to a decreased level of adrenocortical activity commensurate with the lowered metabolic state. When thyroid replacement therapy is administered, the metabolism increases at a greater rate than adrenocortical activity, which can precipitate adrenocortical insufficiency. Therefore, in severe and prolonged hypothyroidism, supplemental adrenocortical steroids may be necessary.

➤*Morphologic hypogonadism and nephrosis:* Rule out morphologic hypogonadism and nephrosis prior to initiating therapy. If hypopituitarism is present, the adrenal deficiency must be corrected prior to starting the drug.

➤*Myxedema:* Patients with myxedema are particularly sensitive to thyroid preparations. Start dosage at a very low level and increase gradually, as acute changes may precipitate adverse cardiovascular events. Myxedema coma therapy requires simultaneous administration of glucocorticoids.

➤*Hyperthyroid effects:* In rare instances, the administration of thyroid hormone may precipitate a hyperthyroid state or may aggravate existing hyperthyroidism.

➤*Pregnancy: Category A.* Thyroid hormones cross the placental barrier to some extent, as evidenced by levels in cord blood of athyreotic fetuses being approximately one-third maternal levels. Transfer of thyroid hormone from the mother to the fetus, however, may not be adequate to prevent in utero hypothyroidism. Clinical experience does not indicate any adverse effect on the fetus when thyroid hormones are administered to a pregnant woman. Do not discontinue thyroid replacement therapy in hypothyroid women during pregnancy.

➤*Lactation:* Minimal amounts of thyroid hormones are excreted in breast milk. Thyroid is not associated with serious adverse reactions. However, exercise caution when thyroid is administered to a nursing woman.

➤*Children:* There is limited experience with liothyronine sodium injection in the pediatric population. Safety and efficacy in pediatric patients have not been established.

Congenital hypothyroidism – Pregnant women provide little or no thyroid hormone to the fetus. The incidence of congenital hypothyroidism is relatively high (1:4,000) and the hypothyroid fetus would not benefit from the small amounts of hormone crossing the placenta. Routine determinations of serum T_4 and/or TSH are strongly advised in neonates in view of the deleterious effects of thyroid deficiency on growth and development.

Initiate treatment immediately upon diagnosis, and maintain for life, unless transient hypothyroidism is suspected; in this case, therapy may be interrupted for 2 to 8 weeks after 3 years of age to reassess the condition. Cessation of therapy is justified in patients who have maintained a normal TSH during those 2 to 8 weeks.

In infants, excessive doses of thyroid hormone preparations may produce craniosynostosis and may adversely affect the tempo of brain maturation and accelerate the bone age with resultant premature closure of the epiphyses and compromised adult stature.

In children, partial loss of hair may be experienced in the first few months of thyroid therapy; this usually is a transient phenomenon that results in later recovery.

Precautions

➤*Monitoring:* Treatment of patients with thyroid hormones requires the periodic assessment of thyroid status by means of appropriate laboratory tests. The TSH suppression test can be used to test the effectiveness of any thyroid preparation, keeping in mind the relative insensitivity of the infant pituitary to the negative feedback effect of thyroid hormones. Serum T_4 levels can be used to test the effectiveness of all thyroid medications except T_3. When the total serum T_4 is low but TSH is normal, a test specific to assess unbound (free) T_4 levels is warranted.

The frequency of TSH monitoring during levothyroxine dose titration depends on the clinical situation, but it is generally recommended at 6- to 8-week intervals until normalization. For patients who have recently initiated levothyroxine therapy and whose serum TSH has normalized or in patients who have had their dosage or brand of levothyroxine changed, measure the serum TSH concentration after 8 to 12 weeks. When the optimum replacement dose has been attained, clinical (physical examination) and biochemical monitoring may be performed every 6 to 12 months, depending on the clinical situation, and whenever there is a change in the patient's status.

The recommended frequency of monitoring of TSH and total or free T_4 in children is as follows: At 2 and 4 weeks after initiation of treatment; every 1 to 2 months during the first year of life; every 2 to 3 months between 1 and 3 years of age; and every 3 to 12 months thereafter until growth is completed. It is recommended that TSH and T_4 levels and a physical examination, if indicated, be performed 2 weeks after any change in levothyroxine dosage.

Specific measurements of T_4 and T_3 by competitive protein binding or radioimmunoassay are not influenced by blood levels of organic or inorganic iodine and have essentially replaced older tests (ie, PBI, BEI, T_4 by column) (see Administration and Dosage).

Persistent clinical and laboratory evidence of hypothyroidism in spite of adequate dosage replacement indicates poor patient compliance, poor absorption, excessive fecal loss, or inactivity of the preparation. Intracellular resistance to thyroid hormone is rare.

➤*Decreased bone mineral density:* In women, long-term levothyroxine therapy has been associated with increased bone resorption, thereby decreasing bone mineral density, especially in postmenopausal women on greater than replacement doses or in women who are receiving suppressive doses of levothyroxine. The increased bone resorption may be associated with increased serum levels and urinary excretion of calcium and phosphorus, elevations in bone alkaline phosphatase, and suppressed serum parathyroid hormone levels. Therefore, it is recommended that patients receiving levothyroxine be given the minimum dose necessary to achieve the desired clinical and biochemical response.

Drug Interactions

Thyroid Hormone Drug Interactions

Precipitant drug	Object drug[a]		Description
Amiodarone Glucocorticoids (eg, dexamethasone ≥ 4 mg/day) Propylthiouracil	Thyroid hormones	⬇	Concurrent use may decrease the peripheral conversion of T_4 to T_3, leading to decreased T_3 levels. However, serum T_4 levels are usually normal but occasionally may be slightly elevated.
Antacids (aluminum and magnesium hydroxides) Bile acid sequestrants (cholestyramine, colestipol) Calcium carbonate Iron salts Sodium polystyrene sulfonate Simethicone Sucralfate	Thyroid hormones	⬇	Concurrent use may reduce the efficacy of the thyroid hormone because of possible binding in the GI tract, preventing absorption. Separate administration by at least 4 hours.
Beta-blockers (eg, propranolol >160 mg/day)	Thyroid hormones	⬇	Concurrent use may decrease the peripheral conversion of T_4 to T_3, leading to decreased T_3 levels. However, serum T_4 levels usually are normal but occasionally may be slightly elevated.
Thyroid hormones	Beta-blockers		The actions of particular beta blockers may be impaired when the hypothyroid patient is converted to the euthyroid state.
Carbamazepine Hydantoins Phenobarbital Rifamycins	Thyroid hormones	⬇	Hepatic degradation of levothyroxine may increase, resulting in increased levothyroxine requirements.
Estrogens, oral contraceptives	Thyroid hormones	⬇	Estrogens increase TBG and may therefore decrease the response to thyroid hormone therapy in patients with a nonfunctioning thyroid gland. An increased thyroid dose may be needed.
Furosemide (> 80 mg IV) Heparin Hydantoins NSAIDs Salicylates (> 2 g/day)	Thyroid hormones	⟷	Administration of these agents with levothyroxine results in an initial transient increase in FT_4. Continued administration results in a decrease in serum T_4 and normal FT_4 and TSH; therefore, patients are clinically euthyroid.
Selective serotonin reuptake inhibitors (eg, sertraline)	Thyroid hormones	⬇	Administration of sertraline in patients stabilized on levothyroxine may result in increased levothroxine requirements.
Tricyclic antidepressants Tetracyclic antidepressants	Thyroid hormones	⬆	Concurrent use of tricyclic/tetracyclic antidepressants and levothyroxine may increase the therapeutic and toxic effects of both drugs, possibly because of increased receptor sensitivity to catecholamines. Toxic effects may include increased risk of cardiac arrhythmias and CNS stimulation.
Thyroid hormones	Tricyclic antidepressants Tetracyclic antidepressants		
Thyroid hormones	Anticoagulants	⬆	The anticoagulant action is increased; a decreased dose may be necessary.
Thyroid hormones	Antidiabetic agents Biguanides Meglitinides Sulfonylureas Thiazolidinediones Insulin	⬇	Initiating thyroid hormones may cause increases in insulin or oral hypoglycemic requirements. Monitor closely.
Thyroid hormones	Digitalis glycosides	⬇	Serum digitalis glycoside levels are reduced in hyperthyroidism or when the hypothyroid patient is converted to the euthyroid state. Therapeutic effects of digitalis glycosides may be reduced.
Thyroid hormones	Growth hormones (somatrem, somatropin)	⬆	Excessive use of thyroid hormones with growth hormones may accelerate epiphyseal closure. However, untreated hypothyroidism may interfere with growth response to growth hormone.
Thyroid hormones	Ketamine	⬆	Concurrent use may produce marked hypertension and tachycardia. Administer with caution.
Thyroid hormones	Radiographic agents	⬇	Thyroid hormones may reduce the uptake of ^{123}I, ^{131}I, ^{99m}TC.
Thyroid hormones	Sympathomimetics	⬆	Concurrent use may increase the effects of either agent. Thyroid hormones may increase the risk of coronary insufficiency when sympathomimetics are given to patients with coronary artery disease. Use with caution.
Sympathomimetics	Thyroid hormones		
Thyroid hormones	Theophyllines	⬆	Decreased theophylline clearance can be expected in hypothyroid patients; clearance returns to normal when euthyroid state is achieved.

[a] ⬆ = Object drug increased ⬇ = Object drug decreased
⟷ = Undetermined clinical effect.

➤*Drug/Lab test interactions:* Consider changes in TBG concentration when interpreting T_4 and T_3 values. In such cases, measure the unbound (free) hormone and/or free T_4 index (FT_4I). Pregnancy, infectious hepatitis, estrogens, estrogen-containing oral contraceptives, and acute intermittent porphyria increase TBG concentrations. Decreases in TBG concentrations are observed in nephrosis, severe hypoproteinemia, severe liver disease, and acromegaly, and after androgen or corticosteroid therapy. Familial hyper- or hypothyroxine binding globulinemias have been described. The incidence of TBG deficiency approximates 1 in 9,000.

Medicinal or dietary iodine interferes with all in vivo tests of radioiodine uptake, producing low uptakes that may not reflect a true decrease in hormone synthesis.

Cytokines: Interferon-α and interleukin-2 – Therapy with interferon-α has been associated with the development of antithyroid microsomal antibodies in 20% of patients and some have transient hypothyroidism, hyperthyroidism, or both. Patients who have antithyroid antibodies before treatment are at higher risk of thyroid dysfunction during treatment. Interleukin-2 has been associated with transient painless thyroiditis in 20% of patients. Interferon-β and -γ have not been reported to cause thyroid dysfunction.

Drugs That May Reduce TSH Secretion

Dopamine/Dopamine agonists Glucocorticoids Octreotide	Use of these agents may result in a transient reduction in TSH secretion when administered at the following doses: Dopamine (≥ 1 mcg/kg/min); glucocorticoids (hydrocortisone ≥ 100 mg/day or equivalent); octreotide (> 100 mcg/day).

Drugs That May Decrease Thyroid Hormone Secretion	
Aminoglutethimide Amiodarone Iodide (including iodine-containing radiographic contrastagents) Lithium Methimazole Propylthiouracil (PTU) Sulfonamides Tolbutamide	Long-term lithium therapy can result in goiter in up to 50% of patients and in subclinical or overt hypothyroidism, each in up to 20% of patients. Oral cholecystographic agents and amiodarone slowly are excreted, producing more prolonged hypothyroidism than parenterally administered iodinated contrast agents. Long-term aminoglutethimide therapy may minimally decrease T_4 and T_3 levels and increase TSH, although all values remain within normal limits in most patients.

Drugs That May Increase Thyroid Hormone Secretion	
Amiodarone Iodide (including iodine-containing radiographic contrast agents)	Iodide and drugs that contain pharmacologic amounts of iodide may cause hyperthyroidism in euthyroid patients with Grave disease previously treated with antithyroid drugs or in euthyroid patients with thyroid autonomy (eg, multinodular goiter or hyperfunctioning thyroid adenoma). Hyperthyroidism may develop over several weeks and may persist for several months after therapy discontinuation. Amiodarone may induce hyperthyroidism by causing thyroiditis.

Drugs That May Alter Serum TBG Concentration	
Drugs that may increase serum TBG concentration	Drugs that may decrease serum TBG concentration
Estrogen-containing oral contraceptives Estrogens (oral) Heroin/Methadone 5-Fluorouracil Mitotane Tamoxifen	Androgens/Anabolic steroids Asparaginase Glucocorticoids Slow-release nicotinic acid

Drugs Associated with Thyroid Hormone and/or TSH Level Alterations by Various Mechanisms	
Chloral hydrate	Nitroprusside
Diazepam	Para-aminosalicylate sodium
Ethionamide	Perphenazine
Lovastatin	Resorcinol (excessive topical use)
Metoclopramide	Thiazide diuretics
6-Mercaptopurine	

➤*Drug/Food interactions:* Consumption of certain foods may affect levothyroxine absorption, thereby necessitating adjustments in dosing. Soybean flour (infant formula), cotton seed meal, walnuts, and dietary fiber may bind and decrease the absorption of levothyroxine from the GI tract.

Adverse Reactions

Adverse reactions other than those indicating hyperthyroidism caused by therapeutic overdosage, initially or during the maintenance period, are rare. Symptoms of overdosage include the following:

➤*Cardiovascular:* Palpitations; tachycardia; arrhythmias; angina; cardiac arrest; increased pulse and blood pressure; CHF; MI.

➤*CNS:* Tremors; headache; nervousness; insomnia; hyperactivity; anxiety, irritability; emotional lability; seizures (rare).

➤*GI:* Diarrhea; vomiting; abdominal cramps.

➤*Hypersensitivity:* Allergic skin reactions (rare). Hypersensitivity reactions to inactive ingredients have occurred in patients treated with thyroid hormone products. These include the following: Urticaria, pruritus, skin rash, flushing, angioedema, various GI symptoms (eg, abdominal pain, nausea, vomiting, diarrhea), fever, arthralgia, serum sickness, and wheezing. Hypersensitivity to levothyroxine itself is not known to occur.

➤*Miscellaneous:* Weight loss; fatigue; increased appetite; menstrual irregularities; excessive sweating; heat intolerance; fever; muscle weakness; dyspnea; hair loss; flushing; decreased bone mineral density; impaired fertility; increase in liver function tests.

Pseudotumor cerebri and slipped capital femoral epiphysis have been reported in children receiving levothyroxine therapy. Overtreatment may result in craniosynostosis in infants and premature closure of the epiphyses in children with resultant compromised adult height.

Liothyronine injection only – Hypotension; phlebitis; twitching.

Overdosage

➤*Acute massive overdosage:* Large doses of antithyroid drugs (eg, methimazole, propylthiouracil) followed in 1 to 2 hours by large doses of iodine may be given to inhibit synthesis and release of thyroid hormones. Glucocorticoids may be given to inhibit the conversion of T_4 to T_3. Because T_4 is highly protein bound, very little drug will be removed by dialysis. Treatment is aimed at reducing GI absorption of the drug and counteracting central and peripheral effects, mainly those of increased sympathetic activity. Refer to General Management of Acute Overdosage. Cardiac glycosides may be indicated if CHF develops. Control fever, hypoglycemia, or fluid loss, if needed. Antiadrenergic agents, particularly propranolol (1 to 3 mg IV over 10 minutes or 80 to 160 mg orally per day), have been used to treat increased sympathetic activity.

➤*Symptoms:* Chronic excessive dosage will produce signs and symptoms of hyperthyroidism (eg, headache, irritability, nervousness, tremor, sweating, increased bowel motility, menstrual irregularities). Angina pectoris, arrhythmia, tachycardia, acute MI, or CHF may be induced or aggravated. In addition, confusion and disorientation may occur. Cerebral embolism, shock, coma, and death have been reported. Seizures have occurred in a child ingesting approximately 18 to 20 mg levothyroxine. Symptoms may not necessarily be evident or may not appear until several days after ingestion of levothyroxine sodium. Massive overdosage may result in symptoms resembling thyroid storm.

➤*Treatment:* Reduce dosage or temporarily discontinue therapy. Reinstitute treatment at a lower dosage. In healthy individuals, normal hypothalamic-pituitary-thyroid axis function is restored in 6 to 8 weeks after thyroid suppression.

Patient Information

Replacement therapy is to be taken for life, except in cases of transient hypothyroidism, usually associated with thyroiditis, and in those receiving a trial of the drug.

Take as a single daily dose, preferably at least 30 minutes before breakfast.

➤*Brand interchange:* Inform patients not to change from one brand of this drug to another without consulting their pharmacist or physician. Products manufactured by different companies may not be equally effective.

Inform patients not to discontinue medication except on the advice of a physician.

Instruct patients to notify their physician if the following symptoms occur: Rapid or irregular heartbeat, chest pain, shortness of breath, leg cramps, headache, nervousness, irritability, sleeplessness, tremors, change in appetite, weight gain or loss, vomiting, diarrhea, excessive sweating, heat intolerance, fever, changes in menstrual periods, hives or skin rash, or any other unusual medical event.

Children my experience partial hair loss in the first few months of therapy, but this is usually a transient phenomenon that results in later recovery.

Not for use as primary or adjunctive therapy in a weight-control program.

Advise patients to notify their physician if they become pregnant while taking thyroid hormones; their dose may need to be changed.

THYROID DESICCATED[a]

Rx	**Armour Thyroid** (Forest)	**Tablets:** 15 mg (¼ gr)[b]	Dextrose. (A TC). Lt. tan. In 100s.
Rx	**Armour Thyroid** (Forest)	**Tablets:** 30 mg (½ gr)[b]	Dextrose. (A TD). Lt. tan. In 100s, 1,000s, 50,000s and UD 100s.
Rx	**Nature-Throid** (Western Research Laboratories)	**Tablets:** 32.4 mg (½ gr)[b]	In 100s.
Rx	**Westhroid** (Western Research Laboratories)		In 100s.
Rx	**Thyroid USP** (Various, eg, URL)	**Tablets:** 32.5 mg (½ gr)[b]	In 100s and 1,000s.
Rx	**Armour Thyroid** (Forest)	**Tablets:** 60 mg (1 gr)[b]	Dextrose. (A TE). Lt. tan. In 100s, 1,000s, 5000s, 50,000s, and UD 100s.
Rx	**Nature-Throid** (Western Research Laboratories)	**Tablets:** 64.8 mg (1 gr)[b]	In 100s.
Rx	**Westhroid** (Western Research Laboratories)		In 100s.
Rx	**Thyroid USP** (Various, eg, URL)	**Tablets:** 65 mg (1 gr)[b]	In 100s and 1,000s.
Rx	**Armour Thyroid** (Forest)	**Tablets:** 90 mg (1½ gr)[b]	Dextrose. (A TJ). Lt. tan. In 100s.
Rx	**Armour Thyroid** (Forest)	**Tablets:** 120 mg (2 gr)[b]	Dextrose. (A TF). Lt. tan. In 100s, 1,000s, 50,000s, and UD 100s.

Thyroid Hormones

THYROID DESICCATED[a]

Rx	**Nature-Throid** (Western Research Laboratories)	**Tablets:** 129.6 mg (2 gr)[b]	In 100s.
Rx	**Westhroid** (Western Research Laboratories)		In 100s.
Rx	**Thyroid USP** (Various, eg, URL)	**Tablets:** 130 mg (2 gr)[b]	In 100s and 1,000s.
Rx	**Armour Thyroid** (Forest)	**Tablets:** 180 mg (3 gr)[b]	Dextrose. (A TG). Lt. tan, scored. In 100s and 1,000s.
Rx	**Nature-Throid** (Western Research Laboratories)	**Tablets:** 194.4 mg (3 gr)[b]	In 100s.
Rx	**Westhroid** (Western Research Laboratories)		In 100s.
Rx	**Thyroid USP** (Various, eg, URL)	**Tablets:** 195 mg (3 gr)[b]	In 100s and 1,000s.
Rx	**Armour Thyroid** (Forest)	**Tablets:** 240 mg (4 gr)[b]	Dextrose. (A TH). Lt. tan. In 100s.
Rx	**Armour Thyroid** (Forest)	**Tablets:** 300 mg (5 gr)[b]	Dextrose. (A TI). Lt. tan, scored. In 100s.
Rx	**Bio-Throid** (Bio-Tech)	**Capsules:** 7.5 mg (⅛ gr)[b]	In 100s and 1,000s.
		15 mg (¼ gr)[b]	In 100s and 1,000s.
		30 mg (½ gr)[b]	In 100s and 1,000s.
		60 mg (1 gr)[b]	In 100s and 1,000s.
		90 mg (1½ gr)[b]	In 100s and 1,000s.
		120 mg (2 gr)[b]	In 100s and 1,000s.
		150 mg (2½ gr)[b]	In 100s and 1,000s.
		180 mg (3 gr)[b]	In 100s and 1,000s.
		240 mg (4 gr)[b]	In 100s and 1,000s.

[a] Porcine derived.

[b] The amounts given in grains are according to the respective manufacturers. The exact equivalent is: 1 gr = 64.8 mg.

THYROID DESICCATED — ORAL

For complete prescribing information, refer to the Thyroid Drugs group monograph.

WARNING

Drugs with thyroid hormone activity, alone or with other therapeutic agents, have been used for the treatment of obesity. In euthyroid patients, doses within the range of daily hormonal requirements are ineffective for weight reduction. Larger doses may produce serious or even life-threatening manifestations of toxicity, particularly when given in association with sympathomimetic amines such as those used for their anorectic effects.

Indications

➤*Hypothyroidism:* As replacement or supplemental therapy in patients with hypothyroidism of any etiology, except transient hypothyroidism during the recovery phase of subacute thyroiditis. This category includes cretinism, myxedema, and ordinary hypothyroidism in patients of any age (children, adults, the elderly), or state (including pregnancy); primary hypothyroidism resulting from functional deficiency, primary atrophy, partial or total absence of thyroid gland, or the effects of surgery, radiation, or drugs, with or without the presence of goiter; and secondary (pituitary) or tertiary (hypothalamic) hypothyroidism.

➤*Pituitary thyroid stimulating hormone (TSH) suppression:* As pituitary TSH suppressants in the treatment or prevention of various types of euthyroid goiters, including thyroid nodules, subacute or chronic lymphocytic thyroiditis (Hashimoto), and multinodular goiter and in the management of thyroid cancer.

➤*Diagnostic agent:* As diagnostic agents in suppression tests to differentiate suspected mild hyperthyroidism or thyroid gland autonomy.

Administration and Dosage

Thyroid USP is composed of desiccated animal porcine thyroid glands. liothyronine (T_3) is approximately 4 times as potent as levothyroxine (T_4) on a microgram for microgram basis. They provide 38 mcg T_4 and 9 mcg T_3 per grain of thyroid.

The dosage of thyroid hormones is determined by the indication and must in every case be individualized according to patient response and laboratory findings.

➤*Hypothyroidism:*

Initial dosage – Institute therapy using low doses, with increments that depend on cardiovascular status. Usual starting dose is 30 mg, with increments of 15 mg every 2 to 3 weeks. Use 15 mg/day in patients with long-standing myxedema, particularly if cardiovascular impairment is suspected. Reduce dosage if angina occurs.

Maintenance dosage – Most patients require 60 to 120 mg/day; failure to respond to 180 mg doses suggests lack of compliance or malabsorption. Adequate therapy usually results in normal TSH and T_4 levels after 2 to 3 weeks of therapy.

Dosage readjustment: Readjust dosage within the first 4 weeks of therapy after proper clinical and laboratory evaluations.

➤*Thyroid cancer:* Larger amounts of thyroid hormone than those used for replacement therapy are required.

➤*Diagnostic agent:* For adults, the usual suppressive dose of T_4 is 1.56 mcg/kg of body weight per day given for 7 to 10 days. These doses usually yield normal serum T_4 and T_3 levels and lack of response to TSH.

➤*Children:* Follow recommendations in the following table. In infants with congenital hypothyroidism, institute therapy with full doses as soon as diagnosis is made.

Recommended Pediatric Dosage for Congenital Hypothyroidism

Age	Dose per day (mg)	Daily dose per kg (mg)
0 to 6 mo	7.5 to 30	2.4 to 6
6 to 12 mo	30 to 45	3.6 to 4.8
1 to 5 y	45 to 60	3 to 3.6
6 to 12 y	60 to 90	2.4 to 3
> 12 y	> 90	1.2 to 1.8

➤*Special populations:* Initiate therapy in low doses (15 to 30 mg) in patients with angina pectoris or the elderly, in whom there is a greater likelihood of occult cardiac disease.

➤*Storage/Stability:* Store at controlled room temperature 15° to 30°C (59° to 86°F) in capped bottles or unbroken plastic strip packing. Dispense in tight, light-resistant containers.

LEVOTHYROXINE SODIUM (T_4; L-thyroxine)

Rx	**Levothyroxine Sodium** (Various, eg, Mylan, Sandoz)	**Tablets:** 0.025 mg	In 100s.
Rx	**Levothroid** (Forest)		(25). Orange, caplet shape. In 100s and 1,000s.
Rx	**Levoxyl** (Jones Pharma)		(25). Orange, oval. In 100s and 1,000s.
Rx	**Synthroid** (Abbott)		Sugar, lactose. (SYNTHROID 25). Orange, scored. In 100s and 1,000s.
Rx	**Thyro-Tabs** (Lloyd[a])		(25). Orange, capsule shape. In 100s and 1,000s.
Rx	**Levothyroxine Sodium** (Various, eg, Mylan, Sandoz)	**Tablets** 0.05 mg	In 100s.
Rx	**Levothroid** (Forest)		(50). White, caplet shape. In 100s and 1,000s.
Rx	**Levoxyl** (Jones Pharma)		(50). White, oval. In 100s and 1,000s.
Rx	**Synthroid** (Abbott)		Sugar, lactose. (SYNTHROID 50). White, scored. In 100s, 1,000s, and UD 100s.
Rx	**Thyro-Tabs** (Lloyd[a])		(50). White, capsule shape. In 100s, 1,000s.

LEVOTHYROXINE SODIUM (T_4; L-thyroxine)

Rx	**Levothyroxine Sodium** (Various, eg, Mylan, Sandoz)	**Tablets:** 0.075 mg	In 100s.
Rx	**Levothroid** (Forest)		(75) Violet, caplet shape. In 100s and 1,000s.
Rx	**Levoxyl** (Jones Pharma)		(75). Purple, oval. In 100s and 1,000s.
Rx	**Synthroid** (Abbott)		Sugar, lactose. (SYNTHROID 75). Violet, scored. In 100s, 1,000s, and UD 100s.
Rx	**Thyro-Tabs** (Lloyd[a])		(75). Violet, capsule shape. In 100s and 1,000s.
Rx	**Levothyroxine Sodium** (Various, eg, Mylan, Sandoz)	**Tablets:** 0.088 mg	In 100s.
Rx	**Levothroid** (Forest)		(88). Mint green, caplet shape. In 100s and 1,000s.
Rx	**Levoxyl** (Jones Pharma)		(88). Olive, oval. In 100s, 1,000s, and UD 100s.
Rx	**Synthroid** (Abbott)		Sugar, lactose. (SYNTHROID 88). Olive, scored. In 100s and 1,000s.
Rx	**Thyro-Tabs** (Lloyd[a])		(88). Rose, capsule shape. In 100s and 1,000s.
Rx	**Unithroid** (Lannett)		Lactose. (JSP 561). Olive, scored. In 100s.
Rx	**Levothyroxine Sodium** (Various, eg, Mylan, Sandoz)	**Tablets:** 0.1 mg	In 100s.
Rx	**Levothroid** (Forest)		(100). Yellow, caplet shape. In 100s and 1,000s.
Rx	**Levoxyl** (Jones Pharma)		(100). Yellow, oval. In 100s and 1,000s.
Rx	**Synthroid** (Abbott)		Sugar, lactose. (SYNTHROID 100). Yellow, scored. In 100s, 1,000s, and UD 100s.
Rx	**Thyro-Tabs** (Lloyd[a])		(100). Yellow, capsule shape. In 100s and 1,000s.
Rx	**Levothyroxine Sodium** (Various, eg, Mylan, Sandoz)	**Tablets:** 0.112 mg	In 100s.
Rx	**Levothroid** (Forest)		(112). Rose, caplet shape. In 100s and 1,000s.
Rx	**Levoxyl** (Jones Pharma)		(112). Rose, oval. In 100s, 1,000s, and UD 100s.
Rx	**Synthroid** (Abbott)		Sugar, lactose. (SYNTHROID 112). Rose, scored. In 100s and 1,000s.
Rx	**Thyro-Tabs** (Lloyd[a])		(112). Mint green, capsule shape. In 100s and 1,000s.
Rx	**Unithroid** (Lannett)		Lactose. (JSP 562). Rose, scored. In 100s.
Rx	**Levothyroxine Sodium** (Various, eg, Mylan, Sandoz)	**Tablets:** 0.125 mg	In 100s.
Rx	**Levothroid** (Forest)		(125). Brown, caplet shape. In 100s and 1,000s.
Rx	**Levoxyl** (Jones Pharma)		(125). Brown, oval. In 100s and 1,000s.
Rx	**Synthroid** (Abbott)		Sugar, lactose. (SYNTHROID 125). Brown, scored. In 100s, 1,000s, and UD 100s.
Rx	**Thyro-Tabs** (Lloyd[a])		(125). Brown, capsule shape. In 100s and 1,000s.
Rx	**Levothyroxine Sodium** (Sandoz)	**Tablets:** 0.137 mg	(GG 137). Turquoise, scored, capsule shape. In 100s.
Rx	**Levoxyl** (Jones Pharma)		(137). Dk blue, oval. In 100s, 1,000s, and UD 100s.
Rx	**Synthroid** (Abbott)		Sugar, lactose. (SYNTHROID 137). Turquoise, scored. In 100s and 1,000s.
Rx	**Levothyroxine Sodium** (Various, eg, Mylan, Sandoz)	**Tablets:** 0.15 mg	In 100s.
Rx	**Levothroid** (Forest)		(150). Blue, caplet shape. In 100s and 1,000s.
Rx	**Levoxyl** (Jones Pharma)		(150). Blue, oval. In 100s and 1,000s.
Rx	**Synthroid** (Abbott)		Sugar, lactose. (SYNTHROID 150). Blue, scored. In 100s, 1,000s, and UD 100s.
Rx	**Thyro-Tabs** (Lloyd[a])		(150). Blue, capsule shape. In 100s and 1,000s.
Rx	**Unithroid** (Lannett)		Lactose. (JSP 520). Blue, scored. In 100s.
Rx	**Levothyroxine Sodium** (Various, eg, Mylan, Sandoz)	**Tablets:** 0.175 mg	In 100s.
Rx	**Levothroid** (Forest)		(175). Lilac, caplet shape. In 100s and 1,000s.
Rx	**Levoxyl** (Jones Pharma)		(175). Turquoise, oval. In 100s, 1,000s, and UD 100s.
Rx	**Synthroid** (Abbott)		Sugar, lactose. (SYNTHROID 175). Lilac, scored. In 100s and 1,000s.
Rx	**Thyro-Tabs** (Lloyd[a])		(175). Lilac, capsule shape. In 100s and 1,000s.
Rx	**Levothyroxine Sodium** (Various, eg, Mylan, Sandoz)	**Tablets:** 0.2 mg	In 100s.
Rx	**Levothroid** (Forest)		(200). Pink, caplet shape. In 100s and 1,000s.
Rx	**Levoxyl** (Jones Pharma)		(200). Pink, oval. In 100s and 1,000s.
Rx	**Synthroid** (Abbott)		Sugar, lactose. (SYNTHROID 200). Pink, scored. In 100s, 1,000s, and UD 100s.
Rx	**Thyro-Tabs** (Lloyd[a])		(200). Pink, capsule shape. In 100s and 1,000s.

LEVOTHYROXINE SODIUM (T_4; L-thyroxine)

Rx	**Levothyroxine Sodium** (Various, eg, Mylan, Sandoz)	**Tablets:** 0.3 mg	In 100s.
Rx	**Levothroid** (Forest)		(300). Green, caplet shape. In 100s and 1,000s.
Rx	**Levoxyl** (Jones Pharma)		(300). Green, oval. In 100s, 1,000s, and UD 100s.
Rx	**Synthroid** (Abbott)		Sugar, lactose. (SYNTHROID 300). Green, scored. In 100s and 1,000s.
Rx	**Thyro-Tabs** (Lloyd[a])		(300). Green, capsule shape. In 100s and 1,000s.
Rx	**Unithroid** (Lannett)		Lactose. (JSP 523). Green. In 100s.
Rx	**Levothyroxine Sodium** (Various, eg, Bedford, McGuff)	**Powder for injection, lyophilized:** 200 mcg	In 10 mL vials.
		500 mcg	In 10 mL vials.

[a] Lloyd, Inc., PO Box 130, Shenandoah, IA 51601; (800) 831-0004.

LEVOTHYROXINE SODIUM — ORAL

For complete and comparative prescribing information, refer to the Thyroid Hormones group monograph.

WARNING

Do not use thyroid hormones, including levothyroxine, either alone or with other therapeutic agents, for the treatment of obesity or for weight loss. In euthyroid patients, doses within the range of daily hormonal requirements are ineffective for weight reduction. Larger doses may produce serious or even life-threatening manifestations of toxicity, particularly when given in association with sympathomimetic amines such as those used for their anorectic effects.

Indications

➤*Hypothyroidism:* As replacement or supplemental therapy in congenital or acquired hypothyroidism of any etiology, except transient hypothyroidism during the recovery phase of subacute thyroiditis. Specific indications include primary (thyroidal), secondary (pituitary), and tertiary (hypothalamic) hypothyroidism and subclinical hypothyroidism. Primary hypothyroidism may result from functional deficiency, primary atrophy, partial or total congenital absence of the thyroid gland, or from the effects of surgery, radiation, or drugs, with or without the presence of goiter.

➤*Pituitary thyrotropin-stimulating hormone (TSH) suppression:* In the treatment or prevention of various types of euthyroid goiters, including thyroid nodules, subacute or chronic lymphocytic thyroiditis (Hashimoto thyroiditis), multinodular goiter and as an adjunct to surgery and radioiodine therapy in the management of thyrotropin-dependent well-differentiated thyroid cancer.

Administration and Dosage

➤*Administration:* Levothyroxine is administered as a single daily dose and should be taken in the morning on an empty stomach, at least 30 minutes to 1 hour before breakfast. Levothyroxine should be taken at least 4 hours apart from drugs that are known to interfere with its absorption (eg, aluminum- and magnesium-containing antacids; hydroxides, such as simethicone; bile acid sequestrants [cholestyramine and colestipol]; calcium carbonate; cation exchange resins [kayexalate]; ferrous sulfate; and sucralfate).

Because of the long half-life of levothyroxine, the peak therapeutic effect at a given dose of levothyroxine may not be attained for 4 to 6 weeks.

➤*Special populations:* Exercise caution when administering levothyroxine to patients with underlying cardiovascular disease, the elderly, and those with concomitant adrenal insufficiency.

➤*Hypothyroidism in adults and in children in whom growth and puberty are complete:* Therapy may begin at full replacement doses in otherwise healthy individuals who are at low risk of coronary artery disease. The average full replacement dosage of levothyroxine is approximately 1.7 mcg/kg/day (eg, 100 to 125 mcg/day for a 70 kg adult). Older patients may require less than 1 mcg/kg/day. Levothyroxine dosages greater than 200 mcg/day are seldom required. An inadequate response to daily dosages greater than or equal to 300 mcg/day is rare and may indicate poor compliance, malabsorption, or drug interactions.

For most patients older than 50 years of age or for patients younger than 50 years of age with underlying cardiac disease, an initial starting dosage of 25 to 50 mcg/day levothyroxine is recommended, with gradual increments in dose at 6- to 8-week intervals, as needed. The recommended starting dosage of levothyroxine in elderly patients with cardiac disease is 12.5 to 25 mcg/day, with gradual dose increments at 4- to 6-week intervals. The levothyroxine dose is generally adjusted in 12.5 to 25 mcg increments until the patient with primary hypothyroidism is clinically euthyroid and the serum TSH has normalized.

In patients with severe hypothyroidism, the recommended initial levothyroxine dosage is 12.5 to 25 mcg/day with increases of 25 mcg/day every 2 to 4 weeks, accompanied by clinical and laboratory assessment, until the TSH level is normalized.

In patients with secondary (pituitary) or tertiary (hypothalamic) hypothyroidism, titrate the levothyroxine dose until the patient is clinically euthyroid and the serum-free T_4 level is restored to the upper half of the normal range.

➤*Pediatric dosage (congenital or acquired hypothyroidism):*

General principles – In patients with congenital hypothyroidism, assess the adequacy of replacement therapy by measuring both serum TSH (using a sensitive assay) and total or free T_4. During the first 3 years of life, the serum total or free T_4 should be maintained at all times in the upper half of the normal range. Failure of the serum T_4 to increase into the upper half of the normal range within 2 weeks of initiation of levothyroxine therapy or of the serum TSH to decrease below 20 mU/L within 4 weeks should alert the physician to the possibility that the child is not receiving adequate therapy. Then make careful inquiry regarding compliance, dose of medication administered, and method of administration prior to raising the dose of levothyroxine.

The recommended frequency of monitoring of TSH and total or free T_4 in children is as follows: at 2 and 4 weeks after the initiation of treatment, every 1 to 2 months during the first year of life, every 2 to 3 months between 1 and 3 years of age, and every 3 to 12 months thereafter until growth is completed. More frequent intervals of monitoring may be necessary if poor compliance is suspected or abnormal values are obtained. It is recommended that TSH and T_4 levels and a physical examination, if indicated, be performed 2 weeks after any change in levothyroxine dosage.

In general, institute levothyroxine therapy at full replacement doses as soon as possible. Delays in diagnosis and institution of therapy may have deleterious effects on the child's intellectual and physical growth and development.

Avoid undertreatment and overtreatment. Undertreatment may result in poor school performance due to impaired concentration and slowed mentation and in reduced adult height. Overtreatment may accelerate the bone age and result in premature epiphyseal closure and compromised adult stature.

Levothyroxine may be administered to infants and children who cannot swallow intact tablets by crushing the tablet and suspending the freshly crushed tablet in a small amount (5 to 10 mL or 1 to 2 teaspoons) of water. This suspension can be administered by spoon or dropper. Do not store the suspension. Do not use foods that decrease absorption of levothyroxine for administering levothyroxine tablets. Soybean flour (infant formula), cotton seed meal, walnuts, and dietary fiber may bind and decrease the absorption of levothyroxine from the GI tract.

Newborns – The recommended starting dosage of levothyroxine in newborn infants is 10 to 15 mcg/kg/day. Consider a lower starting dosage (eg, 25 mcg/day) in infants at risk for cardiac failure, and increase the dose in 4 to 6 weeks as needed based on clinical and laboratory response to treatment. In infants with very low (less than 5 mcg/dL) or undetectable serum T_4 concentrations, the recommended initial starting dosage is 50 mcg/day of levothyroxine.

Infants and children – Levothyroxine therapy is usually initiated at full replacement doses, with the recommended dose per body weight decreasing with age (see the following table). However, in children with chronic or severe hypothyroidism, an initial dosage of 25 mcg/day of levothyroxine is recommended with increments of 25 mcg every 2 to 4 weeks until the desired effect is achieved.

Hyperactivity in an older child can be minimized if the starting dose is one-fourth of the recommended full replacement dose, and the dose is then increased on a weekly basis by an amount equal to one-fourth the full-recommended replacement dose until the full recommended replacement dose is reached.

Levothyroxine Dosing Guidelines for Pediatric Hypothyroidism

Age	Daily dosage per kg body weight[a]
0 to 3 months	10 to 15 mcg/kg/day
3 to 6 months	8 to 10 mcg/kg/day
6 to 12 months	6 to 8 mcg/kg/day
1 to 5 years	5 to 6 mcg/kg/day
6 to 12 years	4 to 5 mcg/kg/day
> 12 years but growth and puberty incomplete	2 to 3 mcg/kg/day
Growth and puberty complete	1.7 mcg/kg/day

[a] Adjust the dosage based on clinical response and laboratory parameters.

LEVOTHYROXINE SODIUM — ORAL

➤*Pregnancy:* Pregnancy may increase levothyroxine requirements.

➤*Subclinical hypothyroidism:* If this condition is treated, a lower levothyroxine dose (eg, 1 mcg/kg/day) than that used for full replacement may be adequate to normalize the serum TSH level. Monitor patients who are not treated yearly for changes in clinical status and thyroid laboratory parameters.

➤*TSH suppression in well-differentiated thyroid cancer and thyroid nodules:* The target level for TSH suppression in these conditions has not been established with controlled studies. In addition, the efficacy of TSH suppression for benign nodular disease is controversial. Therefore, individualize the dose of levothyroxine used for TSH suppression based on the specific disease and the patient being treated.

In the treatment of well-differentiated (papillary and follicular) thyroid cancer, levothyroxine is used as an adjunct to surgery and radioiodine therapy. Generally, TSH is suppressed to less than 0.1 milliunit/L, and this usually requires a levothyroxine dosage greater than 2 mcg/kg/day. However, in patients with high-risk tumors, the target level for TSH suppression may be less than 0.01 milliunit/L.

In the treatment of benign nodules and nontoxic multinodular goiter, TSH is generally suppressed to a higher target (eg, 0.1 to 0.5 milliunit/L for nodules and 0.5 to 1 milliunit/L for multinodular goiter) than that used for the treatment of thyroid cancer. Levothyroxine is contraindicated if the serum TSH is already suppressed due to the risk of precipitating overt thyrotoxicosis. If the serum TSH level is not suppressed, use levothyroxine with caution in conjunction with careful monitoring of thyroid function for evidence of hyperthyroidism and clinical monitoring for potentially associated adverse cardiovascular signs and symptoms of hyperthyroidism.

➤*Myxedema coma:* Myxedema coma is a life-threatening emergency characterized by poor circulation and hypometabolism, and may result in unpredictable absorption of levothyroxine from the GI tract. Therefore, oral thyroid hormone drug products are not recommended to treat this condition. Do not administer thyroid hormone products formulated for IV administration.

➤*Storage/Stability:* Store at 20° to 25°C (68° to 77°F); excursions permitted to 15° to 30°C (59° to 86°F). Protect levothyroxine tablets from light and moisture and dispense in tight, light-resistant containers with child-resistant closure.

LEVOTHYROXINE SODIUM — INJECTION

For complete and comparative prescribing information, refer to the Thyroid Hormones group monograph.

WARNING

Drugs with thyroid hormone activity, alone or together with other therapeutic agents, have been used for the treatment of obesity. In euthyroid patients, doses within the range of daily hormonal requirements are ineffective for weight reduction. Larger doses may produce serious or even life-threatening manifestations of toxicity, particularly when given in association with sympathomimetic amines such as those used for their anorectic effects.

Indications

➤*Hypothyroidism:* As specific replacement therapy for reduced or absent thyroid function of any etiology. Levothyroxine sodium can be used IV whenever a rapid onset of effect is critical, and either IV or IM in hypothyroid patients whenever the oral route is precluded for long periods of time.

Administration and Dosage

➤*Dosage:* Administer by by IM or IV. The initial parenteral dosage should be approximately one-half of the previously established oral dosage of levothyroxine sodium tablets. A daily maintenance dose of 50 to 100 mcg parenterally should suffice to maintain the euthyroid state, once established. Close observation of the patient, with individual adjustment of the dosage as needed, is recommended.

The age and general physical condition of the patient and the severity and duration of hypothyroid symptoms determine the starting dosage and the rate of incremental dosage increase leading to a final maintenance dosage. Clearly it is the physician's judgment of the severity of the disease and closer observation of patient response which determine the rate and extent of dosage increase.

In infants and children, there is great urgency to achieve full thyroid replacement because of the critical importance of thyroid hormone in sustaining growth and maturation. Despite the smaller body size, the dosage needed to sustain a full rate of growth, development and general thriving is higher in the child than in the adult.

Optimal maintenance levels should be adjusted individually to obtain normal serum T_3, T_4, free T_4, index and thyroid-stimulating hormone (TSH) values after several weeks of therapy for hypothyroidism. The patient's clinical status is most important and some patents may be clinically euthyroid with individual laboratory values that are not within normal range (ie, elevated total T_4 with normal T_3). An exception may be seen in congenital hypothyroidism where elevated serum TSH values may persist for the first 2 to 3 years of life despite normalization of free T_4 measurements. In such cases, it generally is recommended that maintenance of normal serum-free T_4 values alone should be considered therapeutically sufficient.

➤*Myxedema coma:* In myxedema coma or stupor, without concomitant severe heart disease, 200 to 500 mcg of levothyroxine sodium may be administered IV as a solution containing 100 mcg/mL. Do not add to other IV fluids. Although the patient may show evidence of increased responsivity within 6 to 8 hours, full therapeutic effect may not be evident until the following day. An additional 100 to 300 mcg or more may be given on the second day if evidence of significant and progressive improvements has not occurred. Levothyroxine sodium produces a predictable increase in the reservoir level of hormone with a 7-day half-life. This usually precludes the need for multiple injections but continued daily administration of lesser amounts parenterally should be maintained until the patient is fully capable of accepting a daily oral dose.

In the presence of concomitant heart disease, the sudden administration of such large doses of levothyroxine sodium IV is clearly not without its cardiovascular risks. Under such circumstances, IV therapy should not be undertaken without weighing the alternative risks of the myxedema coma and the cardiovascular disease. Clinical judgment in this situation may dictate smaller IV doses of levothyroxine sodium.

➤*Monitoring:* Appropriate laboratory tests are beneficial in monitoring thyroid replacement therapy. Although measurements of normal blood levels of thyroxine in patients on oral replacement regimens frequently coincide with clinical impressions of normal thyroid status, higher than normal levels occur occasionally and should not be considered evidence of overdosage per se. In all cases, clinical impressions of the well-being of the patient take precedence over laboratory determination of appropriate individual dosage.

➤*Reconstitution:* Reconstitute the lyophilized levothyroxine sodium by aseptically adding 5 mL of 0.9% Sodium Chloride Injection, USP only. Shake vial to ensure complete mixing. Use immediately after reconstitution. Do not add to other IV fluids. Discard any unused portion.

➤*Storage/Stability:* Store dry product at controlled room temperature 15° to 30°C (59° to 86°F). Protect from light.

LIOTHYRONINE SODIUM (T_3)

Rx	**Cytomel** (Monarch)	**Tablets:** 5 mcg	Sucrose. (JMI D14). White. In 100s.
		25 mcg	Sucrose. (JMI D16). White, scored. In 100s.
		50 mcg	Sucrose. (JMI D17). White, scored. In 100s.
Rx	**Triostat** (Monarch)	**Injection:** 10 mcg/mL	In 1 mL vials.[a]

[a] With 6.8% alcohol, 2.19 mg ammonia (as ammonium hydroxide) per mL.

LIOTHYRONINE SODIUM — ORAL

For complete and comparative prescribing information, refer to the Thyroid Hormones group monograph.

Indications

As replacement or supplemental therapy in patients with hypothyroidism of any etiology, except transient hypothyroidism during the recovery phase of subacute thyroiditis. This category includes cretinism, myxedema and ordinary hypothyroidism in patients of any age (pediatric patients, adults, the elderly), or state (including pregnancy); primary hypothyroidism resulting from functional deficiency, primary atrophy, partial or total absence of thyroid gland, or the effects of surgery, radiation, or drugs, with or without the presence of goiter; and secondary (pituitary) or tertiary (hypothalamic) hypothyroidism. As pituitary thyroid-stimulating hormone (TSH) suppressants, in the treatment or prevention of various types of euthyroid goiters, including thyroid nodules, subacute or chronic lymphocytic thyroiditis (Hashimoto's) and multinodular goiter. As diagnostic agents in suppression tests to differentiate suspected mild hyperthyroidism or thyroid gland autonomy.

Liothyronine sodium tablets can be used in patients allergic to desiccated thyroid or thyroid extract derived from pork or beef.

Administration and Dosage

The dosage of thyroid hormones is determined by the indication and must in every case be individualized according to patient response and laboratory findings.

Liothyronine sodium tablets are intended for oral administration; once-a-day dosage is recommended. Although liothyronine sodium has a rapid cutoff, its metabolic effects persist for a few days following discontinuance.

➤*Mild hypothyroidism:* Recommended starting dosage is 25 mcg daily. Daily dosage then may be increased by up to 25 mcg every 1 or 2 weeks. Usual maintenance dose is 25 to 75 mcg daily.

The rapid onset and dissipation of action of liothyronine sodium (T_3), as compared with levothyroxine sodium (T_4), has led some clinicians to prefer its use in patients who might be more susceptible to the untoward effects of thyroid medication. However, the wide swings in serum T_3 levels that follow

LIOTHYRONINE SODIUM — ORAL

its administration, and the possibility of more pronounced cardiovascular side effects, tend to counterbalance the stated advantages.

Liothyronine sodium tablets may be used in preference to levothyroxine (T_4) during radioisotope scanning procedures, since induction of hypothyroidism in those cases is more abrupt and can be of shorter duration. It may also be preferred when impairment of peripheral conversion of T_4 to T_3 is suspected.

➤*Myxedema:* Recommended starting dosage is 5 mcg daily. This may be increased by 5 to 10 mcg daily every 1 or 2 weeks. When 25 mcg daily is reached, dosage may be increased by 5 to 25 mcg every 1 or 2 weeks until a satisfactory therapeutic response is attained. Usual maintenance dose is 50 to 100 mcg daily.

➤*Congenital hypothyroidism:* Recommended starting dosage is 5 mcg daily, with a 5 mcg increment every 3 to 4 days until the desired response is achieved. Infants a few months old may require only 20 mcg daily for maintenance. At 1 year, 50 mcg daily may be required. Above 3 years, full adult dosage may be necessary.

➤*Simple (nontoxic) goiter:* Recommended starting dosage is 5 mcg daily. This dosage may be increased by 5 to 10 mcg daily every 1 to 2 weeks. When 25 mcg daily is reached, dosage may be increased every week or two by 12.5 or 25 mcg. Usual maintenance dosage is 75 mcg daily.

In the elderly or in pediatric patients, therapy should be started with 5 mcg daily and increased only by 5 mcg increments at the recommended intervals.

When switching a patient to liothyronine sodium tablets from thyroid, L-thyroxine or thyroglobulin, discontinue the other medication, initiate liothyronine sodium at a low dosage, and increase gradually according to the patient's response. When selecting a starting dosage, bear in mind that this drug has a rapid onset of action, and that residual effects of the other thyroid preparation may persist for the first several weeks of therapy.

➤*Thyroid-suppression therapy:* Administration of thyroid hormone in doses higher than those produced physiologically by the gland results in suppression of the production of endogenous hormone. This is the basis for the thyroid-suppression test and is used as an aid in the diagnosis of patients with signs of mild hyperthyroidism in whom baseline laboratory tests appear normal or to demonstrate thyroid gland autonomy in patients with Graves' ophthalmopathy. ^{131}I uptake is determined before and after the administration of the exogenous hormone. A 50% or greater suppression of uptake indicates a normal thyroid-pituitary axis and thus rules out thyroid gland autonomy.

Liothyronine sodium tablets are given in doses of 75 to 100 mcg/day for 7 days, and radioactive iodine uptake is determined before and after administration of the hormone. If thyroid function is under normal control, the radioiodine uptake will drop significantly after treatment. Liothyronine sodium tablets should be administered cautiously to patients in whom there is a strong suspicion of thyroid-gland autonomy, in view of the fact that the exogenous hormone effects will be additive to the endogenous source.

➤*Storage/Stability:* Store between 15° and 30°C (59° and 86°F).

LIOTHYRONINE SODIUM — INJECTION

For complete and comparative prescribing information, refer to the Thyroid Hormones group monograph.

Indications

➤*Myxedema coma/precoma:* Treatment of myxedema coma/precoma.

Liothyronine sodium injection can be used in patients allergic to desiccated thyroid or thyroid extract derived from pork or beef.

Administration and Dosage

➤*Adults:* Myxedema coma is usually precipitated in the hypothyroid patient of long standing by intercurrent illness or drugs such as sedatives and anesthetics and should be considered a medical emergency. Therapy should be directed at the correction of electrolyte disturbances, possible infection, or other intercurrent illness in addition to the administration of IV liothyronine (T_3). Simultaneous glucocorticosteroids are required.

Liothyronine sodium injection (T_3) is for IV administration only. It should not be given IM or subcutaneously.

Initial and subsequent doses of liothyronine sodium injection should be based on continuous monitoring of the patient's clinical status and response to therapy.

Liothyronine sodium injection doses should normally be administered greater than or equal to 4 and less than or equal to 12 hours apart.

Administration of at least 65 mcg/day of IV liothyronine (T_3) in the initial days of therapy was associated with lower mortality.

There is limited clinical experience with IV liothyronine (T_3) at total daily doses exceeding 100 mcg/day.

An initial IV liothyronine sodium injection dose ranging from 25 to 50 mcg is recommended in the emergency treatment of myxedema coma/precoma in adults. In patients with known or suspected cardiovascular disease, an initial dose of 10 to 20 mcg is suggested (see Warnings). However, both the initial dose and subsequent doses should be determined on the basis of continuous monitoring of the patient's clinical condition and response to liothyronine sodium injection therapy. Normally at least 4 hours should be allowed between doses to adequately assess therapeutic response, and no more than 12 hours should elapse between doses to avoid fluctuations in hormone levels. Caution should be exercised in adjusting the dose because of the potential of large changes to precipitate adverse cardiovascular events. Review of the myxedema case reports indicates decreased mortality in patients receiving at least 65 mcg/day in the initial days of treatment. However, there is limited clinical experience at total daily doses above 100 mcg (see Drug Interactions for potential interactions between thyroid hormones and digitalis and vasopressors).

➤*Switching to oral therapy:* Oral therapy should be resumed as soon as the clinical situation has been stabilized and the patient is able to take oral medication. When switching a patient to liothyronine sodium tablets from liothyronine sodium injection, discontinue liothyronine sodium injection, initiate oral therapy at a low dosage, and increase gradually according to the patient's response.

If levothyroxine rather than liothyronine sodium is used in initiating oral therapy, the physician should bear in mind that there is a delay of several days in the onset of levothyroxine activity and that IV therapy should be discontinued gradually.

➤*Storage/Stability:* Store between 2° and 8°C (35° and 46°F).

LIOTRIX

	Product and distributor	Tablet strength (grain)	Content (mcg)[a]		Thyroid equivalent (mg)	How supplied
			T_3	T_4		
Rx	**Thyrolar** (Forest)	¼	3.1	12.5	15	Lactose. (YC). Violet/White. Two-layered. In 100s.
		½	6.25	25	30	Lactose. (YD). Peach/White. Two-layered. In 100s.
		1	12.5	50	60	Lactose. (YE). Pink/White. Two-layered. In 100s.
		2	25	100	120	Lactose. (YF). Green/White. Two-layered. In 100s.
		3	37.5	150	180	Lactose. (YH). Yellow/White. Two-layered. In 100s.

[a] Liothyronine sodium (T_3) is approximately 4 times as potent as levothyroxine (T_4) on a microgram-for-microgram basis.

LIOTRIX — ORAL

For complete prescribing information, refer to the Thyroid Hormones group monograph.

WARNING

Drugs with thyroid hormone activity, alone or with other therapeutic agents have been used for the treatment of obesity. In euthyroid patients, doses within the range of daily hormonal requirements are ineffective for weight reduction. Larger doses may produce serious or even life-threatening manifestations of toxicity, particularly when given in association with sympathomimetic amines such as those used for their anorectic effects.

Indications

➤*Hypothyroidism:* As replacement or supplemental therapy in patients with hypothyroidism of any etiology, except transient hypothyroidism during the recovery phase of subacute thyroiditis. This category includes cretinism, myxedema, and ordinary hypothyroidism in patients of any age (children, adults, the elderly), or state (including pregnancy); primary hypothyroidism resulting from functional deficiency, primary atrophy, partial or total absence of thyroid gland, or the effects of surgery, radiation, or drugs, with or without the presence of goiter; and secondary (pituitary) or tertiary (hypothalamic) hypothyroidism.

➤*Pituitary thyroid stimulating hormone (TSH) suppression:* As pituitary TSH suppressants in the treatment or prevention of various types of euthyroid goiters, including thyroid nodules, subacute or chronic lymphocytic thyroiditis (Hashimoto), and multinodular goiter and in the management of thyroid cancer.

➤*Diagnostic agent:* As diagnostic agents in suppression tests to differentiate suspected mild hyperthyroidism or thyroid gland autonomy.

Administration and Dosage

➤*Dosage equivalents:* Each liotrix 60 mg tablet will usually replace approximately 60 to 65 mg (1 grain) of desiccated thyroid.

Optimal dosage is determined by patient's clinical response and laboratory findings.

➤*Hypothyroidism:*

Initial dosage – Institute therapy using low doses, with increments that depend on cardiovascular status. Usual starting dose is 1 tablet of *Thyrolar ½* with increments of 1 tablet of *Thyrolar ¼* every 2 to 3 weeks. A lower starting dose, 1 tablet/day *Thyrolar ¼* is recommended in patients with long-standing myxedema, particularly if cardiovascular impairment is suspected, in which case extreme caution is recommended. Reduce dosage if angina occurs.

Maintenance dosage – Most patients require 1 tablet *Thyrolar 1* to 1 tablet *Thyrolar 2* per day; failure to respond to 1 tablet *Thyrolar 3* suggests lack of compliance or malabsorption. Maintenance dosages of 1 tablet *Thyrolar 1* to 1 tablet of *Thyrolar 2* per day usually result in normal serum levothyroxine and triiodothyronine levels. Adequate therapy usually results in normal TSH and T_4 levels after 2 to 3 weeks of therapy.

Dosage readjustment: Readjust dosage within the first 4 weeks of therapy after proper clinical and laboratory evaluations including serum levels of T_4 bound and free, and TSH.

➤*Thyroid cancer:* Larger amounts of thyroid hormone than those used for replacement therapy are required. Medullary carcinoma of the thyroid usually is unresponsive to this therapy.

➤*Diagnostic agent:* For adults, the usual suppressive dose of T_4 is 1.56 mcg/kg of body weight per day given for 7 to 10 days. These doses usually yield normal serum T_4 and T_3 levels and lack of response to TSH.

➤*Children:* Follow recommendations in the following table. In infants with congenital hypothyroidism, institute therapy with full doses as soon as diagnosis is made.

Recommended Pediatric Dosage for Congenital Hypothyroidism

Age	Dose per day in mcg		
	T_3/T_4	to	T_3/T_4
0 to 6 mo	3.1/12.5	to	6.25/25
6 to 12 mo	6.25/25	to	9.35/37.5
1 to 5 y	9.35/37.5	to	12.5/50
6 to 12 y	12.5/50	to	18.75/75
Over 12 y			> 18.75/75

➤*Special populations:* In patients with angina pectoris or the elderly, in whom there is a greater likelihood of occult cardiac disease, initiate therapy with low doses (1 tablet of *Thyrolar ¼* or *Thyrolar ½*).

➤*Storage / Stability:* Store at cold temperature between 2° to 8°C (36° to 46°F) in a tight, light-resistant container.

IODINE PRODUCTS

Rx	**Strong Iodine Solution (Lugol's Solution)** (Various, eg, Lannett)	**Solution**: 5% iodine and 10% potassium iodide	In 120 mL, pt and gal.
otc	**ThyroShield** (Fleming)	**Solution**: 65 mg/mL potassium iodide	Parabens, saccharin, sucrose. Black-raspberry flavor. In 30 mL.

IODINE PRODUCTS — ORAL

Indications

Used adjunctively with an antithyroid drug in hyperthyroid patients in preparation for thyroidectomy and to treat thyrotoxic crisis or neonatal thyrotoxicosis.

Thyroid blocking in a radiation emergency.

For use of potassium iodide as an expectorant and for other respiratory tract conditions, see the Iodine Products monograph in the Expectorant section of the Respiratories chapter.

➤*Unlabeled uses:* Potassium iodide (60 mg 3 times daily) has been used effectively in a limited number of patients for Sweet's syndrome (acute febrile neutrophilic dermatosis) in combination with a potent topical steroid, as an alternative to systemic corticosteroids.

Also effective for the treatment of lymphocutaneous sporotrichosis (a dimorphic fungus that typically infects the skin and lymphatic system).

Administration and Dosage

➤*Recommended dietary allowances (RDAs):* The RDA for iodine is 150 mcg for adults.

To prepare hyperthyroid patients for thyroidectomy, administer 2 to 6 drops strong iodine solution 3 times daily for 10 days prior to surgery.

➤*For thyroid blocking in a radiation emergency:* Use only as directed by state or local public health authorities in the event of a radiation emergency. Take for 10 days unless directed otherwise by state or local public health authorities.

Strong iodine solution –

Adults and children (older than 1 year of age): 130 mg daily (crush tablets for small children).

Infants (less than 1 year of age): 65 mg daily.

ThyroShield – Take every 24 hours as directed by public officials. Do not take more than 1 dose in 24 hours.

Adults or children 12 to 18 years of age and at least 150 pounds: Two mL (130 mg) every 24 hours.

Children 12 to 18 years of age and less than 150 pounds or children older than 3 years to 12 years of age: One mL (65 mg) every 24 hours.

Children older than 1 month to 3 years of age: 0.5 mL (32.5 mg) every 24 hours.

Infants from birth to 1 month of age: 0.25 mL (16.25 mg) every 24 hours.

Actions

➤*Pharmacology:* An adequate intake of iodine is necessary for normal thyroid function and the synthesis of thyroid hormones.

Elemental iodine (from the diet or as medication) is reduced in the GI tract and enters the circulation in the form of iodide, which is actively transported and concentrated by the thyroid gland. Hormone synthesis requires the oxidation of iodide and iodination of tyrosyl residues in thyroglobulin to form iodotyrosine precursors. These precursors undergo a "coupling reaction" to yield the active thyroid hormones T_3 and T_4. High concentrations of iodide greatly influence iodine metabolism by the thyroid gland. Large doses of iodides can inhibit T_4 and T_3 synthesis and rapidly inhibit proteolysis of colloid and the release of T_4 and T_3 into the bloodstream.

The effects of iodides are evident within 24 hours; maximum effects are attained after 10 to 15 days of continuous therapy. If administered chronically, therapeutic effects may persist for up to 6 weeks after the crisis has abated.

Contraindications

Hypersensitivity to iodides.

Warnings

➤*Pregnancy: Category D* (potassium iodide). Iodides readily cross the placenta and may cause hypothyroidism and goiter in the fetus or newborn when used long-term or close to term; short-term use (eg, 10 days) may not carry this risk. Administer to pregnant women only if clearly needed.

➤*Lactation:* Iodide is excreted in breast milk; however, the significance to the infant is not known. According to the American Academy of Pediatrics, these agents are not contraindicated in breast-feeding.

Drug Interactions

➤*Lithium carbonate:* Lithium carbonate and iodide preparations may have synergistic hypothyroid activity; concomitant use may result in hypothyroidism.

Adverse Reactions

Possible side effects of potassium iodide include: Skin rashes; swelling of the salivary glands; "iodism" (metallic taste, burning mouth and throat, sore teeth and gums, symptoms of a head cold and sometimes stomach upset and diarrhea); allergic reactions (ie, fever and joint pains, swelling of parts of the face and body and, at times, severe shortness of breath requiring immediate medical attention). Overactivity or underactivity of the thyroid gland or enlargement of the thyroid gland (goiter) may occur rarely.

Overdosage

➤*Acute poisoning:*

Symptoms – Iodine is corrosive, and toxic symptoms are mainly the result of local GI tract irritation. Gastroenteritis, abdominal pain and diarrhea (sometimes bloody) may be seen. Fatalities may occur from circulatory collapse caused by shock, corrosive gastritis or asphyxiation from swelling of the glottis or larynx.

Treatment – Gastric lavage with a soluble starch solution (15 g cornstarch or flour in 500 mL water) is recommended for removing iodine from the stomach. A 1% oral solution of sodium thiosulfate is a specific antidote, as it will reduce iodine to iodide. Milk may help relieve gastric irritation. Correct fluid and electrolyte imbalance, and treat shock if necessary.

➤*Chronic poisoning:* Discontinue use of iodine or iodides. High sodium chloride intake will speed recovery. For iodism characterized by skin or mucous membrane reactions, give cortisone or equivalent corticosteroid 25 to 100 mg every 6 hours orally until symptoms abate.

Patient Information

➤*Strong iodine solution:* Dilute with water or fruit juice to improve taste.

Discontinue use and notify physician if fever, skin rash, metallic taste, swelling of the throat, burning of the mouth and throat, sore gums and teeth, head cold symptoms, severe GI distress or enlargement of the thyroid gland (goiter) occurs.

Antithyroid Agents

Indications

➤*Hyperthyroidism:* Long-term therapy may lead to disease remission. Also used to ameliorate hyperthyroidism in preparation for subtotal thyroidectomy or radioactive iodine therapy.

Propylthiouracil (PTU) and methimazole are also used when thyroidectomy is contraindicated or not advisable.

➤*Unlabeled uses:* PTU (300 mg/day) may be useful in reducing the mortality due to alcoholic liver disease by reducing the hepatic hypermetabolic state induced by alcohol.

Administration and Dosage

In one study, the rate of remission and time to relapse of Grave's disease was significantly increased when antithyroid therapy was given for a prolonged duration (18 months) versus short-term (6 month) treatment. However, the monitoring of thyroid-stimulating antibody values may be a useful guide for shortening the duration of treatment in some patients.

One small study reported that single and divided daily doses of methimazole were equally effective in hyperthyroid patients. Traditionally administered in divided doses, it was suggested that a single daily dose would be effective since methimazole is present in the thyroid for 20 hours and is active for 40 hours despite a serum half-life of 6 to 13 hours. Further study is needed.

Actions

➤*Pharmacology:* PTU and methimazole inhibit the synthesis of thyroid hormones and, thus, are effective in the treatment of hyperthyroidism. They do not inactivate existing thyroxine (T_4) and triiodothyronine (T_3) which are stored in the thyroid or which circulate in the blood, nor do they interfere with the effectiveness of exogenous thyroid hormones. PTU partially inhibits the peripheral conversion of T_4 to T_3.

Both drugs are concentrated in the thyroid gland. Pharmacokinetic data are summarized in the following table:

Various Pharmacokinetic Parameters of Antithyroid Agents

Antithyroid agent	Bioavailability (%)	Protein binding (%)	Transplacental passage	Breast milk levels (M:P)[1]	Half-life (h)	Excreted in urine (%)
Propylthiouracil	80 to 95	75 to 80	Low	Low (0.1)	1 to 2	< 35
Methimazole	80 to 95	0	High	High (1)	6 to 13	< 10

[1] Approximate milk:plasma ratio.

Contraindications

Hypersensitivity to antithyroid drugs; breast-feeding mothers (see Warnings).

Warnings

➤*Hematologic effects:* Agranulocytosis is potentially the most serious side effect of therapy. Instruct patients to report any symptoms of agranulocytosis, such as hay fever, sore throat, skin eruptions, fever, headache or general malaise. In such cases, white blood cell and differential counts should be made to determine whether agranulocytosis has developed. Exercise particular care with patients receiving additional drugs known to cause agranulocytosis. Leukopenia, thrombocytopenia and aplastic anemia (pancytopenia) may also occur. Discontinue the drug in the presence of agranulocytosis, aplastic anemia, hepatitis, fever or exfoliative dermatitis. Monitor the patient's bone marrow function.

One report recommends routine monitoring of the WBC count for at least the first 3 months of therapy, thereby potentially detecting agranulocytosis prior to becoming evident by infection.

➤*Carcinogenesis:* Laboratory animals treated with PTU for more than 1 year have demonstrated thyroid hyperplasia and carcinoma formation. Such animal findings are seen with continuous suppression of thyroid function by sufficient doses of a variety of antithyroid agents, as well as in dietary iodine deficiency, subtotal thyroidectomy, and implantation of autonomous thyrotropic hormone-secreting pituitary tumors. Pituitary adenomas have also been described.

➤*Pregnancy: Category D.* These agents, used judiciously, are effective drugs in hyperthyroidism complicated by pregnancy. Because they readily cross the placenta and can induce goiter and even cretinism in the developing fetus, it is important that a sufficient, but not excessive, dose be given. In many pregnant women, the thyroid dysfunction diminishes as the pregnancy proceeds, thus making a reduction of dose possible. In some instances, these products can be withdrawn 2 or 3 weeks before delivery. PTU can cause fetal harm when administered to a pregnant woman. Approximately 10% will develop neonatal goiter. However, if an antithyroid agent is needed, PTU is preferred because it is less likely than methimazole to cross the placenta and induce fetal/neonatal complications (eg, aplasia cutis).

➤*Lactation:* Postpartum patients receiving antithyroid preparations should not nurse their babies. However, if necessary, the preferred drug is PTU.

➤*Children:* In several case reports, PTU hepatotoxicity has occurred in pediatric patients. Discontinue the drug immediately if signs and symptoms of hepatic dysfunction develop.

Precautions

➤*Monitoring:* Monitor thyroid function tests periodically during therapy. Once clinical evidence of hyperthyroidism has resolved, the finding of an elevated serum TSH indicates that a lower maintenance dose of PTU should be used.

➤*Hemorrhagic effects:* Because PTU may cause hypoprothrombinemia and bleeding, monitor prothrombin time during therapy, especially before surgical procedures.

Drug Interactions

➤*Anticoagulants:* The activity of oral anticoagulants may be potentiated by the anti-vitamin K activity attributed to PTU.

Adverse Reactions

Adverse reactions probably occur in less than 1% of patients. Agranulocytosis is the most serious effect.

➤*CNS:* Paresthesias; neuritis; headache; vertigo; drowsiness; neuropathies; CNS stimulation; depression.

➤*Dermatologic:* Skin rash; urticaria; pruritus; erythema nodosum; skin pigmentation; exfoliative dermatitis; lupus-like syndrome, including splenomegaly, hepatitis, periarteritis and hypoprothrombinemia and bleeding.

➤*GI:* Nausea and vomiting; epigastric distress; loss of taste; sialadenopathy.

➤*Hematologic:* Inhibition of myelopoiesis (agranulocytosis, granulocytopenia and thrombocytopenia); aplastic anemia; hypoprothrombinemia; periarteritis. About 10% of patients with untreated hyperthyroidism have leukopenia (WBC count less than 4,000 per mm^3), often with relative granulocytopenia.

➤*Hepatic:* Jaundice (which may persist for several weeks after discontinuance); hepatitis.

➤*Renal:* Nephritis.

➤*Miscellaneous:* Abnormal hair loss; arthralgia; myalgia; edema; lymphadenopathy; drug fever; interstitial pneumonitis insulin autoimmune syndrome (may result in hypoglycemic coma).

Overdosage

➤*Symptoms:* Nausea; vomiting; epigastric distress; headache; fever; arthralgia; pruritus; edema; pancytopenia. Agranulocytosis is the most serious effect. Rarely, exfoliative dermatitis, hepatitis, neuropathies or CNS stimulation or depression may occur.

➤*Treatment:* Protect the patient's airway and support ventilation and perfusion. Meticulously monitor and maintain, within acceptable limits, the patient's vital signs, blood gases, serum electrolytes, etc. Monitor the patient's bone marrow function. Refer to General Management of Acute Overdosage.

Forced diuresis, peritoneal dialysis, hemodialysis or charcoal hemoperfusion have not been established as beneficial for an overdose of propylthiouracil.

Patient Information

Take at regular intervals around the clock (usually every 8 hours), unless directed otherwise by physician.

Notify physician if fever, sore throat, unusual bleeding or bruising, headache, rash, yellowing of the skin or vomiting occurs.

PROPYLTHIOURACIL (PTU)

Rx	**Propylthiouracil** (Various, eg, Dixon-Shane, Rugby)	**Tablets:** 50 mg	In 100s and 1,000s.

PROPYLTHIOURACIL — ORAL

For complete prescribing information, refer to the Antithyroid Agents group monograph.

Indications

➤*Hyperthyroidism:* Medical treatment of hyperthyroidism. Long-term therapy may lead to remission of the disease. Propylthiouracil may also be used to ameliorate hyperthyroidism in preparation for subtotal thyroidectomy or radioactive iodine therapy. Propylthiouracil is also used when thyroidectomy is contraindicated or not advisable.

➤*Unlabeled uses:* Propylthiouracil 300 mg/day may be useful in reducing the mortality caused by alcoholic liver disease by reducing the hepatic hypermetabolic state induced by alcohol.

Administration and Dosage

The total daily dosage is usually given in 3 equal doses at approximately 8-hour intervals.

➤*Adult:* The initial dosage is 300 mg daily. In patients with severe hyperthyroidism, very large goiters, or both, the beginning dosage usually should be 400 mg daily; an occasional patient will require 600 to 900 mg/daily initially. The usual maintenance dosage is 100 to 150 mg daily.

➤*Pediatric:* For children 6 to 10 years of age, the initial dosage is 50 to 150 mg daily. For pediatric patients 10 years of age and older, the initial dosage is 150 to 300 mg daily. The maintenance dosage is determined by the response of the patient.

Another suggested dosage for children is an initial dosage of 5 to 7 mg/kg/day or 150 to 200 mg/m^2/day in divided doses every 8 hours. The maintenance dosage is ⅓ to ⅔ the initial dose beginning when the patient's euthyroid.

➤*Storage/Stability:* Dispense in a tight, light-resistant container using a child-resistant closure. Store at controlled room temperature 20° to 25°C (68° to 77°F). Protect from light and moisture.

METHIMAZOLE

Rx	**Methimazole** (Par Pharm)	**Tablets:** 5 mg	Lactose. (EM/5). White to off-white. In 100s.
Rx	**Tapazole** (Monarch)		Lactose. (J94). White to off white, scored. In 100s.
Rx	**Methimazole** (Par Pharm)	10 mg	Lactose. (EM/10). White to off-white. In 100s.
Rx	**Tapazole** (Monarch)		Lactose. (J95). White to off white, scored. In 100s.

METHIMAZOLE — ORAL

For complete prescribing information, refer to the Antithyroid Agents group monograph.

Indications

➤*Hyperthyroidism:* Medical treatment of hyperthyroidism. Long-term therapy may lead to remission of the disease. Methimazole may be used to ameliorate hyperthyroidism in preparation for subtotal thyroidectomy or radioactive iodine therapy. Methimazole also is used when thyroidectomy is contraindicated or not advisable.

Administration and Dosage

➤*Approved by the FDA:* March 29, 1999.

➤*Adults:* The initial daily dosage is 15 mg for mild hyperthyroidism, 30 to 40 mg for moderately severe hyperthyroidism, and 60 mg for severe hyperthyroidism, divided into 3 doses at 8-hour intervals. The maintenance dosage is 5 to 15 mg daily.

➤*Children:* Initially, the daily dosage is 0.4 mg/kg of body weight divided into 3 doses and given at 8-hour intervals. The maintenance dosage is approximately one half of the initial dose.

➤*Storage/Stability:* Store at controlled room temperature, 15° to 30°C (59° to 86°F).

SODIUM IODIDE I 131

For Sodium Iodide I 131 prescribing information, see the monograph in the Antineoplastics Chapter.

MECASERMIN RINFABATE (rDNA ORIGIN)

Rx	**Iplex** (Insmed Therapeutic Proteins)	**Injection:** 36 mg per 0.6 mL	Preservative free. 50 mM sodium acetate, 105 mM sodium chloride. In single-dose vials.

MECASERMIN RINFABATE (rDNA ORIGIN) — INJECTION

Indications

➤*Growth failure:* For the treatment of growth failure in children with severe primary insulin-like growth factor-1 (IGF-1) deficiency (primary IGFD) or with growth hormone (GH) gene deletion who have developed neutralizing antibodies to GH.

Mecasermin is not intended for use in subjects with secondary forms of IGF-1 deficiency, such as GH deficiency, malnutrition, hypothyroidism, or chronic treatment with pharmacologic doses of anti-inflammatory steroids. Thyroid and nutritional deficiencies should be corrected before initiating mecasermin.

Mecasermin is not a substitute for GH treatment.

Administration and Dosage

➤*Approved by the FDA:* December 12, 2005.

➤*Dosage:* The dosage and administration should be individualized for each patient. Mecasermin should be administered via subcutaneous injection at an initial dose of 0.5 mg/kg, to be increased into the therapeutic dose range of 1 to 2 mg/kg, given once daily. Mecasermin can be given in the morning or in the evening but should be administered at approximately the same time every day, and the patient should maintain a regular, balanced diet. Mecasermin should not be administered if the patient cannot or will not eat or if they skip a meal. Subsequent doses of mecasermin should not be increased to make up for a missed dose.

In order to establish tolerability to mecasermin, glucose monitoring should be considered at treatment initiation or when a dose has been increased. If frequent symptoms of hypoglycemia or severe hypoglycemia occur, preprandial glucose monitoring should continue. Glucose monitoring is also advised for patients with recent occurrences of asymptomatic or symptomatic hypoglycemia. If evidence of hypoglycemia is present at the time of dosing, the dose should be withheld.

Dose titration/adjustment – Dosage can be titrated up to a maximum of 2 mg/kg daily based on measurement of IGF-1 levels obtained 8 to 18 hours after the previous dose. Treating health care providers should target on-treatment IGF-1 levels of 0 to +2 standard deviation (SD) score for age. Dosage should be adjusted downward in the event of adverse reactions (including hypoglycemia) and/or IGF-1 levels that are greater than or equal to 3 SDs above the normal reference range for IGF-1.

Growth response – Growth response to mecasermin is expected to decrease with time, as seen with other growth-promoting agents. However, failure to increase height velocity during the first year of therapy at least 2 cm/year suggests the need for assessment of compliance and evaluation of other causes of growth failure, such as hypothyroidism, under nutrition, and advanced bone age. Patients with undetectable acid labile subunit (ALS) levels at baseline may require higher doses of mecasermin.

➤*Administration:* Mecasermin is supplied as a single-use, preservative-free solution for subcutaneous injection. Aseptic technique must be followed for administration. Discard any unused portion.

Rotate sites for injection (thigh, abdomen, buttocks, or upper arm). New injections should be given at least 1 inch from previous injection site(s) and never into areas where the skin is tender, bruised, red, hard, or lipodystrophic.

Mecasermin should be administered using sterile, disposable syringes and needles. The syringes should be of small enough volume that the prescribed dose can be withdrawn from the vial with reasonable accuracy.

➤*Storage/Stability:*

Before use – Mecasermin is temperature-sensitive and must be stored frozen at −70°C (−94°F) while in the distribution chain. The patient must be instructed to keep the medication frozen while transferring it to a home freezer (−20°C, −4°F). Frozen (−70°C) mecasermin from the distributor can be transported on dry ice to the patient's home freezer. Mecasermin can be stored frozen up to 2 months at constant temperature (−20°C, −4°F). For use, mecasermin should be removed from the freezer (−20°C, −4°F) and thawed at room temperature (20° to 25°C, 68° to 77°F) for 45 minutes prior to use. The medication must remain in the patient's home freezer until time of use. Do not store in a home freezer that allows contents to thaw during the defrost cycle. Do not use medication if it thaws during transfer or storage, because the stability of the material may be affected.

After thawing – After thawing, allow vial to reach room temperature prior to injection (approximately 45 minutes). The vial should be swirled in a gentle rotary motion to ensure content uniformity. Do not shake. Inspect parenteral drug products visually for particulate matter and discoloration prior to administration whenever solution and container permit. If the solution is cloudy, it may indicate that the drug was previously thawed or exposed to extreme temperatures. If so, it must not be injected. Discard any vial that contains particulate matter or solution that is cloudy or discolored. Use within 1 hour after the vial reaches room temperature. Mecasermin must not be used if it has been at room temperature for more than 2 hours. After removing the dose of mecasermin, discard the vial with any unused portion.

Actions

➤*Pharmacology:* The primary pharmacologic effect of IGF-1 in children is the promotion of linear growth. Secondary pharmacologic actions of IGF-1 include other anabolic effects, insulin sensitization, and insulin-like effects. There are no known direct growth-promoting effects of insulin-like growth factor-binding protein-3 (IGFBP-3). The primary effect of IGFBP-3 in the mecasermin complex is the modulation of IGF-1 action.

In normal human circulation, less than 2% of total IGF-1 exists in the free form. Most circulating IGF-1 is found in association with the GH-dependent binding protein IGFBP-3, and this binary complex further associates with a third serum protein, the GH-dependent ALS, to form a noncovalent ternary complex of approximately 150 kD, which represents the natural physiologic reservoir of IGF-1. The ternary complex consists of 1 molecule each of IGF-1, IGFBP-3, and ALS.

The half-life of IGF-1 in the ternary complex is greater than 12 hours. Proteolytic cleavage of IGFBP-3 and interaction of the ternary complex with proteoglycans have been shown to release IGF-1 from the ternary complex.

➤*Pharmacokinetics:*

Absorption/Distribution – In pediatric patients with severe primary IGFD, 1 mg/kg was administered by subcutaneous injection to 4 patients in a pharmacokinetic substudy of the clinical trial. A summary of the pharmacokinetic parameters for IGF-1 and IGFBP-3, uncorrected for baseline values, is presented in the following table. The assays employed do not distinguish between exogenous and endogenous IGF-1 or IGFBP-3.

Mean (±SD) Pharmacokinetic Parameters in Patients with Primary IGFD Treated with Mecasermin 1 mg/kg (N = 4)

	C_{max} (ng/mL)[a]	T_{max} (h)[b]	AUC_{0-60} (ng h/mL)[c]	Half-life (h)
IGF-1	133 ± 19	11.3 ± 6.2	3,654 ± 237	13.4 ± 2.7
IGFBP-3	1,574 ± 401	19.5 ± 9	62,525 ± 8,352	54.1 ± 31.6

[a] C_{max} = peak plasma concentration.
[b] T_{max} = time to peak plasma concentration.
[c] AUC = area under the curve.

Contraindications

Do not use mecasermin use for growth promotion in patients with closed epiphyses. Mecasermin is contraindicated in the presence of active or suspected neoplasia; discontinue therapy when there is any evidence of active neoplasia. Mecasermin is contraindicated in patients allergic to mecasermin (rhIGF-1/rhIGFBP-3) or any of the excipients in mecasermin. Intravenous (IV) administration of mecasermin is contraindicated.

Warnings

➤*Hypersensitivity reactions:* If sensitivity to mecasermin occurs, discontinue treatment.

As with any exogenous protein administration, local or systemic allergic reactions may occur. Inform parents and patients that such reactions are possible and that if an allergic reaction occurs, interrupt treatment and seek prompt medical attention.

➤*Pregnancy: Category C.*

Animal reproduction studies have not been conducted with mecasermin. Effects of rhIGF-1 on embryofetal development were assessed in rats and rabbits.

Subcutaneous administration of 0.2, 0.5, or 1.25 mg/kg/day rhIGF-1 to rabbits during organogenesis resulted in an increased incidence of fetal loss but no fetal anomalies. Increased early resorptions were observed in rabbits treated with 1.25 mg/kg and increased preimplantation loss was observed (exposure equivalent to greater than or equal to 0.3 times MRHD based on body surface area).

A second rabbit embryofetal development study was conducted to determine the role of hypoglycemia in rhIGF-1 mediated fetal loss. Rabbits were administered subcutaneous dosages of 0, 0.5, and 1.25 mg/kg/day rhIGF-1; 1.25 or 2.5 mg/kg rhIGF-1 plus glucose supplementation; or insulin 2.5 units/kg/day. A comparable degree of hypoglycemia was observed in rabbits treated with 1.25 mg/kg rhIGF-1 alone or insulin 2.5 units/kg. Animals treated with 0.5 mg/kg rhIGF-1 or rhIGF-1 plus glucose maintained normal glucose levels.

Similar to the initial rabbit study, an increase in early fetal resorptions was observed in rabbits treated with 1.25 mg/kg/day rhIGF-1 (2 times the MRHD based on body surface area). This finding was not observed in insulin-treated rabbits despite a comparable degree of drug-induced hypoglycemia. A dose-related increase in postimplantation loss was observed in all rhIGF-1–treated groups (greater than or equal to 0.5 times the MRHD based on body surface area). While the incidence of fetal loss was somewhat reduced in glucose-supplemented rabbits, it was not clearly attributable to drug-induced hypoglycemia because significant fetal loss was still observed in normoglycemic rhIGF-1–treated rabbits.

The effects of mecasermin on a fetus have not been studied. Therefore, there is insufficient medical information to determine whether there are significant risks to a fetus.

➤*Lactation:* It is not known whether this drug is secreted in human milk. Because many drugs are secreted in human milk, exercise caution when administering mecasermin to a breast-feeding woman.

➤*Children:* Mecasermin has not been studied in children younger than 3 years of age with primary IGFD.

MECASERMIN RINFABATE (rDNA ORIGIN) — INJECTION

Precautions

➤*Monitoring:* Consider glucose monitoring at treatment initiation or when a dose has been increased. If frequent symptoms of hypoglycemia or severe hypoglycemia occur, continue preprandial glucose monitoring. Glucose monitoring is also advised for patients with recent occurrences of asymptomatic or symptomatic hypoglycemia.

Give patients periodic examinations to detect potential complications of adenotonsillar enlargement (such as excessive snoring, sleep apnea, chronic middle ear effusions, hearing loss) and administer appropriate treatment if necessary.

Fundoscopic examination is recommended at the initiation of and periodically during the course of mecasermin therapy.

Slipped capital femoral epiphysis and progression of scoliosis can occur in patients who experience rapid growth. During mecasermin treatment, monitor these conditions and other symptoms and signs known to be associated with GH treatment in general.

Since IGF-1 is the main mediator of GH effects and GH may produce acromegalic changes, monitor such changes during mecasermin treatment.

➤*Experienced health care providers:* Therapy with mecasermin should be directed by health care providers experienced in the diagnosis and management of patients with growth disorders.

➤*Use in adults:* Mecasermin has not been studied in adults with primary IGFD.

➤*Hypoglycemia:* Administer mecasermin at approximately the same time every day. Because it has insulin-like hypoglycemic effects, patients should avoid missing meals and should have a balanced diet. Don't administer mecasermin on days when the patient cannot or will not eat. Pay special attention to small children because their oral intake may be inconsistent.

➤*High risk activities:* At the time of initiation of mecasermin therapy and any upward adjustment of dose patients should avoid engaging in any high-risk activities until tolerability has been established (eg, 3 to 5 days).

➤*Lymphoid tissue hypertrophy:* Lymphoid tissue hypertrophy (eg, tonsillar and adenoidal) has been associated with mecasermin.

➤*Intracranial hypertension:* The syndrome of intracranial hypertension, with papilledema, visual changes, headache, and nausea and/or vomiting, may occur during treatment with mecasermin and has been reported in children with growth failure treated with related products (GH, rhIGF-1).

Drug Interactions

None known.

Adverse Reactions

Treatment-emergent adverse reactions were assessed in the clinical study of mecasermin (rDNA origin) injection in children with primary IGFD. In this study, 36 patients had an average exposure of 10.4 months (range, 27 days to 22.5 months), for a total of 374 patient-months. Safety information beyond 1 year of treatment is limited and safety beyond 21 months of treatment has not been established.

➤*Cardiovascular:* Echocardiographic evidence of valvulopathy was observed in a few individuals without associated clinical symptoms. Because of the underlying disease and the lack of a control group, the relationship of the valvular changes to drug treatment cannot be assessed.

➤*CNS:* Headaches were reported in 8 of 36 (22%) patients in the study. One adverse reaction of asymptomatic papilledema was reported. An adverse reaction of increased intracranial pressure and papilledema (possible intracranial hypertension) was also reported, which resolved with revision of a blocked existing ventriculoperitoneal shunt.

➤*Endocrine:* Thyromegaly (5% or more).

➤*GU:* Two patients had ovarian cysts on pelvic ultrasound.

➤*Hematologic/Lymphatic:* Hematuria, iron-deficiency anemia, lymphadenopathy (5% or more).

➤*Hepatic:* Mild elevations in the serum AST and lactate dehydrogenase were found in a significant proportion of patients before and during treatment without treatment discontinuations. Two patients had AST elevations that required temporary interruption of treatment.

Increases in liver and spleen size were noted in several patients on abdominal ultrasound assessments; occasional measurements near the upper limit of normal (ULN) were noted.

One patient had sonographic evidence of hepatomegaly.

Increased transaminases (5% or more).

➤*Local:* Common injection site conditions included erythema, hair growth at the injection sites, and lipohypertrophy.

➤*Metabolic/Nutritional:* Hypoglycemia was reported in 11 of 36 (31%) patients in the study and was generally rated as mild and asymptomatic. Four hypoglycemic episodes were characterized as symptomatic, including 2 cases that required acute intervention.

Hyperglycemia.

➤*Musculoskeletal:* Arthralgia, bone pain, muscular atrophy (5% or more).

➤*Renal:* Increases in kidney size were noted in several patients on abdominal ultrasound assessments; occasional measurements near the ULN were noted. Renal function, as defined by serum creatinine and calculated creatinine clearance, was normal.

➤*Respiratory:* Seven of 36 (19%) patients in the study reported an adverse reaction of tonsillar and/or adenoid hypertrophy, and 2 patients underwent tonsillectomy and/or adenoidectomy.

➤*Immunologic:* By 9 months of treatment, a proportion of patients developed antibodies to the protein complex (90%), rhIGFBP-3 (50%), and/or rhIGF-1 (20%), using assays with varying degrees of sensitivity. No evidence of neutralization of biological activity, such as reduced height velocity, was noted in antibody-positive patients during the first year of mecasermin treatment.

➤*Miscellaneous:* Pain in an extremity (5% or more).

Overdosage

There were no instances of overdosage with mecasermin in the primary IGFD clinical trial.

➤*Symptoms:* Based on the known pharmacological effects of IGF-1, acute overdosage could lead to hypoglycemia. Long-term overdosage could result in signs and/or symptoms of acromegaly.

➤*Treatment:* Treatment of acute overdosage of mecasermin should be directed at reversing hypoglycemia. Mild hypoglycemia can usually be treated with oral glucose or food. If the overdose results in loss of consciousness, treatment with parenteral glucagon or IV glucose may be required.

Patient Information

Instruct patients and/or their caregivers in the safe administration of mecasermin. Because of the possibility of hypoglycemia, patients using mecasermin should be on a regular, balanced diet. Administer mecasermin at the same time every day. Do not administer mecasermin if the patient cannot or will not eat or when a meal is omitted. Institute therapy in accordance with the prescribing health care provider's instructions. The dose of mecasermin should not be increased to make up for a missed dose. If severe or persistent hypoglycemia occurs on treatment, despite adequate food intake, consider mecasermin dose reduction. Educate patients and care givers on how to recognize the signs and symptoms of adverse reactions, particularly hypoglycemia.

Thoroughly instruct patients and/or caregivers in the importance of proper needle disposal. Use a puncture-resistant container for the disposal of used needles and/or syringes (consistent with applicable state requirements). Do not reuse needles and syringes.

MECASERMIN (rDNA ORIGIN)

Rx	**Increlex** (Tercica)	**Injection:** 10 mg/mL	In 40 mL multiple dose vials.[a]

[a] Each vial contains 9 mg/mL benzyl alcohol, 5.84 mg/mL sodium chloride, 2 mg/mL polysorbate 20, and 0.5 M acetate.

MECASERMIN (rDNA ORIGIN) — INJECTION

Indications

➤*Growth failure:* For the long-term treatment of growth failure in children with severe primary insulin-like growth factor-1 (IGF-1) deficiency (primary IGFD) or with growth hormone (GH) gene deletion who have developed neutralizing antibodies to GH. Severe primary IGFD is defined by:

- height standard deviation score less than or equal to −3,
- basal IGF-1 standard deviation score less than or equal to −3, and
- normal or elevated GH.

Severe primary IGFD includes patients with mutations in the GH receptor (GHR), post-GHR signaling pathway, and IGF-1 gene defects; they are not GH deficient; therefore, they cannot be expected to respond adequately to exogenous GH treatment.

Mecasermin is not intended for use in subjects with secondary forms of IGF-1 deficiency, such as GH deficiency, malnutrition, hypothyroidism, or chronic treatment with pharmacologic doses of anti-inflammatory steroids. Correct thyroid and nutritional deficiencies before initiating mecasermin treatment.

Mecasermin is not a substitute for GH treatment.

Administration and Dosage

➤*Approved by the FDA:* August 30, 2005.

Preprandial glucose monitoring should be considered at treatment initiation and until a well-tolerated dose is established. If frequent symptoms of hypoglycemia or severe hypoglycemia occur, preprandial glucose monitoring should continue.

➤*Dosage:* The dosage of mecasermin should be individualized for each patient. The recommended starting dose of mecasermin is 0.04 to 0.08 mg/kg (40 to 80 mcg/kg) twice daily by subcutaneous injection. If well-tolerated for at least 1 week, the dose may be increased by 0.04 mg/kg per dose, to the maximum dose of 0.12 mg/kg given twice daily. Doses greater than 0.12 mg/kg given twice daily have not been evaluated in children with primary IGFD and, because of potential hypoglycemic effects, should not be used. If hypoglycemia occurs with recommended doses, despite adequate food intake, the dose should be reduced. Mecasermin should be administered shortly before or after (approximately 20 minutes) a meal or snack. If the patient is unable to eat shortly before or after a dose for any reason, that

MECASERMIN (rDNA ORIGIN) — INJECTION

dose of mecasermin should be withheld. Subsequent doses of mecasermin should never be increased to make up for 1 or more omitted dose.

➤*Administration:* Mecasermin injection sites should be rotated to a different site with each injection.

Mecasermin should be administered using sterile disposable syringes and needles. The syringes should be of small enough volume that the prescribed dose can be withdrawn from the vial with reasonable accuracy.

➤*Storage/Stability:*

Before opening – Vials of mecasermin are stable when refrigerated (2° to 8°C [35° to 46°F]). Avoid freezing the vials of mecasermin. Protect from direct light. Expiration dates are stated on the labels.

After opening – Vials of mecasermin are stable for 30 days after initial vial entry when stored at 2° to 8°C (35° to 46°F). Avoid freezing the vials of mecasermin. Protect from direct light.

Vial contents should be clear without particulate matter. If the solution is cloudy or contains particulate matter, the contents must not be injected. Mecasermin should not be used after its expiration date. Keep refrigerated and use within 30 days of initial vial entry. Remaining unused material should be discarded.

Actions

➤*Pharmacology:* IGF-1 is the principal hormonal mediator of statural growth. Under normal circumstances, GH binds to its receptor in the liver and other tissues, and stimulates the synthesis/secretion of IGF-1. In target tissues, the type 1 IGF-1 receptor, which is homologous to the insulin receptor, is activated by IGF-1, leading to intracellular signaling, which stimulates multiple processes leading to statural growth. The metabolic actions of IGF-1 are, in part, directed at stimulating the uptake of glucose, fatty acids, and amino acids so that metabolism supports growing tissues.

The following actions have been demonstrated for endogenous human IGF-1:

Tissue growth – 1) Skeletal growth occurs at the cartilage growth plates of the epiphyses of bones where stem cells divide to produce new cartilage cells or chondrocytes. The growth of chondrocytes is under the control of IGF-1 and GH. The chondrocytes become calcified so that new bone is formed, allowing the length of the bones to increase. This results in skeletal growth until the cartilage growth plates fuse at the end of puberty. 2) Cell growth: IGF-1 receptors are present on most types of cells and tissues. IGF-1 has mitogenic activities that lead to an increased number of cells in the body. 3) Organ growth: Treatment of IGF-1 deficient rats with rhIGF-1 results in whole body and organ growth.

Carbohydrate metabolism – IGF-1 suppresses hepatic glucose production and stimulates peripheral glucose utilization and therefore has a hypoglycemic potential. IGF-1 has inhibitory effects on insulin secretion.

➤*Pharmacokinetics:*

Absorption – While the bioavailability of rhIGF-1 after subcutaneous administration in healthy subjects has been reported to be close to 100%, the absolute bioavailability of mecasermin given subcutaneously to subjects with primary IGFD has not been determined.

Distribution – In blood, IGF-1 is bound to 6 IGF binding proteins, with greater than 80% bound as a complex with IGF binding protein 3 (IGFBP-3) and an acid-labile subunit. IGFBP-3 is greatly reduced in subjects with severe primary IGFD, resulting in increased clearance of IGF-1 in these subjects relative to healthy subjects. The total IGF-1 volume of distribution after subcutaneous administration in subjects with severe primary IGFD is estimated to be 0.257 (0.073) L/kg at an mecasermin dose of 0.045 mg/kg, and is estimated to increase as the dose of mecasermin increases.

Metabolism – Both the liver and the kidney have been shown to metabolize IGF-1.

Excretion – The mean terminal half-life after single subcutaneous administration of mecasermin 0.12 mg/kg in pediatric subjects with severe primary IGFD is estimated to be 5.8 hours. Clearance of mecasermin is inversely proportional to IGFBP-3 levels and clearance is estimated to be 0.04 L/h/kg at IGFBP-3 three mcg/mL.

Summary of Mecasermin Single-Dose Pharmacokinetic Parameters[a] in Children[b] with Severe Primary IGFD (0.12 mg/kg SC[c])

	C_{max}[d] (ng/mL)	T_{max}[e] (h)	AUC_{0-8}[f] (h•ng/mL)	$T_{½}$[g] (h)	Vd/F[h] (L/kg)	CL/F[i] (L/h/kg)
n	3	3	3	3	12[j]	12[j]
Mean	234	2	2,932	5.8	0.257	0.0424
CV%[k]	23	0	50	64	28	38

[a] Pharmacokinetic parameters based on baseline adjusted plasma concentrations.
[b] Male/female data combined, ages 12 to 22 years.
[c] SC = subcutaneous injection.
[d] C_{max} = maximum concentration.
[e] T_{max} = time of maximum concentration.
[f] AUC_{0-8} = area under the curve.
[g] $t_{½}$ = half-life.
[h] Vd/F = volume of distribution.
[i] CL/F = systemic clearance.
[j] Data represents 3 subjects each at doses 0.015, 0.03, 0.06, and 0.12 mg/kg SC.
[k] CV% = coefficient of variation in %.

Contraindications

Do not use mecasermin for growth promotion in patients with closed epiphyses. Contraindicated in the presence of active or suspected neoplasia; discontinue therapy if evidence of neoplasia develops.

Intravenous (IV) administration of mecasermin is contraindicated.

Mecasermin should not be used by patients who are allergic to mecasermin (IGF-1) or any of the inactive ingredients in mecasermin.

Warnings

➤*Benzyl alcohol:* Mecasermin contains benzyl alcohol as a preservative. Benzyl alcohol as a preservative has been associated with neurologic toxicity in neonates.

➤*Hypersensitivity reactions:* If sensitivity to mecasermin occurs, discontinue treatment.

➤*Carcinogenesis:* Mecasermin was administered subcutaneously to Sprague Dawley rats at dosages of 0, 0.25, 1, 4, and 10 mg/kg/day for up to 2 years. An increased incidence of adrenal medullary hyperplasia and pheochromocytoma was observed in male rats at dosages of 1 mg/kg/day and above (≥ 1 times the clinical exposure with the maximum recommended human dose [MRHD] based on AUC) and female rats at all dosage levels (≥ 0.3 times the clinical exposure with the MRHD based on AUC). An increased incidence of keratoacanthoma in the skin was observed in male rats at dosages of 4 and 10 mg/kg/day (≥ 4 times the MRHD) and in female rats treated with 10 mg/kg/day (7 times the MRHD based on AUC). An increased incidence of mammary gland carcinoma in both male and female rats was observed in animals treated with 10 mg/kg/day (7 times the MRHD based on AUC). Based on excess mortality secondary to IGF-1 induced hypoglycemia, these skin and mammary tumor findings were only observed at doses that exceeded the maximum tolerated dose (MTD).

➤*Pregnancy:* *Category C.* Embryo-fetal toxicity studies were conducted in Sprague Dawley rats with dosages of 1, 4, and 16 mg/kg/day, and in New Zealand White rabbits with dosages of 0.125, 0.5, and 2 mg/kg/day administered IV. No embryo-fetal developmental abnormalities were observed in rats with dosages up to 16 mg/kg/day (20 times the MRHD based on body surface area [BSA] comparison). In the rabbit study, the no-observed-adverse-effect-level (NOAEL) for maternal toxicity was 2 mg/kg (8 times the MRHD based on BSA) and the NOAEL for fetal toxicity was 0.5 mg/kg (2 times the MRHD based on BSA). Mecasermin displayed no teratogenicity at doses up to 2 mg/kg (8 times the MRHD based on BSA).

The effects of mecasermin on the fetus have not been studied. Therefore, there is insufficient medical information to determine whether there are significant risks to a fetus.

➤*Lactation:* It is not known whether this drug is excreted in human milk. Because many drugs are excreted in human milk, exercise caution when mecasermin is administered to a breast-feeding woman.

➤*Children:* Mecasermin has not been studied in children younger than 2 years of age or in adults.

Precautions

➤*Monitoring:* Consider preprandial glucose monitoring at treatment initiation and until a well-tolerated dose is established. If frequent symptoms of hypoglycemia or severe hypoglycemia occur, continue preprandial glucose monitoring.

Thickening of the soft tissues of the face was observed in several patients and should be monitored during mecasermin treatment.

Slipped capital femoral epiphysis and progression of scoliosis can occur in patients who experience rapid growth. These conditions and other symptoms and signs known to be associated with GH treatment in general should be monitored during mecasermin treatment.

➤*Experienced health care providers:* Treatment with mecasermin should be directed by health care providers who are experienced in the diagnosis and management of patients with growth disorders.

➤*Hypoglycemic effects:* Administer mecasermin shortly before or after a meal or snack, because it has insulin-like hypoglycemic effects. Pay special attention to small children because their oral intake may not be consistent. Do not administer mecasermin when the meal or snack is omitted. Never increase the dose of mecasermin to make up for 1 or more omitted doses. Initiate mecasermin therapy at a low dose and increase the dose only if no hypoglycemia episodes have occurred after at least 7 days of dosing. If severe hypoglycemia or persistent hypoglycemia occurs on treatment despite adequate food intake, consider mecasermin dose reduction.

➤*High-risk activities:* Patients should avoid engaging in any high-risk activities (eg, driving) within 2 to 3 hours after dosing, particularly at the initiation of mecasermin treatment, until a well-tolerated dose of mecasermin has been established.

➤*Lymphoid tissue hypertrophy:* Lymphoid tissue (eg, tonsillar) hypertrophy associated with complications, such as snoring, sleep apnea, and chronic middle-ear effusions, have been reported with the use of mecasermin. Patients should have periodic examinations to rule out such potential complications and receive appropriate treatment if necessary.

➤*Intracranial hypertension (IH):* IH with papilledema, visual changes, headache, nausea, and/or vomiting have been reported in patients treated with mecasermin, as they have been reported with therapeutic GH administration. IH-associated signs and symptoms resolved after interruption of dosing. Funduscopic examination is recommended at the initiation and periodically during the course of mecasermin therapy.

➤*Protein reaction:* As with any exogenous protein administration, local or systemic allergic reactions may occur. Inform parents and patients that such reactions are possible and that if an allergic reaction occurs, treatment should be interrupted and prompt medical attention sought.

MECASERMIN (rDNA ORIGIN) — INJECTION

Drug Interactions

None known.

Adverse Reactions

As with all protein pharmaceuticals, some patients may develop antibodies to mecasermin. Anti-IGF-1 antibodies were present at 1 or more of the periodic assessments in 14 of 23 children with primary IGFD treated for 2 years. However, no clinical consequences of these antibodies were observed (eg, allergic reactions, attenuation of growth).

In clinical studies of 71 subjects with primary IGFD treated for a mean duration of 3.9 years and representing 274 subject-years, no subjects withdrew from any clinical study because of adverse reactions. Adverse reactions considered related to mecasermin treatment that occurred in 5% or more of these study participants are listed by organ class.

➤*Cardiovascular:* Cardiac murmur.

➤*CNS:* Convulsions, dizziness, headache.

➤*GI:* Vomiting.

➤*Hematologic / Lymphatic:* Thymus hypertrophy.

➤*Metabolic / Nutritional:* Hypoglycemia.

➤*Musculoskeletal:* Arthralgia, pain in extremity.

➤*Respiratory:* Snoring, tonsillar hypertrophy.

➤*Special senses:* Abnormal tympanometry, ear pain, ear tube insertion, fluid in middle ear, hypoacusis, otitis media, serous otitis media.

➤*Miscellaneous:* Bruising, lipohypertrophy.

➤*Hypoglycemia:* Hypoglycemia was reported by 30 subjects (42%) at least once during their course of therapy. Most cases of hypoglycemia were mild or moderate in severity. Five subjects had severe hypoglycemia (requiring assistance and treatment) on 1 or more occasion and 4 subjects experienced hypoglycemic seizures/loss of consciousness on 1 or more occasion. Of the 30 subjects reporting hypoglycemia, 14 (47%) had a history of hypoglycemia prior to treatment. The frequency of hypoglycemia was highest in the first month of treatment, and episodes were more frequent in younger children. Symptomatic hypoglycemia was generally avoided when a meal or snack was consumed either shortly (ie, 20 minutes) before or after the administration of mecasermin.

➤*Lymphoid tissue hypertrophy:* Tonsillar hypertrophy was noted in 11 (15%) subjects in the first 1 to 2 years of therapy with lesser tonsillar growth in subsequent years. Tonsillectomy or tonsillectomy/adenoidectomy was performed in 7 subjects; 3 of these had obstructive sleep apnea, which resolved after the procedure in all 3 cases.

➤*Intracranial hypertension:* Intracranial hypertension occurred in 3 subjects. In 2 subjects the events resolved without interruption of mecasermin treatment. Mecasermin treatment was discontinued in the third subject and resumed later at a lower dose without recurrence.

➤*Miscellaneous:* Mild elevations in the serum AST and lactate dehydrogenase (LDH) were found in a significant proportion of patients before and during treatment and no rise in levels of these serum enzymes led to treatment discontinuation. ALT elevations were occasionally noted during treatment. Renal and splenic lengths (measured by ultrasound) increased rapidly on mecasermin treatment during the first years of therapy. This lengthening slowed down subsequently; though in some patients, renal and/or splenic length reached or surpassed the 95th percentile. Renal function (as defined by serum creatinine and calculated creatinine clearance) was normal in all patients, irrespective of renal growth. Elevations in cholesterol and triglycerides to above the upper limit of normal were observed before and during treatment. Echocardiographic evidence of cardiomegaly/valvulopathy was observed in a few individuals without associated clinical symptoms. Because of underlying disease and the lack of control group, the relation of the cardiac changes to drug treatment cannot be assessed.

Thickening of the soft tissues of the face was observed in several patients and should be monitored during mecasermin treatment.

Overdosage

There is no clinical experience with overdosage of mecasermin.

➤*Symptoms:* Based on known pharmacological effects, acute overdosage would be predicted to lead to hypoglycemia. Long-term overdosage may result in signs and symptoms of acromegaly.

➤*Treatment:* Treatment of acute overdose of mecasermin should be directed at reversing hypoglycemia. Oral glucose or food should be consumed. If the overdose results in loss of consciousness, IV glucose or parenteral glucagon may be required to reverse the hypoglycemic effects.

Patient Information

Instruct patients and/or their parents in the safe administration of mecasermin. Give mecasermin shortly before or after (20 minutes on either side of) a meal or snack. Mecasermin should not be administered when the meal or snack is omitted. Never increase the dose of mecasermin to make up for 1 or more omitted doses. Initiate mecasermin therapy at a low dose and increase the dose only if no hypoglycemia episodes have occurred after at least 7 days of dosing. If severe hypoglycemia or persistent hypoglycemia occurs on treatment despite adequate food intake, consider mecasermin dose reduction. Educate patients and caregivers on how to recognize the signs and symptoms of hypoglycemia.

Thoroughly instruct patients and/or parents in the importance of proper needle disposal. Use a puncture-resistant container for the disposal of used needles and/or syringes (consistent with applicable state requirements). Do not reuse needles and syringes.

GROWTH HORMONE

SOMATROPIN

Rx	**Zorbtive** (Serono)	**Powder for injection**: 8.8 mg (≈ 26.4 units)/vial	Sucrose, benzyl alcohol. In 10 mL multi-dose vials with diluent (bacterio-static water for injection).
Rx	**Genotropin Miniquick** (Pharmacia)	**Powder for injection, lyophilized**: 0.2 mg/vial	Preservative free. In single-use syringe with 2-chamber cartridge. In 7s.[a]
		0.4 mg/vial	
		0.6 mg/vial	
		0.8 mg/vial	
		1 mg/vial	
		1.2 mg/vial	
		1.4 mg/vial	
		1.6 mg/vial	
		1.8 mg vial	
		2 mg/vial	
Rx	**Norditropin** (Novo Nordisk)	**Powder for injection, lyophilized:** 4 mg (≈ 12 units)/vial	In vials[b] with diluent.[c]
Rx	**Serostim** (Serono)		Sucrose. In single-use vials with diluent.
Rx	**Nutropin** (Genentech)	**Powder for injection, lyophilized:** 5 mg (≈ 15 units)/vial	In cartons of 2 vials[d] with a 10 mL multiple-dose vial of diluent.[e]
Rx	**Humatrope** (Eli Lilly)		In vials[f] with 5 mL diluent.[g]
Rx	**Serostim** (Serono)		Sucrose. In single-use vials with diluent.
Rx	**Saizen** (Serono)		Sucrose. In vials with diluent.[e]
Rx	**Tev-Tropin** (Gate)		30 mg mannitol. In vials with 5 mL diluent (bacteriostatic 0.9% sodium chloride for injection with benzyl alcohol).
Rx	**Genotropin** (Pharmacia)	**Powder for injection, lyophilized:** 5.8 mg (≈ 17.4 units)/vial	In 5.8 mg *Intra-Mix 2-chamber* cartridge with pressure-release needle and 2-chamber cartridge. In 1s and 5s.[h]
Rx	**Serostim** (Serono)	**Powder for injection, lyophilized:** 6 mg (≈ 18 units)/vial	Sucrose. In single-use vials with diluent.
Rx	**Humatrope** (Eli Lilly)	**Powder for injection, lyophilized:** 6 mg (18 units)/cartridge	In cartridge with prefilled syringe of diluent.[i]

SOMATROPIN

Rx	**Norditropin** (Novo Nordisk)	**Powder for injection, lyophilized:** 8 mg (≈ 24 units)/vial	In vials[b] with diluent.[c]
Rx	**Nutropin** (Genentech)	**Powder for injection, lyophilized:** 10 mg (≈ 30 units)/vial	In cartons of 2 vials[j] with two 10 mL multiple-dose vials of diluent.[e]
Rx	**Humatrope** (Eli Lilly)	**Powder for injection, lyophilized:** 12 mg (36 units)/cartridge	In cartridge with prefilled syringe of diluent.[k]
Rx	**Genotropin** (Pharmacia)	**Powder for injection, lyophilized:** 13.8 mg (≈ 41.4 units)/vial	In *Intra-Mix 2-chamber* cartridge of 1s and 5s.[l]
Rx	**Humatrope** (Eli Lilly)	**Powder for injection, lyophilized:** 24 mg (72 units)/cartridge	In cartridge with prefilled syringe of diluent.[m]
Rx	**Nutropin AQ** (Genentech)	**Injection:** 10 mg (≈ 30 units)/vial	In 2 mL multiple-dose vials (6s).[n]
Rx	**Norditropin** (Novo Nordisk)	**Injection:** 5 mg/1.5 mL	In cartridges.[o]
		Injection: 10 mg/1.5 mL	In cartridges.[o]
		Injection: 15 mg/1.5 mL	In cartridges.[p]
Rx	**Serostim LQ** (Serono)	**Injection:** 6 mg (approximately 18 units) per 0.5 mL	In cartridges (1s or 7s).[q]

[a] With glycine 0.23 mg, mannitol 13.74 mg.
[b] With mannitol 44 mg and glycine 8.8 mg.
[c] With water for injection with 1.5% benzyl alcohol.
[d] With mannitol 45 mg and glycine 1.7 mg.
[e] With Bacteriostatic water for injection with 0.9% benzyl alcohol.
[f] With mannitol 25 mg and glycine 5 mg.
[g] With water for injection with 0.3% Metacresol and 1.7% glycerin.
[h] With mannitol 46.8 mg.
[i] With mannitol 18 mg, glycine 6 mg, water for Injection with 0.3% Metacresol.
[j] With mannitol 90 mg and glycine 3.4 mg.
[k] With mannitol 36 mg, glycine 12 mg, water for injection with 0.3% Metacresol.
[l] With mannitol 46 mg.
[m] With mannitol 72 mg, glycine 24 mg, water for injection with 0.3% Metacresol.
[n] With sodium chloride 17.4 mg, phenol 5 mg, polysorbate 4 mg 20, and sodium citrate 10 mM.
[o] With phenol 4.5 mg and mannitol 60 mg.
[p] With phenol 4.5 mg and mannitol 58 mg.
[q] With 1.02 mg Poloxamer 188, sucrose 40.8 mg, citric acid 1.31 mg.

SOMATROPIN — INJECTION

For complete prescribing information, refer to the Growth Hormone group monograph.

Indications

➤*Genotropin*:

Pediatric patients – For the long-term treatment of pediatric patients who have growth failure due to an inadequate secretion of endogenous growth hormone.

For long-term treatment of pediatric patients who have growth failure due to Prader-Willi syndrome (PWS). The diagnosis of PWS should be confirmed by appropriate genetic testing.

For long-term treatment of growth failure in children born small for gestational age (SGA) who fail to manifest catch-up growth by age 2.

Adult patients – For long-term replacement therapy in adults with growth hormone deficiency (GHD) of either childhood- or adult-onset etiology. GHD should be confirmed by an appropriate growth hormone stimulation test.

➤*Humatrope*:

Pediatric patients – For the long-term treatment of pediatric patients who have growth failure due to an inadequate secretion of normal endogenous growth hormone.

For the treatment of short stature associated with Turner syndrome in patients whose epiphyses are not closed.

For the long-term treatment of idiopathic short stature, also called non-growth hormone-deficient short stature, defined by height SDS less than or equal to −2.25, and associated with growth rates unlikely to permit attainment of adult height in the normal range, in pediatric patients whose epiphyses are not closed and for whom diagnostic evaluation excludes other causes associated with short stature that should be observed or treated by other means.

Adult patients – For replacement of endogenous growth hormone in adults with growth hormone deficiency who meet both of the following 2 criteria:

Adult onset: Patients who have growth hormone deficiency either alone, or with multiple hormone deficiencies (hypopituitarism), as a result of pituitary disease, hypothalamic disease, surgery, radiation therapy, or trauma.

Childhood onset: Patients who were growth hormone-deficient during childhood who have growth hormone deficiency confirmed as an adult before replacement therapy with *Humatrope* is started.

➤*Norditropin*, *Nutropin Depot*, *Tev-Tropin*, and *Saizen*: For the long-term treatment of children with growth failure due to inadequate secretion of endogenous growth hormone.

➤*Nutropin* and *Nutropin AQ*:

Pediatric patients – For the long-term treatment of growth failure due to a lack of adequate endogenous GH secretion.

For the treatment of growth failure associated with chronic renal insufficiency up to the time of renal transplantation. *Nutropin* and *Nutropin AQ* therapy should be used in conjunction with optimal management of chronic renal insufficiency.

For the long-term treatment of short stature associated with Turner syndrome.

Adult patients – For the replacement of endogenous GH in patients with adult GH deficiency who meet both of the following 2 criteria:

1.) Biochemical diagnosis of adult GH deficiency by means of a subnormal response to a standard growth hormone stimulation test (peak GH less than or equal to 5 mcg/L).
2.) Adult onset: Patients who have adult GH deficiency either alone or with multiple hormone deficiencies (hypopituitarism) as a result of pituitary disease, hypothalamic disease, surgery, radiation therapy, or trauma; or childhood onset: Patients who were GH deficient during childhood, confirmed as an adult before replacement therapy with *Nutropin* or *Nutropin AQ* is started.

➤*Serostim*: For the treatment of HIV patients with wasting or cachexia to increase lean body mass and body weight, and improve physical endurance. Concomitant antiretroviral therapy is necessary.

➤*Zorbtive*: For the treatment of short bowel syndrome in patients receiving specialized nutritional support. *Zorbtive* therapy should be used in conjunction with optimal management of short bowel syndrome.

➤*Serostim LQ*: For AIDS wasting or cachexia.

Administration and Dosage

➤*Approved by the FDA:* March 8, 1987.

➤*Genotropin*: Adjust for the individual patient. The weekly dose should be divided into 6 or 7 subcutaneous injections. *Genotropin* may be given in the thigh, buttocks, or abdomen; the site of subcutaneous injections should be rotated daily to help prevent lipoatrophy.

Pediatric growth hormone-deficient patients – 0.16 to 0.24 mg/kg body weight/week.

Pediatric Prader-Willi syndrome patients – 0.24 mg/kg body weight/week.

Pediatric small for gestational age patients – 0.48 mg/kg body weight/week.

Adult growth hormone-deficient patients – The recommended dosage at the start of therapy is not more than 0.04 mg/kg/week. The dose may be increased at 4- to 8-week intervals according to individual patient requirements to a maximum of 0.08 mg/kg/week, depending upon patient tolerance of treatment. Clinical response, side effects, and determination of age-adjusted serum IGF-I may be used as guidance in dose titration. This approach will tend to result in weight-adjusted doses that are larger for women compared with men and smaller for older and obese patients.

Genotropin must not be injected intravenously.

Genotropin is supplied as a powder, filled in a 2-chamber cartridge with the active substance in the front chamber and the diluent in the rear chamber. A reconstitution device is used to co-mix the diluent and the lyophilized powder.

Follow the directions for reconstitution provided with each device. Gently tip the cartridge upside down a few times until the contents are completely dissolved. Do not shake; this may cause denaturation of the active ingredient. For more specific information, see directions accompanying the reconstitution device.

➤*Humatrope*:

Pediatric patients – Dosage and administration schedule should be individualized for each patient. Therapy should not be continued if epiphyseal fusion has occurred. Response to growth hormone therapy tends to decrease with time. However, failure to increase growth rate, particularly during the first year of therapy, should prompt close assessment of compliance and evaluation of other causes of growth failure such as hypothyroidism, undernutrition and advanced bone age.

Growth hormone-deficient pediatric patients: 0.18 mg/kg (0.54 units/kg) of body weight weekly. The maximal replacement weekly dosage is 0.3 mg/kg (0.90 units/kg) of body weight. It should be divided into equal doses given either on 3 alternate days, 6 times per week or daily. The subcutaneous

SOMATROPIN — INJECTION

route of administration is preferable; IM injection is also acceptable. The dosage and administration schedule for *Humatrope* should be individualized for each patient.

Turner syndrome: A weekly dosage of up to 0.375 mg/kg (1.125 units/kg) of body weight administered by subcutaneous injection is recommended. It should be divided into equal doses given either daily or on 3 alternate days.

Patients with idiopathic short stature: A weekly dosage of up to 0.37 mg/kg of body weight administered by subcutaneous injection is recommended. It should be divided into equal doses given 6 to 7 times per week.

Adult patients –

Growth hormone-deficient adult patients: The recommended dosage at the start of therapy is not more than 0.006 mg/kg/day (0.018 units/kg/day) given as a daily subcutaneous injection. The dose may be increased according to individual patient requirements to a maximum of 0.0125 mg/kg/day (0.0375 units/kg/day).

During therapy, dosage should be titrated if required by the occurrence of side effects or to maintain the insulin-like growth factor-I (IGF-I) response below the upper limit of normal IGF-I levels, matched for age and sex. To minimize the occurrence of adverse events in patients with increasing age or excessive body weight, dose reductions may be necessary.

Reconstitution –

Vial: Each 5 mg vial of *Humatrope* should be reconstituted with 1.5 to 5 mL of diluent for *Humatrope*. The diluent should be injected into the vial of *Humatrope* by aiming the stream of liquid against the glass wall. Following reconstitution, the vial should be swirled with a gentle rotary motion until the contents are completely dissolved. Do not shake. The resulting solution should be inspected for clarity. It should be clear. If the solution is cloudy or contains particulate matter, the contents must not be injected.

Cartridge: The *HumatroPen* allows the somatropin dosage volume to be dialed in increments of 0.048 mL per click of dosage knob, and the maximum dosage volume that can be injected is 0.576 mL (based on a 12 click maximum) (see table below for additional information).

Concentration of Reconstituted *Humatrope* Solutions, Incremental Dosage and Maximum Injectable Dose for Each Cartridge

Cartridge	Somatropin concentration	Dose per click of dosage knob	Maximum injectable dose
6 mg	2.08 mg/mL	0.1 mg	1.2 mg
12 mg	4.17 mg/mL	0.2 mg	2.4 mg
24 mg	8.33 mg/mL	0.4 mg	4.8 mg

This cartridge has been designed for use only with the *HumatroPen*. A sterile disposable needle should be used for each administration of *Humatrope*.

➤*Norditropin*: Dosage and schedule for administration must be individualized for each patient. Generally, subcutaneous administration in the evening, 6 to 7 times per week, is recommended. It is recommended to give the injections in the thighs and to vary the injection site on the thigh on a rotating basis. Dosage can be calculated according to body weight.

Generally recommended dosage – 0.024 to 0.034 mg/kg body weight, 6 to 7 times per week by subcutaneous injection.

Norditropin cartridges must be administered using the *Nordipen* injection pen. Each cartridge size has a color-coded corresponding pen which is graduated to deliver the appropriate dose based on the concentration of *Norditropin* in the cartridge.

Norditropin must not be injected if the solution is cloudy or contains particulate matter. Use it only if it is clear and colorless.

Measuring the prescribing dose – 5 mg/1.5 mL, 10 mg/1.5 mL, and 15 mg/1.5 mL *Norditropin* cartridges.

➤*Nutropin* and *Nutropin AQ*: Dosage and administration schedule should be individualized for each patient. Response to growth hormone therapy in pediatric patients tends to decrease with time. However, in pediatric patients failure to increase growth rate, particularly during the first year of therapy, suggests the need for close assessment of compliance and evaluation of other causes of growth failure, such as hypothyroidism, undernutrition, and advanced bone age.

Dosage –

Pediatric growth hormone deficiency: A weekly dosage of up to 0.3 mg/kg of body weight divided into daily subcutaneous injection is recommended. In pubertal patients, a weekly dosage of up to 0.7 mg/kg divided daily may be used.

Adult growth hormone deficiency: The recommended dosage at the start of therapy is not more than 0.006 mg/kg given as a daily subcutaneous injection. The dose may be increased according to individual patient requirements to a maximum of 0.025 mg/kg daily in patients less than 35 years of age and to a maximum of 0.0125 mg/kg daily in patients greater than 35 years of age.

To minimize the occurrence of adverse events in older or overweight patients, lower doses may be necessary. During therapy, dosage should be decreased if required by the occurrence of side effects or excessive IGF-I levels.

Chronic renal insufficiency (CRI): A weekly dosage of up to 0.35 mg/kg of body weight divided into daily subcutaneous injection is recommended. Therapy may be continued up to the time of renal transplantation.

• *Dialysis patients* – Hemodialysis patients should receive their injection at night just prior to going to sleep or at least 3 to 4 hours after their hemodialysis to prevent hematoma formation due to the heparin. Chronic cycling peritoneal dialysis (CCPD) patients should receive their injection in the morning after they have completed dialysis. Chronic ambulatory peritoneal dialysis (CAPD) patients should receive their injection in the evening at the time of the overnight exchange.

Turner syndrome: A weekly dosage of up to 0.375 mg/kg of body weight divided into equal doses 3 to 7 times per week by subcutaneous injection is recommended.

Administration – After the dose has been determined, reconstitute *Nutropin* as follows: Each 5 mg vial should be reconstituted with 1 to 5 ml of bacteriostatic water for injection (benzyl alcohol preserved); or each 10 mg vial should be reconstituted with 1 to 10 ml of bacteriostatic water for injection (benzyl alcohol preserved), only. The pH of *Nutropin* after reconstitution with bacteriostatic water for injection (benzyl alcohol preserved), is approximately 7.4.

Benzyl alcohol as a preservative in bacteriostatic water for injection has been associated with toxicity in newborns. When administering somatropin (rDNA origin) injection to newborns, reconstitute with sterile water for injection. Use only 1 dose per vial and discard the unused portion.

To prepare the *Nutropin* solution, inject the bacteriostatic water for injection (benzyl alcohol preserved), into the *Nutropin* vial, aiming the stream of liquid against the glass wall. Then swirl the product vial with a gentle rotary motion until the contents are completely dissolved. Do not shake. Because somatropin is a protein, shaking can result in a cloudy solution. The *Nutropin* solution should be clear immediately after reconstitution, and the *Nutropin AQ* solution should be clear immediately after removal from the refrigerator. Occasionally, after refrigeration, one may notice that small colorless particles of protein are present in the *Nutropin* and *Nutropin AQ* solutions. This is not unusual for solutions containing proteins. If the solution is cloudy immediately after reconstitution or refrigeration, the contents must not be injected.

Nutropin AQ vial: Before needle insertion, wipe the septum of the *Nutropin AQ* vial or both the *Nutropin* and diluent vials with rubbing alcohol or an antiseptic solution to prevent contamination of the contents by microorganisms that may be introduced by repeated needle insertions. It is recommended that *Nutropin* and *Nutropin AQ* be administered using sterile, disposable syringes and needles. The syringes should be of small enough volume that the prescribed dose can be drawn from the vial with reasonable accuracy.

Nutropin AQ pen cartridge: The *Nutropin AQ* pen cartridge is intended for use only with the *Nutropin AQ* pen. Wipe the septum of the *Nutropin AQ* pen cartridge with rubbing alcohol or an antiseptic solution to prevent contamination of the contents by microorganisms that may be introduced by repeated needle insertions. It is recommended that *Nutropin AQ* be administered using sterile, disposable needles. Follow the directions provided in the *Nutropin AQ* pen instructions for use. The *Nutropin AQ* pen allows for administration of a minimum dose of 0.1 mg to a maximum dose of 4 mg, in 0.1 mg increments.

➤*Nutropin Depot*: Dosage and administration schedule should be individualized for each patient. Response to GH therapy in pediatric patients tends to decrease over time. However in pediatric patients, failure to increase growth rate, particularly during the first year of therapy, suggests the need for close assessment of compliance and evaluation of other causes of growth failure, such as hypothyroidism, under-nutrition, and advanced bone age.

Once-monthly injection – 1.5 mg/kg body weight administered subcutaneously on the same day of each month. Dosages above the recommended once-monthly regimen have not been studied in clinical trials.

Note: Subjects greater than 15 kg will require greater than 1 injection per dose.

Twice-monthly injections – 0.75 mg/kg body weight administered subcutaneously twice each month on the same days of each month (eg, days 1 and 15 of each month). Dosages above the recommended twice-monthly regimen have not been studied in clinical trials.

Note: Subjects greater than 30 kg will require greater than 1 injection per dose.

Number of *Nutropin Depot* Injections per Dose

Patient weight (kg)	0.75 mg/kg twice monthly	1.5 mg/kg once monthly
≤ 15	1	1
> 15 to 30	1	2
> 30 to 45	2	3
> 45 to 60	2	[a]
> 60	3	[a]

[a] Twice monthly dosing recommended.

Preparation of dose – *Nutropin Depot* powder may only be suspended in diluent for *Nutropin Depot* supplied in the kit and administered with the supplied needles.

1.) Using the chart below, determine the volume of diluent needed to suspend *Nutropin Depot*. Withdraw the diluent into a 3 mL syringe using the needle supplied in the kit. Only the diluent supplied in the kit should be used for reconstitution, and any remaining diluent should be discarded.
2.) Inject the diluent into the vial against the vial wall. Swirl the vial vigorously for up to 2 minutes to disperse the powder in the diluent. Mixing is complete when the suspension appears uniform, thick, and milky, and all the powder is fully dispersed. Do not store the vial after reconstitution or the suspension may settle.

SOMATROPIN — INJECTION

3.) Withdraw the required dose. Only 1 vial should be used for each injection. Replace the needle with a new needle from the kit and administer the dose immediately to avoid settling of the suspension in the syringe. Deliver the dose from the syringe at a continuous rate over less than or equal to 5 seconds. Discard unused vial contents as the product contains no preservative. An extra needle has been provided in the kit.

Nutropin Depot Diluent Volume Needed Per Vial	
Vial size (mg somatropin)	Volume of diluent to be added (mL)
13.5	0.8
18	1
22.5	1.2

Note: Because the suspension is viscous and prevents complete withdrawal of the entire vial contents, the vials are overfilled to ensure delivery of the labeled amount of somatropin. Using these diluent volumes for final suspension results in a final concentration of 19 mg/mL somatropin in each vial size.

➤*Saizen*: Dosage and schedule of administration should be individualized for each patient. For the treatment of growth hormone inadequacy, a dosage of 0.06 mg/kg (approximately 0.18 units/kg) administered 3 times per week by subcutaneous or IM injection is recommended.

Treatment with *Saizen* of growth failure due to growth hormone deficiency should be discontinued when the epiphyses are fused. Patients who fail to respond adequately while on *Saizen* therapy should be evaluated to determine the cause of unresponsiveness.

After determining the appropriate patient dose, reconstitute each vial of *Saizen* as follows: 5 mg vial with 1 to 3 mL of bacteriostatic water for injection (benzyl alcohol preserved); 8.8 mg vial with 2 to 3 ml of bacteriostatic water for injection (benzyl alcohol preserved). Approximately 10% mechanical loss can be associated with reconstitution and multi-dose administration.

Benzyl alcohol as a preservative in bacteriostatic water for injection has been associated with toxicity in newborns. When administering to newborns, reconstitute with sterile water for injection. Use only 1 dose per vial and discard the unused portion.

To reconstitute *Saizen*, inject the diluent into the vial of *Saizen*, aiming the liquid against the glass vial wall. Swirl the vial with a gentle rotary motion until contents are dissolved completely. Do not shake. Because *Saizen* growth hormone is a protein, shaking can result in a cloudy solution. The *Saizen* solution should be clear immediately after reconstitution. Do not inject *Saizen* if the reconstituted product is cloudy immediately after reconstitution or refrigeration. Occasionally, after refrigeration, small colorless particles may be present in the *Saizen* solution. This is not unusual for proteins like *Saizen*.

➤*Serostim* and *Serostim LQ*: The usual starting dose is 0.1 mg/kg subcutaneously daily (up to 6 mg). It should be administered subcutaneously daily at bedtime according to the following dosage recommendations:

Serostim Dosing Recommendations	
Weight range	Dose
> 55kg (> 121 lb)	6 mg[a] subcutaneous daily
45 to 55 kg (99 to 121 lb)	5 mg[a] subcutaneous daily
35 to 45 kg (75 to 99 lb)	4 mg[a] subcutaneous daily
< 35 kg (< 75 lb)	0.1 mg/kg subcutaneous daily

[a] Based on an approximate daily dosage of 0.1 mg/kg.

Serostim 4, 5, or 6 mg with sterile water for injection, single-use vials, should be administered to patients requiring 4, 5, or 6 mg daily, respectively, as per the above weight-based dosing table.

Treatment with *Serostim* 0.1 mg/kg every other day was associated with fewer side effects, and resulted in a similar improvement in work output, as compared with *Serostim* 0.1 mg/kg daily. Therefore, a starting dose of *Serostim* 0.1 mg/kg every other day should be considered in patients at increased risk for adverse effects related to recombinant human growth hormone therapy (ie, glucose intolerance). In general, dose reductions (ie, reducing the total daily dose or the number of doses per week) should be considered for side effects potentially related to recombinant human growth hormone therapy, which are unresponsive to symptom-directed treatment.

Most of the effect of *Serostim* on work output and lean body mass was apparent after 12 weeks of treatment. The effect was maintained during an additional 12 weeks of therapy. There are no safety or efficacy data available from controlled studies in which patients were treated with *Serostim* continuously for more than 48 weeks. There are no safety or efficacy data available from controlled trials in which patients were treated intermittently with *Serostim*.

Injection sites should be rotated.

Serostim – Each vial of *Serostim* 4, 5, or 6 mg is reconstituted with 0.5 to 1 mL Sterile Water for Injection.

To reconstitute *Serostim*, inject the diluent into the vial of *Serostim* aiming the liquid against the glass vial wall. Swirl the vial with a gentle rotary motion until contents are dissolved completely. The *Serostim* solution should be clear immediately after reconstitution. Do not inject *Serostim* if the reconstituted product is cloudy immediately after reconstitution.

Serostim LQ – The solution in the cartridge should be allowed to equilibrate to room temperature before administration of the injection. Discard the cartridge after use, even if some drug remains in the cartridge.

➤*Zorbtive*: *Zorbtive* should be administered to patients with short bowel syndrome (SBS) at a dose of approximately 0.1 mg/kg subcutaneously daily to a maximum of 8 mg daily. Administration for more than 4 weeks has not been adequately studied.

Injections should be administered daily for 4 weeks. Changes to concomitant medications should be avoided. Patients and physicians should monitor for adverse events. Treat moderate fluid retention and arthralgias symptomatically or reduce dose by 50%. Discontinue *Zorbtive* for up to 5 days for severe toxicities. Upon resolution of symptoms, resume at 50% of original dose. Permanently discontinue treatment if severe toxicity recurs or does not disappear within 5 days.

Injection sites should be rotated.

Safety and effectiveness in pediatric patients with short bowel syndrome have not been established.

Each vial of *Zorbtive* 4, 5, or 6 mg is reconstituted with 0.5 to 1 mL sterile water for injection. Each vial of *Zorbtive* 8.8 mg is reconstituted in 1 to 2 ml of bacteriostatic water for injection (0.9% benzyl alcohol preserved). See the table below for expected concentration after reconstitution. Approximately 10% mechanical loss can be associated with reconstitution and administration from multidose vials.

Benzyl alcohol as a preservative in bacteriostatic water for injection has been associated with toxicity in newborns. When administering somatropin (rDNA origin) injection to newborns, reconstitute with sterile water for injection. Use only 1 dose per vial and discard the unused portion.

Zorbtive Expected Concentration After Reconstitution (mg/mL)			
	0.5 mL	1 mL	2 mL
4 mg	8	4	-
5 mg	10	5	-
6 mg	12	6	-
8.8 mg	-	8.8	4.4

To reconstitute *Zorbtive*, inject the diluent into the vial of *Zorbtive*, aiming the liquid against the glass vial wall. Swirl the vial with a gentle rotary motion until contents are dissolved completely. The *Zorbtive* solution should be clear immediately after reconstitution. Do not inject *Zorbtive* if the reconstituted product is cloudy immediately after reconstitution (*Zorbtive* 4, 5, 6 mg or 8.8 mg) or after refrigeration (only *Zorbtive* 8.8 mg). The reconstituted *Zorbtive* 8.8 mg can be refrigerated (2° to 8°C [36° to 46°F]) for up to 14 days. Occasionally, after refrigeration, small colorless particles may be present in the *Zorbtive* 8.8 mg solution. This is not unusual for proteins like *Zorbtive*. Allow refrigerated solution to come to room temperature prior to administration. A standard insulin-type subcutaneous syringe is recommended for administration.

➤*Tev-Tropin*: A dosage of up to 0.1 mg/kg (0.3 units/kg) of body weight administered 3 times/week by subcutaneous injection is recommended. The dosage schedule for *Tev-Tropin* should be reconstituted with 1 to 5 mL of bacteriostatic 0.9% sodium chloride for injection, USP (benzyl alcohol preserved). The stream of normal saline should be aimed against the side of the vial to prevent foaming. Swirl the vial with a gentle rotary motion until the contents are completely dissolved and the solution is clear. Do not shake. Because *Tev-Tropin* is a protein, shaking or vigorous mixing will cause the solution to be cloudy. If the resulting solution is cloudy or contains particulate matter, the contents must not be injected.

➤*Storage/Stability:*

Genotropin – Except as noted below, refrigerate at 2° to 8°C (36° to 46°F). Do not freeze. Protect from light.

The 1.5 mg cartridge of *Genotropin* contains a diluent with no preservative. After reconstitution, the cartridge may be refrigerated for up to 24 hours. Use once only and discard any remaining solution.

The 5.8 mg and 13.8 mg cartridges of *Genotropin* contain a diluent with a preservative. Thus, after reconstitution, they may be refrigerated for up to 21 days.

Genotropin Miniquick – Refrigerate prior to dispensing, but may be stored at or below 25°C (77°F) for up to 3 months after dispensing. The diluent has no preservative. After reconstitution, the *Genotropin Miniquick* may be refrigerated for 24 hours before use, the *Genotropin Miniquick* should be used only once and then discarded.

Humatrope – Refrigerate (2° to 8°C [36° to 46°F]) before and after reconstitution. Do not freeze. Store the *HumatroPen*, with the *Humatrope* cartridge attached, in the refrigerator until time of the next injection. Reconstituted *Humatrope* must be used within 28 days. Discard any remaining reconstituted *Humatrope* after 28 days.

Vials:

- *Before reconstitution* – Refrigerate at 2° to 8°C (36° to 46°F). Avoid freezing diluent for *Humatrope*.
- *After reconstitution* – Vials of *Humatrope* are stable for up to 14 days when reconstituted with diluent for *Humatrope* or bacteriostatic water for injection and stored in a refrigerator at 2° to 8°C (36° to 46°F). Avoid freezing the reconstituted vial of *Humatrope*.
- *After reconstitution with sterile water* – Use only 1 dose per *Humatrope* vial and discard the unused portion. If the solution is not used immediately, it must be refrigerated 2° to 8°C (36° to 46°F) and used within 24 hours.

Cartridges:

- *Before reconstitution* – Cartridges of *Humatrope* and diluent for *Humatrope* are stable when refrigerated at 2° to 8°C (36° to 46°F). Avoid freezing diluent for *Humatrope*. Expiration dates are stated on the labels.
- *After reconstitution* – Cartridges of *Humatrope* are stable for up to 28 days when reconstituted with diluent for *Humatrope* and stored in a

SOMATROPIN — INJECTION

refrigerator at 2° to 8°C (36° to 46°F). Store the *HumatroPen* without the needle attached. Avoid freezing the reconstituted cartridge of *Humatrope*.

Norditropin – Refrigerate at 2° to 8°C (36° to 46°F). Do not freeze. Avoid direct light.

After a *Norditropin* cartridge has been inserted into the *NordiPen* injector, it must be stored in the pen in the refrigerator and used within 4 weeks.

Nutropin –

Before reconstitution: Refrigerate at 2° to 8°C (36° to 46°F). Avoid freezing the vials of *Nutropin* and bacteriostatic water for injection (benzyl alcohol preserved).

After reconstitution: Vial contents are stable for 14 days when reconstituted with bacteriostatic water for injection (benzyl alcohol preserved), and stored under refrigeration at 2° to 8°C (36° to 46°F). Store the unused portion of bacteriostatic water for injection (benzyl alcohol preserved) under refrigeration at 2° to 8°C (36° to 46°F). Avoid freezing the reconstituted vial of *Nutropin* and the bacteriostatic water for injection (benzyl alcohol preserved).

Nutropin AQ – Vial contents are stable for 28 days after initial use when stored under refrigeration at 2° to 8°C (36° to 46°F). Avoid freezing the vial of *Nutropin AQ*. The vials and cartridges of *Nutropin AQ* are light sensitive and they should be protected from light. Store the vial and the cartridge refrigerated in a dark place when they are not in use.

Nutropin Depot –

Before suspension: Refrigerate at 2° to 8°C (36° to 46°F). Avoid freezing the vials of *Nutropin Depot* and diluent for *Nutropin Depot*. Do not expose the *Nutropin Depot* vial to temperatures above 25°C (77°F).

After suspension: Because *Nutropin Depot* contains no preservatives, all injections must be given immediately. Do not allow the suspension to settle prior to withdrawal of the dose. Suspended solution cannot be stored or used to suspend another vial of *Nutropin Depot*.

Saizen –

Before reconstitution: Store at room temperature (15° to 30°C [59° to 86°F]).

After reconstitution: When reconstituted with the diluent provided, the reconstituted solution should be stored under refrigeration (2° to 8°C [36° to 46°F]) for up to 14 days. Avoid freezing reconstituted vials.

Serostim –

Before reconstitution: Store at room temperature (15° to 30°C [59° to 86°F]).

After reconstitution with sterile water for injection: The reconstituted solution should be used immediately and any unused portion should be discarded.

Zorbtive –

Before reconstitution: Store at room temperature, (15° to 30°C [59° to 86°F]).

After reconstitution with sterile water for injection: The reconstituted solution should be used immediately and any unused portion should be discarded.

After reconstitution with bacteriostatic water for injection (0.9% benzyl alcohol): The reconstituted solution should be stored under refrigeration (2° to 8°C [36° to 46°F]) for up to 14 days. Avoid freezing reconstituted vials of *Zorbtive*. Store *Serostim LQ* under refrigeration 2° to 8°C (36° to 46°F); protect from light and avoid freezing cartridges.

Tev-Tropin –

Before reconstitution: Refrigerate at 36° to 46 F (2° to 8°C).

After reconstitution: Vials of *Tev-Tropin* are stable for up to 14 days when reconstituted with bacteriostatic 0.9% sodium chloride (normal saline), USP, and stored in a refrigerator at 36° to 46°F (2° to 8°C). Do not freeze the reconstituted solution.

Actions

➤*Pharmacology:*

Tissue growth –

Skeletal growth: Somatropin stimulates skeletal growth in pediatric patients with GHD, PWS, or SGA. The measurable increase in body length after administration of somatropin results from an effect on the epiphyseal plates of long bones. Concentrations of IGF-I, which may play a role in skeletal growth, are generally low in the serum of pediatric patients with GHD, PWS, or SGA, but tend to increase during treatment with somatropin. Elevations in mean serum alkaline phosphatase concentration are also seen.

Cell growth: It has been shown that there are fewer skeletal muscle cells in short-statured pediatric patients who lack endogenous growth hormone as compared with the healthy pediatric population. Treatment with somatropin results in an increase in both the number and size of muscle cells.

Organ growth – GH influences the size of internal organs, including kidneys, and increases red cell mass. Treatment of hypophysectomized or genetic dwarf rats with GH results in organ growth that is proportional to the overall body growth. In healthy rats subjected to nephrectomy-induced uremia, GH promoted skeletal and body growth.

Protein metabolism – Linear growth is facilitated in part by increased cellular protein synthesis. Nitrogen retention, as demonstrated by decreased urinary nitrogen excretion and serum urea nitrogen, follows the initiation of therapy with somatropin.

Carbohydrate metabolism – Pediatric patients with hypopituitarism sometimes experience fasting hypoglycemia that is improved by treatment with somatropin. Large doses of growth hormone may impair glucose tolerance.

Untreated patients with Turner syndrome have an increased incidence of glucose intolerance. Administration of human growth hormone to healthy adults or patients with Turner syndrome resulted in increases in mean serum fasting and postprandial insulin levels although mean values remained in the normal range. In addition, mean fasting and postprandial glucose and hemoglobin A_{1c} levels remained in the normal range.

Lipid metabolism – In GHD patients, administration of somatropin has resulted in lipid mobilization, reduction in body fat stores, and increased plasma fatty acids.

Mineral metabolism – Somatropin induces retention of sodium, potassium, and phosphorus. Serum concentrations of inorganic phosphate are increased in patients with GHD after therapy with somatropin. Serum calcium is not significantly altered by somatropin. Growth hormone could increase calciuria.

Body composition – Adult GHD patients treated with somatropin at the recommended adult dose demonstrate a decrease in fat mass and an increase in lean body mass. When these alterations are coupled with the increase in total body water, the overall effect of somatropin is to modify body composition, an effect that is maintained with continued treatment.

Genotropin – In vitro, preclinical, and clinical tests have demonstrated that *Genotropin* lyophilized powder is therapeutically equivalent to human growth hormone of pituitary origin and achieves similar pharmacokinetic profiles in healthy adults. In pediatric patients who have GHD or PWS, or who were born small for gestational age (SGA), treatment with *Genotropin* stimulates linear growth. In patients with GHD or PWS, treatment with *Genotropin* also normalizes concentrations of IGF-I (insulin-like growth factor-I/somatropin C). In adults with GHD, treatment with *Genotropin* results in reduced fat mass, increased lean body mass, metabolic alterations that include beneficial changes in lipid metabolism, and normalization of IGF-I concentrations.

Humatrope –

Linear growth: Somatropin stimulates linear growth in pediatric patients who lack adequate normal endogenous growth hormone. In vitro, preclinical, and clinical testing have demonstrated that *Humatrope* is therapeutically equivalent to human growth hormone of pituitary origin and achieves equivalent pharmacokinetic profiles in healthy adults. Treatment of growth hormone-deficient pediatric patients and patients with Turner syndrome with somatropin (rDNA) produces increased growth rate and IGF-I (insulin-like growth factor-I/somatomedin-C) concentrations similar to those seen after therapy with human growth hormone of pituitary origin.

Nutropin and *Nutropin AQ* – In vitro and in vivo preclinical and clinical testing have demonstrated that *Nutropin* and *Nutropin AQ* is therapeutically equivalent to pituitary-derived human GH (hGH). Pediatric patients who lack adequate endogenous GH secretion, patients with chronic renal insufficiency, and patients with Turner syndrome that were treated with *Nutropin* resulted in an increase in growth rate and an increase in IGF-I levels similar to that seen with pituitary-derived hGH.

Nutropin Depot – In vivo preclinical and clinical testing has demonstrated that GH stimulates longitudinal bone growth and elevates IGF-I levels.

Serostim – *Serostim* [somatropin (rDNA origin) for injection] is an anabolic and anticatabolic agent which exerts its influence by interacting with specific receptors on a variety of cell types including myocytes, hepatocytes, adipocytes, lymphocytes, and hematopoietic cells. Some, but not all of its effects, are mediated by insulin-like growth factor-I (IGF-I).

HIV-associated wasting or cachexia, which commonly involves involuntary loss of lean body mass or body weight, is a metabolic disorder characterized by abnormalities of intermediary metabolism resulting in weight loss, inappropriate depletion of lean body mass (LBM), and paradoxical preservation of body fat. LBM includes primarily skeletal muscle, organ tissue, blood and blood constituents, and both intracellular and extracellular water. Depletion of LBM results in muscle weakness, organ failure, and death. Unlike nutritional intervention for HIV-associated wasting, in which supplemental calories are converted predominantly to body fat, *Serostim* treatment resulted in a significant increase in LBM and a decrease in fat mass with a significant increase in body weight due to the dominant effect of LBM gain.

Effects on protein, lipid, and carbohydrate metabolism: A 1-week study in 6 patients with HIV-associated wasting has shown that treatment with *Serostim* 0.1 mg/kg/day improved nitrogen balance, increased protein-sparing lipid oxidation, and had little effect on overall carbohydrate metabolism.

Effects on nitrogen and mineral retention: In the 1-week study in 6 patients with HIV-associated wasting, treatment with *Serostim* resulted in the retention of phosphorus, potassium, nitrogen, and sodium. The ratio of retained potassium and nitrogen during *Serostim* therapy was consistent with retention of these elements in lean tissue.

Zorbtive – *Zorbtive* [somatropin (rDNA origin) for injection] is an anabolic and anticatabolic agent which exerts its influence by interacting with specific receptors on a variety of cell types including myocytes, hepatocytes, adipocytes, lymphocytes, and hematopoietic cells. Some, but not all of its effects, are mediated by IGF-I.

Mechanism of action in short bowel syndrome (SBS) patients: Intestinal mucosa contains receptors for growth hormone and for IGF-I, which is known to mediate many of the cellular actions of growth hormone. Thus, the actions of growth hormone on the gut may be direct or mediated via the local or systemic production of IGF.

In human clinical studies the administration of growth hormone has been shown to enhance the transmucosal transport of water, electrolytes, and nutrients.

Nutropin Depot –

Pharmacodynamics: In a 6-month study compared *Nutropin Depot* 0.75 mg/kg every 2 weeks (n = 20) and 1.5 mg/kg every 4 weeks (n = 19).

IGF-I levels peaked between 1.5 and 3.5 days postdose and remained above baseline for approximately 16 to 20 days, confirming GH activity for an extended period. Repeated dosing of *Nutropin Depot* over 6 months showed no progressive accumulation of IGF-I or IGF-binding protein 3 (IGFBP-3).

SOMATROPIN — INJECTION

➤*Pharmacokinetics:*

Absorption –

Genotropin: Following a 0.03 mg/kg subcutaneous injection in the thigh of 1.3 mg/mL *Genotropin* to adult GHD patients, approximately 80% of the dose was systemically available as compared with that available following intravenous dosing. Results were comparable in both male and female patients. Similar bioavailability has been observed in healthy adult male subjects. In healthy adult males, following an subcutaneous injection in the thigh of 0.03 mg/kg, the extent of absorption (AUC) of a concentration of 5.3 mg/mL *Genotropin* was 35% greater than that for 1.3 mg/mL *Genotropin*. The mean (± standard deviation) peak (C_{max}) serum levels were 23 (± 9.4) ng/mL and 17.4 (± 9.2) ng/mL, respectively. In a similar study involving pediatric GHD patients, 5.3 mg/mL *Genotropin* yielded a mean AUC that was 17% greater than that for 1.3 mg/mL *Genotropin*. The mean C_{max} levels were 21 ng/mL and 16.3 ng/mL, respectively. Adult GHD patients received 2 single subcutaneous doses of 0.03 mg/kg of *Genotropin* at a concentration of 1.3 mg/mL, with a 1- to 4-week washout period between injections. Mean C_{max} levels were 12.4 ng/mL (first injection) and 12.2 ng/mL (second injection), achieved at approximately 6 hours after dosing. There are no data on the bioequivalence between the 12 mg/mL formulation and either the 1.3 mg/mL or the 5.3 mg/mL formulations.

Humatrope: *Humatrope* has been studied following IM, subcutaneous, and IV administration in adult volunteers. The absolute bioavailability of *Humatrope* is 75% and 63% after subcutaneous and IM administration, respectively.

Norditropin: An 180-minute IV infusion of *Norditropin* (33 ng/kg/min) was given to 9 GHD patients. A mean (± SD) hGH steady-state serum level of approximately 23.1 (± 15) ng/mL was reached at 150 minutes and a mean clearance rate of approximately 2.3 (± 1.8) mL/min/kg or 139 (± 105) mL/min for hGH was obtained. Following infusion, serum hGH levels had a biexponential decay with a terminal elimination half-life ($t_{½}$) of approximately 21.1 (± 5.1) minutes.

In a study conducted in 18 GHD adult patients, where an subcutaneous dose of 0.024 mg/kg or 3 units/m² was given in the thigh, the mean (± SD) C_{max} values of 13.8 (± 5.8) and 17.1 (± 10) ng/mL were obtained for the 4 and 8 mg *Norditropin* vials, respectively, at approximately 4 to 5 hours post dose. The mean apparent terminal $t_{½}$ values were estimated to be approximately 7 to 10 hours. However, the absolute bioavailability for *Norditropin* after the subcutaneous route of administration is currently not known.

Norditropin cartridge formulation is bioequivalent to *Norditropin* vial formulation.

Nutropin and *Nutropin AQ*: The absolute bioavailability of *Nutropin* and *Nutropin AQ* after subcutaneous administration in healthy adult males has been determined to be 81 ± 20%. The mean terminal $t_{½}$ after subcutaneous administration is significantly longer than that seen after IV administration (2.1 ± 0.43 hours vs 19.5 ± 3.1 minutes) indicating that the subcutaneous absorption of the compound is slow and rate-limiting.

• *Bioequivalence of formulations – Nutropin* has been determined to be bioequivalent to *Nutropin AQ* based on the statistical evaluation of AUC and C_{max}.

Nutropin Depot: In a study of *Nutropin Depot* in pediatric patients with GHD, an subcutaneous dose of 0.75 mg/kg (n = 12) or 1.5 mg/kg (n = 8) was administered. The mean ± SD hGH C_{max} values were 48 ± 26 mcg/L and 90 ± 23 mcg/L, respectively, at 12 to 13 hours postdose. The corresponding $AUC_{0\ to\ 28\ days}$ values were 83 ± 49 mg•day/L and 140 ± 34 mg•day/L, respectively, for the 2 doses. For the 0.75 mg/kg and 1.5 mg/kg doses, the $AUC_{0\ to\ 2\ days}$ accounted for approximately 52 ± 16% and 61 ± 10% of the total $AUC_{0\ to\ 28\ days}$, respectively. Estimates of relative bioavailability in GHD children for a single dose of *Nutropin Depot* ranged from 33% to 38% when compared to a single dose of *Nutropin AQ* in healthy adults, and from 48% to 55% when compared to chronically dosed *Protropin* (somatrem for injection) in GHD children.

Saizen: The absolute bioavailability of recombinant human growth hormone (rhGH) after subcutaneous administration ranges between 70% to 90%.

Serostim and *Zorbtive*: The absolute bioavailability of *Serostim* and *Zorbtive* after subcutaneous administration of a formulation not equivalent to the marketed formulation was determined to be 70% to 90%. The $t_{½}$ (mean ± SD) after subcutaneous administration is significantly longer than that seen after intravenous administration in healthy male volunteers down-regulated with somatostatin (3.94 ± 3.44 hours vs 0.58 ± 0.08 hours), indicating that the subcutaneous absorption of the clinically tested formulation of the compound is slow and rate limiting.

Distribution –

Genotropin: The mean volume of distribution of *Genotropin* following administration to GHD adults was estimated to be 1.3 (± 0.8) L/kg.

Humatrope: The volume of distribution of *Humatrope* after IV injection is about 0.07 L/kg.

Nutropin and *Nutropin AQ*: Animal studies with *Nutropin* and *Nutropin AQ* showed that GH localizes to highly perfused organs, particularly the liver and kidney. The volume of distribution at steady state for *Nutropin* and *Nutropin AQ* in healthy adult males is about 50 mL/kg body weight, approximating the serum volume.

Nutropin Depot: Animal studies with rhGH formulated for daily administration showed that GH localizes to highly perfused organs, particularly the liver and kidney. The volume of distribution at steady state for rhGH formulated for daily administration in healthy adult males is about 50 mL/kg body weight, approximating the serum volume.

Saizen: The mean volume of distribution of rhGH given to healthy volunteers was estimated to be 12 ± 1.08 L.

Serostim and *Zorbtive*: The steady-state volume of distribution (mean ± SD) following IV administration of *Serostim* and *Zorbtive* in healthy volunteers is 12 ± 1.08 L.

Metabolism – The metabolic fate of somatropin involves classical protein catabolism in both the liver and kidneys. In renal cells, at least a portion of the breakdown products is returned to the systemic circulation.

Humatrope: Extensive metabolism studies have not been conducted. The metabolic fate of *Humatrope* involves classical protein catabolism in both the liver and kidneys. In renal cells, at least a portion of the breakdown products of growth hormone is returned to the systemic circulation. In healthy volunteers, mean clearance is 0.14 L/hr/kg. The mean half-life of IV *Humatrope* is 0.36 hours, whereas subcutaneously and intramuscularly administered *Humatrope* have mean half-lives of 3.8 and 4.9 hours, respectively. The longer half-life observed after subcutaneous or IM administration is due to slow absorption from the injection site.

Nutropin, Nutropin AQ and *Nutropin Depot*: Both the liver and kidney have been shown to be important metabolizing organs for GH. Animal studies suggest that the kidney is the dominant organ of clearance. GH is filtered at the glomerulus and reabsorbed in the proximal tubules. It is then cleaved within renal cells into its constituent amino acids, which return to the systemic circulation.

Serostim and *Zorbtive*: Although the liver plays a role in the metabolism of GH, GH is primarily cleaved in the kidney. GH undergoes glomerular filtration and, after cleavage within the renal cells, the peptides and amino acids are returned to the systemic circulation.

Excretion –

Genotropin: The mean terminal half-life of intravenous *Genotropin* in healthy adults is 0.4 hours, whereas subcutaneously administered *Genotropin* has a half-life of 3 hours in GHD adults. The observed difference is due to slow absorption from the subcutaneous injection site.

Saizen: The mean half-life of intravenous somatropin in healthy males is 0.6 hours, whereas subcutaneously and intramuscularly administered somatropin has a half-life of 1.75 and 3.4 hours, respectively. The longer half-life observed after subcutaneous or intramuscular administration is due to slow absorption from the injection site.

Humatrope: Urinary excretion of intact *Humatrope* has not been measured. Small amounts of somatropin have been detected in the urine of pediatric patients following replacement therapy.

Nutropin, Nutropin AQ and *Nutropin Depot*: The mean terminal $t_{½}$ after intravenous administration of rhGH in healthy adult males is estimated to be 19.5 ± 3.1 minutes. Clearance of rhGH after intravenous administration in healthy adults and children is reported to be in the range of 116 to 174 mL/kg/h.

Genotropin: The mean clearance of subcutaneously administered *Genotropin* in 16 GHD adult patients was 0.3 (± 0.11) L/kg/h.

Saizen: The mean clearance of intravenously administered rhGH in 6 healthy male volunteers was 14.6 ± 2.8 L/h.

Serostim and *Zorbtive*: The $t_{½}$ (mean ± SD) in 9 patients with HIV-associated wasting with an average weight of 56.7 ± 6.8 kg, given a fixed dose of 6 mg recombinant hGH (rhGH) subcutaneously was 4.28 ± 2.15 hours. The renal clearance of rhGH after subcutaneous administration in 9 patients with HIV-associated wasting was 0.0015 ± 0.0037 L/hr. No significant accumulation of rhGH appears to occur after 6 weeks of dosing as indicated.

Special populations –

Renal function impairment: Children and adults with chronic renal failure (CRF) and end-stage renal disease (ESRD) tend to have decreased clearance compared to healthy subjects. Endogenous GH production may also increase in some individuals with ESRD. However, no rhGH accumulation has been reported in children with CRF or ESRD dosed with current regimens.

Hepatic function impairment: A reduction in rhGH clearance has been noted in patients with severe liver dysfunction. The clinical significance of this decrease is unknown.

Gender:

• *Nutropin Depot* – Following administration of either 0.75 mg/kg or 1.5 mg/kg *Nutropin Depot*, day 1 GH levels were higher in females compared to males. No relationship was observed between gender and pharmacodynamic marker (IGF-I and IGFBP-3) levels.

• *Serostim* and *Zorbitive* – Biomedical literature indicates that a gender-related difference in the mean clearance of rhGH could exist (clearance of rhGH in males greater than clearance of rhGH in females). However, no gender-based analysis is available in healthy volunteers or patients infected with HIV or short bowel syndrome.

Pharmacokinetic parameters –

Genotropin:

Mean Subcutaneous Pharmacokinetic Parameters in Adult GHD Patients

	Bioavailability (%) (n = 15)	T_{max}[a] (h) (n = 16)	CL/F[b] (L/h × kg) (n = 16)	V_{ss}[c]/F (L/kg) (n = 16)	$T_{½}$[d] (h) (n = 16)
Mean	80.5	5.9	0.3	1.3	3
(± SD[e])	*	(± 1.65)	(± 0.11)	(± 0.8)	(± 1.44)
95% CI[f]	70.5 to 92.1	5 to 6.7	0.2 to 0.4	0.9 to 1.8	2.2 to 3.7

[a] T_{max} = Time of maximum plasma concentration.
[b] CL/F = Plasma clearance.
[c] Vss/F = Volume of distribution.
[d] $T_{½}$ = Terminal half-life.
[e] SD = Standard deviation.
[f] CI = Confidence interval.
* The absolute bioavailability was estimated under the assumption that the log-transformed data follow a normal distribution. The mean and standard deviation of the log-transformed data were mean = 0.22 (± 0.241).

SOMATROPIN — INJECTION

Humatrope:

Summary of Somatropin Parameters in the Healthy Population					
	C_{max}[a] (ng/mL)	T½[b] (h)	$AUC_{0-\infty}$[c] (ng•h/mL)	Cls[d] (L/kg•h)	Vβ[e] (L/kg)
0.02 mg (0.05 units[f])/kg IV					
Mean	415	0.363	156	0.135	0.0703
SD[g]	75	0.053	33	0.029	0.0173
0.1 mg (0.27 units[f])/kg IM					
Mean	53.2	4.93	495	0.215	1.55
SD[g]	25.9	2.66	106	0.047	0.91
0.1 mg (0.27 units[f])/kg subcutaneous					
Mean	63.3	3.81	585	0.179	0.957
SD[g]	18.2	1.4	90	0.028	0.301

[a] C_{max} = Maximum concentration.
[b] T½ = Half-life.
[c] $AUC_{0-\infty}$ = Area under the curve.
[d] Cls = Systemic clearance.
[e] Vβ = Volume of distribution.
[f] Based on previous International Standard of 2.7 units = 1 mg.
[g] SD = Standard deviation.

Nutropin:

Summary of *Nutropin* Pharmacokinetic Parameters in Healthy Adult Males 0.1 mg (Approximately 0.3 units[a])/kg Subcutaneous					
	C_{max}[b] (mcg/L)	T_{max} (h)	T½[c] (h)	$AUC_{0-\infty}$[d] (mcg•h/L)	CL/F_{sc}[e,f] mL/•kg])
Mean[g]	67.2	6.2	2.1	643	158
CV%[h]	29	37	20	12	12

[a] Based on current International Standard of 3 units = 1 mg.
[b] C_{max} = Maximum concentration.
[c] t½ = Half-life.
[d] $AUC_{0-\infty}$ = Area under the curve.
[e] CL/F_{sc} = Systemic clearance.
[f] F_{sc} = SC bioavailability (not determined).
[g] n = 36
[h] CV% = Coefficient of variation in %.

Nutropin AQ:

Summary of *Nutropin AQ* Pharmacokinetic Parameters in Healthy Adult Males 0.1 mg (Approximately 0.3 units[a])/kg Subcutaneous					
	C_{max}[b] (mcg/L)	T_{max} (h)	T½[c] (h)	$AUC_{0-\infty}$[d] (mcg•h/L)	CL/F_{sc}[e,f] mL/•kg])
Mean[g]	71.1	3.9	2.3	677	150
CV%[h]	17	56	18	13	13

[a] Based on current International Standard of 3 units = 1 mg.
[b] C_{max} = Maximum concentration.
[c] t½ = Half-life.
[d] $AUC_{0-\infty}$ = Area under the curve.
[e] CL/F_{sc} = Systemic clearance.
[f] F_{sc} = SC bioavailability (not determined).
[g] n = 36
[h] CV% = Coefficient of variation in %.

Contraindications

Somatropin should not be used for growth promotion in children with closed epiphyses; hypersensitivity to growth hormone; evidence of active malignancy. Antimalignancy treatment must be complete with evidence of remission prior to the institution of therapy.

Growth hormone should not be initiated to treat patients with acute critical illness due to complications following open heart or abdominal surgery, multiple accidental trauma or to patients having acute respiratory failure. Two placebo-controlled clinical trials in non-growth hormone deficient adult patients (n = 522) with these conditions revealed a significant increase in mortality (41.9% vs 19.3%) among somatropin treated patients (doses 5.3 to 8 mg/day) compared to those receiving placebo.

Somatropin injection, when reconstituted with bacteriostatic water for injection (0.9 % benzyl alcohol), should not be used in patients with a known sensitivity to benzyl alcohol.

Somatropin should not be used in hypopituitary children who have evidence of actively growing intracranial tumors. Therapy with somatropin should be discontinued if there is evidence of recurrent tumor growth.

➤*Humatrope*: *Humatrope* should not be reconstituted with the supplied diluent for *Humatrope* for use by patients with a known sensitivity to either metacresol or glycerin.

➤*Genotropin*: In patients with PWS who are severely obese or have severe respiratory impairment.

Warnings

➤*Critical illness:* Growth hormone should not be initiated to treat patients with acute critical illness due to complications following open heart or abdominal surgery, multiple accidental trauma or to patients having acute respiratory failure. Two placebo-controlled clinical trials in non-growth hormone deficient adult patients (n = 522) with these conditions revealed a significant increase in mortality (41.9% vs 19.3%) among somatropin treated patients (doses 5.3 to 8 mg/day) compared to those receiving placebo. The safety of continuing growth hormone treatment in patients receiving replacement doses for approved indications who concurrently develop these illnesses has not been established. Therefore, the potential benefit of treatment continuation with growth hormone in patients having acute critical illnesses should be weighed against the potential risk.

➤*Prader-Willi syndrome:* There have been reports of fatalities with the use of growth hormone in pediatric patients with PWS who had 1 or more of the following risk factors: Severe obesity, history of respiratory impairment or sleep apnea, or unidentified respiratory infection. Male patients with 1 or more of these factors may be at increased risk. Patients with PWS should be evaluated for upper airway obstruction before initiation of treatment with growth hormone. If during treatment with growth hormone patients show signs of upper airway obstruction (including onset of or increased snoring), treatment should be interrupted. All patients with PWS should be evaluated for sleep apnea and monitored if sleep apnea is suspected. All patients with PWS should also have effective weight control and be monitored for signs of respiratory infections, which should be diagnosed as early as possible and treated aggressively.

➤*Norditropen*: *Norditropen* cartridges must be used with their corresponding color-coded *NordiPen* delivery device. A *Norditropen* cartridge must not be inserted into a pen with a different color code.

➤*Hypersensitivity reactions:*

Serostim – Patients should be informed that allergic reactions are possible and that prompt medical attention should be sought if an allergic reaction occurs. None of the 651 study participants with HIV-associated wasting treated with *Serostim* for the first time developed detectable antibodies to growth hormone (greater than 4 pg binding). Patients were not rechallenged.

Humatrope – Do not use the *HumatroPen* injection device and *Humatrope* cartridges if you are allergic to metacresol or glycerin.

If sensitivity to the diluent should occur the vials may be reconstituted with bacteriostatic water for injection or sterile water for injection. When *Humatrope* is used with bacteriostatic water (benzyl alcohol preserved), the solution should be kept refrigerated at 2° to 8°C (36° to 46°F) and used within 14 days. Benzyl alcohol as a preservative in bacteriostatic water for injection has been associated with toxicity in newborns. When administering *Humatrope* to newborns, use the *Humatrope* diluent provided or if the patient is sensitive to the diluent, use sterile water for injection. When *Humatrope* is reconstituted with sterile water for injection in this manner, use only one dose per *Humatrope* vial and discard the unused portion. If the solution is not used immediately, it must be refrigerated (2° to 8°C [36° to 46°F]) and used within 24 hours.

Cartridges should be reconstituted only with the supplied diluent. Cartridges should not be reconstituted with the diluent for *Humatrope* provided with *Humatrope* vials, or with any other solution. Cartridges should not be used if the patient is allergic to metacresol or glycerin.

Nutropin and *Nutropin AQ* – Benzyl alcohol, as a preservative in bacteriostatic water for injection, has been associated with toxicity in newborns. When administering *Nutropin* to newborns, reconstitute with sterile water for injection. Use only 1 dose per *Nutropin* vial and discard the unused portion.

Genotropin – The 5.8 mg and 13.8 mg presentations of *Genotropin* lyophilized powder contain m-cresol as a preservative. These products should not be used by patients with a known sensitivity to this preservative. The 1.5 mg presentation of *Genotropin* is preservative free.

Patients should be informed that allergic reactions are possible and that prompt medical attention should be sought if an allergic reaction occurs.

➤*Elderly:* The safety and efficacy of somatropin (rDNA origin) injection in patients aged 65 years and older has not been evaluated in clinical studies. Elderly patients may be more sensitive to the action of somatropin (rDNA origin) injection and may be more prone to develop adverse reactions.

➤*Pregnancy:*

Humatrope, Tev-Tropin, Norditropin, Nutropin, Nutropin Depot, and *Nutropin AQ* – *Category C.*

Animal reproduction studies have not been conducted with these products. It is also not known whether these products can cause fetal harm when administered to a pregnant woman or can affect reproduction capacity. These products should be given to a pregnant woman only if clearly needed.

Genotropin, Saizen, Zorbtive, Serostim, and *Serostim LQ* – *Category B.*

Reproduction studies carried out with somatropin (rDNA origin) injection at doses of 0.3, 1, and 3.3 mg/kg/day administered subcutaneous in the rat and 0.08, 0.3, and 1.3 mg/kg/day administered intramuscularly in the rabbit (highest doses approximately 24 times and 19 times the recommended human therapeutic levels, respectively, based on body surface area) resulted in decreased maternal body weight gains but were not teratogenic. In rats receiving subcutaneous doses during gametogenesis and up to 7 days of pregnancy, 3.3 mg/kg/day (approximately 24 times human dose) produced anestrus or extended estrus cycles in females and fewer and less motile sperm in males. When given to pregnant female rats (days 1 to 7 of gestation) at 3.3 mg/kg/day a very slight increase in fetal deaths was observed. At 1 mg/kg/day (approximately 7 times human dose) rats showed slightly extended estrus cycles, whereas at 0.3 mg/kg/day no effects were noted.

In perinatal and postnatal studies in rats, somatropin (rDNA origin) injection doses of 0.3, 1, and 3.3 mg/kg/day produced growth-promoting effects in the dams but not in the fetuses. Young rats at the highest dose showed increased weight gain during suckling but the effect was not apparent by 10 weeks of age. No adverse effects were observed on gestation, morphogen-

SOMATROPIN — INJECTION

esis, parturition, lactation, postnatal development, or reproductive capacity of the offsprings due to somatropin (rDNA origin) injection. There are, however, no adequate and well-controlled studies in pregnant women. Because animal reproduction studies are not always predictive of human response, this drug should be used during pregnancy only if clearly needed.

➤*Lactation:* There have been no studies conducted with somatropin (rDNA origin) injection in nursing mothers. It is not known whether this drug is excreted in human milk. Because many drugs are excreted in human milk, caution should be exercised when somatropin (rDNA origin) injection is administered to a nursing woman.

➤*Children:* Safety and efficacy in pediatric patients with HIV have not been established.

Nutropin, Tev-Tropin, Saizen, and *Zorbtive* – Benzyl alcohol as a preservative in bacteriostatic water for injection has been associated with toxicity in newborns. When administering somatropin (rDNA origin) injection to newborns, reconstitute with Sterile Water for Injection. Use only 1 dose/vial and discard the unused portion.

Serostim – In 2 small studies, 11 children with HIV-associated failure to thrive were treated subcutaneously with human growth hormone. In 1 study, 5 children (age range, 6 to 17 years) were treated with 0.04 mg/kg/day for 26 weeks. In a second study, 6 children (age range, 8 to 14 years) were treated with 0.07 mg/kg/day for 4 weeks. Treatment appeared to be well tolerated in both studies. The preliminary data collected on a limited number of patients with HIV-associated failure to thrive appear to be consistent with safety observations in growth hormone-treated adults with AIDS wasting.

Zorbtive – Safety and efficacy have not been established in pediatric patients with short bowel syndrome.

Precautions

➤*Monitoring:* In addition to an evaluation of compliance with the treatment program and of thyroid status, testing for antibodies to human growth hormone should be carried out in any patient who fails to respond to therapy.

Excessive glucocorticoid therapy may prevent optimal response to somatropin. If glucocorticoid replacement therapy is required, the glucocorticoid dosage and compliance should be monitored carefully to avoid either adrenal insufficiency or inhibition of growth-promoting effects.

Therapy with somatropin should be directed by physicians who are experienced in the diagnosis and management of patients with growth hormone deficiency, Turner syndrome, idiopathic short stature, PWS, those who were born small for gestational age (SGA), or adult patients with either childhood-onset or adult-onset GHD. For *Zorbtive*, therapy should be carried out by a physician experienced in the diagnosis and management of short-bowl syndrome.

Hypothyroidism may develop during somatropin therapy. Untreated hypothyroidism will jeopardize the response to growth hormone. Therefore, thyroid hormone determinations should be performed periodically during somatropin administration and thyroid hormone replacement should be initiated when indicated. Bone age should be monitored periodically during somatropin administration especially in patients who are pubertal and/or receiving concomitant thyroid replacement therapy. Under these circumstances, epiphyseal maturation may progress rapidly. Patients with endocrine disorders, including GHD, may have an increased incidence of slipped capital femoral epiphysis. Any child who develops a limp or complains of hip or knee pain during growth hormone therapy should be evaluated.

Intracranial lesions – Patients with preexisting tumors or with growth hormone deficiency secondary to an intracranial lesion should be examined routinely for progression or recurrence of the underlying disease process. In pediatric patients, clinical literature has demonstrated no relationship between somatropin replacement therapy and CNS tumor recurrence. In adults, it is unknown whether there is any relationship between somatropin replacement therapy and CNS tumor recurrence.

Skin lesions – Patients should be monitored carefully for any malignant transformation of skin lesions.

Diabetes – For patients with diabetes mellitus, the insulin dose may require adjustment when somatropin therapy is instituted. Because human growth hormone may induce a state of insulin resistance, patients should be observed for evidence of glucose intolerance. Patients with diabetes or glucose intolerance should be monitored closely during somatropin therapy.

Patients with symptomatic hypoglycemia associated with GHD should be closely monitored.

Thyroid – In patients with hypopituitarism (multiple hormonal deficiencies) standard hormonal replacement therapy should be monitored closely when somatropin therapy is administered. Hypothyroidism may develop during treatment with somatropin, and inadequate treatment of hypothyroidism may prevent optimal response to somatropin.

Injection site – When growth hormone is administered subcutaneous at the same site over a long period of time, tissue atrophy may result. This can be avoided by rotating the injection site.

➤*Slipped capital epiphyses:* Pediatric patients with endocrine disorders, including GHD, may develop slipped capital epiphyses more frequently. Any pediatric patient with the onset of a limp or complaints if hip or knee pain during growth hormone therapy should be evaluated.

➤*Scoliosis:* Growth hormone has not been shown to increase the incidence of scoliosis. Progression of scoliosis can occur in children who experience rapid growth. Because growth hormone increases growth rate, patients with a history of scoliosis who are treated with growth hormone should be monitored for progression of scoliosis. Skeletal abnormalities including scoliosis are commonly seen in untreated Turner syndrome patients.

➤*Post-pubertal patients:* Before continuing treatment as an adult, a post-pubertal GHD patient who received growth hormone replacement therapy in childhood should be reevaluated with proper testing. If continued treatment is appropriate, somatropin should be administered at the reduced dose level recommended for adult GHD patients.

➤*Ear disorders:* Patients with Turner syndrome should be evaluated carefully for otitis media and other ear disorders since these patients have an increased risk of ear or hearing disorders. In a randomized-controlled trial, there was a statistically significant increase, as compared to untreated controls, in otitis media (43% vs 26%) and ear disorders (18% vs 5%) in patients receiving GH. In addition, patients with Turner syndrome should be monitored closely for cardiovascular disorders (eg, stroke, aortic aneurysm, hypertension) as these patients are also at risk for these conditions.

➤*Thyroid disease:* Patients with Turner syndrome have an inherently increased risk of developing autoimmune thyroid disease. Therefore, patients should have periodic thyroid function tests and be treated as indicated.

➤*Intracranial hypertension (IH):* IH with papilledema, visual changes, headache, nausea or vomiting has been reported in a small number of pediatric patients treated with growth hormone products. Symptoms usually occurred within the first 8 weeks of the initiation of growth hormone therapy. In all reported cases, IH-associated signs and symptoms resolved after termination of therapy or a reduction of the growth hormone dose. Funduscopic examination of patients is recommended at the initiation and periodically during the course of growth hormone therapy. Patients with CRI or Turner syndrome may be at increased risk for development of IH.

➤*Epiphyseal closure:* Patients with epiphyseal closure who were treated with growth hormone replacement therapy in childhood should be re-evaluated before continuation of somatropin therapy at the reduced dose level recommended for growth hormone-deficient adults.

➤*Diabetes:*

Nutropin and *Nutropin AQ* –

Because *Nutropin* may reduce insulin sensitivity, patients should be monitored for evidence of glucose intolerance.

Zorbtive – The use of somatropin has been associated with cases of new onset impaired glucose intolerance, new onset type 2 diabetes mellitus and exacerbation of preexisting diabetes mellitus have been reported in patients receiving somatropin. Some patients developed diabetic ketoacidosis and diabetic coma. In some patients, these conditions improved when somatropin was discontinued, while in others the glucose intolerance persisted. Some patients necessitated initiation or adjustment of antidiabetic treatment while on somatropin. Patients with other risk factors for glucose intolerance should be monitored closely during *Zorbtive* therapy.

➤*Weight loss:*

Serostim – *Serostim* [somatropin (rDNA origin) for injection] therapy should be carried out under the regular guidance of a physician who is experienced in the diagnosis and management of HIV infection. Inadequate nutritional intake, malabsorption and hypogonadism, which are common in individuals with HIV infection and which may contribute to catabolism and weight loss, should be diagnosed and treated.

Hyperglycemia may occur in HIV infected individuals due to a variety of reasons. Treatment with *Serostim* 0.1 mg/kg daily and 0.1 mg/kg every other day for 12 weeks were associated with approximately 10 mg/dL and 6 mg/dL increases of mean blood glucose concentration, respectively. The increases occurred early in treatment. Patients with other risk factors for glucose intolerance should be monitored closely during *Serostim* therapy.

➤*Pancreatitis:* Recombinant human growth hormone (rhGH) has been associated with acute pancreatitis.

➤*HIV and growth hormone considerations:* In some experimental systems, recombinant human growth hormone (rhGH) has been shown to potentiate HIV replication in vitro at concentrations ranging from 50 to 250 ng/ml. There was no increase in virus production when the antiretroviral agents, zidovudine, didanosine or lamivudine were added to the culture medium. Additional in vitro studies have shown that rhGH does not interfere with the antiviral activity of zalcitabine or stavudine. In the controlled clinical trials, no significant growth hormone-associated increase in viral burden was observed. However, the protocol required all participants to be on concomitant antiretroviral therapy for the duration of the study. In view of the potential for acceleration of virus replication, it is recommended that HIV patients be maintained on antiretroviral therapy for the duration of *Serostim* treatment.

➤*Lab test abnormalities:* Serum levels of inorganic phosphorus, alkaline phosphatase, and parathyroid hormone (PTH) may increase with GH therapy.

Drug Interactions

➤*CYP-450 system:* Limited published data indicate that growth hormone (GH) treatment increases cytochrome P-450-mediated antipyrine clearance in humans. These data suggest that GH administration may alter the clearance of compounds known to be metabolized by P-450 liver enzymes (eg, corticosteroids, sex steroids, anticonvulsants, cyclosporine). Careful monitoring is advisable when GH is administered in combination with other drugs known to be metabolized by P-450 liver enzymes.

SOMATROPIN — INJECTION

Adverse Reactions

➤*Humatrope:*

Growth-hormone deficient pediatric patients – As with all protein pharmaceuticals, a small percentage of patients may develop antibodies to the protein. During the first 6 months of *Humatrope* therapy in 314 naive patients, only 1.6% developed specific antibodies to *Humatrope* (binding capacity greater that or equal to 0.02 mg/L). None had antibody concentrations which exceeded 2 mg/L. Throughout 8 years of this same study, 2 patients (0.6%) had binding capacity greater than 2 mg/L. Neither patient demonstrated a decrease in growth velocity at or near the time of increased antibody production. It has been reported that growth attenuation from pituitary-derived growth hormone may occur when antibody concentrations are greater than 1.5 mg/L.

In studies with growth hormone-deficient pediatric patients, injection site pain was reported infrequently. A mild and transient edema, which appeared in 2.5% of patients, was observed early during the course of treatment.

Leukemia has been reported in a small number of pediatric patients who have been treated with growth hormone, including growth hormone of pituitary origin as well as of recombinant DNA origin (somatrem and somatropin). The relationship, if any, between leukemia and growth hormone therapy is uncertain.

Turner syndrome patients – In a randomized, concurrent controlled trial, there was a statistically significant increase, in the occurrence of otitis media (43% vs 26%), ear disorders (18% vs 5%) and surgical procedures (45% vs 27%) in patients receiving *Humatrope* compared with untreated control patients (see below). Other adverse events of special interest to Turner syndrome patients were not significantly different between treatment groups (see below). A similar increase in otitis media was observed in an 18 month placebo-controlled trial.

Treatment-Emergent Reactions of Special Interest by Treatment Group in Turner Syndrome

Adverse reaction	Treatment group: Overall	hGH[a]	Untreated[b]	Significance
Total number of patients	136	74	62	
Surgical procedure	50 (36.8%)	33 (44.6%)	17 (27.4%)	P ≤ 0.05
Otitis media	48 (35.3%)	32 (43.2%)	16 (25.8%)	P ≤ 0.05
Ear disorders	16 (11.8%)	13 (17.6%)	3 (4.8%)	P ≤ 0.05
Bone disorder	13 (9.6%)	6 (8.1%)	7 (11.3%)	NS[c]
Edema				
Conjunctival	1 (0.7%)	0	1 (1.6%)	NS
Non-specific	3 (2.2%)	2 (2.7%)	1 (1.6%)	NS
Facial	1 (0.7%)	1 (1.4%)	0	NS
Peripheral	6 (4.4%)	5 (6.8%)	1 (1.6%)	NS
Hyperglycemia	0	0	0	NS
Hyperthyroidism	15 (11%)	10 (13.5%)	5 (8.1%)	NS
Increased nevi[d]	10 (7.4%)	8 (10.8%)	2 (3.2%)	NS
Lymphedema	0	0	0	NS

[a] Dose = 0.3 mg/kg/week.
[b] Open label study.
[c] NS = not significant.
[d] Includes any nevi coded to the following preferred terms: Melanosis, skin hypertrophy, or skin benign neoplasm.

Patients with idiopathic short stature – In the placebo-controlled study, the adverse events associated with *Humatrope* therapy were similar to those observed in other pediatric populations treated with *Humatrope* (see the following table). Mean serum glucose level did not change during *Humatrope* treatment. Mean fasting serum insulin levels increased 10% in the *Humatrope* treatment group at the end of treatment relative to baseline values but remained within the normal reference range. For the same duration of treatment the mean fasting serum insulin levels decreased by 2% in the placebo group. The incidence of above-range values for glucose, insulin, and HbA_{1c} were similar in the growth hormone and placebo-treated groups. No patient developed diabetes mellitus. Consistent with the known mechanism of growth hormone action, *Humatrope*-treated patients had greater mean increases, relative to baseline, in serum insulin-like growth factor-I (IGF-I) than placebo-treated patients at each study observation. However, there was no significant difference between the *Humatrope* and placebo treatment groups in the proportion of patients who had at least one serum IGF-I concentration more than 2 SD above the age- and gender-appropriate mean (*Humatrope*: 9 of 35 patients [26%]; placebo: 7 of 28 patients [25%]).

Nonserious Clinically Significant Treatment-Emergent Adverse Reactions by Treatment Group in Idiopathic Short Stature

Adverse event	Treatment group: *Humatrope*	Placebo
Total number of patients	37	31
Scoliosis	7 (18.9%)	4 (12.9%)
Otitis media	6 (16.2%)	2 (6.5%)
Hyperlipidemia	3 (8.1%)	1 (3.2%)
Gynecomastia	2 (5.4%)	1 (3.2%)
Hypothyroidism	0	2 (6.5%)
Aching joints	0	1 (3.2%)
Hip pain	1 (2.7%)	0
Arthralgia	4 (10.8%)	1 (3.2%)
Arthrosis	4 (10.8%)	2 (6.5%)
Myalgia	9 (24.3%)	4 (12.9%)
Hypertension	1 (2.7%)	0

The adverse reactions observed in the dose-response study (239 patients treated for 2 years) did not indicate a pattern suggestive of a growth hormone dose effect. Among *Humatrope* dose groups, mean fasting blood glucose, mean glycosylated hemoglobin, and the incidence of elevated fasting blood glucose concentrations were similar. One patient developed abnormalities of carbohydrate metabolism (glucose intolerance and high serum HbA_{1c}) on treatment.

Adult patients – In clinical studies in which high doses of *Humatrope* were administered to healthy adult volunteers, the following events occurred infrequently: Headache, localized muscle pain, weakness, mild hyperglycemia, and glucosuria.

In the first 6 months of controlled blinded trials during which patients received either *Humatrope* or placebo, adult onset growth hormone-deficient adults who received *Humatrope* experienced a statistically significant increase in edema (*Humatrope* 17.3% vs placebo 4.4%, P = 0.043) and peripheral edema (11.5% vs 0% respectively, P = 0.017). In patients with adult onset growth hormone deficiency, edema, muscle pain, joint pain, and joint disorder were reported early in therapy and tended to be transient or responsive to dosage titration.

Two of 113 adult onset patients developed carpal tunnel syndrome after beginning maintenance therapy without a low dose (0.00625 mg/kg/day) lead-in phase. Symptoms abated in these patients after dosage reduction.

All treatment-emergent adverse events with greater than or equal to 5% overall incidence during 12 or 18 months of replacement therapy with *Humatrope* are shown below (adult onset patients and childhood onset patients).

Adult patients treated with *Humatrope* who had been diagnosed with growth hormone deficiency in childhood reported side effects less frequently than those with adult onset growth hormone deficiency.

Treatment-Emergent Adverse Reactions with ≥ 5% Overall Incidence in Adult Onset GHD Patients Treated With *Humatrope* for 18 Months Compared to 6 Month Placebo and 12 Month *Humatrope* Exposure

Adverse reaction	18 months exposure [placebo (6 months)/ hGH (12 months)] (n = 46) n	%	18 months hGH exposure (n = 52) n	%
Edema[a]	7	15.2%	11	21.2%
Arthralgia	7	15.2%	9	17.3%
Paresthesia	6	13%	9	17.3%
Myalgia	6	13%	7	13.5%
Pain	6	13%	7	13.5%
Rhinitis	5	10.9%	7	13.5%
Peripheral edema[b]	8	17.4%	6	11.5%
Back pain	5	10.9%	5	9.6%
Headache	5	10.9%	4	7.7%
Hypertension	2	4.3%	4	7.7%
Acne	0	0	3	5.8%
Joint disorder	1	2.2%	3	5.8%
Surgical procedure	1	2.2%	3	5.8%
Flu syndrome	3	6.5%	2	3.9%

[a] P = 0.04 as compared to placebo (6 months).
[b] P = 0.02 as compared to placebo (6 months).

Treatment-Emergent Adverse Reactions With ≥ 5% Overall Incidence in Childhood Onset Growth Hormone Deficient Patients Treated With *Humatrope* for 18 Months vs 6 Month Placebo and 12 Month *Humatrope* Exposure

Adverse reaction	18 months exposure [placebo (6 months)/ hGH (12 months)] (n = 35) n	%	18 months hGH exposure (n = 32) n	%
Flu syndrome	8	22.9%	5	15.6%
AST increased[a]	2	5.7%	4	12.5%
Headache	4	11.4%	3	9.4%

SOMATROPIN — INJECTION

Treatment-Emergent Adverse Reactions With ≥ 5% Overall Incidence in Childhood Onset Growth Hormone Deficient Patients Treated With *Humatrope* for 18 Months vs 6 Month Placebo and 12 Month *Humatrope* Exposure				
	18 months exposure [placebo (6 months)/ hGH (12 months)] (n = 35)		18 months hGH exposure (n = 32)	
Adverse reaction	n	%	n	%
Asthenia	1	2.9%	2	6.3%
Cough increased	0	0%	2	6.3%
Edema	3	8.6%	2	6.3%
Hypesthesia	0	0%	2	6.3%
Myalgia	2	5.7%	2	6.3%
Pain	3	8.6%	2	6.3%
Rhinitis	2	5.7%	2	6.3%
ALT increased	2	5.7%	2	6.3%
Respiratory tract disorder	2	5.7%	1	3.1%
Gastritis	2	5.7%	0	0%
Pharyngitis	5	14.3%	1	3.1%

[a] P = 0.03 as compared to placebo (6 months).

Other adverse drug events that have been reported in growth hormone-treated patients include the following:

Dermatologic – Rare increased growth of preexisting nevi. Patients should be monitored carefully for malignant transformation.

Endocrine – Rare gynecomastia. Rare pancreatitis.

Metabolic – Infrequent, mild and transient peripheral or generalized edema.

Musculoskeletal – Rare carpal tunnel syndrome.

➤*Nutropin* and *Nutropin AQ*: *Nutropin* therapy in adults with GHD of adult onset was associated with an increase of median fasting insulin in the *Nutropin* 0.0125 mg/kg/day group from 9 mcU/mL at baseline to 13 mcU/mL at month 12 with a return to the baseline median after a 3-week post-washout period off GH therapy. In the placebo group there was no change from 8 mcU/mL at baseline to month 12, and after the post-washout the median was 9 mcU/mL. The between-treatment-groups difference in change from baseline to month 12 was significant, $P < 0.0001$. In childhood-onset subjects there was a change of median fasting insulin in the *Nutropin* 0.025 mg/kg/day group from 11 mcU/mL at baseline to 20 mcU/mL at month 12, in the *Nutropin* 0.0125 mg/kg/day group from 8.5 mcU/mL to 11 mcU/mL, and in the placebo group from 7 mcU/mL to 8 mcU/mL. The between-treatment-groups difference for these changes was significant, P = 0.0007.

In subjects with adult-onset GHD there was no between-treatment-group difference in changes from baseline to month 12 in mean HbA_{1c}, P = 0.08. In childhood-onset mean HbA1c increased in the *Nutropin* 0.025 mg/kg/day group from 5.2% at baseline to 5.5% at month 12, and did not change in the *Nutropin* 0.0125 mg/kg/day group from 5.1% at baseline or in the placebo group from 5.3% at baseline. The between-treatment-groups difference was significant, $P = 0.009$.

Patients with growth failure secondary to chronic renal insufficiency should be examined periodically for evidence of progression of renal osteodystrophy. Slipped capital femoral epiphysis or avascular necrosis of the femoral head may be seen in children with advanced renal osteodystrophy, and it is uncertain whether these problems are affected by GH therapy. X-rays of the hip should be obtained prior to initiating GH therapy for CRI patients. Physicians and parents should be alert to the development of a limp or complaints of hip or knee pain in patients treated with *Nutropin*.

As with all protein pharmaceuticals, a small percentage of patients may develop antibodies to the protein. GH antibody binding capacities below 2 mg/L have not been associated with growth attenuation. In some cases when binding capacity exceeds 2 mg/L, growth attenuation has been observed. In clinical studies of pediatric patients that were treated with *Nutropin* for the first time, 0/107 GHD patients, 0/125 CRI patients, and 0/112 Turner syndrome patients screened for antibody production developed antibodies with binding capacities greater than or equal to 2 mg/L at 6 months.

Additional short-term immunologic and renal function studies were carried out in a group of patients with chronic renal insufficiency after approximately 1 year of treatment to detect other potential adverse effects of antibodies to GH. Testing included measurements of C1q, C3, C4, rheumatoid factor, creatinine, creatinine clearance, and BUN. No adverse effects of GH antibodies were noted.

Injection site discomfort has been reported. This is more commonly observed in children switched from another GH product to *Nutropin AQ*. Experience with *Nutropin AQ* in adults is limited.

In studies in patients treated with *Nutropin*, injection site pain was reported infrequently.

Leukemia has been reported in a small number of GHD patients treated with GH. It is uncertain whether this increased risk is related to the pathology of GH deficiency itself, GH therapy, or other associated treatments such as radiation therapy for intracranial tumors. On the basis of current evidence, experts cannot conclude that GH therapy is responsible for these occurrences. The risk to GHD, CRI, or Turner syndrome patients, if any, remains to be established.

Other adverse drug reactions that have been reported in GH-treated patients include the following:

Dermatologic – Rare increased growth of preexisting nevi; patients should be monitored for malignant transformation.

Endocrine – Gynecomastia. Rare pancreatitis.

Metabolic – Mild, transient peripheral edema. In GHD adults, edema or peripheral edema was reported in 41% of GH-treated patients and 25% of placebo-treated patients.

Musculoskeletal – Arthralgias; carpal tunnel syndrome. In GHD adults, arthralgias and other joint disorders were reported in 27% of GH-treated patients and 15% of placebo-treated patients.

➤*Nutropin Depot*: As with all protein pharmaceuticals, patients may develop antibodies to the protein. GH antibody-binding capacities below 2 mg/L have not been associated with growth attenuation. In some cases when binding capacity exceeds 2 mg/L, growth attenuation has been observed. In clinical studies of pediatric patients who were treated with *Nutropin Depot*, 0/138 patients with GHD screened for antibody production developed antibodies with binding capacities greater than or equal to 2 mg/L at any time during a treatment period of up to 17.4 months.

In addition to an evaluation of compliance with the prescribed treatment program and thyroid status, testing for antibodies to GH should be carried out in any patient who fails to respond to therapy.

In studies involving 138 pediatric patients treated with *Nutropin Depot*, the most frequent adverse reactions were injection-site reactions, which occurred in nearly all patients. On average, 2 to 3 injection-site adverse reactions were reported per injection. These reactions included nodules (61% of injections), erythema (53%), pain postinjection (47%), pain during injection (43%), bruising (20%), itching (13%), lipoatrophy (13%), and swelling or puffiness (8%). The intensity of these reactions was generally rated mild to moderate, with pain during injection occasionally rated as severe (7%).

Adverse reactions observed less frequently in the *Nutropin Depot* studies which were considered possibly, probably, or definitely related to the drug by the treating physician (usually occurring 1 to 3 days postdose) included headache (13% of subjects), nausea (8%), lower extremity pain (7%), fever (7%), and vomiting (5%). These symptoms were generally self-limited and well-tolerated. One patient experienced a generalized body rash that was most likely an allergic reaction to *Nutropin Depot*.

Leukemia has been reported in a small number of GHD patients treated with GH. It is uncertain whether this increased risk is related to the pathology of GH deficiency itself, GH therapy, or other associated treatments such as radiation therapy for intracranial tumors. On the basis of current evidence, experts cannot conclude that GH therapy is responsible for these occurrences.

Other adverse drug reactions that have been reported in GH-treated patients include the following:

Dermatologic – Rare increased growth of preexisting nevi; patients should be monitored for malignant transformation.

Endocrine – Gynecomastia.

GI – Rare pancreatitis.

Metabolic – Mild, transient peripheral edema.

Musculoskeletal – Arthralgia, carpal tunnel syndrome. Of these reactions, only edema (less than 1% of patients) and arthralgia (4%) were reported as related to drug in the *Nutropin Depot* studies.

➤*Genotropin*: As with all protein drugs, a small number of patients may develop antibodies to the protein. Growth hormone antibody with binding lower than 2 mg/L has not been associated with growth attenuation. In some cases when binding capacity is greater than 2 mg/L, interference with growth response has been observed.

In 419 pediatric patients evaluated in clinical studies with *Genotropin* lyophilized powder, 244 had been treated previously with *Genotropin* or other growth hormone preparations and 175 had received no previous growth hormone therapy. Antibodies to growth hormone (anti-hGH antibodies) were present in 6 previously treated patients at baseline. Three of the 6 became negative for anti-hGH antibodies during 6 to 12 months of treatment with *Genotropin*. Of the remaining 413 patients, eight (1.9%) developed detectable anti-hGH antibodies during treatment with *Genotropin*; none had an antibody binding capacity greater than 2 mg/L. There was no evidence that the growth response to *Genotropin* was affected in these antibody-positive patients.

In clinical studies with *Genotropin* in pediatric GHD patients, the following events were reported infrequently: Injection site reactions, including pain or burning associated with the injection, fibrosis, nodules, rash, inflammation, pigmentation, or bleeding; lipoatrophy; headache; hematuria; hypothyroidism; and mild hyperglycemia.

Leukemia has been reported in a small number of pediatric patients who have been treated with growth hormone, including growth hormone of pituitary origin and recombinant somatropin. The relationship, if any, between leukemia and growth hormone therapy is uncertain.

In 2 clinical studies with *Genotropin* in pediatric patients with Prader-Willi syndrome, the following drug-related events were reported: Edema, aggressiveness, arthralgia, benign intracranial hypertension, hair loss, headache, and myalgia.

In clinical studies of 273 pediatric patients born small for gestational age treated with *Genotropin*, the following clinically significant events were reported: Mild transient hyperglycemia, 1 patient with benign intracranial

SOMATROPIN — INJECTION

hypertension, 2 patients with central precocious puberty, 2 patients with jaw prominence, and several patients with aggravation of preexisting scoliosis, injection site reactions, and self-limited progression of pigmented nevi. Anti-hGH antibodies were not detected in any of the patients treated with *Genotropin*.

Adverse Reactions Reported by ≥ 5% of 1145 Adult GHD Patients During Clinical Trials of *Genotropin* and Placebo, Grouped by Duration of Treatment

	Double-blind phase		Open-label phase *Genotropin*		
Adverse reaction	Placebo 0 to 6 mo (n = 572)	*Genotropin* 0 to 6 mo (n = 573)	6 to 12 mo (n = 504)	12 to 18 mo (n = 63)	18 to 24 mo (n = 60)
Swelling, peripheral	5.1%	17.5%[a]	5.6%	0%	1.7%
Arthralgia	4.2%	17.3%[a]	6.9%	6.3%	3.3%
Upper respiratory tract infection	14.5%	15.5%	13.1%	15.9%	13.3%
Pain, extremities	5.9%	14.7%[a]	6.7%	1.6%	3.3%
Edema, peripheral	2.6%	10.8%	3%	0%	0%
Paresthesia	1.9%	9.6%[a]	2.2%	3.2%	0%
Headache	7.7%	9.9%	6.2%	0%	0%
Stiffness of extremities	1.6%	7.9%[a]	2.4%	1.6%	0%
Fatigue	3.8%	5.8%	4.6%	6.3%	1.7%
Myalgia	1.6%	4.9%[a]	2%	4.8%	6.7%
Back pain	4.4%	2.8%	3.4%	4.8%	5%

[a] Increased significantly when compared to placebo, P ≤ 0.025: Fisher's Exact Test (one-sided).

In expanded posttrial extension studies, diabetes mellitus developed in 12 of 3,031 patients (0.4%) during treatment with *Genotropin*. All 12 patients had predisposing factors (eg, elevated glycated hemoglobin levels or marked obesity) prior to receiving *Genotropin*. Of the 3031 patients receiving *Genotropin*, 61 (2%) developed symptoms of carpal tunnel syndrome, which lessened after dosage reduction or treatment interruption (52) or surgery (9). Other adverse events that have been reported include generalized edema and hypoesthesia.

➤*Norditropin*: As with all protein drugs, a small percentage of patients may develop antibodies to the protein. Growth hormone antibody with binding capacity lower than 2 mg/L has not been associated with growth attenuation. In some cases, when binding capacity is greater than 2 mg/L, interference with growth response has been observed.

In clinical trials, patients receiving *Norditropin* for up to 12 months have been tested for induction of antibodies and 0/358 patients developed antibodies with binding capacities above 2 mg/L. Among these patients, 165 had previously been treated with other preparations of growth hormone and 193 were previously untreated naive patients.

Because antibodies to somatropin have the potential to inhibit further linear growth, only patients failing to respond to treatment should be tested for antibodies.

The following adverse events have been reported from clinical studies: Headache, localized muscle pain, weakness, mild hyperglycemia, and glucosuria.

Leukemia has been reported in a small number of children who have been treated with growth hormone, including growth hormone of pituitary origin and recombinant somatrem and somatropin. On the basis of current evidence, experts cannot conclude that growth hormone therapy is responsible for these occurrences. If there is any risk to an individual patient, it is minimal.

Fluid retention and peripheral edema may occur.

➤*Saizen*: As with all protein pharmaceuticals, a small percentage of patients may develop antibodies to the protein. Anti-growth hormone (GH) antibody capacities below 2 mg/L have not been associated with growth attenuation. In some cases when binding capacity exceeds 2 mg/L, growth attenuation has been described. In clinical studies with *Saizen* involving 280 patients (204 naive and 76 transfer patients), one patient at 6 months of therapy developed anti-GH antibodies with binding capacities exceeding 2 mg/L. Despite the high binding capacity, these antibodies were not growth attenuating. The patient was subsequently shown to have a hGH-N gene defect. Thus, genetic analysis should be undertaken in any patient in whom anti-GH antibodies with high binding capacities occur. No antibodies against proteins of the host cells were detected in the sera of patients treated up to 5 years. Any patient with well-documented growth hormone deficiency who fails to respond to therapy should be tested for antibodies to human growth hormone and for thyroid status.

In clinical studies in which *Saizen* was administered to growth hormone deficient children, the following events were infrequently seen: Local reactions at the injection site (such as pain, numbness, redness and swelling), hypothyroidism, hypoglycemia, seizures, exacerbation of preexisting psoriasis and disturbances in fluid balance.

Leukemia has been reported in a small number of growth hormone deficient patients treated with growth hormone. It is uncertain whether this increased risk is related to the pathology of growth hormone deficiency itself, growth hormone therapy, or other associated treatments such as radiation therapy for intracranial tumors. So far, epidemiological data fail to confirm the hypothesis of a relationship between growth hormone therapy and leukemia.

➤*Serostim*: No cases of intracranial hypertension (IH) have been observed among patients with AIDS wasting treated with *Serostim*. The syndrome of IH, with papilledema, visual changes, headache, and nausea and/or vomiting has been reported in a small number of children with growth failure treated with growth hormone products. Nevertheless, funduscopic evaluation of patients is recommended at the initiation and periodically during the course of *Serostim* therapy.

Increased tissue turgor (swelling, particularly in the hands and feet) and musculoskeletal discomfort (pain, swelling and/or stiffness) may occur during treatment with *Serostim*, but may resolve spontaneously, with analgesic therapy, or after reducing the frequency of dosing.

Carpal tunnel syndrome may occur during treatment with *Serostim*. If the symptoms of carpal tunnel syndrome do not resolve by decreasing the weekly number of doses of *Serostim*, it is recommended that treatment be discontinued.

In the 12-week, placebo-controlled clinical trial 2, 510 patients were treated with *Serostim*. The most common adverse reactions judged to be associated with *Serostim* were musculoskeletal discomfort and increased tissue turgor (swelling, particularly of the hands or feet), and were more frequently observed when *Serostim* 0.1 mg/kg was administered on a daily basis (see table below). These symptoms were generally rated by investigators as mild to moderate in severity and often subsided with continued treatment or dose reduction. Approximately 23% of patients receiving *Serostim* 0.1 mg/kg daily and 11% of patients receiving 0.1 mg/kg every other day required dose reductions. Discontinuations as a result of adverse events occurred in 10.3% of patients receiving *Serostim* 0.1 mg/kg daily and 6.6% of patients receiving 0.1 mg/kg every other day. The most common reasons for dose reduction and/or drug discontinuation were arthralgia, myalgia, edema, carpal tunnel syndrome, elevated glucose levels, and elevated triglyceride levels.

Clinical adverse events which occurred during the first 12 weeks of study in at least 5% of the patients in any 1 of the 3 treatment groups are listed below by treatment group, without regard to causality assessment.

Controlled Clinical Trial 2: *Serostim* Adverse Reactions

Body system	Placebo Patients (n = 247)	0.1 mg/kg every other day *Serostim* Patients (n = 257)	0.1 mg/kg daily *Serostim* Patients (n = 253)
Musculoskeletal			
Arthralgia	11.3%	24.5%	36.4%
Myalgia	11.7%	17.9%	30.4%
Arthrosis	3.6%	7.8%	10.7%
GI			
Diarrhea	10.1%	10.1%	5.5%
Nausea	4.9%	5.4%	9.1%
Psychiatric			
Insomnia	6.1%	3.9%	5.9%
Respiratory			
Rhinitis	6.5%	5.1%	4%
Upper respiratory tract infection	5.7%	4.3%	3.6%
Bronchitis	5.3%	2.3%	4.7%
Endocrine			
Gynecomastia	0.4%	3.5%	5.5%
CNS			
Paresthesia	4.5%	7.4%	7.9%
Hypesthesia	2.4%	1.6%	5.1%
Metabolic and nutritional			
Edema generalized	1.2%	1.2%	5.9%
Miscellaneous			
Edema peripheral	2.8%	11.3%	26.1%
Headache	9.3%	10.1%	12.6%
Fatigue	4.5%	3.5%	5.1%

Adverse events that occurred in 1% to less than 5% of study participants receiving *Serostim* during the 12-week, placebo-controlled clinical trial 2 are listed below by body system. The list of adverse events has been compiled regardless of causal relationship to *Serostim*.

Cardiovascular – Hypertension, tachycardia.

CNS – Peripheral neuropathy, dizziness, and hypertonia.

Dermatologic – Folliculitis, rash, verruca, and maculopapular rash.

GI – Abdominal pain, anorexia, constipation, dyspepsia, gastroenteritis, and vomiting.

GU – Renal calculus, urinary tract infection.

Male breast neoplasm.

Hematologic/Lymphatic – Lymphadenopathy.

Immunologic – Herpes simplex, moniliasis, and viral infection.

Metabolic/Nutritional – Dependent edema, hypertriglyceridemia, hyperglycemia, and periorbital edema.

Musculoskeletal – Back pain, musculoskeletal pain, and arthropathy.

SOMATROPIN — INJECTION

Ophthalmic – Conjunctivitis.

Psychiatric – Depression, anxiety, and somnolence.

Respiratory – Coughing, sinusitis, pharyngitis, and pneumonia.

Miscellaneous – Rigors, fever, carpal tunnel syndrome, night sweats, edema/face edema, pain, flu-like symptoms, leg pain, chest pain, asthenia. Accident not otherwise specified. During the 12-week, placebo-controlled portion of clinical trial 2, the incidence of hyperglycemia reported as an adverse event was 3.6% for the placebo group, 1.9% for the 0.1 mg/kg every other day group and 3.2% for the 0.1 mg/kg daily group. One case of diabetes mellitus was noted in the 0.1 mg/kg daily group during the first 12-weeks of therapy. In addition, during the extension phase of clinical trial 2, two patients converted from placebo to full dose *Serostim*, and 1 patient converted from placebo to half dose *Serostim*, were discontinued because of the development of diabetes mellitus.

Postmarketing – During postmarketing surveillance, cases of new onset impaired glucose intolerance, new onset type 2 diabetes mellitus and exacerbation of preexisting diabetes mellitus have been reported in patients receiving *Serostim*. Some patients developed diabetic ketoacidosis and diabetic coma. In some patients, these conditions improved when *Serostim* was discontinued, while in others the glucose intolerance persisted. Some patients necessitated initiation or adjustment of antidiabetic treatment while on *Serostim*.

➤*Zorbtive*: Recombinant human growth hormone (rhGH) has been associated with acute pancreatitis.

No cases of intracranial hypertension (IH) have been observed among patients with short bowel syndrome treated with *Zorbtive*. The syndrome of IH, with papilledema, visual changes, headache, and nausea and/or vomiting has been reported in a small number of children with growth failure treated with growth hormone products. Nevertheless, funduscopic evaluation of patients is recommended at the initiation and periodically during the course of *Zorbtive* therapy.

Increased tissue turgor (swelling, particularly in the hands and feet) and musculoskeletal discomfort (pain, swelling and/or stiffness) may occur during treatment with *Zorbtive*, but may resolve spontaneously, with analgesic therapy, or after reducing the frequency of dosing.

Carpal tunnel syndrome may occur during treatment with somatropin. If the symptoms of carpal tunnel syndrome do not resolve by decreasing the dose or frequency of somatropin, it is recommended that treatment be discontinued.

The table below summarizes the number of subjects by system-organ class who experienced an adverse event during the 4-week treatment period of the phase 3 SBS study. To be listed in the table below, an adverse event must have occurred in more than 10% of subjects in any treatment group.

Controlled Trial *Zorbtive* Adverse Reactions: 4-Week Treatment Period

Adverse experiences	SOD [GLN][a] (n = 9) n (%)	rhGH + SOD[a] (n = 16) n (%)	rhGH + SOD][a] (n = 16) n (%)
Total number of subjects with at least 1 adverse reaction	8 (89%)	16 (100%)	16 (100%)
GI	6 (67%)	12 (75%)	12 (75%)
Abdominal pain	1 (11%)	4 (25%)	2 (13%)
Flatulence	2 (22%)	4 (25%)	4 (25%)
Nausea	0 (0)	2 (13%)	5 (31%)
Tenesmus	3 (33%)	1 (6%)	3 (19%)
Vomiting	1 (11%)	3 (19%)	3 (19%)
Hemorrhoids	1 (11%)	1 (6%)	0 (0)
Mouth dry	1 (11%)	1 (6%)	0 (0)
Musculoskeletal	1 (11%)	7 (44%)	7 (44%)
Arthralgia	0 (0)	7 (44%)	5 (31%)
Myalgia	1 (11%)	2 (13%)	0 (0)
Resistance mechanism disorders	4 (44%)	6 (38%)	3 (19%)
Infection	3 (33%)	0 (0)	1 (6%)
Infection bacterial	1 (11%)	3 (19%)	0 (0)
Infection viral	0 (0)	1 (6%)	2 (13%)
Moniliasis	0 (0)	2 (13%)	0 (0)
Application site disorders	1 (11%)	5 (31%)	4 (25%)
Injection site reaction	1 (11%)	3 (19%)	4 (25%)
Injection site pain	0 (0)	5 (31%)	0 (0)
CNS	2 (22%)	4 (25%)	4 (25%)
Dizziness	0 (0)	1 (6%)	2 (13%)
Headache	1 (11%)	1 (6%)	1 (6%)
Hypesthesia	1 (11%)	1 (6%)	1 (6%)
Dermatologic	2 (22%)	4 (25%)	4 (25%)
Rash	0 (0)	1 (6%)	2 (13%)
Pruritus	1 (11%)	0 (0)	1 (6%)
Sweating increased	0 (0)	2 (13%)	0 (0)
Nail disorder	1 (11%)	0 (0)	0 (0)
Respiratory	1 (11%)	1 (6%)	5 (31%)
Rhinitis	1 (11%)	0 (0)	3 (19%)
Metabolic/Nutritional	1 (11%)	3 (19%)	1 (6%)
Dehydration	1 (11%)	3 (19%)	0 (0)
Thirst	1 (11%)	0 (0)	0 (0)
GU	1 (11%)	2 (13%)	1 (6%)
Pyelonephritis	1 (11%)	0 (0)	0 (0)
Psychiatric disorders	2 (22%)	1 (6%)	0 (0)
Depression	2 (22%)	0 (0)	0 (0)
GU, female	1 (11%)	2 (13%)	0 (0)
Breast pain (female)	1 (11%)	1 (6%)	0 (0)
Special senses	0 (0)	0 (0)	2 (13%)
Ear or hearing symptoms	0 (0)	0 (0)	2 (13%)
Miscellaneous	4 (44%)	15 (94%)	15 (94%)
Edema, peripheral	1 (11%)	11 (69%)	13 (81%)
Edema, facial	0 (0)	8 (50%)	7 (44%)
Pain	1 (11%)	3 (19%)	1 (6%)
Chest pain	0 (0)	3 (19%)	0 (0)
Fever	2 (22%)	0 (0)	1 (6%)
Back pain	1 (11%)	1 (6%)	0 (0)
Flu-like disorder	1 (11%)	0 (0)	1 (6%)
Malaise	0 (0)	2 (13%)	0 (0)
Edema, generalized	0 (0)	2 (13%)	0 (0)
Abdomen enlarged	1 (11%)	0 (0)	0 (0)
Allergic reaction	1 (11%)	0 (0)	0 (0)
Rigors (chills)	1 (11%)	0 (0)	0 (0)

[a] SOD] = Specialized oral diet supplemented with glutamine; rhGH + SOD = Human growth hormone plus specialized oral diet; rhGH + SOD] = Human growth hormone plus specialized oral diet supplemented with glutamine.

The table below summarizes the number of subjects by system-organ class who experienced an adverse event during the 12-week follow-up period of the phase 3 SBS study. To be listed in the table below, an adverse event must have occurred in more than 10% of subjects in any treatment group.

Controlled Trial Adverse Events: 12-Week Follow-Up Period

Adverse experiences	SOD][a] (n = 9) n (%)	rhGH + SOD[a] (n = 15) n (%)	rhGH + SOD][a] (n = 16) n (%)
Total number of subjects with at least 1 adverse reaction	7 (78%)	12 (80%)	13 (81%)
GI	3 (33%)	7 (47%)	7 (44%)
Nausea	2 (22%)	3 (20%)	0 (0)
Vomiting	0 (0)	2 (13%)	3 (19%)
Abdominal pain	0 (0)	3 (20%)	1 (6%)
Tenesmus	1 (11%)	0 (0)	3 (19%)
Pancreatitis	1 (11%)	0 (0)	1 (6%)
Constipation	1 (11%)	0 (0)	0 (0)
Crohn disease aggravated	1 (11%)	0 (0)	0 (0)
Gastric ulcer	1 (11%)	0 (0)	0 (0)
Gastrointestinal fistula	1 (11%)	0 (0)	0 (0)
Resistance mechanism disorders	5 (56%)	6 (40%)	5 (31%)
Infection bacterial	3 (33%)	0 (0)	2 (13%)
Infection viral	1 (11%)	3 (20%)	1 (6%)
Infection	1 (11%)	1 (7%)	2 (13%)
Sepsis	0 (0)	3 (20%)	1 (6%)
Respiratory	1 (11%)	2 (13%)	4 (25%)
Rhinitis	0 (0)	1 (7%)	3 (19%)
Laryngitis	1 (11%)	0 (0)	0 (0)
Pharyngitis	1 (11%)	0 (0)	0 (0)
GU, Female	1 (11%)	0 (0)	4 (25%)
Vaginal fungal infection	1 (11%)	0 (0)	0 (0)

SOMATROPIN — INJECTION

Controlled Trial Adverse Events: 12-Week Follow-Up Period			
Adverse experiences	SOD][a] (n = 9) n (%)	rhGH + SOD[a] (n = 15) n (%)	rhGH + SOD][a] (n = 16) n (%)
Dermatologic	1 (11%)	2 (13%)	2 (13%)
Rash	1 (11%)	1 (7%)	0 (0)
Musculoskeletal	0 (0)	2 (13%)	2 (13%)
Arthralgia	0 (0)	2 (13%)	2 (13%)
Psychiatric disorders	1 (11%)	0 (0)	1 (6%)
Depression	1 (11%)	0 (0)	0 (0)
Insomnia	1 (11%)	0 (0)	0 (0)
GU	2 (22%)	0 (0)	0 (0)
Pyelonephritis	1 (11%)	0 (0)	0 (0)
Renal calculus	1 (11%)	0 (0)	0 (0)
Cardiovascular	1 (11%)	0 (0)	0 (0)
Vascular disorder	1 (11%)	0 (0)	0 (0)
Miscellaneous	1 (11%)	4 (27%)	2 (13%)
Application site disorders	1 (11%)	0 (0)	0 (0)
Injection site reaction	1 (11%)	0 (0)	0 (0)
Fatigue	0 (0)	2 (13%)	0 (0)
Fever	1 (11%)	2 (13%)	1 (6%)
Hepatic	1 (11%)	0 (0)	0 (0)
Hepatic function abnormal	1 (11%)	0 (0)	0 (0)

[a] SOD] = Specialized oral diet supplemented with glutamine; rhGH + SOD = Human growth hormone plus specialized oral diet; rhGH + SOD] = Human growth hormone plus specialized oral diet supplemented with glutamine.

Adverse reactions that occurred in 1% to less than 10% of study participants receiving *Zorbtive* in the placebo-controlled clinical efficacy trial are listed below by body system. The list of adverse events has been compiled regardless of causal relationship to *Zorbtive*.

Cardiovascular –
Vascular (extra cardiac): Vasodilatation.
Heart rate and rhythm: Tachycardia.

CNS – Paresthesia, phantom pain, visual field defect.

Dermatologic – Skin disorder, increased sweating, alopecia, bullous eruption.

GI – Melena, rectal hemorrhage, mouth disorder, steatorrhea.

GU – Dysuria, urinary tract infection, abnormal urine.
Female: Breast enlargement, vaginal fungal infection.

Hematologic – Purpura, prothrombin decrease.

Local – Reaction pain, inflammation at injection sites.

Metabolic/Nutritional – Hypomagnesemia.

Musculoskeletal – Arthritis, arthropathy, bursitis, cramps.

Psychiatric – Insomnia.

Respiratory – Bronchospasm, dyspnea, pharyngitis, respiratory tract disorder, respiratory tract infection.

Miscellaneous – Edema, periorbital edema, fungal infection.

The safety profile of patients receiving *Zorbtive* with glutamine was similar to the safety profile of patients receiving *Zorbtive* without glutamine. During the baseline period, 88% of patients receiving *Zorbtive* with glutamine, 88% of patients receiving *Zorbtive* without glutamine, and 78% of patients receiving *Zorbtive* placebo with glutamine reported baseline signs and symptoms (BSS). During the treatment period, 100% of patients receiving *Zorbtive* with and without glutamine reported at least one adverse event, whereas 89% of patients receiving *Zorbtive* placebo with glutamine reported at least 1 adverse event. During the follow-up period 81% of patients receiving *Zorbtive* with glutamine, 80% of patients receiving *Zorbtive* without glutamine and 78% of patients receiving *Zorbtive* placebo with glutamine experienced at least one adverse event. Comparison of the number of serious adverse events before and during treatment demonstrates that this subject population experiences numerous BSSs and adverse events due to their underlying conditions and parenteral nutrition complications. Four subjects (25%) receiving *Zorbtive* without glutamine and 1 subject (11%) in receiving *Zorbtive* placebo with glutamine experienced at least 1 serious adverse event during the treatment period (*Zorbtive* without glutamine: Chest pain, purpura, fungal infection, pharyngitis; *Zorbtive* placebo with glutamine: hemorrhoids). None of the subjects receiving *Zorbtive* with glutamine experienced serious adverse events during the treatment period. During the follow-up period, 3 subjects (19%) receiving *Zorbtive* with glutamine, 5 subjects (33%) receiving *Zorbtive* without glutamine and 3 subjects (33%) receiving *Zorbtive* placebo with glutamine experienced at least 1 serious adverse reaction. There were no deaths in this study.

➤*Tev-Tropin*: None of the patients with anti-GH antibodies in the clinical studies experienced decreased linear growth response to *Tev-Tropin* or any other associated adverse reaction. Growth hormone antibody binding capacities below 2 mg/L have not been associated with growth attenuation. In some cases, when binding capacity exceeds 2 mg/L, growth attenuation has been observed.

In studies of growth hormone-deficient children, headaches occurred infrequently. Injection site reactions (eg, pain, bruise) occurred in 8 of the 164 treated patients.

Leukemia has been reported in a small number of patients treated with other growth hormone products. It is uncertain whether this risk is related to the pathology of growth hormone deficiency itself, growth hormone therapy, or other associated treatments such as radiation therapy for intracranial tumors.

Overdosage

➤*Symptoms:* The recommended dosage of any somatropin (rDNA origin) formulation should not be exceeded. Acute overdosage could lead to fluid retention, headache, nausea, and vomiting. Additionally, acute overdosage could initially lead to hypoglycemia and subsequently to hyperglycemia. Glucose intolerance can occur with overdosage. Long-term overdosage could result in signs and symptoms of gigantism or acromegaly, consistent with the known effects of excess GH.

Genotropin – There is little information on acute or chronic overdosage with *Genotropin* lyophilized powder. Intravenously administered growth hormone has been shown to result in an acute decrease in plasma glucose. Subsequently, hyperglycemia was seen. It is thought that the same effect might occur on rare occasions with a high dosage of *Genotropin* administered subcutaneous. Long-term overdosage may result in signs and symptoms of acromegaly consistent with overproduction of growth hormone.

Patient Information

Patients being treated with growth hormone or their parents should be informed of the potential benefits and risks associated with treatment. Instructions on appropriate use should be given, including a review of the contents of the patient information insert. This information is intended to aid in the safe and effective administration of the medication. It is not a disclosure of all possible adverse or intended effects.

If home use is prescribed, patients or parents should be thoroughly instructed in the importance of proper needle disposal. A puncture resistant container should be used for the disposal of used needles or syringes (consistent with applicable state requirements). Needles and syringes must not be reused.

Patients should be informed that allergic reactions are possible and that prompt medical attention should be sought if an allergic reaction occurs.

Patients should be instructed to rotate injection sites to avoid localized tissue atrophy.

➤*Nutropin and Nutropin AQ:* As with any protein, local or systemic allergic reactions may occur. Parents/patient should be informed that such reactions are possible and that prompt medical attention should be sought if allergic reactions occur.

➤*Genotropin:* Patients and caregivers who will administer *Genotropin* in medically unsupervised situations should receive appropriate training and instruction on the proper use of *Genotropin* from the physician or other suitably qualified health professional.

➤*Humatrope*: It is important to learn the names and functions of the components of the *HumatroPen* and the *Humatrope* Cartridge Kit before injecting yourself or your child. Refer to the *HumatroPen* User Guide for the additional instructions on the use of the *HumatroPen*. Do not reconstitute the drug (mix the diluent with the drug until the drug is dissolved) or inject it until you have been thoroughly trained in the proper techniques by your healthcare professional. Use sterile technique as instructed by your healthcare professional. Dispose of syringes and/or needles after each use in a puncture-resistant container as instructed by your healthcare professional.

Humatrope cartridges are available in 3 different quantities (6, 12, or 24 mg) of *Humatrope*. Make sure that you have the cartridge that your doctor prescribed. Each *Humatrope* cartridge kit contains: One prefilled syringe of diluent for *Humatrope*, one diluent connector, and one cartridge of 6, 12, or 24 mg of *Humatrope*.

POSTERIOR PITUITARY HORMONES

VASOPRESSIN (8-Arginine-Vasopressin)

Rx	**Vasopressin** (Various, eg, American Pharmaceutical Partners, American Regent)	**Injection:** 20 pressor units/mL	With 0.5% chlorobutanol. In 0.5, 1, and 10 mL vials.
Rx	**Pitressin** (Monarch)		With 0.5% chlorobutanol. In 1 mL amps and vials.

VASOPRESSIN — INJECTION

Refer to the general discussion of these products in the Posterior Pituitary Hormones group monograph.

Indications

For prevention and treatment of postoperative abdominal distention, in abdominal roentgenography to dispel interfering gas shadows, and in diabetes insipidus.

➤*Unlabeled uses:* Vasopressin infusions (IV or selective intra-arterial) are used to manage bleeding esophageal varices at a dosage of 0.2 units/min initially, increased to 0.4 units/min if bleeding continues. Maximum recommended dose is 0.9 units/min.

Administration and Dosage

Vasopressin may be administered subcutaneously or intramuscularly.

Ten units of vasopressin (0.5 mL) will usually elicit full physiologic response in adult patients; 5 units will be adequate in many cases. Vasopressin should be given intramuscularly at 3- or 4-hour intervals as needed. The dosage should be proportionately reduced for pediatric patients. (For an additional discussion of dosage, consult the following sections.)

When determining the dose of vasopressin for a given case, the following should be kept in mind.

It is particularly desirable to give a dose not much larger than is just sufficient to elicit the desired physiologic response. Excessive doses may cause undesirable side effects (blanching of the skin, abdominal cramps, nausea) which, though not serious, may be alarming to the patient. Spontaneous recovery from such side effects occurs in a few minutes. It has been found that 1 or 2 glasses of water given at the time vasopressin is administered can reduce such symptoms.

➤*Abdominal distention:* In the average postoperative adult patient, give 5 units (0.25 mL) initially; increase to 10 units (0.5 mL) at subsequent injections if necessary. It is recommended that vasopressin be given intramuscularly and that injections be repeated at 3- or 4-hour intervals as required. Dosage to be reduced proportionately for pediatric patients.

Vasopressin used in this manner will frequently prevent or relieve postoperative distention. These recommendations apply also to distention complicating pneumonia or other acute toxemias.

➤*Abdominal roentgenography:* For the average case, 2 injections of 10 units each (0.5 mL) are suggested. These should be given 2 hours and half an hour, respectively, before films are exposed. Many roentgenologists advise giving an enema prior to the first dose of vasopressin.

➤*Diabetes insipidus:* Vasopressin may be given by injection or administered intranasally on cotton pledgets, by nasal spray, or by dropper. The dose by injection is 5 to 10 units (0.25 to 0.5 mL) repeated 2 or 3 times daily as needed. When vasopressin is administered intranasally by spray or on pledgets, the dosage and interval between treatments must be determined for each patient.

➤*Storage / Stability:* Store between 15° and 25°C (59° and 77°F).

Actions

➤*Pharmacology:* The antidiuretic action of vasopressin is ascribed to increasing reabsorption of water by the renal tubules.

Vasopressin can cause contraction of smooth muscle of the gastrointestinal tract and of all parts of the vascular bed, especially the capillaries, small arterioles, and venules with less effect on the smooth musculature of the large veins. The direct effect on the contractile elements is neither antagonized by adrenergic blocking agents nor prevented by vascular denervation.

➤*Pharmacokinetics:* Following subcutaneous or intramuscular administration of vasopressin injection, the duration of antidiuretic activity is variable but effects are usually maintained for 2 to 8 hours.

The majority of a dose of vasopressin is metabolized and rapidly destroyed in the liver and kidneys. Vasopressin has a plasma half-life of about 10 to 20 minutes. Approximately 5% of a subcutaneous dose of vasopressin is excreted in urine unchanged after 4 hours.

Contraindications

Anaphylaxis or hypersensitivity to the drug or its components.

Warnings

➤*Vascular disease:* This drug should not be used in patients with vascular disease, especially disease of the coronary arteries, except with extreme caution. In such patients, even small doses may precipitate anginal pain, and with larger doses, the possibility of myocardial infarction should be considered.

➤*Water intoxication:* Vasopressin may produce water intoxication. The early signs of drowsiness, listlessness, and headaches should be recognized to prevent terminal coma and convulsions.

➤*Pregnancy: Category C.* Animal reproduction studies have not been conducted with vasopressin. It is also not known whether vasopressin can cause fetal harm when administered to a pregnant woman or can affect reproduction capacity. Vasopressin should be given to a pregnant woman only if clearly needed.

Labor and delivery – Doses of vasopressin sufficient for an antidiuretic effect are not likely to produce tonic uterine contractions that could be deleterious to the fetus or threaten the continuation of the pregnancy.

➤*Lactation:* Exercised caution when vasopressin is administered to a breast-feeding woman.

Precautions

➤*Monitoring:* Electrocardiograms (ECG) and fluid and electrolyte status determinations are recommended at periodic intervals during therapy.

➤*Special risk patients:* Vasopressin should be used cautiously in the presence of epilepsy, migraine, asthma, heart failure, or any state in which a rapid addition to extracellular water may produce hazard for an already overburdened system.

➤*Chronic nephritis:* Chronic nephritis with nitrogen retention contraindicates the use of vasopressin until reasonable nitrogen blood levels have been attained.

Drug Interactions

The following drugs may potentiate the antidiuretic effect of vasopressin when used concurrently: carbamazepine, chlorpropamide, clofibrate, urea, fludrocortisone, tricyclic antidepressants.

The following drugs may decrease the antidiuretic effect of vasopressin when used concurrently: demeclocycline, norepinephrine, lithium, heparin, alcohol.

Ganglionic blocking agents may produce a marked increase in sensitivity to the pressor effects of vasopressin.

Adverse Reactions

Local or systemic allergic reactions may occur in hypersensitive individuals. The following side effects have been reported following the administration of vasopressin.

➤*Cardiovascular:* Cardiac arrest; circumoral pallor; arrhythmias; decreased cardiac output; angina; myocardial ischemia; peripheral vasoconstriction; and gangrene.

➤*CNS:* Tremor; vertigo; "pounding" in head.

➤*Dermatologic:* Sweating; urticaria; cutaneous gangrene.

➤*GI:* Abdominal cramps; nausea; vomiting; passage of gas.

➤*Hypersensitivity:* Anaphylaxis (cardiac arrest and/or shock) has been observed shortly after injection of vasopressin.

➤*Respiratory:* Bronchial constriction.

Overdosage

Water intoxication may be treated with water restriction and temporary withdrawal of vasopressin until polyuria occurs. Severe water intoxication may require osmotic diuresis with mannitol, hypertonic dextrose, or urea alone or with furosemide.

Patient Information

Side effects such as blanching of skin, abdominal cramps, and nausea may be reduced by taking 1 or 2 glasses of water at the time of vasopressin administration. These side effects are usually not serious and probably will disappear within a few minutes.

DESMOPRESSIN ACETATE (1-Deamino-8-D-Arginine Vasopressin)

Rx	**Desmopressin Acetate** (Teva)	**Tablets:** 0.1 mg	Lactose. (93 7316). White to off-white, capsule shape. In 100s.
Rx	**DDAVP** (Aventis)		Lactose. (DDAVP 0.1 rPr). White. In 100s.
Rx	**Desmopressin Acetate** (Teva)	**Tablets:** 0.2 mg	Lactose. (93 7317). White to off-white. In 100s.
Rx	**DDAVP** (Aventis)		Lactose. (DDAVP 0.2 rPr). White. In 100s.
Rx	**Desmopressin Acetate** (Bausch & Lomb)	**Nasal solution:** 0.1 mg/mL (10 mcg/spray)	0.5% chlorobutanol. In 5 mL nasal pump dispenser.
Rx	**DDAVP** (Aventis)	**Nasal solution:** 0.1 mg/mL (0.1 mg equals approximately 400 units arginine vasopressin)	**Nasal spray pump:** 7.5 mg NaCl/mL. In 5 mL bottle with spray pump (50 doses of 10 mcg).[a]
			Rhinal tube delivery system: 9 mg NaCl/mL. In 2.5 mL vials with 2 applicator tubes.[b]
Rx	**Stimate** (Centeon)	**Nasal solution:** 1.5 mg/mL	9 mg NaCl/mL. In 2.5 mL bottle (25 doses of 150 mcg each).[b]
Rx	**Minirin** (Ferring)	**Nasal spray:** 0.1 mg/mL (10 mcg/spray)	In 5 mL (50 doses of 10 mcg).[c]

DESMOPRESSIN ACETATE (1-Deamino-8-D-Arginine Vasopressin)

Rx	**Desmopressin Acetate** (Various, eg, Ferring)	**Injection:** 4 mcg/mL	1 mL single-dose amps and 10 mL multidose vials.
Rx	**DDAVP** (Aventis)		9 mg NaCl/mL. In 1 mL amps and 10 mL multidose vials.[b]

[a] With 1.7 mg citric acid monohydrate, 3 mg disodium phosphate dihydrate, 0.2 mg benzalkonium chloride solution (50%) per mL.

[b] With 5 mg chlorobutanol per mL.

[c] With 5 mg chlorobutanol, 9 mg sodium chloride, and hydrochloric acid per mL.

DESMOPRESSIN ACETATE — ORAL

Refer to the general discussion of these products in the Posterior Pituitary Hormones introduction.

Indications

➤*Central diabetes insipidus:* Desmopressin acetate tablets are indicated as antidiuretic replacement therapy in the management of central diabetes insipidus and for the management of the temporary polyuria and polydipsia following head trauma or surgery in the pituitary region. Desmopressin acetate is ineffective for the treatment of nephrogenic diabetes insipidus.

➤*Primary nocturnal enuresis:* Desmopressin acetate tablets are indicated for the management of primary nocturnal enuresis. Desmopressin may be used alone or as an adjunct to behavioral conditioning or other nonpharmacologic intervention.

Administration and Dosage

➤*Central diabetes insipidus:* The dosage of desmopressin acetate tablets must be determined for each individual patient and adjusted according to the diurnal pattern of response. Response should be estimated by 2 parameters: Adequate duration of sleep and adequate, not excessive, water turnover. Patients previously on intranasal desmopressin therapy should begin tablet therapy 12 hours after the last intranasal dose. During the initial dose titration period, patients should be observed closely and appropriate safety parameters measured to assure adequate response. Patients should be monitored at regular intervals during the course of desmopressin tablet therapy to assure adequate antidiuretic response. Modifications in dosage regimen should be implemented as necessary to assure adequate water turnover.

Adults and children – It is recommended that patients be started on doses of 0.05 mg (½ of the 0.1 mg tablet) 2 times a day and individually adjusted to their optimum therapeutic dose. Most patients in clinical trials found that the optimal dosage range is 0.1 mg to 0.8 mg daily, administered in divided doses. Each dose should be separately adjusted for an adequate diurnal rhythm of water turnover. Total daily dosage should be increased or decreased in the range of 0.1 mg to 1.2 mg divided into 2 or 3 daily doses as needed to obtain adequate antidiuresis. See Children, Warnings for special considerations when administering desmopressin acetate to children who are diabetes insipidus patients.

➤*Primary nocturnal enuresis:* The dosage of desmopressin tablets must be determined for each individual patient and adjusted according to response. Patients previously on intranasal desmopressin therapy can begin tablet therapy the night following (24 hours after) the last intranasal dose. The recommended initial dose for patients at least 6 years of age is 0.2 mg at bedtime. The dose may be titrated up to 0.6 mg to achieve the desired response.

➤*Storage/Stability:* Store at controlled room temperature (20°C to 25°C; 68°F to 77°F). Avoid exposure to excessive heat or light.

Keep out of the reach of children.

Actions

➤*Pharmacology:* Desmopressin tablets contain as active substance, desmopressin acetate, a synthetic analogue of the natural hormone arginine vasopressin.

Contraindications

Hypersensitivity to desmopressin acetate or to any of the components of desmopressin tablets.

Warnings

➤*Fluid/Electrolyte balance:* In very young and elderly patients, in particular, fluid intake should be adjusted downward to decrease the potential occurrence of water intoxication and hyponatremia. Particular attention should be paid to the possibility of the rare occurrence of an extreme decrease in plasma osmolality that may result in seizures which could lead to coma.

➤*Hypersensitivity reactions:* Rare severe allergic reactions have been reported with desmopressin. Anaphylaxis has been reported with IV administration of desmopressin injection, but not with desmopressin tablets.

➤*Pregnancy: Category B.*

There are no adequate and well-controlled studies in pregnant women. Because animal studies are not always predictive of human response, this drug should be used during pregnancy only if clearly needed.

➤*Lactation:* There have been no controlled studies in nursing mothers. A single study in postpartum women demonstrated a marked change in plasma, but little if any change in assayable desmopressin in breast milk following an intranasal dose of 0.01 mg.

It is not known whether the drug is excreted in human milk. Because many drugs are excreted in human milk, caution should be exercised when desmopressin is administered to nursing mothers.

➤*Children:*

Central diabetes insipidus – Desmopressin tablets have been used safely in children at least 4 years of age with diabetes insipidus for periods 44 months or less. In younger children the dose must be individually adjusted in order to prevent an excessive decrease in plasma osmolality leading to hyponatremia and possible convulsions; dosing should start at 0.05 mg (½ of the 0.1 mg tablet). Use of desmopressin tablets in children requires careful fluid intake restrictions to prevent possible hyponatremia and water intoxication.

Primary nocturnal enuresis – Desmopressin tablets have been safely used in children at least 6 years of age with primary nocturnal enuresis for 6 months or less. Some patients respond to a dose of 0.2 mg; however, increasing responses are seen at doses of 0.4 mg and 0.6 mg. No increase in the frequency or severity of adverse reactions or decrease in efficacy was seen with an increased dose or duration. The dose should be individually adjusted to achieve the best results.

Precautions

➤*Monitoring:*

Central diabetes insipidus – Laboratory tests for monitoring the patient with central diabetes insipidus or postsurgical or head trauma-related polyuria and polydipsia include urine volume and osmolality. In some cases, measurements of plasma osmolality may be useful.

Cardiovascular effects – Intranasal formulations of desmopressin acetate at high doses and desmopressin acetate injection have infrequently produced a slight elevation of blood pressure which disappears with a reduction of dosage. Although this effect has not been observed when single oral doses 0.6 mg or less have been administered, the drug should be used with caution in patients with coronary artery insufficiency and/or hypertensive cardiovascular disease, because of a possible rise in blood pressure.

➤*Special risk:* Desmopressin should be used with caution in patients with conditions associated with fluid and electrolyte imbalance, such as cystic fibrosis, since these patients may develop hyponatremia.

Drug Interactions

Desmopressin Drug Interactions

Precipitant drug	Object drug[a]		Description
Desmopressin	Pressor agents	↑	Although desmopressin pressor activity is very low, use large intranasal doses or parenteral doses as large as 0.3 mcg/kg cautiously with other pressor agents. Large doses of desmopressin tablets should be used with other pressor agents only with careful patient monitoring.
Carbamazepine	Desmopressin	↑	Carbamazepine, which potentiates ADH, may potentiate the effects of desmopressin.
Chlorpropamide	Desmopressin	↑	Chlorpropamide, which potentiates ADH, may potentiate the effects of desmopressin.

[a] ↑ = Object drug increased.

Adverse Reactions

Infrequently, large doses of the intranasal formulations of desmopressin and desmopressin injection have produced transient headache, nausea, flushing, and mild abdominal cramps. These symptoms have disappeared with reduction in dosage.

➤*Central diabetes insipidus:* In long-term clinical studies in which patients with diabetes insipidus were followed for periods 44 months or less of desmopressin tablet therapy, transient increases in AST at least 1.5 times the upper limit of normal were occasionally observed. Elevated AST returned to the normal range despite continued use of desmopressin tablets.

➤*Primary nocturnal enuresis:* The only adverse event occurring in at least 3% of patients in controlled clinical trials with desmopressin tablets that was probably, possibly, or remotely related to study drug was headache (4% desmopressin, 3% placebo).

➤*Miscellaneous:* The following adverse events have been reported; however their relationship to desmopressin acetate has not been established: Abnormal thinking, diarrhea, and edema-weight gain.

See Warnings for the possibility of water intoxication and hyponatremia.

Overdosage

➤*Treatment:* In case of overdose, the dose should be reduced, frequency of administration decreased, or the drug withdrawn according to the severity of the condition. There is no known specific antidote for desmopressin. The patient should be observed and treated with appropriate symptomatic therapy.

DESMOPRESSIN ACETATE — INTRANASAL

Refer to the general discussion of these products in the Posterior Pituitary Hormones introduction.

Indications

Before the initial therapeutic administration of intranasal desmopressin acetate, the physician should establish that the patient shows an appropriate change in the coagulation profile following a test dose of intranasal administration of desmopressin acetate nasal spray or rhinal tube.

➤*Stimate* nasal spray:

Hemophilia A – For patients with hemophilia A with Factor VIII coagulant activity levels greater than 5%.

Desmopressin acetate will also stop bleeding in patients with hemophilia A with episodes of spontaneous or trauma-induced injuries such as hemarthroses, IM hematomas, or mucosal bleeding.

Desmopressin is not indicated for the treatment of hemophilia A with Factor VIII coagulant activity levels less than or equal to 5%, or for the treatment of hemophilia B, or in patients who have Factor VIII antibodies.

von Willebrand disease (Type I) – For patients with mild to moderate classic von Willebrand disease (Type I) with Factor VIII levels greater than 5%.

Desmopressin acetate will also stop bleeding in mild to moderate von Willebrand's disease patients with episodes of spontaneous or trauma-induced injuries such as hemarthroses, IM hematomas, mucosal bleeding, or menorrhagia.

Desmopressin acetate nasal spray is not indicated for the treatment of severe classic von Willebrand disease (Type I) and when there is evidence of an abnormal molecular form of Factor VIII antigen (see Warnings).

➤*Rhinal tube and Minirin* and *DDAVP* nasal sprays:

Primary nocturnal enuresis – For the management of primary nocturnal enuresis. The rhinal tube and nasal spray may be used alone or adjunctive to behavioral conditioning or other nonpharmacological intervention. They have been shown to be effective in some cases that are refractory to conventional therapies.

Central cranial diabetes insipidus – As antidiuretic replacement therapy in the management of central cranial diabetes insipidus and for management of the temporary polyuria and polydipsia following head trauma or surgery in the pituitary region. It is ineffective for the treatment of nephrogenic diabetes insipidus.

➤*Unlabeled uses:* Treatment of chronic autonomic failure (eg, nocturnal polyuria, overnight weight loss, morning postural hypotension).

Administration and Dosage

➤*Stimate* nasal spray:

Hemophilia A and von Willebrand's disease (Type I) – Desmopressin acetate (*Stimate*) nasal spray is administered by nasal insufflation, 1 spray per nostril, to provide a total dose of 300 mcg. In patients weighing less than 50 kg, 150 mcg administered as a single spray provided the expected effect on Factor VIII coagulant activity, Factor VIII ristocetin cofactor activity and skin bleeding time. If desmopressin acetate nasal spray is used preoperatively, it should be administered 2 hours prior to the scheduled procedure.

The necessity for repeat administration of desmopressin acetate nasal spray or use of any blood products for hemostasis should be determined by laboratory response as well as the clinical condition of the patient. The tendency toward tachyphylaxis (lessening of response) with repeated administration given more frequently than every 48 hours should be considered in treating each patient.

The nasal spray pump can only deliver doses of 0.1 mL (150 mcg) or multiples of 0.1 mL. If doses other than these are required, desmopressin acetate injection may be used.

The spray pump must be primed prior to the first use. To prime pump, press down 4 times. The bottle should be discarded after 25 doses since the amount delivered thereafter per spray may be substantially less than 150 mcg of drug.

➤*Rhinal tube and Minirin* and *DDAVP* nasal sprays:

Primary nocturnal enuresis – Dosage should be adjusted according to the individual. The recommended initial dose for those 6 years of age and older is 20 mcg or 0.2 mL solution intranasally at bedtime. Adjustment less than or equal to 40 mcg is suggested if the patient does not respond.

Some patients may respond to 10 mcg and adjustment to that lower dose may be done if the patient has shown a response to 20 mcg. It is recommended that one-half of the dose be administered per nostril. Adequately controlled studies with intranasal desmopressin acetate in primary nocturnal enuresis have not been conducted beyond 4 to 8 weeks.

Central cranial diabetes insipidus – Desmopressin acetate nasal spray dosages must be determined for each individual patient and adjusted according to the diurnal pattern of response. Response should be estimated by 2 parameters: Adequate duration of sleep and adequate, not excessive, water turnover. Patients with nasal congestion and blockage have often responded well to intranasal desmopressin acetate. The usual dosage range in adults is 0.1 to 0.4 mL daily, either as a single dose or divided into 2 or 3 doses. Most adults require 0.2 mL daily in 2 divided doses. The morning and evening doses should be separately adjusted for an adequate diurnal rhythm of water turnover. For children aged 3 months to 12 years, the usual dosage range is 0.05 to 0.3 mL daily, either as a single dose or divided into 2 doses. About ¼ to ⅓ of patients can be controlled by a single daily dose of desmopressin acetate administered intranasally.

Nasal spray: The nasal spray pump can only deliver doses of 0.1 mL (10 mcg) or multiples of 0.1 mL. If doses other than these are required, the rhinal tube delivery system may be used.

The spray pump must be primed prior to the first use. To prime pump, press down 4 times. The bottle will now deliver 10 mcg of drug per spray. Discard desmopressin acetate nasal spray after 50 sprays since the amount delivered thereafter per spray may be substantially less than 10 mcg of drug.

Rhinal tube: This drug is administered into the nose through a soft, flexible plastic rhinal tube which has 4 graduation marks on it that measure 0.2, 0.15, 0.1, and 0.05 mL.

➤*Storage/Stability:*

Stimate nasal spray – Keep refrigerated at 2° to 8°C (36° to 46°F). When traveling, product will maintain stability for up to 3 weeks when stored at room temperature, 22°C (72°F).

DDAVP nasal spray – Store at controlled room temperature 20° to 25°C (68° to 77°F). Store bottle in upright position.

Minirin nasal spray – Store refrigerated 2° to 8°C (36° to 46°F). When traveling, closed bottles will maintain stability for 3 weeks when stored at controlled room temperature, 20° to 25°C (68° to 77°F).

Desmopressin acetate rhinal tube – Store refrigerated 2° to 8°C (36° to 46°F). When traveling, closed bottles will maintain stability for 3 weeks when stored at controlled room temperature, 20° to 25°C (68° to 77°F).

Actions

➤*Pharmacology:* Desmopressin is a synthetic analogue of the natural hormone arginine vasopressin.

Stimate nasal spray – One spray or 0.1 mL (150 mcg) of desmopressin acetate nasal spray solution has an antidiuretic activity of approximately 600 units.

Rhinal tube and Minirin and *DDAVP* nasal sprays: One mL (0.1 mg) of intranasal desmopressin acetate has an antidiuretic activity of approximately 400 units; 10 mcg of desmopressin acetate is equivalent to 40 units.

Desmopressin acetate administered intranasally has an antidiuretic effect about one-tenth that of an equivalent dose administered by injection.

Desmopressin acetate has been shown to be more potent than arginine vasopressin in increasing plasma levels of Factor VIII activity in patients with hemophilia and von Willebrand disease Type I.

Dose-response studies were performed in healthy persons using doses of 150 to 450 mcg, administered as 1 to 3 sprays. The response to desmopressin acetate nasal spray is dose-related, with maximal plasma levels of 150% to 250% of initial concentrations achieved for both Factor VIII and von Willebrand factor. The increase is rapid and evident within 30 minutes, reaching a maximum at approximately 1.5 hours.

The change in structure of arginine vasopressin to desmopressin acetate has resulted in a decreased vasopressor action and decreased actions on visceral smooth muscle relative to the enhanced antidiuretic activity, so that clinically effective antidiuretic doses are usually below threshold levels for effects on vascular or visceral smooth muscle.

➤*Pharmacokinetics:*

Absorption – Desmopressin acetate is absorbed rapidly from the nasal mucosa. The bioavailability of desmopressin acetate nasal spray when administered by the intranasal route as a 1.5 mg/mL solution is between 3.3% and 4.1%. The half-life of desmopressin acetate nasal spray is between 3.3 and 3.5 hours, over the range of intranasal doses, 150 to 450 mcg. Plasma concentrations of desmopressin acetate nasal spray were maximal approximately 40 to 45 minutes after dosing.

Excretion – Desmopressin acetate exhibits a biphasic elimination profile, with half-lives of 7.8 and 75.5 minutes for the initial and terminal phases, respectively, in contrast with lysine vasopressin, which has initial and terminal phase half-lives of 2.5 and 14.5 minutes, respectively.

Contraindications

Hypersensitivity to desmopressin acetate or to any of the components of intranasal desmopressin acetate.

Warnings

➤*Water intoxication:* When desmopressin acetate is administered, in particular to pediatric and geriatric patients, fluid intake should be adjusted downward in an effort to decrease the potential occurrence of water intoxication and hyponatremia with accompanying signs and symptoms (headache, nausea/vomiting, decreased serum sodium, and weight gain). Particular attention should be paid to the possibility of the rare occurrence of an extreme decrease in plasma osmolarity that may result in seizures, which could lead to coma.

Patients who do not have need of antidiuretic hormone for its antidiuretic effect, in particular those who are young or elderly, should be cautioned to ingest only enough fluid to satisfy thirst, in order to decrease the potential occurrence of water intoxication and hyponatremia.

➤*von Willebrand disease:* Desmopressin acetate nasal spray should not be used to treat patients with Type IIB von Willebrand disease since platelet aggregation may be induced.

➤*Hypersensitivity reactions:* Severe allergic reactions have been reported rarely. Fatal anaphylaxis has been reported in 1 patient who received desmopressin acetate injection. It is not known whether antibodies to desmopressin acetate are produced after repeated administration.

➤*Elderly:* Clinical studies of intranasal desmopressin acetate did not include sufficient numbers of subjects 65 years of age and older to determine whether they respond differently than younger subjects. However, other postmarketing experience has reported the occurrence of hyponatremia with the use of desmopressin acetate and fluid overload.

DESMOPRESSIN ACETATE — INTRANASAL

Therefore, in elderly patients, fluid intake should be adjusted downward in an effort to decrease the potential occurrence of water intoxication and hyponatremia. Particular attention should be paid to the possibility of the rare occurrence of an extreme decrease in plasma osmolarity that may result in seizures, which could lead to coma.

➤*Pregnancy: Category B.* There are no adequate and well-controlled studies in pregnant women.

➤*Lactation:* There have been no controlled studies in nursing mothers. A single study in postpartum women demonstrated a marked change in plasma, but little if any change in assayable desmopressin acetate in breast milk following an intranasal dose of 10 mcg. It is not known whether this drug is excreted in human milk. Because many drugs are excreted in human milk, caution should be exercised when desmopressin acetate is administered to a nursing woman.

➤*Children:*

Stimate nasal spray – Use in infants and children will require careful fluid intake restriction to prevent possible hyponatremia and water intoxication. Desmopressin acetate nasal spray should not be used in infants younger than 11 months in the treatment of hemophilia A or von Willebrand's disease; safety and efficacy in children between 11 months and 12 years of age has been demonstrated.

Rhinal tube and Minirin and *DDAVP* nasal sprays –

Primary nocturnal enuresis: Intranasal desmopressin acetate has been used in childhood nocturnal enuresis. Short-term (4 to 8 weeks) intranasal desmopressin acetate administration has been shown to be safe and modestly effective in children aged 6 years or older with severe childhood nocturnal enuresis. Adequately controlled studies with desmopressin acetate nasal spray or rhinal tube in primary nocturnal enuresis have not been conducted beyond 4 to 8 weeks. The dose should be individually adjusted to achieve the best results.

Central cranial diabetes insipidus: Intranasal desmopressin acetate has been used in children with diabetes insipidus. Use in infants and children will require careful fluid intake restriction to prevent possible hyponatremia and water intoxication. The dose must be individually adjusted to the patient with attention in the very young to the danger of an extreme decrease in plasma osmolality with resulting convulsions. Dose should start at 0.05 mL or less.

There are reports of an occasional change in response with time, usually greater than 6 months. Some patients may show a decreased responsiveness, others a shortened duration of effect. There is no evidence this effect is due to the development of binding antibodies but may be due to a local inactivation of the peptide.

• *Nasal spray* – Because the spray cannot deliver less than 0.1 mL (10 mcg), smaller doses should be administered using the intranasal delivery system. Do not use the nasal spray in children requiring less than 0.1 mL (10 mcg) per dose.

Precautions

➤*Monitoring:* Although the pressor activity of desmopressin acetate is very low compared to the antidiuretic activity, use of large doses of desmopressin acetate with other pressor agents should only be done with careful patient monitoring.

➤*Cardiovascular effects:* Intranasal desmopressin acetate has infrequently produced changes in blood pressure causing either a slight elevation in blood pressure or a transient fall in blood pressure and a compensatory increase in heart rate. The drug should be used with caution in patients with coronary artery insufficiency and/or hypertensive cardiovascular disease.

➤*Thrombotic events:* There have been rare reports of thrombotic events (thrombosis, acute cerebrovascular thrombosis, acute MI) following desmopressin acetate injection in patients predisposed to thrombus formation. No causality has been determined; however, the drug should be used with caution in these patients.

➤*Nasal mucosa changes:*

Central cranial diabetes insipidus – Since desmopressin acetate nasal spray or rhinal tube is used intranasally, changes in the nasal mucosa such as scarring, edema, or other disease may cause erratic, unreliable absorption in which case desmopressin acetate nasal spray should be discontinued until the nasal problems resolve. For such situations, desmopressin acetate injection should be considered.

Primary nocturnal enuresis – If changes in the nasal mucosa have occurred, unreliable absorption may result. Desmopressin acetate nasal spray or rhinal tube should be discontinued until the nasal problems resolve.

➤*Special risk:* Desmopressin acetate should be used with caution in patients with conditions associated with fluid and electrolyte imbalance, such as cystic fibrosis, because these patients are prone to hyponatremia.

➤*Lab test abnormalities:*

Hemophilia A – Laboratory tests for assessing patient status include levels of Factor VIII coagulant, Factor VIII antigen, and Factor VIII ristocetin cofactor (von Willebrand factor) as well as activated partial thromboplastin time. Factor VIII coagulant activity should be determined before giving desmopressin acetate nasal spray for hemostasis. If Factor VIII coagulant activity is present at less than 5% of normal, desmopressin acetate nasal spray should not be relied on.

von Willebrand's disease – Laboratory tests for assessing patient status include levels of Factor VIII coagulant activity, Factor VIII ristocetin cofactor activity, and Factor VIII von Willebrand factor antigen. The skin bleeding time may be helpful in following these patients. Laboratory tests for following the patient with central cranial diabetes insipidus or postsurgical or head trauma-related polyuria and polydipsia include urine volume and osmolality. In some cases plasma osmolality measurements may be required. For the healthy patient with primary nocturnal enuresis, serum electrolytes should be checked at least once if therapy is continued beyond 7 days.

Drug Interactions

Desmopressin Drug Interactions

Precipitant drug	Object drug[a]		Description
Desmopressin	Pressor agents	↑	Although desmopressin pressor activity is very low, use large intranasal doses or parenteral doses as large as 0.3 mcg/kg cautiously with other pressor agents.
Carbamazepine	Desmopressin	↑	Carbamazepine, which potentiates ADH, may potentiate the effects of desmopressin.
Chlorpropamide	Desmopressin	↑	Chlorpropamide, which potentiates ADH, may potentiate the effects of desmopressin.

[a] ↑ = Object drug increased.

Adverse Reactions

Infrequently, high dosages of intranasal desmopressin acetate have produced transient headache and nausea. Nasal congestion, rhinitis, and flushing have also been reported occasionally along with mild abdominal cramps. These symptoms disappeared with reduction in dosage. Nosebleed, sore throat, cough, and upper respiratory tract infections have also been reported.

Desmopressin acetate injection has infrequently produced changes in blood pressure causing either a slight elevation or a transient fall and a compensatory increase in heart rate. Severe allergic reactions including anaphylaxis have been reported rarely with desmopressin acetate injection.

➤*Stimate* nasal spray: In addition to those listed above, the following have also been reported in clinical trials with desmopressin acetate nasal spray: Somnolence; dizziness; itchy or light-sensitive eyes; insomnia; chills; warm feeling; pain; chest pain; palpitations; tachycardia; dyspepsia; edema; vomiting; agitation; balanitis.

➤*Rhinal tube and Minirin* and *DDAVP* nasal sprays: The following table lists the percent of patients having adverse experiences without regard to relationship to study drug from the pooled pivotal study data for nocturnal enuresis.

Adverse reaction	Placebo (n = 59) %	Desmopressin Acetate 20 mcg (n = 60) %	Desmopressin Acetate 40 mcg (n = 61) %
Abdominal pain	0	2%	2%
Asthenia	0	0	2%
Chills	0	0	2%
Headache	0	2%	5%
Throat pain	2%	0	0
CNS			
Depression	2%	0	0
Dizziness	0	0	3%
Respiratory			
Epistaxis	2%	3%	0
Nostril pain	0	2%	0
Respiratory tract infection	2%	0	0
Rhinitis	2%	8%	3%
Cardiovascular			
Vasodilation	2%	0	0
GI			
GI disorder	0	2%	0
Nausea	0	0	2%
Dermatologic			
Leg rash	2%	0	0
Rash	2%	0	0
Special senses			
Conjunctivitis	0	2%	0
Edema eyes	0	2%	0
Lacrimation disorder	0	0	2%

DESMOPRESSIN ACETATE — INTRANASAL

Overdosage

➤*Treatment:* In cases of overdosage, the dosage should be reduced, frequency of administration decreased, or the drug withdrawn according to the severity of the condition (see Adverse Reactions). There is no known specific antidote for desmopressin acetate or desmopressin acetate nasal spray or rhinal tube.

Patient Information

➤*Stimate* nasal spray: Patients should be informed that the bottle accurately delivers 25 doses of each 150 mcg each. Any solution remaining after 25 doses should be discarded since the amount delivered thereafter may be substantially less than 150 mcg of drug. No attempt should be made to transfer remaining solution to another bottle. Patients should be instructed to read accompanying directions on use of the spray pump carefully before use.

Patients should also be advised that if bleeding is not controlled, the physician should be contacted.

Minirin and *DDAVP* nasal sprays – Patients should be informed that the bottle accurately delivers 50 doses of 10 mcg each. Any solution remaining after 50 doses should be discarded since the amount delivered thereafter may be substantially less than 10 mcg of drug. No attempt should be made to transfer remaining solution to another bottle. Patients should be instructed to read accompanying directions on use of the spray pump carefully before use.

DESMOPRESSIN ACETATE — INJECTION

Refer to the general discussion of these products in the Posterior Pituitary Hormones introduction.

Indications

➤*Hemophilia A:* For patients with hemophilia A with Factor VIII coagulant activity levels more than 5%.

Desmopressin will often maintain hemostasis in patients with hemophilia A during surgical procedures and postoperatively when administered 30 minutes prior to scheduled procedure.

Desmopressin will also stop bleeding in hemophilia A patients with episodes of spontaneous or trauma-induced injuries such as hemarthroses, IM hematomas, or mucosal bleeding.

Desmopressin is not indicated for the treatment of hemophilia A with Factor VIII coagulant activity levels 5% or less, or for the treatment of hemophilia B, or in patients who have Factor VIII antibodies.

In certain clinical situations, it may be justified to try desmopressin in patients with Factor VIII levels between 2% to 5%; however, these patients should be carefully monitored.

➤*von Willebrand Disease (Type I):* For patients with mild to moderate classic von Willebrand disease (Type I) with Factor VIII levels more than 5%. Desmopressin acetate injection will often maintain hemostasis in patients with mild to moderate von Willebrand disease during surgical procedures and postoperatively when administered 30 minutes prior to the scheduled procedure.

Desmopressin will usually stop bleeding in mild to moderate von Willebrand patients with episodes of spontaneous or trauma-induced injuries such as hemarthroses, IM hematomas, or mucosal bleeding.

Those von Willebrand disease patients who are least likely to respond are those with severe homozygous von Willebrand disease with Factor VIII coagulant activity and Factor VIII von Willebrand factor antigen levels less than 1%. Other patients may respond in a variable fashion depending on the type of molecular defect they have. Bleeding time and Factor VIII coagulant activity, ristocetin cofactor activity, and von Willebrand factor antigen should be checked during administration of desmopressin acetate injection to ensure that adequate levels are being achieved.

Desmopressin is not indicated for the treatment of severe classic von Willebrand disease (Type I) and when there is evidence of an abnormal molecular form of Factor VIII antigen (see Warnings).

➤*Diabetes insipidus:* Desmopressin 4 mcg/mL is indicated as antidiuretic replacement therapy in the management of central (cranial) diabetes insipidus and for the management of the temporary polyuria and polydipsia following head trauma or surgery in the pituitary region. Desmopressin is ineffective for the treatment of nephrogenic diabetes insipidus.

Administration and Dosage

➤*Hemophilia A and von Willebrand Disease (Type I):* Desmopressin 4 mcg/mL is administered as an IV infusion at a dose of 0.3 mcg desmopressin acetate/kg body weight diluted in sterile physiological saline and infused slowly over 15 to 30 minutes. In adults and children weighing more than 10 kg, 50 mL of diluent is recommended; in children weighing 10 kg or less, 10 mL of diluent is recommended. Blood pressure and pulse should be monitored during infusion. If desmopressin 4 mcg/mL is used preoperatively, it should be administered 30 minutes prior to the scheduled procedure.

The necessity for repeat administration of desmopressin or use of any blood products for hemostasis should be determined by laboratory response as well as the clinical condition of the patient. The tendency toward tachyphylaxis (lessening of response) with repeated administration given more frequently than every 48 hours should be considered in treating each patient.

➤*Diabetes insipidus:* This formulation is administered subcutaneously or by direct IV injection. Desmopressin 4 mcg/mL dosage must be determined for each patient and adjusted according to the pattern of response. Response should be estimated by 2 parameters: Adequate duration of sleep and adequate, not excessive, water turnover.

The usual dosage range in adults is 0.5 mL (2 mcg) to 1 mL (4 mcg) daily, administered IV or subcutaneously, usually in 2 divided doses. The morning and evening doses should be separately adjusted for an adequate diurnal rhythm of water turnover. For patients who have been controlled on intranasal desmopressin and who must be switched to the injection form, either because of poor intranasal absorption or because of the need for surgery, the comparable antidiuretic dose of the injection is about one-tenth the intranasal dose.

➤*Storage/Stability:* Store refrigerated 2 to 8°C (36 to 46°F). Keep out of the reach of children.

Actions

➤*Pharmacology:* Desmopressin is a synthetic analogue of the natural hormone arginine vasopressin. One mL (4 mcg) of desmopressin has an antidiuretic activity of about 16 units; 1 mcg of desmopressin is equivalent to 4 units.

Desmopressin acetate injection has been shown to be more potent than arginine vasopressin in increasing plasma levels of Factor VIII activity in patients with hemophilia and von Willebrand disease Type I.

Dose-response studies were performed in healthy persons, using doses of 0.1 to 0.4 mcg/kg body weight, infused over a 10-minute period. Maximal dose response occurred at 0.3 to 0.4 mcg/kg. The response to desmopressin of Factor VIII activity and plasminogen activator is dose-related, with maximal plasma levels of 300 to 400 percent of initial concentrations obtained after infusion of 0.4 mcg/kg body weight. The increase is rapid and evident within 30 minutes, reaching a maximum at a point ranging from 90 minutes to 2 hours. The Factor VIII related antigen and ristocetin cofactor activity were also increased to a smaller degree, but still are dose-dependent.

➤*Pharmacokinetics:* The biphasic half-lives of desmopressin acetate injection were 7.8 and 75.5 minutes for the fast and slow phases, respectively, compared with 2.5 and 14.5 minutes for lysine vasopressin, another form of the hormone. As a result, desmopressin acetate injection provides a prompt onset of antidiuretic action with a long duration after each administration.

Contraindications

Known hypersensitivity to desmopressin or to any of the components of desmopressin.

Warnings

Patients who do not have need of antidiuretic hormone for its antidiuretic effect, in particular those who are young or elderly, should be cautioned to ingest only enough fluid to satisfy thirst, in order to decrease the potential occurrence of water intoxication and hyponatremia.

➤*Fluid/Electrolyte balance:* Fluid intake should be adjusted downward, particularly in very young and elderly patients, in order to decrease the potential occurrence of water intoxication and hyponatremia.

➤*Plasma osmolality:* Particular attention should be paid to the possibility of the rare occurrence of an extreme decrease in plasma osmolality that may result in seizures which could lead to coma.

➤*von Willebrand disease:* Desmopressin should not be used to treat patients with Type IIB von Willebrand disease since platelet aggregation may be induced.

➤*Hypersensitivity reactions:* Severe allergic reactions have been reported rarely. Fatal anaphylaxis has been reported in 1 patient who received IV desmopressin. It is not known whether antibodies to desmopressin are produced after repeated injections.

➤*Pregnancy: Category B.*

There are no adequate and well controlled studies in pregnant women. Because animal reproduction studies are not always predictive of human response, this drug should be used during pregnancy only if clearly needed.

➤*Lactation:* There have been no controlled studies in nursing mothers. A single study in postpartum women demonstrated a marked change in plasma, but little if any change in assayable desmopressin acetate injection in breast milk following an intranasal dose of 10 mcg. It is not known whether this drug is excreted in human milk. Because many drugs are excreted in human milk, caution should be exercised when desmopressin acetate injection is administered to a nursing woman.

➤*Children:* Use in infants and children will require careful fluid intake restriction to prevent possible hyponatremia and water intoxication. Desmopressin acetate injection 4 mcg/mL should not be used in infants younger than 3 months of age in the treatment of hemophilia A or von Willebrand disease; safety and efficacy in children younger than 12 years of age with diabetes insipidus have not been established.

Precautions

➤*Monitoring:* Although the pressor activity of desmopressin is very low compared with the antidiuretic activity, use of doses less than or equal to 0.3 mcg/kg of desmopressin with other pressor agents should be done only with careful patient monitoring.

Hemophilia A – In certain clinical situations, it may be justified to try desmopressin in patients with Factor VIII levels between 2% to 5%; however, these patients should be carefully monitored (see Indications).

DESMOPRESSIN ACETATE — INJECTION

Hemophilia A and von Willebrand Disease (Type I) – Blood pressure and pulse should be monitored during infusion (see Indications).

von Willebrand Disease – Laboratory tests for assessing patient status include levels of Factor VIII coagulant activity, Factor VIII ristocetin cofactor activity, and Factor VIII von Willebrand factor antigen. The skin bleeding time may be helpful in following these patients.

Diabetes insipidus – Laboratory tests for monitoring the patient include urine volume and osmolality. In some cases, plasma osmolality may be required.

➤*Hemophilia A:* Laboratory tests for assessing patient status include levels of Factor VIII coagulant, Factor VIII antigen and Factor VIII ristocetin cofactor (von Willebrand factor) as well as activated partial thromboplastin time. Factor VIII coagulant activity should be determined before giving desmopressin acetate injection for hemostasis. If Factor VIII coagulant activity is present at less than 5% of normal, desmopressin acetate injection should not be relied on.

➤*Special risk:* Desmopressin has infrequently produced changes in blood pressure causing either a slight elevation in blood pressure or a transient fall in blood pressure and a compensatory increase in heart rate. The drug should be used with caution in patients with coronary artery insufficiency and/or hypertensive cardiovascular disease.

Desmopressin should be used with caution in patients with conditions associated with fluid and electrolyte imbalance, such as cystic fibrosis, because these patients are prone to hyponatremia.

There have been rare reports of thrombotic events following desmopressin in patients predisposed to thrombus formation. No causality has been determined; however, the drug should be used with caution in these patients.

Drug Interactions

Desmopressin Drug Interactions

Precipitant drug	Object drug[a]		Description
Desmopressin	Pressor agents	↑	Although desmopressin pressor activity is very low, use large intranasal doses or parenteral doses as large as 0.3 mcg/kg cautiously with other pressor agents.

Desmopressin Drug Interactions

Precipitant drug	Object drug[a]		Description
Carbamazepine	Desmopressin	↑	Carbamazepine, which potentiates ADH, may potentiate the effects of desmopressin.
Chlorpropamide	Desmopressin	↑	Chlorpropamide, which potentiates ADH, may potentiate the effects of desmopressin.

[a] ↑ = Object drug increased.

None known. Desmopressin has been used with epsilon aminocaproic acid without adverse effects.

Adverse Reactions

Infrequently, desmopressin has produced transient headache, nausea, mild abdominal cramps, and vulval pain. These symptoms disappeared with reduction in dosage. Occasionally, injection of desmopressin acetate has produced local erythema, swelling, or burning pain. Occasional facial flushing has been reported with the administration of desmopressin. Desmopressin has infrequently produced changes in blood pressure causing either a slight elevation or a transient fall and a compensatory increase in heart rate. Severe allergic reactions including anaphylaxis have been reported rarely with desmopressin.

See Warnings for the possibility of water intoxication and hyponatremia.

There have been rare reports of thrombotic events (acute cerebrovascular thrombosis, acute MI) following desmopressin acetate injection in patients predisposed to thrombus formation.

Overdosage

➤*Treatment:* There is no known specific antidote for desmopressin. In case of overdosage, the dosage should be reduced, frequency of administration decreased, or the drug withdrawn according to the severity of the condition.

VASOPRESSIN RECEPTOR ANTAGONIST

CONIVAPTAN HYDROCHLORIDE

Rx	**Vaprisol** (Astellas)	**Injection:** 5 mg/mL (20 mg)	1.2 g propylene glycol, 0.4 g ethanol. In 4 mL amps.

CONIVAPTAN HYDROCHLORIDE— INJECTION

Indications

➤*Euvolemic hyponatremia:* For the treatment of euvolemic hyponatremia (eg, the syndrome of inappropriate secretion of antidiuretic hormone, or in the setting of hypothyroidism, adrenal insufficiency, pulmonary disorders) in hospitalized patients.

Conivaptan is not indicated for the treatment of patients with congestive heart failure (CHF).

Administration and Dosage

➤*Approved by the FDA:* December 29, 2005

➤*Administration:* For intravenous (IV) use only.

Administration of conivaptan through large veins and changing of the infusion site every 24 hours are recommended to minimize the risk of vascular irritation.

➤*Loading dose:* Conivaptan therapy should begin with a loading dose of 20 mg IV administered over 30 minutes.

➤*Continuous infusion:* The loading dose should be followed by conivaptan 20 mg administered in a continuous IV infusion over 24 hours. Following the initial day of treatment, conivaptan is to be administered for an additional 1 to 3 days in a continuous infusion of 20 mg/day. If serum sodium is not rising at the desired rate, conivaptan may be titrated upward to a dosage of 40 mg daily, again administered in a continuous IV infusion.

The total duration of infusion of conivaptan (after the loading dose) should not exceed 4 days.

➤*Dosage adjustments:* For patients who develop an undesirably rapid rate of rise of serum sodium, conivaptan should be discontinued and serum sodium and neurologic status should be carefully monitored. If the serum sodium continues to rise, conivaptan should not be resumed. If hyponatremia persists or recurs, and the patient has had no evidence of neurologic sequelae of rapid rise in serum sodium, conivaptan may be resumed at a reduced dose.

For patients who develop hypovolemia or hypotension while receiving conivaptan, conivaptan should be discontinued and volume status and vital signs should be frequently monitored. Once the patient is again euvolemic and is no longer hypotensive, conivaptan may be resumed at a reduced dose if the patient remains hyponatremic.

➤*Preparation for administration:*

Compatibility – Conivaptan should be diluted only with 5% dextrose injection.

Conivaptan should not be mixed or administered with Ringer's lactate injection or 0.9% sodium chloride injection. Compatibility with other drugs has not been studied; therefore, conivaptan should not be combined with any other product in the same IV line or bag.

Loading dose – Withdraw 4 mL (20 mg) of conivaptan and add to an infusion bag containing 100 mL of 5% dextrose injection. Gently invert the bag several times to ensure complete mixing of the solution. The contents of the IV bag should be administered over 30 minutes.

Continuous infusion – To prepare a continuous IV infusion containing conivaptan 20 mg, withdraw 4 mL (20 mg) from a single ampule of conivaptan and dilute into an IV bag containing 250 mL of 5% dextrose injection. Gently invert the bag several times to ensure complete mixing of the solution. The contents of the IV bag should be administered over 24 hours.

To prepare a continuous IV infusion containing conivaptan 40 mg, withdraw 4 mL (20 mg) from each of two ampules of conivaptan (8 mL [40 mg] of conivaptan) and dilute into an IV bag containing 250 mL of 5% dextrose injection. Gently invert the bag several times to ensure complete mixing of the solution. The contents of the IV bag should be administered over 24 hours.

The conivaptan ampule is for single use only. Discard unused contents of the ampule.

➤*Storage/Stability:* Store at 25°C (77°F); excursions permitted to 15° to 30°C (59° to 86°F), controlled room temperature. Do not store below 15°C (59°F). Store ampules in their cardboard container and protected from light until ready for use.

Use the diluted solution of conivaptan immediately and complete administration within 24 hours of mixing.

Actions

➤*Pharmacology:* Conivaptan is a dual arginine vasopressin (AVP) antagonist with nanomolar affinity for human V_{1A} and V_2 receptors in vitro. The level of AVP in circulating blood is critical for the regulation of water and electrolyte balance and is usually elevated in both euvolemic and hypervolemic hyponatremia. The AVP effect is mediated through V_2 receptors, which are functionally coupled to aquaporin channels in the apical membrane of the collecting ducts of the kidney. These receptors help to maintain plasma osmolality within the normal range. The predominant pharmacodynamic effect of conivaptan in the treatment of hyponatremia is through its V_2

CONIVAPTAN HYDROCHLORIDE— INJECTION

antagonism of AVP in the renal collecting ducts, an effect that results in aquaresis, or excretion of free water. The pharmacodynamic effects of conivaptan include increased free water excretion (ie, effective water clearance [EWC]) generally accompanied by increased net fluid loss, increased urine output, and decreased urine osmolality. Studies in animal models of hyponatremia showed that conivaptan prevented the occurrence of hyponatremia-related physical signs in rats with the syndrome of inappropriate antidiuretic hormone secretion.

➤*Pharmacokinetics:*

Absorption/Distribution – The pharmacokinetics of conivaptan have been characterized in healthy subjects, special populations, and patients following both oral and IV dosing regimens. The pharmacokinetics of conivaptan following IV infusion (40 to 80 mg/day) and oral administration are nonlinear, and inhibition by conivaptan of its own metabolism seems to be the major factor for the nonlinearity. The intersubject variability of conivaptan pharmacokinetics is high (94% coefficient of variation [CV] in clearance).

The pharmacokinetics of conivaptan and its metabolites were characterized in healthy men administered conivaptan as a 20 mg loading dose (infused over 30 min) followed by a continuous infusion of 40 mg/day for 3 days. Mean C_{max} for conivaptan was 619 ng/mL and occurred at the end of the loading dose. Plasma concentrations reached a minimum at approximately 12 hours after start of the loading dose, then gradually increased over the duration of the infusion to a mean concentration of 188 ng/mL at the end of the infusion.

Conivaptan is extensively bound to human plasma proteins, being 99% bound over the concentration range of approximately 10 to 1,000 ng/mL.

In an open-label safety and efficacy study, the pharmacokinetics of conivaptan were characterized in hypervolemic or euvolemic hyponatremia patients (51 to 89 years of age) receiving conivaptan as a 20 mg loading dose (infused over 30 min) followed by a continuous infusion of 20 or 40 mg/day for 4 days.

The pharmacokinetic parameters are summarized in the table below.

Conivaptan Pharmacokinetic Parameters

Parameter	IV conivaptan 20 mg/day	IV conivaptan 40 mg/day
Conivaptan concentration at the end of loading dose (ng/mL, at 0.5 hours)		
N	12	14
Median (range)	575.8 (144.5 to 764.3)	781.1 (194.5 to 1373.5)
Conivaptan concentration at the end of infusion (ng/mL, at 96 hours)		
N	9	11
Median (range)	107.9 (14.7 to 588.8)	227.5 (4.5 to 1454.1)
Elimination half-life (h)		
N	12	14
Median (range)	6.7 (3.6 to 16.9)	8.6 (4.7 to 25.6)
Clearance (L/h)		
N	12	14
Median (range)	10.1 (2 to 37.6)	9.5 (1.5 to 42.5)

Metabolism/Excretion – CYP3A4 was identified as the sole cytochrome P-450 isozyme responsible for the metabolism of conivaptan. Four metabolites have been identified. The pharmacological activity of the metabolites at V_{1A} and V_2 receptors ranged from approximately 3% to 50% and 50% to 100% that of conivaptan, respectively. The combined exposure of the metabolites following IV administration of conivaptan is approximately 7% that of conivaptan and hence, their contribution to the clinical effect of conivaptan is minimal.

After IV (10 mg) or oral (20 mg) administration of conivaptan in a mass balance study, approximately 83% of the dose was excreted in feces as total radioactivity and 12% in urine over several days of collection. Over the first 24 hours after dosing, approximately 1% of the IV dose was excreted in urine as intact conivaptan.

The mean terminal elimination half-life after conivaptan infusion was 5 hours, and the mean clearance was 15.2 L/h.

Special populations –

Renal function impairment: The effect of renal function impairment on the elimination of conivaptan after IV administration has not been evaluated. However, following administration of oral conivaptan, the AUC for conivaptan was up to 80% higher in patients with renal function impairment (creatinine clearance [Ccr] less than 60 mL/min/1.73 m^2) compared with those with normal renal function. IV conivaptan resulted in higher conivaptan exposure than did oral conivaptan in study subjects without renal function impairment. Exercise caution when administering conivaptan to patients with impaired renal function.

Hepatic function impairment: The effect of hepatic function impairment (including ascites, cirrhosis, or portal hypertension) on the elimination of conivaptan after IV administration has not been systemically evaluated. However, increased systemic exposures after administration of oral conivaptan (up to a mean 2.8-fold increase) have been seen in patients with stable cirrhosis and moderate hepatic impairment. IV conivaptan resulted in higher conivaptan exposure than did oral conivaptan in study subjects without hepatic function impairment. Exercise caution when administering conivaptan to patients with impaired hepatic function.

Elderly: Following a single oral dose of conivaptan (15, 30, or 60 mg), drug exposure (AUC) in elderly men and women (65 to 90 years of age) compared to that seen in young men was similar for the 15 and 30 mg doses but increased nearly 2-fold at the 60 mg dose.

In an open-label study to assess the safety and efficacy of conivaptan, a subset of geriatric hypervolemic or euvolemic hyponatremia patients (67 to 89 years of age) received a 20 mg IV loading dose followed by a 20 mg/day (N = 11) or 40 mg/day (N = 12) IV infusion for 4 days. The median conivaptan plasma concentration in these patients at the end of the loading dose infusion was 628 ng/mL. The median conivaptan plasma concentration at the end of the 4-day continuous infusion was 117 and 258 ng/mL for the 20 and 40 mg/day regimens, respectively.

Children:

Contraindications

In patients with hypovolemic hyponatremia and in those who have hypersensitivity to any of its components. The coadministration of conivaptan with potent CYP3A4 inhibitors such as ketoconazole, itraconazole, clarithromycin, ritonavir, and indinavir, is contraindicated.

Warnings

➤*Renal function impairment:* See Actions for more information.

➤*Hepatic function impairment:* See Actions for more information.

➤*Pregnancy: Category C.* Conivaptan has been shown to have adverse effects on the fetus when given to animals during pregnancy at systemic exposures less than those achieved at a therapeutic dose based on AUC comparisons. There are no adequate and well-controlled studies in pregnant women. Use conivaptan during pregnancy only if the potential benefit justifies the potential risk to the fetus. Apprise the patient of the potential hazard to the fetus.

Conivaptan crosses the placenta and is found in fetal tissue in rats. Fetal tissue levels were less than 10% of maternal plasma concentrations while placental levels were 2.2-fold higher than maternal plasma concentrations indicating that conivaptan can be transferred to the fetus. Conivaptan that is taken up by fetal tissue is slowly cleared, suggesting that fetal accumulation is possible. Milk levels were up to 3 times higher than maternal plasma levels following an IV dose of 1 mg/kg (systemic exposures less than therapeutic based on AUC comparisons).

Labor and delivery – The effect of conivaptan on labor and delivery in humans has not been studied. Conivaptan delayed delivery in rats dosed orally at 10 mg/kg/day by oral gavage (systemic exposures equivalent to the therapeutic dose based on AUC comparisons). Administration of conivaptan at 2.5 mg/kg/day IV increased peripartum pup mortality (systemic exposures were less than the therapeutic dose based on AUC comparisons). These effects may be associated with conivaptan activity on oxytocin receptors in the rat. The relevance to humans is unclear.

➤*Lactation:* It is not known whether conivaptan is excreted in human milk. Because many drugs are excreted in human milk, exercise caution when conivaptan is administered to a lactating woman. Conivaptan is excreted in milk and detected in neonates when given by IV administration to lactating rats. Milk levels of conivaptan in rats reached maximal levels at 1 hour postdose following IV administrations and were up to 3 times greater than maternal plasma levels. Administration of conivaptan at 2.5 mg/kg/day IV increased peripartum pup mortality; systemic exposures were less than the therapeutic dose based on AUC comparisons.

➤*Children:* The safety and efficacy of conivaptan in children have not been studied.

Precautions

➤*Monitoring:* Patients receiving conivaptan must have frequent monitoring of serum sodium, neurologic status, and volume status. An overly rapid rise in serum sodium (greater than 12 mEq/L/24 hours) may result in serious sequelae. Monitor vital signs and volume status frequently in patients who develop hypovolemia or hypotension during therapy.

➤*CHF:* See Indications for more information.

➤*Injection-site reactions:* Conivaptan may cause significant injection site reactions, even with proper dilution and infusion rates. Conivaptan must only be administered when properly prepared and diluted via large veins, and the infusion site should be rotated every 24 hours.

➤*Overly rapid correction of serum sodium:* An overly rapid increase in serum sodium concentration (greater than 12 mEq/L per 24 hours) may result in serious sequelae. In controlled clinical trials of conivaptan, about 9% of patients who received conivaptan in doses of 20 to 40 mg/day IV met laboratory criteria for overly rapid correction of serum sodium, but none of these patients had permanent neurologic sequelae. Although not observed in the clinical studies with conivaptan, osmotic demyelination syndrome has been reported following rapid correction of low serum sodium concentrations.

See Administration and Dosage for more information.

Drug Interactions

➤*CYP3A4:* Conivaptan is a sensitive substrate of CYP3A4. The effect of ketoconazole, a potent CYP3A4 inhibitor, on the pharmacokinetics of conivaptan IV has not been evaluated. Coadministration of oral conivaptan 10 mg with ketoconazole 200 mg resulted in a 4- and 11-fold increase in C_{max} and AUC of conivaptan, respectively.

Coadministration of conivaptan with CYP3A4 inhibitors could lead to an increase in conivaptan concentrations. The consequences of increased conivaptan concentrations are unknown. Concomitant use of conivaptan with potent CYP3A4 inhibitors such as ketoconazole, itraconazole, clarithromycin, ritonavir, and indinavir is contraindicated.

CONIVAPTAN HYDROCHLORIDE— INJECTION

Conivaptan is a potent inhibitor of CYP3A4. The effect of conivaptan on the pharmacokinetics of CYP3A4 substrates has been evaluated with the coadministration of conivaptan with midazolam, simvastatin, and amlodipine. IV conivaptan 40 mg/day increased the mean AUC values by approximately 2- and 3-fold for 1 mg IV or 2 mg oral doses of midazolam, respectively. IV conivaptan 30 mg/day resulted in a 3-fold increase in the AUC of simvastatin. Oral conivaptan 40 mg twice daily resulted in a 2-fold increase in the AUC and half-life of amlodipine.

Conivaptan may increase plasma concentrations of coadministered drugs that are primarily metabolized by CYP3A4. In clinical trials of oral conivaptan, 2 cases of rhabdomyolysis occurred in patients who were also receiving a CYP3A4-metabolized HMG-CoA reductase inhibitor. Closely monitor concomitant use of conivaptan with drugs that are primarily metabolized by CYP3A4 avoid or the combination. If a clinical decision is made to discontinue concomitant medications at recommended doses, allow an appropriate amount of time following the end of conivaptan administration before resuming these medications.

➤*Digoxin:* Coadministration of digoxin 0.5 mg, a P-glycoprotein substrate, with oral conivaptan 40 mg twice daily resulted in a 30% reduction in clearance and a 79% and 43% increase in digoxin C_{max} and AUC values, respectively.

Therefore, if digoxin is administered with conivaptan, the clinician should be alert to the possibility of increases in digoxin levels.

Adverse Reactions

The most common adverse reactions reported with conivaptan administration were infusion site reactions. In studies in patients and healthy volunteers, infusion site reactions occurred in 52.5% of subjects treated with conivaptan 40 mg/day compared to 3.3% in the placebo group. The majority of the reactions were mild and did not lead to discontinuation of drug. However, some serious infusion site reactions did occur, and infusion site reactions were the most common type of adverse event leading to discontinuation of conivaptan.

Conivaptan Adverse Reactions (at least 2%)[a]

Adverse reaction	Placebo N = 61	Conivaptan 40 mg N = 183
Cardiovascular		
Atrial fibrillation	0	5 (2.7%)
Hypertension	0	10 (5.5%)
Hypotension	1 (1.6%)	5 (2.7%)
Orthostatic hypotension	0	10 (5.5%)
Phlebitis	1 (1.6%)	9 (4.9%)
CNS		
Confusional state	1 (1.6%)	7 (3.8%)
Headache	2 (3.3%)	22 (12%)
Insomnia	0	6 (3.3%)
Dermatologic		
Erythema	0	5 (2.7%)
GI		
Constipation	2 (3.3%)	9 (4.9%)
Diarrhea	0	10 (5.5%)
Dry mouth	2 (3.3%)	8 (4.4%)
Nausea	2 (3.3%)	7 (3.8%)
Vomiting	0	12 (6.6%)
GU		
Hematuria	1 (1.6%)	4 (2.2%)
Pollakiuria	0	11 (6%)
Polyuria	0	9 (4.9%)
Urinary tract infection	1 (1.6%)	6 (3.3%)
Hematologic		
Anemia	2 (3.3%)	7 (3.8%)
Local		
Cannula-site reaction	0	10 (5.5%)
Infusion-site erythema	0	9 (4.9%)
Infusion-site pain	1 (1.6%)	14 (7.7%)
Infusion-site phlebitis	0	29 (15.8%)
Infusion-site reaction	0	37 (20.2%)
Infusion-site swelling	1 (1.6%)	5 (2.7%)
Metabolic/Nutritional		
Dehydration	0	4 (2.2%)
Hyperglycemia	0	5 (2.7%)
Hypoglycemia	0	6 (3.3%)
Hypokalemia	1 (1.6%)	18 (9.8%)
Hypomagnesemia	0	4 (2.2%)
Hyponatremia	0	6 (3.3%)
Miscellaneous		
Oral candidiasis	0	4 (2.2%)
Pain	0	4 (2.2%)
Peripheral edema	1 (1.6%)	10 (5.5%)
Pneumonia	0	5 (2.7%)
Pyrexia	0	7 (3.8%)
Thirst	1 (1.6%)	18 (9.8%)

[a] Adapted from MedDRA version 6.0

Overdosage

➤*Symptoms:* Although no data on overdosage in humans are available, conivaptan has been administered as a 20 mg loading dose on day 1 followed by continuous infusion of 80 mg/day for 4 days in hyponatremia patients and up to 120 mg/day for 2 days in CHF patients. No new toxicities were identified at these higher doses, but adverse events related to the pharmacologic activity of conivaptan, (e.g. hypotension and thirst), occurred more frequently at these higher doses.

➤*Treatment:* In case of overdose, based on expected exaggerated pharmacological activity, symptomatic treatment with frequent monitoring of vital signs and close observation of the patient is recommended.

OCTREOTIDE ACETATE

Rx	**Octreotide Acetate** (Sicor)	**Injection:** 0.05 mg/mL	In 1 mL single-dose vials.
Rx	**Sandostatin** (Novartis)		In 1 mL amps.
Rx	**Octreotide Acetate** (Sicor)	**Injection:** 0.1 mg/mL	In 1 mL single-dose vials.
Rx	**Sandostatin** (Novartis)		In 1 mL amps.
Rx	**Octreotide Acetate** (Sicor)	**Injection:** 0.2 mg/mL	In 5 mL multi-dose vials.
Rx	**Sandostatin** (Novartis)		In 5 mL multi-dose vials.
Rx	**Octreotide Acetate** (Sicor)	**Injection:** 0.5 mg/mL	In 1 mL single-dose vials.
Rx	**Sandostatin** (Novartis)		In 1 mL amps.
Rx	**Octreotide Acetate** (Sicor)	**Injection:** 1 mg/mL	In 5 mL multi-dose vials.
Rx	**Sandostatin** (Novartis)		In 5 mL multi-dose vials.
Rx	**Sandostatin LAR Depot** (Novartis)	**Powder for injectable suspension:** 10 mg per 5 mL	In kits w/ 2 mL diluent, 1½" 20-gauge needles and instruction booklet.
		20 mg per 5 mL	In kits w/ 2 mL diluent, 1½" 20-gauge needles and instruction booklet.
		30 mg per 5 mL	In kits w/ 2 mL diluent, 1½" 20-gauge needles and instruction booklet.

OCTREOTIDE ACETATE — INJECTION

Indications

➤*Injection solution:*

Acromegaly – To reduce blood levels of growth hormone and IGF-I (somatomedin C) in acromegaly patients who have had inadequate response to or cannot be treated with surgical resection, pituitary irradiation, and bromocriptine mesylate at maximally tolerated doses. The goal is to achieve normalization of growth hormone and IGF-I (somatomedin C) levels. In patients with acromegaly, octreotide acetate reduces growth hormone to within normal ranges in 50% of patients and reduces IGF-I (somatomedin C) to within normal ranges in 50% to 60% of patients. Since the effects of pituitary irradiation may not become maximal for several years, adjunctive therapy with octreotide acetate to reduce blood levels of growth hormone and IGF-I (somatomedin C) offers potential benefit before the effects of irradiation are manifested.

Carcinoid tumors – For the symptomatic treatment of patients with metastatic carcinoid tumors where it suppresses or inhibits the severe diarrhea and flushing episodes associated with the disease.

Vasoactive intestinal peptide tumors (VIPomas) – For the treatment of the profuse watery diarrhea associated with VIP-secreting tumors.

OCTREOTIDE ACETATE — INJECTION

➤*Injectable suspension:*

Acromegaly – For long-term maintenance therapy in acromegalic patients for whom medical treatment is appropriate and who have been shown to respond to and can tolerate octreotide acetate injection. The goal of treatment in acromegaly is to reduce GH and IGF-1 levels to normal. Octreotide acetate injectable suspension can be used in patients who have had an inadequate response to surgery or in those for whom surgical resection is not an option. It may also be used in patients who have received radiation and have had an inadequate therapeutic response.

Carcinoid tumors – For long-term treatment of the severe diarrhea and flushing episodes associated with metastatic carcinoid tumors in patients in whom initial treatment with octreotide acetate injection has been shown to be effective and tolerated.

VIPomas – For long-term treatment of the profuse watery diarrhea associated with VIP-secreting tumors in patients in whom initial treatment with octreotide acetate injection has been shown to be effective and tolerated.

➤*Unlabeled uses:*

Octreotide is effective in treating the following conditions –

GI fistula: To reduce output from fistulas. Dosage ranges from 50 to 200 mcg every 8 hours.

Variceal bleeding: Dosage ranges from 25 to 50 mcg/h via continuous infusion. Duration is from 18 hours to 5 days.

Diarrheal states: Since octreotide prolongs intestinal transit time, it is beneficial in relieving diarrhea associated with a variety of conditions including: AIDS-related diarrhea (100 to 500 mcg subcutaneously 2 times daily); idiopathic secretory diarrhea; short bowel (ileostomy) syndrome (IV infusion of 25 mcg/hr or subcutaneously 50 mcg twice daily); diabetes; pancreatic cholera syndrome; diarrhea caused by chemotherapy/radiation in cancer patients (50 to 100 mcg subcutaneously 3 times daily for 1 to 3 days).

Pancreatic fistula: To reduce output from pancreatic fistulas. Dosages range from 50 to 200 mcg every 8 hours.

Irritable bowel syndrome: 100 mcg single dose to 125 mcg subcutaneously twice daily.

Dumping syndrome: 50 to 150 mcg/day. Other uses for which octreotide may be beneficial include: Enteric fistula; pancreatitis; pancreatic surgery; glucagonoma; insulinoma; gastrinoma (Zollinger-Ellison syndrome); intestinal obstruction; local radiotherapy; chronic pain management; antineoplastic therapy; decreased insulin requirements in diabetes mellitus; thyrotropin- and TSH-secreting tumors.

Administration and Dosage

➤*Approved by the FDA:* October 21, 1988.

➤*Injection solution:* Administer subcutaneously or IV. Subcutaneous injection is the usual route of administration of octreotide acetate for control of symptoms. Pain with subcutaneous administration may be reduced by using the smallest volume that will deliver the desired dose. Multiple subcutaneous injections at the same site within short periods of time should be avoided. Sites should be rotated in a systematic manner.

Parenteral drug products should be inspected visually for particulate matter and discoloration prior to administration. Do not use if particulates or discoloration are observed. Proper sterile technique should be used in the preparation of parenteral admixtures to minimize the possibility of microbial contamination. Octreotide acetate is not compatible in total parenteral nutrition (TPN) solutions because of the formation of a glycosyl octreotide conjugate, which may decrease the efficacy of the product.

Octreotide acetate is stable in sterile isotonic saline solutions or sterile solutions of dextrose 5% in water for 24 hours. It may be diluted in volumes of 50 to 200 mL and infused IV over 15 to 30 minutes or administered by IV push over 3 minutes. In emergency situations (eg, carcinoid crisis) it may be given by rapid bolus.

The initial dosage is usually 50 mcg administered 2 or 3 times daily. Upward dose titration is frequently required. Dosage information for patients with specific tumors follows.

Acromegaly – Dosage may be initiated at 50 mcg 3 times daily beginning with this low dose may permit adaptation to adverse gastrointestinal effects for patients who will require higher doses. IGF-I (somatomedin C) levels every 2 weeks can be used to guide titration. Alternatively, multiple growth hormone levels at 0 to 8 hours after octreotide acetate administration permit more rapid titration of dose. The goal is to achieve growth hormone levels less than 5 ng/mL or IGF-I (somatomedin C) levels less than 1.9 U/mL in males and less than 2.2 U/mL in females. The dose most commonly found to be effective is 100 mcg 3 times daily, but some patients require less than or equal to 500 mcg 3 times daily for maximum effectiveness. Doses greater than 300 mcg/day seldom result in additional biochemical benefit, and if an increase in dose fails to provide additional benefit, the dose should be reduced. IGF-I (somatomedin C) or growth hormone levels should be reevaluated at 6 month intervals.

Octreotide acetate should be withdrawn yearly for approximately 4 weeks from patients who have received irradiation to assess disease activity. If growth hormone or IGF-I (somatomedin C) levels increase and signs and symptoms recur, octreotide acetate therapy may be resumed.

Carcinoid tumors – The suggested daily dosage during the first 2 weeks of therapy ranges from 100 to 600 mcg/day in 2 to 4 divided doses (mean daily dosage is 300 mcg). In the clinical studies, the median daily maintenance dosage was approximately 450 mcg, but clinical and biochemical benefits were obtained in some patients with as little as 50 mcg, while others required doses less than or equal to 1500 mcg/day. However, experience with doses greater than 750 mcg/day is limited.

VIPomas – Daily dosages of 200 to 300 mcg in 2 to 4 divided doses are recommended during the initial 2 weeks of therapy (range 150 to 750 mcg) to control symptoms of the disease. On an individual basis, dosage may be adjusted to achieve a therapeutic response, but usually doses greater than 450 mcg/day are not required.

➤*Injectable suspension:* Administer under the supervision of a physician. It is important to closely follow the mixing instructions included in the packaging. Administer immediately after mixing. Octreotide acetate injectable suspension should be administered intragluteally at 4-week intervals. Administration at intervals greater than 4 weeks is not recommended because there is no adequate information on whether such patients could be satisfactorily controlled. Deltoid injections are to be avoided because of significant discomfort at the injection site when given in that area. Octreotide acetate injectable suspension should never be administered by the IV or subcutaneous routes.

Acromegaly –

Patients not currently receiving octreotide acetate injection solution: Patients not currently receiving octreotide acetate should begin therapy with octreotide acetate injection given subcutaneously in an initial dose of 50 mcg 3 times daily. Beginning with this low dose may permit adaptation to adverse gastrointestinal effects for patients who require higher doses. Multiple growth hormone (GH) determinations at 0 to 8 hours after a subcutaneous octreotide acetate injection will guide dosage titration. The goal is to attempt to normalize GH and IGF-1 (somatomedin C) levels. Most patients require doses of 100 mcg to 200 mcg 3 times daily for maximum effect but some patients require less than or equal to 500 mcg 3 times daily. Injection sites should be rotated in a systematic manner to avoid irritation.

Although responsiveness of GH to octreotide acetate can be ascertained quickly, patients should be maintained on octreotide acetate injection subcutaneous for greater than or equal to 2 weeks to determine tolerance to octreotide.

Patients who are considered to be "responders" to the drug, based on GH and IGF-1 levels, and who tolerate the drug, can then be switched to octreotide acetate injectable suspension in the dosage scheme described below.

Patients currently receiving octreotide acetate injection solution: Patients currently receiving octreotide acetate injection can be switched directly to octreotide acetate injectable suspension in a dose of 20 mg given IM intragluteally at 4 week intervals for 3 months. (Deltoid injections are to be avoided because of significant discomfort at the injection site when given in that area.) Gluteal injection sites should be alternated to avoid irritation.

At the end of 3 months octreotide acetate injectable suspension dosage may be continued at the same level or increased or decreased based on the following regimen:

- *GH less than or equal to 2.5 ng/mL, IGF-1 normal and clinical symptoms controlled* – Maintain dosage at 20 mg every 4 weeks.
- *GH greater than 2.5 ng/mL, IGF-1 elevated, and clinical symptoms uncontrolled* – Increase dosage to 30 mg every 4 weeks.
- *GH less than or equal to 1 ng/mL, IGF-1 normal and clinical symptoms controlled* – Reduce dosage to 10 mg every 4 weeks.

Patients whose GH, IGF-1, and symptoms are not adequately controlled at a dose of 30 mg may have the dose increased to 40 mg every 4 weeks. Doses greater than 40 mg are not recommended.

Administration of octreotide acetate injectable suspension at intervals greater than 4 weeks is not recommended because there is no adequate information on whether such patients could be satisfactorily controlled.

In patients who have received pituitary irradiation, octreotide acetate injectable suspension should be withdrawn yearly for approximately 8 weeks to assess disease activity. If GH or IGF-1 levels increase and signs and symptoms recur, octreotide acetate injectable suspension therapy may be resumed.

Special populations:

- *Renal failure* – In patients with renal failure requiring dialysis, the half-life of octreotide may be increased, necessitating adjustment of the maintenance dosage.

Carcinoid tumors and VIPomas – Patients not currently receiving octreotide acetate should begin therapy with octreotide acetate injection given subcutaneously. The suggested daily dosage for carcinoid tumors during the first 2 weeks of therapy ranges from 100 to 600 mcg/day in 2 to 4 divided doses (mean daily dosage is 300 mcg). Some patients may require doses less than or equal to 1500 mcg/day. The suggested daily dosage for VIPomas is 200 to 300 mcg in 2 to 4 divided doses (range 150 to 750 mcg); dosage may be adjusted on an individual basis to control symptoms but usually doses greater than 450 mcg/day are not required.

Octreocide acetate injection should be continued for greater than or equal to 2 weeks. Thereafter, patients who are considered "responders" to octreotide acetate and who tolerate the drug may be switched to octreotide acetate injectable suspension in the dosage regimen described under Patients currently receiving octreotide acetate injection.

Patients currently receiving octreotide acetate injection can be switched to octreotide acetate injectable suspension in a dosage of 20 mg given IM intragluteally at 4 week intervals for 2 months. Deltoid injections are to be avoided because of significant discomfort at the injection site when given in that area. Gluteal injection sites should be alternated to avoid irritation. Because of the need for serum octreotide to reach therapeutically effective levels following initial injection of octreotide acetate injectable suspension, carcinoid tumor, and VIPoma patients should continue to receive octreotide acetate injection subcutaneously for greater than or equal to 2 weeks in the same dosage they were taking before the switch. Failure to continue subcutaneous injections for this period may result in exacerbation of symptoms. (Some patients may require 3 or 4 weeks of such therapy.)

After 2 months of a 20 mg dosage of octreotide acetate injectable suspension, dosage may be increased to 30 mg every 4 weeks if symptoms are not adequately controlled. Patients who achieve good control on a 20 mg dose may have their dose lowered to 10 mg for a trial period. If symptoms recur,

OCTREOTIDE ACETATE — INJECTION

dosage should then be increased to 20 mg every 4 weeks. Many patients can, however, be satisfactorily maintained at a 10 mg dosage every 4 weeks. A dose of 10 mg is not recommended as a starting dose, however, because therapeutically effective levels of octreotide are reached more rapidly with a 20 mg dose.

Dosages higher than 30 mg are not recommended because there is no information on their usefulness.

Despite good overall control of symptoms, patients with carcinoid tumors and VIPomas often experience periodic exacerbation of symptoms (regardless of whether they are being maintained on octreotide acetate injection or octreotide acetate injectable suspension). During these periods they may be given octreotide acetate injection subcutaneously for a few days at the dosage they were receiving prior to switch to octreotide acetate injectable suspension. When symptoms are again controlled, the octreotide acetate injection subcutaneous can be discontinued.

Administration of octreotide acetate injectable suspension at intervals greater than 4 weeks is not recommended because there is no adequate information on whether such patients could be adequately controlled.

➤*Storage/Stability:* For prolonged storage, octreotide acetate injection ampuls and multidose vials should be stored at refrigerated temperatures 2° to 8°C (36° to 46°F) and protected from light.

Injection solution – At room temperature, (20° to 30°C; 70° to 86°F), octreotide acetate injection is stable for 14 days if protected from light. The solution can be allowed to come to room temperature prior to administration. Do not warm artificially. After initial use, multiple dose vials should be discarded within 14 days. Ampuls should be opened just prior to administration and the unused portion discarded.

Injectable suspension – Octreotide acetate injectable suspension drug product kit should remain at room temperature for 30 to 60 minutes prior to preparation of the drug suspension. However, after preparation the drug suspension must be administered immediately.

Actions

➤*Pharmacology:* Octreotide acetate exerts pharmacologic actions similar to the natural hormone somatostatin. It is an even more potent inhibitor of growth hormone, glucagon, and insulin than somatostatin. Like somatostatin, it also suppresses LH response to GnRH, decreases splanchnic blood flow, and inhibits release of serotonin, gastrin, vasoactive intestinal peptide, secretin, motilin, and pancreatic polypeptide.

By virtue of these pharmacological actions, octreotide acetate has been used to treat the symptoms associated with metastatic carcinoid tumors (flushing and diarrhea), and vasoactive intestinal peptide (VIP) secreting adenomas (watery diarrhea).

Octreotide acetate substantially reduces growth hormone or IGF-I (somatomedin C) levels in patients with acromegaly.

Single doses of octreotide acetate have been shown to inhibit gallbladder contractility and to decrease bile secretion in healthy volunteers. In controlled clinical trials the incidence of gallstone or biliary sludge formation was markedly increased.

Octreotide acetate suppresses secretion of thyroid-stimulating hormone (TSH).

➤*Pharmacokinetics:*

Absorption – After subcutaneous injection, octreotide is absorbed rapidly and completely from the injection site. Peak concentrations of 5.2 ng/mL (100 mcg dose) were reached 0.4 hours after dosing. Using a specific radioimmunoassay, IV and subcutaneous doses were found to be bioequivalent. Peak concentrations and AUC values were dose proportional after intravenous single doses up to 200 mcg and subcutaneous single doses up to 500 mcg and after subcutaneous multiple doses up to 500 mcg 3 times daily (1,500 mcg/day).

Distribution – In healthy volunteers the distribution of octreotide from plasma was rapid ($t\alpha½$ = 0.2 h), the volume of distribution (V_{dss}) was estimated to be 13.6 L, and the total body clearance ranged from 7 L/h to 10 L/h.

In blood, the distribution into the erythrocytes was found to be negligible and approximately 65% was bound in the plasma in a concentration-independent manner. Binding was mainly to lipoprotein and, to a lesser extent, to albumin.

Metabolism/Excretion – The elimination of octreotide from plasma had an apparent half-life of 1.7 to 1.9 hours compared with 1 to 3 minutes with the natural hormone. The duration of action of octreotide acetate is variable but extends up to 12 hours depending upon the type of tumor. About 32% of the dose is excreted unchanged into the urine. In an elderly population, dose adjustments may be necessary due to a significant increase in the half-life (46%) and a significant decrease in the clearance (26%) of the drug.

Special populations –

Renal function impairment: In patients with renal impairment the elimination of octreotide from plasma was prolonged and total body clearance reduced. In mild renal impairment (Ccr 40 to 60 mL/min) octreotide $t_{½}$ was 2.4 hours and total body clearance was 8.8 L/h, in moderate impairment (Ccr 10 to 39 mL/min) $t_{½}$ was 3 hours and total body clearance 7.3 L/h, and in severely renally impaired patients not requiring dialysis (Ccr less than 10 mL/min) $t_{½}$ was 3.1 hours and total body clearance was 7.6 L/h.

In patients with severe renal failure requiring dialysis, total body clearance was reduced to about half that found in healthy subjects (from approximately 10 L/h to 4.5 L/h).

Liver function impairment: Patients with liver cirrhosis showed prolonged elimination of drug, with octreotide $t_{½}$ increasing to 3.7 hours and total body clearance decreasing to 5.9 L/h, whereas patients with fatty liver disease showed $t_{½}$ increased to 3.4 hours and total body clearance of 8.2 L/h.

Injectable suspension – After a single IM injection of long-acting depot dosage form octreotide acetate injectable suspension in healthy volunteer subjects, the serum octreotide concentration reached a transient initial peak of approximately 0.03 ng/mL/mg within 1 hour after administration progressively declining over the following 3 to 5 days to a nadir of less than 0.01 ng/mL/mg, then slowly increasing and reaching a plateau about 2 to 3 weeks, post injection. Plateau concentrations were maintained over a period of nearly 2 to 3 weeks, showing dose proportional peak concentrations of approximately 0.07 ng/mL/mg. After approximately 6 weeks post injection, octreotide concentration slowly decreased, to less than 0.01 ng/mL/mg by weeks 12 to 13, concomitant with the terminal degradation phase of the polymer matrix of the dosage form. The relative bioavailability of the long-acting release octreotide acetate injectable suspension compared to immediate-release octreotide acetate injection solution given subcutaneously was 60% to 63%.

In patients with acromegaly, the octreotide concentrations after single doses of 10 mg, 20 mg, and 30 mg octreotide acetate injectable suspension were dose proportional. The transient day 1 peak, amounting to 0.3 ng/mL, 0.8 ng/mL, and 1.3 ng/mL, respectively, was followed by plateau concentrations of 0.5 ng/mL, 1.3 ng/mL, and 2 ng/mL, respectively, achieved approximately 3 weeks post injection. These plateau concentrations were maintained for nearly 2 weeks.

Following multiple doses of octreotide acetate injectable suspension given every 4 weeks, steady-state octreotide serum concentrations were achieved after the third injection. Concentrations were dose proportional and higher by a factor of approximately 1.6 to 2 compared to the concentrations after a single dose. The steady-state concentrations were 1.2 ng/mL and 2.1 ng/mL, respectively, at trough and 1.6 ng/mL and 2.6 ng/mL, respectively, at peak with 20 mg and 30 mg octreotide acetate injectable suspension given every 4 weeks. No accumulation of octreotide beyond that expected from the overlapping release profiles occurred over a duration of up to 28 monthly injections of octreotide acetate injectable suspension.

With the long-acting depot formulation octreotide acetate injectable suspension administered IM every 4 weeks, the peak-to-trough variation in octreotide concentrations ranged from 44% to 68%, compared to the 163% to 209% variation encountered with the daily subcutaneous 3 times daily regimen of octreotide acetate injection solution.

In patients with carcinoid tumors, the mean octreotide concentrations after 6 doses of 10 mg, 20 mg, and 30 mg octreotide acetate injectable suspension administered by IM injection every 4 weeks were 1.2 ng/mL, 2.5 ng/mL, and 4.2 ng/mL, respectively. Concentrations were dose proportional and steady-state concentrations were reached after 2 injections of 20 and 30 mg and after 3 injections of 10 mg. In patients with acromegaly, the pharmacokinetics differ somewhat from those in healthy volunteers. A mean peak concentration of 2.8 ng/mL (100 mcg dose) was reached in 0.7 hours after subcutaneous dosing. The volume of distribution (V_{dss}) was estimated to be 21.6 ± 8.5 L and the total body clearance was increased to 18 L/h. The mean percent of the drug bound was 41.2%. The disposition and elimination half-lives were similar to healthy patients.

Contraindications

Sensitivity to this drug or any of its components.

Warnings

➤*Gallbladder and related events:*

Injection solution – Single doses have been shown to inhibit gallbladder contractility and decrease bile secretion in healthy volunteers. In clinical trials with octreotide acetate injection (primarily patients with acromegaly or psoriasis) in patients who had not previously received octreotide, the incidence of biliary tract abnormalities was 63% (27% gallstones, 24% sludge without stones, 12% biliary duct dilatation). The incidence of stones or sludge in patients who received octreotide acetate injection for greater than or equal to 12 months was 52%. The incidence of gallbladder abnormalities did not appear to be related to age, sex, or dose, but was related to duration of exposure. A few patients developed acute cholecystitis, ascending cholangitis, biliary obstruction, cholestatic hepatitis, or pancreatitis during octreotide acetate therapy or following its withdrawal. One patient developed ascending cholangitis during octreotide acetate therapy and died.

Less than 2% of patients treated with octreotide acetate for less than 1 month developed gallstones. Like patients without gallbladder abnormalities, the majority of patients developing gallbladder abnormalities on ultrasound had gastrointestinal symptoms. The symptoms were not specific for gallbladder disease.

Injectable suspension – In clinical trials, 52% of acromegalic patients, most of whom received octreotide acetate injectable suspension for 12 months or longer, developed new biliary abnormalities including gallstones, microlithiasis, sediment, sludge, and dilatation. The incidence of new cholelithiasis was 22%, of which 7% were microstones.

In clinical trials, 62% of malignant carcinoid patients who received octreotide acetate injectable suspension for less than or equal to 18 months developed new biliary abnormalities including gallstones, sludge, and dilatation. New gallstones occurred in a total of 24% of patients. Across all trials, a few patients developed acute cholecystitis, ascending cholangitis, biliary obstruction, cholestatic hepatitis, or pancreatitis during octreotide therapy or following its withdrawal. One patient developed ascending cholangitis during octreotide acetate injection therapy and died. Despite the high incidence of new gallstones in patients receiving octreotide, 1% of patients developed acute symptoms requiring cholecystectomy.

➤*Renal function impairment:*

Injection solution – In patients with renal failure requiring dialysis, the half-life of octreotide may be increased, necessitating adjustment of the maintenance dosage.

OCTREOTIDE ACETATE — INJECTION

➤*Carcinogenesis:* In a 116-week subcutaneous study in rats, a 27% and 12% incidence of injection site sarcomas or squamous cell carcinomas was observed in males and females, respectively, at the highest dose level of 1,250 mcg/kg/day (10 times the human exposure based on body surface area) compared to an incidence of 8% to 10% in the vehicle control groups. The increased incidence of injection site tumors was most probably caused by irritation and the high sensitivity of the rat to repeated subcutaneous injections at the same site. Rotating injection sites would prevent chronic irritation in humans. There have been no reports of injection site tumors in patients treated with octreotide acetate for less than or equal to 5 years. There was also a 15% incidence of uterine adenocarcinomas in the 1,250 mcg/kg/day females compared to 7% in the saline control females and 0% in the vehicle control females. The presence of endometritis coupled with the absence of corpora lutea, the reduction in mammary fibroadenomas, and the presence of uterine dilatation suggest that the uterine tumors were associated with estrogen dominance in the aged female rats, which does not occur in humans.

➤*Pregnancy: Category B.* There are no adequate and well-controlled studies in pregnant women. Because animal reproduction studies are not always predictive of human response, this drug should be used during pregnancy only if clearly needed.

➤*Lactation:* It is not known whether this drug is excreted in human milk. Because many drugs are excreted in milk, caution should be exercised when octreotide acetate is administered to a nursing woman.

➤*Children:* Experience with octreotide acetate in children is limited. Although formal controlled clinical trials have not been performed to evaluate safety and effectiveness in this age group, there are reports of 49 cases in the literature of neonates and infants with congenital hyperinsulinism (also called familial hyperinsulinism [HI], persistent hyperinsulinemic hypoglycemia of infancy [PHHI], or nesidioblastosis) who have received octreotide acetate as an inhibitor of insulin release. The following efficacy and safety information is derived from these 49 patients.

Octreotide acetate has been used to stabilize plasma glucose levels prior to pancreatectomy and to treat recurrent postoperative hypoglycemia. Although most use of octreotide in this setting is short-term, a few reports in the literature have documented longer-term therapy in pediatric patients (2.2 to 5.5 years). Octreotide is an alternative medical treatment to diazoxide for control of hypoglycemia in this disorder. Of 31 pediatric patients who received octreotide acetate as prescribed for congenital hyperinsulinism and for which long-term follow-up was available, octreotide obviated the need for surgery in 3 patients (10%) and was replaced by diazoxide in 4 patients (13%) due to uncontrolled hypoglycemia. Although the remainder of these patients required surgery, there have been a few reports in the literature of patients who have responded to octreotide after failing treatment with surgery or diazoxide. Doses of 3 to 40 mcg/kg/day have been used. At these doses, the majority of side effects were gastrointestinal: Diarrhea, steatorrhea, vomiting, and abdominal distention, each reported in 22% to 35% (n = 11 to 17) of patients. However, they were generally short-lived, with resolution of vomiting and distention in 2 to 4 days, and diarrhea/steatorrhea, within 2 to 4 weeks. Steatorrhea was controlled in most patients with pancreatic enzyme supplements. Poor growth was reported in 37% of patients (n = 7) who received octreotide acetate for 1 to 4.33 years. It was associated with low serum growth hormone or IGF-1 levels in 4 out of 6 patients in whom these parameters were measured. Catch-up growth occurred in 3 out of 3 patients who were followed after octreotide acetate was discontinued. Poor weight gain was reported in 32% of patients (n = 6). Tachyphylaxis was reported in 35% (n = 17) of patients. Asymptomatic gallstones with sludge was reported in 1 infant after 1 year of therapy and was treated with ursodeoxycholic acid. There has been a single report of an infant with nesidioblastosis who experienced a seizure thought to be independent of octreotide acetate therapy. A single death has been reported in a 16-month-old male with enterocutaneous fistula who developed sudden abdominal pain and increased nasogastric drainage and expired 8 hours after receiving a single 100 mcg subcutaneous dose of octreotide acetate.

Precautions

➤*Monitoring:* Growth hormone secreting tumors may sometimes expand and cause serious complications (eg, visual field defects). Therefore, all patients with these tumors should be carefully monitored.

Depressed vitamin B_{12} levels and abnormal Schilling's tests have been observed in some patients receiving octreotide therapy, and monitoring of vitamin B_{12} levels is recommended during chronic octreotide acetate therapy.

In acromegalic patients, 12% developed biochemical hypothyroidism only, 8% developed goiter, and 4% required initiation of thyroid replacement therapy while receiving octreotide acetate. Baseline and periodic assessment of thyroid function (TSH, total or free T_4) is recommended during chronic therapy.

Octreotide has been investigated for the reduction of excessive fluid loss from the GI tract in patients with conditions producing such a loss. If such patients are receiving TPN, serum zinc may rise excessively when the fluid loss is reversed. Patients on TPN and octreotide should have periodic monitoring of zinc levels.

Octreotide acetate alters the balance between the counter-regulatory hormones, insulin, glucagon, and growth hormone, which may result in hypoglycemia or hyperglycemia. Octreotide acetate also suppresses secretion of thyroid-stimulating hormone, which may result in hypothyroidism. Cardiac conduction abnormalities have also occurred during treatment with octreotide acetate. However, the incidence of these adverse events during long-term therapy was determined vigorously only in acromegaly patients who, due to their underlying disease or the subsequent treatment they receive, are at an increased risk for the development of diabetes mellitus, hypothyroidism, and cardiovascular disease. Although the degree to which these abnormalities are related to octreotide acetate therapy is not clear, new abnormalities of glycemic control, thyroid function and ECG developed during octreotide acetate therapy as described below.

Laboratory tests that may be helpful as biochemical markers in determining and following patient response depend on the specific tumor. Based on diagnosis, measurement of the following substances may be useful in monitoring the progress of therapy:

➤*Acromegaly:* Growth hormone, IGF-I (somatomedin C). Responsiveness to octreotide acetate may be evaluated by determining growth hormone levels at 1 to 4 hour intervals for 8 to 12 hours post dose. Alternatively, a single measurement of IGF-I (somatomedin C) level may be made 2 weeks after drug initiation or dosage change.

For patients switched from octreotide acetate injection to octreotide acetate injectable suspension, GH and IGF-1 determinations may be made after 3 monthly injections of octreotide acetate injectable suspension. (Steady-state serum levels of octreotide are reached only after a period of 3 months of monthly injections.) Growth hormone can be determined using the mean of 4 assays taken at 1 hour intervals. Somatomedin C can be determined with a single assay. All GH and IGF-1 determinations should be made 4 weeks after the previous octreotide acetate injectable suspension.

➤*Carcinoid:* 5-HIAA (urinary 5-hydroxyindole acetic acid), plasma serotonin, plasma Substance P.

➤*VIPoma:* VIP (plasma vasoactive intestinal peptide).

Baseline and periodic total or free T_4 measurements should be performed during chronic therapy.

➤*Hypoglycemia or hyperglycemia:* See Adverse Reactions for more information.

The hypoglycemia or hyperglycemia that occurs during octreotide acetate therapy is usually mild, but may result in overt diabetes mellitus or necessitate dose changes in insulin or other hypoglycemic agents. Severe hyperglycemia, subsequent pneumonia, and death following initiation of octreotide acetate therapy was reported in 1 patient with no history of hyperglycemia.

➤*Cardiac effects:* See Adverse Reactions for more information.

In both acromegalic and carcinoid syndrome patients, bradycardia, arrhythmias and conduction abnormalities have been reported during octreotide therapy. Other EKG changes were observed such as QT prolongation, axis shifts, early repolarization, low voltage, R/S transition, early R wave progression, and nonspecific ST-T wave changes. The relationship of these events to octreotide acetate is not established because many of these patients have underlying cardiac disease. Dose adjustments in drugs such as beta blockers that have bradycardia effects may be necessary. In 1 acromegalic patient with severe congestive heart failure, initiation of octreotide acetate injection therapy resulted in worsening of CHF with improvement when drug was discontinued. Confirmation of a drug effect was obtained with a positive rechallenge.

➤*Pancreatitis:* Several cases of pancreatitis have been reported in patients receiving octreotide acetate therapy.

➤*Renal function impairment:* In patients with severe renal failure requiring dialysis, the half-life of octreotide acetate may be increased, necessitating adjustment of the maintenance dosage.

Drug Interactions

Octreotide acetate has been associated with alterations in nutrient absorption, so it may have an effect on absorption of orally administered drugs. Concomitant administration of octreotide acetate with cyclosporine may decrease blood levels of cyclosporine and result in transplant rejection.

Patients receiving insulin, oral hypoglycemic agents, beta blockers, calcium channel blockers, or agents to control fluid and electrolyte balance, may require dose adjustments of these therapeutic agents.

➤*Drug/Food interactions:* Octreotide acetate may alter absorption of dietary fats in some patients.

Adverse Reactions

➤*Cardiovascular:* In acromegalics, sinus bradycardia (less than 50 bpm) developed in 25%; conduction abnormalities occurred in 10% and arrhythmias developed in 9% of patients during octreotide acetate therapy.

Electrocardiograms were performed only in carcinoid patients receiving octreotide acetate injectable suspension. In carcinoid syndrome patients sinus bradycardia developed in 19%; conduction abnormalities occurred in 9%, and arrhythmias developed in 3%. The relationship of these reactions to octreotide acetate is not established because many of these patients have underlying cardiac disease.

➤*Endocrine:* Hypoglycemia and hyperglycemia occurred in 3% and 16% of acromegalic patients, respectively, but only in approximately 1.5% of other patients. Symptoms of hypoglycemia were noted in approximately 2% of patients.

In acromegalics, biochemical hypothyroidism alone occurred in 12% while goiter occurred in 6% during octreotide acetate therapy. In patients without acromegaly, hypothyroidism has only been reported in several isolated patients and goiter has not been reported.

➤*GI:* The most common symptoms are gastrointestinal. The overall incidence of the most frequent of these symptoms in clinical trials of acromegalic patients treated for approximately 1 to 4 years is shown in the table below.

OCTREOTIDE ACETATE — INJECTION

Number (%) of Acromegalic Patients with Common GI Adverse Reactions				
	Octreotide acetate injection solution 3 times daily (n = 114)		Octreotide acetate injectable suspension every 28 days (n = 261)	
Adverse reaction	n	%	n	%
Diarrhea	66	(57.9%)	95	(36.4%)
Abdominal pain or discomfort	50	(43.9%)	76	(29.1%)
Flatulence	15	(13.2%)	67	(25.7%)
Constipation	10	(8.8%)	49	(18.8%)
Nausea	34	(29.8%)	27	(10.3%)
Vomiting	5	(4.4%)	17	(6.5%)

Only 2.6% of the patients on octreotide acetate injection in US clinical trials discontinued therapy due to these symptoms. No acromegalic patient receiving octreotide acetate injectable suspension discontinued therapy for a GI reaction.

In patients receiving octreotide acetate injectable suspension the incidence of diarrhea was dose-related. Diarrhea, abdominal pain, and nausea developed primarily during the first month of treatment with octreotide acetate injectable suspension Thereafter, new cases of these reactions were uncommon. The vast majority of these reactions were mild-to-moderate in severity.

In rare instances gastrointestinal adverse effects may resemble acute intestinal obstruction, with progressive abdominal distention, severe epigastric pain, abdominal tenderness, and guarding.

Dyspepsia, steatorrhea, discoloration of feces, and tenesmus were reported in 4% to 6% of patients.

In a clinical trial of carcinoid syndrome, nausea, abdominal pain, and flatulence were reported in 27% to 38% and constipation or vomiting in 15% to 21% of patients treated with octreotide acetate injectable suspension. Diarrhea was reported as an adverse reaction in 14% of patients but since most of the patients had diarrhea as a symptom of carcinoid syndrome, it is difficult to assess the actual incidence of drug-related diarrhea.

➤*Miscellaneous:* Gallbladder abnormalities, especially stones or biliary sludge, frequently develop in patients on chronic octreotide acetate therapy. Few patients, however, develop acute symptoms requiring cholecystectomy.

Other adverse reactions –
Injection solution: Pain on injection was reported in 7.7%, headache in 6%, and dizziness in 5%. Pancreatitis was also observed.

➤*Injectable suspension:* Gallbladder abnormalities, especially stones or biliary sludge, frequently develop in patients on chronic octreotide therapy. Few patients, however, develop acute symptoms requiring cholecystectomy.

Local – Pain on injection, which is generally mild-to-moderate, and short-lived (usually approximately 1 hour) is dose-related, being reported by 2%, 9%, and 11% of acromegalics receiving doses of 10 mg, 20 mg, and 30 mg, respectively, of octreotide acetate injectable suspension. In carcinoid patients, where a diary was kept, pain at the injection site was reported by approximately 20% to 25% at a 10 mg dose and approximately 30% to 50% at the 20 mg and 30 mg dose.

Other adverse reactions 16% to 20% – Other adverse reactions (relationship to drug not established) in acromegalic or carcinoid syndrome patients receiving octreotide acetate injectable suspension were upper respiratory infection, flu-like symptoms, fatigue, dizziness, headache, malaise, fever, dyspnea, back pain, chest pain, and arthropathy.

➤*Other adverse reactions 5% to 15%:* Other adverse reactions (relationship to drug not established) occurring in an incidence of 5% to 15% in patients receiving octreotide acetate injectable suspension were:

Cardiovascular – Hypertension, peripheral edema, palpitations.

CNS – Paresthesia, hypoesthesia.

Dermatologic – Rash, pruritus, increased sweating.

GI – Dyspepsia, anorexia, hemorrhoids.

GU – Urinary tract infection, renal calculus.

Hematologic – Anemia.

Metabolic/Nutritional – Dehydration, weight decrease.

Musculoskeletal – Myalgia, leg cramps, arthralgia.

Psychiatric – Depression, anxiety, confusion, insomnia.

Respiratory – Coughing, pharyngitis, rhinitis, sinusitis.

Miscellaneous – Asthenia, rigors, earache, allergy, viral infection, otitis media.

➤*Other adverse reactions 1% to 4% :* Other reactions (relationship to drug not established), each observed in 1% to 4% of patients receiving octreotide acetate injection solution, included fatigue, weakness, pruritus, joint pain, backache, urinary tract infection, cold symptoms, flu symptoms, injection site hematoma, bruise, edema, flushing, blurred vision, pollakiuria, fat malabsorption, hair loss, visual disturbance, and depression.

Other reactions (relationship to drug not established), each occurring in an incidence of 1% to 4% in patients receiving octreotide acetate injectable suspension and reported by greater than or equal to 2 patients were:

Cardiovascular – Cardiac failure, angina pectoris, hypertension aggravated, tachycardia, cerebral vascular disorder, phlebitis, hematoma.

CNS – Vertigo, abnormal gait, neuropathy, neuralgia, tremor, dysphonia, hyperkinesia, hypertonia.

Dermatologic – Alopecia, urticaria, acne.

GI – Rectal bleeding, melena, gastritis, gastroenteritis, colitis, gingivitis, taste perversion, stomatitis, glossitis, dry mouth, dysphagia, steatorrhea, diverticulitis.

GU – Incontinence, albuminuria, menstrual irregularities and breast pain in females, impotence in males.

Hepatic – Jaundice.

Metabolic/Nutritional – Hypokalemia, cachexia, gout, hypoproteinemia.

Ophthalmic – Abnormal vision.

Psychiatric – Amnesia, somnolence, nervousness, hallucinations.

Pulmonary – Pulmonary embolism, epistaxis.

Respiratory – Bronchitis, pneumonia, pleural effusion.

Miscellaneous – Injection site inflammation, syncope, ascites, hot flushes, tinnitus, cellulitis, renal abscess, moniliasis, bacterial infection.

➤*Rare adverse reactions:* Other reactions (relationship to drug not established) of potential clinical significance occurring rarely (less than 1%) in clinical trials of octreotide either as octreotide acetate injection or octreotide acetate injectable suspension, or reported postmarketing in patients with acromegaly, carcinoid syndrome, or other disorders include:

Cardiovascular – Aneurysm, myocardial infarction, angina pectoris, aggravated, pulmonary hypertension, cardiac arrest, orthostatic hypotension, atrial fibrillation, arterial thrombosis of the arm.

CNS – Hemiparesis, paresis, convulsions, paranoia, pituitary apoplexy, visual field defect, migraine, aphasia, scotoma, Bell palsy.

Dermatologic – Cellulitis, petechiae, urticaria.

Endocrine – Hypoadrenalism, diabetes insipidus, gynecomastia, galactorrhea.

GI – GI hemorrhage, intestinal obstruction, hepatitis, increase in liver enzymes, fatty liver, peptic/gastric ulcer, gallbladder polyp, appendicitis, pancreatitis.

GU – Lactation and nonpuerperal in females, renal failure, hematuria.

Hematologic – Pancytopenia, thrombocytopenia.

Metabolic/Nutritional – Renal insufficiency, creatinine increased, CK increased, diabetes mellitus.

Musculoskeletal – Raynaud syndrome, arthritis, joint effusion.

Ophthalmic – Glaucoma.

Psychiatric – Suicide attempt, libido decrease.

Respiratory – Pulmonary nodule, status asthmaticus, pneumothorax.

Miscellaneous – Anaphylactoid reactions, including anaphylactic shock, facial edema, generalized edema, abdomen enlarged, malignant hyperpyrexia, deafness, breast carcinoma, basal cell carcinoma, intracranial hemorrhage, retinal vein thrombosis.

➤*Antibodies to octreotide:* Studies to date have shown that antibodies to octreotide develop in less than or equal to 25% of patients treated with octreotide acetate. These antibodies do not influence the degree of efficacy response to octreotide; however, in 2 acromegalic patients who received octreotide acetate injection, the duration of GH suppression following each injection was about twice as long as in patients without antibodies. It has not been determined whether octreotide antibodies will also prolong the duration of GH suppression in patients being treated with octreotide acetate injectable suspension.

Patient Information

Careful instruction in sterile subcutaneous injection technique should be given to the patients and to other persons who may administer octreotide acetate.

➤*Injectable suspension:* Patients with carcinoid tumors and VIPomas should be advised to adhere closely to their scheduled return visits for reinjection in order to minimize exacerbation of symptoms.

Patients with acromegaly should also be urged to adhere to their return visit schedule to help assure steady control of GH and IGF-1 levels.

PEGVISOMANT

Rx	**Somavert** (Pharmacia)	**Powder for injection, lyophilized:** 10 mg (as protein)/vial	In single-dose, sterile glass vial.[a]
		15 mg (as protein)/vial	In single-dose, sterile glass vial.[a]
		20 mg (as protein)/vial	In single-dose, sterile glass vial.[a]

[a] With sterile water for injection and mannitol 36 mg.

PEGVISOMANT — INJECTION

Indications

➤*Acromegaly:* For the treatment of acromegaly in patients who have had an inadequate response to surgery and/or radiation therapy and/or other medical therapies, or for whom these therapies are not appropriate. The goal of treatment is to normalize serum insulin-like growth factor-I (IGF-I) levels.

Administration and Dosage

➤*Approved by the FDA:* March 25, 2003.

➤*Dosage:* A loading dose of 40 mg should be administered subcutaneously under physician supervision. The patient should then be instructed to begin daily subcutaneous injections of 10 mg. Serum IGF-I concentrations should be measured every 4 to 6 weeks, at which time the dosage should be adjusted in 5 mg increments if IGF-I levels are still elevated (or 5 mg decrements if IGF-I levels have decreased below the normal range). While the goals of therapy are to achieve (and then maintain) serum IGF-I concentrations within the age-adjusted normal range and to alleviate the signs and symptoms of acromegaly, titration of dosing should be based on IGF-I levels. It is unknown whether patients who remain symptomatic while achieving normalized IGF-I levels would benefit from increased dosing with pegvisomant.

The maximum daily maintenance dose should not exceed 30 mg.

➤*Reconstitution/Administration:* Pegvisomant is supplied as a lyophilized powder. Each vial of pegvisomant should be reconstituted with 1 mL of the diluent provided in the package (Sterile Water for Injection). Instructions regarding reconstitution and administration are included in the package of pegvisomant and should be closely followed. To prepare the solution, withdraw 1 mL of Sterile Water for Injection and inject it into the vial of pegvisomant, aiming the stream of liquid against the glass wall. Hold the vial between the palms of both hands and gently roll it to dissolve the powder. Do not shake the vial, as this may cause denaturation of pegvisomant. Discard the diluent vial containing the remaining water for injection. After reconstitution, each vial of pegvisomant contains 10, 15, or 20 mg of pegvisomant protein in 1 mL of solution. Parenteral drug products should be inspected visually for particulate matter and discoloration prior to administration. The solution should be clear after reconstitution. If the solution is cloudy, do not inject it. Only 1 dose should be administered from each vial. Pegvisomant should be administered within 6 hours after reconstitution.

➤*Storage/Stability:* Prior to reconstitution, pegvisomant should be stored in a refrigerator at 2° to 8°C (36° to 46°F). Protect from freezing.

After reconstitution, pegvisomant should be administered within 6 hours. Only 1 dose should be administered from each vial.

Actions

➤*Pharmacology:* Pegvisomant selectively binds to growth hormone (GH) receptors on cell surfaces, where it blocks the binding of endogenous GH, and thus interferes with GH signal transduction. Inhibition of GH action results in decreased serum concentrations of insulin-like growth factor-I (IGF-I), as well as other GH-responsive serum proteins, including IGF binding protein-3 (IGFBP-3), and the acid-labile subunit (ALS).

➤*Pharmacokinetics:*

Absorption – Following subcutaneous administration, peak serum pegvisomant concentrations are not generally attained until 33 to 77 hours after administration. The mean extent of absorption of a 20 mg subcutaneous dose was 57%, relative to a 10 mg intravenous dose.

Distribution – The mean apparent volume of distribution of pegvisomant is 7 L (12% coefficient of variation), suggesting that pegvisomant does not distribute extensively into tissues. After a single subcutaneous administration, exposure (C_{max}, AUC) to pegvisomant increases disproportionately with increasing dose. Mean ± SEM serum pegvisomant concentrations after 12 weeks of therapy with daily doses of 10, 15, and 20 mg were 6,600 ± 1330; 16,000 ± 2,200; and 27,000 ± 3,100 ng/mL, respectively.

Metabolism/Excretion – The pegvisomant molecule contains covalently bound polyethylene glycol polymers in order to reduce the clearance rate. Clearance of pegvisomant following multiple doses is lower than seen following a single dose. The mean total body systemic clearance of pegvisomant following multiple doses is estimated to range between 36 to 28 mL/h for subcutaneous doses ranging from 10 to 20 mg/day, respectively. Clearance of pegvisomant was found to increase with body weight. Pegvisomant is eliminated from serum with a mean half-life of approximately 6 days following either single or multiple doses. Less than 1% of administered drug is recovered in the urine over 96 hours. The elimination route of pegvisomant has not been studied in humans.

Contraindications

Hypersensitivity to pegvisomant or any of its components. The stopper on the vial of pegvisomant contains latex.

Warnings

➤*Elderly:* Clinical studies of pegvisomant did not include sufficient numbers of subjects 65 years of age and older to determine whether they respond differently from younger subjects. In general, dose selection for an elderly patient should be cautious, usually starting at the low end of the dosing range, reflecting the greater frequency of decreased hepatic, renal, or cardiac function, and of concomitant disease or other drug therapy.

➤*Pregnancy: Category B.* At the 10 mg/kg/day dose (10 times the maximum human therapeutic dose based on body surface area), a reproducible, slight increase in post-implantation loss was observed in both studies. There are no adequate and well-controlled studies in pregnant women. Because animal reproduction studies are not always predictive of human responses, pegvisomant should be used during pregnancy only if clearly needed.

➤*Lactation:* It is not known whether pegvisomant is excreted in human milk. Because many drugs are excreted in milk, caution should be exercised when pegvisomant is administered to a breast-feeding woman.

➤*Children:* The safety and efficacy of pegvisomant in children have not been established.

Precautions

➤*Monitoring:*

Liver tests (LTs) – Elevations of serum concentrations of alanine aminotransferase (ALT) and aspartate aminotransferase (AST) greater than 10 times the upper limit of normal (ULN) were reported in 2 patients (0.8%) exposed to pegvisomant during premarketing clinical studies. One patient was rechallenged with pegvisomant, and the recurrence of elevated transaminase levels suggested a probable causal relationship between administration of the drug and the elevation in liver enzymes. A liver biopsy performed on the second patient was consistent with chronic hepatitis of unknown etiology. In both patients, the transaminase elevations normalized after discontinuation of the drug.

During the premarketing clinical studies, the incidence of elevations in ALT greater than 3 times but less than or equal to 10 times the ULN in patients treated with pegvisomant and placebo were 1.2% and 2.1%, respectively.

Elevations in ALT and AST levels were not associated with increased levels of serum total bilirubin (TBIL) and alkaline phosphatase (ALP), with the exception of 2 patients with minimal associated increases in ALP levels (ie, less than 3 times ULN). The transaminase elevations did not appear to be related to the dose of pegvisomant administered, generally occurred within 4 to 12 weeks of initiation of therapy, and were not associated with any identifiable biochemical, phenotypic, or genetic predictors.

Baseline serum ALT, AST, TBIL, and ALP levels should be obtained prior to initiating therapy with pegvisomant. The table below lists recommendations regarding initiation of treatment with pegvisomant, based on the results of these liver tests (LTs).

Initiation of Treatment with Pegvisomant Based on Results of Liver Tests

Baseline LT levels	Recommendations
Normal	May treat with pegvisomant. Monitor LTs at monthly intervals during the first 6 months of treatment, quarterly for the next 6 months, and then biannually for the next year.
Elevated, but less than or equal to 3 times ULN	May treat with pegvisomant; however, monitor LTs monthly for at least 1 year after initiation of therapy and then biannually for the next year.
Greater than 3 times ULN	Do not treat with pegvisomant until a comprehensive workup establishes the cause of the patient's liver dysfunction. Determine if cholelithiasis or choledocholithiasis is present, particularly in patients with a history of prior therapy with somatostatin analogs. Based on the workup, consider initiation of therapy with pegvisomant. If the decision is to treat, LTs and clinical symptoms should be monitored very closely.

If a patient develops LT elevations, or any other signs or symptoms of liver dysfunction while receiving pegvisomant, the following patient management is recommended (see table below).

PEGVISOMANT — INJECTION

Continuation of Treatment with Pegvisomant Based on Results of Liver Tests	
LT levels and clinical signs/symptoms	Recommendations
Greater than or equal to 3 but less than 5 times ULN (without signs/symptoms of hepatitis or other liver injury, or increase in serum TBIL)	May continue therapy with pegvisomant. However, monitor LTs weekly to determine if further increases occur (see below). In addition, perform a comprehensive hepatic workup to discern if an alternative cause of liver dysfunction is present.
At least 5 times ULN, or transaminase elevations at least 3 times ULN associated with any increase in serum TBIL (with or without signs/symptoms of hepatitis or other liver injury)	Discontinue pegvisomant immediately. Perform a comprehensive hepatic workup, including serial LTs, to determine if and when serum levels return to normal. If LTsvnormalize (regardless of whether an alternative cause of the liver dysfunction is discovered), consider cautious reinitiation of therapy with pegvisomant, with frequent LT monitoring.
Signs or symptoms suggestive of hepatitis or other liver injury (eg, jaundice, bilirubinuria, fatigue, nausea, vomiting, right upper quadrant pain, ascites, unexplained edema, easy bruisability)	Immediately perform a comprehensive hepatic workup. If liver injury is confirmed, the drug should be discontinued.

➤*Tumor growth:* Tumors that secrete growth hormone (GH) may expand and cause serious complications. Therefore, all patients with these tumors, including those who are receiving pegvisomant, should be carefully monitored with periodic imaging scans of the sella turcica. During clinical studies of pegvisomant, 2 patients manifested progressive tumor growth. Both patients had, at baseline, large globular tumors impinging on the optic chiasm, which had been relatively resistant to previous antiacromegalic therapies. Overall, mean tumor size was unchanged during the course of treatment with pegvisomant in the clinical studies.

➤*Glucose metabolism:* GH opposes the effects of insulin on carbohydrate metabolism by decreasing insulin sensitivity; thus, glucose tolerance may increase in some patients treated with pegvisomant. Although none of the acromegalic patients with diabetes mellitus who were treated with pegvisomant during the clinical studies had clinically relevant hypoglycemia, these patients should be carefully monitored and doses of antidiabetic drugs reduced as necessary.

➤*GH deficiency:* A state of functional GH deficiency may result from administration of pegvisomant, despite the presence of elevated serum GH levels. Therefore, during treatment with pegvisomant, patients should be carefully observed for the clinical signs and symptoms of a GH-deficient state, and serum IGF-I concentrations should be monitored and maintained within the age-adjusted normal range (by adjustment of the dose of pegvisomant).

➤*Lab test abnormalities:*

Liver tests – Recommendations for monitoring LTs are stated above.

IGF-I levels – Treatment with pegvisomant should be evaluated by monitoring serum IGF-I concentrations 4 to 6 weeks after therapy is initiated or any dose adjustments are made and at least every 6 months after IGF-I levels have normalized. The goals of treatment should be to maintain a patient's serum IGF-I concentration within the age-adjusted normal range and to control the signs and symptoms of acromegaly.

GH levels – Pegvisomant interferes with the measurement of serum GH concentrations by commercially available GH assays. Furthermore, even when accurately determined, GH levels usually increase during therapy with pegvisomant. Therefore, treatment with pegvisomant should not be adjusted based on serum GH concentrations.

Drug Interactions

➤*Insulin/Oral hypoglycemic agents:* Acromegalic patients with diabetes mellitus being treated with insulin or oral hypoglycemic agents may require dose reductions of these therapeutic agents after the initiation of therapy with pegvisomant.

➤*Opioids:* In clinical studies, patients on opioids often needed higher serum pegvisomant concentrations to achieve appropriate IGF-I suppression compared with patients not receiving opioids. The mechanism of this interaction is not known.

➤*Drug/Lab test interactions:* Pegvisomant has significant structural similarity to GH, which causes it to cross-react in commercially available GH assays. Because serum concentrations of pegvisomant at therapeutically effective doses are generally 100 to 1,000 times higher than endogenous serum GH levels seen in patients with acromegaly, commercially available GH assays will overestimate true GH levels. Treatment with pegvisomant should therefore not be monitored or adjusted based on serum GH concentrations reported from these assays. Instead, monitoring and dose adjustments should only be based on serum IGF-I levels.

Adverse Reactions

➤*Laboratory changes:* See Precautions for more information. Nine acromegalic patients (9.6%) withdrew from premarketing clinical studies because of adverse reactions, including 2 patients with marked transaminase elevations, 1 patient with lipohypertrophy at the injection sites, and 1 patient with substantial weight gain. The majority of reported adverse reactions were of mild to moderate intensity and limited duration. Most adverse reactions did not appear to be dose dependent.

Number of Patients (%) with Acromegaly Reporting Adverse Reactions in a 12-Week Placebo-Controlled Study with Pegvisomant[a]

Adverse reaction	Pegvisomant 10 mg/day (n = 26)	Pegvisomant 15 mg/day (n = 26)	Pegvisomant 20 mg/day (n = 28)	Placebo (n = 32)
Miscellaneous				
Infection[b]	6 (23%)	0	0	2 (6%)
Pain	2 (8%)	1 (4%)	4 (14%)	2 (6%)
Injection site reaction	2 (8%)	1 (4%)	3 (11%)	0
Accidental injury	2 (8%)	1 (4%)	0	1 (3%)
Back pain	2 (8%)	0	1 (4%)	1 (3%)
Flu syndrome	1 (4%)	3 (12%)	2 (7%)	0
Chest pain	1 (4%)	2 (8%)	0	0
GI				
Abnormal liver function tests	3 (12%)	1 (4%)	1 (4%)	1 (3%)
Diarrhea	1 (4%)	0	4 (14%)	1 (3%)
Nausea	0	2 (8%)	4 (14%)	1 (3%)
CNS				
Dizziness	2 (8%)	1 (4%)	1 (4%)	2 (6%)
Paresthesia	0	0	2 (7%)	2 (6%)
Metabolic/nutritional				
Peripheral edema	2 (8%)	0	1 (4%)	0
Cardiovascular				
Hypertension	0	2 (8%)	0	0
Respiratory				
Sinusitis	2 (8%)	0	1 (4%)	1 (3%)

[a] Table includes only those reactions that were reported in at least 2 patients and at a higher incidence in patients treated with pegvisomant than in patients treated with placebo.

[b] The 6 reactions coded as "infection" in the group treated with pegvisomant 10 mg were reported as cold symptoms (3), upper respiratory tract infection (1), blister (1), and ear infection (1). The 2 reactions in the placebo group were reported as cold symptoms (1) and chest infection (1).

➤*Immunogenicity:* In premarketing clinical studies, approximately 17% of the patients developed low titer, non-neutralizing anti-GH antibodies. Although the presence of these antibodies did not appear to impact the efficacy of pegvisomant, the long-term clinical significance of these antibodies is not known. No assay for anti-pegvisomant antibodies is commercially available for patients receiving pegvisomant.

Overdosage

➤*Symptoms:* In 1 reported incident of acute overdose with pegvisomant during premarketing clinical studies, a patient self-administered 80 mg/day for 7 days. The patient experienced a slight increase in fatigue, had no other complaints, and demonstrated no significant clinical laboratory abnormalities.

➤*Treatment:* Administration of pegvisomant should be discontinued and not resumed until IGF-I levels return to within or above the normal range.

Patient Information

Patients and any other persons who may administer pegvisomant should be carefully instructed by a healthcare professional on how to properly reconstitute and inject the product.

Patients should be informed about the need for serial monitoring of LTs, and told to immediately discontinue therapy and contact their physicians if they become jaundiced. In addition, patients should be made aware that serial IGF-I levels will need to be obtained to allow their physician to properly adjust the dose of pegvisomant.

LARONIDASE

Rx	**Aldurazyme** (BioMarin)	**Injection:** 2.9 mg laronidase per 5 mL	Preservative-free. In 5 mL single-use vials.[a]

[a] Contains 0.1% albumin (human) after dilution. Also contains sodium chloride 43.9 mg, sodium phosphate monbasic monohydrate 63.5 mg, sodium phosphate dibasic heptahydrate 10.7 mg.

LARONIDASE — INJECTION

Indications

➤*Mucopolysaccharidosis I (MPS I):* For patients with Hurler and Hurler-Scheie forms of MPS I and for patients with the Scheie form who have moderate to severe symptoms. The risks and benefits of treating mildly affected patients with the Scheie form have not been established.

Laronidase has been shown to improve pulmonary function and walking capacity. Laronidase has not been evaluated for effects on CNS manifestations of the disorder.

Administration and Dosage

April 30, 2003.

➤*Dosage:* 0.58 mg/kg of body weight administered once-weekly as an intravenous infusion.

➤*Pretreatment:* Pretreatment with antipyretics and/or antihistamines is recommended 60 minutes prior to the start of the infusion.

➤*Administration:* The total volume of the infusion is determined by the patient's body weight and should be delivered over approximately 3 to 4 hours. Patients with a body weight of 20 kg or less should receive a total volume of 100 mL. Patients with a body weight of greater than 20 kg should receive a total volume of 250 mL. The initial infusion rate of 10 mcg/kg/hr may be incrementally increased every 15 minutes during the first hour, as tolerated, until a maximum infusion rate of 200 mcg/kg/hr is reached. The maximum rate is then maintained for the remainder of the infusion (2 to 3 hours).

For Patients Weighing 20 kg or Less	
Total volume of laronidase infusion = 100 mL	
2 mL/h × 15 min (10 mcg/kg/h)	Obtain vital signs, if stable then increase rate to . . .
4 mL/h × 15 min (20 mcg/kg/h)	Obtain vital signs, if stable then increase the rate to . . .
8 mL/h × 15 min (50 mcg/kg/h)	Obtain vital signs, if stable then increase the rate to . . .
16 mL/h × 15 min (100 mcg/kg/h)	Obtain vital signs, if stable then increase the rate to . . .
32 mL/h × approximately 3 h (200 mcg/kg/h)	For the remainder of the infusion.

For Patients Weighing Greater Than 20 kg	
Total volume of laronidase infusion = 250 mL	
5 mL/h × 15 min (10 mcg/kg/h)	Obtain vital signs, if stable then increase the rate to . . .
10 mL/h × 15 min (20 mcg/kg/h)	Obtain vital signs, if stable then increase the rate to . . .
20 mL/h × 15 min (50 mcg/kg/h)	Obtain vital signs, if stable then increase the rate to . . .
40 mL/h × 15 min (100 mcg/kg/h)	Obtain vital signs, if stable then increase the rate to . . .
80 mL/h × approximately 3 h (200 mcg/kg/h)	For the remainder of the infusion.

➤*Preparation:* Each vial of laronidase provides 2.9 mg of laronidase in 5 mL of solution and is intended for single use only. Do not use the vial more than one time. The concentrated solution for infusion must be diluted with 0.1% albumin (human) in 0.9% sodium chloride injection using aseptic techniques. Laronidase should be prepared using PVC containers and administered with a PVC infusion set equipped with an in-line, low protein binding 0.2 micrometer (μm) filter. There is no information on the compatibility of diluted laronidase with glass containers.

➤*Instructions for use (aseptic techniques):*

1.) Determine the number of vials to be diluted based on the individual patient's weight and the recommended dose of 0.58 mg/kg [Patient's weight (kg) × 1 mL/kg of laronidase = Total # mL of laronidase, then Total # of mL of laronidase ÷ 5 mL per Vial = Total # of Vials]. Round up to the nearest whole vial. Remove the required number of vials from the refrigerator to allow them to reach room temperature. Do not heat or microwave vials.
2.) Before withdrawing the laronidase from the vial, visually inspect each vial for particulate matter and discoloration. The laronidase solution should be clear to slightly opalescent and colorless to pale yellow. A few translucent particles may be present. Do not use if the solution is discolored or if there is particulate matter in the solution.
3.) Determine the total volume of the infusion to be used based on the patient's body weight. The total final volume should be either 100 mL (if weight is less than or equal to 20 kg) or 250 mL (if weight is greater than 20 kg).
4.) According to the following instructions, prepare an infusion bag of 0.1% albumin (human) in 0.9% sodium chloride injection. Remove and discard a volume of 0.9% sodium chloride injection equal to the volume of albumin (human) to be added to the infusion bag. Add the appropriate volume of albumin (human) to the infusion bag and gently rotate the infusion bag to ensure proper distribution of the albumin (see table below).
5.) Withdraw and discard a volume of the 0.1% albumin (human) in 0.9% sodium chloride injection from the infusion bag, equal to the volume of laronidase concentrate to be added.
6.) Slowly withdraw the calculated volume of laronidase from the appropriate number of vials using caution to avoid excessive agitation. Do not use a filter needle, as this may cause agitation. Agitation may denature laronidase, rendering it biologically inactive.
7.) Slowly add the laronidase solution to the 0.1% albumin (human) in 0.9% sodium chloride injection using care to avoid agitation of the solutions. Do not use a filter needle.
8.) Gently rotate the infusion bag to ensure proper distribution of laronidase. Do not shake the solution.

Total Volume of Laronidase Infusion	Volume of Albumin (human) 5% to be Added	Volume of Albumin (human) 25% to be Added
100 mL	2 mL	0.4 mL
250 mL	5 mL	1 mL

➤*Compatibility:* Laronidase does not contain any preservatives; therefore after dilution with saline in the infusion bags, any unused product or waste material should be discarded and disposed of in accordance with local requirements.

Laronidase must not be mixed with other medicinal products in the same infusion.

The compatibility of laronidase in solution with other products has not been evaluated.

➤*Storage / Stability:* Store laronidase under refrigeration at 2° to 8°C (36° to 46°F). Do not freeze or shake. Do not use laronidase after the expiration date on the vial. This product contains no preservatives.

The diluted solution should be used immediately. If immediate use is not possible, the diluted solution should be stored refrigerated at 2° to 8°C (36° to 46°F). The in-use storage should not be longer than 36 hours from the time of preparation to completion of administration. Room temperature storage of diluted solution is not recommended.

Actions

➤*Pharmacology:* Mucopolysaccharide storage disorders are caused by the deficiency of specific lysosomal enzymes required for the catabolism of glycosaminoglycans (GAG).

Mucopolysaccharidosis I (MPS I) is characterized by the deficiency of α-L-iduronidase, a lysosomal hydrolase which catalyses the hydrolysis of terminal α-L-iduronic acid residues of dermatan sulfate and heparan sulfate. Reduced or absent α-L-iduronidase activity results in the accumulation of the GAG substrates, dermatan sulfate and heparan sulfate, throughout the body and leads to widespread cellular, tissue, and organ dysfunction.

The rationale of laronidase therapy in MPS I is to provide exogenous enzyme for uptake into lysosomes and increase the catabolism of GAG. Laronidase uptake by cells into lysosomes is most likely mediated by the mannose-6-phosphate-terminated oligosaccharide chains of laronidase binding to specific mannose-6-phosphate receptors.

Because many proteins in the blood are restricted from entry into the central nervous system by the blood brain barrier, effects of intravenously administered laronidase on cells within the central nervous system (CNS) cannot be inferred from activity in sites outside the CNS. The ability of laronidase to cross the blood brain barrier has not been evaluated in animal models or in clinical trials.

➤*Pharmacokinetics:* The pharmacokinetics of laronidase were evaluated in 12 patients with MPS I who received 0.58 mg/kg of laronidase as a 4 hour infusion. After the first, 12th and 26th weekly infusions, the mean maximum plasma concentrations (C_{max}) ranged from 1.2 to 1.7 mcg/mL for the 3 time points. The mean area under the plasma concentration-time curve (AUC_{∞}) ranged from 4.5 to 6.9 mcg•hour/mL. The mean volume of distribution (V_z) ranged from 0.24 to 0.6 L/kg. Mean plasma clearance (CL) ranged from 1.7 to 2.7 mL/min/kg, and the mean elimination half-life ($t_{½}$) ranged from 1.5 to 3.6 hours.

Effects of antibodies – Most patients who received once-weekly infusions of laronidase developed antibodies to laronidase by week 12. Between weeks 1 and 12, increases in plasma clearance of laronidase were observed in some patients which appeared to be proportional to the antibody titer. At week 26, plasma clearance of laronidase was comparable to that at week 1, in spite of the continued and, in some cases, increased titers of antibodies.

Contraindications

There are no known contraindications to the use of laronidase.

Warnings

➤*Hypersensitivity reactions:* Patients treated with laronidase may develop infusion-related hypersensitivity reactions. The most common

LARONIDASE — INJECTION

infusion-related reactions included flushing, fever, headache and rash. Flushing occurred in 5 patients (23%) receiving laronidase; the other reactions were less frequent. All reactions were mild to moderate in severity. In the clinical studies, 1 patient developed an anaphylactic reaction approximately 3 hours after the initiation of the infusion. The reaction consisted of urticaria and airway obstruction. Resuscitation required an emergency tracheostomy. This patient's preexisting MPS I related upper airway obstruction may have contributed to the severity of this reaction.

Some infusion-related reactions may be ameliorated by slowing the rate of infusion or treatment with additional antipyretics and/or antihistamines. If severe hypersensitivity or anaphylactic reactions occur, immediately discontinue the infusion of laronidase and initiate appropriate treatment. Caution should be exercised if epinephrine is being considered for use in patients with MPS I due to the increased prevalence of coronary artery disease in these patients.

The risks and benefits of re-administering laronidase following a severe hypersensitivity or anaphylactic reaction should be considered. Extreme care should be exercised, with appropriate resuscitation measures available, if the decision is made to re-administer the product.

➤*Pregnancy: Category B.* There are no adequate and well-controlled studies in pregnant women. Because animal reproduction studies are not always predictive of human response, laronidase should be used during pregnancy only if clearly needed.

➤*Lactation:* It is not known whether the drug is excreted in human milk. Because many drugs are excreted in human milk, caution should be exercised when laronidase is administered to a nursing woman.

See Patient Information for more information.

➤*Children:* Patients younger than 5 years of age were not included in the clinical studies because of inability to comply with efficacy outcome assessments. It is not known if children younger than 5 respond differently from older children.

Precautions

➤*Pretreatment:* Patients should receive antipyretics and/or antihistamines prior to infusion. If an infusion reaction occurs, regardless of pretreatment, decreasing the infusion rate, temporarily stopping the infusion, and/or administration of additional antipyretics and/or antihistamines may ameliorate the symptoms. If severe hypersensitivity or anaphylactic reactions occur, immediately discontinue the infusion of laronidase and initiate appropriate treatment.

Drug Interactions

No formal drug interaction studies have been conducted.

Adverse Reactions

The most serious adverse reaction reported with laronidase was an anaphylactic reaction consisting of urticaria and airway obstruction, which occurred in 1 patient. Pre-existing upper airway obstruction may have contributed to the severity of the reaction.

The most common adverse reactions associated with laronidase treatment in the clinical studies were upper respiratory tract infection, rash, and injection site reaction.

The most common adverse reactions requiring intervention were infusion-related reactions, particularly flushing. Most infusion-related reactions requiring intervention were ameliorated with slowing of the infusion rate, temporarily stopping the infusion, and/or administering additional antipyretics and/or antihistamines.

The data described below reflect exposure to 0.58 mg/kg of laronidase for 26 weeks in a placebo-controlled double-blind study in 45 patients with MPS I (n = 22 laronidase, and n = 23 placebo). All 45 patients continued into an open-label study of laronidase treatment for an additional 36 weeks. An additional 10 patients participated in a Phase 1 open-label study with continued infusions for up to 3 years. The population in the placebo-controlled study was evenly distributed for gender (n = 23 females and 22 males) and ranged in ages from 6 to 43 years. Of the 45 patients in the placebo-controlled study, 1 was clinically assessed as having Hurler form, 37 Hurler-Scheie, and 7 Scheie. All patients were treated with antipyretics and antihistamines prior to the infusions.

Because clinical trials are conducted under widely varying and controlled conditions, the observed adverse reaction rates may not predict the rates observed in patients in clinical practice.

The following table enumerates adverse reactions and selected laboratory abnormalities that occurred during the placebo-controlled trial in at least 2 patients more in the laronidase group than was observed in the placebo group. Reported adverse reactions have been classified using standard WHOART terms. Observed adverse reactions in the phase 1 study and the open-label treatment period following the controlled study were not different in nature or severity.

Number and (%) of Patients with Adverse Reactions and Selected Laboratory Abnormalities in the Placebo-Controlled Study

Adverse reaction	Placebo (n = 23)	Laronidase (n = 22)
Respiratory system		
Upper respiratory tract infection	4 (17%)	7 (32%)
Body as a whole		
Chest pain	0	2 (9%)
Nervous system		
Hyperreflexia	0	3 (14%)
Paresthesia	1 (4%)	3 (14%)
Skin and appendages		
Rash	5 (22%)	8 (36%)
Resistance mechanism		
Abscess	0	2 (9%)
Liver and biliary system		
Bilirubinemia	0	2 (9%)
Vascular		
Vein disorder	1 (4%)	3 (14%)
Urinary system		
Facial edema	0	2 (9%)
Cardiovascular		
Hypotension	0	2 (9%)
Dependent edema	0	2 (9%)
Vision		
Corneal opacity	0	2 (9%)
Application site		
Injection site pain	0	2 (9%)
Injection site reaction	2 (9%)	4 (18%)
Platelet, bleeding and clotting		
Thrombocytopenia	0	2 (9%)

➤*Infusion-related reactions:* Infusion-related reactions were reported in 7 of 22 patients treated with laronidase. Infusion-related reactions were not significantly different between the laronidase treatment group and the placebo group who received infusions of diluent and all components of laronidase except the laronidase enzyme. The most common infusion-related reactions included flushing, fever, headache and rash. Flushing occurred in 5 patients (23%) receiving laronidase; the other reactions were less frequent. All reactions were mild to moderate in severity. The frequency of infusion-related reactions decreased with continued use during the open-label extended use period. There was 1 case of anaphylaxis during the open-label extension period. The reaction consisted of urticaria and airway obstruction. Resuscitation required an emergency tracheostomy. This patient's preexisting MPS I related upper airway obstruction may have contributed to the severity of this reaction. Less common infusion-related reactions include cough, bronchospasm, dyspnea, urticaria, angioedema and pruritus.

➤*Immunogenicity:* Fifty of 55 patients (91%) treated with laronidase were positive for antibodies to laronidase. The clinical significance of antibodies to laronidase is not known, including the potential for product neutralization.

The data reflect the percentage of patients whose test results were considered positive for antibodies to laronidase using an enzyme-linked immunosorbent assay (ELISA) for laronidase-specific IgG binding antibodies, and are highly dependent on the sensitivity and specificity of the assay. Additionally, the observed incidence of antibodies in an assay may be influenced by several factors including sample handling, timing of sample collection, concomitant medications, and underlying disease. For these reasons, comparison of the incidence of antibodies to laronidase with the incidence of antibodies to other products may be misleading.

Four patients in the controlled study who experienced severe infusion-related reactions were tested for laronidase specific IgE antibodies and complement activation. IgE testing was performed by ELISA and complement activation was measured by the Quidel Enzyme Immunoassay. One of the 4 patients had an anaphylactic reaction consisting of urticaria and airway obstruction and tested positive for both laronidase specific IgE binding antibodies and complement activation.

Other hypersensitivity reactions were also seen in patients receiving laronidase (see Infusion-related reactions).

Overdosage

There is no experience with overdoses of laronidase.

Patient Information

Patients should be informed that a registry for MPS I patients has been established in order to better understand the variability and progression of MPS I disease, and to continue to monitor and evaluate treatments. Patients should be encouraged to participate and advised that their participation may involve long-term follow-up. Information regarding the registry program may be found at http://www.MPSIregistry.com or by calling (800) 745-4447.

GALSULFASE

Rx	**Naglazyme** (BioMarin)	**Solution for Injection:** 1 mg/mL (expressed as protein content)	Preservative-free. In 5 mL single-use vials.[a]

[a] Contains sodium chloride 43.8 mg, sodium phosphate monobasic monohydrate 6.2 mg, sodium phosphate dibasic heptahydrate 1.34 mg, and polysorbate 0.25 mg 80.

GALSULFASE — INJECTION

Indications

➤*Mucopolysaccharidosis VI:* For patients with mucopolysaccharidosis VI (MPS VI; Maroteaux-Lamy syndrome). Galsulfase has been shown to improve walking and stair-climbing capacity.

Administration and Dosage

➤*Approved by the FDA:* May 31, 2005.

➤*Dosage:* 1 mg/kg of body weight administered once weekly as an intravenous (IV) infusion.

➤*Pretreatment:* Pretreatment with antihistamines with or without antipyretics is recommended 30 to 60 minutes prior to the start of the infusion.

➤*Administration:* The total volume of the infusion should be delivered over no less than 4 hours. Galsulfase should be reconstituted in 0.9% sodium chloride injection to a final volume of 250 mL and delivered by controlled IV infusion using an infusion pump. Administer with a polyvinyl chloride (PVC) infusion set equipped with an in-line, low-protein-binding 0.2 mcm filter. The initial infusion rate should be 6 mL/h for the first hour. If the infusion is well tolerated, the rate of infusion may be increased to 80 mL/h for the remaining 3 hours. The infusion time can be extended up to 20 hours if infusion reactions occur.

For patients 20 kg or less who are susceptible to fluid volume overload, consider diluting galsulfase in a volume of 100 mL. The infusion rate (mL/min) should be decreased so that the total infusion duration remains no less than 4 hours.

➤*Preparation:* Each vial of galsulfase provides 5 mg of galsulfase (expressed in protein content) in 5 mL of solution and is intended for single use only. Do not use the vial more than one time. The concentrated solution for infusion must be diluted in 0.9% sodium chloride injection. Galsulfase should be prepared using PVC containers. There is no information on the compatibility of diluted galsulfase with glass containers.

➤*Instructions for use:* Use aseptic technique.

1.) Determine the number of vials to be diluted based on the individual patient's weight and the recommended dose of 1 mg/kg:

Patient's weight (kg) × 1 mL/kg of galsulfase = Total # mL of galsulfase

Total # of mL of galsulfase ÷ 5 mL per vial = Total # of vials

Round to the nearest whole vial. Remove the required number of vials from the refrigerator to allow them to reach room temperature. Do not allow vials to remain at room temperature longer than 24 hours prior to dilution. Do not heat or microwave vials.

1.) Before withdrawing the galsulfase from the vial, visually inspect each vial for particulate matter and discoloration. The galsulfase solution should be clear to slightly opalescent and colorless to pale yellow. A few translucent particles may be present. Do not use if the solution is discolored or if there is particulate matter in the solution.
2.) From a 250 mL infusion bag of 0.9% sodium chloride injection, withdraw and discard a volume equal to the volume of galsulfase to be added. If using a 100 mL infusion bag, this is not necessary.
3.) Slowly withdraw the calculated volume of galsulfase from the appropriate number of vials using caution to avoid excessive agitation. Do not use a filter needle, as this may cause agitation. Agitation may denature galsulfase, rendering it biologically inactive.
4.) Slowly add the galsulfase solution to the 0.9% sodium chloride injection, using care to avoid agitation of the solutions. Do not use a filter needle.
5.) Gently rotate the infusion bag to ensure proper distribution of galsulfase. Do not shake the solution.

➤*Compatibility:* Galsulfase must not be infused with other products in the infusion tubing. The compatibility of galsulfase in solution with other products has not been evaluated.

➤*Storage/Stability:* Store galsulfase under refrigeration at 2° to 8°C (36° to 46°F). Do not freeze or shake. The diluted solution should be used immediately. If immediate use is not possible, the diluted solution should be stored refrigerated at 2° to 8°C (36° to 46°F). Storage after dilution should not exceed 48 hours from the time of preparation to completion of administration. Room temperature storage of diluted solution, other than during infusion, is not recommended.

Galsulfase does not contain preservatives; therefore, after dilution with saline in the infusion bags, any unused product or waste material should be discarded and disposed of in accordance with local requirements.

Actions

➤*Pharmacology:* Mucopolysaccharide storage disorders are caused by the deficiency of specific lysosomal enzymes required for the catabolism of GAG. MPS VI is characterized by the absence or marked reduction in N-acetylgalactosamine 4-sulfatase. The sulfatase activity deficiency results in the accumulation of the GAG substrate dermatan sulfate, throughout the body. This accumulation leads to widespread cellular, tissue, and organ dysfunction. Galsulfase is intended to provide an exogenous enzyme that will be taken up into lysosomes and increase the catabolism of GAG. Galsulfase uptake by cells into lysosomes is most likely mediated by the binding of mannose-phosphate-terminated oligosaccharide chains of galsulfase to specific mannose-6-phosphate receptors.

➤*Pharmacokinetics:* The pharmacokinetic parameters of galsulfase were evaluated in 13 patients with MPS VI who received 1 mg/kg of galsulfase as a 4-hour infusion weekly for 24 weeks. The pharmacokinetic parameters at week 1 and week 24 are shown in the following table.

Galsulfase Pharmacokinetic Parameters (Median, Range)

Pharmacokinetic parameter	Week 1	Week 24
C_{max} (mcg/mL)	0.8 (0.4 to 1.3)	1.5 (0.2 to 5.5)
AUC_{0-t} (h•mcg/mL)[a]	2.3 (1 to 3.5)	4.3 (0.3 to 14.2)
Volume of distribution (mL/kg)	103 (56 to 323)	69 (59 to 2,799)
CL (mL/kg/min)	7.2 (4.7 to 10.5)	3.7 (1.1 to 55.9)
Half-life (min)	9 (6 to 21)	26 (8 to 40)

[a] Area under the plasma galsulfase concentration-time curve from start of infusion to 60 minutes post infusion.

Nearly all patients who receive treatment with galsulfase develop antibodies to galsulfase. Of 30 patients with MPS VI who received weekly galsulfase infusions and had pharmacokinetics evaluated, 29 developed antibodies to galsulfase. Four patients with high antibody titers had decreases in plasma AUC between weeks 1 and 24. One patient with high antibody titers had an increase in plasma AUC between weeks 1 and 24.

Contraindications

None known.

Warnings

➤*Infusion reactions:* Because of the potential for infusion reactions, give patients antihistamines with or without antipyretics prior to infusion. Despite routine pretreatment with antihistamines, infusion reactions, some severe, occurred in 30 of 55 patients treated with galsulfase. Severe symptoms included angioneurotic edema, hypotension, dyspnea, bronchospasm, respiratory distress, apnea, and urticaria. The most common symptoms of infusion reactions included fever, chills/rigors, headache, rash, and mild to moderate urticaria. Nausea, vomiting, elevated blood pressure, retrosternal pain, abdominal pain, malaise, and joint pain were also reported. Initial reactions were observed as late as week 55 of treatment.

Symptoms typically abated with slowing or temporary interruption of the infusion and administration of additional antihistamines, antipyretics, and, occasionally, corticosteroids. Most patients were able to complete their infusions. Subsequent infusions were managed with a slower rate of galsulfase administration, treatment with additional prophylactic antihistamines, and, in the event of a more severe reaction, treatment with prophylactic corticosteroids. Despite these measures, 13 of 30 patients had additional infusion reactions.

If severe infusion reactions occur, immediately discontinue the infusion of galsulfase and initiate appropriate treatment. Consider the risks and benefits of readministering galsulfase following a severe reaction.

No factors were identified that predisposed patients to infusion reactions. There was no association between severity of infusion reactions and titer of antigalsulfase antibodies.

➤*Pregnancy: Category B.* There are no adequate and well-controlled studies in pregnant women. Because animal reproduction studies are not always predictive of human response, use this drug during pregnancy only if clearly needed.

See Patient Information for more information.

➤*Lactation:* It is not known whether galsulfase is excreted in human milk. Because many drugs are excreted in human milk, exercise caution when galsulfase is administered to a breast-feeding woman. Breast-feeding women are encouraged to participate in the clinical surveillance program.

➤*Children:* Safety and efficacy in patients younger than 5 years of age have not been evaluated.

Precautions

➤*Sleep apnea:* Sleep apnea is common in MPS VI patients and antihistamine pretreatment may increase the risk of apneic episodes. Evaluation of airway patency should be considered prior to initiation of treatment. Patients using supplemental oxygen or continuous positive airway pressure (CPAP) during sleep should have these treatments readily available during infusion in the event of an infusion reaction, or extreme drowsiness/sleep induced by antihistamine use.

➤*Acute febrile or respiratory illness:* Consider delaying galsulfase infusions in patients who present with an acute febrile or respiratory illness.

➤*Immunogenicity:* Ninety-eight percent (53/54) of all patients treated with galsulfase developed antigalsulfase immunoglobulin G (IgG) antibodies. Initial evidence of antibody development typically appeared following 4

GALSULFASE — INJECTION

to 8 weeks of treatment. No association was observed between antibody development and urinary GAG levels.

Five patients with high antibody levels had observable differences in pharmacokinetic parameters. Antibodies from 1 patient were analyzed for neutralizing effect and showed evidence of in vitro inhibition of galsulfase activity. Because only 1 patient sample was analyzed for neutralizing activity, the effects of neutralizing antibodies are unclear.

The data reflect the percentage of patients whose test results were considered positive for antibodies to galsulfase using an enzyme-linked immunosorbent assay (ELISA) for galsulfase-specific IgG-binding antibodies, and are highly dependent on the sensitivity and specificity of the assay. Additionally, the observed incidence of antibodies in an assay may be influenced by several factors, including sample handling, timing of sample collection, concomitant medications, and underlying disease. For these reasons, comparison of the incidence of antibodies to galsulfase with the incidence of antibodies to other products may be misleading.

Drug Interactions

No formal drug interaction studies have been conducted.

Adverse Reactions

The most frequent serious adverse reactions related to the use of galsulfase occurred during infusions and included urticaria of the face and neck, bronchospasm, respiratory distress, and apnea.

The most common adverse reactions observed in the clinical studies were headache, fever, arthralgia, vomiting, upper respiratory tract infections, abdominal pain, diarrhea, ear pain, cough, and otitis media.

The most common adverse reactions requiring interventions were infusion-related reactions.

Because clinical trials are conducted under widely varying conditions, the observed adverse reaction rates may not predict the rates observed in patients in clinical practice.

The following table enumerates adverse reactions that were reported during the 6-month placebo-controlled trial and occurred in at least 2 patients more in the reactions group than in the placebo group. Observed adverse reactions in the phase 1, phase 2, and open-label extension studies were not different in nature or severity.

Galsulfase Adverse Reactions		
	Galsulfase (n = 19)	Placebo (n = 20)
Adverse reaction	Number of patients	Number of patients
All	19 (100%)	20 (100%)
Cardiovascular		
Hypertension	2 (11%)	0
GI		
Abdominal pain	10 (53%)	6 (30%)
Gastroenteritis	2 (11%)	0
Respiratory		
Dyspnea	4 (21%)	2 (10%)
Nasal congestion	2 (11%)	0
Pharyngitis	3 (16%)	1 (5%)
Special Senses		
Conjunctivitis	4 (21%)	0
Ear pain	8 (42%)	4 (20%)
Increased corneal opacification	2 (11%)	0
Miscellaneous		
Areflexia	2 (11%)	0
Chest pain	3 (16%)	1 (5%)
Face edema	2 (11%)	0
Malaise	2 (11%)	0
Pain	5 (26%)	1 (5%)
Rigors	4 (21%)	0
Umbilical hernia	2 (11%)	0

Overdosage

There is no experience with overdose of galsulfase.

Patient Information

Inform patients that a clinical surveillance program has been established in order to better understand the variability and progression of the disease in the population as a whole, and to monitor and evaluate long-term treatment effects of galsulfase. The clinical surveillance program will also monitor the effect of galsulfase on pregnant women and their offspring, and determine if galsulfase is excreted in breast milk. Encourage patients to participate and advise them that their participation is voluntary and may involve long-term follow-up. For more information, visit http://www.MPSVI.com or call 1-866-906-6100.

AGALSIDASE BETA

Rx	**Fabrazyme** (Genzyme)	**Powder for injection, lyophilized:** 5.5 mg (5 mg/mL when reconstituted)	Preservative free. In 5 mL single-use vials.[a]
		37 mg (5 mg/mL when reconstituted)	Preservative free. In 20 mL single-use vials.[b]

[a] Contains mannitol 33 mg, sodium phosphate monobasic monohydrate 3 mg, sodium phosphate dibasic heptahydrate 8.8 mg/vial.

[b] Contains mannitol 222 mg, sodium phosphate monobasic monohydrate 20.4 mg, sodium phosphate dibasic heptahydrate 59.2 mg/vial.

AGALSIDASE BETA — INJECTION

Indications

For use in patients with Fabry disease. Agalsidase beta reduces globotriaosylceramide (GL-3) deposition in capillary endothelium of the kidney and certain other cell types.

Administration and Dosage

➤*Approved by the FDA:* Approved April 24, 2003.

➤*Dosage:* 1 mg/kg body weight infused every 2 weeks as an IV infusion.

The initial IV infusion rate should be no more than 0.25 mg/min (15 mg/hr). The infusion rate may be slowed in the event of infusion-associated reactions. After patient tolerance to the infusion is well established, the infusion rate may be increased in increments of 0.05 to 0.08 mg/min (increments of 3 to 5 mg/hr) each subsequent infusion. Thirty-one (31) of 58 (53%) patients have received infusions at rates greater than or equal to 33 mg/hr.

➤*Pretreatment:* Patients should receive antipyretics prior to infusion. If an infusion reaction occurs, regardless of pretreatment, decreasing the infusion rate, temporarily stopping the infusion, or administration of additional antipyretics, antihistamines or steroids may ameliorate the symptoms. Because of the potential for severe infusion reactions, appropriate medical support measures should be readily available when agalsidase beta is administered.

➤*Instructions for use:* Agalsidase beta does not contain any preservatives. Vials are for single-use only. Any unused product should be discarded.

Shaking or agitation of this product should be avoided. Do not use filter needles during the preparation of the infusion.

Reconstitution and dilution (using aseptic technique) – Agalsidase beta vials and diluent should be allowed to reach room temperature prior to reconstitution (approximately 30 minutes). The number of vials needed is based on the patient's body weight (kg) and the recommended dose of 1 mg/kg.

Patient weight (in kg) equals patient dose (in mg).

Patient dose (in mg) divided by 35 mg/vial equals number of vials to reconstitute (if the number of vials includes a fraction, round up to the next whole number).

Example: Patient weight (80 kg) equals patient dose (80 mg). Eighty (80) mg divided by 35 mg/vial equals 2.29 vials; therefore, 3 vials should be reconstituted.

Reconstitute each vial of agalsidase beta by slowly injecting 7.2 mL of sterile water for injection down the inside wall of each vial. Roll and tilt each vial gently. Each vial will yield a 5 mg/mL clear, colorless solution (total extractable amount per vial is 35 mg, 7 mL).

Visually inspect the reconstituted vial for particulate matter and discoloration. Do not use the reconstituted solution if there is particulate matter or if it is discolored.

The reconstituted solution should be further diluted with 0.9% sodium chloride injection to a final total volume of 500 mL. Prior to adding the volume of reconstituted agalsidase beta required for the patient dose, remove an equal volume of 0.9% Sodium Chloride for Injection from the 500 mL infusion bag.

➤*Administration:* Patient dose (in mg) divided by 5 mg/mL equals number of mL of reconstituted agalsidase beta required for patient dose.

Example: Patient dose equals 80 mg. Eighty (80) mg divided by 5 mg/mL equals 16 mL of agalsidase beta.

Slowly withdraw the reconstituted solution from each vial up to the total volume required for the patient dose. Inject the reconstituted agalsidase beta solution directly into the sodium chloride solution. Do not inject in the airspace within the infusion bag. Discard any vial with unused reconstituted solution.

Gently invert infusion bag to mix the solution, avoiding vigorous shaking and agitation.

AGALSIDASE BETA — INJECTION

Agalsidase beta should not be infused in the same intravenous line with other products.

The diluted solution may be filtered through an in-line low protein-binding 0.2 mcm filter during administration.

➤*Storage / Stability:* Store agalsidase beta under refrigeration between 2° to 8°C (36° to 46°F).

Reconstituted and diluted solutions of agalsidase beta should be used immediately. If immediate use is not possible, the reconstituted and diluted solution may be stored for up to 24 hours at 2° to 8°C (36° to 46°F).

Actions

➤*Pharmacology:* Fabry disease is an X-linked genetic disorder of glycosphingolipid metabolism. Deficiency of the lysosomal enzyme α-galactosidase A leads to progressive accumulation of glycosphingolipids, predominantly GL-3, in many body tissues, occurring over a period of years or decades. Clinical manifestations of Fabry disease include renal failure, cardiomyopathy, and cerebrovascular accidents. Accumulation of GL-3 in renal endothelial cells may play a role in renal failure.

Agalsidase beta is intended to provide an exogenous source of α-galactosidase A in Fabry disease patients. Preclinical and clinical studies evaluating a limited number of cell types indicate that agalsidase beta will catalyze the hydrolysis of glycosphingolipids including GL-3.

➤*Pharmacokinetics:* Plasma profiles of agalsidase beta were studied at 0.3, 1 and 3 mg/kg in 15 patients with Fabry disease. The area under the plasma concentration-time curve (AUC_{∞}) and the clearance did not increase proportionately with increasing doses, demonstrating that the enzyme follows nonlinear pharmacokinetics. Terminal half-life was dose independent with a range of 45 to 102 minutes.

In 11 patients with Fabry disease given 1 mg/kg agalsidase beta every 14 days for a total of 11 infusions, the pharmacokinetic responses following repeated dosing fell into 3 categories. In some patients, pharmacokinetic responses were maintained with repeated dosing, whereas in other patients, pharmacokinetic values decreased at infusion 7 relative to baseline and returned to baseline values by infusion 11. In the remaining patients, AUC declined and failed to return to baseline by infusion 11. In these patients, the average AUC was 25% of its initial level. Some patients with elevated titers of antibody to agalsidase were among those with decreased AUC. The development of antibodies to agalsidase did not influence half-life, but reduced both apparent C_{max} and AUC. The long-term consequence of antibody development to the pharmacokinetics of agalsidase has not been established.

Contraindications

No known contraindications.

Warnings

➤*Infusion reactions:* Infusion reactions occurred in many patients treated with agalsidase beta. Some of the reactions were severe. Infusion reactions included fever, rigors, chest tightness, hypertension, hypotension, pruritus, myalgia, dyspnea, urticaria, abdominal pain, and headache. All patients were pretreated with acetaminophen and an antihistamine. Infusion reactions occurred in some patients after receiving antipyretics, antihistamines and oral steroids.

Patients should be given antipyretics prior to infusion. If an infusion reaction occurs, regardless of pretreatment, decreasing the infusion rate, temporarily stopping the infusion, or administration of additional antipyretics, antihistamines or steroids may ameliorate the symptoms. Because of the potential for severe infusion reactions, appropriate medical support measures should be readily available when agalsidase beta is administered.

➤*Pregnancy: Category B.* There are no adequate and well-controlled studies in pregnant women. Because animal reproduction studies are not always predictive of human response, this drug should be used during pregnancy only if clearly needed.

See Patient Information for more information.

Responses in women – Fabry disease is an X-linked genetic disorder. However, some heterozygous women will develop signs and symptoms of Fabry disease due to the variability of the X chromosome inactivation within cells. Generally, the rates of progression of organ impairment are slower than in male Fabry disease patients and severity of signs and symptoms is variable.

➤*Lactation:* It is not known whether agalsidase beta is excreted in human milk. Because many drugs are excreted in human milk, caution should be exercised when agalsidase beta is administered to a breast-feeding woman.

Nursing mothers should be encouraged to enroll in the Fabry registry (see Patient Information).

➤*Children:* The safety and efficacy of agalsidase beta in pediatric patients have not been established.

Precautions

➤*Cardiac function:* Patients with advanced Fabry disease may have compromised cardiac function, which may predispose them to a higher risk of severe complications from infusion reactions. Infusion reactions included fever, rigors, chest tightness, hypertension, hypotension, pruritus, myalgia, dyspnea, urticaria, abdominal pain, and headache. Patients with compromised cardiac function should be monitored closely if the decision is made to administer agalsidase beta.

➤*Immunogenetics:* Most patients develop IgG antibodies to agalsidase beta. Sixty-three (63) of 71 (89%) patients in the clinical studies treated with agalsidase beta have developed antibodies to agalsidase beta. Most patients who develop antibodies do so within the first 3 months of exposure. Some patients developed IgE or skin test reactivity specific to agalsidase beta. Physicians should consider testing for IgE in patients who experienced suspected allergic reactions and consider the risks and benefits of continued treatment in patients with antiagalsidase beta IgE.

Drug Interactions

No drug interaction studies were performed.

Adverse Reactions

The most serious and most common adverse reactions reported with agalsidase beta are infusion reactions. Serious or frequently occurring infusion reactions consisted of 1 or more of the following: Tachycardia, hypertension, throat tightness, chest pain/tightness, dyspnea, fever, chills/rigors, abdominal pain, pruritus, urticaria, nausea, vomiting, lip or ear edema, and rash. Infusion reactions declined in frequency with continued use of agalsidase beta. However, serious infusion reactions may occur after extended durations of agalsidase beta treatment.

Other reported serious adverse events included stroke, pain, ataxia, bradycardia, cardiac arrhythmia, cardiac arrest, decreased cardiac output, vertigo, hypoacousia, and nephrotic syndrome. These adverse events also occur as manifestations of Fabry disease; an alteration in frequency or severity cannot be determined from the small numbers of patients studied.

The data described below reflect exposure of 29 patients to 1 mg/kg agalsidase beta every 2 weeks for 5 months in a placebo-controlled study. All 58 patients continued into an open-label extension study of agalsidase beta treatment for up to 30 additional months. An additional 28 patients received open-label treatment. All patients were treated with antipyretics and antihistamines prior to the infusions.

Because clinical trials are conducted under widely varying and controlled conditions, the observed adverse reaction rates may not predict the rates observed in patients in clinical practice.

The table below enumerates adverse events and selected laboratory abnormalities that occurred during the placebo-controlled trial in at least 2 patients more in the agalsidase beta group than was observed in the placebo group. Reported adverse events have been classified by organ system. Observed adverse events in the Phase ½ study and the open-label treatment period following the controlled study were not different in nature or severity.

Incidence (%) of Adverse Events Occurring in the Placebo-Controlled Study

Adverse event	Placebo (n = 29)	Agalsidase beta (n = 29)
Body as a whole		
Chest pain	3 (10%)	5 (17%)
Fever	5 (17%)	14 (48%)
Pain	3 (10%)	6 (21%)
Pallor	1 (3%)	4 (14%)
Rigors	4 (14%)	15 (52%)
Temperature changed sensation	1 (3%)	5 (17%)
Cardiovascular		
Cardiomegaly	1 (3%)	3 (10%)
Hypertension	0	3 (10%)
Hypotension	2 (7%)	4 (14%)
Edema dependent	1 (3%)	6 (21%)
Central and peripheral nervous system		
Dizziness	2 (7%)	4 (14%)
Headache	11 (38%)	13 (45%)
Paraesthesia	2 (7%)	4 (14%)
GI system		
Dyspepsia	1 (3%)	3 (10%)
Nausea	4 (14%)	8 (28%)
Musculoskeletal system		
Arthrosis	0	3 (10%)
Skeletal pain	0	6 (21%)
Psychiatric		
Anxiety	5 (17%)	8 (28%)
Depression	1 (3%)	3 (10%)
Male reproductive		
Testicular pain	0	2 (7%)
Respiratory system		
Bronchitis	1 (3%)	3 (10%)
Bronchospasm	0	2 (7%)
Laryngitis	0	2 (7%)
Pharyngitis	2 (7%)	8 (28%)
Rhinitis	7 (24%)	11 (38%)
Sinusitis	0	2 (7%)

AGALSIDASE BETA — INJECTION

➤*Immunogenicity:* Sixty-three (63) of 71 (89%) patients in the clinical studies treated with agalsidase beta have developed antibodies to agalsidase beta. Most patients who develop antibodies do so within the first 3 months of exposure. Antibodies to agalsidase beta were purified from 15 patients with high antibody titers (greater than or equal to 12,800) and studied for inhibition of in vitro enzyme activity. Under the conditions of this assay, most of these 15 patients had inhibition of in vitro enzyme activity ranging between 14% to 74% at 1 or more timepoints during the study. No general pattern was seen in individual patient reactivity over time. The clinical significance of binding or inhibitory antibodies to agalsidase beta is not known. In patients followed in the open-label study, reduction of GL-3 in plasma and GL-3 inclusions in superficial skin capillaries was maintained after antibody formation.

The data reflect the percentage of patients whose test results were considered positive for antibodies to agalsidase beta using an ELISA and radioimmunoprecipitation (RIP) assay for antibodies. These results are highly dependent on the sensitivity and specificity of the assay. Additionally, the observed incidence of antibodies in an assay may be influenced by several factors including sample handling, timing of sample collection, concomitant medications, and underlying disease. For these reasons, comparison of the incidence of antibodies to agalsidase beta with the incidence of antibodies to other products may be misleading.

Overdosage

There have been no reports of overdose with agalsidase beta. In clinical trials, patients received doses up to 3 mg/kg body weight.

Patient Information

Patients should be informed that a registry has been established in order to better understand the variability and progression of Fabry disease in the population as a whole and in women, and to monitor and evaluate long-term treatment effects of agalsidase beta. The registry will also monitor the effect of agalsidase beta on pregnant women and their offspring, and determine if agalsidase beta is excreted in breast milk. Patients should be encouraged to participate and advised that their participation is voluntary and may involve long-term follow-up. For more information visit http://www.fabryregistry.com or call (800) 745-4447.

MIGLUSTAT

Rx	**Zavesca** (Actelion)	**Capsules:** 100 mg	Sodium starch glucollate. (OGT 918, 100). White, opaque. Gelatin. In 90s and blister card 18s.

MIGLUSTAT — ORAL

Indications

➤*Gaucher disease:* For the treatment of adult patients with mild to moderate type 1 Gaucher disease for whom enzyme replacement therapy is not a therapeutic option (eg, because of constraints such as allergy, hypersensitivity, or poor venous access).

Administration and Dosage

➤*Approved by the FDA:* July 31, 2003.

➤*Instructions for administration:* Therapy should be directed by physicians who are knowledgeable in the management of Gaucher disease.

➤*Dosage:* One 100 mg capsule administered orally 3 times a day at regular intervals.

It may be necessary to reduce the dose to one 100 mg capsule once or twice a day in some patients if adverse effects such as diarrhea or tremor occur.

➤*Renal function impairment:* In patients with mild renal impairment (adjusted creatinine clearance 50 to 70 mL/min/1.73 m^2), miglustat administration should commence at a dose of 100 mg twice per day. In patients with moderate renal impairment (adjusted creatinine clearance of 30 to 50 mL/min/1.73 m^2), miglustat administration should commence at a dose of one 100 mg capsule per day. Use of miglustat in patients with severe renal impairment (creatinine clearance of less than 30 mL/min/1.73 m^2) is not recommended.

➤*Storage/Stability:* Store at 20° to 25°C (68° to 77°F). Brief exposure to 15° to 30°C (59° to 86°F) permitted.

Actions

➤*Pharmacology:* Miglustat functions as a competitive and reversible inhibitor of the enzyme glucosylceramide synthase, the initial enzyme in a series of reactions which results in the synthesis of most glycosphingolipids. The goal of treatment with miglustat is to reduce the rate of glycosphingolipid biosynthesis so that the amount of glycosphingolipid substrate is reduced to a level which allows the residual activity of the deficient glucocerebrosidase enzyme to be more effective (substrate reduction therapy). In vitro and in vivo studies have shown that miglustat can reduce the synthesis of glucosylceramide-based glycosphingolipids. In clinical trials, miglustat improved liver and spleen volume, as well as hemoglobin concentration and platelet count.

➤*Pharmacokinetics:*

Absorption – After a 100 mg oral dose, the time to maximum observed plasma concentration of miglustat (t_{max}) ranged from 2 to 2.5 hours in Gaucher patients. Plasma concentrations show a biexponential decline, characterized by a short distribution phase and a longer elimination phase. The effective half-life of miglustat is approximately 6 to 7 hours, which predicts that steady-state will be achieved by 1.5 to 2 days following the start of 3 times daily dosing.

Miglustat, dosed at 50 and 100 mg in Gaucher patients, exhibits dose proportional pharmacokinetics. Miglustat's pharmacokinetics were not altered after repeated dosing 3 times daily for up to 12 months.

Coadministration of miglustat with food results in a decrease in the rate of absorption of miglustat (maximum serum concentration [C_{max}] was decreased by 36% and t_{max} delayed 2 hours) but has no statistically significant effect on the extent of absorption of miglustat (area under the plasma concentration curve [AUC] was decreased by 14%).

The mean oral bioavailability of a 100 mg miglustat capsule is about 97% relative to an oral solution administered under fasting conditions.

Distribution – Miglustat does not bind to plasma proteins. Mean apparent volume of distribution of miglustat is 83 to 105 L in Gaucher patients, indicating that miglustat distributes into extravascular tissues.

Excretion – The major route of excretion of miglustat is renal. Miglustat is excreted unchanged in the urine. Renal impairment has a significant effect on the pharmacokinetics of miglustat resulting in increased systemic exposure of miglustat in such patients. There is no evidence that miglustat is metabolized in humans.

Special populations –

Renal function impairment: Limited data in patients with Fabry disease and impaired renal function indicate that clearance (CL/F) of miglustat decreases with decreasing renal function. While the number of subjects with mild and moderate renal impairment was very small, the data suggest an approximate decrease in CL/F of 40% and 60%, respectively, in mild and moderate renal impairment, justifying the need to decrease the dosing of miglustat in such patients dependent upon creatinine clearance levels.

Data in severe renal impairment are limited to 2 patients with creatinine clearances in the range 18 to 29 mL/min and cannot be extrapolated below this range. These data suggest a decrease in CL/F by at least 70% in patients with severe renal impairment. Treatment with miglustat in patients with severe renal impairment is therefore not recommended.

Contraindications

Hypersensitivity to the active substance or any of the excipients; women who are or may become pregnant. If this drug is administered to a woman with reproductive potential, the patient should be apprised of the potential hazard to a fetus.

Warnings

➤*Peripheral neuropathy:* Cases of peripheral neuropathy have been reported in patients treated with miglustat. All patients undergoing miglustat treatment should undergo baseline and repeat neurological evaluations at approximately 6-month intervals. Patients who develop symptoms such as numbness and tingling should have a careful re-assessment of the risk/benefit of miglustat therapy and cessation of treatment may be considered.

➤*Renal function impairment:* Miglustat is known to be substantially excreted by the kidney, and the risk of adverse reactions to this drug may be greater in patients with impaired renal function. The clearance of miglustat is decreased by 40% to 60% in patients with mild to moderate renal impairment, and up to 70% in patients with severe renal impairment. As a result of this, dose reductions are recommended for those patients with mild to moderate renal impairment, the reduction being dependent upon the level of their creatinine clearance adjustment. For those patients with severe renal impairment, treatment with miglustat is not recommended. Because elderly patients are more likely to have decreased renal function, care should be taken in dose selection, and it may be useful to monitor renal function.

➤*Fertility impairment:* Male rats, given 20 mg/kg/day miglustat by (systemic exposure less than the human therapeutic systemic exposure based on body surface area comparisons, mg/m^2) oral gavage 14 days prior to mating, had decreased spermatogenesis with altered sperm morphology and motility and decreased fertility. Decreased spermatogenesis was reversible following 6 weeks of drug withdrawal. A higher doses of 60 mg/kg/day (2 times the human therapeutic systemic exposure based on body surface area comparison, mg/m^2) resulted in seminiferous tubule and testicular atrophy/degeneration.

Female rats were given oral gavage doses of 20, 60, 180 mg/kg/day beginning 14 days before mating and continuing through gestation. Effects observed at 20 mg/kg/day (systemic exposure less than the human therapeutic systemic exposure, based on body surface area comparisons) included decreased corpora lutea, increased postimplantation loss, and decreased live births.

➤*Pregnancy: Category X.*

There are no adequate and well-controlled studies of miglustat in pregnant women. Miglustat should not be used during pregnancy.

Miglustat may cause fetal harm when administered to a pregnant woman. In female rats given miglustat by oral gavage at doses of 20, 60, 180 mg/kg/day beginning 14 days before mating and continuing through gestation day 17 (organogenesis), decreased live births including complete litter loss and decreased fetal weight was observed in the mid- and high-dose groups (sys-

MIGLUSTAT — ORAL

temic exposures greater than or equal to 2 times the human therapeutic systemic exposure based on body surface area comparison). In pregnant rats given miglustat by oral gavage at doses of 20, 60, 180 mg/kg/day from gestation day 6 through lactation (postpartum day 20), dystocia and delayed parturition were observed in the mid- and high-dose groups (systemic exposures greater than or equal to 2 times the human therapeutic systemic exposure, based on body surface area comparison). In addition, decreased live births and pup body weights were observed at greater than 20 mg/kg/day (systemic exposures less than the human therapeutic systemic exposure, based on body surface area comparison).

In pregnant rabbits given miglustat by oral gavage at doses of 15, 30, 45 mg/kg/day during gestation days 6 to 18 (organogenesis), maternal death and decreased body weight gain were observed at 15 mg/kg/day (systemic exposures less than the human therapeutic systemic exposure, based on body surface area comparisons).

Labor and delivery – Studies in pregnant rats exposed to miglustat during gestation through lactation are associated with dystocia and delayed parturition at systemic exposure 2 times the human therapeutic systemic exposure, based on body surface area comparisons.

➤*Lactation:* It is not known whether miglustat is excreted in human milk. Because many drugs are excreted in human milk and because of the potential for serious adverse reactions in nursing infants from miglustat, the drug should not be used in nursing mothers unless the potential benefit justifies the potential risk to the infant. A decision should be made whether to discontinue nursing or discontinue the drug, taking into account the importance of the drug to the lactating woman.

➤*Children:* The safety and efficacy of miglustat have not been evaluated in patients under the age of 18. Treatment with miglustat is associated with diarrhea and weight loss in approximately 85% and up to 65%, respectively, of adult patients. The effects of miglustat on growth and development in children have not been evaluated.

Precautions

➤*Administration:* Therapy should be directed by physicians knowledgeable in the management of patients with Gaucher disease.

➤*Tremor:* Approximately 30% of patients have reported tremor or exacerbation of existing tremor on treatment. These tremors were described as an exaggerated physiological tremor of the hands. Tremor usually began within the first month of therapy and in many cases resolved between 1 to 3 months during treatment. Dose reduction may ameliorate the tremor (usually within days), but discontinuation with treatment may sometimes be required.

➤*Diarrhea and weight loss:* Diarrhea and weight loss were common in clinical studies of patients treated with miglustat; approximately 85% and up to 65% of treated patients, respectively, reported these conditions. Diarrhea appears to be the result of the disaccharidase inhibitory activity of miglustat, with a resultant osmotic diarrhea. It is unclear if weight loss results from the diarrhea and associated gastrointestinal complaints, a decrease in food intake, or a combination of these or other factors. The incidence of diarrhea was noted to decrease over time with continued miglustat treatment, and was noted to result in an increase in the use of antidiarrheal medications, most commonly loperamide. Patients may be instructed to avoid high carbohydrate content foods during treatment with miglustat if they present with diarrhea. The incidence of weight loss was most evident in the first 12 months of treatment.

➤*Male fertility:* Male patients should maintain reliable contraceptive methods while taking miglustat. Studies in the rat have shown that miglustat adversely affects spermatogenesis and sperm parameters, thereby reducing fertility. Until further information is available, it is advised that before seeking to conceive, male patients should cease miglustat and maintain reliable contraceptive methods for 3 months thereafter.

Drug Interactions

➤*Imiglucerase:* While coadministration of miglustat appeared to increase the clearance of imiglucerase by 70%, these results are not conclusive because of the small number of subjects studied and because patients took variable doses of imiglucerase. Combination therapy with imiglucerase and miglustat is not indicated.

Adverse Reactions

➤*Open-label uncontrolled monotherapy trials:* In 2 open-label, uncontrolled monotherapy trials in adult type 1 Gaucher disease patients treated with miglustat at a starting dose of 100 mg 3 times daily (dose range 100 to 200 mg 3 times daily) for 12 months in 28 patients [Study 1], or at a dose of 50 mg 3 times daily for 6 months in 18 patients [Study 2], GI events were observed in more than 80% of patients either at the outset of treatment, or intermittently during treatment. Diarrhea was observed in approximately 85% of patients. Weight loss has been observed in up to 65% of patients.

Adverse Reactions in Greater Than or Equal to 5% of Patients in 2 Open-Label, Uncontrolled Monotherapy Trials of Miglustat

Patients entered in study (n)	Study 1 (starting dose 100 mg 3 times daily)	Study 2 (50 mg 3 times daily)
	28	18
Body system - Preferred term	% of patients reporting	% of patients reporting
CNS		
Dizziness	0%	11%
Headache	21%	22%
Leg cramps	4%	11%
Migraine	0%	6%
Paresthesia	7%	0%
Tremor	11%	11%
GI		
Abdominal pain	18%	50%
Anorexia	7%	0%
Bloating	0%	6%
Diarrhea	89%	89%
Dyspepsia	7%	0%
Epigastric pain not food-related	0%	6%
Flatulence	29%	44%
Nausea	14%	22%
Vomiting	4%	11%
GU, female		
Menstrual disorder	0%	6%
Hematologic		
Thrombocytopenia	7%	6%
Metabolic/Nutritional		
Weight decrease	39%	67%
Ophthalmic		
Visual disturbance	0%	17%
Musculoskeletal		
Cramps	0%	11%

➤*Open-label active-controlled study:*

Adverse Reactions in Greater Than or Equal to 5% of Patients in Open-Label Active Controlled Study

Patients entered in study (n)	Miglustat alone	Imiglucerase alone	Miglustat + imiglucerase
	12	12	12
Body system - Preferred term	% of patients reporting	% of patients reporting	% of patients reporting
CNS			
Dizziness	8%	0%	25%
Gait unsteady	8%	0%	0%
Leg cramps	8%	0%	0%
Numbness localized	0%	0%	8%
Shaking	0%	0%	8%
Tremor	17%	0%	33%
GI			
Abdominal pain	67%	0%	58%
Constipation	8%	0%	25%
Diarrhea	100%	0%	83%
Dry mouth	8%	0%	0%
Flatulence	50%	0%	42%
Nausea	8%	0%	8%
GU, female			
Menstrual irregularity	0%	0%	8%
Metabolic/Nutritional			
Weight decrease	67%	0%	42%
Ophthalmic			
Eye abnormality	0%	0%	8%
Visual disturbance	0%	0%	8%

MIGLUSTAT — ORAL

Adverse Reactions in Greater Than or Equal to 5% of Patients in Open-Label Active Controlled Study			
Patients entered in study (n)	Miglustat alone	Imiglucerase alone	Miglustat + imiglucerase
	12	12	12
Body system - Preferred term	% of patients reporting	% of patients reporting	% of patients reporting
CNS			
Dizziness	8%	0%	25%
Gait unsteady	8%	0%	0%
Leg cramps	8%	0%	0%
Numbness localized	0%	0%	8%
Shaking	0%	0%	8%
Tremor	17%	0%	33%
Psychiatric			
Appetite absent	0%	0%	8%
Jitteriness	0%	0%	8%
Memory loss	8%	0%	0%
Miscellaneous			
Abdominal distension	8%	0%	8%
Abdominal distension gaseous	8%	0%	0%
Back pain	8%	0%	0%
Chills	0%	0%	8%
Heaviness in limbs	8%	0%	0%
Influenza-like symptoms	0%	0%	8%
Pain	0%	8%	8%
Pain legs	0%	0%	8%

Adverse Reactions in Greater Than or Equal to 5% of Patients in Open-Label Active Controlled Study			
Patients entered in study (n)	Miglustat alone	Imiglucerase alone	Miglustat + imiglucerase
	12	12	12
Body system - Preferred term	% of patients reporting	% of patients reporting	% of patients reporting
CNS			
Dizziness	8%	0%	25%
Gait unsteady	8%	0%	0%
Leg cramps	8%	0%	0%
Numbness localized	0%	0%	8%
Shaking	0%	0%	8%
Tremor	17%	0%	33%
Weakness generalized	17%	0%	8%

Overdosage

In the clinical development program for miglustat, no patient experienced an overdose of study drug. However, miglustat has been administered at doses of up to 3,000 mg/day (approximately 10 times the recommended starting dose administered to Gaucher patients) for up to 6 months in human immunodeficiency virus (HIV)-positive patients. Adverse events observed in the HIV studies included granulocytopenia, dizziness, and paresthesia. Leukopenia and neutropenia have also been observed in a similar group of patients receiving 800 mg/day or above.

Patient Information

Patients should be informed of the potential risks and benefits of miglustat and of alternative modes of therapy. Patients should be advised that diarrhea, GI complaints, and weight loss are common side effects of miglustat therapy, and to adhere to dietary instructions. Patients should also be advised to promptly report any numbness, pain, or burning in the hands and feet, and the development of tremor or worsening in an existing tremor.

4-HYDROXYPHENYLPYRUVATE DIOXYGENASE INHIBITOR

NITISINONE

Rx	**Orfadin** (Rare Disease Therapeutics, Inc.)	**Capsules:** 2 mg	NTBC 2 mg. White. In 60s.
		5 mg	NTBC 5 mg. White. In 60s.
		10 mg	NTBC 10 mg. White. In 60s.

NITISINONE — ORAL

Indications

➤*Hereditary tyrosinemia type 1 (HT-1):* Adjunct to dietary reduction of tyrosine and phenylalanine in the treatment of HT-1.

Administration and Dosage

➤*Approved by the FDA:* January 18, 2002.

Treatment with nitisinone should be initiated by a doctor experienced in the treatment of HT-1.

➤*Initial dose:* The dose of nitisinone should be adjusted in each patient. The recommended initial dosage is 1 mg/kg/day divided for morning and evening administration. Since an effect of food is unknown, nitisinone should be taken at least 1 hour before a meal. Because of the long half-life of nitisinone, the total dose may be split unevenly as convenient in order to limit the total number of capsules given at each administration. A nutritionist skilled in managing children with inborn errors of metabolism should be employed to design a low-protein diet deficient in tyrosine and phenylalanine. For young children, capsules may be opened and the contents suspended in a small amount of water, formula, or applesauce immediately before use.

➤*Dose adjustment:* Nitisinone treatment should block the flux through the tyrosine degradation pathway at the level of 4-hydroxyphenylpyruvate dioxygenase. Treatment should lead to normalized porphyrin metabolism (ie, normal erythrocyte porphobilinogen synthase (PBG-S) activity and urine 5-aminolevulinic acid [5-ALA]). Succinylacetone should not be detectable in urine or plasma. If the biochemical parameters (except plasma succinylacetone) are not normalized within 1 month after start of nitisinone treatment, the dosage should be increased to 1.5 mg/kg/day. For plasma succinylacetone, it may take up to 3 months before the level is normalized after the start of nitisinone treatment. Since plasma nitisinone concentration, plasma succinylacetone, urine 5-ALA, and erythrocyte PBG-S activity are not routinely available, it is appropriate during regular monitoring to follow urine succinylacetone, liver function tests, alpha-fetoprotein, and serum tyrosine and phenylalanine levels. However, during the initiation of therapy and during acute exacerbations, it may be necessary to follow more closely all available biochemical parameters. A dosage of 2 mg/kg/day may be needed, especially in infants, once liver function has improved. This dose should be considered as a maximal dose for all patients.

➤*Storage/Stability:* Store refrigerated at 2° to 8° (36° to 46°).

Actions

➤*Pharmacology:* Nitisinone is a competitive inhibitor of 4-hydroxyphenylpyruvate dioxygenase, an enzyme upstream of fumarylacetoacetase (FAH) in the tyrosine catabolic pathway. By inhibiting the normal catabolism of tyrosine in patients with HT-1, nitisinone prevents the accumulation of the catabolic intermediates maleylacetoacetate and fumarylacetoacetate. In patients with HT-1, these catabolic intermediates are converted to the toxic metabolites succinylacetone and succinylacetoacetate, which are responsible for the observed liver and kidney toxicity. Succinylacetone can also inhibit the porphyrin synthesis pathway leading to the accumulation of 5-aminolevulinate, a neurotoxin responsible for the porphyric crises characteristic of HT-1.

Since nitisinone inhibits catabolism of tyrosine, use of this drug can result in elevated plasma levels of this amino acid. Treatment with nitisinone, therefore, requires restriction of the daily intake of tyrosine and phenylalanine to prevent the toxicity associated with elevated plasma levels of tyrosine.

➤*Pharmacokinetics:*

Absorption/Distribution – Nitisinone was greater than 90% bioavailable following oral administration of the labeled compound in rats and was distributed to different organs, particularly the liver and kidney, where radioactivity remained for 7 days after administration. The single-dose pharmacokinetics of nitisinone have been studied in 10 healthy male volunteers 19 to 39 years of age (median age, 32 years). Nitisinone, 1 mg/kg body weight, was administered as a capsule and a liquid. The median time for maximum plasma concentration was 3 hours for the capsule and 15 minutes for the liquid. The capsule and liquid formulation were found to be bioequivalent based on an analysis of area under the plasma concentration-time curve and maximum plasma concentration.

Metabolism – No information on the metabolism of nitisinone in humans is available.

Excretion – Nitisinone was biotransformed in rats and excreted via the urine.

The mean terminal plasma half-life of nitisinone in healthy male volunteers was 54 hours.

Contraindications

None known.

NITISINONE — ORAL

Warnings

➤*High plasma tyrosine levels:* Inadequate restriction of tyrosine and phenylalanine intake can result in elevations in plasma tyrosine. Plasma tyrosine levels should be kept below 500 mcmol/L in order to avoid toxic effects to the eyes (corneal ulcers, corneal opacities, keratitis, conjunctivitis, eye pain, and photophobia), skin (painful hyperkeratotic plaques on the soles and palms), and nervous system (variable degrees of mental retardation and developmental delay). In most patients, eye symptoms were transient, lasting less than 1 week. Six patients had prolonged episodes lasting 16 to 672 days.

➤*Transient thrombocytopenia and leucopenia:* Patients treated with nitisinone and dietary restriction in clinical trials were observed to develop transient thrombocytopenia (3%), leucopenia (3%), or both (1.5%). One patient, who developed both leucopenia and thrombocytopenia, improved after the dose of nitisinone was decreased from 2 to 1 mg/kg. Another patient, who developed thrombocytopenia, had nitisinone stopped for 2 weeks, but platelet values continued to be low for 3 months and slowly returned to normal after 5 months. In all other patients, platelet values and white blood cell counts normalized gradually without documented change in nitisinone dose. No patients developed infections or bleeding as a result of the episodes of leucopenia and thrombocytopenia. Regularly monitor platelet and white blood cell counts during nitisinone therapy.

➤*Elderly:* Clinical studies of nitisinone did not include any subjects 65 years of age or older to determine whether they respond differently from younger subjects. HT-1 is presently a disease of the pediatric population. In general, dose selection for an elderly patient should be cautious, usually starting at the low end of the dosing range, reflecting the greater frequency of decreased hepatic, renal, or cardiac function, and of concomitant disease or other drug therapy in this patient population.

➤*Pregnancy: Category C.* Adequate reproductive toxicity studies have not been conducted with nitisinone. It is not known if nitisinone can cause harm to the fetus if administered to pregnant women. Give nitisinone to a pregnant woman only if clearly needed.

In a single dose-group study in rats given 100 mg/kg/day (12 times the recommended clinical dose based on relative body surface area), reduced litter size, decreased pup weight at birth, and decreased survival of pups after birth were demonstrated.

➤*Lactation:* Although the exposure was not quantified, naive pups that were exposed to nitisinone via breast milk showed signs of ocular toxicity and lower body weight. This suggests that nitisinone is excreted via breast milk in rats. It is not known whether nitisinone is excreted in human milk. Because many drugs are excreted in human milk, exercise caution when nitisinone is administered to a breast-feeding woman.

➤*Children:* Nitisinone has been studied in patients ranging in age from birth to 21.7 years. The median age of enrollment in a study of 207 patients with HT-1 was 9 months.

Precautions

➤*Monitoring:* It is appropriate during regular monitoring to follow urine succinylacetone, liver function tests, alpha-fetoprotein, platelets, white blood cell counts, and serum tyrosine and phenylalanine levels. However, during the initiation of therapy and during acute exacerbations, it may be necessary to follow more closely all available biochemical parameters (eg, plasma nitisinone concentration, plasma succinylacetone levels, urine 5-ALA levels, and erythrocyte PBG-S activity). Regular liver monitoring by imaging (ultrasound, computerized tomography, magnetic resonance imaging) is recommended. Measure serum phosphate as a screening test for patients with renal involvement at risk for secondary hypophosphatemia and rickets. Perform slit-lamp examinations of the eyes before initiation of treatment and during any eye adverse reactions (eg, photophobia, eye pain, signs of inflammation).

➤*Risk of porphyric crises, liver failure, and hepatic neoplasms:* Patients with HT-1 are at increased risk of developing porphyric crises, liver failure, or hepatic neoplasms requiring liver transplantation. These complications of HT-1 were observed in patients treated with nitisinone for a median of 22 months during the clinical trial (liver transplantation, 13%; liver failure, 7%; malignant hepatic neoplasms, 5%; benign hepatic neoplasms, 3%; porphyria, 0.5%). Regular liver monitoring by imaging (ultrasound, computerized tomography, magnetic resonance imaging) and laboratory tests, including serum alpha-fetoprotein concentration, is recommended. An increase in serum alpha-fetoprotein concentration may be a sign of inadequate treatment, but always evaluate patients with increasing alpha-fetoprotein or signs of nodules of the liver during treatment with nitisinone for hepatic malignancy.

➤*General ophthalmologic care:* Perform slit-lamp examination of the eyes before initiation of nitisinone treatment. Patients who develop photophobia, eye pain, or signs of inflammation such as redness, swelling, or burning of the eyes during treatment with nitisinone should undergo slit-lamp reexamination and immediate measurement of the plasma tyrosine concentration. Implement a more restricted diet if the plasma tyrosine level is above 500 mcmol/L. Do not adjust nitisinone dosage in order to lower the plasma tyrosine concentration because the HT-1 metabolic defect may result in deterioration of the patient's clinical condition.

➤*Lab test abnormalities:* Plasma nitisinone concentration, urine and plasma succinylacetone levels, urine 5-ALA levels, and erythrocyte PBG-S activity were used during clinical trials to guide drug dosage. The probability of recurrence of abnormal values of urine succinylacetone was 1% at a nitisinone concentration of 37 mcmol/L (95% confidence interval, 23 to 51 mcmol/L). Assays for plasma nitisinone concentration, plasma succinylacetone, urine 5-ALA, and erythrocyte PBG-S activity are not routinely available in the United States. However, urine succinylacetone levels can be used to guide drug dose adjustment.

Serum alpha-fetoprotein concentrations are generally markedly elevated at the time of diagnosis, and gradually decrease during the course of nitisinone treatment. Increases during therapy may be a sign of inadequate treatment. Promptly evaluate an exponential increase in serum alpha-fetoprotein concentration for potential liver neoplasia.

Drug Interactions

No drug-drug interaction studies have been conducted with nitisinone.

Adverse Reactions

➤*Most frequent adverse reactions:* In a clinical trial of 207 patients treated with nitisinone for HT-1, the most frequent adverse reactions, regardless of causality assessment, occurred in the following organ systems:

Dermatologic – Alopecia, dry skin, exfoliative dermatitis, maculopapular rash, pruritis (1%).

Hematologic/Lymphatic – Leukopenia, thrombocytopenia (3%); epistaxis, porphyria (1%).

Hepatic – Hepatic neoplasm (8%); liver failure (7%).

Special senses – Conjunctivitis, corneal opacity, keratitis, photophobia (2%); blepharitis, cataracts, eye pain (1%).

➤*Adverse reactions occurring in less than 1% of patients:* Adverse reactions that occurred in less than 1% of the patients, regardless of causality assessment, are the following:

Cardiovascular – Cyanosis.

CNS – Brain tumor, encephalopathy, headache, hyperkinesia, nervousness, seizures, somnolence.

GI – Abdominal pain, diarrhea, enanthema, gastritis, gastroenteritis, GI hemorrhage, melena, tooth discoloration.

GU – Amenorrhea.

Hepatic – Elevated hepatic enzymes, hepatic function disorder, liver enlargement.

Metabolic/Nutritional – Dehydration, hypoglycemia, thirst.

Musculoskeletal – Pathologic fracture.

Respiratory – Bronchitis, respiratory insufficiency.

Miscellaneous – Death, infection, otitis, septicemia.

Overdosage

➤*Symptoms:* Accidental ingestion of this drug by individuals eating normal diets not restricted in tyrosine and phenylalanine will result in elevated tyrosine levels. In volunteers given a single 1 mg/kg dose of nitisinone, the plasma tyrosine level reached a maximum of 1,200 mcmol/L from 48 to 120 hours after dosing. After a washout period of 14 days, the mean value of plasma tyrosine was still 808 mcmol/L. Fasted follow-up samples obtained from volunteers several weeks later showed tyrosine values back to normal. Nitisinone was generally well tolerated in these studies. There were no reports of changes in vital signs or laboratory data of any clinical significance. One patient did report sensitivity to sunlight.

Tyrosinemia has been associated with toxicity to eyes, skin, and the nervous system.

➤*Treatment:* No information about specific treatment of overdose is available. Restriction of tyrosine and phenylalanine in the diet should limit toxicity associated with tyrosinemia. Monitor patients for potential adverse reactions.

Patient Information

Advise patients and their caregivers of the need to maintain dietary restriction of tyrosine and phenylalanine when taking nitisinone to treat HT-1.

Advise patients and their caregivers to promptly report unexplained eye symptoms, rash, jaundice, or excessive bleeding.

IMIGLUCERASE

IMIGLUCERASE

Rx	**Cerezyme** (Genzyme)	**Powder for injection, lyophilized**: 212 units (equiv. to a withdrawal dose of 200 units imiglucerase).	Preservative free. In vials.[a]
		424 units (equiv. to a withdrawal dose of 400 units imiglucerase).	Preservative free. In vials.[b]

[a] Contains mannitol 170 mg and sodium citrate 70 mg (trisodium citrate 52 mg, disodium hydrogen citrate 18 mg) per vial.

[b] Contains mannitol 340 mg and sodium citrate 140 mg (trisodium citrate 104 mg, disodium hydrogen citrate 36 mg) per vial.

IMIGLUCERASE — INJECTION

Indications

➤*Gaucher disease:* Imiglucerase is indicated for long-term enzyme replacement therapy for patients with a confirmed diagnosis of Type 1 Gaucher disease that results in 1 or more of the following conditions: anemia, bone disease, hepatomegaly or splenomegaly, and thrombocytopenia.

Administration and Dosage

➤*Approved by the FDA:* May 23, 1994.

➤*Dosage:* Imiglucerase is administered by IV infusion for 1 to 2 hours. Individualize dosage to each patient. Initial dosages range from 2.5 units/kg of body weight 3 times a week to 60 units/kg once every 2 weeks. Sixty units/kg every 2 weeks is the dosage for which the most data are available. Disease severity may dictate initiation of treatment at a relatively high dose or relatively frequent administration. Make dosage adjustments on an individual basis; these may increase or decrease based on achievement of therapeutic goals as assessed by routine comprehensive evaluations of the patient's clinical manifestations.

➤*Reconstitution:* After reconstitution, visually inspect imiglucerase before use. As a protein solution, slight flocculation (described as thin translucent fibers) occasionally occurs after dilution. The diluted solution may be filtered through an in-line, low protein-binding 0.2 mcm filter during administration. Do not use any vials exhibiting opaque particles or discoloration.

On the day of use, after the correct amount of imiglucerase to be administered to the patient has been determined, the appropriate number of vials are each reconstituted with sterile water for injection. The final concentrations and administration volumes are provided in the following table.

Final Imiglucerase Concentrations and Administration Volumes		
	200 unit vial	400 unit vial
Sterile water for reconstitution	5.1 mL	10.2 mL
Final volume of reconstituted product	5.3 mL	10.6 mL
Concentration after reconstitution	40 units/mL	40 units/mL
Withdrawal volume	5 mL	10 mL
Units of enzyme within final volume	200 units	400 units

A nominal 5 mL for the 200-unit vial (10 mL for the 400 unit vial) is withdrawn from each vial. The appropriate amount of imiglucerase for each patient is diluted with 0.9% sodium chloride injection, to a final volume of 100 to 200 mL. Imiglucerase is administered by IV infusion over 1 to 2 hours. Use aseptic techniques when diluting the dose.

Relatively low toxicity, combined with the extended time course of response, allows small dosage adjustments to be made occasionally to avoid discarding partially used bottles. Thus, the dosage administered in individual infusions may be slightly increased or decreased to fully utilize each vial as long as the monthly administered dosage remains substantially unaltered.

➤*Storage / Stability:* Store at 2° to 8°C (36° to 46°F).

Because imiglucerase does not contain any preservative, promptly dilute vials after reconstitution. Do not store for subsequent use. Imiglucerase, after reconstitution, has been shown to be stable for up to 12 hours when stored at room temperature (25°C; 77°F) and at 2° to 8°C (36° to 46°F). Imiglucerase, when diluted, has been shown to be stable for up to 24 hours when stored at 2° to 8°C (36° to 46°F).

Actions

➤*Pharmacology:* Imiglucerase catalyzes the hydrolysis of glucocerebroside to glucose and ceramide. In clinical trials, imiglucerase improved anemia and thrombocytopenia, reduced spleen and liver size, and decreased cachexia to a degree similar to that observed with alglucerase.

➤*Pharmacokinetics:* During 1-hour IV infusions of 4 imiglucerase doses (7.5, 15, 30, 60 units/kg) for injection, steady-state enzymatic activity was achieved within 30 minutes. Following infusion, plasma enzymatic activity declined rapidly with a half-life ranging from 3.6 to 10.4 minutes. Plasma clearance ranged from 9.8 to 20.3 mL/min/kg, (mean ± SD, 14.5 ± 4 mL/min/kg). The volume of distribution corrected for weight ranged from 0.09 to 0.15 L/kg (0.12 ± 0.02 L/kg). These variables do not appear to be influenced by dose or duration of infusion. However, only 1 or 2 patients were studied at each dose level and infusion rate. The pharmacokinetics of imiglucerase do not appear to be different from placental-derived alglucerase.

In patients who developed IgG antibody to imiglucerase, an apparent effect on serum enzyme levels resulted in diminished volume of distribution and clearance and increased elimination half-life compared to patients without antibody.

Contraindications

There are no known contraindications to the use of imiglucerase. Carefully re-evaluate treatment with imiglucerase if there is significant clinical evidence of hypersensitivity to the product.

Warnings

➤*Antibodies:* To date, approximately 15% of patients treated and tested have developed IgG antibody to imiglucerase for injection during the first year of therapy. Patients who developed IgG antibody largely did so within 6 months of treatment and rarely developed antibodies to imiglucerase for injection after 12 months of therapy. Approximately 46% of patients with detectable IgG antibodies experienced symptoms of hypersensitivity.

Patients with antibody to imiglucerase for injection have a higher risk of hypersensitivity reaction. Conversely, not all patients with symptoms of hypersensitivity have detectable IgG antibody. It is suggested that patients be monitored periodically for IgG antibody formation during the first year of treatment.

➤*Hypersensitivity reactions:* Cautiously approach treatment with imiglucerase in patients who have exhibited symptoms of hypersensitivity to the product.

Anaphylactoid reaction has been reported in less than 1% of the patient population. Cautiously conduct further treatment with imiglucerase. Most patients have successfully continued therapy after a reduction in rate of infusion and pretreatment with antihistamines and/or corticosteroids.

➤*Pregnancy: Category C.* Animal reproduction studies have not been conducted with imiglucerase. It also is not known whether imiglucerase causes fetal harm when administered to a pregnant woman, or affects reproductive capacity. Do not administer imiglucerase during pregnancy except when the indication and need are clear and the potential benefit is judged by the health care provider to substantially justify the risk.

➤*Lactation:* It is not known whether this drug is excreted in human milk. Because many drugs are excreted in human milk, exercise caution when imiglucerase is administered to a nursing woman.

➤*Children:* The safety and efficacy of imiglucerase have been established in patients between 2 and 16 years of age. Use of imiglucerase in this age group is supported by evidence from adequate and well-controlled studies of imiglucerase and alglucerase in adults and pediatric patients, with additional data obtained from the medical literature and from long-term postmarketing experience. Imiglucerase has been administered to patients younger than 2 years of age, however, the safety and effectiveness in patients younger than 2 years of age have not been established.

Precautions

➤*Pulmonary hypertension and pneumonia:* In less than 1% of the patient population, pulmonary hypertension and pneumonia also have been observed during treatment with imiglucerase. Pulmonary hypertension and pneumonia are known complications of Gaucher disease, and have been observed in patients receiving and not receiving imiglucerase. No causal relationship with imiglucerase has been established. Evaluate patients with respiratory symptoms in the absence of fever for the presence of pulmonary hypertension.

Therapy with imiglucerase should be directed by health care providers knowledgeable in the management of patients with Gaucher disease.

➤*Prior treatment with alglucerase:* Caution may be advisable in administration of imiglucerase to patients previously treated with alglucerase and who have developed antibody to alglucerase or who have exhibited symptoms of hypersensitivity to alglucerase.

Adverse Reactions

Experience in patients treated with imiglucerase has revealed that approximately 13.8% of patients experienced adverse events that were judged to be related to imiglucerase administration and occurred with an increase in frequency. Some of the adverse events were related to the route of administration. These include discomfort, pruritus, burning, swelling, or sterile abscess at the site of venipuncture. Each of these events were found to occur in less than 1% of the total patient population.

➤*Hypersensitivity:* Symptoms suggestive of hypersensitivity have been noted in approximately 6.6% of patients. Onset of such symptoms has occurred during or shortly after infusions; these symptoms include pruritus, flushing, urticaria, angioedema, chest discomfort, dyspnea, coughing, cyanosis, and hypotension. Anaphylactoid reaction also has been reported. Each of these events occurred in less than 1.5% of the total patient population. Pretreatment with antihistamines and/or corticosteroids and reduced rate of infusion have allowed continued use of imiglucerase in most patients.

➤*Miscellaneous:* Additional adverse reactions that have been reported in approximately 6.5% of patients treated with imiglucerase include nausea, abdominal pain, vomiting, diarrhea, rash, fatigue, headache, fever, dizziness, chills, backache, and tachycardia. Each of these events occurred in less than 1.5% of the total patient population.

Incidence rates cannot be calculated from the spontaneously reported adverse reactions in the postmarketing database. From this database, the most commonly reported adverse events in children (defined as 2 to 12 years of age) included dyspnea, fever, nausea, flushing, vomiting, and coughing, whereas in adolescents (12 to 16 years of age) and in adults (older than 16 years of age) the most commonly reported reactions included headache, pruritis, and rash.

In addition to the adverse reactions that have been observed in patients treated with imiglucerase, the following adverse reactions have been reported for this therapeutic class of drug: Transient peripheral edema and vomiting.

Overdosage

Experience with doses up to 240 units/kg every 2 weeks have been reported. At that dose there have been no reports of obvious toxicity.

ALGLUCOSIDASE ALFA

Rx	**Myozyme** (Genzyme Corporation)	**Powder for injection, lyophilized:** 50 mg	Preservative free. In 20 mL single-use vials.

ALGLUCOSIDASE ALFA — INJECTION

WARNING

Risk of hypersensitivity reactions – Life-threatening anaphylactic reactions, including anaphylactic shock, have been observed in patients during alglucosidase alfa infusion.

Because of the potential for severe infusion reactions, appropriate medical support measures must be readily available when alglucosidase alfa is administered.

Indications

➤*Pompe disease:* For use in patients with Pompe disease (acid alpha-glucosidase deficiency). Alglucosidase alfa has been shown to improve ventilator-free survival in patients with infantile-onset Pompe disease as compared with an untreated historical control, whereas use of alglucosidase alfa in patients with other forms of Pompe disease has not been adequately studied to assure safety and efficacy.

Administration and Dosage

➤*Approved by the FDA:* April 28, 2006.

➤*Recommended dosage:* 20 mg/kg body weight administered every 2 weeks as an intravenous (IV) infusion. The total volume of infusion is determined by the patient's body weight and should be administered over approximately 4 hours.

➤*Infusion rate:* Infusions should be administered in a step-wise manner using an infusion pump. The initial infusion rate should be no more than 1 mg/kg/h. After patient tolerance to the infusion rate is established, the infusion rate may be increased by 2 mg/kg/h every 30 minutes until a maximum rate of 7 mg/kg/h is reached. Vital signs should be obtained at the end of each step. If the patient is stable, alglucosidase alfa may be administered at the maximum rate of 7 mg/kg/h until the infusion is completed. The infusion rate may be slowed and/or temporarily stopped in the event of infusion reactions. See the following table for the infusion rate at each step, expressed as mL/h based on the recommended infusion volume by patient weight.

Alglucosidase Alfa Recommended Infusion Volumes and Rates

Patient weight range (kg)	Total infusion volume (mL)	Step 1 1 mg/kg/h (mL/h)	Step 2 3 mg/kg/h (mL/h)	Step 3 5 mg/kg/h (mL/h)	Step 4 7 mg/kg/h (mL/h)
1.25 to 10	50	3	8	13	18
10.1 to 20	100	5	15	25	35
20.1 to 30	150	8	23	38	53
30.1 to 35	200	10	30	50	70
35.1 to 50	250	13	38	63	88
50.1 to 60	300	15	45	75	105
60.1 to 100	500	25	75	125	175
100.1 to 120	600	30	90	150	210

➤*Reconstitution/Dilution/Administration:* Alglucosidase alfa should be reconstituted, diluted, and administered by a health care provider. Use aseptic technique during preparation. Do not use filter needles during preparation. Determine the number of vials to be reconstituted based on the patient's weight and the recommended dose of 20 mg/kg.

(Patient weight [kg] × dose [mg/kg] = patient dose [in mg])

(Patient dose [in mg] ÷ 50 mg/vial = number of vials to reconstitute)

If the number of vials includes a fraction, round up to the next whole number. Remove the required number of vials from the refrigerator and allow them to reach room temperature prior to reconstitution (approximately 30 minutes).

Reconstitute each alglucosidase alfa vial by slowly injecting 10.3 mL of sterile water for injection to the inside wall of each vial. Each vial will yield 5 mg/mL. The total extractable dose per vial is 50 mg per 10 mL. Avoid forceful impact of the water for injection on the powder and avoid foaming. This is done by slow drop-wise addition of the water for injection down the inside of the vial and not directly onto the lyophilized cake. Tilt and roll each vial gently. Do not invert, swirl, or shake. The reconstituted alglucosidase alfa solution should be protected from light.

Perform an immediate visual inspection on the reconstituted vials for particulate matter and discoloration. If upon immediate inspection opaque particles are observed or if the solution is discolored, do not use. The reconstituted solution may occasionally contain some alglucosidase alfa particles (typically less than 10 in a vial) in the form of thin white strands or translucent fibers subsequent to the initial inspection. This may also happen following dilution for infusion. These particles have been shown to contain alglucosidase alfa and may appear after the initial reconstitution step and increase over time. Studies have shown that these particles are removed via in-line filtration without having a detectable effect on the purity or strength.

Alglucosidase alfa should be diluted in sodium chloride 0.9% for injection immediately after reconstitution, to a final alglucosidase concentration of 0.5 to 4 mg/mL. See the preceding table for the recommended total infusion volume based on patient weight.

Slowly withdraw the reconstituted solution from each vial. Avoid foaming in the syringe. Remove airspace from the infusion bag to minimize particle formation caused by the sensitivity of alglucosidase alfa to air-liquid interfaces. Add the reconstituted alglucosidase alfa solution slowly and directly into the sodium chloride solution. Do not add directly into airspace that may remain within the infusion bag. Avoid foaming in the infusion bag. Gently invert or massage the infusion bag to mix. Do not shake. The diluted solution should be filtered through a 0.2 mcm, low protein-binding, in-line filter during administration to remove any visible particles.

➤*Admixture incompatibility:* Alglucosidase alfa should not be infused in the same IV line with other products.

➤*Storage/Stability:* Refrigerate between 2° to 8°C (36° to 46°F). Do not use alglucosidase alfa after the expiration date on the vial. Alglucosidase alfa does not contain any preservatives. Vials are single-use only. Any unused product should be discarded.

The reconstituted and diluted solution should be administered without delay. If immediate use is not possible, the reconstituted and diluted solution is stable for up to 24 hours at 2° to 8°C (36° to 46°F). Storage of the reconstituted solution at room temperature is not recommended. The reconstituted and diluted alglucosidase alfa solution should be protected from light. Do not freeze or shake.

Actions

➤*Pharmacology:* Pompe disease (glycogenosis type 2, acid maltase deficiency disease) is an inherited disorder of glycogen metabolism caused by the absence or marked deficiency of the lysosomal enzyme acid alpha-glucosidase.

In the infantile-onset form, Pompe disease results in intralysosomal accumulation of glycogen in various tissues, particularly cardiac and skeletal muscles, and hepatic tissues, leading to the development of cardiomyopathy, progressive muscle weakness, and impairment of respiratory function.

In the juvenile- and adult-onset forms, intralysosomal accumulation of glycogen is limited primarily to skeletal muscle, resulting in progressive muscle weakness. Death in all forms is usually related to respiratory failure.

Alglucosidase alfa provides an exogenous source of acid alpha-glucosidase. Binding to mannose-6-phosphate receptors on the cell surface has been shown to occur via carbohydrate groups on the acid alpha-glucosidase molecule, after which it is internalized and transported into lysosomes, where it undergoes proteolytic cleavage that results in increased enzymatic activity. It then exerts enzymatic activity in cleaving glycogen.

➤*Pharmacokinetics:* The pharmacokinetics of alglucosidase alfa were evaluated in 13 patients ranging from 1 month to 7 months of age with infantile-onset Pompe disease who received alglucosidase alfa 20 mg/kg (as an approximate 4-hour infusion) or 40 mg/kg (as an approximate 6.5-hour infusion) every 2 weeks. The measurement of alglucosidase alfa plasma concentration was based on an activity assay using an artificial substrate. Systemic exposure was approximately dose proportional between the 20 and 40 mg/kg doses (see the following table).

Pharmacokinetic Parameters (Mean ± SD[a]) After Single IV Infusion of Alglucosidase Alfa

Pharmacokinetic parameter	20 mg/kg (n = 5)	40 mg/kg (n = 8)
C_{max}[b] (mcg/mL)	162 ± 31	276 ± 64
AUC_{∞}[c] (mcg-h/mL)	811 ± 141	1,781 ± 520
CL[d] (mL/h/kg)	25 ± 4	24 ± 7
V_{ss}[e] (mL/kg)	96 ± 16	119 ± 28
$t_{½}$[f] (h)	2.3 ± 0.4	2.9 ± 0.5

[a] SD = standard deviation.
[b] C_{max} = maximum effective plasma concentration.
[c] AUC_{∞} = area under the plasma concentration time curve.
[d] CL = clearance.
[e] V_{ss} = apparent volume of distribution.
[f] $t_{½}$ = half-life.

The pharmacokinetics of alglucosidase alfa were also evaluated in a separate trial in 14 patients ranging from 6 months to 3.5 years of age with Pompe disease who received alglucosidase alfa 20 mg/kg as an approximate 4-hour infusion every 2 weeks. The pharmacokinetic parameters were similar to those observed for the 20 mg/kg dose group in the trial of patients ranging from 1 month to 7 months of age.

Nineteen of 21 patients who received treatment with alglucosidase alfa and had pharmacokinetics and antibody titer data available at week 12 developed antibodies to alglucosidase alfa. Five patients with antibody titers greater than or equal to 12,800 at week 12 had an average increase in clearance of 50% (range 5% to 90%) from week 1 to week 12. The other 14 patients with antibody titers less than 12,800 at week 12 had similar average clearance values at week 1 and week 12.

Contraindications

None known.

ALGLUCOSIDASE ALFA — INJECTION

Warnings

➤*Cardiac effects:* Cardiac arrhythmia, including ventricular fibrillation, ventricular tachycardia, and bradycardia, resulting in cardiac arrest or death or requiring cardiac resuscitation or defibrillation have been observed in infantile-onset Pompe disease patients with cardiac hypertrophy, associated with the use of general anesthesia for the placement of a central venous catheter intended for alglucosidase alfa infusion. Use caution when administering general anesthesia for the placement of a central venous catheter in infantile-onset Pompe disease patients with cardiac hypertrophy.

➤*Cardiorespiratory failure:* Acute cardiorespiratory failure requiring intubation and inotropic support has been observed after infusion with alglucosidase alfa in 1 infantile-onset Pompe disease patient with underlying cardiac hypertrophy, possibly associated with fluid overload with IV administration of alglucosidase alfa.

➤*Infusion reactions:* Infusion reactions occurred in 20 of 39 (51%) of patients treated with alglucosidase alfa in clinical studies. Some reactions were severe. Severe infusion reactions reported in more than 1 patient in clinical studies and the expanded access program included cyanosis, decreased oxygen saturation, hypotension, pyrexia, and tachycardia. Other infusion reactions reported in more than 1 patient in clinical studies and the expanded access program included agitation, bronchospasm, cough, cyanosis, decreased oxygen saturation, erythema, face edema, feeling hot, flushing, headache, hyperhidrosis, hypertension, hypotension, increased blood pressure, irritability, lacrimation increased, livedo reticularis, nausea, pallor, periorbital edema, pruritus, pyrexia, rash, restlessness, retching, rigors, tachycardia, tachypnea, tremor, urticaria, vomiting, and wheezing. Some patients were pretreated with antihistamines, antipyretics, and/or steroids. Infusion reactions occurred in some patients after receiving antipyretics, antihistamines, or steroids. Infusion reactions may occur at any time during, or up to 2 hours after, the infusion of alglucosidase alfa, and are more likely with higher infusion rates.

Patients with advanced Pompe disease may have compromised cardiac and respiratory function, which may predispose them to a higher risk of severe complications from infusion reactions. Therefore, monitor these patients more closely during administration of alglucosidase alfa.

If an infusion reaction occurs, regardless of pretreatment, decreasing the infusion rate, temporarily stopping the infusion, and/or administration of antihistamines and/or antipyretics may ameliorate the symptoms. If severe infusion reactions occur, consider immediate discontinuation of the administration of alglucosidase alfa and initiate appropriate medical treatment. Because of the potential for severe infusion reactions, make appropriate medical support measures readily available when administering alglucosidase alfa. Treat patients who have experienced infusion reactions with caution when readministering alglucosidase alfa.

➤*Hypersensitivity reactions:* Serious hypersensitivity reactions, including anaphylactic reactions, have been reported during alglucosidase alfa infusion. Some reactions were life-threatening. One patient developed anaphylactic shock during alglucosidase alfa infusion that required life-support measures.

In clinical trials and expanded access programs with alglucosidase alfa, 38 of 280 (approximately 14%) patients treated with alglucosidase alfa have developed infusion reactions that involved at least 2 of 3 body systems: cutaneous, respiratory, or cardiovascular. Cardiovascular reactions included: bradycardia, cyanosis, flushing, hypertension, hypotension, nodal rhythm, pallor, peripheral coldness, rales, tachycardia, and ventricular extrasystoles. Respiratory reactions included: cough, dyspnea, hypoxia, oxygen saturation decreased, respiratory tract irritation, tachypnea, throat tightness, and wheezing/bronchospasm. Cutaneous reactions included: angioneurotic edema, cold sweat, erythema, hyperhidrosis, livedo reticularis, periorbital edema, pruritus, rash, and urticaria. Of these cases, 8 patients experienced severe or significant hypersensitivity reactions.

If severe hypersensitivity or anaphylactic reactions occur, consider immediate discontinuation of the administration of alglucosidase alfa and initiate appropriate medical treatment. Because of the potential for severe infusion reactions, make appropriate medical support measures readily available when administering alglucosidase alfa.

➤*Elderly:* Clinical studies did not include any subjects 65 years of age and older. It is not known whether they respond differently than younger subjects.

➤*Pregnancy: Category B.* A reproduction study has been performed in pregnant mice at dosages up to 40 mg/kg/day (approximately 0.2 times the recommended human biweekly dosage based on body surface area [BSA]) and has revealed no evidence of impaired fertility or harm to the fetus caused by alglucosidase alfa. There are, however, no adequate and well controlled studies in pregnant women. Because animal reproduction studies are not always predictive of human response, only use this drug during pregnancy if clearly needed. Encourage women of childbearing potential to enroll in the Pompe disease patient registry program.

➤*Lactation:* It is not known whether alglucosidase alfa is excreted in human milk. Because many drugs are excreted in human milk, exercise caution when administering alglucosidase alfa to a breast-feeding woman. Encourage breast-feeding women to participate in the Pompe disease registry program.

➤*Children:* Children 1 month to 3.5 years of age at time of first infusion have been treated with alglucosidase alfa in clinical trials. Other open-label clinical trials of alglucosidase alfa have been performed in older children ranging from 2 to 16 years at the initiation of treatment (juvenile-onset Pompe disease); however, the risks and benefits of alglucosidase alfa treatment have not been established in the juvenile-onset Pompe disease population.

Precautions

➤*Monitoring:* Evaluate liver enzymes prior to the initiation of alglucosidase alfa treatment and periodically thereafter. Exercise care in interpreting these tests because aspartate aminotransferase and alanine aminotransferase levels may also be raised as a result of the muscle pathology in patients with Pompe disease.

Monitor vital signs at the end of each infusion rate increase.

➤*Concomitant illness:* Patients with an acute underlying illness at the time of alglucosidase alfa infusion appear to be at greater risk for infusion reactions. Give careful consideration to the patient's clinical status prior to administration of alglucosidase alfa.

➤*Lab test abnormalities:* There are no marketed tests for antibodies against alglucosidase alfa. If testing is warranted, contact the Genzyme Corporation at 1-800-745-4447.

Drug Interactions

No drug interaction studies have been performed.

Adverse Reactions

The following data reflect exposure of 39 Pompe disease patients to alglucosidase alfa 20 or 40 mg/kg administered every other week in 2 separate clinical trials for periods ranging from 1 to 106 weeks (mean, 61 weeks). Patients were 1 month to 3.5 years of age at first treatment. The population was nearly evenly distributed in gender (18 women and 21 men).

Because clinical trials are conducted under more controlled conditions, the observed adverse reaction rates may not predict the rates observed in patients in clinical practice.

The following table enumerates treatment-emergent adverse reactions (regardless of relationship) that occurred in at least 20% of patients treated with alglucosidase alfa in clinical trials. Reported frequencies of adverse reactions have been classified by *Medical Dictionary for Regulatory Activities* terms.

Alglucosidase Alfa Adverse Reactions (≥ 20%)		
Adverse reaction	Number of patients (n = 39)	Number of adverse reactions
Any adverse reaction	39 (100%)	1,859
Cardiovascular	24 (62%)	
Bradycardia	8 (21%)	18
Tachycardia	9 (23%)	31
Dermatologic	32 (82%)	
Diaper dermatitis	14 (36%)	34
Rash	21 (54%)	72
Urticaria	8 (21%)	25
GI	32 (82%)	
Constipation	9 (23%)	14
Diarrhea	24 (62%)	62
Gastroenteritis	16 (41%)	17
Gastroesophageal reflux disease	10 (26%)	13
Vomiting	19 (49%)	62
Hematologic/Lymphatic	17 (44%)	
Anemia	12 (31%)	23
Respiratory	38 (97%)	
Cough	18 (46%)	69
Pharyngitis	14 (36%)	26
Pneumonia	18 (46%)	43
Respiratory distress	13 (33%)	18
Respiratory failure	12 (31%)	24
Tachypnea	9 (23%)	15
Upper respiratory tract infection	17 (44%)	39
Special senses		
Ear infection	13 (33%)	23
Nasopharyngitis	9 (23%)	25
Otitis media	17 (44%)	35
Rhinorrhea	11 (28%)	16
Miscellaneous		
Bronchiolitis	9 (23%)	10
Catheter-related infection	11 (28%)	15
Flushing	8 (21%)	15
General disorders and administration site conditions	38 (97%)	
Infections and infestations	37 (95%)	
Injury, poisoning, and procedural complications	22 (56%)	
Investigations	28 (72%)	

ALGLUCOSIDASE ALFA — INJECTION

Alglucosidase Alfa Adverse Reactions (≥ 20%)		
Adverse reaction	Number of patients (n = 39)	Number of adverse reactions
Oral candidiasis	12 (31%)	20
Oxygen saturation decreased	16 (41%)	44
Postprocedural pain	10 (26%)	20
Pyrexia	36 (92%)	169
Vascular disorders	14 (36%)	

Five additional juvenile-onset Pompe disease patients were evaluated in a single-center, open-label, nonrandomized, uncontrolled, clinical trial. Patients were 5 to 15 years of age, ambulatory (able to walk at least 10 meters in 6 minutes), and not receiving invasive ventilatory support at study entry. All 5 patients received treatment with alglucosidase alfa 20 mg/kg for 26 weeks. The most common treatment-emergent adverse reactions (regardless of causality) observed with alglucosidase alfa treatment in this study were headache, malaise, pharyngitis, rhinitis, and upper abdominal pain.

➤*Cardiorespiratory failure/anaphylactic reactions:* The most serious adverse reactions reported with alglucosidase alfa were cardiorespiratory failure and anaphylactic reactions. Cardiorespiratory failure, possibly associated with fluid overload, was reported in 1 infantile-onset Pompe disease patient; preexisting cardiac hypertrophy likely contributed to the severity of the reaction. Anaphylactic reactions have been reported during alglucosidase alfa infusion.

➤*Immunogenicity:* The majority of patients (34 of 38; 89%) in the 2 clinical trials tested positive for immunoglobulin G (IgG) antibodies to alglucosidase alfa. The data reflect the percentage of patients whose test results were considered positive for antibodies to alglucosidase alfa using an enzyme-linked immunosorbent assay and radioimmunoprecipitation assay for alglucosidase alfa-specific IgG antibodies. Most patients who develop antibodies do so within the first 3 months of exposure. There is evidence to suggest that patients developing sustained titers of at least 12,800 of anti-alglucosidase alfa antibodies may have a poorer clinical response to treatment, or may lose motor function as antibody titers increase. Test patients who have been treated and experience a decrease in motor function for neutralization of enzyme uptake or activity. Five patients with antibody titers of at least 12,800 at week 12 had an average increase in clearance of 50% from week 1 to week 12.

Infusion reactions were reported in 20 of 39 patients (51%) treated with alglucosidase alfa in clinical studies and appear to be more common in antibody-positive patients: 8 of 15 patients with high antibody titers experienced infusion reactions, whereas none of 3 antibody-negative patients experienced infusion reactions.

Approximately 40 patients in clinical trials and expanded access programs have undergone testing for alglucosidase alfa–specific immunoglobulin E (IgE) antibodies. Testing was performed for infusion reactions, especially moderate to severe or recurrent reactions, for which mast-cell activation was suspected. Three of these patients tested positive for alglucosidase alfa specific IgE binding antibodies, 1 of whom experienced an anaphylactic reaction.

➤*Infusion-related reactions:* The most common adverse reactions requiring intervention were infusion-related reactions. Twenty of 39 patients (51%) treated with alglucosidase alfa in clinical studies developed infusion reactions during the infusion or during the 2 hours following infusion. The majority of these reactions were mild to moderate. Infusion reactions reported in more than 1 patient in clinical studies and the expanded access program included agitation, bronchospasm, cough, cyanosis, decreased oxygen saturations, erythema, face edema, feeling hot, flushing, headache, hyperhidrosis, hypertension, hypotension, increased blood pressure, irritability, lacrimation increased, livedo reticularis, nausea, pallor, periorbital edema, pruritus, pyrexia, rash, retching, restlessness, rigors, tachycardia, tachypnea, tremor, urticaria, vomiting, and wheezing. Most infusion-related reactions requiring intervention were ameliorated with slowing of the infusion rate, temporarily stopping the infusion, and/or administration of antipyretics, antihistamines, or steroids.

➤*Most common:* The most common serious treatment-emergent adverse reactions (regardless of relationship) observed in clinical studies with alglucosidase alfa were catheter-related infection, fever, gastroenteritis, pneumonia, respiratory distress, respiratory failure, and respiratory syncytial virus infection.

The most common treatment-emergent adverse reactions (regardless of relationship) were cough, decreased oxygen saturation, diarrhea, fever, gastroenteritis, otitis media, pneumonia, rash, upper respiratory tract infection, and vomiting.

Overdosage

There have been no reports of overdose with alglucosidase alfa. In clinical trials, patients received doses up to 40 mg/kg of body weight.

➤*Animal toxicology:* Results from 2 IV, repeated dose animal toxicology studies using doses of alglucosidase alfa 100 or 200 mg/kg (approximately 1.6 to 3.2 times the recommended human dose based on BSA) in Cynomolgus monkeys to evaluate the possibility of liver accumulation over time showed acid alpha-glucosidase levels above background in liver tissue several days following the last dose; however, no concurrent changes in liver enzymes or histopathology were observed.

Patient Information

Inform patients and their caregivers that a registry for patients with Pompe disease has been established in order to better understand the variability and progression of Pompe disease and to continue to monitor and evaluate treatments. Encourage patients and their caregivers to participate and advise them that their participation may involve long-term follow-up. Information regarding the registry program may be found at http://www.pomperegistry.com or by calling 1-800-745-4447.

CALCITONIN-SALMON

CALCITONIN-SALMON

Rx	**Miacalcin** (Novartis)	**Injection:** 200 units/mL	With phenol. In 2 mL vials.
Rx	**Fortical** (Upsher-Smith)	**Nasal spray:** 200 units/activation (0.09 mL/dose)	Sodium chloride, benzyl alcohol, phenylethyl alcohol. In 3.7 mL metered- dose, glass bottle with pump.
Rx	**Miacalcin** (Novartis)		8.5 mg sodium chloride. In 2 mL metered-dose, glass bottle with pump.

CALCITONIN-SALMON — INJECTION

Indications

➤*Paget disease:* At the present time, effectiveness has been demonstrated principally in patients with moderate to severe disease characterized by polyostotic involvement with elevated serum alkaline phosphatase and urinary hydroxyproline excretion.

➤*Hypercalcemia:* For early treatment of hypercalcemic emergencies, along with other appropriate agents, when a rapid decrease in serum calcium is required, until more specific treatment of the underlying disease can be accomplished. It may also be added to existing therapeutic regimens for hypercalcemia such as intravenous fluids and furosemide, oral phosphate or corticosteroids, or other agents.

➤*Postmenopausal osteoporosis:* For the treatment of postmenopausal osteoporosis in females greater than 5 years postmenopause with low bone mass relative to healthy premenopausal females. Calcitonin-salmon injection should be reserved for patients who refuse or cannot tolerate estrogens or in whom estrogens are contraindicated. Use of calcitonin-salmon injection is recommended in conjunction with adequate calcium and vitamin D intake to prevent the progressive loss of bone mass.

No evidence currently exists to indicate whether or not calcitonin-salmon decreases the risk of vertebral crush fractures or spinal deformity. A recent controlled study, which was discontinued prior to completion because of questions regarding its design and implementation, failed to demonstrate any benefit of salmon calcitonin on fracture rate. No adequate controlled trials have examined the effect of salmon calcitonin injection on vertebral bone mineral density beyond 1 year of treatment. Two (2) placebo-controlled studies with salmon calcitonin have shown an increase in total body calcium at 1 year, followed by a trend to decreasing total body calcium (still above baseline) at 2 years. The minimum effective dose of calcitonin-salmon for prevention of vertebral bone mineral density loss has not been established.

It has been suggested that those postmenopausal patients having increased rates of bone turnover may be more likely to respond to antiresorptive agents such as calcitonin-salmon.

Administration and Dosage

➤*Skin testing:* For patients with suspected sensitivity to calcitonin, skin testing should be considered prior to treatment. Prepare a dilution at 10 units/mL by withdrawing 0.05 mL of the 200 units/mL solution in a tuberculin syringe and filling it to 1 mL with sodium chloride injection. Mix well, discard 0.9 mL and inject intracutaneously 0.1 mL (approximately 1 unit) on the inner aspect of the forearm. Observe the injection site 15 minutes after injection. The appearance of more than mild erythema or wheal constitutes a positive response. Physicians may wish to refer patients who require skin testing to an allergist.

➤*Paget disease:* The recommended starting dose of calcitonin-salmon in Paget's disease is 100 units (0.5 mL) per day administered subcutaneously (preferred for outpatient self-administration) or intramuscularly. Drug effect should be monitored by periodic measurement of serum alkaline phosphatase and 24-hour urinary hydroxyproline (if available) and evaluations of symptoms. A decrease toward normal of the biochemical abnormalities is usually seen, if it is going to occur, within the first few months. Bone pain may also decrease during that time. Improvement of neurologic lesions, when it occurs, requires a longer period of treatment, often more than 1 year.

In many patients, doses of 50 units (0.25 mL) per day or every other day are sufficient to maintain biochemical and clinical improvement. At the present time, however, there are insufficient data to determine whether this reduced dose will have the same effect as the higher dose on forming more normal bone structure. It appears preferable, therefore, to maintain the higher dose in any patient with serious deformity or neurological involvement.

CALCITONIN-SALMON — INJECTION

In any patient with a good response initially who later relapses, either clinically or biochemically, the possibility of antibody formation should be explored. The patient may be tested for antibodies by an appropriate specialized test or evaluated for the possibility of antibody formation by critical clinical evaluation.

Patient compliance should also be assessed in the event of relapse.

In patients who relapse, whether because of antibodies or for unexplained reasons, a dosage increase beyond 100 units/day does not usually appear to elicit an improved response.

➤*Hypercalcemia:* The recommended starting dose of calcitonin-salmon injection, synthetic in hypercalcemia is 4 units/kg body weight every 12 hours by subcutaneous or intramuscular injection. If the response to this dose is not satisfactory after 1 or 2 days, the dose may be increased to 8 units/kg every 12 hours. If the response remains unsatisfactory after 2 more days, the dose may be further increased to a maximum of 8 units/kg every 6 hours. If the volume to be injected exceeds 2 mL, intramuscular injection is preferable and multiple sites of injection should be used.

➤*Postmenopausal osteoporosis:* The minimum effective dose of salmon calcitonin for the prevention of vertebral bone mineral density loss has not been established. Data from a single 1-year placebo-controlled study with salmon calcitonin injection suggested that 100 units (subcutaneously or intramuscularly) every other day might be effective in preserving vertebral bone mineral density. Baseline and interval monitoring of biochemical markers of bone resorption/turnover (eg, fasting AM, second-voided urine hydroxyproline to creatinine ratio) and of bone mineral density may be useful in achieving the minimum effective dose. Patients should also receive supplemental calcium such as calcium carbonate 1.5 g daily and an adequate vitamin D intake (400 units daily). An adequate diet is also essential.

If the volume to be injected exceeds 2 mL, intramuscular injection is preferable and multiple sites of injection should be used.

➤*Storage / Stability:* Store in refrigerator between 2° to 8°C (36° to 46°F).

Actions

➤*Pharmacology:* Calcitonin acts primarily on bone, but direct renal effects and actions on the gastrointestinal tract are also recognized. Calcitonin-salmon appears to have actions essentially identical to calcitonins of mammalian origin, but its potency per mg is greater and it has a longer duration of action. The actions of calcitonin on bone and its role in normal human bone physiology are still incompletely understood.

Bone – Single injections of calcitonin cause a marked transient inhibition of the ongoing bone resorptive process. With prolonged use, there is a persistent, smaller decrease in the rate of bone resorption. Histologically, this is associated with a decreased number of osteoclasts and an apparent decrease in their resorptive activity. Decreased osteocytic resorption may also be involved. There is some evidence that initially bone formation may be augmented by calcitonin through increased osteoblastic activity. However, calcitonin will probably not induce a long-term increase in bone formation.

Animal studies indicate that endogenous calcitonin, primarily through its action on bone, participates with parathyroid hormone in the homeostatic regulation of blood calcium. Thus, high blood calcium levels cause increased secretion of calcitonin which, in turn, inhibits bone resorption. This reduces the transfer of calcium from bone to blood and tends to return blood calcium to the normal level. The importance of this process in humans has not been determined. In healthy adults, who have a relatively low rate of bone resorption, the administration of exogenous calcitonin results in only a slight decrease in serum calcium. In healthy children and in patients with generalized Paget's disease, bone resorption is more rapid and decreases in serum calcium are more pronounced in response to calcitonin.

Paget disease of bone (osteitis deformans) –

Calcitonin-salmon, presumably by an initial blocking effect on bone resorption, causes a decreased rate of bone turnover with a resultant fall in the serum alkaline phosphatase and urinary hydroxyproline excretion in approximately ⅔ of patients treated. These biochemical changes appear to correspond to changes toward more normal bone, as evidenced by a small number of documented examples of:

1.) Radiologic regression of Pagetic lesions,
2.) Improvement of impaired auditory nerve and other neurologic function,
3.) Decreases (measured) in abnormally elevated cardiac output. These improvements occur extremely rarely, if ever, and spontaneously, and are not predictable (elevated cardiac output may disappear over a period of years when the disease slowly enters a sclerotic phase; in the cases treated with calcitonin, however, the decreases were seen in less than 1 year.)

Some patients with Paget disease who have good biochemical or symptomatic responses initially, later relapse. Suggested explanations have included the formation of neutralizing antibodies and the development of secondary hyperparathyroidism, but neither suggestion appears to explain adequately the majority of relapses.

Although the parathyroid hormone levels do appear to rise transiently during each hypocalcemic response to calcitonin, most investigators have been unable to demonstrate persistent hypersecretion of parathyroid hormone in patients treated chronically with calcitonin-salmon.

Circulating antibodies to calcitonin after 2 to 18 months of treatment have been reported in about half of the patients with Paget disease in whom antibody studies were done, but calcitonin treatment remained effective in many of these cases. Occasionally, patients with high antibody titers are found. These patients usually will have suffered a biochemical relapse of Paget disease and are unresponsive to the acute hypocalcemic effects of calcitonin.

Hypercalcemia – In clinical trials, calcitonin-salmon has been shown to lower the elevated serum calcium of patients with carcinoma (with or without demonstrated metastases), multiple myeloma or primary hyperparathyroidism (lesser response). Patients with higher values for serum calcium tend to show greater reduction during calcitonin therapy. The decrease in calcium occurs about 2 hours after the first injection and lasts for about 6 to 8 hours. Calcitonin-salmon given every 12 hours maintained a calcium lowering effect for about 5 to 8 days, the time period evaluated for most patients during the clinical studies. The average reduction of 8-hour post-injection serum calcium during this period was about 9%.

Kidney – Calcitonin increases the excretion of filtered phosphate, calcium, and sodium by decreasing their tubular reabsorption. In some patients, the inhibition of bone resorption by calcitonin is of such magnitude that the consequent reduction of filtered calcium load more than compensates for the decrease in tubular reabsorption of calcium. The result in these patients is a decrease rather than an increase in urinary calcium.

Transient increases in sodium and water excretion may occur after the initial injection of calcitonin. In most patients, these changes return to pretreatment levels with continued therapy.

GI tract – Increasing evidence indicates that calcitonin has significant actions on the gastrointestinal tract. Short-term administration results in marked transient decreases in the volume and acidity of gastric juice and in the volume and the trypsin and amylase content of pancreatic juice. Whether these effects continue to be elicited after each injection of calcitonin during chronic therapy has not been investigated.

➤*Pharmacokinetics:* Peak plasma concentration time for the injection is 16 to 25 minutes.

The metabolism of calcitonin-salmon has not yet been studied clinically. Information from animal studies with calcitonin-salmon and from clinical studies with calcitonins of porcine and human origin suggest that calcitonin-salmon is rapidly metabolized by conversion to smaller inactive fragments, primarily in the kidneys, but also in the blood and peripheral tissues. A small amount of unchanged hormone and its inactive metabolites are excreted in the urine.

It appears that calcitonin-salmon cannot cross the placental barrier and its passage to the cerebrospinal fluid or to breast milk has not been determined.

Contraindications

Clinical allergy to synthetic calcitonin-salmon.

Warnings

➤*Hypersensitivity reactions:* Because calcitonin is protein in nature, the possibility of a systemic allergic reaction exists. Administration of calcitonin-salmon has been reported in a few cases to cause serious allergic-type reactions (eg, bronchospasm, swelling of the tongue or throat, and anaphylactic shock), and in 1 case, death attributed to anaphylaxis. The usual provisions should be made for the emergency treatment of such a reaction should it occur. Allergic reactions should be differentiated from generalized flushing and hypotension.

➤*Carcinogenesis:* The incidence of osteogenic sarcoma is known to be increased in Pagets disease. Pagetic lesions, with or without therapy, may appear by X-ray to progress markedly, possibly with some loss of definition of periosteal margins. Such lesions should be evaluated carefully to differentiate these from osteogenic sarcoma.

An increased incidence of pituitary adenomas has been observed in 1-year toxicity studies in Sprague-Dawley rats administered calcitonin-salmon at dosages of 20 and 80 units/kg/day and in Fisher 344 rats given 80 units/kg/day. The relevance of these findings to humans is unknown.

➤*Pregnancy: Category C.*

Teratogenic – Calcitonin-salmon has been shown to cause a decrease in fetal birth weights in rabbits when given in doses 14 to 56 times the dose recommended for human use. Since calcitonin does not cross the placental barrier, this finding may be due to metabolic effects on the pregnant animal. There are no adequate and well-controlled studies in pregnant women. Calcitonin-salmon injection, synthetic should be used during pregnancy only if the potential benefit justifies the potential risk to the fetus.

➤*Lactation:* It is not known whether this drug is excreted in human milk. As a general rule, nursing should not be undertaken while a patient is on this drug because many drugs are excreted in human milk. Calcitonin has been shown to inhibit lactation in animals.

➤*Children:* Disorders of bone in children referred to as juvenile Paget disease have been reported rarely. The relationship of these disorders to adult Paget disease has not been established and experience with the use of calcitonin in these disorders is very limited. There is no adequate data to support the use of calcitonin-salmon injection, synthetic in children.

Precautions

➤*Hypocalcemic tetany:* The administration of calcitonin possibly could lead to hypocalcemic tetany under special circumstances although no cases have yet been reported. Provisions for parenteral calcium administration should be available during the first several administrations of calcitonin.

➤*Lab test abnormalities:* Periodic examinations of urine sediment of patients on chronic therapy are recommended.

Coarse granular casts and casts containing renal tubular epithelial cells were reported in young adult volunteers at bed rest who were given calcitonin-salmon to study the effect of immobilization on osteoporosis. There was no other evidence of renal abnormality and the urine sediment became normal after calcitonin was stopped. Urine sediment abnormalities have not been reported by other investigators.

Adverse Reactions

➤*Dermatologic:* Local inflammatory reactions at the site of subcutaneous or intramuscular injection have been reported in about 10% of patients.

CALCITONIN-SALMON — INJECTION

Flushing of face or hands occurred in about 2% to 5% of patients. Skin rashes and pruritus of the ear lobes have also been reported.

➤*GI:* Nausea with or without vomiting has been noted in about 10% of patients treated with calcitonin. It is most evident when treatment is first initiated and tends to decrease or disappear with continued administration.

➤*Miscellaneous:* Nocturia, feverish sensation, pain in the eyes, poor appetite, abdominal pain, edema of feet, and salty taste have been reported in patients treated with calcitonin-salmon. Administration of calcitonin-salmon has been reported in a few cases to cause serious allergic-type reactions (eg, bronchospasm, swelling of the tongue or throat, and anaphylactic shock), and in 1 case, death attributed to anaphylaxis. The usual provisions should be made for the emergency treatment of such a reaction should it occur. Allergic reactions should be differentiated from generalized flushing and hypotension.

Overdosage

A dose of 1,000 units subcutaneously may produce nausea and vomiting as the only adverse effects. Doses of 32 units/kg/day for 1 to 2 days demonstrate no other adverse effects.

Data on chronic high dose administration are insufficient to judge toxicity.

Patient Information

Careful instruction in sterile injection technique should be given to the patient, and to other persons who may administer calcitonin-salmon injection, synthetic.

CALCITONIN-SALMON — INTRANASAL

Indications

➤*Postmenopausal osteoporosis:* For the treatment of postmenopausal osteoporosis in females more than 5 years postmenopause with low bone mass relative to healthy premenopausal females. Reserve calcitonin-salmon nasal spray for patients who refuse or cannot tolerate estrogens or in whom estrogens are contraindicated. Use of calcitonin-salmon nasal spray is recommended in conjunction with an adequate calcium (at least 1,000 mg elemental calcium per day) and vitamin D (400 units/day) intake to retard the progressive loss of bone mass. An adequate diet is also essential. The evidence of efficacy is based on increases in spinal bone mineral density observed in clinical trials.

Administration and Dosage

➤*Approved by the FDA:* March 29, 1991.

➤*Dose:* The recommended dose of calcitonin-salmon nasal spray in postmenopausal osteoporotic females is 1 spray (200 units) per day administered intranasally, alternating nostrils daily.

➤*Priming (activation) of pump:* Before the first dose and administration, bring calcitonin-salmon nasal spray to room temperature. To prime the pump, hold the bottle upright and depress the 2 white side arms of the pump toward the bottle until a full spray is produced. The pump is primed once the first full spray is emitted. To administer, carefully place the nozzle into the nostril with the head in the upright position, and firmly depress the pump toward the bottle. Do not prime the pump before each daily dose.

➤*Storage/Stability:* Store unopened bottle(s) in refrigerator between 2° to 8°C (36° to 46°F). Protect from freezing.

Store bottle in use at room temperature between 15° and 30°C (59° to 86°F) in an upright position, for up to 35 days. Each bottle contains at least 30 doses.

Discard all unrefrigerated bottles after 30 days.

Actions

➤*Pharmacology:* Calcitonin acts primarily on bone, but direct renal effects and actions on the GI tract are also recognized. Calcitonin-salmon appears to have actions essentially identical to calcitonins of mammalian origin, but its potency per mg is greater and it has a longer duration of action.

The following information describing the clinical pharmacology of calcitonin has been derived from studies with injectable calcitonin. The mean bioavailability of calcitonin-salmon nasal spray is approximately 3% of that of injectable calcitonin in healthy subjects and, therefore, the conclusions concerning the clinical pharmacology of this preparation may be different.

The actions of calcitonin on bone and its role in normal human bone physiology are still not completely elucidated, although calcitonin receptors have been discovered in osteoclasts and osteoblasts.

Single injections of calcitonin cause a marked transient inhibition of the ongoing bone resorptive process. With prolonged use, there is a persistent, smaller decrease in the rate of bone resorption. Histologically, this is associated with a decreased number of osteoclasts and an apparent decrease in their resorptive activity. In vitro studies have shown that calcitonin-salmon causes inhibition of osteoclast function with loss of the ruffled osteoclast border responsible for resorption of bone. This activity resumes following removal of calcitonin-salmon from the test system. There is some evidence from the in vitro studies that bone formation may be augmented by calcitonin through increased osteoblastic activity.

Animal studies indicate that endogenous calcitonin, primarily through its action on bone, participates with parathyroid hormone in the homeostatic regulation of blood calcium. Thus, high blood calcium levels cause increased secretion of calcitonin that, in turn, inhibits bone resorption. This reduces the transfer of calcium from bone to blood and tends to return blood calcium towards the normal level. The importance of this process in humans has not been determined. In healthy adults who have a relatively low rate of bone resorption, the administration of exogenous calcitonin results in only a slight decrease in serum calcium in the limits of the normal range. In healthy children and in patients with Paget disease in whom bone resorption is more rapid, decreases in serum calcium are more pronounced in response to calcitonin.

Bone biopsy and radial bone mass studies at baseline and after 26 months of daily injectable calcitonin indicate that calcitonin therapy results in formation of normal bone.

Postmenopausal osteoporosis –

Calcitonin-salmon given by the intranasal route has been shown to increase spinal bone mass in postmenopausal women with established osteoporosis but not in early postmenopausal women.

Calcium homeostasis – In 2 clinical studies designed to evaluate the pharmacodynamic response to calcitonin-salmon nasal spray, administration of 100 to 1,600 units to healthy volunteers resulted in rapid and sustained small decreases (but still within the normal range) in both total serum calcium and serum ionized calcium. Single doses greater than 400 units did not produce any further biological response to the drug. The development of hypocalcemia has not been reported in studies in healthy volunteers or postmenopausal females.

Kidney – Studies with injectable calcitonin show increases in the excretion of filtered phosphate, calcium, and sodium by decreasing their tubular reabsorption. Comparable studies have not been carried out with calcitonin-salmon nasal spray.

GI tract – Some evidence from studies with injectable preparations suggest that calcitonin may have significant actions on the GI tract. Short-term administration of injectable calcitonin results in marked transient decreases in the volume and acidity of gastric juice and in the volume and the trypsin and amylase content of pancreatic juice. Whether these effects continue to be elicited after each injection of calcitonin during chronic therapy has not been investigated. These studies have not been conducted with calcitonin-salmon nasal spray.

➤*Pharmacokinetics:*

Absorption/Distribution – The data on bioavailability of calcitonin-salmon nasal spray obtained by various investigators using different methods show great variability. Calcitonin-salmon nasal spray is absorbed rapidly by the nasal mucosa. Peak plasma concentrations of drug appear 31 to 39 minutes after nasal administration compared with 16 to 25 minutes following parenteral dosing. In healthy volunteers approximately 3% (range, 0.3% to 30.6%) of a nasally administered dose is bioavailable compared with the same dose administered by intramuscular (IM) injection.

There is no accumulation of the drug on repeated nasal administration at 10-hour intervals for up to 15 days. Absorption of nasally administered calcitonin has not been studied in postmenopausal women.

Metabolism/Excretion – The half-life of elimination of calcitonin-salmon is calculated to be 43 minutes.

Animal studies suggest that calcitonin is rapidly converted to smaller inactive fragments, primarily in the kidneys but also in the blood and peripheral tissues. A small amount of unchanged hormone and its inactive metabolites are excreted in the urine.

Contraindications

Clinical allergies to calcitonin-salmon.

Warnings

➤*Hypersensitivity reactions:* Because calcitonin is a polypeptide, the possibility of a systemic allergic reaction exists. A few cases of allergic-type reactions have been reported in patients receiving calcitonin-salmon nasal spray, including 1 case of anaphylactic shock, which appears to have been caused by the preservative because the patient could tolerate injectable calcitonin-salmon without incident. With injectable calcitonin-salmon there have been a few reports of serious allergic-type reactions (eg, bronchospasm, swelling of the tongue or throat, anaphylactic shock, and in 1 case death attributed to anaphylaxis). Make the usual provisions for the emergency treatment of such a reaction if it should occur. Allergic reactions should be differentiated from generalized flushing and hypotension.

For patients with suspected sensitivity to calcitonin, consider skin testing prior to treatment utilizing a dilute, sterile solution of calcitonin-salmon synthetic injection. Health care providers may wish to refer patients who require skin testing to an allergist.

➤*Carcinogenesis:* An increased incidence of nonfunctioning pituitary adenomas has been observed in 1-year toxicity studies in Sprague-Dawley and Fischer 344 rats administered subcutaneously calcitonin-salmon at dosages of 80 units/kg/day (16 to 19 times the recommended human parenteral dose and about 130 to 160 times the human intranasal dose based on body surface area). The findings suggest that calcitonin-salmon reduced the latency period for development of pituitary adenomas that do not produce hormones, probably through the perturbation of physiologic processes involved in the evolution of this commonly occurring endocrine lesion in the rat. Although administration of calcitonin-salmon reduces the latency period of the development of nonfunctional proliferative lesions in rats, it did not induce the hyperplastic/neoplastic process.

CALCITONIN-SALMON — INTRANASAL

➤*Pregnancy: Category C.*

Teratogenic – Calcitonin-salmon has been shown to cause a decrease in fetal birth weights in rabbits when given by injection in doses 8 to 33 times the parenteral dose and 70 to 278 times the intranasal dose recommended for human use based on body surface area.

Because calcitonin does not cross the placental barrier, this finding may be due to metabolic effects on the pregnant animal. There are no adequate and well-controlled studies in pregnant women with calcitonin-salmon. Calcitonin-salmon nasal spray is not indicated for use in pregnancy.

➤*Lactation:* It is not known whether this drug is excreted in human milk. As a general rule, a patient should not breastfeed while on this drug because many drugs are excreted in human milk. Calcitonin has been shown to inhibit lactation in animals.

➤*Children:* There are no data to support the use of calcitonin-salmon nasal spray in children. Disorders of bone in children referred to as idiopathic juvenile osteoporosis have been reported rarely. The relationship of these disorders to postmenopausal osteoporosis has not been established and experience with the use of calcitonin in these disorders is very limited.

Precautions

➤*Periodic nasal examinations:* Periodic nasal examinations with visualization of the nasal mucosa, turbinates, septum and mucosal blood vessel status are recommended.

➤*Nasal mucosal alterations:* The development of mucosal alterations or transient nasal conditions occurred in up to 9% of patients who received calcitonin-salmon nasal spray and in up to 12% of patients who received placebo nasal spray in studies in postmenopausal females. The majority of patients (approximately 90%) in whom nasal abnormalities were noted also reported nasally related complaints/symptoms as adverse reactions. Therefore, perform a nasal examination prior to start of treatment with nasal calcitonin and at any time nasal complaints occur.

In all postmenopausal patients treated with calcitonin-salmon nasal spray, the most commonly reported nasal adverse reactions included rhinitis (12%), epistaxis (3.5%), and sinusitis (2.3%). Smoking was shown not to have any contributory effect on the occurrence of nasal adverse events. One patient (0.3%) treated with calcitonin-salmon nasal spray who was receiving 400 units daily developed a small nasal wound. In clinical trials in another disorder (Paget disease), 2.8% of patients developed nasal ulcerations.

If severe ulceration of the nasal mucosa occurs, as indicated by ulcers greater than 1.5 mm in diameter or penetrating below the mucosa, or those associated with heavy bleeding, discontinue calcitonin-salmon nasal spray. Although smaller ulcers often heal without withdrawal of calcitonin-salmon nasal spray, discontinue medication temporarily until healing occurs.

➤*Lab test abnormalities:* Urine sediment abnormalities have not been reported in ambulatory volunteers treated with calcitonin-salmon nasal spray. Coarse granular casts containing renal tubular epithelial cells were reported in young adult volunteers at bed rest who were given injectable calcitonin-salmon to study the effect of immobilization on osteoporosis. There was no evidence of renal abnormality, and the urine sediment became normal after calcitonin was stopped. Consider periodic examinations of urine sediment.

Drug Interactions

Currently, no drug interactions with calcitonin-salmon have been observed. The effects of prior use of diphosphonates in postmenopausal osteoporosis patients have not been assessed; however, in patients with Paget disease prior diphosphonate use appears to reduce the antiresorptive response to calcitonin-salmon nasal spray.

Adverse Reactions

The incidence of adverse reactions reported in studies involving postmenopausal osteoporotic patients chronically exposed to calcitonin-salmon nasal spray (n = 341) and to placebo nasal spray (n = 131) and reported in greater than 3% of calcitonin-salmon nasal spray-treated patients are presented in the following table. Most adverse reactions were mild to moderate in severity. Nasal adverse reactions were most common, with 70% mild, 25% moderate, and 5% severe in nature (placebo rates were 71% mild, 27% moderate, and 2% severe).

Adverse Reactions Occurring in at Least 3% of Postmenopausal Patients Treated Chronically		
	Calcitonin-salmon nasal spray (n = 341)	Placebo (n = 131)
Adverse reaction	% of patients	% of patients
Arthralgia	3.8%	5.3%
Back pain	5%	2.3%
Epistaxis	3.5%	4.6%
Headache	3.2%	4.6%
Rhinitis	12%	6.9%
Symptom of nose[a]	10.6%	16%

[a] Symptom of nose includes nasal crusts, dryness, redness or erythema, nasal sores, irritation, itching, thick feeling, soreness, pallor, infection, stenosis, runny/blocked, small wound, bleeding wound, tenderness, uncomfortable feeling, and sore across bridge of nose.

In addition, the following adverse reactions were reported in fewer than 3% of patients during chronic therapy with calcitonin-salmon nasal spray. Adverse reactions reported in 1% to 3% of patients are identified. The remainder occurred in less than 1% of patients. Other than flushing, nausea, possible allergic reactions, and possible local irritative effects in the respiratory tract, a relationship to calcitonin-salmon nasal spray has not been established.

➤*Cardiovascular:* Angina pectoris (1% to 3%), bundle branch block (less than 1%), hypertension (1% to 3%), myocardial infarction (less than 1%), palpitation (less than 1%), tachycardia (less than 1%).

Vascular – Cerebrovascular accident (less than 1%), flushing (less than 1%), thrombophlebitis (less than 1%).

➤*CNS:* Agitation (less than 1%), dizziness (1% to 3%), migraine (less than 1%), neuralgia (less than 1%), paresthesia (1% to 3%), vertigo (less than 1%).

➤*Dermatologic:* Alopecia (less than 1%), eczema (less than 1%), erythematous rash (1% to 3%), increased sweating (less than 1%), pruritus (less than 1%), skin ulceration (less than 1%).

➤*Endocrine:* Goiter (less than 1%), hyperthyroidism (less than 1%).

➤*GI:* Abdominal pain (1% to 3%), constipation (1% to 3%), diarrhea (1% to 3%), dry mouth (less than 1%), dyspepsia (1% to 3%), flatulence (less than 1%), gastritis (less than 1%), increased appetite (less than 1%), nausea (1% to 3%), vomiting (less than 1%).

➤*Hematologic/Lymphatic:* Anemia (less than 1%), infection (1% to 3%), lymphadenopathy (1% to 3%).

➤*Hepatic:* Cholelithiasis (less than 1%), hepatitis (less than 1%).

➤*Metabolic:* Weight increase (less than 1%).

➤*Musculoskeletal:* Arthritis (less than 1%), arthrosis (1% to 3%), myalgia (1% to 3%), polymyalgia rheumatica (less than 1%), stiffness (less than 1%).

➤*Renal:* Cystitis (1% to 3%), hematuria (less than 1%), pyelonephritis (less than 1%), renal calculus (less than 1%).

➤*Ophthalmic:* Abnormal lacrimation (1% to 3%), blurred vision (less than 1%), conjunctivitis (1% to 3%), vitreous floater (less than 1%).

➤*Psychiatric:* Anorexia (less than 1%), anxiety (less than 1%), depression (1% to 3%); insomnia (less than 1%).

➤*Respiratory:* Bronchitis (less than 1%), bronchospasm (1% to 3%), coughing (less than 1%), dyspnea (less than 1%), pharyngitis (less than 1%), pneumonia (less than 1%), sinusitis (1% to 3%), upper respiratory tract infection (1% to 3%).

➤*Special senses:* Earache (less than 1%), hearing loss (less than 1%), parosmia (less than 1%), taste perversion (less than 1%), thirst (less than 1%), tinnitus (less than 1%).

➤*Miscellaneous:* Fatigue (1% to 3%), fever (less than 1%), influenza-like symptoms (1% to 3%), periorbital edema (less than 1%).

➤*Common adverse reactions associated with the use of injectable calcitonin-salmon vs calcitonin-salmon nasal spray:* Common adverse reactions associated with the use of injectable calcitonin-salmon occurred less frequently in patients treated with calcitonin-salmon nasal spray than in those patients treated with injectable calcitonin. Nausea, with or without vomiting, which occurred in 1.8% of patients treated with the nasal spray (and 1.5% of those receiving placebo nasal spray) occurs in about 10% of patients who take injectable calcitonin-salmon. Flushing, which occurred in less than 1% of patients treated with the nasal spray, occurs in 2% to 5% of patients treated with injectable calcitonin-salmon. Although the administered dosages of injectable and nasal spray calcitonin-salmon are comparable (50 to 100 units daily of injectable versus 200 units daily of nasal spray), the nasal dosage form has a mean bioavailability of about 3% (range 0.3% to 30.6%) and therefore provides less drug to the systemic circulation, possibly accounting for the decrease in frequency of adverse reactions.

Overdosage

No instances of overdose with calcitonin-salmon nasal spray have been reported and no serious adverse reactions have been associated with high doses. There is no known potential for drug abuse for calcitonin-salmon.

Single doses of calcitonin-salmon nasal spray up to 1,600 units, doses up to 800 units/day for 3 days and chronic administration of doses up to 600 units/day have been studied without serious adverse effects. A dose of 1,000 units of calcitonin-salmon injectable solution given subcutaneously may produce nausea and vomiting. A dose of calcitonin-salmon injectable solution of 32 units/kg/day for 1 or 2 days demonstrated no additional adverse effects.

There have been no reports of hypocalcemic tetany. However, the pharmacologic actions of calcitonin-salmon nasal spray suggest that this could occur in overdose. Therefore, provisions for parenteral administration of calcium should be available for the treatment of overdose.

Patient Information

Give careful instructions on pump assembly, priming of the pump, and nasal introduction of calcitonin-salmon nasal spray to the patient. Although instructions for patients are supplied with individual bottles, demonstrate procedures for use to each patient. Patients should notify their doctors if they develop significant nasal irritation.

Advise patients of the following:

- Store new, unassembled bottles in the refrigerator between 2° to 8°C (36° to 46°F).
- Protect the product from freezing.
- Before priming the pump and using a new bottle, allow it to reach room temperature.
- Store bottle in use at room temperature between 15° to 30°C (59° to 86°F) in an upright position, for up to 30 days. Each bottle contains at least 30 doses.

CALCITONIN-SALMON — INTRANASAL

You should keep track of the number of doses used from the bottle. After 30 doses, each spray may not deliver the correct amount of medication, even if the bottle is not completely empty.

CALCIMIMETICS

CINACALCET HYDROCHLORIDE

Rx	**Sensipar** (Amgen)	**Tablets:** 30 mg (as base)	(AMGEN 30). Light-green, oval. Film-coated. In 30s.
		60 mg (as base)	(AMGEN 60). Light-green, oval. Film-coated. In 30s.
		90 mg (as base)	(AMGEN 90). Light-green, oval. Film-coated. In 30s.

CINACALCET HYDROCHLORIDE — ORAL

Indications

➤*Secondary hyperparathyroidism (HPT):* For the treatment of secondary hyperparathyroidism in patients with chronic kidney disease on dialysis.

➤*Hypercalcemia:* For the treatment of hypercalcemia in patients with parathyroid carcinoma.

Administration and Dosage

➤*Approved by the FDA:* March 8, 2004.

Take tablets whole and do not divide. Take with food or shortly after a meal.

Individualize dosage.

➤*Secondary hyperparathyroidism in patients with chronic kidney disease on dialysis:* The recommended starting oral dose of cinacalcet is 30 mg once daily. Measure serum calcium and serum phosphorus within 1 week, and measure iPTH 1 to 4 weeks after initiation or dose adjustment of cinacalcet. Titrate cinacalcet no more frequently than every 2 to 4 weeks through sequential doses of 60, 90, 120, and 180 mg once daily to target iPTH consistent with the NKF-K/DOQI recommendation for chronic kidney disease patients on dialysis of 150 to 300 pg/mL.

Cinacalcet can be used alone or in combination with vitamin D sterols or phosphate binders.

During dose titration, monitor serum calcium levels frequently and if levels decrease below the normal range, take appropriate steps to increase serum calcium levels, such as by providing supplemental calcium, initiating or increasing the dose of calcium-based phosphate binder, initiating or increasing the dose of vitamin D sterols, or temporarily withholding treatment with cinacalcet.

➤*Hypercalcemia:* The recommended starting oral dose of cinacalcet is 30 mg twice daily.

Titrate the dosage of cinacalcet every 2 to 4 weeks through sequential doses of 30 mg twice daily, 60 mg twice daily, 90 mg twice daily, and 90 mg 3 or 4 times daily as necessary to normalize serum calcium levels.

➤*Storage / Stability:* Store at 25°C (77°F); excursions permitted to 15° to 30°C (59° to 86°F).

Actions

➤*Pharmacology:* Reduction in intact parathyroid hormone (iPTH) levels correlated with cinacalcet concentrations in chronic kidney disease patients. The nadir in iPTH level occurs approximately 2 to 6 hours post dose, corresponding with the C_{max} of cinacalcet. After steady state is reached, serum calcium concentrations remain constant over the dosing interval in chronic kidney disease patients.

Secondary hyperparathyroidism in patients with chronic kidney disease is a progressive disease, associated with increases in parathyroid hormone (PTH) levels and derangements in calcium and phosphorus metabolism. Increased PTH stimulates osteoclastic activity resulting in cortical bone resorption and marrow fibrosis. The goals of treatment of secondary hyperparathyroidism are to lower levels of PTH, calcium, and phosphorus in the blood, in order to prevent progressive bone disease and the systemic consequences of disordered mineral metabolism. In chronic kidney disease patients on dialysis with uncontrolled secondary hyperparathyroidism, reductions in PTH are associated with a favorable impact on bone-specific alkaline phosphatase, bone turnover, and bone fibrosis.

The calcium-sensing receptor on the surface of the chief cell of the parathyroid gland is the principal regulator of PTH secretion. Cinacalcet directly lowers PTH levels by increasing the sensitivity of the calcium sensing receptor to extracellular calcium. The reduction in PTH is associated with a concomitant decrease in serum calcium levels.

➤*Pharmacokinetics:*

Absorption / Distribution – After oral administration of cinacalcet, maximum plasma concentration (C_{max}) is achieved in approximately 2 to 6 hours. A food-effect study in healthy volunteers indicated that the C_{max} and area under the curve ($AUC_{(0\text{-inf})}$) were increased 82% and 68%, respectively, when cinacalcet was administered with a high-fat meal compared to fasting. C_{max} and $AUC_{(0\text{-inf})}$ of cinacalcet were increased 65% and 50%, respectively, when cinacalcet was administered with a low-fat meal compared to fasting.

After absorption, cinacalcet concentrations decline in a biphasic fashion with a terminal half-life of 30 to 40 hours. Steady-state drug levels are achieved within 7 days. The mean accumulation ratio is approximately 2 with once-daily oral administration. The median accumulation ratio is approximately 2 to 5 with twice-daily oral administration. The AUC and C_{max} of cinacalcet increase proportionally over the dose range of 30 to 180 mg once daily. The pharmacokinetic profile of cinacalcet does not change over time with once-daily dosing of 30 to 180 mg. The volume of distribution is high (approximately 1,000 L), indicating extensive distribution. Cinacalcet is approximately 93% to 97% bound to plasma protein(s). The ratio of blood cinacalcet concentration to plasma cinacalcet concentration is 0.8 at a blood cinacalcet concentration of 10 ng/mL.

Metabolism / Excretion – Cinacalcet is metabolized by multiple enzymes, primarily CYP3A4, CYP2D6, and CYP1A2. After administration of a 75 mg radiolabeled dose to healthy volunteers, cinacalcet was rapidly and extensively metabolized via: Oxidative N-dealkylation to hydrocinnamic acid and hydroxy-hydrocinnamic acid, which are further metabolized via β-oxidation and glycine conjugation; the oxidative N-dealkylation process also generates metabolites that contain the naphthalene ring; and by oxidation of the naphthalene ring on the parent drug to form dihydrodiols, which are further conjugated with glucuronic acid. The plasma concentrations of the major circulating metabolites including the cinnamic acid derivatives and glucuronidated dihydrodiols markedly exceed parent drug concentrations. The hydrocinnamic acid metabolite was shown to be inactive at concentrations up to 10 mcM in a cell-based assay measuring calcium-receptor activation. The glucuronide conjugates formed after cinacalcet oxidation were shown to have a potency approximately 0.003 times that of cinacalcet in a cell-based assay measuring a calcimimetic response. Renal excretion of metabolites was the primary route of elimination of radioactivity. Approximately 80% of the dose was recovered in the urine and 15% in the feces.

Special populations –

Hepatic function impairment: The disposition of a 50 mg cinacalcet single dose was compared in patients with hepatic impairment and subjects with normal hepatic function. Cinacalcet exposure, $AUC_{(0\text{-inf})}$, was comparable between healthy volunteers and patients with mild hepatic impairment. However, in patients with moderate and severe hepatic impairment (as indicated by the Child-Pugh method), cinacalcet exposures as defined by the $AUC(_{(0\text{-inf})}$ were 2.4 and 4.2 times higher, respectively, than that in healthy patients. The mean half-life of cinacalcet is prolonged by 33% and 70% in patients with moderate and severe hepatic impairment, respectively. Protein binding of cinacalcet is not affected by impaired hepatic function.

Contraindications

Hypersensitivity to any component(s) of this product.

Warnings

➤*Seizures:* In 3 clinical studies of chronic kidney disease patients on dialysis, 5% of the patients in both the cinacalcet and placebo groups reported a history of seizure disorder at baseline. During the trials, seizures (primarily generalized or tonic-clonic) were observed in 1.4% (9/656) of cinacalcet patients and 0.4% (2/470) of placebo-treated patients. Five of the 9 cinacalcet patients had a history of a seizure disorder, and 2 were receiving antiseizure medication at the time of their seizure. Both placebo-treated patients had a history of seizure disorder and were receiving antiseizure medication at the time of their seizure. While the basis for the reported difference in seizure rate is not clear, the threshold for seizures is lowered by significant reductions in serum calcium levels. Therefore, closely monitor serum calcium levels in patients receiving cinacalcet, particularly in patients with a history of a seizure disorder.

➤*Hepatic function impairment:* Cinacalcet exposure as assessed by $AUC_{(0\text{-inf})}$ in patients with moderate and severe hepatic impairment (as indicated by the Child-Pugh method) were 2.4 and 4.2 times higher, respectively, than that in healthy patients. Monitor patients with moderate and severe hepatic impairment throughout treatment with cinacalcet.

➤*Fertility impairment:* Female rats were given oral gavage doses of 5, 25, and 75 mg/kg/day beginning 2 weeks before mating and continuing through gestation day 7. Male rats were given oral doses 4 weeks prior to mating, during mating (3 weeks) and 2 weeks, post-mating. No effects were observed in male or female fertility at 5 and 25 mg/kg/day (exposures up to 3 times those resulting with a human oral dose of 180 mg/day based on AUC comparison). At 75 mg/kg/day, there were slight adverse effects (slight decreases in body weight and food consumption) in males and females.

➤*Pregnancy: Category C.* In pregnant female rats given oral gavage doses of 2, 25, and 50 mg/kg/day during gestation, no teratogenicity was observed at doses up to 50 mg/kg/day (exposure 4 times those resulting with a human oral dose of 180 mg/day based on AUC comparison). Decreased fetal body weights were observed at all doses (less than 1 to 4 times a human oral dose of 180 mg/day based on AUC comparison) in conjunction with maternal toxicity (decreased food consumption and body weight gain).

In pregnant female rabbits given oral gavage doses of 2, 12, and 25 mg/kg/day during gestation no adverse fetal effects were observed (exposures less than with a human oral dose of 180 mg/day based on AUC comparisons). Reductions in maternal food consumption and body weight gain were seen at doses of 12 and 25 mg/kg/day.

In pregnant rats given oral gavage doses of 5, 15, and 25 mg/kg/day during gestation through lactation no adverse fetal or pup (post-weaning) effects

CINACALCET HYDROCHLORIDE — ORAL

were observed at 5 mg/kg/day (exposures less than with a human therapeutic dose of 180 mg/day based on AUC comparisons). Higher doses of 15 and 25 mg/kg/day (exposures 2 to 3 times a human oral dose of 180 mg/day based on AUC comparisons) were accompanied by maternal signs of hypocalcemia (periparturient mortality and early postnatal pup loss), and reductions in postnatal maternal and pup body-weight gain. Cinacalcet has been shown to cross the placental barrier in rabbits.

There are no adequate and well-controlled studies in pregnant women. Use cinacalcet during pregnancy only if the potential benefit justifies the potential risk to the fetus.

➤*Lactation:* Studies in rats have shown that cinacalcet is excreted in the milk with a high milk-to-plasma ratio. It is not known whether this drug is excreted in human milk. Considering these data in rats and because many drugs are excreted in human milk and because of the potential for clinically significant adverse reactions in infants from cinacalcet, decide whether to discontinue nursing or to discontinue the drug, taking into account the importance of the drug to the lactating woman.

➤*Children:* The safety and efficacy of cinacalcet in pediatric patients have not been established.

Precautions

➤*Monitoring:* Closely monitor serum calcium levels in patients receiving cinacalcet.

Patients with chronic kidney disease on dialysis with secondary hyperparathyroidism – Measure serum calcium and serum phosphorus within 1 week, and measure iPTH 1 to 4 weeks after initiation or dose adjustment of cinacalcet. Once the maintenance dose has been established, measure serum calcium and serum phosphorus approximately monthly, and PTH every 1 to 3 months. All iPTH measurements during the cinacalcet trials were obtained using the Nichols IRMA.

In patients with end-stage renal disease, testosterone levels are often below the normal range. In a placebo-controlled trial in patients with chronic kidney disease on dialysis, there were reductions in total and free testosterone in male patients following 6 months of treatment with cinacalcet. Levels of total testosterone decreased by a median of 15.8% in the cinacalcet-treated patients and by 0.6% in the placebo-treated patients. Levels of free testosterone decreased by a median of 31.3% in the cinacalcet-treated patients and by 16.3% in the placebo-treated patients. The clinical significance of these reductions in serum testosterone is unknown.

Patients with parathyroid carcinoma – Serum calcium should be measured within 1 week after initiation or dose adjustment of cinacalcet. Once maintenance dose levels have been established, serum calcium should be measured every 2 months.

➤*Hypocalcemia:* Cinacalcet lowers serum calcium. Therefore, monitor patients carefully for the occurrence of hypocalcemia. Potential manifestations of hypocalcemia include paresthesias, myalgias, cramping, tetany, and convulsions.

Do not initiate cinacalcet treatment if serum calcium is less than the lower limit of the normal range (8.4 mg/dL). Measure serum calcium within 1 week after initiation or dose adjustment of cinacalcet. Once the maintenance dose has been established, measure serum calcium approximately monthly.

If serum calcium falls below 8.4 mg/dL but remains above 7.5 mg/dL, or if symptoms of hypocalcemia occur, use calcium-containing phosphate binders or vitamin D sterols to raise serum calcium. If serum calcium falls below 7.5 mg/dL, or if symptoms of hypocalcemia persist and the dose of vitamin D cannot be increased, withhold administration of cinacalcet until serum calcium levels reach 8 mg/dL, or symptoms of hypocalcemia have resolved. Re-initiate treatment using the next lowest dose of cinacalcet.

In the 26-week studies of patients with chronic kidney disease on dialysis, 66% of patients receiving cinacalcet compared with 25% of patients receiving placebo developed at least 1 serum calcium value less than 8.4 mg/dL. Less than 1% of patients in each group permanently discontinued study drug due to hypocalcemia.

In chronic kidney disease patients with secondary HPT not on dialysis, the long-term safety and efficacy of cinacalcet have not been established. Exploratory investigation indicates that chronic kidney disease patients not on dialysis have an increased risk for hypocalcemia compared to chronic kidney disease patients on dialysis, which may be due to lower baseline calcium levels. In a small, short-term study, in which the median dose of cinacalcet was 30 mg at the completion of the study, 74% of cinacalcet treated patients experienced at least 1 serum calcium value less than 8.4 mg/dL.

➤*Adynamic bone disease:* Adynamic bone disease may develop if iPTH levels are suppressed below 100 pg/mL when assessed using the standard Nichols IRMA. One clinical study evaluated bone histomorphometry in patients treated with cinacalcet for 1 year. Three patients with mild hyperparathyroid bone disease at the beginning of the study developed adynamic bone disease during treatment with cinacalcet. Two of these had iPTH levels below 100 pg/mL at multiple time points during the study. In the three 6-month, phase 3 studies conducted in chronic kidney disease patients on dialysis, 11% of patients treated with cinacalcet had mean iPTH values below 100 pg/mL during the efficacy-assessment phase. If iPTH levels decrease below the NKF-K/DOQI recommended target range (150 to 300 pg/mL) in patients treated with cinacalcet , reduce the dose of cinacalcet or vitamin D sterols or discontinue therapy.

Drug Interactions

➤*Effects cinacalcet on other drugs:*

Drugs metabolized by cytochrome P-450 2D6 (CYP2D6) – Cinacalcet is a strong in vitro inhibitor of CYP2D6. Therefore, dose adjustments of concomitant medications that are predominantly metabolized by CYP2D6 and have a narrow therapeutic index (eg, flecainide, vinblastine, thioridazine, and most tricyclic antidepressants) may be required.

Amitriptyline – Concurrent administration of 25 mg or 100 mg cinacalcet with 50 mg amitriptyline increased amitriptyline exposure and nortriptyline (active metabolite) exposure by approximately 20% in CYP2D6 extensive metabolizers.

➤*Effect of other drugs on cinacalcet:* Cinacalcet is metabolized by multiple cytochrome P-450 enzymes, primarily CYP3A4, CYP2D6, and CYP1A2.

Ketoconazole – Cinacalcet is metabolized in part by CYP3A4. Coadministration of ketoconazole, a strong inhibitor of CYP3A4, increased cinacalcet exposure following a single 90 mg dose of cinacalcet by 2.3- fold. Dose adjustment of cinacalcet may be required and PTH and serum calcium concentrations should be closely monitored if a patient initiates or discontinues therapy with a strong CYP3A4 inhibitor (eg, ketoconazole, erythromycin, itraconazole).

Adverse Reactions

➤*Secondary hyperparathyroidism in patients with chronic kidney disease on dialysis:*

Adverse Reaction Incidence (≥ 5%) in Patients on Dialysis		
Event[a]	Placebo (n = 470) (%)	Cinacalcet (n = 656) (%)
Access infection	4%	5%
Anorexia	4%	6%
Asthenia	4%	7%
Diarrhea	20%	21%
Dizziness	8%	10%
Hypertension	5%	7%
Myalgia	14%	15%
Nausea	19%	31%
Pain chest, non-cardiac	4%	6%
Vomiting	15%	27%

[a] Included are reactions that were reported at a greater incidence in the cinacalcet group than in the placebo group.

The incidence of serious adverse reactions (29% vs 31%) was similar in the cinacalcet and placebo groups, respectively.

➤*12-month experience with cinacalcet:* Two hundred and sixty-six patients from 2 phase 3 studies continued to receive cinacalcet or placebo treatment in a 6-month, double-blind extension study (12-month total treatment duration). The incidence and nature of adverse reactions in this study were similar in the 2 treatment groups, and comparable to those observed in the phase 3 studies.

➤*Parathyroid carcinoma:* The most frequent adverse reactions in this patient group were nausea and vomiting.

Overdosage

➤*Symptoms:* Doses titrated up to 300 mg once daily have been safely administered to patients on dialysis. Overdosage of cinacalcet may lead to hypocalcemia. In the event of overdosage, monitor patients for signs and symptoms of hypocalcemia and take appropriate measures to correct serum calcium levels.

➤*Treatment:* Since cinacalcet is highly protein bound, hemodialysis is not an effective treatment for overdosage of cinacalcet.

Patient Information

Take with food or shortly after a meal. Take tablets whole and do not divide them.

GALLIUM NITRATE

Rx	Ganite (Genta[a])	Injection: 25 mg/mL	Preservative free. In 20 mL single-dose vials.

[a] Genta Incorporated, Berkeley Heights, NJ 07922; (888) TO-GENTA.

GALLIUM NITRATE — INJECTION

WARNING

Concurrent use of gallium nitrate with other potentially nephrotoxic drugs (eg, aminoglycosides, amphotericin B) may increase the risk for developing severe renal insufficiency in patients with cancer-related hypercalcemia. If use of a potentially nephrotoxic drug is indicated during gallium nitrate therapy, gallium nitrate administration should be discontinued and it is recommended that hydration be continued for several days after administration of the potentially nephrotoxic drug. Serum creatinine and urine output should be closely monitored during and subsequent to this period. Gallium nitrate therapy should be discontinued if the serum creatinine level exceeds 2.5 mg/dL.

Indications

➤*Cancer-related hypercalcemia:* For the treatment of clearly symptomatic cancer-related hypercalcemia that has not responded to adequate hydration. In general, patients with a serum calcium (corrected for albumin) less than 12 mg/dL would not be expected to be symptomatic. Mild or asymptomatic hypercalcemia may be treated with conservative measures (ie, saline hydration, with or without diuretics). In the treatment of cancer-related hypercalcemia, it is important first to establish adequate hydration, preferably with intravenous saline, in order to increase the renal excretion of calcium and correct dehydration caused by hypercalcemia.

Administration and Dosage

➤*Approved by the FDA:* January 17, 1991.

➤*Dosage:* The usual recommended dose of gallium nitrate is 200 mg per square meter of body surface area (200 mg/m^2) daily for 5 consecutive days. In patients with mild hypercalcemia and few symptoms, a lower dosage of 100 mg/m^2/day for 5 days may be considered. If serum calcium levels are lowered into the normal range in less than 5 days, treatment may be discontinued early. The daily dose must be administered as an intravenous infusion over 24 hours. The daily dose should be diluted, preferably in 1,000 mL of 0.9% sodium chloride injection or 5% Dextrose injection, for administration as an intravenous infusion over 24 hours. Adequate hydration must be maintained throughout the treatment period, with careful attention to avoid overhydration in patients with compromised cardiovascular status. Controlled studies have not been undertaken to evaluate the safety and effectiveness of retreatment with gallium nitrate.

➤*Storage/Stability:* Store at controlled room temperature 20° to 25°C (68° to 77°F). Contains no preservative. Discard unused portion.

When gallium nitrate is added to either 0.9% Sodium Chloride injection or 5% Dextrose injection, it is stable for 48 hours at room temperature (15° to 30°C [59° to 86°F]) or for 7 days if stored under refrigeration (2° to 8°C [35.6° to 46.4°F]). Parenteral drug products should be inspected visually for particulate matter and discoloration prior to administration whenever solution and container permit.

Actions

➤*Pharmacology:* Gallium nitrate exerts a hypocalcemic effect by inhibiting calcium resorption from bone, possibly by reducing increased bone turnover. Although in vitro and animal studies have been performed to investigate the mechanism of action of gallium nitrate, the precise mechanism for inhibiting calcium resorption has not been determined. No cytotoxic effects were observed on bone cells in drug-treated animals.

➤*Pharmacokinetics:*

Absorption/Distribution – Gallium nitrate was infused at a daily dose of 200 mg/m^2 for 5 (n = 2) or 7 (n = 10) consecutive days to 12 cancer patients. In most patients, apparent steady-state is achieved by 24 to 48 hours. The range of average steady-state plasma levels of gallium observed among 7 fully evaluable patients was between 1,134 and 2,399 ng/mL. The average plasma clearance of gallium (n = 7) following daily infusion of gallium nitrate at a dose of 200 mg/m^2 for 5 or 7 days was 0.15 L/hr/kg (range: 0.12 to 0.2 L/hr/kg). In 1 patient who received daily infusion doses of 100, 150, and 200 mg/m^2, the apparent steady-state levels of gallium did not increase proportionally with an increase in dose.

Metabolism/Excretion – Gallium nitrate is not metabolized either by the liver or the kidney and appears to be significantly excreted via the kidney. Urinary excretion data for a dose of 200 mg/m^2 has not been determined.

Contraindications

Severe renal impairment (serum creatinine greater than 2.5 mg/dL).

Warnings

➤*Nephrotoxic drugs:* Combined use of gallium nitrate with other potentially nephrotoxic drugs (eg, aminoglycosides, amphotericin B) may increase the risk of developing renal insufficiency in patients with cancer-related hypercalcemia.

➤*Renal function impairment:* The hypercalcemic state in cancer patients is commonly associated with impaired renal function. Abnormalities in renal function (elevated BUN and/or serum creatinine) have been observed in clinical trials with gallium nitrate. It is strongly recommended that serum creatinine be monitored during gallium nitrate therapy. Because patients with cancer-related hypercalcemia are frequently dehydrated, it is important that such patients be adequately hydrated with oral and/or intravenous fluids (preferably saline) and that a satisfactory urine output (a urine output of 2 L/day is recommended) be established before therapy with gallium nitrate is started. Adequate hydration should be maintained throughout the treatment period, with careful attention to avoid overhydration in patients with compromised cardiovascular status. Diuretic therapy should not be employed prior to correction of hypovolemia. Gallium nitrate therapy should be discontinued if the serum creatinine level exceeds 2.5 mg/dL.

The use of gallium nitrate in patients with marked renal insufficiency (serum creatinine greater than 2.5 mg/dL) has not been systematically examined. If therapy is undertaken in patients with moderately impaired renal function (serum creatinine 2 to 2.5 mg/dL), frequent monitoring of the patient's renal status is recommended. Treatment should be discontinued if the serum creatinine level exceeds 2.5 mg/dL.

➤*Pregnancy: Category C.* Animal reproduction studies have not been conducted with gallium nitrate. It is also not known whether gallium nitrate can cause fetal harm when administered to a pregnant woman or can affect reproductive capacity. Gallium nitrate should be administered to a pregnant woman only if clearly needed.

➤*Lactation:* It is not known whether gallium nitrate is excreted in human milk. Because of the potential for serious adverse reactions in nursing infants from gallium nitrate, a decision should be made whether to discontinue nursing or discontinue the drug, taking into account the importance of the drug to the mother.

➤*Children:* The safety and efficacy of gallium nitrate in children have not been established.

Precautions

➤*Monitoring:* Renal function (serum creatinine and BUN) and serum calcium must be closely monitored during gallium nitrate therapy. In addition to baseline assessment, the suggested frequency of calcium and phosphorus determinations is daily and twice weekly, respectively. Gallium nitrate should be discontinued if the serum creatinine exceeds 2.5 mg/dL.

➤*Asymptomatic or mild to moderate hypocalcemia:* Asymptomatic or mild to moderate hypocalcemia (6.5 to 8 mg/dL, corrected for serum albumin) occurred in approximately 38% of patients treated with gallium nitrate in the controlled clinical trial. One patient exhibited a positive Chvostek's sign. If hypocalcemia occurs, gallium nitrate therapy should be stopped and short-term calcium therapy may be necessary.

Drug Interactions

The concomitant use of highly nephrotoxic drugs in combination with gallium nitrate may increase the risk for development of renal insufficiency. Available information does not indicate any adverse interaction with diuretics such as furosemide. A symptom complex of dyspnea (associated with interstitial pneumonitis in some instances), mouth soreness, and asthenia has been reported in a small number of multiple myeloma patients receiving low dose (40 mg) gallium nitrate subcutaneously in addition to oral cyclophosphamide and prednisone. The serious nature of the underlying condition of these patients precludes a precise understanding of the relationship of these events to either gallium nitrate treatment alone or with cyclophosphamide.

Adverse Reactions

➤*Cardiovascular:* A decrease in mean systolic and diastolic blood pressure was observed several days after treatment with gallium nitrate in a controlled clinical trial. The decrease in blood pressure was asymptomatic and did not require specific treatment.

➤*Hematologic:* The use of very high doses of gallium nitrate (up to 1,400 mg/m^2) in treating patients for advanced cancer has been associated with anemia, and several patients have received red blood cell transfusions. Because of the serious nature of the underlying illness, it is uncertain that the anemia was caused by gallium nitrate.

➤*Metabolic:* Hypocalcemia may occur after gallium nitrate treatment.

Transient hypophosphatemia of mild-to-moderate degree may occur in up to 79% of hypercalcemic patients following treatment with gallium nitrate. In a controlled clinical trial, 33% of patients had at least 1 serum phosphorus measurement between 1.5 to 2.4 mg/dL, while 46% of patients had at least 1 serum phosphorus value less than 1.5 mg/dL. Patients who develop hypophosphatemia may require oral phosphorus therapy.

Decreased serum bicarbonate, possibly secondary to mild respiratory alkalosis was reported in 40% to 50% of cancer patients treated with gallium nitrate. The cause for this effect is not clear. This effect has been asymptomatic and has not required specific treatment.

➤*Renal:* Adverse renal effects, as demonstrated by rising BUN and creatinine, have been reported in about 12.5% of patients treated with gallium nitrate. In a controlled clinical trial of patients with cancer-related hypercalcemia, 2 patients receiving gallium nitrate and 1 patient receiving calcitonin developed acute renal failure. Due to the serious nature of the patients' underlying conditions, the relationship of these events to the drug was unclear. Gallium nitrate should not be administered to patients with serum creatinine greater than 2.5 mg/dL.

➤*Special senses:* In cancer chemotherapy trials, a small proportion (less than 1%) of patients treated with multiple high doses of gallium nitrate combined with other investigational anticancer drugs, have developed acute optic neuritis. While these patients were critically ill and had received multiple

GALLIUM NITRATE — INJECTION

drugs, a reaction to high-dose gallium nitrate is possible. Most patients had full recovery; however, at least one case of permanent blindness has been reported. One patient with cancer-related hypercalcemia was reported to develop decreased hearing following gallium nitrate administration. Because of the patient's underlying condition and concurrent therapies, the relationship of this event to gallium nitrate administration is unclear. Tinnitus and partial loss of auditory acuity have been reported rarely (less than 1%) in patients who received high-dose gallium nitrate as anticancer treatment.

➤*Miscellaneous:* Other clinical events reported in association with gallium nitrate treatment for cancer as well as cancer-related hypercalcemia include nausea and/or vomiting, tachycardia, lethargy, confusion, dreams and hallucinations, diarrhea, constipation, lower extremity edema, hypothermia, fever, dyspnea, rales and rhonchi, anemia, leukopenia, paresthesia, skin rash, pleural effusion, and pulmonary infiltrates. Due to the serious nature of the underlying condition of these patients, the relationship of these events to therapy with gallium nitrate is unknown. A single case of encephalopathy followed rapidly by coma and death has been reported after treatment in a cancer chemotherapy trial with gallium nitrate 300 mg/m^2/day for 7 days. Treatment with gallium nitrate other than as described in this monograph may be complicated by adverse events not listed.

Overdosage

➤*Symptoms:* Rapid intravenous infusion of gallium nitrate or use of doses higher than recommended (200 mg/m^2) may cause nausea and vomiting and a substantially increased risk of renal insufficiency.

➤*Treatment:* In the event of overdosage, further drug administration should be discontinued, serum calcium should be monitored, and the patient should receive vigorous intravenous hydration, with or without diuretics, for 2 to 3 days. During this time period, renal function and urinary output should be carefully monitored so that fluid intake and output are balanced.

SODIUM PHENYLBUTYRATE

SODIUM PHENYLBUTYRATE

Rx	**Buphenyl** (Ucyclyd Pharma)	**Tablets:** 500 mg	(UCY 500). Off-white, oval. In 250s and 500s.
		Powder: 3.2 g (3 g sodium phenylbutyrate) per tsp	In 500 and 950 mL bottles. Measurers provided.
		9.1 g (8.6 g sodium phenylbutyrate) per tbsp	In 500 and 950 mL bottles. Measurers provided.

SODIUM PHENYLBUTYRATE — ORAL

Indications

➤*Cycle disorders:* Adjunctive therapy in the chronic management of patients with urea cycle disorders involving deficiencies of carbamoyl phosphate synthetase (CPS), ornithine transcarbamoylase (OTC) or argininosuccinic acid synthetase (AAS). It is indicated in all patients with neonatal-onset deficiency (complete enzymatic deficiency, presenting within the first 28 days of life). It is also indicated in patients with late-onset disease (partial enzymatic deficiency, presenting after the first month of life) who have a history of hyperammonemic encephalopathy. It is important that the diagnosis be made early and treatment initiated immediately to improve survival. Any episode of acute hyperammonemia should be treated as a life-threatening emergency.

Administration and Dosage

➤*Tablets:* For oral use only. It is indicated for children weighing more than 20 kg or adults.

Usual dose – 450 to 600 mg/kg/day in patients weighing less than 20 kg, or 9.9 to 13 g/m^2/day in larger patients. Take in equally divided amounts with each meal (eg, three times daily). The safety and efficacy of doses more than 20 g/day (40 tablets) has not been established.

➤*Powder:* For oral use via mouth, gastrostomy or nasogastric tube only. Mix with food (solid or liquid). Avoid acidic beverages. Each level teaspoon dispenses 3.2 g of powder and 3 g of sodium phenylbutyrate. Each level tablespoon dispenses 9.1 g of powder and 8.6 g of sodium phenylbutyrate. Shake lightly before use.

Usual dose – 450 to 600 mg/kg/day in patients weighing less than 20 kg, or 9.9 to 13 g/m^2/day in larger patients. Take in equally divided amounts with each meal or feeding, four to six times daily. The safety and efficacy of doses more than 20 g/day has not been established.

➤*Storage/Stability:* Store at room temperature, 15° to 30°C (59° to 86°F). After opening, keep bottle tightly closed.

Actions

➤*Pharmacology:* Sodium phenylbutyrate is a pro-drug and is rapidly metabolized to phenylacetate. Phenylacetate is a metabolically-active compound that conjugates with glutamine via acetylation to form phenylacetylglutamine. Phenylacetylglutamine is excreted then by the kidneys. On a molar basis, it is comparable to urea (each containing two moles of nitrogen). Therefore, phenylacetylglutamine provides an alternate vehicle for waste nitrogen excretion.

➤*Pharmacokinetics:*

Absorption – Peak plasma levels of phenylbutyrate occur within 1 hour after a single dose of 5 g sodium phenylbutyrate powder with a C_{max} of 195 mcg/ml and for the tablets, a C_{max} of 218 mcg/ml under fasting conditions. The effect of food on phenylbutyrate's absorption is unknown.

Excretion – A majority of the administered compound (approximately 80% to 100%) is excreted by the kidneys within 24 hours as the conjugation product, phenylacetylglutamine. For each gram of sodium phenylbutyrate administered, it is estimated that between 0.12 to 0.15 g of phenylacetylglutamine nitrogen is produced.

Following oral administration of 5 g, measurable plasma levels of phenylbutyrate and phenylacetate were detected 15 and 30 min after dosing, respectively, and phenylacetylglutamine was detected shortly thereafter. The pharmacokinetic parameters for phenylbutyrate for C_{max} (mcg/ml), T_{max} (hours) and elimination half-life were 195, 1 and 0.76 hours, respectively, and for phenylacetate 45.3, 3.55 and 1.29 hours, respectively. The major sites for metabolism are the liver and kidney.

In patients with urea cycle disorders, sodium phenylbutyrate decreases elevated plasma ammonia and glutamine levels. It increases waste nitrogen excretion in the form of phenylacetylglutamine.

Special populations –

Gender: The pharmacokinetic parameters, AUC and C_{max} for both plasma phenylbutyrate and phenylacetate were about 30% to 50% greater in women than in men.

Contraindications

Management of acute hyperammonemia, which is a medical emergency.

Warnings

➤*Fluid retention:* Use with great care, if at all, in patients with CHF or severe renal insufficiency, and in clinical states in which there is sodium retention with edema.

➤*Preexisting neurologic impairment:* Reversal of preexisting neurologic impairment is not likely to occur with treatment, and neurologic deterioration may continue.

➤*Acute hyperammonemic encephalopathy:* Acute hyperammonemic encephalopathy recurred in the majority of patients.

➤*Long-term:* Sodium phenylbutyrate may be required life-long unless orthotopic liver transplantation is elected.

➤*Renal/Hepatic function impairment:* Sodium phenylbutyrate is metabolized in the liver and kidney, and phenylacetylglutamine is primarily excreted by the kidney. Use caution when administering the drug to patients with hepatic or renal insufficiency.

➤*Pregnancy: Category C.* It is not known whether sodium phenylbutyrate can cause fetal harm when administered to a pregnant woman or can affect reproduction capacity. Give sodium phenylbutyrate to a pregnant woman only if clearly needed.

➤*Lactation:* It is not known whether this drug is excreted in breast milk. Because many drugs are excreted in breast milk, exercise caution when administering sodium phenylbutyrate to a breast-feeding woman.

➤*Children:* The use of tablets for neonates, infants, and children 20 kg or less is not recommended (see Administration and Dosage).

Precautions

➤*Monitoring:* Maintain plasma levels of ammonia, arginine, branched-chain amino acids and serum proteins within normal limits, and maintain plasma glutamine at levels less than 1,000 mcmol/L. Periodically monitor serum drug levels of phenylbutyrate and its metabolites, phenylacetate, and phenylacetylglutamine.

Drug Interactions

Sodium Phenylbutyrate Drug Interactions

Precipitant drug	Object drug[a]		Description
Corticosteroids	Sodium phenylbutyrate	⬇	Corticosteroids may cause the breakdown of body protein and increase plasma ammonia levels.
Haloperidol/Valproate	Sodium phenylbutyrate	⬇	Haloperidol/Valproate may cause hyperammonemia.
Probenecid	Sodium phenylbutyrate	⬆	Probenecid is known to inhibit the renal transport of many organic compounds, including hippuric acid, and may affect renal excretion of the conjugation product of sodium phenylbutyrate, as well as its metabolite.

[a] ⬆ = Object drug increased. ⬇ = Object drug decreased.

SODIUM PHENYLBUTYRATE — ORAL

Adverse Reactions

Amenorrhea/menstrual dysfunction (23%); decreased appetite (4%); body odor (probably caused by the metabolite phenylacetate), bad taste or taste aversion (3%).

Other adverse reactions reported in 2% or less of patients:

➤*Cardiovascular:* Arrhythmia, edema (one patient).

➤*CNS:* Depression, neurotoxicity (fatigue, light-headedness, and somnolence; less frequently, disorientation, dysgeusia, exacerbation of a preexisting neuropathy, headache, hypoacusis, and impaired memory). These adverse reactions were mainly mild in severity. The acute onset and reversibility when the phenylacetate infusion was discontinued suggest a drug effect.

➤*GI:* Abdominal pain, constipation, gastritis, nausea, vomiting, rectal bleeding, peptic ulcer disease, pancreatitis (one patient).

➤*Hematologic:* Aplastic anemia, ecchymosis (one patient).

➤*Miscellaneous:* Headache, renal tubular acidosis, rash, syncope, weight gain.

➤*Lab test abnormalities:*

Metabolic – Acidosis (14%); alkalosis, hyperchloremia (7%); hypophosphatemia (6%); hyperuricemia, hyperphosphatemia (2%); hypernatremia, hypokalemia (1%).

Nutritional – Hypoalbuminemia (11%); decreased total protein (3%).

Hepatic – Increased alkaline phosphatase (6%); increased liver transaminases (4%); hyperbilirubinemia (1%).

Hematologic – Anemia (9%); leukopenia, leukocytosis (4%); thrombocytopenia (3%); thrombocytosis (1%).

Overdosage

No adverse experiences have been reported involving overdoses of sodium phenylbutyrate in patients with urea cycle disorders.

➤*Treatment:* In the event of an overdose, discontinue the drug and institute supportive measures. Hemodialysis or peritoneal dialysis may be beneficial.

BETAINE ANHYDROUS

Rx	**Cystadane** (Orphan Medical)	**Powder:** 1 g/1.7 mL	White, granular. In 180 g bottles.

BETAINE ANHYDROUS — ORAL

Indications

➤*Homocystinuria:* Betaine is indicated for the treatment of homocystinuria to decrease elevated homocysteine blood levels. Included within the category of homocystinuria are deficiencies or defects in: 1) Cystathionine beta-synthase (CBS); 2) 5,10–methylenetetrahydrofolate reductase (MTHFR); and 3) cobalamin cofactor metabolism (cbl).

Betaine has been administered concomitantly with vitamin B_6 (pyridoxine), vitamin B_{12} (cyanocobalamin) and folate.

Administration and Dosage

➤*Dosage:* The usual dosage used in adult and pediatric patients is 6 g/day administered orally in divided doses of 3 g twice daily. Dosages of up to 20 g/day have been necessary to control homocysteine levels in some patients. In pediatric patients less than 3 years of age, dosage may be started at 100 mg/kg/day and then increased weekly by 100 mg/kg increments. Dosage in all patients can be gradually increased until plasma homocysteine is undetectable or present only in small amounts.

Measure prescribed amount with the measuring scoop provided (one level 1.7 ml scoop is equal to 1 g of betaine anhydrous powder) and then dissolve in 120 to 180 ml (4 to 6 oz) of water for immediate ingestion.

➤*Storage / Stability:* Store at room temperature, 15° to 30°C (59° to 86°F).

Actions

➤*Pharmacology:* Betaine acts as a methyl group donor in the remethylation of homocysteine to methionine in patients with homocystinuria. As a result, toxic blood levels of homocysteine are reduced in these patients, usually 20% to 80% or less of pre-treatment levels.

Elevated homocysteine blood levels are associated with clinical problems such as cardiovascular thrombosis, osteoporosis, skeletal abnormalities and optic lens dislocation. Plasma levels of homocysteine were decreased in nearly all patients treated with betaine. In observational studies without concurrent controls, clinical improvement was reported by physicians in approximately ¾ of patients taking betaine. Many of these patients were also taking other therapies such as vitamin B_6 (pyridoxine), vitamin B_{12} (cyanocobalamin) and folate with variable biochemical responses. In most cases, adding betaine resulted in a further reduction in homocysteine.

Betaine lowers plasma homocysteine levels in the three types of homocystinuria: Cystathionine beta-synthase (CBS) deficiency; 5,10–methylenetetrahydrofolate reductase (MTHFR) deficiency; and cobalamin cofactor metabolism (cbl) defect.

Betaine has also increased low plasma methionine and S-adenosylmethionine (SAM) levels in patients with MTHFR deficiency and cbl defect.

In CBS-deficient patients, large increases in methionine levels have been observed. However, the increased methionine levels do not appear to have been associated with adverse clinical consequences.

Betaine occurs naturally in the body. It is a metabolite of choline and is present in small amounts in foods (eg, beets, spinach, cereals and seafood).

➤*Pharmacokinetics:* The onset of action is within several days and a steady state in response to dosage is achieved within several weeks. Patients have taken betaine for many years without evidence of tolerance.

Warnings

➤*Pregnancy: Category C.* It is not known whether betaine can cause fetal harm when administered to a pregnant woman or can affect reproductive capacity. Give to a pregnant woman only if clearly needed.

➤*Lactation:* It is not known whether betaine is excreted in breast milk. Its metabolic precursor, choline, occurs at high levels in breast milk. Exercise caution when administering to a nursing woman.

➤*Children:* The majority of case studies of homocystinuria patients treated wih betaine have been pediatric patients. The disorder, in its most severe form, can be manifested within the first months or years of life by lethargy, failure to thrive, developmental delays, seizures or optic lens displacement. Patients have been treated successfully without adverse effects within the first months or years of life with dosages greater than or equal to 6 g/day with resultant biochemical and clinical improvement. However, dosage titration may be preferable in pediatric patients (see Dosage and Administration).

Adverse Reactions

Betaine Anhydrous Adverse Reactions	
Adverse reaction	n = 111
Nausea	2
GI distress	2
Diarrhea	1
Aspirated the powder	1
Caused odor	1
Questionable psychological changes	1
Unspecified problem	1

Overdosage

In an acute toxicology study in rats, death frequently occurred at doses greater than or equal to 10,000 mg/kg.

Patient Information

Shake bottle lightly before removing cap.

Measure with the scoop provided.

One level scoop (1.7 ml) is equivalent to 1 g of betaine anhydrous powder. Measure the number of scoops your physician has prescribed.

Mix with 120 to 180 ml (4 to 6 oz) of water until completely dissolved, then drink immediately.

Always replace the cap tightly after using. Protect from moisture. Do not use if powder does not completely dissolve or gives a colored solution.

CYSTEAMINE BITARTRATE

Rx	**Cystagon** (Mylan)	**Capsules:** 50 mg (as base)	(Cysta 50 Mylan). White. In 100s and 500s.
		150 mg (as base)	(Cystagon 150 Mylan). White. In 100s and 500s.

CYSTEAMINE BITARTRATE — ORAL

Indications

➤*Nephropathic cystinosis:* Management in children and adults.

Administration and Dosage

➤*Approved by the FDA:* August 15, 1994.

➤*Initial dose:* For the management of nephropathic cystinosis, initiate therapy promptly once the diagnosis is confirmed (ie, increased white cell cystine). Start new patients on ¼ to ⅙ of the maintenance dose of cysteamine. The dose should then be raised gradually over 4 to 6 weeks to avoid intolerance.

➤*Maintenance:* The recommended cysteamine maintenance dose for children up to age 12 years is 1.3 g/m^2/day of the free base, given in 4 divided doses. Intact cysteamine capsules should not be administered to children under the age of ≈ 6 years because of the risk of aspiration. Cysteamine capsules may be administered to children under the age of approximately 6 years by sprinkling the capsule contents over food. Patients older than 12 years of age and older than 110 lbs should receive 2 g/day, in 4 divided doses.

When cysteamine is well tolerated, the goal of therapy is to keep leukocyte cystine levels less than 1 nmol/½ cystine/mg protein 5 to 6 hours following administration of cysteamine. Patients with poorer tolerability still receive significant benefit if white cell cystine levels are less than 2 nmol/½ cystine/mg protein. The cysteamine dose can be increased to a maximum of 1.95 g/m^2/day to achieve this level. The dose of 1.95 g/m^2/day has been associated with an increased rate of withdrawal from treatment due to intolerance and an increased incidence of adverse events.

Cystinotic patients taking cysteamine hydrochloride or phosphocysteamine solutions may be transferred to equimolar doses of cysteamine bitartrate capsules.

The recommended maintenance dose of 1.3 g/m^2/day can be approximated by administering cysteamine according to the following table, which takes surface area as well as weight into consideration.

Cysteamine Maintenance Dose	
Weight (lbs)	Cysteamine free base every 6 hours (mg)
0-10	100
11-20	150
21-30	200
31-40	250
41-50	300
51-70	350
71-90	400
91-110	450
> 110	500

Patients older than 12 years of age and more than 110 lbs should receive 2 g/day given in 4 divided doses as a starting maintenance dose. This dose should be reached after 4 to 6 weeks of incremental dosage increases as stated above. The dose should be raised if the leukocyte cystine level remains more than 2 nmol/½ cystine/mg/protein.

Obtain leukocyte cystine measurements, taken 5 to 6 hours after dose administration, for new patients after the maintenance dose is achieved. Patients being transferred from cysteamine hydrochloride or phosphocysteamine solutions to capsules should have their white cell cystine levels measured in 2 weeks, and thereafter every 3 months to assess optimal dosage as described above.

If cysteamine is poorly tolerated initially due to GI tract symptoms or transient skin rashes, temporarily stop therapy, then reinstitute at a lower dose and gradually increase to the proper dose.

Actions

➤*Pharmacology:* Cysteamine is a cystine depleting agent that lowers the cystine content of cells in patients with cystinosis, an inherited defect of lysosomal transport. Cysteamine is an aminothiol that participates within lysosomes in a thiol-disulfide interchange reaction converting cystine into cysteine and cysteine-cysteamine mixed disulfide, both of which can exit the lysosome in patients with cystinosis.

Contraindications

Hypersensitivity to cysteamine or penicillamine.

Warnings

➤*Rash:* If a skin rash develops, withhold cysteamine until the rash clears. Cysteamine may be restarted at a lower dose under close supervision, then slowly titrated to the therapeutic dose. If a severe skin rash develops such as erythema multiforme bullosa or toxic epidermal necrolysis, cysteamine should not be readministered.

➤*CNS symptoms:* CNS symptoms such as seizures, lethargy, somnolence, depression and encephalopathy have been associated with cysteamine. If CNS symptoms develop, carefully evaluate the patient and adjust the dose as necessary. Neurological complications have been described in some cystinotic patients not on cysteamine treatment. This may be a manifestation of the primary disorder. Patients should not engage in hazardous activities until the effects of cysteamine on mental performance are known.

➤*Fertility impairment:* At an oral dose of 375 mg/kg/day (1.7 times the recommended human dose), cysteamine reduced the fertility of rats and offspring survival.

➤*Pregnancy: Category C.* It is not known whether cysteamine can cause fetal harm when administered to a pregnant woman. Use only when clearly needed and when the potential benefits outweigh the potential hazards to the fetus.

➤*Lactation:* It is not known whether cysteamine is excreted in breast milk. Because of the manifested potential of cysteamine for developmental toxicity in suckling rat pups when it was administered to their lactating mothers at an oral dose of 375 mg/kg/day, decide whether to discontinue nursing or to discontinue the drug, taking into account the importance of the drug to the mother.

➤*Children:* The safety and efficacy of cysteamine for cystinotic children have been established. Initiate therapy as soon as the diagnosis of nephropathic cystinosis has been confirmed.

Precautions

➤*Monitoring:* Cysteamine has occasionally been associated with reversible leukopenia and abnormal liver function studies. Therefore, monitor blood counts and liver function studies.

Leukocyte cystine measurements are useful to determine adequate dosage and compliance. When measured 5 to 6 hours after cysteamine administration, the goal should be a level less than 1 nmol/½; cystine/mg protein. In some patients with poorer tolerability for cysteamine, patients may still receive benefit with a white cell cystine level of less than 2 nmol/½; cystine/mg protein. Measurements should be done every 3 months, more frequently when patients are transferred from cysteamine hydrochloride or phosphocysteamine solutions to cysteamine bitartrate.

➤*GI symptoms:* GI symptoms, including nausea, vomiting, anorexia and abdominal pain (sometimes severe), have been associated with cysteamine. If these develop, therapy may have to be interrupted and the dose adjusted. A dose of 1.95 g/m^2/day (approximately 80 to 90 mg/kg/day) was associated with an increased number of withdrawals from treatment because of intolerance and an increased incidence of adverse events.

➤*Concurrent therapy:* Cysteamine can be administered with electrolyte and mineral replacements necessary for management of the Fanconi syndrome as well as vitamin D and thyroid hormone.

Adverse Reactions

In three clinical trials, cysteamine or phosphocysteamine have been administered to 246 children with cystinosis. Causality of side effects is sometimes difficult to determine because adverse effects may result from the underlying disease.

Adverse reactions or intolerance leading to cessation of treatment occurred in 8% of patients in the US studies. Withdrawals due to intolerance, vomiting associated with medication, anorexia, lethargy and fever appeared dose-related, occurring more frequently in those patients receiving 1.95 vs 1.3 g/m^2/day.

The most frequent adverse reactions seen involve the GI (see Precautions) and central nervous systems (see Warnings). These are especially prominent at the initiation of therapy. Temporarily suspending treatment, then gradual reintroduction may be effective in improving tolerance. The most common events (more than 5%) were vomiting (35%), anorexia (31%), fever (22%), diarrhea (16%), lethargy (11%) and rash (7%).

Other adverse reactions are as follows:

➤*CNS:* Somnolence; encephalopathy; headache; seizures; ataxia; confusion; tremor; hyperkinesia; decreased hearing; dizziness; jitteriness.

➤*GI:* Nausea; bad breath; abdominal pain; dyspepsia; constipation; gastroenteritis; duodenitis; duodenal ulceration.

➤*Psychiatric:* Nervousness; abnormal thinking; depression; emotional lability; hallucinations; nightmares.

➤*Miscellaneous:* Abnormal liver function; anemia; leukopenia; dehydration; hypertension; urticaria.

Overdosage

➤*Symptoms:* A single oral dose of 660 mg/kg was lethal to rats. Symptoms of acute toxicity were reduction of motor activity and generalized hemorrhage in the GI tract and kidneys. One case of massive human overdosage has been reported. The patient immediately vomited the drug and did not develop any symptoms.

➤*Treatment:* Should overdose occur, appropriately support the respiratory and cardiovascular systems. No specific antidote is known. Refer to General Management of Acute Overdosage. Hemodialysis may be considered since cysteamine is poorly bound to plasma proteins.

SODIUM BENZOATE AND SODIUM PHENYLACETATE

Rx	**Ammonul** (Ucyclyd Pharma)	**Injection:** sodium benzoate 100 mg and sodium phenylacetate 100 mg per mL	In 50 mL single-use vials.

SODIUM BENZOATE AND SODIUM PHENYLACETATE — INJECTION

Indications

➤*Hyperammonemia:* Adjunctive therapy for the treatment of acute hyperammonemia and associated encephalopathy in patients with deficiencies in enzymes of the urea cycle. In acute neonatal hyperammonemic coma, moderate to severe episodes of hyperammonemic encephalopathy, and episodes of hyperammonemia that fail to respond to an initial course of sodium phenylacetate and sodium benzoate therapy, hemodialysis is the most rapid and effective technique for removing ammonia. In such cases, the coadministration of sodium phenylacetate and sodium benzoate can help prevent the reaccumulation of ammonia by increasing waste nitrogen excretion.

Administration and Dosage

➤*Approved by the FDA:* February 17, 2005.

➤*Administration:* Sodium phenylacetate and sodium benzoate infusion should be started as soon as the diagnosis of hyperammonemia is made.

Administration must be through a central line. Administration through a peripheral line may cause burns.

Sodium phenylacetate and sodium benzoate is administered intravenously (IV) as a loading dose infusion administered over 90 to 120 minutes, followed by an equivalent maintenance dose infusion administered over 24 hours. Sodium phenylacetate and sodium benzoate may not be administered by any other route. Administration of analogous oral drugs (eg, sodium phenylbutyrate) should be terminated prior to sodium phenylacetate and sodium benzoate infusion.

➤*Neonatal hyperammonemic coma:* Hyperammonemic coma (regardless of cause) in the newborn infant should be treated aggressively while the specific diagnosis is pursued.

Hemodialysis – All patients should be promptly hemodialyzed as the procedure of choice using the largest catheters consistent with the patient's size. A target blood flow of 150 mL/min/m^2 may be attained using a 7F catheter. (Ammonia clearance [mL/min] is similar to the blood flow rate [mL/min] through the dialyzer). Clearance of ammonia is approximately 10 times greater by hemodialysis than by peritoneal dialysis or hemofiltration. Exchange transfusion is ineffective in the management of hyperammonemia. Hemodialysis may be repeated until the plasma ammonia level is stable at normal or near normal levels.

➤*Caloric supplementation and protein restriction:* Treatment of hyperammonemia also requires caloric supplementation and restriction of dietary protein. Nonprotein calories should be supplied principally as glucose (8 to 10 mg/kg/min) with *Intralipid* added. Attempts should be made to maintain a caloric intake of more than 80 cal/kg/day.

➤*Dilution:* Sodium phenylacetate and sodium benzoate must be diluted with sterile dextrose injection, 10% (D10W) before administration. The dilution and dosage of sodium phenylacetate and sodium benzoate are determined by weight for neonates, infants, and young children, and by body surface area for larger patients, including older children, adolescents, and adults (see the following table). Maintenance infusions may be continued until elevated plasma ammonia levels have been normalized or the patient can tolerate oral nutrition and medications.

➤*Compatibility:* No compatibility information is presently available for sodium phenylacetate and sodium benzoate infusion solutions except for arginine 10% injection, which may be mixed in the same container as sodium phenylacetate and sodium benzoate. Other infusion solutions and drug products should not be administered together with sodium phenylacetate and sodium benzoate infusion solution. Sodium phenylacetate and sodium benzoate solutions may be prepared in glass and polyvinyl chloride (PVC) containers.

➤*Arginine administration:* IV arginine is an essential component of therapy for patients with carbamyl phosphate synthetase (CPS), ornithine transcarbamylase (OTC), argininosuccinate synthetase (ASS), or argininosuccinate lyase (ASL) deficiency. Because a hyperchloremic acidosis may ensue after high-dose arginine administration, plasma levels of chloride and bicarbonate should be monitored and appropriate amounts of bicarbonate administered.

Pending a specific diagnosis, IV arginine (6 mL/kg of arginine 10% injection over 90 minutes, followed by the same dose over 24 hours) should be given to hyperammonemic infants suspected of having a urea cycle disorder for 2 reasons: 1) infants with deficiencies in enzymes of the urea cycle (apart from arginase deficiency) are usually arginine deficient; 2) hyperammonemia in infants with ASS or ASL deficiency usually respond favorably to arginine administration. If deficiencies of ASS or ASL are excluded as diagnostic possibilities, the IV dose of arginine should be reduced to 2 mL/kg/day.

Sodium Phenylacetate and Sodium Benzoate Dosage Guidelines

Patient population	Components of infusion solution (sodium phenylacetate and sodium benzoate injection must be diluted with sterile dextrose 10% injection at ≥ 25 mL/kg before administration)		Dosage provided		
	Sodium phenylacetate and sodium benzoate injection	Arginine 10% injection	Sodium phenylacetate	Sodium benzoate	Arginine
0 to 20 kg					
Dose	CPS and OTC deficiency				
Loading: Over 90 to 120 min	2.5 mL/kg	2 mL/kg	250 mg/kg	250 mg/kg	200 mg/kg
Maintenance: Over 24 h					
Dose	ASS[a] and ASL deficiency				
Loading: Over 90 to 120 min	2.5 mL/kg	6 mL/kg	250 mg/kg	250 mg/kg	600 mg/kg
Maintenance: Over 24 h					
> 20 kg					
Dose	CPS and OTC deficiency				
Loading: Over 90 to 120 min	55 mL/min^2	2 mL/kg	5.5 g/m^2	5.5 g/m^2	200 mg/kg
Maintenance: Over 24 h					
Dose	ASS[a] and ASL deficiency				
Loading: Over 90 to 120 min	55 mL/m^2	6 mL/kg	5.5 g/m^2	5.5 g/m^2	600 mg/kg
Maintenance: Over 24 h					

[a] ASS patients suspected of having ASS should be infused with sodium phenylacetate and sodium benzoate injection and 600 mg/kg of arginine as a loading dose over a 6-hour infusion period. If the patient is confirmed with ASS, then the loading-dose infusion is administered over 90 minutes.

➤*Converting to oral treatment:* Once elevated ammonia levels have been reduced to the normal range, oral therapy, such as sodium phenylbutyrate, dietary management, and protein restrictions, should be started or reinitiated.

➤*Storage/Stability:* Sodium phenylacetate and sodium benzoate solutions are physically and chemically stable for up to 24 hours at room temperature and room lighting conditions.

Store at 25°C (77°F); excursions permitted to 15° to 30°C (59° to 86°F).

Keep out of the reach of children. This drug is nonpyrogenic.

Actions

➤*Pharmacology:* Sodium phenylacetate and sodium benzoate are metabolically active compounds that can serve as alternatives to urea for the excretion of waste nitrogen. It has been shown that phenylacetylglutamine and hippurate can serve as alternative vehicles to effectively reduce waste nitrogen levels in patients with deficiencies of urea cycle enzymes and, thus, attenuate the risk of ammonia and glutamine-induced neurotoxicity.

Pharmacodynamics – In patients with hyperammonemia caused by deficiencies in enzymes of the urea cycle, sodium phenylacetate and sodium benzoate has been shown to decrease elevated plasma ammonia levels and improve encephalopathy and survival outcome compared with historical controls. These effects are considered to be the result of reduction in nitrogen overload through glutamine and glycine scavenging by sodium phenylacetate and sodium benzoate in combination with appropriate dietary and other supportive measures.

SODIUM BENZOATE AND SODIUM PHENYLACETATE — INJECTION

➤*Pharmacokinetics:*

Absorption/Distribution – The pharmacokinetics of IV administered sodium phenylacetate and sodium benzoate were characterized in healthy adult volunteers. Benzoate and phenylacetate exhibited nonlinear kinetics. Following 90-minute IV infusion, mean area under the curve (AUC_{last}) for benzoate was 20.3, 114.9, 564.6, 562.8, and 1,599.1 mcg/mL after doses of 1, 2, 3.75, 4, and 5.5 g/m^2, respectively. The total clearance decreased from 5.19 to 3.62 L/h/m^2 at the 3.75 and 5.5 g/m^2 doses, respectively.

Similarly, phenylacetate exhibited nonlinear kinetics following the priming dose regimens. AUC_{last} was 175.6, 713.8, 2,040.6, 2,181.6, and 3,829.2 mcg•h/mL following doses of 1, 2, 3.75, 4, and 5.5 g/m^2, respectively. The total clearance decreased from 1.82 to 0.89 mcg•h/mL with increasing dose (3.75 and 4 g/m^2, respectively).

During the sequence of 90-minute priming infusion followed by a 24-hour maintenance infusion, phenylacetate was detected in the plasma at the end of infusion (time to peak concentration [T_{max}] of 2 hours at 3.75 g/m^2), whereas benzoate concentrations declined rapidly (T_{max} of 1.5 hours at 3.75 g/m^2) and were undetectable at 14 and 26 hours following the 3.75 and 4 g/m^2, dose, respectively.

Metabolism/Excretion – A difference in the metabolic rates for phenylacetate and benzoate was noted. The formation of hippurate from benzoate occurred more rapidly than that of phenylacetylglutamine from phenylacetate, and the rate of elimination for hippurate appeared to be more rapid than that of phenylacetylglutamine.

Phenylacetate conjugates with glutamine in the liver and kidneys to form phenylacetylglutamine, via acetylation. Phenylacetylglutamine is excreted by the kidneys via glomerular filtration and tubular secretion. The nitrogen content of phenylacetylglutamine per mole is identical to that of urea (both contain 2 moles of nitrogen). Similarly, preceded by acylation, benzoate conjugates with glycine to form hippuric acid, which is rapidly excreted by the kidneys by glomerular filtration and tubular secretion. One mole of hippuric acid contains 1 mole of waste nitrogen.

Special populations –

Renal function impairment: For effective sodium phenylacetate and sodium benzoate drug therapy, renal clearance of the drug metabolites and subsequently ammonia is required. Closely monitor patients with impaired renal function.

Adult patients with advanced solid tumors: The pharmacokinetics of IV phenylacetate have been reported following administration to adult patients with advanced solid tumors. The decline in serum phenylacetate concentrations following a loading infusion of 150 mg/kg was consistent with saturable enzyme kinetics. Ninety-nine percent of administered phenylacetate was excreted as phenylacetylglutamine.

Contraindications

Hypersensitivity to sodium phenylacetate or sodium benzoate.

Warnings

➤*Acute symptomatic hyperammonemia:* Treat any episode of acute symptomatic hyperammonemia as a life-threatening emergency. Treatment of hyperammonemia may require dialysis, preferably hemodialysis, to remove a large burden of ammonia. Uncontrolled hyperammonemia can rapidly result in brain damage or death, and prompt use of all therapies necessary to reduce ammonia levels is essential.

➤*Appropriate management of hyperammonemia:* Perform management of hyperammonemia caused by inborn errors of metabolism in coordination with medical personnel familiar with these diseases. The severity of the disorder may necessitate the use of hemodialysis combined with nutritional management and medical support. The multidisciplinary nature of the treatment usually requires the facilities of a tertiary or quaternary care center.

➤*Sodium:* Sodium phenylacetate and sodium benzoate contains 30.5 mg of sodium/mL of undiluted product. Use sodium phenylacetate and sodium benzoate with great care, if at all, in patients with congestive heart failure or severe renal insufficiency, and in clinical states in which there is sodium retention with edema. If an adverse reaction does occur, discontinue administration of sodium phenylacetate and sodium benzoate, evaluate the patient, and institute appropriate therapeutic countermeasures.

➤*Extravasation:* Bolus infusion flow rates are relatively high, especially for infants. Extravasation of sodium phenylacetate and sodium benzoate into the perivenous tissues may lead to skin necrosis. If extravasation is suspected, discontinue the infusion and resume at a different infusion site, if necessary. Standard treatment for extravasation can include aspiration of residual drug from the catheter, limb elevation, and intermittent cooling using cold packs. The infusion site must be monitored closely for possible infiltration during drug administration. Do not administer undiluted product.

➤*Renal/Hepatic function impairment:* Because sodium phenylacetate and sodium benzoate are metabolized in the liver and kidney, and because phenylacetylglutamine and hippurate are excreted primarily by the kidney, use caution when administering sodium phenylacetate and sodium benzoate to patients with hepatic or renal function impairment.

➤*Pregnancy: Category C.* Animal reproduction studies have not been conducted with sodium phenylacetate and sodium benzoate. It is not known whether sodium phenylacetate and sodium benzoate can cause fetal harm when administered to a pregnant woman or can affect reproduction capacity. Give sodium phenylacetate and sodium benzoate to a pregnant woman only if clearly needed.

➤*Lactation:* It is not known whether sodium phenylacetate, sodium benzoate, or their conjugation products are excreted in human milk. Because many drugs are excreted in human milk, exercise caution when sodium phenylacetate and sodium benzoate is administered to a breast-feeding woman.

➤*Children:* Sodium phenylacetate and sodium benzoate has been used as a treatment for acute hyperammonemia in pediatric patients, including patients in the early neonatal period.

Precautions

➤*Monitoring:* During and after infusion of sodium phenylacetate and sodium benzoate, ongoing monitoring of neurological status, plasma ammonia levels, clinical laboratory values, and clinical responses are crucial to assess patient response to treatment. The need for other interventions to control hyperammonemia must be considered throughout the course of treatment. Patients with a large ammonia burden or who are not responsive to sodium phenylacetate and sodium benzoate administration require aggressive therapy including hemodialysis.

Because urine potassium loss is enhanced by the excretion of the nonreabsorbable anions, phenylacetylglutamine and hippurate, carefully monitor potassium levels and treat appropriately when necessary. Monitor serum electrolyte levels and maintain them within the normal range.

Because of structural similarities between phenylacetate and benzoate to salicylate, sodium phenylacetate and sodium benzoate may cause side effects typically associated with salicylate overdose, such as hyperventilation and metabolic acidosis. Perform blood chemistry profiles and frequent blood pH and pCO_2 monitoring.

➤*Nausea and vomiting:* Sodium phenylacetate and sodium benzoate infusion has been associated with nausea and vomiting. An antiemetic may be administered during sodium phenylacetate and sodium benzoate infusion.

➤*Loading doses:* Because of prolonged plasma levels achieved by phenylacetate in pharmacokinetic studies, do not administer repeat loading doses of sodium phenylacetate and sodium benzoate.

➤*Corticosteroids:* Use of corticosteroids may cause the breakdown of body protein and, thereby, potentially increase plasma ammonia levels in patients with impaired ability to form urea.

➤*Neurotoxicity:* Neurotoxicity was reported in cancer patients receiving IV phenylacetate, 250 to 300 mg/kg/day for 14 days, repeated at 4-week intervals. Manifestations were predominantly somnolence, fatigue, and light-headedness, with less frequent headaches, dysgeusia, hypoacusis, disorientation, impaired memory, and exacerbation of a preexisting neuropathy. These adverse reactions were mainly mild. The acute onset of symptoms upon initiation of treatment and reversibility of symptoms when the phenylacetate was discontinued suggest a drug effect.

Drug Interactions

Sodium Phenylacetate and Sodium Benzoate Drug Interactions

Precipitant drug	Object drug[a]		Description
Penicillin	Sodium phenylacetate/sodium benzoate	⬇	Some antibiotics such as penicillin may compete with phenylacetylglutamine and hippurate for active secretion by renal tubules, which may affect the overall disposition of the infused drug.
Probenecid	Sodium phenylacetate/sodium benzoate	⬇	Probenecid inhibits renal transport of aminohippuric acid and may affect renal excretion of phenylacetylglutamine.
Valproic acid	Sodium phenylacetate/sodium benzoate	⬇	Valproic acid given to patients with UCDs may exacerbate the condition and antagonize the efficacy of sodium phenylacetate/sodium benzoate.

[a] ⬇ = Object drug decreased.

Adverse Reactions

Sodium Phenylacetate and Benzoate Injection Adverse Reactions (≥ 3%)

Adverse reaction	Patients (n = 316)
Patients with any adverse reaction	163 (52%)
Cardiovascular	
Cardiac disorders	28 (9%)
Hypotension NOS[a]	14 (4%)
Vascular disorders	19 (6%)
CNS	
Agitation	8 (3%)
Brain edema	17 (5%)
CNS disorders	71 (22%)
Coma	10 (3%)
Convulsions NOS	19 (6%)
Mental impairment NOS	18 (6%)
Psychiatric disorders	16 (5%)
Dermatologic	
Skin and subcutaneous tissue disorders	19 (6%)

SODIUM BENZOATE AND SODIUM PHENYLACETATE — INJECTION

Sodium Phenylacetate and Benzoate Injection Adverse Reactions (≥ 3%)	
Adverse reaction	Patients (n = 316)
GI	
Diarrhea NOS	10 (3%)
GI disorders	42 (13%)
Nausea	9 (3%)
Vomiting NOS	29 (12%)
GU	
Renal and urinary disorders	14 (4%)
Urinary tract infection NOS	9 (3%)
Hematologic/Lymphatic	35 (11%)
Anemia NOS	12 (4%)
Disseminated intravascular coagulation	11 (3%)
Metabolic/Nutritional	
Acidosis NOS	8 (3%)
Hyperammonemia	17 (5%)
Hyperglycemia NOS	22 (7%)
Hypocalcemia	8 (3%)
Hypokalemia	23 (7%)
Metabolic acidosis NOS	13 (4%)
Metabolism and nutrition disorders	67 (21%)
Respiratory	
Respiratory distress	9 (3%)
Respiratory, thoracic and mediastinal disorders	47 (15%)
Miscellaneous	
General disorders and administration-site conditions	45 (14%)
Infections	39 (12%)
Injection-site reaction NOS	11 (3%)
Injury, poisoning, and procedural complications	12 (4%)
Investigations	32 (10%)
Pyrexia	17 (5%)

[a] Not otherwise specified.

➤*Clinically important adverse reactions:* Adverse reactions occurred most frequently in the following system organ classes: nervous system disorders (22% of patients), metabolism and nutrition disorders (21% of patients), and respiratory, thoracic, and mediastinal disorders (15% of patients). The most frequently reported adverse reactions were vomiting (9% of patients), hyperglycemia (7% of patients), hypokalemia (7% of patients), convulsions (6% of patients), and mental impairment (6% of patients).

Adverse reactions leading to discontinuation – Adverse reactions leading to study drug discontinuation occurred in 4% of patients. Metabolic acidosis and injection-site reactions each led to discontinuation in 2 patients (less than 1%). Adverse reactions leading to discontinuation in 1 patient included bradycardia, abdominal distension, injection-site extravasation, injection-site hemorrhage, blister, overdose, subdural hematoma, hyperammonemia, hypoglycemia, clonus, coma, increased intracranial pressure, hypercapnia, Kussmaul respiration, respiratory distress, respiratory failure, pruritus, and maculopapular rash.

➤*Less common adverse reactions that could represent drug-induced reactions or are characterized as severe:*

Cardiovascular – Atrial rupture, cardiac or cardiopulmonary arrest/failure, cardiac output decreased, cardiogenic shock, cardiomyopathy, hypertension, pericardial effusion, phlebothrombosis/thrombosis (less than 3%).

CNS – Acute psychosis, aggression, areflexia, ataxia, brain hemorrhage, brain infarction, cerebral atrophy, clonus, confusional state, depressed level of consciousness, encephalopathy, hallucinations, intracranial pressure increased, nerve paralysis, tremor (less than 3%).

Dermatologic – Alopecia, generalized pruritis, rash, urticaria (less than 3%).

GI – GI hemorrhage (less than 3%).

GU – Anuria, renal failure, urinary retention (less than 3%).

Hematologic – Blood carbon dioxide changes, blood pH increased, coagulopathy, pancytopenia, thrombocytopenia (less than 3%).

Hepatic – Cholestasis, hepatic artery stenosis, hepatic failure/hepatotoxicity, jaundice (less than 3%).

Metabolic/Nutritional – Alkalosis, blood glucose changes, dehydration, fluid overload/retention, hyperkalemia, hypernatremia, tetany (less than 3%).

Respiratory – Acute respiratory distress syndrome, pCO_2 changes, dyspnea, hypercapnia, hyperventilation, Kussmaul respiration, pneumonia aspiration, pneumothorax, pulmonary edema, pulmonary hemorrhage, respiratory acidosis or alkalosis, respiratory arrest/failure, respiratory rate increased (less than 3%).

Special senses – Blindness (less than 3%).

Miscellaneous – Acquired hemangioma, asthenia, brain death, brain herniation, chest pain, edema, flushing, hemorrhage, multiorgan failure, neoplasms (benign, malignant, and unspecified), sepsis/septic shock, subdural hematoma (less than 3%).

Overdosage

➤*Symptoms:* Overdosage has been reported during sodium phenylacetate and sodium benzoate treatment in urea cycle-deficient patients. All patients in the uncontrolled open-label study were to be treated at the same dose of sodium phenylacetate and sodium benzoate. However, some patients received more than the dose level specified in the protocol. In 16 of the 64 deaths, the patient received a known overdose of sodium phenylacetate and sodium benzoate. Causes of death in these patients included cardiorespiratory failure/arrest (6 patients), hyperammonemia (3 patients), increased intracranial pressure (2 patients), pneumonitis with septic shock and coagulopathy (1 patient), error in dialysis procedure (1 patient), respiratory failure (1 patient), intractable hypotension and probable sepsis (1 patient), and unknown (1 patient). Additionally, other signs of intoxication may include obtundation (in the absence of hyperammonemia), hyperventilation, a severe compensated metabolic acidosis, perhaps with a respiratory component, large anion gap, hypernatremia and hyperosmolarity, progressive encephalopathy, cardiovascular collapse, and death.

➤*Treatment:* In case of overdose of sodium phenylacetate and sodium benzoate, discontinue the drug and institute appropriate emergency medical monitoring and procedures. In severe cases, the latter may include hemodialysis (procedure of choice) or peritoneal dialysis (when hemodialysis is unavailable).

BROMOCRIPTINE MESYLATE

For complete and comparative prescribing information, see the Bromocriptine mesylate monograph in the Antiparkinson agents group monograph in the CNS chapter.

CABERGOLINE

Rx	**Cabergoline** (Various, eg, Greenstone, Par)	**Tablets:** 0.5 mg	May contain lactose. In 8s.
Rx	**Dostinex** (Pharmacia & Upjohn)		(PU 700). White, scored. Capsule shaped. In bottles of 8.

CABERGOLINE — ORAL

Indications

➤*Hyperprolactinemic disorders:* For the treatment of hyperprolactinemic disorders, either idiopathic or caused by pituitary adenomas.

Administration and Dosage

➤*Approved by the FDA:* December 23, 1996.

➤*Dosage:* The recommended dosage of cabergoline tablets for initiation of therapy is 0.25 mg twice a week. Dosage may be increased by 0.25 mg twice weekly up to a dosage of 1 mg twice a week according to the patient's serum prolactin level.

Dosage increases should not occur more rapidly than every 4 weeks, so that the physician can assess the patient's response to each dosage level. If the patient does not respond adequately, and no additional benefit is observed with higher doses, the lowest dose that achieved maximal response should be used and other therapeutic approaches considered.

After a normal serum prolactin level has been maintained for 6 months, cabergoline may be discontinued, with periodic monitoring of the serum prolactin level to determine whether or when treatment with cabergoline should be reinstituted. The durability of efficacy beyond 24 months of therapy with cabergoline has not been established.

➤*Storage/Stability:* Store at controlled room temperature 20° to 25°C (68° to 77°F) [see USP].

Actions

➤*Pharmacology:* The secretion of prolactin by the anterior pituitary is mainly under hypothalmic inhibitory control, likely exerted through release of dopamine by tuberoinfundibular neurons. Cabergoline is a long-acting dopamine receptor agonist with a high affinity for D_2 receptors. Results of in vitro studies demonstrate that cabergoline exerts a direct inhibitory effect on the secretion of prolactin by rat pituitary lactotrophs. Cabergoline decreased serum prolactin levels in reserpinized rats. Receptor-binding

CABERGOLINE — ORAL

studies indicate that cabergoline has low affinity for dopamine D_1, α_1- and α_2-adrenergic, and 5-HT_1- and 5-HT_2-serotonin receptors.

Pharmacodynamics – Dose response with inhibition of plasma prolactin, onset of maximal effect, and duration of effect has been documented following single cabergoline doses to healthy volunteers (0.05 to 1.5 mg) and hyperprolactinemic patients (0.3 to 1 mg). In volunteers, prolactin inhibition was evident at doses greater than 0.2 mg, while doses greater than or equal to 0.5 mg caused maximal suppression in most subjects. Higher doses produce prolactin suppression in a greater proportion of subjects and with an earlier onset and longer duration of action. In 12 healthy volunteers, 0.5, 1, and 1.5 mg doses resulted in complete prolactin inhibition, with a maximum effect within 3 hours in 92% to 100% of subjects after the 1 and 1.5 mg doses compared with 50% of subjects after the 0.5 mg dose.

In hyperprolactinemic patients (n = 51), the maximal prolactin decrease after a 0.6 mg single dose of cabergoline was comparable to 2.5 mg bromocriptine; however, the duration of effect was markedly longer (14 days vs 24 hours). The time to maximal effect was shorter for bromocriptine than cabergoline (6 hours vs 48 hours).

In 72 healthy volunteers, single or multiple doses (up to 2 mg) of cabergoline resulted in selective inhibition of prolactin with no apparent effect on other anterior pituitary hormones (growth hormone, follicle-stimulating hormone, luteinizing hormone, advenocorticotropic hormone, and thyroid-stimulating hormone) or cortisol.

➤*Pharmacokinetics:*

Absorption – Following single oral doses of 0.5 mg to 1.5 mg given to 12 healthy adult volunteers, mean peak plasma levels of 30 to 70 picograms (pg)/mL of cabergoline were observed within 2 to 3 hours. Over the 0.5-to-7 mg dose range, cabergoline plasma levels appeared to be dose-proportional in 12 healthy adult volunteers and nine adult parkinsonian patients. A repeat-dose study in 12 healthy volunteers suggests that steady-state levels following a once-weekly dosing schedule are expected to be twofold to three-fold higher than after a single dose. The absolute bioavailability of cabergoline is unknown. A significant fraction of the administered dose undergoes a first-pass effect. The elimination half-life of cabergoline estimated from urinary data of 12 healthy subjects ranged between 63 to 69 hours. The prolonged prolactin-lowering effect of cabergoline may be related to its slow elimination and long half-life.

Distribution – In animals, based on total radioactivity, cabergoline (and/or its metabolites) has shown extensive tissue distribution. Radioactivity in the pituitary exceeded that in plasma by greater than 100-fold and was eliminated with a half-life of approximately 60 hours. This finding is consistent with the long-lasting prolactin-lowering effect of the drug. Whole body autoradiography studies in pregnant rats showed no fetal uptake but high levels in the uterine wall. Significant radioactivity (parent plus metabolites) detected in the milk of lactating rats suggests a potential for exposure to nursing infants. The drug is extensively distributed throughout the body. Cabergoline is moderately bound (40% to 42%) to human plasma proteins in a concentration-independent manner. Concomitant dosing of highly protein-bound drugs is unlikely to affect its disposition.

Metabolism – In both animals and humans, cabergoline is extensively metabolized, predominately via hydrolysis of the acylurea bond or the urea moiety. Cytochrome P-450 mediated metabolism appears to be minimal. Cabergoline does not cause enzyme induction and/or inhibition in the rat. Hydrolysis of the acylurea or urea moiety abolishes the prolactin-lowering effect of cabergoline, and major metabolites identified thus far do not contribute to the therapeutic effect.

Excretion – After oral dosing of radioactive cabergoline to five healthy volunteers, approximately 22% and 60% of the dose was excreted within 20 days in the urine and feces, respectively. Less than 4% of the dose was excreted unchanged in the urine. Nonrenal and renal clearances for cabergoline are about 3.2 L/min and 0.08 L/min, respectively. Urinary excretion in hyperprolactinemic patients was similar.

Special populations –

Hepatic function impairment: In 12 patients with mild-to-moderate hepatic dysfunction (Child-Pugh score less than or equal to 10), no effect on mean cabergoline C_{max} or area under the plasma concentration curve (AUC) was observed. However, patients with severe insufficiency (Child-Pugh score greater than 10) show a substantial increase in the mean cabergoline C_{max} and AUC, and thus necessitate caution.

Contraindications

Uncontrolled hypertension; known hypersensitivity to ergot derivatives.

Warnings

➤*Hepatic function impairment:* Because cabergoline is extensively metabolized by the liver, caution should be used, and careful monitoring exercised, when administering cabergoline to patients with hepatic impairment.

➤*Carcinogenesis:* Carcinogenicity studies were conducted in mice and rats with cabergoline given by gavage at doses up to 0.98 mg/kg/day and 0.32 mg/kg/day, respectively. These doses are 7 times and 4 times the maximum recommended human dose calculated on a body surface area basis using total mg/m²/week in rodents and mg/m²/week for a 50 kg human.

There was a slight increase in the incidence of cervical and uterine leiomyomas and uterine leiomyosarcomas in mice. In rats, there was a slight increase in malignant tumors of the cervix and uterus and interstitial cell adenomas. The occurrence of tumors in female rodents may be related to the prolonged suppression of prolactin secretion because prolactin is needed in rodents for the maintenance of the corpus luteum. In the absence of prolactin, the estrogen/progesterone ratio is increased, thereby increasing the risk for uterine tumors. In male rodents, the decrease in serum prolactin levels was associated with an increase in serum luteinizing hormone, which is thought to be a compensatory effect to maintain testicular steroid synthesis. Since these hormonal mechanisms are thought to be species-specific, the relevance of these tumors to humans is not known.

➤*Fertility impairment:* In female rats, a daily dose of 0.003 mg/kg for 2 weeks prior to mating and throughout the mating period inhibited conception. This dose represents approximately 1/28 the maximum recommended human dose calculated on a body surface area basis using total mg/m²/week in rats and mg/m²/week for a 50 kg human.

➤*Elderly:* In general, dose selection for an elderly patient should be cautious, usually starting at the low end of the dosing range, reflecting the greater frequency of decreased hepatic, renal, or cardiac function, and of concomitant disease or other drug therapy.

➤*Pregnancy: Category B.*

Pregnancy-induced hypertension – Dopamine agonists in general should not be used in patients with pregnancy-induced hypertension, for example, preeclampsia and eclampsia, unless the potential benefit is judged to outweigh the possible risk.

Teratogenic – Reproduction studies have been performed with cabergoline in mice, rats, and rabbits administered by gavage.

(Multiples of the maximum recommended human dose in this section are calculated on a body surface area basis using total mg/m²/week for animals and mg/m²/week for a 50 kg human.)

There were maternotoxic effects but no teratogenic effects in mice given cabergoline at doses up to 8 mg/kg/day (approximately 55 times the maximum recommended human dose) during the period of organogenesis.

A dose of 0.012 mg/kg/day (approximately 1/7 the maximum recommended human dose) during the period of organogenesis in rats caused an increase in post-implantation embryofetal losses. These losses could be due to the prolactin inhibitory properties of cabergoline in rats. At daily doses of 0.5 mg/kg/day (approximately 19 times the maximum recommended human dose) during the period of organogenesis in the rabbit, cabergoline caused maternotoxicity characterized by a loss of body weight and decreased food consumption. Doses of 4 mg/kg/day (approximately 150 times the maximum recommended human dose) during the period of organogenesis in the rabbit caused an increased occurrence of various malformations. However, in another study in rabbits, no treatment-related malformations or embryofetotoxicity were observed at doses up to 8 mg/kg/day (approximately 300 times the maximum recommended human dose).

In rats, doses higher than 0.003 mg/kg/day (approximately 1/28 the maximum recommended human dose) from 6 days before parturition and throughout the lactation period inhibited growth and caused death of offspring due to decreased milk secretion.

There are, however, no adequate and well-controlled studies in pregnant women. Because animal reproduction studies are not always predictive of human response, this drug should be used during pregnancy only if clearly needed.

➤*Lactation:* It is not known whether this drug is excreted in human milk. Because many drugs are excreted in human milk and because of the potential for serious adverse reactions in nursing infants from cabergoline, a decision should be made whether to discontinue nursing or to discontinue the drug, taking into account the importance of the drug to the mother. Use of cabergoline for the inhibition or suppression of physiologic lactation is not recommended (see Precautions).

The prolactin-lowering action of cabergoline suggests that it will interfere with lactation. Due to this interference with lactation, cabergoline should not be given to women postpartum who are breastfeeding or who are planning to breastfeed.

➤*Children:* Safety and effectiveness of cabergoline in pediatric patients have not been established.

Precautions

➤*Orthostatic hypotension:* Initial doses higher than 1 mg may produce orthostatic hypotension. Care should be exercised when administering cabergoline with other medications known to lower blood pressure.

➤*Postpartum lactation inhibition or suppression:* Cabergoline is not indicated for the inhibition or suppression of physiologic lactation. Use of bromocriptine, another dopamine agonist for this purpose, has been associated with cases of hypertension, stroke, and seizures.

Drug Interactions

Cabergoline Drug Interactions

Precipitant drug	Object drug[a]		Description
Cabergoline	Antihypertensives	⬆	Additive hypotensive effects may occur when cabergoline is administered with other hypotensive medications. In addition, antihypertensive dosage adjustments may be necessary if antihypertensive medications are administered concurrently with cabergoline.

CABERGOLINE — ORAL

Cabergoline Drug Interactions			
Precipitant drug	Object drug[a]		Description
Dopamine (D_2) antagonists (eg, phenothiazines, butyrophenones, thioxanthenes or metoclopramide)	Cabergoline	⬇	Dopamine (D_2) antagonists may reduce the therapeutic effects of cabergoline. Do not administer with cabergoline.

[a] ⬆ = Object drug increased. ⬇ = Object drug decreased.

Adverse Reactions

In a 4-week, double-blind, placebo-controlled study, treatment consisted of placebo or cabergoline at fixed doses of 0.125, 0.5, 0.75, or 1 mg twice weekly. Doses were halved during the first week. Since a possible dose-related effect was observed for nausea only, the four cabergoline treatment groups have been combined.

Incidence of Reported Adverse Events During the 4-Week, Double-Blind, Placebo-Controlled Trial		
Adverse reaction[a]	Cabergoline (n = 168) 0.125 to 1 mg twice weekly	Placebo (n = 20)
	Number	
GI		
Nausea	45 (27%)	4 (20%)
Constipation	16 (10%)	0
Abdominal pain	9 (5%)	1 (5%)
Dyspepsia	4 (2%)	0
Vomiting	4 (2%)	0
CNS/Peripheral nervous system		
Headache	43 (26%)	5 (25%)
Dizziness	25 (15%)	1 (5%)
Paresthesia	2 (1%)	0
Vertigo	2 (1%)	0
Miscellaneous		
Asthenia	15 (9%)	2 (10%)
Fatigue	12 (7%)	0
Hot flashes	2 (1%)	1 (5%)
Psychiatric		
Somnolence	9 (5%)	1 (5%)
Depression	5 (3%)	1 (5%)
Nervousness	4 (2%)	0
Autonomic nervous system		
Postural hypotension	6 (4%)	0
GU (female)		
Breast pain	2 (1%)	0
Dysmenorrhea	2 (1%)	0
Ophthalmic		
Abnormal vision	2 (1%)	0

[a] Reported at greater than or equal to 1% for cabergoline.

In the 8-week, double-blind period of the comparative trial with bromocriptine, cabergoline (at a dose of 0.5 mg twice weekly) was discontinued because of an adverse event in 4 of 221 patients (2%) while bromocriptine (at a dose of 2.5 mg twice a day) was discontinued in 14 of 231 patients (6%). The most common reasons for discontinuation from cabergoline were headache, nausea and vomiting (3, 2 and 2 patients respectively); the most common reasons for discontinuation from bromocriptine were nausea, vomiting, headache, and dizziness or vertigo (10, 3, 3, and 3 patients respectively).

Incidence of Reported Adverse Events During the 8-Week, Double-Blind Period of the Comparative Trial with Bromocriptine		
Adverse reaction[a]	Cabergoline (n = 221)	Bromocriptine (n = 231)
	Number	
GI		
Nausea	63 (29%)	100 (43%)
Constipation	15 (7%)	21 (9%)
Abdominal pain	12 (5%)	19 (8%)
Dyspepsia	11 (5%)	16 (7%)
Vomiting	9 (4%)	16 (7%)
Dry mouth	5 (2%)	2 (1%)
Diarrhea	4 (2%)	7 (3%)
Flatulence	4 (2%)	3 (1%)
Throat irritation	2 (1%)	0
Toothache	2 (1%)	0
CNS/Peripheral nervous system		
Headache	58 (26%)	62 (27%)
Dizziness	38 (17%)	42 (18%)
Vertigo	9 (4%)	10 (4%)
Paresthesia	5 (2%)	6 (3%)
Miscellaneous		
Asthenia	13 (6%)	15 (6%)
Fatigue	10 (5%)	18 (8%)
Syncope	3 (1%)	3 (1%)
Influenza-like symptoms	2 (1%)	0
Malaise	2 (1%)	0
Periorbital edema	2 (1%)	2 (1%)
Peripheral edema	2 (1%)	1
Psychiatric		
Depression	7 (3%)	5 (2%)
Somnolence	5 (2%)	5 (2%)
Anorexia	3 (1%)	3 (1%)
Anxiety	3 (1%)	3 (1%)
Insomnia	3 (1%)	2 (1%)
Impaired concentration	2 (1%)	1
Nervousness	2 (1%)	5 (2%)
Cardiovascular		
Hot flashes	6 (3%)	3 (1%)
Hypotension	3 (1%)	4 (2%)
Dependent edema	2 (1%)	1
Palpitation	2 (1%)	5 (2%)
GU (female)		
Breast pain	5 (2%)	8 (3%)
Dysmenorrhea	2 (1%)	1
Dermatologic		
Acne	3 (1%)	0
Pruritus	2 (1%)	1
Musculoskeletal		
Pain	4 (2%)	6 (3%)
Arthralgia	2 (1%)	0
Respiratory		
Rhinitis	2 (1%)	9 (4%)
Ophthalmic		
Abnormal vision	2 (1%)	2 (1%)

[a] Reported at greater than or equal to 1% for cabergoline.

Other adverse reactions that were reported at an incidence of less than 1% in the overall clinical studies follow.

➤*Cardiovascular:* Hypotension, syncope, palpitations.

➤*CNS:* Somnolence, nervousness, paresthesia, insomnia, anxiety.

➤*Dermatologic:* Acne, pruritus.

➤*GI:* Dry mouth, flatulence, diarrhea, anorexia.

➤*GU:* Dysmenorrhea, increased libido.

➤*Metabolic/Nutritional:* Weight loss, weight gain.

➤*Respiratory:* Epistaxis, nasal stuffiness.

➤*Special senses:* Abnormal vision.

➤*Miscellaneous:* Facial edema, influenza-like symptoms, malaise. The safety of cabergoline has been evaluated in approximately 1,200 patients with Parkinson disease in controlled and uncontrolled studies at dosages of up to 11.5 mg/day which greatly exceeds the maximum recommended dosage of cabergoline for hyperprolactinemic disorders. In addition to the adverse reactions that occurred in the patients with hyperprolactinemic disorders, the most common adverse reactions in patients with Parkinson disease were dyskinesia, hallucinations, confusion, and peripheral edema. Heart failure, pleural effusion, pulmonary fibrosis, and gastric or duodenal ulcer occurred rarely. One case of constrictive pericarditis has been reported.

CABERGOLINE — ORAL

Overdosage

Overdosage might be expected to produce nasal congestion, syncope, or hallucinations. Measures to support blood pressure should be taken if necessary.

Patient Information

A patient should be instructed to notify her physician if she suspects she is pregnant, becomes pregnant, or intends to become pregnant during therapy. A pregnancy test should be done if there is any suspicion of pregnancy and continuation of treatment should be discussed with her physician.

AGENTS FOR GOUT

In addition to the agents in this section, sulindac and indomethacin (see Nonsteroidal Anti-inflammatory Agents monograph) are indicated for the treatment of gout. See also probenecid and sulfinpyrazone in the Uricosurics section.

Uricosurics

PROBENECID

Rx	**Probenecid** (Various, eg, Geneva, Moore, Parmed, Purepac, Schein, URL)	**Tablets:** 0.5 g	In 100s and 1,000s.

PROBENECID — ORAL

Indications

➤*Hyperuricemia:* For treatment of hyperuricemia associated with gout and gouty arthritis.

➤*Elevation/Prolongation of plasma levels of antibiotics:* As an adjunctive to therapy with penicillin, or with ampicillin, methicillin, oxacillin, cloxacillin, or nafcillin, for elevation and prolongation of plasma levels by whatever route the antibiotic is given.

Administration and Dosage

➤*Gout:* Therapy with probenecid should not be started until acute gouty attack has subsided. However, if an acute attack is precipitated during therapy, probenecid may be continued without changing the dosage, and full therapeutic dosage of colchicine, or other appropriate therapy, should be given to control the acute attack.

Adult – The recommended adult dosage is 250 mg (½ probenecid tablet), twice a day for 1 week, followed by 500 mg (1 tablet) twice a day thereafter. Gastric intolerance may be indicative of overdosage, and may be corrected by decreasing the dosage.

Renal function impairment – Some degree of renal impairment may be present in patients with gout. A daily dosage of 1,000 mg may be adequate. However, if necessary, the daily dosage may be increased by 500 mg increments, every 4 weeks within tolerance (and usually not above 2,000 mg/day) if symptoms of gouty arthritis are not controlled or the 24-hour urate excretion is not above 700 mg. Probenecid may not be effective in chronic renal insufficiency particularly when the glomerular filtration rate is 30 mL/min or less.

Urinary alkalization – As uric acid tends to crystallize out of an acid urine, a liberal fluid intake is recommended, as well as sufficient sodium bicarbonate (3,000 to 7,500 mg/day), or potassium citrate (7,500 mg/day) to maintain an alkaline urine. In these cases when alkali is administered, the acid-base balance of the patient should be watched.

Alkalization of the urine is recommended until the serum urate level returns to normal limits and tophaceous deposits disappear (ie, during the period when urinary excretion of uric acid is at a high level). Thereafter, alkalization of the urine and the usual restriction of purine-producing goods may be somewhat relaxed.

Maintenance therapy – Probenecid should be continued at the dosage that will maintain normal serum urate levels. When acute attacks have been absent for 6 months or more and serum urate levels remain within normal limits, the daily dosage may be decreased by 500 mg every 6 months. The maintenance dosage should not be reduced to the point where serum urate levels tend to rise.

➤*Probenecid and penicillin therapy (general):*

Adults – The recommended dosage is 2,000 mg (4 tablets of probenecid) daily in divided doses. This dosage should be reduced in older patients in whom renal impairment may be present.

Children 2 to 14 years of age –
Initial dose: 25 mg/kg body weight (or 0.7 g/m^2 body surface).
Maintenance dose: 40 mg/kg body weight (or 1.2 g/m^2 body surface) per day, divided into 4 doses. For children weighing more than 50 kg (110 pounds) the adult dosage is recommended.

Probenecid is contraindicated in children under 2 years of age. The PSP excretion test may be used to determine the effectiveness of probenecid in retarding penicillin excretion and maintaining therapeutic levels. The renal clearance of PSP is reduced to about one-fifth the normal rate when dosage of probenecid is adequate.

➤*Penicillin therapy (gonorrhea):*

Probenecid and Penicillin Therapy (Gonorrhea)[a]

Statement	Recommended regimens[b]	Remarks
Uncomplicated gonococcal infection in men and women (urethral, cervical, or rectal)	4.8 million units of aqueous procaine penicillin G[c] IM, in at least 2 doses injected at different sites at 1 visit, plus 1 g probenecid orally just before injections or 3.5 g of ampicillin [c]orally plus 1 g probenecid orally given simultaneously.	Follow-up: Obtain urethral and other appropriate cultures from men, and cervical, anal, and other appropriate cultures from women, 7 to 14 days after completion of treatment.
		Treatment of sexual partners: Persons with known recent exposure to gonorrhea should receive the same treatment as those known to have gonorrhea. Examination and treatment of male sex partners of persons with gonorrhea are essential because of the high prevalence of nonsymptomatic urethral gonococcal infection in such men.
Pharyngeal gonococcal infection in men and women	4.8 million units of aqueous procaine penicillin G[c] IM in at least 2 doses injected at different sites at 1 visit plus 1 g of probenecid just before injections.	Pharyngeal gonococcal infections may be more difficult to treat than anogenital gonorrhea. Posttreatment cultures are essential.
Uncomplicated gonorrhea in pregnant patients	4.8 million units of aqueous procaine penicillin G[c] IM in at least 2 doses injected at different sites at 1 visit, plus 1 g probenecid orally just before injections or 3.5 g ampicillin[c] orally plus 1 g probenecid orally given simultaneously	
Acute gonococcal salpingitis	Outpatients: Aqueous procaine penicillin G[c] or ampicillin[c] with probenecid as for gonorrhea in pregnancy, followed by ampicillin 500 mg[c] 4 times a day for 10 days.	Follow-up of patients with acute salpingitis is essential. All patients should receive repeat pelvic examinations and cultures for *Neisseria gonorrhoeae* after treatment. Examination and appropriate treatment of male sex partners are essential because of the high prevalence of nonsymptomatic urethral gonorrhea in such men.
	Hospitalized patients: See the detailed treatment recommendations in the CDC guidelines.	
Disseminated gonococcal infection (arthritis-dermatitis syndrome)	10 million units of aqueous crystalline penicillin G[c] IV a day for 3 days or until significant clinical improvement occurs. May be followed with ampicillin 500 mg[c] 4 times a day orally to complete 7 days of treatment or 3.5 g ampicillin[c] orally plus 1 g probenecid followed by ampicillin 500 mg[c] 4 times a day for at least 7 days.	

PROBENECID — ORAL

Probenecid and Penicillin Therapy (Gonorrhea)[a]		
Statement	Recommended regimens[b]	Remarks
Gonococcal infection in children	For postpubertal children or those weighing over 45 kg (100 lbs): Use the dosage regimens given above for adults.	See CDC recommendations for detailed information about prevention and treatment of neonatal gonococcal infection and gonococcal ophthalmia.
	Uncomplicated vulvovaginitis and urethritis: Aqueous procaine ponicillin G[c] 75,000 to 10,000 units/kg IM with probenecid 23 mg/kg orally.	

[a] Recommended by Venereal Disease Control Advisory Committee, Center for Disease Control, US Department of Health, Education, and Welfare, Public Health Service (*Morbidity and Mortality Weekly Report*, Vol. 23:341, 342, 347, 348, October 11, 1974).
[b] See CDC recommendations for definition of regimens of choice, alternative regimens, treatment of hypersensitive patients, and other aspects of therapy.
[c] See package circulars of manufacturers for detailed information abut contraindications, warnings, precautions, and adverse reactions.

➤*Note:* Before treating gonococcal infections in patients with suspected primary to secondary syphilis, perform proper diagnostic procedures including darkfield examinations. If concomitant syphilis is suspected, perform monthly serological tests for at least 4 months.

➤*Storage/Stability:*
Pharmacist – Dispense in a well-closed container as defined in the USP. Use child-resistant closure. Store at controlled room temperature 15° to 30°C (59° to 86°F).

Actions

➤*Pharmacology:* Probenecid is a uricosuric and renal tubular-blocking agent. It inhibits the tubular reabsorption of urate, thus increasing the urinary excretion of uric acid and decreasing serum urate levels. Effective uricosuria reduces the miscible urate pool, retards urate deposition, and promotes resorption of urate deposits.

Probenecid inhibits the tubular secretion of penicillin and usually increases penicillin plasma levels by any route the antibiotic is given. A 2- to 4-fold elevation has been demonstrated for various penicillins.

Probenecid has also been reported to inhibit the renal transport of many other compounds including aminohippuric acid (PAH), aminosalicylic acid (PAS), dyphylline, indomethacin, sodium iodomethamate and related iodinated organic acids, 17-ketosteroids, pantothenic acid, phenolsulfonphthalein (PSP), sulfonamides, and sulfonylureas.

Probenecid decreases both hepatic and renal excretion of sulfobromophthalein (BSP). The tubular reabsorption of phosphorus is inhibited in hypoparathyroid but not in euparathyroid individuals.

Probenecid does not influence plasma concentrations of salicylates, nor the excretion of streptomycin, chloramphenicol, chlortetracycline, oxytetracycline or neomycin.

Contraindications

Hypersensitivity to probenecid; children younger than 2 years of age; blood dyscrasias or uric acid kidney stones.

Therapy with probenecid should not be started until an acute gouty attack has subsided.

Warnings

➤*Exacerbation of gout:* Exacerbation of gout following therapy with probenecid may occur; in such cases colchicine or other appropriate therapy is advisable.

➤*Methotrexate:* See Drug Interactions for more information.

➤*Salicylates:* In patients on probenecid the use of salicyates in either small or large doses is contraindicated because it antagonizes the uricosuric action of probenecid.

The biphasic action of salicylates in the renal tubules accounts for the so-called "paradoxical effect" of uricosuric agents. In patients on probenecid who require a mild analgesic agent the use of acetaminophen rather than small doses of salicylates would be preferred.

➤*Hypersensitivity reactions:* The appearance of hypersensitivity reactions requires cessation of therapy with probenecid.

➤*Renal function impairment:* Probenecid has been used in patients with some renal impairment, but dosage requirements may be increased. Probenecid may not be effective in chronic renal insufficiency particularly when the glomerular filtration rate is 30 mL/minute or less. Because of its mechanism of action, probenecid is not recommended in conjunction with a penicillin in the presence of known renal impairment.

➤*Pregnancy: Category B.* Probenecid crosses the placenta and appears in cord blood. It has been used during pregnancy without producing adverse effects in the fetus or in the infant. Use only when clearly needed and when potential benefits outweigh potential hazards to the fetus.

Precautions

➤*Alkalinization of urine:* Hematuria, renal colic, costovertebral pain, and formation of uric acid stones associated with the use of probenecid in gouty patients may be prevented by alkalization of the urine and liberal fluid intake. As uric acid tends to crystallize out of an acid urine, a liberal fluid intake is recommended, as well as sufficient sodium bicarbonate (3,000 to 7,500 mg/day), or potassium citrate (7,500 mg/day) to maintain an alkaline urine. In these cases when alkali is administered, the acid-base balance of the patient should be watched.

➤*Special risk:* Use with caution in patients with a history of peptic ulcer.

Drug Interactions

Probenecid Drug Interactions			
Precipitant drug	Object drug[a]		Description
Probenecid	Acyclovir	↑	Decreased acyclovir renal clearance and increased bioavailability following IV use may occur.
Probenecid	Allopurinol	↑	A beneficial interaction; coadministration may increase the uric acid lowering effect.
Probenecid	Barbiturates	↑	The anesthesia produced by thiopental may be extended or achieved at lower doses.
Probenecid	Benzodiazepines	↑	A more rapid onset or more prolonged benzodiazepine effect may occur.
Probenecid	Clofibrate	↑	Accumulation of clofibric acid (active metabolite of clofibrate) may occur, leading to higher steady-state serum concentrations.
Probenecid	Dapsone	↑	Possible accumulation of dapsone and its metabolites.
Probenecid	Dyphylline	↑	Increased half-life and decreased clearance of dyphylline may occur. This may be beneficial in extending the dyphylline dosing interval.
Probenecid	Methotrexate	↑	Methotrexate's plasma levels, therapeutic effects and toxicity may be enhanced.
Probenecid	NSAIDs	↑	NSAID plasma levels may be increased; toxicity may be enhanced.
Probenecid	Pantothenic acid	↑	Renal transport of pantothenic acid may be inhibited; plasma levels may increase.
Probenecid	Penicillamine	↑	Pharmacologic effects of penicillamine may be attenuated.
Probenecid	Rifampin	↑	Renal transport of rifampin may be inhibited; plasma levels may increase.
Probenecid	Sulfonamides	↑	Renal transport of sulfonamides may be inhibited; plasma levels may increase.
Probenecid	Sulfonylureas	↑	Half-life of sulfonylureas may be increased.
Probenecid	Zidovudine	↑	Increased zidovudine bioavailability may occur; cutaneous eruptions accompanied by systemic symptoms including malaise, myalgia or fever have occurred.
Salicylates	Probenecid	↓	Coadministration may inhibit the uricosuric action of either drug alone.

[a] ↑ = Object drug increased. ↓ = Object drug decreased.

➤*Drug/Lab test interactions:*
Theophylline – Falsely high readings for theophylline have been reported in an in vitro study, using the Schack and Waxler technique, when therapeutic concentrations of theophylline and probenecid were added to human plasma. A reducing substance may appear in the urine of patients receiving probenecid. This disappears with discontinuance of therapy. Suspected glycosuria should be confirmed by using a test specific for glucose.

Adverse Reactions

Headache, GI symptoms (eg, anorexia, nausea, vomiting), urinary frequency, hypersensitivity reactions (including anaphylaxis, dermatitis, pruritus, and fever), sore gums, flushing, dizziness, and anemia have occurred.

PROBENECID — ORAL

In gouty patients, exacerbation of gout and uric acid stones with or without hematuria, renal colic, or costovertebral pain, have been observed. Nephrotic syndrome, hepatic necrosis, and aplastic anemia occur rarely. Hemolytic anemia, which in some instances could be related to genetic deficiency of glucose-6-phosphate dehydrogenase in red blood cells, has been reported.

Patient Information

Avoid taking aspirin or other salicylates that antagonize the effects of probenecid.

Probenecid may cause GI upset and may be taken with food or antacids. If nausea, vomiting or loss of appetite persists, notify physician.

Drink plenty of water, at least 6 to 8 full (8 oz) glasses daily, to prevent development of kidney stones.

SULFINPYRAZONE

Rx	**Sulfinpyrazone** (Various, eg, Barr, Goldline, Rugby)	**Tablets:** 100 mg	In 100s and 500s.
Rx	**Anturane** (Novartis)		White, scored. In 100s.
Rx	**Sulfinpyrazone** (Various, eg, Barr, Goldline, Rugby, Zenith)	**Capsules:** 200 mg	In 100s, 500s and 1,000s.
Rx	**Anturane** (Novartis)		Green. In 100s.

SULFINPYRAZONE — ORAL

Indications

➤*Gouty arthritis:* Sulfinpyrazole is indicated for the treatment of chronic gouty arthritis and intermittent gouty arthritis

➤*Unlabeled uses:* Sulfinpyrazone may decrease the incidence of sudden cardiac death when given to patients 1 to 6 months post-myocardial infarction 300 mg 4 times daily. Sulfinpyrazone may decrease the frequency of systemic embolism in patients with rheumatic mitral stenosis.

A placebo-controlled study of 186 patients with rheumatic mitral stenosis suggested that sulfinpyrazone may decrease the frequency of systemic embolism.

Administration and Dosage

➤*Approved by the FDA:* September 17, 1982.

➤*Initial:* 200 to 400 mg daily in 2 divided doses, with meals or milk, gradually increasing when necessary to full maintenance dosage in 1 week.

➤*Maintenance:* 400 mg daily, given in 2 divided doses, as above. This dosage may be increased to 800 mg daily, if necessary, and may sometimes be reduced to as low as 200 mg daily after the blood urate level has been controlled. Treatment should be continued without interruption even in the presence of acute exacerbations, which can be concomitantly treated with phenylbutazone or colchicine. Patients previously controlled with other uricosuric therapy may be transferred to sulfinpyrazone at full maintenance dosage.

➤*Storage/Stability:* Do not store above 30°C (86°F). Dispense in tight container.

Actions

➤*Pharmacology:* Its pharmacologic activity is the potentiation of the urinary excretion of uric acid. It is useful for reducing the blood urate levels in patients with chronic tophaceous gout and acute intermittent gout, and for promoting the resorption of tophi.

Contraindications

Active peptic ulcer or symptoms of GI inflammation or ulceration; hypersensitivity to phenylbutazone or other pyrazoles, blood dyscrasias, or gouty arthritis.

Warnings

➤*Acute gout attack:* Sulfinpyrazone has minimal anti-inflammatory effect and is not intended for the relief of an acute attack of gout.

In the initial stages of therapy, because of the marked ability of sulfinpyrazone to mobilize urates, acute attacks of gouty arthritis may be precipitated.

➤*Renal function impairment:* Because sulfinpyrazone is a potent uricosuric agent, it may precipitate urolithiasis and renal colic, especially in the initial stages of therapy. For this reason, an adequate fluid intake and alkalinization of the urine are recommended. In cases with significant renal impairment, periodic assessment of renal function is indicated. Occasional cases of renal failure have been reported; but a cause-and-effect relationship has not always been clearly established.

➤*Pregnancy:* It is suggested that sulfinpyrazone be used with caution in pregnant women, weighing the potential risks against the possible benefits.

Studies on the teratogenicity of pyrazole compounds in animals have yielded inconclusive results. Up to the present time, however, there have been no reported cases of human congenital malformation proved to be due to the use of the drug.

➤*Children:* Safety and efficacy in pediatric patients have not been established.

Precautions

➤*Monitoring:* As with all pyrazole compounds, patients receiving sulfinpyrazone should be kept under close medical supervision and periodic blood counts are recommended. It may be administered with care to patients with a history of healed peptic ulcer.

Drug Interactions

➤*Coumarin-type anticoagulants:* Sulfinpyrazone may accentuate the action of coumarin-type anticoagulants and further depress prothrombin activity when these medications are employed simultaneously.

➤*Salicylates:* Salicylates antagonize the uricosuric action of sulfinpyrazone and for this reason their concomitant use is contraindicated in gouty arthritis.

➤*Other drugs:* Recent reports have indicated that sulfinpyrazone potentiates the action of certain sulfonamides, such as sulfadiazine and sulfisoxazole. In addition, other pyrazole compounds (phenylbutazone) have been observed to potentiate the hypoglycemic sulfonylurea agents, as well as insulin. In view of these observations, it is suggested that sulfinpyrazone be used with caution in conjunction with sulfa drugs, the sulfonylurea hypoglycemic agents and insulin.

Sulfinpyrazone Drug Interactions

Precipitant drug	Object drug[a]		Description
Sulfinpyrazone	Acetaminophen	↔	Risk of acetaminophen hepatotoxicity may be increased. Also, therapeutic effects of acetaminophen may be reduced.
Sulfinpyrazone	Anticoagulants, oral	↑	The anticoagulant activity of warfarin will likely be enhanced; hemorrhage could occur.
Sulfinpyrazone	Theophylline	↓	Plasma theophylline clearance may be increased, thus lowering plasma levels.
Sulfinpyrazone	Tolbutamide	↑	Decreased clearance and increased half-life of tolbutamide may occur; hypoglycemia may result. Glyburide was not affected in one study.
Sulfinpyrazone	Verapamil	↓	Increased clearance and decreased bioavailability of verapamil may occur.
Niacin	Sulfinpyrazone	↓	Sulfinpyrazone's uricosuric effect may be reduced.
Salicylates	Sulfinpyrazone	↓	Sulfinpyrazone's uricosuric effect may be suppressed.

[a] ↑ = Object drug increased. ↓ = Object drug decreased. ↔ = Undetermined clinical effect.

Adverse Reactions

➤*Allergic:* Rash has been reported. In most instances, this reaction did not necessitate discontinuance of therapy.

➤*Electrolyte disturbance:* Sulfinpyrazone has not been observed to affect electrolyte balance.

➤*Hematologic:* Blood dyscrasias (anemia, leukopenia, agranulocytosis, thrombocytopenia, and aplastic anemia) have rarely been reported. There has also been a published report associating sulfinpyrazone, administered concomitantly with other drugs including colchicine, with leukemia following long-term treatment of patients with gout. However, the circumstances involved in the two cases reported are such that a cause-and-effect relationship to sulfinpyrazone has not been clearly established.

➤*GI:* The most frequently reported adverse reactions with sulfinpyrazone have been upper GI disturbances. In these patients it is advisable to administer the drug with food, milk, or antacids. Despite this precaution, sulfinpyrazone may aggravate or reactivate peptic ulcer.

Overdosage

➤*Symptoms:* Nausea, vomiting, diarrhea, epigastric pain, ataxia, labored respiration, convulsions, coma. Possible symptoms, seen after overdosage with other pyrazolone derivatives: Anemia, jaundice, ulceration.

➤*Treatment:* No specific antidote. Induce emesis; gastric lavage; supportive treatment (IV glucose infusions, analeptics).

ALLOPURINOL

Rx	**Allopurinol** (Various, eg, Boots, Geneva, Major, Mylan, Parmed, Vangard)	**Tablets**: 100 mg	In 100s, 500s, 1,000s and UD 100s.
Rx	**Zyloprim** (Faro Pharmaceuticals, Inc.)		Lactose. (Zyloprim 100). White, scored. In 100s.
Rx	**Allopurinol** (Various, eg, Boots, Geneva, Major, Mylan, Parmed, Vangard)	**Tablets**: 300 mg	In 100s, 500s, 1,000s and UD 100s.
Rx	**Zyloprim** (Faro Pharmaceuticals, Inc.)		Lactose. (Zyloprim 300). Peach, scored. In 100s and 500s.

ALLOPURINOL — ORAL

For information on allopurinol injection, please refer to the Purine Analogs and Related Agents in the Antineoplastics chapter.

Indications

This is not an innocuous drug. It is not recommended for the treatment of asymptomatic hyperuricemia.

Allopurinol reduces serum and urinary uric acid concentrations. Its use should be individualized for each patient and requires an understanding of its mode of action and pharmacokinetics.

➤*Gout:* The management of patients with signs and symptoms of primary or secondary gout (acute attacks, tophi, joint destruction, uric acid lithiasis, and/or nephropathy).

➤*Malignancies:* The management of patients with leukemia, lymphoma and malignancies who are receiving cancer therapy which causes elevations of serum and urinary uric acid levels. Treatment with allopurinol should be discontinued when the potential for overproduction of uric acid is no longer present.

➤*Calcium oxalate calculi:* The management of patients with recurrent calcium oxalate calculi whose daily uric acid excretion exceeds 800 mg/day in male patients and 750 mg/day in female patients. Therapy in such patients should be carefully assessed initially and reassessed periodically to determine in each case that treatment is beneficial and that the benefits outweigh the risks.

➤*Unlabeled uses:* Allopurinol mouthwash (20 mg in 3% methylcellulose; 1 mg/ml) has been used successfully to prevent fluorouracil-induced stomatitis; 600 mg/day ameliorated the granulocyte suppressant effect of fluorouracil.

Recent studies suggest a role for allopurinol in the prevention of ischemic reperfusion tissue damage; to reduce the incidence of perioperative mortality and postoperative arrhythmias in coronary artery bypass surgery patients (300 mg 12 and 1 hour before surgery); to reduce relapse rates of *H. pylori*-induced duodenal ulcers and treatment of hematemesis from NSAID-induced erosive gastritis (50 mg 4 times daily); to alleviate pain related to acute pancreatitis 50 mg 4 times/day, rectally); to ex vivo preservation and function of organs for liver and kidney transplantation by supplementing preservation solutions with allopurinol; and to reduce rejection episodes in adult cadaver renal transplant recipients by adding low-dose allopurinol 25 mg on alternate days to a triple immunosuppressive regimen of azathioprine/cyclosporine/prednisolone. Allopurinol 20 mg/kg for 15 days has been used successfully against *Leishmania* in the treatment of American cutaneous leishmaniasis and against *Trypanosoma cruzi*; for Chagas' disease (600 to 900 mg/day for 60 days); and as an alternative for patients with epileptic seizures refractory to standard therapy (150 mg/day for children $<$ 20 kg, otherwise 300 mg/day).

Administration and Dosage

➤*Control of gout and hyperuricemia:* The dosage of allopurinol to accomplish full control of gout and to lower serum uric acid to normal or near-normal levels varies with the severity of the disease. The average is 200 to 300 mg/day for patients with mild gout and 400 to 600 mg/day for those with moderately severe tophaceous gout. The appropriate dosage may be administered in divided doses or as a single equivalent dose with the 300 mg tablet. Dosage requirements in excess of 300 mg should be administered in divided doses. The minimal effective dosage is 100 to 200 mg daily and the maximal recommended dosage is 800 mg daily. To reduce the possibility of flare-up of acute gouty attacks, it is recommended that the patient start with a low dose of allopurinol (100 mg daily) and increase at weekly intervals by 100 mg until a serum uric acid level of 6 mg/dl or less is attained but without exceeding the maximal recommended dosage.

➤*Serum uric acid levels:* Normal serum urate levels are usually achieved in 1 to 3 weeks. The upper limit of normal is about 7 mg/dl for men and postmenopausal women and 6 mg/dl for premenopausal women. Too much reliance should not be placed on a single serum uric acid determination since, for technical reasons, estimation of uric acid may be difficult. By selecting the appropriate dosage and, in certain patients, using uricosuric agents concurrently, it is possible to reduce serum uric acid to normal or, if desired, to as low as 2 to 3 mg/dl and keep it there indefinitely.

➤*Concomitant medication therapy:* While adjusting the dosage of allopurinol in patients who are being treated with colchicine and/or anti-inflammatory agents, it is wise to continue the latter therapy until serum uric acid has been normalized and there has been freedom from acute gouty attacks for several months.

➤*Replacement therapy:* In transferring a patient from a uricosuric agent to allopurinol, the dose of the uricosuric agent should be gradually reduced over a period of several weeks and the dose of allopurinol gradually increased to the required dose needed to maintain a normal serum uric acid level.

➤*Hyperuricosuria:* For hyperuricosuric patients, 200 to 300 mg/day in single or divided doses. Adjust dose up or down depending upon the resultant control of the hyperuricosuria based upon subsequent 24-hour urinary urate determination. Patients may also benefit from dietary changes such as reduction of animal protein, sodium, refined sugars, oxalate-rich foods and excessive calcium intake as well as increase in oral fluids and dietary fiber.

It should also be noted that allopurinol is generally better tolerated if taken following meals. A fluid intake sufficient to yield a daily urinary output of at least 2 liters and the maintenance of a neutral or, preferably, slightly alkaline urine are desirable.

The correct size and frequency of dosage for maintaining the serum uric acid just within the normal range is best determined by using the serum uric acid level as an index.

➤*Prevention of uric acid nephropathy during vigorous therapy of neoplastic disease:* For the prevention of uric acid nephropathy during the vigorous therapy of neoplastic disease, treatment with 600 to 800 mg daily for 2 or 3 days is advisable together with a high fluid intake. Otherwise similar considerations to the above recommendations for treating patients with gout govern the regulation of dosage for maintenance purposes in secondary hyperuricemia.

➤*Recurrent calcium oxalate stones:* The dose of allopurinol recommended for management of recurrent calcium oxalate stones in hyperuricosuric patients is 200 to 300 mg/day in divided doses or as the single equivalent. This dose may be adjusted up or down depending upon the resultant control of the hyperuricosuria based upon subsequent 24 hour urinary urate determinations. Clinical experience suggests that patients with recurrent calcium oxalate stones may also benefit from dietary changes such as the reduction of animal protein, sodium, refined sugars, oxalate-rich foods, and excessive calcium intake, as well as an increase in oral fluids and dietary fiber.

➤*Children (6 to 10 years of age):* In secondary hyperuricemia associated with malignancies, children 6 to 10 years of age may be given 300 mg allopurinol daily while those under 6 years are generally given 150 mg daily. The response is evaluated after approximately 48 hours of therapy and a dosage adjustment is made if necessary.

Another suggested dose is 1 mg/kg/day divided every 6 hours, to a maximum of 600 mg/day. After 48 hours of treatment, titrate dose according to serum uric acid levels.

➤*Renal function impairment:* Because allopurinol and its metabolites are primarily eliminated only by the kidneys, accumulation of the drug can occur in renal failure, and the dose of allopurinol should consequently be reduced. With a creatinine clearance of 10 to 20 ml/min, a daily dosage of 200 mg of allopurinol is suitable. When the creatinine clearance is less than 10 ml/min, the daily dosage should not exceed 100 mg. With extreme renal impairment (creatinine clearance less than 3 ml/min) the interval between doses may also need to be lengthened.

➤*Storage / Stability:* Store at 15° to 25°C (59° to 77°F) in a dry place and protect from light.

Actions

➤*Pharmacology:* Allopurinol acts on purine catabolism, without disrupting the biosynthesis of purines. It reduces the production of uric acid by inhibiting the biochemical reactions immediately preceding its formation.

Allopurinol is a structural analog of the natural purine base, hypoxanthine. It is an inhibitor of xanthine oxidase, the enzyme responsible for the conversion of hypoxanthine to xanthine and of xanthine to uric acid, the end product of purine metabolism in man. Allopurinol is metabolized to the corresponding xanthine analog, oxipurinol (alloxanthine), which also is an inhibitor of xanthine oxidase.

It has been shown that reutilization of both hypoxanthine and xanthine for nucleotide and nucleic acid synthesis is markedly enhanced when their oxidations are inhibited by allopurinol and oxipurinol. This reutilization does not disrupt normal nucleic acid anabolism, however, because feedback inhibition is an integral part of purine biosynthesis. As a result of xanthine oxidase inhibition, the serum concentration of hypoxanthine plus xanthine in patients receiving allopurinol for treatment of hyperuricemia is usually in the range of 0.3 to 0.4 mg/dL compared with a normal level of approximately 0.15 mg/dL. A maximum of 0.9 mg/dL of these oxypurines has been reported when the serum urate was lowered to less than 2 mg/dL by high doses of allopurinol. These values are far below the saturation levels at which point their precipitation would be expected to occur (above 7 mg/dL).

Administration of allopurinol generally results in a fall in both serum and urinary uric acid within 2 to 3 days. The degree of this decrease can be manipulated almost at will since it is dose-dependent. A week or more of treatment with allopurinol may be required before its full effects are manifested; likewise, uric acid may return to pretreatment levels slowly (usually after a period of 7 to 10 days following cessation of therapy). This reflects primarily the accumulation and slow clearance of oxipurinol. In some patients a dramatic fall in urinary uric acid excretion may not occur, particularly in those with severe tophaceous gout. It has been postulated that this may be due to the mobilization of urate from tissue deposits as the serum uric acid level begins to fall.

ALLOPURINOL — ORAL

The action of allopurinol differs from that of uricosuric agents, which lower the serum uric acid level by increasing urinary excretion of uric acid. Allopurinol reduces both the serum and urinary uric acid levels by inhibiting the formation of uric acid. The use of allopurinol to block the formation of urates avoids the hazard of increased renal excretion of uric acid posed by uricosuric drugs.

Allopurinol can substantially reduce serum and urinary uric acid levels in previously refractory patients even in the presence of renal damage serious enough to render uricosuric drugs virtually ineffective. Salicylates may be given conjointly for their antirheumatic effect without compromising the action of allopurinol. This is in contrast to the nullifying effect of salicylates on uricosuric drugs.

Allopurinol also inhibits the enzymatic oxidation of mercaptopurine, the sulfur-containing analog of hypoxanthine, to 6-thiouric acid. This oxidation, which is catalyzed by xanthine oxidase, inactivates mercaptopurine. Hence, the inhibition of such oxidation by allopurinol may result in as much as a 75% reduction in the therapeutic dose requirement of mercaptopurine when the two compounds are given together (see Drug Interactions).

➤*Pharmacokinetics:* The renal clearance of hypoxanthine and xanthine is at least 10 times greater than that of uric acid. The increased xanthine and hypoxanthine in the urine have not been accompanied by problems of nephrolithiasis. Xanthine crystalluria has been reported in only three patients. Two of the patients had Lesch-Nyhan syndrome, which is characterized by excessive uric acid production combined with a deficiency of the enzyme, hypoxanthineguanine phosphoribosyltransferase (HGPRTase). This enzyme is required for the conversion of hypoxanthine, xanthine, and guanine to their respective nucleotides. The third patient had lymphosarcoma and produced an extremely large amount of uric acid because of rapid cell lysis during chemotherapy.

Allopurinol is approximately 90% absorbed from the gastrointestinal tract. Peak plasma levels generally occur at 1.5 hours and 4.5 hours for allopurinol and oxipurinol, respectively, and after a single oral dose of 300 mg allopurinol, maximum plasma levels of about 3 mcg/mL of allopurinol and 6.5 mcg/mL of oxipurinol are produced.

Approximately 20% of the ingested allopurinol is excreted in the feces. Because of its rapid oxidation to oxipurinol and a renal clearance rate approximately that of glomerular filtration rate, allopurinol has a plasma half-life of about 1 to 2 hours. Oxipurinol, however, has a longer plasma half-life (approximately 15 hours) and therefore effective xanthine oxidase inhibition is maintained over a 24-hour period with single daily doses of allopurinol. Whereas allopurinol is cleared essentially by glomerular filtration, oxipurinol is reabsorbed in the kidney tubules in a manner similar to the reabsorption of uric acid.

The clearance of oxipurinol is increased by uricosuric drugs, and as a consequence, the addition of a uricosuric agent reduces to some degree the inhibition of xanthine oxidase by oxipurinol and increases to some degree the urinary excretion of uric acid. In practice, the net effect of such combined therapy may be useful in some patients in achieving minimum serum uric acid levels provided the total urinary uric acid load does not exceed the competence of the patient's renal function.

Contraindications

Patients who have developed a severe reaction to allopurinol should not be restarted on the drug.

Warnings

➤*Concomitant medication:* See Drug Interactions for more information.

➤*Drowsiness:* Because of the occasional occurrence of drowsiness, patients should be alerted to the need for due precaution when engaging in activities where alertness is mandatory.

➤*Acute gout attacks:* An increase in acute attacks of gout has been reported during the early stages of administration of allopurinol, even when normal or subnormal serum uric acid levels have been attained. Accordingly, maintenance doses of colchicine generally should be given prophylactically when allopurinol is begun. In addition, it is recommended that the patient start with a low dose of allopurinol (100 mg daily) and increase at weekly intervals by 100 mg until a serum uric acid level of 6 mg/dl or less is attained but without exceeding the maximum recommended dose (800 mg per day). The use of colchicine or anti-inflammatory agents may be required to suppress gouty attacks in some cases. The attacks usually become shorter and less severe after several months of therapy. The mobilization of urates from tissue deposits which cause fluctuations in the serum uric acid levels may be a possible explanation for these episodes. Even with adequate therapy with allopurinol, it may require several months to deplete the uric acid pool sufficiently to achieve control of the acute attacks.

➤*Fluid intake:* A fluid intake sufficient to yield a daily urinary output of at least 2 liters and the maintenance of a neutral or, preferably, slightly alkaline urine are desirable to:

1.) avoid the theoretical possibility of formation of xanthine calculi under the influence of therapy with allopurinol; and
2.) help prevent renal precipitation of urates in patients receiving concomitant uricosuric agents.

➤*Hypersensitivity reactions:* Allopurinol should be discontinued at the first appearance of skin rash or other signs which may indicate an allergic reaction. In some instances a skin rash may be followed by more severe hypersensitivity reactions such as exfoliative, urticarial, and purpuric lesions, as well as Stevens-Johnson syndrome (erythema multiforme exudativum), and/or generalized vasculitis, irreversible hepatotoxicity, and, on rare occasions, death.

➤*Renal function impairment:* The occurrence of hypersensitivity reactions to allopurinol may be increased in patients with decreased renal function receiving thiazide diuretics and allopurinol concurrently. For this reason, in this clinical setting, such combinations should be administered with caution and patients should be observed closely.

Some patients with pre-existing renal disease or poor urate clearance have shown a rise in BUN during administration of allopurinol. Although the mechanism responsible for this has not been established, patients with impaired renal function should be carefully observed during the early stages of administration of allopurinol and the dosage decreased or the drug withdrawn if increased abnormalities in renal function appear and persist.

Renal failure in association with administration of allopurinol has been observed among patients with hyperuricemia secondary to neoplastic diseases. Concurrent conditions such as multiple myeloma and congestive myocardial disease were present among those patients whose renal dysfunction increased after allopurinol was begun. Renal failure is also frequently associated with gouty nephropathy and rarely with hypersensitivity reactions associated with allopurinol. Albuminuria has been observed among patients who developed clinical gout following chronic glomerulonephritis and chronic pyelonephritis.

Patients with decreased renal function require lower doses of allopurinol than those with normal renal function. Lower than recommended doses should be used to initiate therapy in any patients with decreased renal function and they should be observed closely during the early stages of administration of allopurinol. In patients with severely impaired renal function or decreased urate clearance, the half-life of oxipurinol in the plasma is greatly prolonged. Therefore, a dose of 100 mg per day or 300 mg twice a week, or perhaps less, may be sufficient to maintain adequate xanthine oxidase inhibition to reduce serum urate levels.

➤*Hepatic function impairment:* A few cases of reversible clinical hepatotoxicity have been noted in patients taking allopurinol, and in some patients, asymptomatic rises in serum alkaline phosphatase or serum transaminase have been observed. If anorexia, weight loss, or pruritus develop in patients on allopurinol, evaluation of liver function should be part of their diagnostic workup. In patients with pre-existing liver disease, periodic liver function tests are recommended during the early stages of therapy.

➤*Pregnancy:* *Category C.* Reproductive studies have been performed in rats and rabbits at doses up to twenty times the usual human dose (5 mg/kg/day), and it was concluded that there was no impaired fertility or harm to the fetus due to allopurinol. There is a published report of a study in pregnant mice given 50 or 100 mg/kg allopurinol intraperitoneally on gestation days 10 or 13. There were increased numbers of dead fetuses in dams given 100 mg/kg allopurinol but not in those given 50 mg/kg. There were increased numbers of external malformations in fetuses at both doses of allopurinol on gestation day 10 and increased numbers of skeletal malformations in fetuses at both doses on gestation day 13. It cannot be determined whether this represented a fetal effect or an effect secondary to maternal toxicity. There are, however, no adequate or well-controlled studies in pregnant women. Because animal reproduction studies are not always predictive of human response, this drug should be used during pregnancy only if clearly needed.

Experience with allopurinol during human pregnancy has been limited partly because women of reproductive age rarely require treatment with allopurinol. There are two unpublished reports and one published paper of women giving birth to normal offspring after receiving allopurinol during pregnancy.

➤*Lactation:* Allopurinol and oxipurinol have been found in the milk of a mother who was receiving allopurinol. Since the effect of allopurinol on the nursing infant is unknown, caution should be exercised when allopurinol is administered to a nursing woman.

➤*Children:* Allopurinol is rarely indicated for use in children with the exception of those with hyperuricemia secondary to malignancy or to certain rare inborn errors of purine metabolism (see Indications and Administration and Dosage).

Precautions

➤*Monitoring:* The correct dosage and schedule for maintaining the serum uric acid within the normal range is best determined by using the serum uric acid as an index.

In patients with preexisting liver disease, periodic liver function tests are recommended during the early stages of therapy (see Warnings).

Allopurinol and its primary active metabolite, oxipurinol, are eliminated by the kidneys; therefore, changes in renal function have a profound effect on dosage. In patients with decreased renal function or who have concurrent illnesses which can affect renal function such as hypertension and diabetes mellitus, periodic laboratory parameters of renal function, particularly BUN and serum creatinine or creatinine clearance, should be performed and the patient's dosage of allopurinol reassessed.

The prothrombin time should be reassessed periodically in the patients receiving dicumarol who are given allopurinol.

➤*Bone marrow depression:* Bone marrow depression has been reported in patients receiving allopurinol, most of whom received concomitant drugs with the potential for causing this reaction. This has occurred as early as 6 weeks to as long as 6 years after the initiation of therapy of allopurinol. Rarely, a patient may develop varying degrees of bone marrow depression, affecting one or more cell lines, while receiving allopurinol alone.

Drug Interactions

➤*Mercaptopurine, azathioprine:* In patients receiving mercaptopurine or azathioprine, the concomitant administration of 300 to 600 mg of allopurinol per day will require a reduction in dose to approximately one third to one fourth of the usual dose of mercaptopurine or azathioprine. Subse-

ALLOPURINOL — ORAL

quent adjustment of doses of mercaptopurine or azathioprine should be made on the basis of therapeutic response and the appearance of toxic effects.

➤*Thiazide diuretics:* The reports that the concomitant use of allopurinol and thiazide diuretics may contribute to the enhancement of allopurinol toxicity in some patients have been reviewed in an attempt to establish a cause-and-effect relationship and a mechanism of causation. Review of these case reports indicates that the patients were mainly receiving thiazide diuretics for hypertension and that tests to rule out decreased renal function secondary to hypertensive nephropathy were not often performed. In those patients in whom renal insufficiency was documented, however, the recommendation to lower the dose of allopurinol was not followed. Although a causal mechanism and a cause-and-effect relationship have not been established, current evidence suggests that renal function should be monitored in patients on thiazide diuretics and allopurinol even in the absence of renal failure, and dosage levels should be even more conservatively adjusted in those patients on such combined therapy if diminished renal function is detected.

➤*Cytotoxic agents:* Enhanced bone marrow suppression by cyclophosphamide and other cytotoxic agents has been reported among patients with neoplastic disease, except leukemia, in the presence of allopurinol. However, in a well-controlled study of patients with lymphoma on combination therapy, allopurinol did not increase the marrow toxicity of patients treated with cyclophosphamide, doxorubicin, bleomycin, procarbazine, and/or mechlorethamine.

Myelosuppressive effects of cyclophosphamide may be enhanced, possibly increasing the risk of bleeding or infection.

➤*Chlorpropamide:* Chlorpropamide's plasma half-life may be prolonged by allopurinol since allopurinol and chlorpropamide may compete for excretion in the renal tubule. The risk of hypoglycemia secondary to this mechanism may be increased if allopurinol and chlorpropamide are given concomitantly in the presence of renal insufficiency.

➤*Cyclosporine:* Rare reports indicate that cyclosporine levels may be increased during concomitant treatment with allopurinol. Monitoring of cyclosporine levels and possible adjustment of cyclosporine dosage should be considered when these drugs are coadministered.

Allopurinol Drug Interactions

Precipitant drug	Object drug[a]		Description
Allopurinol	Ampicillin, amoxicillin	⬆	The rate of skin rash appears much higher with allopurinol coadministration than with either drug alone.
Allopurinol	Anticoagulants, oral	⬆	Data are conflicting. The anticoagulant action of some agents may be enhanced, but probably not that of warfarin.
Allopurinol	Cyclophosphamide	⬆	Myelosuppressive effects of cyclophosphamide may be enhanced, possibly increasing the risk of bleeding or infection.
Allopurinol	Theophyllines	⬆	Theophylline clearance may be decreased with large allopurinol doses (600 mg/day) leading to increased plasma theophylline levels and possible toxicity.
Allopurinol	Thiopurines	⬆	Clinically significant increases in pharmacologic and toxic effects of oral thiopurines have occurred.
ACE Inhibitors	Allopurinol	⬆	There is possibly a higher risk of hypersensitivity reaction when these agents are coadministered than when each drug is administered alone.
Aluminum salts	Allopurinol	⬇	Pharmacologic effects of allopurinol may be decreased.
Thiazide diuretics	Allopurinol	⬆	Coadministration may increase the incidence of hypersensitivity reactions to allopurinol.
Uricosuric agents	Allopurinol	⬇	Uricosuric agents that increase the excretion of urate are also likely to increase the excretion of oxipurinol and thus lower the degree of inhibition of xanthine oxidase.

[a] ⬆ = Object drug increased. ⬇ = Object drug decreased.

Adverse Reactions

Data upon which the following estimates of incidence of adverse reactions are made are derived from experiences reported in the literature, unpublished clinical trials and voluntary reports since marketing of allopurinol (allopurinol) began. Past experience suggested that the most frequent event following the initiation of allopurinol treatment was an increase in acute attacks of gout (average 6% in early studies). An analysis of current usage suggests that the incidence of acute gouty attacks has diminished to less than 1%. The explanation for this decrease has not been determined but may be due in part to initiating therapy more gradually (see Warnings and Administration and Dosage).

➤*Hypersensitivity:* The most frequent adverse reaction to allopurinol is skin rash. Skin reactions can be severe and sometimes fatal. Therefore, treatment with allopurinol should be discontinued immediately if a rash develops (see Warnings). Some patients with the most severe reaction also had fever, chills, arthralgias, cholestatic jaundice, eosinophilia and mild leukocytosis or leukopenia. Among 55 patients with gout treated with allopurinol for 3 to 34 months (average greater than 1 year) and followed prospectively, Rundles observed that 3% of patients developed a type of drug reaction which was predominantly a pruritic maculopapular skin eruption, sometimes scaly or exfoliative. However, with current usage, skin reactions have been observed less frequently than 1%. The explanation for this decrease is not obvious. The incidence of skin rash may be increased in the presence of renal insufficiency. The frequency of skin rash among patients receiving ampicillin or amoxicillin concurrently with allopurinol has been reported to be increased (see Drug Interactions).

➤*Most common adverse reactions probably causally related:* Early clinical studies and incidence rates from early clinical experience with allopurinol suggested that these adverse reactions were found to occur at a rate of greater than 1%. The most frequent event observed was acute attacks of gout following the initiation of therapy. Analyses of current usage suggest that the incidence of these adverse reactions is now less than 1%. The explanation for this decrease has not been determined, but it may be due to following recommended usage (see Adverse Reactions introduction, Indications, Warnings, and Administration and Dosage).

Dermatologic – Rash; maculopapular rash.

GI – Diarrhea; nausea; alkaline phosphatase increase; AST/ALT increase.

Metabolic/Nutritional – Acute attacks of gout.

➤*Incidence Less Than 1% Probably Causally Related:*

Cardiovascular – Necrotizing angiitis; vasculitis.

CNS – Headache; peripheral neuropathy; neuritis; paresthesia; somnolence.

Dermatologic – Erythema multiforme exudativum (Stevens-Johnson syndrome); toxic epidermal necrolysis (Lyell's syndrome); hypersensitivity vasculitis; purpura; vesicular bullous dermatitis; exfoliative dermatitis; eczematoid dermatitis; pruritus; urticaria; alopecia; onycholysis; lichen planus.

GI – Hyperbilirubinemia; vomiting; intermittent abdominal pain; gastritis; dyspepsia.

GU – Renal failure; uremia (see Warnings).

Hematologic – Thrombocytopenia; eosinophilia; leukocytosis; leukopenia.

Hepatic – Increased alkaline phosphatase, AST and ALT; hepatic necrosis; granulomatous hepatitis; hepatomegaly; cholestatic jaundice.

Musculoskeletal – Myopathy; arthralgias.

Respiratory – Epistaxis.

Special senses – Taste loss/perversion.

Miscellaneous – Ecchymosis; fever.

➤*Incidence less than 1% causal relationship unknown:*

Cardiovascular – Pericarditis; peripheral vascular disease; thrombophlebitis; bradycardia; vasodilation.

CNS – Optic neuritis; confusion; dizziness; vertigo; foot drop; decrease in libido; depression; amnesia; tinnitus; asthenia; insomnia.

Dermatologic – Furunculosis; facial edema; sweating; skin edema.

Endocrine – Infertility (male); hypercalcemia; gynecomastia (male).

GI – Hemorrhagic pancreatitis; GI bleeding; stomatitis; salivary gland swelling; hyperlipidemia; tongue edema; anorexia.

GU – Nephritis; impotence; primary hematuria; albuminuria.

Hematologic/Lymphatic – Aplastic anemia; agranulocytosis; eosinophilic fibrohistiocytic lesion of bone marrow; pancytopenia; prothrombin decrease; anemia; hemolytic anemia; reticulocytosis; lymphadenopathy; lymphocytosis.

Musculoskeletal – Myalgia.

Respiratory – Bronchospasm; asthma; pharyngitis; rhinitis.

Special senses – Cataracts; macular retinitis; iritis; conjunctivitis; amblyopia.

Miscellaneous – Malaise.

Overdosage

In the management of overdosage there is no specific antidote for allopurinol. There has been no clinical experience in the management of a patient who has taken massive amounts of allopurinol. Both allopurinol and oxipurinol are dialyzable; however, the usefulness of hemodialysis or peritoneal dialysis in the management of an overdose of allopurinol is unknown.

Patient Information

Allopurinol is better tolerated if taken with food or milk. A fluid intake, sufficient to yield a daily urinary output of at least 2 L and the maintenance of a neutral or, preferably slightly alkaline urine are desirable. Drink at least 10 to 12 (8 oz) glasses of fluids daily.

Discontinue allopurinol and to consult your doctor immediately at the first sign of a skin rash, painful urination, blood in the urine, irritation of the eyes, or swelling of the lips or mouth.

Continue drug therapy prescribed for gouty attacks since optimal benefit of allopurinol may be delayed for 2 to 6 weeks.

Increase fluid intake during therapy to prevent renal stones.

ALLOPURINOL — ORAL

If a single dose of allopurinol is occasionally forgotten, there is no need to double the dose at the next scheduled time.

There may be certain risks associated with the concomitant use of allopurinol and dicumarol, sulfinpyrazone, mercaptopurine, azathioprine, ampicillin, amoxicillin, and thiazide diuretics, and patients should follow the instructions of their doctor.

Because of the occasional occurrence of drowsiness, patients should take precautions when engaging in activities where alertness is mandatory.

Patients may wish to take allopurinol after meals to minimize gastric irritation.

Use caution when taking large doses of vitamin C; urinary acidification with large doses of vitamin C may increase the possibility of kidney stone formation.

COLCHICINE

Rx	**Colchicine** (Abbott)	**Tablets:** 0.6 mg (1/100 g)	Lactose. Yellow. In 100s
Rx	**Colchicine** (Various, eg, Allscripts, Integrity, Major, Qualitest, URL, Watson, West-ward)		In 30s, 60s, 100s, and 1,000s.
Rx	**Colchicine** (Bedford)	**Injection:** 0.5 mg/mL	In 2 mL vials.

COLCHICINE — ORAL

Indications

➤*Acute gouty arthritis:* Colchicine is specifically indicated for treatment and relief of pain in attacks of acute gouty arthritis. It is also recommended for regular use between attacks as a prophylactic measure, and is often effective in aborting an attack when taken at the first sign of articular discomfort.

➤*Unlabeled uses:* Familial Mediterranean fever (1 to 2 mg/day); for chronic prophylactic therapy to reduce the frequency and severity of painful serositis attacks or as an intermittent short-term therapy to abort an acute attack.

Hepatic cirrhosis (1 mg 5 days weekly).

Primary biliary cirrhosis (0.6 mg twice daily).

Treatment of Behçet disease (0.5 to 1.5 mg/day).

Scleroderma (1 mg/day).

Sweet syndrome (0.5 mg 1 to 3 times daily).

Colchicine also has been used in the treatment of amyloidosis, sarcoid arthritis, acute inflammatory calcific tendonitis, arthritis associated with erythema nodosum, leukemia, adenocarcinoma of the GI tract, mycosis fungoides, and topically to treat intraurethral condyloma acuminata in men.

Prevention of recurrent pericarditis (alone or in combination with steroids or other NSAIDs).

Administration and Dosage

➤*Approved by the FDA:* September 6, 1977.

➤*For acute gouty arthritis:* The usual dose to relieve or abort an attack is 0.6 to 1.2 mg. This dose may be followed by 1 unit of either preparation (0.5 or 0.6 mg) every hour, or 1 or 1.2 mg every 2 hours, until pain is relieved or until diarrhea ensues. Each patient should learn the dose needed and should keep the drug at hand for use at the first sign of an attack. After the initial dose, it is sometimes sufficient to take 0.5 or 0.6 mg every 2 or 3 hours. The drug should be stopped if there is GI discomfort or diarrhea. (Opiates may be needed to control diarrhea.) In subsequent attacks, the patient should be able to judge his medication requirement accurately enough to stop short of his "diarrheal dose." The total amount of colchicine needed to control pain and inflammation during an attack usually ranges from 4 to 8 mg. Articular pain and swelling typically abate within 12 hours and are usually gone in 24 to 48 hours. An interval of 3 days between colchicine courses is advised in order to minimize the possibility of cumulative toxicity.

If corticotropin (ACTH) is administered for treatment of an attack of gouty arthritis, it is recommended that colchicine also be given in doses of at least 1 mg/day, and that the latter be continued for a few days after the hormone is withdrawn.

➤*For prophylaxis during intercritical periods:* To reduce the frequency of paroxysms and lessen their severity, colchicine may be administered continuously. In patients who have less than 1 attack per year, the usual dose is 0.5 or 0.6 mg/day, 3 or 4 days a week. For cases involving more than 1 attack per year, the usual dose is 0.5 or 0.6 mg daily; severe cases may require 2 or three 0.5 mg granules or 0.6 mg tablets daily.

➤*For prophylaxis against attacks of gout in patients undergoing surgery:* In patients with gout, an attack may be precipitated by even a minor surgical procedure. Administer one 0.5 mg granule 3 times a day or one 0.6 mg tablet 3 times daily for 3 days before and 3 days after surgery.

➤*Storage/Stability:* Store below 86°F (30°C).

Actions

➤*Pharmacology:* The exact mechanism of action of colchicine in gout is not completely known, but it involves a reduction in lactic acid production by leukocytes, which results in a decrease in uric acid deposition, and a reduction in phagocytosis, with abatement of the inflammatory response.

Colchicine is not an analgesic, though it relieves pain in acute attacks of gout. It is not a uricosuric agent and will not prevent progression of gout to chronic gouty arthritis. It does have a prophylactic, suppressive effect that helps to reduce the incidence of acute attacks and to relieve the residual pain and mild discomfort that patients with gout occasionally feel.

In man and certain other animals, colchicine can produce a temporary leukopenia that is followed by leukocytosis.

Colchicine has other pharmacologic actions in animals: it alters neuromuscular function, intensifies GI activity by neurogenic stimulation, increases sensitivity to central depressants, heightens response to sympathomimetic compounds, depresses the respiratory center, constricts blood vessels, causes hypertension by central vasomotor stimulation, and lowers body temperature.

➤*Pharmacokinetics:*

Absorption – Colchicine is rapidly absorbed after oral administration.

Distribution – Large amounts of the drug and metabolites enter the intestinal tract in bile and intestinal secretions. Colchicine does not appear to be tightly bound to serum protein; hence, the drug rapidly leaves the blood stream. High concentrations are found in the kidney, liver, and spleen.

Metabolism/Excretion – Colchicine is partially metabolized in the liver. The plasma half-life is about 20 minutes; colchicine has a half-life of about 60 hours in leukocytes. Excretion occurs primarily by biliary and renal routes.

Contraindications

Hypersensitivity to the drug, in those with serious GI, renal, hepatic, or cardiac disorders, and in those with blood dyscrasias.

Warnings

➤*Fertility impairment:* Colchicine arrests cell division in animals and plants. It has adversely affected spermatogenesis in humans and in some animal species under certain conditions.

➤*Pregnancy: Category C.* Colchicine has been shown to be teratogenic in mice when given doses of 1.25 and 1.5 mg/kg and in hamsters when given 10 mg/kg. There are no adequate and well-controlled studies in pregnant women. Use colchicine during pregnancy only if the potential benefit justifies the potential risk to the fetus.

➤*Lactation:* It is not known whether this drug is excreted in human milk. Because many drugs are excreted in human milk, exercise caution when colchicine is administered to a nursing woman.

Precautions

➤*Monitoring:* In patients receiving long-term therapy, perform periodic blood counts.

If nausea, vomiting, or diarrhea occurs, discontinue the drug.

Obtain decreased thrombocyte values during colchicine therapy.

➤*Special risk:* Administer with caution to aged or debilitated patients, and to those with early manifestations of GI, renal, hepatic, cardiac, or hematological disorders.

Colchicine is contraindicated in patients with a known hypersensitivity to the drug, in those with serious GI, renal, hepatic, or cardiac disorders, and in those with blood dyscrasias.

➤*Lab test abnormalities:* Colchicine therapy may cause elevated alkaline phosphatase and AST values.

Drug Interactions

Colchicine is inhibited by acidifying agents.

The action of colchicine is potentiated by alkalinizing agents.

Colchicine may increase sensitivity to the CNS depressants.

Response to sympathomimetic agents may be enhanced by colchicine.

➤*Drug/Lab test interactions:* Colchicine may cause false-positive results when testing urine for RBC or hemoglobin.

Adverse Reactions

Adverse reactions in decreasing order of severity are bone marrow depression, with aplastic anemia, with agranulocytosis, or with thrombocytopenia may occur in patients receiving long-term therapy. Peripheral neuritis, purpura, loss of hair, myopathy, and reversible azoospermia have also been reported.

➤*Dermatologic:* Dermatoses have been reported.

➤*GI:* Diarrhea, nausea, and vomiting may occur with colchicine therapy, especially when maximal doses are necessary for a therapeutic effect. To avoid more serious toxicity, discontinue the drug when these symptoms appear, regardless of whether or not joint pain has been relieved.

➤*Hypersensitivity:* Hypersensitivity reactions may occur infrequently.

COLCHICINE — ORAL

Overdosage

➤*Symptoms:* The onset of toxic effects is usually delayed for several hours or more after the ingestion of an acute overdose. Nausea, vomiting, abdominal pain, and diarrhea occur first. The diarrhea may be bloody due to hemorrhagic gastroenteritis. Burning sensations of the throat, stomach, and skin may be prominent symptoms. Extensive vascular damage may result in shock. Kidney damage, evidenced by hematuria and oliguria, may occur. Muscular weakness may be marked, and ascending paralysis of the central nervous system may develop; the patient usually remains conscious. Delirium and convulsions may occur. Death due to respiratory arrest may result.

Although death from the ingestion of as little as 7 mg has been reported, much larger doses have been survived.

➤*Treatment:* Treatment of colchicine poisoning should begin with gastric lavage and measures to prevent shock. Recent studies appear to support the use of hemodialysis or peritoneal dialysis as part of the treatment of acute overdosage in addition to gastric lavage. Symptomatic and supportive treatment may include atropine and morphine for the relief of abdominal pain, and artificial respiration with oxygen to combat respiratory distress. No specific antidote is known.

Patient Information

Notify physician if skin rash, sore throat, fever, unusual bleeding, bruising, tiredness, weakness, numbness, or tingling occurs.

Discontinue medication as soon as gout pain is relieved or at the first sign of nausea, vomiting, stomach pain, or diarrhea. If symptoms persist, notify the physician.

COLCHICINE — INJECTION

Indications

➤*Gout:* Colchicine is indicated for the treatment of gout. It is effective in relieving the pain of acute attacks, especially if therapy is begun early in the attack and in adequate dosage. Many therapists use colchicine as interval therapy to prevent acute attacks of gout. It has no effect on nongouty arthritis or on uric acid metabolism.

The intravenous use of colchicine is advantageous when a rapid response is desired or when gastrointestinal side effects interfere with oral administration of the medication. Occasionally, intravenous colchicine is effective when the oral preparation is not. After the acute attack has subsided, the patient can usually be given colchicine tablets by mouth.

Administration and Dosage

➤*Administration:* Colchicine injection is for intravenous use only. Severe local irritation occurs if it is administered subcutaneously or intramuscularly.

It is extremely important that the needle be properly positioned in the vein before colchicine is injected. If leakage into surrounding tissue or outside the vein along its course should occur during intravenous administration, considerable irritation and possible tissue damage may follow. There is no specific antidote for the prevention of this irritation. Local application of heat or cold, as well as the administration of analgesics, may afford relief.

The injection should take 2 to 5 minutes for completion. To minimize the risk of extravasation, it is recommended that the injection be made into an established intravenous line into a large vein using normal saline as the intravenous fluid. Colchicine injection should not be diluted with 5% dextrose in water. If a decrease in concentration of colchicine in solution is required, 0.9% sodium chloride injection, which does not contain a bacteriostatic agent, should be used. Solutions that become turbid should not be used.

➤*Acute gouty arthritis:* In the treatment of acute gouty arthritis, the average initial dose of colchicine injection is 2 mg (4 mL). This may be followed by 0.5 mg (1 mL) every 6 hours until a satisfactory response is achieved. In general, the total dosage for the first 24-hour period should not exceed 4 mg (8 mL). Cumulative doses of colchicine above 4 mg have resulted in irreversible multiple organ failure and death. The total dosage for a single course of treatment should not exceed 4 mg. Some clinicians recommend a single intravenous dose of 3 mg, whereas others recommend an initial dose of not more than 1 mg of colchicine intravenously, followed by 0.5 mg once or twice daily if needed.

If pain recurs, it may be necessary to administer a daily dose of 1 to 2 mg (2 to 4 mL) for several days; however, no more colchicine should be given by any route for at least 7 days after a full course of IV therapy (4 mg). Many patients can be transferred to oral colchicine at a dosage similar to that being given intravenously.

➤*Prophylactic/Maintenance of recurrent or chronic gouty arthritis:* In the prophylactic or maintenance therapy of recurrent or chronic gouty arthritis, a dosage of 0.5 to 1 mg (1 to 2 mL) once or twice daily may be used. However, in these cases, oral administration of colchicine is preferable, usually taken in conjunction with a uricosuric agent. If an acute attack of gout occurs while the patient is taking colchicine as maintenance therapy, an alternative drug should be instituted in preference to increasing the dose of colchicine.

➤*Storage/Stability:* Store at controlled room temperature, 15° to 30°C (59° to 86°F).

Actions

➤*Pharmacology:* The mechanism of the relief afforded by colchicine in acute attacks of gouty arthritis is not completely known, but studies on the processes involved in precipitation of an acute attack have helped elucidate how this drug may exert its effects. The drug is not an analgesic, does not relieve other types of pain or inflammation, and is of no value in other types of arthritis. It is not a diuretic and does not influence the renal excretion of uric acid or its level in the blood or the magnitude of the "miscible pool" of uric acid. It also does not alter the solubility of urate in the plasma.

Colchicine is not a uricosuric agent. An acute attack of gout apparently occurs as a result of an inflammatory reaction to crystals of monosodium urate that are deposited in the joint tissue from hyperuric body fluids; the reaction is aggravated as more urate granulocytes that phagocytize the urate crystals. Interference with these processes will prevent the development of an acute attack. Colchicine apparently exerts its effect by reducing the inflammatory response to the deposited crystals and also by diminishing phagocytosis. The deposition of uric acid is favored by an acid pH. In synovial tissues and in leukocytes associated with inflammatory processes, lactic acid production is high; this favors a local decrease in pH that enhances uric acid deposition. Colchicine diminishes lactic acid production by leukocytes both directly and by diminishing phagocytosis, thereby interrupting the cycle of urate crystal deposition and inflammatory response that sustains the acute attack. The oxidation of glucose in phagocytizing as well as in non-phagocytizing leukocytes in vitro is suppressed by colchicine; this suppression may explain the diminished lactic acid production. The precise biochemical step that is affected by colchicine is not yet known. The antimitotic activity of colchicine is unrelated to its effectiveness in the treatment of acute gout, as indicated by the fact that trimethylcolchicinic acid, an analog of colchicine, has no antimitotic activity except in extremely high doses.

Contraindications

Colchicine is contraindicated in patients with gout who also have serious GI, renal, hepatic, or cardiac disorders. Colchicine should not be given in the presence of combined renal and hepatic disease.

Warnings

➤*Pregnancy:* Category D.

Colchicine can cause fetal harm when administered to a pregnant woman. If this drug is used during pregnancy, or if the patient becomes pregnant while taking it, the woman should be apprised the potential hazard to the fetus.

➤*Lactation:* It is not known whether this drug is excreted in human milk. Because many drugs are excreted in human milk, caution should be exercised when colchicine is administered to a nursing woman.

➤*Children:* Safety and efficacy in children have not been established.

Precautions

➤*Mortality related to overdosage:* Cumulative intravenous doses of colchicine above 4 mg have resulted in irreversible multiple organ failure and death (see Administration and Dosage and Overdosage).

➤*Special risk:* Reduction in dosage is indicated if weakness, anorexia, nausea, vomiting, or diarrhea occurs. Rarely, thrombophlebitis occurs at the site of injection. Colchicine should be administered with great caution to aged and debilitated patients, especially those with renal, hepatic, gastrointestinal, or heart disease.

Drug Interactions

Colchicine has been shown to induce reversible malabsorption of vitamin B_{12}, apparently by altering the function of ileal mucosa. The possibility that colchicine may increase response to central nervous system depressants and to sympathomimetic agents is suggested by the results of experiments on animals.

Adverse Reactions

➤*GI:* These consist of abdominal pain, nausea, vomiting, and diarrhea. The diarrhea may be severe. The GI symptoms may occur even though the drug is given intravenously; however, such symptoms are unusual unless the recommended dose is exceeded.

➤*Hematologic:* Prolonged administration may cause bone marrow depression, with agranulocytosis, thrombocytopenia, and aplastic anemia. Peripheral neuritis and depilation have also been reported.

➤*Musculoskeletal:* Myopathy may occur in patients on usual maintenance doses, especially in the presence of renal impairment.

Overdosage

➤*Symptoms:* Symptoms, the onset of which may be delayed, include nausea, vomiting, diarrhea, abdominal pain, hemorrhagic gastroenteritis, and burning pain in the throat, stomach, and skin. Fluid extravasation may lead to shock. Myocardial injury may be accompanied by ST-segment elevation, decreased contractility, and profound shock. Muscle weakness or paralysis may occur and progress to respiratory failure. Hepatocellular damage, renal failure, and lung parenchymal infiltrates may occur and, by the fifth day after overdose, leukopenia, thrombocytopenia, and coagulopathy may also occur. If the patient survives, alopecia and stomatitis may be experienced. There is no clear separation of nontoxic, toxic, and lethal doses of colchicine. The lethal dose of colchicine has been estimated to be 65 mg; however, death has resulted from intravenous doses as small as 7 mg acutely (see Administration and Dosage and Precautions, Special risk). Serum concentrations that may be toxic or lethal are not defined. The intravenous median lethal dose in rats is 1.7 mg/kg.

➤*Treatment:* To obtain up-to-date information about the treatment of overdose, a good resource is your certified regional poison control center. In managing overdosage, consider the possibility of multiple drug overdoses, interaction among drugs, and unusual drug kinetics in your patient.

COLCHICINE — INJECTION

Protect the patient's airway and support ventilation and perfusion. Meticulously monitor and maintain, within acceptable limits, the patient's vital signs, blood gases, serum electrolytes, etc. If colchicine was recently ingested and vomiting has not occurred, perform gastric lavage once the patient is stabilized. Absorption of drugs from the gastrointestinal tract may be decreased by giving activated charcoal, which, in many cases, is more effective than emesis or lavage; consider charcoal instead of or in addition to gastric emptying. Repeated doses of charcoal over time may hasten elimination of some drugs that have been absorbed. Safeguard the patient's airway when employing gastric emptying or charcoal.

Forced diuresis, peritoneal dialysis, hemodialysis, or charcoal hemoperfusion have not been established as beneficial for an overdose of colchicine.

PROBENECID AND COLCHICINE

Rx	**Probenecid and Colchicine** (Various, eg, Ivax, Schein)	**Tablets:** 500 mg probenecid, 0.5 mg colchicine	In 100s and 1,000s.

PROBENECID AND COLCHICINE — ORAL

For complete and comparative prescribing information see the individual probenecid and colchicine monographs.

Indications

For the treatment of chronic gouty arthritis when complicated by frequent, recurrent acute attacks of gout

Administration and Dosage

Do not start therapy with probenecid and colchicine until an acute gouty attack has subsided. However, if an acute attack is precipitated during therapy, probenecid and colchicine may be continued without changing the dosage and additional colchicine or other appropriate therapy given to control the acute attack.

The recommended adult dosage is 1 tablet/day for 1 week followed by 1 tablet twice/day.

EMERGENCY KITS

EMERGENCY KITS

Rx **Cyanide Antidote Package** (Various, eg, Taylor)
- Sodium nitrite, 300 mg in 10 mL (2 amps)
- Sodium thiosulfate, 12.5 g in 50 mL (2 vials)
- Amyl nitrite inhalant, 5 minim/0.3 mL (12 amps)
- Also disposable syringes, stomach tube, tourniquet, and instructions.

EMERGENCY KITS

Indications

➤*Cyanide poisoning:* For treatment of cyanide poisoning.

Administration and Dosage

Personnel should acquire some skill in the proper method of administering the contents of this package prior to an emergency. Cyanide poisoning is rapidly fatal. The patient seldom survives many hours. The prevention of death demands a quick diagnosis and the prompt use of specific antidotes. No valuable time should be lost. Even though the diagnosis is doubtful, institute the recommended therapy immediately. For best results, the physician should be acquainted beforehand with the following steps:

1.) Instruct an assistant how to break an ampule of amyl nitrite, one at a time, in a handkerchief and hold it in front of the patient's mouth for 15 seconds, followed by a rest for 15 seconds. Then reapply until sodium nitrite can be administered. This interrupted schedule is important because continuous use of amyl nitrite may prevent adequate oxygenation.
2.) Discontinue administration of amyl nitrite and inject IV 300 mg (10 mL of a 3% solution) of sodium nitrite at the rate of 2.5 to 5 mL/min. The recommended dose of sodium nitrite for children is 6 to 8 mL/m^2 (approximately 0.2 mL/kg body weight), but is not to exceed 10 mL.
3.) Immediately thereafter, inject 12.5 g (50 mL of a 25% solution) of sodium thiosulfate for adults. The dosage for children is 7 g/m^2 of body surface area, but dosage should not exceed 12.5 g. The same needle and vein may be used.
4.) If the poison was taken by mouth, perform gastric lavage as soon as possible, but this should not delay the treatments outlined above. Lavage may be done concurrently by a third person–a physician or a nurse if one is available. One should take quick action without waiting for positive diagnostic tests.

Watch the patient closely for at least 24 to 48 hours. If signs of poisoning reappear, repeat the injection of both sodium nitrite and sodium thiosulfate, but each in 50% of the original dose. Even if the patient seems perfectly well, the medication may be given for prophylactic purposes 2 hours after the first injections.

If respiration has ceased but the pulse is palpable, apply artificial respiration at once. The purpose is not to revive, per se, but to keep the heart beating. Lay the gauze sponge or handkerchief containing the amyl nitrite over the patient's nose, for it may hasten the resumption of respiratory movements. When signs of breathing appear, promptly inject the above solutions.

Warnings

➤*Methemoglobinemia:* Both sodium nitrite and amyl nitrite in excessive doses induce dangerous methemoglobinemia and can cause death. The amounts found in a single cyanide antidote package are not excessive for an adult. Calculate the doses for children on a surface area or on a weight basis with the dosage adjusted so that excessive methemoglobin is not formed.

DETOXIFICATION AGENTS

Various Detoxification Agents and Their Uses

Drug (trade name)	Toxic/Overdosed substance
Dimercaprol (*BAL In Oil*)	Arsenic, gold, mercury, lead
Deferoxamine mesylate (*Desferal*)	Iron
Dexrazoxane (*Zinecard*)	Doxorubicin-induced cardiomyopathy
Digoxin immune fab (*Digibind, Digifab*)	Digoxin, digitoxin
Edetate calcium disodium (*Calcium Disodium Versenate*)	Lead
Flumazenil (*Romazicon*)	Benzodiazepines
Fomepizole (*Antizol*)	Ethylene glycol, methanol
Mesna (*Mesnex*)	Ifosfamide-induced hemorrhagic cystitis
Methylene blue (Various)	Nitrites
Narcotic antagonists Naloxone (*Narcan*) Nalmefene (*Revex*) Naltrexone (*ReVia*)	Opioids
Physostigmine salicylate (*Antilirium*)	Anticholinergics (including tricyclic antidepressants)
Pralidoxime Cl (*Protopam Cl*)	Organophosphates Anticholinesterases
Sodium thiosulfate (Various)	Cyanide
Succimer (*Chemet*)	Lead
Trientene (*Syprine*)	Copper
Other agents used additionally as antidotes:	
Acetylcysteine (*Mucomyst, Mucosil*)	Acetaminophen
Amyl nitrite, Na Nitrite, Na Thiosulfate (*Cyanide antidote kit*)	Cyanide
Anticholinesterases Pyridostigmine Br (*Mestinon, Regonol*) Neostigmine Br (*Prostigmin*) Edrophonium Cl (*Tensilon*)	Nondepolarizing muscle relaxants
Atropine (Various)	Cholinergic agents: Organophosphates, carbamates, pilocarpine, physostigmine, or choline esters.

Various Detoxification Agents and Their Uses	
Drug (trade name)	Toxic/Overdosed substance
Glucagon	Insulin-induced hypoglycemia, beta blockers
Hydroxocobalamin (Various)	Cyanide poisoning
Leucovorin calcium (*Wellcovorin*)	Folic acid antagonists (eg, methotrexate)
Protamine sulfate (Various)	Heparin
Pyridoxine	Isoniazid
Vitamin K_1 (Various)	Oral anticoagulants

Various Detoxification Agents and Their Uses	
Drug (trade name)	Toxic/Overdosed substance
Nonspecific therapy of overdoses include the following:	
Activated charcoal (Various)	Nonspecific, supportive therapies of overdoses. See also General Management of Acute Overdosage.
Cathartics	
Osmotic diuretics	
Polyethylene glycol electrolyte solution (*GoLYTELY*)	
Syrup of ipecac (Various)	
Urinary acidifiers	
Urinary alkalinizers	

Chelating Agents

TRIENTINE HYDROCHLORIDE

Rx	**Syprine** (Merck)	**Capsules:** 250 mg	(SYPRINE/MSD 661). Light brown. In 100s.

TRIENTINE HYDROCHLORIDE — ORAL

Indications

➤*Wilson disease:* Treatment of patients with Wilson disease who are intolerant of penicillamine.

Administration and Dosage

➤*Approved by the FDA:* November 8, 1985.

➤*Administration:* Take on an empty stomach at least 1 hour before or 2 hours after meals and at least 1 hour apart from any other drug, food, or milk. Swallow the capsules whole and do not open or chew.

➤*Adults:* Initially, 750 to 1,250 mg/day in divided doses 2, 3, or 4 times/day. May increase to a maximum of 2,000 mg/day.

➤*Children 12 years of age and younger:* Initially, 500 to 750 mg/day in divided doses 2, 3, or 4 times/day. May increase to a maximum of 1,500 mg/day.

Increase the daily dose only when the clinical response is not adequate or the concentration of free serum copper is persistently above 20 mcg/dL. Determine optimal long-term maintenance dosage at 6- to 12-month intervals.

➤*Storage/Stability:* Store at 2° to 8°C (36° to 46°F) in a tightly closed container.

Actions

➤*Pharmacology:* Wilson disease (hepatolenticular degeneration) is an inherited metabolic defect resulting in excess copper accumulation, possibly because the liver lacks the mechanism to excrete free copper into the bile. Hepatocytes store excess copper, but when their capacity is exceeded, copper is released into the blood and is taken up into extrahepatic sites. Treat this condition with a low copper diet and chelating agents that bind copper to facilitate its excretion from the body. Trientine is a chelating compound for removal of excess copper from the body.

Contraindications

Hypersensitivity to trientine.

Warnings

➤*Not indicated for the following:* Not indicated for cystinuria; rheumatoid arthritis; biliary cirrhosis.

➤*Patient supervision:* Patients should remain under regular medical supervision throughout the period of drug administration.

➤*Iron deficiency anemia:* Closely monitor patients (especially women) for evidence of iron deficiency anemia.

➤*Elderly:* In general, dose selection should be cautious, usually starting at the low end of the dosing range, reflecting the greater frequency of decreased hepatic, renal, or cardiac function, and of concomitant disease or other drug therapy.

➤*Pregnancy: Category C.* Trientine was teratogenic in rats at doses similar to the human dose. The frequencies of resorptions and fetal abnormalities, including hemorrhage and edema, increased while fetal copper levels decreased. There are no adequate and well-controlled studies in pregnant women. Use during pregnancy only when the potential benefits outweigh the potential hazards to the fetus.

➤*Lactation:* It is not known whether this drug is excreted in breast milk. Exercise caution when administering to a breast-feeding woman.

➤*Children:* Safety and efficacy for use in children have not been established. Trientine has been used clinically in children as young as 6 years of age with no reported adverse effects.

Precautions

➤*Monitoring:* The most reliable index for monitoring treatment is the determination of free copper in the serum, which equals the difference between quantitatively determined total copper and ceruloplasmin-copper. Adequately treated patients will usually have less than 10 mcg free copper/dL of serum.

Therapy may be monitored with a 24-hour urinary copper analysis periodically (ie, every 6 to 12 months). Urine must be collected in copper-free glassware. Because a low copper diet should keep copper absorption down to less than 1 mg/day, the patient probably will be in the desired state of negative copper balance if 0.5 to 1 mg of copper is present in a 24-hour collection of urine.

➤*Hypersensitivity:* There are no reports of hypersensitivity in patients given trientine for Wilson disease. However, there have been reports of asthma, bronchitis, and dermatitis occurring after prolonged environmental exposure in workers who use trientine as a hardener of epoxy resins. Observe patients closely for signs of possible hypersensitivity. Refer to Management of Hypersensitivity Reactions.

Drug Interactions

➤*Mineral supplements:* In general, do not give mineral supplements; they may block the absorption of trientine. However, iron deficiency may develop, especially in children and menstruating or pregnant women, or as a result of the low copper diet recommended for Wilson disease. If necessary, iron may be given in short courses, but because iron and trientine each inhibit absorption of the other, allow 2 hours to elapse between administration of trientine and iron.

➤*Drug/Food interactions:* It is important that trientene be taken on an empty stomach at least 1 hour before or 2 hours after meals and at least 1 hour apart from any other drug, food, or milk. This permits maximum absorption; also, coadministration may inactivate trientine by metal binding in the GI tract.

Adverse Reactions

Iron deficiency, systemic lupus erythematosus, dystonia, muscular spasm, and myasthenia gravis have occurred in patients with Wilson disease who were being treated with trientine.

Trientine is not indicated for treatment of biliary cirrhosis, but in 1 study of 4 patients treated with trientine for primary biliary cirrhosis, the following adverse reactions were reported: Heartburn; epigastric pain and tenderness; thickening, fissuring, and flaking of the skin; hypochromic microcytic anemia; acute gastritis; aphthoid ulcers; abdominal pain; melena; anorexia; malaise; cramps; muscle pain; weakness; rhabdomyolysis. A causal relationship to drug therapy could not be rejected or established.

Overdosage

There is a report of an adult woman who ingested trientine 30 g without apparent ill effects.

Patient Information

Take on an empty stomach at least 1 hour before or 2 hours after meals and at least 1 hour apart from any other drug, food, or milk.

Swallow capsules whole with water. Do not open or chew.

Because of the potential for contact dermatitis, promptly wash any site of exposure to the capsule contents with water.

Take temperature nightly for the first month of treatment, and report any symptoms such as fever or skin eruption.

SUCCIMER (DMSA)

Rx	**Chemet** (Ovation)	**Capsules:** 100 mg	Sucrose. (Chemet 100). White. In 100s.

SUCCIMER — ORAL

Indications

➤*Lead poisoning:* Succimer is indicated for the treatment of lead poisoning in pediatric patients with blood lead levels greater than 45 mcg/dL. Succimer is not indicated for prophylaxis of lead poisoning in a lead-containing environment; the use of succimer should always be accompanied by identification and removal of the source of the lead exposure.

SUCCIMER — ORAL

➤*Unlabeled uses:* Succimer may be beneficial in the treatment of other heavy metal poisonings (eg, mercury, arsenic); further study is needed.

Administration and Dosage

➤*Approved by the FDA:* February 1991.

➤*Dosage:* Start dosage at 10 mg/kg or 350 mg/m^2 every 8 hours for 5 days. Initiation of therapy at higher doses is not recommended (see the following table). Reduce frequency of administration to 10 mg/kg or 350 mg/m^2 every 12 hours (two-thirds of initial daily dosage) for an additional 2 weeks of therapy. A course of treatment lasts 19 days. Repeated courses may be necessary if indicated by weekly monitoring of blood lead concentration. A minimum of 2 weeks between courses is recommended unless blood lead levels indicate the need for more prompt treatment.

Succimer pediatric dosing table

lbs	kg	Dose (mg)[a]	Number of capsules[a]
18 to 35	8 to 15	100	1
36 to 55	16 to 23	200	2
56 to 75	24 to 34	300	3
76 to 100	35 to 44	400	4
> 100	> 45	500	5

[a] To be administered every 8 hours for 5 days, followed by dosing every 12 hours for 14 days.

In young pediatric patients who cannot swallow capsules, succimer can be administered by separating the capsule and sprinkling the medicated beads on a small amount of soft food or putting them in a spoon and following with fruit drink.

Identification of the source of lead in the pediatric patient's environment and its abatement are critical to a successful therapy outcome. Chelation therapy is not a substitute for preventing further exposure to lead and should not be used to permit continued exposure to lead.

Patients who have received calcium EDTA with or without dimercaprol may use succimer for subsequent treatment after an interval of 4 weeks. Data on the concomitant use of succimer with calcium EDTA with or without dimercaprol are not available, and such use is not recommended.

➤*Storage/Stability:* Store between 15° and 25°C (59° and 77°F) and avoid excessive heat.

Actions

➤*Pharmacology:* Succimer is a lead chelator; it forms water-soluble chelates and, consequently, increases the urinary excretion of lead.

➤*Pharmacokinetics:*

Absorption – In a study performed in healthy adult volunteers, after a single dose of ^{14}C-succimer at 16, 32, or 48 mg/kg, absorption was rapid but variable, with peak blood radioactivity levels between 1 and 2 hours.

Metabolism/Excretion – On average, 49% of the radiolabeled dose was excreted: 39% in the feces, 9% in the urine, and 1% as carbon dioxide from the lungs. Since fecal excretion probably represented nonabsorbed drug, most of the absorbed drug was excreted by the kidneys. The apparent elimination half-life of the radiolabeled material in the blood was approximately 2 days.

In other studies of healthy adult volunteers receiving a single oral dose of 10 mg/kg, the chemical analysis of succimer and its metabolites in the urine showed that succimer was rapidly and extensively metabolized. Approximately 25% of the administered dose was excreted in the urine, with the peak blood level and urinary excretion occurring between 2 and 4 hours. Of the total amount of drug eliminated in the urine, approximately 90% was eliminated in altered form as mixed succimer-cysteine disulfides; the remaining 10% was eliminated unchanged. The majority of mixed disulfides consisted of succimer in disulfide linkages with 2 molecules of L-cysteine, the remaining disulfides contained one L-cysteine per succimer molecule.

Contraindications

Allergy to the drug.

Warnings

➤*Lead exposure:* Succimer is not a substitute for effective abatement of lead exposure.

➤*Neutropenia:* Mild-to-moderate neutropenia has been observed in some patients receiving succimer. While a causal relationship to succimer has not been definitely established, neutropenia has been reported with other drugs in the same chemical class. A complete blood count with white blood cell differential and direct platelet counts should be obtained prior to and weekly during treatment with succimer. Therapy should either be withheld or discontinued if the absolute neutrophil count (ANC) is less than 1,200/mcL and the patient is followed closely to document recovery of the ANC to greater than 1,500/mcL or to the patient's baseline neutrophil count. There is limited experience with reexposure in patients who have developed neutropenia. Therefore, such patients should be rechallenged only if the benefit of succimer therapy clearly outweighs the potential risk of another episode of neutropenia and then only with careful patient monitoring.

Patients treated with succimer should be instructed to promptly report any signs of infection. If infection is suspected, the above laboratory tests should be conducted immediately.

➤*Hypersensitivity reactions:* The possibility of allergic or other mucocutaneous reactions to the drug must be borne in mind on readministration (as well as during initial courses). Patients requiring repeated courses of succimer should be monitored during each treatment course. One patient experienced recurrent mucocutaneous vesicular eruptions of increasing severity affecting the oral mucosa, the external urethral meatus and the perianal area on the third, fourth, and fifth courses of the drug. The reaction resolved between courses and upon discontinuation of therapy.

➤*Renal function impairment:* All patients undergoing treatment should be adequately hydrated. Caution should be exercised in using succimer therapy in patients with compromised renal function. Limited data suggests that succimer is dialyzable, but that the lead chelates are not.

➤*Hepatic function impairment:* Transient mild elevations of serum transaminases have been observed in 6% to 10% of patients during the course of succimer therapy. Serum transaminases should be monitored before the start of therapy and at least weekly during therapy. Patients with histories of liver disease should be monitored closely. No data are available regarding the metabolism of succimer in patients with liver disease.

➤*Pregnancy:* Category C.

Teratogenic – Succimer has been shown to be teratogenic and fetotoxic in pregnant mice when given subcutaneously in a dose range of 410 to 1,640 mg/kg/day during the period of organogenesis. There are no adequate and well-controlled studies in pregnant women. Succimer should be used during pregnancy only if the potential benefit justifies the potential risk to the fetus.

➤*Lactation:* It is not known whether this drug is excreted in human milk. Because many drugs and heavy metals are excreted in human milk, nursing mothers requiring succimer therapy should be discouraged from breast-feeding their infants.

➤*Children:* Safety and efficacy in pediatric patients younger than 12 months of age have not been established.

Precautions

➤*Monitoring:* The extent of clinical experience with succimer is limited. Therefore, patients should be carefully observed during treatment.

Neutropenia – See Warnings for more information.

➤*Rebound blood lead levels:* Elevated blood lead levels and associated symptoms may return rapidly after discontinuation of succimer because of redistribution of lead from bone stores to soft tissues and blood. After therapy, patients should be monitored for rebound of blood lead levels, by measuring blood lead levels at least once weekly until stable. However, the severity of lead intoxication (as measured by the initial blood lead level and the rate and degree of rebound of blood lead) should be used as a guide for more frequent blood lead monitoring.

➤*Repeated courses:* Clinical experience with repeated courses is limited. The safety of uninterrupted dosing longer than 3 weeks has not been established, and it is not recommended.

Drug Interactions

Succimer is not known to interact with other drugs, including iron supplements; interactions have not been systematically studied. Concomitant administration of succimer with other chelation therapy, such as calcium EDTA is not recommended.

➤*Drug/Lab test interactions:* Succimer may interfere with serum and urinary laboratory tests. In vitro studies have shown succimer to cause false-positive results for ketones in urine using nitroprusside reagents such as *Ketostix* and falsely decreased measurements of serum uric acid and CPK.

Adverse Reactions

Clinical experience with succimer has been limited. Consequently, the full spectrum and incidence of adverse reactions, including the possibility of hypersensitivity or idiosyncratic reactions, have not been determined. The most common events attributable to succimer (ie, GI symptoms, increases in serum transaminases), have been observed in approximately 10% of patients. Transient mild elevations of serum transaminases have been observed in 6% to 10% of patients during the course of succimer therapy. Rashes, some necessitating discontinuation of therapy, have been reported in approximately 4% of patients. If rash occurs, other causes (eg, measles) should be considered before ascribing the reaction to succimer.

Rechallenge with succimer may be considered if lead levels are high enough to warrant retreatment. One allergic mucocutaneous reaction has been reported on repeated administration of the drug. The patient experienced recurrent mucocutaneous vesicular eruptons of increasing severity affecting the oral mucosa, the external urethral meatus and the perianal area on the third, fourth, and fifth courses of the drug. Mild-to-moderate neutropenia has been observed in some patients receiving succimer. While a causal relationship to succimer has not been definitely established, neutropenia has been reported with other drugs in the same chemical class. The following information presents adverse events reported with the administration of succimer for the treatment of lead and other heavy metal intoxication.

SUCCIMER — ORAL

Incidence of Adverse Reactions in Domestic Studies Regardless of Attribution or Succimer Dosage	Pediatric patients (191)		Adults (134)	
	%	(n)	%	(n)
GI				
Nausea, vomiting, diarrhea, appetite loss, hemorrhoidal symptoms, loose stools, metallic taste in mouth	12%	23	20.9%	28
Metabolic				
Elevated ALT, AST, alkaline phosphatase, elevated serum cholesterol	4.2%	8	10.4%	14
CNS				
Drowsiness, dizziness, sensorimotor neuropathy, sleepiness, paresthesia	1%	2	12.7%	17
Dermatologic				
Papular rash, herpetic rash, rash, mucocutaneous eruptions, pruritus	2.6%	5	11.2%	15
Special senses				
Cloudy film in eye, ears plugged, otitis media, eyes watery	1%	2	3.7%	5
Respiratory				
Sore throat, rhinorrhea, nasal congestion, cough	3.7%	7	0.7%	1
GU				
Decreased urination, voiding difficulty, increased proteinuria	0%		3.7%	5
Cardiovascular				
Arrhythmia	0%		1.8%	2
Hematologic-lymphatic				
Mild-to-moderate neutropenia, increased platelet count, intermittent eosinophilia	0.5%[a]	1	1.5%[a]	2
Musculoskeletal				
Kneecap pain, leg pains	0%		3%	4
Miscellaneous				
Back pain, abdominal cramps, stomach pains, head pain, rib pain, chills, flank pain, fever, flu-like symptoms, heavy head/tired, head cold, headache, moniliasis	5.2%	10	15.7%	21

[a] Does not include neutropenia.

Overdosage

➤*Symptoms:* Doses of 2,300 mg/kg in the rat and 2,400 mg/kg in the mouse produced ataxia, convulsions, labored respiration, and frequently death. No case of overdosage has been reported in humans. Limited data indicate that succimer is dialyzable.

➤*Treatment:* In case of acute overdosage, induction of vomiting or gastric lavage followed by administration of an activated charcoal slurry and appropriate supportive therapy are recommended.

Patient Information

Patients should be instructed to maintain adequate fluid intake. If rash occurs, patients should consult their physicians. Patients should be instructed to promptly report any indication of infection, which may be a sign of neutropenia.

In young pediatric patients unable to swallow capsules, the contents of the capsule can be administered in a small amount of food. Administer by separating the capsule and sprinkling the medicated beads on a small amount of soft food or putting them in a spoon and following with a fruit drink.

DIMERCAPROL

Rx	**BAL In Oil** (Taylor)	**Injection:** 10% (100 mg/mL)	In peanut oil with 20% benzyl benzoate. In 3 mL amps.

DIMERCAPROL — INJECTION

Indications

➤*Poisoning:* Treatment of arsenic, gold, and mercury poisoning. It is indicated in acute lead poisoning when used concomitantly with edetate calcium disodium injection.

Dimercaprol injection is effective for use in acute poisoning by mercury salts if therapy is begun within 1 or 2 hours following ingestion. It is not very effective for chronic mercury poisoning.

Dimercaprol injection is of questionable value in poisoning caused by other heavy metals such as antimony and bismuth.

Administration and Dosage

Administer by deep IM injection only.

Successful treatment depends on beginning injections at the earliest possible moment and on the use of adequate amounts at frequent intervals. Always use other supportive measures in conjunction with dimercaprol injection therapy.

➤*Mild arsenic or gold poisoning:* For mild arsenic or gold poisoning, 2.5 mg/kg of body weight 4 times daily for 2 days, 2 times on the third day, and once daily thereafter for 10 days; for severe arsenic or gold poisoning, 3 mg/kg every 4 hours for 2 days, 4 times on the third day, then twice daily thereafter for 10 days.

➤*Mercury poisoning:* For mercury poisoning, 5 mg/kg initially, followed by 2.5 mg/kg 1 or 2 times daily for 10 days.

➤*Acute lead encephalopathy:* For acute lead encephalopathy, give 4 mg/kg body weight alone in the first dose and administer thereafter at 4-hour intervals in combination with edetate calcium disodium injection at a separate site. For less severe poisoning, reduce the dose to 3 mg/kg after the first dose. Maintain treatment for 2 to 7 days, depending on clinical response.

➤*Storage/Stability:* Store at 15° to 25°C (59° to 77°F). Visually inspect dimercaprol injection for particulate matter and discoloration prior to administration.

Actions

➤*Pharmacology:* The sulfhydryl groups of dimercaprol form complexes with certain heavy metals, thus preventing or reversing the metallic binding of sulfhydryl-containing enzymes. The complex is excreted. The sustained presence of dimercaprol promotes continued excretion of the metallic poisons (arsenic, gold, and mercury). It is also used in combination with edetate calcium disodium injection to promote the excretion of lead.

Contraindications

Dimercaprol injection is contraindicated in most instances of hepatic insufficiency with the exception of postarsenical jaundice. Discontinue the drug or use only with extreme caution if acute renal insufficiency develops during therapy.

Do not use in iron, cadmium, or selenium poisoning, as the resulting dimercaprol-metal complexes are more toxic than the metal alone, especially to the kidneys.

Warnings

➤*Injection site reaction:* There may be local pain at the site of the injection. A reaction apparently peculiar to children is fever which may persist during therapy. It occurs in approximately 30% of children. A transient reduction of the percentage of polymorphonuclear leukocytes may also be observed.

➤*Renal function impairment:* Discontinue dimercaprol injection or use only with extreme caution if acute renal insufficiency develops during therapy.

➤*Hepatic function impairment:* Dimercaprol injection is contraindicated in most instances of hepatic insufficiency, with the exception of postarsenical jaundice.

➤*Pregnancy: Category C.*

Animal reproduction studies have not been conducted with dimercaprol injection. It is also not known whether dimercaprol injection can cause fetal harm when administered to a pregnant woman, or can affect reproduction capacity. Give dimercaprol injection to a pregnant woman only if clearly needed.

➤*Lactation:* It is not known whether this drug is excreted in human milk. However, because many drugs are excreted in human milk, exercise caution when administering dimercaprol injection to a breast-feeding woman.

Precautions

➤*Urinary alkalinization:* Urinary alkalinization is recommended because the dimercaprol-metal complex breaks down easily in an acid medium. Alkaline urine protects the kidney during therapy.

➤*G-6-PD deficiency:* Use with caution in these patients; hemolysis may occur.

DIMERCAPROL — INJECTION

Drug Interactions

➤*Iron:* Do not administer medicinal iron to patients under therapy with dimercaprol injection.

Adverse Reactions

One of the most consistent responses to dimercaprol injection is a rise in blood pressure accompanied by tachycardia. This rise is roughly proportional to the dose administered. Doses larger than those recommended may cause other transitory signs and symptoms in approximate order of frequency as follows: nausea and, in some instances, vomiting; headache; a burning sensation in the lips, mouth, and throat; a feeling of constriction, even pain, in the throat, chest, or hands; conjunctivitis, lacrimation, blepheral spasm, rhinorrhea, and salivation; tingling of the hands; a burning sensation in the penis; sweating of the forehead, hands, and other areas; abdominal pain; and occasional appearance of painful sterile abscesses. Many of the above symptoms are accompanied by a feeling of anxiety, weakness, and unrest and often are relieved by administration of antihistamine.

Overdosage

➤*Symptoms:* Dosage exceeding 5 mg/kg will usually be followed by vomiting, convulsions, and stupor, beginning within 30 minutes and subsiding within 6 hours following injection.

DEFEROXAMINE MESYLATE

Rx	**Deferoxamine Mesylate** (Hospira)	**Powder for injection, lyophilized:** 500 mg	In vials.
Rx	**Desferal** (Novartis)		In vials.
Rx	**Deferoxamine Mesylate** (Hospira)	**Powder for injection, lyophilized:** 2 g	In vials.
Rx	**Desferal** (Novartis)		In vials.

DEFEROXAMINE MESYLATE — INJECTION

Indications

➤*Acute iron intoxication:* An adjunct to standard treatment measures.

➤*Chronic iron overload:* Deferoxamine can promote iron excretion in patients with secondary iron overload from multiple transfusions (as may occur in the treatment of some chronic anemias, including thalassemia). Long-term therapy with deferoxamine slows hepatic iron accumulation; retards or eliminates hepatic fibrosis progression.

➤*Unlabeled uses:* In patients with chronic renal failure, deferoxamine has been used in the treatment of aluminum overload, commonly related to the use of aluminum-contaminated dialysate or ingestion of aluminum-containing phosphorous binding drugs.

Deferoxamine also has been used as a diagnostic test for iron storage disease in patients with normal renal function.

Administration and Dosage

➤*Acute iron intoxication:*

IM – Preferred route; use for all patients not in shock. Initially, 1 g then 500 mg every 4 hours for 2 doses. Subsequently, give 500 mg every 4 to 12 hours based on clinical response. Do not exceed 6 g/day.

IV – Use only in cardiovascular collapse and give by slow infusion. The rate of infusion should not exceed 15 mg/kg/h for the first 1 g administered. Subsequent IV dosing, if needed, must be at a slower rate, not to exceed 125 mg/h.

The reconstituted solution is added to physiologic saline, glucose in water, or lactated Ringer's solution.

Administer an initial dose of 1 g at a rate not to exceed 15 mg/kg/h. This may be followed by 500 mg over 4 hours for 2 doses. Depending on the clinical response, subsequent doses of 500 mg may be administered over 4 to 12 hours. The total amount administered should not exceed 6 g/day.

As soon as possible, stop IV and give IM.

➤*Chronic iron overload:* Individualize dosage.

IM – 500 mg to 1 g/day. Give 2 g IV with, but separate from, each unit of blood. The rate of IV infusion must not exceed 15 mg/kg/h. The total daily dose should not exceed 1 g in the absence of a transfusion, or 6 g even if transfused 3 or more units of blood or packed red blood cells.

SC – 1 to 2 g/day (20 to 40 mg/kg/day) over 8 to 24 hours with continuous mini-infusion pump. Individualize infusion duration. In some patients, iron excretion will be as much after a short infusion (8 to 12 hours) as if the same dose is given over 24 hours.

➤*Children:* Maximum dose is 6 g/24 h.

➤*Preparation:* Deferoxamine is preferably dissolved by adding 5 mL sterile water for injection to each 500 mg vial or 20 mL sterile water for injection to each 2 g vial. The reconstituted deferoxamine solution is isotonic, clear, and colorless to slightly yellowish at the recommended concentration of 10%.

In clinical situations requiring a smaller volume of solution (eg, IM injection), deferoxamine may be dissolved by adding 2 mL sterile water for injection to each 500 mg vial or 8 mL sterile water for injection to each 2 g vial. This concentration may produce a stronger yellow colored solution. Completely dissolve the drug before the solution is withdrawn.

Deferoxamine reconstituted with sterile water for injection is for single use only.

➤*Storage/Stability:* Do not store above 25°C (77°F).

Use the product immediately after reconstitution (commencement of treatment within 3 hours) for microbiological safety. When reconstitution is carried out under validated aseptic conditions (in a sterile laminar flow hood using aseptic technique), the product may be stored at room temperature for a maximum period of 24 hours before use. Do not refrigerate reconstituted solution. Reconstituting desferoxamine in solvents or under conditions other than indicated may result in precipitation. Do not use turbid solutions.

Actions

➤*Pharmacology:* Deferoxamine chelates iron by forming a stable complex that prevents the iron from entering into further chemical reactions. It readily chelates iron from ferritin and hemosiderin but not readily from transferrin; it does not combine with the iron from cytochromes and hemoglobin. One hundred parts by weight can bind approximately 8.5 parts of ferric iron. Does not demonstrably increase electrolyte/trace metal excretion.

➤*Pharmacokinetics:* Deferoxamine is metabolized principally by plasma enzymes, but the pathways have not yet been defined. Iron chelate is excreted renally, giving urine a reddish color. Some is excreted in feces via bile. Elimination half-life is about 6 hours.

Contraindications

Severe renal disease or anuria.

Warnings

➤*Primary hemochromatosis:* Deferoxamine is not indicated for the treatment of primary hemochromatosis because phlebotomy is the method of choice of removing excess iron in this disorder.

➤*Ocular and auditory disturbances:* Ocular and auditory disturbances have been reported when deferoxamine was administered over prolonged periods of time, at high doses, or in patients with low ferritin levels. The ocular disturbances observed have been blurring of vision; cataracts after prolonged administration in chronic iron overload; decreased visual acuity including visual loss, visual defects, scotoma; impaired peripheral, color, and night vision; optic neuritis, cataracts, corneal opacities, and retinal pigmentary abnormalities. The auditory abnormalities reported have been tinnitus and hearing loss including high frequency sensorineural hearing loss. In most cases, ocular and auditory disturbances were reversible upon immediate cessation of treatment.

Visual acuity tests, slit-lamp examinations, funduscopy, and audiometry are recommended periodically in patients treated for prolonged periods of time. Toxicity is more likely to be reversed if symptoms or test abnormalities are detected early.

➤*Acute respiratory distress syndrome:* Acute respiratory distress syndrome, also reported in children, has been described following treatment with excessively high IV doses in patients with acute iron intoxication or thalassemia.

➤*Mutagenesis:* Cytoxicity may occur because deferoxamine has been shown to inhibit DNA synthesis in vitro.

➤*Pregnancy: Category C.* Delayed ossification in mice and skeletal anomalies in rabbits were observed after deferoxamine was administered in daily doses up to 4.5 times the maximum daily human dose. No adverse effects were observed in similar studies in rats. There are no adequate and well-controlled studies in pregnant women. Use deferoxamine during pregnancy only if the potential benefit justifies the potential risk to the fetus.

➤*Lactation:* It is not known whether this drug is excreted in human milk. Exercise caution when deferoxamine is administered to a breast-feeding woman.

➤*Children:* Safety and efficacy in pediatric patients younger than 3 years of age have not been established. Iron mobilization by deferoxamine is relatively poor in patients younger than 3 years of age with relatively little iron overload. Ordinarily, do not give the drug to such patients unless significant iron mobilization (eg, 1 mg or more of iron/day) can be demonstrated.

High doses of deferoxamine and concomitant low ferritin levels also have been associated with growth retardation. After reduction of deferoxamine dose, growth velocity may partially resume to pretreatment rates.

Monitor children receiving deferoxamine for body weight and growth every 3 months.

Precautions

➤*Infections:* Iron overload increases susceptibility of patients to *Yersinia enterocolitica* and *Yersinia pseudotuberculosis* infections. In some rare cases, treatment of deferoxamine has enhanced this susceptibility, resulting in generalized infections by providing this bacteria with a siderophore otherwise missing. In such cases, discontinue deferoxamine treatment until the infection is resolved.

In patients receiving deferoxamine, rare cases of mucormycosis, some with a fatal outcome, have been reported. If any of the suspected signs or symptoms

DEFEROXAMINE MESYLATE — INJECTION

occur, discontinue deferoxamine, carry out mycological tests, and institute appropriate treatment immediately.

➤*Aluminum overload:* In patients with aluminum-related encephalopathy, high doses of deferoxamine may exacerbate neurological dysfunction (seizures), probably owing to an acute increase in circulating aluminum. Deferoxamine may precipitate the onset of dialysis dementia. Treatment with deferoxamine in the presence of aluminum overload may result in decreased serum calcium and aggravation of hyperparathyroidism.

➤*Rapid infusion:* Flushing of the skin, urticaria, hypotension, and shock have occurred in a few patients with rapid IV injection. Therefore, give deferoxamine IM or by slow subcutaneous or IV infusion.

➤*Vitamin C use:* Patients with iron overload usually become vitamin C deficient, probably because iron oxidizes the vitamin. As an adjuvant to iron chelation therapy, vitamin C in doses up to 200 mg for adults may be given in divided doses, starting after an initial month of regular treatment with deferoxamine. Vitamin C increases availability of iron for chelation. In general, 50 mg/day suffices for children under 10 years of age and 100 mg/day for older children. Larger doses of vitamin C fail to produce any additional increase in excretion of iron complex.

In patients with severe chronic iron overload, impairment of cardiac function has been reported following concomitant treatment with deferoxamine and high doses of vitamin C (more than 500 mg/day in adults). The cardiac dysfunction was reversible when vitamin C was discontinued. Take the following precautions when vitamin C and deferoxamine are to be used concomitantly: a) do not give vitamin C supplements to patients with cardiac failure; b) start supplemental vitamin C only after an initial month of regular treatment with deferoxamine; c) give vitamin C only if the patient is receiving deferoxamine regularly, ideally soon after setting up the infusion pump; d) do not exceed the daily vitamin C dose of 200 mg in adults, given in divided doses; e) clinical monitoring of cardiac function is advisable during such combined therapy.

Drug Interactions

Deferoxamine Drug Interactions

Precipitant drug	Object drug[a]		Description
Deferoxamine	Gallium-67	⬇	Imaging results may be distorted because of the rapid urinary excretion of deferoxamine-bound gallium-67. Discontinue deferoxamine 48 hours prior to scintigraphy.
Deferoxamine	Prochlorperazine	⬆	Concurrent use may lead to temporary impairment of consciousness.

[a] ⬆ = Object drug increased. ⬇ = Object drug decreased.

Adverse Reactions

The following adverse reactions have been observed, but there are not enough data to support an estimate of their frequency.

➤*Cardiovascular:* Hypotension, shock, tachycardia.

➤*CNS:* Neurological disturbances including dizziness, peripheral sensory, motor, or mixed neuropathy, paresthesias; exacerbation or precipitation of aluminum-related dialysis encephalopathy (see Precautions).

➤*GI:* Abdominal discomfort, diarrhea, nausea, vomiting.

➤*GU:* Dysuria, impaired renal function (see Contraindications); reddish urine (see Pharmacokinetics).

➤*Hematologic:* Blood dyscrasia (ie, cases of thrombocytopenia and/or leukopenia have been reported. A causal relationship has not been clearly established).

➤*Hypersensitivity:* Anaphylactic reaction with or without shock, angioedema, generalized rash, urticaria.

➤*Local:* Burning, crusting, erythema, eschar, induration, infiltration, local edema, localized irritation, pain, pruritus, swelling, vesicles, wheal formation. Injection site reactions may be associated with systemic allergic reactions.

➤*Musculoskeletal:* Leg cramps have occurred. Growth retardation and bone changes (eg, metaphyseal dysplasia) are common in chelated patients given doses above 60 mg/kg, especially those who begin iron chelation in the first 3 years of life. If doses are kept to 40 mg/kg or below, the risk may be reduced (see Warnings).

➤*Respiratory:* Acute respiratory distress syndrome (with dyspnea, cyanosis, and/or interstitial infiltrates) (see Warnings).

➤*Special senses:* High-frequency sensorineural hearing loss and/or tinnitus are uncommon if dosage guidelines are not exceeded and if dose is reduced when ferritin levels decline. Visual disturbances are rare if dosage guidelines are not exceeded. These may include decreased acuity, blurred vision, loss of vision, dyschromatopsia, night blindness, visual field defects, scotoma, retinopathy (pigmentary degeneration), optic neuritis, and cataracts (see Warnings).

➤*Miscellaneous:* Local injection site reactions may be accompanied by systemic reactions (eg, arthralgia, fever, headache, myalgia, nausea, vomiting, abdominal pain, asthma). Generalized rash has occurred very rarely.

Rare infections with *Yersinia* and mucormycosis have been reported in association with deferoxamine use (see Precautions).

Overdosage

➤*Symptoms:* Inadvertent administration of an overdose or inadvertent IV bolus administration/rapid IV infusion may be associated with hypotension, tachycardia, and GI disturbances; acute but transient loss of vision, aphasia, agitation, headache, nausea, pallor, CNS depression including coma, bradycardia, and acute renal failure have been reported.

➤*Treatment:* There is no specific antidote. Discontinue deferoxamine and undertake appropriate symptomatic measures. Deferoxamine is readily dialyzable.

Patient Information

Patients experiencing dizziness or other nervous system disturbances or impairment of vision or hearing should refrain from driving or operating potentially hazardous machines.

Inform patients that occasionally their urine may show a reddish discoloration.

EDETATE CALCIUM DISODIUM (Calcium EDTA)

Rx	**Calcium Disodium Versenate** (3M Pharm.)	**Injection:** 200 mg/mL	In 5 mL amps.

EDETATE CALCIUM DISODIUM — INJECTION

WARNING

Edetate calcium disodium is capable of producing toxic effects that can be fatal. Lead encephalopathy is relatively rare in adults, but occurs more often in pediatric patients in whom it may be incipient and thus overlooked. The mortality rate in pediatric patients has been high. Patients with lead encephalopathy and cerebral edema may experience a lethal increase in intracranial pressure following, intravenous (IV) infusion, the intramuscular (IM) route is preferred for these patients. In cases where the IV route is necessary, avoid rapid infusion. The dosage schedule should be followed and at no time should the recommended daily dose be exceeded.

Indications

➤*Lead poisoning:* Edetate calcium disodium is indicated for the reduction of blood levels and depot stores of lead in lead poisoning (acute and chronic) and lead encephalopathy, in both pediatric populations and adults. Chelation therapy should not replace effective measures to eliminate or reduce further exposure to lead.

Administration and Dosage

➤*Dosage:* When a source for the lead intoxication has been identified, the patient should be removed from the source, if possible. The recommended dose of edetate calcium disodium for asymptomatic adults and pediatric patients whose blood lead level is less than 70 mcg/dL but greater than 20 mcg/dL (World Health Organization recommended upper allowable level) is 1,000 mg/m^2/day whether given IV or IM.

➤*Lead nephropathy:* For adults with lead nephropathy, the following dosing regimen has been suggested: 500 mg/m^2 every 24 hours for 5 days for patients with serum creatinine levels of 2 to 3 mg/dL, every 48 hours for 3 doses for patients with creatinine levels of 3 to 4 mg/dL, and once weekly for patients with creatinine levels above 4 mg/dL. These regimens may be repeated at 1-month intervals. Edetate calcium disodium, used alone, may aggravate symptoms in patients with very high blood lead levels. When the blood lead level is greater than 70 mcg/dL or clinical symptoms consistent with lead poisoning are present, it is recommended that edetate calcium disodium be used in conjunction with dimercaprol. Please consult published protocols and specialized references for dosage recommendations of combination therapy. Therapy of lead poisoning in adults and pediatric patients with edetate calcium disodium is continued over a period of 5 days. Therapy is then interrupted for 2 to 4 days to allow redistribution of the lead and to prevent severe depletion of zinc and other essential metals. Two courses of treatment are usually employed; however, it depends on severity of the lead toxicity and the patient's tolerance of the drug. Edetate calcium disodium is equally effective whether administered IV or IM. The IM route is used for all patients with overt lead encephalopathy and this route is preferred by some for young pediatric patients. Acutely ill individuals may be dehydrated from vomiting. Since edetate calcium disodium is excreted almost exclusively in the urine, it is very important to establish urine flow with IV fluid administration before the first dose of the chelating agent is given; however, excessive fluid must be avoided in patients with encephalopathy. Once urine flow is established, further IV fluid is restricted to basal water and electrolyte requirements. Administration of edetate calcium disodium should be stopped whenever there is cessation of urine flow in order to avoid unduly high tissue levels of the drug. Edetate calcium disodium must be used in reduced doses in patients with preexisting mild renal disease.

➤*IV administration:* Add the total daily dose of edetate calcium disodium (1,000 mg/m^2/day) to 250 to 500 mL of 5% dextrose or 0.9% sodium chloride injection. The total daily dose should be infused over a period of 8 to 12 hours. Edetate calcium disodium injection is incompatible with 10% dextrose, 10% invert sugar in 0.9% sodium chloride, lactate Ringer's, Ringer's,

EDETATE CALCIUM DISODIUM — INJECTION

one-sixth molar sodium lactate injections, and with injectable amphotericin B and hydralazine hydrochloride.

➤*IM administration:* The total daily dosage (1,000 mg/m²/day) should be divided into equal doses spaced 8 to 12 hours apart. Lidocaine or procaine should be added to the edetate calcium disodium injection to minimize pain at the injection site. The final lidocaine or procaine concentration of 5 mg/mL (0.5%) can be obtained as follows: 0.25 mL of 10% lidocaine solution per 5 mL (entire content of ampul) concentrated edetate calcium disodium; 1 mL of 1% lidocaine or procaine solution per mL of concentrated edetate calcium disodium. When used alone, regardless of method of administration, edetate calcium disodium should not be given at doses larger than those recommended.

➤*Diagnostic test:* Several methods have been described for lead mobilization tests using edetate calcium disodium to assess body stores. These procedures have advantages and disadvantages that should be reviewed in current references. Edetate calcium disodium mobilization tests should not be performed in symptomatic patients and in patients with blood lead levels above 55 mcg/dL for whom appropriate therapy is indicated. Parenteral drugs should be inspected visually for particulate matter and discoloration prior to administration, whenever solution and container permit.

➤*Storage/Stability:* Store at controlled room temperature 15° to 30°C (59° to 86°F).

Actions

➤*Pharmacology:* The pharmacologic effects of edetate calcium disodium are due to the formation of chelates with divalent and trivalent metals. A stable chelate will form with any metal that has the ability to displace calcium from the molecule, a feature shared by lead, zinc, cadmium, manganese, iron, and mercury. The amounts of manganese and iron mobilized are not significant. Copper is not mobilized and mercury is unavailable for chelation because it is too tightly bound to body ligands or it is stored in inaccessible body compartments.

The primary source of lead chelated by edetate calcium disodium is from bone; subsequently, soft-tissue lead is redistributed to bone when chelation is stopped. There is also some reduction in kidney lead levels following chelation therapy. It has been shown in animals that following a single dose of edetate calcium disodium urinary lead output increases, blood lead concentration decreases, but brain lead is significantly increased due to internal redistribution of lead (see Warnings). These data are in agreement with the recent results of others in experimental animals showing that after a 5 day course of treatment there is no net reduction in brain lead.

➤*Pharmacokinetics:*

Absorption – Edetate calcium disodium is poorly absorbed from the GI tract.

Distribution – In blood, all the drug is found in the plasma. Edetate calcium disodium does not appear to penetrate cells; it is distributed primarily in the extracellular fluid with only about 5% of the plasma concentration found in spinal fluid.

Metabolism – Almost none of the compound is metabolized.

Excretion – The half-life of edetate calcium disodium is 20 to 60 minutes. The excretion of calcium by the body is not increased following IV administration of edetate calcium disodium, but the excretion of zinc is considerably increased.

Edetate calcium disodium is excreted primarily by the kidney, with about 50% excreted in 1 hour and over 95% within 24 hours.

Contraindications

Edetate calcium disodium should not be given during periods of anuria, nor to patients with active renal disease or hepatitis.

Warnings

➤*Renal effects:* Edetate calcium disodium may produce the same renal damage as lead poisoning, such as proteinuria and microscopic hematuria. Treatment-induced nephrotoxicity is dose-dependent and may be reduced by ensuring adequate diuresis before therapy begins. Urine flow must be monitored throughout therapy which must be stopped if anuria or severe oliguria develop. The proximal tubule hydropic degeneration usually recovers upon cessation of therapy. Edetate calcium disodium must be used in reduced doses in patients with preexisting mild renal disease. Patients should be monitored for cardiac rhythm irregularities and other ECG changes during IV therapy.

➤*Pregnancy:* Category B.

One reproduction study was performed in rats at doses up to 13 times the human dose and revealed no evidence of impaired fertility or harm to the fetus caused by edetate calcium disodium. Another reproduction study performed in rats at doses up to about 25 to 40 times the human dose revealed evidence of fetal malformations caused by edetate calcium disodium, which were prevented by simultaneous supplementation of dietary zinc. There are, however, no adequate and well-controlled studies in pregnant women. Because animal reproduction studies are not always predictive of human response, this drug should be used during pregnancy only if clearly needed.

Labor and delivery – Edetate calcium disodium has no recognized use during labor and delivery, and its effects during these processes are unknown.

➤*Lactation:* It is not known whether this drug is excreted in human milk. Because many drugs are excreted in human milk, caution should be exercised when edetate calcium disodium is administered to a breast-feeding woman.

➤*Children:* Because lead poisoning occurs in pediatric populations and adults but is frequently more severe in pediatric patients, edetate calcium disodium is used in patients of all ages. The IM route is preferred by some for young pediatric patients. In cases where the IV route is necessary, avoid rapid infusion (see Warning Box). Urine flow must be monitored throughout therapy; edetate calcium disodium therapy must be stopped if anuria or severe oliguria develops. At no time should the recommended daily dosage be exceeded.

Precautions

➤*Monitoring:* Urinalysis and urine sediment, renal and hepatic function and serum electrolyte levels should be checked before each course of therapy and then be monitored daily during therapy in severe cases, and in less serious cases after the second and fifth day of therapy. Therapy must be discontinued at the first sign of renal toxicity. The presence of large renal epithelial cells or increasing number of red blood cells in urinary sediment or greater proteinuria call for immediate stopping of edetate calcium disodium administration. Alkaline phosphatase values are frequently depressed (possibly due to decreased serum zinc levels), but return to normal within 48 hours after cessation of therapy. Elevated erythrocyte protoporphyrin levels (greater than 35 mcg/dL of whole blood) indicate the need to perform a venous blood lead determination. If the whole blood lead concentration is between 25 to 55 mcg/dL a mobilization test can be considered (see Administration and Dosage, Diagnostic test). An elevation of urinary coproporphyrin (adults, greater than 250 mcg/day; pediatric patients under 80 pounds, greater than 75 mcg/day) and elevation of urinary delta aminolevulinic acid (ALA) (adults, greater than 4 mg/day; pediatric patients, greater than 3 mg/ m²/day) are associated with blood lead levels greater than 40 mcg/dL. Urinary coproporphyrin may be falsely negative in terminal patients and in severely iron-depleted pediatric patients who are not regenerating heme. In growing pediatric patients long bone x-rays showing lead lines and abdominal x-rays showing radioopaque material in the abdomen may be of help in estimating the level of exposure to lead.

Drug Interactions

Steroids enhance the renal toxicity of edetate calcium disodium in animals. Edetate calcium disodium interferes with the action of zinc insulin preparations by chelating the zinc.

Adverse Reactions

The following adverse reactions have been associated with the use of edetate calcium disodium:

➤*Allergic:* Histamine-like reactions (sneezing, nasal congestion, lacrimation), rash.

➤*Cardiovascular:* Hypotension, cardiac rhythm irregularities.

➤*CNS:* Tremors, headache, numbness, tingling.

➤*GI:* Cheilosis, nausea, vomiting, anorexia, excessive thirst.

➤*GU:* Glycosuria, proteinuria, microscopic hematuria and large epithelial cells in urinary sediment.

➤*Hematologic:* Transient bone marrow depression, anemia.

➤*Lab test abnormalities:* Mild increases in AST and ALT are common, and return to normal within 48 hours after cessation of therapy.

➤*Metabolic:* Zinc deficiency, hypercalcemia.

➤*Renal:* Acute necrosis of proximal tubules (which may result in fatal nephrosis), infrequent changes in distal tubules and glomeruli.

➤*Miscellaneous:* Pain at IM injection site, fever, chills, malaise, fatigue, myalgia, arthralgia.

Overdosage

➤*Symptoms:* Inadvertent administration of 5 times the recommended dose, infused IV over a 24-hour period, to an asymptomatic 16-month-old patient with a blood lead content of 56 mcg/dL did not cause any ill effects. Edetate calcium disodium can aggravate the symptoms of severe lead poisoning, therefore, most toxic effects (cerebral edema, renal tubular necrosis) appear to be associated with lead poisoning. Because of cerebral edema, a therapeutic dose may be lethal to an adult or a pediatric patient with lead encephalopathy. Higher dosage of edetate calcium disodium may produce a more severe zinc deficiency.

➤*Treatment:* Cerebral edema should be treated with repeated doses of mannitol. Steroids enhance the renal toxicity of edetate calcium disodium in animals and, therefore, are no longer recommended. Zinc levels must be monitored. Good urinary output must be maintained because diuresis will enhance drug elimination. It is not known if edetate calcium disodium is dialyzable.

Patient Information

Patients should be instructed to immediately inform their physician if urine output stops for a period of 12 hours.

PENTETATE ZINC TRISODIUM (Zn-DTPA)

Rx	**Pentetate Zinc Trisodium** (Hameln Pharmaceuticals)	**Solution:** 200 mg/mL	In 5 mL single-use ampules.

PENTETATE ZINC TRISODIUM (Zn-DTPA) — INJECTION

Indications

➤*Radiation contamination:* For treatment of individuals with known or suspected internal contamination with plutonium, americium, or curium to increase the rates of elimination.

Administration and Dosage

➤*Approved by the FDA:* August 11, 2004.

Chelation treatment is most effective if administered within the first 24 hours after internal contamination and should be started as soon as possible after suspected or known internal contamination. However, even when treatment cannot be started right away, give individuals chelation treatment as soon as it becomes available. Chelation treatment is still effective even after time has elapsed following internal contamination; however, the chelating effects of pentetate zinc trisodium are greatest when the radiocontaminants are still circulating or are in interstitial fluids. The efficacy of chelation decreases with time following internal contamination as the radiocontaminants become sequestered in liver and bone.

Individuals should drink plenty of fluids and void frequently to promote dilution of the radioactive chelate in the urine and minimize radiation exposure directly to the bladder.

If internal contamination with radiocontaminants other than plutonium, americium, or curium, or unknown radiocontaminants is suspected, additional therapies may be needed (eg, Prussian blue, potassium iodide).

➤*Intravenous (IV):*

Renal function impairment – Renal impairment may reduce the rate at which chelators remove radiocontaminants from the body. In heavily contaminated patients with renal impairment, use dialysis to increase the rate of elimination. High-efficiency, high-flux dialysis is recommended. Because dialysis fluid will become radioactive, take radiation precautions to protect personnel, other patients, and the general public.

Initial dose – It is preferable to administer pentetate calcium trisodium, if available, as the initial dose during the first 24 hours after internal contamination because pentetate calcium trisodium is more effective than pentetate zinc trisodium during this time period. After 24 hours, pentetate zinc trisodium and pentetate calcium trisodium are equally effective.

Adults and adolescents – A single initial dose of 1 g administered IV.

Children (younger than 12 years of age) – A single initial dose of 14 mg/kg administered IV, not to exceed 1 g.

Maintenance treatment – The duration of chelation treatment depends on the amount of internal contamination and individual response to treatment.

Adults and adolescents: The recommended maintenance dose of pentetate zinc trisodium is 1 g once a day administered IV.

Children (younger than 12 years of age): 14 mg/kg once a day administered IV. The maximum daily dose should not exceed 1 g/day.

➤*Administration:* For inhalation or IV administration. The safety and efficacy of the intramuscular (IM) route of injection have not been established.

IV – The IV route is recommended and should be used if the route of internal contamination is not known or if multiple routes of internal contamination are likely.

Administer pentetate zinc trisodium solution (1 g in 5 mL) either with a slow IV push over a period of 3 to 4 minutes or by IV infusion over 30 minutes diluted in 100 to 250 mL of 5% dextrose in water (D_5W), lactated Ringer's solution, or normal saline.

Inhalation – In individuals whose internal contamination is only by inhalation, administer pentetate zinc trisodium by nebulized inhalation as an alternative route of administration. Dilute pentetate zinc trisodium for nebulization at a 1:1 ratio with sterile water or saline. After nebulization, encourage individuals to avoid swallowing any expectorant. Some individuals may experience respiratory adverse reactions after inhalation therapy. The safety and efficacy of the nebulized route of administration have not been established in the pediatric population.

➤*Storage/Stability:* Store between 15° and 30°C (59° and 86°F).

Actions

➤*Pharmacology:* Pentetate zinc trisodium forms stable chelates with metal ions by exchanging zinc for a metal of greater binding capacity. The radioactive chelates are then excreted by glomerular filtration into the urine. In animal studies, pentetate zinc trisodium forms less stable chelates with uranium and neptunium in vivo, resulting in deposition of these elements in tissues, including the bone. Pentetate zinc trisodium treatments are not expected for uranium and neptunium. Radioactive iodine is not bound by pentetate trisodium.

The efficacy of chelation decreases with time after internal contamination because the transuranium elements become incorporated into the tissues. Give chelation treatment as soon as possible after known or suspected internal contamination with transuranium elements has occurred.

Pentetate zinc trisodium results in minimal depletion of magnesium and manganese.

➤*Pharmacokinetics:*

Absorption – Pentetate zinc trisodium is poorly absorbed in the GI tract. In animal studies, after oral administration, absorption was approximately 5%. In a US Registry of 18 patients who received a single inhaled or IV dose of 1 g, urine data indicate that the inhaled product was absorbed and resulted in a comparable elimination of the radiocontaminant. One study of 2 human subjects who received pentetate calcium trisodium with ^{14}C-DTPA by inhalation revealed approximately 20% absorption from the lungs. Human or animal bioavailability comparisons for pentetate zinc trisodium are not available after administration by inhalation and IV injection.

Distribution – Following IV administration, pentetate zinc trisodium is rapidly distributed throughout the extracellular fluid space. No significant amount of pentetate zinc trisodium penetrates into erythrocytes or other cells. No accumulation of pentetate zinc trisodium in specific organs has been observed. There is little or no binding of the chelating agent by the renal parenchyma.

Metabolism – pentetate zinc trisodium undergoes a minimal amount of metabolic change in the body.

Excretion – Pentetate zinc trisodium is cleared from the plasma in the first few hours after dosing through urinary excretion by glomerular filtration. Renal tubular excretion has not been documented. In stool samples, only a very small amount of radioactivity (less than 3%) was detected.

Special populations –

Renal function impairment: Both pentetate zinc trisodium and its radioactive chelates are excreted by glomerular filtration. Impaired renal function may decrease their rates of elimination and increase the serum half-life of pentetate zinc trisodium.

Contraindications

None known.

Warnings

➤*Exacerbation of asthma:* Nebulized chelation therapy may be associated with exacerbation of asthma. Exercise caution when administering pentetate zinc trisodium by the inhalation route.

➤*Pregnancy:* Category B.

There are no human pregnancy outcome data from which to assess the risk of pentetate zinc trisodium exposure on fetal development. Reproduction studies have been performed in pregnant mice at doses up to 11.5 mmol/kg (31 times the recommended daily dose of 1 g based on body surface area [BSA] adjusted dose) and have revealed no evidence of impaired fertility or harm to the fetus. There was a slight reduction in the average birth weight. Treatment of pregnant women should begin and continue with pentetate zinc trisodium. Use during pregnancy only if clearly needed. Weigh the risk of toxicity from untreated internal radioactive contamination against the risk of pentetate zinc trisodium treatment.

➤*Lactation:* Studies to determine if pentetate zinc trisodium is excreted in breast milk have not been conducted. Radiocontaminants are known to be excreted in breast milk. Women with known or suspected internal contamination with radiocontaminants should not breastfeed, whether or not they are receiving chelation therapy. Take precautions when discarding breast milk.

➤*Children:* The safety and efficacy of pentetate zinc trisodium were established in the adult population and efficacy was extrapolated to the pediatric population for the IV route based on the comparability of pathophysiologic mechanisms. The dose is based on body size adjustment for an IV drug that is renally cleared. The safety and efficacy of the nebulized route of administration have not been established in the pediatric population.

Precautions

➤*Monitoring:* Closely monitor serum electrolytes and essential metals during pentetate zinc trisodium treatment. Mineral or vitamin-plus-mineral supplements may be given as appropriate.

When possible, obtain baseline blood and urine samples (complete blood count [CBC] with differential, blood urea nitrogen [BUN], serum chemistries and electrolytes, urinalysis, and blood and urine radioassays) before initiating treatment.

To establish an elimination curve, obtain a quantitative baseline estimate of the total internalized transuranium elements and measures of radioactivity elimination by appropriate whole-body counting, bioassay (eg, biodosimetry), or fecal/urine sample whenever possible.

During treatment –

- Measure the radioactivity in blood, urine, and fecal samples weekly to monitor the radioactive contaminant elimination rate.
- Monitor CBC with differential, BUN, serum chemistries and electrolytes, and urinalysis measurements regularly.
- Record any adverse reactions from pentetate zinc trisodium.

➤*Endogenous metal depletion:* Treatment over several months with pentetate zinc trisodium could lead to depletion of body stores of endogenous metals (eg, magnesium, manganese). Routinely monitor these elements and, if appropriate, provide mineral or vitamin-plus-mineral supplements.

PENTETATE ZINC TRISODIUM (Zn-DTPA) — INJECTION

➤*Unknown/multiple radiocontaminants:* When an individual is contaminated with multiple radiocontaminants, or when the radiocontaminants are unknown, additional therapies may be needed (eg, Prussian blue, potassium iodide).

➤*Collection of patient treatment data:* To develop long-term response data and information on the risk of developing late malignancy, provide detailed information on patient treatment to the manufacturer. These data should include a record of the radioactive body burden and bioassay results at defined time intervals, a description of measurement methods to facilitate analysis of data, and adverse reactions.

Refer questions regarding the use of pentetate zinc trisodium for the treatment of internal contamination with transuranium elements to the manufacturer.

Drug Interactions

None well documented.

Adverse Reactions

Overall, the presence or absence of adverse reactions was recorded in 310 of 646 individuals. Of these, 19 (6.1%) individuals reported at least 1 adverse reaction. The total number of recorded adverse reactions was 20. Of the 20 adverse reactions, 1 individual treated with pentetate zinc trisodium reported headache, light-headedness, and pelvic pain.

Two individuals experienced cough and/or wheezing with nebulized pentetate calcium trisodium therapy; however, there was no such report of such reactions with nebulized pentetate zinc trisodium.

Patient Information

In individuals with recent internal contamination with plutonium, americium, or curium, pentetate zinc trisodium treatment increases excretion of radioactivity in the urine. Take appropriate safety measures to minimize contamination of others.

When possible, use a toilet instead of a urinal, and flush several times after each use. Completely clean up spilled urine or feces and wash hands thoroughly. If blood or urine comes in contact with clothing or linens, wash them separately.

Drink plenty of fluids and void frequently.

If coughing occurs, carefully dispose of any expectorant. Avoid swallowing the expectorant if possible.

Parents and childcare givers should take extra precaution in handling the urine, feces, and expectorants of children to avoid any additional exposure to either the caregiver or to the child.

Breastfeeding mothers should take extra precaution in disposing of breast milk.

PENTETATE CALCIUM TRISODIUM (Ca-DTPA)

Rx	**Pentetate Calcium Trisodium** (Hameln Pharmaceuticals)	**Injection:** 200 mg/mL	In 5 mL single-use ampules.

PENTETATE CALCIUM TRISODIUM (Ca-DTPA) — INJECTION

Indications

➤*Internal contamination:* Pentetate calcium trisodium is indicated for treatment of individuals with known or suspected internal contamination with plutonium, americium, or curium to increase the rates of elimination.

Administration and Dosage

➤*Approved by the FDA:* August 11, 2004.

The safety and efficacy of the intramuscular (IM) route of injection have not been established.

➤*Dosage:*

Adults and adolescents – A single 1 g initial dose of pentetate calcium trisodium administered intravenously (IV).

Children (younger than 12 years of age) – A single initial dose of 14 mg/kg administered IV, not to exceed 1 g.

Renal function impairment – No dosage adjustment is needed. However, renal impairment may reduce the rate at which chelators remove radiocontaminants from the body. In heavily contaminated patients with renal impairment, dialysis may be used to increase the rate of elimination. High-efficiency, high-flux dialysis is recommended. Because dialysis fluid will become radioactive, radiation precautions must be taken to protect personnel, other patients, and the general public. If pentetate calcium trisodium is not available, proceed with treatment with pentetate zinc trisodium as initial therapy.

➤*Maintenance dosage:* The duration of chelation treatment depends on the amount of internal contamination and individual response to treatment. If additional chelation therapy is indicated after the initial dose, on the next day, it is preferable to switch to pentetate zinc trisodium if available because of the safety concerns associated with prolonged pentetate calcium trisodium use. If pentetate zinc trisodium is not available, treatment may continue with pentetate calcium trisodium; however, give mineral supplements containing zinc concomitantly, as appropriate.

Adults and adolescents – 1 g once daily administered IV.

Children (younger than 12 years of age) – 14 mg/kg once a day administered IV. The maximum daily dose should not exceed 1 g/day.

➤*Administration:*

IV – IV administration of pentetate calcium trisodium is recommended; use if the route of internal contamination is not known or if multiple routes of internal contamination are likely. Administer pentetate calcium trisodium solution (1 g in 5 mL) either with a slow IV push over a period of 3 to 4 minutes or by IV infusion diluted in 100 to 250 mL of 5% dextrose in water (D5W), Ringer's lactate, or normal lactate.

Inhalation – In individuals whose internal contamination is only by inhalation within the preceding 24 hours, pentetate calcium trisodium can be administered by nebulized inhalation as an alternative route of administration. Dilute pentetate calcium trisodium for nebulization at a 1:1 ratio with sterile water or saline. After nebulization, encourage individuals to avoid swallowing any expectorant. Some individuals may experience respiratory adverse reactions after inhalation therapy. The safety and efficacy of the nebulized route of administration have not been established in the pediatric population.

➤*Chelation treatment:* Chelation treatment is most effective if administered within the first 24 hours after internal contamination. Start as soon as possible after suspected or known internal contamination. However, even when treatment cannot be started right away, give individuals chelation treatment as soon as it becomes available. Chelation treatment is effective even after time has elapsed following internal contamination; however, the chelating effects of pentetate calcium trisodium are greatest when radiocontaminants are circulating or are in interstitial fluids. The efficacy of chelation decreases with time following internal contamination as the radiocontaminants become sequestered in liver and bone.

➤*Fluids:* Advise patients to drink plenty of fluids and to void frequently to promote dilution of the radioactive chelate in the urine and minimize radiation exposure directly to the bladder.

➤*Internal contamination with other radiocontaminants:* If internal contamination with radiocontaminants other than plutonium, americium, or curium, or unknown radiocontaminants is suspected, additional therapies may be needed (eg, Prussian blue, potassium iodide).

➤*Handling:* To open the ampule, turn so that the point faces upward and break off the neck with a downward movement. The product may be filtered using a sterile filter if particles are seen subsequent to opening of the ampule.

➤*Storage/Stability:* Store between 15° to 30°C (59° to 86°F).

Actions

➤*Pharmacology:* Pentetate calcium trisodium forms stable chelates with metal ions by exchanging calcium for a metal of greater binding capacity. The radioactive chelates are then excreted by glomerular filtration into the urine. In animal studies, pentetate calcium trisodium forms less stable chelates with uranium and neptunium in vivo resulting in the deposition of these elements in tissues, including the bone. Pentetate calcium trisodium treatments are not expected to be effective for uranium and neptunium. Radioactive iodine is not bound by pentetate trisodium.

Literature and US Registry data in humans indicate that IV administration of pentetate calcium trisodium forms chelates with radioactive contaminants found in the circulation, interstitial fluid, and tissues.

When pentetate calcium trisodium is administered by inhalation within 24 hours of internal radioactive contamination, it can chelate transuranium elements. Expectoration is expected to decrease the amount of radioactive contaminant available for systemic absorption.

The efficacy of chelation decreases with time after internal contamination because the transuranium elements become incorporated into the tissues. Give chelation treatment as soon as possible after known or suspected internal contamination with transuranium elements has occurred.

➤*Pharmacokinetics:*

Absorption – Pentetate calcium trisodium is absorbed poorly in the GI tract. In animal studies, after oral administration, absorption was approximately 5%. In a US Registry of 18 patients who received a single inhaled or IV dose of 1 g, urine data indicate that the inhaled product was absorbed and resulted in a comparable elimination of the radiocontaminant. One study of 2 human subjects that received pentetate calcium trisodium with ^{14}C-DTPA by inhalation revealed approximately 20% absorption from the lungs. Human or animal bioavailability comparisons for pentetate calcium trisodium are not available after administration by inhalation and IV injection.

Distribution – Following IV administration, pentetate calcium trisodium is distributed rapidly throughout the extracellular fluid space. No significant amount of pentetate calcium trisodium penetrates into erythrocytes or other cells. No accumulation of pentetate calcium trisodium in specific organs has been observed. There is little or no binding of the chelating agent by the renal parenchyma.

Metabolism – Pentetate calcium trisodium undergoes a minimal amount of metabolic change in the body.

PENTETATE CALCIUM TRISODIUM (Ca-DTPA) — INJECTION

Studies in animals and humans showed that pentetate calcium trisodium binds endogenous metals of the body (ie, zinc, magnesium, manganese). In an animal study, high doses of pentetate calcium trisodium led to the loss of zinc and manganese mainly from the small intestine, skeleton, pancreas, and testes. Dosing over several days resulted in mobilization or binding of endogenous metals in exchange for calcium and a consequent impairment of metal-controlled or activated systems. The rate and amount of endogenous metal depletion increased with split daily dosing and with the length of treatment. Depletion of these endogenous metals can interfere with necessary mitotic cellular processes. Over longer time periods, depletion of zinc caused by pentetate calcium trisodium therapy may result in transient inhibition of a metalloenzyme-d-aminolevulinic acid dehydrase (ALAD) in the blood and suppressed hematopoiesis.

Excretion – Pentetate calcium trisodium is cleared from the plasma in the first few hours after dosing through urinary excretion by glomerular filtration. Renal tubular excretion has not been documented. In stool samples tested, only a very small amount of radioactivity (less than 3%) was detected.

The plasma retention up to 7 hours postdosing was expressed by the sum of 3 exponential components with average half-lives of 1.4, 14.5, and 94.4 minutes. The level of activity in the plasma was below the limit of detection 24 hours after injection. During the study, no detectable activity was exhaled or excreted in the feces. By 24 hours, cumulative urinary excretion was more than 99% of the injected dose.

Special populations –

Renal function impairment: Pentetate calcium trisodium and its radioactive chelates are excreted by glomerular filtration. Impaired renal function may decrease their rates of elimination and increase the serum half-life of pentetate calcium trisodium.

Contraindications

None known.

Warnings

➤*Endogenous trace metal depletion:* Pentetate calcium trisodium is associated with depletion of endogenous trace metals (eg, zinc, magnesium, manganese). The magnitude of depletion increases with split daily dosing, increasing dose, and increased treatment duration. Only a single initial dose of pentetate calcium trisodium is recommended. If additional chelation therapy is indicated after the initial single dose of pentetate calcium trisodium, it is recommended that therapy be continued with pentetate zinc trisodium. If pentetate zinc trisodium is not available, chelation therapy may continue with pentetate calcium trisodium, but give mineral supplements containing zinc concomitantly, as appropriate.

➤*Asthma exacerbation:* Nebulized chelation therapy may be associated with exacerbation of asthma. Exercise caution when administering pentetate calcium trisodium by the inhalation route.

➤*Pregnancy: Category C.* There are no human pregnancy outcome data from which to assess the risk of pentetate calcium trisodium exposure on fetal development. Pentetate calcium trisodium is believed to be teratogenic based on animal data and because chelation therapy results in the depletion of body stores of zinc which is known to affect deoxyribonucleic acid (DNA) and ribonucleic acid (RNA) synthesis in humans.

In mice, pentetate calcium trisodium has been shown to be teratogenic and embryocidal following 5 daily injections of pentetate calcium trisodium 720 to 2,880 mcmol/kg (2 to 8 times the recommended daily human dose of 1 g based on body surface area [BSA] adjusted dose) given during any period of gestation. The frequency of gross malformations (eg, exencephaly, spina bifida, cleft palate) increased with dose, with higher susceptibility in early- and mid-gestation. Studies of 2 pregnant dogs given daily injections of pentetate calcium trisodium 30 mcmol/kg (approximately half the recommended daily human dose based on BSA) from implantation until parturition showed severe teratogenic effects (especially brain damage).

Multiple doses of pentetate calcium trisodium could result in an increased risk for adverse reproductive outcomes and, thus, are not recommended during pregnancy. Therefore, treatment of pregnant women should begin and continue with pentetate zinc trisodium, if available, except in cases of high internal radioactive contamination. In these cases, consider the risk of immediate and delayed radiation-induced toxicity to the mother and the fetus in comparison with the risk of pentetate calcium trisodium toxicity. Also, because pentetate calcium trisodium is more effective than pentetate zinc trisodium in the first 24 hours after internal contamination, it may be appropriate to use a single dose of pentetate calcium trisodium with vitamin or mineral supplements that contain zinc as the initial treatment.

➤*Lactation:* Studies to determine if pentetate calcium trisodium is excreted in breast milk have not been conducted. Radiocontaminants are known to be excreted in breast milk. Advise women with known or suspected internal contamination with radiocontaminants not to breast-feed, whether or not they are receiving chelation therapy. Take precautions when discarding breast milk.

➤*Children:* The safety and efficacy of pentetate calcium trisodium were established in the adult population, and efficacy was extrapolated to children for the IV route based on the comparability of pathophysiologic mechanisms. The dose is based on body size adjustment for an IV drug that is cleared renally. The safety and efficacy of the nebulized route of administration have not been established in the pediatric population.

➤*Monitoring:* When possible, obtain baseline blood and urine samples (complete blood cell counts [CBC] with differential, serum urea nitrogen, serum chemistries and electrolytes, urinalysis, and blood and urine radioassays) before initiating treatment.

Pentetate calcium trisodium must be given with very careful monitoring of serum zinc and CBC. When appropriate, administer vitamin or mineral supplements that contain zinc.

To establish an elimination curve, obtain a quantitative baseline estimate of the total internalized transuranium element(s) and measures of elimination of radioactivity by appropriate whole-body counting, bioassay (eg, biodosimetry), or fecal/urine sample whenever possible.

Monitoring during treatment –

- Measure the radioactivity in blood, urine, and fecal samples weekly to monitor the radioactive contaminant elimination rate.
- Monitor CBC with differential, serum urea nitrogen, serum chemistries and electrolytes, and urinalysis regularly. If the patient is receiving more than 1 dose of pentetate calcium trisodium, monitor these laboratory tests very carefully and consider mineral supplementation as appropriate.
- Record any adverse reactions from pentetate calcium trisodium.

➤*Fluids:* Advise patients to drink plenty of fluids and void frequently to promote dilution of the radioactive chelate in the urine and minimize radiation exposure directly to the bladder.

➤*Internal contamination with other radiocontaminants:* If internal contamination with radiocontaminants other than plutonium, americium, or curium, or unknown radiocontaminants is suspected, additional therapies may be needed (eg, Prussian blue, potassium iodide).

➤*Collection of patient treatment data:* To develop long-term response data and information on the risk of developing late malignancy, provide detailed information on patient treatment to the manufacturer. In case additional forms are needed, please visit http://www.hameln-pharmaceuticals.com. These data should include a record of the radioactive body burden and bioassay results at defined time intervals, a description of measurement methods to facilitate analysis of data, and adverse reactions.

Refer questions regarding the use of pentetate calcium trisodium for the treatment of internal contamination with transuranium elements to the manufacturer.

➤*Special risk:*

Hemochromatosis – Use pentetate calcium trisodium with caution in individuals with severe hemochromatosis. Deaths have been reported in patients with severe hemochromatosis who received up to 4 times the recommended daily dose by IM injection for more than 1 day. Causal association with these events and the drug has not been established.

None well documented.

Overall, the presence or absence of adverse reactions was recorded in 310 of 646 patients. Of these, 19 (6.1%) reported at least 1 adverse reaction. The total number of recorded adverse reactions was 20. Of the 20 adverse reactions, 18 occurred after treatment with pentetate calcium trisodium. Adverse reactions included allergic reaction, chest pain, dermatitis, diarrhea, headache, injection-site reactions, light-headedness, metallic taste, and nausea. Cough and/or wheezing were experienced by 2 individuals receiving nebulized pentetate calcium trisodium, 1 of whom had a history of asthma.

In the literature, prolonged treatment with pentetate calcium trisodium resulted in depletion of zinc, magnesium, manganese, and, possibly, metalloproteinases.

In previous clinical studies, 3 deaths were reported in patients with severe hemochromatosis who were treated with daily IM pentetate calcium trisodium dosed up to 4 g/day to reduce iron stores. One patient became comatose and died after receiving a total of pentetate calcium trisodium 14 g, and the other 2 died after 2 weeks of daily treatment. Causal association with these events and the drug has not been established.

Patient Information

Radioactive metals are known to be excreted in the urine, feces, and breast milk. In patients with recent internal contamination with plutonium, americium, or curium, pentetate calcium trisodium treatment increases excretion of radioactivity in the urine.

Take appropriate safety measures to minimize contamination of others. When possible, use a toilet instead of a urinal, and flush it several times after each use. Completely clean up spilled urine or feces and wash your hands thoroughly. If blood or urine comes in contact with clothing or linens, wash them separately.

Drink plenty of fluids and void frequently. If patients are coughing, carefully dispose of any expectorant. Avoid swallowing the expectorant if possible.

Parents and caregivers should take extra precaution in handling the urine, feces, and expectorants of children to avoid any additional exposure to either the caregiver or to the child. Breast-feeding mothers should take extra precaution in disposing of breast milk.

Chelating Agents

DEFERASIROX

Rx	Exjade (Novartis)	Tablets for oral suspension: 125 mg	Lactose. (J 125/NVR). Off-white. In 30s.
		250 mg	Lactose. (J 250/NVR). Off-white. In 30s.
		500 mg	Lactose. (J 500/NVR). Off-white. In 30s.

DEFERASIROX — ORAL

Indications

➤*Chronic iron overload:* For the treatment of chronic iron overload due to blood transfusions (transfusional hemosiderosis) in patients 2 years of age and older.

Administration and Dosage

➤*Approved by the FDA:* November 2, 2005.

It is recommended that therapy with deferasirox start when a patient has evidence of chronic iron overload, such as the transfusion of approximately 100 mL/kg of packed red blood cells (approximately 20 units for a 40 kg patient) and a serum ferritin consistently greater than 1,000 mcg/L.

➤*Starting dose:* The recommended initial daily dose is 20 mg/kg body weight.

➤*Maintenance:* After commencing initial therapy, it is recommended that serum ferritin be monitored every month and the dose of deferasirox adjusted if necessary every 3 to 6 months based on serum ferritin trends. Dose adjustments should be made in steps of 5 or 10 mg/kg and should be tailored to the individual patient's response and therapeutic goals (maintenance or reduction of body iron burden). If the serum ferritin falls consistently below 500 mcg/L, consideration should be given to temporarily interrupting therapy. Doses of deferasirox should not exceed 30 mg/kg per day because there is limited experience with doses above this level.

➤*Administration:* Deferasirox should be taken once daily on an empty stomach at least 30 minutes before food, preferably at the same time each day. Tablets should not be chewed or swallowed whole. Deferasirox should not be taken with aluminum-containing antacid products. Doses (mg/kg) should be calculated to the nearest whole tablet. Tablets should be completely dispersed by stirring in water, orange juice, or apple juice until a fine suspension is obtained. Doses of less than 1 g should be dispersed in 3.5 ounces of liquid and doses of greater than 1 g in 7 ounces of liquid. After swallowing the suspension, resuspend any residue in a small volume of liquid and swallow.

➤*Storage/Stability:* Store at 25°C (77°F); excursions are permitted to 15° to 30°C (59° to 86°F). Protect from moisture.

Actions

➤*Pharmacology:* Deferasirox is an orally active chelator that is selective for iron (as Fe^{3+}). It is a tridentate ligand that binds iron with high affinity in a 2:1 ratio. Although deferasirox has very low affinity for zinc and copper, there are variable decreases in the serum concentration of these trace metals after the administration of deferasirox. The clinical significance of these decreases is uncertain.

Pharmacodynamics – Pharmacodynamic effects tested in an iron balance metabolic study showed that deferasirox (10, 20, and 40 mg/kg/day) was able to induce a mean net iron excretion (0.119, 0.329, and 0.445 mg Fe/kg body weight per day, respectively) within the clinically relevant range (0.1 to 0.5 mg/kg/day). Iron excretion was predominantly fecal.

The effect of 20 and 40 mg/kg of deferasirox on QT interval was evaluated in a single-dose, double-blind, randomized, placebo- and active-controlled (moxifloxacin 400 mg), parallel group study in 182 healthy male and female volunteers 18 to 65 years of age. No evidence of prolongation of the QTc interval was observed in this study.

➤*Pharmacokinetics:*

Absorption – Deferasirox is absorbed following oral administration with median times to maximum plasma concentration of about 1.5 to 4 hours. The maximum plasma concentration and AUC of deferasirox increase approximately linearly with dose after single administration and under steady-state conditions. Exposure to deferasirox increased by an accumulation factor of 1.3 to 2.3 after multiple doses. The AUC of deferasirox is 70% compared with an intravenous dose.

Distribution – Deferasirox is highly (approximately 99%) protein bound, almost exclusively to serum albumin. The percentage of deferasirox confined to the blood cells was 5% in humans. The volume of distribution at steady state of deferasirox is 14.37 ± 2.69 L in adults.

Metabolism – Glucuronidation is the main metabolic pathway for deferasirox, with subsequent biliary excretion. Deconjugation of glucuronidates in the intestine and subsequent reabsorption (enterohepatic recycling) is likely to occur. Deferasirox is mainly glucuronidated by UGT1A1 and to a lesser extent UGT1A3. CYP-450-catalyzed (oxidative) metabolism of deferasirox appears to be minor in humans (about 8%). No evidence for induction or inhibition of enzymes at therapeutic doses has been observed.

Excretion – Deferasirox and metabolites are primarily (84% of the dose) excreted in the feces. Renal excretion of deferasirox and metabolites is minimal (8% of the administered dose). The mean elimination half-life ranged from 8 to 16 hours following oral administration.

Special populations –

Hepatic function impairment: Deferasirox is principally excreted by glucuronidation and is minimally (8%) metabolized by oxidative cytochrome P-450 enzymes. Deferasirox has not been studied in patients with hepatic function impairment. Deferasirox treatment has been initiated in patients with baseline liver transaminase levels up to 5 times the upper limit of the normal (ULN) range. The pharmacokinetics of deferasirox were not influenced by such transaminase levels.

Children: Following oral administration of single or multiple doses, systemic exposure of adolescents and children to deferasirox was less than in adults. In children younger than 6 years of age, systemic exposure was about 50% less lower than in adults.

Gender: Females have a moderately lower apparent clearance (by 17.5%) for deferasirox compared with males.

Contraindications

Hypersensitivity to deferasirox or to any other component of deferasirox.

Warnings

➤*Special senses:* Auditory disturbances (eg, high frequency hearing loss, decreased hearing) and ocular disturbances (eg, lens opacities, cataracts, elevations in intraocular pressure, retinal disorders) have been reported at a frequency of less than 1% with deferasirox therapy in the clinical trials. Auditory and ophthalmic testing (including slit lamp examinations and dilated fundoscopy) are recommended before the start of deferasirox treatment and thereafter at regular intervals (every 12 months). If disturbances are noted, consider dose reduction or interruption.

➤*Renal effects:* Deferasirox-treated patients experienced dose-dependent increases in serum creatinine. These increases occurred at a greater frequency compared with deferoxamine-treated patients (38% vs 15%, respectively) in study 1. Most of the creatinine elevations remained within the normal range. Assess serum creatinine before initiating therapy and monitor monthly thereafter. Consider dose reduction, interruption, or discontinuation for elevations in serum creatinine. In the clinical trials, for increases of serum creatinine on 2 consecutive measures (more than 33% in patients older than 15 years of age or more than 33% and greater than the age-appropriate ULN in patients younger than 15 years of age), the daily dose of deferasirox was reduced by 10 mg/kg. Patients with serum creatinine above the ULN were excluded from clinical trials.

In clinical trials, urine protein was measured monthly. Intermittent proteinuria (urine protein/creatinine ratio more than 0.6 mg/mg) occurred in 18.6% of deferasirox-treated patients compared with 7.2% of deferoxamine-treated patients in study 1. Although no patients were discontinued from deferasirox in clinical trials up to 1 year due to proteinuria, close monitoring is recommended. The mechanism and clinical significance of the proteinuria are uncertain.

➤*Hepatic effects:* In study 1, 4 patients discontinued deferasirox because of hepatic abnormalities (drug-induced hepatitis in 2 patients and increased serum transaminases in 2 additional patients). Monitor liver function tests monthly during deferasirox treatment and consider dose modifications for severe or persistent elevations.

➤*Elderly:* Deferasirox did not include sufficient numbers of subjects 65 years of age and older to determine whether they respond differently from younger subjects. Thirty patients 65 years of age and older were included in clinical trials of deferasirox. The majority of these patients had myelodysplastic syndrome (MDS) (MDS, n = 27; other anemias, n = 3). In general, use caution in elderly patients because of the greater frequency of decreased hepatic, renal, or cardiac function, and of concomitant disease or other drug therapy.

➤*Pregnancy: Category B.* Reproduction studies have been performed in pregnant rats at oral dosages up to 100 mg/kg/day (about 0.8 times the recommended human oral dose based on body surface area) and in pregnant rabbits at oral dosages up to 50 mg/kg/day (about 0.8 times the recommended human oral dose based on body surface area). These studies have revealed no evidence of impaired fertility or harm to the fetus because of deferasirox. However, there are no adequate and well-controlled studies in pregnant women. Because animal reproduction studies are not always predictive of human response, use deferasirox during pregnancy only if clearly needed.

➤*Lactation:* It is not known whether deferasirox is excreted in human milk. Deferasirox and its metabolites were excreted in breast milk of rats following a 10 mg/kg dose (about 0.08 times the recommended human oral dose based on body surface area). Because many drugs are excreted in human milk, exercise caution when deferasirox is administered to a breast—feeding woman.

➤*Children:* Of the 700 patients who received deferasirox during clinical trials, 292 were children 2 to younger than 16 years of age with various congenital and acquired anemias, including 52 patients age 2 to younger than 6 years, 121 patients 6 to younger than 12 years of age and 199 patients 12 to younger than 16 years of age. Seventy percent of these patients had beta-thalassemia. Children between 2 to younger than 6 years of age have a systemic exposure to deferasirox approximately 50% of that of adults. However, the safety and efficacy of deferasirox in children was similar to that of adult patients, and younger children responded similarly to older children. The recommended starting dose and dosing modification are the same for children and adults.

DEFERASIROX — ORAL

During the 1 year study, the growth and development were within normal limits.

Precautions

➤*Monitoring:* Measure serum ferritin monthly to assess response to therapy and to evaluate for the possibility of overchelation of iron. If the serum ferritin falls consistently below 500 mcg/L, consider temporarily interrupting therapy with deferasirox. In the clinical studies, the correlation coefficient between the serum ferritin and LIC was 0.63. Therefore, changes in serum ferritin levels may not always reliably reflect changes in LIC.

Assess serum creatinine before initiating therapy and monitor monthly thereafter. Close monitoring of urine protein also is recommended. Monitor liver function tests monthly during deferasirox treatment. Auditory and ophthalmic testing (including slit lamp examinations and dilated funduscopy) are recommended before the start of deferasirox treatment and thereafter at regular intervals (every 12 months).

➤*Rash:* Skin rashes may occur during deferasirox treatment. For rashes of mild to moderate severity, deferasirox may be continued without dose adjustment because the rash often resolves spontaneously. In severe cases, deferasirox may be interrupted. Consider reintroduction at a lower dose with escalation in combination with a short period of oral steroid administration.

Drug Interactions

➤*Aluminum-containing antacids:* The coadministration of deferasirox and aluminum-containing antacid preparations has not been formally studied. Although deferasirox has a lower affinity for aluminum than for iron, do not take deferasirox with aluminum-containing antacid preparations.

➤*Iron chelator therapies:* Do not combine deferasirox with other iron chelator therapies as safety of such combinations has not been established.

➤*Drug/Food interactions:* The bioavailability (AUC) of deferasirox was variably increased when taken with a meal. Take deferasirox on an empty stomach 30 minutes before eating.

Adverse Reactions

A total of 700 patients were treated with deferasirox in therapeutic studies lasting for 48 weeks in adults and children. These 700 patients included 469 with beta-thalassemia, 99 with rare anemias, and 132 with sickle cell disease. Of these patients, 45% were male, 70% were Caucasian, and 292 patients were younger than 16 years of age. In the sickle cell disease population, 89% of patients were black. Four hundred sixty-nine patients (403 beta-thalassemia and 66 rare anemias) were entered into extensions of the original clinical protocols. In ongoing extension studies, median durations of treatment were 85 to 143 weeks.

The following table displays adverse reactions occurring in more than 5% of patients in either treatment group in study 1. Abdominal pain, nausea, vomiting, diarrhea, and skin rashes were the most frequent adverse reactions reported with a suspected relationship to deferasirox.

Deferasirox Adverse Reactions (> 5%)

Adverse reaction	Deferasirox (N = 296)	Deferoxamine (N = 290)
CNS		
Fatigue	18 (6.1%)	14 (4.8%)
Headache	47 (15.9%)	59 (20.3%)
Dermatologic		
Rash	25 (8.4%)	9 (3.1%)
Urticaria	11 (3.7%)	17 (5.9%)
GI		
Abdominal pain	41 (13.9%)	28 (9.7%)
Abdominal pain, upper	23 (7.8%)	15 (5.2%)
Diarrhea	35 (11.8%)	21 (7.2%)
Nausea	31 (10.5%)	14 (4.8%)
Vomiting	30 (10.1%)	28 (9.7%)
Respiratory		
Bronchitis	27 (9.1%)	32 (11%)
Cough	41 (13.9%)	55 (19%)
Respiratory tract infection	28 (9.5%)	23 (7.9%)
Special senses		
Acute tonsillitis	19 (6.4%)	15 (5.2%)
Ear infection	16 (5.4%)	7 (2.4%)
Nasopharyngitis	39 (13.2%)	42 (14.5%)
Pharyngitis	23 (7.8%)	30 (10.3%)
Pharyngolaryngeal pain	31 (10.5%)	43 (14.8%)
Rhinitis	18 (6.1%)	22 (7.6%)
Miscellaneous		
Arthralgia	22 (7.4%)	14 (4.8%)
Back pain	17 (5.7%)	32 (11%)
Creatinine, increased[a]	33 (11.1%)	0 (0%)
Influenza	32 (10.8%)	29 (10%)
Pyrexia	56 (18.9%)	69 (23.8%)

[a] Includes "blood creatinine increased" and "blood creatinine abnormal," which were reported as adverse reactions. Also see the following table.

➤*Most frequent reactions:* The most frequently occurring adverse reactions in the therapeutic trials of deferasirox were diarrhea, vomiting, nausea, headache, abdominal pain, pyrexia, cough, and an increase in serum creatinine. GI symptoms, increases in serum creatinine, and skin rash were dose related.

➤*Lab test abnormalities:* In study 1, 113 patients treated with deferasirox had increases in serum creatinine more than 33% above baseline on 2 separate occasions (see the following table). Twenty-five patients required dose reductions. Increases in serum creatinine appeared to be dose related. Seventeen patients developed elevations in ALT levels more than 5 times the ULN at 2 consecutive visits. Two patients had liver biopsy proven drug-induced hepatitis and both discontinued deferasirox therapy. Two additional patients who did not have elevations in ALT more than 5 times the ULN discontinued deferasirox because of increased ALT. Increases in transaminases did not appear to be dose related.

Deferasirox Increases in Serum Creatinine or ALT

Laboratory parameter	Deferasirox (N = 296)	Deferoxamine (N = 290)
Serum creatinine		
Creatinine > 33% and < ULN at ≥ 2 consecutive postbaseline visits	113 (38.2%)	41 (14.1%)
Creatinine increase > 33% and > ULN at ≥ 2 consecutive postbaseline visits	7 (2.4%)	1 (0.3%)
ALT		
ALT > 5 × ULN at ≥ 2 postbaseline visits	25 (8.4%)	7 (2.4%)
ALT > 5 × ULN at ≥ 2 consecutive postbaseline visits	17 (5.7%)	5 (1.7%)

➤*Discontinuation:* Adverse reactions that led to discontinuations included abnormal liver function tests (2 patients) and drug-induced hepatitis (2 patients), skin rash, glycosuria/proteinuria, Henoch Schönlein purpura, hyperactivity/insomnia, drug fever, and cataract (1 patient each).

➤*Other adverse reactions (0.1% to 1%):* In the overall population of 700 patients, uncommon adverse reactions (0.1% to 1%) included gastritis, edema, sleep disorder, pigmentation disorder, dizziness, anxiety, maculopathy, cholelithiasis, pyrexia, fatigue, pharyngolaryngeal pain, and early cataract and hearing loss. Adverse reactions that most frequently led to dose interruption or dose adjustment were rash, GI disorders, infections, increased serum creatinine, and increased serum transaminases.

Overdosage

➤*Symptoms:* There have been no reports of acute overdose with deferasirox. Single doses up to 80 mg/kg in iron-overloaded beta-thalassemic patients have been tolerated with nausea and diarrhea noted. In healthy volunteers, single doses of up to 40 mg/kg were tolerated.

➤*Treatment:* There is no specific antidote for deferasirox. In case of overdose, induce vomiting gastric lavage.

Patient Information

Advise patients to take deferasirox once daily on an empty stomach at least 30 minutes prior to food, preferably at the same time every day. Tablets should not be chewed or swallowed whole. Patients should completely disperse the tablets first in water, orange juice, or apple juice, and drink the resulting suspension immediately. After swallowing the suspension, patients should resuspend any residue in a small volume of the liquid and swallow.

Caution patients not to take aluminum-containing antacids and deferasirox simultaneously.

Because auditory and ocular disturbances have been reported with deferasirox, patients should have auditory and ophthalmic testing before starting deferasirox treatment and thereafter at regular intervals.

Advise patients experiencing dizziness to exercise caution when driving or operating machinery.

PRUSSIAN BLUE ORAL

Rx	**Radiogardase** (HEYL Chemisch-pharmazeutische Fabrik GmbH & Co.)	**Capsules:** 0.5 g (blue powder in gelatin capsules)	In 30s.

PRUSSIAN BLUE — ORAL

Indications

➤*Internal contamination:* For the treatment of patients with known or suspected internal contamination with radioactive cesium and/or radioactive or non-radioactive thallium to increase their rates of elimination.

Administration and Dosage

➤*Approved by the FDA:* October 2, 2003.

➤*Adults and adolescents:* The recommended dosage of Prussian blue insoluble is 3 g orally 3 times a day.

➤*Children 2 to 12 years of age:* The recommended dosage of Prussian blue insoluble is 1 g orally 3 times a day.

➤*Administration:* In patients who cannot tolerate swallowing large numbers of capsules, the capsules may be opened and mixed with bland food or liquid. This may result in blue discoloration of the mouth and teeth. Prussian blue insoluble capsules may be taken with food to stimulate excretion of cesium or thallium.

➤*Treatment initiation:* Treatment with Prussian blue insoluble should be initiated as soon as possible after contamination is suspected. Contamination should be verified as soon as possible. However, even when treatment cannot be started right away, patients should be given Prussian blue insoluble as soon as it becomes available. Treatment with Prussian blue insoluble is still effective for radioactive cesium contamination even after time has elapsed since exposure.

➤*Treatment for radioactive cesium (^{137}Cs) contamination:* Treatment should continue for a minimum of 30 days and then the patient should be reassessed for the amount of residual whole body radioactivity. The duration of treatment after exposure is dictated by the level of contamination and the judgment of the attending physician. Before, during, and after therapy, pertinent measurements for radioactivity should be made to help determine when to terminate treatment.

During treatment, the radioactivity counts in urine and fecal samples should be measured and recorded weekly to monitor ^{137}Cs elimination rate and the occurrence of any adverse reactions to Prussian blue insoluble (eg, constipation, which can be treated by increasing the amount of fiber in the diet) should be noted.

When the internal radioactivity is substantially decreased, the Prussian blue insoluble dose may be decreased to 1 or 2 g 3 times daily to improve GI tolerance.

➤*Further considerations for radioactive cesium contamination:*

1.) Health professionals should wear appropriate radiation-protective attire and follow procedures at all times. Protect health professionals who are handling patients from unnecessary radiation exposure and monitor health professionals and the area of operation for radiation levels using radiation detection, indication, and computation devices (RADIAC), or thermal luminescent devices (TLD). Control the spread of radiation contamination by establishing patient triage site, patient decontamination area, and a contaminated or dirty material dumpsite. Proper labeling, handling, and disposal of contaminated material needs to be established and followed.
2.) Manage the patient to minimize further injury and to stabilize before external decontamination.
3.) Establish if the patient suffers from a single or combined injury (eg, radiation, burns, trauma, chemical, biological) and whether the contaminant may be internalized. The route of entry of the radiation contaminant needs to be identified and recorded. The route of entry will determine other treatment methods needed (eg, wound debridement, stomach lavage if ingested.) Patients need to be triaged based on their injuries and the level and type of contamination.
4.) A quantitative baseline of the internalized contamination of ^{137}Cs should be obtained by appropriate whole-body counting and/or by bioassay (eg, biodosimetry) or feces/urine sample whenever possible to obtain an estimated internalized radiation contamination of ^{137}Cs, and rate of measured elimination of radiation in the feces in order to establish an elimination curve.

➤*Further considerations for thallium contamination (radioactive and nonradioactive):* General therapy guidelines for thallium contamination should follow the radioactive decontamination procedures listed above for ^{137}Cs, except that there is no need for radiation safety precautions when treating patients contaminated with nonradioactive thallium. For both radioactive and nonradioactive thallium contamination, a quantitative baseline of the internalized thallium contamination should be ascertained by appropriate whole-body counting and/or by bioassay whenever possible.

Patients should also have weekly complete blood counts (CBCs), serum chemistry, and electrolytes while under treatment. The response to other oral medications should be closely monitored.

In cases of severe thallium intoxication, additional types of elimination treatment may be necessary, such as induced emesis followed by gastric intubation and lavage, forced diuresis until urinary thallium excretion is less than 1 mg per 24 hour, charcoal hemoperfusion, which may be useful during the first 48 hours after thallium ingestion (biodistribution phase), and hemodialysis, which has been reported to be effective in thallium intoxication.

➤*Multiple contaminant exposure (radioactive and nonradioactive):* In patients who have contamination with multiple or unknown radioactive isotopes, additional decontamination and treatment procedures may be needed.

➤*Storage / Stability:* Store in the dark at 25°C (77°F); excursions permitted to 15° to 30°C (59° to 86°F).

Actions

➤*Pharmacology:* Prussian blue insoluble ferric(III) hexacyanoferrate(II) is not absorbed through the intact GI wall after oral ingestion. Its clearance from the body depends on the GI tract transit time. Prussian blue insoluble acts by ion-exchange, adsorption, and mechanical trapping within the crystal structure and has a very high affinity for radioactive and non-radioactive cesium and thallium.

Prussian blue insoluble binds cesium and thallium isotopes in the GI tract after these isotopes are ingested or excreted in the bile by the liver, thereby reducing GI reabsorption (enterohepatic circulation). In studies of rats, pigs, and dogs that were internally contaminated with cesium and thallium, the presence of the insoluble complexes in the GI lumen changed the primary elimination route from the kidney to the feces and increased the rate of elimination of these 2 contaminants.

The rate of cesium and thallium elimination was proportional to the duration and dose of Prussian blue insoluble. A radioactive element has a constant rate of disintegration that is reflected by its physical half-life. The rate of element elimination from the body is reflected by its biologic half-life. The combined rate of radiation disintegration and rate of element elimination is reflected by the effective half-life.

Cesium-137 (^{137}Cs) has a physical half-life of 30 years, with a beta energy peak at 174 keV. After entry into the blood, it is distributed uniformly through all body tissues. Approximately 10% of cesium is eliminated rapidly with a biological half-life of 2 days, and 90% is eliminated more slowly, with a biological half-life of 110 days. Less than 1% of the cesium is retained with a longer biological half-life of about 500 days. Cesium follows the movement of potassium and is excreted into the intestine and reabsorbed from the gut into the blood, then to the bile, where it is excreted again into the gut (enterohepatic circulation). Without Prussian blue insoluble treatment, approximately 80% of cesium is excreted through the kidneys and approximately 20% in the feces. Because of cesium's long physical half-life, the rate of radiation elimination is similar to the rate of element elimination from the body.

Thallium-201 (^{201}Tl) has a physical half-life of 3 days with electron and photon emissions, with a gamma energy peak at 167.4 keV. After entry into the blood, thallium is distributed in the kidneys (3%) and all other organs (97%). Nonradioactive thallium, depending on the tissue, has a biological half-life of 8 to 10 days. Thallium also follows the movement of potassium and is excreted by the bile in enterohepatic recirculation. Without Prussian blue insoluble treatment, the fecal to urine excretion ratio of thallium is approximately 2:1.

Based on the mechanisms of action, Prussian blue insoluble may bind to other elements (eg, potassium), and cause electrolyte or other nutritional imbalances.

➤*Pharmacokinetics:*

Absorption – Absorption from multiple doses has not been studied. Food effect studies were not identified in the literature. In animal studies, Prussian blue insoluble was not significantly absorbed.

Excretion – In an animal study (pigs, N= 38), after a single dose of labeled Prussian blue insoluble 40 mg, 99% of the administered Prussian blue dose was excreted unchanged in feces. Food may increase the effectiveness of Prussian blue insoluble by stimulating bile secretion. Food is known to increase bile production and enterohepatic circulation. The increase in enterohepatic circulation may increase the amount of cesium and thallium in the GI lumen, and may increase the amounts available for binding with Prussian blue insoluble.

Renal / Hepatic function impairment – Prussian blue insoluble may be less effective in patients with impaired liver function because of decreased excretion of cesium and thallium in the bile.

Contraindications

None known.

Warnings

➤*Radiation toxicity:* Prussian blue insoluble is administered to decrease radiation exposure. It does not treat the complications of radiation exposure. Patients contaminated with high doses of ^{137}Cs may develop radiation toxicity, including bone marrow suppression with severe neutropenia and thrombocytopenia. Give supportive treatment for radiation toxicity symptoms concomitantly with Prussian blue insoluble treatment.

➤*Contamination with multiple radioactive elements:* In radiological emergencies, the type of elemental exposure may not be known. Prussian blue insoluble may not bind to all radioactive elements, and some radioactive elements may not undergo enterohepatic circulation, which is needed for Prussian blue insoluble binding and elimination. Patients contaminated

PRUSSIAN BLUE — ORAL

with unknown or multiple radioactive elements may require treatment with other agents in addition to Prussian blue insoluble.

➤*Pregnancy: Category C.* Comprehensive animal reproductive studies have not been conducted with Prussian blue insoluble. Since Prussian blue insoluble is not absorbed from the GI tract, effects on the fetus are not expected. In 1 patient who became pregnant 3 years and 8 months after being treated with Prussian blue insoluble for internal contamination with ^{137}Cs (8 mCi), complications or birth defects were not identified in the literature report.

Cesium-137 is known to cross the human placenta. One patient, in Goiânia, was contaminated with 0.005 mCi ^{137}Cs during her fourth month of pregnancy. She was not treated with Prussian blue insoluble. At birth, the concentration of ^{137}Cs was the same in the mother and the infant. Thallium crosses the human placenta. Reported fetal effects in the reviewed literature include fetal death, failure to thrive, alopecia, or in some instances, outwardly normal development. The risk of toxicity from untreated radioactive cesium or thallium exposure is expected to be more than the reproductive toxicity risk of Prussian blue insoluble.

➤*Lactation:* Studies to determine if Prussian blue insoluble is excreted in human milk have not been conducted. Since Prussian blue insoluble is not absorbed from the GI tract, its excretion in milk is highly unlikely. However, cesium and thallium are transmitted from mother to infant in breast milk. Women internally contaminated with cesium or thallium should not breastfeed.

➤*Children:* The safety and efficacy of Prussian blue insoluble and its dosing for children were extrapolated from adult data and supported by pediatric patients who were internally contaminated with ^{137}Cs and treated with Prussian blue insoluble in the Goiânia accident.

Overall, 27 pediatric patients received Prussian blue insoluble in the range of 3 to 10 g/day in divided doses. Prussian blue insoluble treatment reduced the whole-body effective half-life of ^{137}Cs 46% in adolescents and 43% in children ranging from 4 to 12 years of age. In 12 patients for whom the rate of radiation elimination data are available, the rate was similar to that in adults treated with 3 g 3 times daily and in pediatric patients treated with 1 g 3 times daily. By body weight, the dose ranged from 0.32 g/kg in the 12-year-old patient (Prussian blue 10 g daily dose, 31 kg weight) to 0.21 g/kg in the 4-year-old patient (Prussian blue 3 g daily dose, 14 kg weight). Children 2 to 4 years of age are expected to have biliary and GI function that is comparable with the 4-year-old.

There are variations in the developmental maturity of the biliary system and GI tract of neonates and infants (0 to 2 years of age). The dose-related adverse effects of Prussian blue insoluble on an immature GI tract are not known. Dosing in infants and neonates has not been established.

Precautions

➤*Monitoring:* Closely monitor serum electrolytes during Prussian blue insoluble treatment. Prussian blue insoluble may bind to some oral therapeutic drugs. As appropriate, monitor blood levels or clinical response to oral medications.

Patients should also have weekly CBC, serum chemistry, and electrolytes monitored while under treatment.

➤*GI effects:* GI Prussian blue insoluble may cause constipation. Decreased GI motility will slow the transit time of ^{137}Cs bound to Prussian blue insoluble in the GI tract and may increase the radiation absorbed dose to the GI mucosa. Constipation occurring during Prussian blue insoluble treatment may be treated with a fiber-based laxative and/or a high-fiber diet. Use Prussian blue insoluble with caution in patients with disorders associated with decreased GI motility.

➤*Special risk:* Exercise caution when treating patients with preexisting cardiac arrhythmias or electrolyte imbalances. Prussian blue insoluble may bind to some oral therapeutic drugs.

Drug Interactions

Binding to some therapeutic drugs and essential nutrients is possible. The literature contains anecdotal reports of asymptomatic hypokalemia and decreased bioavailability of oral tetracycline. Monitor the serum levels and/or clinical response to critical oral products.

Adverse Reactions

Deaths or serious or severe adverse reactions attributed to Prussian blue insoluble have not been reported.

➤*GI:* Constipation was reported in 10 of 42 patients in the Goiânia accident treated with Prussian blue insoluble. Severity of constipation was mild in 7 patients and moderate in 3 patients. Constipation was successfully treated with a high-fiber diet. Undefined gastric distress was reported in 3 patients treated with Prussian blue insoluble 20 g/day. In these patients, the dose was reduced to 10 g/day for continued treatment.

➤*Lab test abnormalities:* Prussian blue insoluble may bind to electrolytes found in the GI tract. Asymptomatic hypokalemia, with serum potassium levels of 2.5 to 2.9 (normal 3.5 to 5) was reported in 3 of 42 of patients on treatment with Prussian blue insoluble. Exercise caution when treating patients with preexisting cardiac arrhythmias or electrolyte imbalances.

Overdosage

➤*Symptoms:* The clinical effects of overdosing with Prussian blue insoluble are not known. Based on reported adverse reactions and mechanism of action, possible overdose symptoms may include obstipation, obstruction, or severe decrease in electrolytes.

Patient Information

Cesium-137 is excreted in the urine and feces. Take appropriate safety measures to minimize radiation exposure to others. When possible, a toilet should be used instead of a urinal, and it should be flushed several times after each use. Spilled urine or feces should be cleaned up completely, and patients should wash their hands thoroughly. If blood or urine gets onto clothing, such clothing should be washed separately.

Parents and child care givers should take extra precaution in handling the urine and feces of pediatric patients. Care is intended to prevent re-exposure to the adult and pediatric patient.

In patients with constipation, a fiber-based laxative and/or high-fiber diet is recommended during treatment with Prussian blue insoluble. Inform patients taking Prussian blue insoluble that their stools might be blue in color.

In patients who cannot swallow capsules, when the capsules are opened and the contents are mixed with food and eaten, the mouth and teeth might be colored blue.

SODIUM THIOSULFATE

Rx	**Sodium Thiosulfate** (American Regent)	**Injection:** 10% (100 mg/mL) (as pentahydrate)	Preservative-free. In 10 mL single-dose vials.
		25% (250 mg/mL) (as pentahydrate)	Preservative-free. In 50 mL single-dose vials.

SODIUM THIOSULFATE — INJECTION

Indications

➤*Cyanide poisoning:* Sodium thiosulfate is indicated for the treatment of cyanide poisoning.

➤*Unlabeled uses:* Sodium thiosulfate has been used as an antidote for cisplatin-induced nephrotoxicity. It also has been shown to be beneficial for extravasation of significant amounts of cisplatin.

Administration and Dosage

➤*Approved by the FDA:* February 14, 1992.

Death from cyanide poisoning occurs rapidly. Delays in administering the antidote should be avoided.

➤*Slow IV use only:* The dose of sodium thiosulfate whether used alone or in combination with other cyanide antidotes is 12.5 g given IV over approximately 10 minutes. The dosage for children is 7 g/m^2 of body surface area, with a maximum dose of 12.5 g.

➤*Storage/Stability:* Store at controlled room temperature 15° to 30°C (59° to 86°F). Parenteral drug products should be inspected visually for particulate matter and discoloration prior to administration, whenever solution and container permit.

Actions

➤*Pharmacology:* Sodium thiosulfate is used as an antidote for cyanide poisoning. The primary mechanism of cyanide detoxification involves the conversion of cyanide to the thiocyanate ion, which is relatively nontoxic. This reaction involves the enzyme rhodanese (thiosulfate: cyanide sulfurtransferase) that is found in many body tissues, but with the major activity in the liver. The body has the capability to detoxify cyanide, however, the rhodanese enzyme system is slow to respond to large amounts of cyanide. The rhodanese enzyme reaction can be accelerated by supplying an exogenous source of sulfur. This is commonly accomplished by administering sodium thiosulfate. Sodium thiosulfate may be used alone or in combination with nitrite compounds such as amyl nitrite or sodium nitrite.

➤*Pharmacokinetics:* Following IV injection, sodium thiosulfate is distributed throughout the extracellular fluid and is excreted unchanged in the urine. The biological half-life is reported to be 0.65 hours.

Contraindications

None known.

Warnings

➤*Pregnancy: Category C.* Animal reproduction studies have not been conducted with sodium thiosulfate. It is also not known whether sodium thiosulfate can cause fetal harm when administered to a pregnant woman or can affect reproduction capacity. Sodium thiosulfate should be given to a pregnant woman only if clearly needed.

SODIUM THIOSULFATE — INJECTION

Precautions

➤*Monitoring:* Patients should be closely monitored for 24 to 48 hours for symptoms of cyanide poisoning to reappear. In the event symptoms return, sodium thiosulfate administration should be repeated at one-half the original dose.

Sodium thiosulfate is essentially nontoxic. However, studies conducted in dogs, with a constant infusion of sodium thiosulfate, showed hypovolemia that was considered to be caused by an osmotic diuretic effect of sodium thiosulfate.

Adverse Reactions

None known.

SODIUM NITRITE INJECTION

Rx	**Sodium Nitrite** (Hope)	**Injection:** 30 mg/mL	In 10 mL vials.

SODIUM NITRITE — INJECTION

Indications

➤*Cyanide poisoning:* For use with sodium thiosulfate injection and amyl nitrite inhalants in the treatment of cyanide poisoning.

➤*Unlabeled uses:* Hydrogen sulfide poisoning.

Administration and Dosage

Personnel should acquire some skill in the proper method of administering cyanide antidote medications prior to an emergency. Cyanide poisoning is rapidly fatal. The patient seldom survives many hours. The prevention of death demands a quick diagnosis and the prompt use of specific antidotes. No valuable time should be lost. Even though the diagnosis is doubtful, the therapy recommended should be instituted immediately. For best results, the physician should be acquainted beforehand with the following steps:

1.) Instruct an assistant how to break an ampule of amyl nitrite, 1 at a time, in a handkerchief and hold it in front of the patient's mouth for 15 seconds, followed by a rest for 15 seconds. Then reapply until sodium nitrite can be administered. This interrupted schedule is important because continuous use of amyl nitrite may prevent adequate oxygenation.
2.) Discontinue administration of amyl nitrite and inject intravenously 300 mg (10 mL of a 3% solution) of sodium nitrite at the rate of 2.5 to 5 mL/min. The recommended dose of sodium nitrite for children is 6 to 8 mL/m^2 (approximately 0.2 mL/kg of body weight) but is not to exceed 10 mL.
3.) Immediately thereafter, inject 12.5 g (50 mL of a 25% solution) of sodium thiosulfate for adults. The dosage for children is 7 g/m^2 of body surface area, but dosage should not exceed 12.5 g. The same needle and vein may be used.
4.) If the poison was taken by mouth, gastric lavage should be performed as soon as possible, but this should not delay the treatments outlined above. Lavage may be done concurrently by a third person, a physician or a nurse, if one is available. One should take quick action without waiting for positive diagnostic tests.

The patient should be watched closely for at least 24 to 48 hours. If signs of poisoning reappear, injection of both sodium nitrite and sodium thiosulfate should be repeated, but each in one-half of the original dose. Even if the patient seems perfectly well, the medication may be given for prophylactic purposes 2 hours after the first injections.

If respiration has ceased but the pulse is palpable, artificial respiration should be applied at once. The purpose is not to revive, per se, but to keep the heart beating. The gauze sponge or handkerchief continuing the amyl nitrite should be laid over the patient's nose, for it may hasten the resumption of respiration movements. When signs of breathing appear, injection of the above solutions should be made pr omptly.

➤*Storage/Stability:* Store at a controlled room temperature 15° to 30°C (59° to 86°F).

Actions

➤*Pharmacology:* Sodium nitrite reacts with hemoglobin to form methemoglobin. The latter removes cyanide ions from various tissues and couples with them to become cyanmethemoglobin, which has relatively low toxicity. The function of sodium thiosulfate is to convert cyanide to thiocyanate, probably by an enzyme known as rhodanese. The combined mechanism may thus be expressed in a chemical manner:

- $NaNO_2$ + hemoglobin = methemoglobin.
- HCN + methemoglobin = cyanmethemoglobin.
- $Na_2S_2O_3$ + HCN + O = HSCN

The combination of sodium nitrite and sodium thiosulfate is effective therapy against cyanide and hydrocyanic acid poisoning. The 2 substances intravenously injected, 1 after the other (nitrite followed by the thiosulfate) are capable of detoxifying approximately 20 lethal doses of sodium cyanide in dogs and are effective even after respiration has stopped. As long as the heart is still beating, the chances of recovery by utilizing this method are good.

There is not only a summation but also a definite potentiation of action when the nitrite and the thiosulfate are administered together.

Warnings

➤*Methemoglobinemia:* Both sodium nitrite and amyl nitrite in excessive doses induce dangerous methemoglobinemia and can cause death. The dosage recommended is not excessive for an adult. The doses for children should be calculated on a surface area or on a weight basis with the dosage adjusted so that excessive methemoglobulin is not formed.

If signs of excessive methemoglobulin develop (ie, blue skin and mucous membranes, vomiting, shock, and coma), 1% methylene blue solution should be given intravenously. A total dose of 1 to 2 mg/kg of body weight should be administered over a period of 5 to 10 minutes and should be repeated in 1 hour if necessary.

In addition, oxygen inhalation and transfusion of whole fresh blood should be considered.

Precautions

➤*Monitoring:* Nitrites produce significant vasodilation, and rapid administration may result in hypotension. Hypotension may be avoided or lessened by slow administration (eg, IV push over at least 5 minutes) or by diluting the dose in 50 to 100 mL of 5% dextrose in water or normal saline and beginning infusion as a slow drip then increasing to the most rapid rate tolerated. Frequently monitor blood pressure during treatment with sodium nitrite.

Adverse Reactions

Dizziness, flushing, headache, hypotension, methemoglobinemia, nausea, syncope, tachycardia, and vomiting may occur.

NALMEFENE HYDROCHLORIDE

Rx	**Revex** (Ohmeda)	**Injection:** 100 mcg/mL nalmefene base	Blue label.[a] In 1 mL amps.
		1 mg/mL nalmefene base	Green label.[b] In 2 mL amps.

[a] The blue labeled product is for postoperative use.

[b] The green labeled product is for management of overdose.

NALMEFENE HYDROCHLORIDE — INJECTION

Indications

➤*Reversal of opioid effects:* For the complete or partial reversal of opioid drug effects, including respiratory depression, induced by either natural or synthetic opioids.

➤*Opioid overdose:* Management of known or suspected opioid overdose.

➤*Unlabeled uses:* Oral formulation (not available in the US) has been studied in the treatment of pruritis.

Administration and Dosage

➤*Approved by the FDA:* April 17, 1995.

➤*Important information about dosage strengths:* Nalmefene hydrochloride injection is supplied in 2 concentrations that can be identified by their color-coded container labels: A concentration suitable for postoperative use (100 mcg/mL) in a blue-labeled ampule containing 1 mL and a concentration suitable for the management of overdose (1 mg/mL, 10 times as concentrated, 20 times as much drug) in a green-labeled ampule and syringe, both containing 2 mL. Proper steps should be taken to prevent use of the incorrect concentration.

➤*Administration:* Nalmefene hydrochloride injection should be titrated to reverse the undesired effects of opioids. Once adequate reversal has been established, additional administration is not required and may actually be harmful due to unwanted reversal of analgesia or precipitated withdrawal.

➤*Duration of action:* The duration of action of nalmefene hydrochloride injection is as long as most opioid analgesics. The apparent duration of action of nalmefene hydrochloride injection will vary, however, depending on the half-life and plasma concentration of the narcotic being reversed, the presence or absence of other drugs affecting the brain or muscles of respiration, and the dose of nalmefene hydrochloride injection administered. Partially reversing doses of nalmefene hydrochloride injection (1 mcg/kg) lose their effect as the drug is redistributed through the body, and the effects of these low doses may not last more than 30 to 60 minutes in the presence of persistent opioid effects. Fully reversing doses (1 mg/70 kg) have been shown to last many hours in both experimental and clinical studies, but may complicate the management of patients who are in pain, at high cardiovascular risk, or who are physically dependent on opioids.

The recommended doses represent a compromise between a desirable controlled reversal and the need for prompt response and adequate duration of action. Using higher dosages or shorter intervals between incremental doses is likely to increase the incidence and severity of symptoms related to acute withdrawal such as nausea, vomiting, elevated blood pressure, and anxiety.

➤*Patients tolerant to or physically dependent on opioids:* Nalmefene hydrochloride injection may cause acute withdrawal symptoms in individu-

NALMEFENE HYDROCHLORIDE — INJECTION

als who have some degree of tolerance to and dependence on opioids. These patients should be closely observed for symptoms of withdrawal following administration of the initial and subsequent injections of nalmefene hydrochloride injection. Subsequent doses should be administered with intervals of at least 2 to 5 minutes between doses to allow the full effect of each incremental dose of nalmefene hydrochloride injection to be reached.

➤*Recommended doses for reversal of postoperative opioid depression:* Use 100 mcg/mL dosage strength (blue label) and see information following for initial doses.

The goal of treatment with nalmefene hydrochloride injection in the postoperative setting is to achieve reversal of excessive opioid effects without inducing a complete reversal and acute pain. This is best accomplished with an initial dose of 0.25 mcg/kg followed by 0.25 mcg/kg incremental doses at 2- to 5- minute intervals, stopping as soon as the desired degree of opioid reversal is obtained. A cumulative total dose of more than 1 mcg/kg does not provide additional therapeutic effect.

Reversal of Postoperative Opioid Depression

Body weight	mL of nalmefene hydrochloride 100 mcg/mL solution
50 kg	0.125
60 kg	0.15
70 kg	0.175
80 kg	0.2
90 kg	0.225
100 kg	0.25

In cases where the patient is known to be at increased cardiovascular risk, it may be desirable to dilute nalmefene hydrochloride injection 1:1 with saline or sterile water and use smaller initial and incremental doses of 0.1 mcg/kg.

➤*Management of known or suspected opioid overdose:* Use 1 mg/mL dosage strength (green label).

The recommended initial dose of nalmefene hydrochloride injection for non-opioid-dependent patients is 0.5 mg/70 kg. If needed, this may be followed by a second dose of 1 mg/70 kg, 2 to 5 minutes later. If a total dose of 1.5 mg /70 kg has been administered without clinical response, additional nalmefene hydrochloride injection is unlikely to have an effect. Patients should not be given more nalmefene hydrochloride injection than is required to restore the respiratory rate to normal, thus minimizing the likelihood of cardiovascular stress and precipitated withdrawal syndrome.

If there is a reasonable suspicion of opioid dependency, a challenge dose of nalmefene hydrochloride injection 0.1 mg/70 kg should be administered initially. If there is no evidence of withdrawal in 2 minutes, the recommended dosing should be followed.

Nalmefene hydrochloride injection had no effect in cases where opioids were not responsible for sedation and hypoventilation. Therefore, patients should only be treated with nalmefene hydrochloride injection when the likelihood of an opioid overdose is high, based on a history of opioid overdose or the clinical presentation of respiratory depression with concurrent pupillary constriction.

➤*Repeated dosing:* Nalmefene hydrochloride injection is the longest acting of the currently available parenteral opioid antagonists. If recurrence of respiratory depression does occur, the dose should again be titrated to clinical effect using incremental doses to avoid overreversal.

➤*Hepatic and renal disease:* Hepatic disease and renal failure substantially reduce the clearance of nalmefene (see Pharmacokinetics). For single episodes of opioid antagonism, adjustment of nalmefene hydrochloride injection dosage is not required. However, in patients with renal failure, the incremental doses should be delivered slowly (over 60 seconds) to minimize the hypertension and dizziness reported following the abrupt administration of nalmefene to such patients.

➤*Loss of IV access:* Should IV access be lost or not readily obtainable, a pharmacokinetic study has shown that a single dose of nalmefene hydrochloride injection should be effective within 5 to 15 minutes after IM or SC doses of 1 mg (see Pharmacokinetics).

➤*Storage / Stability:* Store at controlled room temperature.

Actions

➤*Pharmacology:* Nalmefene hydrochloride injection prevents or reverses the effects of opioids, including respiratory depression, sedation, and hypotension. Pharmacodynamic studies have shown that nalmefene hydrochloride injection has a longer duration of action than naloxone at fully reversing doses. Nalmefene hydrochloride injection has no opioid agonist activity.

Nalmefene hydrochloride injection is not known to produce respiratory depression, psychotomimetic effects, or pupillary constriction. No pharmacological activity was observed when nalmefene hydrochloride injection was administered in the absence of opioid agonists.

Nalmefene hydrochloride injection has not been shown to produce tolerance, physical dependence, or abuse potential.

Nalmefene hydrochloride injection can produce acute withdrawal symptoms in individuals who are opioid dependent.

➤*Pharmacokinetics:*

Absorption – Nalmefene exhibited dose-proportional pharmacokinetics following IV administration of 0.5 mg to 2 mg.

Mean (CV %) Nalmefene Pharmacokinetic Parameters in Adult Males Following a 1 mg IV Dose

Parameter	Young (n = 18)	Elderly (n = 11)
Age	19 to 32	62 to 80
C_p at 5 minutes (ng/mL)	3.7 (29)	5.8 (38)
V_{dss} (L/kg)	8.6 (19)	8.6 (29)
V_c (L/kg)	3.9 (29)	2.8 (41)
$AUC_{0-\infty}$ (ng•h/mL)	16.6 (27)	17.3 (14)
Terminal t½ (hr)	10.8 (48)	9.4 (49)
Cl_{plasma} (L/h/kg)	0.8 (23)	0.8 (18)

Nalmefene was completely bioavailable following IM or subcutaneous administration in 12 male volunteers relative to IV nalmefene. The relative bioavailabilities of IM and subcutaneous routes of administration were 101.5% ± 8.1% (Mean ± SD) and 99.7% ± 6.9%, respectively. Nalmefene will be administered primarily as an IV bolus, however, nalmefene can be given IM or subcutaneous if venous access cannot be established. While the time to maximum plasma nalmefene concentration was 2.3 ± 1.1 hours following IM, and 1.5 ± 1.2 hours following subcutaneous administrations, therapeutic plasma concentrations are likely to be reached within 5 to 15 minutes after a 1 mg dose in an emergency. Because of the variability in the speed of absorption for IM and subcutaneous dosing, and the inability to titrate to effect, great care should be taken if repeated doses must be given by these routes.

Distribution – Following a 1 mg parenteral dose, nalmefene was rapidly distributed. In a study of brain receptor occupancy, a 1 mg dose of nalmefene blocked more than 80% of brain opioid receptors within 5 minutes after administration. The apparent volumes of distribution centrally (V_c) and at steady-state (V_{dss}) are 3.9 ± 1.1 L/kg and 8.6 ± 1.7 L/kg, respectively. Ultrafiltration studies of nalmefene have demonstrated that 45% (CV 4.1%) is bound to plasma proteins over a concentration range of 0.1 to 2 mcg/mL. An in vitro determination of the distribution of nalmefene in human blood demonstrated that nalmefene distributed 67% (CV 8.7%) into red blood cells and 39% (CV 6.4%) into plasma. The whole blood to plasma ratio was 1.3 (CV 6.6%) over the nominal concentration range in whole blood from 0.376 to 30 ng/mL.

Metabolism – Nalmefene is metabolized by the liver, primarily by glucuronide conjugation, and excreted in the urine. Nalmefene is also metabolized to trace amounts of an N-dealkylated metabolite. Nalmefene glucuronide is inactive and the N-dealkylated metabolite has minimal pharmacological activity. Less than 5% of nalmefene is excreted in the urine unchanged. Seventeen percent (17%) of the nalmefene dose is excreted in the feces. The plasma concentration-time profile in some subjects suggests that nalmefene undergoes enterohepatic recycling.

Excretion – After IV administration of 1 mg nalmefene hydrochloride injection to healthy males (ages 19 to 32), plasma concentrations declined biexponentially with a redistribution and a terminal elimination half-life of 41 ± 34 minutes and 10.8 ± 5.2 hours, respectively. The systemic clearance of nalmefene is 0.8 ± 0.2 L/h/kg and the renal clearance is 0.08 ± 0.04 L/h/kg.

Special populations –

Renal function impairment: There was a statistically significant 27% decrease in plasma clearance of nalmefene in the end-stage renal disease (ESRD) population during interdialysis (0.57 ± 0.2 L/h/kg) and a 25% decreased plasma clearance in the ESRD population during intradialysis (0.59 ± 0.18 L/h/kg) compared to healthy patients (0.79 ± 0.24 L/h/kg). The elimination half-life was prolonged in ESRD patients from 10.2 ± 2.2 hours in healthy patients to 26.1 ± 9.9 hours (see Administration and Dosage).

Hepatic function impairment: Subjects with hepatic disease, when compared to matched healthy controls, had a 28.3% decrease in plasma clearance of nalmefene (0.56 ± 0.21 L/h/kg versus 0.78 ± 0.24 L/h/kg, respectively). Elimination half-life increased from 10.2 ± 2.2 hours to 11.9 ± 2 hours in the hepatically impaired. No dosage adjustment is recommended since nalmefene will be administered as an acute course of therapy.

Elderly: Dose proportionality was observed in nalmefene $AUC_{0-\infty}$ following 0.5 to 2 mg IV administration to elderly male subjects. Following a 1 mg IV nalmefene dose, there were no significant differences between younger (19 to 32 years) and elderly (62 to 80 years) adult male subjects with respect to plasma clearance, steady-state volume of distribution, or half-life. There was an apparent age-related decrease in the central volume of distribution (younger: 3.9 ± 1.1 L/kg, elderly: 2.8 ± 1.1 L/kg) that resulted in a greater initial nalmefene concentration in the elderly group. While initial nalmefene plasma concentrations were transiently higher in the elderly, it would not be anticipated that this population would require dosing adjustment. No clinical adverse events were noted in the elderly following the 1 mg IV nalmefene dose.

Contraindications

Hypersensitivity to the product.

Warnings

➤*Use of nalmefene hydrochloride injection in emergencies:* Nalmefene hydrochloride injection, like all drugs in this class, is not the primary treatment for ventilatory failure. In most emergency settings, treatment with nalmefene hydrochloride injection should follow, not precede, the establishment of a patent airway, ventilatory assistance, administration of oxygen, and establishment of circulatory access.

NALMEFENE HYDROCHLORIDE — INJECTION

➤*Risk of recurrent respiratory depression:* Accidental overdose with long-acting opioids [such as methadone and levo-alpha-acetylmethadol (LAAM)] may result in prolonged respiratory depression. Respiratory depression in both the postoperative and overdose setting may be complex and involve the effects of anesthetic agents, neuromuscular blockers, and other drugs. While nalmefene hydrochloride injection has a longer duration of action than naloxone in fully reversing doses, the physician should be aware that a recurrence of respiratory depression is possible, even after an apparently adequate initial response to nalmefene hydrochloride injection treatment.

Patients treated with nalmefene hydrochloride injection should be observed until, in the opinion of the physician, there is no reasonable risk of recurrent respiratory depression.

➤*Renal function impairment:* See Actions for more information.

➤*Hepatic function impairment:* See Actions for more information.

➤*Elderly:* See Actions for more information.

➤*Pregnancy: Category B.* There are no adequate and well-controlled studies in pregnant women. Because animal reproduction studies are not always predictive of human response, this drug should be used during pregnancy only if clearly needed.

➤*Lactation:* Nalmefene and its metabolites were secreted into rat milk, reaching concentrations approximately 3 times those in plasma at 1 hour and decreasing to about half the corresponding plasma concentrations by 24 hours following bolus administration. As no clinical information is available, caution should be exercised when nalmefene hydrochloride injection is administered to a nursing woman.

➤*Children:* Safety and efficacy of nalmefene hydrochloride injection in children have not been established.

Use in neonates – The safety and effectiveness of nalmefene hydrochloride injection in neonates have not been established in clinical studies. In a preclinical study, nalmefene was administered by subcutaneous injection to rat pups at doses up to 205 mg/m^2/day throughout maternal lactation without producing adverse effects. A preclinical study evaluating the irritancy of the dosage form following arterial and venous administration in animals showed no vascular irritancy.

Nalmefene hydrochloride injection should only be used in the resuscitation of the newborn when, in the opinion of the treating physician, the expected benefits outweigh the risks.

Precautions

➤*Incomplete reversal of buprenorphine:* Preclinical studies have shown that nalmefene at doses up to 10 mg/kg (437 times the maximum recommended human dose) produced incomplete reversal of buprenorphine-induced analgesia in animal models. This appears to be a consequence of a high affinity and slow displacement of buprenorphine from the opioid receptors. Hence, nalmefene hydrochloride injection may not completely reverse buprenorphine-induced respiratory depression.

➤*Special risk:*

Cardiovascular risks with narcotic antagonists – Pulmonary edema, cardiovascular instability, hypotension, hypertension, ventricular tachycardia, and ventricular fibrillation have been reported in connection with opioid reversal in both postoperative and emergency department settings. In many cases, these effects appear to be the result of abrupt reversal of opioid effects.

Although nalmefene hydrochloride injection has been used safely in patients with preexisting cardiac disease, all drugs of this class should be used with caution in patients at high cardiovascular risk or who have received potentially cardiotoxic drugs (see Administration and Dosage).

Risk of precipitated withdrawal – Nalmefene hydrochloride injection, like other opioid antagonists, is known to produce acute withdrawal symptoms and, therefore, should be used with extreme caution in patients with known physical dependence on opioids or following surgery involving high doses of opioids. Imprudent use or excessive doses of opioid antagonists in the postoperative setting has been associated with hypertension, tachycardia, and excessive mortality in patients at high risk for cardiovascular complications.

➤*Drug abuse and dependence:* Nalmefene hydrochloride injection is an opioid antagonist with no agonist activity. It has no demonstrated abuse potential, is not addictive, and is not a controlled substance.

Drug Interactions

Preclinical studies have shown that both flumazenil and nalmefene can induce seizures in animals. The coadministration of both flumazenil and nalmefene produced fewer seizures than expected in a study in rodents, based on the expected effects of each drug alone. Based on these data, an adverse interaction from the coadministration of the 2 drugs is not expected, but physicians should remain aware of the potential risk of seizures from agents in these classes.

Adverse Reactions

Nalmefene was well tolerated and showed no serious toxicity during experimental administration to healthy individuals, even when given at 15 times the highest recommended dose. In a small number of subjects, at doses exceeding the recommended nalmefene hydrochloride injection dose, nalmefene produced symptoms suggestive of reversal of endogenous opioids, such as have been reported for other narcotic antagonist drugs. These symptoms (nausea, chills, myalgia, dysphoria, abdominal cramps, and joint pain) were usually transient and occurred at very low frequency.

Such symptoms of precipitated opioid withdrawal at the recommended clinical doses were seen in both postoperative and overdose patients who were later found to have had histories of covert opioid use. Symptoms of precipitated withdrawal were similar to those seen with other opioid antagonists, were transient following the lower doses used in the postoperative setting, and more prolonged following the administration of the larger doses used in the treatment of overdose.

Tachycardia and nausea following the use of nalmefene in the postoperative setting were reported at the same frequencies as for naloxone at equivalent doses. The risk of both these adverse events was low at doses giving partial opioid reversal and increased with increases in dose. Thus, total doses more than 1 mcg/kg in the postoperative setting and 1.5 mg per 70 kg in the treatment of overdose are not recommended.

Relative Frequencies of Common Adverse Reactions with an Incidence ≥ 1% (all Patients, all Clinical Settings)

Adverse reaction	Nalmefene n = 1127	Naloxone n = 369	Placebo n = 77
Nausea	18%	18%	6%
Vomiting	9%	7%	4%
Tachycardia	5%	8%	
Hypertension	5%	7%	
Postoperative pain	4%	4%	N/A
Fever	3%	4%	
Dizziness	3%	4%	1%
Headache	1%	1%	4%
Chills	1%	1%	
Hypotension	1%	1%	
Vasodilatation	1%	1%	

➤*Incidence less than 1%:* The incidence of adverse reactions was highest in patients who received more than the recommended dose of nalmefene hydrochloride injection.

Cardiovascular – Bradycardia, arrhythmia.

CNS – Somnolence, depression, agitation, nervousness, tremor, confusion, withdrawal syndrome, myoclonus.

Dermatologic – Pruritus.

GI – Diarrhea, pharyngitis, dry mouth.

GU – Urinary retention.

Lab test abnormalities – Transient increases in CPK were reported as adverse events in 0.5% of the postoperative patients studied. These increases were believed to be related to surgery and not believed to be related to the administration of nalmefene hydrochloride injection. Increases in AST were reported as adverse events in 0.3% of the patients receiving either nalmefene or naloxone. The clinical significance of this finding is unknown. No cases of hepatitis or hepatic injury due to either nalmefene or naloxone were observed in the clinical trials.

Overdosage

➤*Symptoms:* IV doses of up to 24 mg of nalmefene, administered to healthy volunteers in the absence of opioid agonists, produced no serious adverse reactions, severe signs or symptoms, or clinically significant laboratory abnormalities. As with all opioid antagonists, use in patients physically dependent on opioids can result in precipitated withdrawal reactions that may result in symptoms that require medical attention.

➤*Treatment:* Treatment of such cases should be symptomatic and supportive. Administration of large amounts of opioids to patients receiving opioid antagonists in an attempt to overcome a full blockade has resulted in adverse respiratory and circulatory reactions.

NALOXONE HYDROCHLORIDE

Rx	**Naloxone hydrochloride** (Various, eg, Hospira, Elkins-Sinn, SoloPak)	**Injection:** 0.4 mg/mL	In 1 mL amps, 1 mL syringes and 1, 2 and 10 mL vials.
Rx	**Narcan** (DuPont Pharm.)		In 1 mL amps and 10 mL vials.[a]
Rx	**Naloxone hydrochloride** (Various, eg, Hospira)	**Neonatal injection:** 0.02 mg/mL	In 2 ml vials.

[a] Available with or without parabens.

NALOXONE HYDROCHLORIDE — INJECTION

Indications

➤*Reversal of opioid effects:* For the complete or partial reversal of narcotic depression, including respiratory depression, induced by opioid including natural and synthetic narcotics, propoxyphene, methadone, nalbuphine, butorphanol and pentazocine.

➤*Opioid overdose:* For the diagnosis of suspected acute opioid overdosage.

➤*Unlabeled uses:* Naloxone has been used to improve circulation in refractory shock. Naloxone has also been used for the reversal of alcoholic coma, dementia of the Alzheimer type and schizophrenia.

Administration and Dosage

Give IV, IM or subcutaneously. The most rapid onset of action is achieved with IV use, which is recommended in emergency situations. Duration of action of some narcotics may exceed that of naloxone. Keep patients under continued surveillance and give repeat doses as necessary.

➤*Adults:*

Narcotic overdose (known or suspected) – Initial dose is 0.4 to 2 mg IV; may repeat IV at 2 to 3 minute intervals. If no response is observed after 10 mg has been administered, question the diagnosis of narcotic-induced or partial narcotic-induced toxicity. IM or subcutaneous administration may be necessary if the IV route is not available.

Postoperative narcotic depression (partial reversal) – Small doses are usually sufficient. Titrate dose according to the patient's response. Excessive dosage may result in significant reversal of analgesia and increase in blood pressure. Similarly, too rapid reversal may induce nausea, vomiting, sweating or circulatory stress.

Initial dose: Inject in increments of 0.1 to 0.2 mg IV at 2 to 3 minute intervals to the desired degree of reversal (ie, adequate ventilation and alertness without significant pain or discomfort).

Repeat dose: Repeat doses may be required within 1 or 2 hr intervals depending on the amount, type (ie, short- or long-acting) and time interval since last administration. Supplemental IM doses have produced a longer lasting effect.

➤*Children:*

Narcotic overdose (known or suspected) – Initial dose is 0.01 mg/kg IV; give a subsequent dose of 0.1 mg/kg if needed. If an IV route is not available, may be given IM or subcutaneously in divided doses. If necessary, dilute with sterile water for injection.

Postoperative narcotic depression – Follow the recommendations and cautions under adult administration guidelines. For initial reversal of respiratory depression, inject in increments of 0.005 to 0.01 mg IV at 2 to 3 minute intervals to desired degree of reversal.

➤*Neonates:*

Narcotic-induced depression – Initial dose is 0.01 mg/kg IV, IM or subcutaneous; may be repeated in accordance with adult administration guidelines.

➤*Intravenous infusion:* Dilute in normal saline or 5% dextrose solutions. The addition of 2 mg in 500 ml of either solution provides a concentration of 0.004 mg/ml. Titrate the administration rate in accordance with the patient's response.

Incompatibilities – Do not mix naloxone with preparations containing bisulfite, metabisulfite, long-chain or high molecular weight anions, or any solution having an alkaline pH. Do not add any drug or chemical agent unless its effect on the chemical and physical stability of the solution has first been established.

➤*Storage/Stability:* Use mixtures within 24 hrs. After 24 hrs, discard unused solution.

Actions

➤*Pharmacology:* The narcotic antagonist naloxone is clinically useful in the reversal of narcotic-induced respiratory depression. Naloxone, a pure narcotic antagonist, will precipitate abstinence syndrome in the presence of narcotic addiction. Because it is devoid of undesirable agonist properties, naloxone is preferred for reversal of narcotic-induced respiratory depression. Naloxone prevents or reverses opioid effects including respiratory depression, sedation and hypotension; it can reverse psychotomimetic and dysphoric effects of agonist-antagonists (eg, pentazocine).

The mechanism of action is not fully understood; evidence suggests that it antagonizes the opioid effects by competing for the same receptor sites. Naloxone is an essentially pure narcotic antagonist, ie, it does not possess "agonistic" or morphine-like properties.

Naloxone does not produce respiratory depression, psychotomimetic effects or pupillary constriction. In the absence of narcotics or agonistic effects of other narcotic antagonists, naloxone exhibits essentially no pharmacologic activity.

➤*Pharmacokinetics:*

Distribution – After parenteral use, naloxone is rapidly distributed in the body. Onset of action of IV naloxone is generally apparent within 2 min; it is only slightly less rapid when given subcutaneously or IM. Duration of action depends upon dose and route. IM use produces a more prolonged effect than IV use. The requirement for repeat doses will also depend upon amount, type and route of the narcotic being antagonized.

Metabolism – Naloxone is metabolized in the liver, primarily by glucuronide conjugation. It is excreted in the urine. The serum of half-life in adults ranged from 30 to 81 minutes (mean 64 ± 12 minutes); in neonates, 3.1 ± 0.5 hours.

Contraindications

Hypersensitivity to these agents.

Warnings

➤*Drug dependence:* Administer cautiously to persons who are known or suspected to be physically dependent on opioids, including newborns of mothers with narcotic dependence. Reversal of narcotic effect will precipitate acute abstinence syndrome.

➤*Repeat administration:* The patient who has satisfactorily responded should be kept under continued surveillance. Administer repeated doses as necessary, because the duration of action of some narcotics may exceed that of the narcotic antagonist.

➤*Respiratory depression:* Not effective against respiratory depression due to nonopioid drugs. Reversal of buprenorphine-induced respiratory depression may be incomplete; if an incomplete response occurs, mechanically assist respiration.

➤*Pregnancy:* *Category B.* No adequate and well controlled studies in pregnant women. Use during pregnancy only when clearly needed.

➤*Lactation:* It is not known whether the drug is excreted in breast milk. Use caution when administering to a nursing woman.

Precautions

➤*Other supportive therapy:* Maintain a free airway and provide artificial respiration, cardiac massage and vasopressor agents; employ when necessary to counteract acute narcotic overdosage.

➤*Cardiovascular effects:* Several instances of hypotension, hypertension, pulmonary edema, ventricular tachycardia and fibrillation have been reported in postoperative patients, most of whom had preexisting cardiovascular disorders or had received other drugs that may have similar adverse cardiovascular effects. A direct cause and effect relationship is not established; use caution in patients with pre-existing cardiac disease or who have received potentially cardiotoxic drugs.

Adverse Reactions

Abrupt reversal of narcotic depression may result in nausea, vomiting, sweating, tachycardia, increased blood pressure and tremulousness.

In postoperative patients, excessive dosage may result in excitement and significant reversal of analgesia, hypotension, hypertension, pulmonary edema and ventricular tachycardia and fibrillation. Seizures have been reported infrequently.

NALTREXONE HYDROCHLORIDE

Rx	**Naltrexone Hydrochloride** (Various, eg, Barr, Eon)	**Tablets:** 50 mg	In 30s, 100s, and 500s.
Rx	**ReVia** (Duramed)	**Tablets:** 50 mg	(ReVia b/275). Beige, round, biconvex, film-coated, scored. In 30s and 100s.

NALTREXONE HYDROCHLORIDE — ORAL

WARNING

Hepatotoxicity – Naltrexone has the capacity to cause hepatocellular injury when given in excessive doses.

Naltrexone is contraindicated in acute hepatitis or liver failure, and its use in patients with active liver disease must be carefully considered in light of its hepatotoxic effects.

The margin of separation between the apparently safe dose of naltrexone and the dose causing hepatic injury appears to be only 5-fold or less. Naltrexone does not appear to be a hepatotoxin at the recommended doses.

Patients should be warned of the risk of hepatic injury and advised to stop the use of naltrexone and seek medical attention if they experience symptoms of acute hepatitis.

Indications

➤*Alcohol dependence:* Treatment of alcohol dependence.

➤*Narcotic addiction:* For the blockade of the effects of exogenously administered opioids. Naltrexone has not been shown to provide any therapeutic benefit except as part of an appropriate plan of management for the addictions.

➤*Unlabeled uses:* Naltrexone has been used in eating disorders and in the treatment of postconcussional syndrome unresponsive to other treatments. To increase patient compliance, a subcutaneous implant is being studied.

Treatment of severe pruritus refractory to traditional treatments. Although most patients experienced improvement in cholestatic pruritus-related symptoms with naltrexone, results are mixed in patients with uremic pruritus.

Administration and Dosage

If there is any question of occult opioid dependence, perform a naloxone challenge test and do not initiate naltrexone therapy until the naloxone challenge is negative.

➤*Treatment of alcoholism:* A dose of 50 mg once daily is recommended for most patients. The placebo-controlled studies that demonstrated the efficacy of naltrexone hydrochloride as an adjunctive treatment of alcoholism used a dose regimen of naltrexone hydrochloride 50 mg once daily for up to 12 weeks. Other dose regimens or durations of therapy were not evaluated in these trials.

A patient is a candidate for treatment with naltrexone if:
- The patient is willing to take a medicine to help with alcohol dependence.
- The patient is opioid free for 7 to 10 days.
- The patient does not have severe or active liver or kidney problems (typical guidelines suggest liver function tests no greater than 3 times the upper limits of normal, and bilirubin normal).
- The patient is not allergic to naltrexone, and no other contraindications are present.

Naltrexone should be considered as only one of many factors determining the success of treatment of alcoholism. Factors associated with a good outcome in the clinical trials with naltrexone were the type, intensity, and duration of treatment; appropriate management of comorbid conditions; use of community-based support groups; and good medication compliance. To achieve the best possible treatment outcome, appropriate compliance-enhancing techniques should be implemented for all components of the treatment program, especially medication compliance.

➤*Treatment of opioid dependence:* Initiate treatment with naltrexone using the following guidelines:

1.) Treatment should not be attempted unless the patient has remained opioid-free for at least 7 to 10 days. Self-reporting of abstinence from opioids in opioid addicts should be verified by analysis of the patient's urine for absence of opioids. The patient should not be manifesting withdrawal signs or reporting withdrawal symptoms.
2.) If there is any question of occult opioid dependence, perform a naloxone challenge test. If signs of opioid withdrawal are still observed following naloxone challenge, treatment with naltrexone should not be attempted. The naloxone challenge can be repeated in 24 hours.
3.) Treatment should be initiated carefully, with an initial dose of 25 mg of naltrexone hydrochloride. If no withdrawal signs occur, the patient may be started on 50 mg a day thereafter.

Naloxone challenge test – The naloxone challenge test should not be performed in a patient showing clinical signs or symptoms of opioid withdrawal, or in a patient whose urine contains opioids. The naloxone challenge test may be administered by either IV or subcutaneous routes.

➤*Intravenous:* Inject 0.2 mg naloxone.

Observe for 30 seconds for signs or symptoms of withdrawal. If no evidence of withdrawal is observed, inject 0.6 mg of naloxone. Observe for an additional 20 minutes.

➤*Subcutaneous:* Administer 0.8 mg naloxone.

Observe for 20 minutes for signs or symptoms of withdrawal.

Note – Individual patients, especially those with opioid dependence, may respond to lower doses of naloxone. In some cases, 0.1 mg IV naloxone has produced a diagnostic response.

➤*Interpretation of the challenge:* Monitor vital signs and observe the patient for signs and symptoms of opioid withdrawal. These may include, but are not limited to nausea, vomiting, dysphoria, yawning, sweating, tearing, rhinorrhea, stuffy nose, craving for opioids, poor appetite, abdominal cramps, sense of fear, skin erythema, disrupted sleep patterns, fidgeting, uneasiness, poor ability to focus, mental lapses, muscle aches or cramps, pupillary dilation, piloerection, fever, changes in blood pressure, pulse or temperature, anxiety, depression, irritability, backache, bone or joint pains, tremors, sensations of skin crawling or fasciculations. If signs or symptoms of withdrawal appear, the test is positive and no additional naloxone should be administered.

Warning – If the test is positive do not initiate naltrexone therapy. Repeat the challenge in 24 hours. If the test is negative, naltrexone therapy may be started if no other contraindications are present. If there is any doubt about the result of the test, hold naltrexone and repeat the challenge in 24 hours.

➤*Alternative dosing schedules:* Once the patient has been started on naltrexone hydrochloride tablets, 50 mg every 24 hours will produce adequate clinical blockade of the actions of parenterally administered opioids (ie, this dose will block the effects of a 25 mg IV heroin challenge). A flexible approach to a dosing regimen may need to be employed in cases of supervised administration. Thus, patients may receive 50 mg of naltrexone hydrochloride every weekday with a 100 mg dose on Saturday, 100 mg every other day, or 150 mg every third day. The degree of blockade produced by naltrexone may be reduced by these extended dosing intervals.

There may be a higher risk of hepatocellular injury with single doses above 50 mg, and use of higher doses and extended dosing intervals should balance the possible risks against the probable benefits.

Patient compliance – Naltrexone should be considered as only 1 of many factors determining the success of treatment. To achieve the best possible treatment outcome, appropriate compliance-enhancing techniques should be implemented for all components of the treatment program, including medication compliance.

➤*Storage/Stability:* Store at controlled room temperature 20° to 25°C (68° to 77°F); excursions permitted between 15° and 30°C (59° to 86°F). Keep tightly closed. Protect from light. Dispense in tight, light-resistant containers with a child-resistant closure, as required.

Actions

➤*Pharmacology:* Naltrexone is a pure opioid antagonist. It markedly attenuates or completely blocks, reversibly, the subjective effects of IV administered opioids.

When coadministered with morphine, on a chronic basis, naltrexone blocks the physical dependence to morphine, heroin and other opioids.

Naltrexone has few, if any, intrinsic actions besides its opioid blocking properties. However, it does produce some pupillary constriction, by an unknown mechanism.

The administration of naltrexone hydrochloride is not associated with the development of tolerance or dependence. In subjects physically dependent on opioids, naltrexone will precipitate withdrawal symptomatology.

Clinical studies indicate that 50 mg of naltrexone hydrochloride will block the pharmacologic effects of 25 mg of IV administered heroin for periods as long as 24 hours. Other data suggest that doubling the dose of naltrexone provides blockade for 48 hours, and tripling the dose of naltrexone provides blockade for about 72 hours.

Naltrexone blocks the effects of opioids by competitive binding (ie, analogous to competitive inhibition of enzymes) at opioid receptors. This makes the blockade produced potentially surmountable, but overcoming full naltrexone blockade by administration of very high doses of opiates has resulted in excessive symptoms of histamine release in experimental subjects.

The mechanism of action of naltrexone in alcoholism is not understood; however, involvement of the endogenous opioid system is suggested by preclinical data. Naltrexone, an opioid receptor antagonist, competitively binds to such receptors and may block the effects of endogenous opioids. Opioid antagonists have been shown to reduce alcohol consumption by animals, and naltrexone has been shown to reduce alcohol consumption in clinical studies.

Naltrexone is not aversive therapy and does not cause a disulfiram-like reaction either as a result of opiate use or ethanol ingestion.

➤*Pharmacokinetics:*

Absorption – Naltrexone is a pure opioid receptor antagonist. Although well-absorbed orally, naltrexone is subject to significant first-pass metabolism with oral bioavailability estimates ranging from 5% to 40%. The activity of naltrexone is believed to be due to both parent and the 6-β-naltrexol metabolite. Naltrexone and 6-β-naltrexol are dose proportional in terms of AUC and C_{max} over the range of 50 to 200 mg and do not accumulate after 100 mg daily doses.

Following oral administration, naltrexone undergoes rapid and nearly complete absorption with approximately 96% of the dose absorbed from the GI tract. Peak plasma levels of both naltrexone and 6-β-naltrexol occur within 1 hour of dosing.

Distribution – The volume of distribution for naltrexone following intravenous administration is estimated to be 1350 L. In vitro tests with human plasma show naltrexone to be 21% bound to plasma proteins over the therapeutic dose range.

Metabolism – The systemic clearance (after IV administration) of naltrexone is −3.5 L/min, which exceeds liver blood flow (−1.2 L/min). This suggests both that naltrexone is a highly extracted drug (greater than 98% metabolized) and that extrahepatic sites of drug metabolism exist. The major metabolite of naltrexone is 6-β-naltrexol. Two other minor metabolites

NALTREXONE HYDROCHLORIDE — ORAL

are 2-hydroxy-3-methoxy-6-β-naltrexol and 2-hydroxy-3-methyl-naltrexone. Naltrexone and its metabolites are also conjugated to form additional metabolic products.

Excretion – Both parent drug and metabolites are excreted primarily by the kidney (53% to 79% of the dose); however, urinary excretion of unchanged naltrexone accounts for less than 2% of an oral dose and fecal excretion is a minor elimination pathway. The mean elimination half-life (t½) values for naltrexone and 6-β-naltrexol are 4 hours and 13 hours, respectively. The renal clearance for naltrexone ranges from 30 to 127 mL/min and suggests that renal elimination is primarily by glomerular filtration. In comparison, the renal clearance for 6-β-naltrexol ranges from 230 to 369 mL/min, suggesting an additional renal tubular secretory mechanism. The urinary excretion of unchanged naltrexone accounts for less than 2% of an oral dose; urinary excretion of unchanged and conjugated 6-β-naltrexol accounts for 43% of an oral dose. The pharmacokinetic profile of naltrexone suggests that naltrexone and its metabolites may undergo enterohepatic recycling.

Contraindications

Patients receiving opioid analgesics; patients currently dependent on opioids, including those currently maintained on opiate agonists (eg, methadone or LAAM (levo-alpha-acetyl-methadol); patients in acute opioid withdrawal; any individual who has failed the naloxone challenge test or who has a positive urine screen for opioids; any individual with acute hepatitis or liver failure; any individual with a history of sensitivity to naltrexone or any other components of this product. It is not known if there is any cross-sensitivity with naloxone or the phenanthrene containing opioids.

Warnings

➤*Hepatoxicity:* Evidence of the hepatotoxic potential of naltrexone is derived primarily from a placebo-controlled study in which naltrexone hydrochloride was administered to obese subjects at a dose approximately 5-fold that recommended for the blockade of opiate receptors (300 mg per day). In that study, 5 of 26 naltrexone recipients developed elevations of serum transaminases (ie, peak ALT values ranging from a low of 121 to a high of 532; or 3 to 19 times their baseline values) after 3 to 8 weeks of treatment. Although the patients involved were generally clinically asymptomatic and the transaminase levels of all patients on whom follow-up was obtained returned to (or toward) baseline values in a matter of weeks, the lack of any transaminase elevations of similar magnitude in any of the 24 placebo patients in the same study is persuasive evidence that naltrexone is a direct (ie, not idiosyncratic) hepatotoxin.

This conclusion is also supported by evidence from other placebo controlled studies in which exposure to naltrexone hydrochloride at doses above the amount recommended for the treatment of alcoholism or opiate blockade (50 mg/day) consistently produced more numerous and more significant elevations of serum transaminases than did placebo. Transaminase elevations in 3 or 9 patients with Alzheimer disease who received naltrexone hydrochloride (at doses up to 300 mg/day) for 5 to 8 weeks in an open clinical trial have been reported.

Although no cases of hepatic failure due to naltrexone administration have ever been reported, physicians are advised to consider this as a possible risk of treatment and to use the same care in prescribing naltrexone as they would other drugs with the potential for causing hepatic injury.

➤*Unintended precipitation of abstinence:* To prevent occurrence of an acute abstinence syndrome, or exacerbation of a preexisting subclinical abstinence syndrome, patients must be opioid-free for a minimum of 7 to 10 days before starting naltrexone. Since the absence of an opioid drug in the urine is often not sufficient proof that a patient is opioid-free, a naloxone challenge should be employed if the prescribing physician feels there is a risk of precipitating a withdrawal reaction following administration of naltrexone.

➤*Attempt to overcome blockade:* While naltrexone is a potent antagonist with a prolonged pharmacologic effect (24 to 72 hours), the blockade produced by naltrexone is surmountable. This is useful in patients who may require analgesia, but poses a potential risk to individuals who attempt, on their own, to overcome the blockade by administering large amounts of exogenous opioids. Indeed, any attempt by a patient to overcome the antagonism by taking opioids is very dangerous and may lead to a fatal overdose. Injury may arise because the plasma concentration of exogenous opioids attained immediately following their acute administration may be sufficient to overcome the competitive receptor blockade. As a consequence, the patient may be in immediate danger of suffering life endangering opioid intoxication (eg, respiratory arrest, circulatory collapse). Patients should be told of the serious consequences of trying to overcome the opiate blockage.

There is also the possibility that a patient who had been treated with naltrexone will respond to lower doses of opioids than previously used, particularly if taken in such a manner that high plasma concentrations remain in the body beyond the time that naltrexone exerts its therapeutic effects. This could result in potentially life-threatening opioid intoxication (respiratory compromise or arrest, circulatory collapse, etc). Patients should be aware that they may be more sensitive to lower doses of opioids after naltrexone treatment is discontinued.

➤*Ultra-rapid opioid withdrawal:* Safe use of naltrexone in rapid opiate detoxification programs has not been established.

➤*Renal function impairment:* Naltrexone and its primary metabolite are excreted primarily in the urine, and caution is recommended in administering the drug to patients with renal impairment.

➤*Hepatic function impairment:* Caution should be exercised when naltrexone hydrochloride is administered to patients with liver disease. An increase in naltrexone AUC of approximately 5- and 10-fold in patients with compensated and decompensated liver cirrhosis, respectively, compared with subjects with normal liver function has been reported. These data also suggest that alterations in naltrexone bioavailability are related to liver disease severity.

➤*Carcinogenesis:* The following statements are based on the results of experiments in mice and rats. The potential carcinogenic effects of the metabolite 6-β-naltrexol are unknown.

In a 2-year carcinogenicity study in rats, there were small increases in the numbers of testicular mesotheliomas in males and tumors of vascular origin in males and females. The incidence of mesothelioma in males given naltrexone at a dietary dose of 100 mg/kg/day (600 mg/m²/day; 16 times the recommended therapeutic dose, based on body surface area) was 6%, compared with a maximum historical incidence of 4%. The incidence of vascular tumors in males and females given dietary doses of 100 mg/kg/day (600 mg/m²/day) was 4%, but only the incidence in females was increased compared with a maximum historical control incidence of 2%. There was no evidence of carcinogenicity in a 2-year dietary study with naltrexone in male and female mice.

➤*Mutagenesis:* The following statements are based on the results of experiments in mice and rats. The potential mutagenic effects of the metabolite 6-β-naltrexol are unknown.

There was limited evidence of a weak genotoxic effect of naltrexone in one gene mutation assay in a mammalian cell line, in the *Drosophila* recessive lethal assay, and in non-specific DNA repair tests with *E. coli*. However, no evidence of genotoxic potential was observed in a range of other in vitro tests, including assays for gene mutation in bacteria, yeast, or in a second mammalian cell line, a chromosomal aberration assay, and an assay for DNA damage in human cells. Naltrexone did not exhibit clastogenicity in an in vivo mouse micronucleus assay.

➤*Fertility impairment:* The following statements are based on the results of experiments in mice and rats. The potential on fertility effects of the metabolite 6-β-naltrexol are unknown.

Naltrexone (100 mg/kg/day [600 mg/m²/day] orally; 16 times the recommended therapeutic dose, based on body surface area) caused a significant increase in pseudopregnancy in the rat. A decrease in the pregnancy rate of mated female rats also occurred. There was no effect on male fertility at this dose level. The relevance of these observations to human fertility is not known.

➤*Pregnancy:* *Category C.*

Statements based on experiments – The following statements are based on the results of experiments in rats. The potential reproductive toxicity of the metabolite 6-β-naltrexol in rats is not known.

Naltrexone increased the incidence of early fetal loss when administered to rats in oral doses greater than or equal to 30 mg/kg/day (180 mg/m²/day; 5 times the recommended therapeutic dose, based on body surface area) and to rabbits at oral doses greater than or equal to 60 mg/kg/day (720 mg/m²/day; 18 times the recommended therapeutic dose, based on body surface area). There was no evidence of teratogenicity when naltrexone was administered orally to rats and rabbits during the period of major organogenesis at doses up to 200 mg/kg/day (32 and 65 times the recommended therapeutic dose, respectively, based on body surface area).

Rats do not form appreciable quantities of the major human metabolite, 6-β-naltrexol; therefore the potential reproductive toxicity of the metabolite in rats is not known.

There are no adequate and well-controlled studies in pregnant women. Naltrexone should be used in pregnancy only when the potential benefit justifies the potential risk to the fetus.

Labor and delivery – Whether or not naltrexone affects the duration of labor and delivery is unknown.

➤*Lactation:* In animal studies, naltrexone and 6-β-naltrexol were excreted in the milk of lactating rats dosed orally with naltrexone. Whether or not naltrexone is excreted in human milk is unknown. Because many drugs are excreted in human milk, caution should be exercised when naltrexone is administered to a nursing woman.

➤*Children:* The safe use of naltrexone in pediatric patients younger than 18 years of age has not been established.

Precautions

➤*Monitoring:* A high index of suspicion for drug-related hepatic injury is critical if the occurrence of liver damage induced by naltrexone is to be detected at the earliest possible time. Evaluations using appropriate batteries of tests to detect liver injury are recommended at a frequency appropriate to the clinical situation and the dose of naltrexone.

➤*When reversal of naltrexone blockade is required:* In an emergency situation in patients receiving fully blocking doses of naltrexone, a suggested plan of management is regional analgesia, conscious sedation with a benzodiazepine, use of nonopioid analgesics or general anesthesia.

In a situation requiring opioid analgesia, the amount of opioid required may be greater than usual, and the resulting respiratory depression may be deeper and more prolonged.

A rapidly acting opioid analgesic which minimizes the duration of respiratory depression is preferred. The amount of analgesic administered should be titrated to the needs of the patient. Non-receptor mediated actions may

NALTREXONE HYDROCHLORIDE — ORAL

occur and should be expected (eg, facial swelling, itching, generalized erythema, bronchoconstriction) presumably due to histamine release.

Irrespective of the drug chosen to reverse naltrexone blockade, the patient should be monitored closely by appropriately trained personnel in a setting equipped and staffed for cardiopulmonary resuscitation.

➤*Accidentally precipitated withdrawal:* Severe opioid withdrawal syndromes precipitated by the accidental ingestion of naltrexone have been reported in opioid-dependent individuals. Symptoms of withdrawal have usually appeared within 5 minutes of ingestion of naltrexone and have lasted for up to 48 hours. Mental status changes including confusion, somnolence and visual hallucinations have occurred. Significant fluid losses from vomiting and diarrhea have required IV fluid administration. In all cases patients were closely monitored and therapy with nonopioid medications was tailored to meet individual requirements.

Use of naltrexone does not eliminate or diminish withdrawal symptoms. If naltrexone is initiated early in the abstinence process, it will not preclude the patient's experience of the full range of signs and symptoms that would be experienced if naltrexone had not been started. Numerous adverse events are known to be associated with withdrawal.

➤*Suicide:* The risk of suicide is known to be increased in patients with substance abuse with or without concomitant depression. This risk is not abated by treatment with naltrexone.

➤*Lab test abnormalities:* Naltrexone does not interfere with thin-layer, gas-liquid, and high pressure liquid chromatographic methods which may be used for the separation and detection of morphine, methadone or quinine in the urine. Naltrexone may or may not interfere with enzymatic methods for the detection of opioids depending on the specificity of the test. Please consult the test manufacturer for specific details.

➤*Drug abuse and dependence:* Naltrexone is a pure opioid antagonist. It does not lead to physical or psychological dependence. Tolerance to the opioid antagonist effect is not known to occur.

Drug Interactions

Studies to evaluate possible interactions between naltrexone and drugs other than opiates have not been performed. Consequently, caution is advised if the concomitant administration of naltrexone and other drugs is required.

The safety and efficacy of concomitant use of naltrexone and disulfiram is unknown, and the concomitant use of 2 potentially hepatotoxic medications is not ordinarily recommended unless the probable benefits outweigh the known risks.

Naltrexone Drug Interactions

Precipitant drug	Object drug[a]		Description
Naltrexone	Opioid-containing products	⬇	Patients taking naltrexone may not benefit from opioid-containing products such as cough/cold and antidiarrheal preparations and opioid analgesics (see Warnings).
Naltrexone	Thioridazine	⬆	Lethargy and somnolence have occurred with concurrent use.

[a] ⬆ = Object drug increased. ⬇ = Object drug decreased.

Adverse Reactions

During 2 randomized, double-blind, placebo-controlled, 12-week trials to evaluate the efficacy of naltrexone as an adjunctive treatment of alcohol dependence, most patients tolerated naltrexone well. In these studies, a total of 93 patients received naltrexone at a dose of 50 mg once daily. Five of these patients discontinued naltrexone because of nausea. No serious adverse events were reported during these 2 trials.

While extensive clinical studies evaluating the use of naltrexone in detoxified, formerly opioid-dependent individuals failed to identify any single, serious untoward risk of naltrexone use, placebo-controlled studies employing up to 5-fold higher doses of naltrexone hydrochloride (up to 300 mg/day) than that recommended for use in opiate receptor blockade have shown that naltrexone causes hepatocellular injury in a substantial proportion of patients exposed at higher doses.

Aside from this finding, and the risk of precipitated opioid withdrawal, available evidence does not incriminate naltrexone, used at any dose, as a cause of any other serious adverse reaction for the patient who is "opioid free." It is critical to recognize that naltrexone can precipitate or exacerbate abstinence signs and symptoms in any individual who is not completely free of exogenous opioids.

Patients with addictive disorders, especially opioid addiction, are at risk for multiple numerous adverse events and abnormal laboratory findings, including liver function abnormalities. Data from both controlled and observational studies suggest that these abnormalities, other than the dose-related hepatotoxicity described above, are not related to the use of naltrexone.

Among opioid-free individuals, naltrexone administration at the recommended dose has not been associated with a predictable profile of serious adverse or untoward events. However, as mentioned above, among individuals using opioids, naltrexone may cause serious withdrawal reactions.

➤*Reported adverse reactions:* Naltrexone has not been shown to cause significant increases in complaints in placebo-controlled trials in patients known to be free of opioids for more than 7 to 10 days. Studies in alcoholic populations and in volunteers in clinical pharmacology studies have suggested that a small fraction of patients may experience an opioid withdrawal-like symptom complex consisting of tearfulness, mild nausea, abdominal cramps, restlessness, bone or joint pain, myalgia, and nasal symptoms. This may represent the unmasking of occult opioid use, or it may represent symptoms attributable to naltrexone. A number of alternative dosing patterns have been recommended to try to reduce the frequency of these complaints.

➤*Alcoholism:* In an open-label safety study with approximately 570 individuals with alcoholism receiving naltrexone, the following new-onset adverse reactions occurred in 2% or more of the patients: Nausea (10%), headache (7%), dizziness (4%), nervousness (4%), fatigue (4%), insomnia (3%), vomiting (3%), anxiety (2%) and somnolence (2%).

Depression, suicidal ideation, and suicidal attempts have been reported in all groups when comparing naltrexone, placebo or controls undergoing treatment for alcoholism.

Rate Ranges of New Onset Reactions

Adverse reaction	Naltrexone	Placebo
Depression	0% to 15%	0% to 17%
Suicide attempt/ideation	0% to 1%	0% to 3%

Although no causal relationship with naltrexone is suspected, physicians should be aware that treatment with naltrexone does not reduce the risk of suicide in these patients.

➤*Opioid addiction (incidence greater than 10%):* The following adverse reactions have been reported both at baseline and during the naltrexone clinical trials in narcotic addiction at an incidence rate of more than 10%: Difficulty sleeping, anxiety, nervousness, abdominal pain/cramps, nausea or vomiting, low energy, joint and muscle pain, and headache.

➤*Opioid addiction (incidence less than 10%):* Loss of appetite, diarrhea, constipation, increased thirst, increased energy, feeling down, irritability, dizziness, skin rash, delayed ejaculation, decreased potency, and chills.

➤*Opioid addiction (incidence less than 1%):*

Cardiovascular – Nosebleeds, phlebitis, edema, increased blood pressure, nonspecific ECG changes, palpitations, tachycardia.

Dermatologic – Oily skin, pruritus, acne, athlete's foot, cold sores, alopecia.

GI – Excessive gas, hemorrhoids, diarrhea, ulcer.

GU – Increased frequency of, or discomfort during, urination; increased or decreased sexual interest.

Musculoskeletal – Painful shoulders, legs or knees, tremors, twitching.

Ophthalmic – Blurred vision, burning, light sensitivity, swollen, aching, strained.

Psychiatric – Depression, paranoia, fatigue, restlessness, confusion, disorientation, hallucinations, nightmares, bad dreams.

Respiratory – Nasal congestion, itching, rhinorrhea, sneezing, sore throat, excess mucus or phlegm, sinus trouble, heavy breathing, hoarseness, cough, shortness of breath.

Special senses – Ears, "clogged", aching, tinnitus.

Miscellaneous – Increased appetite, weight loss, weight gain, yawning, somnolence, fever, dry mouth, head "pounding," inguinal pain, swollen glands, "side" pains, cold feet, "hot spells."

➤*Postmarketing experience:* Data collected from postmarketing use of naltrexone show that most events usually occur early in the course of drug therapy and are transient. It is not always possible to distinguish these occurrences from those signs and symptoms that may result from a withdrawal syndrome. Events that have been reported include anorexia, asthenia, chest pain, fatigue, headache, hot flushes, malaise, changes in blood pressure, agitation, dizziness, hyperkinesia, nausea, vomiting, tremor, abdominal pain, diarrhea, elevations in liver enzymes or bilirubin, hepatic function abnormalities or hepatitis, palpitations, myalgia, anxiety, confusion, euphoria, hallucinations, insomnia, nervousness, somnolence, abnormal thinking, dyspnea, rash, increased sweating, and vision abnormalities.

Depression, suicide, attempted suicide, and suicidal ideation have been reported in the postmarketing experience with naltrexone used in the treatment of opioid dependence. No causal relationship has been demonstrated. In the literature, endogenous opioids have been theorized to contribute to a variety of conditions. In some individuals the use of opioid antagonists has been associated with a change in baseline levels of some hypothalamic, pituitary, adrenal, or gonadal hormones. The clinical significance of such changes is not fully understood.

Adverse events, including withdrawal symptoms and death, have been reported with the use of naltrexone in ultra rapid opiate detoxification programs. The cause of death in these cases is not known.

➤*Lab test abnormalities:* With the exception of liver test abnormalities, result of laboratory tests, like adverse reaction reports, have not shown consistent patterns of abnormalities that can be attributed to treatment with naltrexone.

Idiopathic thrombocytopenic purpura was reported in 1 patient who may have been sensitized to naltrexone in a previous course of treatment with naltrexone. The condition cleared without sequelae after discontinuation of naltrexone and corticosteroid treatment.

NALTREXONE HYDROCHLORIDE — ORAL

Overdosage

➤*Symptoms:* There is limited clinical experience with naltrexone overdosage in humans. In 1 study, subjects who received 800 mg daily naltrexone for up to 1 week showed no evidence of toxicity.

➤*Treatment:* In view of the lack of actual experience in the treatment of naltrexone overdose, patients should be treated symptomatically in a closely supervised environment. Physicians should contact a poison control center for the most up-to-date information.

Patient Information

It is recommended that the prescribing physician relate the following information to patients being treated with naltrexone. You have been prescribed naltrexone as part of the comprehensive treatment for your alcoholism or drug dependence. You should carry identification to alert medical personnel to the fact that you are taking naltrexone. A naltrexone medication card may be obtained from your physician and can be used for this purpose. Carrying the identification card should help to ensure that you can obtain adequate treatment in an emergency. If you require medical treatment, be sure to tell the treating physician that you are receiving naltrexone therapy.

You should take naltrexone as directed by your physician. If you attempt to self-administer heroin or any other opiate drug, in small doses while on naltrexone, you will not perceive any effect. Most important, however, if you attempt to self-administer large doses of heroin or any other opioid (including methadone or LAAM), while on naltrexone, you may die or sustain serious injury including coma.

Naltrexone is well-tolerated in the recommended doses, but may cause liver injury when taken in excess or in people who develop liver disease from other causes. If you develop abdominal pain lasting more than a few days, white bowel movements, dark urine, or yellowing of your eyes, you should stop taking naltrexone immediately and see your doctor as soon as possible.

FLUMAZENIL

Rx	**Flumazenil** (Various, American Pharmaceutical Partners, Apotex, Baxter, Bedford)	**Injection**: 0.1 mg/mL	Parabens, NaCl, EDTA. In 5 and 10 mL vials.
Rx	**Romazicon** (Hoffman-La Roche)		Parabens, EDTA. In 5 and 10 mL vials.

FLUMAZENIL — INJECTION

WARNING

The use of flumazenil has been associated with the occurrence of seizures.

These are most frequent in patients who have been on benzodiazepines for long-term sedation or in overdose cases where patients are showing signs of serious cyclic antidepressant overdose.

Practitioners should individualize the dosage of flumazenil and be prepared to manage seizures.

Indications

➤*Adult patients:* For the complete or partial reversal of the sedative effects of benzodiazepines in cases where general anesthesia has been induced or maintained with benzodiazepines, where sedation has been produced with benzodiazepines for diagnostic and therapeutic procedures, and for the management of benzodiazepine overdose.

➤*Pediatric patients (1 to 17 years of age):* Flumazenil is indicated for the reversal of conscious sedation induced with benzodiazepines.

Administration and Dosage

➤*Approved by the FDA:* December 20, 1991.

➤*Administration:* Flumazenil is recommended for intravenous use only. It is compatible with 5% dextrose in water, lactated ringer's and normal saline solutions. If flumazenil is drawn into a syringe or mixed with any of these solutions, it should be discarded after 24 hours. For optimum sterility, flumazenil should remain in the vial until just before use. As with all parenteral drug products, flumazenil should be inspected visually for particulate matter and discoloration prior to administration, whenever solution and container permit.

To minimize the likelihood of pain at the injection site, flumazenil should be administered through a freely running intravenous infusion into a large vein.

➤*Reversal of conscious sedation:*

Adult patients – For the reversal of the sedative effects of benzodiazepines administered for conscious sedation, the recommended initial dose of flumazenil is 0.2 mg (2 mL) administered intravenously over 15 seconds. If the desired level of consciousness is not obtained after waiting an additional 45 seconds, a further dose of 0.2 mg (2 mL) can be injected and repeated at 60-second intervals where necessary (up to a maximum of 4 additional times) to a maximum total dose of 1 mg (10 mL). The dosage should be individualized based on the patient's response, with most patients responding to doses of 0.6 mg to 1 mg (see Individualization of dosage).

In the event of resedation, repeated dose may be administered at 20-minute intervals as needed. For repeat treatment, no more than 1 mg (given as 0.2 mg/min) should be administered at any one time, and no more than 3 mg should be given in any 1 hour.

It is recommended that flumazenil be administered as the series of small injections described (not as a single bolus injection) to allow the practitioner to control the reversal of sedation to the approximate endpoint desired and to minimize the possibility of adverse effects (see Individualization of dosage).

Pediatric patients – For the reversal of the sedative effects of benzodiazepines administered for conscious sedation in pediatric patients, the recommended initial dose is 0.01 mg/kg (up to 0.2 mg) administered intravenously over 15 seconds. If the desired level of consciousness is not obtained after waiting an additional 45 seconds, further injections of 0.01 mg/kg (up to 0.2 mg) can be administered and repeated at 60-second intervals where necessary (up to a maximum of 4 additional times) to a maximum total dose of 0.05 mg/kg or 1 mg, whichever is lower. The dose should be individualized based on the patient's response. The mean total dose administered in the pediatric clinical trial of flumazenil was 0.65 mg (range, 0.08 mg to 1 mg). Approximately one-half of patients required the maximum of 5 injections.

Resedation occurred in 7 of 60 pediatric patients who were fully alert 10 minutes after the start of flumazenil administration. The safety and efficacy of repeated flumazenil administration in pediatric patients experiencing resedation have not been established.

It is recommended that flumazenil be administered as the series of small injections described (not as a single bolus injection) to allow the practitioner to control the reversal of sedation to the approximate endpoint desired and to minimize the possibility of adverse effects (see Individualization of dosage).

The safety and efficacy of flumazenil in the reversal of conscious sedation in pediatric patients below the age of 1 year have not been established.

➤*Reversal of general anesthesia in adult patients:* For the reversal of the sedative effects of benzodiazepines administered for general anesthesia, the recommended initial dose of flumazenil is 0.2 mg (2 mL) administered intravenously over 15 seconds. If the desired level of consciousness is not obtained after waiting an additional 45 seconds, a further dose of 0.2 mg (2 mL) can be injected and repeated at 60-second intervals where necessary (up to a maximum of 4 additional times) to a maximum total dose of 1 mg (10 mL). The dosage should be individualized based on the patient's response, with most patients responding to doses of 0.6 mg to 1 mg.

In the event of resedation, repeated doses may be administered at 20-minute intervals as needed. For repeat treatment, no more than 1 mg (given as 0.2 mg/min) should be administered at any one time, and no more than 3 mg should be given in any 1 hour.

It is recommended that flumazenil be administered as the series of small injections described (not as a single bolus injection) to allow the practitioner to control the reversal of sedation to the approximate endpoint desired and to minimize the possibility of adverse effects.

➤*Management of suspected benzodiazepine overdose in adult patients:* For initial management of a known or suspected benzodiazepine overdose, the recommended initial dose of flumazenil is 0.2 mg (2 mL) administered intravenously over 30 seconds. If the desired level of consciousness is not obtained after waiting 30 seconds, a further dose of 0.3 mg (3 mL) can be administered over another 30 seconds. Further doses of 0.5 mg (5 mL) can be administered over 30 seconds at 1-minute intervals up to a cumulative dose of 3 mg.

Do not rush the administration of flumazenil. Patients should have a secure airway and intravenous access before administration of the drug and be awakened gradually.

Most patients with a benzodiazepine overdose will respond to a cumulative dose of 1 mg to 3 mg of flumazenil, and doses beyond 3 mg do not reliably produce additional effects. On rare occasions, patients with a partial response at 3 mg may require additional titration up to a total dose of 5 mg (administered slowly in the same manner).

If a patient has not responded 5 minutes after receiving a cumulative dose of 5 mg of flumazenil, the major cause of sedation is likely not to be due to benzodiazepines, and additional flumazenil is likely to have no effect.

In the event of resedation, repeated doses may be given at 20-minute intervals if needed. For repeat treatment, no more than 1 mg (given as 0.5 mg/min) should be given at any one time and no more than 3 mg should be given in any one hour.

➤*Individualization of dosage:*

General principles – The serious adverse effects of flumazenil are related to the reversal of benzodiazepine effects. Using more than the minimally effective dose of flumazenil is tolerated by most patients but may complicate the management of patients who are physically dependent on benzodiazepines or patients who are depending on benzodiazepines for therapeutic effect (such as suppression of seizures in cyclic antidepressant overdose).

In high-risk patients, it is important to administer the smallest amount of flumazenil that is effective. The 1-minute wait between individual doses in the dose-titration recommended for general clinical populations may be too short for high-risk patients. This is because it takes 6 to 10 minutes for any

FLUMAZENIL — INJECTION

single dose of flumazenil to reach full effects. Practitioners should slow the rate of administration of flumazenil administered to high-risk patients as recommended below.

Anesthesia and conscious sedation in adult patients – Flumazenil is well tolerated at the recommended doses in individuals who have no tolerance to (or dependence on) benzodiazepines. The recommended doses and titration rates in anesthesia and conscious sedation (0.2 mg to 1 mg given at 0.2 mg/min) are well tolerated in patients receiving the drug for reversal of a single benzodiazepine exposure in most clinical settings. The major risk will be resedation because the duration of effect of a long-acting (or large dose of a short-acting) benzodiazepine may exceed that of flumazenil. Resedation may be treated by giving a repeat dose at no less than 20-minute intervals. For repeat treatment, no more than 1 mg (at 0.2 mg/min doses) should be given at any one time and no more than 3 mg should be given in any 1 hour.

Overdose in adult patients – The risk of confusion, agitation, emotional lability and perceptual distortion with the doses recommended in patients with benzodiazepine overdose (3 mg to 5 mg administered as 0.5 mg/min) may be greater than that expected with lower doses and slower administration. The recommended doses represent a compromise between desirable slow awakening and the need for prompt response and a persistent effect in the overdose situation. If circumstances permit, the physician may elect to use the 0.2 mg/min titration rate to slowly awaken the patient over 5 to 10 minutes, which may help to reduce signs and symptoms on emergence.

Flumazenil has no effect in cases where benzodiazepines are not responsible for sedation. Once doses of 3 mg to 5 mg have been reached without clinical response, additional flumazenil is likely to have no effect.

Patients tolerant to benzodiazepines – Flumazenil may cause benzodiazepine withdrawal symptoms in individuals who have been taking benzodiazepines long enough to have some degree of tolerance. Patients who had been taking benzodiazepines prior to entry into the flumazenil trials who were given flumazenil in doses over 1 mg, experienced withdrawal-like events 2 to 5 times more frequently than patients who received less than 1 mg.

In patients who may have tolerance to benzodiazepines, as indicated by clinical history or by the need for larger than usual doses of benzodiazepines, slower titration rates of 0.1 mg/min and lower total doses may help reduce the frequency of emergent confusion and agitation. In such cases, special care must be taken to monitor the patients for resedation because of the lower doses of flumazenil used.

Patients physically dependent on benzodiazepines – Flumazenil is known to precipitate withdrawal seizures in patients who are physically dependent on benzodiazepines, even if such dependence was established in a relatively few days of high dose sedation in intensive care unit (ICU) environments. The risk of either seizures or resedation in such cases is high and patients have experienced seizures before regaining consciousness. Flumazenil should be used in such settings with extreme caution, since the use of flumazenil in this situation has not been studied and no information as to dose and rate of titration is available. Flumazenil should be used in such patients only if the potential benefits of using the drug outweigh the risks of precipitated seizures. Physicians are directed to the scientific literature for the most current information in this area.

➤*Storage/Stability:* Store at 25°C (77°F); excursions permitted to 15° to 30°C (59° to 86°F).

Actions

➤*Pharmacology:* Flumazenil, an imidazobenzodiazepine derivative, antagonizes the actions of benzodiazepines on the central nervous system. Flumazenil competitively inhibits the activity at the benzodiazepine recognition site on the GABA/benzodiazepine receptor complex. Flumazenil is a weak partial agonist in some animal models of activity, but has little or no agonist activity in man.

Flumazenil does not antagonize the central nervous system effects of drugs affecting GABA-ergic neurons by means other than the benzodiazepine receptor (including ethanol, barbiturates, or general anesthetics) and does not reverse the effects of opioids.

In animals pretreated with high doses of benzodiazepines over several weeks, flumazenil elicited symptoms of benzodiazepine withdrawal, including seizures. A similar effect was seen in adult human subjects.

Intravenous flumazenil has been shown to antagonize sedation, impairment of recall, psychomotor impairment and ventilatory depression produced by benzodiazepines in healthy human volunteers.

The duration and degree of reversal of benzodiazepine effects are related to the dose and plasma concentrations of flumazenil.

Generally, doses of approximately 0.1 mg to 0.2 mg (corresponding to peak plasma levels of 3 to 6 ng/mL) produce partial antagonism, whereas higher doses of 0.4 to 1 mg (peak plasma levels of 12 to 28 ng/mL) usually produce complete antagonism in patients who have received the usual sedating doses of benzodiazepines. The onset of reversal is usually evident within 1 to 2 minutes after the injection is completed. Eighty percent (80%) response will be reached within 3 minutes, with the peak effect occurring at 6 to 10 minutes. The duration and degree of reversal are related to the plasma concentration of the sedating benzodiazepine as well as the dose of flumazenil given.

In healthy volunteers, flumazenil did not alter intraocular pressure when given alone and reversed the decrease in intraocular pressure seen after administration of midazolam.

➤*Pharmacokinetics:*

Absorption – After IV administration, plasma concentrations of flumazenil follow a 2-exponential decay model. The pharmacokinetics of flumazenil are dose-proportional up to 100 mg.

Distribution – Flumazenil is extensively distributed in the extravascular space with an initial distribution half-life of 4 to 11 minutes and a terminal half-life of 40 to 80 minutes. Peak concentrations of flumazenil are proportional to dose, with an apparent initial volume of distribution of 0.5 L/kg. The volume of distribution at steady-state is 0.9 to 1.1 L/kg. Flumazenil is a weak lipophilic base. Protein binding is approximately 50% and the drug shows no preferential partitioning into red blood cells. Albumin accounts for two thirds of plasma protein binding.

Metabolism – Flumazenil is completely (99%) metabolized. Very little unchanged flumazenil (less than 1%) is found in the urine. The major metabolites of flumazenil identified in urine are the de-ethylated free acid and its glucuronide conjugate. In preclinical studies there was no evidence of pharmacologic activity exhibited by the de-ethylated free acid.

Excretion – Elimination of radiolabeled drug is essentially complete within 72 hours, with 90% to 95% of the radioactivity appearing in urine and 5% to 10% in the feces. Clearance of flumazenil occurs primarily by hepatic metabolism and is dependent on hepatic blood flow. In pharmacokinetic studies of healthy volunteers, total clearance ranged from 0.8 to 1 L/hr/kg.

Special populations –

Children: The pharmacokinetics of flumazenil have been evaluated in 29 pediatric patients ranging in age from 1 to 17 years who had undergone minor surgical procedures. The average doses administered were 0.53 mg (0.044 mg/kg) in patients aged 1 to 5 years, 0.63 mg (0.02 mg/kg) in patients aged 6 to 12 years, and 0.8 mg (0.014 mg/kg) in patients aged 13 to 17 years. Compared to adults, the elimination half-life in pediatric patients was more variable, averaging 40 minutes (range: 20 to 75 minutes). Clearance and volume of distribution, normalized for body weight, were in the same range as those seen in adults, although more variability was seen in the pediatric patients.

Liver function impairment: For patients with moderate liver dysfunction, their mean total clearance is decreased to 40% to 60% and in patients with severe liver dysfunction, it is decreased to 25% of normal value, compared with age-matched healthy subjects. This results in a prolongation of the half-life to 1.3 hours in patients with moderate hepatic impairment and 2.4 hours in severely impaired patients. Caution should be exercised with initial and/or repeated dosing to patients with liver disease.

Food effects – Ingestion of food during an intravenous infusion of the drug results in a 50% increase in clearance, most likely due to the increased hepatic blood flow that accompanies a meal.

Pharmacokinetic parameters –

Pharmacokinetic Parameters Following a 5-Minute Infusion of a Total of 1 mg of Flumazenil Mean (Coefficient of Variation, Range)		
C_{max}(ng/mL)	24	(38%, 11 to 43)
AUC (ng•h/mL)	15	(22%, 10 to 22)
V_{ss} (L/kg)	1	(24%, 0.8 to 1.6)
Cl (L/h/kg	1	(20%, 0.7 to 1.4)
Half-life (min)	54	(21%, 41 to 79)

Contraindications

Hypersensitivity to flumazenil or benzodiazepines; patients who have been given a benzodiazepine for control of a potentially life-threatening condition (eg, control of intracranial pressure or status epilepticus); patients who are showing signs of serious cyclic antidepressant overdose.

Warnings

➤*Risk of seizures:* The reversal of benzodiazepine effects may be associated with the onset of seizures in certain high-risk populations. Possible risk factors for seizures include concurrent major sedative-hypnotic drug withdrawal, recent therapy with repeated doses of parenteral benzodiazepines, myoclonic jerking or seizure activity prior to flumazenil administration in overdose cases, or concurrent cyclic antidepressant poisoning.

Flumazenil is not recommended in cases of serious cyclic antidepressant poisoning, as manifested by motor abnormalities (twitching, rigidity, focal seizure), dysrhythmia (wide QRS, ventricular dysrhythmia, heart block), anticholinergic signs (mydriasis, dry mucosa, hypoperistalsis), and cardiovascular collapse at presentation. In such cases flumazenil should be withheld and the patient should be allowed to remain sedated (with ventilatory and circulatory support as needed) until the signs of antidepressant toxicity have subsided. Treatment with flumazenil has no known benefit to the seriously ill mixed-overdose patient other than reversing sedation and should not be used in cases where seizures (from any cause) are likely.

Most convulsions associated with flumazenil administration require treatment and have been successfully managed with benzodiazepines, phenytoin or barbiturates. Because of the presence of flumazenil, higher than usual doses of benzodiazepines may be required.

➤*Hypoventilation:* Patients who have received flumazenil for the reversal of benzodiazepine effects (after conscious sedation or general anesthesia) should be monitored for resedation, respiratory depression, or other residual benzodiazepine effects for an appropriate period (up to 120 minutes) based on the dose and duration of effect of the benzodiazepine employed.

This is because flumazenil has not been established in patients as an effective treatment for hypoventilation due to benzodiazepine administration. In healthy male volunteers, flumazenil is capable of reversing benzodiazepine-

FLUMAZENIL — INJECTION

induced depression of the ventilatory responses to hypercapnia and hypoxia after a benzodiazepine alone. However, such depression may recur because the ventilatory effects of typical doses of flumazenil (1 mg or less) may wear off before the effects of many benzodiazepines. The effects of flumazenil on ventilatory response following sedation with a benzodiazepine in combination with an opioid are inconsistent and have not been adequately studied. The availability of flumazenil does not diminish the need for prompt detection of hypoventilation and the ability to effectively intervene by establishing an airway and assisting ventilation.

Overdose cases should always be monitored for resedation until the patients are stable and resedation is unlikely.

➤*Hepatic function impairment:* The clearance of flumazenil is reduced to 40% to 60% of healthy in patients with mild to moderate hepatic disease and to 25% of normal in patients with severe hepatic dysfunction. While the dose of flumazenil used for initial reversal of benzodiazepine effects is not affected, repeat doses of the drug in liver disease should be reduced in size or frequency.

➤*Mutagenesis:* No evidence for mutagenicity was noted in the Ames test using 5 different tester strains. Assays for mutagenic potential in *S. cerevisiae* D7 and in Chinese hamster cells were considered to be negative as were blastogenesis assays in vitro in peripheral human lymphocytes and in vivo in a mouse micronucleus assay. Flumazenil caused a slight increase in unscheduled DNA synthesis in rat hepatocyte culture at concentrations that were also cytotoxic; no increase in DNA repair was observed in male mouse germ cells in an in vivo DNA repair assay.

➤*Elderly:* Of the total number of subjects in clinical studies of flumazenil, 248 were 65 years and over. No overall differences in safety or effectiveness were observed between these subjects and younger subjects. Other reported clinical experience has not identified differences in responses between the elderly and younger patients, but greater sensitivity of some older individuals cannot be ruled out.

The pharmacokinetics of flumazenil have been studied in the elderly and are not significantly different from younger patients. Several studies of flumazenil in subjects over the age of 65 years and 1 study in subjects over the age of 80 years suggest that while the doses of benzodiazepine used to induce sedation should be reduced, ordinary doses of flumazenil may be used for reversal.

➤*Pregnancy: Category C.* There are no adequate and well-controlled studies of the use of flumazenil in pregnant women. Flumazenil should be used during pregnancy only if the potential benefit justifies the potential risk to the fetus.

Teratogenic –

In rabbits, embryocidal effects (as evidenced by increased preimplantation and postimplantation losses) were observed at 50 mg/kg or 200 times the human exposure from a maximum recommended intravenous dose of 5 mg. The no-effect dose of 15 mg/kg in rabbits represents 60 times the human exposure.

Nonteratogenic – An animal reproduction study was conducted in rats at oral dosages of 5, 25, and 125 mg/kg/day of flumazenil. Pup survival was decreased during the lactating period, pup liver weight at weaning was increased for the high-dose group (125 mg/kg/day) and incisor eruption and ear opening in the offspring were delayed; the delay in ear opening was associated with a delay in the appearance of the auditory startle response. No treatment-related adverse effects were noted for the other dose groups. Based on the available data from AUC, the effect level (125 mg/kg) represents 120 times the human exposure from 5 mg, the maximum recommended intravenous dose in humans. The no-effect level represents 24 times the human exposure from an intravenous dose of 5 mg.

Labor and delivery – The use of flumazenil to reverse the effects of benzodiazepines used during labor and delivery is not recommended because the effects of the drug in the newborn are unknown.

➤*Lactation:* Caution should be exercised when deciding to administer flumazenil to a breast-feeding woman because it is not known whether flumazenil is excreted in human milk.

➤*Children:* The safety and efficacy of flumazenil have been established in pediatric patients 1 year of age and older. Use of flumazenil in this age group is supported by evidence from adequate and well-controlled studies of flumazenil in adults with additional data from uncontrolled pediatric studies including 1 open-label trial.

The use of flumazenil to reverse the effects of benzodiazepines used for conscious sedation was evaluated in 1 uncontrolled clinical trial involving 107 pediatric patients between the ages of 1 and 17 years. At the doses used, flumazenil's safety was established in this population. Patients received up to 5 injections of 0.01 mg/kg flumazenil up to a maximum total dose of 1 mg at a rate not exceeding 0.2 mg/min.

Of 60 patients who were fully alert at 10 minutes, 7 experienced resedation. Resedation occurred between 19 and 50 minutes after the start of flumazenil administration. None of the patients experienced a return to the baseline level of sedation. All 7 patients were between the ages of 1 and 5 years. The types and frequency of adverse events noted in these pediatric patients were similar to those previously documented in clinical trials with flumazenil to reverse conscious sedation in adults. No patient experienced a serious adverse event attributable to flumazenil.

The safety and efficacy of flumazenil in the reversal of conscious sedation in pediatric patients below the age of 1 year have not been established.

The safety and efficacy of flumazenil have not been established in pediatric patients for reversal of the sedative effects of benzodiazepines used for induction of general anesthesia, for the management of overdose, or for the resuscitation of the newborn, as no well-controlled clinical studies have been performed to determine the risks, benefits, and dosages to be used. However, published anecdotal reports discussing the use of flumazenil in pediatric patients for these indications have reported similar safety profiles and dosing guidelines to those described for the reversal of conscious sedation.

The risks identified in the adult population with flumazenil use also apply to pediatric patients.

Precautions

➤*Return of sedation:* Flumazenil may be expected to improve the alertness of patients recovering from a procedure involving sedation or anesthesia with benzodiazepines, but should not be substituted for an adequate period of postprocedure monitoring. The availability of flumazenil does not reduce the risks associated with the use of large doses of benzodiazepines for sedation.

Patients should be monitored for resedation, respiratory depression or other persistent or recurrent agonist effects for an adequate period of time after administration of flumazenil.

Resedation is least likely in cases where flumazenil is administered to reverse a low dose of a short-acting benzodiazepine (less than 10 mg midazolam). It is most likely in cases where a large single or cumulative dose of a benzodiazepine has been given in the course of a long procedure along with neuromuscular blocking agents and multiple anesthetic agents.

Profound resedation was observed in 1% to 3% of adult patients in the clinical studies. In clinical situations where resedation must be prevented in adult patients, physicians may wish to repeat the initial dose (up to 1 mg of flumazenil given at 0.2 mg/min) at 30 minutes and possibly again at 60 minutes. This dosage schedule, although not studied in clinical trials, was effective in preventing resedation in a pharmacologic study in normal volunteers.

The use of flumazenil to reverse the effects of benzodiazepines used for conscious sedation has been evaluated in 1 open-label clinical trial involving 107 pediatric patients between the ages of 1 and 17 years. This study suggested that pediatric patients who have become fully awake following treatment with flumazenil may experience a recurrence of sedation, especially younger patients (ages 1 to 5). Resedation was experienced in 7 of 60 patients who were fully alert 10 minutes after the start of flumazenil administration. No patient experienced a return to the baseline level of sedation. Mean time to resedation was 25 minutes (range, 19 to 50 minutes). The safety and effectiveness of repeated flumazenil administration in pediatric patients experiencing resedation have not been established.

➤*Use in the ICU:* Flumazenil should be used with caution in the ICU because of the increased risk of unrecognized benzodiazepine dependence in such settings. Flumazenil may produce convulsions in patients physically dependent on benzodiazepines.

Administration of flumazenil to diagnose benzodiazepine-induced sedation in the ICU is not recommended due to the risk of adverse events as described above. In addition, the prognostic significance of a patient's failure to respond to flumazenil in cases confounded by metabolic disorder, traumatic injury, drugs other than benzodiazepines, or any other reasons not associated with benzodiazepine receptor occupancy is unknown.

➤*Use in overdose:* Flumazenil is intended as an adjunct to, not as a substitute for, proper management of airway, assisted breathing, circulatory access and support, internal decontamination by lavage and charcoal, and adequate clinical evaluation.

Necessary measures should be instituted to secure airway, ventilation and intravenous access prior to administering flumazenil. Upon arousal, patients may attempt to withdraw endotracheal tubes or intravenous lines as the result of confusion and agitation following awakening.

➤*Neuromuscular blocking agents:* Flumazenil should not be used until the effects of neuromuscular blockade have been fully reversed.

➤*Psychiatric patients:* Flumazenil has been reported to provoke panic attacks in patients with a history of panic disorder.

➤*Pain on injection:* To minimize the likelihood of pain or inflammation at the injection site, flumazenil should be administered through a freely flowing intravenous infusion into a large vein. Local irritation may occur following extravasation into perivascular tissues.

➤*Respiratory disease:* The primary treatment of patients with serious lung disease who experience serious respiratory depression due to benzodiazepines should be appropriate ventilatory support rather than the administration of flumazenil. Flumazenil is capable of partially reversing benzodiazepine-induced alterations in ventilatory drive in healthy volunteers, but has not been shown to be clinically effective.

➤*Cardiovascular disease:* Flumazenil did not increase the work of the heart when used to reverse benzodiazepines in cardiac patients when given at a rate of 0.1 mg/min in total doses of less than 0.5 mg in studies reported in the clinical literature. Flumazenil alone had no significant effects on cardiovascular parameters when administered to patients with stable ischemic heart disease.

➤*Ambulatory patients:* The effects of flumazenil may wear off before a long-acting benzodiazepine is completely cleared from the body. In general, if a patient shows no signs of sedation within 2 hours after a 1 mg dose of flumazenil, serious resedation at a later time is unlikely. An adequate period of observation must be provided for any patient in whom either long-acting benzodiazepines (such as diazepam) or large doses of short-acting benzodiazepines (such as greater than 10 mg of midazolam) have been used.

➤*Head injury:* Flumazenil should be used with caution in patients with head injury as it may be capable of precipitating convulsions or altering

FLUMAZENIL — INJECTION

cerebral blood flow in patients receiving benzodiazepines. It should be used only by practitioners prepared to manage such complications should they occur.

➤*Use in drug- and alcohol-dependent patients:* Flumazenil should be used with caution in patients with alcoholism and other drug dependencies due to the increased frequency of benzodiazepine tolerance and dependence observed in these patient populations.

Flumazenil is not recommended either as a treatment for benzodiazepine dependence or for the management of protracted benzodiazepine abstinence syndromes, as such use has not been studied.

The administration of flumazenil can precipitate benzodiazepine withdrawal in animals and man. This has been seen in healthy volunteers treated with therapeutic doses of oral lorazepam for up to 2 weeks who exhibited effects such as hot flushes, agitation and tremor when treated with cumulative doses of up to 3 mg doses of flumazenil.

Similar adverse experiences suggestive of flumazenil precipitation of benzodiazepine withdrawal have occurred in some adult patients in clinical trials. Such patients had a short-lived syndrome characterized by dizziness, mild confusion, emotional lability, agitation (with signs and symptoms of anxiety), and mild sensory distortions. This response was dose-related, most common at doses above 1 mg, rarely required treatment other than reassurance and was usually short lived. When required (5 to 10 cases), these patients were successfully treated with usual doses of a barbiturate, a benzodiazepine, or other sedative drug.

Practitioners should assume that flumazenil administration may trigger dose-dependent withdrawal syndromes in patients with established physical dependence on benzodiazepines and may complicate the management of withdrawal syndromes for alcohol, barbiturates, and cross-tolerant sedatives.

➤*Drug abuse and dependence:* Flumazenil acts as a benzodiazepine antagonist, blocks the effects of benzodiazepines in animals and man, antagonizes benzodiazepine reinforcement in animal models, produces dysphoria in healthy subjects, and has had no reported abuse in foreign marketing. Although flumazenil has a benzodiazepine-like structure it does not act as a benzodiazepine agonist in man and is not a controlled substance.

Drug Interactions

Interaction with central nervous system depressants other than benzodiazepines has not been specifically studied; however, no deleterious interactions were seen when flumazenil was administered after narcotics, inhalational anesthetics, muscle relaxants and muscle relaxant antagonists administered in conjunction with sedation or anesthesia. Particular caution is necessary when using flumazenil in cases of mixed drug overdose, since the toxic effects (such as convulsions and cardiac dysrhythmias) of other drugs taken in overdose (especially cyclic antidepressants) may emerge with the reversal of the benzodiazepine effect by flumazenil.

The use of flumazenil is not recommended in epileptic patients who have been receiving benzodiazepine treatment for a prolonged period. Although flumazenil exerts a slight intrinsic anticonvulsant effect, its abrupt suppression of the protective effect of a benzodiazepine agonist can give rise to convulsions in epileptic patients.

Flumazenil blocks the central effects of benzodiazepines by competitive interaction at the receptor level. The effects of nonbenzodiazepine agonists at benzodiazepine receptors, such as zopiclone, triazolopyridazines and others, are also blocked by flumazenil.

Adverse Reactions

Deaths have occurred in patients who received flumazenil in a variety of clinical settings. The majority of deaths occurred in patients with serious underlying disease or in patients who had ingested large amounts of nonbenzodiazepine drugs (usually cyclic antidepressants), as part of an overdose.

Serious adverse events have occurred in all clinical settings, and convulsions are the most common serious adverse events reported. Flumazenil administration has been associated with the onset of convulsions in patients who are relying on benzodiazepine effects to control seizures, are physically dependent on benzodiazepines, or who have ingested large doses of other drugs.

Two of the 446 patients who received flumazenil in controlled clinical trials for the management of a benzodiazepine overdose had cardiac dysrhythmias (1 ventricular tachycardia, 1 junctional tachycardia).

➤*Adverse events in clinical studies:* The following adverse reactions were considered to be related to flumazenil administration (both alone and for the reversal of benzodiazepine effects) and were reported in studies involving 1,875 individuals who received flumazenil in controlled trials. Adverse events most frequently associated with flumazenil alone were limited to dizziness, injection site pain, increased sweating, headache, and abnormal or blurred vision (3% to 9%). Observed percentage reported if greater than 9%.

Cardiovascular – Cutaneous vasodilation (sweating, flushing, hot flushes) (1% to 3%).

GI – Nausea and vomiting (11%).

CNS – Dizziness (vertigo, ataxia) (10%); agitation (anxiety, nervousness, dry mouth, tremor, palpitations, insomnia, dyspnea, hyperventilation) (3% to 9%), and emotional lability (crying abnormal, depersonalization, euphoria, increased tears, depression, dysphoria, paranoia) (1% to 3%).

Special senses – Abnormal vision (visual field defect, diplopia) and paresthesia (sensation abnormal, hypoesthesia).

Miscellaneous – Injection site pain (3% to 9%); fatigue (asthenia, malaise), headache, and injection site reaction (thrombophlebitis, skin abnormality, rash) (1% to 3%).

➤*Less than 1% incidence:* The following adverse events were observed infrequently (less than 1%) in the clinical studies, but were judged as probably related to flumazenil administration and/or reversal of benzodiazepine effects.

CNS – Confusion (difficulty concentrating, delirium), convulsions, and somnolence (stupor).

Special senses – Abnormal hearing (transient hearing impairment, hyperacusis, tinnitus).

➤*Less than 1% incidence; unknown relationship to flumazenil:* The following adverse events occurred with frequencies less than 1% in the clinical trials. Their relationship to flumazenil administration is unknown, but they are included as alerting information for the physician.

Not included in this list is operative site pain that occurred with the same frequency in patients receiving placebo as in patients receiving flumazenil for reversal of sedation following a surgical procedure.

Cardiovascular – Arrhythmia (atrial, nodal, ventricular extrasystoles), bradycardia, tachycardia, hypertension and chest pain.

CNS – Speech disorder (dysphonia, thick tongue).

Miscellaneous – Rigors, shivering, hiccup.

➤*Additional adverse reactions reported during postmarketing experience:* The following events have been reported during postapproval use of flumazenil.

CNS – Fear, panic attacks in patients with a history of panic disorders.

Miscellaneous – Withdrawal symptoms may occur following rapid injection of flumazenil in patients with long-term exposure to benzodiazepines.

Overdosage

➤*Symptoms:* Large intravenous doses of flumazenil, when administered to healthy volunteers in the absence of a benzodiazepine agonist, produced no serious adverse reactions, severe signs or symptoms, or clinically significant laboratory test abnormalities. In clinical studies, most adverse reactions to flumazenil were an extension of the pharmacologic effects of the drug in reversing benzodiazepine effects. Reversal with an excessively high dose of flumazenil may produce anxiety, agitation, increased muscle tone, hyperesthesia and possibly convulsions. Convulsions have been treated with barbiturates, benzodiazepines and phenytoin, generally with prompt resolution of the seizures.

The risk of confusion, agitation, emotional lability and perceptual distortion with the doses recommended in patients with benzodiazepine overdose (3 mg to 5 mg administered as 0.5 mg/min) may be greater than that expected with lower doses and slower administration. The recommended doses represent a compromise between desirable slow awakening and the need for prompt response and a persistent effect in the overdose situation. If circumstances permit, the physician may elect to use the 0.2 mg/min titration rate to slowly awaken the patient over 5 to 10 minutes, which may help to reduce signs and symptoms on emergence.

➤*Treatment:* Flumazenil has no effect in cases where benzodiazepines are not responsible for sedation. Once doses of 3 mg to 5 mg have been reached without clinical response, additional flumazenil is likely to have no effect.

Patient Information

Flumazenil does not consistently reverse amnesia. Patients cannot be expected to remember information told to them in the postprocedure period and instructions given to patients should be reinforced in writing or given to a responsible family member. Physicians are advised to discuss with patients or their guardians, both before surgery and at discharge, that although the patient may feel alert at the time of discharge, the effects of the benzodiazepine may recur. As a result, the patient should be instructed, preferably in writing, that their memory and judgment may be impaired and specifically advised about the following:

1.) Not to engage in any activities requiring complete alertness, and not to operate hazardous machinery or a motor vehicle during the first 24 hours after discharge, and it is certain no residual sedative effects of the benzodiazepine remain.
2.) Not to take any alcohol or nonprescription drugs during the first 24 hours after flumazenil administration or if the effects of the benzodiazepine persist.

PHYSOSTIGMINE SALICYLATE

Rx	**Physostigmine Salicylate** (Taylor)	**Injection:** 1 mg/mL	With 2% benzyl alcohol and 0.1% sodium metabisulfite. In 2 mL ampules.
Rx	**Antilirium** (Forest)		With 2% benzyl alcohol and 0.1% sodium bisulfite. In 2 mL ampules.

PHYSOSTIGMINE SALICYLATE — INJECTION

Indications

➤*Anticholinergic toxicity:* To reverse the effect upon the CNS, caused by clinical or toxic dosages of drugs (including tricyclic antidepressants) capable of producing the anticholinergic syndrome.

➤*Unlabeled uses:* Physostigmine has been used to treat delirium tremens and Alzheimer disease. It may also antagonize diazepam's CNS-depressant effects.

Administration and Dosage

➤*Postanesthesia care:* Administer 0.5 to 1 mg intramuscularly or intravenously. Intravenous administration should be at a slow controlled rate of not more than 1 mg per minute. Dosage may be repealed at intervals of 10 to 30 minutes if desired patient response is not obtained.

➤*Anticholinergic toxicity:* Administer 2 mg intramuscularly or intravenously at slow controlled rate (see above). Dosage may be repeated if life-threatening signs, such as arrhythmia, convulsions or coma occurs.

➤*Pediatric dosage:* Recommended dosage is 0.02 mg/kg, intramuscularly or by slow intravenous injection, no more than 0.5 mg/minute. If the toxic effects persist, and there is no sign of cholinergic effects, the dosage may be repeated at 5 to 10 minute intervals until a therapeutic effect is obtained or a maximum of 2 mg dosage is attained.

In all cases of poisoning, the usual supportive measures should be undertaken.

➤*Storage/Stability:* Store at controlled room temperature 15° to 25°C (59° to 77°F).

Actions

➤*Pharmacology:* Physostigmine salicylate injection is a reversible anticholinesterase which effectively increases the concentration of acetylcholine at the sites of cholinergic transmission. The action of acetylcholine is normally very transient because of its hydrolysis by the enzyme, acetylcholinesterase. Physostigmine salicylate injection inhibits the destructive action of acetylcholinesterase and thereby prolongs and exaggerates the effect of the acetylcholine.

Physostigmine salicylate injection can reverse both central and peripheral anticholinergia. The anticholinergic syndrome has both central and peripheral signs and symptoms. Central toxic effects include anxiety, delirium, disorientation, hallucinations, hyperactivity and seizures. Severe poisoning may produce coma, medullary paralysis and death. Peripheral toxicity is characterized by tachycardia, hyperpyrexia, mydriasis, vasodilation, urinary retention, diminution of GI motility, decrease of secretion in salivary and sweat glands, and loss of secretions in the pharynx, bronchi, and nasal passages.

➤*Pharmacokinetics:*

Absorption – Physostigmine salicylate injection contains a tertiary amine and easily penetrates the blood brain barrier, while an anticholinesterase, such as neostigmine, which has a quaternary ammonium ion is not capable of crossing the barrier. Dramatic reversal of the effects of anticholinergic symptoms can be expected in minutes after the intravenous administration of physostigmine salicylate injection, if the diagnosis is correct and the patient has not suffered anoxia or other insult. The duration of action of physostigmine salicylate injection is relatively short, approximately 45 to 60 minutes.

Metabolism/Excretion – Physostigmine is rapidly hydrolyzed by cholinesterase. Plasma half-life is approximately 1 to 2 hours.

Contraindications

Physostigmine salicylate injection should not be used in the presence of asthma, gangrene, diabetes, cardiovascular disease, mechanical obstruction of the intestine or urogenital tract or any vagotonic state, and in patients receiving choline esters or depolarizing neuromuscular blocking agents (decamethonium, succinylcholine).

For postanesthesia, the concomitant use of atropine with physostigmine salicylate is not recommended, because the atropine antagonizes the action of physostigmine.

Warnings

➤*Discontinue drug:* If excessive symptoms of salivation, emesis, urination and defecation occur, terminate the use of physostigmine salicylate injection. If excessive sweating or nausea occur, reduce the dosage.

➤*Administration rate:* Intravenous administration should be at a slow, controlled rate, no more than 1 mg per minute. Rapid administration can cause bradycardia, hypersalivation leading to respiratory difficulties and possible convulsions.

➤*Cholinergic crisis:* An overdose of physostigmine salicylate injection can cause a cholinergic crisis.

➤*Hypersensitivity reactions:* Because of the possibility of hypersensitivity in an occasional patient, atropine sulfate injection should always be at hand because it is an antagonist and antidote for physostigmine.

➤*Pregnancy:* *Category C.* Transient muscular weakness has been noted in neonates whose mothers were treated with other cholinesterase inhibitors for myasthenia gravis.

Safe use in pregnancy has not been established; therefore, use in pregnant women or women who may become pregnant requires that possible benefits be weighed against possible hazards to the mother and fetus.

➤*Lactation:* Safety for use has not been established; therefore, use in breastfeeding women requires that possible benefits be weighed against possible hazards to the mother and child.

➤*Children:* Reserve for life-threatening situations only.

Precautions

➤*Benzyl alcohol:* Benzyl alcohol, contained in this product as a preservative, has been associated with a fatal "gasping syndrome" in premature infants.

➤*Sulfite sensitivity:* Some of these products contain sodium-bisulfite, a sulfite that may cause allergic-type reactions including anaphylactic symptoms and life-threatening or less severe asthmatic episodes in certain susceptible people. The overall prevalence of sulfite sensitivity in the general population is unknown and probably low. Sulfite sensitivity is seen more frequently in asthmatic or atopic nonasthmatic people than in nonasthmatic people.

Adverse Reactions

Nausea, vomiting and salivation; can be offset by reducing dosage. Bradycardia and convulsions, if IV administration is too rapid.

Overdosage

➤*Symptoms:* Can cause a cholinergic crisis if overdosed.

➤*Treatment:* Appropriate antidote is atropine sulfate.

FOMEPIZOLE (4-Methylpyrazole; 4-MP)

Rx	**Antizol** (Orphan Medical)	**Injection, concentrate:** 1 g/mL	Preservative-free. In 1.5 mL vials.

FOMEPIZOLE (4-Methylpyrazole; 4-MP) — INJECTION

Indications

➤*Ethylene glycol or methanol poisoning:* As an antidote for ethylene glycol (antifreeze) and methanol poisoning or for use in suspected ethylene glycol or methanol ingestion, either alone or in combination with hemodialysis.

Administration and Dosage

➤*Treatment guidelines:* If ethylene glycol or methanol poisoning is left untreated, the natural progression of the poisoning leads to accumulation of toxic metabolites, including glycolic and oxalic acids (ethylene glycol intoxication) and formic acid (methanol intoxication). These metabolites can induce metabolic acidosis, nausea/vomiting, seizures, stupor, coma, calcium oxaluria, acute tubular necrosis, blindness, and death. The diagnosis of these poisonings may be difficult because ethylene glycol or methanol concentrations diminish in the blood as they are metabolized to their respective metabolites. Hence, frequently monitor both ethylene glycol and methanol concentrations and acid-base balance, as determined by serum electrolyte (anion gap) or arterial blood gas analysis, and use to guide treatment.

Treatment consists of blocking the formation of toxic metabolites using inhibitors of alcohol dehydrogenase, such as fomepizole, and correction of metabolic abnormalities. In patients with high ethylene glycol or methanol concentrations (at least 50 mg/dL), significant metabolic acidosis or renal failure, consider hemodialysis to remove ethylene glycol or methanol and the respective toxic metabolites of these alcohols.

Treatment with fomepizole may be discontinued when ethylene glycol or methanol concentrations are undetectable or have been reduced to less than 20 mg/dL, and the patient is asymptomatic with normal pH.

➤*Treatment:* Begin fomepizole treatment immediately upon suspicion of ethylene glycol or methanol ingestion based on patient history or anion gap metabolic acidosis, increased osmolar gap, visual disturbances, oxalate crystals in the urine or a documented serum ethylene glycol or methanol concentration of more than 20 mg/dL.

Administer a loading dose of 15 mg/kg, followed by doses of 10 mg/kg every 12 hours for 4 doses, then 15 mg/kg every 12 hours thereafter until ethylene glycol or methanol concentrations are undetectable or have been reduced to less than 20 mg/dL, and the patient is asymptomatic with normal pH. Administer all doses as a slow IV infusion over 30 minutes.

➤*Hemodialysis:* Consider hemodialysis in addition to fomepizole in the case of renal failure, significant or worsening metabolic acidosis, or a measured ethylene glycol or methanol concentration of at least 50 mg/dL. Dialyze patients to correct metabolic abnormalities and to lower the ethylene glycol concentrations to less than 50 mg/dL.

Fomepizole is dialyzable; increase the frequency of dosing to every 4 hours during hemodialysis.

FOMEPIZOLE (4-Methylpyrazole; 4-MP) — INJECTION

Fomepizole Dosing in Patients Requiring Hemodialysis	
Parameters	Dosing Schedule
At beginning of hemodialysis	
< 6 h since last dose	Do not administer dose.
≥ 6 h since last dose	Administer next scheduled dose.
During hemodialysis	Every 4 h.
At end of hemodialysis	
< 1 h since last dose	Do not administer dose.
1 to 3 h since last dose	Administer ½ of next scheduled dose.
> 3 h since last dose	Administer next scheduled dose.
Maintenance dosing off hemodialysis	Administer next scheduled dose 12 h from last dose.

➤*Preparation:* Using sterile technique, draw the appropriate dose of fomepizole from the vial with a syringe and inject into at least 100 mL of sterile 0.9% sodium chloride injection or dextrose 5% injection. Mix well. Infuse the entire contents of the resulting solution over 30 minutes. Fomepizole, like all parenteral products, should be inspected visually for particulate matter prior to administration. Fomepizole solidifies at temperatures less than 25°C (77°F). If the fomepizole solution has become solid in the vial, liquefy by running the vial under warm water or by holding in the hand. Solidification does not affect the efficacy, safety, or stability of fomepizole.

➤*Storage / Stability:* Store at controlled room temperature, 20° to 25°C (68° to 77°F). Fomepizole diluted in 0.9% sodium chloride injection or dextrose 5% injection remains stable and sterile for at least 24 hours when stored refrigerated or at room temperature. Fomepizole does not contain a preservative. Therefore, maintain sterile conditions and after dilution, do not use after 24 hours. Solutions showing haziness, particulate matter, precipitate, discoloration, or leakage should not be used.

Actions

➤*Pharmacology:* Fomepizole is a competitive inhibitor of alcohol dehydrogenase that catalyzes the oxidation of ethanol to acetaldehyde. Alcohol dehydrogenase also catalyzes the initial steps in the metabolism of ethylene glycol and methanol to their toxic metabolites.

Ethylene glycol is metabolized to glycoaldehyde, which undergoes subsequent sequential oxidations to yield glycolate, glyoxylate, and oxalate. Glycolate and oxalate are the metabolic by-products primarily responsible for the metabolic acidosis and renal damage seen in ethylene glycol toxicosis. The lethal dose of ethylene glycol is approximately 1.4 mL/kg.

Methanol, the main component of windshield wiper fluid, is slowly metabolized via alcohol dehydrogenase to formaldehyde with subsequent oxidation via formaldehyde dehydrogenase to yield formic acid. Formic acid is primarily responsible for the metabolic acidosis and visual disturbances (eg, decreased visual acuity and potential blindness) associated with methanol poisoning. A lethal dose of methanol in humans is approximately 1 to 2 mL/kg.

➤*Pharmacokinetics:*

Absorption / Distribution – After IV infusion, fomepizole rapidly distributes to total body water. The volume of distribution is between 0.6 and 1.02 L/kg. The plasma half-life varies with the dose, even in patients with normal renal function, and has not been calculated. The concentration of fomepizole at which alcohol dehydrogenase is inhibited by 50% in vitro is approximately 0.1 mcmol/L. Fomepizole concentrations in the range of 100 to 300 mcmol/L (8.6 to 24.6 mg/L) have been targeted to ensure adequate plasma concentrations for the effective inhibition of alcohol dehydrogenase.

In healthy volunteers, oral doses of fomepizole (10 to 20 mg/kg) significantly reduced the rate of elimination of moderate doses of ethanol, which is also metabolized through the action of alcohol dehydrogenase (see Drug Interactions.)

Metabolism / Excretion – Only 1% to 3.5% of the administered dose of fomepizole (7 to 20 mg/kg oral and IV) was excreted unchanged in the urine, indicating that metabolism is the major route of elimination. In humans, the primary metabolite of fomepizole is 4-carboxypyrazole (approximately 80% to 85% of administered dose), which is excreted in the urine. With multiple doses, fomepizole rapidly induces its own metabolism via the P-450 system, producing a significant increase in the elimination rate after approximately 30 to 40 hours. After enzyme induction, elimination follows first-order kinetics. Saturable elimination occurs at therapeutic blood concentrations (100 to 300 mcmol/L, 8.2 to 24.6 mg/L).

Contraindications

Documented serious hypersensitivity reaction to fomepizole or other pyrazoles.

Warnings

➤*Fertility impairment:* In rats, fomepizole (110 mg/kg) administered orally for 40 to 42 days resulted in decreased testicular mass (approximately 8% reduction). This dose is approximately 0.6 times the human maximum daily exposure. Reduction was similar for rats treated with either ethanol or fomepizole alone. When fomepizole was given in combination with ethanol, the decrease in testicular mass was significantly greater (approximately 30% reduction) compared with those rats treated exclusively with fomepizole or ethanol.

➤*Elderly:* Safety and effectiveness in elderly patients have not been established.

➤*Pregnancy:* *Category C.* It is not known whether fomepizole can cause fetal harm when administered to pregnant women or can affect reproduction capacity. Give to pregnant women only if clearly needed.

➤*Lactation:* It is not known whether this drug is excreted in breast milk. Exercise caution when fomepizole is administered to a breast-feeding woman.

➤*Children:* Safety and efficacy have not been established.

Precautions

➤*Monitoring:* In addition to specific antidote treatment with fomepizole, patients intoxicated with ethylene glycol or methanol must be managed for metabolic acidosis, acute renal failure (ethylene glycol), adult respiratory distress syndrome, visual disturbances (methanol), and hypocalcemia. Fluid therapy and sodium bicarbonate administration are potential supportive therapies. In addition, potassium and calcium supplementation and oxygen administration are usually necessary. Hemodialysis is necessary in the anuric patient or in patients with severe metabolic acidosis or azotemia (see Administration and Dosage). Assess treatment success by frequent measurements of blood gases, pH, electrolytes, BUN, creatinine, and urinalysis, in addition to other laboratory tests as indicated by individual patient conditions. At frequent intervals throughout the treatment, patients poisoned with ethylene glycol should be monitored for ethylene glycol concentrations in serum and urine, and the presence of urinary oxalate crystals. Similarly, monitor serum methanol concentrations in patients poisoned with methanol.

Because acidosis and electrolyte imbalances can affect the cardiovascular system, perform electrocardiography. In the comatose patient, electroencephalography may also be required. In addition, monitor hepatic enzymes and WBC counts during treatment, as transient increases in serum transaminase concentrations and eosinophilia have been noted with repeated fomepizole dosing.

➤*Administration:* Do not give fomepizole undiluted or by bolus injection. Venous irritation and phlebosclerosis occurred in 2 of 6 healthy volunteers given bolus injections (over 5 minutes) of fomepizole at a concentration of 25 mg/mL.

➤*Allergic reactions:* Minor allergic reactions (mild rash, eosinophilia) have been reported in a few patients receiving fomepizole (see Adverse Reactions). Therefore, monitor patients for signs of allergic reactions.

Drug Interactions

➤*Ethanol:* Oral doses of fomepizole (10 to 20 mg/kg), via alcohol dehydrogenase inhibition, significantly reduced the rate of elimination of ethanol (by approximately 40%) given to healthy volunteers in moderate doses. Similarly, ethanol decreased the rate of elimination of fomepizole (by approximately 50%) by the same mechanism.

Reciprocal interactions may occur with concomitant use of fomepizole and drugs that increase or inhibit the cytochrome P-450 system (eg, carbamazepine, cimetidine, ketoconazole, phenytoin), although this has not been studied.

Adverse Reactions

The most frequent adverse events reported as drug-related or unknown relationship to study drug in the 78 patients and 63 healthy volunteers who received fomepizole were headache (14%), nausea (11%), dizziness, increased drowsiness, and bad taste/metallic taste (6% each). Other adverse events reported in approximately 3% or less of those receiving fomepizole are listed below:

➤*Cardiovascular:* Sinus bradycardia/bradycardia; tachycardia; phlebitis; shock; hypotension; phlebosclerosis.

➤*CNS:* Seizure; vertigo; lightheadedness; nystagmus; agitation; facial flush; anxiety; feeling of drunkenness; strange feeling; decreased environmental awareness.

➤*GI:* Vomiting; diarrhea; dyspepsia; decreased appetite; transient transaminitis; heartburn.

➤*Hematologic / Lymphatic:* Lymphangitis; eosinophilia/hypereosinophilia; disseminated intravascular coagulation; anemia.

➤*Respiratory:* Hiccups; pharyngitis.

➤*Special senses:* Abnormal smell; speech/visual disturbances; roar in ear; transient blurred vision.

➤*Miscellaneous:* Abdominal pain; fever; multiorgan system failure; pain during fomepizole injection; inflammation at injection site; anuria; lumbalgia/backache; hangover; rash; application site reaction.

Overdosage

Nausea, dizziness, and vertigo occurred in healthy volunteers receiving 50 and 100 mg/kg doses of fomepizole (at plasma concentrations of 290 to 520 mcmol/L, 23.8 to 42.6 mg/L). These doses are 3 to 6 times the recommended dose. This dose-dependent CNS effect was short-lived in most subjects and lasted up to 30 hours in 1 subject. Fomepizole is dialyzable, and hemodialysis may be useful in treating cases of overdosage.

PRALIDOXIME CHLORIDE (2-PAM)

Rx	Protopam Chloride (Wyeth-Ayerst)	Powder for injection[a]: 1 g	In 20 mL single-use vials.

[a] Porous cake.

PRALIDOXIME CHLORIDE — INJECTION

Indications

➤*Organophosphate poisoning:* As an antidote in the treatment of poisoning caused by those pesticides and chemicals of the organophosphate class which have anticholinesterase activity.

➤*Anticholinesterase drug overdosage:* The control of overdosage by anticholinesterase drugs used in the treatment of myasthenia gravis.

The principal indications for the use of pralidoxime are muscle weakness and respiratory depression. In severe poisoning, respiratory depression may be caused by muscle weakness.

Administration and Dosage

➤*Approved by the FDA:* March 11, 1964.

➤*Organophosphate poisoning:* Pralidoxime is most effective if administered immediately after poisoning. Generally, little is accomplished if the drug is given more than 36 hours after termination of exposure. When the poison has been ingested, however, exposure may continue for some time due to slow absorption from the lower bowel, and fatal relapses have been reported after initial improvement. Continued administration for several days may be useful in such patients. Close supervision of the patient is indicated for at least 48 to 72 hours. If dermal exposure has occurred, remove clothing and wash the hair and skin thoroughly with sodium bicarbonate or alcohol as soon as possible. Diazepam may be given cautiously if convulsions are not controlled by atropine.

Severe poisoning (coma, cyanosis, respiratory depression) requires intensive management. This includes the removal of secretions, airway management, the correction of acidosis, and hypoxemia.

Give atropine as soon as possible after hypoxemia is improved. Do not give atropine in the presence of significant hypoxia due to the risk of atropine-induced ventricular fibrillation. In adults, atropine may be given IV in doses of 2 to 4 mg. Repeat this at 5- to 10-minute intervals until full atropinization (secretions are inhibited) or signs of atropine toxicity appear (delirium, hyperthermia, muscle twitching).

Maintain some degree of atropinization for at least 48 hours, and until any depressed blood cholinesterase activity is reversed.

Morphine, theophylline, aminophylline, and succinylcholine are contraindicated. Avoid tranquilizers of the reserpine or phenothiazine type.

After the effects of atropine become apparent, pralidoxime may be administered.

Adults – In adults, inject an initial dose of 1 to 2 g of pralidoxime, preferably as an infusion in 100 mL of saline, over a 15- to 30-minute period. If this is not practical or if pulmonary edema is present, give the dose slowly by IV injection as a 5% solution in water over not less than 5 minutes. After about an hour, a second dose of 1 to 2 g will be indicated if muscle weakness has not been relieved. Additional doses may be given cautiously if muscle weakness persists.

In severe cases, especially after ingestion of the poison, it may be desirable to monitor the effect of therapy by ECG because of the possibility of heart block due to the anticholinesterase. Where the poison has been ingested, it is particularly important to take into account the likelihood of continuing absorption from the lower bowel since this constitutes new exposure. In such cases, additional doses of pralidoxime may be needed every 3 to 8 hours. In effect, titrate the patient with pralidoxime as long as signs of poisoning recur. As in all cases of organophosphate poisoning, take care to keep the patient under observation for at least 24 hours.

If convulsions interfere with respiration, they may be controlled by the slow IV injection of diazepam, up to 20 mg in adults.

➤*Anticholinesterase overdose:* As an antagonist to such anticholinesterases as neostigmine, pyridostigmine, and ambenonium, which are used in the treatment of myasthenia gravis, pralidoxime may be given in a dosage of 1 to 2 g by IV followed by increments of 250 mg every 5 minutes.

➤*Renal function impairment:* Because pralidoxime is excreted in the urine, a decrease in renal function will result in increased blood levels of the drug. Thus, reduce the dosage of pralidoxime in the presence of renal insufficiency.

➤*Storage/Stability:* Store at room temperature (approximately 20° to 25°C; 68° to 77°F).

Actions

➤*Pharmacology:* The principal action of pralidoxime is to reactivate cholinesterase (mainly outside of the CNS) which has been inactivated by phosphorylation due to an organophosphate pesticide or related compound. The destruction of accumulated acetylcholine can then proceed, and neuromuscular junctions will again function normally. Pralidoxime also slows the process of aging of phosphorylated cholinesterase to a nonreactivatable form, and detoxifies certain organophosphates by direct chemical reaction. The drug has its most critical effect in relieving paralysis of the muscles of respiration. Because pralidoxime is less effective in relieving depression of the respiratory center, atropine is always required concomitantly to block the effect of accumulated acetylcholine at this site. Pralidoxime relieves muscarinic signs and symptoms, salivation, bronchospasm, etc, but this action is relatively unimportant since atropine is adequate for this purpose.

It has been reported that the supplemental use of oxime cholinesterase reactivators (such as pralidoxime) reduces the incidence and severity of developmental defects in chick embryos exposed to such known teratogens as parathion, bidrin, carbachol, and neostigmine. This protective effect of the oximes was shown to be dose related.

➤*Pharmacokinetics:*

Absorption/Distribution – Pralidoxime is distributed throughout the extracellular water; it is not bound to plasma protein. Consequently, pralidoxime is relatively short acting, and repeated doses may be needed, especially where there is any evidence of continuing absorption of the poison.

The minimum therapeutic concentration of pralidoxime in plasma is 4 mcg/mL; this level is reached in about 16 minutes after a single injection of pralidoxime 600 mg. The apparent half-life of pralidoxime is 74 to 77 minutes.

Excretion – The drug is rapidly excreted in the urine partly unchanged, and partly as a metabolite produced by the liver.

Contraindications

There are no known absolute contraindications for the use of pralidoxime. Relative contraindications include known hypersensitivity to the drug and other situations in which the risk of its use clearly outweighs possible benefit.

Warnings

➤*Phosphorus, inorganic phosphates, organophosphates:* Pralidoxime is not effective in the treatment of poisoning caused by phosphorus, inorganic phosphates, or organophosphates not having anticholinesterase activity.

➤*Carbamate pesticides:* Pralidoxime is not indicated as an antidote for intoxication by pesticides of the carbamate class since it may increase the toxicity of carbaryl.

➤*Renal function impairment:* Because pralidoxime is excreted in the urine, a decrease in renal function will result in increased blood levels of the drug. Thus, reduce the dosage of pralidoxime in the presence of renal insufficiency.

➤*Pregnancy:* Category C.

Teratogenic – Animal reproduction studies have not been conducted with pralidoxime. It is also not known whether pralidoxime can cause fetal harm when administered to a pregnant woman or can affect reproduction capacity. Give pralidoxime to a pregnant woman only if clearly needed.

➤*Lactation:* It is not known whether this drug is excreted in human milk. Because many drugs are excreted in human milk, exercise caution when pralidoxime is administered to a breast-feeding woman.

➤*Children:* Safety and efficacy in pediatric patients have not been established.

Precautions

➤*General information:* Pralidoxime has been very well tolerated in most cases, but it must be remembered that the desperate condition of the organophosphate-poisoned patient will generally mask such minor signs and symptoms as have been noted in healthy subjects.

➤*Injection rate:* IV administration of pralidoxime should be carried out slowly and, preferably, by infusion, since certain side effects, such as tachycardia, laryngospasm, and muscle rigidity, have been attributed in a few cases to a too-rapid rate of injection. Injection rate should not exceed 200 mg/min. If IV administration is not feasible, use IM or subcutaneous injection.

➤*Myasthenia gravis:* Use pralidoxime with great caution in treating organophosphate overdosage in cases of myasthenia gravis since it may precipitate a myasthenic crisis.

➤*Lab test abnormalities:* Institute treatment of organophosphate poisoning without waiting for the results of laboratory tests. Red blood cell, plasma cholinesterase, and urinary paranitrophenol measurements (in the case of parathion exposure) may be helpful in confirming the diagnosis and following the course of the illness. A reduction in red blood cell cholinesterase concentration to below 50% of normal has been seen only with organophosphate ester poisoning.

Drug Interactions

➤*Combination of atropine and pralidoxime:* When atropine and pralidoxime are used together, the signs of atropinization (flushing, mydriasis, tachycardia, dryness of the mouth and nose) may occur earlier than might be expected when atropine is used alone. This is especially true if the total dose of atropine has been large and the administration of pralidoxime has been delayed.

Keep the following precautions in mind in the treatment of anticholinesterase poisoning, although they do not bear directly on the use of pralidoxime: since barbiturates are potentiated by the anticholinesterases, use them cautiously in the treatment of convulsions; avoid morphine, theophylline, aminophylline, succinylcholine, reserpine, and phenothiazine-type tranquilizers in patients with organophosphate poisoning.

PRALIDOXIME CHLORIDE — INJECTION

Adverse Reactions

➤*Combination of atropine and pralidoxime:* When atropine and pralidoxime are used together, the signs of atropinization may occur earlier than might be expected when atropine is used alone. This is especially true if the total dose of atropine has been large and the administration of pralidoxime has been delayed. Excitement and manic behavior immediately following recovery of consciousness have been reported in several cases. However, similar behavior has occurred in cases of organophosphate poisoning that were not treated with pralidoxime.

➤*Lab test abnormalities:* Elevations in AST or ALT enzyme levels were observed in 1 of 6 healthy volunteers given pralidoxime 1,200 mg IM, and in 4 of 6 volunteers given 1,800 mg IM. Levels returned to normal in about 2 weeks. Transient elevations in creatine phosphokinase were observed in all healthy volunteers given the drug. A single IM injection of 330 mg in 1 mL in rabbits caused myonecrosis, inflammation, and hemorrhage.

➤*Local:* 40 to 60 minutes after IM injection, mild to moderate pain may be experienced at the site of injection.

➤*Miscellaneous:* Pralidoxime may cause blurred vision, diplopia and impaired accommodation, dizziness, headache, drowsiness, nausea, tachycardia, increased systolic and diastolic blood pressure, hyperventilation, and muscular weakness when given parenterally to healthy volunteers who have not been exposed to anticholinesterase poisons. In patients, it is very difficult to differentiate the toxic effects produced by atropine or the organophosphate compounds from those of the drug.

Overdosage

➤*Symptoms:* The following have been observed in healthy subjects only: dizziness, blurred vision, diplopia, headache, impaired accommodation, nausea, slight tachycardia. In therapy it has been difficult to differentiate side effects due to the drug from those due to the effects of the poison.

➤*Treatment:* Administer artificial respiration and other supportive therapy as needed.

DIGOXIN IMMUNE FAB (Ovine)

Rx	**Digibind** (GlaxoSmithKline)	**Powder for injection, lyophilized**: 38 mg/vial. Each vial will bind approximately 0.5 mg digoxin.	Sodium chloride 28 mg. Preservative free. In vials.
Rx	**DigiFab** (Savage)	**Powder for injection, lyophilized**: 40 mg/vial. Each vial will bind approximately 0.5 mg digoxin.	Sodium acetate 2 mg. Preservative free. In vials.

DIGOXIN IMMUNE FAB (Ovine) — INJECTION

Indications

For the treatment of life-threatening or potentially life-threatening digoxin toxicity or overdose. *Digibind* also has been successfully used to treat life-threatening digitoxin (not available in the United States) overdose. Digoxin immune Fab is not indicated for milder cases of digitalis toxicity.

Clinical conditions requiring administration include the following:

- Known suicidal or accidental consumption of more than 10 mg of digoxin in previously healthy adults or 4 mg (or more than 0.1 mg/kg [*DigiFab*]) in previously healthy children, or ingestion causing steady-state serum concentrations greater than 10 ng/mL;
- chronic ingestions causing steady-state serum digoxin concentrations exceeding 6 ng/mL in adults or 4 ng/mL in children (*DigiFab*); and
- manifestions of life-threatening toxicity caused by digoxin overdose, including severe ventricular arrhythmias (eg, ventricular tachycardia or fibrillation), progressive bradycardia, and second or third degree heart block not responsive to atropine, serum potassium levels exceeding 5 mEq/L (*Digibind*) or 5.5 mEq/L in adults or 6 mEq/L in children (*DigiFab*) with rapidly progressive signs and symptoms of digoxin toxicity.

Administration and Dosage

The dosage of digoxin immune Fab varies according to the amount of digoxin or digitoxin to be neutralized.

➤*Administration:* Administer IV slowly as an IV infusion over at least 30 minutes. If infusion rate-related reactions occur, stop the infusion and restart at a slower rate. If cardiac arrest is imminent, digoxin can be given as a bolus injection. With bolus injection, an increased incidence of infusion-related reactions may be expected.

It is recommended for *Digibind* to be infused through a 0.22 micron membrane filter to ensure no undissolved particulate matter is administered.

➤*Dosage for acute ingestion of unknown amount:* Twenty vials (760 mg of *Digibind* or 800 mg of *DigiFab*) are adequate to treat most life-threatening ingestions in both adults and children. In small children, it is important to monitor for volume overload. In general, a large dose of digoxin immune Fab has a faster onset of effect, but may enhance the possibility of a febrile reaction. The physician may consider administering 10 vials, observing the patient's response, and following with an additional 10 vials if clinically indicated. Failure of the patient to respond to digoxin immune Fab should alert the physician to the possibility that the clinical problem may not be caused by digitalis toxicity.

➤*Dosage for toxicity during chronic therapy:* In adults, 6 vials (228 mg [*Digibind*] or 240 mg [*DigiFab*]) are usually adequate to reverse most cases of toxicity. This dose can be used in patients who are in acute distress or for whom a serum digoxin or digitoxin concentration is not available. In infants and small children (20 kg or less), a single vial usually should suffice.

➤*Dose determination:* Erroneous calculations may result from inaccurate estimates of the amount of digitalis ingested or absorbed or from nonsteady-state serum digitalis concentrations. Inaccurate serum digitalis concentration measurements are a possible source of error.

Dosage calculations are based on a steady-state volume of distribution of approximately 5 L/kg for digoxin (0.5 L/kg for digitoxin) to convert serum digitalis concentration to the amount of digitalis in the body. Many patients may require higher doses for complete neutralization. Ordinarily, round the doses up to the next whole vial.

If toxicity has not adequately reversed after several hours or appears to recur, readministration of *Digibind* at a dose guided by clinical judgment may be required. If a patient is in need of readministration of *DigiFab* because of recurrent toxicity, or to a new toxic episode that occurs soon after the first episode, measurement of free (unbound) serum digitalis concentrations should be considered because Fab may still be present in the body.

➤*Dosage calculation:* If in any case the dose estimated based on ingested amount differs substantially from that calculated based on the serum digoxin or digitoxin concentration, it may be preferable to use the higher dose estimate.

Acute ingestion of known amount – Each vial will bind approximately 0.5 mg of digoxin (or digitoxin).

$$\text{Dose (in \# of vials)} = \frac{\text{Total digitalis body load (mg)}}{\text{0.5 mg of digitalis bound/vial}}$$

For toxicity from an acute ingestion, total body load in milligrams will be approximately equal to the amount ingested in milligrams for digoxin capsules or digitoxin, or the amount ingested in milligrams multiplied by 0.8 (to account for incomplete absorption) for digoxin tablets.

Approximate Dose for Reversal of a Single Large Digoxin Overdose

Number of digoxin tablets or capsules ingested[a]	Number of vials
25	10
50	20
75	30
100	40
150	60
200	80

[a] 0.25 mg tablets (80% bioavailability); 0.2 mg *Lanoxicaps* capsules (100% bioavailability).

Calculations based on steady-state serum digoxin concentrations – *Adults:* To estimate number of vials for adult patients for whom a steady-state serum digoxin concentration is known, use the following formula:

$$\text{Dose (in \# of vials)} = \frac{\text{(Serum digoxin concentration in ng/mL) (weight in kg)}}{100}$$

Estimates of Fab Fragments (in Number of Vials) From Serum Digoxin Concentration in Adults

Weight (kg)	Serum digoxin concentration (ng/mL)[a] 1	2	4	8	12	16	20
40	0.5 v	1 v	2 v	3 v	5 v	7 v	8 v
60	0.5 v	1 v	3 v	5 v	7 v	10 v	12 v
70	1 v	2 v	3 v	6 v	9 v	11 v	14 v
80	1 v	2 v	3 v	7 v	10 v	13 v	16 v
100	1 v	2 v	4 v	8 v	12 v	16 v	20 v

[a] v = vial

Children:

- *Digibind* – Because infants and small children can have much smaller dosage requirements, reconstitute the 38 mg vial as directed and administer with a tuberculin syringe. For very small doses, dilute the reconstituted vial with 34 mL sterile isotonic saline to achieve 1 mg/mL concentration.

$$\text{Dose (in mg)} = \frac{\text{(Dose [in \# of vials])}}{\text{(38 mg/vial)}}$$

Dose Estimates of *Digibind* from Serum Digoxin Concentration in Infants/Small Children

Weight (kg)	Serum digoxin concentration (ng/mL) 1	2	4	8	12	16	20
1	0.4 mg[a]	1 mg[a]	1.5 mg[a]	3 mg[a]	5 mg	6 mg	8 mg
3	1 mg[a]	2 mg[a]	5 mg	9 mg	14 mg	18 mg	23 mg
5	2 mg[a]	4 mg	8 mg	15 mg	23 mg	30 mg	38 mg
10	4 mg	8 mg	15 mg	30 mg	46 mg	61 mg	76 mg
20	8 mg	15 mg	30 mg	61 mg	91 mg	122 mg	152 mg

[a] Dilution of reconstituted vial to 1 mg/mL may be desirable.

DIGOXIN IMMUNE FAB (Ovine) — INJECTION

• *DigiFab* – Because infants and small children can have much smaller dosage requirements, it is recommended that the 40 mg vial be reconstituted as directed and administered with a tuberculin syringe. For very small doses, a reconstituted vial can be diluted with 36 mL of sterile isotonic saline to achieve a 1 mg/mL concentration.

$$\text{Dose (in mg)} = \frac{\text{(Dose [in \# of vials])}}{\text{(40 mg/vial)}}$$

Dose Estimates of *DigiFab* from Serum Digoxin Concentration in Infants/Small Children

Weight (kg)	Serum digoxin concentration (ng/mL)						
	1	2	4	8	12	16	20
1	0.4 mg[a]	1 mg[a]	1.5 mg[a]	3 mg[a]	5 mg	6.5 mg	8 mg
3	1 mg[a]	2.5 mg[a]	5 mg	10 mg	14 mg	19 mg	24 mg
5	2 mg[a]	4 mg	8 mg	16 mg	24 mg	32 mg	40 mg
10	4 mg	8 mg	16 mg	32 mg	48 mg	64 mg	80 mg
20	8 mg	16 mg	32 mg	64 mg	96 mg	128 mg	160 mg

[1] Dilution of reconstituted vial to 1 mg/mL may be desirable.

➤*Calculations based on steady-state digitoxin concentrations:* The dosage of digoxin immune Fab for digitoxin toxicity can be approximated using the following formula:

$$\text{Dose (in \# of vials)} = \frac{\text{(Serum digitoxin concentration in ng/mL) (weight in kg)}}{1000}$$

➤*Reconstitution:* Dissolve the contents in each vial with 4 mL of Sterile Water for Injection. Mix gently to give a protein concentration of 9.5 mg/mL (*Digibind*) or 10 mg/mL (*DigiFab*). Use reconstituted product promptly. If it is not used immediately, store at 2° to 8°C (36° to 46°F) for up to 4 hours. The reconstituted product may be diluted with sterile isotonic saline to a convenient volume.

➤*Storage/Stability:* Refrigerate at 2° to 8°C (36° to 46°F) for up to 4 hours after reconstitution.

Digibind – Unreconstituted vials can be stored at up to 30°C (86°F) for a total of 30 days.

DigiFab – Do not freeze.

Actions

➤*Pharmacology:* Digoxin immune Fab (ovine) is antigen binding fragments (Fab) derived from specific antidigoxin antibodies produced in sheep. Production involves conjugation of digoxin as a hapten to human albumin. Sheep are immunized with this material to produce antibodies specific for the digoxin molecule. The antibody is papain digested, and digoxin-specific Fab fragments are isolated and purified.

Improvement in signs and symptoms of digitalis intoxication ordinarily begins in 30 minutes or less. Digoxin immune Fab binds molecules of digoxin, making them unavailable for binding at their site of action. The Fab fragment-digoxin complex accumulates in the blood and is excreted by the kidneys. The net effect is to shift the equilibrium away from binding of digoxin to its receptors in the body, thereby reversing its effects.

➤*Pharmacokinetics:* The pharmacokinetic profiles of Fab are similar for both products. The similar volumes of distribution (0.3 L/kg and 0.4 L/kg for *DigiFab* and *Digibind*, respectively) indicate considerable penetration from the circulation into the extracellular space and are consistent with previous reports of ovine Fab distribution, as are the elimination half-life values (15 and 23 hours for *DigiFab* and *Digibind*, respectively). The elimination half-life of 15 to 20 hours in patients with normal renal function appears to be increased up to 10-fold in patients with renal impairment, although volume of distribution remains unaffected.

Contraindications

None known.

Warnings

➤*Allergy to papain or derivatives:* Patients with allergies to papain, chymopapain, other papaya extracts, or the pineapple enzyme bromelain may also be at risk for an allergic reaction to digoxin immune Fab. In addition, it has been noted in the literature that some dust mite allergens and some latex allergens share antigenic structures with papain and patients with these allergies may be allergic to papain. Do not administer digoxin immune Fab to patients with a known history of hypersensitivity to papaya or papain unless the benefits outweigh the risks and appropriate management for anaphylactic reactions is readily available.

➤*Skin testing:*

Digibind – Skin testing for allergy was performed during the clinical investigation of this agent. Only 1 patient developed erythema at the site of skin testing. The patient had no adverse reaction to systemic treatment. Allergy testing is not routinely required before treatment of life-threatening digitalis toxicity because it can delay urgently needed therapy.

Skin testing may be appropriate for high-risk individuals, especially patients with known allergies or those previously treated with digoxin immune Fab. The intradermal skin test can be performed by: 1) Diluting 0.1 mL of reconstituted drug (9.5 mg/mL) in 9.9 mL sterile isotonic saline; 2) injecting 0.1 mL of the 1:100 dilution (9.5 mcg) intradermally and observing for an urticarial wheal surrounded by a zone of erythema. Read the test at 20 minutes.

The scratch test procedure is performed by placing 1 drop of a 1:100 dilution on the skin and making a ¼-inch scratch through the drop with a needle. The area is inspected at 20 minutes for an urticarial wheal surrounded by erythema.

If skin testing causes a systemic reaction, apply a tourniquet above the site of testing and treat anaphylaxis. Avoid further administration of the drug unless its use is absolutely essential; in this case, pretreat the patient with corticosteroids and diphenhydramine and make preparations for treating anaphylaxis.

DigiFab – Skin testing has not proved useful in predicting allergic response to *Digibind*. Because of this and because it may delay urgently needed therapy, skin testing was not performed during the clinical studies of *DigiFab* and is not suggested prior to dosing with this product.

➤*Hypersensitivity reactions:* Allergic reactions have occurred rarely, but consider the possibility of anaphylactic, hypersensitivity, or febrile reactions. If an anaphylactoid reaction occurs, discontinue the drug infusion and initiate appropriate therapy. The need for epinephrine should be balanced against its potential risk in the setting of digitalis toxicity. Refer to Management of Acute Hypersensitivity Reactions.

Patients with known allergies or allergies to sheep protein would be particularly at risk, as would individuals who have previously received antibodies or Fab fragments raised in sheep. Patients with a history of allergy, especially to antibiotics, appear to be at particular risk.

➤*Renal function impairment:* The elimination half-life in renal failure has not been clearly defined. Patients with renal dysfunction have been successfully treated with digoxin immune Fab. There is no evidence to suggest any difference between these patients and patients with normal renal function, but excretion of the Fab fragment-digoxin complex from the body is probably delayed. In patients who are functionally anephric, anticipate failure to clear the Fab fragment-digoxin complex from the blood by glomerular filtration and renal excretion. Whether this would lead to reintoxication by release of newly unbound digoxin into the blood is uncertain. Monitor such patients for a prolonged period for possible recurrence of digitalis toxicity. Monitoring of free (unbound) digoxin concentrations after the administration may be appropriate in order to establish recrudescent toxicity in renal failure patients.

➤*Elderly:* Because elderly patients are more likely to have decreased renal function, it may be useful to monitor renal function and to observe for possible recurrence of toxicity.

➤*Pregnancy: Category C.* It is not known whether this agent can cause fetal harm or affect reproduction capacity. Use only if clearly needed.

➤*Lactation:* It is not known whether this drug is excreted in breast milk. Exercise caution when administering to a breast-feeding mother.

➤*Children:* This agent has been used successfully in infants with no apparent adverse sequelae. Use of this drug in infants should be based on careful consideration of the benefits of the drug balanced against the potential risk involved.

Precautions

➤*Monitoring:* Digoxin immune Fab will interfere with digitalis immunoassay measurements. The standard serum digoxin concentration measurement can be clinically misleading until the Fab fragment is eliminated from the body. Obtain digoxin serum concentrations before digoxin immune Fab or drug administration. These measurements may be difficult to interpret if drawn soon after the last digitalis dose, because at least 6 to 8 hours are required for equilibration of digoxin between serum and tissue. Closely monitor the patient, including temperature, blood pressure, ECG, and potassium concentration during and after drug administration. The total serum digoxin concentration may rise precipitously following administration, but this will be almost entirely bound to the Fab fragment.

Potassium – Severe digitalis intoxication can cause life-threatening elevation in serum potassium concentration by shifting potassium from inside to outside the cell. This can lead to increased renal excretion of potassium. These patients may have hyperkalemia with a total body deficit of potassium. When the effect of digitalis is reversed, potassium shifts back inside the cell with a resulting decline in serum potassium concentration. Hypokalemia may develop rapidly. Monitor serum potassium concentration repeatedly, especially over the first several hours after the drug is given, and cautiously give potassium supplementation when necessary.

➤*Standard intoxication management:* Standard therapy for digitalis intoxication includes withdrawal of the drug, correction of electrolyte disturbances (especially hyperkalemia), acid-base imbalances, hypoxia, and treatment of cardiac arrhythmias. Massive digitalis intoxication can cause hyperkalemia; administration of potassium supplements in the setting of digitalis intoxication may be hazardous.

➤*Digoxin withdrawal:* In a few instances, the condition of those with low cardiac output states and CHF could have been exacerbated by withdrawal of the inotropic effects of digitalis. Patients with atrial fibrillation may develop a rapid ventricular response from withdrawal of the effects of digitalis on the AV node.

Patients with intrinsically poor cardiac function may deteriorate from withdrawal of digoxin. Additional support can be provided by use of IV inotropes (eg, dopamine or dobutamine) or vasodilators. With catecholamines, take care not to aggravate digitalis toxic rhythm disturbances. Do not use other types of digitalis glycosides. Redigitalization should be postponed if possible until the Fab fragments have been eliminated from the body; this may require several days. Patients with impaired renal function may require a week or longer.

DIGOXIN IMMUNE FAB (Ovine) — INJECTION

➤*Immunogenicity:* Prior treatment with digoxin-specific ovine immune Fab carries a theoretical risk of sensitization to ovine serum protein and possible diminution of the efficacy of the drug due to the presence of human antibodies against ovine Fab. Human antibodies to ovine Fab have been reported in some patients receiving *Digibind*; however, to date, there have been no clinical reports of human antiovine immunoglobulin antibodies causing a reduction in binding of ovine digoxin immune Fab or neutralization response to ovine digoxin immune Fab.

Adverse Reactions

Exacerbation of low cardiac output and CHF; hypokalemia; allergic reactions (rarely); rapid ventricular response in patients with atrial fibrillation caused by digoxin withdrawal (see Precautions).

Patient Information

Advise patients to contact their physician immediately if they experience any signs and symptoms of delayed allergic reactions or serum sickness (eg, rash, pruritus, urticaria) after hospital discharge.

ACETYLCYSTEINE (N-Acetylcysteine)

Rx	**Acetylcysteine** (Various, eg, Abbott, American Regent, Mayne)	**Oral solution:** 10%	EDTA. In 4, 10, and 30 mL vials.
Rx	**Mucomyst** (Sandoz)		
Rx	**Acetylcysteine** (Various, eg, Abbott, American Regent, Mayne)	**Oral solution:** 20%	EDTA. In 4, 10, and 30 mL vials.
Rx	**Mucomyst** (Sandoz)		
Rx	**Acetadote** (Cumberland)	**Injection:** 20% (200 mg/mL)	Preservative-free. 0.5 mg/mL EDTA. In 30 mL single-dose vials.

ACETYLCYSTEINE — ORAL

Indications

➤*Acetaminophen overdose:* To prevent or lessen hepatic injury after ingestion of a potentially hepatotoxic quantity of acetaminophen.

It is essential to initiate treatment as soon as possible after the overdose and, in any case, within 24 hours of ingestion.

➤*Mucolytic (oral solution only):* As adjuvant therapy for abnormal, viscid, or inspissated mucus secretions (refer to Acetylcysteine in the Mucolytics section of the Respiratory chapter).

➤*Unlabeled uses:* Although there is conflicting data, some studies support the use of acetylcysteine for the prevention of radiocontrast-induced nephropathy. The oral solution has been administered IV in certain cases. Please contact the Poison Control Center at (800) 222-1222 for further information.

Administration and Dosage

On admission for suspected acetaminophen overdose, draw a serum blood sample at least 4 hours after ingestion to determine the acetaminophen level; this will serve as a basis for determining the need for treatment with acetylcysteine. If the patient presents after 4 hours postingestion, immediately determine the serum acetaminophen sample.

Administer acetylcysteine within 8 hours after acetaminophen ingestion for maximum protection against hepatic injury for patients whose serum acetaminophen levels fall above the "possible" toxicity line on the Rumack-Matthew nomogram. If the time of ingestion is unknown or the serum acetaminophen level is not available, cannot be interpreted, or is not available within the 8-hour time interval from acetaminophen ingestion, immediately administer acetylcysteine if 24 hours or less have elapsed from the reported time of ingestion of an overdose of acetaminophen, regardless of the quantity reported to have been ingested. Do not await results of assays for acetaminophen level before initiating acetylcysteine treatment. Use lavage, ipecac, or activated charcoal as indicated.

The critical ingestion-treatment interval for maximum protection against severe hepatic injury is between 0 and 8 hours. Efficacy diminishes progressively after 8 hours, and treatment initiation between 15 and 24 hours postingestion of acetaminophen yields limited efficacy. However, it does not appear to worsen the condition of patients; therefore, do not withhold treatment because the reported time of ingestion may not be correct.

➤*Oral:* Oral administration requires dilution of 10% or 20% solution with diet cola or other diet soft drinks to a final concentration of 5%. If administered via gastric tube or Miller-Abbott tube, water may be used as the diluent. Freshly prepare the dilutions and use within 1 hour. Remaining undiluted solutions in opened vials can be stored in the refrigerator for up to 96 hours. Regardless of the quantity of acetaminophen reported to have been ingested, immediately administer oral acetylcysteine if 24 hours or less have elapsed from the reported time of ingestion of an acetaminophen overdose.

Oral Acetylcysteine Dosing Guidelines

Dose type	Dose	Frequency	Dilution	Final concentration
Loading dose	140 mg/kg	Once	Dilute with diet cola or other diet soft drinks	5%
Maintenance doses	70 mg/kg	4 hours after loading dose and at 4-hour intervals thereafter for 17 total doses	Dilute with diet cola or other diet soft drinks	5%

If the patient vomits any oral dose within 1 hour of administration, repeat that dose. If the patient is persistently unable to retain the orally administered acetylcysteine, it may be administered by duodenal intubation.

➤*Acetaminophen assays:* The acute ingestion of acetaminophen in quantities of 150 mg/kg or greater may result in hepatic toxicity. However, the reported history of the drug quantity ingested as an overdose often is inaccurate and is not a reliable guide to therapy of the overdose. Therefore, plasma or serum acetaminophen concentrations, determined as early as possible but no sooner than 4 hours following an acute overdose, are essential in assessing the potential risk of hepatoxicity. Acetaminophen levels drawn less than 4 hours postingestion may be misleading. If an assay for acetaminophen cannot be obtained, it is necessary to assume that the overdose is potentially toxic.

➤*Interpretation of acetaminophen assays:* Refer to the nomogram at the end of this section to determine if plasma concentration is in the potentially toxic range.

Interpretation of Nomogram

Predetoxification plasma levels	Hepatic toxicity incidence	Indication
Value falls above the solid black line (probable line)	Probable	Continue with maintenance doses
Value falls above the broken line (possible line)	Possible	Continue with maintenance doses
Value falls below the broken line (possible line)	Unlikely	May discontinue acetylcysteine treatment

➤*Storage/Stability:*

Oral – Store unopened vials at controlled room temperature, 15° to 30°C (59° to 86°F). Use diluted solutions within 1 hour. If only a portion of a vial is used, refrigerate the remaining undiluted portion and use within 96 hours.

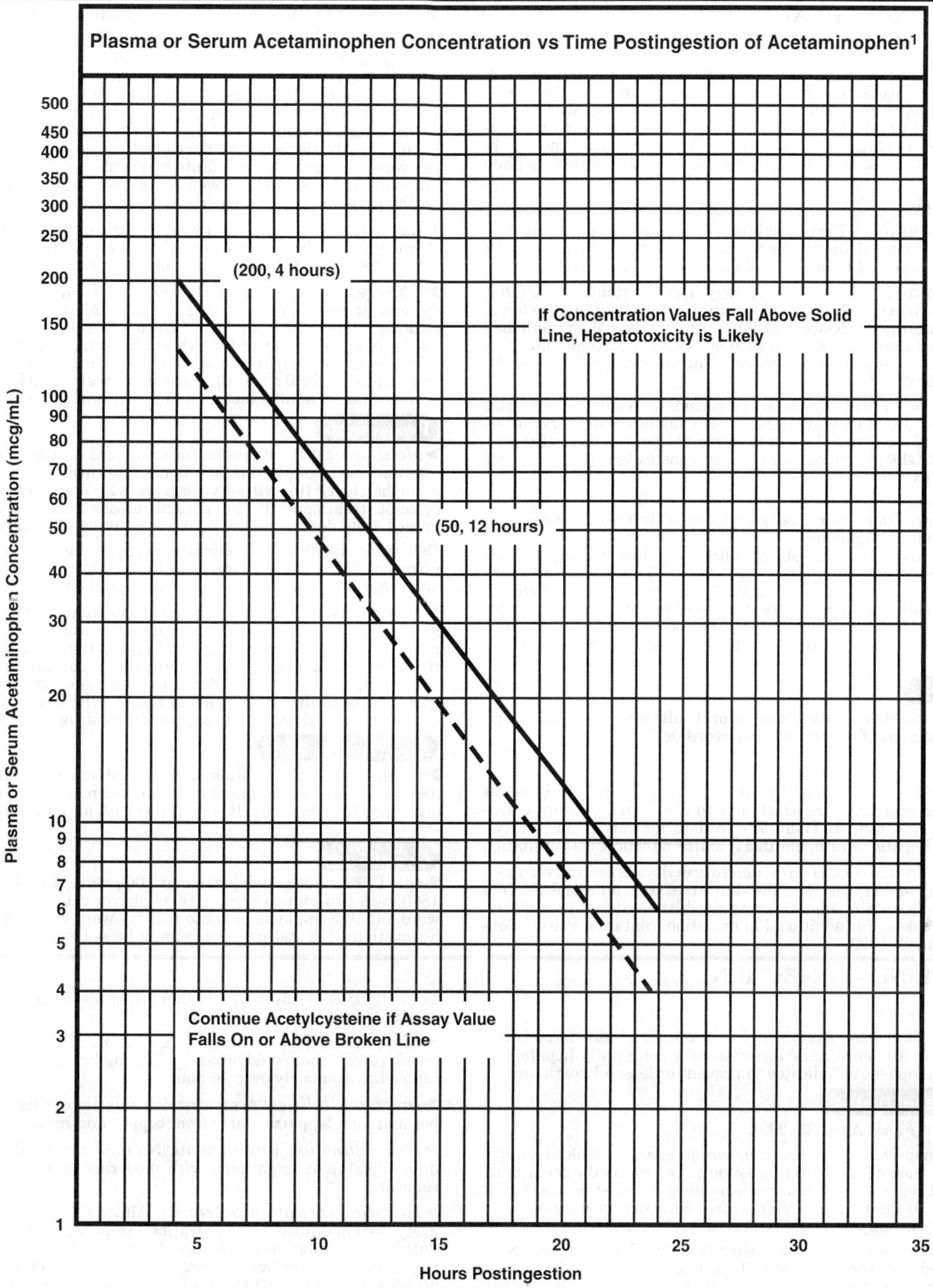

[1] Adapted from Rumack and Matthews. *Pediatrics*. 1975;55:871-876.

ACETYLCYSTEINE — ORAL

Actions

➤*Pharmacology:* Acetylcysteine has been shown to reduce the extent of liver injury following acetaminophen overdose. It is most effective when given early, with benefit seen principally in patients treated within 8 to 10 hours of the overdose. Acetylcysteine likely protects the liver by maintaining or restoring the glutathione levels or by acting as an alternate substrate for conjugation with, and thus detoxification of, the acetaminophen reactive metabolite.

➤*Pharmacokinetics:*

Absorption/Distribution – Bioavailability of oral acetylcysteine is low. The steady-state volume of distribution and the protein binding for IV acetylcysteine were reported to be 0.47 L/kg and 83%, respectively.

Metabolism/Excretion – Acetylcysteine may form cysteine, disulfides, and conjugates in vivo (eg, N, N'-diacetylcysteine, N-acetylcysteine-cysteine, N-acetylcysteine-glutathione, N-acetylcysteine-protein). Based on published data, it was reported that after an oral dose of ^{35}S-acetylcysteine, approximately 22% of total radioactivity was excreted in urine after 24 hours. No metabolites were identified.

After a single IV dose of acetylcysteine, the plasma concentration of total acetylcysteine declined in a polyexponential decay manner with a mean terminal half life ($t_{½}$) of 5.6 hours. The mean clearance for acetylcysteine was reported to be 0.11 L/h/kg and renal clearance constituted approximately 30% of total clearance.

Special populations –

Children: The mean elimination $t_{½}$ of acetylcysteine is longer in newborns (11 hours) than in adults (5.6 hours).

Hepatic function impairment: In subjects with severe liver damage (ie, cirrhosis caused by alcohol [with Child-Pugh score of 7 to 13]) or primary and/or secondary biliary cirrhosis (with Child-Pugh score of 5 to 7), mean $t_{½}$ increased by 80% while mean clearance decreased by 30% compared with control group. The published medical literature does not indicate that the dose of acetylcysteine in patients with hepatic impairment should be reduced.

Contraindications

➤*Oral:* There are no contraindications to oral administration of acetylcysteine in the treatment of acetaminophen overdose.

Warnings

➤*Encephalopathy:* If encephalopathy caused by hepatic failure becomes evident, discontinue acetylcysteine treatment to avoid further administration of nitrogenous substances. There are no data indicating that acetylcysteine influences hepatic failure, but this remains a theoretical possibility.

➤*Hypersensitivity reactions:* If a reaction to acetylcysteine involves more than simply flushing and erythema of the skin, treat it as an anaphylactoid reaction. This usually entails administering antihistaminic drugs and epinephrine in severe cases. For additional information, contact a Poison Control Center at (800) 222-1222.

➤*Mutagenesis:* Acetylcysteine was positive in the in vitro mouse lymphoma cell (L5178Y/TK±) forward mutation test.

➤*Pregnancy: Category B.* In 4 pregnant women with acetaminophen toxicity, oral acetylcysteine was administered at the time of delivery. Acetylcysteine crossed the placenta and was measurable in newborn circulation and cord blood of 3 viable infants following delivery and in cardiac blood of a fourth infant at autopsy (22 weeks gestational age who died 3 hours after birth). No adverse sequelae developed in the 3 viable infants. All mothers recovered and none of the infants had evidence of acetaminophen poisoning. There are no adequate and well-controlled studies in pregnant women. Use during pregnancy only if clearly needed.

➤*Lactation:* It is not known whether this drug is excreted in human milk. Because many drugs are excreted in human milk, exercise caution when administering acetylcysteine to a nursing woman.

➤*Children:* No adverse effects were noted during IV infusion with acetylcysteine at a mean rate of 8.4 mg/kg/h for 24 hours to 10 preterm newborns ranging in gestational age from 25 to 31 weeks and in weight from 500 to 1380 g in one study or in 6 newborns ranging in gestational age from 26 to 30 weeks and in weight from 520 to 1335 g infused with acetylcysteine at 0.1 to 1.3 mg/kg/h for 6 days. Elimination of acetylcysteine was slower in these infants than in adults; mean elimination half life was 11 hours.

Precautions

➤*Monitoring:* On admission for suspected acetaminophen overdose, draw a serum blood sample at least 4 hours after ingestion to determine the acetaminophen level; this will serve as a basis for determining the need for acetylcysteine treatment. If the patient presents after 4 hours postingestion, immediately determine the serum acetaminophen sample.

Determine the AST, ALT, bilirubin, prothrombin time, creatinine, blood urea nitrogen (BUN), blood glucose, and electrolytes in order to monitor hepatic and renal function and electrolyte and fluid balance.

➤*Emesis:* Occasionally, severe and persistent vomiting occurs as a symptom of acute acetaminophen overdose. Treatment with oral acetylcysteine may aggravate the vomiting. Evaluate patients at risk of gastric hemorrhage (eg, esophageal varices, peptic ulcers) concerning the risk of upper GI hemorrhage vs the risk of developing hepatic toxicity; give acetylcysteine treatment accordingly. Dilution of the acetylcysteine minimizes the propensity of oral acetylcysteine to aggravate vomiting.

Adverse Reactions

➤*Oral:* Oral administration of acetylcysteine, especially in the large doses needed to treat acetaminophen overdose, may result in nausea, vomiting, and other GI symptoms. Rash with or without mild fever has been observed rarely.

Overdosage

Single IV doses of acetylcysteine at 1000 mg/kg in mice, 2445 mg/kg in rats, 1500 mg/kg in guinea pigs, 1200 mg/kg in rabbits, and 500 mg/kg in dogs were lethal. Symptoms of acute toxicity were ataxia, convulsions, cyanosis, hypoactivity, labored respiration, and loss of righting reflex.

ACETYLCYSTEINE — INJECTION

Indications

➤*Acetaminophen overdose:* Acetylcysteine injection, administered intravenously within 8 to 10 hours after ingestion of a potentially hepatotoxic quantity of acetaminophen, is indicated to prevent or lessen hepatic injury.

Administration and Dosage

➤*Approved by the FDA:* April 28, 2004.

On admission for suspected acetaminophen overdose, a serum blood sample should be drawn at least 4 hours after ingestion to determine the acetaminophen level and will serve as a basis for determining the need for treatment with acetylcysteine. If the patient presents after 4 hours post-ingestion, the serum acetaminophen sample should be determined immediately.

Acetylcysteine injection should be administered within 8 hours from acetaminophen ingestion for maximal protection against hepatic injury for patients whose serum acetaminophen levels fall above the "possible" toxicity line on the Rumack-Matthew nomogram (line connecting 150 mcg/mL at 4 hours with 50 mcg/mL at 12 hours; see Acetaminophen Assays - Interpretation and methodology section). If the time of ingestion is unknown, or the serum acetaminophen level is not available, cannot be interpreted, or is not available within the 8-hour time interval from acetaminophen ingestion, acetylcysteine injection should be administered immediately if 24 hours or less have elapsed from the reported time of ingestion of an overdose of acetaminophen, regardless of the quantity reported to have been ingested.

The aspartate aminotransferase (AST), alanine aminotransferase (ALT), bilirubin, prothrombin time, creatinine, blood urea nitrogen (BUN), blood glucose, and electrolytes also should be determined in order to monitor hepatic and renal function and electrolyte and fluid balance.

➤*Note:* The critical ingestion-treatment interval for maximal protection against severe hepatic injury is between 0 to 8 hours. Efficacy diminishes progressively after 8 hours and treatment initiation between 15 and 24 hours post ingestion of acetaminophen yields limited efficacy. However, it does not appear to worsen the condition of patients and it should not be withheld, since the reported time of ingestion may not be correct.

➤*The following dosages are recommended for IV administration:* The total dose of acetylcysteine is 300 mg/kg administered over 21 hours.

Loading dose – 150 mg/kg in 200 mL of 5% dextrose, infuse intravenously over 60 minutes.

Maintenance dose – 50 mg/kg in 500 mL of 5% dextrose, infuse intravenously over 4 hours followed by 100 mg/kg in 1,000 mL of 5% dextrose, infuse intravenously over 16 hours.

➤*Incompatibilities:* Acetylcysteine injection is not compatible with rubber and metals, particularly iron, copper and nickel.

➤*Renal function impairment:* No data are available to determine if a dose adjustment in patients with moderate or severe renal impairment is required.

➤*Hepatic function impairment:* Although there was a 3-fold increase in acetylcysteine plasma concentrations in patients with hepatic cirrhosis, no data are available to determine if a dose adjustment in these patients is required. The published medical literature does not indicate that the dose of acetylcysteine in patients with hepatic impairment should be reduced.

➤*Preparation of acetylcysteine for IV administration:* IV administration requires dilution with 5% dextrose. Do not use previously opened vials for IV administration.

Loading dose – Dilute 150 mg/kg in 200 mL of 5% dextrose.

Maintenance dose – 50 mg/kg in 500 mL of 5% dextrose.

Second maintenance dose – 100 mg/kg in 1,000 mL of 5% dextrose.

Dosage guide and preparation –

Acetylcysteine dosage guide by weight (≥ 40 kg)				
Body weight		First	Second	Third
		150 mg/kg in 200 mL 5% Dextrose over 60 minutes	50 mg/kg in 500 mL 5% Dextrose over 4 hours	100 mg/kg in 1,000 mL 5% Dextrose over 16 hours
(kg)	(lb)	Acetylcysteine (mL)	Acetylcysteine (mL)	Acetylcysteine (mL)
100	220	75	25	50
90	198	67.5	22.5	45
80	176	60	20	40

ACETYLCYSTEINE — INJECTION

Acetylcysteine dosage guide by weight (≥ 40 kg)				
Body weight		First	Second	Third
		150 mg/kg in 200 mL 5% Dextrose over 60 minutes	50 mg/kg in 500 mL 5% Dextrose over 4 hours	100 mg/kg in 1,000 mL 5% Dextrose over 16 hours
(kg)	(lb)	Acetylcysteine (mL)	Acetylcysteine (mL)	Acetylcysteine (mL)
70	154	52.5	17.5	35
60	132	45	15	30
50	110	37.5	12.5	25
40	88	30	10	20

Acetylcysteine dosage guide by weight (less than 40 kg)							
Body weight		First		Second		Third	
		150 mg/kg over 60 minutes		50 mg/kg over 4 hours		100 mg/kg over 16 hours	
(kg)	(lb)	Acetylcysteine (mL)	5% Dextrose (mL)	Acetylcysteine (mL)	5% Dextrose (mL)	Acetylcysteine (mL)	5% Dextrose (mL)
30	66	22.5	100	7.5	250	15	500
25	55	18.75	100	6.25	250	12.5	500
20	44	15	60	5	140	10	280
15	33	11.25	45	3.75	105	7.5	210
10	22	7.5	30	2.5	70	5	140

➤*Admixture compatibilities:* Acetylcysteine is hyperosmolar (2,600 mOsm/L) and is compatible with 5% dextrose, ½ normal saline, and water for injection.

➤*Acetaminophen assays, interpretation and methodology:* The acute ingestion of acetaminophen in quantities of 150 mg/kg or greater may result in hepatic toxicity. However, the reported history of the quantity of a drug ingested as an overdose is often inaccurate and is not a reliable guide to therapy of the overdose. Therefore, plasma or serum acetaminophen concentrations, determined as early as possible, but no sooner than 4 hours following an acute overdose, are essential in assessing the potential risk of hepatotoxicity. If an assay for acetaminophen cannot be obtained, it is necessary to assume that the overdose is potentially toxic.

Interpretation of acetaminophen assays –

1.) When results of the plasma acetaminophen assay are available, refer to the nomogram below to determine if plasma concentration is in the potentially toxic range. Values above the line connecting 200 mcg/mL at 4 hours with 50 mcg/mL at 12 hours (probable line) are associated with a probability of hepatic toxicity if an antidote is not administered.
2.) If the predetoxification plasma level is above the line connecting 150 mcg/mL at 4 hours with 37.5 mcg/mL at 12 hours (possible line), continue with maintenance doses of acetylcysteine. It is better to err on the safe side, and thus this line, defining possible toxicity, is plotted 25% below the line, defining probable toxicity.
3.) If the predetoxification plasma level is below the line connecting 150 mcg/mL at 4 hours with 37.5 mcg/mL at 12 hours (possible line), there is minimal risk of hepatic toxicity, and acetylcysteine treatment may be discontinued.

Acetaminophen assay methodology – Suitable assay procedures for measuring acetaminophen levels in plasma are listed below. These methods detect only parent acetaminophen and not conjugated acetaminophen.

Selected techniques (noninclusive): HPLC: Blair D and Rumack BH. *Clin Chem* 1977;23(4):743-5. Howie D, Andriaenssens PI, and Prescott LF. J *Pharm Pharmacol*, 1977;29(4):235-7.

GC: Prescott LF. J *Pharm Pharmacol*, 1971;23(10):807-8.

Colorimetric: Glynn JP and Kendal SE. *Lancet*, 1975;1(May 17):1147-8.

➤*Storage/Stability:* Single-dose vial, preservative-free, discard unused portion.

Stability studies indicate that the reconstituted solution is stable for 24 hours at controlled room temperature.

Store unopened vials at controlled room temperature 20° to 25°C (68° to 77°F).

Actions

➤*Pharmacology:*

Acetaminophen overdose – Acetaminophen is absorbed from the upper gastrointestinal tract with peak plasma levels occurring between 30 and 60 minutes after therapeutic doses and usually within 4 hours following an overdose. It is extensively metabolized in the liver to form principally the sulfate and glucuronide conjugates which are excreted in the urine. A small fraction of an ingested dose is metabolized in the liver by isozyme CYP2E1 of the cytochrome P450 mixed function oxidase enzyme system to form a reactive, potentially toxic, intermediate metabolite. The toxic metabolite preferentially conjugates with hepatic glutathione to form nontoxic cysteine and mercapturic acid derivatives, which are then excreted by the kidney. Recommended therapeutic doses of acetaminophen are not believed to saturate the glucuronide and sulfate conjugation pathways, and therefore are not expected to result in the formation of sufficient reactive metabolite to deplete glutathione stores. However, following ingestion of a large overdose, the glucuronide and sulfate conjugation pathways are saturated resulting in a larger fraction of the drug being metabolized via the cytochrome P450 pathway and therefore, the amount of acetaminophen metabolized to the reactive intermediate increases. The increased formation of the reactive metabolite may deplete the hepatic stores of glutathione with subsequent binding of the metabolite to protein molecules within the hepatocyte resulting in cellular necrosis.

Acetylcysteine IV treatment – Acetylcysteine has been shown to reduce the extent of liver injury following acetaminophen overdose. It is most effective when given early, with benefit seen principally in patients treated within 8 to 10 hours of the overdose. Acetylcysteine likely protects the liver by maintaining or restoring the glutathione levels, or by acting as an alternate substrate for conjugation with, and thus detoxification of, the reactive metabolite.

➤*Pharmacokinetics:*

Distribution – The steady-state volume of distribution (Vd_{ss}) and the protein binding for acetylcysteine were reported to be 0.47 L/kg and 83%, respectively.

Metabolism – Acetylcysteine may form cysteine, disulfides, and conjugates in vivo (N, N′-diacetylcysteine, N-acetylcysteine-cysteine, N-acetylcysteine-glutathione, N-acetylcysteine-protein). Based on published data, it was reported that after an oral dose of ^{35}S-acetylcysteine, about 22% of total radioactivity was excreted in urine after 24 hours. No metabolites were identified.

Excretion – After a single IV dose of acetylcysteine, the plasma concentration of total acetylcysteine declined in a poly-exponential decay manner with a mean terminal half-life ($t_{½}$) of 5.6 hours. The mean clearance for acetylcysteine was reported to be 0.11 L/hr/kg and renal clearance constituted about 30% of total clearance.

Special populations –

Renal function impairment: Pharmacokinetic information is not available in patients with renal impairment.

Hepatic function impairment: In subjects with severe liver damage (ie, cirrhosis due to alcohol with Child-Pugh score of 7 to 13, or primary or secondary biliary cirrhosis with Child-Pugh score of 5 to 7), mean $t_{½}$ increased by 80% while mean CL decreased by 30% compared to control group.

Elderly: Adequate information on acetylcysteine pharmacokinetics in geriatric patients is not available.

Children: The mean elimination $t_{½}$ of acetylcysteine is longer in newborns (11 hours) than in adults (5.6 hours). Pharmacokinetic information is not available in other age groups.

Gender: Adequate information is not available to assess if there are differences in pharmacokinetics (PK) between males and females.

Pregnant women: In 4 pregnant women with acetaminophen toxicity, oral or IV acetylcysteine was administered at the time of delivery. Acetylcysteine was detected in the cord blood of 3 viable infants and in cardiac blood of a fourth infant, sampled at autopsy.

Drug-drug interactions – No drug-drug interaction studies have been conducted.

Contraindications

Acetylcysteine injection is contraindicated in patients with hypersensitivity or previous anaphylactoid reactions to acetylcysteine or any components in the preparation.

Warnings

➤*Hypersensitivity reactions:* Serious anaphylactoid reactions, including death in a patient with asthma, have been reported in patients administered acetylcysteine intravenously.

Acute flushing and erythema of the skin may occur in patients receiving acetylcysteine intravenously. These reactions usually occur 30 to 60 minutes after initiating the infusion and often resolve spontaneously despite continued infusion of acetylcysteine. Anaphylactoid reactions (defined as the occurrence of an acute hypersensitivity reaction during acetylcysteine administration including rash, hypotension, wheezing, and/or shortness of breath) have been observed in patients receiving IV acetylcysteine for acetaminophen overdose and occurred soon after initiation of the infusion. If a reaction to acetylcysteine involves more than simply flushing and erythema of the skin, it should be treated as an anaphylactoid reaction. This usually entails administering antihistaminic drugs as well as epinephrine in severe cases. In addition, the acetylcysteine infusion may be interrupted until treatment of the anaphylactoid symptoms has been initiated and then carefully restarted. If the anaphylactoid reaction returns upon reinitiation of treatment or increases in severity, IV acetylcysteine should be discontinued and alternative patient management should be considered. For additional information, contact the American Association of Poison Control Centers (1-800-222-1222).

➤*Carcinogenesis:* Long-term studies in animals have not been performed to evaluate the carcinogenic potential of acetylcysteine.

➤*Mutagenesis:* Acetylcysteine was not genotoxic in the Ames test or the in vivo mouse micronucleus test. It was, however, positive in the in vitro mouse lymphoma cell (L5178Y/TK±) forward mutation test.

➤*Fertility impairment:* Treatment of male rats with acetylcysteine at an oral dose of 250 mg/kg/day for 15 weeks (compared to the recommended total human IV dose of 300 mg/kg) did not affect the fertility or general reproductive performance.

➤*Elderly:* The clinical studies do not provide a sufficient number of geriatric subjects to determine whether the elderly respond differently.

➤*Pregnancy:* Category B.

Pregnant women – In 4 pregnant women with acetaminophen toxicity, oral or IV acetylcysteine was administered at the time of delivery. Acetyl-

ACETYLCYSTEINE — INJECTION

cysteine crossed the placenta and was measurable in newborn circulation and cord blood of 3 viable infants following delivery and in cardiac blood of a fourth infant at autopsy (22 weeks gestational age who died 3 hours after birth). No adverse sequelae developed in the 3 viable infants. All mothers recovered and none of the infants had evidence of acetaminophen poisoning.

Teratogenic – Teratology studies were performed in rats at oral doses up to 2,000 mg/kg/day and in rabbits at oral doses up to 1,000 mg/kg/day (compared to the recommended total human IV dose of 300 mg/kg) and revealed no evidence of impaired fertility or harm to the fetus due to acetylcysteine. There are, however, no adequate and well-controlled studies in pregnant women. Because animal reproduction studies may not always be predictive of human response, this drug should be used during pregnancy only if clearly needed.

➤*Lactation:* It is not known whether this drug is excreted in human milk. Because many drugs are excreted in human milk, caution should be exercised when acetylcysteine is administered to a nursing woman.

➤*Children:* No adverse effects were noted during IV infusion with acetylcysteine at a mean rate of 8.4 mg/kg/hr for 24 hours to 10 preterm newborns ranging in gestational age from 25 to 31 weeks and in weight from 500 to 1,380 g in 1 study (Study 1) or in 6 newborns ranging in gestational age from 26 to 30 weeks and in weight from 520 to 1,335 g infused with acetylcysteine at 0.1 to 1.3 mg/kg/hr for 6 days (Study 2). Elimination of acetylcysteine was slower in these infants than in adults; mean elimination half-life was 11 hours (Study 1).

Precautions

➤*Special risk:* Acetylcysteine injection should be used with caution in patients with asthma, or where there is a history of bronchospasm.

Drug Interactions

Drug stability and safety of acetylcysteine when mixed with other drugs have not been established.

Adverse Reactions

In the literature the most frequently reported adverse events attributed to IV acetylcysteine administration were rash, urticaria, and pruritus. The frequency of adverse events has been reported to be between 0.2% and 20.8%, and they most commonly occur during the initial loading dose of acetylcysteine.

The incidence of drug-related adverse events occurring within the first 2 hours following acetylcysteine administration reported in a randomized study (Infusion Rate Study) in patients with acetaminophen poisoning is presented in the table below by preferred term. In this study patients were randomized to a 15-minute or a 60-minute loading dose regimen.

Incidence of drug-related adverse events occurring within the first 2 hours following study drug administration by preferred term: Infusion rate study

Treatment group	15 minutes				60 minutes			
Number of patients	(n = 109)				(n = 71)			
Cardiac disorders	5 (5%)				2 (3%)			
Severity:	Unknown	Mild	Moderate	Severe	Unknown	Mild	Moderate	Severe
Tachycardia NOS		4 (4%)	1 (1%)			2 (3%)		
Ear and labyrinth disorders	1 (1%)				0 (0%)			
Severity:	Unknown	Mild	Moderate	Severe	Unknown	Mild	Moderate	Severe
Ear pain			1 (1%)					
Gastro-intestinal disorders	16 (15%)				7 (10%)			
Severity:	Unknown	Mild	Moderate	Severe	Unknown	Mild	Moderate	Severe
Nausea	1 (1%)		6 (6%)			1 (1%)	1 (1%)	
Vomiting NOS		2 (2%)	11 (10%)			2 (3%)	4 (6%)	
General disorders and administration site conditions	1 (1%)				1 (1%)			
Severity:	Unknown	Mild	Moderate	Severe	Unknown	Mild	Moderate	Severe
Chest tightness		1 (1%)						
Feeling hot						1 (1%)		
Immune system disorders	20 (18%)				10 (14%)			
Severity:	Unknown	Mild	Moderate	Severe	Unknown	Mild	Moderate	Severe
Anaphylactoid reaction	2 (2%)	6 (6%)	11 (10%)	1 (1%)		4 (6%)	5 (7%)	1 (1%)
Respiratory, thoracic and mediastinal disorders	2 (2%)				2 (3%)			
Severity:	Unknown	Mild	Moderate	Severe	Unknown	Mild	Moderate	Severe

Incidence of drug-related adverse events occurring within the first 2 hours following study drug administration by preferred term: Infusion rate study

Treatment group	15 minutes				60 minutes			
Number of patients	(n = 109)				(n = 71)			
Pharyngitis			1 (1%)					
Rhinorrhoea		1 (1%)						
Rhonchi						1 (1%)		
Throat tightness						1 (1%)		
Skin and subcutaneous tissue disorders	6 (6%)				5 (7%)			
Severity:	Unknown	Mild	Moderate	Severe	Unknown	Mild	Moderate	Severe
Pruritus		1 (1%)				2 (3%)		
Rash NOS		3 (3%)	2 (2%)			3 (4%)		
Vascular disorders	2 (2%)				3 (4%)			
Severity:	Unknown	Mild	Moderate	Severe	Unknown	Mild	Moderate	Severe
Flushing		1 (1%)	1 (1%)			2 (3%)	1 (1%)	

Adverse events summarized by the Rocky Mountain Poison and Drug Center from 76 published articles in which IV acetylcysteine was administered (acetaminophen overdose and other published uses) are listed with an incidence greater than 1% in the table below. Charcoal, naloxone, and benzodiazepines were administered concomitantly in several of these studies.

Adverse events greater than 1% by body system: Published clinical studies, acetaminophen overdose and other published uses*

Body system classification	Adverse event occurrences	Distribution of all adverse events (%)	Frequency in patients with safety monitoring (n = 2,040)
Miscellaneous			
Urticaria	34	7.96	1.67
Vasodilation and rash	30	7.03	1.47
Vasodilation, rash, and pruritus	42	9.84	2.06
Cardiovascular			
Hypotension	16	3.75	0.78
Syncope	13	3.04	0.64
Vasodilation	28	6.56	1.37
GI			
Dyspepsia	5	1.17	0.24
Nausea	43	10.07	2.11
Vomiting	15	3.51	0.74
CNS			
Abnormal thinking (dysphoria)	8	1.87	0.39
Gait disturbances	5	1.17	0.24
Respiratory			
Bronchospasm	25	5.85	1.23
Coughing	18	4.22	0.88
Dyspnea	11	2.58	0.54
Dermatologic			
Angioedema	33	7.73	1.62
Facial erythema	5	1.17	0.24
Palmar erythema	6	1.41	0.29
Pruritus	5	1.17	0.24
Pruritus and rash	7	1.64	0.34
Rash	21	4.92	1.03
Sweating	6	1.41	0.29
Special senses			
Eye pain	11	2.58	0.54

* Data on file: *Systematic Analysis of Medical Literature Regarding Safety of IV N-acetylcysteine*, Rocky Mountain Poison & Drug Center, Denver Health; 27 December 2001.

Overdosage

Single IV doses of acetylcysteine at 1,000 mg/kg in mice, 2,445 mg/kg in rats, 1,500 mg/kg in guinea pigs, 1,200 mg/kg in rabbits and 500 mg/kg in dogs were lethal. Symptoms of acute toxicity were ataxia, hypoactivity, labored respiration, cyanosis, loss of righting reflex and convulsions.

IPECAC SYRUP

otc	**Ipecac** (Various, eg, Roxane)	**Syrup**	1.5% to 1.75% alcohol. In 15 and 30 mL.
Rx	**Ipecac** (Various, eg, Paddock)	**Syrup**	2% alcohol. In 15 and 30 mL.

IPECAC — ORAL

Indications

➤*Overdose/Poisoning:* Treatment of drug overdose and in certain poisonings.

Administration and Dosage

Ipecac syrup may not work on an empty stomach. Have patient sit upright with head forward before administering dose.

➤*Children (younger than 1 year of age):* 5 to 10 mL, then ½ to 1 glass water. Should *probably* give only with medical supervision. There is controversy over giving to children younger than 1 year of age, although it appears to be safe and effective.

➤*Children older than 1 to 12 years of age):* 15 mL followed by 1 to 2 glasses of water.

➤*Adults:* 15 to 30 mL followed by 3 to 4 glasses of water.

➤*Repeat Dosage:* Repeat dosage (15 mL) once in persons older than one year if vomiting does not occur within 20 to 30 min. If vomiting does not occur within 30 to 45 min after the second dose, perform gastric lavage.

➤*Storage/Stability:* Keep tightly closed at controlled room temperature 15° to 30°C (59° to 86°F).

Actions

➤*Pharmacology:* Ipecac produces vomiting by a local irritant effect on GI mucosa and a central medullary effect (stimulation of chemoreceptor trigger zone). The central effect is caused by emetine and cephaeline, the two alkaloids. An adequate dose causes vomiting within 30 min in more than 90% of patients (average time is less than 20 min).

Contraindications

Semiconscious or unconscious patients. Do not use if strychnine, corrosives such as alkalies and strong acids, or petroleum distillates have been ingested.

Warnings

➤*Special risk: Keep out of reach of children.*

➤*Do not use:* Ordinarily this drug should not be used if strychnine, corrosives such as alkalies (lye) and strong acids, or petroleum distillates such as kerosene, gasoline, coal oil, fuel oil, paint thinner, or cleaning fluid have been ingested.

Do not use in unconscious persons.

➤*Administration:* Do not administer milk with this product.

➤*Syrup/Fluid extract:* Do not confuse ipecac syrup with ipecac fluid extract, which is 14 times stronger and has caused some deaths.

➤*Call an emergency room:* Call an emergency room, poison control center or physician before using; if vomiting does not occur within 30 to 45 minutes after the second dose, perform gastric lavage.

➤*Ipecac Syrup Abuse:* Ipecac syrup abuse may occur in bulimic and anorexic patients. It has been implicated as the causative factor of severe cardiomyopathies, and even death, in several persons with eating disorders who used it regularly to induce vomiting.

➤*Pregnancy: Category C.* It is not known whether the drug can cause harm when administered to a pregnant woman. Minimal systemic absorption is expected when used as directed (see Administration and Dosage).

➤*Lactation:* It is not known whether ipecac alkaloids are excreted in breast milk. Exercise caution if ipecac syrup is used for treatment of a nursing woman.

Precautions

➤*Absorption:* Ipecac syrup can be cardiotoxic if not vomited and allowed to be absorbed. Absorption of emetine may occur and cause heart conduction disturbances, atrial fibrillation or fatal myocarditis.

Drug Interactions

➤*Activated charcoal:* Activated charcoal will absorb ipecac syrup. Do not give activated charcoal until after the patient has vomited, unless directed by a health professional.

Adverse Reactions

Reactions are generally not significant if the dose is not exceeded. Diarrhea (25% in children younger than 3 years of age); drowsiness (20% in children younger than 3 years of age); coughing or choking in association with emesis (less than 4%); mild CNS depression; GI upset (may last several hours after emesis).

Overdosage

➤*Symptoms:* Ipecac is cardiotoxic if absorbed and may cause cardiac conduction disturbances, bradycardia, atrial fibrillation, hypotension, or fatal myocarditis.

➤*Treatment:* Activated charcoal may be given to adsorb ipecac syrup; perform gastric lavage. Support cardiovascular system by symptomatic treatment.

Patient Information

Always consult a physician or poison control center in cases of accidental ingestion.

Give with adequate amounts of water; do not use milk or carbonated beverages. Do not exceed recommended dosage.

CHARCOAL, ACTIVATED

otc	**Activated Charcoal** (Various)	**Powder**	In 15, 30, 40, 120 and 240 g and UD 30 g.
otc	**Activated Charcoal** (Various)	**Liquid:** 208 mg/ml	12.5 g with propylene glycol. In 60 mL bottle. 25 g with propylene glycol. In 120 mL bottle.
otc	**Actidose-Aqua** (Paddock)		25 g in 120 mL suspension. 50 g in 240 mL suspension.
otc	**Actidose with Sorbitol** (Paddock)		25 g in 120 mL suspension with sorbitol. 50 g in 240 mL suspension with sorbitol.
otc	**Liqui-Char** (Jones Medical)		12.5 g in 60 ml bottle, 15 g in 75 mL bottle, 25 g in 120 mL squeeze container, 30 g in 120 mL squeeze container, 50 g in 240 mL squeeze container.
otc	**CharcoAid** (Requa)	**Suspension:** 15 g	Sorbitol. In 120 mL.
		30 g	Sorbitol. In 150 mL.
otc	**CharcoAid 2000** (Requa)	**Liquid:** 15 g	With and without sorbitol. In 120 mL.
		50 g	With and without sorbitol. In 240 mL.
		Granules: 15 g	In 120 mL.

ACTIVATED CHARCOAL — ORAL

Indications

➤*Poisoning:* Activated charcoal liquid is the emergency poison treatment of choice for cases of acute toxic ingestion. Each year, 3 million to 8 million poison exposures occur in the United States. Eighty percent (80%) of these exposures involve healthy, active children under the age of 5 years. Therefore, immediate and effective poison treatment procedures should be at hand in all hospitals and emergency care facilities. Activated charcoal and syrup of ipecac are the prime agents of the treatment process.

➤*Ineffectiveness:* Activated charcoal is ineffective for mineral acids, alkalies and substances insoluble in aqueous acidic solutions. The effectiveness in the lower GI tract of the adsorbent is questionable because passage through the upper tract saturates and deactivates the agent, but drugs adsorbed in the upper tract are not desorbed in the lower intestinal tract.

Administration and Dosage

➤*Administration of activated charcoal:* Preferably to be used at the direction of a physician or poison control center personnel. When administering activated charcoal from a unit-dose bottle, stir thoroughly and shake vigorously the contents of the unit-dose container, and cause the patient to ingest its entire contents. If after administration, a substantial quantity of charcoal remains, add water to the container, shake again, and readminister. When administering activated charcoal from a unit-dose tube, kneed and shake vigorously before using. Carefully cut tip. Administer through a gastric tube or squeeze contents into a glass and have patient drink contents. Milk, ice cream, or sherbet should not be mixed with the charcoal because it will decrease the adsorptive capacity of the activated charcoal. Further, the effectiveness of other medications that may be administered concurrently may be decreased because of the adsorption of the activated charcoal.

ACTIVATED CHARCOAL — ORAL

First, check to ensure that the patient is breathing and remove food or dental work from the mouth so that adequate air can get to the lungs. If the patient is not breathing, administer artificial respiration as the air flow to the lungs must not be impeded. The patient should receive no drugs, coffee, alcohol or carbonated beverages. The patient should be kept warm though not overheated.

When possible, activated charcoal should be administered promptly, preferably within 30 minutes following ingestion of the toxins. To delay treatment longer will permit time for the toxins to permeate the patient's body and so decrease the effectiveness of the charcoal's adsorptive action.

➤*Dosage:*

Activated charcoal in a sorbitol base –

Adults: For adults, the recommended dosage for activated charcoal in a sorbitol base is 50 to 60 g (or the contents of two 25 g or 30 g containers).

Children from 1 to 12 years of age: For children from age 1 to 12 years of age, the recommended dosage is based on the weight of the child.

For children weighing over 32 kg, (71 lbs), the recommended dosage is 50 to 60 g. For children weighing 16 to 32 kg, (38 to 71 lbs), the recommended dosage is 25 to 30 g. For children less than 16 kg, (36 lbs), and for children younger than 1 year of age, activated charcoal in a sorbitol base is not recommended.

Activated charcoal in a sorbitol base is not recommended for multiple-dose activated charcoal therapy because of excessive cathartic action.

Activated charcoal in an aqueous base – A dosage range exists from 5 to 60 g of activated charcoal for optimal therapeutic result. The dosage should be from 8 to 10 times by volume greater than the amount of toxic substance ingested, if that factor is known. If the amount of toxic substance ingested is not known, the amount of activated charcoal in an aqueous base administered should be based upon the weight, size and age of the patient. A dosage of 20 to 30 g should be the minimal dosage for children over 1 year of age and for adults. After the first dose has been administered, additional activated charcoal may be given at the direction of the poison control center or the emergency room physician. However, no damage or harm will occur to the patient if larger than minimal dosage is administered, as the charcoal is readily tolerated by the body and will be eliminated through the intestinal tract.

Actions

➤*Pharmacology:* Activated charcoal adsorbs the toxic substances ingested by forming an effective barrier between any remaining particulate material and the GI mucosa, thus inhibiting any GI absorption. Testing of activated charcoal liquid indicates that the adsorption power of each size of the activated charcoal, when treated with 10% of the alkaloid strychnine sulfate (based on the quantity of charcoal per bottle [eg, 1.5 g of alkaloid to 15 g charcoal]) is not less than 99%. Treatment of the product with dyes (methylene blue) produces similar results. The adsorptive properties of the activated charcoal liquid are slightly decreased during the shelf-life of the product but are still capable of adsorbing at least 99% of the substance tested.

Activated charcoal in a sorbitol base – Sorbitol is hexahydric sugar alcohol which primarily serves as an osmotic cathartic. As a hyperosmotic, cathartic sorbitol produces a hygroscopic action resulting in increased water in the large intestines and increased intraluminal pressure which stimulates catharsis. Catharsis of activated charcoal generally occurs in an average of 1 to 1.5 hours and persists for 8 to 12 hours. The onset of action may be expected to be longer in patients who have ingested toxins which decrease bowel motility such as pharmacologic agents and plants with anticholinergic properties and drugs like narcotics.

Warnings

➤*Activated charcoal in a sorbitol base:* Do not use activated charcoal in a sorbitol base in any person known to have a rare autosomal recessive genetic intolerance to fructose or in patients who are known to be dehydrated. Activated charcoal in a sorbitol base may cause excessive diarrhea.

Precautions

➤*Cathartic effect:* When using activated charcoal in a sorbitol base, be aware that diarrhea may result. Because a profound cathartic effect may occur following use of this product, proper attention should be provided to the patient's fluid and electrolyte needs.

Activated charcoal in a sorbitol base should be used cautiously in patients receiving multiple doses. If activated charcoal in a sorbitol base is used at each dosage interval, profound catharsis may develop, resulting in dehydration and even hypotension.

Adverse Reactions

Activated charcoal will color stool black which may be alarming to patient although medically insignificant.

METHYLENE BLUE

Rx	**Urolene Blue** (Star)	**Tablets:** 65 mg	In 100s and 1,000s.
Rx	**Methylene Blue** (Various, eg, Pasadena)	**Injection:** 10 mg/mL	In 1 and 10 mL amps.

METHYLENE BLUE — ORAL

Indications

Methylene blue is a mild urinary antiseptic and stimulant to mucous surfaces. It has been used as a genitourinary antiseptic in cystitis and urethritis both by internal administration and by irrigation; other bacteriostatic and bactericidal agents have replaced it for this purpose. It is excreted in the urine giving it a blue or greenish color. It is used as a diagnostic agent and indicator dye. Methylene blue is used in the treatment of cyanide poisoning and methemoglobinemia.

Administration and Dosage

1 or 2 tablets 3 times a day after meals with a full glass of water.

Actions

➤*Pharmacology:* Methylene blue is the first dye used as an antiseptic. Its bactericidal properties, however, are very mild, and its present uses center mainly in its oxidation-reduction functions and its tissue-staining property. In relatively high concentration, it oxidizes the ferrous iron of reduced hemoglobin to the ferric state, thereby changing hemoglobin to methemoglobin. In low concentrations, its reduced form appears to increase the speed of the reverse reaction, changing methemoglobin to hemoglobin. Some experiments indicate that methylene blue inhibits amine oxidase in tissues.

Review of the various forms of therapy used to treat kidney stones revealed that all have some deleterious or toxic effect which may preclude their use in some patients. In addition, none of the foregoing agents had the advantage of being chemisorptive, that is absorbing on the crystal surface by chemical rather than physical forces and preventing further crystal growth or agglomeration. Many dyes are known to have this property and the search for a nontoxic, well-tolerated inhibitor of calcium crystallization led to methylene blue. This compound is a direct inhibitor of calcium binding by oxalate and by matrix and, in addition, it reverses intracellular acidosis (such as exists in renal tubular acidosis) by apparent competition with diphosphapyridine nucleotide as a hydrogen receptor.

Contraindications

Use with caution in patients with significant impairment of renal functions, and in patients allergic to methylene blue. Methylene blue is a relatively nontoxic drug and safe to use in most instances.

Warnings

➤*Bladder irritation:* Methylene blue produces no symptoms except occasional irritation of the bladder.

METHYLENE BLUE — INJECTION

Indications

➤*Methemoglobinemia:* Drug-induced methemoglobinemia.

Administration and Dosage

0.1 to 0.2 mL/kg of body weight (0.045 to 0.09 mL/lb of body weight). Inject methylene blue IV very slowly over a period of several minutes.

➤*Storage/Stability:* Store below 40°C (104°F), preferably between 15° to 30°C (59° to 86°F).

Actions

➤*Pharmacology:* Methylene blue will produce 2 opposite actions on hemoglobin. Low concentrations will convert methemoglobin to hemoglobin. High concentrations convert the ferrous iron of reduced hemoglobin to ferric iron which results in the formation of methemoglobin.

Contraindications

Intraspinal injection is contraindicated.

Warnings

➤*Administration:* Methylene blue should not be given by subcutaneous or intrathecal injection.

➤*Pregnancy:* Safety for use in pregnancy has not been established. Use of methylene blue in women of childbearing potential requires that anticipated benefits be weighed against possible hazards.

Precautions

➤*Additional methemoglobin:* Methylene blue must be injected IV very slowly over a period of several minutes to prevent local high concentration of the compound from producing additional methemoglobin. Do not exceed recommended dosage.

Adverse Reactions

Large IV doses of methylene blue produce nausea, abdominal and precordial pain, dizziness, headache, profuse sweating, mental confusion and the formation of methemoglobin.

DIGOXIN

Rx	**Lanoxicaps** (Cardinal Health)	**Capsules**: 0.05 mg	Parabens, sorbitol. (A2C). Red. In 100s.
		0.1 mg	Parabens, sorbitol. (B2C). Yellow. In 100s.
		0.2 mg	Parabens, sorbitol. (C2C). Green. In 100s.
Rx	**Digoxin** (Various, eg, Qualitest)	**Tablets**: 0.125 mg	In 1000s.
Rx	**Lanoxin** (GlaxoWellcome)		Lactose. (Lanoxin Y3B). Yellow, scored. In 30s, 100s, 1000s, 5000s and UD 100s.
Rx	**Digitek** (Bertek Pharm)		Lactose. (B 145). Yellow, round, scored. In 100s, 1000s, and 5000s.
Rx	**Digoxin** (Various, eg, Qualitest)	**Tablets**: 0.25 mg	In 1000s.
Rx	**Lanoxin** (GlaxoWellcome)		Lactose. (Lanoxin X3A). White. In 30s, 100s, 1000s, 5000s and UD 100s.
Rx	**Digitek** (Bertek Pharm)		Lactose. (B 146). White, scored. In 100s, 1000s, and 5000s.
Rx	**Digoxin**[1] (Various, eg, Roxane)	**Elixir, pediatric**: 0.05 mg/mL	In 60 mL and UD 2.5 and 5 mL.
Rx	**Lanoxin** (GlaxoWellcome)		10% alcohol, 0.1% methylparaben. Lime flavor. In 60 mL with calibrated dropper.
Rx	**Digoxin** (Elkins-Sinn)	**Injection**: 0.25 mg/mL	In 2 mL amps.[2]
Rx	**Digoxin** (Various, Hospira, Wyeth-Ayerst)		In 1 and 2 mL *Tubex* or *Carpuject*.[3]
Rx	**Lanoxin** (GlaxoWellcome)		In 2 mL amps.[3]
Rx	**Digoxin Injection, Pediatric** (Abbott)	**Injection, pediatric**: 0.1 mg/mL	In 1 mL amps.[3]
Rx	**Lanoxin** (GlaxoWellcome)		In 1 mL amps.[3]

[1] May contain 10% alcohol.
[2] With 0.1 mL alcohol and 0.4 mL propylene glycol per mL.
[3] With 40% propylene glycol and 10% alcohol.

DIGOXIN — ORAL

Indications

➤*Heart failure:* For the treatment of mild to moderate heart failure. Digoxin increases left ventricular ejection fraction (LVEF) and improves heart failure symptoms as evidenced by exercise capacity and heart failure-related hospitalizations and emergency care, while having no effect on mortality. Where possible, use digoxin with a diuretic and an angiotensin-converting enzyme (ACE) inhibitor, but an optimal order for starting these 3 drugs cannot be specified.

➤*Atrial fibrillation:* Digoxin is indicated for the control of ventricular response rate in patients with chronic atrial fibrillation.

Administration and Dosage

➤*Approved by the FDA:* July 26, 1982 (capsules); September 30, 1997 (tablets); September 6, 1991 (elixir).

➤*Tablets and pediatric elixir:* Recommended dosages of digoxin may require considerable modification because of individual sensitivity of the patient to the drug, the presence of associated conditions, or the use of concurrent medications.

➤*Capsules:* Because of the more complete absorption of digoxin from soft capsules, recommended oral doses are only 80% of those for tablets and elixir.

Because the significance of the higher peak serum concentrations associated with once-daily capsules is not established, divided daily dosing is presently recommended for the following:

1.) Infants and children younger than 10 years of age.
2.) Patients requiring a daily dose of 300 mcg (0.3 mg) or greater.
3.) Patients with histories of digitalis toxicity.
4.) Patients considered likely to become toxic.
5.) Patients in whom compliance is not a problem.

Where compliance is considered a problem, single daily dosing may be appropriate.

➤*Rapid digitalization with a loading dose:*

Tablets – If the patient's clinical response necessitates a change from the calculated loading dose of digoxin, then base calculation of the maintenance dose upon the amount actually given.

A single initial dose of 500 to 750 mcg (0.5 to 0.75 mg) of digoxin tablets usually produces a detectable effect in 0.5 to 2 hours that becomes maximal in 2 to 6 hours. Give additional doses of 125 to 375 mcg (0.125 to 0.375 mg) cautiously at 6- to 8-hour intervals until clinical evidence of an adequate effect is noted. The usual amount of digoxin tablets that a 70 kg patient requires to achieve 8 to 12 mcg/kg peak body stores is 750 to 1,250 mcg (0.75 to 1.25 mg).

Capsules – If the patient's clinical response necessitates a change from the calculated loading dose of digoxin, then base calculation of the maintenance dose upon the amount actually given.

A single initial dose of 400 to 600 mcg (0.4 to 0.6 mg) of digoxin capsules usually produces a detectable effect in 0.5 to 2 hours that becomes maximal in 2 to 6 hours. Additional doses of 100 to 300 mcg (0.1 to 0.3 mg) may be given cautiously at 6- to 8-hour intervals until clinical evidence of an adequate effect is noted. The usual amount of digoxin capsules that a 70 kg patient requires to achieve 8 to 12 mcg/kg peak body stores is 600 to 1,000 mcg (0.6 to 1 mg).

Elixir – Digitalizing and daily maintenance doses for each age group are given below and should provide therapeutic effect with minimum risk of toxicity in most patients with heart failure and normal sinus rhythm. These recommendations assume the presence of healthy renal function.

Usual Digitalizing and Maintenance Dosages for Digoxin Pediatric Elixir in Children with Healthy Renal Function Based on Lean Body Weight

Age	Oral digitalizing[a] dose (mcg/kg)	Daily maintenance dose[b] (mcg/kg)
Premature	20 to 30	20% to 30% of oral digitalizing dose[c]
Full-term	25 to 35	25% to 35% of oral digitalizing dose[c]
1 to 24 months	35 to 60	
2 to 5 years	30 to 40	
5 to 10 years	20 to 35	
Over 10 years	10 to 15	

[a] IV digitalizing doses are 80% of oral digitalizing doses.
[b] Divided daily dosing is recommended for children younger than 10 years of age.
[c] Projected or actual digitalizing dose providing clinical response.

In children with renal disease, carefully titrate digoxin dosing based upon desired clinical response.

Gradual digitalization with a maintenance dose: More gradual digitalization can also be accomplished by beginning an appropriate maintenance dose. The range of percentages provided in the preceding table for the elixir can be used in calculating this dose for patients with normal renal function.

➤*Maintenance dosing:* The dosages of digoxin tablets or capsules used in controlled trials in patients with heart failure have ranged from 125 to 500 mcg (0.125 to 0.5 mg) once daily. In these studies, the digoxin dose has been generally titrated according to the patient's age, lean body weight, and renal function. Therapy is generally initiated at a dosage of 250 mcg (0.25 mg) once daily in patients younger than 70 years of age with good renal function, at a dosage of 125 mcg (0.125 mg) once daily in patients older than age 70 years of age or with impaired renal function, and at a dosage of 62.5 mcg (0.0625 mg) once daily in patients with marked renal impairment. Doses may be increased every 2 weeks according to clinical response.

Tablets –

Usual Daily Maintenance Dose Requirements (Mcg) of Digoxin for Estimated Peak Body Stores of 10 mcg/kg

Corrected Ccr (mL/min per 70 kg)[a]	Lean body weight							Number of days before steady state achieved[b]
	kg	50	60	70	80	90	100	
	lb	110	132	154	176	198	220	
0		62.5[c]	125	125	125	187.5	187.5	22
10		125	125	125	187.5	187.5	187.5	19
20		125	125	187.5	187.5	187.5	250	16
30		125	187.5	187.5	187.5	250	250	14
40		125	187.5	187.5	250	250	250	13
50		187.5	187.5	250	250	250	250	12

DIGOXIN — ORAL

Usual Daily Maintenance Dose Requirements (Mcg) of Digoxin for Estimated Peak Body Stores of 10 mcg/kg

Corrected Ccr (mL/min per 70 kg)[a]		Lean body weight						Number of days before steady state achieved[b]
	kg	50	60	70	80	90	100	
	lb	110	132	154	176	198	220	
60		187.5	187.5	250	250	250	375	11
70		187.5	250	250	250	250	375	10
80		187.5	250	250	250	375	375	9
90		187.5	250	250	250	375	500	8
100		250	250	250	375	375	500	7

[a] Ccr is creatinine clearance, corrected to 70 kg body weight or 1.73 m^2 body surface area. For adults, if only serum creatinine concentrations (Scr) are available, a Ccr (corrected to 70 kg body weight) may be estimated in men as (140 − age)/Scr. For women, multiply this result by 0.85. Note: This equation cannot be used for estimating Ccr in infants or children.
[b] If no loading dose administered.
[c] 62.5 mcg = 0.0625 mg.

Capsules –

Usual Digoxin Capsule Daily Maintenance Dose Requirements (mcg) for Estimated Peak Body Stores of 10 mcg/kg

Corrected Ccr (mL/min per 70 kg)[a]		Lean body weight						Number of days before steady state achieved[b]
	kg	50	60	70	80	90	100	
	lb	110	132	154	176	198	220	
0		50[c]	100	100	100	150	150	22
10		100	100	100	150	150	150	19
20		100	100	150	150	150	200	16
30		100	150	150	150	200	200	14
40		100	150	150	200	200	250	13
50		150	150	200	200	250	250	12
60		150	150	200	200	250	300	11
70		150	200	200	250	250	300	10
80		150	200	200	250	300	300	9
90		150	200	250	250	300	350	8
100		200	200	250	300	300	350	7

[a] Ccr is creatinine clearance, corrected to 70 kg body weight or 1.73 m^2 body surface area. For adults, if only serum creatinine concentrations (Scr) are available, a Ccr (corrected to 70 kg body weight) may be estimated in men as (140 − age)/Scr. For women, multiply this result by 0.85. Note: This equation cannot be used for estimating Ccr in infants or children.
[b] If no loading dose administered.
[c] 50 mcg = 0.05 mg.

In children with renal disease, titrate digoxin carefully based upon clinical response.

It cannot be overemphasized that both the adult and pediatric dosage guidelines provided are based upon average patient response, and substantial individual variation can be expected. Accordingly, base ultimate dosage selection upon clinical assessment of the patient.

➤*Tablets, capsules, and elixir:*

Atrial fibrillation – Peak digoxin body stores larger than the 8 to 12 mcg/kg required for most patients with heart failure and normal sinus rhythm have been used for control of ventricular rate in patients with atrial fibrillation. Titrate doses of digoxin used for the treatment of chronic atrial fibrillation to the minimum dose that achieves the desired ventricular rate control without causing undesirable side effects. Data are not available to establish the appropriate resting or exercise target rates that should be achieved.

➤*Dosage adjustment when changing preparations:* The difference in bioavailability between digoxin injection or capsules and digoxin pediatric elixir or digoxin tablets must be considered when changing patients from one dosage form to another.

Doses of 100 mcg (0.1 mg) and 200 mcg (0.2 mg) of digoxin capsules are approximately equivalent to 125 mcg (0.125 mg) and 250 mcg (0.25 mg) doses of digoxin tablets and pediatric elixir, respectively.

➤*Storage/Stability:*

Tablets, capsules, and elixir – Store at 25°C (77°F); excursions permitted to 15° to 30°C (59° to 86°F) in a dry place and protect from light.

Tablets – Dispense in a tight, light-resistant container.

Actions

➤*Pharmacology:* Digoxin inhibits sodium-potassium ATPase, an enzyme that regulates the quantity of sodium and potassium inside cells. Inhibition of the enzyme leads to an increase in the intracellular concentration of sodium and thus (by stimulation of sodium-calcium exchange) an increase in the intracellular concentration of calcium. The beneficial effects of digoxin result from direct actions on cardiac muscle, as well as indirect actions on the cardiovascular system, mediated by effects on the autonomic nervous system.

Autonomic effects – The autonomic effects include the following:
1.) A vagomimetic action, which is responsible for the effects of digoxin on the sinoatrial and atrioventricular (AV) nodes.
2.) Baroreceptor sensitization, which results in increased afferent inhibitory activity and reduced activity of the sympathetic nervous system and renin-angiotensin system for any given increment in mean arterial pressure.

Pharmacologic consequences – The pharmacologic consequences of these direct and indirect effects are the following:
1.) An increase in the force and velocity of myocardial systolic contraction (positive inotropic action).
2.) A decrease in the degree of activation of the sympathetic nervous system and renin-angiotensin system (neurohormonal deactivating effect).
3.) Slowing of the heart rate and decreased conduction velocity through the AV node (vagomimetic effect).

The effects of digoxin in heart failure are mediated by its positive inotropic and neurohormonal, deactivating effects, whereas the effects of the drug in atrial arrhythmias are related to its vagomimetic actions. In high doses, digoxin increases sympathetic outflow from the CNS. This increase in sympathetic activity may be an important factor in digitalis toxicity.

Hemodynamic – Digoxin produces hemodynamic improvement in patients with heart failure. Short- and long-term therapy with the drug increases cardiac output and lowers pulmonary artery pressure, pulmonary capillary wedge pressure, and systemic vascular resistance. These hemodynamic effects are accompanied by an increase in the LVEF and a decrease in end-systolic and end-diastolic dimensions.

➤*Pharmacokinetics:*

Absorption –

Tablets: Following oral administration, peak serum concentrations of digoxin occur at 1 to 3 hours. Absorption of digoxin from digoxin tablets has been demonstrated to be 60% to 80% complete compared to an identical IV dose of digoxin (absolute bioavailability) or capsules (relative bioavailability). When digoxin tablets are taken after meals, the rate of absorption is slowed, but the total amount of digoxin absorbed is usually unchanged. Comparisons of the systemic availability and equivalent doses for preparation of digoxin are shown in the table below.

Capsules: Absorption of digoxin from digoxin capsules has been demonstrated to be 90% to 100% complete compared with an identical IV dose of digoxin (absolute bioavailability). In comparison, the absolute bioavailability of conventional digoxin tablets has been demonstrated to be 60% to 80%. The enhanced absorption from capsules compared with digoxin tablets and elixir is associated with reduced between patient and within patient variability in steady-state serum concentrations. The peak serum concentrations are higher than those observed after tablets. When digoxin tablets or capsules are taken after meals, the rate of absorption is slowed, but the total amount of digoxin absorbed is usually unchanged. When taken with meals high in bran fiber, however, the amount absorbed from an oral dose may be reduced. Comparisons of the systemic availability and equivalent doses for preparation of digoxin are shown in the following table.

Elixir:

• *Note* – The following data are from studies performed in adults, unless otherwise stated. Absorption of digoxin from digoxin pediatric elixir formulation has been demonstrated to be 70% to 85% complete compared to an identical IV dose of digoxin (absolute bioavailability). When the elixir is taken after meals, the rate of absorption is slowed, but the total amount of digoxin absorbed is usually unchanged.

Tablets, capsules, and elixir: When taken with meals high in bran fiber, however, the amount absorbed from an oral dose may be reduced. Comparisons of the systemic availability and equivalent doses for oral preparations of digoxin are shown in the following table.

Comparisons of the Systemic Availability and Equivalent Doses for Preparations of Digoxin

Product	Absolute bioavailability	Equivalent doses (mcg)[a] among dosage forms			
Digoxin tablets	60% to 80%	62.5	125	250	500
Digoxin pediatric elixir	70% to 85%	62.5	125	250	500
Digoxin capsules	90% to 100%	50	100	200	400
Digoxin injection/IV	100%	50	100	200	400

[a] For example, digoxin 125 mcg tablets equivalent to digoxin 125 mcg pediatric elixir equivalent to digoxin 100 mcg capsules equivalent to digoxin 100 mcg injection/IV.

In some patients, orally administered digoxin is converted to inactive reduction products (eg, dihydrodigoxin) by colonic bacteria in the gut. Data suggest that 1 in 10 patients treated with digoxin tablets will degrade 40% or more of the ingested dose. As a result, certain antibiotics may increase the absorption of digoxin in such patients. Although inactivation of these bacteria by antibiotics is rapid, the serum digoxin concentration will rise at a rate consistent with the elimination half-life of digoxin. The magnitude of rise in serum digoxin concentration relates to the extent of bacterial inactivation, and may be as much as 2-fold in some cases. The phenomenon is minimized with digoxin capsules because they are rapidly absorbed in the upper GI tract.

Distribution – Following drug administration, a 6- to 8-hour tissue-distribution phase is observed. This is followed by a much more gradual

DIGOXIN — ORAL

decline in the serum concentration of the drug, which is dependent on the elimination of digoxin from the body. The peak height and slope of the early portion (absorption/distribution phases) of the serum concentration-time curve are dependent upon the route of administration and the absorption characteristics of the formulation. Clinical evidence indicates that the early high serum concentrations (particularly high for digoxin capsules) do not reflect the concentration of digoxin at its site of action, but that with chronic use, the steady-state postdistribution serum concentrations are in equilibrium with tissue concentrations and correlate with pharmacologic effects. In individual patients, these postdistribution serum concentrations may be useful in evaluating therapeutic and toxic effects.

Digoxin is concentrated in tissues and therefore has a large apparent volume of distribution. Digoxin crosses both the blood-brain barrier and placenta. At delivery, the serum digoxin concentration in the newborn is similar to the serum concentration in the mother. Approximately 25% of digoxin in the plasma is bound to protein. Serum digoxin concentrations are not significantly altered by large changes in fat tissue weight, so that its distribution space correlates best with lean (ie, ideal) body weight, not total body weight.

Metabolism – Only a small percentage (16%) of a dose of digoxin is metabolized. The end metabolites, which include 3 β-digoxigenin, 3-keto-digoxigenin, and their glucuronide and sulfate conjugates, are polar in nature and are postulated to be formed via hydrolysis, oxidation, and conjugation. The metabolism of digoxin is not dependent upon the cytochrome P-450 system, and digoxin is not known to induce or inhibit the cytochrome P-450 system.

Excretion – Elimination of digoxin follows first-order kinetics (that is, the quantity of digoxin eliminated at any time is proportional to the total body content). Following IV administration to healthy volunteers, 50% to 70% of a digoxin dose is excreted unchanged in the urine. Renal excretion of digoxin is proportional to glomerular filtration rate and is largely independent of urine flow. In healthy volunteers (with healthy renal function), digoxin has a half-life of 1.5 to 2 days. The half-life in anuric patients is prolonged to 3.5 to 5 days. Digoxin is not effectively removed from the body by dialysis, exchange transfusion, or during cardiopulmonary bypass because most of the drug is bound to tissue and does not circulate in the blood.

Pharmacodynamic and clinical effects – The times to onset of pharmacologic effect and to peak effect of preparations of digoxin are shown in the following table.

Times to Onset of Pharmacologic Effect and to Peak Effect of Preparations of Digoxin

Product	Time to onset of effect[a]	Time to peak effect[a]
Digoxin tablets	0.5 to 2 hours	2 to 6 hours
Digoxin pediatric elixir	0.5 to 2 hours	2 to 6 hours
Digoxin capsules	0.5 to 2 hours	2 to 6 hours
Digoxin injection/IV	5 to 30 minutes[b]	1 to 4 hours

[a] Documented for ventricular response rate in atrial fibrillation, inotropic effects and electrocardiographic effects.
[b] Depending upon rate of infusion.

Contraindications

Ventricular fibrillation; hypersensitivity to digoxin or to other digitalis preparations.

Warnings

➤*Sinus node disease and AV block:* Because digoxin slows sinoatrial and AV conduction, the drug commonly prolongs the PR interval. The drug may cause severe sinus bradycardia or sinoatrial block in patients with preexisting sinus node disease and may cause advanced or complete heart block in patients with preexisting incomplete AV block. In such patients, give consideration to the insertion of a pacemaker before treatment with digoxin.

➤*Accessory AV pathway (Wolff-Parkinson-White syndrome):* After IV digoxin therapy, some patients with paroxysmal atrial fibrillation or flutter and a coexisting accessory AV pathway have developed increased antegrade conduction across the accessory pathway bypassing the AV node, leading to a very rapid ventricular response or ventricular fibrillation. Unless conduction down the accessory pathway has been blocked (either pharmacologically or by surgery), do not use digoxin in such patients. The treatment of paroxysmal supraventricular tachycardia in such patients is usually direct-current cardioversion.

➤*Use in patients with preserved left ventricular systolic function:* Patients with certain disorders involving heart failure associated with preserved left ventricular ejection fraction may be particularly susceptible to toxicity of the drug. Such disorders include restrictive cardiomyopathy, constrictive pericarditis, amyloid heart disease, and acute cor pulmonale. Patients with idiopathic hypertrophic subaortic stenosis may have worsening of the outflow obstruction due to the inotropic effects of digoxin.

➤*Renal function impairment:* Digoxin is primarily excreted by the kidneys; therefore, patients with impaired renal function require smaller than usual maintenance doses of digoxin. Because of the prolonged elimination half-life, a longer period of time is required to achieve an initial or new steady-state serum concentration in patients with renal impairment than in patients with normal renal function. If appropriate care is not taken to reduce the dose of digoxin, such patients are at high risk for toxicity, and toxic effects will last longer in such patients than in patients with healthy renal function.

➤*Elderly:* The majority of clinical experience gained with digoxin has been in the elderly population. This experience has not identified differences in response or adverse effects between the elderly and younger patients. However, this drug is known to be substantially excreted by the kidney, and the risk of toxic reactions to this drug may be greater in patients with impaired renal function. Because elderly patients are more likely to have decreased renal function, take care in dose selection, which should be based on renal function. It may be useful to monitor renal function.

➤*Pregnancy:* *Category C.*

Teratogenic – Animal reproduction studies have not been conducted with digoxin. It is also not known whether digoxin can cause fetal harm when administered to a pregnant woman or can affect reproductive capacity. Give digoxin to a pregnant woman only if clearly needed.

➤*Lactation:* Studies have shown that digoxin concentrations in the mother's serum and milk are similar. However, the estimated exposure of a nursing infant to digoxin via breast-feeding will be far below the usual infant maintenance dose. Therefore, this amount should have no pharmacologic effect upon the infant. Nevertheless, exercise caution when digoxin is administered to a breast-feeding woman.

➤*Children:* Newborn infants display considerable variability in their tolerance to digoxin. Premature and immature infants are particularly sensitive to the effects of digoxin. Reduce and individualize the dosage of the drug according to their degrees of maturity. Digitalis glycosides can cause poisoning in children due to accidental ingestion.

Precautions

➤*Monitoring:* Patients receiving digoxin should have their serum electrolytes and renal functions (serum creatinine concentrations) assessed periodically; the frequency of assessments will depend on the clinical setting.

➤*Special risk:*

Use in patients with electrolyte disorders – In patients with hypokalemia or hypomagnesemia, toxicity may occur despite serum digoxin concentrations less than 2 ng/mL, because potassium or magnesium depletion sensitizes the myocardium to digoxin. Therefore, it is desirable to maintain normal serum potassium and magnesium concentrations in patients being treated with digoxin. Deficiencies of these electrolytes may result from malnutrition, diarrhea, or prolonged vomiting, as well as the use of the following drugs or procedures: diuretics, amphotericin B, corticosteroids, antacids, dialysis, and mechanical suction of GI secretions.

Hypercalcemia from any cause predisposes the patient to digitalis toxicity. Calcium, particularly when administered rapidly by the IV route, may produce serious arrhythmias in digitalized patients. On the other hand, hypocalcemia can nullify the effects of digoxin in humans; thus, digoxin may be ineffective until serum calcium is restored to normal. These interactions are related to the fact that digoxin affects contractility and excitability of the heart in a manner similar to that of calcium.

Use in thyroid disorders and hypermetabolic states – Hypothyroidism may reduce the requirements for digoxin. Heart failure and/or atrial arrhythmias resulting from hypermetabolic or hyperdynamic states (eg, hyperthyroidism, hypoxia, arteriovenous shunt) are best treated by addressing the underlying condition. Atrial arrhythmias associated with hypermetabolic states are particularly resistant to digoxin treatment. Take care to avoid toxicity if digoxin is used.

Use in patients with acute myocardial infarction – Use digoxin with caution in patients with acute myocardial infarction. The use of inotropic drugs in some patients in this setting may result in undesirable increases in myocardial oxygen demand and ischemia.

Use during electrical cardioversion – It may be desirable to reduce the dose of digoxin for 1 to 2 days prior to electrical cardioversion of atrial fibrillation to avoid the induction of ventricular arrhythmias, but consider the consequences of increasing the ventricular response if digoxin is withdrawn. If digitalis toxicity is suspected, delay elective cardioversion. If it is not prudent to delay cardioversion, select the lowest possible energy level to avoid provoking ventricular arrhythmias.

Drug Interactions

Digoxin Drug Interactions

Precipitant drug	Object drug*		Description
Beta blockers (eg, carvedilol)	Digoxin	⬆	Although beta-blockers and digoxin may be useful in combination to control atrial fibrillation, their additive effects on AV node conduction may result in advanced or complete heart block.
Calcium	Digoxin	⬆	Calcium administered rapidly by the IV route may produce serious arrhythmias in digitalized patients.
Calcium channel blockers (eg, verapamil)	Digoxin	⬆	Although calcium channel blockers and digoxin may be useful in combination to control atrial fibrillation, their additive effects on AV node conduction may result in advanced or complete heart block.

DIGOXIN — ORAL

Digoxin Drug Interactions

Precipitant drug	Object drug*		Description
Succinylcholine	Digoxin	↑	Succinylcholine may cause a sudden extrusion of potassium from muscle cells, thereby causing arrhythmias in digitalized patients.
Sympathomimetics	Digoxin	↑	Concomitant use of digoxin and sympathomimetics increases the risk of cardiac arrhythmias.
Thiazide Diuretics, loop diuretics	Digoxin	↑	Diuretic-induced electrolyte disturbances may predispose to digitalis-induced arrhythmias. Measure plasma levels of potassium and magnesium and supplement low levels. Prevent further losses with dietary sodium restriction or potassium-sparing diuretics.
Thyroid hormones	Digoxin	↓	Thyroid administration to a digitalized, hypothyroid patient may increase the dose requirement of digoxin

* ↑ = Object drug increased. ↓ = Object drug decreased.

➤*Drugs that may increase digoxin:* Potassium-depleting diuretics are a major contributing factor to digitalis toxicity. Quinidine, verapamil, amiodarone, propafenone, indomethacin, itraconazole, alprazolam, and spironolactone raise the serum digoxin concentration due to a reduction in clearance and/or in volume of distribution of the drug, with the implication that digitalis intoxication may result. Erythromycin and clarithromycin (and possibly other macrolide antibiotics) and tetracycline may increase digoxin absorption in patients who inactivate digoxin by bacterial metabolism in the lower intestine, so that digitalis intoxication may result. The risk of this interaction may be reduced if digoxin is given as capsules. Propantheline and diphenoxylate, by decreasing gut motility, may increase digoxin absorption.

➤*Drugs that may decrease digoxin:* Antacids, kaolinpectin, sulfasalazine, neomycin, cholestyramine, certain anticancer drugs, and metoclopramide may interfere with intestinal digoxin absorption, resulting in unexpectedly low serum concentrations. Rifampin may decrease serum digoxin concentration, especially in patients with renal dysfunction, by increasing the nonrenal clearance of digoxin.

➤*Other:* There have been inconsistent reports regarding the effects of other drugs (eg, penicillamine, quinine) on serum digoxin concentration.

Due to the considerable variability of these interactions, individualize the dosage of digoxin when patients receive these medications concurrently. Furthermore, exercise caution when combining a digoxin with any drug that may cause a significant deterioration in renal function, since a decline in glomerular filtration or tubular secretion may impair the excretion of digoxin.

➤*Drug/Lab test interactions:* The use of therapeutic doses of digoxin may cause prolongation of the PR interval and depression of the ST segment on the electrocardiogram. Digoxin may produce false-positive ST-T changes on the electrocardiogram during exercise testing. These electrophysiologic effects reflect an expected effect of the drug and are not indicative of toxicity.

Adverse Reactions

In general, the adverse reactions of digoxin are dose dependent and occur at doses higher than those needed to achieve a therapeutic effect. Hence, adverse reactions are less common when digoxin is used within the recommended dose range or therapeutic serum concentration range and when there is careful attention to concurrent medications and conditions.

Because some patients may be particularly susceptible to side effects with digoxin, always select the dosage of the drug carefully and adjust as the clinical condition of the patient warrants. In the past, when high doses of digoxin were used and little attention was paid to clinical status or concurrent medications, adverse reactions to digoxin were more frequent and severe. Cardiac adverse reactions accounted for about one-half, GI disturbances for about one-fourth, and CNS and other toxicity for about one-fourth of these adverse reactions. However, available evidence suggests that the incidence and severity of digoxin toxicity has decreased substantially in recent years. In recent controlled clinical trials, in patients with predominantly mild to moderate heart failure, the incidence of adverse reactions was comparable in patients taking digoxin and in those taking placebo. In a large mortality trial, the incidence of hospitalization for suspected digoxin toxicity was 2% in patients taking digoxin compared with 0.9% in patients taking placebo. In this trial, the most common manifestations of digoxin toxicity included GI and cardiac disturbances; CNS manifestations were less common.

➤*Adults:*

Cardiovascular – Therapeutic doses of digoxin may cause heart block in patients with preexisting sinoatrial or AV conduction disorders; avoid heart block by adjusting the dose of digoxin. Consider prophylactic use of a cardiac pacemaker if the risk of heart block is considered unacceptable. High doses of digoxin may produce a variety of rhythm disturbances, such as first-degree, second-degree (Wenckebach), or third-degree heart block (including asystole); atrial tachycardia with block; AV dissociation; accelerated junctional (nodal) rhythm; unifocal or multiform ventricular premature contractions (especially bigeminy or trigeminy); ventricular tachycardia; and ventricular fibrillation. Digoxin produces PR prolongation and ST-segment depression, which should not by themselves be considered digoxin toxicity. Cardiac toxicity can also occur at therapeutic doses in patients who have conditions which may alter their sensitivity to digoxin. Such disorders include acute cor pulmonale, amyloid heart disease, constrictive pericarditis, and restrictive cardiomyopathy. Patients with idiopathic hypertrophic subaortic stenosis may have worsening of the outflow obstruction due to the inotropic effects of digoxin.

CNS – Digoxin can produce apathy, confusion, dizziness, headache, mental disturbances (eg, anxiety, depression, delirium, hallucination), visual disturbances (blurred or yellow vision), and weakness.

GI – Digoxin may cause anorexia, diarrhea, nausea, and vomiting. Rarely, the use of digoxin has been associated with abdominal pain, hemorrhagic necrosis of the intestines, and intestinal ischemia.

Miscellaneous – Gynecomastia has been occasionally observed following the prolonged use of digoxin. Thrombocytopenia and maculopapular rash and other skin reactions have been rarely observed. The following table summarizes the incidence of those adverse reactions listed above for patients treated with digoxin tablets or placebo from 2 randomized, double-blind, placebo-controlled withdrawal trials. Patients in these trials were also receiving diuretics with or without ACE inhibitors. These patients had been stable on digoxin, and were randomized to digoxin or placebo. The results shown in the following table reflect the experience in patients following dosage titration with the use of serum digoxin concentrations and careful follow-up. These adverse reactions are consistent with results from a large, placebo-controlled mortality trial (DIG trial) wherein over half the patients were not receiving digoxin prior to enrollment.

Adverse Reactions in 2 Parallel, Double-Blind, Placebo-controlled Withdrawal Trials (Number of Patients Reporting)

Adverse reactions	Digoxin patients (n = 123)	Placebo patients (n = 125)
Cardiovascular		
Heart arrest	1%	1%
Palpitation	1%	4%
Tachycardia	2%	1%
Ventricular extrasystole	1%	1%
CNS		
Dizziness	6%	5%
Headache	4%	4%
Mental disturbances	5%	1%
GI		
Abdominal pain	0%	6%
Anorexia	1%	4%
Diarrhea	4%	1%
Nausea	4%	2%
Vomiting	2%	1%
Miscellaneous		
Death	4%	3%
Rash	2%	1%

➤*Infants and children:* The side effects of digoxin in infants and children differ from those seen in adults in several respects. Although digoxin may produce anorexia, nausea, vomiting, diarrhea, and CNS disturbances in young patients, these are rarely the initial symptoms of overdosage. Rather, the earliest and most frequent manifestation of excessive dosing with digoxin in infants and children is the appearance of cardiac arrhythmias, including sinus bradycardia. In children, the use of digoxin may produce any arrhythmia. The most common are conduction disturbances or supraventricular tachyarrhythmias, such as atrial tachycardia (with or without block) and junctional (nodal) tachycardia. Ventricular arrhythmias are less common. Sinus bradycardia may be a sign of impending digoxin intoxication, especially in infants, even in the absence of first-degree heart block. Any arrhythmia or alteration in cardiac conduction that develops in a child taking digoxin should be assumed to be caused by digoxin, until further evaluation proves otherwise.

Overdosage

➤*Symptoms:* Manifestations of life-threatening toxicity include ventricular tachycardia or ventricular fibrillation, progressive bradyarrhythmias, or heart block. The administration of more than 10 mg of digoxin in a previously healthy adult, or more than 4 mg in a previously healthy child, or a steady-state serum concentration greater than 10 ng/mL often results in cardiac arrest.

➤*Treatment:* Temporarily discontinue digoxin until the adverse reaction resolves. Make every effort to correct factors that may contribute to the adverse reaction (eg, electrolyte disturbances, concurrent medications). Once the adverse reaction has resolved, therapy with digoxin may be reinstituted, following a careful reassessment of dose.

Withdrawal of digoxin may be all that is required to treat the adverse reaction. However, when the primary manifestation of digoxin overdosage is a cardiac arrhythmia, additional therapy may be needed.

If the rhythm disturbance is a symptomatic bradyarrhythmia or heart block, consider the reversal of toxicity with digoxin immune fab (ovine), use of atropine, or insertion of a temporary cardiac pacemaker. However, asymptom-

DIGOXIN — ORAL

atic bradycardia or heart block related to digoxin may require only temporary withdrawal of the drug and cardiac monitoring of the patient.

If the rhythm disturbance is a ventricular arrhythmia, consideration should be given to the correction of electrolyte disorders, particularly if hypokalemia or hypomagnesemia is present. Digoxin immune fab (ovine) is a specific antidote for digoxin and may be used to reverse potentially life-threatening ventricular arrhythmias due to digoxin overdosage.

Make every effort to maintain the serum potassium concentration between 4 and 5.5 mmol/L. Potassium is usually administered orally, but when correction of the arrhythmia is urgent and the serum potassium concentration is low, potassium may be administered cautiously by the IV route. Monitor the electrocardiogram for any evidence of potassium toxicity (eg, peaking of T waves) and observe the effect on the arrhythmia. Potassium salts may be dangerous in patients who manifest bradycardia or heart block due to digoxin (unless primarily related to supraventricular tachycardia) and in the setting of massive digitalis overdosage.

Patients with massive digitalis ingestion should receive large doses of activated charcoal to prevent absorption and bind digoxin in the gut during enteroenteric recirculation. Emesis or gastric lavage may be indicated especially if ingestion has occurred within 30 minutes of the patient's presentation at the hospital. Emesis should not be induced in patients who are obtunded. If a patient presents more than 2 hours after ingestion or already has toxic manifestations, it may be unsafe to induce vomiting or attempt passage of a gastric tube, because such maneuvers may induce an acute vagal episode that can worsen digitalis-related arrhythmias.

Severe digitalis intoxication can cause a massive shift of potassium from inside to outside the cell, leading to life-threatening hyperkalemia. The administration of potassium supplements in the setting of massive intoxication may be hazardous and should be avoided. Hyperkalemia caused by massive digitalis toxicity is best treated with digoxin immune fab (ovine); initial treatment with glucose and insulin may also be required if hyperkalemia itself is acutely life-threatening.

DIGOXIN — INJECTION

Indications

➤*Heart failure:* Treatment of mild to moderate heart failure. Digoxin increases left ventricular ejection fraction and improves heart failure symptoms as evidenced by exercise capacity and heart failure-related hospitalizations and emergency care, while having no effect on mortality. Where possible, use digoxin with a diuretic and an angiotensin-converting enzyme (ACE) inhibitor, but an optimal order for starting these 3 drugs cannot be specified.

➤*Atrial fibrillation:* Digoxin is indicated for the control of ventricular response rate in patients with chronic atrial fibrillation.

Administration and Dosage

➤*Approved by the FDA:* October 24, 1975.

Recommended dosages of digoxin may require considerable modification because of individual sensitivity of the patient to the drug, the presence of associated conditions, or the use of concurrent medications.

Use parenteral administration of digoxin only when the need for rapid digitalization is urgent or when the drug cannot be taken orally. Intramuscular (IM) injection can lead to severe pain at the injection site, thus intravenous (IV) administration is preferred. If the drug must be administered by the IM route, inject it deeply into the muscle and follow with massage.

➤*Adults:* Do not inject more than 500 mcg (2 mL) into a single site.

➤*Children:* Do not inject more than 200 mcg (2 mL) into a single site.

➤*Rapid digitalization with a loading dose:*

Adults –

A single initial IV dose of 400 to 600 mcg (0.4 to 0.6 mg) of digoxin injection usually produces a detectable effect in 5 to 30 minutes that becomes maximal in 1 to 4 hours. Additional doses of 100 to 300 mcg (0.1 to 0.3 mg) may be given cautiously at 6- to 8-hour intervals until clinical evidence of an adequate effect is noted. The usual amount of digoxin injection that a 70 kg patient requires to achieve 8 to 12 mcg/kg peak body stores is 600 to 1,000 mcg (0.6 to 1 mg).

Maintenance dosing in adults:

• *Daily maintenance dose requirements* – The following table provides average daily maintenance dose requirements of digoxin injection for patients with heart failure based upon lean body weight and renal function.

Usual Daily Maintenance Dose Requirements (mcg) of Digoxin Injection for Estimated Peak Body Stores of 10 mcg/kg[a]

Corrected Ccr (mL/min per 70 kg)[b]	Lean body weight							Number of days before steady state achieved[c]
	kg	50	60	70	80	90	100	
	lb	110	132	154	176	198	220	
0		75[d]	75	100	100	125	150	22
10		75	100	100	125	150	150	10
20		100	100	125	150	150	175	16
30		100	125	150	150	175	200	14
40		100	125	150	175	200	225	13
50		125	150	175	200	225	250	12
60		125	150	175	200	225	250	11
70		150	175	200	225	250	275	10
80		150	175	200	250	275	300	9
90		150	200	225	250	300	325	8
100		175	200	250	275	300	350	7

[a] Daily maintenance doses have been rounded to the nearest 25 mcg increment.

[b] Ccr is creatinine clearance, corrected to 70 kg body weight or 1.73 m^2 body surface area. For adults, if only serum creatinine concentrations (Scr) are available, a Ccr (corrected to 70 kg body weight) may be estimated in men as (140 − age)/Scr. For women, this result should be multiplied by 0.85. Note: This equation cannot be used for estimating creatinine clearance in infants or children.

[c] If no loading dose administered.

[d] 75 mcg = 0.075 mg.

Children – Digitalizing and daily maintenance doses for each age group are given in the following table and should provide therapeutic effect with minimum risk of toxicity in most patients with heart failure and normal sinus rhythm.

These recommendations assume the presence of normal renal function.

Administer the loading dose in several portions, with roughly half the total given as the first dose. Give additional fractions of this planned total dose at 4- to 8-hour intervals, with careful assessment of clinical response before each additional dose. If the patient's clinical response necessitates a change from the calculated loading dose of digoxin, then base the calculation of the maintenance dose upon the amount actually given.

Usual Digitalizing and Maintenance Dosages for Digoxin Pediatric Injection in Children with Normal Renal Function Based on Lean Body Weight

Age	IV digitalizing[a] dose (mcg/kg)	Daily IV maintenance dose[b] (mcg/kg)
Premature	15 to 25	20% to 30% of the IV digitalizing dose[c]
Full term	20 to 30	25% to 35% of the IV digitalizing dose[c]
1 to 24 months	30 to 50	
2 to 5 years	25 to 35	
5 to 10 years	15 to 30	
Older than 10 years	8 to 12	

[a] IV digitalizing doses are 80% of oral digitalizing doses.

[b] Divided daily dosing is recommended for children younger than 10 years of age.

[c] Projected or actual digitalizing dose providing clinical response.

In children with renal disease, digoxin dosing must be carefully titrated based on clinical response.

Gradual digitalization with a maintenance dose: Accomplish more gradual digitalization by beginning an appropriate maintenance dose. Use the range of percentages provided above in calculating this dose for patients with normal renal function.

It cannot be overemphasized that these pediatric dosage guidelines are based upon average patient response and substantial individual variation can be expected. Accordingly, base ultimate dosage selection upon clinical assessment of the patient.

➤*Atrial fibrillation:* Peak digoxin body stores larger than the 8 to 12 mcg/kg required for most patients with heart failure and normal sinus rhythm have been used for control of ventricular rate in patients with atrial fibrillation. Doses of digoxin used for the treatment of chronic atrial fibrillation should be titrated to the minimum dose that achieves the desired ventricular rate control without causing undesirable side effects. Data are not available to establish the appropriate resting or exercise target rates that should be achieved.

➤*Dosage adjustment when changing preparations:* Consider the differences in bioavailability between injectable digoxin or digoxin capsules and digoxin pediatric elixir or digoxin tablets when changing patients from 1 dosage form to another.

Adjustments in dosage will seldom be necessary when converting a patient from the IV formulation to capsules.

Doses of 100 mcg (0.1 mg) and 200 mcg (0.2 mg) of digoxin capsules are approximately equivalent to 125 mcg (0.125 mg) and 250 mcg (0.25 mg) doses of digoxin tablets and pediatric elixir, respectively.

➤*Storage/Stability:* Store at 25°C (77°F); excursions permitted to 15° to 30°C (59° to 86°F). Protect from light.

Actions

➤*Pharmacology:*

Mechanism of action – Digoxin inhibits sodium-potassium adenosine triphosphatase (ATPase), an enzyme that regulates the quantity of sodium and potassium inside cells. Inhibition of the enzyme leads to an increase in the intracellular concentration of sodium and thus (by stimulation of sodium-calcium exchange) an increase in the intracellular concentration of calcium. The beneficial effects of digoxin result from direct actions on cardiac muscle, as well as indirect actions on the cardiovascular system mediated by effects on the autonomic nervous system.

DIGOXIN — INJECTION

Autonomic effects: The autonomic effects include the following:
- A vagomimetic action, which is responsible for the effects of digoxin on the sinoatrial and atrioventricular (AV) nodes.
- Baroreceptor sensitization, which results in increased afferent inhibitory activity and reduced activity of the sympathetic nervous system and renin-angiotensin system for any given increment in mean arterial pressure.

Pharmacologic consequences: The pharmacologic consequences of these direct and indirect effects are the following:
- An increase in the force and velocity of myocardial systolic contraction (positive inotropic action).
- A decrease in the degree of activation of the sympathetic nervous system and renin-angiotensin system (neurohormonal deactivating effect).
- Slowing of the heart rate and decreased conduction velocity through the AV node (vagomimetic effect).

The effects of digoxin in heart failure are mediated by its positive inotropic and neurohormonal deactivating effects, whereas the effects of the drug in atrial arrhythmias are related to its vagomimetic actions. In high doses, digoxin increases sympathetic outflow from the CNS. This increase in sympathetic activity may be an important factor in digitalis toxicity.

➤*Pharmacokinetics:*

Absorption – The following data are from studies performed in adults, unless otherwise stated.

Comparisons of the systemic availability and equivalent doses for preparations of digoxin are shown in the following table:

Comparisons of the Systemic Availability and Equivalent Doses for Preparation of Digoxin

Product	Absolute bioavailability	Equivalent doses (mcg)[a] among dosage forms			
Digoxin tablets	60% to 80%	62.5	125	250	500
Digoxin pediatric elixir	70% to 85%	62.5	125	250	500
Digoxin capsules	90% to 100%	50	100	200	400
Digoxin injection/IV	100%	50	100	200	400

[a] For example, digoxin 125 mcg tablets equivalent to digoxin 125 mcg pediatric elixir equivalent to digoxin 100 mcg capsules equivalent to 100 mcg digoxin injection/IV.

Distribution – Following drug administration, a 6- to 8-hour tissue distribution phase is observed. This is followed by a much more gradual decline in the serum concentration of the drug, which is dependent on the elimination of digoxin from the body. The peak height and slope of the early portion (absorption/distribution phases) of the serum concentration-time curve are dependent upon the route of administration and the absorption characteristics of the formulation. Clinical evidence indicates that the early high serum concentrations do not reflect the concentration of digoxin at its site of action, but that with chronic use, the steady-state postdistribution serum concentrations are in equilibrium with tissue concentrations and correlate with pharmacologic effects. In individual patients, these postdistribution serum concentrations may be useful in evaluating therapeutic and toxic effects.

Digoxin is concentrated in tissues and therefore has a large apparent volume of distribution. Digoxin crosses both the blood-brain barrier and the placenta. At delivery, the serum digoxin concentration in the newborn is similar to the serum concentration in the mother. Approximately 25% of digoxin in the plasma is bound to protein. Serum digoxin concentrations are not significantly altered by large changes in fat tissue weight, so that its distribution space correlates best with lean (ie, ideal) body weight, not total body weight.

Metabolism – Only a small percentage (16%) of a dose of digoxin is metabolized. The end metabolites, which include 3 β-digoxigenin, 3-keto-digoxigenin, and their glucuronide and sulfate conjugates, are polar in nature and are postulated to be formed via hydrolysis, oxidation, and conjugation. The metabolism of digoxin is not dependent upon the cytochrome P-450 system, and digoxin is not known to induce or inhibit the cytochrome P-450 system.

Excretion – Elimination of digoxin follows first-order kinetics (ie, the quantity of digoxin eliminated at any time is proportional to the total body content). Following IV administration to healthy volunteers, 50% to 70% of a digoxin dose is excreted unchanged in the urine. Renal excretion of digoxin is proportional to glomerular filtration rate and is largely independent of urine flow. In healthy volunteers with normal renal function, digoxin has a half-life of 1.5 to 2 days. The half-life in anuric patients is prolonged to 3.5 to 5 days. Digoxin is not effectively removed from the body by dialysis, exchange transfusion, or during cardiopulmonary bypass because most of the drug is bound to tissue and does not circulate in the blood.

Special populations –

Renal function impairment:
- *Clearance correlated with renal function* – The clearance of digoxin can be primarily correlated with renal function as indicated by creatinine clearance.

Pharmacodynamic effects – The following are times to onset of pharmacologic effect and peak effect of digoxin preparations, based on ventricular response rate in atrial fibrillation, inotropic effects, and electrocardiographic changes.

Times to Onset of Pharmacologic Effect and to Peak Effect of Preparations of Digoxin

Product	Time to onset of effect[a]	Time to peak effect[a]
Digoxin tablets	0.5 to 2 hours	2 to 6 hours
Digoxin pediatric elixir	0.5 to 2 hours	2 to 6 hours
Digoxin capsules	0.5 to 2 hours	2 to 6 hours
Digoxin injection/IV	5 to 30 minutes[b]	1 to 4 hours

[a] Documented for ventricular response rate in atrial fibrillation, inotropic effects, and electrocardiographic changes.
[b] Depending upon rate of infusion.

Hemodynamic effects – Digoxin produces hemodynamic improvement in patients with heart failure. Short- and long-term therapy with the drug increases cardiac output and lowers pulmonary artery pressure, pulmonary capillary wedge pressure, and systemic vascular resistance. These hemodynamic effects are accompanied by an increase in the left ventricular ejection fraction and a decrease in end-systolic and end-diastolic dimensions.

Contraindications

Ventricular fibrillation; hypersensitivity to digoxin or to other digitalis preparations.

Warnings

➤*Sinus node disease and AV block:* Because digoxin slows sinoatrial and AV conduction, the drug commonly prolongs the PR interval. The drug may cause severe sinus bradycardia or sinoatrial block in patients with preexisting sinus node disease and may cause advanced or complete heart block in patients with preexisting incomplete AV block. In such patients, consider insertion of a pacemaker before treatment with digoxin.

➤*Accessory AV pathway (Wolff-Parkinson-White syndrome):* After IV digoxin therapy, some patients with paroxysmal atrial fibrillation or flutter and a coexisting accessory AV pathway have developed increased antegrade conduction across the accessory pathway bypassing the AV node, leading to a very rapid ventricular response or ventricular fibrillation. Unless conduction down the accessory pathway has been blocked (either pharmacologically or by surgery), digoxin should not be used in such patients. The treatment of paroxysmal supraventricular tachycardia in such patients is usually direct-current cardioversion.

➤*Use in patients with preserved left ventricular systolic function:* Patients with certain disorders involving heart failure associated with preserved left ventricular ejection fraction may be particularly susceptible to toxicity of the drug. Such disorders include restrictive cardiomyopathy, constrictive pericarditis, amyloid heart disease, and acute cor pulmonale. Patients with idiopathic hypertrophic subaortic stenosis may have worsening of the outflow obstruction due to the inotropic effects of digoxin.

➤*Renal function impairment:* Digoxin is primarily excreted by the kidneys; therefore, patients with impaired renal function require smaller than usual maintenance doses of digoxin. Because of the prolonged elimination half-life, a longer period of time is required to achieve an initial or new steady-state serum concentration in patients with renal impairment than in patients with normal renal function. If appropriate care is not taken to reduce the dose of digoxin, such patients are at high risk for toxicity, and toxic effects will last longer in such patients than in patients with normal renal function.

➤*Elderly:* The majority of clinical experience gained with digoxin has been in the elderly population. This experience has not identified differences in response or adverse reactions between the elderly and younger patients. However, this drug is known to be substantially excreted by the kidney, and the risk of toxic reactions to this drug may be greater in patients with impaired renal function. Because elderly patients are more likely to have decreased renal function, take care in dose selection, which should be based on renal function; it may be useful to monitor renal function.

➤*Pregnancy: Category C.*

Teratogenic – Animal reproduction studies have not been conducted with digoxin. It is also not known whether digoxin can cause fetal harm when administered to a pregnant woman or can affect reproductive capacity. Administer digoxin to a pregnant woman only if the benefit to the mother outweighs the risk to the fetus. Give digoxin to a pregnant woman only if clearly needed.

➤*Lactation:* Studies have shown that digoxin concentrations in the mother's serum and milk are similar. However, the estimated exposure of a breast-feeding infant to digoxin via breast-feeding will be far below the usual infant maintenance dose. Therefore, this amount should have no pharmacologic effect upon the infant. Nevertheless, exercise caution when administering digoxin to a breast-feeding woman.

➤*Children:* Newborn infants display considerable variability in their tolerance to digoxin. Premature and immature infants are particularly sensitive to the effects of digoxin, and the dosage of the drug must not only be reduced but must be individualized according to their degree of maturity. Digitalis glycosides can cause poisoning in children due to accidental ingestion.

Precautions

➤*Monitoring:* Patients receiving digoxin should have their serum electrolytes and renal function (serum creatinine concentrations) assessed periodically; the frequency of assessments will depend on the clinical setting.

➤*Use in patients with electrolyte disorders:* In patients with hypokalemia or hypomagnesemia, toxicity may occur despite serum digoxin concen-

DIGOXIN — INJECTION

trations less than 2 ng/mL, because potassium or magnesium depletion sensitizes the myocardium to digoxin. Therefore, it is desirable to maintain normal serum potassium and magnesium concentrations in patients being treated with digoxin. Deficiencies of these electrolytes may result from malnutrition, diarrhea, or prolonged vomiting, as well as the use of the following drugs or procedures: diuretics, amphotericin B, corticosteroids, antacids, dialysis, and mechanical suction of GI secretions.

Hypercalcemia from any cause predisposes the patient to digitalis toxicity. Calcium, particularly when administered rapidly by the IV route, may produce serious arrhythmias in digitalized patients. On the other hand, hypocalcemia can nullify the effects of digoxin in humans; thus, digoxin may be ineffective until serum calcium is restored to normal. These interactions are related to the fact that digoxin affects contractility and excitability of the heart in a manner similar to that of calcium.

➤*Use in thyroid disorders and hypermetabolic states:* Hypothyroidism may reduce the requirements for digoxin. Heart failure and/or atrial arrhythmias resulting from hypermetabolic or hyperdynamic states (eg, hyperthyroidism, hypoxia, or arteriovenous shunt) are best treated by addressing the underlying condition. Atrial arrhythmias associated with hypermetabolic states are particularly resistant to digoxin treatment. Take care to avoid toxicity if digoxin is used.

➤*Use during electrical cardioversion:* It may be desirable to reduce the dose of digoxin for 1 to 2 days prior to electrical cardioversion of atrial fibrillation to avoid the induction of ventricular arrhythmias, but consider the consequences of increasing the ventricular response if digoxin is withdrawn. If digitalis toxicity is suspected, delay elective cardioversion. If it is not prudent to delay cardioversion, select the lowest possible energy level to avoid provoking ventricular arrhythmias.

➤*Special risk:*

Use in patients with acute myocardial infarction – Use digoxin with caution in patients with acute myocardial infarction. The use of inotropic drugs in some patients in this setting may result in undesirable increases in myocardial oxygen demand and ischemia.

Drug Interactions

Digoxin Drug Interactions

Precipitant drug	Object drug*		Description
Beta blockers (eg, carvedilol)	Digoxin	↑	Although beta blockers and digoxin may be useful in combination to control atrial fibrillation, their additive effects on AV node conduction may result in advanced or complete heart block.
Calcium	Digoxin	↑	Calcium administered rapidly by the IV route may produce serious arrhythmias in digitalized patients.
Calcium channel blockers (eg, verapamil)	Digoxin	↑	Although calcium channel blockers and digoxin may be useful in combination to control atrial fibrillation, their additive effects on AV node conduction may result in advanced or complete heart block.
Succinylcholine	Digoxin	↑	Succinylcholine may cause a sudden extrusion of potassium from muscle cells, thereby causing arrhythmias in digitalized patients.
Sympathomimetics	Digoxin	↑	Concomitant use of digoxin and sympathomimetics increases the risk of cardiac arrhythmias.
Thiazide Diuretics, loop diuretics	Digoxin	↑	Diuretic-induced electrolyte disturbances may predispose to digitalis-induced arrhythmias. Measure plasma levels of potassium and magnesium and supplement low levels. Prevent further losses with dietary sodium restriction or potassium-sparing diuretics.
Thyroid hormones	Digoxin	↓	Thyroid administration to a digitalized, hypothyroid patient may increase the dose requirement of digoxin

* ↑ = Object drug increased. ↓ = Object drug decreased.

➤*Drugs that may increase digoxin:* Potassium-depleting diuretics are a major contributing factor to digitalis toxicity. Quinidine, verapamil, amiodarone, propafenone, indomethacin, itraconazole, alprazolam, and spironolactone raise the serum digoxin concentration due to a reduction in clearance and/or volume of distribution of the drug, with the implication that digitalis intoxication may result.

➤*Drugs that may decrease digoxin:* Rifampin may decrease serum digoxin concentration, especially in patients with renal dysfunction, by increasing the nonrenal clearance of digoxin.

➤*Other:* There have been inconsistent reports regarding the effects of other drugs (eg, quinine, penicillamine) on serum digoxin concentration.

Due to the considerable variability of these interactions, individualize dosage of digoxin when patients receive these medications concurrently. Furthermore, exercise caution when combining digoxin with any drug that may cause a significant deterioration in renal function because a decline in glomerular filtration or tubular secretion may impair the excretion of digoxin.

➤*Drug/Lab test interactions:* The use of therapeutic doses of digoxin may cause prolongation of the PR interval and depression of the ST segment on the electrocardiogram. Digoxin may produce false positive ST-T changes on the electrocardiogram during exercise testing. These electrophysiologic effects reflect an expected effect of the drug and are not indicative of toxicity.

Adverse Reactions

In general, the adverse reactions of digoxin are dose dependent and occur at doses higher than those needed to achieve a therapeutic effect. Hence, adverse reactions are less common when digoxin is used within the recommended dose range or therapeutic serum concentration range and when there is careful attention to concurrent medications and conditions.

Because some patients may be particularly susceptible to side effects with digoxin, always select the dosage of the drug carefully and adjust as the clinical condition of the patient warrants. In the past, when high doses of digoxin were used and little attention was paid to clinical status or concurrent medications, adverse reactions to digoxin were more frequent and severe. Cardiac adverse reactions accounted for about one-half, GI disturbances for about one-fourth, and CNS and other toxicity for about one-fourth of these adverse reactions. However, available evidence suggests that the incidence and severity of digoxin toxicity has decreased substantially in recent years. In recent controlled clinical trials, in patients with predominantly mild to moderate heart failure, the incidence of adverse reactions was comparable in patients taking digoxin and in those taking placebo. In a large mortality trial, the incidence of hospitalization for suspected digoxin toxicity was 2% in patients taking digoxin tablets compared with 0.9% in patients taking placebo. In this trial, the most common manifestations of digoxin toxicity included GI and cardiac disturbances; CNS manifestations were less common.

➤*Adults:*

Cardiovascular – Therapeutic doses of digoxin may cause heart block in patients with preexisting sinoatrial or AV conduction disorders; heart block can be avoided by adjusting the dose of digoxin. Prophylactic use of a cardiac pacemaker may be considered if the risk of heart block is considered unacceptable. High doses of digoxin may produce a variety of rhythm disturbances, such as first-degree, second-degree (Wenckebach), or third-degree heart block (including asystole); atrial tachycardia with block; AV dissociation; accelerated junctional (nodal) rhythm; unifocal or multiform ventricular premature contractions (especially bigeminy or trigeminy); ventricular tachycardia; and ventricular fibrillation. Digoxin produces PR prolongation and ST segment depression, which should not by themselves be considered digoxin toxicity. Cardiac toxicity can also occur at therapeutic doses in patients who have conditions which may alter their sensitivities to digoxin (eg, restrictive cardiomyopathy, electrolyte disturbances, hypothyroidism).

CNS – Digoxin can produce visual disturbances (blurred or yellow vision), headache, weakness, dizziness, apathy, confusion, and mental disturbances (eg, anxiety, depression, delirium, hallucination).

GI – Digoxin may cause anorexia, nausea, vomiting, and diarrhea. Rarely, the use of digoxin has been associated with abdominal pain, intestinal ischemia, and hemorrhagic necrosis of the intestines.

Miscellaneous – Gynecomastia has been occasionally observed following the prolonged use of digoxin. Thrombocytopenia and maculopapular rash and other skin reactions have been rarely observed. The following table summarizes the incidence of those adverse reactions listed previously for patients treated with digoxin tablets or placebo from 2 randomized, double-blind, placebo-controlled withdrawal trials. Patients in these trials were also receiving diuretics with or without ACE inhibitors. These patients had been stable on digoxin, and were randomized to digoxin or placebo. The results shown below reflect the experience in patients following dosage titration with the use of serum digoxin concentrations and careful follow-up. These adverse reactions are consistent with results from a large, placebo-controlled mortality trial (DIG trial) wherein over half the patients were not receiving digoxin prior to enrollment.

Adverse Reactions in 2 Parallel, Double-Blind, Placebo-controlled Withdrawal Trials (Number of Patients Reporting)

Adverse reaction	Digoxin patients (n = 123)	Placebo patients (n = 125)
Cardiovascular		
Heart arrest	1%	1%
Palpitation	1%	4%
Tachycardia	2%	1%
Ventricular extrasystole	1%	1%
CNS		
Dizziness	6%	5%
Headache	4%	4%
Mental disturbances	5%	1%

DIGOXIN — INJECTION

Adverse Reactions in 2 Parallel, Double-Blind, Placebo-controlled Withdrawal Trials (Number of Patients Reporting)		
Adverse reaction	Digoxin patients (n = 123)	Placebo patients (n = 125)
GI		
Abdominal pain	0%	6%
Anorexia	1%	4%
Diarrhea	4%	1%
Nausea	4%	2%
Vomiting	2%	1%
Miscellaneous		
Death	4%	3%
Rash	2%	1%

➤*Infants and children:* The side effects of digoxin in infants and children differ from those seen in adults in several respects. Although digoxin may produce anorexia, nausea, vomiting, diarrhea, and CNS disturbances in young patients, these are rarely the initial symptoms of overdosage. Rather, the earliest and most frequent manifestation of excessive dosing with digoxin in infants and children is the appearance of cardiac arrhythmias, including sinus bradycardia. In children, the use of digoxin may produce any arrhythmia. The most common are conduction disturbances or supraventricular tachyarrhythmias, such as atrial tachycardia (with or without block) and junctional (nodal) tachycardia. Ventricular arrhythmias are less common. Sinus bradycardia may be a sign of impending digoxin intoxication, especially in infants, even in the absence of first-degree heart block. Any arrhythmia or alteration in cardiac conduction that develops in a child taking digoxin should be assumed to be caused by digoxin, until further evaluation proves otherwise.

Overdosage

➤*Symptoms:* Manifestations of life-threatening toxicity include ventricular tachycardia or ventricular fibrillation, or progressive bradyarrhythmias or heart block. The administration of more than 10 mg of digoxin in a previously healthy adult, or more than 4 mg in a previously healthy child, or a steady-state serum concentration greater than 10 ng/mL often results in cardiac arrest.

➤*Treatment:* Severe digitalis intoxication can cause a massive shift of potassium from inside to outside the cell, leading to life-threatening hyperkalemia. Avoid the administration of potassium supplements in the setting of massive intoxication because it may be hazardous. Hyperkalemia caused by massive digitalis toxicity is best treated with digoxin immune fab (ovine); initial treatment with glucose and insulin may also be required if hyperkalemia itself is acutely life-threatening.

Temporarily discontinue digoxin until the adverse reaction resolves. Also make every effort to correct factors that may contribute to the adverse reaction (eg, electrolyte disturbances, concurrent medications). Once the adverse reaction has resolved, reinstitute therapy with digoxin, following a careful reassessment of dose.

Withdrawal of digoxin may be all that is required to treat the adverse reaction. However, when the primary manifestation of digoxin overdosage is a cardiac arrhythmia, additional therapy may be needed.

If the rhythm disturbance is a symptomatic bradyarrhythmia or heart block, give consideration to the reversal of toxicity with digoxin immune fab (ovine), the use of atropine, or the insertion of a temporary cardiac pacemaker. However, asymptomatic bradycardia or heart block related to digoxin may require only temporary withdrawal of the drug and cardiac monitoring of the patient.

If the rhythm disturbance is a ventricular arrhythmia, give consideration to the correction of electrolyte disorders, particularly if hypokalemia or hypomagnesemia is present. Digoxin immune fab (ovine) is a specific antidote for digoxin and may be used to reverse potentially life-threatening ventricular arrhythmias due to digoxin overdosage.

Make every effort to maintain the serum potassium concentration between 4 and 5.5 mmol/L. Potassium is usually administered orally, but when correction of the arrhythmia is urgent and the serum potassium concentration is low, potassium may be administered cautiously by the IV route. Monitor the electrocardiogram for any evidence of potassium toxicity (eg, peaking of T waves) and to observe the effect on the arrhythmia. Potassium salts may be dangerous in patients who manifest bradycardia or heart block due to digoxin (unless primarily related to supraventricular tachycardia) and in the setting of massive digitalis overdosage.

Patients with massive digitalis ingestion should receive large doses of activated charcoal to prevent absorption and bind digoxin in the gut during enteroenteric recirculation. Emesis or gastric lavage may be indicated especially if ingestion has occurred within 30 minutes of the patient's presentation at the hospital. Do not induce emesis in patients who are obtunded. If a patient presents more than 2 hours after ingestion or already has toxic manifestations, it may be unsafe to induce vomiting or attempt passage of a gastric tube because such maneuvers may induce an acute vagal episode that can worsen digitalis-related arrhythmias.

INAMRINONE LACTATE

Rx	Inamrinone Lactate (Abbott Hospital)	Injection: 5 mg/mL (as lactate)	In 20 mL amps.[1]

[1] With 0.25 mg/mL sodium metabisulfite.

INAMRINONE — INJECTION

Indications

For the short-term management of congestive heart failure. Because of limited experience and the potential for serious adverse effects (such as thrombocytopenia, arrhythmia, hypotension, chest pain, hepatotoxicity, hypersensitivity reactions, and fever), inamrinone should be used only in patients who can be closely monitored and who have not responded adequately to digitalis, diuretics, or vasodilators. Experience with IV inamrinone in controlled trials does not extend beyond 48 hours of repeated boluses or continuous infusions.

Administration and Dosage

➤*Approved by the FDA:* July 1984.

➤*Loading dose:* Initiate therapy with a 0.75 mg/kg loading dose given slowly over 2 to 3 minutes.

Loading dose determination 0.75 mg/kg (undiluted)										
Patient weight in kg	30	40	50	60	70	80	90	100	110	120
mL of undiluted inamrinone injection	4.5	6	7.5	9	10.5	12	13.5	15	16.5	18

Loading doses of inamrinone injection should be administered as supplied (undiluted). Infusions of inamrinone injection may be administered in normal, or half normal saline solution to a concentration of 1 to 3 mg/mL. Diluted solutions should be used with 24 hours.

Inamrinone injection may be injected into running dextrose (glucose) infusions through a Y-connector or directly into the tubing where preferable.

➤*Maintenance dose:* Continue therapy with a maintenance infusion between 5 and 10 mcg/kg/min.

➤*Rate of infusion:* Based on clinical response, an additional loading dose of 0.75 mg/kg may be given 30 minutes after the initiation of therapy.

The rate of infusion usually ranges from 5 to 10 mcg/kg/min, such that the recommended total daily dose (including loading doses) does not exceed 10 mg/kg. A limited number of patients studied at higher doses support a dosage regimen up to 18 mg/kg/day for shortened durations of therapy.

The following infusion rate table may be used to ensure that the calculations are made correctly.

To use the following table, the concentration of inamrinone infusion solution used must be 2.5 mg/mL (2,500 mcg/mL).

This concentration is prepared by mixing the inamrinone solution with an equal volume of diluent (normal or half normal saline).

➤*Dilution:* To prepare the 2.5 mg/mL concentration recommended for infusion, mix inamrinone with an equal volume of diluent. For example, mix three 20 mL ampuls of inamrinone injection (3 × 20 mL = 60 mL) with 60 mL of diluent for a total volume of 120 mL of the final 2.5 mg/mL solution of inamrinone.

Inamrinone IV Infusion Rate (mL/h) Using 2.5 mg/mL Infusion Concentration										
Patient weight in kg	30	40	50	60	70	80	90	100	110	120
Dosage										
5 mcg/kg/min	4	5	6	7	8	10	11	12	13	14
7.5 mcg/kg/min	5	7	9	11	13	14	16	18	20	22
10 mcg/kg/min	7	10	12	14	17	19	22	24	26	29

Monitoring central venous pressure (CVP) may be valuable in the assessment of hypotension and fluid balance management. Prior correction or adjustment of fluid/electrolytes is essential to obtain satisfactory response with inamrinone.

➤*Incompatibilities:* A chemical interaction occurs slowly over a 24-hour period when the IV solution of inamrinone injection is mixed directly with dextrose (glucose)-containing solutions. Therefore, inamrinone injection should not be diluted with solutions that contain dextrose (glucose) prior to injection.

A chemical interaction occurs immediately, which is evidenced by the formation of a precipitate when furosemide is injected into an IV line of an infusion of inamrinone. Therefore, furosemide should not be administered in IV lines containing inamrinone.

➤*Storage/Stability:* Protect ampuls from light by retaining in carton until time of use. Store at 15° to 30°C (59° to 86°F).

Actions

➤*Pharmacology:* Inamrinone injection is a positive inotropic agent with vasodilator activity, different in structure and mode of action from either digitalis glycosides or catecholamines.

The mechanism of its inotropic and vasodilator effects has not been fully elucidated.

With respect to its inotropic effect, experimental evidence indicates that it is not a beta-adrenergic agonist. It inhibits myocardial cyclic adenosine monophosphate (c-AMP) phosphodiesterase activity and increases cellular levels of c-AMP. Unlike digitalis, it does not inhibit sodium-potassium adenosine triphosphatase activity.

With respect to its vasodilatory activity, inamrinone reduces afterload and preload by its direct relaxant effect on vascular smooth muscle.

➤*Pharmacokinetics:*

Distribution – Following IV bolus (1 to 2 minutes) injection of 0.68 to 1.2 mg/kg to healthy volunteers, inamrinone had a volume of distribution of 1.2 L/kg. Infants and children have a larger volume of distribution.

Inamrinone has been shown in 1 study to be 10% to 22% bound to human plasma protein by ultrafiltration in vitro, and in another study 35% to 49% bound by either ultrafiltration or equilibrium dialysis.

Metabolism/Excretion – Following a distributive phase half-life of about 4.6 minutes in plasma, had a mean apparent first-order terminal elimination half-life of about 3.6 hours. In patients with congestive heart failure receiving infusions of inamrinone the mean apparent first-order terminal elimination half-life was about 5.8 hours. Infants and children have a decreased elimination half-life.

The primary route of excretion in man is via the urine as both inamrinone and several metabolites (N-glycolyl, N-acetate, O-glucuronide and N-glucuronide). In healthy volunteers, approximately 63% of an oral dose of ^{14}C-labeled inamrinone was excreted in the urine over a 96-hour period. In the first 8 hours, 51% of the radioactivity in the urine was inamrinone with 5% as the N-acetate, 8% as the N-glycolate, and less than 5% for each glucuronide. Approximately 18% of the administered dose was excreted in the feces in 72 hours.

In a 24-hour nonradioactive IV study, 10% to 40% of the dose was excreted in urine as unchanged inamrinone with the N-acetyl metabolite representing less than 2% of the dose.

Special populations –

Congestive heart failure: In congestive heart failure patients, after a loading bolus dose, steady-state plasma levels of about 2.4 mcg/mL were able to be maintained by an infusion of 5 to 10 mcg/kg/min. In some congestive heart failure patients, with associated compromised renal and hepatic perfusion, it is possible that plasma levels of inamrinone may rise during the infusion period; therefore, in these patients, it may be necessary to monitor the hemodynamic response or drug level. The principal measures of patient response include cardiac index, pulmonary capillary wedge pressure, central venous pressure, and their relationship to plasma concentrations. Additionally, measurements of blood pressure, urine output, and body weight may prove useful, as may such clinical symptoms as orthopnea, dyspnea, and fatigue.

Contraindications

Hypersensitivity to inamrinone or bisulfites.

Warnings

➤*Mutagenesis:* The mouse micronucleus test (at 7.5 to 10 times the maximum human dose) and the Chinese hamster ovary chromosome aberration assay were positive, indicating both clastogenic potential and suppression of the number of polychromatic erythrocytes. However, the Ames *Salmonella* assay, mouse lymphoma study, and cultured human lymphocyte metaphase analysis were all negative.

➤*Fertility impairment:* The clastogenic effects are in contrast to negative results obtained in the rat male and female fertility studies, and a 3-generation study in rats, both with oral dosing.

Slight prolongation of the rat gestation period was seen in these studies at dose levels of 50 and 100 mg/kg/day. Dystocia occurred in dams receiving 100 mg/kg/day resulting in increased numbers of stillbirths, decreased litter size, and poor pup survival.

➤*Pregnancy: Category C.* In New Zealand white rabbits, inamrinone has been shown to produce fetal skeletal and gross external malformations at oral doses of 16 and 50 mg/kg which were toxic for the rabbit. Studies in French Hy/Cr rabbits using oral doses up to 32 mg/kg/day did not confirm this finding. No malformations were seen in rats receiving inamrinone IV at the maximum dose used, 15 mg/kg/day (approximately the recommended daily IV dose for patients with congestive heart failure). There are no adequate and well-controlled studies in pregnant women. Inamrinone should be used during pregnancy only if the potential benefit justifies the potential risk to the fetus.

➤*Lactation:* Caution should be exercised when inamrinone is administered to nursing women, since it is not known whether it is excreted in human milk.

➤*Children:* Safety and efficacy in pediatric patients have not been established. In preterm infants, short-term use of inamrinone (5 mcg/kg/min) was effective in the management of CHF.

Precautions

➤*Monitoring:* Fluid and electrolyte changes and renal function should be carefully monitored during inamrinone lactate therapy. Improvement in cardiac output with resultant diuresis may necessitate a reduction in the dose of diuretic. Potassium loss due to excessive diuresis may predispose digitalized patients to arrhythmias. Therefore, hypokalemia should be corrected by potassium supplementation in advance of or during inamrinone use.

INAMRINONE — INJECTION

During IV therapy with inamrinone injection, blood pressure and heart rate should be monitored and the rate of infusion slowed or stopped in patients showing excessive decreases in blood pressure.

➤*Pulmonic and/or aortic valvular disease:* Inamrinone injection should not be used in patients with severe aortic or pulmonic valvular disease in lieu of surgical relief of the obstruction. Like other inotropic agents, it may aggravate outflow tract obstruction in hypertrophic subaortic stenosis.

➤*Fluid and electrolyte intake:* Patients who have received vigorous diuretic therapy may have insufficient cardiac-filling pressure to respond adequately to inamrinone injection, in which case, cautious liberalization of fluid and electrolyte intake may be indicated.

➤*Arrhythmias:* Supraventricular and ventricular arrhythmias have been observed in the very high-risk population treated. While inamrinone per se has not been shown to be arrhythmogenic, the potential for arrhythmia, present in congestive heart failure itself, may be increased by any drug or combination of drugs.

➤*Use in acute myocardial infarction:* No clinical trials have been carried out in patients in the acute phase of postmyocardial infarction. Therefore, inamrinone injection is not recommended in these cases.

➤*Sulfite sensitivity:* Some of these products contain sodium metabisulfite, a sulfite that may cause allergic-type reactions including anaphylactic symptoms and life-threatening or less severe asthmatic episodes in certain susceptible people. The overall prevalence of sulfite sensitivity in the general population is unknown and probably low. Sulfite sensitivity is seen more frequently in asthmatic than in nonasthmatic people.

Drug Interactions

In a relatively limited experience, no untoward clinical manifestations have been observed in patients in which inamrinone injection was used concurrently with the following drugs: Digitalis glycosides; lidocaine, quinidine; metoprolol, propranolol; hydralazine, prazosin; isosorbide dinitrate, nitroglycerin; chlorthalidone, ethacrynic acid, furosemide, hydrochlorothiazide, spironolactone; captopril; heparin, warfarin; potassium supplements; insulin; diazepam.

One case report of excessive hypotension has been reported when inamrinone was used concurrently with disopyramide.

Until additional experience is available, concurrent administration with disopyramide should be undertaken with caution.

Adverse Reactions

➤*Cardiovascular:* Cardiovascular adverse reactions reported with inamrinone injection include arrhythmia (3%) and hypotension (1.3%).

➤*GI:* GI adverse reactions reported with inamrinone injection during clinical use included nausea (1.7%), vomiting (0.9%), abdominal pain (0.4%), and anorexia (0.4%).

While GI side effects were seen infrequently with IV therapy, should severe or debilitating ones occur, the physician may wish to reduce dosage or discontinue the drug based on the usual benefit-to-risk considerations.

➤*Hematologic:*

Thrombocytopenia – IV inamrinone injection resulted in platelet count reductions to below 100,000/mm^3 or normal limits in 2.4% of the patients.

It is more common in patients receiving prolonged therapy. To date, in closely monitored clinical trials, in patients whose platelet counts were not allowed to remain depressed, no bleeding phenomena have been observed.

Platelet reduction is dose dependent and appears due to a decrease in platelet survival time. Several patients who developed thrombocytopenia while receiving inamrinone had bone marrow examinations which were normal. There is no evidence relating platelet reduction to immune response or to a platelet-activating factor.

Management of platelet count reductions – Asymptomatic platelet count reduction (to less than 150,000/mm^3) may be reversed within 1 week of a decrease in drug dosage. Further, with no change in drug dosage, the count may stabilize at lower than predrug levels without any clinical sequelae. Predrug platelet counts and frequent platelet counts during therapy are recommended to assist in decisions regarding dosage modifications.

If a platelet count less than 150,000/mm^3 occurs, the following actions may be considered:

- Maintain total daily dose unchanged, since in some cases counts have either stabilized or returned to pretreatment levels.
- Decrease total daily dose.
- Discontinue inamrinone if, in the clinical judgment of the physician, risk exceeds the potential benefit.

➤*Hepatic:* In dogs, at IV doses between 9 and 32 mg/kg/day, inamrinone showed dose-related hepatotoxicity manifested either as enzyme elevation or hepatic cell necrosis or both. Hepatotoxicity has been observed in man following long-term oral dosing and has been observed, in a limited experience (0.2%), following IV administration of inamrinone. There have also been rare reports of enzyme and bilirubin elevation and jaundice.

In clinical experience to date with IV administration, hepatotoxicity has been observed rarely. If acute marked alterations in liver enzymes occur together with clinical symptoms suggesting an idiosyncratic hypersensitivity reaction, inamrinone therapy should be promptly discontinued.

If less than marked enzyme alterations occur without clinical symptoms, these nonspecific changes should be evaluated on an individual basis. The clinician may wish to continue inamrinone, reduce dosage, or discontinue the drug based on the usual benefit/risk considerations.

➤*Hypersensitivity:* There have been reports of several apparent hypersensitivity reactions in patients treated with oral inamrinone for about 2 weeks. Signs and symptoms were variable but included pericarditis, pleuritis and ascites (1 case), myositis with interstitial shadowing on chest x-ray and elevated sedimentation rate (1 case) and vasculitis with nodular pulmonary densities, hypoxemia, and jaundice (1 case). The first patient died, not necessarily of the possible reaction, while the last two resolved with discontinuation of therapy. None of the cases were rechallenged so that attribution to inamrinone is not certain, but possible hypersensitivity reactions should be considered in any patient maintained for a prolonged period on inamrinone.

➤*Miscellaneous:* Additional adverse reactions observed in IV inamrinone clinical studies include fever (0.9%), chest pain (0.2%), and burning at the site of injection (0.2%).

Overdosage

➤*Symptoms:* A death has been reported with a massive accidental overdose (840 mg over 3 hours by initial bolus and infusion) of inamrinone, although causal relation is uncertain. Diligence should be exercised during product preparation and administration.

➤*Treatment:* Doses of inamrinone injection may produce hypotension because of its vasodilator effect. If this occurs, inamrinone administration should be reduced or discontinued. No specific antidote is known, but general measures for circulatory support should be taken.

MILRINONE LACTATE

Rx	**Milrinone Lactate** (Bedford)	**Injection:** 1 mg/mL	47 mg/mL dextrose. In 10, 20, and 50 mL single-dose vials.
Rx	**Primacor** (Sanofi Winthrop)		47 mg anhydrous dextrose. In 10 and 20 mL single-dose vials.
Rx	**Primacor** (Sanofi Winthrop)	**Injection, premixed:** 200 mcg/mL in 5% Dextrose Injection[1]	In 100 mL.

[1] With 0.282 mg/mL lactic acid.

MILRINONE LACTATE — INJECTION

Indications

Milrinone lactate is indicated for the short-term IV treatment of patients with acute decompensated heart failure.

Administration and Dosage

➤*Approved by the FDA:* December 1987.

Milrinone lactate should be administered with a loading dose followed by a continuous infusion (maintenance dose) according to the following guidelines:

➤*Loading dose (50 mcg/kg):* Administer slowly over 10 minutes.

The following table shows the loading dose in milliliters of milrinone lactate (1 mg/mL) by patient body weight (kg).

Loading Dose (mL) Using 1 mg/mL Concentration										
	Patient body weight (kg)									
kg	30	40	50	60	70	80	90	100	110	120
mL	1.5	2	2.5	3	3.5	4	4.5	5	5.5	6

The loading dose may be given undiluted, but diluting to a rounded total volume of 10 or 20 mL (see Maintenance dose for diluents) may simplify the visualization of the injection rate.

➤*Maintenance dose:*

Maintenance Dose			
	Infusion rate	Total daily dose (24 hours)	
Minimum	0.375 mcg/kg/min	0.59 mg/kg	Administer as a continuous IV infusion.
Standard	0.5 mcg/kg/min	0.77 mg/kg	
Maximum	0.75 mcg/kg/min	1.13 mg/kg	

Milrinone lactate drawn from vials should be diluted prior to maintenance dose administration. The diluents that may be used are 0.45% Sodium Chloride Injection USP, 0.9% Sodium Chloride Injection USP, or 5% Dextrose Injection. The table below shows the volume of diluent in milliliters (mL) that must be used to achieve 200 mcg/mL concentration for infusion and the resultant total volumes.

MILRINONE LACTATE — INJECTION

Desired infusion concentration (mcg/mL)	Milrinone 1 mg/mL (mL)	Diluent (mL)	Total volume (mL)
200	10	40	50
200	20	80	100

The infusion rate should be adjusted according to hemodynamic and clinical response. Patients should be closely monitored. In controlled clinical studies, most patients showed an improvement in hemodynamic status as evidenced by increases in cardiac output and reductions in pulmonary capillary wedge pressure.

Dosage may be titrated to the maximum hemodynamic effect and should not exceed 1.13 mg/kg/day. Duration of therapy should depend upon patient responsiveness.

Milrinone Infusion Rate (mL/h) Using 200 mcg/mL Concentration										
Maintenance dose (mcg/kg/min)	Patient body weight (kg)									
	30	40	50	60	70	80	90	100	110	120
0.375	3.4	4.5	5.6	6.8	7.9	9	10.1	11.3	12.4	13.5
0.4	3.6	4.8	6	7.2	8.4	9.6	10.8	12	13.2	14.4
0.5	4.5	6	7.5	9	10.5	12	13.5	15	16.5	18
0.6	5.4	7.2	9	10.8	12.6	14.4	16.2	18	19.8	21.6
0.7	6.3	8.4	10.5	12.6	14.7	16.8	18.9	21	23.1	25.2
0.75	6.8	9	11.3	13.5	15.8	18	20.3	22.5	24.8	27

➤*Dosage adjustment in renally impaired patients:* Data obtained from patients with severe renal impairment (creatinine clearance = 0 to 30 mL/min) but without congestive heart failure have demonstrated that the presence of renal impairment significantly increases the terminal elimination half-life of milrinone lactate. Reductions in infusion rate may be necessary in patients with renal impairment.

Creatinine clearance (mL/min/1.73 m^2)	Infusion rate (mcg/kg/min)
5	0.2
10	0.23
20	0.28
30	0.33
40	0.38
50	0.43

➤*Incompatibilities:* There is an immediate chemical interaction which is evidenced by the formation of a precipitate when furosemide is injected into an IV line of an infusion of milrinone lactate. Therefore, furosemide should not be administered in IV lines containing milrinone lactate.

➤*Storage/Stability:* Discard unused portion after initial use. Store at controlled room temperature 15° to 30°C (59° to 86°F). Avoid freezing. Exposure of pharmaceutical products to heat should be minimized. Avoid excessive heat. Protect from freezing. It is recommended that the flexible containers be stored at room temperature, 25°C (77°F); however, brief exposure up to 40°C (104°F) does not adversely affect the product.

Actions

➤*Pharmacology:* Milrinone lactate is a positive inotrope and vasodilator, with little chronotropic activity different in structure and mode of action from either the digitalis glycosides or catecholamines.

Milrinone lactate, at relevant inotropic and vasorelaxant concentrations, is a selective inhibitor of peak III cyclic adenosine monophosphate (cAMP) phosphodiesterase isozyme in cardiac and vascular muscle. This inhibitory action is consistent with cAMP-mediated increases in intracellular ionized calcium and contractile force in cardiac muscle, as well as with cAMP-dependent contractile protein phosphorylation and relaxation in vascular muscle. Additional experimental evidence also indicates that milrinone lactate is not a beta-adrenergic agonist nor does it inhibit sodium-potassium adenosine triphosphatase activity as do the digitalis glycosides.

Clinical studies in patients with congestive heart failure have shown that milrinone lactate produces dose- and plasma drug concentration-related increases in the maximum rate of increase of left ventricular pressure. Studies in healthy subjects have shown that milrinone lactate produces increases in the slope of the left ventricular pressure-dimension relationship, indicating a direct inotropic effect of the drug. Milrinone lactate also produces dose- and plasma concentration-related increases in forearm blood flow in patients with congestive heart failure, indicating a direct arterial vasodilator activity of the drug.

Both the inotropic and vasodilatory effects have been observed over the therapeutic range of plasma milrinone concentrations of 100 to 300 ng/mL.

In addition to increasing myocardial contractility, milrinone lactate improves diastolic function as evidenced by improvements in left ventricular diastolic relaxation.

Pharmacodynamics – In patients with heart failure due to depressed myocardial function, milrinone lactate produced a prompt dose- and plasma concentration-related increase in cardiac output and decreases in pulmonary capillary wedge pressure and vascular resistance, which were accompanied by mild-to-moderate increases in heart rate. Additionally, there is no increased effect on myocardial oxygen consumption. In uncontrolled studies, hemodynamic improvement during IV therapy with milrinone lactate was accompanied by clinical symptomatic improvement, but the ability of milrinone lactate to relieve symptoms has not been evaluated in controlled clinical trials. The great majority of patients experience improvements in hemodynamic function within 5 to 15 minutes of the initiation of therapy.

In studies in congestive heart failure patients, milrinone lactate, when administered as a loading injection followed by a maintenance infusion, produced significant mean initial increases in cardiac index of 25%, 38%, and 42% at dose regimens of 37.5 mcg/kg/0.375 mcg/kg/min, 50 mcg/kg/0.5 mcg/kg/min, and 75 mcg/kg/0.75 mcg/kg/min, respectively. Over the same range of loading injections and maintenance infusions, pulmonary capillary wedge pressure significantly decreased by 20%, 23%, and 36%, respectively, while systemic vascular resistance significantly decreased by 17%, 21%, and 37%. Mean arterial pressure fell by up to 5% at the 2 lower dose regimens, but by 17% at the highest dose. Patients evaluated for 48 hours maintained improvements in hemodynamic function, with no evidence of diminished response (tachyphylaxis). A smaller number of patients have received infusions of milrinone lactate for periods up to 72 hours without evidence of tachyphylaxis.

The duration of therapy should depend upon patient responsiveness. Patients have been maintained on infusions for up to 5 days.

Milrinone lactate has a favorable inotropic effect in fully digitalized patients without causing signs of glycoside toxicity. Theoretically, in cases of atrial flutter/fibrillation, it is possible that milrinone lactate may increase ventricular response rate because of its slight enhancement of AV node conduction. In these cases, digitalis should be considered prior to the institution of therapy with milrinone lactate.

Improvement in left ventricular function in patients with ischemic heart disease has been observed. The improvement has occurred without inducing symptoms or electrocardiographic signs of myocardial ischemia.

➤*Pharmacokinetics:*

Absorption/Distribution – The steady-state plasma milrinone concentrations after approximately 6 to 12 hours of unchanging maintenance infusion of 0.5 mcg/kg/min are approximately 200 ng/mL. Near maximum favorable effects of milrinone lactate on cardiac output and pulmonary capillary wedge pressure are seen at plasma milrinone concentrations in the 150 to 250 ng/mL range.

Following IV injections of 12.5 to 125 mcg/kg to congestive heart failure patients, milrinone lactate had a volume of distribution of 0.38 L/kg, a mean terminal elimination half-life of 2.3 hours, and a clearance of 0.13 L/kg/h. Following IV infusions of 0.2 to 0.7 mcg/kg/min to congestive heart failure patients, the drug had a volume of distribution of about 0.45 L/kg, a mean terminal elimination half-life of 2.4 hours, and a clearance of 0.14 L/kg/h. These pharmacokinetic parameters were not dose dependent, and the area under the plasma concentration versus time curve following injections was significantly dose dependent.

Milrinone lactate has been shown (by equilibrium dialysis) to be approximately 70% bound to human plasma protein.

Excretion – The primary route of excretion of milrinone lactate in man is via the urine. The major urinary excretions of orally administered milrinone lactate in man are milrinone (83%) and its 0-glucuronide metabolite (12%). Elimination in healthy subjects via the urine is rapid, with approximately 60% recovered within the first 2 hours following dosing and approximately 90% recovered within the first 8 hours following dosing. The mean renal clearance of milrinone lactate is approximately 0.3 L/min, indicative of active secretion.

Contraindications

Hypersensitivity to milrinone.

Warnings

➤*Arrhythmias:* The use of milrinone has been associated with increased frequency of ventricular arrhythmias, including nonsustained ventricular tachycardia. Long-term oral use has been associated with an increased risk of sudden death. Hence, patients receiving milrinone lactate should be observed closely with the use of continuous electrocardiograph monitoring to allow the prompt detection and management of ventricular arrhythmias.

➤*Mutagenesis:* Whereas the Chinese hamster ovary chromosome aberration assay was positive in the presence of a metabolic activation system, results from the Ames test, the mouse lymphoma assay, the micronucleus test, and the in vivo rat bone marrow metaphase analysis indicated an absence of mutagenic potential.

➤*Pregnancy: Category C.*

There are no adequate and well-controlled studies in pregnant women. Milrinone lactate should be used during pregnancy only if the potential benefit justifies the potential risk to the fetus.

➤*Lactation:* Caution should be exercised when milrinone lactate is administered to breast-feeding women, because it is not known whether it is excreted in human milk.

➤*Children:* Safety and efficacy in pediatric patients have not been established.

Precautions

➤*Monitoring:* Patients receiving milrinone lactate should be observed closely with appropriate electrocardiographic equipment. The facility for immediate treatment of potential cardiac events, which may include life-threatening ventricular arrythmias, must be available. The majority of experience with IV milrinone lactate has been in patients receiving digoxin and diuretics. There is no experience in controlled trials with infusions of milrinone lactate for periods exceeding 48 hours.

MILRINONE LACTATE — INJECTION

Fluid and electrolyte changes and renal function should be carefully monitored during therapy with milrinone lactate. Improvement in cardiac output with resultant diuresis may necessitate a reduction in the dose of diuretic. Potassium loss due to excessive diuresis may predispose digitalized patients to arrhythmias. Therefore, hypokalemia should be corrected by potassium supplementation in advance of or during use of milrinone lactate.

During therapy with milrinone lactate, blood pressure and heart rate should be monitored and the rate of infusion slowed or stopped in patients showing excessive decreases in blood pressure.

If prior vigorous diuretic therapy is suspected to have caused significant decreases in cardiac filling pressure, milrinone lactate should be cautiously administered with monitoring of blood pressure, heart rate, and clinical symptomatology.

➤*Arrhythmias:* Supraventricular and ventricular arrhythmias have been observed in the high-risk population treated. In some patients, injections of milrinone lactate and oral milrinone lactate have been shown to increase ventricular ectopy, including nonsustained ventricular tachycardia. The potential for arrhythmia, present in congestive heart failure itself, may be increased by many drugs or combinations of drugs. Patients receiving milrinone lactate should be closely monitored during infusion.

Milrinone lactate produces a slight shortening of AV node conduction time, indicating a potential for an increased ventricular response rate in patients with atrial flutter/fibrillation which is not controlled with digitalis therapy.

➤*Special risk:*

Use in acute myocardial infarction – No clinical studies have been conducted in patients in the acute phase of post myocardial infarction. Until further clinical experience with this class of drugs is gained, milrinone lactate is not recommended in these patients. Milrinone lactate should not be used in patients with severe obstructive aortic or pulmonic valvular disease in lieu of surgical relief of the obstruction. Like other inotropic agents, it may aggravate outflow tract obstruction in hypertrophic subaortic stenosis.

Adverse Reactions

➤*Cardiovascular:* In patients receiving milrinone lactate in phase II and III clinical trials, ventricular arrhythmias were reported in 12.1%: Ventricular ectopic activity, 8.5%; nonsustained ventricular tachycardia, 2.8%; sustained ventricular tachycardia, 1% and ventricular fibrillation, 0.2% (2 patients experienced more than 1 type of arrhythmia). Holter recordings demonstrated that in some patients injection of milrinone lactate increased ventricular ectopy, including nonsustained ventricular tachycardia. Life-threatening arrhythmias were infrequent, and, when present, have been associated with certain underlying factors such as preexisting arrhythmias, metabolic abnormalities (eg, hypokalemia), abnormal digoxin levels and catheter insertion. Milrinone lactate was not shown to be arrhythmogenic in an electrophysiology study. Supraventricular arrhythmias were reported in 3.8% of the patients receiving milrinone lactate. The incidence of both supraventricular and ventricular arrhythmias has not been related to the dose or plasma milrinone concentration.

Other cardiovascular adverse reactions include hypotension, 2.9% and angina/chest pain, 1.2%.

➤*CNS:* Headaches, usually mild to moderate in severity, have been reported in 2.9% of patients receiving milrinone lactate.

➤*Lab test abnormalities:* In the postmarketing experience, liver function test abnormalities have been reported.

➤*Miscellaneous:* Other adverse reactions reported, but not definitely related to the administration of milrinone lactate include hypokalemia, 0.6%; tremor, 0.4%; and thrombocytopenia, 0.4%.

Isolated spontaneous reports of bronchospasm have been received.

Overdosage

➤*Symptoms:* Doses of milrinone lactate may produce hypotension because of its vasodilator effect.

➤*Treatment:* If hypotension occurs, administration of milrinone lactate should be reduced or temporarily discontinued until the patient's condition stabilizes. No specific antidote is known, but general measures for circulatory support should be taken.

ANTIARRHYTHMIC AGENTS

Optimal therapy of cardiac arrhythmias requires documentation, accurate diagnosis and modification of precipitating causes, and if indicated, proper selection and use of antiarrhythmic drugs. Comprehensive information on individual agents is presented in the following monographs.

These drugs are classified according to their effects on the action potential of cardiac cells and their presumed mechanism of action. Although drugs within the same group are similar, that does not imply that another agent within the group would not be more effective or safer in an individual patient.

➤*Group I:* Local anesthetics or membrane-stabilizing agents that depress phase 0.

IA *(quinidine, procainamide, disopyramide)* – Depress phase 0 and prolong the action potential duration.

IB *(tocainide, lidocaine, phenytoin, mexiletine)* – Depress phase 0 slightly and may shorten the action potential duration. Although arrhythmia is not a labeled indication for phenytoin, it is commonly used in treatment of digitalis-induced arrhythmias.

IC *(flecainide, propafenone)* – Marked depression of phase 0. Slight effect on repolarization. Profound slowing of conduction.

Moricizine – A Group I agent that shares some of the characteristics of the Group IA, B and C agents.

➤*Group II (propranolol, esmolol, acebutolol):* Depress phase 4 depolarization.

➤*Group III (bretylium, amiodarone, sotalol):* Produce a prolongation of phase 3 (repolarization).

➤*Group IV (verapamil):* Depresses phase 4 depolarization and lengthen phases 1 and 2 of repolarization.

➤*Digitalis glycosides (digoxin):* Causes a decrease in maximal diastolic potential and action potential duration and increases the slope of phase 4 depolarization.

➤*Adenosine:* Adenosine slows conduction time through the AV node and can interrupt the reentry pathways through the AV node.

➤*Serum drug levels:* Some antiarrhythmic drugs (eg, quinidine) can produce toxic effects that can be easily confused with the symptoms for which the drug has been prescribed. Drug serum levels are important in evaluating toxic or subtherapeutic dosage regimens of most antiarrhythmic drugs. They also aid in monitoring active metabolites (eg, procainamide/NAPA), suspected drug interactions and subtherapeutic response due to drug failure, noncompliance, altered clearance or altered absorption.

➤*Proarrhythmic effects:* Antiarrhythmic agents may cause new or worsened arrhythmias. Such proarrhythmic effects range from an increase in frequency of PVCs to the development of more severe ventricular tachycardia, ventricular fibrillation or torsade de pointes (ie, tachycardia that is more sustained or more rapid), which may lead to death. It is often not possible to distinguish a proarrhythmic effect from the patient's underlying rhythm disorder. It is therefore essential that each patient be evaluated electrocardiographically and clinically prior to and during therapy to determine whether the response to the drug supports continued treatment.

➤*Cardiac arrhythmia suppression trial:* In the National Heart, Lung and Blood Institute's Cardiac Arrhythmia Suppression Trial (CAST), a long-term, multicenter, randomized, double-blind study in patients with asymptomatic non-life-threatening ventricular ectopy who had had a myocardial infarction (MI) more than 6 days but less than 2 years previously, and who demonstrated mild to moderate left ventricular dysfunction, an excessive mortality or nonfatal cardiac arrest rate was seen in patients treated with encainide or flecainide (56/730) compared with that seen in patients assigned to carefully matched placebo treated groups (22/725). This led to discontinuation of those two arms of the trial. In this study, the average duration of treatment with flecainide was 10 months.

The moricizine and placebo arms of the trial were continued in CAST II. In this randomized, double-blind trial, patients with asymptomatic non-life-threatening arrhythmias who had had an MI within 4 to 90 days and left ventricular ejection fraction less than or equal to 0.4 prior to enrollment were evaluated. The average duration of moricizine treatment was 18 months. The study was discontinued because there was no possibility of demonstrating a benefit toward improved survival with moricizine and because of an evolving adverse trend after long-term treatment.

The applicability of these results to other populations (eg, those without recent MI) and to other antiarrhythmic drugs is uncertain, but at present it is prudent (1) to consider any IC agent (especially one documented to provoke new serious arrhythmias) to have a similar risk and (2) to consider the risks of Class IC agents, coupled with the lack of any evidence of improved survival, generally unacceptable in patients without life-threatening ventricular arrhythmias, even if the patients are experiencing unpleasant, but not life-threatening symptoms or signs.

➤*Pharmacokinetics:* The information in the pharmacokinetics table with clinical data and observation can be a valuable tool. However, the information must be used rationally and the data obtained properly (ie, obtaining and analyzing serum level data) to be effective. See individual monographs for more detailed explanations.

Antiarrhythmic Electrophysiology/Electrocardiogram Effects

Antiarrhythmic		Electrophysiology[1]										ECG changes[1]				
		Automaticity		Conduction velocity			Refractory period									
Group	Drug	SA node	Ectopic pacemaker	Atrium	AV node	His-Purkinje	Atrium	AV node	His-Purkinje	Ventricle	Accessory pathways[2]	Heart rate	PR interval	QRS complex	QT_c interval	JT interval
I	Moricizine[3]	0	↓	0	↓	↓	±	0	0	0-↑	↑	0-↑	↑	↑	0	↓
	Quinidine	±	↓	↓	±	↓	↑↑	0-↑[4]	↑↑	↑	↑	±	±	↑	↑	↑
	Procainamide	±	↓	↓	±	↓	↑	0-↑[4]	↑↑	↑	↑↑	±	±	↑	↑	↑
	Disopyramide	±	↓	↓	±	↓	↑↑	0-↑[4]	↑↑	↑	↑	±	±	↑	↑	↑
	Lidocaine	0	↓	—	0	0	0	±	±	±	↑-↓	0	0	0	0-↓	0
	Phenytoin	↓-0	↓	—	0	0	0	±	±	±	—	±	0-↓	0	↓	0
	Tocainide	0-↓	↓	0	0	0	↓	↓	±	↓	↑	0	0	0	0-↓	0
	Mexiletine	↓	↓	0	0	0	0	±	↑	↑	↑	-	0	0	0	0
	Flecainide	↓	↓	↓↓	↓	↓↓	0	0	↑	↑	↑↑	0	↑[5]	↑↑[5]	0-↑[5]	0
	Propafenone	0	↓	0	↓	↓	0	↑	↑	↑	↑	0	↑[5]	↑	0-↑[5]	0
II	Propranolol	↓	↓	±	↓	0-↓	±	↑	0	0	0-↑	↓	0-↑	0	0-↓	0
	Esmolol	↓	↓	±	↓	0-	±	↑	0	0	0-↑	↓	0-↑	0	0-↓	0
	Acebutolol	↓	↓	±	↓	0	±	↑	0	0	0-↑	↓	0-↑	0	0-↓	0
III	Bretylium	↑	↑	0	0	0-↑	0	↓-↑[6]	↑	0-↑	±	0	0	0	0	↑
	Amiodarone	↓	↓	↓	↓	↓	↑	↑	↑	↑	↑	↓	↑	↑	↑↑	↑↑
	Sotalol[7]	↓	↓	0	↓	0	↑↑	↑	↑↑	↑↑	↑	↓	↑	0	↑↑	↑↑
IV	Verapamil	↓	↓	0	↓	0	0	↑	0	0	0	↓	↑	0	0	0
—	Digoxin	0-↓	↑	±	↓	0-↓	±	↑	0	↓	↓-↑	↓	↑	0	↓	↓
—	Adenosine	↓	↓	0	↓	0	0	↑	0	0	0	↑	↑	0	0	—

[1] These values assume therapeutic levels.
[2] Accessory pathways occur in Wolff-Parkinson-White syndrome (preexcitation phenomena) and possibly other abnormal conditions.
[3] Does not belong to any of the 3 subclasses (A, B or C), but does have some properties of each.
[4] Retrograde AV node RP↑; antegrade RP not affected.
[5] Dose-related increases.
[6] Due to a complex balance of direct and indirect autonomic effects.
[7] Has both Group II (beta blocking) and III properties; Class III effects are seen at doses more than 160 mg.

Antiarrhythmic Pharmacokinetics

Antiarrhythmic			Onset (h) (oral)[1]	Duration (h)	Half-life (h)	Protein binding (%)	Excreted unchanged (%)	Therapeutic serum level (mcg/mL)	Toxic serum levels (mcg/mL)
Group		Drug							
I	A	Moricizine	2	10 to 24	1.5 to 3.5[2]	95	< 1	Not applicable	
		Quinidine	0.5	6 to 8	6 to 7	80 to 90	10 to 50	2 to 6	> 8
		Procainamide	0.5	3+	2.5 to 4.7	14 to 23	40 to 70	4 to 8	> 16
		Disopyramide	0.5	6 to 7	4 to 10	20 to 60[3]	40 to 60	2 to 8	> 9
	B	Lidocaine	—	0.25[4]	1 to 2	40 to 80	< 3	1.5 to 6	> 7
		Phenytoin	0.5-1	24+	22 to 36[5]	87 to 93	< 5	10 to 20	> 20
		Tocainide	—	—	11 to 15	10 to 20	28 to 55	4 to 10	> 10
		Mexiletine	—	—	10 to 12	50 to 60	10	0.5 to 2	> 2
	C	Flecainide	—	—	12 to 27	40	30	0.2 to 1	> 1
		Propafenone	—	—	2 to 10[8]	97	< 1	0.06 to 1	—
II		Propranolol	0.5	3 to 5	2 to 3	90 to 95	< 1	0.05 to 0.1	—
		Esmolol	< 5 min	very short	0.15	55	< 2	—	—
		Acebutolol	—	24 to 30	3 to 4	26	15 to 20	—	—
III		Bretylium	—	6 to 8	5 to 10	0 to 8	> 80	0.5 to 1.5	—
		Amiodarone	1 to 3 wks[9]	weeks to months	26 to 107 days	96	negligible	0.5 to 2.5	> 2.5
		Sotalol	—	—	12	0	100	—	—
IV		Verapamil	0.5	6	3 to 7	90	3 to 4	0.08 to 0.3	—
—		Digoxin	0.5 to 2	24+	30 to 40	20 to 25	60	0.5 to 2 ng/mL	> 2.5 ng/mL
—		Adenosine	(34 sec IV)	1 to 2 min	< 10 sec	—	0 (enters body pool)	Not applicable	—

[1] Within 1 to 5 minutes with IV use.
[2] Half-life may be reduced in patients after multiple dosing.
[3] Protein binding is concentration dependent.
[4] Very short after discontinuation of IV infusion.
[5] Half-life increases with increasing dosage.
[6] Half-life 10 to 32 hours in < 10% of patients (slow metabolizers).
[7] Onset of action may occur in 2 to 3 days.

MORICIZINE HYDROCHLORIDE

Rx	**Ethmozine** (Shire)	**Tablets:** 200 mg	Lactose. Lt. green. Film coated. Oval, convex. In 100s and UD 100s.
		250 mg	Lactose. Lt. orange. Film coated. Oval, convex. In 100s and UD 100s.
		300 mg	Lactose. Lt. blue. Film coated. Oval, convex. In 100s and UD 100s.

MORICIZINE HYDROCHLORIDE — ORAL

Refer to the general introductory discussion concerning Antiarrhythmic Agents.

WARNING

Mortality – Moricizine was 1 of 3 antiarrhythmic drugs included in the National Heart Lung and Blood Institute's Cardiac Arrhythmia Suppression Trial (CAST I), a long-term, multicenter, randomized, double-blind study in patients with asymptomatic non-life-threatening ventricular arrhythmias who had a MI more than 6 days, but less than 2 years, previously. An excessive mortality or nonfatal cardiac arrest rate was seen in patients treated with both of the Class IC agents included in the trial, which led to discontinuation of those 2 arms of the trial. Average duration of treatment was 10 months.

The moricizine and placebo arms of the trial were continued in the NHLBI-sponsored CAST II. In this randomized, double-blind trial, patients with asymptomatic non-life-threatening arrhythmias who had an MI within 4 to 90 days and left ventricular ejection fraction 0.4 or less prior to enrollment were evaluated. The average duration of treatment with moricizine in this study was 18 months. The study was discontinued because there was no possibility of demonstrating a benefit toward improved survival with moricizine and because of an evolving adverse trend after long-term treatment, although there was no statistical significance vs placebo.

The applicability of the CAST results to other populations (eg, those without recent MI) is uncertain. Considering the known proarrhythmic properties of moricizine and the lack of evidence of improved survival for any antiarrhythmic drug in patients without life-threatening arrhythmias, it is prudent to reserve the use of moricizine for patients with life-threatening ventricular arrhythmias.

Indications

➤*Ventricular arrhythmias:* For the treatment of documented ventricular arrhythmias, such as sustained ventricular tachycardia, that, in the judgment of the physician are life-threatening. Because of the proarrhythmic effects of morcizine, its use with lesser arrhythmias is generally not recommended. Treatment of patients with asymptomatic ventricular premature contractions should be avoided.

Antiarrhythmic drugs have not been shown to enhance survival in patients with ventricular arrhythmias.

Administration and Dosage

➤*Approved by the FDA:* June 26, 1990.

The dosage of moricizine must be individualized on the basis of antiarrhythmic response and tolerance. Clinical, cardiac rhythm monitoring, electrocardiogram intervals, exercise testing, and/or programmed electrical stimulation testing may be used to guide antiarrhythmic response and dosage adjustment. In general, the patients will be at high risk and should be hospitalized for the initiation of therapy.

➤*Usual adult dosage:* 600 to 900 mg/day, given every 8 hours in 3 equally divided doses. Within this range, the dosage can be adjusted as tolerated, in increments of 150 mg/day at 3-day intervals, until the desired effect is obtained. Patients with life-threatening arrhythmias who exhibit a beneficial response as judged by objective criteria (eg, Holter monitoring, programmed electrical stimulation, exercise testing) can be maintained on chronic moricizine therapy. As the antiarrhythmic effect of moricizine persists for more than 12 hours, some patients whose arrhythmias are well controlled on an every-8- hour regimen may be given the same total daily dose in a every-12-hour regimen to increase convenience and help ensure compliance. When higher doses are used, patients may experience more dizziness and nausea on the every-12-hour regimen.

➤*Hepatic function impairment:* Patients should be started at 600 mg/day or lower and monitored closely, including measurement of ECG intervals, before dosage adjustment.

➤*Renal function impairment:* Patients with significant renal dysfunction should be started at 600 mg/day or lower and monitored closely, including measurement of ECG intervals, before dosage adjustment.

➤*Transfer to moricizine:* Recommendations for transferring patients from another antiarrhythmic to moricizine can be given based on theoretical considerations. Previous antiarrhythmic therapy should be withdrawn for 1 to 2 plasma half-lives before starting moricizine at the recommended dosages. In patients in whom withdrawal of a previous antiarrhythmic is likely to produce life-threatening arrhythmias, hospitalization is recommended.

Moricizine Dosing when Transferring From Other Antiarrhythmics

Other antiarrhythmic	Begin moricizine dosing
Quinidine, disopyramide	6 to 12 hours after last dose
Procainamide	3 to 6 hours after last dose
Encainide, propafenone, tocainide, mexiletine	8 to 12 hours after the last dose
Flecainide	12 to 24 hours after last dose

➤*Storage/Stability:* Store at controlled room temperature 15° to 30°C (59° to 86°F) in a tightly closed, light-resistant container. Keep in carton until dispensed. Protect from light.

Actions

➤*Pharmacology:* Moricizine is a Class I antiarrhythmic agent with potent local anesthetic activity and myocardial membrane stabilizing effects. Moricizine reduces the fast inward current carried by sodium ions.

In isolated dog Purkinje fibers, moricizine shortens phase II and III repolarization, resulting in a decreased action potential duration and effective refractory period. A dose-related decrease in the maximum rate of phase 0 depolarization (V_{max}) occurs without effect on maximum diastolic potential or action potential amplitude. The sinus node and atrial tissue of the dog are not affected.

Although moricizine is chemically related to the neuroleptic phenothiazines, it has no demonstrated central or peripheral dopaminergic activity in animals. Moreover, in patients on chronic moricizine, serum prolactin levels did not increase.

Hemodynamic – In patients with impaired left ventricular function, moricizine has minimal effects on measurements of cardiac performance such as cardiac index, stroke volume index, pulmonary capillary wedge pressure, systemic or pulmonary vascular resistance or ejection fraction, either at rest or during exercise. Moricizine is associated with a small, but consistent increase in resting blood pressure and heart rate. Exercise tolerance in patients with ventricular arrhythmias is unaffected. In patients with a history of congestive heart failure or angina pectoris, exercise duration and rate-pressure product at maximal exercise are unchanged during morcizine administration. Nonetheless, in some cases worsened heart failure in patients with severe underlying heart disease has been attributed to morcizine.

Electrophysiology – Electrophysiology studies in patients with ventricular tachycardia have shown that morcizine, at daily doses of 750 mg and 800 mg, prolongs atrioventricular conduction. Both AV nodal conduction time (AH interval) and His-Purkinje conduction time (HV interval) are prolonged by 10 to 13% and 21 to 26%, respectively. The PR interval is prolonged by 16 to 20% and the QRS by 7 to 18%. Prolongations of 2 to 5% in the corrected QT interval result from widening of the QRS interval, but there is shortening of the JT interval, indicating an absence of significant effect on ventricular repolarization. Intra-atrial conduction or atrial effective refractory periods are not consistently affected; in patients without sinus node dysfunction. Moricizine has minimal effects on sinus cycle length and sinus node recovery time. These effects may be significant in patients with sinus node dysfunction.

➤*Pharmacokinetics:*

Absorption – Following oral administration, morcizine undergoes significant first-pass metabolism resulting in an absolute bioavailability of approximately 38%. Peak plasma concentrations of morcizine are usually reached within 0.5 to 2 hours. Administration 30 minutes after a meal delays the rate of absorption, resulting in lower peak plasma concentrations, but the extent of absorption is not altered. Moricizine plasma levels are proportional to dose over the recommended therapeutic dose range.

Distribution – The apparent volume of distribution after oral administration is very large (greater than or equal to 300 L) and is not significantly related to body weight. Moricizine is approximately 95% bound to human plasma proteins. This binding interaction is independent of morcizine plasma concentration.

Metabolism – The antiarrhythmic and electrophysiologic effects of moricizine are not related in time course or intensity to plasma moricizine concentrations or to the concentrations of any identified metabolite, all of which have short (2 to 3 hours) half-lives. Following single doses of morcizine, there is a prompt prolongation of the PR interval, which becomes normal within 2 hours, consistent with the rapid fall of plasma moricizine. JT interval shortening, however, peaks at about 6 hours and persists for at least 10 hours. Although an effect on VPD rates is seen within 2 hours after dosing, the full effect is seen after 10 to 14 hours and persists in full, when therapy is terminated, for more than 10 hours, after which the effect decays slowly, and is still substantial at 24 hours. This suggests either an unidentified, active, long half-life metabolite or a structural or functional "deep compartment" with slow entry from, and release to, the plasma. The following description of parent compound pharmacokinetics is therefore of uncertain relevance to clinical actions.

Moricizine has been shown to induce its own metabolism. Average morcizine plasma concentrations in patients decrease with multiple dosing. This decrease in plasma levels of parent drug does not appear to affect clinical outcome for patients receiving chronic morcizine therapy.

Excretion – Moricizine undergoes extensive biotransformation. Less than 1% of orally administered morcizine is excreted unchanged in the urine. There are at least 26 metabolites, but no single metabolite has been found to represent as much as 1% of the administered dose, and as stated above, antiarrhythmic response has relatively slow onset and offset. Two metabolites are pharmacologically active in at least one animal model: moricizine sulfoxide and phenothiazine-2-carbamic acid ethyl ester sulfoxide. Each of these metabolites represents a small percentage of the administered dose

MORICIZINE HYDROCHLORIDE — ORAL

(less than 0.6%), is present in lower concentrations in the plasma than the parent drug, and has a plasma elimination half-life of approximately 3 hours.

The plasma half-life of moricizine is 1.5 to 3.5 hours (most values about 2 hours) following single or multiple oral doses in patients with ventricular ectopy. Approximately 56% of the administered dose is excreted in the feces and 39% is excreted in the urine. Some moricizine is also recycled through enterohepatic circulation.

Contraindications

Preexisting second- or third-degree AV block and right bundle branch block when associated with left hemiblock (bifascicular block) unless a pacemaker is present; cardiogenic shock; known hypersensitivity to the drug.

Warnings

➤*Mortality:* Moricizine was 1 of 3 antiarrhythmic drugs included in the National Heart Lung and Blood Institute's Cardiac Arrhythmia Suppression Trial (CAST I), a long-term multicenter, randomized, double-blind study in patients with asymptomatic non-life-threatening ventricular arrhythmias who had had a myocardial infarction more than 6 days, but less than 2 years, previously. An excessive mortality or nonfatal cardiac arrest rate was seen in patients treated with both of the Class IC agents included in the trial, which led to discontinuation of those 2 arms of the trial. The average duration of treatment with these agents was 10 months.

The moricizine and placebo arms of the trial were continued in the NHLBI sponsored CAST II. In this randomized, double-blind trial, patients with asymptomatic non-life-threatening arrhythmias who had had a myocardial infarction within 4 to 90 days and left ventricular ejection fraction less than or equal to 0.4 prior to enrollment were evaluated. The average duration of treatment with morcizine in this study was 18 months. The study was discontinued because there was no possibility of demonstrating a benefit toward improved survival with morcizine and because of an evolving adverse trend after long-term treatment.

The applicability of the CAST results to other populations (eg, those without recent myocardial infarction) is uncertain. Considering the known proarrhythmic properties of morcizine and the lack of evidence of improved survival for any antiarrhythmic drug in patients without life-threatening arrhythmias, the use of moricizine, as well as other antiarrhythmic agents, should be reserved for patients with life-threatening ventricular arrhythmias.

➤*Proarrhythmia:* Like other antiarrhythmic drugs, moricizine can provoke new rhythm disturbances or make existing arrhythmias worse. These proarrhythmic effects can range from an increase in the frequency of VPDs to the development of new or more severe ventricular tachycardia (eg, tachycardia that is more sustained or more resistant to conversion to sinus rhythm) with potentially fatal consequences. It is often not possible to distinguish a proarrhythmic effect from the patient's underlying rhythm disorder, so that the occurrence rates given below must be considered approximations. Note also that drug-induced arrhythmias can generally be identified only when they occur early after starting the drug and when the rhythm can be identified, usually because the patient is being monitored. It is clear from the NIH sponsored CAST (Cardiac Arrhythmia Suppression Trial) that some antiarrhythmic drugs can cause increased sudden death mortality, presumably due to new arrhythmias or asystole that do not appear early after treatment but that represent a sustained increased risk.

Domestic premarketing trials included 1072 patients given morcizine; 397 had baseline lethal arrhythmias (sustained VT or VF and nonsustained VT with hemodynamic symptoms) and 576 had potentially lethal arrhythmias (increased VPDs or NSVT in patients with known structural heart disease, active ischemia, congestive heart failure or an LVEF less than 40% and/or CI less than 2 L/min/m^2). In this population there were 40 (3.7%) identified proarrhythmic events, 26 (2.5%) of which were serious, either fatal (6), new hemodynamically significant sustained VT or VF (4); new sustained VT that was not hemodynamically significant (11) or sustained VT that became syncopal/presyncopal when it had not been before (5). Proarrhythmic effects described as incessant ventricular tachycardia were observed in the postmarketing PES study and in postmarketing adverse event reports.

In general, serious proarrhythmic effects in the domestic premarketing trials were equally common in patients with more and less severe arrhythmias, 2.5% in the patients with baseline lethal arrhythmias vs 2.8% in patients with potentially lethal arrhythmias, although the patients with serious effects were more likely to have a history of sustained VT (38% vs 23%). In the postmarketing comparative PES study, patients treated with morcizine (250 to 300 mg 3 times daily) had a proarrhythmia rate of 14% (8/59).

Five of the 6 fatal proarrhythmic events were in patients with baseline lethal arrhythmias; 4 had prior cardiac arrests. Rates and severity of proarrhythmic events were similar in patients given 600 to 900 mg of morcizine per day and those given higher doses. Patients with proarrhythmic events were more likely than the overall population to have coronary artery disease (85% vs 67%), history of acute myocardial infarction (75% vs 53%), congestive heart failure (60% vs 43%), and cardiomegaly (55% vs 33%). All of the 6 proarrhythmic deaths were in patients with coronary artery disease; 5/6 each had documented acute myocardial infarction, congestive heart failure, and cardiomegaly.

➤*Electrolyte disturbances:* Hypokalemia, hyperkalemia or hypomagnesemia may alter the effects of Class I antiarrhythmic drugs. Electrolyte imbalances should be corrected before administration of morcizine.

➤*Sick sinus syndrome:* Moricizine should be used only with extreme caution in patients with sick sinus syndrome, as it may cause sinus bradycardia, sinus pause or sinus arrest.

➤*Renal function impairment:* Plasma levels of intact moricizine are unchanged in hemodialysis patients, but a significant portion (39%) of moricizine is metabolized and excreted in the urine. Although no identified active metabolite is known to increase in people with renal failure, metabolites of unrecognized importance could be affected. For this reason, moricizine should be administered cautiously in patients with impaired renal function. Patients with significant renal dysfunction should be started on lower doses and monitored for excessive pharmacologic effects, including ECG intervals, before dosage adjustment.

➤*Hepatic function impairment:* Patients with significant liver dysfunction have reduced plasma clearance and an increased half-life of moricizine. Although the precise relationship of morcizine levels to effect is not clear, patients with hepatic disease should be treated with lower doses and closely monitored for excessive pharmacological effects, including effects on ECG intervals, before dosage adjustment. Patients with severe liver disease should be administered morcizine with particular care, if at all.

➤*Carcinogenesis:* In a 24-month mouse study in which moricizine was administered in the feed at concentrations calculated to provide doses ranging up to 320 mg/kg/day, ovarian tubular adenomas and granulosa cell tumors were limited in occurrence to morcizine—treated animals. Although the findings were of borderline statistical significance, or not statistically significant, historical control data indicate that both of these tumors are uncommon in the strain of mouse studied.

In a 24-month study in which moricizine was administered by gavage to rats at doses of 25, 50 and 100 mg/kg/day, Zymbal's Gland Carcinoma was observed in 1 mid-dose and 2 high-dose males. This tumor appears to be uncommon in the strain of rat studied. Rats of both sexes showed a dose-related increase in hepatocellular cholangioma (also described as bile ductile cystadenoma or cystic hyperplasia) along with fatty metamorphosis, possibly due to disruption of hepatic choline utilization for phospholipid biosynthesis. The rat is known to be uniquely sensitive to alteration in choline metabolism.

➤*Pregnancy: Category B.*

There are no adequate and well-controlled studies in pregnant women. Use morcizine during pregnancy only if clearly needed.

Nonteratogenic – In a study in which rats were dosed with moricizine prior to mating, during mating and throughout gestation and lactation, dose levels 3.4 and 6.7 times the maximum recommended human daily dose produced a dose-related decrease in pup and maternal weight gain, possibly related to a larger litter size. In a study in which dosing was begun on day 15 of gestation, moricizine, at a level 6.7 times the maximum recommended human daily dose, produced a retardation in maternal weight gain but no effect on pup growth.

➤*Lactation:* Moricizine is secreted in the milk of laboratory animals and has been reported to be present in human milk. Because of the potential for serious adverse reactions in breast-feeding infants from moricizine, a decision should be made whether to discontinue the drug, taking into account the importance of the drug to the mother.

➤*Children:* The safety and effectiveness of moricizine in children younger than 18 years of age have not been established.

Precautions

➤*Electrocardiographic changes/conduction abnormalities:* Moricizine slows AV nodal and intraventricular conduction, producing dose-related increases in the PR and QRS intervals. In clinical trials, the average increase in the PR interval was 12% and the QRS interval was 14%. Although the QTC interval is increased, this is wholly because of QRS prolongation; the JT interval is shortened, indicating the absence of significant slowing of ventricular repolarization. The degree of lengthening of PR and QRS intervals does not predict efficacy.

In controlled clinical trials and in open studies, the overall incidence of delayed ventricular conduction, including new bundle branch block pattern, was approximately 9.4%. In patients without baseline conduction abnormalities, the frequency of second-degree AV block was 0.2% and third-degree AV block did not occur. In patients with baseline conduction abnormalities, the frequencies of second-degree AV block and third-degree AV block were 0.9% and 1.4%, respectively.

Moricizine therapy was discontinued in 1.6% of patients due to electrocardiographic changes (0.6% due to sinus pause or asystole, 0.2% to AV block, 0.2% to junctional rhythm, 0.4% to intraventricular conduction delay, and 0.2% to wide QRS and/or PR interval).

In patients with pre-existing conduction abnormalities, moricizine therapy should be initiated cautiously. If second- or third-degree AV block occurs, moricizine therapy should be discontinued unless a ventricular pacemaker is in place. When changing the dose of moricizine or adding concomitant medications which may also affect cardiac conduction, patients should be monitored electrocardiographically.

➤*Congestive heart failure:* Most patients with congestive heart failure have tolerated the recommended morcizine daily doses without unusual toxicity or change in effect. Pharmacokinetic differences between morcizine patients with and without congestive heart failure were not apparent. In some cases, worsened heart failure has been attributed to moricizine. Patients with preexisting heart failure should be monitored carefully when moricizine is initiated.

➤*Effects on pacemaker threshold:* The effect of moricizine on the sensing and pacing thresholds of artificial pacemakers has not been sufficiently studied. In such patients, pacing parameters must be monitored, if moricizine is used.

MORICIZINE HYDROCHLORIDE — ORAL

Drug Interactions

Moricizine Drug Interactions

Precipitant Drug	Object Drug*		Comments
Cimetidine	Moricizine	↑	1.4-fold increase in moricizine plasma levels; 49% decrease in clearance. Initiate moricizine at low doses (not more than 600 mg/day).
Digoxin	Moricizine	↑	Additive prolongation of the PR interval, but not with a significant increase in the rate of second- or third-degree AV block. Little change in serum digoxin levels or pharmacokinetics.
Diltiazem	Moricizine	↑	Diltiazem may elevate moricizine concentrations, while moricizine may reduce diltiazem concentrations. Monitor closely.
Moricizine	Diltiazem	↓	
Propranolol	Moricizine	↑	Small additive increase in PR interval; no changes in overall ECG intervals.
Moricizine	Theophylline	↓	Theophylline clearance increased 44% to 66% and plasma half-life decreased 19% to 33% (conventional and sustained-release theophylline).

* ↑ = Object drug increased ↓ = Object drug decreased

➤*Use with other drugs that affect cardiac electrophysiology:* Because of possible additive pharmacologic effects, caution is indicated when moricizine is used with any drug that affects cardiac electrophysiology. Uncontrolled experience in patients indicates no serious adverse interaction during the concomitant use of moricizine and diuretics, vasodilators, antihypertensive drugs, calcium channel blockers, beta-blockers, angiotensin-converting enzyme inhibitors, or warfarin.

Warfarin – Plasma warfarin levels, warfarin pharmacokinetics, and prothrombin times were unaffected during multiple dose moricizine administration to younger, healthy, male subjects in a controlled study. However, there are isolated reports of the need to either increase or decrease warfarin doses after initiation of moricizine. Some patients who were taking warfarin with a stable prothrombin time experienced excessive prolongation of the prothrombin time following the initiation of moricizine. In some cases, liver enzymes also were elevated. Bleeding or bruising may occur. When moricizine is started or stopped in a patient stabilized on warfarin, more frequent prothrombin time monitoring is advisable.

Adverse Reactions

The most serious adverse reaction reported for moricizine is proarrhythmia. This occurred in 3.7% of 1,072 patients with ventricular arrhythmias who received a wide range of doses under a variety of circumstances.

In addition to discontinuations because of proarrhythmias, in controlled clinical trials and in open studies, adverse reactions led to discontinuation of moricizine in 7% of 1,105 patients with ventricular and supraventricular arrhythmias, including 3.2% due to nausea, 1.6% due to ECG abnormalities (principally conduction defects, sinus pause, junctional rhythm, or AV block), 1% due to congestive heart failure and 0.3 to 0.4% due to dizziness, anxiety, drug fever, urinary retention, blurred vision, gastrointestinal upset, rash, and laboratory abnormalities.

The most frequently occurring adverse reactions in the 1,072 patients (including all adverse experiences whether or not considered moricizine-related by the investigator) were dizziness (15.1%), nausea (9.6%), headache (8%), fatigue (5.9%), palpitations (5.8%) and dyspnea (5.7%). Dizziness appears to be related to the size of each dose. In a comparison of 900 mg/day given at 450 mg twice daily or 300 mg 3 times daily, more than 20% of patients experienced dizziness on the twice daily regimen vs 12% on the 3 times daily regimen.

Adverse reactions reported by less than 5%, but in 2% or greater of the patients were sustained ventricular tachycardia, hypesthesias, abdominal pain, dyspepsia, vomiting, sweating, cardiac chest pain, asthenia, nervousness, paresthesias, congestive heart failure, musculoskeletal pain, diarrhea, dry mouth, cardiac death, sleep disorders and blurred vision.

Adverse reactions infrequently reported (in less than 2% of the patients) were as follows:

➤*Cardiovascular:* Hypotension, hypertension, syncope, supraventricular arrhythmias (including atrial fibrillation/flutter), cardiac arrest, bradycardia, pulmonary embolism, myocardial infarction, vasodilation, cerebrovascular events, thrombophlebitis.

➤*CNS:* Tremor, anxiety, depression, euphoria, confusion, somnolence, agitation, seizure, coma, abnormal gait, hallucinations, nystagmus, diplopia, speech disorder, akathisia, loss of memory, ataxia, abnormal coordination, dyskinesia, vertigo, tinnitus.

➤*GU:* Urinary retention or frequency, dysuria, urinary incontinence, kidney pain, impotence, decreased libido.

➤*Respiratory:* Hyperventilation, apnea, asthma, pharyngitis, cough, sinusitis.

➤*GI:* Anorexia, bitter taste, dysphagia, flatulence, ileus.

➤*Miscellaneous:* Drug fever, hypothermia, temperature intolerance, eye pain, rash, pruritus, dry skin, urticaria, swelling of the lips and tongue, periorbital edema. During moricizine therapy, 2 patients developed thrombocytopenia that may have been drug-related. Clinically significant elevations in liver function tests (bilirubin, serum transaminases) and jaundice consistent with hepatitis were rarely reported. Although a cause and effect relationship has not been established, caution is advised in patients who develop unexplained signs of hepatic dysfunction, and consideration should be given to discontinuing therapy.

Three patients developed rechallenge-confirmed drug fever, with 1 patient experiencing an elevation above 39.4°C (103°F) to 40.5°C (105°F), with rigors. Fevers occurred at about 2 weeks in 2 cases, and after 21 weeks in the third. Fevers resolved within 48 hours of discontinuation of moricizine.

Adverse reactions were generally similar in patients over 65 (n = 375) and under 65 (n = 697), although discontinuation of therapy for reasons other than proarrhythmia was more common in older patients (13.9% vs 7.7%). Overall mortality was greater in older patients (9.3% vs 3.9%), but those were not deaths attributed to treatment and the older patients had more serious underlying heart disease.

Incidence (%) of the Most Common Noncardiac Adverse Reactions (Therapy Duration = 1 to 14 Days)

	> 2%		> 2%		> 2%		> 5%		> 5%	
	Moricizine		Placebo		Quinidine		Disopyramide		Propranolol	
Adverse reactions	No.	%	No.	%	No.	%	No.	%	No.	%
Total no. of patients	1,072		618		110		31		24	
Dizziness	121	11.3%	33	5.3%	8	7.3%	-		2	8.3%
Nausea	74	6.9%	18	2.9%	7	6.4%	3	9.7%	-	
Headache	62	5.8%	27	4.4%	-		-		4	16.7%
Pain	41	3.8%	31	5%	6	5.5%	2	6.5%	-	
Dyspnea	41	3.8%	22	3.6%	-		-		-	
Hypesthesia	40	3.7%	-		3	2.7%	-		-	
Fatigue	33	3.1%	16	2.6%	6	5.5%	2	6.5%	3	12.5%
Vomiting	22	2.1%	-		-		-		-	
Dry mouth	-		-		-		11	35.5%	-	
Nervousness	-		-		-		3	9.7%	-	
Blurred vision	-		-		3	2.7%	2	6.5%	3	12.5%
Diarrhea	-		-		25	22.7%	-		-	
Constipation	-		-		-		2	6.5%	-	
Somnolence	-		-		-		-		2	8.3%
Urinary retention	-		-		-		4	12.9%	-	

Overdosage

➤*Symptoms:* Overdosage with moricizine may produce emesis, lethargy, coma, syncope, hypotension, conduction disturbances, exacerbation of congestive heart failure, myocardial infarction, sinus arrest, arrhythmias (including junctional bradycardia, ventricular tachycardia, ventricular fibrillation and asystole), and respiratory failure.

Deaths have occurred after accidental or intentional overdosages of 2,250 and 10,000 mg of moricizine, respectively.

➤*Treatment:* A specific antidote for moricizine has not been identified. In the event of overdosage, treatment should be supportive. Patients should be hospitalized and monitored for cardiac, respiratory and CNS changes. Advanced life support systems, including an intracardiac pacing catheter, should be provided where necessary. Acute overdosage should be treated with appropriate gastric evacuation, and with special care to avoid aspiration. Accidental introduction of moricizine into the lungs of monkeys resulted in rapid arrhythmic death.

IBUTILIDE FUMARATE

Rx	**Corvert** (Pharmacia & Upjohn)	**Solution:** 0.1 mg/mL	In 10 mL vials.

IBUTILIDE FUMARATE — INJECTION

Refer to the general introductory discussion concerning Antiarrhythmic Agents.

WARNING

Life-threatening arrhythmias – Ibutilide fumarate can cause potentially fatal arrythmias, particularly sustained polymorphic ventricular tachycardia usually in association with QT prolongation (torsades de pointes), but sometimes without documented QT prolongation. In registration studies, these arrythmias, which require cardioversion, occurred in 1.7% of treated patients during or within a number of hours of using ibutilide fumarate.

These arrythmias can be reversed if treated promptly. It is essential that ibutilide be administered in a setting of continuous ECG monitoring and by personnel trained in identification and treatment of acute ventricular arrythmias, particularly polymorphic ventricular tachycardia. Patients with atrial fibrillation of more than 2 to 3 days' duration must be adequately anticoagulated, generally for at least 2 weeks.

Appropriate treatment environment –

Choice of patients: Patients with chronic atrial fibrillation have a strong tendency to revert after conversion to sinus rhythm and treatments to maintain sinus rhythm carry risks. Patients to be treated with ibutilide fumarate, therefore, should be carefully selected such that the expected benefits of maintaining sinus rhythm outweigh the immediate risks of ibutilide, and the risks of maintenance therapy, and are likely to offer an advantage compared with alternative management.

Indications

For the rapid conversion of atrial fibrillation or atrial flutter of recent onset to sinus rhythm. Patients with atrial arrhythmias of longer duration are less likely to respond to ibutilide fumarate. The effectiveness of ibutilide has not been determined in patients with arrhythmias of more than 90 days in duration.

Administration and Dosage

➤*Approved by the FDA:* March 1996.

The recommended dose based on controlled trials is outlined below. Ibutilide infusion should be stopped as soon as the presenting arrhythmia is terminated or in the event of sustained or nonsustained ventricular tachycardia, or marked prolongation of QT or QTc.

Recommended Dose of Ibutilide Fumarate Injection

Patient weight	Initial infusion (over 10 minutes)	Second infusion
60 kg (132 lbs) or more	1 vial (1 mg ibutilide fumarate)	If the arrhythmia does not terminate within 10 minutes after the end of the initial infusion, a second 10-minute infusion of equal strength may be administered 10 minutes after completion of the first infusion.
Less than 60 kg (132 lbs)	0.1 mL/kg (0.01 mg/kg ibutilide fumarate)	

See Precautions for more information.

➤*Dilution:* Administer undiluted or diluted in 50 mL of diluent. Ibutilide fumarate may be added to 0.9% Sodium Chloride Injection or 5% Dextrose Injection before infusion. The contents of one 10 mL vial (0.1 mg/mL) may be added to a 50 mL infusion bag to form an admixture of approximately 0.017 mg/mL ibutilide fumarate. Parenteral drug products should be inspected visually for particulate matter and discoloration prior to administration whenever solution and container permit.

➤*Compatibility:* The following diluents are compatible with ibutilide fumarate injection (0.1 mg/mL): 5% Dextrose Injection and 0.9% Sodium Chloride Injection.

The following IV solution containers are compatible with admixtures of ibutilide fumarate injection (0.1 mg/mL): Polyvinyl chloride plastic bags and polyolefin bags.

➤*Storage/Stability:* Store at controlled room temperature 20° to 25°C (68° to 77°F). Store vial in carton until used.

Admixtures of the product, with approved diluents, are chemically and physically stable for 24 hours at room temperature (15° to 30°C; 59° to 86°F) and for 48 hours at refrigerated temperatures (2° to 8°C; 36° to 46°F). Strict adherence to the use of aseptic technique during the preparation of the admixture is recommended in order to maintain sterility.

Actions

➤*Pharmacology:* Ibutilide fumarate injection prolongs action potential duration in isolated adult cardiac myocytes and increases both atrial and ventricular refractoriness in vivo (ie, class III electrophysiologic effects). Voltage clamp studies indicate that ibutilide fumarate, at nanomolar concentrations, delays repolarization by activation of a slow, inward current (predominantly sodium), rather than by blocking outward potassium currents, which is the mechanism by which most other class III antiarrhythmics act. These effects lead to prolongation of atrial and ventricular action potential duration and refractoriness, the predominant electrophysiologic properties of ibutilide fumarate in humans that are thought to be the basis for its antiarrhythmic effect.

➤*Pharmacokinetics:*

Absorption/Distribution – After IV infusion, ibutilide plasma concentrations rapidly decrease in a multiexponential fashion. The pharmacokinetics of ibutilide are highly variable among subjects. Ibutilide has a high systemic plasma clearance that approximates liver blood flow (approximately 29 mL/min/kg), a large steady-state volume of distribution (approximately 11 L/kg) in healthy volunteers, and minimal (approximately 40%) protein binding. Ibutilide is also cleared rapidly and highly distributed in patients being treated for atrial flutter or atrial fibrillation.

The pharmacokinetics of ibutilide are linear with respect to the dose of ibutilide fumarate over the dose range of 0.01 mg/kg to 0.1 mg/kg. The enantiom ers of ibutilide fumarate have pharmacokinetic properties similar to each other and to ibutilide fumarate.

Metabolism/Excretion – In healthy male volunteers, approximately 82% of a 0.01 mg/kg dose of ibutilide fumarate was excreted in the urine (approximately 7% of the dose as unchanged ibutilide) and the remainder (approximately 19%) was recovered in the feces. Ibutilide has a high systemic plasma clearance that approximates liver blood flow (approximately 29 mL/min/kg). The elimination half-life averages approximately 6 hours (range, 2 to 12 hours).

Eight metabolites of ibutilide were detected in metabolic profiling of urine. These metabolites are thought to be formed primarily by ω-oxidation followed by sequential β-oxidation of the heptyl side chain of ibutilide. Of the 8 etabolites, only the ω-hydroxy metabolite possesses class III electrophysiologic properties similar to that of ibutilide in an in vitro isolated rabbit myocardium model. The plasma concentrations of this active metabolite, however, are less than 10% of that of ibutilide.

General pharmacokinetics – The pharmacokinetics of ibutilide are linear with respect to the dose of ibutilide fumarate over the dose range of 0.01 mg/kg to 0.1 mg/kg. The enantiomers of ibutilide fumarate have pharmacokinetic properties similar to each other and to ibutilide fumarate.

Contraindications

Hypersensitivity to ibutilide or any of the other product components.

Warnings

➤*Proarrhythmia:* Like other antiarrhythmic agents, ibutilide fumarate injection can induce or worsen ventricular arrhythmias in some patients. This may have potentially fatal consequences. Torsades de pointes, a polymorphic ventricular tachycardia that develops in the selling of a prolonged QT interval, may occur because of the effect ibutilide fumarate has on cardiac repolarization, but ibutilide fumarate can also cause polymorphic VT in the absence of excessive prolongation of the QT interval. In general, with drugs that prolong the QT interval, the risk of torsades de pointes is thought to increase progressively as the QT interval is prolonged and may be worsened with bradycardia, a varying heart rate, and hypokalemia. In clinical trials conducted in patients with atrial fibrillation and atrial flutter, those with QTc intervals more than 440 msec were not usually allowed to participate, and serum potassium had to be more than 4 mEq/L. Although change in QTc was dose dependent for ibutilide, there was no clear relationship between risk of serious proarrhythmia and dose in clinical studies, possibly due to the small number of events.

➤*Renal/Hepatic function impairment:* Patients with abnormal liver function should be monitored by telemetry for more than the 4-hour period generally recommended.

The safety, efficacy, and pharmacokinetics of ibutilide fumarate have not been established in patients with hepatic or renal dysfunction. However, it is unlikely that dosing adjustments would be necessary in patients with compromised renal or hepatic function based on the following considerations:

- Ibutilide fumarate is indicated for rapid IV therapy (duration less than or equal to 30 minutes) and is dosed to a known, well-defined pharmacologic action (termination of arrhythmia) or to a maximum of two 10-minute infusions.
- Less than 10% of the dose of ibutilide fumarate is excreted unchanged in the urine.
- Drug distribution appears to be one of the primary mechanisms responsible for termination of the pharmacologic effect. Nonetheless, patients with abnormal liver function should be monitored by telemetry for more than the 4–hour period generally recommended.

➤*Pregnancy: Category C.* Ibutilide administered orally was teratogenic (abnormalities included adactyly, interventricular septal defects, and scoliosis) and embryocidal in reproduction studies in rats. On a mg/m^2 basis, corrected for the 3% oral bioavailability, the no adverse effect dose (5 mg/kg/day given orally) was approximately the same as the maximum recommended human dose (MRHD); the teratogenic dose (20 mg/kg/day given orally) was ≈ 4 times the MRHD on a mg/m^2 basis, or 16 times the MRHD on a mg/kg basis. Ibutilide fumarate should not be administered to a pregnant woman unless clinical benefit outweighs potential risk to the fetus.

➤*Lactation:* The excretion of ibutilide into breast milk has not been studied, accordingly, breast-feeding should be discouraged during therapy with ibutilide fumarate.

➤*Children:* Safety and efficacy of ibutilide in children younger than 18 years of age have not been established.

IBUTILIDE FUMARATE — INJECTION

Precautions

➤*Monitoring:* Observe patients with continuous ECG monitoring for at least 4 hours following infusion or until QTc has returned to baseline. Longer monitoring is required if any arrhythmic activity is noted. Skilled personnel and proper equipment, such as a cardioverter/defibrillator, and medication for treatment of sustained ventricular tachycardia, including polymorphic ventricular tachycardia, must be available during administration of ibutilide fumarate and subsequent monitoring of the patient.

➤*Heart block:* Of the 9 (1.5%) ibutilide-treated patients with reports of reversible heart block, 5 had first-degree, 3 had second-degree, and 1 had complete heart block.

Drug Interactions

➤*Antiarrhythmias:* Class IA antiarrhythmic drugs (Vaughan Williams Classification), such as disopyramide, quinidine, and procainamide, and other class III drugs, such as amiodarone and sotalol, should not be given concomitantly with ibutilide fumarate injection or within 4 hours postinfusion because of their potential to prolong refractoriness. In the clinical trials, class I or other class III antiarrhythmic agents were withheld for at least 5 half-lives prior to ibutilide infusion and for 4 hours after dosing, but thereafter were allowed at the physician's discretion.

➤*Other drugs that prolong the QT interval:* The potential for proarrhythmia may increase with the administration of ibutilide fumarate injection to patients who are being treated with drugs that prolong the QT interval, such as phenothiazines, tricyclic antidepressants, tetracyclic antidepressants, and certain antihistamine drugs (H_1 receptor antagonists).

➤*Digoxin:* Supraventricular arrhythmias may mask the cardiotoxicity associated with excessive digoxin levels. Therefore, it is advisable to be particularly cautious in patients whose plasma digoxin levels are above or suspected to be above the usual therapeutic range. Coadministration of digoxin did not have effects on either the safety or efficacy of ibutilide in the clinical trials.

Adverse Reactions

Ibutilide fumarate injection was generally well tolerated in clinical trials. Of the 586 patients with atrial fibrillation or atrial flutter who received ibutilide fumarate in phase 2 or 3 studies, 149 (25%) reported medical events related to the cardiovascular system, including sustained polymorphic ventricular tachycardia (1.7%) and nonsustained polymorphic ventricular tachycardia (2.7%).

Other clinically important adverse events with an uncertain relationship to ibutilide fumarate include the following (0.2% represents 1 patient): Sustained monomorphic ventricular tachycardia (0.2%), nonsustained monomorphic ventricular tachycardia (4.9%), AV block (1.5%), bundle branch block (1.9%), ventricular extrasystoles (5.1%), supraventricular extrasystoles (0.9%), hypotension/postural hypotension (2%), bradycardia/sinus bradycardia (1.2%), nodal arrhythmia (0.7%), congestive heart failure (0.5%), tachycardia/sinus tachycardia/supraventricular tachycardia (2.7%), idioventricular rhythm (0.2%), syncope (0.3%), and renal failure (0.3%). The incidence of those events, except for syncope, was greater in the group treated with ibutilide fumarate than in the placebo group. Another adverse reaction that may be associated with the administration of ibutilide fumarate was nausea, which occurred with a frequency greater than 1% more in ibutilide-treated patients than those treated with placebo.

Treatment-Emergent Medical Events with Frequency of > 1% and Higher than that of Placebo

	Placebo (n = 127)		All ibutilide (n = 586)	
	Patients		Patients	
Event	n	%	n	%
Cardiovascular				
Ventricular extrasystoles	1	0.8%	30	5.1%
Nonsustained monomorphic VT	1	0.8%	29	4.9%
Nonsustained polymorphic VT	-	-	16	2.7%
Hypotension	2	1.6%	12	2%
Bundle branch block	-	-	11	1.9%
Sustained polymorphic VT	-	-	10	1.7%
AV block	1	0.8%	9	1.5%
Hypertension	-	-	7	1.2%
QT segment prolonged	-	-	7	1.2%
Bradycardia	1	0.8%	7	1%
Palpitation	1	0.8%	6	1%
Tachycardia	1	0.8%	16	2.7%
CNS				
Headache	4	3.1%	21	3.6%
GI				
Nausea	1	0.8%	11	1.9%

In the postcardiac surgery study, similar types of medical events were reported. In the 1 mg ibutilide fumarate treatment group (n = 70), 2 patients (2.9%) developed sustained polymorphic ventricular tachycardia and 2 other patients (2.9%) developed nonsustained polymorphic ventricular tachycardia. Polymorphic ventricular tachycardia was not reported in the 73 patients in the 0.5 mg dose group or in the 75 patients in the 0.25 mg dose group.

Overdosage

➤*Symptoms:*

Human experience – In the registration trials with ibutilide fumarate injection, 4 patients were unintentionally overdosed. The largest dose was 3.4 mg administered over 15 minutes. One patient (0.025 mg/kg) developed increased ventricular octopy and monomorphic ventricular tachycardia, another patient (0.032 mg/kg) developed AV block third-degree and nonsustained polymorphic VT, and 2 patients (0.038 and 0.02 mg/kg) had no medical event reports. Based on known pharmacology, the clinical effects of an overdosage with ibutilide could exaggerate the expected prolongation of repolarization seen at usual clinical doses.

➤*Treatment:* Medical events (eg, proarrhythmia, AV block) that occur after the overdosage should be treated with measures appropriate for that condition.

Quinidine

Refer to the general introductory discussion concerning Antiarrhythmic Agents.

Indications

➤*Oral:* Premature atrial, AV junctional and ventricular contractions; paroxysmal atrial (supraventricular) tachycardia; paroxysmal AV junctional rhythm; atrial flutter; paroxysmal and chronic atrial fibrillation; established atrial fibrillation when therapy is appropriate; paroxysmal ventricular tachycardia not associated with complete heart block; maintenance therapy after electrical conversion of atrial fibrillation or flutter.

➤*Parenteral:* When oral therapy is not feasible or when rapid therapeutic effect is required.

Quinidine gluconate – Life-threatening *Plasmodium falciparum* malaria: Unless impossible, start therapy in an intensive care setting with continuous ECG monitoring, frequent blood pressure monitoring and periodic monitoring of parasitemia.

Administration and Dosage

➤*Test dose:* Administer a single 200 mg tablet of quinidine sulfate or 200 mg IM quinidine gluconate to determine whether the patient has an idiosyncratic reaction. Continuously monitor ECG when quinidine is used in large doses.

Adjust the dosage to maintain the plasma concentration between 2 to 6 mcg/mL.

➤*Oral:*

Premature atrial and ventricular contractions – 200 to 300 mg 3 or 4 times daily.

Paroxysmal supraventricular tachycardias – 400 to 600 mg every 2 or 3 hours until the paroxysm is terminated.

Atrial flutter – Administer quinidine after digitalization. Individualize dosage.

Conversion of atrial fibrillation – 200 mg every 2 or 3 hours for 5 to 8 doses, with subsequent daily increases until sinus rhythm is restored or toxic effects occur. Do not exceed a total daily dose of 3 to 4 g in any regimen. Prior to quinidine administration, control the ventricular rate and CHF (if present) with digoxin.

Maintenance therapy – 200 to 300 mg 3 or 4 times daily. Other patients may require larger doses or more frequent administration than the usually recommended schedule. However, institute such an increased dosage only after careful evaluation of the patient, including ECG and quinidine serum level monitoring.

Sustained-release forms – 300 to 600 mg every 8 or 12 hours. Since the rate of absorption from the various sustained release formulations may be markedly different, and since the anhydrous quinidine content is different, do not consider them interchangeable.

➤*Parenteral:* The patient must be under close clinical, ECG and blood pressure monitoring, especially during IV administration to detect any change in rate or rhythm. If the patient's condition is not critical, give quinidine gluconate IM. On the other hand, extreme palpitation, dyspnea, vomiting, and a shock-like state in patients with ventricular tachycardia are signs that IV administration may be required as a lifesaving measure when D-C cardioversion is not available.

IM – In the treatment of acute tachycardia, the initial dose is 600 mg quinidine gluconate. Subsequently, 400 mg quinidine gluconate can be repeated as often as every 2 hours. Determine successive doses by the effect of the preceding dose.

IV – In about 50% of patients who respond successfully to quinidine, the arrhythmia can be terminated by less than or equal to 330 mg quinidine gluconate (or its equivalent in other salts); as much as 500 to 750 mg may be required. Inject slowly. Dilute 10 mL (800 mg) of quinidine gluconate injection to 50 mL with 5% Dextrose Injection. Inject the diluted solution slowly at a rate of 1 mL/min for maximum safety.

Quinidine gluconate – P. falciparum malaria – Two regimens have been empirically shown to be effective, with or without concomitant exchange transfusions. As soon as practical, institute standard oral antiplasmodial therapy.

1.) *Loading,* 15 mg/kg in 250 mL normal saline infused over 4 hours followed by: *Maintenance,* beginning 24 hours after the beginning of the loading dose, 7.5 mg/kg infused over 4 hours, every 8 hours for 7 days or until oral therapy can be instituted.
2.) *Loading,* 10 mg/kg in 250 mL normal saline infused over 1 to 2 hours, followed immediately by: *Maintenance,* 0.02 mg/kg/min for up to 72 hours or until parasitemia decreases to less than 1% or oral therapy can be instituted.

➤*Children:*

The following doses have been suggested –

Oral (quinidine sulfate): 30 mg/kg/24 hours or 900 mg/m^2/24 hours in 5 divided doses.

IV (quinidine gluconate): 2 to 10 mg/kg/dose every 3 to 6 hours as needed; however, this route is not recommended.

Actions

➤*Pharmacology:* Quinidine, a class IA antiarrhythmic, depresses myocardial excitability, conduction velocity and contractility. Therapeutically, it prolongs the effective refractory period and increases conduction time, thereby preventing the reentry phenomenon. In addition, quinidine exerts an indirect anticholinergic effect; it decreases vagal tone and may facilitate conduction in the atrioventricular junction.

➤*Pharmacokinetics:*

Absorption/Distribution – There are differences in the anhydrous quinidine alkaloid content among the various salts. See the following table:

Anhydrous Quinidine Alkaloid Content in Various Salts			
	Quinidine content		Time to peak plasma levels (hours)
Quinidine salts	Active drug	Absorbed	
Quinidine Gluconate	62%	70%	3 to 5
Quinidine Sulfate	83%	73%	1 to 3[a]

[a] 3 to 5 hours for sustained release form.

Quinidine is rapidly absorbed from the GI tract. Maximum effects of quinidine gluconate occur 30 to 90 minutes after IM administration; onset is more rapid after IV administration. Activity persists for ≥ 6 to 8 hours. The average therapeutic serum levels are reported to be 2 to 7 mcg/mL. Toxic reactions may occur at levels from 5 to ≥ 8 mcg/mL. Quinidine is 80% to 90% bound to plasma proteins; the unbound fraction may be significantly increased in patients with hepatic insufficiency. Accumulation occurs in most tissues, except the brain.

Metabolism/Excretion – From 60% to 80% of a dose is metabolized via the liver into several metabolites; the primary metabolites are 3-hydroxyquinidine and 2-oxoquinidinone. Whether or not these or other metabolites have antiarrhythmic activity is unclear and controversial. Quinidine is excreted unchanged (10% to 50%) in the urine within 24 hours. The elimination half-life ranges from 4 to 10 hours in healthy patients, with a mean of 6 to 7 hours. Urinary acidification facilitates quinidine elimination, and alkalinization retards it. In patients with cirrhosis, the elimination half-life may be prolonged and the volume of distribution increased. In congestive heart failure (CHF), total clearance and volume of distribution are decreased. In the elderly, the elimination half-life may be increased. The influence of renal dysfunction on the disposition of quinidine is controversial; volume of distribution and renal clearance may be reduced.

Contraindications

Hypersensitivity or idiosyncrasy to quinidine or other cinchona derivatives manifested by thrombocytopenia, skin eruption or febrile reactions; myasthenia gravis; history of thrombocytopenic purpura associated with quinidine administration; digitalis intoxication manifested by arrhythmias or AV conduction disorders; complete heart block; left bundle branch block or other severe intraventricular conduction defects exhibiting marked QRS widening or bizarre complexes; complete AV block with an AV nodal or idioventricular pacemaker; aberrant ectopic impulses and abnormal rhythms due to escape mechanisms; history of drug-induced torsades de pointes; history of long QT syndrome.

Warnings

➤*Hepatotoxicity:* Occurrences of hepatotoxicity (including granulomatous hepatitis) have been reported due to quinidine hypersensitivity. Unexplained fever or elevation of hepatic enzymes, particularly in the early stages of therapy, warrants consideration. Monitor liver function during the first 4 to 8 weeks of therapy. Discontinuing quinidine usually results in toxicity resolution.

➤*Atrial flutter or fibrillation:* Reversion to sinus rhythm may be preceded by a progressive reduction in degree of AV block to a 1:1 ratio, which results in an extremely rapid ventricular rate. Prior to use in atrial flutter, pretreat with a digitalis preparation.

Although quinidine reduces recurrences of atrial fibrillation after cardioversion, it may be associated with an increase in mortality.

➤*Cardiotoxicity:* Cardiotoxicity (eg, increased PR and QT intervals, 50% widening of QRS complex, ventricular tachyarrhythmias, frequent ventricular ectopic beats or tachycardia) dictates immediate discontinuation of quinidine; closely monitor the ECG. Some specialists recommend quinidine therapy be initiated only in hospitalized patients with ECG monitoring. However, this is generally reserved for patients receiving large doses or who are at high risk.

In susceptible individuals (ie, marginally compensated cardiovascular disease), quinidine may produce clinically important depression of cardiac function such as hypotension, bradycardia or heartblock.

Large oral doses may reduce the arterial pressure by means of peripheral vasodilation. Serious hypotension is more likely with parenteral use.

Use quinidine with extreme caution in incomplete AV block, since complete block and asystole may result. The drug may cause unpredictable dysrhythmias in digitalized patients; use with caution in the presence of digitalis intoxication. Use cautiously in patients with partial bundle branch block, severe CHF and hypotensive states due to the depressant effects of quinidine on myocardial contractility and arterial pressure; usefulness of quinidine is limited unless these conditions are due to or aggravated by the arrhythmia. Consider the potential disadvantages and benefits.

➤*Parenteral therapy:* The dangers of parenteral use of quinidine are increased in the presence of AV block or absence of atrial activity. Administration is more hazardous in patients with extensive myocardial damage. Use of quinidine in digitalis-induced cardiac arrhythmia is extremely dangerous because the cardiac glycoside may already have caused serious impairment of intracardiac conduction system. Too rapid IV administration of as little as 200 mg may precipitate a fall of 40 to 50 mm Hg in arterial pressure. Inject slowly.

➤*Syncope:* Syncope occasionally occurs in patients on long-term quinidine therapy, usually resulting from ventricular tachycardia or fibrillation. It is manifested by sudden loss of consciousness and by polymorphic ventricular tachycardia. This syndrome does not appear to be related to dose or plasma levels but occurs more often with prolonged QT intervals. Syncopal episodes frequently terminate spontaneously or respond to treatment, but are sometimes fatal. Torsades de pointes is often the cause.

➤*Renal, hepatic or cardiac insufficiency:* Use with caution in renal (especially renal tubular acidosis), cardiac or hepatic insufficiency because of potential toxicity.

➤*Hypersensitivity reactions:* Asthma, muscle weakness and infection with fever prior to quinidine administration may mask hypersensitivity reactions to the drug.

Test dose – See Administration and Dosage for more information.

During the first weeks of therapy, although rare, consider hypersensitivity to quinidine including anaphylactoid reactions (eg, angioedema, purpura, acute asthmatic episode, vascular collapse). Refer to Management of Acute Hypersensitivity Reactions.

➤*Pregnancy: Category C.* Quinidine crosses the placenta and achieves fetal serum levels similar to maternal levels. Neonatal thrombocytopenia has occurred after maternal use. Safety for use during pregnancy is not established. Use only when clearly needed and when potential benefits outweigh potential hazards to fetus.

Oxytocic properties – Oxytocic properties are reported with quinidine, as with quinine; clinical significance is not known.

➤*Lactation:* Safety for use in the breast-feeding mother has not been established. Quinidine is excreted into breast milk with a milk:serum ratio of approximately 0.71. Use caution when quinidine is administered to a breast-feeding woman. The American Academy of Pediatrics considers quinidine to be compatible with breast-feeding.

➤*Children:* Safety and efficacy have not been established.

Precautions

➤*Monitoring:* Perform periodic blood counts and liver and kidney function tests. Discontinue use if blood dyscrasias or signs of hepatic or renal disorders occur. Initiate therapy in the hospital and continuously monitor ECG and check quinidine levels. This is generally done when large doses are used or the patient is at increased risk. Frequently measure arterial blood pressure during IV use; discontinue if blood pressure falls significantly.

➤*Vagolytic effects:* Because quinidine has vagolytic activity on the atrium and AV node, administration of cholinergic drugs or use of any other procedure to enhance vagal activity may fail to terminate paroxysmal supraventricular tachycardia.

➤*Potassium balance:* The effect of quinidine is enhanced by potassium and reduced if hypokalemia is present. The risk of drug-induced torsades de pointes is increased by concomitant hypokalemia.

➤*Malaria (P. falciparum):* Dosing schedules known to be effective have been associated with hypotension, increased QRS and corrected QT intervals and cinchonism. Closely monitor ECG and blood pressure.

Drug Interactions

Quinidine Drug Interactions			
Precipitant drug	Object drug*		Description
Amiodarone	Quinidine	↑	Increased quinidine levels may occur with possible production of potentially fatal cardiac dysrhythmias.
Antacids	Quinidine	↑	Certain antacids may increase serum quinidine levels, which may result in toxicity.
Barbiturates	Quinidine	↓	Quinidine serum levels and elimination half-life may be decreased.
Cholinergic drugs	Quinidine	↓	Since quinidine antagonizes the effect of vagal excitation upon the atrium and AV node, concurrent cholinergic agents may result in failure to terminate paroxysmal supraventricular tachycardia.
Cimetidine	Quinidine	↑	Quinidine serum levels may be increased.

Quinidine Drug Interactions

Precipitant drug	Object drug*		Description
Hydantoins	Quinidine	⬇	A decrease in the therapeutic effect of quinidine may occur.
Nifedipine	Quinidine	⬇	Serum levels and actions of quinidine may be lower than predicted by the dosage.
Rifampin	Quinidine	⬇	Increased metabolism of quinidine which may be associated with a reduction in its therapeutic effects.
Sucralfate	Quinidine	⬇	Serum quinidine levels may be reduced, decreasing the therapeutic effects.
Urinary alkalinizers	Quinidine	⬆	Urinary elimination of quinidine is reduced. Serum quinidine levels may be increased accompanied by increased pharmacologic effects.
Verapamil	Quinidine	⬆	Quinidine clearance may be reduced and its half-life prolonged, resulting in hypotension, bradycardia, ventricular tachycardia, AV block and pulmonary edema.
Quinidine	Anticholinergics	⬆	Quinidine exhibits a distinct anticholinergic activity in the myocardial tissues. Concurrent use may cause an additive vagolytic effect.
Quinidine	Anticoagulants	⬆	Anticoagulation may be potentiated; hemorrhage could occur.
Quinidine	Beta-blockers	⬆	Effects of metoprolol or propranolol may be increased in "extensive metabolizers."
Quinidine	Cardiac glycosides (digitoxin, digoxin)	⬆	Plasma levels of the cardiac glycosides are markedly increased. Pharmacologic effects are increased and toxicity may occur.
Quinidine	Disopyramide	⬆	Increased disopyramide levels or decreased quinidine levels may occur.
Disopyramide	Quinidine	⬇	
Quinidine	Nondepolarizing neuromuscular blockers	⬆	Nondepolarizing neuromuscular blocker effects may be enhanced.
Quinidine	Procainamide	⬆	Pharmacologic effects of procainamide may be increased; elevated procainamide and NAPA (major metabolite) plasma levels with toxicity may occur.
Quinidine	Propafenone	⬆	Serum propafenone levels may be increased in rapid extensive metabolizers of the drug (≈ 90% of patients), increasing the pharmacologic effects.
Quinidine	Succinylcholine	⬆	The neuromuscular blockade produced by succinylcholine may be prolonged.
Quinidine	Tricyclic antidepressants	⬆	The clearance of the tricyclic antidepressants may be reduced, possibly resulting in increased pharmacologic effects.

* ⬆ = Object drug increased. ⬇ = Object drug decreased.

➤*Drug/Lab test interactions:* Triamterene and quinidine have similar fluorescence spectra; thus, triamterene will interfere with the fluorescent measurement of quinidine serum levels.

Adverse Reactions

➤*Cardiovascular:* Widening of QRS complex; cardiac asystole; ventricular ectopy; idioventricular rhythms (including ventricular tachycardia and fibrillation and torsades de pointes in some instances); paradoxical tachycardia; arterial embolism; hypotension; ventricular extrasystoles occurring at the rate of one or more every 6 normal beats; prolonged QT interval; complete AV block; ventricular flutter.

Stop use if any of these occur: Increase of more than 25% in duration of QRS complex; disappearance of P waves; restoration of sinus rhythm; decrease in heart rate to 120 bpm in the ECG.

➤*CNS:* Headache; fever; vertigo; apprehension; excitement; confusion; delirium; syncope; dementia; ataxia; depression.

➤*Dermatologic:* Rash; urticaria; cutaneous flushing with intense pruritus; photosensitivity; eczema; exfoliative eruptions; psoriasis; abnormalities of pigmentation.

➤*GI:* The most common reactions seen with quinidine include the following: Nausea; vomiting; abdominal pain; diarrhea; anorexia. These may be preceded by fever.

Rarely, oral quinidine has been associated with esophageal disorders, primarily esophagitis.

➤*Hematologic:* Acute hemolytic anemia; hypoprothrombinemia; thrombocytopenic purpura; agranulocytosis; drug-induced hypoprothrombinemic hemorrhage in patients on chronic anticoagulant therapy; thrombocytopenia; leukocytosis; shift to left in WBC differential; neutropenia.

➤*Hypersensitivity:* Angioedema; acute asthma; vascular collapse; respiratory arrest; hepatic dysfunction, including granulomatous hepatitis; hepatic toxicity; purpura; vasculitis.

➤*Musculoskeletal:* Arthralgia; myalgia.

➤*Ophthalmic:* Mydriasis; blurred vision; disturbed color perception; reduced vision field; photophobia; diplopia; night blindness; scotomata; optic neuritis.

➤*Special senses:* Disturbed hearing (tinnitus, decreased auditory acuity).

➤*Miscellaneous:* Increase in serum skeletal muscle creatine phosphokinase.

Cinchonism – Ringing in the ears; hearing loss; headache; nausea; dizziness; vertigo; light-headedness; disturbed vision. These may appear after a single dose.

Renal/Hepatic – Lupus nephritis; hepatic toxicity, including granulomatous hepatitis; hepatitis.

Lupus erythematosus – Lupus erythematosus has occurred. Symptoms include hepatosplenomegaly/lymphadenopathy and a positive antinuclear antibody test. Symptoms resolve after drug withdrawal.

Overdosage

Severe quinidine intoxication may be associated with depressed mental function, even in hemodynamically stable patients. The patient progresses from lethargy to coma, including respiratory arrest; recurrent generalized motor seizures may occur. The onset of CNS manifestations may be substantially delayed beyond the onset of cardiovascular toxicity; conversely, recovery from coma is often delayed.

➤*Symptoms:*

Cardiovascular – Tachyarrhythmias (sinus tachycardia, ventricular tachycardia, ventricular fibrillation, torsades de pointes); depressed automaticity and conduction (QRS and QTc prolongation, bundle branch block, sinus bradycardia, sinoatrial block, sinus arrest, AV block, ST depression, T inversion); hypotension (depressed contractility and cardiac output, vasodilation); syncope; heart failure.

CNS – Lethargy; confusion; coma; respiratory depression or arrest; seizures; headache; paresthesia; vertigo.

GI – Vomiting; abdominal pain; diarrhea; nausea.

Miscellaneous – Cinchonism; hypokalemia; visual/auditory disturbances; tinnitus; acidosis.

➤*Treatment:* If ingestion of quinidine is recent, gastric lavage, emesis or administration of activated charcoal may reduce absorption. Management of overdosage includes the following: Symptomatic treatment; ECG, blood gases, serum electrolytes and blood pressure monitoring; cardiac pacing, if indicated; acidification of the urine. Avoid alkalinization of the urine. Mechanical ventilation and other supportive measures may be required.

IV infusion of ⅙ molar sodium lactate reportedly reduces the cardiotoxic effects of quinidine. Because marked CNS depression may occur even in the presence of convulsions, do not give CNS depressants. Hypotension may be treated, if necessary, with metaraminol or norepinephrine after adequate fluid volume replacement. Tachydysrhythmias should respond to phenytoin or lidocaine. Hemodialysis has been effective in overdosage but is rarely warranted.

Patient Information

Do not discontinue therapy unless instructed by physician.

May cause GI upset; take with food.

Notify the physician if ringing in the ears, visual disturbances, dizziness, headache, nausea, skin rash, or breathing difficulty occurs.

Do not crush or chew sustained-release tablets.

Quinidine

QUINIDINE SULFATE

Contains 83% anhydrous quinidine alkaloid.

Rx	**Quinidine Sulfate** (Various, eg, Danbury, Eon)	**Tablets:** 200 mg	In 100s and 1000s.
Rx	**Quinidine Sulfate** (Various, eg, Danbury, Eon)	**Tablets:** 300 mg	In 100s and 1000s.
Rx	**Quinidine Sulfate** (Various, eg, Teva)	**Tablets, sustained-release:** 300 mg	In 100s and 250s.

QUINIDINE SULFATE — ORAL

For complete and comparative prescribing information, refer to the Quinidine group monograph.

QUINIDINE GLUCONATE

Contains 62% anhydrous quinidine alkaloid.

Rx	**Quinidine Gluconate** (Various, eg, Geneva)	**Tablets, sustained-release:** 324 mg	In 100s, 250s, and 500s.
Rx	**Quinidine Gluconate** (Lilly)	**Injection:** 80 mg/mL (50 mg/mL quinidine)	In 10 mL multi-dose vials.[1]

[1] With 0.005% EDTA and 0.25% phenol.

QUINIDINE GLUCONATE — INJECTION

For complete and comparative prescribing information, refer to the Quinidine group monograph.

QUINIDINE GLUCONATE — ORAL

For complete and comparative prescribing information, refer to the Quinidine group monograph.

PROCAINAMIDE HYDROCHLORIDE

Rx	**Pronestyl** (Apothecon)	**Tablets**: 375 mg	Tartrazine. (434). Orange. In 100s.
		500 mg	Tartrazine. (435). Red. In 100s.
Rx	**Procainamide HCl**[1] (Various, eg, Teva)	**Tablets, extended-release**: 250 mg	In 100s and 500s.
Rx	**Procainamide HCl**[1] (Various, eg, Teva)	**Tablets, extended-release**: 500 mg	In 100s and 500s.
Rx	**Procainamide HCl**[1] (Various, eg, Teva)	**Tablets, extended-release**: 750 mg	In 100s and 500s.
Rx	**Procanbid**[2] (Monarch)	**Tablets, extended-release**: 500 mg	(PROCANBID 500). White, elliptical. Film-coated. In 60s and UD 100s.
Rx	**Procainamide HCl**[1] (Various, eg, Teva)	**Tablets, extended-release**: 1000 mg	In 100s.
Rx	**Procanbid**[2] (Monarch)		(PROCANBID 1000). Gray, elliptical. Film-coated. In UD 100s.
Rx	**Procainamide HCl** (Various, eg, Ivax)	**Capsules**: 250 mg	May contain parabens. In 100s, 250s, and 1000s.
Rx	**Procainamide HCl** (Various, eg, Ivax)	**Capsules**: 375 mg	May contain parabens. In 100s, 250s, and 1000s.
Rx	**Procainamide HCl** (Various, eg, Ivax)	**Capsules**: 500 mg	May contain parabens. In 100s, 250s, and 1000s.
Rx	**Procainamide HCl** (Various, eg, Hospira)	**Injection**: 500 mg/mL	May contain methylparaben and sodium metabisulfite. In 2 mL vials.

[1] These extended-release tablets are dosed at 6-hour intervals.

[2] These extended-release tablets are dosed at 12-hour intervals.

PROCAINAMIDE HYDROCHLORIDE — ORAL

WARNING

The prolonged administration of procainamide often leads to the development of a positive antinuclear antibody (ANA) test, with or without symptoms of a lupus erythematosus-like syndrome. If a positive ANA titer develops, the benefits versus risks of continued procainamide therapy should be assessed.

Mortality – In the National Heart, Lung and Blood Institute's Cardiac Arrhythmia Suppression Trial (CAST), a long-term, multicentered, randomized, double-blind study in patients with asymptomatic non-life-threatening ventricular arrhythmias who had myocardial infarction more than 6 days but less than 2 years previously, an excessive mortality or nonfatal cardiac arrest rate (7.7%) was seen in patients treated with encainide or flecainide compared with that seen in patients assigned to matched placebo-treated group (3%). The average duration of treatment with onoalnide or flocainide in this study was 10 months.

The applicability of the cast results to other populations (eg, those without recent myocardial infarctions) is uncertain. Considering the known proarrhythmic properties of procainamide and the lack of evidence of improved survival for any antiarrhythmic drug in patients without life-threatening arrhythmias, the use of procainamide as well as other antiarrhythmic agents should be reserved for patients with life-threatening ventricular arrhythmias.

Blood dyscrasias – Agranulocytosis, bone marrow depression, neutropenia, hypoplastic anemia and thrombocytopenia in patients receiving procainamide have been reported at a rate of approximately 0.5%. Most of these patients received procainamide within the recommended dosage range. Fatalities have occurred (with approximately 20% to 25% mortality in reported cases of agranulocytosis). Since most of these events have been noted during the first 12 weeks of therapy, it is recommended that complete blood counts including white cell, differential and platelet counts be performed at weekly intervals for the first 3 months of therapy, and periodically thereafter. Complete blood counts should be performed promptly if the patient develops any signs of infection (such as fever, chills, sore throat or stomatitis), bruising or bleeding. If any of those hematologic disorders are identified, procainamide therapy should be discontinued. Blood counts usually return to normal within 1 month of discontinuation. Caution should be used in patients with preexisting marrow failure or cytopenia of any type.

Indications

For the treatment of documented ventricular arrhythmias, such as sustained ventricular tachycardia, that, in the judgement of the physician, are life-threatening. Because of the proarrythmic effects of procainamide hydrochloride, its use with lesser arrhythmias is generally not recommended. Treatment of patients with asymptomatic ventricular premature contractions should be avoided.

➤*Unlabeled uses:*

Use in children – The following doses of procainamide have been suggested:15 to 50 mg/kg/day divided every 3 to 6 hours. Maximum dose is 4 g/day.

Administration and Dosage

➤*Approved by the FDA:* June 1950.

The oral dose and interval of administration should be adjusted for the individual patient, based on clinical assessment of the degree of underlying myocardial disease, the patient's age, and renal function.

As a general guide, for younger adult patients with normal renal function, an initial total daily oral dose of up to 50 mg/kg of body weight of procainamide hydrochloride capsules or tablets may be used, given in divided doses, every 3 hours, to maintain therapeutic blood levels. For older patients, especially those over 50 years of age, or for patients with renal, hepatic, or cardiac insufficiency, lesser amounts or longer intervals may produce adequate blood levels. The initial daily dose should be divided for administration at 3, 4, or 6 hour intervals as estimated for the patient's needs; then, the dose and interval should be adjusted for the individual.

To Provide up to 50 mg per kg of Body Weight per Day:*	
Patients weighing:	
88 to 110 lb (40 to 50 kg)	250 mg every 3 hours to 500 mg every 6 hours
132 to 154 lb (60 to 70 kg)	375 mg every 3 hours to 750 mg every 6 hours
176 to 198 lb (80 to 90 kg)	500 mg every 3 hours to 1 g every 6 hours
> 220 lb (> 100 kg)	625 mg every 3 hours to 1.25 g every 6 hours

* Initial dosage schedule guide only, to be adjusted for each patient individually, based on age, cardiorenal function, blood level (if available), and clinical response.

➤*Storage/Stability:* Store at controlled room temperature 15° to 30°C (59° to 86°F). Protect from moisture.

Actions

➤*Pharmacology:* Procainamide (PA) increases the effective refractory period of the atria, and to a lesser extent the bundle of His-Purkinje system and ventricles of the heart. It reduces impulse conduction velocity in the atria, His-Purkinje fibers, and ventricular muscle, but has variable effects on the atrioventricular (AV) node, a direct slowing action and a weaker vagolytic effect which may speed AV conduction slightly. Myocardial excitability is reduced in the atria, Purkinje fibers, papillary muscles, and ventricles by an increase in the threshold for excitation, combined with inhibition of ectopic pacemaker activity by retardation of the slow phase of diastolic depolarization, thus decreasing automaticity especially in ectopic sites. Contractility of the undamaged heart is usually not affected by therapeutic concentrations, although slight reduction of cardiac output may occur, and may be significant in the presence of myocardial damage. Therapeutic levels of PA may exert vagolytic effects and produce slight acceleration of heart rate, while high or toxic concentrations may prolong AV conduction time or induce AV block, or even cause abnormal automaticity and spontaneous firing, by unknown mechanisms.

➤*Pharmacokinetics:*

Absorption – Ingested PA is resistant to digestive hydrolysis, and the drug is well absorbed from the entire small intestinal surface, but individual patients vary in their completeness of absorption of PA. Following oral administration of procainamide hydrochloride, plasma PA levels reach about 50% of peak in 30 minutes, 90% at an hour, and peak at about 90 to 120 minutes.

Distribution – About 15% to 20% of PA is reversibly bound to plasma proteins, and considerable amounts are more slowly and reversibly bound to tissues of the heart, liver, lung, and kidney. The apparent volume of distribution eventually reaches about 2 L/kg body weight with a half-time of approximately 5 minutes. While PA has been shown in the dog to cross the blood-brain barrier, it did not concentrate in the brain at levels higher than in plasma. It is not known if PA crosses the placenta. Plasma esterases are far less active in hydrolysis of PA than of procaine. The half-time for elimination of PA is 3 to 4 hours in patients with normal renal function, but reduced creatinine clearance and advancing age each prolong the half-time of elimination of PA.

Metabolism – A significant fraction of the circulating PA may be metabolized in hepatocytes to N-acetylprocainamide (NAPA), ranging from 16% to 21% of an administered dose in "slow acetylators" to 24% to 33% in "fast-acetylators". Since NAPA also has significant antiarrhythmic activity and somewhat slower renal clearance than PA, both hepatic acetylation rate capability and renal function, as well as age, have significant effects on the effective biologic half-time of therapeutic action of administered PA and the NAPA derivative.

Excretion – Trace amounts may be excreted in the urine as free and conjugated p-aminobenzoic acid, 30% to 60% as unchanged PA, and 6% to 52% as the NAPA derivative. Both PA and NAPA are eliminated by active tubular secretion as well as by glomerular filtration. Action of PA on the central nervous system is not prominent, but high plasma concentrations may cause

PROCAINAMIDE HYDROCHLORIDE — ORAL

tremors. While therapeutic plasma levels for PA have been reported to be 3 to 10 mcg/mL, certain patients such as those with sustained ventricular tachycardia, may need higher levels for adequate control. This may justify the increased risk of toxicity. Plasma levels above 10 mcg/mL are increasingly associated with toxic findings, which are seen occasionally in the 10 to 12 mcg/mL range, more often in the 12 to 15 mcg/mL range, and commonly in patients with plasma levels greater than 15 mcg/mL. Overdosage symptoms may result following a single 2 g dose; while 3 g may be dangerous, especially if the patient is a slow acetylator, has decreased renal function, or underlying organic heart disease. Where programmed ventricular stimulation has been used to evaluate efficacy of PA in preventing recurrent ventricular tachyarrythmias, higher plasma levels (mean, 13.6 mcg/mL) of PA were found necessary for adequate control.

Contraindications

➤*Complete heart block:* Procainamide should not be administered to patients with complete heart block because of its effects in suppressing nodal or ventricular pacemakers and the hazard of asystole. It may be difficult to recognize complete heart block in patients with ventricular tachycardia, but if significant slowing of ventricular rate occurs during PA treatment without evidence of AV conduction appearing, PA should be stopped. In cases of second-degree AV block or various types of hemiblock, PA should be avoided or discontinued because of the possibility of increased severity of block, unless the ventricular rate is controlled by an electrical pacemaker.

➤*Idiosyncratic hypersensitivity:* In patients sensitive to procaine or other estertype local anesthetics, cross sensitivity to PA is unlikely; however, it should be borne in mind, and PA should not be used if it produces acute allergic dermatitis, asthma, or anaphylactic symptoms.

➤*Lupus erythematosus:* An established diagnosis of systemic lupus erythematosus is a contraindication to PA therapy, since aggravation of symptoms is highly likely.

➤*Torsades de pointes:* In the unusual ventricular arrhythmia called "les torsades de pointes" (twistings of the points), characterized by alternation of 1 or more ventricular premature beats in the directions of the QRS complexes on ECG in persons with prolonged Q-T and often enhanced U waves, Group 1A antiarrhythmic drugs are contraindicated. Administration of PA in such cases may aggravate this special type of ventricular extrasystole or tachycardia instead of suppressing it.

Warnings

➤*Blood dyscrasias:* Agranulocytosis, bone marrow depression, neutropenia, hypoplastic anemia and thrombocytopenia in patients receiving procainamide hydrochloride have been reported at a rate of approximately 0.5%. Most of these patients received procainamide within the recommended dosage range. Fatalities have occurred (with approximately 20% to 25% mortality in reported cases of agranulocytosis). Since most of these events have been noted during the first 12 weeks of therapy, it is recommended that complete blood counts including white cell, differential and platelet counts be performed at weekly intervals for the first 3 months of therapy, and periodically thereafter. Complete blood counts should be performed promptly if the patient develops any signs of infection (such as fever, chills, sore throat or stomatitis), bruising or bleeding. If any of these hematologic disorders are identified, procainamide therapy should be discontinued. Blood counts usually return to normal within 1 month of discontinuation. Caution should be used in patients with preexisting marrow failure or cytopenia of any type.

➤*Concurrent other antiarrhythmic agents:* Concurrent use of PA with other Group 1A antiarrhythmic agents such as quinidine or disopyramide may produce enhanced prolongation of conduction or depression of contractility and hypotension, especially in patients with cardiac decompensation. Such use should be reserved for patients with serious arrhythmias unresponsive to a single drug and employed only if close observation is possible.

➤*Congestive heart failure:* For patients in congestive heart failure, and those with acute ischemic heart disease or cardiomyopathy, caution should be used in PA therapy, since even slight depression of myocardial contractility may further reduce cardiac output of the damaged heart.

➤*Digitalis intoxication:* Caution should be exercised in the use of procainamide in arrhythmias associated with digitalis intoxication. Procainamide can suppress digitalis-induced arrhythmias; however, if there is concomitant marked disturbance of atrioventricular conduction, additional depression of conduction and ventricular asystole or fibrillation may result. Therefore, use of procainamide should be considered only if discontinuation of digitalis, and therapy with potassium, lidocaine, or phenytoin are ineffective.

➤*First-degree heart block:* Caution should be exercised also if the patient exhibits or develops first-degree heart block while taking PA, and dosage reduction is advised in such cases. If the block persists despite dosage reduction, continuation of PA administration must be evaluated on the basis of current benefit versus risk of increased heart block.

➤*Mortality:* Considering the known proarrhythmic properties of procainamide and the lack of evidence of improved survival for any antiarrhythmic drug in patients without life-threatening arrhythmias, the use of procainamide as well as other antiarrhythmic agents should be reserved for patients with life-threatening ventricular arrhythmias.

➤*Myasthenia gravis:* Patients with myasthenia gravis may show worsening of symptoms from PA due to its procaine-like effect on diminishing acetylcholine release at skeletal muscle motor nerve endings, so that PA administration may be hazardous without optimal adjustment of anticholinesterase medications and other precautions.

➤*Predigitalization for atrial flutter or fibrillation:* Patients with atrial flutter or fibrillation should be cardioverted or digitalized prior to PA administration to avoid enhancement of AV conduction which may result in ventricular rate acceleration beyond tolerable limits. Adequate digitalization reduces but does not eliminate the possibility of sudden increase in ventricular rate as the atrial rate is slowed by PA in these arrhythmias.

➤*Hypersensitivity reactions:* Immediately after initiation of PA therapy, patients should be closely observed for possible hypersensitivity reactions, especially if procaine or local anesthetic sensitivity is suspected, and for muscular weakness if myasthenia gravis is a possibility.

➤*Renal function impairment:* Renal insufficiency may lead to accumulation of high plasma levels from conventional oral doses of PA, with effects similar to those of overdosage, unless dosage is adjusted for the individual patient. Progressive widening of the QRS complex, prolonged Q-T and P-R intervals, lowering of the R and T waves, as well as increasing AV block, may be seen with doses which are excessive for a given patient. Increased ventricular extrasystoles, or even ventricular tachycardia or fibrillation may occur. After IV administration but seldom after oral therapy, transient high plasma levels of PA may induce hypotension, affecting systolic more than diastolic pressures, especially in hypertensive patients. Such high levels may also produce central nervous depression, tremor, and even respiratory depression.

➤*Pregnancy: Category C.*

Teratogenic – Animal reproduction studies have not been conducted with PA. It also is not known whether PA can cause fetal harm when administered to a pregnant woman or can affect reproduction capacity. PA should be given to a pregnant woman only if clearly needed.

➤*Lactation:* Both PA and NAPA are excreted in human milk, and absorbed by the nursing infant. Because of the potential for serious adverse reactions in nursing infants, a decision to discontinue nursing or the drug should be made, taking into account the importance of the drug to the mother.

➤*Children:* Safety and effectiveness in children have not been established.

Precautions

➤*Monitoring:* After a day or so, steady state plasma PA levels are produced following regular oral administration of a given dose of procainamide hydrochloride tablets; procainamide hydrochloride capsules at set intervals, with peak plasma level concentrations of about 90 to 120 minutes after each dose. After achieving and maintaining therapeutic plasma concentrations and satisfactory ECG and clinical responses, continued frequent periodic monitoring of vital signs and ECG is advised. If evidence of QRS widening of greater than 25% or marked prolongation of the Q-T interval occurs, concern for overdosage is advisable if a 50% increase occurs. Elevated serum creatinine or urea nitrogen, reduced creatinine clearance, or history of renal insufficiency, as well as use in older patients (over age 50), provide grounds to anticipate that less than the usual dosage and longer time intervals between doses may suffice, since the urinary elimination of PA and NAPA may be reduced, leading to gradual accumulation beyond normally predicted amounts. If facilities are available for measurement of plasma PA and NAPA, or acetylation capability, individual dose adjustment for optimal therapeutic levels may be easier, but close observation of clinical effectiveness is the most important criterion.

In the longer term, periodic complete blood counts are useful to detect possible idiosyncratic hematologic effects of PA on neutrophil, platelet or red cell homeostasis; agranulocytosis has been reported to occur occasionally in patients on long-term PA therapy. A rising titer of serum ANA may precede clinical symptoms of the lupoid syndrome (see Warning Box and Adverse Reactions). If the lupus erythematosus-like syndrome develops in a patient with recurrent life-threatening arrhythmias not controlled by other agents, corticosteroid suppressive therapy may be used concomitantly with PA. Since the PA-induced lupoid syndrome rarely includes the dangerous pathologic renal changes, PA therapy may not necessarily have to be stopped unless the symptoms of serositis and the possibility of further lupoid effects are of greater risk than the benefit of PA in controlling arrhythmias. Patients with rapid acetylation capability are less likely to develop the lupoid syndrome after prolonged PA therapy.

Laboratory tests such as complete blood count (CBC), ECG, and serum creatinine or urea nitrogen may be indicated, depending on the clinical situation, and periodic rechecking of the CBC and ANA may be helpful in early detection of untoward reactions.

➤*Embolization:* In conversion of atrial fibrillation to normal sinus rhythm by any means, dislodgement of mural thrombi may lead to embolization, which should be kept in mind.

➤*Tartrazine sensitivity:* Procainamide tablets contain FD&C Yellow No. 5 (tartrazine) which may cause allergic-type reactions (including bronchial asthma) in certain susceptible individuals. Although the overall incidence of FD&C Yellow No. 5 (tartrazine) sensitivity in the general population is low, it is frequently seen in patients who also have aspirin hypersensitivity.

Drug Interactions

Procainamide Drug Interactions

Precipitant drug	Object drug*		Description
Amiodarone	Procainamide	↑	Amiodarone may increase procainamide serum concentrations. Monitor procainamide concentrations closely.
Anticholinergics	Procainamide	↑	Coadministration may produce additive antivagal effects on AV conduction. This effect is not as well documented for procainamide as for quinidine.

PROCAINAMIDE HYDROCHLORIDE — ORAL

Procainamide Drug Interactions

Precipitant drug	Object drug*		Description
Antiarrhythmics	Procainamide	↑	Additive effects on the heart may occur with concurrent use of procainamide and other antiarrhythmics (eg, lidocaine, quinidine, disopyramide). Dosage reduction may be necessary (see Warnings). Quinidine also may increase procainamide and NAPA concentrations.
Cimetidine Ranitidine	Procainamide	↑	Cimetidine may increase procainamide serum concentrations because of decreased renal clearance. Avoid this combination, if possible. If cimetidine is necessary, then monitor procainamide concentrations closely and adjust the dose as needed. Large (> 300 mg/day) doses of ranitidine also may have this effect.
Ethanol	Procainamide	↔	The actions of procainamide could be altered, but because the main metabolite (NAPA) is also an antiarrhythmic, specific effects are unclear.
Propranolol	Procainamide	↑	One study showed that propranolol increased procainamide serum concentrations by decreasing the plasma clearance. Another study showed no changes in procainamide clearance.
Quinolones	Procainamide	↑	The risk of life-threatening cardiac arrhythmias, including torsades de pointes, may be increased when procainamide is given with sparfloxacin, gatifloxacin, or moxifloxacin. Sparfloxacin is contraindicated with class IA antiarrhythmics. Also, ofloxacin may increase procainamide concentrations. Monitor concentrations and adjust dose as indicated.
Thioridazine Ziprasidone	Procainamide	↑	Concurrent use may result in synergistic or additive prolongation of the QT_c interval and increase the risk for life-threatening cardiac arrhythmias, including torsades de pointes.
Trimethoprim	Procainamide	↑	Elevated procainamide and NAPA serum levels may occur, possibly resulting in increased pharmacologic effects. Monitor serum concentrations.
Procainamide	Neuromuscular blockers (eg, succinylcholine)	↑	Procainamide may potentiate the neuromuscular blockade produced by agents such as succinylcholine. A reduced dose of the neuromuscular blocker may be required.

* ↑ = Object drug increased. ↔ = Undetermined clinical effect.

➤*Drug/Lab test interactions:* Suprapharmacologic concentrations of lidocaine and meprobamate may inhibit fluorescence of PA and NAPA, and propranolol shows a native fluorescence close to the PA/NAPA peak wavelengths, so that tests which depend on fluorescence measurement may be affected.

Adverse Reactions

➤*Cardiovascular:* Hypotension following oral PA administration is rare. Hypotension and serious disturbances of cardiorhythm such as ventricular asystole or fibrillation are more common after intravenous administration. Second-degree heart block has been reported in 2 of almost 500 patients taking PA orally.

➤*CNS:* Dizziness or giddiness, weakness, mental depression, and psychosis with hallucinations have been reported occasionally.

➤*Dermatologic:* Angioneurotic edema, urticaria, pruritus, flushing, and maculopapular rash have also occurred occasionally.

➤*GI:* Anorexia, nausea, vomiting, abdominal pain, bitter taste, or diarrhea may occur in 3% to 4% of patients taking oral procainamide.

➤*Hematologic:* Neutropenia, thrombocytopenia, or hemolytic anemia may rarely be encountered. Agranulocytosis has occurred after repeated use of PA, and deaths have been reported.

➤*Hepatic:* Elevations of transaminase with and without elevations of alkaline phosphatase and bilirubin have been reported. Some patients have had clinical symptoms (eg, malaise, right upper quadrant pain). Deaths from liver failure have been reported.

➤*Systemic:* A lupus erythematosus-like syndrome of arthralgia, pleural or abdominal pain, and sometimes arthritis, pleural effusion, pericarditis, fever, chills, myalgia, and possibly related hematologic or skin lesions (see below) is fairly common after prolonged PA administration, perhaps more often in patients who are slow acetylators. If a positive ANA titer develops, the benefits versus risks of continued procainamide therapy should be assessed. While some series have been reported less than 1 in 500, others have reported the syndrome in up to 30% of patients on long term oral PA therapy. If discontinuation of PA does not reverse the lupoid symptoms, corticosteroid treatment may be effective.

Overdosage

➤*Symptoms:* Progressive widening of the QRS complex, prolonged QT and PR intervals, lowering of the R and T waves, as well as increasing AV block, may be seen with doses which are excessive for a given patient. Increased ventricular extrasystoles, or even ventricular tachycardia or fibrillation may occur. After IV administration but seldom after oral therapy, transient high plasma levels of PA may induce hypotension, affecting systolic more than diastolic pressures, especially in hypertensive patients. Such high levels may also produce central nervous depression, tremor, and even respiratory depression.

Plasma levels above 10 mcg/mL are increasingly associated with toxic findings, which are seen occasionally in the 10 to 12 mcg/mL range, more often in the 12 to 15 mcg/mL range, and commonly in patients with plasma levels greater than 15 mcg/mL. Overdosage symptoms may result following a single 2 g dose; while 3 g may be dangerous, especially if the patient is a slow acetylator, has decreased renal function, or underlying organic heart disease.

➤*Treatment:* Treatment of overdosage or toxic manifestations includes general supportive measures, close observation, monitoring of vital signs and possibly intravenous pressor agents and mechanical cardiorespiratory support. If available, PA and NAPA plasma levels may be helpful in assessing the potential degree of toxicity and response to therapy. Both PA and NAPA are removed form the circulation by hemodialysis but not peritoneal dialysis. No specific antidote for PA is known.

Patient Information

The physician is advised to explain to the patient that close cooperation in adhering to the prescribed dosage schedule is of great importance in controlling the cardiac arrhythmia safely. The patient should understand clearly that more medication is not necessarily better and may be dangerous, that skipping doses or increasing intervals between doses to suit personal convenience may lead to loss of control of the heart problem, and that "making up" missed doses by doubling up later may be hazardous.

The patient should be encouraged to disclose any history of drug sensitivity, especially to procaine or other local anesthetic agents, or aspirin, and to report any history of kidney disease, congestive heart failure, myasthenia gravis, liver disease, or lupus erythematosus.

The patient should be counseled to report promptly any symptoms of arthralgia, myalgia, fever, chills, skin rash, easy bruising, sore throat or sore mouth, infections, dark urine or icterus, wheezing, muscular weakness, chest or abdominal pain, palpitations, nausea, vomiting, anorexia, diarrhea, hallucinations, dizziness, or depression.

PROCAINAMIDE HYDROCHLORIDE — INJECTION

WARNING

The prolonged administration of procainamide often leads to the development of a positive antinuclear antibody (ANA) test, with or without symptoms of a lupus erythematosus-like syndrome. If a positive ANA titer develops, the benefits versus risks of continued procainamide therapy should be assessed.

Mortality – In the National Heart, Lung and Blood Institute's Cardiac Arrhythmia Suppression Trial (CAST), a long-term, multicenter, randomized, double-blind study in patients with asymptomatic non-life-threatening ventricular arrhythmias who had myocardial infarction more than 6 days but less than 2 years previously, an excessive mortality or nonfatal cardiac arrest rate (7.7%) was seen in patients treated with encainide or flecainide compared with that seen in patients assigned to matched placebo-treated group (3%). The average duration of treatment with onoalnide or flocainide in this study was 10 months.

The applicability of the cast results to other populations (eg, those without recent myocardial infarctions) is uncertain. Considering the known proarrhythmic properties of procainamide and the lack of evidence of improved survival for any antiarrhythmic drug in patients without life-threatening arrhythmias, the use of procainamide as well as other antiarrhythmic agents should be reserved for patients with life-threatening ventricular arrhythmias.

Blood dyscrasias – Agranulocytosis, bone marrow depression, neutropenia, hypoplastic anemia and thrombocytopenia in patients receiving procainamide HCl have been reported at a rate of approximately 0.5%. Most of these patients received procainamide within the recommended dosage range. Fatalities have occurred (with approximately 20 to 25% mortality in reported cases of agranulocytosis). Since most of these events have been noted during the first 12 weeks of therapy, it is recommended that complete blood counts including white cell, differential and platelet counts be performed at weekly intervals for the first 3 months of therapy, and periodically thereafter. Complete blood counts should be performed promptly if the patient develops any signs of infection (such as fever, chills, sore throat or stomatitis), bruising or bleeding. If any of those hematologic disorders are identified, procainamide therapy should be discontinued. Blood counts usually return to normal within 1 month of discontinuation. Caution should be used in patients with preexisting marrow failure or cytopenia of any type.

Indications

For the treatment of documented ventricular arrhythmias, such as sustained ventricular tachycardia, that, in the judgment of the physician, are life-threatening. Because of the proarrhythmic effects of procainamide, its use with lesser arrhythmias is generally not recommended. Treatment of patients with asymptomatic ventricular premature contractions should be avoided.

➤*Unlabeled uses:*

Atrial fibrillation/flutter – Procainamide has been used to convert atrial fibrillation/flutter to sinus rhythm.

Use in children – The following doses of procainamide have been suggested:

IM: 20 to 30 mg/kg/day.

IV: Loading dose is 3 to 6 mg/kg infused over 5 minutes, not to exceed 100 mg/dose. Maintenance dose is 20 to 80 mcg/kg/min as continuous IV infusion; usual maximum is 2 g/day.

For the treatment of hemodynamically stable ventricular tachycardia in children, procainamide (loading dose of 15 mg/kg IV infused over 30 to 60 minutes) may be considered as an alternative agent to amiodarone.

Administration and Dosage

➤*Approved by the FDA:* June 1950.

Intravenous therapy allows most rapid control of serious arrhythmias, including those following myocardial infarction; it should be carried out in circumstances where close observation and monitoring of the patient are possible, such as in hospital or emergency facilities. Intramuscular administration is less apt to produce temporary high plasma levels but therapeutic plasma levels are not obtained as rapidly as with intravenous administration. Oral procainamide dosage forms are preferable for less urgent arrhythmias as well as for long-term maintenance after initial parenteral PA therapy.

Intramuscular administration may be used as an alternative to the oral route for patients with less threatening arrhythmias but who are nauseated or vomiting, who are ordered to receive nothing by mouth preoperatively, or who may have malabsorptive problems. An initial daily dose of 50 mg per kg body weight may be estimated. This amount should be divided into fractional doses of one-eighth to one-quarter to be injected intramuscularly every 3 to 6 hours until oral therapy is possible. If more than 3 injections are given, the physician may wish to assess patient factors such as age and renal function (see below), clinical response, and, if available, blood levels of PA and NAPA in adjusting further doses for that individual. For treatment of arrhythmias associated with anesthesia or surgical operation, the suggested dose is 100 mg to 500 mg by intramuscular injection.

➤*Intravenous administration:* Intravenous administration of procainamide HCl injection should be done cautiously to avoid a possible hypotensive response. If the blood pressure falls 15 mm Hg or more. PA administration should be temporarily discontinued. Electrocardiographic (ECG) monitoring is advisable as well, both for observation of the progress and response of the arrhythmia under treatment, and for early detection of any tendency to excessive widening of the QRS complex, prolongation of the PR interval, or any signs of heart block. Parenteral therapy with PA should be limited to use in hospitals in which monitoring and intensive supportive care are available, or to emergency situations in which equivalent observation and treatment can be provided. Initial arrhythmia control, under blood pressure and ECG monitoring, may usually be accomplished safely within a half-hour by either of the 2 methods which follow.

Direct injection – Direct injection into a vein or into tubing of an established infusion line should be done slowly at a rate not to exceed 50 mg per minute. It is advisable to dilute the 500 mg/mL concentration of procainamide HCl injection prior to intravenous injection to facilitate control of dosage rate. Doses of 100 mg may be administered every 5 minutes at this rate until the arrhythmia is suppressed or until 500 mg has been administered, after which it is advisable to wait 10 minutes or longer to allow for more distribution into tissues before resuming.

Loading infusion – Alternatively, a loading infusion containing 20 mg of procainamide per mL (1 g diluted to 50 mL with 5% Dextrose Injection) may be administered at a constant rate of 1 mL per minute for 25 to 30 minutes to deliver 500 mg to 600 mg of PA. Some effects may be seen after infusion of the first 100 mg or 200 mg; it is unusual to require more than 600 mg to achieve satisfactory antiarrhythmic effects.

The maximum advisable dosage to be given either by repeated bolus injections or such loading infusion is 1 g.

To maintain therapeutic levels, a more dilute intravenous infusion at a concentration of 2 mg/mL is convenient (1 g procainamide injection in 500 mL of 5% Dextrose Injection), and may be administered at 1 mL/min to 3 mL/min. If daily total fluid intake must be limited, a 4 mg/mL concentration (1 g of procainamide HCl injection in 250 mL of 5% Dextrose Injection) administered at 0.5 mL/min to 1.5 mL/min will deliver an equivalent 2 mg to 6 mg/min. The amount needed in a given patient to maintain the therapeutic level should be assessed principally from the clinical response, and will depend upon the patient's weight and age, renal elimination, hepatic acetylation rate, and cardiac status, but should be adjusted for each patient based upon close observation. A maintenance infusion rate of 50 mcg/min/kg body weight to a person with a normal renal PA elimination half time of 3 hours may be expected to produce a plasma level of approximately 6.5 mcg/mL.

Dilutions and Rates for Intravenous Infusions*: Procainamide Injection

	Final concentration	Infusion volume[1]	Procainamide to be added	Infusion rate
Initial loading infusion	20 mg/mL	50 mL	1,000 mg	1 mL/min (for up to 25 to 30 minutes*)
Maintenance infusion	2 mg/mL	500 mL	1,000 mg	1 mL/min to 3 mL/min
	or			
	4 mg/mL	250 mL	1,000 mg	0.5 mL/min to 1.5 mL/min
The maintenance infusion rates are calculated to deliver 2 mg to 6 mg/min, depending on body weight, renal elimination rate, and steady-state plasma level needed to maintain control of the arrhythmia. The 4 mg/mL maintenance concentration may be preferred if total infused volume must be limited.				

[1] All infusions should be made up to final volume with 5% Dextrose Injection.

* The flow rate of any IV procainamide infusion must be monitored closely to avoid transiently high plasma levels and possible hypotension.

Intravenous therapy should be terminated if persistent conduction disturbances or hypotension develop. As soon as the patient's basic cardiac rhythm appears to be stabilized, oral antiarrhythmic maintenance therapy is preferable, if indicated and possible. A period of about 3 to 4 hours (one half time for renal elimination, ordinarily) should elapse after the last intravenous dose before administering the first dose of oral procainamide.

➤*Storage/Stability:* The solutions, which are clear and colorless initially, may develop a slight yellow color in time. This does not indicate a change which should preclude its use, but a solution darker than slightly yellow, or discolored in any other way should not be used.

Store at controlled room temperature 15° to 30°C (59° to 86°F). Do not freeze.

Parenteral drug products should be examined visually for particulate matter and discoloration prior to administration. The solutions, which are clear and colorless initially, may develop a slight yellow color in time.

Actions

➤*Pharmacology:* Procainamide (PA) increases the effective refractory period of the atria, and to a lesser extent the bundle of His-Purkinje system and ventricles of the heart. It reduces impulse conduction velocity in the atria, His-Purkinje fibers, and ventricular muscle, but has variable effects on the atrioventricular (AV) node, a direct slowing action and a weaker vagolytic effect which may speed AV conduction slightly. Myocardial excitability is reduced in the atria, Purkinje fibers, papillary muscles, and ventricles by an increase in the threshold for excitation, combined with inhibition of ectopic pacemaker activity by retardation of the slow phase of diastolic depolarization, thus decreasing automaticity especially in ectopic sites. Contractility of the undamaged heart is usually not affected by therapeutic concentrations, although slight reduction of cardiac output may occur, and may be significant in the presence of myocardial damage. Therapeutic levels of PA may exert vagolytic effects and produce slight acceleration of heart rate, while high or toxic concentrations may prolong AV conduction time or

PROCAINAMIDE HYDROCHLORIDE — INJECTION

induce AV block, or even cause abnormal automaticity and spontaneous firing, by unknown mechanisms.

The electrocardiogram may reflect these effects by showing slight sinus tachycardia (due to the anticholinergic action) and widened QRS complexes and, less regularly, prolonged Q-T and P-R intervals (due to longer systole and slower conduction), as well as some decrease in QRS and T wave amplitude. These direct effects of PA on electrical activity, conduction, responsiveness, excitability and automaticity are characteristic of a Group 1A antiarrhythmic agent, the prototype for which is quinidine; PA effects are very similar. However, PA has weaker vagal blocking action than does quinidine, does not induce alpha-adrenergic blockade, and is less depressing to cardiac contractility.

➤*Pharmacokinetics:*

Absorption/Distribution – Following intramuscular injection, procainamide injection is rapidly absorbed into the bloodstream, and plasma levels peak in 15 to 60 minutes, considerably faster than the orally administered procainamide tablets or capsules which produce peak plasma levels in 90 to 120 minutes. Intravenous administration of procainamide can produce therapeutic procainamide levels within minutes after infusion is started. About 15% to 20% of PA is reversibly bound to plasma proteins, and considerable amounts are more slowly and reversibly bound to tissues of the heart, liver, lung, and kidney. The apparent volume of distribution eventually reaches about 2 L/kg body weight with a half-time of approximately 5 minutes. While PA has been shown in the dog to cross the blood-brain barrier, it did not concentrate in the brain at levels higher than in plasma. It is not known if PA crosses the placenta. Plasma estereses are far less active in hydrolysis of PA than of procaine.

Metabolism/Excretion – The half-time for elimination of PA is 3 to 4 hours in patients with normal renal function, but reduced creatinine clearance and advancing age each prolong the half-time of elimination of PA. A significant fraction of the circulating PA may be metabolized in hepatocytes to N-acetylprocainamide (NAPA), ranging from 16% to 21% of an administered dose in "slow-acetylators" to 24% to 33% in "fast-acetylators". Since NAPA also has significant antiarrhythmic activity and somewhat slower renal clearance than PA, both hepatic acetylation rate capability and renal function, as well as age, have significant effects on the effective biologic half-time of therapeutic action of administered PA and the NAPA derivative. Trace amounts may be excreted in the urine as free and conjugated p-aminobenzoic acid, 30% to 60% as unchanged PA, and 6% to 52% as the NAPA derivative. Both PA and NAPA are eliminated by active tubular secretion as well as by glomerular filtration. Action of PA on the central nervous system is not prominent, but high plasma concentrations may cause tremors. While therapeutic plasma levels for PA have been reported to be 3 mcg/mL to 10 mcg/mL, certain patients such as those with sustained ventricular tachycardia, may need higher levels for adequate control. This may justify the increased risk of toxicity. Plasma levels above 10 mcg/mL are increasingly associated with toxic findings, which are seen occasionally in the 10 mcg/mL to 12 mcg/mL range, more often in the 12 mcg/mL to 15 mcg/mL range, and commonly in patients with plasma levels greater than 15 mcg/mL. Where programmed ventricular stimulation has been used to evaluate efficacy of PA in preventing recurrent ventricular tachyarrhythmias, higher plasma levels (mean, 13.6 mcg/mL) of PA were found necessary for adequate control.

Contraindications

➤*Complete heart block:* Procainamide should not be administered to patients with complete heart block because of its effects in suppressing nodal or ventricular pacemakers and the hazard of asystole. It may be difficult to recognize complete heart block in patients with ventricular tachycardia, but if significant slowing of ventricular rate occurs during PA treatment without evidence of AV conduction appearing, PA should be stopped. In cases of second degree AV block or various types of hemiblock, PA should be avoided or discontinued because of the possibility of increased severity of block, unless the ventricular rate is controlled by an electrical pacemaker.

➤*Idiosyncratic hypersensitivity:* In patients sensitive to procaine or other ester-type local anesthetics, cross sensitivity to PA is unlikely. However, it should be borne in mind, and PA should not be used if it produces acute allergic dermatitis, asthma, or anaphylactic symptoms.

➤*Lupus erythematosus:* An established diagnosis of systemic lupus erythematosus is a contraindication to PA therapy, since aggravation of symptoms is highly likely.

➤*Torsades de pointes:* In the unusual ventricular arrhythmia called "les torsades de pointes" (twistings of the points), characterized by alternation of 1 or more ventricular premature beats in the directions of the QRS complexes on ECG in persons with prolonged Q-T and often enhanced U waves, Group 1A antiarrhythmic drugs are contraindicated. Administration of PA in such cases may aggravate this special type of ventricular extrasystole or tachycardia instead of suppressing it.

Warnings

➤*Mortality:* Considering the known proarrhythmic properties of procainamide and the lack of evidence of improved survival for any antiarrhythmic drug in patients without life-threatening arrhythmias, the use of procainamide as well as other antiarrhythmic agents should be reserved for patients with life-threatening ventricular arrhythmias.

➤*Blood dyscrasias:* Agranulocytosis, bone marrow depression, neutropenia, hypoplastic anemia and thrombocytopenia in patients receiving procainamide have been reported at a rate of approximately 0.5%. Most of these patients received procainamide within the recommended dosage range. Fatalities have occurred (with approximately 20 to 25% mortality in reported cases of agranulocytosis). Since most of these events have been noted during the first 12 weeks of therapy, it is recommended that complete blood counts including white cell, differential and platelet counts be performed at weekly intervals for the first 3 months of therapy, and periodically thereafter. Complete blood counts should be performed promptly if the patient develops any signs of infection (such as fever, chills, sore throat or stomatitis), bruising or bleeding. If any of those hematologic disorders are identified, procainamide therapy should be discontinued. Blood counts usually return to normal within 1 month of discontinuation. Caution should be used in patients with preexisting marrow failure or cytopenia of any type.

➤*Digitalis intoxication:* Caution should be exercised in the use of procainamide in arrhythmias associated with digitalis intoxication. Procainamide can suppress digitalis-induced arrhythmias; however, if there is concomitant marked disturbance of atrioventricular conduction, additional depression of conduction and ventricular asystole or fibrillation may result. Therefore, use of procainamide should be considered only if discontinuation of digitalis, and therapy with potassium, lidocaine, or phenytoin are ineffective.

➤*First degree heart block:* Caution should be exercised also if the patient exhibits or develops first degree heart block while taking PA, and dosage reduction is advised in such cases. If the block persists despite dosage reduction, continuation of PA administration must be evaluated on the basis of current benefit versus risk of increased heart block.

➤*Predigitalization for atrial flutter or fibrillation:* Patients with atrial flutter or fibrillation should be cardioverted or digitalized prior to PA administration to avoid enhancement of AV conduction which may result in ventricular rate acceleration beyond tolerable limits. Adequate digitalization reduces but does not eliminate the possibility of sudden increase in ventricular rate as the atrial rate is slowed by PA in these arrhythmias.

➤*Congestive heart failure:* For patients in congestive heart failure, and those with acute ischemic heart disease or cardiomyopathy, caution should be used in PA therapy, since even slight depression of myocardial contractility may further reduce cardiac output of the damaged heart.

➤*Concurrent use with other antiarrhythmic agents:* Concurrent use of PA with other Group 1A antiarrhythmic agents such as quinidine or disopyramide may produce enhanced prolongation of conduction or depression of contractility and hypotension, especially in patients with cardiac decompensation. Such use should be reserved for patients with serious arrhythmias unresponsive to a single drug and employed only if close observation is possible.

➤*Myasthenia gravis:* Patients with myasthenia gravis may show worsening of symptoms from PA due to its procaine-like effect on diminishing acetylcholine release at skeletal muscle motor nerve endings, so that PA administration may be hazardous without optimal adjustment of anticholinesterase medications and other precautions.

➤*Hypersensitivity reactions:* Immediately after initiation of PA therapy, patients should be closely observed for possible hypersensitivity reactions. In conversion of atrial fibrillation to normal sinus rhythm by any means, dislodgement of mural thrombi may lead to embolization, which should be kept in mind.

➤*Renal function impairment:* Renal insufficiency may lead to accumulation of high plasma levels from conventional doses of PA, with effects similar to those of overdosage, unless dosage is adjusted for the individual patient. Progressive widening of the QRS complex, prolonged Q-T and P-R intervals, lowering of the R and T waves, as well as increasing A-V block, may be seen with doses which are excessive for a given patient. Increased ventricular extrasystoles or even ventricular tachycardia or fibrillation may occur. After intravenous administration but seldom after oral therapy, transient high plasma levels of PA may induce hypotension, affecting systolic more than diastolic pressures, especially in hypertensive patients. Such high levels may also produce central nervous depression, tremor, and even respiratory depression.

➤*Pregnancy: Category C.*

Teratogenic – Animal reproduction studies have not been conducted with PA. It also is not known whether PA can cause fetal harm when administered to a pregnant woman or can affect reproduction capacity. PA should be given to a pregnant woman only if clearly needed.

➤*Lactation:* Both PA and NAPA are excreted in human milk, and absorbed by the breast-feeding infant. Because of the potential for serious adverse reactions in nursing infants, a decision to discontinue breast-feeding or the drug should be made, taking into account the importance of the drug to the mother.

➤*Children:* Safety and effectiveness in pediatric patients have not been established.

Precautions

➤*Monitoring:* Laboratory tests such as complete blood count (CBC), electrocardiogram, and serum creatinine or urea nitrogen may be indicated depending on the clinical situation, and periodic rechecking of the CBC and ANA may be helpful in early detection of untoward reactions.

Blood pressure and ECG monitoring – Blood pressure should be monitored with the patient supine during parenteral, especially intravenous, administration of PA. There is a possibility that relatively high, although transient plasma levels of PA may be attained and cause hypotension before the PA can be distributed from the plasma volume to its full apparent volume of distribution which is approximately 50 times greater. Therefore, caution should be exercised to avoid overly rapid administration of PA. If the blood pressure falls 15 mm Hg or more. PA administration should be temporarily discontinued. Electrocardiographic (ECG) monitoring is advisable as well, both for observation of the progress and response of the arrhythmia under treatment, and for early detection of any tendency to excessive widening of the QRS complex, prolongation of the P-R interval, or any signs of heart block. Parenteral therapy with PA should be limited to use in hospitals in which

PROCAINAMIDE HYDROCHLORIDE — INJECTION

monitoring and intensive supportive care are available, or to emergency situations in which equivalent observation and treatment can be provided.

After achieving and maintaining therapeutic plasma concentrations and satisfactory electrocardiographic and clinical responses, continued frequent periodic monitoring of vital signs and electrocardiograms is advised. If evidence of QRS widening of more than 25% or marked prolongation of the Q-T interval occurs, concern for overdosage is appropriate, and interruption of the PA infusion is advisable if a 50% increase occurs. Elevated serum creatinine or urea nitrogen, reduced creatinine clearance or history of renal insufficiency, as well as use in older patients (over age 50), provide grounds to anticipate that less than the usual dosage or infusion rate may suffice, since the urinary elimination of PA and NAPA may be reduced, leading to gradual accumulation beyond normally predicted amounts. If facilities are available for measurement of plasma PA and NAPA, or acetylation capability, individual dose adjustment for optimal therapeutic levels may be easier, but close observation of clinical effectiveness is the most important criterion.

➤*Special risk:*

Digitalis intoxication – Caution should be exercised in the use of procainamide in arrhythmias associated with digitalis intoxication. Procainamide can suppress digitalis-induced arrhythmias; however, if there is concomitant marked disturbance of atrioventricular conduction, additional depression of conduction and ventricular asystole or fibrillation may result. Therefore, use of procainamide should be considered only if discontinuation of digitalis, and therapy with potassium, lidocaine, or phenytoin are ineffective.

➤*Sulfite sensitivity:* Procainamide HCl injection contains sodium metabisulfite, a sulfite that may cause allergic-type reactions including anaphylactic symptoms and life-threatening or less severe asthmatic episodes in certain susceptible people. The overall prevalence of sulfite sensitivity in the general population is unknown and probably low. Sulfite sensitivity is seen more frequently in asthmatic than in nonasthmatic people.

Drug Interactions

Procainamide Drug Interactions

Precipitant drug	Object drug*		Description
Amiodarone	Procainamide	↑	Amiodarone may increase procainamide serum concentrations. Monitor procainamide concentrations closely.
Anticholinergics	Procainamide	↑	Coadministration may produce additive antivagal effects on AV conduction. This effect is not as well documented for procainamide as for quinidine.
Antiarrhythmics	Procainamide	↑	Additive effects on the heart may occur with concurrent use of procainamide and other antiarrhythmics (eg, lidocaine, quinidine, disopyramide). Dosage reduction may be necessary (see Warnings). Quinidine also may increase procainamide and NAPA concentrations.
Cimetidine Ranitidine	Procainamide	↑	Cimetidine may increase procainamide serum concentrations because of decreased renal clearance. Avoid this combination, if possible. If cimetidine is necessary, then monitor procainamide concentrations closely and adjust the dose as needed. Large (> 300 mg/day) doses of ranitidine also may have this effect.
Ethanol	Procainamide	↔	The actions of procainamide could be altered, but because the main metabolite (NAPA) is also an antiarrhythmic, specific effects are unclear.
Propranolol	Procainamide	↑	One study showed that propranolol increased procainamide serum concentrations by decreasing the plasma clearance. Another study showed no changes in procainamide clearance.
Quinolones	Procainamide	↑	The risk of life-threatening cardiac arrhythmias, including torsades de pointes, may be increased when procainamide is given with sparfloxacin, gatifloxacin, or moxifloxacin. Sparfloxacin is contraindicated with class IA antiarrhythmics. Also, ofloxacin may increase procainamide concentrations. Monitor concentrations and adjust dose as indicated.
Thioridazine Ziprasidone	Procainamide	↑	Concurrent use may result in synergistic or additive prolongation of the QT_c interval and increase the risk for life-threatening cardiac arrhythmias, including torsades de pointes.
Trimethoprim	Procainamide	↑	Elevated procainamide and NAPA serum levels may occur, possibly resulting in increased pharmacologic effects. Monitor serum concentrations.
Procainamide	Neuromuscular blockers (eg, succinylcholine)	↑	Procainamide may potentiate the neuromuscular blockade produced by agents such as succinylcholine. A reduced dose of the neuromuscular blocker may be required.

* ↑ = Object drug increased. ↔ = Undetermined clinical effect.

➤*Drug/Lab test interactions:* Suprapharmacologic concentrations of lidocaine and meprobamate may inhibit fluorescence of PA and NAPA, and propranolol shows a native fluorescence close to the PA/NAPA peak wavelengths, so that tests which depend on fluorescence measurement may be affected.

Adverse Reactions

➤*Cardiovascular:* Hypotension and serious disturbance of cardiorhythm such as ventricular asystole or fibrillation are more common with intravenous administration of PA than with intramuscular administration. Because PA is a peripheral vasodilator in concentrations higher than the usual therapeutic range, transient high plasma levels which may occur especially during intravenous administration may produce temporary but at times severe lowering of blood pressure.

➤*CNS:* Dizziness or giddiness, weakness, mental depression and psychosis with hallucinations have been reported.

➤*Dermatologic:* Angioneurotic edema, urticaria, pruritus, flushing, and maculopapular rash have also occurred.

➤*GI:* Anorexia, nausea, vomiting, abdominal pain, bitter taste or diarrhea may occur in 3% to 4% of patients taking oral procainamide.

➤*Hematologic:* Neutropenia, thrombocytopenia, or hemolytic anemia may rarely be encountered. Agranulocytosis has occurred after repeated use of PA; and deaths have been reported.

➤*Hepatic:* Elevations of transaminase with and without elevations of alkaline phosphatase and bilirubin have been reported. Some patients have had clinical symptoms (eg, malaise, right upper quadrant pain). Deaths from liver failure have been reported.

➤*Miscellaneous:* A lupus erythematosus-like syndrome of arthralgia, pleural or abdominal pain, and sometimes arthritis, pleural effusion, pericarditis, fever, chills, myalgia, and possibly related hematologic or skin lesions (see below) is fairly common after prolonged PA administration, perhaps more often in patients who are slow acetylators.

While some serious have reported less than 1 in 500, others have reported the syndrome in up to 30% of patients on long-term oral PA therapy. If discontinuation of PA does not reverse the lupoid symptoms, corticosteroid treatment may be effective.

Overdosage

➤*Symptoms:* Progressive widening of the QRS complex, prolonged QT and PR intervals, lowering of the R and T waves, as well as increasing A-V block, may be seen with doses which are excessive for a given patient. Increased ventricular extrasystoles or even ventricular tachycardia or fibrillation may occur. After intravenous administration but seldom after oral therapy, transient high plasma levels of PA may induce hypotension, affecting systolic more than diastolic pressures, especially in hypertensive patients. Such high levels may also produce central nervous depression, tremor, and even respiratory depression.

Plasma levels above 10 mcg/mL are increasingly associated with toxic findings, which are seen occasionally in the 10 mcg/mL to 12 mcg/mL range, more often in the 12 mcg/mL to 15 mcg/mL range, and commonly in patients with plasma levels greater than 15 mcg/mL.

➤*Treatment:* Treatment of overdosage or toxic manifestations includes general supportive measures, close observation, monitoring of vital signs and possibly intravenous pressor agents and mechanical cardiorespiratory support if available, PA and NAPA plasma levels may be helpful in assessing the potential degree of toxicity and response to therapy. Both PA and NAPA are removed from the circulation by hemodialysis but not peritoneal dialysis. No specific antidote for PA is known.

Patient Information

The patient should be encouraged to disclose any history of drug sensitivity, especially to procaine or other local anesthetic agents, or aspirin, and to report any history of kidney disease, congestive heart failure, myasthenia gravis, liver disease, or lupus erythematosus.

The patient should be counseled to report any symptoms of arthralgia, myalgia, fever, chills, skin rash, easy bruising, sore throat or sore mouth, infections, dark urine or icterus, wheezing, muscular weakness, chest or abdominal pain, palpitations, nausea, vomiting, anorexia, diarrhea, hallucinations, dizziness, or depression.

DISOPYRAMIDE

Rx	**Disopyramide Phosphate** (Various, eg, Geneva, Tava)	**Capsules:** 100 mg (as phosphate)	In 100s and 500s.
Rx	**Norpace** (Pharmacia)		Lactose. (SEARLE 2752 NORPACE 100 MG). White/Orange. In 100s and 1000s.
Rx	**Disopyramide Phosphate** (Various, eg, Geneva, Teva)	**Capsules:** 150 mg (as phosphate)	In 100s and 500s.
Rx	**Norpace** (Pharmacia)		Lactose. (SEARLE 2762 NORPACE 150 MG). Brown/Orange. In 100s and 1000s.
Rx	**Norpace CR** (Pharmacia)	**Capsules, extended-release:** 100 mg (as phosphate)	Sucrose. (SEARLE 2732 NORPACE CR 100 mg). White/Lt. green. In 100s, 500s, and UD 100s.
Rx	**Disopyramide Phosphate** (Various, eg, Ethex, Geneva)	**Capsules, extended-release:** 150 mg (as phosphate)	In 100s.
Rx	**Norpace CR** (Pharmacia)		Sucrose. (SEARLE 2742 NORPACE CR 150 mg). Brown/Lt. green. In 100s, 500s, and UD 100s.

DISOPYRAMIDE — ORAL

Refer to the general introductory discussion concerning Antiarrhythmic Agents.

WARNING

In the National Heart, Lung, and Blood Institute's Cardiac Arrhythmia Suppression Trial (CAST), a long-term, multicenter, randomized, double-blind study in patients with asymptomatic non-life-threatening ventricular arrhythmias who had an MI more than 6 days but less than 2 years previously, an excessive mortality or nonfatal cardiac arrest rate (7.7%) was seen in patients treated with encainide or flecainide compared with that seen in patients assigned to carefully matched placebo-treated groups (3%). The average duration of treatment with encainide or flecainide in this study was 10 months.

The applicability of the CAST results to other populations (eg, those without recent MI) is uncertain. Considering the known proarrhythmic properties of disopyramide and the lack of evidence of improved survival for any antiarrhythmic drug in patients without life-threatening arrhythmias, the use of disopyramide as well as other antiarrhythmic agents should be reserved for patients with life-threatening ventricular arrhythmias.

Indications

Treatment of documented ventricular arrhythmias (eg, sustained ventricular tachycardia) considered to be life-threatening.

➤*Unlabeled uses:* Disopyramide may be beneficial in the treatment of paroxysmal supraventricular tachycardia.

Administration and Dosage

➤*Approved by the FDA:* 1977.

Individualize dosage. Initiate treatment in the hospital. Do not break or chew extended-release capsules.

➤*Adults:* 400 to 800 mg/day given in divided doses. The recommended dosage for most adults is 600 mg/day given in divided doses. For patients less than 50 kg (110 pounds), give 400 mg/day. Divide the total daily dose and administer every 6 hours in the immediate-release form or every 12 hours in the controlled-release form.

➤*Children:* Divide daily dosage and administer equal doses every 6 hours or at intervals according to patient needs. Closely monitor plasma levels and therapeutic response. Hospitalize patients during initial treatment and start dose titration at the lower end of the ranges provided below:

Suggested Total Daily Disopyramide Dosage in Children[a]

Age (years)	Disopyramide (mg/kg/day)
< 1	10 to 30
1 to 4	10 to 20
4 to 12	10 to 15
12 to 18	6 to 15

[a] Prepare a 1 to 10 mg/mL suspension by adding contents of the immediate-release capsule to cherry syrup, NF. The resulting suspension, when refrigerated, is stable for 1 month; shake thoroughly before measuring dose. Dispense in an amber glass bottle. Do not use the controlled-release form to prepare the solution.

➤*Initial loading dose:* For rapid control of ventricular arrhythmia, give an initial loading dose of 300 mg immediate-release (200 mg for patients less than 50 kg [110 lb]). Therapeutic effects are attained in 30 minutes to 3 hours. If there is no response or no evidence of toxicity within 6 hours of the loading dose, 200 mg every 6 hours may be administered instead of the usual 150 mg. If there is no response within 48 hours, discontinue the drug or carefully monitor subsequent immediate-release doses of 250 or 300 mg every 6 hours.

Do not use the controlled-release form initially if rapid plasma levels are desired.

➤*Severe refractory ventricular tachycardia:* A limited number of patients have tolerated up to 1600 mg/day (400 mg every 6 hours), resulting in plasma levels up to 9 mcg/mL. Hospitalize patients for close evaluation and continuous monitoring.

➤*Cardiomyopathy or possible cardiac decompensation:* Do not administer a loading dose, and limit the initial dosage to 100 mg immediate-release every 6 to 8 hours. Make subsequent dosage adjustments gradually.

➤*Renal/Hepatic function failure:* For patients with moderate renal insufficiency (Ccr greater than 40 mL/min) or hepatic insufficiency, the recommended dosage is 400 mg/day given in divided doses (either 100 mg every 6 hours for immediate release or 200 mg every 12 hours for controlled release).

In severe renal insufficiency (Ccr less than or equal to 40 mL/min), the recommended dosage is 100 mg of immediate-release form given at intervals shown in the following table, with or without an initial loading dose of 150 mg.

Disopyramide (Immediate-release) Dosage in Renal Impairment

Creatinine clearance (mL/min)	Loading dose (mg)	Dose (mg)	Dosage interval (hours)
30 to 40	150	100	8
15 to 30	150	100	12
< 15	150	100	24

➤*Transfer to disopyramide:* Based on theoretical considerations, use the regular maintenance schedule, without a loading dose, 6 to 12 hours after the last dose of quinidine or 3 to 6 hours after the last dose of procainamide. Where withdrawal of quinidine or procainamide is likely to produce life-threatening arrhythmias, consider hospitalization.

When transferring from immediate to controlled release, start maintenance schedule of controlled release 6 hours after the last dose of immediate release.

Actions

➤*Pharmacology:* Disopyramide is a class IA antiarrhythmic agent pharmacologically similar to, but chemically unrelated to, procainamide and quinidine. It decreases the rate of diastolic depolarization (phase 4), decreases the upstroke velocity (phase 0), increases the action potential duration of normal cardiac cells, and prolongs the refractory period (phases 2 and 3). It also decreases the disparity in refractoriness between infarcted and adjacent normally perfused myocardium and does not affect alpha- or beta-adrenergic receptors.

Anticholinergic activity – In vitro anticholinergic activity is approximately 0.06% that of atropine; the usual dose of 150 mg every 6 hours or 300 mg controlled release every 12 hours compares with approximately 0.4 to 0.6 mg of atropine.

Hemodynamic effects – At recommended oral doses, disopyramide rarely produces significant alterations of blood pressure in patients without congestive heart failure. With IV disopyramide (dosage form not available in US), either increases in systolic/diastolic or decreases in systolic blood pressure have occurred depending on the infusion rate and the patient population. IV disopyramide may cause cardiac depression with an approximate mean 10% reduction of cardiac output, which is more pronounced in patients with cardiac dysfunction.

➤*Pharmacokinetics:*

Absorption/Distribution – Following oral administration of immediate-release disopyramide, the drug is rapidly and almost completely (approximately 90%) absorbed. Peak plasma levels usually occur within 2 hours. Therapeutic plasma levels of disopyramide are 2 to 4 mcg/mL. Protein binding is concentration-dependent and varies from 50% to 65%; it is difficult to predict the concentration of the free drug when total drug is measured. After the oral administration of 200 mg disopyramide to 10 cardiac patients with borderline to moderate heart failure, the time to peak serum concentration of 2.3 ± 1.5 hours was increased, and the mean peak serum concentration of 4.8 ± 1.6 mcg/mL was higher than in healthy volunteers.

Immediate-release vs controlled-release: In a crossover study in healthy subjects, the bioavailability of the controlled-release form was similar to that from the immediate-release capsules. With a single 300 mg oral dose, peak disopyramide plasma concentrations of 3.23 ± 0.75 mcg/mL at 2.5 ± 2.3 hours were obtained with two 150 mg immediate-release capsules and 2.22 ± 0.47 mcg/mL at 4.9 ± 1.4 hours with two 150 mg controlled-release capsules. The elimination half-life was 8.31 ± 1.83 hours with the immediate-release capsules and 11.65 ± 4.72 hours with controlled-release capsules. The amount of disopyramide and MND excreted in the urine in 48 hours was 128 and 48 mg, respectively, with the immediate-release capsules and 112 and 33 mg, respectively, with controlled-release capsules.

Following multiple doses, steady-state plasma levels of between 2 and 4 mcg/mL were attained following either 150 mg every 6 hours with immediate-release capsules or 300 mg every 12 hours with controlled-release capsules.

DISOPYRAMIDE — ORAL

Metabolism/Excretion – About 50% is excreted in the urine as the unchanged drug and 30% as metabolites (20% MND). The plasma concentration of MND is approximately one tenth that of disopyramide. The mean plasma half-life is 6.7 hours (range, 4 to 10 hours).

Special populations –

Renal function impairment: A preliminary report of 3 patients on long-term hemodialysis revealed a 45% to 72% reduction in disopyramide half-life during dialysis. In contrast, another study in patients on chronic hemodialysis demonstrated little difference in disopyramide half-life without dialysis (16.8 vs 16.1 hours). Resin and charcoal hemoperfusion were effective in rapidly decreasing disopyramide plasma levels in acute overdosage.

In impaired renal function (creatinine clearance [Ccr] less than 40 mL/min), half-life values ranged from 8 to 18 hours. Therefore, decrease the dose in renal failure to avoid drug accumulation. Altering urinary pH does not affect plasma half-life.

Contraindications

Cardiogenic shock; preexisting second- or third-degree AV block (if no pacemaker is present); congenital QT prolongation; hypersensitivity to disopyramide.

Warnings

➤*Mortality:* Considering the known proarrhythmic properties of disopyramide and the lack of evidence of improved survival for any antiarrhythmic drug in patients without life-threatening arrhythmias, the use of disopyramide as well as other antiarrhythmic agents should be reserved for patients with life-threatening ventricular arrhythmias.

➤*Proarrhythmic effects:* Because of the proarrhythmic effects, use with lesser arrhythmias is generally not recommended.

➤*Asymptomatic ventricular premature contractions:* Avoid treatment of patients with this condition.

➤*Survival:* Antiarrhythmic drugs have not been shown to enhance survival in patients with ventricular arrhythmias.

➤*Negative inotropic properties:*

Heart failure/hypotension – May cause or aggravate CHF or produce severe hypotension, especially in patients with primary cardiomyopathy or inadequately compensated CHF. Do not use in patients with uncompensated or marginally compensated CHF or hypotension unless secondary to cardiac arrhythmia. Treat patients with a history of heart failure with careful attention to the maintenance of cardiac function, including optimal digitalization. If hypotension occurs or CHF worsens, discontinue use; restart at a lower dosage after adequate cardiac compensation has been established.

Do not give a loading dose to patients with myocarditis or other cardiomyopathy; closely monitor initial dosage and subsequent adjustments.

QRS widening – Although unusual, QRS widening (more than 25%) may occur; discontinue use in such cases.

QT_c prolongation – QT_c prolongation and worsening of the arrhythmia, including ventricular tachycardia and fibrillation, may occur. Patients who have QT prolongation in response to quinidine may be at particular risk. As with other Type IA antiarrhythmics, disopyramide has been associated with torsade de pointes. If QT prolongation more than 25% is observed and if ectopy continues, monitor closely and consider discontinuing the drug.

➤*Atrial tachyarrhythmias:* Digitalize patients with atrial flutter or fibrillation prior to administration to ensure that enhancement of AV conduction does not increase ventricular rate beyond acceptable limits.

➤*Conduction abnormalities:* Use caution in patients with sick sinus syndrome, Wolff-Parkinson-White (WPW), syndrome or bundle branch block.

➤*Heart block:* If first degree heart block develops, reduce dosage. If the block persists, drug continuation must depend upon the benefit compared to the risk of higher degrees of heart block. Development of second- or third-degree AV block or unifascicular, bifascicular, or trifascicular block requires discontinuation of therapy, unless ventricular rate is controlled by a ventricular pacemaker.

➤*Concomitant antiarrhythmic therapy:* Reserve concomitant use of disopyramide with other class IA or class IC antiarrhythmics or propranolol for life-threatening arrhythmias unresponsive to a single agent. Such use may produce serious negative inotropic effects or may excessively prolong conduction, particularly in patients with cardiac decompensation.

➤*Hypoglycemia:* Reported in rare instances. Monitor blood glucose levels in patients with CHF, chronic malnutrition, hepatic or renal disease, and in those taking drugs which could compromise normal glucoregulatory mechanisms in the absence of food (eg, beta-adrenoceptor blockers, alcohol).

➤*Anticholinergic activity:* Do not use in patients with urinary retention, glaucoma, or myasthenia gravis unless adequate overriding measures are taken. Urinary retention may occur in either sex, but males with benign prostatic hypertrophy are at particular risk. In patients with a family history of glaucoma, measure intraocular pressure before initiating therapy. Use with special care in patients with myasthenia gravis, because disopyramide could precipitate a myasthenic crisis.

➤*Renal function impairment:* Reduce dosage in impaired renal function. Carefully monitor ECG for prolongation of PR interval, evidence of QRS widening or other signs of overdosage. The controlled-release form is not recommended for patients with severe renal insufficiency (Ccr less than or equal to 40 mL/min).

➤*Hepatic function impairment:* Hepatic function impairment increases plasma half-life; therefore, reduce dosage in such patients. Carefully monitor the ECG. Patients with cardiac dysfunction have a higher potential for hepatic impairment.

➤*Pregnancy: Category C.* Disopyramide was associated with decreased numbers of implantation sites and decreased growth and survival of pups when administered to pregnant rats at 250 mg/kg/day (≥ 20 times the usual daily human dose), a level at which weight gain and food consumption of dams were also reduced. Increased resorption rates were reported in rabbits at 60 mg/kg/day (≥ 5 times the usual daily human dose). At a maternal concentration of 2.3 mg/L disopyramide, the fetal cord concentration is 0.9 mg/L. Well-controlled studies have not been performed in pregnant women and experience is limited. Use only when clearly needed and when the potential benefits outweigh the potential hazards to the fetus. Disopyramide has been found in human fetal blood. Disopyramide may stimulate contractions of the pregnant uterus.

➤*Lactation:* Disopyramide has been detected in breast milk at a concentration not exceeding that in maternal plasma. Therefore, decide whether to discontinue breast-feeding or to discontinue the drug taking into account the importance of the drug to the mother.

➤*Children:* Safety and efficacy have not been established.

Precautions

➤*Potassium imbalance:* Disopyramide may be ineffective in *hypo*kalemia and its toxic effects may be enhanced in *hyper*kalemia. Correct any potassium deficit before instituting therapy.

Drug Interactions

➤*CYP 450 system:* In vitro metabolic studies indicate that disopyramide is metabolized by CYP3A4; inhibitors of this system (eg, erythromycin, clarithromycin) may elevate plasma levels of disopyramide.

Disopyramide Drug Interactions

Precipitant drug	Object drug*		Description
Antiarrhythmics	Disopyramide	↑	Other antiarrhythmics (eg, procainamide, lidocaine) have been used with disopyramide; however, widening of the QRS complex or QT prolongation may occur.
Beta-blockers	Disopyramide	↔	This interaction is difficult to predict. Disopyramide clearance may be decreased; other adverse effects (eg, sinus bradycardia, hypotension) may occur. Others report no occurrence of synergistic or additive negative inotropic effects.
Cisapride	Disopyramide	↑	The risk of life-threatening cardiac arrhythmias, including torsades de pointes, may be increased due to possibly additive prolongation of the QT interval.
Disopyramide	Cisapride		
Clarithromycin Erythromycin	Disopyramide	↑	Increased disopyramide plasma levels may occur. Arrhythmias and increased QTc intervals have occurred.
Fluoroquinolones	Disopyramide	↑	The risk of life-threatening cardiac arrhythmias, including torsades de pointes, may be increased. Sparfloxacin is contraindicated and gatifloxacin, levofloxacin, and moxifloxacin should be avoided in patients receiving disopyramide.
Hydantoins	Disopyramide	↓	Disopyramide serum levels, half-life and bioavailability may be decreased; anticholinergic effects may be enhanced. Effects may persist for several days after hydantoin withdrawal.
Quinidine	Disopyramide	↑	Concurrent use may result in increased disopyramide serum levels and decreased quinidine levels. This may result in disopyramide toxicity or decreased response to quinidine.
Disopyramide	Quinidine	↓	
Rifampin	Disopyramide	↓	Disopyramide serum levels may be decreased.
Thioridazine Ziprasidone	Disopyramide	↑	The risk of life-threatening cardiac arrhythmias, including torsades de pointes, may be increased. Coadministration is contraindicated.

DISOPYRAMIDE — ORAL

Disopyramide Drug Interactions			
Precipitant drug	Object drug*		Description
Verapamil	Disopyramide	↔	Until data on this interaction are available, it is recommended that disopyramide not be administered within 48 hours before or 24 hours after verapamil.
Disopyramide	Anticoagulants	⬇	Decreased prothrombin time after disopyramide discontinuation may occur. However, this may be due to a hemodynamic effect and not an interaction.
Disopyramide	Digoxin	⬆	Although serum digoxin levels may be increased, a clinically significant interaction appears unlikely. A beneficial interaction has also been suggested.

* ⬆ = Object drug increased. ⬇ = Object drug decreased. ↔ = Undetermined clinical effect.

Adverse Reactions

The most serious adverse reactions are hypotension and CHF. The most common reactions are anticholinergic and dose-dependent. These may be transitory, but may be persistent or severe. Urinary retention is the most serious anticholinergic effect.

➤*Cardiovascular:* Hypotension with or without CHF, increased CHF, edema, weight gain, cardiac conduction disturbances, shortness of breath, syncope, chest pain (1% to 3%); AV block (less than 1%). There have been reports of severe myocardial depression (with hypotension and an increase in venous pressure) and unexplained severe epigastric pain following standard oral doses.

➤*CNS:* Dizziness, fatigue, headache (3% to 9%); nervousness (1% to 3%); depression, insomnia (less than 1%); acute psychosis (rare, prompt reversal when therapy discontinued).

➤*Dermatologic:* Generalized rash, dermatoses, itching (1% to 3%).

➤*GI:* Dry mouth (32%); nausea, pain, bloating, gas (3% to 9%); anorexia, diarrhea, vomiting (1% to 3%); elevated liver enzymes (less than 1%); reversible cholestatic jaundice.

➤*GU:* Urinary hesitancy (14%); constipation (11%); urinary retention, frequency and urgency (3% to 9%); impotence (1% to 3%); dysuria, elevated creatinine (less than 1%).

➤*Hematologic:* Decreased hemoglobin, hematocrit (less than 1%); thrombocytopenia, reversible agranulocytosis (rare).

➤*Musculoskeletal:* Muscle weakness, malaise, aches/pain (3% to 9%);

➤*Special senses:* Blurred vision, dry nose, eyes and throat (3% to 9%).

➤*Miscellaneous:* Hypokalemia, elevated cholesterol and triglycerides (1% to 3%); numbness, tingling, elevated BUN (less than 1%); hypoglycemia; fever and respiratory difficulty; gynecomastia (rare); anaphylactoid reactions; lupus erythematosus symptoms (most cases occurred in patients who had been switched to disopyramide from procainamide after developing symptoms).

Overdosage

➤*Symptoms:* Overdose may be followed by apnea, loss of consciousness, cardiac arrhythmias, loss of spontaneous respiration and death. Toxic plasma levels produce excessive widening of the QRS complex and QT interval, worsening of CHF, hypotension, varying conduction disturbances, bradycardia, and finally, asystole. Anticholinergic effects may also be observed.

➤*Treatment:* Prompt, vigorous treatment is necessary even in the absence of symptoms. Such treatment may be lifesaving and may include gastric lavage followed by activated charcoal by mouth or stomach tube.

Administration of isoproterenol, dopamine, cardiac glycosides, diuretics, intra-aortic balloon counterpulsation, mechanical ventilation, hemodialysis or charcoal hemoperfusion may be used. Monitor ECG.

If progressive AV block develops, implement endocardial pacing. In case of impaired renal function, measures to increase the GFR may reduce the toxicity. Altering urinary pH does not affect plasma half-life or the amount of disopyramide excreted in the urine.

Anticholinergic effects can be reversed with neostigmine.

Refer also to General Management of Acute Overdosage.

Patient Information

May cause dry mouth, difficult urination, dizziness, breathing difficulty, constipation or blurred vision. Notify physician if symptoms persist, but do not discontinue unless instructed to do so by physician.

Do not break or chew extended-release capsules.

FLECAINIDE ACETATE

Rx	**Flecainide** (Various, eg, Mylan, Par)	**Tablets:** 50 mg	In 100s.
Rx	**Tambocor** (3M Pharm.)		(TR 50 3M). White. In 100s and UD 100s.
Rx	**Flecainide** (Various, eg, Mylan, Par)	**Tablets:** 100 mg	In 100s.
Rx	**Tambocor** (3M Pharm.)		(TR 100 3M). White, scored. In 100s and UD 100s.
Rx	**Flecainide** (Various, eg, Mylan, Par)	**Tablets:** 150 mg	In 100s.
Rx	**Tambocor** (3M Pharm.)		(TR 150 3M). White, scored. Oval. In 100s.

FLECAINIDE ACETATE — ORAL

Refer to the general introductory discussion concerning Antiarrhythmic Agents.

WARNING

Mortality – Flecainide was included in the National Heart Lung and Blood Institute's Cardiac Arrhythmia Suppression Trial (CAST), a long-term, multicenter, randomized, double-blind study in patients with asymptomatic non-life-threatening ventricular arrhythmias who had an MI more than 6 days but less than 2 years previously. An excessive mortality or non-fatal cardiac arrest rate was seen in patients treated with flecainide compared with that seen in patients assigned to a carefully matched placebo-treated group. This rate was 5.1% for flecainide and 2.3% for the matched placebo. The average duration of treatment with flecainide in this study was 10 months.

The applicability of the CAST results to other populations (eg, those without recent MI) is uncertain, but at present, it is prudent to consider the risks of Class IC agents (including flecainide), coupled with the lack of any evidence of improved survival, generally unacceptable in patients without life-threatening ventricular arrhythmias, even if the patients are experiencing unpleasant, but not life-threatening, symptoms or signs.

Ventricular proarrhythmic effects in patients with atrial fibrillation/flutter – A review of the world literature revealed reports of 568 patients treated with oral flecainide for paroxysmal atrial fibrillation/flutter (PAF). Ventricular tachycardia was experienced in 0.4% of these patients. Of 19 patients in the literature with chronic atrial fibrillation (CAF), 10.5% experienced ventricular tachycardia (VT) or ventricular fibrillation (VF). Flecainide is not recommended for use in patients with CAF. Case reports of ventricular proarrhythmic effects in patients treated with flecainide for atrial fibrillation/flutter have included increased premature ventricular contractions (PVCs), VT, VF, and death.

WARNING (cont.)

As with other Class I agents, patients treated with flecainide for atrial flutter have been reported with 1:1 atrioventricular conduction due to slowing the atrial rate. A paradoxical increase in the ventricular rate also may occur in patients with atrial fibrillation who receive flecainide. Concomitant negative chronotropic therapy such as digoxin or beta-blockers may lower the risk of this complication.

Indications

For the prevention of PAF associated with disabling symptoms and paroxysmal supraventricular tachycardias (PSVT), including atrioventricular nodal reentrant tachycardia, atrioventricular reentrant tachycardia and other supraventricular tachycardias of unspecified mechanism associated with disabling symptoms in patients without structural heart disease.

Prevention of documented life-threatening ventricular arrhythmias, such as sustained ventricular tachycardia.

Administration and Dosage

➤*Approved by the FDA:* 1985.

For patients with sustained ventricular tachycardia, initiate therapy in the hospital and monitor rhythm.

Flecainide has a long half-life (12 to 27 hours). Steady-state plasma levels in normal renal and hepatic function may not be achieved until 3 to 5 days of therapy at a given dose. Therefore, do not increase dosage more frequently than once every 4 days, since optimal effect may not be achieved during the first 2 to 3 days of therapy.

An occasional patient not adequately controlled by (or intolerant of) a dose given at 12 hour intervals may be dosed at 8 hour intervals.

Once the arrhythmia is controlled, it may be possible to reduce the dose, as necessary, to minimize side effects or effects on conduction.

➤*PSVT and PAF:* The recommended starting dose is 50 mg every 12 hours. Doses may be increased in increments of 50 mg twice daily every

FLECAINIDE ACETATE — ORAL

4 days until efficacy is achieved. For PAF patients, a substantial increase in efficacy without a substantial increase in discontinuation for adverse experiences may be achieved by increasing the flecainide dose from 50 to 100 mg twice daily. The maximum recommended dose for patients with paroxysmal supraventricular arrhythmias is 300 mg/day.

➤*Sustained ventricular tachycardia:*

Initial dose – 100 mg every 12 hours. Increase in 50 mg increments twice daily every 4 days until effective. Most patients do not require more than 150 mg every 12 hours (300 mg/day). Maximum dose is 400 mg/day.

Use of higher initial doses and more rapid dosage adjustments have resulted in an increased incidence of proarrhythmic events and CHF, particularly during the first few days of dosing. Therefore, a loading dose is not recommended.

➤*CHF or MI:* Use cautiously in patients with a history of CHF or myocardial dysfunction.

➤*Renal impairment:* In severe renal impairment (Ccr ≤ 35 mL/min/1.73 m^2), the initial dosage is 100 mg once daily (or 50 mg twice daily). Frequent plasma level monitoring is required to guide dosage adjustments. In patients with less severe renal disease, initial dosage is 100 mg every 12 hours. Increase dosage cautiously at intervals more than 4 days, observing the patient closely for signs of adverse cardiac effects or other toxicity. It may take more than 4 days before a new steady-state plasma level is reached following a dosage change. Monitor plasma levels to guide dosage adjustments (see below).

➤*Transfer to flecainide:* Theoretically, when transferring patients from another antiarrhythmic to flecainide, allow at least 2 to 4 plasma half-lives to elapse for the drug being discontinued before starting flecainide at the usual dosage. Consider hospitalization of patients in whom withdrawal of a previous antiarrhythmic is likely to produce life-threatening arrhythmias.

➤*Administration with amiodarone:* When flecainide is given in the presence of amiodarone, reduce the usual flecainide dose by 50% and monitor the patient closely for adverse effects. Plasma level monitoring is strongly recommended to guide dosage with such combination therapy.

Actions

➤*Pharmacology:* Flecainide has local anesthetic activity and belongs to the membrane stabilizing (Class I) group of antiarrhythmic agents; it has electrophysiologic effects characteristic of the IC class of antiarrhythmics.

Hemodynamic effects – Flecainide does not usually alter heart rate, although bradycardia and tachycardia have been reported occasionally.

Decreases in ejection fraction, consistent with a negative inotropic effect, have been observed after a single dose of 200 to 250 mg; both increases and decreases in ejection fraction have been encountered during multidose therapy at usual therapeutic doses.

➤*Pharmacokinetics:*

Absorption/Distribution – Oral absorption is nearly complete. Peak plasma levels are attained at about 3 hours (range, 1 to 6 hours). Flecainide does not undergo significant first-pass effect.

The plasma half-life averages 20 hours (range, 12 to 27 hours) after multiple oral doses. Steady-state levels are approached in 3 to 5 days; once at steady-state, no accumulation occurs during chronic therapy. Over the usual therapeutic range, plasma levels are approximately proportional to dose.

In patients with congestive heart failure (CHF; NYHA class III), the rate of flecainide elimination from plasma (mean half-life, 19 hours) is moderately slower than for healthy subjects (mean half-life, 14 hours).

Plasma protein binding is about 40% and is independent of plasma drug level over the range of 0.015 to about 3.4 mcg/mL.

Metabolism/Excretion – In vitro metabolic studies have confirmed that cytochrome P450 2D6 is involved in the metabolism of flecainide. About 30% of a single oral dose (range, 10% to 50%) is excreted in urine unchanged. The two major urinary metabolites are meta-O-dealkylated flecainide (active, but ≈ ⅕ as potent) and the meta-O-dealkylated lactam (inactive). These two metabolites (primarily conjugated) account for most of the remaining portion of the dose. Several minor metabolites (≤ 3%) are also found in urine; 5% is excreted in feces.

Special populations –

Renal function impairment: Flecainide elimination depends on renal function. With increasing renal impairment, the extent of unchanged drug in urine is reduced and the half-life is prolonged. There is no simple relationship between creatinine clearance and the rate of flecainide elimination from plasma.

Hemodialysis removes only approximately 1% of an oral dose as unchanged flecainide.

Contraindications

Preexisting second- or third-degree AV block, right bundle branch block when associated with a left hemiblock (bifascicular block), unless a pacemaker is present to sustain the cardiac rhythm if complete heart block occurs; recent MI; presence of cardiogenic shock; hypersensitivity to the drug.

Warnings

➤*Mortality:* Flecainide was included in the National Heart Lung and Blood Institute's Cardiac Arrhythmia Suppression Trial (CAST), a long-term multicenter, randomized, double-blind study in patients with asymptomatic non-life-threatening ventricular arrhythmias who had an MI more than 6 days, but less than 2 years previously. An excessive mortality or nonfatal cardiac arrest rate was seen in patients treated with flecainide compared with that seen in a carefully matched placebo-treated group. This rate was 16/315 (5.1%) for flecainide and 7/309 (2.3%) for its matched placebo. The average duration of treatment was 10 months.

As with other antiarrhythmics, there is no evidence that flecainide favorably affects survival or the incidence of sudden death.

➤*Ventricular proarrhythmic effects in patients with atrial fibrillation/flutter:* A review of the world literature revealed reports of 568 patients treated with oral flecainide for paroxysmal atrial fibrillation/flutter (PAF). Ventricular tachycardia was experienced in 0.4% (2/568) of these patients. Of 19 patients in the literature with chronic atrial fibrillation (CAF), 10.5% (2) experienced VT or VF. Flecainide is not recommended for use in patients with chronic atrial fibrillation. Case reports of ventricular proarrhythmic effects in patients treated with flecainide for atrial fibrillation/flutter have included increased PVCs, VT, VF and death.

As with other class I agents, patients treated with flecainide for atrial flutter have been reported with 1:1 atrioventricular conduction because of slowing the atrial rate. A paradoxical increase in the ventricular rate also may occur in patients with atrial fibrillation who receive flecainide. Concomitant negative chronotropic therapy such as digoxin or beta-blockers may lower the risk of this complication.

➤*Non-life-threatening ventricular arrhythmias:* The applicability of the CAST results to other populations (eg, those without recent infarction) is uncertain, but at present it is prudent to consider the risks of Class IC agents, coupled with the lack of any evidence of improved survival, generally unacceptable in patients whose ventricular arrhythmias are not life-threatening, even if the patients are experiencing unpleasant but not life-threatening symptoms or signs.

➤*Proarrhythmic effects:* Flecainide can cause new or worsened arrhythmias. Such proarrhythmic effects range from an increase in frequency of PVCs to the development of more severe ventricular tachycardia (eg, tachycardia that is more sustained or more resistant to conversion to sinus rhythm, with potentially fatal consequences. Three-fourths of proarrhythmic events were new or worsened ventricular tachyarrhythmias, the remainder being increased frequency of PVCs or new supraventricular arrhythmias.

The relatively high frequency of proarrhythmic events in patients with sustained ventricular tachycardia and serious underlying heart disease, and the need for titration and monitoring, requires that therapy of patients with sustained ventricular tachycardia be started in the hospital.

➤*Sick sinus syndrome:* Use only with extreme caution; the drug may cause sinus bradycardia, sinus pause or sinus arrest. The frequency probably increases with higher trough plasma levels, especially when they exceed 1 mcg/mL.

➤*Heart failure:* Flecainide has a negative inotropic effect and may cause or worsen CHF, particularly in patients with cardiomyopathy, preexisting severe heart failure (NYHA functional class III or IV) or low ejection fractions (< 30%). In patients with supraventricular arrhythmias, new or worsened CHF developed in 0.4% of patients. In patients with sustained ventricular tachycardia during a mean duration of 7.9 months of flecainide therapy, 6.3% developed new CHF. In patients with sustained ventricular tachycardia and a history of CHF in a mean duration of 5.4 months of therapy, 25.7% developed worsened CHF. Exacerbation of preexisting CHF occurred more commonly in studies including patients with Class III or IV failure than in studies which excluded such patients. Use cautiously in patients with a history of CHF or myocardial dysfunction. The initial dosage should be no more than 100 mg twice daily; monitor patients carefully. Give close attention to maintenance of cardiac function, including optimal digitalis, diuretic or other therapy. Where CHF has developed or worsened during treatment, the time of onset has ranged from a few hours to several months after starting therapy. Some patients who develop reduced myocardial function while on flecainide can continue with adjustment of digitalis or diuretics; others may require dosage reduction or discontinuation of flecainide. When feasible, monitor plasma flecainide levels. Keep trough plasma levels less than 0.7 to 1 mcg/mL.

➤*Cardiac conduction:* Flecainide slows cardiac conduction in most patients to produce dose-related increases in PR, QRS and QT intervals.

➤*Electrolyte disturbance:* Hypokalemia or hyperkalemia may alter the effects of Class I antiarrhythmic drugs. Correct preexisting hypokalemia or hyperkalemia before administration.

➤*Effects on pacemaker thresholds:* Flecainide increases endocardial pacing thresholds and may suppress ventricular escape rhythms. Effects are reversible if flecainide is discontinued. Use with caution in patients with permanent pacemakers or temporary pacing electrodes. Do not administer to patients with existing poor thresholds or nonprogrammable pacemakers unless suitable pacing rescue is available.

Determine the pacing threshold in patients with pacemakers prior to instituting therapy, after 1 week of administration and at regular intervals thereafter. Generally, threshold changes are within the range of multiprogrammable pacemakers, and a doubling of either voltage or pulse width is usually sufficient to regain capture.

➤*Urinary pH:* Flecainide elimination is altered by urinary pH; alkalinization (as may occur in rare conditions such as renal tubular acidosis or strict vegetarian diet) decreases, and acidification increases flecainide renal excretion. These alterations in pH (outside a range of pH 5 to 7) may produce toxic or subtherapeutic plasma levels.

➤*Hepatic function impairment:* Because flecainide elimination from plasma can be markedly slower in patients with significant hepatic impairment, do not use in such patients unless the potential benefits outweigh the risks. If used, frequent and early plasma level monitoring is required to

FLECAINIDE ACETATE — ORAL

guide dosage; make dosage increases very cautiously when plasma levels have plateaued (after more than 4 days).

➤*Elderly:* From age 20 to 80, plasma levels are only slightly higher with advancing age; flecainide elimination from plasma is somewhat slower in elderly subjects than in younger subjects. Patients up to age 80 and above have been safely treated with usual doses.

➤*Pregnancy: Category C.* Flecainide had teratogenic and embryotoxic effects in one breed of rabbit when given in doses up to 35 mg/kg/day. There are no adequate and well controlled studies in pregnant women. Use during pregnancy only if potential benefits outweigh potential hazards to the fetus.

➤*Lactation:* Flecainide is excreted in breast milk in concentrations as high as 4 times (with average levels about 2.5 times) corresponding plasma levels; assuming a maternal plasma level at the top of the therapeutic range (1 mcg/mL), the calculated daily dose to a breast-feeding infant (assuming about 700 mL breast milk over 24 hours) would be less than 3 mg. Because of the drug's potential for serious adverse effects in infants, determine whether to discontinue nursing or discontinue the drug, taking into account the importance of the drug to the mother.

➤*Children:* Safety and efficacy for use in children younger than 18 years of age have not been established.

In pediatric patients with structural heart disease, flecainide has been associated with cardiac arrest and sudden death. Flecainide should be started in the hospital with rhythm monitoring. Any use of flecainide in children should be directly supervised by a cardiologist skilled in the treatment of arrhythmias in children.

Precautions

➤*Monitoring:* The majority of patients treated successfully had trough plasma levels between 0.2 and 1 mcg/mL. The probability of adverse experiences, especially cardiac, may increase with higher trough plasma levels, especially levels more than 1 mcg/mL. Monitor trough plasma levels periodically, especially in patients with severe or moderate chronic renal failure or severe hepatic disease and CHF, as drug elimination may be slower.

Drug Interactions

➤*CYP450 system:* Drugs that inhibit CYP2D6 (such as quinidine) may increase the plasma concentrations of flecainide in patients who are on chronic flecainide therapy, especially if these patients are extensive metabolizers.

Flecainide Drug Interactions

Precipitant drug	Object drug*		Description
Amiodarone	Flecainide	↑	Flecainide plasma levels may be increased.
Cimetidine	Flecainide	↑	Flecainide plasma levels and half-life may be increased.
Cisapride	Flecainide	↑	The risk of life-threatening cardiac arrhythmias, including torsades de pointes, may be increased due to possibly additive prolongation of the QT interval.
Flecainide	Cisapride		
Disopyramide	Flecainide	↑	Disopyramide has negative inotropic properties; do not use with flecainide unless benefits outweigh risks.
Propranolol	Flecainide	↑	Flecainide and propranolol levels were increased in healthy subjects. Negative inotropic effects were additive; effects on PR interval were less than additive.
Flecainide	Propranolol	↑	
Ritonavir	Flecainide	↑	Coadministration may produce large increases in serum flecainide concentrations. Ritonavir is contraindicated in patients receiving flecainide.
Urinary acidifiers	Flecainide	↓	Alterations in urinary excretion and plasma elimination of flecainide occur with changes in urinary pH (acidic urine increases elimination and decreases bioavailability; alkaline urine decreases elimination and increases bioavailability).
Urinary alkalinizers	Flecainide	↑	

Flecainide Drug Interactions

Precipitant drug	Object drug*		Description
Verapamil	Flecainide	↑	Verapamil has negative inotropic properties; do not use with flecainide unless benefits outweigh risks.
Flecainide	Digoxin	↑	Digoxin's absorption, peak concentration and bioavailability may be increased.

* ↑ = Object drug increased. ↓ = Object drug decreased.

➤*Drug/Food interactions:* Milk may inhibit absorption in infants. A reduction in flecainide dosage should be considered when milk is removed from the diet of infants.

Adverse Reactions

Most frequent – Dizziness (18.9%), including light-headedness, faintness, unsteadiness and near syncope; dyspnea (10.3%); headache (9.6%); nausea (8.9%); fatigue (7.7%); palpitation (6.1%); chest pain (5.4%); asthenia (4.9%); tremor (4.7%); constipation (4.4%); edema (3.5%); abdominal pain (3.3%).

➤*Cardiovascular:* New or worsened arrhythmias; episodes of unresuscitatable VT or ventricular fibrillation (cardiac arrest); new or worsened CHF; second-degree (0.5%) or third-degree (0.4%) AV block; sinus bradycardia, sinus pause or sinus arrest (1.2%); tachycardia (1% to 3%); angina pectoris, bradycardia, hypertension, hypotension (less than 1%).

In post-MI patients with asymptomatic PVCs and nonsustained ventricular tachycardia, flecainide therapy was associated with a 5.1% rate of death and nonfatal cardiac arrest, compared with a 2.3% rate in a matched placebo group.

➤*CNS:* Hypesthesia, paresthesia, paresis, ataxia, flushing, increased sweating, vertigo, syncope, somnolence, tinnitus, anxiety, insomnia, depression, malaise (1% to 3%); twitching, weakness, convulsions, neuropathy, speech disorder, stupor, amnesia, confusion, euphoria, depersonalization, morbid dreams, apathy (less than 1%).

➤*Dermatologic:* Rash (1% to 3%); urticaria, exfoliative dermatitis, pruritus, alopecia (less than 1%).

➤*GI:* Vomiting, diarrhea, dyspepsia, anorexia (1% to 3%); flatulence, change in taste, dry mouth (less than 1%).

➤*GU:* Impotence, decreased libido, polyuria, urinary retention (less than 1%).

➤*Hematologic:* Leukopenia, thrombocytopenia (less than 1%).

➤*Ophthalmic:* Visual disturbances including blurred vision, difficulty in focusing, spots before eyes (15.9%); diplopia (1% to 3%); eye pain/irritation, photophobia, nystagmus (less than 1%).

➤*Miscellaneous:* Fever (1% to 3%); swollen lips, tongue and mouth, arthralgia, bronchospasm, myalgia (less than 1%).

Overdosage

➤*Symptoms:* Animal studies suggest that the following events might occur with overdosage: Lengthening of the PR interval; increase in the QRS duration, QT interval and amplitude of the T wave; reduction in heart rate and myocardial contractility; conduction disturbances; hypotension; death from respiratory failure or asystole.

➤*Treatment:* Treatment should be supportive and may include the following: Removal of unabsorbed drug from the GI tract (charcoal instillation appears to be effective in lowering flecainide plasma concentrations, even after an interval of 90 minutes from ingestion of flecainide); inotropic agents or cardiac stimulants such as dopamine, dobutamine or isoproterenol; mechanical ventilation; circulatory assists such as intra-aortic balloon pumping; transvenous pacing in the event of conduction block. Because of the drug's long plasma half-life (12 to 27 hours) and the possibility of nonlinear elimination kinetics at very high doses, these supportive treatments may need to be continued for extended periods of time. Since flecainide elimination is much slower when urine is very alkaline (pH ≥ 8), theoretically, acidification of urine to promote drug excretion may be beneficial in overdose cases with very alkaline urine. There is no evidence that acidification from normal urinary pH increases excretion. Hemodialysis is not effective. Refer to General Management of Acute Overdosage.

Patient Information

Take as prescribed; serious heart disturbances can result from missing doses, and serious side effects can result from increasing or decreasing doses without supervision.

MEXILETINE HYDROCHLORIDE

Rx	**Mexitil** (Boehringer Ingelheim)	**Capsules:** 150 mg	(BI 66). Red and caramel. In 100s and UD 100s.
		200 mg	(BI 67). Red. In 100s and UD 100s.
		250 mg	(BI 68). Red and aqua. In 100s and UD 100s.

MEXILETINE HYDROCHLORIDE — ORAL

Refer to the general introductory discussion concerning Antiarrhythmic Agents.

Indications

For the treatment of documented ventricular arrhythmias, such as sustained ventricular tachycardia, that, in the judgment of the physician, are life-threatening. Because of the proarrhythmic effects of mexiletine, its use with lesser arrhythmias is generally not recommended. Treatment of patients with asymptomatic ventricular premature contractions should be avoided.

Initiation of mexiletine treatment, as with other antiarrhythmic agents used to treat life-threatening arrhythmias, should be carried out in the hospital.

➤*Unlabeled uses:* The use of prophylactic mexiletine may significantly reduce the incidence of ventricular tachycardia and other ventricular arrhythmias in the acute phase of MI. However, mortality may not be reduced.

Treatment of diabetic neuropathy refractory to traditional therapies.

Administration and Dosage

➤*Approved by the FDA:* December 30, 1985.

The dosage of mexiletine must be individualized on the basis of response and tolerance, both of which are dose related. Administration with food or antacid is recommended. Initiate mexiletine therapy with 200 mg every 8 hours when rapid control of arrhythmia is not essential. A minimum of 2 to 3 days between dose adjustments is recommended. Dose may be adjusted in 50 or 100 mg increments up or down.

As with any antiarrhythmic drug, clinical and electrocardiographic evaluation (including Holter monitoring if necessary for evaluation) are needed to determine whether the desired antiarrhythmic effect has been obtained and to guide titration and dose adjustment.

Satisfactory control can be achieved in most patients by 200 to 300 mg given every 8 hours with food or antacid. If satisfactory response has not been achieved at 300 mg every 8 hours, and the patient tolerates mexiletine well, a dose of 400 mg every 8 hours may be tried. As the severity of CNS side effects increases with total daily dose, the dose should not exceed 1,200 mg/day.

➤*Loading dose:* When rapid control of ventricular arrhythmia is essential, an initial loading dose of 400 mg of mexiletine may be administered, followed by a 200 mg dose in 8 hours. Onset of therapeutic effect is usually observed within 30 minutes to 2 hours.

➤*Every 12-hour dosage schedule:* Some patients responding to mexiletine may be transferred to a 12-hour dosage schedule to improve convenience and compliance. If adequate suppression is achieved on a mexiletine dose of 300 mg or less every 8 hours, the same total daily dose may be given in divided doses every 12 hours while monitoring carefully the degree of suppression of ventricular ectopy. This dose may be adjusted up to a maximum of 450 mg every 12 hours to achieve the desired response.

➤*Transferring to mexiletine:* The following dosage schedule, based on theoretical considerations rather than experimental data, is suggested for transferring patients from other Class I oral antiarrhythmic agents to mexiletine:

Mexiletine treatment may be initiated with a 200 mg dose, and titrated to response as described above, 6 to 12 hours after the last dose of quinidine sulfate, 3 to 6 hours after the last dose of procainamide, 6 to 12 hours after the last dose of disopryramide or 8 to 12 hours after the last dose of tocainide.

In patients in whom withdrawal of the previous antiarrhythmic agent is likely to produce life-threatening arrhythmias, hospitalization of the patient is recommended.

When transferring from lidocaine to mexiletine, the lidocaine infusion should be stopped when the first oral dose of mexiletine is administered. The infusion line should be left open until suppression of the arrhythmia appears to be satisfactorily maintained. Consideration should be given to the similarity of the adverse effects of lidocaine and mexiletine and the possibility that they may be additive.

➤*Renal function impairment:* In general, patients with renal failure will require the usual doses of mexiletine. Patients with severe liver disease, however, may require lower doses and must be monitored closely. Similarly, marked, right-sided congestive heart failure can reduce hepatic metabolism and reduce the needed dose. Plasma level may also be affected by certain concomitant drugs.

➤*Storage/Stability:* Store at controlled room temperature 20° to 25°C (68° to 77°F).

Actions

➤*Pharmacology:* Mexiletine is a local anesthetic, antiarrhythmic agent, structurally similar to lidocaine, but orally active. In animal studies, mexiletine has been shown to be effective in the suppression of induced ventricular arrhythmias, including those induced by glycoside toxicity and coronary artery ligation. Mexiletine, like lidocaine, inhibits the inward sodium current, thus reducing the rate of rise of the action potential, Phase 0. Mexiletine decreased the effective refractory period (ERP) in Purkinje fibers. The decrease in ERP was of lesser magnitude than the decrease in action potential duration (APD), with a resulting increase in the ERP/APD ratio.

➤*Pharmacokinetics:*

Absorption – Mexiletine is well absorbed (approximately 90%) from the GI tract. Unlike lidocaine, its first-pass metabolism is low. Peak blood levels are reached in 2 to 3 hours.

The absorption rate of mexiletine is reduced in clinical situations such as acute myocardial infarction in which gastric emptying time is increased. Narcotics, atropine and magnesium-aluminum hydroxide have also been reported to slow the absorption of mexiletine. Metoclopramide has been reported to accelerate absorption.

Distribution – Mexiletine is 50% to 60% bound to plasma protein, with a volume of distribution of 5 to 7 L/kg.

Metabolism – Mexiletine is metabolized in the liver.

Several metabolites of mexiletine have shown minimal antiarrhythmic activity in animal models. The most active is the minor metabolite N-methylmexiletine, which is less than 20% as potent as mexiletine. The urinary excretion of N-methylmexiletine in man is less than 0.5%. Thus the therapeutic activity of mexiletine is due to the parent compound.

Excretion – Approximately 10% is excreted unchanged by the kidney. While urinary pH does not normally have much influence on elimination, marked changes in urinary pH influence the rate of excretion: acidification accelerates excretion, while alkalinization retards it.

In healthy subjects, the plasma elimination half-life of mexiletine is approximately 10 to 12 hours.

Mexiletine plasma levels of at least 0.5 mcg/mL are generally required for therapeutic response. An increase in the frequency of CNS adverse effects has been observed when plasma levels exceed 2 mcg/mL. Thus the therapeutic range is approximately 0.5 to 2 mcg/mL. Plasma levels within the therapeutic range can be attained with either 3 times daily or twice-daily dosing but peak to trough differences are greater with the latter regimen, creating the possibility of adverse effects at peak and arrhythmic escape at trough. Nevertheless, some patients may be transferred successfully to the twice-daily regimen. If adequate suppression is achieved on a mexiletine dose of 300 mg or less every 8 hours, the same total daily dose may be given in divided doses every 12 hours while monitoring carefully the degree of suppression of ventricular ectopy. This dose may be adjusted up to a maximum of 450 mg every 12 hours to achieve the desired response.

Special populations –

Renal function impairment: Consistent with the limited renal elimination of mexiletine, little change in the half-life has been detected in patients with reduced renal function. In 8 patients with creatinine clearance less than 10 mL/min, the mean plasma elimination half-life was 15.7 hours; in 7 patients with creatinine clearance between 11 to 40 mL/min, the mean half-life was 13.4 hours.

Hepatic function impairment: Hepatic impairment prolongs the elimination half-life of mexiletine. In 8 patients with moderate to severe liver disease, the mean half-life was approximately 25 hours.

Contraindications

Cardiogenic shock or preexisting second- or third-degree AV block (if no pacemaker is present).

Warnings

➤*Mortality:* Considering the known proarrhythmic properties of mexiletine and the lack of evidence of improved survival for any antiarrhythmic drug in patients without life-threatening arrhythmias, the use of mexiletine as well as other antiarrhythmic agents should be reserved for patients with life-threatening ventricular arrhythmia.

➤*Proarrhythmia:* Like other antiarrhythmics, mexiletine can cause worsening of arrhythmias. This has been uncommon in patients with less serious arrhythmias (frequent premature beats or nonsustained ventricular tachycardia), but is of greater concern in patients with life-threatening arrhythmias such as sustained ventricular tachycardia. In patients with such arrhythmias subjected to programmed electrical stimulation or to exercise provocation, 10% to 15% of patients had exacerbation of the arrhythmia, a rate not greater than that of other agents.

➤*Urinary pH:* Concurrent drug therapy or dietary regimens which may markedly alter urinary pH should be avoided during mexiletine therapy. The minor fluctuations in urinary pH associated with normal diet do not affect the excretion of mexiletine.

➤*Blood dyscrasias:* Among 10,867 patients treated with mexiletine in the compassionate-use program, marked leukopenia (neutrophils less than 1,000/mm^3) or agranulocytosis were seen in 0.06%, and milder depressions of leukocytes were seen in 0.08%, and thrombocytopenia was observed in 0.16%. Many of these patients were seriously ill and receiving concomitant medications with known hematologic adverse effects. Rechallenge with mexiletine in several cases was negative. Marked leukopenia or agranulocytosis did not occur in any patient receiving mexiletine alone; 5 of the 6 cases of agranulocytosis were associated with procainamide (sustained-release preparations in 4) and 1 with vinblastine. If significant hematologic changes are observed, the patient should be evaluated carefully, and, if warranted, mexiletine should be discontinued. Blood counts usually return to normal within 1 month of discontinuation.

➤*Hepatic effects:*

Acute liver injury – In postmarketing experience, abnormal liver function tests have been reported some in the first few weeks of therapy with mexiletine. Most of these have been observed in the setting of congestive heart failure or ischemia, and their relationship to mexiletine has not been established.

AST elevation and liver injury – In 3-month controlled trials, elevations of AST greater than 3 times the upper limit of normal occurred in about 1% of both mexiletine-treated and control patients. Approximately 2% of patients in the mexiletine compassionate use program had elevations of AST greater than or equal to 3 times the upper limit of normal. These elevations frequently occurred in association with identifiable clinical events and

MEXILETINE HYDROCHLORIDE — ORAL

therapeutic measures such as congestive heart failure, acute myocardial infarction, blood transfusions and other medications. These elevations were often asymptomatic and transient, usually not associated with elevated bilirubin levels and usually did not require discontinuation of therapy. Marked elevations of AST (greater than 1000 U/L) were seen before death in 4 patients with end-stage cardiac disease (severe congestive heart failure, cardiogenic shock).

Rare instances of severe liver injury, including hepatic necrosis, have been reported in association with mexiletine treatment. It is recommended that patients in whom an abnormal liver test has occurred, or who have signs or symptoms suggesting liver dysfunction, be evaluated carefully. If persistent or worsening elevation of hepatic enzymes is detected, consideration should be given to discontinuing therapy.

➤*Pregnancy: Category C.*

Teratogenic – Reproduction studies performed with mexiletine in rats, mice and rabbits at doses up to 4 times the maximum human oral dose (24 mg/kg in a 50 kg patient) revealed no evidence of teratogenicity or impaired fertility but did show an increase in fetal resorption. There are no adequate and well-controlled studies in pregnant women; this drug should be used in pregnancy only if the potential benefit justifies the potential risk to the fetus.

➤*Lactation:* Mexiletine appears in human milk in concentrations similar to those observed in plasma. Therefore, if the use of mexiletine is deemed essential, an alternative method of infant feeding should be considered.

➤*Children:* Safety and efficacy in the pediatric population have not been established.

Precautions

➤*Monitoring:* Because mexiletine is metabolized in the liver, and hepatic impairment has been reported to prolong the elimination half-life of mexiletine, patients with liver disease should be followed carefully while receiving mexiletine. The same caution should be observed in patients with hepatic dysfunction secondary to congestive heart failure.

➤*Seizures:* Convulsions (seizures) did not occur in mexiletine controlled clinical trials. In the compassionate-use program, convulsions were reported in about 2 of 1,000 patients. Twenty-eight percent (28%) of these patients discontinued therapy. Convulsions were reported in patients with and without a history of seizures. Mexiletine should be used with caution in patients with known seizure disorder.

➤*Special risk:* If a ventricular pacemaker is operative, patients with second- or third-degree heart block may be treated with mexiletine if monitored continuously. A limited number of patients (45 of 475 in controlled clinical trials) with preexisting first-degree AV block were treated with mexiletine; none of these patients developed second- or third-degree AV block. Caution should be exercised when it is used in such patients or in patients with preexisting sinus node dysfunction or intraventricular conduction abnormalities.

Mexiletine should be used with caution in patients with hypotension and severe congestive heart failure because of the potential for aggravating these conditions.

Drug Interactions

➤*CYP450 system:* Because mexiletine is a substrate for CYP2D6 and CYP1A2, inhibition or induction of either of these enzymes would be expected to alter mexiletine concentrations.

Mexiletine Drug Interactions

Precipitant drug	Object drug*		Description
Aluminum-Magnesium Hydroxide Atropine Narcotics	Mexiletine	↓	Mexiletine absorption may be slowed.
Cimetidine	Mexiletine	↔	Cimetidine may increase or decrease mexiletine plasma levels.
Fluvoxamine	Mexiletine	↑	The clearance of mexiletine was decreased by 38% following coadministration with fluvoxamine, a CYP1A2 inhibitor.
Hydantoins	Mexiletine	↓	Increased mexiletine clearance leading to lower steady-state plasma levels may occur.
Metoclopramide	Mexiletine	↑	Mexiletine absorption may be accelerated.
Propafenone	Mexiletine	↑	Mexiletine plasma concentrations may be elevated in extensive metabolizers due to propafenone inhibiting the metabolism (CYP2D6) of mexiletine. When mexiletine is initiated, slowly titrate the dose.
Rifampin	Mexiletine	↓	Increased mexiletine clearance leading to lower steady-state plasma levels may occur.
Urinary acidifiers	Mexiletine	↓	Renal clearance of mexiletine is related to urinary pH. In acidic urine, mexiletine clearance may be increased.
Urinary alkalinizers	Mexiletine	↑	Renal clearance of mexiletine is related to urinary pH. In alkaline urine, mexiletine clearance may be decreased.
Mexiletine	Caffeine	↑	Clearance of caffeine may be decreased by 50%
Mexiletine	Theophylline	↑	Serum theophylline levels may be increased; increased pharmacologic and toxic effects may occur.

* ↑ = Object drug increased. ↓ = Object drug decreased. ↔ = Undetermined clinical effect.

Adverse Reactions

Mexiletine commonly produces reversible GI and nervous system adverse reactions but is otherwise well tolerated. Mexiletine has been evaluated in 483 patients in 1- and 3-month controlled studies and in over 10,000 patients in a large, compassionate-use program. Dosages in the controlled studies ranged from 600 to 1200 mg/day; some patients (8%) in the compassionate-use program were treated with higher daily doses (1600 to 3200 mg/day). In the 3-month controlled trials comparing mexiletine to quinidine, procainamide and disopyramide, the most frequent adverse reactions were upper GI distress (41%), light-headedness (10.5%), tremor (12.6%) and coordination difficulties (10.2%). Similar frequency and incidence were observed in the 1-month placebo-controlled trial. Although these reactions were generally not serious, and were dose related and reversible with a reduction in dosage, by taking the drug with food or antacid or by therapy discontinuation, they led to therapy discontinuation in 40% of patients in the controlled trials.

Comparative Incidence (%) of Adverse Reactions Among Patients Treated with Mexiletine and Placebo in the 4-Week, Double-Blind Crossover Trial

	Mexiletine (n = 53)	Placebo (n = 49)
Cardiovascular		
Palpitations	7.5%	10.2%
Chest pain	7.5%	4.1%
Increased ventricular arrhythmia/PVCs	1.9%	—
CNS		
Dizziness/light-headedness	26.4%	14.3%
Tremor	13.2%	—
Nervousness	11.3%	6.1%
Coordination difficulties	9.4%	—
Changes in sleep habits	7.5%	16.3%
Paresthesias/numbness	3.8%	2%
Weakness	1.9%	4.1%
Fatigue	1.9%	2%
Tinnitus	1.9%	4.1%
Confusion/Clouded sensorium	1.9%	2%
GI		
Nausea/vomiting/heartburn	39.6%	6.1%
Miscellaneous		
Blurred vision/visual disturbances	7.5%	2%
Dyspnea/respiratory	5.7%	10.2%
Headache	7.5%	6.1%
Nonspecific edema	3.8%	—
Rash	3.8%	2%

Comparative Incidence (%) of Adverse Reactions Among Patients Treated with Mexiletine or Control Drugs in the 12-week Double-Blind Trials (≥ 1%)

	Mexiletine (n = 430)	Quinidine (n = 262)	Procainamide (n = 78)	Disopyramide (n = 69)
Cardiovascular				
Palpitations	4.3%	4.6%	1.3%	5.8%
Chest pain	2.6%	3.4%	1.3%	2.9%
Angina/angina-like pain	1.7%	1.9%	2.6%	2.9%
Increased ventricular arrhythmias/PVCs	1%	2.7%	2.6%	—
CNS				
Dizziness/light-headedness	18.9%	14.1%	14.1%	2.9%
Tremor	13.2%	2.3%	3.8%	1.4%
Coordination difficulties	9.7%	1.1%	1.3%	

MEXILETINE HYDROCHLORIDE — ORAL

Comparative Incidence (%) of Adverse Reactions Among Patients Treated with Mexiletine or Control Drugs in the 12-week Double-Blind Trials (≥ 1%)

	Mexiletine (n = 430)	Quinidine (n = 262)	Procainamide (n = 78)	Disopyramide (n = 69)
Changes in sleep habits	7.1%	2.7%	11.5%	8.7%
Weakness	5%	5.3%	7.7%	2.9%
Nervousness	5%	1.9%	6.4%	5.8%
Fatigue	3.8%	5.7%	5.1%	1.4%
Speech difficulties	2.6%	0.4%	—	—
Confusion/ Clouded sensorium	2.6%	—	3.8%	—
Paresthesias/ numbness	2.4%	2.3%	2.6%	—
Tinnitus	2.4%	1.5%	—	—
Depression	2.4%	1.1%	1.3%	1.4%
GI				
Nausea/ vomiting/ heartburn	39.3%	21.4%	33.3%	14.5%
Diarrhea	5.2%	33.2%	2.6%	8.7%
Constipation	4%	—	6.4%	11.6%
Changes in appetite	2.6%	1.9%	—	—
Abdominal pain/ cramps/ discomfort	1.2%	1.5%	—	1.4%
Miscellaneous				
Blurred vision/ Visual disturbances	5.7%	3.1%	5.1%	7.2%
Headache	5.7%	6.9%	7.7%	4.3%
Rash	4.2%	3.8%	10.3%	1.4%
Dyspnea/ respiratory	3.3%	3.1%	5.1%	2.9%
Dry mouth	2.8%	1.9%	5.1%	14.5%
Arthralgia	1.7%	2.3%	5.1%	1.4%
Fever	1.2%	3.1%	2.6%	—

➤*Less than 1%:* Syncope, edema, hot flashes, hypertension, short-term memory loss, loss of consciousness, other psychological changes, diaphoresis, urinary hesitancy/retention, malaise, impotence/decreased libido, pharyngitis, congestive heart failure.

➤*Treatment under compassionate-use circumstances:* An additional group of over 10,000 patients has been treated in a program allowing administration of mexiletine under compassionate-use circumstances. These patients were seriously ill, with the large majority on multiple drug therapy. Twenty-four percent (24%) of the patients continued in the program for 1 year or longer. Adverse reactions leading to therapy discontinuation occurred in 15% of patients (usually upper GI system or nervous system effects). In general, the more common adverse reactions were similar to those in the controlled trials. Less common adverse events possibly related to mexiletine use include the following:

Cardiovascular – Syncope and hypotension, each about 6 in 1000; bradycardia, about 4 in 1000; angina/angina-like pain, about 3 in 1000; edema, atrioventricular block/conduction disturbances and hot flashes, each about 2 in 1000; atrial arrhythmias, hypertension and cardiogenic shock, each about 1 in 1000.

CNS – Short-term memory loss, about 9 in 1000 patients; hallucinations and other psychological changes, each about 3 in 1000; psychosis and convulsions/seizures, each about 2 in 1000; loss of consciousness, about 6 in 10,000.

Dermatologic – Rare cases of exfoliative dermatitis and Stevens-Johnson syndrome with mexiletine treatment have been reported.

GI – Dysphagia, about 2 in 1000; peptic ulcer, about 8 in 10,000; upper GI bleeding, about 7 in 10,000; esophageal ulceration, about 1 in 10,000. Rare cases of severe hepatitis/acute hepatic necrosis.

Hematologic – Blood dyscrasias were not seen in the controlled trials but did occur among 10,867 patients treated with mexiletine in the compassionate-use program.

Myelofibrosis was reported in 2 patients in the compassionate-use program: 1 was receiving long-term thiotepa therapy, and the other had pretreatment myeloid abnormalities.

Lab test abnormalities – Abnormal liver function tests, about 5 in 1,000 patients; positive ANA and thrombocytopenia, each about 2 in 1,000; leukopenia (including neutropenia and agranulocytosis), about 1 in 1,000; myelofibrosis, about 2 in 10,000 patients.

Miscellaneous – Diaphoresis, about 6 in 1,000; altered taste, about 5 in 1,000; salivary changes, hair loss and impotence/decreased libido, each about 4 in 1000; malaise, about 3 in 1,000; urinary hesitancy/retention, each about 2 in 1,000; hiccups, dry skin, laryngeal and pharyngeal changes and changes in oral mucous membranes, each about 1 in 1,000; SLE syndrome, about 4 in 10,000.

➤*Postmarketing:* In postmarketing experience, there have been isolated, spontaneous reports of pulmonary changes including pulmonary fibrosis during mexiletine therapy with or without other drugs or diseases that are known to produce pulmonary toxicity. A causal relationship to mexiletine therapy has not been established. In addition, there have been isolated reports of exacerbation of congestive heart failure in patients with preexisting compromised ventricular function. There have been rare reports of pancreatitis associated with mexiletine treatment.

Overdosage

➤*Symptoms:* Clinical findings associated with mexiletine overdosage have included nausea, hypotension, sinus bradycardia, paresthesia, seizures, bundle branch block, AV heart block, asystole, ventricular tachyarrythmia, including ventricular fibrillation, cardiovascular collapse and coma. The lowest known dose in a fatality case was 4.4 g, with postmortem serum mexiletine level of 34 to 37 mcg/mL. Patients have recovered from ingestion of 4 to 18 g of mexiletine.

➤*Treatment:* There is no specific antidote for mexiletine. Management of mexiletine overdosage includes general supportive measures, close observation and monitoring of vital signs. In addition, the use of pharmacologic interventions (eg, pressor agents, atropine, anticonvulsants) or transvenous cardiac pacing is suggested, depending on the patient's clinical condition.

Patient Information

Take medication with food or an antacid.

Adverse effects such as nausea, vomiting, heartburn, diarrhea, constipation, dizziness, tremor, nervousness, coordination difficulties, changes in sleep habits, headache, visual disturbances, tingling/numbness, weakness, ringing in the ears and palpitations/chest pain may occur. Notify physician if they become bothersome.

Notify physician if signs of liver injury or blood cell damage occur, such as unexplained general tiredness, jaundice, fever or sore throat.

Avoid changes in diet that could drastically acidify or alkalinize the urine.

PROPAFENONE HYDROCHLORIDE

Rx	**Propafenone** (Various, eg, Watson)	**Tablets:** 150 mg	In 100s and 500s.
Rx	**Rythmol** (Reliant)		(150). White, scored. Film coated. In 100s and UD 100s.
Rx	**Propafenone** (Various, eg, Watson)	225 mg	In 100s and 500s.
Rx	**Rythmol** (Reliant)		(225). Tan, scored. Film coated. In 100s and UD 100s.
Rx	**Propafenone** (Various, eg, Ethex, Mutual, URL)	300 mg	In 100s.
Rx	**Rythmol** (Reliant)		(300). White, scored. Film coated. In 100s and UD 100s.
Rx	**Rythmol SR** (Reliant)	**Capsules, extended-release:** 225 mg	(a 225). White. In 100s.
		325 mg	(a 325). White. In 100s.
		425 mg	(a 425). White. In 100s.

PROPAFENONE HYDROCHLORIDE — ORAL

Refer to the general introductory discussion concerning Antiarrhythmic Agents.

WARNING

In the National Heart, Lung, and Blood Institute's Cardiac Arrhythmia Suppression Trial (CAST), a long-term, multicenter, randomized, double-blind study in patients with asymptomatic non-life-threatening ventricular arrhythmias who had an MI more than 6 days but less than 2 years previously, an increased rate of death or reversed cardiac arrest rate (7.7%) was seen in patients treated with encainide or flecainide (Class 1C antiarrhythmics) compared with that seen in patients assigned to placebo (3%). The average duration of treatment with encainide or flecainide in this study was 10 months.

The applicability of the CAST results to other populations (eg, those without recent MI) or other antiarrhythmic drugs is uncertain, but at present, it is prudent to consider any 1C antiarrhythmic to have a significant risk in patients with structural heart disease. Given the lack of any evidence that these drugs improve survival, antiarrhythmic agents should generally be avoided in patients with nonlife-threatening ventricular arrhythmias, even if the patients are experiencing unpleasant, but not life-threatening symptoms or signs.

Indications

➤*Atrial fibrillation/flutter:*

Immediate-release (IR) – To prolong the time to recurrence of paroxysmal atrial fibrillation/flutter associated with disabling symptoms in patients without structural heart disease.

Some patients with atrial flutter treated with propafenone have developed 1:1 conduction, producing an increase in ventricular rate. Concomitant treatment with drugs that increase the functional AV refractory period is recommended.

Extended-release (ER) – To prolong the time to recurrence of symptomatic atrial fibrillation in patients with structural heart disease.

➤*Paroxysmal supraventricular tachycardia (PSVT) (IR only):* To prolong the time to recurrence of PSVT associated with disabling symptoms in patients without structural heart disease.

➤*Ventricular arrhythmias (IR only):* For the treatment of ventricular arrhythmias, such as sustained ventricular tachycardia, that are life-threatening. Because of the proarrhythmic effects of propafenone, its use with lesser ventricular arrhythmias is not recommended, even if patients are symptomatic, and reserve any use of the drug for patients in whom the potential benefits outweigh the risks.

Propafenone, like other antiarrhythmic drugs, has not been shown to enhance survival in patients with ventricular or atrial arrhythmias.

Administration and Dosage

➤*Approved by the FDA:* 1989.

➤*IR:* Individually titrate on the basis of response and tolerance. Initiate with 150 mg every 8 hours (450 mg/day). Dosage may be increased at a minimum of 3- to 4-day intervals to 225 mg every 8 hours (675 mg/day) and, if necessary, to 300 mg every 8 hours (900 mg/day). The safety and efficacy of dosages exceeding 900 mg/day have not been established. In those patients in whom significant widening of the QRS complex or second- or third-degree AV block occurs, consider dose reduction.

As with other antiarrhythmics, in the elderly or patients with marked previous myocardial damage, increase dose more gradually during initial treatment phase.

➤*ER:* Individually titrate on the basis of response and tolerance. Therapy should be initiated with 225 mg given every 12 hours. Dosage may be increased at a minimum of 5-day intervals to 325 mg given every 12 hours. If additional therapeutic effect is needed, the dose may be increased to 425 mg given every 12 hours.

In patients with hepatic function impairment or having significant widening of the QRS complex or second or third degree AV block, dose reduction should be considered.

The SR capsules can be taken with or without food. Do not crush or further divide the contents of the capsule.

Actions

➤*Pharmacology:* Propafenone is a Class IC antiarrhythmic with local anesthetic effects and direct stabilizing action on myocardial membranes. Propafenone's electrophysiologic effect manifests itself in a reduction of upstroke velocity (Phase 0) of the monophasic action potential. In Purkinje fibers, and to a lesser extent myocardial fibers, propafenone reduces fast inward current carried by sodium ions. Diastolic excitability threshold is increased and effective refractory period prolonged. Propafenone reduces spontaneous automaticity and depresses triggered activity.

➤*Pharmacokinetics:*

Absorption/Distribution – Propafenone is nearly completely absorbed after oral administration with peak plasma levels occurring approximately 3.5 hours after administration in most individuals. It exhibits extensive first-pass metabolism resulting in a dose-dependent and dosage-form-dependent absolute bioavailability (eg, a 150 mg tablet had absolute bioavailability of 3.4%, a 300 mg tablet 10.6% and 300 mg solution 21.4%). Bioavailability increases further at doses above those recommended. Propafenone follows a nonlinear pharmacokinetic disposition presumably due to saturation of first-pass hepatic metabolism as the liver is exposed to higher concentrations of propafenone and shows a very high degree of interindividual variability. For example, for a threefold increase in daily dose from 300 to 900 mg/day, there is a tenfold increase in steady-state plasma concentration.

Metabolism/Excretion – There are two genetically determined patterns of propafenone metabolism. In more than 90% of patients, the drug is rapidly and extensively metabolized with an elimination half-life of 2 to 10 hours. These patients metabolize propafenone into two active metabolites: 5-hydroxypropafenone (formed by CYP2D6) and N-depropylpropafenone (formed by CYP3A4 and CYP1A2). In vitro, these metabolites have antiarrhythmic activity comparable to propafenone, but in man they both are usually present in concentrations less than 20% of propafenone. Nine additional metabolites have been identified, most in only trace amounts. The saturable hydroxylation pathway is responsible for the nonlinear pharmacokinetic disposition.

In fewer than 10% of patients, propafenone metabolism is slower because the 5-hydroxy metabolite is not formed or is minimally formed. The estimated propafenone elimination half-life ranges from 10 to 32 hours. In these patients, the N-depropylpropafenone is present in quantities comparable to the levels measured in extensive metabolizers. In slow metabolizers, propafenone pharmacokinetics are linear.

There are significant differences in plasma concentrations of propafenone in slow and extensive metabolizers, the former achieving concentrations 1.5 to 2 times those of the extensive metabolizers at daily doses of 675 to 900 mg/day. At low doses the differences are greater, with slow metabolizers attaining concentrations more than 5 times those of extensive metabolizers. Because the difference decreases at high doses and is mitigated by the lack of the active 5-hydroxy metabolite in the slow metabolizers, and because steady-state conditions are achieved after 4 to 5 days of dosing, the recommended dosing regimen is the same for all patients. Titrate dosage carefully with close attention to clinical and ECG evidence of toxicity. In addition, the beta-blocking action of propafenone appears to be enhanced in slow metabolizers.

Special populations –

Hepatic function impairment: Bioavailability increases and the clearance of propafenone is reduced and the elimination half-life increased in patients with significant hepatic dysfunction (see Warnings).

Contraindications

Uncontrolled CHF; cardiogenic shock; sinoatrial, AV and intraventricular disorders of impulse generation or conduction (eg, sick sinus node syndrome, AV block) in the absence of an artificial pacemaker; bradycardia; marked hypotension; bronchospastic disorders; manifest electrolyte imbalance; hypersensitivity to the drug.

Warnings

➤*Mortality:* See the Warning box for more information.

➤*Proarrhythmic effects:* Propafenone, like other antiarrhythmic agents, may cause new or worsened arrhythmias. Such proarrhythmic effects range from an increase in frequency of PVCs to the development of more severe ventricular tachycardia, ventricular fibrillation or torsades de pointes (ie, tachycardia that is more sustained or more rapid), which may lead to fatal consequences. It may also worsen premature ventricular contractions or supraventricular arrhythmias, and it may prolong the QT interval. It is therefore essential that each patient be evaluated electrocardiographically and clinically prior to, and during therapy to determine whether response to propafenone supports continued use. Because propafenone prolongs the QRS interval in the electrocardiogram, changes in the QT interval are difficult to interpret.

➤*Non-life-threatening arrhythmias:* Use of propafenone is not recommended in patients with less severe ventricular arrhythmias, even if the patients are symptomatic.

➤*Survival:* There is no evidence from controlled trials that the use of propafenone favorably affects survival or the incidence of sudden death.

➤*Nonallergic bronchospasm (eg, chronic bronchitis, emphysema):* In general, these patients should not receive propafenone or other agents with beta-adrenergic blocking activity.

➤*Congestive heart failure (CHF):* New or worsened CHF has occurred in 3.7% of patients with ventricular arrhythmia; of those, 0.9% were probably or definitely related to propafenone. Of the patients with CHF probably related to propafenone, 80% had preexisting heart failure and 85% had coronary artery disease. CHF attributable to propafenone developed rarely (less than 0.2%) in patients who had no previous history of CHF.

As propafenone exerts both beta blockade and a (dose-related) negative inotropic effect on cardiac muscle, patients with CHF should be fully compensated before receiving propafenone. If CHF worsens, discontinue propafenone unless CHF is due to the cardiac arrhythmia and, if indicated, restart at a lower dosage only after adequate cardiac compensation has been established.

➤*Conduction disturbances:* Propafenone slows AV conduction and also causes first degree AV block. Average PR interval prolongation and increases in QRS duration are closely correlated with dosage increases and concomitant increases in propafenone plasma concentrations. The incidence of first-, second- and third-degree AV block observed in 2127 ventricular arrhythmia patients was 2.5%, 0.6% and 0.2%, respectively. Development of second- or third-degree AV block requires a reduction in dosage or discontinuation of propafenone. Bundle branch block (1.2%) and intraventricular conduction delay (1.1%) have occurred in patients receiving propafenone. Bradycardia has also occurred (1.5%). Experience in patients with sick sinus node syndrome is limited and these patients should not be treated with propafenone.

PROPAFENONE HYDROCHLORIDE — ORAL

Propafenone should not be given to patients with atrioventricular and intraventricular conduction defects in the absence of a pacemaker (see Contraindications).

➤*Effects on pacemaker threshold:* Pacing and sensing thresholds of artificial pacemakers may be altered. Monitor and program pacemakers accordingly during therapy.

➤*Hematologic disturbances:* Agranulocytosis (fever, chills, weakness, and neutropenia) has been reported in patients receiving propafenone. Generally, the agranulocytosis occurred within the first 2 months of propafenone therapy and upon discontinuation of therapy, the white count usually normalized by 14 days. Unexplained fever and/or decrease in white cell count, particularly during the first 3 months of therapy, warrants consideration of possible agranulocytosis/granulocytopenia. Instruct patients to promptly report the development of any signs of infection such as fever, sore throat or chills.

➤*Renal function impairment:* A considerable percentage of propafenone metabolites (18.5% to 38% of the dose/48 hours) are excreted in the urine. Administer cautiously to patients with impaired renal function. Carefully monitor for signs of overdosage.

➤*Hepatic function impairment:* Propafenone is highly metabolized by the liver; administer cautiously to patients with impaired hepatic function. Severe liver dysfunction increases the bioavailability of propafenone to approximately 70%, compared to 3% to 40% for patients with normal liver function; the mean half-life is approximately 9 hours. The dose of propafenone should be approximately 20% to 30% of the dose given to patients with normal hepatic function. Carefully monitor for excessive pharmacological effects.

➤*Fertility impairment:* IV propafenone decreases spermatogenesis in rabbits, dogs and monkeys. These effects were reversible, were not found following oral dosing and were seen only at lethal or sublethal dose levels.

➤*Elderly:* Because of the possible increased risk of impaired hepatic or renal function in this age group, use with caution. The effective dose may be lower in these patients.

➤*Pregnancy: Category C.* Propafenone is embryotoxic in rabbits and rats when given in doses 3 and 6 times, respectively, the maximum recommended human dose. There are no adequate and well controlled studies in pregnant women. Use during pregnancy only if the potential benefit justifies the potential risk to the fetus.

➤*Lactation:* Propafenone is excreted in breast milk. Decide whether to discontinue nursing or to discontinue the drug, taking into account the importance of the drug to the mother.

➤*Children:* The safety and efficacy of propafenone in children have not been established.

Precautions

➤*Elevated ANA titers:* Positive ANA titers have occurred. They have been reversible upon cessation of treatment and may disappear even with continued therapy. These laboratory findings were usually not associated with clinical symptoms, but there is one case of drug-induced lupus erythematosus (positive rechallenge); it resolved completely upon therapy discontinuation. Carefully evaluate patients who develop an abnormal ANA test and, if persistent or worsening elevation of ANA titers is detected, consider discontinuing therapy.

➤*Renal/Hepatic changes:* Renal changes have been observed in the rat following 6 months of oral administration of propafenone at doses of 180 and 360 mg/kg/day (2 to 4 times the maximum recommended human dose). Both inflammatory and noninflammatory changes in the renal tubules with accompanying interstitial nephritis were observed. These lesions were reversible in that they were not found in rats treated at these dosage levels and allowed to recover for 6 weeks. Fatty degenerative changes of the liver were found in rats following chronic administration of propafenone at dose levels 3 times the maximum recommended human dose.

➤*Neuromuscular dysfunction:* Exacerbation of myasthenia gravis has been reported during propafenone therapy.

Drug Interactions

➤*CYP-450 system:* Drugs that inhibit CYP2D6, CYP1A2, and CYP3A4 might lead to increased plasma levels of propafenone. When propafenone is administered with inhibitors of these enzymes, closely monitor patients and adjust dose accordingly.

Propafenone Drug Interactions			
Precipitant drug	Object drug *		Description
Anesthetics, local	Propafenone	↑	Concurrent use (ie, during pacemaker implantations, surgery or dental use) may increase the risks of CNS side effects.
Cimetidine	Propafenone	↑	The maximum propafenone concentration may be increased, possibly resulting in increased pharmacologic effects.
Cisapride	Propafenone	↑	The risk of life-threatening cardiac arrhythmias, including torsades de pointes, may be increased due to possibly additive prolongation of the QT interval.
Propafenone	Cisapride		
Quinidine	Propafenone	↑	Serum propafenone levels may be increased in rapid, extensive metabolizers of the drug, possibly increasing the pharmacologic effects.
Rifamycins	Propafenone	↓	Increased propafenone clearance may occur, resulting in decreased plasma levels and a possible loss of therapeutic effect.
Ritonavir	Propafenone	↑	Coadministration may produce large increases in serum propafenone concentrations. Ritonavir is contraindicated in patients receiving propafenone.
SSRIs (eg, fluoxetine)	Propafenone	↑	Plasma propafenone levels may be elevated. Certain SSRIs may inhibit the metabolism (CYP2D6) of propafenone.
Propafenone	Anticoagulants	↑	Increased warfarin plasma levels and prothrombin time may occur.
Propafenone	Beta-blockers	↑	The plasma levels and pharmacologic effects of beta blockers metabolized by the liver may be increased.
Propafenone	Cyclosporine	↑	Increased whole blood cyclosporine trough levels and decreased renal function may occur.
Propafenone	Desipramine	↑	Coadministration may result in elevated serum desipramine levels.
Propafenone	Digoxin	↑	Serum digoxin levels may be increased, resulting in toxicity.
Propafenone	Mexiletine	↑	Mexiletine plasma concentrations may be elevated in extensive metabolizers due to propafenone inhibiting the metabolism (CYP2D6) of mexiletine.
Propafenone	Theophylline	↑	Propafenone may increase theophylline concentrations, possibly resulting in toxicity.

* ↑ = Object drug increased. ↓ = Object drug decreased.

➤*Drug/Food interactions:* Although food increased the peak blood level and bioavailability of propafenone in a single dose study, food did not change bioavailability significantly during multiple dose administration.

Adverse Reactions

Propafenone Adverse Reactions (%)[a]							
	Incidence by total daily dose					Incidence vs placebo	
Adverse reaction	450 mg (n = 1430)	600 mg (n = 1337)	≥ 900 mg (n = 1333)	Total incidence (n = 2127)	% of patients who discontinued	Propafenone (n = 247)	Placebo (n = 111)
Cardiovascular							
Angina	1.7	2.1	3.2	4.6	0.5	1.2	—
Atrial fibrillation	0.7	0.7	0.5	1.2	0.4	—	—
AV block, first-degree	0.8	1.2	2.1	2.5	0.3	4.5	0.9
AV block, second-degree	—	—	—	—	—	1.2	—
Bradycardia	0.5	0.8	1.1	1.5	0.5	—	—
Bundle branch block	0.3	0.7	1	1.2	0.5	1.2	—
Chest pain	0.5	0.7	1.4	1.8	0.2	—	—
CHF	0.8	2.2	2.6	3.7	1.4	—	—
Hypotension	0.1	0.5	1	1.1	0.4	—	—
Intraventricular conduction delay	0.2	0.7	0.9	1.1	0.1	4	—
Palpitations	0.6	1.6	2.6	3.4	0.5	2.4	0.9
Proarrhythmia	2	2.1	2.9	4.7	4.7	1.2	—
PVCs	0.6	0.6	1.1	1.5	0.1	—	—
QRS duration, increased	0.5	0.9	1.7	1.9	0.5	—	—
Syncope	0.8	1.3	1.4	2.2	0.7	—	—
Ventricular tachycardia	1.4	1.6	2.9	3.4	1.2	—	—

PROPAFENONE HYDROCHLORIDE — ORAL

Propafenone Adverse Reactions (%)[a]

Adverse reaction	Incidence by total daily dose			Total incidence (n = 2127)	% of patients who discontinued	Incidence vs placebo	
	450 mg (n = 1430)	600 mg (n = 1337)	≥ 900 mg (n = 1333)			Propafenone (n = 247)	Placebo (n = 111)
CNS							
Anorexia	0.5	0.7	1.6	1.7	0.4	1.6	0.9
Anxiety	0.7	0.5	0.9	1.5	0.6	2	1.8
Ataxia	0.3	0.6	1.5	1.6	0.2	—	—
Dizziness	3.6	6.6	11	12.5	2.4	6.5	5.4
Drowsiness	0.6	0.5	0.7	1.2	0.2	—	—
Fatigue	1.8	2.8	4.1	6	1	—	—
Headache	1.5	2.5	2.8	4.5	1	4.5	4.5
Insomnia	0.3	1.3	0.7	1.5	0.3	—	—
Loss of balance	—	—	—	—	—	1.2	—
Tremor	0.3	0.8	1.1	1.4	0.3	—	—
GI							
Abdominal pain/ cramps	0.8	0.9	1.1	1.7	0.4	—	—
Constipation	2	4.1	5.3	7.2	0.5	4	—
Diarrhea	0.5	1.6	1.7	2.5	0.6	1.2	0.9
Dry mouth	0.9	1	1.4	2.4	0.2	2	0.9
Dyspepsia	1.3	1.7	2.5	3.4	0.9	—	—
Flatulence	0.3	0.7	0.9	1.2	0.1	1.2	—
Nausea/vomiting	2.4	6.1	8.9	10.7	3.4	2.8	0.9
Unusual taste	2.5	4.9	6.3	8.8	0.7	7.3	0.9
Other							
Blurred vision	0.6	2.4	3.1	3.8	0.8	2	0.9
Diaphoresis	0.6	0.4	1.1	1.4	0.3	—	—
Dyspnea	2.2	2.3	3.6	5.3	1.6	2	2.7
Edema	0.6	0.4	1	1.4	0.2	—	—
Pain, joints	0.2	0.4	0.9	1	0.1	—	—
Rash	0.6	1.4	1.9	2.6	0.8	—	—
Weakness	0.6	1.6	1.7	2.4	0.7	—	—

[a] Data are pooled from separate studies and are not necessarily comparable.

Adverse reactions occur most frequently in the GI, cardiovascular and CNS. About 20% of patients discontinued treatment due to adverse reactions. The most common events were dizziness, unusual taste, first-degree AV block, intraventricular conduction delay, nausea or vomiting and constipation. Headache was common, but not increased compared to placebo.

The most common adverse reactions appeared to be dose-related, especially dizziness, nausea or vomiting, unusual taste, constipation and blurred vision. Some less common reactions may also have been dose-related, such as first degree AV block, CHF, dyspepsia and weakness.

In addition to the reactions listed in the table, the following adverse reactions were reported (< 1%) either in clinical trials or in marketing experience (causal relationship not determined).

➤*Cardiovascular:* Atrial flutter; AV dissociation; cardiac arrest; flushing; hot flashes; sick sinus syndrome; sinus pause or arrest; supraventricular tachycardia; prolongation of the PR and QRS intervals.

➤*CNS:* Abnormal dreams, speech or vision; apnea; coma; confusion; depression; memory loss; numbness; paresthesias; psychosis/mania; seizures (0.3%); tinnitus; unusual smell sensation; vertigo.

➤*GI:* Cholestasis (0.1%); elevated liver enzymes (alkaline phosphatase, serum transaminases) (0.2%); gastroenteritis, hepatitis (0.03%). A number of patients with liver abnormalities associated with propafenone therapy have been reported in postmarketing experience. Some appeared due to hepatocellular injury, some were cholestatic and some showed a mixed picture.

➤*Hematologic:* Agranulocytosis; anemia; bruising; granulocytopenia; increased bleeding time; leukopenia; purpura; thrombocytopenia.

➤*Miscellaneous:* Alopecia; eye irritation; hyponatremia/inappropriate ADH secretion; impotence; increased glucose; kidney failure; positive ANA (0.7%); lupus erythematosus; muscle cramps; muscle weakness; nephrotic syndrome; pain; pruritus.

Overdosage

➤*Symptoms:* The following symptoms are usually most severe within 3 hours of ingestion may include hypotension, somnolence, bradycardia, intra-atrial and intraventricular conduction disturbances, and rarely convulsions and high grade ventricular arrhythmias.

➤*Treatment:* Defibrillation as well as infusion of dopamine and isoproterenol have been effective in controlling rhythm and blood pressure. Convulsions have been alleviated with IV diazepam. General supportive measures such as ventilatory assistance and cardiopulmonary resuscitation may be necessary. Refer to General Management of Acute Overdosage. Hemodialysis does not appear to alter drug clearance.

Patient Information

Palpitations, chest pain, blurred or abnormal vision, or difficult breathing may occur. Notify the physician if these become bothersome.

Notify the physician if signs of infection develop such as fever, sore throat, chills or unusual bruising or bleeding.

Be aware of signs of overdosage or toxicity such as hypotension, excessive drowsiness, decreased heart rate or abnormal heartbeat.

BRETYLIUM TOSYLATE

Rx	**Bretylium Tosylate in 5% Dextrose** (Various, eg, Abbott)	**Injection:** 2 mg/mL (500 mg/vial)	In 250 mL vials.
		4 mg/mL (1000 mg/vial)	In 250 mL vials.
Rx	**Bretylium Tosylate** (Various)	**Injection:** 50 mg/mL	In 10 mL amps, vials and syringes.

BRETYLIUM TOSYLATE — INJECTION

Refer to the general introductory discussion concerning Antiarrhythmic Agents.

WARNING

Patients should be kept in the supine position until tolerance to the hypotensive effect of bretylium develops. Tolerance occurs unpredictably but may be present after several days.

Indications

Prophylaxis and therapy of ventricular fibrillation.

Treatment of life-threatening ventricular arrhythmias, such as ventricular tachycardia, that have failed to respond to adequate doses of a first-line antiarrhythmic agent, such as lidocaine.

➤*Unlabeled uses:* Bretylium is a second-line agent following lidocaine in the protocol for advanced cardiac life support during CPR. For resistant VF and VT (after lidocaine, defibrillation, and procainamide failures), give bretylium 5 to 10 mg/kg IV; repeat as needed up to 30 mg/kg; use a bolus every 15 to 30 minutes, infusion 1 to 2 mg/min. For life-threatening arrhythmia use an undiluted infusion of 1 g per 250 mL.

Administration and Dosage

Use of bretylium tosylate should be limited to intensive care units, coronary care units or other facilities where equipment and personnel for constant monitoring of cardiac arrhythmias and blood pressure are available.

Following injection of bretylium tosylate there may be a delay of 20 minutes to 2 hours in the onset of antiarrhythmic action, although it appears to act within minutes in ventricular fibrillation. The delay in effect appears to be longer after intramuscular than after intravenous injection.

Bretylium tosylate is to be used clinically only for treatment of life-threatening ventricular arrhythmias under constant electrocardiographic monitoring. The clinical use of bretylium tosylate is for short-term use only.

Patient should either be kept supine during the course of bretylium tosylate therapy or be closely observed for postural hypotension. The optimal dose schedule for parenteral administration of bretylium tosylate has not been determined. There is comparatively little experience with dosages greater than 40 mg/kg/day, although such doses have been used without apparent adverse effects. The following schedule is suggested.

➤*For immediately life-threatening ventricular arrhythmias such as ventricular fibrillation of hemodynamically unstable ventricular tachycardia:* Administer undiluted bretylium tosylate injection at a dosage of 5 mg/kg of body weight by rapid intravenous injection. Other usual cardiopulmonary resuscitative procedures, including electrical cardioversion, should be employed prior to and following the injection in accordance with good medical practice. If ventricular fibrillation persists, the dosage may be increased to 10 mg/kg and repeated as necessary.

For continuous suppression, dilute bretylium tosylate injection with Dextrose Injection or Sodium Chloride Injection using the data below and administer the diluted solution as a constant infusion of 1 to 2 mg bretylium tosylate per minute. When administering bretylium tosylate (or any potent medication) by continuous intravenous infusion, it is advisable to use a precision volume control device. An alternative maintenance schedule is to infuse the diluted solution at a dosage of 5 to 10 mg bretylium per kg body weight, over a period greater than 8 minutes, every 6 hours. More rapid infusion may cause nausea and vomiting.

➤*Other ventricular arrhythmias:*

Intravenous use – Bretylium tosylate injection must be diluted as described above before intravenous use. Administer the diluted solution at a dosage of 5 to 10 mg bretylium tosylate per kg of body weight by intravenous infusion over a period greater than 8 minutes. More rapid infusion may cause nausea and vomiting. Subsequent doses may be given at 1- to 2-hour intervals if the arrhythmia persists.

BRETYLIUM TOSYLATE — INJECTION

For maintenance therapy, the same dosage may be administered every 6 hours, or a constant infusion of 1 to 2 mg bretylium tosylate per minute may be given. (See following table.)

Suggested Bretylium Tosylate Admixture Dilutions and Administration Rates for Continuous Infusion Maintenance Therapy Arranged in Descending Order of Concentration

Preparation				Administration		
Amount of bretylium tosylate	Volume of IV fluid*	Final volume	Final concentration (mg/mL)	Dose mg/min	Microdrops per min	mL/h
2 g (40 mL)	500 mL	540 mL	3.7	1	16	16
1 g (20 mL)	250 mL	270 mL	3.7	1.5	24	24
				2	32	32
1 g (20 mL)	500 mL	520 mL	1.9	1	32	32
500 mg (10 mL)	250 mL	260 mL	1.9	1.5	47	47
				2	63	63
For fluid-restricted patients:						
500 mg (10 mL)	50 mL	60 mL	8.3	1	7	7
				1.5	11	11
				2	14	14

* IV fluid may be either Dextrose Injection or Sodium Chloride Injection. This table does not consider the overfill volume present in the IV fluids.

Dilution for IV use: Each vial/syringe of bretylium tosylate injection should be diluted with a minimum of 50 mL of Dextrose Injection or Sodium Chloride Injection prior to IV use. Rapid intravenous administration may cause severe nausea and vomiting. Therefore, the diluted solution should be infused over a period more than 8 minutes. However, in treating existing ventricular fibrillation bretylium tosylate should be given as rapidly as possible and may be given without dilution.

Intramuscular injection – Do not dilute bretylium tosylate prior to intramuscular injection. Inject 5 to 10 mg bretylium tosylate per kg of body weight. Subsequent doses may be given at 1- to 2-hour intervals if the arrhythmia persists. Thereafter maintain the same dosage every 6 to 8 hours.

Intramuscular injection should not be made directly into or near a major nerve, and the site of injection should be varied on repeated injection. No more than 5 mL should be injected intramuscularly in one site.

As soon as possible, and when indicated, patients should be changed to an oral antiarrhythmic agent for maintenance therapy.

Use various sites for IM injection: When injected IM, not more than 5 mL should be given in a site, and injection sites should be varied since repeated intramuscular injection into the same site may cause atrophy and necrosis of muscle tissue, fibrosis, vascular degeneration and inflammatory changes.

➤*Renal function impairment:* Because bretylium is excreted principally via the kidney, the dosage interval should be increased in patients with impaired renal function.

➤*Storage/Stability:* Inspect parenteral drug products visually for particulate matter and discoloration prior to administration whenever solution and container permit.

Actions

➤*Pharmacology:* Bretylium is a bromobenzyl quaternary ammonium compound which selectively accumulates in sympathetic ganglia and their postganglionic adrenergic neurons where it inhibits norepinephrine release by depressing adrenergic nerve terminal excitability.

Bretylium also suppresses ventricular fibrillation and ventricular arrhythmias. The mechanisms of the antifibrillatory and antiarrhythmic actions of bretylium are not established. In efforts to define these mechanisms, the following electrophysiologic actions of bretylium tosylate have been demonstrated in animal experiments:

1.) Increase in ventricular fibrillation threshold.
2.) Increase in action potential duration and effective refractory period without changes in heart rate.
3.) Little effect on the rate of rise or amplitude of the cardiac action potential (Phase 0) or in resting membrane potential (Phase 4) in normal myocardium. However, when cell injury slows the rate of rise, decreases amplitude, and lowers resting membrane potential, bretylium transiently restores these parameters toward normal.
4.) In canine hearts with infarcted areas bretylium decreases the disparity in action potential duration between normal and infarcted regions.
5.) Increase in impulse formation and spontaneous firing rate of pacemaker tissue as well as increased ventricular conduction velocity.

➤*Pharmacokinetics:*

Excretion – Bretylium is eliminated intact by the kidneys. No metabolites have been identified following administration of bretylium tosylate in man and laboratory animals. In man, approximately 70% to 80% of a ^{14}C-labeled intramuscular dose is excreted in the urine during the first 24 hours, with an additional 10% excreted over the next 3 days.

The terminal half-life in 4 healthy volunteers averaged 7.8 ± 0.6 hours (range, 6.9 to 8.1). In 1 patient with a creatinine clearance of 21 mL/min•1.73 m^2, the half-life was 16 hours. In 1 patient with a creatinine clearance of 1 mL/min•1.73 m^2 the half-life was 31.5 hours. During hemodialysis, this patient's arterial and venous bretylium tosylate concentrations declined rapidly, resulting in a half-life of 13 hours. During dialysis there was a 2-fold increase in total bretylium clearance.

Contraindications

There are no contraindications to use in treatment of ventricular fibrillation or life-threatening refractory ventricular arrhythmias.

Warnings

➤*Hypotension:* Administration of bretylium tosylate regularly results in postural hypotension, subjectively recognized by dizziness, lightheadedness, vertigo or faintness. Some degree of hypotension is present in about 50% of patients while they are supine. Hypotension may occur at doses lower than those needed to suppress arrhythmias.

Hypotension with supine systolic pressure greater than 75 mmHg need not be treated unless there are associated symptoms. If supine systolic pressure falls below 75 mmHg, an infusion of dopamine or norepinephrine may be used to raise blood pressure. When catecholamines are administered, a dilute solution should be employed and blood pressure monitored closely because the pressor effects of the catecholamines are enhanced by bretylium. Volume expansion with blood or plasma and correction of dehydration should be carried out where appropriate.

➤*Transient hypertension and increased frequency of arrhythmias:* Due to the initial release of norepinephrine from adrenergic postganglionic nerve terminals by bretylium tosylate, transient hypertension or increased frequency of premature ventricular contractions and other arrhythmias may occur in some patients.

➤*Hyperthermia:* In a small number of patients, hyperthermia, characterized by temperature in excess of 41.1°C (106°F), has been reported in association with bretylium tosylate administration. Temperature rise can begin within 1 hour or later after administration of drug, and reach a peak within 1 to 3 days. If hyperthermia is suspected or diagnosed, bretylium should be discontinued and appropriate treatment instituted immediately.

➤*Pregnancy: Category C.*

Animal reproduction studies have not been conducted with bretylium tosylate. It is also not known whether bretylium tosylate can cause harm when administered to a pregnant woman or can affect reproduction capacity. Bretylium tosylate should be given to pregnant women only if clearly needed.

➤*Children:* The safety and efficacy of this drug in children has not been established. Bretylium tosylate has been administered to a limited number of pediatric patients, but such use has been inadequate to define fully proper dosage and limitations for use.

Precautions

➤*Patients with fixed cardiac output:* In patients with fixed cardiac output (ie, severe aortic stenosis or severe pulmonary hypertension), bretylium tosylate should be avoided since severe hypotension may result from a fall in peripheral resistance without a compensatory increase in cardiac output. If survival is threatened by the arrhythmia, bretylium tosylate may be used but vasoconstrictive catecholamines should be given promptly if severe hypotension occurs.

Drug Interactions

Bretylium Drug Interactions

Precipitant drug	Object drug*		Description
Bretylium	Catecholamines	↑	The pressor effects of catecholamines (eg, dopamine, norepinephrine) are enhanced by bretylium. When catecholamines are administered, use dilute solutions and closely monitor blood pressure (see Warnings).
Bretylium	Digoxin	↑	Digitalis toxicity may be aggravated by the initial release of norepinephrine caused by bretylium. When a life-threatening cardiac arrhythmia occurs, use bretylium only if the etiology of the arrhythmia does not appear to be digitalis toxicity and if other antiarrhythmic drugs are not effective. Avoid simultaneous initiation of therapy.

* ↑ = Object drug increased

Adverse Reactions

Hypotension and postural hypotension have been the most frequently reported adverse reactions. Nausea and vomiting occurred in about 3% of patients primarily when bretylium tosylate was administered rapidly by the intravenous route (see Precautions). Vertigo, dizziness, lightheadedness and syncope, which sometimes accompanied postural hypotension, were reported in about 7 patients in 1000.

➤*Cardiovascular:* Bradycardia, increased frequency of premature ventricular contractions, transitory hypertension, initial increase in arrhythmias, precipitation of anginal attacks, and sensation of substernal pressure have also been reported in a small number of patients (ie, ≈ 1 to 2 patients in 1,000).

BRETYLIUM TOSYLATE — INJECTION

➤*Miscellaneous:* Renal dysfunction, diarrhea, abdominal pain, hiccups, erythematous macular rash, flushing, confusion, paranoid psychosis, emotional lability, lethargy, generalized tenderness, anxiety, shortness of breath, diaphoresis, nasal stuffiness and mild conjunctivitis have been reported in about 1 patient in 1000. Hyperthermia has also been reported. The relationship of bretylium tosylate administration to these reactions has not been clearly established.

Overdosage

➤*Symptoms:* In the presence of life-threatening arrhythmias, underdosage with bretylium probably presents a greater risk to the patient than potential overdosage. However, 1 case of accidental overdose has been reported in which a rapidly injected intravenous bolus of 30 mg/kg was given instead of an intended 10 mg/kg dose during an episode of ventricular tachycardia. Marked hypertension resulted, followed by protracted refractory hypotension. The patient expired 18 hours later in asystole, complicated by renal failure and aspiration pneumonitis. Bretylium serum levels were 8000 ng/mL. The exaggerated hemodynamic response was attributed to the rapid injection of a very large dose while some effective circulation was still present. Neither the total dose nor the serum levels observed in this patient are in themselves associated with toxicity. Total doses of 30 mg/kg are not unusual and do not cause toxicity when given incrementally during cardiopulmonary resuscitation procedures. Similarly, patients maintained on chronic bretylium therapy have had documented serum levels of 12,000 ng/mL. These levels were achieved after sequential dosage increases over time with no apparent ill effects.

➤*Treatment:* If bretylium tosylate is overdosed and symptoms of toxicity develop, administration of nitroprusside or another short-acting intravenous antihypertensive agent should be considered for the treatment of the hypertensive response. Long-acting drugs that might potentiate the subsequent hypotensive effects of bretylium should not be used. Hypotension should be treated with appropriate fluid therapy and pressor agents such as dopamine or norepinephrine. Dialysis is probably not useful in the treatment of bretylium tosylate overdose.

AMIODARONE HYDROCHLORIDE

Rx	**Pacerone** (Upsher Smith)	**Tablets**: 100 mg	Lactose. (P US 144). In 30s and UD 100s.
Rx	**Amiodarone HCl** (Various, eg, Eon Labs, Teva)	**Tablets**: 200 mg	In 60s, 100s, 250s, 500s, and UD 100s.
Rx	**Cordarone** (Wyeth-Ayerst)		Lactose. (C 200 WYETH 4188). Pink, scored, convex. In 60s and UD 100s.
Rx	**Pacerone** (Upsher Smith)		Lactose. (P_{200} U-S 0147). Pink, scored. In 60s, 90s, 500s, and UD 100s.
Rx	**Pacerone** (Upsher Smith)	**Tablets**: 400 mg	Lactose. (P_{400} 01 45). Light yellow, oval, scored. In 30s, 100s, 500s, and UD 100s.
Rx	**Amiodarone HCl** (Various, eg, American Pharm Partners, Faulding)	**Injection**: 50 mg/mL	May contain benzyl alcohol. In 3 mL vials and amps.
Rx	**Cordarone** (Wyeth-Ayerst)		20.2 mg/mL benzyl alcohol. In 3 mL amps.

AMIODARONE HYDROCHLORIDE — ORAL

Refer to the general introductory discussion concerning Antiarrhythmic Agents.

WARNING

Life-threatening arrhythmias – Amiodarone is intended for use only in patients with the indicated life-threatening arrhythmias because its use is accompanied by substantial toxicity.

Potentially fatal toxicities – Amiodarone has several potentially fatal toxicities, the most important of which is pulmonary toxicity (hypersensitivity pneumonitis or interstitial/alveolar pneumonitis) that has resulted in clinically manifest disease at rates as high as 10% to 17% in some series of patients with ventricular arrhythmias given doses around 400 mg/day, and as abnormal diffusion capacity without symptoms in a much higher percentage of patients. Pulmonary toxicity has been fatal approximately 10% of the time. Liver injury is common with amiodarone, but is usually mild and evidenced only by abnormal liver enzymes. Overt liver disease can occur, however, and has been fatal in a few cases. Like other antiarrhythmics, amiodarone can exacerbate the arrhythmia, eg, by making the arrhythmia less well tolerated or more difficult to reverse. This has occurred in 2% to 5% of patients in various series, and significant heart block or sinus bradycardia has been seen in 2% to 5%. All of these events should be manageable in the proper clinical setting in most cases. Although the frequency of such proarrhythmic events does not appear greater with amiodarone than with many other agents used in this population, the effects are prolonged when they occur.

High-risk patients – Even in patients at high risk of arrhythmic death, in whom the toxicity of amiodarone is an acceptable risk, amiodarone poses major management problems that could be life-threatening in a population at risk of sudden death, so that every effort should be made to utilize alternative agents first.

The difficulty of using amiodarone effectively and safely itself poses a significant risk to patients. Patients with the indicated arrhythmias must be hospitalized while the loading dose of amiodarone is given, and a response generally requires at least one week, usually two or more. Because absorption and elimination are variable, maintenance-dose selection is difficult, and it is not unusual to require dosage decrease or discontinuation of treatment. In a retrospective survey of 192 patients with ventricular tachyarrhythmias, 84 required dose reduction and 18 required at least temporary discontinuation because of adverse effects, and several series have reported 15% to 20% overall frequencies of discontinuation due to adverse reactions. The time at which a previously controlled life-threatening arrhythmia will recur after discontinuation or dose adjustment is unpredictable, ranging from weeks to months. The patient is obviously at great risk during this time and may need prolonged hospitalization. Attempts to substitute other antiarrhythmic agents when amiodarone must be stopped will be made difficult by the gradually, but unpredictably, changing amiodarone body burden. A similar problem exists when amiodarone is not effective; it still poses the risk of an interaction with whatever subsequent treatment is tried.

Indications

➤*Ventricular arrhythmias:* Only for the treatment of the following documented, life-threatening recurrent ventricular arrhythmias when these have not responded to documented adequate doses of other available antiarrhythmics or when alternative agents could not be tolerated:

1.) Recurrent ventricular fibrillation.
2.) Recurrent hemodynamically unstable ventricular tachycardia.

➤*Unlabeled uses:* Amiodarone has shown effectiveness for conversion of atrial fibrillation and maintenance of sinus rhythm. It also appears to be useful in treating supraventricular tachycardia.

Administration and Dosage

➤*Approved by the FDA:* December 27, 1985.

➤*Administration:* In order to ensure that an antiarrhythmic effect will be observed without waiting several months, loading doses are required. A uniform, optimal dosage schedule for administration of amiodarone has not been determined. Because of the food effect on absorption, amiodarone should be administered consistently with regard to meals.

➤*Life-threatening ventricular arrhythmias (eg, ventricular fibrillation or hemodynamically unstable ventricular tachycardia):*

Amiodarone Oral Dosage Suggestions			
	Loading dose (daily)	Adjustment and maintenance dose (daily)	
Ventricular arrhythmias	1 to 3 wk	≈ 1 mo	usual maintenance
	800 to 1,600 mg	600 to 800 mg	400 mg

Close monitoring of the patient is indicated during the loading phase, particularly until risk of recurrent ventricular tachycardia or fibrillation has abated. Because of the serious nature of the arrhythmia and the lack of predictable time course of effect, loading should be performed in a hospital setting. Loading doses of 800 to 1,600 mg/day are required for 1 to 3 weeks (occasionally longer) until initial therapeutic response occurs. (Administration of amiodarone in divided doses with meals is suggested for total daily doses of 1,000 mg or higher, or when gastrointestinal intolerance occurs.) If side effects become excessive, the dose should be reduced. Elimination of recurrence of ventricular fibrillation and tachycardia usually occurs within 1 to 3 weeks, along with reduction in complex and total ventricular ectopic beats.

➤*Dosage titration / adjustment:* Individual patient titration is suggested according to the following guidelines. Upon starting amiodarone therapy, an attempt should be made to gradually discontinue prior antiarrhythmic drugs. When adequate arrhythmia control is achieved, or if side effects become prominent, amiodarone dose should be reduced to 600 to 800 mg/day for one month and then to the maintenance dose, usually 400 mg/day. Some patients may require larger maintenance doses, up to 600 mg/day, and some can be controlled on lower doses. Amiodarone may be administered as a single daily dose, or in patients with severe gastrointestinal intolerance as a twice-daily dose. In each patient, the chronic maintenance dose should be determined according to antiarrhythmic effect as assessed by symptoms, Holter recordings, and/or programmed electrical stimulation and by patient tolerance. Plasma concentrations may be helpful in evaluating nonresponsiveness or unexpectedly severe toxicity.

The lowest effective dose should be used to prevent the occurrence of side effects. In all instances, the physician must be guided by the severity of the individual patient's arrhythmia and response to therapy.

When dosage adjustments are necessary, the patient should be closely monitored for an extended period of time because of the long and variable half-life of amiodarone and the difficulty in predicting the time required to attain a new steady-state level of drug.

AMIODARONE HYDROCHLORIDE — ORAL

➤*Storage/Stability:* Keep tightly closed. Store at room temperature, approximately 25°C (77°F). Protect from light. Dispense in a light-resistant, tight container. Use carton to protect contents from light.

Actions

➤*Pharmacology:* In animals, amiodarone is effective in the prevention or suppression of experimentally induced arrhythmias. The antiarrhythmic effect of amiodarone may be due to at least two major properties:

1.) a prolongation of the myocardial cell-action potential duration and refractory period; and
2.) noncompetitive alpha- and beta-adrenergic inhibition.

Amiodarone prolongs the duration of the action potential of all cardiac fibers while causing minimal reduction of dV/dt (maximal upstroke velocity of the action potential). The refractory period is prolonged in all cardiac tissues. Amiodarone increases the cardiac refractory period without influencing resting membrane potential, except in automatic cells where the slope of the prepotential is reduced, generally reducing automaticity. These electrophysiologic effects are reflected in a decreased sinus rate of 15% to 20%, increased PR and QT intervals of about 10%, the development of U-waves, and changes in T-wave contour. These changes should not require discontinuation of amiodarone as they are evidence of its pharmacological action, although amiodarone can cause marked sinus bradycardia or sinus arrest and heart block. On rare occasions, QT prolongation has been associated with worsening of arrhythmia.

➤*Pharmacokinetics:*

Absorption – Following oral administration in man, amiodarone is slowly and variably absorbed. The bioavailability of amiodarone is approximately 50%, but has varied between 35% and 65% in various studies. Maximum plasma concentrations are attained 3 to 7 hours after a single dose. Despite this, the onset of action may occur in 2 to 3 days, but more commonly takes 1 to 3 weeks, even with loading doses. Plasma concentrations with chronic dosing at 100 to 600 mg/day are approximately dose proportional, with a mean 0.5 mg/L increase for each 100 mg/day. These means, however, include considerable individual variability.

Although electrophysiologic effects, such as prolongation of QTc, can be seen within hours after a parenteral dose of amiodarone, effects on abnormal rhythms are not seen before 2 to 3 days and usually require 1 to 3 weeks, even when a loading dose is used. There may be a continued increase in effect for longer periods still. There is evidence that the time to effect is shorter when a loading-dose regimen is used.

Food effects: See Drug Interactions for more information.

Distribution – Amiodarone has a very large but variable volume of distribution, averaging about 60 L/kg, because of extensive accumulation in various sites, especially adipose tissue and highly perfused organs, such as the liver, lung, and spleen. One major metabolite of amiodarone, desethylamiodarone (DEA), has been identified in man; it accumulates to an even greater extent in almost all tissues.

Amiodarone and its metabolite have a limited transplacental transfer of approximately 10% to 50%. The parent drug and its metabolite have been detected in breast milk.

Amiodarone is highly protein-bound (approximately 96%).

Metabolism – DEA is the major metabolite of amiodarone. No data are available on the activity of DEA in humans, but in animals, it has significant electrophysiologic and antiarrhythmic effects generally similar to amiodarone itself. DEA's precise role and contribution to the antiarrhythmic activity of oral amiodarone are not certain. The development of maximal ventricular class III effects after oral amiodarone administration in humans correlates more closely with DEA accumulation over time than with amiodarone accumulation.

Excretion – Amiodarone is eliminated primarily by hepatic metabolism and biliary excretion and there is negligible excretion of amiodarone or DEA in urine. Neither amiodarone nor DEA is dialyzable.

In clinical studies of 2 to 7 days, clearance of amiodarone after intravenous administration in patients with VT and VF ranged between 220 and 440 mL/hr/kg.

Following single dose administration in 12 healthy subjects, amiodarone exhibited multicompartmental pharmacokinetics with a mean apparent plasma terminal elimination half-life of 58 days (range, 15 to 142 days) for amiodarone and 36 days (range, 14 to 75 days) for the active metabolite (DEA). In patients, following discontinuation of chronic oral therapy, amiodarone has been shown to have a biphasic elimination with an initial one-half reduction of plasma levels after 2.5 to 10 days. A much slower terminal plasma-elimination phase shows a half-life of the parent compound ranging from 26 to 107 days, with a mean of approximately 53 days and most patients in the 40- to 55-day range. In the absence of a loading dose period, steady-state plasma concentrations, at constant oral dosing, would therefore be reached between 130 and 535 days, with an average of 265 days. For the metabolite, the mean plasma-elimination half-life was approximately 61 days. These data probably reflect an initial elimination of drug from well-perfused tissue (the 2.5- to 10-day half-life phase), followed by a terminal phase representing extremely slow elimination from poorly perfused tissue compartments such as fat.

The considerable intersubject variation in both phases of elimination, as well as uncertainty as to what compartment is critical to drug effect, requires attention to individual responses once arrhythmia control is achieved with loading doses because the correct maintenance dose is determined, in part, by the elimination rates. Base daily maintenance doses of amiodarone on individual patient requirements.

Consistent with the slow rate of elimination, antiarrhythmic effects persist for weeks or months after amiodarone is discontinued, but the time of recurrence is variable and unpredictable. In general, when the drug is resumed after recurrence of the arrhythmia, control is established relatively rapidly compared to the initial response, presumably because tissue stores were not wholly depleted at the time of recurrence.

Special populations –

Elderly: Normal subjects older than 65 years of age show lower clearances (about 100 mL/hr/kg) than younger subjects (about 150 mL/h/kg) and an increase in t½ of DEA is prolonged. Although no dosage adjustment for patients with renal, hepatic, or cardiac abnormalities has been defined during chronic treatment with amiodarone, close clinical monitoring is prudent for elderly patients and those with severe left ventricular dysfunction.

Contraindications

Severe sinus-node dysfunction, causing marked sinus bradycardia; second- and third-degree atrioventricular block; and when episodes of bradycardia have caused syncope (except when used in conjunction with a pacemaker).

Hypersensitivity to the drug or to any of its components, including iodine.

Warnings

➤*Life-threatening arrhythmias:* See the Warning box for more information.

➤*High-risk patients:* See the Warning box for more information.

➤*Pulmonary disorders:*

Pulmonary toxicity – There have been postmarketing reports of acute-onset (days to weeks) pulmonary injury in patients treated with oral amiodarone with or without initial IV therapy. Findings have included pulmonary infiltrates on X-ray, bronchospasm, wheezing, fever, dyspnea, cough, hemoptysis, and hypoxia. Some cases have progressed to respiratory failure and/or death.

Amiodarone may cause a clinical syndrome of cough and progressive dyspnea accompanied by functional, radiographic, gallium-scan, and pathological data consistent with pulmonary toxicity, the frequency of which varies from 2% to 7% in most published reports, but is as high as 10% to 17% in some reports. Therefore, when amiodarone therapy is initiated, a baseline chest X-ray and pulmonary-function tests, including diffusion capacity, should be performed. The patient should return for a history, physical exam, and chest X-ray every 3 to 6 months.

In a patient receiving amiodarone, any new respiratory symptoms should suggest the possibility of pulmonary toxicity, and the history, physical exam, chest X-ray, and pulmonary function tests (with diffusion capacity) should be repeated and evaluated. A 15% decrease in diffusion capacity has a high sensitivity but only a moderate specificity for pulmonary toxicity; as the decrease in diffusion capacity approaches 30%, the sensitivity decreases but the specificity increases. A gallium scan also may be performed as part of the diagnostic workup.

Fatalities, secondary to pulmonary toxicity, have occurred in approximately 10% of cases. However, in patients with life-threatening arrhythmias, discontinuation of amiodarone therapy due to suspected drug-induced pulmonary toxicity should be undertaken with caution, as the most common cause of death in these patients is sudden cardiac death. Therefore, every effort should be made to rule out other causes of respiratory impairment (ie, congestive heart failure with Swan-Ganz catheterization if necessary, respiratory infection, pulmonary embolism, malignancy, etc.) before discontinuing amiodarone in these patients. In addition, bronchoalveolar lavage, transbronchial lung biopsy and/or open lung biopsy may be necessary to confirm the diagnosis, especially in those cases where no acceptable alternative therapy is available.

Pulmonary toxicity secondary to amiodarone seems to result from either indirect or direct toxicity as represented by hypersensitivity pneumonitis or interstitial/alveolar pneumonitis, respectively.

Patients with preexisting pulmonary disease have a poorer prognosis if pulmonary toxicity develops.

Hypersensitivity pneumonitis – Hypersensitivity pneumonitis usually appears earlier in the course of therapy, and rechallenging these patients with amiodarone results in a more rapid recurrence of greater severity.

Bronchoalveolar lavage is the procedure of choice to confirm this diagnosis, which can be made when a T suppressor/cytotoxic (CD8-positive) lymphocytosis is noted. Steroid therapy should be instituted and amiodarone therapy discontinued in these patients.

If a diagnosis of amiodarone-induced hypersensitivity pneumonitis is made, amiodarone should be discontinued, and treatment with steroids should be instituted.

Interstitial/alveolar pneumonitis – Interstitial/alveolar pneumonitis may result from the release of oxygen radicals and/or phospholipidosis and is characterized by findings of diffuse alveolar damage, interstitial pneumonitis or fibrosis in lung biopsy specimens.

Phospholipidosis (foamy cells, foamy macrophages) due to inhibition of phospholipase, will be present in most cases of amiodarone-induced pulmonary toxicity; however, these changes also are present in approximately 50% of all patients on amiodarone therapy. These cells should be used as markers of therapy, but not as evidence of toxicity. A diagnosis of amiodarone-induced interstitial/alveolar pneumonitis should lead, at a minimum, to dose reduction or, preferably, to withdrawal of the amiodarone to establish reversibility, especially if other acceptable antiarrhythmic therapies are available. Where these measures have been instituted, a reduction in symptoms of amiodarone-induced pulmonary toxicity was usually noted within the first week, and a clinical improvement was greatest in the first two to three weeks. Chest X-ray changes usually resolve within two to four months. According to some experts, steroids may prove beneficial. Prednisone in doses of 40 to 60 mg/day or equivalent doses of other steroids have been given and tapered over the course of several weeks depending upon the condition of the patient. In some cases rechallenge with amiodarone at a lower

AMIODARONE HYDROCHLORIDE — ORAL

dose has not resulted in return of toxicity. Recent reports suggest that the use of lower loading and maintenance doses of amiodarone are associated with a decreased incidence of amiodarone-induced pulmonary toxicity.

If a diagnosis of amiodarone-induced interstitial/alveolar pneumonitis is made, steroid therapy should be instituted and, preferably, amiodarone discontinued or, at a minimum, reduced in dosage. Some cases of amiodarone-induced interstitial/alveolar pneumonitis may resolve following a reduction in amiodarone dosage in conjunction with the administration of steroids. In some patients, rechallenge at a lower dose has not resulted in return of interstitial/alveolar pneumonitis; however, in some patients (perhaps because of severe alveolar damage) the pulmonary lesions have not been reversible.

➤*Cardiac effects:*

Proarrhythmia – Amiodarone, like other antiarrhythmics, can cause serious exacerbation of the presenting arrhythmia, a risk that may be enhanced by the presence of concomitant antiarrhythmics. Exacerbation has been reported in about 2% to 5% in most series, and has included new ventricular fibrillation, incessant ventricular tachycardia, increased resistance to cardioversion, and polymorphic ventricular tachycardia associated with QTc prolongation (Torsade de Pointes [TdP]). In addition, amiodarone has caused symptomatic bradycardia or sinus arrest with suppression of escape foci in 2% to 4% of patients.

See Drug Interactions for more information.

The need to coadminister amiodarone with any other drug known to prolong the QTc interval must be based on a careful assessment of the potential risks and benefits of doing so for each patient. A careful assessment of the potential risks and benefits of doing so for each patient. A careful assessment of the potential risks and benefits of administering amiodarone must be made in patients with thyroid dysfunction due to the possibility of arrhythmia breakthrough or exacerbation of arrhythmia in these patients.

➤*Hepatic effects:* Elevations of hepatic enzyme levels are seen frequently in patients exposed to amiodarone and in most cases are asymptomatic. If the increase exceeds three times normal, or doubles in a patient with an elevated baseline, discontinuation of amiodarone or dosage reduction should be considered. In a few cases in which biopsy has been done, the histology has resembled that of alcoholic hepatitis or cirrhosis. Hepatic failure has been a rare cause of death in patients treated with amiodarone.

➤*Ophthalmologic effects:* Cases of optic neuropathy and/or optic neuritis, usually resulting in visual impairment, have been reported in patients treated with amiodarone. In some cases, visual impairment has progressed to permanent blindness. Optic neuropathy and/or neuritis may occur at any time following initiation of therapy. A causal relationship to the drug has not been clearly established. If symptoms of visual impairment appear, such as changes in visual acuity and decreases in peripheral vision, prompt ophthalmic examination is recommended. Appearance of optic neuropathy and/or neuritis calls for reevaluation of amiodarone therapy. The risks and complications of antiarrhythmic therapy with amiodarone must be weighed against its benefits in patients whose lives are threatened by cardiac arrhythmias. Regular ophthalmic examination, including fundoscopy and slit-lamp examination, is recommended during administration of amiodarone.

Corneal microdeposits appear in the majority of adults treated with amiodarone. They are usually discernible only by slit-lamp examination, but give rise to symptoms such as visual halos or blurred vision in as many as 10% of patients. Corneal microdeposits are reversible upon reduction of dose or termination of treatment. Asymptomatic microdeposits alone are not a reason to reduce dose or discontinue treatment.

➤*Carcinogenesis:* Amiodarone was associated with a statistically significant, dose-related increase in the incidence of thyroid tumors (follicular adenoma and/or carcinoma) in rats. The incidence of thyroid tumors was greater than control even at the lowest dose level tested, ie, 5 mg/kg/day (approximately 0.08 times the maximum recommended human maintenance dose; 600 mg in a 50 kg patient [dose compared on a body surface area basis]).

➤*Fertility impairment:* In a study in which oral amiodarone was administered to male and female rats, beginning 9 weeks prior to mating, reduced fertility was observed at a dose level of 90 mg/kg/day (approximately 1.4 times the maximum recommended human maintenance dose; 600 mg in a 50 kg patient [dose compared on a body surface area basis]).

➤*Elderly:* Clinical studies of amiodarone did not include sufficient numbers of subjects 65 years of age and older to determine whether they respond differently from younger subjects. Other reported clinical experience has not identified differences in responses between the elderly and younger patients. In general, dose selection for an elderly patient should be cautious, usually starting at the low end of the dosing range, reflecting the greater frequency of decreased hepatic, renal, or cardiac function, and of concomitant disease or other drug therapy.

➤*Pregnancy: Category D.* Amiodarone can cause fetal harm when administered to a pregnant woman. Although amiodarone use during pregnancy is uncommon, there have been a small number of published reports of congenital goiter/hypothyroidism and hyperthyroidism. If amiodarone is administered during pregnancy, or if the patient becomes pregnant while taking amiodarone, the patient should be apprised of the potential hazard to the fetus.

In general, amiodarone should be used during pregnancy only if the potential benefit to the mother justifies the unknown risk to the fetus.

➤*Lactation:* Amiodarone and one of its major metabolites, desethylamiodarone (DEA), are excreted in human milk, suggesting that breast-feeding could expose the nursing infant to a significant dose of the drug. Nursing offspring of lactating rats administered amiodarone have been shown to be less viable and have reduced body-weight gains. Therefore, when amiodarone therapy is indicated, the mother should be advised to discontinue nursing.

➤*Children:* The safety and effectiveness of amiodarone in pediatric patients have not been established; therefore, its use in pediatric patients is not recommended.

Precautions

➤*Monitoring:* Perform baseline chest x-rays and pulmonary function tests, including diffusion capacity before therapy initiation. Repeat a history, physical exam, and chest x-ray every 3 to 6 months.

Monitor thyroid function at baseline and periodically during therapy, particularly in the elderly and in any patient with a history of thyroid nodules, goiter, or other thyroid dysfunction.

Perform regular ophthalmic examination, including fundoscopy and slit-lamp examination, during administration of amiodarone.

Monitor liver enzymes on a regular basis.

Closely monitor FiO_2 and the determinants of oxygen delivery to the tissues (eg, SaO_2, PaO_2) in patients on amiodarone.

➤*Electrolyte disturbances:* Since antiarrhythmic drugs may be ineffective or may be arrhythmogenic in patients with hypokalemia, any potassium or magnesium deficiency should be corrected before instituting amiodarone therapy. Use caution when coadministering amiodarone with drugs which may induce hypokalemia and/or hypomagnesemia.

➤*CNS effects:* Chronic administration of oral amiodarone in rare instances may lead to the development of peripheral neuropathy that may resolve when amiodarone is discontinued, but this resolution has been slow and incomplete.

➤*Thyroid abnormalities:* Amiodarone inhibits peripheral conversion of thyroxine (T_4) to triiodothyronine (T_3) and may cause increased thyroxine levels, decreased T_3 levels, and increased levels of inactive reverse T_3 (rT_3) in clinically euthyroid patients. It is also a potential source of large amounts of inorganic iodine. Because of its release of inorganic iodine, or perhaps for other reasons, amiodarone can cause either hypothyroidism or hyperthyroidism. Thyroid function should be monitored prior to treatment and periodically thereafter, particularly in elderly patients, and in any patient with a history of thyroid nodules, goiter, or other thyroid dysfunction. Because of the slow elimination of amiodarone and its metabolites, high plasma iodide levels, altered thyroid function, and abnormal thyroid function tests may persist for several weeks or even months following amiodarone tablets withdrawal.

Hypothyroidism – Hypothyroidism has been reported in 2% to 4% of patients in most series, but in 8% to 10% in some series. This condition may be identified by relevant clinical symptoms and particularly by elevated serum thyroid-stimulating hormone (TSH) levels. In some clinically hypothyroid amiodarone-treated patients, free thyroxine index values may be normal. Hypothyroidism is best managed by amiodarone dose reduction and/or thyroid hormone supplement. However, therapy must be individualized, and it may be necessary to discontinue amiodarone in some patients.

Hyperthyroidism – Hyperthyroidism occurs in about 2% of patients receiving amiodarone, but the incidence may be higher among patients with prior inadequate dietary iodine intake. Amiodarone-induced hyperthyroidism usually poses a greater hazard to the patient than hypothyroidism because of the possibility of arrhythmia breakthrough or aggravation, which may result in death . In fact, if any new signs of arrhythmia appear, the possibility of hyperthyroidism should be considered. Hyperthyroidism is best identified by relevant clinical symptoms and signs, accompanied usually by abnormally elevated levels of serum T_3 radioimmunoassay (RIA), and further elevations of serum T_4, and a subnormal serum TSH level (using a sufficiently sensitive TSH assay). The finding of a flat TSH response to a thyroid-releasing hormone (TRH) is confirmatory of hyperthyroidism and may be sought in equivocal cases. Since arrhythmia breakthroughs may accompany amiodarone-induced hyperthyroidism, aggressive medical treatment is indicated, including, if possible, dose reduction or withdrawal of amiodarone.

The institution of antithyroid drugs, beta-adrenergic blockers and/or temporary corticosteroid therapy may be necessary. The action of antithyroid drugs may be especially delayed in amiodarone-induced thyrotoxicosis because of substantial quantities of preformed thyroid hormones stored in the gland. Radioactive iodine therapy is contraindicated because of the low radioiodine uptake associated with amiodarone-induced hyperthyroidism. Experience with thyroid surgery in this setting is extremely limited, and this form of therapy runs the theoretical risk of inducing thyroid storm. Amiodarone-induced hyperthyroidism may be followed by a transient period of hypothyroidism.

➤*Surgery:*

Hypotension post-bypass – Rare occurrences of hypotension upon discontinuation of cardiopulmonary bypass during open-heart surgery in patients receiving amiodarone have been reported. The relationship of this event to amiodarone therapy is unknown.

Volatile anesthetic agents – Close perioperative monitoring is recommended in patients undergoing general anesthetic who are on amiodarone therapy as they may be more sensitive to the myocardial depressant and conduction effects of halogenated inhalational anesthetics.

➤*Lab test abnormalities:* Elevations in liver enzymes (AST and ALT) can occur. Liver enzymes in patients on relatively high maintenance doses should be monitored on a regular basis. Persistent significant elevations in the liver enzymes or hepatomegaly should alert the physician to consider reducing the maintenance dose of amiodarone or discontinuing therapy. Amiodarone alters the results of thyroid function tests, causing an increase

AMIODARONE HYDROCHLORIDE — ORAL

in serum T_4 and serum reverse T_3, and a decline in serum T_3 levels. Despite these biochemical changes, most patients remain clinically euthyroid.

➤*Photosensitivity:* Amiodarone has induced photosensitization in about 10% of patients; some protection may be afforded by the use of sun-barrier creams or protective clothing. During long-term treatment, a blue-gray discoloration of the exposed skin may occur. The risk may be increased in patients of fair complexion or those with excessive sun exposure, and may be related to cumulative dose and duration of therapy.

Drug Interactions

Amiodarone Drug Interactions

Precipitant drug	Object drug*		Description
Amiodarone	Antiarrhythmics (eg, quinidine, procainamide, disopyramide, flecainide)	↑	Amiodarone may increase serum concentrations of these antiarrhythmics. Reduce dose of antiarrhythmic with coadministration.
Amiodarone	Anticoagulants (eg, warfarin)	↑	Prothrombin time (PT) may increase. Potentiation of anticoagulant response is almost always seen in patients receiving amiodarone and can result in serious or fatal bleeding. A 30% to 50% anticoagulant dose reduction is typically required. Onset is 3 to 4 days and may persist for months after amiodarone discontinuation. Closely monitor PT.
Amiodarone	Beta blockers (eg, propranolol)	↑	Effects of beta blockers eliminated by hepatic metabolism may be increased. Because amiodarone has weak beta blocking activity, concomitant use can increase risk of hypotension and bradycardia.
Amiodarone	Calcium channel blockers (eg, verapamil, diltiazem)	↑	Amiodarone inhibits AV conduction and decreases myocardial contractility; increased risk of AV block with verapamil or diltiazem or hypotension with any calcium blocker may occur.
Amiodarone	Cardiac glycosides (eg, digoxin, digitoxin)	↑	Amiodarone taken concomitantly with digoxin increases the serum digoxin concentrations by 70% after one day. Reduce the dose of digitalis by 50% or discontinue.
Amiodarone	Cisapride	↑	Risk of life-threatening cardiac arrhythmias, including torsades de pointes, may be increased because of possibly additive prolongation of the QT interval.
Amiodarone	Cyclosporine	↑	Concomitant use has produced persistently elevated plasma cyclosporine levels resulting in elevated creatinine despite reduction in dose of cyclosporine.
Amiodarone	Dextromethorphan	↑	Chronic use (> 2 weeks) of amiodarone administration impairs metabolism of dextromethorphan.
Amiodarone	Fentanyl	↑	May cause hypotension, bradycardia, decreased cardiac output.
Amiodarone	HMG-CoA reductase inhibitors (eg, simvastatin)	↑	Simvastatin in combination with amiodarone has been associated with reports of myopathy/rhabdomyolysis.
Amiodarone	Hydantoins (eg, phenytoin)	↑	Chronic use (> 2 weeks) of amiodarone impairs metabolism of phenytoin. Increased hydantoin concentrations with symptoms of toxicity may occur. Also, amiodarone serum levels may be decreased.
Hydantoins (eg, phenytoin)	Amiodarone	↓	
Amiodarone	Lidocaine	↑	Sinus bradycardia has been reported with oral amiodarone in combination with lidocaine for local anesthesia. Seizure, associated with increased lidocaine concentrations, has been reported with concomitant administration of IV amiodarone.
Amiodarone	Methotrexate	↑	Chronic use (> 2 weeks) of amiodarone impairs metabolism of methotrexate. Methotrexate toxicity may be increased.
Amiodarone	Theophylline	↑	Increased theophylline levels with toxicity may occur. Effects may not be seen for ≥ 1 week of concomitant therapy and may persist for an extended period after amiodarone discontinuation.
Amiodarone	Thioridazine	↑	The risk of life-threatening cardiac arrhythmias, including torsades de pointes, may be increased.
Amiodarone	Vardenafil	↑	The risk of life-threatening cardiac arrhythmias, including torsades de pointes, may be increased.
Amiodarone	Ziprasidone	↑	The risk of life-threatening cardiac arrhythmias, including torsades de pointes, may be increased.
Azole antifungals (eg, itraconazole)	Amiodarone	↑	The risk of life-threatening cardiac arrhythmias, including torsades de pointes, may be increased.
Cholestyramine	Amiodarone	↓	Increased enterohepatic elimination of amiodarone and reduced serum levels and half-life may occur.
Cimetidine	Amiodarone	↑	Increased serum amiodarone levels may occur.
Fluoroquinolones (eg, sparfloxacin)	Amiodarone	↑	The risk of life-threatening cardiac arrhythmias, including torsades de pointes, may be increased.
Macrolide antibiotics (eg, azithromycin)	Amiodarone	↑	The risk of life-threatening cardiac arrhythmias, including torsades de pointes, may be increased.
Protease inhibitors Ritonavir Indinavir Nelfinavir Atazanavir	Amiodarone	↑	Large increases in amiodarone concentrations may occur, increasing the risk of amiodarone toxicity.
Rifamycins (eg, rifampin)	Amiodarone	↓	Serum concentrations of amiodarone and its active metabolite may be decreased, reducing its pharmacologic effect.
St. John's Wort	Amiodarone	↓	St. John's wort induces CYP3A4 reducing amiodarone levels.

* ↑ = Object drug increased. ↓ = Object drug decreased.

➤*Drug/Lab test interactions:* Amiodarone alters the results of thyroid function tests, causing an increase in serum T_4 and serum reverse T_3 levels and a decline in serum T_3 levels. Despite these biochemical changes, most patients remain clinically euthyroid. Elevations in liver enzymes (ALT and AST) can occur.

➤*Drug/Food interactions:* After a high-fat meal and an overnight fast, the AUC and C_{max} increased by 2.3 and 3.8 times, respectively, in the presence of food. Food also increased the rate of absorption of amiodarone, decreasing the time to T_{max} by 37%. The AUC and C_{max} metabolite DEA increased by 55% and 32%, respectively, in the presence of food. Because of the food effect on absorption, amiodarone should be administered consistently with regard to meals.

Grapefruit juice inhibits metabolism of oral amiodarone in the intestinal mucosa, resulting in increased amiodarone AUC by 50% and C_{max} by 84%, and decreased DEA to unquantifiable concentrations.

Adverse Reactions

Adverse reactions have been very common in virtually all series of patients treated with amiodarone for ventricular arrhythmias with relatively large doses of drug (400 mg/day and above), occurring in about three-fourths of all patients and causing discontinuation in 7% to 18%. The most serious reactions are pulmonary toxicity, exacerbation of arrhythmia, and rare serious liver injury (see Warnings), but other adverse effects constitute important problems. They are often reversible with dose reduction or cessation of amiodarone treatment. Most of the adverse effects appear to become more frequent with continued treatment beyond six months, although rates appear to remain relatively constant beyond one year. The time and dose relationships of adverse effects are under continued study.

In surveys of almost 5,000 patients treated in open U.S. studies and in published reports of treatment with amiodarone, the adverse reactions most frequently requiring discontinuation of drug included pulmonary infiltrates or fibrosis, paroxysmal ventricular tachycardia, congestive heart failure, and elevation of liver enzymes. Other symptoms causing discontinuations less often included visual disturbances, solar dermatitis, blue skin discoloration, hyperthyroidism, and hypothyroidism.

AMIODARONE HYDROCHLORIDE — ORAL

➤*Cardiovascular:* Cardiovascular adverse reactions, other than exacerbation of the arrhythmias, include the uncommon occurrence of congestive heart failure (3%) and bradycardia. Bradycardia usually responds to dosage reduction but may require a pacemaker for control. CHF rarely requires drug discontinuation. Cardiac conduction abnormalities occur infrequently and are reversible on discontinuation of drug.

Cardiac arrhythmias, congestive heart failure, SA node dysfunction (1% to 3%); cardiac conduction abnormalities, hypotension (less than 1%).

➤*CNS:* Neurologic problems are extremely common, occurring in 20% to 40% of patients and including malaise and fatigue, tremor and involuntary movements, poor coordination and gait, and peripheral neuropathy; they are rarely a reason to stop therapy and may respond to dose reductions or discontinuation.

Abnormal gait/ataxia, dizziness, lack of coordination, malaise and fatigue, paresthesias, tremor/abnormal involuntary movements (4% to 9%); decreased libido, headache, insomnia, sleep disturbances (1% to 3%).

➤*Dermatologic:* Dermatologic adverse reactions occur in about 15% of patients, with photosensitivity being most common (about 10%). Sunscreen and protection from sun exposure may be helpful, and drug discontinuation is not usually necessary. Prolonged exposure to amiodarone occasionally results in a blue-gray pigmentation. This is slowly and occasionally incompletely reversible on discontinuation of drug but is of cosmetic importance only.

Solar dermatitis/photosensitivity (4% to 9%); alopecia, blue skin discoloration, rash, spontaneous ecchymosis, (less than 1%).

➤*Endocrine:* Hyperthyroidism, hypothyroidism (1% to 3%).

➤*GI:* Gastrointestinal complaints, most commonly anorexia, constipation, nausea, and vomiting, occur in about 25% of patients but rarely require discontinuation of drug. These commonly occur during high-dose administration (ie, loading dose) and usually respond to dose reduction or divided doses.

Nausea, vomiting (10% to 33%); anorexia, constipation (4% to 9%); abdominal pain (1% to 3%).

➤*Hepatic:* Abnormal liver function tests (4% to 9%); nonspecific hepatic disorders (1% to 3%).

➤*Ophthalmic:* Ophthalmic abnormalities including optic neuropathy and/or optic neuritis, in some cases progressing to permanent blindness, corneal degeneration, eye discomfort, lens opacities, macular degeneration, papilledema, photosensitivity, and scotoma, and have been reported.

Asymptomatic corneal microdeposits are present in virtually all adult patients who have been on the drug for more than 6 months. Some patients develop eye symptoms of dry eyes, halos, and photophobia. Vision is rarely affected and drug discontinuation is rarely needed.

Visual disturbances (4% to 9%).

➤*Respiratory:* Fibrosis, pulmonary inflammation (4% to 9%).

➤*Miscellaneous:* Abnormal salivation, abnormal taste and smell, coagulation abnormalities, edema, flushing (1% to 3%).

➤*Postmarketing reports:*

Cardiovascular – Sinus arrest.

CNS – Confusional state, delirium, disorientation, hallucination, pseudotumor cerebri.

Dermatologic – Erythema multiforme, exfoliative dermatitis, pruritus, Stevens-Johnson syndrome, toxic epidermal necrolysis (sometimes fatal).

GU – Epididymitis, impotence.

Hematologic – Aplastic anemia, hemolytic anemia, neutropenia, pancytopenia, thrombocytopenia.

Hepatic – Cholestatic hepatitis, cirrhosis, hepatitis.

Musculoskeletal – Myopathy, muscle weakness, rhabdomyolysis.

Respiratory – Bronchiolitis obliterans organizing pneumonia (possibly fatal), bronchospasm, cough, dyspnea, hemoptysis, hypoxia, pleuritis, possibly fatal respiratory disorders (including distress, failure, arrest, and ARDS), pulmonary infiltrates, wheezing.

Miscellaneous – Angioedema, fever, pancreatitis, syndrome of inappropriate antidiuretic hormone secretion (SIADH), vasculitis.

Overdosage

➤*Symptoms:* There have been cases, some fatal, of amiodarone overdose.

➤*Treatment:* In addition to general supportive measures, the patient's cardiac rhythm and blood pressure should be monitored, and if bradycardia ensues, a beta-adrenergic agonist or a pacemaker may be used. Hypotension with inadequate tissue perfusion should be treated with positive inotropic and/or vasopressor agents. Neither amiodarone nor its metabolite is dialyzable.

Patient Information

Instruct patients to not drink grapefruit juice during treatment with amiodarone tablets. Grapefruit juice affects how amiodarone is absorbed in the stomach.

Instruct patients to avoid exposing their skin to the sun or sun lamps. Amiodarone can cause a photosensitive reaction. Instruct patients to wear sunblock cream or protective clothing when out in the sun.

Advise women to avoid pregnancy while on amiodarone tablets, because it may harm the fetus.

Instruct women not to breast-feed while taking amiodarone tablets, because it may pass into their milk and can harm the baby.

AMIODARONE HYDROCHLORIDE — INJECTION

Indications

➤*Ventricular arrhythmias:* For initiation of treatment and prophylaxis of frequently recurring ventricular fibrillation and hemodynamically unstable ventricular tachycardia in patients refractory to other therapy. Amiodarone injection also can be used to treat patients with ventricular tachycardia (VT)/ventricular fibrillation (VF) for whom oral amiodarone is indicated, but who are unable to take oral medication. During or after treatment with amiodarone injection, patients may be transferred to oral amiodarone therapy.

Amiodarone injection should be used for acute treatment until the patient's ventricular arrhythmias are stabilized. Most patients will require this therapy for 48 to 96 hours, but amiodarone injection may be safely administered for longer periods if necessary.

➤*Unlabeled uses:* Amiodarone has shown effectiveness for conversion of atrial fibrillation and atrial flutter and maintenance of sinus rhythm. It also appears to be useful in treating supraventricular tachycardia, and IV amiodarone has shown effectiveness in the treatment of AV nodal reentry tachycardia.

Administration and Dosage

➤*Approved by the FDA:* August 3, 1995.

Amiodarone shows considerable interindividual variation in response. Thus, although a starting dose adequate to suppress life-threatening arrhythmias is needed, close monitoring with adjustment of dose as needed is essential. The recommended starting dose of amiodarone injection is about 1000 mg over the first 24 hours of therapy, delivered by the following infusion regimen:

Amiodarone IV dose recommendations (first 24 h)		
Loading infusions	First rapid:	150 mg over the first 10 min (15 mg/min). Add 3 mL of amiodarone IV (150 mg) to 100 mL D_5W (concentration = 1.5 mg/mL). Infuse 100 mL over 10 min.
	Followed by slow:	360 mg over the next 6 h (1 mg/min). Add 18 mL of amiodarone IV (900 mg) to 500 mL D_5W (concentration = 1.8 mg/mL).
Maintenance infusion		540 mg over the remaining 18 hours (0.5 mg/min). Decrease the rate of the slow loading infusion to 0.5 mg/min.

After the first 24 hours, the maintenance infusion rate of 0.5 mg/min (720 mg per 24 hours) should be continued utilizing a concentration of 1 to 6 mg/mL (amiodarone injection concentrations greater than 2 mg/mL should be administered via a central venous catheter). In the event of breakthrough episodes of VF or hemodynamically unstable VT, 150 mg supplemental infusions of amiodarone injection mixed in 100 mL of D_5W may be administered. Such infusions should be administered over 10 minutes to minimize the potential for hypotension. The rate of the maintenance infusion may be increased to achieve effective arrhythmia suppression.

The first 24-hour dose may be individualized for each patient; however, in controlled clinical trials, mean daily doses above 2,100 mg were associated with an increased risk of hypotension. The initial infusion rate should not exceed 30 mg/min.

Based on the experience from clinical studies of amiodarone injection, a maintenance infusion of up to 0.5 mg/min can be cautiously continued for 2 to 3 weeks regardless of the patient's age, renal function, or left ventricular function. There has been limited experience in patients receiving amiodarone injection for longer than 3 weeks.

➤*Administration:* The surface properties of solutions containing injectable amiodarone are altered such that the drop size may be reduced. This reduction may lead to underdosage of the patient by up to 30% if drop counter infusion sets are used. Amiodarone injection must be delivered by a volumetric infusion pump.

Amiodarone injection should, whenever possible, be administered through a central venous catheter dedicated to that purpose. An in-line filter should be used during administration.

Amiodarone injection concentrations greater than 3 mg/mL in D_5W have been associated with a high incidence of peripheral vein phlebitis; however, concentrations of less than or equal to 2.5 mg/mL appear to be less irritating. Therefore, for infusions longer than 1 hour, amiodarone injection concentrations should not exceed 2 mg/mL unless a central venous catheter is used.

AMIODARONE HYDROCHLORIDE — INJECTION

➤*Admixture incompatibility:* Amiodarone injection in D_5W is incompatible with the drugs shown in the table below.

Amiodarone Y-site injection incompatibility			
Drug	Vehicle	Amiodarone concentration	Comments
Aminophylline	D_5W	4 mg/mL	Precipitate
Cefamandole nafate	D_5W	4 mg/mL	Precipitate
Cefazolin sodium	D_5W	4 mg/mL	Precipitate
Mezlocillin sodium	D_5W	4 mg/mL	Precipitate
Heparin sodium	D_5W	-	Precipitate
Sodium bicarbonate	D_5W	3 mg/mL	Precipitate

➤*IV to oral transition:* Patients whose arrhythmias have been suppressed by amiodarone injection may be switched to oral amiodarone. The optimal dose for changing from intravenous to oral administration of amiodarone will depend on the dose of amiodarone injection already administered, as well as the bioavailability of oral amiodarone. When changing to oral amiodarone therapy, clinical monitoring is recommended, particularly for elderly patients.

Amiodarone Recommendations for oral dosage after IV infusion	
Duration of amiodarone IV infusion[a]	Initial daily dose of oral amiodarone
Less than 1 wk	800 to 1,600 mg
1 to 3 wk	600 to 800 mg
Greater than 3 wk[b]	400 mg

[a] Assuming 720 mg/day infusion (0.5 mg/min).
[b] Amiodarone IV is not intended for maintenance treatment.

➤*Storage/Stability:* Store at room temperature, 15° to 25°C (59° to 77°F). Protect from light and excessive heat. Use carton to protect contents from light until used.

Amiodarone injection infusions exceeding 2 hours must be administered in glass or polyolefin bottles containing D_5W. Use of evacuated glass containers for admixing amiodarone injection is not recommended as incompatibility with a buffer in the container may cause precipitation.

It is well known that amiodarone adsorbs to polyvinyl chloride (PVC) tubing and the clinical trial dose administration schedule was designed to account for this adsorption. All of the clinical trials were conducted using PVC tubing and its use is therefore recommended. The concentrations and rates of infusion provided above reflect doses identified in these studies. It is important that the recommended infusion regimen be followed closely.

Amiodarone injection has been found to leach out plasticizers, including DEHP [di-(2-ethylhexyl) phthalate] from intravenous tubing (including PVC tubing). The degree of leaching increases when infusing amiodarone injection at higher concentrations and lower flow rates than provided above.

Amiodarone injection does not need to be protected from light during administration.

Amiodarone Solution Stability			
Solution	Concentration (mg/mL)	Container	Comments
5% dextrose in water (D_5W)	1 to 6	PVC	Physically compatible, with amiodarone loss less than 10% at 2 h at room temperature.
5% dextrose in water (D_5W)	1 to 6	Polyolefin, glass	Physically compatible, with no amiodarone loss at 24 h at room temperature.

Actions

➤*Pharmacology:* Amiodarone is generally considered a class III antiarrhythmic drug, but it possesses electrophysiologic characteristics of all four Vaughan Williams classes. Like class I drugs, amiodarone blocks sodium channels at rapid pacing frequencies, and like class II drugs, it exerts a noncompetitive antisympathetic action. One of its main effects, with prolonged administration, is to lengthen the cardiac action potential, a class III effect. The negative chronotropic effect of amiodarone in nodal tissues is similar to the effect of class IV drugs. In addition to blocking sodium channels, amiodarone blocks myocardial potassium channels, which contributes to slowing of conduction and prolongation of refractoriness. The antisympathetic action and the block of calcium and potassium channels are responsible for the negative dromotropic effects on the sinus node and for the slowing of conduction and prolongation of refractoriness in the atrioventricular (AV) node. Its vasodilatory action can decrease cardiac workload and consequently myocardial oxygen consumption.

Administration of amiodarone injection prolongs intranodal conduction (Atrial-His, AH) and refractoriness of the atrioventricular node (ERP AVN), but has little or no effect on sinus cycle length (SCL), refractoriness of the right atrium and right ventricle (ERP RA and ERP RV), repolarization (QTc), intraventricular conduction (QRS), and infranodal conduction (His-ventricular, HV). A comparison of the electrophysiologic effects of amiodarone IV and oral amiodarone is shown in the table below.

Effects of IV and Oral Amiodarone on Electrophysiologic Parameters								
Formulation	SCL	QRS	QTc	AH	HV	ERP RA	ERP RV	ERP AVN
IV	↔[a]	↔	↔	↑	↔	↔	↔	↑
Oral	↑	↔	↑	↑	↔	↑	↑	↑

[a] No change.

At higher doses (greater than 10 mg/kg) of amiodarone injection, prolongation of the ERP RV and modest prolongation of the QRS have been seen. These differences between oral and intravenous administration suggest that the initial acute effects of amiodarone injection may be predominantly focused on the AV node, causing an intranodal conduction delay and increased nodal refractoriness due to slow channel blockade (class IV activity) and noncompetitive adrenergic antagonism (class II activity).

Pharmacodynamics – Amiodarone injection has been reported to produce negative inotropic and vasodilatory effects in animals and humans. In clinical studies of patients with refractory VF or hemodynamically unstable VT, treatment-emergent, drug-related hypotension occurred in 288 of 1836 patients (16%) treated with amiodarone injection. No correlations were seen between the baseline ejection fraction and the occurrence of clinically significant hypotension during infusion of amiodarone injection.

➤*Pharmacokinetics:*

Absorption/Distribution – Amiodarone exhibits complex disposition characteristics after intravenous administration. Peak serum concentrations after single 5 mg/kg 15-minute intravenous infusions in healthy subjects range between 5 and 41 mg/L. Peak concentrations after 10-minute infusions of 150 mg amiodarone injection in patients with ventricular fibrillation (VF) or hemodynamically unstable ventricular tachycardia (VT) range between 7 and 26 mg/L. Due to rapid distribution, serum concentrations decline to 10% of peak values within 30 to 45 minutes after the end of the infusion. In clinical trials, after 48 hours of continued infusions (125, 500, or 1000 mg/day) plus supplemental (150 mg) infusions (for recurrent arrhythmias), amiodarone mean serum concentrations between 0.7 to 1.4 mg/L were observed (n = 260).

There is no established relationship between drug concentration and therapeutic response for short-term intravenous use. Steady-state amiodarone concentrations of 1 to 2.5 mg/L have been associated with antiarrhythmic effects and acceptable toxicity following chronic oral amiodarone therapy.

The following table summarizes the mean ranges of pharmacokinetic parameters of amiodarone reported in single dose IV (5 mg/kg over 15 min) studies of healthy subjects.

Pharmacokinetic Profile after Amiodarone Injection Administration				
Drug	Clearance (mL/h/kg)	V_c[a] (L/kg)	V_{ss}[a] (L/kg)	t½ (days)
Amiodarone	90 to 158	0.2	40 to 84	20 to 47
Desethylamiodarone	197 to 290	—	68 to 168	≥ AMI t½

Metabolism/Excretion – N-desethylamiodarone (DEA) is the major active metabolite of amiodarone in humans. DEA serum concentrations above 0.05 mg/L are not usually seen until after several days of continuous infusion but with prolonged therapy reach approximately the same concentration as amiodarone. The enzymes responsible for the N-deethylation are believed to be the cytochrome P450 3A (CYP3A) subfamily, principally CYP3A4. This isozyme is present in both the liver and intestines. The highly variable systemic availability of oral amiodarone may be attributed potentially to large interindividual variability in CYP3A4 activity.

Since grapefruit juice is known to inhibit CYP3A4-mediated metabolism of oral amiodarone in the intestinal mucosa, resulting in increased plasma levels of amiodarone; grapefruit juice should not be taken during treatment with oral amiodarone.

Amiodarone is eliminated primarily by hepatic metabolism and biliary excretion and there is negligible excretion of amiodarone or DEA in urine. Neither amiodarone nor DEA is dialyzable. Amiodarone and DEA cross the placenta and both appear in breast milk.

Desethylamiodarone clearance and volume involve an unknown biotransformation factor.

In clinical studies of 2 to 7 days, clearance of amiodarone after intravenous administration in patients with VT and VF ranged between 220 and 440 mL/hr/kg.

Special populations –

Hepatic function impairment: After a single dose of amiodarone injection in cirrhotic patients, significantly lower C_{max} and average concentration values are seen for DEA, but mean amiodarone levels are unchanged.

Elderly: Healthy subjects older than 65 years of age show lower clearances (about 100 mL/h/kg) than younger subjects (about 150 mL/h/kg) and an increase in t½ from about 20 to 47 days.

Severe left ventricular dysfunction: In patients with severe left ventricular dysfunction, the pharmacokinetics of amiodarone are not significantly altered but the terminal disposition t½ of DEA is prolonged.

Contraindications

Hypersensitivity to any of the components of amiodarone injection, including iodine; or cardiogenic shock; marked sinus bradycardia; second- or third-degree AV block unless a functioning pacemaker is available.

Warnings

➤*Hypotension:* Hypotension is the most common adverse effect seen with amiodarone injection. In clinical trials, treatment-emergent, drug-related hypotension was reported as an adverse effect in 288 (16%) of 1,836 patients

AMIODARONE HYDROCHLORIDE — INJECTION

treated with amiodarone injection. Clinically significant hypotension during infusions was seen most often in the first several hours of treatment and was not dose related, but appeared to be related to the rate of infusion. Hypotension necessitating alterations in amiodarone injection therapy was reported in 3% of patients, with permanent discontinuation required in less than 2% of patients.

Initially treat by slowing the infusion; additional standard therapy may be needed, including the following: vasopressor drugs, positive inotropic agents, and volume expansion. Monitor the initial rate of infusion closely; do not let it exceed that prescribed.

In some cases, hypotension may be refractory resulting in fatal outcome.

➤*Cardiac effects:*

Bradycardia and AV block – Drug-related bradycardia occurred in 90 (4.9%) of 1,836 patients in clinical trials while they were receiving amiodarone injection for life-threatening VT/VF; it was not dose-related. Treat bradycardia by slowing the infusion rate or discontinuing amiodarone injection. In some patients, inserting a pacemaker is required. Despite such measures, bradycardia was progressive and terminal in 1 patient during the controlled trials. Treat patients with a known predisposition to bradycardia or AV block with amiodarone injection in a setting where a temporary pacemaker is available.

Proarrhythmia – Like all antiarrhythmic agents, amiodarone injection may cause a worsening of existing arrhythmias or precipitate a new arrhythmia. Proarrhythmia, primarily torsades de pointes, has been associated with prolongation by amiodarone injection of the QTc interval to 500 ms or greater. Although QTc prolongation occurred frequently in patients receiving amiodarone injection, torsades de pointes or new-onset VF occurred infrequently (less than 2%). Monitor patients for QTc prolongation during infusion with amiodarone injection. Reserve combination of amiodarone with other antiarrhythmic therapy that prolongs the QTc for patients with life-threatening ventricular arrhythmias who are incompletely responsive to a single agent.

See Drug Interactions for more information.

The need to coadminister amiodarone with any other drug known to prolong the QTc interval must be based on a careful assessment of the potential risks and benefits of doing so for each patient.

A careful assessment of the potential risks and benefits of administering amiodarone injection must be made in patients with thyroid dysfunction due to the possibility of arrhythmia breakthrough or exacerbation of arrhythmia, which may result in death, in these patients.

➤*Long-term use:* See Precautions for more information.

➤*Carcinogenesis:* No carcinogenicity studies were conducted with amiodarone injection. However, oral amiodarone caused a statistically significant, dose-related increase in the incidence of thyroid tumors (follicular adenoma and/or carcinoma) in rats. The incidence of thyroid tumors in rats was greater than the incidence in controls even at the lowest dose level tested ie, 5 mg/kg/day (approximately 0.08 times the maximum recommended human maintenance dose; 600 mg in a 50 kg patient [dose compared on a body surface area basis]).

➤*Fertility impairment:* No fertility studies were conducted with amiodarone injection. However, in a study in which amiodarone was orally administered to male and female rats, beginning at 9 weeks prior to mating, reduced fertility was observed at a dose level of 90 mg/kg/day (approximately 1.4 times the maximum recommended human maintenance dose; 600 mg in a 50 kg patient [dose compared on a body surface area basis]).

➤*Elderly:* In general, dose selection for an elderly patient should be cautious, usually starting at the low end of the dosing range, reflecting the greater frequency of decreased hepatic, renal, or cardiac function, and of concomitant disease or other drug therapy.

➤*Pregnancy: Category D.* Although oral amiodarone use during pregnancy is uncommon, there have been a small number of published reports of congenital goiter/hypothyroidism and hyperthyroidism. If amiodarone injection is administered during pregnancy, apprise the patient of the potential hazard to the fetus.

Only use amiodarone injection during pregnancy if the potential benefit to the mother justifies the risk to the fetus.

➤*Lactation:* Amiodarone and 1 of its major metabolites, desethylamiodarone (DEA), are excreted in human milk, suggesting that breast-feeding could expose the nursing infant to a significant dose of the drug. Nursing offspring of lactating rats administered amiodarone have demonstrated reduced viability and reduced body weight gains. Weigh the risk of exposing the infant to amiodarone against the potential benefit of arrhythmia suppression in the mother. Advise the mother to discontinue nursing.

➤*Children:* The safety and efficacy of amiodarone in the pediatric population have not been established; therefore, its use in pediatric patients is not recommended.

See Precautions for more information.

Precautions

➤*Monitoring:* Monitor for hypotension, especially during the first few hours of infusion. Monitor for QTc prolongation during infusion with amiodarone injection. Close perioperative monitoring is recommended in patients undergoing general anesthesia who are on amiodarone therapy.

Monitor thyroid function at baseline and periodically during therapy, particularly in the elderly and in any patient with a history of thyroid nodules, goiter, or other thyroid dysfunction.

Monitor liver enzymes on a regular basis.

Closely monitor FiO_2 and the determinants of oxygen delivery to the tissues (eg, SaO_2, PaO_2) in patients on amiodarone.

➤*Hepatic effects:* Elevations of blood hepatic enzyme values (alanine aminotransferase [ALT], aspartate aminotransferase [AST], and gamma-glutamyl transferase [GGT]) are seen commonly in patients with immediately life-threatening VT/VF. Interpreting elevated AST activity can be difficult because the values may be elevated in patients who have had recent myocardial infarction, congestive heart failure, or multiple electrical defibrillations. Approximately 54% of patients receiving amiodarone injection in clinical studies had baseline liver enzyme elevations, and 13% had clinically significant elevations. In 81% of patients with both baseline and on-therapy data available, the liver enzyme elevations either improved during therapy or remained at baseline levels. Baseline abnormalities in hepatic enzymes are not a contraindication to treatment.

Rare cases of fatal hepatocellular necrosis after treatment with amiodarone injection have been reported. Two patients, one 28 years of age and the other 60 years of age, were treated for atrial arrhythmias with an initial infusion of 1500 mg over 5 hours, a rate much higher than recommended. Both patients developed hepatic and renal failure within 24 hours after the start of amiodarone injection treatment and died on day 14 and day 4, respectively. Because these episodes of hepatic necrosis may have been due to the rapid rate of infusion with possible rate-related hypotension, closely monitor the initial rate of infusion and do not let it exceed that prescribed.

In patients with life-threatening arrhythmias, weigh the potential risk of hepatic injury against the potential benefit of amiodarone injection therapy, but carefully monitor patients receiving amiodarone injection for evidence of progressive hepatic injury. Give consideration to reducing the rate of administration or withdrawing amiodarone injection in such cases.

➤*Pulmonary disorders:*

Pulmonary toxicity – There have been postmarketing reports of acute-onset (days to weeks) pulmonary injury in patients treated with amiodarone IV. Findings have included pulmonary infiltrates on X-ray, bronchospasm, wheezing, fever, dyspnea, cough, hemoptysis, and hypoxia. Some cases have progressed to respiratory failure and/or death.

Adult respiratory distress syndrome (ARDS) – Two percent (2%) of patients were reported to have ARDS during clinical studies involving 48 hours of therapy. ARDS is a disorder characterized by bilateral, diffuse pulmonary infiltrates with pulmonary edema and varying degrees of respiratory insufficiency. The clinical and radiographic picture can arise after a variety of lung injuries, such as those resulting from trauma, shock, prolonged cardiopulmonary resuscitation, and aspiration pneumonia, conditions present in many of the patients enrolled in the clinical studies. There have been postmarketing reports of ARDS in amiodarone IV patients. Amiodarone IV may play a role in causing or exacerbating pulmonary disorders in those patients.

Postoperatively, occurrences of ARDS have been reported in patients receiving oral amiodarone therapy who have undergone either cardiac or noncardiac surgery. Although patients usually respond well to vigorous respiratory therapy, in rare instances the outcome has been fatal. Until further studies have been performed, it is recommended that FiO_2 and the determinants of oxygen delivery to the tissues (eg, SaO_2, PaO_2) be closely monitored in patients on amiodarone.

Pulmonary fibrosis – Only 1 of more than 1,000 patients treated with amiodarone injection in clinical studies developed pulmonary fibrosis. In that patient, the condition was diagnosed 3 months after treatment with amiodarone injection, during which time she received oral amiodarone. Pulmonary toxicity is a well-recognized complication of long-term amiodarone use.

➤*Surgery:* Close perioperative monitoring is recommended in patients undergoing general anesthesia who are on amiodarone therapy as they may be more sensitive to the myocardial depressant and conduction effects of halogenated inhalational anesthetics.

➤*Benzyl alcohol:* Benzyl alcohol, contained in some of these products as a preservative, has been associated with a fatal "gasping syndrome" in premature infants.

➤*Electrolyte disturbances:* Patients with hypokalemia or hypomagnesemia should have the condition corrected whenever possible before being treated with amiodarone injection, as these disorders can exaggerate the degree of QTc prolongation and increase the potential for torsades de pointes. Give special attention to electrolyte and acid-base balance in patients experiencing severe or prolonged diarrhea or in patients receiving concomitant diuretics.

Drug Interactions

Amiodarone Drug Interactions

Precipitant drug	Object drug[a]		Description
Amiodarone	Antiarrhythmics (eg, quinidine, procainamide, disopyramide, flecainide)	↑	Amiodarone may increase serum concentrations of these antiarrhythmics. Monitor patients closely. Reduce dose of antiarrhythmic with coadministration.

AMIODARONE HYDROCHLORIDE — INJECTION

Amiodarone Drug Interactions

Precipitant drug	Object drug[a]		Description
Amiodarone	Anticoagulants (eg, warfarin)	↑	Prothrombin time (PT) may increase. Potentiation of anticoagulant response is almost always seen in patients receiving amiodarone and can result in serious or fatal bleeding. A 30% to 50% anticoagulant dose reduction is typically required. Onset is 3 to 4 days and may persist for months after amiodarone discontinuation. Closely monitor PT.
Amiodarone	Beta blockers (eg, propranolol)	↑	Effects of beta blockers eliminated by hepatic metabolism may be increased. Because amiodarone has weak beta blocking activity, concomitant use can increase risk of hypotension and bradycardia.
Amiodarone	Cardiac glycosides (eg, digoxin, digitoxin)	↑	Amiodarone taken concomitantly with digoxin increases the serum digoxin concentration by 70% after 1 day. Reduce dose of digitalis therapy by 50% or discontinue.
Amiodarone	Calcium channel blockers (eg, verapamil, diltiazem)	↑	Amiodarone inhibits AV conduction and decreases myocardial contractility; increased risk of AV block with verapamil or diltiazem or hypotension with any calcium blocker may occur.
Amiodarone	Cisapride	↑	Risk of life-threatening cardiac arrhythmias, including torsades de pointes, may be increased because of possibly additive prolongation of the QT interval.
Amiodarone	Cyclosporine	↑	Concomitant use has produced persistently elevated plasma cyclosporine levels resulting in elevated creatinine despite reduction in dose of cyclosporine.
Amiodarone	Dextromethorphan	↑	Chronic use (> 2 weeks) of amiodarone impairs metabolism of dextromethorphan.
Amiodarone	Disopyramide	↑	Increases QT prolongation and possible arrhythmias.
Amiodarone	Fentanyl	↑	May cause hypotension, bradycardia, decreased cardiac output.
Amiodarone	HMG-CoA reductase inhibitors (eg, simvastatin)	↑	Simvastatin in combination with amiodarone has been associated with reports of myopathy/rhabdomyolysis.
Amiodarone	Hydantoins (eg, phenytoin)	↑	Chronic use (> 2 weeks) of amiodarone impairs metabolism of phenytoin. Increased hydantoin concentrations with symptoms of toxicity may occur. Also, amiodarone serum levels may be decreased.
Hydantoins (eg, phenytoin)	Amiodarone	↓	
Amiodarone	Lidocaine	↑	Sinus bradycardia has been reported with oral amiodarone in combination with lidocaine for local anesthesia. Seizure, associated with increased lidocaine concentrations, has been reported with concomitant administration of IV amiodarone.
Amiodarone	Methotrexate	↑	Chronic use (> 2 weeks) of amiodarone impairs metabolism of methotrexate.
Amiodarone	Theophylline	↑	Increased theophylline levels with toxicity may occur. Effects may not be seen for ≥ 1 week of concomitant therapy and may persist for an extended period after amiodarone discontinuation.
Amiodarone	Thioridazine	↑	The risk of life-threatening cardiac arrhythmias, including torsades de pointes, may be increased.
Azole antifungals (eg, itraconazole)	Amiodarone	↑	The risk of life-threatening cardiac arrhythmias, including torsades de pointes, may be increased.
Cholestyramine	Amiodarone	↓	Increased enterohepatic elimination of amiodarone and reduced serum levels and half-life may occur.
Cimetidine	Amiodarone	↑	Increased serum amiodarone levels may occur.
Fluoroquinolones (eg, sparfloxacin)	Amiodarone	↑	The risk of life-threatening cardiac arrhythmias, including torsades de pointes, may be increased.
Macrolide antibiotics (eg, azithromycin)	Amiodarone	↑	The risk of life-threatening cardiac arrhythmias, including torsades de pointes, may be increased.
Protease inhibitors Ritonavir Indinavir Nelfinavir Atazanavir	Amiodarone	↑	Large increases in amiodarone concentrations may occur, increasing the risk of amiodarone toxicity.
Rifamycins (eg, rifampin)	Amiodarone	↓	Serum concentrations of amiodarone and its active metabolite may be decreased, reducing its pharmacologic effect.
St. John's Wort	Amiodarone	↓	St. John's wort induces CYP3A4 reducing amiodarone levels.

[a] ↑ = Object drug increased. ↓ = Object drug decreased.

➤*Drug/food interactions:* Grapefruit juice inhibits metabolism of oral amiodarone in the intestinal mucosa, resulting in increased amiodarone AUC by 50% and C_{max} by 84%, and decreased DEA to unquantifiable concentrations. Consider this information when changing from intravenous amiodarone to oral amiodarone.

Adverse Reactions

The most important treatment-emergent adverse effects were hypotension, asystole/cardiac arrest/electromechanical dissociation (EMD), cardiogenic shock, congestive heart failure, bradycardia, liver function test abnormalities, VT, and AV block. Overall, treatment was discontinued for about 9% of the patients because of adverse effects. The most common adverse effects leading to discontinuation of amiodarone injection therapy were hypotension (1.6%), asystole/cardiac arrest/EMD (1.2%), VT (1.1%), and cardiogenic shock (1%).

IV Amiodarone Adverse Reactions (%)

Adverse reaction	Controlled studies (n = 814)	Open-label studies (n = 1,022)	Total (n = 1,836)
Cardiovascular			
Bradycardia	49 (6%)	41 (4%)	90 (4.9%)
Congestive heart failure	18 (2.2%)	21 (2%)	39 (2.1%)
Heart arrest	29 (3.5%)	26 (2.5%)	55 (2.9%)
Hypotension	165 (20.2%)	123 (12%)	288 (15.6%)
Ventricular tachycardia	15 (1.8%)	30 (2.9%)	45 (2.4%)
GI			
Liver function tests abnormal	35 (4.2%)	29 (2.8%)	64 (3.4%)
Nausea	29 (3.5%)	43 (4.2%)	72 (3.9%)
Miscellaneous			
Fever	24 (2.9%)	13 (1.2%)	37 (2%)

➤*IV Adverse reactions:* Other treatment-emergent possibly drug-related adverse events reported in less than 2% of patients receiving amiodarone injection in the manufacturer's controlled and uncontrolled studies included the following:

Cardiovascular – Atrial fibrillation, nodal arrhythmia, prolonged QT interval, sinus bradycardia, VF.

GI – Diarrhea, vomiting.

Hepatic – Increased ALT, increased AST.

Respiratory – Lung edema, respiratory disorder.

Miscellaneous – Abnormal kidney function, shock, Stevens-Johnson syndrome, thrombocytopenia.

➤*Postmarketing:*

Cardiovascular – Hypotension (sometimes fatal), sinus arrest.

CNS – Pseudotumor cerebri.

Dermatologic – Erythema multiforme, exfoliative dermatitis, toxic epidermal necrolysis.

Hematologic – Neutropenia, pancytopenia.

AMIODARONE HYDROCHLORIDE — INJECTION

Respiratory – Bronchospasm, cough, dyspnea, hemoptysis, hypoxia, possibly fatal respiratory disorders (including distress, failure, arrest, and ARDS), pulmonary infiltrates, wheezing.

Miscellaneous – Anaphylactic/anaphylactoid reaction (including shock), angioedema, fever, syndrome of inappropriate antidiuretic hormone secretion (SIADH).

Local – Cellulitis, edema, erythema, necrosis, pain, phlebitis, pigment changes, skin sloughing, thrombophlebitis, and venous thrombosis.

Overdosage

➤*Symptoms:* Effects of an inadvertent overdose of amiodarone injection include hypotension, cardiogenic shock, bradycardia, AV block, and hepatotoxicity.

There have been cases, some fatal, of amiodarone overdose.

➤*Treatment:* Treat hypotension and cardiogenic shock by slowing the infusion rate or with standard therapy: Vasopressor drugs, positive inotropic agents, and volume expansion. Bradycardia and AV block may require temporary pacing. Closely monitor hepatic enzyme concentrations. Amiodarone is not dialyzable.

ADENOSINE

Rx	**Adenosine** (Various, eg, Baxter, Bedford, Sicor)	**Injection:** 3 mg/mL	NaCl 9 mg/mL. Preservative free. In 2 and 4 mL vials and 2 mL disposable syringes.
Rx	**Adenocard** (Fujisawa)		NaCl 9 mg/mL. Preservative free. In 2 mL vials and 2 and 5 mL syringes.

ADENOSINE — INJECTION

Indications

➤*Paroxysmal supraventricular tachycardia (PSVT):* Conversion to sinus rhythm of PSVT, including that associated with accessory bypass tracts (Wolff-Parkinson-White [W-P-W] syndrome). When clinically advisable, attempt appropriate vagal maneuvers (eg, Valsalva maneuver) prior to use.

➤*Unlabeled uses:* Adenosine has been used in the noninvasive assessment of patients with suspected coronary artery disease in conjunction with ^{201}thallium tomography; results are similar to assessment with IV dipyridamole.

Administration and Dosage

➤*Approved by the FDA:* October 1989.

For rapid bolus IV use only. To be certain the solution reaches the systemic circulation, administer either directly into a vein or, if given into an IV line, as proximal as possible and follow with a rapid saline flush.

➤*Adult:*

Initial dose – 6 mg as a rapid IV bolus (administered over a 1 to 2 second period).

Repeat administration – If the first dose does not result in elimination of the supraventricular tachycardia within 1 to 2 minutes, give 12 mg as a rapid IV bolus. Repeat 12 mg dose a second time if required.

➤*Children:* The dosages used in neonates, infants, children, and adolescents were equivalent to those administered to adults on a weight basis.

Less than 50 kg –

Initial dose: 0.05 to 0.1 mg/kg as a rapid IV bolus given either centrally or peripherally. A saline flush should follow.

Repeat administration: If conversion of PSVT does not occur within 1 to 2 minutes, additional bolus injections of adenosine can be administered at incrementally higher doses, increasing the amount given by 0.05 to 0.1 mg/kg. Follow each bolus with a saline flush. Continue this process until sinus rhythm is established or a maximum single dose of 0.3 mg/kg is used.

Greater than or equal to 50 kg – Administer the adult dose.

Doses more than 12 mg are not recommended.

➤*Storage/Stability:* Store at room temperature 15° to 30°C (59° to 86°F). Do not refrigerate because crystallization may occur. If this occurs, let crystals warm to room temperature. The solution must be clear at the time of use. Discard unused portion.

Actions

➤*Pharmacology:* Adenosine slows conduction time through the AV node, can interrupt the re-entry pathways through the AV node, and can restore normal sinus rhythm in patients with PSVT, including PSVT associated with W-P-W syndrome.

Adenosine is antagonized competitively by methylxanthines such as caffeine and theophylline and potentiated by blockers of nucleoside transport such as dipyridamole. Adenosine is not blocked by atropine.

The usual IV bolus dose of 6 or 12 mg will not have systemic hemodynamic effects. When larger doses are given by infusion, adenosine decreases blood pressure by decreasing peripheral resistance.

➤*Pharmacokinetics:* IV adenosine is rapidly removed from the circulation. Following an IV bolus, adenosine is taken up by erythrocytes and vascular endothelial cells. Adenosine is primarily metabolized to inosine and adenosine monophosphate (AMP). Half-life of AMP is estimated to be less than 10 seconds.

Contraindications

Second- or third-degree AV block (except in patients with a functioning artificial pacemaker); sinus node disease, such as sick sinus syndrome or symptomatic bradycardia (except in patients with a functioning artificial pacemaker); known hypersensitivity to adenosine.

Warnings

➤*Heart block:* Adenosine decreases conduction through the AV node and may produce a short-lasting first-, second- or third-degree heart block. Institute appropriate therapy as needed. Patients who develop high-level block on 1 dose of adenosine should not be given additional doses. Because of the very short half-life, these effects are generally self-limiting.

Transient or prolonged episodes of asystole have been reported with fatal outcomes in some cases. Rarely, ventricular fibrillation has been reported following adenosine administration, including resuscitated and fatal events. In most instances, these cases were associated with the concomitant use of digoxin and, less frequently, with digoxin and verapamil. Although no causal relationship or drug-drug interaction has been established, use adenosine with caution in patients receiving digoxin or digoxin and verapamil in combination. Appropriate resuscitative measures should be made available.

➤*Arrhythmias:* At the time of conversion to normal sinus rhythm, a variety of new rhythms may appear on the ECG. They generally last only a few seconds without intervention and may take the form of premature ventricular contractions, atrial premature contractions, sinus bradycardia, sinus tachycardia, skipped beats, and varying degrees of AV nodal block. Such findings were seen in 55% of patients.

➤*Treatment of other arrhythmias:* Adenosine is not effective in converting rhythms other than PSVT, such as atrial flutter, atrial fibrillation, or ventricular tachycardia to normal sinus rhythm. Use in such patients has not resulted in adverse consequences.

➤*Ventricular response:* In the presence of atrial flutter or atrial fibrillation, a transient modest slowing of ventricular response may occur immediately following use.

➤*Bronchoconstriction:* Adenosine administered by inhalation has been reported to cause bronchoconstriction in asthmatic patients, presumably due to mast cell degranulation and histamine release. These effects have not been observed in normal subjects. Adenosine has been administered to a limited number of patients with asthma and mild to moderate exacerbation of their symptoms has been reported. Respiratory compromise has occurred using adenosine infusion in patients with obstructive pulmonary disease. Use adenosine with caution in patients with obstructive lung disease not associated with bronchoconstriction (eg, emphysema, bronchitis) and avoid use in patients with bronchoconstriction or bronchospasm (eg, asthma). Discontinue adenosine in any patient who develops severe respiratory difficulties.

➤*Mutagenesis:* Adenosine, like other nucleosides at millimolar concentrations present for several doubling times of cells in culture, is known to produce a variety of chromosomal alterations.

➤*Elderly:* Use adenosine with caution in geriatric patients because this population may have a diminished cardiac function, nodal dysfunction, concomitant diseases, or drug therapy that may alter hemodynamic function and produce severe bradycardia or AV block.

➤*Pregnancy: Category C.* Because adenosine is a naturally occurring material, widely dispersed throughout the body, no fetal effects would be anticipated. However, because it is not known whether the drug can cause fetal harm when administered to pregnant women, use during pregnancy only if clearly needed.

Drug Interactions

Adenosine Drug Interactions

Precipitant drug	Object drug*		Description
Carbamazepine	Adenosine	↑	Carbamazepine may increase the degree of heart block produced by other agents. As the primary effect of adenosine is to decrease conduction through the AV node, higher degrees of heart block may be produced in the presence of carbamazepine.
Dipyridamole	Adenosine	↑	The effects of adenosine are potentiated. Thus, smaller doses of adenosine may be effective in the presence of dipyridamole.
Methylxanthines (eg, caffeine, theophylline)	Adenosine	↓	The effects of adenosine are antagonized. In the presence of methylxanthines, larger doses of adenosine may be required or adenosine may be ineffective.

ADENOSINE — INJECTION

Adenosine Drug Interactions			
Precipitant drug	Object drug*		Description
Adenosine	Digoxin Verapamil	↑	The use of adenosine with digoxin and verapamil may rarely be associated with ventricular fibrillation.

* ↑ = Object drug increased. ↓ = Object drug decreased.

Adverse Reactions

➤*Cardiovascular:* Facial flushing (18%); headache (2%); sweating, palpitations, chest pain, hypotension (less than 1%); prolonged asystole; ventricular fibrillation; ventricular tachycardia; transient increase in blood pressure; bradycardia; atrial fibrillation (postmarket).

➤*CNS:* Light-headedness (2%); dizziness, tingling in arms, numbness (1%); apprehension, blurred vision, burning sensation, heaviness in arms, neck/back pain (less than 1%).

➤*GI:* Nausea (3%); metallic taste, tightness in throat, pressure in groin (less than 1%).

➤*Respiratory:* Shortness of breath/dyspnea (12%); chest pressure (7%); hyperventilation, head pressure (less than 1%); bronchospasm (postmarket).

Overdosage

Adverse effects are generally rapidly self-limiting. Individualize treatment of prolonged adverse effects and direct toward the specific effect. Methylxanthines are competitive antagonists of adenosine (see Drug Interactions). Refer to General Management of Acute Overdosage.

DOFETILIDE

Rx	**Tikosyn** (Pfizer)	**Capsules:** 125 mcg	(TKN 125 PFIZER). Light orange/white. In 14s, 60s, and UD 40s.
		250 mcg	(TKN 250 PFIZER). Peach. In 14s, 60s, and UD 40s.
		500 mcg	(TKN 500 PFIZER). Peach/white. In 14s, 60s, and UD 40s.

DOFETILIDE — ORAL

WARNING

To minimize the risk of induced arrhythmia, patients initiated or re-initiated on dofetilide should be placed for a minimum of 3 days in a facility that can provide calculations of creatinine clearance, continuous electrocardiographic monitoring, and cardiac resuscitation. For detailed instructions regarding dose selection, see Administration and Dosage. Dofetilide is available only to hospitals and prescribers who have received appropriate dofetilide dosing and treatment initiation education.

Indications

➤*Maintenance of normal sinus rhythm (delay in AF/AFI recurrence):* Maintenance of normal sinus rhythm (delay in time to recurrence of atrial fibrillation/atrial flutter [AF/AFl]) in patients with atrial fibrillation/atrial flutter of more than 1 week duration who have been converted to normal sinus rhythm. Because dofetilide can cause life threatening ventricular arrhythmias, it should be reserved for patients in whom atrial fibrillation/atrial flutter is highly symptomatic.

➤*Conversion of atrial fibrillation/flutter:* Conversion of atrial fibrillation and atrial flutter to normal sinus rhythm.

➤*Unlabeled uses:* Ventricular arrhythmias (inconclusive data).

Administration and Dosage

➤*Approved by the FDA:* October 1, 1999.

Therapy with dofetilide must be initiated (and, if necessary, reinitiated) in a setting that provides continuous electrocardiographic (ECG) monitoring and in the presence of personnel trained in the management of serious ventricular arrhythmias. Patients should continue to be monitored in this way for a minimum of 3 days. Additionally, patients should not be discharged within 12 hours of electrical or pharmacological conversion to normal sinus rhythm.

The dose of dofetilide must be individualized according to calculated creatinine clearance and QTc. (QT interval should be used if the heart rate is less than 60 beats per minute. There are no data on use of dofetilide when the heart rate is less than 50 beats per minute.) The usual recommended dose of dofetilide is 500 mcg twice daily, as modified by the dosing algorithm described below. For consideration of a lower dose, see Special considerations below.

Patients with atrial fibrillation should be anticoagulated according to usual medical practice prior to electrical or pharmacological cardioversion. Anticoagulant therapy may be continued after cardioversion according to usual medical practice for the treatment of people with AF. Hypokalemia should be corrected before initiation of dofetilide therapy.

Patients to be discharged on dofetilide therapy from an inpatient setting as described above must have an adequate supply of dofetilide, at the patient's individualized dose, to allow uninterrupted dosing until the patient receives the first outpatient supply.

Dofetilide is distributed only to those hospitals and other appropriate institutions confirmed to have received applicable dosing and treatment initiation education programs. Inpatient and subsequent outpatient discharge and refill prescriptions are filled only upon confirmation that the prescribing physician has received applicable dosing and treatment initiation education programs. For this purpose, a list for use by pharmacists is maintained containing hospitals and physicians who have received one of the education programs.

➤*Instructions for individualized dose initiation:*

Initiation of dofetilide therapy –

Step 1. Electrocardiographic assessment: Prior to administration of the first dose, the QTc must be determined using an average of 5 to 10 beats. If the QTc is more than 440 msec (500 msec in patients with ventricular conduction abnormalities), dofetilide is contraindicated. If heart rate is less than 60 beats per minute, QT interval should be used. Patients with heart rates less than 50 beats per minute have not been studied.

Step 2. Calculation of creatinine clearance: Prior to the administration of the first dose, the patient's creatinine clearance must be calculated.

When serum creatinine is given in mcmol/L, divide the value by 88.4 (1 mg/dL = 88.4 mcmol/L).

Step 3. Starting dose: The starting dose of dofetilide is determined as follows:

Calculated Creatinine Clearance	Dofetilide Dose
> 60 mL/min	500 mcg twice daily
40 to 60 mL/min	250 mcg twice daily
20 to < 40 mL/min	125 mcg twice daily
< 20 mL/min	Dofetilide is contraindicated in these patients.

Step 4.: Administer the adjusted dofetilide dose and begin continuous ECG monitoring.

Step 5.: At 2 to 3 hours after administering the first dose of dofetilide, determine the QTc. If the QTc has increased by more than 15% compared with the baseline established in Step 1 or if the QTc is more than 500 msec (550 msec in patients with ventricular conduction abnormalities), subsequent dosing should be adjusted as follows:

If the starting dose based on creatinine clearance is:	Then the adjusted dose (for QTc prolongation) is:
500 mcg twice daily	250 mcg twice daily
250 mcg twice daily	125 mcg twice daily
125 mcg twice daily	125 mcg once daily

Step 6.: At 2 to 3 hours after each subsequent dose of dofetilide, determine the QTc (for in-hospital doses 2 to 5). No further down titration of dofetilide based on QTc is recommended.

• *Note* – If at any time after the second dose of dofetilide is given, the QTc is more than 500 msec (550 msec in patients with ventricular conduction abnormalities), dofetilide should be discontinued.

Step 7.: Patients are to be continuously monitored by ECG for a minimum of 3 days, or for a minimum of 12 hours after electrical or pharmacological conversion to normal sinus rhythm, whichever is greater.

Maintenance of dofetilide therapy – Renal function and QTc should be reevaluated every 3 months or as medically warranted. If QTc exceeds 500 milliseconds (550 msec in patients with ventricular conduction abnormalities), dofetilide therapy should be discontinued and patients should be carefully monitored until QTc returns to baseline levels. If renal function deteriorates, adjust dose as described in Initiation of dofetilide therapy, Step 3.

➤*Special considerations:*

Consideration of a dose lower than that determined by the algorithm – The dosing algorithm shown above should be used to determine the individualized dose of dofetilide. In clinical trials, the highest dose of 500 mcg twice daily of dofetilide as modified by the dosing algorithm led to greater effectiveness than lower doses of 125 or 250 mcg twice daily as modified by the dosing algorithm. The risk of torsade de pointes, however, is related to dose as well as to patient characteristics. Physicians, in consultation with their patients, may therefore in some cases choose doses lower than determined by the algorithm. It is critically important that if at any time this lower dose is increased, the patient needs to be rehospitalized for 3 days. Previous toleration of higher doses does not eliminate the need for rehospitalization. The maximum recommended dose in patients with a calculated creatinine clearance more than 60 mL/min is 500 mcg twice daily; doses more than 500 mcg twice daily have been associated with an increased incidence of torsade de pointes.

DOFETILIDE — ORAL

A patient who misses a dose should not double the next dose. The next dose should be taken at the usual time.

Cardioversion – If patients do not convert to normal sinus rhythm within 24 hours of initiation of dofetilide therapy, electrical conversion should be considered. Patients continuing on dofetilide after successful electrical cardioversion should continue to be monitored by electrocardiography for 12 hours post cardioversion, or a minimum of 3 days after initiation of dofetilide therapy, whichever is greater.

Switch to dofetilide from Class I or other Class III antiarrhythmic therapy – Before initiating dofetilide therapy, previous antiarrhythmic therapy should be withdrawn under careful monitoring for a minimum of 3 plasma half-lives. Because of the unpredictable pharmacokinetics of amiodarone, dofetilide should not be initiated following amiodarone therapy until amiodarone plasma levels are below 0.3 mcg/mL or until amiodarone has been withdrawn for at least 3 months.

Stopping dofetilide prior to administration of potentially interacting drugs – If dofetilide needs to be discontinued to allow dosing of other potentially interacting drug(s), a washout period of at least 2 days should be followed before starting the other drug(s).

➤*Storage / Stability:* Store at controlled room temperature, 15° to 30°C (59° to 86°F). Protect from moisture and humidity. Dispense in tight containers.

Actions

➤*Pharmacology:* Dofetilide shows Vaughan Williams Class III antiarrhythmic activity. The mechanism of action is blockade of the cardiac ion channel carrying the rapid component of the delayed rectifier potassium current, I_{Kr}. At concentrations covering several orders of magnitude, dofetilide blocks only I_{Kr} with no relevant block of the other repolarizing potassium currents (eg, I_{Ks}, I_{K1}). At clinically relevant concentrations, dofetilide has no effect on sodium channels (associated with Class I effect), adrenergic alpha receptors, or adrenergic beta receptors.

➤*Pharmacokinetics:*

Absorption / Distribution – The oral bioavailability of dofetilide is more than 90%, with maximal plasma concentrations occurring at about 2 to 3 hours in the fasted state. Oral bioavailability is unaffected by food or antacid. The terminal half life of dofetilide is approximately 10 hours; steady state plasma concentrations are attained within 2 to 3 days, with an accumulation index of 1.5 to 2. Plasma concentrations are dose proportional. Plasma protein binding of dofetilide is 60% to 70%, is independent of plasma concentration, and is unaffected by renal impairment. Volume of distribution is 3 L/kg.

Metabolism / Excretion – Approximately 80% of a single dose of dofetilide is excreted in urine, of which approximately 80% is excreted as unchanged dofetilide with the remaining 20% consisting of inactive or minimally active metabolites. Renal elimination involves both glomerular filtration and active tubular secretion (via the cation transport system, a process that can be inhibited by cimetidine, trimethoprim, prochlorperazine, megestrol and ketoconazole). In vitro studies with human liver microsomes show that dofetilide can be metabolized by CYP3A4, but it has a low affinity for this isoenzyme. Metabolites are formed by N-dealkylation and N-oxidation. There are no quantifiable metabolites circulating in plasma, but 5 metabolites have been identified in urine.

Special populations –

Renal function impairment: In volunteers with varying degrees of renal impairment and patients with arrhythmias, the clearance of dofetilide decreases with decreasing creatinine clearance. As a result, and as seen in clinical studies, the half-life of dofetilide is longer in patients with lower creatinine clearances. Because increase in QT interval and the risk of ventricular arrhythmias are directly related to plasma concentrations of dofetilide, dosage adjustment based on calculated creatinine clearance is critically important. Patients with severe renal impairment (creatinine clearance less than 20 mL/min) were not included in clinical or pharmacokinetic studies.

Contraindications

Congenital or acquired long QT syndromes. Dofetilide should not be used in patients with a baseline QT interval or QTc more than 440 msec (500 msec in patients with ventricular conduction abnormalities).

Severe renal impairment (calculated creatinine clearance less than 20 mL/min).

Concomitant use with verapamil or the cation transport system inhibitors cimetidine, trimethoprim (alone or in combination with sulfamethoxazole) or ketoconazole; other known inhibitors of the renal cation transport system such as prochlorperazine and megestrol should not be used in patients on dofetilide.

Hypersensitivity to the drug.

Warnings

➤*Ventricular arrhythmia:* Dofetilide can cause serious ventricular arrhythmias, primarily torsade de pointes (TdP) type ventricular tachycardia, a polymorphic ventricular tachycardia associated with QT interval prolongation. QT interval prolongation is directly related to dofetilide plasma concentration. Factors such as reduced creatinine clearance or certain dofetilide drug interactions will increase dofetilide plasma concentration. The risk of TdP can be reduced by controlling the plasma concentration through adjustment of the initial dofetilide dose according to creatinine clearance and by monitoring the ECG for excessive increases in the QT interval.

Treatment with dofetilide must therefore be started only in patients placed for a minimum of 3 days in a facility that can provide electrocardiographic monitoring and in the presence of personnel trained in the management of serious ventricular arrhythmias. Calculation of the creatinine clearance for all patients must precede administration of the first dose of dofetilide. For detailed instructions regarding dose selection, see Administration and Dosage.

The risk of dofetilide-induced ventricular arrhythmia was assessed in 3 ways in clinical studies:

1.) by description of the QT interval and its relation to the dose and plasma concentration of dofetilide;
2.) by observing the frequency of TdP in dofetilide-treated patients according to dose;
3.) by observing the overall mortality rate in patients with atrial fibrillation and in patients with structural heart disease.

Relation of QT interval to dose – The QT interval increases linearly with increasing dofetilide dose.

Frequency of torsade de pointes –

Summary of Torsade de Pointes in Patients Randomized to Dofetilide by Dose; Patients with Supraventricular Arrhythmias

	Dofetilide dose				
	< 250 mcg twice daily	250 mcg twice daily	> 250 to 500 mcg twice daily	> 500 mcg twice daily	All doses
Number of patients	217	388	703	38	1,346
Torsade de pointes	0	1 (0.3%)	6 (0.9%)	4 (10.5%)	11 (0.8%)

Incidence of Torsade de Pointes before and after Introduction of Dosing According to Renal Function

	Total	Before	After
Population	n/N %	n/N %	n/N %
Supraventricular arrhythmias	11/1,346 (0.8%)	6/193 (3.1%)	5/1,153 (0.4%)
DIAMOND CHF	25/762 (3.3%)	7/148 (4.7%)	18/614 (2.9%)
DIAMOND MI	7/749 (0.9%)	3/101 (3%)	4/648 (0.6%)
DIAMOND AF	4/249 (1.6%)	0/43 (0%)	4/206 (1.9%)

The majority of the episodes of TdP occurred within the first 3 days of dofetilide therapy (10/11 events in the studies of patients with supraventricular arrhythmias; 19/25 and 4/7 events in DIAMOND CHF and DIAMOND MI, respectively; 2/4 events in the DIAMOND AF subpopulation).

Mortality – In a pooled survival analysis of patients in the supraventricular arrhythmia population (low prevalence of structural heart disease), deaths occurred in 0.9% (12/1346) of patients receiving dofetilide and 0.4% (3/677) in the placebo group. Adjusted for duration of therapy, primary diagnosis, age, gender, and prevalence of structural heart disease, the point estimate of the hazard ratio for the pooled studies (dofetilide/placebo) was 1.1 (95% CI: 0.3, 4.3). The DIAMOND CHF and MI trials examined mortality in patients with structural heart disease (ejection fraction less than or equal to 35%). In these large, double-blind studies, deaths occurred in 36% (541/1511) of dofetilide patients and 37% (560/1517) of placebo patients. In an analysis of 506 DIAMOND patients with atrial fibrillation/flutter at baseline, 1-year mortality on dofetilide was 31% vs 32% on placebo.

Because of the small number of events, an excess mortality due to dofetilide cannot be ruled out with confidence in the pooled survival analysis of placebo-controlled trials in patients with supraventricular arrhythmias. However, it is reassuring that in 2 large placebo-controlled mortality studies in patients with significant heart disease (DIAMOND CHF/MI), there were no more deaths in dofetilide-treated patients than in patients given placebo.

➤*Women:* Female patients constituted 32% of the patients in the placebo-controlled trials of dofetilide. As with other drugs that cause torsade de pointes, dofetilide was associated with a greater risk of torsade de pointes in female patients than in male patients. During the dofetilide clinical development program the risk of torsade de pointes in females was approximately 3 times the risk in males. Unlike torsade de pointes, the incidence of other ventricular arrhythmias was similar in female patients receiving dofetilide and patients receiving placebo. Although no study specifically investigated this risk, in post-hoc analyses, no increased mortality was observed in females on dofetilide compared with females on placebo.

➤*Renal function impairment:* The overall systemic clearance of dofetilide is decreased and plasma concentration increased with decreasing creatinine clearance. The dose of dofetilide must be adjusted based on creatinine clearance. Patients undergoing dialysis were not included in clinical studies, and appropriate dosing recommendations for these patients are unknown. There is no information about the effectiveness of hemodialysis in removing dofetilide from plasma.

➤*Hepatic function impairment:* After adjustment for creatinine clearance, no additional dose adjustment is required for patients with mild or moderate hepatic impairment. Patients with severe hepatic impairment have not been studied. Dofetilide should be used with particular caution in these patients.

➤*Fertility impairment:* There was no effect on mating or fertility when dofetilide was administered to male and female rats at doses as high as 1 mg/kg/day, a dose that would be expected to provide a mean dofetilide $AUC_{(0\text{-}24h)}$ about 3 times the maximum likely human AUC. Increased inci-

DOFETILIDE — ORAL

dences of testicular atrophy and epididymal oligospermia and a reduction in testicular weight were, however, observed in other studies in rats. Reduced testicular weight and increased incidence of testicular atrophy were also consistent findings in dogs and mice. The no effect doses for these findings in chronic administration studies in these 3 species (3, 0.1 and 6 mg/kg/day) were associated with mean dofetilide AUCs that were about 4, 1.3 and 3 times the maximum likely human AUC, respectively.

➤*Elderly:* Because elderly patients are more likely to have decreased renal function with a reduced creatinine clearance, care must be taken in dose selection.

➤*Pregnancy: Category C.* Dofetilide has been shown to adversely affect in utero growth and survival of rats and mice when orally administered during organogenesis at doses of 2 or more mg/kg/day. Other than an increased incidence of nonossified fifth metacarpal, and the occurrence of hydroureter and hydronephroses at doses as low as 1 mg/kg/day in the rat, structural anomalies associated with drug treatment were not observed in either species at doses below 2 mg/kg/day. The clearest drug-effect associations were for sternebral and vertebral anomalies in both species; cleft palate, adactyly, levocardia, dilation of cerebral ventricles, hydroureter, hydronephroses, and unossified metacarpal in the rat; and increased incidence of unossified calcaneum in the mouse. The "no observed adverse effect dose" in both species was 0.5 mg/kg/day. The mean dofetilide $AUCs_{(0\text{-}24h)}$ at this dose in the rat and mouse are estimated to be about equal to the maximum likely human AUC and about half the likely human AUC, respectively. There are no adequate and well controlled studies in pregnant women. Therefore, dofetilide should only be administered to pregnant women where the benefit to the patient justifies the potential risk to the fetus.

➤*Lactation:* There is no information on the presence of dofetilide in breast milk. Patients should be advised not to breast-feed an infant if they are taking dofetilide.

➤*Children:* The safety and effectiveness of dofetilide in children (younger than 18 years old) has not been established.

Precautions

➤*Cardiac conduction disturbances:* Animal and human studies have not shown any adverse effects of dofetilide on conduction velocity. No effect on AV nodal conduction following dofetilide treatment was noted in healthy volunteers and in patients with first-degree heart block. Patients with sick sinus syndrome or with second— or third-degree heart block were not included in the Phase 3 clinical trials unless a functioning pacemaker was present. Dofetilide has been used safely in conjunction with pacemakers (53 patients in DIAMOND studies, 136 in trials in patients with ventricular and supraventricular arrhythmias).

Drug Interactions

Because there is a linear relationship between dofetilide plasma concentration and QTc, concomitant drugs that interfere with the metabolism or renal elimination of dofetilide may increase the risk of arrhythmia (torsade de pointes). Dofetilide is metabolized to a small degree by the CYP3A4 isoenzyme of the cytochrome P450 system and an inhibitor of this system could increase systemic dofetilide exposure. More important, dofetilide is eliminated by cationic renal secretion, and 3 inhibitors of this process have been shown to increase systemic dofetilide exposure. The magnitude of the effect on renal elimination by cimetidine, trimethoprim and ketoconazole (all contraindicated concomitant uses with dofetilide) suggests that all renal cation transport inhibitors should be contraindicated.

➤*Potential drug interactions:* Dofetilide is eliminated in the kidney by cationic secretion. Inhibitors of renal cationic secretion are contraindicated with dofetilide. In addition, drugs that are actively secreted via this route (eg, triamterene, metformin, amiloride) should be coadministered with care as they might increase dofetilide levels.

Dofetilide is metabolized to a small extent by the CYP3A4 isoenzyme of the cytochrome P450 system. Inhibitors of the CYP3A4 isoenzyme could increase systemic dofetilide exposure. Inhibitors of this isoenzyme (eg, macrolide antibiotics, azole antifungal agents, protease inhibitors, serotonin reuptake inhibitors, amiodarone, cannabinoids, diltiazem, grapefruit juice, nefazodone, norfloxacin, quinine, zafirlukast) should be cautiously coadministered with dofetilide as they can potentially increase dofetilide levels. Dofetilide is not an inhibitor of CYP3A4 nor of other cytochrome P450 isoenzymes (eg, CYP2C9, CYP2D6) and is not expected to increase levels of drugs metabolized by CYP3A4.

Dofetilide Drug Interactions

Precipitant	Object[a]		Description
Amiloride Metformin Megestrol Prochlorperazine Triamterene	Dofetilide	↑	Inhibitors of dofetilide elimination of renal cationic secretion are contraindicated. Use caution when coadministering drugs actively secreted via cationic secretion as they might increase dofetilide levels.
Antiarrhythmic agents (Class I or Class III)	Dofetilide	↑	Withhold Class I or Class III antiarrhythmic agents for ≥ 3 plasma half-lives prior to dofetilide dosing.
Bepridil Certain oral macrolides Cisapride Phenothiazines Tricyclic antidepressants	Dofetilide	↑	Administration of drugs that prolong the QT interval have not been studied in conjunction with dofetilide administration and are not recommended for coadministration.
Cimetidine	Dofetilide	↑	Concomitant use of cimetidine is contraindicated. Cimetidine increased dofetilide plasma levels by 58%. Use omeprazole, ranitidine, or antacids as an alternative to cimetidine.
Digoxin	Dofetilide	↔	A higher occurrence of torsades de pointes was associated in patients concomitantly administered digoxin with dofetilide.
Ketoconazole	Dofetilide	↑	Concomitant use of ketoconazole is contraindicated. Ketoconazole increased dofetilide C_{max} and AUC by 53% and 41% in males and 97% and 69% in females, respectively.
Potassium-depleting diuretics	Dofetilide	↑	Hypokalemia or hypomagnesemia may occur with administration of potassium-depleting diuretics, increasing the potential for torsades de pointes. Potassium levels should be within normal range prior to administration of dofetilide and maintained in the normal range during dofetilide administration.
Trimethoprim Trimethoprim/sulfamethoxazole	Dofetilide	↑	Concomitant use of trimethoprim alone or in combination with sulfamethoxazole is contraindicated. Coadministration increased dofetilide AUC by 103% and C_{max} by 93%
Verapamil	Dofetilide	↑	Concomitant use of verapamil is contraindicated. Dofetilide peak plasma concentrations increased by 42% when coadministered with verapamil, although overall exposure to dofetilide was not significantly increased. Concomitant administration was associated with a higher occurrence of torsades de pointes.

[a] ↑ = Object drug increased. ↔ = Undetermined clinical effect.

➤*Drug/Food interactions:* Grapefruit juice can potentially increase dofetilide levels.

Adverse Reactions

In studies of patients with supraventricular arrhythmias a total of 1,346 and 677 patients were exposed to dofetilide and placebo for 551 and 207 patient years, respectively. A total of 8.7% of patients in the dofetilide groups were discontinued from clinical trials due to adverse events compared to 8% in the placebo groups. The most frequent reason for discontinuation (greater than 1%) was ventricular tachycardia (2% on dofetilide vs 1.3% on placebo). The most frequent adverse events were headache, chest pain, and dizziness.

➤*Serious arrhythmias and conduction disturbances:* Torsade de pointes is the only arrhythmia that showed a dose-response relationship to dofetilide treatment. It did not occur in placebo-treated patients. The incidence of torsade de pointes in patients with supraventricular arrhythmias was 0.8% (11 of 1,346). The incidence of torsade de pointes in patients who were dosed according to the recommended dosing regimen was 0.8% (4 of 525).

DOFETILIDE — ORAL

Incidence of Serious Arrhythmias and Conduction Disturbances in Patients with Supraventricular Arrhythmias					
	Dofetilide dose				Placebo
Arrhythmia event	< 250 mcg twice daily (n = 217)	250 mcg twice daily (n = 388)	> 250 to 500 mcg twice daily (n = 703)	> 500 mcg twice daily (n = 38)	(n = 677)
Ventricular arrhythmias[a,b]	3.7%	2.6%	3.4%	15.8%	2.7%
Ventricular fibrillation	0%	0.3%	0.4%	2.6%	0.1%
Ventricular tachycardia[b]	3.7%	2.6%	3.3%	13.2%	2.5%
Torsade de pointes	0%	0.3%	0.9%	10.5%	0%
Various forms of block					
AV block	0.9%	1.5%	0.4%	0%	0.3%
Bundle branch block	0%	0.5%	0.1%	0%	0.1%
Heart block	0%	0.5%	0.1%	0%	0.1%

[a] Patients with more than 1 arrhythmia are counted only once in this category.
[b] Ventricular arrhythmias and ventricular tachycardia include all cases of torsade de pointes.

In the DIAMOND trials a total of 1511 patients were exposed to dofetilide for 1757 patient years. The incidence of torsade de pointes was 3.3% in CHF patients and 0.9% in patients with a recent MI.

Incidence of Serious Arrhythmias and Conduction Disturbances in Patients with AF at Entry to the DIAMOND Studies		
	Dofetilide (n = 249)	Placebo (n = 257)
Ventricular arrhythmias[a,b]	14.5%	13.6%
Ventricular fibrillation	4.8%	3.1%
Ventricular tachycardia[b]	12.4%	11.3%
Torsade de pointes	1.6%	0%
Various forms of block		
AV block	0.8%	2.7%
(Left) bundle branch block	0%	0.4%
Heart block	1.2%	0.8%

[a] Patients with more than 1 arrhythmia are counted only once in this category.
[b] Ventricular arrhythmias and ventricular tachycardia include all cases of torsade de pointes.

➤*Other adverse reactions:*

Frequency of Adverse Events Occurring at 2% on Dofetilide, and Numerically More Frequently on Dofetilide than Placebo in Patients with Supraventricular Arrhythmias		
Adverse event	Dofetilide	Placebo
Headache	11%	9%
Chest pain	10%	7%
Dizziness	8%	6%
Respiratory tract infection	7%	5%
Dyspnea	6%	5%
Nausea	5%	4%
Flu syndrome	4%	2%
Insomnia	4%	3%
Accidental injury	3%	1%
Back pain	3%	2%
Procedure (medical/surgical/ health service)	3%	2%
Diarrhea	3%	2%
Rash	3%	2%
Abdominal pain	3%	2%

Adverse events reported at a rate more than 2% but no more frequently on dofetilide than on placebo were angina pectoris, anxiety, arthralgia, asthenia, atrial fibrillation, complications (application, injection, incision, insertion, or device), hypertension, pain, palpitation, peripheral edema, supraventricular tachycardia, sweating, urinary tract infection, and ventricular tachycardia.

The following adverse events have been reported with a frequency of less than or equal to 2% and numerically more frequently with dofetilide than placebo in patients with supraventricular arrhythmias: angioedema, bradycardia, cerebral ischemia, cerebrovascular accident, edema, facial paralysis, flaccid paralysis, heart arrest, increased cough, liver damage, migraine, myocardial infarct, paralysis, paresthesia, sudden death, and syncope.

The incidences of clinically significant laboratory test abnormalities in patients with supraventricular arrhythmias were similar for patients on dofetilide and those on placebo. No clinically relevant effects were noted in serum alkaline phosphatase, serum GGT, LDH, AST, ALT, total bilirubin, total protein, blood urea nitrogen, creatinine, serum electrolytes (calcium, chloride, glucose, magnesium, potassium, sodium) or creatine kinase. Similarly, no clinically relevant effects were observed in hematologic parameters.

In the DIAMOND population, adverse events other than those related to the postinfarction and heart failure patient population were generally similar to those seen in the supraventricular arrhythmia groups.

Overdosage

➤*Symptoms:* Dofetilide overdose was rare in clinical studies; there were two reported cases of dofetilide overdose in the oral clinical program. One patient received very high multiples of the recommended dose (28 capsules), was treated with gastric aspiration 30 minutes later, and experienced no events. One patient inadvertently received two 500 mcg doses 1 hour apart and experienced ventricular fibrillation and cardiac arrest 2 hours after the second dose.

In the supraventricular arrhythmia population only 38 patients received doses greater than 500 mcg twice daily, all of whom received 750 mcg twice daily irrespective of creatinine clearance. In this very small patient population the incidence of torsade de pointes was 10.5% (4/38 patients), and the incidence of new ventricular fibrillation was 2.6% (1/38 patients).

➤*Treatment:* There is no known antidote to dofetilide; treatment of overdose should therefore be symptomatic and supportive. The most prominent manifestation of overdosage is likely to be excessive prolongation of the QT interval.

In cases of overdose cardiac monitoring should be initiated. Charcoal slurry may be given soon after overdosing but has been useful only when given within 15 minutes of dofetilide administration. Treatment of torsade de pointes or overdose may include administration of isoproterenol infusion, with or without cardiac pacing. Administration of intravenous magnesium sulfate may be effective in the management of torsade de pointes. Close medical monitoring and supervision should continue until the QT interval returns to normal levels.

Isoproterenol infusion into anesthetized dogs with cardiac pacing rapidly attenuates the dofetilide-induced prolongation of atrial and ventricular effective refractory periods in a dose-dependent manner. Magnesium sulfate, administered prophylactically either intravenously or orally in a dog model, was effective in the prevention of dofetilide-induced torsade de pointes ventricular tachycardia. Similarly, in man, intravenous magnesium sulfate may terminate torsade de pointes, irrespective of cause.

Patient Information

Prior to initiation of dofetilide therapy, the patient should be advised to read the patient package insert and reread it each time therapy is renewed in case the patient's status has changed. The patient should be fully instructed on the need for compliance with the recommended dosing of dofetilide and the potential for drug interactions, and the need for periodic monitoring of QTc and renal function to minimize the risk of serious abnormal rhythms.

➤*Medications and supplements:* Assessment of patients' medication history should include all over-the-counter, prescription and herbal/natural preparations with emphasis on preparations that may affect the pharmacokinetics of dofetilide such as cimetidine (see Contraindications), trimethoprim alone or in combination with sulfamethoxazole (see Contraindications), prochlorperazine (see Contraindications), megestrol (see Contraindications), ketoconazole (see Contraindications), other cardiovascular drugs (especially verapamil - see Contraindications), phenothiazines, and tricyclic antidepressants (see Warnings). If a patient is taking dofetilide and requires antiulcer therapy, omeprazole, ranitidine or antacids (aluminum and magnesium hydroxides) should be used as alternatives to cimetidine, as these agents have no effect on the pharmacokinetics of dofetilide. Patients should be instructed to notify their health care providers of any change in over-the-counter, prescription or supplement use. If a patient is hospitalized or is prescribed a new medication for any condition, the patient must inform the health care provider of ongoing dofetilide therapy. Patients should also check with their health care provider and/or pharmacist prior to taking a new over-the-counter preparation.

➤*Electrolyte imbalance:* If patients experience symptoms that may be associated with altered electrolyte balance, such as excessive or prolonged diarrhea, sweating, vomiting, loss of appetite, or thirst, these conditions should immediately be reported to their health care provider.

➤*Dosing schedule:* Patients should be instructed not to double the next dose if a dose is missed. The next dose should be taken at the usual time.

LIDOCAINE HYDROCHLORIDE

Refer to the general introductory discussion concerning Antiarrhythmic Agents. For prescribing information, see the Lidocaine Hydrochloride monograph in the CNS chapter.

CALCIUM CHANNEL BLOCKING AGENTS

Indications

Calcium Channel Blocking Agents – Summary of Indications[a]

Indications (✔ = labeled; X = unlabeled)	Amlodipine	Diltiazem	Diltiazem SR	Diltiazem ER	Diltiazem IV	Felodipine	Isradipine	Nicardipine	Nicardipine SR	Nicardipine IV	Nifedipine	Nifedipine ER	Nimodipine	Nisoldipine	Verapamil	Verapamil SR	Verapamil ER	Verapamil IV
Angina pectoris																		
Vasospastic	✔	✔		✔							✔	✔[b]			✔		✔[c]	
Chronic stable	✔	✔		✔				✔			✔	✔[b]			✔		✔[c]	
Unstable															✔		✔[c]	
Hypertension	✔		✔	✔		✔	✔	✔	✔	✔		✔		✔	✔	✔	✔	
Subarachnoid hemorrhage													✔					
Atrial fibrillation/flutter					✔													✔
Paroxysmal supraventricular tachycardia					✔										✔[d]			✔
Unlabeled uses																		
Prevention of migraine headaches		X													X			
Pulmonary hypertension	X	X				X					X							
Raynaud's phenomenon	X	X				X	X				X							
Preterm labor											X							
Hypertrophic cardiomyopathy															X			

[a] For more detailed information, see the information below and individual drug monographs.
[b] Except *Adalat CC*.
[c] *Covera-HS* only.
[d] For prophylaxis of repetitive paroxysmal supraventricular tachycardia.

➤*Vasospastic (Prinzmetal's or variant) angina (amlodipine, diltiazem immediate-release [IR] and extended-release [ER], nifedipine IR and ER [except Adalat CC]*, verapamil IR and ER [*Covera-HS* only]): Treatment of spontaneous coronary artery spasm presenting as Prinzmetal's variant angina (resting angina with ST segment elevation during attacks).

➤*Chronic stable (classic effort-associated) angina (amlodipine, diltiazem IR and ER, nicardipine, nifedipine IR and ER [except Adalat CC]*, verapamil IR and ER [*Covera-HS* only]): For the treatment of chronic stable angina, alone or in combination with other antianginals.

➤*Unstable angina at rest:* Verapamil IR and ER (*Covera-HS* only).

➤*Hypertension:* Amlodipine, diltiazem sustained-release (SR) and ER, felodipine, isradipine, nicardipine IR and SR, nicardipine IV, nifedipine ER, nisoldipine, and oral verapamil.

➤*Subarachnoid hemorrhage (SAH) (nimodipine only):* For the improvement of neurological outcome by reducing the incidence and severity of ischemic deficits in patients with subarachnoid hemorrhage from ruptured intracranial berry aneurysms regardless of their post-ictus neurological condition (ie, Hunt and Hess Grades I to V).

➤*Paroxysmal supraventricular tachycardias (PSVT) (diltiazem IV and verapamil IV):* Rapid conversion of PSVT to sinus rhythm.

➤*Prophylaxis of repetitive PSVT:* Verapamil IR.

➤*Atrial fibrillation / flutter (diltiazem IV and verapamil IV):* For temporary control of rapid ventricular rate in atrial fibrillation or atrial flutter.

Actions

➤*Pharmacology:* In specialized automatic and conducting cells in the heart, calcium is involved in genesis of action potential. In contractile cells of the myocardium, it links excitation to contraction and controls energy storage and use. Systemic and coronary arteries are influenced by movement of calcium across cell membranes of vascular smooth muscle. Contractile processes of cardiac and vascular smooth muscle depend upon movement of extracellular calcium ions into these cells through specific ion channels.

The calcium channel blockers (ie, slow channel blockers, calcium antagonists), share the ability to inhibit movement of calcium ions across the cell membrane. The effects on the cardiovascular system include depression of mechanical contraction of myocardial and smooth muscle and depression of both impulse formation (automaticity) and conduction velocity. Calcium channel blockers are classified by structure as follows: Diphenylalkylamines – **verapamil**; benzothiazepines – **diltiazem**; dihydropyridines – **amlodipine, felodipine, isradipine, nicardipine, nifedipine, nimodipine, nisoldipine**.

Although these agents are similar in that they all act on the slow (calcium) channel, they have different degrees of selectivity in their effects on vascular smooth muscle, myocardium, or specialized conduction and pacemaker tissues. The resulting clinical effects depend on the direct activity of the drug, reflex physiological responses (primarily β-adrenergic response to vasodilation), and the patient's cardiovascular status. This heterogeneity of the calcium blockers, in part, determines their clinical application and the different side effects produced by each agent.

In animals, **nimodipine** had a greater effect on cerebral arteries than on other arteries, possibly because it is highly lipophilic. While studies show a favorable effect on severity of neurological deficits caused by cerebral vasospasm following SAH, there is no arteriographic evidence that the drug prevents or relieves spasm of these arteries. Therefore, the actual mechanism of action is unknown.

Hemodynamic – (See Pharmacokinetics table.) These agents dilate the coronary arteries and arterioles in normal and ischemic regions and inhibit coronary artery spasm. This increases myocardial oxygen delivery in patients with coronary artery spasm and vasospastic (Prinzmetal's or variant) angina.

The drugs reduce arterial blood pressure at rest and with exercise by dilating peripheral arterioles and reducing total peripheral resistance (afterload) against which the heart works. This reduces myocardial energy consumption and oxygen requirements and probably accounts for the efficacy in chronic stable angina.

These agents exhibit a negative inotropic effect, but this is rare because of reflex responses to vasodilation. In patients with normal ventricular function, there may be a small increase in cardiac index without major effects on ejection fraction or left ventricular end diastolic pressure or volume (LVEDP or LVEDV).Usual **verapamil** IV doses may slightly increase left ventricular filling pressure. Acute worsening of heart failure may be seen when **verapamil** is used in moderate to severe cardiac dysfunction. In patients with impaired ventricular function, most acute studies have shown some increase in ejection fraction and reduction in left ventricular filling pressure. **Nicardipine** use in coronary artery disease and normal or moderately abnormal left ventricular function significantly increased ejection fraction and cardiac output with no significant change or a small decrease in LVEDP. Administration of a single dose of **nisoldipine** leads to decreased systemic vascular resistance and blood pressure with a transient increase in heart rate.

Electrophysiology – **Verapamil** slows AV conduction and prolongs the effective refractory period (ERP) within the AV node in a rate-related manner, thus reducing ventricular rate because of atrial flutter or atrial fibrillation. By interrupting re-entry at the AV node, verapamil can restore normal sinus rhythm in patients with PSVT, including Wolff-Parkinson-White (W-P-W) syndrome. It can interfere with sinus node impulse generation and induce sinus arrest or sinoatrial block in patients with sick sinus syndrome. AV block can occur in patients without pre-existing conduction defects. Verapamil decreases the frequency of episodes of PSVT. Verapamil may shorten the antegrade ERP of the accessory bypass tracts. It does not alter the normal atrial action potential or intraventricular conduction time, but it depresses amplitude, velocity of depolarization, and conduction in depressed atrial fibers.

Patients with supraventricular tachycardia convert to normal sinus rhythm within 10 minutes after verapamil IV (approximately 60% to 80%). About 70% of patients with atrial flutter or fibrillation with a fast ventricular rate respond with a decrease in heart rate of at least 20%. Conversion of atrial flutter or fibrillation to sinus rhythm is uncommon (about 10%) after verapamil and may reflect the spontaneous conversion rate. Slowing of the ventricular rate in patients with atrial fibrillation/flutter lasts 30 to 60 minutes after a single injection.

Because a small fraction (less than 1%) of patients treated with verapamil have life-threatening adverse responses, the initial use of verapamil injection should, if possible, be in a treatment setting with monitoring and resuscitation facilities, including D.C.-cardioversion capability. As familiarity with the patient's response is gained, use in an office setting may be acceptable.

Diltiazem decreases SA and AV conduction in isolated tissues. Diltiazem IV in doses of 20 mg prolongs AH conduction time and AV node functional and effective refractory periods by approximately 20%. Diltiazem-associated prolongation of the AH interval is not more pronounced in patients with first-degree heart block. In patients with sick sinus syndrome, diltiazem significantly prolongs sinus cycle length (up to 50%).

➤*Pharmacokinetics:*

Calcium Channel Blocking Agents: Pharmacokinetics[a]

	Parameters	Amlodipine	Diltiazem	Felodipine	Isradipine	Nicardipine	Nifedipine	Nimodipine	Nisoldipine	Verapamil
Pharmacokinetics	Extent of absorption (oral) (%)	nd	nd	≈ 100	90-95	≈ 100	100	nd	nd	> 90
	Absolute bioavailability (oral) (%)	64-90	40	≈ 20	15-24	≈ 35	45-75 (IR) 84-89 (ER)	≈ 13	≈ 5	20-35 (IR)
	Volume of distribution	nd	≈ 305 L (IV)	10 L/kg	3 L/kg	8.3 L/kg (IV)	nd	nd	nd	nd
	T_{max} (h)	6-12	2-4 (IR) 10-14 (ER) 6-11 (SR)	2.5-5	1.5 (IR) 7-18 (CR)	0.5-2 (IR) 1-4 (SR)	0.5 (IR) 6 (ER)	1	6-12	1-2 (IR) ≈ 11 (ER) ≈ 7-9 (SR)
	Protein binding (%)	93	70-80	> 99	95	> 95	92-98	> 95	> 99	≈ 90
	Metabolism	Hepatic	Hepatic	Hepatic	Hepatic	Hepatic	Hepatic	Hepatic	Hepatic	Hepatic
	Major metabolites	90% converted to inactive	Desacetyl-diltiazem[b]	6 inactive	Mono acids and cyclic lactone[c]	nd	Inactive	Numerous, inactive	5 major urinary metabolites	Norverapamil[d]
	Half-life, elimination (h)	30-50	3-4.5 (IR) 4-9.5 (ER) 5-7 (SR) ≈ 3.4 (IV)	11-16	8	2-4	≈ 2 (IR) ≈ 7 (ER)	≈ 8-9[e]	7-12	2.8-7.4[f] 4.5-12[g] ≈ 12 (SR) 2-5 (IV)
	Clearance, systemic	nd	≈ 65 L/h (IV)	≈ 0.8 L/min	1.4 L/min	0.4 L/h•kg (IV)	nd	nd	nd	nd
	Excreted unchanged in urine (%)	10	2-4	±	0	< 1	< 0.1	< 1	trace	3-4
	Excreted in urine (%)	nd	nd	70	60-65	60 (oral) 49 (IV)	60-80	nd	60-80	≈ 70
	Excreted in feces (%)	nd	nd	10	25-30	35 (oral) 43 (IV)	15	nd	nd	≥ 16
ECG Changes	Heart rate	±	0-↓	↑↑	↑	↑↑	0-↑		±	±
	QRS complex	0	nd	0	0	0	nd		0	nd
	PR interval	0	↑	0	0	0	nd		0	↑
	QT interval	0	nd	0	↑	↑	nd		0	nd
Hemodynamics	Myocardial contractility	0-↓	0-↓	0-↓	↓	0-↓	0-↓	na	0-↓	↓↓
	Cardiac output/index	↑	0-↑	nd	↑	↑↑	↑		nd	±
	Peripheral vascular resistance	↓↓	↓↓[h]	↓↓[h]	↓↓	↓↓↓	↓↓↓		↓↓	↓↓

[a] ↑↑↑ or ↓↓↓ = pronounced effect; ↑↑ or ↓↓ = moderate effect; ↑ or ↓ = slight effect; ± = negligible amount or effect; nd = no data; na = not applicable.
[b] 25% to 50% as potent a coronary vasodilator as diltiazem; plasma levels are 10% to 20% of the parent drug.
[c] Of 6 metabolites identified, accounting for > 75%.
[d] Major metabolite; cardiovascular activity is ≈ 20% that of verapamil.
[e] Earlier elimination rates are much more rapid, equivalent to a half-life of 1 to 2 hours.
[f] After single doses.
[g] After repetitive doses.
[h] Dose-related.

Contraindications

Hypersensitivity to the drug; in patients with known hypersensitivity to dihydropyridine calcium channel blockers (**nisoldipine**); sick sinus syndrome or second- or third-degree AV block except with a functioning pacemaker, hypotension less than 90 mmHg systolic (**diltiazem**, and **verapamil**).

➤*Diltiazem:* Acute MI and pulmonary congestion documented by x-ray on admission.

Injectable –
- Sick sinus syndrome except in the presence of a functioning ventricular pacemaker.
- Second- or third-degree AV block except in the presence of a functioning ventricular pacemaker.
- Severe hypotension or cardiogenic shock.
- Hypersensitivity to the drug.
- IV diltiazem and IV beta-blockers should not be administered together or in close proximity (within a few hours).
- Atrial fibrillation or atrial flutter associated with an accessory bypass tract such as in W-P-W syndrome or short PR syndrome.
- Initial use of injectable forms of diltiazem should be, if possible, in a setting where monitoring and resuscitation capabilities, including DC cardioversion/defibrillation, are present. Once familiarity of the patient's response is established, use in an office setting may be acceptable.
- Ventricular tachycardia.
- In newborns, because of the presence of benzyl alcohol (*Cardizem Lyo-Ject Syringe* only).

➤*Nicardipine:* Advanced aortic stenosis.

➤*Verapamil:* Severe left ventricular dysfunction; cardiogenic shock and severe CHF, unless secondary to a supraventricular tachycardia amenable to verapamil therapy, and in patients with atrial flutter or atrial fibrillation and an accessory bypass tract.

Verapamil IV –

- Severe hypotension or cardiogenic shock.
- Second- or third-degree AV block (except in patients with a functioning artificial ventricular pacemaker).
- Sick sinus syndrome (except in patients with a functioning artificial ventricular pacemaker).
- Severe CHF (unless secondary to a supraventricular tachycardia amenable to verapamil therapy).
- IV β-adrenergic blocking agents. IV verapamil and IV beta-adrenergic blocking drugs should not be administered in close proximity to each other (within a few hours) because both may have a depressant effect on myocardial contractility and AV conduction (see Drug Interactions).
- Patients with atrial flutter or atrial fibrillation and an accessory bypass tract (eg, W-P-W, Lown-Ganong-Levine [L-G-L] syndromes) are at risk to develop ventricular tachyarrhythmia, including ventricular fibrillation if verapamil is administered. Therefore, the use of verapamil in these patients is contraindicated.
- Ventricular tachycardia. Patients with wide-complex ventricular tachycardia (QRS greater than or equal to 0.12 sec) can result in marked hemodynamic deterioration and ventricular fibrillation.
- Known hypersensitivity.

Warnings

➤*Hypotension:* Hypotension, usually modest and well tolerated, occasionally may occur during initial titration or with dosage increases, and may be more common in patients taking concomitant β-blockers. Hypotensive episodes may be caused by excess vasodilation induced by **nifedipine** or by direct cardiopressor effects of **verapamil** and **diltiazem**. Nifedipine has the greatest effect on vascular smooth muscle; therefore, incidence of adverse reactions resulting from vasodilation (eg, headache, flushing) is greater. Because **amlodipine**-induced hypotension is gradual in onset, acute hypotension rarely has been reported. Nonetheless, exercise caution when administering amlodipine as with any other peripheral vasodilator, particularly in patients with severe aortic stenosis.

Systolic pressure less than 90 mmHg or diastolic pressure less than 60 mmHg was seen in 5% to 10% of patients with supraventricular tachycardia and in about 10% of the patients with atrial flutter/fibrillation who were given IV **verapamil**.

Carefully monitor blood pressure during initial administration and titration. Closely observe patients already taking antihypertensives.

➤*CHF:* CHF has developed rarely, usually in patients receiving a β-blocker, after beginning **nifedipine**. Patients with tight aortic stenosis may be at greater risk, as the unloading effect would be of less benefit to these patients because of their fixed impedance to flow across the aortic valve.

Isradipine – Exercise caution when using isradipine in CHF, particularly in combination with a beta-blocker.

Nisoldipine – Exercise caution when using nisoldipine in patients with heart failure or compromised ventricular function, particularly in combination with a beta-blocker.

Verapamil – Verapamil has a negative inotropic effect that is usually compensated by its afterload reduction (decreased systemic vascular resistance) properties without a net impairment of ventricular performance. In clinical studies with oral **verapamil**, 1.8% developed CHF or pulmonary edema. Avoid verapamil in patients with severe left ventricular dysfunction (ie, ejection fraction less than 30%) or moderate to severe symptoms of cardiac failure and in patients with any degree of ventricular dysfunction if they are receiving a β-adrenergic blocker. Control patients with milder ventricular dysfunction, if possible, with digitalis or diuretics before verapamil treatment.

Use **diltiazem**, **nicardipine**, **nisoldipine**, **felodipine**, and **amlodipine** with caution in CHF patients.

➤*Cardiac conduction:* **Verapamil** IV slows AV nodal conduction and SA nodes; it rarely produces second- or third-degree AV block, bradycardia, and in extreme cases, asystole. This is more likely to occur in patients with sick sinus syndrome (which is more common in older patients). Asystole in patients other than those with sick sinus syndrome is usually of short duration (a few seconds or less), with spontaneous return to AV nodal or normal sinus rhythm.

Oral **verapamil** may lead to first-degree AV block and transient bradycardia, sometimes accompanied by nodal escape rhythms. PR-interval prolongation is correlated with verapamil plasma concentrations especially during the early titration phase of therapy. Higher degrees of AV block are infrequent (0.8%). Marked first-degree block or progressive development to second- or third-degree AV block requires dose reduction or discontinuation of verapamil and institution of appropriate therapy, depending on the clinical situation.

Patients with atrial flutter/fibrillation and an accessory AV pathway may develop increased antegrade conduction, producing a very rapid ventricular response or ventricular fibrillation after receiving IV verapamil (or digitalis). Although a risk of this occurring with oral verapamil has not been established, such patients receiving oral verapamil may be at risk and its use in these patients is contraindicated (see Contraindications). Treatment is usually D.C. cardioversion.

Diltiazem prolongs AV node refractory periods without significantly prolonging sinus node recovery time, except in sick sinus syndrome. This may rarely result in abnormally slow heart rates (particularly in sick sinus syndrome) or second- or third-degree AV block. Concomitant use with β-adrenergic blockers or digitalis may be additive on cardiac conduction. A patient with Prinzmetal's angina developed periods of asystole (2 to 5 seconds) after 60 mg diltiazem. If high-degree AV block occurs in sinus rhythm, discontinue diltiazem IV and institute appropriate supportive measures.

➤*Premature ventricular contractions (PVCs):* During conversion or marked reduction in ventricular rate, benign complexes of unusual appearance (sometimes resembling PVCs) may occur after **verapamil** IV. Similar complexes of no clinical significance occur during spontaneous conversion of supraventricular tachycardia after D.C. cardioversion and other therapy. These complexes appear to have no clinical significance.

➤*Hypertrophic cardiomyopathy:* Serious adverse effects were seen in 120 patients with hypertrophic cardiomyopathy (most refractory or intolerant to propranolol) who received oral **verapamil** at doses up to 720 mg/day. Three patients died with pulmonary edema; all had severe left ventricular outflow obstruction and a history of left ventricular dysfunction. Eight had pulmonary edema or severe hypotension; most had abnormally high (greater than 20 mmHg) pulmonary wedge pressure and a marked left ventricular outflow obstruction. Coadministration of quinidine preceded the severe hypotension in 3 of the 8 patients (2 of whom developed pulmonary edema). Sinus bradycardia occurred in 11%, second-degree AV block in 4% and sinus arrest in 2%. Most adverse effects responded to dose reduction; discontinuation of verapamil was rare.

➤*Antiplatelet effects:* Calcium channel blockers, alone and with aspirin, have caused inhibition of platelet function. Episodes of bruising, petechiae, and bleeding have occurred.

Nifedipine – Decreases platelet aggregation in vitro. Limited clinical studies have demonstrated a moderate but statistically significant decrease in platelet aggregation and increase in bleeding time in some patients. This is thought to be a function of inhibition of calcium transport across the platelet membrane.

➤*Withdrawal syndrome:* Abrupt withdrawal of calcium channel blockers may cause increased frequency and duration of chest pain. The rebound angina is probably the result of the increased flow of calcium into cells causing coronary arteries to spasm. Gradually taper the dose under medical supervision. Results of other studies do not support the occurrence of a withdrawal syndrome; however, caution is still warranted when discontinuing these agents.

➤*β-blocker withdrawal:* Patients recently withdrawn from β-blockers may develop a withdrawal syndrome with increased angina, probably related to increased sensitivity to catecholamines. Initiation of **nifedipine** will not prevent this occurrence and might exacerbate it by provoking reflex catecholamine release. Taper β-blockers rather than stopping them abruptly before beginning nifedipine.

Nicardipine – Gradually reduce β-blocker dose over 8 to 10 days with coadministration.

➤*Hepatic function impairment:* Patients with hepatic impairment (liver cirrhosis) have a longer disposition half-life and higher bioavailability of **nifedipine** than healthy volunteers. Protein binding may be greatly reduced in patients with renal or hepatic impairment.

Because **verapamil** is highly metabolized by the liver, it should be administered cautiously to patients with impaired hepatic function. Severe liver dysfunction prolongs the elimination half-life of verapamil to about 14 to 16 hours; therefore, administer approximately 30% of the dose given to patients with normal liver function to these patients. Carefully monitor for abnormal prolongation of the PR interval or other signs of excessive pharmacologic effects.

Bioavailability of nifedipine is increased in hepatic cirrhosis. With **nifedipine** IV, half-life and volume of distribution are increased and plasma protein binding is decreased. Carefully monitor for abnormal prolongation of the PR interval and other signs of excessive pharmacologic effects.

Because **amlodipine**, **diltiazem**, **nicardipine**, **felodipine**, **nisoldipine**, and **nimodipine** are extensively metabolized by the liver, use with caution in impaired hepatic function or reduced hepatic blood flow. In severe liver disease, elevated nicardipine blood levels (4-fold increase in AUC) and prolonged half-life (19 hours) occurred; patients on nimodipine had an approximately doubled maximum drug concentration. Consider decreasing the dose of calcium channel blockers and monitor drug response (ie, blood pressure, PR interval) in cirrhosis patients.

➤*Renal function impairment:* The pharmacokinetics of **diltiazem** in patients with impaired renal function are similar to the pharmacokinetic profile of patients with normal renal function. However, caution is still advised. About 70% of a dose of **verapamil** is excreted as metabolites in the urine. Administer verapamil cautiously to patients with impaired renal function. Carefully monitor these patients for abnormal prolongation of the PR interval or other signs of overdosage (see Overdosage). Effects of single IV doses should not increase, although duration may be prolonged.

Nicardipine – Mean plasma concentrations, AUC, and maximum concentration were approximately 2-fold higher in patients with mild renal impairment. Doses must be adjusted.

Nifedipine – Although nifedipine has been used safely in patients with renal dysfunction and has exerted a beneficial effect in certain cases, rare, reversible elevations in BUN and serum creatinine have occurred in patients with pre-existing chronic renal insufficiency. The relationship to therapy is uncertain in most cases but probable in some.

➤*Increased angina:* About 7% of patients developed increased frequency, duration or severity of angina on starting **nicardipine** or at the time of dosage increases. Rarely, patients, particularly those who have severe obstructive coronary artery disease have developed increased frequency, duration, or severity of angina or acute MI on starting **nifedipine** or at the time of dosage increase. The mechanism of these effects have not been established.

➤*Increased intracranial pressure:* **Verapamil** IV has increased intracranial pressure in patients with supratentorial tumors at the time of anesthesia induction. Use with caution and perform appropriate monitoring.

➤*Duchenne's muscular dystrophy:* **Verapamil** may decrease neuromuscular transmission in patients with Duchenne's muscular dystrophy, and prolong recovery from the neuromuscular blocking agent vecuronium. It may be necessary to decrease dosage of verapamil when administering it to patients with attenuated neuromuscular transmission. Verapamil IV can precipitate respiratory muscle failure in these patients; therefore, use with caution.

➤*Carcinogenesis:* Rats treated with **nicardipine** showed a dose-dependent increase in thyroid hyperplasia and neoplasia (follicular adenoma carcinoma), possibly linked to a nicardipine-induced reduction in plasma thyroxine levels with a consequent increase in thyroid stimulating hormone (TSH) plasma levels. In rats given **nimodipine**, a higher incidence of adenocarcinoma of the uterus and Leydig-cell adenoma of testes occurred. In rats given **isradipine** or **felodipine**, there were dose-dependent increases in benign Leydig cell tumors and testicular hyperplasia.

➤*Elderly:* Make dose selection for an elderly patient with caution, usually starting at the low end of the dosing range, reflecting the greater frequency of decreased hepatic, renal, or cardiac function and of concomitant disease or other drug therapy.

➤*Pregnancy: Category C.* Teratogenic and embryotoxic effects have been demonstrated in small animals, usually at doses higher than the usual human dosage. There are no well-controlled studies in pregnant women. Use during pregnancy only when clearly needed and when potential benefits outweigh potential hazards to the fetus.

Amlodipine – Significantly decreased litter size (by about 50%) and significantly increased the number of intrauterine deaths (about 5-fold) in rats administered 10 mg/kg amlodipine for 14 days before mating and throughout mating and gestation. Gestation period and duration of labor is also prolonged.

Diltiazem – Doses given at 4 to 10 times the human dose resulted in embryo and fetal death and skeletal abnormalities; incidence of stillbirths was increased at 20 or more times the human dose.

Felodipine – In rabbits, doses 0.8 to 8 times the maximum dosage resulted in digital anomalies (dose-related) in the fetuses, and a prolongation of parturition with difficult labor and increased frequency of fetal and early postnatal deaths occurred in rats. Significant enlargement of the mammary glands also occurred in pregnant rabbits.

Isradipine – There was a significant reduction in maternal weight gain in rats with a dose 150 times the maximum recommended human dose (MRHD). Decrements in maternal body weight gain and increased fetal resorptions occurred in rabbits following doses 2.5, 7.5, and 25 times the MRHD. Also, reduced maternal body weight gain during late pregnancy in rats was associated with reduced birth weights and decreased peri- and postnatal pup survival.

Nicardipine – Nicardipine was embryocidal in animals at 150 mg/kg/day but not 25 to 50 times the human dose. However, dystocia, reduced birth weights, reduced neonatal survival, and reduced neonatal weight gain occurred at 50 times the human dose.

Nifedipine – Nifedipine administration was associated with a variety of embryotoxic, placentotoxic, and fetotoxic effects, including stunted fetuses (rats, mice, rabbits), rib deformities (mice), cleft palate (mice), small placentas, and underdeveloped chorionic villi (monkeys), embryonic and fetal deaths (rats, mice, rabbits), and prolonged pregnancy/decreased neonatal survival (rats; not evaluated on other species). On a mg/kg basis, all of the doses associated with teratogenic, embryotoxic, or fetotoxic effects in animals were higher (3.5 to 42 times) than the MRHD of 120 mg/day. The doses associated with placentotoxic effect in monkeys were equivalent to or lower than the MRHD on a mg/m^2 basis.

Nimodipine – In animals, nimodipine has resulted in malformations and stunted fetuses at doses of 1 and 10 mg/kg/day but not at 3 mg/kg/day in 1 study. Doses of 30 to 100 mg/kg/day resulted in stunted fetuses, stillbirths, and higher incidences of skeletal variation.

Nisoldipine – Nisoldipine was fetotoxic but not teratogenic in rats and rabbits at doses resulting in maternal toxicity (reduced maternal body weight gain). In pregnant rats, increased fetal resorption (postimplantation loss) was observed at 100 mg/kg/day and decreased fetal weight was observed at both 30 and 100 mg/kg/day. These doses are, respectively, about 5 and 16 times the MRHD when compared on a mg/m^2 basis. In pregnant rabbits, decreased fetal and placental weights were observed at a dose of 30 mg/kg/day, about 10 times the MRHD when compared on a mg/m^2 basis. In a study in which pregnant monkeys (both treated and control) had high rates of abortion and mortality, the only surviving fetus from a group exposed to a maternal dose of 100 mg nisoldipine/kg/day (about 30 times the MRHD when compared on a mg/m^2 basis) presented with forelimb and vertebral abnormalities not previously seen in control monkeys of the same strain.

Verapamil, oral – Oral verapamil in rats with doses 1.5 and 6 times the human dose was embryocidal and retarded fetal growth and development, probably due to reduced weight gains in dams. Verapamil crosses the placenta and can be detected in umbilical vein blood at delivery.

➤*Lactation:* **Verapamil**, **diltiazem**, and **nifedipine** are excreted in breast milk. One report suggests that diltiazem concentrations in breast milk may approximate serum levels. Significant concentrations of **nicardipine** and **nimodipine** appear in maternal milk of rats. It is not known if nimodipine, **isradipine**, **amlodipine**, **nisoldipine**, or **felodipine** are excreted in breast milk. Discontinue nursing while taking amlodipine, diltiazem, nicardipine, verapamil, or nimodipine. If using felodipine, isradipine, nifedipine, or nisoldipine, decide whether to discontinue nursing or discontinue the drug, taking into account the importance of the drug to the mother.

➤*Children:* Safety and efficacy of oral **verapamil**, **diltiazem**, **felodipine**, **amlodipine**, **nicardipine**, **nifedipine**, **nisoldipine**, and **isradipine** have not been established. Use of *Procardia* in the pediatric population is not recommended.

Controlled studies of IV **verapamil** have not been conducted in pediatric patients, but uncontrolled experience indicates that results of treatment are similar to those in adults. Patients under 6 months of age may not respond to IV verapamil; this resistance may be related to a developmental difference of AV node responsiveness. However, in rare instances, severe hemodynamic side effects, some of them fatal, have occurred following IV verapamil administration in neonates and infants. Therefore, use caution when administering verapamil to this group of pediatric patients. The most commonly used single doses in patients up to 12 months of age have ranged from 0.1 to 0.2 mg/kg of body weight, while in patients 1 to 15 years of age, the most commonly used single doses ranged from 0.1 to 0.3 mg/kg of body weight. Most of the patients received the lower dose of 0.1 mg/kg once, but in some cases, the dose was repeated once or twice every 10 to 30 minutes.

Precautions

➤*Acute hepatic injury:* In rare instances, symptoms consistent with acute hepatic injury, as well as significant elevations in enzymes such as alkaline phosphatase, CPK, LDH, AST, and ALT have occurred with oral **diltiazem** and **nifedipine**. The potential for acute hepatic injury exists following administration of IV diltiazem. These were reversible on drug discontinuation. Drug relationship was uncertain in most cases, but probable in some. These laboratory abnormalities rarely have been associated with clinical symptoms; however, cholestasis with or without jaundice has occurred with nifedipine. Rare instances of allergic hepatitis also occurred with nifedipine.

Elevations of transaminases with and without concomitant elevations in alkaline phosphatase and bilirubin have occurred with **verapamil**. Elevations sometimes have been transient and may disappear with continued verapamil treatment. Several cases of hepatocellular injury related to verapamil have been proven by rechallenge; half of these cases had clinical symptoms (malaise, fever, or right upper quadrant pain) in addition to elevations of AST, ALT, and alkaline phosphatase. Periodically monitor liver function in patients treated with verapamil.

Isolated cases of elevated LDH, alkaline phosphatase, and ALT levels have occurred rarely with **nimodipine.**

➤*Edema:* Mild to moderate peripheral edema, typically associated with arterial vasodilation and not caused by left ventricular dysfunction, occurs in 10% to about 30% of patients receiving **nifedipine**. It occurs primarily in the lower extremities and usually responds to diuretic therapy. With patients whose angina is complicated by CHF, differentiate this peripheral edema from the effects of increasing left ventricular dysfunction.

Peripheral edema, generally mild and not associated with generalized fluid retention, may occur with **felodipine** within 2 to 3 weeks of therapy initiation. The incidence is both age- and dose-dependent, with frequency ranging from about 10% in patients under 50 years of age taking 5 mg/day to about 30% in patients over 60 years of age taking 20 mg/day.

Drug Interactions

➤*CYP450:* CYP3A4 has a major role in the metabolism of all the calcium channel blockers. Inducers and inhibitors of CYP3A4 can affect the metabolism of the dihydropyridines as well as **verapamil** and **diltiazem**. In general, diltiazem and verapamil inhibit other CYP3A4 substrates (eg, midazolam, carbamazepine), whereas the dihydropyridines do not.

Calcium Channel Blocker Drug Interactions

Precipitant drug	Object drug[a]		Description
Amiodarone	Calcium channel blockers– Diltiazem, verapamil	↑	Coadministration may result in cardiotoxicity with bradycardia and decreased cardiac output. Monitor closely.
Azole antifungals	Calcium channel blockers– Nisoldipine	↑	Serum nisoldipine concentrations may be elevated. If coadministration cannot be avoided, observe clinical response, monitor cardiovascular status, and adjust nisoldipine dose accordingly.
Azole antifungals– Itraconazole	Calcium channel blockers– Felodipine, isradipine, nifedipine	↑	Serum concentrations of the calcium channel blocker may be increased. Observe clinical response, monitor cardiovascular status, and adjust calcium channel blocker dose accordingly.
Barbiturates	Calcium channel blockers– Felodipine, nifedipine, verapamil	↓	Pharmacologic effects of the calcium channel blocker may be decreased.

Calcium Channel Blocker Drug Interactions			
Precipitant drug	Object drug[a]		Description
Beta-blockers	Calcium channel blockers	↑	Coadministration may cause additive or synergistic effects. Diltiazem, isradipine, nicardipine, nifedipine, and verapamil may inhibit the metabolism of certain beta-blockers. Monitor cardiac function and adjust dosages as needed.
Calcium channel blockers–Diltiazem, isradipine, nicardipine, nifedipine, verapamil	Beta-blockers		
Calcium salts	Calcium channel blockers–Verapamil	↓	Clinical effects and toxicities of verapamil may be reversed by calcium.
Carbamazepine, Oxcarbazepine	Calcium channel blockers–Felodipine	↓	Pharmacologic effects of felodipine may be decreased. Patients may require higher doses of felodipine.
Cisapride	Calcium channel blockers–Nifedipine	↑	Cisapride may increase nifedipine serum concentrations. Monitor closely and adjust dose of nifedipine as needed.
Cyclosporine	Calcium channel blockers–Nifedipine, felodipine	↑	Pharmacologic and toxic effects of nifedipine or felodipine may be increased. Cyclosporine levels and toxicity may be increased when given concurrently with diltiazem, felodipine, nicardipine, or verapamil. However, verapamil may be nephroprotective when given before cyclosporine. Monitor cyclosporine levels and adjust the dose as needed.
Calcium channel blockers–Diltiazem, felodipine, nicardipine, verapamil	Cyclosporine		
Erythromycin	Calcium channel blockers–Felodipine	↑	Coadministration may increase the effects of felodipine. Monitor cardiovascular status closely and adjust felodipine dose as needed.
H_2 antagonists–Cimetidine, ranitidine	Calcium channel blockers–Diltiazem, felodipine, isradipine, nicardipine, nifedipine, nimodipine, nisoldipine, verapamil	↑	Serum concentrations of the calcium channel blocker may be increased when given concurrently with cimetidine. Ranitidine also has been shown to affect diltiazem concentrations. Monitor cardiovascular status closely. Adjust dose as needed.
Hydantoins (eg, phenytoin)	Calcium channel blockers–Felodipine, nisoldipine, verapamil	↓	The pharmacologic effects of the calcium channel blocker may be decreased. Monitor cardiovascular status closely. Adjust dose as needed.
Melatonin	Calcium channel blockers–Nifedipine	↓	Concurrent use may decrease the antihypertensive effects of nifedipine.
Nafcillin	Calcium channel blockers–Nifedipine	↓	Nafcillin administration results in a large reduction in the plasma concentration of nifedipine; loss of efficacy is likely to result. Nafcillin would be expected to reduce the plasma concentrations of other calcium channel blockers as well. Avoid coadministration.
Quinupristin/Dalfopristin	Calcium channel blockers–Nifedipine	↑	Concurrent use may increase the plasma concentration of nifedipine. The metabolism of other calcium channel blockers would likely be reduced by quinupristin/dalfopristin.
Rifampin	Calcium channel blockers–Diltiazem, isradipine, nicardipine, nifedipine, verapamil	↓	Coadministration may decrease the therapeutic effects of the calcium channel blocker. Monitor cardiovascular status closely. Adjust dose as needed.
St. John's Wort	Calcium channel blockers–Nifedipine	↓	Coadministration may reduce the plasma concentration of nifedipine. The metabolism of other calcium channel blockers would likely be increased by St. John's Wort as well.
Valproic acid	Calcium channel blockers–Nimodipine	↑	Valproic acid increases the AUC of nimodipine with no effect on the elimination half-life. Monitor closely.
Calcium channel blockers	Anesthetics	↑	Calcium channel blockers may potentiate the cardiac effects and vascular dilation associated with anesthetics. Severe hypotension has been reported during fentanyl anesthesia with concomitant use of a beta blocker and a calcium channel blocker. Titrate doses carefully.
Calcium channel blockers–Verapamil	Antiarrhythmic agents–Disopyramide, flecainide	↑	Concomitant use of verapamil and flecainide may have additive effects. Until data on possible interactions between verapamil and disopyramide are obtained, the manufacturer recommends not administering disopyramide within 48 h before or 24 h after verapamil administration.
Calcium channel blockers–Verapamil	Antineoplastics-Doxorubicin	↑	Verapamil appears to increase doxorubicin serum concentrations.
Antineoplastics	Calcium channel blockers–Verapamil	↓	The absorption of verapamil can be reduced by the cyclophosphamide, oncovin, procarbazine, prednisone (COPP) and the vindesine, adriamycin, cisplatin (VAC) drug regimens.
Calcium channel blockers–Diltiazem, verapamil	Benzodiazepines–Midazolam, triazolam	↑	Effects of certain benzodiazepines may be increased.
Calcium channel blockers–Diltiazem, verapamil	Buspirone	↑	Coadministration may increase the effects of buspirone. Monitor closely and adjust buspirone dose as needed.
Calcium channel blockers–Diltiazem, verapamil	Carbamazepine	↑	Serum carbamazepine concentrations may be increased. Monitor serum levels and adjust dosage as necessary.
Calcium channel blockers–Nifedipine	Calcium channel blockers–Diltiazem	↑	Diltiazem increases nifedipine plasma concentrations and nifedipine increases diltiazem plasma concentrations.
Calcium channel blockers–Diltiazem	Calcium channel blockers–Nifedipine		
Calcium channel blockers–Diltiazem, nifedipine, verapamil	Digoxin	↑	Serum digoxin concentrations may be elevated, causing increased toxicity. Coadministration with diltiazem or nifedipine has produced conflicting reports. Monitor digoxin levels and adjust the dose as needed.
Calcium channel blockers–Verapamil	Dofetilide	↑	Concurrent use may increase dofetilide plasma concentration with increased risk of ventricular arrhythmias. Coadministration is contraindicated.
Calcium channel blockers–Verapamil	Ethanol	↑	Verapamil may cause increased and prolonged CNS effects of ethanol.
Calcium channel blockers–Diltiazem, verapamil	HMG-CoA reductase inhibitors	↑	Plasma concentrations of certain HMG-CoA reductase inhibitors (eg, atorvastatin) may be elevated. If coadministration cannot be avoided, administer a conservative dose of the HMG-CoA reductase inhibitor.
Calcium channel blockers–Isradipine	Lovastatin	↓	Plasma concentrations of lovastatin may be reduced, decreasing pharmacologic effect. Monitor clinical response and adjust therapy as needed.

Calcium Channel Blocker Drug Interactions

Precipitant drug	Object drug[a]		Description
Calcium channel blockers– Diltiazem, verapamil	Imipramine	↑	Coadministration increases imipramine serum concentrations.
Calcium channel blockers– Diltiazem, verapamil	Lithium	↑↓	Coadministration with verapamil has caused a reduction in lithium levels and toxicity. Coadministration with diltiazem has caused neurotoxicity.
Calcium channel blockers– Diltiazem	Methylprednisolone	↑	Pharmacologic and toxic effects of methylprednisolone may be increased.
Calcium channel blockers– Diltiazem	Moricizine	↑	Concurrent use may increase moricizine concentrations, while moricizine may decrease diltiazem concentrations.
Moricizine	Calcium channel blockers– Diltiazem	↓	
Calcium channel blockers– Verapamil	Nondepolarizing muscle relaxants	↑	Nondepolarizing muscle relaxant effects may be enhanced. Respiratory depression may be prolonged. Avoid concurrent use if possible.
Calcium channel blockers– Verapamil	Prazosin	↑	Concurrent use may increase serum prazosin concentrations and may increase the sensitivity to prazosin-induced postural hypotension.
Calcium channel blockers– Diltiazem, verapamil	Quinidine	↑	Coadministration may increase the therapeutic and adverse effects of quinidine. Use quinidine with verapamil only when no other alternative exists. Closely monitor quinidine serum levels and cardiac effects. Quinidine decreased the AUC of nisoldipine by 26% but not the peak concentration.
Quinidine	Calcium channel blockers– Nisoldipine	↓	
Calcium channel blockers– Nifedipine	Quinidine	↓	Serum levels and actions of quinidine may be decreased. Serum concentrations and actions of nifedipine may be increased.
Quinidine	Calcium channel blockers– Nifedipine	↑	
Calcium channel blockers– Diltiazem, verapamil	Sirolimus	↑	Coadministration may increase sirolimus plasma concentrations.
Calcium channel blockers– Diltiazem, nifedipine, verapamil	Tacrolimus	↑	Tacrolimus levels may be elevated, increasing toxicity. Monitor serum levels and adjust dosage as needed.
Calcium channel blockers– Diltiazem, verapamil	Theophyllines	↑	Pharmacologic and toxic effects of theophyllines may be increased. Monitor serum levels and adjust dosage as needed.
Calcium channel blockers– Nifedipine	Vincristine	↑	Vincristine levels may be elevated, possibly increasing toxicity.

[a] ↑ = Object drug increased. ↓ = Object drug decreased.

➤*Drug/Food interactions:* Grapefruit juice may increase the serum concentrations of **felodipine**, **nicardipine**, **nifedipine**, **nisoldipine**, **verapamil**, and possibly **amlodipine**.

Diltiazem – Administration of certain diltiazem ER products with a high-fat breakfast increased AUC and C_{max}.

Felodipine – When administered with either a high fat or carbohydrate diet, felodipine C_{max} is increased by approximately 60%; AUC is unchanged. Coadministration with grapefruit juice resulted in more than a 2-fold increase in the AUC and C_{max} but no prolongation in the half-life of felodipine.

Isradipine – Administration with food significantly increases isradipine's time to peak by about an hour but has no effect on the AUC. Food has been shown to decrease the extent of bioavailability of isradipine CR by up to 25%.

Nicardipine – When nicardipine was administered 1 or 3 hours after a high-fat meal, the mean C_{max} and AUC were lower (20% to 30%) than when given to fasting subjects. When nicardipine SR was administered with a high-fat breakfast, mean C_{max} was 45% lower, AUC was 25% lower, and trough levels were 75% higher than when given in the fasting state.

Nifedipine – When *Adalat CC* was given immediately after a high-fat meal in healthy volunteers, there was an average increase of 60% in the peak plasma concentration, a prolongation in the time to peak concentration, but no significant change in the AUC. Coadministration of nifedipine with grapefruit juice resulted in up to a 2-fold increase in AUC and C_{max}. Avoid coadministration.

Nimodipine – Nimodipine administration following a standard breakfast resulted in a 68% lower peak plasma concentration and 38% lower bioavailability relative to dosing under fasted conditions.

Nisoldipine – Food with a high-fat content had a pronounced effect on the release of nisoldipine from the coat-core formulation and resulted in a significant increase in C_{max} by up to 300%. However, total exposure was decreased about 25%, presumably because more of the drug was released proximally. Avoid concomitant intake of a high-fat meal with nisoldipine ER. Do not administer nisoldipine with grapefruit juice, as this has been shown to result in a mean increase in C_{max} of about 3-fold (ranging up to 7-fold) and AUC of almost 2-fold (ranging up to 5-fold).

Verapamil – Administration of verapamil SR with food produced decreased AUC but a narrower peak-to-trough ratio.

Adverse Reactions

Calcium Channel Blocker Adverse Reactions (%)[a]

	Adverse Reactions	Amlodipine	Diltiazem Oral (IV)[b]	Felodipine	Isradipine[b]	Nicardipine Oral (IV)[b]	Nifedipine[b]	Nimodipine	Nisoldipine	Verapamil Oral (IV)[b]
Cardiovascular	Angina/Angina pectoris		< 2	0.5-1.5		†	≤ 1			≤ 1
	Angina increased					5.6[c]	≤ 1			
	Arrhythmia	≤ 1	< 2 (1[d])	0.5-1.5			≤ 1			
	Arrhythmia, ventricular		< 1				< 0.5			
	Atrial fibrillation	≤ 1	1.4		≤ 1		< 1		≤ 1	
	AV block (1°, 2°, or 3°)		≤ 7.6 (< 1)			(†)			≤ 1	0.8-1.7
	Bradycardia	≤ 1	≤ 6 (< 1)				< 1	≤ 1		1.4 (1.2)
	Chest pain	≤ 1	< 1	0.5-1.5	≤ 2.7	(0.7)	≤ 3		2	≤ 1
	CHF		< 2 (< 1)					< 1	≤ 1	1.8
	Edema	1.8-14.6[e]	≤ 6 (< 1)		3.5-35.9[c]	0.6-1	10-30[c]	≤ 1.2[c]		1.7-3
	ECG abnormalities		≤ 4.1			0.6 (1.4)		≤ 1.4		2
	Facial edema			0.5-1.5			≤ 1		≤ 1	
	Hypertension		< 1			(0.7)		< 1	≤ 1	1.7
	Hypotension	≤ 1	< 2	0.5-1.5	≤ 1	† (5.6)	< 1	≤ 8.1[c]	≤ 1	0.7-2.5
	Hypotension, postural	≤ 1	< 1			≤ 0.9 (1.4)	< 1		≤ 1	0.4
	Hypotension, symptomatic		(3.2)							(1.5)
	MI		< 1	0.5-1.5	≤ 1				< 1	< 1
	Palpitations	0.7-4.5[c]	≤ 2	0.4-2.5	1-5.1[c]	2.8-4.1	≤ 7	< 1	3	≤ 1
	Peripheral edema		2-15 (4.3)	2-17.4		(†)	7-29[c]		7-29[c]	3.7
	Sinus bradycardia		< 1							
	Supraventricular tachycardia					(0.7)			≤ 1	
	Syncope	≤ 1	< 2 (< 1)	0.5-1.5	≤ 1	0.8 (0.7)	≤ 1		≤ 1	≤ 1
	Tachycardia	≤ 1	< 2	0.5-1.5	≤ 3.4	0.8-3.4 (3.5)	≤ 1	≤ 1.4		
	Vasculitis	≤ 1								≤ 1
	Vasodilation		≤ 3			4.7-5.5 (0.7)			4	
	Ventricular extrasystoles	≤ 0.1	≤ 2			† (1.4)			≤ 1	
	Ventricular tachycardia	≤ 1	(< 1)			† (0.7)				
CNS	Abnormal dreams	≤ 1	< 2			0.4			≤ 1	
	Amnesia	≤ 0.1	< 2						≤ 1	
	Anxiety/Anxiety disorders	≤ 1		0.5-1.5		†	≤ 1		≤ 1	
	Asthenia	1-2	≤ 4 (< 1)	2.2-3.9		0.9-5.8 (0.7)	≤ 4			2
	Ataxia	≤ 0.1					≤ 1		≤ 1	
	Confusion					† (†)	< 1		≤ 1	≤ 1
	Depression	≤ 1	< 2	0.5-1.5	≤ 1	†	≤ 1	≤ 1.4	≤ 1	(†)
	Dizziness/Lightheadedness	≤ 3.4[c]	≤ 10 (< 1)	2.7-3.7	3.4-8	1.6-6.9 (1.4)	4-27	< 1	3-10[c]	3-4.7 (1.2)
	Drowsiness				≤ 1					
	Equilibrium disturbances						≤ 2			≤ 1
	Fatigue/Lethargy	4.5[c]			≤ 8.5[c]		4-5.9			1.7-4.5
	Headache	7.3	≤ 12 (< 1)	10.6-14.7	10.3-22	6.2-8.2	10-23	≤ 4.1[c]	22	2.2-12.1 (1.2)
	Hypesthesia	≤ 1				(0.7)	≤ 1		≤ 1	
	Insomnia	≤ 1	< 2	0.5-1.5	≤ 1	0.6	< 3		≤ 1	≤ 1
	Malaise	≤ 1	< 1			0.6	≤ 1		≤ 1	
	Migraine	≤ 0.1					< 1		≤ 1	
	Nervousness	≤ 1	≤ 2	0.5-1.5	≤ 1	0.6	≤ 7		≤ 1	
	Paresthesia	≤ 1	< 2 (< 1)	1.2-1.6	≤ 1	1 (0.7)	≤ 3		≤ 1	≤ 1
	Shakiness/Jitteriness						≤ 2			≤ 1
	Sleep disturbances						≤ 2			1.4
	Somnolence	1.3-1.6[e]	< 2	0.5-1.5		1.1-1.4	< 3		≤ 1	≤ 1
	Tremor	≤ 1	< 2			0.6	≤ 8		≤ 1	
	Vertigo	≤ 1	< 1			†	≤ 3		≤ 1	(†)
	Weakness				≤ 1.2		10-12			

Calcium Channel Blocker Adverse Reactions (%)[a]

	Adverse Reactions	Amlodipine	Diltiazem Oral (IV)[b]	Felodipine	Isradipine[b]	Nicardipine Oral (IV)[b]	Nifedipine[b]	Nimodipine	Nisoldipine	Verapamil Oral (IV)[b]
Dermatologic	Acne							≤ 1.4	≤ 1	
	Dermatitis	≤ 0.1	≤ 1				≤ 2			
	Erythema multiforme	≤ 1	< 1							≤ 1
	Hair loss	≤ 0.1	†				≤ 1		≤ 1	≤ 1
	Injection site reactions		(3.9)			(1.4)				
	Leukocytoclastic vasculitis		†	0.5						
	Pruritus	1-2	< 2 (< 1)		≤ 1		< 3	< 1	≤ 1	
	Rash	1-2	≤ 2	0.2-2	≤ 2.6	0.4-1.2	≤ 3	≤ 2.4	≤ 2	≤ 2.4
	Rash maculopapular	≤ 1							≤ 1	
	Stevens-Johnson syndrome		†				< 0.5			≤ 1
	Urticaria	≤ 0.1	< 1	0.5-1.5	≤ 1		≤ 2		≤ 1	≤ 1 (†)
GI	Abdominal discomfort	1.6	1	0.5-1.5	≤ 5.1	(0.7)	< 3			(0.6)
	Abdominal distention		≤ 2		1.2					
	Acid regurgitation			0.5-1.5						
	Anorexia	≤ 1	< 2						≤ 1	
	Appetite increase	≤ 0.1							≤ 1	
	Constipation	≤ 1	≤ 3.6 (< 1)	0.3-1.5	≤ 3.8	0.6	≤ 3.3			3.9-11.7
	Diarrhea	≤ 1	≤ 2	0.5-1.5	≤ 3.4		< 3	≤ 4.2	≤ 1	≤ 2.4
	Dry mouth	≤ 1	< 2 (< 1)	0.5-1.5	≤ 1	0.4-1.4	< 3		≤ 1	≤ 1
	Dysgeusia	≤ 0.1	< 2				≤ 1		≤ 1	
	Dysphagia	≤ 1							≤ 1	
	Dyspepsia	1-2	≤ 6	0.5-3.9		0.8-1.5 (†)	< 3		≤ 1	2.5-2.7
	Flatulence	≤ 1	< 1	0.5-1.5			< 3		≤ 1	
	Gastritis	≤ 0.1							≤ 1	
	GI distress									≤ 1
	GI hemorrhage		< 1				< 1	< 1	≤ 1	
	Gingival hyperplasia	≤ 1	†	< 0.5			≤ 1		≤ 1	≤ 1
	Nausea	2.9[c]	≤ 2.2 (< 1)	1-1.7	1-5.1	1.9-2.2 (4.9)	2-11	0.6-1.4	2	1.7-2.7 (0.9)
	Thirst	≤ 1	< 2							
	Vomiting	≤ 1	≤ 2 (< 1)	0.5-1.5	≤ 1.3	0.4-0.6 (4.9)	≤ 1	< 1		
GU	Decreased libido			0.5-1.5	≤ 1		≤ 1		≤ 1	
	Dysuria	≤ 0.1		0.5-1.5			≤ 1		≤ 1	
	Gynecomastia		< 2	0.5-1.5			< 0.5		≤ 1	
	Hematuria					(0.7)	≤ 1		≤ 1	
	Impotence		≤ 2	0.5-1.5	≤ 1	†	≤ 3		≤ 1	≤ 1
	Nocturia	≤ 1	< 2		≤ 1	0.4	≤ 1		≤ 1	
	Polyuria	≤ 1	< 2	0.5-1.5		(1.4)	< 3			
	Sexual difficulties	≤ 2	< 2				≤ 2			
	Urinary frequency	≤ 1		0.5-1.5	1.3-3.4	≤ 0.6 (†)	≤ 3		≤ 1	≤ 1
Hematologic	Anemia			0.5-1.5			< 0.5	< 1	≤ 1	
	Ecchymosis								≤ 1	≤ 1
	Leukopenia	≤ 1	†		≤ 1		< 0.5		≤ 1	
	Petechiae		< 2						≤ 1	
	Purpura	≤ 1	< 1				≤ 1			≤ 1
	Thrombocytopenia	≤ 1	†			(†)	< 0.5	< 1		
Musculoskeletal	Arthralgia	≤ 1	1.4	0.5-1.5		†	< 3		≤ 1	≤ 1
	Arthritis						< 1		≤ 1	
	Back pain	≤ 1	1.7-2.9	0.5-1.5			≤ 1			
	Hypertonia	≤ 0.1	< 1			(†)	≤ 1		≤ 1	
	Leg cramps				≤ 1		≤ 3		≤ 1	
	Leg pain			0.5-1.5			≤ 3			
	Muscle cramps	1-2	< 2	0.5-1.5			≤ 8	≤ 1.4		≤ 1
	Myalgia	≤ 1	≤ 2.3	0.5-1.5		1	≤ 1		≤ 1	1.1
	Neck pain		< 1			(†)	< 1			
	Rigors	≤ 1					≤ 1			

Calcium Channel Blocker Adverse Reactions (%)[a]										
	Adverse Reactions	Amlodipine	Diltiazem Oral (IV)[b]	Felodipine	Isradipine[b]	Nicardipine Oral (IV)[b]	Nifedipine[b]	Nimodipine	Nisoldipine	Verapamil Oral (IV)[b]
Respiratory	Bronchitis		≤ 4	0.5-1.5						
	Cough	≤ 0.1		0.8-1.7	≤ 1		≤ 6			
	Cough increased		1-3				< 1		≤ 1	
	Dyspnea	1-2	≤ 6 (< 1)	0.5-1.5	≤ 3.4	0.6 (0.7)	≤ 6	≤ 1.2	≤ 1	1.4
	Epistaxis	≤ 1	< 2	0.5-1.5			≤ 3		≤ 1	
	Nasal congestion		< 2				≤ 6			
	Pharyngitis		1.4-6	0.5-1.5			< 1		≤ 5	3
	Respiratory disorder		< 1			(†)	≤ 1			
	Respiratory infection			0.5-1.5			≤ 1			
	Rhinitis	≤ 0.1	≤ 9.6			†			≤ 1	2.7
	Sinusitis		2	0.5-1.5		†	≤ 1		≤ 3	3
	Upper respiratory infection			0.7-3.9			≤ 1			5.4
	Wheezing						6	< 1		
Special senses	Abnormal vision	≤ 1				†	≤ 1		≤ 1	
	Amblyopia		(< 1)				< 1		≤ 1	
	Blurred vision		< 1			†	≤ 2			≤ 1
	Conjunctivitis	≤ 1				(†)			≤ 1	
	Tinnitus	≤ 1	< 2			† (†)	≤ 1		≤ 1	≤ 1
Miscellaneous	Accidental injury		< 1.3							1.5
	Angioedema	≤ 1		0.5-1.5			≤ 0.5			
	Chills						≤ 2		≤ 1	
	Fever		< 1			(†)	≤ 2		≤ 1	
	Flu-like illness/syndrome/ symptoms		≤ 2.3	0.5-1.5					≤ 1	3.7
	Flushing	0.7-4.5[e]	≤ 3 (1.7)	3.9-6.9	1.2-5.1[c]	5.6-9.7	≤ 25	≤ 2.1		0.6-0.8
	Gout		1-2				≤ 1		≤ 1	
	Hot flashes					†	≤ 1			
	Hyperglycemia	≤ 1	< 2							
	Infection		≤ 6			†				12.1
	Pain	≤ 1	≤ 6			0.6	< 3			
	Sore throat					†	6			
	Sweating		< 1 (< 1)			(1.4)	≤ 2	< 1	≤ 1	≤ 1
	Sweating increased	≤ 1				0.6	≤ 1			(†)
	Weight gain	≤ 1	< 2				≤ 1		≤ 1	
	Weight loss						< 1		≤ 1	

[a] Data are pooled from separate studies and are not necessarily comparable.
[b] Includes data for SR/ER form.
[c] Dose-related.
[d] Functional rhythm or isorhythmic dissociation.
[e] Dose-related and higher in females.
† Occurs, no incidence reported.

In addition to the adverse effects listed in the table, the following have been reported:

Amlodipine – Peripheral ischemia, peripheral neuropathy, rash erythematous, pancreatitis, micturition disorder, postural dizziness, depersonalization, allergic reaction, hot flushes, arthrosis, diplopia, eye pain (less than or equal to 1%); cardiac failure, pulse irregularity, skin discoloration/dryness, twitching, cold/clammy skin, apathy, agitation, loose stools, parosmia, muscle weakness, abnormal visual accommodation, xerophthalmia (less than or equal to 0.1%).

Diltiazem – Asymptomatic hypotension (1.3%); bundle branch block, hallucination, personality change, photosensitivity, gait abnormalities, crystalluria, osteoarticular pain, neck rigidity, hyperuricemia, albuminuria (less than 2%); arthrosis (1%); eye irritation, pallor, phlebitis, tooth disorder, eructation, skin hypertrophy (nevus), cystitis, kidney calculus, dysmenorrhea, pyelonephritis, urinary tract infection, eye hemorrhage, ophthalmitis, otitis media, sinus pause, sinus node dysfunction, ventricular fibrillation, kidney failure, respiratory distress, contact dermatitis, stomach ulcers, colitis, neuropathy, myocardial ischemia, vaginitis, prostate disease, bursitis, bone pain, lymphadenopathy, ear pain, bigeminal extrasystole, asystole, atrial flutter (less than 1%).

Felodipine – Sneezing (less than or equal to 1.6%); rhinorrhea (0.2% to 1.6%); premature beats, irritability, erythema, urinary urgency, visual disturbances, influenza, arm/foot/hip/knee pain, contusion (0.5% to 1.5%); warm sensation (less than or equal to 1.5%).

Isradipine – Foot cramps, shortness of breath, ventricular fibrillation, numbness, tingling, transient ischemic attack, stroke, hyperhidrosis, visual disturbance, throat discomfort (less than or equal to 1%).

Nicardipine – Pedal edema (4.4% to 8%); hemopericardium, hypokalemia, intracranial hemorrhage, injection site pain (0.7%); ST segment depression, inverted T wave, deep-vein thrombophlebitis, hypophosphatemia, ear disorder, allergic reaction, peripheral vascular disorder, hyperkinesia, atypical chest pain (rare).

Nifedipine – Giddiness (27%); heat sensation (4% to 25%); muscle tremor (8%); heartburn (11%); mood changes (less than or equal to 7%); transient hypotension (5%); abdominal cramps, joint stiffness; muscle inflammation, chest congestion (less than or equal to 2%); periorbital edema, eructation, GI reflux, melena, abnormal lacrimation, breast pain (less than or equal to 1%); cellulitis, pelvic pain, cardiac arrest, extrasystole, phlebitis, cutaneous angiectases, esophagitis, lymphadenopathy, rales, diplopia, kidney calculus, breast engorgement (less than 1%); erythromelalgia, allergenic hepatitis, arthritis with ANA (+), transient blindness, exfoliative dermatitis, toxic epidermal necrolysis, paranoia, psychiatric disturbances (less than 0.5%). Very rarely, therapy was associated with an increase in anginal pain, possibly caused by associated hypotension. Transient unilateral loss of vision also occurred.

In a subgroup of approximately 250 patients with a diagnosis of CHF as well as angina pectoris (about 10% of the total patient population), dizziness or lightheadedness, peripheral edema, headache, or flushing each occurred in 1 in 8 patients. Hypotension occurred in about 1 in 20 patients. Syncope occurred in approximately 1 patient in 250. MI or symptoms of CHF each occurred in about 1 patient in 15. Atrial or ventricular dysrhythmias each occurred in approximately 1 patient in 150.

Nimodipine – GI symptoms (less than or equal to 2.4%); rebound vasospasm, jaundice, hyponatremia, disseminated intravascular coagulation, deep-vein thrombosis, neurological deterioration, phenytoin toxicity, decreased platelet count, hepatitis, hematoma (less than 1%).

Nisoldipine – Cellulitis, cerebrovascular accident, jugular venous distension, systolic ejection murmur, venous insufficiency, colitis, glossitis, hepatomegaly, melena, mouth ulceration, diabetes mellitus, thyroiditis, hypokalemia, increased serum creatine kinase, increased nonprotein nitrogen, myasthenia, myositis, blepharitis, ear pain, glaucoma, itchy eyes, keratoconjunctivitis, otitis media, retinal detachment, watery eyes, temporary unilateral loss of vision, vitreous floater, increased BUN and serum creatinine, vaginal hemorrhage, vaginitis, tenosynovitis, abnormal thinking, cerebral ischemia, end inspiratory wheeze and fine rales, laryngitis, pleural effusion, dry skin, herpes simplex, herpes zoster, pustular rash, skin discoloration, skin ulcer, fungal dermatitis, exfoliative dermatitis, T wave abnormalities on ECG (flattening, inversion, nonspecific changes), asthma (less than or equal to 1%); chest tightness (rare).

Verapamil – Allergy aggravated (less than or equal to 2%); ankle edema (1.4%); pulmonary edema (1.8%); severe tachycardia (1%); atrioventricular dissociation, claudication, cerebrovascular accident, psychotic symptoms, exanthema, hyperkeratosis, macules, galactorrhea/hyperprolactinemia, spotty menstruation, bruising (less than or equal to 1%); broncho/laryngeal spasm, itch (rare); rotary nystagmus, sleepiness, muscle fatigue, seizures during injection (occasional); respiratory failure (low frequency).

In clinical trials related to the control of ventricular response in digitalized patients who had atrial fibrillation or flutter, ventricular rates below 50 at rest occurred in 15% of patients and asymptomatic hypotension occurred in 5% of patients.

➤*Lab test abnormalities:* Rare, usually transient, but occasionally significant elevations of enzymes such as alkaline phosphatase, CPK, LDH, AST, and ALT have occurred with **diltiazem** and **nifedipine** (see Precautions). **Felodipine** patients experienced an ALT increase of 0.5% to 1.5%. Positive direct Coombs' test with or without hemolytic anemia has occurred with **nifedipine**. Abnormal liver function test (1.2%), isolated cases of decreased platelet counts (0.3%), and elevated nonfasting serum glucose, LDH (0.4%), alkaline phosphatase (0.2%), and ALT (0.2%) have occurred rarely with **nimodipine**. Abnormal liver function tests have occurred with **nisoldipine**, elevated liver function tests have occurred with **isradipine**, elevated liver enzymes occurred with **verapamil** (1.4%), and abnormal liver chemistries were reported with **nicardipine**.

➤*Postmarketing experience:*

Amlodipine – Jaundice and hepatic enzyme elevations (mostly consistent with cholestasis or hepatitis), in some cases severe enough to require hospitalization, have been reported in association with use of amlodipine.

Diltiazem – Infrequently reported postmarketing events include the following: Allergic reactions; alopecia; asystole; angioedema; erythema multiforme; Stevens-Johnson syndrome; toxic epidermal necrolysis; extrapyramidal symptoms; gingival hyperplasia; hemolytic anemia; increased bleeding time; leukopenia; purpura; retinopathy; thrombocytopenia; generalized rash; leukocytoclastic vasculitis; exfoliative dermatitis.

Nifedipine – There have been rare reports of the following: Toxic epidermal necrolysis; exfoliative dermatitis; Stevens-Johnson syndrome; and photosensitivity reactions.

Nisoldipine – Systemic hypersensitivity reaction has been reported very rarely, which may include 1 or more of the following: Angioedema, shortness of breath, tachycardia, chest tightness, hypotension, rash.

Overdosage

➤*Symptoms:* Symptoms of overdosage include marked and prolonged hypotension and bradycardia, both of which may result in decreased cardiac output. Junctional rhythms and second- or third-degree AV block may be seen. Death has occurred. Toxic **diltiazem** blood levels in man are not known, but there have been 29 reports of diltiazem overdose in doses ranging from less than 1 to 10.8 g. Sixteen of these reports involved multiple drug ingestion.

Ingestion of 900 mg of **nifedipine** IR and 4800 mg **nifedipine** ER in 2 patients resulted in dizziness, palpitations, flushing, nervousness, loss of consciousness, nausea, vomiting, generalized edema, and profound hypotension. One patient had sinus bradycardia and varying degrees of AV block. Both patients recovered. Significant hyperglycemia was seen initially in the nifedipine IR patient, but plasma glucose levels rapidly normalized without further treatment.

One patient ingested 250 mg **amlodipine** and was asymptomatic. Another patient ingested 120 mg, underwent gastric lavage, and remained normotensive. A third patient took 105 mg and had hypotension (90/50 mmHg), which normalized following plasma expansion. A 19 month old ingested 30 mg (2 mg/kg) and had no evidence of hypotension but had a heart rate of 180 bpm.

➤*Treatment:* If the patient is seen shortly after oral ingestion, employ lavage, activated charcoal, and cathartics. Treatment is supportive. Refer to General Management of Acute Overdosage. Beta-adrenergic agonists and IV calcium have been used effectively. Treat cardiac failure with inotropic agents (isoproterenol, dopamine, or dobutamine) and diuretics. In patients with hypertrophic cardiomyopathy, use α-adrenergic agents (phenylephrine HCl or metaraminol bitartrate) to maintain blood pressure; avoid isoproterenol and norepinephrine. Monitor cardiac and respiratory function; elevate the extremities. Because these agents are highly protein bound, dialysis is not likely to help. Verapamil cannot be removed by hemodialysis.

Calcium Channel Blocker Overdosage: Suggested Treatment of Acute Cardiovascular Adverse Reactions[a]

Adverse reaction	Proven effective treatment[b]	Supportive treatment
Symptomatic hypotension requiring treatment	Dopamine Calcium chloride Isoproterenol HCl Metaraminol bitartrate Norepinephrine bitartrate	IV fluids Trendelenburg position
Bradycardia, AV block, h asystole	Atropine Calcium chloride Cardiac pacing Isoproterenol HCl Norepinephrine bitartrate	IV fluids
Rapid ventricular rate (caused by antegrade conduction in flutter/fibrillation with W-P-W or L-G-L syndromes)	D.C. cardioversion Lidocaine Procainamide	IV fluids

[a] Actual treatment and dosage should depend on the severity of the clinical situation and the judgment and experience of the treating physician.
[b] Drug therapy is administered IV.

Patient Information

Notify physician if any of the following occur: Irregular heart beat, shortness of breath, swelling of the hands and feet, pronounced dizziness, constipation, nausea, or hypotension.

➤*Diltiazem (Dilacor XR):* Swallow whole; do not open, crush, or chew.

➤*Felodipine:* Swallow whole; do not crush or chew.

Mild gingival hyperplasia has occurred; good dental hygiene decreases its incidence and severity.

➤*Isradipine:* Swallow controlled-release tablets whole. Do not chew, divide, or crush. The empty tablet shell is eliminated in the stool.

➤*Nifedipine ER:* Swallow whole; do not chew, divide, or crush. Take *Adalat CC* on an empty stomach. An empty tablet may appear in the stool; this is no cause for concern.

➤*Nisoldipine:* Nisoldipine is an extended-release tablet; swallow whole. Do not chew, divide, or crush the tablet. Do not administer with a high-fat meal. Grapefruit juice, which has been shown to increase significantly the bioavailability of nisoldipine and other dihydropyridine-type calcium channel blockers, should not be taken with nisoldipine.

➤*Verapamil ER / SR:* Do not crush or chew the contents of the pellet-filled capsule. When the sprinkle method of administration is prescribed, explain to patients the details of proper technique. Swallow *Covera-HS* tablets whole; do not break, crush, or chew. The patient should not be concerned if they occasionally observe this outer shell in their stool as it passes from the body.

NISOLDIPINE

Rx	**Sular** (First Horizon)	**Tablets, extended-release**: 10 mg	Lactose. (891 ZENECA 10). Oyster. Film-coated. In 100s.
		20 mg	Lactose. (892 ZENECA 20). Yellow cream. Film-coated. In 100s and UD 100s.
		30 mg	Lactose. (893 ZENECA 30). Mustard. Film-coated. In 100s and UD 100s.
		40 mg	Lactose. (894 ZENECA 40). Burnt orange. Film-coated. In 100s.

NISOLDIPINE — ORAL

For complete and comparative prescribing information, refer to the Calcium Channel Blockers group monograph.

Indications

➤*Hypertension:* Treatment of hypertension. It may be used alone or in combination with other antihypertensive agents.

Administration and Dosage

➤*Approved by the FDA:* February 2, 1995.

➤*Dosage:* The dosage of nisoldipine must be adjusted to each patient's needs. Therapy usually should be initiated with 20 mg orally once daily, then increased by 10 mg per week or longer intervals to attain adequate control of blood pressure. Usual maintenance dosage is 20 to 40 mg once daily. Blood pressure response increases over the 10 to 60 mg daily dose range, but adverse event rates also increase. Doses beyond 60 mg once daily are not recommended. Nisoldipine has been used safely with diuretics, ACE inhibitors, and beta-blocking agents.

➤*Elderly / hepatic function impairment:* Patients over age 65, or patients with impaired liver function are expected to develop higher plasma concentrations of nisoldipine. Their blood pressure should be monitored closely during any dosage adjustment. A starting dose not exceeding 10 mg daily is recommended in these patient groups.

➤*Administration:* Nisoldipine tablets should be administered orally once daily. Administration with a high-fat meal can lead to excessive peak drug concentration and should be avoided. Grapefruit products should be avoided before and after dosing. Nisoldipine is an extended-release dosage form and tablets should be swallowed whole, not bitten, divided or crushed.

➤*Storage / Stability:* Protect from light and moisture. Store at controlled room temperature, 20° to 25°C (68° to 77°F) Dispense in tight, light-resistant containers.

NIFEDIPINE

Rx	**Nifedipine** (Mylan)	**Tablets, extended-release**: 30 mg	In 100s and 300s.
Rx	**Adalat CC** (Schering)		Lactose. (30 ADALAT CC). Pink. Film-coated. In 100s, 1,000s, and UD 100s.
Rx	**Afeditab CR** (Watson)		(ELN 30). Brick red. In 100s.
Rx	**Nifediac CC** (Teva)		(B 30). Mustard yellow. Film coated. In 100s, 300s, and 1000s.
Rx	**Nifedical XL** (Teva)		Lactose. (B 30). Reddish brown. Film-coated. In 100s and 300s.
Rx	**Procardia XL** (Pfizer)		(PROCARDIA XL 30). Rose pink. Film-coated. In 100s, 300s, 5000s, and UD 100s.
Rx	**Nifedipine** (Mylan)	**Tablets, extended-release**: 60 mg	In 100s and 300s.
Rx	**Adalat CC** (Schering)		Lactose. (60 ADALAT CC). Salmon. Film-coated. In 100s, 1,000s, and UD 100s.
Rx	**Afeditab CR** (Watson)		(ELN 60). Brick red. In 100s.
Rx	**Nifediac CC** (Teva)		Lactose. (B 60). Mustard yellow. Film coated. In 100s, 300s, and 1000s.
Rx	**Nifedical XL** (Teva)		Lactose. (B 60). Reddish brown. Film-coated. In 100s and 300s.
Rx	**Procardia XL** (Pfizer)		(PROCARDIA XL 60). Rose pink. Film-coated. In 100s, 300s, 5000s, and UD 100s.
Rx	**Nifedipine** (Mylan)	**Tablets, extended-release**: 90 mg	In 100s.
Rx	**Adalat CC** (Schering)		Lactose. (90 ADALAT CC). Dark red. Film-coated. In 100s and UD 100s.
Rx	**Nifediac CC** (Teva)		Lactose. (B 90). Yellow. Film coated. In 100s.
Rx	**Procardia XL** (Pfizer)		(PROCARDIA XL 90). Rose pink. Film-coated. In 100s and UD 100s.
Rx	**Nifedipine** (Various, eg, Purepac)	**Capsules**: 10 mg	May be liquid-filled. In 100s and 300s.
Rx	**Procardia** (Pfizer)		Liquid-filled. Saccharin. (PROCARDIA PFIZER 260). Orange. In 100s and 300s.
Rx	**Nifedipine** (Various, eg, Major, Purepac)	**Capsules**: 20 mg	May be liquid-filled. In 100s and 300s.
Rx	**Procardia** (Pfizer)		Liquid-filled. (PROCARDIA 20 PFIZER 261). Orange. In 100s.

NIFEDIPINE — ORAL

For complete and comparative prescribing information, refer to the Calcium Channel Blockers group monograph.

Indications

➤*Vasospastic angina (except Adalat CC, Afeditab CR, Nifediac CC):* For the management of vasospastic angina confirmed by any of the following criteria: 1) classical pattern of angina at rest accompanied by ST segment elevation; 2) angina or coronary artery spasm provoked by ergonovine; or 3) angiographically demonstrated coronary artery spasm. In patients who have had angiography, the presence of significant fixed obstructive disease is not incompatible with the diagnosis of vasospastic angina, provided that the above criteria are satisfied. Also may be used when clinical presentation suggests a vasospastic component, but where vasospasm has not been confirmed (eg, where pain has a variable threshold on exertion, or in unstable angina where electrocardiographic findings are compatible with intermittent vasospasm, or when angina is refractory to nitrates or adequate doses of beta-blockers).

➤*Chronic stable angina (except Adalat CC, Afeditab CR, Nifediac CC):* Classic effort-associated angina without vasospasm in patients who remain symptomatic despite adequate doses of beta blockers or organic nitrates or who cannot tolerate those agents.

➤*Hypertension (extended-release only):* May be used alone or in combination with other antihypertensive agents.

➤*Unlabeled uses:* Topical nifedipine (not commercially available in the US) has been shown to be beneficial in the treatment of anal fissures.

Administration and Dosage

Individualize dosage. Excessive doses can result in hypotension. Avoid coadministration of nifedipine with grapefruit juice.

➤*Capsules:*

Dosage – 10 mg 3 times/day; swallow whole. Usual range is 10 to 20 mg 3 times/day. Some patients, especially those with coronary artery spasm, respond only to higher doses, more frequent administration, or both. In such patients, 20 to 30 mg 3 or 4 times/day may be effective. Doses above 120 mg/day are rarely necessary. More than 180 mg/day is not recommended.

Titrate throughout 7 to 14 days to assess response to each dose level; monitor blood pressure before proceeding to higher doses. If symptoms warrant, titrate more rapidly, but assess frequently based on physical activity level, attack frequency, and sublingual nitroglycerin consumption. Increase dose from 10 to 20 mg 3 times/day, and then 30 mg 3 times/day throughout 3 days.

Hospitalized patients – In hospitalized patients under close observation, the dose may be increased in 10 mg increments throughout 4- to 6-hour periods as required to control pain and arrhythmias caused by ischemia. A single dose should rarely exceed 30 mg.

➤*Tablets, extended-release:* Take care when dispensing nifedipine to assure the extended-release doseform has been prescribed. Swallow whole; do not bite or divide tablet.

Procardia XL and Nifedical XL – 30 or 60 mg once daily. Titrate over a 7- to 14-day period. Titration may proceed more rapidly if the patient is frequently assessed. Titration to doses above 120 mg is not recommended.

Angina patients maintained on the nifedipine capsule formulation may be switched to the extended-release tablet at the nearest equivalent total daily dose. Experience with doses greater than 90 mg in angina is limited; therefore, use with caution and only when clinically warranted.

Adalat CC, Afeditab CR, Nifediac CC (hypertension) – Administer once daily on an empty stomach. In general, titrate over a 7- to 14-day period, starting with 30 mg once daily. Base upward titration on therapeutic efficacy and safety. Usual maintenance dose is 30 to 60 mg once daily. Titration to doses above 90 mg/day is not recommended.

➤*Discontinuation:* No "rebound effect" has been observed upon discontinuation of nifedipine. However, if discontinuation of nifedipine is necessary, sound clinical practice suggests the dosage be decreased gradually with close physician supervision.

➤*Coadministration with other antianginal drugs:* Sublingual nitroglycerin may be taken as required for the control of acute manifestations of angina, particularly during nifedipine titration. Coadministration of nifedipine with beta blockers or long-acting nitrates is usually well tolerated, but there have been occasional reports suggesting that the combination, especially with beta blockers, may increase the likelihood of congestive heart failure, severe hypotension or exacerbation of angina.

➤*Storage/Stability:*

Capsules – Store at controlled room temperature 15° to 25°C (59° to 77°F). Protect from light, moisture, and humidity. Prevent freezing; capsules may be liquid-filled. Replace cap tightly after each opening.

Tablets – Store below 30°C (86°F). Protect from moisture and humidity.

NICARDIPINE HYDROCHLORIDE

Rx	**Nicardipine hydrochloride** (Various, eg Mylan)	**Capsules**: 20 mg	In 90s and 500s.
Rx	**Cardene** (Roche)		(CARDENE 20 mg ROCHE). White. In 100s and 500s.
Rx	**Nicardipine HCl** (Various, eg Mylan)	**Capsules**: 30 mg	In 90s and 500s.
Rx	**Cardene** (Roche)		(CARDENE 30 mg ROCHE). Lt. blue. In 100s and 500s.
Rx	**Cardene SR** (Roche)	**Capsules, sustained-release**: 30 mg	Lactose. (CARDENE SR 30 mg ROCHE). Pink. In 60s and 200s.
		45 mg	Lactose. (CARDENE SR 45 mg ROCHE). Powder blue. In 60s and 200s.
		60 mg	Lactose. (CARDENE SR 60 mg ROCHE). Light blue/white. In 60s.
Rx	**Cardene I.V.** (ESP Pharma)[1]	**Injection**: 2.5 mg/mL	48 mg sorbitol. In 10 mL amps.

[1] ESP Pharma, Inc., 2035 Lincoln Highway, Suite 2150, Edison, NJ 08817; (866) 437-7742; http://www.esppharma.com

NICARDIPINE HYDROCHLORIDE — ORAL

For complete and comparative prescribing information, refer to the Calcium Channel Blockers group monograph.

Indications

➤*Immediate-release capsules:*

Stable angina – Management of patients with chronic stable angina (effort-associated angina). Nicardipine may be used alone or in combination with beta-blockers.

Hypertension – Treatment of hypertension. Nicardipine may be used alone or in combination with other antihypertensive drugs.

➤*Sustained-release capsules:* Treatment of hypertension. Nicardipine sustained release may be used alone or in combination with other antihypertensive drugs.

Administration and Dosage

➤*Approved by the FDA:* December 21, 1988.

➤*Immediate-release capsules:*

Angina – The dose should be individually titrated for each patient beginning with 20 mg 3 times daily. Doses in the range of 20 to 40 mg 3 times a day have been shown to be effective. At least 3 days should be allowed before increasing the nicardipine dose to ensure achievement of steady-state plasma drug concentrations.

Concomitant use with other antianginal agents: Sublingual nitroglycerin (NTG) may be taken as required to abort acute anginal attacks during nicardipine therapy.

• *Prophylactic nitrate therapy* – Nicardipine may be safely coadministered with short- and long-acting nitrates.

• *Beta-blockers* – Nicardipine may be safely coadministered with beta-blockers. The combination is well tolerated.

➤*Hypertension:*

Immediate-release capsules – The dose of nicardipine should be individually adjusted according to the blood pressure response beginning with 20 mg 3 times daily. The effective doses in clinical trials have ranged from 20 mg to 40 mg 3 times daily. The maximum blood pressure lowering effect occurs approximately 1 to 2 hours after dosing. To assess the adequacy of blood pressure response, the blood pressure should be measured at trough (8 hours after dosing). Because of the prominent peak effects of nicardipine, blood pressure should be measured 1 to 2 hours after dosing, particularly during initiation of therapy. Because of prominent effects at the time of peak blood levels, initial titration should be performed with measurements of blood pressure at peak effect (1 to 2 hours after dosing) and just before the next dose. At least 3 days should be allowed before increasing the nicardipine dose to ensure achievement of steady state plasma drug concentrations.

Sustained-release capsules – The dose of nicardipine sustained release should be individually adjusted according to the blood pressure response beginning with 30 mg 2 times daily. The effective doses in clinical trials have ranged from 30 mg to 60 mg 2 times daily. The maximum blood pressure lowering effect at steady state is sustained from 2 hours until 6 hours after dosing. When initiating therapy or upon increasing dose, blood pressure should be measured 2 to 4 hours after the first dose or dose increase, as well as at the end of a dosing interval.

The total daily dose of immediate-release nicardipine may not be a useful guide to judging the effective dose of nicardipine sustained release. Patients currently receiving immediate-release nicardipine may be titrated with nicardipine sustained release starting at their current total daily dose of immediate-release nicardipine and then reexamined to assess the adequacy of blood pressure control.

➤*Concomitant use with other antihypertensive agents:*

Diuretics – Nicardipine may be safely coadministered with thiazide diuretics.

Beta-blockers – Nicardipine may be safely coadministered with beta blockers.

➤*Renal function impairment:*

Immediate-release capsules – Although there is no evidence that nicardipine impairs renal function, careful dose titration beginning with 20 mg 3 times daily is advised. When nicardipine 20 mg or 30 mg 3 times daily was given to hypertensive patients with mild renal impairment, mean plasma concentrations, AUC and C_{max} were approximately 2-fold higher in renally impaired patients than in healthy controls. Doses in these patients must be adjusted.

Sustained-release capsules – Although there is no evidence that nicardipine sustained release impairs renal function, careful dose titration beginning with 30 mg nicardipine sustained release twice daily is advised. When nicardipine 45 mg sustained-release 2 times a day was given to hypertensive patients with moderate renal impairment, mean AUC and C_{max} values were approximately 2-fold to 3-fold higher than in patients with mild renal impairment. Doses in these patients must be adjusted. Mean AUC and C_{max} values were similar in patients with mildly impaired renal function and normal volunteers.

➤*Hepatic function impairment:*

Immediate-release capsules – Nicardipine should be administered cautiously in patients with severely impaired hepatic function. A suggested starting dose of 20 mg twice a day is advised with individual titration based on clinical findings maintaining the twice a day schedule.

Sustained-release capsules – Since the liver is the major site of biotransformation and since nicardipine is subject to first pass metabolism, the drug should be used with caution in patients having impaired liver function or reduced hepatic blood flow. Patients with severe liver disease developed elevated blood levels (4-fold increase in AUC) and prolonged half-life (19 hours) of nicardipine. Nicardipine sustained release has not been studied in patients with severe liver impairment.

➤*Congestive heart failure:* Caution is advised when titrating nicardipine dosage in patients with congestive heart failure.

➤*Storage/Stability:* Store bottles at 15° to 30°C (59° to 86°F) and dispense in light-resistant containers, such as the manufacturer's original container.

NICARDIPINE HYDROCHLORIDE — INJECTION

For complete and comparative prescribing information, refer to the Calcium Channel Blockers group monograph.

Indications

➤*Hypertension:* Nicardipine IV is indicated for the short-term treatment of hypertension when oral therapy is not feasible or not desirable. For prolonged control of blood pressure, transfer patients to oral medication as soon as their clinical conditions permit.

Administration and Dosage

➤*Approved by the FDA:* January 30, 1992.

Nicardipine IV is intended for intravenous use. Dosage must be individualized depending upon the severity of hypertension and the response of the patient during dosing.

Blood pressure should be monitored both during and after the infusion; too rapid or excessive reduction in either systolic or diastolic blood pressure during parenteral treatment should be avoided.

➤*Preparation:* Ampuls must be diluted before infusion.

Dilution – Nicardipine IV is administered by slow continuous infusion at a concentration of 0.1 mg/mL. Each ampul (25 mg) should be diluted with 240 mL of compatible intravenous fluid (see below), resulting in 250 mL of solution at a concentration of 0.1 mg/mL.

Nicardipine IV has been found to be compatible and stable in glass or polyvinyl chloride containers for 24 hours at controlled room temperature with:

1.) Dextrose (5%) Injection, USP
2.) Dextrose (5%) and Sodium Chloride (0.45%) Injection, USP
3.) Dextrose (5%) and Sodium Chloride (0.9%) Injection, USP
4.) Dextrose (5%) with 40 mEq Potassium, USP
5.) Sodium Chloride (0.45%) Injection, USP
6.) Sodium Chloride (0.9%) Injection, USP

Nicardipine IV is not compatible with sodium bicarbonate (5%) injection or Ringer's lactate injection.

The diluted solution is stable for 24 hours at room temperature.

➤*Dosage:*

As a substitute for oral nicardipine therapy – The intravenous infusion rate required to produce an average plasma concentration equivalent to a given oral dose at steady state is given in the following table:

Oral Nicardipine Dose	Equivalent IV Infusion Rate
20 mg every 8 hours	0.5 mg/h
30 mg every 8 hours	1.2 mg/h
40 mg every 8 hours	2.2 mg/h

For initiation of therapy in a drug-free patient – The time course of blood pressure decrease is dependent on the initial rate of infusion and the frequency of dosage adjustment.

Nicardipine IV is administered by slow continuous infusion at a concentration of 0.1 mg/mL. With constant infusion, blood pressure begins to fall within minutes. It reaches about 50% of its ultimate decrease in about 45 minutes and does not reach final steady state for about 50 hours.

When treating acute hypertensive episodes in patients with chronic hypertension, discontinuation of infusion is followed by a 50% offset of action in 30 ± 7 minutes but plasma levels of drug and gradually decreasing antihypertensive effects exist for about 50 hours.

Titration: For gradual reduction in blood pressure, initiate therapy at 50 mL/h (5 mg/h). If desired blood pressure reduction is not achieved at this dose, the infusion rate may be increased by 25 mL/h (2.5 mg/h) every 15 minutes up to a maximum of 150 mL/h (15 mg/h), until desired blood pressure reduction is achieved.

For more rapid blood pressure reduction, initiate therapy at 50 mL/hr (5 mg/h). If desired blood pressure reduction is not achieved at this dose, the infusion rate may be increased by 25 mL/hr (2.5 mg/h) every 5 minutes up to a maximum of 150 mL/h (15 mg/h), until desired blood pressure reduction is achieved. Following achievement of the blood pressure goal, the infusion rate should be decreased to 30 mL/h (3 mg/h).

Maintenance: The rate of infusion should be adjusted as needed to maintain desired response.

➤*Conditions requiring infusion adjustment:*

Hypotension or tachycardia – If there is concern of impending hypotension or tachycardia, the infusion should be discontinued. When blood pressure has stabilized, infusion of nicardipine IV may be restarted at low doses such as 30 to 50 mL/hr (3 to 5 mg/hr) and adjusted to maintain desired blood pressure.

NICARDIPINE HYDROCHLORIDE — INJECTION

Infusion site changes – Nicardipine IV should be continued as long as blood pressure control is needed. The infusion site should be changed every 12 hours if administered via peripheral vein.

Impaired cardiac, hepatic, or renal function – Caution is advised when titrating nicardipine IV in patients with congestive heart failure or impaired hepatic or renal function.

➤*Transfer to oral antihypertensive agents:* If treatment includes transfer to an oral antihypertensive agent other than nicardipine capsules, therapy should generally be initiated upon discontinuation of nicardipine IV. If nicardipine IV capsules are to be used, the first dose of a 3–times-daily regimen should be administered 1 hour prior to discontinuation of the infusion.

➤*Storage/Stability:* Store at controlled room temperature, 20° to 25°C (68° to 77°F).

Freezing does not adversely affect the product, but exposure to elevated temperatures should be avoided.

Protect from light. Store ampuls in carton until used.

As with all parenteral drugs, nicardipine IV should be inspected visually for particulate matter and discoloration prior to administration, whenever solution and container permit. Nicardipine IV is normally light yellow in color.

ISRADIPINE

Rx	**DynaCirc CR** (Reliant)	**Tablets, controlled-release:** 5 mg	(DynaCirc CR 5). Lt. pink. Film-coated. In 30s and 100s.
		10 mg	(DynaCirc CR 10). Beige. Film-coated. In 30s and 100s.
Rx	**DynaCirc** (Reliant)	**Capsules:** 2.5 mg[1]	Lactose. (DynaCirc 2.5). White. In 60s and 100s.
		5 mg[1]	Lactose. (DynaCirc 5). Lt. pink. In 60s and 100s.

[1] May contain benzyl alcohol and parabens.

ISRADIPINE — ORAL

For complete and comparative prescribing information, refer to the Calcium Channel Blockers group monograph.

Indications

➤*Hypertension:* Management of hypertension. It may be used alone or concurrently with thiazide-type diuretics.

Administration and Dosage

➤*Approved by the FDA:* December 1990.

➤*Controlled-release tablets:* The dosage of isradipine controlled-release tablets should be individualized. The recommended initial dose of isradipine is 5 mg once-daily as monotherapy or in combination with a thiazide diuretic. An antihypertensive response usually occurs within 2 hours, with the peak antihypertensive response occurring 8 to 10 hours post-dose; blood pressure reduction is maintained for at least 24 hours following drug administration. If necessary, the dose may be adjusted in increments of 5 mg at 2- to 4-week intervals up to a maximum dose of 20 mg/day. Adverse experiences are increased in frequency above 10 mg/day.

Isradipine controlled-release tablets should be swallowed whole and should not be bitten or divided.

Elderly/hepatic/renal function impairment – The bioavailability (increased AUC) of immediate-release isradipine is increased in elderly patients (above 65 years of age), patients with hepatic functional impairment, and patients with mild renal impairment. Ordinarily, a starting dose of isradipine 5 mg once daily should be used in these patients.

➤*Capsules:* The dosage of isradipine should be individualized. The recommended initial dose of isradipine is 2.5 mg twice a day alone or in combination with a thiazide diuretic. An antihypertensive response usually occurs within 2 to 3 hours. Maximal response may require 2 to 4 weeks. If a satisfactory reduction in blood pressure does not occur after this period, the dose may be adjusted in increments of 5 mg/day at 2- to 4-week intervals up to a maximum of 20 mg/day. Most patients, however, show no additional response to doses above 10 mg/day, and adverse effects are increased in frequency above 10 mg/day.

Elderly/hepatic/renal function impairment – The bioavailability of isradipine (increased AUC) is increased in elderly patients (above 65 years of age), patients with hepatic functional impairment, and patients with mild renal impairment. Ordinarily, the starting dose should still be 2.5 mg twice a day in these patients.

➤*Storage/Stability:* Below 30°C (86°F) in a tight container, protected from moisture, humidity, and light.

NIMODIPINE

Rx	**Nimotop** (Bayer)	**Capsules, liquid-filled:** 30 mg	(NIMOTOP). Ivory. In UD 30s and 100s.

NIMODIPINE — ORAL

For complete and comparative prescribing information, refer to the Calcium Channel Blockers group monograph.

WARNING

Do not administer nimodipine IV or by other parenteral routes. Deaths and serious, life-threatening adverse reactions have occurred when the contents of nimodipine capsules have been injected parenterally.

Indications

Nimodipine is indicated for the improvement of neurological outcome by reducing the incidence and severity of ischemic deficits in patients with subarachnoid hemorrhage from ruptured intracranial berry aneurysms regardless of their postictus neurological condition (ie, Hunt and Hess Grades I to V).

Administration and Dosage

➤*Approved by the FDA:* December, 1988.

Nimodipine is given orally in the form of ivory-colored, soft gelatin 30 mg capsules for subarachnoid hemorrhage.

The oral dose is 60 mg (two 30 mg capsules) every 4 hours for 21 consecutive days, preferably not less than 1 hour before or 2 hours after meals. Oral nimodipine therapy should commence within 96 hours of the subarachnoid hemorrhage.

If the capsule cannot be swallowed (eg, at the time of surgery, or if the patient is unconscious) a hole should be made in both ends of the capsule with an 18-gauge needle, and the contents of the capsule extracted into a syringe. The contents should then be emptied into the patient's in situ nasogastric tube and washed down the tube with 30 mL of normal saline (0.9%).

The contents of nimodipine capsules must not be administered by IV injection or other parenteral routes.

➤*Hepatic function impairment:* Patients with hepatic cirrhosis have substantially reduced clearance and approximately doubled C_{max}. Dosage should be reduced to 30 mg every 4 hours, with close monitoring of blood pressure and heart rate.

➤*Storage/Stability:* Store the capsules in the manufacturer's original foil package at 25°C (77°F); excursions are permitted to 15° to 30°C (59° to 86°F). Capsules should be protected from light and freezing.

FELODIPINE

Rx	**Plendil** (AstraZeneca)	**Tablets, extended release:** 2.5 mg	Lactose. (PLENDIL 450). Sage green. In 30s, 100s, and UD 100s.
		5 mg	Lactose. (PLENDIL 451). Lt. red-brown. In 30s, 100s, and UD 100s.
		10 mg	Lactose. (PLENDIL 452). Red-brown. In 30s, 100s, and UD 100s.

FELODIPINE — ORAL

For complete and comparative prescribing information, refer to the Calcium Channel Blockers group monograph.

Indications

➤*Hypertension:* For the treatment of hypertension. Felodipine may be used alone or concomitantly with other antihypertensive agents.

Administration and Dosage

➤*Approved by the FDA:* August 1991.

➤*Dosage:* The recommended starting dose is 5 mg once daily. Depending on the patient's response, the dosage can be decreased to 2.5 mg or increased to 10 mg once daily. These adjustments generally should occur at intervals of not less than 2 weeks. The recommended dosage range is 2.5 to 10 mg once daily. In clinical trials, doses above 10 mg daily increased blood pressure (BP) response but a large increase in the rate of peripheral edema and other vasodilatory adverse events. Modification of the recommended dosage usually is not required in renal impairment.

Take without food or with a light meal. Swallow whole; do not crush or chew.

➤*Elderly:* Patients over 65 years are likely to develop higher plasma felodipine concentrations. In general, dose selection for an elderly patient should be cautious, usually starting at the low end of the dosing range (2.5 mg daily). Closely monitor BP during dosage adjustment.

➤*Hepatic function impairment:* Patients with impaired liver function may have elevated plasma drug concentrations and may respond to lower doses; closely monitor BP during dosage adjustment of felodipine.

➤*Storage/Stability:* Store below 30°C (86°F). Keep container tightly closed. Protect from light.

AMLODIPINE

Rx	**Norvasc** (Pfizer)	**Tablets**: 2.5 mg	(NORVASC 2.5). White, diamond shape. In 90s and 100s.
Rx	**Amvaz** (Reddy)		(R 176). Off-white. In 90s and 500s.
Rx	**Norvasc** (Pfizer)	**Tablets**: 5 mg	(NORVASC 5). White, elongated octagon. In 90s, 100s, 300s, and UD 100s.
Rx	**Amvaz** (Reddy)		(R 177). White to off-white. In 90s, 500s, and UD 7s.
Rx	**Norvasc** (Pfizer)	**Tablets**: 10 mg	(NORVASC 10). White. In 90s, 100s, and UD 100s.
Rx	**Amvaz** (Reddy)		(R 178). White to off-white, oval. In 90s, 500s, and UD 7s.

AMLODIPINE BESYLATE — ORAL

For complete and comparative prescribing information, refer to the Calcium Channel Blockers group monograph.

Indications

➤*Hypertension:* For the treatment of hypertension. It may be used alone or in combination with other antihypertensive agents.

➤*Chronic stable angina:* For the treatment of chronic stable angina. Amlodipine may be used alone or in combination with other antianginal agents.

➤*Vasospastic angina (Prinzmetal's or variant angina):* For the treatment of confirmed or suspected vasospastic angina. Amlodipine may be used as monotherapy or in combination with other antianginal drugs.

Administration and Dosage

➤*Approved by the FDA:* July 31, 1992.

➤*Hypertension:* The usual initial antihypertensive oral dose of amlodipine is 5 mg once daily with a maximum dose of 10 mg once daily. Small, fragile, or elderly individuals, or patients with hepatic insufficiency may be started on 2.5 mg once daily, and this dose may be used when adding amlodipine to other antihypertensive therapy.

Dosage should be adjusted according to each patient's need. In general, titration should proceed over 7 to 14 days so that the physician can fully assess the patient's response to each dose level. Titration may proceed more rapidly, however, if clinically warranted, provided the patient is assessed frequently.

➤*Chronic stable or vasospastic angina:* The recommended dose for chronic stable or vasospastic angina is 5 to 10 mg, with the lower dose suggested in the elderly and in patients with hepatic insufficiency. Most patients will require 10 mg for adequate effect.

➤*Storage/Stability:* Store bottles at controlled room temperature, 15° to 30°C (59° to 86°F) and dispense in tight, light-resistant containers.

DILTIAZEM HYDROCHLORIDE

Rx	**Diltiazem HCl** (Various, eg, Mylan, Teva)	**Tablets**: 30 mg	May contain lactose or methylparaben. In 100s, 500s, and 1000s.
Rx	**Cardizem** (Biovail)		Lactose, methylparaben. (MARION 1771). Green. In 100s, 500s and UD 100s.
Rx	**Diltiazem HCl** (Various, eg, Mylan, Teva, Watson)	**Tablets**: 60 mg	May contain lactose or methylparaben. In 100s, 500s, and 1000s.
Rx	**Cardizem** (Biovail)		Lactose, methylparaben. (MARION 17 72). Yellow, scored. In 100s, 500s, and UD 100s.
Rx	**Diltiazem HCl** (Various, eg, Mylan, Teva, Watson)	**Tablets**: 90 mg	May contain lactose or methylparaben. In 100s, 500s, and 1000s.
Rx	**Cardizem** (Biovail)		Lactose, methylparaben. (CARDIZEM 90 mg). Green, scored. In 100s and UD 100s.
Rx	**Diltiazem HCl** (Various, eg, Mylan, Teva, Watson)	**Tablets**: 120 mg	May contain lactose or methylparaben. In 100s, 500s, and 1000s.
Rx	**Cardizem** (Biovail)		Lactose, methylparaben. (CARDIZEM 120 mg). Yellow, scored. In 100s and UD 100s.
Rx	**Cardizem LA** (Biovail)	**Tablets, extended-release:** 120 mg	Sucrose. (B 120 mg). White, capsule-shaped. In 7s, 30s, 90s, and 1000s.
		180 mg	Sucrose. (B 180 mg). White, capsule-shaped. In 7s, 30s, 90s, and 1000s.
		240 mg	Sucrose. (B 240 mg). White, capsule-shaped. In 7s, 30s, 90s, and 1000s.
		300 mg	Sucrose. (B 300 mg). White, capsule-shaped. In 7s, 30s, 90s, and 1000s.
		360 mg	Sucrose. (B 360 mg). White, capsule-shaped. In 7s, 30s, 90s, and 1000s.
		420 mg	Sucrose. (B 420 mg). White, capsule-shaped. In 7s, 30s, 90s, and 1000s.
Rx	**Diltiazem HCl Extended Release** (Various, eg, Mylan, Teva)	**Capsules, extended-release:**[a] 60 mg	May contain sucrose or sugar spheres. In 100s.
Rx	**Diltiazem HCl Extended Release** (Various, eg, Mylan, Teva)	**Capsules, extended-release:**[a] 90 mg	May contain sucrose or sugar spheres. In 100s.
Rx	**Diltiazem HCl Extended Release** (Various, eg, Mylan, Purepac, Teva)	**Capsules, extended-release:**[a] 120 mg	May contain sucrose or sugar spheres. In 30s, 90s, 100s, 500s, and 1000s.
Rx	**Cardizem CD** (Biovail)		Sucrose. (cardizem CD 120 mg). Lt. turquoise blue. In 30s, 90s, and UD 100s.
Rx	**Cartia XT** (Andrx)		Sucrose. (Andrx 597 120 mg). White/Orange. In 30s, 90s, 500s, and 1000s.
Rx	**Dilacor XR** (Watson)		(A Dilacor XR 120 mg). Pink/Flesh. In 100s and 500s.
Rx	**Dilt-XR** (Apotex)		(APO 014). Orange opaque/white. In 100s.
Rx	**Diltia XT** (Andrx)		Lactose. (Andrx 548 120 mg). White. In 100s, 500s, and 1000s.
Rx	**Taztia XT** (Andrx)		(ANDRX 696 120 mg). Pink. In 30s and 90s.
Rx	**Tiazac** (Forest)		Sucrose. (Tiazac 120). Lavender. In 7s, 30s, 90s, and 1000s.

DILTIAZEM HYDROCHLORIDE

Rx	**Diltiazem HCl Extended Release** (Various, eg, Purepac, Teva)	**Capsules, extended-release:**[a] 180 mg	May contain sucrose or sugar spheres. In 30s, 90s, 100s, 500s, and 1000s.
Rx	**Cardizem CD** (Biovail)		Sucrose. (cardizem CD 180 mg). Lt. turquoise blue/Blue. In 30s, 90s, and UD 100s.
Rx	**Cartia XT** (Andrx)		Sucrose. (Andrx 598 180 mg). Yellow/Orange. In 30s, 90s, 500s, and 1000s.
Rx	**Dilacor XR** (Watson)		(A Dilacor XR 180 mg). Lavender/Flesh. In 100s and 500s.
Rx	**Dilt-XR** (Apotex)		(APO 015). Bright orange opaque/white. In 100s.
Rx	**Diltia XT** (Andrx)		Lactose. (Andrx 549 180 mg). Gray/White. In 100s, 500s, and 1000s.
Rx	**Taztia XT** (Andrx)		(ANDRX 697 180 mg). Lt. blue/Buff. In 30s and 90s.
Rx	**Tiazac** (Forest)		Sucrose. (Tiazac 180). White/Blue-green. In 7s, 30s, 90s, and 1000s.
Rx	**Diltiazem HCl Extended Release** (Various, eg, Purepac, Teva)	**Capsules, extended-release:**[a] 240 mg	May contain sucrose or sugar spheres. In 30s, 90s, 100s, 500s, and 1000s.
Rx	**Cardizem CD** (Biovail)		Sucrose. (cardizem CD 240 mg). Blue. In 30s, 90s, and UD 100s.
Rx	**Cartia XT** (Andrx)		Sucrose. (Andrx 599 240 mg). Lt. brown/Orange. In 30s, 90s, 500s, and 1000s.
Rx	**Dilacor XR** (Watson)		(A Dilacor XR 240 mg). Lt. blue/Flesh. In 100s and 500s.
Rx	**Dilt-XR** (Apotex)		(APO 016). Brown opaque/white. In 100s.
Rx	**Diltia XT** (Andrx)		Lactose. (Andrx 550 240 mg). Gray. In 100s, 500s, and 1000s.
Rx	**Taztia XT** (Andrx)		(ANDRX 698 240 mg). Pink/Lt. blue. In 30s and 90s.
Rx	**Tiazac** (Forest)		Sucrose. (Tiazac 240). Blue-green/Lavender. In 7s, 30s, 90s, and 1000s.
Rx	**Diltiazem HCl Extended Release** (Various, eg, Purepac, Teva)	**Capsules, extended-release:**[a] 300 mg	May contain sucrose or sugar spheres. In 30s, 90s, 500s, and 1000s.
Rx	**Cardizem CD** (Biovail)		Sucrose. (cardizem CD 300 mg). Lt. gray/Blue. In 30s, 90s, and UD 100s.
Rx	**Cartia XT** (Andrx)		Sucrose. (Andrx 600 300 mg). Orange. In 30s, 90s, 500s, and 1000s.
Rx	**Taztia XT** (Andrx)		(ANDRX 699 300 mg). Pink/Buff. In 30s and 90s.
Rx	**Tiazac** (Forest)		Sucrose. (Tiazac 300). White/Lavender. In 7s, 30s, 90s, and 1000s.
Rx	**Diltiazem HCl** (Various, eg, Inwood)	**Capsules, extended-release:**[a] 360 mg	In 90s.
Rx	**Cardizem CD** (Biovail)		Sucrose. (cardizem CD 360 mg). Lt. blue/White. In 90s.
Rx	**Taztia XT** (Andrx)		(ANDRX 700 360 mg). Lt. blue. In 30s and 90s.
Rx	**Tiazac** (Forest)		Sucrose. (Tiazac 360). Blue-green. In 7s, 30s, 90s, and 1000s.
Rx	**Tiazac** (Forest)	**Capsules, extended-release:**[a] 420 mg	Sucrose. (Tiazac 420). White. In 7s, 30s, 90s, and 1000s.
Rx	**Diltiazem HCl** (Various, eg, Apotex, Baxter, Bedford, Bertek)	**Injection:** 5 mg/mL	In 5, 10, and 25 mL vials.
Rx	**Cardizem** (Biovail)		In 5 and 10 mL single-use vials.
Rx	**Cardizem** (Biovail)	**Powder for injection:** 25 mg	Single-use containers. Carton of 6 *Lyo-Ject* syringes with diluent.

[a] Note: The terms "extended-release" and "sustained-release" sometimes are used interchangeably.

DILTIAZEM HYDROCHLORIDE — ORAL

For complete and comparative prescribing information, refer to the Calcium Channel Blockers group monograph.

Indications

➤*Extended-release capsules and tablets:* For the treatment of hypertension. It may be used alone or in combination with other antihypertensive medications.

➤*Extended-release capsules and immediate-release tablets:* For the management of chronic stable angina and angina due to coronary artery spasm.

➤*Extended-release tablets:* For the management of chronic stable angina.

➤*Unlabeled uses:* Used topically (2% gel, cream, or ointment) in treatment of anal fissures (reduction of pain and bleeding, promotion of healing).

Administration and Dosage

➤*Approved by the FDA:* 1982.

➤*Extended-release capsules and tablets:* Patients controlled on diltiazem alone or in combination with other medications may be switched to diltiazem extended-release capsules or tablets at the nearest equivalent total daily dose. Higher doses of extended-release diltiazem may be needed in some patients. Closely monitor patients. Subsequent titration to higher or lower doses may be necessary and should be initiated as clinically warranted. There is limited general clinical experience with doses above 360 mg, but the safety and efficacy of doses as high as 540 mg have been studied in clinical trials. The incidence of adverse reactions increases as the dose increases with first-degree atrioventricular (AV) block, dizziness, and sinus bradycardia bearing the strongest relationship to dose.

Hypertension – Dosage needs to be adjusted by titration to individual patient needs. When used as monotherapy, reasonable starting doses are 180 to 240 mg once daily, although some patients may respond to lower doses. Maximum antihypertensive effect is usually observed by 14 days of chronic therapy; therefore, schedule dosage adjustments accordingly. The dosage range for extended-release tablets studied in clinical trials was 120 to 540 mg once daily. Individual patients may respond to higher doses of extended-release capsules up to 480 mg once daily. For the extended-release tablets, the dosage may be titrated to a maximum of 540 mg daily.

Extended-release tablets: Diltiazem extended-release tablets are intended for once-daily administration. The tablets should be swallowed whole and not chewed or crushed.

Diltiazem extended-release tablets should be taken about the same time once each day either in the morning or at bedtime. Consider the time of dosing when making dose adjustments based on trough effects.

Angina –

Extended-release capsules: Adjust dosages for the treatment of angina to each patient's needs, starting with a dose of 120 or 180 mg once daily. Individual patients may respond to higher doses of up to 480 mg once daily. When necessary, titration may be carried out over a 7- to 14-day period.

Extended-release tablets: Individualize dosage for treatment of angina based on response. The initial dose of 180 mg once daily may be increased at intervals of 7 to 14 days if adequate response is not obtained. Extended-release tablet doses above 360 mg appear to confer no additional benefit.

Diltiazem extended-release tablets can be given once daily, either in the evening or in the morning. The tablets should be swallowed whole and not chewed or crushed.

➤*Exertional angina pectoris due to atherosclerotic coronary artery disease or angina pectoris at rest due to coronary artery spasm:*

Immediate-release tablets – Dosage must be adjusted to each patient's needs. Starting with 30 mg 4 times daily, before meals and at bedtime, dosage should be increased gradually (given in divided doses 3 or 4 times daily) at 1- to 2-day intervals until optimum response is obtained. Although individual patients may respond to any dosage level, the average optimum dosage range appears to be 180 to 360 mg/day. There are no available data concerning dosage requirements in patients with impaired renal or hepatic function. If the drug must be used in such patients, titrate with particular caution.

➤*Concomitant use with other cardiovascular agents:*

Sublingual nitroglycerin – May be taken as required to abort acute anginal attacks during diltiazem therapy.

Prophylactic nitrate therapy – Diltiazem may be safely coadministered with short- and long-acting nitrates.

Beta-blockers – Controlled and uncontrolled domestic studies suggest that concomitant use of diltiazem and beta-blockers is usually well tolerated, but

DILTIAZEM HYDROCHLORIDE — ORAL

available data are not sufficient to predict the effects of concomitant treatment in patients with left ventricular dysfunction or cardiac conduction abnormalities.

Administration of diltiazem concomitantly with propranolol in 5 healthy volunteers resulted in increased propranolol levels in all subjects and bioavailability of propranolol was increased approximately 50%. In vitro, propranolol appears to be displaced from its binding sites by diltiazem. If combination therapy is initiated or withdrawn in conjunction with propranolol, an adjustment in the propranolol dose may be warranted.

Antihypertensives –

Extended-release formulations: Diltiazem has an additive antihypertensive effect when used with other antihypertensive agents. Therefore, the dosage of diltiazem or the concomitant antihypertensives may need to be adjusted when adding one to the other.

➤*Tiazac*: Hypertensive or anginal patients who are treated with other formulations of diltiazem can safely be switched to *Tiazac* capsules at the nearest equivalent total daily dose. Subsequent titration to higher or lower doses may, however, be necessary and should be initiated as clinically indicated.

Sprinkling the capsule contents on food – *Tiazac* extended-release capsules may also be administered by carefully opening the capsule and sprinkling the capsule contents on a spoonful of applesauce. The applesauce should be swallowed immediately without chewing and followed with a glass of cool water to ensure complete swallowing of the capsule contents. The applesauce should not be hot, and it should be soft enough to be swallowed without chewing. Use any capsule contents/applesauce mixture immediately and do not store for future use. Subdividing the contents of the extended-release capsule is not recommended.

➤*Storage/Stability:* Dispense in a tight, light-resistant container. Store at 25°C (77°F); excursions permitted to 15° to 30°C (59° to 86°F). Avoid excessive humidity and temperatures above 30°C (86°F).

DILTIAZEM HYDROCHLORIDE — INJECTION

For complete and comparative prescribing information, refer to the Calcium Channel Blockers group monograph.

Indications

➤*Atrial fibrillation or atrial flutter:* Temporary control of rapid ventricular rate in atrial fibrillation or atrial flutter. It should not be used in patients with atrial fibrillation or atrial flutter associated with an accessory bypass tract such as in Wolff-Parkinson-White (WPW) syndrome or short PR syndrome.

In addition, diltiazem single-use solution for injection or diltiazem single-use syringe are indicated for the following:

➤*Paroxysmal supraventricular tachycardia:* Rapid conversion of paroxysmal supraventricular tachycardias (PSVTs) to sinus rhythm. This includes AV nodal reentrant tachycardias and reciprocating tachycardias associated with an extranodal accessory pathway such as the WPW syndrome or short PR syndrome. Unless otherwise contraindicated, appropriate vagal maneuvers should be attempted prior to administration of diltiazem single-use solution for injection or diltiazem single-use syringe.

The use of diltiazem single-use syringe, diltiazem single-use solution, or diltiazem powder for reconstitution should be undertaken with caution when the patient is compromised hemodynamically or is taking other drugs that decrease any or all of the following: Peripheral resistance, myocardial filling, myocardial contractility, or electrical impulse propagation in the myocardium.

Administration and Dosage

➤*Approved by the FDA:* 1982.

➤*Direct IV single injections (bolus):* The initial dose of diltiazem single-use solution for injection or diltiazem single-use syringe should be 0.25 mg/kg actual body weight as a bolus administered over 2 minutes (20 mg is a reasonable dose for the average patient). If response is inadequate, a second dose may be administered after 15 minutes. The second bolus dose of diltiazem single-use solution for injection or diltiazem single-use syringe should be 0.35 mg/kg actual body weight administered over 2 minutes (25 mg is a reasonable dose for the average patient). Subsequent IV bolus doses should be individualized for each patient. Patients with low body weights should be dosed on a mg/kg basis. Some patients may respond to an initial dose of 0.15 mg/kg, although duration of action may be shorter. Experience with this dose is limited.

➤*Continuous IV infusion:* Mix thoroughly. Use within 24 hours. Keep refrigerated until use. For continued reduction of the heart rate (up to 24 hours) in patients with atrial fibrillation or atrial flutter, an IV infusion of diltiazem single-use solution for injection, diltiazem single-use syringe, or diltiazem powder for reconstitution may be administered. (For reconstitution of diltiazem single-use syringe or diltiazem powder for reconstitution, see instructions contained within packaging.) Immediately following bolus administration of 20 mg (0.25 mg/kg) or 25 mg (0.35 mg/kg) diltiazem single-use solution for injection or diltiazem single-use syringe, and reduction of heart rate, begin an IV infusion of diltiazem single-use solution for injection, diltiazem single-use syringe, or diltiazem powder for reconstitution. The recommended initial infusion rate of diltiazem single-use solution for injection, diltiazem single-use syringe, or diltiazem powder for reconstitution is 10 mg/h. Some patients may maintain response to an initial rate of 5 mg/h. The infusion rate may be increased in 5 mg/h increments up to 15 mg/h as needed, if further reduction in heart rate is required. The infusion may be maintained for up to 24 hours.

Diltiazem shows dose-dependent, nonlinear pharmacokinetics. Duration of infusion longer than 24 hours and infusion rates greater than 15 mg/h have not been studied. Therefore, infusion duration exceeding 24 hours and infusion rates exceeding 15 mg/h are not recommended.

Dilution –

Preparation: To prepare diltiazem single-use solution for injection, diltiazem single-use syringe, or diltiazem powder for reconstitution for continuous IV infusion, aseptically transfer the appropriate quantity (see paragraphs below) of diltiazem to the desired volume of either Normal Saline, D5W, or D5W/0.45% NaCl. Mix thoroughly. Keep diluted diltiazem single-use solution for injection refrigerated until use. Diluted diltiazem single-use syringe and diltiazem powder for reconstitution may be stored at room temperature 15° to 30°C (59° to 86°F). Use within 24 hours. Keep refrigerated until use.

Diluent volume	Quantity of diltiazem injection to add	Final concentration	Administration dose*	Infusion rate
100 mL	125 mg (25 mL)	1 mg/mL	10 mg/h	10 mL/h
			15 mg/h	15 mL/h
250 mL	250 mg (50 mL)	0.83 mg/mL	10 mg/h	12 mL/h
			15 mg/h	18 mL/h
500 mL	250 mg (50 mL)	0.45 mg/mL	10 mg/h	22 mL/h
			15 mg/h	33 mL/h

* 5 mg/h may be appropriate for some patients.

Compatibility – Diltiazem single-use solution for injection, diltiazem single-use syringe, and diltiazem powder for reconstitution were tested for compatibility with 3 commonly used IV fluids at a maximal concentration of 1 mg diltiazem per milliliter. Diltiazem single-use solution for injection, diltiazem single-use syringe, and diltiazem powder for reconstitution were found to be physically compatible and chemically stable in the following parenteral solutions for at least 24 hours when stored in glass (diltiazem single-use solution for injection/diltiazem single-use syringe only) or polyvinylchloride (PVC) bags at controlled room temperature 15° to 30°C (59° to 86°F) or under refrigeration 2° to 8°C (36° to 46°F).

1.) Dextrose (5%) injection.
2.) Sodium chloride (0.9%) injection.
3.) Dextrose (5%) and sodium chloride (0.45%) injection.

Physical incompatibilities – Because of potential physical incompatibilities, it is recommended that diltiazem single-use solution for injection, diltiazem single-use syringe, or diltiazem powder for reconstitution not be mixed with any other drugs in the same container. If possible, it is recommended that diltiazem single-use solution for injection, diltiazem single-use syringe, or diltiazem powder for reconstitution not be coinfused in the same IV line. Parenteral drug products should be inspected visually for particulate matter and discoloration prior to administration whenever solution and container permit.

➤*Diltiazem single-use solution for injection/diltiazem single-use syringe:* Physical incompatibilities (precipitate formation or cloudiness) were observed when diltiazem single-use solution for injection or diltiazem single-use syringe was infused in the same IV line with the following drugs: Acetazolamide, acyclovir, aminophylline, ampicillin, ampicillin sodium/sulbactam sodium, cefamandole, cefoperazone, diazepam, furosemide, hydrocortisone sodium succinate, insulin, (regular: 100 U/mL), methylprednisolone sodium succinate, mezlocillin, nafcillin, phenytoin, rifampin, and sodium bicarbonate.

Diltiazem single-use syringe was found to be compatible with insulin (regular, 100 units/mL).

➤*Diltiazem powder for reconstitution:* Physical incompatibilities (precipitate formation or cloudiness) were observed when diltiazem powder for reconstitution at a concentration of 1 mg/mL diluted in normal saline was infused in the same IV line with the following drugs: Acetazolamide, acyclovir, cefoperazone sodium, diazepam, furosemide, phenytoin, and rifampin.

Diltiazem powder for reconstitution at a concentration of 1 mg/mL diluted in normal saline was infused in the same IV line and was found to be compatible with the following drugs: aminophylline, ampicillin sodium, ampicillin sodium/sulbactam sodium, cefamandole, hydrocortisone sodium succinate, regular insulin (100 units/mL), methylprednisolone sodium succinate, mezlocillin sodium, nafcillin sodium, and sodium bicarbonate.

➤*Transition to further antiarrhythmic therapy:* Transition to other antiarrhythmic agents following administration of diltiazem single-use solution for injection is generally safe. However, reference should be made to the respective agent manufacturer's package insert for information relative to dosage and administration.

In controlled clinical trials, therapy with antiarrhythmic agents to maintain reduced heart rate in atrial fibrillation or atrial flutter or for prophylaxis of PSVT was generally started within 3 hours after bolus administration of diltiazem single-use solution for injection. These antiarrhythmic agents were IV or oral digoxin, class 1 antiarrhythmics (eg, quinidine, procainamide), calcium channel blockers, and oral beta-blockers.

DILTIAZEM HYDROCHLORIDE — INJECTION

Experience in the use of antiarrhythmic agents following maintenance infusion of diltiazem single-use solution for injection is limited. Patients should be dosed on an individual basis and reference should be made to the respective manufacturer's monograph for information relative to dosage and administration.

➤*Storage/Stability:*

Diltiazem single-use solution for injection – Store product under refrigeration 2° to 8°C (36° to 46°F). Do not freeze. May be stored at room temperature for up to 1 month. Destroy after 1 month at room temperature. Single-use containers. Discard unused portion.

Diltiazem single-use syringe – Product is to be stored at room temperature 15° to 30°C (59° to 86°F). Do not freeze. Reconstituted material is stable for 24 hours at controlled room temperature. Single-use containers. Discard unused portion.

Diltiazem powder for reconstitution – Product is to be stored at room temperature 15° to 30°C (59° to 86°F). Do not freeze. Reconstituted material is stable for 24 hours at controlled room temperature. Single-use vial.

VERAPAMIL HYDROCHLORIDE

Rx	**Verapamil Hydrochloride** (Various, eg, Geneva, Major, Watson)	**Tablets:** 40 mg	May contain lactose. In 30s, 100s, 500s, and 1000s.
Rx	**Calan** (Searle)		Lactose. (CALAN 40). Pink. Film-coated. In 100s.
Rx	**Verapamil Hydrochloride** (Various, eg, Geneva, Ivax, Major, Mylan, Watson)	**Tablets:** 80 mg	May contain lactose. In 100s, 250s, 500s, 1000s, 7000s, and UD 100s.
Rx	**Calan** (Searle)		Lactose. (CALAN 80). Peach, oval, scored. Film-coated. In 100s, 500s, and 1000s.
Rx	**Verapamil Hydrochloride** (Various, eg, Geneva, Ivax, Major, Mylan, Watson)	**Tablets:** 120 mg	May contain lactose. In 100s, 250s, 500s, 1000s, 4000s, and UD 100s.
Rx	**Calan** (Searle)		Lactose. (CALAN 120). Brown, oval, scored. Film-coated. In 100s and 1000s.
Rx	**Verapamil Hydrochloride Extended Release** (Various, eg, Ivax, Mylan)	**Tablets, extended-release:**[1] 120 mg	In 100s.
Rx	**Verapamil Hydrochloride Extended Release** (Various, eg, Ivax, Mylan)	**Tablets, extended-release:**[1] 180 mg	In 100s and 500s.
Rx	**Covera-HS** (Searle)		(COVERA-HS 2011). Lavender. Film coated. In 100s and UD 100s.
Rx	**Verapamil Hydrochloride Extended Release** (Various, eg, Ivax, Mylan)	**Tablets, extended-release:**[1] 240 mg	In 100s and 500s.
Rx	**Covera-HS** (Searle)		(COVERA-HS 2021). Pale yellow. Film-coated. In 100s and UD 100s.
Rx	**Calan SR** (Searle)	**Tablets, sustained-release:**[1] 120 mg	(CALAN SR 120). Lt. violet, oval. Film-coated. In 100s and UD 100s.
Rx	**Isoptin SR** (Abbott)		(KNOLL 120 SR). Lt. violet, oval. Film-coated. In 100s.
Rx	**Calan SR** (Searle)	**Tablets, sustained-release:**[1] 180 mg	(CALAN SR 180). Lt. pink, oval, scored. Film-coated. In 100s and UD 100s.
Rx	**Isoptin SR** (Abbott)		(ISOPTIN SR 180 MG). Lt. pink, oval, scored. Film-coated. In 100s.
Rx	**Calan SR** (Searle)	**Tablets, sustained-release:**[1] 240 mg	(CALAN SR 240). Lt. green, capsule shape, scored. Film-coated. In 100s, 500s, and UD 100s.
Rx	**Isoptin SR** (Abbott)		(ISOPTIN SR). Lt. green, capsule shape, scored. Film-coated. In 100s and 500s.
Rx	**Verapamil Hydrochloride Extended Release** (Various, eg, Mylan, Teva, UDL)	**Capsules, extended-release:**[1] 120 mg	May be pellet-filled. May contain sugar. In 100s, 500s, and UD 100s.
		180 mg	May be pellet-filled. May contain sugar. In 100s, 500s, and UD 100s.
		240 mg	May be pellet-filled. May contain sugar. In 100s, 500s, and UD 80s.
Rx	**Verelan PM** (Schwarz Pharma)	**Capsules, extended-release:**[1] 100 mg	Sugar. (SCHWARZ 4085/100 mg). White/Amethyst. In 100s.
		200 mg	Sugar. (SCHWARz 4086 200 mg). Amethyst. In 100s.
		300 mg	Sugar. (SCHWARz 4087 300 mg). Lavender/Amethyst. In 100s.
Rx	**Verelan** (Schwarz Pharma)	**Capsules, sustained-release:**[1] 120 mg	Pellet-filled. Sugar, parabens. (SCHWARZ 2490 VERELAN 120 mg). Yellow. In 100s.
		180 mg	Pellet-filled. Sugar, parabens. (SCHWARZ 2489 VERELAN 180 mg). Lt. gray/yellow. In 100s.
		240 mg	Pellet-filled. Sugar, parabens. (SCHWARz 2491 VERELAN 240 mg). Dk. blue/yellow. In 100s.
		360 mg	Pellet-filled. Sugar, parabens. (SCHWARz 2495 VERELAN 360 mg). Lavender/Yellow. In 100s.
Rx	**Verapamil Hydrochloride** (Various, eg, American Regent, Hospira)	**Injection:** 2.5 mg/mL	May contain sodium chloride. In 2 and 4 mL vials, amps, and syringes. Also in 2 mL fill in single-use, 2 mL *Carpuject* syringe; and 2 mL fill in single-use 2 mL *Carpuject Interlink* syringe.

[1] Note: The terms "extended-release" and "sustained-release" sometimes are used interchangeably.

VERAPAMIL HYDROCHLORIDE — ORAL

For complete and comparative prescribing information, refer to the Calcium Channel Blockers group monograph.

Indications

➤*Immediate-release:*

Angina – Treatment of vasospastic (Prinzmetal's variant), chronic stable (classic effort-associated) and unstable (crescendo, preinfarction) angina.

Arrhythmias – With digitalis to control ventricular rate at rest and during stress in chronic atrial flutter or fibrillation. May use for prophylaxis of repetitive paroxysmal supraventricular tachycardia (PSVT).

Hypertension – Treatment of essential hypertension.

➤*Sustained-release/Extended-release:* For management of hypertension and angina (*Covera-HS* only).

Administration and Dosage

➤*Approved by the FDA:* March 8, 1982.

Avoid verapamil in patients with severe left ventricular dysfunction (eg, ejection fractions less than 30%) or moderate to severe symptoms of cardiac failure and in patients with any degree of ventricular dysfunction if they are receiving a beta-adrenergic blocker. If possible, control patients with milder ventricular dysfunction with optimum doses of digitalis or diuretics before verapamil treatment.

Individualize dosage. Do not exceed 480 mg/day; safety and efficacy are not established. Half-life increases during chronic use; maximum response may be delayed.

➤*Immediate-release:*

Angina – Usual dose is 80 to 120 mg 3 times/day. However, 40 mg 3 times a day may be warranted in patients who have increased response to verapamil (eg, decreased hepatic function, elderly). Base upward titration on safety and efficacy evaluated approximately 8 hours after dosing. Dosage may be increased daily (eg, unstable angina) or weekly until optimum clinical response is obtained.

VERAPAMIL HYDROCHLORIDE — ORAL

Arrhythmias – Dosage range in digitalized patients with chronic atrial fibrillation is 240 to 320 mg/day in divided doses 3 or 4 times/day. Dosage range for prophylaxis of PSVT (nondigitalized patients) is 240 to 480 mg/day in divided doses 3 or 4 times/day. Maximum effects will be apparent during the first 48 hours of therapy.

Hypertension – The usual initial monotherapy dose is 80 mg 3 times/day (240 mg/day). Daily dosages of 360 and 480 mg have been used, but there is no evidence that dosages beyond 360 mg provide added effect. Consider beginning titration at 40 mg 3 times/day in patients who might respond to lower doses (eg, elderly people or those of small stature). Antihypertensive effects are evident within the first week of therapy. Base upward titration on therapeutic efficacy, assessed at the end of the dosing interval.

➤*Extended-release:* Individualize the dose by titration. When administered at bedtime, office evaluation of blood pressure (BP) during morning and early afternoon hours is essentially a measure of peak effect. The usual evaluation of trough effect, which sometimes might be needed to evaluate the appropriateness of any given dose, would be just prior to bedtime. Swallow whole; do not chew, break, or crush the tablets.

Capsules – The usual daily dose is 240 mg once daily in the morning. However, initial doses of 120 mg/day may be warranted in patients who may have an increased response to verapamil (eg, elderly people, those of small stature). Base upward titration on therapeutic efficacy and safety evaluated approximately 24 hours after dosing. The antihypertensive effects of extended-release verapamil are evident within the first week of therapy.

If adequate response is not obtained with 120 mg verapamil, the dose may be titrated upward in the following manner:

180 mg in the morning,
240 mg in the morning,
360 mg in the morning,
480 mg in the morning.

Tablets – Initiate therapy with 180 mg given in the morning. Lower initial doses of 120 mg/day may be warranted in patients who may have an increased response to verapamil (eg, elderly people or those of small stature). Base upward titration on therapeutic efficacy and safety evaluated weekly and approximately 24 hours after the previous dose. The antihypertensive effects of extended-release verapamil tablets are evident within the first week of therapy.

If adequate response is not obtained with 180 mg verapamil extended-release tablets, the dose may be titrated upward in the following manner:

240 mg each morning,
180 mg each morning plus 180 mg each evening; or 240 mg each morning plus 120 mg each evening,
240 mg every 12 hours.

Covera-HS tablets – Initiate therapy with 180 mg/day at bedtime. Clinical trials explored dose ranges between 180 and 540 mg given at bedtime and found effects to persist throughout the dosing interval.

If an adequate response is not obtained with 180 mg, the dose may be titrated upward in the following manner:

240 mg each evening,
360 mg each evening (2 × 180 mg),
480 mg each evening (2 × 240 mg).

Verelan PM – Usual daily dose is 200 mg/day at bedtime. In rare instances, initial doses of 100 mg/day may be warranted in patients who have an increased response to verapamil (eg, impaired or hepatic function, elderly, people of small stature). Base upward titration on safety and efficacy evaluated approximately 24 hours after dosing. Antihypertensive effects are evident within the first week of therapy.

If an adequate response is not obtained with 200 mg, the dose may be titrated upward in the following manner:

300 each evening,
400 mg each evening (2 × 200 mg).

➤*Sustained-release:* Individualize the dose by titration. Dose of 120 mg/day may be warranted in patients who may have increased response (eg, elderly or people of small stature). Antihypertensive effects are evident within the first week. When switching from the immediate-release formulation, total daily dose (in mg) may remain the same.

Calan SR and Isoptin SR – Initiate therapy with 180 mg given in the morning with food. Base upward titration on safety and efficacy evaluated weekly and approximately 24 hours after the previous dose.

Sustained release characteristics are not altered when the tablet is divided in half.

If adequate response is not obtained with 180 mg, the dose may be titrated upward in the following manner:

240 each morning,
180 mg each morning plus 180 each evening, or 240 mg each morning plus 120 mg each evening,
240 mg every 12 hours.

Verelan – Usual daily dose is 240 mg once daily in the morning. Base upward titration on safety and efficacy evaluated approximately 24 hours after dosing.

If adequate response is not obtained with 120 mg, the dose may be titrated upward in the following manner:

180 mg in the morning,
240 mg in the morning,
360 mg in the morning,
480 mg in the morning.

Pellet-filled capsules – Do not chew or crush the contents of the capsule. Pellet-filled capsules also may be administered by carefully opening the capsule and sprinkling the pellets on a spoonful of applesauce. Swallow the applesauce immediately without chewing and follow with a glass of cool water to ensure complete swallowing of the pellets. The applesauce used should not be hot, and it should be soft enough to be swallowed without chewing. Use any pellet/applesauce mixture immediately and do not store for future use. Subdividing the contents of the capsule is not recommended.

➤*Concomitant therapy:* Concomitant therapy with oral beta-adrenergic blocking agents may be beneficial in certain patients with chronic stable angina or hypertension, but available information is not sufficient to predict with confidence the effects of concurrent treatment in patients with left ventricular dysfunction or cardiac conduction abnormalities.

➤*Storage/Stability:* Store at controlled room temperature 15° to 30°C (59° to 86°F). Protect from light.

Extended-release tablets (Covera-HS, Verelan) – Store at controlled room temperature 20° to 25°C (68° to 77°F).

Oral – Dispense in tight, light-resistant container. Protect from moisture.

VERAPAMIL HYDROCHLORIDE — INJECTION

For complete and comparative prescribing information, refer to the Calcium Channel Blockers group monograph.

Indications

➤*Supraventricular tachycardia:* Rapid conversion to sinus rhythm of paroxysmal supraventricular tachycardias, including those associated with accessory bypass tracts (Wolff-Parkinson-White [W-P-W] and Lown-Ganong-Levine [L-G-L] syndromes). When clinically advisable, attempt appropriate vagal maneuvers (eg, Valsalva maneuver) prior to verapamil administration.

➤*Atrial flutter of fibrillation:* Temporary control of rapid ventricular rate in atrial flutter or atrial fibrillation except when the atrial flutter or atrial fibrillation are associated with accessory bypass tracts (Wolff-Parkinson-White [W-P-W]and Lown-Ganong-Levine [L-G-L] syndromes).

Administration and Dosage

➤*Approved by the FDA:* September 10, 1984.

For IV use only. Give verapamil injection as a slow IV injection over at least a 2-minute period of time under continuous electrocardiographic (ECG) and blood pressure monitoring. The recommended IV doses of verapamil injection are as follows:

➤*Adult:*

Initial dose – 5 to 10 mg (0.075 to 0.15 mg/kg body weight) given as an IV bolus over at least 2 minutes.

Repeat dose – 10 mg (0.15 mg/kg body weight) 30 minutes after the first dose if the initial response is not adequate. An optimal interval for subsequent IV doses has not been determined, and should be individualized for each patient.

Elderly – Administer the dose over at least 3 minutes to minimize the risk of untoward drug effects.

➤*Children:*

Initial dose –

0 to 1 year: Administer 0.1 to 0.2 mg/kg body weight (usual single dose range, 0.75 to 2 mg) as an IV bolus over at least 2 minutes under continuous ECG monitoring.

1 to 15 years: Administer 0.1 to 0.3 mg/kg body weight (usual single dose range, 2 to 5 mg) as an IV bolus over at least 2 minutes. Do not exceed 5 mg.

Repeat dose –

0 to 1 year: Administer 0.1 to 0.2 mg/kg body weight (usual single dose range, 0.75 to 2 mg) 30 minutes after the first dose if the initial response is not adequate (under continuous ECG monitoring). An optimal interval for subsequent IV doses has not been determined, and should be individualized for each patient.

1 to 15 years: Administer 0.1 to 0.3 mg/kg body weight (usual single dose range, 2 to 5 mg) 30 minutes after the first dose if the initial response is not adequate. Do not exceed 10 mg as a single dose. An optimal interval for subsequent IV doses has not been determined, and should be individualized for each patient.

➤*Note:* Visually inspect parenteral drug products for particulate matter and discoloration prior to administration, whenever solution and container permit.

Verapamil is physically compatible and chemically stable for at least 24 hours at 25°C (77°F) protected from light in most common large volume parenteral solutions. Avoid admixing verapamil injection with albumin, amphotericin B, hydralazine hydrochloride and trimethoprim with sulfamethoxazole. Verapamil injection will precipitate in any solution with a pH above 6.

Single-dose vials – Use only if solution is clear and vial seal is intact. Discard unused amount of solution immediately following withdrawal of any portion of contents. For stability reasons, this product is not recommended for dilution with sodium lactate injection in polyvinyl chloride bags.

➤*Storage/Stability:* Store at controlled room temperature 15° to 30°C (59° to 86°F). Protect from light.

Indications

➤*Amyl nitrite:* For the rapid relief of angina pectoris. The effect of amyl nitrite appears within 30 seconds and lasts for approximately 3 to 5 minutes.

➤*Isosorbide dinitrate:*

Tablets, extended-release (ER) tablets, and sustained-release (SR) capsules – For the prevention of angina pectoris caused by coronary artery disease (CAD). The onset of action of immediate- and controlled-release oral isosorbide dinitrate is not sufficiently rapid for these products to be useful in aborting an acute anginal episode.

Sublingual tablets – For the prevention and treatment of angina pectoris caused by CAD. However, because the onset of action of sublingual isosorbide dinitrate is significantly slower than that of sublingual nitroglycerin, sublingual isosorbide dinitrate is not the drug of first choice for abortion of an acute anginal episode.

➤*Isosorbide mononitrate:*

Tablets, ER tablets – For the treatment (*Monoket* only) and prevention of angina pectoris caused by CAD. The onset of action of immediate- and controlled-release oral isosorbide mononitrate is not sufficiently rapid for these products to be useful in aborting an acute anginal episode.

➤*Nitroglycerin:*

Lingual spray, sublingual tablets – For the acute relief of an attack or prophylaxis of angina pectoris caused by CAD.

ER capsules, ointment, transdermal patch – For the prevention of angina pectoris caused by CAD. The onset of action of transdermal and oral nitroglycerin is not sufficiently rapid for this product to be useful in aborting an acute attack.

Intravenous (IV) – For the treatment of perioperative hypertension; for control of congestive heart failure (CHF) in the setting of acute myocardial infarction (MI); for the treatment of angina pectoris in patients who have not responded to sublingual nitroglycerin and beta-blockers; for induction of intraoperative hypotension.

➤*Unlabeled uses:*

Isosorbide dinitrate, oral – Used with hydralazine to increase survival among black patients with advanced heart failure; for the treatment of acute angle-closure glaucoma in emergency situations, not intended for long-term management; achalasia.

Isosorbide mononitrate, oral – Used in combination with nadolol to prevent recurrent variceal bleeding.

Nitroglycerin, IV – For the management of acute MI; treatment of hypertensive emergencies; used in combination with vasopressin to treat variceal bleeding; cocaine-induced acute coronary syndrome; management of Prinzmetal angina that occurs in patients without coronary heart disease.

Nitroglycerin, sublingual – For the management of acute MI; management of Prinzmetal angina that occurs in patients without coronary heart disease.

Nitroglycerin, topical – For the management of acute MI; treatment of chronic anal fissure pain; erectile dysfunction; Raynaud disease; management of Prinzmetal angina that occurs in patients without coronary heart disease.

Actions

➤*Pharmacology:* The principal pharmacological action of nitrates is relaxation of the vascular smooth muscle and consequent dilation of peripheral arteries and especially the veins. Dilation of the veins promotes peripheral pooling of blood and decreases venous return to the heart, thereby reducing left ventricular end-diastolic pressure and pulmonary capillary wedge pressure (preload). Arteriolar relaxation reduces systemic vascular resistance, systolic arterial pressure, and mean arterial pressure (afterload). Dilation of the coronary arteries also occurs. The relative importance of preload reduction, afterload reduction, and coronary dilation remains undefined.

Therapeutic doses of **nitroglycerin** may reduce systolic, diastolic, and mean arterial blood pressure. Effective coronary perfusion pressure is usually maintained but can be compromised if blood pressure falls excessively or increased heart rate decreases diastolic filling time. Heart rate is usually slightly increased, presumably because of a compensatory response to the fall in blood pressure. Cardiac index may be increased, decreased, or unchanged. Myocardial oxygen consumption or demand (as measured by the pressure-rate product, tension-time index, and stroke-work index) is decreased and a more favorable supply-demand ratio can be achieved. Patients with elevated left ventricular filling pressures and increased systemic vascular resistance in association with a depressed cardiac index are likely to experience an improvement in cardiac index. In contrast, when filling pressures and cardiac index are normal, cardiac index may be slightly reduced following nitroglycerin administration.

Nitroglycerin forms free radical nitric oxide (NO), which activates guanylate cyclase, resulting in an increase of guanosine 3'5' monophosphate (cyclic GMP) in smooth muscle and other tissues. These events lead to dephosphorylation of myosin light chains, which regulate the contractile state in smooth muscle and result in vasodilation.

Amyl nitrite causes a nonspecific relaxation of smooth muscle with the most prominent actions occurring in vascular smooth muscle. This effect on vascular smooth muscle results in coronary vasodilation and decreased systemic vascular resistance and left ventricular preload and afterload. Myocardial ischemia is relieved in patients with angina pectoris, with an abatement of chest pain and possibly other related symptoms.

➤*Pharmacokinetics:*

Amyl nitrite –

Absorption: Amyl nitrite vapors are absorbed rapidly through the pulmonary alveoli, manifesting therapeutic effect within 1 minute after inhalation.

Metabolism: The drug is metabolized rapidly, probably by hydrolytic denitration.

Elimination: Approximately one third of inhaled amyl nitrite is excreted in the urine.

Isosorbide dinitrate –

Absorption: Absorption of isosorbide dinitrate after oral dosing is nearly complete but bioavailability is highly variable (10% to 90%). Maximum serum levels are reached approximately 1 hour after ingestion. The average bioavailability of isosorbide dinitrate is approximately 25%; most studies have observed progressive increases in bioavailability during chronic therapy.

Distribution: The volume of distribution of isosorbide dinitrate is 2 to 4 L/kg, and this volume is cleared at a rate of 2 to 4 L/min; therefore, half-life in serum is approximately 1 hour.

Metabolism: Isosorbide dinitrate has extensive first-pass metabolism in the liver. Clearance is affected primarily by denitration to the 2-mononitrate (15% to 25%) and the 5-mononitrate (75% to 85%). Both metabolites have biological activity, especially the 5-mononitrate. The 5-mononitrate is cleared from the serum by denitration to isosorbide, glucuronidation to the 5-mononitrate glucuronide, and denitration/hydration to sorbitol. The 2-mononitrate has been less well studied, but it appears to participate in the same metabolic pathways.

Elimination: Isosorbide dinitrate has an overall elimination half-life of approximately 5 hours.

Isosorbide mononitrate –

Absorption: After oral administration of isosorbide mononitrate, T_{max} is achieved in 30 to 60 minutes, with an absolute bioavailability of approximately 100%.

Distribution: The volume of distribution of isosorbide mononitrate is approximately 0.6 L/kg; less than 5% is bound to plasma protein and distributed into blood cells and saliva.

Metabolism: Isosorbide mononitrate is primarily metabolized by the liver but is not subject to first-pass metabolism. It is cleared from the serum by denitration to isosorbide, glucuronidation to the mononitrate, and denitration/hydration to sorbitol. None of the metabolites are vasoactive.

Elimination: The overall elimination half-life is approximately 5 hours; 96% of the dose is excreted in the urine within 5 days and 1% eliminated in the feces. Renal clearance accounts for about 4% of total body clearance. The rate of clearance is the same in healthy young adults, in patients with various degrees of renal, hepatic, or cardiac dysfunction, and in the elderly.

Isosorbide Mononitrate Pharmacokinetic Parameters

Parameter	Single-dose studies		Multiple-dose studies	
	Isosorbide mononitrate 60 mg	Isosorbide mononitrate ER tablets 60 mg	Isosorbide mononitrate ER tablets 60 mg	Isosorbide mononitrate ER tablets 120 mg
C_{max} (ng/mL)	1,242 to 1,534	424 to 541	557 to 572	1,151 to 1,180
T_{max} (h)	0.6 to 0.7	3.1 to 4.5	2.9 to 4.2	3.1 to 3.2
AUC (ng•h/mL)	8,189 to 8,313	5,990 to 7,452	6,625 to 7,555	14,241 to 16,800
t½ (h)	4.8 to 5.1	6.3 to 6.6	6.2 to 6.3	6.2 to 6.4
Cl/F (mL/min)	120 to 122	151 to 187	132 to 151	119 to 140

Food effects: See Drug Interactions for more information. Isosorbide mononitrate is significantly removed from the blood during hemodialysis; however, an additional dose to compensate for drug lost is not necessary. In patients undergoing continuous ambulatory peritoneal dialysis, blood levels are similar to patients not on dialysis.

Nitroglycerin lingual spray –

Absorption: In a pharmacokinetic study when a single dose of nitroglycerin 0.8 mg lingual spray was administered to healthy volunteers (n = 24), the mean C_{max} and T_{max} were 1,041 pg/mL•min and 7.5 minutes, respectively. Additionally, in these subjects the mean AUC was 12,769 pg/mL•min.

Nitroglycerin sublingual –

Absorption: Nitroglycerin is rapidly absorbed following sublingual administration. Mean peak plasma concentrations occur at a mean time of approximately 6 to 7 minutes postdose. Maximal drug concentration (C_{max}) and area under the curve (AUC) increase dose proportionally following nitroglycerin 0.3 to 0.6 mg sublingual tablets. The absolute bioavailability is approximately 40% but tends to be variable because of factors influencing drug absorption, such as sublingual hydration and mucosal metabolism.

Mean peak 1,2- and 1,3-dinitroglycerin plasma concentrations occur at approximately 15 minutes postdose.

Mean Nitroglycerin (SD) Values

Parameter	2 × 0.3 mg *Nitrostat* tablets	1 × 0.6 mg *Nitrostat* tablets
C_{max} (ng/mL)	2.3 (1.7)	2.1 (1.5)
T_{max} (min)	6.4 (2.5)	7.2 (3.2)
$AUC_{(0-\infty)}$ (min)	14.9 (8.2)	14.9 (11.4)
t½ (min)	2.8 (1.1)	2.6 (0.6)

Distribution: At plasma concentrations between 50 and 500 ng/mL, the binding of nitroglycerin to plasma proteins is approximately 60%, while that of 1,2-dinitroglycerin and 1,3-dinitroglycerin is 60% and 30%, respectively.

Metabolism: Nitroglycerin is rapidly metabolized to dinitrates and mononitrates. A liver reductase enzyme is of primary importance in the metabolism of nitroglycerin to glycerol dinitrate and mononitrate metabolites and ultimately to glycerol and organic nitrate. Known sites of extrahepatic metabolism include red blood cells and vascular walls. The 1,2- and 1,3-dinitroglycerin metabolites have been reported to possess approximately 2% and 10% of the pharmacological activity of nitroglycerin. Glycerol mononitrate metabolites of nitroglycerin are biologically inactive.

Elimination: Nitroglycerin plasma concentrations decrease rapidly with a mean elimination half-life of 2 to 3 minutes (range, 1.5 to 7.5 minutes). Clearance (13.6 L/min) greatly exceeds hepatic blood flow. Metabolism is the primary route of drug elimination. The elimination half-life of 1,2- and 1,3-dinitroglycerin is 36 and 32 minutes, respectively.

Nitroglycerin ER –

Absorption: The maximum achievable daily duration of antianginal effect from nitroglycerin ER capsules is approximately 12 hours. Controlled trials of multiple-dose oral nitroglycerin have shown statistically significant antianginal efficacy 2.5 to 4 hours after a dose when oral nitroglycerin had been administered 4 times a day for 2 weeks or 3 times a day for 1 week.

Distribution: The volume of distribution of nitroglycerin is approximately 3 L/kg.

Metabolism: The first products in the metabolism of nitroglycerin are inorganic nitrate and the 1,2- and 1,3-dinitroglycerols. The dinitrates are less effective vasodilators than nitroglycerin, but they are longer lived in the serum and their net contribution to the overall effect of chronic nitroglycerin regimens is not known. The dinitrates are further metabolized to (nonvasoactive) mononitrates and, ultimately, to glycerol and carbon dioxide. Known sites of extrahepatic metabolism include red blood cells and vascular walls.

Elimination: Nitroglycerin is cleared at extremely rapid rates, with a resulting serum half-life of approximately 3 minutes. The observed clearance rates (close to 1 L/kg/min) greatly exceed hepatic blood flow.

Nitroglycerin transdermal, ointment –

Absorption: In healthy volunteers, steady-state plasma concentrations of nitroglycerin are reached in approximately 2 hours after application of the patch and are maintained for the duration of wearing the system (observations have been limited to 24 hours). The onset of action of transdermal nitroglycerin is not sufficiently rapid for it to be useful in aborting an acute anginal episode. It is reasonable to believe that the rate of nitroglycerin absorption from patches may vary with the site of application, but this relationship has not been adequately studied. Nitroglycerin levels rise to steady state within about 1 hour after nitroglycerin ointment application.

Distribution: The volume of distribution of nitroglycerin is approximately 3 L/kg.

Metabolism: The first products in the metabolism of nitroglycerin are inorganic nitrate and the 1,2- and 1,3-dinitroglycerols. The dinitrates are less effective vasodilators than nitroglycerin, but they are longer lived in the serum and their net contribution to the overall effect of chronic nitroglycerin regimens is not known. The dinitrates are further metabolized to (nonvasoactive) mononitrates and, ultimately, to glycerol and carbon dioxide. Known sites of extrahepatic metabolism include red blood cells and vascular walls.

Elimination: Nitroglycerin is cleared at extremely rapid rates, with a resulting serum half-life of approximately 3 minutes. The observed clearance rates (close to 1 L/kg/min) greatly exceed hepatic blood flow. Upon removal of the nitroglycerin transdermal patch, the plasma concentration declines, with a half-life of approximately 1 hour. After removal of ointment, levels wane with a half-life of approximately half an hour.

Nitroglycerin IV –

Absorption: The pharmacokinetic results from clinical trials with the IV formulation are consistent with results from other trials with other formulations of nitroglycerin and other nitrates.

Distribution: The volume of distribution of nitroglycerin is approximately 3 L/kg.

Metabolism: The first products in the metabolism of nitroglycerin are inorganic nitrate and the 1,2- and 1,3-dinitroglycerols. The dinitrates are less effective vasodilators than nitroglycerin, but they are longer lived in the serum and their net contribution to the overall effect of chronic nitroglycerin regimens is not known. The dinitrates are further metabolized to (nonvasoactive) mononitrates and, ultimately, to glycerol and carbon dioxide. Known sites of extrahepatic metabolism include red blood cells and vascular walls.

Elimination: Continuous IV nitroglycerin lost almost all of its hemodynamic effect after 48 hours. Nitroglycerin is cleared at extremely rapid rates, with a resulting serum half-life of approximately 3 minutes. The observed clearance rates (close to 1 L/kg/min) greatly exceed hepatic blood flow.

Contraindications

➤*Amyl nitrite:* Patients with glaucoma, recent head trauma, cerebral hemorrhage, and pregnancy.

➤*Isosorbide dinitrate:* Allergic reactions to isosorbide dinitrate or any of its ingredients.

➤*Isosorbide mononitrate:* Hypersensitivity or idiosyncratic reactions to other nitrates or nitrites.

➤*Nitroglycerin:* Allergic reactions to organic nitrates.

Patients who are using certain drugs for erectile dysfunction (eg, sildenafil citrate), because these drugs have been shown to potentiate the hypotensive effects of organic nitrates (sublingual tablets, lingual spray, transdermal).

Allergy to the adhesives used in the transdermal patches (transdermal).

Patients with early MI, severe anemia, increased intracranial pressure, known hypersensitivity to nitroglycerin (sublingual tablets).

Patients with pericardial tamponade, restrictive cardiomyopathy, constrictive pericarditis, solutions containing dextrose in patients with known allergy to corn or corn products (IV).

Warnings

➤*Phosphodiesterase inhibitors:* See Drug Interactions for more information.

➤*Acute MI and/or CHF:* The benefits of nitrates (other than **nitroglycerin in dextrose**) in patients with acute MI or CHF have not been established. If electing to use these products, use careful clinical and hemodynamic monitoring to avoid the hazards of hypotension and tachycardia. Because the effects of **isosorbide mononitrate** and **isosorbide dinitrate** are so difficult to terminate rapidly, these products are not recommended in these settings.

➤*Arcing:* Do not discharge a cardioverter/defibrillator through a paddle electrode that overlies a **nitroglycerin transdermal** system patch. The arcing that may be seen in this situation is harmless in itself, but it may be associated with local current concentration that can cause damage to the paddles and burns to the patient.

➤*Polyvinyl chloride (PVC) tubing:* Because of the problem of nitroglycerin absorption by PVC tubing, use nitroglycerin IV with the least absorptive infusion tubing (ie, non-PVC tubing) available.

➤*IV filters:* Some in-line IV filters also absorb **nitroglycerin**; avoid these filters.

➤*Hemolysis/Pseudoagglutination:* Do not administer solutions containing dextrose without electrolytes through the same administration set as blood because this may result in pseudoagglutination or hemolysis.

➤*Electrolyte concentrations:* The IV administration of solutions may cause fluid overloading, resulting in dilution of serum electrolyte concentrations, overhydration, and congested states of pulmonary edema. The risk of dilutional states is inversely proportional to the electrolyte concentration in the injections. The risk of solute overload causing congested states with peripheral and pulmonary edema is directly proportional to the electrolyte concentration of the injections.

➤*Postural hypotension:* Transient episodes of dizziness, weakness, syncope, or other signs of cerebral ischemia caused by postural hypotension may develop following inhalation of **amyl nitrite**, particularly if the patient is standing immobile. This effect may be more frequent in patients who also have consumed alcohol. To hasten recovery, use measures that facilitate venous return (eg, head-low posture, deep breathing, movement of extremities).

➤*Flammability:* **Amyl nitrite** is very flammable. Do not use where it would become ignited.

➤*Carcinogenesis:* Animal carcinogenicity studies with **nitroglycerin** products have not been performed. Rats receiving up to 434 mg/kg/day of dietary nitroglycerin for 2 years developed dose-related fibrotic and neoplastic changes in the liver, including carcinomas, and interstitial cell tumors in the testes. At high doses, the incidence of hepatocellular carcinomas was 48% in males and 33% in females versus 0% in the controls, and incidences of testicular tumors were 52% versus 8% in controls.

➤*Elderly:* Clinical experience for organic nitrates reported in the literature identified a potential for severe hypotension and increased sensitivity to nitrates in the elderly. Nitrate therapy may aggravate the angina caused by hypertrophic cardiomyopathy, particularly in the elderly.

Elderly patients may have reduced baroreceptor function and may develop severe orthostatic hypotension when vasodilators are used. Use **isosorbide mononitrate ER** tablets with caution in elderly patients who may be volume depleted, on multiple medications, or who are already hypotensive. Hypotension induced by isosorbide mononitrate may be accompanied by paradoxical bradycardia and increased angina pectoris.

Use caution in dose selection for an elderly patient, usually starting at the low end of the dosing range, reflecting the greater frequency of decreased hepatic, renal, or cardiac function, and of concomitant disease or other drug therapy.

➤*Pregnancy:* *Category C* (**nitroglycerin, isosorbide dinitrate, isosorbide mononitrate** [ie, *ISMO*], **amyl nitrite**); *Category B* (**isosorbide mononitrate ER** [ie, *Imdur*], isosorbide mononitrate [ie, *Monoket*]).

Amyl nitrite can cause fetal harm to the fetus when it is administered to a pregnant woman because it significantly reduces systemic blood pressure and blood flow on the maternal side of the placenta.

There are no adequate and well-controlled studies in pregnant women with nitroglycerin. It is not known whether nitroglycerin can cause fetal harm when administered to a pregnant woman or can affect reproductive capacity. Give nitroglycerin to a pregnant woman only if clearly needed.

At oral doses 35 and 150 times the maximum recommended human daily dose, isosorbide dinitrate has been shown to cause a dose-related increase in embryotoxicity (increase in mummified pups) in rabbits.

➤*Lactation:* It is not known whether nitrates are excreted in human milk. Because many drugs are excreted in human milk, exercise caution when administering nitrates to a breast-feeding woman.

➤*Children:* Safety and efficacy in children have not been established.

Precautions

➤*Angina:* Nitrate therapy may aggravate angina caused by hypertrophic cardiomyopathy.

➤*Tolerance:* Use only the smallest dose required for effective relief of the acute anginal attack. Excessive use of **sublingual nitroglycerin** may lead to the development of tolerance. In industrial workers who have had long-term exposure to unknown (presumably high) doses of organic nitrates, tolerance clearly occurs. As tolerance to other forms of nitroglycerin develops, the effects of sublingual nitroglycerin on exercise tolerance, although still observable, is blunted.

Tolerance to **amyl nitrite** may develop with repeated use of the drug for prolonged periods of time. Tolerance may be minimized by beginning with the smallest effective dose and alternating the drug with another coronary vasodilator.

➤*Severe hypotension:* Severe hypotension, particularly with upright posture, may occur with small doses of nitrates; therefore, use these drugs with caution in patients who may be volume depleted or who are already hypotensive. Hypotension induced by **nitroglycerin** may be accompanied by paradoxical bradycardia and increased angina pectoris.

➤*Withdrawal:* Chest pain, acute MI, and even sudden death have occurred during temporary withdrawal of nitrates from industrial workers who have had long-term exposure to unknown doses of organic nitrates, demonstrating the existence of true physical dependence.

➤*Nitrate-free interval:* Several clinical trials of nitroglycerin in patients with angina pectoris have evaluated regimens that incorporated a 10- to 12-hour nitrate-free interval. In some of these trials, an increase in the frequency of anginal attacks during the nitrate-free interval was observed in a small number of patients. In one trial, patients had decreased exercise tolerance at the end of the nitrate-free interval. Hemodynamic rebound has been observed rarely; on the other hand, few studies were designed that rebound, if it had occurred, would have been detected. The importance of these findings to the routine clinical use of nitrates is unknown.

➤*Fluid load:* Lower concentrations of **nitroglycerin IV** and **nitroglycerin in dextrose injection** increase the potential precision of dosing, but these concentrations increase the total fluid volume that must be delivered to patients. Total fluid load may be a dominant consideration in patients with compromised function of the heart, liver, and/or kidneys.

➤*Nitroglycerin infusions:* Administer nitroglycerin IV and nitroglycerin in dextrose infusions only via an infusion pump that can maintain a constant infusion rate. Intracoronary injection of nitroglycerin IV and nitroglycerin in dextrose infusions has not been studied.

➤*Diabetes mellitus:* Use solutions containing dextrose with caution in patients with known subclinical or overt diabetes mellitus.

➤*Methemoglobinemia:* See Overdose for more information.

➤*Discontinuation:* Discontinue **sublingual nitroglycerin** if blurring of vision or drying of the mouth occurs. Excessive dosages of nitroglycerin may produce severe headaches.

➤*Drug abuse and dependence:* Volatile nitrites, including **amyl nitrite**, are abused for sexual stimulation, with headache as a common side effect. Tolerance to nitrites can develop; conditions and duration have not been established.

Drug Interactions

Nitrate Drug Interactions

Precipitant drug	Object drug*		Description
Alcohol	Nitrates	↑	Severe hypotension and cardiovascular collapse may occur.
Aspirin	Nitrates	↑	The vasodilatory and hemodynamic effects of nitrates may be enhanced by coadministration of aspirin.
Phosphodiesterase inhibitors (eg, sildenafil, tadalafil, vardenafil)	Nitrates	↑	Phosphodiesterase inhibitors have been shown to potentiate the hypotensive effects of organic nitrates. Concomitant use is contraindicated.
Vasodilators	Nitrates	↑	Additive hypotension may occur.
Nitrates	Antihypertensives Beta-blockers Calcium channel blockers	↑	Possible additive hypotension may occur. Marked orthostatic hypotension may occur with coadministration with calcium channel blockers. Dose adjustments of either class may be necessary.
Nitrates	Nondepolarizing muscle relaxants (eg, pancuronium)	↑	Nitrates may potentiate the actions of pancuronium, possibly resulting in profound and severe respiratory depression.
Nitrates	Phenothiazines	↑	Possible additive hypotension may occur. Dose adjustment of either class of agent may be necessary.
Nitrates, IV	Heparin	↓	Nitroglycerin IV reduces the anticoagulant effect of heparin; monitor aPTT in patients receiving these drugs concomitantly and adjust heparin dose as needed.
Nitrates, long-acting	Nitrates, sublingual	↓	A decrease in therapeutic effect of sublingual nitroglycerin may result from use of long-acting nitrates.
Nitrates, oral	Dihydroergotamine	↑	Oral administration of nitroglycerin markedly decreases the first-pass metabolism of dihydroergotamine and subsequently increases its oral bioavailability. Ergotamine is known to precipitate angina pectoris. Therefore, patients receiving sublingual nitroglycerin should avoid ergotamine and related drugs or be monitored for symptoms of ergotism if this is not possible.
Nitroglycerin	Alteplase	↓	Nitroglycerin administration decreases the thrombolytic effect of alteplase. Avoid concurrent use.

* ↑ = Object drug increased. ↓ = Object drug decreased.

➤*Drug/Lab test interactions:* Nitrates and nitrites may interfere with the *Zlatkis-Zak* color reaction causing falsely low readings in serum cholesterol determinations.

Because of the propylene glycol content of **nitroglycerin IV**, serum triglyceride assays that rely on glycerol oxidase may give falsely elevated results in patients receiving this medication.

➤*Drug/Food interactions:* Concomitant food intake may decrease the rate (increase in T_{max}) but not the extent (AUC) of absorption of **isosorbide mononitrate**.

Adverse Reactions

➤*Amyl nitrite:* Mild transitory headache, dizziness, and flushing of the face are common with the use of amyl nitrite. The following adverse reactions may occur in susceptible patients: cold sweat, hypotension, involuntary passing of urine and feces, nausea, pallor, restlessness, syncope, tachycardia, vomiting, weakness. Excessively high doses of amyl nitrite administered chronically may cause methemoglobinemia.

➤*Isosorbide mononitrate tablets:*

Cardiovascular – Cardiovascular disorder, chest pain (1% or more); acute MI, angina pectoris, apoplexy, arrhythmias, atrial fibrillation, bradycardia, edema, hypertension, hypotension, pallor, palpitations, postural hypotension, premature ventricular contractions, supraventricular tachycardia, syncope, tachycardia (less than 1%).

CNS – Dizziness, emotional lability, fatigue, headache (1% or more); agitation, anxiety, confusion, depression, hypesthesia, hypokinesia, impaired concentration, insomnia, nervousness, nightmares, restlessness, tremor, vertigo (less than 1%).

Dermatologic – Pruritus, rash (1% or more); sweating (less than 1%).

GI – Abdominal pain, diarrhea, nausea, vomiting (1% or more); anorexia, decreased weight, dry mouth, dyspepsia, tenesmus, thirst, tooth disorder (less than 1%).

GU – Dysuria, impotence, prostatic disorder, urinary frequency (less than 1%).

Musculoskeletal – Arthralgia, muscle cramps (less than 1%).

Respiratory – Increased cough, upper respiratory tract infection (1% or more); asthma, dyspnea, sinusitis (less than 1%).

Miscellaneous – Allergic reaction, flushing, pain (1% or more); amblyopia, asthenia, back pain, bitter taste, blurred vision, cold sweat, diplopia, increased appetite, malaise, neck pain, neck stiffness, paresthesia, rigors, susurrus aurium (less than 1%).

➤*Isosorbide mononitrate ER tablets:*

Cardiovascular – Angina pectoris aggravated, arrhythmia, arrhythmia atrial, atrial fibrillation, bradycardia, bundle branch block, cardiac failure, extrasystole, heart murmur, heart sound abnormal, hypertension, hypotension, MI, palpitation, Q-wave abnormality, tachycardia, ventricular tachycardia (5% or less); syncope (postmarketing).

CNS – Dizziness, headache (more than 5%); anxiety, concentration impaired, confusion, decreased libido, depression, dizziness, fatigue, headache, hypesthesia, insomnia, migraine, nervousness, neuritis, paroniria, paresis, paresthesia, somnolence, tremor, vertigo (5% or less).

Dermatologic – Acne, hair texture abnormal, increased sweating, pruritus, rash, skin nodule (5% or less).

GI – Abdominal pain, constipation, diarrhea, dry mouth, dyspepsia, flatulence, gastric ulcer, gastritis, glossitis, hemorrhagic gastric ulcer, hemorrhoids, loose stools, melena, nausea, vomiting (5% or less).

GU – Atrophic vaginitis, breast pain, impotence, polyuria, renal calculus, urinary tract infection (5% or less).

Hematologic – Hypochromic anemia, purpura, thrombocytopenia (5% or less).

Hepatic – ALT increase, AST increase (5% or less).

Metabolic/Nutritional – Edema, hyperuricemia, hypokalemia (5% or less).

Musculoskeletal – Arthralgia, frozen shoulder, muscle weakness, musculoskeletal pain, myalgia, myositis, tendon disorder, torticollis (5% or less).

Respiratory – Bronchitis, bronchospasm, coughing, dyspnea, increased sputum, nasal congestion, pharyngitis, pneumonia, pulmonary infiltration, rales, rhinitis, sinusitis (5% or less).

Special senses – Conjunctivitis, earache, photophobia, tinnitus, tympanic membrane perforation, vision abnormal (5% or less).

Miscellaneous – Asthenia, back pain, bacterial infection, chest pain, fever, flu-like symptoms, flushing, hot flushes, intermittent claudication, leg ulcer, malaise, moniliasis, ptosis, rigors, varicose vein, viral infection (5% or less).

➤*Nitroglycerin lingual spray:* Adverse reactions to oral nitroglycerin dosage forms, particularly headache and hypotension, are generally dose-related. In clinical trials at various doses of nitroglycerin, the following adverse reactions have been observed: headache which may be severe and persistent, is the most commonly reported side effect of nitroglycerin with an incidence of about 50% in some studies. Cutaneous vasodilation with flushing may occur. Transient episodes of dizziness and weakness as well as other signs of cerebral ischemia associated with postural hypotension may occasionally develop. Occasionally, an individual may exhibit marked sensitivity to the hypotensive effects of nitrates and severe responses (collapse, nausea, pallor, perspiration, restlessness, vomiting, and weakness) may occur even with therapeutic doses. Drug rash and/or exfoliative dermatitis have been reported in patients receiving nitrate therapy. Nausea and vomiting are uncommon.

More than 2% – Dizziness, headache, paresthesia.

2% or less – Abdominal pain, asthenia, dyspnea, peripheral edema, pharyngitis, rhinitis, vasodilation.

➤*Nitroglycerin sublingual:* Headache which may be severe and persistent may occur immediately after use. Dizziness, palpitation, vertigo, weakness, and other manifestations of postural hypotension may develop occasionally, particularly in erect, immobile patients. Marked sensitivity to the hypotensive effects of nitrates (manifested by collapse, diaphoresis, nausea, pallor, vomiting, and weakness) may occur at therapeutic doses. Syncope caused by nitrate vasodilation has been reported. Drug rash, exfoliative dermatitis, and flushing have been reported in patients receiving nitrate therapy.

➤*Nitroglycerin ointment, transdermal, IV, ER capsules, and isosorbide dinitrate:* Adverse reactions to nitroglycerin and isosorbide dinitrate are generally dose related, and almost all of these reactions are the result of the activity of these drugs as vasodilators. Headache, which may be severe, is the most commonly reported side effect. Headache may be recurrent with each daily dose, especially at higher doses. Transient episodes of light-headedness, occasionally related to blood pressure changes, also may occur. Hypotension occurs infrequently, but in some patients it may be severe enough to warrant discontinuation of therapy. Syncope, crescendo angina, and rebound hypertension have been reported but are uncommon.

Allergic reactions to nitroglycerin are also uncommon, and the great majority of those reported have been cases of contact dermatitis or fixed drug eruptions in patients receiving nitroglycerin ointment or patch. There have been a few reports of anaphylactoid reactions; these reactions can probably occur in patients receiving nitroglycerin by any route.

Application-site irritation may occur with transdermal nitroglycerin but is rarely severe. The most frequent adverse reactions with transdermal nitroglycerin were as follows: headache (63%); light-headedness (6%); hypotension and/or syncope (4%); increased angina (2%).

Overdosage

➤*Symptoms:* The ill effects of nitrate overdose are generally the result of the capacity of nitrates to induce vasodilation, venous pooling, reduced cardiac output, and hypotension. These hemodynamic changes may have protean manifestations, including increased intracranial pressure, with any or all of the following; persistent throbbing headache, confusion, and moderate fever; vertigo; palpitations; visual disturbances; nausea and vomiting (possibly with colic and even bloody diarrhea); syncope (especially in the upright posture); air hunger and dyspnea, later followed by reduced ventilatory effort; diaphoresis, with the skin either flushed or cold or clammy; heart block and bradycardia; paralysis; coma; seizures; and death.

Inhaled doses of 5 to 10 drops of **amyl nitrite** may cause violent flushing of the face, accompanied by a feeling of imminent bursting of the head and very excessive heart action. The inhalation of larger amounts may produce a feeling of suffocation and muscular weakness. Symptoms comparable to shock may be produced (eg, incontinence, nausea, pallor, restlessness, sweating, syncope, vomiting, weakness) attributable to pooling of blood in the postarteriolar vessels and failure of the venous blood to return to the heart.

Methemoglobinemia – Methemoglobinemia has been reported in patients receiving other organic nitrates. Certainly, nitrate ions liberated during metabolism of nitrates can oxidize hemoglobin into methemoglobin. However, even in patients totally without cytochrome b_5 reductase activity and assuming that the nitrate moiety of the nitrate is quantitatively applied to oxidation of hemoglobin, approximately 2 mg/kg of **isosorbide mononitrate** or 1 mg/kg of **nitroglycerin** or **isosorbide dinitrate** should be required before any of these patients manifests clinically significant (10% or more) methemoglobinemia. In patients with normal reductase function, significant production of methemoglobin should require larger doses of the nitrate. In one study in which 36 patients received 2 to 4 weeks of continuous nitroglycerin therapy at 3.1 to 4.4 mg/h, the average methemoglobin level measured was 0.2%; this was comparable with that observed in parallel patients who received placebo.

Notwithstanding these observations, there are case reports of significant methemoglobinemia in association with moderate overdoses of organic nitrates. None of the affected patients were thought to be unusually susceptible.

➤*Treatment:* Dialysis is known to be ineffective in removing **isosorbide mononitrate** from the body. No specific antagonist to the vasodilator effects of nitrates is known, and no intervention has been subject to controlled study as a therapy of nitrate overdose. Because the hypotension associated with nitrate overdose is the result of venodilation and arterial hypovolemia, direct prudent therapy in this situation toward an increase in central fluid volume. Passive elevation of the patient's legs may be sufficient, but IV infusion of normal saline or similar fluid also may be necessary.

In patients with renal disease or CHF, therapy resulting in central volume expansion may be hazardous. Treatment of nitrate overdose in these patients may be subtle and difficult and invasive monitoring may be required.

Measures that facilitate venous return, such as head-low posture, deep breathing, and movement of extremities, may be used. The use of epinephrine aggravates the shock-like reaction. Inject methylene blue for treatment of severe methemoglobinemia with dyspnea. For treating cyanide poisoning, methylene blue is contraindicated where nitrites cause iatrogenic methemoglobinemia.

Patient Information

Instruct patients to carefully follow the prescribed schedule of dosing.

Instruct patients to take oral nitrates on an empty stomach with a glass of water.

Daily headaches sometimes accompany treatment with nitrates. In patients who get these headaches, the headaches are a marker of the activity of the drug. Instruct patients to resist the temptation to avoid headaches by altering the schedule of their treatment with nitrates because loss of headache is likely to be associated with simultaneous loss of antianginal efficacy.

Treatment with nitrates may be associated with light-headedness on standing, especially just after rising from a recumbent or seated position. This effect may be more frequent in patients who have also consumed alcohol. Aspirin or acetaminophen often successfully relieves nitrate-induced headaches with no deleterious effect on antianginal efficacy.

Instruct patients not to take nitrate products with certain drugs taken for erectile dysfunction (phosphodiesterase inhibitors) because of the risk of dangerously lowering their blood pressure.

Inform patients that the antianginal efficacy of **isosorbide mononitrate** or **isosorbide dinitrate** is strongly related to its dosing regimen and to carefully follow the prescribed schedule of dosing. For most patients taking isosorbide mononitrate ER tablets, this can be accomplished by taking the dose on arising. For most patients taking isosorbide mononitrate IR tablets, this can be accomplished by taking the first dose on awakening and the second dose 7 hours later.

Keep tablets and capsules in original container. Keep container closed tightly.

➤*Brand interchange:* Instruct patients not to change from one brand of this drug to another without consulting their pharmacist or health care provider. Products manufactured by different companies may not be equally effective.

➤*Amyl nitrite inhalant:* Instruct patients to use when lying down only. Amyl nitrite is highly flammable; advise patients not to use where it might be ignited. Advise patients to use amyl nitrite in a well-ventilated room.

➤*ER tablets, capsules:* Instruct patients to swallow whole and not chew. Not for sublingual use.

➤*Lingual spray:* Instruct patients to spray onto or under tongue. Instruct patients not to inhale spray.

➤*Sublingual tablets:* Instruct patients to dissolve tablet under tongue and not swallow. A lack of burning or stinging sensation does not indicate a loss of potency. Advise patients to use when seated and to take at the first sign of an anginal attack before severe pain develops. If angina is not relieved in 5 minutes, instruct patients to dissolve a second tablet under the tongue. If pain is not relieved within another 5 minutes, instruct patients to dissolve a third tablet. If pain continues or intensifies, advise patients to notify their health care provider immediately or report to the nearest emergency room.

Instruct patients to keep **nitroglycerin** in original glass container, tightly capped, and to discard the cotton once the bottle is opened.

➤*Transdermal patches:* Patient instructions are available with products. Advise patients that there is enough residual **nitroglycerin** in discarded patches that they are a potential hazard to children and pets. Instruct patients to use caution when discarding.

➤*Ointment:* Patient instructions are available with products. Instruct patients to spread a thin layer on skin using applicator or dose-measuring papers. Instruct patients not to use fingers and to not rub or massage. Instruct patients to keep tube tightly closed.

AMYL NITRITE

Rx	**Amyl Nitrite** (Various, eg, James Alexander)	**Inhalant:** 0.3 mL	Covered glass capsules. In 12s.

AMYL NITRITE — INHALATIONAL

For complete prescribing information, refer to the Nitrates group monograph.

Indications

➤*Angina pectoris:* For the rapid relief of angina pectoris. The effect of amyl nitrite appears within 30 seconds and lasts for approximately 3 to 5 minutes.

Administration and Dosage

With the patient in recumbent or seated position, a capsule of amyl nitrite is held away from the face, crushed between the fingers, and held under the patient's nose. Two to 6 inhalations of the vapors from the capsule are usually sufficient to promptly produce therapeutic effects. Caution is recommended to avoid inhalation of the drug when it is administered by someone other than the patient. If necessary, the dose may be repeated in 3 to 5 minutes.

➤*Storage/Stability:* Store in a cool place, 2° to 8°C (36° to 46°F). Contents are flammable; protect from light.

ISOSORBIDE DINITRATE, ORAL

Rx	**Isosorbide Dinitrate** (Various, eg, IVAX Pharm, Major, Par, Sandoz, West-Ward)	**Tablets:** 5 mg	In 100s, 500s, 1,000s, and UD 100s.
Rx	**Isordil Titradose** (Wyeth)		Lactose. (WYETH 4152). Pink, scored. In 100s and 1,000s.
Rx	**Isosorbide Dinitrate** (Various, eg, IVAX Pharm, Major, Par, Sandoz, UDL, West-Ward)	**Tablets:** 10 mg	In 100s, 500s, 1,000s and UD 100s.
Rx	**Isordil Titradose** (Wyeth)		Lactose. (WYETH 4153). White, scored. In 100s and 1,000s.
Rx	**Isosorbide Dinitrate** (Various, eg, IVAX Pharm, Major, Par, Sandoz, UDL, URL, West-Ward)	**Tablets:** 20 mg	In 100s, 1,000s, and UD 100s.
Rx	**Isordil Titradose** (Wyeth)		Lactose. (WYETH 4154). Green, scored. In 100s and 500s.
Rx	**Isosorbide Dinitrate** (Various, eg, Imiren, Par)	**Tablets:** 30 mg	In 100s, 500s, 1,000s, and UD 100s.
Rx	**Isordil Titradose** (Wyeth)		Lactose. (WYETH 4159). Blue, scored. In 100s.
Rx	**Isordil Titradose** (Wyeth)	**Tablets:** 40 mg	Lactose. (WYETH 4192). Lt. green, scored. In 100s.
Rx	**Isochron** (Forest)	**Tablets, extended-release:** 40 mg	Lactose. (IL/3613). Peach colored, scored. In 100s.
Rx	**Isosorbide Dinitrate** (Various, eg, Qualitest, West-Ward)	**Tablets, sublingual:** 2.5 mg	May contain lactose. In 100s, 1,000s, and UD 100s.
Rx	**Isosorbide Dinitrate** (Various, eg, Qualitest, West-Ward)	**Tablets, sublingual:** 5 mg	May contain lactose. In 100s, 1,000s, and UD 100s.
Rx	**Dilatrate-SR** (Schwarz Pharma)	**Capsules, sustained-release:** 40 mg	Lactose, sucrose. (Schwarz 0920). Pink, opaque. In 100s.

ISOSORBIDE DINITRATE — ORAL

For complete and comparative prescribing information, refer to the Nitrates group monograph.

Indications

➤*Angina pectoris:* For the treatment (sublingual tablets only) and prevention of angina pectoris caused by coronary artery disease. The onset of action of oral isosorbide dinitrate is not sufficiently rapid for this product to be useful in aborting an acute anginal episode.

➤*Unlabeled uses:* Used with hydralazine to increase survival among black patients with advanced heart failure; for the treatment of acute angle-closure glaucoma in emergency situations, not intended for long-term management; achalasia.

Administration and Dosage

➤*Tablets:* Initial dose is 5 to 20 mg 2 or 3 times daily. For maintenance therapy, 10 to 40 mg 2 or 3 times daily is recommended. A daily dose-free interval of at least 14 hours is advisable to minimize tolerance.

➤*Tablets, sublingual:* Usual starting dose is 2.5 to 5 mg. Titrate upward until angina is relieved or side effects limit the dose. Every dosing regimen for isosorbide dinitrate must provide a daily dose-free interval to minimize the development of tolerance; one of the daily dose-free intervals must be longer than 14 hours.

Do not crush or chew sublingual tablets.

Acute prophylaxis – A patient anticipating activity likely to cause angina should take 1 sublingual tablet (2.5 to 5 mg) approximately 15 minutes before the activity is expected to begin. Isosorbide dinitrate sublingual tablets may be used to abort an acute anginal episode, but its use is recommended only in patients who fail to respond to sublingual nitroglycerin.

➤*Tablets, extended-release and capsules, sustained-release:* The initial dose is 40 mg; maintenance dose is 40 to 80 mg every 8 to 12 hours. Do not crush or chew these preparations.

Tolerance – Tolerance to these agents may develop. Consider administering the short-acting preparations 2 or 3 times daily (last dose no later than 7 pm) and the sustained-release preparations once daily or twice daily at 8 am and 2 pm (see Precautions).

➤*Storage/Stability:*

Tablets – Store at room temperature, approximately 25°C (77°). Protect from light. Keep bottles tightly closed. Dispense in a light-resistant, tight container.

Tablets, extended-release – Store at 25°C (77°); excursions permitted to 15° to 30°C (59° to 86°F). Dispense in well-closed container.

Tablets, sublingual – Store at controlled room temperature 15° to 30°C (59° to 86°F). Protect from light and moisture. Dispense in a tight, light-resistant container.

Capsules, sustained-release – Store at controlled room temperature 15° to 30°C (59° to 86°F) in a dry place.

ISOSORBIDE MONONITRATE, ORAL

Rx	**Isosorbide Mononitrate** (Various, eg, Kremers Urban, Purepac, Schwarz Pharma)	**Tablets:** 10 mg	May contain lactose. In 100s.
Rx	**Monoket** (Schwarz Pharma)		Lactose. (10 SCHWARZ 610). White, scored. In 100s.
Rx	**ISMO** (Wyeth)	**Tablets:** 20 mg	Lactose. (ISMO 20). Orange, scored. Film coated. In 100s and UD 100s.
Rx	**Isosorbide Mononitrate** (Various, eg, Kremers Urban, Purepac, Schwarz Pharma, Teva)		May contain lactose. In 100s and 500s.
Rx	**Monoket** (Schwarz Pharma)		Lactose. (20 SCHWARZ 620). White, scored. In 100s, 180s, and UD 100s.
Rx	**Isosorbide Mononitrate** (Various, eg, Ethex, Kremers Urban)	**Tablets, extended-release:** 30 mg	May contain lactose. In 100s and 1,000s.
Rx	**Imdur** (Key)		(IMDUR 30). Rose colored, scored. In 100s and UD 100s.

ISOSORBIDE MONONITRATE, ORAL

Rx	**Isosorbide Mononitrate** (Various, eg, Ethex, Kremers Urban)	**Tablets, extended-release**: 60 mg	May contain lactose. In 100s and 1,000s.
Rx	**Imdur** (Key)		(IMDUR 60). Yellow, scored. In 100s and UD 100s.
Rx	**Isosorbide Mononitrate** (Various, eg, Ethex, Kremers Urban)	**Tablets, extended-release**: 120 mg	May contain lactose. In 100s and 1,000s.
Rx	**Imdur** (Key)		(IMDUR 120). White. In 100s and UD 100s.

ISOSORBIDE MONONITRATE — ORAL

For complete and comparative prescribing information, refer to the Nitrates group monograph.

Indications

➤*Angina pectoris:* For the treatment (*Monoket* only) and prevention of angina pectoris caused by coronary artery disease. The onset of action of oral isosorbide mononitrate is not sufficiently rapid for this product to be useful in aborting an acute angina episode.

➤*Unlabeled uses:* Used in combination with nadolol to prevent recurrent variceal bleeding.

Administration and Dosage

➤*Approved by the FDA:* December 1991.

➤*Tablets:* 20 mg twice daily, with the 2 doses given 7 hours apart. A starting dose of 5 mg (½ tablet of the 10 mg dosing strength) may be appropriate for people of particularly small stature, but should be increased to at least 10 mg by the second or third day of therapy. Suggested regimen is to give first dose on awakening and second dose 7 hours later. The asymmetric (2 doses, 7 hours apart) dosing regimen provides a daily nitrate-free interval to minimize the development of tolerance.

➤*Tablets, extended-release:* Initially, 30 mg (given as a single 30 mg tablet or one half of a 60 mg tablet) or 60 mg (given as a single tablet) once daily. After several days, the dosage may be increased to 120 mg (given as a single 120 mg tablet or as two 60 mg tablets) once daily. Rarely, 240 mg may be required. Suggested regimen is to give daily dose in the morning on arising. Do not crush or chew extended-release tablets, and swallow them together with a half glassful of fluid.

➤*Storage/Stability:*

Tablets – Store at controlled room temperature 15° to 30°C (59° to 86°F). Keep tightly closed.

Tablets, extended-release – Store at 25°C (77°F); excursions permitted to 15° to 30°C (59° to 86°F). Protect from excessive moisture.

NITROGLYCERIN, INTRAVENOUS

Rx	**Nitroglycerin** (Various, eg, American Regent)	**Solution for injection**[a]: 5 mg/mL	In 5 and 10 mL single-dose vials.
Rx	**Nitroglycerin in 5% Dextrose** (Various, eg, Abbott, Baxter)	**Injection**: 100 mcg/mL	In 250 and 500 mL glass containers.
		200 mcg/mL	In 250 and 500 mL glass containers.
		400 mcg/mL	In 250 and 500 mL glass containers.

[a] Requires dilution.

NITROGLYCERIN — INJECTION

For complete and comparative prescribing information, refer to the Nitrates group monograph.

Indications

➤*Angina pectoris:* For the treatment of angina pectoris in patients who have not responded to sublingual nitroglycerin and beta-blockers.

➤*Congestive heart failure (CHF):* For control of CHF in the setting of acute myocardial infarction (MI).

➤*Intraoperative hypotension:* For induction of intraoperative hypotension.

➤*Perioperative hypertension:* For the treatment of perioperative hypertension.

➤*Unlabeled uses:* For the management of an acute MI; treatment of hypertensive emergencies; used in combination with vasopressin to treat variceal bleeding; cocaine-induced acute coronary syndrome; management of Prinzmetal angina that occurs in patients without coronary heart disease.

Administration and Dosage

➤*Dosage requirements:* Dosage is affected by the type of container and administration set used. The usual starting adult dose in clinical studies using polyvinyl chloride (PVC) administration sets was 25 mcg/min. When using a nonabsorbing infusion set, the initial dosage should be 5 mcg/min delivered through an infusion pump capable of exact and constant delivery of the drug. Adjust subsequent titration to the clinical situation, with dose increments becoming more cautious as partial response is seen. Initial titration should be in 5 mcg/min increments, with increases every 3 to 5 minutes until some response is noted. If no response occurs at 20 mcg/min, increments of 10 and even 20 mcg/min can be used. Once a partial blood pressure response is observed, reduce the dose and lengthen the interval between increments.

Some patients with normal or low left ventricular filling pressure or pulmonary capillary wedge pressure (PCWP) (eg, angina patients without other complications) may be hypersensitive to the effects of nitroglycerin and may respond fully to doses as small as 5 mcg/min. Titrate carefully and monitor closely.

There is no fixed optimum dose. Because of variations in the responsiveness of individual patients to the drug, titrate each patient to the desired level of hemodynamic function. Continuously monitor physiologic parameters (eg, blood pressure, heart rate) and other measurements (eg, PCWP) to achieve correct dose. Maintain adequate systemic blood and coronary perfusion pressures.

➤*Preparation of infusion:* Not for direct intravenous (IV) injection. Nitroglycerin for injection is a concentrated potent drug that must be diluted prior to its infusion. Invert the glass parenteral bottle several times to assure uniform dilution of the nitroglycerin.

Initial dilution – Transfer the contents of 1 nitroglycerin vial (containing nitroglycerin 25 or 50 mg) into a 500 mL glass bottle of either 5% dextrose or 0.9% sodium chloride. This yields a final concentration of 50 mcg/mL or 100 mcg/mL. Diluting nitroglycerin 5 mg into 100 mL will also yield a final concentration of 50 mcg/mL.

After the initial dosage titration, the concentration of the solution may be increased, if necessary, to limit fluids given to the patient. The nitroglycerin concentration should not exceed 400 mcg/mL.

Maintenance dilution – It is important to consider the fluid requirements of the patient as well as the expected duration of infusion in selecting the appropriate dilution of nitroglycerin injection.

➤*Nitroglycerin for injection dilution table:* Each milliliter of nitroglycerin contains nitroglycerin 5 mg.

Total contents: each 5 mL vial contains nitroglycerin 25 mg; each 10 mL vial contains nitroglycerin 50 mg.

Nitroglycerin Dilution				
Milliliters of nitroglycerin injection		Final concentration		
		100 mcg/mL	200 mcg/mL	400 mcg/mL
Volume	mg	up to	up to	up to
5 mL	25 mg	250 mL	125 mL	—
10 mL	50 mg	500 mL	250 mL	125 mL
20 mL	100 mg	1,000 mL	500 mL	250 mL
40 mL	200 mg	—	1,000 mL	500 mL

➤*Administration sets:* Use only with glass IV bottles and administration set provided. Total amount of nitroglycerin (20% to 60%) in the final diluted solution for infusion could be adsorbed by PVC tubing of IV administration sets in general use. Greater adsorption occurs with low flow rates, high concentrations, and long tubing. Although the rate of loss is highest during early administration (when flow rates are lowest), the loss is neither constant nor self-limiting; consequently, no simple calculation or correction can convert theoretical infusion rate (based on concentration of solution) to actual delivery rate. Manufacturers have developed non-PVC infusion tubing in which nitroglycerin loss is less than 5%. Use IV sets provided by manufacturers or use similar infusion sets.

➤*Change in nitroglycerin concentration:* If the concentration is adjusted, it is imperative to flush or replace the infusion set before a new concentration is used. If the set was not flushed or replaced, it could take minutes to hours, depending upon the flow rate and the dead space of the set, for the new concentration to reach the patient.

NITROGLYCERIN — INJECTION

➤*Flow rates:*

Nitroglycerin for injection –

Flow Rate (microdrops/min = mL/h)			
	Solution Concentration (mcg/mL)		
Dose (mcg/min)	100	200	400
5	3	—	—
10	6	3	—
15	9	—	—
20	12	6	3
30	18	9	—
40	24	12	6
60	36	18	9
80	48	24	12
120	72	36	18
160	96	48	24
240	—	72	36
320	—	96	48
480	—	—	72
640	—	—	96

Premixed nitroglycerin with dextrose –

Necessary Flow Rates (mL/h)[a]			
Desired dose (mcg/min)	Solution concentration (mcg/mL)		
	100	200	400
5	3	1.5	0.8
10	6	3	1.5
15	9	4.5	2.3

Necessary Flow Rates (mL/h)[a]			
Desired dose (mcg/min)	Solution concentration (mcg/mL)		
	100	200	400
20	12	6	3
30	18	9	4.5
40	24	12	6
50	30	15	7.5
60	36	18	9
80	48	24	12
100	60	30	15
120	72	36	18
140	84	42	21
160	96	48	24
180	108	54	27
200	120	60	30
240	144	72	36
280	168	84	42
320	192	96	48
500	300	150	75

[a] With a set that produces 60 drops/mL, 1 mL/h = 1 drop/min.

➤*Admixture incompatibilities:* Nitroglycerin for injection and nitroglycerin in 5% dextrose should not be mixed with other drugs.

➤*Storage/Stability:*

Nitroglycerin for injection – Store at controlled room temperature 15° to 30°C (59° to 86°F). Discard unused portion. Protect from freezing and light.

Premixed nitroglycerin with dextrose – Store at room temperature (25°C); however, brief exposure up to 40°C does not adversely affect the product. Avoid excessive heat and protect from freezing.

NITROGLYCERIN, ORAL

Rx	**Nitroglycerin** (Various, eg, Glenmark, Konec, Pliva)	**Tablets, sublingual**: 0.3 mg (1/200 grain)	May contain lactose. In 100s.
Rx	**NitroQuick** (Ethex)		Lactose. In 100s.
Rx	**Nitrostat** (Parke-Davis)		Lactose. (N 3). White. In 100s.
Rx	**NitroTab** (Able)		Lactose. In 100s.
Rx	**Nitroglycerin** (Various, eg, Glenmark, Konec, Pliva)	**Tablets, sublingual**: 0.4 mg (1/150 grain)	May contain lactose. In 25s and 100s.
Rx	**NitroQuick** (Ethex)		Lactose. In 25s and 100s.
Rx	**Nitrostat** (Parke-Davis)		Lactose. (N 4). White. In 25s and 100s.
Rx	**NitroTab** (Able)		Lactose. In 25s and 100s.
Rx	**Nitroglycerin** (Various, eg, Glenmark, Konec, Pliva)	**Tablets, sublingual**: 0.6 mg (1/100 grain)	May contain lactose. In 100s.
Rx	**NitroQuick** (Ethex)		Lactose. In 100s.
Rx	**Nitrostat** (Parke-Davis)		Lactose. (N 6). White. In 100s.
Rx	**NitroTab** (Able)		Lactose. In 100s.
Rx	**Nitroglycerin** (Various, eg, Dixon-Shane, Goldline, Major, Moore, Rugby, URL, Vitarino)	**Capsules, extended-release**: 2.5 mg	In 60s, 100s, and UD 60s and 100s.
Rx	**Nitro-Time** (Time-Cap Labs)		Lactose, sucrose. (TCL-1221). Pink/clear. In 60s, 90s, and 100s.
Rx	**Nitroglycerin** (Various, eg, Dixon-Shane, Goldline, Major, Moore, Rugby, URL, Vitarine)	**Capsules, extended-release**: 6.5 mg	In 60s, 100s, and UD 100s.
Rx	**Nitro-Time** (Time-Cap Labs)		Lactose, sucrose. (TCL-1222). Blue/yellow. In 60s, 90s, and 100s.
Rx	**Nitroglycerin** (Various, eg, Dixon-Shane, Major, Moore, Rugby, URL, Vitarine)	**Capsules, extended-release**: 9 mg	In 30s, 60s, 100s, and UD 100s.
Rx	**Nitro-Time** (Time-Cap Labs)		Lactose, sucrose. (TCL-1223). Green/yellow. In 60s, 90s, and 100s.
Rx	**Nitrolingual** (First Horizon)	**Aerosol spray, lingual**: 0.4 mg/metered dose	Alcohol 20%, peppermint oil. In 4.9 and 12 g (60 and 200 metered doses).

NITROGLYCERIN — ORAL

For complete and comparative prescribing information, refer to the Nitrates group monograph.

Indications

➤*Angina pectoris:* For acute relief of an attack (sublingual tablets, lingual spray only) or prophylaxis of angina pectoris caused by coronary artery disease.

The onset of action of nitroglycerin extended-release capsules is not sufficiently rapid for this product to be useful in aborting an acute anginal episode.

➤*Unlabeled uses:*

Nitroglycerin sublingual – For the management of an acute myocardial infarction (MI); management of Prinzmetal angina that occurs in patients without coronary heart disease.

Administration and Dosage

➤*Tablets, sublingual:* Dissolve 1 tablet under tongue or in buccal pouch (between cheek and gum) at first sign of an acute anginal attack. Dose may be repeated approximately every 5 minutes until relief is obtained. Take no more than 3 tablets in a 15-minute period. If pain continues, prompt medical

NITROGLYCERIN — ORAL

attention is recommended. May be used prophylactically 5 to 10 minutes prior to engaging in activities that might precipitate an acute attack. Do not swallow tablet.

The patient should rest during administration, preferably in the sitting position.

➤*Capsules, extended-release:* The usual starting dose is 2.5 to 6.5 mg, 3 or 4 times daily. Titrate upward to an effective dose until side effects limit the dose. Upward dose titration in these increments 2 to 4 times daily over a period of days or weeks can be attempted. In studies, doses as high as 26 mg given 4 times daily have been effective.

Give the smallest effective dose 2 to 4 times daily. Monitor blood pressure at initiation of therapy or with dosage change.

Capsules must be swallowed; not for chewing or sublingual use.

➤*Aerosol spray:*

Dosage – At the onset of attack, spray 1 or 2 metered doses onto or under the tongue. No more than 3 metered doses are recommended within a 15-minute period. If chest pain persists, prompt medical attention is recommended. May be used prophylactically 5 to 10 minutes prior to engaging in activities that might precipitate an acute attack.

Administration – During application the patient should rest, ideally in the sitting position. The container should be held vertically with the valve head uppermost and the spray orifice as close to the mouth as possible. The dose should preferably be sprayed onto the tongue by pressing the button firmly and the mouth should be closed immediately after each dose. Do not inhale spray. The medication should not be expectorated or the mouth rinsed for 5 to 10 minutes following administration. Instruct patients to familiarize themselves with the position of the spray orifice, which can be identified by the finger rest on top of the valve, in order to facilitate orientation for administration at night.

➤*Storage / Stability:*

Tablets, sublingual – Store at controlled room temperature 25°C (77°F); excursions permitted to 15° to 30°C (59° to 86°F). Protect from moisture.

Capsules, extended-release – Store at controlled room temperature 15° to 30°C (59° to 86°F). Dispense in a tight container.

Aerosol spray – Store at 25°C (77°F); excursions permitted to 15° to 30°C (59° to 86°F).

NITROGLYCERIN TOPICAL

Rx	**Nitroglycerin** (Various, eg, DHS)	**Ointment**: 2%	In 30 and 60 g tubes.
Rx	**Nitro-Bid** (E Fougera)		Lactose. In a lanolin-white petrolatum base. In 30 and 60 g tubes and UD 1 g.

[a] Various systems have the same release rates but variable surface areas and nitroglycerin contents.

NITROGLYCERIN — TOPICAL

For complete and comparative prescribing information, refer to the Nitrates group monograph.

Indications

➤*Angina pectoris:* For the prevention of angina pectoris caused by coronary artery disease. The onset of action of nitroglycerin ointment is not sufficiently rapid for this product to be useful in aborting an acute attack.

➤*Unlabeled uses:* Used topically in the treatment of anal fissures in children.

For the management of an acute myocardial infarction (MI); treatment of chronic anal fissure pain; erectile dysfunction; Raynaud disease; management of Prinzmetal angina that occurs in patients without coronary heart disease.

Administration and Dosage

➤*Usual therapeutic dose:* Apply 2 daily ½ inch (7.5 mg) doses, 1 applied on rising in the morning and 1 applied 6 hours later. The dose can be doubled and even doubled again in patients tolerating this dose but failing to respond to it.

➤*Administration:* Each tube of ointment is supplied with a pad of ruled, impermeable paper applicators. To apply the ointment using 1 of the applicators, place the applicator on a flat surface, printed side down. Squeeze the necessary amount of ointment from the tube onto the applicator, place the applicator (ointment side down) on the desired area of the skin, and tape the applicator into place.

➤*Storage / Stability:* Store at controlled room temperature at 15° to 30°C (59° to 86°F). Close tightly immediately after use.

NITROGLYCERIN TRANSDERMAL

Rx	**Nitroglycerin Transdermal** (Mylan)	**Transdermal patch**: 0.1 mg/h	4 cm^2 surface area. In 30s.
Rx	**Minitran** (3M)	**Transdermal patch**: 0.1 mg/h (9 mg total nitroglycerin)	3.3 cm^2 surface area. In 30s.
Rx	**Nitro-Dur** (Key)	**Transdermal patch**: 0.1 mg/h (20 mg total nitroglycerin)	5 cm^2 surface area. In 30s and UD 30s.
Rx	**Nitroglycerin Transdermal** (Various, eg, Hercon Labs, Major, Mylan)	**Transdermal patch**: 0.2 mg/h (16 to 62.5 mg[a] total nitroglycerin)	6 to 10 cm^2 surface area.[a] In 30s.
Rx	**Minitran** (3M)	**Transdermal patch**: 0.2 mg/h (18 mg total nitroglycerin)	6.7 cm^2 surface area. In 30s.
Rx	**Nitrek** (Bertek)	**Transdermal patch**: 0.2 mg/h (22.4 mg total nitroglycerin)	8 cm^2 surface area. In 30s.
Rx	**Nitro-Dur** (Key)	**Transdermal patch**: 0.2 mg/h (40 mg total nitroglycerin)	10 cm^2 surface area. In 30s and UD 30s.
Rx	**Nitro-Dur** (Key)	**Transdermal patch**: 0.3 mg/h (60 mg total nitroglycerin)	15 cm^2 surface area. In 30s and UD 30s.
Rx	**Nitroglycerin Transdermal** (Various, eg, Hercon Labs, Major, Mylan)	**Transdermal patch**: 0.4 mg/h (32 to 125 mg[a] total nitroglycerin)	13 to 20 cm^2 surface area.[a] In 30s.
Rx	**Minitran** (3M)	**Transdermal patch**: 0.4 mg/h (36 mg total nitroglycerin)	13.3 cm^2 surface area. In 30s.
Rx	**Nitrek** (Bertek)	**Transdermal patch**: 0.4 mg/h (44.8 mg total nitroglycerin)	16 cm^2 surface area. In 30s.
Rx	**Nitro-Dur** (Key)	**Transdermal patch**: 0.4 mg/h (80 mg total nitroglycerin)	20 cm^2 surface area. In 30s and UD 30s.
Rx	**Nitroglycerin Transdermal** (Various, eg, Hercon Labs, Major, Mylan)	**Transdermal patch**: 0.6 mg/h (75 to 187.5 mg[a] total nitroglycerin)	20 to 30 cm^2 surface area.[a] In 30s.
Rx	**Minitran** (3M)	**Transdermal patch**: 0.6 mg/h (54 mg total nitroglycerin)	20 cm^2 surface area. In 30s.
Rx	**Nitrek** (Bertek)	**Transdermal patch**: 0.6 mg/h (67.2 mg total nitroglycerin)	24 cm^2 surface area. In 30s.
Rx	**Nitro-Dur** (Key)	**Transdermal patch**: 0.6 mg/h (120 mg total nitroglycerin)	30 cm^2 surface area. In 30s and UD 30s.
Rx	**Nitro-Dur** (Key)	**Transdermal patch**: 0.8 mg/h (160 mg total nitroglycerin)	40 cm^2 surface area. In 30s and UD 30s.

[a] Various systems have the same release rates but variable surface areas and nitroglycerin contents.

Nitrates

NITROGLYCERIN — TRANSDERMAL

For complete and comparative prescribing information, refer to the Nitrates group monograph.

Indications

➤*Angina pectoris:* For the prevention of angina pectoris caused by coronary artery disease. The onset of action of transdermal nitroglycerin is not sufficiently rapid for this product to be useful in aborting an acute attack.

➤*Unlabeled uses:* For the management of an acute myocardial infarction (MI); treatment of chronic anal fissure pain; erectile dysfunction; Raynaud disease; management of Prinzmetal angina that occurs in patients without coronary heart disease.

Administration and Dosage

➤*Application of system:* Apply once daily to a skin site free of hair and not subject to excessive movement. Do not apply to distal parts of extremities such as below the knee or elbow. The chest is the preferred site. Avoid areas with cuts or irritations. Do not apply the patch immediately after showering or bathing; it is best to wait until the skin is completely dry. After applying the patch, wash hands to remove any drug. Once the patch is securely on, contact with water (eg, bathing, swimming, showering) will not affect the patch. In the unlikely event that a patch falls off, discard it and put a new one on a different skin site.

➤*Starting dose:* 0.2 to 0.4 mg/h. Doses between 0.4 and 0.8 mg/h have shown continued effectiveness for 10 to 12 hours daily for at least 1 month of intermittent administration. Although the minimum nitrate-free interval has not been defined, data show that a nitrate-free interval of 10 to 12 hours is sufficient. Thus, an appropriate dosing schedule would include a daily "patch-on" period of 12 to 14 hours and a "patch-off" period of 10 to 12 hours. Tolerance is a major factor limiting efficacy when the system is used continuously for more than 12 hours each day.

➤*Storage/Stability:* Store at controlled room temperature 15° to 30°C (59° to 86°F). Avoid extremes of temperature and/or humidity. Do not refrigerate. Do not store outside of the protective package. Apply immediately upon removal from package.

Peripheral Vasodilators

ISOXSUPRINE HYDROCHLORIDE

Rx	**Isoxsuprine HCl** (Various)	**Tablets**: 10 mg	In 60s, 100s, 500s, 1000s and UD 100s.
Rx	**Vasodilan** (Mead Johnson)		(10 MJ 543). In 100s, 1000s and UD 1000s.
Rx	**Voxsuprine** (Major)		In 100s, 250s, 1000s and UD 100s.
Rx	**Isoxsuprine HCl** (Various)	**Tablets**: 20 mg	In 60s, 100s, 500s, 1000s and UD 100s.
Rx	**Vasodilan** (Mead Johnson)		(20 MJ 544). In 100s and 1000s.
Rx	**Voxsuprine** (Major)		In 100s, 250s, 1000s and UD 100s.

ISOXSUPRINE HYDROCHLORIDE — ORAL

For complete prescribing information, refer to the Antihypertensives Treatment Guidelines in the Appendix.

Indications

➤*"Possibly effective":* For relief of symptoms associated with cerebral vascular insufficiency; peripheral vascular disease of arteriosclerosis obliterans, thromboangiitis obliterans (Buerger disease) and Raynaud disease.

➤*Unlabeled uses:* Isoxsuprine has been used in the treatment of dysmenorrhea and threatened premature labor, but efficacy has not been established.

Administration and Dosage

10 to 20 mg 3 or 4 times daily.

Actions

➤*Pharmacology:* Isoxsuprine is a vasodilator that acts primarily on blood vessels within skeletal muscle. In healthy subjects, resting blood flow in skeletal muscle is increased; cutaneous blood flow is usually not affected. Isoxsuprine is an alpha-adrenoreceptor antagonist with beta-adrenoreceptor stimulating properties; however, vasodilation is not blocked by propranolol. Isoxsuprine may act directly on vascular smooth muscle. The drug also causes cardiac stimulation (increased contractility, heart rate and cardiac output) and uterine relaxation. At high doses, it lowers blood viscosity and inhibits platelet aggregation.

Contraindications

Immediately postpartum; in the presence of arterial bleeding.

Warnings

➤*Rash:* If rash appears, discontinue use. A causal relationship is not established.

➤*Pregnancy:* *Category C.* There are no reports of isoxsuprine causing congenital defects. Hypotension, hypocalcemia, hypoglycemia, ileus, tachycardia and death have occurred when cord serum levels are more than 10 ng/mL.

Pulmonary edema has been reported in mothers treated with beta-stimulants. Isoxsuprine is neither approved nor recommended for the treatment of premature labor.

Adverse Reactions

➤*Cardiovascular:* Hypotension; tachycardia; chest pain.

➤*GI:* Nausea; vomiting; abdominal distress.

➤*Miscellaneous:* Dizziness; weakness; severe rash.

Patient Information

May cause palpitations or skin rash. Notify physician if these symptoms become particularly bothersome.

If dizziness (orthostatic hypotension) occurs, avoid sudden changes in posture.

PAPAVERINE HYDROCHLORIDE

Rx	**Papaverine HCl** (Various, eg, Eon, Qualitest, Time-Cap Labs)	**Capsules, extended release**: 150 mg	In 100s, 500s, and 1000s.
Rx	**Papaverine HCl** (Various)	**Injection**: 30 mg/mL	In 2 mL vials and 10 mL multiple-dose vials.

PAPAVERINE HYDROCHLORIDE — ORAL

For more information, refer to the Antihypertensives Treatment Guidelines in the Appendix.

Indications

➤*Ischemia:* For relief of cerebral and peripheral ischemia associated with arterial spasm and myocardial ischemia complicated by arrhythmias.

Administration and Dosage

➤*Dosage:* One capsule every 12 hours. In difficult cases, administration may be increased to 1 capsule every 8 hours or 2 capsules every 12 hours.

Store at controlled room temperature, 15° to 30°C (59° to 86°F). Dispense in tight, light resistant containers.

PAPAVERINE HYDROCHLORIDE — INJECTION

For more information, refer to the Antihypertensives Treatment Guidelines in the Appendix.

Indications

Papaverine is recommended in various conditions accompanied by spasm of smooth muscle, such as vascular spasm associated with acute MI (coronary occlusion), angina pectoris, peripheral and pulmonary embolism, peripheral vascular disease in which there is a vasospastic element, or certain cerebral angiospastic states; and visceral spasm, as in ureteral, biliary, or gastrointestinal colic.

Administration and Dosage

Papaverine may be administered intravenously or intramuscularly. The intravenous route is recommended when an immediate effect is desired, but the drug must be injected slowly over the course of 1 or 2 minutes to avoid uncomfortable or alarming side effects.

Parenteral administration of papaverine in doses of 1 to 4 mL is repeated every 3 hours as indicated. In the treatment of cardiac extrasystoles, 2 doses may be given 10 minutes apart.

➤*Incompatibilities:* Papaverine injection should not be added to Ringer's lactate injection, because precipitation would result.

➤*Storage/Stability:* Store at controlled room temperature 15° to 30°C (59° to 86°F). Protect from light. Retain in carton until time of use.

Actions

➤*Pharmacology:* The most characteristic effect of papaverine is relaxation of the tonus of all smooth muscle, especially when it has been spasmodically

PAPAVERINE HYDROCHLORIDE — INJECTION

contracted. Papaverine apparently acts directly on the muscle itself. This relaxation is noted in the vascular system and bronchial musculature and in the gastrointestinal, biliary, and urinary tracts.

The main actions of papaverine are exerted on cardiac and smooth muscle. Papaverine relaxes various smooth muscles, especially those of larger arteries; this relaxation may be prominent if spasm exists. The antispasmodic effect is a direct one and unrelated to muscle innervation, and the muscle still responds to drugs and other stimuli causing contraction. Papaverine has minimal actions on the CNS, although very large doses tend to produce some sedation and sleepiness in some patients. In certain circumstances, mild respiratory stimulation can be observed, but this is therapeutically inconsequential. Papaverine stimulates respiration by acting on carotid and aortic body chemoreceptors.

Papaverine relaxes the smooth musculature of the larger blood vessels, including the coronary, cerebral, peripheral, and pulmonary arteries. This action is particularly evident when such vessels are in spasm, induced reflexly or by drugs, and it provides the basis for the clinical use of papaverine in peripheral or pulmonary arterial embolism.

Experimentally in dogs, the alkaloid has been shown to cause fairly marked and long-lasting coronary vasodilatation and an increase in coronary blood flow. However, it also appears to have a direct inotropic effect and, when increased mechanical activity coincides with decreased systemic pressure, increases in coronary blood flow may not be sufficient to prevent brief periods of hypoxic myocardial depression.

➤*Pharmacokinetics:*

Absorption – Papaverine is effective by all routes of administration. A considerable fraction of the drug localizes in fat depots and in the liver, with the remainder being distributed throughout the body.

Distribution – About 90% of the drug is bound to plasma protein. Although estimates of its biologic half-life vary widely, reasonably constant plasma levels can be maintained with oral administration at 6-hour intervals.

Metabolism – It is metabolized in the liver.

Excretion – The drug is excreted in the urine in an inactive form.

Contraindications

IV injection of papaverine is contraindicated in the presence of complete atrioventricular heart block. When conduction is depressed, the drug may produce transient ectopic rhythms of ventricular origin, either premature beats or paroxysmal tachycardia.

Papaverine is not indicated for the treatment of impotence by intracorporeal injection. The intracorporeal injection of papaverine has been reported to have resulted in persistent priapism requiring medical and surgical intervention.

Warnings

➤*Cardiac:* Large doses can depress AV and intraventricular conduction and thereby produce serious arrhythmias. When conduction is depressed, it may produce transient ectopy of ventricular origin, either premature beats or paroxysmal tachycardia.

➤*Hepatic effects:* Chronic hepatitis, as evidenced by an increase in serum bilirubin and serum glutamic transaminase, has been reported in 3 cases following long-term papaverine therapy. One patient had jaundice, and another had abnormal liver function on biopsy.

The medication should be discontinued if hepatic hypersensitivity with GI symptoms, jaundice, or eosinophilia becomes evident or if liver function test values become altered.

➤*Pregnancy: Category C.* No teratogenic effects were observed in rats when papaverine was administered subcutaneously as a single agent. It is not known whether papaverine can cause fetal harm when administered to a pregnant woman or can affect reproduction capacity.

➤*Lactation:* It is not known whether this drug is excreted in human milk. Because many drugs are excreted in human milk, caution should be exercised when papaverine is administered to a breast-feeding woman.

➤*Children:* Safety and efficacy for use in children have not been established.

Precautions

➤*Special risk:* Use with caution in patients with glaucoma.

➤*Drug abuse and dependence:* Drug dependence resulting from the abuse of many of the selective depressants, including papaverine, has been reported.

Drug Interactions

➤*Levodopa:* Loss of control of Parkinson disease may occur following the introduction of papaverine. Although the mechanism is unknown, papaverine may block dopamine receptors in the striatum.

Adverse Reactions

The following adverse reactions have been reported: general discomfort, nausea, abdominal discomfort, anorexia, constipation or diarrhea, skin rash, malaise, vertigo, headache, intensive flushing of the face, perspiration, increase in the depth of respiration, increase in heart rate, a slight rise in blood pressure, and excessive sedation.

Hepatitis, probably related to an immune mechanism, has been reported infrequently. Rarely, this has progressed to cirrhosis.

Overdosage

➤*Symptoms:* The symptoms of toxicity from papaverine often result from vasomotor instability and include nausea, vomiting, weakness, central nervous system depression, nystagmus, diplopia, diaphoresis, flushing, dizziness, and sinus tachycardia. In large overdoses, papaverine is a potent inhibitor of cellular respiration and a weak calcium antagonist. Following an oral overdose of 15 g, metabolic acidosis with hyperventilation, hyperglycemia, and hypokalemia have been reported. No information on toxic serum concentrations is available.

➤*Treatment:* To obtain up-to-date information about the treatment of overdose, a good resource is your certified regional poison control center. In managing overdosage, consider the possibility of multiple drug overdoses, interaction among drugs, and unusual drug kinetics in your patient.

Protect the patient's airway and support ventilation and perfusion. Meticulously monitor vital signs, blood gases, blood chemistry values, and other variables.

If convulsions occur, consider diazepam, phenytoin, or phenobarbital. If the seizures are refractory, general anesthesia with thiopental or halothane and paralysis with a neuromuscular blocking agent may be necessary.

For hypotension, consider intravenous fluids, elevation of the legs, and an inotropic vasopressor, such as dopamine or norepinephrine (levarterenol). Theoretically, calcium gluconate may be helpful in treating some of the toxic cardiovascular effects of papaverine; monitor the ECG and plasma calcium concentrations.

Forced diuresis, peritoneal dialysis, hemodialysis, or charcoal hemoperfusion have not been established as beneficial for an overdose of papaverine.

HYDRALAZINE HYDROCHLORIDE

Rx	**Hydralazine** (Various, eg, Camall, Goldline, Rugby, Schein)	**Tablets:** 10 mg	In 100s, 1000s and UD 100s.
Rx	**Apresoline** (Novartis)		Lactose. Yellow. In 100s and 1200s.
Rx	**Hydralazine** (Various, eg, Camall, Goldline, Rugby)	**Tablets:** 25 mg	In 100s, 1000s and UD 100s.
Rx	**Apresoline** (Novartis)		Blue. In 100s and 1000s.
Rx	**Hydralazine** (Various, eg, Camall, Goldline, Rugby)	**Tablets:** 50 mg	In 100s, 1000s and UD 100s.
Rx	**Apresoline** (Novartis)		Lactose. Light blue. In 100s and 1000s.
Rx	**Hydralazine** (Various, eg, Camall, Goldline, Rugby)	**Tablets:** 100 mg	In 100s and 1000s.
Rx	**Apresoline** (Novartis)		Tartrazine. Peach. In 100s.
Rx	**Hydralazine** (Solopak)	**Injection:** 20 mg per mL	In 1 mL vials.

HYDRALAZINE HYDROCHLORIDE — ORAL

For more information, refer to the Antihypertensives Treatment Guidelines in the Appendix.

Indications

Essential hypertension, alone or as an adjunct.

➤*Unlabeled uses:* Hydralazine in doses up to 800 mg 3 times daily has been effective in reducing afterload in the treatment of congestive heart failure (CHF) and severe aortic insufficiency and after valve replacement.

Administration and Dosage

Initiate therapy in gradually increasing dosages; adjust according to individual response. Start with 10 mg 4 times daily for the first 2 to 4 days, increase to 25 mg 4 times daily for the balance of the first week. For the second and subsequent weeks, increase dosage to 50 mg 4 times daily. For maintenance, adjust dosage to the lowest effective levels.

The incidence of toxic reactions, particularly the LE cell syndrome, is high in the group of patients receiving large doses of hydralazine hydrochloride.

In a few resistant patients, up to 300 mg of hydralazine hydrochloride daily may be required for a significant antihypertensive effect. In such cases, a lower dosage of hydralazine hydrochloride combined with a thiazide or reserpine or a beta-blocker may be considered. However, when combining therapy, individual titration is essential to ensure the lowest possible therapeutic dose of each drug.

➤*Children:* Safety and efficacy in pediatric patients have not been established in controlled clinical trials; although, there is experience with the use of hydralazine in these patients. The usual recommended oral starting dos-

HYDRALAZINE HYDROCHLORIDE — ORAL

age is 0.75 mg/kg of body weight daily in 4 divided doses. Dosage may be increased gradually over the next 3 to 4 weeks to a maximum of 7.5 mg/kg or 200 mg daily.

➤*Storage/Stability:* Do not store above 30°C (86°F).

Dispense in tight, light-resistant container.

Actions

➤*Pharmacology:* Although the precise mechanism of action of hydralazine is not fully understood, the major effects are on the cardiovascular system. Hydralazine apparently lowers blood pressure by exerting a peripheral, vasodilating effect through a direct relaxation of vascular smooth muscle. Hydralazine, by altering cellular calcium metabolism, interferes with the calcium movements within the vascular smooth muscle that are responsible for initiating or maintaining the contractile state.

The peripheral, vasodilating effect of hydralazine results in decreased arterial blood pressure (diastolic more than systolic); decreased peripheral vascular resistance; and an increased heart rate, stroke volume, and cardiac output. The preferential dilatation of arterioles, as compared to veins, minimizes postural hypotension and promotes the increase in cardiac output. Hydralazine usually increases renin activity in plasma, presumably as a result of increased secretion of renin by the renal juxtaglomerular cells in response to reflex sympathetic discharge. This increase in renin activity leads to the production of angiotensin II, which then causes stimulation of aldosterone and consequent sodium reabsorption. Hydralazine also maintains or increases renal and cerebral blood flow.

➤*Pharmacokinetics:*

Absorption/Distribution – Hydralazine is rapidly absorbed after oral administration, and peak plasma levels are reached at 1 to 2 hours. Plasma levels of apparent hydralazine decline with a half-life of 3 to 7 hours. Binding to human plasma protein is 87%. Plasma levels of hydralazine vary widely among individuals. Hydralazine is subject to polymorphic acetylation; slow acetylators generally have higher plasma levels of hydralazine and require lower doses to maintain control of blood pressure.

Metabolism/Excretion – Hydralazine undergoes extensive hepatic metabolism; it is excreted mainly in the form of metabolites in the urine.

Contraindications

Hypersensitivity to hydralazine; coronary artery disease; mitral valvular rheumatic heart disease.

Warnings

➤*Systemic erythematosus-like symptoms:* In a few patients, hydralazine may produce a clinical picture simulating systemic lupus erythematosus, including glomerulonephritis. In such patients, hydralazine should be discontinued unless the benefit-to-risk determination requires continued antihypertensive therapy with this drug. Symptoms and signs usually regress when the drug is discontinued, but residua have been detected many years later. Long-term treatment with steroids may be necessary.

➤*Carcinogenesis:* In a lifetime study in Swiss albino mice, there was a statistically significant increase in the incidence of lung tumors (adenomas and adenocarcinomas) of both male and female mice given hydralazine continuously in their drinking water at a dosage of about 250 mg/kg/day (about 80 times the maximum recommended human dose). In a 2-year carcinogenicity study of rats given hydralazine by gavage at dose levels of 15, 30, and 60 mg/kg/day ($\approx$ 5 to 20 times the recommended human daily dosage), microscopic examination of the liver revealed a small, but statistically significant, increase in benign neoplastic nodules in male and female rats from the high-dose group and in female rats from the intermediate-dose group. Benign interstitial cell tumors of the testes were also significantly increased in male rats from the high-dose group. The tumors observed are common in aged rats, and a significantly increased incidence was not observed until 18 months of treatment.

➤*Mutagenesis:* Hydralazine was shown to be mutagenic in bacterial systems (gene mutation and DNA repair) and in 1 of 2 rats and 1 rabbit hepatocyte in vitro DNA repair studies. Additional in vivo and in vitro studies, using lymphoma cells, germinal cells, and fibroblasts from mice, bone marrow cells from Chinese hamsters, and fibroblasts from human cell lines, did not demonstrate any mutagenic potential for hydralazine.

➤*Pregnancy: Category C.* Animal studies indicate that hydralazine is teratogenic in mice at 20 to 30 times the maximum daily human dose of 200 to 300 mg and possibly in rabbits at 10 to 15 times the maximum daily human dose, but that it is nonteratogenic in rats. Teratogenic effects observed were cleft palate and malformations of facial and cranial bones.

There are no adequate and well-controlled studies in pregnant women. Although clinical experience does not include any positive evidence of adverse effects on the human fetus, hydralazine should be used during pregnancy only if the expected benefit justifies the potential risk to the fetus.

➤*Lactation:* Hydralazine has been shown to be excreted in breast milk. Because many drugs are excreted in human milk, caution should be exercised when hydralazine is administered to a breast-feeding woman.

➤*Children:* Safety and efficacy in pediatric patients have not been established in controlled clinical trials; although, there is experience with the use of hydralazine in these patients. The usual recommended oral starting dosage is 0.75 mg/kg of body weight daily in 4 divided doses. Dosage may be increased gradually over the next 3 to 4 weeks to a maximum of 7.5 mg/kg or 200 mg daily.

Precautions

➤*Monitoring:* Complete blood counts and antinuclear antibody titer determinations are indicated before and periodically during prolonged therapy with hydralazine, even though the patient is asymptomatic. These studies are also indicated if the patient develops arthralgia, fever, chest pain, continued malaise, or other unexplained signs or symptoms.

A positive antinuclear antibody titer requires that the physician carefully weigh the implications of the test results against the benefits to be derived from antihypertensive therapy with hydralazine.

➤*Peripheral neuritis:* Peripheral neuritis, evidenced by paresthesia, numbness, and tingling, has been observed. Published evidence suggests an antipyridoxine effect, and that pyridoxine should be added to the regimen if symptoms develop.

➤*Cardiovascular effects:* Myocardial stimulation produced by hydralazine hydrochloride can cause anginal attacks and ECG changes of myocardial ischemia. The drug has been implicated in the production of myocardial infarction (MI). It must, therefore, be used with caution in patients with suspected coronary artery disease.

The "hyperdynamic" circulation caused by hydralazine hydrochloride may accentuate specific cardiovascular inadequacies. For example, hydralazine hydrochloride may increase pulmonary artery pressure in patients with mitral valvular disease. The drug may reduce the pressor responses to epinephrine. Postural hypotension may result from hydralazine hydrochloride but is less common than with ganglionic-blocking agents. It should be used with caution in patients with cerebral vascular accidents.

➤*Renal effects:* In hypertensive patients with healthy kidneys who are treated with hydralazine hydrochloride, there is evidence of increased renal blood flow and a maintenance of glomerular filtration rate. In some instances where control values were below normal, improved renal function has been noted after administration of hydralazine hydrochloride. However, as with any antihypertensive agent, hydralazine hydrochloride should be used with caution in patients with advanced renal damage.

➤*Tartrazine sensitivity:* Some of these products may contain FD&C Yellow No. 5 (tartrazine), which may cause allergic-type reactions (including bronchial asthma) in certain susceptible individuals. Although the overall incidence of FD&C Yellow No. 5 (tartrazine) sensitivity in the general population is low, it is frequently seen in patients who are also hypersensitive to aspirin.

Drug Interactions

Hydralazine Drug Interactions

Precipitant drug	Object drug*		Description
Beta blockers Metoprolol Propranolol	Hydralazine	⬆	Serum levels of either drug may be increased by concurrent use.
Hydralazine	Beta blockers Metoprolol Propranolol	⬆	
Indomethacin	Hydralazine	⬇	The pharmacologic effects of hydralazine may be decreased.

* ⬆ = Object drug increased. ⬇ = Object drug decreased.

MAO inhibitors should be used with caution in patients receiving hydralazine.

When other potent parenteral antihypertensive drugs, such as diazoxide, are used in combination with hydralazine, patients should be continuously observed for several hours for any excessive fall in blood pressure. Profound hypotensive episodes may occur when diazoxide injection and hydralazine hydrochloride are used concomitantly.

➤*Drug/Food interactions:* Administration of hydralazine with food results in higher plasma levels.

Adverse Reactions

Adverse reactions with hydralazine hydrochloride are usually reversible when dosage is reduced. However, in some cases it may be necessary to discontinue the drug.

The following adverse reactions have been observed, but there has not been enough systematic collection of data to support an estimate of their frequency.

➤*Common:*

Miscellaneous – Headache, anorexia, nausea, vomiting, diarrhea, palpitations, tachycardia, angina pectoris.

➤*Less frequent:*

Cardiovascular – Hypotension, paradoxical pressor response, edema.

CNS – Peripheral neuritis, evidenced by paresthesia, numbness, and tingling; dizziness; tremors; muscle cramps; psychotic reactions characterized by depression, disorientation, or anxiety.

GI – Constipation and paralytic ileus.

GU – Difficulty in urination.

Hematologic – Blood dyscrasias, consisting of reduction in hemoglobin and red cell count; leukopenia; agranulocytosis; purpura; lymphadenopathy; splenomegaly.

Hypersensitivity – Rash, urticaria, pruritus, fever, chills, arthralgia, eosinophilia, and, rarely, hepatitis.

HYDRALAZINE HYDROCHLORIDE — ORAL

Respiratory – Dyspnea.

Miscellaneous – Nasal congestion, flushing, lacrimation, conjunctivitis.

Overdosage

➤*Highest known dose survived:* Adults, 10 g orally.

➤*Symptoms:* Signs and symptoms of overdosage include hypotension, tachycardia, headache, and generalized skin flushing.

Complications can include myocardial ischemia and subsequent MI, cardiac arrhythmia, and profound shock.

➤*Treatment:* There is no specific antidote.

The gastric contents should be evacuated, taking adequate precautions against aspiration and for protection of the airway. An activated charcoal slurry may be instilled if conditions permit. These manipulations may have to be omitted or carried out after cardiovascular status has been stabilized, since they might precipitate cardiac arrhythmias or increase the depth of shock.

Support of the cardiovascular system is of primary importance. Shock should be treated with plasma expanders. If possible, vasopressors should not be given, but if a vasopressor is required, care should be taken not to precipitate or aggravate cardiac arrhythmia. Tachycardia responds to beta blockers. Digitalization may be necessary, and renal function should be monitored and supported as required.

No experience has been reported with extracorporeal or peritoneal dialysis.

Patient Information

Patients should be informed of possible side effects and advised to take the medication regularly and continuously as directed.

HYDRALAZINE HYDROCHLORIDE — INJECTION

For more information, refer to the Antihypertensives Treatment Guidelines in the Appendix.

Indications

Severe essential hypertension when the drug cannot be given orally or when there is an urgent need to lower blood pressure.

➤*Unlabeled uses:* Hydralazine in doses up to 800 mg 3 times daily has been effective in reducing afterload in the treatment of congestive heart failure (CHF), severe aortic insufficiency and after valve replacement.

Administration and Dosage

➤*Approved by the FDA:* June 30, 1997.

When there is urgent need, therapy in the hospitalized patient may be initiated intramuscularly or as a rapid intravenous bolus injection directly into the vein. Hydralazine hydrochloride injection should be used only when the drug cannot be given orally. The usual dose is 20 to 40 mg, repeated as necessary.

Certain patients (especially those with marked renal damage) may require a lower dose. Blood pressure should be checked frequently. It may begin to fall within a few minutes after injection, with the average maximal decrease occurring in 10 to 80 minutes. In cases where there has been increased intracranial pressure, lowering the blood pressure may increase cerebral ischemia. Most patients can be transferred to oral hydralazine hydrochloride within 24 to 48 hours.

The product should be used immediately after the vial is opened. It should not be added to infusion solutions. Hydralazine injection may discolor upon contact with metal; discolored solutions should be discarded.

➤*Storage/Stability:* Store between 15° to 30°C (59° to 86°F).

Actions

➤*Pharmacology:* Although the precise mechanism of action of hydralazine is not fully understood, the major effects are on the cardiovascular system. Hydralazine apparently lowers blood pressure by exerting a peripheral vasodilating effect through a direct relaxation of vascular smooth muscle. Hydralazine, by altering cellular calcium metabolism, interferes with the calcium movements within the vascular smooth muscle that are responsible for initiating or maintaining the contractile state.

The peripheral vasodilating effect of hydralazine results in decreased arterial blood pressure (diastolic more than systolic); decreased peripheral vascular resistance; and an increased heart rate, stroke volume, and cardiac output. The preferential dilatation of arterioles, as compared to veins, minimizes postural hypotension and promotes the increase in cardiac output. Hydralazine usually increases renin activity in plasma, presumably as a result of increased secretion of renin by the renal juxtaglomerular cells in response to reflex sympathetic discharge. This increase in renin activity leads to the production of angiotensin II, which then causes stimulation of aldosterone and consequent sodium reabsorption. Hydralazine also maintains or increases renal and cerebral blood flow.

The average maximal decrease in blood pressure usually occurs 10 to 80 minutes after administration of hydralazine injection. No other pharmacokinetic data on hydralazine injection are available.

Contraindications

Hypersensitivity to hydralazine; coronary artery disease; mitral valvular rheumatic heart disease.

Warnings

➤*Systemic lupus erythematosus-like symptoms:* In a few patients hydralazine may produce a clinical picture simulating systemic lupus erythematosus including glomerulonephritis. In such patients hydralazine should be discontinued unless the benefit-to-risk determination requires continued antihypertensive therapy with this drug. Symptoms and signs usually regress when the drug is discontinued but residua have been detected many years later. Long-term treatment with steroids may be necessary.

➤*Carcinogenesis:* In a lifetime study in Swiss albino mice, there was a statistically significant increase in the incidence of lung tumors (adenomas and adenocarcinomas) of both male and female mice given hydralazine continuously in their drinking water at a dosage of about 250 mg/kg/day (about 80 times the maximum recommended human dose). In a 2-year carcinogenicity study of rats given hydralazine by gavage at dose levels of 15, 30, and 60 mg/kg/day (approximately 5 to 20 times the recommended human daily dosage), microscopic examination of the liver revealed a small, but statistically significant, increase in benign neoplastic nodules in male and female rats from the high-dose group and in female rats from the intermediate-dose group. Benign interstitial cell tumors of the testes were also significantly increased in male rats from the high-dose group. The tumors observed are common in aged rats and a significantly increased incidence was not observed until 18 months of treatment. The extent to which these findings indicate a risk to man is uncertain. While long-term clinical observation has not suggested that human cancer is associated with hydralazine use, epidemiologic studies have so far been insufficient to arrive at any conclusions.

➤*Mutagenesis:* Hydralazine was shown to be mutagenic in bacterial systems (Gene Mutation and DNA Repair) and in one of two rats and one rabbit hepatocyte in vitro DNA repair studies.

➤*Pregnancy: Category C.*

Teratogenic – Animal studies indicate that hydralazine is teratogenic in mice at 20 to 30 times the maximum daily human dose of 200 to 300 mg and possibly in rabbits at 10 to 15 times the maximum daily human dose, but that it is nonteratogenic in rats. Teratogenic effects observed were cleft palate and malformations of facial and cranial bones.

There are no adequate and well-controlled studies in pregnant women. Although clinical experience does not include any positive evidence of adverse effects on the human fetus, hydralazine should be used during pregnancy only if the expected benefit justifies the potential risk to the fetus.

➤*Lactation:* It is not known whether this drug is excreted in human milk. Because many drugs are excreted in human milk, caution should be exercised when hydralazine injection is administered to a breast-feeding woman.

➤*Children:* Safety and efficacy in pediatric patients have not been established in controlled clinical trials, although there is experience with the use of hydralazine hydrochloride in children. The usual recommended parenteral dosage, administered intramuscularly or intravenously, is 1.7 to 3.5 mg/kg of body weight daily, divided into 4 to 6 doses.

Precautions

➤*Monitoring:* Complete blood counts and antinuclear antibody titer determinations are indicated before and periodically during prolonged therapy with hydralazine even though the patient is asymptomatic. These studies are also indicated if the patient develops arthralgia, fever, chest pain, continued malaise, or other unexplained signs or symptoms.

A positive antinuclear antibody titer requires that the physician carefully weigh the implications of the test results against the benefits to be derived from antihypertensive therapy with hydralazine hydrochloride.

Blood dyscrasias, consisting of reduction in hemoglobin and red cell count, leukopenia, agranulocytosis, and purpura, have been reported. If such abnormalities develop, therapy should be discontinued.

➤*Cardiovascular changes:* Myocardial stimulation produced by hydralazine can cause anginal attacks and ECG changes of myocardial ischemia. The drug has been implicated in the production of myocardial infarction. It must, therefore, be used with caution in patients with suspected coronary artery disease.

The "hyperdynamic" circulation caused by hydralazine may accentuate specific cardiovascular inadequacies. For example, hydralazine may increase pulmonary artery pressure in patients with mitral valvular disease. The drug may reduce the pressor responses to epinephrine. Postural hypotension may result from hydralazine but is less common than with ganglionic blocking agents. It should be used with caution in patients with cerebral vascular accidents.

➤*Renal effects:* In hypertensive patients with normal kidneys who are treated with hydralazine, there is evidence of increased renal blood flow and a maintenance of glomerular filtration rate. In some instances where control values were below normal, improved renal function has been noted after administration of hydralazine. However, as with any antihypertensive agent, hydralazine should be used with caution in patients with advanced renal damage.

Peripheral neuritis – Peripheral neuritis, evidenced by paresthesia, numbness, and tingling, has been observed. Published evidence suggests an antipyridoxine effect, and that pyridoxine should be added to the regimen if symptoms develop.

HYDRALAZINE HYDROCHLORIDE — INJECTION

Drug Interactions

Hydralazine Drug Interactions			
Precipitant drug	Object drug*		Description
Beta-blockers Metoprolol Propranolol	Hydralazine	↑	Serum levels of either drug may be increased by concurrent use.
Hydralazine	Beta-blockers Metoprolol Propranolol	↑	
Indomethacin	Hydralazine	↓	The pharmacologic effects of hydralazine may be decreased.

* ↑ = Object drug increased. ↓ = Object drug decreased.

MAO inhibitors should be used with caution in patients receiving hydralazine.

When other potent parenteral antihypertensive drugs, such as diazoxide, are used in combination with hydralazine, patients should be continuously observed for several hours for any excessive fall in blood pressure. Profound hypotensive episodes may occur when diazoxide injection and hydralazine injection are used concomitantly.

Adverse Reactions

Adverse reactions with hydralazine hydrochloride are usually reversible when dosage is reduced. However, in some cases it may be necessary to discontinue the drug.

The following adverse reactions have been observed, but there has not been enough systematic collection of data to support an estimate of their frequency.

➤*Common:*

Miscellaneous – Headache, anorexia, nausea, vomiting, diarrhea, palpitations, tachycardia, angina pectoris.

➤*Less frequent:*

Cardiovascular – Hypotension, paradoxical pressor response, edema.

CNS – Peripheral neuritis, evidenced by paresthesia, numbness, and tingling; dizziness; tremors; muscle cramps; psychotic reactions characterized by depression, disorientation, or anxiety.

GI – Constipation, paralytic ileus.

GU – Difficulty in urination.

Hematologic – Blood dyscrasias, consisting of reduction in hemoglobin and red cell count, leukopenia, agranulocytosis, purpura; lymphadenopathy; splenomegaly.

Hypersensitivity – Rash, urticaria, pruritus, fever, chills, arthralgia, eosinophilia, and, rarely, hepatitis.

Respiratory – Dyspnea.

Miscellaneous – Nasal congestion, flushing, lacrimation, conjunctivitis.

Overdosage

➤*Highest known dose survived:* Adults, 10 g orally.

➤*Symptoms:* Signs and symptoms of overdosage include hypotension, tachycardia, headache, and generalized skin flushing.

Complications can include myocardial ischemia and subsequent myocardial infarction, cardiac arrhythmia, and profound shock.

➤*Treatment:* There is no specific antidote.

Support of the cardiovascular system is of primary importance. Shock should be treated with plasma expanders. If possible, vasopressors should not be given, but if a vasopressor is required, care should be taken not to precipitate or aggravate cardiac arrhythmia. Tachycardia responds to beta blockers. Digitalization may be necessary, and renal function should be monitored and supported as required.

No experience has been reported with extracorporeal or peritoneal dialysis.

MINOXIDIL

Rx	**Minoxidil** (Various, eg, Elkins-Sinn, PAR, Southwood, URL, Watson)	**Tablets:** 2.5 mg	In 100s, 500s, and 1000s.
Rx	**Minoxidil** (Various, eg, Major, PAR, Southwood, URL, Watson)	**Tablets:** 10 mg	In 100s, 500s and 1000s.

MINOXIDIL — ORAL

For complete prescribing information, refer to the Antihypertensives Treatment Guidelines in the Appendix.

WARNING

Minoxidil may produce serious adverse effects. It can cause pericardial effusion, occasionally progressing to tamponade, and it can exacerbate angina pectoris. Reserve for hypertensive patients who do not respond adequately to maximum therapeutic doses of a diuretic and 2 other antihypertensive agents.

In experimental animals, minoxidil caused several kinds of myocardial lesions and other adverse cardiac effects.

Administer under close supervision, usually concomitantly with a beta -adrenergic blocking agent, to prevent tachycardia and increased myocardial workload. Usually, it must be given with a diuretic, frequently one acting in the ascending limb of the loop of Henle to prevent serious fluid accumulation. When first administering minoxidil, hospitalize and monitor patients with malignant hypertension and those already receiving guanethidine to avoid too rapid or large orthostatic decreases in blood pressure.

Indications

➤*Severe hypertension:* Severe hypertension that is symptomatic or associated with target organ damage, and is not manageable with maximum therapeutic doses of a diuretic plus 2 other antihypertensives. Use in milder degrees of hypertension is not recommended because the benefit-risk ratio in such patients has not been defined.

➤*Alopecia androgenetica (topical only):* Topical minoxidil is used for the treatment of male pattern baldness (alopecia androgenetica) of the vertex of the scalp (see Minoxidil Topical Solution monograph in the Dermatological Agents chapter). Use of the tablets, in any formulation, to promote hair growth is not an approved use. Effects of extemporaneous formulations and dosages have not been shown to be safe and effective.

Administration and Dosage

➤*Approved by the FDA:* October 1979.

➤*Adults and children (over 12 years of age):* Initial dosage is 5 mg/day as a single dose. Daily dosage can be increased to 10, 20, then 40 mg in single or divided doses if required. Effective range is usually 10 to 40 mg/day. Maximum dosage is 100 mg/day.

➤*Children (younger than 12 years of age):* Initial dosage is 0.2 mg/kg/day as a single dose. Dose may be increased in 50 to 100% increments until optimum blood pressure control is achieved. Effective range is usually 0.25 to 1 mg/kg/day. Maximum dosage is 50 mg daily. Experience in children is limited, particularly in infants; monitor closely. Titrate carefully for optimal effects.

➤*Dose frequency:* The magnitude of within-day fluctuation of arterial pressure during therapy is directly proportional to the extent of pressure reduction. If supine diastolic pressure has been reduced less than 30 mm Hg, administer the drug only once a day; if reduced more than 30 mm Hg, divide the daily dosage into 2 equal parts.

➤*Dosage adjustment intervals:* Must be carefully titrated and adjusted at 3-day intervals or more because full response to a given dose is not attained until then. If more rapid management is required, adjustments can be made every 6 hours with careful monitoring.

➤*Concomitant drug therapy:*

Diuretics – Use minoxidil with a diuretic in patients relying on renal function for maintaining salt and water balance. Diuretics have been used at the following dosages when starting minoxidil therapy: hydrochlorothiazide (50 mg twice daily) or other thiazides at equally effective doses; chlorthalidone (50 to 100 mg/day); furosemide (40 mg twice daily). If excessive salt and water retention results in a weight gain of more than 2.3 kg (5 lb), change diuretic therapy to furosemide. In furosemide-treated patients, increase dosage in accordance with their needs.

Beta-blockers/Other sympathetic nervous system suppressants – When beginning therapy, the β-blocker dosage should be equal to 80 to 160 mg/day propranolol in divided doses. If β-blockers are contraindicated, use methyldopa 250 to 750 mg twice daily; give for at least 24 hours before starting minoxidil due to delay in onset. Clonidine may also be used to prevent tachycardia induced by minoxidil; usual dosage is 0.1 to 0.2 mg twice daily.

Sympathetic nervous system suppressants may not completely prevent a heart rate increase, but usually prevent tachycardia. Typically, patients receiving a β-blocker prior to minoxidil have bradycardia; expect an increase in heart rate toward normal when minoxidil is added. Simultaneous treatment with minoxidil and a β-blocker or other sympathetic nervous system suppressant causes little change in heart rate, since their opposing cardiac effects usually nullify each other.

➤*Storage/Stability:* Store minoxidil at controlled room temperature of 15° to 30°C (59° to 86°F).

Actions

➤*Pharmacology:* Minoxidil is a direct-acting peripheral vasodilator. It does not interfere with vasomotor reflexes; therefore, it does not produce orthostatic hypotension. The drug does not affect CNS function.

Because it causes peripheral vasodilation, minoxidil elicits a reduction of peripheral arteriolar resistance. This action, with the associated fall in blood pressure, triggers sympathetic, vagal inhibitory, and renal homeostatic mechanisms, including an increase in renin secretion, which leads to increased cardiac rate and output, and salt and water retention. These

MINOXIDIL — ORAL

adverse effects can usually be minimized by coadministration of a diuretic and a beta-adrenergic-blocking agent or other sympathetic nervous system suppressant.

Antihypertensive effects – Minoxidil reduces elevated systolic and diastolic blood pressure by decreasing peripheral vascular resistance. The blood pressure response to minoxidil is dose-related and proportional to the extent of hypertension. In humans, forearm and renal vascular resistance decline; forearm blood flow increases while renal blood flow and glomerular filtration rate (GFR) are preserved.

When used in severely hypertensive patients resistant to other therapy, frequently with an accompanying diuretic and β-adrenergic blocker, minoxidil decreased the blood pressure and reversed encephalopathy and retinopathy. The drug reduced supine diastolic blood pressure by 20 mm Hg, or by 90 mm Hg or less in approximately 75% of the patients studied.

➤*Pharmacokinetics:*

Absorption/Distribution – Minoxidil is not protein bound and is at least 90% absorbed from the GI tract. Plasma levels of the parent drug reach a maximum within the first hour and decline rapidly thereafter.

Onset/Duration: The extent and time course of blood pressure reduction by minoxidil do not correspond closely to its plasma concentration. After an effective single oral dose, blood pressure usually starts to decline within 30 minutes, reaches a minimum between 2 and 3 hours and recovers at a linear rate of about 30% per day. The total duration of effect is approximately 75 hours.

When minoxidil is administered chronically once or twice a day, the time required to achieve maximum effect on blood pressure is inversely related to the size of the dose. Thus, maximum effect is achieved on 10 mg/day within 7 days, on 20 mg/day within 5 days, and on 40 mg/day within 3 days.

Metabolism/Excretion – Predominantly by conjugation with glucuronic acid, 90% is metabolized. Metabolites exert much less pharmacologic effect than minoxidil itself; all are excreted principally in the urine. Renal clearance corresponds to the GFR. Minoxidil and its metabolites are hemodialyzable. Average plasma half-life is 4.2 hours.

Contraindications

Hypersensitivity to any component of the product; pheochromocytoma (because the drug may stimulate secretion of catecholamines from the tumor through its antihypertensive action).

Warnings

➤*Mild hypertension:* Because of potential for serious adverse effects, use in milder degrees of hypertension is not recommended; benefit-risk ratio in such patients is not defined.

➤*Cardiac lesions:*

Animal toxicology – Minoxidil has produced cardiac lesions in animals in general, including grossly visible hemorrhagic lesions of the atrium, epicardium, endocardium, and walls of small arteries and arterioles; necrosis of papillary muscles and subendocardial areas of left ventricle. Cardiac hypertrophy and dilation occurred but was partly reversed by diuretics in monkeys, suggesting increased heart weight may be related to fluid overload. In a 1-year dog study, serosanguinous pericardial fluid was noted.

Human toxicology – Autopsies of 150 patients who died from various causes who had also received minoxidil did not reveal right atrial or other hemorrhagic pathology of the kind seen in dogs. Instances of necrotic areas in papillary muscles were seen, but occurred in the presence of known pre-existing ischemic heart disease and did not appear different from or more common than lesions in patients never exposed to minoxidil.

➤*ECG changes:* Rarely, a large negative amplitude of the T wave may encroach upon the ST segment, but the ST segment is not independently altered. These changes usually disappear with continuance of treatment and revert to the pretreatment state if therapy is discontinued. No symptoms, alterations in blood cell counts or plasma enzyme concentrations, or signs of myocardial damage have been noted. Long-term treatment of patients manifesting such changes has provided no evidence of deteriorating cardiac function. At present, the changes appear to be nonspecific and without identifiable clinical significance.

➤*Fluid and electrolyte balance:* Monitor fluid and electrolyte balance and body weight. Give with a diuretic to prevent fluid retention and possible CHF; a loop diuretic is usually required. If used without a diuretic, retention of several hundred mEq salt and corresponding volumes of water can occur in a few days, leading to increased plasma and interstitial fluid volume and local or generalized edema. Diuretics alone or with restricted salt intake usually minimize fluid retention, but reversible edema developed in approximately 10% of nondialysis patients so treated. Ascites has also occurred. Diuretic effectiveness is limited by impaired renal function. Condition of patients with pre-existing CHF occasionally deteriorates due to fluid retention, but because of the fall in blood pressure (afterload reduction), more than twice as many improve than worsen.

Refractory fluid retention rarely requires discontinuation of minoxidil. Under close medical supervision, it may be possible to resolve refractory salt retention by discontinuing the drug for 1 or 2 days, and then resuming treatment in conjunction with vigorous diuretic therapy.

➤*Tachycardia/Angina:* Minoxidil increases heart rate; this can be prevented by coadministration of a β-adrenergic blocking drug or other sympathetic nervous system suppressants (eg, clonidine, methyldopa). The ability of β-adrenergic blocking agents to minimize papillary muscle lesions in animals is further reason for such concomitant use.

In addition, angina may worsen or appear for the first time during treatment, probably because of the increased oxygen demands associated with increased heart rate and cardiac output. This can usually be prevented by sympathetic blockade or β-adrenergic blocking drugs.

➤*Pericardial effusion:* Occasionally with tamponade, it has occurred in about 3% of treated patients not on dialysis, especially those with inadequate or compromised renal function. Many cases were associated with connective tissue disease, the uremic syndrome, CHF, or fluid retention, but were instances in which these potential causes of effusion were not present. Observe patients closely for signs of pericardial disorder. Perform echocardiographic studies if suspicion arises. More vigorous diuretic therapy, dialysis, pericardiocentesis, or surgery may be required. If the effusion persists, consider drug withdrawal.

➤*Hazard of rapid control of blood pressure:* Too rapid control of very severe blood pressure elevation can precipitate syncope, cerebrovascular accidents, MI, and ischemia of special sense organs with resulting decrease or loss of vision or hearing. Patients with compromised circulation or cryoglobulinemia may also suffer ischemic episodes of affected organs. Although such events have not been unequivocally associated with minoxidil use, experience is limited.

Hospitalize any patient with malignant hypertension during initial treatment to assure that blood pressure is not falling more rapidly than intended.

➤*Hemodilution:* Hematocrit, hemoglobin, and erythrocyte count usually fall about 7% initially and then recover to pretreatment levels.

➤*Hypersensitivity reactions:* Manifested as a skin rash, hypersensitivity reactions occur in fewer than 1% of patients and rare reports of bullous eruptions and Stevens-Johnson syndrome. Deciding whether the drug should be discontinued depends on treatment alternatives.

➤*Renal function impairment:* Renal failure or dialysis patients may require smaller doses; closely supervise to prevent precipitation of cardiac failure or exacerbation of renal failure.

➤*Carcinogenesis:* Dietary administration of minoxidil to mice for up to 2 years was associated with an increased incidence of malignant lymphomas in females at all dose levels (10, 25, and 63 mg/kg/day) and an increased incidence of hepatic nodules in males (63 mg/kg/day). There was no effect of dietary minoxidil on the incidence of malignant liver tumors.

➤*Fertility impairment:* In rats given 1 or 5 times the maximum recommended human dose, there was a dose-dependent reduction in conception rate.

➤*Elderly:* Clinical studies did not include sufficient numbers of subjects 65 years of age and older to determine whether they respond differently from younger subjects. Other reported clinical experience has not identified differences in responses between elderly and younger patients. In general, dose selection for an elderly patient should be cautious, usually starting at the low end of the dosing range, reflecting the greater frequency of decreased hepatic, renal, or cardiac function, and of concomitant disease or other drug therapy.

➤*Pregnancy: Category C.* Minoxidil reduced conception rate and increased fetal absorption in small animals when administered at 5 times the human dose. There are no adequate and well-controlled studies in pregnant women. Use only when clearly needed and when potential benefits outweigh potential hazards to the fetus.

➤*Lactation:* Safety for use in the breast-feeding mother has not been established. Minoxidil is excreted in breast milk; do not breast-feed while taking minoxidil.

➤*Children:* Use in children is limited, particularly in infants. The recommendations under Administration and Dosage are only a rough guide; careful titration is essential.

Precautions

➤*Monitoring:* Monitor initially and periodically thereafter body weight, blood pressure, fluid, and electrolyte balance; signs and symptoms of pericardial effusion; ECG changes; CBC; alkaline phosphatase; renal function tests.

Repeat tests that are abnormal at initiation of minoxidil therapy (eg, urinalysis, renal function tests, ECG, chest x-ray, echocardiogram) to ascertain whether improvement or deterioration is occurring under therapy. Initially, perform such tests frequently, at 1- to 3-month intervals, and as stabilization occurs, at 6- to 12-month intervals.

➤*Myocardial infarction:* Minoxidil has not been used in patients who have had an MI within the preceding month. A reduction in arterial pressure with the drug might further limit blood flow to the myocardium, although this might be compensated by decreased oxygen demand because of lower blood pressure.

➤*Hypertrichosis:* Elongation, thickening, and enhanced pigmentation of fine body hair develops within 3- to 6-weeks after starting therapy in approximately 80% of patients. It is usually first noticed on the temples, between the eyebrows, between the hairline and the eyebrows, or in the sideburn area of the upper lateral cheek, later extending to the back, arms, legs, and scalp. Upon discontinuation of the drug, new hair growth stops, but 1- to 6-months may be required for restoration to pretreatment appearance.

No endocrine abnormalities have been found to explain the abnormal hair growth; thus, it is hypertrichosis without virilism. Inform patients (especially children and women) about this effect before therapy.

Drug Interactions

➤*Guanethidine:* Although minoxidil does not cause orthostatic hypotension, use in patients on guanethidine can result in profound orthostatic

MINOXIDIL — ORAL

effects. If possible, discontinue guanethidine well before minoxidil is instituted. If this is not possible, start minoxidil in the hospital and institutionalize the patient until severity of effects are no longer present or the patient has learned to avoid activities that provoke them.

Adverse Reactions

➤*Cardiovascular:* Pericardial effusion and occasionally with tamponade (3%). Changes in direction and magnitude of T waves occur (approximately 60%).

➤*GI:* Nausea; vomiting.

➤*Hematologic:* Initially, hematocrit, hemoglobin, and erythrocyte count usually fall about 7%, and then recover to pretreatment levels. Thrombocytopenia and leukopenia (WBC fewer than 3,000/mm³) have been reported rarely.

➤*Hypersensitivity:* Rashes including bullous eruptions (rare) and Stevens-Johnson syndrome. (See Warnings.)

➤*Lab test abnormalities:* Alkaline phosphatase increased varyingly without other evidence of liver or bone abnormality. Serum creatinine increased an average of 6% and BUN slightly more, but later declined to pretreatment levels.

➤*Miscellaneous:* Temporary edema (7%); breast tenderness (fewer than 1%).

Hypertrichosis – Elongation, thickening, and enhanced pigmentation of fine body hair develops within 3 to 6 weeks of starting therapy in approximately 80% of patients.

Overdosage

➤*Symptoms:* Exaggerated hypotension is likely in association with residual sympathetic nervous system blockade from previous therapy (guanethidine-like effects or alpha-adrenergic blockade), which prevents compensatory maintenance of blood pressure.

➤*Treatment:* Administer normal saline IV to maintain blood pressure and facilitate urine formation. Avoid sympathomimetics (eg, norepinephrine, epinephrine) with excessive cardiac stimulating action. Phenylephrine, angiotensin II, vasopressin, and dopamine reverse hypotension due to minoxidil, but use only in underperfusion of a vital organ.

Radioimmunoassay can determine plasma concentration. However, due to blood level variations, it is difficult to establish a warning level. At 100 mg/day, peak blood levels of 1,641 and 2,441 ng/mL were seen in two patients. Regard an increase greater than 2,000 ng/mL as overdosage unless the patient has taken no more than the maximum dose.

Patient Information

Patient package insert is available with product.

Minoxidil is usually taken with at least 2 other antihypertensive medications. Take all medications as prescribed; do not discontinue any except on advice of physician.

Enhanced growth and darkening of fine body hair (approximately 80% of patients) may occur; however, do not stop medication without consulting physician.

Notify physician immediately if any of the following occur: Heart rate increase of 20 bpm or more over normal; rapid weight gain of more than 5 pounds (2.3 kg); unusual swelling of extremities, face, or abdomen; breathing difficulty, especially when lying down; new or aggravated angina symptoms (chest, arm, or shoulder pain); severe indigestion; dizziness, lightheadedness, or fainting.

Nausea or vomiting may occur.

EPOPROSTENOL SODIUM (PGI_2; PGX; Prostacyclin)

Rx	**Flolan** (GlaxoWellcome)	**Powder for reconstitution:** 0.5 mg	Mannitol, NaCl. In 17 mL.
		1.5 mg	Mannitol, NaCl. In 17 mL.

EPOPROSTENOL SODIUM — INJECTION

For more information, refer to the Antihypertensives Treatment Guidelines in the Appendix.

Indications

For the long-term intravenous treatment of primary pulmonary hypertension and pulmonary hypertension associated with the scleroderma spectrum of disease in NYHA Class III and Class IV patients who do not respond adequately to conventional therapy.

Administration and Dosage

➤*Approved by the FDA:* September 20, 1995.

➤*Dosage:* Administer continuous chronic infusion of epoprostenol through a central venous catheter. Temporary peripheral IV infusion may be used until central access is established. Initiate chronic infusion of epoprostenol at 2 ng/kg/min, and increase in increments of 2 ng/kg/min every 15 minutes or longer until dose-limiting pharmacologic effects are elicited or until a tolerance limit to the drug is established and further increases in the infusion rate are not clinically warranted. If dose-limiting pharmacologic effects occur, then decrease the infusion rate to an appropriate chronic infusion rate whereby the pharmacologic effects of epoprostenol are tolerated.

In clinical trials, the most common dose-limiting adverse reactions were nausea, vomiting, hypotension, sepsis, headache, abdominal pain, or respiratory disorder (most treatment-limiting adverse reactions were not serious). If the initial infusion rate of 2 ng/kg/min is not tolerated, identify a lower dose which is tolerated by the patient.

➤*Dosage adjustments:* Base changes in the chronic infusion rate on persistence, recurrence, or worsening of the patient's symptoms of pulmonary hypertension and the occurrence of adverse events due to excessive doses of epoprostenol. In general, expect increases in dose from the initial chronic dose.

Consider increments in dose if symptoms of pulmonary hypertension persist or recur after improving. Increase the infusion by 1 to 2 ng/kg/min increments at intervals sufficient to allow assessment of clinical response; these intervals should be at least 15 minutes. In clinical trials, incremental increases in dose occurred at intervals of 24 to 48 hours or longer. Following establishment of a new chronic infusion rate, observe the patient, and monitor standing and supine blood pressure and heart rate for several hours to ensure that the new dose is tolerated.

During chronic infusion, the occurrence of dose-limiting pharmacological events may necessitate a decrease in infusion rate, but the adverse event may occasionally resolve without dosage adjustment. Make dosage decreases gradually in 2 ng/kg/min decrements every 15 minutes or longer until the dose-limiting effects resolve. Avoid abrupt withdrawal of epoprostenol or sudden large reductions in infusion rates. Except in life-threatening situations (eg, unconsciousness, collapse), adjust infusion rates of epoprostenol only under the direction of a physician.

In patients receiving lung transplants, doses of epoprostenol were tapered after the initiation of cardiopulmonary bypass.

➤*Administration:* Epoprostenol is administered by continuous IV infusion via a central venous catheter using an ambulatory infusion pump. During initiation of treatment, epoprostenol may be administered peripherally.

To facilitate extended use at ambient temperatures exceeding 25°C (77°F), a cold pouch with frozen gel packs was used in clinical trials. The cold pouches and gel packs used in clinical trials were obtained from Palco Labs, Palo Alto, California. Any cold pouch used must be capable of maintaining the temperature of reconstituted epoprostenol between 2° and 8°C (35.6° and 46.4°F) for 12 hours.

➤*Reconstitution:* Epoprostenol is stable only when reconstituted with sterile diluent for epoprostenol. Epoprostenol must not be reconstituted or mixed with any other parenteral medications or solutions prior to or during administration.

Select a concentration for the solution of epoprostenol which is compatible with the infusion pump being used with respect to minimum and maximum flow rates, reservoir capacity, and the infusion pump criteria listed above. Epoprostenol, when administered chronically, should be prepared in a drug delivery reservoir appropriate for the infusion pump with a total reservoir volume of at least 100 mL. Prepare epoprostenol using 2 vials of sterile diluent for epoprostenol for use during a 24-hour period.

Reconstitution and Dilution Instructions

To make 100 mL of solution with final concentration (ng/mL) of:	Directions
3,000 ng/mL	Dissolve contents of one 0.5 mg vial with 5 mL of sterile diluent for epoprostenol. Withdraw 3 mL and add to sufficient sterile diluent for epoprostenol to make a total of 100 mL.
5,000 ng/mL	Dissolve contents of one 0.5 mg vial with 5 mL of sterile diluent for epoprostenol. Withdraw entire vial contents and add sufficient sterile diluent for epoprostenol to make a total of 100 mL.
10,000 ng/mL	Dissolve contents of two 0.5 mg vials each with 5 mL of sterile diluent for epoprostenol. Withdraw entire vial contents and add sufficient sterile diluent for epoprostenol to make a total of 100 mL.
15,000 ng/mL[a]	Dissolve contents of one 1.5 mg vial with 5 mL of sterile diluent for epoprostenol. Withdraw entire vial contents and add sufficient sterile diluent for epoprostenol to make a total of 100 mL.

[a] Higher concentrations may be required for patients who receive epoprostenol long-term.

EPOPROSTENOL SODIUM — INJECTION

Generally, 3,000 ng/mL and 10,000 ng/mL are satisfactory concentrations to deliver between 2 to 16 ng/kg/min in adults. Concentrations higher than 15,000 ng/mL may be required for patients who receive epoprostenol long-term. Infusion rates may be calculated using the following formula:

$$\text{Infusion Rate (mL/h)} = \frac{[\text{Dose (ng/kg/min)} \times \text{Weight (kg)} \times 60]}{\text{Final Concentration (ng/mL)}}$$

The following tables provide infusion delivery rates for doses up to 16 ng/kg/min based upon patient weight, drug delivery rate, and concentration of the solution of epoprostenol to be used. These tables may be used to select the most appropriate concentration of epoprostenol that will result in an infusion rate between the minimum and maximum flow rates of the infusion pump, and which will allow the desired duration of infusion from a given reservoir volume. Higher infusion rates, and therefore, more concentrated solutions may be necessary with long-term administration of epoprostenol.

Infusion Rates for Epoprostenol at a Concentration of 3,000 ng/mL

Patient weight (kg)	Dose or drug delivery rate (ng/kg/min)							
	2	4	6	8	10	12	14	16
	Infusion delivery rate (mL/h)							
10	-	-	1.2	1.6	2	2.4	2.8	3.2
20	-	1.6	2.4	3.2	4	4.8	5.6	6.4
30	1.2	2.4	3.6	4.8	6	7.2	8.4	9.6
40	1.6	3.2	4.8	6.4	8	9.6	11.2	12.8
50	2	4	6	8	10	12	14	16
60	2.4	4.8	7.2	9.6	12	14.4	16.8	19.2
70	2.8	5.6	8.4	11.2	14	16.8	19.6	22.4
80	3.2	6.4	9.6	12.8	16	19.2	22.4	25.6
90	3.6	7.2	10.8	14.4	18	21.6	25.2	28.8
100	4	8	12	16	20	24	28	32

Infusion Rates for Epoprostenol at a Concentration of 5,000 ng/mL

Patient weight (kg)	Dose or drug delivery rate (ng/kg/min)							
	2	4	6	8	10	12	14	16
	Infusion delivery rate (mL/h)							
10	-	-	-	1	1.2	1.4	1.7	1.9
20	-	1	1.4	1.9	2.4	2.9	3.4	3.8
30	-	1.4	2.2	2.9	3.6	4.3	5	5.8
40	1	1.9	2.9	3.8	4.8	5.8	6.7	7.7
50	1.2	2.4	3.6	4.8	6	7.2	8.4	9.6
60	1.4	2.9	4.3	5.8	7.2	8.6	10.1	11.5
70	1.7	3.4	5	6.7	8.4	10.1	11.8	13.4
80	1.9	3.8	5.8	7.7	9.6	11.5	13.4	15.4
90	2.2	4.3	6.5	8.6	10.8	13	15.1	17.3
100	2.4	4.8	7.2	9.6	12	14.4	16.8	19.2

Infusion Rates for Epoprostenol at a Concentration of 10,000 ng/mL

Patient weight (kg)	Dose or drug delivery rate (ng/kg/min)						
	4	6	8	10	12	14	16
	Infusion delivery rate (mL/h)						
20	-	-	1	1.2	1.4	1.7	1.9
30	-	1.1	1.4	1.8	2.2	2.5	2.9
40	1	1.4	1.9	2.4	2.9	3.4	3.8
50	1.2	1.8	2.4	3	3.6	4.2	4.8
60	1.4	2.2	2.9	3.6	4.3	5	5.8
70	1.7	2.5	3.4	4.2	5	5.9	6.7
80	1.9	2.9	3.8	4.8	5.8	6.7	7.7
90	2.2	3.2	4.3	5.4	6.5	7.6	8.6
100	2.4	3.6	4.8	6	7.2	8.4	9.6

Infusion Rates for Epoprostenol at a Concentration of 15,000 ng/mL

Patient weight (kg)	Dose or drug delivery rate (ng/kg/min)						
	4	6	8	10	12	14	16
	Infusion delivery rate (mL/h)						
30	-	-	1	1.2	1.4	1.7	1.9
40	-	1	1.3	1.6	1.9	2.2	2.6
50	-	1.2	1.6	2	2.4	2.8	3.2
60	1	1.4	1.9	2.4	2.9	3.4	3.8
70	1.1	1.7	2.2	2.8	3.4	3.9	4.5
80	1.3	1.9	2.6	3.2	3.8	4.5	5.1
90	1.4	2.2	2.9	3.6	4.3	5	5.8
100	1.6	2.4	3.2	4	4.8	5.6	6.4

➤*Storage/Stability:* Unopened vials of epoprostenol are stable until the date indicated on the package when stored at 15° to 25°C (59° to 77°F) and protected from light in the carton. Unopened vials of sterile diluent for epoprostenol are stable until the date indicated on the package when stored at 15° to 25°C (59° to 77°F).

Prior to use, reconstituted solutions of epoprostenol must be protected from light and must be refrigerated at 2° to 8°C (36° to 46°F) if not used immediately. Do not freeze reconstituted solutions of epoprostenol. Discard any reconstituted solution that has been frozen. Discard any reconstituted solution if it has been refrigerated for more than 48 hours.

During use, a single reservoir of reconstituted solution of epoprostenol can be administered at room temperature for a total duration of 8 hours, or it can be used with a cold pouch and administered up to 24 hours with the use of 2 frozen 6 oz gel packs in a cold pouch. When stored or in use, reconstituted epoprostenol must be insulated from temperatures greater than 25°C (77°F) and less than 0°C (32°F), and must not be exposed to direct sunlight.

Prior to use at room temperature, 15° to 25°C (59° to 77°F), reconstituted solutions of epoprostenol may be stored refrigerated at 2° to 8°C (36° to 46°F) for no longer than 40 hours. When administered at room temperature, reconstituted solutions may be used for no longer than 8 hours. This 48-hour period allows the patient to reconstitute a 2-day supply (200 mL) of epoprostenol. Each 100 mL daily supply may be divided into 3 equal portions. Two of the portions are stored refrigerated at 2° to 8°C (36° to 46°F) until they are used.

Prior to infusion with the use of a cold pouch, solutions may be stored refrigerated at 2° to 8°C (36° to 46°F) for up to 24 hours. When a cold pouch is employed during the infusion, reconstituted solutions of epoprostenol may be used for no longer than 24 hours. Change the gel packs every 12 hours. Reconstituted solutions may be kept at 2° to 8°C (36° to 46°F), either in refrigerated storage or in a cold pouch or a combination of the two, for no more than 48 hours.

Visually inspect parenteral drug products for particulate matter and discoloration prior to administration whenever solution and container permit. If either occurs, do not administer epoprostenol.

Store the vials of epoprostenol at 15° to 25°C (59° to 77°F). Protect from light.

Store the vials of sterile diluent for epoprostenol at 15° to 25°C (59° to 77°F). Do not freeze.

Actions

➤*Pharmacology:* Epoprostenol has 2 major pharmacological actions: Direct vasodilation of pulmonary and systemic arterial vascular beds, and inhibition of platelet aggregation. In animals, the vasodilatory effects reduce right and left ventricular afterload and increase cardiac output and stroke volume. The effect of epoprostenol on heart rate in animals varies with dose. At low doses, there is vagally mediated bradycardia, but at higher doses, epoprostenol causes reflex tachycardia in response to direct vasodilation and hypotension. No major effects on cardiac conduction have been observed. Additional pharmacologic effects of epoprostenol in animals include bronchodilation, inhibition of gastric acid secretion, and decreased gastric emptying.

➤*Pharmacokinetics:* Epoprostenol is rapidly hydrolyzed at neutral pH in blood and is also subject to enzymatic degradation. Animal studies using tritium-labelled epoprostenol have indicated a high clearance (93 mL/min/kg), small volume of distribution (357 mL/kg), and a short half-life (2.7 minutes). During infusions in animals, steady-state plasma concentrations of tritium-labelled epoprostenol were reached within 15 minutes and were proportional to infusion rates.

No available chemical assay is sufficiently sensitive and specific to assess the in vivo human pharmacokinetics of epoprostenol. The in vitro half-life of epoprostenol in human blood at 37°C (98.6°F), and pH 7.4 is approximately 6 minutes; the in vivo half-life of epoprostenol in humans is therefore expected to be no greater than 6 minutes. The in vitro pharmacologic half-life of epoprostenol in human plasma, based on inhibition of platelet aggregation, was similar for males (n = 954) and females (n = 1,024).

Tritium-labelled epoprostenol has been administered to humans in order to identify the metabolic products of epoprostenol. Epoprostenol is metabolized to 2 primary metabolites: 6-keto-$PGF_{1\alpha}$ (formed by spontaneous degradation) and 6,15-diketo-13,14-dihydro-$PGF_{1\alpha}$ (enzymatically formed), both of which have pharmacological activity orders of magnitude less than epoprostenol in animal test systems. The recovery of radioactivity in urine and feces over a 1-week period was 82% and 4% of the administered dose, respectively. Fourteen additional minor metabolites have been isolated from urine, indicating that epoprostenol is extensively metabolized in humans.

Contraindications

A large study evaluating the effect of epoprostenol on survival in NYHA Class III and IV patients with CHF due to severe left ventricular systolic dysfunction was terminated after an interim analysis of 471 patients revealed a higher mortality in patients receiving epoprostenol plus conventional therapy than in those receiving conventional therapy alone. The

EPOPROSTENOL SODIUM — INJECTION

chronic use of epoprostenol in patients with congestive heart failure due to severe left ventricular systolic dysfunction is therefore contraindicated.

Some patients with pulmonary hypertension have developed pulmonary edema during dose initiation, which may be associated with pulmonary veno-occlusive disease. Do not use epoprostenol chronically in patients who develop pulmonary edema during dose initiation.

Epoprostenol is also contraindicated in patients with known hypersensitivity to the drug or to structurally related compounds.

Warnings

➤*Abrupt withdrawal:* Abrupt withdrawal (including interruptions in drug delivery) or sudden large reductions in dosage of epoprostenol may result in symptoms associated with rebound pulmonary hypertension, including dyspnea, dizziness, and asthenia. In clinical trials, one Class III PPH patient's death was judged attributable to the interruption of epoprostenol. Avoid abrupt withdrawal.

➤*Sepsis:* During long-term follow-up in the clinical trial of PPH, sepsis was reported at least once in 14% of patients and occurred at a rate of 0.32 infections/patient per year in patients treated with epoprostenol. This rate was higher than reported in patients using chronic indwelling central venous catheters to administer parenteral nutrition, but lower than reported in oncology patients using these catheters.

➤*Elderly:* Clinical studies of epoprostenol in pulmonary hypertension did not include sufficient numbers of subjects aged 65 and over to determine whether they respond differently from younger patients. Other reported clinical experience has not identified differences in responses between the elderly and younger patients. In general, dose selection for an elderly patient should be cautious, usually starting at the low end of the dosing range, reflecting the greater frequency of decreased hepatic, renal, or cardiac function and of concomitant disease or other drug therapy.

➤*Pregnancy: Category B.*

There are no adequate and well-controlled studies in pregnant women. Because animal reproduction studies are not always predictive of human response, use during pregnancy only if clearly needed.

➤*Lactation:* It is not known whether this drug is excreted in human milk. Because many drugs are excreted in human milk, exercise caution when epoprostenol is administered to a breast-feeding woman.

➤*Children:* Safety and efficacy in children have not been established.

Precautions

➤*Monitoring:* Based on clinical trials, the acute hemodynamic response to epoprostenol did not correlate well with improvement in exercise tolerance or survival during chronic use of epoprostenol. Adjust dosage of epoprostenol during chronic use at the first sign of recurrence or worsening of symptoms attributable to pulmonary hypertension or the occurrence of adverse events associated with epoprostenol. Following dosage adjustments, closely monitor standing and supine blood pressure and heart rate for several hours.

➤*Experienced clinicians:* Epoprostenol should be used only by clinicians experienced in the diagnosis and treatment of pulmonary hypertension. The diagnosis of PPH or PH/SSD should be carefully established.

Epoprostenol is a potent pulmonary and systemic vasodilator. Dose initiation with epoprostenol must be performed in a setting with adequate personnel and equipment for physiologic monitoring and emergency care. Dose initiation in controlled PPH clinical trials was performed during right heart catheterization. In uncontrolled PPH and controlled PH/SSD clinical trials, dose initiation was performed without cardiac catheterization. Carefully weigh the risk of cardiac catheterization in patients with pulmonary hypertension should be carefully weighed against the potential benefits. During dose initiation, asymptomatic increases in pulmonary artery pressure coincident with increases in cardiac output occurred rarely. In such cases, consider dose reduction, but such an increase does not imply that chronic treatment is contraindicated.

➤*Permanent IV catheter:* During chronic use, epoprostenol is delivered continuously on an ambulatory basis through a permanent indwelling central venous catheter. Unless contraindicated, administer anticoagulant therapy to PPH and PH/SSD patients receiving epoprostenol to reduce the risk of pulmonary thromboembolism or systemic embolism through a patent foramen ovale. In order to reduce the risk of infection, aseptic technique must be used in the reconstitution and administration of epoprostenol as well as in routine catheter care. Because epoprostenol is metabolized rapidly, even brief interruptions in the delivery of epoprostenol may result in symptoms associated with rebound pulmonary hypertension including dyspnea, dizziness, and asthenia. Base the decision to initiate therapy with epoprostenol upon the understanding that there is a high likelihood that IV therapy with epoprostenol will be needed for prolonged periods, possibly years, and carefully consider the patient's ability to accept and care for a permanent IV catheter and infusion pump.

Drug Interactions

Epoprostenol Drug Interactions

Precipitant drug	Object drug[a]		Description
Epoprostenol	Diuretics Vasodilators	↑	Coadministration could cause additional reductions in blood pressure.
Epoprostenol	Antiplatelet agents Anticoagulants	↑	Coadministration can increase the risk of bleeding, although this did not occur in clinical trials.

[a] ↑ = Object drug increased.

In a pharmacokinetic substudy in patients with congestive heart failure receiving furosemide or digoxin in whom therapy with epoprostenol was initiated, apparent oral clearance values for furosemide (n = 23) and digoxin (n = 30) were decreased by 13% and 15%, respectively, on the second day of therapy and had returned to baseline values by day 87. The change in furosemide clearance value is not likely to be clinically significant. However, patients on digoxin may show elevations of digoxin concentrations after initiation of therapy with epoprostenol, which may be clinically significant in patients prone to digoxin toxicity.

Adverse Reactions

➤*Adverse reactions during dose initiation and escalation:* During early clinical trials, epoprostenol was increased in 2 ng/kg/min increments until the patients developed symptomatic intolerance. The most common adverse events and the adverse events that limited further increases in dose were generally related to the major pharmacologic effect of epoprostenol, vasodilation. The most common dose-limiting adverse events (occurring in greater than or equal to 1% of patients) were nausea, vomiting, headache, hypotension, and flushing, but also include chest pain, anxiety, dizziness, bradycardia, dyspnea, abdominal pain, musculoskeletal pain, and tachycardia.

Adverse Reactions During Dose Initiation and Escalation

Adverse reactions occurring in ≥ 1% of patients	Epoprostenol (n = 391)
Abdominal pain	5%
Anxiety, nervousness, agitation	11%
Back pain	2%
Bradycardia	5%
Chest pain	11%
Dizziness	8%
Dyspnea	2%
Dyspepsia	1%
Flushing	58%
Headache	49%
Hypesthesia/Paresthesia	1%
Hypotension	16%
Musculoskeletal pain	3%
Nausea/Vomiting	32%
Sweating	1%
Tachycardia	1%

➤*Adverse reactions during chronic administration:* Interpretation of adverse events is complicated by the clinical features of PPH and PH/SSD, which are similar to some of the pharmacologic effects of epoprostenol (eg, dizziness, syncope). Adverse events probably related to the underlying disease include dyspnea, fatigue, chest pain, edema, hypoxia, right ventricular failure, and pallor. Several adverse events, on the other hand, can clearly be attributed to epoprostenol. These include headache, jaw pain, flushing, diarrhea, nausea and vomiting, flu-like symptoms, and anxiety/nervousness.

➤*Adverse reactions during chronic administration for PPH:* In an effort to separate the adverse effects of the drug from the adverse effects of the underlying disease, the table below lists adverse events that occurred at a rate at least 10% different in the 2 groups in controlled trials for PPH.

Adverse Reactions Regardless of Attribution Occurring in Patients with PPH with ≥ 10% Difference between Epoprostenol and Conventional Therapy Alone

Adverse reaction	Epoprostenol (n = 52)	Conventional therapy (n = 54)
Occurrence more common with epoprostenol		
Cardiovascular		
Flushing	42%	2%
Tachycardia	35%	24%
CNS		
Anxiety/nervousness/tremor	21%	9%
Dizziness	83%	70%
Headache	83%	33%

EPOPROSTENOL SODIUM — INJECTION

Adverse Reactions Regardless of Attribution Occurring in Patients with PPH with ≥ 10% Difference between Epoprostenol and Conventional Therapy Alone		
Adverse reaction	Epoprostenol (n = 52)	Conventional therapy (n = 54)
Occurrence more common with epoprostenol		
Hypesthesia, hyperesthesia, paresthesia	12%	2%
GI		
Diarrhea	37%	6%
Nausea/vomiting	67%	48%
Musculoskeletal		
Jaw pain	54%	0%
Myalgia	44%	31%
Nonspecific musculoskeletal pain	35%	15%
Miscellaneous		
Chills/fever/sepsis/flu-like symptoms	25%	11%
Occurrence more common with conventional therapy		
Cardiovascular		
Heart failure	31%	52%
Shock	0%	13%
Syncope	13%	24%
Respiratory		
Hypoxia	25%	37%

Thrombocytopenia has been reported during uncontrolled clinical trials in patients receiving epoprostenol. The following table lists additional adverse events reported in PPH patients receiving epoprostenol plus conventional therapy or conventional therapy alone during controlled clinical trials.

Adverse Reactions Regardless of Attribution Occurring in Patients with PPH with < 10% Difference Between Epoprostenol and Conventional Therapy Alone		
Adverse reaction	Epoprostenol (n = 52)	Conventional therapy (n = 54)
Cardiovascular		
Angina pectoris	19%	20%
Arrhythmia	27%	20%
Bradycardia	15%	9%
Cerebrovascular accident	4%	0%
Cyanosis	31%	39%
Hemorrhage	19%	11%
Hypotension	27%	31%
Myocardial ischemia	2%	6%
Pallor	21%	30%
Palpitation	63%	61%
Supraventricular tachycardia	8%	0%
CNS		
Confusion	6%	11%
Convulsion	4%	0%
Depression	37%	44%
Insomnia	4%	4%
Dermatologic		
Pruritus	4%	0%
Rash	10%	13%
Sweating	15%	20%
GI		
Abdominal pain	27%	31%
Anorexia	25%	30%
Ascites	12%	17%
Constipation	6%	2%
Metabolic		
Edema	60%	63%
Hypokalemia	6%	4%
Weight gain	6%	4%
Weight reduction	27%	24%
Musculoskeletal		
Arthralgia	6%	0%
Bone pain	0%	4%
Chest pain	67%	65%
Respiratory		
Cough increase	38%	46%
Dyspnea	90%	85%
Epistaxis	4%	2%
Pleural effusion	4%	2%
Special senses		
Amblyopia	8%	4%
Vision abnormality	4%	0%
Miscellaneous		
Asthenia	87%	81%

➤*Adverse events during chronic administration for PH/SSD:* In an effort to separate the adverse reactions of the drug from the adverse effects of the underlying disease, the table below lists adverse events that occurred at a rate at least 10% different in the 2 groups in controlled trial for patients with PH/SSD.

Adverse Reactions Regardless of Attribution Occurring in Patients with PH/SSD with ≥ 10% Difference between Epoprostenol and Conventional Therapy Alone		
Adverse reaction	Epoprostenol (n = 56)	Conventional therapy (n = 55)
Occurrence more common with epoprostenol		
Cardiovascular		
Flushing	23%	0%
Hypotension	13%	0%
CNS		
Headache	46%	5%
Dermatologic		
Eczema/rash/urticaria	25%	4%
Skin ulcer	39%	24%
GI		
Anorexia	66%	47%
Diarrhea	50%	5%
Nausea/vomiting	41%	16%
Musculoskeletal		
Jaw pain	75%	0%
Pain/neck pain/arthralgia	84%	65%
Occurrence more common with conventional therapy		
Cardiovascular		
Cyanosis	54%	80%
Pallor	32%	53%
Syncope	7%	20%
CNS		
Dizziness	59%	76%
GI		
Ascites	23%	33%
Esophageal reflux/gastritis	61%	73%
Metabolic		
Weight decrease	45%	56%
Respiratory		
Hypoxis	55%	65%

The following table lists additional adverse reactions reported in PH/SSD patients receiving epoprostenol plus conventional therapy or conventional therapy alone during controlled clinical trials.

Adverse Events Regardless of Attribution Occurring in Patients with PH/SSD with < 10% Difference Between Epoprostenol and Conventional Therapy Alone		
Adverse reaction[a]	Epoprostenol (n = 56)	Conventional therapy (n = 55)
Cardiovascular		
Heart failure/heart failure right	11%	13%
Myocardial infarction	4%	0%
Palpitation	63%	71%
Shock	5%	5%
Tachycardia	43%	42%
Vascular disorder	95%	89%
Vascular disorder peripheral	96%	100%
CNS		
Anxiety/hyperkinesia/nervousness/tremor	7%	5%
Depression/depression psychotic	13%	4%
Hyperesthesia/hypesthesia/paresthesia	5%	0%

EPOPROSTENOL SODIUM — INJECTION

Adverse Events Regardless of Attribution Occurring in Patients with PH/SSD with < 10% Difference Between Epoprostenol and Conventional Therapy Alone

Adverse reaction[a]	Epoprostenol (n = 56)	Conventional therapy (n = 55)
Insomnia	9%	0%
Somnolence	4%	2%
Dermatologic		
Collagen disease	82%	84%
Pruritus	4%	2%
Sweat	41%	36%
GI		
Abdominal enlargement	4%	0%
Abdominal pain	14%	7%
Constipation	4%	2%
Flatulence	5%	4%
Hematologic/Lymphatic		
Thrombocytopenia	4%	0%
GU		
Hematuria	5%	0%
Urinary tract infection	7%	0%
Metabolic		
Edema/edema peripheral/edema genital	79%	87%
Hypercalcemia	48%	51%
Hyperkalemia	4%	0%
Thirst	0%	4%
Musculoskeletal		
Arthritis	52%	45%
Back pain	13%	5%
Chest pain	52%	45%
Leg cramps	5%	7%
Respiratory		
Cough increase	82%	82%
Dyspnea	100%	100%
Epistaxis	9%	7%
Pharyngitis	5%	2%
Pleural effusion	7%	0%
Pneumonia	5%	0%
Pneumothorax	4%	0%
Pulmonary edema	4%	2%
Respiratory disorder	7%	4%
Sinusitis	4%	4%
Miscellaneous		
Asthenia	100%	98%
Chills/fever/sepsis/flu-like symptoms	13%	11%
Hemorrhage/hemorrhage injection site/ hemorrhage rectal	11%	2%
Infection/rhinitis	21%	20%

[a] Adverse events which occurred in at least 2 patients in either treatment group.

Although the relationship to epoprostenol administration has not been established, pulmonary embolism has been reported in several patients taking epoprostenol and there have been reports of hepatic failure.

➤*Adverse events attributable to the drug delivery system:* Chronic infusions of epoprostenol are delivered using a small, portable infusion pump through an indwelling central venous catheter. During controlled PPH trials of up to 12 weeks duration, up to 21% of patients reported a local infection and up to 13% of patients reported pain at the injection site. During a controlled PH/SSD trial of 12 weeks' duration, 14% of patients reported a local infection and 9% of patients reported pain at the injection site. During long-term follow-up in the clinical trial of PPH, sepsis was reported at least once in 14% of patients and occurred at a rate of 0.32 infections per patient per year in patients treated with epoprostenol. This rate was higher than reported in patients using chronic indwelling central venous catheters to administer parenteral nutrition, but lower than reported in oncology patients using these catheters. Malfunctions in the delivery system resulting in an inadvertent bolus of or a reduction in epoprostenol were associated with symptoms related to excess or insufficient epoprostenol, respectively (see Adverse events during chronic administration).

➤*Postmarketing:* In addition to adverse reactions reported from clinical trials, the following events have been identified during postapproval use of epoprostenol. Because they are reported voluntarily from a population of unknown size, estimates of frequency cannot be made. These events have been chosen for inclusion due to a combination of their seriousness, frequency of reporting, or potential causal connection to epoprostenol injection.

Endocrine – Hyperthyroidism.

Hematologic/Lymphatic – Anemia, hypersplenism, pancytopenia, splenomegaly.

Overdosage

➤*Symptoms:* Signs and symptoms of excessive doses of epoprostenol during clinical trials are the expected dose-limiting pharmacologic effects of epoprostenol, including flushing, headache, hypotension, tachycardia, nausea, vomiting, and diarrhea. Treatment will ordinarily require dose reduction of epoprostenol.

➤*Treatment:* One patient with secondary pulmonary hypertension accidentally received 50 mL of an unspecified concentration of epoprostenol. The patient vomited and became unconscious with an initially unrecordable blood pressure. Epoprostenol was discontinued and the patient regained consciousness within seconds. In clinical practice, fatal occurrences of hypoxemia, hypotension, and respiratory arrest have been reported following overdosage of epoprostenol.

Single IV doses of epoprostenol at 10 and 50 mg/kg (2,703 and 27,027 times the recommended acute phase human dose based on body surface area) were lethal to mice and rats, respectively. Symptoms of acute toxicity were hypoactivity, ataxia, loss of righting reflex, deep slow breathing, and hypothermia.

Patient Information

Patients receiving epoprostenol sodium should receive the following information: Epoprostenol sodium must be reconstituted only with sterile diluent for epoprostenol sodium. Epoprostenol sodium is infused continuously through a permanent indwelling central venous catheter via a small, portable infusion pump. Thus, therapy with epoprostenol sodium requires commitment by the patient to drug reconstitution, drug administration, and care of the permanent central venous catheter. Sterile technique must be adhered to in preparing the drug and in the care of the catheter, and even brief interruptions in the delivery of epoprostenol sodium may result in rapid symptomatic deterioration. A patient's decision to receive epoprostenol sodium should be based upon the understanding that there is a high likelihood that therapy with epoprostenol sodium will be needed for prolonged periods, possibly years. The patient's ability to accept and care for a permanent intravenous catheter and infusion pump should also be carefully considered.

TREPROSTINIL SODIUM

Rx	**Remodulin** (United Therapeutics)	**Injection:** 1 mg/mL	Sodium chloride 5.3 mg. In 20 mL multi-use vials.
		2.5 mg/mL	Sodium chloride 5.3 mg. In 20 mL multi-use vials.
		5 mg/mL	Sodium chloride 5.3 mg. In 20 mL multi-use vials.
		10 mg/mL	Sodium chloride 4 mg. In 20 mL multi-use vials.

TREPROSTINIL SODIUM — INJECTION

Indications

➤*Pulmonary arterial hypertension (PAH):* Treprostinil is indicated as a continuous subcutaneous or intravenous (IV) infusion (for those not able to tolerate a subcutaneous infusion) for the treatment of PAH in patients with New York Heart Association (NYHA) Class II to IV symptoms to diminish symptoms associated with exercise.

➤*Clinical deterioration during transition from epoprostenol:* Treprostinil is indicated to diminish the rate of clinical deterioration in patients requiring transition from epoprostenol.

Administration and Dosage

➤*Approved by the FDA:* May 21, 2002.

Treprostinil can be administered as supplied or diluted for IV infusion with sterile water for injection or 0.9% sodium chloride injection prior to administration.

➤*Initial dose:* Treprostinil is administered by continuous infusion. Treprostinil is preferably infused subcutaneously, but can be administered by a central IV line if the subcutaneous route is not tolerated because of severe site pain or reaction. The infusion rate is initiated at 1.25 ng/kg/min. If this initial dose cannot be tolerated because of systemic effects, the infusion rate should be reduced to 0.625 ng/kg/min.

➤*Dosage adjustments:* The goal of chronic dosage adjustments is to establish a dose at which PAH symptoms are improved, while minimizing excessive pharmacologic effects of treprostinil (eg, headache, nausea, emesis, restlessness, anxiety, infusion-site pain or reaction).

The infusion rate should be increased in increments of no more than 1.25 ng/kg/min per week for the first 4 weeks and then no more than 2.5 ng/kg/min per week for the remaining duration of infusion, depending on clinical response. There is little experience with doses greater than 40 ng/kg/min. Abrupt cessation of infusion should be avoided. Abrupt withdrawal or sudden large reductions in dosage of treprostinil may result in worsening of PAH symptoms and should be avoided.

TREPROSTINIL SODIUM — INJECTION

➤*Hepatic function impairment:* In patients with mild or moderate hepatic insufficiency, decrease the initial dose of treprostinil to 0.625 ng/kg/min ideal body weight; increase cautiously. Treprostinil has not been studied in patients with severe hepatic insufficiency.

➤*Administration:*

Subcutaneous infusion – Treprostinil is administered subcutaneously by continuous infusion, via a self-inserted subcutaneous catheter, using an infusion pump designed for subcutaneous drug delivery. To avoid potential interruptions in drug delivery, the patient must have immediate access to a backup infusion pump and subcutaneous infusion sets. The ambulatory infusion pump used to administer treprostinil should be small and lightweight; be adjustable to approximately 0.002 mL/h; have occlusion/no delivery, low battery, programming error and motor malfunction alarms; have delivery accuracy of ± 6% or better; and be positive pressure driven. The reservoir should be made of polyvinyl chloride, polypropylene, or glass.

For subcutaneous infusion, treprostinil is delivered without further dilution at a calculated subcutaneous infusion rate (mL/h) based on a patient's dose (ng/kg/min), weight (kg), and the vial strength (mg/mL) of treprostinil being used. During use, a single reservoir (syringe) of undiluted treprostinil can be administered up to 72 hours at 37°C (98.6°F). The subcutaneous infusion rate is calculated using the following formula:

$$\text{SC infusion rate (mL/h)} = \frac{\text{dose (ng/kg/min)} \times \text{weight (kg)} \times 0.00006}{\text{treprostinil vial strength (mg/mL)}}$$

In the above formula, conversion factor of 0.00006 = 60 min/hour × 0.000001 mg/ng.

IV infusion – Treprostinil must be diluted with either sterile water for injection or 0.9% sodium chloride injection and is administered IV by continuous infusion, via a surgically placed indwelling central venous catheter, using an infusion pump designed for IV drug delivery. To avoid potential interruptions in drug delivery, the patient must have immediate access to a backup infusion pump and infusion sets. The ambulatory infusion pump used to administer treprostinil should be small and lightweight; have occlusion/no delivery, low battery, programming error and motor malfunction alarms; have delivery accuracy of ±6% or better of the hourly dose; and be positive pressure driven. The reservoir should be made of polyvinyl chloride, polypropylene, or glass.

Diluted treprostinil has been shown to be stable at ambient temperature for up to 48 hours at concentrations as low as 0.004 mg/mL (4,000 ng/mL).

When using an appropriate infusion pump and reservoir, a predetermined IV infusion rate should first be selected to allow for a desired infusion period length of up to 48 hours between system changeovers. Typical IV infusion system reservoirs have volumes of 50 or 100 mL. With this selected IV infusion rate (mL/h) and the patient's dose (ng/kg/min) and weight (kg), the diluted IV treprostinil concentration (mg/mL) can be calculated using the following formula:

$$\text{Step 1: Diluted IV treprostinil concentration (mg/mL)} = \frac{\text{dose (ng/kg/min)} \times \text{weight (kg)} \times 0.00006}{\text{IV infusion rate (mL/h)}}$$

The amount of treprostinil injection needed to make the required diluted IV treprostinil concentration for the given reservoir size can then be calculated using the following formula:

$$\text{Step 2: Amount of treprostinil injection (mL)} = \frac{\text{diluted IV treprostinil concentration (mg/mL)}}{\text{treprostinil vial strength (mg/mL)}} \times \text{total volume of diluted treprostinil solution in reservoir (mL)}$$

The calculated amount of treprostinil injection is then added to the reservoir along with the sufficient volume of diluent (sterile water for injection or 0.9% sodium chloride injection) to achieve the desired total volume in the reservoir.

In patients requiring transition from epoprostenol – Transition from epoprostenol to treprostinil is accomplished by initiating the infusion of treprostinil and increasing it, while simultaneously reducing the dose of intravenous epoprostenol. The transition to treprostinil should take place in a hospital with constant observation of response (e.g., walk distance and signs and symptoms of disease progression). During the transition, treprostinil is initiated at a recommended dose of 10% of the current epoprostenol dose, and then escalated as the epoprostenol dose is decreased.

Patients are individually titrated to a dose that allows transition from epoprostenol therapy to treprostinil while balancing prostacylin-limiting adverse events. Increases in the patient's symptoms of PAH should be first treated with increases in the dose of treprostinil. Side effects normally associated with prostacylin and prostacylin analogs are to be first treated by decreasing the dose of epoprostenol.

Recommended Transition Dose Changes

Step	Epoprostenol Dose	Treprostinil Dose
1	Unchanged	10% starting epoprostenol dose
2	80% epoprostenol dose	30% starting epoprostenol dose
3	60% epoprostenol dose	50% starting epoprostenol dose
4	40% epoprostenol dose	70% starting epoprostenol dose
5	20% epoprostenol dose	90% starting epoprostenol dose
6	5% epoprostenol dose	110% starting epoprostenol dose
7	0	110% starting epoprostenol dose + additional 5–10% increments as needed

➤*Storage/Stability:* Unopened vials of treprostinil are stable until the date indicated when stored at 15° to 25°C (59° to 77°F). Store at 25°C (77°F), with excursions permitted to 15° to 30°C (59° to 86°F).

During use, a single reservoir (syringe) of undiluted treprostinil can be administered up to 72 hours at 37°C (98.6°F). Diluted treprostinil solution can be administered up to 48 hours at 37°C (98.6°F) when diluted to concentrations as low as 0.004 mg/mL in sterile water for injection or 0.9% sodium chloride injection. A single vial of treprostinil should be used for no more than 30 days after the initial introduction into the vial.

Actions

➤*Pharmacology:* The major pharmacologic actions of treprostinil are direct vasodilation of pulmonary and systemic arterial vascular beds and inhibition of platelet aggregation. In animals, the vasodilatory effects reduce right and left ventricular afterload and increase cardiac output and stroke volume. Other studies have shown that treprostinil causes a dose-related negative inotropic and lusitropic effect. No major effects on cardiac conduction have been observed.

➤*Pharmacokinetics:*

Absorption – Treprostinil is relatively rapidly and completely absorbed after subcutaneous infusion, with an absolute bioavailability approximating 100%. Steady-state concentrations occurred in approximately 10 hours. Concentrations in patients treated with an average dose of 9.3 ng/kg/min were approximately 2 mcg/L.

Distribution – The volume of distribution of the drug in the central compartment is approximately 14 L per 70 kg ideal body weight. Treprostinil at in vitro concentrations ranging from 330 to 10,000 mcg/L was 91% bound to human plasma protein.

Metabolism – Treprostinil is substantially metabolized by the liver, but the precise enzymes responsible are unknown. Five metabolites have been described (HU1 through HU5). The biological activity and metabolic fate of these metabolites are unknown. The chemical structure of HU1 is unknown. HU5 is the glucuronide conjugate of treprostinil. The other metabolites are formed by oxidation of the 3-hydroxyoctyl side chain (HU2) and subsequent additional oxidation (HU3) or dehydration (HU4). Based on the results of in vitro human hepatic cytochrome P-450 studies, treprostinil does not inhibit CYP 1A2, 2C9, 2C19, 2D6, 2E1, or 3A. Whether treprostinil induces these enzymes has not been studied.

Excretion – The elimination of treprostinil is biphasic, with a terminal half-life of approximately 4 hours. Approximately 79% of an administered dose is excreted in the urine as unchanged drug (4%) and as the identified metabolites (64%). Approximately 13% of a dose is excreted in the feces. Systemic clearance is approximately 30 L/h for a 70 kg ideal body weight person.

Special populations –

Hepatic function impairment: In patients with portopulmonary hypertension and mild (n = 4) or moderate (n = 5) hepatic insufficiency, treprostinil at a subcutaneous dose of 10 ng/kg/min for 150 minutes had a C_{max} that was increased 2- and 4-fold, respectively, and an AUC $_{0\text{-}\infty}$ that was increased 3- and 5-fold, respectively, compared with healthy subjects. Clearance in patients with hepatic insufficiency was reduced by up to 80% compared with healthy adults.

In patients with mild or moderate hepatic insufficiency, decrease the initial dose of treprostinil to 0.625 ng/kg/min ideal body weight; increase cautiously. Treprostinil has not been studied in patients with severe hepatic insufficiency. The pharmacokinetics of continuous subcutaneous treprostinil are linear over the dose range of 1.25 to 22.5 ng/kg/min (corresponding to plasma concentrations of about 0.03 to 8 mcg/L) and can be described by a 2-compartment model. Dose proportionality at infusion rates greater than 22.5 ng/kg/min has not been studied.

Subcutaneous and IV administration of treprostinil demonstrated bioequivalence at steady state at a dose of 10 ng/kg/min.

Contraindications

Known hypersensitivity to the drug or to structurally related compounds.

Warnings

➤*Route of administration:* Treprostinil is indicated for subcutaneous or IV use only.

➤*Renal/Hepatic function impairment:* Use caution in patients with hepatic or renal impairment.

See Administration and Dosage for more information.

➤*Elderly:* Clinical studies of treprostinil did not include sufficient numbers of patients 65 years of age and older to determine whether they respond differently from younger patients. In general, use caution in dose selection for an elderly patient, reflecting the greater frequency of decreased hepatic, renal, or cardiac function, and of concomitant disease or other drug therapy.

TREPROSTINIL SODIUM — INJECTION

➤*Pregnancy: Category B.*

In pregnant rabbits, effects of continuous, subcutaneous infusions of treprostinil during organogenesis were limited to an increased incidence of fetal skeletal variations (bilateral full rib or right rudimentary rib on lumbar 1) associated with maternal toxicity (reduction in body weight and food consumption) at an infusion rate of treprostinil 150 ng/kg/min (about 41 times the starting human rate of infusion, on a ng/m^2 basis, and 5 times the average rate used in clinical trials).

Because animal reproduction studies are not always predictive of human response, use treprostinil during pregnancy only if clearly needed.

➤*Lactation:* It is not known whether treprostinil is excreted in human milk or absorbed systemically after ingestion. Because many drugs are excreted in human milk, exercise caution when treprostinil is administered to breast-feeding women.

➤*Children:* Safety and efficacy in pediatric patients have not been established. Clinical studies of treprostinil did not include sufficient numbers of patients 16 years of age and younger to determine whether they respond differently from older patients. In general, use caution in dose selection.

Precautions

➤*Administration:* Treprostinil should be used only by clinicians experienced in the diagnosis and treatment of PAH.

Treprostinil is a potent pulmonary and systemic vasodilator. Initiation of treprostinil must be performed in a setting with adequate personnel and equipment for physiological monitoring and emergency care. Therapy with treprostinil may be used for prolonged periods; carefully consider the patient's ability to administer injection and care for an infusion system.

➤*Dosage adjustments:* Increase the dose for lack of improvement in, or worsening of, symptoms and decrease it for excessive pharmacologic effects or for unacceptable infusion-site symptoms (ie, headache, nausea, emesis, restlessness, anxiety, infusion-site pain or reaction).

Abrupt withdrawal or sudden large reductions in dosage of treprostinil may result in worsening of PAH symptoms and should be avoided.

Drug Interactions

Reduction in blood pressure caused by treprostinil may be exacerbated by drugs that by themselves alter blood pressure, such as diuretics, antihypertensive agents, or vasodilators. Because treprostinil inhibits platelet aggregation, there is also a potential for increased risk of bleeding, particularly among patients maintained on anticoagulants.

Adverse Reactions

Patients receiving treprostinil as a subcutaneous infusion reported a wide range of adverse reactions, many potentially related to the underlying disease (eg, dyspnea, fatigue, chest pain, right ventricular heart failure, pallor). During clinical trials with subcutaneous infusion of treprostinil, infusion-site pain and reaction were the most common adverse reactions among those treated with treprostinil. Infusion-site reaction was defined as any local adverse reaction other than pain or bleeding/bruising at the infusion site and included symptoms such as erythema, induration, or rash. Infusion-site reactions were sometimes severe and could lead to discontinuation of treatment.

Treprostinil Subcutaneous Infusion-Site Adverse Reactions

	Reaction		Pain	
Adverse reaction	Placebo	Treprostinil	Placebo	Treprostinil
Severe	1%	38%	2%	39%
Requiring narcotics[a]	NA[b]	NA[b]	1%	32%
Leading to discontinuation	0%	3%	0%	7%

[a] Based on prescriptions for narcotics, not actual use.
[b] Medications used to treat infusion-site pain were not distinguished from those used to treat site reactions.

Other adverse reactions included diarrhea, jaw pain, edema, vasodilation, and nausea, and these are generally considered to be related to the pharmacologic effects of treprostinil, whether administered subcutaneously or IV.

Adverse reactions during chronic dosing – The following table lists adverse reactions that occurred at a rate of at least 3% and were more frequent in patients treated with subcutaneous treprostinil than with placebo in controlled trials in PAH.

Subcutaneous Treprostinil Adverse Reactions

Adverse reaction	Treprostinil (n = 236)	Placebo (n = 233)
CNS		
Dizziness	9%	8%
Headache	27%	23%
Dermatologic		
Pruritus	8%	6%
Rash	14%	11%
GI		
Diarrhea	25%	16%
Nausea	22%	18%
Miscellaneous		
Edema	9%	3%
Hypotension	4%	2%
Infusion-site pain	85%	27%
Infusion-site reaction	83%	27%
Jaw pain	13%	5%
Vasodilation	11%	5%

Reported adverse reactions (at least 3%) are included except those too general to be informative, and those not plausibly attributable to the use of the drug, because they were associated with the condition being treated or are very common in the treated population.

Adverse reactions attributable to the drug-delivery system – In controlled studies of treprostinil administered subcutaneously, there were no reports of infection related to the drug-delivery system. There were 187 infusion system complications reported in 28% of patients (23% treprostinil, 33% placebo); 173 (93%) were pump related and 14 (7%) related to the infusion set. Eight of these patients (4 treprostinil; 4 placebo) reported nonserious adverse reactions resulting from infusion-system complications. Adverse reactions resulting from problems with the delivery systems were typically related to either symptoms of excess treprostinil (eg, nausea) or return of PAH symptoms (eg, dyspnea). These events were generally resolved by correcting the delivery system pump or infusion-set problem (eg, replacing the syringe or battery, reprogramming the pump, straightening a crimped infusion line). Adverse reactions resulting from problems with the delivery system did not lead to clinical instability or rapid deterioration.

There are no controlled clinical studies with treprostinil administered IV. Among the subjects (N = 38) treated for 12 weeks in an open-label study, 2 patients had either line infections or sepsis. Other reactions potentially related to the mode of infusion include arm swelling, hematoma, pain, and paresthesias.

Overdosage

➤*Symptoms:* Signs and symptoms of overdose with treprostinil during clinical trials are extensions of its dose-limiting pharmacologic effects and include diarrhea, flushing, headache, hypotension, nausea, and vomiting. In controlled clinical trials, 7 patients received some level of overdose; in open-label follow-on treatment, 7 additional patients received an overdose. These occurrences resulted from accidental bolus administration of treprostinil, errors in pump programmed rate of administration, and prescription of an incorrect dose. In only 2 cases did excess delivery of treprostinil produce an event of substantial hemodynamic concern (hypotension, near-syncope).

➤*Treatment:* Most events were self-limiting and resolved with reduction or withholding of treprostinil.

Patient Information

Treprostinil is infused continuously through a subcutaneous or surgically placed indwelling central venous catheter, via an infusion pump. Therapy with treprostinil will be needed for prolonged periods, possibly years. Carefully consider the patient's ability to accept and care for a catheter and to use an infusion pump.

In order to reduce the risk of infection, aseptic technique must be used in the preparation and administration of treprostinil. Additionally, inform patients that subsequent disease management may require the initiation of an alternative IV prostacyclin therapy, epoprostenol sodium.

PERIPHERAL VASODILATOR COMBINATIONS

Rx	**Lipo-Nicin/100 mg** (ICN Pharm)	**Tablets:** 100 mg niacin, 75 mg niacinamide, 150 mg vitamin C, 25 mg B_1, 2 mg B_2 and 10 mg B_6. *Dose: 1 tablet daily.*	Blue. In 100s.
Rx	**Lipo-Nicin/300 mg** (ICN Pharm)	**Capsules, timed release:** 300 mg niacin, 150 mg vitamin C, 25 mg B_1, 2 mg B_2 and 10 mg B_6. *Dose: 1 capsule daily.*	Clear. In 100s.

PERIPHERAL VASODILATOR COMBINATIONS

In these combinations: *NIACIN* (see Vitamins monograph) is used for its vasodilating action.

Human B-Type Natriuretic Peptide

NESIRITIDE

Rx	**Natrecor** (Scios)	**Powder for injection, lyophilized:** 1.5 mg	Mannitol. In single-use vials.

NESIRITIDE — INJECTION

Indications

➤*Congestive heart failure:* For the intravenous treatment of patients with acutely decompensated congestive heart failure who have dyspnea at rest or with minimal activity. In this population, the use of nesiritide reduced pulmonary capillary wedge pressure and improved dyspnea.

Administration and Dosage

➤*Approved by the FDA:* August 10, 2001.

Nesiritide is for intravenous (IV) use only. There is limited experience with administering nesiritide for longer than 48 hours. Blood pressure should be monitored closely during nesiritide administration.

If hypotension occurs during the administration of nesiritide, the dose should be reduced or discontinued and other measures to support blood pressure should be started (IV fluids, changes in body position). In the vasodilation in the management of acute congestive heart failure (VMAC) trial, when symptomatic hypotension occurred, nesiritide was discontinued and subsequently could be restarted at a dose that was reduced by 30% (with no bolus administration) once the patient was stabilized. Because hypotension caused by nesiritide may be prolonged (up to hours), a period of observation may be necessary before restarting the drug.

➤*Dosing instructions:* The recommended dose of nesiritide is an IV bolus of 2 mcg/kg followed by a continuous infusion at a dose of 0.01 mcg/kg/min. Nesiritide should not be initiated at a dose that is above the recommended dose.

Prime the IV tubing with an infusion of 25 mL prior to connecting to the patient's vascular access port and prior to administering the bolus or starting the infusion.

Bolus followed by infusion – After preparation of the infusion bag, as described previously, withdraw the bolus volume (see data below) from the nesiritide infusion bag, and administer it over approximately 60 seconds through an IV port in the tubing. Immediately following the administration of the bolus, infuse nesiritide at a flow rate of 0.1 mL/kg/hr. This will deliver a nesiritide infusion dose of 0.01 mcg/kg/min.

To calculate the appropriate bolus volume and infusion flow rate to deliver a 0.01-mcg/kg/min dose, use the following formulas (or refer to the following dosing data).

Bolus volume:

$$\text{Bolus volume (mL)} = 0.33 \times \text{Patient weight (kg)}$$

Infusion flow rate:

$$\text{Infusion flow rate (mL/hr)} = 0.1 \times \text{Patient weight (kg)}$$

Nesiritide weight-adjusted bolus volume and infusion flow rate (2 mcg/kg bolus followed by a 0.01 mcg/kg/min dose)

Patient weight (kg)	Volume of bolus (mL)	Rate of infusion (mL/h)
60	20	6
70	23.3	7
80	26.7	8
90	30	9
100	33.3	10
110	36.7	11

➤*Dose adjustments:* The dose-limiting side effect of nesiritide is hypotension. Do not initiate nesiritide at a dose that is higher than the recommended dose of a 2 mcg/kg bolus followed by an infusion of 0.01 mcg/kg/min. In the VMAC trial there was limited experience with increasing the dose of nesiritide above the recommended dose (23 patients, all of whom had central hemodynamic monitoring). In those patients, the infusion dose of nesiritide was increased by 0.005 mcg/kg/min (preceded by a bolus of 1 mcg/kg), no more frequently than every 3 hours up to a maximum dose of 0.03 mcg/kg/min. Nesiritide should not be titrated at frequent intervals as is done with other IV agents that have a shorter half-life.

➤*Chemical/physical interactions:* Nesiritide is physically or chemically incompatible with injectable formulations of heparin, insulin, ethacrynate sodium, bumetamide, enalaprilat, hydralazine, and furosemide. These drugs should not be co-administered as infusions with nesiritide through the same IV catheter. The preservative sodium metabisulfite is incompatible with nesiritide. Injectable drugs that contain sodium metabisulfite should not be administered in the same infusion line as nesiritide. The catheter must be flushed between administration of nesiritide and incompatible drugs.

Nesiritide binds to heparin and therefore could bind to the heparin lining of a heparin-coated catheter, decreasing the amount of nesiritide delivered to the patient for some period of time. Therefore, nesiritide must not be administered through a central heparin-coated catheter. Concomitant administration of a heparin infusion through a separate catheter is acceptable.

➤*Storage/Stability:* Store nesiritide at controlled room temperature (20° to 25°C; 68° to 77°F); excursions permitted to 15° to 30°C (59° to 86°F; see USP controlled room temperature), or refrigerated (2° to 8°C; 36° to 46°F). Keep in carton until time of use.

Reconstituted vials of nesiritide may be left at controlled room temperature (20° to 25°C; 68° to 77°F) as per United States Pharmacopeia (USP) or may be refrigerated (2° to 8°C; 36° to 46°F) for up to 24 hours.

Actions

➤*Pharmacology:* Human BNP binds to the particulate guanylate cyclase receptor of vascular smooth muscle and endothelial cells, leading to increased intracellular concentrations of guanosine 3'5'-cyclic monophosphate (cGMP) and smooth muscle cell relaxation. Cyclic GMP serves as a second messenger to dilate veins and arteries. Nesiritide has been shown to relax isolated human arterial and venous tissue preparations that were precontracted with either endothelin-1 or the alpha-adrenergic agonist, phenylephrine.

In human studies, nesiritide produced dose-dependent reductions in pulmonary capillary wedge pressure (PCWP) and systemic arterial pressure in patients with heart failure.

➤*Pharmacokinetics:*

Absorption – The recommended dosing regimen of nesiritide is a 2 mcg/kg IV bolus followed by an intravenous infusion dose of 0.01 mcg/kg/min. With this dosing regimen, 60% of the 3-hour effect on PCWP reduction is achieved within 15 minutes after the bolus, reaching 95% of the 3-hour effect within 1 hour. Approximately 70% of the 3-hour effect on SBP reduction is reached within 15 minutes. The pharmacodynamic (PD) half-life of the onset and offset of the hemodynamic effect of nesiritide is longer than what the PK half-life of 18 minutes would predict. For example, in patients who developed symptomatic hypotension in the VMAC trial, half of the recovery of SBP toward the baseline value after discontinuation or reduction of the dose of nesiritide was observed in about 60 minutes. When higher doses of nesiritide were infused, the duration of hypotension was sometimes several hours.

Distribution – In patients with congestive heart failure (CHF), nesiritide administered intravenously by infusion or bolus exhibits biphasic disposition from the plasma.

In these patients, the mean volume of distribution of the central compartment (Vc) of nesiritide was estimated to be 0.073 L/kg, the mean steady-state volume of distribution (V_{ss}) was 0.19 L/kg, and the mean clearance (CL) was approximately 9.2 mL/min/kg. At steady state, plasma BNP levels increase from baseline endogenous levels by approximately 3- to 6-fold with nesiritide infusion doses ranging from 0.01 to 0.03 mcg/kg/min.

Excretion – The mean terminal elimination half-life ($t_{½}$) of nesiritide is approximately 18 minutes and was associated with approximately ⅔ of the area-under-the-curve (AUC). The mean initial elimination phase was estimated to be approximately 2 minutes.

Human BNP is cleared from the circulation via the following 3 independent mechanisms, in order of decreasing importance:

1.) Binding to cell surface clearance receptors with subsequent cellular internalization and lysosomal proteolysis.
2.) Proteolytic cleavage of the peptide by endopeptidases, such as neutral endopeptidase, which are present on the vascular lumenal surface.
3.) Renal filtration.

Contraindications

Hypersensitivity to any components of the product. Nesiritide should not be used as primary therapy for patients with cardiogenic shock or in patients with a systolic blood pressure less than 90 mm Hg.

Warnings

➤*Low cardiac filling pressures:* Administration of nesiritide should be avoided in patients suspected of having, or known to have, low cardiac filling pressures.

➤*Cardiovascular:* Nesiritide may cause hypotension. In the VMAC trial, in patients given the recommended dose (2 mcg/kg bolus followed by a 0.01 mcg/kg/min infusion) or the adjustable dose, the incidence of symptomatic hypotension in the first 24 hours was similar for nesiritide (4%) and IV nitroglycerin (5%). When hypotension occurred, however, the duration of symptomatic hypotension was longer with nesiritide (mean duration was 2.2 hours) than with nitroglycerin (mean duration was 0.7 hours). In earlier trials, when nesiritide was initiated at doses greater than the 2 mcg/kg bolus followed by a 0.01 mcg/kg/min infusion (ie, 0.015 and 0.030 mcg/kg/min preceded by a small bolus), there were more hypotensive episodes and these episodes were of greater intensity and duration. They were also more often symptomatic or more likely to require medical intervention. Nesiritide should be administered only in settings where blood pressure can be monitored closely, and the dose of nesiritide should be reduced or the drug discontinued in patients who develop hypotension. The rate of symptomatic hypotension may be increased in patients with a blood pressure less than 100 mmHg at baseline, and nesiritide should be used cautiously in these patients. The potential for hypotension may be increased by combining nesiritide with other drugs that may cause hypotension. For example, in the VMAC trial in patients treated with either nesiritide or nitroglycerin therapy, the frequency of symptomatic hypotension in patients who received an oral ACE inhibitor was 6%, compared with a frequency of symptomatic hypotension of 1% in patients who did not receive an oral ACE inhibitor.

NESIRITIDE — INJECTION

➤*Renal effects:* Nesiritide may affect renal function in susceptible individuals. In patients with severe heart failure whose renal function may depend on the activity of the renin-angiotensin-aldosterone system, treatment with nesiritide may be associated with azotemia. When nesiritide was initiated at doses more than 0.01 mcg/kg/min (0.015 and 0.030 mcg/kg/min), there was an increased rate of elevated serum creatinine over baseline compared with standard therapies, although the rate of acute renal failure and need for dialysis was not increased. In the 30-day follow-up period in the VMAC trial, 5 patients in the nitroglycerin group (2%) and 9 patients in the nesiritide group (3%) required first-time dialysis.

➤*Hypersensitivity reactions:* Parenteral administration of protein pharmaceuticals or *E. coli*-derived products should be attended by appropriate precautions in case of an allergic or untoward reaction. No serious allergic or anaphylactic reactions have been reported with nesiritide.

➤*Pregnancy: Category C.*

Animal reproductive studies have not been conducted with nesiritide. It is also not known whether nesiritide can cause fetal harm when administered to pregnant women or can affect reproductive capacity. Nesiritide should be used during pregnancy only if the potential benefit justifies any possible risk to the fetus.

➤*Lactation:* It is not known whether this drug is excreted in human milk. Therefore, caution should be exercised when nesiritide is administered to a breast-feeding woman.

➤*Children:* The safety and efficacy of nesiritide in children have not been established.

Precautions

➤*Special risk:* Nesiritide is not recommended for patients for whom vasodilating agents are not appropriate, such as patients with significant valvular stenosis, restrictive or obstructive cardiomyopathy, constrictive pericarditis, pericardial tamponade, or other conditions in which cardiac output is dependent upon venous return, or for patients suspected to have low cardiac filling pressures.

Drug Interactions

None known.

Adverse Reactions

Adverse reactions that occurred with at least a 3% frequency during the first 24 hours of nesiritide infusion are shown in the following table.

Nesiritide Adverse Reactions (≥ 3%)

	VMAC Trial		Other Long Infusion Trials		
	Nitroglycerin	Nesiritide Recommended dose	Control*	Nesiritide mcg/kg/min 0.015	Nesiritide mcg/kg/min 0.03
Adverse Reaction	(n = 216)	(n = 273)	(n = 256)	(n = 253)	(n = 246)
Cardiovascular					
Hypotension	25 (12%)	31 (11%)	20 (8%)	56 (22%)	87 (35%)
Symptomatic hypotension	10 (5%)	12 (4%)	8 (3%)	28 (11%)	42 (17%)
Asymptomatic hypotension	17 (8%)	23 (8%)	13 (5%)	31 (12%)	49 (20%)
Ventricular tachycardia (VT)	11 (5%)	9 (3%)	25 (10%)	25 (10%)	10 (4%)
Non-sustained VT	11 (5%)	9 (3%)	23 (9%)	24 (9%)	9 (4%)
Ventricular extrasystoles	2 (1%)	7 (3%)	15 (6%)	10 (4%)	9 (4%)
Angina pectoris	5 (2%)	5 (2%)	6 (2%)	14 (6%)	6 (2%)
Bradycardia	1 (< 1%)	3 (1%)	1 (< 1%)	8 (3%)	13 (5%)
CNS					
Insomnia	9 (4%)	6 (2%)	7 (3%)	15 (6%)	15 (6%)
Dizziness	4 (2%)	7 (3%)	7 (3%)	16 (6%)	12 (5%)
Anxiety	6 (3%)	8 (3%)	2 (1%)	8 (3%)	4 (2%)
GI					
Nausea	13 (6%)	10 (4%)	12 (5%)	24 (9%)	33 (13%)
Vomiting	4 (2%)	4 (1%)	2 (1%)	6 (2%)	10 (4%)
Miscellaneous					
Headache	44 (20%)	21 (8%)	23 (9%)	23 (9%)	17 (7%)
Abdominal pain	11 (5%)	4 (1%)	10 (4%)	6 (2%)	8 (3%)
Back pain	7 (3%)	10 (4%)	4 (2%)	5 (2%)	3 (1%)

* Includes dobutamine, milrinone, nitroglycerin, placebo, dopamine, nitroprusside, or amrinone.

➤*Other adverse reactions that occurred in at least 1%:* Adverse reactions that are not listed in the above table that occurred in at least 1% of patients who received any of the above nesiritide doses included:

Miscellaneous – Tachycardia, atrial fibrillation, AV node conduction abnormalities, catheter pain, fever, injection site reaction, confusion, paresthesia, somnolence, tremor, increased cough, hemoptysis, apnea, increased creatinine, sweating, pruritus, rash, leg cramps, amblyopia, anemia. All reported events (at least 1%) are included except those already listed, those too general to be informative, and those not reasonably associated with the use of the drug because they were associated with the condition being treated or are very common in the treated population.

➤*Placebo and active-controlled clinical trials:*

Cardiovascular – In placebo and active-controlled clinical trials, nesiritide has not been associated with an increase in atrial or ventricular tachyarrhythmias. In placebo-controlled trials, the incidence of VT in both nesiritide and placebo patients was 2%. In the PRECEDENT (prospective randomized evaluation of cardiac ectopy with dobutamine or nesiritide therapy) trial, the effects of nesiritide (n = 163) and dobutamine (n = 83) on the provocation or aggravation of existing ventricular arrhythmias in patients with decompensated CHF was compared using Holter monitoring. Treatment with nesiritide (0.015 and 0.03 mcg/kg/min without an initial bolus) for 24 hours did not aggravate preexisting VT or the frequency of premature ventricular beats, compared to a baseline 24-hour holter tape.

➤*Effect on mortality:* In the VMAC trial, the mortality rates at 6 months in the patients receiving nesiritide and nitroglycerin were 25.1% (95% confidence interval, 20.0% to 30.5%) and 20.8% (95% confidence interval, 15.5% to 26.5%), respectively. In all controlled trials combined, the mortality rates for nesiritide and active control (including nitroglycerin, dobutamine, nitroprusside, milrinone, amrinone, and dopamine) patients were 21.5% and 21.7%, respectively.

➤*Lab test abnormalities:* In the PRECEDENT trial, the incidence of elevations in serum creatinine to more than 0.5 mg/dL above baseline through day 14 was higher in the nesiritide 0.015 mcg/kg/min group (17%) and the nesiritide 0.03 mcg/kg/min group (19%) than with standard therapy (11%). In the VMAC trial, through day 30, the incidence of elevations in creatinine to more than 0.5 mg/dL above baseline was 28% and 21% in the nesiritide (2 mcg/kg bolus followed by 0.01 mcg/kg/min) and nitroglycerin groups, respectively.

Overdosage

No data are available with respect to overdosage in humans. The expected reaction would be excessive hypotension, which should be treated with drug discontinuation or reduction and appropriate measures.

Endothelin Receptor Antagonist

BOSENTAN

Rx	Tracleer (Actelion Pharm.)	Tablets: 62.5 mg	(62.5). Orange/White. Film-coated. In 60s.
		125 mg	(125). Orange/White. Film-coated. In 60s.

BOSENTAN — ORAL

WARNING

Potential liver injury – Bosentan causes at least a 3-fold (upper limit of normal [ULN]) elevation of liver aminotransferases (ALT and AST) in about 11% of patients, accompanied by elevated bilirubin in a small number of cases. Because these changes are a marker for potential serious liver injury, serum aminotransferase levels must be measured prior to initiation of treatment and then monthly. To date, in a setting of close monitoring, elevations have been reversible, within a few days to 9 weeks, either spontaneously or after dose reduction or discontinuation, and without sequelae.

Elevations in aminotransferases require close attention. Avoid using bosentan in patients with elevated aminotransferases (greater than 3 times ULN) at baseline because monitoring liver injury may be more difficult. If liver aminotransferase elevations are accompanied by clinical symptoms of liver injury (eg, abdominal pain, fever, jaundice, nausea, unusual lethargy or fatigue, vomiting) or increases in bilirubin greater than or equal to 2 times ULN, stop treatment. There is no experience with the reintroduction of bosentan in these circumstances.

Contraindication –

Pregnancy: Bosentan is very likely to produce major birth defects if used by pregnant women; this effect has been seen consistently when it is administered to animals. Therefore, pregnancy must be excluded before the start of treatment with bosentan and prevented thereafter by the use of a reliable method of contraception. Do not use hormonal contraceptives, including oral, injectable, transdermal, and implantable contraceptives, as the sole means of contraception because these may not be effective in patients receiving bosentan. Therefore, effective contraception through additional forms of contraception must be practiced. Obtain monthly pregnancy tests.

Because of potential liver injury and in an effort to make the chance of fetal exposure to bosentan as small as possible, bosentan may be prescribed only through the bosentan access program by calling 1-866-228-3546. Adverse reactions also can be reported directly via this number.

Indications

➤*Pulmonary arterial hypertension (PAH):* Bosentan is indicated for the treatment of PAH in patients with World Health Organization Class III or IV symptoms, to improve exercise ability and decrease the rate of clinical worsening.

➤*Unlabeled uses:* Prevention of digital ulcers in systemic sclerosis.

Administration and Dosage

➤*Approved by the FDA:* November 20, 2001.

➤*Dosage:* Bosentan treatment should be initiated at a dosage of 62.5 mg twice daily for 4 weeks and then increased to the maintenance dosage of 125 mg twice daily. Dosages above 125 mg twice daily did not appear to confer additional benefit sufficient to offset the increased risk of liver injury.

Tablets should be administered morning and evening with or without food.

Dosage Adjustment and Monitoring in Patients Developing Aminotransferase Abnormalities with Bosentan

ALT/AST levels	Treatment and monitoring recommendations
> 3 and ≤ 5 × ULN	Confirm by another aminotransferase test. If confirmed, reduce the daily dose or interrupt treatment and monitor aminotransferase levels at least every 2 weeks. If the aminotransferase levels return to pretreatment values, continue or reintroduce the treatment as appropriate.
> 5 and ≤ 8 × ULN	Confirm by another aminotransferase test. If confirmed, stop treatment and monitor aminotransferase levels at least every 2 weeks. Once the aminotransferase levels return to pretreatment values, consider reintroduction of the treatment.
> 8 × ULN	Treatments should be stopped and reintroduction of bosentan should not be considered. There is no experience with the reintroduction of bosentan in these circumstances.

➤*Reintroduction:* If bosentan is reintroduced it should be at the starting dose; aminotransferase levels should be checked within 3 days and thereafter according to the recommendations in the preceding table.

If liver aminotransferase elevations are accompanied by clinical symptoms of liver injury (eg, abdominal pain, fever, jaundice, nausea, unusual lethargy or fatigue, vomiting) or increases in bilirubin greater than or equal to 2 times ULN, treatment should be stopped. There is no experience with the reintroduction of bosentan in these circumstances.

➤*Women of childbearing potential:* Bosentan treatment should only be initiated in women of childbearing potential following a negative pregnancy test and only in those who practice adequate contraception that does not rely solely upon hormonal contraceptives, including oral, injectable, transdermal, or implantable contraceptives. Input from a gynecologist or similar expert on adequate contraception should be sought as needed. Urine or serum pregnancy tests should be obtained monthly in women of childbearing potential taking bosentan.

➤*Hepatic function impairment:* Because there is in vivo and in vitro evidence that the main route of excretion of bosentan is biliary, liver impairment could be expected to increase exposure (maximum serum concentration [C_{max}]), area under the curve of bosentan. Mild liver impairment was shown not to impact the pharmacokinetics of bosentan. The influence of moderate or severe liver impairment on the pharmacokinetics of bosentan has not been evaluated. There are no specific data to guide dosing in hepatically impaired patients; caution should be exercised in patients with mildly impaired liver function. Bosentan should generally be avoided in patients with moderate or severe hepatic function impairment.

➤*Patients with low body weight:* In patients with a body weight below 40 kg but who are older than 12 years of age, the recommended initial and maintenance dosage is 62.5 mg twice daily.

➤*Treatment discontinuation:* There is limited experience with abrupt discontinuation of bosentan. No evidence for acute rebound has been observed. Nevertheless, to avoid the potential for clinical deterioration, gradual dosage reduction (62.5 mg twice daily for 3 to 7 days) should be considered.

➤*Storage/Stability:* Store at 20° to 25°C (68° to 77°F). Excursions are permitted between 15° and 30°C (59° and 86°F).

Actions

➤*Pharmacology:* Endothelin-1 (ET-1) is a neurohormone, the effects of which are mediated by binding to ET_A and ET_B receptors in the endothelium and vascular smooth muscle. ET-1 concentrations are elevated in plasma and lung tissue of patients with PAH, suggesting a pathogenic role for ET-1 in this disease. Bosentan is a specific and competitive antagonist at endothelin receptor types ET_A and ET_B. Bosentan has a slightly higher affinity for ET_A receptors than for ET_B receptors.

➤*Pharmacokinetics:*

Absorption/Distribution – After oral administration, C_{max} of bosentan are attained within 3 to 5 hours in healthy adult subjects. The exposure to bosentan after intravenous (IV) and oral administration is approximately 2-fold greater in adult patients with PAH than in healthy adult subjects. Steady state is reached within 3 to 5 days.

The absolute bioavailability of bosentan in healthy volunteers is about 50% and is unaffected by food. The volume of distribution is about 18 L. Bosentan is highly bound (greater than 98%) to plasma proteins, mainly albumin. Bosentan does not penetrate into erythrocytes.

Metabolism/Excretion – Bosentan has 3 metabolites, 1 of which is pharmacologically active and may contribute 10% to 20% of the effect of bosentan. Bosentan is an inducer of CYP2C9 and CYP3A4 and possibly also of CYP2C19. Total clearance after a single IV dose is about 8 L/h. Upon multiple oral dosing, plasma concentrations decrease gradually to 50% to 65% of those seen after single-dose administration, probably the effect of autoinduction of the metabolizing liver enzymes. Bosentan is eliminated by biliary excretion following metabolism in the liver. Less than 3% of an administered oral dose is recovered in urine.

The terminal elimination half-life is about 5 hours in healthy adult subjects.

Special populations –

Renal function impairment: In patients with severe renal function impairment (creatinine clearance, 15 to 30 mL/min), plasma concentrations of bosentan were essentially unchanged and plasma concentrations of the 3 metabolites were increased approximately 2-fold compared with people with healthy renal function. These differences do not appear to be clinically important.

Hepatic function impairment: In vitro and in vivo evidence showing extensive hepatic metabolism of bosentan suggests that liver impairment would significantly increase exposure of bosentan. In a study comparing 8 patients with mild liver impairment (as indicated by the Child-Pugh method) to 8 controls, the single- and multiple-dose pharmacokinetics of bosentan were not altered in patients with mild hepatic function impairment. The influence of moderate or severe liver impairment on the pharmacokinetics of bosentan has not been evaluated. Generally, avoid using bosentan in patients with moderate or severe liver abnormalities and/or elevated aminotransferases greater than 3 times ULN.

Contraindications

Bosentan is very likely to produce major birth defects if used by pregnant women, as this effect has been seen consistently when it is administered to animals.

See Warning box and Warnings for more information.

BOSENTAN — ORAL

➤*Cyclosporine A:* Coadministration of cyclosporine A and bosentan resulted in markedly increased plasma concentrations of bosentan. Therefore, concomitant use of bosentan and cyclosporine A is contraindicated.

➤*Glyburide:* An increased risk of liver enzyme elevations was observed in patients receiving glyburide concomitantly with bosentan. Therefore, coadministration of glyburide and bosentan is contraindicated.

➤*Hypersensitivity:* Bosentan is also contraindicated in patients who are hypersensitive to bosentan or any component of the medication.

Warnings

➤*Hepatotoxicity:* Elevations in ALT or AST by more than 3 times the ULN were observed in 11% of bosentan-treated patients (n = 658) compared with 2% of placebo-treated patients (n = 280). Three-fold increases were seen in 12% of 95 PAH patients on 125 mg twice daily and 14% of 70 PAH patients on 250 mg twice daily. Eight-fold increases were seen in 2% of PAH patients on 125 mg twice daily and 7% of PAH patients on 250 mg twice daily. Bilirubin increases to greater than or equal to 3 times ULN were associated with aminotransferase increases in 2 of 658 (0.3%) of patients treated with bosentan.

The combination of hepatocellular injury (increases in aminotransferases of greater than 3 times ULN) and increases in total bilirubin (greater than or equal to 3 times ULN) is a marker for potential serious liver injury.

Elevations of AST and/or ALT associated with bosentan are dose dependent, occur both early and late in treatment, usually progress slowly, are typically asymptomatic, and to date have been reversible after treatment interruption or cessation. These aminotransferase elevations may reverse spontaneously while continuing treatment with bosentan.

Liver aminotransferase levels must be measured prior to initiation of treatment and then monthly. If elevated aminotransferase levels are seen, initiate changes in monitoring and treatment. If liver aminotransferase elevations are accompanied by clinical symptoms of liver injury (eg, abdominal pain, fever, jaundice, nausea, unusual lethargy or fatigue, vomiting) or increases in bilirubin greater than or equal to 2 times ULN, stop treatment. There is no experience with the reintroduction of bosentan in these circumstances.

➤*Hepatic function impairment:* Liver aminotransferase levels must be measured prior to initiation of treatment and then monthly. Generally, avoid using bosentan in patients with moderate to severe liver impairment. In addition, generally, avoid using bosentan in patients with elevated aminotransferases (greater than 3 times ULN) because monitoring liver injury in these patients may be more difficult.

There are no specific data to guide dosing in hepatically impaired patients; exercise caution in patients with mildly impaired liver function.

➤*Carcinogenesis:* Two years of dietary administration of bosentan to mice produced an increased incidence of hepatocellular adenomas and carcinomas in males at dosages as low as 450 mg/kg/day (about 8 times the maximum recommended human oral dose [MRHD] of 125 mg twice daily, on a mg/m^2 basis). In the same study, dosages greater than 2,000 mg/kg/day (about 32 times the MRHD) were associated with an increased incidence of colon adenomas in both males and females. In rats, dietary administration of bosentan for 2 years was associated with an increased incidence of brain astrocytomas in males at dosages as low as 500 mg/kg/day (about 16 times the MRHD).

➤*Fertility impairment:* Many endothelin receptor antagonists have profound effects on the histology and function of the testes in animals. These drugs have been shown to induce atrophy of the seminiferous tubules of the testes and to reduce sperm counts and male fertility in rats when administered for longer than 10 weeks. Where studied, testicular tubular atrophy and decreases in male fertility observed with endothelin receptor antagonists appear irreversible.

An increased incidence of testicular tubular atrophy was observed in rats given bosentan orally at dosages as low as 125 mg/kg/day (about 4 times the MRHD and the lowest doses tested) for 2 years but not at dosages as high as 1,500 mg/kg/day (about 50 times the MRHD) for 6 months. Effects on sperm count and motility were evaluated only in the much shorter duration fertility studies in which males had been exposed to the drug for 4 to 6 weeks.

➤*Pregnancy: Category X.*

Teratogenic – Bosentan is expected to cause fetal harm if administered to pregnant women. Bosentan was teratogenic in rats given oral dosages greater than or equal to 60 mg/kg/day (twice the MRHD of 125 mg, twice daily, on a mg/m^2 basis). In an embryo-fetal toxicity study in rats, bosentan showed dose-dependent teratogenic effects, including malformations of the head, mouth, face, and large blood vessels. Bosentan increased stillbirths and pup mortality at oral dosages of 60 and 300 mg/kg/day (2 and 10 times, respectively, the MRHD on a mg/m^2 basis). Although birth defects were not observed in rabbits given oral dosages of up to 1,500 mg/kg/day, plasma concentrations of bosentan in rabbits were lower than those reached in the rat. The similarity of malformations induced by bosentan and those observed in endothelin-1 knockout mice and in animals treated with other endothelin receptor antagonists indicates that teratogenicity is a class effect of these drugs. There are no data on the use of bosentan in pregnant women.

Exclude pregnancy before the start of treatment with bosentan and prevent thereafter by use of reliable contraception. It has been demonstrated that hormonal contraceptives, including oral, injectable, transdermal, and implantable contraceptives, may not be reliable in the presence of bosentan; do not use as the sole contraceptive method in patients receiving bosentan. Therefore, effective contraception through additional forms of contraception must be practiced. Seek input from a gynecologist or similar expert on adequate contraception as needed.

Start bosentan only in patients known not to be pregnant. For women of childbearing potential, do not issue a prescription for bosentan unless the patient assures that she is not sexually active or provides negative results from a urine or serum pregnancy test performed during the first 5 days of a normal menstrual period and at least 11 days after the last unprotected act of sexual intercourse.

Obtain follow-up urine or serum pregnancy tests monthly in women of childbearing potential taking bosentan. Advise the patient that if there is any delay in onset of menses or any other reason to suspect pregnancy, she must notify the health care provider immediately for pregnancy testing. If the pregnancy test is positive, the health care provider and patient must discuss the risk to the pregnancy and to the fetus.

➤*Lactation:* It is not known whether this drug is excreted in human milk. Because many drugs are excreted in human milk, breast-feeding while taking bosentan is not recommended.

➤*Children:* Safety and efficacy in children have not been established.

Precautions

➤*Monitoring:* Obtain monthly follow-up urine or serum pregnancy tests in women of childbearing potential taking bosentan.

Liver aminotransferase levels must be measured prior to initiation of treatment and then monthly. If elevated aminotransferase levels are seen, changes in monitoring and treatment must be initiated.

Monitor hemoglobin levels after 1 and 3 months of treatment and then every 3 months.

➤*Hematologic changes:* Treatment with bosentan caused a dose-related decrease in hemoglobin and hematocrit. Monitor hemoglobin levels after 1 and 3 months of treatment and then every 3 months. The overall mean decrease in hemoglobin concentration for bosentan-treated patients was 0.9 g/dL (change to end of treatment). Most of this decrease of hemoglobin concentration was detected during the first few weeks of bosentan treatment and hemoglobin levels stabilized by 4 to 12 weeks of bosentan treatment. In placebo-controlled studies of all uses of bosentan, marked decreases in hemoglobin (greater than 15% decrease from baseline resulting in values less than 11 g/dL) were observed in 6% of bosentan-treated patients and 3% of placebo-treated patients. In patients with PAH treated with dosages of 125 and 250 mg twice daily, marked decreases in hemoglobin occurred in 3% compared with 1% in placebo-treated patients.

A decrease in hemoglobin concentration by at least 1 g/dL was observed in 57% of bosentan-treated patients as compared with 29% of placebo-treated patients. In 80% of those patients whose hemoglobin decreased by at least 1 g/dL, the decrease occurred during the first 6 weeks of bosentan treatment.

During the course of treatment the hemoglobin concentration remained within normal limits in 68% of bosentan-treated patients compared with 76% of placebo patients. The explanation for the change in hemoglobin is not known, but it does not appear to be hemorrhage or hemolysis.

It is recommended that hemoglobin concentrations be checked after 1 and 3 months, and every 3 months thereafter. If a marked decrease in hemoglobin concentration occurs, undertake further evaluation to determine the cause and need for specific treatment.

➤*Fluid retention:* In a placebo-controlled trial of patients with severe chronic heart failure (CHF), there was an increased incidence of hospitalization for CHF associated with weight gain and increased leg edema during the first 4 to 8 weeks of treatment with bosentan. In addition, there have been numerous postmarketing reports of fluid retention in patients with pulmonary hypertension, occurring within weeks after starting bosentan. Patients required intervention with a diuretic, fluid management, or hospitalization for decompensating heart failure.

Drug Interactions

➤*CYP-450 system:* Bosentan is metabolized by CYP2C9 and CYP3A4. Inhibition of these isoenzymes may increase the plasma concentration of bosentan. Bosentan is an inducer of CYP3A4 and CYP2C9. Consequently, plasma concentrations of drugs metabolized by these 2 isoenzymes will be decreased when bosentan is coadministered. Bosentan had no relevant inhibitory effect on any CYP isoenzymes tested (CYP1A2, CYP2C9, CYP2C19, CYP2D6, CYP3A4). Consequently, bosentan is not expected to increase the plasma concentrations of drugs metabolized by these enzymes.

Bosentan Drug Interactions

Precipitant drug	Object drug[a]		Description
Cyclosporine A	Bosentan	↑	Coadministration increased bosentan trough concentrations ≈ 30-fold and steady-state concentrations 3- to 4-fold. Cyclosporine A plasma concentrations decreased ≈ 50%. Coadministration is contraindicated.
Bosentan	Cyclosporine A	↓	

BOSENTAN — ORAL

Bosentan Drug Interactions			
Precipitant drug	Object drug[a]		Description
Glyburide	Bosentan	⬇	Glyburide plasma concentrations were decreased ≈ 40% when administered with bosentan, whereas the plasma concentrations of bosentan were also decreased ≈ 30%. However, coadministration is contraindicated because an increased risk of elevated liver enzymes was also observed in patients receiving concomitant therapy.
Bosentan	Glyburide		
Ketoconazole	Bosentan	⬆	Coadministration increased bosentan plasma concentrations ≈ 2-fold. No dosage adjustment is necessary, but consider increased effects of bosentan.
Tacrolimus	Bosentan	⬆	Although not studied in humans, coadministration resulted in markedly increased plasma concentrations of bosentan in animals. Exercise caution.
Bosentan	Hormonal contraceptives (including oral, transdermal, injectable, and implantable)	⬇	There is a possibility of contraception failure when bosentan is coadministered. Women should not rely on hormonal contraception alone when taking bosentan.
Bosentan	Statins (eg, atorvastatin, lovastatin, simvastatin)	⬇	The plasma concentrations of simvastatin and its metabolite decreased ≈ 50% when coadministered with bosentan. Bosentan is also expected to reduce plasma concentrations of other statins significantly metabolized by CYP3A4 (ie, atorvastatin, lovastatin). Monitor cholesterol levels and adjust statin dose accordingly.
Bosentan	Warfarin	⬇	Coadministration decreased the plasma concentrations of S-warfarin and R-warfarin 29% and 38%, respectively. Clinically relevant changes in INR or warfarin dose were not seen in patients with PAH during clinical trials.

[a] ⬆ = Object drug increased. ⬇ = Object drug decreased.

Adverse Reactions

Treatment discontinuation – Treatment discontinuation because of adverse reactions other than those related to pulmonary hypertension during the clinical trials in patients with PAH were more frequent on bosentan (5%; 8 of 165 patients) than on placebo (3%; 2 of 80 patients). In this database the only cause of discontinuations greater than 1% and occurring more often on bosentan was abnormal liver function.

➤*Adverse reactions (greater than or equal to 3%):*

Bosentan Adverse Reactions (≥ 3%)[a]				
	Bosentan (n = 165)		Placebo (n = 80)	
Adverse reaction	Number	%	Number	%
Cardiovascular				
Hypotension	11	7%	3	4%
Palpitations	8	5%	1	1%
CNS				
Fatigue	6	4%	1	1%
Headache	36	22%	16	20%
Dermatologic				
Flushing	15	9%	4	5%
Pruritus	6	4%	0	0%
GI				
Abnormal hepatic function	14	8%	2	3%
Dyspepsia	7	4%	0	0%
Metabolic				
Edema	7	4%	2	3%
Edema, lower limb	13	8%	4	5%
Respiratory				
Nasopharyngitis	18	11%	6	8%

[a] Note: Only adverse reactions with onset from start of treatment to 1 calendar day after end of treatment are included. All reported reactions (at least 3%) are included except those too general to be informative, and those not reasonably associated with the use of the drug because they were associated with the condition being treated or are very common in the treated population.

➤*Placebo-controlled studies:* In placebo-controlled studies of bosentan in PAH and for other diseases (primarily chronic heart failure), a total of 677 patients were treated with bosentan at daily doses ranging from 100 to 2,000 mg and 288 patients were treated with placebo. The duration of treatment ranged from 4 weeks to 6 months. For the adverse reactions that occurred in greater than or equal to 3% of bosentan-treated patients, the only ones that occurred more frequently on bosentan than on placebo (greater than or equal to 2% difference) were headache (16% vs 13%), flushing (7% vs 2%), abnormal hepatic function (6% vs 2%), leg edema (5% vs 1%), and anemia (3% vs 1%).

➤*Postmarketing:* Hypersensitivity, rash.

➤*Lab test abnormalities:*

Increased liver aminotransferases – Bosentan causes at least 3-fold (ULN) elevation of liver aminotransferases (ALT and AST) in about 11% of patients, accompanied by elevated bilirubin in a small number of cases. Because these changes are a marker for potential serious liver injury, serum aminotransferase levels must be measured prior to initiation of treatment and then monthly. To date, in a setting of close monitoring, elevations have been reversible, within a few days to 9 weeks, either spontaneously or after dose reduction or discontinuation, and without sequelae.

See Warning Box and Warnings for more information.

Decreased hemoglobin and hematocrit – Treatment with bosentan caused a dose-related decrease in hemoglobin and hematocrit. Monitor hemoglobin levels after 1 and 3 months of treatment and then every 3 months. The overall mean decrease in hemoglobin concentration for bosentan-treated patients was 0.9 g/dL (change to end of treatment). Most of this decrease of hemoglobin concentration was detected during the first few weeks of bosentan treatment and hemoglobin levels stabilized by 4 to 12 weeks of bosentan treatment.

See Precautions for more information.

➤*Long-term treatment:* The long-term follow-up of the patients who were treated with bosentan in the 2 pivotal studies and their open-label extensions (N = 235) shows that 93% and 84% of patients were still alive at 1 and 2 years, respectively, after the start of treatment with bosentan. These estimates may be influenced by the presence of epoprostenol treatment, which was administered to 43 of 235 patients. Without a control group, these data must be interpreted cautiously and cannot be interpreted as an improvement in survival.

Overdosage

➤*Symptoms:* Bosentan has been given as a single dose of up to 2,400 mg in healthy volunteers, or up to 2,000 mg/day for 2 months in patients, without any major clinical consequences. The most common adverse reaction was headache of mild to moderate intensity. In the cyclosporine A interaction study, in which dosages of 500 and 1,000 mg twice daily of bosentan were given concomitantly with cyclosporine A, trough plasma concentrations of bosentan increased 30-fold, resulting in severe headache, nausea, and vomiting, but no serious adverse reactions. Mild decreases in blood pressure and increases in heart rate were observed.

➤*Treatment:* There is no specific experience of overdosage with bosentan beyond the doses described. Massive overdosage may result in pronounced hypotension requiring active cardiovascular support.

Patient Information

Advise patients to consult the bosentan medication guide on the safe use of bosentan.

Discuss with the patient the importance of monthly monitoring of serum aminotransferases and urine or serum pregnancy testing and of avoidance of pregnancy. Discuss options for effective contraception and measures to prevent pregnancy with women. Seek input from a gynecologist or similar expert on adequate contraception as needed.

ILOPROST INHALATIONAL

Rx	**Ventavis** (CoTherix)	**Solution for inhalation:** 10 mcg/mL	Preservative-free. In 1 and 2 mL single-dose ampules.

ILOPROST INHALATIONAL

Indications

➤*Pulmonary arterial hypertension:* For the treatment of pulmonary arterial hypertension (World Health Organization [WHO] group I) in patients with New York Heart Association (NYHA) class III or IV symptoms. In controlled trials, it improved a composite endpoint consisting of exercise tolerance, symptoms (NYHA class), and lack of deterioration.

➤*Unlabeled uses:* Intravenous (IV) administration of iloprost for the treatment of severe Raynaud phenomenon associated with systemic sclerosis.

Administration and Dosage

➤*Approved by the FDA:* December 29, 2004.

Iloprost is intended to be inhaled using the *I-neb AAD System* or the *Prodose AAD* system. The first inhaled dose should be 2.5 mcg (as delivered at the mouthpiece). If this dose is well tolerated, increase dosing to 5 mcg and maintain that dose. Take iloprost 6 to 9 times/day (no more than every 2 hours) during waking hours, according to individual need and tolerability. The maximum daily dose evaluated in clinical studies was 45 mcg (5 mcg 9 times/day).

Each inhalation treatment requires 1 single-use ampule. The 2 mL single-use ampule delivers 20 mcg to the medication chamber of either of the AAD delivery systems. The 2 mL must be used with the *Prodose AAD System* and may be used with the *I-neb AAD System*. The 1 mL ampule delivers 10 mcg to the medication chamber and must be used only with the *I-neb AAD System*. Both the 2 mL and the 1 mL ampules deliver a nominal dose of either 2.5 or 5 mcg at the mouthpiece.

To avoid potential interruptions in drug delivery caused by equipment malfunctions, the patient should have easy access to a backup *Prodose AAD* system.

➤*Administration:* For each inhalation session, transfer the entire contents of 1 opened ampule of iloprost into either the *I-neb AAD System* or *Prodose AAD* system medication chamber 2 mL amp only immediately before use. After each inhalation session, discard any solution remaining in the medication chamber. Use of the remaining solution will result in unpredictable dosing. Follow the manufacturer's instructions for cleaning the *I-neb AAD System* or the *Prodose AAD* system components after each dose administration.

➤*Preparation for administration:*

1.) With one hand, hold the bottom of the ampule with the blue dot facing away from the body.
2.) With the other hand, wrap the included rubber pad around the entire ampule.
3.) Using thumbs, break open the neck of the ampule by snapping the top toward the body.
4.) Transfer the entire contents of the ampule into the medication chamber of the *I-neb AAD System* or *Prodose AAD System*.
5.) Safely dispose of the open ampule, out of the reach of children and as instructed by a health care provider.
6.) Follow the instructions provided by the drug manufacturer for administration of the iloprost dose and maintenance of the *I-neb AAD System* or *Prodose AAD System*.

Mixing with other medications – Direct mixing of iloprost with other medications in the *I-neb AAD System* or *Prodose AAD Systemhas* not been evaluated.

➤*Alternative treatments:* Use of iloprost with other approved treatments for pulmonary hypertension has not been studied. If patients deteriorate while on this treatment, consider alternative treatments. Several patients whose status deteriorated while on iloprost were successfully switched to IV epoprostenol.

➤*Storage/Stability:* Store at 20° to 25°C (68° to 77°F); excursions permitted to 15° to 30°C (59° to 86°F).

Actions

➤*Pharmacology:* Iloprost is a synthetic analog of prostacyclin PGI_2. Iloprost dilates systemic and pulmonary arterial vascular beds. It also affects platelet aggregation; however, the relevance of this effect to the treatment of pulmonary hypertension is unknown. The 2 diastereoisomers of iloprost differ in their potency in dilating blood vessels, with the 4S isomer substantially more potent than the 4R isomer.

➤*Pharmacokinetics:*

Absorption – Iloprost administered IV has linear pharmacokinetics over the dose range of 1 to 3 ng/kg/min.

The absolute bioavailability of inhaled iloprost has not been determined. Following inhalation of iloprost (5 mcg), patients with pulmonary hypertension have iloprost peak serum levels of approximately 150 pg/mL. Iloprost was generally not detectable in the plasma 30 minutes to 1 hour after inhalation.

Distribution – Following IV infusion, the apparent steady-state volume of distribution was 0.7 to 0.8 L/kg in healthy subjects. Iloprost is approximately 60% protein bound, mainly to albumin, and this ratio is concentration independent in the range of 30 to 3,000 pg/mL.

Metabolism/Excretion – Clearance in healthy subjects was approximately 20 mL/min/kg. Iloprost is metabolized principally via beta-oxidation of the carboxyl side chain. The main metabolite is tetranor-iloprost, which is found in the urine in free and conjugated form.

In vitro studies reveal that cytochrome P-450-dependent metabolism plays only a minor role in the biotransformation of iloprost. IV and oral [^{3}H]-iloprost showed that recovery of total radioactivity more than 14 hours postdose was 81%, with 68% and 12% recoveries in urine and feces, respectively.

The half-life of iloprost is 20 to 30 minutes.

Special populations –

Hepatic function impairment: In an IV iloprost study in patients with liver cirrhosis, the mean clearance in Child-Pugh class B subjects was approximately 10 mL/min/kg (half that of healthy patients). Following oral administration, the mean area under the curve ($AUC_{0\text{-}8h}$) in Child-Pugh class B patients was 1,725 pg•h/mL compared with 117 pg•h/mL in healthy subjects receiving the same oral iloprost dose. In Child-Pugh class A subjects, the mean $AUC_{0\text{-}8h}$ was 639 pg•h/mL. Although exposure increased with hepatic impairment, there was no effect on half-life.

Renal function impairment: In a study with IV infusion of iloprost in patients with end-stage renal failure requiring intermittent dialysis treatment, the mean $AUC_{0\text{-}4h}$ was 230 pg•h/mL compared with 54 pg•h/mL in patients with renal failure not requiring intermittent dialysis and 48 pg•h/mL in healthy patients. The half-life was similar in both groups.

Contraindications

None known.

Warnings

➤*Administration:* Iloprost is intended for inhalation administration only via the *I-neb AAD System* or *Prodose AAD System*, a pulmonary drug delivery device. It has not been studied with any other nebulizers.

➤*Syncope:* Because of the risk of syncope, monitor vital signs while initiating iloprost. In patients with low systemic blood pressure, take care to avoid further hypotension. Do not initiate iloprost in patients with systolic blood pressure less than 85 mm Hg. Be alert to the presence of concomitant conditions or drugs that might increase the risk of syncope. Syncope can also occur in association with pulmonary arterial hypertension, particularly in association with physical exertion. The occurrence of exertional syncope may reflect a therapeutic gap or insufficient efficacy; consider the need to adjust dose or change therapy.

➤*Pulmonary edema:* If signs of pulmonary edema occur when inhaled iloprost is administered in patients with pulmonary hypertension, stop the treatment immediately. This may be a sign of pulmonary venous hypotension.

➤*Renal function impairment:* Dose adjustment is not required in patients not on dialysis. Use caution in treating patients on dialysis.

➤*Hepatic function impairment:* Because iloprost elimination is reduced in patients with impaired liver function, exercise caution during iloprost therapy in patients with at least Child-Pugh class B hepatic impairment.

➤*Elderly:* Dose selection for an elderly patient should be cautious, usually starting at the low end of the dosing range, reflecting the greater frequency of decreased hepatic, renal, or cardiac function and of concomitant disease or other drug therapy.

➤*Pregnancy: Category C.* Studies in pregnant Han-Wistar rats, continuous IV administration of iloprost at a dosage of 0.01 mg/kg/day (serum levels not available) led to shortened digits of the thoracic extremity in fetuses and pups. However, in gravid Sprague-Dawley rats, iloprost clathrate (13% iloprost) significantly increased the number of nonviable fetuses at a maternally toxic oral dosage of 250 mg/kg/day and in Han-Wistar rats was found to be embryolethal in 15 of 44 litters at an IV dosage of 1 mg/kg/day. There are no adequate and well-controlled studies in pregnant women. Use during pregnancy only if the potential benefit justifies the potential risk to the fetus.

➤*Lactation:* It is not known whether iloprost is excreted in human milk. In studies with Han-Wistar rats, higher mortality was observed in pups of lactating dams receiving iloprost IV at 1 mg/kg/day. In Sprague-Dawley rats, higher mortality was also observed in nursing pups at a maternally toxic oral dosage of 250 mg/kg/day of iloprost clathrate (13% iloprost by weight). Because many drugs are excreted in human milk and because of the potential for serious adverse reactions in breast-feeding infants from iloprost, decide whether to discontinue breast-feeding or the drug, taking into account the importance of the drug to the mother.

➤*Children:* Safety and efficacy in children have not been established.

Precautions

➤*Monitoring:* Because of the risk of syncope, monitor vital signs while initiating iloprost. Do not initiate iloprost in patients with systolic blood pressure less than 85 mm Hg.

➤*Contact with iloprost solution:* Do not allow iloprost solution to come into contact with the skin or eyes; avoid oral ingestion of iloprost solution.

➤*Special risk:* Iloprost has not been studied in patients with pulmonary hypertension, which increases mean AUC in otherwise healthy patients.

ILOPROST INHALATIONAL

Iloprost has not been evaluated in patients with chronic obstructive pulmonary disease (COPD), severe asthma, or acute pulmonary infections.

Drug Interactions

➤*Vasodilators/Antihypertensive agents:* Iloprost has the potential to increase the hypotensive effect of vasodilators and antihypertensive agents.

➤*Anticoagulants:* Iloprost inhibits platelet function; there is a potential for increased risk of bleeding.

Adverse Reactions

The following table shows adverse reactions reported by at least 4 iloprost patients and reported at least 3% more frequently for iloprost patients than placebo patients in the 12-week, placebo-controlled study.

Iloprost Adverse Reactions

Adverse reaction	Iloprost (n = 101)	Placebo (n = 102)
Cardiovascular		
Hypotension	11%	6%
Palpitations	7%	4%
Syncope	8%	5%
Vasodilation (flushing)	27%	9%
CNS		
Headache	30%	20%
Insomnia	8%	2%
GI		
Nausea	13%	8%
Vomiting	7%	2%
Lab test abnormalities		
Abnormal lab test	7%	3%
Increased alkaline phosphatase	6%	1%
Increased gamma-glutamyltransferase (GGT)	6%	3%
Respiratory		
Hemoptysis	5%	2%
Increased cough	39%	26%
Pneumonia	4%	1%
Miscellaneous		
Back pain	7%	3%
Flu syndrome	14%	10%
Muscle cramps	6%	3%
Tongue pain	4%	0%
Trismus	12%	3%

Serious adverse reactions reported with the use of inhaled iloprost and not shown in the previous table include chest pain, congestive heart failure, dyspnea, kidney failure, peripheral edema, and supraventricular tachycardia.

➤*Adverse reactions with higher doses:* In a study in healthy volunteers (n = 160), inhaled doses of iloprost solution were given every 2 hours, beginning with 5 mcg and increasing up to 20 mcg for a total of 6 dose inhalations (total cumulative dose of 70 mcg) or up to the highest dose tolerated in a subgroup of 40 volunteers. There were 13 subjects (32%) who failed to reach the highest scheduled dose (20 mcg). Five were unable to increase the dose because of mild to moderate transient chest pain/discomfort/tightness, usually accompanied by headache, nausea, and dizziness. The remaining 8 subjects discontinued for other reasons.

Overdosage

➤*Symptoms:* In clinical trials of iloprost, no case of overdose was reported. Signs and symptoms to be anticipated are extensions of the dose-limiting pharmacological effects, including diarrhea, flushing, headache, hypotension, nausea, and vomiting.

➤*Treatment:* A specific antidote is not known. Interruption of the inhalation session, monitoring, and symptomatic measures are recommended.

Patient Information

Advise patients receiving iloprost to use the drug only as prescribed with the *I-neb AAD System* or *Prodose AAD System*, a pulmonary drug-delivery device, following the manufacturer's instructions. Train patients in proper administration techniques, including dosing frequency, ampule dispensing, *I-neb AAD System* or *Prodose AAD System* operation, and equipment cleaning.

Advise patients that they may have a fall in blood pressure with iloprost, so they may become dizzy or even faint. They should stand up slowly when they get out of a chair or bed. If fainting gets worse, patients should consult their doctors about dose adjustment.

Advise patients that iloprost should be inhaled at intervals of not less than 2 hours and that the acute benefits of iloprost may not last 2 hours.

Patients should avoid oral ingestion or skin contact of iloprost solution.

The most common side effects with iloprost include reddening of the face caused by dilation of blood vessels (flushing), increased cough, low blood pressure (hypotension), headache, nausea, spasms of the jaw muscles that cause trouble opening your mouth, and fainting (syncope).

Patients should not put any other medicines in the *I-neb AAD System* or *Prodose AAD System* while using iloprost.

VASODILATOR COMBINATIONS

Rx	**BiDil** (NitroMed[a])	**Tablets:** 20 mg isosorbide dinitrate/ 37.5 mg hydralazine hydrochloride	Lactose. (N 20). Orange, scored. Film-coated. In 180s.

[a] NitroMed, Inc., 15 Ingram Boulevard, Lavergne, TN 37086; (781) 266-4186.

VASODILATOR COMBINATIONS — ORAL

For additional prescribing information, refer to the Nitrates group monograph and the Hydralazine individual monograph.

Indications

➤*Heart failure:* For the treatment of heart failure as an adjunct to standard therapy in self-identified black patients to improve survival, to prolong time to hospitalization for heart failure, and to improve patient-reported functional status. There is little experience in patients with the New York Heart Association class IV heart failure.

Administration and Dosage

➤*Approved by the FDA:* June 23, 2005.

One tablet 3 times a day; may be titrated to a maximum tolerated dose not to exceed 2 tablets 3 times a day.

Although titration can be rapid (3 to 5 days), some patients may experience side effects and may take longer to reach their maximum tolerated dose. The dosage may be decreased to as little as one-half tablet 3 times a day if intolerable side effects occur. Efforts should be made to titrate up as soon as side effects subside.

➤*Storage/Stability:* Store at 25°C (77°F), excursions permitted to 15° to 30°C (59° to 86°F). Protect from light. Dispense in a light-resistant, tight container.

WARNING

Atenolol, metoprolol, nadolol, propranolol, timolol – There have been reports of exacerbation of angina and, in some cases, myocardial infarction and ventricular arrythmias, following abrupt discontinuance of beta-adrenergic blocking agents therapy. Therefore, when discontinuance of beta-adrenergic blocking agents is planned, gradually reduce the dosage over at least a few weeks, and caution the patient against interruption or cessation of therapy without a physician's advice. If beta-adrenergic blocking agents therapy is interrupted and exacerbation of angina occurs or acute coronary insufficiency develops, it is usually advisable to promptly reinstitute beta-adrenergic blocking agents therapy and take other measures appropriate for the management of angina pectoris. Because coronary artery disease may be unrecognized, it may be prudent to follow the above advice in patients who are given beta-adrenergic blocking agents for other indications.

Sotalol – To minimize the risk of induced arrhythmia, place patients initiated or reinitiated on sotalol or sotalol AF for a minimum of 3 days (on their maintenance dose) in a facility that can provide cardiac resuscitation, continuous electrocardiographic monitoring, and calculations of creatinine clearance. For detailed instructions regarding dose selection and special cautions for people with renal impairment, see Administration and Dosage.

Do not substitute sotalol for sotalol AF because of significant differences in labeling (eg, patient package insert, dosing administration, safety administration).

Indications

➤*Hypertension (all except esmolol and sotalol):* Used alone as initial drug choice or in combination with other drugs, particularly a thiazide diuretic. Not indicated for treatment of hypertensive emergencies.

➤*Angina pectoris (nadolol, propranolol, atenolol, metoprolol):* Long-term management.

➤*Hypertrophic subaortic stenosis (propranolol):* Useful in managing exertional or other stress-induced angina, palpitations, and syncope. Improves exercise performance. Efficacy appears to be caused by reduction of elevated outflow pressure gradient that is exacerbated by beta receptor stimulation. Clinical improvement may be temporary.

➤*Cardiac arrhythmias (acebutolol, esmolol, propranolol, sotalol):* Use acebutolol for ventricular premature beats only. Use sotalol for documented life-threatening ventricular arrhythmias, such as sustained ventricular tachycardia.

Supraventricular arrhythmias (propranolol) – Paroxysmal atrial tachycardias, particularly those arrhythmias induced by catecholamines or digitalis or associated with the Wolff-Parkinson-White syndrome); persistent sinus tachycardia that is noncompensatory and impairs the well-being of the patient.

Tachycardias and arrhythmias caused by thyrotoxicosis when they cause distress or increased hazard and when immediate effect is necessary as adjunctive, short-term (2 to 4 weeks) therapy. May be used with, but not in place of, specific therapy.

Persistent atrial extrasystoles that impair the well-being of the patient and do not respond to conventional measures. Atrial flutter and fibrillation when ventricular rate cannot be controlled by digitalis alone, or when digitalis is contraindicated.

Supraventricular tachycardia (esmolol) – Rapid control of ventricular rate in patients with atrial fibrillation or atrial flutter in perioperative, postoperative, or other emergent circumstances in which short-term control of ventricular rate with a short-acting agent is desirable.

Sinus tachycardia (esmolol) – Noncompensatory sinus tachycardia in which the rapid heart rate requires intervention. Esmolol is not intended for use in chronic settings where transfer to another agent is anticipated.

Intraoperative and postoperative tachycardia and hypertension (esmolol) – Treatment of tachycardia and hypertension that may occur during induction and tracheal intubation, during surgery, on emergence from anesthesia, and in the postoperative period, when in the physician's judgment such specific intervention is indicated.

Ventricular tachycardias (propranolol) – In ventricular tachycardias, with the exception of those induced by catecholamines or digitalis, propranolol is not the drug of first choice. In critical situations when cardioversion techniques or other drugs are not indicated or are ineffective, propranolol may be considered.

Persistent premature ventricular extrasystoles that impair the well-being of the patient and do not respond to conventional measures.

Tachyarrhythmias of digitalis intoxication (propranolol) – If it is persistent following discontinuation of digitalis and correction of electrolyte abnormalities, tachyarrhythmias are usually reversible with oral propranolol. Severe bradycardia may occur. Reserve IV propranolol for life-threatening arrhythmias. Temporary maintenance with oral therapy may be indicated.

Resistant tachyarrhythmias caused by excessive catecholamine action during anesthesia (propranolol) – All general inhalation anesthetics produce some degree of myocardial depression; therefore, use propranolol with extreme caution.

Maintenance of normal sinus rhythm (sotalol) – In patients with highly symptomatic atrial fibrillation/atrial flutter (AFIB/AFL) who are currently in sinus rhythm (*Betapace AF* only).

➤*MI (propranolol, timolol):* Indicated in clinically stable patients who have survived the acute phase of an MI to reduce cardiovascular mortality and risk of reinfarction. Initiate treatment within 1 to 4 weeks after infarction.

Metoprolol and atenolol – Both are also indicated in the treatment of hemodynamically stable patients with definite or suspected acute MI. Treatment can be initiated as soon as the patient's clinical condition allows or within 3 to 10 days of the acute event.

➤*CHF (metoprolol):* Treatment of stable, symptomatic (NYHA Class II or III) heart failure of ischemic, hypertensive, or cardiomyopathic origin (*Toprol-XL* 25 mg only). Studied in patients already receiving ACE inhibitors, diuretics, and, in the majority of cases, digitalis. In this population, *Toprol-XL* decreased the rate of mortality plus hospitalization, largely through a reduction in cardiovascular mortality and hospitalizations for heart failure.

➤*Pheochromocytoma (propranolol):* After primary treatment with an alpha-adrenergic blocking agent has been instituted, propranolol may be useful as adjunctive therapy if the control of tachycardia becomes necessary before or during surgery.

With inoperable or metastatic pheochromocytoma, propranolol may be useful as an adjunct to the management of symptoms caused by excessive beta receptor stimulation.

➤*Migraine (propranolol, timolol):* For the prophylaxis of common migraine headache.

➤*Essential tremor (propranolol):* For the management of familial or hereditary essential tremor consisting of involuntary, rhythmic, and oscillatory movements. Propranolol causes a reduction in the tremor amplitude but not in the tremor frequency. It is not indicated for the treatment of tremor associated with Parkinsonism.

➤*Unlabeled uses:* The agents listed have been evaluated for use in the following conditions:

Akathisia (antipsychotic-induced) – Propranolol (30 to 120 mg/day), metoprolol (50 to 400 mg/day).

Atrial fibrillation (rapid heart rate control) – Metoprolol (2.5 to 5 mg IV bolus over 2 minutes, up to 3 doses).

Atrial fibrillation (maintenance heart rate control) – Metoprolol (25 to 100 mg twice daily).

Angina (stable) – Acebutolol, bisoprolol.

Angina (unstable) – Atenolol (5 mg over 5 minutes IV, up to 3 doses; 25 to 100 mg/day orally), esmolol (500 mcg/kg bolus and infusion of 10 to 200 mcg/kg/minute), metoprolol (5 mg over 5 minutes IV, up to 3 doses; 25 to 100 mg twice daily orally).

CHF (stable) – Immediate-release metoprolol (initial dose of 12.5 mg twice daily, increase to up to 50 mg twice daily), bisoprolol (initial dose of 2.5 mg daily, increase to up to 10 mg daily).

Generalized anxiety disorder – Propranolol (initial dose of 10 mg twice daily; maximum daily dose is 360 mg).

Hypertensive crises – Esmolol (loading dose of 500 mcg/kg over 1 minute, followed by infusion at 25 to 50 mcg/kg/min, which may be increased by 25 mcg/kg/min every 10 to 20 minutes until the desired response is obtained; maximum dose is 300 mcg/kg/min).

Hyperthyroidism adjunctive therapy – Propranolol and nadolol may provide symptomatic improvement until euthyroid state is achieved.

Migraine prophylaxis – Atenolol (50 to 200 mg/day), metoprolol (100 to 200 mg/day), and nadolol (40 to 240 mg/day).

Parkinsonian tremor – Propranolol SR (initial dose of 60 mg in the morning; may be increased up to 160 mg/day); nadolol.

Prevention of variceal bleeding caused by portal hypertension – Propranolol (initial dose of 40 mg twice daily; average maintenance dose is 160 mg/day), nadolol (80 mg/day), atenolol, timolol, metoprolol.

Beta-Adrenergic Blocking Agents

Beta-Adrenergic Blocking Agents – Summary of Indications[1]

Indications ✓= labeled x = unlabeled	Acebutolol	Atenolol	Betaxolol	Bisoprolol	Esmolol	Metoprolol[2]	Nadolol	Penbutolol	Pindolol	Propranolol[2]	Sotalol	Timolol
Hypertension	✓	✓	✓	✓		✓	✓	✓	✓	✓		✓
Angina pectoris		✓				✓	✓			✓		
Cardiac arrhythmias												
Supraventricular arrhythmias/tachycardias					✓					✓		
Sinus tachycardia					✓							
Intraoperative and postoperative tachycardia and hypertension					✓							
Ventricular arrhythmias/tachycardias										✓	✓[3]	
Premature ventricular contractions (PVCs)	✓											
Digitalis-induced tachyarrhythmias										✓		
Resistant tachyarrhythmias (during anesthesia)										✓		
Atrial ectopy						x						
Maintenance of normal sinus rhythm											✓	
MI		✓				✓				✓		✓
CHF (stable)[4]				x		✓[5]						
Pheochromocytoma										✓		
Migraine prophylaxis		x				x	x			✓		✓
Hypertrophic subaortic stenosis										✓		
Parkinsonian tremors							x			x[6]		
Akathisia, antipsychotic-induced						x				x		
Variceal bleeding in portal hypertension		x				x	x			x		x
Atrial fibrillation												
Rapid heart rate control						x						
Maintenance heart rate control						x						
Generalized anxiety disorder										x		
Angina												
Stable	x			x								
Unstable		x			x	x						

[1] For more detailed information, see preceding Indications and individual monographs.
[2] Includes long-acting formulation.
[3] Not *Betapace AF*.
[4] See Precautions or Warnings.
[5] *Toprol-XL* 25 mg only.
[6] Sustained-release only.

Actions

➤*Pharmacology:*

Pharmacologic/Pharmacokinetic Properties of Beta-Adrenergic Blocking Agents

0 – none + – low ++ – moderate +++ – high Drug	Adrenergic-receptor blocking activity	Membrane stabilizing activity	Intrinsic sympathomimetic activity	Lipid solubility	Extent of absorption (%)	Absolute oral bioavailability (%)	Half-life (hrs)	Protein binding (%)	Metabolism/Excretion
Acebutolol	β_1[1]	+[2]	+	Low	90	20-60	3-4	26	Hepatic; renal excretion 30% to 40%; nonrenal excretion 50% to 60% (bile; intestinal wall)
Atenolol	β_1[1]	0	0	Low	50	50-60	6-7	6-16	≈ 50% excreted unchanged in feces
Betaxolol	β_1[1]	+	0	Low	≈ 100	89	14-22	≈ 50	Hepatic; > 80% recovered in urine, 15% unchanged
Bisoprolol	β_1[1]	0	0	Low	≥ 90	80	9-12	≈ 30	≈ 50% excreted unchanged in urine, remainder as inactive metabolites; < 2% excreted in feces.
Esmolol	β_1[1]	0	0	Low	na[3]	na[3]	0.15	55	Rapid metabolism by esterases in cytosol of red blood cells
Metoprolol	β_1[1]	0[2]	0	Moderate	≈ 100	40-50	3-7	12	Hepatic; renal excretion, < 5% unchanged
Metoprolol, long-acting						77[4]			
Nadolol	β_1 β_2	0	0	Low	30	30-50	20-24	30	Urine, unchanged
Penbutolol	β_1 β_2	0	+	High	≈ 100	≈ 100	≈ 5	80-98	Hepatic (conjugation, oxidation); renal excretion of metabolites (17% as conjugate)
Pindolol	β_1 β_2	0	+++	Low	> 95	≈ 100	3-4[5]	40	Urinary excretion of metabolites (60% to 65%) and unchanged drug (35% to 40%)
Propranolol	β_1 β_2	++	0	High	< 90	30	3-5	90	Hepatic; < 1% excreted unchanged in urine
Propranolol, long-acting						9-18	8-11		
Sotalol	β_1 β_2	0	0	Low	nd[6]	90-100	12	0	Not metabolized; excreted unchanged in urine
Timolol	β_1 β_2	0	0	Low to moderate	90	75	4	< 10	Hepatic; urinary excretion of metabolites and unchanged drug

[1] Inhibits β_2 receptors (bronchial and vascular) at higher doses.
[2] Detectable only at doses much greater than required for beta blockade.
[3] Not applicable (available IV only).
[4] Average bioavailability; not absolute.
[5] In elderly hypertensive patients with normal renal function, t½ variable: 7 to 15 hours.
[6] No data.

Beta-Adrenergic Blocking Agents

Beta-adrenergic receptor blocking agents compete with beta-adrenergic agonists for available beta receptor sites. Propranolol, nadolol, timolol, penbutolol, sotalol, and pindolol inhibit both the β_1 receptors (located chiefly in myocardium, kidney, and eye) and β_2 receptors (located chiefly in adipose tissue, pancreas, liver, and smooth and skeletal muscle), inhibiting the chronotropic, inotropic, and vasodilator responses to β-adrenergic stimulation. Metoprolol, acebutolol, bisoprolol, esmolol, betaxolol, and atenolol are cardioselective and preferentially inhibit β_1 receptors.

Propranolol and, to a lesser extent, acebutolol and betaxolol, exert a quinidine-like (anesthetic) membrane action (membrane stabilizing activity; MSA), which affects cardiac action potential. Pindolol, penbutolol, and acebutolol have intrinsic sympathomimetic activity (ISA) in therapeutic dosage ranges. ISA or partial agonist activity is mediated directly at adrenergic receptor sites and may be blocked by other β antagonists. ISA is manifested by a smaller reduction in resting cardiac output and resting heart rate (4 to 8 beats per minute [BPM]) than is seen with drugs lacking ISA; clinical significance has not been evaluated and there is no evidence that exercise cardiac output is less affected by pindolol.

➤*Pharmacokinetics:*

Absorption – Systemic bioavailability following oral administration of metoprolol, acebutolol, timolol, and propranolol is low because of significant first-pass hepatic metabolism. Pindolol and sotalol have no significant first-pass effect; first-pass metabolism of bisoprolol is ≈ 20%. Ingestion with food enhances the bioavailability of propranolol and metoprolol, and reduces the absorption of sotalol; this effect is not noted with nadolol, pindolol, bisoprolol, or betaxolol.

Distribution – There is no simple correlation between dose or plasma level and therapeutic effect; the dose-sensitivity range observed in clinical practice is wide because sympathetic tone varies widely among individuals. There is no reliable test to estimate sympathetic tone or to determine whether total β-blockade has been achieved; proper dosage requires titration. There appear to be significant correlations between acebutolol plasma levels and both the reduction in resting heart rate and the percent of β-blockade of exercise-induced tachycardia.

Metoprolol and propranolol readily enter the CNS. Because of their high water solubility, sotalol, acebutolol, nadolol, and atenolol do not pass the blood-brain barrier; these drugs may have a lower incidence of CNS side effects.

Contraindications

Sinus bradycardia; greater than first-degree heart block; cardiogenic shock; CHF unless secondary to a tachyarrhythmia treatable with beta-blockers; overt cardiac failure; hypersensitivity to beta-blocking agents.

➤*Acebutolol:* Persistently severe bradycardia.

➤*Propranolol, nadolol, timolol, penbutolol, sotalol, and pindolol:* Bronchial asthma, including severe chronic obstructive pulmonary disease.

➤*Metoprolol:* Treatment of MI in patients with a heart rate less than 45 BPM; significant heart block greater than first-degree (PR interval greater than or equal to 0.24 sec); systolic blood pressure less than 100 mm Hg; moderate to severe cardiac failure.

➤*Sotalol:* Congenital or acquired long QT syndromes.

Warnings

➤*Mortality:* The National Heart Lung and Blood Institute conducted the Cardiac Arrhythmia Suppression Trial (CAST-I), a long-term, multicenter, randomized, double-blind study in patients with asymptomatic non-life-threatening ventricular ectopy who had an MI > 6 days but < 2 years previously. An excessive mortality or nonfatal cardiac arrest was seen in patients treated with encainide or flecainide (56/730) compared with that seen in patients assigned to matched placebo-treated groups (22/725), and a similar excess has been seen with moricizine. The average duration of treatment with encainide or flecainide in this study was 10 months.

CAST-II originally was designed as a blinded, randomized trial divided into a 14-day exposure phase to evaluate the risk of initiating treatment with moricizine after MI, and a long-term phase to evaluate survival after MI. The study was stopped early because the first 14-day period of treatment with moricizine after MI was associated with excess mortality, as compared with no treatment or placebo. As with the antiarrhythmic agents used in CAST-I, the use of moricizine to reduce mortality after MI is not only ineffective, but also harmful.

The applicability of these results to other populations (eg, those without recent MI) and to other than Class I antiarrhythmic agents is uncertain. **Sotalol** is devoid of Class I effects, and in a large controlled trial in patients with a recent MI who did not necessarily have ventricular arrhythmias, sotalol did not produce increased mortality at doses up to 320 mg/day. Conversely, in the large postinfarction study using a nontitrated initial dose of 320 mg once daily and in a second small randomized trial in high-risk postinfarction patients treated with high doses (320 mg twice daily), there have been suggestions of an excess of early sudden deaths.

➤*Proarrhythmia:* Like other antiarrhythmic agents, sotalol can provoke new or worsened ventricular arrhythmias in some patients, including sustained ventricular tachycardia or ventricular fibrillation, with potentially fatal consequences. Because of its effect on cardiac repolarization (QTc interval prolongation), torsades de pointes (a polymorphic ventricular tachycardia with prolongation of the QT interval and a shifting electrical axis) is the most common form of proarrhythmia associated with sotalol, occurring in about 4% of high-risk (history of sustained ventricular tachycardia/ventricular fibrillation [VT/VF]) patients. The risk of torsades de pointes progressively increases with prolongation of the QT interval and is worsened also by reduction in heart rate and reduction in serum potassium.

Overall, 4.3% of patients experienced a new or worsened ventricular arrhythmia. Of this 4.3%, there was new or worsened sustained ventricular tachycardia in approximately 1% of patients and torsades de pointes in 2.4%. Additionally, in approximately 1% of patients, deaths were considered possibly drug-related and may have been associated with proarrhythmic events. In patients with a history of sustained ventricular tachycardia, the incidence of torsades de pointes was 4% and worsened VT approximately 1%; in patients with other, less serious, ventricular and supraventricular arrhythmias, the incidence of torsades de pointes was 1% and 1.4%, respectively. Torsade de pointes arrhythmias were dose related.

In addition to dose and presence of sustained VT, other risk factors for torsades de pointes were gender (females had a higher incidence), excessive prolongation of the QTc interval, and history of cardiomegaly or CHF. Patients with sustained ventricular tachycardia and a history of CHF appear to have the highest risk for serious proarrhythmia (7%). Of the patients experiencing torsades de pointes, ≈ ⅔ spontaneously reverted to their baseline rhythm. The others were either converted electrically (D/C cardioversion or overdrive pacing) or treated with other drugs. Although **sotalol** therapy was discontinued in most patients experiencing torsades de pointes, 17% were continued on a lower dose. Nonetheless, use with particular caution if the QTc is > 500 msec on-therapy and give serious consideration to reducing the dose or discontinuing therapy when the QTc exceeds 550 msec. However, because of the multiple risk factors associated with torsades de pointes, exercise caution regardless of the QTc interval.

Proarrhythmic events must be anticipated not only on initiating sotalol therapy, but with every upward dose adjustment. Proarrhythmic events most often occur within 7 days of initiating therapy or of an increase in dose; 75% of serious proarrhythmias (torsades de pointes and worsened VT) occurred within 7 days of initiating therapy, while 60% of such events occurred within 3 days of initiation or a dosage change. Initiating therapy at 80 mg twice daily with gradual upward dose titration and appropriate evaluations for efficacy and safety prior to dose escalation, should reduce the risk of proarrhythmia. Avoiding excessive accumulation of sotalol in patients with diminished renal function, by appropriate dose reduction, should also reduce the risk of proarrhythmia.

➤*Cardiac failure:* Sympathetic stimulation is a vital component supporting circulatory function in CHF, and beta-blockade carries the potential hazard of further depressing myocardial contractility and precipitating more severe failure. Administer cautiously in hypertensive patients who have CHF controlled by digitalis and diuretics. Beta-blockers do not abolish the inotropic action of digitalis on heart muscle. Digitalis and beta-blockers slow AV conduction. If cardiac failure persists, withdraw beta-blocker therapy.

Although cardiac failure rarely occurs in properly selected patients, advise patients to consult a physician at the first sign or symptom of impending CHF or unexplained respiratory symptoms.

In patients without a history of cardiac failure, continued myocardial depression can lead to cardiac failure. At the first sign or symptom of impending cardiac failure, fully digitalize patients or treat with diuretics and closely observe the response. If cardiac failure continues, withdraw therapy (gradually, if possible).

Studies suggest that in certain patients with CHF, beta blockers may result in symptomatic and hemodynamic improvements. β_1 selective agents are the drugs of choice; start with a low dose and titrate upward. They should not be used as routine therapy nor for acute heart failure. In these studies, most patients had idiopathic dilated cardiomyopathy. Further study is needed to identify patients most likely to benefit from therapy as well as the appropriate drug.

➤*Wolff-Parkinson-White syndrome:* In several cases, the tachycardia was replaced by a severe bradycardia requiring a demand pacemaker after **propranolol** administration with as little as 5 mg.

➤*Abrupt withdrawal:* The occurrence of a β-blocker withdrawal syndrome is controversial. However, hypersensitivity to catecholamines has been observed in patients withdrawn from β-blocker therapy. Exacerbation of angina, MI, ventricular arrhythmias, and death have occurred after abrupt discontinuation of therapy. When discontinuing chronically administered β-blocking agents, particularly in patients with ischemic heart disease, reduce dosage gradually over 1 to 2 weeks and carefully monitor the patient. If therapy with an alternative β-adrenergic blocker is desired, the patient may be transferred directly to comparable doses of another agent without interrupting β-blocking therapy. If angina markedly worsens or acute coronary insufficiency develops, reinstitute administration promptly, at least temporarily, and employ other measures to manage unstable angina.

Because coronary artery disease may be unrecognized, do not discontinue therapy abruptly, even in patients treated only for hypertension, as abrupt withdrawal may result in transient symptoms (eg, tremulousness, sweating, palpitations, headache, malaise).

It has been suggested that β-adrenergic blockers may be discontinued abruptly during acute MI if indicated because the withdrawal phenomenon is not a major clinical problem in these patients.

➤*Peripheral vascular disease:* Treatment with β-antagonists reduces cardiac output and can precipitate or aggravate the symptoms of arterial insufficiency in patients with peripheral or mesenteric vascular disease. Exercise caution with such patients and observe closely for evidence of progression of arterial obstruction.

➤*Nonallergic bronchospasm (eg, chronic bronchitis, emphysema):* In general, do not administer β-blockers to patients with bronchospastic diseases. Administer **nadolol**, **timolol**, **penbutolol**, **propranolol**, **sotalol**, and **pindolol** with caution, because they may block bronchodilation produced by endogenous or exogenous catecholamine stimulation of β_2 receptors.

Because of their relative β_1 selectivity, low doses of **metoprolol**, **acebutolol**, **betaxalol**, **bisoprolol**, and **atenolol** may be used with caution in patients with bronchospastic disease who do not respond to, or cannot tolerate, other antihypertensive treatment. Because β_1 selectivity is not absolute, use the lowest possible dose of a β_2-stimulating agent. It may be advisable initially to administer in smaller divided doses, instead of larger doses twice daily, to avoid the higher plasma levels associated with the longer dosing interval. **Esmolol** may also be used with caution in patients with asthma if an IV agent is required.

Because it is unknown to what extent β_2-stimulating agents may exacerbate myocardial ischemia and the extent of infarction, β-blockers should not be used prophylactically. If bronchospasm not related to CHF occurs, discontinue β-blockers. A theophylline derivative or a β_2 agonist may be administered cautiously, depending on the clinical condition of the patient. Both theophylline derivatives and β_2 agonists may produce serious cardiac arrhythmias.

➤*Bradycardia:*
Metoprolol – Metoprolol produces a decrease in sinus heart rate in most patients; this decrease is greatest among patients with high initial heart rates and least among patients with low initial heart rates. Acute MI (particularly inferior infarction) may, in itself, produce significant lowering of the sinus rate. If the sinus rate decreases to < 40 BPM, particularly if associated with lowered cardiac output, give IV atropine (0.25 to 0.5 mg). If treatment with atropine is not successful, discontinue metoprolol and consider cautious administration of isoproterenol or installation of a cardiac pacemaker.

➤*Pheochromocytoma:* It is hazardous to use **propranolol** or **atenolol** unless α-adrenergic blocking drugs are already in use, because this would predispose to serious blood pressure elevation. Blocking only the peripheral dilator (β) action of epinephrine leaves its constrictor (α) action unopposed. In the event of hemorrhage or shock, there is a disadvantage in having both β and α blockade; the combination prevents the increase in heart rate and peripheral vasoconstriction needed to maintain blood pressure.

➤*Sinus bradycardia (heart rate < 50 bpm):* This occurred in 13% of patients receiving **sotalol** in clinical trials, and led to discontinuation in about 3%. Bradycardia itself increases risk of torsades de pointes. Sinus pause, sinus arrest, and sinus node dysfunction occur in less than 1% of patients. Incidence of 2nd- or 3rd- degree AV block is approximately 1%.

➤*Electrolyte disturbances:* Do not use **sotalol** in patients with hypokalemia or hypomagnesemia prior to correction of imbalance, as these conditions can exaggerate the degree of QT prolongation and increase the potential for torsades de pointes. Give special attention to electrolyte and acid-base balance in patients experiencing severe or prolonged diarrhea or patients receiving concomitant diuretic drugs.

➤*Hypotension:* If hypotension (systolic blood pressure ≤ 90 mmHg) occurs, discontinue drug and carefully assess patient's hemodynamic status and extent of myocardial damage. Invasive monitoring of central venous, pulmonary capillary wedge, and arterial pressures may be required. Institute fluids, positive inotropic agents, balloon counterpulsation or other appropriate therapy. If hypotension is associated with sinus bradycardia or AV block, direct treatment at reversing these.

In clinical trials, 20% to 50% of patients treated with **esmolol** have had hypotension, generally defined as systolic pressure < 90 mmHg or diastolic pressure < 50 mmHg. About 12% of the patients have been symptomatic (mainly diaphoresis or dizziness). Hypotension can occur at any dose, but is dose-related; therefore, doses > 200 mcg/kg/min are not recommended. Closely monitor patients, especially if pretreatment blood pressure is low. Decrease of dose or termination of infusion reverses hypotension, usually within 30 minutes.

➤*Anaphylaxis:* Anaphylaxis has occurred and may include symptoms such as profound hypotension, bradycardia with or without AV nodal block, severe sustained bronchospasm, hives, and angioedema. Deaths have occurred. Refer to Management of Acute Hypersensitivity Reactions.However, patients have been resistant to conventional therapy, especially epinephrine. Aggressive therapy may be required.

➤*Anesthesia and major surgery:* Necessity, or desirability, of withdrawing β-blockers prior to major surgery is controversial. β-blockade impairs the heart's ability to respond to β-adrenergically mediated reflex stimuli. While this might help prevent arrhythmic response, risk of excessive myocardial depression during general anesthesia may be enhanced, and difficulty restarting and maintaining heart beat has occurred. If β-blockers are withdrawn, allow several days between the last dose and anesthesia. If treatment is continued, take particular care when using anesthetics that depress the myocardium, such as ether, cyclopropane and trichlorethylene; use the lowest possible β-blocker doses. Others may recommend withdrawal of β-blockers well before surgery takes place.

In the event of emergency surgery, effects of β-blockers can be reversed by β-receptor agonists (eg, isoproterenol, dopamine, dobutamine, norepinephrine).

➤*AV block:* **Metoprolol** slows AV conduction and may produce significant first (PR interval greater than or equal to 0.26 sec), second, or third-degree heart block. Acute MI also produces heart block.

If heart block occurs, discontinue metoprolol and give IV atropine (0.25 to 0.5 mg). If treatment with atropine is not successful, consider cautious administration of isoproterenol or installation of a cardiac pacemaker.

➤*Sick sinus syndrome:* Use **sotalol** only with extreme caution in patients with sick sinus syndrome associated with symptomatic arrhythmias because it may cause sinus bradycardia, sinus pauses, or sinus arrest.

➤*Concomitant use of calcium channel blockers (atenolol):* Bradycardia and heart block can occur and the left ventricular end diastolic pressure can rise when beta-blockers are administered with verapamil or diltiazem. Patients with preexisting conduction abnormalities or left ventricular dysfunction are particularly susceptible.

➤*Recent acute MI (sotalol):* Sotalol can be used safely and effectively in the long-term treatment of life-threatening ventricular arrhythmias following an MI. However, experience in the use of sotalol to treat cardiac arrhythmias in the early phase of recovery from acute MI is limited and at least at high initial doses is not reassuring. In the first 2 weeks post-MI, caution is advised and careful dose titration is especially important, particularly in patients with markedly impaired ventricular function.

➤*Intraoperative and postoperative tachycardia and hypertension:* Do not use esmolol as the treatment for hypertension in patients in whom the increased blood pressure is primarily caused by the vasoconstriction associated with hypothermia.

➤*Renal/Hepatic function impairment:* Use with caution. **Timolol**'s half-life is essentially unchanged in moderate renal insufficiency; however, marked hypotensive responses have been seen in patients with marked renal impairment undergoing dialysis. Dosage reduction may be necessary in impaired renal or hepatic function.

Because **nadolol**, **sotalol**, and **atenolol** are eliminated primarily by the kidney, half-life increases in renal failure; dosage adjustments are necessary.**Bisoprolol**'s half-life is increased in patients with creatinine clearance less than 40 mL/min and in cirrhosis; adjust dosage. Although **acebutolol** is excreted through the GI tract, the active metabolite, diacetolol, is eliminated primarily by the kidney; reduce daily acebutolol dose. Administer **esmolol** with caution in impaired renal function because its acid metabolite is primarily excreted unchanged by the kidney. Elimination half-life of the acid metabolite was prolonged 10-fold and plasma level was considerably elevated in end-stage renal disease. Poor renal function has only minor effects on **pindolol** clearance, but poor hepatic function may cause pindolol blood levels to increase substantially. Expect **penbutolol** conjugate accumulation upon multiple dosing in renal insufficiency. **Metoprolol**'s systemic availability and half-life in renal failure do not differ significantly from those in normal subjects; dosage reduction is usually not needed. **Betaxolol** is primarily metabolized in the liver to metabolites that are inactive and then excreted by the kidneys; clearance is somewhat reduced in patients with renal failure but little changed in patients with hepatic disease. Reduce dosage in patients with severe renal impairment and those on dialysis; dosage reductions have not routinely been necessary in hepatic insufficiency.

➤*Pregnancy: Category D* (**atenolol**). Atenolol can cause fetal harm when administered to a pregnant woman. Atenolol crosses the placental barrier and appears in cord blood. Administration of atenolol, starting in the second trimester of pregnancy, has been associated with the birth of infants that are small for gestational age. No studies have been performed on the use of atenolol in the first trimester and the possibility of fetal injury cannot be excluded.

Category C (**betaxolol**, **esmolol**, **metoprolol**, **nadolol**, **timolol**, **propranolol**, **penbutolol**, **bisoprolol**). Embryotoxic effects have been demonstrated in animals at doses 5 to 600 times higher than the maximum recommended doses in humans.

Category B (**acebutolol**, **pindolol**, **sotalol**). Acebutolol and its major metabolite, diacetolol, cross the placenta. Neonates of mothers who received acebutolol during pregnancy have reduced birth weight and decreased blood pressure and heart rate. Sotalol crosses the placenta and is found in amniotic fluid; subnormal birth weight has occurred.

Safety for use during pregnancy has not been established. Use only when clearly needed and when the potential benefits outweigh the potential hazards to the fetus.

Although cases of teratogenicity in humans have not been reported, problems have occurred during delivery. These include the following: Neonatal bradycardia, hypoglycemia and apnea, low Apgar scores, maternal and fetal bradycardia, hypothermia, oliguria, poor peripheral perfusion, and small birth weight infants (caused by chronic therapy). Some of the effects on the neonate may last up to 72 hours postpartum.

➤*Lactation:* **Propranolol**, **pindolol**, **timolol**, **sotalol**, **betaxalol**, and **nadolol** are excreted in breast milk. **Acebutolol** and diacetolol (its major metabolite) appear in breast milk with a milk:plasma ratio of 7.1 and 12.2, respectively. **Metoprolol** is excreted in breast milk in very small quantities; an infant consuming 1 L of breast milk would receive a dose of < 1 mg of the drug. **Atenolol** is excreted in breast milk at a ratio of 1.5 to 6.8. In one patient, the peak atenolol milk:plasma ratio was 3.6 and the estimated infant dose (maternal dose, 100 mg/day) was 0.13 mg/feeding (75 mL). Another infant developed cyanosis and 2 incidences of bradycardia following maternal atenolol ingestion (100 mg/day). Small amounts of **bisoprolol** (< 2% of the dose) are detected in the breast milk of rats; it is not known if it is excreted in human breast milk. Betaxolol is excreted in sufficient amounts to have pharmacological effects in the infant. It is not known if **penbutolol**, or **esmolol** are excreted in breast milk. Nursing should not be undertaken by mothers receiving these drugs.

➤*Children:* Safety and efficacy for use in children have not been established.

IV administration of **propranolol** is not recommended in children; however, oral propranolol has been used (see Administration and Dosage).

Precautions

➤*Diabetes/Hypoglycemia:* β-adrenergic blockade may blunt premonitory signs and symptoms (eg, pulse rate, tachycardia, blood pressure changes) of acute hypoglycemia, but other manifestations such as dizziness and sweating may not be significantly affected. Hypoglycemic attacks may be accompanied by a precipitous elevation of blood pressure in patients on **propranolol**. Nonselective β-blockers may potentiate insulin-induced hypoglycemia. This is less likely with cardioselective agents. **Atenolol** does not potentiate insulin-induced hypoglycemia and, unlike nonselective β-blockers, does not delay recovery of blood glucose to normal levels.

Use with caution in diabetic patients, especially those with labile diabetes. β blockade reduces the release of insulin in response to hyperglycemia; it may be necessary to adjust the dose of antidiabetic drugs.

Propranolol therapy, particularly in infants and children, diabetic or not, has been associated with hypoglycemia, especially during fasting as in preparation for surgery. Hypoglycemia also has been found after this type of drug therapy and prolonged physical exertion and has occurred in renal insufficiency, both during dialysis and sporadically, in patients on propranolol.

➤*Thyrotoxicosis:* β-adrenergic blockers may mask clinical signs (eg, tachycardia) of developing or continuing hyperthyroidism. Abrupt withdrawal may exacerbate symptoms of hyperthyroidism, including thyroid storm; therefore, monitor closely and withdraw the drug slowly.

Propranolol may change thyroid-function tests, increasing T_4 and reverse T_3, and decreasing T_3.

➤*Serum lipid concentrations:* Although study results conflict, β-blockers may alter serum lipids including an increase in the concentration of total triglycerides, total cholesterol and LDL and VLDL cholesterol, and a decrease in the concentration of HDL cholesterol; however, this finding is not clinically significant. Other studies suggest **pindolol** does not significantly alter serum lipid concentrations and **acebutolol** actually lowers total and LDL cholesterol levels; **bisoprolol** did not significantly alter total cholesterol and triglycerides. Further studies are needed.

➤*Muscle weakness:* Beta-blockade has potentiated muscle weakness consistent with certain myasthenic symptoms (eg, diplopia, ptosis, generalized weakness). **Timolol** rarely increased muscle weakness in some patients with myasthenia gravis or myasthenic symptoms.

Drug Interactions

Beta-Blocker Drug Interactions

Precipitant drug	Object drug*		Description
Aluminum salts Barbiturates Calcium salts Cholestyramine Colestipol Penicillins (ampicillin) Rifampin	β-blockers	⬇	The bioavailability and plasma levels of certain β-blockers may be decreased by these agents, possibly resulting in a decreased pharmacologic effect.
Calcium channel blockers	β-blockers	⬆	Pharmacologic effects of β-blockers as well as nifedipine and verapamil may be synergistic or additive. Diltiazem and nicardipine may decrease the metabolism of certain beta blockers, thus increasing the pharmacologic effects.
Cimetidine	β-blockers Metoprolol Propranolol	⬆	Pharmacokinetic parameters of β-blockers metabolized by cytochrome P450 may be altered by cimetidine; pharmacodynamic effects may be increased.
Contraceptives, oral	β-blockers	⬆	Bioavailability and plasma levels of certain β-blockers may be increased.
Diphenhydramine	β-blockers	⬆	Diphenhydramine may increase plasma concentrations and cardiovascular effects of certain β-blockers through inhibition of CYP2D6-mediated metabolism.
Flecainide	β-blockers	⬆	The bioavailability of either agent may be increased, possibly increasing the pharmacologic effects.
β-blockers	Flecainide		
Haloperidol	β-blockers Propranolol	⬆	Pharmacologic effects (hypotensive episodes) of both drugs may be increased.
β-blockers Propranolol	Haloperidol		
Hydralazine	β-blockers Metoprolol Propranolol	⬆	Serum levels and, hence, pharmacologic effects of β-blockers and hydralazine may be enhanced.
β-blockers Metoprolol Propranolol	Hydralazine		
Hydroxychloroquine	β-blockers	⬆	Plasma concentrations and cardiovascular effects of certain β-blockers may be increased because hydroxychloroquine inhibits the CYP2D6-mediated β-blocker metabolism.
Loop diuretics	β-blockers Propranolol	⬆	Propranolol plasma levels and cardiovascular effects may be enhanced. Atenolol was not affected.
MAO inhibitors	β-blockers Metoprolol Nadolol	⬆	Bradycardia may develop during concurrent use.
NSAIDs Salicylates Sulfinpyrazone	β-blockers	⬇	NSAIDs, salicylates, and sulfinpyrazone may inhibit the synthesis of prostaglandins involved in the antihypertensive activity of β-blockers.
Phenothiazines	β-blockers Propranolol	⬆	Propranolol bioavailability and plasma levels and phenothiazine plasma levels may be increased, possibly resulting in increased effects.
β-blockers Propranolol	Phenothiazines		
Propafenone	β-blockers Metoprolol Propranolol	⬆	Plasma levels of β-blockers metabolized by the liver may be increased.
Quinidine	β-blockers	⬆	Plasma β-blocker levels may be increased in "extensive metabolizers," possibly resulting in increased effects.
Quinolones Ciprofloxacin	β-blockers	⬆	Bioavailability of β-blockers metabolized by cytochrome P450 may be increased.
SSRIs	β-blockers Metoprolol Propranolol	⬆	Certain SSRIs may inhibit the metabolism (CYP2D6) of certain β-blockers, leading to excessive β-blockade.
Thioamines	β-blockers Metoprolol Propranolol	⬆	The pharmacokinetics of the β-blockers may be altered, increasing the pharmacologic effects.
Thyroid hormones	β-blockers Metoprolol Propranolol	⬇	The actions of certain β-blockers may be impaired when the hypothyroid patient is converted to the euthyroid state.
β-blockers Propranolol	Anticoagulants	⬆	Propranolol may increase the anticoagulant effect of warfarin.
β-blockers Metoprolol Propranolol	Benzodiazepines	⬆	Effects of certain benzodiazepines may be increased by lipophilic β-blockers. Atenolol does not interact.
β-blockers	Clonidine	⬆	Life-threatening and fatal increases in blood pressure have occurred after discontinuation of clonidine in patients receiving a β-blocker or after simultaneous withdrawal.
β-blockers	Disopyramide	⬌	Difficult to predict; disopyramide clearance may be decreased; adverse effects may occur (eg, sinus bradycardia, hypotension) or there may be no occurrence of negative synergistic or additive negative inotropic effects.
β-blockers	Epinephrine	⬆	Nonselective β-blockade allows alpha receptor effects of epinephrine to predominate. Increasing vascular resistance leads to initial hypertensive episode followed by bradycardia.

Beta-Blocker Drug Interactions			
Precipitant drug	Object drug*		Description
β-blockers	Ergot alkaloids	↑	Peripheral ischemia manifested by cold extremities, possible peripheral gangrene may develop due to ergot alkaloid-mediated vasoconstriction and β-blocker-mediated blockade of peripheral $β_2$ receptors, allowing for unopposed ergot action.
β-blockers Propranolol	Gabapentin	↑	Gabapentin adverse reactions may be increased.
β-blockers	Lidocaine	↑	Increased lidocaine levels may occur, resulting in toxicity.
β-blockers	Nondepolarizing muscle relaxants	↔	β-blockers may potentiate, counteract, delay, or have no effect on the actions of the nondepolarizing muscle relaxants.
β-blockers	Prazosin	↑	Concurrent administration may increase the postural hypotension produced by prazosin.
β-blockers	Sulfonylureas	↓	Hypoglycemic effects of sulfonylureas may be attenuated.
β-blockers Nonselective	Theophylline	↔	Reduced elimination of theophylline may occur. Pharmacologic antagonism can also be expected, thus reducing the effects of one or both agents. Cardioselective agents may be preferred.

* ↑ = Object drug increased. ↓ = Object drug decreased.
↔ = Undetermined clinical effect.

➤*Drug/Lab test interactions:* These agents may produce hypoglycemia and interfere with **glucose** or **insulin** tolerance tests. **Propranolol** and **betaxolol** may interfere with the glaucoma screening test because of a reduction in intraocular pressure.

➤*Drug/Food interactions:* Food enhances the bioavailability of **metoprolol** and **propranolol**; food does not enhance the bioavailability of **nadolol, bisoprolol**, or **pindolol**. The rate of **penbutolol** absorption is slowed by the presence of food; however, extent of absorption is not appreciably affected. **Sotalol** absorption is reduced ≈ 20% by a standard meal.

Adverse Reactions

Most adverse effects are mild and transient and rarely require withdrawal of therapy.

➤*Cardiovascular:* Bradycardia; torsades de pointes and other serious new ventricular arrhythmias (see Warnings); cardiovascular disorder; automatic implantable cardioverter/defibrillator (AICD) discharge; development of mitral regurgitation; cardiac reinfarction; total cardiac arrest; nonfatal cardiac arrest; cardiogenic shock; development of ventricular septal defect; chest pain; hypertension; hypotension (including asymptomatic and orthostatic); peripheral ischemia; flushing; worsening of angina and arterial insufficiency; shortness of breath; peripheral vascular insufficiency (cold extremities, paresthesia of hands); arterial insufficiency; claudication (including intermittent); heart failure; CHF; sinoatrial block; cerebral vascular accident; edema; pulmonary edema; vasodilation; presyncope and syncope; tachycardia (including ventricular); palpitations; conduction disturbances; first-, second- and third-degree heart block; intensification of AV block; abnormal ECG; bundle branch block plus major axis deviation; supraventricular tachycardia (including atrial fibrillation and flutter); angina pectoris; AV block; MI; thrombosis; cerebrovascular disorder; leg cramps; thrombophlebitis; disturbance rhythm atrial; disturbance rhythm subjective; diaphoresis; proarrhythmia; peripheral vascular disorder.

➤*CNS:* Dizziness; vertigo; tiredness/fatigue; headache; mental depression (lassitude, weakness); peripheral neuropathy; paralysis; paresthesias; hypesthesia; hyperesthesia; lethargy; anxiety; nervousness; diminished concentration/memory; somnolence; restlessness; insomnia; sleep disturbances; nightmares; bizarre or many dreams; sedation; change in behavior; altered consciousness; mood change; slightly clouded sensorium; incoordination; reversible mental depression progressing to catatonia; hallucinations; an acute reversible syndrome characterized by disorientation of time and place, short-term memory loss, emotional lability, decreased performance on neuropsychometrics, slurred speech, tinnitus and lightheadedness; increase in signs and symptoms of myasthenia gravis; ataxia; neuralgia; neuropathy; numbness; stupor; abnormal thinking; amnesia; impaired concentration; confusion; seizures; local weakness; stroke.

It has been suggested that the more lipophilic the β-blocker, the higher the CNS penetration and subsequent incidence of adverse CNS effects. These effects may improve or disappear when a less lipophilic agent is substituted.

➤*Dermatologic:* Rash; pruritus; skin irritation; increased pigmentation; sweating/hyperhidrosis; alopecia (including reversible); dry skin; psoriasis (often reversible); acne; eczema; flushing; exfoliative dermatitis; peripheral skin necrosis; psoriasiform rash or exacerbation of psoriasis; erythematous rash; hypertrichosis; skin disorders; erythema, skin discoloration; burning at infusion site; thrombophlebitis; local skin necrosis; cutaneous vasculitis.

➤*Endocrine:* Hyperglycemia; hypoglycemia; unstable diabetes.

➤*GI:* Gastric/epigastric pain; flatulence; gastritis; constipation; nausea; diarrhea; colon problem; dry mouth; vomiting; heartburn; appetite disorder; anorexia; bloating; abdominal discomfort/pain; mesenteric arterial thrombosis; ischemic colitis; retroperitoneal fibrosis; hepatomegaly; dyspepsia; taste distortion; elevated liver enzymes (see Lab Test Abnormalities); elevated bilirubin; acute hepatitis with jaundice; GI disorder; increased appetite; mouth ulceration; rectal disorders; dysphagia; abnormal taste; taste loss; abdominal distension; taste perversion; digestive tract disorders; taste abnormalities; indigestion.

➤*GU:* Sexual dysfunction; impotence or decreased libido; dysuria; nocturia; pollakiuria; urinary retention or frequency; urinary tract infection; cystitis; renal colic; GU disorder; renal failure; cystitis; micturition disorder; oliguria; proteinuria; abnormal renal function; renal pain; menstrual disorders; prostatitis.

➤*Hematologic:* Agranulocytosis; nonthrombocytopenic or thrombocytopenic purpura; bleeding; thrombocytopenia; eosinophilia; leukopenia; pulmonary emboli; hyperlipidemia; anemia; leukocytosis; lymphadenopathy; purpura.

➤*Hypersensitivity:* Pharyngitis; photosensitivity reaction; erythematous rash; fever combined with aching and sore throat; laryngospasm; respiratory distress; angioedema; anaphylaxis (see Warnings).

➤*Lab test abnormalities:* **Propranolol** may elevate blood urea levels in patients with severe heart disease. **Propranolol** and **metoprolol** may cause elevated serum transaminase, alkaline phosphatase, and LDH. **Timolol** may produce slight increases in BUN, serum potassium, and serum uric acid, and slight decreases in hemoglobin and hematocrit and HDL cholesterol; however, these alterations are not progressive and are not associated with clinical manifestations. Increases in liver function tests have been reported.

Minor persistent elevations in AST and ALT have occurred in 7% of patients treated with **pindolol**, but progressive elevations were not observed and liver injury has not been reported. Alkaline phosphatase, LDH, and uric acid are also elevated on rare occasions. The significance of this is unknown. Elevations of AST and ALT of 1 to 2 times normal have occurred with **bisoprolol** (3.9% to 6.2%). Small increases in uric acid, creatinine, BUN, serum potassium, glucose, and phosphorus, and decreases in WBC and platelets have also occurred, although they were generally not of clinical importance. Liver abnormalities (increased AST and ALT) have occurred in a small number of patients receiving **acebutolol**.

The development of antinuclear antibodies (ANA) has been associated with β-blocker therapy. Symptoms of arthralgia and myalgias were infrequent and reversed upon drug discontinuation.

➤*Musculoskeletal:* Joint pain; arthralgia; muscle cramps/pain; back/neck pain; arthritis; twitching/tremor; localized pain; extremity pain; myalgia; pain; shoulder pain; joint disorder; arthropathy; tendonitis; chest pain; muscle cramps.

➤*Ophthalmic:* Eye irritation/discomfort; visual disturbances; dry/burning eyes; blurred vision; conjunctivitis; ocular pain/pressure; abnormal lacrimation; ptosis; eye disorder; abnormal vision; blepharitis; ocular hemorrhage; iritis; cataract; scotoma; diplopia.

➤*Respiratory:* Bronchospasm; dyspnea; cough; bronchial obstruction; rales; wheeziness; nasal stuffiness; pharyngitis; rhonchi; laryngospasm with respiratory distress; asthma; rhinitis; sinusitis; pulmonary problem; upper respiratory tract problem; cold symptoms; flu symptoms; bronchitis; lung disorder; cough; epistaxis; pneumonia; tracheobronchitis.

➤*Miscellaneous:* Facial swelling; weight gain; weight loss; decreased exercise tolerance; lupus syndrome and lupus-like reactions; Peyronie's disease; Raynaud's phenomenon; speech disorder; rigors; earache; gout; asthenia; malaise; infection; fever; death; tinnitus; injury; salivation; sweating; allergy; breast pain; breast fibroadenosis; labyrinth disorders; deafness; acidosis; diabetes; hypercholesterolemia; hyperglycemia; hyperkalemia; hyperlipemia; hyperuricemia; hypokalemia; thirst; cold sensation; systemic lupus erythmatosus (rarely); speech disorder; midscapular pain; pemphigoid rash; hypertensive reaction in patients with pheochromocytoma.

Overdosage

➤*Symptoms:* Bradycardia, hypotension, low-output cardiac failure, and cardiogenic shock are the most common effects of beta-blocker intoxication.

Cardiovascular – Asystole; tachycardia (partial agonists); prolonged QT interval (sotalol); prolonged QRS complex (membrane-stabilizing agents); ventricular dysrhythmias (membrane-stabilizing agents, sotalol); hypotension; hypertension (partial agonists); bradycardia; AV block.

CNS – Seizures; coma; depressed level of consciousness.

GI – Mesenteric ischemia; esophageal spasms.

Metabolic – Hyperkalemia; hypoglycemia.

Respiratory – Apnea; cyanosis; respiratory depression; bronchospasm.

Miscellaneous – Renal failure.

➤*Treatment:* Perform evaluation of the "ABCs" (airway, breathing, and circulation) as well as rapid assessment of serum glucose levels with correction of hypoglycemia using IV glucagon. Early ventilatory control is essential in addition to chest radiography, serum electrolytes, and arterial blood gases. Administer activated charcoal to all patients and perform gastric lavage in patients who present within 1 to 2 hours after ingestion. In patients who ingest sustained-release preparations, consider whole-bowel irrigation with polyethylene glycol solution. Treat seizures with initial administration of benzodiazepines. Use barbiturates if benzodiazepines are ineffective. **Atenolol**, **acebutolol**, **sotalol**, and **nadolol** are the only beta-blockers that can successfully be removed by hemodialysis. Although rare, bronchospasm should be treated with β-agonists. Parenteral ephinephrine may be required in severe cases. See Management of Acute Overdosage.

Other treatments for cardiovascular complications include the following:

1.) *Catecholamine agents:* Epinephrine had the greatest effect of all agents. High-dose isoproterenol and dopamine also have been used for β-blocker toxicity.
2.) *Phosphodiesterase inhibitors:* A positive inotropic effect without an increase in myocardial oxygen demand has been shown in the canine model using amrinone. Milrinone, aminophylline, and theophylline also have been employed for β-blocker toxicity.
3.) *Atropine:* Atropine is the least effective agent in the treatment of β-blocker toxicity, although it is the most frequently used. The lack of effect of a 1 mg dose of atropine may be diagnostic for β-blocker poisoning.
4.) *Pacing:* External cardiac pacing or transvenous pacing is often attempted to treat β-blocker-induced bradycardia; however, it may be ineffective. Overdrive pacing may be necessary in cases of torsades de pointes associated with sotalol intoxification.
5.) *Intra-aortic balloon pump:* If other measures fail, insertion of an intra-aortic balloon pump may restore perfusion.

Patient Information

Do not discontinue medication abruptly, except on advice of physician. Sudden cessation of therapy may precipitate or exacerbate angina.

Consult pharmacist or physician before using other products that may contain α-adrenergic stimulants (eg, nasal decongestants, *otc* cold preparations).

Notify physician if symptoms of CHF occur (eg, difficult breathing, especially on exertion or when lying down; night cough; swelling of the extremities).

Notify physician if any of the following occur: Slow pulse rate, dizziness, lightheadedness, confusion or depression, skin rash, fever, sore throat, unusual bleeding or bruising.

May produce drowsiness, dizziness, lightheadedness, blurred vision; patient should observe caution while driving or performing other tasks requiring alertness, coordination, or physical dexterity.

➤*Diabetics:* These agents may mask signs of hypoglycemia or alter blood glucose levels.

➤*Propranolol and metoprolol:* Food may enhance bioavailability; take at the same time each day.

➤*Nadolol, pindolol, acebutolol, atenolol, bisoprolol, betaxolol, and penbutolol:* May be taken without regard to meals.

➤*Sotalol:* Food may reduce absorption. Take on an empty stomach.

ATENOLOL

Rx	**Atenolol** (Various, eg, Geneva, ESI Lederle, Mutual, Mylan, Teva, UDL, URL)	**Tablets:** 25 mg	In 100s, 500s, 1000s, *Robot Ready* 25s, and UD 100s.
Rx	**Tenormin** (AstraZeneca)		(T 107). White. In 100s.
Rx	**Atenolol** (Various, eg, Danbury, ESI Lederle, Mutual, Mylan, Schein, Teva, URL)	**Tablets:** 50 mg	In 100s and 1000s.
Rx	**Tenormin** (AstraZeneca)		(Tenormin 105). White, scored. In 100s, 1000s, and UD 100s.
Rx	**Atenolol** (Various, eg, Danbury, ESI Lederle, Mutual, Mylan, Schein, Teva, URL)	**Tablets:** 100 mg	In 100s and 1000s.
Rx	**Tenormin** (AstraZeneca)		(Tenormin 101). White. In 100s and UD 100s.
Rx	**Tenormin** (AstraZeneca)	**Injection:** 5 mg	In 10 mL ampules.

ATENOLOL — ORAL

For complete and comparative prescribing information, refer to the Beta-Adrenergic Blocking Agents group monograph.

WARNING

Advise patients with coronary artery disease who are being treated with atenolol against abrupt discontinuation of therapy. Severe exacerbation of angina and the occurrence of myocardial infarction and ventricular arrhythmias have been reported in angina patients following the abrupt discontinuation of therapy with beta-blockers. The last two complications may occur with or without preceding exacerbation of the angina pectoris. As with other beta-blockers, when discontinuation of atenolol is planned, observe the patient carefully and advise the patient to limit physical activity to a minimum. If the angina worsens or acute coronary insufficiency develops, it is recommended that atenolol be promptly reinstituted, at least temporarily. Because coronary artery disease is common and may be unrecognized, it may be prudent not to discontinue atenolol therapy abruptly, even in patients treated only for hypertension.

Indications

➤ *Hypertension:* Management of hypertension. They may be used alone or concomitantly with other antihypertensive agents, particularly with a thiazide-type diuretic.

➤*Angina pectoris due to coronary atherosclerosis:* Long-term management of patients with angina pectoris.

➤*Acute MI:* Management of hemodynamically stable patients with definite or suspected acute MI to reduce cardiovascular mortality. Treatment can be initiated as soon as the patient's clinical condition allows. In general, there is no basis for treating patients like those who were excluded from the ISIS-1 trial (blood pressure less than 100 mm Hg systolic, heart rate more than 50 bpm) or have other reasons to avoid beta blockade. As noted above, some subgroups (eg, elderly patients with systolic blood pressure below 120 mm Hg) seemed less likely to benefit.

➤*Unlabeled uses:*

Migraine prophylaxis – Atenolol 50 to 200 mg/day.

Angina (unstable) – Atenolol 25 to 100 mg/day.

Prevention of variceal bleeding caused by portal hypertension – Atenolol may be useful for this condition. Atenolol 50 mg/day, started 72 hours before coronary artery bypass operations, appears effective in reducing the incidence of supraventricular arrhythmias.

Administration and Dosage

➤*Approved by the FDA:* August 1981.

➤*Hypertension:* The initial dose of atenolol is 50 mg given as 1 tablet a day either alone or added to diuretic therapy. The full effect of this dose will usually be seen within 1 to 2 weeks. If an optimal response is not achieved, the dosage should be increased to atenolol 100 mg given as 1 tablet a day. Increasing the dosage beyond 100 mg a day is unlikely to produce any further benefit.

Atenolol may be used alone or concomitantly with other antihypertensive agents including thiazide-type diuretics, hydralazine, prazosin, and alpha-methyldopa.

➤*Angina pectoris:* The initial dose of atenolol is 50 mg given as 1 tablet a day. If an optimal response is not achieved within 1 week, the dosage should be increased to atenolol 100 mg given as 1 tablet a day. Some patients may require a dosage of 200 mg once a day for optimal effect.

Twenty-four-hour control with once daily dosing is achieved by giving doses larger than necessary to achieve an immediate maximum effect. The maximum early effect on exercise tolerance occurs with doses of 50 to 100 mg, but at these doses the effect at 24 hours is attenuated, averaging approximately 50% to 75% of that observed with once a day oral doses of 200 mg.

➤*Acute MI:* In patients with definite or suspected acute MI, treatment with atenolol IV injection should be initiated as soon as possible after the patient's arrival in the hospital and after eligibility is established. Such treatment should be initiated in a coronary care or similar unit immediately after the patient's hemodynamic condition has stabilized. Treatment should begin with the IV administration of atenolol 5 mg over 5 minutes followed by another 5 mg IV injection 10 minutes later. Atenolol IV injection should be administered under carefully controlled conditions including monitoring of blood pressure, heart rate, and electrocardiogram. Dilutions of atenolol IV injection in Dextrose Injection, Sodium Chloride Injection, or Dextrose and Sodium Chloride Injection may be used. These admixtures are stable for 48 hours if they are not used immediately.

In patients who tolerate the full IV dose (10 mg), atenolol tablets 50 mg should be initiated 10 minutes after the last IV dose followed by another 50 mg oral dose 12 hours later. Thereafter, atenolol can be given orally either 100 mg once daily or 50 mg twice a day for a further 6 to 9 days or until discharge from the hospital. If bradycardia or hypotension requiring treatment or any other untoward effects occur, atenolol should be discontinued (see full monograph prior to initiating therapy with atenolol tablets).

Data from other beta blocker trials suggest that if there is any question concerning the use of IV beta blocker or clinical estimate that there is a contraindication, the IV beta blocker may be eliminated and patients fulfilling the safety criteria may be given atenolol tablets 50 mg twice daily or 100 mg once a day for at least 7 days (if the IV dosing is excluded).

Although the demonstration of efficacy of atenolol is based entirely on data from the first 7 postinfarction days, data from other beta blocker trials suggest that treatment with beta blockers that are effective in the postinfarction setting may be continued for 1 to 3 years if there are no contraindications.

Atenolol is an additional treatment to standard coronary care unit therapy.

➤*Elderly patients or patients with renal impairment:* Atenolol is excreted by the kidneys; consequently dosage should be adjusted in cases of severe impairment of renal function. Some reduction in dosage may also be

ATENOLOL — ORAL

appropriate for the elderly, since decreased kidney function is a physiologic consequence of aging. Atenolol excretion would be expected to decrease with advancing age.

No significant accumulation of atenolol occurs until creatinine clearance falls below 35 mL/min/1.73 m². Accumulation of atenolol and prolongation of its half-life were studied in subjects with creatinine clearance between 5 and 105 mL/min. Peak plasma levels were significantly increased in subjects with creatinine clearances less than 30 mL/min.

The following maximum oral dosages are recommended for elderly, renally impaired patients and for patients with renal impairment due to other causes:

Creatinine clearance (mL/min/1.73 m²)	Atenolol elimination half-life (h)	Maximum dosage
15 to 35	16 to 27	50 mg daily
< 15	> 27	25 mg daily

Some renally impaired or elderly patients being treated for hypertension may require a lower starting dose of atenolol: 25 mg given as 1 tablet a day. If this 25 mg dose is used, assessment of efficacy must be made carefully. This should include measurement of blood pressure just prior to the next dose ("trough" blood pressure) to ensure that the treatment effect is present for a full 24 hours.

Although a similar dosage reduction may be considered for elderly or renally impaired patients being treated for indications other than hypertension, data are not available for these patient populations.

Patients on hemodialysis should be given 25 or 50 mg after each dialysis; this should be done under hospital supervision as marked falls in blood pressure can occur.

➤*Cessation of therapy in patients with angina pectoris:* If withdrawal of atenolol therapy is planned, it should be achieved gradually and patients should be carefully observed and advised to limit physical activity to a minimum.

➤*Storage/Stability:* Store at controlled room temperature, 20° to 25°C (68° to 77°F). Dispense in a well-closed, light- and child-resistant containers.

ATENOLOL — INJECTION

For complete and comparative prescribing information, refer to the Beta-Adrenergic Blocking Agents group monograph.

WARNING

Advise patients with coronary artery disease who are being treated with atenolol against abrupt discontinuation of therapy. Severe exacerbation of angina and the occurrence of myocardial infarction and ventricular arrhythmias have been reported in angina patients following the abrupt discontinuation of therapy with beta-blockers. The last two complications may occur with or without preceding exacerbation of the angina pectoris. As with other beta-blockers, when discontinuation of atenolol is planned, carefully observe the patient and advise the patient to limit physical activity to a minimum. If the angina worsens or acute coronary insufficiency develops, it is recommended that atenolol be promptly reinstituted, at least temporarily. Because coronary artery disease is common and may be unrecognized, it may be prudent not to discontinue atenolol therapy abruptly even in patients treated only for hypertension.

Indications

➤*Acute myocardial infarction:* Management of hemodynamically stable patients with definite or suspected acute myocardial infarction to reduce cardiovascular mortality. Treatment can be initiated as soon as the patient's clinical condition allows. Such treatment should be initiated in a coronary care or similar unit immediately after the patient's hemodynamic condition has stabilized. In general, there is no basis for treating patients like those who were excluded from the ISIS-1 trial (blood pressure less than 100 mmHg systolic, heart rate less than 50 bpm) or have other reasons to avoid beta blockade. As noted above, some subgroups (eg, elderly patients with systolic blood pressure below 120 mmHg) seemed less likely to benefit.

Administration and Dosage

➤*Approved by the FDA:* August 1981.

➤*Acute myocardial infarction:* In patients with definite or suspected acute myocardial infarction, treatment with atenolol IV injection should be initiated as soon as possible after the patient's arrival in the hospital and after eligibility is established. Such treatment should be initiated in a coronary care or similar unit immediately after the patient's hemodynamic condition has stabilized. Treatment should begin with the IV administration of 5 mg atenolol over 5 minutes followed by another 5 mg IV injection 10 minutes later. Atenolol IV injection should be administered under carefully controlled conditions including monitoring of blood pressure, heart rate, and electrocardiogram. Dilutions of atenolol IV injection in Dextrose Injection, Sodium Chloride Injection, or Sodium Chloride and Dextrose Injection may be used. These admixtures are stable for 48 hours if they are not used immediately.

In patients who tolerate the full IV dose (10 mg), atenolol tablets 50 mg should be initiated 10 minutes after the last IV dose followed by another 50 mg oral dose 12 hours later. Thereafter, atenolol can be given orally either 100 mg once daily or 50 mg twice a day for a further 6 to 9 days or until discharge from the hospital. If bradycardia or hypotension requiring treatment or any other untoward effects occur, atenolol should be discontinued (see full prescribing information prior to initiating therapy with atenolol tablets.)

Data from other beta-blocker trials suggest that if there is any question concerning the use of IV beta blocker or clinical estimate that there is a contraindication, the IV beta blocker may be eliminated and patients fulfilling the safety criteria may be given atenolol tablets 50 mg twice daily or 100 mg once a day for at least 7 days (if the IV dosing is excluded).

Although the demonstration of efficacy of atenolol is based entirely on data from the first 7 postinfarction days, data from other beta blockers trials suggest that treatment with beta blockers that are effective in the postinfarction setting may be continued for 1 to 3 years if there are no contraindications.

Atenolol is an additional treatment to standard coronary care unit therapy.

➤*Patients with renal impairment:* Since atenolol is excreted via the kidneys, dosage should be adjusted in cases of severe impairment of renal function. No significant accumulation of atenolol occurs until creatinine clearance falls below 35 mL/min/1.73 m² (normal range is 100 to 150 mL/min/1.73 m²); therefore oral atenolol doses should be reduced in patients with creatinine clearance less than 35 mL/min/1.73 m².

Patients on hemodialysis should be given 50 mg after each dialysis; this should be done under hospital supervision as marked falls in blood pressure can occur.

➤*Cessation of therapy:* If withdrawal of atenolol therapy is planned, it should be achieved gradually over a period of about 2 weeks. Patients should be carefully observed and advised to limit physical activity to a minimum.

Parenteral drug products should be inspected visually for particulate matter and discoloration prior to administration, whenever solution and container permit.

➤*Storage/Stability:* Protect from light. Keep ampules in outer packaging until time of use. Store at controlled room temperature 20° to 25°C (68° to 77°F) .

ESMOLOL HYDROCHLORIDE

Rx	**Esmolol** (Baxter)	**Injection:** 10 mg/mL	Preservative free. In 10 mL vials.
Rx	**Brevibloc** (Baxter)		In 10 mL vials.
Rx	**Brevibloc Double Strength** (Baxter)	**Injection:** 20 mg/mL	Preservative free. In ready-to-use 5 mL vials and 100 mL bags.
Rx	**Brevibloc** (Baxter)	**Injection:** 250 mg/mL	25% alcohol. In 10 mL amps.[1]

[1] With 25% propylene glycol.

ESMOLOL HYDROCHLORIDE — INJECTION

For complete and comparative prescribing information, refer to the Beta-Adrenergic Blocking Agents group monograph.

Indications

➤*Supraventricular tachycardia:* For the rapid control of ventricular rate in patients with atrial fibrillation or atrial flutter in perioperative, postoperative, or other emergent circumstances where short-term control of ventricular rate with a short-acting agent is desirable. Esmolol hydrochloride is also indicated in noncompensatory sinus tachycardia where, in the physician's judgment, the rapid heart rate requires specific intervention. Esmolol hydrochloride is not intended for use in chronic settings where transfer to another agent is anticipated.

➤*Intraoperative and postoperative tachycardia or hypertension:* For the treatment of tachycardia and hypertension that occur during induction and tracheal intubation, during surgery, on emergence from anesthesia, and in the postoperative period, when in the physician's judgment such specific intervention is considered indicated.

Use of esmolol hydrochloride to prevent such events is not recommended.

➤*Unlabeled uses:* For unstable angina, 2 to 24 mg/min as a continuous infusion.

Administration and Dosage

➤*Approved by the FDA:* December 31, 1986.

➤*2,500 mg ampul:* The following is a suggested administration for supraventricular tachycardia based on patient weight for both the 1-minute loading infusion (at 500 mcg/kg/min) and the 4-minute maintenance infusion (at

ESMOLOL HYDROCHLORIDE — INJECTION

50/100/150/200/250/300 mcg/kg/min). Drug dilution: Five g esmolol in 500 mL diluent = 10 mg/mL.

Dosage in supraventricular tachycardia								
		1 minute loading infusion (mcg/kg/min)	4 minute maintenance infusion (mcg/kg/min)					
		500	50	100	150	200	250	300
Suggested administration for supraventricular tachycardia. Drug dilution: 5 g esmolol in 500 mL diluent = 10 mg/mL								
Patient wt		Infusion rates (mL/min)	Infusion rates (mL/h)					
lbs	kg							
110	50	2.5	15	30	45	60	75	90
121	55	2.75	16.5	33	49.5	66	82.5	99
132	60	3	18	36	54	72	90	108
143	65	3.25	19.5	39	58.5	78	97.5	117
154	70	3.5	21	42	63	84	105	126
165	75	3.75	22.5	45	67.5	90	112.5	135
176	80	4	24	48	72	96	120	144
187	85	4.25	25.5	51	76.5	102	127.5	153
198	90	4.5	27	54	81	108	135	162
209	95	4.75	28.5	57	85.5	114	142.5	171
220	100	5	30	60	90	120	150	180
231	105	5.25	31.5	63	94.5	126	157.5	189
242	110	5.5	33	66	99	132	165	198

➤*Dilution:* Aseptically prepare a 10 mg/mL infusion by adding two 2,500 mg ampuls to a 500 mL container or one 2500 mg ampul to a 250 mL container of a compatible intravenous solution listed below. (Remove overage prior to dilution as appropriate.) This yields a final concentration of 10 mg/mL. The diluted solution is stable for at least 24 hours at room temperature. Note: Concentrations of esmolol hydrochloride greater than 10 mg/mL are likely to produce irritation on continued infusion. Infusion concentrations of 20 mg/mL were associated with more serious venous irritation, including thrombophlebitis, than concentrations of 10 mg/mL. Extravasation of 20 mg/mL may lead to a serious local reaction and possible skin necrosis. Concentrations greater than 10 mg/mL or infusion into small veins or through a butterfly catheter should be avoided. Esmolol hydrochloride has, however, been well tolerated when administered via a central vein.

The 2,500 mg ampul is not for direct intravenous injection. This dosage form is a concentrated, potent drug which must be diluted prior to its infusion. Esmolol hydrochloride should not be admixed with sodium bicarbonate. Esmolol hydrochloride should not be mixed with other drugs prior to dilution in a suitable intravenous fluid. (See compatibility section below.)

➤*100 mg vial:* This dosage form is prediluted to provide a ready-to-use 10 mg/mL concentration recommended for esmolol hydrochloride intravenous administration. It may be used to administer the appropriate esmolol hydrochloride loading dosage infusions by hand-held syringe while the maintenance infusion is being prepared.

When using the 100 mg vial, a loading dose of 0.5 mg/kg/min for a 70 kg patient would be 3.5 mL.

➤*Supraventricular tachycardia:* Dosage needs to be titrated, using ventricular rate as the guide.

An initial loading dose of 0.5 mg/kg (500 mcg/kg) infused over a minute duration followed by a maintenance infusion of 0.05 mg/kg/min 50 mcg/kg/min) for the next 4 minutes is recommended. This should give a rough guide with respect to the responsiveness of ventricular rate.

After the 4 minutes of initial maintenance infusion (total treatment duration being 5 minutes), depending upon the desired ventricular response, the maintenance infusion may be continued at 0.05 mg/kg/min or increased step-wise (eg, 0.1 mg/kg/min, 0.15 mg/kg/min to a maximum of 0.2 mg/kg/min) with each step being maintained for 4 or more minutes.

If more rapid slowing of ventricular response is imperative, the 0.5 mg/kg loading dose infused over a 1-minute period may be repeated, followed by a maintenance infusion of 0.1 mg/kg/min for 4 minutes. Then, depending upon ventricular rate, another (and final) loading dose of 0.5 mg/kg/min infused over a 1 minute period may be administered followed by a maintenance infusion of 0.15 mg/kg/min. If needed, after 4 minutes of the 0.15 mg/kg/min maintenance infusion, the maintenance infusion may be increased to a maximum of 0.2 mg/kg/min.

In the absence of loading doses, constant infusion of a single concentration of esmolol reaches pharmacokinetic and pharmacodynamic steady-state in about 30 minutes. Maintenance infusions (with or without loading doses) may be continued for as long as 24 hours.

The following information summarizes the above and assumes that 3 loading doses (the maximum recommended) are infused over 1 minute and incremental maintenance doses are required after each loading dose. There should be no fourth loading dose, but the maintenance dose may be incremented 1 more time.

In the treatment of supraventricular tachycardia, responses to esmolol hydrochloride usually (over 95%) occur within the range of 50 to 200 mcg/kg/min (0.05 to 0.2 mg/kg/min). The average effective dosage is approximately 100 mcg/kg/min (0.1 mg/kg/min) although dosages as low as 25 mcg/kg/min (0.025 mg/kg/min) have been adequate in some patients. Dosages as high as 300 mcg/kg/min (0.3 mg/kg/min) have been used, but these provide little added effect and an increased rate of adverse effects, and are not recommended. Dosage of esmolol hydrochloride in supraventricular tachycardia must be individualized by titration in which each step consists of a loading dosage followed by a maintenance dosage.

To initiate treatment of a patient with supraventricular tachycardia, administer a loading infusion of 500 mcg/kg/min (0.5 mg/kg/min) over 1 minute followed by a 4 minute maintenance infusion of 50 mcg/kg/min (0.05 mg/kg/min). If an adequate therapeutic effect is observed over the 5 minutes of drug administration, maintain the maintenance infusion dosage with periodic adjustments up or down as needed. If an adequate therapeutic effect is not observed, the same loading dosage is repeated over 1 minute followed by an increased maintenance infusion rate of 100 mcg/kg/min (0.1 mg/kg/min).

Continue titration procedure as above, repeating the original loading infusion of 500 mcg/kg/min (0.5 mg/kg/min) over 1 minute, but increasing the maintenance infusion rate over the subsequent 4 minutes by 50 mcg/kg/min (0.05 mg/kg/min) increments. As the desired heart rate or blood pressure is approached, omit subsequent loading doses and titrate the maintenance dosage up or down to endpoint. Also, if desired, increase the interval between steps from 5 to 10 minutes.

As the desired heart rate or end point is approached, the loading infusion may be omitted and the maintenance infusion titrated to 300 mcg/kg/min (0.3 mg/kg/min) or downward as appropriate. Maintenance dosage above 200 mcg/kg/min (0.2 mg/kg/min) have not been shown to have significantly increased benefits. The interval between titration steps may be increased from 20 minutes to 24 hours, maintenance dose titrated to heart rate or other clinical end point.

This specific dosage regimen has not been studied intraoperatively and, because of the time required for titration, may not be optimal for intraoperative use.

The safety of dosages above 300 mcg/kg/min (0.3 mg/kg/min) has not been studied.

In the event of an adverse reaction, the dosage of esmolol hydrochloride may be reduced or discontinued. If a local infusion site reaction develops, an alternate infusion site should be used and caution should be taken to prevent extravasation. The use of butterfly needles should be avoided.

Abrupt cessation of esmolol hydrochloride in patients has not been reported to produce the withdrawal effects which may occur with abrupt withdrawal of beta blockers following chronic use in coronary artery disease (CAD) patients. However, caution should still be used in abruptly discontinuing infusions of esmolol hydrochloride in CAD patients.

After achieving an adequate control of the heart rate and a stable clinical status in patients with supraventricular tachycardia, transition to alternative antiarrhythmic agents such as propranolol, digoxin, or verapamil may be accomplished. A recommended guideline for such a transition is given below but the physician should carefully consider the labeling instructions for the alternative agent selected.

Alternative agent	Dosage
Propranolol hydrochloride	10 to 20 mg every 4 to 6 hours
Digoxin	0.125 to 0.5 mg every 6 hours (oral or IV)
Verapamil	80 mg every 6 hours

The dosage of esmolol hydrochloride should be reduced as follows:

1.) Thirty (30) minutes following the first dose of the alternative agent, reduce the infusion rate of esmolol hydrochloride by one-half (50%).
2.) Following the second dose of the alternative agent, monitor the patient's response and if satisfactory control is maintained for the first hour, discontinue esmolol hydrochloride.

The use of infusions of esmolol hydrochloride up to 24 hours has been well documented; in addition, limited data from 24 to 48 hours (n = 48) indicate that esmolol hydrochloride is well tolerated up to 48 hours.

➤*Intraoperative and postoperative tachycardia or hypertension:* In the intraoperative and postoperative settings it is not always advisable to slowly titrate the dose of esmolol hydrochloride to a therapeutic effect. Therefore, 2 dosing options are presented: Immediate control dosing and a gradual control when the physician has time to titrate.

Immediate control – For intraoperative treatment of tachycardia or hypertension give an 80 mg (approximately 1 mg/kg) bolus dose over 30 seconds followed by a 150 mcg/kg/min infusion, if necessary. Adjust the infusion rate as required up to 300 mcg/kg/min to maintain desired heart rate or blood pressure.

Gradual control – For postoperative tachycardia and hypertension, the dosing schedule is the same as that used in supraventricular tachycardia. To initiate treatment, administer a loading dosage infusion of 500 mcg/kg/min of esmolol hydrochloride for 1 minute followed by a 4 minute maintenance infusion of 50 mcg/kg/min. If an adequate therapeutic effect is not observed within 5 minutes, repeat the same loading dosage and follow with a maintenance infusion increased to 100 mcg/kg/min (see Supraventricular tachycardia).

Note: Higher dosages (250 to 300 mcg/kg/min) may be required for adequate control of blood pressure than those required for the treatment of

ESMOLOL HYDROCHLORIDE — INJECTION

atrial fibrillation, flutter and sinus tachycardia. One third of the postoperative hypertensive patients required these higher doses.

Parenteral drug products should be inspected visually for particulate matter and discoloration prior to administration, whenever solution and container permit.

➤*Directions for use of esmolol hydrochloride premixed injection and esmolol hydrochloride premixed injection double strength:* This dosage form is prediluted to 100 or 250 mL to provide a ready-to-use, iso-osmotic solution of 20 or 10 mg/mL esmolol hydrochloride in sodium chloride. Do not introduce additives to esmolol hydrochloride premixed injection or esmolol hydrochloride premixed injection double strength. See directions for use of the premixed bag for additional information.

➤*Directions for use of the premixed bag:* Esmolol hydrochloride premixed injection and esmolol hydrochloride premixed injection, double strength are provided in 250 mL and 100 mL *Intra Via* bags, which are ready-to-use, non-latex, non-PVC bags with 2 PVC ports, a medication port and a delivery port. In the case of esmolol hydrochloride premixed injection, the medication port is to be used only for withdrawing an initial bolus from the bag; the medication withdrawal port is not intended for repeat bolus administration. Use aseptic technique when withdrawing the bolus dose. Do not add any additional medications to esmolol hydrochloride premixed injection. Each bag is for single-patient use only and contains no preservative. It is advised that once the drug has been withdrawn from esmolol hydrochloride premixed injection, the bag should be used within 24 hours, with any unused portion discarded.

The esmolol hydrochloride premixed injection contains esmolol hydrochloride at a concentration of 10 mg/mL. When using a 10 mg/mL concentration, a loading dose of 0.5 mg/kg infused over 1 minute period of time, for a 70 kg patient, is 3.5 mL. The loading dose can be removed from the medication port of the premixed bag.

The esmolol hydrochloride premixed injection double strength contains esmolol hydrochloride at a concentration of 20 mg/mL. When using a 20 mg/mL concentration, a loading dose of 0.5 mg/kg infused over 1 minute period of time, for a 70 kg patient, is 1.75 mL. The loading dose can be removed from the medication port of the premixed bag.

Caution – Do not use plastic containers in series connections. Such use could result in an embolism due to residual air being drawn from the primary container before administration of the fluid from the secondary container is completed.

To open – Do not remove unit from overwrap until ready to use. Do not use if overwrap has been previously opened or damaged. The overwrap is a moisture barrier. The inner bag maintains sterility of the solution.

Tear overwrap at notch and remove premixed bag. Some opacity of the plastic due to moisture absorption during the sterilization process may be observed. This is normal and does not affect the solution quality or safety. The opacity will diminish gradually.

Check for minute leaks by squeezing the inner bag firmly. If leaks are found, discard solution as sterility may be impaired. Do not use unless the solution is clear, colorless to light yellow, and the seal is intact.

Fill out the patient information label supplied and apply to the inner bag.

Do not introduce additives to esmolol hydrochloride premixed injection or esmolol hydrochloride premixed injection-double strength.

Preparation for intravenous administration (use aseptic technique) –
1.) Suspend premixed bag from eyelet support.
2.) Remove plastic protector from delivery port at bottom of bag.
3.) Attach administration set. Refer to complete directions accompanying set.

➤*Directions for use of the 10 mL ready-to-use vial (10 mg/mL) and double strength injection 5 mL ready-to-use vial (20 mg/mL):* This dosage form is prediluted to provide a ready-to-use, iso-osmotic solution of either 10 or 20 mg/mL esmolol hydrochloride in sodium chloride recommended for esmolol hydrochloride intravenous administration. It may be used to administer the appropriate esmolol hydrochloride loading dosage infusions by hand-held syringe while the maintenance infusion is being prepared.

The 10 mL double strength ready-to-use vial contains esmolol hydrochloride at a concentration of 10 mg/mL. When using a 10 mg/mL concentration, a loading dose of 0.5 mg/kg infused over 1 minute period of time, for a 70 kg patient is 3.5 mL.

The 5 mL ready-to-use vial contains esmolol hydrochloride at a concentration of 20 mg/mL. When using a 20 mg/mL concentration, a loading dose of 0.5 mg/kg infused over 1 minute period of time, for a 70 kg patient is 1.75 mL.

➤*Directions for use of the esmolol hydrochloride concentrate 10 mL ampul (250 mg/mL):* The 2,500 mg ampul is not for direct intravenous injection. This dosage form is a concentrated, potent drug which must be diluted prior to its infusion. Esmolol hydrochloride should not be admixed with sodium bicarbonate. Esmolol hydrochloride should not be mixed with other drugs prior to dilution in a suitable intravenous fluid. (See compatibility section below.)

Dilution – Aseptically prepare a 10 mg/mL infusion by adding two 2,500 mg ampuls to a 500 mL container or one 2,500 mg ampul to a 250 mL container of a compatible intravenous solution listed below. (Remove overage prior to dilution as appropriate.) This yields a final concentration of 10 mg/mL. The diluted solution is stable for at least 24 hours at room temperature. Note: Concentrations of esmolol hydrochloride greater than 10 mg/mL are likely to produce irritation on continued infusion. Esmolol hydrochloride has, however, been well tolerated when administered via a central vein.

➤*Compatibility with commonly used intravenous fluids:* Esmolol hydrochloride injection was tested for compatibility with 10 commonly used intravenous fluids at a final concentration of 10 mg esmolol hydrochloride per mL. Esmolol hydrochloride injection was found to be compatible with the following solutions and was stable for at least 24 hours at controlled room temperature or under refrigeration:
1.) Dextrose (5%) Injection.
2.) Dextrose (5%) in Lactated Ringer's Injection.
3.) Dextrose (5%) in Ringer's Injection.
4.) Dextrose (5%) and Sodium Chloride (0.45%) Injection.
5.) Dextrose (5%) and Sodium Chloride (0.9%) Injection.
6.) Lactated Ringer's Injection.
7.) Potassium Chloride (40 mEq/L) in Dextrose (5%) Injection.
8.) Sodium Chloride (0.45%) Injection.
9.) Sodium Chloride (0.9%) Injection.

Esmolol injection is not compatible with sodium bicarbonate (5%) injection.

➤*Storage/Stability:* Store at 25°C (77°F). Excursions permitted to 15° to 30°C (59° to 86°F). Protect from freezing. Avoid excessive heat.

BETAXOLOL HYDROCHLORIDE

Rx	Kerlone (Sanofi)	Tablets: 10 mg	Lactose. (KERLONE 10). White, scored. Film-coated. In 100s.
		20 mg	Lactose. (KERLONE 20 β). White. Film-coated. In 100s.

BETAXOLOL HYDROCHLORIDE — ORAL

For complete and comparative prescribing information, refer to the Beta-Adrenergic Blocking Agents group monograph.

Indications

Management of hypertension. It may be used alone or concomitantly with other antihypertensive agents, particularly thiazide diuretics.

Administration and Dosage

➤*Approved by the FDA:* October 27, 1989.

The initial dose of betaxolol hydrochloride in hypertension is ordinarily 10 mg once daily either alone or added to diuretic therapy. The full antihypertensive effect is usually seen within 7 to 14 days. If the desired response is not achieved the dose can be doubled after 7 to 14 days. Increasing the dose beyond 20 mg has not been shown to produce a statistically significant additional antihypertensive effect; but the 40 mg dose has been studied and is well tolerated. An increased effect (reduction) on heart rate should be anticipated with increasing dosage. If monotherapy with betaxolol does not produce the desired response, the addition of a diuretic agent or other antihypertensive should be considered (see Drug Interactions).

➤*Concomitant therapy:* Nifedipine, chlorthalidone, and hydrochlorothrozide have been coadministered with betaxolol and have not altered its pharmacokinetics. Calcium antagonists may be used in combination with beta-adrenergic blocking agents when heart function is normal, but should be avoided in patients with impaired cardiac function. Catecholamine-depleting drugs may have an additive effect when given with beta-blocking agentts. Use with caution.

➤*Dosage adjustments for specific patients:*

Patients with renal failure –

In patients with severe renal impairment and those undergoing dialysis the initial dose of betaxolol is 5 mg once daily. If the desired response is not achieved, dosage may be increased by 5 mg/day increments every 2 weeks to a maximum dose of 20 mg/day.

Elderly patients – Consideration should be given to reduction in the starting dose to 5 mg in elderly patients. These patients are especially prone to beta blocker-induced bradycardia, which appears to be dose related and sometimes responds to reductions in dose.

Cessation of therapy – If withdrawal of betaxolol therapy is planned, it should be achieved gradually over a period of about 2 weeks. Patients should be carefully observed and advised to limit physical activity to a minimum.

➤*Storage/Stability:* Store between 15° to 25°C (59° to 77°F).

PENBUTOLOL SULFATE

Rx	**Levatol** (Schwarz Pharma)	**Tablets:** 20 mg	(RC22). Yellow, scored, capsule shape. In 100s.

PENBUTOLOL — ORAL

For complete and comparative prescribing information, refer to the Beta-Adrenergic Blocking Agents group monograph.

Indications

Penbutolol is indicated in the treatment of mild to moderate arterial hypertension. It may be used alone or in combination with other antihypertensive agents, especially thiazide-type diuretics.

Administration and Dosage

The usual starting and maintenance dose of penbutolol, used alone or in combination with other antihypertensive agents, such as thiazide-type diuretics, is 20 mg given once daily.

Doses of 40 mg and 80 mg have been well-tolerated but have not been shown to give a greater antihypertensive effect. The full effect of a 20- or 40-mg dose is seen by the end of 2 weeks. A dose of 10 mg also lowers blood pressure, but the full effect is not seen for 4 to 6 weeks.

➤*Storage/Stability:* Store at controlled room temperature 15° to 30°C (59° to 86°F). Keep tightly closed and protect from light.

CARTEOLOL HYDROCHLORIDE

Rx	**Cartrol** (Abbott)	**Tablets:** 2.5 mg	Lactose. Gray. In 100s.
		5 mg	Lactose. White. In 100s.

CARTEOLOL HYDROCHLORIDE — ORAL

For complete and comparative prescribing information, refer to the Beta-Adrenergic Blocking Agents group monograph.

Indications

Carteolol hydrochloride is indicated in the management of hypertension. It may be used alone or in combination with other antihypertensive agents, especially thiazide diuretics. Preliminary data indicate that carteolol does not have a favorable effect on arrhythmias.

Administration and Dosage

➤*Approved by the FDA:* December 28, 1988.

Dosage must be individualized. The initial dose of carteolol hydrochloride is 2.5 mg given as a single daily oral dose either alone or added to diuretic therapy. If an adequate response is not achieved, the dose can be gradually increased to 5 mg and 10 mg as single daily doses. Increasing the dose above 10 mg/day is unlikely to produce further substantial benefits and, in fact, may decrease the response. The usual maintenance dose of carteolol is 2.5 or 5 mg once daily.

➤*Dosage adjustment in renal impairment:* Carteolol is excreted principally by the kidneys. When administering carteolol hydrochloride to patients with renal impairment, the dosage regimen should be adjusted individually by the physician. Guidelines for dose interval adjustment based upon creatinine clearance (mL/h) are listed below:

- For Ccr greater than 60 mL/h, the dosage interval is every 24 hours.
- For Ccr 20 to 60 mL/h, the dosage interval is every 48 hours.
- For Ccr less than 20 mL/h, the dosage interval is every 72 hours.

➤*Storage/Stability:* Store under controlled room temperature, 15° to 30°C (59° to 86°F).

BISOPROLOL FUMARATE

Rx	**Bisoprolol Fumarate** (Eon)	**Tablets:** 5 mg	In 30s and 100s.
Rx	**Zebeta** (Barr)		(B1 LL). Pink, scored, heart shape, biconvex. Film-coated. In 30s.
Rx	**Bisoprolol Fumarate** (Eon)	10 mg	In 30s and 100s.
Rx	**Zebeta** (Barr)		(B3 LL). White, heart shape, biconvex. Film-coated. In 30s.

BISOPROLOL FUMARATE — ORAL

For complete and comparative prescribing information, refer to the Beta-Adrenergic Blocking Agents group monograph.

Indications

➤*Hypertension:* Used alone or in combination with other antihypertensive agents.

Administration and Dosage

➤*Approved by the FDA:* July 31, 1992.

Individualize dosage. May be given without regard to meals.

➤*Initial dose:* 5 mg once daily. In some patients, 2.5 mg may be appropriate. If the antihypertensive effect of 5 mg is inadequate, the dose may be increased to 10 mg and then, if necessary, to 20 mg once daily.

➤*Renal/Hepatic function impairment:* In patients with renal dysfunction (creatinine clearance < 40 mL/min) or hepatic impairment (hepatitis or cirrhosis), use an initial daily dose of 2.5 mg and use caution in dose titration. Since limited data suggest that bisoprolol is not dialyzable, drug replacement is not necessary in patients undergoing hemodialysis.

➤*Storage/Stability:* Store at controlled room temperature 20° to 25°C (68° to 77°F), protected from moisture. Dispense in tight containers as defined in the USP.

PINDOLOL

Rx	**Pindolol** (Various, eg, Mutual, Mylan, URL, Watson)	**Tablets:** 5 mg	In 100s, 500s, and 1000s.
Rx	**Visken** (Novartis)		(Visken 5 V). White, heart shape. In 100s.
Rx	**Pindolol** (Various, eg, Mutual, Mylan, URL, Watson)	**Tablets:** 10 mg	In 100s, 500s, and 1000s.
Rx	**Visken** (Novartis)		(Visken 10 V). White, heart shape. In 100s.

PINDOLOL — ORAL

For complete and comparative prescribing information, refer to the Beta-Adrenergic Blocking Agents group monograph.

Indications

Pindolol tablets are indicated in the management of hypertension. They may be used alone or concomitantly with other antihypertensive agents, particularly with a thiazide-type diuretic.

Administration and Dosage

➤*Approved by the FDA:* September 3, 1982.

The dosage of pindolol should be individualized. The recommended initial dose of pindolol is 5 mg twice daily alone or in combination with other antihypertensive agents. An antihypertensive response usually occurs within the first week of treatment. Maximal response, however, may take as long as or occasionally longer than 2 weeks. If a satisfactory reduction in blood pressure does not occur within 3 to 4 weeks, the dose may be adjusted in increments of 10 mg/day at these intervals up to a maximum of 60 mg/day.

➤*Storage/Stability:* Store at controlled room temperature 15° to 30° C (59° to 86°F). Protect from light. Dispense in a tight, light-resistant container using a child-resistant closure.

METOPROLOL

Rx	**Metoprolol Tartrate** (Various, eg, Caraco, Mylan)	**Tablets:** 25 mg	In 30s, 90s, 100s, and 1000s.
Rx	**Metoprolol Tartrate** (Various, eg, Mylan, Qualitest, Teva, URL, Watson)	**Tablets:** 50 mg	In 100s and 1000s.
Rx	**Lopressor** (Novartis)		Lactose. (GEIGY 51 51). Pink, scored, capsule shape, biconvex. In 100s, 1000s, and UD 100s.
Rx	**Metoprolol Tartrate** (Various, eg, Mylan, Qualitest, Teva, URL, Watson)	**Tablets:** 100 mg	In 100s and 1000s.
Rx	**Lopressor** (Novartis)		Lactose. (GEIGY 71 71). Light blue, scored, capsule shape, biconvex. In 100s and 1000s.
Rx	**Toprol XL** (AstraZeneca)	**Tablets, extended-release:** 25 mg (23.75 mg metoprolol succinate equivalent to 25 mg metoprolol tartrate)	(AB). White, scored, oval, biconvex. Film-coated. In 100s.
		50 mg (47.5 mg metoprolol succinate equivalent to 50 mg metoprolol tartrate)	(A mo). White, scored, biconvex. Film-coated. In 100s.
		100 mg (95 mg metoprolol succinate equivalent to 100 mg metoprolol tartrate)	(A ms). White, scored, biconvex. Film-coated. In 100s.
		200 mg (190 mg metoprolol succinate equivalent to 200 mg metoprolol tartrate)	(A my). White, scored, oval, biconvex. Film-coated. In 100s.
Rx	**Metoprolol Tartrate** (Hospira)	**Injection:** 1 mg/mL	In amps and *Carpuject* sterile cartridge units with Luer-Lock.
Rx	**Lopressor** (Novartis)		In 5 mL amps.

METOPROLOL TARTRATE — ORAL

For complete and comparative prescribing information, refer to the Beta-Adrenergic Blocking Agents group monograph.

WARNING

Ischemic heart disease – Following abrupt cessation of therapy with certain beta-blocking agents, exacerbations of angina pectoris and, in some cases, myocardial infarction have occurred. When discontinuing chronically administered metoprolol tartrate, particularly in patients with ischemic heart disease, gradually reduce the dosage over a period of 1 to 2 weeks and carefully monitor the patient. If angina markedly worsens or acute coronary insufficiency develops, reinstate metoprolol tartrate administration promptly, at least temporarily, and take other measures appropriate for the management of unstable angina. Warn patients against interruption or discontinuation of therapy without the physician's advice. Because coronary artery disease is common and may be unrecognized, it may be prudent not to discontinue metoprolol tartrate therapy abruptly, even in patients treated only for hypertension.

Indications

➤*Hypertension:* For the treatment of hypertension. May be used alone or in combination with other antihypertensive agents.

➤*Angina pectoris:* Long-term treatment of angina pectoris.

➤*Myocardial infarction:* Treatment of hemodynamically stable patients with definite or suspected acute myocardial infarction to reduce cardiovascular mortality. Treatment with intravenous metoprolol tartrate can be initiated as soon as the patient's clinical condition allows. Alternatively, treatment can begin within 3 to 10 days of the acute event.

Administration and Dosage

➤*Approved by the FDA:* August 1978.

The dosage of metoprolol tartrate should be individualized. Metoprolol tartrate should be taken with or immediately following meals.

➤*Hypertension:* The usual initial dosage is 100 mg daily in single or divided doses, whether used alone or added to a diuretic. The dosage may be increased at weekly (or longer) intervals until optimum blood pressure reduction is achieved. In general, the maximum effect of any given dosage level will be apparent after 1 week of therapy. The effective dosage range is 100 to 450 mg/day. Dosages above 450 mg/day have not been studied. While once-daily dosing is effective and can maintain a reduction in blood pressure throughout the day, lower doses (especially 100 mg) may not maintain a full effect at the end of the 24-hour period, and larger or more frequent daily doses may be required. This can be evaluated by measuring blood pressure near the end of the dosing interval to determine whether satisfactory control is being maintained throughout the day. Beta-1 selectivity diminishes as the dose of metoprolol tartrate is increased.

➤*Angina pectoris:* The usual initial dosage is 100 mg daily, given in 2 divided doses. The dosage may be gradually increased at weekly intervals until optimum clinical response has been obtained or there is pronounced slowing of the heart rate. The effective dosage range is 100 to 400 mg/day. Dosages above 400 mg/day have not been studied. If treatment is to be discontinued, the dosage should be reduced gradually over a period of 1 to 2 weeks.

➤*Myocardial infarction:*

Early treatment – During the early phase of definite or suspected acute myocardial infarction, treatment with metoprolol tartrate can be initiated as soon as possible after the patient's arrival in the hospital. Such treatment should be initiated in a coronary care or similar unit immediately after the patient's hemodynamic condition has stabilized.

Treatment in this early phase should begin with the intravenous administration of 3 bolus injections of 5 mg of metoprolol tartrate each; the injections should be given at approximately 2-minute intervals. During the intravenous administration of metoprolol tartrate, blood pressure, heart rate, and electrocardiogram should be carefully monitored.

In patients who tolerate the full intravenous dose (15 mg), metoprolol tartrate tablets, 50 mg every 6 hours, should be initiated 15 minutes after the last intravenous dose and continued for 48 hours. Thereafter, patients should receive a maintenance dosage of 100 mg twice daily (see Late treatment).

Patients who appear not to tolerate the full intravenous dose should be started on metoprolol tartrate tablets either 25 mg or 50 mg every 6 hours (depending on the degree of intolerance) 15 minutes after the last intravenous dose or as soon as their clinical condition allows. In patients with severe intolerance, treatment with metoprolol tartrate should be discontinued.

Late treatment – Patients with contraindications to treatment during the early phase of suspected or definite myocardial infarction, patients who appear not to tolerate the full early treatment, and patients in whom the physician wishes to delay therapy for any other reason should be started on metoprolol tartrate tablets, 100 mg twice daily, as soon as their clinical condition allows. Therapy should be continued for at least 3 months. Although the efficacy of metoprolol tartrate beyond 3 months has not been conclusively established, data from studies with other beta blockers suggest that treatment should be continued for 1 to 3 years.

➤*Storage/Stability:* Store between 15° to 30°C (59° to 86°F). Protect from moisture. Dispense in tight, light-resistant container.

METOPROLOL SUCCINATE — ORAL

For complete and comparative prescribing information, refer to the Beta-Adrenergic Blocking Agents group monograph.

WARNING

Ischemic heart disease – Following abrupt cessation of therapy with certain beta-blocking agents, exacerbations of angina pectoris and, in some cases, myocardial infarction have occurred. When discontinuing chronically administered metoprolol, particularly in patients with ischemic heart disease, gradually reduce the dosage over a period of 1 to 2 weeks and carefully monitor the patient. If angina markedly worsens or acute coronary insufficiency develops, reinstate metoprolol administration promptly, at least temporarily, and take other measures appropriate for the management of unstable angina. Warn patients against interruption or discontinuation of therapy without the physician's advice. Because coronary artery disease is common and may be unrecognized, it may be prudent not to discontinue metoprolol therapy abruptly, even in patients treated only for hypertension.

Indications

➤*Hypertension:* Treatment of hypertension. They may be used alone or in combination with other antihypertensive agents.

➤*Angina pectoris:* Long-term treatment of angina pectoris.

➤*Heart failure:* Treatment of stable, symptomatic (NYHA class II or III) heart failure of ischemic, hypertensive, or cardiomyopathic origin. It was studied in patients already receiving ACE inhibitors, diuretics, and, in the majority of cases, digitalis. In this population, metoprolol succinate extended-release tablets decreased the rate of mortality plus hospitalization, largely through a reduction in cardiovascular mortality and hospitalizations for heart failure.

Administration and Dosage

➤*Approved by the FDA:* August 1978.

An extended-release tablet intended for once-daily administration. When switching from immediate-release metoprolol tablet to metoprolol succinate extended-release, the same total daily dose of metoprolol succinate should be used.

As with immediate-release metoprolol, dosages of extended-release metoprolol succinate should be individualized and titration may be needed in some patients.

Metoprolol succinate extended-release tablets are scored and can be divided; however, the whole or half tablet should be swallowed whole and not chewed or crushed.

➤*Hypertension:* The usual initial dosage is 50 to 100 mg daily in a single dose, whether used alone or added to a diuretic. The dosage may be increased at weekly (or longer) intervals until optimum blood pressure reduction is achieved. In general, the maximum effect of any given dosage level will be apparent after 1 week of therapy. Dosages above 400 mg/day have not been studied.

➤*Angina pectoris:* The dosage of extended-release metoprolol succinate should be individualized. The usual initial dosage is 100 mg daily, given in a single dose. The dosage may be gradually increased at weekly intervals until optimum clinical response has been obtained or there is a pronounced slowing of the heart rate. Dosages above 400 mg/day have not been studied. If treatment is to be discontinued, the dosage should be reduced gradually over a period of 1 to 2 weeks.

➤*Heart failure:* Dosage must be individualized and closely monitored during up-titration. Prior to initiation of extended-release metoprolol succinate, the dosing of diuretics, ACE inhibitors, and digitalis (if used) should be stabilized. The recommended starting dose of extended-release metoprolol succinate is 25 mg once daily for 2 weeks in patients with NYHA class II heart failure and 12.5 mg once daily in patients with more severe heart failure. The dose should then be doubled every 2 weeks to the highest dosage level tolerated by the patient or up to 200 mg of extended-release metoprolol succinate. If transient worsening of heart failure occurs, it may be treated with increased doses of diuretics, and it may also be necessary to lower the dose of extended-release metoprolol succinate or temporarily discontinue it. The dose of extended-release metoprolol succinate should not be increased until symptoms of worsening heart failure have been stabilized. Initial difficulty with titration should not preclude later attempts to introduce extended-release metoprolol succinate. If heart failure patients experience symptomatic bradycardia, the dose of extended-release metoprolol succinate should be reduced.

➤*Storage / Stability:* Store at 25°C (77°F). Excursions permitted to 15° to 30°C (59° to 86°F) (see USP controlled room temperature).

METOPROLOL TARTRATE — INJECTION

For complete and comparative prescribing information, refer to the Beta-Adrenergic Blocking Agents group monograph.

WARNING

Ischemic heart disease – Following abrupt cessation of therapy with certain beta-blocking agents, exacerbations of angina pectoris and, in some cases, myocardial infarction have occurred. When discontinuing chronically administered metoprolol, particularly in patients with ischemic heart disease, gradually reduce the dosage over a period of 1 to 2 weeks and carefully monitor the patient. If angina markedly worsens or acute coronary insufficiency develops, reinstate metoprolol administration promptly, at least temporarily, and take other measures appropriate for the management of unstable angina. Warn patients against interruption or discontinuation of therapy without the physician's advice. Because coronary artery disease is common and may be unrecognized, it may be prudent not to discontinue metoprolol therapy abruptly, even in patients treated only for hypertension.

Indications

➤*Myocardial infarction:* Treatment of hemodynamically stable patients with definite or suspected acute myocardial infarction to reduce cardiovascular mortality. Treatment with intravenous metoprolol tartrate can be initiated as soon as the patient's clinical condition allows. Alternatively, treatment can begin within 3 to 10 days of the acute event.

Administration and Dosage

➤*Approved by the FDA:* August 1978.

➤*Myocardial infarction:*

Early treatment – During the early phase of definite or suspected acute myocardial infarction, treatment with metoprolol tartrate can be initiated as soon as possible after the patient's arrival in the hospital. Such treatment should be initiated in a coronary care or similar unit immediately after the patient's hemodynamic condition has stabilized.

Treatment in this early phase should begin with the intravenous administration of 3 bolus injections of 5 mg of metoprolol tartrate each; the injections should be given at approximately 2-minute intervals. During the intravenous administration of metoprolol tartrate, blood pressure, heart rate, and electrocardiogram should be carefully monitored.

In patients who tolerate the full intravenous dose (15 mg), metoprolol tartrate tablets, 50 mg every 6 hours, should be initiated 15 minutes after the last intravenous dose and continued for 48 hours. Thereafter, patients should receive a maintenance dosage of 100 mg twice daily (see Late treatment).

Patients who appear not to tolerate the full intravenous dose should be started on metoprolol tartrate tablets either 25 mg or 50 mg every 6 hours (depending on the degree of intolerance) 15 minutes after the last intravenous dose or as soon as their clinical condition allows. In patients with severe intolerance, treatment with metoprolol tartrate should be discontinued.

Late treatment – Patients with contraindications to treatment during the early phase of suspected or definite myocardial infarction, patients who appear not to tolerate the full early treatment, and patients in whom the physician wishes to delay therapy for any other reason should be started on metoprolol tartrate tablets, 100 mg twice daily, as soon as their clinical condition allows. Therapy should be continued for at least 3 months. Although the efficacy of metoprolol tartrate beyond 3 months has not been conclusively established, data from studies with other beta blockers suggest that treatment should be continued for 1 to 3 years.

➤*Storage / Stability:* Do not store above 30°C (86°F). Protect from light.

TIMOLOL MALEATE

Rx	**Timolol Maleate** (Various, eg, Mylan)	**Tablets:** 5 mg	In 100s.
Rx	**Blocadren** (Merck)		(MSD 59 BLOCADREN). Light blue. In 100s.
Rx	**Timolol Maleate** (Various, eg, Mylan)	**Tablets:** 10 mg	In 100s.
Rx	**Timolol Maleate** (Various, eg, Mylan)	**Tablets:** 20 mg	In 100s.
Rx	**Blocadren** (Merck)		(MSD 437 BLOCADREN). Light blue, scored, capsule shape. In 100s.

TIMOLOL MALEATE — ORAL

For complete and comparative prescribing information, refer to the Beta-Adrenergic Blocking Agents group monograph.

WARNING

Exacerbation of ischemic heart disease following abrupt withdrawal – Hypersensitivity to catecholamines has been observed in patients withdrawn from beta-blocker therapy; exacerbation of angina and, in some cases, myocardial infarction have occurred after abrupt discontinuation of such therapy. When discontinuing chronically administered timolol, particularly in patients with ischemic heart disease, gradually reduce the dosage over a period of one to two weeks and carefully monitor the patient. If angina markedly worsens or acute coronary insufficiency develops, reinstitute timolol administration promptly, at least temporarily, and take other measures appropriate for the management of unstable angina. Warn patients against interruption of discontinuation of therapy without the physician's advice. Because coronary artery disease is common and may be unrecognized, it may be prudent not to discontinue timolol therapy abruptly, even in patients treated only for hypertension.

Indications

➤*Hypertension:* Treatment of hypertension. It may be used alone or in combination with other antihypertensive agents, especially thiazide-type diuretics.

➤*Myocardial infarction:* In patients who have survived the acute phase of myocardial infarction, and are clinically stable, to reduce cardiovascular mortality and the risk of reinfarction.

➤*Migraine:* Prophylaxis of migraine headache.

Administration and Dosage

➤*Approved by the FDA:* August, 1978.

➤*Hypertension:* The usual initial dosage of timolol maleate is 10 mg twice a day, whether used alone or added to diuretic therapy. Dosage may be increased or decreased depending on heart rate and blood pressure response. The usual total maintenance dosage is 20 to 40 mg/day. Increases in dosage to a maximum of 60 mg/day divided into 2 doses may be necessary. There should be an interval of at least 7 days between increases in dosages. Timolol maleate may be used with a thiazide diuretic or with other antihypertensive agents. Patients should be observed carefully during initiation of such concomitant therapy.

➤*Myocardial infarction:* The recommended dosage for long-term prophylactic use in patients who have survived the acute phase of a myocardial infarction is 10 mg given twice daily.

➤*Migraine:* The usual initial dosage of timolol maleate is 10 mg twice a day. During maintenance therapy, the 20 mg daily dosage may be administered as a single dose. Total daily dosage may be increased to a maximum of 30 mg, given in divided doses, or decreased to 10 mg once per day, depending on clinical response and tolerability. If a satisfactory response is not obtained after 6 to 8 weeks use of the maximum daily dosage, therapy with timolol maleate should be discontinued.

➤*Storage/Stability:* Store at controlled room temperature, 15° to 30°C (59° to 86°F). Keep container tightly closed. Protect from light.

SOTALOL HYDROCHLORIDE

Rx	**Sotalol HCl** (Various, eg, Eon, Global, Par, Teva)	**Tablets:** 80 mg	Lactose. In 100s, 500s, and 1000s.
Rx	**Betapace** (Berlex)		Lactose. (Betapace 80 mg). Light blue, scored, capsule shape. In 100s and UD 100s.
Rx	**Sotalol HCl** (Various, eg, Eon, Global, Par, Teva)	**Tablets:** 120 mg	Lactose. In 100s, 500s, and 1000s.
Rx	**Betapace** (Berlex)		Lactose. (Betapace 120 mg). Light blue, scored, capsule shape. In 100s and UD 100s.
Rx	**Sotalol HCl** (Various, eg, Eon, Global, Par, Teva)	**Tablets:** 160 mg	Lactose. In 100s, 500s, and 1000s.
Rx	**Betapace** (Berlex)		Lactose. (Betapace 160 mg). Light blue, scored, capsule shape. In 100s and UD 100s.
Rx	**Sotalol HCl** (Various, eg, Eon, Global, Par, Teva)	**Tablets:** 240 mg	Lactose. In 100s, 500s, and 1000s.
Rx	**Betapace** (Berlex)		Lactose. (Betapace 240 mg). Light blue, scored, capsule shape. In 100s and UD 100s.
Rx	**Sotalol HCl AF** (Apotex)	**Tablets:** 80 mg	(APO AF 80). White to off-white, capsule shape, scored. In 100s.
Rx	**Betapace AF** (Berlex)		Lactose. (80 mg/BERLEX). White, scored, capsule shape. In UD 60s and 100s.
Rx	**Sotalol HCl AF** (Apotex)	**Tablets:** 120 mg	(APO AF 120). White to off-white, capsule shape, scored. In 100s.
Rx	**Betapace AF** (Berlex)		Lactose. (120 mg/BERLEX). White, scored, capsule shape. In UD 60s and 100s.
Rx	**Sotalol HCl AF** (Apotex)	**Tablets:** 160 mg	(APO AF 160). White to off-white, capsule shape, scored. In 100s.
Rx	**Betapace AF** (Berlex)		Lactose. (160 mg/BERLEX). White, scored, capsule shape. In UD 60s and 100s.

SOTALOL HYDROCHLORIDE — ORAL

For complete prescribing information, refer to the Beta-Adrenergic Blocking Agents group monograph.

WARNING

To minimize the risk of induced arrhythmia, place patients initiated or reinitiated on sotalol AF or sotalol for a minimum of 3 days (on their maintenance dose) in a facility that can provide cardiac resuscitation, continuous electrocardiographic (ECG) monitoring, and calculations of creatinine clearance. Calculate creatinine clearance prior to dosing. Do not substitute sotalol for sotalol AF because of significant differences in labeling (ie, patient package insert, dosing administration, safety information).

Indications

➤*Betapace:* Oral *Betapace* (sotalol) is indicated for the treatment of documented ventricular arrhythmias, such as sustained ventricular tachycardia, that in the judgment of the physician are life-threatening. Because of the proarrhythmic effects of sotalol, including a 1.5% to 2% rate of torsade de pointes or new ventricular tachycardia (VT)/ventricular fibrillation (VF) in patients with either nonsustained ventricular tachycardia (NSVT) or supraventricular arrhythmias, its use in patients with less severe arrhythmias, even if the patients are symptomatic, is generally not recommended. Treatment of patients with asymptomatic ventricular premature contractions should be avoided.

Initiation of sotalol treatment or increasing doses, as with other antiarrhythmic agents used to treat life-threatening arrhythmias, should be carried out in the hospital. The response to treatment should then be evaluated by a suitable method (eg, PES or Holter monitoring) prior to continuing the patient on chronic therapy. Various approaches have been used to determine the response to antiarrhythmic therapy, including sotalol.

In the Electrophysiologic Study Versus Electrocardiographic Monitoring Trial (ESVEM) trial, response by Holter monitoring was tentatively defined as 100% suppression of ventricular tachycardia, 90% suppression of nonsustained VT, 80% suppression of paired ventricular premature contractions (VPCs), and 75% suppression of total VPCs in patients who had at least 10 VPCs/hour at baseline; this tentative response was confirmed if VT lasting 5 or more beats was not observed during treadmill exercise testing using a standard Bruce protocol. The programmed electrical stimulation (PES) protocol utilized a maximum of 3 extra stimuli at 3 pacing cycle lengths and 2 right ventricular pacing sites. Response by PES was defined as prevention of induction of the following:

1.) Monomorphic VT lasting over 15 seconds.
2.) Nonsustained polymorphic VT containing more than 15 beats of monomorphic VT in patients with a history of monomorphic VT.
3.) Polymorphic VT or VF greater than 15 beats in patients with VF or a history of aborted sudden death without monomorphic VT.
4.) Two episodes of polymorphic VT or VF of greater than 15 beats in a patient presenting with monomorphic VT. Sustained VT or NSVT producing hypotension during the final treadmill test was considered a drug failure.

In a multicenter, open-label, long-term study of sotalol in patients with life-threatening ventricular arrhythmias that had proven refractory to other antiarrhythmic medications, response by Holter monitoring was defined as in ESVEM. Response by PES was defined as noninducibility of sustained VT by at least double extrastimuli delivered at a pacing cycle length of 400

SOTALOL HYDROCHLORIDE — ORAL

msec. Overall survival and arrhythmia recurrence rates in this study were similar to those seen in ESVEM, although there was no comparative group to allow a definitive assessment of outcome.

Antiarrhythmic drugs have not been shown to enhance survival in patients with ventricular arrhythmias.

➤*Betapace AF*: *Betapace AF* is indicated for the maintenance of normal sinus rhythm [delay in time to recurrence of atrial fibrillation/atrial flutter (AFIB/AFL)] in patients with symptomatic AFIB/AFL who are currently in sinus rhythm. Because *Betapace AF* can cause life-threatening ventricular arrhythmias, it should be reserved for patients in whom AFIB/AFL is highly symptomatic. Patients with paroxysmal AFIB whose AFIB/AFL that is easily reversed (by Valsalva maneuver, for example) should usually not be given *Betapace AF*.

In general, antiarrhythmic therapy for AFIB/AFL aims to prolong the time in normal sinus rhythm. Recurrence is expected in some patients.

Sotalol is also indicated for the treatment of documented life-threatening ventricular arrhythmias and is marketed under the trade name *Betapace* (sotalol HCl). *Betapace*, however, must not be substituted for *Betapace AF* because of significant differences in labeling.

Administration and Dosage

➤*Approved by the FDA:* October 30, 1992.

➤*Betapace*: As with other antiarrhythmic agents, sotalol should be initiated and doses increased in a hospital with facilities for cardiac rhythm monitoring and assessment. Sotalol should be administered only after appropriate clinical assessment, and the dosage of sotalol must be individualized for each patient on the basis of therapeutic response and tolerance. Proarrhythmic reactions can occur not only at initiation of therapy, but also with each upward dosage adjustment.

Dosage of sotalol should be adjusted gradually, allowing 3 days between dosing increments in order to attain steady-state plasma concentrations, and to allow monitoring of QT intervals. Graded dose adjustment will help prevent the usage of doses which are higher than necessary to control the arrhythmia. The recommended initial dose is 80 mg twice daily. This dose may be increased, if necessary, after appropriate evaluation to 240 or 320 mg/day (120 to 160 mg twice daily). In most patients, a therapeutic response is obtained at a total daily dose of 160 to 320 mg/day, given in 2 or 3 divided doses. Some patients with life-threatening refractory ventricular arrhythmias may require doses as high as 480 to 640 mg/day; however, these doses should only be prescribed when the potential benefit outweighs the increased risk of adverse reactions, in particular proarrhythmia. Because of the long terminal elimination half-life of sotalol dosing on more than a twice-daily regimen is usually not necessary.

Dosage in renal impairment – Because sotalol is excreted predominantly in urine and its terminal elimination half-life is prolonged in conditions of renal impairment, the dosing interval (time between divided doses) of sotalol should be modified (when creatinine clearance is lower than 60 mL/min) according to the following table.

Creatinine clearance mL/min	Dosing* interval (hours)
> 60 mL/min	12 hours
30 to 59 mL/min	24 hours
10 to 29 mL/min	36 to 48 hours
< 10 mL/min	Dose should be individualized.

* The initial dose of 80 mg and subsequent doses should be administered at these intervals. See following paragraph for dosage escalations.

Because the terminal elimination half-life of sotalol HCl is increased in patients with renal impairment, a longer duration of dosing is required to reach steady-state. Dose escalations in renal impairment should be done after administration of at least 5 to 6 doses at appropriate intervals (see above).

Extreme caution should be exercised in the use of sotalol in patients with renal failure undergoing hemodialysis. The half-life of sotalol is prolonged (up to 69 hours) in anuric patients. Sotalol, however, can be partly removed by dialysis with subsequent partial rebound in concentrations when dialysis is completed. Both safety (heart rate, QT interval) and efficacy (arrhythmia control) must be closely monitored.

Pediatrics: The use of sotalol in pediatric patients with renal impairment has not been investigated. Sotalol elimination is predominantly via the kidney in the unchanged form. Use of sotalol in any age group with decreased renal function should be at lower doses or at increased intervals between doses. Monitoring of heart rate and QTc is more important and it will take much longer to reach steady-state with any dose and/or frequency of administration.

Transfer to sotalol – Before starting sotalol, previous antiarrhythmic therapy should generally be withdrawn under careful monitoring for a minimum of 2 to 3 plasma half-lives if the patient's clinical condition permits. Treatment has been initiated in some patients receiving IV lidocaine without ill effect. After discontinuation of amiodarone, sotalol should not be initiated until the QT interval is normalized.

➤*Betapace AF*:

Administration and dosage in adults – Therapy with *Betapace AF* must be initiated (and, if necessary, titrated) in a setting that provides continuous electrocardiographic (ECG) monitoring and in the presence of personnel trained in the management of serious ventricular arrhythmias. Patients should continue to be monitored in this way for a minimum of 3 days on the maintenance dose. In addition, patients should not be discharged within 12 hours of electrical or pharmacological conversion to normal sinus rhythm.

The QT interval is used to determine patient eligibility for *Betapace AF* treatment and for monitoring safety during treatment. The baseline QT interval must be less than or equal to 450 msec in order for a patient to be started on *Betapace AF* therapy. During initiation and titration, the QT interval should be monitored 2 to 4 hours after each dose. If the QT interval prolongs to 500 msec or greater, the dose must be reduced or the drug discontinued.

The dose of *Betapace AF* must be individualized according to calculated creatinine clearance. In patients with a creatinine clearance greater than 60 mL/min *Betapace AF* is administered twice daily while in those with a creatinine clearance between 40 and 60 mL/min, the dose is administered once daily. In patients with a creatinine clearance less than 40 mL/min *Betapace AF* is contraindicated. The recommended initial dose of *Betapace AF* is 80 mg and is initiated as shown in the dosing algorithm described below. The 80 mg dose can be titrated upward to 120 mg during initial hospitalization or after discharge on 80 mg in the event of recurrence, by rehospitalization and repeating the same steps used during the initiation of therapy (see Upward titration of dose).

Patients with atrial fibrillation should be anticoagulated according to usual medical practice. Hypokalemia should be corrected before initiation of *Betapace AF* therapy.

Patients to be discharged on *Betapace AF* therapy from an in-patient setting should have an adequate supply of *Betapace AF*, to allow uninterrupted therapy until the patient can fill a *Betapace AF* prescription.

Initiation of Betapace AF therapy:

- *Step 1* –
  Electrocardiographic assessment: Prior to administration of the first dose, the QT interval must be determined using an average of 5 beats. If the baseline QT is greater than 450 msec (JT greater than or equal to 330 msec if QRS over 100 msec), *Betapace AF* is contraindicated.
- *Step 2* –
  Calculation of creatinine clearance: Prior to the administration of the first dose, the patient's creatinine clearance should be calculated using the following formula:

Male

Ccr (male) = (140 - age) × body weight in kg/72 × serum creatinine (mg/dL).

Female

Ccr (female) = (140 - age) × body weight in kg × 0.85/72 × serum creatinine (mg/dL).

When serum creatinine is given in mcmol/L, divide the value by 88.4 (1 mg/dL = 88.4 mcmol/L).

- *Step 3* –
  Starting dose: The starting dose of *Betapace AF* is 80 mg twice daily if the creatinine clearance is greater than 60 mL/min, and 80 mg once daily if the creatinine clearance is 40 to 60 mL/min. If the creatinine clearance is less than 40 mL/min *Betapace AF* is contraindicated.
- *Step 4* – Administer the appropriate daily dose of *Betapace AF* and begin continuous ECG monitoring with QT interval measurements 2 to 4 hours after each dose.
- *Step 5* – If the 80 mg dose level is tolerated and the QT interval remains less than 500 msec after at least 3 days (after 5 or 6 doses if patient receiving once-daily dosing), the patient can be discharged. Alternatively, during hospitalization, the dose can be increased to 120 mg twice daily and the patient followed for 3 days on this dose (followed for 5 or 6 doses if patient receiving once-daily doses).

Upward titration of dose: If the 80 mg dose level (given twice daily or once daily depending upon the creatinine clearance) does not reduce the frequency of relapses of AFIB/AFL and is tolerated without excessive QT-interval prolongation (ie, greater than or equal to 520 msec), the dose level may be increased to 120 mg (twice daily or once daily depending upon the creatinine clearance). As proarrhythmic reactions can occur not only at initiation of therapy, but also with each upward dosage adjustment, steps 2 through 5 used during initiation of *Betapace AF* therapy should be followed when increasing the dose level. In the US multicenter dose-response study, the 120 mg dose (twice daily or once daily) was found to be the most effective in prolonging the time to ECG documented symptomatic recurrence of AFIB/AFL. If the 120 mg dose does not reduce the frequency of early relapse of AFIB/AFL and is tolerated without excessive QT interval prolongation (greater than or equal to 520 msec), an increase to 160 mg (twice daily or once daily depending upon the creatinine clearance), can be considered. Steps 2 through 5 used during the initiation of therapy should be used again to introduce such an increase.

Maintenance of Betapace AF therapy: Renal function and QT should be reevaluated regularly if medically warranted. If QT is 520 msec or greater (JT 430 msec or greater if QRS is greater than 100 msec), the dose of *Betapace AF* therapy should be reduced and patients should be carefully monitored until QT returns to less than 520 msec. If the QT interval is greater than or equal to 520 msec while on the lowest maintenance dose level (80 mg) the drug should be discontinued. If renal function deteriorates, reduce the daily dose in half by administering the drug once daily (see Step 3, Initiation of *Betapace AF* therapy).

Special considerations: The maximum recommended dose in patients with a calculated creatinine clearance greater than 60 mL/min is 160 mg twice daily, doses greater than 160 mg twice daily have been associated with an increased incidence of torsade de pointes and are not recommended.

SOTALOL HYDROCHLORIDE — ORAL

A patient who misses a dose should not double the next dose. The next dose should be taken at the usual time.

Administration and dosage in children – As in adults the following precautionary measures should be considered when initiating sotalol treatment in children: Initiation of treatment in the hospital after appropriate clinical assessment; individualized regimen as appropriate; gradual increase of doses if required; careful assessment of therapeutic response and tolerability; and frequent monitoring of the QTc interval and heart rate.

For children aged about 2 years and older: For children aged about 2 years and older, with normal renal function, doses normalized for body surface area are appropriate for both initial and incremental dosing. Since the Class III potency in children is not very different from that in adults, reaching plasma concentrations that occur within the adult dose range is an appropriate guide. From pediatric pharmacokinetic data the following is recommended.

For initiation of treatment, 30 mg/m^2 3 times a day (90 mg/m^2 total daily dose) is approximately equivalent to the initial 160 mg total daily dose for adults. Subsequent titration to a maximum of 60 mg/m^2 (approximately equivalent to the 360 mg total daily dose for adults) can then occur. Titration should be guided by clinical response, heart rate and QTc, with increased dosing being preferably carried out in-hospital. At least 36 hours should be allowed between dose increments to attain steady-state plasma concentrations of sotalol in patients with age-adjusted normal renal function.

For children aged about 2 years or younger: For children aged about 2 years or younger, the above pediatric dosage should be reduced by a factor that depends heavily upon age, age plotted on a logarithmic scale in months.

For a child aged 20 months, the dosing suggested for children with normal renal function aged 2 years or greater should be multiplied by about 0.97; the initial starting dose would be (30 × 0.97) = 29.1 mg/m^2, administered 3 times daily. For a child aged 1 month, the starting dose should be multiplied by 0.68; the initial starting dose would be (30 × 0.68) = 20 mg/m^2, administered 3 times daily. For a child aged about 1 week, the initial starting dose should be multiplied by 0.3; the starting dose would be (30 × 0.3) = 9 mg/m^2. Similar calculations should be made for increased doses as titration proceeds. Since the half-life of sotalol decreases with decreasing age (below about 2 years), time to steady-state will also increase. Thus, in neonates the time to steady-state may be as long as a week or longer.

In all children, individualization of dosage is required. As in adults *Betapace* (sotalol HCl) should be used with particular caution in children if the QTc is greater than 500 msec on therapy and serious consideration should be given to reducing the dose or discontinuing therapy when QTc exceeds 550 msec.

The use of *Betapace AF* (sotalol) in children with renal impairment has not been investigated. Sotalol elimination is predominantly via the kidney in the unchanged form. Use of sotalol in any age group with decreased renal function should be at lower doses or at increased intervals between doses. Monitoring of heart rate and QTc is more important and it will take much longer to reach steady-state with any dose or frequency of administration.

Transfer to Betapace AF from Betapace – Patients with a history of symptomatic AFIB/AFL who are currently receiving *Betapace* for the maintenance of normal sinus should be transferred to *Betapace AF* because of the significant differences in labeling (ie, patient package insert, dosing administration, and safety information).

Transfer to Betapace AF from other antiarrhythmic agents – Before starting *Betapace AF*, previous antiarrhythmic therapy should generally be withdrawn under careful monitoring for a minimum of 2 to 3 plasma half-lives if the patient's clinical condition permits. Treatment has been initiated in some patients receiving IV lidocaine without ill effect. After discontinuation of amiodarone, *Betapace AF* should not be initiated until the QT interval is normalized.

Preparation of extemporaneous oral solution – *Betapace* syrup 5 mg/mL can be compounded using Simple Syrup containing 0.1% sodium benzoate (syrup, NF) as follows:

1.) Measure 120 mL of Simple Syrup.
2.) Transfer the syrup to a 6-ounce amber plastic (polyethylene terephthalate [PET]) prescription bottle. Note: An oversized bottle is used to allow for a headspace, so that there will be more effective mixing during shaking of the bottle.
3.) Add 5 *Betapace* 120 mg tablets to the bottle. These tablets are added intact; it is not necessary to crush the tablets. Note: The addition of the tablets can also be done first. The tablets can also be crushed if preferred. If the tablets are crushed, care should be taken to transfer the entire quantity of tablet powder into the bottle containing the syrup.
4.) Shake the bottle to wet the entire surface of the tablets. If the tablets have been crushed, shake the bottle until the endpoint is achieved.
5.) Allow the tablets to hydrate for approximately 2 hours.
6.) After at least 2 hours have elapsed, shake the bottle intermittently over the course of at least another 2 hours until the tablets are completely disintegrated. Note: The tablets can be allowed to hydrate overnight to simplify the disintegration process.

The end point is achieved when a dispersion of fine particles in the syrup is obtained.

This compounding procedure results in a solution containing 5 mg/mL of sotalol HCl. The fine solid particles are the water-insoluble inactive ingredients of the tablets.

This extemporaneously prepared oral solution of sotalol HCl (with suspended inactive particles) must be shaken well prior to administration. This is to ensure that the amount of inactive solid particles per dose remains constant throughout the duration of use.

➤*Storage / Stability:* Dispense in a tight, light-resistant container using a child-resistant closure.

Betapace – Store at controlled room temperature, between 15° to 30°C (59° to 86°F).

Betapace AF – Store at 25°C (77°F); excursions permitted to 15° to 30°C (59° to 86°F).

Stability of suspension – Stability studies indicate that the suspension is stable when stored at controlled room temperature (15° to 30°C; 59° to 86°F) and ambient humidity for 3 months.

ACEBUTOLOL HYDROCHLORIDE

Rx	**Acebutolol HCl** (Various, eg, Mylan, Watson)	**Capsules:** 200 mg	In 100s and 1000s.
Rx	**Sectral** (ESP Pharma)		(Wyeth 4177 Sectral 200). Purple/orange. In 100s and *Redipak* 100s.
Rx	**Acebutolol HCl** (Various, eg, ESI Lederle, Mylan, Watson)	**Capsules:** 400 mg	In 100s and 1000s.
	Sectral (ESP Pharma)		(Wyeth 4179 Sectral 400). Brown/orange. In 100s.

ACEBUTOLOL HYDROCHLORIDE — ORAL

For complete and comparative prescribing information, refer to the Beta-Adrenergic Blocking Agents group monograph.

Indications

➤*Hypertension:* Management of hypertension in adults. It may be used alone or in combination with other antihypertensive agents, especially thiazide-type diuretics.

➤*Ventricular arrhythmias:* Management of ventricular premature beats; it reduces the total number of premature beats, as well as the number of paired and multiform ventricular ectopic beats, and R-on-T beats.

Administration and Dosage

➤*Approved by the FDA:* December 28, 1984.

➤*Hypertension:* The initial dosage of acebutolol in uncomplicated, mild to moderate hypertension is 400 mg. This can be given as a single daily dose, but in occasional patients, twice-daily dosing may be required for adequate 24-hour blood pressure control. An optimal response is usually achieved with dosages of 400 to 800 mg/day; although, some patients have been maintained on as little as 200 mg/day. Patients with more severe hypertension or who have demonstrated inadequate control may respond to a total of 1200 mg daily (administered twice daily), or to the addition of a second antihypertensive agent. Beta-1 selectivity diminishes as dosage is increased.

➤*Ventricular arrhythmia:* The usual initial dose of acebutolol HCl is 400 mg daily given as 200 mg twice daily. Dosage should be increased gradually until an optimal clinical response is obtained, generally at 600 to 1200 mg/day. If treatment is to be discontinued, the dosage should be reduced gradually over a period of about 2 weeks.

➤*Use in older patients:* Older patients have an approximately 2-fold increase in bioavailability and may require lower maintenance doses. Doses greater than 800 mg/day should be avoided in the elderly.

➤*Storage / Stability:* Store at room temperature, approximately 25°C (77°F). Keep tightly closed. Protect from light. Dispense in a light-resistant, tight container.

NADOLOL

Rx	**Nadolol** (Various, eg, Apothecon, Mylan, UDL)	**Tablets:** 20 mg	In 100s and UD 100s.
Rx	**Corgard** (Monarch)		(CORGARD 20 BL 232). Scored. In 100s and *Unimatic* 100s.
Rx	**Nadolol** (Various, eg, Apothecon, Mylan, UDL, Zenith)	**Tablets:** 40 mg	In 100s, 1000s, and UD 100s.
Rx	**Corgard** (Monarch)		(CORGARD 40 BL 208). Scored. In 100s, 1000s, and *Unimatic* 100s.

NADOLOL

Rx	**Nadolol** (Various, eg, Apothecon, Mylan, UDL, Zenith)	**Tablets:** 80 mg	In 30s, 100s, 500s, 1000s, and UD 100s.
Rx	**Corgard** (Monarch)		(CORGARD 80 BL 241). Scored. In 100s, 1000s, and *Unimatic* 100s.
Rx	**Nadolol** (Various, eg, Apothecon, Zenith)	**Tablets:** 120 mg	In 100s, 500s, and 1000s.
Rx	**Corgard** (Monarch)		(CORGARD 120 MG BL 208). Scored. In 100s and 1000s.
Rx	**Nadolol** (Various, eg, Apothecon, Zenith)	**Tablets:** 160 mg	In 100s, 500s, and 1000s.
Rx	**Corgard** (Monarch)		(246). Scored. In 100s.

NADOLOL — ORAL

For complete and comparative prescribing information, refer to the Beta-Adrenergic Blocking Agents group monograph.

WARNING

Exacerbation of ischemic heart disease following abrupt withdrawal – Hypersensitivity to catecholamines has been observed in patients withdrawn from beta-blocker therapy; exacerbation of angina and, in some cases, myocardial infarction have occurred after abrupt discontinuation of such therapy. When discontinuing chronically administered nadolol, particularly in patients with ischemic heart disease, gradually reduce the dosage over a period of one to two weeks and carefully monitor the patient. If angina markedly worsens or acute coronary insufficiency develops, reinstitute nadolol administration promptly, at least temporarily, and take other measures appropriate for the management of unstable angina. Warn patients against interruption or discontinuation of therapy without the physician's advice. Because coronary artery disease is common and may be unrecognized, it may be prudent not to discontinue nadolol therapy abruptly, even in patients treated only for hypertension.

Indications

➤*Angina pectoris:* Nadolol is indicated for the long-term management of patients with angina pectoris.

➤*Hypertension:* Nadolol is indicated in the management of hypertension; it may be used alone or in combination with other antihypertensive agents, especially thiazide diuretics.

Administration and Dosage

➤*Approved by the FDA:* December 1979.

Dosage must be individualized. Nadolol may be administered without regard to meals.

➤*Angina pectoris:* The usual initial dose is 40 mg nadolol once daily. Dosage may be gradually increased in 40 to 80 mg increments at 3 to 7 day intervals until optimum clinical response is obtained or there is pronounced slowing of the heart rate. The usual maintenance dose is 40 or 80 mg administered once daily. Doses up to 160 or 240 mg administered once daily may be needed.

The usefulness and safety in angina pectoris of dosages exceeding 240 mg/day have not been established. If treatment is to be discontinued, reduce the dosage gradually over a period of 1 to 2 weeks.

➤*Hypertension:* The usual initial dose is 40 mg nadolol once daily, whether it is used alone or in addition to diuretic therapy. Dosage may be gradually increased in 40 to 80 mg increments until optimum blood pressure reduction is achieved. The usual maintenance dose is 40 or 80 mg administered once daily. Doses up to 240 or 320 mg administered once daily may be needed.

➤*Renal function impairment:* Absorbed nadolol is excreted principally by the kidneys and, although nonrenal elimination does occur, dosage adjustments are necessary in patients with renal impairment. The following dose intervals are recommended:

If the Ccr is greater than 50 mL/min per 1.73 m^2, then a dosage interval of 24 hours is recommended.

If the creatinine clearance is 31 to 50 mL/min per 1.73 m^2, then a dosage interval of 24 to 36 hours is recommended.

If the creatinine clearance is 10 to 30 mL/min per 1.73 m^2, then a dosage interval of 24 to 48 hours is recommended.

If the creatinine clearance is less than 10 mL/min per 1.73 m^2, then a dosage interval of 40 to 60 hours is recommended.

➤*Storage/Stability:* Store at controlled room temperature 15° to 30°C (59° to 86°F). Protect from light. Dispense in a tight, light-resistant container using a child-resistant closure.

PROPRANOLOL HYDROCHLORIDE

Rx	**Propranolol HCl** (Various, eg, Mylan, Schein, Watson)	**Tablets:** 10 mg	In 100s, 500s, 1000s, 5000s, and UD 100s.
Rx	**Inderal** (Wyeth-Ayerst)		(I INDERAL 10). Orange, scored, hexagonal. In 100s, 1000s, 5000s, and UD 100s.
Rx	**Propranolol HCl** (Various, eg, Mylan, Schein, Watson)	**Tablets:** 20 mg	In 100s, 500s, 1000s, 5000s, and UD 100s.
Rx	**Inderal** (Wyeth-Ayerst)		(I INDERAL 20). Blue, scored, hexagonal. In 100s, 1000s, 5000s, and UD 100s.
Rx	**Propranolol HCl** (Various, eg, Mylan, Schein, Watson)	**Tablets:** 40 mg	In 100s, 500s, 1000s, 5000s, and UD 100s.
Rx	**Inderal** (Wyeth-Ayerst)		(I INDERAL 40). Green, scored, hexagonal. In 100s, 1000s, 5000s, and UD 100s.
Rx	**Propranolol HCl** (Various, eg, Mylan, Watson)	**Tablets:** 60 mg	In 100s, 500s, and UD 100s.
Rx	**Inderal** (Wyeth-Ayerst)		(I INDERAL 60). Pink, scored, hexagonal. In 100s and 1000s.
Rx	**Propranolol HCl** (Various, eg, Mylan, Schein)	**Tablets:** 80 mg	In 100s, 500s, 1000s, and UD 100s.
Rx	**Inderal** (Wyeth-Ayerst)		(I INDERAL 80). Yellow, scored, hexagonal. In 100s, 1000s, and 5000s.
Rx	**Propranolol HCl** (Various, eg, Qualitest, Watson)	**Tablets:** 90 mg	In 100s and 500s.
Rx	**Propranolol HCl** (Various, eg, ESI Lederle)	**Capsules, extended-release:** 60 mg	In 100s and 1000s.
Rx	**Inderal LA** (Wyeth-Ayerst)		(INDERAL LA 60). White/light blue. In 100s and 1000s.
Rx	**Propranolol HCl** (Various, eg, ESI Lederle)	**Capsules, extended-release:** 80 mg	In 100s and 1000s.
Rx	**Inderal LA** (Wyeth-Ayerst)		(INDERAL LA 80). Light blue. In 100s, 1000s, and UD 100s.
Rx	**InnoPran XL** (Reliant)		Sugar spheres. (80 RD201). Gray/White. In 30s, 100s, 500s, and UD 100s.
Rx	**Propranolol HCl** (Various, eg, ESI Lederle)	**Capsules, extended-release:** 120 mg	In 100s and 1000s.
Rx	**Inderal LA** (Wyeth-Ayerst)		(INDERAL LA 120). Light blue/Dark blue. In 100s, 1000s, and UD 100s.
Rx	**InnoPran XL** (Reliant)		Sugar spheres. (120 RD201). Gray/off-white. In 30s, 100s, 500s, and UD 100s.
Rx	**Propranolol HCl** (Various, eg, ESI Lederle)	**Capsules, extended-release:** 160 mg	In 100s.
Rx	**Inderal LA** (Wyeth-Ayerst)		(INDERAL LA 160). Dark blue. In 100s, 1000s, and UD 100s.
Rx sf	**Propranolol HCl** (Roxane)	**Solution, oral:** 4 mg/mL	Parabens, saccharin, sorbitol. Dye free. Strawberry-mint flavor. In 500 mL and UD 5 mL patient cups (40s).
		8 mg/mL	Parabens, saccharin, sorbitol. Dye free. Strawberry-mint flavor. In 500 mL.

PROPRANOLOL HYDROCHLORIDE

Rx sf	**Propranolol Intensol** (Roxane)	**Oral solution, concentrated:** 80 mg/mL	Alcohol and dye free. In 30 mL with dropper.
Rx	**Propranolol HCl** (Various, eg, Bedford)	**Injection:** 1 mg/mL	In 1 mL vials.
Rx	**Inderal** (Wyeth-Ayerst)		In 1 mL amps.

PROPRANOLOL HYDROCHLORIDE — ORAL

WARNING

Angina pectoris – There have been reports of exacerbation of angina and, in some cases, myocardial infarction, following abrupt discontinuance of propranolol therapy. Therefore, when discontinuance of propranolol is planned, the dosage should be gradually reduced over at least a few weeks, and the patient should be cautioned against interruption or cessation of therapy without a physician's advice. If propranolol therapy is interrupted and exacerbation of angina occurs, it is usually advisable to reinstitute propranolol therapy and take other measures appropriate for the management of angina pectoris. Because coronary artery disease may be unrecognized, it may be prudent to follow the above advice in patients considered at risk of having occult atherosclerotic heart disease who are given propranolol for other indications.

Indications

➤*Immediate-release tablets, oral solution, and sustained-release capsules:*

Hypertension – Management of hypertension. It may be used alone or used in combination with other antihypertensive agents, particularly a thiazide diuretic. Propranolol is not indicated in the management of hypertensive emergencies.

Angina pectoris due to coronary atherosclerosis – Long-term management of patients with angina pectoris.

Migraine – Prophylaxis of common migraine headache. The efficacy of propranolol in the treatment of a migraine attack that has started has not been established and propranolol is not indicated for such use.

Hypertrophic subaortic stenosis – Management of hypertrophic subaortic stenosis, especially for treatment of exertional or other stress-induced angina, palpitations, and syncope. Propranolol also improves exercise performance. The effectiveness of propranolol in this disease appears to be due to a reduction of the elevated outflow pressure gradient which is exacerbated by beta-receptor stimulation. Clinical improvement may be temporary.

➤*Immediate-release tablets and oral solution:*

Cardiac arrhythmias –

Supraventricular arrhythmias: Paroxysmal atrial tachycardias, particularly those arrhythmias induced by catecholamines or digitalis or associated with the Wolff-Parkinson-White syndrome. Beta-adrenergic blockade in patients with Wolff-Parkinson-White syndrome and tachycardia has been associated with severe bradycardia requiring treatment with a pacemaker. In 1 case, this resulted after an initial dose of 5 mg propranolol.

Persistent sinus tachycardia which is non-compensatory and impairs the well-being of the patient.

Tachycardias and arrhythmias due to thyrotoxicosis when causing distress or increased hazard and when immediate effect is necessary as adjunctive, short-term (2 to 4 weeks) therapy. May be used with, but not in place of, specific therapy.

Persistent atrial extrasystoles which impair the well-being of the patient and do not respond to conventional measures.

Atrial flutter and fibrillation when ventricular rate cannot be controlled by digitalis alone, or when digitalis is contraindicated.

Ventricular tachycardias: Ventricular arrhythmias do not respond to propranolol as predictably as do the supraventricular arrhythmias, but propranolol may be useful for persistent premature ventricular extrasystoles which do not respond to conventional measures and impair the well-being of the patient.

Tachyarrhythmias of digitalis intoxication: If digitalis-induced tachyarrhythmias persist following discontinuance of digitalis and correction of electrolyte abnormalities, they are usually reversible with oral propranolol. Severe bradycardia may occur. Intravenous propranolol is reserved for life-threatening arrhythmias. Temporary maintenance with oral therapy may be indicated.

Resistant tachyarrhythmias due to excessive catecholamine action during anesthesia: Tachyarrhythmias due to excessive catecholamine action during anesthesia may sometimes arise because of release of endogenous catecholamines or administration of catecholamines. When usual measures fail in such arrythmias, propranolol may be given intravenously to abolish them. All general inhalation anesthetics produce some degree of myocardial depression. Therefore, when propranolol HCl is used to treat arrhythmias during anesthesia, it should be used with extreme caution and constant ECG and central venous pressure monitoring.

Myocardial infarction – Propranolol is indicated to reduce cardiovascular mortality in patients who have survived the acute phase of myocardial infarction and are clinically stable.

Essential tremor – Propranolol is indicated in the management of familial or hereditary essential tremor. Familial or essential tremor consists of involuntary, rhythmic, oscillatory movements, usually limited to the upper limbs. It is absent at rest but occurs when the limb is held in a fixed posture or position against gravity and during active movement. Propranolol causes a reduction in the tremor amplitude but not in the tremor frequency. Propranolol is not indicated for the treatment of tremor associated with parkinsonism.

Pheochromocytoma – After primary treatment with an alpha-adrenergic blocking agent has been instituted, propranolol HCl may be useful as adjunctive therapy if the control of tachycardia becomes necessary before or during surgery. It is hazardous to use propranolol HCl unless alpha-adrenergic blocking drugs are already in use, since this would predispose patients to serious blood pressure elevation. Blocking only the peripheral dilator (beta) action of epinephrine leaves its constrictor (alpha) action unopposed. In the event of hemorrhage or shock, there is a disadvantage in having both beta and alpha blockade since the combination prevents the increase in heart rate and peripheral vasoconstriction needed to maintain blood pressure.

With inoperable or metastatic pheochromocytoma, propranolol HCl may be useful as an adjunct to the management of symptoms due to excessive beta-receptor stimulation.

➤*Extended-release capsules:*

Hypertension – Propranolol extended-release is indicated in the management of hypertension; it may be used alone or in combination with other antihypertensive agents.

Administration and Dosage

➤*Approved by the FDA:* November 1967.

The dosage range for propranolol is different for each indication, and varies between formulations.

➤*Immediate-release tablets and oral solution:*

Hypertension – Dosage must be individualized.

The usual initial dosage is 40 mg propranolol HCl twice daily, whether used alone or added to a diuretic. Dosage may be increased gradually until adequate blood pressure control is achieved. The usual maintenance dosage is 120 to 240 mg per day. In some instances a dosage of 640 mg may be required. The time needed for full hypertensive response to a given dosage is variable and may range from a few days to several weeks.

While twice-daily dosing is effective and can maintain a reduction in blood pressure throughout the day, some patients, especially when lower doses are used, may experience a modest rise in blood pressure toward the end of the 12-hour dosing interval. This can be evaluated by measuring blood pressure near the end of the dosing interval to determine whether satisfactory control is being maintained throughout the day. If control is not adequate, a larger dose, or 3-times-daily may achieve better control.

Angina pectoris – Dosage must be individualized.

Total daily doses of 80 to 320 mg when administered orally, twice a day, 3 times a day or 4 times a day, have been shown to increase exercise tolerance to reduce ischemic change in the ECG. If treatment is to be discontinued, reduce dosage gradually over a period of several weeks.

Arrhythmias – 10 to 30 mg 3 or 4 times daily before meals and at bedtime.

Myocardial infarction – The recommended daily dosage is 180 mg to 240 mg per day in divided doses. Although a 3-times-daily regimen was used in the Beta Blocker Heart Attack Trial and a 4-times-daily regimen in the Norwegian Multicenter Trial, there is a reasonable basis for the use of either a 3-times-daily or a twice-daily regimen. The effectiveness and safety of daily dosages greater than 240 mg for prevention of cardiac mortality have not been established. However, higher dosages may be needed to effectively treat coexisting diseases such as angina or hypertension (see above).

Migraine – Dosage must be individualized.

The initial oral dose is 80 mg propranolol HCl daily in divided doses. The usual effective dose range is 160 to 240 mg per day. The dosage may be increased gradually to achieve optimal migraine prophylaxis. If a satisfactory response is not obtained within 4 to 6 weeks after reaching the maximum dose, propranolol therapy should be discontinued. It may be advisable to withdraw the drug gradually over a period of several weeks.

Essential tremor – Dosage must be individualized.

The initial dosage is 40 mg propranolol HCl twice daily. Optimum reduction of essential tremor is usually achieved with a dose of 120 mg per day. Occasionally, it may be necessary to administer 240 to 320 mg per day.

Hypertrophic subaortic stenosis – 20 to 40 mg 3 or 4 times daily before meals and at bedtime.

Pheochromocytoma –

Preoperatively: 60 mg daily in divided doses for 3 days prior to surgery, concomitantly with an alpha-adrenergic blocking agent.

Management of inoperable tumor: 30 mg daily in divided doses.

Use in pediatric patients – Oral dosage for treating hypertension requires individual titration beginning with a 1 mg/kg (body weight) per day dosage regimen (ie, 0.5 mg/kg twice daily).

PROPRANOLOL HYDROCHLORIDE — ORAL

The usual pediatric dosage range is 2 to 4 mg/kg/day in 2 equally divided doses (ie, 1 mg/kg twice daily to 2 mg/kg twice daily). Pediatric dosage calculated by weight (recommended) generally produces propranolol plasma levels in a therapeutic range similar to that in adults. On the other hand, pediatric doses calculated on the basis of body surface area (not recommended) usually result in plasma levels above the mean adult therapeutic range. Doses above 16 mg/kg/day should not be used in pediatric patients. If treatment with propranolol is to be discontinued, a gradually decreasing dose titration over a 7- to 14-day period is necessary.

➤*Concentrated oral solution:*

Proper use of concentrated oral solution, 80 mg – Propranolol concentrated oral solution, 80 mg is a concentrated oral solution as compared to standard oral liquid medications. It is recommended that the propranolol HCl concentrated oral solution be mixed with liquid or semi-solid food such as water, juices, soda or soda-like beverages, applesauce, and puddings.

Use only the calibrated dropper provided with this product. Draw into the dropper the amount prescribed for a single dose. Then squeeze the dropper contents into a liquid or semi-solid food. Stir the liquid or food gently for a few seconds. The propranolol formulation blends quickly and completely. The entire amount of the mixture, of drug and liquid or drug and food, should be consumed immediately. Do not store for future use.

➤*Sustained-release capsules:* Propranolol sustained-release capsules provide propranolol HCl in a sustained-release capsule for administration once daily. If patients are switched from propranolol HCl tablets to propranolol sustained-release capsules, care should be taken to ensure that the desired therapeutic effect is maintained. Propranolol sustained-release capsules should not be considered a simple mg-for-mg substitute for propranolol tablets. Propranolol sustained-release capsules have different kinetics and produce lower blood levels. Retitration may be necessary, especially to maintain effectiveness at the end of the 24-hour dosing interval.

Hypertension – Dosage must be individualized. The usual initial dosage is 80 mg once daily, whether used alone or added to a diuretic. The dosage may be increased to 120 mg once daily or higher until adequate blood pressure control is achieved. The usual maintenance dosage is 120 to 160 mg once daily. In some instances, a dosage of 640 mg may be required. The time needed for full hypertensive response to a given dosage is variable and may range from a few days to several weeks.

Angina pectoris – Dosage must be individualized. Starting with 80 mg once daily, dosage should be gradually increased at 3- to 7-day intervals until optimal response is obtained. Although individual patients may respond at any dosage level, the average optimal dosage appears to be 160 mg once daily. In angina pectoris, the value and safety of dosage exceeding 320 mg per day have not been established.

If treatment is to be discontinued, reduce dosage gradually over a period of a few weeks.

Migraine – Dosage must be individualized. The initial oral dose is 80 mg once daily. The usual effective dose range is 160 to 240 mg once daily. The dosage may be increased gradually to achieve optimal migraine prophylaxis. If a satisfactory response is not obtained within 4 to 6 weeks after reaching the maximal dose, therapy should be discontinued. It may be advisable to withdraw the drug gradually over a period of several weeks.

Hypertrophic subaortic stenosis – 80 to 160 mg once daily.

Pediatric dose – At this time the data on the use of the drug in this age group are too limited to permit adequate directions for use.

➤*Extended-release capsules:* Propranolol HCl extended release should be administered once daily at bedtime (approximately 10 pm) and should be taken consistently either on an empty stomach or with food. The starting dose is 80 mg but dosage should be individualized and titration may be needed to a dose of 120 mg. In the clinical trial, doses of propranolol HCl extended-release above 120 mg had no additional effects on blood pressure. The time needed for full antihypertensive response is variable, but is usually achieved within 2 to 3 weeks.

➤*Storage / Stability:*

Immediate-release tablets – Store at controlled room temperature, 20° to 25°C (68° to 77°F). Dispense in a well-closed, light-resistant container with a child-resistant closure.

Oral solution – Store at controlled room temperature, 15° to 30°C (59° to 86°F).

Sustained-release capsules – Store at room temperature (20° to 25°C; 68° to 77°F).

Protect from light, moisture, freezing, and excessive heat.

Dispense in a tight, light-resistant container.

Use carton to protect contents from light.

Extended-release capsules – Store at 25°C (77°F); excursions permitted to 15° to 30°C (59° to 86°F) in a tightly closed container. The unit dose packaging should be stored in the carton.

PROPRANOLOL HYDROCHLORIDE — INJECTION

For complete and comparative prescribing information, refer to the Beta-Adrenergic Blocking Agents group monograph.

WARNING

Angina pectoris – There have been reports of exacerbation of angina and, in some cases, myocardial infarction, following abrupt discontinuance of propranolol therapy. Therefore, when discontinuance of propranolol is planned, gradually reduce the dosage over at least a few weeks, and caution the patient against interruption or cessation of therapy without a physician's advice. If propranolol therapy is interrupted and exacerbation of angina occurs, it is usually advisable to reinstitute propranolol therapy and take other measures appropriate for the management of angina pectoris. Because coronary artery disease may be unrecognized, it may be prudent to follow the above advice in patients considered at risk of having occult atherosclerotic heart disease who are given propranolol for other indications.

Indications

➤*Cardiac arrhythmias:* Supraventricular, ventricular, tachyarrhythmias of digitalis intoxication, and resistant tachyarrhythmias caused by excessive catecholamine action during anesthesia.

➤*MI:* For treatment of MI.

➤*Hypertrophic subaortic stenosis:* Especially for treatment of exertional or other stress-induced angina, palpitations, and syncope.

➤*Pheochromocytoma:* As adjunctive therapy following primary treatment with an alpha-adrenergic blocker.

➤*Hypertension:* Used alone or in combination with other antihypertensive agents.

➤*Migraine prophylaxis:* For prophylaxis of migraines.

➤*Angina pectoris:* When caused by coronary atherosclerosis.

➤*Essential tremor:* Familial or hereditary.

Administration and Dosage

➤*Approved by the FDA:* November 1967.

Reserve IV use for life-threatening arrhythmias or those occurring under anesthesia.

➤*Usual dose:* 1 to 3 mg under careful monitoring (eg, central venous pressure, ECG). Do not exceed 1 mg/min to avoid lowering blood pressure and causing cardiac standstill. Allow sufficient time for the drug to reach site of action, particularly when slow circulation is present. If necessary, give a second dose after 2 minutes. Thereafter, do not give additional drug in < 4 hours. Do not give additional propranolol after the desired alteration in rate and/or rhythm is achieved. Transfer to oral therapy as soon as possible. IV use has not been evaluated adequately in managing hypertensive emergencies.

➤*Pediatrics:* IV use is not recommended; however, an unlabeled dose of 0.01 to 0.1 mg/kg/dose to a maximum of 1 mg/dose by slow infusion over 5 minutes has been used for arrhythmias.

➤*Storage / Stability:* Store at controlled room temperature, 20° to 25°C (68° to 77°F). Protect from freezing and excessive heat.

LABETALOL HYDROCHLORIDE

Rx	**Labetalol hydrochloride** (Various, eg, Apothecon, Eon, Ivax, Mutual, UDL, URL, Watson)	**Tablets:** 100 mg	In 30s, 100s, 250s, 500s, and 1000s.
Rx	**Trandate** (Faro Pharmaceuticals, Inc.)		(Trandate 100). Lt. orange, scored. Film-coated. In 100s, 500s, and UD 100s.
Rx	**Labetalol HCl** (Various, eg, Apothecon, Eon, Ivax, Mutual, UDL, URL, Watson)	**Tablets:** 200 mg	In 30s, 100s, 250s, 500s, and 1000s.
Rx	**Trandate** (Faro Pharmaceuticals, Inc.)		(Trandate 200). White, scored. Film-coated. In 100s, 500s, and UD 100s.
Rx	**Labetalol HCl** (Various, eg, Apothecon, Eon, Ivax, Mutual, Teva, URL, Watson)	**Tablets:** 300 mg	In 30s, 100s, 250s, 500s, and 1000s.
Rx	**Trandate** (Faro Pharmaceuticals, Inc.)		(Trandate 300). Peach, scored. Film-coated. In 100s, 500s, and UD 100s.

Alpha/Beta-Adrenergic Blocking Agents

LABETALOL HYDROCHLORIDE

Rx	**Labetalol HCl** (Various, eg, Apothecon, Bedford Labs)	**Injection:** 5 mg/mL[1]	Dextrose, EDTA, parabens. In 20 and 40 mL multidose vials.
Rx	**Normodyne** (Key)		Dextrose, EDTA, parabens. In 20 mL multidose vials and 4 and 8 mL prefilled syringes.
Rx	**Trandate** (Faro Pharmaceuticals, Inc.)		In 20 and 40 mL multidose vials.

[1] With 0.1 mg EDTA and 0.8 mg methylparaben and 0.1 mg propylparaben.

LABETALOL HYDROCHLORIDE — ORAL

Indications

➤*Hypertension:* Management of hypertension. Labetalol tablets may be used alone or in combination with other antihypertensive agents, especially thiazide and loop diuretics.

➤*Unlabeled uses:* Labetalol has effectively lowered blood pressure and relieved symptoms in patients with pheochromocytoma; higher IV doses may be required. However, paradoxical hypertensive responses have occurred; therefore, use caution when administering labetalol. Labetalol has been used to treat clonidine withdrawal hypertension.

Administration and Dosage

Dosage must be individualized. The recommended initial dosage is 100 mg twice daily whether used alone or added to a diuretic regimen. After 2 or 3 days, using standing blood pressure as an indicator, dosage may be titrated in increments of 100 mg twice a day every 2 or 3 days. The usual maintenance dosage of labetalol is between 200 and 400 mg twice daily.

Because the full antihypertensive effect of labetalol is usually seen within the first 1 to 3 hours of the initial dose or dose increment, the assurance of a lack of an exaggerated hypotensive response can be clinically established in the office setting. The antihypertensive effects of continued dosing can be measured at subsequent visits, approximately 12 hours after a dose, to determine whether further titration is necessary.

Patients with severe hypertension may require from 1,200 to 2,400 mg/day, with or without thiazide diuretics. If side effects (principally nausea or dizziness) occur with these doses administered twice daily, the same total daily dose administered 3 times daily may improve tolerability and facilitate further titration. Titration increments should not exceed 200 mg twice daily.

When a diuretic is added, an additive antihypertensive effect can be expected. In some cases this may necessitate a labetalol dosage adjustment. As with most antihypertensive drugs, optimal dosages of labetalol tablets are usually lower in patients also receiving a diuretic.

When transferring patients from other antihypertensive drugs, labetalol tablets should be introduced as recommended and the dosage of the existing therapy progressively decreased.

➤*Elderly patients:* As in the general patient population, labetalol therapy may be initiated at 100 mg twice daily and titrated upwards in increments of 100 mg twice a day as required for control of blood pressure. Since some elderly patients eliminate labetalol more slowly, however, adequate control of blood pressure may be achieved at a lower maintenance dosage compared to the general population. The majority of elderly patients will require between 100 and 200 mg twice a day.

➤*Storage/Stability:* Labetalol tablets should be stored between 2° and 30°C (36° and 86°F). Labetalol tablets in the unit dose boxes should be protected from excessive moisture.

Actions

➤*Pharmacology:* Labetalol combines both selective, competitive, alpha-1-adrenergic blocking and nonselective, competitive, beta-adrenergic blocking activity in a single substance. In man, the ratios of alpha- to beta-blockade have been estimated to be approximately 1:3 and 1:7 following oral and IV administration, respectively. Beta-2-agonist activity has been demonstrated in animals with minimal beta-1-agonist (ISA) activity detected. In animals, at doses greater than those required for alpha- or beta-adrenergic blockage, a membrane-stabilizing effect has been demonstrated.

➤*Pharmacokinetics:*

Absorption – Labetalol is completely absorbed from the GI tract with peak plasma levels occurring 1 to 2 hours after oral administration. The relative bioavailability of labetalol tablets compared to an oral solution is 100%. The absolute bioavailability (fraction of drug reaching systemic circulation) of labetalol when compared to an IV infusion is 25%; this is due to extensive "first-pass" metabolism. Despite "first-pass" metabolism, there is a linear relationship between oral doses of 100 to 3000 mg and peak plasma levels. The absolute bioavailability of labetalol is increased when administered with food.

The plasma half-life of labetalol following oral administration is about 6 to 8 hours. Steady-state plasma levels of labetalol during repetitive dosing are reached by about the third day of dosing. In patients with decreased hepatic or renal function, the elimination half-life of labetalol is not altered; however, the relative bioavailability in hepatically impaired patients is increased due to decreased "first-pass" metabolism.

Metabolism/Excretion – The metabolism of labetalol is mainly through conjugation to glucuronide metabolites. These metabolites are present in plasma and are excreted in the urine and, via the bile, into the feces. Approximately 55% to 60% of a dose appears in the urine as conjugates or unchanged labetalol within the first 24 hours of dosing.

Labetalol has been shown to cross the placental barrier in humans. Only negligible amounts of the drug crossed the blood-brain barrier in animal studies. Labetalol is approximately 50% protein bound. Neither hemodialysis nor peritoneal dialysis removes a significant amount of labetalol from the general circulation (less than 1%).

Elderly patients: Some pharmacokinetic studies indicate that the elimination of labetalol is reduced in elderly patients. Therefore, although elderly patients may initiate therapy at the currently recommended dosage of 100 mg twice a day, elderly patients will generally require lower maintenance dosages than nonelderly patients.

Contraindications

Bronchial asthma, overt cardiac failure, greater-than-first-degree heart block, cardiogenic shock, severe bradycardia, other conditions associated with severe and prolonged hypotension, and hypersensitivity to any component of the product.

Beta-blockers, even those with apparent cardioselectivity, should not be used in patients with a history of obstructive airway disease, including asthma.

Warnings

➤*Hepatic injury:* Severe hepatocellular injury, confirmed by rechallenge in at least 1 case, occurs rarely with labetalol therapy. The hepatic injury is usually reversible, but hepatic necrosis and death have been reported. Injury has occurred after both short- and long-term treatment and may be slowly progressive despite minimal symptomatology. Similar hepatic events have been reported with a related research compound, dilevalol, including 2 deaths. Dilevalol is 1 of the 4 isomers of labetalol. Thus, for patients taking labetalol, periodic determination of suitable hepatic laboratory tests would be appropriate. Appropriate laboratory testing should be done at the first symptom/sign of liver dysfunction (eg, pruritus, dark urine, persistent anorexia, jaundice, right upper quadrant tenderness, or unexplained "flu-like" symptoms). If the patient has laboratory evidence of liver injury or jaundice, labetalol should be stopped and not restarted.

➤*Cardiac failure:* Sympathetic stimulation is a vital component supporting circulatory function in congestive heart failure. Beta blockade carries a potential hazard of further depressing myocardial contractility and precipitating more severe failure. Although beta-blockers should be avoided in overt congestive heart failure, if necessary, labetalol can be used with caution in patients with a history of heart failure who are well compensated. Congestive heart failure has been observed in patients receiving labetalol. Labetalol HCl does not abolish the inotropic action of digitalis on heart muscle.

➤*In patients without a history of cardiac failure:* In patients with latent cardiac insufficiency, continued depression of the myocardium with beta-blocking agents over a period of time can, in some cases, lead to cardiac failure. At the first sign or symptom of impending cardiac failure, patients should be fully digitalized or be given a diuretic, and the response should be observed closely. If cardiac failure continues despite adequate digitalization and diuretic, therapy with labetalol tablets should be withdrawn (gradually, if possible).

➤*Exacerbation of ischemic heart disease following abrupt withdrawal:* Angina pectoris has not been reported upon labetalol discontinuation. However, hypersensitivity to catecholamines has been observed in patients withdrawn from beta blocker therapy; exacerbation of angina and, in some cases, myocardial infarction have occurred after abrupt discontinuation of such therapy. When discontinuing chronically administered labetalol tablets, particularly in patients with ischemic heart disease, the dosage should be gradually reduced over a period of 1 to 2 weeks and the patient should be carefully monitored. If angina markedly worsens or acute coronary insufficiency develops, therapy with labetalol tablets should be reinstituted promptly, at least temporarily, and other measures appropriate for the management of unstable angina should be taken. Patients should be warned against interruption or discontinuation of therapy without the physician's advice. Because coronary artery disease is common and may be unrecognized, it may be prudent not to discontinue therapy with labetalol tablets abruptly in patients being treated for hypertension.

➤*Nonallergic bronchospasm (eg, chronic bronchitis and emphysema):* Patients with bronchospastic disease should, in general, not receive beta blockers. Labetalol tablets may be used with caution, however, in patients who do not respond to, or cannot tolerate, other antihypertensive agents. It is prudent, if labetalol tablets are used, to use the smallest effective dose, so that inhibition of endogenous or exogenous beta agonists is minimized.

➤*Pheochromocytoma:* Labetalol has been shown to be effective in lowering blood pressure and relieving symptoms in patients with pheochromocytoma. However, paradoxical hypertensive responses have been reported in a few patients with this tumor; therefore, use caution when administering labetalol to patients with pheochromocytoma.

➤*Diabetes mellitus and hypoglycemia:* Beta-adrenergic blockade may prevent the appearance of premonitory signs and symptoms (eg, tachycardia) of acute hypoglycemia. This is especially important with labile diabet-

LABETALOL HYDROCHLORIDE — ORAL

ics. Beta-blockade also reduces the release of insulin in response to hyperglycemia; it may therefore be necessary to adjust the dose of antidiabetic drugs.

➤*Major surgery:* The necessity or desirability of withdrawing beta-blocking therapy before major surgery is controversial. Protracted severe hypotension and difficulty in restarting or maintaining a heartbeat have been reported with beta blockers. The effect of labetalol's alpha-adrenergic activity has not been evaluated in this setting.

➤*Hepatic function impairment:* Labetalol tablets should be used with caution in patients with impaired hepatic function since metabolism of the drug may be diminished.

➤*Elderly:* As in the general population, some elderly patients (60 years of age and older) have experienced orthostatic hypotension, dizziness, or lightheadedness during treatment with labetalol. Because elderly patients are generally more likely than younger patients to experience orthostatic symptoms, they should be cautioned about the possibility of such side effects during treatment with labetalol.

➤*Pregnancy: Category C.*

Teratogenic – Teratogenic studies were performed with labetalol in rats and rabbits at oral doses up to approximately 6 and 4 times the maximum recommended human dose (MRHD), respectively. No reproducible evidence of fetal malformations was observed. Increased fetal resorptions were seen in both species at doses approximating the MRHD. A teratology study performed with labetalol in rabbits at IV doses up to 1.7 times the MRHD revealed no evidence of drug-related harm to the fetus. There are no adequate and well-controlled studies in pregnant women. Labetalol should be used during pregnancy only if the potential benefit justifies the potential risk to the fetus.

Nonteratogenic – Hypotension, bradycardia, hypoglycemia, and respiratory depression have been reported in infants of mothers who were treated with labetalol for hypertension during pregnancy. Oral administration of labetalol to rats during late gestation through weaning at doses of 2 to 4 times the MRHD caused a decrease in neonatal survival.

Labor and delivery – Labetalol given to pregnant women with hypertension did not appear to affect the usual course of labor and delivery.

➤*Lactation:* Small amounts of labetalol (approximately 0.004% of the maternal dose) are excreted in human milk. Caution should be exercised when labetalol tablets are administered to a breast-feeding woman.

➤*Children:* Safety and efficacy in children have not been established.

Precautions

➤*Monitoring:* As with any new drug given over prolonged periods, laboratory parameters should be observed over regular intervals. In patients with concomitant illnesses, such as impaired renal function, appropriate tests should be done to monitor these conditions.

Drug Interactions

➤*Tricyclic antidepressants:* In 1 survey, 2.3% of patients taking labetalol in combination with tricyclic antidepressants experienced tremor, as compared to 0.7% reported to occur with labetalol alone. The contribution of each of the treatments to this adverse reaction is unknown, but the possibility of a drug interaction cannot be excluded.

➤*Beta-agonists:* Drugs possessing beta-blocking properties can blunt the bronchodilator effect of beta-receptor agonist drugs in patients with bronchospasm; therefore, doses greater than the normal antiasthmatic dose of beta agonist bronchodilator drugs may be required.

➤*Cimetidine:* Cimetidine has been shown to increase the bioavailability of labetalol. Since this could be explained either by enhanced absorption or by an alteration of hepatic metabolism of labetalol, special care should be used in establishing the dose required for blood pressure control in such patients.

➤*Halothane:* Synergism has been shown between halothane anesthesia and intravenously administered labetalol. During controlled hypotensive anesthesia using labetalol in association with halothane, high concentrations (3% or above) of halothane should not be used because the degree of hypotension will be increased and because of the possibility of a large reduction in cardiac output and an increase in central venous pressure. The anesthesiologist should be informed when a patient is receiving labetalol.

➤*Nitroglycerin:* Labetalol blunts the reflex tachycardia produced by nitroglycerin without preventing its hypotensive effect. If labetalol is used with nitroglycerin in patients with angina pectoris, additional antihypertensive effects may occur.

➤*Calcium channel blockers:* Care should be taken if labetalol is used concomitantly with calcium antagonists of the verapamil type.

➤*Risk of anaphylactic reaction:* While taking beta-blockers, patients with a history of severe anaphylactic reaction to a variety of allergens may be more reactive to repeated challenge, either accidental, diagnostic, or therapeutic. Such patients may be unresponsive to the usual doses of epinephrine used to treat allergic reaction.

➤*Drug/Lab test interactions:* The presence of labetalol metabolites in the urine may result in falsely elevated levels of urinary catecholamines, metanephrine, normetanephrine, and vanillylmandelic acid when measured by fluorimetric or photometric methods. In screening patients suspected of having a pheochromocytoma and being treated with labetalol, a specific method, such as a high performance liquid chromatographic assay with solid phase extraction (eg, *J Chromatogr* 385:241,1987) should be employed in determining levels of catecholamines.

Labetalol has also been reported to produce a false-positive test for amphetamine when screening urine for the presence of drugs using the commercially available assay methods *Toxi-Lab A* (thin-layer chromatographic assay) and *Emit-d.a.u.* (radioenzymatic assay). When patients being treated with labetalol have a positive urine test for amphetamine using these techniques, confirmation should be made by using more specific methods, such as a gas chromatographic mass spectrometer technique.

Adverse Reactions

Most adverse effects are mild and transient and occur early in the course of treatment. In controlled clinical trials of 3 to 4 months' duration, discontinuation of labetalol tablets due to 1 or more adverse effects was required in 7% of all patients. In these same trials, other agents with solely beta-blocking activity used in the control groups led to discontinuation in 8% to 10% of patients, and a centrally acting alpha agonist led to discontinuation in 30% of patients.

The incidence rates of adverse reactions listed in the following table were derived from multicenter, controlled clinical trials comparing labetalol, placebo, metoprolol, and propranolol over treatment periods of 3 and 4 months. Where the frequency of adverse effects for labetalol and placebo is similar, causal relationship is uncertain. The rates are based on adverse reactions considered probably drug related by the investigator. If all reports are considered, the rates are somewhat higher (eg, dizziness, 20%; nausea, 14%; fatigue, 11%), but the overall conclusions are unchanged.

Adverse reaction	Labetalol (n = 227) %	Placebo (n = 98) %	Propranolol (n = 84) %	Metoprolol (n = 49) %
Autonomic nervous system				
Nasal stuffiness	3%	0%	0%	0%
Ejaculation failure	2%	0%	0%	0%
Impotence	1%	0%	1%	3%
Increased sweating	< 1%	0%	0%	0%
Cardiovascular				
Edema	1%	0%	0%	0%
Postural hypotension	1%	0%	0%	0%
Bradycardia	0%	0%	5%	12%
CNS				
Dizziness	11%	3%	4%	4%
Paresthesia	< 1%	0%	0%	0%
Drowsiness	< 1%	2%	2%	2%
Dermatologic				
Rash	1%	0%	0%	0%
Gastrointestinal				
Nausea	6%	1%	1%	2%
Vomiting	< 1%	0%	0%	0%
Dyspepsia	3%	1%	1%	0%
Abdominal pain	0%	0%	1%	2%
Diarrhea	< 1%	0%	2%	0%
Taste distortion	1%	0%	0%	0%
Respiratory				
Dyspnea	2%	0%	1%	2%
Special senses				
Vertigo	2%	1%	0%	0%
Vision abnormality	1%	0%	0%	0%
Miscellaneous				
Fatigue	5%	0%	12%	12%
Asthenia	1%	1%	1%	0%
Headache	2%	1%	1%	2%

The adverse effects were reported spontaneously and are representative of the incidence of adverse effects that may be observed in a properly selected hypertensive patient population, ie, a group excluding patients with bronchospastic disease, overt congestive heart failure, or other contraindications to beta blocker therapy.

Clinical trials also included studies utilizing daily doses up to 2400 mg in more severely hypertensive patients. Certain of the side effects increased with increasing dose, as shown in the following table that depicts the entire US therapeutic trials data base for adverse reactions that are clearly or possibly dose related.

LABETALOL HYDROCHLORIDE — ORAL

Labetalol Adverse Reaction According to Dose									
Daily dose (mg)	200	300	400	600	800	900	1,200	1,600	2,400
Number of patients	522	181	606	608	503	117	411	242	175
Dizziness (%)	2%	3%	3%	3%	5%	1%	9%	13%	16%
Fatigue	2%	1%	4%	4%	5%	3%	7%	6%	10%
Nausea	< 1%	0%	1%	2%	4%	0%	7%	11%	19%
Vomiting	0%	0%	< 1%	< 1%	< 1%	0%	1%	2%	3%
Dyspepsia	1%	0%	2%	1%	1%	0%	2%	2%	4%
Paresthesia	2%	0%	2%	2%	1%	1%	2%	5%	5%
Nasal stuffiness	1%	1%	2%	2%	2%	2%	4%	5%	6%
Ejaculation failure	0%	2%	1%	2%	3%	0%	4%	3%	5%
Impotence	1%	1%	1%	1%	2%	4%	3%	4%	3%
Edema	1%	0%	1%	1%	1%	0%	1%	2%	2%

In addition, a number of other less common adverse events have been reported.

➤*Cardiovascular:* Hypotension, and rarely, syncope, bradycardia, heart block.

➤*CNS:* Paresthesia, most frequently described as scalp tingling. In most cases, it was mild and transient and usually occurred at the beginning of treatment.

➤*Dermatologic:* Rashes of various types, such as generalized maculopapular, lichenoid, urticarial, bullous lichen planus, psoriaform, and facial erythema; Peyronie's disease; reversible alopecia.

➤*GU:* Difficulty in micturition, including acute urinary bladder retention.

➤*Hepatic:* Hepatic necrosis, hepatitis, cholestatic jaundice, elevated liver function tests.

➤*Hypersensitivity:* Rare reports of hypersensitivity (eg, rash, urticaria, pruritus, angioedema, dyspnea) and anaphylactoid reactions.

➤*Immunologic:* Antimitochondrial antibodies.

➤*Musculoskeletal:* Muscle cramps, toxic myopathy.

➤*Ophthalmic:* Dry eyes.

➤*Respiratory:* Bronchospasm.

➤*Miscellaneous:* Fever. Systemic lupus erythematosus, positive antinuclear factor.

➤*Lab test abnormalities:* There have been reversible increases of serum transaminases in 4% of patients treated with labetalol and tested and, more rarely, reversible increases in blood urea.

Overdosage

➤*Symptoms:* Overdosage with labetalol causes excessive hypotension that is posture sensitive and, sometimes, excessive bradycardia. Patients should be placed supine and their legs raised if necessary to improve the blood supply to the brain. If overdosage with labetalol follows oral ingestion, gastric lavage or pharmacologically induced emesis (using syrup of ipecac) may be useful for removal of the drug shortly after ingestion. The following additional measures should be employed if necessary.

➤*Treatment:*

Excessive bradycardia – Administer atropine or epinephrine.

Cardiac failure – Administer a digitalis glycoside and a diuretic. Dopamine or dobutamine may also be useful.

Hypotension – Administer vasopressors (eg, norepinephrine). There is pharmacologic evidence that norepinephrine may be the drug of choice.

Bronchospasm – Administer epinephrine or an aerosolized beta-2-agonist.

Seizures – Administer diazepam. In severe beta-blocker overdose resulting in hypotension or bradycardia, glucagon has been shown to be effective when administered in large doses (5 to 10 mg rapidly over 30 seconds, followed by continuous infusion of 5 mg per hour that can be reduced as the patient improves).

Neither hemodialysis nor peritoneal dialysis removes a significant amount of labetalol from the general circulation (less than 1%).

Patient Information

As with all drugs with beta-blocking activity, certain advice to patients being treated with labetalol is warranted. This information is intended to aid in the safe and effective use of this medication. It is not a disclosure of all possible adverse or intended effects. While no incident of the abrupt withdrawal phenomenon (exacerbation of angina pectoris) has been reported with labetalol, dosing with labetalol tablets should not be interrupted or discontinued without a physician's advice. Patients being treated with labetalol tablets should consult a physician at any signs or symptoms of impending cardiac failure or hepatic dysfunction. Also, mild transient scalp tingling may occur, usually when treatment with labetalol tablets is initiated.

LABETALOL HYDROCHLORIDE — INJECTION

Indications

➤*Severe hypertension:* For control of blood pressure in severe hypertension.

Administration and Dosage

➤*Approved by the FDA:* August 1, 1984.

Labetalol hydrochloride injection is intended for IV use in hospitalized patients. Dosage must be individualized depending upon the severity of hypertension and the response of the patient during dosing.

Patients should always be kept in a supine position during the period of IV drug administration. A substantial fall in blood pressure on standing should be expected in these patients. The patient's ability to tolerate an upright position should be established before permitting any ambulation, such as using toilet facilities.

Either of 2 methods of administration of labetalol hydrochloride injection may be used: Repeated IV injections or slow continuous infusion.

➤*Repeated IV injection:* Initially, labetalol hydrochloride injection should be given in a dose of 20 mg labetalol hydrochloride (which corresponds to 0.25 mg/kg for an 80 kg patient) by slow IV injection over a 2-minute period.

Immediately before the injection and at 5 and 10 minutes after injection, supine blood pressure should be measured to evaluate response. Additional injections of 40 mg or 80 mg can be given at 10-minute intervals until a desired supine blood pressure is achieved or a total of 300 mg labetalol hydrochloride has been injected. The maximum effect usually occurs within 5 minutes of each injection.

➤*Slow continuous infusion:* Labetalol hydrochloride injection is prepared for IV continuous infusion by diluting the contents with commonly used IV fluids (see below). Examples of methods of preparing the infusion solution are as follows:

The contents of either two 20 mL vials (40 mL), or one 40 mL vial, are added to 160 mL of a commonly used IV fluid such that the resultant 200 mL of solution contains 200 mg of labetalol hydrochloride, 1 mg/mL. The diluted solution should be administered at a rate of 2 mL/min to deliver 2 mg/min.

Alternatively, the contents of either two 20 mL vials (40 mL), or one 40 mL vial, of labetalol hydrochloride injection are added to 250 mL of a commonly used IV fluid. The resultant solution will contain 200 mg of labetalol hydrochloride, approximately 2 mg per 3 mL. The diluted solution should be administered at a rate of 3 mL/min to deliver approximately 2 mg/min.

The rate of infusion of the diluted solution may be adjusted according to the blood pressure response, at the discretion of the physician. To facilitate a desired rate of infusion, the diluted solution can be infused using a controlled administration mechanism (eg, graduated burette, mechanically driven infusion pump).

Since the half-life of labetalol is 5 to 8 hours, steady-state blood levels (in the face of a constant rate of infusion) would not be reached during the usual infusion time period. The infusion should be continued until a satisfactory response is obtained and should then be stopped and oral labetalol hydrochloride started (see below). The effective IV dose is usually in the range of 50 to 200 mg. A total dose of up to 300 mg may be required in some patients.

➤*Blood pressure monitoring:* The blood pressure should be monitored during and after completion of the infusion or IV injections. Rapid or excessive falls in either systolic or diastolic blood pressure during IV treatment should be avoided. In patients with excessive systolic hypertension, the decrease in systolic pressure should be used as indicator of effectiveness in addition to the response of the diastolic pressure.

➤*Initiation of dosing with labetalol hydrochloride tablets:* Subsequent oral dosing with labetalol hydrochloride tablets should begin when it has been established that the supine diastolic blood pressure has begun to rise. The recommended initial dose is 200 mg, followed in 6 to 12 hours by an additional dose of 200 or 400 mg, depending on the blood pressure response. Thereafter, inpatient titration with labetalol hydrochloride tablets may proceed as follows:

LABETALOL HYDROCHLORIDE — INJECTION

Inpatient Titration Instructions	
Regimen	Daily dose[a]
200 mg twice a day	400 mg
400 mg twice a day	800 mg
800 mg twice a day	1,600 mg
1200 mg twice a day	2,400 mg

[a] If needed, the total daily dose may be given in 3 divided doses.

While in the hospital, the dosage of labetalol hydrochloride tablets may be increased at 1-day intervals to achieve the desired blood pressure reduction.

The recommended initial dosage is 100 mg twice daily whether used alone or added to a diuretic regimen. After 2 or 3 days, using standing blood pressure as an indicator, dosage may be titrated in increments of 100 mg twice a day every 2 or 3 days. The usual maintenance dosage of labetalol hydrochloride is between 200 and 400 mg twice daily.

➤*Compatibility with commonly used IV fluids:* Parenteral drug products should be inspected visually for particulate matter and discoloration prior to administration, where solution and container permit.

Labetalol injection was tested for compatibility with commonly used IV fluids at final concentrations of 1.25 to 3.75 mg labetalol hydrochloride per mL of mixture. Labetalol injection was found to be compatible with and stable (for 24 hours refrigerated or at room temperature) in mixtures with the following solutions: Ringers Injection; Lactated Ringers Injection; 5% Dextrose and Ringers Injection; 5% Lactated Ringers and 5% Dextrose Injection; 5% Dextrose Injection; 0.9% Sodium Chloride Injection; 5% Dextrose and 0.2% Sodium Chloride Injection; 2.5% Dextrose and 0.45% Sodium Chloride Injection; 5% Dextrose and 0.9% Sodium Chloride Injection; 5% Dextrose and 0.33% Sodium Chloride Injection.

Labetalol injection was not compatible with 5% Sodium Bicarbonate Injection. Care should be taken when administering alkaline drugs, including furosemide, in combination with labetalol. Compatibility should be ensured prior to administering these drugs together.

➤*Storage/Stability:* Store between 2° and 30°C (36° and 86°F). Protect from freezing and light.

Actions

➤*Pharmacology:* Labetalol combines both selective, competitive alpha-1-adrenergic-blocking and nonselective, competitive beta-adrenergic-blocking activity in a single substance. In man, the ratios of alpha- to beta-blockade have been estimated to be approximately 1:3 and 1:7 following oral and IV administration, respectively. Beta-2-agonist activity has been demonstrated in animals with minimal beta-1-agonist (ISA) activity detected. In animals, at doses greater than those required for alpha- or beta-adrenergic blockade, a membrane-stabilizing effect has been demonstrated.

➤*Pharmacokinetics:*

Distribution – Labetalol has been shown to cross the placental barrier in humans. Only negligible amounts of the drug crossed the blood-brain barrier in animal studies. Labetalol is approximately 50% protein bound. Neither hemodialysis nor peritoneal dialysis removes a significant amount of labetalol from the general circulation (less than 1%).

Metabolism/Excretion – Following IV infusion, the elimination half-life is about 5.5 hours, and the total body clearance is approximately 33 mL/min/kg. The plasma half-life of labetalol following oral administration is about 6 to 8 hours. In patients with decreased hepatic or renal function, the elimination half-life of labetalol is not altered; however, the relative bioavailability in hepatically impaired patients is increased due to decreased "first-pass" metabolism.

The metabolism of labetalol is mainly through conjugation to glucuronide metabolites. These metabolites are present in plasma and are excreted in the urine and, via the bile, into the feces. Approximately 55% to 60% of a dose appears in the urine as conjugates or unchanged labetalol within the first 24 hours of dosing.

Contraindications

Bronchial asthma, overt cardiac failure, greater than first-degree heart block, cardiogenic shock, severe bradycardia, other conditions associated with severe and prolonged hypotension, hypersensitivity to any component of the product.

Beta-blockers, even those with apparent cardioselectivity, should not be used in patients with a history of obstructive airway disease, including asthma.

Warnings

➤*Cardiac failure:* Sympathetic stimulation is a vital component supporting circulatory function in congestive heart failure. Beta blockade carries a potential hazard of further depressing myocardial contractility and precipitating more severe failure. Although beta blockers should be avoided in overt congestive heart failure, if necessary, labetalol can be used with caution in patients with a history of heart failure who are well compensated. Congestive heart failure has been observed in patients receiving labetalol. Labetalol does not abolish the inotropic action of digitalis on heart muscle.

Patients without histories of cardiac failure – In patients with latent cardiac insufficiency, continued depression of the myocardium with beta-blocking agents over a period of time can lead, in some cases, to cardiac failure. At the first sign or symptom of impending cardiac failure, patients should be fully digitalized or be given a diuretic, and the response observed closely. If cardiac failure continues, despite adequate digitalization and diuretic, labetalol therapy should be withdrawn (gradually if possible).

➤*Ischemic heart disease:* Angina pectoris has not been reported upon labetalol discontinuation. However, following abrupt cessation of therapy with some beta-blocking agents in patients with coronary artery disease, exacerbations of angina pectoris and, in some cases, myocardial infarction have been reported. Therefore, such patients should be cautioned against interruption of therapy without the physician's advice. Even in the absence of overt angina pectoris, when discontinuation of labetalol is planned, the patient should be carefully observed and should be advised to limit physical activity. If angina markedly worsens or acute coronary insufficiency develops, labetalol administration should be reinstituted promptly, at least temporarily, and other measures appropriate for the management of unstable angina should be taken.

➤*Nonallergic bronchospasm (eg, chronic bronchitis, emphysema):* Since labetalol injection at the usual IV therapeutic doses has not been studied in patients with nonallergic bronchospastic disease, it should not be used in such patients.

➤*Pheochromocytoma:* IV labetalol has been shown to be effective in lowering the blood pressure and relieving symptoms in patients with pheochromocytoma; higher than usual doses may be required. However, paradoxical hypertensive responses have been reported in a few patients with this tumor; therefore, use caution when administering labetalol to patients with pheochromocytoma.

➤*Diabetes mellitus and hypoglycemia:* Beta-adrenergic blockade may prevent the appearance of premonitory signs and symptoms (eg, tachycardia) of acute hypoglycemia. This is especially important with labile diabetics. Beta blockade also reduces the release of insulin in response to hyperglycemia; it may therefore be necessary to adjust the dose of antidiabetic drugs.

➤*Major surgery:* The necessity or desirability of withdrawing beta-blocking therapy prior to major surgery is controversial. Protracted severe hypotension and difficulty in restarting or maintaining a heartbeat have been reported with beta-blockers. The effect of labetalol's alpha-adrenergic activity has not been evaluated in this setting.

Several deaths have occurred when labetalol injection was used during surgery (including when used in cases to control bleeding).

➤*Rapid decreases of blood pressure:* Caution must be observed when reducing severely elevated blood pressure. Although such findings have not been reported with IV labetalol, a number of adverse reactions, including cerebral infarction, optic nerve infarction, angina, and ischemic changes in the electrocardiogram, have been reported with other agents when severely elevated blood pressure was reduced over time courses of several hours to as long as 1 or 2 days. The desired blood pressure lowering should therefore be achieved over as long a period of time as is compatible with the patient's status.

➤*Hepatic effects:* Severe hepatocellular injury, confirmed by rechallenge in at least 1 case, occurs rarely with labetalol therapy. The hepatic injury is usually reversible, but hepatic necrosis and death have been reported. Injury has occurred after both short- and long-term treatment and may be slowly progressive despite minimal symptomatology. Similar hepatic events have been reported with a related compound, dilevalol HCl, including 2 deaths. Dilevalol hydrochloride is 1 of the 4 isomers of labetalol hydrochloride. Thus, for patients taking labetalol, periodic determination of suitable hepatic laboratory tests would be appropriate. Laboratory testing should also be done at the very first symptom or sign of liver dysfunction (eg, pruritus, dark urine, persistent anorexia, jaundice, right upper quadrant tenderness, unexplained "flu-like" symptoms). If the patient has jaundice or laboratory evidence of liver injury, labetalol should be stopped and not restarted.

➤*Hypersensitivity reactions:* While taking beta-blockers, patients with histories of severe anaphylactic reactions to a variety of allergens may be more reactive to repeated challenge, either accidental, diagnostic, or therapeutic. Such patients may be unresponsive to the usual doses of epinephrine used to treat allergic reactions.

➤*Hepatic function impairment:* Use labetalol injection with caution in patients with impaired hepatic function since metabolism of the drug may be diminished.

➤*Pregnancy:* Category C.

Teratogenic – Teratogenic studies have been performed with labetalol in rats and rabbits at oral doses up to approximately 6 and 4 times the maximum recommended human dose (MRHD), respectively. No reproducible evidence of fetal malformations was observed. Increased fetal resorptions were seen in both species at doses approximating the MRHD. A teratology study performed with labetalol in rabbits at IV doses up to 1.7 times the MRHD revealed no evidence of drug-related harm to the fetus. There are no adequate and well-controlled studies in pregnant women. Labetalol should be used during pregnancy only if the potential benefit justifies the potential risk to the fetus.

Nonteratogenic – Hypotension, bradycardia, hypoglycemia, and respiratory depression have been reported in infants of mothers who were treated with labetalol for hypertension during pregnancy. Oral administration of labetalol to rats during late gestation through weaning at doses of 2 to 4 times the MRHD caused a decrease in neonatal survival.

Labor and delivery – Labetalol given to pregnant women with hypertension did not appear to affect the usual course of labor and delivery.

LABETALOL HYDROCHLORIDE — INJECTION

➤*Lactation:* Small amounts of labetalol (approximately 0.004% of the maternal dose) are excreted in human milk. Caution should be exercised when labetalol injection is administered to a breast-feeding woman.

➤*Children:* Safety and efficacy in pediatric patients have not been established.

Precautions

➤*Monitoring:* Routine laboratory tests are ordinarily not required before or after IV labetalol. In patients with concomitant illnesses, such as impaired renal function, appropriate tests should be done to monitor these conditions.

➤*Following coronary artery bypass surgery:* In 1 uncontrolled study, patients with low cardiac indices and elevated systemic vascular resistance following IV labetalol experienced significant declines in cardiac output with little change in systemic vascular resistance. One of these patients developed hypotension following labetalol HCl treatment. Therefore, use of labetalol should be avoided in such patients.

➤*High-dose labetalol:* Administration of up to 3 g/day as an infusion for up to 2 to 3 days has been anecdotally reported; several patients experienced hypotension or bradycardia.

➤*Hypotension:* Symptomatic postural hypotension (incidence, 58%) is likely to occur if patients are tilted or allowed to assume the upright position within 3 hours of receiving labetalol injection. Therefore, the patient's ability to tolerate an upright position should be established before permitting any ambulation.

Drug Interactions

➤*Other antihypertensive agents:* Because labetalol injection may be administered to patients already being treated with other medications, including other antihypertensive agents, careful monitoring of these patients is necessary to detect and treat promptly any undesired effect from concomitant administration.

➤*Tricyclic antidepressants:* In 1 survey, 2.3% of patients taking labetalol orally in combination with tricyclic antidepressants experienced tremor compared with 0.7% reported to occur with labetalol alone. The contribution of each of the treatments to this adverse reaction is unknown but the possibility of a drug interaction cannot be excluded.

➤*Beta-agonist bronchodilators:* Drugs possessing beta-blocking properties can blunt the bronchodilator effect of beta-receptor agonist drugs in patients with bronchospasm; therefore, doses greater than the normal antiasthmatic dose of beta-agonist bronchodilator drugs may be required.

➤*Halothane:* Synergism has been shown between halothane anesthesia and IV labetalol. During controlled hypotensive anesthesia using labetalol in association with halothane, high concentrations (3% or above) of halothane should not be used because the degree of hypotension will be increased and because of the possibility of a large reduction in cardiac output and an increase in central venous pressure. The anesthesiologist should be informed when a patient is receiving labetalol.

➤*Nitroglycerin:* Labetalol blunts the reflex tachycardia produced by nitroglycerin without preventing its hypotensive effect. If labetalol hydrochloride is used with nitroglycerin in patients with angina pectoris, additional antihypertensive effects may occur.

➤*Calcium-channel blockers:* Care should be taken if labetalol is used concomitantly with calcium antagonists of the verapamil type.

➤*Furosemide:* When drug products that are alkaline, such as furosemide, have been administered in combination with labetalol, a white precipitate has been noted. Therefore, these drugs should not be administered in the same infusion line.

➤*Drug/Lab test interactions:* The presence of labetalol metabolites in the urine may result in falsely elevated levels of urinary catecholamines, metanephrine, normetanephrine, and vanillylmandelic acid (VMA) when measured by fluorimetric or photometric methods. In screening patients suspected of having a pheochromocytoma and being treated with labetalol, a specific method, such as a high-performance liquid chromatographic assay with solid phase extraction should be employed in determining levels of catecholamines.

Labetalol has also been reported to produce a false-positive test for amphetamine when screening urine for the presence of drugs using the commercially available assay methods *Toxi-Lab A* (thin-layer chromatographic assay) and *Emit-d.a.u.* (radioenzymatic assay). When patients being treated with labetalol have a positive urine test for amphetamine using these techniques, confirmation should be made by using more specific methods, such as a gas chromatographic-mass spectrometer technique.

Adverse Reactions

Labetalol injection is usually well tolerated. Most adverse reactions have been mild and transient, and in controlled trials involving 92 patients did not require labetalol withdrawal. Symptomatic postural hypotension (incidence, 58%) is likely to occur if patients are tilted or allowed to assume the upright position within 3 hours of receiving labetalol hydrochloride injection. Moderate hypotension occurred in 1 of 100 patients while supine. Increased sweating was noted in 1 of 100 patients, and flushing occurred in 1 of 100 patients.

The following also were reported with labetalol HCl injection with the incidence per 100 patients noted:

➤*Cardiovascular:* Ventricular arrhythmia in 1.

➤*CNS:* Dizziness in 9; tingling of the scalp/skin in 7; hypoesthesia (numbness) and vertigo, 1 each.

➤*Dermatologic:* Pruritus in 1.

➤*GI:* Nausea in 13; vomiting in 4; dyspepsia and taste distortion, 1 each.

➤*Metabolic:* Transient increases in blood urea nitrogen and serum creatinine levels occurred in 8 of 100 patients; these were associated with drops in blood pressure, generally patients with prior renal insufficiency.

➤*Psychiatric:* Somnolence/yawning in 3.

➤*Respiratory:* Wheezing in 1.

Overdosage

➤*Treatment:* Overdosage with labetalol hydrochloride injection causes excessive hypotension that is posture-sensitive, and sometimes, excessive bradycardia. Patients should be placed supine and their legs raised if necessary to improve the blood supply to the brain. If overdosage with labetalol follows oral ingestion, gastric lavage or pharmacologically induced emesis (using syrup of ipecac) may be useful for removal of the drug shortly after ingestion. The following additional measures should be employed if necessary:

Excessive bradycardia – Administer atropine or epinephrine.

Cardiac failure – Administer a digitalis glycoside and a diuretic. Dopamine or dobutamine may also be useful.

Hypotension – Administer vasopressors (eg, norepinephrine). There is pharmacological evidence that norepinephrine may be the drug of choice.

Bronchospasm – Administer epinephrine or an aerosolized beta-2 agonist.

Seizures – Administer diazepam.

Other – In severe beta-blocker overdose resulting in hypotension or bradycardia, glucagon has been shown to be effective when administered in large doses (5 to 10 mg rapidly over 30 seconds, followed by continuous infusion of 5 mg/hr that can be reduced as the patient improves).

Neither hemodialysis nor peritoneal dialysis removes a significant amount of labetalol from the general circulation (less than 1%).

Patient Information

The following information is intended to aid in the safe and effective use of this medication. It is not a disclosure of all possible adverse or intended effects. During and immediately following (for up to 3 hours) labetalol injection, the patient should remain supine. Subsequently, the patient should be advised on how to proceed gradually to become ambulatory, and should be observed at the time of first ambulation.

When the patient is started on labetalol hydrochloride tablets, following adequate control of blood pressure with labetalol injection, appropriate directions for titration of dosage should be provided.

As with all drugs with beta-blocking activity, certain advice to patients being treated with labetalol is warranted: While no incident of the abrupt withdrawal phenomenon (exacerbation of angina pectoris) has been reported with labetalol, dosing with labetalol tablets should not be interrupted or discontinued without a physician's advice. Patients being treated with labetalol tablets should consult a physician at any signs or symptoms of impending cardiac failure or hepatic dysfunction. Also, transient scalp tingling may occur, usually when treatment with labetalol tablets is initiated.

CARVEDILOL

Rx	**Coreg** (GlaxoSmithKline)	**Tablets:** 3.125 mg	Lactose, sucrose. (39 SB). White, oval. Film-coated. In 100s.
		6.25 mg	Lactose, sucrose. (4140 SB). White, oval. Film-coated. In 100s.
		12.5 mg	Lactose, sucrose. (4141 SB). White, oval. Film-coated. In 100s.
		25 mg	Lactose, sucrose. (4142 SB). White, oval. Film-coated. In 100s.

CARVEDILOL — ORAL

Indications

➤*Congestive heart failure:* Treatment of mild to severe heart failure of ischemic or cardiomyopathic origin, usually in addition to diuretics, ACE inhibitor, and digitalis, to increase survival and, also, to reduce the risk of hospitalization.

➤*Left ventricular dysfunction following myocardial infarction:* To reduce cardiovascular mortality in clinically stable patients who have survived the acute phase of a myocardial infarction and have a left ventricular ejection fraction of less than or equal to 40% (with or without symptomatic heart failure).

CARVEDILOL — ORAL

➤*Hypertension:* Management of essential hypertension. It can be used alone or in combination with other antihypertensive agents, especially thiazide-type diuretics.

➤*Unlabeled uses:* Carvedilol appears to be beneficial in the treatment of the following conditions: angina pectoris (25 to 50 mg twice daily); idiopathic cardiomyopathy (6.25 to 25 mg twice daily).

Administration and Dosage

➤*Approved by the FDA:* September 14, 1995.

➤*Congestive heart failure:* Dosage must be individualized and closely monitored by a physician during up-titration. Prior to initiation of carvedilol, it is recommended that fluid retention be minimized. The recommended starting dose of carvedilol is 3.125 mg twice daily for 2 weeks. Patients who tolerate a dose of 3.125 mg twice daily may have their dose increased to 6.25, 12.5 and 25 mg twice daily over successive intervals of at least 2 weeks. Patients should be maintained on lower doses if higher doses are not tolerated. A maximum dose of 50 mg twice daily has been administered to patients with mild-to-moderate heart failure weighing over 85 kg (187 lbs).

Patients should be advised that initiation of treatment and (to a lesser extent) dosage increases may be associated with transient symptoms of dizziness or lightheadedness (and rarely syncope) within the first hour after dosing. Thus during these periods they should avoid situations such as driving or hazardous tasks, where symptoms could result in injury. In addition, carvedilol should be taken with food to slow the rate of absorption. Vasodilatory symptoms often do not require treatment, but it may be useful to separate the time of dosing of carvedilol from that of the ACE inhibitor or to reduce temporarily the dose of the ACE inhibitor. The dose of carvedilol should not be increased until symptoms of worsening heart failure or vasodilation have been stabilized.

Fluid retention (with or without transient worsening heart failure symptoms) should be treated by an increase in the dose of diuretics.

The dose of carvedilol should be reduced if patients experience bradycardia (heart rate less than 55 beats/min).

Episodes of dizziness or fluid retention during initiation of carvedilol can generally be managed without discontinuation of treatment and do not preclude subsequent successful titration of, or a favorable response to, carvedilol.

➤*Left ventricular dysfunction following myocardial infarction:* Dosage must be individualized and monitored during up-titration. Treatment with carvedilol may be started as an inpatient or outpatient and should be started after the patient is hemodynamically stable and fluid retention has been minimized. It is recommended that carvedilol be started at 6.25 mg twice daily and increased after 3 to 10 days, based on tolerability to 12.5 mg twice daily, then again to the target dose of 25 mg twice daily. A lower starting dose may be used (3.125 mg twice daily) or, the rate of up-titration may be slowed if clinically indicated (eg, due to low blood pressure or heart rate, or fluid retention). Patients should be maintained on lower doses if higher doses are not tolerated. The recommended dosing regimen need not be altered in patients who received treatment with an IV or oral β-blocker during the acute phase of the myocardial infarction.

➤*Hypertension:* Dosage must be individualized. The recommended starting dose of carvedilol is 6.25 mg twice daily. If this dose is tolerated, using standing systolic pressure measured about 1 hour after dosing as a guide, the dose should be maintained for 7 to 14 days, and then increased to 12.5 mg twice daily if needed, based on trough blood pressure, again using standing systolic pressure 1 hour after dosing as a guide for tolerance. This dose should also be maintained for 7 to 14 days and can then be adjusted upward to 25 mg twice daily if tolerated and needed. The full antihypertensive effect of carvedilol is seen within 7 to 14 days. Total daily dose should not exceed 50 mg. Carvedilol should be taken with food to slow the rate of absorption and reduce the incidence of orthostatic effects.

Addition of a diuretic to carvedilol, or carvedilol to a diuretic can be expected to produce additive effects and exaggerate the orthostatic component of carvedilol action.

➤*Anesthesia and major surgery:* If carvedilol treatment is to be continued perioperatively, particular care should be taken when anesthetic agents which depress myocardial function, such as ether, cyclopropane, and trichloroethylene, are used.

For excessive bradycardia – Atropine, 2 mg IV.

To support cardiovascular function – Glucagon, 5 to 10 mg IV rapidly over 30 seconds, followed by a continuous infusion of 5 mg/hour; sympathomimetics (dobutamine, isoprenaline, adrenaline) at doses according to body weight and effect.

➤*Hepatic function impairment:* Carvedilol should not be given to patients with severe hepatic function impairment.

➤*Storage/Stability:* Store below 30°C (86°F). Protect from moisture. Dispense in a tight, light-resistant container.

Actions

➤*Pharmacology:* Carvedilol is a racemic mixture in which nonselective beta-adrenoreceptor blocking activity is present in the S(−) enantiomer and alpha-adrenergic blocking activity is present in both R(+) and S(−) enantiomers at equal potency. Carvedilol has no intrinsic sympathomimetic activity.

➤*Pharmacokinetics:*

Absorption/Distribution – Carvedilol is rapidly and extensively absorbed following oral administration, with absolute bioavailability of approximately 25% to 35% due to a significant degree of first-pass metabolism. Following oral administration, the apparent mean terminal elimination half-life of carvedilol generally ranges from 7 to 10 hours. Plasma concentrations achieved are proportional to the oral dose administered. When administered with food, the rate of absorption is slowed, as evidenced by a delay in the time to reach peak plasma levels, with no significant difference in extent of bioavailability. Taking carvedilol with food should minimize the risk of orthostatic hypotension.

Carvedilol is more than 98% bound to plasma proteins, primarily with albumin. The plasma-protein binding is independent of concentration over the therapeutic range. Carvedilol is a basic, lipophilic compound with a steady-state volume of distribution of approximately 115 L, indicating substantial distribution into extravascular tissues. Plasma clearance ranges from 500 to 700 mL/min.

Metabolism/Excretion – Carvedilol is extensively metabolized. Following oral administration of radiolabeled carvedilol to healthy volunteers, carvedilol accounted for only about 7% of the total radioactivity in plasma as measured by area under the curve (AUC). Less than 2% of the dose was excreted unchanged in the urine. Carvedilol is metabolized primarily by aromatic ring oxidation and glucuronidation. The oxidative metabolites are further metabolized by conjugation via glucuronidation and sulfation. The metabolites of carvedilol are excreted primarily via the bile into the feces. Demethylation and hydroxylation at the phenol ring produce 3 active metabolites with β-receptor blocking activity. Based on preclinical studies, the 4′-hydroxyphenyl metabolite is approximately 13 times more potent than carvedilol for β-blockade.

Compared with carvedilol, the 3 active metabolites exhibit weak vasodilating activity. Plasma concentrations of the active metabolites are about one-tenth of those observed for carvedilol and have pharmacokinetics similar to the parent.

Carvedilol undergoes stereoselective first-pass metabolism with plasma levels of R(+)-carvedilol approximately 2 to 3 times higher than S(−)-carvedilol following oral administration in healthy subjects. The mean apparent terminal elimination half-lives for R(+)-carvedilol range from 5 to 9 hours compared with 7 to 11 hours for the S(−)-enantiomer.

The primary P-450 enzymes responsible for the metabolism of both R(+) and S(−)-carvedilol in human liver microsomes were CYP2D6 and CYP2C9 and to a lesser extent CYP3A4, 2C19, 1A2, and 2E1. CYP2D6 is thought to be the major enzyme in the 4′- and 5′-hydroxylation of carvedilol, with a potential contribution from 3A4. CYP2C9 is thought to be of primary importance in the O-methylation pathway of S(−)-carvedilol.

Carvedilol is subject to the effects of genetic polymorphism with poor metabolizers of debrisoquin (a marker for cytochrome P-450 2D6) exhibiting 2- to 3-fold higher plasma concentrations of R(+)-carvedilol compared to extensive metabolizers. In contrast, plasma levels of S(−)-carvedilol are increased only about 20% to 25% in poor metabolizers, indicating this enantiomer is metabolized to a lesser extent by cytochrome P450 2D6 than R(+)-carvedilol. The pharmacokinetics of carvedilol do not appear to be different in poor metabolizers of S-mephenytoin (patients deficient in cytochrome P-450 2C19).

Special populations –

Renal function impairment: Although carvedilol is metabolized primarily by the liver, plasma concentrations of carvedilol have been reported to be increased in patients with renal impairment. Based on mean AUC data, approximately 40% to 50% higher plasma concentrations of carvedilol were observed in hypertensive patients with moderate to severe renal impairment compared to a control group of hypertensive patients with normal renal function. However, the ranges of AUC values were similar for both groups. Changes in mean peak plasma levels were less pronounced, approximately 12% to 26% higher in patients with impaired renal function.

Consistent with its high degree of plasma protein binding, carvedilol does not appear to be cleared significantly by hemodialysis.

Hepatic function impairment: Compared with healthy subjects, patients with cirrhotic liver disease exhibit significantly higher concentrations of carvedilol (approximately 4- to 7-fold) following single-dose therapy.

Elderly: Plasma levels of carvedilol average about 50% higher in the elderly compared with younger subjects.

Congestive heart failure: Steady-state plasma concentrations of carvedilol and its enantiomers increased proportionally over the 6.25 to 50 mg dose range in patients with congestive heart failure. Compared with healthy subjects, congestive heart failure patients had increased mean AUC and C_{max} values for carvedilol and its enantiomers, with up to 50% to 100% higher values observed in 6 patients with NYHA class IV heart failure. The mean apparent terminal elimination half-life for carvedilol was similar to that observed in healthy subjects.

Contraindications

Bronchial asthma (2 cases of death from status asthmaticus have been reported in patients receiving single doses of carvedilol) or related bronchospastic conditions, second- or third-degree AV block, sick sinus syndrome or severe bradycardia (unless a permanent pacemaker is in place); cardiogenic shock or decompensated heart failure requiring the use of intravenous inotropic therapy (such patients should first be weaned from IV therapy before initiating carvedilol); clinically manifest hepatic function impairment; hypersensitivity to the drug.

Warnings

➤*Cessation of therapy with carvedilol:* Patients with coronary artery disease, who are being treated with carvedilol, should be advised against abrupt discontinuation of therapy. Severe exacerbation of angina and the occurrence of myocardial infarction and ventricular arrhythmias have been reported in angina patients following the abrupt discontinuation of therapy

CARVEDILOL — ORAL

with beta-blockers. The last 2 complications may occur with or without preceding exacerbation of the angina pectoris. As with other beta-blockers, when discontinuation of carvedilol is planned, the patients should be carefully observed and advised to limit physical activity to a minimum. Carvedilol should be discontinued over 1 to 2 weeks whenever possible. If the angina worsens or acute coronary insufficiency develops, it is recommended that carvedilol be promptly reinstituted, at least temporarily. Because coronary artery disease is common and may be unrecognized, it may be prudent not to discontinue carvedilol therapy abruptly even in patients treated only for hypertension or heart failure.

➤*Hypotension and postural hypotension:* Hypotension and postural hypotension occurred in 9.7% and syncope in 3.4% of congestive heart failure patients receiving carvedilol compared to 3.6% and 2.5% of placebo patients, respectively. The risk for these events was highest during the first 30 days of dosing, corresponding to the up-titration period and was a cause for discontinuation of therapy in 0.7% of carvedilol patients, compared to 0.4% of placebo patients. In a long-term, placebo-controlled trial in severe heart failure (COPERNICUS), hypotension and postural hypotension occurred in 15.1% and syncope in 2.9% of heart failure patients receiving carvedilol compared to 8.7% and 2.3% of placebo patients, respectively. These events were a cause for discontinuation of therapy in 1.1% of carvedilol patients, compared to 0.8% of placebo patients.

Postural hypotension occurred in 1.8% and syncope in 0.1% of hypertensive patients, primarily following the initial dose or at the time of dose increase and was a cause for discontinuation of therapy in 1% of patients.

In the CAPRICORN study of survivors of an acute myocardial infarction, hypotension or postural hypotension occurred in 20.2% of patients receiving carvedilol compared to 12.6% of placebo patients. Syncope was reported in 3.9% and 1.9% of patients, respectively. These events were a cause for discontinuation of therapy in 2.5% of patients receiving carvedilol, compared to 0.2% of placebo patients.

➤*Peripheral vascular disease:* Beta-blockers can precipitate or aggravate symptoms of arterial insufficiency in patients with peripheral vascular disease. Caution should be exercised in such individuals.

➤*Anesthesia and major surgery:* If carvedilol treatment is to be continued perioperatively, particular care should be taken when anesthetic agents which depress myocardial function, such as ether, cyclopropane, and trichloroethylene, are used.

See Administration and Dosage for more information.

➤*Diabetes and hypoglycemia:* Beta-blockers may mask some of the manifestations of hypoglycemia, particularly tachycardia. Nonselective beta-blockers may potentiate insulin-induced hypoglycemia and delay recovery of serum glucose levels. Patients subject to spontaneous hypoglycemia, or diabetic patients receiving insulin or oral hypoglycemic agents, should be cautioned about these possibilities and carvedilol should be used with caution. In congestive heart failure patients, there is a risk of worsening hyperglycemia.

➤*Thyrotoxicosis:* Beta-adrenergic blockade may mask clinical signs of hyperthyroidism, such as tachycardia. Abrupt withdrawal of beta-blockade may be followed by an exacerbation of the symptoms of hyperthyroidism or may precipitate thyroid storm.

➤*Pheochromocytoma:* In patients with pheochromocytoma, an alpha-blocking agent should be initiated prior to the use of any beta-blocking agent. Although carvedilol has both alpha- and beta-blocking pharmacologic activities, there has been no experience with its use in this condition. Therefore, caution should be taken in the administration of carvedilol to patients suspected of having pheochromocytoma.

➤*Cardiac failure:* Worsening cardiac failure or fluid retention may occur during up-titration of carvedilol. If such symptoms occur, diuretics should be increased and the carvedilol dose should not be advanced until clinical stability resumes. Occasionally it is necessary to lower the carvedilol dose or temporarily discontinue it. Such episodes do not preclude subsequent successful titration of carvedilol. In a placebo-controlled trial of patients with severe heart failure, worsening heart failure during the first 3 months was reported to a similar degree with carvedilol and with placebo. When treatment was maintained beyond 3 months, worsening heart failure was reported less frequently in patients treated with carvedilol than with placebo. Worsening heart failure observed during long-term therapy is more likely to be related to the patients' underlying disease than to treatment with carvedilol.

➤*Prinzmetal's variant angina:* Agents with nonselective beta-blocking activity may provoke chest pain in patients with Prinzmetal's variant angina. There has been no clinical experience with carvedilol in these patients although the alpha-blocking activity may prevent such symptoms. However, caution should be taken in the administration of carvedilol to patients suspected of having Prinzmetal's variant angina.

➤*Renal effects:* Rarely, use of carvedilol in patients with congestive heart failure has resulted in deterioration of renal function. Patients at risk appear to be those with low blood pressure (systolic BP less than 100 mm Hg), ischemic heart disease and diffuse vascular disease, or underlying renal insufficiency. Renal function has returned to baseline when carvedilol was stopped. In patients with these risk factors it is recommended that renal function be monitored during up-titration of carvedilol and the drug discontinued or dosage reduced if worsening of renal function occurs.

➤*Hepatic effects:* At the first symptom/sign of liver dysfunction (eg, pruritus, dark urine, persistent anorexia, jaundice, right upper quadrant tenderness, or unexplained "flu-like" symptoms), laboratory testing should be performed. If the patient has laboratory evidence of liver injury or jaundice, carvedilol should be stopped and not restarted.

➤*Hypersensitivity reactions:* While taking beta-blockers, patients with a history of severe anaphylactic reaction to a variety of allergens may be more reactive to repeated challenge, either accidental, diagnostic or therapeutic. Such patients may be unresponsive to the usual doses of epinephrine used to treat allergic reaction.

➤*Fertility impairment:* At doses greater than or equal to 200 mg/kg/day (greater than or equal to 32 times the MRHD as mg/m^2) carvedilol was toxic to adult rats (sedation, reduced weight gain) and was associated with a reduced number of successful matings, prolonged mating time, significantly fewer corpora lutea and implants per dam and complete resorption of 18% of the litters. The no-observed-effect dose level for overt toxicity and impairment of fertility was 60 mg/kg/day (10 times the MRHD as mg/m^2).

➤*Pregnancy:* *Category C.*

Teratogenic – Studies performed in pregnant rats and rabbits given carvedilol revealed increased post-implantation loss in rats at doses of 300 mg/kg/day (50 times the MRHD as mg/m^2) and in rabbits at doses of 75 mg/kg/day (25 times the MRHD as mg/m^2). In the rats, there was also a decrease in fetal body weight at the maternally toxic dose of 300 mg/kg/day (50 times the MRHD as mg/m^2), which was accompanied by an elevation in the frequency of fetuses with delayed skeletal development (missing or stunted 13th rib). In rats the no-observed-effect level for developmental toxicity was 60 mg/kg/day (10 times the MRHD as mg/m^2); in rabbits it was 15 mg/kg/day (5 times the MRHD as mg/m^2). There are no adequate and well-controlled studies in pregnant women. Carvedilol should be used during pregnancy only if the potential benefit justifies the potential risk to the fetus.

➤*Lactation:* It is not known whether this drug is excreted in human milk. Studies in rats have shown that carvedilol or its metabolites (as well as other β-blockers) cross the placental barrier and are excreted in breast milk. There was increased mortality at 1 week post-partum in neonates from rats treated with 60 mg/kg/day (10 times the MRHD as mg/m^2) and above during the last trimester through day 22 of lactation. Because many drugs are excreted in human milk and because of the potential for serious adverse reactions in nursing infants from β-blockers, especially bradycardia, a decision should be made whether to discontinue nursing or to discontinue the drug, taking into account the importance of the drug to the mother. The effects of other α- and β-blocking agents have included perinatal and neonatal distress.

➤*Children:* Safety and efficacy in patients less than 18 years of age have not been established.

Precautions

➤*Abrupt discontinuation:* Because carvedilol has beta-blocking activity, it should not be discontinued abruptly, particularly in patients with ischemic heart disease. Instead, it should be discontinued over 1 to 2 weeks.

➤*Bradycardia / syncope:* In clinical trials, carvedilol caused bradycardia in about 2% of hypertensive patients and 9% of congestive heart failure patients, and 6.5% of myocardial infarction patients with left ventricular dysfunction. If pulse rate drops below 55 beats/min, the dosage should be reduced.

To decrease the likelihood of syncope or excessive hypotension, treatment should be initiated with 3.125 mg twice daily for congestive heart failure patients and 6.25 mg twice daily for hypertensive patients and survivors of an acute myocardial infarction with left ventricular dysfunction. Dosage should then be increased slowly and the drug should be taken with food. During initiation of therapy, the patient should be cautioned to avoid situations such as driving or hazardous tasks, where injury could result should syncope occur.

➤*Hyperglycemia:* In congestive heart failure patients with diabetes, carvedilol therapy may lead to worsening hyperglycemia, which responds to intensification of hypoglycemic therapy. It is recommended that blood glucose be monitored when carvedilol dosing is initiated, adjusted, or discontinued.

➤*Nonallergic bronchospasm (eg, chronic bronchitis and emphysema):* Patients with bronchospastic disease should, in general, not receive beta-blockers. Carvedilol may be used with caution, however, in patients who do not respond to, or cannot tolerate, other antihypertensive agents. It is prudent, if carvedilol is used, to use the smallest effective dose, so that inhibition of endogenous or exogenous beta-agonists is minimized.

In clinical trials of patients with congestive heart failure, patients with bronchospastic disease were enrolled if they did not require oral or inhaled medication to treat their bronchospastic disease. In such patients, it is recommended that carvedilol be used with caution. The dosing recommendations should be followed closely and the dose should be lowered if any evidence of bronchospasm is observed during up-titration.

➤*Lab test abnormalities:* Reversible elevations in serum transaminases (ALT or AST) have been observed during treatment with carvedilol. Rates of transaminase elevations (2 to 3 times the upper limit of normal) observed during controlled clinical trials have generally been similar between patients treated with carvedilol and those treated with placebo. However, transaminase elevations, confirmed by rechallenge, have been observed with carvedilol. In a long-term, placebo-controlled trial in severe heart failure, patients treated with carvedilol had lower values for hepatic transaminases than patients treated with placebo, possibly because carvedilol-induced improvements in cardiac function led to less hepatic congestion or improved hepatic blood flow.

CARVEDILOL — ORAL

Drug Interactions

➤*CYP-450:* Because carvedilol undergoes substantial oxidative metabolism, the metabolism and pharmacokinetics of carvedilol may be affected by induction or inhibition of cytochrome P450 enzymes.

Interactions of carvedilol with strong inhibitors of CYP2D6 (eg, quinidine, fluoxetine, paroxetine, propafenone) have not been studied, but these drugs would be expected to increase blood levels of the R(+) enantiomer of carvedilol. Retrospective analysis of side effects in clinical trials showed that poor 2D6 metabolizers had a higher rate of dizziness during up-titration, presumably resulting from vasodilating effects of the higher concentrations of the alpha-blocking R(+) enantiomer.

Carvedilol Drug Interactions

Precipitant drug	Object drug*		Description
Carvedilol	Antidiabetic agents	⬆	Agents with beta-blocking properties may enhance the blood sugar-reducing effect of insulin and oral hypoglycemics. In patients taking insulin or oral hypoglycemics, regular monitoring of blood glucose is recommended.
Carvedilol	Calcium channel blockers (diltiazem, verapamil)	⬆	Isolated cases of conduction disturbance (rarely with hemodynamic compromise) have been observed when carvedilol is coadministered with diltiazem. As with other agents with beta-blocking properties, if carvedilol is to be administered orally with calcium channel blockers of the verapamil or diltiazem type, it is recommended that ECG and BP be monitored.
Carvedilol	Catecholamine-depleting agents (eg, reserpine)	⬆	Closely observe patients taking agents with beta-blocking properties and a drug that can deplete catecholamines for signs of hypotension or severe bradycardia.
Carvedilol	Clonidine	⬆	Coadministration of clonidine with agents with beta-blocking properties may potentiate BP and heart-rate-lowering effects. When concomitant treatment with agents with beta-blocking properties and clonidine is to be terminated, discontinue the beta-blocking agent first. Clonidine therapy can then be discontinued several days later by gradually decreasing the dosage.
Carvedilol	Cyclosporine	⬆	Coadministration of carvedilol and cyclosporine may cause an increase in mean trough cyclosporine concentrations. Monitor cyclosporine concentrations closely after carvedilol initiation and adjust cyclosporine dose as appropriate.
Carvedilol	Digoxin	⬆	Digoxin concentrations are increased by ≈ 15% during concurrent use. Therefore, increased monitoring of digoxin is recommended when initiating, adjusting, or discontinuing carvedilol.
Cimetidine	Carvedilol	⬆	Cimetidine increased carvedilol AUC by ≈ 30% but caused no change in C_{max}.
Rifampin	Carvedilol	⬇	Rifampin reduced AUC and C_{max} of carvedilol by ≈ 70%.
SSRIs (eg, fluoxetine, paroxetine)	Carvedilol	⬆	Certain selective serotonin reuptake inhibitors (SSRIs) may inhibit metabolism of some beta blockers; possible excessive beta blockade (bradycardia) may occur. Monitor cardiac function during coadministration.
Diphenhydramine	Carvedilol	⬆	Diphenhydramine may inhibit carvedilol metabolism, resulting in increased plasma concentrations and cardiovascular effects of carvedilol.
Carvedilol	Disopyramide	⬆	Clearance of disopyramide may be decreased by carvedilol, resulting in increased adverse effects (eg, sinus bradycardia, hypotension). Monitor patients closely during coadministration.
Hydroxychloroquine	Carvedilol	⬆	Hydroxychloroquine may inhibit metabolism of carvedilol, resulting in increased plasma concentrations and cardiovascular effects. Monitor patients when hydroxychloroquine is started or stopped.

* ⬆ = Object drug increased. ⬇ = Object drug decreased.

Adverse Reactions

➤*Congestive heart failure:* Carvedilol has been evaluated for safety in congestive heart failure in more than 3,000 patients worldwide of whom 2,100 participated in placebo-controlled clinical trials. Approximately 60% of the total treated population received carvedilol for at least 6 months and 30% received carvedilol for at least 12 months. Both in US clinical trials comparing carvedilol in daily doses up to 100 mg (n = 765) to placebo (n = 437), and in a multinational clinical trial in severe heart failure (COPERNICUS) that compared carvedilol in daily doses up to 50 mg (n = 1,156) with placebo (n = 1,133), discontinuation rates for adverse experiences were similar in carvedilol and placebo patients. In these databases, the only cause of discontinuation greater than 1%, and occurring more often on carvedilol was dizziness (1.3% on carvedilol, 0.6% on placebo in the COPERNICUS trial).

The following table shows adverse reactions reported in patients with mild to moderate heart failure enrolled in US placebo-controlled clinical trials, and with severe heart failure enrolled in the COPERNICUS trial. Shown are adverse events that occurred more frequently in drug-treated patients than placebo-treated patients with an incidence of greater than 3% in patients treated with carvedilol regardless of causality. Median study medication exposure was 6.3 months for both carvedilol and placebo patients in the trials of mild to moderate heart failure, and 10.4 months in the trial of severe heart failure patients.

Carvedilol Adverse Reactions (% Occurrence)

Adverse reactions	Mild to moderate HF Carvedilol (n = 765)	Mild to moderate HF Placebo (n = 437)	Severe heart failure Carvedilol (n = 1,156)	Severe heart failure Placebo (n = 1,133)
Cardiovascular				
Angina pectoris	2%	3%	6%	4%
Bradycardia	9%	1%	10%	3%
Hypotension	9%	3%	14%	8%
Syncope	3%	3%	8%	5%
CNS				
Dizziness	32%	19%	24%	17%
Headache	8%	7%	5%	3%
GI				
Diarrhea	12%	6%	5%	3%
Nausea	9%	5%	4%	3%
Vomiting	6%	4%	1%	2%
Metabolic				
BUN increased	6%	5%	-	-
Hypercholesterolemia	4%	3%	1%	1%
Hyperglycemia	12%	8%	5%	3%
NPN increased	6%	5%	-	-
Peripheral edema	2%	1%	7%	6%
Weight increase	10%	7%	12%	11%
Musculoskeletal				
Arthralgia	6%	5%	1%	1%
Respiratory				
Increased cough	8%	9%	5%	4%
Rales	4%	4%	4%	2%
Special senses				
Abnormal vision	5%	2%	-	-
Miscellaneous				
Asthenia	7%	7%	11%	9%
Dependent edema	4%	2%	-	-
Digoxin level increased	5%	4%	2%	1%
Fatigue	24%	22%	-	-
Generalized edema	5%	3%	6%	5%

CARVEDILOL — ORAL

Cardiac failure and dyspnea were also reported in these studies, but the rates were equal or greater in patients who received placebo.

➤*Other adverse reactions:* The following adverse reactions were reported with a frequency of greater than 1% but less than or equal to 3% and more frequently with carvedilol in US placebo-controlled trials in patients with mild to moderate heart failure, or in patients with severe heart failure in the COPERNICUS trial.

Cardiovascular – Fluid overload, postural hypotension, aggravated angina pectoris, AV block, palpitation, hypertension.

CNS – Hypesthesia, vertigo, paresthesia.

GI – Melena, periodontitis.

GU –
Male: Impotence.

Hematologic – Prothrombin decreased, purpura, thrombocytopenia.

Hepatic – ALT increased, AST increased.

Immunologic – Infection.

Metabolic/Nutritional – Hyperuricemia, hypoglycemia, hyponatremia, increased alkaline phosphatase, glycosuria, hypervolemia, diabetes mellitus, increased GGT, weight loss, hyperkalemia, increased creatinine.

Musculoskeletal – Muscle cramps.

Psychiatric – Somnolence.

Renal – Renal insufficiency, albuminuria, hematuria.

Special senses – Blurred vision.

Miscellaneous – Allergy, malaise, hypovolemia, fever, leg edema.

The following adverse reaction has been reported in postmarketing experience: Reports of aplastic anemia have been rare and received only when carvedilol was administered concomitantly with other medications associated with the event.

➤*Left ventricular dysfunction following myocardial infarction:* The most common adverse reactions reported with carvedilol in the CAPRICORN trial were consistent with the profile of the drug in the US heart failure trials and the COPERNICUS trial. The only additional adverse events reported in CAPRICORN in greater than 3% of the patients and more commonly on carvedilol were dyspnea, anemia, and lung edema. The following adverse events were reported with a frequency of greater than 1% but less than or equal to 3% and more frequently with carvedilol: Flu syndrome, cerebrovascular accident, peripheral vascular disorder, hypotonia, depression, gastrointestinal pain, arthritis, and gout. The overall rates of discontinuations due to adverse events were similar in both groups of patients. In this database, the only cause of discontinuation greater than 1%, and occurring more often on carvedilol was hypotension (1.5% on carvedilol, 0.2% on placebo).

➤*Hypertension:*

Adverse Reactions in US Placebo-Controlled Hypertension Trials Incidence ≥ 1%, Regardless of Causality

	Adverse reactions	
	Carvedilol (n = 1,142)	Placebo (n = 462)
	% occurrence	% occurrence
Cardiovascular		
Bradycardia	2%	-
Postural hypotension	2%	-
Peripheral edema	1%	-
CNS		
Dizziness	6%	5%
Insomnia	2%	1%
GI		
Diarrhea	2%	1%
Hematologic		
Thrombocytopenia	1%	-
Metabolic		
Hypertriglyceridemia	1%	-

Dyspnea and fatigue were also reported in these studies, but the rates were equal or greater in patients who received placebo.

➤*Possibly or probably drug-related adverse reactions (incidence greater than 0.1% to less than or equal to 1%):* The following adverse reactions were reported as possibly or probably related in worldwide open or controlled trials with carvedilol in patients with hypertension or congestive heart failure.

Cardiovascular – Peripheral ischemia, tachycardia.

CNS – Hypokinesia.

Dermatologic – Pruritus, erythematous rash, maculopapular rash, psoriaform rash, photosensitivity reaction.

GI – Bilirubinemia, increased hepatic enzymes (0.2% of hypertension patients and 0.4% of congestive heart failure patients were discontinued from therapy because of increases in hepatic enzymes.

GU – Decreased libido (men).

Hematologic – Anemia, leukopenia.

Metabolic/Nutritional – Hypokalemia, hypertriglyceridemia.

Psychiatric – Nervousness, sleep disorder, aggravated depression, impaired concentration, abnormal thinking, paroniria, emotional lability.

Respiratory – Asthma.

See Contraindications for more information.

Special senses – Tinnitus.

Miscellaneous – Dry mouth, increased sweating, increased micturition frequency. The following reactions were reported in less than or equal to 0.1% of patients and are potentially important:

Complete AV block, bundle branch block, myocardial ischemia, cerebrovascular disorder, convulsions, migraine, neuralgia, paresis, anaphylactoid reaction, alopecia, exfoliative dermatitis, amnesia, GI hemorrhage, bronchospasm, pulmonary edema, decreased hearing, respiratory alkalosis, increased BUN, decreased HDL, pancytopenia, and atypical lymphocytes.

Overdosage

➤*Symptoms:* Overdosage may cause severe hypotension, bradycardia, cardiac insufficiency, cardiogenic shock, and cardiac arrest. Respiratory problems, bronchospasms, vomiting, lapses of consciousness, and generalized seizures may also occur.

Cases of overdosage with carvedilol alone or in combination with other drugs have been reported. Quantities ingested in some cases exceeded 1000 mg. Symptoms experienced included low blood pressure and heart rate. Standard supportive treatment was provided and individuals recovered.

➤*Treatment:* The patient should be placed in a supine position and, where necessary, kept under observation and treated under intensive-care conditions. Gastric lavage or pharmacologically induced emesis may be used shortly after ingestion. The following agents may be administered

For excessive bradycardia – Atropine, 2 mg IV.

To support cardiovascular function – Glucagon, 5 to 10 mg IV rapidly over 30 seconds, followed by a continuous infusion of 5 mg/hour; sympathomimetics (dobutamine, isoprenaline, adrenaline) at doses according to body weight and effect.

If peripheral vasodilation dominates, it may be necessary to administer adrenaline or noradrenaline with continuous monitoring of circulatory conditions. For therapy-resistant bradycardia, pacemaker therapy should be performed. For bronchospasm, β-sympathomimetics (as aerosol or IV) or aminophylline IV should be given. In the event of seizures, slow IV injection of diazepam or clonazepam is recommended.

In the event of severe intoxication where there are symptoms of shock, treatment with antidotes must be continued for a sufficiently long period of time consistent with the 7- to 10-hour half-life of carvedilol.

Patient Information

Patients taking carvedilol should not interrupt or discontinue using carvedilol without a physician's advice.

Congestive heart failure patients should consult their physician if they experience signs or symptoms of worsening heart failure such as weight gain or increasing shortness of breath. They may experience a drop in blood pressure when standing, resulting in dizziness and, rarely, fainting. Patients should sit or lie down when these symptoms of lowered blood pressure occur.

If patients experience dizziness or fatigue, they should avoid driving or hazardous tasks.

They should consult a physician if they experience dizziness or faintness, in case the dosage should be adjusted.

They should take carvedilol with food.

Diabetic patients should report any changes in blood sugar levels to their physician.

Contact lens wearers may experience decreased lacrimation.

METHYLDOPA AND METHYLDOPATE HYDROCHLORIDE

Rx	**Methyldopa** (Various, eg, Ivax, Mylan)	**Tablets:** 250 mg methyldopa	May contain EDTA. In 100s, 500s, 1000s, and UD 100s.
Rx	**Methyldopa** (Various, eg, Ivax, Mylan)	**Tablets:** 500 mg methyldopa	May contain EDTA. In 100s, 500s, and UD 100s.
Rx	**Methyldopate HCl** (Various, eg, Abbott, American Regent)	**Injection:** 50 mg methyldopate HCl/mL	May contain sulfites,[1] EDTA. In single-dose vials and *ADD-vantage* vials.

[1] Refer to individual product package insert for sulfite content.

METHYLDOPA AND METHYLDOPATE HYDROCHLORIDE

Indications

➤*Hypertension:* Treatment of hypertension.

➤*Hypertensive crises:* Methyldopate may be used to initiate treatment of hypertensive crises; however, because of its slow onset of action, other agents may be preferred for rapid reduction of blood pressure (BP).

➤*Unlabeled uses:* Hypertension in pregnancy.

Administration and Dosage

➤*Oral:*

Adults –

Initial therapy: 250 mg 2 or 3 times/day in the first 48 hours. Adjust dosage at intervals of not less than 2 days until an adequate response is achieved. To minimize sedation, increase dosage in the evening. By adjustment of dosage, morning hypotension may be prevented without sacrificing control of afternoon blood pressure.

Maintenance therapy: 500 mg to 2 g/day in 2 to 4 doses. The maximum recommended daily dosage is 3 g. Once an effective dosage range is attained, a smooth blood pressure response occurs in most patients in 12 to 24 hours.

Children – Individualize dosage. Initial oral dosage is based on 10 mg/kg/day in 2 to 4 doses. The maximum daily dosage is 65 mg/kg or 3 g, whichever is less.

Concomitant drug therapy – When methyldopa is given with antihypertensives other than thiazides, limit the initial dosage to 500 mg/day in divided doses; when added to a thiazide, the dosage of thiazide need not be changed.

➤*IV:* Add the desired dose to 100 mL of 5% dextrose or give in 5% dextrose injection in a concentration of 10 mg/mL. Administer over 30 to 60 minutes. When control has been obtained, substitute oral therapy starting with the same parenteral dosage schedule.

Adults – 250 to 500 mg every 6 hours as required (maximum 1 g every 6 hours).

Children – 20 to 40 mg/kg/day in divided doses every 6 hours. The maximum daily dosage is 65 mg/kg or 3 g, whichever is less.

➤*Tolerance:* Tolerance may occur, usually between the second and third month of therapy. Adding a diuretic or increasing the dosage of methyldopa frequently restores blood pressure control. A thiazide is recommended if therapy was not started with a thiazide or if effective control of blood pressure cannot be maintained on 2 g/day methyldopa.

➤*Discontinuation:* Methyldopa has a relatively short duration of action; therefore, withdrawal is followed by return of hypertension, usually within 48 hours. This is not complicated by a overshoot of BP.

➤*Renal function impairment:* Methyldopa is largely excreted by the kidneys; patients with impaired renal function may respond to smaller doses.

➤*Storage/Stability:* Store tablets and vials at controlled room temperature (15° to 30°C [59° to 86°F]). Dispense tablets in a well-closed container; use child-resistant closure.

Actions

➤*Pharmacology:* The mechanism of action of methyldopa has not been conclusively demonstrated but is probably because of the drug's metabolism to alpha-methylnorepinephrine, which lowers arterial pressure by the stimulation of central inhibitory alpha-adrenergic receptors, false neurotransmission, and/or reduction of plasma renin activity. Methyldopa causes a net reduction in tissue concentrations of serotonin, dopamine, norepinephrine, and epinephrine.

Methyldopa reduces standing and supine BP. It usually produces highly effective lowering of supine pressure with infrequent symptomatic postural hypotension. Exercise hypotension and diurnal BP variations rarely occur.

Methyldopate hydrochloride, the ethyl ester of methyldopa hydrochloride, is pharmacologically equivalent.

➤*Pharmacokinetics:*

Absorption/Distribution – Following oral administration, methyldopa is variably absorbed. The mean bioavailability is approximately 50%. Methyldopa crosses the blood-brain barrier and is converted in the CNS to active alpha-methylnoradrenaline. Methyldopa crosses the placental barrier and appears in cord blood and breast milk. A decrease in BP occurs within 4 to 6 hours following IV or oral administration and lasts 10 to 16 hours or 12 to 24 hours, respectively.

Metabolism/Excretion – Methyldopa is extensively metabolized. Approximately 17% of a dose of methyldopate HCl appears in plasma as free methyldopa. The average T_{max} is 2 hours. The total volume of distribution is about 0.6 L/kg. Approximately 70% (oral) and approximately 49% (IV) of the drug that is absorbed is excreted in the urine as methyldopa and its mono-O-sulfate conjugate. The renal clearance is approximately 130 mL/min (oral) and approximately 156 mL/min (IV) in healthy subjects and is diminished in renal insufficiency. After oral doses, excretion is essentially complete in 36 hours. Biphasic elimination occurs after IV and oral administration; the half-life of the alpha-phase is approximately 0.21 hours and the beta-phase approximately 1.28 hours in healthy subjects. Methyldopa is less than 20% bound to plasma proteins. The drug is removed by dialysis.

Contraindications

Active hepatic disease, such as acute hepatitis or active cirrhosis; if previous methyldopa therapy has been associated with liver disorders; coadministration with monoamine oxidase inhibitors (MAOIs); hypersensitivity to any component of these formulations, including sulfites.

Warnings

➤*Positive Coombs' test/hemolytic anemia:* It is important to recognize that a positive Coombs' test, hemolytic anemia, and liver disorders may occur with methyldopa therapy. The rare occurrences of hemolytic anemia or liver disorders could lead to potentially fatal complications unless properly recognized and managed.

With prolonged therapy, 10% to 20% of patients develop a positive direct Coombs' test, usually between 6 and 12 months of therapy. The lowest incidence reported was at a dosage of 1 g/day or less. This is associated rarely with hemolytic anemia, which could lead to potentially fatal complications and is difficult to predict. Prior existence or development of a positive direct Coombs' test is not a contraindication to methyldopa, but if it develops during therapy, determine whether hemolytic anemia exists and whether the positive Coombs' test may be a problem. For example, in addition to a positive direct Coombs' test there is less often a positive indirect Coombs' test that may interfere with cross-matching of blood.

See Precautions for more information.

When methyldopa produces a positive Coombs' test alone or with hemolytic anemia, the red cell is usually coated with IgG gamma globulin. The positive Coombs' test may not revert to normal until weeks to months after methyldopa is stopped.

➤*Blood transfusions:* Should the need for transfusion arise in a patient receiving methyldopa, perform both a direct and indirect Coombs' test. In the absence of hemolytic anemia, usually only the direct Coombs' test will be positive. A positive direct Coombs' test alone will not interfere with typing or cross-matching. If the indirect Coombs' test is also positive, problems may arise in the major cross-match and the assistance of a hematologist or transfusion expert will be needed.

➤*Edema/Weight gain:* Some patients taking methyldopa experience clinical edema or weight gain, which may be controlled by use of a diuretic. Do not continue methyldopa if edema progresses or signs of heart failure appear.

➤*Hepatic toxicity:* Fever has occasionally occurred within the first 3 weeks of therapy, sometimes associated with eosinophilia or abnormalities in 1 or more liver function tests (eg, alkaline phosphatase, AST, ALT, bilirubin, prothrombin time). Jaundice with or without fever may occur, usually within the first 2 to 3 months of therapy. In some patients, the findings are consistent with cholestasis. In others, the findings are consistent with hepatitis and hepatocellular injury. Fatal hepatic necrosis has been reported rarely. These hepatic changes may represent hypersensitivity reactions. If fever, abnormalities in liver function tests or jaundice appear, discontinue therapy; temperature and abnormalities in liver function revert to normal when the drug is discontinued. Do not reinstitute methyldopa in such patients.

The incidence of severe cytotoxic injury is estimated to be less than 0.1% to 0.5%.

➤*Hematologic disorders:* Rarely, a reversible reduction of the white blood cell (WBC) count with a primary effect on granulocytes has been seen but promptly returns to normal upon drug discontinuation. Rare cases of granulocytopenia have been reported. WBC returned to normal after drug discontinuation. Reversible thrombocytopenia occurs rarely.

➤*Renal function impairment:* Methyldopa and its metabolites accumulate in renal failure. There is a marked accumulation of unidentified metabolites in renal failure patients, which may explain the strong and prolonged hypotensive action of methyldopa in these patients.

Hypertension has recurred occasionally after dialysis in patients given methyldopa because the drug is removed by this procedure.

➤*Hepatic function impairment:* Use with caution in patients with previous liver disease or dysfunction.

➤*Elderly:* Syncope in older patients may be related to an increased sensitivity and advanced arteriosclerotic vascular disease. This may be avoided with lower doses.

➤*Pregnancy:* *Category B* (oral). *Category C* (IV). Methyldopa crosses the placenta and achieves fetal concentrations similar to the maternal serum. No unusual adverse reactions or obvious teratogenic effects have been reported despite rather wide use during pregnancy. Neonates born to mothers receiving methyldopa have demonstrated a decreased systolic blood pressure of 4 to 5 mm Hg for 2 days after delivery, compared with controls.

Published reports of the use of methyldopa during all trimesters indicate that if this drug is used during pregnancy, the possibility of fetal harm appears remote. Use only when clearly needed and when potential benefits outweigh the potential hazards to the fetus.

➤*Lactation:* Methyldopa is excreted in breast milk in small amounts. After 750 to 2,000 mg/day, milk levels of free and conjugated methyldopa ranged from 0.1 to 0.9 mcg/mL. The American Academy of Pediatrics considers methyldopa to be compatible with breastfeeding.

➤*Children:* See Administration and Dosage.

Precautions

➤*Monitoring:* Blood count, Coombs' tests, and liver function tests are recommended before initiating therapy and at periodic intervals. Perform periodic determinations of hepatic function, particularly during the first 6 to 12 weeks of therapy or when an unexplained fever occurs.

METHYLDOPA AND METHYLDOPATE HYDROCHLORIDE

➤*Paradoxical pressor response:* This has been reported with IV administration of methyldopate HCl.

➤*Involuntary choreoathetotic movements:* Involuntary choreoathetotic movements have been observed rarely in patients with severe bilateral cerebrovascular disease. Should these occur, discontinue methyldopa therapy.

➤*Sedation:* Usually transient, sedation may occur during initial therapy or whenever the dose is increased.

➤*Urine discoloration:* Rarely, when urine is exposed to air after voiding, it may darken because of breakdown of methyldopa or its metabolites.

➤*Sulfite sensitivity:* Some of these products contain sulfites that may cause allergic-type reactions, including anaphylactic symptoms and life-threatening or less severe asthmatic episodes in certain susceptible persons. The overall prevalence of sulfite sensitivity in the general population is unknown and probably low; it is seen more frequently in asthmatic than in nonasthmatic people.

Drug Interactions

Methyldopa Drug Interactions

Precipitant drug	Object drug*		Description
Methyldopa	Anesthetics	↑	Reduced doses of anesthetics may be required. Hypotension during anesthesia can be controlled by vasopressors because adrenergic receptors remain sensitive.
Methyldopa	Haloperidol	↑	Methyldopa may potentiate the antipsychotic effects of haloperidol or the combination may produce psychosis.
Methyldopa	Levodopa	↑	Blood-pressure-lowering effects of methyldopa may be potentiated by levodopa. Central effects of levodopa in Parkinson's disease may be potentiated by methyldopa.
Levodopa	Methyldopa	↑	
Methyldopa	Lithium	↑	Lithium toxicity characterized by GI symptoms, polyuria, muscle weakness, lethargy, and tremor has been reported following methyldopa coadministration.
Methyldopa	MAOIs	↑	Metabolites of methyldopa stimulate release of endogenous catecholamines that are usually metabolized by MAOIs, thereby leading to excessive sympathetic stimulation. Coadministration is contraindicated.
Methyldopa	Phenothiazines	↑	Serious elevations in blood pressure may occur.
Methyldopa	Sympathomimetics	↑	Methyldopa may potentiate the pressor effects of sympathomimetics and lead to hypertension.
Beta-blockers, nonselective (eg, propranolol)	Methyldopa	↑	Nonselective beta blockers and methyldopa rarely may cause a hypertensive crisis.
Ferrous sulfate or gluconate	Methyldopa	↓	A decrease in the bioavailability of methyldopa when it is ingested with ferrous sulfate or ferrous gluconate has been demonstrated.

* ↑ = Object drug increased. ↓ = Object drug decreased.

➤*Drug/Lab test interactions:* Methyldopa may interfere with tests for the following: Urinary uric acid by phosphotungstate method; serum creatinine by alkaline picrate method; AST by colorimetric methods. Interference with spectrophotometric methods for AST analysis is not reported.

Because methyldopa causes fluorescence in urine samples at the same wave lengths as catecholamines, falsely high levels of urinary catecholamines may occur and will interfere with the diagnosis of pheochromocytoma. Methyldopa does not interfere with measurement of vanillylmandelic acid (VMA) by methods converting VMA to vanillin.

Adverse Reactions

➤*Cardiovascular:* Bradycardia; prolonged carotid sinus hypersensitivity; aggravation of angina pectoris; CHF; paradoxical pressor response with IV use; pericarditis; myocarditis; vasculitis; orthostatic hypotension; edema and weight gain usually relieved by a diuretic. Discontinue methyldopa if edema progresses or signs of heart failure appear.

➤*CNS:* Sedation, usually transient, may occur during initial therapy or whenever the dose is increased; headache, asthenia, or weakness (may be early, transient symptoms); dizziness; lightheadedness; symptoms of cerebrovascular insufficiency; paresthesias; parkinsonism; Bell palsy; decreased mental acuity; involuntary choreoathetotic movements; psychic disturbances, including nightmares and reversible mild psychoses or depression.

➤*Dermatologic:* Rash; toxic epidermal necrolysis.

➤*Endocrine:* Breast enlargement; gynecomastia; lactation; hyperprolactinemia; amenorrhea.

➤*GI:* Nausea; vomiting; distention; constipation; flatus; diarrhea; colitis; dry mouth; sore or "black" tongue; pancreatitis; sialoadenitis.

➤*GU:* Impotence; decreased libido.

➤*Hematologic:* Positive Coombs' test, hemolytic anemia (see Warnings); bone marrow depression; leukopenia; granulocytopenia; thrombocytopenia; eosinophilia; positive tests for antinuclear antibody, lupus erythematosus cells, and rheumatoid factor.

➤*Hepatic:* Abnormal liver function tests; jaundice; hepatitis, liver disorders (see Warnings).

➤*Hypersensitivity:* Drug-related fever; lupus-like syndrome.

➤*Miscellaneous:* Nasal stuffiness; rise in BUN; arthralgia with or without joint swelling; myalgia.

Overdosage

➤*Symptoms:* Sedation; acute hypotension; weakness; bradycardia; dizziness; lightheadedness; constipation; distention; flatus; diarrhea; nausea; vomiting and other responses attributable to brain and GI malfunction.

➤*Treatment:* Employ gastric lavage or emesis and general supportive measures when ingestion is recent. When ingestion has been earlier, infusions may be helpful to promote urinary excretion. Otherwise, management includes special attention to cardiac rate and output, blood volume, electrolyte imbalance, paralytic ileus, urinary function, and cerebral activity. Refer to General Management of Acute Overdosage. Sympathomimetic drugs (eg, norepinephrine, epinephrine, metaraminol bitartrate) may be indicated. In severe cases, consider hemodialysis.

CLONIDINE HYDROCHLORIDE — ORAL

Rx	**Clonidine** (Various, eg, Geneva, Mylan, UDL)	**Tablets:** 0.1 mg	In 100s, 500s, 1000s and UD 100s.
Rx	**Catapres** (Boehringer Ingelheim)		(BI-6). Tan, scored. In 100s, 1000s and UD 100s.
Rx	**Clonidine** (Various, eg, Geneva, Mylan, UDL)	**Tablets:** 0.2 mg	In 100s, 500s, 1000s and UD 100s.
Rx	**Catapres** (Boehringer Ingelheim)		(BI-7). Orange, scored. In 100s, 1000s and UD 100s.
Rx	**Clonidine** (Various, eg, Geneva, Mylan, UDL)	**Tablets:** 0.3 mg	In 100s and UD 100s.
Rx	**Catapres** (Boehringer Ingelheim)		(BI-11). Peach, scored. In 100s.

CLONIDINE HYDROCHLORIDE — ORAL

For complete prescribing information, refer to the Antihypertensives Treatment Guidelines in the Appendix.

Indications

Treatment of hypertension. Clonidine may be employed alone or concomitantly with other antihypertensive agents.

➤*Unlabeled uses:* Reduction of hot flashes.

Alcohol withdrawal – 300 to 600 mcg every 6 hours.

Atrial fibrillation – 75 mcg oral single dose or twice daily; alone or with digoxin.

Attention deficit hyperactivity disorder – 5 mcg/kg/day for 8 weeks.

Constitutional growth delay in children – 37.5 to 150 mcg/m²/day.

Gilles de la Tourette's syndrome – 150 to 200 mcg/day.

Hyperhidrosis – 250 mcg 3 to 5 times/day.

CLONIDINE HYDROCHLORIDE — ORAL

Hypertensive "urgencies" (diastolic more than 120 mmHg) – Initially 100 to 200 mcg, followed by 50 to 100 mcg/hour to a maximum of 800 mcg.

Methadone/opiate detoxification – 15 to 16 mcg/kg/day.

Pheochromocytoma diagnosis (overnight clonidine suppression test) – 300 mcg.

Postherpetic neuralgia – 200 mcg/day.

Psychosis in schizophrenic patients – Less than or equal to 900 mcg/day.

Restless leg syndrome – 100 to 300 mcg/day; up to 900 mcg/day.

Ulcerative colitis – 300 mcg 3 times a day.

Unlabeled route of administation – Sublingual clonidine, using a dosage of 200 to 400 mcg/day, may be effective in hypertensive paients unable to take oral medication. Onset ocurs within 30 to 60 minutes and blood pressure appears to be maintained on a twice-daily regimen.

Administration and Dosage

➤*Adults:* The dose of clonidine hydrochloride must be adjusted according to the patient's individual blood pressure response. The following is a general guide to its administration.

Initial dose – 0.1 mg tablet twice daily (morning and bedtime). Elderly patients may benefit from a lower initial dose.

➤*Maintenance dose:* Further increments of 0.1 mg per day may be made at weekly intervals if necessary until the desired response is achieved. Taking the larger portion of the oral daily dose at bedtime may minimize transient adjustment effects of dry mouth and drowsiness. The therapeutic doses most commonly employed have ranged from 0.2 mg to 0.6 mg per day given in divided doses. Studies have indicated that 2.4 mg is the maximum effective daily dose, but doses as high as this have rarely been employed.

➤*Renal function impairment:* Dosage must be adjusted according to the degree of impairment, and patients should be carefully monitored. Since only a minimal amount of clonidine is removed during routine hemodialysis, there is no need to give supplemental clonidine following dialysis.

➤*Storage/Stability:* Store below 30°C (86°F). Dispense in tight, light-resistant container.

Actions

➤*Pharmacology:* Clonidine stimulates alpha-adrenoreceptors in the brain stem. This action results in reduced sympathetic outflow from the CNS and in decreases in peripheral resistance, renal vascular resistance, heart rate, and blood pressure. Clonidine hydrochloride acts relatively rapidly. The patient's blood pressure declines within 30 to 60 minutes after an oral dose, the maximum decrease occurring within 2 to 4 hours. Renal blood flow and glomerular filtration rate remain essentially unchanged. Normal postural reflexes are intact; therefore, orthostatic symptoms are mild and infrequent.

Acute studies with clonidine hydrochloride in humans have demonstrated a moderate reduction (15% to 20%) of cardiac output in the supine position with no change in the peripheral resistance: at a 45° tilt there is a smaller reduction in cardiac output and a decrease of peripheral resistance. During long-term therapy, cardiac output tends to return to control values, while peripheral resistance remains decreased. Slowing of the pulse rate has been observed in most patients given clonidine, but the drug does not alter normal hemodynamic response to exercise.

Tolerance to the antihypertensive effect may develop in some patients, necessitating a reevaluation of therapy.

Other studies in patients have provided evidence of a reduction in plasma renin activity and in the excretion of aldosterone and catecholamines. The exact relationship of these pharmacologic actions to the antihypertensive effect of clonidine has not been fully elucidated.

Clonidine acutely stimulates growth hormone release in both children and adults, but does not produce a chronic elevation of growth hormone with long-term use.

➤*Pharmacokinetics:* The plasma level of clonidine peaks in ≈ 3 to 5 hours and the plasma half-life ranges from 12 to 16 hours. The half-life increases up to 41 hours in patients with severe impairment of renal function. Following oral administration about 40% to 60% of the absorbed dose is recovered in the urine as unchanged drug in 24 hours. About 50% of the absorbed dose is metabolized in the liver.

Contraindications

Known hypersensitivity to clonidine.

Warnings

➤*Withdrawal:* Patients should be instructed not to discontinue therapy without consulting their physician. Sudden cessation of clonidine treatment has, in some cases, resulted in symptoms such as nervousness, agitation, headache, and tremor accompanied or followed by a rapid rise in blood pressure and elevated catecholamine concentrations in the plasma. The likelihood of such reactions to discontinuation of clonidine therapy appears to be greater after administration of higher doses or continuation of concomitant betablocker treatment; special caution is therefore advised in these situations. Rare instances of hypertensive encephalopathy, cerebrovascular accidents and death have been reported after clonidine withdrawal. When discontinuing therapy with clonidine hydrochloride, the physician should reduce the dose gradually over 2 to 4 days to avoid withdrawal symptomatology.

An excessive rise in blood pressure following discontinuation of clonidine hydrochloride therapy can be reversed by administration of oral clonidine hydrochloride or by IV phentolamine. If therapy is to be discontinued in patients receiving a beta-blocker and clonidine concurrently, the beta-blocker should be withdrawn several days before the gradual discontinuation of clonidine hydrochloride.

➤*Hypersensitivity reactions:* In patients who have developed localized contact sensitization to clonidine, continuation of transdermal clonidine hydrochloride or substitution of oral clonidine hydrochloride therapy may be associated with the development of a generalized skin rash.

In patients who develop an allergic reaction to transdermal clonidine hydrochloride, substitution of oral clonidine hydrochloride may also elicit an allergic reaction (including generalized rash, urticaria, or angioedema).

➤*Fertility impairment:* Fertility of male or female rats was unaffected by clonidine doses as high as 150 mcg/kg (approximately 3 times MRDHD). In a separate experiment, fertility of female rats appeared to be affected at dose levels of 500 to 2000 mcg/kg (10 to 40 times the oral MRDHD on a mg/kg basis; 2 to 8 times the MRDHD on a mg/m^2 basis).

➤*Pregnancy: Category C.*

Teratogenic –

In rats, doses as low as ⅓ the oral MRDHD (1⁄15 the MRDHD on a mg/m^2 basis) of clonidine were associated with increased resorptions in a study in which dams were treated continuously from 2 months prior to mating. Increased resorptions were not associated with treatment at the same time or at higher dose levels (up to 3 times the oral MRDHD) when the dams were treated on gestation days 6 to 15. Increases in resorption were observed at much higher dose levels (40 times the oral MRDHD on a mg/kg basis; 4 to 8 times the MRDHD on a mg/m^2 basis) in mice and rats treated on gestation days 1 to 14 (lowest dose employed in the study was 500 mcg/kg).

No adequate, well-controlled studies have been conducted in pregnant women. Because animal reproduction studies are not always predictive of human response, this drug should be used during pregnancy only if clearly needed.

➤*Lactation:* As clonidine hydrochloride is excreted in human milk, caution should be exercised when clonidine hydrochloride is administered to a breast-feeding woman.

➤*Children:* Safety and efficacy in pediatric patients below the age of 12 years have not been established.

Because children commonly have GI illnesses that lead to vomiting, they may be particularly susceptible to hypertensive episodes resulting from abrupt inability to take medication.

Precautions

➤*Perioperative use:* Administration of clonidine hydrochloride should be continued to within 4 hours of surgery and resumed as soon as possible thereafter. Blood pressure should be carefully monitored during surgery and additional measures to control blood pressure should be available if required.

➤*Ophthalmologic effects:* In several studies with oral clonidine hydrochloride, a dose-dependent increase in the incidence and severity of spontaneous retinal degeneration was seen in albino rats treated for 6 months or longer. Tissue distribution studies in dogs and monkeys showed a concentration of clonidine in the choroid.

In combination with amitriptyline, clonidine hydrochloride administration led to the development of corneal lesions in rats within 5 days.

➤*Special risk:* Clonidine hydrochloride should be used with caution in patients with severe coronary insufficiency, conduction disturbances, recent myocardial infarction, cerebrovascular disease or chronic renal failure.

➤*Hazardous tasks:* Patients who engage in potentially hazardous activities, such as operating machinery or driving, should be advised of a possible sedative effect of clonidine. They should also be informed that this sedative effect may be increased by concomitant use of alcohol, barbiturates, or other sedating drugs.

Drug Interactions

Clonidine Drug Interactions

Precipitant drug	Object drug*		Description
Clonidine	Levodopa	⬇	The effectiveness of levodopa may be reduced.
Beta-adrenergic blocking agents	Clonidine	⬆	Attenuation or reversal of antihypertensive effect and potentially life-threatening increases in blood pressure.
Prazosin	Clonidine	⬇	The antihypertensive effectiveness of clonidine may be decreased.
Tricyclic antidepressants	Clonidine	⬇	Tricyclic antidepressants may block antihypertensive effects of clonidine and possibly life-threatening elevations in blood pressure may occur.
Verapamil	Clonidine	⬆	Synergistic pharmacologic and toxic effects, possibly causing atrioventricular (AV) block and severe hypotension.

* ⬆ = Object drug increased. ⬇ = Object drug decreased.

CLONIDINE HYDROCHLORIDE — ORAL

➤*Amitriptyline:* Amitriptyline in combination with clonidine enhances the manifestation of corneal lesions in rats.

➤*Sedating drugs:* Clonidine may potentiate the CNS-depressive effects of alcohol, barbiturates or other sedating drugs. If a patient receiving clonidine hydrochloride is also taking tricyclic antidepressants, the hypotensive effect of clonidine may be reduced, necessitating an increase in the clonidine dose.

➤*Digitalis, calcium channel blockers, beta-blockers:* Due to a potential for additive effects such as bradycardia and AV block, caution is warranted in patients receiving clonidine concomitantly with agents known to affect sinus node function or AV nodal conduction (eg digitalis, calcium channel blockers, beta-blockers).

Adverse Reactions

Most adverse reactions are mild and tend to diminish with continued therapy. The most frequent (which appear to be dose related) are dry mouth, occurring in about 40 of 100 patients; drowsiness, about 33 in 100; dizziness, about 16 in 100; constipation and sedation, each about 10 in 100.

The following less frequent adverse experiences have also been reported in patients receiving clonidine hydrochloride USP, but in many cases patients were receiving concomitant medication and a causal relationship has not been established.

➤*Cardiovascular:* Orthostatic symptoms, about 3 in 100 patients; palpitations and tachycardia, and bradycardia, each about 5 in 1000. Syncope, Raynaud's phenomenon, congestive heart failure, and electrocardiographic abnormalities (ie, sinus node arrest, functional bradycardia, high degree AV block and arrhythmias) have been reported rarely. Rare cases of sinus bradycardia and atrioventricular block have been reported, both with and without the use of concomitant digitalis.

➤*CNS:* Nervousness and agitation, about 3 in 100 patients; mental depression, about 1 in 100 and insomnia, about 5 in 1000. Other behavioral changes, vivid dreams or nightmares, restlessness, anxiety, visual and auditory hallucinations and delirium have rarely been reported.

➤*Dermatologic:* Rash, about 1 in 100 patients; pruritus, about 7 in 1000; hives, angioneurotic edema and urticaria, about 5 in 1000; alopecia, about 2 in 1000.

➤*GI:* Nausea and vomiting, about 5 in 100 patients; anorexia and malaise, each about 1 in 100; mild transient abnormalities in liver function tests, about 1 in 100; hepatitis, parotitis, constipation, pseudo-obstruction, and abdominal pain, rarely.

➤*GU:* Decreased sexual activity, impotence and loss of libido, about 3 in 100 patients; nocturia, about 1 in 100; difficulty in micturition, about 2 in 1000; urinary retention, about 1 in 1000.

➤*Hematologic:* Thrombocytopenia, rarely.

➤*Metabolic:* Weight gain, about 1 in 100 patients; gynecomastia, about 1 in 1000; transient elevation of blood glucose or serum creatine phosphokinase, rarely.

➤*Musculoskeletal:* Muscle or joint pain, about 6 in 1000 and leg cramps, about 3 in 1000.

➤*Ophthalmic:* Dryness of the eyes, burning of the eyes and blurred vision were reported.

➤*Special senses:* Dryness of the nasal mucosa was rarely reported.

➤*Miscellaneous:* Weakness, about 10 in 100 patients; fatigue, about 4 in 100; headache and withdrawal syndrome each about 1 in 100. Also reported were pallor; a weakly positive Coombs' test; increased sensitivity to alcohol; and fever.

Overdosage

➤*Symptoms:* Hypertension may develop early and may be followed by hypotension, bradycardia, respiratory depression, hypothermia, drowsiness, decreased or absent reflexes, weakness, irritability and miosis. The frequency of CNS depression may be higher in children than adults. Large overdoses may result in reversible cardiac conduction defects or dysrhythmias, apnea, coma and seizures. Signs and symptoms of overdose generally occur within 30 minutes to 2 hours after exposure. As little as 0.1 mg of clonidine has produced signs of toxicity in children.

The largest overdose reported to date involved a 28-year-old man who ingested 100 mg of clonidine hydrochloride powder. This patient developed hypertension followed by hypotension, bradycardia, apnea, hallucinations, semicoma, and premature ventricular contractions. The patient fully recovered after intensive treatment. Plasma clonidine levels were 60 ng/mL after 1 hour, 190 ng/mL after 1.5 hours, 370 ng/mL after 2 hours, and 120 ng/mL after 5.5 and 6.5 hours. In mice and rats, the oral LD_{50} of clonidine is 206 and 465 mg/kg, respectively.

➤*Treatment:* There is no specific antidote for clonidine overdosage. Clonidine overdosage may result in the rapid development of CNS depression; therefore, induction of vomiting with ipecac syrup is not recommended. Gastric lavage may be indicated following recent or large ingestions. Administration of activated charcoal or a cathartic may be beneficial. Supportive care may include atropine sulfate for bradycardia, IV fluids or vasopressor agents for hypotension and vasodilators for hypertension. Naloxone may be a useful adjunct for the management of clonidine-induced respiratory depression, hypotension or coma; blood pressure should be monitored because the administration of naloxone has occasionally resulted in paradoxical hypertension. Tolazoline administration has yielded inconsistent results and is not recommended as first-line therapy. Dialysis is not likely to significantly enhance the elimination of clonidine.

Patient Information

Patients should be cautioned against interruption of clonidine hydrochloride therapy without their physician's advice.

CLONIDINE HYDROCHLORIDE— TRANSDERMAL

	Product/Distributor	Release Rate (mg/24 h)	Surface Area (cm²)	Total Clonidine Content (mg)	How Supplied
Rx	**Catapres-TTS-1** (Boehringer Ingelheim)	0.1	3.5	2.5	Mineral oil. In 12s.
Rx	**Catapres-TTS-2** (Boehringer Ingelheim)	0.2	7	5	Mineral oil. In 12s.
Rx	**Catapres-TTS-3** (Boehringer Ingelheim)	0.3	10.5	7.5	Mineral oil. In 4s.

CLONIDINE — TRANSDERMAL

Indications

Treatment of hypertension. It may be employed alone or concomitantly with other antihypertensive agents.

➤*Unlabeled uses:*

Cyclosporine-associated nephrotoxicity – 100 to 200 mcg/day transdermal.

Diabetic diarrhea – 100 to 600 mcg every 12 hours or 300 mcg/24-hour patch (1 to 2 patches/week).

Hot flushes – 100 mcg/24–hour patch every 7 days.

Smoking cessation facilitation – 150 to 400 mcg/day or 200 mcg per 24–hour patch.

Administration and Dosage

Apply transdermal clonidine once every 7 days to a hairless area of intact skin on the upper outer arm or chest. Each new application of clonidine transdermal should be on a different skin site from the previous location. If the system loosens during 7-day wearing, the adhesive overlay should be applied directly over the system to ensure good adhesion. There have been rare reports of the need for patch changes prior to 7 days to maintain blood pressure control.

To initiate therapy, clonidine transdermal dosage should be titrated according to individual therapeutic requirements, starting with the 0.1 mg clonidine transdermal system. If after 1 or 2 weeks the desired reduction in blood pressure is not achieved, increase the dosage by adding another 0.1 mg clonidine transdermal system or changing to a larger system. An increase in dosage above two 0.3 mg clonidine transdermal systems is usually not associated with additional efficacy.

When substituting clonidine transdermal for oral clonidine or for other antihypertensive drugs, physicians should be aware that the antihypertensive effect of clonidine transdermal may not commence until 2 to 3 days after initial application. Therefore, gradual reduction of prior drug dosage is advised. Some or all previous antihypertensive treatment may have to be continued, particularly in patients with more severe forms of hypertension.

➤*Renal function impairment:* Dosage must be adjusted according to the degree of impairment, and patients should be carefully monitored. Since only a minimal amount of clonidine is removed during routine hemodialysis, there is no need to give supplemental clonidine following dialysis.

➤*Storage / Stability:* Store below 30°C (86°F).

Actions

➤*Pharmacology:* Clonidine stimulates alpha-adrenoreceptors in the brain stem. This action results in reduced sympathetic outflow from the central nervous system and in decreases in peripheral resistance, renal vascular resistance, heart rate, and blood pressure. Renal blood flow and glomerular filtration rate remain essentially unchanged. Normal postural reflexes are intact; therefore, orthostatic symptoms are mild and infrequent.

Acute studies with clonidine hydrochloride in humans have demonstrated a moderate reduction (15% to 20%) of cardiac output in the supine position with no change in the peripheral resistance; at a 45° tilt there is a smaller reduction in cardiac output and a decrease of peripheral resistance.

During long-term therapy, cardiac output tends to return to control values, while peripheral resistance remains decreased. Slowing of the pulse rate has been observed in most patients given clonidine, but the drug does not alter normal hemodynamic responses to exercise.

Tolerance to the antihypertensive effect may develop in some patients, necessitating a reevaluation of therapy.

Other studies in patients have provided evidence of a reduction in plasma resin activity and in the excretion of aldosterone and catecholamines. The exact relationship of these pharmacologic actions to the antihypertensive effect of clonidine has not been fully elucidated.

CLONIDINE — TRANSDERMAL

Clonidine acutely stimulates the release of growth hormone in children as well as adults but does not produce a chronic elevation of growth hormone with long-term use.

➤*Pharmacokinetics:* The plasma half-life of clonidine is 12.7 ± 7 hours. Following oral administration, about 40% to 60% of the absorbed dose is recovered in the urine as unchanged drug within 24 hours. The remainder of the absorbed dose is metabolized in the liver.

Contraindications

Hypersensitivity to clonidine or any component of the therapeutic system.

Warnings

➤*Withdrawal:* Patients should be instructed not to discontinue therapy without consulting their physician. Sudden cessation of clonidine treatment has, in some cases, resulted in symptoms such as nervousness, agitation, headache, and confusion accompanied or followed by a rapid rise in blood pressure and elevated catecholamine concentrations in the plasma. The likelihood of such reactions to discontinuation of clonidine therapy appears to be greater after administration of higher doses or continuation of concomitant betablocker treatment and special caution is therefore advised in these situations. Rare instances of hypertensive encephalopathy, cerebrovascular accidents and death have been reported after clonidine withdrawal. When discontinuing clonidine transdermal therapy, the physician should reduce the dose gradually over 2 to 4 days to avoid withdrawal symptomatology.

An excessive rise in blood pressure following discontinuation of clonidine transdermal therapy can be reversed by administration of oral clonidine hydrochloride or by intravenous phentolamine. If therapy is to be discontinued in patients receiving a betablocker and clonidine concurrently, the betablocker should be withdrawn several days before the gradual discontinuation of clonidine transdermal.

➤*Fertility impairment:* Fertility of male and female rats was unaffected by clonidine doses as high as 150 mcg/kg (≈ 3 times the MRDHD). In a separate experiment, fertility of female rats appeared to be affected at dose levels of 500 to 2000 mcg/kg (10 to 40 times the oral MRDHD on a mg/kg basis; 2 to 8 times the MRDHD on a mg/m^2 basis).

➤*Pregnancy:* *Category C.*

Teratogenic –

In rats, doses as low as ⅓ the oral MRDHD (1⁄15 the MRDHD on a mg/m^2 basis) of clonidine were associated with increased resorptions in a study in which dams were treated continuously from 2 months prior to mating. Increased resorptions were not associated with treatment at the same or at higher dose levels (up to 3 times the oral MRDHD) when the dams were treated on gestation days 6 to 15. Increases in resorption were observed at much higher dose levels (40 times the oral MRDHD on a mg/kg basis; 4 to 8 times the MRDHD on a mg/m^2 basis) in mice and rats treated on gestation days 1 to 14 (lowest dose employed in the study was 500 mcg/kg).

No adequate well-controlled studies have been conducted in pregnant women. Because animal reproduction studies are not always predictive of human response, this drug should be used during pregnancy only if clearly needed.

➤*Lactation:* As clonidine is excreted in human milk, caution should be exercised when clonidine transdermal is administered to a breast-feeding woman.

➤*Children:* Safety and effectiveness in pediatric patients below the age of 12 have not been established (see Withdrawal).

Precautions

➤*Skin rash:* In patients who have developed localized contact sensitization to clonidine transdermal, continuation of clonidine transdermal or substitution of oral clonidine hydrochloride therapy may be associated with development of a generalized skin rash.

In patients who develop an allergic reaction to clonidine transdermal, substitution of oral clonidine hydrochloride may also elicit an allergic reaction (including generalized rash, urticaria, or angioedema).

➤*Perioperative use:* Clonidine transdermal therapy should not be interrupted during the surgical period. Blood pressure should be carefully monitored during surgery and additional measures to control blood pressure should be available if required. Physicians considering starting clonidine transdermal therapy during the perioperative period must be aware that therapeutic plasma clonidine levels are not achieved until 2 to 3 days after initial application of clonidine transdermal (see Administration and Dosage).

➤*Defibrillation or cardioversion:* The transdermal clonidine systems should be removed before attempting defibrillation or cardioversion because of the potential for altered electrical conductivity which may increase the risk of arcing, a phenomenon associated with the use of defibrillators.

➤*Ophthalmologic effects:* In several studies with oral clonidine hydrochloride, a dose-dependent increase in the incidence and severity of spontaneous retinal degeneration was seen in albino rats treated for 6 months or longer. Tissue distribution studies in dogs and monkeys showed a concentration of clonidine in the choroid.

In view of the retinal degeneration seen in rats, eye examinations were performed during clinical trials in 908 patients before, and periodically after, the start of clonidine therapy. In 353 of these 908 patients, the eye examinations were carried out over periods of 24 months or longer. Except for some dryness of the eyes, no drug-related abnormal ophthalmological findings were recorded and, according to specialized tests such as electroetinography and macular dazzle, retinal function was unchanged.

In combination with amitriptyline, clonidine hydrochloride administration led to the development of corneal lesions in rats within 5 days.

➤*Special risk:* Clonidine transdermal should be used with caution in patients with severe coronary insufficiency, conduction disturbances, recent MI, cerebrovascular disease, or chronic renal failure.

In rare instances, loss of blood pressure control has been reported in patients using clonidine transdermal according to the instructions for use.

Drug Interactions

Clonidine Drug Interactions

Precipitant drug	Object drug*		Description
Clonidine	Levodopa	⬇	The effectiveness of levodopa may be reduced.
Beta-adrenergic blocking agents	Clonidine	⬆	Attenuation or reversal of antihypertensive effect and potentially life-threatening increases in blood pressure.
Prazosin	Clonidine	⬇	The antihypertensive effectiveness of clonidine may be decreased.
Tricyclic antidepressants	Clonidine	⬇	Tricyclic antidepressants may block antihypertensive effects of clonidine and possibly life-threatening elevations in blood pressure may occur.
Verapamil	Clonidine	⬆	Synergistic pharmacologic and toxic effects, possibly causing atrioventricular (AV) block and severe hypotension.

* ⬆ = Object drug increased. ⬇ = Object drug decreased.

➤*Amitriptyline:* Amitriptyline, in combination with clonidine enhances the manifestation of corneal lesions in rats.

➤*Sedating drugs:* Clonidine may potentiate the CNS-depressive effects of alcohol, barbiturates or other sedating drugs. If a patient receiving clonidine is also taking tricyclic antidepressants, the hypotensive effect of clonidine may be reduced, necessitating an increase in the clonidine dose.

➤*Digitalis, calcium channel blockers, beta-blockers:* Due to a potential for additive effects such as bradycardia and AV block, caution is warranted in patients receiving clonidine concomitantly with agents known to affect sinus node function or AV nodal conduction (eg, digitalis, calcium channel blockers, beta-blockers).

Adverse Reactions

Most systemic adverse effects during clonidine transdermal therapy have been mild and have tended to diminish with continued therapy. In a 3-month multiclinic trial of clonidine transdermal in 101 hypertensive patients, the systemic adverse reactions were: dry mouth (25 patients) and drowsiness (12), fatigue (6), headache (5), lethargy and sedation (3 each), insomnia, dizziness, impotence/sexual dysfunction, dry throat (2 each) and constipation, nausea, change in taste and nervousness (1 each).

In the above mentioned 3-month controlled clinical trial, as well as other uncontrolled clinical trials, the most frequent adverse reactions were dermatological and are described below.

In the 3-month trial, 51 of the 101 patients had localized skin reactions such as erythema (26 patients) and/or pruritus, particularly after using an adhesive overlay throughout the 7-day dosage interval. Allergic contact sensitization to clonidine transdermal was observed in 5 patients. Other skin reactions were localized vesiculation (7 patients), hyperpigmentation (5), edema (3), excoriation (3), burning (3), papulas (1), throbbing (1), blanching (1), and a generalized macular rash (1).

In additional clinical experience, contact dermatitis resulting in treatment discontinuation was observed in 128 of 673 patients (about 19 in 100) after a mean duration of treatment of 37 weeks. The incidence of contact dermatitis was about 34 in 100 among white women, about 18 in 100 in white men, about 14 in 100 in black women, and ≈ 8 in 100 in black men. Analysis of skin reaction data showed that the risk of having to discontinue clonidine transdermal treatment because of contact dermatitis was greatest between treatment weeks 6 and 26, although sensitivity may develop either earlier or later in treatment.

In a large-scale clinical acceptability and safety study by 451 physicians in a total of 3539 patients, other allergic reactions were recorded for which a causal relationship to clonidine transdermal was not established; maculopapular rash (10 cases); urticaria (2 cases); and angioedema of the face (2 cases), which also affected the tongue in one of the patients.

➤*Postmarketing:* Other adverse effects reported since the drug has been marketed are listed below by body system. In this setting, an incidence or causal relationship cannot always be accurately determined. However, none of the events listed below occurred in a frequency more than 0.5%.

Cardiovascular – Congestive heart failure; cerebrovascular accident; electrocardiographic abnormalities (i.e., bradycardia, sick sinus syndrome disturbances and arrhythmias); chest pain; orthostatic symptoms; syncope, increases in blood pressure; sinus bradycardia and atrioventricular block

CLONIDINE — TRANSDERMAL

with and without the use of concomitant digitalis; Raynaud's phenomenon; tachycardia; bradycardia; and palpitations.

Dermatologic – Angioneurotic edema; localized or generalized rash; hives; urticaria; contact dermatitis; pruritus; alopecia; and localized hypo- or hyperpigmentation.

GI – Anorexia and vomiting.

GU – Difficult micturition; loss of libido; and decreased sexual activity.

Metabolic – Gynecomastia or breast enlargement and weight gain.

Musculoskeletal – Muscle or joint pain; and leg cramps.

Ophthalmic – Blurred vision; burning of the eyes and dryness of the eyes.

Psychiatric – Delirium; mental depression; visual and auditory hallucinations; localized numbness; vivid dreams or nightmares; restlessness; anxiety; agitation; irritability; other behavioral changes; and drowsiness.

Miscellaneous – Fever; malaise; weakness; and pallor; and withdrawal syndrome.

Overdosage

➤*Symptoms:* Hypertension may develop early and may be followed by hypotension, bradycardia, respiratory depression, hypothermia, drowsiness, decreased or absent reflexes, weakness, irritability and miosis. The frequency of CNS depression may be higher in children than adults. Large overdoses may result in reversible cardiac conduction defects or arrhythmias, apnea, coma and seizures. Signs and symptoms of overdose generally occur within 30 minutes to 2 hours after exposure. As little as 0.1 mg of clonidine has produced signs of toxicity in children.

If symptoms of poisoning occur following dermal exposure, remove all clonidine transdermal systems. After their removal, the plasma clonidine levels will persist for about 8 hours, then decline slowly over a period of several days. Rare cases of clonidine transdermal poisoning due to accidental or deliberate mouthing or ingestion of the patch have been reported, many of them involving children.

The largest overdose reported to date, involved a 28-year-old male who ingested 100 mg of clonidine hydrochloride powder. This patient developed hypertension followed by hypotension, bradycardia, apnea, hallucinations, semicoma, and premature ventricular contractions. The patient fully recovered after intensive treatment. Plasma clonidine levels were 60 ng/mL after 1 hour, 190 ng/mL after 1.5 hours, 370 ng/mL after 2 hours, and 120 ng/mL after 5.5 and 6.5 hours. In mice and rats, the oral LD_{50} of clonidine is 206 and 465 mg/kg, respectively.

➤*Treatment:* There is no specific antidote for clonidine overdosage. Ipecac syrup-induced vomiting and gastric lavage would not be expected to remove significant amounts of clonidine following dermal exposure. If the patch is ingested, whole bowel irrigation may be considered and the administration of activated charcoal or cathartic may be beneficial. Supportive care may include atropine sulfate for bradycardia, intravenous fluids or vasopressor agents for hypotension and vasodilators for hypertension. Naloxone may be a useful adjunct for the management of clonidine-induced respiratory depression, hypotension and/or coma; blood pressure should be monitored since the administration of naloxone has occasionally resulted in paradoxical hypertension. Totazoline administration has yielded inconsistent results and is not recommended as first-line therapy. Dialysis is not likely to significantly enhance the elimination of clonidine.

Patient Information

Patients should be cautioned against interruption of clonidine transdermal therapy without their physician's advice.

Patients who engage in potentially hazardous activities, such as operating machinery or driving, should be advised of a possible sedative effect of clonidine. They should also be informed that this sedative effect may be increased by concomitant use of alcohol, barbiturates, or other sedating drugs.

Patients should be instructed to consult their physicians promptly about the possible need to remove the patch if they observe moderate to severe localized erythema or vesicle formation at the site of application or generalized skin rash.

If a patient experiences isolated, mild localized skin irritation before completing 7 days of use, the system may be removed and replaced with a new system applied to a fresh skin site.

If the system should begin to loosen from the skin after application, the patient should be instructed to place the adhesive overlay directly over the system to ensure adhesion during its 7-day use.

Used clonidine transdermal patches contain a substantial amount of their initial drug content which may be harmful to infants and children if accidentally applied or ingested. Therefore, patients should be cautioned to keep both used and unused clonidine transdermal patches out of the reach of children. After use, clonidine transdermal should be folded in half with the adhesive sides together and discarded away from children's reach.

Instructions for use, storage and disposal of the system are provided in each box of clonidine transdermal.

GUANFACINE HYDROCHLORIDE

Rx	**Tenex** (ESP Pharma[1])	**Tablets:** 1 mg	Lactose. (1 AHR Tenex). Light pink. Diamond shape. In 100s, 500s and *Dis-Co* 100s.
		2 mg	Lactose. (2 AHR Tenex). Yellow. Diamond shape. In 100s.

[1] ESP Pharma, Inc., 2035 Lincoln Highway, Suite 2150, Edison, NJ 08817; (866) 437–7742; http://www.esppharma.com.

GUANFACINE HYDROCHLORIDE — ORAL

Indications

Management of hypertension. Guanfacine hydrochloride may be given alone or in combination with other antihypertensive agents, especially thiazide-type diuretics.

➤*Unlabeled uses:* Guanfacine (0.03 to 1.5 mg/day) may be beneficial in ameliorating withdrawal symptoms when discontinuing heroin usage.

In a small study, guanfacine (1 mg/day for 12 weeks) significantly reduced the frequency of migraine headache and reduced nausea and vomiting.

Treatment of attention deficit hyperactivity disorder (ADHD).

Administration and Dosage

➤*Approved by the FDA:* October 27, 1986.

The recommended initial dose of guanfacine hydrochloride when given in combination with another antihypertensive drug is 1 mg daily given at bedtime to minimize somnolence. If after 3 to 4 weeks of therapy, 1 mg does not give a satisfactory result, a dose of 2 mg may be given, although most of the effect of guanfacine is seen at 1 mg. Higher daily doses have been used, but adverse reactions increase significantly with doses above 3 mg/day.

The frequency of rebound hypertension is low, but it can occur. When rebound occurs, it does so after 2 to 4 days, which is delayed compared with clonidine hydrochloride. This is consistent with the longer half-life of guanfacine. In most cases, after abrupt withdrawal of guanfacine, blood pressure returns to pretreatment levels slowly (within 2 to 4 days) without ill effects.

➤*Storage/Stability:* Store at controlled room temperature 15° to 30°C (59° to 86°F). Dispense in tight, child- and light-resistant container.

Actions

➤*Pharmacology:* Guanfacine hydrochloride is an orally active antihypertensive agent whose principal mechanism of action appears to be stimulation of central α_2-adrenergic receptors. By stimulating these receptors, guanfacine reduces sympathetic nerve impulses from the vasomotor center to the heart and blood vessels. This results in a decrease in peripheral vascular resistance and a reduction in heart rate.

➤*Pharmacokinetics:*

Absorption/Distribution – Relative to an IV dose of 3 mg, the absolute oral bioavailability of guanfacine is about 80%. Peak plasma concentrations occur from 1 to 4 hours with an average of 2.6 hours after single oral doses or at steady state.

The area under the concentration-time curve (AUC) increases linearly with the dose.

The drug is approximately 70% bound to plasma proteins, independent of drug concentration.

The whole body volume of distribution is high (a mean of 6.3 L/kg), which suggests a high distribution of drug to the tissues.

Metabolism/Excretion – In individuals with healthy renal function, the average elimination half-life is approximately 17 hours (range, 10 to 30 hours). Younger patients tend to have shorter elimination half-lives (13 to 14 hours) while older patients tend to have half-lives at the upper end of the range. Steady-state blood levels were attained within 4 days in most subjects.

In individuals with healthy renal function, guanfacine and its metabolites are excreted primarily in the urine. Approximately 50% (40% to 75%) of the dose is eliminated in the urine as unchanged drug; the remainder is eliminated mostly as conjugates of metabolites produced by oxidative metabolism of the aromatic ring.

The guanfacine-to-creatinine clearance ratio is greater than 1, which would suggest that tubular secretion of drug occurs.

Special populations –

Renal function impairment: The clearance of guanfacine in patients with varying degrees of renal insufficiency is reduced, but plasma levels of drug are only slightly increased compared to patients with healthy renal function. When prescribing for patients with renal impairment, the low end of the dosing range should be used. Patients on dialysis also can be given usual doses of guanfacine as the drug is poorly dialyzed.

Contraindications

Hypersensitivity to guanfacine hydrochloride.

GUANFACINE HYDROCHLORIDE — ORAL

Warnings

➤*Elderly:* In general, dose selection for an elderly patient should be cautious, usually starting at the low end of the dosing range, reflecting the greater frequency of decreased hepatic, renal or cardiac function, and of concomitant disease or other drug therapy.

➤*Pregnancy: Category B.*

Administration of guanfacine to rats at 70 times the maximum recommended human dose and to rabbits at 20 times the maximum recommended human dose resulted in no evidence of harm to the fetus. Higher doses (100 and 200 times the maximum recommended human dose in rabbits and rats, respectively) were associated with reduced fetal survival and maternal toxicity. Rat experiments have shown that guanfacine crosses the placenta.

There are, however, no adequate and well-controlled studies in pregnant women. Because animal reproduction studies are not always predictive of human response, this drug should be used during pregnancy only if clearly needed.

Labor and delivery – Guanfacine is not recommended in the treatment of acute hypertension associated with toxemia of pregnancy. There is no information available on the effects of guanfacine on the course of labor and delivery.

➤*Lactation:* It is not known whether guanfacine is excreted in human milk. Because many drugs are excreted in human milk, caution should be exercised when guanfacine hydrochloride is administered to a breast-feeding woman. Experiments with rats have shown that guanfacine is excreted in the milk.

➤*Children:* Safety and efficacy in children under 12 years of age have not been demonstrated. Therefore, the use of guanfacine in this age group is not recommended.

There have been spontaneous postmarketing reports of mania and aggressive behavioral changes in children with attention deficit hyperactivity disorder (ADHD) receiving guanfacine. The reported cases were from a single center. All patients had medical or family risk factors for bipolar disorder. All patients recovered upon discontinuation of guanfacine hydrochloride.

Precautions

➤*Sedation:* Guanfacine, like other orally active central alpha-2-adrenergic agonists, causes sedation or drowsiness, especially when beginning therapy. These symptoms are dose related. When guanfacine is used with other centrally active depressants (such as phenothiazines, barbiturates, or benzodiazepines), the potential for additive sedative effects should be considered.

➤*Rebound:* Abrupt cessation of therapy with orally active central α_2-adrenergic agonists may be associated with increases (from depressed on-therapy levels) in plasma and urinary catecholamines, symptoms of "nervousness and anxiety" and, less commonly, increases in blood pressure to levels significantly greater than those prior to therapy.

➤*Special risk:* Like other antihypertensive agents, guanfacine should be used with caution in patients with severe coronary insufficiency, recent myocardial infarction, cerebrovascular disease or chronic renal or hepatic failure.

➤*Hazardous tasks:* Patients who receive guanfacine should be advised to exercise caution when operating dangerous machinery or driving motor vehicles until it is determined that they do not become drowsy or dizzy from the medication.

Drug Interactions

➤*Other CNS-depressant drugs:* The potential for increased sedation when guanfacine is given with other CNS-depressant drugs should be appreciated.

➤*CYP-450 enzyme inducers:* The administration of guanfacine concomitantly with a known microsomal enzyme inducer (phenobarbital or phenytoin) to 2 patients with renal impairment reportedly resulted in significant reductions in elimination half-life and plasma concentration. In such cases, therefore, more frequent dosing may be required to achieve or maintain the desired hypotensive response. Further, if guanfacine is to be discontinued in such patients, careful tapering of the dosage may be necessary in order to avoid rebound phenomena (see Rebound above).

Adverse Reactions

Adverse reactions noted with guanfacine are similar to those of other drugs of the central α_2-adrenoreceptor agonist class were as follows: dry mouth, sedation (somnolence), weakness (asthenia), dizziness, constipation, and impotence. While the reactions are common, most are mild and tend to disappear on continued dosing.

Skin rash with exfoliation has been reported in a few cases; although clear cause-and-effect relationships to guanfacine could not be established, should a rash occur, guanfacine should be discontinued and the patient monitored appropriately.

Guanfacine Dose-response Monotherapy Study

Adverse reaction	Placebo (n = 59)	0.5 mg (n = 60)	1 mg (n = 61)	2 mg (n = 60)	3 mg (n = 59)
Asthenia	0%	2%	3%	7%	3%
Constipation	0%	2%	0%	5%	15%
Dizziness	8%	12%	2%	8%	15%
Dry mouth	0%	10%	10%	42%	54%
Fatigue	2%	2%	5%	8%	10%
Headache	8%	13%	7%	5%	3%
Impotence	0%	0%	0%	7%	3%
Somnolence	8%	5%	10%	13%	39%

The percent of patients who dropped out because of adverse reactions are shown in the following table for each dosage group.

	Placebo	0.5 mg	1 mg	2 mg	3 mg
Percent dropouts	0%	2%	5%	13%	32%

The most common reasons for dropouts among patients who received guanfacine were dry mouth, somnolence, dizziness, fatigue, weakness, and constipation.

➤*Combination therapy with chlorthalidone:* In a 12-week, placebo-controlled, dose-response study of guanfacine administered with 25 mg chlorthalidone at bedtime, the frequency of the most commonly observed adverse reactions showed a clear dose relationship from 0.5 to 3 mg as follows:

Guanfacine/Chlorthalidone Dose-response Study

Adverse reactions	Placebo (n = 73)	0.5 mg (n = 72)	1 mg (n = 72)	2 mg (n = 72)	3 mg (n = 72)
Asthenia	0 (0%)	2 (3%)	0 (0%)	2 (2%)	7 (10%)
Constipation	0 (0%)	0 (0%)	0 (0%)	1 (1%)	1 (1%)
Dizziness	2 (2%)	1 (1%)	3 (4%)	6 (8%)	3 (4%)
Dry mouth	5 (7%)	4 (5%)	6 (8%)	8 (11%)	20 (28%)
Fatigue	3 (3%)	2 (3%)	2 (3%)	5 (6%)	3 (4%)
Headache	3 (4%)	4 (3%)	3 (4%)	1 (1%)	2 (2%)
Impotence	1 (1%)	1 (0%)	0 (0%)	1 (1%)	3 (4%)
Somnolence	1 (1%)	3 (4%)	0 (0%)	1 (1%)	10 (14%)

There were 41 premature terminations because of adverse reactions in this study. The percent of patients who dropped out and the dose at which the dropout occurred were as follows:

Dose	Placebo	0.5 mg	1 mg	2 mg	3 mg
Percent dropouts	6.9%	4.2%	3.2%	6.9%	8.3%

Reasons for dropouts among patients who received guanfacine were somnolence, headache, weakness, dry mouth, dizziness, impotence, insomnia, constipation, syncope, urinary incontinence, conjunctivitis, paresthesia, and dermatitis.

In a second 12-week, placebo-controlled, combination therapy study in which the dose could be adjusted upward to 3 mg per day in 1 mg increments at 3-week intervals (ie, a setting more similar to ordinary clinical use) the most commonly recorded reactions were dry mouth, 47%; constipation, 16%; fatigue, 12%; somnolence, 10%; asthenia, 6%; dizziness, 6%; headache, 4%; and insomnia, 4%.

Reasons for dropouts among patients who received guanfacine were somnolence, dry mouth, dizziness, impotence, constipation, confusion, depression, and palpitations.

➤*Comparison with clonidine:* In the clonidine/guanfacine comparison, the most common adverse reactions noted were as follows:

Guanfacine vs Clonidine Adverse Reactions

Adverse reactions	Guanfacine (n = 279)	Clonidine (n = 278)
Constipation	10%	5%
Dizziness	11%	8%
Dry mouth	30%	37%
Fatigue	9%	8%
Headache	4%	4%
Insomnia	4%	3%
Somnolence	21%	35%

➤*Adverse reactions (3% or less):* Adverse reactions occurring in 3% or less of patients in the 3 controlled trials of guanfacine with a diuretic were the following:

Cardiovascular – Bradycardia, palpitations, substernal pain.

CNS – Amnesia, confusion, depression, insomnia, libido decrease.

Dermatologic – Dermatitis, pruritus, purpura, sweating.

GI – Abdominal pain, diarrhea, dyspepsia, dysphagia, nausea.

GU – Testicular disorder, urinary incontinence.

Musculoskeletal – Leg cramps, hypokinesia.

GUANFACINE HYDROCHLORIDE — ORAL

Ophthalmic – Conjunctivitis, iritis, vision disturbance.

Respiratory – Dyspnea.

Special senses – Rhinitis, taste perversion, tinnitus.

Miscellaneous – Malaise, paresthesia, paresis.

➤*Adverse reactions in an open-label trial of 1 year:* Adverse reaction reports tend to decrease over time. In an open-label trial of 1 year's duration, 580 hypertensive subjects were given guanfacine, titrated to achieve goal blood pressure, alone (51%), with diuretic (38%), with beta blocker (3%), with diuretic plus beta blocker (6%), or with diuretic plus vasodilator (2%). The mean daily dose of guanfacine reached was 4.7 mg.

Adverse reaction	Incidence of adverse reactions at any time during the study (n = 580)	Incidence of adverse reactions at end of 1 year (n = 580)
Dry mouth	60%	15%
Drowsiness	33%	6%
Dizziness	15%	1%
Constipation	14%	3%
Weakness	5%	1%
Headache	4%	0.2%
Insomnia	5%	0%

➤*Dropouts due to adverse effects in the 1-year trial:* There were 52 (8.9%) dropouts due to adverse effects in this 1-year trial. The causes were as follows: Dry mouth (n = 20), weakness (n = 12), constipation (n = 7), somnolence (n = 3), nausea (n = 3), orthostatic hypotension (n = 2), insomnia (n = 1), rash (n = 1), nightmares (n = 1), headache (n = 1), and depression (n = 1).

➤*Postmarketing:* An open-label postmarketing study involving 21,718 patients was conducted to assess the safety of guanfacine hydrochloride 1 mg/day given at bedtime for 28 days. Guanfacine was administered with or without other antihypertensive agents. Adverse events reported in the postmarketing study at an incidence greater than 1% included dry mouth, dizziness, somnolence, fatigue, headache and nausea. The most commonly reported adverse events in this study were the same as those observed in controlled clinical trials.

➤*Less frequent, possibly guanfacine-related events observed in the postmarketing study or reported spontaneously include:*

Cardiovascular – Bradycardia, palpitations, syncope, tachycardia.

CNS – Paresthesias, vertigo.

Agitation, anxiety, confusion, depression, insomnia, nervousness.

Dermatologic – Alopecia, dermatitis, exfoliative dermatitis, pruritus, rash.

GI – Abdominal pain, constipation, diarrhea, dyspepsia.

GU – Nocturia, urinary frequency.
Males: Impotence.

Hepatic – Abnormal liver function tests.

Musculoskeletal – Arthralgia, leg cramps, leg pain, myalgia.

Ophthalmic – Blurred vision.

Respiratory – Dyspnea.

Special senses – Alterations in taste.

Miscellaneous – Asthenia, chest pain, edema, malaise, tremor.

➤*Rare and serious disorders:* Rare, serious disorders with no definitive cause and effect relationship to guanfacine have been reported spontaneously or in the postmarketing study. These events include acute renal failure, cardiac fibrillation, cerebrovascular accident, congestive heart failure, heart block, and myocardial infarction.

Overdosage

➤*Symptoms:* Drowsiness, lethargy, bradycardia and hypotension have been observed following overdose with guanfacine.

A 25-year-old female intentionally ingested 60 mg. She presented with severe drowsiness and bradycardia of 45 beats/minute. Gastric lavage was performed and an infusion of isoproterenol (0.8 mg in 12 hours) was administered. She recovered quickly and without sequelae.

A 28-year-old female who ingested 30 to 40 mg developed only lethargy, was treated with activated charcoal and a cathartic, was monitored for 24 hours, and was discharged in good health.

A 2-year-old male weighing 12 kg, who ingested up to 4 mg of guanfacine, developed lethargy. Gastric lavage (followed by activated charcoal and sorbitol slurry via NG tube) removed some tablet fragments within 2 hours after ingestion, and vital signs were normal. During 24-hour observation in ICU, systolic pressure was 58 and heart rate 70 at 16 hours postingestion. No intervention was required, and the child was discharged fully recovered the next day.

➤*Treatment:* Gastric lavage and supportive therapy as appropriate. Guanfacine is not dialyzable in clinically significant amounts (2.4%).

Patient Information

Patients who receive guanfacine should be advised to exercise caution when operating dangerous machinery or driving motor vehicles until it is determined that they do not become drowsy or dizzy from the medication. Patients should be warned that their tolerance for alcohol and other CNS depressants may be diminished. Patients should be advised not to discontinue therapy abruptly.

GUANABENZ ACETATE

Rx	**Guanabenz Acetate** (Various, eg, Ivax, Watson)	**Tablets:** 4 mg	In 100s and 500s.
Rx	**Wytensin** (Wyeth-Ayerst)		(Wyeth 73/W4). Orange. In 100s, 500s and Redipak 100s.
Rx	**Guanabenz Acetate** (Various, eg, Ivax, Watson)	8 mg	In 100s and 500s.
Rx	**Wytensin** (Wyeth-Ayerst)		(Wyeth 74/W8). Gray, scored. In 100s.

GUANABENZ ACETATE — ORAL

Indications

➤*Hypertension:* Treatment of hypertension. It may be employed alone or in combination with a thiazide diuretic.

Administration and Dosage

➤*Approved by the FDA:* September 7, 1982.

Dosage with guanabenz acetate tablets should be individualized. A starting dose of 4 mg twice a day is recommended, whether guanabenz is used alone or with a thiazide diuretic. Dosage may be increased in increments of 4 to 8 mg/day every 1 to 2 weeks, depending on the patient's response. The maximum dose studied to date has been 32 mg twice daily, but doses as high as this are rarely needed.

Actions

➤*Pharmacology:* Guanabenz acetate is an orally active central alpha-2-adrenergic agonist. Its antihypertensive action appears to be mediated via stimulation of central alpha adrenergic receptors, resulting in a decrease of sympathetic outflow from the brain at the bulbar level to the peripheral circulatory system.

➤*Pharmacokinetics:* In human studies, approximately 75% of an orally administered dose of guanabenz acetate is absorbed and metabolized with less than 1% of unchanged drug recovered from the urine. Peak plasma concentrations of unchanged drug occur between 2 and 5 hours after a single oral dose. The average half-life for guanabenz is ≈ 6 hours. The site or sites of metabolism of guanabenz have not been determined. The effect of meals on the absorption of guanabenz acetate tablets has not been studied.

Contraindications

Sensitivity to the drug.

Warnings

➤*Renal function impairment:* The disposition of orally administered guanabenz acetate is altered modestly in patients with renal impairment. Guanabenz half-life is prolonged and clearance decreased, more so in patients on hemodialysis. The clinical significance of these findings is unknown.

➤*Mutagenesis:* In the *Salmonella* microsome mutagenicity (Ames) test system, guanabenz at 200 to 500 mcg per plate or at 30 to 50 mcg/mL in suspension gave dose-related increases in the number of mutants in 1 (TA 1537) of 5 *Salmonella typhimurium* strains with or without inclusion of rat liver microsomes.

➤*Fertility impairment:* Reproductive studies showed a decreased pregnancy rate in rats administered high oral doses (9.6 mg/kg) of guanabenz acetate, suggesting an impairment of fertility. The fertility of treated males (9.6 mg/kg) may also have been affected, as suggested by the decreased pregnancy rate of their mates even though the females received guanabenz only during the last third of pregnancy.

➤*Pregnancy: Category C.*

Teratogenic – Guanabenz acetate may have adverse effects on the fetus when administered to pregnant women. A teratology study in mice has indicated a possible increase in skeletal abnormalities when guanabenz acetate is given orally at doses of 3 to 6 times the maximum recommended human dose of 1 mg/kg. These abnormalities, principally costal and vertebral, were not noted in similar studies in rats and rabbits. However, increased fetal loss has been observed after oral guanabenz acetate administration to pregnant rats (14 mg/kg) and rabbits (20 mg/kg). Reproductive studies of guanabenz in rats have shown slightly decreased live-birth indices, decreased fetal survival rate, and decreased pup body weight at oral doses of 6.4 and 9.6 mg/kg. There are no adequate, well-controlled studies in pregnant women.

GUANABENZ ACETATE — ORAL

Guanabenz should be used during pregnancy only if the potential benefit justifies the potential risk to the fetus.

➤*Lactation:* Because no information is available on the excretion of guanabenz in human milk, it should not be administered to breast-feeding mothers.

➤*Children:* The safety and efficacy of guanabenz acetate in children younger than 12 years of age have not been demonstrated. Therefore, its use in this age group cannot be recommended at this time.

Precautions

➤*Monitoring:* Careful monitoring of blood pressure during guanabenz dose titration is suggested in patients with coexisting hypertension, coexisting chronic hepatic dysfunction, or renal impairment.

➤*Sedation:* Guanabenz causes sedation or drowsiness in a large fraction of patients. When guanabenz is used with centrally-active depressants, such as phenothiazines, barbiturates, and benzodiazepines, the potential for additive sedative effects should be considered.

➤*Vascular insufficiency:* Guanabenz, like other antihypertensive agents, should be used with caution in patients with severe coronary insufficiency, recent MI, cerebrovascular disease, or severe hepatic or renal failure.

➤*Rebound:* Sudden cessation of therapy with central alpha agonists like guanabenz may rarely result in "overshoot" hypertension and more commonly produces an increase in serum catecholamines and subjective symptomatology.

➤*Hazardous tasks:* Patients who receive guanabenz should be advised to exercise caution when operating dangerous machinery or driving motor vehicles until it is determined that they do not become drowsy or dizzy from the medication (see Patient Information).

Drug Interactions

Guanabenz has not been demonstrated to cause any drug interactions when administered with other drugs, such as digitalis, diuretics, analgesics, anxiolytics, and anti-inflammatory or anti-infective agents, in clinical trials. However, the potential for increased sedation when guanabenz is administered concomitantly with CNS-depressant drugs should be noted.

Adverse Reactions

The following table shows the incidence of adverse effects, occurring in 5% or more of patients in a study comparing guanabenz acetate to placebo, at a starting dose of 8 mg twice daily.

Most Common Guanabenz Adverse Reactions

Adverse reaction	Placebo (%) (n = 102)	Guanabenz acetate (%) (n = 109)
Dizziness	7	17
Drowsiness or sedation	12	39
Dry mouth	7	28
Headache	6	5
Weakness	7	10

In other controlled clinical trials at the starting dose of 16 mg/day in 476 patients, the incidence of dry mouth was slightly higher (38%) and that of dizziness was slightly lower (12%), but the incidence of the most frequent adverse effects was similar to the placebo-controlled trial.

Although these side effects were not serious, they led to discontinuation of treatment approximately 15% of the time. In more recent studies using an initial dose of 8 mg/day in 274 patients, the incidence of drowsiness or sedation was lower, approximately 20%.

Other adverse effects were reported during clinical trials with guanabenz but are not clearly distinguishable from placebo effects and occurred with a frequency of less than or equal to 3%:

➤*Cardiovascular:* Chest pain, edema, arrhythmias, palpitations.

In very rare instances atrioventricular dysfunction, up to and including complete AV block, has been caused by guanabenz.

➤*CNS:* Anxiety, ataxia; depression; sleep disturbances.

➤*GI:* Nausea; epigastric pain; diarrhea; vomiting; constipation; abdominal discomfort.

➤*GU:* Urinary frequency; disturbances of sexual function (decreased libido; impotence).

➤*Dermatologic:* Rash; pruritus.

➤*Musculoskeletal:* Aches in extremities; muscle aches.

➤*Respiratory:* Dyspnea.

➤*Special senses:* Blurring of vision; nasal congestion.

➤*Miscellaneous:* Gynecomastia; taste disorders.

Overdosage

➤*Symptoms:* Accidental ingestion of guanabenz caused hypotension, somnolence, lethargy, irritability, miosis, and bradycardia in 2 children aged 1 and 3 years. Gastric lavage and administration of pressor substances, fluids, atropine, ipecac and oral activated charcoal resulted in complete and uneventful recovery within 12 hours in both patients.

➤*Treatment:* Because experience with accidental overdosage is limited, the suggested treatment is mainly supportive while the drug is being eliminated from the body and until the patient is no longer symptomatic. Vital signs and fluid balance should be carefully monitored. An adequate airway should be maintained and, if indicated, assisted respiration instituted. There is no data available on the dialyzability of guanabenz.

Patient Information

Patients who receive guanabenz should be advised to exercise caution when operating dangerous machinery or driving motor vehicles until it is determined that they do not become drowsy or dizzy from the medication. Patients should be warned that their tolerance for alcohol and other CNS depressants may be diminished. Patients should be advised not to discontinue therapy abruptly.

RESERPINE

Rx	**Reserpine** (Various, eg, Eon, Moore, Rugby)	**Tablets:** 0.1 mg	In 100s, 1000s and 5000s.
Rx	**Reserpine** (Various, eg, Eon, Moore, Rugby, URL)	**Tablets:** 0.25 mg	In 100s, 1000s and 5000s.

RESERPINE — ORAL

Indications

➤*Hypertension:* Mild essential hypertension.

Adjunctive therapy with other antihypertensive agents in more severe forms of hypertension.

➤*Psychotic states:* Relief of symptoms in agitated psychotic states (eg, schizophrenia), primarily in those individuals unable to tolerate phenothiazine derivatives or in those who also require antihypertensive medication.

Administration and Dosage

➤*Hypertension:* In the average patient not receiving other antihypertensive agents, the usual initial dosage is 0.5 mg daily for 1 or 2 weeks. For maintenance, reduce to 0.1 to 0.25 mg daily. Use higher dosages cautiously because occurrence of serious mental depression and other side affects may increase considerably.

➤*Psychiatric disorders:* The usual initial dosage is 0.5 mg daily, but may range from 0.1 to 1 mg. Adjust dosage upward or downward according to the patient's response.

➤*Children:* Reserpine is not recommended for use in children. If it is be used in treating a child, the usual recommended starting dose is 20 mcg/kg daily. The maximum recommended dose is 0.25 mg (total) daily.

Actions

➤*Pharmacology:* Reserpine depletes stores of catecholamine and 5-hydroxytryptamine in many organs, including the brain and adrenal medulla. Most of its pharmacological effects have been attributed to this action. Depletion is slower and less complete in the adrenal medulla than in other tissues. The depression of sympathetic nerve function results in a decreased heart rate and a lowering of arterial blood pressure. The sedative and tranquilizing properties of reserpine are thought to be related to depletion of catecholamine and 5-hydroxytryptamine from the brain.

➤*Pharmacokinetics:* Reserpine is characterized by slow onset of action and sustained effects. Both cardiovascular and CNS effects may persist for a period of time following withdrawal of the drug.

Mean maximum plasma levels of 1.54 ng/mL were attained after a median of 3.5 hours in six healthy subjects receiving a single oral 1 mg dose. Bioavailability was ≈ 50% of that of a corresponding IV dose. Plasma levels of reserpine after IV administration declined with a mean half-life of 33 hours. Reserpine is extensively bound (96%) to plasma proteins. No definitive studies on the metabolism of reserpine have been made.

Contraindications

Hypersensitivity; mental depression or history of mental depression (especially with suicidal tendencies); active peptic ulcer; ulcerative colitis; patients receiving electroconvulsive therapy.

Warnings

➤*Depression:* Exercise extreme caution in treating patients with a history of mental depression. Reserpine may cause mental depression. Recognition of depression may be difficult, because this condition may often be disguised by somatic complaints (masked depression). Discontinue the drug at first signs of depression (eg, despondency, early morning insomnia, loss of appe-

RESERPINE — ORAL

tite, impotence or self-deprecation). Drug-induced depression may persist for several months after drug withdrawal and may be severe enough to result in suicide.

➤*Ulcers:* Since reserpine increases GI motility and secretion, use cautiously in patients with a history of peptic ulcer, ulcerative colitis or gallstones (biliary colic may be precipitated).

➤*Cardiovascular effects:* Preoperative withdrawal of reserpine does not assure that circulatory instability will not occur. It is important that the anesthesiologist be aware of the patient's drug intake and consider this in the overall management, since hypotension has occurred in patients receiving reserpine. Anticholinergic or adrenergic drugs (eg, metaraminol, norepinephrine) have been employed to treat adverse vagocirculatory effects.

➤*Renal function impairment:* Exercise caution when treating hypertensive patients with renal insufficiency, since they adjust poorly to lowered blood pressure levels.

➤*Carcinogenesis:* Reserpine is an animal tumorigen, causing an increased incidence of mammary fibroadenomas in female mice, malignant tumors of the seminal vesicles in male mice and malignant adrenal medullary tumors in male rats. The breast neoplasms are thought to be related to reserpine's prolactin-elevating effect. The extent to which these findings indicate a risk to humans is uncertain. Tissue culture experiments show that about 33% of human breast tumors are prolactin-dependent, a factor of considerable importance if the use of the drug is contemplated in a patient with previously detected breast cancer. The possibility of an increased risk of breast cancer in reserpine users has been studied extensively; however, no firm conclusion has emerged. Although a few epidemiologic studies have suggested a slightly increased risk (less than two-fold in all studies except one in women who have used reserpine), other studies of generally similar design have not confirmed this.

➤*Pregnancy:* Category C. There are no adequate and well controlled studies of reserpine in pregnant women. Reserpine crosses the placental barrier. Increased respiratory tract secretions, nasal congestion, cyanosis and anorexia may occur in neonates of reserpine-treated mothers. Use during pregnancy only if the potential benefit justifies the potential risk to the fetus.

➤*Lactation:* Reserpine is excreted in breast milk. Increased respiratory tract secretions, nasal congestion, cyanosis and anorexia may occur in breastfed infants. Because of the potential for adverse reactions in nursing infants and the potential for tumorigenicity, decide whether to discontinue nursing or to discontinue the drug, taking into account the importance of the drug to the mother.

➤*Children:* Safety and efficacy have not been established by means of controlled clinical trials, although there is experience with the use of reserpine in children. Because of adverse effects such as emotional depression and lability, sedation and stuffy nose, reserpine is not usually recommended as a Step-2 drug in the treatment of hypertension in children.

Drug Interactions

Reserpine Drug Interactions

Precipitant drug	Object drug*		Description
MAO inhibitors	Reserpine	⟷	Avoid MAO inhibitors or use with extreme caution.
Tricyclic antidepressants	Reserpine	↓	Concurrent use may decrease the antihypertensive effect of reserpine.
Reserpine	Digitalis glycosides Quinidine	↑	Use reserpine cautiously with digitalis and quinidine, since cardiac arrhythmias have occurred.
Reserpine	Sympathomimetics, direct-acting	↑	Closely monitor concurrent use of reserpine and direct- or indirect-acting sympathomimetics. The action of direct-acting amines (eg, epinephrine, isoproterenol, phenylephrine, metaraminol) may be prolonged when given to patients taking reserpine. The action of indirect-acting amines (eg, ephedrine, tyramine, amphetamines) is inhibited.
	Sympathomimetics, indirect-acting	↓	

* ↑ = Object drug increased. ↓ = Object drug decreased. ⟷ = Undetermined clinical effect.

Adverse Reactions

The following adverse reactions are listed in decreasing order of severity, not frequency.

➤*Cardiovascular:* Arrhythmias (particularly when used concurrently with digitalis or quinidine); syncope; angina-like symptoms; bradycardia; edema.

➤*CNS:* Parkinsonian syndrome and other extrapyramidal tract symptoms (rare); dizziness; headache; paradoxical anxiety; depression; nervousness; nightmares; dull sensorium; drowsiness.

➤*GI:* Vomiting; diarrhea; nausea; anorexia; dryness of mouth; hypersecretion.

➤*GU:* Pseudolactation; impotence; dysuria; gynecomastia; decreased libido; breast engorgement.

➤*Respiratory:* Dyspnea; epistaxis; nasal congestion.

➤*Special senses:* Deafness; optic atrophy; glaucoma; uveitis; conjunctival injection.

➤*Miscellaneous:* Hypersensitivity reactions: Purpura, rash, pruritus; weight gain; muscular aches.

Overdosage

➤*Symptoms:* No deaths due to acute poisoning with reserpine have been reported.

Highest known doses survived – Children, 1,000 mg (age and sex not specified), young children, 200 mg (20-month-old boy). The clinical picture of acute poisoning is characterized chiefly by signs and symptoms due to the reflex parasympathomimetic effect of reserpine.

Impairment of consciousness may occur and may range from drowsiness to coma, depending on the severity of overdosage. Flushing of the skin, conjunctival injection and pupillary constriction are to be expected. Hypotension, hypothermia, central respiratory depression and bradycardia may develop in cases of severe overdosage. Increased salivary secretion, gastric secretion and diarrhea also may occur.

➤*Treatment:* There is no specific antidote. Evacuate stomach contents, taking adequate precautions against aspiration and for protection of the airway. Activated charcoal slurry should be instilled.

Treat the effects of reserpine overdosage symptomatically. If hypotension is severe enough to require treatment with a vasopressor, use one having a direct action upon vascular smooth muscle (eg, phenylephrine, norepinephrine, metaraminol). Since reserpine is long-acting, observe the patient carefully for at least 72 hours, and administer treatment as required.

Patient Information

Inform patients of possible side effects and advise them to take the medication regularly and continuously as directed.

ALPHA-1-ADRENERGIC BLOCKERS

Indications

➤*Hypertension:* For the treatment of hypertension, alone or in combination with other antihypertensive agents (except **tamsulosin**).

➤*Benign prostatic hyperplasia (BPH):*

Terazosin – Treatment of symptomatic BPH.

Doxazosin – Treatment of urinary outflow obstruction and obstructive symptoms (hesitation, intermittency, dribbling, weak urinary stream, incomplete emptying of the bladder) and irritative symptoms (nocturia, daytime frequency, urgency, burning) associated with BPH.

Tamsulosin – Treatment of the signs and symptoms of BPH.

➤*Unlabeled uses:*

Prazosin – Treatment of BPH.

Terazosin – Symptomatic treatment of chronic abacterial prostatitis.

Actions

➤*Pharmacology:* **Doxazosin**, **prazosin**, and **terazosin** selectively block alpha-1-adrenergic receptors. This blockade causes a reduction in systemic vascular resistance, thus causing an antihypertensive effect. The degree of smooth muscle tone in the prostate and bladder neck is mediated by the alpha-1-adrenergic receptor, which is present in high density in the prostatic stroma, prostatic capsule, and bladder neck. Blockade of the alpha-1-adrenergic receptor decreases urethral resistance and may relieve the obstruction and improve urine flow and BPH symptoms.

Tamsulosin selectively inhibits the alpha-1A-adrenergic receptor. Approximately 70% of the alpha-1-adrenergic receptors in human prostate are of the alpha-1A subtype. Tamsulosin is not intended for use as an antihypertensive drug.

Doxazosin causes maximum reductions in blood pressure 2 to 6 hours after dosing, which is associated with a small increase in standing heart rate. Doxazosin has a greater effect on blood pressure and heart rate in the standing position.

Prazosin lowers blood pressure in the supine and standing positions. This effect is most pronounced on the diastolic blood pressure. The antihypertensive action usually is not accompanied by a reflex tachycardia.

Terazosin decreases blood pressure gradually within 15 minutes following oral administration. Terazosin treatment in normotensive men with BPH did not result in a clinically significant blood pressure-lowering effect.

ALPHA-1-ADRENERGIC BLOCKERS

➤*Pharmacokinetics:*

Special populations –

Hepatic function impairment: Administration of a single dose of doxazosin 2 mg to patients with cirrhosis (Child-Pugh Class A) showed a 40% increase in exposure to **doxazosin**.

Elderly: In patients 70 years of age and older taking **terazosin**, plasma clearance decreased by 31.7%, compared with younger patients. For **tamsulosin**, a 40% higher AUC in those 55 to 75 years of age was seen compared with younger subjects. Enterohepatic recycling of **doxazosin** is suggested by secondary peaking of plasma concentrations. Plasma elimination of doxazosin is biphasic. After morning dosing of doxazosin, the AUC was 11% less than after evening dosing and the time to peak concentration after evening dosing occurred significantly later than after morning dosing (5.6 vs 3.5 hours).

Terazosin undergoes minimal hepatic first-pass metabolism and nearly all the circulating dose is in the form of the parent drug.

The mean steady-state apparent volume of distribution of **tamsulosin** after IV administration was 16 L, which is suggestive of distribution into extracellular fluids in the body. Tamsulosin is widely distributed to most tissues. The cytochrome P450 enzymes that primarily catalyze the Phase I metabolism of tamsulosin have not been conclusively identified. The metabolites of tamsulosin undergo extensive conjugation to glucuronide or sulfate prior to renal excretion.

Pharmacokinetics of Alpha-1-Adrenergic Blockers

Parameter	Prazosin	Terazosin	Doxazosin	Tamsulosin
Oral bioavailability	nd	nd	≈ 65%	> 90% (fasting state)
T_{max}	≈ 3 h	≈ 1 h	≈ 2 to 3 h	4 to 5 h (fasting state) 6 to 7 h (fed state)
Protein binding	High	90% to 94%	≈ 98%	94% to 99%[a]
Metabolism	Extensively metabolized, primarily by demethylation and conjugation	nd	First-pass metabolism; extensively metabolized by the liver, mainly by O-demethylation or hydroxylation	CYP450
Half-life, elimination	2 to 3 h	≈ 12 h	≈ 22 h	9 to 15 h
Excretion	Bile and feces	Urine (≈ 40%)[b] Feces (≈ 60%)[c]	Urine (≈ 9%) Feces (≈ 63%)[d]	Urine (76%) Feces (21%)

nd = no data.
[a] Primarily bound to alpha-1-acid glycoprotein.
[b] Approximately 10% of an oral dose is excreted as parent drug in the urine.
[c] Approximately 20% of an oral dose is excreted as parent drug in the feces.
[d] 4.8% of the dose is excreted as unchanged drug in the feces and a trace amount is excreted in the urine as unchanged drug.

Contraindications

Hypersensitivity to quinazolines (eg, **doxazosin**, **prazosin**, **tamsulosin**, **terazosin**) or to any components of the products.

Warnings

➤*"First-dose" effect and orthostatic hypotension:* **Prazosin**, **terazosin**, **doxazosin**, and **tamsulosin**, like other α-adrenergic blocking agents, can cause marked hypotension (especially postural hypotension) and syncope with sudden loss of consciousness with the first few doses. Anticipate a similar effect if therapy is interrupted for more than a few doses, if dosage is increased rapidly, or if another antihypertensive drug is introduced. Syncope is due to an excessive postural hypotensive effect, although the syncopal episode has occasionally been preceded by severe supraventricular tachycardia with heart rates of 120 to 160 beats per minute.

The "first-dose" phenomenon may be minimized by limiting the initial dose to 1 mg of **terazosin** or **prazosin** (given at bedtime) or **doxazosin**. Slowly increase dosage of these drugs. Add additional antihypertensives with caution. Caution patients to avoid situations where injury could result should syncope occur during initiation of therapy. Hypotension may develop in patients also receiving a β-adrenergic blocker.

If syncope occurs, place patient in recumbent position and treat supportively. More common than loss of consciousness are dizziness and lightheadedness.

Syncopal episodes have usually occurred within 30 to 90 minutes of the initial dose of **prazosin**; the incidence is approximately 1% with an initial dose of 2 mg or greater. Syncope occurred in about 1% of **terazosin** patients and was not necessarily associated with early doses. There is evidence that the orthostatic effect of terazosin is greater, even in chronic use, shortly after dosing. Syncope occurred in 0.7% of **doxazosin** patients with dose titration every 1 to 2 weeks; none of these events were reported at the starting dose of 1 mg and 1.2% occurred at 16 mg/day. Other symptoms of lowered blood pressure (eg, dizziness, lightheadedness palpitations) are more common, occurring in approximately 28% of terazosin patients and up to 23% of doxazosin patients (approximately 2% of doxazosin patients discontinued therapy).

➤*Priapism:* Rarely (probably less frequently than once in every several thousand patients), alpha-$_1$ antagonists have been associated with priapism (painful penile erection, sustained for hours and unrelieved by sexual intercourse or masturbation). Because this condition can lead to permanent impotence if not promptly treated, patients must be advised about the seriousness of the condition.

➤*Hepatic function impairment:* Administer **doxazosin** with caution to patients with evidence of impaired hepatic function or to patients receiving drugs known to influence hepatic metabolism.

➤*Fertility impairment:* Reduced fertility occurred in male rats treated with **doxazosin** 20 mg/kg/day. The effect was reversible within 2 weeks of drug withdrawal. Nine of 39 male rats failed to sire a litter after **terazosin** 30 to 120 mg/kg/day. Testicular atrophy also has occurred in rats and dogs receiving terazosin or **prazosin**. Studies in rats revealed significantly reduced fertility in males dosed with single or multiple daily doses of 300 mg/kg/day of **tamsulosin** (AUC exposure in rats about 50 times the human exposure with the maximum therapeutic dose). The effects on fertility were reversible, showing improvement by 3 days after a single dose and 4 weeks after multiple dosing. Effects on fertility in males were completely reversed within 9 weeks of discontinuation of multiple dosing. Multiple doses of 10 and 100 mg/kg/day tamsulosin (⅕ and 16 times the anticipated human AUC exposure) did not significantly alter fertility in male rats. Studies in female rats revealed significant reductions in fertility after single or multiple dosing with 300 mg/kg/day of the R-isomer or racemic mixture of tamsulosin, respectively.

➤*Pregnancy: Category C*(**prazosin**, **terazosin**, **doxazosin**). *Category B* (**tamsulosin**). A doxazosin dosage of 82 mg/kg/day in rabbits was associated with reduced fetal survival. In rats, maternal doxazosin doses 8 times the human AUC exposure (12 mg/day) delayed postnatal development. Terazosin doses 280 times the maximum recommended human dose in rats resulted in fetal resorptions; increased fetal resorptions, decreased fetal weight, and increased number of supernumerary ribs occurred with doses 60 times the maximum recommended human dose. Significantly more rat pups died in the group dosed with terazosin (more than 75 times the maximum recommended human dose) vs controls.

There are no adequate and well-controlled studies in pregnant women. Safety for use during pregnancy has not been established. Use only when clearly needed and when the potential benefits outweigh the potential hazards to the fetus. **Tamsulosin** is not indicated for use in women.

➤*Lactation:* **Doxazosin** accumulates in breast milk of lactating rats following a single 1 mg/kg dose with a maximum concentration about 20 times greater than the maternal plasma concentration. It is not known whether **terazosin** or **tamsulosin** are excreted in breast milk. Tamsulosin is not indicated for use in women. **Prazosin** is excreted in small amounts in breast milk. Exercise caution when administering these drugs to a nursing woman.

➤*Children:* Safety and efficacy for use in children have not been established.

Precautions

➤*Hemodilution:* Small but statistically significant decreases in hematocrit, hemoglobin, white blood cells, total protein, and albumin were observed in controlled clinical trials with **terazosin**. These laboratory findings suggest the possibility of hemodilution.

➤*Leukopenia/Neutropenia:* In hypertensive patients receiving **doxazosin**, mean WBC and neutrophil counts were decreased by 2.4% and 1%, respectively, compared with placebo, a phenomenon seen with other alpha blocking drugs. In BPH patients, the incidence of clinically significant WBC abnormalities was 0.4%. No patients became symptomatic as a result of the low counts. WBCs and neutrophil counts returned to normal after drug discontinuation.

➤*Weight gain:* There was a tendency for patients to gain weight during **terazosin** therapy. In placebo-controlled monotherapy trials, male and female patients receiving terazosin gained a mean of 0.8 and 1 kg, respectively, compared with losses of 0.1 and 0.5 kg, respectively, in the placebo group. Patients receiving **doxazosin** gained a mean of 0.6 kg compared with a mean loss of 0.1 kg for placebo patients.

➤*Cholesterol:* During controlled clinical studies, patients receiving **terazosin** monotherapy had a small but statistically significant decrease (3%) in total cholesterol and the combined LDL and VLDL fractions. No significant changes were observed in HDL fraction and triglycerides. In clinical trials involving normocholesterolemic patients, **doxazosin** reduced total serum cholesterol by 2% to 3% and LDL by 4%, and increased HDL to total cholesterol ratio by 4%. The clinical significance is unknown.

➤*Cardiotoxicity:* An increased incidence of myocardial necrosis or fibrosis occurred in rats and mice following 6 to 18 months of **doxazosin** 40 to 80 mg/kg/day. There is no evidence that similar lesions occur in humans.

➤*Prostatic cancer:* Carcinoma of the prostate and BPH cause many of the same symptoms and frequently co-exist. Therefore, examine patients thought to have BPH prior to starting **terazosin** therapy to rule out prostate carcinoma.

ALPHA-1-ADRENERGIC BLOCKERS

Drug Interactions

Alpha-1-Antiadrenergic Blocker Drug Interactions

Precipitant drug	Object drug*		Description
Alcohol	Alpha-1-adrenergic blockers	⬆	Coadministration may cause increased risk of hypotension. Advise patients to avoid alcohol.
Beta blockers	Alpha-1-adrenergic blockers Prazosin	⬆	Beta-blockers may enhance the acute postural hypotensive reaction following the first dose of prazosin; terazosin and doxazosin have been combined with beta blockers with no adverse reaction.
Cimetidine	Alpha-1-adrenergic blockers Tamsulosin	⬆	Cimetidine decreased the clearance of tamsulosin 26% and increased the AUC 44%. Use with caution.
Indomethacin	Alpha-1-adrenergic blockers Prazosin	⬇	The antihypertensive action of prazosin may be decreased. No interaction occurred in patients receiving doxazosin, terazosin, and NSAIDs.
Verapamil	Alpha-1-adrenergic blockers Prazosin Terazosin	⬆	Verapamil appears to increase serum prazosin levels and may increase the sensitivity to prazosin-induced postural hypotension. Verapamil increased terazosin AUC 24%, C_{max} 25%, and C_{min} 32% and decreased T_{max} 0.5 h.
Alpha$_1$-adrenergic blockers Prazosin	Clonidine	⬇	The antihypertensive effect of clonidine may be decreased.

* ⬆ = Object drug increased. ⬇ = Object drug decreased.

➤*Drug/Lab test interactions:* In a study of 5 patients given **prazosin** 12 to 24 mg/day for 10 to 14 days, there was an average increase of 42% in the urinary metabolite of norepinephrine and an average increase in urinary vanillylmandelic acid (VMA) of 17%. Therefore, false-positive results may occur in screening tests for pheochromocytoma in patients who are being treated with **prazosin**. If an elevated VMA is found, discontinue prazosin and retest the patient after 1 month.

Doxazosin and **terazosin** do not affect plasma concentrations of prostate specific antigen (PSA) in patients treated for up to 3 years (doxazosin), 2 years (terazosin), or 1 year (**tamsulosin**).

➤*Drug/Food interactions:* Administration of **terazosin** capsules immediately after meals delayed T_{max} by about 40 minutes. For **tamsulosin**, the T_{max} is reached by 4 to 5 hours under fasting conditions and by 6 to 7 hours after administration with food. Taking tamsulosin under fasted conditions results in a 30% increase in AUC and 40% to 70% increase in C_{max} compared with fed conditions.

Adverse Reactions

Alpha-1-Adrenergic Blocker Adverse Reactions (%)[a]

	Hypertension			BPH			
Adverse Reaction	Prazosin	Terazosin	Doxazosin	Terazosin	Doxazosin	Tamsulosin 0.4 mg	Tamsulosin 0.8 mg
Cardiovascular							
Palpitations	5.3	4.3	2	0.9	1.2	-	-
Postural hypotension/ hypotension	1 to 4	1.3	0.3 to 1	0.6 to 3.9	0.3 to 1.7	0.2	0.4
Tachycardia	< 1	1.9	0.3	-	0.9	-	-
Arrhythmia	-	≥ 1	1	-	-	-	-
Chest pain	-	≥ 1	2	-	1.2	4	4.1
Vasodilation	-	≥ 1	-	-	-	-	-
Syncope	1 to 4	-	0.5 to 1	0.6	0.5	0.2	0.4
Peripheral ischemia	-	-	0.3	-	-	-	-
Angina pectoris	-	-	< 0.5	-	0.6	-	-
CNS							
Depression	1 to 4	0.3	1	-	-	-	-
Dizziness	10.3	19.3	19	9.1	15.6[b]	14.9	17.1
Decreased libido/ sexual dysfunction	-	0.6	2	-	0.8	1	2
Nervousness	1 to 4	2.3	2	-	-	-	-
Paresthesia	< 1	2.9	1	-	-	-	-
Somnolence	-	5.4	5	3.6	3	3	4.3
Anxiety	-	≥ 1	-	-	1.1	-	-
Insomnia	-	≥ 1	1	-	1.2	2.4	1.4
Asthenia	≈ 7	11.3[c]	1 to 12	7.4[c]	-	7.8	8.5
Fatigue	-	-	-	-	8	-	-
Drowsiness	7.6	-	-	-	-	-	-
Ataxia	-	-	1	-	-	-	-
Hypertonia	-	-	1	-	-	-	-
Hallucinations	< 1	-	-	-	-	-	-
Kinetic disorders	-	-	1	-	-	-	-
Dermatologic							
Pruritus	< 1	≥ 1	1	-	-	-	-
Rash	1 to 4	≥ 1	1	-	-	-	-
Sweating	-	≥ 1	0.5 to 1	-	1.1	-	-
Alopecia/Lichen planus	< 1	-	< 0.5	-	-	-	-
GI							
Nausea	4.9	4.4	3	1.7	1.5	2.6	3.9
Vomiting	1 to 4	≥ 1	≤ 2	-	1.4	-	-
Dry mouth	1 to 4	≥ 1	-	-	-	-	-
Diarrhea	1 to 4	≥ 1	2	-	2.3	6.2	4.3
Constipation	1 to 4	≥ 1	1	-	-	-	-
Abdominal discomfort/pain	< 1	≥ 1	0	-	2.4	-	-
Flatulence	-	≥ 1	1	-	-	-	-
Liver function abnormalities	< 1	-	-	-	-	-	-
Pancreatitis	< 1	-	-	-	-	-	-
Tooth disorder	-	-	-	-	-	1.2	2

ALPHA-1-ADRENERGIC BLOCKERS

Alpha-1-Adrenergic Blocker Adverse Reactions (%)[a]							
	Hypertension			BPH			
Adverse Reaction	Prazosin	Terazosin	Doxazosin	Terazosin	Doxazosin	Tamsulosin 0.4 mg	Tamsulosin 0.8 mg
Dyspepsia	-	≥ 1	1	-	1.7	-	-
GU							
Impotence	< 1	1.2	-	1.6	1.1	-	-
Urinary frequency	1 to 4	≥ 1	0	-	-	-	-
Urinary tract infection	-	≥ 1	-	1.3	1.4	-	-
Incontinence	< 1	≥ 1[4]	1	-	-	-	-
Polyuria	-	-	2		-	-	-
Priapism	< 1	-	-	-	-	-	-
Abnormal ejaculation	-	-	-	-	-	8.4	18.1
Dysuria	-	-	-	-	0.5	-	-
Musculoskeletal							
Shoulder/Neck/Back/ Extremity pain	-	1 to 3.5	-	-	-	7	8.3
Arthritis, joint disorder/ muscle pain, gout, cramps	-	≥ 1	1	-	-	-	-
Arthralgia	< 1	≥ 1	1	-	-	-	-
Myalgia	-	≥ 1	1	-	-	-	-
Muscle weakness	-	-	1	-	-	-	-
Respiratory							
Dyspnea	1 to 4	3.1	1	1.7	2.6	-	-
Nasal congestion	1 to 4	5.9	-	1.9	-	-	-
Sinusitis	-	2.6	< 0.5	-	-	2.2	3.7
Bronchitis/Cold symptoms/ bronchospasm	-	≥ 1	< 0.5	-		-	-
Epistaxis	1 to 4	≥ 1	1	-	-	-	-
Flu symptoms	-	≥ 1	< 0.5	2.4	1.1	-	-
Increased cough	-	≥ 1	< 0.5	-	-	3.4	4.5
Pharyngitis/Rhinitis	-	≥ 1	< 0.5/3	1.9	< 0.5	5.8/13.1	5.1/17.9
Special senses							
Blurred vision/ amblyopia	1 to 4	1.6	-	1.3	-	-	-
Abnormal vision	-	≥ 1	2	0.6	1.4	-	-
Conjunctivitis, reddened sclera/eye pain	1 to 4	≥ 1	1	-	-	-	-
Tinnitus	< 1	≥ 1	1	-	-	-	-
Vertigo	1 to 4	-	2	1.4	-	0.6	1
Amblyopia	-	-	-	1.3	-	0.2	2
Miscellaneous							
Headache	7.8	16.2	14	4.9	9.9	19.3	21.1
Edema	1 to 4	0.9	4	-	2.7	-	-
Peripheral edema	-	5.5	-	0.9	-	-	-
Weight gain	-	0.5	0.5 to 1	0.5	-	-	-
Facial edema	-	≥ 1	1	-	-	-	-
Fever	< 1	≥ 1	< 0.5	-	-	-	-
Flushing	-	-	1	-	-	-	-
Diaphoresis	< 1	-	-	-	-	-	-
Positive ANA titer	< 1	-	-	-	-	-	-
Infection	-	-	< 0.5	-	-	9	10.8
Pain	-	-	2	-	2	-	-
Lack of energy	6.9	-	-	-	-	-	-
Weakness	6.5	-	-	-	-	-	-
Fatigue/Malaise	-	-	12	-	-	-	-
Gout	-	≥ 1	-	-	-	-	-

[a] Data are pooled from separate studies and are not necessarily comparable.
[b] Includes vertigo.
[c] Includes weakness, tiredness, lassitude, and fatigue.
[d] Primarily reported in postmenopausal women.

➤*Doxazosin (hypertension):*

Cardiovascular – MI, cerebrovascular accident (fewer than 0.5%).

CNS – Hypesthesia, agitation (0.5% to 1%); paresis, tremor, twitching, confusion, migraine, impaired concentration, paroniria, amnesia, emotional lability, abnormal thinking, depersonalization (fewer than 0.5%).

Dermatologic – Dry skin, eczema (fewer than 0.5%).

GI – Increased appetite, anorexia, fecal incontinence, gastroenteritis (fewer than 0.5%).

GU – Breast pain, renal calculus (fewer than 0.5%).

Hematologic – Lymphadenopathy, purpura (fewer than 0.5%).

Metabolic/Nutritional – Thirst, gout, hypokalemia (fewer than 0.5%).

Special senses – Parosmia, earache, taste perversion, photophobia, abnormal lacrimation (fewer than 0.5%).

Miscellaneous – Pallor, hot flushes, fever/rigors, decreased weight (fewer than 0.5%).

➤*Postmarketing:*

Cardiovascular –
Prazosin: Angina pectoris, hypotension, bradycardia.

CNS –
Prazosin: Flushing, insomnia.

GU –
Doxazosin: Priapism, gynecomastia, hematuria, micturition disorder, micturition frequency, nocturia.

Hematologic –
Doxazosin: Leukopenia, thrombocytopenia.

Hepatic –
Doxazosin: Hepatitis, hepatitis cholestatic.

Miscellaneous –
Doxazosin: Allergic reaction, urticaria, bronchospasm aggravated, vomiting, hypesthesia, bradycardia.
Prazosin: Allergic reaction, asthenia, malaise, pain, gynecomastia, urticaria, vasculitis, eye pain.
Tamsulosin: Allergic-type reactions (eg, skin rash, pruritus, angioedema of the tongue, lips, and face, urticaria) have been reported with positive rechallenge in some cases; priapism (rare); palpitations, constipation, vomiting (infrequent).
Terazosin: Allergic reactions, including anaphylaxis; priapism; thrombocytopenia; atrial fibrillation.

ALPHA-1-ADRENERGIC BLOCKERS

Overdosage

➤*Symptoms:* Accidental ingestion of at least 50 mg **prazosin** in a 2-year-old child produced profound drowsiness and depressed reflexes. No decrease in blood pressure was noted. Recovery was uneventful.

Several cases of **doxazosin** overdose have been reported (doses ranging from 1 to 40 mg in children and 60 to 70 mg in adults). All children made full recoveries. One adult developed hypotension that responded to fluid therapy. The other adult (with chronic renal failure, epilepsy, and depression) died; death was attributed to a grand mal seizure resulting from hypotension. The most likely manifestation of overdosage would be hypotension.

One patient reported an overdose of thirty 0.4 mg **tamsulosin** capsules. Following the ingestion of the capsules, the patient reported a severe headache.

➤*Treatment:* Restore blood pressure and normalize heart rate by keeping the patient supine. Treat shock with volume expanders. If necessary, use vasopressors and monitor and support renal function. These drugs are highly protein bound; dialysis may not be of benefit. Refer to General Management of Acute Overdosage.

Patient Information

Inform patients of the possibility of syncopal and orthostatic symptoms, especially at the initiation of therapy. Avoid driving or hazardous tasks for 12 to 24 hours after the first dose, after a dosage increase, and after interruption of therapy when treatment is resumed. Use caution when rising from a sitting or lying position. If dizziness or palpitations are bothersome, contact the physician for possible dose adjustment. These effects also may occur if patients drink alcohol, stand for long periods of time, or exercise, or if the weather is hot.

Drowsiness or somnolence may occur. Use caution when driving or operating heavy machinery.

Advise patients about the possibility of priapism as a result of treatment with alpha-$_1$ antagonists. Let patients know that this adverse event is very rare. If they experience priapism, advise them to bring it to immediate medical attention because, if not treated promptly, it can lead to permanent erectile dysfunction (impotence).

Advise patients not to crush, chew, or open **tamsulosin** capsules.

PRAZOSIN HYDROCHLORIDE

Rx	**Prazosin HCl** (Various, eg, Ivax)	**Capsules:** 1 mg (as base)	In 100s, 250s, 500s, and 1000s.
Rx	**Minipress** (Pfizer)		(431). White. In 250s.
Rx	**Prazosin HCl** (Various, eg, Ivax)	**Capsules:** 2 mg (as base)	In 100s, 250s, 500s, and 1000s.
Rx	**Minipress** (Pfizer)		(437). Pink/white. In 250s.
Rx	**Prazosin HCl** (Various, eg, Ivax)	**Capsules:** 5 mg (as base)	In 100s, 250s, and 500s.
Rx	**Minipress** (Pfizer)		(438). Blue/white. In 250s.

PRAZOSIN HYDROCHLORIDE — ORAL

For complete and comparative prescribing information, refer to the Alpha-1-Adrenergic Blockers group monograph.

Indications

➤*Hypertension:* Treatment of hypertension. It can be used alone or in combination with other antihypertensive drugs such as diuretics or beta-adrenergic-blocking agents.

Administration and Dosage

The dose of prazosin hydrochloride should be adjusted according to the patient's individual blood pressure response. The following is a guide to its administration:

➤*Initial dose:* 1 mg 2 or 3 times a day. Syncopal episodes have usually occurred within 30 to 90 minutes of the initial dose of the drug; occasionally they have been reported in association with rapid dosage increases or the introduction of another antihypertensive drug into the regimen of a patient taking high doses of prazosin. The incidence of syncopal episodes is approximately 1% in patients given an initial dose of 2 mg or greater. Clinical trials conducted during the investigational phase of this drug suggest that syncopal episodes can be minimized by limiting the initial dose of the drug to 1 mg, by subsequently increasing the dosage slowly, and by introducing any additional antihypertensive drugs into the patient's regimen with caution.

➤*Maintenance dose:* Dosage may be slowly increased to a total daily dose of 20 mg given in divided doses. The therapeutic dosages most commonly employed have ranged from 6 mg to 15 mg daily given in divided doses. Doses higher than 20 mg usually do not increase efficacy; however, a few patients may benefit from further increases up to a daily dose of 40 mg given in divided doses. After initial titration some patients can be maintained adequately on a twice daily dosage regimen.

➤*Use with other drugs:* When adding a diuretic or other antihypertensive agent, the dose of prazosin HCl should be reduced to 1 mg or 2 mg 3 times a day and retitration then carried out.

➤*Storage/Stability:* Store at controlled room temperature 15° to 30°C (59° to 86°F). Protect from moisture and light. Dispense in a tight, light-resistant container using a child-resistant closure.

TERAZOSIN HYDROCHLORIDE

Rx	**Terazosin HCl** (Geneva)	**Tablets:** 1 mg (as base)	In 100s and 1000s.
		2 mg (as base)	In 100s and 1000s.
		5 mg (as base)	In 100s and 1000s.
		10 mg (as base)	In 100s and 1000s.
Rx	**Terazosin HCl** (Various, eg, Apotex, Geneva, Teva)	**Capsules:** 1 mg (as base)	May contain lactose. In 100s and 500s.
Rx	**Hytrin** (Abbott)		Parabens. (HH). Grey. In 100s and UD 100s.
Rx	**Terazosin HCl** (Various, eg, Apotex, Geneva, Teva)	2 mg (as base)	May contain lactose. In 100s and 500s.
Rx	**Hytrin** (Abbott)		Parabens. (HY). Yellow. In 100s and UD 100s.
Rx	**Terazosin HCl** (Various, eg, Apotex, Geneva, Teva)	5 mg (as base)	May contain lactose. In 100s and 500s.
Rx	**Hytrin** (Abbott)		Parabens. (HK). Red. In 100s and UD 100s.
Rx	**Terazosin HCl** (Various, eg, Apotex, Geneva, Teva)	10 mg (as base)	May contain lactose. In 100s and 500s.
Rx	**Hytrin** (Abbott)		Parabens. (HN). Blue. In 100s. and UD 100s

TERAZOSIN HYDROCHLORIDE — ORAL

For complete and comparative prescribing information, refer to the Alpha-1-Adrenergic Blockers group monograph.

Indications

➤*Benign prostatic hyperplasia (BPH):* Treatment of symptomatic benign prostatic hyperplasia (BPH). There is a rapid response, with approximately 70% of patients experiencing an increase in urinary flow and improvement in symptoms of BPH when treated with terazosin. The long-term effects of terazosin on the incidence of surgery, acute urinary obstruction, or other complications of BPH are yet to be determined.

➤*Hypertension:* Treatment of hypertension. It can be used alone or in combination with other antihypertensive agents such as diuretics or beta-adrenergic-blocking agents.

Administration and Dosage

If terazosin administration is discontinued for several days, therapy should be reinstituted using the initial dosing regimen.

➤*Benign prostatic hyperplasia:*

Initial dose – 1 mg at bedtime is the starting dose for all patients, and this dose should not be exceeded as an initial dose. Patients should be closely monitored during initial administration in order to minimize the risk of severe hypotensive response.

Subsequent doses – The dose should be increased in a stepwise fashion to 2, 5, or 10 mg once daily to achieve the desired improvement of symptoms or flow rates. Doses of 10 mg once daily are generally required for the clinical response. Therefore, treatment with 10 mg for a minimum of 4 to 6 weeks may be required to assess whether a beneficial response has been achieved. Some patients may not achieve a clinical response despite appropriate titration. Although some additional patients responded at a 20 mg daily dose, there was an insufficient number of patients studied to draw definitive conclusions about this dose. There are insufficient data to support the use of higher doses for those patients who show inadequate or no response to 20 mg daily. If terazosin HCl administration is discontinued for several days or longer, therapy should be reinstituted using the initial dosing regimen.

Use with other drugs – Caution should be observed when terazosin HCl is administered concomitantly with other antihypertensive agents, especially the calcium channel blocker verapamil, to avoid the possibility of developing significant hypotension. When using terazosin HCl and other antihypertensive agents concomitantly, dosage reduction and retitration of either agent may be necessary.

➤*Hypertension:* The dose of terazosin and the dose interval (12 or 24 hours) should be adjusted according to the patient's individual blood pressure response. The following is a guide to its administration:

Initial dose – 1 mg at bedtime is the starting dose for all patients, and this dose should not be exceeded. This initial dosing regimen should be strictly observed to minimize the potential for severe hypotensive effects.

Subsequent doses – The dose may be slowly increased to achieve the desired blood pressure response. The usual recommended dose range is 1 to 5 mg administered once a day; however, some patients may benefit from doses as high as 20 mg/day. Doses over 20 mg do not appear to provide further blood pressure effect and doses over 40 mg have not been studied. Blood pressure should be monitored at the end of the dosing interval to ensure control is maintained throughout the interval. It may also be helpful to measure blood pressure 2 to 3 hours after dosing to see if the maximum and minimum responses are similar, and to evaluate symptoms such as dizziness or palpitations, which can result from excessive hypotensive response. If response is substantially diminished at 24 hours an increased dose or use of a twice daily regimen can be considered. If terazosin HCl administration is discontinued for several days or longer, therapy should be reinstituted using the initial dosing regimen. In clinical trials, except for the initial dose, the dose was given in the morning.

➤*Storage/Stability:* Store at controlled room temperature 15° to 30°C (59° to 86°F). Protect from light and moisture. Dispense in a tight, light-resistant container using a child-resistant closure.

DOXAZOSIN MESYLATE

Rx	**Doxazosin Mesylate** (Various, eg, Apotex, Ethex, Ivax, Mylan, Teva)	**Tablets:** 1 mg (as base)	May contain lactose. In 100s, 500s, 1000s, and UD 100s.
Rx	**Cardura** (Pfizer)		Lactose. (Cardura 1 mg). White. In 100s and UD 100s.
Rx	**Doxazosin Mesylate** (Various, eg, Apotex, Ethex, Ivax, Mylan, Teva)	**Tablets:** 2 mg (as base)	May contain lactose. In 100s, 500s, 1000s, and UD 100s.
Rx	**Cardura** (Pfizer)		Lactose. (Cardura 2 mg). Yellow. In 100s and UD 100s.
Rx	**Doxazosin Mesylate** (Various, eg, Apotex, Ethex, Ivax, Mylan, Teva)	**Tablets:** 4 mg (as base)	May contain lactose. In 100s, 500s, 1000s, and UD 100s.
Rx	**Cardura** (Pfizer)		Lactose. (Cardura 4 mg). Orange. In 100s and UD 100s.
Rx	**Doxazosin Mesylate** (Various, eg, Apotex, Ethex, Ivax, Mylan, Teva)	**Tablets:** 8 mg (as base)	May contain lactose. In 100s, 500s, 1000s, and UD 100s.
Rx	**Cardura** (Pfizer)		Lactose. (Cardura 8 mg). Green. In 100s and UD 100s.

DOXAZOSIN MESYLATE — ORAL

For complete and comparative prescribing information, refer to the Alpha-1-Adrenergic Blockers group monograph.

Indications

➤*Benign prostatic hyperplasia (BPH):* Treatment of both the urinary outflow obstruction and obstructive and irritative symptoms associated with BPH: Obstructive symptoms (hesitation, intermittency, dribbling, weak urinary stream, incomplete emptying of the bladder), and irritative symptoms (nocturia, daytime frequency, urgency, burning). Doxazosin mesylate may be used in all BPH patients whether hypertensive or normotensive. In patients with hypertension and BPH, both conditions were effectively treated with doxazosin mesylate monotherapy. Doxazosin mesylate provides rapid improvement in symptoms and urinary flow rate in 66% to 71% of patients. Sustained improvements with doxazosin mesylate were seen in patients treated for up to 14 weeks in double-blind studies and up to 2 years in open-label studies.

➤*Hypertension:* Treatment of hypertension. Doxazosin mesylate may be used alone or in combination with diuretics, beta-adrenergic blocking agents, calcium channel blockers or angiotensin-converting enzyme inhibitors.

Administration and Dosage

➤*Approved by the FDA:* November 2, 1990.

➤*Dosage must be individualized:* The initial dosage of doxazosin mesylate in patients with hypertension or BPH is 1 mg given once daily in the morning or evening. This starting dose is intended to minimize the frequency of postural hypotension and first dose syncope associated with doxazosin mesylate. Postural effects are most likely to occur between 2 and 6 hours after a dose. Therefore blood pressure measurements should be taken during this time period after the first dose and with each increase in dose. If doxazosin mesylate administration is discontinued for several days, therapy should be restarted using the initial dosing regimen.

➤*Benign prostatic hyperplasia:* The initial dosage of doxazosin mesylate is 1 mg, given once daily in the morning or evening. Depending on the individual patient's urodynamics and BPH symptomatology, dosage may then be increased to 2 mg and thereafter to 4 mg and 8 mg once daily, the maximum recommended dose for BPH. The recommended titration interval is 1 to 2 weeks. Blood pressure should be evaluated routinely in these patients.

➤*Hypertension:* The initial dosage of doxazosin mesylate is 1 mg given once daily. Depending on the individual patient's standing blood pressure response (based on measurements taken at 2 to 6 hours post-dose and 24 hours post-dose), dosage may then be increased to 2 mg, and thereafter if necessary to 4 mg, 8 mg, and 16 mg to achieve the desired reduction in blood pressure. Increases in dose beyond 4 mg increase the likelihood of excessive postural effects including syncope, postural dizziness/vertigo, and postural hypotension. At a titrated dose of 16 mg once daily the frequency of postural effects is about 12% compared with 3% for placebo.

➤*Storage/Stability:* Store at controlled room temperature 15° to 30°C (59° to 86°F).

TAMSULOSIN HYDROCHLORIDE

Rx	**Flomax** (Abbott)	**Capsules:** 0.4 mg	(Flomax 0.4 mg BI 58). Olive green/orange. In 100s and 1,000s.

TAMSULOSIN HYDROCHLORIDE — ORAL

For complete and comparative prescribing information, refer to the Alpha-1-Adrenergic Blockers group monograph.

Indications

➤*Benign prostatic hyperplasia (BPH):* Treatment of the signs and symptoms of benign prostatic hyperplasia (BPH). Tamsulosin capsules are not indicated for the treatment of hypertension.

➤*Unlabeled uses:* Used as adjunctive therapy in the management of ureteral stones.

Administration and Dosage

➤*Approved by the FDA:* April 15, 1997.

Tamsulosin capsules 0.4 mg once daily is recommended as the dose for the treatment of the signs and symptoms of BPH. It should be administered approximately 30 minutes following the same meal each day.

For those patients who fail to respond to the 0.4 mg dose after 2 to 4 weeks of dosing, the dose of tamsulosin capsules can be increased to 0.8 mg once daily. If tamsulosin capsules administration is discontinued or interrupted for several days at either the 0.4 mg or 0.8 mg dose, therapy should be started again with the 0.4 mg once daily dose.

➤*Storage/Stability:* Store at controlled room temperature 20° to 25°C (68° to 77°F).

ALFUZOSIN HYDROCHLORIDE

Rx	**Uroxatral** (Sanofi-Syntholabo)	**Tablets, extended-release:** 10 mg	Mannitol. (X10). White, yellow. In 30s. 100s, and UD 100s.

ALFUZOSIN HYDROCHLORIDE — ORAL

For complete and comparative prescribing information, refer to the Alpha-1-Adrenergic Blockers group monograph.

Indications

➤*Benign prostatic hyperplasia:* Treatment of the signs and symptoms of benign prostatic hyperplasia.

Administration and Dosage

➤*Approved by the FDA:* June 12, 2003.

The recommended dosage is one 10 mg alfuzosin hydrochloride extended-release tablet daily to be taken immediately after the same meal each day. The tablets should not be chewed or crushed.

➤*Storage/Stability:* Store at 25°C (77°F); excursions permitted to 15° to 30°C (59° to 86°F). Protect from light and moisture. Keep alfuzosin hydrochloride extended-release tablets out of reach of children.

MECAMYLAMINE HYDROCHLORIDE

Rx	**Inversine** (Targacept)	**Tablets:** 2.5 mg	Lactose, talc. (LBS01). Yellow. In 100s.

MECAMYLAMINE HYDROCHLORIDE — ORAL

Refer to the general discussion of these products in the Antihypertensives Treatment Guidelines in the Appendix.

Indications

➤*Essential and/or malignant hypertension:* For the management of moderately severe to severe essential hypertension and in uncomplicated cases of malignant hypertension.

Administration and Dosage

➤*Approved by the FDA:* October 28, 2002.

➤*Dosage:* Therapy is usually started with 2.5 mg twice daily. Determine the initial dosage by blood pressure readings in the erect position at the time of maximal drug effect, as well as by other signs and symptoms of orthostatic hypotension. Adjust dosage in increments of 2.5 mg at intervals of no less than 2 days until the desired blood pressure response occurs (a dosage just under that which causes signs of mild postural hypotension).

The average total daily dosage is 25 mg, usually in 3 divided doses. However, as little as 2.5 mg/day may be sufficient. A range of 2 to 4 or more doses may be required in severe cases when smooth control is difficult to obtain. In severe or urgent cases, larger increments at smaller intervals may be needed. Partial tolerance may develop, requiring an increase in daily dosage.

Administration after meals may cause a more gradual absorption and smoother control of excessively high blood pressure. The timing of doses in relation to meals should be consistent. Because blood pressure response to antihypertensive drugs is increased in the early morning, give the larger dose at noon and perhaps in the evening. The morning dose should be relatively small or may be omitted.

➤*Maintenance dosage:* Regulate the effective maintenance dosage by blood pressure readings in the erect position and by limiting the dosage to that which causes slight faintness or dizziness in the erect position. If the patient or a relative can use a sphygmomanometer or another blood-pressure monitoring device, the patient may be given instructions to reduce or omit a dose if readings fall below a designated level or if faintness or light-headedness occurs. However, the patient should not institute any changes without consulting a physician.

➤*Concomitant antihypertensive therapy:* Reduce the dosage of other agents, as well as that of mecamylamine, to avoid excessive hypotension. However, continue thiazides in their usual dosage, while decreasing mecamylamine at least 50%.

➤*Storage/Stability:* Store at 25°C (77°F); excursions permitted to 15° to 30°C (59° to 86°F).

Actions

➤*Pharmacology:* Mecamylamine reduces blood pressure in both normotensive and hypertensive individuals. It has a gradual onset of action (0.5 to 2 hours) and a long lasting effect (usually 6 to 12 hours or more). A small oral dosage often produces a smooth and predictable reduction of blood pressure. Although this antihypertensive effect is predominantly orthostatic, the supine blood pressure is also significantly reduced.

➤*Pharmacokinetics:*

Absorption – Mecamylamine is almost completely absorbed from the gastrointestinal tract, resulting in consistent lowering of blood pressure in most patients with hypertensive cardiovascular disease.

Distribution – Mecamylamine crosses the blood-brain and placental barriers.

Excretion – Mecamylamine is excreted slowly in the urine in the unchanged form. The rate of its renal elimination is influenced markedly by urinary pH. Alkalinization of the urine reduces, and acidification promotes, renal excretion of mecamylamine.

Contraindications

Mecamylamine should not be used in mild, moderate, labile hypertension and may prove unsuitable in uncooperative patients. It is contraindicated in coronary insufficiency or recent myocardial infarction.

Mecamylamine should be given with great discretion, if at all, when renal insufficiency is manifested by a rising or elevated BUN. The drug is contraindicated in uremia. Patients receiving antibiotics and sulfonamides should generally not be treated with ganglion blockers. Other contraindications are glaucoma, organic pyloric stenosis or hypersensitivity to the product.

Warnings

➤*CNS effects:* Mecamylamine, a secondary amine, readily penetrates into the brain and may produce CNS effects. Tremor, choreiform movements, mental aberrations, and convulsions may occur rarely. These have occurred most often when large doses of mecamylamine HCl were used, especially in patients with cerebral or renal insufficiency.

➤*Discontinuation of therapy:* When ganglion blockers or other potent antihypertensive drugs are discontinued suddenly, hypertensive levels return. In patients with malignant hypertension and others, this may occur abruptly and may cause fatal cerebral vascular accidents or acute congestive heart failure. Withdraw mecamylamine HCl gradually and substitute other antihypertensive therapy, if necessary. However, the effects of mecamylamine HCl can last hours to days after therapy is discontinued.

➤*Renal function impairment:* Evaluate the patient's condition, particularly renal and cardiovascular function. Give with great discretion, if at all, when renal insufficiency is manifested by a rising or elevated BUN. When renal, cerebral, or coronary blood flow is deficient, avoid any additional impairment that might result from hypotension.

➤*Pregnancy: Category C.* Animal reproduction studies have not been conducted with mecamylamine. It is not known whether mecamylamine can cause fetal harm when given to a pregnant woman or can affect reproductive capacity. Administer to a pregnant woman only if clearly needed.

➤*Lactation:* Because of the potential for serious adverse reactions in breast-feeding infants from mecamylamine, decide whether to discontinue breast-feeding or the drug, taking into account the importance of the drug to the mother.

➤*Children:* Safety and efficacy in children have not been established.

Precautions

➤*Monitoring:* Evaluate the patient's condition carefully, particularly renal and cardiovascular function. When renal, cerebral, or coronary blood flow is deficient, any additional impairment, which might result from added hypotension, must be avoided.

The action of mecamylamine HCl may be potentiated by excessive heat, fever, infection, hemorrhage, pregnancy, anesthesia, surgery, vigorous exercise, other antihypertensive drugs, alcohol, and salt depletion as a result of diminished intake or increased excretion caused by diarrhea, vomiting, excessive sweating, or diuretics.

During therapy with mecamylamine HCl, do not restrict sodium intake but, if necessary, adjust the dosage of the ganglion blocker.

Because urinary retention may occur in patients on ganglion blockers, use caution in patients with prostatic hypertrophy, bladder neck obstruction, and urethral stricture.

➤*Special risk:* Frequent loose bowel movements with abdominal distention and decreased borborygmi may be the first signs of paralytic ileus. If these are present, discontinue mecamylamine HCl immediately and take remedial steps.

Use caution in patients with marked cerebral and coronary arteriosclerosis or after a recent cerebral accident.

Drug Interactions

➤*Antibiotics and sulfonamides:* In general, do not treat patients receiving antibiotics and sulfonamides with ganglion blockers.

➤*Anesthesia, other antihypertensives, alcohol:* The action of mecamylamine HCl may be potentiated by anesthesia, other antihypertensive drugs, and alcohol.

Other antihypertensives – When mecamylamine is given with other antihypertensive drugs, reduce the dosage of these other agents, as well as that of mecamylamine, to avoid excessive hypotension. However, continue thiazides in their usual dosage, while decreasing mecamylamine at least 50%.

Adverse Reactions

The following adverse reactions have been reported and within each category are listed in order of decreasing severity.

➤*Cardiovascular:* Orthostatic dizziness and syncope, postural hypotension.

➤*CNS:* Convulsions, choreiform movements, mental aberrations, tremor, and paresthesias.

➤*GI:* Ileus, constipation (sometimes preceded by small, frequent liquid stools), vomiting, nausea, anorexia, glossitis and dryness of mouth.

➤*GU:* Urinary retention, impotence, decreased libido.

➤*Respiratory:* Interstitial pulmonary edema and fibrosis.

➤*Special senses:* Blurred vision, dilated pupils.

➤*Miscellaneous:* Weakness, fatigue, sedation.

Overdosage

➤*Symptoms:* Signs of overdosage include hypotension (which may progress to peripheral vascular collapse), postural hypotension, nausea, vomiting, diarrhea, constipation, paralytic ileus, urinary retention, dizziness, anxiety, dry mouth, mydriasis, blurred vision, or palpitations. A rise in intraocular pressure may occur.

➤*Treatment:* Pressor amines may be used to counteract excessive hypotension. Because patients being treated with ganglion blockers are more than normally reactive to pressor amines, small doses of the latter are recommended to avoid excessive response.

Patient Information

Take after meals. Use consistent timing of doses in relation to meals.

Mecamylamine may cause dizziness, light-headedness, or fainting, especially when rising from a lying or sitting position. This effect may be increased by alcoholic beverages, exercise, or during hot weather. Getting up slowly may help alleviate such a reaction.

WARNING

Pregnancy – When used in pregnancy during the second and third trimesters, angiotensin-converting enzyme inhibitors (ACEIs) can cause injury to and even death in the developing fetus. When pregnancy is detected, discontinue the ACEI as soon as possible. Refer to the general discussion of these products in the Antihypertensives Introduction.

Indications

Refer to individual monographs for specific indications.

ACEI Indications

Indications	Benazepril	Captopril	Enalapril	Enalaprilat	Fosinopril	Lisinopril	Moexipril	Perindopril	Quinapril	Ramipril	Trandolapril
Hypertension	✓	✓	✓	✓	✓	✓	✓	✓	✓	✓	✓
Heart failure		✓	✓		✓	✓			✓	✓[a]	✓[a]
Left ventricular dysfunction, post-MI		✓									✓
Left ventricular dysfunction, asymptomatic			✓								
Improve survival post-MI						✓					
Reduce risk of MI, stroke, and death from cardiovascular causes										✓	
Diabetic nephropathy		✓									

[a] Following MI.

➤*Hypertension:* The ACEIs are effective alone and in combination with other antihypertensives, especially thiazide-type diuretics. Blood pressure-lowering effects of ACEIs and thiazides are approximately additive.

Per JNC 7 guidelines†, use thiazide-type diuretics as initial therapy for most patients with hypertension, either alone or in combination with 1 or the other classes (eg, ACEIs).

➤*Heart failure:* **Captopril**, **enalapril**, **fosinopril**, **lisinopril**, and **quinapril** are indicated in the treatment of (congestive) heart failure, usually in combination with diuretics and/or digitalis. **Ramipril** and **trandolapril** are indicated in stable patients who are symptomatic from CHF within the first few days after sustaining acute MI.

➤*Left ventricular dysfunction:* **Enalapril** is indicated to treat clinically stable asymptomatic patients with left ventricular dysfunction (ejection fraction 35% or less). It has been shown to decrease the rate of developing overt heart failure and decrease the incidence of hospitalization for heart failure.

Captopril is indicated to improve survival following MI in clinically stable patients with left ventricular dysfunction manifested as an ejection fraction of 40% or less and to reduce the incidence of overt heart failure and subsequent hospitalizations for CHF in these patients.

Trandolapril is indicated in stable patients who have evidence of left ventricular systolic dysfunction (identified by wall motion abnormalities).

➤*MI:* **Lisinopril** is indicated in the treatment of hemodynamically stable patients within 24 hours of acute MI to improve survival.

➤*Reduction in risk of MI, stroke, and death from cardiovascular causes:* **Ramipril** is indicated in patients 55 years of age or older who are at high risk of developing a major cardiovascular event because of a history of coronary artery disease, stroke, peripheral vascular disease, or diabetes that is accompanied by at least 1 other cardiovascular risk factor (eg, hypertension, elevated total cholesterol levels, low HDL levels, cigarette smoking, documented microalbuminuria), to reduce the risk of MI, stroke, or death from cardiovascular causes.

➤*Diabetic nephropathy:* **Captopril** is indicated for the treatment of diabetic nephropathy (proteinuria over 500 mg/day) in patients with type 1 insulin-dependent diabetes mellitus and retinopathy. Captopril decreases the rate of progression of renal insufficiency and development of serious adverse clinical outcomes (death or need for renal transplantation or dialysis).

➤*Unlabeled uses:*

JNC 7 guidelines – Per JNC 7 guidelines, ACEIs have been shown in clinical trials to be beneficial in the following: Heart failure, post MI, high coronary disease risk, diabetes, chronic kidney disease, and recurrent stroke prevention.

Stroke prevention – **Perindopril**, alone and in combination with a diuretic, has been shown to reduce the risk of stroke among hypertensive and nonhypertensive individuals with a history of stroke or transient ischemic attack.

Migraine prophylaxis – One clinical study showed **lisinopril** to be effective as a prophylactic treatment of migraine.

Diabetic nephropathy – Other ACEIs (eg, **enalapril**, **ramipril**) have been shown to be effective in the treatment of diabetic nephropathy in normotensive patients.

Nondiabetic nephropathy – **Ramipril** and **benazepril** have shown favorable effects on the progression of nondiabetic nephropathy.

Bartter syndrome – ACEIs may be of benefit in the management of Bartter syndrome.

Renovascular hypertension – ACEIs have shown effectiveness in the treatment of renovascular hypertension.

Hypertensive emergencies/urgencies – **Enalaprilat** (1.25 mg IV over 5 minutes every 6 hours; titrate by 1.25 mg increments up to a maximum dose of 5 mg) may be useful in the management of hypertensive emergencies. **Captopril** (25 to 50 mg at 1- or 2-hour intervals) may be useful for hypertensive urgencies.

Scleroderma renal crisis – Prompt treatment of scleroderma renal crisis with ACEIs may reverse acute renal failure.

Hypertension in children (**Captopril**) – For infants, consider initial captopril doses of 0.15 to 0.3 mg/kg/dose followed by upward titration as needed. For children, consider initial doses of 0.3 to 0.5 mg/kg/dose given every 8 hours, followed by upward titration as needed. The maximum captopril dose is 6 mg/kg/day in divided doses.

Actions

➤*Pharmacology:* The ACEIs appear to act primarily through suppression of the renin-angiotensin-aldosterone system. Based on chemical structure, they can be classified into 3 groups: Sulfhydryl-containing (**captopril**); dicarbocyl-containing (**enalapril**, **lisinopril**, **benazepril**, **quinapril**, **moexipril**, **perindopril**, **trandolapril**, **ramipril**); and phosphorus-containing (**fosinopril**).

Synthesized by the kidneys, renin is released into the circulation where it acts on angiotensinogen to produce angiotensin I, a relatively inactive decapeptide. Angiotensin I is then converted by the angiotensin-converting enzyme (ACE) to angiotensin II, a potent endogenous vasoconstrictor that also stimulates aldosterone secretion from the adrenal cortex, contributing to sodium and fluid retention. ACEIs prevent the conversion of angiotensin I to angiotensin II by inhibiting ACE; they do not alter pressor responses to other agents.

Inhibiting ACE results in decreased plasma angiotensin II and increased plasma renin activity (PRA), the latter resulting from loss of negative feedback on renin release caused by reduction in angiotensin II. This leads to decreased aldosterone secretion, resulting in small increases in serum potassium along with sodium and fluid loss.

Increased prostaglandin synthesis also may play a role in the antihypertensive action of ACEI. ACE is identical to bradykininase (kininase II); thus, ACEIs can increase bradykinin levels. Because bradykinin stimulates prostaglandin biosynthesis, these peptides may contribute to the pharmacological effects of ACEIs.

The ACEIs produce a reduction of peripheral arterial resistance in hypertensive patients, an increase in cardiac output, and little or no change in heart rate. Renal blood flow increases, but glomerular filtration rate (GFR) is usually unchanged.

Blood pressure reduction may be progressive. To achieve maximal effects, several weeks of therapy may be required. Blood pressure-lowering effects of ACEIs and thiazide-type diuretics are additive, but captopril and β-blockers have a less than additive effect. Standing and supine blood pressures are lowered to about the same extent. Orthostatic effects and tachycardia are infrequent but may occur in volume- or salt-depleted patients. Abrupt withdrawal is not associated with a rapid increase in blood pressure.

The ACEIs are antihypertensive even in low-renin hypertensives. They are antihypertensive in all races studied, but black hypertensives (usually low-renin hypertensives) show a smaller average response to monotherapy than nonblacks.

Some ACEIs have demonstrated a beneficial effect on the severity of heart failure and an improvement in maximal exercise tolerance in patients with heart failure. In these patients, ACEIs significantly decrease peripheral (systemic vascular) resistance, blood pressure (afterload), pulmonary capillary wedge pressure (preload), and pulmonary vascular resistance, and increase cardiac output and exercise tolerance time. These effects occur after the first dose and persist for the duration of therapy.

➤*Pharmacokinetics:*

Absorption/Distribution – The presence of food in the GI tract reduces the absorption of **captopril** by about 30% to 40%. Food intake also reduces **moexipril** C_{max} 70% to 80% and AUC 40% to 50%. Therefore, take captopril and moexipril 1 hour before meals (see Drug Interactions).

† Chobanian AV, Bakris GI, Black HR, et al, and the National High Blood Pressure Education Program Coordinating Committee. The Seventh Report of the Joint National Committee on Prevention, Detection, Evaluation, and Treatment of High Blood Pressure: the JNC 7 report. *JAMA*. 2003;289:2560-2572. http://www.nhlbi.nih.gov/guidelines/hypertension/express.pdf

Animal studies indicate that **benazepril** (and metabolites), **enalapril**, **lisinopril**, captopril, and **perindopril** cross the blood-brain barrier poorly, if at all. **Enalaprilat**, **fosinopril**/fosinoprilat, and **quinapril** do not cross the blood-brain barrier.

Metabolism/Excretion – With the exception of **captopril** and **lisinopril**, most of the ACEIs are prodrugs that are rapidly converted to their active metabolites following oral administration.

The effective half-lives for accumulation are as follows: 10 to 11 hours for benazeprilat, 11 hours for enalaprilat, 11.5 hours for fosinoprilat, 12 hours for lisinopril, 12 hours for moexiprilat, and 3 hours for quinaprilat.

Special populations –

Renal function impairment:

• *Benazepril* – In patients with Ccr 30 mL/min or less, peak benazeprilat levels and the initial (alpha phase) half-life increase, and the time to steady state may be delayed. In patients with renal failure, biliary clearance may compensate to an extent.

• *Captopril* – Excretion rates are reduced and retention of captopril occurs in patients with impaired renal function. Captopril can be removed by hemodialysis.

• *Enalapril/Enalaprilat* – With GFR of 30 mL/min or less, peak and trough enalaprilat levels increase, T_{max} increases, and time to steady state may be delayed. Enalaprilat is dialyzable at the rate of 62 mL/min.

• *Fosinopril* – In patients with end-stage renal disease (Ccr less than 10 mL/min), the total body clearance of fosinoprilat is approximately one half of that in patients with normal renal function. Fosinopril is not well dialyzed.

• *Lisinopril* – Impaired renal function (GFR less than 30 mL/min) decreases lisinopril elimination, increases peak and trough levels, increases T_{max}, and time to attain steady state is prolonged. Lisinopril can be removed by hemodialysis.

• *Moexipril* – The effective elimination half-life and AUC of moexipril and moexiprilat are increased with decreasing renal function. At Ccr in the range of 10 to 40 mL/min, the half-life of moexiprilat is increased by a factor of 3 to 4.

• *Perindopril* – Perindoprilat AUC increases with decreasing renal function. At Ccr of 30 to 80 mL/min, AUC is about double that of 100 mL/min. When Ccr drops below 30 mL/min, AUC increases more markedly. Perindopril dialysis clearance ranges from 41.7 to 76.7 mL/min and perindoprilat dialysis clearance ranges from 37.4 to 91 mL/min.

• *Quinapril* – The half-life of quinaprilat increases as Ccr decreases. There is a linear correlation between plasma quinaprilat clearance and Ccr. Chronic hemodialysis or continuous ambulatory peritoneal dialysis has little or no effect on the elimination of quinapril and quinaprilat.

• *Ramipril* – In patients with Ccr less than 40 mL/min, peak levels of ramiprilat are approximately doubled, and trough levels may be as much as 5 times higher. In multiple dose regimens, the ramiprilat AUC is 3 to 4 times as large as it is in patients with normal renal function.

• *Trandolapril* – The plasma concentrations of trandolapril and trandolaprilat are approximately 2-fold greater and renal clearance is reduced by about 85% in patients with Ccr below 30 mL/min and in patients on hemodialysis.

Hepatic function impairment:

• *Fosinopril* – In patients with hepatic insufficiency (alcoholic or biliary cirrhosis), the rate of hydrolysis of fosinopril may be slowed. The apparent total body clearance of fosinoprilat is approximately one half of that in patients with normal hepatic function.

• *Moexipril* – In patients with mild to moderate cirrhosis given single 15 mg doses, the C_{max} of moexipril was increased by about 50% and the AUC increased by about 120%, while the C_{max} for moexiprilat was decreased by about 50% and the AUC increase by about 300%.

• *Perindopril* – The bioavailability of perindoprilat is increased, and plasma concentrations were about 50% higher than those with normal liver function.

• *Quinapril* – Quinaprilat concentrations are reduced in patients with alcoholic cirrhosis because of impaired deesterification of quinapril.

• *Ramipril* – The metabolism of ramipril to ramiprilat appears to be slowed, and plasma ramipril levels are increased about 3-fold.

• *Trandolapril* – Following oral administration in patients with mild to moderate alcoholic cirrhosis, plasma concentrations of trandolapril and trandolaprilat were, respectively, 9- and 2-fold greater than in healthy subjects, but inhibition of ACE activity was not affected.

Elderly:

• *Lisinopril* – Older patients have (approximately doubled) higher blood levels and AUC than younger patients.

• *Moexipril* – The AUC and C_{max} of moexiprilat is about 30% greater than in younger subjects.

• *Perindopril* – Plasma concentrations of perindopril and perindoprilat in patients older than 70 years of age are approximately twice those observed in younger patients.

• *Quinapril* – Elimination of quinaprilat may be reduced in patients 65 years of age and older.

• *Ramipril* – Peak ramiprilat levels and AUC are higher in older patients.

• *Trandolapril* – The plasma concentration of trandolapril is increased in elderly hypertensive patients, but the plasma concentration of trandolaprilat and inhibition of ACE activity are similar in elderly and young hypertensive patients.

Heart failure:

• *Fosinopril* – The effective half-life of fosinoprilat was 14 hours.

• *Perindopril* – Perindoprilat clearance is reduced in CHF patients, resulting in 40% higher-dose interval AUC.

• *Quinapril* – Elimination of quinaprilat may be reduced in patients with heart failure.

Pharmacokinetics of the Active Moieties of ACEIs

ACEI	Onset (h)	Peak effect (h)	Duration (h)	Bioavailability (%)	T_{max} (h)	Protein binding	Effect of food on absorption	Active metabolite	Elimination half-life (h)	Routes of elimination
Benazepril	1	2-4	24	≥ 37	0.5-1 (1-4)[a,b]	≈ 96.7% (≈ 95.3%)[a]	slows absorption	benazeprilat		renal (20%)[a] bile (11%-12%)[a]
Captopril	≤ 0.5	1-1.5	6-10 (dose-related)	≥ 75	1	≈ 25%-30%	absorption reduced by ≈ 30%-40%		< 2	renal (> 95%)
Enalapril	1	4-6	≥ 24	≈ 60	1 (3-4)[a]		none	enalaprilat		renal feces
Enalaprilat	0.25	1-4	≈ 6	na			na			renal (> 90%)
Fosinopril	1	2-6	24	≈ 36	3	99.4%[a]	slows absorption	fosinoprilat	≈ 12[a]	renal (≈ 50%) feces (≈ 50%)
Lisinopril	1	6	24	≈ 25	7	none	none			renal (100%)
Moexipril	≈ 1	3-6	24	≈ 13	≈ 1.5[a]	≈ 50%[a]	markedly reduced	moexiprilat	2-9[a]	renal (13%) feces (53%)
Perindopril				≈ 75	≈ 1 (3-7)[a]	≈ 60% (10%-20%)[a]	reduces bioavailability of metabolite	perindoprilat	≈ 0.8-1 (3-10)[a]	renal
Quinapril	≤ 1	2-4	24	≥ 60	1 (≈ 2)[a]	≈ 97%	moderately reduced	quinaprilat	≈ 2[a]	renal
Ramipril	1-2	3-6	24	≥ 50-60	1 (2-4)[a]	≈ 73% (≈ 56%)[a]	slows absorption	ramiprilat	9-18[a]	renal (60%) feces (40%)
Trandolapril		4-8	24	≈ 10 (70)[a]	1 (4-10)[a]	≈ 80%	slows absorption	trandolaprilat	≈ 6 (10)[a]	renal (≈ 33%) feces (≈ 66%)

[a] Active metabolite.

[b] 1 to 2 hours in fasting state and 2 to 4 hours in nonfasting state.

Contraindications

Hypersensitivity to these products and in patients with a history of angioedema related to previous treatment with an ACEI; in patients with hereditary or idiopathic angioedema (**enalapril**, **enalaprilat**, **lisinopril**).

Warnings

➤*Hematologic effects:* Neutropenia (less than 1,000/mm³) with myeloid hypoplasia resulted from use of **captopril**. About half of the neutropenic patients developed systemic or oral cavity infections or other features of agranulocytosis. The risk of neutropenia is dependent on the patient's clinical status. In hypertension with normal renal function (serum creatinine less than 1.6 mg/dL, no collagen vascular disease [eg, systemic lupus erythematosus, scleroderma]), neutropenia occurred in 1 patient in more than 8,600 exposed. In patients with some degree of renal failure (serum creatinine at least 1.6 mg/dL) but no collagen vascular disease, the risk of neutropenia was about 1 in 500. Daily doses of captopril were relatively high. Concomitant allopurinol and captopril have been associated with neutropenia. In collagen vascular diseases and impaired renal function, neutropenia has occurred in 3.7% of patients. In heart failure, the same risk factors for neutropenia appear present; about half of cases had serum creatinine at least 1.6 mg/dL, and more than 75% also were on procainamide.

Neutropenia usually has been detected within 3 months after captopril initiation. Bone marrow examinations consistently showed myeloid hypoplasia, frequently accompanied by erythroid hypoplasia and decreased numbers of megakaryocytes (eg, hypoplastic bone marrow, pancytopenia); anemia and thrombocytopenia were sometimes seen. In general, neutrophils returned to normal about 2 weeks after captopril was discontinued; serious infections were limited to clinically complex patients. About 13% of neutropenia cases were fatal, but almost all were in patients with serious illness having collagen vascular disease, renal failure, heart failure, immunosuppressant therapy, or a combination of these factors. Discontinuation of captopril and other drugs has generally led to prompt return of the normal WBC count; upon confirmation of neutropenia, withdraw the drug and closely observe the patient.

Neutropenia/leukopenia/agranulocytosis has occurred rarely with **enalapril** or **lisinopril** and in 1 patient on **quinapril**; a causal relationship cannot be excluded. Data are insufficient to show that **moexipril**, **perindopril**, **ramipril**, **benazepril**, **trandolapril**, or **fosinopril** do not cause agranulocytosis at similar rates. Periodically monitor WBC counts.

➤*Anaphylactoid and possibly related reactions:* Presumably because ACEIs affect the metabolism of eicosanoids and polypeptides, including endogenous bradykinin, patients receiving ACEIs may be subject to a variety of adverse reactions, some of them serious.

Angioedema – Angioedema has occurred in patients treated with ACEIs. It may occur at any time during treatment with **enalapril** (0.2%); **captopril**, **lisinopril**, **perindopril**, **quinapril** (0.1%); **trandolapril** (0.13%); **benazepril** (about 0.5%); **moexipril** (less than 0.5%); **ramipril** (0.3%); or **fosinopril** (0.2% to 1%). Angioedema of the face, extremities, lips, mucous membranes, tongue, glottis, or larynx has occurred. In instances where swelling has been confined to the face and lips, the condition has generally resolved without treatment, although antihistamines have been useful in relieving symptoms. Angioedema associated with laryngeal edema may be fatal. If laryngeal stridor or angioedema of the face, tongue, larynx, or glottis occurs and appears likely to cause airway obstruction, discontinue treatment and institute appropriate therapy (eg, epinephrine solution 1:1000 SC) immediately. Use with extreme caution in patients with hereditary angioedema (caused by a deficiency of C1 esterase inhibitor). Intestinal angioedema has been reported in patients treated with ACEIs. These patients presented with abdominal pain (with or without nausea or vomiting); in some cases there was no history of facial angioedema and C1 esterase levels were normal. The angioedema was diagnosed by procedures including abdominal CT scan or ultrasound, or at surgery, and symptoms resolved after stopping the ACE inhibitor. Include intestinal angioedema in the differential diagnosis of patients on ACE inhibitors presenting with abdominal pain. Symptoms resolved after stopping ACEIs. Patients with a history of angioedema unrelated to ACEI therapy may be at increased risk of angioedema while receiving an ACEI. Black patients receiving ACE inhibitor monotherapy have been reported to have a higher incidence of angioedema compared with nonblacks.

Anaphylactoid reactions during desensitization – Two patients undergoing desensitizing treatment with hymenoptera venom while receiving ACEIs sustained life-threatening anaphylactoid reactions. In the same patients, these reactions were avoided when ACEIs were temporarily withheld, but they reappeared upon inadvertent rechallenge.

Anaphylactoid reactions during membrane exposure – Anaphylactoid reactions have been reported in patients dialyzed with high-flux membranes and treated concomitantly with an ACEI. In such patients, immediately stop dialysis and initiate aggressive therapy for anaphylactoid reactions. Symptoms have not been relieved by antihistamines in these situations. Consider a different type of dialysis membrane or a different class of medication. Anaphylactoid reactions also have occurred in patients undergoing low-density lipoprotein apheresis with dextran sulfate absorption.

➤*Proteinuria:* Total urinary proteins of more than 1 g/day were seen in about 0.7% of **captopril** patients. About 90% of affected patients showed evidence of prior renal disease or received relatively high doses of captopril (more than 150 mg/day) or both. Nephrotic syndrome occurred in approximately one fifth of these cases. In most cases, proteinuria cleared within 6 months, regardless of whether captopril was continued; creatinine and BUN were seldom altered.

➤*Hypotension:*

First-dose effect – ACEIs may cause a profound fall in blood pressure following the first dose. Excessive hypotension is rare in uncomplicated hypertensive patients, but is possible with ACEI use in severely salt/volume depleted people such as those treated vigorously with diuretics or patients on dialysis. Patients at risk for excessive hypotension, sometimes associated with oliguria and/or progressive azotemia, and rarely with acute renal failure and/or death, include those with the following conditions or characteristics: Heart failure, hyponatremia, high-dose diuretic therapy, recent intensive diuresis or increase in diuretic dose, renal dialysis, or severe volume and/or salt depletion. Correct volume and/or salt depletion before initiating treatment. Excessive perspiration, dehydration, vomiting, and/or diarrhea may also lead to an excessive fall in blood pressure because of reduction in fluid volume.

Minimize the possibility of hypotension either by discontinuing the diuretic or by increasing salt intake about 1 week prior to initiating ACEIs, or initiate with small doses. Alternatively, provide medical supervision for at least 2 hours after the initial dose and until blood pressure has stabilized for at least an additional hour.

A transient hypotensive response is not a contraindication for further doses of these agents, which usually can be given without difficulty once the blood pressure has stabilized. If excessive hypotension occurs, place patient in supine position and, if necessary, give normal saline IV. A dose reduction or discontinuation of the ACEI or concomitant diuretic may be necessary.

Heart failure – In heart failure where the blood pressure was either normal or low, transient decreases in mean blood pressure more than 20% occurred in about half of patients taking **captopril**. Transient hypotension may occur after the first several doses. This effect is usually well tolerated, and it is asymptomatic or produces brief, mild lightheadedness. It rarely has been associated with arrhythmia or conduction defects. Start therapy under close medical supervision. Follow patients closely for the first 2 weeks and whenever the dose of ACEI or diuretic is increased. Also follow patients with ischemic heart, aortic stenosis, or cerebrovascular disease in whom an excessive fall in blood pressure could result in MI or cerebrovascular accident.

Hypotension is not a reason to discontinue the ACEI. Some decrease in systemic blood pressure is common and desirable in heart failure. The magnitude of the decrease is greatest early in treatment, stabilizes within 1 to 2 weeks, and generally returns to pretreatment levels without a decrease in efficacy within 2 months.

Acute MI – In a study, patients with an acute MI had a higher incidence of persistent hypotension (systolic blood pressure less than 90 mm Hg for more than 1 hour) when treated with **lisinopril**. Treatment must not be initiated in acute MI patients at risk of further serious hemodynamic deterioration after treatment with a vasodilator (eg, systolic blood pressure of 100 mm Hg or lower) or cardiogenic shock.

➤*Hepatic failure:* Rarely ACEIs have been associated with a syndrome that starts with cholestatic jaundice and progresses to fulminant hepatic necrosis and (sometimes) death. The mechanism of this syndrome is not understood. Patients receiving ACEIs who develop jaundice or marked elevations of hepatic enzymes should discontinue the ACEI and receive appropriate medical follow-up.

➤*Renal function impairment:* Some hypertensive patients with unilateral or bilateral renal artery stenosis have developed increases in BUN and serum creatinine after reduction of blood pressure (20% of patients with **enalapril**). Monitor renal function in such patients during the first few weeks of therapy. Dosage reduction and/or discontinuation of the ACEI and/or diuretic may be required. For some patients, it may not be possible to normalize blood pressure and maintain adequate renal perfusion.

About 20% of heart failure patients develop stable elevations of BUN and serum creatinine more than 20% above normal or baseline with long-term **captopril**. Less than 5% of patients, generally those with severe pre-existing renal disease, require treatment discontinuation; subsequent improvement probably relies on the severity of underlying renal disease.

In patients with severe CHF whose renal function may depend on the activity of the renin-angiotensin-aldosterone system, treatment with ACEIs may be associated with oliguria and/or progressive azotemia and, rarely, with acute renal failure and/or death.

Some hypertensive or heart failure patients with no apparent pre-existing renal vascular disease have developed increases in BUN and serum creatinine; these are usually minor and transient, especially when the ACEI was given with a diuretic. This is more likely to occur in patients with pre-existing renal impairment. Dosage adjustment and/or discontinuation of the diuretic and/or ACEI may be required. However, captopril has shown renal protective effects in hypertensive patients with some renal dysfunction.

Impaired renal function decreases **lisinopril** elimination, which is excreted principally through the kidneys, but this decrease becomes clinically important only when the GFR is less than 30 mL/min. The elimination half-life of quinaprilat increases as creatinine clearance decreases. Dosage adjustment may be necessary for **quinapril**, **benazepril**, **ramipril**, **captopril**, **trandolapril**, **moexipril**, **enalapril**, **perindopril**, and **lisinopril**. Impaired renal function decreases total clearance of fosinoprilat and approximately doubles the AUC. However, in general, no dosing adjustment is needed (see Pharmacokinetics).

➤*Hepatic function impairment:* Patients with impaired liver function could develop markedly elevated plasma levels of unchanged **fosinopril**, **moexipril**, or **ramipril**. No formal pharmacokinetic studies with ramipril have been done in hypertensive patients with impaired liver function. In patients with alcoholic or biliary cirrhosis, the rate, but not extent, of fosinopril hydrolysis was reduced; the total body clearance of fosinoprilat was decreased and AUC approximately doubled. Quinaprilat concentrations are reduced in patients with alcoholic cirrhosis caused by impaired deesterification of **quinapril**. Consider lower **trandolapril** doses in patients with mild to moderate alcoholic cirrhosis; plasma concentrations of trandolapril and trandolaprilat were increased. Perindoprilat plasma concentrations may be elevated.

➤*Elderly:* Elderly patients may have higher blood levels and AUC of **lisinopril**, ramiprilat, **perindopril**, quinaprilat, and moexiprilat. This may relate to decreased renal function rather than to age itself. No overall differences in effectiveness or safety were observed between elderly patients receiving **trandolapril**, **fosinopril**, or **benazepril**; however, greater sensitivity of some older individuals cannot be ruled out.

➤*Pregnancy: Category C* (first trimester); *Category D* (second and third trimesters). ACEIs can cause fetal and neonatal morbidity and death when administered to pregnant women. Several dozen cases have been reported in the world literature. When pregnancy is detected, discontinue ACEIs as soon as possible.

The use of ACEIs during the second and third trimesters of pregnancy has been associated with fetal and neonatal injury, including hypotension, neonatal skull hypoplasia, anuria, reversible or irreversible renal failure, and death. Oligohydramnios also has occurred, presumably resulting from decreased fetal renal function; oligohydramnios in this setting has been associated with fetal limb contractures, craniofacial deformation, and hypoplastic lung development. Prematurity, intrauterine growth retardation, and patent ductus arteriosus also have been reported, although it is not clear whether these occurrences were caused by the ACEI exposure.

These adverse effects do not appear to have resulted from intrauterine ACEI exposure that has been limited to the first trimester. Inform mothers whose embryos and fetuses are exposed to ACEIs only during the first trimester. Nonetheless, when patients become pregnant, make every effort to discontinue the use of the ACEI as soon as possible.

Rarely (probably less often than 1 in every 1000 pregnancies), no alternative to ACEIs will be found. In these rare cases, apprise the mother of the potential hazards to the fetus, and perform serial ultrasound examinations to assess the intra-amniotic environment.

If oligohydramnios is observed, discontinue the ACEI unless it is considered lifesaving for the mother. Contraction stress testing, a non-stress test, or biophysical profiling may be appropriate, depending on the week of pregnancy. However, patients and physicians should be aware that oligohydramnios may not appear until after the fetus has sustained irreversible injury.

Closely observe infants with histories of in utero exposure to ACEIs for hypotension, oliguria, and hyperkalemia. If oliguria occurs, direct attention toward support of blood pressure and renal perfusion. Exchange transfusion or dialysis may be required as a means of reversing hypotension or substituting for disordered renal function. Some of these agents may be removed from neonatal circulation by exchange transfusion or dialysis (see Overdosage); however, limited experience has not shown that such removal is central to the treatment of these infants.

➤*Lactation:* Several ACEIs have been detected in breast milk. Do not administer **trandolapril**, **captopril**, **benazepril**, **fosinopril**, **enalapril**, **quinapril**, or **ramipril** to nursing mothers. It is not known whether **lisinopril**, **moexipril**, or **perindopril** are excreted in breast milk. Because of the potential for serious adverse effects, exercise caution when these drugs are administered to nursing women. Decide whether to discontinue nursing or discontinue the drug, taking into account the importance of the drug to the mother.

➤*Children:* Safety and efficacy have not been established. However, there is limited experience with the use of **captopril** in children. Dosage, on a weight basis, was comparable to or less than that used in adults. Infants, especially newborns, may be more susceptible to the adverse hemodynamic effects of captopril. Excessive, prolonged, and unpredictable decreases in blood pressure and associated complications, including oliguria and seizures, have occurred. Use captopril in children only when other measures for controlling blood pressure have not been effective.

Antihypertensive effects of **enalapril** have been established in hypertensive pediatric patients 1 month to 16 years of age and with **lisinopril** in patients 6 to 16 years of age. Enalapril and lisinopril are not recommended in neonates and in pediatric patients with GFR less than 30 mL/min/1.73 m^2, because no data is available.

Precautions

➤*Monitoring:* Patients with impaired renal function should have WBCs and differential counts monitored prior to starting treatment and at approximately 2-week intervals for about 3 months, then periodically. Consider periodic monitoring of WBCs in patients with collagen vascular disease and renal disease.

➤*Hyperkalemia:* Elevated serum potassium (at least 0.5 mEq/L greater than the upper limit of normal) was observed in 0.4% of hypertensive patients given **trandolapril**; 1.4% with **perindopril**; about 1% of hypertensive patients given **benazepril**, **enalapril**, **ramipril**, or **moexipril**; about 2% of patients receiving **lisinopril** or **quinapril**, about 2.6% of hypertensive patients given **fosinopril**, and about 4.8% of CHF patients given lisinopril. In most cases, these were resolved despite continued therapy. Hyperkalemia was a cause of therapy discontinuation in 0.28% of hypertensive patients on enalapril, about 0.1% with lisinopril and fosinopril, less than 0.1% with quinapril, no patients on ramipril and trandolapril, 2% of type 1 diabetics with proteinuria receiving **captopril**, 0.6% of heart failure patients on lisinopril, and 0.1% of MI patients on lisinopril. Risk factors for development of hyperkalemia may include renal insufficiency, diabetes mellitus, and concomitant use of agents that increase serum potassium (eg, potassium-sparing diuretics, potassium supplements, and/or potassium containing salt substitutes).

➤*Valvular stenosis:* Theoretically, patients with aortic stenosis might be at risk of decreased coronary perfusion when treated with vasodilators, because they do not develop as much afterload reduction as others. Use with caution in patients with obstruction in the outflow tract of the left ventricle (eg, aortic stenosis, hypertrophic cardiomyopathy).

➤*Surgery/Anesthesia:* In patients undergoing major surgery or during anesthesia with agents that produce hypotension, ACEIs will block angiotensin II formation secondary to compensatory renin release. Hypotension can be corrected by volume expansion.

➤*Cough:* Chronic cough has occurred with the use of all ACEIs, presumably caused by the inhibition of the degradation of endogenous bradykinin. Characteristically, the cough is nonproductive, persistent, and resolves within 1 to 7 days (but can take as long as 2 weeks) after therapy discontinuation. Consider ACEI-induced cough as part of the differential diagnosis of cough.

The cough appears to have a higher incidence in women. The incidence of cough, although still reported as 0.5% to 3% by some manufacturers, appears to range from 5% to 25% and has been reported to be as high as 39%, resulting in discontinuation rates as high as 15%. The use of sulindac, diclofenac, indomethacin, nifedipine, cromolyn, or nebulized bupivacaine may be effective in managing cough; although, this is only based on a small number of patients. Further study is needed.

➤*Photosensitivity:* Photosensitization may occur; therefore, caution patients to take protective measures (ie, sunscreens, protective clothing) against exposure to ultraviolet light or sunlight until tolerance is determined.

Drug Interactions

ACEI Drug Interactions

Precipitant drug	Object drug*		Description
Antacids (eg, aluminum and magnesium hydroxide, simethicone)	ACEIs	↓	Bioavailability of ACEIs may be decreased. May be more likely with **captopril** and **fosinopril**. Separate the administration times by 1 to 2 hours if an interaction is suspected.
Capsaicin	ACEIs	↑	Capsaicin may cause or exacerbate coughing associated with ACEI treatment and vice versa.
Diuretics	ACEIs	↑	Possible excessive reduction in blood pressure, especially in those patients with intravascular volume depletion, can occur. Consider discontinuing the diuretic or increasing salt intake prior to initiation of treatment with an ACEI. If this is not possible, consider reduction of initial ACEI dose.
Iron salts	ACEIs Captopril	↓	Oral iron preparations may reduce captopril blood levels. Separate administration by at least 2 hours.
NSAIDS (eg, indomethacin, aspirin)	ACEIs	↓	This combination reduced hypotensive effects of ACEIs. More prominent in low-renin or volume-dependent hypertensive patients; concomitant use may further deteriorate renal function.
Rifampin	ACEIs Enalapril	↓	Pharmacologic effects of enalapril may be decreased.
ACEIs Captopril	Allopurinol	↑	A higher risk of hypersensitivity reaction is possible when these drugs are given concurrently.
ACEIs	Digoxin	↑↓	Plasma levels of digoxin may be increased or decreased, possibly because of altered renal clearance. Monitor digoxin plasma levels.
ACEIs	Diuretics (eg, loop diuretics)	↓	The effects of loop diuretics may be decreased; possible inhibition of angiotensin II production by the ACEI.
ACEIs	Lithium	↑	Increased serum lithium levels and symptoms of toxicity may occur; monitor lithium levels frequently.
ACEIs	Hypoglycemic agents/insulin	↑	Rarely, hypoglycemia has been reported during concomitant therapy. Monitor symptoms of hypoglycemia during initiation of therapy.
ACEIs	Potassium preparations/ Potassium-sparing diuretics	↑	Coadministration may result in elevated serum potassium concentrations. Use with caution; monitor potassium levels and renal function frequently.
ACEIs Quinapril	Tetracycline	↓	Tetracycline absorption was reduced 28% to 37%, possibly caused by the high magnesium content of quinapril tablets.

* ↑ = Object drug increased. ↓ = Object drug decreased.

➤*Drug/Lab test interactions:* **Captopril** may cause a false-positive urine test for acetone.

Fosinopril may cause a false-low measurement of serum digoxin levels with the *Digi-Tab RIA Kit for Digoxin*. Other kits, such as the *Coat-A-Count RIA Kit*, may be used.

➤*Drug/Food interactions:* Food significantly reduces the absorption of **captopril** 30% to 40%. Administer captopril 1 hour before meals. Food intake reduces the C_{max} and AUC of **moexipril** about 70% and 40%, respectively, after a low-fat breakfast and 80% and 50%, respectively, after a high-fat breakfast; take moexipril in the fasting state and administer 1 hour before meals. Food reduces the biotransformation of **perindopril** to the active metabolite perindoprilat by approximately 43%, resulting in a reduction in the plasma ACE inhibition curve of approximately 20%. The rate and extent of **quinapril** absorption are diminished moderately (about 25% to 30%) when administered during a high-fat meal. The rate, but not extent, of **ramipril**, **fosinopril**, and **trandolapril** absorption is reduced by food. Food does not reduce the GI absorption of **benazepril**, **enalapril**, and **lisinopril**.

Adverse Reactions

Adverse Reactions Shared by the ACEIs[a] (%)

✓ = Reported; no incidence given.

Adverse reactions	Benazepril	Captopril	Enalapril/ Enalaprilat	Fosinopril	Lisinopril	Moexipril	Perindopril	Quinapril	Ramipril	Trandolapril
Cardiovascular										
Angina pectoris	< 1	0.2-0.3	1.5	0.2-1		< 1		< 0.5	< 1-3	
Bradycardia			0.5-1	0.4-1	0.3-1				< 1	0.3-4.7
Cardiac arrest		✓[b]	0.5-1	✓	0.3-1		✓		< 1	
Cerebrovascular accident		✓[b]	0.5-1	0.2-1	0.3-1	< 1	0.2	< 0.5	< 1	
Chest pain		1	2.1	0.2-2.2	3.4	> 1	2.4	2.4	< 1	0.3-1
Hypotension[c]	0.3	✓	0.9-6.7	0.2-4.4	1.2-9.7	0.51	0.3-1	2.9	0.5-11	0.3-11
MI		0.2-0.3	0.5- 1.2	0.2-1	0.3-1	< 1	0.3-1	< 0.5	< 1	
Orthostatic hypotension/effects	0.4	✓[b]	1.2-2.2	≤ 1.2-1.9	0.3- 1.2	0.51	0.3-1	< 0.5	2	
Palpitations	< 1	1	0.5-1	0.2-1	0.3-1	< 1	0.9-1.1	0.5-1	< 1	0.3-1
Peripheral edema	< 1				0.3-1	> 1				
Rhythm disturbances		✓[b]	0.5-1	≤ 0.2-1.4		< 1		< 0.5		
Tachycardia		1	0.5-1	0.4-1	0.3-1			0.5-1	< 1	
CNS										
Anxiety	< 1					< 1	0.3-1		< 1	0.3-1
Ataxia		✓[b]	0.5-1		0.3-1					
Confusion		✓[b]	0.5-1	0.2-1	0.3-1					
Depression		✓[b]	0.5-1	0.4-1			2	0.5-1	< 1	
Dizziness	3.6		0.5-7.9	1.6-11.9	5.4-11.8	4.3	8.2	3.9-7.7	1.9-4	1.3-23
Fatigue	2.4		0.5-3	≥ 1	2.5	2.4		2.6	2	
Headache	6.2		1.8-5.2	≥ 1	4.4-5.7	> 1	23.8	1.7		
Insomnia/Sleep disturbances	< 1		0.5-1	0.2-1	0.3-1	< 1	2.5	0.5-1	< 1	0.3-1
Malaise					0.3-1	< 1	0.3-1	0.5-1	< 1	
Nervousness	< 1	✓[b]	0.5-1		0.3-1	< 1	1.1	0.5-1	< 1	
Paresthesias	< 1		0.5-1	0.2-1	0.3-1		2.3	0.5-1	< 1	0.3-1
Peripheral edema	< 1					> 1				
Somnolence/Drowsiness	1.6	✓[b]	0.5-1	0.2-1	0.3-1	< 1	1.3	0.5-1	< 1	0.3-1
Vertigo			1.6	0.2-1	0.2		0.3-1	0.5-1	< 1-2	0.3-1
Dermatologic										
Alopecia	< 1		0.5-1		0.3-1	< 1		0.5-1		
Diaphoresis/Sweating	< 1		0.5-1	0.2-1	0.3-1	< 1	0.3-1	0.5-1	< 1	
Erythema multiforme		✓[b]	0.5-1				0.3-1		< 1	
Exfoliative dermatitis		✓[b]	0.5-1	✓			✓	< 0.5		
Flushing	< 1	0.2-0.5	0.5-1	0.2-1	0.3-1	1.6				0.3-1
Pemphigus/Pemphigoid	< 1	✓	0.5-1		0.3-1			0.5-1		0.3-1
Photosensitivity	< 1	✓	0.5-1	0.2-1	0.3-1	< 1		< 0.5	< 1	
Pruritus	< 1	2	0.5-1	0.2-1	< 1		0.3-1	0.5-1	< 1	0.3-1
Rash	< 1	4-7	0.5-1.4	0.2-1	0.01-1.7	1.6	2.3	1.4	< 1	0.3-1
Stevens-Johnson syndrome	< 1	✓[b]	0.5-1		rare				< 1	
Toxic epidermal necrolysis			0.5-1		rare				< 1	
Urticaria			0.5-1	0.2-1	0.3-1	< 1		< 1	< 1	
GI										
Abdominal pain			1.6	0.2-1	2.2	< 1	2.7	1	< 1	0.3-1
Anorexia			0.5-1						< 1	
Constipation	< 1		0.5-1	0.2-1	0.3-1	< 1	0.3-1	0.5-1	< 1	0.3-1
Diarrhea			1.4-2.1	> 1	2.7-3.7	3.1	4.3	1.7	≤ 1	0.3-1
Dry mouth			0.5-1	0.2-1	0.3-1	< 1	0.3-1	0.5-1	< 1	
Dysgeusia		2-4								
Dyspepsia		✓[b]	0.5-1		0.3-1	> 1	0.3-1.9	< 0.5	< 1	0.3-6.4
Hepatitis		✓[b]	0.5-1	0.2-1	0.3-1	< 1		< 0.5	< 1	
Nausea	1.3		1.3-1.4	1.2-2.2	2	> 1	2.3	2.4	2	
Pancreatitis	< 1	✓[b]	0.5-1	0.2-1	0.3-1	< 1	✓	< 0.5	< 1	0.3-1
Vomiting	< 1		1.3	1.2-2.2	0.3-1.1	< 1	1.5	2.4	2	0.3-1

Adverse Reactions Shared by the ACEIs[a] (%)

✓ = Reported; no incidence given.

Adverse reactions	Benazepril	Captopril	Enalapril/ Enalaprilat	Fosinopril	Lisinopril	Moexipril	Perindopril	Quinapril	Ramipril	Trandolapril
GU										
Decreased libido	< 1			0.2-1	0.4					0.3-1
Impotence	< 1	✓[b]	0.5-1		1			0.5-1	< 1	0.3-1
Oliguria		0.1-0.2	0.5-1		0.3-1	< 1				
UTI	< 1		1.3		0.3-1		2.8	0.5-1		
Musculoskeletal										
Arthralgia	< 1	✓	✓	0.2-1	0.3-1	< 1	0.3-1	0.5-1	< 1	
Arthritis	< 1		✓	✓	0.3-1		1		< 1	
Muscle cramps			0.5-1	0.2-1	0.5					0.3-1
Myalgia	< 1	✓[b]	✓	0.2-1	0.3-1	1.3	0.3-1.1		< 1	4.7
Respiratory										
Asthma	< 1	✓	0.5-1		0.3-1					
Bronchitis	< 1		1.3		0.3-1		0.3-1			
Bronchospasm		✓[b]	0.5-1	0.2-1	0.3-1	< 1				
Cough[d]	1.2	0.5-2	1.3-2.2	2.2-9.7	0.5-3.5	6.1	6-12	2-4.3	8	1.9-35
Dyspnea	< 1		1.3	≥ 1	0.3-1	< 1	0.3-1		< 1	0.3-1
Pharyngitis				0.2-1	0.3-1	1.8	3.3	0.5-1		
Rhinitis		✓[b]		0.2-1	0.3-1	> 1	4.8			
Sinusitis	< 1			0.2-1	0.3-1	> 1	0.6-5.2			
Upper respiratory tract infection			0.5-1	2.2	1.5-2.1	> 1	8.6		✓	0.3-1
Miscellaneous										
Anemia[e]	✓	≤ 0.2		✓	0.3-1	< 1		< 0.5	< 1	
Angioedema[c]	0.5	0.1	✓	0.2-1	0.1	< 1	0.1	0.1	0.3	0.13
Asthenia	< 1	✓[b]	1.1-1.6		1.3		7.9		2	3.3
Blurred vision		✓[b]	0.5-1		0.3-1					
Eosinophilia		✓	✓	✓	0.3-1				< 1	
Fever		✓	0.5-1	0.4-1	0.3-1		0.3-1.5		< 1	
Syncope	0.1	✓[b]	0.5-2.2	0.2-1	0.3-1.8	0.51	0.3-1	0.5-1	< 1-2	5.9
Tinnitus			0.5-1	0.2-1	0.3-1	< 1	1.5		< 1	
Vasculitis		✓	✓		0.3-1		✓		< 1	

[a] Data are pooled from separate studies and are not necessarily comparable. Data included for both hypertension and heart failure indications.
[b] Postmarketing.
[c] See Warnings or Precautions.
[d] See Precautions. Although still reported at 0.5% to 3% by some manufacturers, the incidence appears to range from 5% to 25% and has been reported to be as high as 39%.
[e] Including aplastic and hemolytic.

➤*Cardiovascular:*

Benazepril – Postural dizziness (1.5%); postural hypotension (0.4%); ECG changes (rare).

Captopril – Raynaud syndrome, CHF (0.2% to 0.3%).

Enalapril – Pulmonary embolism and infarction, pulmonary edema, atrial fibrillation, Raynaud phenomenon (0.5 to 1%).

Fosinopril – Hypertensive crisis, claudication, hypertension, conduction disorder, cerebral infarction, sudden death, cardiorespiratory arrest, shock, transient ischemic attacks (0.2% to 1%).

Lisinopril – Ventricular/atrial tachycardia; pulmonary embolism, premature ventricular contractions, pulmonary infarction, paroxysmal nocturnal dyspnea, decreased blood pressure, chest discomfort, atrial fibrillation, arrhythmias, transient ischemic attack (0.3 to 1%); postinfarction angina (0.3%).

Perindopril – Abnormal ECG (1.8%); ventricular extrasystole, vasodilation, abnormal conduction, heart murmur (0.3% to 1%).

Quinapril – Vasodilation (0.5% to 1%); heart failure, hypertensive crisis, cardiogenic shock (less than 0.5%).

Ramipril – CHF, arrhythmia, transient ischemic attack (less than 1%).

Trandolapril – Stroke (3.3%); cardiogenic shock (3.8%); first-degree AV block (0.3% to 1%).

➤*CNS:*

Enalapril – Peripheral neuropathy, dream abnormality, dysesthesia (0.5% to 1%).

Fosinopril – Memory disturbance, tremor, mood change, numbness, behavior change (0.2% to 1%).

Lisinopril – Stroke, memory impairment, tremor, irritability, hypersomnia, peripheral neuropathy, spasm (0.3% to 1%).

Moexipril – Mood changes (less than 1%).

Perindopril – Migraine, amnesia, psychosexual disorder (0.3% to 1%).

Ramipril – Amnesia, convulsions, hearing loss, neuralgia, neuropathy, tremor, vision disturbances (less than 1%); angioneurotic edema (0.3%).

➤*Dermatologic:*

Benazepril – Dermatitis (less than 1%).

Captopril – Rash, often with pruritus and sometimes with fever, arthralgia, and eosinophilia occurred in 4 to 7 of 100 patients, usually during the first 4 weeks of therapy. It is usually maculopapular and rarely urticarial. The rash is usually mild and disappears within a few days of dosage reduction, short-term treatment with an antihistaminic agent, and/or discontinuing therapy; remission may occur even if captopril is continued. Between 7% and 10% of patients with rash have shown an eosinophilia and/or positive ANA titers. Pallor (0.2% to 0.5%).

Enalapril – Herpes zoster (0.5% to 1%).

Lisinopril – Erythema, herpes zoster, skin lesions, skin infections (0.3% to 1%).

Perindopril – Skin infection, tinea, dry skin, erythema, fever blisters (0.3% to 1%); purpura (0.1%).

Quinapril – Dermatopolymyositis (less than 0.5%).

Ramipril – Purpura, onycholysis (less than 1%).

➤*GI:*

Benazepril – Gastritis, melena (less than 1%).

Captopril – Weight loss may be associated with taste loss; taste impairment is reversible and usually self-limited (2 to 3 months) even with continuous administration (2% to 4%).

Enalapril – Hepatic failure, stomatitis, ileus, taste alterations, melena, glossitis (0.5% to 1%).

Fosinopril – Dysphagia, abdominal distention, flatulence, heartburn, appetite/weight change, hepatomegaly (0.2% to 1%); hepatic failure, jaundice (hepatocellular or cholestatic).

Lisinopril – Flatulence, gastritis, heartburn, GI cramps, weight loss/gain, taste disturbances, hepatocellular/cholestatic jaundice (0.3% to 1%).

Moexipril – Appetite/weight change, taste alterations (less than 1%).

Perindopril – Flatulence (1%); dry mucous membranes, appetite increased, gastroenteritis (0.3% to 1%).

Quinapril – GI hemorrhage (less than 0.5%); flatulence, dry throat (0.5% to 1%).

Ramipril – Abdominal pain occurs sometimes with enzyme changes suggesting pancreatitis; dysphagia, gastroenteritis, increased salivation, taste disturbance (less than 1%).

Trandolapril – Gastritis (4.2%); abdominal distention (0.3% to 1%).

➤*Hematologic:* Small decreases in hemoglobin and/or hematocrit have been attributed to many ACEIs but are rarely of clinical importance unless another cause of anemia coexists.

Benazepril – Thrombocytopenia, hemolytic anemia, leukopenia (less than 1%).

Captopril – Neutropenia/agranulocytosis). Cases of anemia, thrombocytopenia, and pancytopenia have been reported.

Enalapril – Neutropenia, thrombocytopenia, bone marrow suppression (0.5% to 1%); hemolytic anemia, including cases of hemolysis in patients with G-6-PD deficiency, has been reported.

Fosinopril – Lymphadenopathy (0.2% to 1%); neutropenia, leukopenia.

Lisinopril – Rare cases of bone marrow depression, hemolytic anemia, leukopenia/neutropenia, thrombocytopenia.

Perindopril – Hematoma, ecchymosis (0.3% to 1%); leukopenia, neutropenia (0.1%).

Quinapril – Hemolytic anemia, agranulocytosis, thrombocytopenia (less than 0.5%).

Ramipril – Pancytopenia, hemolytic anemia, thrombocytopenia (less than 1%); leukopenia (rare).

Trandolapril – Decreased leukocytes, decreased neutrophils, low lymphocytes, thrombocytopenia (0.3% to 1%).

➤*Lab test abnormalities:* Hyperkalemia; hyponatremia, elevated liver transaminases and serum bilirubin.

Benazepril – Elevations in uric acid and blood glucose.

Captopril – Elevation of alkaline phosphatase.

Fosinopril – Elevations of LDH and alkaline phosphatase.

Moexipril – Elevations of uric acid (rare).

Perindopril – Triglyceride increase (1.3%); potassium decrease, uric acid increase, alkaline phosphatase increase, cholesterol increase, glucose increase (0.3% to 1%).

Ramipril – Elevations of uric acid and blood glucose (rare).

Trandolapril – Elevated serum uric acid (15%).

➤*Respiratory:* Eosinophilic pneumonitis has been attributed to many ACEIs.

Enalapril – Rhinorrhea, sore throat, hoarseness, pulmonary infiltrates (0.5% to 1%).

Fosinopril – Pleuritic chest pain, tracheobronchitis, abnormal breathing, sinus abnormalities (0.4% to 1%); laryngitis/hoarseness, epistaxis (0.2% to 1%); a symptom-complex of cough, bronchospasm, and eosinophilia has been observed in 2 patients.

Lisinopril – Common cold (1.1%); nasal congestion (0.4%); influenza (0.3%); malignant lung neoplasms, hemoptysis, pulmonary infiltrates, pleural effusion, wheezing, orthopnea, painful respiration, epistaxis, laryngitis, rhinorrhea, pneumonia, pharyngeal pain (0.3% to 1%).

Perindopril – Posterior nasal drip, rhinorrhea, throat disorder, sneezing, epistaxis, hoarseness (0.3% to 1%); pulmonary fibrosis (less than 0.1%).

Trandolapril – Epistaxis, throat inflammation (0.3% to 1%).

➤*Renal:* Elevation, usually transient and minor, in serum creatinine and BUN).

Benazepril – Proteinuria (rare; see Warnings).

Captopril – Proteinuria (1%; see Warnings); renal insufficiency, renal failure, nephrotic syndrome, polyuria, urinary frequency (0.1% to 0.2%).

Enalapril – Renal failure, renal dysfunction (0.5% to 1%).

Fosinopril – Renal insufficiency, urinary frequency, abnormal urination, kidney pain (0.2% to 1%).

Lisinopril – Renal dysfunction (2%); acute renal failure, anuria, uremia, progressive azotemia, pyelonephritis, dysuria (0.3% to 1%).

Moexipril – Urinary frequency (more than 1%); renal insufficiency (less than 1%).

Perindopril – Proteinuria (1% to 1.5%); kidney stone, urinary frequency, urinary retention, hematuria (0.3% to 1%).

Quinapril – Acute renal failure, worsening renal failure (less than 0.5%).

Ramipril – Abnormal kidney function (1%); proteinuria (rare).

➤*Miscellaneous:* Anaphylactoid reactions have occurred (see Warnings). A symptom complex has occurred and may include the following: Positive ANA, elevated ESR, arthralgia, arthritis, myalgia/myositis, fever, interstitial nephritis, vasculitis, rash, eosinophilia, serositis, leukocytosis, photosensitivity, other dermatologic manifestations.

Benazepril – Hypertonia, infection (less than 1%).

Enalapril – Anosmia, conjunctivitis, dry eyes, tearing, flank pain, gynecomastia, myalgia, myositis, serositis (0.5% to 1%).

Fosinopril – Musculoskeletal pain (0.2% to 3.3%); weakness (1.4%); edema, vision/taste disturbance, eye irritation, sexual dysfunction, hyperhidrosis, fall, gout, influenza, cold sensation, pain, swelling/weakness of extremities, abnormal vocalization, abnormal urination, kidney pain, weight gain, muscle ache (0.2% to 1%).

Lisinopril – Neck/hip/leg/knee/arm/joint/shoulder/low back pain, gout, lumbago, fluid overload, dehydration, diabetes mellitus, chills, virus infection, pain, pelvic/flank pain, edema, facial edema, visual loss, diplopia, photophobia, breast pain (0.3% to 1%).

Moexipril – Flu syndrome (3.1%); pain, urinary frequency (more than 1%).

Quinapril – Back pain (0.5% to 1.2%); amblyopia, viral infections, edema (0.5% to 1%); agranulocytosis (less than 0.5%).

Perindopril – Back pain (5.8% or less); low extremity pain (4.7%); edema (3.9%); injury (2.3%); viral infection (0.3% to 3.4%); upper extremity pain (0.2% to 2.8%); hypertonia (0.2% to 2.7%); seasonal allergy (2%); ear infection (1.3% or less); neck pain, male sexual dysfunction (1.4%); joint pain, menstrual disorder (1.1%); pain, cold/hot sensation, chills, fluid retention, facial edema, vaginitis, flank pain, gout, conjunctivitis, earache (0.3% to 1%).

Ramipril – Flu syndrome, edema, epistaxis, weight gain, hypoglycemia (less than 1%).

Trandolapril – Hypocalcemia (4.7%); intermittent claudication (3.8%); edema, extremity pain, gout (0.3% to 1%).

Postmarketing –

Captopril: Anaphylactoid reactions; gynecomastia; cerebrovascular insufficiency; bullous pemphigus; glossitis; jaundice; hepatitis, including rare cases of necrosis; cholestasis; symptomatic hyponatremia; myasthenia; eosinophilic pneumonitis.

Overdosage

➤*Symptoms:* Hypotension is most common. Systolic blood pressures of 95 and 80 mm Hg have occurred following **lisinopril** and **captopril** overdoses, respectively. One reported case of **perindopril** overdose developed hypothermia and circulatory arrest, then died following ingestion of up to 180 mg.

➤*Treatment:* Treatment includes usual supportive measures. Refer to General Management of Acute Overdosage. The primary concern is correction of hypotension. Volume expansion with an IV infusion of normal saline is the treatment of choice to restore blood pressure.

Captopril, **enalaprilat**, trandolaprilat, **lisinopril**, and **perindopril** may be removed by hemodialysis. There are inadequate data concerning the efficacy of removing captopril by hemodialysis in neonates and children. Enalaprilat has been removed from neonatal circulation by peritoneal dialysis. **Benazepril** is only slightly dialyzable, but dialysis might be considered in overdosed patients with severely impaired renal function. It is not known if **ramipril**, **moexipril**, or ramiprilat are removed by hemodialysis. Hemodialysis and peritoneal dialysis have little effect on the elimination of **fosinoprilat**, **quinapril**, and quinaprilat. Use caution with concurrent use of ACEIs and polyacrylonitrile dialyzers because of the possibility of severe, sudden, and sometimes fatal reactions. Stop the dialysis immediately and begin measures to treat anaphylactoid reactions.

Patient Information

Apprise female patients of childbearing age about the consequences of second and third trimester exposure to ACEIs and that these consequences do not appear to have resulted from intrauterine ACEI exposure limited to the first trimester. Ask these patients to report pregnancies to their physicians as soon as possible.

Take **captopril** and **moexipril** 1 hour before meals.

Stop taking the drug and notify physician if any of the following occurs: sore throat, fever, swelling of hands or feet, irregular heartbeat, chest pains, signs of angioedema (eg, swelling of face, eyes, lips, tongue, difficulty swallowing or breathing, hoarseness).

Excessive perspiration, dehydration, vomiting, and diarrhea may lead to a fall in blood pressure.

May cause dizziness, fainting, or lightheadedness, especially during the first days of therapy; avoid sudden changes in posture. If actual syncope occurs, discontinue drug until physician has been contacted. Heart failure patients should avoid rapid increases in physical activity.

May cause rash or impaired taste perception. Notify physician if these persist.

Do not use potassium supplements or salt substitutes containing potassium without consulting a physician.

A persistent dry cough may occur and usually does not subside unless the medication is stopped. If this effect becomes bothersome, consult a physician.

Advise patients planning to undergo any surgery and/or anesthesia to inform their physician that they are taking an ACEI that has a long duration of action.

BENAZEPRIL HYDROCHLORIDE

Rx	**Benazepril HCl** (Various, eg, Ivax, Teva)	**Tablets:** 5 mg	May contain lactose, maltodextrin. In 100s, 500s, and 1,000s.
	Lotensin (Novartis)		Lactose, castor oil. (LOTENSIN 5). Light yellow. In 90s, 100s, and UD 100s.
	Benazepril HCl (Various, eg, Ivax, Teva)	10 mg	May contain lactose, maltodextrin. In 100s, 500s, 1,000s, 2,500s, 5,000s, and UD 100s.
	Lotensin (Novartis)		Lactose, castor oil. (LOTENSIN 10). Dark yellow. In 90s, 100s, and UD 100s.
	Benazepril HCl (Various, eg, Ivax, Teva)	20 mg	May contain lactose, maltodextrin. In 100s, 500s, 1,000s, 2,500s, 5,000s, and UD 100s.
	Lotensin (Novartis)		Lactose, castor oil. (LOTENSIN 20). Pink. In 90s, 100s, and UD 100s.
	Benazepril HCl (Various, eg, Ivax, Teva)	40 mg	May contain lactose, maltodextrin. In 100s, 500s, 1,000s, 2,500s, 5,000s, and UD 100s.
	Lotensin (Novartis)		Lactose. (LOTENSIN 40). Dark rose. In 90s, 100s, and UD 100s.

BENAZEPRIL — ORAL

For complete and comparative prescribing information, refer to the Angiotensin-Converting Enzyme Inhibitors group monograph.

WARNING

Use in pregnancy – When used in pregnancy during the second and third trimesters, angiotension-converting enzyme (ACE) inhibitors can cause injury and even death to the developing fetus. When pregnancy is detected, discontinue benazepril as soon as possible.

Indications

➤*Hypertension:* Benazepril is indicated for the treatment of hypertension. It may be used alone or in combination with thiazide diuretics.

➤*Unlabeled uses:* Nondiabetic neuropathy; per Joint National Committee on the Prevention, Detection, Evaluation, and Treatment of High Blood Pressure (JNC) guidelines, ACE inhibitors have been shown in clinical trials to be beneficial in heart failure, post myocardial infarction (MI), high coronary disease risk, diabetes, chronic kidney disease, and recurrent stroke prevention.

Administration and Dosage

➤*Approved by the FDA:* June 25, 1991.

➤*Hypertension:*

Adults – The recommended initial dosage for patients not receiving a diuretic is 10 mg/day. The usual maintenance dosage range is 20 to 40 mg/day administered as a single dose or 2 equally divided doses. A dose of 80 mg gives an increased response, but experience with this dose is limited. The divided regimen was more effective in controlling trough (predosing) blood pressure than the same dose given as a once-daily regimen. Base dosage adjustment on measurement of peak (2 to 6 hours after dosing) and trough responses. If a once-daily regimen does not give adequate trough response, consider an increase in dosage or divided administration. If blood pressure is not controlled with benazepril alone, a diuretic can be added.

Total daily doses above 80 mg have not been evaluated.

Coadministration of benazepril with potassium supplements, potassium salt substitutes, or potassium-sparing diuretics can lead to increases of serum potassium.

In patients who are currently being treated with a diuretic, symptomatic hypotension occasionally can occur following the initial dose of benazepril. To reduce the likelihood of hypotension, if possible, discontinue the diuretic 2 to 3 days prior to beginning therapy with benazepril. Then, if blood pressure is not controlled with benazepril alone, do not resume diuretic therapy.

If the diuretic cannot be discontinued, use an initial dose of benazepril 5 mg to avoid excessive hypotension.

Children 6 years of age and older – In children, dosages of benazepril between 0.1 and 0.6 mg/kg once daily have been studied, and doses greater than 0.1 mg/kg were shown to reduce blood pressure. Based on this, the recommended starting dosage of benazepril is 0.2 mg/kg once per day as monotherapy. Doses above 0.6 mg/kg (or in excess of 40 mg daily) have not been studied in pediatric patients.

For pediatric patients who cannot swallow tablets or for whom the calculated dosage (mg/kg) does not correspond to the available tablet strengths for benazepril, follow the suspension preparation instructions to administer benazepril as a suspension.

Treatment with benazepril is not advised for children younger than 6 years of age and in pediatric patients with glomerular filtration rate less than 30 mL, as there are insufficient data available to support a dosing recommendation in these groups.

➤*Renal function impairment:* For patients with a creatinine clearance less than 30 mL/min per 1.73 m^2 (serum creatinine greater than 3 mg/dL), the recommended initial dosage is benazepril 5 mg once daily. Dosage may be titrated upward until blood pressure is controlled or to a maximum total daily dose of 40 mg.

➤*Storage/Stability:* Do not store the tablets above 30°C (86°F). Protect the tablets from moisture.

Dispense in tight container.

Refrigerate the suspension at 2° to 8°C (36° to 46°F); it can be stored for up to 30 days in the PET bottle with a child-resistant screw-cap closure. Shake the suspension before each use.

CAPTOPRIL

Rx	**Captopril** (Various, eg, Geneva, Mylan, Teva, UDL, Watson, West-Ward)	**Tablets:** 12.5 mg	In 100s, 500s, 1000s, 5000s, UD 100s, and blister 600s.
Rx	**Capoten** (Par)		Lactose. White, oval. In 100s and UD 100s.
Rx	**Captopril** (Various, eg, Geneva, Mylan, Teva, UDL, Watson, West-Ward)	**Tablets:** 25 mg	In 100s, 500s, 1000s, 5000s, UD 100s, and blister 600s.
Rx	**Capoten** (Par)		Lactose. White, rounded square, quadrisected. In 100s, 1000s, and UD 100s.
Rx	**Captopril** (Various, eg, Geneva, Mylan, Teva, UDL, Watson, West-Ward)	**Tablets:** 50 mg	In 100s, 500s, 1000s, 5000s, UD 100s, and blister 600s.
Rx	**Capoten** (Par)		Lactose. White, oval. In 100s, 1000s, and UD 100s.
Rx	**Captopril** (Various, eg, Geneva, Mylan, Teva, UDL, Watson, West-Ward)	**Tablets:** 100 mg	In 100s, 500s,1000s, UD 100s, and blister 600s.
Rx	**Capoten** (Par)		Lactose. White, oval. In 100s.

CAPTOPRIL — ORAL

For complete and comparative prescribing information, refer to the Angiotensin-Converting Enzyme Inhibitors group monograph.

WARNING

Pregnancy – When used in pregnancy during the second and third trimesters, angiotensin-converting enzyme (ACE) inhibitors can cause injury and even death to the developing fetus. When pregnancy is detected, captopril should be discontinued as soon as possible.

Indications

➤*Hypertension:* Captopril is indicated for the treatment of hypertension.

Captopril tablets may be used as initial therapy for patients with normal renal function, in whom the risk is relatively low. In patients with impaired renal function, particularly those with collagen vascular disease, captopril should be reserved for hypertensive patients who have either developed unacceptable side effects on other drugs, or have failed to respond satisfactorily to drug combinations.

Captopril is effective alone and in combination with other antihypertensive agents, especially thiazide diuretics. The blood pressure-lowering effects of captopril and thiazides are approximately additive.

CAPTOPRIL — ORAL

➤*Heart failure:* Captopril is indicated in the treatment of congestive heart failure usually in combination with diuretics and digitalis. The beneficial effect of captopril in heart failure does not require the presence of digitalis; however, most controlled clinical trial experience with captopril has been in patients receiving digitalis, as well as diuretic treatment.

➤*Left ventricular dysfunction after myocardial infarction:* Captopril is indicated to improve survival following myocardial infarction in clinically stable patients with left ventricular dysfunction manifested as an ejection fraction less than 40% and to reduce the incidence of overt heart failure and subsequent hospitalizations for congestive heart failure in these patients.

In considering use of captopril, it should be noted that in controlled clinical trials, ACE inhibitors have an effect on blood pressure that is less in black patients than in nonblack patients.

Administration and Dosage

Captopril tablets should be taken 1 hour before meals. Dosage must be individualized.

➤*Hypertension:* Initiation of therapy requires consideration of recent antihypertensive drug treatment, the extent of blood pressure elevation, salt restriction, and other clinical circumstances. If possible, discontinue the patient's previous antihypertensive drug regimen for 1 week before starting captopril.

The initial dose of captopril is 25 mg twice daily or 3 times daily. If satisfactory reduction of blood pressure has not been achieved after 1 or 2 weeks, the dose may be increased to 50 mg twice daily or 3 times daily. Concomitant sodium restriction may be beneficial when captopril is used alone.

The dose of captopril in hypertension usually does not exceed 50 mg 3 times daily. Therefore, if the blood pressure has not been satisfactorily controlled after 1 to 2 weeks at this dose (and the patient is not already receiving a diuretic), a modest dose of a thiazide-type diuretic (eg, hydrochlorothiazide, 25 mg daily), should be added. The diuretic dose may be increased at 1- to 2-week intervals until its highest usual antihypertensive dose is reached.

If captopril is being started in a patient already receiving a diuretic, therapy should be initiated under close medical supervision, with dosage and titration of captopril as noted above.

If further blood pressure reduction is required, the dose of captopril may be increased to 100 mg twice daily or 3 times daily and then, if necessary, to 150 mg twice daily or 3 times daily (while continuing the diuretic). The usual dose range is 25 to 150 mg twice daily or 3 times daily. A maximum daily dose of 450 mg captopril should not be exceeded.

For patients with severe hypertension (eg, accelerated or malignant hypertension), when temporary discontinuation of current antihypertensive therapy is not practical or desirable, or when prompt titration to more normotensive blood pressure levels is indicated, diuretic should be continued but other current antihypertensive medication stopped and captopril dosage promptly initiated at 25 mg twice daily or 3 times daily, under close medical supervision.

When necessitated by the patient's clinical condition, the daily dose of captopril may be increased every 24 hours or less under continuous medical supervision until a satisfactory blood pressure response is obtained or the maximum dose of captopril is reached. In this regimen, addition of a more potent diuretic (eg, furosemide, may also be indicated).

Beta-blockers may also be used in conjunction with captopril therapy, but the effects of the 2 drugs are less than additive.

➤*Heart failure:* Initiation of therapy requires consideration of recent diuretic therapy and the possibility of severe salt/volume depletion. In patients with either normal or low blood pressure, who have been vigorously treated with diuretics and who may be hyponatremic and/or hypovolemic, a starting dose of 6.25 or 12.5 mg 3 times daily may minimize the magnitude or duration of the hypotensive effect; for these patients, titration to the usual daily dosage can then occur within the next several days.

For most patients the usual initial daily dosage is 25 mg 3 times daily. After a dose of 50 mg 3 times daily is reached, further increases in dosage should be delayed, where possible, for at least 2 weeks to determine if a satisfactory response occurs. Most patients studied have had a satisfactory clinical improvement at 50 or 100 mg 3 times daily. A maximum daily dose of captopril 450 mg should not be exceeded.

Captopril should generally be used in conjunction with a diuretic and digitalis. Captopril therapy must be initiated under very close medical supervision.

➤*Left ventricular dysfunction after myocardial infarction:* The recommended dose for long-term use in patients following a myocardial infarction is a target maintenance dose of 50 mg 3 times daily.

Therapy may be initiated as early as 3 days following a myocardial infarction. After a single dose of 6.25 mg, captopril therapy should be initiated at 12.5 mg 3 times daily. Captopril should then be increased to 25 mg 3 times daily during the next several days and to a target dose of 50 mg 3 times daily over the next several weeks as tolerated.

Captopril may be used in patients treated with other postmyocardial infarction therapies (eg, thrombolytics, aspirin, beta-blockers).

➤*Renal function impairment:* Because captopril is excreted primarily by the kidneys, excretion rates are reduced in patients with impaired renal function. These patients will take longer to reach steady-state captopril levels and will reach higher steady-state levels for a given daily dose than patients with normal renal function. Therefore, these patients may respond to smaller or less frequent doses.

Accordingly, for patients with significant renal impairment, initial daily dosage of captopril should be reduced, and smaller increments utilized for titration, which should be quite slow (1- to 2-week intervals). After the desired therapeutic effect has been achieved, the dose should be slowly back-titrated to determine the minimal effective dose. When concomitant diuretic therapy is required, a loop diuretic (eg, furosemide), rather than a thiazide diuretic, is preferred in patients with severe renal impairment.

➤*Storage/Stability:* Store at controlled room temperature 15° to 30°C (59° to 86°F). Keep bottles tightly closed (protect from moisture).

ENALAPRIL MALEATE

Rx	**Enalapril Maleate** (Various, eg, Geneva, Mylan, Teva, Watson)	**Tablets:** 2.5 mg	In 100s and 1000s.
Rx	**Vasotec** (Biovail)		Lactose. (VASOTEC MSD 14). Yellow, barrel-shape, scored. In 100s, 1000s, 10,000s, unit-of-use 90s, and UD 100s.
Rx	**Enalapril Maleate** (Various, eg, Geneva, Mylan, Teva, Watson)	**Tablets:** 5 mg	In 100s and 1000s.
Rx	**Vasotec** (Biovail)		Lactose. (MSD 712 VASOTEC). White, barrel-shape, scored. In 100s, 1000s,10,000s, unit-of-use 90s, and UD 100s.
Rx	**Enalapril Maleate** (Various, eg, Geneva, Mylan, Teva, Watson)	**Tablets:** 10 mg	In 100s and 1000s.
Rx	**Vasotec** (Biovail)		Lactose. (MSD 713 VASOTEC). Salmon, barrel-shape. In 100s, 1000s, 10,000s, unit-of-use 90s, and UD 100s.
Rx	**Enalapril Maleate** (Various, eg, Geneva, Mylan, Teva, Watson)	**Tablets:** 20 mg	In 100s and 1000s.
Rx	**Vasotec** (Biovail)		Lactose. (MSD 714 VASOTEC). Peach, barrel-shape. In 100s, 1000s, 10,000s, unit-of-use 90s, and UD 100s.
Rx	**Enalaprilat** (Various, eg, Hospira, Baxter, Bedford	**Injection:** 1.25 mg enalaprilat/mL	In 1 and 2 mL vials.

ENALAPRIL MALEATE — ORAL

For complete and comparative prescribing information, refer to the Angiotensin-Converting Enzyme Inhibitors group monograph.

WARNING

Use in pregnancy – When used in pregnancy during the second and third trimesters, ACE inhibitors can cause injury and even death to the developing fetus. When pregnancy is detected, enalapril maleate should be discontinued as soon as possible.

Indications

➤*Hypertension:* Enalapril maleate is indicated for the treatment of hypertension.

Enalapril maleate is effective alone or in combination with other antihypertensive agents, especially thiazide-type diuretics. The blood pressure-lowering effects of enalapril maleate and thiazides are approximately additive.

➤*Heart failure:* Enalapril maleate is indicated for the treatment of symptomatic congestive heart failure, usually in combination with diuretics and digitalis. In these patients enalapril maleate improves symptoms, increases survival, and decreases the frequency of hospitalization.

➤*Asymptomatic left ventricular dysfunction:* In clinically stable asymptomatic patients with left ventricular dysfunction (ejection fraction less than or equal to 35%), enalapril maleate decreases the rate of development of overt heart failure and decreases the incidence of hospitalization for heart failure.

ENALAPRIL MALEATE — ORAL

Administration and Dosage

➤*Approved by the FDA:* December 24, 1985.

➤*Hypertension:* In patients who are currently being treated with a diuretic, symptomatic hypotension occasionally may occur following the initial dose of enalapril maleate. The diuretic should, if possible, be discontinued for 2 to 3 days before beginning therapy with enalapril maleate to reduce the likelihood of hypotension. If the patient's blood pressure is not controlled with enalapril maleate alone, diuretic therapy may be resumed. Patients at risk for excessive hypotension, sometimes associated with oliguria or progressive azotemia, and rarely with acute renal failure or death, include those with the following conditions or characteristics: Heart failure, hyponatremia, high dose diuretic therapy, recent intensive diuresis or increase in diuretic dose, renal dialysis, or severe volume or salt depletion of any etiology. It may be advisable to eliminate the diuretic (except in patients with heart failure), reduce the diuretic dose or increase salt intake cautiously before initiating therapy with enalapril maleate in patients at risk for excessive hypotension who are able to tolerate such adjustments. In patients at risk for excessive hypotension, therapy should be started under very close medical supervision and such patients should be followed closely for the first 2 weeks of treatment and whenever the dose of enalapril or diuretic is increased. Similar considerations may apply to patients with ischemic heart or cerebrovascular disease, in whom an excessive fall in blood pressure could result in a myocardial infarction or cerebrovascular accident.

If the diuretic cannot be discontinued an initial dose of 2.5 mg should be used under medical supervision for at least 2 hours and until blood pressure has stabilized for at least an additional hour.

The recommended initial dose in patients not on diuretics is 5 mg once a day. Dosage should be adjusted according to blood pressure response. The usual dosage range is 10 to 40 mg/day administered in a single dose or 2 divided doses. In some patients treated once daily, the antihypertensive effect may diminish toward the end of the dosing interval. In such patients, an increase in dosage or twice-daily administration should be considered. If blood pressure is not controlled with enalapril maleate alone, a diuretic may be added.

Coadministration of enalapril maleate with potassium supplements, potassium salt substitutes, or potassium-sparing diuretics may lead to increases of serum potassium. Risk factors for the development of hyperkalemia include renal insufficiency, diabetes mellitus, and the concomitant use of potassium-sparing diuretics, potassium supplements or potassium-containing salt substitutes, which should be used cautiously, if at all, with enalapril maleate.

➤*Dosage adjustment in hypertensive patients with renal impairment:* The usual dose of enalapril is recommended for patients with a creatinine clearance greater than 30 mL/min (serum creatinine of up to approximately 3 mg/dL). For patients with creatinine clearance less than or equal to 30 mL/min (serum creatinine greater than or equal to 3 mg/dL), the first dose is 2.5 mg once daily. The dosage may be titrated upward until blood pressure is controlled or to a maximum of 40 mg daily.

Renal status	Creatinine clearance mL/min	Initial dose mg/day
Normal renal function	> 80 mL/min	5 mg
Mild impairment	≤ 80 to 30 mL/min	5 mg
Moderate to severe impairment	≤ 30 mL/min	2.5 mg
Dialysis patients[a]	-	2.5 mg on dialysis day[b]

[a] Anaphylactoid reactions have been reported in patients dialyzed with high-flux membranes and treated concomitantly with an ACE inhibitor. Anaphylactoid reactions have also been reported in patients undergoing low-density lipoprotein apheresis with dextran sulfate absorption.
[b] Dosage on nondialysis days should be adjusted depending on the blood pressure response.

➤*Heart failure:* Enalapril maleate is indicated for the treatment of symptomatic heart failure, usually in combination with diuretics and digitalis. In the placebo-controlled studies that demonstrated improved survival, patients were titrated as tolerated up to 40 mg, administered in 2 divided doses.

The recommended initial dose is 2.5 mg. The recommended dosing range is 2.5 to 20 mg given twice a day. Doses should be titrated upward, as tolerated, over a period of a few days or weeks. The maximum daily dose administered in clinical trials was 40 mg in divided doses.

After the initial dose of enalapril maleate tablet, the patient should be observed under medical supervision for at least 2 hours and until blood pressure has stabilized for at least an additional hour. If possible, the dose of any concomitant diuretic should be reduced which may diminish the likelihood of hypotension. The appearance of hypotension after the initial dose of enalapril maleate does not preclude subsequent careful dose titration with the drug, following effective management of the hypotension.

➤*Asymptomatic left ventricular dysfunction:* In the trial that demonstrated efficacy, patients were started on 2.5 mg twice daily and were titrated as tolerated to the targeted daily dose of 20 mg (in divided doses).

➤*Dosage adjustment in patients with heart failure and renal impairment or hyponatremia:* In patients with heart failure who have hyponatremia (serum sodium less than 130 mEq/L) or with serum creatinine greater than 1.6 mg/dL, therapy should be initiated at 2.5 mg daily under close medical supervision (see Heart failure). The dose may be increased to 2.5 mg twice daily, then 5 mg twice daily and higher as needed, usually at intervals of 4 days or more if at the time of dosage adjustment there is not excessive hypotension or significant deterioration of renal function. The maximum daily dose is 40 mg.

➤*Pediatric hypertensive patients:* The usual recommended starting dose is 0.08 mg/kg (up to 5 mg) once daily. Dosage should be adjusted according to blood pressure response. Doses above 0.58 mg/kg (or in excess of 40 mg) have not been studied in pediatric patients.

Enalapril is not recommended in neonates or in pediatric patients with glomerular filtration rate less than 30 mL/min per 1.73 m^2, as no data are available.

➤*Storage/Stability:* Store at 15° to 30°C (59° to 86°F). Avoid transient temperatures above 50°C (122°F). Protect from moisture. Dispense in a tight container. Use child-resistant closure (as required).

Dispense in a tight container if product package is subdivided.

The suspension should be refrigerated at 2° to 8°C (36° to 46°F) and can be stored for up to 30 days. Shake the suspension before each use.

ENALAPRILAT — INJECTION

For complete and comparative prescribing information, refer to the Angiotensin-Converting Enzyme Inhibitors group monograph.

WARNING

Use in pregnancy – When used in pregnancy during the second and third trimesters, angiotensin-converting enzyme (ACE) inhibitors can cause injury and even death to the developing fetus. When pregnancy is detected, discontinue enalaprilat as soon as possible.

Indications

➤*Hypertension:* Enalaprilat is indicated for the treatment of hypertension when oral therapy is not practical.

Administration and Dosage

➤*Approved by the FDA:* 1985.

For intravenous (IV) administration only.

➤*Hypertension:* The dosage in hypertension is 1.25 mg every 6 hours administered IV over a 5-minute period. A clinical response is usually seen within 15 minutes. Peak effects after the first dose may not occur for up to 4 hours after dosing. The peak effects of the second and subsequent doses may exceed those of the first.

No dosage regimen for enalaprilat has been clearly demonstrated to be more effective in treating hypertension than 1.25 mg every 6 hours. However, in controlled clinical studies in hypertension, doses as high as 5 mg every 6 hours were well tolerated for up to 36 hours. There has been inadequate experience with dosages greater than 20 mg/day.

In studies of patients with hypertension, enalaprilat has not been administered for periods longer than 48 hours. In other studies, patients have received enalaprilat for as long as 7 days.

The dosage for patients being converted to enalaprilat from oral therapy for hypertension with enalapril maleate is 1.25 mg every 6 hours. For conversion from IV to oral therapy, the recommended initial dose of enalapril maleate is 5 mg once a day with subsequent dosage adjustments as necessary.

➤*Patients on diuretic therapy:* For patients on diuretic therapy, the recommended starting dose for hypertension is 0.625 mg administered IV over a 5-minute period (see Patients at risk of excessive hypotension). A clinical response is usually seen within 15 minutes. Peak effects after the first dose may not occur for up to 4 hours after dosing, although most of the effect is usually apparent within the first hour. If there is an inadequate clinical response after 1 hour, the 0.625 mg dose may be repeated. Additional doses of 1.25 mg may be administered at 6-hour intervals.

For conversion from IV to oral therapy, the recommended initial dosage of enalapril maleate for patients who have responded to 0.625 mg of enalaprilat every 6 hours is 2.5 mg once a day with subsequent dosage adjustment as necessary.

➤*Dosage adjustment in renal impairment:* The usual dosage of 1.25 mg of enalaprilat every 6 hours is recommended for patients with a creatinine clearance greater than 30 mL/min (serum creatinine of up to approximately 3 mg/dL). For patients with creatinine clearance 30 mL/min or less (serum creatinine to 3 mg/dL) or less, the initial dose is 0.625 mg.

If there is an inadequate clinical response after 1 hour, the 0.625 mg dose may be repeated. Additional doses of 1.25 mg may be administered at 6-hour intervals.

ENALAPRILAT — INJECTION

For dialysis patients, see the following information on patients at risk of excessive hypotension.

For conversion from IV to oral therapy, the recommended initial dosage of enalapril maleate is 5 mg once a day for patients with creatinine clearance greater than 30 mL/min and 2.5 mg once daily for patients with creatinine clearance 30 mL/min or less. Dosage should then be adjusted according to blood pressure response.

➤*Patients at risk of excessive hypotension:* Hypertensive patients at risk of excessive hypotension include those with the following concurrent conditions or characteristics: heart failure, hyponatremia, high dose diuretic therapy, recent intensive diuresis or increase in diuretic dose, renal dialysis, or severe volume or salt depletion of any etiology. Single doses of enalaprilat as low as 0.2 mg have produced excessive hypotension in normotensive patients with these diagnoses. Because of the potential for an extreme hypotensive response in these patients, therapy should be started under very close medical supervision. The starting dose should be no greater than 0.625 mg administered IV over a period of no less than 5 minutes and preferably longer (up to 1 hour).

Closely follow patients whenever the dose of enalaprilat is adjusted or diuretic is increased.

➤*Administration:* Administer enalaprilat as a slow IV infusion, as indicated previously. It may be administered as provided or diluted with up to 50 mL of a compatible diluent.

Visually inspect parenteral drug products for particulate matter and discoloration prior to use whenever solution and container permit.

➤*Compatibility and stability:* Enalaprilat as supplied and mixed with the following IV diluents has been found to maintain full activity for 24 hours at room temperature:

1.) 5% dextrose injection
2.) 0.9% sodium chloride injection
3.) 0.9% sodium chloride injection in 5% dextrose
4.) 5% dextrose in Ringer's lactate injection
5.) McGaw Isolyte E.

➤*Storage/Stability:* Store below 30°C (86°F). Store at 25°C (77°F), excursions permitted to 15° to 30°C (59° to 86°F).

FOSINOPRIL SODIUM

Rx	**Fosinopril Sodium** (Teva)	**Tablets:** 10 mg	Isopropyl alcohol, lactose. (9 3 72 22). White to off-white, rectangular, scored. In 90s and 1000s.
Rx	**Monopril** (Bristol-Myers Squibb)		Lactose. (BMS MONOPRIL 10). White to off-white, biconvex flat-end, diamond shape, scored. In 90s and 1000s.
Rx	**Fosinopril Sodium** (Teva)	**Tablets:** 20 mg	Isopropyl alcohol, lactose. (93 7223). White to off-white, capsule shape, scored. In 90s and 1000s.
Rx	**Monopril** (Bristol-Myers Squibb)		Lactose. (BMS MONOPRIL 20). White to off-white, oval. In 90s, 1000s, and UD 100s.
Rx	**Fosinopril Sodium** (Teva)	**Tablets:** 40 mg	Isopropyl alcohol, lactose. (93 7224). White to off-white, round, scored. In 90s and 1000s.
Rx	**Monopril** (Bristol-Myers Squibb)		Lactose. (BMS MONOPRIL 40). White to off-white, biconvex hexagonal. In 90s.

FOSINOPRIL SODIUM — ORAL

For complete prescribing information, refer to the Angiotensin-Converting Enzyme Inhibitors group monograph.

WARNING

Use in pregnancy – When used in pregnancy during the second and third trimesters, angiotensin-converting enzyme (ACE) inhibitors can cause injury and even death to the developing fetus. When pregnancy is detected, discontinue fosinopril as soon as possible.

Indications

➤*Hypertension:* Fosinopril is indicated for the treatment of hypertension. It may be used alone or in combination with thiazide diuretics.

➤*Heart failure:* Fosinopril is indicated in the management of heart failure as adjunctive therapy when added to conventional therapy, including diuretics with or without digitalis.

Administration and Dosage

➤*Approved by the FDA:* 1991.

➤*Hypertension:* The recommended initial dosage of fosinopril is 10 mg once a day, both as monotherapy and when the drug is added to a diuretic. Dosage should then be adjusted according to blood pressure response at peak (2 to 6 hours) and trough (about 24 hours after dosing) blood levels. The usual dosage range needed to maintain a response at trough is 20 to 40 mg, but some patients appear to have a further response to 80 mg. In some patients treated with once daily dosing, the antihypertensive effect may diminish toward the end of the dosing interval. If trough response is inadequate, consider dividing the daily dose. If blood pressure is not adequately controlled with fosinopril alone, a diuretic may be added.

Administration of fosinopril with potassium supplements, potassium salt substitutes, or potassium-sparing diuretics can lead to increases of serum potassium. Administer cautiously, if at all, with fosinopril.

In patients who are currently being treated with a diuretic, symptomatic hypotension occasionally can occur following the initial dose of fosinopril. To reduce the likelihood of hypotension, discontinue the diuretic, if possible, 2 to 3 days prior to beginning therapy with fosinopril. Then, if blood pressure is not controlled with fosinopril alone, resume diuretic therapy. If diuretic therapy cannot be discontinued, use an initial dose of 10 mg of fosinopril with careful medical supervision for several hours and until blood pressure has stabilized.

➤*Heart failure:* Digitalis is not required for fosinopril to manifest improvements in exercise tolerance and symptoms. Most placebo-controlled clinical trial experience has been with both digitalis and diuretics present as background therapy.

The usual starting dosage of fosinopril is 10 mg once daily. Following the initial dose of fosinopril, the patient should be observed under medical supervision for at least 2 hours for the presence of hypotension or orthostasis and, if present, until blood pressure stabilizes. An initial dose of 5 mg is preferred in heart failure patients with moderate to severe renal failure or those who have been vigorously diuresed.

Dosage should be increased, over a several week period, to a dose that is maximal and tolerated but not exceeding 40 mg once daily. The usual effective dosage range is 20 to 40 mg once daily.

The appearance of hypotension, orthostasis, or azotemia early in dose titration should not preclude further careful dose titration. Consider reducing the dose of concomitant diuretic.

Renal function impairment – In patients with impaired renal function, the total body clearance of fosinoprilat is approximately 50% slower than in patients with healthy renal function. Since hepatobiliary elimination partially compensates for diminished renal elimination, the total body clearance of fosinoprilat does not differ appreciably with any degree of renal impairment (creatinine clearances less than 80 mL/min per 1.73 m^2), including end-stage renal failure (creatinine clearance less than 10 mL/min per 1.73 m^2). This relative constancy of body clearance of active fosinoprilat, resulting from the dual route of elimination, permits use of the usual dose in patients with any degree of renal impairment.

➤*Storage/Stability:* Store at 25°C (77°F); excursions permitted to 15° to 30°C (59° to 86°F). Protect from moisture by keeping bottle tightly closed.

LISINOPRIL

Rx	**Lisinopril** (Various, eg, Apotex, Geneva, Mylan, Teva, Watson)	**Tablets:** 2.5 mg	In 100s, 500s, and 1000s.
Rx	**Prinivil** (Merck)		Mannitol. (MSD 15). White, flat-faced, beveled edge. In unit-of-use 30s, 100s, and UD 100s.
Rx	**Zestril** (AstraZeneca)		Mannitol. (ZESTRIL 2½ 135). White. In 100s.
Rx	**Lisinopril** (Various, eg, Apotex, Geneva, Mylan, Teva, Watson)	**Tablets:** 5 mg	In 100s and 1000s.
Rx	**Prinivil** (Merck)		Mannitol. (MSD 19 PRINIVIL). White, shield shape, scored. In 1000s, 10,000s, unit-of-use 90s and 100s, UD 100s, and blister pack 31s.
Rx	**Zestril** (AstraZeneca)		Mannitol. (ZESTRIL 130). Pink, capsule shape, bisected. In 100s and UD 100s.

LISINOPRIL

Rx	**Lisinopril** (Various, eg, Apotex, Geneva, Mylan, Teva, Watson)	**Tablets:** 10 mg	In 100s and 1000s.
Rx	**Prinivil** (Merck)		Mannitol. (MSD 106 PRINIVIL). Light yellow, shield shape. In 1000s, 10,000s, unit-of-use 30s, 90s, 100s, UD 100s, and blister pack 31s.
Rx	**Zestril** (AstraZeneca)		Mannitol. (ZESTRIL 10 131). Pink. In 100s and UD 100s.
Rx	**Lisinopril** (Various, eg, Apotex, Geneva, Mylan, Teva, Watson)	**Tablets:** 20 mg	In 100s and 1000s.
Rx	**Prinivil** (Merck)		Mannitol. (MSD 207 PRINIVIL). Peach, shield shape. In 1000s, 10,000s, unit-of-use 30s, 90s, and 100s, UD 100s, and blister pack 31s.
Rx	**Zestril** (AstraZeneca)		Mannitol. (ZESTRIL 20 132). Red. In 100s and UD 100s.
Rx	**Lisinopril** (Various, eg, Apotex, Geneva, Mylan, Teva, Watson)	**Tablets:** 30 mg	In 100s, 500s, and 1000s.
Rx	**Zestril** (AstraZeneca)		Mannitol. (ZESTRIL 30 133). Red. In 100s.
Rx	**Lisinopril** (Various, eg, Apotex, Geneva, Mylan, Teva, Watson)	**Tablets:** 40 mg	In 100s, 500s, 1000s, and UD 100s.
Rx	**Prinivil** (Merck)		Mannitol. (MSD 237 Prinivil). Rose red, shield shape. In unit-of-use 100s.
Rx	**Zestril** (AstraZeneca)		Mannitol. (ZESTRIL 40 134). Yellow. In 100s.

LISINOPRIL — ORAL

For complete and comparative prescribing information, refer to the Angiotensin-Converting Enzyme Inhibitors group monograph.

WARNING

Use in pregnancy – When used in pregnancy during the second and third trimesters, angiotensin-converting enzyme (ACE) inhibitors can cause injury and even death to the developing fetus. When pregnancy is detected, lisinopril should be discontinued as soon as possible.

The use of ACE inhibitors during the second and third trimesters of pregnancy has been associated with fetal and neonatal injury, including hypotension, neonatal skull hypoplasia, anuria, reversible or irreversible renal failure, and death. Oligohydramnios has also been reported, presumably resulting from decreased fetal renal function; oligohydramnios in this setting has been associated with fetal limb contractures, craniofacial deformation, and hypoplastic lung development. Prematurity, intrauterine growth retardation, and patent ductus arteriosus have also been reported, although it is not clear whether these occurrences were due to the ACE inhibitor exposure.

Indications

➤*Hypertension:* Lisinopril is indicated for the treatment of hypertension. It may be used alone as initial therapy or concomitantly with other classes of antihypertensive agents.

➤*Heart failure:* Lisinopril is indicated as adjunctive therapy in the management of heart failure in patients who are not responding adequately to diuretics and digitalis.

➤*Acute MI:* Lisinopril is indicated for the treatment of hemodynamically stable patients within 24 hours of acute MI, to improve survival. Patients should receive, as appropriate, the standard recommended treatments such as thrombolytics, aspirin, and beta blockers.

Administration and Dosage

➤*Approved by the FDA:* 1987.

➤*Hypertension:*

Initial therapy – In patients with uncomplicated essential hypertension not on diuretic therapy, the recommended initial dose is 10 mg once a day. Dosage should be adjusted according to blood pressure response. The usual dosage range is 20 to 40 mg/day administered in a single daily dose. The antihypertensive effect may diminish toward the end of the dosing interval regardless of the administered dose, but most commonly with a dose of 10 mg/day. This can be evaluated by measuring blood pressure just prior to dosing to determine whether satisfactory control is being maintained for 24 hours. If it is not, an increase in dose should be considered. Doses up to 80 mg have been used but do not appear to give a greater effect. If blood pressure is not controlled with lisinopril alone, a low dose of a diuretic may be added. Hydrochlorothiazide 12.5 mg has been shown to provide an additive effect. After the addition of a diuretic, it may be possible to reduce the dose of lisinopril.

➤*Diuretic-treated patients:* In hypertensive patients who are currently being treated with a diuretic, symptomatic hypotension may occur occasionally following the initial dose of lisinopril. The diuretic should be discontinued, if possible, for 2 to 3 days before beginning therapy with lisinopril to reduce the likelihood of hypotension. It may be advisable to eliminate the diuretic (except in patients with heart failure), reduce the diuretic dose or increase salt intake cautiously before initiating therapy with lisinopril in patients at risk for excessive hypotension who are able to tolerate such adjustments. The dosage of lisinopril should be adjusted according to blood pressure response. If the patient's blood pressure is not controlled with lisinopril alone, diuretic therapy may be resumed as described above.

If the diuretic cannot be discontinued, an initial dose of 5 mg should be used under medical supervision for at least 2 hours and until blood pressure has stabilized for at least an additional hour. When a diuretic is added to the therapy of a patient receiving lisinopril, an additional antihypertensive effect is usually observed. Studies with ACE inhibitors in combination with diuretics indicate that the dose of the ACE inhibitor can be reduced when it is given with a diuretic.

Concomitant administration of lisinopril with potassium supplements, potassium salt substitutes, or potassium-sparing diuretics may lead to increases of serum potassium. Therefore, if concomitant use of these agents is indicated because of demonstrated hypokalemia, they should be used with caution and with frequent monitoring of serum potassium. Potassium-sparing agents should generally not be used in patients with heart failure who are receiving lisinopril.

➤*Renal function impairment:* The usual dose of lisinopril (10 mg) is recommended for patients with a creatinine clearance greater than 30 mL/min (serum creatinine of up to approximately 3 mg/dL). For patients with creatinine clearance greater than or equal to 10 mL/min but less than or equal to 30 mL/min (serum creatinine greater than or equal to 3 mg/dL), the first dose is 5 mg once daily. For patients with creatinine clearance less than 10 mL/min (usually on hemodialysis), the recommended initial dose is 2.5 mg (dosage or dosing interval should be adjusted depending on the blood pressure response). The dosage may be titrated upward until blood pressure is controlled or to a maximum of 40 mg daily.

Lisinopril Dosage in Renal Imparment

Renal status	Creatinine clearance (mL/min)	Initial dose (mg/day)
Normal renal function to mild impairment	> 30 mL/min	10 mg/day
Moderate-to-severe renal impairment	≥ 10 mL/min ≤ 30 mL/min	5 mg/day
Dialysis patients*	< 10 mL/min	2.5 mg/day**

* See Warnings, Anaphylactoid reactions during membrane exposure.
** Dosage or dosing interval should be adjusted depending on the blood pressure response.

➤*Heart failure:* Lisinopril is indicated as adjunctive therapy with diuretics and digitalis. The recommended starting dose is 5 mg once a day. When initiating treatment with lisinopril in patients with heart failure, the initial dose should be administered under medical observation, especially in those patients with low blood pressure (systolic blood pressure less than 100 mm Hg). The mean peak blood pressure lowering occurs 6 to 8 hours after dosing. Observation should continue until blood pressure is stable. The concomitant diuretic dose should be reduced, if possible, to help minimize hypovolemia which may contribute to hypotension. The appearance of hypotension after the initial dose of lisinopril does not preclude subsequent careful dose titration with the drug, following effective management of the hypotension.

The usual effective dosage range is 5 to 40 mg/day, administered as a single daily dose. The dose of lisinopril can be increased by increments of no greater than 10 mg, at intervals of no less than 2 weeks to the highest tolerated dose, up to a maximum of 40 mg daily. Dose adjustment should be based on the clinical response of individual patients.

Dosage adjustment in heart failure and renal function impairment or hyponatremia – In patients with heart failure who have hyponatremia (serum sodium less than 130 mEq/L) or moderate-to-severe renal impairment (creatinine clearance less than or equal to 30 mL/min or serum creatinine greater than 3 mg/dL), therapy with lisinopril should be initiated at a dose of 2.5 mg once a day under close medical supervision. In patients with severe congestive heart failure whose renal function may depend on the activity of the renin-angiotensin-aldosterone system, treatment with angiotensin-converting enzyme inhibitors, including lisinopril, may be associated with oliguria or progressive azotemia and rarely with acute renal failure or death.

➤*Acute MI:* In hemodynamically stable patients within 24 hours of the onset of symptoms of acute MI, the first dose of lisinopril is 5 mg given orally, followed by 5 mg after 24 hours, 10 mg after 48 hours and then 10 mg of lisinopril once daily. Dosing should continue for 6 weeks. Patients should

LISINOPRIL — ORAL

receive, as appropriate, the standard recommended treatments such as thrombolytics, aspirin and beta blockers.

Patients with a low systolic blood pressure (less than or equal to 120 mm Hg) when treatment is started or during the first 3 days after the infarct should be given a lower 2.5 mg oral dose of lisinopril. Patients with acute MI in the Gruppo Italiano per lo Studio della Sopravvienza nell'Infarto Miocardico (GISSI-3) study had a higher (9% vs 3.7%) incidence of persistent hypotension (systolic blood pressure less than 90 mm Hg for greater than 1 hour) when treated with lisinopril. Treatment with lisinopril must not be initiated in acute MI patients at risk of further serious hemodynamic deterioration after treatment with a vasodilator (eg, systolic blood pressure of less than or equal to 100 mm Hg) or cardiogenic shock. If hypotension occurs (systolic blood pressure less than or equal to 100 mm Hg) a daily maintenance dose of 5 mg may be given with temporary reductions to 2.5 mg if needed. If prolonged hypotension occurs (systolic blood pressure less than 90 mm Hg for greater than 1 hour) lisinopril should be withdrawn. For patients who develop symptoms of heart failure, see above.

Dosage in patients with MI with renal function impairment – In acute MI, treatment with lisinopril should be initiated with caution in patients with evidence of renal dysfunction, defined as serum creatinine concentration greater than 2 mg/dL. No evaluation of dosage adjustment in MI patients with severe renal impairment has been performed.

➤*Elderly:* In general, blood pressure response and adverse experiences were similar in younger and older patients given similar doses of lisinopril. Pharmacokinetic studies, however, indicate that maximum blood levels and area under the plasma concentration-time curve (AUC) are doubled in older patients, so that dosage adjustments should be made with particular caution.

➤*Children greater than or equal to 6 years of age:* The usual recommended starting dose is 0.07 mg/kg once daily (up to 5 mg total). Dosage should be adjusted according to blood pressure response. Doses above 0.61 mg/kg (or in excess of 40 mg) have not been studied in pediatric patients.

Lisinopril is not recommend in pediatric patients under 6 years of age or in pediatric patients with glomerular filtration rate less than 30 mL/min/1.73 min^2.

➤*Storage / Stability:* Store at controlled room temperature, 20° to 25°C (68° to 77°F), and protect from moisture. Dispense in a tight container.

MOEXIPRIL HYDROCHLORIDE

Rx	**Univasc** (Schwarz Pharma)	**Tablets:** 7.5 mg	Lactose. (707 SP 7.5). Pink, scored. Film-coated. In 100s and unit-of-use 90s.
		15 mg	Lactose. (715 SP 15). Salmon, scored. Film-coated. In 100s and unit-of-use 90s.

MOEXIPRIL HYDROCHLORIDE — ORAL

For complete and comparative prescribing information, refer to the Angiotensin-Converting Enzyme Inhibitors group monograph.

Indications

➤*Hypertension:* Moexipril hydrochloride is indicated for treatment of patients with hypertension. It may be used alone or in combination with thiazide diuretics.

Administration and Dosage

➤*Approved by the FDA:* April 19, 1995.

➤*Hypertension:* The recommended initial dose of moexipril in patients not receiving diuretics is 7.5 mg, 1 hour prior to meals, once daily. Dosage should be adjusted according to blood pressure response. The antihypertensive effect of moexipril may diminish towards the end of the dosing interval. Blood pressure should, therefore, be measured just prior to dosing to determine whether satisfactory blood pressure control is obtained. If control is not adequate, increased dose or divided dosing can be tried. The recommended dose range is 7.5 to 30 mg daily, administered in 1 or 2 divided doses 1 hour before meals. Total daily doses above 60 mg a day have not been studied in hypertensive patients.

In patients who are currently being treated with a diuretic, symptomatic hypotension may occasionally occur following the initial dose of moexipril. The diuretic should, if possible, be discontinued for 2 to 3 days before therapy with moexipril is begun, to reduce the likelihood of hypotension. If the patient's blood pressure is not controlled with moexipril alone, diuretic therapy may then be reinstituted. If diuretic therapy cannot be discontinued, an initial dose of 3.75 mg of moexipril should be used with medical supervision until blood pressure has stabilized.

➤*Dosage in renal impairment:* For patients with a creatinine clearance less than or equal to 40 mL/min/1.73 m_2, an initial dose of 3.75 mg once daily should be given cautiously. Doses may be titrated upward to a maximum daily dose of 15 mg.

➤*Storage / Stability:* Store, tightly closed, at controlled room temperature. Protect from excessive moisture.

If product package is subdivided, dispense in tight containers.

PERINDOPRIL ERBUMINE

Rx	**Aceon** (Solvay Pharm)	**Tablets:** 2 mg	Lactose. (ACN 2 SLV SLV). White, oblong, scored. In 100s.
		4 mg	Lactose. (ACN 4 SLV SLV). Pink, oblong, scored. In 100s.
		8 mg	Lactose. (ACN 8 SLV SLV). Salmon, oblong, scored. In 100s.

PERINDOPRIL ERBUMINE — ORAL

For complete and comparative prescribing information, refer to the Angiotensin-Converting Enzyme Inhibitors group monograph.

WARNING

Pregnancy – When used in pregnancy during the second and third trimesters, angiotensin-converting enzyme (ACE) inhibitors can cause injury and even death to the developing fetus. When pregnancy is detected, discontinue perindopril as soon as possible.

Indications

➤*Hypertension:* Perindopril is indicated for the treatment of patients with essential hypertension. Perindopril may be used alone or given with other classes of antihypertensives, especially thiazide diuretics.

In considering use of perindopril, note that in controlled trials ACE inhibitors have an effect on blood pressure that is less in black patients than in nonblack patients. In addition, note that black patients receiving ACE inhibitor monotherapy have been reported to have a higher incidence of angioedema compared with nonblack patients.

➤*Stable coronary artery disease (CAD):* Perindopril is indicated in patients with stable CAD to reduce the risk of cardiovascular mortality or nonfatal myocardial infarction (MI). Perindopril can be used with conventional treatment for management of CAD, such as antiplatelet, antihypertensive, or lipid-lowering therapy.

Administration and Dosage

➤*Approved by the FDA:* December 30, 1993.

➤*Hypertension:*

Uncomplicated hypertensive patients – In patients with essential hypertension, the recommended initial dosage is 4 mg once a day. The dosage may be titrated upward until blood pressure, when measured just before the next dose, is controlled, or to a maximum of 16 mg/day. The usual maintenance dose range is 4 to 8 mg administered as a single daily dose. Perindopril may also be administered in 2 divided doses. When once-daily dosing was compared with twice-daily dosing in clinical studies, the twice-daily regimen was generally slightly superior, but not by more than approximately 0.5 to 1 mm Hg.

Stable CAD – In patients with stable CAD, perindopril should be given at an initial dose of 4 mg once daily for 2 weeks, and then increased as tolerated, to a maintenance dosage of 8 mg once daily. In elderly patients (70 years of age and older), perindopril should be given as a 2 mg dose once daily in the first week, followed by 4 mg once daily in the second week, and 8 mg once daily for maintenance dosage, if tolerated.

Elderly – As in younger patients, the recommended initial dosages of perindopril for the elderly (older than 65 years of age) is 4 mg daily in 1 or 2 divided doses. The daily dosage may be titrated upward until blood pressure, when measured just before the next dose, is controlled, but experience with perindopril is limited in the elderly at doses exceeding 8 mg. Doses greater than 8 mg should be administered with caution and under close medical supervision.

Concomitant diuretics – If blood pressure is not adequately controlled with perindopril alone, a diuretic may be added. In patients currently being treated with a diuretic, symptomatic hypotension occasionally can occur following the initial dose of perindopril. To reduce the likelihood of such reaction, the diuretic should be discontinued, if possible, 2 to 3 days prior to beginning perindopril therapy. Then, if blood pressure is not controlled with perindopril alone, the diuretic should be resumed.

If the diuretic cannot be discontinued, an initial dosage of 2 to 4 mg daily in 1 or 2 divided doses should be used with careful medical supervision for several hours and until blood pressure has stabilized. The dosage should be titrated as previously described.

After the first dose of perindopril, the patient should be followed closely for the first 2 weeks of treatment and whenever the dose of perindopril and/or diuretics is increased. In patients who are currently being treated with a diuretic, symptomatic hypotension occasionally can occur following the initial dose of perindopril. To reduce the likelihood of hypotension, the dose of diuretic, if possible, can be adjusted, which may diminish the likelihood of hypotension. The appearance of hypotension after the initial dose of perin-

PERINDOPRIL ERBUMINE — ORAL

dopril does not preclude subsequent careful dose titration with the drug, following effective management of the hypotension.

Renal function impairment – Kinetic data indicate that perindoprilat elimination is decreased in renally impaired patients, with a marked increase in accumulation when creatinine clearance (Ccr) drops below 30 mL/min. In such patients (Ccr less than 30 mL/min), safety and efficacy of perindopril have not been established. For patients with lesser degrees of impairment (Ccr greater than 30 mL/min), the initial dosage should be 2 mg/day and dosage should not exceed 8 mg/day because of limited clinical experience. During dialysis, perindopril is removed with the same clearance as in patients with normal renal function.

➤*Storage/Stability:* Store at controlled room temperature (20° to 25°C [68° to 77°F]). Protect from moisture.

QUINAPRIL HYDROCHLORIDE

Rx	**Quinapril Hydrochloride** (Various, eg, Greenstone, Mylan, Par, Teva)	**Tablets:** 5 mg	May contain lactose. In 90s and 500s.
Rx	**Accupril** (Pfizer)		Lactose. (PD 527 5). Brown, elliptical, scored. Film-coated. In 90s and UD 100s.
Rx	**Quinapril Hydrochloride** (Various, eg, Greenstone, Mylan, Par, Teva)	**Tablets:** 10 mg	May contain lactose. In 90s and 500s.
Rx	**Accupril** (Pfizer)		Lactose. (PD 530 10). Brown, triangular. Film-coated. In 90s and UD 100s.
Rx	**Quinapril Hydrochloride** (Various, eg, Greenstone, Mylan, Par, Teva)	**Tablets:** 20 mg	May contain lactose. In 90s and 500s.
	Accupril (Pfizer)		Lactose. (PD 532 20). Brown. Film-coated. In 90s and UD 100s.
Rx	**Quinapril Hydrochloride** (Various, eg, Greenstone, Mylan, Par, Teva)	**Tablets:** 40 mg	May contain lactose. In 90s and 500s.
Rx	**Accupril** (Pfizer)		Lactose. (PD 535 40). Brown, elliptical. Film-coated. In 90s.

QUINAPRIL HYDROCHLORIDE — ORAL

For complete and comparative prescribing information, refer to the Angiotensin-Converting Enzyme Inhibitors group monograph.

WARNING

Use in pregnancy – When used in pregnancy during the second and third trimesters, ACE inhibitors can cause injury and even death to the developing fetus. When pregnancy is detected, quinapril should be discontinued as soon as possible.

Indications

➤*Hypertension:* Quinapril is indicated for the treatment of hypertension. It may be used alone or in combination with thiazide diuretics.

➤*Heart failure:* Quinapril is indicated in the management of heart failure as adjunctive therapy when added to conventional therapy including diuretics or digitalis. In using quinapril, consideration should be given to the fact that another angiotensin-converting enzyme (ACE) inhibitor, captopril, has caused agranulocytosis, particularly in patients with renal impairment or collagen vascular disease. Available data are insufficient to show that quinapril does not have a similar risk.

Administration and Dosage

➤*Approved by the FDA:* November 19, 1991.

➤*Hypertension:*

Monotherapy – The recommended initial dosage of quinapril in patients not on diuretics is 10 or 20 mg once daily. Dosage should be adjusted according to blood pressure response measured at peak (2 to 6 hours after dosing) and trough (predosing). Generally, dosage adjustments should be made at intervals of at least 2 weeks. Most patients have required dosages of 20, 40, or 80 mg/day, given as a single dose or in 2 equally divided doses. In some patients treated once daily, the antihypertensive effect may diminish toward the end of the dosing interval. In such patients an increase in dosage or twice-daily administration may be warranted. In general, doses of 40 to 80 mg and divided doses give a somewhat greater effect at the end of the dosing interval.

Concomitant diuretics – If blood pressure is not adequately controlled with quinapril monotherapy, a diuretic may be added. In patients who are currently being treated with a diuretic, symptomatic hypotension occasionally can occur following the initial dose of quinapril. To reduce the likelihood of hypotension, the diuretic should, if possible, be discontinued 2 to 3 days prior to beginning therapy with quinapril. Then, if blood pressure is not controlled with quinapril alone, diuretic therapy should be resumed.

If the diuretic cannot be discontinued, an initial dose of 5 mg quinapril should be used with careful medical supervision for several hours and until blood pressure has stabilized.

The dosage should subsequently be titrated (as described above) to the optimal response.

Renal function impairment – Kinetic data indicate that the apparent elimination half-life of quinapril increases as creatinine clearance decreases. Recommended starting doses, based on clinical and pharmacokinetic data from patients with renal impairment, are as follows:

Creatinine clearance	Maximum recommended initial dose
> 60 mL/min	10 mg
30 to 60 mL/min	5 mg
10 to 30 mL/min	2.5 mg
< 10 mL/min	Insufficient data for dosage recommendation.

Patients should subsequently have their dosage titrated (as described above) to the optimal response.

Elderly (65 years of age and older) – The recommended initial dosage of quinapril in elderly patients is 10 mg given once daily followed by titration (as described above) to the optimal response.

➤*Heart failure:* Quinapril is indicated as adjunctive therapy when added to conventional therapy including diuretics or digitalis. The recommended starting dose is 5 mg twice daily. This dose may improve symptoms of heart failure, but increases in exercise duration have generally required higher doses. Therefore, if the initial dosage of quinapril is well tolerated, patients should then be titrated at weekly intervals until an effective dose, usually 20 to 40 mg daily given in 2 equally divided doses, is reached or undesirable hypotension, orthostatis, or azotemia prohibit reaching this dose.

Following the initial dose of quinapril, the patient should be observed under medical supervision for at least 2 hours for the presence of hypotension or orthostatis and, if present, until blood pressure stabilizes. The appearance of hypotension, orthostasis, or azotemia early in dose titration should not preclude further careful dose titration. Consideration should be given to reducing the dose of concomitant diuretics.

➤*Dose adjustments in patients with heart failure and renal impairment or hyponatremia:* Pharmacokinetic data indicate that quinapril elimination is dependent on level of renal function. In patients with heart failure and renal impairment, the recommended initial dose of quinapril is 5 mg in patients with a creatinine clearance greater than 30 mL/min and 2.5 mg in patients with a creatinine clearance of 10 to 30 mL/min. There is insufficient data for dosage recommendation in patients with a creatinine clearance less than 10 mL/min. If the initial dose is well tolerated, quinapril may be administered the following day as a twice daily regimen. In the absence of excessive hypotension or significant deterioration of renal function, the dose may be increased at weekly intervals based on clinical and hemodynamic response.

➤*Storage/Stability:* Store at controlled room temperature 15° to 30°C (59° to 86°F). Protect from light.

RAMIPRIL

Rx	**Altace** (Monarch)	**Capsules:** 1.25 mg	Gelatin. Yellow. In 100s and UD 100s.
		2.5 mg	Gelatin. Orange. In 100s, 500s, 1000s, UD 100s, and bulk pack 5000s.
		5 mg	Gelatin. Red. In 100s, 500s, 1000s, UD 100s, and bulk pack 5000s.
		10 mg	Gelatin. Blue. In 100s, 500s, and 1000s.

RAMIPRIL — ORAL

For complete and comparative prescribing information, refer to the Angiotensin-Converting Enzyme Inhibitors group monograph.

WARNING

Use in pregnancy – When used in pregnancy during the second and third trimesters, angiotensin-converting enzyme (ACE) inhibitors can cause injury and even death to the developing fetus. When pregnancy is detected, ramipril should be discontinued as soon as possible.

Indications

➤*Reduction in risk of myocardial infarction, stroke, and death from cardiovascular causes:* Ramipril is indicated in patients 55 years or older at high risks of developing major cardiovascular events because of a history of coronary artery disease, stroke, peripheral vascular disease, or diabetes that is accompanied by at least 1 other cardiovascular risk factor (eg, hypertension, elevated total cholesterol levels, low HDL levels, cigarette smoking, documented microalbuminuria) to reduce the risk of myocardial infarction, stroke, or death from cardiovascular causes. Ramipril can be used in addition to other needed treatments (such as antihypertensive, antiplatelet or lipid-lowering therapy).

➤*Hypertension:* Ramipril is indicated for the treatment of hypertension. It may be used alone or in combination with thiazide diuretics. In using ramipril, consideration should be given to the fact that another ACE inhibitor, captopril, has caused agranulocytosis, particularly in patients with renal impairment or collagen-vascular disease. Available data are insufficient to show that ramipril does not have a similar risk.

➤*Heart failure postmyocardial infarction:* Ramipril is indicated in stable patients who have demonstrated clinical signs of congestive heart failure within the first few days after sustaining acute myocardial infarction (MI). Administration of ramipril to such patients has been shown to decrease the risk of death (principally cardiovascular death) and to decrease the risks of failure-related hospitalization and progression to severe/resistant heart failure.

Administration and Dosage

➤*Approved by the FDA:* 1991.

Blood-pressure decreases associated with any dose of ramipril depend, in part, on the presence or absence of volume depletion (eg, past and current diuretic use) or the presence or absence of renal artery stenosis. If such circumstances are suspected to be present, the initial starting dose should be 1.25 mg once daily.

➤*Reduction in risk of myocardial infarction, stroke, and death from cardiovascular causes:* Ramipril should be given at an initial dose of 2.5 mg (once a day) for 1 week, 5 mg (once a day) for the next 3 weeks, and then increased as tolerated, to a maintenance dose of 10 mg (once a day). If the patient is hypertensive or recently postmyocardial infarction, it can also be given as a divided dose.

➤*Hypertension:* The recommended initial dose for patients not receiving a diuretic is 2.5 mg once a day. Dosage should be adjusted according to the blood-pressure response. The usual maintenance dosage range is 2.5 to 20 mg/day administered as a single dose or in 2 equally divided doses. In some patients treated once daily, the antihypertensive effect may diminish toward the end of the dosing interval. In such patients, an increase in dosage or twice-daily administration should be considered. If blood pressure is not controlled with ramipril alone, a diuretic can be added.

➤*Heart failure post-myocardial infarction:* For the treatment of postinfarction patients who have shown signs of congestive failure, the recommended starting dose of ramipril is 2.5 mg twice daily (5 mg/day). A patient who becomes hypotensive at this dose may be switched to 1.25 mg twice daily, but all patients should then be titrated (as tolerated) toward a target dose of 5 mg twice daily, with dose increases being about 3 weeks apart.

After the initial dose of ramipril, the patient should be observed under medical supervision for 2 hours or more and until blood pressure has stabilized for at least an additional hour. If possible, the dose of any concomitant diuretic should be reduced which may diminish the likelihood of hypotension. The appearance of hypotension after the initial dose of ramipril does not preclude subsequent careful dose titration with the drug, following effective management of the hypotension.

The ramipril capsule is usually swallowed whole. The ramipril capsule can also be opened and the contents sprinkled on a small amount (approximately 4 oz) of applesauce or mixed in 4 oz (120 mL) of water or apple juice. To be sure that ramipril is not lost when such a mixture is used, the mixture should be consumed in its entirety. The described mixtures can be prepared and stored for up to 24 hours at room temperature or up to 48 hours under refrigeration.

Coadministration of ramipril with potassium supplements, potassium salt substitutes, or potassium-sparing diuretics can lead to increases of serum potassium.

In patients who are currently being treated with a diuretic, symptomatic hypotension occasionally can occur following the initial dose of ramipril. To reduce the likelihood of hypotension, the diuretic should, if possible, be discontinued 2 to 3 days prior to beginning therapy with ramipril. Then, if blood pressure is not controlled with ramipril alone, diuretic therapy should be resumed.

If the diuretic cannot be discontinued, an initial dose of 1.25 mg ramipril should be used to avoid excess hypotension.

➤*Dosage adjustment in renal function impairment:* In patients with creatinine clearance less than 40 mL/min per 1.73 m^2 (serum creatinine approximately greater than 2.5 mg/dL) doses only 25% of those normally used should be expected to induce full therapeutic levels of ramiprilat.

Hypertension – For patients with hypertension and renal impairment, the recommended initial dose is 1.25 mg ramipril once daily. Dosage may be titrated upward until blood pressure is controlled or to a maximum total daily dose of 5 mg.

Heart failure post-myocardial infarction – For patients with heart failure and renal impairment, the recommended initial dose is 1.25 mg ramipril once daily. The dose may be increased to 1.25 mg twice daily and up to a maximum dose of 2.5 mg twice daily depending upon clinical response and tolerability.

➤*Storage / Stability:* Store at controlled room temperature (15° to 30°C; 59° to 86°F). Dispense in well-closed container with safety closure.

TRANDOLAPRIL

Rx	**Mavik** (Abbott)	**Tablets:** 1 mg	Lactose. (FT). Salmon, scored. In 100s and UD 100s.
		2 mg	Lactose. (FX). Yellow. In 100s and UD 100s.
		4 mg	Lactose. (FZ). Rose. In 100s and UD 100s.

TRANDOLAPRIL — ORAL

For complete and comparative prescribing information, refer to the Angiotensin-Converting Enzyme Inhibitors group monograph.

WARNING

Use in pregnancy – When used in pregnancy during the second and third trimesters, ACE inhibitors can cause injury and even death to the developing fetus. When pregnancy is detected, trandolapril should be discontinued as soon as possible. See Warnings, Pregnancy.

Indications

➤*Hypertension:* Trandolapril is indicated for the treatment of hypertension. It may be used alone or in combination with other antihypertensive medication such as hydrochlorothiazide.

➤*Heart failure post myocardial infarction or left-ventricular dysfunction post myocardial infarction:* Trandolapril is indicated in stable patients who have evidence of left-ventricular systolic dysfunction (identified by wall motion abnormalities) or who are symptomatic from congestive heart failure within the first few days after sustaining acute myocardial infarction. Administration of trandolapril to white patients has been shown to decrease the risk of death (principally cardiovascular death) and to decrease the risk of heart failure-related hospitalization.

Administration and Dosage

➤*Approved by the FDA:* April 26, 1996.

➤*Hypertension:* The recommended initial dosage of trandolapril for patients not receiving a diuretic is 1 mg once daily in nonblack patients and 2 mg in black patients. Dosage should be adjusted according to the blood pressure response. Generally, dosage adjustments should be made at intervals of at least 1 week. Most patients have required dosages of 2 to 4 mg once daily. There is little clinical experience with doses above 8 mg.

Patients inadequately treated with once-daily dosing at 4 mg may be treated with twice-daily dosing. If blood pressure is not adequately controlled with trandolapril monotherapy, a diuretic may be added.

In patients who are currently being treated with a diuretic, symptomatic hypotension occasionally can occur following the initial dose of trandolapril. To reduce the likelihood of hypotension, the diuretic should, if possible, be discontinued 2 to 3 days prior to beginning therapy with trandolapril. Then, if blood pressure is not controlled with trandolapril alone, diuretic therapy should be resumed. If the diuretic cannot be discontinued, an initial dose of 0.5 mg trandolapril should be used with careful medical supervision for several hours until blood pressure has stabilized. The dosage should subsequently be titrated (as described above) to the optimal response.

Coadministration of trandolapril with potassium supplements, potassium salt substitutes, or potassium-sparing diuretics can lead to increases of serum potassium.

➤*Heart failure post myocardial infarction or left-ventricular dysfunction post myocardial infarction:* The recommended starting dose is 1 mg, once daily. Following the initial dose, all patients should be titrated (as tolerated) toward a target dose of 4 mg, once daily. If a 4 mg dose is not tolerated, patients can continue therapy with the greatest tolerated dose.

TRANDOLAPRIL — ORAL

➤*Dosage adjustment in renal impairment or hepatic cirrhosis:* For patients with a creatinine clearance less than 30 mL/min, or with hepatic cirrhosis, the recommended starting dose, based on clinical and pharmacokinetic data, is 0.5 mg daily. Patients should subsequently have their dosage titrated (as described above) to the optimal response.

➤*Storage/Stability:* Store at controlled room temperature: 20° to 25°C (68° to 77°F).

Angiotensin II Receptor Antagonists

WARNING

When used in pregnancy during the second and third trimesters, drugs that act directly on the renin-angiotensin system can cause injury and even death to the developing fetus. When pregnancy is detected, discontinue angiotensin II receptor antagonists (AIIRAs) as soon as possible.

Indications

➤*Hypertension:* For the treatment of hypertension, alone or in combination with other antihypertensive agents.

➤*Nephropathy in type 2 diabetics (losartan and irbesartan):* For the treatment of diabetic nephropathy with an elevated serum creatinine and proteinuria (urinary albumin to creatinine ratio 300 mg/g or more with losartan; greater than 300 mg/day with irbesartan) in patients with type 2 diabetes and a history of hypertension. In this population, losartan and irbesartan reduce the rate of progression of nephropathy as measured by the occurrence of doubling of serum creatinine or end stage renal disease (need for dialysis or renal transplantation).

➤*Heart failure (valsartan):* For the treatment of heart failure (NYHA class II to IV) in patients who are intolerant of angiotensin-converting enzyme inhibitors (ACEIs).

➤*Hypertension with left ventricular hypertrophy (losartan):* To reduce the risk of stroke in patients with hypertension and left ventricular hypertrophy, but there is evidence that this benefit does not apply to black patients.

Actions

➤*Pharmacology:* **Candesartan**, **eprosartan**, **irbesartan**, **losartan**, **olmesartan**, **telmisartan**, and **valsartan** are angiotensin II receptor (type AT_1) antagonists. Angiotensin II (formed from angiotensin I in a reaction catalyzed by angiotensin-converting enzyme [ACE; kininase II]) is a potent vasoconstrictor, the primary vasoactive hormone of the renin-angiotensin system, and an important component in the pathophysiology of hypertension. Its effects are vasoconstriction, stimulation of synthesis and release of aldosterone, cardiac stimulation, and renal re-absorption of sodium. AIIRAs block the vasoconstrictor and aldosterone-secreting effects of angiotensin II by selectively blocking the binding of angiotensin II to the AT_1 receptor in many tissues (eg, vascular smooth muscle, adrenal gland). There is also an AT_2 receptor in many tissues, but it is not known to be associated with cardiovascular homeostasis. AIIRAs have much greater affinity (greater than 10,000-fold, candesartan; 1000 times greater, eprosartan; greater than 8500-fold, irbesartan; approximately 1000-fold, losartan; greater than 12,500-fold, olmesartan; greater than 3000-fold, telmisartan; approximately 20,000-fold, valsartan) for the AT_1 than for the AT_2 receptor and do not exhibit any agonist activity. In vitro binding studies indicate that losartan is a reversible, competitive inhibitor of the AT_1 receptor. The active metabolite is 10 to 40 times more potent by weight than losartan and appears to be a reversible, non-competitive inhibitor of the AT_1 receptor. The primary metabolite of valsartan is essentially inactive with an affinity for the AT_1 receptor approximately 1/200 of valsartan itself.

AIIRAs do not inhibit ACE (kininase II, the enzyme that converts angiotensin I to angiotensin II and degrades bradykinin), nor do they bind to or block other hormone receptors or ion channels known to be important in cardiovascular regulation.

AIIRAs inhibit the pressor effect of angiotensin II (as well as angiotensin I) infusions. Removal of the negative feedback of angiotensin II causes a 2- to 3-fold rise in plasma renin activity and a consequent rise in angiotensin II plasma concentration in hypertensive patients. The resulting increased plasma renin activity and angiotensin II circulating levels are insufficient to alter the effects of AIIRAs on blood pressure. AIIRAs do not affect the response to bradykinin, whereas ACE inhibitors do increase the response. AIIRAs have very little effect on serum potassium. There was a small uricosuric effect with losartan leading to a minimal decrease in serum uric acid (mean decrease less than 0.4 mg/dL) during chronic oral administration.

➤*Pharmacokinetics:*

Angiotensin II Antagonist Pharmacokinetics

Parameters	Candesartan	Eprosartan	Irbesartan	Losartan (metabolite)[a]	Olmesartan	Telmisartan	Valsartan
Bioavailability	≈ 15%	≈ 13%	60% to 80%	≈ 33%	≈ 26%	42%/58% (40 mg/160 mg)	≈ 25%
Food effect (AUC/C_{max})	no effect	↓< 25%	no effect	↓10%/↓14%	no effect	↓6%/↓20% (40 mg AUC/ 160 mg AUC)	↓40%/↓50%
Plasma bound	> 99%	≈ 98%	90%	98.7% (99.8%)	99%	> 99.5%	95%
T_{max}	3 to 4 h	1 to 2 h	1.5 to 2 h	1 h (3 to 4 h)	1 to 2 h	0.5 to 1 h	2 to 4 h
Volume of distribution	0.13 L/kg	308 L	53 to 93 L	≈ 34 L (≈ 12 L)	≈ 17L	≈ 500 L	17 L[b]
Converted to metabolites	minor	minor	< 20%	≈ 14%	none	≈ 11%	≈ 20%
Metabolism	O-deethylation	glucuronidation	CYP2C9	CYP2C9; CYP3A4	none	conjugation	unknown
Terminal half-life	≈ 9 hr	5 to 9 h	11 to 15 h	≈ 2 h (6 to 9 h)	≈ 13 h	≈ 24 h	≈ 6 h[b]
Total plasma clearance	0.37 mL/min/kg	≈ 130 mL/min[b]	157 to 176 mL/min	≈ 600 mL/min (≈ 50 mL/min)	1.3 L/h	> 800 mL/min	≈ 2 L/h[b]
Renal clearance	0.19 mL/min/kg	≈30 to 40 mL/min	3 to 3.5 mL/min	≈ 75 mL/min (≈ 25 mL/min)	0.6 L/h	nd[c]	≈ 0.62 L/h[b]
Recovered in the urine	≈ 33%	≈ 7%	≈ 20%	≈ 45/≈ 35% (IV/oral)	35% to 50%	0.91%/ 0.49% (IV/oral)	≈ 13%
Recovered in the feces	≈ 67%	≈ 90%	≈ 80%	≈ 50/≈ 60% (IV/oral)	50% to 65%	> 97%	≈ 83%

[a] Active.
[b] IV dosing.
[c] nd = no data

AIIRAs do not accumulate in plasma upon repeated once-daily dosing.

Losartan undergoes substantial first-pass metabolism and is converted to an active carboxylic acid metabolite (14% of dose) that is responsible for most of the angiotensin II receptor antagonism. Cytochrome P-450 2C9 and 3A4 isozymes are involved in losartan's biotransformation.

The enzyme(s) responsible for **valsartan** metabolism have not been identified but do seem to be cytochrome P-450 isozymes.

In vitro studies of **irbesartan** oxidation by cytochrome P-450 isoenzymes indicated irbesartan was oxidized primarily by 2C9; metabolism by 3A4 was negligible. Irbesartan was neither metabolized by, nor did it substantially induce or inhibit, isoenzymes commonly associated with drug metabolism (1A1, 1A2, 2A6, 2B6, 2D6, 2E1). There was no induction or inhibition of 3A4.

Telmisartan is metabolized by conjugation to form a pharmacologically inactive acylglucuronide; the glucuronide of the parent compound is the only metabolite that has been identified in human plasma and urine. After a single dose, the glucuronide represents approximately 11% of the measured radioactivity in plasma. The cytochrome P450 isoenzymes are not involved in the metabolism of telmisartan.

Candesartan is rapidly and completely bioactivated by ester hydrolysis during absorption from the GI tract to candesartan, a selective AT_1 subtype angiotensin II receptor antagonist. Candesartan is mainly excreted unchanged in urine and feces (via bile). It undergoes minor hepatic metabolism by O-deethylation to an inactive metabolite. Candesartan and its inactive metabolite do not accumulate in serum upon repeated once-daily dosing.

Olmesartan shows linear pharmacokinetics following single oral doses of up to 320 mg and multiple oral doses of up to 80 mg. Steady-state levels are achieved within 3 to 5 days, and no accumulation in plasma occurs with once-daily dosing. Following the rapid and complete conversion of olmesartan medoxomil to olmesartan during absorption, there is virtually no further metabolism of olmesartan. Olmesartan crossed the blood-brain barrier poorly, if at all. It passed across the placental barrier in rats and was distributed to the fetus. It was distributed to milk at low levels in rats.

Absolute bioavailability following a single 300 mg oral dose of **eprosartan** is approximately 13%. Eprosartan plasma concentrations peak at 1 to 2 hours after an oral dose in the fasted state. Plasma concentrations of eprosartan increase in a slightly less than dose-proportional manner over the 100 to 800 mg dose range. The terminal elimination half-life following oral administration is typically 5 to 9 hours.

Contraindications

Hypersensitivity to any component of these products.

Warnings

➤*Hypotension/volume- or salt-depleted patients:* In patients who are intravascularly volume depleted (eg, those treated with diuretics), symptomatic hypotension may occur. Correct these conditions prior to administration or start treatment under close medical supervision with a reduced dose.

If hypotension occurs, place the patient in the supine position and, if necessary, give an IV infusion of normal saline. A transient hypotensive response is not a contraindication to further treatment, which usually can be continued once the blood pressure has stabilized.

➤*Race:* **Losartan** was effective in reducing blood pressure regardless of race, although the effect was somewhat less in black patients (usually a low-renin population).In healthy black subjects, **irbesartan** AUC values were approximately 25% greater than in white subjects; there were no differences in C_{max} values.

➤*Gender:* Plasma concentrations of **telmisartan** are generally 2 to 3 times higher in women than in men. However, in clinical trials, no significant increases in blood pressure response or in the incidence of orthostatic hypotension were found in women. No dosage adjustment is necessary.

➤*Cough:* In trials where **valsartan** was compared with an ACE inhibitor with or without placebo, the incidence of dry cough was significantly greater in the ACE inhibitor group (7.9%) than in the groups who received valsartan (2.6%) or placebo (1.5%). In patients who had dry cough when previously receiving ACE inhibitors, the incidences of cough in patients who received AIIRAs, hydrochlorothiazide, or lisinopril were approximately 20%, approximately 19%, and 69%, respectively.

There was no significant difference in the incidence of cough between **losartan**, **olmesartan**, **eprosartan**, or **telmisartan** and placebo.**Irbesartan** use was not associated with an increased incidence of dry cough, as is typically associated with ACE inhibitor use.

➤*Renal function impairment:* As a consequence of inhibiting the renin-angiotensin-aldosterone system, changes in renal function may be anticipated in susceptible individuals. In patients whose renal function may depend on the activity of the renin-angiotensin-aldosterone system (eg, patients with severe CHF), treatment with ACE inhibitors and angiotensin receptor antagonists has been associated with oliguria or progressive azotemia and rarely, with acute renal failure or death. In studies of ACE inhibitors in patients with unilateral or bilateral renal artery stenosis, increases in serum creatinine or BUN have been reported. AIIRAs would be expected to behave similarly. In some patients, these effects were reversible upon discontinuation of therapy. No dosage adjustment is necessary for patients with renal impairment unless they are volume-depleted.

Losartan – Plasma concentrations of losartan are not altered in patients with Ccr above 30 mL/min. In patients with lower Ccr, AUCs are about 50% greater and they are doubled in hemodialysis patients. Plasma concentrations of the active metabolite are not significantly altered in patients with renal impairment or in hemodialysis patients.

Valsartan – There is no apparent correlation between renal function (measured by Ccr) and exposure (measured by AUC) to valsartan in patients with different degrees of renal impairment. Consequently, dose adjustment is not required in patients with mild to moderate renal dysfunction. No studies have been performed in patients with severe impairment of renal function (Ccr less than 10 mL/min).Valsartan is not removed from plasma by hemodialysis. In the case of severe renal disease, exercise care with valsartan dosing.

In a 4-day trial of valsartan in 12 patients with unilateral renal artery stenosis, no significant increases in serum creatinine or BUN were observed. There has been no long-term use of valsartan in patients with unilateral or bilateral renal artery stenosis, but anticipate an effect similar to that seen with ACE inhibitors.

Irbesartan – The pharmacokinetics of irbesartan are not altered in patients with renal impairment or in patients on hemodialysis. Irbesartan is not removed by hemodialysis.

Candesartan – In hypertensive patients with renal insufficiency, serum concentrations of candesartan were elevated. After repeated dosing, the AUC and C_{max} were approximately doubled in patients with severe renal impairment (Ccr less than 30 mL/min/1.73 m^2) compared with patients with normal kidney function. The pharmacokinetics of candesartan in hypertensive patients undergoing hemodialysis are similar to those in hypertensive patients with severe renal impairment. Candesartan cannot be removed by hemodialysis. No initial dosage adjustment is necessary in patients with renal insufficiency.

Telmisartan – Renal excretion does not contribute to telmisartan clearance. Based on modest experience in patients with mild-to-moderate renal impairment (Ccr of 30 to 80 mL/min, mean clearance approximately 50 mL/min), no dosage adjustment is necessary in patients with decreased renal function. Telmisartan is not removed from blood by hemofiltration.

Eprosartan – Following administration of 600 mg once daily, there was an almost 2-fold increase in AUC and a 50% and 30% increase in C_{max} in moderate and severe renal impairment. The unbound eprosartan fractions increased by 35% and 59% in patients with moderate and severe renal impairment. No initial dosing adjustment is generally necessary in patients with moderate and severe renal impairment, with maximum dose not exceeding 600 mg daily. Eprosartan was poorly removed by hemodialysis (CL_{HD} less than 1 L/h).

➤*Hepatic function impairment:*

Candesartan – No differences in the pharmacokinetics were observed in patients with mild to moderate chronic liver disease. No initial dosage adjustment is necessary in patients with mild hepatic disease.

Irbesartan – The pharmacokinetics of irbesartan following repeated oral administration were not significantly affected in patients with mild to moderate cirrhosis of the liver. No dosage adjustment is necessary in patients with hepatic insufficiency.

Losartan – Following administration in patients with mild to moderate alcoholic cirrhosis of the liver, plasma concentrations of losartan and its active metabolite were, respectively, 5 times and about 1.7 times those in young male volunteers. Compared with healthy subjects, the total plasma clearance in patients with hepatic insufficiency was about 50% lower and the oral bioavailability was about 2 times higher. A lower starting dose is recommended for patients with a history of hepatic impairment.

Based on pharmacokinetic data that demonstrate significantly increased plasma concentrations of losartan in cirrhotic patients, consider a lower dose for patients with impaired hepatic function.

Olmesartan – Increases in $AUC_{0-\infty}$ and C_{max} were observed in patients with moderate hepatic impairment compared with those in matched controls, with an increase in AUC of about 60%.

Telmisartan – As the majority of telmisartan is eliminated by biliary excretion, patients with biliary obstructive disorders or hepatic insufficiency can be expected to have reduced clearance. Use telmisartan with caution in these patients. In patients with hepatic insufficiency, plasma concentrations of telmisartan are increased, and absolute bioavailability approaches 100%.

Valsartan – On average, patients with mild to moderate chronic liver disease have twice the exposure (measured by AUC values) to valsartan of healthy volunteers (matched by age, sex, and weight). In general, no dosage adjustment is needed in patients with mild to moderate liver disease. However, exercise care in this patient population.

As the majority of valsartan is eliminated in the bile, patients with mild to moderate hepatic impairment, including patients with biliary obstructive disorders, showed lower valsartan clearance (higher AUCs). Exercise care in administering valsartan to these patients.

Eprosartan – Eprosartan AUC (but not C_{max}) values increased, on average, by approximately 40% in men with decreased hepatic function compared with healthy men after a single 100 mg oral dose of eprosartan. The extent of eprosartan plasma protein binding was not influenced by hepatic dysfunction. No dosage adjustment is necessary for patients with hepatic impairment.

➤*Carcinogenesis:* Female rats given the highest dose (270 mg/kg/day) of **losartan** had a slightly higher incidence of pancreatic acinar adenoma.

➤*Fertility impairment:* The administration of toxic dosage levels of **losartan** in female rats was associated with a significant decrease in the number of corpora lutea/female, implants/female, and live fetuses/female at C-section. At 100 mg/kg/day only a decrease in the number of corpora lutea/female was observed. Fertility and reproductive performance in male rats were not affected.

➤*Elderly:* No dosage adjustment is necessary when initiating AIIRAs in the elderly. No overall differences in effectiveness or safety of **candesartan**, **irbesartan**, **losartan**, **olmesartan**, **eprosartan**, or **telmisartan** were observed between elderly patients and younger patients, but greater sensitivity of some older individuals cannot be ruled out.

Based on the pooled data from randomized trials, the decrease in diastolic blood pressure and systolic blood pressure with eprosartan was slightly less in patients 65 years of age and older compared with younger patients. Adverse experiences were similar in younger and older patients.

➤*Pregnancy: Category C* (first trimester); *Category D* (second and third trimesters).

Fetal/Neonatal morbidity/mortality – Drugs that act directly on the renin-angiotensin system can cause fetal and neonatal morbidity and death when administered to pregnant women. Several dozen cases have been reported in patients who were taking ACE inhibitors. When pregnancy is detected, discontinue AIIRAs as soon as possible.

The use of drugs that act directly on the renin-angiotensin system during the second and third trimesters of pregnancy has been associated with fetal and neonatal injury, including hypotension, neonatal skull hypoplasia, anuria, reversible or irreversible renal failure, and death. Oligohydramnios has also been reported, presumably resulting from decreased fetal renal function; oligohydramnios, in this setting, has been associated with fetal limb contractures, craniofacial deformation, and hypoplastic lung development. Prematurity, intrauterine growth retardation, and patent ductus arteriosus have also occurred, although it is not clear whether these occurrences were caused by exposure to the drug. These adverse effects do not appear to have resulted from intrauterine drug exposure in the first trimester.

Inform mothers whose embryos and fetuses are exposed to an AIIRA only during the first trimester. Nonetheless, when patients become pregnant, physicians should have the patient discontinue the use of AIIRAs as soon as possible.

Rarely (probably less often than once in every 1000 pregnancies), no alternative to an AIIRA will be found. In these rare cases, apprise the mother of the potential hazards to her fetus, and perform serial ultrasound examinations to assess the intra-amniotic environment.

If oligohydramnios is observed, discontinue the drug unless it is considered lifesaving for the mother. Contraction stress testing (CST), a non-stress test (NST), or biophysical profiling (BPP) may be appropriate, depending on the week of pregnancy. However, patients and physicians should be aware that oligohydramnios may not appear until after the fetus has sustained irreversible injury.

Closely observe infants with histories of in utero exposure to an AIIRA for hypotension, oliguria, and hyperkalemia. If oliguria occurs, direct attention toward support of blood pressure and renal perfusion. Exchange transfusion or dialysis may be required as means of reversing hypotension or substituting for disordered renal function.

Candesartan – Oral doses of 10 mg/kg/day or greater of candesartan administered to pregnant rats during late gestation and continued through lactation were associated with reduced survival and an increased incidence of hydronephrosis in the offspring. The 10 mg/kg/day dose in rats is approximately 2.8 times the maximum recommended human dose (MRHD) of 32 mg on a mg/m^2 basis (comparison assumes human body weight of 50 kg). Candesartan given to pregnant rabbits at an oral dose of 3 mg/kg/day (approximately 1.7 times the MRHD on a mg/m^2 basis) caused maternal toxicity (decreased body weight and death) but, in surviving dams, had no adverse effects on fetal survival, fetal weight, or external, visceral, or skeletal development. No maternal toxicity or adverse effects on fetal development were observed when oral doses up to 1000 mg/kg/day of candesartan (approximately 138 times the MRHD on a mg/m^2 basis) were administered to pregnant mice.

Eprosartan – Eprosartan has been shown to produce maternal and fetal toxicities (maternal and fetal mortality, low maternal body weight and food consumption, resorptions, abortions, and litter loss) in pregnant rabbits given oral doses as low as 10 mg/kg/day of eprosartan. No maternal or fetal adverse effects were observed at 3 mg/kg/day; this oral dose yielded a systemic exposure (AUC) to unbound eprosartan 0.8 times that achieved in humans given 400 mg twice daily. No adverse effects on in utero or postnatal development and maturation of offspring were observed when eprosartan was administered to pregnant rats at oral doses up to 1000 mg/kg/day of eprosartan (the 1000 mg/kg/day dose in nonpregnant rats yielded systemic exposure to unbound eprosartan approximately 0.6 times the exposure achieved in humans given 400 mg twice daily).

Irbesartan – When pregnant rats were dosed with irbesartan from day 0 to day 20 of gestation (oral doses of 50, 180, and 650 mg/kg/day), increased incidences of renal pelvic cavitation, hydroureter, or absence of renal papilla were observed in fetuses at doses of at least 50 mg/kg/day (approximately equivalent to the MRHD, 300 mg/day, on a body surface area basis). Subcutaneous edema was observed in fetuses at doses of at least 180 mg/kg/day (about 4 times the MRHD on a body surface area basis). As these abnormalities were not observed in rats in which irbesartan exposure (oral doses of 50, 150, and 450 mg/kg/day) was limited to gestation days 6 to 15, they appear to reflect late gestational effects of the drug. In pregnant rabbits, oral doses of 30 mg/kg/day of irbesartan were associated with maternal mortality and abortion. Surviving females receiving this dose (about 1.5 times the MRHD on a body surface area basis) had a slight increase in early resorptions and a corresponding decrease in live fetuses. Irbesartan was found to cross the placental barrier in rats and rabbits.

Radioactivity was present in the rat and rabbit fetus during late gestation and in rat milk following oral doses of radiolabeled irbesartan.

Losartan – Losartan has been shown to produce adverse effects in rat fetuses and neonates, including decreased body weight, delayed physical and behavioral development, mortality, and renal toxicity. With the exception of neonatal weight gain (which was affected at doses as low as 10 mg/kg/day), doses associated with these effects exceeded 25 mg/kg/day (approximately 3 times the MRHD of 100 mg on a mg/m^2 basis). These findings are attributed to drug exposure in late gestation and during lactation. Significant levels of losartan and its active metabolite were shown to be present in rat fetal plasma during late gestation and in rat milk.

Telmisartan – In rabbits, embryolethality associated with maternal toxicity (reduced body weight gain and food consumption) was observed at 45 mg/kg/day of telmisartan (about 6.4 times the MRHD of 80 mg on a mg/m^2 basis). In rats, maternally toxic (reduction in body weight gain and food consumption) telmisartan doses of 15 mg/kg/day (about 1.9 times the MRHD on a mg/m^2 basis), administered during late gestation and lactation, were observed to produce adverse effects in neonates, including reduced viability, low birth weight, delayed maturation, and decreased weight gain. Telmisartan has been shown to be present in rat fetuses during late gestation and in rat milk. The no-observed-effect doses for developmental toxicity in rats and rabbits, 5 and 15 mg/kg/day, respectively, are about 0.64 and 3.7 times, on a mg/m^2 basis, the MRHD of telmisartan (80 mg/day).

➤*Lactation:* AIIRAs were present in rat milk. It is not known if AIIRAs are excreted in human breast milk. Because of the potential for adverse effects on the nursing infant, decide whether to discontinue nursing or discontinue the drug, taking into account the importance of the drug to the mother.

➤*Children:* Safety and efficacy have not been established.

Precautions

➤*Potassium supplements:* Tell patients receiving **losartan** not to use potassium supplements or salt substitutes containing potassium without consulting the prescribing physician.

➤*Lab test abnormalities:*

Liver function tests – Occasional elevations (more than 150% in **valsartan**-treated patients) of liver enzymes or serum bilirubin have occurred.Three patients (less than 0.1%) treated with valsartan discontinued treatment for elevated liver chemistries.Minor elevations of ALT, AST, and alkaline phosphatase occurred for comparable percentages of patients taking **eprosartan** or placebo in controlled clinical trials.

Creatinine/Blood urea nitrogen (BUN) – Minor increases in BUN or serum creatinine were observed infrequently with **candesartan**, in less than 0.1% of patients with essential hypertension treated with **losartan** alone, in 0.8% of patients taking **valsartan**, less than 0.7% with **irbesartan**, and 0.6% and 1.3%, respectively, of patients taking **eprosartan**. At least a 0.5 mg/dL rise in creatinine was observed in 0.4% of **telmisartan** patients compared with 0.3% of placebo patients.

Hemoglobin and hematocrit – A greater than 2 g/dL decrease in hemoglobin was observed in 0.8% of **telmisartan** patients compared with 0.3% of placebo patients. No patients discontinued therapy because of anemia.

Small decreases in hemoglobin and hematocrit occurred frequently in patients treated with **losartan** alone but were rarely of clinical importance.

Decreases of more than 20% in hemoglobin and hematocrit were observed in 0.4% and 0.8%, respectively, of **valsartan** patients, vs 0.1% and 0.1% with placebo. One valsartan patient discontinued treatment for microcytic anemia. Neutropenia was observed in 1.9% of patients treated with valsartan and 0.8% of patients treated with placebo.

Mean decreases in hemoglobin of 0.2 g/dL were observed in 0.2% of patients receiving **irbesartan**. Neutropenia (less than 1000 cells/mm^3) occurred at similar frequencies (0.3%).

Small decreases in hemoglobin and hematocrit (mean decreases of approximately 0.2 g/dL and 0.5 volume percent, respectively) were observed in patients treated with **candesartan** alone but were rarely of clinical importance. Anemia, leukopenia, and thrombocytopenia were associated with withdrawal of 1 patient each from clinical trials.

A greater than 20% decrease in hemoglobin was observed in 0.1% of patients taking **eprosartan**. Leukopenia (WBC count of up to 3×10^3/mm^3) occurred in 0.3% of patients taking eprosartan and in 0.3% of patients given placebo in controlled clinical trials. Neutropenia (neutrophil count of up to 1.5×10^3/mm^3) occurred in 1.3% of patients taking eprosartan and in 1.4% of patients given placebo in controlled clinical trials. Thrombocytopenia (platelet count of up to 100×10^9/L) occurred in 0.3% of patients taking eprosartan (1 patient) and in no patient given placebo in controlled clinical trials. Four patients receiving eprosartan in clinical trials were withdrawn for thrombocytopenia.

Small decreases in hemoglobin and hematocrit (mean decreases of approximately 0.3 g/dL and 0.3 volume percent, respectively) were observed with **olmesartan**.

Serum potassium – Increases of more than 20% in serum potassium were observed in 4.4% of **valsartan**-treated patients vs 2.9% of placebo-treated patients.

A small increase (mean increase of 0.1 mEq/L) was observed in patients treated with **candesartan** alone but was rarely of clinical importance. One patient from a CHF trial was withdrawn for hyperkalemia (serum potassium, 7.5 mEq/L). This patient was also receiving spironolactone.

A potassium value of at least 5.6 mmol/L occurred in 0.9% of patients taking **eprosartan** and 0.3% of patients given placebo in controlled clinical trials. One patient was withdrawn from clinical trials for hyperkalemia and 3 for hypokalemia.

Hyperuricemia – Hyperuricemia was rarely found (0.6% with **candesartan** vs 0.5% with placebo).

Drug Interactions

Angiotensin II Receptor Antagonist Drug Interactions

Precipitant drug	Object drug[a]		Description
Cimetidine	Losartan	↑	Coadministration led to an increase of ≈ 18% in AUC of losartan but did not affect the pharmacokinetics of its active metabolite.
Fluconazole	Losartan	↑	Fluconazole may inhibit the metabolism of losartan (CYP2C9), causing increased antihypertensive and adverse effects. Fluconazole did not affect the pharmacokinetics of eprosartan.
Indomethacin	Losartan	↓	The hypotensive effect of losartan may be reduced.
Phenobarbital	Losartan	↓	Coadministration led to a reduction of ≈ 20% in the AUC of losartan and its active metabolite.
Rifamycins	Losartan	↓	Rifamycins may increase the metabolism of losartan, thereby decreasing antihypertensive effects.
Telmisartan	Digoxin	↑	Median increases in digoxin peak plasma concentration (49%) and in trough concentration (20%) were seen with coadministration.

Angiotensin II Receptor Antagonist Drug Interactions			
Precipitant drug	Object drug[a]		Description
Telmisartan	Warfarin	↔	Telmisartan administered for 10 days slightly decreased the mean warfarin trough plasma concentration; this decrease did not result in a change in the International Normalized Ratio.

[a] ↑ = Object drug increased. ↓ = Object drug decreased. ↔ = Undetermined clinical effect.

➤*CYP450:* In vitro studies show significant inhibition of the formation of the active metabolite of **losartan** by inhibitors of cytochrome P450 3A4 (eg, ketoconazole, troleandomycin) or P450 2C9 (sulfaphenazole). The pharmacodynamic consequences of concomitant use of losartan and these inhibitors have not been examined.

In vitro studies show significant inhibition of the formation of oxidized **irbesartan** metabolites with the known cytochrome CYP2C9 substrates/inhibitors, tolbutamide, and nifedipine. However, clinical consequences were negligible.

➤*Potassium:* As with other drugs that block angiotensin II or its effects, concomitant use of potassium-sparing diuretics (eg, spironolactone, triamterene, amiloride), potassium supplements, or salt substitutes containing potassium may lead to increases in serum potassium.

➤*Drug/Food interactions:* A meal has only minor effects on **losartan** AUC or on the AUC of the metabolite (about 10% decrease). Food decreases **valsartan**'s C_{max} by 50% and its AUC by 40%. Food slightly reduces the bioavailability of **telmisartan**, with an AUC reduction of about 6% with the 40 mg tablet and about 20% after a 160 mg dose. Food does not affect the bioavailability of **irbesartan**, **olmesartan**, or **candesartan**. Administering **eprosartan** with food delays absorption and causes variable changes (less than 25%) in C_{max} and AUC values that do not appear clinically important.

Adverse Reactions

In general, treatment with AIIRAs is well tolerated. In controlled clinical trials, discontinuation of therapy because of adverse reactions was required in 2.3% of patients treated with **losartan** or **valsartan**, 2.4% with **olmesartan** and **candesartan**, 2.8% with **telmisartan**, 3.3% with **irbesartan**, and 4% with **eprosartan** vs 3.7%, 2%, 2.7%, 3.4%, 6.1%, 4.5%, and 6.5%, respectively, given placebo.

Angiotensin II Receptor Antagonist Adverse Reactions (%)[a]

Adverse reaction	Candesartan (n = 2350)	Eprosartan (n = 1202)	Irbesartan (n = 1965)	Losartan (n = 1075)	Olmesartan (n = 3278)	Telmisartan (n = 1455)	Valsartan (n = 2316)
CNS							
Dizziness	4	≥ 1	≥ 1	3.5	3	1	> 1
Insomnia	-	< 1	-	1.4	> 0.5	> 0.3	> 0.2
Headache	≥ 1	≥ 1	≥ 1	≥ 1	> 1	1	> 1
Fatigue	> 1	2	4	-	> 0.5	1	2
Anxiety/Nervousness	≥ 0.5	< 1	≥ 1	< 1	-	> 0.3	> 0.2
Depression	≥ 0.5	1	< 1	< 1	-	> 0.3	-
GI							
Diarrhea	> 1	≥ 1	3	2.4	> 1	3	> 1
Dyspepsia/Heartburn	≥ 0.5	≥ 1	2	1.3	> 0.5	1	> 0.2
Nausea/Vomiting	> 1	< 1	≥ 1	≥ 1	-	1	> 1
Abdominal pain	> 1	2	≥ 1	≥ 1	> 0.5	1	2
Musculoskeletal							
Arthralgia	> 1	2	-	< 1	> 0.5	> 0.3	> 1
Pain[b]	3	< 1	≥ 1	1 to 1.8	> 1	1 to 3	> 0.2
Muscle cramp	-	-	-	1.1	-	-	> 0.2
Myalgia	≥ 0.5	≥ 1	-	1	> 0.5	1	> 0.2
Trauma	-	-	2	-	-	-	-
Respiratory							
Upper respiratory tract infection	6	8	9	7.9	> 1	7	> 1
Cough[c]	> 1	4	2.8	3.4	-	1	> 1
Nasal congestion	-	-	-	2	-	-	-
Sinus disorder	-	-	≥ 1	1.5	-	-	-
Sinusitis	> 1	≥ 1	-	1	> 1	3	> 1
Pharyngitis	2	4	≥ 1	≥ 1	> 1	1	> 1
Rhinitis	2	4	≥ 1	< 1	> 1	> 0.3	> 1
Influenza/Influenza-like symptoms	-	< 1	≥ 1	< 1	> 1	1	-
Bronchitis	> 1	≥ 1	-	< 1	> 1	> 0.3	-
Miscellaneous							
Viral infection	-	2	-	-	-	-	3
Edema	-	≥ 1	≥ 1	≥ 1	-	-	> 1
Chest pain	> 1	≥ 1	≥ 1	≥ 1	> 0.5	1	-
Rash	≥ 0.5	< 1	≥ 1	< 1	> 0.5	> 0.3	> 0.2
Tachycardia	≥ 0.5	< 1	≥ 1	< 1	> 0.5	> 0.3	-
Urinary tract infection	-	4	≥ 1	< 1	> 0.5	1	-
Peripheral edema	> 1	-	-	-	> 0.5	1	-
Albuminuria	> 1	< 1	-	-	-	-	-
Hypertension	-	-	-	-	-	1	-
Hypertriglyceridemia	≥ 0.5	1	-	-	> 1	-	-
Creatine phosphokinase increased	≥ 0.5	< 1	-	-	> 1	-	-
Hyperglycemia	≥ 0.5	< 1	-	-	> 1	-	-
Hematuria	≥ 0.5	< 1	-	-	> 1	-	-
Inflicted injury	-	2	-	-	> 1	-	-

[a] Data are pooled from separate studies and are not necessarily comparable.
[b] This includes back and leg pain.
[c] See Warnings.

➤*Candesartan:*

Cardiovascular – Palpitation (at least 0.5%).

CNS – Paresthesia, vertigo, somnolence (at least 0.5%).

Metabolic/Nutritional – Hyperuricemia (at least 0.5%).

Miscellaneous – Asthenia, fever, epistaxis, dyspnea, sweating increased, gastroenteritis (at least 0.5%).

Other reported events observed less frequently included angina pectoris, MI, and angioedema.

Adverse reactions occurred at about the same rates in men and women, older and younger patients, and black and nonblack patients.

Postmarketing experience: Abnormal hepatic function, hepatitis, neutropenia, leukopenia, agranulocytosis, pruritus, urticaria.

➤*Eprosartan:*

Cardiovascular – Angina pectoris, bradycardia, abnormal ECG, specific abnormal ECG, extrasystoles, atrial fibrillation, hypotension (including orthostatic hypotension), palpitations (less than 1%).

CNS – Ataxia, migraine, neuritis, nervousness, paresthesia, somnolence, tremor, vertigo (less than 1%).

Dermatologic – Eczema, furunculosis, pruritus, maculopapular rash, increased sweating (less than 1%).

GI – Anorexia, constipation, dry mouth, esophagitis, flatulence, gastritis, gastroenteritis, gingivitis, periodontitis, toothache (less than 1%).

GU – Cystitis, micturition frequency, polyuria, renal calculus, urinary incontinence (less than 1%).

Hematologic – Anemia, purpura (less than 1%).

Hepatic – Increased ALT and AST (less than 1%).

Metabolic/Nutritional – Diabetes mellitus, glycosuria, gout, hypercholesterolemia, hyperkalemia, hypokalemia, hyponatremia (less than 1%).

Musculoskeletal – Arthritis, aggravated arthritis, arthrosis, skeletal pain, tendinitis (less than 1%).

Respiratory – Asthma, epistaxis (less than 1%).

Special senses – Conjunctivitis, abnormal vision, xerophthalmia, tinnitus (less than 1%).

Miscellaneous – Alcohol intolerance, asthenia, substernal chest pain, peripheral edema, fever, hot flushes, malaise, rigors, herpes simplex, otitis externa, otitis media, leg cramps, peripheral ischemia (less than 1%).

Facial edema was reported in 5 patients receiving eprosartan. Angioedema has been reported with other AIIRAs.

➤*Irbesartan:*

Cardiovascular – Flushing, hypertension, cardiac murmur, MI, angina pectoris, arrhythmic/conduction disorder, cardio-respiratory arrest, heart failure, hypertensive crisis (less than 1%).

CNS – Sleep disturbance, numbness, somnolence, emotional disturbance, paresthesia, tremor, transient ischemic attack, cerebrovascular accident (less than 1%).

Dermatologic – Pruritus, dermatitis, ecchymosis, face erythema, urticaria (less than 1%).

Endocrine – Sexual dysfunction, libido change, gout (less than 1%).

GI – Constipation, oral lesion, gastroenteritis, flatulence, abdominal distention (less than 1%).

GU – Abnormal urination, prostate disorder (less than 1%).

Musculoskeletal – Extremity swelling, muscle cramp, arthritis, muscle ache, musculoskeletal chest pain, joint stiffness, bursitis, muscle weakness (less than 1%).

Respiratory – Epistaxis, tracheobronchitis, congestion, pulmonary congestion, dyspnea, wheezing (less than 1%).

Special senses – Vision disturbance, hearing abnormality, ear infection, ear pain, conjunctivitis, other eye disturbance, eyelid abnormality, ear abnormality (less than 1%).

Miscellaneous – Fever, chills, facial edema, upper extremity edema (less than 1%).

The incidence of hypotension or orthostatic hypotension was low in irbesartan-treated patients (0.4%), unrelated to dosage, and similar to the incidence among placebo-treated patients (0.2%). Dizziness, syncope, and vertigo were reported with equal or less frequency in patients receiving irbesartan compared with placebo.

Postmarketing: Urticaria, angioedema (involving swelling of the face, lips, pharynx, or tongue), increased liver function tests, jaundice. Hyperkalemia has been reported rarely.

➤*Losartan:*

Cardiovascular – Angina pectoris, second degree AV block, CVA, hypotension, MI, arrhythmias including atrial fibrillation, palpitation, sinus bradycardia, ventricular tachycardia, ventricular fibrillation (less than 1%).

CNS – Anxiety disorder, ataxia, confusion, dream abnormality, hypesthesia, decreased libido, memory impairment, migraine, paresthesia, peripheral neuropathy, panic disorder, sleep disorder, somnolence, tremor, vertigo (less than 1%).

Dermatologic – Alopecia, dermatitis, dry skin, ecchymosis, erythema, flushing, photosensitivity, pruritus, sweating, urticaria (less than 1%).

GI – Anorexia, constipation, dental pain, dry mouth, flatulence, gastritis (less than 1%).

GU – Impotence, nocturia, urinary frequency (less than 1%).

Musculoskeletal – Arm pain, hip pain, joint swelling, knee pain, shoulder pain, stiffness, arthritis, fibromyalgia, muscle weakness (less than 1%).

Respiratory – Dyspnea, pharyngeal discomfort, epistaxis, respiratory congestion (less than 1%).

Special senses – Blurred vision, burning/stinging in the eye, conjunctivitis, taste perversion, tinnitus, decrease in visual acuity (less than 1%).

Miscellaneous – Asthenia/fatigue (at least 1%); facial edema, fever, orthostatic effects, syncope, anemia, gout (less than 1%).

A patient with known hypersensitivity to aspirin and penicillin, when treated with losartan, was withdrawn from the study because of swelling of the lips and eyelids and facial rash, reported as angioedema, which returned to normal 5 days after therapy was discontinued.

Superficial peeling of palms and hemolysis was reported in 1 subject.

Postmarketing experience: Hepatitis (rare); dry cough (including positive rechallenges), hyperkalemia, hyponatremia. Angioedema, including swelling of the larynx and glottis, causing airway obstruction or swelling of the face, lips, pharynx, or tongue has been reported rarely in patients treated with losartan; some of these patients previously experienced angioedema with other drugs including ACE inhibitors. Vasculitis, including Henoch-Schönlein purpura, has been reported. Anaphylactic reactions have been reported.

➤*Olmesartan:*

GI – Gastroenteritis, nausea (greater than 0.5%).

Metabolic/Nutritional – Hypercholesterolemia, hyperlipemia, hyperuricemia (greater than 0.5%).

Musculoskeletal – Arthritis, skeletal pain (greater than 0.5%).

Miscellaneous – Pain, vertigo (greater than 0.5%).

Facial edema was reported in 5 patients receiving olmesartan. Angioedema has been reported with other AIIRAs.

➤*Telmisartan:*

Cardiovascular – Palpitation, dependent edema, angina pectoris, leg edema, abnormal ECG (more than 0.3%).

CNS – Somnolence, migraine, vertigo, paresthesia, involuntary muscle contractions, hypesthesia (greater than 0.3%).

Dermatologic – Dermatitis, eczema, pruritus (greater than 0.3%).

GI – Flatulence, constipation, gastritis, vomiting, dry mouth, hemorrhoids, gastroenteritis, enteritis, gastroesophageal reflux, toothache, nonspecific GI disorders (greater than 0.3%).

GU – Micturition frequency, cystitis (greater than 0.3%).

Metabolic – Gout, hypercholesterolemia, diabetes mellitus (greater than 0.3%).

Musculoskeletal – Arthritis, leg cramps (greater than 0.3%).

Respiratory – Asthma, dyspnea, epistaxis (greater than 0.3%).

Special senses – Abnormal vision, conjunctivitis, tinnitus, earache (greater than 0.3%).

Miscellaneous – Impotence, increased sweating, flushing, allergy, fever, leg pain, malaise, infection, fungal infection, abscess, otitis media, cerebrovascular disorder (greater than 0.3%).

A single case of angioedema was reported (among a total of 3781 patients treated with telmisartan).

➤*Valsartan:*

CNS – Paresthesia, somnolence (greater than 0.2%).

GU – Constipation, dry mouth, flatulence (greater than 0.2%).

Miscellaneous – Allergic reaction, asthenia, palpitations, dyspnea, vertigo, impotence, pruritus (greater than 0.2%).

Other reported events seen less frequently in clinical trials included chest pain, syncope, anorexia, vomiting, and angioedema.

Dose-related orthostatic effects were seen in less than 1% of patients. An increase in the incidence of dizziness was observed in patients treated with 320 mg valsartan (8%) compared with 10 to 160 mg (2% to 4%).

Postmarketing experience: Hepatitis (very rare), elevated liver enzymes, angioedema (rare), impaired renal function, hyperkalemia, alopecia.

Overdosage

Limited data are available. The most likely manifestation of overdosage with an AIIRA would be hypotension, dizziness, and tachycardia; bradycardia could occur from parasympathetic (vagal) stimulation. If symptomatic hypotension should occur, institute supportive treatment. Refer to General Management of Acute Overdosage. AIIRAs cannot be removed by hemodialysis.

Patient Information

Tell patients of childbearing age about the consequences of second- and third-trimester exposure to drugs that act on the renin-angiotensin system, and tell them that these consequences do not appear to have resulted from intrauterine drug exposure that has been limited to the first trimester. Ask these patients to report pregnancies to their physicians as soon as possible.

LOSARTAN POTASSIUM ORAL

Rx	**Cozaar** (Merck)	**Tablets:** 25 mg	Lactose, 2.12 mg potassium. (MRK 951). Lt. green, teardrop shape. Film-coated. In 1000s, unit-of-use 90s and 100s, and UD 100s.
		50 mg	Lactose, 4.24 mg potassium. (MRK 952 COZAAR). Green, teardrop shape. Film-coated. In 1000s, unit-of-use 30s, 90s, and 100s, and UD 100s.
		100 mg	Lactose, 8.48 mg potassium. (960 MRK). Dk. green, teardrop shape. Film-coated. In 1000s, unit-of-use 30s, 90s, and 100s, and UD 100s.

LOSARTAN POTASSIUM — ORAL

For complete and comparative prescribing information, refer to the Angiotensin II Receptor Antagonists group monograph.

WARNING

When used in pregnancy during the second and third trimesters, drugs that act directly on the remin-angiotensin system can cause injury and even death to the developing fetus. When pregnancy is detected, losartan should be discontinued as soon as possible.

Indications

➤*Hypertension:* Losartan is indicated for the treatment of hypertension. It may be used alone or in combination with other antihypertensive agents, including diuretics.

➤*Hypertensive patients with left ventricular hypertrophy:* Losartan is indicated to reduce the risk of stroke in patients with hypertension and left ventricular hypertrophy, but there is evidence that this benefit does not apply to black patients. In the Losartan Intervention For End point reduction in hypertension (LIFE) study, black patients treated with atenolol were at lower risk of experiencing the primary composite end point compared with black patients treated with losartan. In the subgroup of black patients (n = 533; 6% of the LIFE study patients), there were 29 primary end points among 263 patients on atenolol (11%, 26 per 1,000 patient-years) and 46 primary end points among 270 patients (17%, 42 per 1,000 patient-years) on losartan. This finding could not be explained on the basis of differences in the populations other than race or on any imbalances between treatment groups. In addition, blood pressure reductions in both treatment groups were consistent between black and nonblack patients. Given the difficulty in interpreting subset differences in large trials, it cannot be known whether the observed difference is the result of chance. However, the LIFE study provides no evidence that the benefits of losartan potassium on reducing the risk of cardiovascular events in hypertensive patients with left ventricular hypertrophy apply to black patients.

➤*Nephropathy in type 2 diabetes patients:* Losartan is indicated for the treatment of diabetic nephropathy with an elevated serum creatinine and proteinuria (urinary albumin to creatinine ratio greater than or equal to 300 mg/g) in patients with type 2 diabetes and a history of hypertension. In this population, losartan reduces the rate of progression of nephropathy as measured by the occurrence of doubling of serum creatinine or end stage renal disease (need for dialysis or renal transplantation).

Administration and Dosage

➤*Approved by the FDA:* April 14, 1995.

Losartan may be administered with other antihypertensive agents.

Losartan may be administered with or without food.

➤*Adult hypertension:* Dosing must be individualized. The usual starting dosage of losartan is 50 mg once daily, with 25 mg used in patients with possible depletion of intravascular volume (eg, patients treated with diuretics) and patients with a history of hepatic impairment. In patients who are intravascularly volume-depleted (eg, those treated with diuretics), symptomatic hypotension may occur after initiation of therapy with losartan. Correct these conditions prior to administration of losartan potassium, or a lower starting dose should be used. Losartan can be administered once or twice daily with total daily doses ranging from 25 to 100 mg.

If the antihypertensive effect measured at trough using once-a-day dosing is inadequate, a twice-a-day regimen at the same total daily dose or an increase in dose may give a more satisfactory response. The effect of losartan is substantially present within 1 week, but in some studies the maximal effect occurred in 3 to 6 weeks.

If blood pressure is not controlled by losartan alone, a low dose of a diuretic may be added. Hydrochlorothiazide has been shown to have an additive effect. Addition of a low dose of hydrochlorothiazide (12.5 mg) to losartan 50 mg once daily resulted in placebo-adjusted blood pressure reductions of 15.5/9.2 mm Hg.

No initial dosage adjustment is necessary for elderly patients or for patients with renal impairment, including patients on dialysis.

➤*Pediatric hypertensive patients 6 years of age and older:* The usual recommended starting dosage is 0.7 mg/kg once daily (up to 50 mg total) administered as a tablet or suspension. Dosage should be adjusted according to blood pressure response. Doses above 1.4 mg/kg (or in excess of 100 mg) daily have not been studied in pediatric patients.

Losartan is not recommended in pediatric patients younger than 6 years of age or in pediatric patients with glomerular filtration rate less than 30 mL/min per 1.73 m^2.

Preparation of suspension (for 200 mL of a 2.5 mg/mL suspension) – Add 10 mL of purified water to an 8 ounce (240 mL) amber polyethylene terephthalate (PET) bottle containing ten 50 mg losartan tablets. Immediately shake for at least 2 minutes. Let the concentrate stand for 1 hour and then shake for 1 minute to disperse the tablet contents. Separately prepare a 50/50 volumetric mixture of *Ora-Plus* and *Ora-Sweet SF*. Add 190 mL of the 50/50 *Ora-Plus/Ora-Sweet SF*™ mixture to the tablet and water slurry in the PET bottle and shake for 1 minute to disperse the ingredients. The suspension should be refrigerated at 2° to 8°C (36° to 46°F) and can be stored for up to 4 weeks. Shake the suspension prior to each use and return promptly to the refrigerator.

➤*Hypertensive patients with left ventricular hypertrophy:* The usual starting dosage is 50 mg of losartan potassium once daily. Hydrochlorothiazide 12.5 mg daily should be added or the dose of losartan potassium should be increased to 100 mg once daily followed by an increase in hydrochlorothiazide to 25 mg once daily based on blood pressure response.

➤*Nephropathy in type 2 diabetic patients:* The usual starting dose is 50 mg once daily. The dose should be increased to 100 mg once daily based on blood pressure response. Losartan may be administered with insulin and other commonly used hypoglycemic agents (eg, sulfonylureas, glitazones, glucosidase inhibitors).

➤*Storage/Stability:* Store at 25°C (77°F); excursions permitted to 15° to 30°C (59° to 86°F). Keep container tightly closed. Protect from light.

VALSARTAN

Rx	**Diovan** (Novartis)	**Tablets:** 40 mg	(NVR DO). Yellow. Scored. In 30s and UD 100s.
		80 mg	(NVR DV). Pale red, almond shape. In 90s and UD 100s.
		160 mg	(NVR DX). Gray-orange, almond shape. In 90s and UD 100s.
		320 mg	(NVR DXL). Dark grayish violet, almond shape. In 90s and UD 100s.

VALSARTAN — ORAL

For complete and comparative prescribing information, refer to the Angiotensin II Receptor Antagonists group monograph.

WARNING

Use in pregnancy – When used in pregnancy during the second and third trimesters, drugs that act directly on the renin-angiotensin system can cause injury and even death to the developing fetus. When pregnancy is detected, discontinue valsartan as soon as possible. The use of drugs that act directly on the renin-angiotensin system during the second and third trimesters of pregnancy has been associated with fetal and neonatal injury, including hypotension, neonatal skull hypoplasia, anuria, reversible or irreversible renal failure, and death. Oligohydramnios has also been reported, presumably resulting from decreased fetal renal function; oligohydramnios in this setting has been associated with fetal limb contractures, craniofacial deformation, and hypoplastic lung development. Prematurity, intrauterine growth retardation, and patent ductus arteriosus have also been reported, although it is not clear whether these occurrences were due to exposure to the drug.

Indications

➤*Hypertension:* Valsartan is indicated for the treatment of hypertension. It may be used alone or in combination with other antihypertensive agents.

➤*Heart failure:* Valsartan is indicated for the treatment of heart failure (New York Heart Association [NYHA] class II to IV). In a controlled clinical trial, valsartan significantly reduced hospitalizations for heart failure. There is no evidence that valsartan provides added benefits when it is used with an adequate dose of an angiotensin-converting enzyme (ACE) inhibitor.

➤*Postmyocardial infarction:* In clinically stable patients with left ventricular failure or left ventricular dysfunction following myocardial infarction, valsartan is indicated to reduce cardiovascular mortality.

Administration and Dosage

➤*Approved by the FDA:* December 23, 1996.

➤*Hypertension:* The recommended starting dosage of valsartan is 80 or 160 mg once daily when used as monotherapy in patients who are not volume-depleted. Patients requiring greater reductions may be started at a higher dose. Valsartan may be used over a dose range of 80 to 320 mg daily.

The antihypertensive effect is substantially present within 2 weeks and maximal reduction is generally attained after 4 weeks. If additional antihypertensive effect is required, the dosage may be increased to a maximum of 320 mg or a diuretic may be added. The addition of a diuretic has a greater effect than dose increases beyond 80 mg.

Valsartan may be administered with other antihypertensive agents.

Valsartan may be administered with or without food.

➤*Heart failure:* The recommended starting dosage of valsartan is 40 mg twice daily. Uptitration to 80 and 160 mg twice daily should be done to the highest dose, as tolerated by the patient. Consider reducing the dose of concomitant diuretics. The maximum daily dose administered in clinical trials is 320 mg in divided doses.

➤*Postmyocardial infarction:* Valsartan may be initiated as early as 12 hours after a myocardial infarction (MI). The recommended starting dosage of valsartan is 20 mg twice daily. Patients may be uptitrated within 7 days to 40 mg twice daily, with subsequent titrations to a target maintenance dosage of 160 mg twice daily, as tolerated by the patient. If symptom-

VALSARTAN — ORAL

atic hypotension or renal dysfunction occur, consider a dosage reduction. Valsartan may be given with other standard postmyocardial infarction treatment, including thrombolytics, aspirin, beta-blockers, and statins.

➤*Storage/Stability:* Protect from moisture.

Dispense in a tight container.

Store tablets at 25°C (77°F); excursions permitted to 15° to 30°C (59° to 86°F).

IRBESARTAN

Rx	**Avapro** (Bristol-Myers Squibb Sanofi-Synthelabo Partnership)	**Tablets:** 75 mg	Lactose. (2771). White to off-white, oval. In 30s and 90s.
		150 mg	Lactose. (2772). White to off-white, oval. In 30s, 90s, 500s, and UD 100s.
		300 mg	Lactose. (2773). White to off-white, oval. In 30s, 90s, and 500s.

IRBESARTAN — ORAL

For complete and comparative prescribing information, refer to the Angiotensin II Receptor Antagonists group monograph.

WARNING

When used in pregnancy during the second and third trimesters, drugs that act directly on the renin-angiotensin system can cause injury and even death to the developing fetus. When pregnancy is detected, irbesartan should be discontinued as soon as possible.

Indications

➤*Hypertension:* Irbesartan is indicated for the treatment of hypertension; it may be used alone or in combination with other antihypertensive agents.

➤*Nephropathy in type 2 diabetic patients:* Irbesartan is indicated for the treatment of diabetic nephropathy with an elevated serum creatinine and proteinuria (greater than 300 mg/day) in patients with type 2 diabetes and hypertension. In this population, irbesartan reduces the rate of progression of nephropathy as measured by the occurrence of doubling of serum creatinine or endstage renal disease (need for dialysis or renal transplantation).

Administration and Dosage

➤*Approved by the FDA:* September 30, 1997.

Irbesartan may be administered with other antihypertensive agents.

Irbesartan may be administered with or without food.

No dosage adjustment is necessary in elderly patients, or in patients with hepatic impairment or mild to severe renal impairment.

In controlled trials, the addition of irbesartan to hydrochlorothiazide doses of 6.25, 12.5, or 25 mg produced further dose-related reductions in blood pressure similar to those achieved with the same monotherapy dose of irbesartan.

➤*Hypertension:* The recommended initial dose of irbesartan is 150 mg once daily. Patients requiring further reduction in blood pressure should be titrated to 300 mg once daily.

A low dose of a diuretic may be added if blood pressure is not controlled by irbesartan alone. Hydrochlorothiazide has been shown to have an additive effect. Patients not adequately treated by the maximum dose of 300 mg once daily are unlikely to derive additional benefit from a higher dose or twice-daily dosing.

➤*Nephropathy in type 2 diabetic patients:* The recommended target maintenance dose is 300 mg once daily. There are no data on the clinical effects of lower doses of irbesartan on diabetic nephropathy.

➤*Pediatric patients:*

Children younger than 6 years – Safety and effectiveness have not been established.

Children 6 to 12 years – Pharmacokinetic parameters in pediatric subjects (age 6 to 16, n = 21) were comparable with adults. At doses up to 150 mg daily for 4 weeks, irbesartan was well tolerated in hypertensive children and adolescents. Blood pressure reductions were comparable to adults receiving 150 mg daily; however, greater sensitivity in some patients cannot be ruled out. An initial dose of 75 mg once daily is reasonable. Patients requiring further reduction in blood pressure should be titrated to 150 mg once daily.

Adolescent patients 13 to 16 years – Pharmacokinetic parameters in pediatric subjects (age 6 to 16, n = 21) were comparable with adults. At doses up to 150 mg daily for 4 weeks, irbesartan was well tolerated in hypertensive children and adolescents. Blood pressure reductions were comparable to adults receiving 150 mg daily; however, greater sensitivity in some patients cannot be ruled out. An initial dose of 150 mg once daily is reasonable. Patients requiring further reduction in blood pressure should be titrated to 300 mg once daily. Higher doses are not recommended.

➤*Volume- and salt-depleted patients:* Excessive reduction of blood pressure was rarely seen in patients with uncomplicated hypertension treated with irbesartan (less than 0.1%). Initiation of antihypertensive therapy may cause symptomatic hypotension in patients with intravascular volume or sodium depletion, (eg, in patients treated vigorously with diuretics or in patients on dialysis). Such volume depletion should be corrected prior to administration of antihypertensive therapy, or a low starting dose of irbesartan should be used, and the patient should be monitored closely. A lower initial dose of irbesartan (75 mg) is recommended in patients with depletion of intravascular volume or salt (eg, patients treated vigorously with diuretics or on hemodialysis).

➤*Storage/Stability:* Store at a temperature between 15° and 30°C (59° and 86°F).

CANDESARTAN CILEXETIL

Rx	**Atacand** (AstraZeneca)	**Tablets:** 4 mg	Lactose. (ACF 004). White to off-white. In unit-of-use 30s.
		8 mg	Lactose. (ACG 008). Lt. pink. In unit-of-use 30s.
		16 mg	Lactose. (ACH 016). Pink. In unit-of-use 30s and 90s and UD 100s.
		32 mg	Lactose. (ACL 032). Pink. In unit-of-use 30s and 90s and UD 100s.

CANDESARTAN CILEXETIL — ORAL

For complete and comparative prescribing information, refer to the Angiotensin II Receptor Antagonists group monograph.

WARNING

Use in pregnancy – When used in pregnancy during the second and third trimesters, drugs that act directly on the renin-angiotensin system can cause injury and even death to the developing fetus. When pregnancy is detected, discontinue candesartan as soon as possible. Drugs that act directly on the renin-angiotensin system can cause fetal and neonatal morbidity and death when administered to pregnant women.

Indications

➤*Hypertension:* Candesartan is indicated for the treatment of hypertension. It may be used alone or in combination with other antihypertensive agents.

➤*Heart failure:* Candesartan is indicated for the treatment of heart failure (New York Heart Association [NYHA] class II to IV and ejection fraction up to 40%) to reduce the risk of death from cardiovascular causes and reduce hospitalizations for heart failure.

Administration and Dosage

➤*Approved by the FDA:* June 4, 1998.

Candesartan may be administered with or without food.

➤*Hypertension:* Dosage must be individualized. Blood pressure response is dose related over the range of 2 to 32 mg. The usual recommended starting dosage of candesartan is 16 mg once daily when it is used as monotherapy in patients who are not volume depleted. Candesartan can be administered once or twice daily with total daily doses ranging from 8 to 32 mg. Larger doses do not appear to have a greater effect, and there is relatively little experience with such doses. Most of the antihypertensive effect is present within 2 weeks, and maximal blood pressure reduction is generally obtained within 4 to 6 weeks of treatment with candesartan. If blood pressure is not controlled by candesartan alone, a diuretic may be added. Candesartan may be administered with other antihypertensive agents.

➤*Heart failure:* The recommended initial dosage for treating heart failure is 4 mg once daily. The target dosage is 32 mg once daily, which is achieved by doubling the dose at approximately 2-week intervals, as tolerated by the patient.

➤*Hepatic function impairment:* No initial dosage adjustment is necessary for patients with mildly impaired hepatic function. In patients with moderate hepatic impairment, consider initiating candesartan at a lower dose.

➤*Volume-depleted patients:* For patients with possible depletion of intravascular volume (eg, patients treated with diuretics, particularly those with impaired renal function), initiate candesartan under close medical supervision and consider administering a lower dose.

➤*Storage/Stability:* Store at 25°C (77°F); excursions permitted to 15° to 30°C (59° to 86°F). Keep the container tightly closed.

Angiotensin II Receptor Antagonists

TELMISARTAN

Rx	**Micardis** (Boehringer Ingelheim)	**Tablets:** 20 mg	Sorbitol. (50H). White. In blister pack 28s.
		40 mg	Sorbitol. (51H). White, oblong. In blister pack 28s.
		80 mg	Sorbitol. (52H). White, oblong. In blister pack 28s.

TELMISARTAN — ORAL

For complete and comparative prescribing information, refer to the Angiotensin II Receptor Antagonists group monograph.

WARNING

Use in pregnancy – When used in pregnancy during the second and third trimesters, drugs that act directly on the renin-angiotensin system can cause injury and even death to the developing fetus. When pregnancy is detected, telmisartan tablets should be discontinued as soon as possible.

Indications

➤*Hypertension:* Telmisartan is indicated for the treatment of hypertension. It may be used alone or in combination with other antihypertensive agents.

Administration and Dosage

➤*Approved by the FDA:* November 10, 1998

➤*Hypertension:* Individualize dosage. The usual starting dose is 40 mg once daily. Blood pressure response is dose related over the range of 20 to 80 mg. May be administered with or without food. May be administered with other antihypertensive agents. Most of the antihypertensive effect is apparent within 2 weeks; maximal reduction is generally attained after 4 weeks. When additional blood pressure reduction beyond that achieved with 80 mg is required, a diuretic may be added.

➤*Storage/Stability:* Store at 25°C (77°F); excursions permitted to 15° to 30°C (59° to 86°F). Tablets should not be removed from blisters until immediately before administration.

EPROSARTAN MESYLATE

Rx	**Teveten** (Biovail)	**Tablets:** 600 mg	Lactose. (SOLVAY 5046). White, capsule shape. Film-coated. In 100s.

EPROSARTAN MESYLATE — ORAL

For complete and comparative prescribing information, refer to the Angiotensin II Receptor Antagonists group monograph.

WARNING

Use in pregnancy – When used in pregnancy during the second and third trimesters, drugs that act directly on the renin-angiotensin system can cause injury and even death to the developing fetus. When pregnancy is detected, eprosartan mesylate tablets should be discontinued as soon as possible.

Indications

➤*Hypertension:* Eprosartan mesylate tablets are indicated for the treatment of hypertension. It may be used alone or in combination with other antihypertensives such as diuretics and calcium channel blockers.

Administration and Dosage

➤*Approved by the FDA:* October 22, 1999.

➤*Hypertension:* The usual recommended starting dose of eprosartan mesylate tablets is 600 mg once daily when used as monotherapy in patients who are not volume depleted. Eprosartan mesylate tablets can be administered once or twice daily with total daily doses ranging from 400 to 800 mg. There is limited experience with doses beyond 800 mg/day.

If the antihypertensive effect measured at trough using once-daily dosing is inadequate, a twice-a-day regimen at the same total daily dose or an increase in dose may give a more satisfactory response. Achievement of maximum blood pressure reduction in most patients may take 2 to 3 weeks.

Eprosartan mesylate tablets may be used in combination with other antihypertensive agents such as thiazide diuretics or calcium channel blockers if additional blood pressure-lowering effect is required. Discontinuation of treatment with eprosartan does not lead to a rapid rebound increase in blood pressure.

➤*Elderly, hepatically impaired or renally impaired patients:* No initial dosing adjustment is generally necessary for elderly or hepatically impaired patients or those with renal impairment. No initial dosing adjustment is generally necessary in patients with moderate and severe renal impairment, with maximum dose not exceeding 600 mg daily.

Eprosartan mesylate tablets may be taken with or without food.

➤*Storage/Stability:* Store at controlled room temperature 20° to 25°C (68° to 77°F).

OLMESARTAN MEDOXOMIL

Rx	**Benicar** (Sankyo Pharma)	**Tablets:** 5 mg	Lactose. (Sankyo C12). Yellow. Film-coated. In 30s.
		20 mg	Lactose. (Sankyo C14). White. Film-coated. In 30s, 90s, and blister card 100s.
		40 mg	Lactose. (Sankyo C15). White, oval. Film-coated. In 30s, 90s, and blister card 100s.

OLMESARTAN MEDOXOMIL — ORAL

For complete and comparative prescribing information, refer to the Angiotensin II Receptor Antagonists group monograph.

WARNING

Use in pregnancy – When used in pregnancy during the second and third trimesters, drugs that act directly on the renin-angiotensin system can cause injury and even death to the developing fetus. When pregnancy is detected, olmesartan medoxomil should be discontinued as soon as possible.

Indications

➤*Hypertension:* Olmesartan medoxomil is indicated for the treatment of hypertension. It may be used alone or in combination with other antihypertensive agents.

Administration and Dosage

➤*Approved by the FDA:* April 25, 2002.

➤*Hypertension:* Dosage must be individualized. The usual recommended starting dose of olmesartan medoxomil is 20 mg once daily when used as monotherapy in patients who are not volume-contracted. For patients requiring further reduction in blood pressure after 2 weeks of therapy, the dose of olmesartan medoxomil may be increased to 40 mg. Doses above 40 mg do not appear to have greater effect. Twice-daily dosing offers no advantage over the same total dose given once daily.

➤*Special populations:* No initial dosage adjustment is recommended for elderly patients, for patients with moderate to marked renal impairment (creatinine clearance less than 40 mL/min) or with moderate to marked hepatic dysfunction. For patients with possible depletion of intravascular volume (eg, patients treated with diuretics, particularly those with impaired renal function), olmesartan medoxomil should be initiated under close medical supervision, and consideration should be given to use of a lower starting dose. If hypotension occurs, the patient should be placed in the supine position and, if necessary, given an IV infusion of normal saline. A transient hypotensive response is not a contraindication to further treatment, which usually can be continued without difficulty once the blood pressure has stabilized.

Olmesartan medoxomil may be administered with or without food.

If blood pressure is not controlled by olmesartan medoxomil alone, a diuretic may be added. Olmesartan medoxomil may be administered with other antihypertensive agents.

➤*Storage/Stability:* Store at 20° to 25°C (68° to 77°F).

Selective Aldosterone Receptor Antagonists

EPLERENONE ORAL

Rx	**Inspra** (Pfizer)	**Tablets:** 25 mg	Lactose. (Pfizer NSR/25). Yellow, diamond shape. Film-coated. In 30s, 90s, and unit doses.
		50 mg	Lactose. (Pfizer NSR/50). Yellow, diamond shape. Film-coated. In 30s and 90s.

EPLERENONE — ORAL

Indications

➤*Congestive heart failure (CHF) post-myocardial infarction (MI):* Eplerenone is indicated to improve survival of stable patients with left ventricular systolic dysfunction (ejection fraction less than or equal to 40%) and clinical evidence of CHF after an acute MI.

➤*Hypertension:* Eplerenone is indicated for the treatment of hypertension. Eplerenone may be used alone or in combination with other antihypertensive agents.

➤*Unlabeled uses:* Possible therapy used alone or in combination with an angiotensin-converting enzyme (ACE) inhibitor for reducing left ventricular hypertrophy (LVH); as adjunctive therapy to reduce microalbuminuria in diabetic hypertensive patients.

Administration and Dosage

➤*Approved by the FDA:* September 30, 2002.

➤*CHF post-MI:* The recommended dosage of eplerenone is 50 mg once daily. Initiate treatment at 25 mg once daily and titrate to the target dosage of 50 mg once daily, preferably within 4 weeks as tolerated by the patient. Administer eplerenone with or without food.

Dosage Adjustment in CHF

Serum potassium (mEq/L)	Action	Dosage adjustment
< 5	Increase	25 mg every other day to 25 mg daily; 25 mg daily to 50 mg daily
5 to 5.4	Maintain	No adjustment
5.5 to 5.9	Decrease	50 mg to 25 mg daily; 25 mg daily to 25 mg every other day; 25 mg every other day to withhold
≥ 6	Withhold	

Following withholding eplerenone due to serum potassium greater than or equal to 6 mEq/L, eplerenone can be restarted at a dosage of 25 mg every other day when serum potassium levels have fallen below 5.5 mEq/L.

Measure serum potassium before initiating eplerenone therapy, within the first week and at 1 month after the start of treatment or dosage adjustment. Assess serum potassium periodically thereafter. Factors such as patient characteristics and serum potassium levels may indicate that additional monitoring is appropriate. In the eplerenone post-acute myocardial infarction heart failure efficacy and survival study (EPHESUS), the majority of hyperkalemia was observed within the first 3 months after randomization. Adjust the dosage based on the serum potassium level and as shown in the previous table.

➤*Hypertension:* Use eplerenone alone or in combination with other antihypertensive agents. The recommended starting dosage of eplerenone is 50 mg administered once daily. The full therapeutic effect of eplerenone is apparent within 4 weeks. For patients with an inadequate blood pressure response to 50 mg once daily, increase the dosage of eplerenone to 50 mg twice daily. Higher dosages of eplerenone are not recommended either because they have no greater effect on blood pressure than 100 mg or because they are associated with an increased risk of hyperkalemia.

No adjustment of the starting dose is recommended for the elderly or for patients with mild to moderate hepatic impairment. For patients receiving weak CYP3A4 inhibitors, such as erythromycin, saquinavir, verapamil, and fluconazole, reduce the starting dosage to 25 mg once daily.

➤*Storage / Stability:* Store at 25°C (77°F); excursions permitted to 15° to 30°C (59° to 86°F).

Actions

➤*Pharmacology:* Eplerenone binds to the mineralocorticoid receptor and blocks the binding of aldosterone, a component of the renin-angiotensin-aldosterone-system (RAAS). Aldosterone synthesis, which occurs primarily in the adrenal gland, is modulated by multiple factors, including angiotensin II and non-RAAS mediators such as corticotropin and potassium. Aldosterone binds to mineralocorticoid receptors in both epithelial (eg, kidney) and nonepithelial (eg, heart, blood vessels, brain) tissues and increases blood pressure through induction of sodium reabsorption and possibly other mechanisms.

Eplerenone has been shown to produce sustained increases in plasma renin and serum aldosterone, consistent with inhibition of the negative regulatory feedback of aldosterone on renin secretion. The resulting increased plasma renin activity and aldosterone circulating levels do not overcome the effect of eplerenone.

Eplerenone selectively binds to recombinant human mineralocorticoid receptors compared with its binding to recombinant human glucocorticoid, progesterone, and androgen receptors.

➤*Pharmacokinetics:*

Absorption – Absorption is not affected by food.

Mean peak plasma concentrations of eplerenone are reached approximately 1.5 hours following oral administration. The absolute bioavailability of eplerenone is unknown. Both peak plasma levels (C_{max}) and area under the curve (AUC) are dose proportional over doses of 25 to 100 mg and less than proportional at doses above 100 mg.

Distribution – The plasma protein binding of eplerenone is about 50% and is primarily bound to alpha-1 acid glycoproteins. The apparent volume of distribution at steady state ranged from 43 to 90 L. Eplerenone does not preferentially bind to red blood cells. Inhibitors of CYP3A4 (eg, ketoconazole, saquinavir) increase blood levels of eplerenone.

Metabolism – Eplerenone metabolism is primarily mediated via CYP3A4. No active metabolites of eplerenone have been identified in human plasma. Eplerenone is cleared predominantly by cytochrome P-450 (CYP) 3A4 metabolism, with an elimination half-life of 4 to 6 hours. Steady state is reached within 2 days.

Excretion – Less than 5% of an eplerenone dose is recovered as unchanged drug in the urine and feces. Following a single oral dose of radiolabeled drug, approximately 32% of the dose was excreted in the feces and approximately 67% was excreted in the urine. The elimination half-life of eplerenone is approximately 4 to 6 hours. The apparent plasma clearance is approximately 10 L/h.

Special populations –

Renal function impairment: The pharmacokinetics of eplerenone were evaluated in patients with varying degrees of renal impairment and in patients undergoing hemodialysis. Compared with control subjects, steady-state AUC and C_{max} were increased by 38% and 24%, respectively, in patients with severe renal function impairment and were decreased by 26% and 3%, respectively, in patients undergoing hemodialysis. No correlation was observed between plasma clearance of eplerenone and creatinine clearance. Eplerenone is not removed by hemodialysis.

Hepatic function impairment: The pharmacokinetics of eplerenone 400 mg have been investigated in patients with moderate (Child-Pugh class B) hepatic function impairment and compared with healthy subjects. Steady-state C_{max} and AUC of eplerenone were increased by 3.6% and 42%, respectively.

Elderly: The pharmacokinetics of eplerenone at a dosage of 100 mg once daily have been investigated in the elderly (65 years of age and older).

At steady state, elderly subjects had increases in C_{max} (22%) and AUC (45%) compared with younger subjects (18 to 45 years of age).

Gender: The pharmacokinetics of eplerenone at a dosage of 100 mg once daily have been investigated in men and women.

The pharmacokinetics of eplerenone did not differ significantly between men and women.

Race: The pharmacokinetics of eplerenone at a dosage of 100 mg once daily have been investigated in black patients.

At steady state, C_{max} was 19% lower and AUC was 26% lower in black patients.

Heart failure: The pharmacokinetics of eplerenone 50 mg were evaluated in 8 patients with heart failure (New York Heart Association [NYHA] classification II-IV), and 8 matched (gender, age, weight) healthy controls. Compared with the controls, steady state AUC and C_{max} in patients with stable heart failure were 38% and 30% higher, respectively.

Pharmacokinetic drug-drug interactions – Drug-drug interaction studies were conducted with a dose of eplerenone 100 mg.

Eplerenone is metabolized primarily by CYP3A4. A potent inhibitor of CYP3A4 (ketoconazole) caused increased exposure of about 5-fold, while less potent CYP3A4 inhibitors (erythromycin, saquinavir, verapamil, and fluconazole) gave approximately 2-fold increases. Grapefruit juice caused only a small increase (about 25%) in exposure.

Contraindications

Eplerenone is contraindicated in all patients with the following:

1.) Serum potassium greater than 5.5 mEq/L at initiation.
2.) Creatinine clearance less than or equal to 30 mL/min.
3.) Concomitant use with the following potent CYP3A4 inhibitors: clarithromycin, itraconazole, ketoconazole, nefazodone, nelfinavir, ritonavir, and troleandomycin. Do not use eplerenone with other drugs noted to be potent CYP3A4 inhibitors.

➤*Hypertension:* Eplerenone is also contraindicated for the treatment of hypertension in patients with the following:

1.) Type 2 diabetes with microalbuminuria.
2.) Serum creatinine greater than 2 mg/dL in men or greater than 1.8 mg/dL in women.
3.) Creatinine clearance less than 50 mL/min.
4.) Concomitant use of potassium supplements or potassium-sparing diuretics (amiloride, spironolactone, or triamterene).

Warnings

➤*Hyperkalemia:* The principal risk of eplerenone is hyperkalemia. Hyperkalemia can cause serious, sometimes fatal, arrhythmias. Patients who develop hyperkalemia (greater than 5.5 mEq/L) may still benefit from eplerenone with proper dose adjustment. Minimize hyperkalemia by patient selection, avoidance of certain concomitant treatments, and periodic monitoring until the effect of eplerenone has been established. Dose reduction of eplerenone has been shown to decrease potassium levels.

Treat patients with CHF post-MI who have serum creatinine levels greater than 2 mg/dL (men) or greater than 1.8 mg/dL (women) or creatinine clearance less than or equal to 50 mL/min with caution. The rates of hyperkalemia increased with declining renal function.

Treat diabetic patients with CHF post-MI, including those with proteinuria, with caution. The subset of patients in EPHESUS with both diabetes and proteinuria on the baseline urinalysis had increased rates of hyperkalemia.

EPLERENONE — ORAL

➤*Renal function impairment:* Eplerenone is contraindicated in patients with serum potassium greater than 5.5 mEq/L at initiation and/or creatinine clearance less than or equal to 30 mL/min.

➤*Carcinogenesis:* There was no drug-related tumor response in heterozygous P53-deficient mice when tested for 6 months at dosages up to 1,000 mg/kg/day (systemic AUC exposures up to 9 times the exposure in humans receiving the 100 mg/day therapeutic dosage). Statistically significant increases in benign thyroid tumors were observed after 2 years in both male and female rats when administered eplerenone 250 mg/kg/day (highest dosage tested) and in male rats only at 75 mg/kg/day. These dosages provided systemic AUC exposures approximately 2 to 12 times higher than the average human therapeutic exposure at 100 mg/day. Repeat dose administration of eplerenone to rats increases the hepatic conjugation and clearance of thyroxin, which results in increased levels of thyrotropin (TSH) by a compensatory mechanism. Drugs that have produced thyroid tumors by this rodent-specific mechanism have not shown a similar effect in humans.

➤*Mutagenesis:* Eplerenone was nongenotoxic in a battery of assays including in vitro bacterial mutagenesis (Ames test in *Salmonella* spp. and *Escherichia coli*), in vitro mammalian cell mutagenesis (mouse lymphoma cells), in vitro chromosomal aberration (Chinese hamster ovary cells), in vivo rat bone marrow micronucleus formation, and in vivo/ex vivo unscheduled DNA synthesis in rat liver.

➤*Fertility impairment:* Male rats treated with eplerenone at 1,000 mg/kg/day for 10 weeks (AUC 17 times that at the 100 mg/day human therapeutic dosage) had decreased weights of seminal vesicles and epididymides and slightly decreased fertility. Dogs administered eplerenone at dosages of 15 mg/kg/day and higher (AUC 5 times that at the 100 mg/day human therapeutic dosage) had dosage-related prostate atrophy. The prostate atrophy was reversible after daily treatment for 1 year at 100 mg/kg/day. Dogs with prostate atrophy showed no decline in libido, sexual performance, or semen quality. Testicular weight and histology were not affected by eplerenone in any test animal species at any dosage.

➤*Elderly:*

Data from CHF post-MI trials – Of the total number of patients in EPHESUS, 3,340 (50%) were 65 years of age and older, while 1,326 (20%) were 75 years of age and older. Patients older than 75 years of age did not appear to benefit from the use of eplerenone. No differences in the overall incidence of adverse reactions were observed between elderly and younger patients. However, due to age-related decreases in creatinine clearance, the incidence of laboratory-documented hyperkalemia was increased in patients 65 years of age and older.

Data from hypertension trials – Of the total number of subjects in clinical hypertension studies of eplerenone, 1,123 (23%) were 65 years of age and older, while 212 (4%) were 75 years of age and older. No overall differences in safety or efficacy were observed between elderly subjects and younger subjects.

➤*Pregnancy: Category B.* There are no adequate and well-controlled studies in pregnant women. Use eplerenone during pregnancy only if the potential benefit justifies the potential risk to the fetus.

Teratogenic – Embryo-fetal development studies were conducted with dosages up to 1,000 mg/kg/day in rats and 300 mg/kg/day in rabbits (exposures up to 32 and 31 times the human AUC for the 100 mg/day therapeutic dosage, respectively). No teratogenic effects were seen in rats or rabbits, although decreased body weight in maternal rabbits and increased rabbit fetal resorptions and postimplantation loss were observed at the highest administered dosage. Because animal reproduction studies are not always predictive of human response, use eplerenone during pregnancy only if clearly needed.

➤*Lactation:* The concentration of eplerenone in human breast milk after oral administration is unknown. However preclinical data show that eplerenone and/or metabolites are present in rat breast milk (0.85:1 [milk:plasma] AUC ratio) obtained after a single oral dose. Peak concentrations in plasma and milk were obtained from 0.5 to 1 hour after dosing. Rat pups exposed by this route developed normally. Because many drugs are excreted in human milk and because of the unknown potential for adverse reactions on the breast-feeding infant, make a decision whether to discontinue breast-feeding or discontinue the drug, taking into account the importance of the drug to the mother.

➤*Children:* The safety and efficacy of eplerenone have not been established in children.

Drug Interactions

➤*Inhibitors of CYP450 3A4:* Eplerenone metabolism is predominantly mediated via CYP3A4. A pharmacokinetic study evaluating the administration of a single dose of eplerenone 100 mg with ketoconazole 200 mg twice daily, a potent inhibitor of the CYP3A4 pathway, showed a 1.7-fold increase in C_{max} of eplerenone and a 5.4-fold increase in AUC of eplerenone. Do not use eplerenone with drugs described as strong inhibitors of CYP3A4 in their labeling.

➤*Administration with other CYP3A4 inhibitors:* Administration of eplerenone with other CYP3A4 inhibitors (eg, erythromycin 500 mg twice daily, verapamil 240 mg daily, saquinavir 1,200 mg 3 times daily, fluconazole 200 mg daily) resulted in increases in C_{max} of eplerenone ranging from 1.4- to 1.6-fold and AUC from 2- to 2.9-fold.

➤*Angiotensin-converting enzyme (ACE) inhibitors and angiotensin II receptor antagonists:*

Data from CHF post-MI studies – In EPHESUS, 3,020 (91%) patients receiving eplerenone 25 to 50 mg also received ACE inhibitors or angiotensin II receptor antagonists. Rates of patients with maximum potassium levels greater than 5.5 mEq/L were similar regardless of the use of ACE inhibitors or angiotensin II receptor antagonists.

Data from hypertension studies – In clinical studies of patients with hypertension, the addition of eplerenone 50 to 100 mg to ACE inhibitors and angiotensin II receptor antagonists increased mean serum potassium slightly (about 0.09 to 0.13 mEq/L). In a study in diabetics with microalbuminuria eplerenone 200 mg combined with the ACE inhibitor enalapril 10 mg increased the frequency of hyperkalemia (serum potassium greater than 5.5 mEq/L) from 17% on enalapril alone to 38%.

➤*Lithium:* A drug interaction study of eplerenone with lithium has not been conducted. Lithium toxicity has been reported in patients receiving lithium concomitantly with diuretics and ACE inhibitors. Monitor serum lithium levels frequently if eplerenone is coadministered with lithium.

➤*Nonsteroidal anti-inflammatory drugs (NSAIDs):* A drug interaction study of eplerenone with an NSAID has not been conducted. The administration of other potassium-sparing antihypertensives with NSAIDs has been shown to reduce the antihypertensive effect in some patients and result in severe hyperkalemia in patients with impaired renal function. Therefore, when eplerenone and NSAIDs are used concomitantly, observe patients to determine whether the desired effect on blood pressure is obtained.

Eplerenone Drug Interactions

Precipitant drug	Object drug*		Description
ACE inhibitors Angiotensin II antagonists	Eplerenone	↑	Increased risk of hyperkalemia with coadministration.
CYP3A4 inhibitors	Eplerenone	↑	Coadministration of potent inhibitors (eg, ketoconazole) resulted in increased exposure of about 5-fold; less potent inhibitors yielded about a 2-fold increase (see Administration and Dosage and Contraindications).
NSAIDs	Eplerenone	↑↓	Coadministration of NSAIDs with other potassium-sparing antihypertensives may cause decreased antihypertensive effect and results in severe hyperkalemia in patients with impaired renal function.
St. John's wort	Eplerenone	↓	Approximately 30% decrease in eplerenone AUC.
Eplerenone	Lithium	↑	Coadministration of lithium with diuretics and ACE inhibitors may lead to lithium toxicity; frequently monitor serum lithium levels if coadministered with eplerenone.

* ↑ = Object drug increased. ↓ = Object drug decreased.

➤*Drug/Food interactions:* Coadministration with grapefruit juice produced a small increase (about 25%) in exposure.

Adverse Reactions

➤*Data from CHF post-MI trials:* In EPHESUS, safety was evaluated in 3,307 patients treated with eplerenone and 3,301 placebo-treated patients. The overall incidence of adverse reactions reported with eplerenone (78.9%) was similar to placebo (79.5%). Adverse reactions occurred at a similar rate regardless of age, gender, or race. Patients discontinued treatment due to an adverse reaction at similar rates in either treatment group (4.4% eplerenone vs 4.3% placebo).

Adverse reactions that occurred more frequently in patients treated with eplerenone than placebo were hyperkalemia (3.4% vs 2%) and increased creatinine (2.4% vs 1.5%). Discontinuations due to hyperkalemia or abnormal renal function were less than 1% in both groups. Hypokalemia occurred less frequently in patients treated with eplerenone (0.6% vs 1.6%).

The rates of sex hormone-related adverse reactions are shown in the following table.

Rates of Sex Hormone-Related Adverse Reactions in EPHESUS

	Rates in men			Rates in women
	Gynecomastia	Mastodynia	Either	Abnormal vaginal bleeding
Eplerenone	0.4%	0.1%	0.5%	0.4%
Placebo	0.5%	0.1%	0.6%	0.4%

➤*Data from hypertension trials:* Eplerenone has been evaluated for safety in 3,091 patients treated for hypertension. A total of 690 patients were treated for over 6 months, and 106 patients were treated for over 1 year.

In placebo-controlled studies, the overall rates of adverse reactions were 47% with eplerenone and 45% with placebo. Adverse reactions occurred at a similar rate regardless of age, gender, or race. Therapy was discontinued due to an adverse reaction in 3% of patients treated with eplerenone and 3% of patients given placebo. The most common reasons for discontinuation of eplerenone were headache, dizziness, angina pectoris/MI, and increased gamma-glutamyl-transferase (GGT). The adverse reactions that were reported at a rate of at least 1% of patients and at a higher rate in patients treated with eplerenone in daily doses of 25 to 400 mg versus placebo are shown in the following table.

EPLERENONE — ORAL

Rates (%) of Adverse Reactions Occurring in Placebo-Controlled Hypertension Studies in ≥ 1% of Patients Treated with Eplerenone (25 to 400 mg) and at a More Frequent Rate than in Placebo-Treated Patients		
Adverse reaction	Eplerenone (n = 945)	Placebo (n = 372)
CNS		
Dizziness	3%	2%
GI		
Abdominal pain	1%	0%
Diarrhea	2%	1%
GU		
Albuminuria	1%	0%
Metabolic		
Hypercholesterolemia	1%	0%
Hypertriglyceridemia	1%	0%
Respiratory		
Coughing	2%	1%
Miscellaneous		
Fatigue	2%	1%
Influenza-like symptoms	2%	1%

Note – Adverse reactions that are too general to be informative or are very common in the treated population are excluded.

Gynecomastia and abnormal vaginal bleeding were reported with eplerenone but not with placebo. The rates of these sex hormone-related adverse reactions are shown in the following table. The rates increased slightly with increasing duration of therapy. In females, abnormal vaginal bleeding was also reported in 0.8% of patients on antihypertensive medications (other than spironolactone) in active-control arms of the studies with eplerenone.

Rates of Sex Hormone-Related Adverse Reactions with Eplerenone in Hypertension Clinical Studies				
	Rates in men			Rates in women
	Gynecomastia	Mastodynia	Either	Abnormal vaginal bleeding
All controlled studies	0.5%	0.8%	1%	0.6%
Controlled studies lasting ≥ 6 months	0.7%	1.3%	1.6%	0.8%
Open-label, long-term study	1%	0.3%	1%	2.1%

➤*Clinical laboratory test findings:*

Data from CHF post-MI trials –

Creatinine: Increases of more than 0.5 mg/dL were reported for 6.5% of patients administered eplerenone and for 4.9% of placebo-treated patients.

Potassium: In EPHESUS, the frequency of patients with changes in potassium (less than 3.5 mEq/L or greater than 5.5 mEq/L or greater than or equal to 6 mEq/L) receiving eplerenone compared with placebo are displayed in the following table.

Hypokalemia (< 3.5 mEq/L) or Hyperkalemia (> 5.5 or ≥ 6 mEq/L) in EPHESUS (%)		
Potassium (mEq/L)	Eplerenone (n = 3,251)	Placebo (n = 3,237)
< 3.5	273 (8.4%)	424 (13.1%)
> 5.5	508 (15.6%)	363 (11.2%)
≥ 6	180 (5.5%)	126 (3.9%)

The following table shows the rates of hyperkalemia in EPHESUS as assessed by baseline renal function (creatinine clearance).

Rates of Hyperkalemia (> 5.5 mEq/L) in EPHESUS by Baseline Creatinine Clearance[a]		
Baseline creatinine clearance	Eplerenone	Placebo
≤ 30 mL/min	31.5%	22.6%
31 to 50 mL/min	24.1%	12.7%
51 to 70 mL/min	16.9%	13.1%
> 70 mL/min	10.8%	8.7%

[a] Estimated using the Cockroft-Gault formula.

The following table shows the rates of hyperkalemia in EPHESUS as assessed by 2 baseline characteristics: presence/absence of proteinuria from baseline urinalysis and presence/absence of diabetes.

Rates of Hyperkalemia (> 5.5 mEq/L) in Ephesus by Proteinuria and History of Diabetes[a]		
	Eplerenone	Placebo
Proteinuria, no diabetes	16%	11%
Diabetes, no proteinuria	18%	13%
Proteinuria and diabetes	26%	16%

[a] Diabetes assessed as positive medical history at baseline; proteinuria assessed by positive dipstick urinalysis at baseline.

Data from hypertension trials –

Potassium: In placebo-controlled fixed-dose studies, the mean increases in serum potassium were dose related and are shown in the following table along with the frequencies of values greater than 5.5 mEq/L.

Changes in Serum Potassium in the Placebo-Controlled, Fixed-Dose Studies Hypertension Studies of Eplerenone			
Daily dosage	n	Mean change mEq/L	% > 5.5 mEq/L
Placebo	194	0	1
25	97	0.08	0
50	245	0.14	0
100	193	0.09	1
200	139	0.19	1
400	104	0.36	8.7

Patients with both type 2 diabetes and microalbuminuria are at increased risk of developing persistent hyperkalemia. In a study in such patients taking eplerenone 200 mg, the frequencies of maximum serum potassium levels greater than 5.5 mEq/L were 33% with eplerenone given alone and 38% when eplerenone was given with enalapril.

Rates of hyperkalemia increased with decreasing renal function. In all studies serum potassium elevations greater than 5.5 mEq/L were observed in 10.4% of patients treated with eplerenone with baseline calculated creatinine clearance less than 70 mL/min, 5.6% of patients with baseline creatinine clearance of 70 to 100 mL/min, and 2.6% of patients with baseline creatinine clearance of greater than 100 mL/min.

Sodium: Serum sodium decreased in a dose-related manner. Mean decreases ranged from 0.7 mEq/L at 50 mg daily to 1.7 meq/L at 400 mg daily. Decreases in sodium (less than 135 mEq/L) were reported for 2.3% of patients administered eplerenone and 0.6% of placebo-treated patients.

Triglycerides – Serum triglycerides increased in a dose-related manner. Mean increases ranged from 7.1 mg/dL at 50 mg daily to 26.6 mg/dL at 400 mg daily. Increases in triglycerides (above 252 mg/dL) were reported for 15% of patients administered eplerenone and 12% of placebo-treated patients.

Cholesterol – Serum cholesterol increased in a dose-related manner. Mean changes ranged from a decrease of 0.4 mg/dL at 50 mg daily to an increase of 11.6 mg/dL at 400 mg daily. Increases in serum cholesterol values greater than 200 mg/dL were reported for 0.3% of patients administered eplerenone and 0% of placebo-treated patients.

Liver function tests – Serum ALT and GGT increased in a dose-related manner. Mean increases ranged from 0.8 units/L at 50 mg daily to 4.8 units/L at 400 mg daily for ALT and 3.1 units/L at 50 mg daily to 11.3 units/L at 400 mg daily for GGT. Increases in ALT levels greater than 120 units/L (3 times the upper limit of normal [ULN]) were reported for 15 of 2,259 patients administered eplerenone and 1 of 351 placebo-treated patients. Increases in ALT levels greater than 200 units/L (5 times the ULN) were reported for 5 of 2,259 of patients administered eplerenone and 1 of 351 placebo-treated patients. Increases of ALT greater than 120 units/L and bilirubin greater than 1.2 mg/dL were reported in 1 of 2,259 patients administered eplerenone and 0 of 351 placebo-treated patients. Hepatic failure was not reported in patients receiving eplerenone.

Serum urea nitrogen / creatinine – Serum creatinine increased in a dose-related manner. Mean increases ranged from 0.01 mg/dL at 50 mg daily to 0.03 mg/dL at 400 mg daily. Increases in serum urea nitrogen to greater than 30 mg/dL and serum creatinine to greater than 2 mg/dL were reported for 0.5% and 0.2%, respectively, of patients administered eplerenone and 0% of placebo-treated patients.

Uric acid – Increases in uric acid to greater than 9 mg/dL were reported in 0.3% of patients administered eplerenone and 0% of placebo-treated patients.

Overdosage

No cases of human overdosage with eplerenone have been reported. Lethality was not observed in mice, rats, or dogs after single oral doses that provided C_{max} exposures at least 25 times higher than in humans receiving eplerenone 100 mg/day. Dogs showed emesis, salivation, and tremors at a C_{max} 41 times the human therapeutic C_{max}, progressing to sedation and convulsions at higher exposures.

The most likely manifestation of human overdosage would be anticipated to be hypotension or hyperkalemia. Eplerenone cannot be removed by hemodialysis. Eplerenone has been shown to bind extensively to charcoal. If symptomatic hypotension occurs, institute supportive treatment. If hyperkalemia develops, initiate standard treatment.

Patient Information

Inform patients receiving eplerenone not to use potassium supplements, salt substitutes containing potassium, or contraindicated drugs without consulting their doctors.

ANTIHYPERTENSIVE COMBINATIONS

Content given per capsule or tablet.

	Product and Distributor	Diuretic	Other Content	How Supplied
Rx	**Renese-R Tablets** (Pfizer)	2 mg polythiazide	0.25 mg reserpine	Lactose. (Pfizer 446). Blue, scored. In 100s and 1000s.
Rx	**Chlorothiazide/Reserpine Tablets** (Various, eg, Mylan)	500 mg chlorothiazide	0.125 mg reserpine	In 100s.
Rx	**Chloroserpine Tablets** (Rugby)	250 mg chlorothiazide	0.125 mg reserpine	In 100s and 1000s.
Rx	**Hydrochlorothiazide/Reserpine Tablets** (Various)	50 mg hydrochlorothiazide	0.125 mg reserpine	In 100s and 1000s.
Rx	**Hydro-Serp Tablets** (Rugby)			In 1000s.
Rx	**Hydroserpine #2 Tablets** (Various, eg, Rugby)			In 100s, 250s, 400s and 1000s.
Rx	**Hydrochlorothiazide/Reserpine Tablets** (Various)	25 mg hydrochlorothiazide	0.125 mg reserpine	In 100s and 1000s.
Rx	**Hydroserpine #1 Tablets** (Various, eg, Rugby)			In 100s and 1000s.
Rx	**Salutensin-Demi** (Shire)	25 mg hydroflumethiazide	0.125 mg reserpine	Lactose, sucrose. Yellow. In 100s.
Rx	**Salutensin Tablets** (Roberts)	50 mg hydroflumethiazide	0.125 mg reserpine	Lactose, sucrose. (BL S1)Green. In 100s and 1000s.
Rx	**Diutensen-R Tablets** (Wallace)	2.5 mg methyclothiazide	0.1 mg reserpine	White, pink. Mottled. In 100s, 500s and 5000s.
Rx	**Metatensin #4 Tablets** (Hoechst Marion Roussel)	4 mg trichlormethiazide	0.1 mg reserpine	Lactose. (Merrell 65) Lavender. In 100s.
Rx	**Rauwolfia/Bendroflumethiazide Tablets** (Various, eg, Rugby)	4 mg bendroflumethiazide	50 mg powdered rauwolfia serpentina	In 100s.
Rx	**Rauzide Tablets** (B-M Squibb)			In 100s.
Rx	**Hydrap-ES Tablets** (Parmed)	15 mg hydrochlorothiazide	0.1 mg reserpine 25 mg hydralazine HCl	(CC124). Salmon pink. In 100s, 500s, 1000s.
Rx	**Ser-Ap-Es Tablets** (Novartis)			Lactose, sucrose. (71). Salmon pink. In 100s and 1000s.
Rx	**Tri-Hydroserpine Tablets** (Rugby)			In 100s and 1000s.
Rx	**Hydrochlorothiazide/Hydralazine Caps** (Various, eg, Moore, Zenith-Goldline)	50 mg hydrochlorothiazide	50 mg hydralazine HCl	In 100s, 500s and 1000s.
Rx	**Apresazide 50/50 Capsules** (Novartis)			Parabens. Pink, white. In 100s.
Rx	**Hydrochlorothiazide/Hydralazine Caps** (Various, eg, Moore, Zenith-Goldline)	25 mg hydrochlorothiazide	25 mg hydralazine HCl	In 100s, 500s and 1000s.
Rx	**Apresazide 25/25 Capsules** (Novartis)			Parabens. Lt. blue, white. In 100s.
Rx	**Atenolol/Chlorthalidone Tablets** (Various, eg, Zenith-Goldline)	25 mg chlorthalidone	100 mg atenolol	In 50s, 100s, 250s, 500s, and 1000s.
Rx	**Tenoretic 100 Tablets** (Zeneca)			(ICI 117). White, scored. In 100s.
Rx	**Atenolol/Chlorthalidone Tablets** (Various, eg, Zenith-Goldline)	25 mg chlorthalidone	50 mg atenolol	In 50s, 100s, 250s, 500s, and 1000s.
Rx	**Tenoretic 50 Tablets** (Zeneca)			(ICI 115). White, scored. In 100s.
Rx	**Corzide Tablets 80/5** (Monarch)	5 mg bendroflumethiazide	80 mg nadolol	Lactose. (CORZIDE 80/5 BL 284). In 100s.
Rx	**Corzide Tablets 40/5** (Monarch)	5 mg bendroflumethiazide	40 mg nadolol	Lactose. (CORZIDE 40/5 BL 283). In 100s.
Rx	**Bisoprolol Fumarate and Hydrochlorothiazide Tablets** (Various, eg, ESI Lederle, Mylan, Purepac, Ivax)	6.25 mg hydrochlorothiazide	2.5 mg bisoprolol fumarate	In 100s, 500s, and 1000s.
	Ziac Tablets (Barr			(LL B 12). In 30s and 100s.
Rx	**Bisoprolol Fumarate and Hydrochlorothiazide Tablets** (Various, eg, ESI Lederle, Mylan, Purepac, Ivax)	6.25 mg hydrochlorothiazide	5 mg bisoprolol fumarate	In 100s, 500s, and 1000s.
	Ziac Tablets (Barr			(LL B 13). In 30s and 100s.
Rx	**Bisoprolol Fumarate and Hydrochlorothiazide Tablets** (Various, eg, ESI Lederle, Mylan, Purepac, Ivax)	6.25 mg hydrochlorothiazide	10 mg bisoprolol fumarate	In 30s, 100s, 500s, and 1000s.
	Ziac Tablets (Barr)			(LL B 14). In 30s.
Rx	**Timolide 10-25 Tablets** (Merck)	25 mg hydrochlorothiazide	10 mg timolol maleate	(TIMOLIDE MSD 67). In 100s.
Rx	**Propranolol/Hydrochlorothiazide Tablets** (Various, eg, Mylan)	25 mg hydrochlorothiazide	80 mg propranolol HCl	In 100s and 1000s.
Rx	**Propranolol/Hydrochlorothiazide Tablets** (Various, eg, Mylan)	25 mg hydrochlorothiazide	40 mg propranolol HCl	In 100s.
Rx	**Inderide 40/25 Tablets** (Wyeth-Ayerst)			Lactose. (Inderide 40/25). In 100s, 1000s and UD 100s.
Rx	**Methyldopa and Hydrochlorothiazide Tablets** (Various, eg, Rugby)	50 mg hydrochlorothiazide	500 mg methyldopa	In 100s, 250s, and 500s.
Rx	**Aldoril D50 Tablets** (Merck)			(MSD 935 ALDORIL). White. Oval. Film coated. In 100s.
Rx	**Methyldopa/Hydrochlorothiazide Tablets** (Various, eg, Rugby)	30 mg hydrochlorothiazide	500 mg methyldopa	In 100s, 250s and 500s.
Rx	**Aldoril D30 Tablets** (Merck)			(MSD 694 ALDORIL). Salmon. Oval. Film coated. In 100s.

ANTIHYPERTENSIVE COMBINATIONS

	Product and Distributor	Diuretic	Other Content	How Supplied
Rx	**Methyldopa/Hydrochlorothiazide Tablets** (Various, eg, Goldline, Mylan, Rugby)	25 mg hydrochlorothiazide	250 mg methyldopa	In 100s, 500s, 1000s and UD 100s.
Rx	**Aldoril-25 Tablets** (Merck)			(MSD 456 ALDORIL). White. Film coated. In 100s, 1000s and UD 100s.
Rx	**Methyldopa/Hydrochlorothiazide Tablets** (Various, eg, Mylan, Zenith-Goldline)	15 mg hydrochlorothiazide	250 mg methyldopa	In 100s, 500s, 1000s and UD 100s.
Rx	**Aldoril-15 Tablets** (Merck)			(MSD 423 ALDORIL). Salmon. Film coated. In 100s and 1000s.
Rx	**Metoprolol Tartrate/Hydrochlorothiazide Tablets** (Mylan)	50 mg hydrochlorothiazide	100 mg metoprolol tartrate	Lactose. (M 445). Peach, capsule shape, scored. In 100s and 500s.
Rx	**Lopressor HCT 100/50 Tablets** (Novartis)			Lactose, sucrose. (GEIGY 73 73). White, yellow, scored. Capsule shape. In 100s.
Rx	**Metoprolol Tartrate/Hydrochlorothiazide Tablets** (Mylan)	25 mg hydrochlorothiazide	100 mg metoprolol tartrate	Lactose. (M 434). Peach, oval, scored. In 100s and 500s.
Rx	**Lopressor HCT 100/25 Tablets** (Novartis)			Lactose, sucrose. (GEIGY 53 53). White, pink, scored. Capsule shape. In 100s.
Rx	**Metoprolol Tartrate/Hydrochlorothiazide Tablets** (Mylan)	25 mg hydrochlorothiazide	50 mg metoprolol tartrate	Lactose. (M 424). Peach, scored. In 100s and 500s.
Rx	**Lopressor HCT 50/25 Tablets** (Novartis)			Lactose, sucrose. (GEIGY 35 35). White, blue, scored. Capsule shape. In 100s.
Rx	**Captopril and Hydrochlorothiazide Tablets** (Teva)	25 mg hydrochlorothiazide	50 mg captopril	In 100s and 1000s.
Rx	**Capozide 50/25 Tablets** (B-M Squibb)			(CAPOZIDE 50/25). Peach. Biconvex, oval. In 100s.
Rx	**Captopril and Hydrochlorothiazide Tablets** (Teva)	25 mg hydrochlorothiazide	25 mg captopril	In 100s and 1000s.
Rx	**Capozide 25/25 Tablets** (B-M Squibb)			(CAPOZIDE 25/25). Peach, scored. Biconvex, square. In 100s.
Rx	**Captopril and Hydrochlorothiazide Tablets** (Teva)	15 mg hydrochlorothiazide	50 mg captopril	In 100s and 1000s.
Rx	**Capozide 50/15 Tablets** (B-M Squibb)			(CAPOZIDE 50/15). White, orange, mottled, scored. Oval. In 100s.
Rx	**Captopril and Hydrochlorothiazide Tablets** (Teva)	15 mg hydrochlorothiazide	25 mg captopril	In 100s and 1000s.
Rx	**Capozide 25/15 Tablets** (B-M Squibb)			(CAPOZIDE 25/15). White, orange, mottled, scored. Biconvex, square. In 100s.
Rx	**Benazepril HCl/Hydrochlorothiazide** (Sandoz)	25 mg hydrochlorothiazide	20 mg benazepril	Castor oil, lactose. (GG 367). Red. In 100s.
Rx	**Lotensin HCT Tablets 20/25** (Novartis)			Lactose. (LOTENSIN HCT 75 75). Red, scored. Oblong. In 100s and *Accu-Pak* 100s.
Rx	**Benazepril HCl/Hydrochlorothiazide** (Sandoz)	12.5 mg hydrochlorothiazide	20 mg benazepril	Castor oil, lactose. (GG 366). Grayish-violet. In 100s.
Rx	**Lotensin HCT Tablets 20/12.5** (Novartis)			Lactose. (LOTENSIN HCT 74 74) Grayish-violet, scored. Oblong. In 100s and *Accu-Pak* 100s.
Rx	**Benazepril HCl/Hydrochlorothiazide** (Sandoz)	12.5 mg hydrochlorothiazide	10 mg benazepril	Castor oil, lactose. (GG 365). Light pink. In 100s.
Rx	**Lotensin HCT Tablets 10/12.5** (Novartis)			Lactose. (LOTENSIN HCT 72 72) Lt. pink, scored. Oblong. In 100s and *Accu-Pak* 100s.
Rx	**Quinapril Hydrochloride/Hydrochlorothiazide Tablets** (Greenstone)	12.5 mg hydrochlorothiazide	10 mg quinapril HCl	Lactose. (G 222). Pink, scored, elliptical. Film-coated. In 90s.
Rx	**Accuretic** (Parke-Davis)			Lactose. (PD 222). Pink, scored elliptical, biconvex. Film-coated. In 30s.
Rx	**Quinaretic Tablets** (Amide)			(A238). Peach, oval. Film-coated. In 30s, 100s, and 500s.
Rx	**Quinapril Hydrochloride/Hydrochlorothiazide Tablets** (Greenstone)	12.5 mg hydrochlorothiazide	20 mg quinapril HCl	Lactose. (G 220). Pink, scored, triangular. Film-coated. In 90s.
Rx	**Accuretic** (Parke-Davis)			Lactose. (PD 220). Pink, scored triangular. Film-coated. In 30s.
Rx	**Quinaretic Tablets** (Amide)			(A239). Peach, triangular. Film-coated. In 30s, 100s, and 500s.
Rx	**Quinapril Hydrochloride/Hydrochlorothiazide Tablets** (Greenstone)	25 mg hydrochlorothiazide	20 mg quinapril HCl	Lactose. (G 223). Pink. Film-coated. In 90s.
Rx	**Accuretic** (Parke-Davis)			Lactose. (PD 223). Pink, scored round, biconvex. Film-coated. In 30s.
Rx	**Quinaretic Tablets** (Amide)			(A240). Peach. Film-coated. In 30s, 100s, and 500s.
Rx	**Teveten HCT** (Biovail)	12.5 mg hydrochlorothiazide	600 mg eprosartan	Lactose. (SOLVAY 5147). Butterscotch, capsule shape. Film-coated. In 100s.
Rx	**Teveten HCT** (Biovail)	25 mg hydrochlorothiazide	600 mg eprosartan	Lactose. (SOLVAY 5150). Brick red, capsule shape. Film-coated. In 100s.

ANTIHYPERTENSIVE COMBINATIONS

	Product and Distributor	Diuretic	Other Content	How Supplied
Rx	**Avalide Tablets** (Bristol-Myers Squibb)	12.5 mg hydrochlorothiazide	150 mg irbesartan	Lactose. (2775). Peach, biconvex. Oval. In 30s, 90s, 500s, and blister pack 100s.
		12.5 mg hydrochlorothiazide	300 mg irbesartan	Lactose. (2776). Peach, biconvex. Oval. In 30s, 90s, 500s, and blister pack 100s.
		25 mg hydrochlorothiazide	300 mg irbesartan	Lactose. (2788). Pink, biconvex. Oval. Film coated. In 30s and 90s.
Rx	**Micardis HCT Tablets** (Boehringer Ingelheim)	12.5 mg hydrochlorothiazide	40 mg telmisartan	Sorbitol, lactose. (H4). Bilayered (red and white, possibly with red specks), oblong. In blister pack 30s.
		12.5 mg hydrochlorothiazide	80 mg telmisartan	Sorbitol, lactose. (H8). Bilayered (red and white, possibly with red specks), oblong. In blister pack 30s.
		25 mg hydrochlorothiazide	80 mg telmisartan	Sorbitol, lactose. (H9). Bilayered (yellow and white, possibly with yellow specks), oblong. In blister pack 30s.
Rx	**Benazepril HCl/Hydrochlorothiazide** (Sandoz)	6.25 mg hydrochlorothiazide	5 mg benazepril	Lactose. (GG 364). White. In 100s.
Rx	**Lotensin HCT Tablets 5/6.25** (Novartis)			Lactose. (C-G 57LOTENSIN HCT 57 57). White, scored. Oblong. In 100s and *Accu-Pak* 100s.
Rx	**Enalapril Maleate/Hydrochlorothiazide Tablets** (Eon)	25 mg hydrochlorothiazide	10 mg enalapril maleate	Lactose. (E 172). Salmon. In 100s and 1000s.
Rx	**Vaseretic 10-25 Tablets** (Biovail)			(VASERETIC MSD 720). Red. In 100s.
Rx	**Enalapril Maleate/Hydrochlorothiazide Tablets** (Eon)	12.5 mg hydrochlorothiazide	5 mg enalapril maleate	Lactose. (E 151). Green. In 100s and 1000s.
Rx	**Vaseretic 5-12.5 Tablets** (Biovail)			Lactose. (MSD 173). Square-capsule shape. In unit-of-use 100s.
Rx	**Lisinopril/Hydrochlorothiazide Tablets** (Various, eg, Geneva, Ivax)	25 mg hydrochlorothiazide	20 mg lisinopril	In 100s, 500s, 1000s, and UD 100s.
Rx	**Prinzide 25 Tablets** (Merck)			(MSD 142 PRINZIDE). In 30s and 100s.
Rx	**Zestoretic Tablets** (Zeneca)			(Stuart 145 Zestoretic). Peach. Biconvex. In 100s.
Rx	**Lisinopril/Hydrochlorothiazide Tablets** (Various, eg, Geneva, Ivax)	12.5 mg hydrochlorothiazide	20 mg lisinopril	In 100s, 500s, 1000s, and UD 100s.
Rx	**Prinzide 12.5 Tablets** (Merck)			(MSD 140 PRINZIDE). In 30s and 100s.
Rx	**Zestoretic Tablets** (Zeneca)			(Stuart 142 Zestoretic). White. Biconvex. In 100s.
Rx	**Lisinopril/Hydrochlorothiazide Tablets** (Various, eg, Geneva, Ivax)	12.5 mg hydrochlorothiazide	10 mg lisinopril	In 100s, 500s, 1000s, and UD 100s.
Rx	**Prinzide Tablets** (Merck)			(MSD 145 PRINZIDE). In 30s and 100s.
Rx	**Zestoretic Tablets** (Zeneca)			(Stuart 141). Peach. Biconvex. In 100s.
Rx	**Clorpres Tablets** (Bertek)	15 mg chlorthalidone	0.3 mg clonidine HCl	(M72). Yellow, scored. In 100s.
Rx	**Combipres 0.3 Tablets** (Boehringer Ingelheim)			Lactose, parabens. (BI 10). White, scored. Oval. In 100s.
Rx	**Clorpres Tablets** (Bertek)	15 mg chlorthalidone	0.2 mg clonidine HCl	(M27). Yellow, scored. In 100s.
Rx	**Combipres 0.2 Tablets** (Boehringer Ingelheim)			Lactose, parabens. (BI 9). Blue, scored. Oval. In 100s and 1000s.
Rx	**Clorpres Tablets** (Bertek)	15 mg chlorthalidone	0.1 mg clonidine HCl	(M1). Yellow, scored. In 100s.
Rx	**Combipres 0.1 Tablets** (Boehringer Ingelheim)			Lactose, parabens. (BI 8). Pink, scored. Oval. In 100s and 1000s.
Rx	**Minizide 5 Capsules** (Pfizer)	0.5 mg polythiazide	5 mg prazosin HCl	(436). Blue-green, blue. In 100s.
Rx	**Minizide 2 Capsules** (Pfizer)	0.5 mg polythiazide	2 mg prazosin HCl	(432). Blue-green, pink. In 100s.
Rx	**Minizide 1 Capsules** (Pfizer)	0.5 mg polythiazide	1 mg prazosin HCl	(430). Blue-green. In 100s.
Rx	**Hyzaar Tablets** (Merck)	12.5 mg hydrochlorothiazide	50 mg losartan potassium	4.24 mg potassium, lactose. (MRK 717 HYZAAR). Yellow. Teardrop shape. Film coated. In 30s, 90s, 100s and UD 100s.
		12.5 mg hydrochlorothiazide	100 mg losartan potassium	8.48 mg potassium, lactose. (745). White, oval. In 30s, 90s, 1,000s, 5,000s, and UD 100s.
		25 mg hydrochlorothiazide	100 mg losartan potassium	8.48 mg potassium, lactose. (MRK 747 HYZAAR). Lt. yellow. Teardrop shape. Film-coated. In unit-of-use 30s and 100s and UD 100s.

ANTIHYPERTENSIVE COMBINATIONS

	Product and Distributor	Diuretic	Other Content	How Supplied
Rx	**Lotrel Capsules** (Novartis)		2.5 mg amlodipine, 10 mg benazepril HCl	(LOTREL 2255). White/gold bands. In 100s.
			5 mg amlodipine, 10 mg benazepril HCl	(LOTREL 2260). Lt. brown/white bands. In 100s.
			5 mg amlodipine, 20 mg benazepril HCl	(LOTREL 2265). Pink/white bands. In 100s.
			10 mg amlodipine, 20 mg benazepril HCl	Lactose. (Lotrel 0364). Purple. In 100s.
Rx	**Lexxel Extended-Release Tablets** (Astra Pharm)		5 mg enalapril maleate, 2.5 mg felodipine	Lactose. (LEXXEL2, 5-2.5). White, biconvex. Film-coated. In unit-of-use 30s and UD 100s.
			5 mg enalapril maleate, 5 mg felodipine	Lactose. (LEXXEL 1, 5-5). White biconvex. Film-coated. In unit-of-use 30s, 100s and UD 100s.
Rx	**Uniretic Tablets** (Schwarz)	25 mg hydrochlorothiazide	15 mg moexipril HCl	Lactose. (725 S P). In 100s.
		12.5 mg hydrochlorothiazide	15 mg moexipril HCl	(720 SP). White, oval, scored. Film coated. In 100s.
		12.5 mg hydrochlorothiazide	7.5 mg moexipril	Lactose. (712 S P). In 100s.
Rx	**Diovan HCT Tablets** (Novartis)	12.5 mg hydrochlorothiazide	80 mg valsartan	(CG HGH). Lt. orange. Talc. In 100s, 4000s, and UD 100s.
		12.5 mg hydrochlorothiazide	160 mg valsartan	(CG HHH). Dk. red. Talc. In 100s, 4000s, and UD 100s.
		25 mg hydrochlorothiazide	160 mg valsartan	Talc. (NVR HXH). Brown orange, ovaloid. In 100s and UD 100s.
Rx	**Benicar HCT** (Sankyo Pharma)	12.5 mg hydrochlorothiazide	20 mg olmesartan medoxomil	Lactose. (Sankyo C22). Reddish-yellow. Film-coated. In 30s, 90s, 1000s, and blister cards of 10.
		12.5 mg hydrochlorothiazide	40 mg olmesartan medoxomil	Lactose. (Sankyo C23). Reddish-yellow, oval. Film-coated. In 30s, 90s, 1000s, and blister cards of 10.
		25 mg hydrochlorothiazide	40 mg olmesartan medoxomil	Lactose. (Sankyo C25). Pink, oval. Film-coated. In 30s, 90s, 1000s, and blister cards of 10.
Rx	**Atacand HCT** (AstraZeneca)	12.5 mg hydrochlorothiazide	16 mg candesartan cilexetil	Lactose. (ACS 162). Peach, oval. Biconvex. In 1000s, UD 100s, and unit-of-use 30s and 90s.
		12.5 mg hydrochlorothiazide	32 mg candesartan cilexetil	Lactose. (ACJ 322). Yellow, oval. Biconvex. In 1000s, UD 100s, and unit-of-use 30s and 90s.
Rx	**Tarka Tablets** (Abbott)		1 mg trandolapril/240 mg verapamil	Lactose. (242 TARKA). White, oval, flim-coated. In 100s.
			2 mg trandolapril/180 mg verapamil	Lactose. (182 TARKA). Pink, oval, film-coated. In 100s.
			2 mg trandolapril/240 mg verapamil	Lactose. (242 TARKA). Gold, oval. Film-coated. In 100s.
			4 mg trandolapril/240 mg verapamil	Lactose. (244). Reddish-brown, oval, film-coated. In 100s.
Rx	**Fosinopril Sodium and Hydrochlorothiazide Tablets** (Ranbaxy)	12.5 mg hydrochlorothiazide	10 mg fosinopril sodium	Lactose. (RC 3). White to off-white. In 30s, 100s, and 1,000s.
Rx	**Monopril-HCT Tablets** (Bristol-Myers Squibb)			Lactose. (1492). Peach. In 100s.
Rx	**Fosinopril Sodium and Hydrochlorothiazide Tablets** (Ranbaxy)	12.5 mg hydrochlorothiazide	20 mg fosinopril sodium	Lactose. (RC 4). White to off-white. In 30s, 100s, and 1,000s.
Rx	**Monopril-HCT Tablets** (Bristol-Myers Squibb)			Lactose. (1493). Peach, bisected. In 100s.

PHENTOLAMINE

Rx	**Phentolamine Mesylate for Injection** (Bedford)	**Powder for Injection:** 5 mg (as mesylate)	Mannitol. In 2 mL vials.

PHENTOLAMINE MESYLATE— INJECTION

Indications

➤*Hypertensive episodes in patients with pheochromocytoma:* Phentolamine mesylate for injection is indicated for the prevention or control of hypertensive episodes that may occur in a patient with pheochromocytoma as a result of stress or manipulation during preoperative preparation and surgical excision.

➤*Prevention or treatment of dermal necrosis from norepinephrine extravasation:* Phentolamine mesylate for injection is indicated for the prevention or treatment of dermal necrosis and sloughing following IV administration or extravasation of norepinephrine.

➤*Pheochromocytoma diagnosis:* Phentolamine mesylate for injection is also indicated for the diagnosis of pheochromocytoma by the phentolamine blocking test.

➤*Unlabeled uses:* Phentolamine has been used to treat hypertensive crises secondary to MAO inhibitor/sympathomimetic amine interactions and rebound hypertension on withdrawal of clonidine, propranolol, or other antihypertensives. It has also been used in combination with papaverine as an intracavernous injection for impotence.

Administration and Dosage

➤*Approved by the FDA:* March 11, 1998.

➤*Prevention or control of hypertensive episodes in the patient with pheochromocytoma:* For preopertative reduction of elevated blood pressure, 5 mg of phentolamine mesylate (1 mg for children) is injected intravenously or intramuscularly 1 or 2 hours before surgery, and repeated if necessary.

During surgery, phentolamine mesylate (5 mg for adults, 1 mg for children) is administered intravenously as indicated, to help prevent or control paroxysms of hypertension, tachycardia, respiratory depression, convulsions, or other effects of epinephrine intoxication. (Postoperatively, norepinephrine may be given to control the hypotension that commonly follows complete removal of a pheochromocytoma.)

Prevention or treatment of dermal necrosis and sloughing following intravenous administration or extravasation of norepinephrine.

➤*Prevention:* Ten (10) mg of phentolamine mesylate is added to each liter of solution containing norepinephrine. The pressor effect of norepinephrine is not affected.

➤*Treatment:* 5 to 10 mg of phentolamine mesylate in 10 mL of saline is injected into the area of extravasation within 12 hours.

➤*Diagnosis of pheochromocytoma (phentolamine blocking test):* The test is most reliable in detecting pheochromocytoma in patients with sustained hypertension and least reliable in those with paroxysmal hypertension. False-positive tests may occur in patients with hypertension without pheochromocytoma.

The dose for adults is 5 mg; the dose for children is 1 mg.

➤*Storage/Stability:* Store at controlled room temperature, 15° to 30°C (59° to 86°F).

The reconstituted solution should be used upon preparation and should not be stored.

Actions

➤*Pharmacology:* Phentolamine mesylate produces an alpha-adrenergic block of relatively short duration. It also has direct, but less marked, positive inotropic and chronotropic effects on cardiac muscle and vasodilator effects on vascular smooth muscle.

➤*Pharmacokinetics:*

Metabolism/Excretion – Phentolamine has a half-life in the blood of 19 minutes following IV administration. Approximately 13% of a single IV dose appears in the urine as unchanged drug.

Contraindications

Myocardial infarction, history of MI, coronary insufficiency, angina, or other evidence suggestive of coronary artery disease; hypersensitivity to phentolamine or related compounds.

Warnings

➤*Cardiovascular events:* Myocardial infarction, cerebrovascular spasm, and cerebrovascular occlusion have been reported to occur following the administration of phentolamine, usually in association with marked hypotensive episodes.

Tachycardia and cardiac arrhythmias may occur with the use of phentolamine or other alpha-adrenergic blocking agents. When possible, administration of cardiac glycosides should be deferred until cardiac rhythm returns to normal.

➤*Not drug of choice for diagnosis of pheochromocytoma:* For screening tests in patients with hypertension, the generally available urinary assay of catecholamines or other biochemical assays have largely replaced the phentolamine and other pharmacological tests for reasons of accuracy and safety. None of the chemical or pharmacological tests is infallible in the diagnosis of pheochromocytoma. The phentolamine-blocking test is not the procedure of choice and should be reserved for cases in which additional confirmatory evidence is necessary and the relative risks involved in conducting the test have been considered.

➤*Pregnancy: Category C.*

Teratogenic – Administration of phentolamine to pregnant rats and mice at oral doses 24 to 30 times the usual daily human dose (based on a 60 kg human) resulted in slightly decreased growth and slight skeletal immaturity of the fetuses. Immaturity was manifested by increased incidence of incomplete or unossified calcanei and phalangeal nuclei of the hind limb and of incompletely ossified sternebrae. At oral doses 60 times the usual daily human dose (based on a 60 kg human), a slightly lower rate of implantation was found in the rat. Phentolamine did not affect embryonic or fetal development in the rabbit at oral doses 20 times the usual daily human dose (based on a 60 kg human). No teratogenic or embryotoxic effects were observed in the rat, mouse, or rabbit studies.

There are no adequate and well-controlled studies in pregnant women. Phentolamine should be used during pregnancy only if the potential benefit justifies the potential risk to the fetus.

➤*Lactation:* It is not known whether this drug is excreted in human milk. Because many drugs are excreted in human milk and because of the potential for serious adverse reactions in nursing infants from phentolamine, a decision should be made whether to discontinue nursing or to discontinue the drug, taking into account the importance of the drug to the mother.

➤*Children:* See Administration and Dosage.

Adverse Reactions

Acute and prolonged hypotensive episodes, tachycardia, and cardiac arrhythmias have been reported. In addition, weakness, dizziness, flushing, orthostatic hypotension, nasal stuffiness, nausea, vomiting, and diarrhea may occur.

Overdosage

➤*Symptoms:* Overdosage with phentolamine is characterized chiefly by cardiovascular disturbances, such as arrhythmias, tachycardia, hypotension, and possibly shock. In addition, the following might occur: Excitation, headache, sweating, pupillary contraction, visual disturbances; nausea, vomiting, diarrhea; hypoglycemia.

Acute toxicity – No deaths due to acute poisoning with phentolamine have been reported. Oral LD_{50}, mice 1000 mg/kg; rats 1250 mg/kg.

➤*Treatment:* There is no specific antidote.

A decrease in blood pressure to dangerous levels or other evidence of shock-like conditions should be treated vigorously and promptly. The patient's legs should be kept raised and a plasma expander should be administered. If necessary, intravenous infusion or norepinephrine, titrated to maintain blood pressure at the normotensive level, and all available supportive measures should be included. Epinephrine should not be used, since it may cause a paradoxical reduction in blood pressure.

PHENOXYBENZAMINE HYDROCHLORIDE ORAL

Rx	**Dibenzyline** (Wellspring)	**Capsules:** 10 mg	(SKF E33). Red. In 100s

PHENOXYBENZAMINE HYDROCHLORIDE— ORAL

Indications

➤*Pheochromocytoma:* Pheochromocytoma, to control episodes of hypertension and sweating. If tachycardia is excessive, it may be necessary to use a beta-blocking agent concomitantly.

Administration and Dosage

➤*Pheochromocytoma:* Initially, phenoxybenzamine hydrochloride 10 mg twice a day. Dosage should be increased every other day, usually to 20 to 40 mg 2 or 3 times a day, until an optimal dosage is obtained, as judged by blood pressure control.

The dosage should be adjusted to fit the needs of each patient. Small initial doses should be slowly increased until the desired effect is obtained or the side effects from blockade become troublesome. After each increase, the patient should be observed on that level before instituting another increase. The dosage should be carried to a point where symptomatic relief or objective improvement are obtained, but not so high that the side effects from blockade become troublesome.

➤*Storage/Stability:* Store between 15° and 30°C (59° and 86°F).

Actions

➤*Pharmacology:* Phenoxybenzamine hydrochloride is a long-acting, adrenergic, alpha-receptor blocking agent which can produce and maintain chemical sympathectomy by oral administration. It increases blood flow to the skin, mucosa and abdominal viscera, and lowers both supine and erect blood pressures. It has no effect on the parasympathetic system.

PHENOXYBENZAMINE HYDROCHLORIDE— ORAL

➤*Pharmacokinetics:*

Absorption / Distribution – Twenty percent to 30% of orally administered phenoxybenzamine appears to be absorbed in the active form.

The half-life of orally administered phenoxybenzamine hydrochloride is not known; however, the half-life of IV administered drug is ≈ 24 hours. Demonstrable effects with IV administration persist for at least 3 to 4 days, and the effects of daily administration are cumulative for nearly a week.

Contraindications

Conditions where a fall in blood pressure may be undesirable.

Warnings

➤*Hypotension:* Phenoxybenzamine-induced alpha-adrenergic blockade leaves beta-adrenergic receptors unopposed. Compounds that stimulate both types of receptors may therefore produce an exaggerated hypotensive response and tachycardia.

➤*Mutagenesis:* Phenoxybenzamine hydrochloride has shown in vitro mutagenic activity in the Ames test and in the mouse lymphoma assay; it has not shown mutagenic activity in the micronucleus test in mice. In rats and mice repeated intraperitoneal administration of phenoxybenzamine hydrochloride resulted in peritoneal sarcomas. Chronic oral dosing in rats has produced malignant tumors in the GI tract. The majority of these tumors were found in the nonglandular stomach of the rats.

In chronic oral studies in rats, ulcerative or erosive gastritis of the glandular stomach occurred which was probably drug related.

➤*Pregnancy:* Category C.

Teratogenic – Adequate reproductive studies have not been performed with phenoxybenzamine hydrochloride. It is also not known whether phenoxybenzamine hydrochloride can cause fetal harm when administered to a pregnant woman. Phenoxybenzamine should be given to a pregnant woman only if clearly needed.

➤*Lactation:* It is not known whether this drug is excreted in human milk. Because many drugs are excreted in human milk, and because of the potential for serious adverse reactions from phenoxybenzamine hydrochloride, a decision should be made whether to discontinue breast-feeding or the drug, taking into account the importance of the drug to the mother.

➤*Children:* Safety and efficacy in children have not been established.

Precautions

➤*Special risk:* Administer with caution in patients with marked cerebral or coronary arteriosclerosis or renal damage. Adrenergic-blocking effect may aggravate symptoms of respiratory infections.

Drug Interactions

Phenoxybenzamine hydrochloride may interact with compounds that stimulate both alpha- and beta-adrenergic receptors (ie, epinephrine) to produce an exaggerated hypotensive response and tachycardia.

Phenoxybenzamine blocks hyperthermia production by levarterenol and blocks hypothermia production by reserpine.

Adverse Reactions

The following adverse reactions have been observed, but there are insufficient data to support an estimate of their frequency.

➤*CNS:*

Autonomic nervous system – Postural hypotension, tachycardia, inhibition of ejaculation, nasal congestion, miosis.

➤*Miscellaneous:* GI irritation, drowsiness, fatigue.

These so-called side effects are actually evidence of adrenergic blockade and vary according to the degree of blockade.

Overdosage

➤*Symptoms:* These are largely the result of block of the sympathetic nervous system and of the circulating epinephrine. They may include the following: postural hypotension resulting in dizziness or fainting; tachycardia, particularly postural; vomiting; lethargy; shock.

➤*Treatment:* When symptoms and signs of overdosage exist, discontinue the drug. Treatment of circulatory failure, if present, is a prime consideration. In cases of mild overdosage, recumbent position with legs elevated usually restores cerebral circulation. In the more severe cases, the usual measures to combat shock should be instituted. Usual pressor agents are not effective. Epinephrine is contraindicated because it stimulates both alpha and beta receptors; since alpha receptors are blocked, the net effect of epinephrine administration is vasodilation and a further drop in blood pressure (epinephrine reversal).

The patient may have to be kept flat for 24 hours or more in the case of overdose, as the effect of the drug is prolonged. Leg bandages and an abdominal binder may shorten the period of disability.

IV infusion of levarterenol bitartrate may be used to combat severe hypotensive reactions, because it stimulates alpha receptors primarily. Although phenoxybenzamine hydrochloride is an alpha-adrenergic blocking agent, a sufficient dose of levarterenol bitartrate will overcome this effect.

The oral LD_{50} for phenoxybenzamine is approximately 2,000 mg/kg in rats and approximately 500 mg/kg in guinea pigs.

METYROSINE

Rx	**Demser** (MSD)	**Capsules:** 250 mg	(MSD 690 DEMSER). Two-tone blue. In 100s.

METYROSINE — ORAL

Indications

Metyrosine is indicated in the treatment of patients with pheochromocytoma for:

1.) Preoperative preparation of patients for surgery.
2.) Management of patients when surgery is contraindicated.
3.) Chronic treatment of patients with malignant pheochromocytoma.

Administration and Dosage

The recommended initial dosage of metyrosine for adults and children 12 years of age and older is 250 mg orally 4 times daily. This may be increased by 250 mg to 500 mg every day to a maximum of 4 g/day in divided doses. When used for preoperative preparation, the optimally effective dosage of metyrosine should be given for at least 5 to 7 days.

Optimally effective dosages of metyrosine usually are between 2 and 3 g/day, and the dose should be titrated by monitoring clinical symptoms and catecholamine excretion. In patients who are hypertensive, dosage should be titrated to achieve normalization of blood pressure and control of clinical symptoms. In patients who are usually normotensive, dosage should be titrated to the amount that will reduce urinary metanephrines and/or vanillylmandelic acid by 50% or more.

If patients are not adequately controlled by the use of metyrosine, an alpha-adrenergic blocking agent (phenoxybenzamine) should be added.

➤*Children:* Use of metyrosine in children younger than 12 years of age has been limited and a dosage schedule for this age group cannot be given.

Actions

➤*Pharmacology:* Metyrosine inhibits tyrosine hydroxylase, which catalyzes the first transformation in catecholamine biosynthesis (ie, the conversion of tyrosine to dihydroxyphenylalanine [DOPA]). Because the first step is also the rate-limiting step, blockade of tyrosine hydroxylase activity results in decreased endogenous levels of catecholamines, usually measured as decreased urinary excretion of catecholamines and their metabolites.

In patients with pheochromocytoma, who produce excessive amounts of norepinephrine and epinephrine, administration of 1 to 4 g of metyrosine per day has reduced catecholamine biosynthesis from approximately 35% to 80% as measured by the total excretion of catecholamines and their metabolites (metanephrine and vanillylmandelic acid). The maximum biochemical effect usually occurs within 2 to 3 days, and the urinary concentration of catecholamines and their metabolites usually returns to pretreatment levels within 3 to 4 days after metyrosine is discontinued. In some patients the total excretion of catecholamines and catecholamine metabolites may be lowered to normal or near normal levels (less than 10 mg per 24 hours). In most patients the duration of treatment has been 2 to 8 weeks, but several patients have received metyrosine for periods of 1 to 10 years.

Most patients with pheochromocytoma treated with metyrosine experience decreased frequency and severity of hypertensive attacks with their associated headache, nausea, sweating, and tachycardia. In patients who respond, blood pressure decreases progressively during the first 2 days of therapy with metyrosine; after withdrawal, blood pressure usually increases gradually to pretreatment values within 2 to 3 days.

➤*Pharmacokinetics:* Metyrosine is well absorbed from the GI tract. From 53% to 88% (mean 69%) was recovered in the urine as unchanged drug following maintenance oral doses of 600 to 4,000 mg per 24 hours in patients with pheochromocytoma or essential hypertension. Less than 1% of the dose was recovered as catechol metabolites. These metabolites are probably not present in sufficient amounts to contribute to the biochemical effects of metyrosine. The quantities excreted, however, are sufficient to interfere with accurate determination of urinary catecholamines determined by routine techniques.

Plasma half-life of metyrosine determined over an 8-hour period after single oral doses was 3 to 3.7 hours in 3 patients.

Contraindications

Known hypersensitivity to this compound.

Warnings

➤*Maintain fluid volume during and after surgery:* When metyrosine is used preoperatively, alone or especially in combination with alpha-adrenergic blocking drugs, adequate intravascular volume must be maintained intraoperatively (especially after tumor removal) and postoperatively to avoid hypotension and decreased perfusion of vital organs resulting from vasodilatation and expanded volume capacity. Following tumor removal, large volumes of plasma may be needed to maintain blood pressure and central venous pressure within the normal range.

In addition, life-threatening arrhythmias may occur during anesthesia and surgery, and may require treatment with a beta-blocker or lidocaine. During surgery, patients should have continuous monitoring of blood pressure and electrocardiogram.

➤*Intraoperative effects:* While the preoperative use of metyrosine in patients with pheochromocytoma is thought to decrease intraoperative problems with blood pressure control, metyrosine does not eliminate the danger

METYROSINE — ORAL

of hypertensive crises or arrhythmias during manipulation of the tumor, and the alpha-adrenergic blocking drug, phentolamine, may be needed.

➤*Interaction with alcohol:* Metyrosine may add to the sedative effects of alcohol and other CNS depressants (eg, hypnotics, sedatives, tranquilizers).

➤*Long-term use:* The total human experience with the drug is quite limited and few patients have been studied long-term. Chronic animal studies have not been carried out. Therefore, suitable laboratory tests should be carried out periodically in patients requiring prolonged use of metyrosine and caution should be observed in patients with impaired hepatic or renal function.

➤*Pregnancy: Category C.* Animal reproduction studies have not been conducted with metyrosine. It is also not known whether metyrosine can cause fetal harm when administered to a pregnant woman or can affect reproduction capacity. Metyrosine should be given to a pregnant woman only if clearly needed.

➤*Lactation:* It is not known whether metyrosine is excreted in human milk. Because many drugs are excreted in human milk, caution should be exercised when metyrosine is administered to a nursing woman.

➤*Children:* Safety and efficacy in children younger than 12 years of age have not been established.

Precautions

➤*Metyrosine crystalluria:* Crystalluria and urolithiasis have been found in dogs treated with metyrosine at doses similar to those used in humans, and crystalluria has also been observed in a few patients. To minimize the risk of crystalluria, patients should be urged to maintain water intake sufficient to achieve a daily urine volume of more than 2,000 mL, particularly when doses more than 2 g/day are given. Routine examination of the urine should be carried out. Metyrosine will crystallize as needles or rods. If metyrosine crystalluria occurs, fluid intake should be increased further. If crystalluria persists, the dosage should be reduced or the drug discontinued.

➤*Hazardous tasks:* When receiving metyrosine, patients should be warned about engaging in activities requiring mental alertness and motor coordination, such as driving a motor vehicle or operating machinery. metyrosine may have additive sedative effects with alcohol and other CNS depressants (eg, hypnotics, sedatives, tranquilizers).

Drug Interactions

Caution should be observed in administering metyrosine to patients receiving phenothiazines or haloperidol because the extrapyramidal effects of these drugs can be expected to be potentiated by inhibition of catecholamine synthesis.

Concurrent use of metyrosine with alcohol or other CNS depressants can increase their sedative effects.

➤*Drug/Lab test interactions:* Spurious increases in urinary catecholamines may be observed in patients receiving metyrosine due to the presence of metabolites of the drug.

Adverse Reactions

➤*CNS:*

Sedation – The most common adverse reaction to metyrosine is moderate to severe sedation, which has been observed in almost all patients. It occurs at both low and high dosages. Sedative effects begin within the first 24 hours of therapy, are maximal after 2 to 3 days, and tend to wane during the next few days. Sedation usually is not obvious after 1 week unless the dosage is increased, but at dosages more than 2,000 mg/day some degree of sedation or fatigue may persist.

In most patients who experience sedation, temporary changes in sleep pattern occur following withdrawal of the drug. Changes consist of insomnia that may last for 2 or 3 days and feelings of increased alertness and ambition. Even patients who do not experience sedation while on metyrosine may report symptoms of psychic stimulation when the drug is discontinued.

Extrapyramidal signs – Extrapyramidal signs such as drooling, speech difficulty, and tremor have been reported in ≈ 10% of patients. These occasionally have been accompanied by trismus and frank parkinsonism.

Anxiety and psychic disturbances – Anxiety and psychic disturbances such as depression, hallucinations, disorientation, and confusion may occur. These effects seem to be dose dependent and may disappear with reduction of dosage.

➤*GI:* Diarrhea occurs in approximately 10% of patients and may be severe. Antidiarrheal agents may be required if continuation of metyrosine is necessary.

➤*Miscellaneous:* Infrequently, slight swelling of the breast, galactorrhea, nasal stuffiness, decreased salivation, dry mouth, headache, nausea, vomiting, abdominal pain, and impotence or failure of ejaculation may occur. Crystalluria and transient dysuria and hematuria have been observed in a few patients. Hematologic disorders (including eosinophilia, anemia, thrombocytopenia, and thrombocytosis), increased AST levels, peripheral edema, and hypersensitivity reactions such as urticaria and pharyngeal edema have been reported rarely.

Overdosage

➤*Symptoms:* Signs of metyrosine overdosage include those central nervous system effects observed in some patients even at low dosages.

At doses exceeding 2,000 mg/day, some degree of sedation or feeling of fatigue may persist. Doses of 2,000 to 4,000 mg/day can result in anxiety or agitated depression, neuromuscular effects (including fine tremor of the hands, gross tremor of the trunk, tightening of the jaw with trismus), diarrhea, and decreased salivation with dry mouth.

➤*Treatment:* Reduction of drug dose or cessation of treatment results in the disappearance of these symptoms.

The acute toxicity of metyrosine was 442 mg/kg and 752 mg/kg in the female mouse and rat respectively.

Patient Information

Patients should be advised to maintain a liberal fluid intake.

When receiving metyrosine, patients should be warned about engaging in activities requiring mental alertness and motor coordination, such as driving a motor vehicle or operating machinery. metyrosine may have additive sedative effects with alcohol and other CNS depressants (eg, hypnotics, sedatives, tranquilizers).

NITROPRUSSIDE SODIUM

Rx	**Sodium Nitroprusside** (Elkins-Sinn)	**Powder for Injection:** 50 mg per vial	In single dose 5 mL vials.
Rx	**Nitropress** (Abbott)		In single dose 2 mL Fliptop Vials.

NITROPRUSSIDE SODIUM— INJECTION

WARNING

After reconstitution, nitroprusside is not suitable for direct injection. The reconstituted solution must be further diluted in 5% Dextrose Injection before infusion.

Nitroprusside can cause precipitous decreases in blood pressure. In patients not properly monitored, these decreases can lead to irreversible ischemic injuries or death. Use only when available equipment and personnel allow blood pressure to be continuously monitored.

Except when used briefly or at low (less than 2 mcg/kg/min) infusion rates, nitroprusside injection gives rise to important quantities of cyanide ion, which can reach toxic, potentially lethal levels. The usual dose rate is 0.5 to 10 mcg/kg/min, but infusion at the maximum dose rates should never last more than 10 minutes. If blood pressure has not been adequately controlled after 10 minutes of infusion at the maximum rate, terminate administration immediately.

Although acid-base balance and venous oxygen concentration should be monitored and may indicate cyanide toxicity, these laboratory tests provide imperfect guidance.

Indications

➤*Hypertensive crises:* Immediate reduction of blood pressure of patients in hypertensive crises. Administer concomitant longer-acting antihypertensive medication so that the duration of treatment with nitroprusside can be minimized.

➤*Bleeding reduction during surgery:* Production of controlled hypotension in order to reduce bleeding during surgery.

➤*Acute congestive heart failure (CHF):* For use in acute congestive heart failure.

➤*Unlabeled uses:* Myocardial infarction with coadministration of dopamine; left ventricular failure with coadministration of oxygen, morphine and a loop diuretic.

Administration and Dosage

➤*Reconstitution:* Dissolve the contents of a 50 mg vial in 2 to 3 mL Dextrose in Water or Sterile Water for Injection. Depending on the desired concentration, the initially reconstituted solution containing 50 mg must be further diluted in 250 to 1,000 mL 5% Dextrose Injection.

➤*Verification of the chemical integrity of the product:* Nitroprusside solution can be inactivated by reactions with trace contaminants. Products of these reactions are often blue, green or red, much brighter than the faint brownish color of unreacted nitroprusside. Do not use discolored solutions, or solutions with particulate matter visible.

➤*Admixture compatibility:* Esmolol and nitroprusside are compatible for at least 24 hours in 5% Dextrose Injection at room temperature and protected from light.

➤*CHF:* Nitroprusside can be titrated by increasing the infusion rate until measured cardiac output is no longer increasing, systemic blood pressure cannot be further reduced without compromising the perfusion of vital organs or the maximum recommended infusion rate has been reached, whichever comes earliest.

➤*Avoidance of excessive hypotension:* While the average effective rate in adults and children is about 3 mcg/kg/min, some patients will become dangerously hypotensive when they receive nitroprusside at this rate. Therefore, start at a very low rate (0.3 mcg/kg/min), with gradual upward titration every few minutes until the desired effect is achieved or the maximum recommended infusion rate (10 mcg/kg/min) has been reached.

Because nitroprusside's hypotensive effect is very rapid in onset and in dissipation, small variations in infusion rate can lead to wide, undesirable variations in blood pressure. Do not infuse through ordinary IV apparatus regulated only by gravity and mechanical clamps. Use only an infusion pump, preferably a volumetric pump.

Because nitroprusside can induce essentially unlimited blood pressure reduction, the blood pressure of a patient receiving this drug must be continuously monitored, using either a continually reinflated sphygmomanometer or (preferably) an intra-arterial pressure sensor.

➤*Infusion rates:* The following table shows the infusion rates for adults and children of various weights corresponding to the recommended initial and maximal doses (0.3 mcg/kg/min and 10 mcg/kg/min, respectively). Some of the listed infusion rates are so slow or so rapid as to be impractical, and these practicalities must be considered when the concentration to be used is selected. Note that when the concentration used in a given patient is changed, the tubing is still filled with a solution at the previous concentration.

Infusion Rates to Achieve Initial (0.3 mcg/kg/min) and Maximal (10 mcg/kg/min) Dosing of Nitroprusside

Patient weight		Nitroprusside concentration					
		200 mcg/mL Infusion rate (mL/h)		100 mcg/mL Infusion rate (mL/h)		50 mcg/mL Infusion rate (mL/h)	
kg	lbs	Initial	Maximal	Initial	Maximal	Initial	Maximal
10	22	1	30	2	60	4	120
20	44	2	60	4	120	7	240
30	66	3	90	5	180	11	360
40	88	4	120	7	240	14	480
50	110	5	150	9	300	18	600
60	132	5	180	11	360	22	720
70	154	6	210	13	420	25	840
80	176	7	240	14	480	29	960
90	198	8	270	16	540	32	1,080
100	220	9	300	18	600	36	1,200

➤*Avoidance of cyanide toxicity:* When more than 500 mcg/kg nitroprusside is administered faster than 2 mcg/kg/min, cyanide is generated faster than the unaided patient can eliminate it.

➤*Consideration of methemoglobinemia and thiocyanate toxicity:* Rare patients receiving more than 10 mg/kg of nitroprusside will develop methemoglobinemia; other patients, especially those with impaired renal function, will predictably develop thiocyanate toxicity after prolonged, rapid infusions. Test patients for these toxicities.

➤*Storage/Stability:* Protect the diluted solution from light by promptly wrapping with the supplied opaque sleeve, aluminum foil or other opaque material. It is not necessary to cover the infusion drip chamber or the tubing.

Store at room temperature 15° to 30°C (59° to 86°F).

If properly protected from light, the freshly reconstituted and diluted solution is stable for 24 hours.

Actions

➤*Pharmacology:* Nitroprusside is a potent IV antihypertensive agent. The principal pharmacological action of nitroprusside is relaxation of vascular smooth muscle and consequent dilation of peripheral arteries and veins. Other smooth muscle (eg, uterus, duodenum) is not affected. Nitroprusside is more active on veins than on arteries, but this selectivity is much less marked than that of nitroglycerin. Dilation of the veins promotes peripheral pooling of blood and decreases venous return to the heart, thereby reducing left ventricular end-diastolic pressure and pulmonary capillary wedge pressure (preload). Arteriolar relaxation reduces systemic vascular resistance, systolic arterial pressure and mean arterial pressure (afterload). Dilation of the coronary arteries also occurs.

In association with the decrease in blood pressure, nitroprusside administered IV to hypertensive and normotensive patients produces slight increases in heart rate and a variable effect on cardiac output. In hypertensive patients, moderate doses induce renal vasodilation roughly proportional to the decrease in systemic blood pressure, so there is no appreciable change in renal blood flow or glomerular filtration rate.

In normotensive subjects, acute reduction of mean arterial pressure to 60 to 75 mm Hg by infusion of nitroprusside caused a significant increase in renin activity. In the same study, 10 renovascular-hypertensive patients given nitroprusside had significant increases in renin release from the involved kidney at mean arterial pressures of 90 to 137 mm Hg.

The hypotensive effect of nitroprusside is seen within 1 to 2 minutes after the start of an adequate infusion, and it dissipates almost as rapidly after an infusion is discontinued. The effect is augmented by ganglionic blocking agents and inhaled anesthetics.

➤*Pharmacokinetics:*

Absorption/Distribution – Infused nitroprusside is rapidly distributed to a volume that is approximately coextensive with the extracellular space. The drug is cleared from this volume by intraerythrocytic reaction with hemoglobin (HgB), and nitroprusside's resulting circulatory half-life is about 2 minutes.

Metabolism/Excretion – The products of the nitroprusside/HgB reaction are cyanmethemoglobin (cyanmetHgB) and cyanide ion (CN^-). Safe use of nitroprusside injection must be guided by knowledge of the further metabo-

NITROPRUSSIDE SODIUM— INJECTION

lism of these products. The essential features of nitroprusside metabolism are: One molecule of nitroprusside is metabolized by combination with HgB to produce one molecule of cyanmethemoglobin and four CN^- ions; methemoglobin, obtained from HgB, can sequester cyanide as cyanmethemoglobin; thiosulfate reacts with cyanide to produce thiocyanate (SCN^-); thiocyanate is eliminated in the urine; cyanide, not otherwise removed, binds to cytochromes; cyanide is much more toxic than methemoglobin or thiocyanate.

When the Fe^{+++} of cytochromes is bound to cyanide, the cytochromes are unable to participate in oxidative metabolism. In this situation, cells may be able to provide for their energy needs by utilizing anaerobic pathways, but they thereby generate an increasing body burden of lactic acid. Other cells may be unable to utilize these alternate pathways, and they may die hypoxic deaths.

When CN^- is infused or generated within the bloodstream, essentially all of it is bound to methemoglobin until intraerythrocytic methemoglobin has been saturated. At healthy steady state, most people have < 1% of their HgB in the form of methemoglobin. Nitroprusside metabolism can lead to methemoglobin formation (a) through dissociation of cyanmethemeglobin formed in the original reaction of nitroprusside with HgB and (b) by direct oxidation of HgB by the released nitroso group. Relatively large quantities of nitroprusside, however, are required to produce significant methemoglobinemia.

When thiosulfate is supplied only by normal physiologic mechanisms, conversion of CN^- to SCN^- generally proceeds at about 1 mcg/kg/min. This rate of CN^- clearance corresponds to steady-state processing of a nitroprusside infusion of slightly more than 2 mcg/kg/min. CN^- accumulates when nitroprusside infusions exceed this rate.

In patients with normal renal function, clearance of SCN^- is primarily renal, with a half-life of about 3 days. In renal failure, the half-life can be doubled or tripled.

Contraindications

Treatment of compensatory hypertension, where the primary hemodynamic lesion is aortic coarctation or arteriovenous shunting; to produce hypotension during surgery in patients with known inadequate cerebral circulation or in moribund patients (A.S.A. Class 5E) coming to emergency surgery; patients with congenital (Leber's) optic atrophy or with tobacco amblyopia (these rare conditions are probably associated with defective or absent rhodanese and patients with unusually high cyanide/thiocyanate ratios); acute CHF associated with reduced peripheral vascular resistance such as high-output heart failure that may be seen in endotoxic sepsis.

Warnings

➤*Excessive hypotension:* Small transient excesses in the infusion rate of nitroprusside can result in excessive hypotension, sometimes to levels so low as to compromise the perfusion of vital organs. These hemodynamic changes may lead to a variety of associated symptoms. Nitroprusside-induced hypotension will be self-limited within 1 to 10 minutes after discontinuation of the infusion; during these few minutes, it may be helpful to put the patient into a head-down (Trendelenburg) position to maximize venous return. If hypotension persists more than a few minutes after discontinuation of the infusion, nitroprusside is not the cause, and the true cause must be sought.

➤*Cyanide toxicity:* Nitroprusside infusions at rates more than 2 mcg/kg/min generate CN^- faster than the body can normally dispose of it. (When sodium thiosulfate is given, the body's capacity for CN^- elimination is greatly increased.) Methemoglobin normally present in the body can buffer a certain amount of CN^-, but the capacity of this system is exhausted by the CN^- produced from nitroprusside 500 mcg/kg. This amount of nitroprusside is administered in less than 1 hour when the drug is administered at 10 mcg/kg/min (the maximum recommended rate). Thereafter, the toxic effects of CN^- may be rapid, serious and even lethal.

The true rates of clinically important cyanide toxicity cannot be assessed from spontaneous reports or published data. Most patients reported to have experienced such toxicity have received relatively prolonged infusions, and the only patients whose deaths have been unequivocally attributed to nitroprusside-induced cyanide toxicity have been patients who had received nitroprusside infusions at rates much greater than those now recommended (30 to 120 mcg/kg/min). Elevated cyanide levels, metabolic acidosis and marked clinical deterioration, however, have occasionally been reported in patients who received infusions at recommended rates for only a few hours and even, in one case, for only 35 minutes. In some of these cases, infusion of sodium thiosulfate caused dramatic clinical improvement, supporting the diagnosis of cyanide toxicity.

Cyanide toxicity may manifest itself as venous hyperoxemia with bright red venous blood, as cells become unable to extract the oxygen delivered to them; metabolic (lactic) acidosis; air hunger; confusion; death. Cyanide toxicity due to causes other than nitroprusside has been associated with angina pectoris and myocardial infarction, ataxia, seizures and stroke, and other diffuse ischemic damage.

➤*Hypertensive patients:* Hypertensive patients and patients concomitantly receiving other antihypertensive medications may be more sensitive to the effects of nitroprusside.

➤*Methemoglobinemia:* Nitroprusside infusions can cause sequestration of hemoglobin as methemoglobin. The back-conversion process is normally rapid, and clinically significant methemoglobinemia (more than 10%) is only seen rarely. Even patients congenitally incapable of back-converting methemoglobin should demonstrate 10% methemoglobinemia only after they have received about 10 mg/kg nitroprusside; a patient receiving nitroprusside at the maximum recommended rate (10 mcg/kg/min) would take more than 16 hours to reach this total accumulated dose.

Methemoglobin levels can be measured by most clinical laboratories. Suspect the diagnosis in patients who have received more than 10 mg/kg of nitroprusside and who exhibit signs of impaired oxygen delivery despite adequate cardiac output and adequate arterial pO_2. Classically, methemoglobinemic blood is described as chocolate brown, without color change on exposure to air.

When methemoglobinemia is diagnosed, the treatment of choice is 1 to 2 mg/kg of methylene blue, administered IV over several minutes. In patients likely to have substantial amounts of cyanide bound to methemoglobin as cyanmethemoglobin, treatment of methemoglobinemia with methylene blue must be undertaken with extreme caution.

➤*Thiocyanate toxicity:* Most of the cyanide produced during metabolism of nitroprusside is eliminated in the form of thiocyanate. When cyanide elimination is accelerated by the coinfusion of thiosulfate, thiocyanate production is increased. Thiocyanate is mildly neurotoxic (eg, tinnitus, miosis, hyperreflexia) at serum levels of 1 mmol/L (60 mg/L). Thiocyanate toxicity is life-threatening when levels are 3 or 4 times higher (200 mg/L).

The steady-state thiocyanate level after prolonged infusions of nitroprusside is increased with increased infusion rate, and the half-time of accumulation is 3 to 4 days. To keep the steady-state thiocyanate level < 1 mmol/L, a prolonged infusion should not be more rapid than 3 mcg/kg/min; in anuric patients, the corresponding limit is just 1 mcg/kg/min. When prolonged infusions are more rapid than these, measure thiocyanate levels daily.

Physiologic maneuvers (eg, those that alter the pH of the urine) are not known to increase the elimination of thiocyanate. Thiocyanate clearance rates during dialysis, on the other hand, can approach the blood flow rate of the dialyzer.

Thiocyanate interferes with iodine uptake by the thyroid.

➤*Hepatic function impairment:* Because cyanide is metabolized by hepatic enzymes, it may accumulate in patients with severe liver impairment. Therefore, use with caution in patients with hepatic insufficiency.

➤*Elderly:* Use special caution because elderly patients may be more sensitive to the hypotensive effects of the drug.

➤*Pregnancy: Category C.* In 3 studies in pregnant ewes, nitroprusside crossed the placental barrier. Fetal cyanide levels were dose-related to maternal levels of nitroprusside. The metabolic transformation of nitroprusside given to pregnant ewes led to fatal levels of cyanide in the fetuses. The infusion of 25 mcg/kg/min nitroprusside for 1 hour in pregnant ewes resulted in the death of all fetuses. There are no adequate or well controlled studies in pregnant women. It is not known whether nitroprusside can cause fetal harm when administered to a pregnant woman or can affect reproductive capacity. Give to a pregnant woman only if clearly needed.

The effects of administering sodium thiosulfate in pregnancy, either by itself or as a co-infusion with sodium nitroprusside, are completely unknown.

➤*Lactation:* It is not known whether nitroprusside and its metabolites are excreted in breast milk. Because of the potential for serious adverse reactions in nursing infants, decide whether to discontinue breast-feeding or the drug, taking into account the importance of the drug to the mother.

➤*Children:* See Administration and Dosage.

Precautions

➤*Monitoring:* The cyanide-level assay is technically difficult, and cyanide levels in body fluids other than packed red blood cells are difficult to interpret. Cyanide toxicity will lead to lactic acidosis and venous hyperoxemia, but these findings may not be present until more than 1 hour after the cyanide capacity of the body's red-cell mass has been exhausted.

➤*Intracranial pressure:* Like other vasodilators, nitroprusside can cause increases in intracranial pressure. In patients whose intracranial pressure is already elevated, use only with extreme caution.

➤*Anesthesia:* When nitroprusside (or any other vasodilator) is used for controlled hypotension during anesthesia, the patient's capacity to compensate for anemia and hypovolemia may be diminished. If possible, correct preexisting anemia and hypovolemia prior to use.

Hypotensive anesthetic techniques may also cause abnormalities of the pulmonary ventilation/perfusion ratio. Patients intolerant of these abnormalities may require a higher fraction of inspired oxygen.

Exercise extreme caution in patients who are especially poor surgical risks (A.S.A. Classes 4 and 4E).

Adverse Reactions

➤*Cardiovascular:* Bradycardia; ECG changes; tachycardia.

➤*Hematologic:* Decreased platelet aggregation; methemoglobinemia.

➤*Miscellaneous:* Thiocyanate toxicity; flushing; venous streaking; irritation at the infusion site; rash; hypothyroidism; ileus; increased intracranial pressure).

Rapid blood pressure reduction – Abdominal pain, apprehension, diaphoresis, dizziness, headache, muscle twitching, nausea, palpitations, restlessness, retching and retrosternal discomfort have been noted when the blood pressure was reduced too rapidly. Symptoms quickly disappeared when the infusion was slowed or discontinued, and they did not reappear with a continued (or resumed) slower infusion.

Overdosage

➤*Symptoms:* Toxicity has occurred at doses well below the recommended maximum infusion rate of 10 mcg/kg/min. Overdosage of nitroprusside can be manifested as excessive hypotension, cyanide toxicity or as thiocyanate toxicity.

The acute IV mean lethal doses (LD_{50}) of nitroprusside in rabbits, dogs, mice and rats are 2.8, 5, 8.4 and 11.2 mg/kg, respectively.

NITROPRUSSIDE SODIUM— INJECTION

➤*Treatment:* Measure cyanide levels and blood gases for venous hyperoxemia or acidosis. Acidosis may not appear until more than 1 hour after the appearance of dangerous cyanide levels; do not wait for laboratory tests. Reasonable suspicion of cyanide toxicity is adequate grounds for initiation of treatment.

Treatment of cyanide toxicity consists of: Discontinuing the administration of nitroprusside; providing a buffer for cyanide by using sodium nitrite to convert as much HgB into methemoglobin as the patient can safely tolerate; and then infusing sodium thiosulfate in sufficient quantity to convert the cyanide into thiocyanate.

The medications for treatment are contained in commercially available cyanide antidote kits. Alternatively, discrete stocks of medications can be used. Hemodialysis is ineffective in removal of cyanide, but it will eliminate most thiocyanate.

Antidote kits – Cyanide antidote kits contain both amyl nitrite and sodium nitrite for induction of methemoglobinemia. The amyl nitrite is supplied in the form of inhalant ampules, for use where IV administration of sodium nitrite may be delayed. In a patient who already has a patent IV line, use of amyl nitrite confers no benefit that is not provided by infusion of sodium nitrite.

Nitrite-thiosulfate regimen – Sodium nitrite is available in a 3% solution; inject 4 to 6 mg/kg (about 0.2 mL/kg) over 2 to 4 minutes. This dose converts about 10% of the patient's HgB into methemoglobin; this level of methemoglobinemia is not associated with any important hazard of its own. The nitrite infusion may cause transient vasodilation and hypotension, and this hypotension must, if it occurs, be routinely managed.

Immediately after infusion of the sodium nitrite, infuse sodium thiosulfate. This agent is available in 10% and 25% solutions, and the recommended dose is 150 to 200 mg/kg; a typical adult dose is 50 mL of the 25% solution. Thiosulfate treatment of an acutely cyanide-toxic patient will raise thiocyanate levels, but not to a dangerous degree.

The nitrite-thiosulfate regimen may be repeated, at half the original doses, after 2 hours.

Hydroxocobalamin – No concrete guidelines have been developed for hydroxocobalamin.

Prophylactically during surgery: Doses of 25 mg/h for 4 hours.

Treatment: A dose of 4 to 5 g of hydroxocobalamin alone, or a combination of 8 g of sodium thiosulfate and 4 g of hydroxocobalamin.

DIAZOXIDE, PARENTERAL

Rx	**Hyperstat IV** (Schering)	**Injection:** 15 mg/mL	In 20 mL amps.

DIAZOXIDE — PARENTERAL

Indications

➤*Severe hypertension:* Emergency reduction of blood pressure; short-term use in severe, nonmalignant and malignant hypertension in hospitalized adults and in acute severe hypertension in hospitalized children when an urgent decrease of diastolic pressure is required. Institute treatment with oral agents as soon as the hypertensive emergency is controlled.

Administration and Dosage

Diazoxide injection was originally recommended for use by bolus administration of 300 mg. However, recent studies have shown that minibolus administration is as effective in reducing blood pressure, and therefore, it is the recommended dosage.

During and immediately following injection, the patient should remain supine. Administer only into a peripheral vein. The dose is given IV in less than 30 seconds. Do not give IM, subcutaneously or into body cavities. The solution's alkalinity is irritating to tissue; avoid extravasation. Subcutaneous administration has produced inflammation and pain without subsequent necrosis. If subcutaneous leakage occurs, treat with warm compresses and rest.

➤*Adults:* Administer undiluted and rapidly by IV injections of 1 to 3 mg/kg, up to a maximum of 150 mg in a single injection. This dose may be repeated at 5 to 15 minute intervals until a satisfactory reduction in blood pressure has been achieved (diastolic pressure less than 100 mmHg).

This method of administration of diazoxide is as effective as bolus administration of 300 mg, but usually reduces blood pressure more gradually, perhaps lessening the circulatory and neurological risks associated with acute hypotension.

➤*Repeated administration:* Repeated administration at intervals of 4 to 24 hours will usually maintain the blood pressure below pretreatment levels until oral antihypertensive medication can be instituted. Adjust the interval between injections by the duration of the response to each injection. It is usually unnecessary to continue treatment for more than 4 to 5 days; do not use for more than 10 days.

➤*Concomitant diuretic therapy:* Because repeated administration can lead to sodium and water retention, a diuretic may be necessary for maximal blood pressure reduction and to avoid congestive failure.

➤*Storage/Stability:* Protect from light/freezing. Store between 2° to 30°C (36° to 86°F).

Actions

➤*Pharmacology:* Diazoxide, a nondiuretic antihypertensive, is structurally related to the thiazides. It promptly reduces blood pressure by relaxing smooth muscle in the peripheral arterioles. Increases in heart rate and in cardiac output occur as blood pressure is reduced. Coronary blood flow is maintained. Renal blood flow is increased after an initial decrease. Transient hyperglycemia occurs in the majority of patients.

➤*Pharmacokinetics:* Diazoxide is extensively bound to serum protein (more than 90%) and may therefore displace other highly protein-bound agents. The plasma half-life is 28 ± 8.3 hours. The duration of antihypertensive effect varies, but is generally less than 12 hours.

Generally, hypotensive effects begin within 1 min, maximum effects occurring within 2 to 5 min. Blood pressure increases gradually over the next 20 minutes, and then more slowly over the next 3 to 15 hours .

Contraindications

Treatment of compensatory hypertension, such as that associated with aortic coarctation or arteriovenous shunt; dissecting aortic aneurysm; hypersensitivity to diazoxide, thiazides or to other sulfonamide derivatives.

Warnings

➤*Myocardial lesions in animals:* Diazoxide IV in dogs induces subendocardial necrosis and necrosis of papillary muscles. These lesions, which are also produced by other vasodilators (eg, hydralazine, minoxidil) and catecholamines, are presumed to be related to anoxia from reflex tachycardia and decreased blood pressure.

➤*Rapid decrease in blood pressure:* Observe caution when reducing severely elevated blood pressure. Use only the 150 mg minibolus. The 300 mg IV dose of diazoxide is less predictable and less controllable and has been associated with angina and with myocardial and cerebral infarction. Optic nerve infarction was reported when a 100 mmHg reduction in diastolic pressure occurred over 10 minutes following a single 300 mg bolus. In one prospective trial conducted in patients with severe hypertension and coexistent coronary artery disease, a 50% incidence of ischemic changes in the ECG was observed following single 300 mg bolus injections of diazoxide. Achieve the desired blood pressure over as long a period of time as is compatible. At least several hours and preferably 1 or 2 days is tentatively recommended.

Improved safety with equal efficacy can be achieved by giving diazoxide as a minibolus dose until diastolic blood pressure less than 100 mmHg is achieved. If hypotension severe enough to require therapy results, it usually responds to the Trendelenberg maneuver. If necessary, administer sympathomimetics such as dopamine or norepinephrine. Special attention is required in diabetes mellitus and if salt and water retention present serious problems.

Transient hyperglycemia occurs in the majority of patients, but usually requires treatment only in patients with diabetes mellitus; it will respond to the usual management including insulin. Monitor blood glucose levels, especially in patients with diabetes and in those requiring multiple injections of diazoxide. Cataracts have been observed in a few animals receiving repeated daily doses of IV diazoxide.

➤*Fluid and electrolyte balance:* Diazoxide causes sodium retention; repeat injections may precipitate edema and CHF. This retention responds to diuretic agents if adequate renal function exists. Coadministered thiazides may potentiate diazoxide's antihypertensive, hyperglycemic and hyperuricemic actions. Increased extracellular fluid volume may cause treatment failure in nonresponsive patients.

➤*Pheochromocytoma:* Diazoxide is ineffective against hypertension due to pheochromocytoma.

➤*Pregnancy: Category C.* Safety for use is not established. Diazoxide crosses the placenta and appears in cord blood. It reduces fetal or pup survival, and reduces fetal growth in rats, rabbits and dogs at daily doses of 30, 21 or 10 mg/kg, respectively. In rats treated at term, doses of 10 mg/kg or more prolonged parturition.

If given prior to delivery, it may produce fetal or neonatal hyperbilirubinemia, thrombocytopenia, altered carbohydrate metabolism and other adverse reactions.

Labor and delivery – Not for use during pregnancy. IV administration during labor may stop uterine contractions, requiring administration of an oxytocic agent. An episode of maternal hypotension and fetal bradycardia occurred in a patient in labor who received both reserpine and hydralazine prior to administration of diazoxide. Neonatal hyperglycemia following intrapartum use of diazoxide IV occurred.

➤*Lactation:* Information is not available concerning the passage of diazoxide in breast milk. Decide whether to discontinue breast-feeding or the drug, taking into account the importance of the drug to the mother.

Precautions

➤*Monitoring:* Diazoxide requires close and frequent blood pressure monitoring; it may cause hypotension, requiring treatment with sympathomimetic drugs. Use diazoxide primarily in the hospital and where facilities exist to treat such untoward reactions.

Monitor the blood pressure closely until it has stabilized. Thereafter, hourly measurements will indicate any unusual response. Further decreases in blood pressure at 30 minutes or more after injection may be due to causes other than diazoxide. Have the patient remain recumbent for at least 1 hour after injection. In ambulatory patients, measure the blood pressure with the patient standing before ending surveillance.

DIAZOXIDE — PARENTERAL

Perform appropriate diagnostic laboratory tests prior to, during and following diazoxide injection. Tests include: Hematologic (hematocrit, hemoglobin, white blood cell and platelet counts); metabolic (glucose, uric acid, total protein, albumin); electrolyte (sodium, potassium) and osmolality; renal function (creatinine, urine-protein); ECG.

➤*Special risk:* Use with care in patients with impaired cerebral or cardiac circulation, in whom abrupt reductions in blood pressure might be detrimental or in whom mild tachycardia or decreased blood perfusion may be deleterious. Avoid prolonged hypotension so as not to aggravate preexisting renal failure.

Drug Interactions

Because diazoxide is highly protein bound, it can be expected to displace other highly protein-bound agents (eg, warfarin), resulting in higher blood levels of these agents.

Diazoxide (Parenteral) Drug Interactions

Precipitant drug	Object drug[a]		Description
Diazoxide	Hydantoins	⬇	Serum hydantoin levels may be decreased, possibly resulting in decreased anticonvulsant action.
Diazoxide	Sulfonylureas	⬇	Addition of diazoxide to sulfonylurea therapy could destabilize the patient, resulting in hyperglycemia.
Thiazide diuretics	Diazoxide	⬆	Coadministration may potentiate the hyperuricemic and antihypertensive effects of diazoxide.

[a] ⬆ = Object drug increased. ⬇ = Object drug decreased.

➤*Drug/Lab test interactions:* Hyperglycemic and hyperuricemic effects of diazoxide preclude assessment of these metabolic states. Increased renin secretion, IgG concentrations and decreased cortisol secretion have occurred. Diazoxide inhibits glucagon-stimulated insulin release and will cause a false-negative insulin response to glucagon.

Adverse Reactions

The following adverse reactions were reported with rapid IV bolus administration of 300 mg diazoxide. The currently recommended minibolus dosing regimen may result in similar adverse reactions, but with less frequency and severity. The most common adverse reactions were hypotension (7%); nausea, vomiting (4%); dizziness, weakness (2%). Additional adverse reactions were as follows:

➤*Cardiovascular:* Sodium and water retention after repeated injections, especially important in patients with impaired cardiac reserve; hypotension to shock levels; myocardial ischemia, usually transient and manifested by angina, atrial and ventricular arrhythmias and marked ECG changes, but occasionally leading to myocardial infarction; optic nerve infarction following too rapid decrease in severely elevated blood pressure; supraventricular tachycardia; palpitations; bradycardia; chest discomfort or nonanginal chest tightness.

➤*CNS:* Cerebral ischemia, usually transient, but occasionally leading to infarction and manifested by unconsciousness, convulsions, paralysis, confusion or focal neurological deficit such as numbness of the hands; vasodilative phenomena (eg, orthostatic hypotension), sweating, flushing and generalized or localized sensations of warmth; transient neurological findings secondary to alteration in regional blood flow to the brain, such as headache (sometimes throbbing), dizziness, lightheadedness, sleepiness (also reported as lethargy, somnolence or drowsiness), euphoria or "funny feeling," ringing in the ears and momentary hearing loss; weakness of short duration; apprehension; anxiety; malaise; blurred vision.

➤*GI:* Acute pancreatitis (rare); nausea; vomiting; abdominal discomfort; anorexia; alterations in taste; parotid swelling; salivation; dry mouth; ileus; constipation; diarrhea.

➤*Miscellaneous:* Hyperglycemia in diabetic patients after repeated injections; hyperosmolar coma in an infant; transient hyperglycemia in nondiabetic patients; transient retention of nitrogenous wastes; respiratory findings secondary to smooth muscle relaxation, such as dyspnea, cough and choking sensation; warmth or pain along injected vein; cellulitis without sloughing or phlebitis at injection site of extravasation; back pain and increased nocturia; lacrimation; hypersensitivity reactions; papilledema induced by plasma volume expansion secondary to the administration of diazoxide in a patient who had received 11 injections (300 mg/dose) over a 22 day period; transient cataract in an infant; hirsutism; decreased libido.

Overdosage

Overdosage may cause hypotension that can usually be controlled with the Trendelenburg maneuver. If necessary, sympathomimetic agents, such as dopamine or norepinephrine, may be administered. Failure of blood pressure to rise in response to such agents suggests that the hypotension may not have been caused by diazoxide. Excessive hyperglycemia will respond to conventional therapy of hyperglycemia. Diazoxide may be removed from blood by hemodialysis.

FENOLDOPAM MESYLATE

Rx	**Corlopam** (Hospira)	**Injection, concentrate:** 10 mg/mL	In 1 and 2 mL single-dose ampules.[a]
Rx	**Fenoldopam Mesylate** (Baxter)	**Injection:** 10 mg/mL	In 1 and 2 mL single-dose ampules.[b]

[a] With 1 mg sodium metabisulfite.

[b] With sodium metabisulfite.

FENOLDOPAM — INJECTION

Indications

➤*Severe hypertension:*

Adults – For the in-hospital, short-term (up to 48 hours) management of severe hypertension when rapid, but quickly reversible, emergency reduction of blood pressure is clinically indicated, including malignant hypertension with deteriorating end-organ function. Transition to oral therapy with another agent can begin at any time after blood pressure is stable during fenoldopam infusion.

Children: For the in-hosptial, short-term (up to 4 hours) reduction in blood pressure.

Administration and Dosage

➤*Approved by the FDA:* September 23, 1997.

➤*Severe hypertension:*

Adults – The optimal magnitude and rate of blood pressure reduction in acutely hypertensive patients have not been rigorously determined, but, in general, both delayed and too-rapid decreases appear undesirable in sick patients. An initial fenoldopam dose that produces the desired magnitude and rate of blood pressure reduction in a given clinical situation may be chosen from the following table. Doses less than 0.1 mcg/kg/min have very modest effects and appear only marginally useful in this population. In general, as the initial dosage increases, there is a greater and more rapid blood pressure reduction. However, lower initial dosages (0.03 to 0.1 mcg/kg/min) titrated slowly have been associated with less reflex tachycardia than have higher initial dosages (greater than or equal to 0.3 mcg/kg/min). In clinical trials, dosages from 0.01 to 1.6 mcg/kg/min have been studied. Most of the effect of a given infusion rate is attained in 15 minutes.

Pharmacodynamic Effects of Fenoldopam in Adult Hypertensive Emergency Patients

Time point and pharmacodynamic parameters	Drug dosage (mcg/kg/min) 0.01 (n = 25)	0.03 (n = 24)	0.1 (n = 22)	0.3 (n = 23)
Preinfusion baseline				
Systolic blood pressure – mean ± standard error (SE)	210 ± 21	208 ± 26	205 ± 24	211 ± 17
Diastolic blood pressure – mean ± SE	136 ± 16	135 ± 11	133 ± 14	136 ± 15
Heart rate – mean ± SE	87 ± 20	84 ± 14	81 ± 19	80 ± 14
15 minutes of infusion[a]				
Systolic blood pressure	−5 ± 4	−7 ± 4	−16 ± 4	−19 ± 4
Diastolic blood pressure	−5 ± 3	−8 ± 3	−12 ± 2	−21 ± 2
Heart rate	−2 ± 3	+1 ± 1	+2 ± 1	+11 ± 2
30 minutes of infusion[a]				
Systolic blood pressure	−6 ± 4	−11 ± 4	−21 ± 3	−16 ± 4
Diastolic blood pressure	−10 ± 3	−12 ± 3	−17 ± 3	−20 ± 2
Heart rate	−2 ± 3	−1 ± 1	+3 ± 2	+12 ± 3
1 hour of infusion[a]				
Systolic blood pressure	−5 ± 3	−9 ± 4	−19 ± 4	−22 ± 4
Diastolic blood pressure	−8 ± 3	−13 ± 3	−18 ± 2	−23 ± 2
Heart rate	−1 ± 3	0 ± 2	+3 ± 2	+11 ± 3
4 hours of infusion[a]				
Systolic blood pressure	−14 ± 4	−20 ± 5	−23 ± 4	−37 ± 4
Diastolic blood pressure	−12 ± 3	−18 ± 3	−21 ± 3	−29 ± 3
Heart rate	−2 ± 4	0 ± 2	+4 ± 2	+11 ± 2

[a] Mean change from baseline ± SE.

Administration: Fenoldopam should be administered by continuous intravenous (IV) infusion. A bolus dose should not be used. Hypotension and rapid decreases of blood pressure should be avoided. The initial dose should be titrated upward or downward, no more frequently than every 15 minutes

FENOLDOPAM — INJECTION

(and less frequently as goal pressure is approached) to achieve the desired therapeutic effect. The recommended increments for titration are 0.05 to 0.1 mcg/kg/min.

Use of a calibrated, mechanical infusion pump is recommended for proper control of infusion rate during fenoldopam infusion. In clinical trials, fenoldopam treatment was safely performed without the need for intra-arterial blood pressure monitoring; blood pressure and heart rate were monitored at frequent intervals, typically every 15 minutes. Frequent blood pressure monitoring is recommended.

The fenoldopam infusion can be abruptly discontinued or gradually tapered prior to discontinuation. Oral antihypertensive agents can be added during fenoldopam infusion or following its discontinuation. Patients in controlled clinical trials have received IV fenoldopam for as long as 48 hours.

➤*Children:* Fenoldopam should be administered IV by a continuous infusion pump appropriate for the delivery of low infusion rates. Monitoring of blood pressure should be continuous, usually by way of an intra-arterial line. Heart rate should also be continuously monitored. In the clinical trial, the usual starting dosage was 0.2 mcg/kg/min with an effect on mean arterial pressure (MAP) evident within 5 minutes. At a constant infusion rate, the effect was maximal after 20 to 25 minutes. Increased dosages of up to 0.3 to 0.5 mcg/kg/min every 20 to 30 minutes were generally well tolerated. Tachycardia without further decrease in MAP occurred at dosages greater than 0.8 mcg/kg/min. Upon discontinuation of the fenoldopam infusion after an average of 4 hours of therapy, blood pressure and heart rate returned to near baseline within 30 minutes.

Pharmacodynamic Effects of Fenoldopam in Children Baseline Mean and Mean Change ± SE

	Drug Dosage (mcg/kg/min)				
	Placebo (n = 16)	0.05 (n = 15[a])	0.2 (n = 16)	0.8 (n = 15)	3.2 (n = 15)
Preinfusion baseline					
MAP	81 ± 4	77 ± 5	75 ± 4	88 ± 6	74 ± 4
Systolic blood pressure	108 ± 5	103 ± 6	104 ± 6	117 ± 7	98 ± 4
Diastolic blood pressure	62 ± 4	61 ± 4	57 ± 3	69 ± 6	56 ± 3
Heart rate	106 ± 8	110 ± 7	119 ± 7	125 ± 6	122 ± 6
Change at 5 minutes of infusion					
MAP	4 ± 2	3 ± 3	−2 ± 2	−3 ± 3	−6 ± 3
Systolic blood pressure	5 ± 3	3 ± 3	−2 ± 3	−5 ± 3	−8 ± 3
Diastolic blood pressure	4 ± 2	6 ± 2	−1 ± 2	−2 ± 2	−4 ± 2
Heart rate	2 ± 3	−2 ± 3	−1 ± 3	4 ± 3	−2 ± 3
Change at 30 minutes of infusion (LOCF[b])					
MAP	0 ± 3	−1 ± 3	−2 ± 3	−10 ± 3	−10 ± 3
Systolic blood pressure	−3 ± 4	0 ± 4	−3± 4	−12 ± 4	−10 ± 4
Diastolic blood pressure	0 ± 3	1 ± 3	−2 ± 3	−8 ± 3	−6 ± 3
Heart rate	−6 ± 4	−4 ± 4	5 ± 4	7 ± 4	14 ± 4

[a] For MAP, n = 14; otherwise, n = 15.
[b] Dropouts were accounted for using the Last Observation Carried Forward (LOCF) method of analysis.

➤*Preparation of infusion solution:*

Warning – Contents of ampules must be diluted before infusion. Each ampule is for single use only.

Adults –

Dilution: The fenoldopam injection ampule concentrate must be diluted in 0.9% sodium chloride injection or 5% dextrose injection using the following dilution schedule:

Dilution of Fenoldopam for Adults

mL of concentrate (mg of drug)	Added to	Final concentration
4 mL (40 mg)	1,000 mL	40 mcg/mL
2 mL (20 mg)	500 mL	40 mcg/mL
1 mL (10 mg)	250 mL	40 mcg/mL

Infusion rates: The drug dose rate must be individualized according to body weight and according to the desired rapidity and extent of pharmacodynamic effect. The following table provides the calculated infusion volume in mL/h for a range of doses and body weights. The infusion should be administered using a calibrated mechanical infusion pump that can accurately and reliably deliver the desired infusion rate.

Fenoldopam Infusion Rates (mL/h) for Adults (> 40 kg)

Body weight (kg)	Infusion rate 0.025 (mcg/kg/min)	0.05 (mcg/kg/min)	0.1 (mcg/kg/min)	0.2 (mcg/kg/min)	0.3 (mcg/kg/min)	0.5 (mcg/kg/min)	0.8 (mcg/kg/min)	1 (mcg/kg/min)	1.2 (mcg/kg/min)	1.4 (mcg/kg/min)	1.6 (mcg/kg/min)
	Infusion rates (mL/h) of 40 mcg/mL solution										
40	1.5	3	6	12	18	30	48	60	72	84	96
50	1.9	3.8	7.5	15	22.5	37.5	60	75	90	105	120
60	2.3	4.5	9	18	27	45	72	90	108	126	144
70	2.6	5.3	10.5	21	31.5	52.5	84	105	126	147	168
80	3	6	12	24	36	60	96	120	144	158	192
90	3.4	6.8	13.5	27	40.5	67.5	108	135	162	189	216
100	3.8	7.5	15	30	45	75	120	150	180	210	240
110	4.1	8.3	16.5	33	49.5	82.5	132	165	198	231	264
120	4.5	9	18	36	54	90	144	180	216	252	288
130	4.9	9.8	19.5	39	58.5	97.5	156	195	234	273	312
140	5.3	10.5	21	42	63	105	168	210	252	294	336
150	5.6	11.3	22.5	45	67.5	112.5	180	225	270	315	360

Children –

Dilution:

Dilution of Fenoldopam for Children

mL of concentrate (mg of drug)	Added to	Final concentration
3 mL (30 mg)	500 mL	60 mcg/mL
1.5 mL (15 mg)	250 mL	60 mcg/mL
0.6 mL (6 mg)	100 mL	60 mcg/mL

Infusion rates – The following table provides the calculated infusion volume in mL/h for a range of drug doses and body weights. The infusion should be administered using a calibrated mechanical infusion pump that can accurately and reliably deliver the desired infusion rate. Because low flow rates (eg, < 0.5 mL/h) may not be practical and because of volume overload, it may be necessary to increase the concentration of fenoldopam in the infused solutions.

Fenoldopam Infusion Rates for Children Between 5 and 70 kg

Body Weight (kg)	Infusion rate 0.2 mcg/kg/min	0.5 mcg/kg/min	0.8 mcg/kg/min	1 mcg/kg/min	1.2 mcg/kg/min
	Infusion rates (mL/h) of 60 mcg/mL solution				
5	1	2.5	4	5	6
10	2	5	8	10	12
20	4	10	16	20	24
30	6	15	24	30	36
40	8	20	32	40	48
50	10	25	40	50	60
60	12	30	48	60	72
70	14	35	56	70	84

FENOLDOPAM — INJECTION

Parenteral drug products should be inspected visually for particulate matter and discoloration prior to administration whenever solution and container permit. If particulate matter or cloudiness is observed, the drug should be discarded.

➤*Storage/Stability:* Store at 2° to 30°C (35.6° to 86°F). The diluted solution is stable under normal ambient light and temperature conditions for at least 24 hours. Diluted solution that is not used within 24 hours of preparation should be discarded.

Actions

➤*Pharmacology:* Fenoldopam is a rapidly acting vasodilator. It is an agonist for D_1-like dopamine receptors and binds with moderate affinity to α_2-adrenoceptors. It has no significant affinity for D_2-like receptors, alpha-1 and beta adrenoceptors, 5-HT_1 and 5-HT_2 receptors, or muscarinic receptors. Fenoldopam is a racemic mixture with the R-isomer responsible for the biological activity. The R-isomer has approximately 250-fold higher affinity for D_1-like receptors than does the S-isomer. In nonclinical studies, fenoldopam had no agonist effect on presynaptic D_2-like dopamine receptors, or alpha- or beta-adrenoceptors, nor did it affect angiotensin-converting enzyme (ACE) activity. Fenoldopam may increase norepinephrine plasma concentration.

In animals, fenoldopam has vasodilating effects in coronary, renal, mesenteric, and peripheral arteries. All vascular beds, however, do not respond uniformly to fenoldopam. Vasodilating effects have been demonstrated in renal efferent and afferent arterioles.

➤*Pharmacokinetics:*

Absorption/Distribution –

Adults: Fenoldopam administered as a constant infusion at dosages of 0.01 to 1.6 mcg/kg/min produced steady-state plasma concentrations that were proportional to infusion rates. Steady-state concentrations are attained in about 20 minutes (4 half-lives). The steady-state plasma concentrations of fenoldopam, at comparable infusion rates, were similar in normotensive patients and in patients with mild-to-moderate hypertension or hypertensive emergencies.

Children: In children 1 month to 12 years of age, steady-state fenoldopam plasma concentrations were proportional to dosage (0.05 to 3.2 mcg/kg/min). The elimination half-life and clearance were 3 to 5 minutes and 3 L/h/kg, respectively. In radiolabeled studies in rats, no more than 0.005% of fenoldopam crossed the blood-brain barrier.

Metabolism/Excretion – Radiolabeled studies show that about 90% of infused fenoldopam is eliminated in urine, 10% in feces. Elimination is largely by conjugation, without participation of cytochrome P-450 enzymes. The principal routes of conjugation are methylation, glucuronidation, and sulfation. Only 4% of the administered dose is excreted unchanged. Animal data indicate that the metabolites are inactive. The elimination half-life was about 5 minutes in mild to moderate hypertensive patients, with little difference between the R (active) and S isomers.

Contraindications

None known.

Warnings

➤*Carcinogenesis:* In a 24-month study, mice treated orally with fenoldopam at 12.5, 25, or 50 mg/kg/day, reduced to 25 mg/kg/day on day 209 of study, showed no increase above controls in the incidence of neoplasms. Female mice in the highest dose group had an increased incidence and degree of severity of a fibro-osseous lesion of the sternum compared with control or low-dose animals. Compared with controls, female mice in the middle- and upper-dose groups had a higher incidence and degree of severity of chronic nephritis. These pathologic lesions were not seen in male mice treated with fenoldopam.

In a 24-month study, rats treated orally with fenoldopam at 5, 10, or 20 mg/kg/day, with the mid- and high-dose groups increased to 15 or 25 mg/kg/day, respectively, on day 372 of the study, showed no increase above controls in the incidence or type of neoplasms. Compared with the controls, rats in the mid- and high-dose groups had a higher incidence of hyperplasia of collecting duct epithelium at the tip of the renal papilla.

➤*Mutagenesis:* Fenoldopam did not induce bacterial gene mutation in the Ames test or mammalian gene mutation in the Chinese hamster ovary (CHO) cell assay. In the in vitro chromosomal aberration assay with CHO cells, fenoldopam was associated with statistically significant and dose-dependent increases in chromosomal aberrations, and in the proportion of aberrant metaphases. However, no chromosomal damage was seen in the in vivo mice micronucleus or bone marrow assays.

➤*Elderly:* Clinical studies of fenoldopam did not include sufficient numbers of subjects 65 years of age and older to determine whether they respond differently from younger subjects. Other reported clinical experience has not identified differences in responses between the elderly and younger patients. In general, dose selection for an elderly patient should be cautious, usually starting at the low end of the dosing range, reflecting the greater frequency of decreased hepatic, renal, or cardiac function, and of concomitant disease or other drug therapy.

➤*Pregnancy: Category B.* Oral reproduction studies have been performed in rats and rabbits at dosages of 12.5 to 200 mg/kg/day and 6.25 to 25 mg/kg/day, respectively. Studies have revealed maternal toxicity at the highest doses tested but no evidence of impaired fertility or harm to the fetus due to fenoldopam. However, there are no adequate and well-controlled studies in pregnant women. Since animal reproduction studies are not always predictive of human response, use fenoldopam in pregnancy only if clearly needed.

➤*Lactation:* Fenoldopam is excreted in milk in rats. It is not known whether this drug is excreted in human milk. Because many drugs are excreted in human milk, exercise caution when fenoldopam is administered to a breast-feeding woman.

➤*Children:* Antihypertensive effects of fenoldopam have been studied in children younger than 1 month of age (at least 2 kg or full term) to 12 years of age requiring blood pressure reduction.

Clinical studies of fenoldopam did not include subjects 12 to 16 years of age to determine if they respond differently from younger subjects or adults. The pharmacokinetics of fenoldopam are independent of age when corrected for body weight. Consider the patient's clinical condition and concomitant drug therapy when making a dose selection for patients 12 to 16 years of age.

Precautions

➤*Monitoring:* Monitor blood pressure and heart rate at frequent intervals, typically every 15 minutes to avoid hypotension and rapid decreases of blood pressure. In children, continuously monitor blood pressure by way of an intra-arterial line. Monitor electrolytes every 6 hours.

➤*Intraocular pressure:* In a clinical study of 12 patients with open-angle glaucoma or ocular hypertension (mean baseline intraocular pressure was 29.2 mm Hg with a range of 22 to 33 mm Hg), infusion of fenoldopam at escalating doses ranging from 0.05 to 0.5 mcg/kg/min over a 3.5-hour period caused a dose-dependent increase in intraocular pressure (IOP). At the peak effect, the IOP was raised by a mean of 6.5 mm Hg (range −2 to +8.5 mm Hg, corrected for placebo effect). Upon discontinuation of the fenoldopam infusion, the IOP returned to baseline values within 2 hours. Undertake fenoldopam administration to patients with glaucoma or intraocular hypertension with caution.

➤*Tachycardia:* Fenoldopam causes a dose-related tachycardia, particularly with infusion rates above 0.1 mcg/kg/min. Tachycardia in adults diminishes over time but remains substantial at higher doses. Tachycardia in children persists for at least 4 hours at dosages greater than 0.8 mcg/kg/min.

➤*Hypotension:* Fenoldopam may occasionally produce symptomatic hypotension, and close monitoring of blood pressure during administration is essential. It is particularly important to avoid systemic hypotension when administering the drug to patients who have sustained an acute cerebral infarction or hemorrhage. In children, fenoldopam was only administered to patients with an indwelling intra-arterial line.

➤*Hypokalemia:* Decreases in serum potassium occasionally to values below 3 mEq/L were observed after less than 6 hours of fenoldopam infusion. It is not clear if the hypokalemia reflects a pressure natriuresis with enhanced potassium-sodium exchange or a direct drug effect. During clinical trials, electrolytes were monitored at intervals of 6 hours. Hypokalemia was treated with either oral or IV potassium supplementation. Patient management should include appropriate attention to serum electrolytes.

➤*Sulfite sensitivity:* Contains sodium metabisulfite, a sulfite that may cause allergic-type reactions including anaphylactic symptoms and life-threatening or less severe asthmatic episodes in certain susceptible people. The overall prevalence of sulfite sensitivity in the general population is unknown and probably low. Sulfite sensitivity is seen more frequently in asthmatic than in nonasthmatic people.

Drug Interactions

➤*Drug interactions with beta-blockers:* Avoid concomitant use of fenoldopam with beta-blockers. If the drugs are used together, exercise caution because unexpected hypotension could result from beta-blocker inhibition of the sympathetic reflex response to fenoldopam.

Adverse Reactions

➤*Adults:* Fenoldopam causes a dose-related fall in blood pressure and increase in heart rate. In controlled clinical studies of severe hypertension in patients with end-organ damage, 3% (4/137) of patients withdrew because of excessive falls in blood pressure. Increased heart rate could, in theory, lead to ischemic cardiac events or worsened heart failure, although these events have not been observed. The most common events reported as associated with fenoldopam use are headache, cutaneous dilation (flushing), nausea, and hypotension, each reported in greater than 5% of patients.

➤*Cardiovascular:*

Tachycardia – See Precautions for more information.

Hypotension – See Precautions for more information.

➤*Adverse reactions in hypertensive adult patients:* Adverse reactions occurring more than once in any dosing group (once if potentially important or plausibly drug related) in the fixed-dose constant-infusion studies are presented in the following table by infusion-rate group. There was no clear dose relationship, except possibly for headache, nausea, and flushing.

FENOLDOPAM — INJECTION

Fenoldopam Adverse Reactions[a] in Adults

	Adverse reaction	Fenoldopam dosage (mcg/kg/min)					
		Placebo (n = 7)	0.01 (n = 26)	0.03 to 0.04 (n = 31)	0.1 (n = 28)	0. 3 to 0.4 (n = 29)	0.6 to 0.8 (n = 11)
Cardiovascular	ST-T abnormalities (primarily T-wave inversion)	0	2	4	0	1	0
	Flushing	0	0	0	0	1	3
	Hypotension [b]	0	0	0	2	0	2
	Postural hypotension	0	2	0	0	0	0
	Tachycardia [b]	0	0	0	0	0	2
CNS	Headache	1	5	4	7	8	6
	Nervousness/ Anxiety	0	0	1	0	0	2
	Insomnia	0	2	0	0	0	0
	Dizziness	0	1	1	2	2	0
GI	Nausea	0	3	0	3	5	4
	Vomiting	0	2	0	2	1	2
	Abdominal pain/ fullness	0	2	0	0	2	1
	Constipation	0	0	0	0	0	2
	Diarrhea	0	0	0	0	2	0
Metabolic/ Nutritional	Increased creatinine[b]	0	0	2	0	0	0
	Hypokalemia [b]	0	2	2	0	1	0

Fenoldopam Adverse Reactions[a] in Adults

	Adverse reaction	Fenoldopam dosage (mcg/kg/min)					
		Placebo (n = 7)	0.01 (n = 26)	0.03 to 0.04 (n = 31)	0.1 (n = 28)	0. 3 to 0.4 (n = 29)	0.6 to 0.8 (n = 11)
Miscellaneous	Back pain	0	1	0	1	2	2
	Injection site reaction	0	1	3	0	3	2
	Nasal congestion	0	0	0	0	0	2
	Sweating	0	0	0	1	1	2
	Urinary tract infection	0	2	0	1	0	0

[a] Includes events reported by 2 or more patients receiving fenoldopam treatment across all dose groups.
[b] Investigator defined; no protocol definition.

➤*Additional adverse reactions (0.5% to 5%):*

Cardiovascular – Angina pectoris, bradycardia, extrasystoles, heart failure, ischemic heart disease, myocardial infarction, palpitations.

Hematologic / Lymphatic – Bleeding, leukocytosis.

Metabolic – Elevated lactate dehydrogenase, elevated serum glucose, elevated serum urea nitrogen (BUN), elevated transaminase.

Respiratory – Dyspnea, upper respiratory tract disorder.

Miscellaneous – Limb cramp, nonspecific chest pain, oliguria, pyrexia.

Children – In children, the most common adverse reactions reported during short-term administration in controlled trials (30 minutes) were hypotension and tachycardia. However, because of the short exposure, there is limited experience with defining adverse reactions in children. The long-term effects of fenoldopam on growth and development have not been studied.

Overdosage

➤*Symptoms:* Intentional fenoldopam overdosage has not been reported. The most likely reaction would be excessive hypotension.

➤*Treatment:* Treat excessive hypotension with drug discontinuation and appropriate supportive measures.

Patient Information

This product contains sulfite, which can cause allergic reactions in certain individuals (eg, asthma patients).

Before taking this medicine, tell your health care provider if you have glaucoma or increased pressure in the eye, or if you are taking beta-blockers.

ANTIHYPERLIPIDEMIC AGENTS

Lowering cholesterol levels can arrest or reverse in all vascular beds and can significantly decrease the morbidity and mortality associated with atherosclerosis. Each 10% reduction in cholesterol levels is associated with an approximate 20% to 30% reduction in the incidence of coronary heart disease. Hyperlipidemia, particularly elevated serum cholesterol and low-density lipoprotein (LDL) levels, is a risk factor in the development of atherosclerotic cardiovascular disease.

Individually assess potential benefits and risks of therapy. The cornerstone of treatment in primary hyperlipidemia is diet restriction and weight reduction. Limit or eliminate alcohol intake. Use drug therapy in conjunction with diet and after maximal efforts to control serum lipids by diet alone prove unsatisfactory, when tolerance to or compliance with diet is poor, or when hyperlipidemia is severe and risk of complications is high. Treat contributory diseases such as hypothyroidism or diabetes mellitus.

Elevated blood cholesterol levels are a major cause of coronary artery disease. Lowering these levels (specifically, LDL cholesterol) will reduce the risk of heart attacks caused by coronary heart disease (CHD).

➤*Risk factors:* Positive risk factors for CHD (other than high LDL) include: age (men 45 years of age and older; women 55 years of age and older or women who go through premature menopause without estrogen replacement therapy); family history of premature CHD; smoking; hypertension (greater than 140/90 mmHg); low HDL cholesterol (less than 35 mg/dL); obesity (greater than 30% overweight); and diabetes mellitus. Physical inactivity is not listed but should also be considered.

➤*Negative:* Negative risk factors include: High HDL cholesterol (greater than or equal to 60 mg/dL); subtract one risk factor if the patient's HDL is at this level.

All Americans (except children younger than 2 years old) should adopt a diet that reduces total dietary fat, decreases intake of saturated fat, increases intake of polyunsaturated fat, and reduces daily cholesterol intake to less than or equal to 250 to 300 mg.

The following treatments guidelines are provided by the National Cholesterol Education Program Expert Panel on Detection, Evaluation and Treatment of High Blood Cholesterol in Adults 20 years of age and older.

Classification of Total and HDL-Cholesterol Levels (Adults ≥ 20 years of Age)

Level (mg/dL) (mmol/L)	Classification
< 200 (5.2)	desirable
200 to 239 (5.2 to 6.2)	borderline high
≥ 240 (6.2)	high
HDL < 35 (0.9)	low

1.) Total blood cholesterol less than 200 mg/dL: HDL greater than or equal to 35 mg/dL, repeat total cholesterol and HDL measurements within 5 years or with physical exam; provide education on general population eating pattern, physical activity, and risk factor education. HDL less than 35 mg/dL, do lipoprotein analysis; base further action on LDL levels.
2.) Total blood cholesterol 200 to 239 mg/dL: HDL greater than or equal to 35 mg/dL and less than 2 risk factors, provide information on dietary modification, physical activity, and risk factor reduction; reevaluate in 1 to 2 years, repeat total and HDL cholesterol measurements, and reinforce nutrition and physical activity education. HDL less than 35 mg/dL or greater than or equal to 2 risk factors, analyze lipoprotein; base further action on LDL levels.
3.) Total blood cholesterol greater than or equal to 240 mg/dL: Analyze lipoprotein; base further action on LDL levels.

Classification of LDL-Cholesterol Levels

Level (mg/dL) (mmol/L)	Classification
< 130 (3.4)	desirable
130 to 159 (3.4 to 4.1)	borderline high
≥ 160 (4.1)	high

1.) LDL greater than or equal to 160 mg/dL without CHD and with less than 2 risk factors: Dietary treatment.
2.) LDL greater than or equal to 130 mg/dL without CHD and with greater than or equal to 2 risk factors: Dietary treatment.
3.) LDL greater than or equal to 190 mg/dL without CHD and with less than 2 other risk factors, or LDL greater than or equal to 160 mg/dL without CHD and with greater than or equal to 2 other risk factors: Drug treatment.

➤*Hyperlipidemias:* Elevation of serum cholesterol, triglycerides, or both is characteristic of hyperlipidemias. Differentiation of the specific biochemical abnormality requires identification of specific lipoprotein fractions in the serum. Lipoproteins transport serum lipids and are identified by their density and electrophoretic mobility. Chylomicrons are the largest and least dense of the lipoproteins, followed in order of increasing density and decreasing size by very low density lipoproteins (VLDL or pre-β), intermediate low density lipoproteins (ILDL or broad-β), low density lipoproteins (LDL or β) and high density lipoproteins (HDL or α). Triglycerides are transported primarily by chylomicrons and VLDL; the predominant cholesterol transporting lipoprotein is LDL.

Elevations and treatment associated with each type of hyperlipidemia follow:

Hyperlipidemias and Their Treatment[1]

Hyperlipidemia type	I	IIa	IIb	III	IV	V
Lipids						
Cholesterol	N-⇧	↑	↑	N-↑	N-⇧	N-↑
Triglycerides	↑	N	↑	N-↑	↑	↑
Lipoproteins						
Chylomicrons	↑	N	N	N	N	↑
VLDL (pre-β)	N-⇧	N-↓	↑	N-⇧	↑	↑
ILDL (broad-β)[2]				↑		
LDL (β)	↓	↑	↑	↑	N-⇩	↓
HDL (α)	↓	N	N	N	N-⇩	↓
Treatment	Diet	Diet HMG-CoA reductase inhibitors Bile acid sequestrants Nicotinic acid	Diet HMG-CoA reductase inhibitors Bile acid sequestrants[3] Gemfibrozil[4] Nicotinic acid	Diet Nicotinic acid Gemfibrozil	Diet Gemfibrozil Nicotinic acid Fenofibrate	Diet Gemfibrozil Nicotinic acid[5] Fenofibrate

[1] N = normal ↑ = increase ↓ = decrease ⇧ = slight increase ⇩ = slight decrease
[2] An abnormal lipoprotein.
[3] Particularly useful if hypercholesterolemia predominates.
[4] In patients with inadequate response to weight loss, bile acid sequestrants, nicotinic acid.
[5] Norethindrone acetate (women) and oxandrolone (men) are effective, but use is not FDA-approved.

The following table summarizes the effects of the various antihyperlipidemic drugs on serum lipids and lipoproteins:

Antihyperlipidemic Drug Effects[1]

	Lipids		Lipoproteins		
Drug	Cholesterol	Triglycerides	VLDL (pre-β)	LDL (β)	HDL
Atorvastatin	↓	↓	↓	↓	↑
Cerivastatin	↓	↓	↓	↓	↑
Cholestyramine	↓	→↑	→↑	↓	→↑
Colestipol	↓	→↑	↑	↓	→↑
Fenofibrate	↓	↓	↓	↑	↑
Fluvastatin	↓	↓	↓	↓	↑
Gemfibrozil	↓	↓	↓	→↓	↑
Lovastatin	↓	↓	↓	↓	↑
Nicotinic acid	↓	↓	↓	↓	↑
Pravastatin	↓	↓	↓	↓	↑
Simvastatin	↓	↓	↓	↓	↑

[1] ↓ = decrease ↑ = increase → = unchanged

➤*General considerations:*

1.) Define the type of hyperlipoproteinemia, and establish baseline serum cholesterol and triglyceride levels.
2.) Institute a trial of diet, weight reduction and physical activity, which are extremely important elements of therapy for high blood cholesterol. Remind patients to restrict their dietary intake of cholesterol and saturated fats and to adhere to prescribed dietary regimens. Drug therapy does not reduce the importance of adhering to diet.
3.) Carefully monitor the patient during treatment, including serum cholesterol and triglyceride levels.
4.) Consider failure of cholesterol level to fall or a significant rise in triglyceride level as indications to discontinue medication.

➤*Dietary treatment:* Reducing elevated cholesterol levels and maintaining adequate nutrition is the aim of dietary therapy. Step I and Step II diets are specifically designed to progressively reduce saturated fatty acids and cholesterol intake and promote weight loss in overweight individuals by eliminating excess total calories and increasing physical activity.

Step I – Total fat intake less than or equal to 30% of calories; saturated fatty acid intake less than 8% to 10% of calories; cholesterol intake less than 300 mg/day. Measure serum total cholesterol and adherence to diet at 4 to 6 weeks and at 3 months. If cholesterol and LDL level goals are met, monitor quarterly the first year and twice a year thereafter. If response is insufficient, proceed to Step II.

Step II – Saturated fatty acid intake less than 7% of calories; cholesterol intake less than 200 mg/day. Measure serum total cholesterol and adherence to diet at 4 to 6 weeks and at 3 months. Begin long-term monitoring if goal has been met. Consider drug therapy if goal has not been attained. Carry out intensive diet therapy and counseling for greater than or equal to 6 months before starting drug therapy. Continue dietary treatment during drug treatment.

➤*Drug treatment:* **Cholestyramine** and **colestipol** are used to lower cholesterol. HMG-CoA reductase inhibitors, **gemfibrozil**, **nicotinic acid**, and **fenofibrate** are used to lower both cholesterol and triglycerides. Gemfibrozil and fenofibrate lower serum triglycerides much more effectively than cholesterol levels. When both cholesterol and triglycerides are elevated, treatment of the hypertriglyceridemia should take precedence. When hypercholesterolemia is treated first, an exacerbation of the hypertriglyceridemia may occur. Serum cholesterol often falls to normal levels without specific therapy following treatment of the hypertriglyceridemia.

First choice – Drugs of first choice include HMG-CoA reductase inhibitors, gemfibrozil or nicotinic acid. Measure LDL-cholesterol levels at 4 to 6 weeks and at 3 months. The target LDL level for treatment is less than or equal to 130 mg/dL. If the response is adequate, monitor every 4 months; if inadequate, switch to another agent or use a combination of 2 drugs. Refer patients who fail to respond to combination therapy to a lipid disorder specialist.

Estrogen – Estrogen replacement therapy can be considered in postmenopausal women with high serum cholesterol because estrogens have been shown to reduce total and LDL- and raise HDL-cholesterol levels.

Combination therapy – Because drug therapy of different hyperlipoproteinemias involves different mechanisms and pharmacologic actions, consider a combined drug regimen in stubborn cases. However, experience with combination therapy is limited. The coadministration of a bile acid sequestrant with either nicotinic acid or an HMG-CoA reductase inhibitor can lower LDL-cholesterol levels by greater than or equal to 40% to 50%. Use HMG-CoA reductase inhibitors and gemfibrozil concomitantly with caution because of the risks of myopathy, rhabdomyolysis and acute renal failure.

Bile Acid Sequestrants

Refer to general discussions on these agents in Antihyperlipidemic Agents Introduction.

Indications

➤*Hyperlipidemia:* Adjunctive therapy to diet for the reduction of elevated serum cholesterol in patients with primary hypercholesterolemia (elevated low-density lipoprotein [LDL]) who do not respond adequately to diet.

These agents may lower LDL cholesterol in patients who also have hypertriglyceridemia, but they are not indicated where hypertriglyceridemia is the abnormality of most concern.

Bile acid sequestrants may raise serum triglyceride levels and are not recommended as monotherapy in patients with triglyceride levels higher than 400 mg/dL or in patients with familial dysbetalipoproteinemia. They may be used as monotherapy in patients with triglyceride levels less than 200 mg/dL. Per the National Cholesterol Education Program (NCEP) Third Report, bile acid sequestrants should be considered as LDL-lowering therapy in patients with moderately elevated LDL cholesterol; women who are considering pregnancy and have elevated LDL cholesterol; patients who need only modest reductions in their LDL cholesterol level to reach their target goal; and for use as combination therapy with an HMG-CoA reductase inhibitor in patients with very high LDL cholesterol levels.

➤*Pruritus (cholestyramine only):* Relief of pruritus associated with partial biliary obstruction. Cholestyramine has been shown to have a variable effect on serum cholesterol in these patients.

➤*Unlabeled uses:*

Cholestyramine – Postvagotomy diarrhea.

Colestipol – Relief of pruritus associated with partial biliary obstruction (including primary biliary cirrhosis and various other forms of bile stasis).

Cholestyramine and colestipol – Binds to the toxin produced by *Clostridium difficile*; bile salt-mediated diarrhea; adjunctive treatment for hyperthyroidism; digitalis toxicity (see Cardiac Glycosides monograph); hyperoxaluria.

Administration and Dosage

Mix dry granules with liquid. Swallow tablets whole.

Cholesterol reduction should occur during the first month of therapy. Continue therapy to sustain cholesterol reduction. If adequate reduction is not attained, discontinue therapy.

➤*Concomitant therapy:* Evidence suggests that the cholesterol-lowering effects of these agents and an HMG-CoA reductase inhibitor are additive. Additive effects on LDL cholesterol also are seen with combined cholestyramine and nicotinic acid therapy.

Actions

➤*Pharmacology:* Cholesterol is the major, and probably sole, precursor of bile acids. During normal digestion, bile acids are secreted via the bile from the liver and gallbladder into the intestines to emulsify the fat and lipid materials in food, thus facilitating absorption. A major portion of the bile acids secreted is reabsorbed from the intestines and returned via the portal circulation to the liver, which completes the enterohepatic cycle.

Bile-acid-sequestering resins bind bile acids in the intestine to form an insoluble complex that is excreted in the feces. This results in a partial removal of bile acids from the enterohepatic circulation, preventing their absorption. Because these agents are anion-exchange resins, the chloride anions of the resin are replaced by other anions. These agents are hydrophilic but insoluble in water. They remain unchanged in the GI tract and are not absorbed.

The increased fecal loss of bile acids leads to an increased oxidation of cholesterol to bile acids. This results in an increased number of LDL receptors, increased hepatic uptake of LDL, decreased beta lipoprotein or LDL serum levels, and decreased serum cholesterol levels. Although bile-acid-sequestering resins produce an increase in the hepatic synthesis of cholesterol, serum cholesterol levels fall. Plasma cholesterol levels fall secondary to an increased rate of clearance of cholesterol-rich lipoproteins from the plasma. Serum triglyceride levels may increase or remain unchanged in treated patients.

The decline in serum cholesterol is usually evident within 1 month. When the resins are discontinued, serum cholesterol levels usually return to baseline within 1 month. Determine serum cholesterol levels periodically.

In patients with partial biliary obstruction, reduction of serum bile acid levels by **cholestyramine** reduces bile acid deposits in the dermal tissues with a resultant decrease in pruritus.

➤*Pharmacokinetics:*

Absorption – Bile acid sequestrants are hydrophilic but virtually water insoluble (99.75%), not hydrolyzed by digestive enzymes, and not absorbed.

Excretion – After administration of 1.9 g of **colesevelam** twice per day for 28 days, an average of 0.05% of a single dose was excreted in the urine. For **colestipol**, administration of 20 g per day for 60 days, less than 0.17% of a single dose was excreted in the urine.

Contraindications

Hypersensitivity to bile acid sequestering resins or any components of the products; complete biliary obstruction (cholestyramine only); bowel obstruction (colesevelam only).

Warnings

➤*Phenylketonurics:* Some products may contain phenylalanine. See individual monographs.

➤*Powder / Granules:* Avoid accidental inhalation or esophageal distress; do not take dry. Mix with fluids before ingesting.

➤*Calcified material:* Calcified material has been observed in the biliary tree and the gall bladder; however, this may be due to liver disease and not drug-related. One patient experienced biliary colic on each of 3 occasions on which he took **cholestyramine**. Another patient, diagnosed with an acute abdominal symptom complex, showed a "pasty mass" in the transverse colon on x-ray.

➤*Carcinogenesis:* The incidence of intestinal tumors in studies was higher in **cholestyramine**-treated rats than in controls. The total incidence of fatal and nonfatal neoplasms was similar in both treatment groups. Various alimentary system cancers were more prevalent with **cholestyramine**.

In a 104-week carcinogenicity study with **colesevelam** in rats, a statistically significant increase in the incidence of pancreatic acinar cell adenoma was seen in male rats at dosages higher than 1.2 g/kg/day (approximately 20 times the maximum human dosage, based on body weight, mg/kg). A statistically significant increase in thyroid C-cell adenoma was seen in female rats at 2.4 g/kg/day (approximately 40 times the maximum human dosage, based on body weight, mg/kg).

➤*Pregnancy: Category B* (**colesevelam**). *Category C* (**cholestyramine/colestipol**). These agents are not absorbed systemically, and are not expected to cause fetal harm when administered during pregnancy in recommended doses. There are no adequate and well-controlled studies in pregnant women, and the known interference with fat-soluble vitamin absorption may be detrimental even with supplementation. No adverse fetal effects were observed when **cholestyramine** was used for the treatment of cholestasis of pregnancy. Weigh the potential benefits against the risks.

➤*Lactation:* Exercise caution when administering to a breast-feeding woman. The possible lack of proper vitamin absorption may have an effect on breast-feeding infants.

➤*Children:*

Cholestyramine – Dosage schedules have not been established. Standard texts list a usual pediatric dosage of anhydrous cholestyramine resin 240 mg/kg/day in 2 to 3 divided doses, normally not to exceed 8 g/day with dose titration based on response and tolerance. In calculating pediatric dosages, anhydrous cholestyramine resin 80 mg is contained in 110 mg of *Prevalite*; anhydrous cholestyramine 44.4 mg is contained in 100 mg of *Questran*; and anhydrous cholestyramine 62.7 mg is contained in 100 mg of *Questran Light*. The effects of long-term administration and efficacy in maintaining lowered cholesterol levels are unknown.

Colestipol and colesevelam – Safety and efficacy have not been established.

Precautions

➤*Monitoring:* Determine serum cholesterol levels at baseline, then frequently during the first few months of therapy and periodically thereafter. Periodically measure serum triglyceride levels to detect significant changes.

➤*Diet:* Before instituting therapy, vigorously attempt to control serum cholesterol with an appropriate dietary regimen and weight reduction.

➤*Thyroid function:* While there have been no reports of hypothyroidism induced in individuals with normal thyroid function, the theoretical possibility exists, particularly in patients with limited thyroid reserve.

➤*Contributing diseases:* Prior to initiating therapy, investigate and treat diseases contributing to increased blood cholesterol (eg, alcoholism, diabetes mellitus, dysproteinemias, hypothyroidism, nephrotic syndrome, obstructive liver disease, other drug therapy).

➤*Malabsorption:* Because they sequester bile acids, these resins may interfere with normal fat absorption and digestion and may prevent absorption of fat-soluble vitamins such as A, D, K, and folic acid.

Chronic use may increase bleeding tendencies due to hypoprothrombinemia associated with vitamin K deficiency. This usually responds promptly to parenteral vitamin K_1; prevent recurrences by giving oral vitamin K_1.

➤*Reduced folate:* Reduction of serum or red cell folate has been reported over long-term administration of **cholestyramine**. Consider supplementation with folic acid.

➤*Hyperchloremic acidosis:* Prolonged use of chloride anion-exchange resins may cause hyperchloremic acidosis, especially for younger and smaller patients in which relative dosage may be higher.

➤*GI disorders:* The safety and efficacy of colesevelam in patients with dysphagia, swallowing disorders, severe GI motility disorders, or major GI tract surgery have not be established. Use with caution.

➤*Constipation:* These agents may produce or severely worsen preexisting constipation. Fecal impaction may occur and hemorrhoids may be aggravated. Avoid constipation in patients with symptomatic coronary artery disease. Most instances of constipation are mild, transient, and controlled with standard treatment. Some patients require decreased dosage or discontinuation of therapy.

Gradually increase the dosage to minimize the risk of developing fecal impaction. Encourage increased fluid intake and inclusion of additional dietary fiber to alleviate constipation; a stool softener may be added if needed.

Colestipol tablets – In patients with preexisting constipation, the starting dosage should be 2 g once or twice daily.

Colestipol and cholestyramine oral suspension – In patients with preexisting constipation, the starting dosage is 1 packet or 1 scoop once daily for 5 to 7 days, increasing to twice daily with monitoring of constipation and of serum lipoproteins, at least twice, 4 to 6 weeks apart.

Drug Interactions

Bile Acid Sequestrant (BAS) Drug Interactions

Precipitant drug	Object drug*		Description
BAS	Anticoagulants	⬇	Cholestyramine may decrease anticoagulant effect; separate the administration of these agents.
BAS	Mycophenolate	⬇	≈ 40% decrease in the area under the curve (AUC) by cholestyramine.
BAS	Thyroid hormones	⬇	Possible loss of efficacy of thyroid and potential hypothyroidism with concurrent cholestyramine. Separate administration by 6 h.
BAS	Verapamil, sustained-release	⬇	Colesevelam decreased the maximum plasma concentration (C_{max}) and AUC of sustained-release verapamil by approximately 31% and 11%, respectively.

Bile Acid Sequestrant (BAS) Drug Interactions			
Precipitant drug	Object drug*		Description
BAS	Vitamins A, D, E, K, folic acid	⬇	Malabsorption may occur during administration of bile acid sequestrants (see Precautions).

* ⬇ = Object drug decreased.

For cholestyramine and colestipol, binding in the GI tract may delay or reduce the absorption of concomitant oral medication. Take other drugs at least 1 hour before or 4 to 6 hours after these agents. Discontinuation of a resin could pose a hazard if a potentially toxic, significantly bound drug has been titrated to a maintenance level while on the resin.

Cholestyramine and Colestipol Drug Interactions (Decreased Serum Levels or GI Absorption)		
Corticosteroids	HMG-CoA reductase inhibitors	Phosphate supplements
Digitalis glycosides	Hydrocortisone	Propranolol
Doxepin	Imipramine	Tetracyclines
Estrogens/progestins	NSAIDs	Thiazide diuretics
Furosemide	Penicillin G	Ursodiol
Gemfibrozil	Phenobarbital	Valproic acid
Glipizide		

Adverse Reactions

➤*Colesevelam:*

Colesevelam Adverse Reactions (> 2%)		
Adverse reaction	Placebo (n = 258)	Colesevelam only (n = 807)
CNS		
Asthenia	2	4
Headache	8	6
GI		
Abdominal pain	5	5
Constipation	7	11
Diarrhea	7	5
Dyspepsia	3	8
Flatulence	14	12
Nausea	4	4
Musculoskeletal		
Back pain	6	3
Myalgia	0	2
Respiratory		
Cough increased	2	2
Pharyngitis	2	3
Rhinitis	3	3
Sinusitis	4	2
Miscellaneous		
Accidental injury	3	4
Flu syndrome	3	3
Infection	13	10
Pain	7	5

➤*Cholestyramine/colestipol:*

Cardiovascular – Chest pain, angina, tachycardia (colestipol); syncope (cholestyramine).

CNS – Dizziness, fatigue, headache (eg, migraine, sinus).
Cholestyramine: Anxiety, drowsiness, femoral nerve pain, paresthesia, tinnitus, vertigo.
Colestipol: Insomnia, light-headedness, weakness.

GI –
Cholestyramine/Colestipol: Abdominal discomfort/pain/cramping, aggravated or bleeding hemorrhoids, anorexia, blood in the stool, constipation, diarrhea, intestinal gas (bloating and flatulence), nausea, vomiting.
Colestipol: Heartburn, indigestion, loose stools; cholecystitis, cholelithiasis, peptic ulceration. (rare).
Cholestyramine: Bleeding from known duodenal ulcer, diverticulitis, dyspepsia, dysphagia, eructation, hiccups, pancreatitis, rectal pain, steatorrhea, sour taste, ulcer attack; rare reports of intestinal obstruction, including 2 deaths, in pediatric patients. Occasional calcified material has been observed in the biliary tree, including calcification of the gallbladder; however, this may be a manifestation of liver disease and not drug related (see Warnings). One patient experienced biliary colic on 3 occasions; one patient was diagnosed with acute abdominal symptom complex and was found to have a "pasty mass" in the transverse colon on x-ray.

Hematologic – Anemia, ecchymosis, increased prothrombin time (cholestyramine).

Hypersensitivity –
Cholestyramine: Asthma, shortness of breath, urticaria, wheezing.
Colestipol: Rash; dermatitis, urticaria (rare).

Musculoskeletal – Aches and pains in the extremities, arthritis, backache, muscle/joint pains.

Renal – Burnt odor to urine, diuresis, dysuria, hematuria (cholestyramine).

Miscellaneous –
Colestipol: Shortness of breath, swelling of hands or feet.
Cholestyramine: Bleeding tendencies due to hypoprothrombinemia (vitamin K deficiency); edema; dental bleeding; dental caries; erosion of tooth enamel; hyperchloremic acidosis in children (see Precautions); rash and irritation of the skin, tongue, and perianal area; increased libido; osteoporosis; swollen glands; tooth discoloration; uveitis; vitamin A (1 case of night blindness) and D deficiencies; weight loss/gain.

Lab test abnormalities –
Colestipol: Transient, modest elevations of AST, ALT, and alkaline phosphatase.
Cholestyramine: Liver function abnormalities.

Overdosage

The main potential harm is GI tract obstruction. Location and degree of obstruction and status of gut motility determine treatment. Overdosage has been reported in a patient taking 150% of the maximum recommended daily dose of **cholestyramine** for several weeks; no ill effects were reported.

Patient Information

Instruct patients not to take the powder in dry form but to mix with beverages, highly fluid soups, cereals, or pulpy fruits (see Administration and Dosage in individual monographs).

Instruct patients to swallow **colestipol** tablets whole 1 at a time and not to cut, crush, or chew.

Medication may interfere with absorption of concomitant drugs. Advise patients to take other drugs 1 hour before or 4 to 6 hours after **cholestyramine**, **colestipol**, or **colesevelam** (see Drug Interactions).

Constipation, flatulence, nausea, and heartburn may occur and may disappear with continued therapy. Advise patients to notify health care provider if these effects become bothersome or if unusual bleeding (eg, from the gums or rectum) occurs.

Sipping or holding the resin suspension in the mouth for prolonged periods may lead to changes in the surface of the teeth, resulting in discoloration, erosion of enamel, or decay; instruct patients to maintain good oral hygiene.

Instruct patient to inform health care provider if pregnant, planning to become pregnant, or breastfeeding.

CHOLESTYRAMINE

Rx	**Cholestyramine** (Various, eg, Eon, Novopharm)	**Powder for oral suspension**: anhydrous cholestyramine resin 4 g per 9 g powder	May contain sucrose, sorbitol. In 9 g packets (42s and 60s) and 378 g cans.
Rx	**Questran** (Par)		Sucrose. In 9 g packets (60s) and 378 g cans.
Rx	**Cholestyramine Light** (Various, eg, Eon, Novopharm)	**Powder for oral suspension**: anhydrous cholestyramine resin 4 g per 5.7 g powder	May contain aspartame. In 5 and 5.7 g packets (60s) and 210, 231, and 239 g cans.
Rx	**Prevalite** (Upsher Smith)	**Powder for oral suspension**: anhydrous cholestyramine resin 4 g per 5.5 g powder	Aspartame, phenylalanine 14.1 mg per 5.5 g. Orange flavor. In 5.5 g packets (42s and 60s) and 231 g cans (42 doses).
Rx	**Questran Light** (Par)	**Powder for oral suspension**: anhydrous cholestyramine resin 4 g per 6.4 g powder	Maltodextrin, aspartame, phenylalanine 28.1 mg per 6.4 g. Orange vanilla flavor. In 6.4 g packets (60s) and 268 g cans.

CHOLESTYRAMINE — ORAL

For complete and comparative prescribing information, refer to the Bile Acid Sequestrants group monograph.

Indications

➤*Hyperlipidemia:* Adjunctive therapy to diet for reduction of elevated serum cholesterol in patients with primary hypercholesterolemia (elevated low-density lipoprotein [LDL] cholesterol) who do not respond adequately to diet. May be useful to lower LDL cholesterol in patients who also have hypertriglyceridemia, but it is not indicated where hypertriglyceridemia is the abnormality of most concern.

➤*Pruritus:* Relief of pruritus associated with partial biliary obstruction.

➤*Unlabeled uses:* Binds to the toxin produced by *Clostridium difficile*; bile salt-mediated and postvagotomy diarrhea; digitalis toxicity (see Cardiac Glycosides monograph); adjunctive treatment for hyperthyroidism; hyperoxaluria.

CHOLESTYRAMINE — ORAL

Administration and Dosage

➤*Approved by the FDA:* August 3, 1973.

➤*Adults:* 4 g (1 packet or 1 full scoop) 1 to 2 times daily. Individualize dosage.

➤*Children:* Although an optimal dosage schedule has not been established, standard texts list a usual pediatric dosage of 240 mg/kg/day of anhydrous cholestyramine resin in 2 to 3 divided doses, normally not to exceed 8 g/day with dosage titration based on response and tolerance.

When calculating pediatric doses, anhydrous cholestyramine resin 80 mg is contained in 110 mg of *Prevalite*, 44.4 mg in 100 mg of *Questran* powder, and 62.7 mg in 100 mg of *Questran Light*.

The effects of long-term drug administration and effect in maintaining lowered cholesterol levels in pediatric patients are unknown.

➤*Preparation of powder:* Mix the contents of 1 powder packet or 1 level scoopful with 60 to 180 mL (2 to 6 fl oz) water or noncarbonated beverage. Stir to uniform consistency and drink. Do not take in dry form. Always mix with water or other fluids, highly fluid soups, or pulpy fruits, such as applesauce or crushed pineapple.

➤*Maintenance dose:* 2 to 4 packets or full scoops daily (anhydrous cholestyramine resin 8 to 16 g) divided into 2 doses. Increase dose gradually, with periodic assessment of lipid/lipoprotein levels at intervals of at least 4 weeks. Although the recommended dosing schedule is twice daily, cholestyramine may be administered in 1 to 6 doses/day.

➤*Maximum dose:* 6 packets or scoopfuls (anhydrous cholestyramine resin 24 g) per day.

➤*Administration:* Recommended administration time is at mealtime; this may be modified to avoid interference with absorption of concomitant medications.

➤*Concomitant medications:* Because cholestyramine resin may bind other drugs given concurrently, it is recommended that patients take other drugs at least 1 hour before or 4 to 6 hours after (or at as large an interval as possible) cholestyramine to avoid impeding their absorption.

➤*Constipation:*

Oral suspension – In patients with preexisting constipation, the starting dosage should be 1 packet or 1 scoop once daily for 5 to 7 days, increasing to twice daily with monitoring of constipation and of serum lipoproteins, at least twice, 4 to 6 weeks apart.

➤*Storage/Stability:* Store at controlled room temperature, 15° to 30°C (59° to 86°F).

COLESEVELAM HYDROCHLORIDE

Rx	**WelChol** (Sankyo Pharma)	**Tablets:** 625 mg	(Sankyo C01). Off-white, film-coated. In 180s and 540s.

COLESEVELAM HYDROCHLORIDE — ORAL

For complete and comparative prescribing information, refer to the Bile Acid Sequestrants group monograph.

Indications

➤*Hyperlipidemia:* Adjunctive therapy to diet and exercise and used alone or in combination with an HMG-CoA reductase inhibitor to reduce elevated low-density lipoprotein (LDL) cholesterol in patients with primary hypercholesterolemia (Fredrickson type IIa).

Administration and Dosage

➤*Approved by the FDA:* May 30, 2000.

Take with a liquid.

➤*Monotherapy:* Starting dosage is 3 tablets taken twice daily with meals or 6 tablets once daily with a meal. The dose can be increased to 7 tablets depending on desired therapeutic effect.

➤*Combination therapy:* For maximum therapeutic effect in combination with an HMG-CoA reductase inhibitor, the recommended dosage of colesevelam is 3 tablets taken twice daily with meals or 6 tablets taken once daily with a meal. Dosages of 4 to 6 tablets/day have been shown to be safe and effective when coadministered with an HMG-CoA reductase inhibitor or when the 2 drugs are dosed apart.

➤*Storage/Stability:* Store at room temperature (25°C; 77°F); excursions permitted to 15° to 30°C (59° to 86°F). Protect from moisture. Brief exposure to 40°C (104°F) does not adversely affect the product.

COLESTIPOL HYDROCHLORIDE

Rx	**Colestid** (Pharmacia)	**Tablets:** 1 g	(U). Yellow, elliptical. In 120s and 500s.
		Granules for oral suspension: colestipol hydrochloride 5 g per 7.5 g granules	Unflavored: In 300 and 500 g bottles and 5 g packets (30s and 90s). Flavored: Aspartame, mannitol. Orange flavor. In 450 g bottles (60 doses) and 7.5 g packets (60s).

COLESTIPOL HYDROCHLORIDE — ORAL

For complete and comparative prescribing information, refer to the Bile Acid Sequestrants group monograph.

Indications

➤*Hyperlipidemia:* Adjunctive therapy to diet for the reduction of elevated serum total and low-density lipoprotein (LDL) cholesterol in patients with primary hypercholesterolemia (elevated LDL cholesterol) who do not respond adequately to diet.

Generally, colestipol has no clinically significant effect on serum triglycerides, but with its use, triglyceride levels may be raised in some patients.

➤*Unlabeled uses:* Treatment of digitalis toxicity (see Cardiac Glycosides monograph); hyperoxaluria; diarrhea due to bile acids; adjunctive treatment for hyperthyroidism; relief of pruritus associated with partial biliary obstruction (including primary biliary cirrhosis and various other forms of bile stasis); binds to the toxin produced by *Clostridium difficile*.

Administration and Dosage

➤*Approved by the FDA:* April 4, 1977.

➤*Granules:*

Adults – 5 to 30 g/day (1 to 6 packets or level scoopfuls) given once daily or in divided doses. The starting dosage is 5 g once or twice daily with a daily increment of 5 g at 1- or 2-month intervals.

Preparation of granules – Mix in liquids, soups, cereals, or pulpy fruits (eg, crushed pineapple, pears, peaches). Do not take dry. Add the prescribed amount to a glassful (90 mL or more) of liquid; stir until completely mixed. A heavy or pulpy juice may minimize complaints about consistency. Colestipol will not dissolve. It may also be mixed with carbonated beverages slowly stirred in a large glass; however, this mixture may be associated with GI complaints. Rinse glass with a small amount of additional beverage to ensure that all the medication is taken.

➤*Tablets:* 2 to 16 g/day given once or in divided doses. The starting dosage is 2 g once or twice daily. Dosage increases of 2 g, once or twice daily, should occur at 1- or 2-month intervals. Periodically assess lipid/lipoprotein levels. If the desired effect is not obtained at recommended dose, consider combined therapy or alternate treatment.

➤*Administration:* Swallow tablets whole, 1 at a time; do not cut, chew, or crush. The tablets may be taken with plenty of water or other appropriate fluids.

➤*Concomitant medications:* Patients should take other drugs at least 1 hour before or 4 hours after colestipol to minimize possible interference with its absorption.

➤*Constipation:*

Tablets – In patients with preexisting constipation, the starting dosage should be 2 g once or twice a day.

Oral suspension – In patients with preexisting constipation, the starting dosage should be 1 packet or 1 scoop once daily for 5 to 7 days, increasing to twice daily with monitoring of constipation and of serum lipoproteins, at least twice, 4 to 6 weeks apart.

➤*Storage/Stability:* Store at controlled room temperature 20° to 25°C (68° to 77°F).

HMG-CoA Reductase Inhibitors

Refer to the general discussion of these products in the Antihyperlipidemic Agents Introduction.

Indications

Refer to individual product monographs for specific indications.

➤*Antihyperlipidemics:* Use HMG-CoA reductase inhibitors in addition to a diet restricted in saturated fat and cholesterol when diet and other nonpharmacological therapies alone have produced inadequate responses.

HMG-CoA Reductase Inhibitor Indications

Indication	Atorvastatin	Fluvastatin	Lovastatin	Pravastatin	Rosuvastatin	Simvastatin
Heterozygous familial hypercholesterolemia in adolescents	✓		✓[a]	✓		✓
Homozygous familial hyperlipidemia	✓				✓	✓
Hypertriglyceridemia[b]	✓[c]			✓[c]	✓[c]	✓[c]
Mixed dyslipidemia	✓[d]	✓[d]	✓[d,e]	✓[d]	✓[d]	✓[d]
Primary dysbetalipoproteinemia	✓[f]			✓[f]		✓[f]
Primary hypercholesterolemia	✓[g]	✓[g]	✓[g]	✓[g]	✓[g]	✓[g]
Primary prevention of coronary events			✓	✓		✓
Secondary prevention of cardiovascular event(s)		✓	✓	✓		✓

[a] Immediate-release only.
[b] Not indicated in hypertriglyceridemia patients with low or normal LDL despite elevated total cholesterol.
[c] Includes Fredrickson type IV.
[d] Includes Fredrickson types IIa and IIb.
[e] Extended-release only.
[f] Includes Fredrickson type III.
[g] Includes heterozygous familial and nonfamilial hypercholesterolemia.

Before initiating treatment with HMG-CoA reductase inhibitors, exclude secondary causes of hypercholesterolemia (eg, poorly controlled hypothyroidism, nephrotic syndrome, dysproteinemias, obstructive liver disease, other drug therapy, alcoholism). Perform a lipid profile to measure total cholesterol (total-C), LDL cholesterol (LDL-C), HDL cholesterol (HDL-C), and triglycerides (TG). Estimate LDL-C in patients with TG less than 400 mg/dL (less than 4.5 mmol/L) using the following equation: LDL-C = total-C − (⅕TG + HDL-C). Determine LDL-C by ultracentrifugation for patients with TG greater than 400 mg/dL because this equation is less accurate.

Actions

➤*Pharmacology:* These agents, also referred to as the statins, competitively inhibit 3-hydroxy-3-methyl-glutaryl-coenzyme A (HMG-CoA) reductase, the enzyme that catalyzes the conversion of HMG-CoA to mevalonate. This conversion is an early rate-limiting step in cholesterol biosynthesis. By inhibiting this enzyme, statins markedly reduce plasma concentrations of LDL and total cholesterol and to a lesser extent Apo-B and triglycerides and increase levels of HDL cholesterol. The mechanism of the LDL-lowering effect may involve both reduction of VLDL concentration and induction of the LDL receptor, leading to reduced production and/or increased catabolism of LDL. **Lovastatin** and **simvastatin** are inactive lactone prodrugs that are rapidly hydrolyzed to their active beta-hydroxyacid forms. The other statins are administered in their active forms.

These agents are highly effective in reducing total cholesterol and LDL in heterozygous familial and nonfamilial forms of hypercholesterolemia and mixed hyperlipidemia. A marked response was seen within 1 to 2 weeks, and the maximum therapeutic response occurred within 4 to 6 weeks. The response was maintained during therapy. In studies of some agents, single daily doses given in the evening were more effective than in the morning, perhaps because cholesterol is synthesized mainly at night.

➤*Pharmacokinetics:*

Pharmacokinetics of HMG-CoA Reductase Inhibitors

Drug	Bioavailability	Excretion	t½ (h)	Major metabolites	Protein binding	Effects of renal/hepatic impairment
Atorvastatin	≈ 14% absolute bioavailability; first-pass metabolism (CYP3A4)	< 2% (urine)	≈ 14[a]	Metabolized to ortho- and parahydroxylated derivatives (activity equivalent to parent)	≥ 98%	Plasma levels not affected by renal disease; markedly increased with chronic alcoholic liver disease.
Fluvastatin	98% absorbed; absolute bioavailability 24%; saturable first-pass metabolism (CYP2C9); mean relative bioavailibility is ≈ 29% for XR[b] compared with IR[c]	≈ 5% (urine) ≈ 90% (feces)	< 3 (IR) ≈ 9 (XR)	Hydroxylated metabolites (active, do not circulate systemically)	98%	Potential drug accumulation with hepatic insufficiency.
Lovastatin	≈ 30% absorbed; extensive first-pass metabolism (CYP3A4); < 5% of oral dose reaches general circulation as active inhibitors; bioavailability for XR was 190% compared with IR	10% (urine) 83% (feces)	3 to 4 (IR)	Beta-hydroxyacid; 6′-hydroxy derivative; 2 additional active metabolites	> 95%	Increased plasma concentration with severe renal disease.
Pravastatin	34% absorbed; absolute bioavailability 17%; extensive first-pass metabolism; plasma levels may not correlate with efficacy	≈ 20% (urine) 70% (feces)	77[d]	Major degradation product: 3α-hydroxy isomeric metabolite (1/10 to 1/40 activity of parent)	≈ 50%	Potential drug accumulation with renal or hepatic insufficiency. Mean AUC varied 18-fold in cirrhotic patients and peak values varied 47-fold.
Rosuvastatin	absolute biovailabilty ≈ 20%; not extensively metabolized (≈ 10%; CYP2C9)	90% (feces)	19	N-desmethyl rosuvastatin (≈ ⅙ to ½ activity of parent)	88%	Increased plasma concentrations with severe renal impairment and hepatic disease.
Simvastatin	≈ 85% absorbed; extensive first-pass metabolism (CYP3A4); < 5% of oral dose reaches general circulation	13% (urine) 60% (feces)	—	Beta-hydroxyacid; 6′-hydroxy, 6′-hydroxymethyl, 6′-exomethylene derivatives	≈ 95%	Higher systemic exposure may occur in hepatic and severe renal insufficiency.

[a] For unmetabolized atorvastatin only. The t½ is 20 to 30 hours for the active metabolites.
[b] XR = extended-release.
[c] IR = immediate-release.
[d] Parent plus metabolites.

Contraindications

Hypersensitivity to any component of these products; active liver disease or unexplained persistent elevated liver function tests; pregnancy, lactation (see Warnings).

Warnings

➤*Skeletal muscle effects:* All statins have been associated with myalgia, myopathy (ie, muscle pain, tenderness, or weakness with creatine phosphokinase [CPK] values above 10 times the ULN), and rhabdomyolysis. Uncomplicated myalgia has been reported with drugs in this class. Myopathy sometimes takes the form of rhabdomyolysis with or without acute renal failure secondary to myoglobinuria, and rare fatalities have occurred. Factors that may predispose patients to myopathy with HMG-CoA reductase inhibitors include advanced age (65 years of age or older), hypothyroidism, and renal insufficiency. The risk of myopathy/rhabdomyolysis is dose related and also increases when statins are given concomitantly with other drugs that inhibit their metabolism (eg, cyclosporine, erythromycin, or azole antifungals) or other drugs that can cause myopathy when given alone (eg, fibrates or lipid-lowering doses of niacin). Generally avoid concomitant use of these agents with statins. If combination use is being considered, carefully weigh the benefit against the potential risks of these combinations. For dosage adjustments refer to individual product monographs. See also Drug Interactions.

Consider myopathy in any patient with diffuse myalgias, muscle tenderness or weakness, and/or marked CPK elevation. Advise patients to promptly report muscle pain, tenderness, or weakness, particularly with malaise or fever. Discontinue the drug if markedly elevated CPK levels occur or if myopathy is diagnosed or suspected.

Consider temporarily withholding or discontinuing drug therapy in any patient with an acute, serious condition suggestive of a myopathy or with a risk factor predisposing them to the development of renal failure secondary to rhabdomyolysis, including the following: Severe acute infection; sepsis; hypotension; major surgery; trauma; severe metabolic, endocrine, or electrolyte disorders; uncontrolled seizures.

➤*Endocrine effects:* Statins interfere with cholesterol synthesis and lower circulating cholesterol levels and, as such, might theoretically blunt adrenal or gonadal steroid hormone production. Small declines in total testosterone with no commensurate elevation in LH have been noted with the use of **fluvastatin. Pravastatin** showed inconsistent results with regard to possible effects on basal steroid hormone levels; **atorvastatin**, **lovastatin**, **rosuvastatin**, and **simvastatin** did not reduce basal plasma cortisol concentration or basal plasma testosterone concentration or impair adrenal reserve. Appropriately evaluate patients who display clinical evidence of endocrine dysfunction. Exercise caution when administering HMG-CoA reductase inhibitors with drugs that affect steroid levels or activity, such as ketoconazole, spironolactone, and cimetidine.

➤*CNS effects:* In animals, CNS vascular lesions characterized by perivascular hemorrhage, edema, mononuclear cell infiltration of perivascular spaces and other similar CNS vascular lesions have been observed with drugs in this class.

➤*Hyperlipidemia, secondary causes:* Prior to initiating therapy, exclude secondary causes of hyperlipidemia (eg, poorly controlled hypothyroidism, nephrotic syndrome, dysproteinemias, obstructive liver disease, other drug therapy, alcoholism) and measure total-C, HDL-C, and triglycerides.

➤*Hypersensitivity reactions:* An apparent hypersensitivity syndrome has occurred rarely with drugs in this class. Refer to Management of Acute Hypersensitivity Reactions.

➤*Renal function impairment:* A single 20 mg dose of **pravastatin** was given to patients with varying degrees of renal impairment. Although no effect on pravastatin or its 3α-hydroxy-isomeric metabolite was observed, a small increase in mean AUC values and half-life was seen for the inactive hydroxylation metabolite. Closely monitor patients with renal impairment. Higher systemic exposure of **simvastatin** may occur in severe renal insufficiency. Plasma concentrations after a single dose of **lovastatin** were approximately 2-fold higher in patients with severe renal insufficiency. Plasma concentrations of **rosuvastatin** increased to a clinically significant extent (about 3-fold) in patients with severe renal impairment. Consider a dose reduction for patients on 40 mg rosuvastatin therapy with unexplained persistent proteinuria during routine urinalysis testing.

➤*Hepatic function impairment:* Use with caution in patients who consume substantial quantities of alcohol, who have a history of liver disease, or have signs suggestive of liver disease. Active liver disease or unexplained persistent transaminase elevations are contraindications for the use of HMG-CoA reductase inhibitors.

Marked persistent increases (greater than 3 times ULN occurring on 2 or more occasions) in serum transaminases have occurred. The incidence of these abnormalities with **lovastatin** was 0.1%, 0.9%, and 1.5% for 20, 40, and 80 mg, respectively. The incidence of these abnormalities with **rosuvastatin** was 0.4%, 0%, 0%, and 0.1% for 5, 10, 20, and 40 mg respectively. The incidence of these abnormalities with **fluvastatin** was 0.2%, 1.5%, and 2.7% with 20, 40, and 80 mg, respectively. The incidence of these abnormalities with **pravastatin** was less than 1.2%. The incidence of these abnormalities with simvastatin was 0.9% and 2.1% for 40 and 80 mg, respectively. The incidence of these abnormalities with **atorvastatin** was 0.2%, 0.2%, 0.6% and 2.3% for 10, 20, 40 and 80 mg, respectively. When the drug was interrupted or discontinued or the dosage was reduced, transaminase levels usually fell slowly to pretreatment levels. In pravastatin-treated patients, abnormalities did not appear to be related to treatment duration and were not associated with cholestasis.

For **lovastatin** it is recommended that liver function tests (LFTs) be performed before the initiation of treatment, 6 and 12 weeks after initiation of therapy or elevation in dose, and periodically (eg, semiannually) thereafter. For **rosuvastatin**, **fluvastatin**, and **atorvastatin**, it is recommended that LFTs be performed prior to and at 12 weeks following both the initiation of therapy and any elevation in dose, and periodically (eg, semiannually) thereafter. For **pravastatin** and **simvastatin**, perform LFTs prior to the initiation of therapy, prior to elevation of dose, and when otherwise clinically indicated. For patients titrated to the 80 mg dose of simvastatin, perform LFTs prior to titration, 3 months after titration to the 80 mg dose, and periodically thereafter (eg, semiannually) for the first year of treatment. Liver enzyme changes generally occur in the first 3 months of treatment with atorvastatin, fluvastatin, or rosuvastatin and within 3 to 12 months of starting lovastatin or simvastatin. Monitor patients who develop increased transaminase levels until the abnormalities resolve. If an increase in ALT or AST greater than 3 times ULN persists, reduce dose or withdraw therapy.

➤*Carcinogenesis:* Significantly increased incidence of uterine stromal polyps was observed in female rats given 80 mg/kg/day **rosuvastatin**. In mice, increased incidence of hepatocellular adenoma and carcinoma was observed at 200 mg/kg/day.

In mice, a statistically significant increase in the incidence of hepatocellular carcinomas and adenomas was observed at **lovastatin** doses of 500 mg/kg/day. In addition, an increase in the incidence of papilloma in nonglandular stomach mucosa was seen in mice.

Rats given **pravastatin** doses of 100 mg/kg showed an increased incidence of hepatocellular carcinomas in males (approximately 12 times the human dose of 80 mg based on body surface area). In mice, 250 and 500 mg/kg resulted in a significant increase in the incidence of lung adenomas in treated females (approximately 15- and 23-times the human dose of 80 mg based on AUC, respectively).

In mice receiving **simvastatin** (25, 100, and 400 mg/kg/day), the incidence of liver carcinoma and adenoma and lung adenoma was significantly increased. In female rats receiving simvastatin at levels approximately 11 times higher than in humans given 80 mg simvastatin based on AUC, there was a statistically significant increase in thyroid follicular adenomas.

In rats given **fluvastatin** doses of 6, 9, and 18 to 24 mg/kg/day (approximately 9 to 35 times the mean human drug levels after a 40 mg dose), a low incidence of forestomach squamous papillomas and 1 forestomach carcinoma was considered to reflect prolonged hyperplasia induced by direct contact exposure to fluvastatin rather than to systemic effects. An increased incidence of thyroid follicular cell adenomas and carcinomas occurred in males after 18 to 24 mg/kg/day. In contrast with other HMG-CoA reductase inhibitors, no hepatic adenomas or carcinomas were observed.

The carcinogenicity study with fluvastatin conducted in mice at dose levels of 0.3, 15, and 30 mg/kg/day revealed, as in rats, a statistically significant increase in forestomach squamous cell papillomas in males and females at 30 mg/kg/day and females at 15 mg/kg/day. These treatment levels represented plasma drug levels of approximately 0.05, 2, and 7 times the mean human plasma drug concentration after a 40 mg oral dose.

In rats at dose levels of 10, 30, and 100 mg/kg/day of **atorvastatin**, 2 rare muscle tumors were found in high-dose females. In one, there was a rhabdomyosarcoma and, in another, there was a fibrosarcoma. A study in mice given 100, 200, or 400 mg/kg/day found a significant increase in liver adenomas in high-dose males and liver carcinomas in high-dose females.

➤*Fertility impairment:* Drug-related testicular atrophy, decreased spermatogenesis, spermatocytic degeneration, and giant cell formation were seen in dogs given **lovastatin** 20 mg/kg/day and in dogs given **simvastatin** 10 mg/kg/day.

There was decreased fertility in male rats treated with simvastatin 25 mg/kg for 34 weeks.

Spermatidic giant cells were seen in testicles of dogs treated with **rosuvastatin** 30 mg/kg/day. This effect also was seen in monkeys as well as vacuolation of seminiferous tubular epithelium with doses of 30 mg/kg/day.

There was aplasia and aspermia in the epididymis of 2 of 10 rats treated with 100 mg/kg/day of **atorvastatin** for 3 months (16 times the human AUC at the 80 mg dose); testis weights were significantly lower at 30 and 100 mg/kg and epididymal weight was lower at 100 mg/kg. Male rats given 100 mg/kg/day for 11 weeks prior to mating had decreased sperm motility, spermatid head concentration, and increased abnormal sperm. Atorvastatin caused no adverse effects on semen parameters, or reproductive organ histopathology in dogs given doses of 10, 40, or 120 mg/kg for 2 years.

Seminal vesicles and testes were small in hamsters treated with **fluvastatin** for 3 months at 20 mg/kg/day (approximately 3 times the 40 mg human daily dose based on surface area, mg/m^2). There was tubular degeneration and aspermatogenesis in testes as well as vesiculitis of seminal vesicles. Vesiculitis of seminal vesicles and edema of the testes were also seen in rats treated for 2 years at 18 mg/kg/day (approximately 4 times the human C_{max} achieved with a 40 mg daily dose).

➤*Elderly:* For the general patient population, plasma concentrations of **fluvastatin** do not vary either as a function of age or gender, but in patients older than 70 years of age, the AUC of **lovastatin** immediate-release, **simvastatin**, and **pravastatin** is increased. Elderly patients (65 years of age and older) demonstrated a greater treatment response to LDL-C, total-C, and LDL/HDL ratio than patients younger than 65 years of age with fluvastatin. The safety and efficacy of **atorvastatin**, **rosuvastatin**, and lovastatin extended-release in patients 70 years of age and older were similar to those of patients younger than 70 years of age.

➤*Pregnancy: Category X.* Contraindicated during pregnancy. Congenital anomalies and/or skeletal malformations have occurred in animals. There are no data in pregnant women. However, because HMG-CoA reductase inhibitors can decrease synthesis of cholesterol and possibly other products of the cholesterol biosynthesis pathway, they may cause fetal harm when given to pregnant women. Give to women of childbearing age only if they are highly unlikely to conceive and have been informed of potential hazards. If a patient becomes pregnant while on the drug, immediately discontinue the drug and apprise her of the potential hazard to the fetus.

➤*Lactation:* **Atorvastatin** is excreted in the milk of rats and is likely to be excreted in breast milk; it is not known whether **lovastatin**, **simvastatin**, and **rosuvastatin** are excreted in breast milk;a small amount of **pravastatin** is excreted in breast milk; **fluvastatin** is present in breast milk in a 2:1 ratio (milk:plasma). Because of the potential for serious adverse reactions in nursing infants, caution women taking these drugs not to nurse their infants.

➤*Children:* **Atorvastatin**, **simvastatin**, and **lovastatin** are indicated for treatment of patients 10 to 17 years of age with heterozygous familial hypercholesterolemia.**Pravastatin** is indicated for the treatment of patients 8 to 18 years of age with heterozygous familial hypercholesterolemia. Safety and efficacy have not been established for atorvastatin, simvastatin, and lovastatin in prepubertal patients and patients younger than 10 years of age. Safety and efficacy have not been established in patients younger than 8 years of age for pravastatin. Safety and efficacy have not been established in patients younger than 18 years of age for **fluvastatin**. Safety and efficacy of **rosuvastatin** have not been established in pediatric patients.

Precautions

➤*Monitoring:* For **lovastatin**, perform LFTs before initiating therapy, at 6 and 12 weeks after initiation of therapy or after dose elevation, and periodically thereafter (approximately 6-month intervals). For **rosuvastatin**, **fluvastatin**, and **atorvastatin**, it is recommended that LFTs be performed prior to and at 12 weeks following both the initiation of therapy and any elevation in dose, and periodically (eg, semiannually) thereafter. For **pravastatin** and **simvastatin**, perform LFTs prior to the initiation of therapy, prior to elevation of dose, and when otherwise clinically indicated. For patients titrated to the 80 mg dose of simvastatin, perform LFTs prior to titration, 3 months after titration to the 80 mg dose, and periodically thereafter (eg, semiannually) for the first year of treatment. Pay special attention to patients who develop elevated serum transaminase levels. If transaminase levels progress, particularly if they rise to 3 times the ULN and are persistent, discontinue the drug.

Because HMG-CoA reductase inhibitors may increase CPK and transaminase levels, consider this in the differential diagnosis of chest pain in patients treated with these agents.

➤*Diet:* Before instituting therapy, attempt to control hypercholesterolemia with diet, exercise, and weight reduction in obese patients. Treat underlying medical problems.

➤*Ophthalmologic effects:* There was a high prevalence of baseline lenticular opacities in the patient population included in the early clinical trials with **lovastatin**. During these trials, new opacities appeared in both the lovastatin and placebo groups. There was no clinically significant change in visual acuity in the patients who had new opacities reported nor was any patient, including those with opacities noted at baseline, discontinued from therapy because of a decrease in visual acuity.

A 3-year, double-blind study found no clinically significant differences between lovastatin and placebo groups in the incidence, type, or progression of lenticular opacities.

➤*Homozygous familial hypercholesterolemia:* HMG-CoA reductase inhibitors are reported to be less effective in patients with rare homozygous familial hypercholesterolemia, possibly because these patients have few functional LDL receptors.

Drug Interactions

➤*CYP450 system:* **Atorvastatin**, **lovastatin**, and **simvastatin** are primarily metabolized by CYP3A4; they may interact with CYP3A4 inhibitors (eg, itraconazole, erythromycin, protease inhibitors, nefazodone, cyclosporine) thereby increasing the risk of myopathy by reducing the elimination of the HMG-CoA reductase inhibitors.

Fluvastatin is primarily metabolized by CYP2C9; it may interact with CYP2C9 inhibitors. Data indicate that **pravastatin** and **rosuvastatin** are not metabolized by CYP3A4 to a clinically significant extent.

➤*Drugs that may cause myopathy:* The risk of myopathy is increased by the following lipid-lowering drugs that can cause myopathy when given alone: Gemfibrozil, other fibrates, and niacin (at least 1 g/day).

HMG-CoA Reductase Inhibitor Drug Interactions

Precipitant drug	Object drug*		Description
Amiodarone	HMG-CoA reductase inhibitors Lovastatin Simvastatin	↑	Increased risk of myopathy with concomitant use. See Administration and Dosage of the individual monographs for dosing recommendations.
Antacids	HMG-CoA reductase inhibitors Rosuvastatin Atorvastatin	↓	Coadministration with *Maalox TC* suspension decreased **atorvastatin** levels by ≈ 35%; LDL-C reduction was not altered. Coadministration of **rosuvastatin** and an aluminum/magnesium combination antacid decreased rosuvastatin levels by 54%. Administer antacids at least 2 hours after rosuvastatin.
Azole antifungals (eg, itraconazole ketoconazole)	HMG-CoA reductase inhibitors	↑	Coadministration increased **lovastatin** levels ≈ 20-fold in healthy volunteers. Temporarily interrupt or consider reducing the dose of HMG-CoA reductase inhibitors if systemic azole antifungals are needed. The risk of myopathy is increased. **Pravastatin** and **rosuvastatin** levels are affected the least.
Bile acid sequestrants (BAS) (eg, colestipol, cholestyramine)	HMG-CoA reductase inhibitors	↓	The HMG-CoA reductase inhibitor may adsorb to the BAS, reducing the GI absorption of the HMG-CoA reductase inhibitor. A decrease in **pravastatin** (40% to 50%) and **lovastatin** bioavailability may occur. Take pravastatin 1 hour before or 4 hours after BAS. Coadministration of cholestyramine with **fluvastatin** resulted in decreased AUC and C_{max}. Take fluvastatin 4 hours after cholestyramine. Plasma levels of **atorvastatin** decreased ≈ 25% with coadministration with colestipol.
Cimetidine Ranitidine Omeprazole	HMG-CoA reductase inhibitors Fluvastatin	↑	Coadministration results in a significant increase in fluvastatin C_{max} (43% to 70%) and AUC (24% to 33%), with an 18% to 23% decrease in plasma clearance.
Cyclosporine	HMG-CoA reductase inhibitors Rosuvastatin	↑	Concurrent administration increases risk of severe myopathy or rhabdomyolysis. If coadministration cannot be avoided, consider decreasing HMG-CoA reductase inhibitor dose. See Administration and Dosage of the individual monographs for dosing information.
Diltiazem	HMG-CoA reductase inhibitors Atorvastatin Lovastatin Simvastatin	↑	Coadministration may result in elevated plasma levels of the HMG-CoA reductase inhibitor, increasing the risk of myopathy.
Fibric acid derivatives (eg, gemfibrozil)	HMG-CoA reductase inhibitors	↑	Severe myopathy or rhabdomyolysis reported with **lovastatin.** Urinary excretion and protein binding of **pravastatin** may be decreased. Avoid concurrent use. Coadministration increases the risk of myopathy. Concurrent use of gemfibrozil with pravastatin is not recommended. See Administration and Dosage of the individual monographs for dosing recommendations.
Glyburide	HMG-CoA reductase inhibitors Fluvastatin	↑	Coadministration increased glyburide C_{max}, AUC, and half life approximately 50%, 69%, and 121%, respectively. Coadministration also led to an increase in fluvastatin C_{max} and AUC by 44% and 51%, respectively. Monitor patients.
HMG-CoA reductase inhibitors Fluvastatin	Glyburide		
Isradipine	HMG-CoA reductase inhibitors Lovastatin	↓	Isradipine may increase clearance of lovastatin and its metabolites by increasing hepatic blood flow.
Macrolides Erythromycin Clarithromycin	HMG-CoA reductase inhibitors Atorvastatin Lovastatin Simvastatin	↑	Coadministration increases the risk of severe myopathy or rhabdomyolysis. **Atorvastatin** plasma levels increased by ≈ 40%.
Nefazodone	HMG-CoA reductase inhibitors Atorvastatin Lovastatin Simvastatin	↑	Increased risk of myopathy with concomitant use.
Niacin (nicotinic acid)	HMG-CoA reductase inhibitors	↑	Concurrent administration increases risk of severe myopathy or rhabdomyolysis.

HMG-CoA Reductase Inhibitor Drug Interactions

Precipitant drug	Object drug*		Description
Amiodarone	HMG-CoA reductase inhibitors Lovastatin Simvastatin	↑	Increased risk of myopathy with concomitant use. See Administration and Dosage of the individual monographs for dosing recommendations.
Phenytoin	HMG-CoA reductase inhibitors Fluvastatin	↑	A single dose of extended release phenytoin 300 mg increased mean steady-state fluvastatin C_{max} by 27% and AUC by 40% and fluvastatin increased the mean phenytoin C_{max} by 5% and AUC by 20%. Monitor patients.
HMG-CoA reductase inhibitors Fluvastatin	Phenytoin		
Propranolol	HMG-CoA reductase inhibitors Simvastatin	↔	Coadministration resulted in a significant decrease in simvastatin C_{max}, but no change in AUC.
Protease Inhibitors (eg, nelfinavir, ritonavir)	HMG-CoA reductase inhibitors Atorvastatin Lovastatin Simvastatin	↑	Concomitant use may result in elevated plasma levels, increasing the risk of myopathy. Nelfinavir is contraindicated in patients taking lovastatin or simvastatin.
Protease Inhibitors Ritonavir Saquinavir	HMG-CoA reductase inhibitors Pravastatin	↓	Concomitant use may result in decreased pravastatin plasma levels, possibly decreasing efficacy.
Rifampin	HMG-CoA reductase inhibitors Fluvastatin Simvastatin	↓	Coadministration may cause a decrease in fluvastatin C_{max} and AUC and an increase in plasma clearance.
St. John's wort	HMG-CoA reductase inhibitors Lovastatin Simvastatin	↓	Coadministration may result in decreased HMG-CoA reductase inhibitor plasma levels, possibly decreasing efficacy.
Verapamil	HMG-CoA reductase inhibitors Atorvastatin Lovastatin Simvastatin	↑	Increased risk of myopathy with concomitant use. See Administration and Dosage of the individual monographs for dosing recommendations.
HMG-CoA reductase inhibitors Fluvastatin	Diclofenac	↑	Coadministration increased the mean diclofenac C_{max} and AUC by 60% and 25%, respectively.
HMG-CoA reductase inhibitors Atorvastatin Fluvastatin Simvastatin	Digoxin	↑	Slight elevation in digoxin levels possible. Concomitant multiple doses of **atorvastatin** and digoxin increased steady-state digoxin levels by ≈ 20%. A 40 mg **fluvastatin** dose demonstrated an 11% increase in digoxin C_{max} and a slight increase in digoxin urinary clearance. Monitor digoxin patients appropriately.
HMG-CoA reductase inhibitors Atorvastatin Rosuvastatin	Oral contraceptives	↑	Coadministration with atorvastatin increased AUC for norethindrone and ethinyl estradiol by ≈ 30% and 20%, respectively.
HMG-CoA reductase inhibitors Fluvastatin Lovastatin Rosuvastatin Simvastatin	Warfarin	↑	Increased INR has been demonstrated with concomitant use of lovastatin, simvastatin, rosuvastatin, and fluvastatin. Bleeding also has been reported in a few patients concomitantly receiving lovastatin. Atorvastatin and pravastatin had no clinically significant effect on PT when given with warfarin.

* ↑ = Object drug increased. ↓ = Object drug decreased. ↔ = Undetermined clinical effect.

➤*Drug/Food interactions:* Administration of **rosuvastatin** with food decreased the rate of drug absorption by 20% as assessed by C_{max} but there was no effect on the extent of absorption as assessed by AUC. Rosuvastatin may be given with or without food.

Under fasting conditions, **lovastatin** levels are approximately ⅔ of those found when given immediately after meals; take lovastatin with meals.

Food reduces systemic bioavailability of **pravastatin**, but lipid-lowering effects of the drug are similar when taken with, or 1 hour prior to, meals; pravastatin may be taken without regard to meals.

Simvastatin levels are similar when administered in a fasting state or with food; simvastatin may be taken without regard to meals.

No therapeutic differences were evident when **fluvastatin** was administered with food compared with 4 hours postprandially. Fluvastatin may be taken without regard to meals.

LDL-C reduction is similar whether **atorvastatin** is given with or without food anytime of day. Plasma atorvastatin concentrations are lower (approximately 30% for C_{max} and AUC) following evening drug administration compared with morning. Food decreases the rate and extent of drug absorption by approximately 25% and 9%, respectively.

Grapefruit juice – Coadministration with large quantities of grapefruit juice (at least 1 quart daily) may result in increased plasma levels of lovastatin, simvastatin, or atorvastatin, increasing the risk of myopathy. Avoid concurrent use.

Adverse Reactions

These agents are generally well tolerated; adverse reactions are usually mild and transient.

In placebo-controlled trials, more than 2% of **atorvastatin**-treated patients, 1% of **fluvastatin**-treated patients, and 1.7% of **pravastatin**-treated patients discontinued treatment because of adverse events; the most common reasons for discontinuation of pravastatin were asymptomatic serum transaminase increases and mild, nonspecific GI complaints.

HMG-CoA Reductase Inhibitor Adverse Reactions (%)[a]

Adverse reaction	Atorvastatin	Fluvastatin[b]	Lovastatin[b]	Pravastatin[c]	Rosuvastatin (n = 744)	Simvastatin
CNS						
Asthenia	2.2 to 3.8	—	1.2 to 3	—	2.7	1.6
Depression	< 2	—	—	—	≥ 2	—
Dizziness	≥ 2	1.9 to 2.2	0.5 to 2	3.3	≥ 2	—
Headache	2.5 to 16.7	4.7 to 8.9	2.1 to 7	6.2	5.5	3.5
Insomnia	≥ 2	0.9 to 2.7	0.5 to 1	< 1	≥ 2	—
Paresthesia	< 2	—	0.5 to 1	< 1	≥ 2	—
GI						
Abdominal pain/cramps	2.1 to 3.8	3.7 to 4.9	2 to 2.5	5.4	≥ 2	0.9 to 3.2
Acid regurgitation	—	—	0.5 to 1	—	—	—
Constipation	1.1 to 2.5	2.3 to 3.1	2 to 3.5	4	≥ 2	2.3
Diarrhea	2.7 to 5.3	3.5 to 4.9	2.2 to 3	6.2	3.4	0.5 to 1.9
Dry mouth	—	—	0.5 to 1	—	—	—
Dysgeusia	—	—	0.8	—	—	—
Dyspepsia	1.3 to 2.8	3.5 to 7.9	1 to 1.6	—	3.4	1.1
Flatulence	1.1 to 2.8	1.4 to 2.6	3.7 to 4.5	3.3	≥ 1	0.9 to 1.9
Gastroenteritis	< 2	—	—	—	≥ 2	—
Heartburn	—	—	1.6	2.9	—	—
Nausea/Vomiting	≥ 2/< 2	2.5 to 3.2	1.9 to 2.5/0.5 to 1	7.3	3.4/≥ 1	0.4 to 1.3
Tooth disorder	—	1.4 to 2.1	—	—	≥ 1	—
GU						
Urinary abnormality	—	—	—	2.4	—	—
Urinary tract infection	≥ 2	1.6 to 2.7	2 to 3	—	2.3	—
Musculoskeletal						
Arthralgia	2 to 5.1	1.3 to 4	0.5 to 1	—	≥ 2	—
Arthritis	≥ 2	1.3 to 2.1	—	—	≥ 2	—
Back pain	1.1 to 3.8	5.7	5	—	2.6	—
Leg pain	< 2	—	0.5 to 1	—	—	—
Localized pain	—	—	0.5 to 1	10	—	—
Muscle cramps/ pain	—	—	0.6 to 1.1	—	—	—
Myalgia	1.3 to 5.6	3.8 to 5	1.8 to 3	2.7	2.8	1.2
Shoulder pain	—	—	0.5 to 1	—	—	—
Respiratory						
Bronchitis	≥ 2	1.8 to 7.6	—	—	≥ 2	—
Common cold		—	—	7	—	—
Cough	—	1.9 to 2.4	—	2.6	≥ 2	—
Pharyngitis	1.3 to 2.5	2.4 to 3.8	—	—	—	—
Rhinitis	≥ 2	1.5 to 4.7	—	4	2.2	—
Sinusitis	2.5 to 6.4	2.6 to 3.5	4 to 6	—	2	—
Upper respiratory tract infection	—	12.5 to 16.2	—	—	—	2.1
Miscellaneous						
Accidental trauma	1.3 to 4.2	4.2 to 5.1	4 to 6	—	≥ 2	—
Allergy	0.9 to 2.8	1 to 2.3	—	< 1	—	—
Alopecia	< 2	—	0.5 to 1	< 1	—	—
Blurred vision/eye irritation	—	—	0.9 to 1.2	—	—	—
Chest pain	≥ 2	—	0.5 to 1	3.7	≥ 2	—
Fatigue	—	1.6 to 2.7	—	3.8	—	—
Flu syndrome	2.2 to 3.2	5.1 to 7.1	5	2.4	2.3	—
Hypertension	< 2	—	—	—	≥ 2	—
Infection	2.8 to 10.3	—	11 to 16	—	≥ 2	—
Pain	—	—	3 to 5	—	≥ 2	—
Peripheral edema	≥ 2	—	—	—	≥ 2	—
Rash/pruritus	1.1 to 3.9/< 2	1.6 to 2.3	0.8 to 1.3/0.5 to 1	4/< 1	≥ 2/≥ 1	0.6/0.5

[a] All events. Data are pooled from separate studies and are not necessarily comparable.
[b] Immediate-release and extended-release combined.
[c] Includes short-term and long-term studies.

The following adverse effects have also been reported with drugs in this class (includes postmarketing).

➤*Cardiovascular:* Angina pectoris; arrhythmia; palpitation; phlebitis; postural hypotension; syncope; vasodilation.

➤*CNS:* Abnormal dreams; anxiety; dysfunction of certain cranial nerves (eg, alteration of taste, impairment of extraocular movement, facial paresis); emotional lability; facial paralysis; hyperkinesia; hypertonia; hypesthesia; incoordination; memory loss; migraine; peripheral nerve palsy; peripheral neuropathy; psychic disturbances; somnolence; torticollis; tremor; vertigo.

➤*Dermatologic:* Acne; contact dermatitis; eczema; seborrhea; skin ulcer; sweating; urticaria; various skin changes (eg, nodules, discoloration, dryness of skin/mucous membranes, changes in hair/nails).

➤*GI:* Anorexia; biliary pain; cheilitis; cholestatic jaundice; cirrhosis; colitis; duodenal ulcer; dysphagia; enteritis; eructation; esophagitis; fatty change in liver; fulminant hepatic necrosis; gastritis; glossitis; gum hemorrhage; hemorrhage; hepatitis, including chronic active hepatitis; hepatoma; increased appetite; melena; pancreatitis; periodontal abscess; rectal mouth ulceration; stomach ulcer; stomatitis; tenesmus; ulcerative stomach.

➤*GU:* Abnormal ejaculation; albuminuria; breast enlargement; cystitis; dysuria; epididymitis; erectile dysfunction; fibrocystic breast; gynecomastia; hematuria; impotence; kidney calculus; loss of libido; metrorrhagia; nocturia; nephritis; renal failure; urinary frequency, incontinence, retention, and urgency; vaginal or uterine hemorrhage.

➤*Hematologic/Lymphatic:* Anemia; ecchymosis; lymphadenopathy; petechiae; thrombocytopenia.

➤*Hypersensitivity:* An apparent hypersensitivity syndrome has been reported rarely including 1 or more of the following features: Anaphylaxis; angioedema; arthritis; asthenia; chills; dermatomyositis; dyspnea; eosinophilia; erythema multiforme (eg, Stevens-Johnson syndrome); erythrocyte sedimentation rate (ESR) increase; fever; flushing; hemolytic anemia; leukopenia; lupus erythematosus-like syndrome; malaise; photosensitivity; polymyalgia rheumatica; positive antinuclear antibody (ANA); purpura; thrombocytopenia; toxic epidermal necrolysis; urticaria; vasculitis.

➤*Metabolic/Nutritional:* Diabetes mellitus; gout; hyperglycemia; hypoglycemia; increased CPK; weight gain.

➤*Musculoskeletal:* Bursitis; myalgia; myasthenia; myopathy; myositis; pathological fracture; rhabdomyolysis (see Warnings); tendinous contracture; tenosynovitis.

➤*Ophthalmic:* Amblyopia; dry eyes; eye hemorrhage; glaucoma; ophthalmoplegia; progression of cataracts (lens opacities; see Precautions); refraction disorder.

➤*Respiratory:* Asthma; dyspnea; epistaxis; pneumonia.

➤*Special senses:* Deafness; parosmia; taste loss; taste perversion; tinnitus.

➤*Miscellaneous:* Face edema; fever; generalized edema; malaise; neck rigidity; neck pain; pelvic pain; photosensitivity reaction.

➤*Lab test abnormalities:* Alkaline phosphatase and bilirubin; CPK (11% with **lovastatin**, levels at least twice normal); γ-glutamyl transpeptidase; increased serum transaminases (AST, ALT); liver function test abnormalities; thyroid function test abnormalities.

Overdosage

➤*Symptoms:* Five healthy volunteers received up to 200 mg **lovastatin** as a single dose without clinically significant adverse events. A few cases of accidental overdosage have been reported; no patients had any specific symptoms, and all recovered without sequelae. Maximum dose was 5 to 6 g.

The maximum single oral dose of **fluvastatin** capsules received by healthy volunteers was 80 mg. No clinically significant adverse experiences were seen at this dose. The maximum dose administered with an extended-release formulation was 640 mg for 2 weeks. This dose was not well tolerated and produced a variety of GI complaints and an increase in transaminase values.

A few cases of overdosage with **simvastatin** have occurred; no patients had any specific symptoms; all recovered without sequelae. The maximum dose taken was 3.6 g.

➤*Treatment:* Treat symptomatically and institute supportive measures as required. Refer to General Management of Acute Overdosage. The dialyzability of these agents and their metabolites is unknown.

There is no specific treatment for HMG-CoA reductase inhibitor overdosage. Because of extensive drug binding to plasma proteins, hemodialysis is not expected to significantly enhance atorvastatin clearance. Hemodialysis does not significantly enhance rosuvastatin clearance.

Patient Information

May cause photosensitivity (sensitivity to sunlight). Avoid prolonged exposure to the sun and other ultraviolet light. Use sunscreens and wear protective clothing until tolerance is determined.

If patient becomes pregnant, discontinue the drug immediately to avoid harmful effects in the developing fetus.

Promptly report unexplained muscle pain, tenderness, or weakness, especially if accompanied by fever or malaise.

Follow dietary and exercise recommendations.

Take **lovastatin** with meals; **fluvastatin**, **pravastatin**, **simvastatin**, **atorvastatin**, and **rosuvastatin** may be taken without regard to meals.

Advise patients to swallow lovastatin ER tablets whole; do not chew, crush, or cut.

When patients are taking rosuvastatin with an aluminum and magnesium hydroxide combination antacid, advise the patient to take the antacid at least 2 hours after rosuvastatin administration.

Advise patients to inform a physician of any medications they are taking before taking any new ones.

LOVASTATIN (Mevinolin)

Rx	**Lovastatin** (Various, eg, Eon, Mylan, Purepac, Teva)	**Tablets**: 10 mg	May contain lactose. In 30s, 60s, 100s, 500s, and 1000s.
Rx	**Mevacor** (Merck)		Lactose. (MSD 730 MEVACOR). Peach, octagonal. In unit-of-use 60s.
Rx	**Lovastatin** (Various, eg, Eon, Mylan, Purepac, Teva)	**Tablets**: 20 mg	May contain lactose. In 30s, 60s, 90s, 100s, 500s, and 1000s.
Rx	**Mevacor** (Merck)		Lactose. (MSD 731 MEVACOR). Lt. blue, octagonal. In 1000s, 10,000s, unit-of-use 60s and 90s, and UD 100s.
Rx	**Lovastatin** (Various, eg, Eon, Mylan, Purepac, Teva)	**Tablets**: 40 mg	May contain lactose. In 30s, 60s, 90s, 100s, 500s, and 1000s.
Rx	**Mevacor** (Merck)		Lactose. (MSD 732 MEVACOR). Green, octagonal. In 1000s, 10,000s, and unit-of-use 60s and 90s.
Rx	**Altoprev** (Andrx)	**Tablets, extended-release**: 10 mg	Sugar, lactose. (10). Dk. orange. In 30s.
		20 mg	Sugar, lactose. (20). Orange. In 30s.
		40 mg	Sugar, lactose. (40). Peach. In 30s.
		60 mg	Sugar, lactose. (60). Lt. peach. In 30s.

LOVASTATIN — ORAL

For complete and comparative prescribing information, refer to the HMG-CoA Reductase Inhibitors group monograph.

Indications

Therapy with lovastatin should be a component of multiple-risk factor intervention in those individuals with dyslipidemia at risk for atherosclerotic vascular disease. Lovastatin should be used in addition to a diet restricted in saturated fat and cholesterol as part of a treatment strategy to lower total cholesterol (total-C) and low-density lipoprotein cholesterol (LDL-C) to target levels when the response to diet and other nonpharmacological measures alone has been inadequate to reduce risk.

➤*Primary prevention of coronary heart disease (CHD):* In individuals without symptomatic cardiovascular disease, average to moderately elevated total-C and LDL-C, and below average high-density lipoprotein cholesterol (HDL-C), lovastatin is indicated to reduce the risk of the following: Myocardial infarction (MI); unstable angina; coronary revascularization procedures.

➤*Coronary heart disease:* Lovastatin is indicated to slow the progression of coronary atherosclerosis in patients with coronary heart disease as part of a treatment strategy to lower total-C and LDL-C to target levels.

➤*Hypercholesterolemia:* Therapy with lipid-altering agents should be a component of multiple-risk factor intervention in those individuals at significantly increased risk for atherosclerotic vascular disease due to hypercholesterolemia. Lovastatin is indicated as an adjunct to diet for the reduction of elevated total-C and LDL-C levels in patients with primary hypercholesterolemia (types IIa and IIb), when the response to diet restricted in saturated fat and cholesterol and to other nonpharmacological measures alone has been inadequate.

Extended-release tablets – Lovastatin is indicated as an adjunct to diet for the reduction of elevated total-C, LDL-C, Apo B, and TG, and to increase HDL-C in patients with primary hypercholesterolemia (heterozygous familial and non-familial) and mixed dyslipidemia (Fredrickson types IIa and IIb, see information below) when the response to diet restricted in saturated fat and cholesterol and to other non-pharmacological measures alone has been inadequate.

Administration and Dosage

➤*Approved by the FDA:* August 13, 1987.

The patient should be placed on a standard cholesterol-lowering diet before receiving lovastatin and should continue on this diet during treatment with lovastatin.

➤*Immediate-release tablets:* Lovastatin immediate-release tablets should be given with meals.

Adults – The usual recommended starting dose is 20 mg once a day given with the evening meal. The recommended dosing range is 10 to 80 mg/day in single or 2 divided doses; the maximum recommended dose is 80 mg/day. Doses should be individualized according to the recommended goal of therapy. Patients requiring reductions in LDL-C of 20% or more to achieve their goal should be started on 20 mg/day of lovastatin. A starting dose of 10 mg may be considered for patients requiring smaller reductions. Adjustments should be made at intervals of 4 weeks or more.

Cholesterol levels should be monitored periodically and consideration should be given to reducing the dosage of lovastatin if cholesterol levels fall significantly below the targeted range.

Adolescent patients (10 to 17 years of age) with heterozygous familial hypercholesterolemia – The recommended dosing range is 10 to 40 mg/day; the maximum recommended dose is 40 mg/day. Doses should be individualized according to the recommended goal of therapy. Patients requiring reductions in LDL-C of 20% or more to achieve their goal should be started on 20 mg/day of lovastatin. A starting dose of 10 mg may be considered for patients requiring smaller reductions. Adjustments should be made at intervals of 4 weeks or more.

➤*Extended-release tablets:* The usual recommended starting dose is 20, 40, or 60 mg once daily given in the evening at bedtime. The recommended dosing range is 10 to 60 mg/day, in single doses. Doses should be individualized according to the recommended goal of therapy. A starting dose of 10 mg may be considered for patients requiring smaller reductions. Adjustments should be made at intervals of 4 weeks or more.

The extended-release tablets should be swallowed whole and not crushed, chewed, or cut.

Monitor cholesterol levels periodically and consider reducing the dosage of the extended-release tablets if cholesterol levels fall significantly below the targeted range.

➤*Dosage in patients taking cyclosporine:* In patients taking cyclosporine concomitantly with lovastatin immediate- or extended-release, therapy should begin with 10 mg of lovastatin and should not exceed 20 mg/day.

➤*Dosage in patients taking amiodarone or verapamil:* In patients taking amiodarone or verapamil concomitantly with lovastatin immediate- or extended-release, the dose should not exceed 40 mg/day.

➤*Concomitant lipid-lowering therapy:* Lovastatin is effective alone or when used concomitantly with bile-acid sequestrants. If lovastatin is used in combination with gemfibrozil, other fibrates, or lipid-lowering doses (greater than or equal to 1 g/day) of niacin, the dose of lovastatin should not exceed 20 mg/day.

LOVASTATIN — ORAL

Extended-release tablets – Use of lovastatin extended-release tablets with fibrates or niacin should generally be avoided. However, if lovastatin extended-release tablets are used in combination with fibrates or niacin, the dose of lovastatin extended-release should generally not exceed 20 mg.

➤*Dosage in renal function impairment:* In patients with severe renal insufficiency (Ccr less than 30 mL/min), dosage increases above 20 mg/day should be carefully considered and, if deemed necessary, implemented cautiously.

➤*Storage / Stability:*

Immediate-release tablets – Store between 5° to 30°C (41° to 86°F). Lovastatin tablets must be protected from light and stored in a well-closed, light-resistant container.

Extended-release tablets – Store at controlled room temperature 20° to 25°C (68° to 77°F). Avoid excessive heat and humidity.

SIMVASTATIN

Rx	**Zocor** (Merck)	**Tablets:** 5 mg	Lactose. (MSD 726 ZOCOR). Buff, shield shape. Film-coated. In 1000s, unit-of-use 30s, 60s, and 90s, and UD 100s.
		10 mg	Lactose. (MSD 735 ZOCOR). Peach, shield shape. Film-coated. In 1000s, 10,000s, unit-of-use 30s and 90s, and UD 100s.
		20 mg	Lactose. (MSD 740 ZOCOR). Tan, shield shape. Film-coated. In 1000s, 10,000s, unit-of-use 30s, 60s, and 90s, and UD 100s.
		40 mg	Lactose. (MSD 749 ZOCOR). Brick red, shield shape. Film-coated. In 1000s, unit-of-use 30s, 60s, and 90s, and UD 100s.
		80 mg	Lactose. (543 80). Brick red, capsule shape. Film-coated. In 1000s, unit-of-use 30s, 60s, and 90s, and UD 100s.

SIMVASTATIN— ORAL

For complete and comparative prescribing information, refer to the HMG-CoA Reductase Inhibitors group monograph.

Indications

➤*Adolescents 10 to 17 years of age with heterozygous familial hypercholesterolemia:* As an adjunct to diet to reduce total and LDL cholesterol and Apo-B levels in adolescent boys and girls who are at least 1 year postmenarche, 10 to 17 years of age, with heterozygous familial hypercholesterolemia if after an adequate trial of diet therapy LDL cholesterol remains 190 mg/dL or greater or LDL cholesterol remains 160 mg/dL or greater and there is a positive family history of premature cardiovascular disease or 2 or more other cardiovascular disease risk factors are present in the adolescent patient.

➤*Hyperlipidemia:* To reduce elevated total and LDL cholesterol, Apo-B, and triglyceride levels; to increase HDL cholesterol in patients with primary hypercholesterolemia (heterozygous familial and nonfamilial) and mixed dyslipidemia (Fredrickson types IIa and IIb); treatment of hypertriglyceridemia (Fredrickson type IV hyperlipidemia); primary dysbetalipoproteinemia (Fredrickson type III hyperlipidemia); to reduce total and LDL cholesterol in homozygous familial hypercholesterolemia as an adjunct to other lipid-lowering treatments (eg, LDL apheresis) or if such treatments are unavailable.

➤*Primary and secondary prevention of coronary events:* In patients at high risk of coronary events because of existing coronary heart disease, diabetes, peripheral vessel disease, history of stroke or other cerebrovascular disease, to reduce the risk of total mortality by reducing coronary death; to reduce the risk of nonfatal MI and stroke; to reduce the need for coronary and noncoronary revascularization procedures.

Administration and Dosage

➤*Approved by the FDA:* December 23, 1991.

Place patient on a standard cholesterol-lowering diet. In patients with CHD or at high risk of CHD, simvastatin can be started simultaneously with diet. Individualize the dosage according to the goals of therapy and the patient's response.

➤*Dose:* The recommended usual starting dose is 20 to 40 mg once a day in the evening. For patients at high risk for a CHD event because of existing CHD, diabetes, peripheral vessel disease, history of stroke or other cerebrovascular disease, the recommended starting dose is 40 mg/day. Perform lipid determinations after 4 weeks of therapy and periodically thereafter.

➤*Homozygous familial hypercholesterolemia:* The recommended dosage is 40 mg/day in the evening or 80 mg/day in 3 divided doses of 20 mg, 20 mg, and an evening dose of 40 mg. Use simvastatin as an adjunct to other lipid-lowering treatments (eg, LDL apheresis) in these patients or if such treatments are unavailable.

➤*Adolescents 10 to 17 years of age with heterozygous familial hypercholesterolemia:* Usual recommended starting dose is 10 mg once a day in the evening. The recommended dosing range is 10 to 40 mg/day; maximum dose is 40 mg/day. Individualize dose according to recommended goal of therapy. Adjust at intervals of 4 weeks or more.

➤*Concomitant cyclosporine:* In patients taking cyclosporine concomitantly with simvastatin, begin therapy with 5 mg/day; do not exceed 10 mg/day.

➤*Concomitant amiodarone or verapamil:* In patients taking amiodarone or verapamil concomitantly with simvastatin, the dose should not exceed 20 mg/day.

➤*Concomitant lipid-lowering therapy:* Simvastatin is effective alone or when used concomitantly with bile acid sequestrants. The combined use of simvastatin with gemfibrozil should be avoided unless the benefit of further alteration in lipid levels is likely to outweigh the increased risk of this drug combination. However, if simvastatin is used in combination with gemfibrozil, the dose of simvastatin generally should not exceed 10 mg/day. Use with caution with other fibrates or lipid-lowering doses (1 g/day or more) of niacin.

➤*Renal function impairment:* Exercise caution when simvastatin is administered to patients with severe renal insufficiency. Initiate therapy in such patients with 5 mg/day and monitor closely.

➤*Storage / Stability:* Store between 5° and 30°C (41° and 86°F).

PRAVASTATIN SODIUM

Rx	**Pravachol** (Bristol-Myers Squibb)	**Tablets:** 10 mg	Lactose. (P PRAVACHOL 10). Pink-to-peach, rectangular. In 90s.
		20 mg	Lactose. (P PRAVACHOL 20). Yellow, rectangular. In 90s, 1000s, and UD 100s.
		40 mg	Lactose, FD & C Blue No 1. (P PRAVACHOL 40). Green, rectangular. In 90s and UD 100s.
		80 mg	Lactose. (BMS 80). Yellow, oval. In 90s and 500s.

PRAVASTATIN SODIUM— ORAL

For complete and comparative prescribing information, refer to the HMG-CoA Reductase Inhibitors group monograph.

Indications

➤*Primary prevention of coronary events:* In hypercholesterolemic patients without clinically evident coronary heart disease (CHD), to reduce the risk of MI; to reduce the risk of undergoing myocardial revascularization procedures; to reduce the risk of cardiovascular mortality with no increase in death from noncardiovascular causes.

➤*Secondary prevention of cardiovascular events:* In patients with clinically evident CHD, to reduce the risk of total mortality by reducing coronary death, MI, undergoing myocardial revascularization procedures, stroke, and stroke/transient ischemic attack, and slow the progression of coronary atherosclerosis.

➤*Hyperlipidemia:* As an adjunct to diet for the reduction of elevated total and LDL cholesterol, Apo-B, and triglyceride levels and to increase HDL cholesterol in patients with primary hypercholesterolemia and mixed dyslipidemia (Fredrickson types IIa and IIb). As adjunctive therapy to diet for the treatment of patients with elevated serum triglyceride levels (Fredrickson type IV). For the treatment of patients with primary dysbetalipoproteinemia (Fredrickson type III) who do not respond adequately to diet.

➤*Adolescents (8 years of age and older) with heterozygous familial hypercholesterolemia:* As an adjunct to diet and lifestyle modification for treatment of heterozygous familial hypercholesterolemia in children and adolescents 8 years of age and older if after an adequate trial of diet LDL-C remains 190 mg/dL or greater or LDL-C remains 160 mg/dL or greater AND there is a positive family history of premature cardiovascular disease or 2 or more other CVD risk factors are present in the patient.

Administration and Dosage

➤*Approved by the FDA:* October 31, 1991.

Place the patient on a standard cholesterol-lowering diet before starting pravastatin, and continue on this diet during treatment.

Pravastatin can be administered as a single dose at any time of the day, with or without food. Because the maximal effect of a given dose is seen within

PRAVASTATIN SODIUM— ORAL

4 weeks, perform periodic lipid determinations at this time and adjust dosage according to the patient's response to therapy and established treatment guidelines.

➤*Adults:* The recommended starting dose is 40 mg once/day. If a daily dose of 40 mg does not achieve desired cholesterol levels, 80 mg once/day is recommended.

➤*Pediatric patients:*

Children 8 to 13 years of age – 20 mg once daily. Doses greater than 20 mg have not been studied in this patient population.

Adolescents 14 to 18 years of age – The recommended starting dose is 40 mg once daily. Doses greater than 40 mg have not been studied in this patient population. Re-evaluate children and adolescents treated with pravastatin in adulthood and make appropriate changes to their cholesterol-lowering regimen to achieve adult goals for LDL-C.

➤*Concomitant immunosuppressants:* In patients taking immunosuppressive drugs such as cyclosporine concomitantly with pravastatin, begin therapy with pravastatin 10 mg once/day at bedtime and titrate to higher doses with caution. Most patients treated with this combination received a maximum pravastatin dose of 20 mg/day.

➤*Concomitant lipid-lowering therapy:* The lipid-lowering effects of pravastatin on total and LDL cholesterol are enhanced when combined with a bile acid binding resin. When administering a bile acid binding resin (eg, cholestyramine, colestipol) and pravastatin, give pravastatin either 1 hour or more before or at least 4 hours following the resin. Avoid the combined use of pravastatin and fibrates unless the benefit of further alterations in lipid levels is likely to outweigh the increased risk of this drug combination.

➤*Renal/Hepatic function impairment:* Use a starting dose of 10 mg/day in significant renal or hepatic function impairment.

➤*Storage/Stability:* Store at 25°C (77°F); excursions permitted to 15° to 30°C (59° to 86°F). Keep tightly closed; protect from light and moisture.

ROSUVASTATIN CALCIUM

Rx	**Crestor** (AstraZeneca)	**Tablets:** 5 mg (as base)	Lactose. (ZD4522 5). Yellow. In 90s.
		10 mg (as base)	Lactose. (ZD4522 10). Pink. In 90s and UD 100s.
		20 mg (as base)	Lactose. (ZD4522 20). Pink. In 90s and UD 100s.
		40 mg (as base)	Lactose. (ZD4522 40). Pink, oval. In 30s and UD 100s.

ROSUVASTATIN CALCIUM — ORAL

For complete and comparative prescribing information, refer to the HMG-CoA Reductase Inhibitors group monograph.

Indications

Rosuvastatin calcium is indicated:

1.) As an adjunct to diet to reduce elevated total cholesterol (total-C), low-density lipoprotein cholesterol (LDL-C), apolipoprotein B (ApoB), non-high-density lipoprotein cholesterol (HDL-C), and triglyceride (TG) levels and to increase HDL-C in patients with primary hypercholesterolemia (heterozygous familial and nonfamilial) and mixed dyslipidemia (Fredrickson Type IIa and IIb).
2.) As an adjunct to diet for the treatment of patients with elevated serum TG levels (Fredrickson type IV).
3.) To reduce LDL-C, total-C, and ApoB in patients with homozygous familial hypercholesterolemia as an adjunct to other lipid-lowering treatments (eg, LDL apheresis) or if such treatments are unavailable.

Administration and Dosage

➤*Approved by the FDA:* August 13, 2003.

The patient should be placed on a standard cholesterol-lowering diet before receiving rosuvastatin calcium and should continue on this diet during treatment. Rosuvastatin calcium can be administered as a single dose at any time of day, with or without food.

➤*Hypercholesterolemia (heterozygous familial and nonfamilial) and mixed dyslipidemia (Fredrickson type IIa and IIb):* The dose range for rosuvastatin calcium is 5 to 40 mg once daily. Therapy with rosuvastatin calcium should be individualized according to goal of therapy and response. The usual recommended starting dose of rosuvastatin calcium is 10 mg once daily. Initiation of therapy with 5 mg once daily may be considered for patients requiring less aggressive LDL-C reductions or who have predisposing factors for myopathy. Factors that may predispose patients to myopathy with HMG-CoA reductase inhibitors include advanced age (greater than or equal to 65 years of age), hypothyroidism, and renal insufficiency. The incidence of myopathy increased at doses of rosuvastatin above the recommended dosage range. For patients with marked hypercholesterolemia (LDL-C greater than 190 mg/dL) and aggressive lipid targets, a 20 mg starting dose may be considered. The 40 mg dose of rosuvastatin calcium should be reserved for those patients who have not achieved goal LDL-C at 20 mg. After initiation, or upon titration of rosuvastatin calcium, lipid levels should be analyzed within 2 to 4 weeks and dosage adjusted accordingly.

➤*Homozygous familial hypercholesterolemia:* The recommended starting dose of rosuvastatin calcium is 20 mg once daily in patients with homozygous FH. The maximum recommended daily dose is 40 mg. Rosuvastatin calcium should be used in these patients as an adjunct to other lipid-lowering treatments (eg, LDL apheresis) or if such treatments are unavailable. Response to therapy should be estimated from preapheresis LDL-C levels.

➤*Dosage in patients taking cyclosporine:* In patients taking cyclosporine, therapy should be limited to rosuvastatin calcium 5 mg once daily.

➤*Concomitant lipid-lowering therapy:* The effect of rosuvastatin calcium on LDL-C and total-C may be enhanced when used in combination with a bile acid-binding resin. If rosuvastatin calcium is used in combination with gemfibrozil, the dose of rosuvastatin calcium should be limited to 10 mg once daily.

➤*Dosage in patients with renal insufficiency:* No modification of dosage is necessary for patients with mild to moderate renal insufficiency. For patients with severe renal impairment (Ccr less than 30 mL/min per 1.73 m^2) not on hemodialysis, dosing of rosuvastatin calcium should be started at 5 mg once daily and not to exceed 10 mg once daily.

➤*Special populations:*

- Rosuvastatin should be prescribed with caution in patients with predisposing factors for myopathy, such as renal impairment, advanced age, and hypothyroidism.
- Patients should be advised to promptly report unexplained muscle pain, tenderness, or weakness, particularly if accompanied by malaise or fever. Rosuvastatin therapy should be discontinued if markedly elevated CK levels occur or myopathy is diagnosed or suspected.
- The risk of myopathy during treatment with rosuvastatin may be increased with concurrent administration of other lipid-lowering therapies or cyclosporine. The benefit of further alterations in lipid levels by the combined use of rosuvastatin with fibrates or niacin should be carefully weighed against the potential risks of this combination. Combination therapy with rosuvastatin and gemfibrozil should generally be avoided.
- The risk of myopathy during treatment with rosuvastatin may be increased in circumstances which increase rosuvastatin drug levels.
- Rosuvastatin therapy should also be temporarily withheld in any patient with an acute, serious condition suggestive of myopathy or predisposing to the development of renal failure secondary to rhabdomyolysis (eg, sepsis, hypotension, major surgery, trauma, severe metabolic, endocrine, and electrolyte disorders, or uncontrolled seizures).

➤*Storage/Stability:* Store at controlled room temperature, 20° to 25°C (68° to 77°F). Protect from moisture.

FLUVASTATIN SODIUM

Rx	**Lescol** (Novartis)	**Capsules:** 20 mg (as base)	Benzyl alcohol, parabens, EDTA. (20 LESCOL). Brown/Light brown. In 30s and 100s.
		40 mg (as base)	Benzyl alcohol, parabens, EDTA. (40 LESCOL). Brown/Gold. In 30s and 100s.
Rx	**Lescol XL** (Novartis)	**Tablets, extended-release:** 80 mg (as base)	(Lescol XL 80). Yellow. Film-coated. In 30s and 100s.

FLUVASTATIN SODIUM — ORAL

For complete and comparative prescribing information, refer to the HMG-CoA Reductase Inhibitors group monograph.

Indications

Therapy with lipid-altering agents should be used in addition to a diet restricted in saturated fat and cholesterol.

➤*Hypercholesterolemia (heterozygous familial and nonfamilial) and mixed dyslipidemia:* Fluvastatin sodium capsules and extended-release tablets are indicated to reduce elevated total cholesterol (Total-C), low-density lipoprotein cholesterol (LDL), triglycerides (TG), and apolipoprotein B (Apo B) levels, and to increase high-density lipoprotein cholesterol (HDL) in patients with primary hypercholesterolemia and mixed dyslipid-

FLUVASTATIN SODIUM — ORAL

emia (Fredrickson Type IIa and IIb) whose response to dietary restriction of saturated fat and cholesterol and other nonpharmacological measures has not been adequate.

➤*Secondary prevention of coronary events:* In patients with coronary heart disease, fluvastatin sodium capsules and extended-release tablets are indicated to reduce the risk of undergoing coronary revascularization procedures.

➤*Atherosclerosis:* Fluvastatin sodium capsules and extended-release tablets are also indicated to slow the progression of coronary atherosclerosis in patients with coronary heart disease as part of a treatment strategy to lower total and LDL cholesterol to target levels.

Administration and Dosage

➤*Approved by the FDA:* December 31, 1993.

The patient should be placed on a standard cholesterol-lowering diet before receiving fluvastatin sodium and should continue on this diet during treatment with fluvastatin sodium.

For patients requiring LDL reduction to a goal of greater than or equal to 25%, the recommended starting dose is 40 mg as 1 capsule, 80 mg as 1 fluvastatin sodium extended-release tablet administered as a single dose in the evening or 80 mg in divided doses of the 40 mg capsule given twice daily. For patients requiring LDL reduction to a goal of less than 25%, a starting dose of 20 mg may be used. The recommended dosing range is 20 to 80 mg/day. Fluvastatin sodium capsules or extended-release tablets may be taken without regard to meals, since there are no apparent differences in the lipid-lowering effects of fluvastatin sodium administered with the evening meal or 4 hours after the evening meal. Since the maximal reductions in LDL of a given dose are seen within 4 weeks, periodic lipid determinations should be performed and dosage adjustment made according to the patient's response to therapy and established treatment guidelines. The therapeutic effect of fluvastatin sodium capsules or extended-release tablets is maintained with prolonged administration.

➤*Concomitant therapy:* Lipid-lowering effects on total cholesterol and LDL cholesterol are additive when fluvastatin sodium is combined with a bile-acid binding resin or niacin. When administering a bile-acid resin (eg, cholestyramine) and fluvastatin sodium, fluvastatin sodium should be administered at bedtime, at least 2 hours following the resin to avoid a significant interaction due to drug binding to resin. Myopathy and rhabdomyolysis (with or without acute renal failure) have been reported when another HMG-CoA reductase inhibitor was used in combination with immunosuppressive drugs, gemfibrozil, erythromycin, or lipid-lowering doses of nicotinic acid. Concomitant therapy with HMG-CoA reductase inhibitors and these agents is generally not recommended.

➤*Dosage in renal function impairment:* Because fluvastatin sodium is cleared hepatically with less than 6% of the administered dose excreted into the urine, dose adjustments for mild to moderate renal impairment are not necessary. Fluvastatin has not been studied at doses greater than 40 mg in patients with severe renal impairment; therefore caution should be exercised when treating such patients at higher doses.

➤*Storage/Stability:* Store at 25°C (77°F); excursions permitted to 15° to 30°C (59° to 86°F). Dispense in a tight container. Protect from light.

ATORVASTATIN CALCIUM

Rx	**Lipitor** (Pfizer)	**Tablets**: 10 mg (as base)	Lactose. (PD 155 10). White, elliptical. Film-coated. In 90s, 5,000s, and UD 100s.
		20 mg (as base)	Lactose. (PD 156 20). White, elliptical. Film-coated. In 90s, 5,000s, and UD 100s.
		40 mg (as base)	Lactose. (PD 157 40). White, elliptical. Film-coated. In 90s and 500s.
		80 mg (as base)	Lactose. (PD 158 80). White, elliptical. Film-coated. In 90s and 500s.

ATORVASTATIN CALCIUM — ORAL

For complete and comparative prescribing information, refer to the HMG-CoA Reductase Inhibitors group monograph.

Indications

➤*Heterozygous familial hypercholesterolemia in children 10 to 17 years of age:* As an adjunct to diet to reduce total cholesterol (total-C), low-density lipoprotein cholesterol (LDL-C), and apolipoprotein B (apo B) levels in boys and postmenarchal girls, 10 to 17 years of age with heterozygous familial hypercholesterolemia if, after an adequate trial of diet therapy, LDL-C remains 190 mg/dL or greater or LDL-C remains 160 mg/dL or greater and there is a positive family history of premature cardiovascular disease or 2 or more other cardiovascular disease risk factors are present in the pediatric patient.

➤*Homozygous familial hypercholesterolemia:* To reduce total-C and LDL-C in patients with homozygous familial hypercholesterolemia as an adjunct to other lipid-lowering treatments (eg, LDL apheresis) or if such treatments are unavailable.

➤*Hypercholesterolemia (heterozygous familial and nonfamilial) and mixed dyslipidemia (Frederickson types IIa and IIb):* As an adjunct to diet to reduce elevated total-C, LDL-C, apo B, and triglyceride levels, and to increase high-density lipoprotein cholesterol (HDL-C) in patients with primary hypercholesterolemia (heterozygous familial and nonfamilial) and mixed dyslipidemia (Frederickson types IIa and IIb).

➤*Hyperlipoproteinemia type III:* For the treatment of patients with primary hyperlipoproteinemia type III who do not respond adequately to diet.

➤*Hypertriglyceridemia:* As an adjunct to diet for the treatment of patients with elevated serum triglyceride levels (Frederickson type IV).

➤*Prevention of cardiovascular disease:* In adult patients without clinically evident coronary heart disease, but with multiple risk factors for coronary heart disease, such as age, smoking, hypertension, low HDL-C, or a family history of early coronary heart disease, atorvastatin is indicated to reduce the risk of myocardial infarction (MI) and stroke, and to reduce the risk for revascularization procedures and angina.

In patients with type 2 diabetes and without clinically evident coronary heart disease, but with multiple risk factors for coronary heart disease, such as retinopathy, albuminuria, smoking, or hypertension, atorvastatin is indicated to reduce the risk of MI and stroke.

➤*National Cholesterol Education Program (NCEP) guidelines:* Therapy with lipid-altering agents should be a component of multiple-risk-factor intervention in individuals at increased risk for atherosclerotic vascular disease caused by hypercholesterolemia. Use lipid-altering agents, in addition to a diet restricted in saturated fat and cholesterol, only when the response to diet and other nonpharmacological measures has been inadequate (see the following NCEP guidelines).

NCEP Treatment Guidelines: LDL-C Goals and Cutpoints for Therapeutic Lifestyle Changes and Drug Therapy in Different Risk Categories

Risk category	LDL-C goal (mg/dL)	LDL level at which to initiate therapeutic lifestyle changes (mg/dL)	LDL level at which to consider drug therapy (mg/dL)
Coronary heart disease or coronary heart disease risk equivalents (10-year risk > 20%)	< 100	≥ 100	≥ 130 (100 to 129: drug optional)[a]
≥ 2 risk factors (10-year risk ≤ 20%)	< 130	≥ 130	10-year risk 10% to 20%: ≥ 130; 10-year risk < 10%: ≥ 160
0 to 1 risk factor[b]	< 160	≥ 160	≥ 190 (160 to 189: LDL-lowering drug optional)

[a] Some authorities recommend use of LDL-lowering drugs in this category if an LDL-C level of < 100 mg/dL cannot be achieved by therapeutic lifestyle changes. Others prefer use of drugs that primarily modify triglycerides and HDL-C (eg, nicotinic acid, fibrate). Clinical judgement also may call for deferring drug therapy in this subcategory.

[b] Almost all people with 0 to 1 risk factor have 10-year risk < 10%; thus, 10-year risk assessment in people with 0 to 1 risk factor is not necessary.

After the LDL-C goal has been achieved, if the triglyceride level is still greater than or equal to 200 mg/dL, non–HDL-C (total-C minus HDL-C) becomes a secondary target of therapy. Non–HDL-C goals are set 30 mg/dL higher than LDL-C goals for each risk category.

NCEP classification for children – The NCEP classification of cholesterol levels in pediatric patients with a familial history of hypercholesterolemia or premature cardiovascular disease is summarized in the following table:

NCEP Classification of Cholesterol Levels in Children

Category	Total-C (mg/dL)	LDL-C (mg/dL)
Acceptable	< 170	< 110
Borderline	170 to 199	110 to 129
High	≥ 200	≥ 130

Administration and Dosage

➤*Approved by the FDA:* December 17, 1996.

➤*Diet:* The patient should be placed on a standard cholesterol-lowering diet before receiving atorvastatin and should continue on this diet during treatment with atorvastatin.

HMG-CoA Reductase Inhibitors

ATORVASTATIN CALCIUM — ORAL

➤*Heterozygous familial hypercholesterolemia in children 10 to 17 years of age:* The recommended starting dosage of atorvastatin is 10 mg/day; the maximum recommended dosage is 20 mg/day (doses greater than 20 mg have not been studied in this patient population). Doses should be individualized according to the recommended goal of therapy. Adjustments should be made at intervals of 4 weeks or more.

➤*Homozygous familial hypercholesterolemia:* The dosage of atorvastatin in patients with homozygous familial hypercholesterolemia is 10 to 80 mg daily. Atorvastatin should be used as an adjunct to other lipid-lowering treatments (eg, LDL apheresis) in these patients or if such treatments are unavailable.

➤*Hypercholesterolemia (heterozygous familial and nonfamilial) and mixed dyslipidemia (Fredrickson types IIa and IIb):* The recommended starting dosage of atorvastatin is 10 or 20 mg once daily. Patients who require a large reduction in LDL-C (more than 45%) may be started at 40 mg once daily. The dosage range is 10 to 80 mg once daily. Atorvastatin can be administered as a single dose at any time of the day, with or without food. The starting dose and maintenance doses of atorvastatin should be individualized according to patient characteristics such as goal of therapy and response. After initiation and/or upon titration of atorvastatin, lipid levels should be analyzed within 2 to 4 weeks and dosage adjusted accordingly.

Because the goal of treatment is to lower LDL-C, the NCEP recommends that LDL-C levels be used to initiate and assess treatment response. Only if LDL-C levels are not available should total-C be used to monitor therapy.

➤*Concomitant therapy:* Atorvastatin may be used in combination with a bile acid-binding resin for additive effect. The combination of 3-hydroxy-3-methylgluatryl coenzyme A (HMG-CoA) reductase inhibitors and fibrates (eg, gemfibrozil) should generally be avoided.

The risk of myopathy during treatment with drugs in this class is increased with coadministration of fibric acid derivatives, cyclosporine, erythromycin, niacin, or azole antifungals. Health care providers considering combined therapy with atorvastatin and fibric acid derivatives, erythromycin, immunosuppressive drugs, azole antifungals, or lipid-lowering doses of niacin should carefully weigh the potential benefits and risks and carefully monitor patients for any signs or symptoms of muscle pain, tenderness, or weakness, particularly during the initial months of therapy and during any periods of upward dosage titration of either drug. Periodic creatine phosphokinase (CPK) determinations may be considered in such situations, but there is no assurance that such monitoring will prevent the occurrence of severe myopathy.

➤*Storage/Stability:* Store at controlled room temperature 20° to 25°C (68° to 77°F).

Fibric Acid Derivatives

GEMFIBROZIL

Rx	**Gemfibrozil** (Various, eg, Apotex, Mylan, UDL, Warner Chilcott)	**Tablets**: 600 mg	In 60s, 500s, blister pack 25s, and UD 100s.
Rx	**Lopid** (Parke-Davis)		(LOPID P-D 737). Parabens. White, scored, elliptical. Film coated. In 60s, 500s, and UD 100s.

GEMFIBROZIL — ORAL

Refer to the general discussion of these products in the Antihyperlipidemic Agents Introduction.

Indications

➤*Hypertriglyceridemia :* Gemfibrozil is indicated as adjunctive therapy to diet for treatment of adult patients with very high elevations of serum triglyceride levels (types IV and V hyperlipidemia) who present a risk of pancreatitis and who do not respond adequately to a determined dietary effort to control them. Patients who present such risk typically have serum triglycerides over 2000 mg/dL and have elevations of very low-density lipoproteins (VLDL) cholesterol and fasting chylomicrons (type V hyperlipidemia). Subjects who consistently have total serum or plasma triglycerides less than 1000 mg/dL are unlikely to present a risk of pancreatitis. Gemfibrozil therapy may be considered for those subjects with triglyceride elevations between 1000 and 2000 mg/dL who have a history of pancreatitis or of recurrent abdominal pain typical of pancreatitis. It is recognized that some type IV patients with triglycerides less than 1000 mg/dL may, through dietary or alcoholic indiscretion, convert to a type V pattern with massive triglyceride elevations accompanying fasting chylomicronemia, but the influence of gemfibrozil therapy on the risk of pancreatitis in such situations has not been adequately studied. Drug therapy is not indicated for patients with type I hyperlipoproteinemia, who have elevations of chylomicrons and plasma triglycerides, but who have normal levels of VLDL. Inspection of plasma refrigerated for 14 hours is helpful in distinguishing types I, IV, and V hyperlipoproteinemia.

➤*Prevention of cardiovascular disease:* Gemfibrozil is indicated as adjunctive therapy to diet for reducing the risk of developing coronary heart disease only in type IIb patients without history of or symptoms of existing coronary heart disease who have had an inadequate response to weight loss, dietary therapy, exercise, and other pharmacologic agents (such as bile acid sequestrants and nicotinic acid, known to reduce low-density lipoprotein [LDL] and raise high-density lipoprotein [HDL] cholesterol) and who have the following triad of lipid abnormalities: Low HDL cholesterol levels in addition to elevated LDL cholesterol and elevated triglycerides. The National Cholesterol Education Program has defined a serum HDL cholesterol value that is consistently less than 35 mg/dL as constituting an independent risk factor for coronary heart disease. Patients with significantly elevated triglycerides should be closely observed when treated with gemfibrozil. In some patients with high triglyceride levels, treatment with gemfibrozil is associated with a significant increase in LDL cholesterol. Because of potential toxicity such as malignancy, gallbladder disease, abdominal pain leading to appendectomy, and other abdominal surgeries, an increased incidence in noncoronary mortality, and the 44% relative increase during the trial period in age-adjusted all-cause mortality seen with the chemically and pharmacologically related drug, clofibrate, the potential benefit of gemfibrozil in treating type IIa patients with elevations of LDL cholesterol only is not likely to outweigh the risks. Gemfibrozil is also not indicated for the treatment of patients with low HDL cholesterol as their only lipid abnormality.

The initial treatment for dyslipidemia is dietary therapy specific for the type of lipoprotein abnormality. Excess body weight and excess alcohol intake may be important factors in hypertriglyceridemia and should be managed prior to any drug therapy. Physical exercise can be an important ancillary measure, and has been associated with rises in HDL cholesterol. Diseases contributory to hyperlipidemia, such as hypothyroidism or diabetes mellitus, should be looked for and adequately treated. Estrogen therapy is sometimes associated with massive rises in plasma triglycerides, especially in subjects with familial hypertriglyceridemia. In such cases, discontinuation of estrogen therapy may obviate the need for specific drug therapy of hypertriglyceridemia. The use of drugs should be considered only when reasonable attempts have been made to obtain satisfactory results with nondrug methods. If the decision is made to use drugs, the patient should be instructed that this does not reduce the importance of adhering to diet.

Administration and Dosage

➤*Approved by the FDA:* September 27, 1993.

The recommended dose for adults is 1200 mg administered in 2 divided doses 30 minutes before the morning and evening meal.

Actions

➤*Pharmacology:* The mechanism of action of gemfibrozil has not been definitely established. In man, gemfibrozil has been shown to inhibit peripheral lipolysis and to decrease the hepatic extraction of free fatty acids, thus reducing hepatic triglyceride production. Gemfibrozil inhibits synthesis and increases clearance of VLDL carrier apolipoprotein B, leading to a decrease in VLDL production.

➤*Pharmacokinetics:*

Absorption/Distribution – Gemfibrozil is well absorbed from the GI tract after oral administration. Peak plasma levels occur in 1 to 2 hours with a plasma half-life of 1.5 hours following multiple doses. Gemfibrozil is completely absorbed after oral administration of gemfibrozil tablets, reaching peak plasma concentrations 1 to 2 hours after dosing. Gemfibrozil pharmacokinetics are affected by the timing of meals relative to time of dosing. In 1 study, both the rate and extent of absorption of the drug were significantly increased when administered 0.5 hour before meals. Average AUC was reduced by 14% to 44% when gemfibrozil was administered after meals compared to 0.5 hour before meals. In a subsequent study, rate of absorption of gemfibrozil was maximum when administered 0.5 hour before meals with the C_{max} 50% to 60% greater than when given either with meals or fasting. In this study, there were no significant effects on AUC of timing of dose relative to meals.

Gemfibrozil is highly bound to plasma proteins and there is potential for displacement interactions with other drugs such as with HMG-CoA-reductase inhibitors and anticoagulants.

Metabolism – Gemfibrozil mainly undergoes oxidation of a ring methyl group to successively form a hydroxymethyl and a carboxyl metabolite.

Excretion – Approximately 70% of the administered human dose is excreted in the urine, mostly as the glucuronide conjugate, with less than 2% excreted as unchanged gemfibrozil. Six percent (6%) of the dose is accounted for in the feces.

Contraindications

Hepatic or severe renal dysfunction, including primary biliary cirrhosis; preexisting gallbladder disease; hypersensitivity to gemfibrozil.

Combination therapy of gemfibrozil with cerivastatin is contraindicated in patients due to the increased risk of myopathy and rhabdomyolysis.

Warnings

➤*Gallstones:* A gallstone prevalence substudy of 450 Helsinki Heart Study participants showed a trend toward a greater prevalence of gallstones during the study within the gemfibrozil treatment group (7.5% vs 4.9% for the placebo group, a 55% excess for the gemfibrozil group). A trend toward a greater incidence of gallbladder surgery was observed for the gemfibrozil group (17 vs 11 subjects, a 54% excess). This result did not differ statistically from the increased incidence of cholecystectomy observed in the WHO study in the group treated with clofibrate. Both clofibrate and gemfibrozil may

GEMFIBROZIL — ORAL

increase cholesterol excretion into the bile leading to cholelithiasis. If cholelithiasis is suspected, gallbladder studies are indicated. Gemfibrozil therapy should be discontinued if gallstones are found.

Because a reduction of mortality from coronary heart disease has not been demonstrated and because liver and interstitial cell testicular tumors were increased in rats, gemfibrozil should be administered only to those patients described in Indications. If a significant serum lipid response is not obtained, gemfibrozil should be discontinued.

➤*Concomitant anticoagulants:* Caution should be exercised when anticoagulants are given in conjunction with gemfibrozil. The dosage of the anticoagulant should be reduced to maintain the prothrombin time at the desired level to prevent bleeding complications. Frequent prothrombin determinations are advisable until it has been definitely determined that the prothrombin level has stabilized.

➤*Skeletal muscle effects:* Concomitant therapy with gemfibrozil and an HMG-CoA reductase inhibitor is associated with an increased risk of skeletal muscle toxicity manifested as rhabdomyolysis, markedly elevated creatine kinase (CPK) levels and myoglobinuria, leading in a high proportion of cases to acute renal failure and death. Because of an observed marked increased risk of myopathy and rhabdomyolysis, the specific combination of gemfibrozil and cerivastatin is absolutely contraindicated. In patients who have had an unsatisfactory lipid response to either drug alone, the benefit of combined therapy with gemfibrozil and HMG-CoA reductase inhibitors other than cerivastatin does not outweigh the risks of severe myopathy, rhabdomyolysis, and acute renal failure. The use of fibrates alone, including gemfibrozil, may occasionally be associated with myositis. Patients receiving gemfibrozil and complaining of muscle pain, tenderness, or weakness should have prompt medical evaluation for myositis, including serum creatine kinase level determination. If myositis is suspected or diagnosed, gemfibrozil therapy should be withdrawn.

➤*Cataracts:* Subcapsular bilateral cataracts occurred in 10% and unilateral in 6.3% of male rats treated with gemfibrozil at 10 times the human dose.

➤*Renal function impairment:* There have been reports of worsening renal insufficiency upon the addition of gemfibrozil therapy in individuals with baseline plasma creatinine greater than 2 mg/dL. In such patients, the use of alternative therapy should be considered against the risks and benefits of a lower dose of gemfibrozil.

➤*Hepatic function impairment:* Abnormal liver function tests have been observed occasionally during gemfibrozil administration, including elevations of AST, ALT, LDH, bilirubin, and alkaline phosphatase. These are usually reversible when gemfibrozil is discontinued. Therefore, periodic liver function studies are recommended and gemfibrozil therapy should be terminated if abnormalities persist.

➤*Carcinogenesis:* Long-term studies have been conducted in rats at 0.2 and 1.3 times the human exposure (based on AUC). The incidence of benign liver nodules and liver carcinomas was significantly increased in high-dose male rats. The incidence of liver carcinomas increased also in low-dose males, but this increase was not statistically significant (P = 0.1). Male rats had a dose-related and statistically significant increase of benign Leydig-cell tumors. The higher dose female rats had a significant increase in the combined incidence of benign and malignant liver neoplasms. Long-term studies have been conducted in mice at 0.1 and 0.7 times the human exposure (based on AUC). There were no statistically significant differences from controls in the incidence of liver tumors, but the doses tested were lower than those shown to be carcinogenic with other fibrates.

➤*Mutagenesis:* Electron microscopy studies have demonstrated a florid hepatic peroxisome proliferation following gemfibrozil administration to the male rat. An adequate study to test for peroxisome proliferation has not been done in humans but changes in peroxisome morphology have been observed. Peroxisome proliferation has been shown to occur in humans with either of 2 other drugs of the fibrate class when liver biopsies were compared before and after treatment in the same individual.

➤*Fertility impairment:* Administration of approximately 2 times the human dose (based on surface area) to male rats for 10 weeks resulted in a dose-related decrease of fertility. Subsequent studies demonstrated that this effect was reversed after a drug-free period of about 8 weeks, and it was not transmitted to the offspring.

➤*Pregnancy: Category C.* Gemfibrozil has been shown to produce adverse effects in rats and rabbits at doses between 0.5 and 3 times the human dose (based on surface area). There are no adequate and well-controlled studies in pregnant women. Gemfibrozil should be used during pregnancy only if the potential benefit justifies the potential risk to the fetus. Administration of gemfibrozil to female rats at 2 times the human dose (based on surface area) before and throughout gestation caused a dose-related decrease in conception rate and, at the high dose, an increase in stillborns and a slight reduction in pup weight during lactation. There were also dose-related increased skeletal variations. Anophthalmia occurred, but rarely.

Administration of 0.6 and 2 times the human dose (based on surface area) of gemfibrozil to female rats from gestation day 15 through weaning caused dose-related decreases in birth weight and suppressions of pup growth during lactation.

Administration of 1 and 3 times the human dose (based on surface area) of gemfibrozil to female rabbits during organogenesis caused a dose-related decrease in litter size and, at the high dose, an increased incidence of parietal bone variations.

➤*Lactation:* It is not known whether this drug is excreted in human milk. Because many drugs are excreted in human milk and because of the potential for tumorigenicity shown for gemfibrozil in animal studies, a decision should be made whether to discontinue nursing or to discontinue the drug, taking into account the importance of the drug to the mother.

➤*Children:* Safety and efficacy in children have not been established.

Precautions

➤*Monitoring:*

Initial therapy – Laboratory studies should be done to ascertain that the lipid levels are consistently abnormal. Before instituting gemfibrozil therapy, every attempt should be made to control serum lipids with appropriate diet, exercise, weight loss in obese patients, and control of any medical problems such as diabetes mellitus and hypothyroidism that are contributing to the lipid abnormalities.

Continued therapy – Periodic determination of serum lipids should be obtained, and the drug withdrawn if lipid response is inadequate after 3 months of therapy.

Hepatic function – Abnormal liver function tests have been observed occasionally during gemfibrozil administration, including elevations of AST, ALT, LDH, bilirubin, and alkaline phosphatase. These are usually reversible when gemfibrozil is discontinued. Periodic liver function studies are recommended and gemfibrozil therapy should be terminated if abnormalities persist.

➤*Lab test abnormalities:* Mild hemoglobin, hematocrit, and white blood cell decreases have been observed in occasional patients following initiation of gemfibrozil therapy. However, these levels stabilize during long-term administration. Rarely, severe anemia, leukopenia, thrombocytopenia, and bone marrow hypoplasia have been reported. Therefore, periodic blood counts are recommended during the first 12 months of gemfibrozil administration.

Drug Interactions

Gemfibrozil Drug Interactions

Precipitant drug	Object drug[a]		Description
Gemfibrozil	Anticoagulants	↑	Gemfibrozil may enhance the pharmacologic effects of these agents. If this combination cannot be avoided, observe for signs of bleeding and monitor prothrombin time.
Gemfibrozil	Cyclosporine	↓	Pharmacologic effect may be decreased. Monitor whole blood cyclosporine concentrations. Adjust the dose of cyclosporine as indicated and observe the patient for signs of toxicity or rejection when gemfibrozil therapy is stopped or started.
Gemfibrozil	HMG-CoA reductase inhibitors	↑	Rhabdomyolysis has been associated with the administration of HMG-CoA reductase inhibitors and gemfibrozil. If combined use cannot be evaded, frequently monitor for symptoms and signs of rhabdomyolysis and myopathy.
Gemfibrozil	Sulfonylureas	↑	Increased hypoglycemic effects may occur. Monitor blood glucose levels when gemfibrozil is stopped or started from the treatment regimen. Adjust glyburide dose accordingly.

[a] ↑ = Object drug increased. ↓ = Object drug decreased.

Adverse Reactions

In the double-blind, controlled phase of the primary prevention component of the Helsinki Heart Study, 2046 patients received gemfibrozil for up to 5 years. In that study, the following adverse reactions were statistically more frequent in subjects in the gemfibrozil group:

Adverse reaction	Gemfibrozil (n = 2046)	Placebo (n = 2035)
	Frequency in percent of subjects	
GI reactions	34.2%	23.8%
Dyspepsia	19.6%	11.9%
Abdominal pain	9.8%	5.6%
Acute appendicitis (histologically confirmed in most cases)	1.2%	0.6%
Atrial fibrillation	0.7%	0.1%
Adverse reactions reported by > 1% of subjects, but without a significant difference between groups		
Diarrhea	7.2%	6.5%
Fatigue	3.8%	3.5%

GEMFIBROZIL — ORAL

Adverse reaction	Gemfibrozil (n = 2046)	Placebo (n = 2035)
	Frequency in percent of subjects	
Nausea/vomiting	2.5%	2.1%
Eczema	1.9%	1.2%
Rash	1.7%	1.3%
Vertigo	1.5%	1.3%
Constipation	1.4%	1.3%
Headache	1.2%	1.1%

➤*Gallbladder surgery:* Gallbladder surgery was performed in 0.9% of gemfibrozil and 0.5% of placebo subjects in the primary prevention component, a 64% excess, which is not statistically different from the excess of gallbladder surgery observed in the clofibrate compared to the placebo group of the WHO study. Gallbladder surgery was also performed more frequently in the gemfibrozil group compared to placebo (1.9% vs 0.3%, $P = 0.07$) in the secondary prevention component. A statistically significant increase in appendectomy in the gemfibrozil group was seen also in the secondary prevention component (6 on gemfibrozil vs 0 on placebo, $P = 0.014$).

Nervous system and special senses adverse reactions were more common in the gemfibrozil group. These included hypesthesia, paresthesias, and taste perversion. Other adverse reactions that were more common among gemfibrozil treatment group subjects but where a causal relationship was not established include cataracts, peripheral vascular disease, and intracerebral hemorrhage.

From other studies it seems probable that gemfibrozil is causally related to the occurrence of musculoskeletal symptoms, and to abnormal liver function tests and hematologic changes.

Reports of viral and bacterial infections (eg, common cold, cough, urinary tract infections) were more common in gemfibrozil treated patients in other controlled clinical trials of 805 patients. Additional adverse reactions that have been reported for gemfibrozil are listed below by system. These are categorized according to whether a causal relationship to treatment with gemfibrozil is probable or not established.

➤*Adverse events in which a causal relationship to treatment with gemfibrozil is probable:*

CNS – Dizziness; somnolence; paresthesia; peripheral neuritis; decreased libido; depression; headache.

Dermatologic – Exfoliative dermatitis; rash; dermatitis; pruritus.

GI – Cholestatic jaundice.

GU – Impotence.

Hematologic – Anemia; leukopenia; bone marrow hypoplasia; eosinophilia.

Hypersensitivity – Angioedema; laryngeal edema; urticaria.

Lab test abnormalities – Increased creatine phosphokinase; increased bilirubin; increased liver transaminases (AST, ALT); increased alkaline phosphatase.

Musculoskeletal – Myopathy; myasthenia; myalgia; painful extremities; arthralgia; synovitis; rhabdomyolysis (see Warnings).

Ophthalmic – Blurred vision.

➤*Adverse events in which a causal relationship to treatment with gemfibrozil has not been established:*

Cardiovascular – Extrasystoles.

CNS – Confusion; convulsions; syncope.

Dermatologic – Alopecia; photosensitivity.

GI – Pancreatitis; hepatoma; colitis.

GU – Decreased male fertility; renal dysfunction.

Hematologic – Thrombocytopenia.

Hypersensitivity – Anaphylaxis; Lupus-like syndrome; vasculitis.

Lab test abnormalities – Positive antinuclear antibody.

Ophthalmic – Retinal edema.

Miscellaneous – Weight loss.

Overdosage

➤*Symptoms:* There have been reported cases of overdosage with gemfibrozil. In one case, a 7-year-old child recovered after ingesting up to 9 g of gemfibrozil. Symptoms reported with overdosage were abdominal cramps, abnormal liver function tests, diarrhea, increased CPK, joint and muscle pain, nausea and vomiting.

➤*Treatment:* Symptomatic supportive measures should be taken if an overdose occurs.

FENOFIBRATE

Rx	**Tricor** (Abbott)	**Tablets:** 48 mg	Lactose, sucrose. (FI). Yellow. In 90s.
Rx	**Triglide** (First Horizon)	**Tablets:** 50 mg	Lactose. (FH 50). Off-white. In 90s.
Rx	**Lofibra** (Gate)	**Tablets:** 54 mg	Lactose. (93 7330). Yellow. Film coated. In 90s.
Rx	**Tricor** (Abbott)	**Tablets:** 145 mg	Lactose, sucrose. (FO). White. In 90s.
Rx	**Lofibra** (Gate)	**Tablets:** 160 mg	Lactose. (93 7331). White to off-white, oval. Film coated. In 90s.
Rx	**Triglide** (First Horizon)		Lactose. (FH 160). Off-white. In 90s.
Rx	**Antara** (Reliant)	**Capsules:** 43 mg (micronized fenofibrate)	Sugar spheres. (43 ANTARA). Lt. green/white to off-white. In 30s and 100s.
Rx	**Lofibra** (Gate)	**Capsules:** 67 mg (micronized fenofibrate)	Lactose. (Lofibra 67 mg Gate 322). Opaque pink. In 100s.
Rx	**Antara** (Reliant)	**Capsules:** 130 mg (micronized fenofibrate)	Sugar spheres. (130 ANTARA). Dk. green/white. In 30s and 100s.
Rx	**Lofibra** (Gate)	**Capsules:** 134 mg (micronized fenofibrate)	Lactose. (Lofibra 134 mg Gate 323). Opaque lt. blue. In 100s.
		200 mg (micronized fenofibrate)	Lactose. (Lofibra 200 mg Gate 324). Opaque orange. In 100s.

FENOFIBRATE — ORAL

Refer to the general discussion of these agents in the Antihyperlipidemic Agents introduction.

Indications

➤*Hypercholesterolemia:* Adjunctive therapy to diet for the reduction of low-density lipoprotein cholesterol (LDL-C), total cholesterol, triglycerides, and apolipoprotein B and to increase high-density lipoprotein cholesterol (HDL-C) in adult patients with primary hypercholesterolemia or mixed dyslipidemia (Fredrickson types IIa and IIb). Use lipid-altering agents in addition to a diet restricted in saturated fat and cholesterol when response to diet and nonpharmacological interventions alone has been inadequate.

Drug therapy is not indicated for patients with type I hyperlipoproteinemia who have elevations of chylomicrons and plasma triglycerides, but normal levels of very low-density lipoprotein (VLDL). Inspection of plasma refrigerated for 14 hours is helpful in distinguishing types I, IV, and V hyperlipoproteinemia.

➤*Hypertriglyceridemia:* Adjunctive therapy to diet for treatment of adult patients with hypertriglyceridemia (Fredrickson types IV and V hyperlipidemia). Improving glycemic control in diabetic patients showing fasting chylomicronemia will usually reduce fasting triglycerides and eliminate chylomicronemia, thereby obviating the need for pharmacologic intervention.

Markedly elevated levels of serum triglycerides (eg, more than 2,000 mg/dL) may increase the risk of developing pancreatitis. The effect of fenofibrate therapy on reducing this risk has not been adequately studied.

➤*National Cholesterol Education Program Guidelines:*

National Cholesterol Education Program Guidelines

Risk category	LDL goal (mg/dL)	LDL level at which to initiate therapeutic lifestyle changes (mg/dL)	LDL level at which to consider drug therapy (mg/dL)
CHD[a] or CHD risk equivalents (10-year risk > 20%)	< 100	≥ 100	≥ 130 (100 to 129: drug optional)[b]
2 + risk factors (10-year risk ≤ 20%)	< 130	≥ 130	10-year risk 10% to 20%: ≥ 130 10-year risk < 10%: ≥ 160
0 to 1 risk factor[c]	< 160	≥ 160	≥ 190 (160 to 189: LDL-lowering drug optional)

[a] CHD = coronary heart disease.
[b] Some authorities recommend use of LDL-lowering drugs in this category if an LDL-C level of less than 100 mg/dL cannot be achieved by therapeutic lifestyle changes. Others prefer use of drugs that primarily modify triglycerides and HDL-C (eg, nicotinic acid, fibrates). Clinical judgment also may call for deferring drug therapy in this subcategory.
[c] Almost all people with 0 to 1 risk factor have 10-year risk less than 10%; thus, 10-year risk assessment in people with 0 to 1 risk factor is not necessary.

FENOFIBRATE — ORAL

After the LDL-C goal has been achieved, if the triglyceride levels are still higher than 200 mg/dL, non-HDL-C (total-C minus HDL-C) becomes the secondary target of therapy. Non-HDL-C goals are set 30 mg/dL higher than LDL-C goals for each risk category.

➤*Unlabeled uses:* Treatment of hyperuricemia.

Administration and Dosage

➤*Approved by the FDA:* February 13, 1998.

Patients should be placed on an appropriate lipid-lowering diet before receiving fenofibrate and should continue this diet during treatment. Give capsules and tablets with meals, optimizing the bioavailability of the medication. *Antara* and *Tricor* can be given without regard to meals.

➤*Dosage:* Individualize dosage according to patient response and adjust if necessary following repeat lipid determinations at 4- to 8-week intervals. Monitor lipid levels periodically and consider reducing the dose of fenofibrate if lipid levels fall significantly below the targeted range. Withdraw therapy in patients who do not have an adequate response after 2 months of treatment with the maximum recommended dose.

Fenofibrate Dosing Recommendations

Dosing regimen	*Antara*	*Lofibra* tablets[a]	*Lofibra* capsules[a]	*Tricor*	*Triglide*
Primary hypercholesterolemia or mixed hyperlipidemia	Initial dosage: 130 mg/day	Initial dosage: 160 mg/day	Initial dosage: 200 mg/day	Initial dosage: 145 mg/day	Initial dosage: 160 mg/day
Hypertriglyceridemia	Initial dosage: 43 to 130 mg/day	Initial dosage: 54 to 160 mg/day	Initial dosage: 67 to 200 mg/day	Initial dosage: 48 to 145 mg/day	Initial dosage: 50 to 160 mg/day
	Max dosage: 130 mg/day	Max dosage: 160 mg/day	Max dosage: 200 mg/day	Max dosage: 145 mg/day	Max dosage: 160 mg/day
Renal function impairment	Initial dosage: 43 mg/day	Initial dosage: 54 mg/day	Initial dosage: 67 mg/day	Initial dosage: 48 mg/day	Initial dosage: 50 mg/day
Elderly	Initial dosage: 43 mg/day	Initial dosage: 54 mg/day	Initial dosage: 67 mg/day	Initial dosage: 48 mg/day	Initial dosage: 50 mg/day

[a] Taken with meals.

➤*Nonpharmacologic therapy:* The initial treatment for dyslipidemia is dietary therapy specific for the type of lipoprotein abnormality. Excess body weight and excess alcoholic intake may be important factors in hypertriglyceridemia and should be addressed prior to any drug therapy. Physical exercise can be an important ancillary measure.

Consider the use of drugs only when reasonable attempts have been made to obtain satisfactory results with nondrug methods. If the decision is made to use drugs, instruct the patient that drug therapy does not reduce the importance of adhering to diet.

➤*Renal function impairment:* See the preceding table. Increase dose only after evaluation of the effects on renal function and lipid levels.

➤*Storage/Stability:* Store at controlled room temperature, 20° to 25°C (68° to 77°F); excursions permitted to 15° to 30° C (59° to 86°F). Dispense in a tightly closed container. Keep out of the reach of children. Protect from moisture.

Actions

➤*Pharmacology:* Fenofibric acid, the active metabolite of fenofibrate, produces reductions in total cholesterol, LDL-C, apolipoprotein B, total triglycerides, and triglyceride-rich lipoprotein in treated patients. In addition, treatment with fenofibrate results in increases in HDL and apoproteins apoAI and apoAII.

Through its mechanism of activating the peroxisome proliferator activated receptor α (PPARα), fenofibrate increases lipolysis and elimination of triglyceride-rich particles from plasma by activating lipoprotein lipase and reducing production of apoprotein C-III (an inhibitor of lipoprotein lipase activity). The resulting fall in triglycerides produces an alteration in the size and composition of LDL from small, dense particles (which are thought to be atherogenic because of their susceptibility to oxidation), to large buoyant particles. These larger particles have a greater affinity for cholesterol receptors and are catabolized rapidly.

Activation of PPARα also induces an increase in the synthesis of apoproteins, A-I, A-II, and HDL-C.

Fenofibrate also reduces serum uric acid levels in hyperuricemic and healthy individuals by increasing the urinary excretion of uric acid.

➤*Pharmacokinetics:*

Absorption/Distribution – Fenofibrate is well absorbed from the GI tract; absorption of micronized fenofibrate is increased when administered with food. Peak plasma levels of fenofibric acid occur within 4 to 8 hours (depending on product) after administration, and steady-state plasma levels are achieved within 5 to 7 days of dosing. Accumulation following multiple doses does not occur. Serum protein binding is approximately 99%.

Metabolism – Fenofibrate is rapidly hydrolyzed by esterases to the active metabolite, fenofibric acid; no unchanged fenofibrate is detected in plasma. Fenofibric acid is primarily conjugated with glucuronic acid and then excreted in urine. A small amount of fenofibric acid is reduced at the carbonyl moiety to a benzhydrol metabolite, which is, in turn, conjugated with glucuronic acid and excreted in urine.

Excretion – Fenofibrate is eliminated with a half-life of 20 to 23 hours, allowing once-daily administration. It is mainly excreted in urine in the form of metabolites, primarily fenofibric acid and fenofibric acid glucuronide; about 60% of the dose appears in urine and 25% in feces.

Contraindications

Hepatic or severe renal dysfunction, including primary biliary cirrhosis; unexplained, persistent liver function abnormality; preexisting gallbladder disease (see Warnings); hypersensitivity to fenofibrate.

Warnings

➤*Hepatic effects:* Fenofibrate is associated with increases in serum transaminase (AST or ALT). Increases to more than 3 times the upper limit of normal (ULN) occurred in 5.3% of patients taking fenofibrate.

When transaminase determinations were followed after discontinuation of treatment or during continued treatment, a return to normal limits was usually observed. In an 8-week dose-ranging study, the incidence of ALT or AST elevations to at least 3 times the ULN was 13% in patients receiving dosages equivalent to 134 to 200 mg/day (*Lofibra*, micronized), 107 to 160 mg/day (*Lofibra*), 87 to 130 mg/day (*Antara*), or 96 to 145 mg/day (*Tricor*) and was 0% in those receiving dosages equivalent to 43 mg (*Antara*), 54 mg (*Lofibra*), 67 mg (*Lofibra*, micronized) or less, or placebo. Hepatocellular, chronic active, and cholestatic hepatitis associated with fenofibrate therapy have been reported after exposures of weeks to several years. In extremely rare cases, cirrhosis has been reported in association with chronic active hepatitis. Perform regular periodic monitoring of liver function and discontinue therapy if enzyme levels persist above 3 times the ULN (see Precautions).

➤*Diabetic patients:* Improving glycemic control in diabetic patients showing fasting chylomicronemia will usually reduce fasting triglycerides and eliminate chylomicronemia, thereby obviating the need for pharmacologic intervention.

➤*Cholelithiasis:* Fenofibrate, like clofibrate and gemfibrozil, may increase cholesterol excretion into the bile, leading to cholelithiasis. If cholelithiasis is suspected, gallbladder studies are indicated. Discontinue therapy if gallstones are found.

➤*Hypersensitivity reactions:* Acute hypersensitivity reactions, including severe skin rashes requiring patient hospitalization and treatment with steroids, have occurred very rarely during treatment with fenofibrate, including rare spontaneous reports of Stevens-Johnson syndrome and toxic epidermal necrolysis. Urticaria was seen in 1.1% versus 0% and rash in 1.4% versus 0.8% of fenofibrate and placebo patients, respectively, in controlled trials. Refer to Management of Acute Hypersensitivity Reactions.

➤*Renal function impairment:* In patients with creatinine clearance (Ccr) less than 50 mL/min, the rate of clearance of fenofibric acid was greatly reduced, and it accumulated during chronic dosage. However, in patients with Ccr 50 to 90 mL/min, the oral clearance and the oral volume of distribution of fenofibric acid are increased compared with healthy adults (2.1 L/h and 95 L vs 1.1 L/h and 30 L, respectively). Therefore, minimize the dosage in patients who have Ccr less than 50 mL/min.

➤*Carcinogenesis:* The incidence of liver carcinoma, pancreatic carcinomas, pancreatic adenomas, and benign testicular interstitial cell tumors was increased in 24-month rat studies at doses from 0.3 to 6 times the maximum recommended human dose.

A comparative carcinogenicity study was done in rats comparing 3 drugs: fenofibrate (10 and 60 or 70 mg/kg), clofibrate (400 mg/kg), and gemfibrozil (250 mg/kg). Pancreatic acinar adenomas were increased in males and females on fenofibrate; hepatocellular carcinoma and pancreatic acinar adenomas were increased in males and hepatic neoplastic nodules in females treated with clofibrate; hepatic neoplastic nodules were increased in males and females treated with gemfibrozil while testicular interstitial cell tumors were increased in males on all 3 drugs.

In a 21-month study in mice at doses of 10, 45, and 200 mg/kg (approximately 0.2, 0.7, and 3 times the maximum recommended human dose on the basis of mg/m^2 surface area), there were statistically significant increases in liver carcinoma at 3 times the maximum recommended human dose in males and females. In a second 18-month study at the same doses, there was a significant increase in liver carcinoma in male mice and liver adenoma in female mice at 3 times the maximum recommended human dose.

Electron microscopy studies have demonstrated peroxisomal proliferation following fenofibrate administration to the rat. An adequate study to test for peroxisome proliferation in humans has not been done, but changes in peroxisome morphology and numbers have been observed in humans after treatment with other members of the fibrate class when liver biopsies were compared before and after treatment in the same individual.

➤*Elderly:* Fenofibric acid is known to be substantially excreted by the kidney, and the risk of adverse reactions to this drug may be greater in patients with impaired renal function. Because elderly patients are more likely to have decreased renal function, take care in dose selection.

➤*Pregnancy: Category C.* Fenofibrate is embryocidal and teratogenic in rats when given in doses 7 to 10 times the maximum recommended human dose and embryocidal in rabbits when given at 9 times the maximum recommended human dose. There are no adequate and well-controlled studies in pregnant women. Use during pregnancy only if the potential benefit justifies the potential risk to the fetus.

Administration of 9 times the maximum recommended human dose of fenofibrate to female rats before and throughout gestation caused 100% of dams to delay delivery and resulted in a 60% increase in postimplantation loss, a decrease in litter size, a decrease in birth weight, a 40% survival of pups at

FENOFIBRATE — ORAL

birth, a 4% survival of pups as neonates, and a 0% survival of pups to weaning, and an increase in spina bifida.

Administration of 10 times the maximum recommended human dose to female rats on days 6 to 15 of gestation caused an increase in gross, visceral, and skeletal findings in fetuses (domed head/hunched shoulders/rounded body/abnormal chest, kyphosis, stunted fetuses, elongated sternal ribs, malformed sternebrae, extra foramen in palatine, misshapen vertebrae, supernumerary ribs).

Administration of 7 times the maximum recommended human dose to female rats from day 15 of gestation through weaning caused a delay in delivery, a 40% decrease in live births, a 75% decrease in neonatal survival, and decreases in pup weight, at birth as well as on days 4 and 21 postpartum.

Administration of 9 and 18 times the maximum recommended human dose to female rabbits caused abortions in 10% of dams at 9 times and 25% of dams at 18 times the maximum recommended human dose and death of 7% of fetuses at 18 times the maximum recommended human dose.

➤*Lactation:* Do not use fenofibrate in breast-feeding mothers. Because of the potential for tumorigenicity seen in animal studies, decide whether to discontinue breast-feeding or the drug.

➤*Children:* Safety and efficacy in children have not been established.

Precautions

➤*Monitoring:* Obtain periodic determination of serum lipids during initial therapy in order to establish the lowest effective dose of fenofibrate. Withdraw therapy in patients who do not have an adequate response after 2 months of treatment with the maximum recommended dose. Perform liver function tests regularly, including serum ALT for the duration of therapy with fenofibrate; discontinue therapy if enzyme levels persist above 3 times the normal limit. Periodic blood counts also are recommended during the first 12 months of fenofibrate administration.

➤*Pancreatitis:* Pancreatitis has been reported in patients taking fenofibrate, gemfibrozil, and clofibrate. This occurrence may represent a failure of efficacy in patients with severe hypertriglyceridemia, a direct drug effect, or a secondary phenomenon mediated through biliary tract stone or sludge formation with obstruction of the common bile duct.

➤*Skeletal muscle effects:* The use of fibrates alone, including fenofibrate, may occasionally be associated with myopathy. Treatment with drugs of the fibrate class has been associated on rare occasions with rhabdomyolysis, usually in patients with impaired renal function. Consider myopathy in any patient with diffuse myalgias, muscle tenderness or weakness, and/or marked elevations of creatine phosphokinase (CPK) levels.

Assess CPK levels in patients reporting these symptoms and discontinue therapy if markedly elevated CPK levels occur or myopathy is diagnosed.

➤*Initial therapy:* Ascertain that lipid levels are consistently abnormal before instituting fenofibrate therapy. Make every attempt to control serum lipids with appropriate diet, exercise, weight loss in obese patients, and control of any medical problems (eg, diabetes mellitus, hypothyroidism) that are contributing to the lipid abnormalities. If possible, discontinue or change medications known to exacerbate hypertriglyceridemia (eg, beta-blockers, thiazides, estrogens) prior to consideration of triglyceride-lowering drug therapy.

➤*Hematologic changes:* Mild to moderate hemoglobin, hematocrit, and white blood cell decreases have been observed in patients following initiation of fenofibrate therapy. However, these levels stabilize during long-term administration. Extremely rare spontaneous reports of thrombocytopenia and agranulocytosis have been received during postmarketing surveillance outside of the United States. Periodic blood counts are recommended during the first 12 months of fenofibrate administration.

Drug Interactions

Fenofibrate Drug Interactions

Precipitant drug	Object drug*		Description
Bile acid sequestrants	Fenofibrate	⬇	Because bile acid sequestrants may bind other drugs given concurrently, patients should take fenofibrate at least 1 hour before or 4 to 6 hours after a bile acid binding resin to avoid impeding its absorption.
Fenofibrate	Anticoagulants, oral	⬆	Potentiation of coumarin-type anticoagulants has been observed with prolongation of the prothrombin time/international normalized ratio (PT/INR). Frequent PT/INR determinations and anticoagulant dosage reduction are advisable.
Fenofibrate	Cyclosporine	⬆	Coadministration may lead to increased risk of nephrotoxicity. Carefully consider the benefits and risks of using fenofibrate with immunosuppressants and other potentially nephrotoxic agents, and employ the lowest effective dose.
Fenofibrate	HMG-CoA reductase inhibitors	⬆	The combined use of fenofibrate and HMG-CoA reductase inhibitors has been associated with rhabdomyolysis, marked elevated creatine kinase (CK) levels, and myoglobinuria, leading in a high proportion of cases to acute renal failure. Avoid this drug combination unless the benefit of further alterations in lipid levels is likely to outweigh the increased risk of this drug combination.

* ⬆ = Object drug increased. ⬇ = Object drug decreased.

➤*Drug/Food interactions:* The absorption of micronized fenofibrate is increased when administered with food, compared with fasting conditions.

Adverse Reactions

Adverse reactions led to discontinuation of treatment in 5% of patients treated with fenofibrate and in 3% treated with placebo. Increases in liver function tests were the most frequent events causing discontinuation (1.6%) of fenofibrate treatment.

Fenofibrate Adverse Reactions (%)

Adverse reaction	Fenofibrate[a] (n = 439)	Placebo (n = 365)
GI		
Abdominal pain	4.6%	4.4%
Constipation	2.1%	1.4%
Diarrhea	2.3%	4.1%
Nausea	2.3%	1.9%
Lab test abnormalities		
ALT increased	3%	1.6%
AST increased	3.4%[b]	0.5%
CPK increased	3%	1.4%
Liver function tests abnormal	7.5%[b]	1.4%
Respiratory		
Respiratory disorder	6.2%	5.5%
Rhinitis	2.3%	1.1%
Miscellaneous		
Asthenia	2.1%	3%
Back pain	3.4%	2.5%
Flu syndrome	2.1%	2.7%
Headache	3.2%	2.7%

[a] Dose equivalent to *Antara* 130 mg, *Lofibra* 200 mg, *Tricor* 145 mg.
[b] Significantly different from placebo.

The following are additional adverse reactions reported by at least 3 patients in placebo-controlled trials or reported in other controlled or open trials, regardless of causality.

➤*Cardiovascular:* Abnormal electrocardiogram; angina pectoris; arrhythmia; atrial fibrillation; cardiovascular disorder; coronary artery disorder; extrasystoles; hypertension; hypotension; migraine; myocardial infarction; palpitation; peripheral vascular disorder; phlebitis; tachycardia; varicose vein; vascular disorder; vasodilation; ventricular extrasystoles.

➤*CNS:* Anxiety; decreased libido; depression; dizziness; dry mouth; hypertonia; insomnia; nervousness; neuralgia; paresthesia; somnolence; vertigo.

➤*Dermatologic:* Acne; alopecia; contact dermatitis; eczema; fungal dermatitis; herpes simplex; herpes zoster; maculopapular rash; nail disorder; pruritus; rash; skin disorder; skin ulcer; sweating; urticaria.

➤*GI:* Anorexia; cholecystitis; cholelithiasis; colitis; diarrhea; duodenal ulcer; dyspepsia; eructation; esophagitis; flatulence; gastritis; gastroenteritis; GI disorder; increased appetite; increased gamma glutamyl transpeptidase; liver fatty deposit; nausea; nausea/vomiting; peptic ulcer; rectal disorder; rectal hemorrhage; tooth disorder; vomiting.

➤*GU:* Abnormal kidney function; cystitis; dysuria; gynecomastia; prostatic disorder; unintended pregnancy; urinary frequency; urolithiasis; vaginal moniliasis.

FENOFIBRATE — ORAL

➤*Hematologic/Lymphatic:* Anemia; ecchymosis; eosinophilia; leukopenia; lymphadenopathy; thrombocytopenia.

➤*Metabolic/Nutritional:* Creatinine increased; edema; gout; hyperuricemia; hypoglycemia; peripheral edema; weight gain; weight loss.

➤*Musculoskeletal:* Arthralgia; arthritis; arthrosis; bursitis; joint disorder; leg cramps; myalgia; myasthenia; myositis; tenosynovitis.

➤*Respiratory:* Allergic pulmonary alveolitis; asthma; bronchitis; cough increased; dyspnea; laryngitis; pharyngitis; pneumonia; sinusitis.

➤*Special senses:* Abnormal vision; amblyopia; cataract specified; conjunctivitis; ear pain; eye disorder; otitis media; refraction disorder.

➤*Miscellaneous:* Accidental injury; allergic reaction; chest pain; cyst; diabetes mellitus; fever; hernia; infection; malaise; pain (unspecified); photosensitivity reaction.

Overdosage

If indicated, elimination of unabsorbed drug should be achieved by gastric lavage; observe usual precautions to maintain the airway. Because fenofibrate is highly bound to plasma proteins, do not consider hemodialysis. Refer to General Management of Acute Overdosage.

Patient Information

Advise patients to promptly report unexplained muscle pain, tenderness, or weakness, particularly if accompanied by malaise or fever.

NIACIN (Nicotinic acid)

For complete prescribing information, refer to the Niacin monograph in the Nutrients and Nutritionals Agents chapter.

EZETIMIBE

Rx	**Zetia** (Merck/Schering-Plough)	**Tablets**: 10 mg	Lactose. (414). Capsule shape. In 30s, 90s, 500s, and UD 100s.

EZETIMIBE — ORAL

Indications

➤*Primary hypercholesterolemia:*

Monotherapy – As adjunctive therapy to diet for the reduction of elevated total cholesterol (total-C), low density lipoprotein cholesterol (LDL-C), and apolipoprotein B (APOB) in patients with primary (heterozygous familial and nonfamilial) hypercholesterolemia.

Combination therapy with hydroxymethyl glutaryl coenzyme A (HMG-CoA) reductase inhibitors – In combination with an HMG-CoA reductase inhibitor as adjunctive therapy to diet for the reduction of elevated total-C, LDL-C, and APOB in patients with primary (heterozygous familial and nonfamilial) hypercholesterolemia.

➤*Mixed hyperlipidemia:*

Combination therapy with fenofibrate – In combination with fenofibrate as adjunctive therapy to diet for the reduction of total-C, LDL-C, APOB, and non-high-density lipoprotein cholesterol (non-HDL-C) in patients with mixed hyperlipidemia.

➤*Homozygous familial hypercholesterolemia (HoFH):* The combination of ezetimibe and atorvastatin or simvastatin is indicated for the reduction of elevated total-C and LDL-C levels in patients with HoFH, as an adjunct to other lipid-lowering treatments (eg, LDL apheresis) or if such treatments are unavailable.

➤*Homozygous sitosterolemia:* As adjunctive therapy to diet for the reduction of elevated sitosterol and campesterol levels in patients with homozygous familial sitosterolemia.

Administration and Dosage

➤*Approved by the FDA:* October 25, 2002.

The patient should be placed on a standard cholesterol-lowering diet before receiving ezetimibe and should continue on this diet during treatment with ezetimibe.

➤*Dosage:* 10 mg once daily. Ezetimibe can be administered with or without food.

➤*Coadministration with HMG-CoA reductase inhibitors or fenofibrate:* Ezetimibe may be administered with an HMG-CoA reductase inhibitor (in patients with primary hypercholesterolemia) or with fenofibrate (in patients with mixed hyperlipidemia) for incremental effect. For convenience, the daily dose of ezetimibe may be taken at the same time as the HMG-CoA reductase inhibitor or fenofibrate, according to the dosing recommendations for the respective medications.

➤*Coadministration with bile acid sequestrants:* Dosing of ezetimibe should occur either greater than or equal to 2 hours before or greater than or equal to 4 hours after administration of a bile acid sequestrant.

➤*Hepatic function impairment:* No dosage adjustment is necessary in patients with mild hepatic function impairment. Because of the unknown effects of the increased exposure to ezetimibe in patients with moderate or severe hepatic function impairment, ezetimibe is not recommended in these patients.

➤*Storage/Stability:* Store at 25°C (77°F); excursions permitted to 15° to 30°C (59° to 86°F). Protect from moisture.

Actions

➤*Pharmacology:* Ezetimibe has a mechanism of action that differs from those of other classes of cholesterol-reducing compounds (HMG-CoA reductase inhibitors, bile acid sequestrants [resin], fibric acid derivatives, and plant stanols).

Ezetimibe does not inhibit cholesterol synthesis in the liver, or increase bile acid excretion. Instead, ezetimibe localizes and appears to act at the brush border of the small intestine and inhibits the absorption of cholesterol, leading to a decrease in the delivery of intestinal cholesterol to the liver. This causes a reduction of hepatic cholesterol stores and an increase in clearance of cholesterol from the blood; this distinct mechanism is complementary to that of HMG-CoA reductase inhibitors.

➤*Pharmacokinetics:*

Absorption – After oral administration, ezetimibe is absorbed and extensively conjugated to a pharmacologically active phenolic glucuronide (ezetimibe-glucuronide). After a single dose of ezetimibe 10 mg to fasted adults, mean ezetimibe peak plasma concentrations (C_{max}) of 3.4 to 5.5 ng/mL were attained within 4 to 12 hours (t_{max}). Ezetimibe-glucuronide mean C_{max} values of 45 to 71 ng/mL were achieved between 1 and 2 hours (t_{max}). There was no substantial deviation from dose proportionality between 5 and 20 mg. The absolute bioavailability of ezetimibe cannot be determined, as the compound is virtually insoluble in aqueous media suitable for injection. Ezetimibe has variable bioavailability; the coefficient of variation, based on intersubject variability, was 35% to 60% for AUC values.

Effect of food on oral absorption: Concomitant food administration (high fat or non-fat meals) had no effect on the extent of absorption of ezetimibe when administered as ezetimibe 10 mg tablets. The C_{max} value of ezetimibe was increased by 38% with consumption of high fat meals. Ezetimibe can be administered with or without food.

Distribution – Ezetimibe and ezetimibe-glucuronide are highly bound (greater than 90%) to human plasma proteins.

Metabolism/Excretion – Ezetimibe is primarily metabolized in the small intestine and liver via glucuronide conjugation (a phase II reaction) with subsequent biliary and renal excretion. Minimal oxidative metabolism (a phase I reaction) has been observed in all species evaluated.

In humans, ezetimibe is rapidly metabolized to ezetimibe-glucuronide. Ezetimibe and ezetimibe-glucuronide are the major drug-derived compounds detected in plasma, constituting approximately 10% to 20% and 80% to 90% of the total drug in plasma, respectively. Both ezetimibe and ezetimibe-glucuronide are slowly eliminated from plasma with a half-life of approximately 22 hours for both ezetimibe and ezetimibe-glucuronide. Plasma concentration-time profiles exhibit multiple peaks, suggesting enterohepatic recycling.

Following oral administration of ^{14}C-ezetimibe (20 mg) to human subjects, total ezetimibe (ezetimibe + ezetimibe-glucuronide) accounted for approximately 93% of the total radioactivity in plasma. After 48 hours, there were no detectable levels of radioactivity in the plasma.

Approximately 78% and 11% of the administered radioactivity were recovered in the feces and urine, respectively, over a 10-day collection period. Ezetimibe was the major component in feces and accounted for 69% of the administered dose, while ezetimibe-glucuronide was the major component in urine and accounted for 9% of the administered dose.

Special populations –

Renal function impairment: After a single 10 mg dose of ezetimibe in patients with severe renal disease (n = 8; mean Ccr less than or equal to 30 mL/min/1.73 m^2), the mean AUC values for total ezetimibe, ezetimibe-glucuronide, and ezetimibe were increased approximately 1.5-fold, compared to healthy subjects (n = 9).

Hepatic function impairment: After a single dose of ezetimibe 10 mg, the mean area under the curve (AUC) for total ezetimibe was increased approximately 1.7-fold in patients with mild hepatic insufficiency (Child-Pugh score 5 to 6), compared to healthy subjects. The mean AUC values for total ezetimibe and ezetimibe were increased approximately 3- to 4- fold and 5- to 6-fold, respectively, in patients with moderate (Child-Pugh score 7 to 9) or severe hepatic impairment (Child-Pugh score 10 to 15). In a 14-day, multiple-dose study (10 mg daily) in patients with moderate hepatic insufficiency, the mean AUC values for total ezetimibe and ezetimibe were increased approximately 4-fold on Day 1 and Day 14 compared to healthy subjects. Due to the unknown effects of the increased exposure to ezetimibe in patients with moderate or severe hepatic insufficiency, ezetimibe is not recommended in these patients.

Elderly: In a multiple-dose study with ezetimibe given 10 mg once daily for 10 days, plasma concentrations for total ezetimibe were about 2-fold higher in older (greater than or equal to 65 years) healthy subjects compared to younger subjects.

Gender: In a multiple-dose study with ezetimibe given 10 mg once daily for 10 days, plasma concentrations for total ezetimibe were slightly higher (less than 20%) in women than in men.

Drug interactions –

Gemfibrozil: In a study of 12 healthy adult men, coadministration of gemfibrozil (600 mg twice daily) significantly increased the oral bioavailability of total ezetimibe by a factor of 1.7. Ezetimibe (10 mg once daily) did not significantly affect the bioavailability of gemfibrozil.

Antacids: In a study of 12 healthy adults, a single dose of antacid (aluminum hydroxide and magnesium hydroxide 20 mL) administration had no significant effect on the oral bioavailability of total ezetimibe, ezetimibe-glucuronide, or ezetimibe based on AUC values. The C_{max} value of total ezetimibe was decreased by 30%.

Cholestyramine: In a study of 40 healthy hypercholesterolemic (LDL-C greater than or equal to 130 mg/dL) adult subjects, concomitant cholestyramine (4 g twice daily) administration decreased the mean AUC values of total ezetimibe and ezetimibe approximately 55% and 80%, respectively.

Contraindications

Hypersensitivity to any component of this medication.

The combination of ezetimibe with an HMG-CoA reductase inhibitor is contraindicated in patients with active liver disease or unexplained persistent elevations in serum transaminases.

All HMG-CoA reductase inhibitors are contraindicated in pregnant and nursing women. When ezetimibe is administered with an HMG-CoA reductase inhibitor in a woman of childbearing potential, refer to the pregnancy category and product labeling for the HMG-CoA reductase inhibitor.

Warnings

➤*Hepatic function impairment:* In controlled clinical monotherapy studies, the incidence of consecutive elevations (greater than or equal to 3 times the upper limit of normal [ULN]) in serum transaminases was similar between ezetimibe (0.5%) and placebo (0.3%).

Due to the unknown effects of the increased exposure to ezetimibe in patients with moderate or severe hepatic insufficiency, ezetimibe is not recommended in these patients.

EZETIMIBE — ORAL

➤*Elderly:* Of the patients who received ezetimibe in clinical studies, 948 were 65 and older (this included 206 who were 75 and older). The effectiveness and safety of ezetimibe were similar between these patients and younger subjects. Greater sensitivity of some older individuals cannot be ruled out.

➤*Pregnancy: Category C.* There are no adequate and well-controlled studies of ezetimibe in pregnant women. Ezetimibe should be used during pregnancy only if the potential benefit justifies the risk to the fetus.

In oral (gavage) embryo-fetal development studies of ezetimibe conducted in rats and rabbits during organogenesis, there was no evidence of embryolethal effects at the doses tested (250, 500, 1000 mg/kg/day). In rats, increased incidences of common fetal skeletal findings (extra pair of thoracic ribs, unossified cervical vertebral centra, shortened ribs) were observed at 1000 mg/kg/day (approximately 10 times the human exposure at 10 mg daily based on $AUC_{0\text{-}24h}$ for total ezetimibe). In rabbits treated with ezetimibe, an increased incidence of extra thoracic ribs was observed at 1,000 mg/kg/day (150 times the human exposure at 10 mg daily based on $AUC_{0\text{-}24h}$ for total ezetimibe). Ezetimibe crossed the placenta when pregnant rats and rabbits were given multiple oral doses.

Multiple dose studies of ezetimibe given in combination with HMG-CoA reductase inhibitors (statins) in rats and rabbits during organogenesis result in higher ezetimibe and statin exposures. Reproductive findings occur at lower doses in combination therapy compared to monotherapy.

All HMG-CoA reductase inhibitors are contraindicated in pregnant and nursing women. When ezetimibe is administered with an HMG-CoA reductase inhibitor in a woman of childbearing potential, refer to the pregnancy category and package labeling for the HMG-CoA reductase inhibitor.

The effects of ezetimibe on labor and delivery in pregnant women are unknown.

➤*Lactation:* In rat studies, exposure to total ezetimibe in breast-feeding pups was up to half of that observed in maternal plasma. It is not known whether ezetimibe is excreted into human breast milk; therefore, ezetimibe should not be used in breast-feeding mothers unless the potential benefit justifies the potential risk to the infant.

➤*Children:* The pharmacokinetics of ezetimibe in adolescents (10 to 18 years) have been shown to be similar to that in adults. Treatment experience with ezetimibe in the pediatric population is limited to 4 patients (9 to 17 years) in the sitosterolemia study and 5 patients (11 to 17 years) in the HoFH study. Treatment with ezetimibe in children (less than 10 years) is not recommended.

Precautions

➤*Skeletal muscle:* In clinical trials, there was no excess of myopathy or rhabdomyolysis associated with ezetimibe compared with the relevant control arm (placebo or HMG-CoA reductase inhibitor alone). However, myopathy and rhabdomyolysis are known adverse reactions to HMG-CoA reductase inhibitors and other lipid-lowering drugs. In clinical trials, the incidence of CPK greater than 10 times ULN was 0.2% for ezetimibe vs 0.1% for placebo, and 0.1% for ezetimibe coadministered with an HMG-CoA reductase inhibitor vs 0.4% for HMG-CoA reductase inhibitors alone.

Drug Interactions

Ezetimibe Drug Interactions

Precipitant drug	Object drug[a]		Description
Antacids	Ezetimibe	⬇	Administration of an aluminum- and magnesium-containing antacid decreased the C_{max} of ezetimibe 30% but had no significant effect on the AUC.
Cholestyramine	Ezetimibe	⬇	Coadministration decreased the mean AUC of ezetimibe ≈ 55%. The incremental LDL-C reduction caused by adding ezetimibe to cholestyramine may be reduced.
Fibric acid derivatives Fenofibrate Gemfibrozil	Ezetimibe	⬆	Coadministration of ezetimibe with fenofibrate or gemfibrozil increased the total ezetimibe concentration 1.5- and 1.7-fold, respectively. Because fibrates may increase cholesterol excretion into the bile, leading to cholelithiasis, and ezetimibe was shown in animal studies to increase cholesterol in the gallbladder bile, concomitant use is not recommended until use in patients is studied.
Cyclosporine	Ezetimibe	⬆	Total ezetimibe level increased 12-fold in 1 transplant patient receiving multiple medications, including cyclosporine. Monitor closely.

[a] ⬆ = Object drug increased. ⬇ = Object drug decreased.

➤*Drug/Food interactions:* Coadministration with food (high-fat or nonfat meals) had no effect on the extent of absorption of ezetimibe when administered as ezetimibe 10 mg tablets. The C_{max} value of ezetimibe was increased 38% with consumption of high-fat meals. Ezetimibe may be administered with or without food.

Adverse Reactions

Ezetimibe has been evaluated for safety in more than 4,700 patients in clinical trials. Clinical studies of ezetimibe (administered alone or with an HMG-CoA reductase inhibitor) demonstrated that ezetimibe was generally well tolerated. The overall incidence of adverse events reported with ezetimibe was similar to that reported with placebo, and the discontinuation rate due to adverse events was also similar for ezetimibe and placebo.

➤*Monotherapy:* Adverse effects reported in greater than or equal to 2% of patients treated with ezetimibe and at an incidence greater than placebo in placebo-controlled studies of ezetimibe, regardless of causality assessment, are shown in the following table.

Clinical Adverse Events Occurring in ≥ 2% of Patients Treated with Ezetimibe and at an Incidence Greater Than Placebo, Regardless of Causality[1]

Body system/ organ class adverse event	Placebo (%) (n = 795)	Ezetimibe 10 mg (%) (n = 1,691)
GI		
Abdominal pain	2.8%	3%
Diarrhea	3%	3.7%
Infection and infestations		
Viral infection	1.8%	2.2%
Pharyngitis	2.1%	2.3%
Sinusitis	2.8%	3.6%
Musculoskeletal		
Arthralgia	3.4%	3.8%
Back pain	3.9%	4.1%
Respiratory		
Coughing	2.1%	2.3%
Miscellaneous		
Fatigue	1.8%	2.2%

[1] Includes patients who received placebo or ezetimibe alone.

The frequency of less common adverse events was comparable between ezetimibe and placebo.

➤*Combination with an HMG-CoA reductase inhibitor:* Ezetimibe has been evaluated for safety in combination studies in more than 2000 patients.

In general, adverse experiences were similar between ezetimibe administered with HMG-CoA reductase inhibitors and HMG-CoA reductase inhibitors alone. However, the frequency of increased transaminases was slightly higher in patients receiving ezetimibe administered with HMG-CoA reductase inhibitors than in patients treated with HMG-CoA reductase inhibitors alone.

Clinical adverse experiences reported in greater than or equal to 2% of patients and at an incidence greater than placebo in four placebo-controlled trials where ezetimibe was administered alone or initiated concurrently with various HMG-CoA reductase inhibitors, regardless of causality assessment, are shown in the following table.

Clinical Adverse Events Occurring in ≥ 2% of Patients and at an Incidence Greater than Placebo, Regardless of Causality, in Ezetimibe/Statin Combination Studies[2]

Body system/ organ class adverse event	Placebo (%) (n = 259)	Ezetimibe 10 mg (%) (n = 262)	All statins[3](%) (n = 936)	Ezetimibe + all statins[3] (%) (n = 925)
GI				
Abdominal pain	2.3%	2.7%	3.1%	3.5%
Infection and infestations				
Pharyngitis	1.9%	3.1%	2.5%	2.3%
Sinusitis	1.9%	4.6%	3.6%	3.5%
Upper respiratory tract infection	10.8%	13%	13.6%	11.8%
Musculoskeletal				
Arthralgia	2.3%	3.8%	4.3%	3.4%
Back pain	3.5%	3.4%	3.7%	4.3%
Myalgia	4.6%	5%	4.1%	4.5%
Diarrhea	1.5%	3.4%	2.9%	2.8%
Miscellaneous				
Chest pain	1.2%	3.4%	2%	1.8%
Dizziness	1.2%	2.7%	1.4%	1.8%
Fatigue	1.9%	1.9%	1.4%	2.8%
Headache	5.4%	8%	7.3%	6.3%

[2] Includes 4 placebo-controlled combination studies in which ezetimibe was initiated concurrently with an HMG-CoA reductase inhibitor.
[3] All statins = all doses of all HMG-CoA reductase inhibitors.

Overdosage

No cases of overdosage with ezetimibe have been reported. Administration of ezetimibe 50 mg/day to 15 subjects for up to 14 days was generally well tolerated. In the event of an overdose, symptomatic and supportive measures should be employed.

AMLODIPINE BESYLATE/ATORVASTATIN CALCIUM

Rx	**Caduet** (Pfizer)	**Tablets:** 2.5 mg amlodipine besylate/10 mg atorvastatin calcium (as base)	Calcium carbonate. (Pfizer CDT 251). White. Film coated. In 30s.
		2.5 mg amlodipine besylate/20 mg atorvastatin calcium (as base)	Calcium carbonate. (Pfizer CDT 252). White. Film coated. In 30s.
		2.5 mg amlodipine besylate/40 mg atorvastatin calcium (as base)	Calcium carbonate. (Pfizer CDT 254). White. Film coated. In 30s.
		5 mg amlodipine besylate/10 mg atorvastatin calcium (as base)	Calcium carbonate. (Pfizer CDT 051). White. Film coated. In 30s.
		5 mg amlodipine besylate/20 mg atorvastatin calcium (as base)	Calcium carbonate. (Pfizer CDT 052). White. Film coated. In 30s.
		5 mg amlodipine besylate/40 mg atorvastatin calcium (as base)	Calcium carbonate. (Pfizer CDT 054). White. Film coated. In 30s.
		5 mg amlodipine besylate/80 mg atorvastatin calcium (as base)	Calcium carbonate. (Pfizer CDT 058). White. Film coated. In 30s.
		10 mg amlodipine besylate/10 mg atorvastatin calcium (as base)	Calcium carbonate. (Pfizer CDT 101). Blue. Film coated. In 30s.
		10 mg amlodipine besylate/20 mg atorvastatin calcium (as base)	Calcium carbonate. (Pfizer CDT 102). Blue. Film coated. In 30s.
		10 mg amlodipine besylate/40 mg atorvastatin calcium (as base)	Calcium carbonate. (Pfizer CDT 104). Blue. Film coated. In 30s.
		10 mg amlodipine besylate/80 mg atorvastatin calcium (as base)	Calcium carbonate. (Pfizer CDT 108). Blue. Film coated. In 30s.

AMLODIPINE BESYLATE/ATORVASTATIN CALCIUM — ORAL

For additional prescribing information, refer to the individual monographs for Amlodipine and Atorvastatin Calcium.

Indications

Indicated in patients for whom treatment with both amlodipine and atorvastatin is appropriate.

➤*Amlodipine:* For the treatment of hypertension, chronic stable angina, and confirmed or suspected vasospastic angina (Prinzmetal or Variant angina).

➤*Atorvastatin:* As an adjunct to diet to reduce elevated total-cholesterol (C), LDL-C, apo B, and triglyceride (TG) levels and to increase HDL-C in patients with primary hypercholesterolemia (heterozygous familial and non-familial) and mixed dyslipidemia (Fredrickson types IIa and IIb); as an adjunct to diet for the treatment of patients with elevated serum TG levels (Fredrickson type IV); for the treatment of patients with primary dysbetalipoproteinemia (Fredrickson type III); to reduce total-C and LDL-C in patients with homozygous familial hypercholesterolemia as an adjunct to other lipid-lowering treatments (eg, LDL apheresis) or if such treatments are unavailable; to reduce total-C, LDL-C, and apo B levels in boys and post-menarchal girls (10 to 17 years of age with heterozygous familial hypercholesterolemia).

Administration and Dosage

➤*Approved by the FDA:* January 30, 2004.

Individualize dosage. Lipid-altering agents should be used in addition to a diet restricted in saturated fat and cholesterol, only when the response to diet and other nonpharmacological measures has been inadequate.

Amlodipine/Atorvastatin may be substituted for its individually titrated components. Patients may be given the equivalent dose of amlodipine/atorvastatin or a dose of amlodipine/atorvastatin with increased amounts of amlodipine, atorvastatin, or both for additional antianginal effects, blood pressure lowering, or lipid-lowering effect.

As initial therapy for one indication and continuation of treatment of the other, the recommended starting dose of amlodipine/atorvastatin should be selected based on the continuation of the component being used and the recommended starting dose of the added monotherapy. The maximum dose of the amlodipine component is 10 mg once daily. The maximum dose of the atorvastatin component is 80 mg/day.

➤*Concomitant therapy:* Atorvastatin may be used in combination with a bile acid-binding resin for additive effect. The combination of HMG-CoA reductase inhibitors and fibrates generally should be avoided.

➤*Storage/Stability:* Store at 25°C (77°F); excursions permitted to 15° to 30°C (59° to 86°F).

NIACIN (EXTENDED RELEASE)/LOVASTATIN

Rx	**Advicor** (Kos)	**Tablets:** 500/20 mg	(KOS 502). Lt. yellow, capsule shape. In 30s, 90s, and 180s.
		1000/20 mg	(KOS 1002). Dk. pink/lt. purple, capsule shape. In 30s, 90s, and 180s.

NIACIN (EXTENDED RELEASE)/LOVASTATIN — ORAL

Refer to the general discussion of these products in the Antihyperlipidemic Agents Introduction.

Indications

➤*Primary hypercholesterolemia/mixed dyslipidemia:* For the treatment of primary hypercholesterolemia (heterozygous familial and nonfamilial) and mixed dyslipidemia (Frederickson Types IIa and IIb) in the following: Patients treated with lovastatin who require further TG-lowering or HDL-raising who may benefit from having niacin added to their regimen; patients treated with niacin who require further LDL-lowering who may benefit from having lovastatin added to their regimen.

Administration and Dosage

The usual recommended starting dose for extended-release niacin tablets is 500 mg at bedtime. Niacin extended-release tablets must be titrated and the dose should not be increased by more than 500 mg every 4 weeks up to a maximum dose of 2000 mg/day, to reduce the incidence and severity of side effects. Patients already receiving a stable dose of niacin extended-release tablets may be switched directly to a niacin-equivalent dose of niacin extended-release/lovastatin tablets.

The usual recommended starting dose of lovastatin is 20 mg once/day. Make dose adjustments at intervals of 4 weeks or more. Patients already receiving a stable dose of lovastatin may receive concomitant dosage titration with niacin extended-release tablets, and switch to niacin extended-release/lovastatin tablets once a stable dose of niacin extended-release tablets has been reached.

Flushing of the skin may be reduced in frequency or severity by pretreatment with aspirin (taken up to approximately 30 minutes prior to niacin extended-release/lovastatin tablets dose) or other nonsteroidal anti-inflammatory drugs. Flushing, pruritus, and GI distress also are greatly reduced by slowly increasing the dose of niacin and avoiding administration on an empty stomach.

Equivalent doses of niacin extended-release/lovastatin tablets may be substituted for equivalent doses of niacin extended-release tablets but should not be substituted for other modified-release (sustained- or timed-release) niacin preparations or immediate-release (crystalline) niacin preparations. Patients previously receiving niacin products other than niacin extended-release tablets should be started on niacin extended-release tablets with the recommended niacin extended-release tablets titration schedule, and the dose should subsequently be individualized based on patient response.

Take niacin extended-release/lovastatin tablets at bedtime, with a low-fat snack, and individualize dose according to patient response.

Take whole; do not break, chew, or crush before swallowing. Do not increase the dose by more than 500 mg/day (based on the niacin extended release component) every 4 weeks. The lowest dose of niacin extended-release/lovastatin tablets is 500/20 mg. Doses greater than 2000/40 mg/day are not recommended. If therapy is discontinued for an extended period (greater than 7 days), begin reinstitution of therapy with the lowest dose.

➤*Storage/Stability:* Store at room temperature (20° to 25°C; 68° to 77°F).

EZETIMIBE/SIMVASTATIN

Rx	**Vytorin** (Merck/Schering-Plough)	**Tablets:** 10 mg ezetimibe/10 mg simvastatin	(311). White to off-white, capsule shape. In 30s, 90s, 1000s, and UD 100s.
		10 mg ezetimibe/20 mg simvastatin	(312). White to off-white, capsule shape. In 30s, 90s, 1000s, and UD 100s.
		10 mg ezetimibe/40 mg simvastatin	(313). White to off-white, capsule shape. In 30s, 90s, 500s, UD 50s.
		10 mg ezetimibe/80 mg simvastatin	(315). White to off-white, capsule shape. In 30s, 90s, 500s, and UD 50s.

EZETIMIBE/SIMVASTATIN — ORAL

Indications

➤*Primary hypercholesterolemia:* Adjunctive therapy to diet for reducing elevated total-C, LDL-C, Apo B, TG, and non-HDL-C, and increasing HDL-C in patients with primary (heterozygous familial and non-familial) hypercholesterolemia or mixed hyperlipidemia.

➤*Homozygous familial hypercholesterolemia (HoFH):* For reducing elevated total-C and LDL-C in patients with homozygous familial hypercholesterolemia, as an adjunct to other lipid-lowering treatments (eg, LDL apheresis) or if such treatments are unavailable.

Administration and Dosage

➤*Approved by the FDA:* July 26, 2004

Place the patient on a standard cholesterol-lowering diet before the patient receives ezetimibe and simvastatin. The patient should continue on this diet during treatment with ezetimibe and simvastatin. Individualize the dosage according to the baseline LDL-C level, the recommended goal of therapy, and the patient's response. Take ezetimibe and simvastatin as a single daily dose in the evening, with or without food.

➤*Dose:* The dosage range is 10 mg ezetimibe/10 mg simvastatin daily through 10 ezetimibe/80 mg simvastatin daily. The recommended usual starting dose is 10 mg ezetimibe/20 mg simvastatin daily. Initiation of therapy with 10 mg ezetimibe/10 mg simvastatin daily may be considered for patients requiring less aggressive LDL-C reductions. Patients who require a larger reduction in LDL-C (greater than 55%) may be started at 10 mg ezetimibe/40 mg simvastatin daily. After initiation or titration or ezetimibe and simvastatin, lipid levels may be analyzed after 2 or more weeks and dosage adjusted, if needed.

➤*Homozygous familial hypercholesterolemia:* The recommended dosage for patients with homozygous familial hypercholesterolemia is 10 mg ezetimibe/40 mg simvastatin daily or 10 ezetimibe/80 mg simvastatin daily in the evening. Use ezetimibe and simvastatin as an adjunct to other lipid-lowering treatments (eg, LDL apheresis) in these patients or if such treatments are unavailable.

➤*Hepatic function impairment:* Use is not recommended in patients with moderate or severe hepatic insufficiency. No dosage adjustment is necessary in patients with mild hepatic insufficiency.

➤*Renal function impairment:* For patients with severe renal insufficiency, do not start ezetimibe and simvastatin unless the patient has already tolerated treatment with simvastatin at a dose of 5 mg or higher. Exercise caution when ezetimibe and simvastatin is administered to these patients, and monitor them closely.

➤*Concomitant bile acid sequestrants:* Give ezetimibe and simvastatin either 2 hours or more before or 4 hours or more after administration of a bile acid sequestrant.

➤*Concomitant cyclosporine or danazol:* Exercise caution when initiating ezetimibe and simvastatin in the setting of cyclosporine. In patients taking cyclosporine or danazol, do not start ezetimibe and simvastatin unless the patient has already tolerated treatment with simvastatin at a dose of 5 mg or higher. Do not exceed 10 mg ezetimibe/10 mg simvastatin daily.

➤*Concomitant amiodarone or verapamil:* In patients taking amiodarone or verapamil concomitantly with ezetimibe and simvastatin, do not exceed 10 mg ezetimibe/20 mg simvastatin daily.

➤*Storage/Stability:* Store at 20° to 25°C (68° to 77°F). Keep container tightly closed.

VASOPRESSORS USED IN SHOCK

➤*Shock:* Shock is a state of inadequate tissue perfusion. It can be caused by, or cause, a decreased supply of, or an increased demand for, oxygen and nutrients. The imbalance between supply and demand interferes with normal cellular function. Widespread cellular dysfunction can result in death. Inadequate tissue perfusion can occur even if cardiac output, peripheral resistance, and other factors that determine blood pressure (eg, blood volume) are normal or elevated. Therefore, hypotension need not be present for the patient to be in shock.

Shock produces various physiologic responses. Some, such as lactic acidosis, occur as a direct result of tissue hypoperfusion. Others, such as catecholamine release, also serve to compensate for the absolute or relative reduction in tissue perfusion. The systemic responses to shock can be beneficial in the early stages and classically consist of an increase in circulating catecholamines, vasodilation, and increased vascular permeability. These early responses produce a "hyperdynamic" state, which may be referred to as "warm" shock, so named because blood flow to the skin and extremities is still maintained. If left uncorrected, however, these responses become counterproductive and contribute to the relentless progression of the shock state. Profound vascular decompensation occurs, which is associated with a further loss of blood flow to the vital organs, skin, and extremities. Thus, more advanced shock is "cold" shock.

➤*Clinical manifestations:* Clinical manifestations of shock are variable and nonspecific. In addition, underlying or concurrent disease states, drug therapy, and patient age may alter the response to hypoperfusion. Signs and symptoms of shock include:

Skin – Pallor, cyanosis, cold and clammy, sweating.

CNS – Agitation, confusion, disorientation, coma.

Cardiovascular – Tachycardia, arrhythmias, wide pulse pressure, gallop rhythm, hypotension.

Pulmonary – Tachypnea, pulmonary edema.

Renal – Oliguria (< 0.5 mL/kg/hr).

Metabolic – Acidosis, hypoglycemia or hyperglycemia.

➤*Causes:* The causes of shock are varied. Despite the etiology, advanced shock tends to follow a common clinical course. However, identifying the underlying cause may assist in the selection of general supportive therapy and is essential for selecting specific therapy.

➤*Types of shock:*

Hypovolemic shock – Hypovolemic shock occurs when intravascular volume is reduced by > 15% to 25%. The volume loss can be absolute (eg, hemorrhage, fluid loss due to burns, diarrhea or vomiting, excess diuresis, diabetes) or relative (eg, sequestration of body fluids, capillary leak).

Cardiogenic shock – Cardiogenic shock occurs when the heart is unable to deliver an adequate cardiac output to maintain vital organ perfusion. This can be caused by an acute MI, sustained ventricular arrhythmias, severe cardiomyopathy, or CHF.

Septic shock – Septic shock occurs as a result of circulatory insufficiency associated with overwhelming infection.

Obstructive shock – Obstructive shock occurs when obstruction of blood flow results in inadequate tissue perfusion. Massive pulmonary embolism, pericardial tamponade, restrictive pericarditis, and severe cardiac valve dysfunction can reduce blood flow enough to produce shock.

Neurogenic shock – An uncommon form of shock that occurs as a result of blockade of neurohumoral outflow. The neurohumoral blockade may be induced by pharmacologic agents (eg, spinal anesthesia) or by direct injury to the spinal cord.

Other causes of shock – Other causes include anaphylaxis, hypoglycemia, hypothyroidism and hypoadrenalism (ie, Addison disease).

➤*Management:* Management of shock is aimed at providing basic life support (eg, airway, breathing, circulation) while attempting to correct the underlying cause. Antibiotics, inotropes, hormones (eg, insulin, thyroid) and other agents may be used to treat the underlying disease states in the shock patient. However, initial pharmacologic interventions are primarily aimed at supporting the circulation.

Blood pressure is a function of the peripheral vascular resistance and the cardiac output. Cardiac output is determined by the heart rate and stroke volume. The stroke volume is a function of the contractile state of the heart and the volume of blood in the ventricle available to be pumped out (ie, preload). Manipulation of any of these parameters can produce a change in blood pressure.

Fluids – Relative or absolute volume depletion occurs in most shock states, especially in the early or "warm" phase in which vasodilation is prominent. Adequate volume repletion is necessary to maintain cardiac output, urine flow, and the integrity of the microcirculation. Attempts to support the circulation with vasopressors or inotropes will be unsuccessful if the intravascular volume is depleted.

The choice of fluids is probably irrelevant in the early stages. Although whole blood might be preferred for the patient with hemorrhagic shock, the delay in availability of blood products often negates any advantage. There is no clear superiority of crystalloids or colloids in emergency fluid resuscitation. Hydroxyethyl starch and the dextrans are also suitable plasma volume expanders.

Vasopressors – Sympathomimetic agents are used in shock to treat hypoperfusion in normovolemic patients and in patients unresponsive to whole blood or plasma volume expanders. These agents increase myocardial contractility, constrict capacitance vessels, and dilate resistance vessels. In cardiogenic shock or advanced shock from other causes associated with a low cardiac output, they may be combined with vasodilators (eg, nitroprusside, nitroglycerin) to maintain blood pressure while the vasodilator improves myocardial performance. Nitroprusside is used to reduce preload and afterload and improve cardiac output. Nitroglycerin directly relaxes the venous vasculature and decreases preload.

Pharmacology – Sympathomimetic agents produce α-adrenergic stimulation (vasoconstriction), β_1-adrenergic stimulation (increase myocardial contractility, heart rate, automaticity, and AV conduction), and β_2-adrenergic activity (peripheral vasodilation). Dopamine also causes vasodilation of the renal and mesenteric, cerebral and coronary beds by dopaminergic receptor activation. Adrenergic agents are useful in improving hemodynamic status by improving myocardial contractility and increasing heart rate, which results in increased cardiac output. Peripheral resistance is increased by vasoconstriction. Increased cardiac output and increased peripheral resistance increase blood pressure. The relative activity and predominance of these actions result in a number of hemodynamic responses which may affect coronary perfusion, renal perfusion, cardiac output, total peripheral resistance and blood pressure. These actions are summarized in the Sites of Action/Hemodynamic Response table. The actual response of an individual patient will depend largely on clinical status at time of administration.

Other drugs – A number of other drug classes have been used as supportive therapy in shock patients. However, with the exception of vasodilator treatment of cardiogenic shock, none of these treatments appear superior to vasopressor therapy. These drugs include: Opiate antagonists, prostaglandin inhibitors, corticosteroids, and thyrotropin-releasing hormone.

Monitoring – The monitoring of shock patients and their response to drugs requires special vigilance. Monitor heart rate, blood pressure, and ECG continuously. Record urine output and fluid intake frequently. Due to rapid and life-threatening changes that can occur in the hemodynamically unstable patient, optimal drug selection, dose titration, and management is probably best achieved with the use of invasive hemodynamic monitoring. Monitoring of central venous pressures via a central venous catheter will provide an estimation of the patient's fluid status by approximating the diastolic pressure of the right ventricle. When warranted, additional hemodynamic data can be obtained through the use of a pulmonary artery catheter (ie, Swan-Ganz). Changes in the pulmonary artery wedge pressure (a measure of left ventricular end diastolic volume), cardiac output, and peripheral vascular resistance can be monitored and therapy adjusted accordingly.

Administration – Administration should only be via the IV route using a large-bore, free-flowing IV in the antecubital vein or a central vein because of unpredictable absorption. Small IVs in the extremities are both unreliable and unsafe for vasopressor administration. Frequent monitoring of the IV sites for extravasation injury is essential when vasopressor agents are being used.

Prolonged, high-dose therapy – Prolonged, high-dose therapy can produce cyanosis and tissue necrosis of distal extremities. The principle of using the lowest dose that produces an adequate response for the shortest period of time is very important when using these agents.

Plasma volume depletion – Prolonged use of vasopressors may result in plasma volume depletion; this should be corrected by appropriate fluid and electrolyte replacement therapy. If plasma volumes are not corrected, hypotension may recur when these drugs are discontinued. Blood pressure may be maintained at the risk of severe peripheral vasoconstriction with diminution in blood flow and tissue perfusion.

Acidosis – Acidosis lessens the response to vasopressors; therefore, correct acidosis if it exists or develops during the course of vasopressor therapy.

Avoid continuous IV therapy – Acute tolerance develops during continuous IV administration. High concentration/low volume (250 mL) vasopressor solutions administered with the aid of an infusion control device allows for maximum dosing flexibility since fluids and drugs can be regulated independently, and the development of tolerance is minimized.

Effects of Vasopressors Used in Shock

+++ pronounced effect
++ *moderate effect*
+ *slight effect*
0 *no effect*
↑ *increase*
↓ *decrease*

		SITES OF ACTION				HEMODYNAMIC RESPONSE			
		HEART		BLOOD VESSELS					
		Contractility (Inotropic) β_1	SA Node Rate (Chronotropic) β_1	Vasoconstriction α	Vasodilatation β_2	Renal Perfusion	Cardiac Output	Total Peripheral Resistance	Blood Pressure
⇧ Pressors	Isoproterenol	+++	+++	0	+++	↑[1] or ↓[2]	↑	↓	↑[3]↓[4]
	Dobutamine	+++	0 to +[5]	0 to +[5]	+	0	↑	↓	↑
	Dopamine	+++	+ to ++[5]	+ to +++[5]	0 to +[6]	↑[5]	↑	↓[5] or ↑	0 to ↑
⇧	Epinephrine	+++	+++	+++[5]	++[5]	↓	↑	↓	↑[3]↓[4]
Mixed	Norepinephrine	++	++[7]	+++	0	↓	0 or ↓	↑	↑
	Ephedrine	++	++	+	0 to +	↓	↑	↑ or ↓	↑
⇩	Mephentermine	+	+	+	++	↑ or ↓	↑	0 to ↑	↑
	Metaraminol	+	+	++	0	↓	↓	↑	↑
Inotropic	Methoxamine	0	0[7]	+++	0	↓	0 or ↓	↑	↑
⇩	Phenylephrine	0	0[7]	+++	0	↓	↓	↑	↑

[1] Cardiogenic or septicemic shock.
[2] Normotensive patient.
[3] Systolic effect.
[4] Diastolic effect.
[5] Effects are dose dependent.
[6] Dilates renal and splanchnic beds via dopaminergic effect at doses < 10 mcg/kg/min.
[7] Decreased heart rate may result from reflex mechanisms.

Common Dilutions and Infusion Rates for Selected Drugs Used in Shock

Drug	Usual Dilution for IV Infusion	Infusion Rate
Isoproterenol	2 mg (10 mL) in 500 mL D5W (4 mcg/mL) or 1 mg (5 mL) in 250 mL D5W	5 mcg/min
Dobutamine	250 mg in 250 to 500 mL NS or D5W (500 to 1000 mcg/mL)	2.5 to 15 mcg/kg/min
Dopamine	200 to 800 mg in 250 to 500 mL NS or D5W (400 to 3200 mcg/mL)	Low dose – 2.5 to 10 mcg/kg/min High dose – 20 to 50 mcg/kg/min
Norepinephrine	4 mg in 250 mL of D5W (16 mcg/mL)	Initial: 8 to 12 mcg/min Maintenance: 2 to 4 mcg/min

ISOPROTERENOL HYDROCHLORIDE

Rx	**Isoproterenol** (Various, eg, Abbott)	**Injection:** 1:5000 solution (0.2 mg/mL)[1]	In 5 and 10 mL vials.
Rx	**Isuprel** (Sanofi Winthrop)		In 1 and 5 mL amps.
Rx	**Isuprel** (Sanofi Winthrop)	**Injection:** 1:50,000 (0.02 mg/mL)[1]	In 10 mL w/needle.

[1] With sodium metabisulfite.

ISOPROTERENOL HYDROCHLORIDE — INJECTION

Refer to the general discussion of these products in the Vasopressors Used in Shock group monograph.

Indications

Isoproterenol hydrochloride injection is indicated:

- For mild or transient episodes of heart block that do not require electric shock or pacemaker therapy.
- For serious episodes of heart block and Adams-Stokes attacks (except when caused by ventricular tachycardia or fibrillation).
- For use in cardiac arrest until electric shock or pacemaker therapy, the treatments of choice, is available.
- For bronchospasm occurring during anesthesia.
- As an adjunct to fluid and electrolyte replacement therapy and the use of other drugs and procedures in the treatment of hypovolemic and septic shock, low cardiac output (hypoperfusion) states, congestive heart failure, and cardiogenic shock.

Administration and Dosage

Isoproterenol hydrochloride injection should generally be started at the lowest recommended dose and the rate of administration gradually increased if necessary while carefully monitoring the patient. Isoproterenol hydrochloride injection 1:50,000 is administered by intravenous (IV) injection. Isoproterenol hydrochloride injection 1:5000 is suitable only for addition to a large volume IV solution single-dose container to prepare a dilute concentration for slow IV infusion.

Recommended Dosage for Adults with Heart Block, Adams-Stokes Attacks, and Cardiac Arrest

Route of administration	Preparation of dilution	Initial dose	Subsequent dose range*
Bolus IV injection	Dilute 1 mL (0.2 mg) of 1:5000 solution to 10 mL with sodium chloride injection or 5% dextrose injection or	0.02 mg to 0.06 mg (1 mL to 3 mL of diluted solution)	0.01 to 0.2 mg (0.5 mL to 10 mL of diluted solution)
	Use 1:50,000 solution undiluted	0.02 mg to 0.06 mg (1 mL to 3 mL)	
IV infusion	Dilute 10 mL (2 mg) of 1:5000 solution in 500 mL of 5% dextrose injection	5 mcg/min (1.25 mL of diluted solution per minute)	

* Subsequent dosage and method of administration depend on the ventricular rate and the rapidity with which the cardiac pacemaker can take over when the drug is gradually withdrawn.

There are no well-controlled studies in children to establish appropriate dosing; however, the American Heart Association recommends an initial infusion rate of 0.1 mcg/kg/min, with the usual range being 0.1 mcg/kg/min to 1 mcg/kg/min.

ISOPROTERENOL HYDROCHLORIDE — INJECTION

Recommended Dosage for Adults with Shock and Hypoperfusion States		
Route of administration	Preparation of dilution[1]	Infusion rate[2]
IV infusion	Dilute 5 mL (1 mg) of 1:5000 solution in 500 mL of 5% dextrose injection	0.5 mcg to 5 mcg per minute (0.25 mL to 2.5 mL of diluted solution)

[1] Concentrations up to 10 times greater have been used when limitation of volume is essential.

[2] Rates over 30 mcg per minute have been used in advanced stages of shock. The rate of infusion should be adjusted on the basis of heart rate, central venous pressure, systemic blood pressure, and urine flow. If the heart rate exceeds 110 beats per minute, it may be advisable to decrease or temporarily discontinue the infusion.

Recommended Dosage for Adults with Bronchospasm Occurring During Anesthesia			
Route of administration	Preparation of dilution	Initial dose	Subsequent dose
Bolus IV injection	Dilute 1 mL (0.2 mg) of 1:5000 solution to 10 mL with sodium chloride injection or 5% dextrose injection or	0.01 mg to 0.02 mg (0.5 mL to 1 mL of diluted solution)	The initial dose may be repeated when necessary.
	Use 1:50,000 solution undiluted	0.01 mg to 0.02 mg (0.5 mL to 1 mL)	

Adequacy and safety of intravenous isoproterenol in children are not established. Based on published literature, the initial dose of intravenous isoproterenol used in children is not established. Based on published literature, the initial dose of intravenous isoproterenol used in children (7 to 19 years of age) ranges between 0.05 to 0.17 mcg/kg/min, which is increased gradually by 0.1 to 0.2 mcg/kg/min at intervals of 15 to 20 minutes, titrated to clinical response; maximum dose ranging between 1.3 to 2.7 mcg/kg/min has been used. In children generally, postoperative cardiac patients with bradycardia require lower doses (0.029 ± 0.002 mcg/kg/min) of intravenous isoproterenol than asthma patients (0.5 ± 0.21 mcg/kg/min).

➤*Storage/Stability:* Store at controlled room temperature 15° to 30°C (59° to 86°F).

Protect from light. Retain in carton until time of use. Do not use the injection if its color is pinkish or darker than slightly yellow or if it contains a precipitate.

Actions

➤*Pharmacology:* Isoproterenol is a potent nonselective beta-adrenergic agonist with very low affinity for alpha-adrenergic receptors. IV infusion of isoproterenol in man lowers peripheral vascular resistance, primarily in skeletal muscle but also in renal and mesenteric vascular beds. Diastolic pressure falls. Renal blood flow is decreased in normotensive subjects but is increased markedly in shock. Systolic blood pressure may remain unchanged or rise although mean arterial pressure typically falls. Cardiac output is increased because of the positive inotropic and chronotropic effects of the drug in the face of diminished peripheral vascular resistance. The cardiac effects of isoproterenol may lead to palpitations, sinus tachycardia, and more serious arrhythmias; large doses of isoproterenol may cause myocardial necrosis in animals.

➤*Pharmacokinetics:* Isoproterenol is readily absorbed when given parenterally or as an aerosol. It is metabolized primarily in the liver and other tissues by catechol-O-methyl transferase (COMT). Isoproterenol is a relatively poor substrate for monoamine oxidase (MAO) and is not taken up by sympathetic neurons to the same extent as are epinephrine and norepinephrine. The duration of action of isoproterenol may therefore be longer than that of epinephrine, but is still brief.

Contraindications

Tachyarrhythmias; tachycardia or heart block caused by digitalis intoxication; ventricular arrhythmias which require inotropic therapy; and angina pectoris.

Warnings

➤*Use following an MI:* Isoproterenol hydrochloride injection, by increasing myocardial oxygen requirements while decreasing effective coronary perfusion, may have a deleterious effect on the injured or failing heart. Most experts discourage its use as the initial agent in treating cardiogenic shock following myocardial infarction. However, when a low arterial pressure has been elevated by other means, isoproterenol hydrochloride injection may produce beneficial hemodynamic and metabolic effects.

In a few patients, presumably with organic disease of the AV node and its branches, isoproterenol hydrochloride injection has paradoxically been reported to worsen heart block or to precipitate Adams-Stokes attacks during normal sinus rhythm or transient heart block.

There are case reports of occasional fatal cardiac dysrhythmia and myocardial necrosis at autopsy as a result of intravenous isoproterenol. ECG changes and serum CPK-MB level elevation consistent with transient myocardial ischemia and abnormal echocardiographic findings suggestive of myocardial dysfunction have been documented with the use of intravenous isoproterenol hydrochloride infusion for the treatment of severe asthma exacerbations in children. Care should be taken to ensure that oxygen is always administered during isoproterenol infusions in patients with asthma. Heart rate, blood pressure, arrhythmias and evidence of myocardial ischemia by ECG should be monitored. Arterial blood gases should also be monitored carefully and PaO_2 maintained above 60 torr. Where ECG suggests myocardial ischemia, cardiac enzymes including cardiac-specific CPK-MB isoenzyme levels should be determined.

➤*Pregnancy:* *Category C.*

Animal reproduction studies have not been conducted with isoproterenol hydrochloride. It is also not known whether isoproterenol hydrochloride can cause fetal harm when administered to a pregnant woman or can affect reproduction capacity. Isoproterenol hydrochloride should be given to a pregnant woman only if clearly needed.

➤*Lactation:* It is not known whether this drug is excreted in human milk. Because many drugs are excreted in human milk, caution should be exercised when isoproterenol hydrochloride injection is administered to a nursing woman.

➤*Children:* The safety and effectiveness of isoproterenol hydrochloride in pediatric patients have not been established.

Precautions

➤*Monitoring:* In addition to the routine monitoring of systemic blood pressure, heart rate, urine flow, and the electrocardiograph, the response to therapy should also be monitored by frequent determination of the central venous pressure and blood gases. Patients in shock should be closely observed during isoproterenol hydrochloride injection administration. If the heart rate exceeds 110 beats per minute, it may be advisable to decrease the infusion rate or temporarily discontinue the infusion. Determinations of cardiac output and circulation time may also be helpful. Appropriate measures should be taken to ensure adequate ventilation. Careful attention should be paid to acid-base balance and to the correction of electrolyte disturbances. In cases of shock associated with bacteremia, suitable antimicrobial therapy is, of course, imperative.

Suggested minimal precautions while infusing isoproterenol hydrochloride continuously include careful monitoring of blood pressure and pulse, ECG monitoring of heart rate, arrhythmias, and evidence of myocardial ischemia, and where ECG evidence suggests myocardial ischemia, daily determination of cardiac enzymes including the more specific CPK-MB isoenzyme, monitoring arterial pH and blood gases carefully and maintaining PaO_2 above 60 torr by administration of supplemental oxygen.

➤*Lowest recommended dose:* Isoproterenol hydrochloride injection should generally be started at the lowest recommended dose. This may be gradually increased, if necessary, while carefully monitoring the patient. Doses sufficient to increase the heart rate to more than 130 beats per minute may increase the likelihood of inducing ventricular arrhythmias. Such increases in heart rate will also tend to increase cardiac work and oxygen requirements which may adversely affect the failing heart or the heart with a significant degree of arteriosclerosis.

➤*Special populations:* Particular caution is necessary in administering isoproterenol hydrochloride injection to patients with coronary artery disease, coronary insufficiency, diabetes, hyperthyroidism, and sensitivity to sympathomimetic amines.

➤*Volume expanders:* Adequate filling of the intravascular compartment by suitable volume expanders of primary importance in most cases of shock, and should precede the administration of vasoactive drugs. In patients with normal cardiac function, determination of central venous pressure is a reliable guide during volume replacement. If evidence of hypoperfusion persists after adequate volume replacement, isoproterenol hydrochloride injection may be given.

➤*Sulfite sensitivity:* Contains sodium metabisulfite, a sulfite that may cause allergic-type reactions including anaphylactic symptoms and life-threatening or less severe asthmatic episodes in certain susceptible people. The overall prevalence of sulfite sensitivity in the general population is unknown and probably low. Sulfite sensitivity is seen more frequently in asthmatic than in nonasthmatic people.

Drug Interactions

Isoproterenol Drug Interactions			
Precipitant drug	Object drug *		Description
Bretylium	Isoproterenol	↑	Bretylium potentiates the action of vasopressors on adrenergic receptors, possibly resulting in arrhythmias.
Guanethidine	Isoproterenol	↑	Guanethidine may increase the pressor response of the direct-acting vasopressors, possibly resulting in severe hypertension.
Halogenated hydrocarbon anesthetics	Isoproterenol	↑	Halogenated hydrocarbon anesthetics may sensitize the myocardium to the effects of catecholamines. Use of vasopressors may lead to serious arrhythmias; use with caution.

ISOPROTERENOL HYDROCHLORIDE — INJECTION

Isoproterenol Drug Interactions			
Precipitant drug	Object drug *		Description
Oxytocic drugs	Isoproterenol	↑	In obstetrics, if vasopressor drugs are used either to correct hypotension or added to the local anesthetic solution, some oxytocic drugs may cause severe persistent hypertension.
Tricyclic antidepressants	Isoproterenol	↑	The pressor response of the direct-acting vasopressors may be potentiated by these agents; use with caution.

* ↑ = Object drug increased.

➤*Epinephrine:* Isoproterenol injection and epinephrine should not be administered simultaneously because both drugs are direct cardiac stimulants and their combined effects may induce serious arrhythmias. The drugs may, however, be administered alternately provided a proper interval has elapsed between doses.

➤*Inhalation anesthetics:* Isoproterenol injection should be used with caution, if at all, when potent inhalational anesthetics such as halothane are employed because of potential to sensitize the myocardium to effects of sympathomimetic amines.

➤*IV methylxanthines and IV steroids:* Cautions should be maintained when using continuous IV isoproterenol hydrochloride infusions in conjunction with intravenous methyl xanthines (aminophylline, theophylline) and intravenous corticosteroids. The use of isoproterenol hydrochloride with aminophylline and corticosteroids may be additive in cardiotoxic properties and can lead to myocardial necrosis and death. Severe cardiac symptoms of sympathetic overactivation (ie, hypertension, tachycardia, arrhythmias, seizures, myocardial ischemia, and fatal myocardial necrosis) have been reported.

Adverse Reactions

The following reactions to isoproterenol hydrochloride injection have been reported:

➤*Cardiovascular:* Tachycardia, palpitations, angina, Adams-Stokes attacks, pulmonary edema, hypertension, hypotension, ventricular arrhythmias, tachyarrhythmias.

In a few patients, presumably with organic disease of the AV node and its branches, isoproterenol hydrochloride injection has been reported to precipitate Adams-Stokes seizures during normal sinus rhythm or transient heart block.

➤*CNS:* Nervousness, headache, dizziness.

➤*Miscellaneous:* Flushing of the skin, sweating, mild tremors, weakness. The following reactions to isoproterenol hydrochloride have been reported in healthy adult controls undergoing upright tilt testing:

Symptoms	Patients (n = 15)	Control group I (n = 13)	Control group II (n = 9)
Warmth	87%	93%	78%
Diaphoresis	87%	77%	56%
Dizziness	80%	77%	56%
Pallor	40%	69%	78%
Visual blurring*	33%	77%	56%
Nausea	40%	39%	22%
Shakiness	20%	8%	22%
Weakness	27%	15%	0%
Headache	33%	8%	0%
Dyspnea	29%	15%	0%

* $P = 0.03$ (difference between patients vs controls).

Overdosage

The acute toxicity of isoproterenol hydrochloride in animals is much less than that of epinephrine. Excessive doses in animals or man can cause a striking drop in blood pressure, and repeated large doses in animals may result in cardiac enlargement and focal myocarditis.

Cardiotoxicity is quite common with use of intravenous isoproterenol infusions. Cardiotoxicity is characterized by ventricular tachyarrhythmias frequently culminating in ventricular fibrillation and sudden death and is associated histologically with well-defined areas of myocardial necrosis.

Cardiotoxicity is highly associated with elevation of CPK-MB isoenzyme levels and ECG abnormalities which should be looked for. There is reason to suspect that there may be a subgroup of patients with asthma who are at increased risk when receiving both beta-adrenergic agonists and methyl xanthines. Risk factors for cardiotoxicity with isoproterenol hydrochloride infusions during treatment of severe asthma include the presence of hypercapnia (Pco_2 greater than 50 mmHg), acidosis (pH less than 7.3) and/or concomitant use of other medications such as corticosteroids or particularly aminophylline and methyl xanthines which may potentiate the cardiotoxic effects of isoproterenol.

In case of accidental overdosage as evidenced mainly by tachycardia or other arrhythmias, palpitations, angina, hypotension, or hypertension, reduce rate of administration or discontinue isoproterenol hydrochloride injection until patient's condition stabilizes. Blood pressure, pulse, respiration, and EKG should be monitored.

It is not known whether isoproterenol hydrochloride is dialyzable.

The oral LD_{50} of isoproterenol hydrochloride in mice is 3,850 mg/kg ± 1,190 mg/kg of pure drug in solution.

DOBUTAMINE

Rx	**Dobutamine hydrochloride** (Various, eg, Hospira)	**Injection:** 12.5 mg/mL	May contain sulfites. In 20 mL vials.

DOBUTAMINE — INJECTION

Refer to the general discussion of these products in the Vasopressors Used in Shock group monograph.

Indications

➤*Cardiac decompensations:* Dobutamine is indicated when parenteral therapy is necessary for inotropic support in the short-term treatment of adults with cardiac decompensation due to depressed contractility resulting either from organic heart disease or from cardiac surgical procedures. Experience with intravenous dobutamine in controlled trials does not extend beyond 48 hours of repeated boluses or continuous infusions.

➤*Unlabeled uses:* Doses of dobutamine 2 and 7.75 mcg/kg/min infused for 10 minutes each have been used investigationally in 12 children with congenital heart disease undergoing diagnostic cardiac catheterization. The drug appears effective in augmenting cardiovascular function in children, and no adverse effects were noted.

Administration and Dosage

➤*Approved by the FDA:* October 19, 1993.

➤*Rate of administration:* The rate of infusion needed to increase cardiac output usually ranges from 2.5 to 10 mcg/kg/min. On rare occasions, infusion rates up to 40 mcg/kg/min have been required. A metering device is recommended for controlling the rate of drug administration.

Adjust rate of administration and duration of therapy according to patient response, as determined by heart rate, presence of ectopic activity, blood pressure, urine flow, and, when possible, measurement of central venous or pulmonary wedge pressure and cardiac output.

Concentrations up to 5000 mcg/mL have been administered (250 mg/50 mL). Determine the final volume administered by the fluid requirements of the patient.

Infusion Rates of Various Dilutions of Dobutamine			
Desired Delivery Rate (mcg/kg/min)	Infusion Rate (mL/kg/min)		
	250 mcg/mL	500 mcg/mL	1000 mcg/mL
2.5	0.01	0.005	0.0025
5	0.02	0.01	0.005
7.5	0.03	0.015	0.0075
10	0.04	0.02	0.01
12.5	0.05	0.025	0.0125
15	0.06	0.03	0.015

➤*Preparation and stability:* At the time of administration, dobutamine must be further diluted in an IV container to at least a 50 mL solution using one of the following intravenous solutions as a diluent: 5% Dextrose Injection, 5% Dextrose and 0.45% Sodium Chloride Injection, 5% Dextrose and 0.9% Sodium Chloride Injection, 10% Dextrose Injection, *Isolyte M* with 5% Dextrose Injection, Lactated Ringer's Injection, 5% Dextrose in Ringer's Lactate Injection, *Normosol-M* in D5W, 20% *Osmitrol* in Water for Injection, 0.9% Sodium Chloride Injection, or Sodium Lactate Injection. Intravenous solutions should be used within 24 hours.

➤*Storage/Stability:* Store at controlled room temperature, 15° to 30°C (59° to 86°F).

Actions

➤*Pharmacology:* Dobutamine is a direct-acting inotropic agent whose primary activity results from stimulation of the β receptors of the heart while producing comparatively mild chronotropic, hypertensive, arrhythmogenic, and vasodilative effects. It does not cause the release of endogenous norepinephrine, as does dopamine. In animal studies, dobutamine produces less increase in heart rate and less decrease in peripheral vascular resistance for a given inotropic effect than does isoproterenol.

In patients with depressed cardiac function, both dobutamine and isoproterenol increase the cardiac output to a similar degree. In the case of dobutamine, this increase is usually not accompanied by marked increases in

DOBUTAMINE — INJECTION

heart rate (although tachycardia is occasionally observed), and the cardiac stroke volume is usually increased. In contrast, isoproterenol increases the cardiac index primarily by increasing the heart rate while stroke volume changes little or declines.

The effective infusion rate of dobutamine varies widely from patient to patient, and titration is always necessary. At least in pediatric patients, dobutamine-induced increases in cardiac output and systemic pressure are generally seen, in any given patient, at lower infusion rates than those that cause substantial tachycardia.

➤*Pharmacokinetics:*

Absorption/Distribution – The onset of action of dobutamine is within 1 to 2 minutes; however, as much as 10 minutes may be required to obtain the peak effect of a particular infusion rate.

Metabolism – The plasma half-life of dobutamine in humans is 2 minutes. The principal routes of metabolism are methylation of the catechol and conjugation.

Excretion – In human urine, the major excretion products are the conjugates of dobutamine and 3-O-methyl dobutamine. The 3-O-methyl derivative of dobutamine is inactive.

Contraindications

Idiopathic hypertrophic subaortic stenosis; previous manifestations of hypersensitivity to dobutamine.

Warnings

➤*Increase in heart rate or blood pressure:* Dobutamine may cause a marked increase in heart rate or blood pressure, especially systolic pressure. Approximately 10% of adult patients in clinical studies have had rate increases of 30 beats/minute or more, and about 7.5% have had a 50 mmHg or greater increase in systolic pressure. Usually, reduction of dosage promptly reverses these effects. Because dobutamine facilitates atrioventricular conduction, patients with atrial fibrillation are at risk of developing rapid ventricular response. In patients who have atrial fibrillation with rapid ventricular response, a digitalis preparation should be used prior to institution of therapy with dobutamine. Patients with preexisting hypertension appear to face an increased risk of developing an exaggerated pressor response.

➤*Ectopic activity:* Dobutamine may precipitate or exacerbate ventricular ectopic activity, but it rarely has caused ventricular tachycardia.

➤*Hypersensitivity reactions:* Reactions suggestive of hypersensitivity associated with administration of dobutamine including skin rash, fever, eosinophilia, and bronchospasm, have been reported occasionally.

➤*Carcinogenesis:* Studies to evaluate the carcinogenic potential of dobutamine have not been conducted.

➤*Mutagenesis:* Studies to evaluate the mutagenic potential of dobutamine have not been conducted.

➤*Fertility impairment:* Studies to evaluate the potential of dobutamine to affect fertility, have not been conducted.

➤*Pregnancy: Category B.*

Teratogenic – There are, however, no adequate and well-controlled studies in pregnant women. Because animal reproduction studies are not always predictive of human response, this drug should be used during pregnancy only if clearly needed.

➤*Lactation:* It is not known whether this drug is excreted in human milk. Because many drugs are excreted in human milk, caution should be exercised when dobutamine is administered to a nursing woman. If a mother requires dobutamine treatment, breastfeeding should be discontinued for the duration of the treatment.

➤*Children:* Dobutamine has been shown to increase cardiac output and systemic pressure in pediatric patients of every age group. In premature neonates, however, dobutamine is less effective than dopamine in raising systemic blood pressure without causing undue tachycardia, and dobutamine has not been shown to provide any added benefit when given to such infants already receiving optimal infusions of dopamine.

Precautions

➤*Monitoring:* During the administration of dobutamine, as with any adrenergic agent, ECG, and blood pressure should be continuously monitored. In addition, pulmonary wedge pressure and cardiac output should be monitored whenever possible to aid in the safe and effective infusion of dobutamine.

➤*Special risk:*

Hypovolemia – Hypovolemia should be corrected with suitable volume expanders before treatment with dobutamine is instituted.

Use following acute myocardial infarction (MI) – Clinical experience with dobutamine following MI has been insufficient to establish the safety of the drug for this use. There is concern that any agent that increases contractile force and heart rate may increase the size of an infarction by intensifying ischemia, but it is not known whether dobutamine does so.

➤*Lab test abnormalities:* Dobutamine, like other β_2-agonists, can produce a mild reduction in serum potassium concentration, rarely to hypokalemic levels. Accordingly, consideration should be given to monitoring serum potassium.

➤*Sulfite sensitivity:* Dobutamine contains sodium bisulfite, a sulfite that may cause allergic-type reactions, including anaphylactic symptoms and life-threatening or less severe asthmatic episodes, in certain susceptible people. The overall prevalence of sulfite sensitivity in the general population is unknown and probably low. Sulfite sensitivity is seen more frequently in asthmatic than in nonasthmatic people.

Drug Interactions

Dobutamine Drug Interactions

Precipitant drug	Object drug*		Description
Bretylium	Dobutamine	↑	Bretylium may potentiate the action of vasopressors on adrenergic receptors, possibly resulting in arrhythmias.
Guanethidine	Dobutamine	↑	Guanethidine may increase the pressor response of the direct-acting vasopressors, possibly resulting in severe hypertension.
Halogenated hydrocarbon anesthetics	Dobutamine	↑	Halogenated hydrocarbon anesthetics may sensitize the myocardium to the effects of catecholamines. Use of vasopressors may lead to serious arrhythmias; use with extreme caution.
Oxytocic drugs	Dobutamine	↑	In obstetrics, if vasopressor drugs are used either to correct hypotension or added to local anesthetic solutions, some oxytocic drugs may cause severe persistent hypertension.
Tricyclic antidepressants	Dobutamine	↑	The pressor response of the direct-acting vasopressors may be potentiated by these agents; use with caution.

* ↑ = Object drug increased.

➤*Beta-blockers:* Animal studies indicate that dobutamine may be ineffective if the patient has recently received a β-blocking drug. In such a case, the peripheral vascular resistance may increase.

➤*Nitroprusside:* Preliminary studies indicate that the concomitant use of dobutamine and nitroprusside results in a higher cardiac output and, usually, a lower pulmonary wedge pressure than when either drug is used alone.

Adverse Reactions

➤*Cardiovascular:*

Increased heart rate, blood pressure, and ventricular ectopic activity – A 10 to 20 mm Hg increase in systolic blood pressure and an increase in heart rate of 5 to 15 beats/minute have been noted in most patients (see Warnings regarding exaggerated chronotropic and pressor effects). Approximately 5% of patients have had increased premature ventricular beats during infusions. These effects are dose related.

Hypotension – Precipitous decreases in blood pressure have occasionally been described in association with dobutamine therapy. Decreasing the dose or discontinuing the infusion typically results in rapid return of blood pressure to baseline values. In rare cases, however, intervention may be required and reversibility may not be immediate.

➤*Lab test abnormalities:* Isolated cases of thrombocytopenia have been reported.

Administration of dobutamine, like other catecholamines, can produce a mild reduction in serum potassium concentration, rarely to hypokalemic levels.

➤*Local:*

Reactions at sites of IV infusion – Phlebitis has occasionally been reported. Local inflammatory changes have been described following inadvertent infiltration. Isolated cases of cutaneous necrosis (destruction of skin tissue) have been reported.

➤*Miscellaneous:*

Uncommon effects – The following adverse effects have been reported in 1% to 3% of patients: nausea, headache, anginal pain, nonspecific chest pain, palpitations, and shortness of breath.

Overdosage

➤*Symptoms:* Overdoses of dobutamine have been reported rarely. The following is provided to serve as a guide if such an overdose is encountered.

Toxicity from dobutamine is usually due to excessive cardiac β-receptor stimulation. The duration of action of dobutamine is generally short ($t_{1/2}$ = 2 minutes) because it is rapidly metabolized by catechol-0-methyltranferase. The symptoms of toxicity may include anorexia, nausea, vomiting, tremor, anxiety, palpitations, headache, shortness of breath, and anginal and nonspecific chest pain. The positive inotropic and chronotropic effects of dobutamine on the myocardium may cause hypertension, tachyarrhythmias, myocardial ischemia, and ventricular fibrillation. Hypotension may result from vasodilation.

➤*Treatment:* To obtain up-to-date information about the treatment of overdose, a good resource is your certified regional poison control center. In managing overdosage, consider the possibility of multiple drug overdoses, interaction among drugs, and unusual drug kinetics in your patient.

The initial actions to be taken in a dobutamine overdose are discontinuing administration, establishing an airway, and ensuring oxygenation and ven-

DOBUTAMINE — INJECTION

tilation. Resuscitative measures should be initiated promptly. Severe ventricular tachyarrhythmias may be successfully treated with propranolol or lidocaine. Hypertension usually responds to a reduction in dose or discontinuation of therapy.

Protect the patient's airway and support ventilation and perfusion. If needed, meticulously monitor and maintain, within acceptable limits, the patient's vital signs, blood gases, serum electrolytes, etc.

If the product is ingested, unpredictable absorption may occur from the mouth and the GI tract. Absorption of drugs from the GI tract may be decreased by giving activated charcoal, which, in many cases, is more effective than emesis or lavage; consider charcoal instead of or in addition to gastric emptying. Repeated doses of charcoal over time may hasten elimination of some drugs that have been absorbed. Safeguard the patient's airway when employing gastric emptying or charcoal.

Forced diuresis, peritoneal dialysis, hemodialysis, or charcoal hemoperfusion have not been established as beneficial for an overdose of dobutamine.

DOPAMINE HYDROCHLORIDE

Rx	**Dopamine Hydrochloride** (Various, eg, American Regent, Astra, ESI)	**Injection:** 40 mg/mL	In 5 mL amps, 5, 10 and 20 mL vials and 5 and 10 mL syringes.
Rx	**Dopamine Hydrochloride** (Abbott)		In 5 mL and 10 mL Pintop vials, Fliptop vials and additive syringes.[1]
Rx	**Dopamine Hydrochloride** (Various, eg, American Regent, Astra, ESI)	**Injection:** 80 mg/mL	In 5 mL amps; 5 and 20 mL vials and 10 mL syringes.
Rx	**Dopamine Hydrochloride** (Abbott)		In 10 mL vials.[1]
Rx	**Dopamine Hydrochloride** (Various)	**Injection:** 160 mg/mL	In 5 mL vials.
Rx	**Dopamine Hydrochloride in 5% Dextrose** (Various, eg, Baxter, Hospira)	**Injection:** 80 mg/100 mL (0.8 mg/mL)[2]	In 250 and 500 mL.
		160 mg/100 mL (1.6 mg/mL)[2]	In 250 and 500 mL.
		320 mg/100 mL (3.2 mg/mL)[2]	In 250 mL.

[1] With 9 mg sodium metabisulfite.
[2] With 50 mg sodium metabisulfite.

DOPAMINE HYDROCHLORIDE — INJECTION

Refer to the general discussion of these products in the Vasopressors Used in Shock group monograph.

WARNING

Antidote for peripheral ischemia – To prevent sloughing and necrosis in ischemic areas, the area should be infiltrated as soon as possible with 10 to 15 mL of saline solution containing 5 to 10 mg of phentolamine, an adrenergic blocking agent. A syringe with a fine hypodermic needle should be used, and the solution liberally infiltrated throughout the ischemic area. Sympathetic blockade with phentolamine causes immediate and conspicuous local hyperemic changes if the area is infiltrated within 12 hours. Therefore, phentolamine should be given as soon as possible after the extravasation is noted.

Indications

➤*Hemodynamic imbalances:* Dopamine is indicated for the correction of hemodynamic imbalances present in the shock syndrome due to myocardial infarctions, trauma, endotoxic septicemia, open heart surgery, renal failure, and chronic cardiac decompensation as in congestive failure.

➤*Poor perfusion of vital organs:* Urine flow appears to be one of the better diagnostic signs by which adequacy of vital organ perfusion can be monitored. Nevertheless, the physician should also observe the patient for signs of reversal of confusion of comatose condition. Loss of pallor, increase in toe temperature, and/or adequacy of nail bed capillary filling may also be used as indices of adequate dosage. Clinical studies have shown that when dopamine is administered before urine flow has diminished to levels approximating 0.3 mL/min, prognosis is more favorable. Nevertheless, in a number of oliguric or anuric patients, administration of dopamine has resulted in an increase in urine flow which in some cases reached normal levels. Dopamine may also increase urine flow in patients whose output is within normal limits and thus may be of value in reducing the degree of preexisting fluid accumulation. It should be noted that at doses above those optimal for the individual patient urine flow may decrease, necessitating reduction of dosage. Concurrent administration of dopamine and diuretic agents may produce an additive or potentiating effect.

➤*Low cardiac output:* Increased cardiac output is related to the direct inotropic effect of dopamine on the myocardium. Increased cardiac output at low or moderate doses appears to be related to a favorable prognosis. Increase in cardiac output has been associated with either static or decreased systemic vascular resistance (SVR). Static or decreased SVR associated with low or moderate increments in cardiac output is believed to be a reflection of differential effects on specific vascular beds with increased resistance in peripheral beds (eg, femoral) and concomitant decreases in mesenteric and renal vascular beds. Redistribution of blood flow parallels these changes so that an increase in cardiac output is accompanied by an increase in mesenteric and renal blood flow. In many instances the renal fraction of the total cardiac output has been found to increase. The increase in cardiac output produced by dopamine is not associated with substantial decreases in systemic vascular resistance as may occur with isoproterenol.

➤*Hypotension:* Hypotension due to inadequate cardiac output can be managed by administration of low to moderate doses of dopamine, which have little effect on SVR. At high therapeutic doses, the alpha adrenergic activity of dopamine becomes more prominent and thus may correct hypotension due to diminished SVR. As in the case of other circulatory decompensation states, prognosis is better in patients whose blood pressure and urine flow have not undergone profound deterioration. Therefore, it is suggested that the physician administer dopamine as soon as a definite trend toward decreased systolic and diastolic pressure becomes evident.

➤*Unlabeled uses:* Chronic obstructive pulmonary disease (COPD) (4 mcg/kg/min); congestive heart failure (CHF) (2 to 5 mcg/kg/min); respiratory distress syndrome (RDS) in infants (starting at 5 mcg/kg/min).

Administration and Dosage

➤*Approved by the FDA:* February 4, 1982.

This is a potent drug. It must be diluted before administration to patient.

Do not add dopamine injection to sodium bicarbonate or other alkaline IV solutions, since the drug is inactivated in alkaline solution.

Mixing of dopamine with alteplase in the same container should be avoided as visible particulate matter has been observed.

It is recommended that dopamine not be added to amphotericin B solutions because amphotericin B is physically unstable in dopamine-containing solutions.

➤*Storage/Stability:* Store at controlled room temperature 15° to 30°C (59° to 86°F).

Dopamine has been found to be stable for a minimum of 24 hours after dilution in the sterile IV solutions listed above. However, as with all IV admixtures, dilution should be made just prior to administration.

Actions

➤*Pharmacology:* Dopamine is a natural catecholamine formed by the decarboxylation of 3,4-dihydroxyphenylalanine (DOPA). It is a precursor to norepinephrine in noradrenergic nerves and is also a neurotransmitter in certain areas of the central nervous system, especially in the nigrostriatal tract, and in a few peripheral sympathetic nerves.

Dopamine produces positive chronotropic and inotropic effects on the myocardium, resulting in increased heart rate and cardiac contractility. This is accomplished directly by exerting an agonist action on beta-adrenoceptors and indirectly by causing release of norepinephrine from storage sites in sympathetic nerve endings.

➤*Pharmacokinetics:*

Absorption/Distribution – Dopamine's onset of action occurs within 5 minutes of intravenous administration, and with dopamine's plasma half-life of about 2 minutes, the duration of action is less than 10 minutes. If monoamine oxidase (MAO) inhibitors are present, however, the duration may increase to 1 hour. The drug is widely distributed in the body but does not cross the blood-brain barrier to a significant extent.

Metabolism/Excretion – Dopamine is metabolized in the liver, kidney, and plasma by MAO and catechol-O-methyltransferase to the inactive compounds homovanillic acid (HVA) and 3,4-dihydroxyphenylacetic acid. About 25% of the dose is taken up into specialized neurosecretory vesicles (the adrenergic nerve terminals), where it is hydroxylated to form norepinephrine. It has been reported that about 80% of the drug is excreted in the urine within 24 hours, primarily as HVA and its sulfate and glucuronide conjugates and as 3,4-dihydroxyphenylacetic acid. A very small portion is excreted unchanged.

Contraindications

Pheochromocytoma; uncorrected tachyarrhythmias; ventricular fibrillation.

Warnings

➤*Weaning:* When discontinuing the infusion, it may be necessary to gradually decrease the dose of dopamine while expanding blood volume with IV fluids, since sudden cessation may result in marked hypotension.

Do not add dopamine to any alkaline diluent solution, since the drug is inactivated in alkaline solution.

Patients who have been treated with MAO inhibitors prior to the administration of dopamine will require substantially reduced dosage. Because dopamine is metabolized by monoamine oxidase, inhibition of this enzyme prolongs and potentiates the effect of dopamine. Patients who have been treated with MAO inhibitors within 2 to 3 weeks prior to the administration

DOPAMINE HYDROCHLORIDE — INJECTION

of dopamine should receive initial doses of dopamine not greater than one-tenth (1/10 of the usual dose.

➤*Mutagenesis:* Dopamine at doses approaching maximal solubility shows no clear genotoxic potential in the Ames test. Although there was a reproducible dose-dependent increase in the number of revertant colonies with strains TA100 and TA98, both with and without metabolic activation, the small increase was considered inconclusive evidence of mutagenicity. In the L5178Y $TK^{+/-}$ mouse lymphoma assay, dopamine at the highest concentrations used of 750 mcg/mL without metabolic activation, and 3000 mcg/mL with activation, was toxic and associated with increases in mutant frequencies when compared to untreated and solvent controls; at the lower concentrations no increases over controls were noted.

➤*Pregnancy: Category C.*

Teratogenic – Teratogenicity studies in rats and rabbits at dopamine dosages up to 6 mg/kg/day IV during organogenesis produced no detectable teratogenic or embryotoxic effects, although maternal toxicity consisting of mortalities, decrease body weight gain, and pharmacotoxic signs were observed in rats. In a published study, dopamine administered at 10 mg/kg subcutaneously for 30 days, markedly prolonged metestrus and increased mean pituitary and ovary weights in female rats. Similar administration to pregnant rats throughout gestation or for 5 days starting on gestation day 10 or 15 resulted in decreased body weight gains, increased mortalities and slight increases in cataract formation among the offspring. There are no adequate and well-controlled studies in pregnant women, and it is not known if dopamine hydrochloride crosses the placental barrier. Dopamine should be used during pregnancy only if the potential benefit justifies the potential risk to the fetus.

Labor and delivery – In obstetrics, if vasopressor drugs are used to correct hypotension or are added to a local anesthetic solution the interaction with some oxytocic drugs may cause severe hypertension.

➤*Lactation:* It is not known whether this drug is excreted in human milk. Because many drugs are excreted in human milk, caution should be exercised when dopamine is administered to a breast-feeding mother.

➤*Children:* Safety and effectiveness in children have not been established. Dopamine HCl has been used in a limited number of pediatric patients, but such use has been inadequate to fully define proper dosage and limitations for use. Peripheral gangrene has been reported in neonates and children.

Precautions

➤*Monitoring:* Close monitoring of these indices (urine flow, cardiac output and blood pressure) during dopamine infusion is necessary as in the case of any adrenergic agent.

➤*Hypovolemia:* Prior to treatment with dopamine, hypovolemia should be fully corrected, if possible with either whole blood or plasma as indicated. Monitoring of central venous pressure of left ventricular filling pressure may be helpful in detecting and treating hypovolemia.

➤*Hypoxia, hypercapnia, acidosis:* These conditions which may also reduce the effectiveness and/or increase the incidence of adverse effects of dopamine, must be identified and corrected prior to, or concurrently with administration of dopamine.

➤*Ventricular arrhythmias:* If an increased number of ectopic beats are observed, the dose should be reduced if possible.

➤*Decreased pulse pressure:* If a disproportionate rise in the diastolic pressure (ie, a marked decrease in the pulse pressure) is observed in patients receiving dopamine, the infusion rate should be decreased and the patient observed carefully for further evidence of predominant vasoconstrictor activity, unless such an effect is desired.

➤*Hypotension:* At lower infusion rates, if hypotension occurs, the infusion rate should be rapidly increased until adequate blood pressure is obtained. If hypotension persists, dopamine should be discontinued and a more potent vasoconstrictor agent such as norepinephrine should be administered.

➤*Extravasation:* Dopamine should be infused into a large vein whenever possible to prevent the possibility of extravasation into tissue adjacent to the infusion site. Extravasation may cause necrosis and sloughing of surrounding tissue. Large veins of the antecubital fossa are preferred to veins in the dorsum of the hand or ankle. Less suitable infusion sites should be used only if the patient's condition requires immediate attention. The physician should switch to more suitable sites as rapidly as possible. The infusion site should be continuously monitored for free flow.

➤*Occlusive vascular disease:* Patients with a history of occlusive vascular disease (eg, atherosclerosis, arterial embolism, and Raynaud's disease, cold injury, diabetic endarteritis, and Buerger disease) should be closely monitored for any changes in color or temperature of the skin in the extremities. If a change in skin color or temperature occurs and is thought to be the result of compromised circulation to the extremities, the benefits of continued dopamine infusion should be weighed against the risk of possible necrosis. This condition may be reversed by either decreasing or discontinuing the rate of infusion.

➤*Sulfite sensitivity:* Some of these products contain sodium metabisulfite, a sulfite that may cause allergic-type reactions including anaphylactic symptoms and life-threatening or less severe asthmatic episodes in certain susceptible people. The overall prevalence of sulfite sensitivity in the general population is unknown, and probably low. Sulfite sensitivity is seen more frequently in asthmatic than in nonasthmatic people.

Drug Interactions

Dopamine Drug Interactions			
Precipitant drug	Object drug*		Description
Dopamine	Guanethidine	⬇	The antihypertensive effects of guanethidine may be partially or totally reversed by the mixed-acting sympathomimetics.
Halogenated hydrocarbon anesthetics	Dopamine	⬆	Halogenated hydrocarbon anesthetics may sensitize the myocardium to the effects of catecholamines. Use of vasopressors may lead to serious arrhythmias; use with extreme caution.
Monoamine oxidase inhibitors (MAOIs)	Dopamine	⬆	MAOIs increase the pressor response to dopamine by 6- to 20-fold. Dopamine is metabolized by MAOIs, and inhibition of this enzyme prolongs and potentiates the effect of dopamine. This interaction also may occur with furazolidone, an antimicrobial with MAOI activity. Avoid these combinations; if given inadvertently and hypertension occurs, administer phentolamine.
Oxytocic drugs	Dopamine	⬆	In obstetrics, if vasopressor drugs are used to correct hypotension or are added to the local anesthetic solution, some oxytocics may cause severe persistent hypertension.
Dopamine	Phenytoin	⬇	Concomitant infusion of dopamine has been reported to lead to seizures, severe hypotension, and bradycardia. If necessary, discontinue phenytoin and provide supportive treatment.
Tricyclic antidepressants	Dopamine	⬇	The pressor response of the mixed-acting vasopressors may be decreased by these agents; a higher dose of the sympathomimetic may be necessary.

* ⬆ = Object drug increased. ⬇ = Object drug decreased.

➤*Halogenated hydrocarbon anesthetics:* Cyclopropane or halogenated hydrocarbon anesthetics increase cardiac autonomic irritability and may sensitize the myocardium to the action of certain intravenously administered catecholamines, such as dopamine. The interaction appears to be related both to pressor activity and to the beta-adrenergic-stimulating properties of these catecholamines, and may produce ventricular arrhythmias. Therefore, extreme caution should be exercised when administering dopamine to patients receiving cyclopropane or halogenated hydrocarbon anesthetics. Results of studies in animals indicate that dopamine induced ventricular arrhythmias during anesthesia can be reversed by propranolol.

➤*MAO inhibitors:* Because dopamine is metabolized by monoamine oxidase, inhibition of this enzyme prolongs and potentiates the effect of dopamine. Patients who have been treated with MAO inhibitors within 2 to 3 weeks prior to the administration of dopamine should receive initial doses of dopamine not greater than one-tenth (1/10 of the usual dose.

➤*Dopamine and diuretics:* Coadministration of low-dose dopamine and diuretic agents may produce an additive or potentiating effect on urine flow.

➤*Beta-blockers/alpha-adrenergic blocking agents:* Cardiac effects of dopamine are antagonized by beta-adrenergic blocking agents, such as propranolol and metroprolol. The peripheral vasoconstriction caused by high doses of dopamine is antagonized by alpha-adrenergic blocking agents. Dopamine-induced renal and mesenteric vasodilation is not antagonized by either alpha- or beta-adrenergic blocking agents.

➤*Haloperidol and phenothiazines:* Butyrophenones (such as haloperidol) and phenothiazines can suppress the dopaminergic renal and mesenteric vasodilation induced with low-dose dopamine infusion.

➤*Vasopressors, ergonovine, oxytocics:* The concomitant use of vasopressors, vasoconstrictive agents (such as ergonovine) and some oxytocic drugs may result in severe hypertension.

Adverse Reactions

The following adverse reactions have been observed, but there are not enough data to support an estimate of their frequency.

➤*Cardiovascular:* Ventricular arrhythmia (at very high doses), ectopic beats, tachycardia, anginal pain, palpitation, cardiac conduction abnormalities, widened QRS complex, bradycardia, hypotension, hypertension, vasoconstriction.

DOPAMINE HYDROCHLORIDE — INJECTION

➤*CNS:* Headache, anxiety.

➤*Dermatologic:* Piloerection.

➤*GI:* Nausea, vomiting.

➤*Metabolic/Nutritional:* Azotemia.

➤*Respiratory:* Dyspnea.

➤*Miscellaneous:* Gangrene of the extremities has occurred when moderate to high doses were administered for prolonged periods or in patients with occlusive vascular disease receiving low doses of dopamine.

A few cases of peripheral cyanosis have been reported.

Overdosage

➤*Treatment:* In case of accidental overdosage, as evidenced by excessive blood pressure elevation, reduce rate of administration or temporarily discontinue dopamine until patient's condition stabilizes. Since the duration of action of dopamine is quite short, no additional remedial measures are usually necessary. If these measures fail to stabilize the patient's condition, use of the short-acting alpha adrenergic blocking agent, phentolamine, should be considered.

EPINEPHRINE

Rx	**Epinephrine** (Abbott)	**Solution:** 1:1000 (1 mg/mL)	In 1 mL amps[1]
Rx	**EpiPen** (Dey)		In 0.3 mL single-dose auto-injectors.[2]
Rx	**Adrenalin Chloride** (Monarch)	**Solution:** 1:1000 (1 mg/mL as HCl)	In 1 mL amps[3] and 30 mL *Steri-vials*.[4]
Rx	**EpiPen Jr** (Dey)	**Solution:** 1:2000 (0.5 mg/mL)	In 0.3 mL single-dose auto-injectors.[2]
Rx	**Epinephrine** (Abbott)	**Solution:** 1:10,000 (0.1 mg/mL)	In 10 mL single-dose *Abboject* prefilled syringes with either 18-G 3.5 inch or 21-G 1.5 inch needles, in 10 mL single-dose *Abboject* prefilled *LifeShield* syringes,[5] and in 10 mL vials.
Rx	**Adrenalin Chloride Solution** (Monarch)	**Solution for inhalation:** 1:100 (10 mg/mL as HCl) solution	In 7.5 mL.[6]
Rx	**Adrenalin Chloride Solution** (Monarch)	**Topical solution:** 1:1000 (1 mg/mL as HCl) solution	In 30 mL.[7]
otc	**microNefrin** (Bird)	**Solution for inhalation:** 2.25% racepinephrine HCl (1.125% epinephrine base)	In 15 and 30 mL.[8]
otc	**Nephron** (Nephron)		In 15 mL.[8]
otc	**S2** (Nephron)		In 15 mL.[8]
otc	**Epinephrine Mist** (Various, eg, Alpharma, Major)	**Aerosol:** 0.22 mg epinephrine/spray	May contain alcohol. In 15 mL.
otc	**Primatene Mist** (Wyeth Consumer Healthcare)		34% alcohol. In 15 mL w/mouthpiece or 15 and 22.5 mL refills.
Rx	**Epinephrine** (Various, eg, Abbott, American Regent)	**Injection:** 1:1000 (1 mg/mL as HCl) solution	May contain sodium metabisulfite. In 1 mL amps.
Rx	**Adrenalin Chloride Solution** (Monarch)		In 1 mL amps[9] and 30 mL *Steri-vials*.[10]
Rx	**Epinephrine** (Abbott)	**Injection:** 1:10,000 (0.1 mg/mL) solution	In 10 mL prefilled syringe.[9]

[1] With 0.9 mg sodium metabisulfite and 9 mg sodium chloride per mL.
[2] With 0.5 mg sodium metabisulfite and 1.8 mg sodium chloride.
[3] With not more than 0.1% sodium bisulfite.
[4] With 0.5% chlorobutanol and not more than 0.15% sodium bisulfite.
[5] With 0.46 mg sodium metabisulfite and 8.16 mg sodium chloride per mL.
[6] With benzethonium chloride and 0.2% sodium bisulfite.
[7] With chlorobutanol and 0.15% sodium bisulfite.
[8] With sodium bisulfite, potassium metabisulfite, chlorobutanol, benzoic acid, and propylene glycol.
[9] With sodium bisulfite.
[10] With sodium bisulfite and chlorobutanol.

EPINEPHRINE — INHALATION

Refer to the general discussion of these products in the Vasopressors Used in Shock group monograph. See also Bronchodilators in the Respiratory Agents chapter and Agents for Glaucoma in the Ophthalmic and Otic Agents chapter.

Indications

➤*Bronchial asthma (Rx and OTC):* For temporary relief of shortness of breath, tightness of chest, and wheezing due to bronchial asthma. The inhalation of epinephrine solution 1:100 eases breathing for asthma patients by reducing spasms of bronchial muscles.

Administration and Dosage

➤*Rx:* For relief of bronchial congestion in asthma, epinephrine solution 1:100 should be applied with a glass or plastic nebulizer capable of delivering a very fine spray, and which will work with a very small amount of solution.

Approximately 10 drops (not more) of epinephrine solution 1:100 are placed in the reservoir of the nebulizer, the nozzle of which is placed just inside the partially opened mouth. As the bulb is squeezed once or twice, the patient inhales deeply, drawing the vaporized solution into the lungs. Treatment should be started at the first symptoms. Rinsing the mouth with water immediately after using epinephrine solution 1:100 will help prevent the sensation of dryness of mouth and throat, which may otherwise follow.

Adults and children 4 years of age and older – Inhalation dosage for adults, children, and adolescents 4 years of age and older is 1 to 3 inhalations not more often than every 3 hours. The use of this product by children and adolescents should be supervised by an adult.

Children younger than 4 years of age – Consult a physician.

When the nebulizer contains any liquid and is not in use, it should be stoppered and kept in an upright position. Because of oxidation, epinephrine solution 1:100 will turn pink to brown when exposed to air. Light, heat, alkalies, and certain metals (eg, copper, iron, zinc) will also promote deterioration. A discolored inhalation solution or one containing a precipitate should not be used.

➤*OTC:*

Adults and children 4 years of age and older – Start with 1 inhalation, then wait at least 1 minute. If not relieved, use once more. Do not use again for at least 3 hours.

Children younger than 4 years of age – Consult a doctor.

The use of this product by children should be supervised by an adult.

Each inhalation delivers 0.22 mg of epinephrine.

➤*Storage/Stability:* Do not use the inhalation solution if it is pinkish or darker than slightly yellow or if it contains a precipitate.

Rx – Store between 15° and 25°C (59° and 77°F). Protect from light and freezing.

OTC – Store at room temperature 15° and 30°C (59° and 86°F).

Contents under pressure. Do not puncture or throw container into incinerator. Using or storing near open flame or heating above 49°C (120°F) may cause bursting.

Warnings

➤*Proper diagnosis:* Do not use this product unless a diagnosis of asthma has been made by a physician.

➤*Hypodermic injection:* Epinephrine solution 1:100 is supplied for use by oral (not nasal) inhalation only. Because of the relatively high concentration, epinephrine solution 1:100 is not suitable for hypodermic injection.

➤*Symptomatic relief:* Do not continue to use this product, but seek medical assistance immediately, if symptoms are not relieved within 20 minutes or become worse.

➤*Excessive use:* Do not use this product more frequently or at higher doses than recommended unless directed by a physician. Excessive use may cause nervousness and rapid heart beat and possibly, adverse effects on the heart.

➤*Pregnancy:* As with any drug, if you are pregnant, seek the advice of a health professional before using this product.

➤*Lactation:* As with any drug, if you are breast-feeding a baby, seek the advice of a health professional before using this product.

➤*Children:* Keep this and all drugs out of the reach of children. In case of accidental overdose, seek professional assistance or contact a poison control center immediately.

Precautions

➤*Special risk:* Do not use this product if you have heart disease, high blood pressure, thyroid disease, or difficulty in urination due to enlargement of the prostate gland unless directed by a physician.

Do not use this product if you have ever been hospitalized for asthma or if you are taking any prescription drug for asthma unless directed by a physician.

EPINEPHRINE — INHALATION

Drug Interactions

Epinephrine Drug Interactions			
Precipitant drug	Object drug *		Description
Alpha-adrenergic blockers (eg, phentolamine)	Epinephrine	⬇	The vasoconstricting and hypertensive effects are antagonized by alpha-adrenergic blocking drugs.
Beta-adrenergic blockers, nonspecific	Epinephrine	⬆	Coadministration allows alpha-receptor effects of epinephrine to predominate, causing hypertension and reflex bradycardia.
Cardiac glycosides	Epinephrine	⬆	Cardiac glycosides may sensitize the myocardium to the actions of sympathomimetics.
Chlorpromazine	Epinephrine	⬇	Chlorpromazine may reverse the pressor effects of epinephrine.
Diuretic drugs	Epinephrine	⬇	Diuretic agents may decrease vascular response to pressor drugs such as epinephrine.
Furazolidone	Epinephrine	⬆	Furazolidone may increase the pressor sensitivity to epinephrine, possibly resulting in hypertension. Avoid coadministration if possible.
Halogenated hydrocarbon anesthetics, cyclopropane	Epinephrine	⬆	Halogenated hydrocarbon anesthetics and cyclopropane may sensitize the myocardium to the effects of epinephrine and may lead to serious arrhythmias; use with extreme caution.
Levothyroxine Antihistamines (eg, chlorpheniramine, tripelennamine, diphenhydramine)	Epinephrine	⬆	The pressor response of the direct-acting vasopressors may be potentiated by these agents; use with caution.
Monoamine oxidase inhibitors (MAOIs)	Epinephrine	⬆	Although coadministration of an MAOI with an indirect- or mixed-acting sympathomimetic may cause severe headache, hypertension, high fever, and hypertensive crisis, direct-acting sympathomimetics (eg, epinephrine) appear to interact minimally.
Methyldopa	Epinephrine	⬆	Coadministration may result in increased pressor response, possibly resulting in hypertension.
Oxytocic drugs	Epinephrine	⬆	Coadministration may result in hypertension.
Reserpine	Epinephrine	⬆	Reserpine may potentiate the pressor response of epinephrine, resulting in hypertension.
Sympathomimetic drugs (eg, isoproterenol)	Epinephrine	⬆	Do not coadminister epinephrine with other sympathomimetic drugs because of possible additive effects and increased toxicity. Combined effects may induce serious cardiac arrhythmias. They may be administered alternately when the preceding effect of other such drugs has subsided.
Tricyclic antidepressants	Epinephrine	⬆	The pressor response of the direct-acting vasopressors may be potentiated by these agents; use with caution.
Epinephrine	Guanethidine	⬇	Epinephrine may antagonize the effects of guanethidine, resulting in decreased antihypertensive effect and requiring increased dosage of guanethidine.

* ⬆ = Object drug increased. ⬇ = Object drug decreased.

Do not use this product if you are presently taking a prescription drug for high blood pressure or depression without first consulting your physician.

➤*MAOIs:* Do not use this product if you are now taking a prescription monoamine oxidase inhibitor (MAOI) (certain drugs for depression, psychiatric, emotional conditions, or Parkinsons disease), or for weeks after stopping MAOI drug. If you are uncertain whether your prescription drug contains an MAOI, consult a health professional before taking this product.

Patient Information

➤*OTC:*

Directions for use of mouthpiece – The mouthpiece, which is enclosed in the *Primatene Mist* 15 mL (not the refill size), should be used for inhalation only with *Primatene Mist*.

Take plastic cap off mouthpiece. (For refills, use mouthpiece from previous purchase.)

Care of mouthpiece: The *Primatene Mist* mouthpiece should be washed once a day with hot, soapy water, rinsed thoroughly, and dried with a clean, lint-free cloth.

If the unit becomes clogged and fails to spray, please write and send the clogged unit to: Whitehall-Robins Healthcare, PO Box 26609, Richmond, VA 23261-6609.

EPINEPHRINE — INJECTION

Refer to the general discussion of these products in the Vasopressors Used in Shock group monograph. See also Bronchodilators in the Respiratory Agents chapter and Agents for Glaucoma in the Ophthalmic and Otic Agents chapter.

Indications

➤*1:1,000:* Epinephrine is used to relieve respiratory distress due to bronchospasm, to provide rapid relief of hypersensitivity reactions to drugs and other allergens, and to prolong the action of anesthetics. Its cardiac effects may be of use in restoring cardiac rhythm in cardiac arrest due to various causes, but it is not used in cardiac failure or in hemorrhagic, traumatic, or cardiogenic shock.

Epinephrine is used as a hemostatic agent. It is also used in treating mucosal congestion of hay fever, rhinitis, and acute sinusitis; to relieve bronchial asthmatic paroxysms; in syncope due to complete heart block or carotid sinus hypersensitivity; for symptomatic relief of serum sickness, urticaria, angioneurotic edema; for resuscitation in cardiac arrest following anesthetic accidents; in simple (open-angle) glaucoma; for relaxation of uterine musculature and to inhibit uterine contractions. Epinephrine injection can be utilized to prolong the action of anesthetics used in local and regional anesthesia.

➤*1:1,000 (auto-injector) and 1:2,000 (auto-injector):* Epinephrine by auto-injector is indicated in the emergency treatment of allergic reactions (anaphylaxis) to insect stings or bites, foods, drugs, and other allergens, as well as idiopathic or exercise-induced anaphylaxis. The epinephrine auto-injectors are intended for immediate self-administration by a person with a history of an anaphylactic reaction. Such reactions may occur within minutes after exposure and consist of flushing, apprehension, syncope, tachycardia, thready or unobtainable pulse associated with a fall in blood pressure, convulsions, vomiting, diarrhea and abdominal cramps, involuntary voiding, wheezing, dyspnea due to largyngeal spasm, pruritus, rashes, urticaria, or angioedema. The epinephrine auto-injectors are designed as emergency supportive therapy only and are not replacements or substitutes for immediate medical or hospital care.

➤*1:10,000:* Epinephrine injection is indicated for IV injection in the following:

1.) Treatment of acute hypersensitivity (anaphylactoid reactions to drugs, animal serums and other allergens).
2.) Treatment of acute asthmatic attacks to relieve bronchospasm not controlled by inhalation or subcutaneous administration of other solutions of the drug.
3.) Treatment and prophylaxis of cardiac arrest and attacks of transitory atrioventricular (AV) heart block with syncopal seizures (Stokes-Adams syndrome).

In acute attacks of ventricular standstill, physical measures should be applied first. When external cardiac compression and attempts to restore the circulation by electrical defibrillation or use of a pacemaker fail, intracardiac puncture, and intramyocardial injection of epinephrine may be effective.

➤*Unlabeled uses:* Endoscopic injection therapy with epinephrine or a mixture of epinephrine and saline has been shown to be a safe and effective hemostatic option in the management of acute lower GI bleeding.

Administration and Dosage

Do not remove ampules from carton until ready to use. Do not use the injection if its color is pinkish or darker than slightly yellow or if it contains a precipitate.

Do not administer unless solution is clear and container is intact. Discard unused portion.

Epinephrine is readily destroyed by alkalies and oxidizing agents. In the latter category are oxygen, chlorine, bromine, iodine, permanganates, chromates, nitrites, and salts of easily reducible metals, especially iron.

➤*Subcutaneously or intramuscularly:*

1:1,000 – 0.2 to 1 mL (mg). Start with a small dose and increase if required.
Note: The subcutaneous is the preferred route of administration. If given intramuscularly, injection into the buttocks should be avoided.

EPINEPHRINE — INJECTION

For bronchial asthma in pediatric patients, administer 0.01 mL/kg or 0.3 mL/m^2 to a maximum of 0.5 mL subcutaneously, repeated every 4 hours if required.

Neonates may be given a dose of 0.01 mg per kg of body weight; for the infant, 0.05 mg is an adequate initial dose, and this may be repeated at 20- to 30-minute intervals in the management of asthma attacks.

For bronchial asthma and certain allergic manifestations (eg, angioedema, urticeria, serum sickness, anaphylactic shock), use epinephrine subcutaneously.

➤*IV:* The adult IV dose for hypersensitivity reactions or to relieve bronchospasm usually ranges from 0.1 to 0.25 mg (1 to 2.5 mL of 1:10,000 solution) injected slowly. Neonates may be given a dose of 0.01 mg/kg of body weight; for the infant 0.05 mg is an adequate initial dose, and this may be repeated at 20- to 30-minute intervals in the management of asthma attacks.

1:10,000 – Epinephrine injection (1:10,000) is administered by IV injection or, in cardiac arrest, by intracardiac injection into the left ventricular chamber or via endotracheal tube directly into the bronchial tree.

➤*Epinephrine auto-injectors:* Usual epinephrine adult dose for allergic emergencies is 0.3 mg. For pediatric use, the appropriate dosage may be 0.15 or 0.3 mg, depending upon the body weight of the patient. A dosage of 0.01 mg per kg body weight is recommended. Epinephrine auto-injector (1:2,000), which provides a dosage of 0.15 mg, may be more appropriate for patients weighing less than 30 kg. However, the prescribing physician has the option of prescribing more or less than these amounts, based on careful assessment of each individual patient and recognizing the life-threatening nature of the reactions for which this drug is being prescribed. The physician should consider using other forms of injectable epinephrine if doses lower than 0.15 mg are felt to be necessary.

Each epinephrine auto-injector contains a single dose of epinephrine. With severe persistent anaphylaxis, repeat injections with an additional epinephrine auto-injector may be necessary.

➤*Cardiac resuscitation:*

1:1000 – A dose of 0.5 mL (0.5 mg) diluted to 10 mL with sodium chloride injection can be administered intravenously or intracardially to restore myocardial contractility.

Intracardiac injection should only be administered by personnel well trained in the technique, if there has not been sufficient time to establish an IV route.

External cardiac massage should follow intracardial administration to permit the drug to enter coronary circulation. The drug should be used secondarily to unsuccessful attempts with physical or electromechanical methods.

1:10,000 – Epinephrine injection is administered by intravenous injection or in cardiac arrest, by intracardiac injection into the left ventricular chamber or via endotracheal tube directly into the bronchial tree.

In cardiac arrest, 0.5 to 1 mg (5 to 10 mL of 1:10,000 solution) may be given. During a resuscitation effort, 0.5 mg (5 mL) should be administered IV every 5 minutes.

Intracardiac injection should only be administered by personnel well trained in the technique, if there has not been sufficient time to establish an IV route. The intracardiac dose usually ranges from 0.3 to 0.5 mg (3 to 5 mL of 1:10,000 solution).

Alternatively, if the patient has been intubated, epinephrine can be injected via the endotracheal tube directly into the bronchial tree at the same dosage as for IV injection. It is rapidly absorbed through the lung capillary bed.

➤*Intraspinal use:* Usual dose is 0.2 to 0.4 mL added to anesthetic spinal use with local anesthetic. Epinephrine 1:100,000 to 1:20,000 is the usual concentration employed with local anesthetics.

➤*Ophthalmologic use:*

1:1,000 – Ophthalmologic use (for producing conjunctival decongestion, to control hemorrhage, produce myariasis and reduce intraocular pressure)—Use a concentration of 1:10,000 to 1:1,000.

➤*Regional anesthesia:* A final concentration of 1:200,000 of epinephrine injection is recommended for infiltration injection, nerve block, caudal or other epidural blocks. From 0.3 to 0.4 mg of epinephrine (0.3 to 0.4 mL of 1:1,000 solution) may be mixed with spinal anesthetic agents.

➤*Storage/Stability:* Store at controlled room temperature 15° to 30°C (59° to 86°F).

Protect from light.

Epinephrine deteriorates rapidly on exposure to air or light, turning pink from oxidation to adrenochrome and brown from the formation of melanin. Solutions which show evidence of discoloration should be replaced.

Auto-injectors – Epinephrine is light sensitive, and should be stored in the tube provided. Store in a dark place at room temperature (15° to 30°C; 59° to 86°F). Do not refrigerate. Contains no latex.

Actions

➤*Pharmacology:* Epinephrine is a sympathomimetic drug. It activates an adrenergic receptive mechanism on effector cells and imitates all actions of the sympathetic nervous system except those on the arteries of the face and sweat glands. The actions of epinephrine resemble the effects of stimulation of adrenergic nerves. To a variable degree it acts on both alpha and beta receptor sites of sympathetic effector cells, and is the most potent alpha receptor activator. Its most prominent actions are on the beta receptors of the heart, vascular and other smooth muscle. When given by rapid IV injection, it produces a rapid rise in blood pressure, mainly systolic, by:

1.) Direct stimulation of cardiac muscle which increases the strength of ventricular contraction.
2.) Increasing the heart rate.
3.) Constriction of the arterioles in the skin, mucosa and splanchnic areas of the circulation.

When given by slow IV injection, epinephrine usually produces only a moderate rise in systolic and a fall in diastolic pressure. Although some increases in pulse pressure occurs, there is usually no great elevation in mean blood pressure. Accordingly, the compensatory reflex mechanisms that come into play with a pronounced increase in blood pressure do not antagonize the direct cardiac actions of epinephrine as much as with catecholamines that have a predominant action on alpha receptors.

Total peripheral resistance decreases by action of epinephrine on beta receptors of the skeletal muscle vasculature and blood flow is thereby enhanced. Usually this vasodilator effect of the drug on the circulation predominates so that the modest rise in systolic pressure which follows slow injection or absorption is mainly the result of direct cardiac stimulation and increase in cardiac output. In some instances peripheral resistance is not altered or may even rise owing to a greater ratio of alpha to beta activity in different vascular areas.

Epinephrine relaxes the smooth muscles of the bronchi and iris and is a physiologic antagonist of histamine. The drug also produces an increase in blood sugar and glycogenolysis in the liver.

➤*Pharmacokinetics:*

Absorption/Distribution – IV injection produces an immediate and intensified response. Following IV injection, epinephrine disappears rapidly from the bloodstream.

Metabolism/Excretion – The large portion of injection doses is excreted in the urine as inactivated compounds. The remainder is excreted in the urine as unchanged or conjugated compounds.

The drug becomes fixed in the tissues and is rapidly inactivated chiefly by enzymatic transformation in the liver and other tissues to metanephrine or normetanephrine, either of which is subsequently conjugated and excreted in the urine in the form of sulfates and glucuronides. Either sequence results in the formation of 3-methoxy-4-hydroxy-mandelic acid (vanillylmandelic acid: VMA) which also is detectable in the urine.

Contraindications

In patients with known hypersensitivities to sympathomimetic amines.

In narrow-angle (congestive) glaucoma, shock (nonanaphylactic), during general anesthesia and halogenated hydrocarbons or cyclopropane and in individuals with organic brain damage. Epinephrine is also contraindicated with local anesthesia of certain areas (fingers, toes) because of the danger of vasoconstriction producing sloughing of tissue; in labor because it may delay the second stage; in cardiac dilatation and coronary insufficiency.

Except as diluted for admixture with local anesthetics to reduce absorption and prolong action, epinephrine should not ordinarily be used in those cases where vasopressor drugs may be contraindicated (eg, in thyrotoxicosis, diabetes, in obstetrics when maternal blood pressure is in excess of 130/80 and in hypertension and other cardiovascular disorders.

There are no absolute contraindications to the use of epinephrine in a life-threatening situation.

Warnings

➤*Light exposure:* Epinephrine injection is subject to oxidation and should be protected against exposure to light and stored in light-resistant containers.

➤*Special risk populations:* Administer this medication with caution to those with cardiovascular disease, hypertension, diabetes, or hyperthyroidism; to psychoneurotic individuals; and to pregnant women.

Patients with long-standing bronchial asthma and emphysema who have developed degenerative heart disease should be administered the drug with extreme caution.

➤*Overdosage:* Overdosage or inadvertent IV injection of epinephrine may result in angina pectoris, aortic rupture, or cerebral hemorrhage, resulting from the sharp rise in blood pressure.

➤*Fatality:* Fatalities may also result from pulmonary edema because of the peripheral constriction and cardiac stimulation produced. Rapidly acting vasodilators such as nitrites, or alpha-blocking agents may counteract the marked pressor effects of epinephrine.

➤*Arrhythmias:* Epinephrine may induce potentially serious cardiac arrhythmias in patients not suffering from heart disease and in patients with organic heart disease or who are receiving drugs that sensitize the myocardium.

➤*Epinephrine auto-injectors:* Accidental injection into the hands or feet may result in loss of blood flow to the affected area and should be avoided. If there is an accidental injection into these areas, advise the patient to go immediately to the nearest emergency room for treatment. Epinephrine auto-injectors should only be injected into the anterolateral aspect of the thigh.

➤*Renal function impairment:* Parenterally administered epinephrine initially may produce constriction of renal blood vessels and decrease urine formation.

➤*Elderly:* Administer with caution to elderly patients.

EPINEPHRINE — INJECTION

➤*Pregnancy:* Category C.

Epinephrine has been shown to be teratogenic in rats when given in doses about 25 times the human dose. There are no adequate and well-controlled studies in pregnant women. It is also not known whether epinephrine can cause fetal harm when administered to a pregnant woman or can affect reproduction capacity. Epinephrine should be given to a pregnant woman only if clearly needed and if anticipated benefits outweigh possible hazards.

Labor and delivery – Parenteral administration of epinephrine if used to support blood pressure during low or other spinal anesthesia for delivery can cause acceleration of fetal heart rate and should not be used in obstetrics when maternal blood pressure exceeds 130/80.

➤*Children:* Epinephrine may be given safely to pediatric patients at a dosage appropriate to body weight.

Precautions

➤*Special risk:* Although epinephrine can produce ventricular fibrillation, its actions in restoring electrical activity in asystole and in enhancing defibrillation of the fibrillating ventricle are well documented. The drug, however, should be used with caution in patients with ventricular fibrillation.

Epinephrine should be used cautiously in patients with hyperthyroidism, hypertension and cardiac arrhythmias. All vasopressors should be used cautiously in patients taking monoamine oxidase (MAO) inhibitors.

Epinephrine is ordinarily administered with extreme caution to patients who have heart disease.

Epinephrine auto-injectors – Some patients may be at greater risk of developing adverse reactions after epinephrine administration. These include the following: Hyperthyroid individuals, individuals with cardiovascular disease, hypertension, or diabetes, elderly individuals, pregnant women, pediatric patients under 30 kg (66 lbs) body weight using *EpiPen* and pediatric patients under 15 kg (33 lbs) body weight using *EpiPen Jr.*

Despite these concerns, epinephrine is essential for the treatment of anaphylaxis. Therefore, patients with these conditions, or any other person who might be in a position to administer epinephrine auto-injectors to patients experiencing anaphylaxis should be carefully instructed in regard to the circumstances under which this lifesaving medication should be used.

1:10,000 – In patients with prefibrillatory rhythm, IV epinephrine must be used judiciously with extreme caution because of its excitatory action on the heart. Since the myocardium is sensitized to this action of the drug by many anesthetic agents, epinephrine may convert asystole to ventricular fibrillation if used in the treatment of anesthetic cardiac accidents.

➤*Sulfite sensitivity:*

1:1000 – Epinephrine is the preferred treatment for serious allergic or other emergency situations, even though these products may contain sodium metabisulfite, a sulfite that may in other products cause allergic-type reactions, including anaphylactic symptoms or life-threatening or less severe asthmatic episodes in certain susceptible persons. The alternatives to using epinephrine in a life-threatening situation may not be satisfactory. The presence of a sulfite in this product should not deter administration of the drug for treatment of serious allergic or other emergency situations.

Drug Interactions

Epinephrine Drug Interactions

Precipitant drug	Object drug *		Description
Alpha-adrenergic blockers (eg, phentolamine)	Epinephrine	⬇	The vasoconstricting and hypertensive effects are antagonized by alpha-adrenergic blocking drugs.
Beta-adrenergic blockers, nonspecific	Epinephrine	⬆	Coadministration allows alpha-receptor effects of epinephrine to predominate, causing hypertension and reflex bradycardia.
Cardiac glycosides	Epinephrine	⬆	Cardiac glycosides may sensitize the myocardium to the actions of sympathomimetics.
Chlorpromazine	Epinephrine	⬇	Chlorpromazine may reverse the pressor effects of epinephrine.
Diuretic drugs	Epinephrine	⬇	Diuretic agents may decrease vascular response to pressor drugs such as epinephrine.
Furazolidone	Epinephrine	⬆	Furazolidone may increase the pressor sensitivity to epinephrine, possibly resulting in hypertension. Avoid coadministration if possible.
Halogenated hydrocarbon anesthetics, cyclopropane	Epinephrine	⬆	Halogenated hydrocarbon anesthetics and cyclopropane may sensitize the myocardium to the effects of epinephrine and may lead to serious arrhythmias; use with extreme caution.
Levothyroxine Antihistamines (eg, chlorpheniramine, tripelennamine, diphenhydramine)	Epinephrine	⬆	The pressor response of the direct-acting vasopressors may be potentiated by these agents; use with caution.
Monoamine oxidase inhibitors (MAOIs)	Epinephrine	⬆	Although coadministration of an MAOI with an indirect- or mixed-acting sympathomimetic may cause severe headache, hypertension, high fever, and hypertensive crisis, direct-acting sympathomimetics (eg, epinephrine) appear to interact minimally.
Methyldopa	Epinephrine	⬆	Coadministration may result in increased pressor response, possibly resulting in hypertension.
Oxytocic drugs	Epinephrine	⬆	Coadministration may result in hypertension.
Reserpine	Epinephrine	⬆	Reserpine may potentiate the pressor response of epinephrine, resulting in hypertension.
Sympathomimetic drugs (eg, isoproterenol)	Epinephrine	⬆	Do not coadminister epinephrine with other sympathomimetic drugs because of possible additive effects and increased toxicity. Combined effects may induce serious cardiac arrhythmias. They may be administered alternately when the preceding effect of other such drugs has subsided.
Tricyclic antidepressants	Epinephrine	⬆	The pressor response of the direct-acting vasopressors may be potentiated by these agents; use with caution.
Epinephrine	Guanethidine	⬇	Epinephrine may antagonize the effects of guanethidine, resulting in decreased antihypertensive effect and requiring increased dosage of guanethidine.

* ⬆ = Object drug increased. ⬇ = Object drug decreased.

➤*Digitalis glycosides and diuretic agents:* Use of epinephrine with excessive doses of digitalis, mercurial diuretics, quinidine, or other drugs that sensitize the heart to arrhythmias is not recommended. Anginal pain may be induced when coronary insufficiency is present.

➤*Drug/Lab test interactions:*

Non-interaction – Sodium chloride added to render the solution isotonic for injection of the active ingredient is present in amounts insufficient to affect serum electrolyte balance of sodium (Na^+) and chloride (Cl^-)ions.

Adverse Reactions

➤*Transient and minor side effects:* Transient and minor side effects of anxiety, headache, fear, and palpitations occur only with systemic therapeutic doses, especially in hyperthyroid individuals. Adverse effects such as cardiac arrhythmias and excessive rise in blood pressure may occur with systemic therapeutic doses or with inadvertent overdosage. Repeated local injections can result in necrosis at sites of injection from vascular constriction. "Epinephrine-fastness" can occur with prolonged use.

➤*Other adverse reactions:* Other adverse reactions include cerebral hemorrhage, hemiplegia, subarachnoid hemorrhage, anginal pain in patients with angina pectoris, anxiety, restlessness, headache, tremor, weakness, dizziness, pallor and respiratory difficulty. Such reactions are unlikely when epinephrine is diluted to 1:200,000 for injection with local anesthetic agents.

➤*Epinephrine auto-injectors:* Side effects of epinephrine may include palpitations, tachycardia, sweating, nausea and vomiting, respiratory difficulty, pallor, dizziness, weakness, tremor, headache, apprehension, nervousness and anxiety.

Cardiac arrhythmias may follow administration of epinephrine.

Overdosage

➤*Symptoms:* Erroneous administration of large doses of epinephrine may lead to precordial distress, vomiting, headache, dyspnea, as well as unusually elevated blood pressure.

Overdosage or inadvertent intravascular injection of epinephrine may cause cerebral hemorrhage resulting from a sharp rise in blood pressure. Fatalities may also result from pulmonary edema because of peripheral vascular constriction together with cardiac stimulation.

➤*Treatment:* Toxic effects of overdosage can be counteracted by injection of an alpha-adrenergic blocker and a beta-adrenergic blocker. In the event of a sharp rise in blood pressure, rapid-acting vasodilators such as the nitrites,

EPINEPHRINE — INJECTION

or alpha-adrenergic-blocking agents can be given to counteract the marked pressor effect of large doses of epinephrine.

Patient Information

Epinephrine is essential for the treatment of anaphylaxis. Patients with histories of severe allergic reactions (anaphylaxis) to insect stings or bites, foods, drugs, and other allergens, as well as idiopathic and exercise-induced anaphylaxis should be carefully instructed about the circumstances under which this lifesaving medication should be used. It must be clearly determined that the patient is at risk of future anaphylaxis, since the following risks may be associated with epinephrine administration.

EPINEPHRINE — TOPICAL

Refer to the general discussion of these products in the Vasopressors Used in Shock group monograph. See also Bronchodilators in the Respiratory Agents chapter and Agents for Glaucoma in the Ophthalmic and Otic Agents chapter.

Indications

➤*Nasal decongestant:* For use as a nasal decongestant.

Administration and Dosage

Apply locally as drops or spray or with a sterile swab, as required. See product labeling for dilution instructions.

NOREPINEPHRINE BITARTRATE (Levarterenol)

Rx	**Norepinephrine Bitartrate** (Abbott)	**Injection:** 1 mg (as base)/mL	In 4 mL amps.[1]
Rx	**Levophed** (Abbott)		In 4 mL amps.[2]

[1] Contains 0.46 mg sodium metabisulfite and 8.2 mg sodium chloride.

[2] Contains ≤ 2 mg metabisulfite.

NOREPINEPHRINE BITARTRATE — INJECTION

Refer to the general discussion of these products in the Vasopressors Used in Shock group monograph.

WARNING

Antidote for extravasation ischemia – To prevent sloughing and necrosis in areas in which extravasation has taken place, the area should be infiltrated as soon as possible with 10 mL to 15 mL of saline solution containing from 5 mg to 10 mg of phentolamine, an adrenergic blocking agent. A syringe with a fine hypodermic needle should be used, with the solution being infiltrated liberally throughout the area, which is easily identified by its cold, hard, and pallid appearance. Sympathetic blockade with phentolamine causes immediate and conspicuous local hyperemic changes if the area is infiltrated within 12 hours. Therefore, phentolamine should be given as soon as possible after the extravasation is noted.

Indications

➤*Blood pressure control in acute hypotensive states:* For blood pressure control in certain acute hypotensive states (eg, pheochromocytomectomy, sympathectomy, poliomyelitis, spinal anesthesia, MI, septicemia, blood transfusion, and drug reactions).

➤*Cardiac arrest:* As an adjunct in the treatment of cardiac arrest and profound hypotension.

Administration and Dosage

Norepinephrine bitartrate is a concentrated, potent drug which must be diluted in dextrose containing solutions prior to infusion. An infusion of norepinephrine bitartrate should be given into a large vein.

➤*Restoration of blood pressure in acute hypotensive states:* Blood volume depletion should always be corrected as fully as possible before any vasopressor is administered. When, as an emergency measure, intraaortic pressures must be maintained to prevent cerebral or coronary artery ischemia, norepinephrine bitartrate can be administered before and concurrently with blood volume replacement.

Average dosage – Add a 4 mL ampul (4 mg) of norepinephrine bitartrate to 1000 mL of a 5% dextrose containing solution. Each mL of this dilution contains 4 mcg of the base of norepinephrine bitartrate. Give this solution by IV infusion. Insert a plastic IV catheter through a suitable bore needle well advanced centrally into the vein and securely fixed with adhesive tape, avoiding, if possible, a catheter tie-in technique as this promotes stasis. An IV drip chamber or other suitable metering device is essential to permit an accurate estimation of the rate of flow in drops per minute. After observing the response to an initial dose of 2 mL to 3 mL (from 8 mcg to 12 mcg of base) per minute, adjust the rate of flow to establish and maintain a low normal blood pressure (usually 80 mm Hg to 100 mm Hg systolic) sufficient to maintain the circulation to vital organs. In previously hypertensive patients, it is recommended that the blood pressure should be raised no more than 40 mm Hg below the preexisting systolic pressure. The average maintenance dose ranges from 0.5 mL to 1 mL per min (from 2 mcg to 4 mcg of base).

High dosage – Great individual variation occurs in the dose required to attain and maintain an adequate blood pressure. In all cases, dosage of norepinephrine bitartrate should be titrated according to the response of the patient. Occasionally much larger or even enormous daily doses (as high as 68 mg base or 17 ampuls) may be necessary if the patient remains hypotensive, but occult blood volume depletion should always be suspected and corrected when present. Central venous pressure monitoring is usually helpful in detecting and treating this situation.

Fluid intake – The degree of dilution depends on clinical fluid volume requirements. If large volumes of fluid (dextrose) are needed at a flow rate that would involve an excessive dose of the pressor agent per unit of time, a solution more dilute than 4 mcg per mL should be used. On the other hand, when large volumes of fluid are clinically undesirable, a concentration more than 4 mcg/mL may be necessary.

Duration of therapy – The infusion should be continued until adequate blood pressure and tissue perfusion are maintained without therapy. Infusions of norepinephrine bitartrate should be reduced gradually, avoiding abrupt withdrawal. In some of the reported cases of vascular collapse due to acute MI, treatment was required for up to 6 days.

➤*Adjunctive treatment in cardiac arrest:* Infusions of norepinephrine bitartrate are usually administered by IV during cardiac resuscitation to restore and maintain an adequate blood pressure after an effective heartbeat and ventilation have been established by other means. Norepinephrine bitartrate's powerful beta-adrenergic stimulating action is also thought to increase the strength and effectiveness of systolic contractions once they occur.

Average dosage – To maintain systemic blood pressure during the management of cardiac arrest, norepinephrine bitartrate is used in the same manner as described under restoration of blood pressure in acute hypotensive states.

Do not use the solution if its color is pinkish or darker than slightly yellow or if it contains a precipitate.

Avoid contact with iron salts, alkalis, or oxidizing agents.

➤*Storage/Stability:* Store at 25°C (77°F); excursions permitted to 15° to 30°C (59° to 86°F).

Protect from light.

Actions

➤*Pharmacology:* Norepinephrine bitartrate functions as a peripheral vasoconstrictor (alpha-adrenergic action) and as an inotropic stimulator of the heart and dilator of coronary arteries (beta-adrenergic action).

Contraindications

➤*Emergency use only:* Norepinephrine bitartrate should not be given to patients who are hypotensive from blood volume deficits except as an emergency measure to maintain coronary and cerebral artery perfusion until blood volume replacement therapy can be completed. If norepinephrine bitartrate is continuously administered to maintain blood pressure in the absence of blood volume replacement, the following may occur: Severe peripheral and visceral vasoconstriction, decreased renal perfusion and urine output, poor systemic blood flow despite "normal" blood pressure, tissue hypoxia, and lactate acidosis.

➤*Mesenteric or peripheral vascular thrombosis:* Norepinephrine bitartrate should also not be given to patients with mesenteric or peripheral vascular thrombosis (because of the risk of increasing ischemia and extending the area of infarction) unless, in the opinion of the attending physician, the administration of norepinephrine bitartrate is necessary as a lifesaving procedure.

Cardiac arrhythmias may result from the use of norepinephrine bitartrate injection in patients with profound hypoxia or hypercarbia.

Cyclopropane and halothane anesthetics increase cardiac autonomic irritability and therefore seem to sensitize the myocardium to the action of IV administered epinephrine or norepinephrine. Hence, the use of norepinephrine bitartrate injection during cyclopropane and halothane anesthesia is generally considered contraindicated because of the risk of producing ventricular tachycardia or fibrillation.

Warnings

See Drug Interactions for more information.

➤*Elderly:* Clinical studies of norepinephrine bitartrate did not include sufficient numbers of patients aged 65 and over to determine whether they respond differently from younger subjects. Other reported clinical experience has not identified differences in responses between the elderly and younger patients. In general, dose selection for an elderly patient should be cautious, usually starting at the low end of the dosing range, reflecting the greater frequency of decreased hepatic, renal, or cardiac function, and of concomitant disease or other drug therapy.

Norepinephrine bitartrate injection infusions should not be administered into the veins in the leg in elderly patients.

➤*Pregnancy: Category C.*

Animal reproduction studies have not been conducted with norepinephrine bitartrate. It is also not known whether norepinephrine bitartrate can cause

NOREPINEPHRINE BITARTRATE — INJECTION

fetal harm when administered to a pregnant woman or can affect reproduction capacity. Norepinephrine bitartrate should be given to a pregnant woman only if clearly needed.

➤*Lactation:* It is not known whether this drug is excreted in human milk. Because many drugs are excreted in human milk, caution should be exercised when norepinephrine bitartrate is administered to a breast-feeding woman.

➤*Children:* Safety and effectiveness in pediatric patients have not been established.

Precautions

➤*Monitoring:* Because of the potency of norepinephrine bitartrate and because of varying response to pressor substances, the possibility always exists that dangerously high blood pressure may be produced with overdoses of this pressor agent. It is desirable, therefore, to record the blood pressure every 2 minutes from the time administration is started until the desired blood pressure is obtained, then every 5 minutes if administration is to be continued.

The rate of flow must be watched constantly, and the patient should never be left unattended while receiving norepinephrine bitartrate injection. Headache may be a symptom of hypertension due to overdosage.

➤*Site of infusion:* Whenever possible, infusions of norepinephrine bitartrate injection should be given into a large vein, particularly an antecubital vein because, when administered into this vein, the risk of necrosis of the overlying skin from prolonged vasoconstriction is apparently very slight. Some authors have indicated that the femoral vein is also an acceptable route of administration. A catheter tie-in technique should be avoided, if possible, since the obstruction to blood flow around the tubing may cause stasis and increased local concentration of the drug. Occlusive vascular diseases (eg, atherosclerosis, arteriosclerosis, diabetic endarteritis, Buerger's disease) are more likely to occur in the lower than in the upper extremity. Therefore, one should avoid the veins of the leg in elderly patients or in those suffering from such disorders. Gangrene has been reported in a lower extremity when infusions of norepinephrine bitartrate injection were given in an ankle vein.

➤*Extravasation:* The infusion site should be checked frequently for free flow. Care should be taken to avoid extravasation of norepinephrine bitartrate injection into the tissues, as local necrosis might ensue due to the vasoconstrictive action of the drug. Blanching along the course of the infused vein, sometimes without obvious extravasation, has been attributed to vasa vasorum constriction with increased permeability of the vein wall, permitting some leakage.

This also may progress on rare occasions to superficial slough, particularly during infusion into leg veins in elderly patients or in those suffering from obliterative vascular disease. Hence, if blanching occurs, consideration should be given to the advisability of changing the infusion site at intervals to allow the effects of local vasoconstriction to subside.

➤*Sulfite sensitivity:* Norepinephrine bitartrate injection contains sodium metabisulfite, a sulfite that may cause allergic-type reactions including anaphylactic symptoms and life-threatening or less severe asthmatic episodes in certain susceptible people. The overall prevalence of sulfite sensitivity in the general population is unknown. Sulfite sensitivity is seen more frequently in asthmatic than in nonasthmatic people.

Drug Interactions

➤*Cyclopropane and halothane anesthetics:* Cyclopropane and halothane anesthetics increase cardiac autonomic irritability and therefore seem to sensitize the myocardium to the action of IV administered epinephrine or norepinephrine. Hence, the use of norepinephrine bitartrate injection during cyclopropane and halothane anesthesia is generally considered contraindicated because of the risk of producing ventricular tachycardia or fibrillation. The same type of cardiac arrhythmias may result from the use of norepinephrine bitartrate injection in patients with profound hypoxia or hypercarbia.

➤*MAO inhibitors (MAOIs):* Norepinephrine bitartrate injection should be used with extreme caution in patients receiving monoamine oxidase inhibitors (MAOI) or antidepressants of the triptyline or imipramine types, because severe, prolonged hypertension may result.

Adverse Reactions

➤*Cardiovascular:* Bradycardia, probably as a reflex result of a rise in blood pressure, arrhythmias.

➤*CNS:* Anxiety, transient headache.

➤*Dermatologic:* Extravasation necrosis at injection site.

➤*Respiratory:* Respiratory difficulty.

➤*Miscellaneous:* Ischemic injury due to potent vasoconstrictor action and tissue hypoxia.

➤*Prolonged administration or overdosage:* Prolonged administration of any potent vasopressor may result in plasma volume depletion which should be continuously corrected by appropriate fluid and electrolyte replacement therapy. If plasma volumes are not corrected, hypotension may recur when norepinephrine bitartrate injection is discontinued, or blood pressure may be maintained at the risk of severe peripheral and visceral vasoconstriction (eg, decreased renal perfusion) with diminution in blood flow and tissue perfusion with subsequent tissue hypoxia and lactic acidosis and possible ischemic injury. Gangrene of extremities has been rarely reported.

Hypersensitivity – Overdoses or conventional doses in hypersensitive persons (eg, hyperthyroid patients) cause severe hypertension with violent headache, photophobia, stabbing retrosternal pain, pallor, intense sweating, and vomiting.

Overdosage

Overdosage with norepinephrine bitartrate may result in headache, severe hypertension, reflex bradycardia, marked increase in peripheral resistance, and decreased cardiac output. In case of accidental overdosage, as evidenced by excessive blood pressure elevation, discontinue norepinephrine bitartrate injection until the condition of the patient stabilizes.

EPHEDRINE

otc	**Ephedrine Sulfate** (West-Ward)	**Capsules:** 25 mg	In 100s.
Rx	**Ephedrine Sulfate** (Various, eg, UDL)	**Injection:** 50 mg/mL	In 1 mL single-dose vials
Rx	**Ephedrine Sulfate** (Hospira)		Preservative free. In 1 mL single-dose amps.

EPHEDRINE SULFATE— ORAL

Refer to the general discussion of these products in the Vasopressors Used in Shock group monograph and the Sympathomimetic Bronchodilator group monograph in the Respiratory Agents chapter.

Indications

➤*Asthma:* Oral ephedrine is indicated for temporary relief of shortness of breath, tightness of chest, wheezing, and for easing breathing in bronchial asthma.

Administration and Dosage

➤*Oral:*

Adults and children 12 years of age and older – 12.5 to 25 mg every 4 hours, not to exceed 150 mg in 24 hours.

Children younger than 12 years of age – For use in children younger than 12 years of age, consult a physician.

EPHEDRINE SULFATE — INJECTION

Refer to the general discussion of these products in the Vasopressors Used in Shock group monographand the Sympathomimetic Bronchodilator group monograph in the Respiratory Agents chapter.

Indications

➤*Allergic disorders:* Treatment of allergic disorders, such as bronchial asthma. The drug has long been used as a pressor agent, particularly during spinal anesthesia when hypotension frequently occurs. In Stokes-Adams syndrome with complete heart block, ephedrine has a value similar to that of epinephrine. It is indicated as a CNS stimulant in narcolepsy and depressive states. It is also used in myasthenia gravis.

Administration and Dosage

➤*Adults:* The usual parenteral dose is 25 to 50 mg given subcutaneously or IM. Intravenously, 5 to 25 mg may be administered slowly, repeated in 5 to 10 minutes, if necessary.

➤*Children:* The usual subcutaneous or IM dose is 0.5 mg/kg of body weight or 16.7 mg/m^2 of body surface every 4 to 6 hours.

➤*Storage/Stability:* Store at controlled room temperature 15° to 25°C (59° to 77°F). Protect from light.

Actions

➤*Pharmacology:* Ephedrine sulfate is a potent sympathomimetic that stimulates both α and β receptors and has clinical uses related to both actions. Its peripheral actions, which it owes in part to the release of norepinephrine, simulate responses that are obtained when adrenergic nerves are stimulated. These include an increase in blood pressure, stimulation of heart muscle, constriction of arterioles, relaxation of the smooth muscle of the bronchi and gastrointestinal tract, and dilation of the pupils. In the bladder, relaxation of the detrusor muscle is not prominent, but the tone of the trigone and vesicle sphincter is increased.

Ephedrine sulfate also has a potent effect on the CNS. It stimulates the cerebral cortex and subcortical centers, which accounts for its use in narcolepsy.

The cardiovascular responses reported in man include moderate tachycardia, unchanged or augmented stroke volume, enhanced cardiac output, variable alterations in peripheral resistance and usually a rise in blood pressure. The action of ephedrine is more prominent on the heart than on the blood vessels. Ephedrine sulfate increases the flow of coronary, cerebral and muscle blood.

EPHEDRINE SULFATE — INJECTION

In patients with myasthenia gravis, administration of ephedrine sulfate injection, USP produces a real but modest increase in motor power. The exact mechanism by which ephedrine sulfate affects skeletal muscle contractions is unknown.

Contraindications

Allergic reactions to ephedrine sulfate are rare. The hypersensitivity, if known, is a specific contraindication. Patients hypersensitive to other sympathomimetics may also be hypersensitive to ephedrine sulfate.

Warnings

➤*Pregnancy: Category C.* Animal reproduction studies have not been conducted with ephedrine sulfate injection, USP. Also, it is not known whether the drug can cause fetal harm when administered to a pregnant woman or can affect reproduction capacity. Ephedrine sulfate injection, USP should be given to a pregnant woman only if clearly indicated.

It is not known what effect ephedrine sulfate injection, USP may have on the newborn or on the child's later growth and development when the drug is administered to the mother just before or during labor.

➤*Lactation:* Ephedrine sulfate is excreted in breast milk. Use by breastfeeding mothers is not recommended because of the higher than usual risks for infants.

Precautions

➤*Special risk:* Special care should be used when administering ephedrine sulfate injection to patients with heart disease, angina pectoris, diabetes, hyperthyroidism, prostatic hypertrophy or hypertension and to patients receiving digitalis. Prolonged use may produce a syndrome resembling an anxiety state. Tolerance to ephedrine sulfate may develop, but temporary discontinuance to the drug restores its original effectiveness.

➤*Drug abuse and dependence:* Prolonged abuse of ephedrine sulfate injection can lead to symptoms of paranoid schizophrenia. When this occurs, patients exhibit such physical signs as tachycardia, poor nutrition and hygiene, fever, cold sweat and dilated pupils.

Some measure of tolerance may develop with prolonged or excessive use but addiction does not occur. Temporary cessation of medication and subsequent readministration restores its effectiveness.

Drug Interactions

➤*General anesthetics and digitalis glycosides:* Concurrent use of ephedrine sulfate with general anesthetics, especially cyclopropane or halogenated hydrocarbons or digitalis glycosides may cause cardiac arrhythmias, since these medications may sensitize the myocardium to the effects of ephedrine sulfate.

➤*Guanethidine, bethanidine, debrisoquin:* Therapeutic doses of ephedrine sulfate can inhibit the hypotensive effect of guanethidine, bethanidine, and debrisoquin by displacing the adrenergic blockers from their site of action in the sympathetic neurons. The effect in man is seen as a relative or a complete blockade of the antihypertensive drug by a sudden rise in blood pressure. Concomitant use of ephedrine sulfate injection, USP and oxytocics may cause severe hypotension.

➤*MAOIs:* Monoamine oxidase inhibitors may potentiate the pressor effect of ephedrine sulfate, possibly resulting in a hypertensive crisis. Ephedrine sulfate injection should not be administered during or within 14 days following the administration of MAO inhibitors.

Adverse Reactions

With large doses of ephedrine sulfate most patients will experience nervousness, insomnia, vertigo, headache, tachycardia, palpitation and sweating. Some patients have nausea, vomiting and anorexia. Vesical sphincter spasm may occur and result in difficult and painful urination. Urinary retention may develop in males with prostatism.

Precordial pain and cardiac arrhythmias may occur following administration of ephedrine sulfate injection.

Overdosage

➤*Symptoms:* The principal manifestation of ephedrine sulfate poisoning is convulsions. In acute poisoning the following signs and symptoms may occur: nausea, vomiting, chills, cyanosis, irritability, nervousness, fever, suicidal behavior, tachycardia, dilated pupils, blurred vision, opisthotonos, spasms, convulsions, pulmonary edema, gasping respirations, coma and respiratory failure. Initially, the patient may have hypertension, followed later by hypotension accompanied by anuria.

➤*Treatment:* If respirations are shallow or cyanosis is present, artificial respiration should be administered. Vasopressors are contraindicated. In cardiovascular collapse blood pressure should be maintained.

Antidote – For hypertension, 5 mg phentolamine mesylate diluted in saline may be administered slowly intravenously, or 100 mg may be given orally. Convulsions may be controlled by diazepam or paraldehyde. Cool applications and dexamethasone 1 mg/kg, administered slowly intravenously, may control pyrexia.

METARAMINOL

Rx	**Aramine** (Merck)	**Injection:** 10 mg per mL (1%, as bitartrate)	In 10 mL vials.[1]

[1] With 0.15% methylparaben, 0.02% propylparaben and 0.2% sodium bisulfite.

METARAMINOL — INJECTION

Refer to the general discussion of these products in the Vasopressors Used in Shock group monograph.

Indications

➤*Prevention and treatment of acute hypotensive states occurring with spinal anesthesia:* Prevention and treatment of the acute hypotensive state occurring with spinal anesthesia.

➤*Hypotension due to hemorrhage:* Adjunctive treatment of hypotension due to hemorrhage, reactions to medications, surgical complications, and shock associated with brain damage due to trauma or tumor.

Administration and Dosage

➤*Approved by the FDA:* December 22, 1987.

Metaraminol may be given IM, subcutaneously, or IV, depending on the nature and severity of the indication.

Allow at least 10 minutes to elapse before increasing the dose because the maximum effect is not immediately apparent. When the vasopressor is discontinued, observe the patient carefully as the effect of the drug tapers off; so that therapy can be reinitiated promptly if the blood pressure falls too rapidly. The response to vasopressors may be poor in patients with coexistent shock and acidosis. When indicated, established methods of shock management should be used, such as blood or fluid replacement.

➤*IM or subcutaneous injection:*

Prevention of hypotension – The recommended dose is 2 to 10 mg (0.2 to 1 mL). As with other agents given subcutaneously only the preferred sites of injection, as set forth in standard texts, should be used.

➤*IV infusion:*

Adjunctive treatment of hypotension – The recommended dose is 15 to 100 mg (1.5 to 10 mL) in 500 mL of Sodium Chloride Injection or 5% Dextrose Injection, adjusting the rate of infusion to maintain the blood pressure at the desired level. Higher concentrations of metaraminol, 150 to 500 mg per 500 mL of infusion fluid, have been used.

If the patient needs more saline or dextrose solution at a rate of flow that would provide an excessive dose of the vasopressor, the recommended volume of infusion fluid (500 mL) should be increased accordingly. Metaraminol may also be added to less than 500 mL of infusion fluid if a smaller volume is desired.

➤*Compatibility information:* In addition to Sodium Chloride Injection and Dextrose Injection 5%, the following infusion solutions were found physically and chemically compatible with injection metaraminol when 5 mL of metaraminol injection, 10 mg/mL (metaraminol equivalent), was added to 500 mL of infusion solution: Ringer's Injection, Lactated Ringer's Injection, Dextran 6% in Saline, *Normosol-R* pH 7.4, and *Normosol-M* in D5-W.

➤*Direct IV injection:* In severe shock, when time is of great importance, this agent should be given by direct IV injection. The suggested dose is 0.5 to 5 mg (0.05 to 0.5 mL), followed by an infusion of 15 to 100 mg (1.5 to 10 mL) in 500 mL of infusion fluid as described previously.

Vials may be sterilized by autoclaving or by immersion in a sterilizing solution.

➤*Storage/Stability:* Protect from light. Store container in carton until contents have been used. Avoid storage at temperatures below −20°C (−4°F) and above 40°C (104°F).

Actions

➤*Pharmacology:* The pressor effect of metaraminol begins in 1 to 2 minutes after IV infusion, in about 10 minutes after IM injection, and in 5 to 20 minutes after SC injection. The effect lasts from about 20 minutes to 1 hour. Metaraminol has a positive inotropic effect on the heart and a peripheral vasoconstrictor action.

Renal, coronary, and cerebral blood flow are a function of perfusion pressure and regional resistance. In patients with insufficient or failing vasoconstriction, there is additional advantage to the peripheral action of metaraminol, but in most patients with shock, vasoconstriction is adequate and any further increase is unnecessary. Blood flow to vital organs may decrease with metaraminol if regional resistance increases excessively.

The pressor effect of metaraminol is decreased but not reversed by alpha-adrenergic-blocking agents. Primary or secondary fall in blood pressure and tachyphylactic response to repeated use are uncommon.

Contraindications

Use of metaraminol with cyclopropane or halothane anesthesia should be avoided, unless clinical circumstances demand such use.

Hypersensitivity to any component of this product, including sulfites.

Warnings

See Drug Interactions for more information.

➤*Pregnancy: Category C.* Animal reproduction studies have not been conducted with metaraminol. It is not known whether metaraminol can cause fetal harm when given to a pregnant woman or can affect reproduction capacity. Metaraminol should be given to a pregnant woman only if clearly needed.

METARAMINOL — INJECTION

➤*Lactation:* It is not known whether this drug is secreted in human milk. Because many drugs are secreted in human milk, caution should be exercised when metaraminol is given to a nursing woman.

➤*Children:* Safety and efficacy in pediatric patients have not been established.

Precautions

➤*Hypertensive response:* Caution should be used to avoid excessive blood pressure response. Rapidly induced hypertensive responses have been reported to cause acute pulmonary edema, arrhythmias, cerebral hemorrhage, or cardiac arrest.

With the prolonged action of metaraminol, a cumulative effect is possible. If there is an excessive vasopressor response, there may be a prolonged elevation of blood pressure even after discontinuation of therapy.

When vasopressor amines are used for long periods, the resulting vasoconstriction may prevent adequate expansion of circulating volume and may cause perpetuation of shock. There is evidence that plasma volume may be reduced in all types of shock, and that the measurement of central venous pressure is useful in assessing the adequacy of the circulating blood volume. Therefore, blood or plasma volume expanders should be used when the principal reason for hypotension or shock is decreased circulating volume.

➤*Special risk:* Patients with cirrhosis should be treated with caution, with adequate restoration of electrolytes if diuresis ensues. Fatal ventricular arrhythmia was reported in 1 patient with Laennec's cirrhosis while receiving metaraminol bitartrate. In several instances, ventricular extrasystoles that appeared during infusion of this vasopressor subsided promptly when the rate of infusion was reduced.

Because of its vasoconstrictor effect, metaraminol should be given with caution in heart or thyroid disease, hypertension, or diabetes. Sympathomimetic amines may provoke a relapse in patients with a history of malaria.

➤*Sulfite sensitivity:* Metaraminol contains sodium bisulfite, a sulfite that may cause allergic-type reactions including anaphylactic symptoms and life-threatening or less severe asthmatic episodes in certain susceptible people. The overall prevalence of sulfite sensitivity in the general population is unknown and probably low. Sulfite sensitivity is seen more frequently in asthmatic than in nonasthmatic people.

Drug Interactions

Metaraminol Drug Interactions

Precipitant drug	Object drug*		Description
Metaraminol	Guanethidine	⬇	The antihypertensive effects of guanethidine may be partially or totally reversed by the mixed-acting sympathomimetics.
Digitalis glycosides	Metaraminol	⬆	Use metaraminol with caution in digitalized patients, because the combination of digitalis and sympathomimetic amines may cause ectopic arrhythmias.
Halogenated hydrocarbon anesthetics	Metaraminol	⬆	Halogenated hydrocarbon anesthetics may sensitize the myocardium to the effects of catecholamines. Use of vasopressors may lead to serious arrhythmias; use with extreme caution.
Monoamine oxidase (MAO) inhibitors	Metaraminol	⬆	MAOIs increase the pressor response to mixed-acting vasopressors. Possible hypertensive crisis and intracranial hemorrhage may occur. This interaction may also occur with furazolidone, an antimicrobial with MAO inhibitor activity. Avoid this combination; if given inadvertently and hypertension occurs, administer phentolamine.
Oxytocic drugs	Metaraminol	⬆	If vasopressor drugs are used in obstetrics to correct hypotension or added to the local anesthetic solution, some oxytocic drugs may cause severe persistent hypertension.
Tricyclic antidepressants	Metaraminol	⬇	The pressor response of the mixed-acting vasopressors may be decreased by these agents; a higher dose of the sympathomimetic may be necessary.

* ⬆ = Object drug increased. ⬇ = Object drug decreased.

Adverse Reactions

Sympathomimetic amines, including metaraminol, may cause sinus or ventricular tachycardia, or other arrhythmias, especially in patients with myocardial infarction.

In patients with a history of malaria, these compounds may provoke a relapse.

Abscess formation, tissue necrosis, or sloughing rarely may follow the use of metaraminol. In choosing the site of injection, it is important to avoid those areas recognized as not suitable for use of any pressor agent and to discontinue the infusion immediately if infiltration or thrombosis occurs. Although the physician may be forced by the urgent nature of the patient's condition to choose injection sites that are not recognized as suitable, the physician should, when possible, use the preferred areas of injection. The larger veins of the antecubital fossa or the thigh are preferred to veins in the dorsum of the hand or ankle veins, particularly in patients with peripheral vascular disease, diabetes mellitus, Buerger's disease, or conditions with coexistent hypercoagulability.

Overdosage

➤*Symptoms:* Overdosage may result in severe hypertension, accompanied by headache, constricting sensation in the chest, nausea, vomiting, euphoria, diaphoresis, pulmonary edema, tachycardia, bradycardia, sinus arrhythmia, atrial or ventricular arrhythmias, cerebral hemorrhage, myocardial infarction, cardiac arrest or convulsions.

The oral LD_{50} in the rat and mouse is 240 mg/kg and 99 mg/kg, respectively.

➤*Treatment:* Should an excessive elevation of blood pressure occur, it may be immediately relieved by a sympatholytic agent (eg, phentolamine). An appropriate antiarrhythmic agent may also be required.

PHENYLEPHRINE HYDROCHLORIDE

Rx	**Phenylephrine hydrochloride** (Various, eg, American Regent)	**Injection:** 1% (10 mg/mL)	In 1 and 5 mL vials.
Rx	**Neo-Synephrine** (Sanofi Winthrop)		In 1 mL Uni-Nest amps.[1]

[1] With sodium bisulfite.

PHENYLEPHRINE HYDROCHLORIDE — INJECTION

Refer to the general discussion of these products in the Vasopressors Used in Shock group monograph.

WARNING

Physicians should completely familiarize themselves with the complete contents of this monograph before prescribing phenylephrine injection.

Indications

➤*Blood pressure maintenance:* Maintenance of an adequate level of blood pressure during spinal and inhalation anesthesia and for the treatment of vascular failure in shock, shock-like states and drug-induced hypotension or hypersensitivity. It is also employed to overcome paroxysmal supraventricular tachycardia, to prolong spinal anesthesia, and as a vasoconstrictor in regional analgesia.

Administration and Dosage

Phenylephrine injection is generally injected subcutaneously, IM, slowly IV, or in dilute solution as a continuous IV infusion. In patients with paroxysmal supraventricular tachycardia and, if indicated, in case of emergency, phenylephrine injection is administered directly IV. The dose should be adjusted according to the pressor response.

Dosage calculations

Dose required	Use phenylephrine injection 1%
10 mg	1 mL
5 mg	0.5 mL
1 mg	0.1 mL

For convenience in intermittent IV administration, dilute 1 mL phenylephrine injection 1% with 9 mL of Sterile Water for Injection to yield 0.1% phenylephrine injection.

Dose required	Use diluted phenylephrine injection 0.1%
0.1 mg	0.1 mL
0.2 mg	0.2 mL
0.5 mg	0.5 mL

PHENYLEPHRINE HYDROCHLORIDE — INJECTION

➤*Mild or moderate hypotension:*

Subcutaneously or IM – The usual dose is from 2 to 5 mg. The range is from 1 to 10 mg. The initial dose should not exceed 5 mg.

IV – The usual dose is 0.2 mg. The range is from 0.1 to 0.5 mg. The initial dose should not exceed 0.5 mg. Injections should not be repeated more often than every 10 to 15 minutes. A 5 mg IM dose should raise blood pressure for 1 to 2 hours. A 0.5 mg IV dose should elevate the blood pressure for about 15 minutes.

➤*Severe hypotension and shock (including drug-related hypotension):* Blood-volume depletion should always be corrected as fully as possible before any vasopressor is administered. When, as an emergency measure, intraaortic pressures must be maintained to prevent cerebral or coronary artery ischemia, phenylephrine can be administered before and concurrently with blood-volume replacement.

Hypotension and occasionally severe shock may result from overdosage or idiosyncrasy following the administration of certain drugs, especially adrenergic- and ganglionic-blocking agents, rauwolfia and veratrum alkaloids, and phenothiazine tranquilizers. Patients who receive a phenothiazine derivative as preoperative medication are especially susceptible to these reactions. As an adjunct in the management of such episodes, phenylephrine injection is a suitable agent for restoring blood pressure.

Higher initial and maintenance doses of phenylephrine are required in patients with persistent or untreated severe hypotension or shock. Hypotension produced by powerful, peripheral, adrenergic-blocking agents, chlorpromazine, or pheochromocytomectomy may also require more intensive therapy.

➤*Continuous infusion:* Add 10 mg of the drug (1 mL of 1% solution) to 500 mL of Dextrose Injection or Sodium Chloride Injection (providing a 1:50,000 solution). To raise the blood pressure rapidly, start the infusion at about 100 mcg to 180 mcg/min (based on 20 drops/mL, this would be 100 to 180 drops/min). When the blood pressure is stabilized (at a low normal level for the individual), a maintenance rate of 40 to 60 mcg/min usually suffices (based on 20 drops/mL, this would be 40 to 60 drops/min). If the drop size of the infusion system varies from the 20 drops/mL, the dose must be adjusted accordingly.

If a prompt initial pressor response is not obtained, additional increments of phenylephrine (10 mg or more) are added to the infusion bottle. The rate of flow is then adjusted until the desired blood-pressure level is obtained. In some cases, a more potent vasopressor, such as norepinephrine bitartrate, may be required. Hypertension should be avoided. The blood pressure should be checked frequently. Headache or bradycardia may indicate hypertension. Arrhythmias are rare.

➤*Spinal anesthesia-hypotension:* Routine parenteral use of phenylephrine has been recommended for the prophylaxis and treatment of hypotension during spinal anesthesia. It is best administered SC or IM 3 or 4 minutes before injection of the spinal anesthetic. The total requirement for high anesthetic levels is usually 3 mg, and for lower levels, 2 mg. For hypotensive emergencies during spinal anesthesia, phenylephrine may be injected IV, using an initial dose of 0.2 mg. Any subsequent dose should not exceed the previous dose by more than 0.1 to 0.2 mg, and no more than 0.5 mg should be administered in a single dose.

To combat hypotension during spinal anesthesia in children, a dose of 0.5 to 1 mg per 25 pounds body weight, administered SC or IM, is recommended.

➤*Prolongation of spinal anesthesia:* The addition of 2 to 5 mg of phenylephrine to the anesthetic solution increases the duration of motor block by as much as approximately 50% without any increase in the incidence of complications such as nausea, vomiting or blood pressure disturbances.

➤*Vasoconstrictor for regional analgesia:* Concentrations about 10 times those employed when epinephrine is used as a vasoconstrictor are recommended. The optimum strength is 1:20,000 (made by adding 1 mg of phenylephrine to every 20 mL of local anesthetic solution). Some pressor responses can be expected when 2 mg or more are injected.

➤*Paroxysmal supraventricular tachycardia:* Rapid IV injection (within 20 to 30 seconds) is recommended. The initial dose should not exceed 0.5 mg, and subsequent doses, which are determined by the initial blood pressure response, should not exceed the preceding dose by more than 0.1 to 0.2 mg and should never exceed 1 mg.

Parenteral drug products should be inspected visually for particulate matter and discoloration prior to administration, whenever solution and container permit.

➤*Storage/Stability:* Store at controlled room temperature 15° to 30°C (59° to 86°F). Protect from light. Keep covered in carton until time of use. For single use only. Discard unused portion.

Actions

➤*Pharmacology:* Phenylephrine is a powerful postsynaptic, alpha-receptor stimulant with little effect on the beta receptors of the heart. In therapeutic doses, it produces little if any stimulation of either the spinal cord or cerebrum. A singular advantage of this drug is the fact that repeated injections produce comparable effects.

Contraindications

Severe hypertension or ventricular tachycardia; hypersensitivity to phenylephrine or to any of the components.

Warnings

➤*Pregnancy:* Category C.

Teratogenic – Animal reproduction studies have not been conducted with phenylephrine. It is also not known whether phenylephrine can cause fetal harm when administered to a pregnant woman or can affect reproduction capacity. Phenylephrine should be given to a pregnant woman only if clearly needed.

Labor and delivery – If vasopressor drugs are either used to correct hypotension or added to the local anesthetic solution, the obstetrician should be cautioned that some oxytocic drugs may cause severe persistent hypertension and that even a rupture of a cerebral blood vessel may occur during the postpartum period (see Warnings).

➤*Lactation:* It is not known whether this drug is excreted in human milk. Because many drugs are excreted in human milk, caution should be exercised when phenylephrine is administered to a breast-feeding woman.

➤*Children:* To combat hypotension during spinal anesthesia in children, a dose of 0.5 to 1 mg per 25 pounds of body weight, administered subcutaneously, or IM, is recommended.

Precautions

➤*Special risk:* Use only with extreme caution in elderly patients or in patients with hyperthyroidism, bradycardia, partial heart block, myocardial disease or severe arteriosclerosis.

➤*Sulfite sensitivity:* Some of these products contain sodium metabisulfite, a sulfite that may cause allergic-type reactions including anaphylactic symptoms and life-threatening or less severe asthmatic episodes in certain susceptible people. The overall prevalence of sulfite sensitivity in the general population is unknown and probably low. Sulfite sensitivity is seen more frequently in asthmatic than in nonasthmatic people.

Drug Interactions

➤*Vasopressors:* Vasopressors, particularly metaraminol, may cause serious cardiac arrhythmias during halothane anesthesia and therefore should be used only with great caution or not at all.

If used in conjunction with oxytocic drugs, the pressor effect of sympathomimetic pressor amines is potentiated. The pressor effect of sympathomimetic pressor amines is markedly potentiated in patients receiving monamine oxidase inhibitors (MAOIs). Therefore, when initiating pressor therapy in these patients, the initial dose should be small and used with due caution. The pressor response of adrenergic agents may also be potentiated by tricyclic antidepressants. The obstetrician should be warned that some oxytocic drugs may cause severe persistent hypertension and that even a rupture of a cerebral blood vessel may occur during the postpartum period.

➤*MAO inhibitors:* The pressor effect of sympathomimetic pressor amines is markedly potentiated in patients receiving monoamine oxidase inhibitors (MAOI). Therefore, when initiating pressor therapy in these patients, the initial dose should be small and used with due caution. The pressor response of adrenergic agents may also be potentiated by tricyclic antidepressants.

Adverse Reactions

Headache, reflex bradycardia, excitability, restlessness and rarely arrhythmias.

Overdosage

The oral LD_{50} in the rat is 350 mg/kg, in the mouse 120 mg/kg.

➤*Symptoms:* Overdosage may induce ventricular extrasystoles and short paroxysms of ventricular tachycardia, a sensation of fullness in the head and tingling of the extremities.

➤*Treatment:* Should an excessive elevation of blood pressure occur, it may be immediately relieved by an alpha-adrenergic-blocking agent (eg, phentolamine).

MIDODRINE HYDROCHLORIDE

Rx	**Midodrine Hydrochloride** (Global)	**Tablets:** 2.5 mg	(G 421). White. In 100s, 500s, and 1,000s.
Rx	**ProAmatine** (Shire)		(RPC 2.5 003). White, scored. In 100s.
Rx	**Midodrine Hydrochloride** (Global)	**Tablets:** 5 mg	(G 422). Lt. orange. In 100s, 500s, and 1,000s.
Rx	**ProAmatine** (Shire)		(RPC 5 004). Orange, scored. In 100s.
Rx	**ProAmatine** (Shire)	**Tablets:** 10 mg	(RPC 10 007). Blue, scored. In 100s.

MIDODRINE HYDROCHLORIDE — ORAL

WARNING

Because midodrine can cause marked elevation of supine blood pressure, it should be used in patients whose lives are considerably impaired despite standard clinical care. The indication for use of midodrine in the treatment of symptomatic orthostatic hypotension is based primarily on a change in a surrogate marker of effectiveness, an increase in systolic blood pressure measured 1 minute after standing, a surrogate marker considered likely to correspond to a clinical benefit. At present, however, clinical benefits of midodrine, principally improved ability to carry out activities of daily living, have not been verified.

Indications

➤*Orthostatic hypotension:* Treatment of symptomatic orthostatic hypotension. Because midodrine can cause marked elevation of supine blood pressure (BP greater than 200 mmHg systolic), it should be used in patients whose lives are considerably impaired despite standard clinical care, including nonpharmacologic treatment (such as support stockings), fluid expansion, and lifestyle alterations. The indication is based on midodrine's effect on increases in 1-minute standing systolic blood pressure, a surrogate marker considered likely to correspond to a clinical benefit. At present however, clinical benefits of midodrine principally improved ability to perform life activities have not been established. Further clinical trials are underway to verify and describe the clinical benefits of midodrine.

After initiation of treatment, midodrine should be continued only for patients who report significant symptomatic improvement.

➤*Unlabeled uses:* Management of urinary incontinence (2.5 to 5 mg 2 to 3 times a day).

Administration and Dosage

➤*Approved by the FDA:* September 6, 1996.

The recommended dose of midodrine is 10 mg 3 times daily. Dosing should take place during the daytime hours when the patient needs to be upright, pursuing the activities of daily living. A suggested dosing schedule of approximately 4-hour intervals is as follows: shortly before, or upon arising in the morning, midday, and late afternoon (not later than 6 pm). Doses may be given in 3-hour intervals, if required, to control symptoms, but not more frequently. Single doses as high as 20 mg have been given to patients, but severe and persistent systolic supine hypertension occurs at a high rate (approximately 45%) at this dose. In order to reduce the potential for supine hypertension during sleep, midodrine should not be given after the evening meal or less than 4 hours before bedtime. Total daily doses greater than 30 mg have been tolerated by some patients, but their safety and usefulness have not been studied systematically or established. Because of the risk of supine hypertension, midodrine should be continued only in patients who appear to attain symptomatic improvement during initial treatment.

See Precautions for more information.

➤*Renal function impairment:* Because desglymidodrine is excreted renally, dosing in patients with abnormal renal function should be cautious; although this has not been systematically studied, it is recommended that treatment of these patients be initiated using 2.5 mg doses.

➤*Storage/Stability:* Store at 25°C (77°F). Excursions permitted to 15° to 30°C (59° to 86°F); see USP controlled room temperature.

Actions

➤*Pharmacology:* Midodrine forms an active metabolite, desglymidodrine, that is an alpha-1 agonist, and exerts its actions via activation of the alpha-adrenergic receptors of the arteriolar and venous vasculature, producing an increase in vascular tone and elevation of blood pressure. Desglymidodrine does not stimulate cardiac beta-adrenergic receptors. Desglymidodrine diffuses poorly across the blood-brain barrier, and is therefore not associated with effects on the central nervous system.

➤*Pharmacokinetics:*

Absorption/Distribution – Midodrine is a prodrug (ie, the therapeutic effect of orally administered midodrine is due to the major metabolite desglymidodrine) formed by deglycination of midodrine. After oral administration, midodrine is rapidly absorbed. The plasma levels of the prodrug peak after about half an hour, and decline with a half-life of approximately 25 minutes, while the metabolite reaches peak blood concentrations about 1 to 2 hours after a dose of midodrine and has a half-life of about 3 to 4 hours. The absolute bioavailability of midodrine (measured as desglymidodrine) is 93%. The bioavailability of desglymidodrine is not affected by food. Approximately the same amount of desglymidodrine is formed after intravenous and oral administration of midodrine. Neither midodrine nor desglymidodrine is bound to plasma proteins to any significant extent.

Metabolism – Thorough metabolic studies have not been conducted, but it appears that deglycination of midodrine to deglymidodrine takes place in many tissues, and both compounds are metabolized in part by the liver. Neither midodrine nor desglymidodrine is a substrate for monoamine oxidase.

Excretion – Renal elimination of midodrine is insignificant. The renal clearance of desglymidodrine is of the order of 385 mL/min, most, about 80%, by active renal secretion. The actual mechanism of active secretion has not been studied, but it is possible that it occurs by the base-secreting pathway responsible for the secretion of several other drugs that are bases.

Contraindications

Severe organic heart disease, acute renal disease, urinary retention, pheochromocytoma, thyrotoxicosis, persistent and excessive supine hypertension.

Warnings

➤*Supine hypertension:* The most potentially serious adverse reaction associated with midodrine therapy is marked elevation of supine arterial blood pressure (supine hypertension). Systolic pressure of about 200 mmHg were seen overall in about 13.4% of patients given 10 mg of midodrine. Systolic elevations of this degree were most likely to be observed in patients with relatively elevated pretreatment systolic blood pressures (mean, 170 mmHg). There is no experience in patients with initial supine systolic pressure above 180 mmHg, as those patients were excluded from the clinical trials. Use of midodrine in such patients is not recommended. Sitting blood pressures were also elevated by midodrine therapy. It is essential to monitor supine and sitting blood pressures in patients maintained on midodrine.

➤*Renal function impairment:* Midodrine use has not been studied in patients with renal impairment. Because desglymidodrine is eliminated via the kidneys, and higher blood levels would be expected in such patients, midodrine should be used with caution in patients with renal impairment, with a starting dose of 2.5 mg. Renal function should be assessed prior to initial use of midodrine.

➤*Hepatic function impairment:* Midodrine use has not been studied in patients with hepatic impairment. Midodrine should be used with caution in patients with hepatic impairment, as the liver has a role in the metabolism of midodrine.

➤*Pregnancy:* *Category C.*

Midodrine increased the rate of embryo resorption, reduced fetal body weight in rats and rabbits, and decreased fetal survival in rabbits when given in doses 13 (rat) and 7 (rabbit) times the maximum human dose based on body surface area (mg/m^2). There are no adequate and well-controlled studies in pregnant women. Midodrine should be used during pregnancy only if the potential benefit justifies the potential risk to the fetus. No teratogenic effects have been observed in studies in rats and rabbits.

➤*Lactation:* It is not known whether this drug is excreted in human milk. Because many drugs are excreted in human milk, caution should be exercised when midodrine is administered to a breast-feeding woman.

➤*Children:* Safety and efficacy in pediatric patients have not been established.

Precautions

➤*Monitoring:* Blood pressure should be monitored carefully when midodrine is used concomitantly with other agents that cause vasoconstriction (eg, phenylephrine, ephedrine, dihydroergotamine, phenylpropanolamine, pseudoephedrine).

Because desglymidodrine is eliminated by the kidneys and the liver has a role in its metabolism, evaluation of the patient should include assessment of renal and hepatic function prior to initiating therapy and subsequently, as appropriate.

➤*Potential for supine and sitting hypertension:* The potential for supine and sitting hypertension should be evaluated at the beginning of midodrine therapy. Supine hypertension can often be controlled by preventing the patient from becoming fully supine (ie, sleeping with the head of the bed elevated). The patient should be cautioned to report symptoms of supine hypertension immediately. Symptoms may include cardiac awareness, pounding in the ears, headache, blurred vision, etc. The patient should be advised to discontinue the medication immediately if supine hypertension persists.

➤*Slight slowing of the heart rate:* A slight slowing of the heart rate may occur after administration of midodrine, primarily due to vagal reflex. Caution should be exercised when midodrine is used concomitantly with cardiac glycosides (eg, digitalis), psychopharmacologic agents, beta blockers or other agents that directly or indirectly reduce heart rate. Patients who experience any signs or symptoms suggesting bradycardia (pulse slowing, increased dizziness, syncope, cardiac awareness) should be advised to discontinue midodrine and should be reevaluated.

➤*Special risk:*

Patients with urinary retention problems – Use cautiously in patients with urinary retention problems, as desglymidodrine acts on the alpha-adrenergic receptors of the bladder neck.

Orthostatic hypotensive patients – Use with caution in orthostatic hypotensive patients who are also diabetic, as well as those with a history of visual problems who are also taking fludrocortisone acetate, which is known to cause an increase in intraocular pressure and glaucoma.

Drug Interactions

Midodrine Drug Interactions

Precipitant drug	Object drug*		Description
Alpha-adrenergic blocking agent (eg, prazosin, terazosin, doxazosin)	Midodrine	⬇	Alpha-adrenergic antagonist agents can antagonize the effects of midodrine.
Metformin, H_2 antagonists, procainamide, triamterene, flecainide, quinidine	Midodrine	⟷	There may be a potential for interactions with these drugs.

MIDODRINE HYDROCHLORIDE — ORAL

Midodrine Drug Interactions			
Precipitant drug	Object drug*		Description
Phenylephrine, pseudoephedrine, ephedrine, dihydroergotamine	Midodrine	↑	The use of drugs that stimulate alpha-adrenergic agonists may enhance or potentiate the pressor effects of midodrine.
Midodrine	Cardiac glycosides, psychopharmacologics, beta-blockers	↑	When coadministered with midodrine, cardiac glycosides, psychopharmacologic agents, or beta-blockers may enhance or precipitate bradycardia, A-V block, or arrhythmia (see Precautions).
Midodrine	Steroid therapy (eg, fludrocortisone)	↑	Concomitant use may increase the risk of supine hypertension. Reduce the dose of fludrocortisone or decrease the salt intake prior to initiation of treatment with midodrine. Fludrocortisone also causes an increase in intraocular pressure and glaucoma (see Precautions).

* ↑ = Object drug increased. ↓ = Object drug decreased. ↔ = Undetermined clinical effect.

Adverse Reactions

Most frequent adverse reactions – Supine and sitting hypertension; paresthesia and pruritus, mainly of the scalp; goosebumps; chills; urinary urge; urinary retention and urinary frequency.

The frequency of these reactions in a 3-week placebo-controlled trial is shown in the following table:

Adverse reactions				
	Placebo (n = 88)		Midodrine (n = 82)	
Reaction	Number of reports	Percent of patients	Number of reports	Percent of patients
Total number of reports	22		77	
Paresthesia[1]	4	4.5%	15	18.3%
Piloerection	0	0%	11	13.4%
Dysuria[2]	0	0%	11	13.4%
Pruritus[3]	2	2.3%	10	12.2%
Supine hypertension[4]	0	0%	6	7.3%
Chills	0	0%	4	4.9%
Pain[5]	0	0%	4	4.9%
Rash	1	1.1%	2	2.4%

[1] Includes hyperesthesia and scalp paresthesia.
[2] Includes dysuria (1), increased urinary frequency (2), impaired urination (1), urinary retention (5), urinary urgency (2).
[3] Includes scalp pruritus.
[4] Includes patients who experienced an increase in supine hypertension.
[5] Includes abdominal pain and pain increase.

Less frequent adverse reactions – Headache; feeling of pressure/fullness in the head; vasodilation/flushing face; confusion/thinking abnormality; dry mouth; nervousness/anxiety, and rash.

Other adverse reactions (rare) – Visual field defect; dizziness; skin hyperesthesia; insomnia; somnolence; erythema multiforme; canker sore; dry skin; dysuria; impaired urination; asthenia; backache; pyrosis; nausea; gastrointestinal distress; flatulence, and leg cramps.

Most potentially serious adverse reaction – Supine hypertension. The feelings of paresthesia, pruritus, piloerection and chills are pilomotor reactions associated with the action of midodrine on the alpha-adrenergic receptors of the hair follicles. Feelings of urinary urgency, retention, and frequency are associated with the action of midodrine on the alpha-receptors of the bladder neck.

Overdosage

➤*Symptoms:* Symptoms of overdose could include hypertension, piloerection (goosebumps), a sensation of coldness and urinary retention. There are 2 reported cases of overdosage with midodrine, both in young males. One patient ingested midodrine drops, 250 mg, experienced systolic blood pressure greater than 200 mmHg, was treated with an IV injection of 20 mg of phentolamine, and was discharged the same night without any complaints. The other patient ingested 205 mg of midodrine (41 [5 mg] tablets), and was found lethargic and unable to talk, unresponsive to voice but responsive to painful stimuli, hypertensive and bradycardic. Gastric lavage was performed, and the patient recovered fully by the next day without sequelae.

The single doses that would be associated with symptoms of overdosage or would be potentially life-threatening are unknown. The oral LD_{50} is approximately 30 to 50 mg/kg in rats, 675 mg/kg in mice, and 125 to 160 mg/kg in dogs.

➤*Treatment:* Desglymidodrine is dialyzable.

Recommended general treatment, based on the pharmacology of the drug, includes induced emesis and administration of alpha-sympatholytic drugs (eg, phentolamine).

Patient Information

Patients should be told that certain agents in over-the-counter products, such as cold remedies and diet aids, can elevate blood pressure, and therefore, should be used cautiously with midodrine, as they may enhance or potentiate the pressor effects of midodrine. These agents include phenylephrine, pseudoephedrine, ephedrine, and phenylpropanolamine. Patients should also be made aware of the possibility of supine hypertension. They should be told to avoid taking their dose if they are to be supine for any length of time (ie, they should take their last daily dose of midodrine 3 to 4 hours before bedtime to minimize nighttime supine hypertension).

POTASSIUM REMOVING RESINS

SODIUM POLYSTYRENE SULFONATE

Rx	**SPS** (Carolina Medical Products Co.)	**Suspension**: 15 g per 60 mL. Sodium content 1.5 g (65 mEq).	With 21.5 mL sorbitol solution (equivalent to 20 g sorbitol) and 0.3% alcohol per 60 mL, propylene glycol, sodium saccharin and methyl- and propylparabens. Cherry flavor. In 120, 480 mL, and UD 60 mL.
Rx	**Sodium Polystyrene Sulfonate** (Roxane)	**Suspension**: 15 g per 60 mL.	With 14.1 g sorbitol and 0.1% alcohol per 60 mL. In 60, 120, 200, and 500 mL.
Rx	**Kayexalate** (Sanofi Winthrop)	**Powder**: Finely powdered sodium polystyrene sulfonate. Sodium content ≈ 100 mg (4.1 mEq) per g.	In 1 lb jars.
Rx	**Kionex** (Paddock)	**Powder**: Finely ground sodium polystyrene sulfonate (4 level tsp = ≈ 15 g). Sodium content ≈ 100 mg (4.1 mEq) per g.	In 454 g.

SODIUM POLYSTYRENE SULFONATE

Indications

➤*Hyperkalemia:* For treatment of hyperkalemia.

Administration and Dosage

➤*Approved by the FDA:* December 8, 1982.

➤*Oral administration:*

Sodium polystyrene sulfonate suspension – The average daily adult dose is 15 g (60 mL) to 60 g (240 mL) of suspension. This is best provided by administering 15 g (60 mL) of sodium polystyrene sulfonate suspension 1 to 4 times daily. Each 60 mL of sodium polystyrene sulfonate suspension contains 1500 mg (65 mEq) of sodium. Since the in vivo efficiency of sodium-potassium exchange resins is approximately 33%, about one-third of the resin's actual sodium content is being delivered to the body.

Sodium polystyrene sulfonate powder – Suspension of this drug should be freshly prepared from powder and not stored beyond 24 hours.

The average daily adult dose of the resin is 15 to 60 g. This is best provided by administering 15 g (≈ 4 level teaspoons) of sodium polystyrene sulfonate 1 to 4 times daily. One gram of sodium polystyrene sulfonate contains 4.1 mEq of sodium; one level teaspoon contains approximately 3.5 g of sodium polystyrene sulfonate and 15 mEq of sodium. (A heaping teaspoon may contain as much as 10 g to 12 g of sodium polystyrene sulfonate.) Since the in

SODIUM POLYSTYRENE SULFONATE

vivo efficiency of sodium-potassium exchange resins is ≈ 33%, about one-third of the resin's actual sodium content is being delivered to the body.

Each dose should be given as a suspension in a small quantity of water or, for greater palatability, in syrup. The amount of fluid usually ranges from 20 mL to 100 mL, depending on the dose, or may be simply determined by allowing 3 to 4 mL per gram of resin. Sorbitol may be administered in order to combat constipation. In smaller children and infants, lower doses should be employed by using as a guide a rate of 1 mEq of potassium per gram of resin as the basis of calculation.

The suspension may be introduced into the stomach through a plastic tube and, if desired, given with a diet appropriate for a patient in renal failure.

➤*Rectal administration:* The suspension may also be given, although with less effective results, as a retention enema for adults of 30 g (120 mL) to 50 g (200 mL) every 6 hours. The enema should be retained as long as possible and followed by a cleansing enema.

After an initial cleansing enema, a soft, large size (French 28) rubber tube is inserted into the rectum for a distance of 20 cm, with the tip well into the sigmoid colon and taped in place. The suspension is introduced at body temperature by gravity. The suspension is flushed with 50 or 100 mL of fluid, following which the tube is clamped and left in place. If back leakage occurs, the hips are elevated on pillows or a knee-chest position is taken temporarily. The suspension is kept in the sigmoid colon for several hours, if possible. Then the colon is irrigated with a nonsodium-containing solution at body temperature in order to remove the resin. Two quarts of flushing solution may be necessary. The returns are drained constantly through a Y tube connection. Particular attention should be paid to this cleansing enema when sorbitol has been used.

The intensity and duration of therapy depend upon the severity and resistance of hyperkalemia.

➤*Storage/Stability:* Sodium polystyrene sulfonate should not be heated for to do so may alter the exchange properties of the resin. Shake well before using. Dispense in a tight container.

Store at controlled room temperature, 15° to 30°C (59° to 86°F).

Actions

➤*Pharmacology:* As the resin passes along the intestine or is retained in the colon after administration by enema, the sodium ions are partially released and are replaced by potassium ions. For the most part, this action occurs in the large intestine, which excretes potassium ions to a greater degree than does the small intestine. The efficiency of this process is limited and unpredictably variable. It commonly approximates the order of 33%, but the range is so large that definite indices of electrolyte balance must be clearly monitored. Metabolic data are unavailable.

Contraindications

Hypokalemia; hypersensitivity to sodium polystyrene sulfonate.

Warnings

➤*Alternative therapy in severe hyperkalemia:* Since the effective lowering of serum potassium with sodium polystyrene sulfonate may take hours to days, treatment with this drug alone may be insufficient to rapidly correct severe hyperkalemia associated with states of rapid tissue breakdown (eg, burns and renal failure) or hyperkalemia so marked as to constitute a medical emergency. Therefore, other definite measures, including dialysis, should always be considered and may be imperative.

➤*Hypokalemia:* Serious potassium deficiency can occur from sodium polystyrene sulfonate therapy. The effect must be carefully controlled by frequent serum potassium determinations within each 24–hour period. Since intracellular potassium deficiency is not always reflected by serum potassium levels, the level at which treatment with sodium polystyrene sulfonate should be discontinued must be determined individually for each patient. Important aids in making this determination are the patient's clinical condition and electrocardiogram. Early clinical signs of severe hypokalemia include a pattern of irritable confusion and delayed thought processes. Electrocardiographically, severe hypokalemia is often associated with a lengthened Q-T interval, widening, flattening, or inversion of the T wave, and prominent U waves. Also, cardiac arrhythmias may occur, such as premature atrial, nodal, and ventricular contractions, and supraventricular and ventricular tachycardias. The toxic effects of digitalis are likely to be exaggerated. Marked hypokalemia can also be manifested by severe muscle weakness, at times extending into frank paralysis.

➤*Electrolyte disturbances:* Like all cation-exchange resins, sodium polystyrene sulfonate is not totally selective (for potassium) in its actions, and small amounts of other cations such as magnesium and calcium can also be lost during treatment. Accordingly, patients receiving sodium polystyrene sulfonate should be monitored for all applicable electrolyte disturbances.

➤*Systemic alkalosis:* Systemic alkalosis has been reported after cation-exchange resins were administered orally in combination with nonabsorbable cation-donating antacids and laxatives such as magnesium hydroxide and aluminum carbonate. Magnesium hydroxide should not be administered with sodium polystyrene sulfonate. One case of grand mal seizure has been reported in a patient with chronic hypocalcemia of renal failure who was given sodium polystyrene sulfonate with magnesium hydroxide as a laxative (see Drug Interactions).

➤*Pregnancy: Category C.* Animal reproduction studies have not been conducted with sodium polystyrene sulfonate. It is also not known whether sodium polystyrene sulfonate can cause fetal harm when administered to a pregnant woman or can affect reproduction capacity. Sodium polystyrene sulfonate should be given to a pregnant woman only if clearly needed.

➤*Lactation:* It is not known whether this drug is excreted in human milk. Because many drugs are excreted in human milk, caution should be exercised when sodium polystyrene sulfonate is administered to a nursing woman.

Precautions

➤*Sodium:* Caution is advised when sodium polystyrene sulfonate is administered to patients who cannot tolerate even a small increase in sodium loads (ie, severe congestive heart failure, severe hypertension, or marked edema). In such instances compensatory restriction of sodium intake from other sources may be indicated.

➤*Constipation:* If constipation occurs, patients should be treated with sorbitol (from 10 to 20 mL of 70% syrup every 2 hours or as needed to produce 1 to 2 watery stools daily) a measure which also reduces any tendency to fecal impaction.

Drug Interactions

➤*Antacids:* The simultaneous oral administration of sodium polystyrene sulfonate with nonabsorbable cation-donating antacids and laxatives may reduce the resin's potassium exchange capability.

Systemic alkalosis has been reported after cation-exchange resins were administered orally in combination with nonabsorbable cation-donating antacids and laxatives such as magnesium hydroxide and aluminum carbonate. Magnesium hydroxide should not be administered with sodium polystyrene sulfonate. One case of grand mal seizure has been reported in a patient with chronic hypocalcemia of renal failure who was given sodium polystyrene sulfonate with magnesium hydroxide as a laxative. Intestinal obstruction due to concretions of aluminum hydroxide when used in combination with sodium polystyrene sulfonate has been reported.

➤*Digitalis:* The toxic effects of digitalis on the heart, especially various ventricular arrhythmias and A-V nodal dissociation, are likely to be exaggerated by hypokalemia, even in the face of serum digoxin concentrations in the "normal range".

Adverse Reactions

Sodium polystyrene sulfonate may cause some degree of gastric irritation. Anorexia, nausea, vomiting, and constipation may occur especially if high doses are given. Also, hypokalemia, hypocalcemia, and significant sodium retention may occur. Occasionally diarrhea develops. Large doses in elderly individuals may cause fecal impaction. This effect may be obviated through usage of the resin in enemas as described under Administration and Dosage. Rare instances of colonic necrosis have been reported. Intestinal obstruction due to concretions of aluminum hydroxide, when used in combination with sodium polystyrene sulfonate, has been reported.

EDETATE DISODIUM

EDETATE DISODIUM

Rx	**Edetate Disodium** (Various, eg, McGuff, Schein)	**Injection:** 150 mg/mL	In 20 mL vials.
Rx	**Endrate** (Abbott)		In 20 mL amps.

EDETATE DISODIUM — INJECTION

WARNING

Use of this drug is recommended only when the severity of the clinical condition justifies the aggressive measures associated with this type of therapy.

Indications

➤*Hypercalcemia:* Emergency treatment of hypercalcemia.

➤*Ventricular arrhythmias:* Control of ventricular arrhythmias associated with digitalis toxicity.

➤*Unlabeled uses:*

Chelation treatment – Chelation treatment is not indicated for atherosclerotic vascular diseases. Although it has been advocated for these diseases (eg, coronary artery disease, cerebrovascular disease, peripheral vascular disease) based on the theory of decalcification of atherosclerotic plaques, both the proposed explanations of pathogenesis and mechanism of action are suspect. In addition, edetate disodium (EDTA) is not innocuous. The medical community generally agrees that chelation therapy is not an acceptable treatment for atherosclerotic vascular diseases.

Administration and Dosage

➤*Adults:* Administer 50 mg/kg/day to a maximum dose of 3 g in 24 hours. Dissolve dose in 500 mL of 5% Dextrose Injection or 0.9% Sodium Chloride Injection. Infuse over ≥ 3 hours and do not exceed the patient's cardiac

EDETATE DISODIUM — INJECTION

reserve. A suggested regimen includes five consecutive daily doses followed by 2 days without medication; repeat this regimen as necessary, up to 15 doses.

➤*Children:* Administer 40 mg/kg/day (18 mg/lb/day) to a maximum dose of 70 mg/kg/day. Dissolve in a sufficient volume of 5% Dextrose Injection or 0.9% Sodium Chloride Injection to bring the final concentration to not more than 3%. Infuse over ≥ 3 hours; do not exceed the patient's cardiac reserve.

➤*Storage/Stability:* Store at room temperature.

Actions

➤*Pharmacokinetics:* EDTA forms chelates with many divalent and trivalent metals. Because of its affinity for calcium, EDTA will lower serum calcium levels during IV infusion. Slow infusion may cause mobilization of extracirculatory calcium stores. The chelate formed is excreted in the urine. EDTA exerts a negative inotropic effect on the heart.

Additionally, EDTA forms chelates with other polyvalent metals, thus increasing urinary excretion of magnesium, zinc and other trace elements. It does not chelate with potassium, but may reduce the serum level; increased potassium excretion may occur.

Contraindications

Anuria; hypersensitivity to any component of the preparation.

Warnings

➤*Rapid IV infusion:* Rapid IV infusion or a high serum concentration of EDTA may cause a precipitous drop in serum calcium and may result in death. Toxicity depends on total dosage and rate of administration. Do not exceed recommended dosage and rates of administration.

➤*Dilution:* Dilution before infusion is necessary because of EDTA's irritant effect on the tissues and because of the danger of serious side effects.

➤*Calcium:* The oxalate method of determining serum calcium tends to give low readings in the presence of EDTA; modification (eg, acidifying the sample) or use of a different method may be required for accuracy. The least interference will be noted immediately before a subsequent dose is administered.

➤*Hypokalemia:* Use with caution in patients with clinical or subclinical potassium deficiency; monitor serum potassium levels and ECG changes.

➤*Diabetics:* Blood sugar and insulin requirements may be lower in insulin-dependent diabetics.

➤*Hypomagnesemia:* Consider the possibility of hypomagnesemia during prolonged therapy.

➤*Renal function impairment:* Prior to treatment, assess renal excretory function; perform periodic BUN and creatinine determinations and daily urinalysis during treatment.

➤*Pregnancy: Category C.* Safety for use during pregnancy has not been established. Use only when clearly needed and when the potential benefits outweigh the potential hazards to the fetus.

➤*Lactation:* Safety for use during breastfeeding has not been established.

Precautions

➤*Monitoring:* Because of the possibility of inducing an electrolyte imbalance during treatment, perform appropriate laboratory determinations to evaluate cardiac status. Repeat as often as clinically indicated, particularly in patients with ventricular arrhythmia and those with a history of seizures or intracranial lesions. If clinical evidence suggests any disturbance of liver function during treatment, perform appropriate laboratory determinations; withdraw drug if required.

➤*Postural hypotension:* After infusion, have the patient remain supine for a short time because of the possibility of postural hypotension.

➤*Cardiac effects:* Consider the possibility of an adverse effect on myocardial contractility when administering the drug to patients with heart disease. Use this drug cautiously in patients with limited cardiac reserve or incipient congestive failure.

Adverse Reactions

➤*CNS:* Transient circumoral paresthesia, numbness and headache.

➤*GI:* Nausea, vomiting and diarrhea (fairly common).

➤*Miscellaneous:* Transient drop in systolic and diastolic blood pressure; thrombophlebitis; febrile reactions; hyperuricemia; anemia; exfoliative dermatitis; other toxic skin and mucous membrane reactions. Nephrotoxicity and damage to the reticuloendothelial system with hemorrhagic tendencies have been reported with excessive dosages.

Overdosage

Because EDTA may produce a precipitous drop in serum calcium, have an IV calcium salt (such as calcium gluconate) available. Exercise extreme caution in the use of IV calcium in the treatment of tetany, especially in digitalized patients, because the action of the drug and the replacement of calcium ions may produce a reversal of the desired digitalis effect.

CARDIOPLEGIC SOLUTIONS

CARDIOPLEGIC SOLUTION

Rx	**Plegisol** (Abbott)	**Solution:** 17.6 mg calcium chloride dihydrate, 325.3 mg magnesium chloride hexahydrate, 119.3 mg potassium chloride and 643 mg sodium chloride per 100 mL (approx. 260 mOsm/L)	In single-dose 1000 mL flexible plastic container.

CARDIOPLEGIC SOLUTION

Indications

With ischemia and hypothermia, induces cardiac arrest during open heart surgery.

Administration and Dosage

The following information is a guide:

Following institution of cardiopulmonary bypass at perfusate temperatures of 28° to 30°C, (82° to 86°F) and cross-clamping of the ascending aorta, administer the buffered solution by rapid infusion into the aortic root. The initial rate of infusion may be 300 mL/m²/minute (about 540 mL/min in a 1.8 meter, 70 kg adult with 1.8 square meters of surface area) given for 2 to 4 minutes. Concurrent external cooling (regional hypothermia of the pericardium) may be accomplished by instilling a refrigerated (4°C) physiologic solution such as *Normosol-R* (balanced electrolyte replacement solution) or Ringer's Injection into the chest cavity. If myocardial electromechanical activity persists or recurs, the solution may be reinfused at a rate of 300 mL/m²/min for 2 minutes. Repeat every 20 to 30 minutes or sooner if myocardial temperature rises above 15° to 20°C or returning cardiac activity is observed. The regional hypothermia solution around the heart also may be replenished continuously or periodically in order to maintain adequate hypothermia. Suction may be used to remove warmed infusates. An implanted thermistor probe may be used to monitor myocardial temperature.

The volumes of solution instilled into the aortic root may vary depending on the duration or type of open heart surgical procedure.

➤*Preparation of solution:* The solution contains no preservatives and is intended only for a single operative procedure. After adjusting pH with sodium bicarbonate, extemporaneous alternative buffering is not recommended. Discard the unused portion.

Add 10 mL (840 mg) of 8.4% Sodium Bicarbonate Injection (10 mEq each of sodium and bicarbonate) to each 1000 mL of the cardioplegic solution just prior to administration to adjust pH to approximately 7.8 when measured at room temperature. Use of any other Sodium Bicarbonate Injection may not achieve this pH due to the varying pH's of Sodium Bicarbonate Injections. Cool the buffered solution with added sodium bicarbonate to 4°C prior to administration and use within 24 hours of mixing.

➤*Admixture incompatibility:* Additives may be incompatible. Consult with pharmacist, if possible. When introducing additives, use aseptic technique, mix thoroughly and do not store.

➤*Storage/Stability:* Store at 25°C (77°F); however, brief exposure up to 40°C (104°F) does not adversely affect the product. Protect from freezing and extreme heat.

Actions

➤*Pharmacology:* Cardioplegic solution with added sodium bicarbonate, when cooled and instilled into the coronary artery vasculature, causes prompt arrest of cardiac electromechanical activity, combats intracellular ion losses and buffers ischemic acidosis. When used with hypothermia and ischemia, the action may be characterized as cold ischemic potassium-induced cardioplegia. This provides a quiet, relaxed heart and bloodless field of operation. The component electrolytes and their physiologic effects are listed below:

➤*Pharmacokinetics:*

Calcium (Ca^{++}) ion – Maintains integrity of cell membrane to ensure against calcium paradox during reperfusion.

Magnesium (Mg^{++}) ion – May help stabilize the myocardial membrane by inhibiting a myosin phosphorylase, which protects adenosine triphosphate (ATP) reserves for postischemic activity. The protective effects of magnesium and potassium are additive.

Potassium (K^{++}) ion – Causes prompt cessation of mechanical myocardial contractile activity. The immediacy of the arrest thus preserves energy supplies for postischemic contractile activity in diastole.

Chloride (Cl^-) and sodium (Na^+) ions – Sodium is essential to maintain ionic integrity of myocardial tissue. Chloride ions maintain the electroneutrality of the solution and have no specific role in the production of cardiac arrest.

Bicarbonate (HCO_3^-) anion – Acts as a buffer to render the solution slightly alkaline and compensate for the metabolic acidosis that accompanies ischemia.

Contraindications

Do not administer without the addition of 8.4% Sodium Bicarbonate Injection.

CARDIOPLEGIC SOLUTION

Not for IV injection; only for instillation into cardiac vasculature.

Warnings

➤*Intended use:* Only those trained to perform open heart surgery should use this solution. It is intended only for use during cardiopulmonary bypass when the coronary circulation is isolated from the systemic circulation.

➤*Right heart venting:* Right heart venting is recommended. If large volumes of cardioplegic solution are infused and allowed to return to the heart lung machine without any venting from the right heart, plasma magnesium and potassium levels may rise. Development of severe hypotension and metabolic acidosis while on bypass has occurred when large volumes (8 to 10 L) of solution are instilled and allowed to enter the pump and then the systemic circulation.

➤*Pregnancy: Category C.* Safety for use during pregnancy has not been established. Use only when clearly needed and when the potential benefits outweigh the potential hazards to the fetus.

Precautions

➤*Monitoring:* Monitor myocardial temperature during surgery to maintain hypothermia.

Continuous ECG monitoring of myocardial activity during the procedure is essential.

Appropriate equipment to defibrillate the heart following cardioplegia and inotropic agents during postoperative recovery should be readily available.

➤*Do not administer:* Do not administer unless solution is clear and container is undamaged.

Adverse Reactions

Potential hazards of open heart surgery include myocardial infarction, ECG abnormalities and arrhythmias, including ventricular fibrillation. Spontaneous recovery may be delayed or absent when circulation is restored. Defibrillation by electric shock may be required to restore normal cardiac function.

Overdosage

Overzealous instillation may result in unnecessary dilatation of the myocardial vasculature and leakage into the perivascular myocardium, possibly causing tissue edema.

AGENTS FOR PATENT DUCTUS ARTERIOSUS

ALPROSTADIL (Prostaglandin E_1; PGE_1)

Rx	**Prostin VR Pediatric** (Upjohn)	**Injection**: 500 mcg/mL[1]	In 1 mL amps.

[1] In 1 mL dehydrated alcohol.

ALPROSTADIL — INJECTION

WARNING

Apnea is experienced by about 10% to 12% of neonates with congenital heart defects treated with alprostadil pediatric sterile solution. Apnea is most often seen in neonates weighing less than 2 kg at birth and usually appears during the first hour of drug infusion. Therefore, monitor respiratory status throughout treatment, and use alprostadil pediatric injection where ventilatory assistance is immediately available.

Indications

➤*Patent ductus arteriosus:* For palliative, not definitive, therapy to temporarily maintain the patency of the ductus arteriosus until corrective or palliative surgery can be performed in neonates who have congenital heart defects and who depend upon the patent ductus for survival. Such congenital heart defects include pulmonary atresia, pulmonary stenosis, tricuspid atresia, tetralogy of Fallot, interruption of the aortic arch, coarctation of the aorta, or transposition of the great vessels, with or without other defects.

Administration and Dosage

➤*Administration:* The preferred route of administration for alprostadil pediatric sterile solution is continuous IV infusion into a large vein. Alternatively, alprostadil pediatric injection may be administered through an umbilical artery catheter placed at the ductal opening. Increases in blood pO_2 (torr) have been the same in neonates who received the drug by either route of administration.

Alprostadil pediatric sterile solution must be diluted before it is administered.

➤*Dosage:* Begin infusion with 0.05 to 0.1 mcg alprostadil per kg of body weight per minute. A starting dose of 0.1 mcg/kg of body weight per minute is the recommended starting dose based on clinical studies; however, adequate clinical response has been reported using a starting dose of 0.05 mcg/kg of body weight per minute. After a therapeutic response is achieved (increased pO_2 in infants with restricted pulmonary blood flow or increased systemic blood pressure and blood pH in infants with restricted systemic blood flow), reduce the infusion rate to provide the lowest possible dosage that maintains the response. This may be accomplished by reducing the dosage from 0.1 to 0.05 to 0.025 to 0.01 mcg/kg of body weight per minute. If response to 0.05 mcg/kg of body weight per minute is inadequate, dosage can be increased up to 0.4 mcg/kg of body weight per minute; although, in general, higher infusion rates do not produce greater effects.

➤*Dilution instructions:* To prepare infusion solutions, dilute 1 mL of alprostadil pediatric sterile solution with sodium chloride injection or dextrose injection. Undiluted alprostadil pediatric sterile solution may interact with the plastic sidewalls of volumetric infusion chambers, causing a change in the appearance of the chamber and creating a hazy solution. Should this occur, the solution and the volumetric infusion chamber should be replaced.

When using a volumetric infusion chamber, the appropriate amount of IV infusion solution should be added to the chamber first. The undiluted alprostadil pediatric sterile solution should then be added to the IV infusion solution, avoiding direct contact of the undiluted solution with the walls of the volumetric infusion chamber.

Dilute to volumes appropriate for the pump delivery system available. Prepare fresh infusion solutions every 24 hours. Discard any solution more than 24 hours old.

Sample Dilutions and Infusion Rates to Provide a Dosage of 0.1 mcg/kg of Body Weight per Minute

Add 1 ampule (500 mcg) alprostadil to:	Approximate concentration of resulting solution (mcg/mL)	Infusion rate (mL/min/kg of body weight)
250 mL	2	0.05
100 mL	5	0.02
50 mL	10	0.01
25 mL	20	0.005

Example – To provide 0.1 mcg/kg of body weight per minute to an infant weighing 2.8 kg using a solution of 1 ampule alprostadil pediatric injection in 100 mL of saline or dextrose: Infusion rate = 0.02 mL/min/kg × 2.8 kg = 0.056 mL/min or 3.36 mL/h.

➤*Storage/Stability:* Store alprostadil pediatric sterile solution in a refrigerator at 2° to 8°C (36° to 46°F).

Actions

➤*Pharmacology:* Alprostadil (prostaglandin E_1) is one of a family of naturally occurring acidic lipids with various pharmacologic effects. Vasodilation, inhibition of platelet aggregation, and stimulation of intestinal and uterine smooth muscle are among the most notable of these effects. IV doses of 1 to 10 mcg of alprostadil per kg of body weight lower the blood pressure in mammals by decreasing peripheral resistance. Reflex increases in cardiac output and rate accompany the reduction in blood pressure.

Smooth muscle of the ductus arteriosus is especially sensitive to alprostadil, and strips of lamb ductus markedly relax in the presence of the drug. In addition, administration of alprostadil reopened the closing ductus of newborn rats, rabbits, and lambs. These observations led to the investigation of alprostadil in infants who had congenital defects which restricted the pulmonary or systemic blood flow and who depended on a patent ductus arteriosus for adequate blood oxygenation and lower body perfusion.

In infants with restricted pulmonary blood flow, about 50% responded to alprostadil infusion with at least a 10 torr increase in blood pO_2 (mean increase about 14 torr and mean increase in oxygen saturation about 23%). In general, patients who responded best had low pretreatment blood pO_2 and were 4 days old or less.

In infants with restricted systemic blood flow, alprostadil often increased pH in those having acidosis, increased systemic blood pressure, and decreased the ratio of pulmonary artery pressure to aortic pressure.

➤*Pharmacokinetics:*

Metabolism/Excretion – Alprostadil must be infused continuously because it is very rapidly metabolized. As much as 80% of the circulating alprostadil may be metabolized in 1 pass through the lungs, primarily by β- and ω- oxidation. The metabolites are excreted primarily by the kidney, and excretion is essentially complete within 24 hours after administration. No unchanged alprostadil has been found in the urine, and there is no evidence of tissue retention of alprostadil or its metabolites.

Contraindications

None known.

Warnings

➤*Apnea:* Apnea is experienced by about 10% to 12% of neonates with congenital heart defects treated with alprostadil pediatric sterile solution. Apnea is most often seen in neonates weighing less than 2 kg at birth and usually appears during the first hour of drug infusion. Therefore, monitor

ALPROSTADIL — INJECTION

respiratory status throughout treatment, and use alprostadil pediatric injection where ventilatory assistance is immediately available.

➤*Gastric outlet obstruction:* The administration of alprostadil pediatric injection to neonates may result in gastric outlet obstruction secondary to antral hyperplasia. This effect appears to be related to duration of therapy and cumulative dose of the drug. Closely monitor neonates receiving alprostadil pediatric injection at recommended doses for more than 120 hours for evidence of antral hyperplasia and gastric outlet obstruction.

➤*Duration of infusion:* Infuse alprostadil pediatric injection for the shortest time and at the lowest dose that will produce the desired effects. Weigh the risks of long-term infusion of alprostadil pediatric injection against the possible benefits that critically ill infants may derive from its administration.

Precautions

➤*Monitoring:* In all neonates, monitor arterial pressure intermittently by umbilical artery catheter, auscultation, or with a Doppler transducer. Should arterial pressure fall significantly, decrease the rate of infusion immediately.

In infants with restricted pulmonary blood flow, measure efficacy of alprostadil pediatric injection by monitoring improvement in blood oxygenation. In infants with restricted systemic blood flow, measure efficacy by monitoring improvement of systemic blood pressure and blood pH.

➤*Skeletal effects:* Cortical proliferation of the long bones, first observed in dogs, has also been observed in infants during long-term infusions of alprostadil. The cortical proliferation in infants regressed after withdrawal of the drug.

➤*Causes of death unrelated to ductus arteriosus:* In infants treated with alprostadil pediatric injection at the usual doses for 10 hours to 12 days, and who died of causes unrelated to ductus structural weakness, tissue sections of the ductus and pulmonary arteries have shown intimal lacerations, a decrease in medial muscularity and disruption of the medial and internal elastic lamina. Localized and aneurysmal dilatations and vessel wall edema also were seen compared to a series of pathological specimens from infants not treated with alprostadil pediatric injection. The incidence of such structural alterations has not been defined.

➤*Hematologic effects:* Because alprostadil inhibits platelet aggregation, use alprostadil pediatric injection cautiously in neonates with bleeding tendencies.

➤*Respiratory distress syndrome:* Do not use alprostadil pediatric injection in neonates with respiratory distress syndrome. A differential diagnosis should be made between respiratory distress syndrome (hyaline membrane disease) and cyanotic heart disease (restricted pulmonary blood flow). If full diagnostic facilities are not immediately available, cyanosis (pO_2 less than 40 torr) and restricted pulmonary blood flow apparent on an x-ray are appropriate indicators of congenital heart defects.

Drug Interactions

None known.

Adverse Reactions

➤*Cardiovascular:* The most common cardiovascular adverse reactions reported have been flushing in about 10% of patients (more common after intraarterial dosing), bradycardia in about 7%, hypotension in about 4%, tachycardia in about 3%, cardiac arrest in about 1%, and edema in about 1%. The following reactions have been reported in less than 1% of the patients: Congestive heart failure, hyperemia, second degree heart block, shock, spasm of the right ventricle infundibulum, supraventricular tachycardia, and ventricular fibrillation.

➤*CNS:* Apnea has been reported in about 12% of the neonates treated. Other common adverse reactions reported have been fever in about 14% of the patients treated and seizures in about 4%. The following reactions have been reported in less than 1% of the patients: Cerebral bleeding, hyperextension of the neck, hyperirritability, hypothermia, jitteriness, lethargy, and stiffness.

➤*GI:* The most common GI adverse reaction reported has been diarrhea in about 2% of the patients. The following reactions have been reported in less than 1% of the patients: gastric regurgitation and hyperbilirubinemia.

➤*GU:* Anuria and hematuria have been reported in less than 1% of the patients.

➤*Hematologic:* The most common hematologic event reported has been disseminated intravascular coagulation in about 1% of the patients. The following events have been reported in less than 1% of the patients: anemia, bleeding, and thrombocytopenia.

➤*Musculoskeletal:* Cortical proliferation of the long bones has been reported.

➤*Respiratory:* The following reactions have been reported in less than 1% of the patients: Bradypnea, bronchial wheezing, hypercapnia, respiratory depression, respiratory distress, and tachypnea.

➤*Miscellaneous:* Sepsis has been reported in about 2% of the patients. Peritonitis has been reported in less than 1% of the patients. Hypokalemia has been reported in about 1%, and hypoglycemia and hyperkalemia have been reported in less than 1% of the patients.

Overdosage

➤*Symptoms:* Apnea, bradycardia, pyrexia, hypotension, and flushing may be signs of drug overdosage.

➤*Treatment:* If apnea or bradycardia occurs, discontinue the infusion, and provide appropriate medical treatment. Use caution in restarting the infusion. If pyrexia or hypotension occurs, reduce the infusion rate until these symptoms subside. Flushing is usually a result of incorrect intraarterial catheter placement, and the catheter should be repositioned.

INDOMETHACIN SODIUM TRIHYDRATE

Rx	**Indocin I.V.** (Merck)	**Powder for Injection:** 1 mg (as sodium trihydrate)	In single dose vials.

INDOMETHACIN SODIUM TRIHYDRATE — INJECTION

For information on oral indomethacin, see Nonsteroidal Anti-inflammatory Agents.

Indications

➤*Patent ductus arteriosus:* To close a hemodynamically significant patent ductus arteriosus in premature infants weighing between 500 and 1,750 g when after 48 hours usual medical management (eg, fluid restriction, diuretics, digitalis, respiratory support) is ineffective. Clear-cut clinical evidence of a hemodynamically significant patent ductus arteriosus should be present, such as respiratory distress, a continuous murmur, a hyperactive precordium, cardiomegaly, and pulmonary plethora on chest x-ray.

➤*Unlabeled uses:* Indomethacin IV has been used prophylactically to reduce the incidence of symptomatic patent ductus arteriosus in premature infants with a high probability of developing this condition; a single dose of 0.2 mg/kg 24 hours after birth has been used. However, no study has shown a significant decrease in neonatal morbidity.

Administration and Dosage

➤*Approved by the FDA:* March 18, 1987.

➤*Administration:* For IV administration only.

The drug should be administered carefully to avoid extravascular injection or leakage as the solution may be irritating to tissue.

➤*Dosage:* Dosage recommendations for closure of the ductus arteriosus depends on the age of the infant at the time of therapy. A course of therapy is defined as 3 IV doses of indomethacin sodium trihydrate IV given at 12 to 24 hour intervals, with careful attention to urinary output. If anuria or marked oliguria (urinary output less than 0.6 mL/kg/hr) is evident at the scheduled time of the second or third dose of indomethacin sodium trihydrate IV, no additional doses should be given until laboratory studies indicate that renal function has returned to normal.

Dosage according to age at first dose is as follows:

Age at 1st dose	Dosage (mg/kg)		
Less than 48 hours	1st (0.2)	2nd (0.1)	3rd (0.1)
2 to 7 days	0.2	0.2	0.2
Over 7 days	0.2	0.25	0.25

If the ductus arteriosus closes or is significantly reduced in size after an interval of 48 hours or more from completion of the first course of indomethacin sodium trihydrate IV, no further doses are necessary. If the ductus arteriosus reopens, a second course of 1 to 3 doses may be given, each dose separated by a 12 to 24 hour interval as described above.

If the neonate remains unresponsive to therapy with indomethacin sodium trihydrate IV after 2 courses, surgery may be necessary for closure of the ductus arteriosus. If severe adverse reactions occur, stop the drug.

➤*Preparation of solution:* The solution should be prepared only with 1 to 2 mL of preservative-free sterile Sodium Chloride Injection, 0.9% or preservative-free Sterile Water for Injection. Benzyl alcohol as a preservative has been associated with toxicity in neonates. Therefore, all diluents should be preservative-free. If 1 mL of diluent is used, the concentration of indomethacin in the solution will equal approximately 0.1 mg per 0.1 mL; if 2 mL of diluent are used, the concentration of the solution will equal approximately 0.05 mg per 0.1 mL. Any unused portion of the solution should be discarded because there is no preservative contained in the vial. A fresh solution should be prepared just prior to each administration. Once reconstituted, the indomethacin solution may be injected intravenously. While the optimal rate of injection has not been established, published literature suggests an infusion rate over 20 to 30 minutes.

Further dilution with IV infusion solutions is not recommended. Indomethacin sodium trihydrate IV is not buffered, and reconstitution with solutions at pH values less than 6 may result in precipitation of the insoluble indomethacin free acid moiety.

➤*Storage/Stability:* Store below 30°C (86°F). Protect from light. Store container in carton until contents have been used.

INDOMETHACIN SODIUM TRIHYDRATE — INJECTION

Actions

➤*Pharmacology:* Although the exact mechanism of action through which indomethacin causes closure of a patent ductus arteriosus is not known, it is believed to be through inhibition of prostaglandin synthesis. Indomethacin has been shown to be a potent inhibitor of prostaglandin synthesis, both in vitro and in vivo. In human newborns with certain congenital heart malformations, PGE 1 dilates the ductus arteriosus. In fetal and newborn lambs, E type prostaglandins have also been shown to maintain the patency of the ductus, and as in human newborns, indomethacin causes its constriction.

Studies in healthy young animals and in premature infants with patent ductus arteriosus indicated that, after the first dose of IV indomethacin, there was a transient reduction in cerebral blood flow velocity and cerebral blood flow. Similar decreases in mesenteric blood flow and velocity have been observed. The clinical significance of these effects has not been established.

➤*Pharmacokinetics:*

Absorption/Distribution – The disposition of indomethacin following IV administration (0.2 mg/kg) in preterm neonates with patent ductus arteriosus has not been extensively evaluated. Even though the plasma half-life of indomethacin was variable among premature infants, it was shown to vary inversely with postnatal age and weight. In one study, of 28 neonates who could be evaluated, the plasma half-life in those less than 7 days old averaged 20 hours (range: 3 to 60 hours, n = 18). In neonates over 7 days, the mean plasma half-life of indomethacin was 12 hours (range: 4 to 38 hours, n = 10). Grouping the neonates by weight, mean plasma half-life in those weighing less than 1000 g was 21 hours (range: 9 to 60 hours, n = 10); in those neonates weighing greater than 1000 g, the mean plasma half-life was 15 hours (range: 3 to 52 hours, n = 18).

In adults, approximately 99% of indomethacin is bound to protein in plasma over the expected range of therapeutic plasma concentrations. The percent bound in neonates has not been studied. In controlled trials in premature infants, however, no evidence of bilirubin displacement has been observed as evidenced by increased incidence of bilirubin encephalopathy (kernicterus). Indomethacin has been found to cross the blood-brain barrier and the placenta.

Metabolism/Excretion – Following IV administration in adults, indomethacin is eliminated via renal excretion, metabolism, and biliary excretion. Indomethacin undergoes appreciable enterohepatic circulation. The mean plasma half-life of indomethacin is 4.5 hours. In the absence of enterohepatic circulation, it is 90 minutes.

Contraindications

Contraindicated in neonates with proven or suspected infection that is untreated; neonates who are bleeding, especially those with active intracranial hemorrhage or GI bleeding; neonates with thrombocytopenia; neonates with coagulation defects; neonates with or who are suspected of having necrotizing enterocolitis; neonates with significant impairment of renal function; neonates with congenital heart disease in whom patency of the ductus arteriosus is necessary for satisfactory pulmonary or systemic blood flow (eg, pulmonary atresia, severe tetralogy of Fallot, severe coarctation of the aorta).

Warnings

➤*GI effects:* In the collaborative study, major GI bleeding was no more common in those neonates receiving indomethacin than in those neonates on placebo. However, minor GI bleeding (ie, chemical detection of blood in the stool) was more commonly noted in those neonates treated with indomethacin. Severe GI effects have been reported in adults with various arthritic disorders treated chronically with oral indomethacin (for further information, see monograph for indomethacin sodium trihydrate capsules).

➤*CNS effects:* Prematurity per se, is associated with an increased incidence of spontaneous intraventricular hemorrhage. Because indomethacin may inhibit platelet aggregation, the potential for intraventricular bleeding may be increased. However, in the large multicenter study of indomethacin sodium trihydrate IV, the incidence of intraventricular hemorrhage in neonates treated with indomethacin sodium trihydrate IV was not significantly higher than in the control neonates.

➤*Renal effects:* Indomethacin sodium trihydrate IV may cause significant reduction in urine output (greater than or equal to 50%) with concomitant elevations of blood urea nitrogen and creatinine, and reductions in glomerular filtration rate and creatinine clearance. These effects in most neonates are transient, disappearing with cessation of therapy with indomethacin sodium trihydrate IV. However, because adequate renal function can depend upon renal prostaglandin synthesis, indomethacin sodium trihydrate IV may precipitate renal insufficiency, including acute renal failure, especially in neonates with other conditions that may adversely affect renal function (eg, extracellular volume depletion from any cause, congestive heart failure, sepsis, concomitant use of any nephrotoxic drug, hepatic dysfunction). When significant suppression of urine volume occurs after a dose of indomethacin sodium trihydrate IV, no additional dose should be given until the urine output returns to normal levels.

Because renal function may be reduced by indomethacin sodium trihydrate IV, consideration should be given to reduction in dosage of those medications that rely on adequate renal function for their elimination.

➤*Hepatic effects:* Severe hepatic reactions have been reported in adults treated chronically with oral indomethacin for arthritic disorders (for further information, see monograph for indomethacin sodium trihydrate capsules). If clinical signs and symptoms consistent with liver disease develop in the neonate, or if systemic manifestations occur, indomethacin sodium trihydrate IV should be discontinued.

➤*Pregnancy:* In rats and mice, oral indomethacin 4 mg/kg/day given during the last 3 days of gestation caused a decrease in maternal weight gain and some maternal and fetal deaths. An increased incidence of neuronal necrosis in the diencephalon in the live-born fetuses was observed. At 2 mg/kg/day, no increase in neuronal necrosis was observed as compared to the control groups. Administration of 0.5 or 4 mg/kg/day during the first 3 days of life did not cause an increase in neuronal necrosis at either dose level.

Pregnant rats, given 2 mg/kg/day and 4 mg/kg/day during the last trimester of gestation, delivered offspring whose pulmonary blood vessels were both reduced in number and excessively muscularized. These findings are similar to those observed in the syndrome of persistent pulmonary hypertension of the neonate.

Precautions

➤*Monitoring:* Indomethacin sodium trihydrate IV in preterm infants may suppress water excretion to a greater extent than sodium excretion. When this occurs, a significant reduction in serum sodium values (ie, hyponatremia) may result. Neonates should have serum electrolyte determinations done during therapy with indomethacin sodium trihydrate IV. Renal function and serum electrolytes should be monitored. Since renal function may be reduced by indomethacin sodium trihydrate IV, consideration should be given to reduction in dosage of those medications that rely on adequate renal function for their elimination. If anuria or marked oliguria (urinary output less than 0.6 mL/kg/h) is evident at the scheduled time of the second or third dose of indomethacin sodium trihydrate IV, no additional doses should be given until laboratory studies indicate that renal function has returned to normal.

➤*Infection:* Indomethacin sodium trihydrate may mask the usual signs and symptoms of infection. Therefore, the physician must be continually on the alert for this and should use the drug with extra care in the presence of existing controlled infection.

➤*Platelet aggregation:* Indomethacin sodium trihydrate IV may inhibit platelet aggregation. In one small study, platelet aggregation was grossly abnormal after indomethacin therapy (given orally to premature infants to close the ductus arteriosus). Platelet aggregation returned to normal by the tenth day. Premature infants should be observed for signs of bleeding.

Drug Interactions

➤*Digitalis:* Because the half-life of digitalis (given frequently to preterm infants with patent ductus arteriosus and associated cardiac failure) may be prolonged when given concomitantly with indomethacin, the neonate should be observed closely; frequent ECGs and serum digitalis levels may be required to prevent or detect digitalis toxicity early.

➤*Aminoglycosides :* In one study of premature infants treated with indomethacin sodium trihydrate IV and also receiving either gentamicin or amikacin, both peak and trough levels of these aminoglycosides were significantly elevated.

➤*Furosemide:* Therapy with indomethacin may blunt the natriuretic effect of furosemide. This response has been attributed to inhibition of prostaglandin synthesis by nonsteroidal anti-inflammatory drugs. In a study of 19 premature infants with patent ductus arteriosus treated with either indomethacin sodium trihydrate IV alone or a combination of indomethacin sodium trihydrate IV and furosemide, results showed that neonates receiving both indomethacin sodium trihydrate IV and furosemide had significantly higher urinary output, higher levels of sodium and chloride excretion, and higher glomerular filtration rates than did those receiving indomethacin sodium trihydrate IV alone. In this study, the data suggested that therapy with furosemide helped to maintain renal function in the premature infant when indomethacin sodium trihydrate IV was added to the treatment of patent ductus arteriosus.

Adverse Reactions

In a double-blind, placebo-controlled trial of 405 premature infants weighing less than or equal to 1750 g with evidence of large ductal shunting, in those neonates treated with indomethacin (n = 206), there was a statistically significantly greater incidence of bleeding problems, including gross or microscopic bleeding into the GI tract, oozing from the skin after needle stick, pulmonary hemorrhage, and disseminated intravascular coagulopathy. There was no statistically significant difference between treatment groups with reference to intracranial hemorrhage.

The neonates treated with indomethacin sodium trihydrate also has a significantly higher incidence of transient oliguria and elevations of serum creatinine (greater than or equal to 1.8 mg/dL) than did the neonates treated with placebo.

The incidences of retrolental fibroplasia (grades 3 and 4) and pneumothorax in neonates treated with indomethacin sodium trihydrate IV were not greater than in placebo controls and were statistically significantly lower than in surgically treated neonates.

The following additional adverse reactions in neonates have been reported from the collaborative study, anecdotal case reports, from other studies using rectal, oral, or IV indomethacin for treatment of patent ductus arteriosus or in marketed use. The rates are calculated from a database that contains experience of 849 indomethacin-treated neonates reported in the medical literature, regardless of the route of administration. One-year follow-up is available on 175 neonates and shows no long-term sequelae that could be attributed to indomethacin. In controlled clinical studies, only electrolyte imbalance and renal dysfunction (of the reactions listed below) occurred statistically significantly more frequently after indomethacin sodium trihydrate IV than after placebo. Reactions marked with a single asterisk (*) occurred in 3% to 9% of indomethacin-treated neonates; those marked with a double asterisk (**) occurred in 3% to 9% of both indomethacin- and placebo-treated neonates. Unmarked reactions occurred in less than 3% of neonates.

INDOMETHACIN SODIUM TRIHYDRATE — INJECTION

➤*Cardiovascular:* Intracranial bleeding**; pulmonary hypertension.

➤*GI:* GI bleeding*; vomiting; abdominal distention; transient ileus; localized perforation(s) of the small and/or large intestines.

➤*Hematologic:* Decreased platelet aggregation.

Indomethacin sodium trihydrate IV may inhibit platelet aggregation. In one small study, platelet aggregation was grossly abnormal after indomethacin therapy (given orally to premature infants to close the ductus arteriosus). Platelet aggregation returned to normal by the tenth day. Premature infants should be observed for signs of bleeding.

➤*Metabolic:* Hyponatremia*; elevated serum potassium*; reduction in blood sugar, including hypoglycemia, increased weight gain (fluid retention).

➤*Renal:* Renal dysfunction in 41% of neonates, including greater than or equal to 1 of the following: Reduced urinary output; reduced urine sodium, chloride, or potassium, urine osmolality, free water clearance, or glomerular filtration rate; elevated serum creatinine or BUN; uremia.

➤*Additional adverse reactions:* The following adverse reactions have been reported in neonates treated with indomethacin, however, a causal relationship to therapy with indomethacin IV has not been established.

Cardiovascular – Bradycardia.

GI – Necrotizing enterocolitis.

Hematologic – Disseminated intravascular coagulation.

Ophthalmic – Retrolental fibroplasia**.

Metabolic – Acidosis/alkalosis.

Respiratory – Apnea; exacerbation of preexisting pulmonary infection.

Patient Information

Because renal function may be reduced by indomethacin sodium trihydrate IV, consideration should be given to reduction in dosage of those medications that rely on adequate renal function for their elimination.

SCLEROSING AGENTS

Indications

➤*Varicose veins:* Treatment of small, uncomplicated varicose veins of the lower extremities.

Sclerosing agents may be useful as a supplement to venous ligation to obliterate residual varicosed veins or in patients who have conditions which increase the risk of surgery. Ineffective sclerotherapy may decrease the potential success of later surgery.

➤*Morrhuate sodium:* This has been used for the treatment of internal hemorrhoids; there is no substantial evidence for this indication.

➤*Unlabeled uses:* Sclerosing agents have been used to treat esophageal varices, introduced via a flexible fiberoptic esophagoscope.

Actions

➤*Pharmacology:* These agents are mild sclerosing drugs used in the treatment of varicose veins. They produce their effect by irritation and inflammation of the venous intimal endothelium and formation of a thrombus. This blood clot occludes the injected vein and fibrous tissue develops, resulting in the obliteration of the vein.

Morrhuate sodium is a mixture of the sodium salts of the saturated and unsaturated fatty acids of cod liver oil.

Contraindications

Hypersensitivity to any component of these drugs; acute superficial thrombophlebitis; underlying arterial disease; varicosities caused by abdominal and pelvic tumors; uncontrolled diabetes mellitus; sepsis; blood dyscrasia; thyrotoxicosis; tuberculosis; neoplasms; asthma; acute respiratory or skin diseases; any condition which causes the patient to be bedridden; extensive injection treatment in patients who are severely debilitated or senile; an unusual local reaction at the injection site or any systemic reaction; persistent occlusion of deep veins.

Delay treatment if there is any acute local or systemic infection, including infected ulcers.

Do not use if there is significant valvular or deep venous incompetence.

Warnings

➤*Hypersensitivity reactions:* Anaphylactoid and allergic reactions have occurred. Anaphylactoid reactions may occur within a few minutes after the injection and are most likely to occur when therapy is reinstituted after several weeks. Refer to Management of Acute Hypersensitivity Reactions.

➤*Pregnancy:* Safety for use during pregnancy has not been established. Use only when clearly needed and when the potential benefits outweigh the potential hazards to the fetus.

Precautions

➤*Deep vein thrombosis:* Do not undertake sclerotherapy for the treatment of varicosities unless valvular competency and deep vein patency and competency are determined. Perform the Trendelenburg test, Perthes' test and angiography. Because of the danger of extension of thrombosis into the deep veins, perform a thorough preinjection evaluation for valvular competence and slowly inject a small amount (not more than 2 mL) of the preparation into the varicosity. Necrosis may result from direct injection of sclerosing agents.

➤*Initial treatment:* Initially treat most patients with symptomatic primary varicosed veins with compression stockings. If this treatment is inadequate, surgery may be required.

➤*Administration:* For IV use only. Inadvertent intra-arterial injection may result in severe ischemic damage.

Adverse Reactions

➤*CNS:* Drowsiness and headache may occur rarely with morrhuate.

➤*Hypersensitivity:* Dizziness; weakness; vascular collapse; asthma; respiratory depression; GI disturbances (ie, nausea and vomiting); urticaria (rare).

➤*Local:* Burning; cramping sensations; urticaria; tissue sloughing and necrosis may occur with extravasation (morrhuate).

➤*Respiratory:* Pulmonary embolism has occurred.

➤*Miscellaneous:* Postoperative sloughing can occur.

ETHANOLAMINE OLEATE

Rx	**Ethamolin** (Questcor)	**Injection:** 5%	In 2 mL amps.[1]

[1] With 2% benzyl alcohol.

ETHANOLAMINE OLEATE — INJECTION

Refer to the general discussion of these products in the Sclerosing Agents group monograph.

Indications

➤*Esophageal varices:* Ethanolamine oleate injection is indicated for the treatment of patients with esophageal varices that have recently bled, to prevent rebleeding.

Ethanolamine oleate is not indicated for the treatment of patients with esophageal varices that have not bled. There is no evidence that treatment of this population decreases the likelihood of bleeding.

Administration and Dosage

➤*Dosage:* Local ethanolamine oleate injection sclerotherapy of esophageal varices should be performed by physicians who are familiar with an acceptable technique. The usual IV dose is 1.5 to 5 mL per varix. The maximum dose per treatment session should not exceed 20 mL. Patients with significant liver dysfunction (Child class C) or concomitant cardiopulmonary disease should usually receive less than the recommended maximum dose. Submucosal injections are not recommended as they are reportedly more likely to result in ulceration at the site of injection.

To obliterate the varix, injections may be made at the time of the acute bleeding episode and then after 1 week, 6 weeks, 3 months, and 6 months as indicated.

Parenteral drug products should be inspected visually for particulate matter and discoloration before administration whenever solution and container permit.

➤*Storage / Stability:* Store at controlled room temperature, 15° to 30°C (59° to 86°F). Protect from light.

Actions

➤*Pharmacology:* When injected IV, ethanolamine oleate injection acts primarily by irritation of the intimal endothelium of the vein and produces a sterile dose-related inflammatory response. This results in fibrosis and possible occlusion of the vein. Ethanolamine oleate injection also rapidly diffuses through the venous wall and produces a dose-related extravascular inflammatory reaction.

The oleic acid component of the ethanolamine oleate injection is responsible for the inflammatory response, and may also activate coagulation in vivo by release of tissue factor and activation of Hageman factor. The ethanolamine component, however, may inhibit fibrin clot formation by chelating calcium, so that a procoagulant action of ethanolamine oleate has not been demonstrated.

After injection, ethanolamine oleate disappears from the injection site within 5 minutes via the portal vein. When volumes larger than 20 mL are injected, some ethanolamine oleate also flows into the azygos vein through the periesophageal vein. In human autopsy studies it was found that within 4 days after injection there is neutrophil infiltration of the esophageal wall and hemorrhage within 6 days. Granulation tissue is first seen at 10 days, red thrombi obliterating the varices by 20 days, and sclerosis of the varices by 2.5 months. The time course of these findings suggests that sclerosis of esophageal varices will be a delayed rather than an immediate effect of the drug.

The minimum lethal dose of ethanolamine oleate injection administered IV to rabbits is 130 mg/kg.

ETHANOLAMINE OLEATE — INJECTION

In dogs, ethanolamine oleate injected into the right atrium at a dose of 1 mL/kg over 1 minute has been shown to increase extravascular lung water. The maximum recommended human dose is 20 mL, or 0.4 mL/kg for a 50 kg person. The concentration of ethanolamine oleate reaching the lung in human treatment will be less than in the dog studies, but pleural effusions, pulmonary edema, pulmonary infiltration and pneumonitis have been reported in clinical trials, and minimizing the total per session dose, especially in patients with concomitant cardiopulmonary disease, is recommended.

Contraindications

Known hypersensitivity to ethanolamine, oleic acid, or ethanolamine oleate.

Warnings

➤*Varicosities of the leg:* The practice of injecting varicosities of the leg with ethanolamine oleate injection is not supported by adequately controlled clinical trials. Therefore, such use is not recommended.

➤*Hypersensitivity reactions:* Fatal anaphylactic shock was reported following injection of a larger than normal volume of ethanolamine oleate injection into a man who had a known allergic disposition. Although there are only 3 known reports of anaphylaxis, the possibility of an anaphylactic reaction should be kept in mind, and the physician should be prepared to treat it appropriately. In extreme emergencies, 0.25 mL of a 1:1000 IV solution of epinephrine (0.25 mg) should be used and allergic reactions should be controlled with antihistamines.

➤*Renal function impairment:* Acute renal failure with spontaneous recovery followed injection of 15 to 20 mL of ethanolamine oleate injection into 2 women.

➤*Elderly:* Fatal aspiration pneumonia has occurred in elderly patients undergoing esophageal variceal sclerotherapy with ethanolamine oleate injection. This adverse event appears to be procedure related rather than drug related, but as aspiration of blood or stomach contents is not uncommon in patients with bleeding esophageal varices, special precautions should be taken to prevent its occurrence, especially in the elderly and critically ill subjects.

➤*Pregnancy: Category C.*

Ethanolamine oleate injection should be used in pregnant women only when clearly needed.

Teratogenic – Animal reproduction studies have not been conducted with ethanolamine oleate injection. It is also not known whether ethanolamine oleate injection can cause fetal harm when administered to a pregnant woman or can affect reproduction capacity. Ethanolamine oleate injection should be given to a pregnant woman only if clearly needed.

➤*Lactation:* It is not known whether this drug is excreted in human milk. Because many drugs are excreted in human milk, caution should be exercised when ethanolamine oleate injection is administered to a nursing woman.

➤*Children:* Safety and efficacy in pediatric patients have not been established.

Precautions

➤*Severe injection necrosis:* The physician should bear in mind that severe injection necrosis may result from direct injection of sclerosing agents, especially if excessive volumes are used. At least 1 fatal case of extensive esophageal necrosis and death has been reported. The drug should be administered by physicians who are familiar with an acceptable injection technique.

➤*Child class C:* Patients in Child class C are more likely to develop esophageal ulceration than those in classes A and B. Complications of ulceration, necrosis, and delayed esophageal perforation appear to occur more frequently when ethanolamine oleate injection is injected submucosally. This route is not recommended.

➤*Cardiorespiratory disease:* In patients with concomitant cardiorespiratory disease, careful monitoring and minimization of the total dose per session is recommended.

Adverse Reactions

The reported frequency of complications/adverse events per injection session was 13%. The most common complications were pleural effusion/infiltration (2.1%), esophageal ulcer (2.1%), pyrexia (1.8%), retrosternal pain (1.6%), esophageal stricture (1.3%), and pneumonia (1.2%).

➤*Local:* Other adverse local esophageal reactions have also been reported at rates of 0.1% to 0.4%, including esophagitis, tearing of the esophagus, sloughing of the mucosa overlying the injected varix, ulceration, stricture, necrosis, periesophageal abscess and perforation. These complications appear to be dependent upon the dose and the patient's clinical state.

➤*Miscellaneous:* Bacteremia has been observed in patients following injection of esophageal varices with ethanolamine oleate. Pyrexia and retrosternal pain are not infrequently observed during the postinjection period. Fatal aspiration pneumonia has occurred in patients with esophageal varices who underwent ethanolamine oleate injection sclerotherapy. Anaphylactic shock and acute renal failure with spontaneous recovery have occurred. A case of disseminated intravascular coagulation has been reported.

Spinal cord paralysis due to occlusion of the anterior spinal artery has been reported in 1 child 8 hours after ethanolamine oleate sclerotherapy.

Overdosage

➤*Symptoms:* Overdosage of ethanolamine oleate injection can result in severe intramural necrosis of the esophagus. Complications resulting from such overdosage have resulted in death.

SODIUM TETRADECYL SULFATE

Rx	**Sotradecol** (Bioniche Pharma)	**Injection:** 10 mg/mL	Benzyl alcohol 0.02 mL. In 2 mL vials.
		30 mg/mL	Benzyl alcohol 0.02 mL. In 2 mL vials.

SODIUM TETRADECYL SULFATE — INJECTION

Indications

➤*Varicose veins:* Sodium tetradecyl sulfate is indicated in the treatment of small uncomplicated varicose veins of the lower extremities that show simple dilation with competent valves. Consider the benefit-to-risk ratio in selected patients who are at great surgical risks.

➤*Unlabeled uses:* Bleeding esophageal varices.

Administration and Dosage

➤*Approved by the FDA:* January 29, 1988.

➤*Dosage:* Sodium tetradecyl sulfate injection is for intravenous (IV) use only. The strength of solution required depends on the size and degree of varicosity. In general, the 1% solution will be found most useful with the 3% solution preferred for larger varicosities. Keep the dose small, using 0.5 to 2 mL (preferably 1 mL maximum) for each injection, and do not exceed the maximum 10 mL single treatment.

➤*Incompatibilities:* Do not include heparin in the same syringe as sodium tetradecyl sulfate because they are incompatible.

➤*Storage/Stability:* Store at 20° to 25°C (68° to 77°F).

Visually inspect parenteral drug products for particulate matter and discoloration prior to administration. Do not use if precipitated or discolored.

Actions

➤*Pharmacology:* Sodium tetradecyl sulfate is a sclerosing agent. IV injection causes intima inflammation and thrombus formation. This usually occludes the injected vein. Subsequent formation of fibrous tissue results in partial or complete vein obliteration that may or may not be permanent.

Contraindications

Sodium tetradecyl sulfate is contraindicated in previous hypersensitivity reactions to the drug; in acute superficial thrombophlebitis; valvular or deep vein incompetence; huge superficial veins with wide open communications to deeper veins; phlebitis migrans; acute cellulitis; allergic conditions; acute infections; varicosities caused by abdominal and pelvic tumors (unless the tumor has been removed); bedridden patients; uncontrolled systemic diseases, such as diabetes, toxic hyperthyroidism, tuberculosis, asthma, neoplasm, sepsis, blood dyscrasias, and acute respiratory or skin diseases.

Warnings

➤*Administration:* Sodium tetradecyl sulfate should be administered only by a health care provider familiar with venous anatomy, the diagnosis and treatment of conditions affecting the venous system, and proper injection technique. Severe adverse local reactions, including tissue necrosis, may occur following extravasation; therefore, extreme care in IV needle placement and use of the minimal effective volume at each injection site are important.

➤*Deep vein thrombosis/pulmonary embolism:* Because of the danger of thrombosis extension into the deep venous system, carry out thorough preinjection evaluation for valvular competency and slowly inject a small amount (not over 2 mL) of the preparation into the varicosity. Deep venous patency must be determined by angiography or noninvasive testing, such as duplex ultrasound. Venous sclerotherapy should not be undertaken if tests, such as Trendelenberg, Perthes, and angiography, show significant valvular or deep venous incompetence.

The development of deep vein thrombosis and pulmonary embolism have been reported following sclerotherapy treatment of superficial varicosities. Patients should have posttreatment follow-up of sufficient duration to assess for the development of deep vein thrombosis. Embolism may occur as long as 4 weeks after injection of sodium tetradecyl sulfate. Adequate posttreatment compression may decrease the incidence of deep vein thrombosis.

➤*Hypersensitivity reactions:* Emergency resuscitation equipment should be immediately available. Allergic reactions, including fatal anaphylaxis, have been reported. As a precaution against anaphylactic shock, it is recommended that sodium tetradecyl sulfate 0.5 mL be injected into a varicosity, followed by observation of the patient for several hours before administration of a second or larger dose. Keep the possibility of an anaphylactic reaction in mind, and be prepared to treat it appropriately.

➤*Pregnancy: Category C.* Animal reproduction studies have not been conducted with sodium tetradecyl sulfate. It also is not known whether sodium tetradecyl sulfate can cause fetal harm when administered to a pregnant

SODIUM TETRADECYL SULFATE — INJECTION

woman or can affect reproduction capacity. Administer sodium tetradecyl sulfate to a pregnant woman only if clearly needed and the benefits outweigh the risks.

➤*Lactation:* It is not known whether this drug is excreted in human milk. Because many drugs are excreted in human milk, exercise caution when sodium tetradecyl sulfate is administered to a breastfeeding woman.

➤*Children:* Safety and efficacy in children have not been established.

Precautions

➤*Arterial disease:* Exercise extreme caution in the presence of underlying arterial disease, such as marked peripheral arteriosclerosis or thromboangiitis obliterans (Buerger disease).

➤*Benzyl alcohol:* Benzyl alcohol, contained in this product as a preservative, has been associated with an increased incidence of neurological and other complications in premature infants that are sometimes fatal.

Drug Interactions

➤*Antiovulatory drugs:* No well-controlled studies have been performed in patients taking antiovulatory agents (eg, oral contraceptives). Use judgment and evaluate any patient taking antiovulatory drugs prior to initiating treatment with sodium tetradecyl sulfate.

Adverse Reactions

➤*Hypersensitivity:* Allergic reactions, such as hives, asthma, hay fever, and anaphylactic shock, have been reported. Mild systemic reactions that have been reported include headache, nausea, and vomiting.

At least 6 deaths have been reported with the use of sodium tetradecyl sulfate. Four cases of anaphylactic shock leading to death have been reported in patients who received sodium tetradecyl sulfate. One of these 4 patients reported a history of asthma, a contraindication to the administration of sodium tetradecyl sulfate.

➤*Local:* Local reactions consisting of pain, urticaria, or ulceration may occur at the site of injection. A permanent discoloration may remain along the path of the sclerosed vein segment. Sloughing and necrosis of tissue may occur following extravasation of the drug.

➤*Miscellaneous:* One death has been reported in a patient who received sodium tetradecyl sulfate and who had been receiving an antiovulatory agent. Another death (fatal pulmonary embolism) has been reported in a 36-year-old woman treated with sodium tetradecyl acetate and who was not taking oral contraceptives.

Overdosage

The IV LD_{50} of sodium tetradecyl sulfate in mice was reported to be 90 ± 5 mg/kg.

In rats, the acute IV LD_{50} of sodium tetradecyl sulfate was estimated to be between 72 and 108 mg/kg.

Purified sodium tetradecyl sulfate was found to have an LD_{50} of 2 g/kg when administered orally by stomach tube as a 25% aqueous solution to rats. In rats given 0.15 g/kg in drinking water for 30 days, no appreciable toxicity was seen, although some growth inhibition was discernible.

MORRHUATE SODIUM

Rx	**Morrhuate Sodium** (Pasadena Research Labs)	**Injection**: 50 mg/mL	In 30 mL multiple use vials.
Rx	**Scleromate** (Glenwood)		In 5 mL amps, 10 mL vials, 10 mL fill in 20 mL vials.

MORRHUATE SODIUM — INJECTION

Complete prescribing information for these products begins in the Sclerosing Agents group monograph.

Administration and Dosage

➤*To determine possible sensitivity:* 0.25 to 1 mL of 5% injection into a varicosity 24 hours before administration of a large dose.

➤*Usual adult dose for obliteration of small or medium veins:* 50 to 100 mg (1 to 2 mL). *For large veins:* 150 to 250 mg (3 to 5 mL). The drug may be given as multiple injections at one time or in single doses. Therapy may be repeated at 5 to 7 day intervals, according to the patient's response.

Following injection, the vein promptly becomes hard and swollen for 2 to 4 inches, depending on the size and response of the vein. After 24 hours, the vein is hard and slightly tender to the touch (with little or no periphlebitis). The skin around the injection becomes light-bronze; this color usually disappears quickly. An aching sensation and feeling of stiffness usually occurs and lasts approximately 48 hours.

➤*Administration:* When small veins are injected, or the injection solution is cold, or when solid matter has separated in the solution, warm the ampul or vial by immersing in hot water. The solution should become clear on warming; use only a clear solution that contains no solid matter. Because the solution froths easily, use a large bore needle to fill the syringe; however, use a small bore needle for the injection.

For IV use only. Avoid extravasation. Dosage depends on the size and degree of varicosity.

➤*Storage / Stability:* Store below 40°C (104°F); refrigerate preferably between 15° and 30°C (59° and 86°F).

MISCELLANEOUS ANTIANGINAL AGENTS

RANOLAZINE

Rx	**Ranexa** (CV Therapeutics[a])	**Tablets, extended-release**: 500 mg	(CVT 500). Lt. orange, oblong. Film coated. In 500s and unit-of-use 60s.

[a] CV Therapeutics, Inc., 3172 Porter Dr., Palo Alto, CA 94304; (650) 384-8500; http://www.cvt.com

RANOLAZINE — ORAL

Indications

➤*Chronic angina:* For the treatment of chronic angina. Because ranolazine prolongs the QT interval, reserve its use for patients who have not achieved an adequate response with other antianginal drugs. Use ranolazine in combination with amlodipine, beta-blockers, or nitrates.

The effect on angina rate or exercise tolerance appeared to be smaller in women than men.

Administration and Dosage

➤*Approved by the FDA:* January 27, 2006.

➤*Adults:* Ranolazine dosing should be initiated at 500 mg twice daily and increased to 1,000 mg twice daily as needed, based on clinical symptoms. The maximum recommended daily dose of ranolazine is 1,000 mg twice daily.

➤*Administration:* Ranolazine may be taken with or without meals. Ranolazine should be swallowed whole and not crushed, broken, or chewed.

➤*Dosage adjustments:* Dose adjustments of ranolazine are generally not required on the basis of age or gender, or in patients with congestive heart failure (CHF; New York Heart Association [NYHA] class I to IV) or diabetes mellitus.

➤*Concomitant therapy:* See Drug Interactions for more information.

➤*Storage / Stability:* Store at 25°C (77°F); excursions are permitted to 15° to 30°C (59° to 86°F).

Actions

➤*Pharmacology:* Ranolazine has antianginal and anti-ischemic effects that do not depend upon reductions in heart rate or blood pressure. The mechanism of action of ranolazine is unknown. It does not increase the rate-pressure product, a measure of myocardial work, at maximal exercise.

Pharmacodynamic effects –

Hemodynamic effects: See Precautions for more information.

Electrocardiogram (ECG) effects: See Warnings for more information.

➤*Pharmacokinetics:*

Absorption / Distribution – The absorption of ranolazine is highly variable. For example, at a dosage of 1,000 mg twice daily, the mean steady-state maximum effective plasma concentration (C_{max}) was 2,569 ng/mL; 95% of C_{max} values were between 420 and 6,080 ng/mL. The pharmacokinetics of the (+) R and (−) S-enantiomers of ranolazine are similar in healthy volunteers. Steady state is generally achieved within 3 days of twice daily dosing with ranolazine. At steady state over the dosage range 500 to 1,000 mg twice daily, C_{max} and area under the plasma concentration-time curve $(AUC)_{0-\tau}$ increase slightly more than proportionally to dose, 2.2- and 2.4-fold, respectively. With twice daily dosing, the peak/trough ratio of the ranolazine plasma concentration is 1.6 to 3.

After oral administration of ranolazine, peak plasma concentrations of ranolazine are reached between 2 and 5 hours. After oral administration of ^{14}C-ranolazine as a solution, 73% of the dose is systemically available as ranolazine or metabolites. The bioavailability of ranolazine from *Ranexa* relative to that from a solution of ranolazine is 76%. Over the concentration range of 0.25 to 10 mcg/mL, ranolazine is approximately 62% bound to human plasma proteins.

Food effect: Food (high-fat breakfast) has no important effect on the C_{max} and AUC of ranolazine. Therefore, ranolazine may be taken without regard to meals.

Metabolism / Excretion – The apparent terminal half-life of ranolazine is 7 hours. Following a single oral dose of ranolazine solution, approximately 75% of the dose is excreted in urine and 25% in feces. Ranolazine is metabolized rapidly and extensively in the liver and intestine; less than 5% is excreted unchanged in urine and feces. The pharmacologic activity of the metabolites has not been well characterized. After dosing to steady state with 500 to 1,500 mg twice daily, the 4 most abundant metabolites in plasma

RANOLAZINE — ORAL

have AUC values ranging from about 5% to 33% that of ranolazine, and display apparent half-lives ranging from 6 to 22 hours. Ranolazine is metabolized mainly by CYP3A and to a lesser extent by CYP2D6.

Special populations –

Renal function impairment: In a pharmacokinetic study in patients with varying degrees of renal function impairment, ranolazine plasma levels appeared to increase about 50%. The pharmacokinetics of ranolazine in patients on dialysis have not been assessed. In 6 subjects with severe renal function impairment on ranolazine 500 mg twice daily, mean diastolic blood pressure increased approximately 10 to 15 mm Hg.

Hepatic function impairment: The disposition of ranolazine administered in a dosage of 500 mg twice daily was studied in 16 subjects with mild or moderate hepatic function impairment and 16 healthy volunteers. The plasma concentrations of ranolazine were increased in the subjects with mild (Child-Pugh class A) and moderate (Child Pugh class B) liver impairment by factors of 1.3 and 1.6, respectively, relative to the healthy volunteers. In the same study, patients with mild and moderate hepatic function impairment had increases in QTc that were larger than those of normal subjects at the same plasma ranolazine level.

Contraindications

Ranolazine is contraindicated in patients with preexisting QT prolongation, with hepatic function impairment (Child-Pugh classes A [mild], B [moderate], or C [severe]), on QT-prolonging drugs, and on potent and moderately potent CYP3A inhibitors (eg, diltiazem).

Warnings

➤*QT prolongation:* Ranolazine has been shown to prolong the QTc interval in a dose-related manner. While the clinical significance of the QTc prolongation in the case of ranolazine is unknown, other drugs with this potential have been associated with torsades de pointes–type arrhythmias and sudden death.

With repeat dosing, the mean effect on QTc of ranolazine 1,000 mg twice daily, at T_{max}, is about 6 msec. However, in 5% of the population the prolongation of QTc is 15 msec. Age, CHF NYHA class I to IV, diabetes, gender, heart rate, race, and weight have no significant effect on the relationship between ranolazine plasma level and increase in QTc. The relationship between ranolazine levels and QTc remains linear over a concentration range up to 4-fold greater than the concentrations produced by 1,000 mg twice daily, and is not affected by changes in heart rate. Do not use dosages higher than 1,000 mg twice daily.

There are no studies examining the effects of ranolazine in patients with preexisting QT prolongation or receiving other QT prolonging drugs. Because of possible additive effects on the QT interval, avoid ranolazine use in patients with known QT prolongation (eg, congenital long QT syndrome, uncorrected hypokalemia), patients with known history of ventricular tachycardia, and patients receiving drugs that prolong the QTc interval, such as class Ia (eg, quinidine) and class III (eg, dofetilide, sotalol) antiarrhythmics and antipsychotics (eg, thioridazine, ziprasidone).

➤*Tumor promotion:* A published study reported that ranolazine promoted tumor formation and progression to malignancy when given to transgenic adenomatous polyposis coli (APC) (min/+) mice at a dosage of 30 mg/kg twice daily. The clinical significance of this finding is unclear.

➤*Hepatic function impairment:* Because the QTc-prolonging effect is increased approximately 3-fold in patients with hepatic dysfunction, ranolazine is contraindicated in patients with mild, moderate, or severe liver disease.

➤*Elderly:* Of the chronic angina patients treated with ranolazine in controlled studies, 496 (48%) were 65 years of age and older, and 114 (11%) were 75 years of age and older. No overall differences in efficacy were observed between older and younger patients. There were no differences in safety for patients 65 years of age and older compared with younger patients, but patients 75 years of age and older on ranolazine, compared with placebo, appeared to have a higher incidence of adverse reactions, serious adverse reactions, and drug discontinuations because of adverse reactions. In controlled ranolazine studies, the placebo-subtracted incidence of any adverse reaction in patients 75 years of age and older treated with ranolazine was 23%, and 11% discontinued ranolazine because of unacceptable adverse reactions. In CARISA and ERICA, the most commonly reported placebo-subtracted adverse reactions in patients 75 years of age and older on ranolazine included constipation (19%), nausea (6%), and dizziness (6%). In general, use caution when selecting dose for an elderly patient, usually starting at the low end of the dosing range, reflecting the greater frequency of decreased cardiac, hepatic, or renal function, and of concomitant disease or other drug therapy.

➤*Pregnancy: Category C.* There are no adequate studies assessing the effect of ranolazine on the developing fetus. There are no adequate and well-controlled studies in pregnant women. Use ranolazine during pregnancy only when the potential benefit to the patient justifies the potential risk to the fetus.

➤*Lactation:* It is not known whether ranolazine is excreted in human milk. Because many drugs are excreted in human milk and because of the potential for serious adverse reactions from ranolazine in breast-feeding infants, decide whether to discontinue breast-feeding or ranolazine, taking into account the importance of the drug to the mother.

➤*Children:* Safety and efficacy in children have not been established.

Precautions

➤*Monitoring:* Regularly monitor blood pressure after initiation of ranolazine in patients with severe renal function impairment. Obtain baseline and follow-up ECGs to evaluate effects on QT interval.

➤*Renal function impairment:* Ranolazine increases blood pressure by about 15 mm Hg in patients with severe renal function impairment. Regularly monitor blood pressure after initiation of ranolazine in such patients.

➤*Lab test abnormalities:* See Adverse Reactions for more information.

Transient eosinophilia was observed infrequently on ranolazine. Small mean decreases in hematocrit (1.2%) also were observed on ranolazine in controlled studies; however, there was no evidence of occult fecal blood loss.

➤*Drug abuse and dependence:* Ranolazine does not have any potential for abuse or dependence.

Drug Interactions

➤*CYP-450 system:* In vitro studies indicate that ranolazine is a P-gp substrate. Inhibitors of P-gp may increase the absorption of ranolazine. Exercise caution when coadministering ranolazine and P-gp inhibitors such as ritonavir and cyclosporine.

In vitro studies indicate that ranolazine and its O-demethylated metabolite are inhibitors of CYP3A and CYP2D6. Ranolazine and its most abundant metabolites are not known to inhibit the metabolism of substrates for CYP1A2, 2C9, 2C19, or 2E1 in human liver microsomes, suggesting that ranolazine is unlikely to alter the pharmacokinetics of drugs metabolized by these enzymes.

Ranolazine is primarily metabolized by CYP3A. Avoid using ranolazine with potent or moderately potent inhibitors of CYP3A because coadministration will increase ranolazine plasma levels and QTc prolongation. These inhibitors include ketoconazole and other azole antifungals, diltiazem, grapefruit juice or grapefruit-containing products, HIV protease inhibitors, macrolide antibiotics, and verapamil.

The inhibitory effects of ranolazine on CYP2D6 have been evaluated in extensive metabolizers of dextromethorphan. The study showed that ranolazine and/or metabolites partially inhibit CYP2D6. Concomitant use of ranolazine with other drugs metabolized by CYP2D6, such as tricyclic antidepressants and antipsychotics, has not been formally studied, but lower doses of the other drug than usually prescribed may be required in the presence of ranolazine. No dose adjustment of ranolazine is necessary when it is coadministered with drugs inhibiting CYP2D6.

Ranolazine Drug Interactions

Precipitant drug	Object drug[a]		Description
Diltiazem	Ranolazine	↑	Diltiazem causes dose-dependent mean increases in average ranolazine steady-state concentrations of about 1.8- to 2.3-fold. Concomitant use is not recommended.
Ketoconazole	Ranolazine	↑	Ketoconazole increases average steady-state plasma concentrations of ranolazine 3.2-fold. Do not use ranolazine during treatment with ketoconazole.
Macrolide antibiotics (eg, erythromycin)	Ranolazine	↑	Concomitant use may increase ranolazine plasma levels and QTc prolongation. Avoid coadministration.
Paroxetine	Ranolazine	↑	Paroxetine increases average steady-state plasma concentrations of ranolazine 1.2-fold.
Protease inhibitors (eg, ritonavir)	Ranolazine	↑	Concomitant use may increase ranolazine plasma levels and QTc prolongation. Avoid coadministration.
QT-prolonging drugs (eg, quinidine, sotalol, thioridazine, ziprasidone)	Ranolazine	↑	Concurrent use of ranolazine and QT prolonging drugs is contraindicated.
Verapamil	Ranolazine	↑	Verapamil increases ranolazine steady-state plasma concentrations about 2-fold. Concomitant use is not recommended.
Ranolazine	Digoxin	↑	Coadministration of ranolazine and digoxin results in a 1.5-fold elevation of digoxin plasma concentrations. May need to reduce digoxin dose.
Ranolazine	Simvastatin	↑	Coadministration of ranolazine and simvastatin results in about a 2-fold increase in plasma concentrations of simvastatin and its active metabolites. May need to reduce simvastatin dose.

[a] ↑ = Object drug increased.

RANOLAZINE — ORAL

➤*Drug/Food interactions:*

Grapefruit – Concomitant use may increase ranolazine plasma levels and QTc prolongation. Avoid coadministration.

Adverse Reactions

In controlled clinical trials of angina patients, the most frequently reported treatment-emergent adverse reactions (greater than 4%), occurring more often with ranolazine than placebo, were dizziness (6.2%), headache (5.5%), constipation (4.5%), and nausea (4.4%). In open-label, long-term treatment studies, a similar adverse reaction profile was observed in patients treated with ranolazine.

About 6% of patients discontinued treatment with ranolazine because of an adverse reaction in controlled studies in angina patients compared with about 3% on placebo. The most common adverse reactions that led to discontinuation more frequently on ranolazine than placebo were dizziness (1.3% vs 0.1%) and nausea (1% vs 0%), asthenia, constipation, and headache (each about 0.5% vs 0%).

Small, reversible elevations in serum creatinine and BUN levels have been observed in clinical studies with ranolazine. These elevations were observed without evidence of renal toxicity.

The most commonly observed treatment-emergent adverse reactions for chronic angina patients from CARISA and ERICA that occurred more frequently with ranolazine than placebo are shown in the following table.

Ranolazine Adverse Reactions (≥ 2%)

Adverse reactions	Placebo (n = 552)	Ranolazine[a] (n = 835)
CNS		
Dizziness	12 (2%)	41 (5%)
Headache	11 (2%)	22 (3%)
GI		
Constipation	9 (2%)	63 (8%)
Nausea	5 (1%)	33 (4%)

[a] Dosages include 500 mg twice daily, 750 mg twice daily, and 1,000 mg twice daily.

Ranolazine Incidence of Dizziness and Syncope

Adverse reactions	Placebo (n = 552)	Ranolazine 750 mg twice daily (n = 279)	Ranolazine 1,000 mg twice daily (n = 556)
Dizziness	12 (2%)	10 (4%)	31 (6%)
Syncope	0	0	4 (0.7%)

➤*Adverse reactions occurring among all ranolazine-treated patients with chronic angina:* A total of 2,018 patients with chronic angina were treated with ranolazine in controlled clinical trials.

The following additional adverse reactions occurred at an incidence of greater than 0.5% to less than 2% in patients treated with ranolazine and were more frequent than the incidence observed in placebo-treated patients.

➤*Cardiovascular:* Palpitations.

➤*GI:* Abdominal pain, dry mouth, vomiting.

➤*Respiratory:* Dyspnea.

➤*Special senses:* Tinnitus, vertigo.

➤*Miscellaneous:* Peripheral edema.

Other rarer (0.5% or less) but potentially medically important adverse reactions observed more frequently with ranolazine than placebo treatment in controlled studies included: blurred vision, bradycardia, hematuria, hypesthesia, hypotension, orthostatic hypotension, paresthesia, tremor.

Overdosage

➤*Symptoms:* In the event of overdose, the expected symptoms would be confusion, diplopia, dizziness, nausea/vomiting, and paresthesia. Syncope with prolonged loss of consciousness may develop.

➤*Treatment:* Because the QTc interval increases with ranolazine plasma concentration, continuous ECG monitoring may be warranted in the event of overdose. If required, initiate general supportive measures. Because ranolazine is about 62% bound to plasma proteins, complete clearance of ranolazine by hemodialysis is not likely.

PHENAZOPYRIDINE HCl (Phenylazo Diamino Pyridine HCl)

otc	**Azo-Standard** (Alcon)	**Tablets:** 95 mg	(W). In 30s.
otc	**Prodium** (Breckenridge)		In 12s and 30s.
Rx	**Phenazopyridine Hydrochloride** (Various, eg, Moore, Parmed, URL)	**Tablets:** 100 mg	In 100s, 1,000s, and UD 100s.
otc	**Baridium** (Pfeiffer)		In 32s.
Rx	**Geridium** (Goldline)		Burgundy. Sugar coated. In 100s and 1,000s.
Rx	**Pyridiate** (Rugby)		In 100s.
Rx	**Pyridium** (Parke-Davis)		Sucrose, lactose. (WC 180). Maroon. In 100s, 1,000s, and UD 100s.
Rx	**Urogesic** (Edwards)		In 100s.
Rx	**UTI Relief** (Consumers Choice Systems)	**Tablets:** 97.2 mg	In 12s.
Rx	**Phenazopyridine Hydrochloride** (Various, eg, Moore, Parmed, URL)	**Tablets:** 200 mg	In 100s, 1,000s, and UD 100s.
Rx	**Geridium** (Goldline)		Burgundy. Sugar coated. In 100s.
Rx	**Pyridium** (Parke-Davis)		Sucrose, lactose. (P-D 181). Maroon. In 100s, 1,000s, and UD 100s.

PHENAZOPYRIDINE HYDROCHLORIDE — ORAL

Urinary analgesics in combination with urinary anti-infectives are listed in the Anti-Infectives chapter.

Indications

Phenazopyridine HCl is indicated for the symptomatic relief of pain, burning, urgency, frequency, and other discomforts arising from irritation of the lower urinary tract mucosa caused by infection, trauma, surgery, endoscopic procedures, or the passage of sounds or catheters. The use of phenazopyridine HCl for relief of symptoms should not delay definitive diagnosis and treatment of causative conditions. Because it provides only symptomatic relief, prompt appropriate treatment of the cause of pain must be instituted and phenazopyridine HCl should be discontinued when symptoms are controlled.

The analgesic action may reduce or eliminate the need for systemic analgesics or narcotics. It is, however, compatible with antibacterial therapy and can help to relieve pain and discomfort during the interval before antibacterial therapy controls the infection. Treatment of a urinary tract infection with phenazopyridine HCl should not exceed 2 days because there is a lack of evidence that the combined administration of phenazopyridine HCl and an antibacterial provides greater benefit than administration of the antibacterial alone after 2 days.

Administration and Dosage

When used concomitantly with an antibacterial agent for the treatment of a urinary tract infection (UTI), the administration of phenazopyridine HCl should not exceed 2 days.

➤*Adults:*

100 mg tablets – Adult dosage is 2 tablets 3 times/day after meals.

200 mg tablets – Adult dosage is 1 tablet 3 times/day after meals.

➤*Children (6 to 12 years of age):* 12 mg/kg/day divided into 3 oral doses for 2 days.

➤*Storage/Stability:* Store at controlled room temperature 15° to 30°C (59° to 86°F).

Actions

➤*Pharmacology:* Phenazopyridine HCl is excreted in the urine where it exerts a topical analgesic effect on the mucosa of the urinary tract. This action helps to relieve pain, burning, urgency, and frequency. The precise mechanism of action is not known. Phenazopyridine is compatible with antibacterial therapy and can help relieve pain and discomfort before antibacterial therapy controls the infection.

➤*Pharmacokinetics:*

Excretion – The pharmacokinetic properties of phenazopyridine HCl have not been determined. Phenazopyridine HCl is rapidly excreted by the kidneys, with as much as 65% of an oral dose being excreted unchanged in the urine.

Contraindications

Phenazopyridine HCl should not be used in patients who have previously exhibited hypersensitivity to it. The use of phenazopyridine HCl is contraindicated in patients with renal insufficiency.

Warnings

➤*Carcinogenesis:* Long-term administration of phenazopyridine HCl has induced neoplasia in rats (large intestine) and mice (liver). Although no association between phenazopyridine HCl and human neoplasia has been reported, adequate epidemiological studies along these lines have not been conducted.

➤*Elderly:* A yellowish tinge of the skin or sclera may indicate accumulation due to impaired renal excretion and the need to discontinue therapy. The decline in renal function associated with advanced age should be kept in mind.

➤*Pregnancy: Category B.* Reproduction studies have been performed in rats at doses up to 50 mg/kg/day and have revealed no evidence of impaired fertility or harm to the fetus due to phenazopyridine HCl. There are, however, no adequate and well controlled studies in pregnant women. Because animal reproduction studies are not always predictive of human response, this drug should be used during pregnancy only if clearly needed.

➤*Lactation:* No information is available on the appearance of phenazopyridine HCl, or its metabolites in human milk.

➤*Children:* Do not give to children younger than 12 years of age unless directed by physician.

Precautions

➤*Skin/sclera discoloration:* A yellowish tinge of the skin or sclera may indicate accumulation due to impaired renal excretion and the need to discontinue therapy. The decline in renal function associated with advanced age should be kept in mind.

➤*Duration of therapy:* Treatment of a urinary tract infection (UTI) with phenazopyridine should not exceed 2 days because there is a lack of evidence that the combined administration of phenazopyridine and an antibacterial provides greater benefit than administration of the antibacterial alone after 2 days.

Patients should be informed that phenazopyridine HCl produces a reddish-orange discoloration of the urine and may stain fabric. This is not abnormal and represents no cause for alarm.

Staining of contact lenses has been reported.

➤*Lab test abnormalities:* Due to its properties as an azo dye, phenazopyridine HCl may interfere with urinalysis based on spectrometry or color reactions.

Adverse Reactions

Headache; rash; pruritus; occasional gastrointestinal disturbance. An anaphylactoid-like reaction has been described. Methemoglobinemia, hemolytic anemia, renal and hepatic toxicity have been described, usually at overdosage levels.

Staining of contact lenses has been reported.

Overdosage

➤*Symptoms:* Exceeding the recommended dose in patients with good renal function or administering the usual dose to patients with impaired renal function (common in elderly patients) may lead to increased serum levels and toxic reactions. Methemoglobinemia generally follows a massive, acute overdose. Oxidative Heinz body hemolytic anemia may also occur, and "bite cells" (degmacytes) may be present in a chronic overdosage situation. Red blood cell G-6-PD deficiency may predispose to hemolysis. Renal and hepatic impairment and occasional failure, usually due to hypersensitivity, may also occur.

➤*Treatment:* Methylene blue, 1 to 2 mg/kg/body weight intravenously or ascorbic acid 100 to 200 mg, given orally should cause prompt reduction of the methemoglobinemia and disappearance of the cyanosis which is an aid in diagnosis.

Patient Information

Phenazopyridine HCl may cause GI upset; take after meals.

Phenazopyridine HCl produces an orange to red color in the urine and may stain fabric. This is not abnormal and represents no cause for alarm. Staining of contact lenses has also occurred.

Do not use long term to treat undiagnosed urinary tract pain. This drug treats painful symptoms but not the source or cause of the pain.

PENTOSAN POLYSULFATE SODIUM

Rx	**Elmiron** (Baker Norton)	**Capsule:** 100 mg	(BNP7600). White. In 100s.

PENTOSAN POLYSULFATE SODIUM — ORAL

Indications

For the relief of bladder pain or discomfort associated with interstitial cystitis.

Administration and Dosage

➤*Approved by the FDA:* September 26, 1996.

The recommended dose of pentosan polysulfate sodium is 300 mg/day taken as one 100 mg capsule orally 3 times daily. The capsules should be taken with water at least 1 hour before meals or 2 hours after meals.

Patients receiving pentosan polysulfate sodium should be reassessed after 3 months. If improvement has not occurred and if limiting adverse events are not present, pentosan polysulfate sodium may be continued for another 3 months.

The clinical value and risks of continued treatment in patients whose pain has not improved by 6 months is not known.

➤*Storage / Stability:* Store at controlled room temperature 15° to 30° C (59° to 86°F).

Actions

➤*Pharmacology:* Pentosan polysulfate sodium is a low molecular weight heparin-like compound. It has anticoagulant and fibrinolytic effects. The mechanism of action of pentosan polysulfate sodium in interstitial cystitis is not known.

Pharmacodynamics – The mechanism by which pentosan polysulfate sodium achieves its effects in patients is unknown. In preliminary clinical models, pentosan polysulfate sodium adhered to the bladder wall mucosal membrane. The drug may act as a buffer to control cell permeability preventing irritating solutes in the urine from reaching the cells.

➤*Pharmacokinetics:*

Absorption – In preliminary clinical studies with different doses of radiolabeled pentosan polysulfate sodium, absorption was ≈ 3% of the administered dose (n = 3).

Food effects: The effect of food on absorption of pentosan polysulfate sodium is not known. In clinical trials, pentosan polysulfate sodium was administered with water 1 hour before or 2 hours after meals.

Distribution – Preclinical studies with parenterally administered radiolabeled pentosan polysulfate sodium showed distribution to the uroepithelium of the genitourinary tract with lesser amounts found in the liver, spleen, lung, skin, periosteum, and bone marrow. Erythrocyte penetration is low in animals.

Metabolism – Preliminary literature studies of metabolism in 5 healthy volunteers with radiolabeled drug suggest that 68% of the dose, at about 1 hour after IV administration, undergoes partial desulfation in the liver and spleen. In another study of 3 healthy volunteers, partial depolymerization occurs in the kidney. Both the desulfation and depolymerization can be saturated with continued dosing.

Excretion – In preliminary clinical studies in 8 healthy male volunteers, the elimination half-life of pentosan polysulfate sodium had a mean value at 24 hours after IV injection of 40 mg.

The elimination half-life in urine following orally administered radiolabeled pentosan polysulfate sodium was determined to be 4.8 hours for the unchanged drug.

In preliminary human studies in 3 healthy male volunteers, after single doses of radiolabeled drug, urinary excretion averaged 3.5% of the administered dose. After multiple doses of pentosan polysulfate sodium, urine excretion of radioactivity averaged 11% of the administered dose.

Further analyses of the urinary fraction obtained after repeated dosing showed that about 3% of the dose may be unchanged pentosan polysulfate sodium.

Contraindications

Hypersensitivity to the drug, structurally related compounds, or excipients.

Warnings

➤*Hepatic function impairment:* Pentosan polysulfate sodium is desulfated by both the liver and the spleen. The extent to which hepatic insufficiency or splenic disorders may increase the bioavailability of the parent or active metabolites of pentosan polysulfate sodium is not known. Caution should be exercised when using pentosan polysulfate sodium in these patients.

Mildly (< 2.5 × normal) elevated transaminase, alkaline phosphatase, gamma-glutamyl transpeptidase, and lactic dehydrogenase occurred in 1.2% of patients. The increases usually appeared 3 to 12 months after the start of pentosan polysulfate sodium therapy, and were not associated with jaundice or other clinical signs or symptoms. These abnormalities are usually transient, may remain essentially unchanged, or may rarely progress with continued use. Increases in PTT and PT (< 1% for both) or thrombocytopenia (0.2%) were noted.

➤*Pregnancy: Category B.* Reproduction studies have been performed in mice and rats with intravenous daily doses of 15 mg/kg, and in rabbits with 7.5 mg/kg. These doses are 0.42 and 0.14 times the daily oral human doses of pentosan polysulfate sodium when normalized to body surface area. These studies did not reveal evidence of impaired fertility or harm to the fetus from pentosan polysulfate sodium. Direct in vitro bathing of cultured mouse embryos with pentosan polysulfate sodium (PPS) at a concentration of 1 mg/mL may cause reversible limb bud abnormalities. Adequate and well controlled studies have not been performed in pregnant women. Because animal studies are not always predictive of human response, this drug should be used in pregnancy only if clearly needed.

➤*Lactation:* It is not known whether this drug is excreted in human milk. Because many drugs are excreted in human milk, caution should be exercised when pentosan polysulfate sodium is administered to a nursing woman.

➤*Children:* Safety and effectiveness in pediatric patients below the age of 16 years have not been established.

Precautions

Pentosan polysulfate sodium is a weak anticoagulant (1/15 the activity of heparin). Bleeding complications of ecchymosis, epistaxis, and gum hemorrhage have been reported (see Adverse Reactions). Patients undergoing invasive procedures or having signs/symptoms of underlying coagulopathy or other increased risk of bleeding (due to other therapies such as coumarin anticoagulants, heparin, t-PA, streptokinase, or high dose aspirin) should be evaluated for hemorrhage. Patients with diseases such as aneurysms, thrombocytopenia, hemophilia, gastrointestinal ulcerations, polyps, or diverticula should be carefully evaluated before starting pentosan polysulfate sodium.

A similar product that was given subcutaneously, sublingually, or intramuscularly (and not initially metabolized by the liver) is associated with delayed immunoallergic thrombocytopenia with symptoms of thrombosis and hemorrhage. Caution should be exercised when using pentosan polysulfate sodium in patients who have a history of heparin induced thrombocytopenia.

Alopecia is associated with pentosan polysulfate sodium and with heparin products. In clinical trials of pentosan polysulfate sodium, alopecia could begin within the first 4 weeks of treatment. Ninety-seven percent (97%) of the cases of alopecia reported were alopecia areata, limited to a single area on the scalp.

➤*Lab test abnormalities:* Pentosan polysulfate sodium did not affect prothrombin time (PT) or partial thromboplastin time (PTT) up to 1200 mg per day in 24 healthy male subjects treated for 8 days. Pentosan polysulfate sodium also inhibits the generation of factor Xa in plasma and inhibits thrombin-induced platelet aggregation in human platelet rich plasma ex vivo. (See Warnings for additional information.)

Drug Interactions

Not studied.

Adverse Reactions

Pentosan polysulfate sodium was evaluated in clinical trials in a total of 2627 patients (2343 women, 262 men, 22 unknown) with a mean age of 47 [range 18 to 88 with 581 (22%) over 60 years of age]. Of the 2627 patients, 128 patients were in a 3–month trial and the remaining 2499 patients were in a long term unblinded trial.

Deaths occurred in 6/2627 (0.2%) patients who received the drug over a period of 3 to 75 months. The deaths appear to be related to other concurrent illnesses or procedures, except in one patient for whom the cause was not known.

Serious adverse events occurred in 33/2627 (1.3%) patients. Two patients had severe abdominal pain or diarrhea and dehydration that required hospitalization. Because there was not a control group of patients with interstitial cystitis who were concurrently evaluated, it is difficult to determine which events are associated with pentosan polysulfate sodium and which events are associated with concurrent illness, medicine, or other factors.

Adverse Reactions in Placebo-Controlled Clinical Trials of Pentosan Polysulfate Sodium 100 mg 3 Times a Day for 3 Months

Body system/adverse reaction		Pentosan polysulfate sodium (n = 128)	Placebo (n = 130)
CNS	Overall number of patients*	3	5
	Insomnia	1	0
	Headache	1	3
	Severe emotional lability/ depression	2	1
	Nystagmus/dizziness	1	1
	Hyperkinesia	1	1
GI	Overall number of patients*	7	7
	Nausea	3	3
	Diarrhea	3	6
	Dyspepsia	1	0
	Jaundice	0	1
	Vomiting	0	2
Dermatologic/allergic	Overall number of patients*	2	4
	Rash	0	2

PENTOSAN POLYSULFATE SODIUM — ORAL

Adverse Reactions in Placebo-Controlled Clinical Trials of Pentosan Polysulfate Sodium 100 mg 3 Times a Day for 3 Months			
Body system/adverse reaction		Pentosan polysulfate sodium (n = 128)	Placebo (n = 130)
	Pruritus	0	2
	Lacrimation	1	1
	Rhinitis	1	1
	Increased sweating	1	0
Miscellaneous	Overall number of patients*	1	3
	Amenorrhea	0	1
	Arthralgia	0	1
	Vaginitis	1	1
Total reactions		17	27
Total number of patients reporting adverse reactions		13	19

* Within a body system, the individual reactions do not sum to equal overall number of patients because a patient may have more than one reaction.

The adverse events described below were reported in an unblinded clinical trial of 2499 interstitial cystitis patients treated with pentosan polysulfate sodium. Of the original 2499 patients, 1192 (48%) received pentosan polysulfate sodium for 3 months; 892 (36%) received pentosan polysulfate sodium for 6 months; and 598 (24%) received pentosan polysulfate sodium for one year, 355 (14%) received pentosan polysulfate sodium for 2 years, and 145 (6%) for 4 years.

➤*Frequency (1 to 4%):*

Miscellaneous – Alopecia (4%), diarrhea (4%), nausea (4%), headache (3%), rash (3%), dyspepsia (2%), abdominal pain (2%), liver function abnormalities (1%), dizziness (1%).

➤*Frequency (≤1%):* The adverse events described below were reported in an unblinded clinical trial of 2499 interstitial cystitis patients treated with pentosan polysulfate sodium. Of the original 2499 patients, 1192 (48%) received pentosan polysulfate sodium for 3 months; 892 (36%) received pentosan polysulfate sodium for 6 months; and 598 (24%) received pentosan polysulfate sodium for one year, 355 (14%) received pentosan polysulfate sodium for 2 years, and 145 (6%) for 4 years.

Dermatologic – Pruritus, urticaria.

GI – Vomiting, mouth ulcer, colitis, esophagitis, gastritis, flatulence, constipation, anorexia, gum hemorrhage.

Hematologic – Anemia, ecchymosis, increased prothrombin time, increased partial thromboplastin time, leukopenia, thrombocytopenia.

Hypersensitivity – Allergic reaction, photosensitivity.

Respiratory – Pharyngitis, rhinitis, epistaxis, dyspnea.

Special senses – Conjunctivitis, tinnitus, optic neuritis, amblyopia, retinal hemorrhage.

Overdosage

Overdose has not been reported. Based upon the pharmacodynamics of the drug, toxicity is likely to be reflected as anticoagulation, bleeding, thrombocytopenia, liver function abnormalities, and gastric distress. (See Pharmacokinetics, Warnings, and Precautions.) In the event of acute overdosage, the patient should be given gastric lavage if possible, carefully observed and given symptomatic and supportive treatment.

Patient Information

Patients should take the drug as prescribed, in the dosage prescribed, and no more frequently than prescribed. Patients should be reminded that pentosan polysulfate sodium has a weak anticoagulant effect. This effect may increase bleeding times.

DIMETHYL SULFOXIDE (DMSO)

Rx	**Dimethyl Sulfoxide** (Bioniche)	**Solution**: 50% aqueous solution	In 50 mL.
Rx	**Rimso-50** (Research Industries)		In 50 mL.

DIMETHYL SULFOXIDE — SOLUTION

Indications

For the symptomatic relief of patients with interstitial cystitis. Dimethyl sulfoxide has not been approved as being safe and effective for any other indication. There is no clinical evidence of effectiveness of dimethyl sulfoxide in the treatment of bacterial infections of the urinary tract.

Administration and Dosage

Instillation of 50 ml of dimethyl sulfoxide directly into the bladder may be accomplished by catheter or aseptic syringe and allowed to remain for 15 minutes. Application of an analgesic lubricant gel such as lidocaine jelly to the urethra is suggested prior to insertion of the catheter to avoid spasm. The medication is expelled by spontaneous voiding. It is recommended that the treatment be repeated every two weeks until maximum symptomatic relief is obtained. Thereafter, time intervals between therapy may be increased appropriately.

Administration of oral analgesic medication or suppositories containing belladonna and opium prior to the instillation of dimethyl sulfoxide can reduce bladder spasm.

In patients with severe interstitial cystitis with very sensitive bladders, the initial treatment, and possibly the second and third (depending on patient response) should be done under anesthesia. (Saddle block has been suggested.)

Dimethyl sulfoxide should not be given IM or IV.

➤*Storage / Stability:* Protect from strong light. Store at room temperature (59° to 86°F) (15° to 30°C). Do not autoclave.

Actions

➤*Pharmacology:* Dimethyl sulfoxide is metabolized in man by oxidation to dimethyl sulfone or by reduction to dimethyl sulfide. Dimethyl sulfoxide and dimethyl sulfone are excreted in the urine and feces. Dimethyl sulfide is eliminated through the breath and skin and is responsible for the characteristic odor from patients on dimethyl sulfoxide medication. Dimethyl sulfone can persist in serum for longer than two weeks after a single intravesical instillation. No residual accumulation of dimethyl sulfoxide has occurred in man or lower animals who have received treatment for protracted periods of time. Following topical application, dimethyl sulfoxide is absorbed and generally distributed in the tissues and body fluids.

Contraindications

None known.

Warnings

➤*Hypersensitivity reactions:* Dimethyl sulfoxide can initiate the liberation of histamine and there has been occasional hypersensitivity reaction with topical administration of dimethyl sulfoxide. This hypersensitivity has been reported in one patient receiving intravesical dimethyl sulfoxide. The physician should be cognizant of this possibility in prescribing dimethyl sulfoxide. If anaphylactoid symptoms develop, appropriate therapy should be instituted.

➤*Pregnancy: Category C.* Dimethyl sulfoxide caused teratogenic responses in hamsters, rats and mice when administered intraperitoneally at high doses (2.5-12 g/kg). Oral or topical doses of dimethyl sulfoxide did not cause problems of reproduction in rats, mice and hamsters. Topical doses (5 g/kg first two days, then 2.5 g/kg - last eight days) produced terata in rabbits, but in another study, topical doses of 1.1 gm/kg days 3 through 16 of gestation failed to produce any abnormalities. There are no adequate and well controlled studies in pregnant women. Dimethyl sulfoxide should be used during pregnancy only if the potential benefit justifies the potential risk to the fetus.

➤*Lactation:* It is not known whether this drug is excreted in human milk. Because many drugs are excreted in human milk, caution should be exercised when dimethyl sulfoxide is administered to a nursing woman.

➤*Children:* Safety and effectiveness in children have not been established.

Precautions

Changes in the refractive index and lens opacities have been seen in monkeys, dogs and rabbits given high doses of dimethyl sulfoxide chronically. Since lens changes were noted in animals, full eye evaluations, including slit lamp examinations, are recommended prior to and periodically during treatment.

Approximately every six months, patients receiving dimethyl sulfoxide should have a biochemical screening, particularly liver and renal function tests and complete blood count.

Intravesical instillation of dimethyl sulfoxide may be harmful to patients with urinary tract malignancy because of dimethyl sulfoxide-induced vasodilation.

Some data indicate that dimethyl sulfoxide potentiates other concomitantly administered medications.

➤*Drug abuse and dependence:* None known.

Adverse Reactions

A garlic-like taste may be noted by the patient within a few minutes after instillation of dimethyl sulfoxide. This taste may last several hours and because of the presence of metabolites, an odor on the breath and skin may remain for 72 hours.

Transient chemical cystitis has been noted following instillation of dimethyl sulfoxide.

The patient may experience moderately severe discomfort on administration. Usually this becomes less prominent with repeated administration.

Overdosage

The oral LD_{50} of dimethyl sulfoxide in the dog is greater than 10 g/kg. It is improbable that this dosage level could be obtained with intravesical instillation of dimethyl sulfoxide in the patient.

In case of accidental oral ingestion, specific measures should be taken to induce emesis. Additional measures which may be considered are gastric lavage, activated charcoal and forced diuresis.

DIMETHYL SULFOXIDE — SOLUTION

Patient Information

Dimethyl sulfoxide is a sterile solution of 50% dimethyl sulfoxide (DMSO) and 50% water that has been approved by the U.S. Food and Drug Administration for use in the symptomatic relief of patients with interstitial cystitis.

Dimethyl sulfoxide will be instilled in the bladder on an inpatient or outpatient basis, which will be determined by your physician.

Some data indicate that dimethyl sulfoxide could change the effectiveness of any medication(s) that you may be presently receiving. Be sure to mention the name and dosage of all medications you are taking to your physician before a dimethyl sulfoxide instillation.

A garlic-like taste may be noted by the patient within a few minutes after instillation of dimethyl sulfoxide. This taste may last several hours. An odor on the breath and skin may be present and remain for up to 72 hours.

Some patients may experience discomfort on administration of the drug. Usually this becomes less prominent with repeated administration.

If you are pregnant or nursing, ask your physician about the advisability of using dimethyl sulfoxide.

Some eye changes have been observed in animals treated with DMSO in large doses for prolonged periods. Therefore your doctor may want you to have eye evaluations, including slit lamp examinations prior to and periodically during treatment.

INTERSTITIAL CYSTITIS COMBINATIONS

Rx	**Phenazopyridine Plus** (Breckenridge)	**Tablets:** 150 mg phenazopyridine hydrochloride, 0.3 mg hyoscyamine hydrobromide, 15 mg butabarbital	(B-251). Dk brown. In 30s.
Rx	**Pyridium Plus** (Warner Chilcott)		Lactose. (WC 182). Dk maroon. In 30s.
Rx	**Trellium Plus** (Breckenridge)		(B-251). Dk brown. In 30s.

INTERSTITIAL CYSTITIS COMBINATIONS — ORAL

For complete prescribing information, refer to the Phenazopyridine Hydrochloride individual monograph, the Gastrointestinal Anticholinergic/Antispasmodic group monograph, and the Barbiturates group monograph.

Indications

For the symptomatic relief of pain, burning, frequency, urgency, and dysuria, particularly when accompanied by the detrusor muscle spasm and apprehension.

These symptoms may arise from infection, trauma, surgery, endoscopic procedures, or the passage of sounds or catheters.

Therapy does not interfere with antibacterial therapy and can help relieve symptoms of pain and discomfort before definitive treatment is effective. The use for symptomatic relief should not delay definitive diagnosis and treatment. Treatment of a urinary tract infection with this product should not exceed 2 days because there is a lack of evidence that the combined administration of phenazopyridine hydrochloride and an antibacterial provides greater benefit than administration of the antibacterial alone after 2 days.

In the absence of infection, this product may be the only medication required.

Administration and Dosage

➤*Adults:* One tablet 4 times a day (after meals and at bedtime).

When used concomitantly with an antibacterial agent for the treatment of a urinary tract infection, administration should not exceed 2 days.

➤*Storage/Stability:* Store at 25°C (77°F); excursions permitted to 15° to 30°C (59° to 86°F). Dispense in a tight, light-resistant container.

CELLULOSE SODIUM PHOSPHATE

CELLULOSE SODIUM PHOSPHATE

Rx	**Calcibind** (Mission)	**Powder:** Inorganic phosphate content 31% to 36% and sodium content ≈ 11%	In 300 g bulk powder.

CELLULOSE SODIUM PHOSPHATE — ORAL

Indications

Cellulose sodium phosphate (CSP) is indicated only for absorptive hypercalciuria Type I with recurrent calcium oxalate or calcium in phosphate nephrolithiasis. Appropriate use of CSP substantially reduces the incidence of new stone formation in these patients. Causes of hypercalciuria other than hyperabsorption cannot be expected to respond to CSP. Treatment with CSP is not needed for absorptive hypercalciuria Type II because dietary calcium restriction provides adequate treatment. In patients without hyperabsorption of calcium, CSP would be expected to cause excessive parathyroid hormone secretion and possible hyperparathyroid bone disease.

Absorptive hypercalciuria Type I is characterized by

1.) recurrent passage or formation of calcium oxalate and/or calcium phosphate renal stones,
2.) no evidence of bone disease,
3.) normal serum calcium and phosphorus,
4.) increased intestinal calcium absorption,
5.) hypercalciuria,
6.) normal urinary calcium during fasting,
7.) normal parathyroid function,
8.) lack of renal "leak" or excessive skeletal mobilization of calculi. Minimal diagnostic tests include serum calcium and phosphorus, parathyroid hormone (PTH) level obtained before breakfast, 24-hour urinary calcium on a diet restricted in calcium and sodium, and a fasting urinary excretion of calcium.

The diagnosis of absorptive hypercalciuria Type I can be made if there is: a) recurrent calcium nephrolithiasis without clinical evidence of bone disease, b) normal serum calcium and phosphorus (borderline values should be repeated), c) 24-hour urinary calcium greater than 200 mg/day on a diet of 400 mg calcium and 100 mEq sodium/day, d) normal serum immunoreactive PTH, and e) normal fasting urinary calcium. A definite diagnosis requires, in addition, evidence of high intestinal calcium absorption (eg, urinary calcium greater than 0.2 mg/mg creatinine after oral load of 1 g calcium.)

Administration and Dosage

➤*Approved by the FDA:* December 28, 1982.

The amount of dietary calcium bound depends upon actual mixing of CSP with a meal. Consequently, CSP should be taken with a meal; the amount of dietary calcium bound by CSP is considerably reduced when CSP is administered more than 1 hour after a meal. Both the initial and maintenance doses of CSP are based on measurements of 24-hour urinary calcium excretion. The recommended initial dose of CSP is 15 g/day (5 g with each meal) in patients with urinary calcium greater than 300 mg/day (on moderate calcium-restricted diet, ie, avoidance of dairy products). When urinary calcium declines to less than 150 mg/day, the dosage of CSP should be reduced to 10 g/day (5 g with supper, 2.5 g each with remaining meal). Patients with controlled urinary calcium on moderate calcium-restricted diet of less than 300 mg/day (but greater than 200 mg/day) should begin on CSP 10 g/day.

The following general measures should be imposed during CSP therapy. A moderate calcium intake is recommended, by avoidance of dairy products. A moderate dietary oxalate restriction should be imposed by discouraging ingestion of spinach (and similar dark greens), rhubarb, chocolate and brewed tea. Vitamin C supplementation should be denied because of its potential metabolism to oxalate. A high sodium intake should be discouraged by advising avoidance of "salty" foods and salt shakers, in an attempt to achieve an intake of less than 150 mEq/day. Fluid intake should be encouraged to achieve a minimum urine output of 2 L/day.

The dose of oral magnesium supplements, given as magnesium gluconate, depends upon the dose of CSP. Those receiving 15 g of CSP/day should take 1.5 g of magnesium gluconate before breakfast and again at bedtime (separately from CSP). Those taking 10 g of CSP/day should take 1 gram of magnesium gluconate twice a day. To avoid binding of magnesium by CSP, supplemental magnesium should be given at least 1 hour before or after a dose of CSP.

It is recommended that each dose of CSP (in the powder form) be suspended in a glass of water, soft drink or fruit juice, and ingested within ½ hour of the meal. It should not be given with magnesium gluconate.

➤*Storage/Stability:* Store under refrigeration at 2° to 8°C (36° to 46°F).

Actions

➤*Pharmacology:* CSP alters urinary composition of calcium, magnesium, phosphate and oxalate by affecting their absorption in the intestinal tract. When it is given orally with meals, CSP binds dietary and secreted calcium, and reduces urinary calcium by approximately 50 mg/5 g of CSP. It also binds dietary Mg and lowers urinary Mg. Oral magnesium supplementation given separately from CSP partly overcomes this effect.

CSP administration increases urinary phosphorus (P) and oxalate. The usual rise in urinary P of 150 to 250 mg/15 g CSP largely reflects the hydrolysis of 7% to 30% of CSP in the intestinal tract and absorption of released P. An increase in urinary oxalate occurs. Since CSP binds divalent cations, the cations are not available to complex oxalate and thereby limit its absorption. The rise in urinary oxalate may be largely prevented by moderate dietary oxalate restriction and the use of a modest dose of CSP (10 to 15 g/day).

The marked reduction in urinary calcium with only slightly increased urinary phosphorus and oxalate leads to a reduction in urinary saturation and propensity for spontaneous nucleation of calcium oxalate and calcium phosphate (brushite).

CSP does not apparently alter the metabolism of trace metals, since it does not significantly change the serum concentration of copper, zinc or iron.

Contraindications

CSP is contraindicated in

1.) primary or secondary hyperparathyroidism, including renal hypercalciuria (renal calcium leak),
2.) hypomagnesemic states (serum magnesium less than 1.5 mg/dL),
3.) bone disease (osteoporosis, osteomalacia, osteitis),
4.) hypocalcemic states (eg, hypoparathyroidism, intestinal malabsorption),
5.) normal or low intestinal absorption and renal excretion of calcium,
6.) enteric hyperoxaluria. It should not be used in patients with high fasting urinary calcium or hypophosphatemia, unless a high skeletal mobilization of calcium can be excluded.

CELLULOSE SODIUM PHOSPHATE — ORAL

Warnings

In patients with congestive heart failure or ascites, sodium contained in CSP (35 to 48 mEq exchangeable sodium/15 g CSP) may represent a hazard.

➤*Carcinogenesis:* No long-term studies were conducted to determine the carcinogenic potential of CSP.

➤*Mutagenesis:* No long-term studies were conducted to determine the mutagenic potential of CSP.

➤*Fertility impairment:* No long-term studies were conducted to determine the potential of CSP to impair fertility.

➤*Pregnancy: Category C.*

Animal reproduction studies have not been conducted with CSP. It is also not known whether CSP can cause fetal harm when administered to a pregnant woman or can affect reproduction capacity. However, because of the increased requirement of dietary calcium in pregnant women, CSP should be given to pregnant women only if clearly needed.

➤*Children:* Because of the increased requirement for dietary calcium in growing children, the use of CSP in children less than 16 years of age is not recommended.

Precautions

By inhibiting intestinal calcium absorption, CSP may stimulate parathyroid function leading to hyperparathyroid hormone levels. CSP treatment has been shown to maintain parathyroid function within normal limits, if it is used only in patients with absorptive hypercalciuria Type I (increased intestinal calcium restricted diet), at a dosage just sufficient to restore normal calcium absorption but not sufficient to cause subnormal absorption.

The following additional complications may potentially develop during long-term use of CSP: Hyperoxaluria and hypomagnesiuria, which would negate the beneficial effect of hypocalciuria on new stone formation; magnesium depletion, depletion of trace metals (copper, zinc, iron). All of these effects may be minimized by restricting the use of CSP to absorptive hypercalciuria Type I only, and by taking precautionary measures (see Administration and Dosage) and by monitoring serum calcium, magnesium, copper, zinc, iron, parathyroid hormone, and complete blood count every 3 to 6 months. Absorptive hypercalciuria Type I is characterized by

1.) recurrent passage or formation of calcium oxalate and/or calcium phosphate renal stones,
2.) no evidence of bone disease,
3.) normal serum calcium and phosphorus,
4.) increased intestinal calcium absorption,
5.) hypercalciuria,
6.) normal urinary calcium during fasting,
7.) normal parathyroid function,
8.) lack of renal "leak" or excessive skeletal mobilization of calculi.A moderate calcium intake is recommended, by avoidance of dairy products. A moderate dietary oxalate restriction should be imposed by discouraging ingestion of spinach (and similar dark greens), rhubarb, chocolate and brewed tea. Vitamin C supplementation should be denied because of its potential metabolism to oxalate. A high sodium intake should be discouraged by advising avoidance of "salty" foods and salt shakers, in an attempt to achieve an intake of less than 150 mEq/day. Fluid intake should be encouraged to achieve a minimum urine output of 2 L/day. Borderline values for parathyroid hormone and calcium should be repeated promptly. Serum PTH should be obtained at least once between the first 2 weeks to 3 months of treatment and the treatment should be adjusted or stopped if a rise in serum PTH above normal appears. If there is an inadequate hypocalciuric response to CSP treatment (a reduction in urinary calcium of less than 30 mg/5 g of CSP), while patients are maintained on moderate calcium and sodium restriction, the treatment may be considered ineffective and should be stopped. Cessation of treatment should be considered if urinary oxalate exceeds 55 mg/day on moderate dietary oxalate restriction.

Adverse Reactions

Some patients may have gastrointestinal complaints, manifested by poor taste of the drug, loose bowel movements, diarrhea or dyspepsia.

IMPOTENCE AGENTS

ALPROSTADIL (Prostaglandin E_1; PGE_1)

Rx	**Caverject** (Pharmacia & Upjohn)	**Injection, aqueous**: 10 mcg/mL	In 1 mL ampules and kit.[a]
		20 mcg/mL	In 1 mL ampules and kit.[a]
		40 mcg/2 mL	In 2 mL ampules and kit.[a]
Rx	**Caverject** (Pharmacia & Upjohn)	**Powder for injection, lyophilized**: 5 mcg/mL (after reconstitution)	With 8.4 mg benzyl alcohol and lactose. In vials with diluent syringes.
		10 mcg/mL (after reconstitution)	With 8.4 mg benzyl alcohol and lactose. In vials and vials with diluent syringes.
		20 mcg/mL (after reconstitution)	With 8.4 mg benzyl alcohol and lactose. In vials and vials with diluent syringes.
		40 mcg/mL (after reconstitution)	With 8.4 mg benzyl alcohol and lactose. In vials with diluent syringes.
Rx	**Caverject Impulse** (Pharmacia & Upjohn)	**Powder for injection, lyophilized**: 10 mcg/0.5 mL (after reconstitution)[b]	With 4.45 mg benzyl alcohol and lactose. In blister tray.[c]
		20 mcg/0.5 mL (after reconstitution)[d]	With 4.45 mg benzyl alcohol and lactose. In blister tray.[c]
Rx	**Edex** (Schwarz Pharma)	**Powder for injection, lyophilized**: 5 mcg/mL (after reconstitution)	Lactose. In single-dose vials and kit.[e]
		10 mcg/mL (after reconstitution)	Lactose. In single-dose vials and kit.[e]
		20 mcg/mL (after reconstitution)	Lactose. In single-dose vials and kit.[e]
		40 mcg/mL (after reconstitution)	Lactose. In single-dose vials and kit.[e]
Rx	**Muse** (Vivus)	**Pellet**: 125 mcg	In individual foil pouches.
		250 mcg	In individual foil pouches.
		500 mcg	In individual foil pouches.
		1000 mcg	In individual foil pouches.

[a] Kit contains 2 mL *Luer-lock* syringe, 2 one-half inch needles (one 27-gauge and one 30-gauge), alcohol swab.
[b] Amounts can be delivered in increments of 10 mcg/0.5 mL, 2.5 mcg/0.125 mL, 5 mcg/0.25 mL, or 7.5 mcg/0.375 mL.
[c] Blister tray contains 1 dual chamber syringe system, 1 needle, 2 alcohol swabs.
[d] Amounts can be delivered in increments of 20 mcg/0.5 mL, 5 mcg/0.125 mL, 10 mcg/0.25 mL, or 15 mcg/0.375 mL.
[e] Kit contains prefilled syringe (with 1.2 mL of 0.9% sodium chloride), plunger rod, 2 one-half inch needles (one 27-gauge and one 30-gauge), 2 alcohol swabs, tape.

ALPROSTADIL — INTRACAVERNOSAL

For information on the use of alprostadil for patent ductus arteriosus, refer to the specific monograph in the Cardiovasculars chapter.

Indications

➤*Erectile dysfunction:* For the treatment of erectile dysfunction due to neurogenic, vasculogenic, psychogenic, or mixed etiology.

May be a useful adjunct to other diagnostic tests in the diagnosis of erectile dysfunction.

Administration and Dosage

➤*Approved by the FDA:* July 6, 1995.

Advise the patient not to exceed the optimum alprostadil dose which was determined in the doctor's office. In general, always use the lowest possible effective dose.

➤*Caverject* formulations: Individualize the dose of intracavernosal alprostadil for each patient by careful titration under supervision by the physician. In clinical studies, patients were treated with alprostadil sterile powder in doses ranging from 0.2 to 140 mcg; however, since 99% of patients received doses of 60 mcg or less, doses of greater than 60 mcg are not recommended. In clinical studies, over 80% of patients experienced an erection sufficient for sexual intercourse after intracavernosal injection of alprostadil.

➤*Edex* dual-chamber cartridge: The dosage range of *Edex* sterile powder for the treatment of erectile dysfunction is 1 to 40 mcg. Give the intracavernosal injection over a 5- to 10-second interval. In a study with a dose range of 1 to 20 mcg of *Edex* sterile powder, the mean dose was 10.7 mcg at the end of the dose titration period. In 2 studies with a dose range of 1 to 40 mcg of *Edex* sterile powder, the mean dose was 21.9 mcg at the end of the dose titration period. Doses greater than 40 mcg have not been studied.

➤*Aqueous solution and sterile powder:* A ½-inch, 27- to 30-gauge needle is generally recommended.

➤*Caverject* dual-chamber system: The 10 mcg strength is designed to deliver a minimum dose of 2.5 mcg and a maximum dose of 10 mcg. The 20 mcg strength is designed to deliver a minimum dose of 5 mcg and a maximum dose of 20 mcg. Because the *Caverject* dual-chamber system is designed to deliver doses of 2.5 mcg or greater (see General procedures for solution preparation), alprostadil sterile powder or alprostadil aqueous solution for injection may be used for an initial dose of 1.25 mcg. Determine the

ALPROSTADIL — INTRACAVERNOSAL

most suitable formulation of alprostadil for the individual patient (ie, alprostadil dual-chamber system, alprostadil sterile powder, or alprostadil aqueous solution for injection).

➤*Initial titration in physician's office:*

Erectile dysfunction of vasculogenic, psychogenic, or mixed etiology – Initiate dosage titration at 2.5 mcg of alprostadil. If there is a partial response, the dose may be increased by 2.5 mcg to a dose of 5 mcg and then in increments of 5 to 10 mcg, depending upon erectile response, until the dose that produces an erection suitable for intercourse and not exceeding a duration of 1 hour is reached. If there is no response to the initial 2.5 mcg dose, the second dose may be increased to 7.5 mcg, followed by increments of 5 to 10 mcg. The patient must stay in the physician's office until complete detumescence occurs. If there is no response, then the next higher dose may be given within 1 hour. If there is a response, then there should be at least a 1-day interval before the next dose is given.

Erectile dysfunction of pure neurogenic etiology (spinal cord injury) – Initiate dose titration at 1.25 mcg of alprostadil. The dose may be increased by 1.25 mcg to a dose of 2.5 mcg, followed by an increment of 2.5 mcg to a dose of 5 mcg, and then in 5 mcg increments until the dose that produces an erection suitable for intercourse and not exceeding a duration of 1 hour is reached. The patient must stay in the physician's office until complete detumescence occurs. If there is no response, then the next higher dose may be given within 1 hour. If there is a response, then there should be at least a 1-day interval before the next dose is given.

➤*Maintenance therapy:*

Aqueous solution and sterile powder –

Two needles are provided: A ½ inch, 27-gauge needle and a ½ inch, 30-gauge needle.

Caverject dual-chamber system – Alprostadil dual chamber system in the 10 mcg strength is designed to deliver a minimum dose of 2.5 mcg and a maximum dose of 10 mcg. Alprostadil dual chamber system in the 20 mcg strength is designed to deliver a minimum dose of 5 mcg and a maximum dose of 20 mcg. Determine the most suitable formulation of alprostadil for the individual patient (ie, alprostadil dual-chamber system, alprostadil sterile powder, or alprostadil aqueous solution for injection). The first injections of alprostadil must be done at the physician's office by medically trained personnel. Self-injection therapy by the patient can be started only after the patient is properly instructed and well trained in the self-injection technique.

The physician should make a careful assessment of the patient's skills and competence with this procedure. The intracavernosal injection must be done under sterile conditions. The site of injection is usually along the dorsolateral aspect of the proximal third of the penis. Avoid visible veins. Alternate the side of the penis that is injected and the site of injection; cleanse the injection site with an alcohol swab.

The dose of alprostadil that is selected for self-injection treatment should provide the patient with an erection that is satisfactory for sexual intercourse and that is maintained for no longer than 1 hour. If the duration of erection is longer than 1 hour, reduce the dose of alprostadil. Use the lowest effective dose at home. Initiate self-injection therapy for use at home at the dose that was determined in the physician's office; however, make dose adjustment, if required (up to 57% of patients in 1 clinical study), only after consultation with the physician. Adjust the dose in accordance with the titration guidelines described above. The efficacy of alprostadil for long-term use of up to 6 months has been documented in an uncontrolled, self-injection study. The mean dose of alprostadil at the end of 6 months was 20.7 mcg in this study.

Exercise careful and continuous follow-up of the patient while in the self-injection program. This is especially true for the initial self-injections, since adjustments in the dose of alprostadil may be needed. The recommended frequency of injection is no more than 3 times weekly, with at least 24 hours between each dose.

All formulations of intracavernosal alprostadil are intended for single use only and should be discarded after use. Instruct the user in the proper disposal of the injection materials (eg, device, syringes, needles, ampoule or reconstituted vial).

While on self-injection treatment, it is recommended that the patient visit the prescribing physician's office every 3 months. At that time, assess the efficacy and safety of the therapy, and the dose of alprostadil, if needed.

➤*Alprostadil as an adjunct to the diagnosis of erectile dysfunction:* In the simplest diagnostic test for erectile dysfunction (pharmacologic testing), patients are monitored for the occurrence of an erection after an intracavernosal injection of alprostadil. Extensions of this testing are the use of alprostadil as an adjunct to laboratory investigations, such as duplex or Doppler imaging, ^{133}Xenon washout tests, radioisotope penogram, and penile arteriography, to allow visualization and assessment of penile vasculature. For any of these tests, use a single dose of alprostadil that induces an erection with firm rigidity.

➤*General procedure for dose or solution preparation:*

Aqueous solution – Alprostadil aqueous solution injection is packaged in a 1 mL polyethylene ampule containing 10.2 or 20.2 mcg per mL of alprostadil, depending on ampule strength. The deliverable amount of alprostadil is 10 or 20 mcg/mL because approximately 0.2 mcg is lost due to adsorption to the syringe during administration. Alprostadil injection is also available in 2 mL ampules containing 40.4 mcg per 2 mL (20.2 mcg/mL) of alprostadil. The deliverable amount of alprostadil is 40 mcg per 2 mL (20 mcg/mL) because approximately 0.4 mcg is lost due to adsorption to the syringe during administration. To prepare a dose for administration, remove the ampule from the foil wrapping. Allow the ampule contents to warm to room temperature. The ampule should not be cool to the touch. Do not immerse in water. Do not microwave.

Shake the ampule vigorously for at least 30 seconds. Next, hold the shorter tab closest to the neck of the ampule and shake it downward with a quick snap to clear any solution from the neck. Holding the ampule by the edges, twist the top of the ampule and lift upward to remove it. Make sure the open end of the ampule does not touch your hands or any other surface. After opening the ampule, immediately transfer the solution to a syringe and use promptly. Visually inspect parenteral drug products for particulate matter and discoloration prior to administration whenever the solution and container permit.

Caution: Do not reuse any remaining alprostadil solution due to the possibility of bacterial contamination.

Caverject sterile powder – Alprostadil sterile powder for injection is packaged in a 5 mL glass vial. Bacteriostatic water for injection or sterile water, both preserved with benzyl alcohol 0.945% w/v, must be used as the diluent for reconstitution. After reconstitution with 1 mL of diluent, the volume of the resulting solution is 1.13 mL. One mL of this solution will contain 5.4, 10.5, 20.5 or 41.1 mcg of alprostadil depending on vial strength, 172 mg of lactose, 47 mcg of sodium citrate and 8.4 mg of benzyl alcohol. The deliverable amount of alprostadil is 5, 10, 20, or 40 mcg per mL because approximately 0.4 mcg for the 5 mcg strength, 0.5 mcg for the 10 and 20 mcg strengths, and 1.1 mcg for the 40 mcg strength is lost due to adsorption to the vial and syringe. After reconstitution, use the solution of alprostadil within 24 hours when stored at or below 25°C (77°F) and do not refrigerate or freeze. Visually inspect parenteral drug products for particulate matter and discoloration prior to administration whenever the solution and container permit.

Caverject dual-chamber system – Alprostadil dual-chamber system consists of a disposable, single-dose, dual-chamber syringe system. The system includes a glass cartridge, which contains sterile, freeze-dried alprostadil in the front chamber and sterile bacteriostatic water for injection in the rear chamber. Following proper reconstitution instructions, the 10 mcg strength syringe can deliver up to 0.5 mL of solution. Each 0.5 mL of solution contains 10 mcg of alprostadil, 324.7 mcg of alpha cyclodextrin, 45.4 mg of lactose, 23.5 mcg of sodium citrate, and 4.45 mg of benzyl alcohol. The delivery device can be set to deliver a solution volume of 0.125, 0.25, 0.375, or 0.5 mL to enable administration of 2.5, 5, 7.5, or 10 mcg of alprostadil. Following proper reconstitution instructions, the 20 mcg strength syringe can deliver up to 0.5 mL of solution. Each 0.5 mL of solution contains 20 mcg of alprostadil, 649.3 mcg of alpha cyclodextrin, 45.4 mg of lactose, 23.5 mcg of sodium citrate, and 4.45 mg of benzyl alcohol. The delivery device can be set to deliver a solution volume of 0.125, 0.25, 0.375, or 0.5 mL to enable administration of 5, 10, 15, or 20 mcg of alprostadil. After reconstitution, use the solution of alprostadil within 24 hours when stored at or below 25°C (77°F). Visually inspect parenteral drug products for particulate matter and discoloration prior to administration whenever the solution and container permit. Do not use if particulate matter or discoloration are present. Following a single use, properly discard the injection device and any remaining solution.

Edex dual-chamber cartridge – The *Edex* injection device is used to reconstitute the single-dose, dual-chamber cartridge. The plunger is used to force the sterile 0.9% sodium chloride (1.075 mL) in 1 chamber into the chamber containing alprostadil. After reconstitution, the *Edex* injection device is used to administer the intracavernosal injection of alprostadil. The reusable *Edex* injection device is for use only with the cartridges and needles included in the *Edex* cartridge packs.

Prepare the *Edex* solution immediately before use. Do not administer unless solution is clear. Do not add any drugs or solutions to the *Edex* solution. Discard any unused solution remaining in the cartridge. Do not store the reconstituted solution.

The *Edex* cartridge contains a solid layer or lyophilized cake of dry white powder approximately 3/8" in thickness for the cartridge. A normal cake may appear cracked or crumbled. If the cartridge is damaged, the cake may shrink in size. Do not use the cartridge if it appears damaged or the cake is substantially reduced in size.

➤*Storage/Stability:*

Aqueous solution – Store alprostadil injection frozen at −20° to −10°C (−4° to 14°F) until dispensed. After dispensing, store in a freezer at −20° to −10°C (−4° to 14°F) for up to 3 months. During this 3-month period, alprostadil injection may be moved to and kept in a refrigerator at 2° to 8°C (36° to 46°F) for up to 7 days. Once refrigerated, use within 7 days or discard; do not refreeze. Once removed from the foil wrapping, use the solution in the ampule immediately after allowing it to warm to room temperature or discard it. Use open ampules of alprostadil injection immediately and do not store them.

Caverject sterile powder – Store the 40 mcg strength at 2° to 8°C (36° to 46°F) until dispensed. After dispensing, the alprostadil 40 mcg strength may be stored at or below 25°C (77°F) for 3 months or until expiration date, whichever occurs first.

When reconstituted and used as directed, the deliverable amount of alprostadil is 5, 10, 20 or 40 mcg, respectively. Use the reconstituted solution within 24 hours when stored at or below 25°C (77°F) and do not refrigerate or freeze. Use only the accompanying diluent or bacteriostatic water for injection with benzyl alcohol when reconstituting alprostadil sterile powder.

Caverject dual-chamber system – Store the unreconstituted product at 25°C (77°F); excursions permitted to 15° to 30°C (59° to 86°F).

When reconstituted and used as directed, the deliverable amount for the 10 mcg strength is 10 mcg per 0.5 mL or an increment of 10 mcg per 0.5 mL, 2.5 mcg per 0.125 mL, 5 mcg per 0.25 mL, or 7.5 mcg per 0.375 mL of alprostadil, and the deliverable amount for the 20 mcg strength is 20 mcg per 0.5 mL or an increment of 20 mcg per 0.5 mL, 5 mcg per 0.125 mL, 10 mcg per 0.25 mL, or 15 mcg per 0.375 mL of alprostadil. Use the reconstituted solution within 24 hours when stored at or below 25°C (77°F).

Edex cartridge: Store at 25°C (77°F); excursions permitted between 15° and 30°C (59° to 86°F).

ALPROSTADIL — INTRACAVERNOSAL

When the cartridge is placed into the *Edex* injection device and reconstituted, the deliverable amount of alprostadil in each mL is 10, 20, or 40 mcg, respectively. The cartridge is supplied in a package.

Actions

➤*Pharmacology:* Alprostadil (PGE_1) is 1 of the prostaglandins, a family of naturally occurring acidic lipids with various pharmacological effects. Endogenous PGE_1 is derived from dihomo-gamma-linolenic acid, a fatty acid found within the phospholipids of cellular membranes. As an endogenous substance, PGE_1 exerts its biological effects either directly or indirectly by regulating and modifying the synthesis and effects of other hormones and mediators.

Alprostadil is a smooth muscle relaxant. Precontracted isolated preparations of the human corpus cavernosum, corpus spongiosum, and cavernous artery are relaxed by alprostadil. Alprostadil has been shown to bind to specific receptors in human penile tissue. Two types of receptors that differ in their PGE_1-binding affinity have been identified. The binding of alprostadil to its receptors is accompanied by an increase in intracellular cAMP levels. Human cavernous smooth muscle cells respond to alprostadil by releasing intracellular calcium into the surrounding medium. Smooth muscle relaxation is associated with a reduction of cytoplasmic free calcium concentration. Alprostadil also attenuates presynaptic noradrenaline release in the corpus cavernosum, which is essential for the maintenance of a flaccid and nonerect penis.

Alprostadil has a wide variety of pharmacological actions; vasodilation and inhibition of platelet aggregation are among the most notable of these effects. In most animal species tested, alprostadil relaxed retractor penis and corpus cavernosum urethrae in vitro. Alprostadil also relaxed isolated preparations of human corpus cavernosum and spongiosum, as well as cavernous arterial segments contracted by either noradrenaline or $PGF_{2\alpha}$ in vitro. In pigtail monkeys (*Macaca nemestrina*), alprostadil increased cavernous arterial blood flow in vivo. The degree and duration of cavernous smooth muscle relaxation in this animal model was dose dependent.

Alprostadil induces erection by relaxation of trabecular smooth muscle and by dilation of cavernosal arteries. This leads to expansion of lacunar spaces and entrapment of blood by compressing the venules against the tunica albuginea, a process referred to as the corporal veno-occlusive mechanism.

➤*Pharmacokinetics:*

Absorption – For the treatment of erectile dysfunction, alprostadil is administered by injection into the corpora cavernosa. The absolute bioavailability of alprostadil estimated from systemic exposure was about 98% as compared to the same dose given by a short-term IV infusion.

Edex: After intracavernosal injection of 20 mcg of *Edex* in 24 patients with erectile dysfunction, mean systemic plasma concentrations of PGE_1 increased from baseline of 0.8 ± 0.6 pg/mL to a peak (C_{max}) of 16.8 ± 18.9 pg/mL (corrected for baseline) within 2 to 5 minutes and dropped to endogenous plasma levels within 2 hours (see the following table). The absolute bioavailability of alprostadil estimated from systemic exposure was about 98% as compared to the same dose given by a short-term IV infusion.

Distribution – After intracavernosal injection of 20 mcg of alprostadil in 24 patients with erectile dysfunction, mean systemic plasma concentrations of PGE_1 increased from baseline of 0.8 ± 0.6 pg/mL to a peak (C_{max}) of 16.8 ± 18.9 pg/mL (corrected for baseline) within 2 to 5 minutes and dropped to endogenous plasma levels within 2 hours.

Plasma levels of PGE_1 were measured using a radioimmunoassay method. PGE_1 is bound in plasma primarily to albumin (81% bound) and, to a lesser extent, α-globulin IV-4 fraction (55% bound). No significant binding to erythrocytes or white blood cells was observed.

Edex: The volume of distribution for PGE_1 was not estimated. Approximately 93% of PGE_1 found in plasma is protein bound.

Metabolism – PGE_1 is metabolized in the corpus cavernosum after intracavernosal administration. PGE_1 entering the systemic circulation is rapidly and extensively metabolized in the lungs with a first-pass pulmonary elimination of 60% to 90% of PGE_1. Enzymatic oxidation of the C15-hydroxy group followed by reduction of the C13, 14-double bond produces the primary metabolites, 15-keto-PGE_1, 15-keto-PGE_0, and PGE_0. 15-keto-PGE_1 has only been detected in vitro in homogenized lung preparations, whereas 15-keto-PEG_0 and PGE_0 have been measured in plasma. Unlike the 15-keto metabolites, which are less pharmacologically active than the parent compound, PGE_0 is similar in potency to PGE_1 in vitro using isolated animal organs.

After intracavernosal injection of 20 mcg of alprostadil to 24 patients with erectile dysfunction, mean systemic plasma 15-keto-PGE_0 levels increased within 7 minutes from endogenous levels of 12.9 ± 11.8 pg/mL to a C_{max} of 421 ± 337 pg/mL (corrected for baseline), followed by a decrease to baseline levels in several hours. Mean systemic plasma PGE_0 levels increased within 20 minutes from endogenous levels of 0.6 ± 0.5 pg/mL to a C_{max} of 3.9 ± 2.3 pg/mL (corrected for baseline), followed by a decrease to baseline levels in several hours.

Excretion – After further degradation of PGE_1 by beta and omega oxidation, the main metabolites are excreted primarily in urine (88%) and feces (12%) over 72 hours, and total excretion is essentially complete (92%) within 24 hours after administration. No unchanged PGE_1 has been found in the urine, and there is no evidence of tissue retention of PGE_1 and its metabolites. After intracavernosal injection of 20 mcg of alprostadil in patients with erectile dysfunction, the terminal half-lives ($t_{½}$) of 15-keto-PGE_0 and PGE_0 were calculated to be 40.9 ± 16.5 minutes and 63.2 ± 31.1 minutes, respectively. The terminal half-life of PGE_1 in healthy volunteers was calculated to be around 9 to 11 minutes, which is consistent with that reported in the literature (8 minutes).

Mean total body clearance of PGE_1 in patients with erectile dysfunction was calculated to be around 115 L/min after an IV infusion of 20 mcg alprostadil. The above value exceed cardiac output, indicating extensive and rapid elimination of PGE_1 in the lungs or blood.

Special populations –

Renal function impairment: In a study in symptomatic subjects with end-stage renal disease undergoing hemodialysis and age/weight/sex-matched healthy volunteers, 120 mcg of alprostadil was administered by IV infusion over 2 hours. The mean C_{max} value of PGE_1 in renally impaired patients was 37% lower as compared to that in healthy volunteers, whereas mean C_{max} values of 15-keto-PGE_0 and PGE_0 in these patients increased 104% and 145% respectively as compared to those in healthy volunteers. The terminal half-lives of PGE_1, PGE_0, and 15-keto-PGE_0 and plasma albumin levels were similar in these patients vs healthy volunteers. The mechanism responsible for the observed discrepancies between renally impaired subjects and healthy volunteers is not known.

Hepatic function impairment: In a study in symptomatic subjects with impaired hepatic function and age/weight/sex matched healthy volunteers, 120 mcg of alprostadil was administered by IV infusion over 2 hours. The mean C_{max} value of PGE_1 in hepatically impaired patients was 96% higher than in healthy volunteers. Mean C_{max} values of both 15-keto-PGE_0 and PGE_0 increased 65% as compared to those in healthy volunteers. Due to the fact that PGE_1 is primarily metabolized in the lung, the observed differences between hepatically impaired subjects and healthy volunteers were not anticipated; the mechanism responsible for the observed discrepancies is not known.

Pulmonary disease: The pulmonary extraction of alprostadil following intravascular administration was reduced by 15% (66 ± 3.2% vs 78 ± 2.4%) in patients with ARDS compared with a control group of patients with normal respiratory function who were undergoing cardiopulmonary bypass surgery. Pulmonary clearance was found to vary as a function of cardiac output and pulmonary intrinsic clearance in a group of 14 patients with ARDS or at risk of developing ARDS following trauma or sepsis. In this study, the extraction efficiency of alprostadil ranged from subnormal (11%) to normal (90%), with an overall mean of 67%.

Edex – After reconstitution, PGE_1 immediately dissociates from the α-cyclodextrin inclusion; the in vivo disposition of both components occurs independently after administration. After IV infusion of radiolabeled α-cyclodextrin to healthy volunteers, the radiolabeled components were rapidly eliminated within 24 hours, urine accounting for 81% to 83% of radioactivity and feces for 0.1%. There was no evidence of significant accumulation of radiolabeled α-cyclodextrin in the body even after 7 days of repeated IV injection. After intracavernosal administration in monkeys, radiolabeled α-cyclodextrin was rapidly distributed from the injection site, with less than 0.1% of the dose remaining in the penis 1 hour after administration. There was no evidence of tissue retention of radiolabeled α-cyclodextrin in monkeys.

Contraindications

Hypersensitivities to the drug or other prostaglandins; patients who have conditions that might predispose them to priapism, such as sickle cell anemia or trait, multiple myeloma, or leukemia; patients with anatomical deformations of the penis, such as angulation, cavernosal fibrosis, or Peyronie's disease; patients with penile implants; men for whom sexual activity is inadvisable or contraindicated.

Alprostadil is intended for use in adult men only. Alprostadil is not indicated for use in women, children, or newborns.

Warnings

➤*Priapism and prolonged erection:* Prolonged erection, defined as erection lasting greater than 4 to less than or equal to 6 hours in duration, occurred in 4% of 1,861 patients treated up to 18 months in studies of alprostadil sterile powder. The incidence of priapism (erections lasting greater than 6 hours in duration) was 0.4% with the same length of use. Pharmacologic intervention or aspiration of blood from the corpora cavernosum was performed in 2 of the 7 patients with priapism. To minimize the chances of prolonged erection or priapism, titrate alprostadil injection slowly to the lowest effective dose. Instruct the patient to immediately report to his prescribing physician, or, if unavailable, to seek immediate medical assistance for any erection that persists longer than 4 hours. If priapism is not treated immediately, penile tissue damage and permanent loss of potency may result. Treat priapism according to established medical practice.

Edex – Prolonged erections greater than 4 hours in duration occurred in 4% of all patients treated up to 24 months. The incidence of priapism (erections greater than 6 hours in duration) was less than 1% with long-term use for up to 24 months. In the majority of cases, spontaneous detumescence occurred. Pharmacologic intervention or aspiration of blood from the corpora was necessary in 1.6% of 311 patients with prolonged erections/priapism.

➤*Elderly:* Of the approximately 1,065 patients who entered the in-office dose-titration period in clinical studies, 25% were 65 and older. In clinical studies, geriatric patients required, on average, higher minimally effective doses and had higher rates of lack of effect (optimum dose not determined). Overall differences in safety were not observed between these geriatric patients and younger patients. Dose and titrate geriatric patients according to the same recommendations as younger patients, and always use the lowest possible effective dose.

This drug is known to be substantially excreted by the kidney, and the risk of toxic reactions to this drug may be greater in patients with impaired renal function. Because elderly patients are more likely to have decreased renal function, take care in dose selection, and it may be useful to monitor renal function.

➤*Pregnancy:* Alprostadil is not indicated for use in women.

➤*Lactation:* Alprostadil is not indicated for use in women.

➤*Children:* Alprostadil is not indicated for use in pediatric patients.

ALPROSTADIL — INTRACAVERNOSAL

Precautions

➤*Monitoring:* Regular follow-up of patients, with careful examination of the penis at the start of therapy and at regular intervals (eg, 3 months), is strongly recommended to detect signs of penile fibrosis. Discontinue treatment with alprostadil in patients who develop penile angulation, cavernosal fibrosis, or Peyronie's disease. Treatment can be resumed if the penile abnormality subsides.

➤*Penile fibrosis:* The overall incidence of penile fibrosis, including Peyronie's disease, reported in clinical studies with alprostadil was 3%. In 1 self-injection clinical study where duration of use was up to 18 months, the incidence of fibrosis was 7.8%.

➤*Hypotension:* Intracavernosal injections of alprostadil can lead to increased peripheral blood levels of PGE_1 and its metabolites, especially in those patients with significant corpora cavernosa venous leakage. Increased peripheral blood levels of PGE_1 and its metabolites may lead to hypotension or dizziness.

➤*Anticoagulants:* See Drug Interactions for more information.

➤*Other medical causes:* Diagnose and treat underlying treatable medical causes of erectile dysfunction prior to initiation of therapy with alprostadil.

➤*Vasoactive agents:* The safety and efficacy of combinations of alprostadil and other vasoactive agents have not been systematically studied. Therefore, the use of such combinations is not recommended.

➤*Bleeding disorder:* After injection of the alprostadil solution, compression of the injection site for 5 minutes, or until bleeding stops, is necessary. Patients on anticoagulants, such as warfarin or heparin, may have increased propensity for bleeding after intracavernosal injection.

➤*Caverject* dual-chamber system: Alprostadil dual-chamber system is designed for one use only. Following a single use, properly discard the injection device and any remaining solution.

Alprostadil dual-chamber system uses a superfine (29-gauge) needle. As with all superfine needles, the possibility of needle breakage exists. Careful instruction in proper handling and injection techniques may minimize the potential for needle breakage.

Drug Interactions

Alprostadil Drug Interactions

Precipitant drug	Object drug*		Description
Alprostadil	Anticoagulants	⬆	Patients on anticoagulants (eg, warfarin, heparin) may have increased propensity for bleeding after intracavernosal injection. Coadministration with heparin resulted in a 140% and 120% increase in PTT and TT, respectively. Use caution with coadministration.
Alprostadil	Vasoactive agents	⟷	The safety and efficacy of combinations of alprostadil and other vasoactive agents have not been systematically studied. Therefore, the use of such combinations is not recommended.

* ⬆ = Object drug increased. ⟷ = Undetermined clinical effect.

Adverse Reactions

➤*Local adverse reactions:* The following local adverse reaction information was derived from controlled and uncontrolled studies, including an uncontrolled 18-month safety study.

Local adverse reactions reported by ≥ 1% of patients treated with alprostadil injection for up to 18 months[a]

Event	Alprostadil injection (n = 1,861)
Injection site ecchymosis	2%
Injection site hematoma	3%
Penis disorder[b]	3%
Penile edema	1%
Penile fibrosis[c]	3%
Penile pain	37%
Penile rash	1%
Prolonged erection	4%

[a] Except for penile pain (2%), no significant local adverse reactions were reported by 294 patients who received 1 to 3 injections of placebo.
[b] Includes numbness, yeast infection, irritation, sensitivity, phimosis, pruritus, erythema, venous leak, penile skin tear, strange feeling of penis, discoloration of penile head, itch at tip of penis.
[c] The overall incidence of penile fibrosis, including Peyronie's disease, reported in clinical studies with alprostadil was 3%. In 1 self-injection clinical study where duration of use was up to 18 months, the incidence of fibrosis was 7.8%. Regular follow-up of patients, with careful examination of the penis, is strongly recommended to detect signs of penile fibrosis. Treatment with alprostadil should be discontinued in patients who develop penile angulation, cavernosal fibrosis, or Peyronie's disease.

➤*Penile pain:* Penile pain after intracavernosal administration of alprostadil was reported at least once by 37% of patients in clinical studies of up to 18 months in duration. In the majority of the cases, penile pain was rated mild or moderate in intensity. Three percent (3%) of patients discontinued treatment because of penile pain. The frequency of penile pain was 2% in 294 patients who received 1 to 3 injections of placebo.

➤*Prolonged erection/priapism:* In clinical trials, prolonged erection was defined as an erection that lasted for 4 to 6 hours; priapism was defined as erection that lasted 6 hours or longer. The frequency of prolonged erection after intracavernosal administration of alprostadil was 4%, while the frequency of priapism was 0.4%. In the majority of cases, spontaneous detumescence occurred.

See Warnings for more information.

➤*Hematoma/ecchymosis:* The frequency of hematoma and ecchymosis was 3% and 2%, respectively. In most cases, hematoma/ecchymosis was judged to be a complication of a faulty injection technique. Accordingly, proper instruction of the patient in self-injection is of importance to minimize the potential of hematoma/ecchymosis.

The following local adverse reactions were reported by less than 1% of patients after injection of alprostadil: Balanitis; injection site hemorrhage; injection site inflammation; injection site itching; injection site swelling; injection site edema; urethral bleeding; penile warmth; numbness; yeast infection; irritation; sensitivity; phimosis; pruritus; erythema; venous leak; painful erection; and abnormal ejaculation.

➤*Systemic adverse events:* The following systemic adverse event information was derived from controlled and uncontrolled studies, including an uncontrolled 18-month safety study.

Alprostadil Adverse Reactions (≥ 1%)[a]

Adverse reaction	Alprostadil (n = 1,861)
Cardiovascular	
Hypertension	2%
CNS	
Dizziness	1%
Headache	2%
GU	
Prostatic disorder[b]	2%
Musculoskeletal	
Back pain	1%
Respiratory	
Cough	1%
Flu syndrome	2%
Nasal congestion	1%
Sinusitis	2%
Upper respiratory tract infection	4%
Miscellaneous	
Localized pain[c]	2%
Trauma[d]	2%

[a] No significant adverse events were reported by 294 patients who received 1 to 3 injections of placebo.
[b] Prostatitis, pain, hypertrophy, enlargement.
[c] Pain in various anatomical structures other than injection site.
[d] Injuries, fractures, abrasions, lacerations, dislocations.

The following systemic events, which were reported for less than 1% of patients in clinical studies, were judged by investigators to be possibly related to use of alprostadil: Testicular pain, scrotal disorder, scrotal edema, hematuria, testicular disorder, impaired urination, urinary frequency, urinary urgency, pelvic pain, hypotension, vasodilation, peripheral vascular disorder, supraventricular extrasystoles, vasovagal reactions, hypesthesia, nongeneralized weakness, diaphoresis, rash, nonapplication site pruritus, skin neoplasm, nausea, dry mouth, increased serum creatinine, leg cramps, and mydriasis.

Hemodynamic changes, manifested as decreases in blood pressure and increases in pulse rate, were observed during clinical studies, principally at doses above 20 mcg and above 30 mcg of alprostadil, respectively, and appeared to be dose-dependent. However, these changes were usually clinically unimportant; only 3 patients discontinued the treatment because of symptomatic hypotension.

➤*Needle breakage:* During postmarketing surveillance, needle breakage requiring surgical extraction has been reported with the administration of alprostadil sterile powder. Careful instruction in proper patient handling and injection techniques may minimize the potential of needle breakage.

➤*Caverject* dual-chamber system vs sterile powder: The safety of alprostadil dual-chamber system was evaluated in a study that compared the formulation of alprostadil for injection contained in the alprostadil dual-chamber system with the formulation contained in alprostadil sterile powder. The doses used by the 87 patients in this crossover study were the same for both formulations. The number and type of events reported for alprostadil dual-chamber system were consistent between formulations in this study and in other controlled and uncontrolled studies with alprostadil sterile powder.

➤*Edex* dual-chamber cartridge: *Edex*, administered by intracavernosal injection in doses ranging from 1 to 40 mcg per injection for periods up to 24 months, has been evaluated in clinical trials for safety in over 1,065 patients with erectile dysfunction. Discontinuation of therapy due to a side effect in clinical trials was required in approximately 9% of patients treated with *Edex*, and less than 1% of patients treated with placebo.

Local – The following local adverse reactions were reported in studies including 1,065 patients treated with *Edex* for up to 2 years.

Penile pain: With use of up to 24 months, penile pain was reported at least once by 29% of patients during injection, 35% of patients during erection,

ALPROSTADIL — INTRACAVERNOSAL

and 30% of patients after erection. On a per injection basis, 15% of injections were associated with penile pain. Penile pain was judged by patients to be mild in intensity for 80% of painful injections, moderate in intensity for 16% of painful injections, and severe in intensity for 4% of painful injections. The frequency of penile pain reports decreased over time; 41% of the patients experienced pain during the first 2 months and 3% of the patients experienced pain during months 21 to 24. In placebo-controlled studies, penile pain was reported by 31% of patients after *Edex* and by 9% of patients after placebo injection.

Prolonged erection/priapism: Prolonged erections greater than 4 hours in duration occurred in 4% of all patients treated up to 24 months. In placebo-controlled studies, 3% of patients treated with *Edex* and less than 1% of patients treated with placebo reported prolonged erections greater than 4 hours. The incidence of priapism (erections greater than 6 hours in duration) was less than 1% with long-term use for up to 24 months. In the majority of cases, spontaneous detumescence occurred. A higher incidence of prolonged erections was found in younger patients (less than 40 years), nondiabetic patients, and patients treated with psychogenic etiology of erectile dysfunction.

Hematoma/ecchymosis: In patients treated with *Edex* for up to 24 months, local bleeding, hematoma, and ecchymosis were observed in 15%, 5%, and 4% of patients, respectively. In placebo-controlled studies, the frequency of local bleeding was 6% with injection of *Edex* and 3% with injection of placebo. In most cases, these reactions were attributed to faulty injection technique.

Alprostadil Local Adverse Reactions (≥ 1%)[a]

Local reaction	*Edex* (n = 1,065) n (%)
Penile pain after erection	317 (30%)
Penile pain during injection	305 (29%)
Penile pain during erection	368 (35%)
Penile pain (other)[b]	116 (11%)
Prolonged erection	
> 4 to ≤ 6 hours	44 (4%)
> 6 hours	6 (< 1%)
Bleeding	158 (15%)
Cavernous body fibrosis	20 (2%)
Ecchymosis	44 (4%)
Erythema	17 (2%)
Faulty injection technique[c]	59 (6%)
Hematoma	56 (5%)
Penile angulation	72 (7%)
Penis disorder	28 (3%)
Penile fibrosis	52 (5%)
Peyronie's disease	11 (1%)

[a] Protocol numbers KU-620-001, KU-620-002, KU-620-003, F-8653.
[b] Penile pain reported without an association to injection site or erection, such as pain in penis and scrotum, pain in glans penis, and burning penile pain.
[c] Examples include injection into glans penis, urethra, or subcutaneously.

Hemodynamic changes – Hemodynamic changes, manifested as increases or decreases in blood pressure and pulse rate, were observed during clinical studies but did not appear to be dose dependent. Four patients (less than 1%) reported clinical symptoms of hypotension such as dizziness or syncope.

***Edex* Adverse Reactions (≥ 1%)**

Adverse reaction	*Edex* (n = 1,065)
Cardiovascular	
Abnormal ECG	12 (1%)
Hypertension	17 (2%)
Myocardial infarction	13 (1%)
Dermatologic	
Skin disorder	14 (1%)
GU	
Inguinal hernia	11 (1%)
Prostate disorder	15 (1%)
Testicular pain	13 (1%)
Metabolic/nutritional	
Hypercholesterolemia	12 (1%)
Hyperglycemia	12 (1%)
Hypertriglyceridemia	17 (2%)
Musculoskeletal	
Back pain	23 (2%)
Leg pain	13 (1%)
Respiratory	
Sinusitis	14 (1%)
Upper respiratory tract infection	58 (5%)
Special senses	
Abnormal vision	11 (1%)
Miscellaneous	
Headache	20 (2%)
Infection	18 (2%)
Influenza-like symptoms	35 (3%)
Pain	16 (2%)

Overdosage

➤*Edex*: Limited data are available in regard to *Edex* overdose in humans. Systemic reactions are uncommon with intracavernosal injection of *Edex*. Hypotension occurred in less than 1% of patients treated with *Edex*.

A single dose rising tolerance study in healthy volunteers indicated that single IV doses of alprostadil from 1 to 120 mcg were well tolerated. Beginning with a 40 mcg bolus IV dose, the frequency of drug-related systemic adverse events increased in a dose-dependent manner, characterized mainly by facial flushing.

➤*Symptoms:* The primary symptom of an overdose is a prolonged erection or priapism.

➤*Treatment:* Because of the potential for tissue hypoxia and possible necrosis, it is strongly recommended to treat an erection lasting more than 6 hours. The patient is strongly encouraged to go to the nearest emergency room if his personal physician is not available.

Overdosage was not observed in clinical trials with alprostadil. If intracavernous overdose of alprostadil occurs, the patient should be under medical supervision until any systemic effects have resolved or until penile detumescence has occurred. Symptomatic treatment of any systemic symptoms would be appropriate.

Patient Information

To ensure safe and effective use of alprostadil, thoroughly instruct and train the patient in the self-injection technique before he begins intracavernosal treatment with alprostadil at home. Establish the desirable dose in the physician's office.

Instruct the patient not to reuse or to share needles, syringes, or cartridges. As with all prescription medicines, the patient should not allow anyone else to use his medicine.

The dose of alprostadil that is established in the physician's office should not be changed by the patient without consulting the physician. The patient may expect an erection to occur within 5 to 20 minutes. A standard treatment goal is to produce an erection lasting no longer than 1 hour. Generally, do not use alprostadil more than 3 times per week, with at least 24 hours between each use.

Patients should be aware of possible side effects of therapy with alprostadil; the most frequently occurring is penile pain after injection, usually mild to moderate in severity. A potentially serious adverse reaction with intracavernosal therapy is priapism. Accordingly, instruct the patient to contact the physician's office immediately or, if unavailable, to seek immediate medical assistance if an erection persists for longer than 4 hours.

The patient should report any penile pain that was not present before or that increased in intensity, as well as the occurrence of nodules or hard tissue in the penis to his physician as soon as possible. As with any intravenous injection, an infection is a possibility. Instruct patients to report to the physician any penile redness, swelling, tenderness, or curvature of the erect penis. The patient must visit the physician's office for regular checkups for assessment of the therapeutic benefit and safety of treatment with alprostadil.

Individuals who are sexually active should be counseled about the protective measures that are necessary to guard against the spread of sexually transmitted diseases, including the human immunodeficiency virus (HIV). Use of intracavernosal alprostadil offers no protection from the transmission of sexually transmitted or bloodborne diseases. The injection of alprostadil can induce a small amount of bleeding at the site of injection. In patients infected with bloodborne diseases, this could increase the risk of transmission of bloodborne diseases between partners.

➤*Aqueous solution:* Instruct the patient to transfer the solution from the pharmacy to his home freezer or refrigerator as soon as possible. Brief (2 hours or less) exposure to conditions as warm as 25°C (77°F) will not harm the product.

Discard any ampule containing sterile solution with precipitates or discoloration. The ampule is designed for 1 use only and should be discarded after withdrawal of proper volume of the solution. Properly discard needles after use; do not reuse or share with other persons. Patient instructions for administration are included in each package of alprostadil.

➤*Caverject* sterile powder: Carefully follow the instructions for preparation of the solution of alprostadil sterile powder for intracavernosal injection. Discard vials with precipitates or discoloration. The reconstituted vial is designed for 1 use only and should be discarded after withdrawal of proper volume of the solution. Do not shake the content of the reconstituted vial. Properly discard the needle after use; do not reuse or share with other persons. Patient instructions for administration are included in each package of alprostadil sterile powder.

➤*Caverject* dual-chamber system: Discard any reconstituted solution with precipitates or discoloration. The alprostadil dual-chamber syringe system is designed for 1 use only and should be discarded after use. Properly discard the device and the needle after use.

➤*Edex* dual-chamber cartridge: Carefully follow the instructions for the preparation of the *Edex* solution. The reconstituted solution may initially appear cloudy due to small air bubbles. Do not use the solution if it remains cloudy, contains precipitates, or is discolored. Gently mix the reconstituted solution. Do not shake it. A patient information pamphlet is included in each package of *Edex* kits and cartridges.

Use *Edex* immediately after reconstitution. The patient should follow the instructions in the patient information pamphlet to limit the possibility of bacterial contamination. The reconstituted cartridge is designed for 1 use only and should be discarded after use.

The *Edex* cartridge contains a solid layer or lyophilized of dry white powder approximately 3/16" in thickness for the vial and 3/8" in thickness for the

ALPROSTADIL — INTRACAVERNOSAL

cartridge. A normal cake may appear cracked or crumbled. If the vial or cartridge is damaged, the cake may shrink in size. Do not use the vial or cartridge if they appear damaged or if the cake is substantially reduced in size.

If the dosage prescribed is less than 1 mL of *Edex* solution, excess solution will be expelled through the needle as the plunger is pushed and the upper rim of the top stopper reaches the correct volume mark for the prescribed dose. Properly discard the needle after use; do not reuse or share with other persons.

The dose of *Edex* that is established in the physician's office should not be changed by the patient without consulting the physician. The patient may expect an erection to occur within 5 to 20 minutes. A standard treatment goal is to produce an erection lasting no longer than 1 hour. Do not use *Edex* more than 3 times per week, with at least 24 hours between each use.

➤*Note:* Use of intracavernosal alprostadil offers no protection from the transmission of sexually transmitted diseases. Counsel individuals who use alprostadil about the protective measures that are necessary to guard against the spread of sexually transmitted diseases, including the human immunodeficiency virus (HIV).

The injection of alprostadil can induce a small amount of bleeding at the site of injection. In patients infected with bloodborne diseases, this could increase the risk of transmission of bloodborne diseases between partners.

ALPROSTADIL — UROGENITAL

For information on the use of alprostadil for patent ductus arteriosus, refer to the specific monograph in the Cardiovasculars chapter.

Indications

➤*Erectile dysfunction:* For the treatment of erectile dysfunction. Studies that established benefit demonstrated improvements in success rates for sexual intercourse compared with similarly administered placebo.

Administration and Dosage

➤*Approved by the FDA:* November 19, 1996.

Alprostadil urethral suppository is a transurethral delivery system available in 4 dosage strengths: 125 mcg, 250 mcg, 500 mcg, and 1000 mcg. Alprostadil urethral suppository should be administered as needed to achieve an erection. The onset of effect is within 5 to 10 minutes after administration. The duration of effect is approximately 30 to 60 minutes. However, the actual duration will vary from patient to patient. Each patient should be instructed by a medical professional on proper technique for administering alprostadil urethral suppository prior to self-administration. The maximum frequency of use is no more than 2 systems per 24-hour period.

➤*Initiation of therapy:* Dose titration should be undertaken under the supervision of a physician to test a patient's responsiveness to alprostadil urethral suppository, to demonstrate proper administration technique (see detailed instructions for alprostadil urethral suppository administration in patient package insert), and to monitor for evidence of hypotension. Patients should be individually titrated to the lowest dose that is sufficient for sexual intercourse. The lower doses of alprostadil urethral suppository (125 mcg or 250 mcg) are recommended for initial dosing. If necessary, the dose should be increased (or decreased) on separate occasions in a step wise manner until the patient achieves an erection that is sufficient for sexual intercourse.

➤*Home treatment regimen:* Alprostadil urethral suppository should be used as needed to achieve an erection. The maximum frequency of use is 2 administrations per 24-hour period. Each alprostadil urethral suppository is for single use only and should be properly discarded after use.

➤*Storage / Stability:* Store unopened foil pouches in a refrigerator at 2° to 8°C (36° to 46°F). Do not expose alprostadil urethral suppository to temperatures above 30°C (86°F). Alprostadil urethral suppository may be kept at room temperature (below 30°C or 86°F) for up to 14 days prior to use.

Actions

➤*Pharmacology:* Prostaglandin E1 is a naturally occurring acidic lipid that is synthesized from fatty acid precursors by most mammalian tissues and has a variety of pharmacologic effects. Human seminal fluid is a rich source of prostaglandins, including PGE_1 and PGE_2, and the total concentration of prostaglandins in ejaculate has been estimated to be approximately 100 to 200 mcg/mL. In vitro, alprostadil (PGE_1) has been shown to cause dose-dependent smooth muscle relaxation in isolated corpus cavernosum and corpus spongiosum preparations. Additionally, vasodilation has been demonstrated in isolated cavernosal artery segments that were precontracted with either norepinephrine or prostaglandin $F_{2}\alpha$. When alprostadil was injected into the corpus cavernosum of pigtail monkeys in vivo, dose-dependent increases in cavernosal artery blood flow were observed.

In human studies using Doppler duplex ultrasonography, intraurethral administration of 500 mcg of alprostadil resulted in an increase in cavernosal artery diameter and a 5- to 10-fold increase in peak systolic flow velocities. These results suggest that intraurethral alprostadil is absorbed from the urethra, transported throughout the erectile bodies by communicating vessels between the corpus spongiosum and corpora cavernosa, and able to induce vasodilation of the targeted vascular beds.

The vasodilatory effects of alprostadil on the cavernosal arteries and the trabecular smooth muscle of the corpora cavernosa result in rapid arterial inflow and expansion of the lacunar spaces within the corpora. As the expanded corporal sinusoids are compressed against the tunica albuginea, venous outflow through subtunical vessels is impeded and penile rigidity develops. This process is referred to as the corporal veno-occlusive mechanism.

The most notable systemic effects of alprostadil are vasodilation, inhibition of platelet aggregation, and stimulation of intestinal and uterine smooth muscle. Intravenous doses of 1 to 10 mcg/kg of body weight lower blood pressure in mammals by decreasing peripheral resistance. Reflex increases in cardiac output and heart rate may accompany these effects.

➤*Pharmacokinetics:*

Absorption – About 80% of alprostadil administered by alprostadil urethral suppository is absorbed within 10 minutes and is rapidly cleared from the systemic circulation by the lungs, leaving barely detectable systemic blood levels.

Alprostadil urethral suppository is designed to deliver alprostadil directly to the urethral lining for transfer via the corpus spongiosum to the corpora cavernosa. Intraurethral administration of alprostadil urethral suppository is preceded by urination, and the residual urine disperses the medicated pellet, permitting alprostadil to be absorbed by the urethral mucosa. The transurethral absorption of alprostadil after alprostadil urethral suppository administration is biphasic. Initial absorption is rapid, with approximately 80% of an administered dose absorbed within 10 minutes. The mean time to the maximum plasma PGE_1 concentration after a 1000 mcg intraurethral dose of alprostadil urethral suppository is approximately 16 minutes.

In 10 healthy human volunteers, endogenous PGE_1 levels in the ejaculate averaged 31 mcg (range 0 to 161 mcg). In these same volunteers, an average of 123 mcg of additional PGE_1 (range 30 to 369 mcg) was present in the ejaculate obtained 10 minutes after the highest dose (1000 mcg) of alprostadil urethral suppository. The mean total endogenous PGE content (PGE_1, PGE_2, 19-OH-PGE_1, and 19-OH-PGE_2) of the ejaculate in these subjects was 444 mcg (range 0 to 1423 mcg).

Distribution – Following alprostadil urethral suppository administration, alprostadil is absorbed from the urethral mucosa into the corpus spongiosum. A portion of the administered dose is transported to the corpora cavernosa through collateral vessels, while the remainder passes into the pelvic venous circulation through veins draining the corpus spongiosum. The half-life of alprostadil in humans is short, varying between 30 seconds and 10 minutes, depending on the body compartment in which it is measured and the physiological status of the subject. Nearly all of the alprostadil entering the central venous circulation is removed in a single pass through the lungs; thus peripheral venous plasma levels of PGE_1 are low or undetectable (less than 2 pg/mL) after alprostadil urethral suppository administration. The mean maximum plasma PGE_1 concentration following intraurethral administration of the highest dose of alprostadil urethral suppository (1000 mcg) was barely detectable (11.4 pg/mL). In a study of 14 subjects, the plasma PGE_1 level was shown to be undetachable within 60 minutes of alprostadil urethral suppository administration in most subjects.

Metabolism – Alprostadil is rapidly metabolized locally by enzymatic oxidation of the 15-hydroxyl group to 15-keto-PGE_1. The enzyme catalyzing this process has been isolated from many tissues in the lower genito-urinary tract including the urethra, prostate, and corpus cavernosum. 15-keto-PGE_1 retains little (1% to 2%) of the biological activity of PGE_1. 15-keto-PGE_1 is rapidly reduced at the C_{13}-C_{14} position to form the most abundant metabolite in plasma, 13,14-dihydro,15-keto PGE_1 (DHK-PGE_1), which is biologically inactive. The majority of DHK-PGE_1 is further metabolized to smaller prostaglandin remnants that are cleared primarily by the kidney and liver. Between 60% and 90% of PGE_1 has been shown to be metabolized after 1 pass through the pulmonary capillary beds.

Excretion – After intravenous administration of tritium-labeled alprostadil in man, labeled drug disappears rapidly from the blood in the first 10 minutes, and by 1 hour radioactivity in the blood reaches a low level. The metabolites of alprostadil are excreted primarily by the kidney, with approximately 90% of an administered intravenous dose excreted in the urine within 24 hours of dosing. The remainder is excreted in the feces. There is no evidence of tissue retention of alprostadil or its metabolites following intravenous administration.

Special populations –

Pulmonary disease: The near-complete pulmonary first-pass metabolism of PGE_1 is the primary factor influencing the systemic pharmacokinetics of alprostadil urethral suppository and is a reason that peripheral venous plasma levels of PGE_1 are low or undetectable (less than 2 pg/mL) following alprostadil urethral suppository administration.

Patients with pulmonary disease therefore may have a reduced capacity to clear the drug. In patients with the adult respiratory distress syndrome (ARDS), pulmonary extraction of intravascularly administered alprostadil was reduced by approximately 15% compared to a control group of patients with normal respiratory function (66 ± 3.2% vs 78 ± 2.4%).

Contraindications

Hypersensitivity to alprostadil; in patients with urethral stricture, balanitis (inflammation/infection of the glans of the penis), severe hypospadias and curvature, and in patients with acute or chronic urethritis; in patients who are prone to venous thrombosis or who have a hyperviscosity syndrome and are therefore at increased risk of priapism (rigid erection lasting 6 or more hours). Alprostadil urethral suppository should not be used in men for whom sexual activity is inadvisable (see General Precautions) or for sexual intercourse with a pregnant woman unless the couple uses a condom barrier.

Warnings

➤*Hypotension / Syncope:* Because of the potential for symptomatic hypotension and syncope, which occurred in 3% and 0.4%, respectively, of patients during in-clinic dosing, alprostadil urethral suppository titration should be carried out under medical supervision. During post-marketing surveillance syncope occurring within one hour of administration has been reported. Patients should be cautioned to avoid activities, such as driving or hazardous tasks, where injury could result if hypotension or syncope were to occur after alprostadil urethral suppository administration.

ALPROSTADIL — UROGENITAL

➤*Mutagenesis:* Alprostadil concentrations increased chromosomal aberrations above control incidence in the in vitro Chinese hamster ovary chromosomal aberration assay.

➤*Pregnancy: Category C.* Alprostadil has been shown to be embryo toxic (decreased fetal weight) when administered as a subcutaneous bolus to pregnant rats at doses as low as 500 mcg/kg/day. Doses of 2000 mcg/kg/day resulted in increased resorptions, reduced numbers of live fetuses, increased incidences of visceral and skeletal variations (primarily left umbilical artery and generalized reduction in ossification of the entire skeleton) and gross visceral and skeletal malformations (primarily edema, hydrocephaly, anophthalmia/microphthalmia, and skeletal anomalies). The latter dose produced maternal toxicity (ataxia, lethargy, diarrhea, and retarded body weight gain). When administered by continuous intravenous infusion, evidence of embryotoxicity (decreased fetal weight gain and increased incidence of hydroureter) was observed at 2000 mcg/kg/day, a dose that was also associated with a decrease in maternal weight gain. Intravaginal administration of up to 4000 mcg/day of alprostadil to pregnant rabbits (1100 mcg/kg/day or about 12.5 times the maximum recommended daily dose adjusted for body surface area) resulted in no evidence of harm to the fetus. Alprostadil urethral suppository should not be used for sexual intercourse with a pregnant woman unless the couple uses a condom barrier.

➤*Lactation:* Not indicated for use in newborns, children, or women.

➤*Children:* Not indicated for use in newborns or children.

Precautions

➤*Medical history/physical exam:* A complete medical history and physical examination should be undertaken to exclude reversible causes of erectile dysfunction prior to the initiation of alprostadil urethral suppository therapy. In addition, underlying disorders that might preclude the use of alprostadil urethral suppository (see Contraindications) should be sought.

➤*Cardiovascular effects:* During in-clinic dosing, patients should be monitored for symptoms of hypotension, and the lowest effective dose of alprostadil urethral suppository should be prescribed.

➤*Hematologic effects:* Patients administering alprostadil urethral suppository improperly may be at risk of urethral abrasion resulting in minor bleeding or spotting. Patients on anticoagulant therapy or with bleeding disorders may be at higher risk of bleeding. Patients on anticoagulant therapy have been safely treated with alprostadil urethral suppository; however, the risk/benefit ratio in these patients should be considered prior to prescribing alprostadil urethral suppository.

➤*Resumption of sexual activity:* Sexual intercourse is considered a vigorous physical activity, and it increases heart rate as well as cardiac work. Physicians may want to examine the cardiac fitness of patients prior to treating erectile dysfunction.

➤*Priapism and prolonged erection:* In clinical trials of alprostadil urethral suppository, priapism (rigid erection lasting more than 6 hours) and prolonged erection (rigid erection between 4 and 6 hours) were reported infrequently (less than 0.1% and 0.3% of patients, respectively). Nevertheless, these events are a potential risk of pharmacologic therapy and can cause penile injury. Physicians should lower the dose or consider discontinuing alprostadil urethral suppository treatment in any patient who develops priapism or prolonged erection.

Drug Interactions

Because there are low or undetectable (less than 2 pg/mL) amounts of alprostadil found in the peripheral venous circulation following alprostadil urethral suppository administration, systemic drug-drug interactions with alprostadil urethral suppository are unlikely. The presence of medications in the circulation that attenuate erectile function, however, may influence the response to alprostadil urethral suppository.

Adverse Reactions

➤*In-clinic titration:* In the 2 largest double-blind, parallel, placebo-controlled trials, 1511 patients received alprostadil urethral suppository at least 1 time in the clinic setting. The most frequently reported drug-related side effects during in-clinic titration included pain in the penis (36%), urethra (13%), or testes (5%). These discomforts were most commonly reported as mild and transient, but about 7% of patients withdrew at this stage because of adverse events. Urethral bleeding/spotting and other minor abrasions to the urethra were reported in approximately 3% of patients. Symptomatic lowering of blood pressure (hypotension) occurred in 3% of patients. Dizziness was reported in 4% of patients. Syncope (fainting) was reported by 0.4% of patients.

➤*Home treatment:* Nine hundred ninety-six patients (66% of those who began titration) were studied during the home treatment portion of 2 phase III placebo-controlled studies. Fewer than 2% of patients discontinued from these studies primarily because of adverse events. The following information summarizes the frequency of adverse events reported by patients using alprostadil urethral suppository or placebo.

Alprostadil Adverse Reactions (≥ 2%)

Adverse reaction	Alprostadil urethral suppository (n = 486)	Placebo (n = 511)
GU		
Penile pain	32%	3%
Urethral burning	12%	4%
Minor urethral bleeding/spotting	5%	1%
Testicular pain	5%	1%
CNS		
Dizziness	2%	< 1%
Miscellaneous		
Flu symptoms	4%	2%
Headache	3%	2%
Pain	3%	1%
Accidental injury	3%	2%
Back pain	2%	1%
Pelvic pain	2%	< 1%
Respiratory		
Rhinitis	2%	< 1%
Infection	3%	2%

➤*Female partner adverse events:* The most common drug-related adverse event reported by female partners during placebo-controlled clinical studies was vaginal burning/itching, reported by 5.8% of partners of patients on active vs 0.8% of partners of patients on placebo. It is unknown whether this adverse event experienced by female partners was a result of the medication or a result of resuming sexual intercourse, which occurred much more frequently in partners of patients on active medication.

Overdosage

Overdosage has not been reported with alprostadil urethral suppository. Overdosage with alprostadil urethral suppository may result in hypotension, persistent penile pain, and possibly priapism (rigid erection lasting greater than or equal to 6 hours). Priapism can result in permanent worsening of erectile function. Patients suspected of overdosage who develop these symptoms should be kept under medical supervision until systemic or local symptoms have resolved.

Patient Information

Patients should be informed that alprostadil urethral suppository offers no protection from the transmission of sexually transmitted diseases. Patients and partners who use alprostadil urethral suppository need to be counseled about the protective measures that are necessary to guard against the spread of sexually transmitted agents, including the human immunodeficiency virus (HIV).

Although unreported in clinical trials, there is the possibility that an overdosage of alprostadil urethral suppository can cause priapism, a painful erection of the penis sustained for hours and unrelieved by sexual intercourse or masturbation. This condition is serious and, if untreated, it can lead to permanent inability to have an erection. Patients who experience a prolonged erection should seek prompt medical attention.

Patients should be instructed how to administer alprostadil urethral suppository. A patient package insert must be given to each patient at the initiation of alprostadil urethral suppository therapy.

➤*Information for partners:* Partners of patients using alprostadil urethral suppository should be informed that alprostadil urethral suppository offers no protection from the transmission of sexually transmitted diseases. Patients and partners who use alprostadil urethral suppository should be counseled about the protective measures that are necessary to guard against the spread of sexually transmitted agents, including the human immunodeficiency virus (HIV). Human semen contains PGE_1, but additional amounts may be present from alprostadil urethral suppository administration (see Pharmacokinetics). Partners who have experienced an extended period of sexual abstinence should be encouraged to seek advice from a healthcare professional prior to resuming sexual intercourse. The use of a water-based lubricant may facilitate vaginal penetration.

It is recommended that couples using alprostadil urethral suppository employ adequate contraception if the female partner is of childbearing potential. There is no information on the effects on early pregnancy of PGE_1 at the levels received by female partners. Alprostadil urethral suppository has no contraceptive properties. Alprostadil urethral suppository should not be used if the female partner is pregnant, unless the couple uses a condom barrier.

YOHIMBINE HYDROCHLORIDE

Rx	**Yohimbine HCl** (Various, eg, Eon)	**Tablets:** 5.4 mg	May contain lactose. In 100s, 500s, and 1000s.
Rx	**Aphrodyne** (Star)		(APHRODYNE). Aqua, scored. In 100s and 1000s.
Rx	**Yocon** (Glenwood)		In 100s and 1000s.

YOHIMBINE HYDROCHLORIDE — ORAL

Indications

Yohimbine has no FDA sanctioned indications.

➤*Unlabeled uses:* Sympatholytic and mydriatic. It may have activity as an aphrodisiac.

Impotence – Impotence has been successfully treated with yohimbine in male patients with vascular or diabetic origins and psychogenic origins (18 mg/day).

Orthostatic hypotension – Orthostatic hypotension may be favorably affected by yohimbine.

Administration and Dosage

➤*Male erectile impotence:* Experimental dosage has been 1 tablet (5.4 mg) 3 times/day. Occasional side effects reported with this dosage are nausea, dizziness, or nervousness. If side effects occur, reduce to one-half tablet 3 times/day, followed by gradual increases to 1 tablet 3 times/day. Results of therapy greater than 10 weeks are not known.

Store at controlled room temperature 15° to 30° C (59° to 86° F).

Actions

➤*Pharmacology:* Yohimbine, an indolalkylamine alkaloid, has chemical similarity to reserpine. It is the principal alkaloid of the bark of the *Corynanthe yohimbi* tree and also is found in *Rauwolfia serpentina* (L) Benth.

Yohimbine blocks presynaptic α_2-adrenergic receptors. Its peripheral autonomic nervous system effect is to increase parasympathetic (cholinergic) and decrease sympathetic (adrenergic) activity. In male sexual performance, erection is linked to cholinergic activity and α_2-adrenergic blockade, which theoretically results in increased penile blood inflow, decreased outflow, or both. Yohimbine exerts a stimulating action on mood and may increase anxiety. Such actions appear to require high doses. Yohimbine has a mild antidiuretic action, probably via stimulation of hypothalmic centers and release of posterior pituitary hormone.

Its action on peripheral blood vessels resembles that of reserpine, though it is weaker and of shorter duration. The drug reportedly exerts no significant influence on cardiac stimulation.

➤*Pharmacokinetics:*

Absorption/Distribution – Oral absorption appears to be extremely rapid, with a mean T_{max} of less than 1 hour. The low bioavailability of approximately 30% is thought to be caused by first-pass metabolism rather than poor absorption. The mean distribution half-life is less than 30 minutes, and the mean apparent volume of distribution ranged from 24.6 to 226 L. Approximately 82% of yohimbine is bound to plasma proteins.

Metabolism/Excretion – Yohimbine undergoes extensive first-pass metabolism that results in poor but highly variable bioavailability. It also undergoes extensive biotransformation in the liver and extrahepatic sites, and at least 2 hydroxylated metabolites have been identified. After single-dose administration, the terminal half-life of yohimbine is 0.25 to 2.5 hours. The active metabolite (11-hydroxy-yohimbine) has a longer elimination half-life of 6 hours. Less than 1% of the yohimbine dose is recovered in the urine as unchanged drug.

Contraindications

Renal disease; hypersensitivity to any component.

Warnings

➤*Special risk patients:* Not for use in geriatric, psychiatric, or cardiorenal patients with a history of gastric or duodenal ulcer. Generally, not for use in females.

➤*Pregnancy:* Do not use during pregnancy.

➤*Children:* Do not use in children.

Drug Interactions

➤*Antidepressants:* Do not use with yohimbine.

Adverse Reactions

Yohimbine readily penetrates the CNS and produces a complex pattern of responses in lower doses than those required to produce peripheral α-adrenergic blockade. These include antidiuresis and central excitation including elevated blood pressure and heart rate, increased motor activity, nervousness, irritability, and tremor. Dizziness, nausea, headache, and skin flushing have been reported.

Overdosage

Yohimbine may be toxic if ingested in high doses. The drug causes severe hypotension, abdominal distress, and weakness. Larger doses may cause CNS stimulation and paralysis.

Phosphodiesterase Type 5 Inhibitors

Indications

➤*Erectile dysfunction (except Revatio)*: For the treatment of erectile dysfunction.

➤*Pulmonary arterial hypertension (Revatio only)*: For the treatment of pulmonary arterial hypertension (World Health Organization [WHO] Group I) to improve exercise ability.

➤*Unlabeled uses:* The use of **sildenafil** in women with sexual dysfunction has been evaluated in small clinical trials. The results are mixed, with many studies unable to demonstrate efficacy.

Actions

➤*Pharmacology:* **Sildenafil**, **tadalafil**, and **vardenafil** are selective inhibitors of phosphodiesterase type 5 (PDE5). The physiologic mechanism of penile erection involves release of nitric oxide (NO) in the corpus cavernosum during sexual stimulation. NO activates the enzyme guanylate cyclase, resulting in increased synthesis of cyclic guanosine monophosphate (cGMP) in the smooth muscle cells of the corpus cavernosum. The cGMP, in turn, triggers smooth muscle relaxation, allowing increased blood flow into the penis, resulting in erection. Sildenafil, tadalafil, and vardenafil enhance the effects of NO by inhibiting PDE5 that is responsible for the degradation of cGMP in the smooth muscle cells of the corpus cavernosum. Because sexual stimulation is required to initiate the local release of NO, the inhibition of PDE5 by sildenafil, tadalafil, or vardenafil has no effect in the absence of sexual stimulation.

PDE5 also is found in lower concentrations in other tissues, including platelets, vascular and visceral smooth muscle, and skeletal muscle. In these tissues, inhibition of PDE5 may be the basis for the enhanced platelet antiaggregatory activity of NO, inhibition of platelet thrombus formation, and peripheral arterial-venous dilation.

Sildenafil – Sildenafil is also an inhibitor of cGMP PDE5 in the smooth muscle of the pulmonary vasculature, where PDE5 is responsible for degradation of cGMP. Sildenafil, therefore, increases cGMP within pulmonary vascular smooth muscle cells, resulting in relaxation. In patients with pulmonary hypertension, this can lead to vasodilation of the pulmonary vascular bed, and, to a lesser degree, vasodilation in the systemic circulation.

Sildenafil is more potent on PDE5 than on other known phosphodiesterases (more than 10-fold for PDE6, more than 80-fold for PDE1, more than 700-fold for PDE2, PDE3, PDE4, PDE7, PDE8, PDE9, PDE10, and PDE11). The approximate 4,000-fold selectivity for PDE5 versus PDE3 is important because PDE3 is involved in the control of cardiac contractility. Sildenafil is only about 10-fold as potent for PDE5 compared with PDE6, an enzyme found in the retina. This lower selectivity is thought to be the basis for abnormalities related to color vision observed with higher doses or plasma levels.

Tadalafil – In vitro studies have shown that the effect of tadalafil is more potent on PDE5 than on other phosphodiesterases. These studies have shown that tadalafil is more than 10,000-fold more potent for PDE5 than for PDE1, PDE2, PDE4, and PDE7 enzymes, which are found in the heart, brain, blood vessels, liver, leukocytes, skeletal muscle, and other organs. Tadalafil is more than 10,000-fold more potent for PDE5 than for PDE3, an enzyme found in the heart and blood vessels. Additionally, tadalafil is 700-fold more potent for PDE5 than for PDE6, which is found in the retina and is responsible for phototransduction. Tadalafil is more than 9,000-fold more potent for PDE5 than for PDE8, PDE9, PDE10, and 14-fold more potent for PDE5 than for PDE11A1, an enzyme found in human skeletal muscle. Tadalafil inhibits human recombinant PDE11A1 activity at concentrations within the therapeutic range. The physiological role and clinical consequence of PDE11 inhibition in humans have not been defined.

Vardenafil – The inhibitory effect of vardenafil is more selective on PDE5 than for other known phosphodiesterases (more than 15-fold relative to PDE6, more than 130-fold relative to PDE1, more than 300-fold relative to PDE11, and more than 1,000-fold relative to PDE2, PDE3, PDE4, PDE7, PDE8, PDE9, and PDE10).

Effects on blood pressure (BP) –

Sildenafil: Single oral doses of sildenafil 100 mg produced a mean maximum decrease of 8.4/5.5 mm Hg in healthy volunteers. The decrease in BP was most notable approximately 1 to 2 hours after dosing and was not different than placebo at 8 hours. Similar effects on BP were noted with sildenafil 25, 50, and 100 mg. Larger effects were recorded among patients receiving concomitant nitrates.

Vardenafil: In a clinical pharmacology study of patients with erectile dysfunction, single doses of vardenafil 20 mg caused a mean maximum decrease in supine BP of 7 mm Hg systolic and 8 mm Hg diastolic (compared with placebo), accompanied by a mean maximum increase in heart rate of 4 beats/minute. The maximum decrease in BP occurred between 1 and 4 hours after dosing. Following multiple dosing for 31 days, similar BP responses were observed on day 31 as on day 1.

➤*Pharmacokinetics:*

Absorption/Distribution –

Phosphodiesterase Type 5 Inhibitor Pharmacokinetics

Parameters	Sildenafil	Tadalafil	Vardenafil
Bioavailability	≈ 40%	Not determined	≈ 15%
T_{max}	0.5 to 2 h (median, 1 h)[a]	0.5 to 6 h (median, 2 h)[b]	0.5 to 2 h (median, 1 h)[c]
Effect of food (high-fat meal)	C_{max} reduced 29% T_{max} increased 1 h	No effect	C_{max} reduced 18% to 50%
Onset of action	≈ 30 min	≈ 30 min	≈ 20 min[d]
Maximum effect	no data	no data	45 to 90 min[d]
Duration of action	≥ 4 h	36 h	< 5 h
Volume of distribution[e]	105 L	≈ 63 L	208 L

Phosphodiesterase Type 5 Inhibitor Pharmacokinetics			
Parameters	Sildenafil	Tadalafil	Vardenafil
Protein binding[f]	≈ 96%	94%	≈ 95%
Metabolism	CYP3A4 (major) CYP2C9 (minor)	CYP3A4	CYP3A4 (major) CYP3A5, CYP2C isoforms (minor)
Active metabolite	Yes[g]	No	Yes[h]
Terminal half-life	≈ 4 h	17.5 h	4 to 5 h
Excretion	Feces (≈ 80%) Urine (≈ 13%)	Feces (≈ 61%) Urine (≈ 36%)	Feces (≈ 91% to 95%) Urine (≈ 2% to 6%)
Clearance	no data	2.5 L/h	56 L/h

[a] Oral dosing in the fasted state.
[b] Single oral dose.
[c] Single oral dose of 20 mg; fasted state.
[d] Based on animal studies.
[e] At steady state.
[f] For parent drug and major circulating metabolite.
[g] Accounts for approximately 20% of sildenafil's pharmacologic activity.
[h] Accounts for approximately 7% of vardenafil's pharmacologic activity.

Sildenafil and **vardenafil** are rapidly absorbed. The pharmacokinetics of sildenafil and vardenafil are dose-proportional over the recommended dose range. Protein binding for both drugs is independent of total drug concentrations.

Based on measurements of sildenafil in semen of healthy volunteers 90 minutes after dosing, less than 0.001% of the administered dose may appear in the semen of patients. Following a single vardenafil 20 mg oral dose in healthy volunteers, a mean of 0.00018% of the administered dose was obtained in semen 90 minutes after dosing. Less than 0.0005% of the administered **tadalafil** dose appeared in the semen of healthy subjects.

Metabolism/Excretion – **Sildenafil**, **tadalafil**, and **vardenafil** are cleared predominantly by the CYP3A4 (major route), 3A5 (minor route; vardenafil), and CYP2C9 (minor route; sildenafil and vardenafil) hepatic microsomal isoenzymes. Sildenafil is converted into an active metabolite by N-desmethylation and is further metabolized. This metabolite has a PDE selectivity profile similar to sildenafil and an in vitro potency for PDE5 approximately 50% of the parent drug. Plasma concentrations of this metabolite are approximately 40% of those seen for sildenafil, so that the metabolite accounts for approximately 20% of sildenafil's pharmacologic effects. However, in patients with pulmonary arterial hypertension, the ratio of the metabolite to sildenafil is higher. Both sildenafil and the metabolite have terminal half-lives of approximately 4 hours. The major circulating metabolite of vardenafil, M1, results from desethylation at the piperazine moiety of vardenafil. M1 is subject to further metabolism. The plasma concentration of M1 is approximately 26% that of the parent compound. M1 accounts for approximately 7% of total pharmacologic activity. Tadalafil is predominantly metabolized by CYP3A4 to a catechol metabolite. The catechol metabolite undergoes extensive methylation and glucuronidation to form the methylcatechol and methylcatechol glucuronide conjugate, respectively. The major circulating metabolite is the methylcatechol glucuronide. In vitro data suggests that metabolites are not expected to be pharmacologically active at observed metabolite concentrations.

Special populations –

Renal function impairment: In volunteers with severe renal impairment (creatinine clearance [Ccr] 30 mL/min or less), **sildenafil** clearance was reduced, resulting in approximately double the area under the curve (AUC) and C_{max}, compared with age-matched volunteers with no renal impairment. In the moderate (Ccr 30 to 50 mL/min) or severe (Ccr less than 30 mL/min) renal impairment groups, the AUC of **vardenafil** was 20% to 30% higher compared with that observed in a control group with normal (Ccr greater than 80 mL/min) renal function. In studies using single-dose **tadalafil** (5 to 10 mg), tadalafil AUC doubled in subjects with mild (Ccr 51 to 80 mL/min) or moderate (Ccr 31 to 50 mL/min) renal insufficiency. In subjects with end-stage renal disease on hemodialysis, there was a 2-fold increase in C_{max} and 2.7- to 4.1-fold increase in AUC following single-dose administration of tadalafil 10 or 20 mg.

Hepatic function impairment: In volunteers with hepatic cirrhosis (Child-Pugh class A and B), **sildenafil** clearance was reduced, resulting in increases in AUC (84%) and C_{max} (47%), compared with age-matched volunteers with no hepatic impairment. In volunteers with mild hepatic impairment (Child-Pugh class A), the C_{max} and AUC following a **vardenafil** 10 mg dose were increased by 22% and 17%, respectively, compared with healthy control subjects. In volunteers with moderate hepatic impairment (Child-Pugh class B), the C_{max} and AUC following a vardenafil 10 mg dose were increased by 130% and 160%, respectively, compared with healthy control subjects.

Elderly: Healthy elderly volunteers (65 years of age and older) had a reduced clearance of **sildenafil**, with free plasma concentrations approximately 40% greater than those seen in healthy younger volunteers (18 to 45 years of age). In a study of healthy elderly (65 years of age and older) and younger (18 to 45 years of age) men, mean C_{max} and AUC of **vardenafil** were 34% and 52% higher, respectively, in elderly men. Healthy elderly men (65 years of age and older) had a lower oral clearance of **tadalafil**, resulting in a 25% higher AUC with no effect on C_{max} relative to that observed in healthy subjects 19 to 45 years of age.

Pulmonary hypertension: In patients with pulmonary hypertension, the average steady-state concentrations were 20% to 50% higher when compared with those of healthy volunteers. There was also a doubling of C_{min} levels compared with healthy volunteers. Both findings suggest a lower clearance and/or a higher oral bioavailability of **sildenafil** in patients with pulmonary hypertension compared with healthy volunteers.

Contraindications

Hypersensitivity to any component of the tablet; administration with nitrates (either regularly and/or intermittently) and NO donors because of the potentiation of hypotension (see Drug Interactions).

Warnings

➤*Priapism and prolonged erection:* Prolonged erections lasting longer than 4 hours and priapism (painful erections longer than 6 hours in duration) have been reported infrequently for this class of compounds. In the event of an erection that persists longer than 4 hours, whether painful or not, advise the patient to seek immediate medical assistance. If priapism is not treated immediately, penile tissue damage and permanent loss of potency may result.

Use with caution in patients who have conditions that might predispose them to priapism (eg, sickle cell anemia, multiple myeloma, leukemia) or in patients with anatomical deformation of the penis (eg, angulation, cavernosal fibrosis, Peyronie disease).

➤*Cardiovascular effects:* There is a potential for cardiac risk associated with sexual activity. Treatments for erectile dysfunction, including these agents, generally should not be used in men for whom sexual activity is inadvisable because of their underlying cardiovascular status. Consider the cardiovascular status of patients to determine whether patients with underlying cardiovascular disease could be adversely affected by vasodilatory effects (eg, transient decreases in BP) of these drugs, especially in combination with sexual activity.

Patients with the following underlying conditions can be particularly sensitive to the actions of vasodilators, including **sildenafil**, **tadalafil**, and **vardenafil**: those with left ventricular outflow obstruction (eg, aortic stenosis, idiopathic hypertrophic subaortic stenosis) and those with severely impaired autonomic control of BP.

There are no controlled clinical data on the safety or efficacy of sildenafil in patients who have suffered a myocardial infarction (MI), stroke, or life-threatening arrhythmia within the last 6 months; patients with resting hypotension (BP lower than 90/50 mm Hg) or hypertension (BP higher than 170/110 mm Hg); patients with cardiac failure (*Viagra* only) or coronary artery disease causing unstable angina; patients with retinitis pigmentosa; or patients on bosentan therapy (*Revatio* only). Use caution when prescribing sildenafil in these groups. Use of vardenafil is not recommended in the patients listed above and in severe hepatic impairment (Child-Pugh class C) and end-stage renal disease requiring dialysis.

The following groups of patients with cardiovascular disease were not included in clinical safety and efficacy trials for tadalafil, and, therefore, the use of tadalafil is not recommended in these groups until further information is available:

- Patients with an MI within the previous 90 days
- patients with unstable angina or angina occurring during sexual intercourse
- patients with New York Heart Association class 2 or greater heart failure in the last 6 months
- patients with uncontrolled arrhythmias, hypotension (BP lower than 90/50 mm Hg), or uncontrolled hypertension (BP higher than 170/100 mm Hg)
- patients with a stroke within the previous 6 months
- patients with known hereditary degenerative retinal disorders, including retinitis pigmentosa.

Sildenafil/Tadalafil – Serious cardiovascular, cerebrovascular, and vascular events, including MI, sudden cardiac death, ventricular arrhythmia, cerebrovascular hemorrhage, transient ischemic attack, hypertension, subarachnoid and intracerebral hemorrhages, and pulmonary hemorrhage have been reported postmarketing in temporal association with sildenafil. Most of these patients had preexisting cardiovascular risk factors. Many of these events were reported to occur during or shortly after sexual activity, and a few were reported to occur shortly after the use of sildenafil without sexual activity. Others were reported to have occurred hours to days after sildenafil use and sexual activity. It is not possible to determine whether these events are directly related to sildenafil, to sexual activity, to the patient's underlying cardiovascular disease, to a combination of these factors, or to other factors.

Tadalafil – The effect of a single dose of tadalafil 100 mg on the QT interval was evaluated at the time of peak tadalafil concentration in a randomized, double-blind, placebo- and active (IV ibutilide)-controlled crossover study in 90 healthy men 18 to 53 years of age. The mean change in QTc (Fridérica QT correction) for tadalafil, relative to placebo, was 3.5 msec. The mean change in QTc (individual QT correction) for tadalafil, relative to placebo, was 2.8 msec. In this study, the mean increase in heart rate associated with a tadalafil 100 mg dose compared with placebo was 3.1 beats/minute.

Vardenafil –

Congenital or acquired QT prolongation: In a study of the effects of vardenafil on QT interval in 59 healthy men, therapeutic (10 mg) and supratherapeutic (80 mg) doses of vardenafil and the active control moxifloxacin (400 mg) produced similar increases in QTc interval. Consider this observation in clinical decisions when prescribing vardenafil. Patients with congenital QT prolongation and those taking class IA (eg, quinidine, procainamide) or class III (eg, amiodarone, sotalol) antiarrhythmic medications should avoid using vardenafil.

➤*Renal function impairment:* In volunteers with severe renal impairment (Ccr 30 mL/min or less), **sildenafil** clearance was reduced, resulting in approximately double the AUC and C_{max}. Consider an initial sildenafil 25 mg dose in these patients. There are no clinical data on the safety or efficacy of **vardenafil** in patients with end-stage renal disease requiring dialysis, and, therefore, its use is not recommended.

Limit **tadalafil** to 5 mg not more than once daily in patients with severe renal insufficiency or end-stage renal disease. The starting dose in patients with a moderate degree of renal insufficiency should be 5 mg not more than once daily, and the maximum dose should be limited to 10 mg not more than once every 48 hours. No dose adjustment is required in patients with mild renal insufficiency.

In patients with moderate (Ccr 30 to 50 mL/min) to severe (Ccr less than 30 mL/min) renal impairment, the AUC of vardenafil was 20% to 30% higher compared with that observed in a control group with normal renal function (Ccr more than 80 mL/min). No dosage adjustment for vardenafil is required.

➤*Hepatic function impairment:* In volunteers with hepatic cirrhosis, **sildenafil** clearance was reduced, resulting in increases in AUC (84%) and C_{max} (47%). Consider an initial sildenafil 25 mg dose in these patients. In patients with mild or moderate hepatic impairment, do not exceed a **tadalafil** 10 mg dose. Because of insufficient information in patients with severe hepatic impairment, use of tadalafil in these patients is not recommended. In volunteers with mild hepatic impairment (Child-Pugh class A), the C_{max} and AUC following a **vardenafil** 10 mg dose were increased by 22% and 17%, respectively, compared with healthy control subjects. In volunteers with moderate hepatic impairment (Child-Pugh class B), the C_{max} and AUC following a vardenafil 10 mg dose were increased by 130% and 160%, respectively, compared with healthy control subjects. Consequently, a starting dose of 5 mg is recommended for patients with moderate hepatic impairment, and the maximum dose should not exceed 10 mg. Vardenafil has not been evaluated in patients with severe (Child-Pugh class C) hepatic impairment and its use is not recommended in these patients.

➤*Fertility impairment:* In beagle dogs given **tadalafil** daily for 3 to 12 months, there was treatment-related, nonreversible degeneration and atrophy of the seminiferous tubular epithelium in the testes in 20% to 100% of the dogs that resulted in a decrease in spermatogenesis in 40% to 75% of the dogs at doses of 10 mg/kg/day or more.

➤*Elderly:* Healthy elderly volunteers (65 years of age and older) had reduced **sildenafil** clearance with free plasma concentrations approximately 40% greater than those in healthy younger volunteers 18 to 45 years of age. Consider an initial sildenafil 25 mg dose in these patients. Healthy male elderly subjects (65 years of age and older) had a lower oral clearance of **tadalafil**, resulting in a 25% higher AUC with no effect on C_{max} relative to that observed in healthy subjects 19 to 45 years of age. In a study of healthy elderly (65 years of age and older) and younger (18 to 45 years of age) men, mean C_{max} and AUC of **vardenafil** were 34% and 52% higher, respectively, in elderly men. Consequently, consider a lower starting dose of vardenafil (5 mg) in patients 65 years of age and older.

➤*Pregnancy: Category B.* These agents for erectile dysfunction are not indicated for use in women. There are no adequate and well-controlled studies of these agents in pregnant women. **Tadalafil** and/or its metabolites cross the placenta, resulting in fetal exposure in rats. In a rat prenatal and postnatal development study at doses of tadalafil 60, 200, and 1,000 mg/kg, there was a reduction in postnatal survival of pups. Retarded physical development of pups in the absence of maternal effects was observed following maternal exposure to **vardenafil** 1 and 8 mg/kg, possibly because of vasodilation and/or secretion of the drug into milk. The number of living pups born to rats exposed pre- and postnatally was reduced at 60 mg/kg/day.

➤*Lactation:* These agents for erectile dysfunction are not indicated for use in women. **Tadalafil** and/or its metabolites were secreted into the milk of lactating rats at concentrations approximately 2.4-fold greater than found in the plasma. **Vardenafil** was secreted into the milk of lactating rats at concentrations approximately 10-fold greater than found in plasma. Following a single oral dose of 3 mg/kg, 3.3% of the administered dose was excreted into the milk within 24 hours. It is not known if the drugs are excreted in human breast milk.

➤*Children:* These agents for erectile dysfunction are not indicated for use in newborns or children.

Safety and efficacy of **sildenafil** in pediatric pulmonary hypertension patients have not been established.

Precautions

➤*Erectile dysfunction:* Undertake thorough medical history and physical examination to diagnose erectile dysfunction, determine potential underlying causes, and identify appropriate treatment.

The safety and efficacy of combinations of **sildenafil**, **tadalafil**, or **vardenafil** with other treatments for erectile dysfunction have not been studied. Therefore, the use of such combinations is not recommended.

➤*Deformation of penis:* Use these agents with caution in patients with anatomical deformation of the penis (eg, angulation, cavernosal fibrosis, Peyronie disease) or in patients who have conditions that may predispose them to priapism (eg, sickle cell anemia, multiple myeloma, leukemia).

➤*Hematologic effects:* **Sildenafil**, **tadalafil**, or **vardenafil** have no effect on bleeding time when taken alone or with aspirin. In vitro studies with human platelets indicate that sildenafil potentiates the antiaggregatory effect of sodium nitroprusside (a NO donor). In rabbits, the combination of heparin and sildenafil had an additive effect on bleeding time, but this interaction has not been studied in humans. There is no safety information on the administration of sildenafil, tadalafil, or vardenafil to patients with bleeding disorders or active peptic ulceration.

The incidence of epistaxis was higher in patients with pulmonary arterial hypertension secondary to connective tissue disease (sildenafil 13%, placebo 0%) than in primary pulmonary hypertension patients (sildenafil 3%, placebo 2%). The incidence of epistaxis was also higher in sildenafil-treated patients with concomitant oral vitamin K antagonists (9% vs 2% in those not treated with concomitant vitamin K antagonists).

➤*Visual disturbances:* Single oral doses of PDE inhibitors have demonstrated transient, dose-related impairment of color discrimination (blue/green), with peak effects near the time of peak plasma levels. The findings were most evident 1 hour after administration, diminishing but still present 6 hours after administration. This finding is consistent with the inhibition of PDE6, which is involved in phototransduction in the retina. An evaluation of visual function of **sildenafil** up to 200 mg and **tadalafil** 40 mg revealed no effects on visual acuity, intraocular pressure, or pupillometry. In a single-dose study of 25 healthy men, **vardenafil** 40 mg, twice the maximum daily recommended dose, did not alter visual acuity, intraocular pressure, or fundoscopic and slit-lamp findings.

➤*Retinitis pigmentosa:* A minority of patients with retinitis pigmentosa have genetic disorders of retinal phosphodiesterases. There is no safety information on the administration of **sildenafil**, **tadalafil**, or **vardenafil** to patients with known hereditary degenerative retinal disorders, including retinitis pigmentosa. Therefore, use is not recommended.

Drug Interactions

➤*CYP450 system:* PDE5 inhibitors are metabolized principally by the cytochrome P-450 (CYP) isoforms 3A4 (major route), 3A5 (major route; **vardenafil**), and 2C9 (minor route; **sildenafil**, vardenafil). Therefore, inhibitors of these isoenzymes may increase PDE5 inhibitor concentrations and inducers of these isoenzymes (eg, carbamazepine, phenytoin, phenobarbital) may decrease PDE5 inhibitor concentrations. See Administration and Dosage sections of the individual monographs for dosing recommendations.

➤*Alpha-blockers:* Caution is advised when PDE5 inhibitors are coadministered with alpha-blockers. PDE5 inhibitors and alpha-adrenergic blocking agents are both vasodilators with BP-lowering effects. When vasodilators are used in combination, an additive effect on BP may be anticipated. In some patients, concomitant use of these 2 drug classes can lower BP significantly, leading to symptomatic hypotension (eg, fainting). Give consideration to the following:

- Patients should be stable on alpha-blocker therapy prior to initiating a PDE5 inhibitor. Patients who demonstrate hemodynamic instability on alpha-blocker therapy alone are at increased risk of symptomatic hypotension with concomitant use of PDE5 inhibitors.
- In those patients who are stable on alpha-blocker therapy, initiate PDE5 inhibitors at the lowest recommended starting dose.
- In those patients already taking an optimized dose of a PDE5 inhibitor, initiate alpha-blocker therapy at the lowest dose. Stepwise increases in alpha-blocker dose may be associated with further lowering of BP in patients taking a PDE5 inhibitor.
- Safety of combined use of PDE5 inhibitors and alpha-blockers may be affected by other variables, including intravascular volume depletion and other antihypertensive drugs.

PDE5 Inhibitor Drug Interactions

Precipitant drug	Object drug[a]		Description
Alcohol	PDE5 inhibitors	⬆	Alcohol and PDE5 inhibitors are mild systemic vasodilators. Substantial consumption of alcohol in combination with a PDE5 inhibitor may produce decreases in BP, postural dizziness, and orthostatic hypotension.
Alpha-blockers (eg, doxazosin, terazosin)	PDE5 inhibitors	⬆	Coadministration of a PDE5 inhibitor with an alpha-blocker may cause BP to be significantly lowered. Dose modifications may be required (see Administration and Dosage).
PDE5 inhibitors	Alpha-blockers (eg, doxazosin, terazosin)		
Amlodipine	PDE5 inhibitors Sildenafil Tadalafil	⬆	Coadministration of sildenafil and amlodipine produced an additional mean reduction in BP of 8/7 mm Hg. Amlodipine administered with tadalafil reduced mean supine systolic/diastolic BP by 3/2 mm Hg.
PDE5 inhibitors Sildenafil Tadalafil	Amlodipine		
Angiotensin II receptor blockers	PDE5 inhibitors Tadalafil	⬆	Coadministration of tadalafil and an angiotensin II receptor blocker produced a mean reduction in supine BP of 8/4 mm Hg.
PDE5 inhibitors Tadalafil	Angiotensin II receptor blockers		
Antacids	PDE5 inhibitors Tadalafil	⬇	Simultaneous administration of tadalafil with an antacid (magnesium hydroxide/aluminum hydroxide) reduced the rate of tadalafil absorption without altering the AUC.

PDE5 Inhibitor Drug Interactions			
Precipitant drug	Object drug[a]		Description
Azole antifungals (eg, ketoconazole, itraconazole)	PDE5 inhibitors	↑	Ketoconazole and itraconazole are CYP3A4 inhibitors and therefore would reduce the PDE5 inhibitor clearance. Coadministration of vardenafil with ketoconazole produced a 10-fold increase in vardenafil AUC and a 4-fold increase in C_{max}. Dose adjustments are recommended (see Administration and Dosage).
Beta-blockers, (nonspecific)	PDE5 inhibitors Sildenafil	↑	The AUC of sildenafil's active metabolite, N-desmethyl sildenafil, was increased 102% by nonspecific beta-blockers. This effect is not expected to be of clinical consequence.
Bosentan	PDE5 inhibitors Sildenafil	↓	Coadministration of bosentan and sildenafil resulted in a decrease in sildenafil AUC by 63% and C_{max} by 55%. Sildenafil (at steady state) increased bosentan AUC by 50% and C_{max} by 42%.
PDE5 inhibitors Sildenafil	Bosentan	↑	
Cimetidine	PDE5 inhibitors Sildenafil	↑	Coadministration yielded a 56% increase in sildenafil plasma concentrations.
Diuretics	PDE5 inhibitors Sildenafil Tadalafil	↑	The AUC of sildenafil's active metabolite, N-desmethyl sildenafil, was increased 62% by loop diuretics and potassium-sparing diuretics. This effect is not expected to be of clinical consequence. Coadministration of tadalafil with a thiazide diuretic caused a decrease in BP.
Enalapril	PDE5 inhibitors Tadalafil	↑	Coadministration of tadalafil and enalapril produced a mean reduction in supine BP of 4/1 mm Hg.
PDE5 inhibitors Tadalafil	Enalapril		
Macrolides (eg, erythromycin)	PDE5 inhibitors	↑	Coadministration of sildenafil and erythromycin (CYP3A4 inhibitor) resulted in a 182% increase in sildenafil systemic exposure. Erythromycin produced a 4-fold increase in vardenafil AUC and a 3-fold increase in C_{max}. Also consider interactions with clarithromycin and troleandomycin.
Metoprolol	PDE5 inhibitors Tadalafil	↑	Coadministration of tadalafil and metoprolol produced a mean reduction in supine BP of 5/3 mm Hg.
PDE5 inhibitors Tadalafil	Metoprolol		
Nifedipine	PDE5 inhibitors Vardenafil	↑	Coadministration of vardenafil and nifedipine produced an additional mean reduction in supine BP of 6/5 mm Hg.
PDE5 inhibitors Vardenafil	Nifedipine		
Nitrates (eg, isosorbide dinitrate, nitroglycerin)	PDE5 inhibitors	↑	Concomitant use is contraindicated. PDE5 inhibitors potentiate the vasodilatory effect of circulating nitric oxide, resulting in a significant and potentially fatal drop in BP.
PDE5 inhibitors	Nitrates (eg, isosorbide dinitrate, nitroglycerin)		
Protease inhibitors (eg, ritonavir, indinavir, saquinavir)	PDE5 inhibitors	↑	When coadministered with a protease inhibitor, the PDE5 inhibitor plasma concentrations may be substantially elevated, resulting in severe and potentially fatal hypotension. Dose modifications are recommended (see Administration and Dosage). Concomitant use of vardenafil with ritonavir or indinavir may lead to a decrease in the protease inhibitor plasma concentration.
PDE5 inhibitors Vardenafil	Protease inhibitors (ie, ritonavir, indinavir)	↓	
Rifampin	PDE5 inhibitors Sildenafil Tadalafil	↓	Rifampin and other CYP3A4 inducers increase sildenafil and tadalafil clearance.
Tacrolimus	PDE5 inhibitors Sildenafil	↑	Sildenafil plasma concentrations may be elevated, increasing risk of side effects.
PDE5 inhibitors Sildenafil	Anticoagulants (vitamin K-dependent)	↑	In pulmonary arterial hypertension patients, the concomitant use of vitamin K antagonists and sildenafil resulted in a greater incidence of bleeding (primarily epistaxis).

[a] ↑ = Object drug increased. ↓ = Object drug decreased.

➤*Drug/Food interactions:* Although specific interactions have not been studied, grapefruit juice (CYP3A4 inhibitor) would likely increase PDE5 inhibitor exposure. When taken with a high-fat meal, the rate of **sildenafil** absorption is reduced, with a mean delay in T_{max} of 60 minutes and a mean reduction in C_{max} of 29%. High-fat meals caused a reduction in **vardenafil** C_{max} by 18% to 50%.

Adverse Reactions

➤*Erectile dysfunction:*

Phosphodiesterase Type 5 Inhibitors Adverse Reactions (%)[a]					
	Sildenafil	Vardenafil	Tadalafil		
Adverse reaction	(n = 734)[b]	(n = 2,203)[c]	5 mg (N = 151)	10 mg (N = 394)	20 mg (N = 635)
CNS					
Dizziness	2%	2%	—	—	—
Headache	16%	15%	11%	11%	15%
GI					
Diarrhea	3%	< 2%	—	—	—
Dyspepsia	7%	4%	4%	8%	10%
Nausea	—	2%	—	—	—
Respiratory					
Nasal congestion	4%	—	2%	3%	3%
Rhinitis	—	9%	—	—	—
Sinusitis	< 2%	3%	—	—	—
Miscellaneous					
Abnormal vision[d]	3%	< 2%	—	—	—
Accidental injury	< 2%	3%	—	—	—
Back pain	> 2%[e]	2%	3%	5%	6%
Flu syndrome	> 2%[e]	3%			
Flushing[f]	10%	11%	2%	3%	3%
Increased creatine kinase	—	2%	—	—	—
Limb pain	—	—	1%	3%	3%
Myalgia	< 2%	< 2%	1%	4%	3%
Rash	2%	< 2%	—	—	—
Urinary tract infection	3%	—	—	—	—

[a] Data are pooled from separate studies and are not necessarily comparable.
[b] As needed flexible-dose studies.
[c] Fixed and flexible-dose studies. Flexible-dose studies started all patients at vardenafil 10 mg and allowed a decrease in dose to 5 mg or increase in dose to 20 mg based on side effects and efficacy.
[d] Mild and transient, predominantly color tinge to vision but also increased sensitivity to light or blurred vision. Only 1 patient discontinued because of abnormal vision.
[e] Incidence is equally common with placebo.
[f] The term flushing includes facial flushing and flushing. In fixed-dose studies, dyspepsia (17%) and abnormal vision (11%) were more common at the **sildenafil** 100 mg dose than at lower doses.

Placebo-controlled trials suggested a dose effect in the incidence of some adverse reactions (headache, flushing, dyspepsia, nausea, rhinitis) over the **vardenafil** 5, 10, and 20 mg doses.

The following adverse reactions were reported in less than 2% of patients.

Cardiovascular – Angina pectoris, chest pain, hypotension, palpitation, postural hypotension, syncope, tachycardia, abnormal electrocardiogram, AV block, cardiac arrest, cardiomyopathy, cerebral thrombosis, heart failure, myocardial ischemia, hypertension, MI.

CNS – Hypesthesia, insomnia, paresthesia, somnolence, vertigo, abnormal dreams, ataxia, depression, hypertonia, migraine, neuralgia, neuropathy, reflexes decreased, tremor, dizziness.

Dermatologic – Pruritus, sweating, contact dermatitis, exfoliative dermatitis, herpes simplex, photosensitivity reaction, skin ulcer, urticaria, rash.

GI – Abnormal liver function tests, dry mouth, dysphagia, esophagitis, gastritis, vomiting, abdominal pain, colitis, gastroenteritis, gingivitis, glossitis, rectal hemorrhage, stomatitis, diarrhea, gamma-glutamyl transpeptidase (GGTP) increased, gastroesophageal reflux, loose stools, nausea, upper abdominal pain.

GU – Abnormal ejaculation, anorgasmia, breast enlargement, cystitis, genital edema, nocturia, urinary frequency, urinary incontinence, erection increased, spontaneous penile erection, priapism (including prolonged or painful erections).

Hematologic – Anemia, leukopenia.

Metabolic/Nutritional – Edema, gout, hyperglycemia, hypernatremia, hyperuricemia, hypoglycemia reaction, peripheral edema, thirst, unstable diabetes.

Musculoskeletal –

Sildenafil: Arthritis, arthrosis, bone pain, myasthenia, synovitis, tendon rupture, tenosynovitis, arthralgia, neck pain.

Tadalafil: In tadalafil clinical pharmacology trials, back pain or myalgia generally occurred 12 to 24 hours after dosing and typically resolved within 48 hours. The back pain/myalgia associated with tadalafil treatment was characterized by diffuse bilateral lower lumbar, gluteal, thigh, or thoracolumbar muscular discomfort and was exacerbated by recumbancy. In general, pain was reported as mild or moderate in severity and resolved without medical treatment, but severe back pain was reported infrequently (less than 5% of all reports). When medical treatment was necessary, acetaminophen or nonsteroidal anti-inflammatory drugs were generally effective; however, in a small percentage of subjects who required treatment, a mild narcotic (eg, codeine) was used. Overall, approximately 0.5% of all tadalafil-treated subjects discontinued treatment as a consequence of back pain/myalgia. Diagnostic testing, including measures for inflammation, muscle injury, or renal damage revealed no evidence of medically significant underlying pathology.

Respiratory – Dyspnea, pharyngitis, asthma, bronchitis, cough increased, laryngitis, sputum increased, epistaxis.

Special senses – Conjunctivitis, eye pain, cataract, deafness, dry eyes, ear pain, eye hemorrhage, mydriasis, photophobia, tinnitus, blurred vision, conjunctival hyperemia, eyelid swelling, lacrimation increased, changes in color vision, chromatopsia, dim vision, glaucoma, watery eyes.

Miscellaneous – Asthenia, face edema, pain, accidental fall, allergic reaction, chills, shock, anaphylactic reaction (including laryngeal edema).

Postmarketing – Nonarteritic anterior ischemic optic neuropathy (NAION), a cause of decreased vision including permanent loss of vision, has been reported rarely postmarketing in temporal association with the use of PDE5 inhibitors. Most, but not all, of these patients had underlying anatomic or vascular risk factors for developing NAION, including but not necessarily limited to: low cup or disc ratio ("crowded disc"), age older than 50 years, diabetes, hypertension, coronary artery disease, hyperlipidemia, and smoking. It is not possible to determine whether these events are related directly to the use of PDE5 inhibitors, to the patient's underlying vascular risk factors or anatomical defects, to a combination of these factors, or to other factors.

Sildenafil: Anxiety, diplopia, epistaxis, hematuria, increased intraocular pressure, ocular burning, ocular redness or bloodshot appearance, ocular swelling/pressure, paramacular edema, priapism, prolonged erection, retinal vascular disease or bleeding, seizure, temporary vision loss/decreased vision, vitreous detachment/traction.

Tadalafil: Hypersensitivity reactions including exfoliative dermatitis, Stevens-Johnson syndrome, urticaria; priapism; retinal vein occlusion; visual field defects (see also Warnings).

Vardenafil: Visual disturbances, including vision loss (temporary or permanent), such as visual field defect, retinal vein occlusion, and reduced visual acuity, also have been reported rarely in postmarketing experience. It is not possible to determine whether these reactions are related directly to the use of vardenafil.

➤*Pulmonary arterial hypertension:*

Sildenafil Adverse Reactions in Pulmonary Arterial Hypertension Clinical Trial (≥ 3%)

Adverse reaction	Sildenafil 20 mg 3 times daily (n = 69)	Placebo (n = 70)
CNS		
Headache	46%	39%
Insomnia	7%	1%
GI		
Diarrhea, not otherwise specified	9%	6%
Dyspepsia	13%	7%
Gastritis not otherwise specified	3%	0%
Respiratory		
Dyspnea exacerbated	7%	3%
Rhinitis not otherwise specified	4%	0%
Sinusitis	3%	0%
Miscellaneous		
Epistaxis	9%	1%
Erythema	6%	1%
Flushing	10%	4%
Myalgia	7%	4%
Paresthesia	3%	0%
Pyrexia	6%	3%

At doses higher than the recommended 20 mg 3 times daily dose, there was a greater incidence of some adverse reactions including diarrhea, flushing, myalgia, and visual disturbances. Visual disturbances were identified as mild and transient, and were predominantly color-tinge to vision but also included increased sensitivity to light or blurred vision.

In the pivotal study, the incidence of retinal hemorrhage at the recommended sildenafil 20 mg 3 times daily dose was 1.4% versus 0% placebo and for all sildenafil doses studied was 1.9% versus 0% placebo. The incidence of eye hemorrhage at both the recommended dose and at all doses studied was 1.4% for sildenafil versus 1.4% for placebo. The patients experiencing these events had risk factors for hemorrhage including concurrent anticoagulant therapy.

Overdosage

➤*Symptoms:* In studies with healthy volunteers of single **sildenafil** doses up to 800 mg, adverse reactions were similar to those seen at lower doses, but incidence rates were increased. The maximum dose of **vardenafil** for which human data are available is a single 120 mg dose administered to 8 healthy men. The majority of these subjects experienced reversible back pain/myalgia and/or abnormal vision. Single **tadalafil** doses up to 500 mg have been given to healthy subjects, and multiple daily doses up to 100 mg have been given to patients. Adverse reactions were similar to those seen at lower doses.

➤*Treatment:* In cases of overdose, adopt standard supportive measures as required. Refer to General Management of Acute Overdosage. Renal dialysis is not expected to accelerate clearance as these drugs are highly bound to plasma proteins and are not significantly eliminated in urine.

Patient Information

Discuss with patients the contraindication of these agents with concurrent organic nitrates. Concomitant use with nitrates could cause BP to suddenly drop to an unsafe level, resulting in dizziness, syncope, or even heart attack or stroke.

Discuss with patients the potential for **tadalafil** to augment the BP-lowering effect of alpha-blockers and antihypertensive medications.

Discuss with patients the potential cardiac risk of sexual activity in patients with preexisting cardiovascular risk factors. Advise patients who experience symptoms (eg, angina pectoris, dizziness, nausea) upon initiation of sexual activity to refrain from further activity and discuss the episode with their physician.

Advise patients to stop use of all PDE5 inhibitors and to seek medical attention in the event of a sudden loss of vision in 1 or both eyes. Such an event may be a sign of NAION, a cause of decreased vision, including permanent loss of vision that has been reported rarely postmarketing in temporal association with the use of all PDE5 inhibitors. It is not possible to determine whether these events are related directly to the use of PDE5 inhibitors or other factors. Also discuss with patients the increased risk of NAION in individuals who have already experienced NAION in 1 eye, including whether such individuals could be adversely affected by use of vasodilators such as PDE5 inhibitors.

These agents offer no protection against sexually transmitted diseases. Consider counseling patients about the protective measures necessary to guard against sexually transmitted diseases, including HIV.

Advise patients that these agents have no effect in the absence of sexual stimulation. Sexual stimulation is required for an erection to occur after taking these agents.

Warn patients to seek immediate medical attention if erections last for longer than 4 hours.

Advise patients to contact the prescribing physician if new medications that may interact with these agents are prescribed by another health care provider.

Inform patients that substantial consumption of alcohol (eg, 5 units or greater) in combination with a PDE5 inhibitor can increase the potential for orthostatic signs and symptoms, including increase in heart rate, decrease in standing BP, dizziness, and headache.

SILDENAFIL CITRATE

Rx	**Revatio** (Pfizer)	**Tablets:** 20 mg	Lactose (RVT20). White. Film-coated. In 90s.
Rx	**Viagra** (Pfizer)	**Tablets:** 25 mg	Lactose. (VGR25 PFIZER). Blue, rounded-diamond shape. Film-coated. In 30s.
		50 mg	Lactose. (VGR50 PFIZER). Blue, rounded-diamond shape. Film-coated. In 30s and 100s.
		100 mg	Lactose. (VGR100 PFIZER). Blue, rounded-diamond shape. Film-coated. In 30s and 100s.

SILDENAFIL CITRATE — ORAL

For complete and comparative prescribing information, refer to the Phosphodiesterase Type 5 Inhibitors group monograph.

Indications

➤*Pulmonary arterial hypertension (Revatio* only): For the treatment of pulmonary arterial hypertension (World Health Organization Group 1) to improve exercise ability.

➤*Erectile dysfunction (Viagra* only): For the treatment of erectile dysfunction.

➤*Unlabeled uses:* Treatment of antidepressant/antipsychotic–induced sexual dysfunction. The use of sildenafil in women with sexual dysfunction has been evaluated in small clinical trials. The results are quite mixed, with may studies unable to demonstrate efficacy.

Administration and Dosage

➤*Approved by the FDA:* March 27, 1998.

➤*Dosage:*

Pulmonary arterial hypertension – 20 mg 3 times daily. Sildenafil tablets should be taken approximately 4 to 6 hours apart, with or without food. In the clinical trial, no greater efficacy was achieved with the use of higher doses. Treatment with doses higher than 20 mg 3 times daily is not recommended. Dosages lower than 20 mg 3 times daily were not tested. Whether dosages lower than 20 mg 3 times daily are effective is not known.

Erectile dysfunction – 50 mg taken, as needed, approximately 1 hour before sexual activity. However, sildenafil citrate may be taken anywhere from 4 hours to 0.5 hour before sexual activity. Based on effectiveness and toleration, the dose may be increased to a maximum recommended dose of 100 mg or decreased to 25 mg. The maximum recommended dosing frequency is once per day.

➤*Concomitant use with nitrates:* Sildenafil citrate was shown to potentiate the hypotensive effects of nitrates and its administration in patients who use nitric oxide donors or nitrates in any form is therefore contraindicated.

➤*Concomitant use with alpha-blockers:* Simultaneous administration of sildenafil doses above 25 mg and an alpha-blocker may lead to symptomatic hypotension in some patients. Doses of 50 mg or 100 mg of sildenafil should not be taken within 4 hours of alpha-blocker administration. A 25 mg dose of sildenafil may be taken at any time.

➤*Storage/Stability:* Store at 25°C (77°F); excursions permitted to 15° to 30°C (59° to 86°F).

TADALAFIL

Rx	**Cialis** (Lilly)	**Tablets:** 5 mg	Lactose. (C 5). Yellow, almond shape. Film-coated. In 30s.
		10 mg	Lactose. (C 10). Yellow, almond shape. Film-coated. In 30s.
		20 mg	Lactose. (C 20). Yellow, almond shape. Film-coated. In 30s.

TADALAFIL — ORAL

For complete prescribing information, refer to the Phosphodiesterase Type 5 Inhibitors group monograph.

Indications

➤*Erectile dysfunction:* For the treatment of erectile dysfunction.

Administration and Dosage

➤*Approved by the FDA:* November 21, 2003.

➤*Dosage:* 10 mg taken prior to anticipated sexual activity. The dose may be increased to 20 mg or decreased to 5 mg based on individual efficacy and tolerability. The maximum recommended dosing frequency is once per day in most patients. Tadalafil may be taken without regard to food.

➤*Renal function impairment:* No dose adjustment is required in patients with mild renal insufficiency. For patients with moderate (creatinine clearance [Ccr] 31 to 50 mL/min) renal insufficiency, a starting dose of 5 mg not more than once daily is recommended, and the maximum dose should be limited to 10 mg not more than once every 48 hours. For patients with severe (Ccr less than 30 mL/min) renal insufficiency on hemodialysis, the maximum recommended dose is 5 mg.

➤*Hepatic function impairment:* For patients with mild or moderate degrees of hepatic impairment (Child-Pugh class A or B), the dose of tadalafil should not exceed 10 mg once daily. In patients with severe hepatic impairment (Child-Pugh class C), the use of tadalafil is not recommended.

➤*Storage/Stability:* Store at 25°C (77°F); excursions permitted to 15° to 30°C (59° to 86°F). Keep out of the reach of children.

VARDENAFIL HYDROCHLORIDE

Rx	**Levitra** (Bayer)	**Tablets:** 2.5 mg	(BAYER 2.5). Orange, round. Film-coated. In 30s.
		5 mg	(BAYER 5). Orange, round. Film-coated. In 30s.
		10 mg	(BAYER 10). Orange, round. Film-coated. In 30s.
		20 mg	(BAYER 20). Orange, round. Film-coated. In 30s.

VARDENAFIL HYDROCHLORIDE — ORAL

For complete prescribing information, refer to the Phosphodiesterase Type 5 Inhibitors group monograph.

Indications

➤*Erectile dysfunction:* For the treatment of erectile dysfunction.

Administration and Dosage

➤*Approved by the FDA:* August 19, 2003.

10 mg, taken orally approximately 60 minutes before sexual activity. The dose may be increased to a maximum recommended dose of 20 mg or decreased to 5 mg based on efficacy and side effects. The maximum recommended dosing frequency is once daily. Vardenafil can be taken with or without food. Sexual stimulation is required for response to treatment.

➤*Elderly:* A starting dose of vardenafil 5 mg should be considered in patients 65 years of age and older.

➤*Hepatic function impairment:* For patients with mild hepatic function impairment (Child-Pugh class A), no dosage adjustment of vardenafil is required. Vardenafil clearance is reduced in patients with moderate hepatic function impairment (Child-Pugh class B), and a starting dose of vardenafil 5 mg is recommended. The maximum dose in patients with moderate hepatic function impairment should not exceed 10 mg. Vardenafil has not been evaluated in patients with severe hepatic function impairment (Child-Pugh class C).

➤*Concomitant medications:* The dosage of vardenafil may require adjustment in patients receiving certain CYP3A4 inhibitors (eg, erythromycin, indinavir, itraconazole, ketoconazole, ritonavir). For ritonavir, a single dose of vardenafil 2.5 mg should not be exceeded in a 72-hour period. For indinavir, ketoconazole 400 mg daily, and itraconazole 400 mg daily, a single dose of vardenafil 2.5 mg should not be exceeded in a 24-hour period. For ketoconazole 200 mg daily, itraconazole 200 mg daily, and erythromycin, a single dose of vardenafil 5 mg should not be exceeded in a 24-hour period. For alpha-blockers, caution is advised when phosphodiesterase type 5 (PDE5) inhibitors, including vardenafil, are used concomitantly with alpha-blockers because of the potential for an additive effect on blood pressure. In some patients, concomitant use of these 2 drug classes can lower blood pressure significantly leading to symptomatic hypotension (eg, fainting). Concomitant treatment should be initiated only if the patient is stable on alpha-blocker therapy. In those patients who are stable on alpha-blocker therapy, vardenafil should be initiated at a dose of 5 mg (2.5 mg when used concomitantly with certain CYP3A4 inhibitors.

➤*Storage/Stability:* Store at 25°C (77°F); excursions permitted to 15° to 30°C (59° to 86°F).

ACETOHYDROXAMIC ACID

Rx	**Lithostat** (Mission)	**Tablets:** 250 mg	(Mission MPC 500). White. In unit-of-use 100s.

ACETOHYDROXAMIC ACID — ORAL

Indications

➤*Chronic urea-splitting urinary infection:* Adjunctive therapy in patients with chronic urea-splitting urinary infection. Acetohydroxamic acid is intended to decrease urinary ammonia and alkalinity, but it should not be used in lieu of curative surgical treatment (for patients with stones) or antimicrobial treatment. Long-term treatment with acetohydroxamic acid may be warranted to maintain urease inhibition as long as urea-splitting infection is present. Experience with acetohydroxamic acid does not go beyond 7 years. A patient monograph should be distributed to each patient who receives acetohydroxamic acid.

Administration and Dosage

➤*Approved by the FDA:* May 31, 1983.

➤*Adults:* Acetohydroxamic acid should be administered orally, 1 tablet 3 to 4 times a day in a total daily dose of 10 to 15 mg/kg/day. The recommended starting dose is 12 mg/kg/day, administered at 6- to 8-hour intervals at a time when the stomach is empty. The maximum daily dose should be no more than 1.5 g, regardless of body weight.

➤*Children:* In children an initial dose of 10 mg/kg/day is recommended. Close monitoring of the patient's clinical condition and hematologic status is recommended. Titration of the dose to higher or lower levels may be required to obtain an optimum therapeutic effect or to reduce the risk of side effects.

➤*Renal function impairment:* The dosage should be reduced in patients with reduced renal function. Patients whose serum creatinine is greater than 1.8 mg/dL should take no more than 1 g/day; such patients should be dosed at 12-hour intervals. Further reductions in dosage to prevent the accumulation of toxic concentrations in the blood may also be desirable. Insufficient data exists to accurately characterize the optimum dose or dose interval in patients with moderate degrees of renal insufficiency.

Patients with advanced renal insufficiency (ie, serum creatinine greater than 2.5 mg/dL) should not be treated with acetohydroxamic acid. The risk of accumulation of toxic blood levels of acetohydroxamic acid seems to be greater than the chances for a beneficial effect in such patients.

➤*Storage / Stability:* Acetohydroxamic acid should be stored in a dry place at room temperature, 15° to 30°C (59° to 86°F). Container should be closed tightly.

Actions

➤*Pharmacology:* Acetohydroxamic acid reversibly inhibits the bacterial enzyme urease, thereby inhibiting the hydrolysis of urea and production of ammonia in urine infected with urea-splitting organisms. The reduced ammonia levels and decreased pH enhance the effectiveness of antimicrobial agents and allow an increased cure rate of these infections.

➤*Pharmacokinetics:*

Absorption / Distribution – Acetohydroxamic acid is well absorbed from the gastrointestinal tract after oral administration; peak blood levels occur from 0.25 to 1 hour after dosing. The compound is distributed throughout body water, and there is no known binding to any tissue. Acetohydroxamic acid chelates with dietary iron within the gut. This reaction may interfere with absorption of acetohydroxamic acid and with iron. Concomitant hypochromic anemia should be treated with intramuscular iron.

Metabolism / Excretion – In rodents, the metabolic fate of acetohydroxamic acid is well known; 55% is excreted unchanged in urine, 25% is excreted as acetamide or acetate and 7% is excreted by the lungs as carbon dioxide. Less than 1% is excreted in the feces. Approximately 5% of the administered dose is unaccounted for. In rodents, acetohydroxamic acid shows a dose-related change in pharmacokinetics; with increasing dose, there is an increase in the half-life and an increase in the percent of the administered dose recovered in urine as unchanged acetohydroxamic acid.

Pharmacokinetics in man are generally similar to rodents including the dose-related increase in half-life, but they are not as well characterized as in the rodent. Thirty-six to sixty-five percent (36% to 65%) of the oral dosage is excreted unchanged in the urine. It is unaltered acetohydroxamic acid in the urine that provides the therapeutic effect, but the precise concentration of acetohydroxamic acid in urine that is necessary to inhibit urease is incompletely delineated. Therapeutic benefit may be obtained from concentrations as low as 8 mcg/mL; higher concentrations (ie, 30 mcg/mL) are expected to provide more complete inhibition of urease. The plasma half-life of acetohydroxamic acid is approximately 5 to 10 hours in subjects with normal renal function and is prolonged in patients with reduced renal function.

Urinary infections – Acetohydroxamic acid has been evaluated clinically in patients with urea-splitting urinary infections, often accompanied by struvite stone disease, that were recalcitrant to other forms of medical and surgical management. In these clinical trials, acetohydroxamic acid reduced the pathologically elevated urinary ammonia and pH levels that result from the hydrolysis of urea by the enzyme, urease.

Acetohydroxamic acid does not acidify urine directly nor does it have a direct antibacterial effect. The usefulness of reducing ammonia levels and decreasing urinary pH is suggested by single (not yet replicated) clinical trials in which urease inhibition allowed successful antibiotic treatment of urea-splitting *Proteus* infections after surgical removal of struvite stones in patients not cured by 3 months of antibacterial treatment alone, and reduced the rate of stone growth in patients who were not candidates for surgical removal of stones.

Contraindications

Patients whose physical state and disease are amenable to definitive surgery and appropriate antimicrobial agents; patients whose urine is infected by nonurease-producing organisms; patients whose urinary infections can be controlled by culture-specific oral antimicrobial agents; patients whose renal function is poor (ie, serum creatinine greater than 2.5 mg/dL or creatinine clearance less than 20 mL/min); female patients who do not evidence a satisfactory method of contraception; patients who are pregnant (see Warnings).

Warnings

➤*Coombs negative hemolytic anemia:* A Coombs negative hemolytic anemia has occurred in patients receiving acetohydroxamic acid. Gastrointestinal upset characterized by nausea, vomiting, anorexia, and generalized malaise has accompanied the most severe forms of hemolytic anemia. Approximately 15% of patients receiving acetohydroxamic acid have had only laboratory findings of an anemia. However, most patients developed a mild reticulocytosis. The untoward reactions have reverted to normal following cessation of treatment. A complete blood count, including a reticulocyte count, is recommended after 2 weeks of treatment. If the reticulocyte count exceeds 6%, a reduced dosage should be entertained. A CBC and reticulocyte count are recommended at 3-month intervals for the duration of treatment.

➤*Renal function impairment:* Since acetohydroxamic acid is eliminated primarily by the kidneys, patients with significantly impaired renal function should be closely monitored, and a reduction of daily dose may be needed to avoid excessive drug accumulation (see Administration and Dosage).

➤*Hepatic function impairment:* Abnormalities of liver function have not been reported to date. However, a chloro-benzene derivative of acetohydroxamic acid caused significant liver dysfunction in an unrelated study. Therefore, close monitoring of liver function is recommended (see Carcinogenesis for discussion of possible hepatic carcinogenesis).

➤*Carcinogenesis:* Well-controlled, long-term animal studies that identify the carcinogenic potential of acetohydroxamic acid treatment have not been conducted. Acetamide, a metabolite of acetohydroxamic acid, has been shown to cause hepatocellular carcinoma in rats at oral doses 1500 times the human dose.

➤*Mutagenesis:* Acetohydroxamic acid is cytotoxic and was positive for mutagenicity in the Ames test.

➤*Pregnancy: Category X.*

Acetohydroxamic acid may cause fetal harm when administered to a pregnant woman. Acetohydroxamic acid was teratogenic (retarded or clubbed rear leg at 750 mg/kg and above and exencephaly and encephalocele at 1500 mg/kg) when given intraperitoneally to rats. Acetohydroxamic acid is contraindicated in women who are or may become pregnant. If this drug is used during pregnancy, or if the patient becomes pregnant while taking this drug, the patient should be informed of the potential hazard to the fetus.

➤*Lactation:* It is not known whether acetohydroxamic acid is secreted in human milk. Because many drugs are excreted in human milk, and because of the potential for serious adverse reactions in nursing infants from acetohydroxamic acid, a decision should be made whether to discontinue nursing or the drug, taking into account the significance of the drug to the mother's well-being.

➤*Children:* Children with chronic, recalcitrant, urea-splitting urinary infection may benefit from treatment with acetohydroxamic acid. However, detailed studies involving dosage and dose intervals in children have not been established. Children have tolerated a dose of 10 mg/kg/day, taken in 2 or 3 divided doses, satisfactorily for periods up to 1 year. Close monitoring of such patients is mandatory.

Precautions

➤*Hematologic effects:* Bone marrow depression (leukopenia, anemia, and thrombocytopenia) has occurred in experimental animals receiving large doses of acetohydroxamic acid, but has not been seen in man to date. Acetohydroxamic acid is a known inhibitor of DNA synthesis and also chelates metals, notably iron. Its bone marrow suppressant effect is probably related to its ability to inhibit DNA synthesis, but anemia could also be related to depletion of iron stores. To date, the only clinical effect noted has been hemolysis, with a decrease in the circulating red blood cells, hemoglobin and hematocrit. Abnormalities in platelet or white blood cell count have not been noted. However, clinical monitoring of the platelet and white cell count is recommended.

Drug Interactions

AHA Drug Interactions

Precipitant drug	Object drug*		Description
Alcoholic beverages	AHA	↑	Alcoholic beverages taken with AHA have caused rash
AHA	Heavy metals	↓	AHA chelates heavy metals, notably iron. The absorption of iron and AHA from the intestinal lumen may be reduced when both drugs are taken concomitantly. When iron is indicated, administer IM.

* ↑ = Object drug increased. ↓ = Object drug decreased.

ACETOHYDROXAMIC ACID — ORAL

Acetohydroxamic acid has been used concomitantly with insulin, oral and parenteral antibiotics, and progestational agents. No clinically significant interactions have been noted, but until wider clinical experience is obtained, acetohydroxamic acid should be used with caution in patients receiving other therapeutic agents.

➤*Drug/Food interactions:* Acetohydroxamic acid taken in association with alcoholic beverages has resulted in a rash (see Adverse Reactions).

Adverse Reactions

Experience with acetohydroxamic acid is limited. About 150 patients have been treated, most for periods of more than a year.

Adverse reactions have occurred in up to 30% of the patients receiving acetohydroxamic acid. In some instances the reactions were symptomatic; in others only changes in laboratory parameters were noted. Adverse reactions seem to be more prevalent in patients with preexisting thrombophlebitis or phlebothrombosis or in patients with advanced degrees of renal insufficiency. The risk of adverse reactions is highest during the first year of treatment. Chronic treatment does not seem to increase the risk nor the severity of adverse reactions.

The following reactions have been reported:

➤*Cardiovascular:* Superficial phlebitis involving the lower extremities has occurred in several patients on acetohydroxamic acid during the early (phase II) clinical trials. Several of the affected patients had had phlebitic episodes prior to treatment. One patient developed deep vein thrombosis of the lower extremities. The patient with phlebothrombosis had an associated traumatic injury to the groin. It is unclear whether the phlebitis was related to or exacerbated by treatment with acetohydroxamic acid. No patient in the 3 year controlled (phase III) clinical trial developed phlebitis. In all instances these vascular abnormalities returned to normal following appropriate medical therapy. Embolic phenomena have been reported in 3 patients taking acetohydroxamic acid in the phase II trial. The phlebitis and emboli resolved following discontinuation of acetohydroxamic acid and implementation of appropriate medical therapy. Several patients have resumed treatment with acetohydroxamic acid without ill effect. Palpitations have also been reported in patients taking acetohydroxamic acid.

➤*CNS:* Mild headaches are commonly reported (about 30%) during the first 48 hours of treatment. These headaches are mild, responsive to oral salicylate-type analgesics, and usually disappear spontaneously. The headaches have not been associated with vertigo, tinnitus, or visual or auditory abnormalities. Tremulousness and nervousness have also been reported.

➤*Dermatologic:* A nonpruritic, macular skin rash has occurred in the upper extremities and on the face of several patients taking acetohydroxamic acid on a long-term basis, usually when acetohydroxamic acid has been taken concomitantly with alcoholic beverages, but in a few patients in the absence of alcohol consumption. The rash commonly appears 30 to 45 minutes after ingestion of alcoholic beverages; it characteristically disappears spontaneously in 30 to 60 minutes. The rash may be associated with a general sensation of warmth. In some patients the rash is sufficiently severe to warrant discontinuation of treatment, but most patients have continued treatment, avoiding alcohol or using smaller quantities of it. Alopecia has also been reported in patients taking acetohydroxamic acid.

➤*GI:* Gastrointestinal symptoms, nausea, vomiting, anorexia, and malaise have occurred in 20% to 25% of patients. In most patients the symptoms were mild, transitory, and did not result in interruption of treatment. Approximately 3% of patients developed a hemolytic anemia of sufficient magnitude to warrant interruption in treatment; several of these patients also had symptoms of gastrointestinal upset.

➤*Hematologic:* Approximately 15% of patients have had laboratory findings characteristic of a hemolytic anemia. A mild reticulocytosis (5% to 6%) without anemia, is even more prevalent. The laboratory findings are occasionally accompanied by systemic symptoms such as malaise, lethargy and fatigue, and gastrointestinal symptoms. Symptoms and laboratory findings have invariably improved following cessation of treatment with acetohydroxamic acid. The hematological abnormalities are more prevalent in patients with advanced renal failure.

➤*Psychiatric:* Depression, anxiety, nervousness, and tremulousness have been observed in approximately 20% of patients taking acetohydroxamic acid. In most patients the symptoms were mild and transitory, but in about 6% of patients the symptoms were sufficiently distressing to warrant interruption or discontinuation of treatment.

➤*Respiratory:* No symptoms have been reported. Radiographic evidence of small pulmonary emboli has been seen in three patients with phlebitis in their lower legs.

Overdosage

➤*Symptoms:* Acute deliberate overdosage in man has not occurred, but would be expected to induce the following symptoms: Anorexia, malaise, lethargy, diminished sense of well-being, tremulousness, anxiety, nausea and vomiting. Laboratory findings are likely to include an elevated reticulocyte count and a severe hemolytic reaction requiring hospitalization, symptomatic treatment, and possibly blood transfusions. Concomitant reduction in platelets or white blood cells should be anticipated.

Milder overdosages resulting in hemolysis have occurred in an occasional patient with reduced renal function after several weeks or months of continuous treatment.

The acute LD_{50} of acetohydroxamic acid in animals (rats) is 4.8 g/kg.

➤*Treatment:* Recommended treatment for an overdosage reaction consists of cessation of treatment, close monitoring of hematologic status, symptomatic treatment, and blood transfusions as required by the clinical circumstances. The drug is probably dialyzable, but this property has not been tested clinically.

Patient Information

Advise patients that the daily dosage of acetohydroxamic acid is important to the proper treatment of their condition. Advise patients to report any unusual side effects to their health care provider.

GENITOURINARY IRRIGANTS

NEOMYCIN AND POLYMYXIN B IRRIGANT

Rx	**Neosporin G.U. Irrigant** (GlaxoWellcome)	**Solution:** 40 mg neomycin (as sulfate) and 200,000 units polymyxin B sulfate/ml	In 1 ml amps (10s and 50s) and 20 ml multidose vials.[a]

[a] With methylparaben.

NEOMYCIN AND POLYMYXIN B — IRRIGATION

Indications

➤*Urinary bladder irrigant:* Continuous irrigant or rinse for short-term use (up to 10 days) in the urinary bladder of abacteriuric patients to help prevent bacteriuria and gram-negative rod bacteremia associated with the use of indwelling catheters.

Administration and Dosage

Not for injection.

For use with catheter systems permitting continuous irrigation of the urinary bladder: Add 1 ml irrigant to 1 L isotonic saline solution. Connect the container to the inflow lumen of the three-way catheter. Connect the outflow lumen via a sterile disposable plastic tube to a disposable plastic collection bag.

Adjust flow rate to 1 L/24 hours. If the patient's urine output exceeds 2 L/day, increase flow rate to 2 L/24 hours.

The rinse of the bladder must be continuous. Do not interrupt the inflow or rinse solution for more than a few minutes.

Actions

➤*Pharmacology:* Polymyxin B sulfate is bactericidal to most gram-negative bacilli, particularly against *Pseudomonas* infections. Neomycin sulfate is bactericidal against a wide range of gram-negative organisms including *Proteus vulgaris* and gram-positive organisms. When used topically, these drugs are rarely irritating.

Contraindications

Hypersensitivity to any component.

Precautions

➤*Recent UT surgery:* Safety and efficacy have not been established for use in patients with recent lower urinary tract surgery.

➤*Neomycin toxicity:* Neomycin is nephrotoxic and ototoxic, particularly when given parenterally in higher than recommended doses. Cases of nephrotoxicity or ototoxicity have been reported following its topical use for extensive burns and wound irrigation. Although the possibility of these reactions is remote with use of the minimal amount in bladder irrigations, such reactions may occur if irrigations are continued beyond the recommended maximum of 10 days; observe caution.

➤*Superinfection:* Use of antibiotics (especially prolonged or repeated therapy) may result in bacterial or fungal overgrowth of nonsusceptible organisms. Such overgrowth may lead to a secondary infection. Appropriate measures should be taken if superinfection occurs.

Adverse Reactions

The prevalence of neomycin hypersensitivity has increased; however, topical application to mucous membranes rarely results in local or systemic reactions.

CITRIC ACID, GLUCONO-DELTA-LACTONE AND MAGNESIUM CARBONATE IRRIGANT (Hemiacidrin)

Rx	**Renacidin** (Guardian)	**Powder for Solution:** 156 to 171 g citric acid (anhydrous), 21 to 30 g d-gluconic acid (as lactone) w/75 to 87 g purified magnesium hydroxycarbonate, 9 to 15 g magnesium acid citrate, 2 to 6 g Ca (as carbonate) and 17 to 21 g water (combined & free)/300 g bottle	In 150 g.
		Solution: 6.602 g citric acid (anhydrous), 0.198 g glucono-delta-lactone, 3.177 g magnesium carbonate and 0.023 g benzoic acid/100 ml	In 500 ml.

CITRIC ACID, GLUCONO-DELTA-LACTONE AND MAGNESIUM CARBONATE (Hemiacidrin) — IRRIGATION

Indications

➤*Solution:* Local irrigation for dissolution of renal calculi composed of apatite (a calcium carbonate-phosphate compound) or struvite (magnesium ammonium phosphates) in patients who are not candidates for surgical removal of the calculi.

As adjunctive therapy to dissolve residual apatite or struvite calculi and fragments after surgery or to achieve partial dissolution of renal calculi to facilitate surgical removal.

For dissolution of bladder calculi of the struvite or apatite variety by local intermittent irrigation through a urethral catheter or cystostomy catheter as an alternative or adjunct to surgical procedures.

For use as an intermittent irrigating solution to prevent or minimize encrustations of indwelling urinary tract catheters.

➤*Powder for solution:* For use in preparing solutions for irrigating indwelling urethral catheters and the urinary bladder, to dissolve or prevent formation of calcifications.

➤*Unlabeled uses:* Hemiacidrin has been used as a renal pelvis irrigation, with meticulous attention to intrapelvic pressure and urosepsis.

Administration and Dosage

➤*Solution:*

Renal calculi – It is essential that patients be free from urinary tract infections prior to initiating chemolytic therapy. A nephrostomy tube is placed at surgery or percutaneously to permit lavage of the calculi. A single catheter may be sufficient if the calculus is not obstructing the ureter or ureteropelvic junction. In patients with an obstructed ureter, a retrograde catheter can be placed through the ureter to the renal pelvis via a cystoscope. This second catheter is used to irrigate the calculus while the percutaneous nephrostomy tube is used for drainage. Pressure measurements are made under fluoroscopy to assure that 2 to 3 ml/min can be infused without causing pain, pyelovenous or pyelotubular backflow or manometric evidence of elevated pressure within the collecting system. For postoperative patients, irrigation should not be started before the fourth or fifth postoperative day. Irrigation of the renal pelvis is begun with sterile saline only after a sterile urine has been demonstrated. The saline is infused at a rate of 60 ml/hr initially, and the rate is increased until pain or an elevated pressure (25 cm H_2O) appears, or until a maximum flow rate of 120 ml/hr is achieved. Inspect the site of insertion for leakage. If leakage occurs, the irrigation is discontinued temporarily to allow for complete healing around the nephrostomy tube.

If no leakage or flank pain occurs, start irrigation with hemiacidrin with a flow rate equal to maximum rate achieved with the saline solution. Place a clamp on the inflow tube and instruct patients and nursing personnel to stop the irrigating solution whenever pain develops. Nursing personnel who are responsible for performing the irrigation must be instructed concerning location of the nephrostomy tube(s) and direction of flow of irrigating solution to ensure against misconnection of inflowing and egress tubes. Perform nephrostomograms periodically to assure proper placement of catheter tip and to assess efficacy. If stones fail to change size after several days of adequate irrigation, discontinue the procedure.

Upon demonstration of complete dissolution of the calculus, the inflow tube is clamped and left in place for a few days to ensure that no obstruction exists, after which time the nephrostomy tube is removed.

Bladder calculi – Chemolysis of bladder calculi is used as an alternative to cystoscopic or surgical removal of the stones in patients who refuse surgery or cystoscopic removal or in whom these procedures constitute an unwarranted risk. Following appropriate studies to evaluate possible vesicoureteral reflux, 30 ml of hemiacidrin is instilled through a urinary catheter into the bladder and the catheter is clamped for 30 to 60 minutes. The clamp is then released and the bladder is drained. This is repeated 4 to 6 times a day. A continuous drip through a 3-way Foley catheter is an alternative means of dissolving bladder stones. In the presence of bladder spasm and associated high pressure reflux, all precautions required for irrigation of the renal pelvis must be observed.

Indwelling urinary tract catheter encrustation – Periodic instillation of hemiacidrin is indicated to minimize or prevent encrustation of indwelling catheters which frequently results in plugging of the catheter and discomfort to the patient. This is accomplished by instilling 30 ml of the solution through the catheter and then clamping the catheter for 10 minutes, after which the clamp is removed to allow drainage of the bladder. This process is repeated 3 times a day.

➤*Powder for solution:* Irrigating indwelling catheters – Administer as a 10% solution (sterile) in distilled water. Irrigation is carried out with 30 to 60 ml 2 to 3 times daily by means of a rubber syringe.

➤*Preparation of the solution:* Always add powder to the water; do not add water to the powder when preparing solutions.

Dissolve the contents of one 300 g bottle in 3000 ml of sterile distilled water, or any smaller quantity of powder in the proportionately smaller amount of water. Since powder may be reactive upon addition to water, add slowly to the water, with constant agitation, in a container larger than that which the amount of solution actually requires. Do not stopper or cap the container during preparation. Thoroughly mix the solution for as long as possible (up to 15 to 20 minutes). This can be achieved through the use of a mechanical mixer where available. Solutions often vary in color from almost colorless to a definite clear yellow solution.

After thorough mixing, filter the solution through a coarse filter to remove any undissolved matter. Alternatively, if desired, allow the solution to stand and decant. (A 10% solution was filtered after 24 hours and the residue dried at 105°C for 8 hours, then weighed. The weight of the residue equalled 0.008% of the solution.)

The residue which may be noted on a filter consists primarily of the insolubles present in the original magnesium hydroxycarbonate, which has about 0.03% to 0.05% acid insolubles in the form of a small amount of silica (or calcium, as the silicate) and iron oxides which remain undissolved when the solution is prepared. It may be yellow or even brown or black in color.

➤*Storage / Stability:*

Solution – Minimize exposure of hemiacidrin to heat or cold. Store at controlled room temperature (15° to 30°C; 59° to 86°F). Avoid excessive heat or cold (keep from freezing). Brief exposure to temperatures of up to 40°C (104°F) or temperatures down to 5°C (41°F) does not adversely affect the product.

Actions

➤*Pharmacology:* The action of hemiacidrin on susceptible apatite calculi results from an exchange of magnesium from the irrigating solution for the insoluble calcium contained in the stone matrix or calcification. The magnesium salts thereby formed are soluble in the gluconocitrate irrigating solution resulting in the dissolution of the calculus. Struvite calculi are composed mainly of magnesium ammonium phosphates which are solubilized by hemiacidrin due to its acidic pH.

Hemiacidrin is not effective for dissolution of calcium oxalate, uric acid or cysteine stones.

Contraindications

➤*Solution:* Urinary tract infections (see Warnings); presence of demonstrable urinary tract extravasation.

➤*Powder for solution:* Biliary calculi; therapy or preventive therapy above the ureteral-vesical junction, therefore contraindicated for use with ureteral catheters, nephrostomy or pyelostomy tubes or renal lavage for dissolving calculi.

Warnings

➤*Urinary tract infection:* Stop the drug immediately if patient develops fever, urinary tract infection, signs and symptoms consistent with urinary tract infection, persistent flank pain, or if hypermagnesemia or elevated serum creatinine develops.

Urea-splitting bacteria reside within struvite and apatite stones which therefore serve as a source of infection. Dissolution therapy with hemiacidrin in the presence of an infected urinary tract may lead to sepsis and death. Obtain urine specimens for culture prior to initiating chemolytic therapy of the renal pelvis. Institute appropriate antibiotic therapy to treat any infection detected. A sterile urine must be present prior to initiating therapy. An infected stone can serve as a continual source for infection; therefore, continue antibiotic therapy throughout the course of dissolution therapy.

➤*Severe hypermagnesemia:* Severe hypermagnesemia has occurred. Use caution when irrigating the renal pelvis of patients with impaired renal function. Observe patients for early signs and symptoms of hypermagnesemia including nausea, lethargy, confusion and hypotension. Severe hypermagnesemia may result in hyporeflexia, dyspnea, apnea, coma, cardiac arrest and subsequent death. Monitor serum magnesium levels and evaluate deep tendon reflexes. Treatment of hypermagnesemia should include discontinuation of hemiacidrin followed by therapy with IV calcium gluconate, fluids and diuresis in severe cases.

➤*Not indicated:* Not indicated for dissolution of calcium oxalate, uric acid or cysteine calculi.

➤*Pregnancy: Category C.* It is not known whether hemiacidrin can cause fetal harm when administered to a pregnant woman or can affect reproduction capacity. Give to a pregnant woman only if clearly needed.

➤*Lactation:* Magnesium is known to be excreted into breast milk. However, it is not known whether hemiacidrin is excreted in breast milk. Exercise caution when hemiacidrin is administered to a nursing woman.

Precautions

➤*Vesicoureteral reflux:* Vesicoureteral reflux frequently occurs in patients with indwelling urethral or cystostomy catheters. Cystogram prior to initiation of hemiacidrin is essential for such patients. If reflux is demonstrated, all precautions recommended for renal pelvis irrigation must be taken.

➤*Catheter care:* Hospitalization is prolonged for days to weeks when chemolytic therapy is used in lieu of, or following, surgery. Reserve this therapy for selected patients. Care must be taken during chemolysis of renal calculi with hemiacidrin to maintain the patency of the irrigating catheter. Calculus fragments and debris may obstruct the outflow catheter. Continued irrigation under those circumstances leads to increased intrapelvic pressure with a danger of tissue damage or absorption of the irrigating solution. Catheter outflow blockage may be prevented by flushing the catheter with saline and repositioning of the catheter. Frequent monitoring of the system should be performed by a nurse, an aide or any person with sufficient skills to be able to detect any problems with the patency of the catheter. At the first sign of obstruction, discontinue the irrigation and disconnect the system.

➤*Intrapelvic pressures:* Intrapelvic pressures must be maintained at or below 25 cm of water. The preferred method of pressure control is the insertion of an open Y connection pop-off valve into the infusion line allowing immediate decompression if pressure exceeds 25 cm of water. An alternative method has been proposed to direct or stop the flow of the irrigating solution to prevent increased intrapelvic pressure: Placement of a pinch clamp on the inflow line which can be used by the patient or nurse to stop the irrigation at the first sign of flank pain. However, extreme caution must be taken when

CITRIC ACID, GLUCONO-DELTA-LACTONE AND MAGNESIUM CARBONATE (Hemiacidrin) — IRRIGATION

relying on cooperation of the patient. Patients may not be sufficiently alert to detect signs and symptoms of outflow obstruction. This is especially true in elderly patients, sedated patients or those with severe neurological dysfunction with varying degrees of sensory loss or motor paralysis.

➤*Monitoring:* Throughout the course of therapy, monitor patients to ensure safety. Obtain serum creatinine phosphate and magnesium every few days. Collect urine specimens for culture and antibacterial sensitivity every 3 days or less and at the first sign of fever. Stop the irrigation if any culture exhibits growth and initiate appropriate antibacterial therapy. The irrigation may be started again after a course of antibacterial therapy upon demonstration of a sterile urine. Struvite calculi frequently contain bacteria within the stone; therefore, continue antibacterial therapy throughout the course of dissolution therapy. Hypermagnesemia or an elevated serum creatinine level are indications to halt the irrigation until they return to pre-irrigation levels. Evidence of severe urothelial edema on X-ray is also an indication for temporarily halting the irrigation until the complication resolves.

Drug Interactions

➤*Magnesium-containing medications:* Concurrent use may contribute to production of hypermagnesemia and is not recommended.

Adverse Reactions

Solution – The most common adverse reaction in selected case series is transient flank pain which occurs in most patients. Additional reactions include: Urothelial ulceration or edema (13%); fever (20% but up to 40% in some case series); urinary tract infection, back pain, dysuria, transient hematuria, nausea, hypermagnesemia, hyperphosphatemia, elevated serum creatinine, candidiasis, bladder irritability (1% to 10%); septicemia, ileus, vomiting, thrombophlebitis (less than 1%). Death from sepsis has occurred.

Powder for solution – Occasional temporary pain or burning sensation from this procedure; discontinue use if this occurs.

Hexitol Irrigants

Indications

In transurethral prostatic resection or other transurethral surgical procedures.

Administration and Dosage

Do not use unless solution is clear and seal unbroken. Use as required for irrigation.

➤*Storage/Stability:* Promptly use the contents of opened containers; discard unused portions of the solution. Do not warm above 66°C (150°F). Protect from freezing and avoid storage at temperatures above 40°C (104°F).

Actions

➤*Pharmacology:* Hexitol irrigants are nonelectrolytic and nonhemolytic urologic irrigation solutions. The amount of solution absorbed intravascularly during transurethral prostatic surgery is variable and depends primarily on the extent and duration of the surgery. Mannitol is confined to the extracellular space, only slightly metabolized, rapidly excreted in the urine and is, therefore, an effective osmotic diuretic. The sorbitol-containing products will be metabolized to carbon dioxide (70%) and dextrose (30%) or excreted by the kidneys.

Contraindications

Anuria; injection.

Warnings

➤*Special risk:* Use caution in significant cardiopulmonary or renal dysfunction (see Precautions).

➤*Systemic effects:* Irrigating fluids used during transurethral prostatectomy may enter the systemic circulation in relatively large volumes. Therefore, the irrigation solution must be considered as a systemic drug. The osmotic diuresis it may produce can significantly alter cardiopulmonary and renal dynamics.

➤*Diabetes mellitus:* Hyperglycemia from metabolism of sorbitol may occur in patients with diabetes mellitus.

➤*Sorbitol solution:* Use with caution in patients unable to metabolize sorbitol rapidly enough to avoid the development of hyperosmolar states.

Precautions

➤*Cardiovascular effects:* Carefully evaluate cardiovascular status of the patient, particularly one with cardiac disease, before and during transurethral prostatic resection when mannitol irrigant is used. The quantity of fluid absorbed into systemic circulation may cause expansion of extracellular fluid, leading to fulminating CHF.

➤*Fluid and electrolyte balance:* Systemic absorption of the solutions may cause a shift of sodium-free intracellular fluid into the extracellular compartment, lowering serum sodium concentration and aggravating any preexisting hyponatremia.

A significant diuresis resulting from the irrigating solution may obscure and intensify inadequate hydration or hypovolemia. Excessive loss of water and electrolytes may lead to hypernatremia.

Adverse Reactions

Since significant systemic absorption occurs, the potential for systemic effects must be considered. The following effects have been noted from intravenous infusion:

➤*Cardiovascular:* Pulmonary congestion; hypotension; tachycardia; angina-like pains; thrombophlebitis.

➤*Electrolyte disturbance:* Acidosis; electrolyte loss; marked diuresis; urinary retention; edema; dry mouth; thirst; dehydration.

➤*Miscellaneous:* Blurred vision; convulsions; nausea; vomiting; rhinitis; chills; vertigo; backache; urticaria; diarrhea.

Additional reactions associated with sorbitol solution include slight increases in postoperative serum glucose and inhibition of intestinal absorption of vitamin B_{12}.

MANNITOL

For mannitol prescribing information, see the Hexitol Irrigants group mono and the Mannitol monograph in the Osmotic Diuretics.

SORBITOL IRRIGATION

Rx	**Sorbitol** (Kendall McGaw)	**Solution:** 3.3% (183 mOsm/L)	In 2000 ml.
Rx	**Sorbitol** (Travenol)	**Solution:** 3% (165 mOsm/L)	In 1500 and 3000 ml.

SORBITOL — IRRIGATION

For complete and comparative prescribing information, refer to the Hexitol Irrigants group monograph.

MANNITOL AND SORBITOL

Rx	**Sorbitol-Mannitol** (Abbott)	**Solution:** 0.54 g mannitol and 2.7 g sorbitol/100 ml (178 mOsm/L)	In 1500 and 3000 ml.

MANNITOL AND SORBITOL — IRRIGATION

For complete and comparative prescribing information, refer to the Hexitol Irrigants group monograph.

SUBY'S SOLUTION G

Rx	**Suby's Solution G** (Various, eg, Abbott, Travenol)	**Solution:** 3.24 g citric acid (monohydrate), 0.43 g sodium carbonate (anhydrous) and 0.38 g magnesium oxide (anhydrous) per 100 ml	In 1000 ml.

SUBY'S SOLUTION G — IRRIGATION

Indications

To dissolve phosphatic calculi or incrustations in the bladder and urethra; to irrigate the bladder and urethra with an acidic solution.

Administration and Dosage

Not for IV, SC or IM injection.

Administer 1 to 3 liters daily by intermittent irrigation or by tidal instillation and drainage to allow continuous irrigation of the bladder for periods of several hours. Intermittent irrigation of the bladder (after the manner of intermittent peritoneal dialysis) may be preferred to promote more prolonged contact of the irrigation with bladder stones; tidal (continuous in and out flow) irrigation may be less efficient and require larger amounts of irrigation fluid.

Use contents of opened container promptly to minimize the possibility of bacterial growth or pyrogen formation. Do not use solution unless clear and seal is intact. Discard unused portion.

Contraindications

Do not use in presence of fulminating bladder infections, bleeding, ulcerations or other open wounds.

Not for injection into body tissue.

Not for irrigation during transurethral surgical procedures.

These solutions are conductive; do not use in the presence of electrical instrumentation.

Warnings

➤*Administration:* For use in irrigation of the lower urinary tract only.

➤*Pyelonephritis:* Not recommended for dissolving phosphate calculi in the renal pelvis because of the risk of creating back pressure that may reactivate an existing pyelonephritis.

➤*Do not use:* Do not use solution to replace other indicated measures including correction of underlying metabolic disorders, surgical intervention and treatment of infection.

➤*Pregnancy: Category C.* It is not known whether this irrigation solution can cause fetal harm when given to a pregnant woman or can affect reproduction capacity. Administer to a pregnant woman only if clearly needed.

Precautions

➤*Reflux:* Avoid reflux of the solution up the ureters into the renal pelvis. Repeated or continuous use may cause bleeding. Solution is irritating to urethra; after each treatment, irrigate with sterile saline or water.

➤*Sudden death:* Four cases of sudden death were reported during lavage therapy with a similarly acting solution. The autopsy indicated that calcium phosphate sludge resulting from dissolving stone is a severe irritant to the renal pelvis and is probably absorbed to some degree as evidenced by a terminal serum phosphorus of three times the normal level in one case. Disintegration of calculi into phosphate sludge by acids might form a variety of toxic compounds in small quantities. Since pyelonephritis accompanies renal calculus disease in many cases, pyelorenal backflow of chemicals may aggravate the infectious process causing progression to a severe toxemia.

Adverse Reactions

Discomfort or pain due to bladder irritation during irrigation. In the presence of undetected mucosal lesions, irrigation may initiate bleeding from the bladder.

ACETIC ACID FOR IRRIGATION

Rx	**Acetic Acid for Irrigation** (Various, eg, Abbott, Baxter, Kendall McGaw)	**Solution:** 0.25%	In 250, 500 and 1000 ml.

ACETIC ACID — IRRIGATION

Indications

For bladder irrigation.

GLYCINE (AMINOACETIC ACID) FOR IRRIGATION

Rx	**Glycine for Irrigation** (Various, eg, Hospira, Baxter, Kendall McGaw)	**Solution:** 1.5%	In 1500, 2000, 3000, 4000 and 5000 ml.

GLYCINE — IRRIGATION

Indications

Glycine irrigation 1.5% is indicated for use as irrigating fluid during transurethral prostatic resection and other transurethral surgical procedures.

Administration and Dosage

Glycine irrigation 1.5% should be administered only by transurethral instillation with appropriate urologic instrumentation. A disposable irrigation set should be used. The total volume of solution used for irrigation is solely at the discretion of the surgeon.

Height of container(s) above the operating table in excess of 60 cm (approximately 2 ft.) has been reported to increase intravascular absorption of the irrigating fluid.

➤*Incompatibilities:* Additives may be incompatible. Consult with pharmacist, if available. When introducing additives, use aseptic technique, mix thoroughly and do not store.

➤*Storage/Stability:* Exposure of pharmaceutical products to heat should be minimized. Avoid excessive heat. Protect from freezing. It is recommended that the product be stored at room temperature (25°C; 77°F).

Do not heat container over 66°C (150°F).

Parenteral drug products should be inspected visually for particulate matter and discoloration prior to administration, whenever solution container permits.

SODIUM CHLORIDE FOR IRRIGATION

Rx	**Sodium Chloride for Irrigation** (Various, eg, Abbott, Baxter, Kendall McGaw)	**Solution (Isotonic):** 0.9%	In 150, 250, 500, 1000, 1500, 2000 and 4000 ml.
Rx	**Sodium Chloride for Irrigation** (Various, eg, Abbott, Baxter)	**Solution (Hypotonic):** 0.45%	In 500, 1000 and 1500 ml.

SODIUM CHLORIDE — IRRIGATION

For sodium chloride prescribing information, see the Sodium Chloride monograph in the IV Nutritional Electrolytes section.

STERILE WATER FOR IRRIGATION

Rx	**Sterile Water for Irrigation** (Various, eg, Abbott, Baxter, Kendall McGaw)	In 250, 500, 1000, 2000 and 4000 ml.

STERILE WATER — IRRIGATION

Indications

For use as an irrigating solution.

CYSTINE-DEPLETING AGENTS

CYSTEAMINE BITARTRATE

Refer to the Cysteamine bitartrate monograph in the Endocrine Metabolic Agents chapter for full prescribing information.

TIOPRONIN

Rx	**Thiola** (Mission)	**Tablets:** 100 mg	(Mission SS 121). White. Sugar coated. In 100s.

TIOPRONIN — ORAL

Indications

➤*Kidney stones:* For the prevention of cystine (kidney) stone formation in patients with severe homozygous cystinuria with urinary cystine greater than 500 mg/day, who are resistant to treatment with conservative measures of high fluid intake, alkali and diet modification, or who have adverse reactions to d-penicillamine.

Administration and Dosage

➤*Approved by the FDA:* August 11, 1988.

It is recommended that a conservative treatment program should be attempted first. At least 3 L of fluid (ten 10 oz. glassfuls) should be provided, including 2 glasses with each meal and at bedtime. The patients should be expected to awake at night to urinate; they should drink 2 more glasses of fluids before returning to bed. Additional fluids should be consumed if there is excessive sweating or intestinal fluid loss. A minimum urine output of 2 L/day on a consistent basis should be sought. A modest amount of alkali should be provided in order to maintain urinary pH at a high normal range (6.5 to 7). Potassium alkali are advantageous over sodium alkali, because they do not cause hypercalciuria and are less likely to cause the complication of calcium stones.

Excessive alkali therapy is not advisable. When urinary pH increases above 7 with alkali therapy, the complication of calcium phosphate nephrolithiasis may ensue because of the enhanced urinary supersaturation of hydroxyapatite in an alkaline environment.

In patients who continue to form cystine stones on the above conservative program, tiopronin may be added to the treatment program. Tiopronin may also be substituted for d-penicillamine in patients who have developed toxicity to the latter drug. In both situations, the conservative treatment program should be continued.

The dose of tiopronin should not be arbitrary but should be based on that amount required to reduce urinary cystine concentration to below its solubility limit (generally less than 250 mg/L). The extent of the decline in cystine excretion is generally dependent on the tiopronin dosage.

Tiopronin may be begun at a dosage of 800 mg/day in adult patients with cystine stones. In a multiclinic trial, average dose of tiopronin was about 1000 mg/day. However, some patients require a smaller dose. In children, initial dosage may be based on 15 mg/kg/day. Urinary cystine should be measured at 1 month after tiopronin treatment, and every 3 months thereafter. Tiopronin dosage should be readjusted depending on the urinary cystine value. Whenever possible, tiopronin should be given in divided doses 3 times/day at least 1 hour before or 2 hours after meals.

In patients who had shown severe toxicity to d-penicillamine, tiopronin might be begun at a lower dosage.

➤*Storage / Stability:* Store at 25°C (77°F); excursions permitted to 15° to 30°C (59° to 86°F).

Actions

➤*Pharmacology:* Tiopronin is an active reducing agent which undergoes thiol-disulfide exchange with cystine to form a mixed disulfide of Thiola-cysteine.

From this reaction, a water-soluble mixed disulfide is formed and the amount of sparingly soluble cystine is reduced.

➤*Pharmacokinetics:* When tiopronin is given orally, up to 48% of dose appears in urine during the first 4 hours and up to 78% by 72 hours. Thus, in patients with cystinuria, sufficient amount of tiopronin or its active metabolites could appear in urine to react with cystine, lowering cystine excretion.

The decrement in urinary cystine produced by tiopronin is generally proportional to the dose. A reduction in urinary cystine of 250 to 350 mg/day at a tiopronin dosage of 1 g/day, and a decline of approximately 500 mg/day at a dosage of 2 g/day, might be expected. Tiopronin causes a sustained reduction in cystine excretion without apparent loss of effectiveness. Tiopronin has a rapid onset and offset of action, showing a fall in cystine excretion on the first day of administration and a rise on the first day of drug withdrawal.

Contraindications

The use of tiopronin during pregnancy is contraindicated, except in those with severe cystinuria where the anticipated benefit of inhibited stone formation clearly outweighs possible hazards of treatment (see Warnings).

Tiopronin should not be begun again in patients with a history of developing agranulocytosis, aplastic anemia or thrombocytopenia on this medication.

Mothers maintained on tiopronin treatment should not nurse their infants.

Warnings

Despite apparent lower toxicity of tiopronin, tiopronin may potentially cause all the serious adverse reactions reported for d-penicillamine. Thus, although no death has been reported to result directly from tiopronin treatment, a fatal outcome from tiopronin is possible, as has been reported with d-penicillamine therapy from such complications as aplastic anemia, agranulocytosis, thrombocytopenia, Goodpasture's syndrome or myasthenia gravis.

➤*Hematologic effects:* Leukopenia of the granulocytic series may develop without eosinophilia. Thrombocytopenia may be immunologic in origin or occur on an idiosyncratic basis. The reduction in peripheral blood white count to less than 3500/mm^3 or in platelet count to below 100,000 mm^3 mandates cessation of therapy. Patients should be instructed to report promptly the occurrence of any symptom or sign of these hematological abnormalities, such as fever, sore throat, chills, bleeding or easy bruisability.

➤*Proteinuria:* Proteinuria, sometimes sufficiently severe to cause nephrotic syndrome, may develop from membranous glomerulopathy. A close observation of affected patients is mandatory.

➤*Complications:* The following complications, though rare, have been reported during d-penicillamine therapy and could occur during tiopronin treatment. When there are abnormal urinary findings associated with hemoptysis and pulmonary infiltrates suggestive of Goodpasture's syndrome, tiopronin treatment should be stopped. Appearance of myasthenic syndrome or myasthenia gravis requires cessation of treatment. When pemphigus-type reactions develop, tiopronin therapy should be stopped. Steroid treatment may be necessary.

➤*Fertility impairment:* High doses of tiopronin in experimental animals have been shown to interfere with maintenance of pregnancy and viability of the fetus.

➤*Pregnancy: Category C.* D-penicillamine has been shown to cause skeletal defects and cleft palates in the fetus when given to pregnant rats at 10 times the dose recommended for human use. A similar teratogenicity might be expected for tiopronin although no such findings could be related to the drug in studies in mice and rats at doses up to 10 times the highest recommended human dose. There are no adequate and well-controlled studies in pregnant women. Tiopronin should be used during pregnancy only if the potential benefit justifies potential risk to the fetus.

➤*Lactation:* Because tiopronin may be excreted in milk and because of the potential serious adverse reactions of nursing infants from tiopronin, mothers taking tiopronin should not nurse their infants.

➤*Children:* Safety and effectiveness below the age of 9 years have not been established.

Precautions

➤*Monitoring:* To help monitor potential complications, the following tests are recommended: peripheral blood counts, direct platelet count, hemoglobin, serum albumin, liver function tests, 24-hour urinary protein and routine urinalysis at 3– to 6–month intervals during treatment. In order to assess effect on stone disease, urinary cystine analysis should be monitored frequently during the first 6 months when the optimum dose schedule is being determined, and at 6-month intervals thereafter. Abdominal roentogenogram (KUB) is advised on a yearly basis to monitor the size and appearance/disappearance of stone(s).

➤*Complications:* Patients should be advised of the potential development of complications and to report promptly the occurrence of any symptom or sign of them.

Adverse Reactions

Some patients may develop drug fever, usually during the first month of therapy. Tiopronin treatment should be discontinued until the fever subsides. It may be reinstated at a small dose, with a gradual increase in dosage until the desired level is achieved.

A generalized rash (erythematous, maculopapular or morbilliform) accompanied by pruritus may develop during the first few months of treatment. It may be controlled by antihistamine therapy, typically recedes when tiopronin treatment is discontinued, and seldom recurs when tiopronin treatment is restarted at a lower dosage. Less commonly, rash may appear late in the course of treatment (of more than 6 months). Located usually in the trunk, the late rash is associated with intense pruritus, recedes slowly after discontinuing treatment, and usually recurs upon resumption of treatment.

A drug reaction simulating lupus erythematous, manifested by fever, arthralgia and lymphadenopathy may develop. It may be associated with a positive antinuclear antibody test, but not necessarily with nephropathy. It may require discontinuance of tiopronin treatment.

A reduction in taste perception may develop. It is believed to be the result of chelation of trace metals by tiopronin. Hypogeusia is often self-limiting.

Unlike during d-penicillamine therapy, vitamin B_6 deficiency is uncommonly associated with tiopronin treatment.

Some patients may complain of wrinkling and friability of skin. This complication usually occurs after long-term treatment, and is believed to result from the effect of tiopronin on collagen.

A multiclinic trial involving 66 cystinuric patients in the United States indicated that tiopronin is associated with fewer or less severe adverse reactions than d-penicillamine. Among those who had to stop taking d-penicillamine due to toxicity, 64.7% could take tiopronin. In those without history of d-penicillamine treatment, only 5.9% developed reactions of sufficient severity to require tiopronin withdrawal. A review of available literature supports the findings from this trial.

Despite this apparent reduced toxicity to tiopronin relative to d-penicillamine, tiopronin treatment may potentially be associated with all the adverse reactions reported with d-penicillamine. They include:

➤*CNS:* Myasthenic syndrome in about 1 in 50 patients.

➤*Dermatologic:* Pharyngitis, oral ulcers, rash, ecchymosis, pruritus, urticaria, warts, skin wrinkling, pemphigus, elastosis perforans serpiginosa in about 1 in 6 patients.

TIOPRONIN — ORAL

➤*GI:* Nausea, emesis, diarrhea or softstools, anorexia, abdominal pain, bloating or flatus in about 1 in 6 patients.

➤*Hematologic:* Increased bleeding, anemia, leukopenia, thrombocytopenia, eosinophilia in about 1 in 25 patients.

➤*Hepatic:* Jaundice and abnormal liver function tests have been reported during tiopronin therapy for non-cystinuric conditions. A direct cause and effect relationship, based upon these foreign reports, has not been established. Although such complications were not encountered in the small multi-center trials in the United States, patients should be carefully monitored and if any abnormalities are noted, the drug should be discontinued and the patient treated by appropriate measures.

➤*Hypersensitivity:* Laryngeal edema, dyspnea, respiratory distress, fever, chills, arthralgia, weakness, fatigue, myalgia, adenopathy in about 1 in 25 patients.

➤*Pulmonary:* Bronchiolitis, hemoptysis, pulmonary infiltrates, dyspnea in about 1 in 50 patients.

➤*Renal:* Proteinuria, nephrotic syndrome, hematuria in about 1 in 20 patients.

➤*Special senses:* Impairment in taste and smell in about 1 in 25 patients. These reactions are more likely to develop during tiopronin therapy among patients who had previously shown toxicity to d-penicillamine.

In patients who had previously manifested adverse reactions to d-penicillamine, adverse reactions to tiopronin are more likely to occur than in patients who took tiopronin for the first time. A close supervision with a careful monitoring of potential side effects is mandatory during tiopronin treatment. Patients should be told to report promptly any symptoms suggesting toxicity. The treatment with tiopronin should be stopped if severe toxicity develops.

PENICILLAMINE

Rx	**Cuprimine** (Merck)	**Capsules:** 125 mg	Lactose. (MSD 672). Opaque yellow and gray. In 100s.
		250 mg	Lactose. (MSD 602). Ivory. In 100s.
Rx	**Depen** (Wallace)	**Tablets, titratable:** 250 mg	Lactose, EDTA. (37-4401). White. Scored. Oval. In 100s.

PENICILLAMINE — ORAL

WARNING

Physicians planning to use penicillamine should thoroughly familiarize themselves with its toxicity, special dosage considerations, and therapeutic benefits. Penicillamine should never be used casually. Each patient should remain constantly under the close supervision of the physician. Patients should be warned to report promptly any symptoms suggesting toxicity.

Indications

For the treatment of Wilson's disease, cystinuria, and in patients with severe, active rheumatoid arthritis who have failed to respond to an adequate trial of conventional therapy.

➤*Rheumatoid arthritis:* Because penicillamine can cause severe adverse reactions, restrict its use in rheumatoid arthritis to patients who have severe, active disease and who have failed to respond to an adequate trial of conventional therapy. Even then, carefully consider the benefit-to-risk ratio. Use other measures, such as rest, physiotherapy, salicylates, and corticosteroids, when indicated, in conjunction with penicillamine.

Administration and Dosage

➤*Administration:* In all patients receiving penicillamine, it is important that penicillamine be given on an empty stomach, at least 1 hour before meals or 2 hours after meals, and at least 1 hour apart from any other drug, food, or milk. Because penicillamine increases the requirement for pyridoxine, patients may require a daily supplement of pyridoxine.

➤*Wilson's disease:* Optimal dosage can be determined by measurement of urinary copper excretion and the determination of free copper in the serum. The urine must be collected in copper-free glassware, and should be quantitatively analyzed for copper before and soon after initiation of therapy with penicillamine.

Determination of 24-hour urinary copper excretion is of greatest value in the first week of therapy with penicillamine. In the absence of any drug reaction, continue a dose between 0.75 and 1.5 g that results in an initial 24-hour cupriuresis of over 2 mg for about 3 months, by which time the most reliable method of monitoring maintenance treatment is the determination of free copper in the serum. This equals the difference between quantitatively determined total copper and ceruloplasmin-copper. Adequately treated patients will usually have less than 10 mcg free copper/dL of serum. It is seldom necessary to exceed a dosage of 2 g/day. If the patient is intolerant to therapy with penicillamine, alternative treatment is trientine hydrochloride.

In patients who cannot tolerate as much as 1 g/day initially, initiating dosage with 250 mg/day, and increasing gradually to the requisite amount, gives closer control of the effects of the drug and may help to reduce the incidence of adverse reactions.

➤*Cystinuria:* It is recommended that penicillamine be used along with conventional therapy. By reducing urinary cystine, it decreases crystalluria and stone formation. In some instances, it has been reported to decrease the size of, and even to dissolve, stones already formed.

The usual dosage of penicillamine in the treatment of cystinuria is 2 g/day for adults, with a range of 1 to 4 g/day. For pediatric patients, dosage can be based on 30 mg/kg/day. Divide the total daily amount into 4 doses. If 4 equal doses are not feasible, give the larger portion at bedtime. If adverse reactions necessitate a reduction in dosage, it is important to retain the bedtime dose.

Initiating dosage with 250 mg/day, and increasing gradually to the requisite amount, gives closer control of the effects of the drug and may help to reduce the incidence of adverse reactions.

In addition to taking penicillamine, patients should drink copiously. It is especially important to drink about a pint of fluid at bedtime and another pint once during the night when urine is more concentrated and more acid than during the day. The greater the fluid intake, the lower the required dosage of penicillamine.

Dosage must be individualized to an amount that limits cystine excretion to 100 to 200 mg/day in those with no history of stones, and below 100 mg/day in those who have had stone formation and/or pain. Thus, in determining dosage, the inherent tubular defect, the patient's size, age, and rate of growth, and his diet and water intake all must be taken into consideration.

The standard nitroprusside cyanide test has been reported useful as a qualitative measure of the effective dose: Add 2 mL of freshly prepared 5% sodium cyanide to 5 mL of a 24-hour aliquot of protein-free urine and let stand 10 minutes. Add 5 drops of freshly prepared 5% sodium nitroprusside and mix. Cystine will turn the mixture magenta. If the result is negative, it can be assumed that cystine excretion is less than 100 mg/g creatinine.

Although penicillamine is rarely excreted unchanged, it also will turn the mixture magenta. If there is any question as to which substance is causing the reaction, a ferric chloride test can be done to eliminate doubt: Add 3% ferric chloride dropwise to the urine. Penicillamine will turn the urine an immediate and quickly fading blue. Cystine will not produce any change in appearance.

➤*Rheumatoid arthritis:* The principal rule of treatment with penicillamine in rheumatoid arthritis is patience. The onset of therapeutic response is typically delayed. Two or 3 months may be required before the first evidence of a clinical response is noted.

When treatment with penicillamine has been interrupted because of adverse reactions or other reasons, reintroduce the drug cautiously by starting with a lower dosage and increasing slowly.

Initial therapy – The currently recommended dosage regimen in rheumatoid arthritis begins with a single daily dose of 125 mg or 250 mg which is thereafter increased at 1- to 3-month intervals, by 125 mg or 250 mg/day, as patient response and tolerance indicate. If a satisfactory remission of symptoms is achieved, continue the dose associated with the remission. If there is no improvement and there are no signs of potentially serious toxicity after 2 to 3 months of treatment with doses of 500 to 750 mg/day, increases of 250 mg/day at 2- to 3-month intervals may be continued until a satisfactory remission occurs or signs of toxicity develop. If there is no discernible improvement after 3 to 4 months of treatment with 1,000 to 1,500 mg penicillamine/day, it may be assumed the patient will not respond and penicillamine should be discontinued.

Maintenance therapy – The maintenance dosage of penicillamine must be individualized, and may require adjustment during the course of treatment. Many patients respond satisfactorily to a dosage within the 500 to 750 mg/day range. Some need less.

Changes in maintenance dosage levels may not be reflected clinically or in the erythrocyte sedimentation rate for 2 to 3 months after each dosage adjustment.

Some patients will subsequently require an increase in the maintenance dosage to achieve maximal disease suppression. In those patients who do respond, but who evidence incomplete suppression of their disease after the first 6 to 9 months of treatment, the daily dosage of penicillamine may be increased by 125 mg or 250 mg/day at 3-month intervals. It is unusual in current practice to employ a dosage in excess of 1 g/day, but up to 1.5 g/day has sometimes been required.

Management of exacerbations – During the course of treatment, some patients may experience an exacerbation of disease activity following an initial good response. These may be self-limited and can subside within 12 weeks. They are usually controlled by the addition of nonsteroidal anti-inflammatory drugs, and only if the patient has demonstrated a true "escape" phenomenon (as evidenced by failure of the flare to subside within this time period) should an increase in the maintenance dose ordinarily be considered.

In the rheumatoid patient, migratory polyarthralgia due to penicillamine is extremely difficult to differentiate from an exacerbation of the rheumatoid arthritis. Discontinuance or a substantial reduction in dosage of penicillamine for up to several weeks will usually determine which of these processes is responsible for the arthralgia.

Duration of therapy – The optimum duration of therapy with penicillamine in rheumatoid arthritis has not been determined. If the patient has been in remission for 6 months or more, a gradual, stepwise dosage reduction in decrements of 125 mg or 250 mg/day at approximately 3-month intervals may be attempted.

PENICILLAMINE — ORAL

Concomitant drug therapy – Do not use penicillamine in patients who are receiving gold therapy, antimalarial or cytotoxic drugs, oxyphenbutazone, or phenylbutazone. Other measures, such as salicylates, other nonsteroidal anti-inflammatory drugs, or systemic corticosteroids, may be continued when penicillamine is initiated. After improvement commences, analgesic and anti-inflammatory drugs may be slowly discontinued as symptoms permit. Steroid withdrawal must be done gradually, and many months of treatment with penicillamine may be required before steroids can be completely eliminated.

Dosage frequency – Based on clinical experience dosages up to 500 mg/day can be given as a single daily dose. Administer dosages in excess of 500 mg/day in divided doses.

➤*Storage / Stability:* Keep container tightly closed.

Actions

➤*Pharmacology:* Penicillamine is a chelating agent recommended for the removal of excess copper in patients with Wilson's disease. From in vitro studies which indicate that 1 atom of copper combines with 2 molecules of penicillamine, it would appear that 1 g of penicillamine should be followed by the excretion of about 200 mg of copper; however, the actual amount excreted is about 1% of this.

Penicillamine also reduces excess cystine excretion in cystinuria. This is done, at least in part, by disulfide interchange between penicillamine and cystine, resulting in formation of penicillamine-cysteine disulfide, a substance that is much more soluble than cystine and is excreted readily.

Penicillamine interferes with the formation of cross-links between tropocollagen molecules and cleaves them when newly formed.

The mechanism of action of penicillamine in rheumatoid arthritis is unknown although it appears to suppress disease activity. Unlike cytotoxic immunosuppressants, penicillamine markedly lowers IgM rheumatoid factor but produces no significant depression in absolute levels of serum immunoglobulins. Also unlike cytotoxic immunosuppressants which act on both, penicillamine in vitro depresses T-cell activity but not B-cell activity.

In vitro, penicillamine dissociates macroglobulins (rheumatoid factor) although the relationship of the activity to its effect in rheumatoid arthritis is not known.

In rheumatoid arthritis, the onset of therapeutic response to penicillamine may not be seen for 2 or 3 months. In those patients who respond, however, the first evidence of suppression of symptoms such as pain, tenderness, and swelling is generally apparent within 3 months. The optimum duration of therapy has not been determined. If remissions occur, they may last from months to years, but usually require continued treatment.

In all patients receiving penicillamine, it is important that penicillamine be given on an empty stomach, at least 1 hour before meals or 2 hours after meals, and at least 1 hour apart from any other drug, food, or milk. This permits maximum absorption and reduces the likelihood of inactivation by metal binding in the gastrointestinal tract.

➤*Pharmacokinetics:*

Absorption – Penicillamine is absorbed rapidly but incompletely (40% to 70%) from the gastrointestinal tract, with wide interindividual variations. Food, antacids, and iron reduce absorption of the drug. The peak plasma concentration of penicillamine occurs 1 to 3 hours after ingestion; it is approximately 1 to 2 mg/L after an oral dose of 250 mg. The drug appears in the plasma as free penicillamine, penicillamine disulfide, and cysteine-penicillamine disulfide. When prolonged treatment is stopped, there is a slow elimination phase lasting 4 to 6 days.

More than 80% of plasma penicillamine is bound to proteins. The drug also binds to erythrocytes and macrophages.

Metabolism / Excretion – A small fraction of the dose is metabolized in the liver to s-methyl-D-penicillamine. Drug excretion is primarily renal, mainly as disulfides.

Contraindications

Except for the treatment of Wilson's disease or certain cases of cystinuria, use of penicillamine during pregnancy is contraindicated.

Although breast milk studies have not been reported in animals or humans, mothers on therapy with penicillamine should not nurse their infants.

Patients with a history of penicillamine-related aplastic anemia or agranulocytosis should not be restarted on penicillamine.

Because of its potential for causing renal damage, penicillamine should not be administered to rheumatoid arthritis patients with a history or other evidence of renal insufficiency.

Warnings

➤*Fatalities:* The use of penicillamine has been associated with fatalities due to certain diseases such as aplastic anemia, agranulocytosis, thrombocytopenia, Goodpasture's syndrome, and myasthenia gravis.

➤*Hematologic effects:* Leukopenia and thrombocytopenia have been reported to occur in up to 5% of patients during penicillamine therapy. Leukopenia is of the granulocytic series and may or may not be associated with an increase in eosinophils. A confirmed reduction in WBC below 3,500/mm^3 mandates discontinuance of penicillamine therapy. Thrombocytopenia may be on an idiosyncratic basis, with decreased or absent megakaryocytes in the marrow, when it is part of an aplastic anemia. In other cases the thrombocytopenia is presumably on an immune basis since the number of megakaryocytes in the marrow has been reported to be normal or sometimes increased. The development of a platelet count below 100,000/mm^3, even in the absence of clinical bleeding, requires at least temporary cessation of penicillamine therapy. A progressive fall in either platelet count or WBC in 3 successive determinations, even though values are still within the normal range, likewise requires at least temporary cessation.

➤*Goodpasture's syndrome:* Goodpasture's syndrome has occurred rarely. The development of abnormal urinary findings associated with hemoptysis and pulmonary infiltrates on x-ray requires immediate cessation of penicillamine.

➤*Obliterative bronchiolitis:* Obliterative bronchiolitis has been reported rarely. Caution the patient to report immediately pulmonary symptoms such as exertional dyspnea, unexplained cough or wheezing. Pulmonary function studies should be considered at that time.

➤*CNS effects:* Onset of new neurologic symptoms has been reported with penicillamine. Occasionally, neurologic symptoms become worse during initiation of therapy with penicillamine. Myasthenic syndrome sometimes progressing to myasthenia gravis has been reported. Ptosis and diplopia, with weakness of the extraocular muscles, are often early signs of myasthenia. In the majority of cases, symptoms of myasthenia have receded after withdrawal of penicillamine.

➤*Pemphigus vulgaris:* Most of the various forms of pemphigus have occurred during treatment with penicillamine. Pemphigus vulgaris and pemphigus foliaceus are reported most frequently, usually as a late complication of therapy. The seborrhea-like characteristics of pemphigus foliaceus may obscure an early diagnosis. When pemphigus is suspected, discontinue penicillamine. Treatment has consisted of high doses of corticosteroids alone or, in some cases, concomitantly with an immunosuppressant. Treatment may be required for only a few weeks or months, but may need to be continued for more than a year.

➤*Administration:* Once instituted for Wilson's disease or cystinuria, treatment with penicillamine should, as a rule, be continued on a daily basis. Interruptions for even a few days have been followed by sensitivity reactions after reinstitution of therapy.

➤*Hypersensitivity reactions:* Observe the skin and mucous membranes for allergic reactions. Early and late rashes have occurred. Early rash occurs during the first few months of treatment and is more common. It is usually a generalized pruritic, erythematous, maculopapular, or morbilliform rash and resembles the allergic rash seen with other drugs. Early rash usually disappears within days after stopping penicillamine and seldom recurs when the drug is restarted at a lower dosage. Pruritus and early rash may often be controlled by the concomitant administration of antihistamines. Less commonly, a late rash may be seen, usually after 6 months or more of treatment, and requires discontinuation of penicillamine. It is usually on the trunk, is accompanied by intense pruritus, and is usually unresponsive to topical corticosteroid therapy. Late rash may take weeks to disappear after penicillamine is stopped and usually recurs if the drug is restarted.

The appearance of a drug eruption accompanied by fever, arthralgia, lymphadenopathy, or other allergic manifestations usually requires discontinuation of penicillamine.

➤*Renal function impairment:* Proteinuria and/or hematuria may develop during therapy and may be warning signs of membranous glomerulopathy which can progress to a nephrotic syndrome. Close observation of these patients is essential. In some patients the proteinuria disappears with continued therapy; in others, penicillamine must be discontinued. When a patient develops proteinuria or hematuria, the physician must ascertain whether it is a sign of drug-induced glomerulopathy or is unrelated to penicillamine.

Rheumatoid arthritis patients who develop moderate degrees of proteinuria may be continued cautiously on penicillamine therapy, provided that quantitative 24-hour urinary protein determinations are obtained at intervals of 1 to 2 weeks. Do not increase the penicillamine dosage under these circumstances. Proteinuria which exceeds 1 g per 24 hours, or proteinuria which is progressively increasing, requires either discontinuance of the drug or a reduction in the dosage. In some patients, proteinuria has been reported to clear following reduction in dosage.

In rheumatoid arthritis patients, penicillamine should be discontinued if unexplained gross hematuria or persistent microscopic hematuria develops.

In patients with Wilson's disease or cystinuria, the risks of continued penicillamine therapy in patients manifesting potentially serious urinary abnormalities must be weighed against the expected therapeutic benefits.

Up to 1 year or more may be required for any urinary abnormalities to disappear after penicillamine has been discontinued.

➤*Carcinogenesis:* Long-term animal carcinogenicity studies have not been done with penicillamine. There is a report that 5 of 10 autoimmune disease-prone NZB hybrid mice developed lymphocytic leukemia after a 6-month intraperitoneal treatment with a dose of 400 mg/kg penicillamine 5 days per week.

➤*Pregnancy:* Penicillamine has been shown to be teratogenic in rats when given in doses 6 times higher than the highest dose recommended for human use. Skeletal defects, cleft palates and fetal toxicity (resorptions) have been reported.

There are no controlled studies on the use of penicillamine in pregnant women. Although normal outcomes have been reported, characteristic congenital cutis laxa and associated birth defects have been reported in infants born of mothers who received therapy with penicillamine during pregnancy. Use penicillamine in women of childbearing potential only when the expected benefits outweigh the possible hazards. Apprise women on therapy with penicillamine who are of childbearing potential of this risk. Advise them to report promptly any missed menstrual periods or other indications of possible pregnancy, and to follow closely for early recognition of pregnancy.

See Contraindications for more information.

Wilson's disease – Reported experience shows that continued treatment with penicillamine throughout pregnancy protects the mother against

PENICILLAMINE — ORAL

relapse of the Wilson's disease, and that discontinuation of penicillamine has deleterious effects on the mother.

If penicillamine is administered during pregnancy to patients with Wilson's disease, it is recommended that the daily dosage be limited to 750 mg. If cesarean section is planned, reduce the daily dose to 250 mg, but not lower, for the last 6 weeks of pregnancy and postoperatively until wound healing is complete.

Cystinuria – If possible, do not give penicillamine during pregnancy to women with cystinuria. There are reports of women with cystinuria on therapy with penicillamine who gave birth to infants with generalized connective tissue defects who died following abdominal surgery. If stones continue to form in these patients, the benefits of therapy to the mother must be evaluated against the risk to the fetus.

Rheumatoid arthritis – Do not administer penicillamine to rheumatoid arthritis patients who are pregnant, and discontinue the drug promptly in patients in whom pregnancy is suspected or diagnosed.

There is a report that a woman with rheumatoid arthritis treated with less than 1 g a day of penicillamine during pregnancy gave birth (cesarean delivery) to an infant with growth retardation, flattened face with broad nasal bridge, low set ears, short neck with loose skin folds, and unusually lax body skin.

➤*Lactation:* Although breast milk studies have not been reported in animals or humans, mothers on therapy with penicillamine should not nurse their infants.

➤*Children:* The efficacy of penicillamine in juvenile rheumatoid arthritis has not been established.

Precautions

➤*Monitoring:* Because of the potential for serious hematological and renal adverse reactions to occur at any time, routine urinalysis, white and differential blood cell count, hemoglobin determination, and direct platelet count must be done twice weekly, together with monitoring of the patient's skin, lymph nodes and body temperature, during the first month of therapy, every 2 weeks for the next 5 months, and monthly thereafter. Patients should be instructed to report promptly the development of signs and symptoms of granulocytopenia and/or thrombocytopenia such as fever, sore throat, chills, bruising, or bleeding. The above laboratory studies should then be promptly repeated.

When penicillamine is used in cystinuria, an annual x-ray for renal stones is advised. Cystine stones form rapidly, sometimes in 6 months.

Because of rare reports of intrahepatic cholestasis and toxic hepatitis, liver function tests are recommended every 6 months for the duration of therapy. In Wilson's disease, these are recommended every 3 months, at least during the first year of treatment.

➤*Drug fever:* Some patients may experience drug fever, a marked febrile response to penicillamine, usually in the second to third week following initiation of therapy. Drug fever may sometimes be accompanied by a macular cutaneous eruption.

In the case of drug fever in patients with Wilson's disease or cystinuria, temporarily discontinue penicillamine until the reaction subsides. Then reinstitute penicillamine with a small dose that is gradually increased until the desired dosage is attained. Systemic steroid therapy may be necessary, and is usually helpful, in such patients in whom drug fever and rash develop several times.

In the case of drug fever in rheumatoid arthritis patients, because other treatments are available, discontinue penicillamine and try another therapeutic alternative. Experience indicates that the febrile reaction will recur in a very high percentage of patients upon readministration of penicillamine.

➤*Antibody development:* Certain patients will develop a positive antinuclear antibody (ANA) test and some of these may show a lupus erythematosus-like syndrome similar to drug-induced lupus associated with other drugs. The lupus erythematosus-like syndrome is not associated with hypocomplementemia and may be present without nephropathy. The development of a positive ANA test does not mandate discontinuance of the drug; however, be alert to the possibility that a lupus erythematosus-like syndrome may develop in the future.

➤*Oral ulcerations:* Some patients may develop oral ulcerations which in some cases have the appearance of aphthous stomatitis. The stomatitis usually recurs on rechallenge but often clears on a lower dosage. Although rare, cheilosis, glossitis and gingivostomatitis have also been reported. These oral lesions are frequently dose-related and may preclude further increase in penicillamine dosage or require discontinuation of the drug.

➤*Hypogeusia:* Hypogeusia (a blunting or diminution in taste perception) has occurred in some patients. This may last 2 to 3 months or more and may develop into a total loss of taste; however, it is usually self-limited despite continued penicillamine treatment. Such taste impairment is rare in patients with Wilson's disease.

➤*Concomitant medications:* See Drug Interactions for more information.

➤*Cross-sensitivity:* Patients who are allergic to penicillin may theoretically have cross-sensitivity to penicillamine. The possibility of reactions from contamination of penicillamine by trace amounts of penicillin has been eliminated now that penicillamine is being produced synthetically rather than as a degradation product of penicillin.

➤*Vitamin supplementation:* Give patients with Wilson's disease or cystinuria 25 mg/day pyridoxine during therapy, since penicillamine increases the requirement for this vitamin. Patients also may receive benefit from a multivitamin preparation, although there is no evidence that deficiency of any vitamin other than pyridoxine is associated with penicillamine. In Wilson's disease, multivitamin preparations must be copper-free.

Rheumatoid arthritis patients whose nutrition is impaired should also be given a daily supplement of pyridoxine. Do not give mineral supplements because they may block the response to penicillamine.

Iron deficiency may develop, especially in pediatric patients and in menstruating women. In Wilson's disease, this may be a result of adding the effects of the low copper diet, which is probably also low in iron, and the penicillamine to the effects of blood loss or growth. In cystinuria, a low methionine diet may contribute to iron deficiency, since it is necessarily low in protein. If necessary, iron may be given in short courses, but a period of 2 hours should elapse between administration of penicillamine and iron, since oral iron has been shown to reduce the effects of penicillamine.

➤*Collagen and elastin effects:* Penicillamine causes an increase in the amount of soluble collagen. In the rat this results in inhibition of normal healing and also a decrease in tensile strength of intact skin. In man this may be the cause of increased skin friability at sites especially subject to pressure or trauma, such as shoulders, elbows, knees, toes, and buttocks. Extravasations of blood may occur and may appear as purpuric areas, with external bleeding if the skin is broken, or as vesicles containing dark blood. Neither type is progressive. There is no apparent association with bleeding elsewhere in the body and no associated coagulation defect has been found. Therapy with penicillamine may be continued in the presence of these lesions. They may not recur if dosage is reduced. Other reported effects probably due to the action of penicillamine on collagen are excessive wrinkling of the skin and development of small, white papules at venipuncture and surgical sites.

The effects of penicillamine on collagen and elastin make it advisable to consider a reduction in dosage to 250 mg/day, when surgery is contemplated. Delay reinstitution of full therapy until wound healing is complete.

Drug Interactions

Penicillamine Drug Interactions

Precipitant drug	Object drug*		Description
Penicillamine	Digoxin	⬇	Digoxin serum levels may be reduced, possibly decreasing its pharmacological effects. The digoxin dose may need to be increased.
Penicillamine	Gold therapy, antimalarial or cytotoxic drugs, oxyphenbutazone or pheylbutazone	⬆	Do not use these drugs in patients who are concurrently receiving penicillamine. These drugs are associated with similar serious hematologic and renal reactions.
Penicillamine	Gold salts	⬆	Patients who have had **gold salt** therapy discontinued due to a major toxic reaction may be at greater risk of serious adverse reactions with penicillamine, but not necessarily of the same type. However, this is controversial.
Antacids	Penicillamine	⬇	The absorption of penicillamine is decreased by 66% with coadministration of antacids.
Iron salts	Penicillamine	⬇	The absorption of penicillamine is decreased by 35% with coadministration of iron salts.

* ⬆ = Object drug increased. ⬇ = Object drug decreased.

➤*Drug/Food interactions:* The absorption of penicillamine is decreased by 52% when taken with food.

Adverse Reactions

Penicillamine is a drug with a high incidence of untoward reactions, some of which are potentially fatal. Therefore, it is mandatory that patients receiving penicillamine therapy remain under close medical supervision throughout the period of drug administration.

Reported incidences (%) for the most commonly occurring adverse reactions in rheumatoid arthritis patients are noted, based on 17 representative clinical trials reported in the literature (1,270 patients).

➤*Allergic:* Generalized pruritus, early and late rashes (5%), pemphigus, and drug eruptions which may be accompanied by fever, arthralgia, or lymphadenopathy have occurred. Some patients may show a lupus erythematosus-like syndrome similar to drug-induced lupus produced by other pharmacological agents.

Urticaria and exfoliative dermatitis have occurred.

Thyroiditis has been reported; hypoglycemia in association with anti-insulin antibodies has been reported. These reactions are extremely rare.

Some patients may develop a migratory polyarthralgia, often with objective synovitis.

➤*CNS:* Tinnitus, optic neuritis and peripheral sensory and motor neuropathies (including polyradiculoneuropathy [ie, Guillain-Barré syndrome]) have been reported. Muscular weakness may or may not occur with the peripheral neuropathies. Visual and psychic disturbances; mental disorders; and agitation and anxiety have been reported.

PENICILLAMINE — ORAL

➤*GI:* Anorexia, epigastric pain, nausea, vomiting, or occasional diarrhea may occur (17%).

Isolated cases of reactivated peptic ulcer have occurred, as have hepatic dysfunction including hepatic failure, and pancreatitis. Intrahepatic cholestasis and toxic hepatitis have been reported rarely. There have been a few reports of increased serum alkaline phosphatase, lactic dehydrogenase, and positive cephalin flocculation and thymol turbidity tests.

Some patients may report a blunting, diminution, or total loss of taste perception (12%); or may develop oral ulcerations. Although rare, cheilosis, glossitis, and gingivostomatitis have been reported.

Gastrointestinal side effects are usually reversible following cessation of therapy.

➤*Hematologic:* Penicillamine can cause bone marrow depression. Leukopenia (2%) and thrombocytopenia (4%) have occurred. Fatalities have been reported as a result of thrombocytopenia, agranulocytosis, aplastic anemia, and sideroblastic anemia.

Thrombotic thrombocytopenic purpura, hemolytic anemia, red cell aplasia, monocytosis, leukocytosis, eosinophilia, and thrombocytosis have also been reported.

➤*Renal:* Patients on penicillamine therapy may develop proteinuria (6%) and/or hematuria which, in some, may progress to the development of the nephrotic syndrome as a result of an immune complex membranous glomerulopathy. Renal failure has been reported.

➤*Miscellaneous:*

Neuromuscular – Myasthenia gravis; dystonia. Adverse reactions that have been reported rarely include thrombophlebitis; hyperpyrexia; falling hair or alopecia; lichen planus; polymyositis; dermatomyositis; mammary hyperplasia; elastosis perforans serpiginosa; toxic epidermal necrolysis; anetoderma (cutaneous macular atrophy); and Goodpasture's syndrome, a severe and ultimately fatal glomerulonephritis associated with intra-alveolar hemorrhage. Vasculitis, including fatal renal vasculitis, has also been reported. Allergic alveolitis, obliterative bronchiolitis, interstitial pneumonitis and pulmonary fibrosis have been reported in patients with severe rheumatoid arthritis, some of whom were receiving penicillamine. Bronchial asthma also has been reported.

Increased skin friability, excessive wrinkling of skin, and development of small white papules at venipuncture and surgical sites have been reported; yellow nail syndrome.

The chelating action of the drug may cause increased excretion of other heavy metals such as zinc, mercury and lead.

There have been reports associating penicillamine with leukemia. However, circumstances involved in these reports are such that a cause and effect relationship to the drug has not been established.

URINARY ALKALINIZERS

Urinary alkalinizing agents are bases or salts of bases that increase the excretion of free base in the urine, effectively raising the urinary pH.

Used to correct acidosis in renal tubular disorders and to minimize uric acid crystallization as adjuvants to uricosuric agents in gout. Urine alkalinization increases solubility of sulfonamides and the renal elimination of phenobarbital.

SODIUM BICARBONATE

For oral sodium bicarbonate prescribing information, see the monograph in the Systemic Alkalinizer section . For information on parenteral sodium bicarbonate, refer to the monograph in the Nutrients and Nutritionals chapter. Also see the Antacids group monograph.

POTASSIUM CITRATE

Rx	**Urocit-K** (Mission)	**Tablets:** 5 mEq	(Mission MPC 600). In 100s.
		10 mEq	In 100s.

POTASSIUM CITRATE — ORAL

For complete prescribing information on citrate and citric acid, see monograph in the Nutrients and Nutritionals chapter.

Indications

For the management of renal tubular acidosis (RTA) with calcium stones, hypocitraturic calcium oxalate nephrolithiasis of any etiology, and uric acid lithiasis with or without calcium stones.

Administration and Dosage

➤*Approved by the FDA:* August 30, 1985.

Treatment with potassium citrate should be added to a regimen that limits salt intake (avoidance of foods with high salt content and of added salt at the table) and encourages high fluid intake (urine volume should be at least 2 L/day).

➤*Dosage:* The objective of treatment with potassium citrate is to provide a sufficient dosage to restore normal urinary citrate (greater than 320 mg/day and as close to the normal mean of 640 mg/day as possible), and to increase urinary pH to a level of 6 to 7.

- Potassium citrate should be dosed according to the level of measured urinary citrate: For severe hypocitraturia (measured citrate level less than 150 mg/day) the dosage of potassium citrate is 60 mEq/day in divided dosage (20 mEq 3 times/day or 15 mEq 4 times/day with meals or within 30 minutes after meals).
- For mild to moderate hypocitraturia (measured citrate level greater than 150 mg/day) the dosage of potassium citrate is 30 mEq/day in divided dosage (10 mEq 3 times/day with meals or within 30 minutes after meals).
- Twenty four-hour urinary citrate and/or urinary pH measurements should be used to determine the adequacy of the initial dosage and to evaluate the effectiveness of any dosage change.
- Urinary citrate and/or pH should be measured every 4 months.
- Dosages of potassium citrate greater than 100 mEq/day have not been studied and should be avoided.

➤*Hypocitraturia:* In patients with severe hypocitraturia (urinary citrate of less than 150 mg/day), therapy should be initiated at a dosage of 60 mEq/day (20 mEq 3 times/day or 15 mEq 4 times/day with meals or within 30 minutes after meals or bedtime snack). In patients with mild to moderate hypocitraturia (greater than 150 mg/day), potassium citrate should be initiated at a dosage of 30 mEq/day (10 mEq 3 times/day with meals). Twenty-four hour urinary citrate and/or urinary pH measurements should be used to determine the adequacy of the initial dosage and to evaluate the effectiveness of any dosage change. In addition, urinary citrate and/or pH should be measured every 4 months.

➤*Storage / Stability:* Store in a cool, dry place.

POTASSIUM CITRATE COMBINATIONS

Rx	**Citrolith** (Beach Pharm.)	**Tablets:** 50 mg potassium citrate and 950 mg sodium citrate	(Beach 1136). In 100s & 500s.
Rx	**Polycitra** (Willen)	**Syrup:** 550 mg potassium citrate, 500 mg sodium citrate, 334 mg citric acid/5 ml. (1 mEq K, 1 mEq Na per ml; equiv. to 2 mEq bicarbonate)	Alcohol free. In 120 and 480 ml.
Rx *sf*	**Polycitra-LC** (Willen)	**Solution:** 550 mg K citrate, 500 mg sodium citrate, 334 mg citric acid/5 ml. (1 mEq K, 1 mEq Na per ml; equiv. to 2 mEq bicarbonate)	Alcohol free. In 120 and 480 ml.
Rx *sf*	**Polycitra-K** (Willen)	**Solution:** 1100 mg potassium citrate, 334 mg citric acid/5 ml. (2 mEq K/ml; equiv. to 2 mEq bicarbonate)	Alcohol free. In 120 and 480 ml.
		Crystals for Reconstitution: 3300 mg K citrate, 1002 mg citric acid per UD packet (equiv. to 30 mEq bicarb.)	Alcohol free. In single dose packets.

POTASSIUM CITRATE COMBINATIONS — ORAL

For complete prescribing information on citrate and citric acid, see monograph in the Nutrients and Nutritionals chapter.

Administration and Dosage

➤*Liquids:* 15 to 20 ml 4 times daily usually maintains a urinary pH of 7 to 7.6 for 24 hours; 10 to 15 ml 4 times daily usually maintains a urinary pH of 6.5 to 7.4.

Adults – 15 to 30 ml 4 times daily, after meals and at bedtime, diluted with water.

Children – 5 to 15 ml 4 times daily, after meals and at bedtime, diluted with water.

➤*Tablets:* 1 to 4 tablets with a full glass of water, after meals and at bedtime.

SODIUM CITRATE AND CITRIC ACID SOLUTION (Shohl's Solution, Modified)

Rx sf	**Sodium Citrate/Citric Acid** (Pharmaceutical Associates)	**Solution:** 500 mg sodium citrate/334 mg citric acid per 5 ml (1 mEq sodium equiv. to 1 mEq bicarbonate/ml)	In 473 mL.
Rx sf	**Bicitra** (Alza Corp.)		Grape flavored. In 120 and 473 ml and UD 15 and 30 ml.
Rx	**Oracit** (Carolina Medical Products)	**Solution:** 490 mg sodium citrate/640 mg citric acid per 5 ml (1 mEq sodium equiv. to 1 mEq bicarbonate/ml)	In 500 ml and UD 15 and 30 ml.

SODIUM CITRATE AND CITRIC ACID SOLUTION (Shohl's Solution, Modified) — ORAL

Administration and Dosage

➤*Systemic alkalinization:*

Adults – 10 to 30 ml diluted in 30 to 90 ml water, after meals and at bedtime.

Children (older than 2 years of age) – 5 to 15 ml diluted in 30 to 90 ml water, after meals and at bedtime. Consult physician for use in children younger than 2 years of age.

➤*Neutralizing buffer:* 15 ml diluted in 15 ml water, as a single dose.

URINARY ACIDIFIERS

ASCORBIC ACID

For information on the use of ascorbic acid as a urinary acidifier, see the vitamin C monograph in the Nutritional Agents chapter.

Acid Phosphates

Indications

To acidify the urine and lower urinary calcium concentration.

Increases the antibacterial activity of methenamine.

Reduces odor and rash caused by ammoniacal urine.

Contraindications

Renal insufficiency (less than 30% of normal), infected magnesium ammonium phosphate stones, hyperphosphatemia and hyperkalemia. Also use with caution if potassium regulation is desired. Use sodium acid phosphate cautiously in patients on sodium restriction.

Warnings

➤*Concurrent potassium supplementation:* Consider potassium content of these products. Decrease supplemental potassium dosage to avoid hyperkalemia.

➤*Pregnancy: Category C.* Safe use during pregnancy is not established. Use only when clearly needed and when potential benefits outweigh potential hazards to the fetus.

➤*Lactation:* Safety for use in the nursing mother has not been established. It is not known whether this drug is excreted in breast milk. Exercise caution when administering to a nursing woman.

Precautions

➤*Special risk:* Cardiac disease (particularly digitalized patients), Addison's disease, acute dehydration, severe renal insufficiency or chronic renal disease, extensive tissue breakdown (such as severe burns), myotonia congenita, cardiac failure, cirrhosis of the liver or severe hepatic disease, peripheral and pulmonary edema, hypernatremia, hypertension, toxemia of pregnancy, hypoparathyroidism, acute pancreatitis and rickets.

➤*Lab test abnormalities:* Carefully monitor renal function and serum electrolytes (calcium, phosphorus, potassium) at periodic intervals during phosphate therapy if required. High serum phosphate levels increase incidence of extraskeletal calcification.

Drug Interactions

Acid Phosphate Drug Interactions

Precipitant drug	Object drug*		Description
Acid phosphates	Salicylates	↑	Acidified urine reduces excretion of salicylates and may lead to salicylate toxicity.
Antacids	Acid phosphates	↓	Antacids containing magnesium, calcium or aluminum in conjunction with phosphate preparations may bind the phosphate and prevent absorption.
Antihypertensives; Corticosteroids	Acid phosphates	↑	Antihypertensives, especially diazoxide, guanethidine, hydralazine, methyldopa or rauwolfia alkaloids; or corticosteroids, especially mineralocorticoids or corticotropin; used concurrently with sodium phosphate may result in hypernatremia.
Potassium-containing medications	Acid phosphates	↑	Potassium-containing medications or potassium-sparing diuretics may cause hyperkalemia when used concurrently with potassium salts. Perform periodic serum potassium level determinations.

* ↑ = Object drug increased. ↓ = Object drug decreased.

Adverse Reactions

Mild laxation may occur; it usually subsides with dosage reduction. If it persists, discontinue use. Abdominal discomfort, diarrhea, nausea and vomiting may occur.

Less frequent – Fast or irregular heartbeat, dizziness, headache, mental confusion, seizures, weakness or heaviness of legs, unusual tiredness, muscle cramps, numbness, tingling, pain or weakness in hands or feet, numbness or tingling around lips, shortness of breath or troubled breathing, swelling of feet or legs, unusual weight gain, low urine output, thirst, bone and joint pain.

Patient Information

Notify physician if abdominal pain, nausea or vomiting occurs.

Warn patients with kidney stones of the possibility of passing old stones when phosphate therapy is started.

Advise patients to avoid antacids containing aluminum, calcium or magnesium which may prevent phosphate absorption.

To assure against GI injury associated with oral ingestion of concentrated potassium salt preparations, instruct patients to dissolve tablets completely in an appropriate amount of water before taking.

POTASSIUM ACID PHOSPHATE

Rx	**K-Phos Original** (Beach)	**Tablets:** 500 mg (contains 3.7 mEq potassium)	Sodium free. (Beach 1111). White, scored. In 100s and 500s.

POTASSIUM ACID PHOSPHATE — ORAL

For complete prescribing information, refer to the Acid Phosphates group monograph.

Indications

➤*Elevated urinary pH:* For use in patients with elevated urinary pH. Potassium acid phosphate helps keep calcium soluble and reduces odor and rash caused by ammoniacal urine. Also, by acidifying the urine, it increases the antibacterial activity of methenamine mandelate and methenamine hippurate.

Administration and Dosage

➤*Dosage:* Two tablets dissolved in 6 to 8 oz of water 4 times daily with meals and at bedtime. For best results, let the tablets soak in water for 2 to 5 minutes, or more if necessary, and stir. If any tablet particles remain undissolved, they may be crushed and stirred vigorously to speed dissolution.

➤*Storage/Stability:* Keep tightly closed. Store at controlled room temperature, 20° to 25°C (68° to 77°F).

POTASSIUM ACID PHOSPHATE AND SODIUM ACID PHOSPHATE

Rx	**K-Phos Neutral** (Beach)	**Tablets**: 852 mg dibasic sodium phosphate anhydrous, 155 mg monobasic potassium phosphate and 130 mg monobasic sodium phosphate monohydrate (contains 1.1 mEq potassium and 13.0 mEq sodium)	(Beach 1125). White, film coated. In 100s and 500s.
Rx	**K-Phos M.F.** (Beach)	**Tablets**: 155 mg potassium acid phosphate and 350 mg sodium acid phosphate (contains 1.1 mEq potassium and 2.9 mEq sodium)	(Beach 1135). White, scored. In 100s and 500s.
Rx	**K-Phos No. 2** (Beach)	**Tablets**: 305 mg potassium acid phosphate and 700 mg sodium acid phosphate (contains 2.3 mEq potassium and 5.8 mEq sodium)	(Beach 1134). Brown. In 100s and 500s.

POTASSIUM ACID PHOSPHATE AND SODIUM ACID PHOSPHATE — ORAL

For complete prescribing information, refer to the Acid Phosphates group monograph.

Administration and Dosage

1 to 2 tablets 4 times daily with a full glass of water. When the urine is difficult to acidify, administer 1 tablet every 2 hours. Do not exceed 8 tablets in 24 hours.

In addition to the GI anticholinergics (refer to the Gastrointestinal Agents chapter), many of which are recommended for urologic conditions, the following agents are indicated specifically for urologic disorders. Urinary anticholinergics in combination with urinary anti-infective agents are listed in the Anti-Infectives, Systemic chapter. Urinary anticholinergics in combination with urinary analgesics also are available.

FLAVOXATE HYDROCHLORIDE

Rx	**Flavoxate** (Global)	**Tablets**: 100 mg	(G 181). Off-white. Film-coated. In 100s.
Rx	**Urispas** (Ortho-McNeil)		Castor oil. (URISPAS SKF). White. Film-coated. In UD 100s.

FLAVOXATE HYDROCHLORIDE — ORAL

Indications

For symptomatic relief of dysuria, urgency, nocturia, suprapubic pain, frequency and incontinence as may occur in cystitis, prostatitis, urethritis, urethrocystitis/urethrotrigonitis. Flavoxate hydrochloride is not indicated for definitive treatment, but is compatible with drugs used for the treatment of urinary tract infections.

Administration and Dosage

➤*Adults and children older than 12 years of age:* One or two 100 mg tablets 3 or 4 times a day. With improvement of symptoms, the dose may be reduced. This drug cannot be recommended for infants and children younger than 12 years of age because safety and efficacy have not been demonstrated in this age group.

➤*Storage/Stability:* Store between 15° and 30°C (59° and 86°F).

Actions

➤*Pharmacology:* Flavoxate hydrochloride counteracts smooth muscle spasm of the urinary tract and exerts its effect directly on the muscle.

➤*Pharmacokinetics:* In a single study of 11 healthy male subjects, the time to onset of action was 55 minutes. The peak effect was observed at 112 minutes.

Fifty-seven percent of the flavoxate HCl was excreted in the urine within 24 hours.

Contraindications

Pyloric or duodenal obstruction, obstructive intestinal lesions or ileus, achalasia, GI hemorrhage and obstructive uropathies of the lower urinary tract.

Warnings

➤*Glaucoma:* Give cautiously to patients with suspected glaucoma.

➤*Pregnancy:* *Category B.*

Reproduction studies have been performed in rats and rabbits at doses up to 34 times the human dose and revealed no evidence of impaired fertility or harm to the fetus due to flavoxate HCl. There are, however, no well-controlled studies in pregnant women. Because animal reproduction studies are not always predictive of human response, this drug should be used during pregnancy only if clearly needed.

➤*Lactation:* It is not known whether this drug is excreted in human milk. Because many drugs are excreted in human milk, caution should be exercised when flavoxate HCl is administered to a nursing woman.

➤*Children:* Safety and efficacy in children younger than 12 years of age have not been established.

Precautions

➤*Hazardous tasks:* Patients should be informed that if drowsiness and blurred vision occur, they should not operate a motor vehicle or machinery or participate in activities where alertness is required.

Adverse Reactions

➤*Allergic:* Urticaria and other dermatoses, eosinophilia and hyperpyrexia.

➤*Cardiovascular:* Tachycardia and palpitation.

➤*CNS:* Vertigo, headache, mental confusion, especially in the elderly, drowsiness, nervousness.

➤*GI:* Nausea, vomiting, dry mouth.

➤*Hematologic:* Leukopenia (1 case which was reversible upon discontinuation of the drug).

➤*Ophthalmic:* Increased ocular tension, blurred vision, disturbance in eye accommodation.

➤*Renal:* Dysuria.

Overdosage

The oral LD_{50} for flavoxate HCl in rats is 4273 mg/kg. The oral LD_{50} for flavoxate HCl in mice is 1837 mg/kg.

➤*Treatment:* It is not known whether flavoxate HCI is dialyzable.

Patient Information

Patients should be informed that if drowsiness and blurred vision occur, they should not operate a motor vehicle or machinery or participate in activities where alertness is required.

OXYBUTYNIN CHLORIDE

Rx	**Oxybutynin Chloride** (Various, eg, Dixon-Shane, Goldline, Pliva, Sidmak, UDL, Watson)	**Tablets**: 5 mg	In 100s, 500s, 1000s, blister pack 25s, and UD 100s.
Rx	**Ditropan** (ALZA)		Lactose. (DITROPAN 92 00). Blue, scored. In 100s, 1000s, and UD 100s.
Rx	**Ditropan XL** (ALZA)	**Tablets, extended-release**: 5 mg	Lactose. (5 XL). Pale yellow. In 100s.
		10 mg	Lactose. (10 XL). Pink. In 100s.
		15 mg	Lactose. (15 XL). Gray. In 100s.
Rx	**Oxybutynin Chloride** (Various, eg, Apotex, Cypress, Morton Grove)	**Syrup**: 5 mg/5 mL	In 473 mL.
Rx	**Ditropan** (ALZA)		Sorbitol, sucrose, methylparaben. In 473 mL.
Rx	**Oxytrol** (Watson)	**Transdermal system**: 36 mg of oxybutynin delivering 3.9 mg oxybutynin per day.	(OXYTROL). 39 cm^2 system. In patient calendar boxes of 8 systems.

OXYBUTYNIN CHLORIDE — ORAL

Indications

➤*Tablets and syrup:* For the relief of symptoms of bladder instability associated with voiding in patients with uninhibited neurogenic or reflex neurogenic bladder (ie, urgency, frequency, urinary leakage, urge incontinence, dysuria).

➤*Extended-release tablets:* For the treatment of overactive bladder with symptoms of urge urinary incontinence, urgency, and frequency.

Oxybutynin chloride is also indicated in the treatment of pediatric patients aged 6 years and older with symptoms of detrusor overactivity associated with a neurological condition (eg, spina bifida).

Administration and Dosage

➤*Tablets:*

Adults – One 5 mg tablet 2 to 3 times daily. The maximum recommended dose is one 5 mg tablet 4 times daily. A lower starting dose of 2.5 mg 2 or 3 times a day is recommended for the frail elderly.

Children (older than 5 years of age) – One 5 mg tablet twice daily. The maximum recommended dose is one 5 mg tablet 3 times daily.

➤*Syrup:*

Adults – 1 teaspoon (5 mg/5 mL) syrup 2 to 3 times daily. The maximum recommended dose is 1 teaspoon (5 mg/5 mL) syrup 4 times daily. A lower starting dose of 2.5 mg 2 or 3 times a day is recommended for the frail elderly.

Children (older than 5 years of age) – 1 teaspoon (5 mg/5 mL) syrup 2 times a day. The maximum recommended dose is 1 teaspoon (5 mg/5 mL) syrup 3 times a day.

➤*Extended-release tablets:* Oxybutynin chloride extended-release tablets must be swallowed whole with the aid of liquids, and must not be chewed, divided, or crushed. May be administered with or without food.

Adults – 5 mg once daily. Dosage may be adjusted in 5 mg increments to achieve a balance of efficacy and tolerability (up to a maximum of 30 mg/day). In general, dosage adjustment may proceed at approximately weekly intervals.

Children (6 years of age and older) – 5 mg once daily. Dosage may be adjusted in 5 mg increments to achieve a balance of efficacy and tolerability (up to a maximum of 20 mg/day).

OXYBUTYNIN CHLORIDE — ORAL

➤*Storage/Stability:*

Tablets and syrup – Store at controlled room temperature 15° to 30°C (59° to 86°F). Dispense in tight, light-resistant container.

Extended-release tablets – Store at 25°C (77°F); excursions permitted to 15° to 30°C (59° to 86°F). Protect from moisture and humidity.

Actions

➤*Pharmacology:* Oxybutynin chloride exerts a direct antispasmodic effect on smooth muscle and inhibits the muscarinic action of acetylcholine on smooth muscle. Oxybutynin chloride exhibits only one-fifth of the anticholinergic activity of atropine on the rabbit detrusor muscle, but 4 to 10 times the antispasmodic activity. No blocking effects occur at skeletal neuromuscular junctions or autonomic ganglia (antinicotinic effects).

Oxybutynin chloride relaxes bladder smooth muscle. In patients with conditions characterized by involuntary bladder contractions, cystometric studies have demonstrated that oxybutynin increases bladder (vesical) capacity, diminishes the frequency of uninhibited contractions of the detrusor muscle, and delays the initial desire to void. Oxybutynin thus decreases urgency and the frequency of both incontinent episodes and voluntary urination.

Antimuscarinic activity resides predominately in the R-isomer. A metabolite, desethyloxybutynin, has pharmacological activity similar to that of oxybutynin in in vitro studies.

➤*Pharmacokinetics:*

Absorption –

Tablets and syrup: Following oral administration, oxybutynin is rapidly absorbed achieving C_{max} within an hour, following which plasma concentration decreases with an effective half-life of approximately 2 to 3 hours. The absolute bioavailability of oxybutynin is reported to be about 6% (range 1.6% to 10.9%) for both the tablet and syrup. Wide interindividual variation in pharmacokinetic parameters is evident following oral administration of oxybutynin.

The mean pharmacokinetic parameters for R- and S-oxybutynin are summarized below. The plasma concentration-time profiles for R- and S-oxybutynin are similar in shape.

Mean (SD) R- and S-Oxybutynin Pharmacokinetic Parameters Following 3 Doses of Oxybutynin Chloride 5 mg Administered Every 8 Hours (n = 23)

Parameters (units)	R-oxybutynin	S-oxybutynin
C_{max} (ng/mL)	3.6 (2.2)	7.8 (4.1)
t_{max} (hr)	0.89 (0.34)	0.65 (0.32)
AUC_t (ng•hr/mL)	22.6 (11.3)	35 (17.3)
AUC_{inf} (ng•hr/mL)	24.3 (12.3)	37.3 (18.7)

Oxybutynin chloride steady-state pharmacokinetics was also studied in 23 pediatric patients with detrusor overactivity associated with a neurological condition (eg, spina bifida). These pediatric patients were on oxybutynin chloride tablets (n = 11) with total daily dose ranging from 7.5 mg to 15 mg (0.22 to 0.53 mg/kg) or oxybutynin chloride syrup (n = 12) with total daily dose ranging from 5 mg to 22.5 mg (0.26 to 0.75 mg/kg). Overall, most patients (86.9%) were taking a total daily oxybutynin chloride dose between 10 mg and 15 mg. Sparse sampling technique was used to obtain serum samples. When all available data are normalized to an equivalent of 5 mg twice daily oxybutynin chloride, the mean pharmacokinetic parameters derived for R- and S-oxybutynin and R- and S-desethyloxybutynin are summarized below for tablet and syrup. The plasma-time concentration profile for R- and S-oxybutynin are similar in shape.

Mean ± SD R- and S-Oxybutynin and R- and S-Desethyloxybutynin Pharmacokinetic Parameters in Children 5 to 15 Years of Age Following Administration of 7.5 to 15 mg Total Daily Dose of Oxybutynin Chloride Tablets (n = 11)

All available data normalized to an equivalent of oxybutynin chloride tablets 5 mg 2 times a day or 3 times a day at steady rates				
	R-oxybutynin	S-oxybutynin	R-desethyl-oxybutynin	S-desethyl-oxybutynin
C_{max}* (ng/mL)	6.1 ± 3.2	10.1 ± 7.5	55.4 ± 17.9	28.2 ± 10
t_{max} (hr)	1	1	2	2
AUC** (ng•hr/mL)	19.8 ± 7.4	28.4 ± 12.7	238.8 ± 77.6	119.5 ± 50.7

* Reflects C_{max} for pooled data. ** $AUC_{0\text{-end of dosing interval}}$.

Mean ± SD R- and S-Oxybutynin and R- and S-Desethyloxybutynin Pharmacokinetic Parameters in Children 5 to 15 Years of Age Following Administration of 5 to 22.5 mg Total Daily Dose of Oxybutynin Chloride Syrup (n = 12)

All available data normalized to an equivalent of oxybutynin chloride syrup 5 mg 2 times a day or 3 times a day at steady rates				
	R-oxybutynin	S-oxybutynin	R-desethyl-oxybutynin	S-desethyl-oxybutynin
C_{max}* (ng/mL)	5.7 ± 6.2	7.3 ± 7.3	54.2 ± 34	27.8 ± 20.7
t_{max} (hr)	1	1	1	1
AUC** (ng•hr/mL)	16.3 ± 17.1	20.2 ± 20.8	209.1 ± 174.2	99.1 ± 87.5

* Reflects C_{max} for pooled data. ** $AUC_{0\text{-end of dosing interval}}$.

Extended-release tablets: Following the first dose of oxybutynin chloride extended-release tablets, oxybutynin plasma concentrations rise for 4 to 6 hours; thereafter steady concentrations are maintained for up to 24 hours, minimizing fluctuations between peak and trough concentrations associated with oxybutynin.

The relative bioavailabilities of R- and S-oxybutynin from oxybutynin chloride extended-release tablets are 156% and 187%, respectively, compared with oxybutynin. The mean pharmacokinetic parameters for R- and S-oxybutynin are summarized below. The plasma concentration-time profiles for R- and S-oxybutynin are similar in shape.

Mean (SD) R- and S-Oxybutynin Pharmacokinetic Parameters Following a Single Dose of Oxybutynin Chloride 10 mg Extended-Release Tablets (n = 43)

Parameters (units)	R-oxybutynin	S-oxybutynin
C_{max} (ng/mL)	1 (0.6)	1.8 (1)
t_{max} (hr)	12.7 (5.4)	11.8 (5.3)
$t_{½}$ (hr)	13.2 (6.2)	12.4 (6.1)
$AUC_{(0-48)}$ (ng•hr/mL)	18.4 (10.3)	34.2 (16.9)
AUC_{inf} (ng•hr/mL)	21.3 (12.2)	39.5 (21.2)

Steady-state oxybutynin plasma concentrations are achieved by day 3 of repeated oxybutynin chloride extended-release tablet dosing, with no observed drug accumulation or change in oxybutynin and desethyloxybutynin pharmacokinetic parameters.

Oxybutynin chloride steady-state pharmacokinetics was studied in 19 children aged 5 to 15 years with detrusor overactivity associated with a neurological condition (eg, spina bifida). The children were on oxybutynin chloride total daily dose ranging from 5 to 20 mg (0.1 to 0.77 mg/kg). Sparse sampling technique was used to obtain serum samples. When all available data are normalized to an equivalent of 5 mg per day oxybutynin chloride, the mean pharmacokinetic parameters derived for R- and S-oxybutynin and R- and S-desethyloxybutynin are summarized below. The plasma-time concentration profiles for R- and S-oxybutynin are similar in shape.

Mean ± SD R- and S-Oxybutynin and R- and S-Desethyloxybutynin Pharmacokinetic Parameters in Children 5 to 15 Years of Age Following Administration of 5 to 20 mg Oxybutynin Chloride Extended-Release Tablets Once Daily (n = 19)

All available data normalized to an equivalent of oxybutynin chloride extended-release tablets 5 mg once daily				
	R-oxybutynin	S-oxybutynin	R-desethyl-oxybutynin	S- desethyl-oxybutynin
C_{max} (ng/mL)	0.7 ± 0.4	1.3 ± 0.8	7.8 ± 3.7	4.2 ± 2.3
t_{max} (hr)	5	5	5	5
AUC (ng•hr/mL)	12.8 ± 7	23.7 ± 14.4	125.1 ± 66.7	73.6 ± 47.7

Mean steady state (±SD) R-oxybutynin plasma concentrations following administration of 5 to 20 mg oxybutynin chloride once daily in children aged 5 to 15. Plot represents all available data normalized to an equivalent of oxybutynin chloride 5 mg once daily.

- *Food effects* –

Tablets and syrup: Data in the literature suggests that oxybutynin chloride solution coadministered with food resulted in a slight delay in absorption and an increase in its bioavailability by 25% (n = 18).

Extended-release tablets: The rate and extent of absorption and metabolism of oxybutynin chloride are similar under fed and fasted conditions.

Distribution – Plasma concentrations of oxybutynin decline biexponentially following IV or oral administration. The volume of distribution is 193 L after IV administration of 5 mg oxybutynin chloride.

Metabolism – Oxybutynin chloride is metabolized primarily by the cytochrome P450 enzyme systems, particularly CYP3A4 found mostly in the liver and gut wall. Its metabolic products include phenylcyclohexyl-glycolic acid, which is pharmacologically inactive, and desethyloxybutynin, which is pharmacologically active.

Extended-release tablets: Following oxybutynin chloride extended-release tablet administration, plasma concentrations of R- and S-desethyloxybutynin are 73% and 92%, respectively, of concentrations observed with oxybutynin.

Excretion – Oxybutynin chloride is extensively metabolized by the liver, with less than 0.1% of the administered dose excreted unchanged in the urine. Also, less than 0.1% of the administered dose is excreted as the metabolite desethyloxybutynin.

OXYBUTYNIN CHLORIDE — ORAL

Contraindications

Urinary retention, gastric retention and other severe decreased GI motility conditions, uncontrolled narrow-angle glaucoma and in patients who are at risk for these conditions; hypersensitivity to the drug substance or other components of the product.

Warnings

➤*Renal function impairment:*

Extended-release tablets – Oxybutynin chloride extended-release tablets should be used with caution in patients with renal impairment. There is no experience with the use of oxybutynin chloride extended-release tablets in patients with renal insufficiency.

➤*Hepatic function impairment:*

Extended-release tablets – There is no experience with the use of oxybutynin chloride extended-release tablets in patients with hepatic insufficiency. Oxybutynin chloride extended-release tablets should be used with caution in patients with hepatic impairment.

➤*Elderly:*

Tablets and syrup – Clinical studies of oxybutynin chloride did not include sufficient numbers of subjects 65 years of age and older to determine whether they respond differently from younger patients. Other reported clinical experience has not identified differences in responses between healthy elderly and younger patients; however, a lower initial starting dose of 2.5 mg given 2 or 3 times a day has been recommended for the frail elderly due to a prolongation of the elimination half-life from 2 to 3 hours to 5 hours. In general, dose selection for an elderly patient should be cautious, usually starting at the low end of the dosing range, reflecting the greater frequency of decreased hepatic, renal or cardiac function, and of concomitant disease or other drug therapy.

➤*Pregnancy: Category B.*

The safety of oxybutynin chloride administration to women who are or who may become pregnant has not been established. Therefore, oxybutynin chloride should not be given to pregnant women unless, in the judgment of the physician, the probable clinical benefits outweigh the possible hazards.

➤*Lactation:* It is not known whether oxybutynin chloride is excreted in human milk. Because many drugs are excreted in human milk, caution should be exercised when oxybutynin chloride is administered to a nursing woman.

➤*Children:*

Tablets and syrup – The safety and efficacy of oxybutynin chloride administration have been demonstrated for children 5 years of age or older. However, as there is insufficient clinical data for children younger than 5 years of age, oxybutynin chloride is not recommended for this age group.

Extended-release tablets – The safety and efficacy of oxybutynin chloride were studied in 60 children in a 24-week, open-label trial. Patients were aged 6 to 15 years, all had symptoms of detrusor overactivity in association with a neurological condition (eg, spina bifida), all used clean intermittent catheterization, and all were current users of oxybutynin chloride. Study results demonstrated that administration of oxybutynin chloride 5 to 20 mg/day was associated with an increase from baseline in mean urine volume per catheterization from 108 mL to 136 mL, an increase from baseline in mean urine volume after morning awakening from 148 mL to 189 mL, and an increase from baseline in the mean percentage of catheterizations without a leaking episode from 34% to 51%.

Urodynamic results were consistent with clinical results. Administration of oxybutynin chloride resulted in an increase from baseline in mean maximum cystometric capacity from 185 mL to 254 mL, a decrease from baseline in mean detrusor pressure at maximum cystometric capacity from 44 cm H_2O to 33 cm H_2O, and a reduction in the percentage of patients demonstrating uninhibited detrusor contractions (of at least 15 cm H_2O) from 60% to 28%.

Oxybutynin chloride is not recommended in pediatric patients who can not swallow the tablet whole without chewing, dividing, or crushing, or in children under the age of 6 years.

Precautions

➤*Urinary retention:* Oxybutynin chloride should be administered with caution to patients with clinically significant bladder outflow obstruction because of the risk of urinary retention. Oxybutynin chloride is contraindicated in patients with urinary retention and in patients who are at risk for urinary retention.

➤*Gastrointestinal disorders:* Oxybutynin chloride should be administered with caution to patients with gastrointestinal obstructive disorders because of the risk of gastric retention. Oxybutynin chloride is contraindicated in patients with gastric retention and other severe decreased gastrointestinal motility conditions and in patients at risk for these conditions.

Oxybutynin chloride like other anticholinergic drugs, may decrease gastrointestinal motility and should be used with caution in patients with conditions such as ulcerative colitis, and intestinal atony.

Oxybutynin chloride should be used with caution in patients who have gastroesophageal reflux or who are concurrently taking drugs (such as bisphosphonates) that can cause or exacerbate esophagitis.

Extended-release tablets – As with any other nondeformable material, caution should be used when administering oxybutynin chloride extended-release tablets to patients with preexisting severe gastrointestinal narrowing (pathologic or iatrogenic). There have been rare reports of obstructive symptoms in patients with known strictures in association with the ingestion of other drugs in nondeformable controlled-release formulations.

➤*Special risk:*

Tablets and syrup – Oxybutynin chloride should be used with caution in the frail elderly, in patients with hepatic or renal impairment, and in patients with myasthenia gravis. Oxybutynin chloride may aggravate the symptoms of hyperthyroidism, coronary heart disease, congestive heart failure, cardiac arrhythmias, hiatal hernia, tachycardia, hypertension, myasthenia gravis, and prostatic hypertrophy. Administration of oxybutynin chloride to patients with ulcerative colitis may suppress intestinal motility to the point of producing a paralytic ileus and precipitate or aggravate toxic megacolon, a serious complication of the disease.

Extended-release tablets – Oxybutynin chloride should be used with caution in patients with hepatic or renal impairment and in patients with myasthenia gravis due to the risk of symptom aggravation.

Drug Interactions

Oxybutynin Drug Interactions

Precipitant drug	Object drug*		Description
Oxybutynin	Anticholinergic agents	↑	Concomitant use may increase the frequency and/or severity of anticholinergic-like effects. Anticholinergic agents may potentially alter the absorption of some concomitantly administered drugs because of anticholinergic effects on GI motility.
Anticholinergic agents	Oxybutynin		
Oxybutynin	Beta blockers Atenolol	↑	The bioavailability of atenolol may be increased. If an increase in beta blockade is suspected, tailoring the beta blocker dose downward may be necessary.
Oxybutynin	Digoxin	↑	Serum levels of digoxin administered as slow-dissolution oral tablets may be increased and actions enhanced. Serum level monitoring may assist in tailoring dosage. Problems may be avoided with use of digoxin elixir or capsules.
Oxybutynin	Haloperidol	↔	Effects are variable. Use oxybutynin only when clearly needed. Routinely monitor these patients; discontinue anticholinergic or tailor haloperidol if necessary.
Oxybutynin	Phenothiazines	↓	Pharmacologic/therapeutic actions of phenothiazines may be decreased by anticholinergics. Tailor the phenothiazine dose as needed.
Amantadine	Oxybutynin	↑	Anticholinergic side effects may be increased. Decrease the dose of oxybutynin during coadministration. Monitor patient response and adjust the dose accordingly.

* ↑ = Object drug increased. ↓ = Object drug decreased. ↔ = Undetermined clinical effect.

➤*Tablets and syrup:* Mean oxybutynin chloride plasma concentrations were approximately 3- to 4-fold higher when oxybutynin chloride was administered with ketoconazole, a potent CYP3A4 inhibitor.

➤*Extended-release tablets:* Mean oxybutynin chloride plasma concentrations were approximately 2-fold higher when oxybutynin was administered with ketoconazole, a potent CYP3A4 inhibitor.

Other inhibitors of the cytochrome P450 3A4 enzyme system, such as antimycotic agents (eg, itraconazole and miconazole) or macrolide antibiotics (eg, erythromycin and clarithromycin), may alter oxybutynin mean pharmacokinetic parameters (ie, C_{max} and AUC). The clinical relevance of such potential interactions is not known. Caution should be used when such drugs are coadministered.

Adverse Reactions

➤*Tablets and syrup:* The safety and efficacy of oxybutynin chloride was evaluated in a total of 199 patients in 3 clinical trials comparing oxybutynin chloride with oxybutynin chloride extended-release (see below). These participants were treated with oxybutynin chloride 5 to 20 mg/day for up to 6 weeks. The table below shows the incidence of adverse events judged by investigator to be at least possibly related to treatment and reported by at least 5% of patients.

Oxybutynin Adverse Reactions (> 5%)

Adverse reaction	Oxybutynin chloride (5 to 20 mg/day) (n = 199)
General	
Abdominal pain	6.5%
Headache	6%

OXYBUTYNIN CHLORIDE — ORAL

Oxybutynin Adverse Reactions (> 5%)	
Adverse reaction	Oxybutynin chloride (5 to 20 mg/day) (n = 199)
GI	
Dry mouth	71.4%
Constipation	12.6%
Nausea	10.1%
Dyspepsia	7%
Diarrhea	5%
CNS	
Dizziness	15.6%
Somnolence	12.6%
Special senses	
Blurred vision	9%
GU	
Impaired urination	10.6%
Increased post void residuals	5%
Urinary tract infection	5%

The most common adverse events reported by patients receiving oxybutynin chloride 5 to 20 mg/day were the expected side effects of anticholinergic agents. The incidence of dry mouth was dose-related.

In addition, the following adverse events were reported by 2% to less than 5% of patients using oxybutynin chloride (5 to 20 mg/day) in all studies.

Cardiovascular – Palpitation.

CNS – Insomnia, nervousness, confusion.

Dermatologic – Dry skin.

Metabolic/Nutritional – Peripheral edema.

Special senses – Dry eyes, taste perversion.

Miscellaneous – Asthenia, dry nasal and sinus mucous membranes.

Other adverse events that have been reported include tachycardia, hallucinations, cycloplegia, mydriasis, impotence, suppression of lactation, vasodilatation, rash, decreased gastrointestinal motility, flatulence, urinary retention, convulsions, and decreased sweating.

➤*Symptoms associated with the use of other anticholinergic drugs:* Following administration of oxybutynin chloride, the symptoms that can be associated with the use of other anticholinergic drugs may occur:

Cardiovascular – Palpitations, tachycardia, vasodilatation.

CNS – Asthenia, dizziness, drowsiness, hallucinations, insomnia, restlessness.

Dermatologic – Decreased sweating, rash.

GI – Constipation, decreased gastrointestinal motility, dry mouth, nausea.

GU – Urinary hesitance and retention.

Ophthalmic – Amblyopia, cycloplegia, decreased lacrimation, mydriasis.

Miscellaneous – Impotence, suppression of lactation.

➤*Extended-release tablets:* The safety and efficacy of oxybutynin chloride extended-release tablets was evaluated in a total of 580 participants who received oxybutynin chloride extended-release tablets in clinical trials (429 patients, 151 healthy volunteers). These participants were treated with 5 to 30 mg/day for up to 4.5 months. Safety information is provided for 429 patients from 3 controlled clinical studies and one open label study. The adverse reactions are reported regardless of causality.

Oxybutynin Adverse Reactions (≥ 5%)	
Adverse reaction	Oxybutynin chloride 5 to 30 mg/day (n = 429)
Miscellaneous	
Headache	9.8%
Asthenia	6.8%
Pain	6.8%
GI	
Dry mouth	60.8%
Constipation	13.1%
Diarrhea	9.1%
Nausea	8.9%
Dyspepsia	6.8%
CNS	
Somnolence	11.9%
Dizziness	6.3%
Respiratory	
Rhinitis	5.6%
Special senses	
Blurred vision	7.7%
Dry eyes	6.1%
GU	
Urinary tract infection	5.1%

The most common adverse reactions reported by patients receiving 5 to 30 mg/day oxybutynin chloride extended-release tablets were the expected side effects of anticholinergic agents. The incidence of dry mouth was dose-related.

The discontinuation rate for all adverse reactions was 6.8%. The most frequent adverse reaction causing early discontinuation of study medication was nausea (1.9%), while discontinuation due to dry mouth was 1.2%.

➤*Adverse reactions were reported by 2% to less than 5% of patients using oxybutynin chloride extended-release tablets (5 to 30 mg/day):*
Cardiovascular – Hypertension, palpitation, vasodilatation.

CNS – Insomnia, nervousness, confusion.

Dermatologic – Dry skin, rash.

GI – Flatulence, gastroesophageal reflux.

GU – Impaired urination (hesitancy), increased post void residual volume, urinary retention, cystitis.

Musculoskeletal – Arthritis.

Respiratory – Upper respiratory tract infection, cough, sinusitis, bronchitis, pharyngitis.

Miscellaneous – Abdominal pain, dry nasal and sinus mucous membranes, accidental injury, back pain, flu syndrome.

Other adverse reactions have been reported with oxybutynin chloride: Tachycardia, hallucinations, cycloplegia, mydriasis, impotence, and suppression of lactation.

Additional rare adverse events reported from worldwide postmarketing experience with oxybutynin chloride include peripheral edema, cardiac arrhythmia, tachycardia, hallucinations, convulsions, and impotence.

Additional adverse events reported with some other oxybutynin chloride formulations include cycloplegia, mydriasis, and suppression of lactation.

Overdosage

➤*Tablets and syrup:*
Symptoms – Overdosage with oxybutynin chloride has been associated with anticholinergic effects including central nervous system excitation (eg, restlessness, tremor, irritability, convulsions, delirium, hallucinations), flushing, fever, dehydration, cardiac arrhythmia, vomiting, and urinary retention. Other symptoms may include hypotension or hypertension, respiratory failure, paralysis, and coma.

Ingestion of 100 mg oxybutynin chloride in association with alcohol has been reported in a 13-year-old boy who experienced memory loss, and a 34 year old woman who developed stupor, followed by disorientation and agitation on awakening, dilated pupils, dry skin, cardiac arrhythmia, and retention of urine. Both patients fully recovered with symptomatic treatment.

Treatment – Treatment should be symptomatic and supportive. Activated charcoal may be administered as well as a cathartic.

➤*Extended-release tablets:* The continuous release of oxybutynin from oxybutynin chloride extended-release tablets should be considered in the treatment of overdosage. Patients should be monitored for at least 24 hours. Treatment should be symptomatic and supportive. Activated charcoal as well as a cathartic may be administered.

Overdosage with oxybutynin chloride has been associated with anticholinergic effects including CNS excitation, flushing, fever, dehydration, cardiac arrhythmia, vomiting, and urinary retention.

Ingestion of 100 mg oxybutynin chloride in association with alcohol has been reported in a 13-year-old boy who experienced memory loss, and a 34-year-old woman who developed stupor, followed by disorientation and agitation on awakening, dilated pupils, dry skin, cardiac arrhythmia, and retention of urine. Both patients fully recovered with symptomatic treatment.

Patient Information

Patients should be informed that heat prostration (fever and heat stroke due to decreased sweating) can occur when anticholinergics such as oxybutynin chloride are administered in the presence of high environmental temperature.

Because anticholinergic agents such as oxybutynin chloride may produce drowsiness (somnolence) or blurred vision, patients should be advised to exercise caution.

Patients should be informed that alcohol may enhance the drowsiness caused by anticholinergic agents such as oxybutynin chloride.

Patients should be informed that oxybutynin chloride extended-release tablets should be swallowed whole with the aid of liquids. Patients should not chew, divide, or crush tablets. The medication is contained within a nonabsorbable shell designed to release the drug at a controlled rate. The tablet shell is eliminated from the body; patients should not be concerned if they occasionally notice in their stool something that looks like a tablet.

OXYBUTYNIN — TRANSDERMAL

Indications

➤*Overactive bladder:* For the treatment of overactive bladder with symptoms of urge urinary incontinence, urgency, and frequency.

Administration and Dosage

➤*Approved by the FDA:* February 26, 2003.

➤*Administration:* Oxybutynin transdermal system should be applied to dry, intact skin on the abdomen, hip, or buttock. A new application site should be selected with each new system to avoid reapplication to the same site within 7 days.

➤*Dosage:* One 3.9 mg/day system applied twice weekly (every 3 to 4 days).

➤*Storage/Stability:* Store at 25°C (77°F); excursions permitted to 15° to 30°C (59° to 86°F). Protect from moisture and humidity. Do not store outside the sealed pouch. Apply immediately after removal from the protective pouch. Discard used oxybutynin transdermal system in household trash in a manner that prevents accidental application or ingestion by children, pets, or others.

Actions

➤*Pharmacology:* The free base form of oxybutynin is pharmacologically equivalent to oxybutynin hydrochloride. Oxybutynin acts as a competitive antagonist of acetylcholine at postganglionic muscarinic receptors, resulting in relaxation of bladder smooth muscle. In patients with conditions characterized by involuntary detrusor contractions, cystometric studies have demonstrated that oxybutynin increases maximum urinary bladder capacity and increases the volume to first detrusor contraction. Oxybutynin thus decreases urinary urgency and the frequency of both incontinence episodes and voluntary urination.

Oxybutynin is a racemic (50:50) mixture of R- and S-isomers. Antimuscarinic activity resides predominantly in the R-isomer. The active metabolite, N-desethyloxybutynin, has pharmacological activity on the human detrusor muscle that is similar to that of oxybutynin in in vitro studies.

➤*Pharmacokinetics:*

Absorption – Oxybutynin is transported across intact skin and into the systemic circulation by passive diffusion across the stratum corneum. The average daily dose of oxybutynin absorbed from the 39 cm^2 oxybutynin transdermal system is 3.9 mg. The average (SD) nominal dose, 0.1 (0.02) mg oxybutynin per cm^2 surface area, was obtained from analysis of residual oxybutynin content of systems worn over a continuous 4-day period during 303 separate occasions in 76 healthy volunteers. Following application of the first oxybutynin transdermal system 3.9 mg/day system, oxybutynin plasma concentration increases for approximately 24 to 48 hours, reaching average maximum concentrations of 3 to 4 ng/mL. Thereafter, steady concentrations are maintained for up to 96 hours. Absorption of oxybutynin is bioequivalent when oxybutynin transdermal system is applied to the abdomen, buttocks, or hip. Average plasma concentrations were measured during a randomized, crossover study of the 3 recommended application sites in 24 healthy men and women.

Steady-state conditions are reached during the second oxybutynin transdermal system application. Average steady-state plasma concentrations were 3.1 ng/mL for oxybutynin and 3.8 ng/mL for N-desethyloxybutynin. The following information provides a summary of pharmacokinetic parameters of oxybutynin in healthy volunteers after single and multiple applications of oxybutynin transdermal system.

Mean (SD) oxybutynin pharmacokinetic parameters from single and multiple dose studies in healthy men and women volunteers after application of oxybutynin transdermal system on abdomen: Single and multiple dose studies in healthy men and women volunteers reported the following mean (SD) oxybutynin pharmacokinetic parameters after abdominal application of the oxybutynin transdermal system: For the first single dose study, the C_{max} was 3 (0.8) ng/mL, the median t_{max} was 48 hours, and the AUC_{inf} was 245 (59) ng/mL•hr. For the second single dose study, the C_{max} was 3.4 (1.1) ng/mL, the median t_{max} was 36 hours, and the AUC_{inf} was 279 (99) ng/mL•hr. For the first multiple dose study, the C_{max} was 6.6 (2.4) ng/mL, the median t_{max} was 10 hours, the C_{avg} was 4.2 (1.1) and the $AUC_{0\text{-}96}$ was 408 (108) ng/mL•hr. For the second multiple dose study, the C_{max} was 4.2 (1) ng/mL, the median t_{max} was 28 hours, the C_{avg} was 3.1 (0.7) and the $AUC_{0\text{-}84}$ was 259 (57) ng/mL•hr.

Distribution – Oxybutynin is widely distributed in body tissues following systemic absorption. The volume of distribution was estimated to be 193 L after intravenous administration of 5 mg oxybutynin chloride.

Metabolism – Oxybutynin is metabolized primarily by the cytochrome P450 enzyme systems, particularly CYP3A4, found mostly in the liver and gut wall. Metabolites include phenylcyclohexylglycolic acid, which is pharmacologically inactive, and N-desethyloxybutynin, which is pharmacologically active.

After oral administration of oxybutynin, presystemic first-pass metabolism results in an oral bioavailability of approximately 6% and higher plasma concentration of the N-desethyl metabolite compared to oxybutynin. The plasma concentration AUC ratio of N-desethyl metabolite to parent compound following a single 5 mg oral dose of oxybutynin chloride was 11.9:1.

Transdermal administration of oxybutynin bypasses the first-pass gastrointestinal and hepatic metabolism, reducing the formation of the N-desethyl metabolite. Only small amounts of CYP3A4 are found in skin, limiting presystemic metabolism during transdermal absorption. The resulting plasma concentration AUC ratio of N-desethyl metabolite to parent compound following multiple oxybutynin transdermal system applications was 1.3:1.

Following intravenous administration, the elimination half-life of oxybutynin is approximately 2 hours. Following removal of oxybutynin transdermal system, plasma concentrations of oxybutynin and N-desethyloxybutynin decline with an apparent half-life of approximately 7 to 8 hours.

Excretion – Oxybutynin is extensively metabolized by the liver, with less than 0.1% of the administered dose excreted unchanged in the urine. Also, less than 0.1% of the administered dose is excreted as the metabolite N-desethyloxybutynin.

Special populations –

Race: Japanese volunteers demonstrated a somewhat lower metabolism of oxybutynin to N-desethyloxybutynin compared to white volunteers.

Contraindications

Urinary retention, gastric retention, or uncontrolled narrow-angle glaucoma and in patients who are at risk for these conditions; hypersensitivity to oxybutynin or other components of the product.

Warnings

➤*Renal/Hepatic function impairment:* Use with caution in patients with hepatic or renal impairment.

➤*Elderly:* Of the total number of patients in the clinical studies of oxybutynin transdermal system, 49% were 65 and over. No overall differences in safety or effectiveness were observed between these subjects and younger subjects, and other reported clinical experience has not identified differences in response between elderly and younger patients, but greater sensitivity of some older individuals cannot be ruled out.

➤*Pregnancy: Category B.*

Teratogenic –

The safety of oxybutynin transdermal system administration to women who are or who may become pregnant has not been established. Therefore, oxybutynin transdermal system should not be given to pregnant women unless, in the judgment of the physician, the probable clinical benefits outweigh the possible hazards.

➤*Lactation:* It is not known whether oxybutynin is excreted in human milk. Because many drugs are excreted in human milk, caution should be exercised when oxybutynin transdermal system is administered to a nursing woman.

➤*Children:* Safety and efficacy have not been established.

Precautions

➤*Urinary retention:* Oxybutynin transdermal system should be administered with caution to patients with clinically significant bladder outflow obstruction because of the risk of urinary retention. Oxybutynin is contraindicated in patients with urinary retention.

➤*Gastrointestinal disorders:* Oxybutynin transdermal system should be administered with caution to patients with gastrointestinal obstructive disorders because of the risk of gastric retention. Oxybutynin is contraindicated in patients with gastric retention.

Oxybutynin transdermal system, like other anticholinergic drugs, may decrease gastrointestinal motility and should be used with caution in patients with conditions such as ulcerative colitis, intestinal atony, and myasthenia gravis. Oxybutynin transdermal system should be used with caution in patients who have gastroesophageal reflux or who are concurrently taking drugs (such as bisphosphonates) that can cause or exacerbate esophagitis.

Drug Interactions

Oxybutynin Drug Interactions

Precipitant drug	Object drug*		Description
Oxybutynin	Anticholinergic agents	↑	Concomitant use may increase the frequency and/or severity of anticholinergic-like effects. Anticholinergic agents may potentially alter the absorption of some concomitantly administered drugs because of anticholinergic effects on GI motility.
Anticholinergic agents	Oxybutynin		
Oxybutynin	Beta blockers Atenolol	↑	The bioavailability of atenolol may be increased. If an increase in beta blockade is suspected, tailoring the beta blocker dose downward may be necessary.
Oxybutynin	Digoxin	↑	Serum levels of digoxin administered as slow-dissolution oral tablets may be increased and actions enhanced. Serum level monitoring may assist in tailoring dosage. Problems may be avoided with use of digoxin elixir or capsules.
Oxybutynin	Haloperidol	↔	Effects are variable. Use oxybutynin only when clearly needed. Routinely monitor these patients; discontinue anticholinergic or tailor haloperidol if necessary.

OXYBUTYNIN — TRANSDERMAL

Oxybutynin Drug Interactions			
Precipitant drug	Object drug*		Description
Oxybutynin	Phenothiazines	⬇	Pharmacologic/therapeutic actions of phenothiazines may be decreased by anticholinergics. Tailor the phenothiazine dose as needed.
Amantadine	Oxybutynin	⬆	Anticholinergic side effects may be increased. Decrease the dose of oxybutynin during coadministration. Monitor patient response and adjust the dose accordingly.

* ⬆ = Object drug increased. ⬇ = Object drug decreased. ⬌ = Undetermined clinical effect.

Adverse Reactions

Oxybutynin Adverse Reactions (≥ 2%) (Study 1)				
Adverse reaction*	Placebo (n = 132)		Oxybutynin transdermal system (3.9 mg/day) (n = 125)	
Application site pruritus	n = 8	6.1%	n = 21	16.8%
Dry mouth	n = 11	8.3%	n = 12	9.6%
Application site erythema	n = 3	2.3%	n = 7	5.6%
Application site vesicles	n = 0	0%	n = 4	3.2%
Diarrhea	n = 3	2.3%	n = 4	3.2%
Dysuria	n = 0	0%	n = 3	2.4%

* Includes adverse reactions judged by the investigator as possibly, probably, or definitely treatment-related.

Oxybutynin Adverse Reactions (≥ 2%) (Study 2)				
Adverse reaction*	Placebo (n = 117)		Oxybutynin transdermal system (3.9 mg/day) (n = 121)	
Application site pruritus	n = 5	4.3%	n = 17	14%
Application site erythema	n = 2	1.7%	n = 10	8.3%
Dry mouth	n = 2	1.7%	n = 5	4.1%
Constipation	n = 0	0%	n = 4	3.3%
Application site rash	n = 1	0.9%	n = 4	3.3%
Application site macules	n = 0	0%	n = 3	2.5%
Abnormal vision	n = 0	0%	n = 3	2.5%

* Includes adverse reactions judged by the investigator as possibly, probably, or definitely treatment-related.

Other adverse reactions reported by greater than 1% of oxybutynin transdermal system-treated patients, and judged by the investigator to be possibly, probably or definitely related to treatment include: Abdominal pain, nausea, flatulence, fatigue, somnolence, headache, flushing, rash, application site burning and back pain.

Most treatment-related adverse reactions were described as mild or moderate in intensity. Severe application site reactions were reported by 6.4% of oxybutynin transdermal system-treated patients in study 1 and by 5% of oxybutynin transdermal system-treated patients in study 2.

Treatment-related adverse reactions that resulted in discontinuation were reported by 11.2% of oxybutynin transdermal system-treated patients in study 1 and 10.7% of oxybutynin transdermal system-treated patients in study 2. Most of these were secondary to application site reaction. In the 2 pivotal studies, no patient discontinued oxybutynin transdermal system treatment due to dry mouth.

In the open-label extension, the most common treatment-related adverse reactions were: Application site pruritus, application site erythema, and dry mouth.

Overdosage

Plasma concentration of oxybutynin declines within 1 to 2 hours after removal of transdermal system(s). Patients should be monitored until symptoms resolve.

➤*Symptoms:* Overdosage with oxybutynin has been associated with anticholinergic effects including CNS excitation, flushing, fever, dehydration, cardiac arrhythmia, vomiting, and urinary retention. Ingestion of 100 mg oral oxybutynin chloride in association with alcohol has been reported in a 13-year-old boy who experienced memory loss, and in a 34-year-old woman who developed stupor, followed by disorientation and agitation on awakening, dilated pupils, dry skin, cardiac arrhythmia, and retention of urine.

➤*Treatment:* Both patients recovered fully with symptomatic treatment.

TOLTERODINE TARTRATE

Rx	**Detrol** (Pfizer)	**Tablets:** 1 mg	(TO). White. Film-coated. In 60s, 500s, and UD 140s.
		2 mg	(DT). White. Film-coated. In 60s, 500s, and UD 140s.
Rx	**Detrol LA** (Pfizer)	**Capsules, extended-release:** 2 mg	Sucrose. (2). Blue-green. In 30s, 90s, 500s, and UD blister 100s.
		4 mg	Sucrose. (4). Blue. In 30s, 90s, 500s, and UD blister 100s.

TOLTERODINE TARTRATE — ORAL

Indications

➤*Overactive bladder:* For the treatment of patients with an overactive bladder with symptoms of urge urinary incontinence, urgency, and frequency.

Administration and Dosage

➤*Approved by the FDA:* March 25, 1998.

➤*Immediate-release tablets:* 2 mg twice daily. Lower the dose to 1 mg twice daily based on individual response and tolerability. For patients with significantly reduced hepatic or renal function or who are currently taking drugs that are potent inhibitors of CYP3A4, the recommended dose of tolterodine is 1 mg twice daily.

➤*Extended-release capsules:* 4 mg/day. Tolterodine extended-release capsules should be taken once daily with liquids and swallowed whole. Lower the dose to 2 mg daily based on individual response and tolerability; however, limited efficacy data is available for 2 mg tolterodine extended-release capsules.

For patients with significantly reduced hepatic or renal function or who are currently taking drugs that are potent inhibitors of CYP3A4, the recommended dose of tolterodine extended-release capsules is 2 mg daily.

➤*Storage/Stability:* Store at controlled room temperature 25°C (77°F); excursions permitted to 15° to 30°C (59° to 86°F).

Extended-release capsules – Protect from light.

Actions

➤*Pharmacology:* Tolterodine is a competitive muscarinic receptor antagonist. Both urinary bladder contraction and salivation are mediated via cholinergic muscarinic receptors.

After oral administration, tolterodine is metabolized in the liver, resulting in the formation of the 5-hydroxymethyl derivative, a major pharmacologically active metabolite. The 5-hydroxymethyl metabolite, which exhibits an antimuscarinic activity similar to that of tolterodine, contributes significantly to the therapeutic effect. Both tolterodine and the 5-hydroxymethyl metabolite exhibit a high specificity for muscarinic receptors, since both show negligible activity or affinity for other neurotransmitter receptors and other potential cellular targets, such as calcium channels.

Tolterodine has a pronounced effect on bladder function. Effects on urodynamic parameters before and 1 and 5 hours after a single 6.4 mg dose of immediate-release tolterodine were determined in healthy volunteers. The main effects of tolterodine at 1 and 5 hours were an increase in residual urine, reflecting an incomplete emptying of the bladder, and a decrease in detrusor pressure. These findings are consistent with antimuscarinic action on the lower urinary tract.

➤*Pharmacokinetics:*

Absorption –

Immediate-release tablets: In a study of ^{14}C-tolterodine in healthy volunteers who received a 5 mg oral dose, at least 77% of the radiolabeled dose was absorbed. Immediate-release tolterodine is rapidly absorbed, and maximum serum concentrations (C_{max}) typically occur within 1 to 2 hours after dose administration. C_{max} and area under the concentration-time curve (AUC) determined after dosage of immediate-release tolterodine are dose proportional over the range of 1 to 4 mg.

• *Effect of food* – Food intake increases the bioavailability of tolterodine (average increase 53%), but does not affect the levels of the 5-hydroxymethyl metabolite in extensive metabolizers. This change is not expected to be a safety concern, and adjustment of dose is not needed.

Extended-release capsules: In a study with ^{14}C-tolterodine solution in healthy volunteers who received a 5 mg oral dose, at least 77% of the radiolabeled dose was absorbed. C_{max} and area under the concentration-time curve (AUC) determined after dosage of immediate-release tolterodine are dose proportional over the range of 1 to 4 mg. Based on the sum of unbound serum concentrations of tolterodine and the 5-hydroxymethyl metabolite ("active moiety"), the AUC of 4 mg/day extended-release tolterodine is equivalent to 4 mg (2 mg twice daily) immediate-release tolterodine. C_{max} and C_{min} levels of extended-release tolterodine are about 75% and 150% of

TOLTERODINE TARTRATE — ORAL

immediate-release tolterodine, respectively. Maximum serum concentrations of extended-release tolterodine are observed 2 to 6 hours after dose administration.

Distribution – Tolterodine is highly bound to plasma proteins, primarily α_1-acid glycoprotein. Unbound concentrations of tolterodine average 3.7% ± 0.13% over the concentration range achieved in clinical studies. The 5-hydroxymethyl metabolite is not extensively protein bound, with unbound fraction concentrations averaging 36% ± 4%. The blood-to-serum ratio of tolterodine and the 5-hydroxymethyl metabolite averages 0.6 and 0.8, respectively, indicating that these compounds do not distribute extensively into erythrocytes. The volume of distribution of tolterodine following administration of a 1.28 mg IV dose is 113 ± 26.7 L.

Metabolism – Tolterodine is extensively metabolized by the liver following oral dosing. The primary metabolic route involves the oxidation of the 5-methyl group and is mediated by the cytochrome P450 2D6 (CYP2D6) and leads to the formation of a pharmacologically active 5-hydroxymethyl metabolite. Further metabolism leads to formation of the 5-carboxylic acid and N-dealkylated 5-carboxylic acid metabolites, which account for 51% ± 14% and 29% ± 6.3% of the metabolites recovered in the urine, respectively.

Variability in metabolism: A subset (about 7%) of the white population is devoid of CYP2D6, the enzyme responsible for the formation of the 5-hydroxymethyl metabolite of tolterodine. The identified pathway of metabolism for these individuals ("poor metabolizers") is dealkylation via cytochrome P450 3A4 (CYP3A4) to N-dealkylated tolterodine. The remainder of the population is referred to as "extensive metabolizers." Pharmacokinetic studies revealed that tolterodine is metabolized at a slower rate in poor metabolizers than in extensive metabolizers; this results in significantly higher serum concentrations of tolterodine and in negligible concentrations of the 5-hydroxymethyl metabolite.

• *Immediate-release tablets* – Because of differences in the protein-binding characteristics of tolterodine and the 5-hydroxymethyl metabolite, the sum of unbound serum concentrations of tolterodine and the 5-hydroxymethyl metabolite is similar in extensive and poor metabolizers at steady state. Since tolterodine and the 5-hydroxymethyl metabolite have similar antimuscarinic effects, the net activity of tolterodine immediate-release tablets is expected to be similar in extensive and poor metabolizers.

Excretion – Following administration of a 5 mg oral dose of ^{14}C-tolterodine to healthy volunteers, 77% of radioactivity was recovered in urine and 17% was recovered in feces in 7 days. Less than 1% (less than 2.5% in poor metabolizers) of the dose was recovered as intact tolterodine, and 5% to 14% (less than 1% in poor metabolizers) was recovered as the active 5-hydroxymethyl metabolite.

Immediate-release tablets: Most of the radioactivity was recovered within the first 24 hours, which is consistent with the apparent half-life of tolterodine: 1.9 to 3.7 hours in pharmacokinetic studies.

A summary of mean (± standard deviation) pharmacokinetic parameters of immediate-release tolterodine and the 5-hydroxymethyl metabolite in extensive and poor metabolizers is provided in the following tables. These data were obtained following single and multiple doses of 4 mg tolterodine administered twice daily to 16 healthy male volunteers (8 extensive metabolizers, 8 poor metabolizers).

Summary of Mean (± SD) Pharmacokinetic Parameters of Tolterodine and Its Active Metabolite (5-hydroxymethyl Metabolite) in Healthy Volunteers[a]

	Tolterodine					5-hydroxymethyl metabolite			
Phenotype (CYP2D6)	t_{max} (hr)	C_{max}[b] (mcg/L)	C_{avg}[b] (mcg/L)	t½ (hr)	CL/F (L/hr)	t_{max} (hr)	C_{max}[b] (mcg/L)	C_{avg}[b] (mcg/L)	t½ (hr)
Single dose									
EM	1.6 ± 1.5	1.6 ± 1.2	0.5 ± 0.35	2 ± 0.7	534 ± 697	1.8 ± 1.4	1.8 ± 0.7	0.62 ± 0.26	3.1 ± 0.7
PM	1.4 ± 0.5	10 ± 4.9	8.3 ± 4.3	6.5 ± 1.6	17 ± 7.3	NA	NA	NA	NA
Multiple dose									
EM	1.2 ± 0.5	2.6 ± 2.8	0.58 ± 0.54	2.2 ± 0.4	415 ± 377	1.2 ± 0.5	2.4 ± 1.3	0.92 ± 0.46	2.9 ± 0.4
PM	1.9 ± 1	19 ± 7.5	12 ± 5.1	9.6 ± 1.5	11 ± 4.2	NA	NA	NA	NA

[a] C_{max} = Maximum plasma concentration; t_{max} = time of occurrence of C_{max}; C_{avg} = Average plasma concentration; t½ = Terminal elimination half-life; CL/F = Apparent oral clearance; EM = Extensive metabolizers; PM = Poor metabolizers.
[b] Parameter was dose-normalized from 4 mg to 2 mg.

Extended-release capsules: A summary of mean (± standard deviation) pharmacokinetic parameters of extended-release tolterodine and the 5-hydroxymethyl metabolite in extensive and poor metabolizers is provided in the table below. These data were obtained following single and multiple doses of extended-release tolterodine administered daily to 17 healthy male volunteers (13 extensive metabolizers, 4 poor metabolizers).

Summary of Mean (± SD) Pharmacokinetic Parameters of Extended-Release Tolterodine and Its Active Metabolite (5-hydroxymethyl Metabolite) in Healthy Volunteers[a]

	Tolterodine				5-hydroxymethyl metabolite			
	t_{max}[b] (hr)	C_{max} (mcg/L)	C_{avg} (mcg/L)	t½ (hr)	t_{max}[b] (hr)	C_{max} (mcg/L)	C_{avg} (mcg/L)	t½ (hr)
Single dose 4 mg[c]								
EM	4 (2 to 6)	1.3 (0.8)	0.8 (0.57)	8.4 (3.2)	4 (3 to 6)	1.6 (0.5)	1 (0.32)	8.8 (5.9)
Multiple dose 4 mg								
EM	4 (2 to 6)	3.4 (4.9)	1.7 (2.8)	6.9 (3.5)	4 (2 to 6)	2.7 (0.9)	1.4 (0.6)	9.9 (4)
PM	4 (3 to 6)	19 (16)	13 (11)	18 (16)	NA	NA	NA	NA

[a] C_{max} = Maximum plasma concentration; t_{max} = Time of occurrence of C_{max}; C_{avg} = Average plasma concentration; t½ = Terminal elimination half-life; CL/F = Apparent oral clearance.
[b] Data presented as median (range).
[c] Parameter dose-normalized from 8 to 4 mg for the single-dose data.

Special populations –

Renal function impairment:

• *Immediate-release tablets* – Renal impairment can significantly alter the disposition of immediate-release tolterodine and its metabolites. In a study conducted in patients with creatinine clearance between 10 and 30 mL/min, immediate-release tolterodine and the 5-hydroxymethyl metabolite levels were approximately 2 to 3 fold higher in patients with renal impairment than in healthy volunteers. Exposure levels of other metabolites of tolterodine (eg, tolterodine acid, N-dealkylated tolterodine acid, N-dealkylated tolterodine, and N-dealkylated hydroxylated tolterodine) were significantly higher (10- to 30-fold) in renally impaired patients as compared with the healthy volunteers. The recommended dosage for patients with significantly reduced renal function is 1 mg tolterodine twice daily.

• *Extended-release capsules* – Renal impairment can significantly alter the disposition of immediate-release tolterodine and its metabolites. In a study conducted in patients with creatinine clearance between 10 and 30 mL/min, immediate-release tolterodine and the 5-hydroxymethyl metabolite levels were approximately 2- to 3-fold higher in patients with renal impairment than in healthy volunteers. Exposure levels of other metabolites of tolterodine (eg, tolterodine acid, N-dealkylated tolterodine acid, N-dealkylated tolterodine and N-dealkylated hydroxy tolterodine) were significantly higher (10- to 30-fold) in renally impaired patients as compared to the healthy volunteers. The recommended dose for patients with significantly reduced renal function is 2 mg/day tolterodine.

Hepatic function impairment: Liver impairment can significantly alter the disposition of immediate-release tolterodine. In a study conducted in cirrhotic patients, the elimination half-life of immediate-release tolterodine was longer in cirrhotic patients (mean, 7.8 hours) than in healthy, younger and elderly volunteers (mean, 2 to 4 hours). The clearance of orally administered tolterodine was substantially lower in cirrhotic patients (1 ± 1.7 L/hr/kg) than in healthy volunteers (5.7 ± 3.8 L/hr/kg). The recommended dose for patients with significantly reduced hepatic function is 1 mg immediate-release tolterodine twice daily or 2 mg/day extended-release tolterodine.

Children:

• *Extended-release capsules* –

The pharmacokinetics of tolterodine extended-release capsules have been evaluated in pediatric patients ranging in age from 11 to 15 years. The dose-plasma concentration relationship was linear over the range of doses assessed. Parent/metabolite ratios differed according to CYP2D6 metabolizer status: Extensive metabolizers had low serum concentrations of tolterodine and high concentrations of the active 5-hydroxymethyl metabolite, while poor metabolizers had high concentrations of tolterodine and negligible active metabolite concentrations.

Contraindications

Urinary retention, gastric retention, or uncontrolled narrow-angle glaucoma; hypersensitivity to the drug or its ingredients.

Warnings

➤*Renal/Hepatic function impairment:*

Immediate-release tablets – For patients with significantly reduced hepatic function or renal function, the recommended dose of tolterodine is 1 mg twice daily.

Extended-release capsules – For patients with significantly reduced hepatic function or renal function, the recommended dose is 2 mg/day extended-release tolterodine.

➤*Pregnancy: Category C.*

When given at doses of 30 to 40 mg/kg/day, tolterodine has been shown to be embryolethal and reduce fetal weight, and increase the incidence of fetal abnormalities (cleft palate, digital abnormalities, intra-abdominal hemorrhage, and various skeletal abnormalities, primarily reduced ossification) in mice. At these doses, the AUC values were about 20- to 25-fold higher than in humans. Rabbits treated subcutaneously at a dose of 0.8 mg/kg/day achieved an AUC of 100 mcg•hr/L, which is about 3-fold higher than that resulting from the human dose. This dose did not result in any embryotoxicity or teratogenicity. There are no studies of tolterodine in pregnant women. Therefore, only use tolterodine during pregnancy if the potential benefit for the mother justifies the potential risk for the fetus.

TOLTERODINE TARTRATE — ORAL

➤*Lactation:* Tolterodine is excreted into the milk in mice. Offspring of female mice treated with tolterodine 20 mg/kg/day during the lactation period had slightly reduced body-weight gain. The offspring regained the weight during the maturation phase. It is not known whether tolterodine is excreted in human milk; therefore, do not administer tolterodine during nursing. Decide whether to discontinue nursing or to discontinue tolterodine in nursing mothers.

➤*Children:* Safety and efficacy have not been established.

Extended-release capsules – A total of 710 pediatric patients (486 on extended-release tolterodine, 224 on placebo) 5 to 10 years of age with urinary frequency and urge incontinence were studied in two phase 3 randomized, placebo-controlled, double-blind, 12-week studies. The percentage of patients with urinary tract infections was higher in patients treated with extended-release tolterodine (6.6%) compared with patients who received placebo (4.5%). Aggressive, abnormal, and hyperactive behavior and attention disorders occurred in 2.9% of children treated with extended-release tolterodine compared with 0.9% of children treated with placebo.

Precautions

➤*Risk of urinary retention and gastric retention:* Administer tolterodine with caution to patients with clinically significant bladder outflow obstruction because of the risk of urinary retention and to patients with GI obstructive disorders, such as pyloric stenosis, because of the risk of gastric retention.

➤*Controlled narrow-angle glaucoma:* Use tolterodine with caution in patients being treated for narrow-angle glaucoma.

Drug Interactions

➤*CYP3A4 inhibitors:* Ketoconazole, an inhibitor of the drug metabolizing enzyme CYP3A4, significantly increased plasma concentrations of tolterodine when coadministered to subjects who were poor metabolizers. For patients receiving ketoconazole or other potent CYP3A4 inhibitors such as other azole antifungals (eg, itraconazole, miconazole) or macrolide antibiotics (eg, erythromycin, clarithromycin), or cyclosporine or vinblastine, the recommended dose is 1 mg twice daily of immediate-release tolterodine or 2 mg/day extended-release tolterodine.

Adverse Reactions

➤*Immediate-release tablets:* The phase 2 and 3 clinical trial program for tolterodine included 3,071 patients who were treated with tolterodine (n = 2,133) or placebo (n = 938). The patients were treated with 1, 2, 4, or 8 mg/day for up to 12 months. No differences in the safety profile of tolterodine were identified based on age, gender, race, or metabolism.

The data described below reflect exposure to 2 mg tolterodine twice daily in 986 patients and to placebo in 683 patients exposed for 12 weeks in 5 phase 3, controlled clinical studies. Because clinical trials are conducted under widely varying conditions, adverse reaction rates observed in the clinical trials of a drug cannot be directly compared with rates in the clinical trials of another drug and may not reflect the rates observed in practice. The adverse reaction information from clinical trials does, however, provide a basis for identifying the adverse reactions that appear to be related to drug use and approximating rates.

Sixty-six percent (66%) of patients receiving 2 mg tolterodine twice daily reported adverse reactions versus 56% of placebo patients. The most common adverse reactions reported by patients receiving tolterodine were dry mouth, headache, constipation, vertigo/dizziness, and abdominal pain. Dry mouth, constipation, abnormal vision (accommodation abnormalities), urinary retention, and xerophthalmia are expected side effects of antimuscarinic agents.

Dry mouth was the most frequently reported adverse reaction for patients treated with 2 mg tolterodine twice daily in the phase 3 clinical studies, occurring in 34.8% of patients treated with tolterodine and 9.8% of placebo-treated patients. One percent (1%) of patients treated with tolterodine discontinued treatment due to dry mouth.

The frequency of discontinuation due to adverse reactions was highest during the first 4 weeks of treatment. Seven percent (7%) of patients treated with tolterodine 2 mg twice daily discontinued treatment due to adverse reactions verses 6% of placebo patients. The most common adverse reactions leading to discontinuation were dizziness and headache.

Three percent (3%) of patients treated with 2 mg tolterodine twice daily reported a serious adverse reaction versus 4% of placebo patients. Significant ECG changes in QT and QTc have not been demonstrated in clinical-study patients treated with tolterodine 2 mg twice daily. The table below lists the adverse reactions reported in 1% or more of the patients treated with 2 mg tolterodine twice daily in the 12-week studies. The adverse reactions are reported regardless of causality.

Tolterodine Adverse Reactions[a] (> 1%)

Body system	Adverse reaction	% Tolterodine (n = 986)	% Placebo (n = 683)
Autonomic nervous	Accommodation abnormal	2%	1%
	Dry mouth	35%	10%
CNS	Vertigo/dizziness	5%	3%
Dermatologic	Dry skin	1%	0%
GI	Abdominal pain	5%	3%
	Constipation	7%	4%
	Diarrhea	4%	3%
	Dyspepsia	4%	1%
GU	Dysuria	2%	1%
Metabolic/ nutritional	Weight gain	1%	0%
Musculoskeletal	Arthralgia	2%	1%
Psychiatric	Somnolence	3%	2%
Special senses	Xerophthalmia	3%	2%
Miscellaneous	Chest pain	2%	1%
	Fatigue	4%	3%
	Headache	7%	5%
	Infection	1%	0%
	Influenza-like symptoms	3%	2%

[a] In nearest integer.

➤*Extended-release capsules:* The phase 2 and 3 clinical trial program for tolterodine extended-release capsules included 1,073 patients who were treated with tolterodine extended-release capsules (n = 537) or placebo (n = 536). The patients were treated with 2, 4, 6, or 8 mg/day for up to 15 months. Because clinical trials are conducted under widely varying conditions, adverse reaction rates observed in the clinical trials of a drug cannot be directly compared with rates in the clinical trials of another drug and may not reflect the rates observed in practice. The adverse reaction information from clinical trials does, however, provide a basis for identifying the adverse reactions that appear to be related to drug use and for approximating rates. The data described below reflect exposure to 4 mg extended-release tolterodine capsules once daily every morning in 505 patients and to placebo in 507 patients exposed for 12 weeks in the phase 3, controlled clinical study.

Adverse reactions were reported in 52% (n = 263) of patients receiving tolterodine extended-release capsules and in 49% (n = 247) of patients receiving placebo. The most common adverse reactions reported by patients receiving tolterodine extended-release capsules were dry mouth, headache, constipation, and abdominal pain. Dry mouth was the most frequently reported adverse reaction for patients treated with tolterodine extended-release capsules, occurring in 23.4% of patients treated with tolterodine extended-release capsules and 7.7% of placebo-treated patients. Dry mouth, constipation, abnormal vision (accommodation abnormalities), urinary retention, and dry eyes are expected side effects of antimuscarinic agents. A serious adverse reaction was reported by 1.4% (n = 7) of patients receiving tolterodine extended-release capsules and by 3.6% (n = 18) of patients receiving placebo.

The frequency of discontinuation due to adverse reactions was highest during the first 4 weeks of treatment. Similar percentages of patients treated with tolterodine extended-release capsules or placebo discontinued treatment due to adverse reactions. Treatment was discontinued due to adverse reactions and dry mouth was reported as an adverse reaction in 2.4% (n = 12) of patients treated with tolterodine extended-release capsules and in 1.2% (n = 6) of patients treated with placebo.

The table below lists the adverse reactions reported in greater than or equal to 1% of patients treated with 4 mg tolterodine extended-release capsules once daily in the 12-week study. The adverse reactions were reported regardless of causality.

Tolterodine Adverse Reactions[a] (≥ 1%)

Body system	Adverse reaction	% Tolterodine extended-release capsules (n = 505)	% Placebo (n = 507)
Autonomic nervous system	Dry mouth	23%	8%
CNS	Dizziness	2%	1%
GI	Abdominal pain	4%	2%
	Constipation	6%	4%
	Dyspepsia	3%	1%
GU	Dysuria	1%	0%
Psychiatric	Anxiety	1%	0%
	Somnolence	3%	2%
Respiratory	Sinusitis	2%	1%
Special senses	Abnormal vision	1%	0%
	Xerophthalmia	3%	2%
Miscellaneous	Fatigue	2%	1%
	Headache	6%	4%

[a] In nearest integer.

➤*Postmarketing:* The following events have been reported in association with tolterodine use in clinical practice: Anaphylactoid reactions, including angioedema; tachycardia; palpitations; peripheral edema; and hallucinations. Because these spontaneously reported reactions are from the worldwide postmarketing experience, the frequency of reactions and the role of tolterodine in their causation cannot be reliably determined.

Overdosage

A 27-month-old child who ingested 5 to 7 immediate-release tablets of 2 mg tolterodine was treated with a suspension of activated charcoal and was hospitalized overnight with symptoms of dry mouth. The child fully recovered.

TOLTERODINE TARTRATE — ORAL

➤*Treatment:* Overdosage with tolterodine immediate-release tablets or extended-release capsules can potentially result in severe central anticholinergic effects and should be treated accordingly.

ECG monitoring is recommended in the event of overdosage. In dogs, changes in the QT interval (slight prolongation of 10% to 20%) were observed at a suprapharmacologic dose of 4.5 mg/kg, which is about 68 times higher than the recommended human dose. In clinical trials of healthy volunteers and patients, QT interval prolongation was not observed with immediate-release tolterodine at doses up to 4 mg twice daily of tolterodine (higher doses were not evaluated).

Patient Information

Inform patients that antimuscarinic agents such as tolterodine may produce blurred vision, dizziness, or drowsiness.

TROSPIUM CHLORIDE

Rx	**Sanctura** (Odyssey, Indevus)	**Tablets:** 20 mg	Lactose, sucrose. Brownish yellow, biconvex. Glossy-coated. In 60s, 500s, and blister 14s.

TROSPIUM CHLORIDE — ORAL

Indications

➤*Overactive bladder:* For the treatment of overactive bladder with symptoms of urge urinary incontinence, urgency, and urinary frequency.

Administration and Dosage

➤*Approved by the FDA:* May 28, 2004.

The recommended dose is 20 mg twice daily. Trospium should be dosed at least 1 hour before meals or given on an empty stomach.

➤*Renal function impairment:* For patients with severe renal impairment (creatinine clearance [Ccr] less than 30 mL/min), the recommended dose is 20 mg once daily at bedtime.

➤*Elderly:* In geriatric patients 75 years of age or older, dose may be titrated down to 20 mg once daily based upon tolerability.

➤*Storage/Stability:* Store at controlled room temperature 20° to 25°C (68° to 77°F).

Actions

➤*Pharmacology:* Trospium is an antispasmodic, antimuscarinic agent.

Trospium antagonizes the effect of acetylcholine on muscarinic receptors in cholinergically innervated organs. Its parasympatholytic action reduces the tonus of smooth muscle in the bladder. Receptor assays showed that trospium has negligible affinity for nicotinic receptors as compared with muscarinic receptors at concentrations obtained from therapeutic doses.

Pharmacodynamics – Placebo-controlled studies employing urodynamic variables were conducted in patients with conditions characterized by involuntary detrusor contractions. The results demonstrate that trospium increases maximum cystometric bladder capacity and volume at first detrusor contraction.

➤*Pharmacokinetics:*

Absorption – After oral administration, less than 10% of the dose is absorbed. Mean absolute bioavailability of a 20 mg dose is 9.6% (range, 4% to 16.1%). Peak plasma concentrations (C_{max}) occur between 5 to 6 hours post-dose. Mean C_{max} increases greater than dose-proportionally; a 3-fold and 4-fold increase in C_{max} was observed for dose increases from 20 to 40 mg and from 20 to 60 mg, respectively. AUC exhibits dose linearity for single doses up to 60 mg. Trospium exhibits diurnal variability in exposure with a decrease in C_{max} and AUC of up to 59% and 33%, respectively, for evening relative to morning doses.

Effect of food: Administration with a high fat meal resulted in reduced absorption, with AUC and C_{max} values 70% to 80% lower than those obtained when trospium was administered while fasting. Therefore, it is recommended that trospium should be taken at least 1 hour prior to meals or on an empty stomach.

Distribution – Protein binding ranged from 50% to 85% when therapeutic concentration levels (0.5 to 50 ng/mL) were incubated with human serum in vitro.

The ^{3}H-trospium ratio of plasma to whole blood was 1.6:1. This ratio indicates that the majority of ^{3}H-trospium is distributed in plasma. The apparent volume of distribution for a 20 mg oral dose is 395 (± 140) L.

Metabolism – The metabolic pathway of trospium in humans has not been fully defined. Of the 10% of the dose absorbed, metabolites account for approximately 40% of the excreted dose following oral administration. The major metabolic pathway is hypothesized as ester hydrolysis with subsequent conjugation of benzylic acid to form azoniaspironortropanol with glucuronic acid. Cytochrome P450 is not expected to contribute significantly to the elimination of trospium. In vitro data from human liver microsomes investigating the inhibitory effect of trospium on seven cytochrome P450 isoenzyme substrates (CYP1A2, 2A6, 2C9, 2C19, 2D6, 2E1, and 3A4) suggest a lack of inhibition at clinically relevant concentrations of trospium.

Excretion – The plasma half-life for trospium following oral administration is approximately 20 hours. After administration of oral ^{14}C-trospium chloride, the majority of the dose (85.2%) was recovered in feces and a smaller amount (5.8% of the dose) was recovered in urine; 60% of the radioactivity excreted in urine was unchanged trospium.

The mean renal clearance for trospium (29.07 L/hr) is 4-fold higher than average glomerular filtration rate, indicating that active tubular secretion is a major route of elimination for trospium. There may be competition for elimination with other compounds that are also renally eliminated. Carefully monitor patients receiving such drugs.

Special populations –

Renal function impairment: Severe renal impairment significantly altered the disposition of trospium. A 4.5-fold and 2-fold increase in mean $AUC_{0-\infty}$ and C_{max}, respectively, and the appearance of an additional elimination phase with a long half-life (approximately 33 hours) was detected in patients with severe renal insufficiency (Ccr less than 30 mL/min) compared with healthy, nearly age-matched subjects. The different pharmacokinetic behavior of trospium in patients with severe renal insufficiency necessitates adjustment of dosage frequency. The pharmacokinetics of trospium have not been studied in people with moderate or mild renal impairment (Ccr ranging from 30 to 80 mL/min).

Hepatic function impairment: There is no information regarding the effect of severe hepatic impairment on exposure to trospium. Maximum trospium concentration (C_{max}) increased 12% and 63% in subjects with mild and moderate hepatic impairment, respectively, compared with healthy subjects. Mean area under the plasma concentration-time curve (AUC) was similar. Use caution when administering trospium to patients with moderate and severe hepatic dysfunction. Use caution when administering trospium in patients with moderate or severe hepatic dysfunction.

Elderly: Age did not appear to significantly affect the pharmacokinetics of trospium; however, increased anticholinergic side effects unrelated to drug exposure were observed in patients 75 years of age or older.

Gender: Studies comparing the pharmacokinetics in different genders had conflicting results. When a single 40 mg trospium dose was administered to 16 elderly subjects, exposure was 45% lower in elderly women compared to elderly men. When 20 mg trospium was dosed twice daily for 4 days to 6 elderly men and 6 elderly women (60 to 75 years), AUC and C_{max} were 26% and 68% higher, respectively, in women without hormone replacement therapy than in men.

Contraindications

Urinary retention, gastric retention, or uncontrolled narrow-angle glaucoma and in patients who are at risk for these conditions; hypersensitivity to the drug or its ingredients.

Warnings

➤*Renal function impairment:* See Administration and Dosage for more information.

➤*Hepatic function impairment:* Use caution when administering trospium in patients with moderate or severe hepatic dysfunction.

➤*Elderly:* Of the 591 patients with overactive bladder who received treatment with trospium in the 2 US, placebo-controlled, efficacy and safety studies, 249 patients (42%) were 65 years of age and older. Eighty-eight trospium-treated patients (15%) were 75 years of age and older.

In these 2 studies, the incidence of commonly reported anticholinergic adverse events in patients treated with trospium (including dry mouth, constipation, dyspepsia, urinary tract infection, and urinary retention) was higher in patients 75 years of age and older as compared with younger patients. This effect may be related to an enhanced sensitivity to anticholinergic agents in this patient population. Therefore, based upon tolerability, the dose frequency of trospium may be reduced to 20 mg once daily in patients 75 years of age and older.

➤*Pregnancy: Category C.*

Trospium has been shown to cause maternal toxicity in rats and a decrease in fetal survival in rats administered approximately 10 times the expected clinical exposure (AUC). The no effect levels for maternal and fetal toxicity were approximately equivalent to the expected clinical exposure in rats, and about 5 to 6 times the expected clinical exposure in rabbits. No malformations or developmental delays were observed. There are no adequate and well-controlled studies in pregnant women. Use trospium during pregnancy only if the potential benefit justifies the potential risk to the fetus.

➤*Lactation:* Trospium (2 mg/kg orally and 50 mcg/kg IV) was excreted, to a limited extent (less than 1%), into the milk of lactating rats. The activity observed in the milk was primarily from the parent compound. It is not known whether this drug is excreted in human milk. Because many drugs are excreted in human milk, exercise caution when trospium is administered to a nursing woman. Use trospium during lactation only if the potential benefit justifies the potential risk to the child.

➤*Children:* Safety and efficacy have not been established.

Precautions

➤*Risk of urinary retention:* Administer trospium with caution to patients with clinically significant bladder outflow obstruction because of the risk of urinary retention.

➤*Decreased GI motility:* Administer trospium with caution to patients with GI obstructive disorders because of the risk of gastric retention. Trospium, like other anticholinergic drugs, may decrease GI motility; use with caution in patients with conditions such as ulcerative colitis, intestinal atony, and myasthenia gravis.

TROSPIUM CHLORIDE — ORAL

➤*Controlled narrow-angle glaucoma:* In patients being treated for narrow-angle glaucoma, use trospium only if the potential benefits outweigh the risks, and, in that circumstance, only with careful monitoring.

Drug Interactions

The concomitant use of trospium with other anticholinergic agents that produce dry mouth, constipation, and other anticholinergic pharmacological effects may increase the frequency and/or severity of such effects. Anticholinergic agents may potentially alter the absorption of some concomitantly administered drugs due to anticholinergic effects on GI motility.

➤*Drugs eliminated by active tubular secretion:* Although studies to assess drug-drug interactions with trospium have not been conducted, trospium has the potential for pharmacokinetic interactions with other drugs that are eliminated by active tubular secretion (eg, digoxin, procainamide, pancuronium, morphine, vancomycin, metformin, tenofovir). Coadministration of trospium with drugs that are eliminated by active renal tubular secretion may increase the serum concentration of trospium and/or the coadministered drug due to competition for this elimination pathway. Carefully monitor patients receiving such drugs.

Adverse Reactions

The 2 most common adverse events reported by patients receiving 20 mg trospium twice daily were dry mouth and constipation. The single most frequently reported adverse event for trospium, dry mouth, occurred in 20.1% of trospium treated patients and 5.8% of patients receiving placebo. In the 2 phase 3 US studies, dry mouth led to discontinuation in 1.9% of patients treated with 20 mg trospium twice daily. For the patients who reported dry mouth, most had their first occurrence of the event within the first month of treatment.

Trospium Adverse Reactions (≥ 1%)

Adverse reaction	Placebo (n = 590)	Trospium 20 mg twice daily (n = 591)
CNS		
Headache	12 (2%)	25 (4.2%)
GI		
Abdominal pain upper	7 (1.2%)	9 (1.5%)
Constipation	27 (4.6%)	57 (9.6%)
Constipation aggravated	5 (0.8%)	8 (1.4%)
Dry mouth	34 (5.8%)	119 (20.1%)
Dyspepsia	2 (0.3%)	7 (1.2%)
Flatulence	5 (0.8%)	7 (1.2%)
GU		
Urinary retention	2 (0.3%)	7 (1.2%)
Ophthalmic		
Dry eyes (not otherwise specified)	2 (0.3%)	7 (1.2%)
Miscellaneous		
Fatigue	8 (1.4%)	11 (1.9%)

Other adverse events from the phase 3, US, placebo-controlled trials judged possibly related to treatment with trospium by the investigator, occurring in greater than or equal to 0.5% of trospium-treated patients, and more common with trospium than placebo are tachycardia (not otherwise specified), vision blurred, abdominal distension, vomiting (not otherwise specified), dysgeusia, dry throat, and dry skin.

During controlled clinical studies, 1 event of angioneurotic edema was reported.

➤*Postmarketing:* Additional spontaneous adverse events, regardless of relationship to drug, reported from marketing experience with trospium include the following: anaphylactic reaction, chest pain, gastritis, hallucinations and delirium, "hypertensive crisis," palpitations, rhabdomyolysis, Stevens-Johnson syndrome, supraventricular tachycardia, syncope, vision abnormal.

Overdosage

➤*Symptoms:* Overdosage with trospium may result in severe anticholinergic effects.

A baby 7 months of age experienced tachycardia and mydriasis after administration of a single dose of trospium 10 mg given by a sibling. The baby's weight was reported as 5 kg. Following admission into the hospital and about 1 hour after ingestion of the trospium, medicinal charcoal was administered for detoxification. While hospitalized, the baby experienced mydriasis and tachycardia up to 230 bpm. Therapeutic intervention was not deemed necessary. The baby was discharged as completely recovered the following day.

➤*Treatment:* Treatment should be provided according to symptoms and supportive care. In the event of overdosage, ECG monitoring is recommended.

Patient Information

Inform patients that anticholinergic agents, such as trospium, may produce clinically significant adverse reactions related to anticholinergic pharmacological activity. For example, heat prostration (fever and heat stroke due to decreased sweating) can occur when anticholinergics such as trospium are used in a hot environment. Because anticholinergics such as trospium may also produce dizziness or blurred vision, advise patients to exercise caution. Inform patients that alcohol may enhance the drowsiness caused by anticholinergic agents.

Take trospium 1 hour prior to meals or on an empty stomach. If a dose is skipped, advise patients to take the next dose 1 hour prior to their next meal.

SOLIFENACIN SUCCINATE

Rx	**Vesicare** (GlaxoSmithKline)	**Tablets:** 5 mg	(VESIcare 150). Lt. yellow, round. Film-coated. In 30s, 90s, and UD 100s.
		10 mg	(VESIcare 151). Lt. pink, round. Film-coated. In 30s, 90s, and UD 100s.

SOLIFENACIN SUCCINATE — ORAL

Indications

➤*Overactive bladder:* For the treatment of overactive bladder with symptoms of urge urinary incontinence, urgency, and urinary frequency.

Administration and Dosage

➤*Approved by the FDA:* November 19, 2004.

➤*Dosage:* 5 mg once daily. If the 5 mg dose is well tolerated, the dose may be increased to 10 mg once daily.

➤*Administration:* Take solifenacin with liquids and swallow whole. Administer solifenacin with or without food.

➤*Renal function impairment:* For patients with severe renal impairment (creatinine clearance less than 30 mL/min), a daily dose of solifenacin greater than 5 mg is not recommended.

➤*Hepatic function impairment:* For patients with moderate hepatic impairment (Child-Pugh B), a daily dose of solifenacin greater than 5 mg is not recommended. Use of solifenacin in patients with severe hepatic impairment (Child Pugh C) is not recommended.

➤*Dose adjustment with CYP3A4 inhibitors:* When administered with therapeutic doses of ketoconazole or other potent CYP3A4 inhibitors, a daily dose of solifenacin greater than 5 mg is not recommended.

➤*Storage / Stability:* Store at 25°C (77°F) with excursions permitted from 15° to 30°C (59° to 86°F).

Actions

➤*Pharmacology:* Solifenacin is a competitive muscarinic receptor antagonist. Muscarinic receptors play an important role in several major cholinergically mediated functions, including contractions of urinary bladder smooth muscle and stimulation of salivary secretion.

➤*Pharmacokinetics:*

Absorption – After oral administration of solifenacin to healthy volunteers, peak plasma levels (C_{max}) of solifenacin are reached within 3 to 8 hours after administration, and at steady state ranged from 32.3 to 62.9 ng/mL for the 5 and 10 mg solifenacin tablets, respectively. The absolute bioavailability of solifenacin is approximately 90%, and plasma concentrations of solifenacin are proportional to the dose administered.

Distribution – Solifenacin is approximately 98% (in vivo) bound to human plasma proteins, principally to α_1-acid glycoprotein. Solifenacin is highly distributed to non-CNS tissues, having a mean steady-state volume of distribution of 600 L.

Metabolism – Solifenacin is extensively metabolized in the liver. The primary pathway for elimination is by way of CYP3A4; however, alternate metabolic pathways exist. The primary metabolic routes of solifenacin are through N-oxidation of the quinuclidin ring and 4R-hydroxylation of tetrahydroisoquinoline ring. One pharmacologically active metabolite (4R-hydroxy solifenacin), occurring at low concentrations and unlikely to contribute significantly to clinical activity, and 3 pharmacologically inactive metabolites (N-glucuronide and the N-oxide and 4R-hydroxy-N-oxide of solifenacin) have been found in human plasma after oral dosing.

Excretion – Following the administration of ^{14}C-solifenacin succinate 10 mg to healthy volunteers, 69.2% of the radioactivity was recovered in the urine and 22.5% in the feces over 26 days. Less than 15% (as mean value) of the dose was recovered in the urine as intact solifenacin. The major metabolites identified in urine were N-oxide of solifenacin, 4R-hydroxy solifenacin, and 4R-hydroxy-N-oxide of solifenacin, and in feces 4R-hydroxy solifenacin. The elimination half-life of solifenacin following chronic dosing is approximately 45 to 68 hours.

Special populations –

Renal function impairment: Use solifenacin with caution in patients with renal impairment. There is a 2.1-fold increase in AUC and 1.6-fold increase in $t_{½}$ of solifenacin in patients with severe renal impairment. Doses of solifenacin greater than 5 mg are not recommended in patients with severe renal impairment (Ccr less than 30 mL/min).

Hepatic function impairment: Use solifenacin with caution in patients with reduced hepatic function. There is a 2-fold increase in the $t_{½}$ and 35% increase in AUC of solifenacin in patients with moderate hepatic impairment. Doses of solifenacin greater than 5 mg are not recommended in

SOLIFENACIN SUCCINATE — ORAL

patients with moderate hepatic impairment (Child-Pugh B). Solifenacin is not recommended for patients with severe hepatic impairment (Child-Pugh C).

Elderly: Multiple-dose studies of solifenacin in elderly volunteers (65 to 80 years of age) showed that C_{max}, AUC, and t½ values were 20% to 25% higher as compared with the younger volunteers (18 to 55 years of age).

Contraindications

Urinary retention, gastric retention, uncontrolled narrow-angle glaucoma, and hypersensitivity to the drug substance or other components of the product.

Warnings

➤*Renal function impairment:* Use solifenacin with caution in patients with reduced renal function.

See Administration and Dosage for more information.

➤*Hepatic function impairment:* Use solifenacin with caution in patients with reduced hepatic function.

See Administration and Dosage for more information.

➤*Pregnancy:* Category C.

Reproduction studies have been performed in mice, rats, and rabbits. After oral administration of ^{14}C-solifenacin to pregnant mice, drug-related material has been shown to cross the placental barrier. No embryotoxicity or teratogenicity was observed in mice treated with 30 mg/kg/day (1.2 times exposure at the MRHD). Administration of solifenacin to pregnant mice, at doses of 100 mg/kg and greater (3.6 times exposure at the MRHD), during the major period of organ development resulted in reduced fetal body weights. Administration of 250 mg/kg (7.9 times exposure at the MRHD) to pregnant mice resulted in an increased incidence of cleft palate. In utero and lactational exposures to maternal doses of solifenacin of 100 mg/kg/day and greater (3.6 times exposure at the MRHD) resulted in reduced peripartum and postnatal survival, reductions in body weight gain, and delayed physical development (eye opening and vaginal patency). An increase in the percentage of male offspring was also observed in litters from offspring exposed to maternal doses of 250 mg/kg/day. No embryotoxic effects were observed in rats at up to 50 mg/kg/day (less than 1 times exposure at the MRHD) or in rabbits at up to 50 mg/kg/day (1.8 times exposure at the MRHD). There are no adequate and well-controlled studies in pregnant women. Because animal reproduction studies are not always predictive of human response, use solifenacin during pregnancy only if the potential benefit justifies the potential risk to the fetus.

➤*Lactation:* After oral administration of ^{14}C-solifenacin to lactating mice, radioactivity was detected in maternal milk. There were no adverse observations in mice treated with 30 mg/kg/day (1.2 times exposure at the MRHD). Pups of female mice treated with 100 mg/kg/day (3.6 times exposure at the MRHD) or greater revealed reduced body weights, postpartum pup mortality, or delays in the onset of reflex and physical development during the lactation period.

It is not known whether solifenacin is excreted in human milk. Because many drugs are excreted in human milk, do not administer solifenacin during breastfeeding. A decision should be made whether to discontinue breastfeeding or to discontinue solifenacin in breastfeeding mothers.

➤*Children:* Safety and efficacy have not been established.

Precautions

➤*Bladder outflow obstruction:* As with other anticholinergic drugs, administer solifenacin with caution to patients with clinically significant bladder outflow obstruction because of the risk of urinary retention.

➤*GI obstructive disorders and decreased GI motility:* As with other anticholinergics, use solifenacin with caution in patients with decreased GI motility.

➤*Controlled narrow-angle glaucoma:* Use solifenacin with caution in patients being treated for narrow-angle glaucoma. Solifenacin is contraindicated in patients with uncontrolled narrow-angle glaucoma.

➤*Patients with congenital or acquired QT prolongation:* In a study of the effect of solifenacin on the QT interval in 76 healthy women, the QT prolonging effect appeared less with solifenacin 10 mg than with 30 mg (3 times the maximum recommended dose), and the effect of solifenacin 30 mg did not appear as large as that of the positive control moxifloxacin at its therapeutic dose. Consider this observation in clinical decisions to prescribe solifenacin for patients with a known history of QT prolongation or patients who are taking medications known to prolong the QT interval.

Drug Interactions

➤*P450 system:* In vitro drug metabolism studies have shown that solifenacin is a substrate of CYP3A4. Inducers or inhibitors of CYP3A4 may alter solifenacin pharmacokinetics.

Following the administration of solifenacin 10 mg in the presence of ketoconazole 400 mg, a potent inhibitor of CYP3A4, the mean C_{max} and AUC of solifenacin increased 1.5- and 2.7-fold, respectively. Therefore, it is recommended not to exceed a 5 mg daily dose of solifenacin when administered with therapeutic doses of ketoconazole or other potent CYP3A4 inhibitors.

Adverse Reactions

Solifenacin has been evaluated for safety in 1,811 patients in randomized, placebo-controlled trials. Expected side effects of antimuscarinic agents are dry mouth, constipation, blurred vision (accommodation abnormalities), urinary retention, and dry eyes. The most common adverse events reported in patients treated with solifenacin were dry mouth and constipation, and the incidence of these side effects was higher in the 10 mg compared with the 5 mg dose group. In the four 12-week, double-blind clinical trials, there were 3 intestinal serious adverse events in patients, all treated with solifenacin 10 mg (1 fecal impaction, 1 colonic obstruction, and 1 intestinal obstruction). The overall rate of serious adverse events in the double-blind trials was 2%. Angioneurotic edema has been reported in 1 patient taking solifenacin 5 mg. Compared with 12 weeks of treatment with solifenacin, the incidence and severity of adverse events were similar in patients who remained on the drug for up to 12 months. The most frequent reason for discontinuation because of an adverse event was dry mouth (1.5%). The table below lists adverse events, regardless of causality, that were reported in randomized, placebo-controlled trials at an incidence greater than placebo and in 1% or more of patients treated with solifenacin 5 or 10 mg once daily for up to 12 weeks.

Solifenacin Adverse Events

Adverse reaction	Placebo (%)	Solifenacin 5 mg (%)	Solifenacin 10 mg (%)
Number of patients	1,216	578	1,233
Number of patients with treatment-emergent adverse events	634	265	773
CNS			
Dizziness	1.8%	1.9%	1.8%
GI			
Abdominal pain, upper	1%	1.9%	1.2%
Constipation	2.9%	5.4%	13.4%
Dry mouth	4.2%	10.9%	27.6%
Dyspepsia	1%	1.4%	3.9%
Nausea	2%	1.7%	3.3%
Vomiting	0.9%	0.2%	1.1%
GU			
Urinary retention	0.6%	0	1.4%
Urinary tract infection	2.8%	2.8%	4.8%
Psychiatric			
Depression	0.8%	1.2%	0.8%
Respiratory			
Cough	0.2%	0.2%	1.1%
Special senses			
Dry eyes	0.6%	0.3%	1.6%
Vision blurred	1.8%	3.8%	4.8%
Vascular			
Hypertension	0.6%	1.4%	0.5%
Miscellaneous			
Edema, lower limb	0.7%	0.3%	1.1%
Fatigue	1.1%	1%	2.1%
Influenza	1.3%	2.2%	0.9%
Pharyngitis	1%	0.3%	1.1%

Overdosage

➤*Symptoms:*

Acute – Overdosage with solifenacin can potentially result in severe anticholinergic effects and should be treated accordingly. The highest solifenacin dose given to human volunteers was a single 100 mg dose.

Chronic – Intolerable anticholinergic side effects (fixed and dilated pupils, blurred vision, failure of heel-to-toe exam, tremors, and dry skin) occurred on day 3 in healthy volunteers taking 50 mg daily (5 times the maximum recommended therapeutic dose) and resolved within 7 days following discontinuation of drug.

➤*Treatment:* No cases of acute overdosage have been reported, but in the event of overdose with solifenacin, treat with gastric lavage and appropriate supportive measures.

Patient Information

Inform patients that antimuscarinic agents such as solifenacin have been associated with constipation and blurred vision. Advise patients to contact their physician if they experience severe abdominal pain or become constipated for 3 or more days. Because solifenacin may cause blurred vision, advise patients to exercise caution in decisions to engage in potentially dangerous activities until the drug's effect on the patient's vision has been determined. Heat prostration (caused by decreased sweating) can occur when anticholinergic drugs, such as solifenacin, are used in a hot environment. Patients should read the patient leaflet before starting therapy with solifenacin.

DARIFENACIN HYDROBROMIDE

Rx	**Enablex** (Novartis)	**Tablets, extended-release:** 7.5 mg	Lactose. (DF 7.5). White. In 30s, 90s, and UD 100s.
		15 mg	Lactose. (DF 15). Lt. peach. In 30s, 90s, and UD 100s.

DARIFENACIN HYDROBROMIDE — ORAL

Indications

➤*Overactive bladder:* For the treatment of overactive bladder with symptoms of urge urinary incontinence, urgency, and frequency.

Administration and Dosage

➤*Approved by the FDA:* December 22, 2004.

➤*Dosage:* The recommended starting dose is 7.5 mg once daily. Based upon individual response, the dose may be increased to 15 mg once daily, as early as 2 weeks after starting therapy. Take darifenacin extended-release tablets once daily with liquid. Take with or without food. Swallow whole; do not chew, divide, or crush.

➤*Hepatic function impairment:* For patients with moderate hepatic impairment, the daily dose of darifenacin should not exceed 7.5 mg. Darifenacin is not recommended for use in patients with severe hepatic impairment.

➤*Coadministration with CYP450 inhibitors:* See Drug Interactions for more information.

➤*Storage/Stability:* Store at 25°C (77°F); excursions permitted to 15° to 30°C (59° to 86°F). Protect from light. Keep away from children.

Actions

➤*Pharmacology:* Darifenacin is a competitive muscarinic receptor antagonist. Muscarinic receptors play an important role in several major cholinergically mediated functions, including contractions of the urinary bladder smooth muscle and stimulation of salivary secretion.

In vitro studies using human recombinant muscarinic receptor subtypes show that darifenacin has greater affinity for the M_3 receptor than for the other known muscarinic receptors (9- and 12-fold greater affinity for M_3 compared with M_1 and M_5, respectively, and 59-fold greater affinity for M_3 compared with both M_2 and M_4). M_3 receptors are involved in contraction of human bladder and GI smooth muscle, saliva production, and iris sphincter function. Adverse drug effects, such as dry mouth, constipation, and abnormal vision, may be mediated through effects on M_3 receptors in these organs.

Pharmacodynamics – In 3 cystometric studies performed in patients with involuntary detrusor contractions, increased bladder capacity was demonstrated by an increased volume threshold for unstable contractions and diminished frequency of unstable detrusor contractions after darifenacin extended-release tablet treatment. These findings are consistent with an antimuscarinic action on the urinary bladder.

➤*Pharmacokinetics:*

Absorption – The mean oral bioavailability of darifenacin in EMs at steady state is estimated to be 15% and 19% for 7.5 and 15 mg tablets, respectively.

After oral administration of darifenacin to healthy volunteers, peak plasma concentrations of darifenacin are reached approximately 7 hours after multiple dosing; steady state plasma concentrations are achieved by the sixth day of dosing.

Mean (SD) Steady State Pharmacokinetic Parameters From Darifenacin 7.5 mg and 15 mg Extended-Release Tablets Based On Pooled Data By Predicted CYP2D6 Phenotype

	Darifenacin 7.5 mg (N = 68 EM, 5 PM)					Darifenacin 15 mg (N = 102 EM, 17 PM)				
	AUC_{24} (ng•h/mL)	C_{max} (ng/mL)	C_{avg} (ng/mL)	T_{max} (h)	t½ (h)	AUC_{24} (ng•h/mL)	C_{max} (ng/mL)	C_{avg} (ng/mL)	T_{max} (h)	t½ (h)
EM	29.24 (15.47)	2.01 (1.04)	1.22 (0.64)	6.49 (4.19)	12.43 (5.64)[a]	88.9 (67.87)	5.76 (4.24)	3.7 (2.83)	7.61 (5.06)	12.05 (12.37)[b]
PM	67.56 (13.13)	4.27 (0.98)	2.81 (0.55)	5.2 (1.79)	19.95[c]	157.71 (77.08)	9.99 (5.09)	6.58 (3.22)	6.71 (3.58)	7.4[d]

[a] N = 25 [b] N = 8 [c] N = 2 [d] N = 1

Distribution – Darifenacin is approximately 98% bound to plasma proteins (primarily to alpha-1-acid glycoprotein). The steady-state volume of distribution (Vss) is estimated to be 163 L.

Metabolism – Darifenacin is extensively metabolized by the liver following oral dosing.

Metabolism is mediated by cytochrome P450 enzymes CYP2D6 and CYP3A4. The 3 main metabolic routes are as follows
1.) monohydroxylation in the dihydrobenzofuran ring
2.) dihydrobenzofuran ring opening
3.) N-dealkylation of the pyrrolidine nitrogen

The initial products of the hydroxylation and N-dealkylation pathways are the major circulating metabolites, but they are unlikely to contribute significantly to the overall clinical effect of darifenacin.

A subset of individuals (approximately 7% white and 2% black) are PMs of CYP2D6 metabolized drugs. Individuals with normal CYP2D6 activity are referred to as EMs. The metabolism of darifenacin in PMs will be principally mediated via CYP3A4. The darifenacin ratios (PM:EM) for C_{max} and area under the curve (AUC) following darifenacin 15 mg once-daily at steady state were 1.9 and 1.7, respectively.

Excretion – Following administration of an oral dose of ^{14}C-darifenacin solution to healthy volunteers, approximately 60% of the radioactivity was recovered in the urine and 40% in the feces. Only a small percentage of the excreted dose was unchanged darifenacin (3%). Estimated darifenacin clearance is 40 L/h for EMs and 32 L/h for PMs. The elimination half-life of darifenacin following chronic dosing is approximately 13 to 19 hours.

Special populations –

Hepatic function impairment: The daily dose of darifenacin should not exceed 7.5 mg once daily for patients with moderate hepatic impairment (Child-Pugh B). No dose adjustment is recommended for patients with mild hepatic impairment (Child-Pugh A).

Darifenacin pharmacokinetics were investigated in subjects with mild (Child-Pugh A) or moderate (Child-Pugh B) impairment of hepatic function given darifenacin 15 mg once daily to steady state. Mild hepatic impairment had no effect on the pharmacokinetics of darifenacin. However, protein binding of darifenacin was affected by moderate hepatic impairment. After adjusting for plasma protein binding, unbound darifenacin exposure was estimated to be 4.7-fold higher in subjects with moderate hepatic impairment than subjects with normal hepatic function. Subjects with severe hepatic impairment (Child-Pugh C) have not been studied; therefore, darifenacin is not recommended for use in these patients.

Elderly: No dose adjustment is recommended for the elderly. A population pharmacokinetic analysis of patient data indicated a trend for clearance of darifenacin to decrease with age (6% per decade relative to a median age of 44). Following administration of darifenacin 15 mg once daily, darifenacin exposure at steady state was approximately 12% to 19% higher in volunteers between 45 and 65 years of age compared with younger volunteers aged 18 to 44 years of age.

Gender: No dose adjustment is recommended based on gender. Pharmacokinetic parameters were calculated for 22 male and 25 female healthy volunteers. Darifenacin C_{max} and AUC at steady state were approximately 57% to 79% and 61% to 73% higher in females than in males, respectively.

Contraindications

Urinary retention, gastric retention, or uncontrolled narrow-angle glaucoma and in patients who are at risk for these conditions; hypersensitivity to the drug or its ingredients.

Warnings

➤*Hepatic function impairment:* See Administration and Dosage for more information.

➤*Pregnancy: Category C.* Darifenacin was not teratogenic in rats and rabbits at doses up to 50 and 30 mg/kg/day, respectively. At the dose of 50 mg/kg in rats, there was a delay in the ossification of the sacral and caudal vertebrae that was not observed at 10 mg/kg (approximately 13 times the AUC of free plasma concentration at MRHD). Exposure in this study at 50 mg/kg corresponds to approximately 59 times the AUC of free plasma concentration at MRHD. Dystocia was observed in dams at 10 mg/kg/day (17 times the AUC of free plasma concentration at MRHD). Slight developmental delays were observed in pups at this dose. At 3 mg/kg/day (5 times the AUC of free plasma concentration at MRHD), there were no effects on dams or pups. At the dose of 30 mg/kg in rabbits, darifenacin was shown to increase post-implantation loss but not at 10 mg/kg (9 times the AUC of free plasma concentration at MRHD). Exposure to unbound drug at 30 mg/kg in this study corresponds to approximately 28 times the AUC at MRHD. In rabbits, dilated ureter and/or kidney pelvis was observed in offspring at 30 mg/kg/day and one case was observed at 10 mg/kg/day along with urinary bladder dilation consistent with pharmacological action of darifenacin. No effect was observed at 3 mg/kg/day (2.8 times the AUC of free plasma concentration at MRHD). There are no studies of darifenacin in pregnant women. Because animal reproduction studies are not always predictive of human response, use darifenacin during pregnancy only if the benefit to the mother outweighs the potential risk to the fetus.

➤*Lactation:* Darifenacin is excreted into the milk of rats. It is not known whether darifenacin is excreted into human milk. Use caution before administering darifenacin to a breast-feeding woman.

➤*Children:* The safety and efficacy of darifenacin in pediatric patients have not been established.

Precautions

➤*Controlled narrow-angle glaucoma:* Use darifenacin with caution in patients being treated for narrow-angle glaucoma and only where the potential benefits outweigh the risks.

➤*Decreased GI motility:* Administer darifenacin with caution to patients with GI obstructive disorders because of the risk of gastric retention. Darifenacin, like other anticholinergic drugs, may decrease GI motility; use with caution in patients with conditions such as severe constipation, ulcerative colitis, and myasthenia gravis.

➤*Risk of urinary retention:* Administer darifenacin extended-release tablets with caution to patients with clinically significant bladder outflow obstruction because of the risk of urinary retention.

DARIFENACIN HYDROBROMIDE — ORAL

Drug Interactions

Darifenacin Drug Interactions			
Precipitant Drug	Object Drug[a]		Description
Moderate CYP3A4 inhibitors (eg, diltiazem, erythromycin, fluconazole, verapamil)	Darifenacin	↑	Darifenacin levels may be increased; no dosing adjustments are recommended.
Potent CYP3A4 inhibitors (eg, clarithromycin, itraconazole, ketoconazole, nefazodone, protease inhibitors [eg, nelfinavir, ritonavir])	Darifenacin	↑	Darifenacin levels may be increased; darifenacin should not exceed 7.5 mg when coadministered with potent CYP3A4 inhibitors.
Darifenacin	Anticholinergic drugs	↑	Additive anticholinergic adverse effects may occur.
Darifenacin	CYP2D6 substrates (eg, flecainide, thioridazine, tricyclic antidepressants [eg, desipramine, imipramine])	↑	Use caution when darifenacin is used with drugs metabolized by CYP2D6 and that have a narrow therapeutic window. The mean C_{max} and AUC of imipramine were increased 57% and 70%, respectively, in the presence of steady state darifenacin 30 mg once daily; active metabolite of imipramine, desipramine increased 3.6-fold.
Darifenacin	Digoxin	↑	Darifenacin 30 mg daily coadministered with digoxin 0.25 mg at steady state resulted in 16% increase in digoxin; monitor digoxin.

[a] ↑ = Object drug increased.

Adverse Reactions

During the clinical development of darifenacin extended-release tablets, a total of 7,363 patients and volunteers were treated with doses of darifenacin from 3.75 to 75 mg once daily.

The safety of darifenacin was evaluated in phase II and III controlled clinical trials in a total of 8,830 patients, 6,001 of whom were treated with darifenacin. Of this total, 1,069 patients participated in three 12-week, phase III, fixed-dose efficacy and safety studies. Of this total, 337 and 334 patients received darifenacin 7.5 and 15 mg daily, respectively. In all long-term trials combined, 1,216 and 672 patients received treatment with darifenacin for at least 24 and 52 weeks, respectively.

In all placebo-controlled trials combined, the incidence of serious adverse reactions for 7.5 mg, 15 mg, and placebo was similar.

In all fixed-dose phase III studies combined, 3.3% of patients treated with darifenacin discontinued because of all adverse reactions versus 2.6% in placebo. Dry mouth leading to study discontinuation occurred in 0%, 0.9%, and 0% of patients treated with darifenacin 7.5 mg daily, darifenacin 15 mg daily, and placebo respectively. Constipation leading to study discontinuation occurred in 0.6%, 1.2%, and 0.3% of patients treated with darifenacin 7.5 mg daily, darifenacin 15 mg daily, and placebo, respectively.

The table below lists the adverse reactions reported (regardless of causality) in 2% or more of patients treated with 7.5 or 15 mg darifenacin extended-release tablets and greater than placebo in the 3 fixed-dose, placebo-controlled phase III studies (studies 1, 2, and 3). Adverse reactions were reported by 54% and 66% of patients receiving 7.5 and 15 mg once daily darifenacin extended-release tablets, respectively, and by 49% of patients receiving placebo. In these studies, the most frequently reported adverse reactions were dry mouth and constipation. The majority of adverse reactions in darifenacin-treated subjects were mild or moderate in severity and most occurred during the first 2 weeks of treatment.

Darifenacin Adverse Reactions[a] (≥ 2%) (Studies 1, 2, and 3)			
	Percentage of Subjects With Adverse Reaction (%)		
Adverse reaction	Darifenacin 7.5 mg (N = 337)	Darifenacin 15 mg (N = 334)	Placebo (N = 388)
CNS			
Dizziness	0.9	2.1	1.3
GI			
Abdominal pain	2.4	3.9	0.5
Constipation	14.8	21.3	6.2
Diarrhea	2.1	0.9	1.8
Dry mouth	20.2	35.3	8.2
Dyspepsia	2.7	8.4	2.6
Nausea	2.7	1.5	1.5
GU			
Urinary tract infection	4.7	4.5	2.6
Ophthalmic			
Dry eyes	1.5	2.1	0.5
Miscellaneous			
Asthenia	1.5	2.7	1.3

[a] Regardless of causality.

Other adverse reactions reported, regardless of causality, by at least 1% of darifenacin patients in either the 7.5 or 15 mg once-daily darifenacin dose groups in these fixed-dose, placebo-controlled phase III studies include the following: abnormal vision, accidental injury, arthralgia, back pain, bronchitis, dry skin, flu syndrome, hypertension, pain, peripheral edema, pharyngitis, pruritus, rash, rhinitis, sinusitis, urinary tract disorder, vaginitis, vomiting, and weight gain.

Study 4 was a 12-week, placebo-controlled, dose-titration regimen study in which darifenacin was administered in accordance with dosing recommendations. All patients initially received placebo or darifenacin 7.5 mg daily, and after 2 weeks, patients and physicians were allowed to adjust upward to darifenacin 15 mg if needed. In this study, the most commonly reported adverse reactions also were constipation and dry mouth. The incidence of discontinuation because of all adverse reactions was 3.1% and 6.7% for placebo and for darifenacin, respectively.

Darifenacin Adverse Reactions[a] (More than 3%) (Study 4)		
Adverse reaction	Darifenacin 7.5 mg per 15 mg (N = 268)	Placebo (N = 127)
CNS		
Headache	18 (6.7%)	7 (5.5%)
GI		
Constipation	56 (20.9%)	10 (7.9%)
Dry mouth	50 (18.7%)	11 (8.7%)
Dyspepsia	12 (4.5%)	2 (1.6%)
Nausea	11 (4.1%)	2 (1.6%)
GU		
Urinary tract infection	10 (3.7%)	4 (3.1%)
Miscellaneous		
Accidental injury	8 (3%)	3 (2.4%)
Flu syndrome	8 (3%)	3 (2.4%)

[a] Regardless of causality.

➤*GI:* Constipation was reported as a serious adverse reaction in 6 patients in the darifenacin phase I to III clinical trials, including 1 patient with benign prostatic hypertrophy (BPH), one overactive bladder (OAB) patient taking darifenacin 30 mg daily, and only one OAB patient taking the recommended doses. The latter patient was hospitalized for investigation with colonoscopy after reporting 9 months of chronic constipation that was reported as being moderate in severity.

➤*GU:* Acute urinary retention (AUR) requiring treatment was reported in a total of 16 patients in the darifenacin phase I to III clinical trials. Of these 16 cases, 7 were reported as serious adverse reactions, including 1 patient with detrusor hyperreflexia secondary to a stroke, 1 patient with BPH, 1 patient with irritable bowel syndrome (IBS), and 4 OAB patients taking darifenacin 30 mg daily. Of the remaining 9 cases, none were reported as serious adverse reactions. Three occurred in OAB patients taking the recommended doses, and 2 of these required bladder catheterization for 1 to 2 days.

Overdosage

➤*Symptoms:* Overdosage with antimuscarinic agents, including darifenacin extended-release tablets can result in severe antimuscarinic effects.

➤*Treatment:* Treatment should be symptomatic and supportive. In the event of overdosage, ECG monitoring is recommended. Darifenacin has been administered in clinical trials at doses up to 75 mg (5 times the maximum therapeutic dose) and signs of overdose were limited to abnormal vision.

Patient Information

Inform patients that anticholinergic agents, such as darifenacin, may produce clinically significant adverse events related to anticholinergic pharmacological activity including constipation, urinary retention, and blurred vision. Heat prostration (caused by decreased sweating) can occur when anticholinergics such as darifenacin are used in a hot environment.

Because anticholinergics, such as darifenacin, may produce dizziness or blurred vision, advise patients to exercise caution in decisions to engage in potentially dangerous activities until the drug's effects have been determined.

DARIFENACIN HYDROBROMIDE — ORAL

Advise patients to read the patient information leaflet before starting therapy with darifenacin.

Instruct patients that darifenacin may be taken with or without food. Darifenacin should be taken once daily with liquid.

Advise patients to swallow darifenacin tablets whole and not to chew, crush, or divide the tablets.

Inform patients that dry mouth may occur.

URINARY CHOLINERGICS

BETHANECHOL CHLORIDE

Rx	**Bethanechol Chloride** (Various, eg, Goldline, Ivax, Qualitest, UDL)	**Tablets:** 5 mg	In 100s, 1000s, and UD 100s.
Rx	**Bethanechol Chloride** (Various, eg, Goldline, Ivax, Qualitest, UDL)	10 mg	In 100s, 250s, 1000s, and UD 100s.
Rx	**Bethanechol Chloride** (Various, eg, Goldline, Ivax, Qualitest, UDL)	25 mg	In 100s, 250s, 1000s, and UD 100s.
Rx	**Urecholine** (Odyssey)		Lactose. (OP 704). Yellow, scored. In 100s.
Rx	**Bethanechol Chloride** (Various, eg, Goldline, Ivax, Qualitest, UDL)	50 mg	In 100s, 500s, 1000s, and UD 100s.

BETHANECHOL CHLORIDE — ORAL

Indications

➤*Urinary retention:* For the treatment of acute postoperative and postpartum nonobstructive (functional) urinary retention and for neurogenic atony of the urinary bladder with retention.

➤*Unlabeled uses:* In adults for treatment and diagnosis of reflux esophagitis. In infants and children, an oral dosage has been used for gastroesophageal reflux.

Administration and Dosage

➤*Approved by the FDA:* May 29, 1984.

Preferably, give the drug when the stomach is empty. If taken soon after eating, nausea and vomiting may occur.

The usual adult dosage is 10 to 50 mg 3 or 4 times a day. The minimum effective dose is determined by giving 5 or 10 mg initially and repeating the same amount at hourly intervals until satisfactory response occurs or until a maximum of 50 mg has been given. The effects of the drug sometimes appear within 30 minutes and usually within 60 to 90 minutes. The drug's effects persist for about 1 hour.

The effects of the drug can be abolished promptly by atropine.

➤*Storage/Stability:* Dispense in a tight container. Store at 20° to 25°C (68° to 77°F).

Actions

➤*Pharmacology:* Bethanechol chloride acts principally by producing the effects of stimulation of the parasympathetic nervous system. It increases the tone of the detrusor urinae muscle, usually producing a contraction sufficiently strong to initiate micturition and empty the bladder. It stimulates gastric motility, increases gastric tone, and often restores impaired rhythmic peristalsis.

Stimulation of the parasympathetic nervous system releases acetylcholine at the nerve endings. When spontaneous stimulation is reduced and therapeutic intervention is required, acetylcholine can be given, but it is rapidly hydrolyzed by cholinesterase, and its effects are transient. Bethanechol chloride is not destroyed by cholinesterase and its effects are more prolonged than those of acetylcholine.

Effects on the GI and urinary tracts sometimes appear within 30 minutes after oral administration of bethanechol chloride, but more often 60 to 90 minutes are required to reach maximum effectiveness. Following oral administration, the usual duration of action of bethanechol is 1 hour, although large doses (300 to 400 mg) have been reported to produce effects for up to 6 hours. SC injection produces a more intense action on bladder muscle than does oral administration of the drug.

Because of the selective action of bethanechol, nicotinic symptoms of cholinergic stimulation are usually absent or minimal when orally or subcutaneously administered in therapeutic doses, while muscarinic effects are prominent. Muscarinic effects usually occur within 5 to 15 minutes after SC injection, reach a maximum in 15 to 30 minutes, and disappear within 2 hours. Doses that stimulate micturition and defecation and increase peristalsis do not ordinarily stimulate ganglia or voluntary muscles. Therapeutic test doses in healthy human subjects have little effect on heart rate, blood pressure, or peripheral circulation.

➤*Pharmacokinetics:* Bethanechol chloride does not cross the blood-brain barrier because of its charged quaternary amine moiety. The metabolic fate and mode of excretion of the drug have not been elucidated.

Contraindications

Hypersensitivity to bethanechol chloride, hyperthyroidism, peptic ulcer, latent or active bronchial asthma, pronounced bradycardia or hypotension, vasomotor instability, coronary artery disease, epilepsy, and parkinsonism.

Bethanechol chloride should not be employed when the strength or integrity of the GI or bladder wall is in question, or in the presence of mechanical obstruction; when increased muscular activity of the GI tract or urinary bladder might prove harmful, as following recent urinary bladder surgery, GI resection and anastomosis, or when there is possible GI obstruction; in bladder neck obstruction, spastic GI disturbances, acute inflammatory lesions of the GI tract, or peritonitis; or in marked vagotonia.

Warnings

➤*Pregnancy: Category C.* Animal reproduction studies have not been conducted with bethanechol chloride. It is also not known whether bethanechol chloride can cause fetal harm when administered to a pregnant woman or can affect reproduction capacity. Bethanechol chloride should be given to a pregnant woman only if clearly needed.

➤*Lactation:* It is not known whether this drug is excreted in human milk. Because many drugs are excreted in human milk and because of the potential for serious adverse reactions from bethanechol chloride in nursing infants, a decision should be made whether to discontinue nursing or to discontinue the drug, taking into account the importance of the drug to the mother.

➤*Children:* Safety and efficacy in children have not been established.

Precautions

➤*Reflex infection:* In urinary retention, if the sphincter fails to relax as bethanechol chloride contracts the bladder, urine may be forced up the ureter into the kidney pelvis. If there is bacteriuria, this may cause reflux infection.

➤*Tartrazine sensitivity:* Some of these products contain tartrazine, which may cause allergic-type reactions (including bronchial asthma) in susceptible individuals. Although the incidence of sensitivity is low, it is frequently seen in patients who also have aspirin hypersensitivity.

Drug Interactions

Bethanechol Drug Interactions

Precipitant drug	Object drug*		Description
Cholinergic drugs	Bethanechol	↑	Additive effects may occur, particularly with cholinesterase inhibitors.
Ganglionic blocking compounds	Bethanechol	↑	A critical fall in blood pressure may occur that is usually preceded by severe abdominal symptoms.
Quinidine Procainamide	Bethanechol	↓	Quinidine or procainamide may antagonize cholinergic effects of bethanechol.

* ↑ = Object drug increased. ↓ = Object drug decreased.

Adverse Reactions

➤*Cardiovascular:* A fall in blood pressure with reflex tachycardia; vasomotor response.

➤*CNS:* Headache.

➤*Dermatologic:* Flushing producing a feeling of warmth; sensation of heat about the face; sweating.

➤*GI:* Abdominal cramps or discomfort; colicky pain; nausea and belching; diarrhea; borborygmi (rumbling/gurgling of stomach); salivation.

➤*Renal:* Urinary urgency.

➤*Respiratory:* Bronchial constriction; asthmatic attacks.

➤*Special senses:* Lacrimation; miosis.

➤*Miscellaneous:* Malaise.

➤*Casual relationship unknown:*
CNS – Seizures.

Overdosage

➤*Symptoms:* Early signs of overdosage are abdominal discomfort, salivation, flushing of the skin (hot feeling), sweating, nausea, and vomiting.

The oral LD_{50} of bethanechol chloride is 1510 mg/kg in the mouse.

➤*Treatment:* Atropine sulfate is a specific antidote. The recommended dose for adults is 0.6 mg. Repeat doses can be given every 2 hours, according to clinical response. The recommended dosage in infants and children up to 12 years of age is 0.01 mg/kg (to a maximum single dose of 0.4 mg) repeated every 2 hours as needed until the desired effect is obtained, or adverse effects of atropine preclude further usage. SC injection of atropine is preferred except in emergencies when the IV route may be employed.

Patient Information

Bethanechol chloride tablets should preferably be taken 1 hour before or 2 hours after meals to avoid nausea or vomiting. If taken soon after eating, nausea and vomiting may occur.

BETHANECHOL CHLORIDE — ORAL

Dizziness, lightheadedness or fainting may occur, especially when getting up from a lying or sitting position.

May cause abdominal discomfort, salivation, sweating, or flushing; notify physician if these effects are pronounced.

NEOSTIGMINE METHYLSULFATE

Refer to the Neostigmine methylsulfate monograph in the CNS chapter for full prescribing information.

PHOSPHATE BINDERS

SEVELAMER HYDROCHLORIDE

Rx	**Renagel** (Genzyme)	**Tablets:** 400 mg	(RENAGEL 400). Oval. Film-coated. In 360s.
		800 mg	(RENAGEL 800). Oval. Film-coated. In 180s

SEVELAMER — ORAL

Indications

➤*Hyperphosphatemia:* For the control of serum phosphorus in patients with chronic kidney disease (CKD) on hemodialysis. The safety and efficacy of sevelamer in patients not on hemodialysis have not been studied. In hemodialysis patients, sevelamer decreases the incidence of hypercalcemic episodes relative to patients on calcium acetate treatment.

➤*Unlabeled uses:* Treatment of hyperuricemia in patients undergoing hemodialysis.

Administration and Dosage

➤*Approved by the FDA:* October 30, 1998.

➤*Administration:* Because the contents of sevelamer expand in water, tablets must be swallowed intact and not crushed, chewed, broken into pieces, or taken apart prior to administration.

➤*Patients not taking a phosphate binder:* Based on serum phosphorus level, the recommended starting dosage of sevelamer is 800 to 1,600 mg, which can be administered as 1 to 2 sevelamer 800 mg tablets or 2 to 4 sevelamer 400 mg tablets, with each meal. The following table provides recommended starting dosages of sevelamer for patients not taking a phosphate binder.

Sevelamer Starting Dosage for Patients Not Taking a Phosphate Binder

Serum phosphorus	Sevelamer 800 mg	Sevelamer 400 mg
> 5.5 and < 7.5 mg/dL	1 tablet 3 times daily with meals	2 tablets 3 times daily with meals
≥ 7.5 and < 9 mg/dL	2 tablets 3 times daily with meals	3 tablets 3 times daily with meals
≥ 9 mg/dL	2 tablets 3 times daily with meals	4 tablets 3 times daily with meals

➤*Patients switching from calcium acetate:* In a study in 84 end-stage renal disease (ESRD) patients on hemodialysis, a similar reduction in serum phosphorus was seen with equivalent doses (mg for mg) of sevelamer (capsule formulation) and calcium acetate. The following table gives recommended starting dosages of sevelamer based on a patient's current calcium acetate dose.

Starting Dosage for Patients Switching from Calcium Acetate to Sevelamer

Calcium acetate 667 mg (tablets per meal)	Sevelamer 800 mg (tablets per meal)	Sevelamer 400 mg (tablets per meal)
1 tablet	1 tablet	2 tablets
2 tablets	2 tablets	3 tablets
3 tablets	3 tablets	5 tablets

➤*Dose titration:* Adjust dosage based on the serum phosphorus concentration with a goal of lowering serum phosphorus to 5.5 mg/dL or less. The dosage may be increased or decreased by 1 tablet per meal at 2-week intervals as necessary. Below is a dosage titration guideline. The average dosage in a phase 3 trial designed to lower serum phosphorus to 5 mg/dL or less was approximately 3 sevelamer 800 mg tablets per meal. The maximum average daily sevelamer dose studied was 13 g.

Sevelamer Dosage Titration Guideline

Serum phosphorus	Sevelamer dosage
> 5.5 mg/dL	Increase 1 tablet per meal at 2-week intervals
3.5 to 5.5 mg/dL	Maintain current dosage
< 3.5 mg/dL	Decrease 1 tablet per meal

➤*Storage/Stability:* Store at 25°C (77°F). Excursions permitted to 15° to 30°C (59° to 86°F). Protect from moisture.

Actions

➤*Pharmacology:* Patients with ESRD retain phosphorus and can develop hyperphosphatemia. High serum phosphorus can precipitate serum calcium, resulting in ectopic calcification. When the product of serum calcium and phosphorus concentrations (Ca × P) exceeds 55 mg²/dL², there is an increased risk that ectopic calcification will occur. Hyperphosphatemia plays a role in the development of secondary hyperparathyroidism in renal impairment. An increase in parathyroid hormone (PTH) levels is characteristic of patients with chronic renal failure. Increased levels of PTH can lead to osteitis fibrosa, a bone disease. A decrease in serum phosphorus may decrease serum PTH levels.

Treatment of hyperphosphatemia includes reduction in dietary intake of phosphate, inhibition of intestinal phosphate absorption with phosphate binders, and removal of phosphate with dialysis. Sevelamer taken with meals has been shown to decrease serum phosphorus concentrations in patients with ESRD on hemodialysis. Sevelamer does not contain aluminum or other metals and does not cause aluminum intoxication.

Sevelamer treatment also results in a lowering of low-density lipoprotein (LDL) and total serum cholesterol levels.

➤*Pharmacokinetics:* A mass balance study using ^{14}C-sevelamer hydrochloride in 16 healthy male and female volunteers showed that sevelamer is not systemically absorbed. No absorption studies have been performed in patients with renal disease.

Contraindications

Hypophosphatemia or bowel obstruction; hypersensitivity to sevelamer or any of its constituents.

Warnings

➤*Carcinogenesis:* Standard lifetime carcinogenicity bioassays were conducted in mice and rats. Rats were given sevelamer by diet at 0.3, 1, and 3 g/kg/day. There was an increased incidence of urinary bladder transitional cell papilloma in male rats (3 g/kg/day) at exposures 2 times the maximum human oral dose of 13 g, based on a comparison of relative body surface area. Mice received mean dietary dosages of 0.8, 3, and 9 g/kg/day. Increased incidence of tumors was not observed in mice at exposures up to 3 times the maximum human oral dose of 13 g, based on comparison of relative body surface area.

➤*Mutagenesis:* In an in vitro mammalian cytogenetics test with metabolic activation, sevelamer caused a statistically significant increase in the number of structural chromosome aberrations. Sevelamer was not mutagenic in the Ames bacterial mutation assay.

➤*Pregnancy: Category C.* In pregnant rats given dietary dosages of 0.5, 1.5, and 4.5 g/kg/day during organogenesis, reduced or irregular ossification of fetal bones, probably because of a reduced absorption of fat-soluble vitamin D occurred in the mid- and high-dosage groups (exposures less than the maximum human dose of 13 g, based on a comparison of relative body surface area). In pregnant rabbits given oral dosages of 100, 500, and 1,000 mg/kg/day by gavage during organogenesis, an increased incidence of early resorptions occurred at exposures 2 times the maximum human dose of 13 g based on a comparison of relative body surface area. Requirements for vitamins and other nutrients are increased in pregnancy. The effect of sevelamer on the absorption of vitamins and other nutrients has not been studied in pregnant women.

➤*Children:* The safety and efficacy of sevelamer has not been established in pediatric patients.

Precautions

➤*Monitoring:* Sevelamer does not contain calcium or alkali supplementation; monitor serum calcium, bicarbonate, and chloride levels.

➤*GI disorders:* The safety and efficacy of sevelamer in patients with dysphagia, swallowing disorders, severe GI motility disorders, or major GI tract surgery have not been established. Consequently, exercise caution when sevelamer is used in patients with these GI disorders.

➤*Vitamin deficiencies:* In preclinical studies in rats and dogs, sevelamer reduced vitamin D, E, K, and folic acid levels at doses of 6 to 100 times the recommended human dose. In clinical trials, there was no evidence of reduction in serum levels of vitamins, with the exception of a 1-year clinical trial in which sevelamer treatment was associated with reduction of 25-hydroxyvitamin D (normal range, 10 to 55 mcg/mL) from 39 ± 22 mcg/mL to 34 ± 22 mcg/mL ($P < 0.01$). Most (approximately 75%) patients in sevelamer clinical trials received vitamin supplements, which is typical of patients on hemodialysis.

Drug Interactions

When administering any other oral medication where a reduction in the bioavailability of that medication would have a clinically significant effect on safety or efficacy, administer the drug at least 1 hour before or 3 hours after sevelamer, or consider monitoring blood levels of the drug. Patients taking antiarrhythmic and antiseizure medications were excluded from the clinical

SEVELAMER — ORAL

trials. Take special precautions when prescribing sevelamer to patients taking these medications.

Adverse Reactions

In a placebo-controlled study with a treatment duration of 2 weeks, the adverse reactions reported for sevelamer capsules (n = 24) were similar to those reported for placebo (n = 12). In a crossover study with treatment durations of 8 weeks each, the adverse reactions reported for sevelamer capsules (n = 82) were similar to those reported for calcium acetate (n = 82) and included headache, infection, pain, hypertension, hypotension, thrombosis, diarrhea, dyspepsia, vomiting, and cough increased. In a parallel design study with treatment duration of 52 weeks, adverse reactions reported for sevelamer tablets (n = 99) were similar to those reported for calcium (calcium acetate and calcium carbonate) (n = 101) (see the following table).

Sevelamer Adverse Reactions		
Adverse reaction	Sevelamer (n = 99)	Calcium acetate (n = 101)
Cardiovascular		
Hypertension	10.1%	5.9%
CNS		
Headache	9.1%	15.8%
Dermatologic		
Pruritus	13.1%	9.9%
GI		
Constipation	8.1%	11.9%
Diarrhea	19.2%	22.8%
Dyspepsia	16.2%	6.9%
Nausea	20.2%	19.8%
Vomiting	22.2%	21.8%
Musculoskeletal		
Arthralgia	12.1%	17.8%
Pain in limb	13.1%	14.9%
Respiratory		
Bronchitis	11.1%	12.9%
Cough	7.1%	12.9%
Dyspnea	10.1%	16.8%
Nasopharyngitis	14.1%	7.9%
Upper respiratory tract infection	5.1%	10.9%
Miscellaneous		
Back pain	4%	17.8%
Mechanical complication of implant	6.1%	10.9%
Pyrexia	5.1%	10.9%

In the parallel design study, the major reason for dropout in the sevelamer group was GI adverse reactions. In a long-term, open-label extension trial, adverse reactions possibly related to sevelamer capsules that were not dose-related included the following: constipation (2%), diarrhea (4%), flatulence (4%), dyspepsia (5%), and nausea (7%).

➤*Postmarketing:* During postmarketing experience, the following adverse reactions have been reported in patients receiving sevelamer although no direct relationship to sevelamer could be established: abdominal pain, pruritis, rash.

Overdosage

Sevelamer has been given to healthy volunteers in dosages of up to 14 g/day for 8 days with no adverse reactions. Sevelamer has been given in average dosages up to 13 g/day to hemodialysis patients. There are no reported overdosages with sevelamer. Because sevelamer is not absorbed, the risk of systemic toxicity is low.

Patient Information

Inform patients to take sevelamer with meals and adhere to their prescribed diets. Give instructions on concomitant medications that should be dosed apart from sevelamer. Because the contents of sevelamer expand in water, tablets must be swallowed intact and not crushed, chewed, broken into pieces, or taken apart prior to administration.

LANTHANUM CARBONATE

Rx	**Fosrenol** (Shire)	**Tablets, chewable:** 250 mg	(S405 250). White to off-white, flat, beveled. In 90s.
		500 mg	(S405 500). White to off-white, flat, beveled. In 90s.
		750 mg	(S405 750). White to off-white, flat, beveled. In 90s.
		1,000 mg	(S405 1000). White to off-white, flat, beveled. In 90s.

LANTHANUM CARBONATE — ORAL

Indications

➤*Phosphate reduction:* To reduce serum phosphate in patients with end-stage renal disease (ESRD).

Administration and Dosage

➤*Approved by the FDA:* October 26, 2004.

➤*Dosage:* Divide the total daily dose of lanthanum and take with meals. The recommended initial total daily dose of lanthanum is 750 to 1,500 mg. Titrate the dose every 2 to 3 weeks until an acceptable serum phosphate level is reached. Monitor serum phosphate levels as needed during dose titration and on a regular basis thereafter.

In clinical studies of ESRD patients, lanthanum doses up to 3,750 mg were evaluated. Most patients required a total daily dose between 1,500 and 3,000 mg to reduce plasma phosphate levels to less than 6 mg/dL. Doses were generally titrated in increments of 750 mg/day.

➤*Administration:* Chew tablets completely before swallowing. Do not swallow intact tablets.

➤*Storage/Stability:* Store at 25°C (77°F); excursions permitted to 15° to 30°C (59° to 86°F). Protect from moisture.

Actions

➤*Pharmacology:* Patients with ESRD can develop hyperphosphatemia that may be associated with secondary hyperparathyroidism and elevated calcium phosphate product. Elevated calcium phosphate product increases the risk of ectopic calcification. Treatment of hyperphosphatemia usually includes all of the following: reduction in dietary intake of phosphate, removal of phosphate by dialysis, and inhibition of intestinal phosphate absorption with phosphate binders.

Pharmacodynamics – Lanthanum dissociates in the acid environment of the upper GI tract to release lanthanum ions that bind dietary phosphate released from food during digestion. Lanthanum inhibits absorption of phosphate by forming highly insoluble lanthanum phosphate complexes, consequently reducing serum phosphate and calcium phosphate product.

In vitro studies have shown that in the physiologically relevant pH range of 3 to 5 in gastric fluid, lanthanum binds approximately 97% of the available phosphate when lanthanum is present in a 2-fold molar excess to phosphate. In order to bind dietary phosphate efficiently, administer lanthanum with or immediately after a meal.

➤*Pharmacokinetics:*

Absorption/Distribution – Following single-dose or multiple-dose oral administration of lanthanum to healthy subjects, the concentration of lanthanum in plasma was very low (bioavailability less than 0.002%). Following oral administration in ESRD patients, the mean lanthanum C_{max} was 1 ng/mL. During long-term administration (52 weeks) in ESRD patients, the mean lanthanum concentration in plasma was approximately 0.6 ng/mL. There was minimal increase in plasma lanthanum concentrations with increasing doses within the therapeutic dose range. The effect of food on the bioavailability of lanthanum has not been evaluated, but the timing of food intake relative to lanthanum administration (during and 30 minutes after food intake) has a negligible effect on the systemic level of lanthanum.

In vitro, lanthanum is highly bound (more than 99%) to human plasma proteins, including human serum albumin, α1-acid glycoprotein, and transferrin. Binding to erythrocytes in vivo is negligible in rats.

In 105 bone biopsies from patients treated with lanthanum for up to 4.5 years, rising levels of lanthanum were noted over time. Estimates of elimination half-life from bone ranged from 2 to 3.6 years. Steady-state bone concentrations were not reached during the period studied.

In studies in mice, rats, and dogs, lanthanum concentrations in many tissues increased over time and were several orders of magnitude higher than plasma concentrations (particularly in the GI tract, bone, and liver). Steady-state tissue concentrations in bone and liver were achieved in dogs between 4 and 26 weeks. Relatively high levels of lanthanum remained in these tissues for longer than 6 months after cessation of dosing in dogs. There is no evidence from animal studies that lanthanum crosses the blood-brain barrier.

Metabolism/Excretion – Lanthanum is not metabolized and is not a substrate of CYP450. In vitro metabolic inhibition studies showed that lanthanum at concentrations of 10 and 40 mcg/mL does not have relevant inhibitory effects on any of the CYP450 isoenzymes tested (1A2, 2C9/10, 2C19, 2D6, and 3A4/5). Lanthanum was cleared from plasma following discontinuation of therapy with an elimination half-life of 53 hours.

No information is available regarding the mass balance of lanthanum in humans after oral administration. In rats and dogs, the mean recovery of lanthanum after an oral dose was approximately 99% and 94%, respectively, and was essentially all from feces. Biliary excretion is the predominant route of elimination for circulating lanthanum in rats. In healthy volunteers administered intravenous (IV) lanthanum as the soluble chloride salt (120 mcg), renal clearance was less than 2% of total plasma clearance. Quantifiable amounts of lanthanum were not measured in the dialysate of treated ESRD patients.

LANTHANUM CARBONATE — ORAL

Contraindications

None known.

Warnings

➤*Carcinogenesis:* In the mouse, oral administration of lanthanum for up to 99 weeks at a dosage of 1,500 mg/kg/day (1.3 times the MRHD) was associated with an increased incidence of glandular stomach adenomas in male mice.

➤*Pregnancy:* *Category C.* No adequate and well-controlled studies have been conducted in pregnant women. The effect of lanthanum on the absorption of vitamins and other nutrients has not been studied in pregnant women. Lanthanum is not recommended for use during pregnancy.

In pregnant rabbits, oral administration of lanthanum at 1,500 mg/kg/day (5 times the MRHD) was associated with a reduction in maternal body weight gain and food consumption, increased postimplantation loss, reduced fetal weights, and delayed fetal ossification. Lanthanum administered to rats from implantation through lactation at 2,000 mg/kg/day (3.4 times the MRHD) caused delayed eye opening, reduction in body weight gain, and delayed sexual development (preputial separation and vaginal opening) of the offspring.

➤*Lactation:* It is not known whether lanthanum is excreted in human milk. Because many drugs are excreted in human milk, exercise caution when lanthanum is administered to a nursing woman.

➤*Children:* While growth abnormalities were not identified in long-term animal studies, lanthanum was deposited into developing bone, including growth plate. The consequences of such deposition in developing bone in pediatric patients are unknown. Therefore, the use of lanthanum in this population is not recommended.

Precautions

➤*Long-term effects:* There were no differences in the rates of fracture or mortality in patients treated with lanthanum compared with alternative therapy for up to 3 years. The duration of treatment exposure and time of observation in the clinical program are too short to conclude that lanthanum does not affect the risk of fracture or mortality beyond 3 years.

➤*Special risk:* Patients with acute peptic ulcer, ulcerative colitis, Crohn disease, or bowel obstruction were not included in lanthanum clinical studies. Use this drug with caution in patients with these conditions.

Drug Interactions

An in vitro study showed no evidence that lanthanum forms insoluble complexes with warfarin, digoxin, furosemide, phenytoin, metoprolol, and enalapril in simulated gastric fluid. However, it is recommended that compounds known to interact with antacids not be taken within 2 hours of dosing with lanthanum.

Adverse Reactions

The most common adverse reactions for lanthanum were GI events, such as nausea and vomiting, and they generally abated over time with continued dosing.

In double-blind, placebo-controlled studies where a total of 180 and 95 ESRD patients were randomized to lanthanum and placebo, respectively, for 4 to 6 weeks of treatment, the most common reactions that were more frequent (5% difference or more) in the lanthanum group were abdominal pain, dialysis graft occlusion, nausea, and vomiting (see the following table).

Lanthanum Adverse Reactions

Adverse reaction	Lanthanum (N = 180)	Placebo (N = 95)
GI		
Abdominal pain	5%	0%
Nausea	11%	5%
Vomiting	9%	4%
Miscellaneous		
Dialysis graft occlusion	8%	1%

The safety of lanthanum was studied in 2 long-term clinical trials that included 1,215 patients treated with lanthanum and 943 patients with alternative therapy. Fourteen percent of patients in these comparative, open-label studies discontinued therapy in the lanthanum-treated group because of adverse reactions. GI adverse reactions, such as nausea, diarrhea, and vomiting, were the most common type of event leading to discontinuation.

The most common adverse reactions (5% or more in either treatment group) in both the long-term (2 year), open-label, active-controlled study of lanthanum vs alternative therapy (study A) and the 6-month, comparative study of lanthanum vs calcium carbonate (study B) are shown in the following table. Study A events have been adjusted for mean exposure differences between treatment groups (with a mean exposure of 0.9 years on lanthanum and 1.3 years on alternative therapy). The adjustment for mean exposure was achieved by multiplying the observed adverse reaction rates in the alternative therapy group by 0.71.

Lanthanum Adverse Reactions (≥ 5%)

	Study A		Study B	
Adverse reaction	Lanthanum (N = 682)	Alternative therapy adjusted rates (N = 676)	Lanthanum (N = 533)	Calcium carbonate (N = 267)
Cardiovascular				
Hypotension	16%	17%	8%	9%
CNS				
Headache	21%	20%	5%	6%
GI				
Abdominal pain	17%	17%	5%	3%
Constipation	14%	13%	6%	7%
Diarrhea	23%	22%	13%	10%
Nausea	36%	28%	16%	13%
Vomiting	26%	21%	18%	11%
Metabolic				
Hypercalcemia	4%	8%	0%	20%
Respiratory				
Bronchitis	5%	6%	5%	6%
Rhinitis	5%	7%	7%	6%
Miscellaneous				
Dialysis graft complication	26%	25%	3%	5%
Dialysis graft occlusion	21%	20%	4%	6%

Overdosage

There is no experience with lanthanum overdosage. Lanthanum was not acutely toxic in animals by the oral route. No deaths and no adverse effects occurred in mice, rats, or dogs after single oral doses of 2,000 mg/kg. In clinical trials, daily lanthanum doses up to 4,718 mg were well tolerated in healthy adults when administered with food, with the exception of GI symptoms. Given the topical activity of lanthanum in the gut, and the excretion in feces of the majority of the dose, supportive therapy is recommended for overdosage.

Patient Information

Instruct patients to take lanthanum tablets with or immediately after meals. Tablets should be chewed completely before swallowing; intact tablets should not be swallowed.

VAGINAL PREPARATIONS

Vaginal Antifungal Agents

Indications

➤*Candidiasis:* Local treatment of vulvovaginal candidiasis (eg, moniliasis, vaginal yeast infection).

Actions

➤*Pharmacology:* Treatment of vaginal candidiasis (moniliasis) is complicated by a high recurrence rate because of the ubiquitous nature of *Candida albicans* and non-albicans species of *Candida*. Predisposing factors include diabetes, antibiotics, pregnancy, corticosteroids, oral contraceptives containing 75 to 150 mcg of estrogen, intrauterine devices, and decreased host immunity (eg, HIV).

Agents approved for local treatment of vulvovaginal candidiasis include **nystatin** (a polyene antibiotic), the imidazoles (**butoconazole**, **clotrimazole**, **miconazole**, **tioconazole**), and **terconazole** (a triazole derivative).

Nystatin and imidazoles – Nystatin and imidazoles bind to sterols in the cell membrane of the fungus with a resultant change in membrane permeability allowing leakage of intracellular components.

Terconazole – Terconazole's exact pharmacologic mode of action is uncertain. It may exert antifungal activity by disruption of normal fungal cell membrane permeability.

➤*Pharmacokinetics:*

Butoconazole – Approximately 1.7% is absorbed after vaginal administration. Peak plasma levels (13.6 to 18.6 ng/mL) of the drug and its metabolites were attained between 12 and 24 hours.

Terconazole – Following daily intravaginal administration of 0.8% terconazole 40 mg (0.8% cream × 5 g) for 7 days to healthy humans, plasma concentrations were low and gradually rose to a daily peak (mean of 5.9 ng/mL) at 6.6 hours. Following oral (30 mg) administration of terconazole, the harmonic half-life of elimination from the blood for the parent terconazole was 6.9 hours (range, 4 to 11.3). Terconazole is extensively metabolized. In vitro, terconazole is highly protein bound (94.9%) and the degree of binding is independent of the drug concentration.

Nystatin – Nystatin is not absorbed from intact skin or mucous membranes.

➤*Microbiology:* **Miconazole** is active against susceptible strains of *Trichophyton* spp., *Epidermophyton* spp., *Candida albicans*, and *Microsporum* spp. **Clotrimazole**, **tioconazole**, **nystatin**, **terconazole**, and **butoconazole** are active against *Candida* spp. (*Candida albicans*). Other pathogens commonly associated with vulvovaginitis (*Trichomonas* and *Gardnerella vaginalis*) do not respond to these antifungal agents.

Contraindications

Hypersensitivity to specific drug or component of the product.

Warnings

➤*Diagnosis:* It is important that vaginal infections be differentiated, as bacterial vaginosis, trichomoniasis, and vulvovaginal candidiasis may produce common symptoms. The diagnosis of vulvovaginitis (*Trichomonas vaginalis* and *Haemophilus vaginalis*) may be confirmed prior to therapy by KOH smears or cultures. This does not apply to *otc* use of these agents, which requires self-diagnosis by the patient.

➤*OTC products:*

Other conditions – If abdominal pain, fever, or offensive-smelling vaginal discharge is present, do not use these products. If there is no improvement within 3 to 7 days, stop using these products. Consult a doctor, a condition more serious than a yeast infection may be present.

Vaginal itch / discomfort – Patients should consult a physician before using these products if it is their first experience with vaginal itch and discomfort.

Recurrent infections – For patients with frequently recurrent candidal vaginitis, it is important to consider factors that predispose to infection. The discontinuation of oral contraceptives decreases the frequency of yeast vaginitis for many women. Eliminating nylon and tight-fitting garments can also be helpful. Many diabetic patients with poor glycemic control have recurring yeast vaginitis. Patients with recurrent yeast vaginitis should be tested for HIV.

➤*Pregnancy: Category A* – **nystatin**; *Category B* – **clotrimazole, nystatin**†; *Category C* – **butoconazole, terconazole, miconazole.** During pregnancy, use of a vaginal applicator may be contraindicated; manual insertion of vaginal tablets may be preferred. Use only on advice of physician.

Because small amounts of these drugs may be absorbed from the vagina, use during the first trimester only when essential. Use of **butoconazole** during the second and third trimesters has been approved. Possible exposure of the fetus through direct transfer of **terconazole** from an irritated vagina to the fetus by diffusion across amniotic membranes may occur.

➤*Lactation:* Because nystatin is poorly absorbed, if at all, serum and milk levels would not occur with **nystatin**. It is not known whether the other drugs are excreted in breast milk. Safety for use during lactation has not been established. Exercise caution or temporarily discontinue nursing during administration.

Terconazole – Because of the potential for adverse reactions in nursing infants from terconazole, decide whether to discontinue nursing or to discontinue the drug, taking into account the importance of the drug to the mother.

➤*Children:* Safety and efficacy have not been established with **butoconazole, terconazole, nystatin,** and **miconazole** (*Monistat Dual-Pak* only). Safety and efficacy have not been established in children younger than 12 years of age with **clotrimazole, tioconazole,** and **miconazole**.

Precautions

➤*For vaginal use only:* Do not use creams in mouth or eyes.

➤*Irritation:* If irritation, sensitization, fever, chills, or flu-like symptoms occur, discontinue use.

➤*Chronic or recurrent candidiasis:* Chronic or recurrent candidiasis may be a symptom of unrecognized diabetes mellitus or a damaged immune system (including HIV infection). A persistently resistant infection may actually be caused by reinfection; evaluate sources of reinfection.

➤*Refractory patients:* If there is lack of response, repeat microbiological studies to confirm diagnosis and rule out other pathogens before reinstituting antifungal therapy.

Drug Interactions

➤*Miconazole:* Concomitant use of warfarin and miconazole intravaginal cream or suppository may cause an increase in PT, INR, and bleeding. Monitor appropriately.

Adverse Reactions

Irritation; sensitization; vulvovaginal burning.

Clotrimazole – Skin irritation with symptoms of redness, itching, burning, blistering, peeling, urticaria, or skin fissures.

Miconazole – Burning, irritation, pruritus, discharge, edema, and pain have occurred at the administration site. Other adverse reactions include GI cramping, nausea, and headache. Genital erythema, vaginal tenderness, dysuria, allergic reaction, dry mouth, flatulence, perianal burning, pelvic cramping, rash, urticaria, skin irritation, periorbital edema, and conjunctival pruritus occurred in less than 1% of patients in trials.

Butoconazole – Vulvar/vaginal burning, itching, soreness and swelling, pelvic or abdominal pain or cramping, or a combination of 2 or more of these symptoms.

Terconazole – Headache (21% to 26%); dysmenorrhea (6%); pain of the female genitalia (5%); body pain (2.1%); abdominal pain (3.4%); fever (1% to 1.7%); chills (0.4%); vulvovaginal burning (5.2%); itching (2.3%); irritation (3.1%). Most frequent reason for discontinuing therapy was vulvovaginal itching (0.6% to 0.7%).

Photosensitivity reactions may occur following repeated dermal application under conditions of filtered artificial ultraviolet light.

Tioconazole – Vaginal swelling or redness; difficult or burning urination; headache; abdominal pain/cramping; upper respiratory tract infection.

Patient Information

Patient instructions are enclosed with product. Patients should carefully read *otc* product labeling.

Open applicator just prior to administration to prevent contamination. Clean reusable applicators after use with mild soap solution and rinse thoroughly with water.

Insert high into the vagina (except during pregnancy).

Complete full course of therapy. Use continuously, even during menstrual period.

Notify physician if burning or irritation, skin rash, or hives occur.

Refrain from sexual intercourse.

Use sanitary napkin or minipad to prevent staining of clothing. Do not use a tampon.

The base used in some of these formulations may interact with (weaken) certain latex products such as condoms, diaphragms, or vaginal spermicides. Concurrent use (within 72 hours) is not recommended. The effect is temporary and occurs only during treatment.

CLOTRIMAZOLE

otc	**Clotrimazole** (Various, eg, Taro)	**Vaginal suppositories:** 200 mg	In 3s with applicator.
otc	**Gyne-Lotrimin 3** (Schering-Plough)		In 3s with applicator.
otc	**Clotrimazole** (Various, eg, Taro)	**Vaginal cream:** 2%	In 21 g tube with 3 disposable applicators.
otc	**Gyne-Lotrimin 3** (Schering-Plough)		Benzyl alcohol. In 21 g tube with 3 disposable applicators.
otc	**Clotrimazole** (Various, eg, Alpharma, Major, Warrick)	**Vaginal cream:** 1%	In 15, 30, and 45 g with applicator(s).
otc	**Mycelex-7** (Bayer)		Benzyl alcohol, cetostearyl alcohol. In 45 g with 1 applicator or 45 g with 7 disposable applicators.
otc	**Gyne-Lotrimin 7** (Schering-Plough)		In 45 g with 1 applicator, 45 g with 7 applicators, or 45 g with 7 prefilled applicators.
otc	**Mycelex-7 Combination Pack** (Bayer)	**Vaginal suppositories:** 100 mg	Lactose, povidone. In 7s with applicator.
		Topical cream: 1%	Benzyl alcohol, cetostearyl alcohol. Polysorbate 80. In 7 g tubes.
otc	**Clotrimazole Combination Pack** (Various, eg, Taro)	**Vaginal suppositories:** 200 mg	In 3s with applicator.
		Topical cream: 1%	In tubes.
otc	**Gyne-Lotrimin 3 Combination Pack** (Schering-Plough)	**Vaginal suppositories:** 200 mg	Lactose. In 3s with applicator.
		Topical cream: 1%	Benzyl alcohol, cetyl stearyl alcohol. In 7 g tubes.

† Briggs GG, et al. *Drugs in Pregnancy and Lactation* 5th ed.

CLOTRIMAZOLE — VAGINAL

Refer to the general discussion of these products in the Vaginal Antifungal agents group monograph. For information on oral and topical clotrimazole, refer to individual monographs.

Indications

For the treatment of vaginal yeast (candidiasis) infections and for the relief of external vulvar itching and irritation associated with vaginal yeast infections.

Administration and Dosage

Do not use in girls under 12 years of age. Do not use in the eyes or mouth. For vaginal use only.

➤*Vaginal suppositories:* Unwrap 1 insert, place it in the applicator, and use the applicator to place the insert high into the vagina, preferably at bedtime.

100 mg – Repeat this procedure daily for 7 consecutive days.

200 mg – Repeat this procedure daily for 3 consecutive days.

➤*Vaginal cream:*

Intravaginal –

1%: Insert 1 applicatorful per day, preferably at bedtime, for 7 consecutive days.

2%: Insert 1 applicatorful per day, preferably at bedtime, for 3 consecutive days.

Topical 1% cream – For relief of external vulvar itching, squeeze a small amount of clotrimazole cream onto your finger and gently spread the cream onto the irritated area of the vulva. Use once or twice a day for up to 7 days as needed to relieve external vulvar itching. The cream should not be used for vulvar itching due to causes other than a yeast infection.

➤*Storage/Stability:* Store at room temperature 15° to 30°C (59° to 86°F). Avoid excessive heat above 30°C (86°F). Avoid freezing. Keep out of the reach of children.

MICONAZOLE NITRATE

otc	**Monistat-7** (Personal Products)	**Vaginal suppositories**: 100 mg	In 7s with applicator.
otc	**Miconazole 7** (Rugby)		Hydrogenated vegetable oil base. In 7s with applicator.
otc	**Monistat** (Personal Products)	**Topical cream**: 2%	In 9 g tubes.
otc	**Miconazole Nitrate** (Various, eg, Alpharma, E. Fougera, G & W Labs, Major, Rugby, Taro)	**Vaginal cream**: 2%	In 15, 30, and 45 g with applicator(s).
otc	**Femizol-M** (Lake Consumer Products)		In 45 g with applicator.
otc	**Monistat 7** (Personal Products)		In 35 and 45 g tubes with 1 applicator or 7 *Ultraslim* disposable applicators, or in 7 prefilled applicators with 5 g cream.
otc	**Monistat 3** (Personal Products)		In 3 prefilled applicators.
Rx	**Monistat 1 Combination Pack** (Personal Products)	**Vaginal suppositories**: 1200 mg	Glycerin, mineral oil, petrolatum. In 1s with applicator.
		Topical cream: 2%	Steryl and cetyl alcohol. In 9 g tubes.
otc	**M-Zole 3 Combination Pack** (Alpharma)	**Vaginal suppositories**: 200 mg	Hydrogenated vegetable oil. In 3s with reusable applicator or 3 disposable applicators.
		Topical cream: 2%	In 9 g tubes.
otc	**Monistat 3 Combination Pack** (Personal Products)	**Vaginal suppositories**: 200 mg	In 3s with 1 reusable applicator or 3 disposable applicators.
		Topical cream: 2%	In tubes.
otc	**Vagistat-3 Combination Pack** (Bristol-Myers Squibb)	**Vaginal suppositories**: 200 mg	Hydrogenated vegetable oil. In 3s with 3 disposable applicators.
		Topical cream: 2%	Mineral oil. In 9 g tube.
otc	**Monistat 7 Combination Pack** (Personal Products)	**Vaginal suppositories**: 100 mg	In 7s with 1 applicator.
		Topical cream: 2%	In tubes.
otc	**M-Zole 7 Dual Pack** (Alpharma)	**Vaginal suppositories**: 100 mg	Mineral oil. In 7s with 1 applicator.
		Topical cream: 2%	In 9 g tubes.

MICONAZOLE NITRATE — VAGINAL

Refer to the general discussion of these products in the Vaginal Antifungal Agents group monograph. For information on topical miconazole, refer to the monograph in the Dermatologicals chapter.

Indications

➤*Suppositories:* For the treatment of vulvovaginal candidiasis (moniliasis).

➤*Cream:* For the relief of external vulvar itching and irritation associated with a yeast infection.

Administration and Dosage

➤*Suppositories:* Insert 1 suppository intravaginally once daily at bedtime for 1 day (1200 mg), 3 consecutive days (200 mg), or 7 consecutive days (100 mg).

➤*Cream:*

Intravaginal – Insert 1 applicatorful intravaginally once daily at bedtime for 3 to 7 days.

Topical – Apply to affected areas twice daily (morning and evening) for up to 7 days or as needed.

Repeat course if necessary, after ruling out other pathogens.

➤*Storage/Stability:* Store at 15° to 30°C (59° to 86°F).

TIOCONAZOLE

otc	**Vagistat-1** (Bristol-Myers Squibb)	**Vaginal ointment**: 6.5%	White petrolatum. In 300 mg prefilled, single-dose applicator.
otc	**Monistat 1** (Personal Products)		In 4.6 g prefilled, single-dose applicator.

TIOCONAZOLE — VAGINAL

Refer to the general discussion of these products in the Vaginal Antifungal Agents group monograph.

Indications

➤*Candidiasis:* For the treatment of recurrent vaginal yeast infections (candidiasis).

Administration and Dosage

➤*For best results when treating infection:* Use this product at bedtime, even during your menstrual period for full course of treatment.

Dry the genital area thoroughly after a shower, bath or swim. Change out of a wet bathing suit or damp clothes as soon as possible. A dry area is less likely to lead to the overgrowth of yeast.

Wear cotton underwear and loose-fitting clothes.

Wipe from front to back after bowel movement or after urination.

Do not douche, because douching may wash the drug out of the vagina.

Do not use tampons, because they remove some of the drug from the vagina. Use deodorant-free sanitary napkins or pads as needed.

Do not use spermicides, as they may interfere with tioconazole.

Do not have vaginal intercourse while using tioconazole.

Do not scratch the skin outside the vagina. Scratching can cause more irritation and can spread the infection.

➤*Storage/Stability:* Store at controlled room temperature 15° to 30°C (59° to 86°F). Keep this and all drugs out of the reach of children.

Vaginal Antifungal Agents

NYSTATIN

Rx	**Nystatin** (Various, eg, Goldline)	**Vaginal tablets:** 100,000 units	In 15s and 30s with applicator(s).

NYSTATIN — VAGINAL

Refer to the general discussion of these products in the Vaginal Antifungal Agents group monograph. For information on oral nystatin suspension and troches for oral candidiasis, oral nystatin tablets for intestinal candidiasis, and topical nystatin, refer to the individual monographs.

Indications

➤*Yeast infections:* For the treatment of vulvovaginal candidiasis (moniliasis).

Administration and Dosage

The usual dosage is 1 tablet inserted high in the vagina by means of applicator daily for 2 weeks.

Symptomatic relief may occur in a few days; continue full course of treatment.

➤*Storage/Stability:* Store at 15° to 30°C (59° to 86°F).

TERCONAZOLE VAGINAL

Rx	**Terconazole** (Various, eg, Taro, Watson)	**Vaginal cream:** 0.4%	Alcohols. In 45 g tubes.
Rx	**Terazol 7** (Ortho-McNeil)		Cetyl alcohol, stearyl alcohol. In 45 g tube with 1 measured-dose applicator.
Rx	**Terconazole** (Various, eg, Taro, Watson)	**Vaginal cream:** 0.8%	Alcohols. In 20 g tubes.
Rx	**Terazol 3** (Ortho-McNeil)		In 20 g tube with measured-dose applicator.
Rx	**Zazole** (PharmaDerm)		Alcohols. In 20 g tube with measured-dose applicator.
Rx	**Terconazole** (Perrigo)	**Vaginal suppositories:** 80 mg	Coconut oil/palm kernel oil. White to off-white, elliptically shaped. In 2.5 g. In 3s with applicator.
Rx	**Terazol 3** (Ortho-McNeil)		Coconut oil/palm kernel oil. White to off-white, eliptically shaped. In 2.5 g. In 3s.

TERCONAZOLE — VAGINAL

Refer to the general discussion of these products in the Vaginal Antifungal Agents group monograph.

Indications

➤*Candidiasis:* For the local treatment of vulvovaginal candidiasis (moniliasis). As terconazole is effective only for vulvovaginitis caused by the genus *Candida*, the diagnosis should be confirmed by KOH smears or cultures.

Administration and Dosage

➤*Approved by the FDA:* December 31, 1987.

➤*Dosage:* 1 full 5 g applicator (20 mg terconazole for 0.4% vaginal cream; 40 mg terconazole for 0.8% vaginal cream) or 1 terconazole vaginal suppository (80 mg) should be administered intravaginally once daily at bedtime for 3 consecutive days. Before prescribing another course of therapy, the diagnosis should be reconfirmed by smears or cultures and other pathogens commonly associated with vulvovaginitis ruled out. The therapeutic effect of terconazole is not affected by menstruation.

➤*Storage/Stability:* Store at controlled room temperature 15° to 30°C (59° to 86°F).

BUTOCONAZOLE NITRATE VAGINAL

Rx	**Gynazole•1** (Ther-Rx)	**Vaginal cream:** 2%	EDTA, parabens, mineral oil. In 5 g prefilled, single-dose applicator (1s).
otc	**Mycelex-3** (Bayer)		Cetyl and stearyl alcohol, parabens, mineral oil. In 3 prefilled, single-dose applicators, or in 20 g with 3 disposable applicators.

BUTOCONAZOLE NITRATE — VAGINAL

Refer to the general discussion of these products in the Vaginal Antifungal Agents group monograph.

Indications

➤*Candidiasis:* For the local treatment of vulvovaginal candidiasis (infections caused by *Candida*). The diagnosis may be confirmed by KOH smears or cultures.

Administration and Dosage

➤*Approved by the FDA:* December 21, 1995.

➤*Rx formulation:* The recommended dose of butoconazole nitrate is 1 applicatorful of cream (approximately 5 g of the cream) intravaginally. This amount of cream contains approximately 100 mg of butoconazole nitrate.

➤*OTC formulation:*

- Before using, read the educational pamphlet enclosed with the package.
- Do not use in females under 12 years of age.
- Insert 1 applicator full of cream into the vagina for 3 consecutive days, preferably at bedtime.
- Dispose of applicator after use.

➤*Storage/Stability:*

Rx formulation – Store at 25°C (77°F); excursions permitted to 15° to 30°C (59° to 86°F). Avoid heat above 30°C (86°F).

OTC formulation – Avoid excessive heat above 30°C (86°F) and avoid freezing.

Miscellaneous Anti-infectives

CLINDAMYCIN PHOSPHATE INTRAVAGINAL

Rx	**Clindamycin Phosphate** (Greenstone)	**Cream:** 2%	Benzyl alcohol, cetostearyl alcohol, mineral oil. In 40 g tube with 7 disposable applicators.
Rx	**Cleocin** (Pfizer)		Benzyl alcohol, cetostearyl alcohol, mineral oil. In 40 g tube with 7 disposable applicators.
Rx	**ClindaMax** (PharmaDerm)		Benzyl alcohol, cetostearyl alcohol, mineral oil. In 40 g tube with 7 disposable applicators.
Rx	**Clindesse** (KV Pharma)		EDTA, mineral oil, parabens. In carton of 1 single-dose prefilled disposable applicator.
Rx	**Cleocin** (Pfizer)	**Suppositories:** 100 mg (as base)	In cartons of 3 with applicator.

CLINDAMYCIN PHOSPHATE — VAGINAL

Indications

➤*Bacterial vaginosis:* For the treatment of bacterial vaginosis (formerly referred to as *Haemophilus* vaginitis, *Gardnerella* vaginitis, nonspecific vaginitis, *Corynebacterium* vaginitis, or anaerobic vaginosis) in nonpregnant women.

Cleocin and ClindaMax creams only – Clindamycin cream can be used to treat pregnant women during the second and third trimester.

Administration and Dosage

➤*Cream:* One applicatorful (5 g containing approximately 100 mg clindamycin) intravaginally, preferably at bedtime, for 3 or 7 consecutive days in nonpregnant women and for 7 consecutive days in pregnant women (*Cleocin, ClindaMax*); a single applicatorful (approximately 5 g of vaginal cream containing approximately 100 mg clindamycin phosphate) administered once intravaginally at anytime of the day (*Clindesse*).

➤*Suppositories:* One suppository (containing clindamycin equivalent to 100 mg clindamycin/2.5 g suppository) intravaginally/day, preferably at bedtime, for 3 consecutive days.

➤*Storage/Stability:*

Cream – Store at controlled room temperature 20° to 25°C (68° to 77°F). Protect from freezing.

CLINDAMYCIN PHOSPHATE — VAGINAL

Suppositories – Store at 25°C (77°F); excursions permitted to 15° to 30°C (59° to 86°F). Avoid heat over 30°C (86°F) and high humidity.

Actions

➤*Pharmacology:* Clindamycin is a water soluble ester of the semi-synthetic antibiotic produced by a 7(S)-chloro-substitution of the 7(R)-hydroxyl group of the parent antibiotic lincomycin. Clindamycin inhibits bacterial protein synthesis at the level of the bacterial ribosome. The antibiotic binds preferentially to the 50S ribosomal subunit and affects the process of peptide chain initiation. Although clindamycin is inactive in vitro, rapid in vivo hydrolysis converts this compound to the antibacterially active clindamycin.

➤*Pharmacokinetics:*

Cream – Following a once-daily intravaginal dose of 100 mg clindamycin vaginal cream administered to 6 healthy female volunteers for 7 days, approximately 5% of the administered dose was absorbed systemically. The peak serum clindamycin concentration averaged 18 and 25 ng/mL on day 1 and day 7, respectively. These peak concentrations were attained approximately 10 hours postdosing.

Following a once-daily intravaginal dose of 100 mg clindamycin vaginal cream administered for 7 consecutive days to 5 women with bacterial vaginosis, absorption was slower and less variable than that observed in healthy females. Approximately 5% of the dose was absorbed systemically. The peak serum clindamycin concentration averaged 13 and 16 ng/mL on day 1 and day 7, respectively. These peak concentrations were attained approximately 14 hours postdosing.

There was little or no systemic accumulation of clindamycin after repeated vaginal dosing of clindamycin vaginal cream. The systemic half life was 1.5 to 2.6 hours.

Suppositories – Systemic absorption of clindamycin was estimated following an intravaginal dose of 1 clindamycin suppository (equivalent to 100 mg clindamycin) administered once daily to 11 healthy female volunteers for 3 days. Approximately 30% of the administered dose was absorbed systemically on day 3 of dosing based on AUC. The mean AUC following day 3 of the suppository dosing was 3.2 mcg•h/mL. The C_{max} observed on day 3 of the suppository dosing averaged 0.27 mcg/mL and was observed approximately 5 hours after dosing. The mean apparent elimination half life after the suppository dosing was 11 hours and is considered to be limited by the absorption rate.

➤*Microbiology:* Clindamycin is active in vitro against most strains of the following organisms that have been reported to be associated with bacterial vaginosis: *Bacteroides* spp., *Gardnerella vaginalis*; *Mobiluncus* spp.; *Mycoplasma hominis*; *Peptostreptococcus* spp.

Contraindications

Hypersensitivity to clindamycin, lincomycin, or any components of the products; regional enteritis; ulcerative colitis; "antibiotic-associated" colitis.

Warnings

➤*Pseudomembranous colitis:* Pseudomembranous colitis has been reported with nearly all antibacterial agents, including clindamycin, and may range in severity from mild to life-threatening. Orally and parenterally administered clindamycin has been associated with severe colitis that may end fatally. Diarrhea, bloody diarrhea, and colitis (including pseudomembranous colitis) have been reported with the use of orally and parenterally administered clindamycin as well as with topical (dermal) formulations of clindamycin. Therefore, it is important to consider this diagnosis in patients who present with diarrhea subsequent to the administration of clindamycin, even when administered by the vaginal route, because approximately 5% (cream) and 30% (suppository) of the clindamycin dose is systemically absorbed from the vagina.

Treatment with antibacterial agents alters the normal flora of the colon and may permit overgrowth of clostridia. Studies indicate that a toxin produced by *Clostridium difficile* is a primary cause of "antibiotic-associated" colitis.

After the diagnosis of pseudomembranous colitis has been established, initiate therapeutic measures. Mild cases of pseudomembranous colitis usually respond to discontinuation of the drug alone. In moderate to severe cases, give consideration to management with fluids and electrolytes, protein supplementation, and treatment with an antibacterial drug clinically effective against *C. difficile* colitis.

Onset of pseudomembranous colitis symptoms may occur during or after antimicrobial treatment.

➤*Mineral oil / oleaginous base:* The cream contains mineral oil and the suppositories contain an oleaginous base, both which can weaken latex or rubber products such as condoms or vaginal contraceptive diaphragms. Use of such products within 72 hours (*Cleocin*) or 5 days (*Clindesse*) following treatment with clindamycin is not recommended.

➤*Diagnosis:* A clinical diagnosis of bacterial vaginosis is usually defined by the presence of a homogeneous vaginal discharge that has a pH of greater than 4.5, emits a "fishy" amine odor when mixed with a 10% KOH solution, and contains clue cells on microscopic examination. Gram's stain results consistent with a diagnosis of bacterial vaginosis include markedly reduced or absent *Lactobacillus* morphology, predominance of *Gardnerella* morphotype, and absent or few white blood cells.

Rule out other pathogens commonly associated with vulvovaginitis (eg, *Trichomonas vaginalis*, *Chlamydia trachomatis*, *Neisseria gonorrhoeae*, *Candida albicans*, and herpes simplex virus).

➤*Pregnancy: Category B.* Clindamycin cream has been studied in pregnant women during the second trimester. In women treated for 7 days, abnormal labor was reported in 1.1% of patients who received clindamycin cream compared with 0.5% of patients who received placebo. There are no adequate and well-controlled studies in pregnant women during the first trimester of pregnancy treated with clindamycin cream; there are no adequate and well-controlled studies in pregnant women treated with clindamycin suppositories. Use during pregnancy only if clearly needed.

➤*Lactation:* It is not known if clindamycin is excreted in breast milk following the use of vaginally administered clindamycin. However, clindamycin has been detected in breast milk after oral or parenteral administration. Because of the potential for serious adverse reactions in nursing infants, decide whether to discontinue nursing or discontinue the drug, taking into account the importance of the drug to the mother.

➤*Children:* Safety and efficacy in children have not been established.

Precautions

➤*For intravaginal use only:* Avoid contact with the eyes. Clindamycin contains ingredients that will cause burning and irritation of the eye. In the event of accidental contact, rinse the eye with copious amounts of cool tap water.

➤*Overgrowth of nonsusceptible organisms:* The use of clindamycin may result in the overgrowth of nonsusceptible organisms, particularly yeasts, in the vagina. In studies using clindamycin suppositories, treatment-related moniliasis was reported in 2.7% of women patients and vaginitis in 3.6%. In women who received clindamycin cream treatment for 3 days, *C. albicans* was reported in 8.8% and vaginitis in 9% of patients; in the 7-day treatment, *C. albicans* was detected in 10.5% and vaginitis in 10.7% of patients.

Drug Interactions

➤*Neuromuscular blocking agents:* Clindamycin has been shown to have neuromuscular blocking properties that may enhance the action of other neuromuscular blocking agents; use with caution in patients receiving such agents.

Adverse Reactions

➤*Cream:*

Nonpregnant women – In clinical trials involving nonpregnant women, 1.8% of 600 patients who received treatment with clindamycin cream for 3 days and 2.7% of 1325 patients who received treatment for 7 days discontinued therapy because of drug-related adverse events. Medical events judged to be related, probably related, possibly related, or of unknown relationship to vaginally administered clindamycin cream were reported for 20.7% of the patients receiving treatment for 3 days and 21.3% of the patients receiving treatment for 7 days.

Clindamycin Adverse Reactions (≥ 1%)

Adverse reaction	Clindamycin cream 3 day (n = 600)	Clindamycin cream 7 day (n = 1325)
GU		
Trichomonal vaginitis	0	1.3
Vaginal moniliasis	7.7	10.4
Vulvovaginal disorder	3.2	5.3
Vulvovaginitis	6	4.4
Miscellaneous		
Moniliasis (body)	1.3	0.2

Other adverse events (less than 1%):
- *CNS* – Dizziness, headache, vertigo.
- *Dermatologic* – Erythema, maculopapular rash, moniliasis, pruritus (nonapplication site), rash, urticaria.
- *GI* – Abdominal cramps, constipation, diarrhea, dyspepsia, flatulence, generalized abdominal pain, GI disorder, localized abdominal pain, nausea, vomiting.
- *GU* – Endometriosis, menstrual disorder, metrorrhagia, urinary tract infection, vaginal discharge, vaginal pain, vaginitis/vaginal infection.
- *Respiratory* – Epistaxis.
- *Miscellaneous* – Allergic reaction, bacterial infection, fungal infection, halitosis, hyperthyroidism, inflammatory swelling, taste perversion.

Pregnant women – In a clinical trial involving pregnant women during the second trimester, 1.7% of 180 patients who received treatment for 7 days discontinued therapy because of drug-related adverse events. Medical events judged to be related, probably related, possibly related, or of unknown relationship to vaginally administered clindamycin cream were reported for 22.8% of pregnant patients.

Clindamycin Adverse Reactions (≥ 1%)

Adverse reaction	Clindamycin cream 7 day (n = 180)	Placebo 7 day (n = 184)
GU		
Abnormal labor	1.1	0.5
Vaginal moniliasis	13.3	7.1
Vulvovaginal disorder	6.7	7.1
Miscellaneous		
Fungal infection	1.7	0
Pruritus, nonapplication site	1.1	0

CLINDAMYCIN PHOSPHATE — VAGINAL

Other adverse events (less than 1%):
- *Dermatologic* – Erythema, pruritus (topical application site).
- *GU* – Dysuria, metrorrhagia, trichomonal vaginitis, vaginal pain.
- *Miscellaneous* – Upper respiratory infection.

➤*Suppositories:* In clinical trials involving nonpregnant women, 3 of 589 (0.5%) patients who received treatment with clindamycin suppositories discontinued therapy because of drug-related adverse events. Adverse events judged to have a reasonable possibility of having been caused by clindamycin suppositories were reported for 10.5% of patients. Events reported by 1% or more of patients receiving clindamycin suppositories were as follows:

GU – Vulvovaginal disorder (3.4%), vaginal pain (1.9%), vaginal moniliasis (1.5%).

Miscellaneous – Fungal infection (1%).

Other adverse events (less than 1%) –
Dermatologic: Application-site pain, application-site pruritus, nonapplication-site pruritus, rash.
GI: Abdominal cramps, diarrhea, localized abdominal pain, nausea, vomiting.
GU: Dysuria, menstrual disorder, pyelonephritis, vaginal discharge, vaginitis/vaginal infection.
Miscellaneous: Fever, flank pain, generalized pain, headache, localized edema, moniliasis.

➤*Other clindamycin formulations:* Clindamycin vaginal cream and suppositories afford minimal peak serum levels and systemic exposure of clindamycin compared with 100 mg oral clindamycin dosing. Although these lower levels of exposure are less likely to produce the common reactions seen with oral clindamycin, the possibility of these and other reactions cannot be excluded presently. Refer to the Clindamycin and Lincomycin monographs in the Anti-Infectives chapter.

Overdosage

Vaginally applied cream or suppositories could be absorbed in sufficient amounts to produce systemic effects.

Patient Information

Instruct patients not to engage in vaginal intercourse or use other vaginal products (eg, tampons, douches) during treatment with this product.

Advise patients that the cream contains mineral oil and the suppositories contain an oleaginous base, both which can weaken latex or rubber products such as condoms or vaginal contraceptive diaphragms. Use of such products within 72 hours following treatment with clindamycin is not recommended.

METRONIDAZOLE

Rx	**MetroGel-Vaginal** (3M)	**Gel:** 0.75%	EDTA, parabens. In 70 g tube with 5 applicators.

METRONIDAZOLE — VAGINAL

Metronidazole is also available for topical and systemic use. For further information, refer to the individual monographs in the Anti-infectives chapter and the Dermatological Agents chapter.

Indications

➤*Bacterial vaginosis:* For the treatment of bacterial vaginosis (formerly referred to as *Haemophilus* vaginitis, *Gardnerella* vaginitis, nonspecific vaginitis, *Corynebacterium* vaginitis, or anaerobic vaginosis).

Administration and Dosage

One applicatorful (approximately 5 g containing approximately 37.5 mg metronidazole) intravaginally once or twice daily for 5 days. For once-a-day dosing, administer at bedtime.

➤*Storage/Stability:* Store at controlled room temperature 15° to 30°C (59° to 86°F). Protect from freezing.

Actions

➤*Pharmacology:* Metronidazole, a member of the imidazole class, is classified therapeutically as an antiprotozoal and antibacterial agent. The intracellular target of action of metronidazole on anaerobes are largely unknown. The 5-nitro group of metronidazole is reduced by metabolically active anaerobes, and studies have demonstrated that the reduced form of the drug interacts with bacterial DNA. However, it is not clear whether interaction with DNA alone is an important component in the bactericidal action of metronidazole.

➤*Pharmacokinetics:* A single intravaginal 5 g dose of metronidazole vaginal gel (equivalent to 37.5 mg metronidazole) to 12 healthy subjects resulted in a mean maximum serum metronidazole concentration of 237 ng/mL (range, 152 to 368 ng/mL). This is approximately 2% of the mean maximum serum metronidazole concentration reported in the same subjects administered a single oral 500 mg dose of metronidazole (mean C_{max} = 12,785 ng/mL; range, 10,013 to 17,400 ng/mL). These peak concentrations were obtained 6 to 12 hours after dosing with metronidazole vaginal gel and 1 to 3 hours after dosing with oral metronidazole.

The extent of exposure (AUC) of metronidazole, when administered as a single intravaginal 5 g dose was approximately 4% of the AUC of a single oral 500 mg dose (4977 ng•h/mL and approximately 125,000 ng•h/mL, respectively). When administered vaginally, absorption was approximately half that of an equivalent oral dose.

Patients with bacterial vaginosis – Single and multiple 5 g doses of metronidazole vaginal gel to 4 patients with bacterial vaginosis resulted in a mean maximum serum metronidazole concentration of 214 ng/mL on day 1 and 294 ng/mL on day 5. Steady-state metronidazole serum concentrations following oral dosages of 400 to 500 mg twice daily have been reported to range from 6000 to 20,000 ng/mL.

➤*Microbiology:* Metronidazole is active in vitro against most strains of the following organisms that have been reported to be associated with bacterial vaginosis: *Bacteroides* sp.; *Gardnerella vaginalis*; *Mobiluncus* sp.; *Peptostreptococcus* sp.

Contraindications

Hypersensitivity to metronidazole, parabens, or other ingredients of the formulation or other nitroimidazole derivatives.

Warnings

➤*Convulsive seizures and peripheral neuropathy:* Convulsive seizures and peripheral neuropathy, the latter characterized mainly by numbness or paresthesia of an extremity, have been reported in patients treated with oral or IV metronidazole. The appearance of abnormal neurologic signs demands the prompt discontinuation of metronidazole vaginal gel therapy. Administer with caution to patients with CNS diseases.

➤*Psychotic reactions:* Psychotic reactions have been reported in alcoholic patients who were using oral metronidazole and disulfiram concurrently. Do not administer metronidazole vaginal gel to patients who have taken disulfiram within the last 2 weeks.

➤*Diagnosis:* A clinical diagnosis of bacterial vaginosis is usually defined by the presence of a homogeneous vaginal discharge that has a pH of greater than 4.5, emits a "fishy" amine odor when mixed with a 10% KOH solution, and contains clue cells on microscopic examination. Gram's stain results consistent with a diagnosis of bacterial vaginosis include markedly reduced or absent *Lactobacillus* morphology, predominance of *Gardnerella* morphotype, and absent or few white blood cells.

Rule out other pathogens commonly associated with vulvovaginitis (eg, *Trichomonas vaginalis*, *Chlamydia trachomatis*, *Neisseria gonorrheae*, *Candida albicans*, herpes simplex virus).

➤*Hepatic function impairment:* Patients with severe hepatic disease metabolize metronidazole slowly. This results in the accumulation of metronidazole and its metabolites in the plasma. Accordingly, administer metronidazole vaginal gel cautiously in these patients.

➤*Carcinogenesis:* Metronidazole has shown evidence of carcinogenic activity in a number of studies involving chronic oral administration in mice and rats.

➤*Pregnancy: Category B.* Metronidazole crosses the placental barrier and rapidly enters the fetal circulation. There are no adequate and well-controlled studies in pregnant women. Use during pregnancy only if clearly needed.

➤*Lactation:* Specific studies of metronidazole levels in breast milk following intravaginally administered metronidazole have not been performed. However, metronidazole is secreted in breast milk in concentrations similar to those found in plasma following oral administration. Decide whether to discontinue nursing or to discontinue the drug, taking into account the importance of the drug to the mother.

➤*Children:* Safety and efficacy in children have not been established.

Precautions

➤*Vaginal candidiasis:* Known or previously unrecognized vaginal candidiasis may present more prominent symptoms during metronidazole vaginal gel therapy; approximately 6% to 10% of patients developed symptomatic *Candida* vaginitis during or immediately after therapy.

➤*For intravaginal use only:* Avoid contact with the eyes. Metronidazole vaginal gel contains ingredients that may cause burning and irritation of the eye. In the event of accidental contact with the eye, rinse with copious amounts of cool tap water.

Drug Interactions

Metronidazole Vaginal Gel Interactions

Precipitant drug	Object drug*		Description
Cimetidine	Metronidazole	↑	Use of cimetidine with oral metronidazole may prolong the half-life and decrease plasma clearance of metronidazole. Consider this possibility with the vaginal gel.
Metronidazole	Anticoagulants	↑	Oral metronidazole may potentiate the anticoagulant effect of warfarin, resulting in a prolongation of prothrombin time. Consider this possibility with the vaginal gel.

METRONIDAZOLE — VAGINAL

Metronidazole Vaginal Gel Interactions			
Precipitant drug	Object drug*		Description
Metronidazole	Disulfiram	↑	Concurrent use may result in acute psychosis or a confusional state. Do not administer vaginal gel to patients who have taken disulfiram within the last 2 weeks.
Metronidazole	Ethanol	↑	Disulfiram-like reaction to alcohol has occurred with oral metronidazole. Consider the possibility of such a reaction with the vaginal gel.
Metronidazole	Lithium	↑	In patients stabilized on relatively high doses of lithium, short-term oral metronidazole therapy has been associated with elevation of serum lithium levels and, in a few cases, signs of lithium toxicity. Consider this possibility with the vaginal gel.

* ↑ = Object drug increased.

➤*Drug/Lab test interactions:* Metronidazole may interfere with certain types of determinations of serum chemistry values, such as AST, ALT, LDH, triglycerides, and glucose hexokinase; values of zero may be observed.

Adverse Reactions

In a randomized, single-blind clinical trial of 505 nonpregnant women who received metronidazole vaginal gel once or twice/day, 2 patients (1 from each regimen) discontinued therapy early because of drug-related adverse events. One patient discontinued the drug because of moderate abdominal cramping and loose stools, while the other patient discontinued the drug because of mild vaginal burning. These symptoms resolved after discontinuation of the drug.

Medical events judged to be related, probably related, or possibly related to administration of metronidazole vaginal gel once or twice/day were reported for 39% (195/505) of patients.

➤*CNS:* Headache (5%); dizziness (2%); depression, fatigue (less than 1%).

➤*Dermatologic:* Generalized itching or rash (less than 1%).

➤*GI:* GI discomfort (7%); nausea and/or vomiting (4%); unusual taste (2%); decreased appetite, diarrhea/loose stools (1%); abdominal bloating/gas, dry mouth, thirst (less than 1%).

➤*GU:* Vaginal discharge (12%); symptomatic *Candida* cervicitis/vaginitis (10%); vulva/vaginal irritative symptoms (9%); pelvic discomfort (3%); darkened urine (less than 1%).

➤*Miscellaneous:* Unspecified cramping (1%).

Other metronidazole formulations – Other effects that have been reported in association with the use of topical (dermal) formulations of metronidazole include skin irritation, transient skin erythema, and mild skin dryness and burning (2% or less).

Metronidazole vaginal gel affords minimal peak serum levels and systemic exposure of metronidazole compared with 500 mg oral dosing. Although these lower levels of exposure are less likely to produce the common reactions seen with oral metronidazole, the possibility of these and other reactions cannot be excluded. Refer to the Metronidazole Oral monograph in the Anti-Infectives chapter.

Overdosage

Vaginally applied metronidazole gel could be absorbed in sufficient amounts to produce systemic effects (see Warnings).

Patient Information

Caution patients about drinking alcohol while being treated with metronidazole vaginal gel. While blood levels are significantly lower than with usual doses of oral metronidazole, a possible interaction with alcohol cannot be excluded.

Instruct patients not to engage in vaginal intercourse during treatment with this product.

Advise patients that this medicine is to be used intravaginally only.

MISCELLANEOUS VAGINAL PREPARATIONS

otc	**Lubrin** (Kenwood/Bradley)	**Inserts**: Caprylic/capric triglyceride, glycerin *Indication*: Prolonged lubrication for sexual intercourse. *Dosage*: 1 intravaginally 5 to 30 minutes before intercourse. Allow 5 to 10 minutes for insert to dissolve.	In 5s and 12s.
otc	**Vaginex** (Quality Health)	**Cream**: Tripelennamine HCl *Indication*: Temporary relief of external vaginal irritation. *Dosage*: Apply externally 3 or 4 times a day.	In 30 and 300 g.
otc	**Astroglide** (BioFilm)	**Gel**: Glycerin, propylene glycol, parabens *Indication*: Vaginal lubricant. *Dosage*: Apply externally or internally.	In 66.5 ml bottle and 5 ml travel packets.
otc	**Lubricating Jelly** (Taro)	**Jelly**: Glycerin, propylene glycol *Indication*: Provides additional vaginal moisture. *Dosage*: Apply as needed.	In 60 and 125 g.
otc	**K-Y** (Johnson & Johnson)	**Jelly**: Glycerin, hydroxyethyl cellulose, methylparaben *Indication*: Vaginal lubricant *Dosage*: Apply as needed.	Sterile or regular. In 12, 60 and 120 g.
otc	**Surgel** (Ulmer)	**Gel**: Propylene glycol, glycerin *Indication*: Vaginal lubricant.	In 120 and 240 ml and 1 gal.
Rx	**Fem pH** (Pharmics)	**Vaginal jelly**: 0.9% glacial acetic acid, 0.025% oxyquinoline sulfate, glycerin, lactic acid, PEG 4500 *Indication*: Adjunctive therapy when restoration and maintenance of vaginal acidity is desirable *Dosage*: 1 applicatorful administered intravaginally morning and evening.	In 50 g with applicator.
otc	**Trimo-San** (Cooper Surgical[a])	**Jelly**: 0.025% oxyquinoline sulfate, 0.7% sodium borate, 0.1% sodium lauryl sulfate, glycerin, methylparaben *Indication*: Controls odor-causing bacteria. Helps maintain normal vaginal pH 4. *Dosage*: ½ applicator 2 or 3 times per week.	In 120 g with applicator.
Rx	**Amino-Cerv pH 5.5** (Milex)	**Cream**: 8.34% urea, 0.5% sodium propionate, 0.83% methionine, 0.35% cystine, 0.83% inositol *Indications*: Treatment of mild cervicitis and postpartum cervicitis/cervical tears, postconization and for postsurgical procedures. *Dosage*: See manufacturer's information.	Water miscible base. In 82.5 g with applicator. Buffered to pH 5.5 in water-miscible creme base.
otc	**Yeast X** (Fleet)	**Suppositories**: Pulsatilla 28× *Indication*: Relieves vaginal irritation, itching and burning. *Dosage*: One suppository daily as needed.	In 12s with applicator.
otc	**Norforms** (Fleet)	**Suppositories**: PEG-18, PEG-32, PEG-20 stearate, methylparaben *Indication*: Feminine deodorant. *Dosage*: One suppository daily as needed.	In 12s and 24s with applicator.
otc	**Moist Again** (Lake)	**Gel**: Aloe vera, EDTA, methylparaben, glycerin *Indication*: Vaginal lubricant. *Dosage*: Apply as needed.	In 70.8 g.
otc	**H-R Lubricating Jelly** (Carter-Wallace)	**Jelly**: Hydroxypropyl, methylcellulose, parabens *Indication*: Vaginal lubricant. *Dosage*: Apply as needed.	In 150 g.
otc	**Acid Jelly** (Hope Pharmaceuticals)	**Jelly**: 0.025% oxyquinoline sulfate, 0.7% ricinoleic acid, 0.921% glacial acetic acid, 5% glycerin, propylparaben *Indication*: As adjunctive therapy in those cases where restoration and maintenance of vaginal acidity is desirable. *Dosage*: 1 applicatorful, morning and evening.	In 85 g with applicator.
otc	**Vagi•Gard Maximum Strength** (Lake)	**Cream**: 20% benzocaine, 3% resorcinol, methylparaben, sodium sulfite, EDTA, mineral oil *Indication*: Relieves external vaginal irritation, itching and burning. *Dosage*: Apply externally 3 to 4 times/day.	In 45 g.
otc	**Vagi•Gard Advanced Sensitive Formula** (Lake)	**Cream**: 5% benzocaine, 2% resorcinol, methylparaben, sodium sulfite, EDTA, mineral oil *Indication*: Relieves external vaginal irritation, itching and burning. *Dosage*: Apply externally 3 to 4 times/day.	In 45 g.
otc	**UTI Feminine Hygiene Pack** (Consumers Choice Systems)	**Kit**: *Indication*: For temporary relief of minor irritations and burning. *Dosage*: Apply to the affected area ≤ 3 to 4 times daily.	
		Wipes: Polysorbate 20, EDTA, methylparaben.	In 20s.
		Cream: Oat beta glucan, aloe. Cetyl alcohol, cetearyl alcohol, EDTA, parabens.	In 15 g.
otc	**Yeast•Gard** (Lake)	**Suppositories**: Pulsatilla 28×, *Candida albicans* 28× *Indication*: Relieves vaginal irritation, itching and burning. *Dosage*: One suppository daily for 7 days.	In 15s with applicator.
otc	**WHF Lubricating Gel** (Lake)	**Gel**: Chlorhexidine gluconate, methylparaben, glycerin *Indication*: Relieves vaginal dryness. *Dosage*: Apply as needed.	In 113.4 g tube and 3 g individual packets.
otc	**Massengill Feminine Cleansing Wash** (SmithKline Beecham)	**Liquid**: Sodium laureth sulfate, sodium oleth sulfate, magnesium oleth sulfate, PEG-120 methyl glucose dioleate, parabens *Indication*: Vaginal cleansing. *Dosage*: Apply externally.	In 240 ml.
otc	**Vagisil** (Combe)	**Powder**: Cornstarch, aloe, mineral oil, magnesium stearate, silica, benzethonium chloride, fragrance *Indication*: Absorbs moisture. *Dosage*: Apply externally.	In 198 and 312 g.
otc	**Maxilube** (Mission)	**Jelly**: Water, silicone oil, glycerin, carbomer 934, triethanolamine, sodium lauryl sulfate, parabens *Indication*: Vaginal lubricant.	In 90 and 150 g.

[a] Cooper Surgical, 95 Corporate Drive, Trumbull, CT, 06611; 1-(800) 243-2974; fax 1-(800) 262-0105.

DOUCHE PRODUCTS

otc	**Massengill Douche** (SK-Beecham)	**Powder:** Ammonium alum, phenol, methyl salicylate, eucalyptus oil, menthol, thymol, PEG-8	In 120, 240, 480 and 660 g jar and UD Packettes (10s and 12s).
otc	**Trichotine Douche** (Reed & Carnrick)	**Powder:** Sodium lauryl sulfate, sodium perborate, monohydrate silica	In 150 and 360 g.
Rx	**Vagisec Douche** (Schmid)	**Solution:** Polyoxyethylene nonyl phenol, EDTA	In 120 ml.
otc	**Trichotine Douche** (Reed & Carnrick)	**Solution:** Sodium lauryl sulfate, sodium borate, 8% SD alcohol 23-A, EDTA	In 120 and 240 ml.
otc	**Massengill Baking Soda Freshness** (SK-Beecham)	**Solution:** Sodium bicarbonate	In 180 ml.
otc	**Yeast-Gard Medicated Douche** (Lake)	**Concentrate:** 10% povidone-iodine	In 240 ml.
otc	**Massengill Medicated Douche w/Cepticin** (SK-Beecham)	**Liquid concentrate:** 12% povidone-iodine	In 120 and 240 ml.
otc	**Yeast-Gard Medicated Disposable Douche Premix** (Lake Pharm)	**Solution:** Octoxynol-9, lactic acid, sodium lactate, sodium benzoate, aloe vera	In 180 ml twin-pack.
otc	**Massengill Medicated Disposable Douche w/Cepticin** (SK-Beecham)	**Solution:** 10% povidone-iodine (0.30% when diluted)	In 5 ml vial w/180 ml bottle of sanitized water.
otc	**Summer's Eve Medicated Disposable Douche** (Fleet)	**Solution:** 0.30% povidone-iodine when reconstituted	In 135 ml (1s and 2s).
otc	**Yeast-Gard Medicated Disposable Douche** (Lake)		In 180 ml twin-pack w/two 5.4 ml medicated douche concentrate packets.
otc	**Summer's Eve Disposable Douche** (Fleet)	**Solution, regular:** Citric acid, sodium benzoate	In 135 ml (1s, 2s and 4s).
		Solution, scented: Citric acid, octoxynol 9, sodium benzoate, EDTA	In herbal, musk and white flowers scents. In 135 ml (1s, 2s and 4s).
otc	**Summer's Eve Post–Menstrual Disposable Douche** (Fleet)	**Solution:** Sodium lauryl sulfate, parabens, monosodium and disodium phosphates, EDTA	In 135 ml (2s).
otc	**Feminique Disposable Douche** (Schmid)	**Solution:** Vinegar	In 180 ml (2s).
otc	**Massengill Disposable Douche** (SK-Beecham)		In 180 ml.
otc	**Massengill Vinegar & Water Extra Mild** (SK-Beecham)		Preservative free. In 180 ml.
otc	**Summer's Eve Disposable Douche** (Fleet)		In 135 ml (1s and 2s).
otc	**Summer's Eve Disposable Douche Extra Cleansing** (Fleet)	**Solution:** Vinegar, sodium chloride, benzoic acid	In 135 ml (1s, 2s and 4s).
otc	**Massengill Vinegar & Water Extra Cleansing with Puraclean** (SK-Beecham)	**Solution:** Vinegar, cetylpyridinium chloride, diazolidinyl urea, EDTA	In 180 ml.

DOUCHE PRODUCTS — VAGINAL

Indications

Vaginal douches are for general cleansing of the vaginal and perineal areas; for deodorizing; for relief of itching, burning and edema; for removing vaginal secretions or discharge or for altering vaginal acidity.

➤*Povidone-iodine, cetylpyridinium chloride, eucalyptol, menthol, oxyquinoline sulfate, phenol, sodium perborate, and thymol:* Povidone-iodine, cetylpyridinium chloride, eucalyptol, menthol, oxyquinoline sulfate, phenol, sodium perborate, and thymol may have antiseptic or germicidal activity.

Povidine-iodine also relieves minor irritation. It may be absorbed from the vagina; advise patients with thyroid disorders and pregnant patients to avoid iodine-containing douches.

➤*Eucalyptol, menthol, phenol, methyl salicylate, and thymol:* Eucalyptol, menthol, phenol, methyl salicylate, and thymol are counterirritants used for their anesthetic or antipruritic effects.

➤*Ammonium alum:* Ammonium alum is an astringent that reduces local edema and inflammation; high concentrations can be irritating.

➤*Docusate sodium, octoxynol 9, alkyl aryl sulfonate, sodium lauryl sulfate, and benzalkonium chloride:* Docusate sodium, octoxynol 9, alkyl aryl sulfonate, sodium lauryl sulfate, and benzalkonium chloride are surfactants that facilitate douche spread over vaginal mucosa.

➤*Sodium perborate, sodium bicarbonate, lactic acid, sodium acetate, and citric acid:* Sodium perborate, sodium bicarbonate, lactic acid, sodium acetate, and citric acid affect pH.

Patient Information

Consult manufacturers' recommendations for proper dilution and use of these products.

Vaginal douches are not contraceptive agents.

Douche no sooner than 6 hours after use of a vaginal spermicide.

If irritation occurs, discontinue use.

If infection or disease is suspected, consult physician.

Actions

➤*Pharmacology:* Topical contraceptive agents provide spermicidal action, which is generally reliable when properly used, either in conjunction with a vaginal diaphragm or as the sole method of contraception. These agents are generally less effective than oral contraceptives. To minimize the potential for conception, follow directions for use carefully.

Condom use and STD – The CDC advises the use of condoms to prevent sexually transmitted diseases (STD). If used properly, condoms help prevent infection by *Chlamydia trachomatis, Ureaplasma urealyticum, Trichomonas vaginalis, Candida albicans*, herpes simplex 1 and 2 (when lesions are on penis or female genital area), human papilloma virus, *Treponema pallidum, Haemophilus ducreyi* and AIDS.

Nonoxynol 9 – Nonoxynol 9 helps to inhibit a variety of sexually transmissible organisms, including those responsible for gonorrhea, chlamydial infection, candidiasis, genital herpes, syphilis, trichomoniasis and AIDS.

The following table gives ranges of pregnancy rates reported for various means of contraception. Efficacy in most cases depends greatly upon degree of compliance and user reliability. No other contraceptive drug or device except levonorgestrel implant and medroxyprogesterone injection approaches the efficacy of the combined oral contraceptives.

Pregnancy Rates for Various Means of Contraception (%)[1]

Method of contraception	Lowest expected[2]	Typical[3]
Oral Contraceptives		3
Combined	0.1	nd[4]
Progestin only	0.5	nd
Mechanical/Chemical		
Levonorgestrel implant	0.2	0.2
Medroxyprogesterone injection	0.3	0.3
IUD		
Progesterone	2	nd
Copper T 380A	0.8	nd
Condom		
Without spermicide	2	12
With spermicide[5]	1.8	4-6
Spermicide alone	3	21
Diaphragm (with spermicidal cream or gel)	6	18
Female condom	2-4	12-25
Periodic abstinence (ie, rhythm; all methods)	1-9	20
Sterility		
Vasectomy	0.1	0.15
Tubal ligation	0.2	0.4
No contraception	85	85

[1] During first year of continuous use.
[2] Best guess of percentage expected to experience an accidental pregnancy among couples who initiate a method and use it consistently and correctly.
[3] A "typical" couple who initiates a method and experiences an accidental pregnancy.
[4] nd = no data.
[5] Used as a separate product (not in condom package).

Warnings

➤*Sensitivity:* Should sensitivity to the ingredients or irritation of the vagina or penis develop, discontinue use and consult your physician.

➤*Pregnancy:* Controversy surrounds the relationship between the use of vaginal spermicides during pregnancy and congenital malformations. One 1981 study has suggested an association between vaginal spermicides and congenital anomalies (eg, limb-reduction deformities, neoplasms, chromosomal abnormalities). However, many other studies do not support these findings and several of the authors of the 1981 study agree that a causal association is unlikely. The FDA concurs with the Advisory Committee on Fertility and Maternal Health Drugs that there is currently no need for a labeling revision of spermicidal products.

Patient Information

Consult manufacturers' recommendations for proper use of these products. The following general principles should be noted:

Apply at least 10 minutes, but not more than 1 hour before intercourse to ensure effectiveness.

Apply high in the vagina, near the cervix.

Reapply prior to each time intercourse takes place.

Allow suppositories adequate time to disperse.

Do not douche for 6 to 8 hours after intercourse. Premature douching may dilute the spermicide, remove few sperm and may propel sperm into the uterus.

MISCELLANEOUS SPERMICIDES

otc	**Delfen Contraceptive** (Advanced Care)	**Vaginal Foam:** 12.5% nonoxynol 9	In 20 g w/applicator and 42 g refills.
otc	**Conceptrol Disposable Contraceptive** (Advanced Care)	**Vaginal Gel:** 4% nonoxynol 9	In 2.7 g prefilled applications (6s and 10s).
otc	**Semicid** (Whitehall)	**Suppositories:** 100 mg nonoxynol 9	Methylparaben. In 9s and 18s.
otc	**VCF** (Apothecus)	**Vaginal Film:** 28% nonoxynol 9	Glycerin, alcohol. In 3s, 6s and 12s.

For complete prescribing information, see the Spermicides group monograph.

SPERMICIDES USED WITH A VAGINAL DIAPHRAGM

otc	**Gynol II Contraceptive** (Advanced Care)	**Gel:** 2% nonoxynol 9	In 75 g w/applicator and 75 and 114 g refills.
otc	**Shur-Seal** (Milex)	**Gel:** 2% nonoxynol 9	In 24 UD gel paks.
otc	**K-Y Plus** (Johnson & Johnson)	**Gel:** 2.2% nonoxynol 9	Methylparaben. In 113 g.
otc	**Advantage 24** (Women's Health Institute)	**Gel:** 3.5% nonoxynol 9	Mineral oil, glycerin, parabens, palm oil, sorbic acid. In 3s and 6s (1.5 g each) with applicators.
otc	**Gynol II Extra Strength Contraceptive** (Advanced Care)	**Jelly:** 3% nonoxynol 9	In 75 g and 114 g.

SPERMICIDES USED WITH A VAGINAL DIAPHRAGM

For complete prescribing information, see the Spermicides group monograph.

Administration and Dosage

The following products are for use in conjunction with a vaginal diaphragm.

SPERMICIDE-CONTAINING CONDOMS

otc	**Excita Extra** (Schmid)	**Condom:** 8% nonoxynol 9	Ribbed. In 3s, 12s and 36s.
otc	**Sheik Elite** (Schmid)		In 3s, 12s. 24s and 36s

SPERMICIDE-CONTAINING CONDOMS

For complete prescribing information, see the Spermicides group monograph.

Actions

➤*Pharmacology:* A latex condom with a lubricant containing the spermicide nonoxynol 9. The combination of barrier protection combined with the spermicide improves contraceptive effectiveness over traditional condoms.

Indications

➤*Edema:* Adjunctive therapy in edema associated with congestive heart failure (CHF), hepatic cirrhosis, and corticosteroid and estrogen therapy. Useful in edema caused by renal dysfunction (eg, nephrotic syndrome, acute glomerulonephritis, chronic renal failure).

Indapamide – Indapamide alone is indicated for edema associated with CHF.

Metolazone, rapidly acting (Mykrox) – Metolazone, rapidly acting (*Mykrox*) has not been evaluated for the treatment of CHF or fluid retention caused by renal or hepatic disease, and the correct dosage for these conditions and other edematous states has not been established. Because a safe and effective diuretic dose has not been established, do not use *Mykrox* when diuresis is desired.

➤*Hypertension:* As the sole therapeutic agent or to enhance other antihypertensive drugs in more severe forms of hypertension.

➤*Unlabeled uses:*

Calcium nephrolithiasis – Thiazide diuretics have been used alone and in combination with amiloride or allopurinol to prevent formation and recurrence of calcium nephrolithiasis in hypercalciuric and normal calciuric patients. Thiazides correct hypercalciuria, reduce urinary saturation, enhance inhibitor activity against spontaneous nucleation of calcium oxalate and brushite, and restore normal parathyroid function and intestinal calcium absorption. Doses of hydrochlorothiazide 50 or 100 mg daily, trichloromethiazide 4 mg/day, chlorthalidone 50 mg/day, and indapamide 2.5 mg/day have been used.

Osteoporosis – Thiazide diuretics may be useful in reducing the incidence of osteoporosis in postmenopausal women, alone or in combination with calcium or estrogen. Further studies are necessary to confirm this use. Although data conflict, use of thiazides in older patients may be associated with a reduced risk of hip fracture.

Diabetes insipidus – Thiazide diuretics reduce urine volume by 30% to 50%. They constitute the mainstay of therapy for nephrogenic diabetes insipidus.

Administration and Dosage

➤*Edema:* Intermittent therapy may be advantageous. With administration every other day, or on a 3- to 5-day per week schedule, electrolyte imbalance is less likely.

➤*Hypertension:* Reduce dosage of other agents as soon as thiazides are added to the regimen to prevent excessive hypotension. As blood pressure falls, a further reduction in dosage may be necessary.

➤*Renal function impairment:* If the patient has a creatinine clearance (Ccr) less than 40 to 50 mL/min, a glomerular filtration rate (GFR) less than 25 mL/min or is not responsive to thiazides, a loop diuretic may be more effective. **Metolazone** is the only thiazide-like diuretic that may produce diuresis in patients with GFR less than 20 mL/min. Indapamide may also be effective in patients with renal function impairment.

➤*Coadministration:* Concurrent metolazone and furosemide (and probably other loop diuretics) have been used in the management of patients refractory to furosemide or other diuretics administered alone because of their synergistic effect on diuresis (see Drug Interactions). Metolazone 2.5 to 10 mg is added to the therapy, and the dose is doubled every 24 hours until the desired response is achieved. Decrease the furosemide dose if synergism occurs with the first dose of metolazone. Hydrochlorothiazide 50 mg may be used and may be safer because of its shorter action. This effect also has been noted with other thiazides in combination with other loop diuretics.

Actions

➤*Pharmacology:* Thiazide diuretics increase the urinary excretion of sodium and chloride in approximately equivalent amounts. They inhibit reabsorption of sodium and chloride in the cortical thick ascending limb of the loop of Henle and the early distal tubules. Many of these compounds possess some degree of carbonic anhydrase inhibition activity (metolazone has no activity) because of the sulfonamide moiety; however, this is unlikely to be encountered clinically. Other common actions include increased potassium and bicarbonate excretion, decreased calcium excretion, and uric acid retention. At maximal therapeutic dosages all thiazides are approximately equal in diuretic efficacy, but metolazone may be more effective in patients with impaired renal function. Metolazone (a quinazoline derivative), chlorthalidone (a phthalimidine derivative), and indapamide (an indoline) are included here because of their structural and pharmacological similarities to the thiazides.

The exact antihypertensive mechanism of the thiazides is unknown, although sodium depletion appears to be of primary importance. During initial therapy, cardiac output decreases and extracellular volume diminishes. With chronic therapy, cardiac output normalizes, peripheral vascular resistance falls, and there is a persistent small reduction in extracellular volume.

In hypertensive patients, daily doses of indapamide have no appreciable cardiac inotropic or chronotropic effect, and little or no effect on GFR or renal plasma flow. The drug decreases peripheral resistance, with little or no effect on cardiac output, rate or rhythm. Indapamide had an antihypertensive effect in patients with varying degrees of renal impairment, although in general, diuretic effects declined as renal function decreased.

➤*Pharmacokinetics:* The antihypertensive action requires several days to produce effects. Administration for up to 2 to 4 weeks is usually required for optimal therapeutic effect. The duration of the antihypertensive effect of the thiazides is sufficiently long to adequately control blood pressure with a single daily dose. Despite extensive use of diuretics, pharmacokinetic data are limited. It is important to emphasize the lack of relationship between plasma levels and diuretic effect.

Pharmacokinetics of Thiazides and Related Diuretics

Diuretic	Onset (h)	Peak (h)	Duration (h)	Equivalent dose (mg)	Percent absorbed	Half-life (h)
Bendroflumethiazide	2	4	16 to 12	5	≈ 100	3 to 3.9
Chlorothiazide	2[a]	4[a]	16 to 12	500	10 to 21[b]	0.75 to 2
Chlorthalidone	2 to 3	2 to 6	24 to 72	50	64[b]	40
Hydrochlorothiazide	2	4 to 6	16 to 12	50	65 to 75	5.6 to 14.8
Indapamide	1 to 2	within 2	up to 36	2.5	93	≈ 14
Methyclothiazide	2	6	24	5	nd[c]	nd[c]
Metolazone[d]	1	2	12 to 24	5	65	nd[c]
Trichlormethiazide	2	6	24	2	nd[c]	2.3 to 7.3

[a] Following IV use, onset of action is 15 minutes; peak occurs in 30 minutes.
[b] Bioavailability may be dose-dependent.
[c] nd = No data.
[d] *Mykrox*: Peak plasma concentrations reached in 2 to 4 h, t½ approximately 14 h.

Contraindications

Anuria; renal decompensation; hypersensitivity to thiazides or related diuretics or sulfonamide-derived drugs; hepatic coma or precoma (**metolazone**).

Warnings

➤*Parenteral use:* Use IV **chlorothiazide** only when patients are unable to take oral medication or in an emergency. In infants and children, IV use is not recommended.

Avoid simultaneous administration of chlorothiazide with whole blood or its derivatives.

➤*Lupus erythematosus:* Lupus erythematosus exacerbation or activation has occurred.

➤*Hypersensitivity reactions:* Hypersensitivity reactions may occur in patients with or without a history of allergy or bronchial asthma; cross-sensitivity with sulfonamides may also occur. Have epinephrine 1:1,000 immediately available. Refer to Management of Acute Hypersensitivity Reactions.

➤*Renal function impairment:* Use with caution in severe renal disease because these agents may precipitate azotemia. Cumulative effects of the drug may develop in patients with impaired renal function. Monitor renal function periodically. If progressive renal impairment becomes evident, indicated by a rising nonprotein nitrogen (NPN) or BUN, consider withholding or discontinuing therapy. If the patient has a Ccr less than 40 to 50 mL/min, a GFR less than 25 mL/min or is not responsive to thiazides, a loop diuretic may be more effective. **Metolazone** is the only thiazide-like diuretic that may produce diuresis in patients with GFR less than 20 mL/min. Indapamide may also be useful in patients with impaired renal function.

➤*Hepatic function impairment:* Use with caution because minor alterations of fluid and electrolyte balance may precipitate hepatic coma.

➤*Pregnancy: Category B* (**chlorothiazide, chlorthalidone, hydrochlorothiazide, indapamide, metolazone**); *Category C* (**bendroflumethiazide, methyclothiazide, trichlormethiazide**). Routine use during normal pregnancy is inappropriate. Diuretics decrease plasma volume and can decrease placental perfusion. Diuretics do not prevent development of toxemia, nor are they useful in the treatment of toxemia.

Thiazides are indicated in pregnancy when edema is due to pathologic causes, just as they are in the absence of pregnancy. Dependent edema in pregnancy, resulting from restriction of venous return by the gravid uterus, is not properly treated by the use of diuretics. In rare instances, hypervolemia during normal pregnancy results in edema that may cause extreme discomfort that is not relieved by rest; a short course of diuretics may provide relief.

Thiazides cross the placental barrier and appear in cord blood. Use only when clearly needed and when potential benefits outweigh the potential hazards to the fetus. These hazards include fetal or neonatal jaundice, thrombocytopenia, hemolytic anemia, electrolyte imbalances and hypoglycemia.

➤*Lactation:* Thiazides may appear in breast milk. **Chlorthalidone** has a low milk to plasma ratio of 0.05. Discontinue breast-feeding or the drug, taking into account the importance of the drug to the mother.

➤*Children:* **Bendroflumethiazide, chlorthalidone, hydrochlorothiazide, methyclothiazide, metolazone, trichlormethiazide** – Safety and efficacy have not been established. **Metolazone** is not recommended for use in children. In infants and children, IV use of **chlorothiazide** has been limited and is generally not recommended.

Precautions

➤*Monitoring:* Perform initial and periodic determinations of serum electrolytes, BUN, uric acid, and glucose. Observe patients for clinical signs of fluid or electrolyte imbalance (eg, hyponatremia, hypochloremic alkalosis, hypokalemia, hypomagnesemia, changes in serum and urinary calcium).

➤*Fluid/electrolyte balance:* Serum and urine electrolyte determinations are particularly important in patients vomiting excessively or receiving parenteral fluids, in patients subject to electrolyte imbalance (including those with heart failure, kidney disease and cirrhosis), and in patients on a salt restricted diet. Warning signs of imbalance include the following: dry mouth, thirst, weakness, lethargy, drowsiness, restlessness, muscle pains or cramps, confusion, seizures, muscular fatigue, hypotension, oliguria, tachycardia, and GI disturbances.

Hypokalemia – Hypokalemia may develop (with consequent weakness, cramps, cardiac dysrhythmias) during concomitant corticosteroids, ACTH and especially with brisk diuresis, with severe liver disease or cirrhosis, vomiting or diarrhea, or after prolonged therapy. Inadequate oral electrolyte intake also contributes to hypokalemia. Hypokalemia may cause cardiac arrhythmias and sensitize or exaggerate the heart's response to toxic effects of digitalis (eg, increased ventricular irritability). Avoid or treat hypokalemia by using potassium-sparing diuretics, potassium supplements, or foods with high potassium content. Hypokalemia is a particular hazard in digitalized patients, or patients who have or have had a ventricular arrhythmia; dangerous or fatal arrhythmias may be precipitated. Hypokalemia is dose-related.

Hyponatremia/Hypochloremia – A chloride deficit is generally mild and usually does not require specific treatment, except in extraordinary circumstances (as in liver or renal disease). However, treatment of metabolic or hypochloremic alkalosis may require chloride replacement. Dilutional hyponatremia may occur in edematous patients in hot weather; appropriate therapy is water restriction, rather than salt administration, except in rare life-threatening instances. Thiazide-induced hyponatremia has been associated with death and neurologic damage in elderly patients. CNS manifestations include seizures, coma, and extensor-plantar response. Infrequently, severe hyponatremia accompanied by hypokalemia has occurred with recommended **indapamide** doses, primarily in elderly women.

Rarely, the rapid onset of severe hyponatremia or hypokalemia has occurred following initial doses of thiazide and non-thiazide diuretics. When symptoms consistent with electrolyte imbalance appear rapidly, discontinue the drug and initiate supportive measures immediately. Parenteral electrolytes may be required.

Hypomagnesemia – Thiazide diuretics have been shown to increase urinary excretion of magnesium, resulting in hypomagnesemia.

Hypercalcemia – Calcium excretion may be decreased by thiazide diuretics. Thiazides may cause a slight intermittent elevation of serum calcium in the absence of calcium metabolism disorders. Serum calcium levels return to normal upon discontinuation. Pathologic changes in the parathyroid glands with hypercalcemia and hypophosphatemia may occur in a few patients on prolonged thiazide therapy. Marked hypercalcemia may be evidence of hidden hyperparathyroidism. Common complications of hyperparathyroidism, such as renal lithiasis, bone resorption, and peptic ulceration, are not seen. Discontinue thiazides before performing parathyroid function tests.

➤*Glucose tolerance:* Hyperglycemia may occur with thiazide diuretics. Insulin or oral hypoglycemic agent dosage requirements in diabetic patients may be altered. Latent diabetes mellitus may become manifest during thiazide diuretic administration; diabetic complications may occur. Monitor serum glucose concentrations (see Drug Interactions). Administration time (ie, morning vs evening) may influence glucose tolerance; in a small study, blood glucose levels were higher when trichlormethiazide was taken in the evening.

➤*Hyperuricemia:* Hyperuricemia may occur or acute gout may be precipitated in certain patients receiving thiazides, even in those patients without a history of gouty attacks. Hyperuricemia with infrequent gouty attacks may occur in patients with a history of gout. Monitor serum uric acid concentrations periodically during treatment. One report suggests that it is not necessary to lower uric acid levels with pharmacologic measures in patients receiving thiazide diuretics who are without renal damage or history of gout. Serum uric acid increased by an average of 1 mg/dL in patients on **indapamide**.

➤*Post-sympathectomy:* Antihypertensive effects may be enhanced in the postsympathectomy patient.

➤*Lipids:* Use thiazides with caution in patients with moderate or high cholesterol concentrations and in patients with elevated triglyceride levels. Thiazides may cause increased concentrations of total serum cholesterol, total triglycerides, and low-density lipoproteins (LDL) (but not high-density lipoproteins [HDL]) in some patients, although these appear to return to pretreatment levels with long-term therapy. **Indapamide** does not appear to increase serum cholesterol.

➤*Photosensitivity:* Photosensitization may occur; therefore, caution patients to take protective measures (eg, sunscreens, protective clothing) against exposure to ultraviolet light and/or sunlight until tolerance is determined.

➤*Tartrazine sensitivity:* Some of these products contain tartrazine (FD&C yellow #5), which may cause allergic-type reactions (including bronchial asthma) in susceptible individuals. Although the incidence of sensitivity is low, it is frequently seen in patients who also have aspirin hypersensitivity. Specific products containing tartrazine are identified in the product listings.

Drug Interactions

Thiazides and Related Diuretic Drug Interactions

Precipitant drug	Object drug[a]		Description
Thiazides	Allopurinol	↑	Concurrent use may increase the incidence of hypersensitivity reactions to allopurinol.
Thiazides	Anesthetics	↑	Effects of these drugs may be potentiated by thiazide administration; dosage adjustments may be required. Monitor and correct fluid and electrolyte imbalance prior to surgery if feasible.
Thiazides	Anticoagulants	↓	Anticoagulant effects may be diminished.
Thiazides	Antigout agents	↓	Because thiazide diuretics may raise blood uric acid levels, dosage adjustment of antigout agents may be necessary.
Thiazides	Antineoplastics	↑	Thiazides may prolong antineoplastic-induced leukopenia.
Thiazides	Calcium salts	↑	Hypercalcemia resulting from renal tubular reabsorption or bone release of calcium may be amplified by exogenous calcium.
Thiazides	Diazoxide	↑	Hyperglycemia, often with symptoms and similar to frank diabetes, may occur.
Thiazides	Digitalis glycosides	↑	Diuretic-induced hypokalemia and hypomagnesemia may precipitate digitalis-induced arrhythmias.
Thiazides	Lithium	↑	Thiazides may induce lithium toxicity by decreasing its renal excretion. However, they have been used together for therapeutic reasons and can be coadministered safely with close lithium level monitoring.
Thiazides	Loop diuretics	↑	Both groups have synergistic effects that may result in profound diuresis and serious electrolyte abnormalities. Certain combinations have been used therapeutically in patients refractory to furosemide (see Administration and Dosage).
Thiazides	Methyldopa	↑	There have been rare occurrences of hemolytic anemia with concomitant use.
Thiazides	Nondepolarizing muscle relaxants	↑	Neuromuscular-blocking effects may be increased; respiratory depression may be prolonged.
Thiazides	Sulfonylureas insulin	↓	Thiazides increase fasting blood glucose and may decrease sulfonylurea hypoglycemia. Hyponatremia also may occur. The dosage may need to be adjusted.
Thiazides	Vitamin D	↑	The biological actions of vitamin D may be enhanced. Hypercalcemia could manifest.
Amphotericin B, Corticosteroids	Thiazides	↑	Electrolyte depletion may be intensified, particularly hypokalemia. Monitor potassium levels.
Anticholinergics	Thiazides	↑	Anticholinergics may substantially increase thiazide diuretic absorption.
Bile acid sequestrants (cholestyramine, colestipol)	Thiazides	↓	Bile acid sequestrants bind thiazides and reduce their absorption from the GI tract up to 85%. Thiazides should be given ≥ 2 hours before the resin.
Methenamines	Thiazides	↓	Possible decreased effectiveness of thiazides because of the alkalinization of urine.

Thiazides and Related Diuretic Drug Interactions			
Precipitant drug	Object drug[a]		Description
NSAIDs	Thiazides	⬇	Some NSAIDs (particularly indomethacin) may reduce the diuretic, natriuretic, and antihypertensive effects of thiazide diuretics. Observe closely to determine if the desired diuretic effects are obtained. Sulindac may enhance the diuretic effect.

[a] ⬆ = Object drug increased. ⬇ = Object drug decreased

➤*Drug/Lab test interactions:* Thiazides may decrease serum protein-bound iodine (PBI) levels without signs of thyroid disturbance. Thiazides also may cause diagnostic interference of serum electrolyte levels, blood and urine glucose levels (usually only in patients with a predisposition to glucose intolerance), serum bilirubin levels (by displacement from albumin binding), and serum uric acid levels. In uremic patients, serum magnesium levels may be increased. **Bendroflumethiazide** and **trichlormethiazide** may interfere with the **phenolsulfonphthalein test** because of decreased excretion. In the **phentolamine** and **tyramine tests**, bendroflumethiazide may produce false-negative and trichlormethiazide may produce false-positive results.

Adverse Reactions

Adverse Reactions of Thiazides and Related Diuretics								
Adverse reaction	Bendroflumethiazide	Chlorothiazide	Chlorthalidone	Hydrochlorothiazide	Indapamide	Methyclothiazide	Metolazone	Trichlormethiazide
Cardiovascular								
Hypotension		✓						
Orthostatic hypotension	✓	✓		✓	< 5%	✓	< 2%[a]	✓
Palpitations					< 5%		< 2%[b]	✓
CNS								
Anxiety					≥ 5%		< 2%[c]	
Blurred vision (may be transient)	✓	✓		✓	< 5%	✓	✓[c]	
Depression					< 5%		< 2%[b]	✓
Dizziness/Lightheadedness	✓	✓	✓	✓	≥ 5%	✓	10%[b]	✓
Drowsiness					< 5%		✓[c]	✓
Fatigue/Lethargy/Malaise/Lassitude					≥ 5%		4%[b]	✓
Headache	✓	✓	✓	✓	≥ 5%	✓	9%[b]	✓
Nervousness					≥ 5%		< 2%[c]	
Paresthesias	✓	✓	✓	✓		✓	✓[c]	✓
Restlessness/Insomnia	✓	✓	✓	✓	< 5%	✓	✓[c]	✓
Vertigo	✓	✓	✓	✓	< 5%	✓	✓[c]	✓
Weakness	✓	✓	✓	✓	≥ 5%	✓	< 2%[b]	✓
Xanthopsia	✓	✓	✓	✓		✓		✓
Dermatologic								
Alopecia		✓[e]		✓				
Anaphylactic reactions	✓	✓		✓[d]		✓		
Erythema multiforme, Stevens-Johnson syndrome		✓[e]		✓		✓		
Exfoliative dermatitis/ toxic epidermal necrolysis	✓	✓[e]	✓	✓				
Fever	✓	✓		✓		✓		
Necrotizing angiitis, vasculitis, cutaneous vasculitis	✓	✓	✓	✓	< 5%	✓	✓[b]	✓
Photosensitivity/Photosensitivity dermatitis	✓	✓	✓	✓		✓	✓[c]	✓
Pruritus	✓				< 5%		< 2%[a]	
Purpura	✓	✓	✓	✓		✓	✓[c]	✓
Rash	✓	✓	✓	✓	< 5%	✓	< 2%[b]	✓
Urticaria	✓	✓	✓	✓		✓	✓[c]	✓
GI								
Abdominal pain/cramping/bloating	✓	✓	✓	✓	< 5%	✓	< 2%[b]	✓
Anorexia	✓	✓	✓	✓	< 5%	✓	✓[c]	✓
Constipation	✓	✓	✓	✓	< 5%	✓	< 2%[b]	✓
Diarrhea	✓	✓	✓	✓	< 5%	✓	< 2%[b]	✓
Dry mouth					< 5%		< 2%[a]	✓
Gastric irritation/epigastric distress	✓	✓	✓	✓	< 5%	✓		✓
Hepatitis	✓						✓[c]	
Jaundice (intrahepatic/cholestatic)	✓	✓	✓	✓		✓	✓[c]	✓
Nausea	✓	✓	✓	✓	< 5%	✓	< 2%[b]	✓
Pancreatitis	✓	✓	✓	✓		✓	✓[c]	✓
Sialadenitis	✓	✓		✓		✓		
Vomiting	✓	✓	✓	✓	< 5%	✓	< 2%[b]	✓
GU								
Impotence/Reduced libido	✓	✓	✓	✓	< 5%	✓	< 2%[b]	✓
Interstitial nephritis		✓		✓				
Nocturia					< 5%		< 2%[a]	
Renal failure/dysfunction		✓		✓				
Hematologic								
Agranulocytosis	✓	✓	✓	✓		✓	✓[c]	✓
Aplastic/Hypoplastic anemia	✓	✓	✓	✓		✓	✓[c]	✓
Hemolytic anemia	✓	✓		✓		✓		
Leukopenia	✓	✓	✓	✓		✓	✓[c]	✓
Thrombocytopenia	✓	✓	✓	✓		✓		✓
Metabolic								
Electrolyte imbalance		✓		✓		✓		
Glycosuria	✓	✓	✓	✓	< 5%	✓	✓[c]	✓
Hyperglycemia	✓	✓	✓	✓	< 5%	✓	✓[c]	
Hyperuricemia	✓	✓	✓	✓	< 5%	✓		✓
Miscellaneous								
Muscle cramp/spasm	✓	✓	✓	✓	≥ 5%	✓	6%[b]	
Respiratory distress (including pneumonitis/pulmonary edema)	✓	✓						

[a] Rapidly acting doseform only.
[b] Percentage of occurrence refers to rapidly acting doseform; however, this adverse reaction also occurred with the slow-acting doseform.
[c] Slow-acting doseform only.
[d] Possibly with life-threatening anaphylactic shock.
[e] IV doseform.

Whenever adverse reactions are moderate or severe, reducing the thiazide dosage or withdrawing therapy will generally reverse the effect.

➤*Cardiovascular:*

Hydrochlorothiazide – Allergic myocarditis.

Indapamide – Premature ventricular contractions, irregular heartbeat (less than 5%).

Metolazone –
Rapidly acting: Chest pain, precordial pain (3%); cold extremities, edema (less than 2%).
Slow-acting: Venous thrombosis, chest pain, excessive volume depletion, hemoconcentration.

➤*CNS:*

Indapamide – Loss of energy, numbness of extremities, tension, irritability, agitation (greater than 5%); tingling of extremities (less than 5%).

Metolazone –
Slow-acting: Syncope, neuropathy.
Rapidly acting: Weird feeling, neuropathy (less than 2%).

➤*GI:* Cholecystitis (possible increased risk in patients with gallstones).

Metolazone –
Rapidly acting: Bitter taste (less than 2%).

➤*GU:*

Bendroflumethiazide – Allergic glomerulonephritis.

Chlorothiazide IV – Hematuria.

Indapamide – Frequent urination, polyuria (less than 5%).

➤*Dermatologic:*

Bendroflumethiazide – Ecchymosis.

Indapamide – Hives (less than 5%).

Metolazone –
Rapidly acting: Dry skin (less than 2%).

Trichlormethiazide – Lichenoid dermatitis.

➤*Musculoskeletal:*

Metolazone – Joint pain; back pain (rapidly acting; less than 2%); swelling (slow-acting).

➤*Respiratory:*

Indapamide – Rhinorrhea (less than 5%).

Metolazone –
Rapidly acting: Cough, epistaxis, sinus congestion, sore throat (less than 2%).

Trichlormethiazide – Dyspnea.

➤*Miscellaneous:* Neutropenia.

Bendroflumethiazide – Metabolic acidosis in diabetics.

Indapamide – Flushing, weight loss (less than 5%).

Methyclothiazide – Inappropriate antidiuretic hormone (ADH) secretion.

Metolazone –
Slow-acting: Chills, acute gouty attack.
Rapidly acting: Eye itching, tinnitus (less than 2%).

➤*Lab test abnormalities:* Hypercalcemia, hypokalemia, hyponatremia; hypomagnesemia, hypochloremia, hypochloremic alkalosis, hypophosphatemia, increase in BUN, elevation of creatinine, decreased serum PBI levels.

Clinical hypokalemia – Clinical hypokalemia occurred in 3% and 7% of patients given **indapamide** 2.5 and 5 mg, respectively.

Increases in plasma levels of total cholesterol, triglycerides, and LDL cholesterol have been associated with thiazide diuretics (see Precautions).

Fluid/electrolyte imbalance – There are isolated reports of nonedematous individuals developing severe fluid and electrolyte derangements after only brief exposure to normal doses of thiazides. This condition usually is manifested as severe dilutional hyponatremia, hypokalemia and hypochloremia. It may be because of inappropriately increased ADH secretion and appears to be idiosyncratic. Potassium replacement is apparently the most important therapy along with removal of the offending drug.

Overdosage

➤*Symptoms:* Changes caused by plasma volume depletion (eg, orthostatic hypotension, dizziness, drowsiness, syncope, electrolyte abnormalities, hemoconcentration, hemodynamic changes); signs of potassium deficiency (eg, confusion, dizziness, muscular weakness, GI disturbances); nausea; vomiting. In severe instances, hypotension and depressed respiration may occur. Lethargy of varying degrees may progress to coma within a few hours, with minimal depression of respiration and cardiovascular function and without significant serum electrolyte changes or dehydration. GI irritation and hypermotility, temporary BUN elevation, CNS effects, cardiac abnormalities, and seizures also have been reported, especially in patients with compromised renal function.

➤*Treatment:* Perform gastric lavage or induce emesis; give activated charcoal. Prevent aspiration. Avoid cathartics because electrolyte and fluid loss may be enhanced. GI effects are usually of short duration, but may require symptomatic treatment. Monitor serum electrolyte levels and renal function. Maintain hydration, electrolyte balance, respiration and cardiovascular-renal function. Asymptomatic hyperuricemia usually responds to fluids, but if clinical gout is suspected, indomethacin may be started. Support respiration and cardiac circulation if hypotension and depressed respiration occur. Refer to General Management of Acute Overdosage. Dialysis is unlikely to be effective.

Patient Information

May cause GI upset; may be taken with food or milk.

Drug will initially increase urination, which should subside after a few weeks; advise patients to take early during the day or as directed.

Advise patients to notify health care provider if muscle pain, weakness or cramps, nausea, vomiting, restlessness, excessive thirst, tiredness, drowsiness, increased heart rate or pulse, diarrhea, or dizziness occurs.

May cause photosensitivity (sensitivity to sunlight). Advise patients to avoid prolonged exposure to the sun and other ultraviolet light. Instruct them to use sunscreens and wear protective clothing until tolerance is determined.

May increase blood sugar levels in patients with diabetes.

Patients should not drink alcohol or take other medications without health care provider's approval; this includes nonprescription medicines for appetite control, asthma, colds, cough, hay fever, or sinus.

Advise patients to not interrupt, discontinue, or adjust the dose even if feeling well and to follow health care provider's instructions regarding missed doses.

May cause gout attacks. Instruct patients to contact health care provider if significant sudden joint pain occurs.

CHLOROTHIAZIDE

Rx	**Chlorothiazide** (Various, eg, Major, Mylan)	**Tablets:** 250 mg	In 100s and 250s.
Rx	**Diuril** (Merck)		Lactose. (MSD 214). White, scored. In 100s and 1000s.
Rx	**Chlorothiazide** (Various, eg, Goldline, Mylan)	**Tablets:** 500 mg	In 100s, 500s, 1000s and UD 100s.
Rx	**Diurigen** (Goldline)		In 100s and 1000s.
Rx	**Diuril** (Merck)		Lactose. (MSD 432). White, scored. In 100s, 1000s, 5000s and UD 100s.
Rx	**Diuril** (Merck)	**Oral Suspension:** 250 mg per 5 mL	0.5% alcohol, saccharin, 0.12% methylparaben, 0.02% propylparaben, 0.1% benzoic acid, sucrose. In 237 mL.
Rx	**Diuril** (Merck)	**Powder for Injection, lyophilized:** 500 mg (as sodium)	0.25 g mannitol. In 20 mL vials.

CHLOROTHIAZIDE — ORAL

For complete and comparative prescribing information, refer to the Thiazides and Related Diuretics group monograph.

Indications

➤*Edema:* As adjunctive therapy in edema associated with congestive heart failure, hepatic cirrhosis, and corticosteroid and estrogen therapy.

Chlorothiazide has also been found useful in edema due to various forms of renal dysfunction such as nephrotic syndrome, acute glomerulonephritis, and chronic renal failure.

➤*Hypertension:* Management of hypertension either as the sole therapeutic agent or to enhance the effectiveness of other antihypertensive drugs in the more severe forms of hypertension.

➤*Unlabeled uses:* Calcium nephrolithiasis; osteoporosis; diabetes insipidus.

Administration and Dosage

➤*Approved by the FDA:* October 1957.

➤*Edema:* The usual adult dosage is 0.5 to 1 g once or twice a day. Many patients with edema respond to intermittent therapy (ie, administration on alternate days or on 3 to 5 days each week). With an intermittent schedule, excessive response and the resulting undesirable electrolyte imbalance are less likely to occur.

➤*Control of hypertension:* The usual adult starting dosage is 0.5 or 1 g a day as a single or divided dose. Dosage is increased or decreased according to blood pressure response. Rarely, some patients may require up to 2 g a day in divided doses.

CHLOROTHIAZIDE — ORAL

➤*Infants and children:*

Diuresis and control of hypertension – The usual pediatric dosage is 10 to 20 mg/kg (5 to 10 mg/lb) per day in single or 2 divided doses, not to exceed 375 mg/day (2.5 to 7.5 mL or ½ to 1½ teaspoonfuls of the oral suspension daily) in infants up to 2 years of age or 1 g/day in children 2 to 12 years of age. In infants less than 6 months of age, doses up to 30 mg/kg (15 mg/lb) per day in 2 divided doses may be required.

➤*Storage/Stability:*

Tablets – Keep container tightly closed. Protect from moisture, freezing (−20°C; −4°F), and store at room temperature (15° to 30°C; 59° to 86°F). Protect from light. Dispense in a tight, light-resistant container using a child-resistant closure.

Oral suspension – Keep container tightly closed. Protect from freezing (−20°C; −4°F). Store at room temperature (15° to 30°C; 59° to 86°F).

CHLOROTHIAZIDE — INJECTION

For complete and comparative prescribing information, refer to the Thiazides and Related Diuretics group monograph.

Administration and Dosage

➤*Adults:*

Edema – 0.5 to 1 g once or twice a day, orally or IV. Reserve IV route for patients unable to take oral medication or for emergency situations.

Many patients with edema respond to intermittent therapy (administration on alternate days or on 3 to 5 days each week). With an intermittent schedule, excessive response and undesirable electrolyte imbalance are less likely to occur.

Hypertension (oral forms only) – Starting dose is 0.5 to 1 g/day as a single or divided dose. Adjust dosage according to the blood pressure response. Rarely, some patients may require up to 2 g/day in divided doses.

➤*Infants and children:* IV use is not generally recommended.

➤*Preparation of parenteral solution:* Add 18 ml of sterile water for injection to the vial to prepare an isotonic solution. Never add less than 18 ml. Discard unused solution after 24 hours. The solution is compatible with dextrose or sodium chloride solutions for IV infusion. Avoid simultaneous administration with whole blood or its derivatives. Extravasation must be rigidly avoided. Do not give SC or IM.

HYDROCHLOROTHIAZIDE

Rx	**Hydrochlorothiazide** (Various, eg, Major, Schein, Zenith)	**Tablets:** 25 mg	In 30s, 100s, 500s, 1000s, 5000s, UD 32s and UD 100s.
Rx	**HydroDIURIL** (Merck)		Lactose. (MSD 42). Peach, scored. In 100s and 1000s.
Rx	**Hydro-Par** (Parmed)		Peach, scored. In 1000s.
Rx	**Hydrochlorothiazide** (Various, eg, Danbury, Schein, Zenith)	**Tablets:** 50 mg	In 30s, 100s, 500s, 1000s, 5000s and UD 100s.
Rx	**Ezide** (Econo Med)		In 100s and 1000s.
Rx	**Hydro-Par** (Parmed)		In 1000s and 5000s.
Rx	**Hydrochlorothiazide** (Various, eg, Schein)	**Tablets:** 100 mg	In 30s, 100s, 250s, 500s, 1000s and UD 100s.
Rx	**Hydrochlorothiazide** (Various, eg, Mylan, Watson)	**Capsules:** 12.5 mg	In 100s and 500s.
Rx	**Microzide Capsules** (Watson)		Lactose. (Microzide 12.5). Light teal/teal. In 100s.

HYDROCHLOROTHIAZIDE — ORAL

For complete and comparative prescribing information, refer to the Thiazides and Related Diuretics group monograph.

Indications

➤*Hypertension:* Management of hypertension either as the sole therapeutic agent, or in combination with other antihypertensives. Unlike potassium-sparing combination diuretic products, hydrochlorothiazide may be used in those patients in whom the development of hyperkalemia cannot be risked, including patients taking ACE inhibitors.

Hydrochlorothiazide is indicated in the management of hypertension either as the sole therapeutic agent or to enhance the effectiveness of other antihypertensive drugs in the more severe forms of hypertension.

➤*Edema:* Adjunctive therapy in edema associated with congestive heart failure, hepatic cirrhosis, and corticosteroid and estrogen therapy.

Hydrochlorothiazide has also been found useful in edema due to various forms of renal dysfunction such as nephrotic syndrome, acute glomerulonephritis, and chronic renal failure.

Administration and Dosage

➤*Capsules:*

Hypertension – The adult initial dose of hydrochlorothiazide is one capsule given once daily whether given alone or in combination with other antihypertensives. Total daily doses greater than 50 mg are not recommended.

➤*Tablets:*

Adults –

Edema: The usual adult dosage is 25 to 100 mg daily as a single or divided dose. Many patients with edema respond to intermittent therapy, ie, administration on alternate days or on 3 to 5 days each week. With an intermittent schedule, excessive response and the resulting undesirable electrolyte imbalance are less likely to occur.

Hypertension: The usual initial dose in adults is 25 mg daily given as a single dose. The dose may be increased to 50 mg daily, given as a single or two divided doses. Doses above 50 mg are often associated with marked reductions in serum potassium (see Precautions).

Patients usually do not require doses in excess of 50 mg of hydrochlorothiazide daily when used concomitantly with other antihypertensive agents.

Infants and children –

For diuresis and for control of hypertension: The usual pediatric dosage is 0.5 to 1 mg per pound (1 to 2 mg/kg) per day in single or 2 divided doses, not to exceed 37.5 mg/day in infants up to 2 years of age or 100 mg/day in children 2 to 12 years of age. In infants less than 6 months of age, doses up to 1.5 mg per pound (3 mg/kg) per day in 2 divided doses may be required (see Warnings, Children).

➤*Storage/Stability:* Keep container tightly closed. Protect from light, moisture, freezing, −20°C (−4°F) and store at room temperature, 15° to 30°C (59° to 86°F).

BENDROFLUMETHIAZIDE

Rx	**Naturetin** (Princeton)	**Tablets:** 5 mg	(606). Green, scored. In 100s.
		10 mg	(618). Orange, scored. In 100s.

BENDROFLUMETHIAZIDE — ORAL

For complete and comparative prescribing information, see Thiazides and Related Diuretics group monograph.

Indications

➤*Edema:* Adjunctive therapy in edema associated with congestive heart failure, hepatic cirrhosis, and corticosteroid and estrogen therapy.

Bendroflumethiazide has also been found useful in edema due to various forms of renal dysfunction, such as nephrotic syndrome, acute glomerulonephritis, and chronic renal failure.

➤*Hypertension:* Management of hypertension either as the sole therapeutic agent or to enhance the effectiveness of other antihypertensive drugs in the more severe forms of hypertension.

➤*Unlabeled uses:* Osteoporosis; diabetes insipidus.

Administration and Dosage

➤*Diuretic:* 5 mg once daily, preferably given in the morning. To initiate therapy, doses up to 20 mg may be given once daily or divided into 2 doses. A single daily dose of 2.5 to 5 mg should suffice for maintenance.

Alternatively, intermittent therapy may be advantageous in many patients. By administering the preparation every other day or on a 3- to 5-day per week schedule, electrolyte imbalance is less likely to occur; however, the possibility still exists.

➤*Antihypertensive:* The suggested initial dosage is 5 to 20 mg daily. Maintenance dosage may range from 2.5 to 15 mg per day depending on the individual response of the patient. When the diuretic is used with other antihypertensive agents, lower maintenance doses for each drug are usually sufficient.

➤*Storage/Stability:* Dispense in tight containers. Store at room temperature; avoid excessive heat.

METHYCLOTHIAZIDE

Rx	**Methyclothiazide** (Various, eg, Schein, Zenith)	**Tablets:** 2.5 mg	In 100s and 1000s.
Rx	**Methyclothiazide** (Various, eg, Geneva, Parmed, Zenith)	**Tablets:** 5 mg	In 1000s.
Rx	**Enduron** (Abbott)		(Enduron). Salmon. Square. In 100s, 1000s, 5000s and *Abbo-Pac* 100s.

METHYCLOTHIAZIDE — ORAL

For complete and comparative prescribing information, see Thiazides and Related Diuretics group monograph.

Indications

➤*Hypertension:* Management of hypertension, either as the sole therapeutic agent or to enhance the effect of other antihypertensive drugs in the more severe forms of hypertension.

➤*Edema:* Adjunctive therapy in edema associated with congestive heart failure, hepatic cirrhosis, and corticosteroid and estrogen therapy.

Methyclothiazide tablets have also been found useful in edema due to various forms of renal dysfunction such as the nephrotic syndrome, acute glomerulonephritis, and chronic renal failure.

Administration and Dosage

➤*Approved by the FDA:* June 3, 1982.

➤*Edematous conditions:* The usual adult dose ranges from 2.5 to 10 mg once daily. Maximum effective single dose is 10 mg; larger single doses do not accomplish greater diuresis, and are not recommended.

➤*Hypertension:* 2.5 to 5 mg once daily. If control of blood pressure is not satisfactory after 8 to 12 weeks of therapy with 5 mg once daily, another antihypertensive drug should be added. Increasing the dosage of methyclothiazide will usually not result in further lowering of blood pressure.

Methyclothiazide may be either employed alone for mild-to-moderate hypertension or concurrently with other antihypertensive drugs in the management of more severe forms of hypertension. Combined therapy may provide adequate control of hypertension with lower dosage of the component drugs and fewer or less severe side effects. An enhanced response frequently follows its concurrent administration with deserpidine so that dosage of both drugs may be reduced.

When other antihypertensive agents are to be added to the regimen, this should be accomplished gradually. Ganglionic-blocking agents should be given at only half the usual dose because their effect is potentiated by pretreatment with methyclothiazide tablets.

➤*Storage/Stability:* Store below 30°C (86°F).

INDAPAMIDE

Rx	**Indapamide** (Various, eg, Major, Mylan, Purepac, Teva, Watson, Zenith)	**Tablets:** 1.25 mg	In 100s, 500s, and 1000s.
Rx	**Lozol** (Rhone-Poulenc Rorer)		(R 7). Orange. Octagonal. Film coated. In 100s.
Rx	**Lozol** (Rhone-Poulenc Rorer)	2.5 mg	(R 8). White. Octagonal. Film coated. In 100s, 1000s and UD 100s.

INDAPAMIDE — ORAL

For complete and comparative prescribing information, see Thiazides and Related Diuretics group monograph.

Indications

➤*Hypertension:* For the treatment of hypertension, alone or in combination with other antihypertensive drugs.

➤*Edema of congestive heart failure:* For the treatment of salt and fluid retention associated with congestive heart failure.

Administration and Dosage

➤*Approved by the FDA:* July 6, 1983.

➤*Hypertension:* 1.25 mg as a single daily dose taken in the morning. If the response to 1.25 mg is not satisfactory after 4 weeks, the daily dose may be increased to 2.5 mg taken once daily. If the response to 2.5 mg is not satisfactory after 4 weeks, the daily dose may be increased to 5 mg taken once daily, but adding another antihypertensive should be considered.

➤*Edema of congestive heart failure:* 2.5 mg as a single daily dose taken in the morning. If the response to 2.5 mg is not satisfactory after 1 week, the daily dose may be increased to 5 mg taken once daily.

In general, doses of greater than or equal to 5 mg have not appeared to provide additional effects on blood pressure or heart failure, but are associated with a greater degree of hypokalemia. There is minimal clinical trial experience in patients with doses greater than 5 mg once a day.

➤*Concomitant use with other antihypertensives:* If the antihypertensive response to indapamide is insufficient, indapamide may be combined with other antihypertensive drugs, with careful monitoring of blood pressure. It is recommended that the usual dose of other agents be reduced by 50% during initial combination therapy. As the blood pressure response becomes evident, further dosage adjustments may be necessary.

➤*Storage/Stability:* Keep tightly closed. Store at controlled room temperature 15° to 30°C (59° to 86°F). Avoid excessive heat. This product should be dispensed in a tight container with a child-resistant cap.

METOLAZONE

Rx	**Metolazone** (Various, eg, Eon, Mylan)	**Tablets:** 2.5 mg	In 100s and 1000s.
Rx	**Zaroxolyn** (Fisons)		(2 1/2 Zaroxolyn). Pink. In 100s, 1000s and UD 100s.
Rx	**Metolazone** (Various, eg, Eon)	**Tablets:** 5 mg	In 100s.
Rx	**Zaroxolyn** (Fisons)		(5 Zaroxolyn). Blue. In 100s, 1000s and UD 100s.
Rx	**Metolazone** (Various, eg, Eon)	**Tablets:** 10 mg	In 100s.
Rx	**Zaroxolyn** (Fisons)		(10 Zaroxolyn). Yellow. In 100s, 1000s and UD 100s.

METOLAZONE — ORAL

For complete and comparative prescribing information, refer to the Thiazides and Related Diuretics group monograph.

WARNING

Do not interchange – Do not interchange *Zaroxolyn* tablets and other formulations of metolazone that share its slow and incomplete bioavailability.

Indications

➤*Hypertension:* For the treatment of hypertension, alone or in combination with other antihypertensive drugs of a different class.

➤*Salt and water retention:* For the treatment of salt and water retention, including the following: edema accompanying congestive heart failure; edema accompanying renal diseases, including the nephrotic syndrome and states of diminished renal function.

➤*Unlabeled uses:* Osteoporosis; diabetes insipidus.

Administration and Dosage

➤*Dosage:* A single daily dose is recommended. Titrate therapy to gain an initial therapeutic response and to determine the minimal dose possible to maintain the desired therapeutic response.

Usual single daily dosage schedules – Suitable initial dosages will usually fall in the ranges given.

Edema of cardiac failure: 5 to 20 mg once daily.
Edema of renal disease: 5 to 20 mg once daily.
Mild to moderate essential hypertension: 2.5 mg to 5 mg once daily.

Treatment of edematous states – The time interval required for the initial dosage to produce an effect may vary. Diuresis and saluresis usually begin within 1 hour and persist for greater than or equal to 24 hours. When a desired therapeutic effect has been obtained, it may be advisable to reduce the dose if possible. The daily dose depends on the severity of the patient's

METOLAZONE — ORAL

condition, sodium intake, and responsiveness. Base a decision to change the daily dose on the results of thorough clinical and laboratory evaluations. If antihypertensive drugs or diuretics are given concurrently with metolazone tablets, more careful dosage adjustment may be necessary. For patients who tend to experience paroxysmal nocturnal dyspnea, it may be advisable to employ a larger dose to ensure prolongation of diuresis and saluresis for a full 24-hour period.

Treatment of hypertension – The time interval required for the initial dosage regimen to show effect may vary from 3 or 4 days to 3 to 6 weeks in the treatment of elevated blood pressure. Adjust doses at appropriate intervals to achieve maximum therapeutic effect.

➤*Storage/Stability:* Store at 20° to 25°C (68° to 77°F). Protect from light. Dispense in a tight, light-resistant container using a child-resistant closure.

CHLORTHALIDONE

Rx	**Thalitone** (Monarch)	**Tablets**: 15 mg	Lactose. (M 024). White. Kidney shaped. In 100s.
Rx	**Chlorthalidone** (Various, eg, Geneva, Goldline)	**Tablets**: 25 mg	In 100s, 1000s.
Rx	**Chlorthalidone** (Various, eg, Geneva, Goldline, Major, Schein)	**Tablets**: 50 mg	In 100s, 250s, and 1000s.
Rx	**Chlorthalidone** (Various, eg, Goldline, Schein)	**Tablets**: 100 mg	In 100s, 500s and 1000s.
Rx	**Hygroton** (RPR)		(RPR 21). White, scored. In 100s.

CHLORTHALIDONE — ORAL

For complete and comparative prescribing information, refer to the Thiazides and Related Diuretics group monograph.

Indications

➤*Hypertension:* Management of hypertension either alone or in combination with other antihypertensive drugs.

➤*Edema:* Adjunctive therapy in edema associated with congestive heart failure, hepatic cirrhosis, and corticosteroid and estrogen therapy.

Chlorthalidone has also been found useful in edema due to various forms of renal dysfunction such as nephrotic syndrome, acute glomerulonephritis, and chronic renal failure.

Administration and Dosage

➤*Hypertension:* Therapy in most patients should be initiated with a single daily dose of 15 mg. If the response is insufficient after a suitable trial, the dosage may be increased to 30 mg and then to a single daily dose of 45 to 50 mg. If additional control is required, the addition of a second antihypertensive drug is recommended. Increases in serum uric acid and decreases in serum potassium are dose-related over the 15 to 50 mg/day range and beyond.

➤*Edema:*

Initiation – Adults, initially 30 to 60 mg daily or 60 mg on alternate days. Some patients may require 90 to 120 mg at these intervals or up to 120 mg daily. Dosages above this level, however, do not usually produce a greater response.

Maintenance – Maintenance doses may often be lower than initial doses and should be adjusted according to the individual patient. Effectiveness is well sustained during continued use.

➤*Storage/Stability:* Store below 30°C (86°F).

WARNING

These agents are potent diuretics; excess amounts can lead to a profound diuresis with water and electrolyte depletion. Careful medical supervision is required and dosage must be individualized.

Indications

➤*Edema:* Edema associated with CHF, hepatic cirrhosis and renal disease, including the nephrotic syndrome. Particularly useful when greater diuretic potential is desired.

Parenteral administration is indicated when a rapid onset of diuresis is desired (eg, acute pulmonary edema), when GI absorption is impaired or when oral use is not practical for any reason. As soon as it is practical, replace with oral therapy.

➤*Hypertension (furosemide, oral; torsemide, oral):* Alone or in combination with other antihypertensive drugs. Hypertensive patients who are inadequately controlled with thiazides may not be adequately controlled with furosemide alone.

➤*Ethacrynic acid: Ascites:* Short-term management of ascites due to malignancy, idiopathic edema and lymphedema.

Congenital heart disease, nephrotic syndrome – Short-term management of hospitalized pediatric patients, other than infants.

Pulmonary edema, acute – Adjunctive therapy.

➤*Unlabeled uses:* Ethacrynic acid is being investigated for the treatment of glaucoma; a single injection into the eye may reduce intraocular pressure for a week or more. Further study is needed.

Bumetanide 1 mg may be beneficial in the treatment of adult nocturia; it is not effective in males with prostatic hypertrophy.

Administration and Dosage

Individualize therapy. Reserve parenteral use for when oral medication is not practical or in emergency situations. Replace with oral therapy as soon as practical.

➤*Concomitant administration:* Concurrent metolazone and furosemide have been used in the management of patients refractory to furosemide or other diuretics due to their synergistic effect on diuresis. Metolazone 2.5 to 10 mg is added to the therapy, and the dose is doubled every 24 hours until the desired response is achieved. Decrease the furosemide dose if the synergism occurs with the first dose of metolazone. Hydrochlorothiazide (50 mg) may be used and may be safer because of its shorter action. This effect has also been noted with other thiazides in combination with other loop diuretics.

Actions

➤*Pharmacology:* Furosemide and ethacrynic acid inhibit primarily reabsorption of sodium and chloride, not only in proximal and distal tubules, but also the loop of Henle. High efficacy is largely due to unique site of action. Action on distal tubule is independent of any inhibitory effect on carbonic anhydrase or aldosterone.

In contrast, bumetanide is more chloruretic than natriuretic and may have an additional action in the proximal tubule; it does not appear to act on the distal tubule.

Torsemide acts from within the lumen of the thick ascending portion of the loop of Henle, where it inhibits the $Na^+/K^+/2Cl^-$-carrier system; effects in other segments of the nephron have not been demonstrated. Diuretic activity thus correlates better with the rate of drug excretion in urine than with the blood concentration. Torsemide increases the urinary excretion of sodium, chloride, and water, but does not significantly alter glomerular filtration rate, renal plasma flow or acid-base balance.

Because ethacrynic acid inhibits the reabsorption of filtered sodium to a much greater proportion than most other diuretics, it may be effective in many patients with significant degrees of renal insufficiency.

➤*Pharmacokinetics:* These agents are metabolized and excreted primarily through the urine. Protein binding of these agents exceeds 90%. Furosemide is metabolized approximately 30% to 40%, and its urinary excretion is 60% to 70%. Significantly more furosemide is excreted in urine after IV injection than after the tablet or oral solution. Recent evidence suggests that furosemide glucuronide is the only, or at least the major, biotransformation product of furosemide.

Oral administration of bumetanide revealed that 81% was excreted in urine, 45% of it as unchanged drug. Bumetanide increases potassium excretion in a dose-related fashion; it also decreases uric acid excretion and increases serum uric acid. Urinary and biliary metabolites are formed by oxidation of the N-butyl side chain. Biliary excretion of bumetanide amounted to only 2% of the administered dose.

Torsemide is cleared from the circulation by both hepatic metabolism (approximately 80% of total clearance) and excretion into the urine (approximately 20% of total clearance). The major metabolite in humans is the carboxylic acid derivative, which is biologically inactive. Two of the lesser metabolites possess some diuretic activity, but for practical purposes metabolism terminates the action of the drug. Most renal clearance occurs via active secretion of the drug by the proximal tubules into tubular urine. Simultaneous food intake delays the time to C_{max} by about 30 minutes, but overall bioavailability and diuretic activity are unchanged.

Pharmacokinetic Parameters of the Loop Diuretics								
Diuretic	Bioavailability (%)	Half-life (min)	Onset of action (min)	Peak (min)	Duration (hr)	Dosage (mg)	Relative potency	Doses/day
Furosemide								
Oral	60-64[1]	≈ 120[2]	within 60	60-120[4]	6-8	20-80	1	1-2
IV or IM			within 5[3]	30	2	20-40	1	
Ethacrynic acid								
Oral	≈100	60	within 30	120	6-8	50-100	0.6-0.8	1-2
IV			within 5	15-30	2	50	0.6-0.8	1-2
Bumetanide								
Oral	72-96	60-90[5]	30-60	60-120	4-6	0.5-2	≈ 40	1
IV			within minutes	15-30	0.5-1	0.5-1	≈ 40	1-3
Torsemide								
Oral	≈ 80	210	within 60	60-120	6-8	5-20	2-4	1
IV			within 10	within 60	6-8	5-20	2-4	1

[1] Decreased in uremia and nephrosis.
[2] Prolonged in renal failure, uremia and in neonates.
[3] Somewhat delayed after IM administration.
[4] Decreased in CHF.
[5] Prolonged in renal disease.

Contraindications

Anuria; hypersensitivity to these compounds or to sulfonylureas; infants (ethacrynic acid); patients with hepatic coma or in states of severe electrolyte depletion until the condition is improved or corrected (bumetanide).

Warnings

➤*Dehydration:* Excessive diuresis may result in dehydration and reduction in blood volume with circulatory collapse and the possibility of vascular thrombosis and embolism, particularly in elderly patients.

➤*Hepatic cirrhosis and ascites:* In these patients, sudden alterations of electrolyte balance may precipitate hepatic encephalopathy and coma. Do not institute therapy until the basic condition is improved. Initiate therapy in the hospital with small doses and careful monitoring. Supplemental potassium chloride and, if required, an aldosterone antagonist help to prevent hypokalemia and metabolic alkalosis.

➤*Ototoxicity:* Tinnitus, reversible and irreversible hearing impairment, deafness and vertigo with a sense of fullness in the ears have been reported. Deafness is usually reversible and of short duration (1 to 24 hours); however, irreversible hearing impairment has occurred. Usually, ototoxicity is associated with rapid injection, with severe renal impairment, with doses several times the usual dose and with concurrent use with other ototoxic drugs.

➤*Systemic lupus erythematosus:* Systemic lupus erythematosus may be exacerbated or activated.

➤*Diarrhea:* In a few patients, ethacrynic acid has produced severe, watery diarrhea. If this occurs, discontinue the drug and do not readminister.

Because of the amount of sorbitol in the **furosemide** solution vehicle, the possibility of diarrhea, especially in children, exists when higher dosages are given.

Thrombocytopenia – Since there have been rare spontaneous reports of thrombocytopenia with **bumetanide**, observe regularly for possible occurrence.

➤*Hypersensitivity reactions:* Patients with known sulfonamide sensitivity may show allergic reactions to **furosemide**, **torsemide** or **bumetanide**. Bumetanide use following instances of allergic reactions to furosemide suggests a lack of cross-sensitivity. Refer to Management of Acute Hypersensitivity Reactions.

➤*Renal function impairment:* If increasing azotemia, oliguria or reversible increases in BUN or creatinine occur during treatment of severe progressive renal disease, discontinue therapy.

If high-dose parenteral **furosemide** therapy is used, controlled IV infusion is advisable. For adults, an infusion rate less than or equal to 4 mg/min has been used.

➤*Pregnancy: Category B* (ethacrynic acid, torsemide); *Category C* (furosemide, bumetanide). There are no adequate and well controlled studies in pregnant women. Use only when clearly needed and when the potential benefits outweigh the potential hazards to the fetus.

Furosemide – Furosemide caused unexplained maternal deaths and abortions in rabbits when 25 to 100 mg/kg (2 to 8 times the maximum recommended human dose) was administered. No pregnant rabbits survived a dose of 100 mg/kg. Data indicate that fetal lethality can precede maternal deaths. Studies in mice and rabbits showed an increased incidence of fetal hydronephrosis. Since furosemide may increase the incidence of patent ductus arteriosus in preterm infants with respiratory-distress syndrome (see Children), use caution when administering before delivery.

Bumetanide – Bumetanide appears to be nonteratogenic, but has a slight embryocidal effect in rats when given in doses of 3400 times the maximum human therapeutic dose and in rabbits at doses of 3.4 times the maximum human therapeutic dose. In rabbits, a decrease in litter size and an increase in resorption rate were noted at oral doses 3.4 to 10 times the maximum human therapeutic dose.

Torsemide – Fetal and maternal toxicity (decrease in average body weight, increase in fetal resorption and delayed fetal ossification) occurred in rabbits and rats.

➤*Lactation:* **Furosemide** appears in breast milk; such transfer of **ethacrynic acid**, **torsemide** and **bumetanide** is unknown. Because of the potential for adverse reactions in nursing infants, decide whether to discontinue nursing or to discontinue the drug, taking into account the importance of the drug to the mother.

➤*Children:* Safety and efficacy for use of **torsemide** in children, **bumetanide** in children younger than 18 years old, and **ethacrynic acid** in infants (oral) and children (IV) have not been established.

Furosemide – Furosemide stimulates renal synthesis of prostaglandin E_2 and may increase the incidence of patent ductus arteriosus when given in the first few weeks of life, to premature infants with respiratory-distress syndrome. Renal calcifications (from barely visible on x–ray to staghorn) have occurred in some severely premature infants treated with IV furosemide for edema due to patent ductus arteriosus and hyaline membrane disease. Concurrent use of chlorothiazide has reportedly decreased hypercalciuria and dissolved some calculi.

Precautions

➤*Monitoring:* Observe for blood dyscrasias, liver or kidney damage or idiosyncratic reactions. Perform frequent serum electrolyte, calcium, glucose, uric acid, CO_2, creatinine and BUN determinations during the first few months of therapy and periodically thereafter (see Electrolyte imbalance and Laboratory test abnormalities).

➤*Cardiovascular effects:* Too vigorous a diuresis, as evidenced by rapid and excessive weight loss, may induce an acute hypotensive episode. In elderly cardiac patients, avoid rapid contraction of plasma volume and the resultant hemoconcentration to prevent thromboembolic episodes, such as cerebral vascular thromboses and pulmonary emboli.

➤*Electrolyte imbalance:* Electrolyte imbalance may occur, especially in patients receiving high doses with restricted salt intake. Perform periodic determinations of serum electrolytes. Observe patients for signs of fluid or electrolyte imbalance (eg, hyponatremia, hypochloremic alkalosis, hypokalemia, hypomagnesemia, hypocalcemia). Digitalis therapy may exaggerate metabolic effects of hypokalemia with reference to myocardial activity. Serum and urine electrolyte determinations are important in patients who are vomiting excessively, in patients who are receiving parenteral fluids, corticosteroids or ACTH, during brisk diuresis or when cirrhosis is present. Warning signs are dryness of mouth, thirst, anorexia, weakness, lethargy, drowsiness, restlessness, muscle pains or cramps, muscle fatigue, tetany (rarely), hypotension, oliguria, tachycardia, arrhythmia and GI disturbances (eg, nausea/vomiting).

Profound electrolyte and water loss may be avoided by weighing the patient periodically, adjusting dosage, initiating treatment with small doses and using the drugs intermittently. When excessive diuresis occurs, withdraw the drugs until homeostasis is restored. If excessive electrolyte loss occurs, reduce dosage or withdraw the drug temporarily.

Hypokalemia – Hypokalemia prevention requires particular attention to the following: Patients receiving digitalis and diuretics for CHF, hepatic cirrhosis and ascites; in aldosterone excess with normal renal function; potassium-losing nephropathy; certain diarrheal states; or where hypokalemia is an added risk to the patient (eg, history of ventricular arrhythmias).

Possible drug-related deaths occurred with **ethacrynic acid** in critically ill patients refractory to other diuretics. There are two categories: Patients with severe myocardial disease who received digitalis and developed acute hypokalemia with fatal arrhythmia; or patients with severely decompensated hepatic cirrhosis with ascites, with or without encephalopathy, who had electrolyte imbalances and died because of intensification of the electrolyte defect. Liberalization of salt intake and supplementary potassium are often necessary.

Hypomagnesemia – Loop diuretics increase the urinary excretion of magnesium.

Hypocalcemia – Serum calcium levels may be lowered (rare cases of tetany have occurred).

➤*Gastric hemorrhage:* **Ethacrynic acid** may increase the risk of gastric hemorrhage associated with corticosteroid treatment.

➤*Hyperuricemia:* Asymptomatic hyperuricemia can occur, and rarely, gout may be precipitated. Reversible elevations of BUN may be seen, usually in association with dehydration, particularly in patients with renal insufficiency. Serum creatinine may also be increased.

➤*Glucose:* Increases in blood glucose and alterations in glucose tolerance tests (fasting and 2 hour postprandial sugar) have been observed. Rare cases of precipitation of diabetes mellitus have occurred. Although these effects have not been reported with **bumetanide**, the possibility of an effect on glucose metabolism exists.

➤*Lipids:* Increases in LDL and total cholesterol and triglycerides with minor decreases in HDL cholesterol may occur.

➤*Photosensitivity:* Photosensitization (photoallergy or phototoxicity) may occur; therefore, caution patients to take protective measures (ie, sunscreens, protective clothing) against exposure to sunlight or ultraviolet light (eg, tanning beds) until tolerance is determined.

Drug Interactions

Loop Diuretic Drug Interactions

Precipitant drug	Object drug*		Description
Loop diuretics	Aminoglycosides	↑	Auditory toxicity appears to be increased with concurrent use. Hearing loss of varying degrees may occur.
Loop diuretics	Anticoagulants	↑	Anticoagulant activity may be enhanced.
Loop diuretics Furosemide	Beta blockers Propranolol	↑	Plasma levels of propranolol may be increased.
Loop diuretics	Chloral hydrate	↑	Although rare, transient diaphoresis, hot flashes, hypertension, tachycardia, weakness and nausea may occur with concurrent use.
Loop diuretics	Digitalis glycosides	↑	Diuretic-induced electrolyte disturbances may predispose to digitalis-induced arrhythmias.
Loop diuretics	Lithium	↑	Possible increased plasma lithium levels and toxicity.
Loop diuretics	Nondepolarizing muscle relaxants	↔	The actions of the muscle relaxants may be antagonized or potentiated, perhaps dependent on the loop diuretic dosage.
Loop diuretics	Sulfonylureas	↓	Loop diuretics may decrease glucose tolerance, resulting in hyperglycemia in patients previously well controlled on sulfonylureas.
Loop diuretics	Theophyllines	↔	The actions of theophyllines may be altered, enhanced or inhibited.
Charcoal	Loop diuretics Furosemide	↓	Charcoal can reduce the absorption of furosemide. Depending on the clinical situation, this will reduce its effectiveness or toxicity.
Cisplatin	Loop diuretics	↑	Additive ototoxicity may occur.
Clofibrate	Loop diuretics Furosemide	↑	An exaggerated diuretic response may occur.
Hydantoins Phenytoin	Loop diuretics Furosemide	↓	Hydantoins may reduce the diuretic effects of furosemide.
NSAIDs	Loop diuretics	↓	Effects of the loop diuretics may be decreased.
Probenecid	Loop diuretics	↓	The actions of the loop diuretics may be reduced.
Salicylates	Loop diuretics	↓	The diuretic response may be impaired in patients with cirrhosis and ascites.
Thiazide diuretics	Loop diuretics	↑	Both groups have synergistic effects that may result in profound diuresis and serious electrolyte abnormalities (see Administration and Dosage).

* ↑ = Object drug increased. ↓ = Object drug decreased. ↔= Undetermined clinical effect.

➤*Drug/Food interactions:* The bioavailability of **furosemide** is decreased and its degree of diuresis reduced when administered with food.

Adverse Reactions

➤*Furosemide:*

GI – Anorexia; nausea; vomiting; diarrhea; oral and gastric irritation; cramping; constipation; pancreatitis; jaundice; ischemic hepatitis.

CNS – Vertigo; headache; blurred vision; hearing loss; dizziness; paresthesia; xanthopsia; restlessness; fever.

Hematologic – Anemia; leukopenia; purpura; aplastic anemia; thrombocytopenia; agranulocytosis.

Dermatologic – Photosensitivity; urticaria; pruritus; necrotizing angiitis (vasculitis, cutaneous vasculitis); interstitial nephritis; exfoliative dermatitis; erythema multiforme; rash; occasionally, local irritation and pain with parenteral use.

Cardiovascular – Orthostatic hypotension; thrombophlebitis; chronic aortitis.

Miscellaneous – Glycosuria; muscle spasm; weakness; urinary bladder spasm; hyperuricemia; hyperglycemia.

➤*Ethacrynic acid:*

GI – Anorexia; nausea; vomiting; diarrhea; pancreatitis (acute); jaundice; discomfort; pain; sudden watery, profuse diarrhea; GI bleeding; dysphagia.

Hematologic – Severe neutropenia has occurred in a few critically ill patients also receiving agents known to produce this effect. Rare instances of Henoch-Schoenlein purpura have occurred in patients with rheumatic heart disease. Thrombocytopenia; agranulocytosis.

Miscellaneous – Fever; chills; hematuria; apprehension; confusion; fatigue; malaise; acute gout; sense of fullness in the ears; abnormal liver function tests in seriously ill patients on multiple drug therapy that included ethacrynic acid (rare); vertigo; headache; blurred vision; tinnitus; hearing loss (irreversible); rash; occasionally, local irritation and pain have occurred with parenteral use; hyperuricemia; hyperglycemia. Acute symptomatic hypoglycemia with convulsions occurred in two uremic patients who received doses above those recommended.

➤*Bumetanide:*

CNS – Asterixis; encephalopathy with preexisting liver disease; impaired hearing; ear discomfort; vertigo; headache; dizziness.

GI – Upset stomach; dry mouth; nausea; vomiting; diarrhea; pain.

GU – Premature ejaculation; difficulty maintaining erection; renal failure.

Musculoskeletal – Weakness; arthritic pain; pain; muscle cramps; fatigue.

Cardiovascular – Hypotension; ECG changes; chest pain.

Miscellaneous – Hives; pruritus; itching; dehydration; sweating; hyperventilation; nipple tenderness; rash; thrombocytopenia.

Lab test abnormalities – Diuresis rarely (less than or equal to 1%) accompanied by changes in LDH, total serum bilirubin, serum proteins, AST, ALT, alkaline phosphatase, cholesterol and creatinine clearance; deviations in hemoglobin, prothrombin time, hematocrit, WBC, platelet counts and differential counts; increases in urinary glucose and protein; hyperuricemia; hypochloremia; hypokalemia; azotemia; hyponatremia; increased serum creatinine; hyperglycemia; variations in phosphorus, CO_2 content, bicarbonate and calcium (see Precautions).

➤*Torsemide:*

CNS – Headache (7.3%); dizziness (3.2%); asthenia (2%); insomnia (1.2%); nervousness (1.1%); syncope.

GI – Diarrhea (2%); constipation, nausea (1.8%); dyspepsia (1.6%); edema (1.1%); GI hemorrhage; rectal bleeding.

Cardiovascular – ECG abnormality (2%); sore throat (1.6%); chest pain (1.2%); atrial fibrillation; hypotension; ventricular tachycardia; shunt thrombosis.

Respiratory – Rhinitis (2.8%); cough increase (2%).

Musculoskeletal – arthralgia (1.8%); myalgia (1.6%).

Lab test abnormalities – Hyperglycemia; hyperuricemia; hypokalemia; hypovolemia.

Miscellaneous – Excessive urination (6.7%); rash.

Overdosage

➤*Symptoms:* Acute profound water loss, volume and electrolyte depletion, dehydration, reduction of blood volume, and circulatory collapse with a possibility of vascular thrombosis and embolism. Electrolyte depletion may be manifested by weakness, dizziness, mental confusion, anorexia, lethargy, vomiting and cramps.

➤*Treatment:* Replace fluid and electrolyte losses by careful monitoring of the urine and electrolyte output and serum electrolyte levels. Assure adequate drainage in urinary bladder outlet obstruction (such as prostatic hypertrophy). Hemodialysis does not accelerate furosemide or torsemide elimination. Induce emesis or perform gastric lavage. If required, give oxygen or artificial respiration. Treatment includes supportive measures. Refer to General Management of Acute Overdosage.

Patient Information

May cause GI upset; take with food or milk (see Drug Interactions). Torsemide may be given without regard to meals.

Drug will increase urination; take early in the day.

Notify physician if muscle weakness, cramps, nausea or dizziness occurs.

Orthostatic hypotension may occur; get up slowly.

➤*Diabetes mellitus patients:* May increase blood glucose levels, affecting urine glucose tests.

➤*Photosensitivity:* Photosensitivity may occur in some patients. Caution patients to take protective measures (ie, sunscreens, protective clothing) against exposure to ultraviolet light or sunlight.

➤*Hypertensive patients:* Hypertensive patients should avoid medications that may increase blood pressure, including *otc* products for appetite suppression and cold symptoms.

FUROSEMIDE

Rx	**Furosemide** (Various, eg, Danbury, Geneva, Major, Mylan, Parmed, Roxane, Schein, Zenith)	**Tablets:** 20 mg	In 100s, 500s, 1000s and UD 100s.
Rx	**Lasix** (Aventis)		Lactose. (Lasix Hoechst). White. Oval. In 100s, 500s, 1000s and UD 100s.
Rx	**Furosemide** (Various, eg, Danbury, Geneva, Major, Mylan, Parmed, Roxane, Schein, Zenith)	**Tablets:** 40 mg	In 60s, 100s, 500s and 1000s and UD 100s.
Rx	**Lasix** (Aventis)		Lactose. (Lasix 40). White, scored. In 500s, 1000s, UD 100s and unit-of-use 100s.
Rx	**Furosemide** (Various, eg, Danbury, Geneva, Mylan, Parmed, Roxane, Schein)	**Tablets:** 80 mg	In 100s, 500s, 1000s and UD 100s.
Rx	**Lasix** (Aventis)		Lactose. (Lasix 80). White. In 50s, 500s and UD 100s.
Rx	**Furosemide** (Various, eg, Geneva, Roxane)	**Oral Solution:** 10 mg/ml	In 60 and 120 ml.
Rx	**Furosemide** (Roxane)	**Oral Solution:** 40 mg/5 ml	Pineapple/peach flavor. In 500 ml and UD 5 & 10 ml.
Rx	**Furosemide** (Various, eg, American Regent, Sanofi Winthrop)	**Injection:** 10 mg/ml	In 10 ml and 2, 4, and 10 ml single-dose vials.

FUROSEMIDE — ORAL

For complete and comparative prescribing information, refer to the Loop Diuretics group monograph.

WARNING

Furosemide is a potent diuretic which, if given in excessive amounts, can lead to a profound diuresis with water and electrolyte depletion. Therefore, careful medical supervision is required and dose and schedule must be adjusted to the individual patient's needs (see Administration and Dosage).

Indications

➤*Edema:* Furosemide is indicated in adult and pediatric patients for the treatment of edema associated with congestive heart failure, cirrhosis of the liver, and renal disease, including the nephrotic syndrome. Furosemide is particularly useful when an agent with greater diuretic potential is desired.

➤*Hypertension:* Oral furosemide may be used in adults for the treatment of hypertension alone or in combination with other antihypertensive agents. Hypertensive patients who cannot be adequately controlled with thiazides will probably also not be adequately controlled with furosemide alone.

Administration and Dosage

➤*Approved by the FDA:* July 27, 1982.

➤*Edema:*

Adults – The usual initial dose of furosemide is 20 to 80 mg given as a single dose. Ordinarily a prompt diuresis ensues. If needed, the same dose can be administered 6 to 8 hours later or the dose may be increased. The dose may be raised by 20 to 40 mg and given not sooner than 6 to 8 hours after the previous dose until the desired diuretic effect has been obtained. This individually determined single dose should then be given once or twice daily. The dose of furosemide may be carefully titrated up to 600 mg/day in patients with clinically severe edematous states.

Edema may be most efficiently and safely mobilized by giving furosemide on 2 to 4 consecutive days each week.

When doses exceeding 80 mg/day are given for prolonged periods, careful clinical observations and laboratory monitoring are particularly advisable (See Precautions, Laboratory Tests).

Children – The usual initial dose of oral furosemide in pediatric patients is 2 mg/kg body weight, given as a single dose. If the diuretic response is not satisfactory after the initial dose, dosage may be increased by 1 or 2 mg/kg no sooner than 6 to 8 hours after the previous dose. Doses greater than 6 mg/kg body weight are not recommended.

For maintenance therapy in pediatric patients, the dose should be adjusted to the minimum effective level.

For ease of administration, and to allow maximum flexibility in dosing, the use of furosemide oral solution is suggested.

Furosemide oral solution: For ease of administration, and to allow maximum flexibility in dosing, the use of furosemide oral solution is suggested in pediatric patients.

➤*Hypertension:* Therapy should be individualized according to the patient's response to gain maximal therapeutic response and to determine the minimal dose needed to maintain that therapeutic response.

Adults – The usual initial dose of furosemide for hypertension is 80 mg, usually divided into 40 mg twice a day. Dosage should then be adjusted according to response. If response is not satisfactory, add other antihypertensive agents.

Changes in blood pressure must be carefully monitored when furosemide is used with other antihypertensive drugs, especially during initial therapy. To prevent excessive drop in blood pressure, the dosage of other agents should be reduced by at least 50 percent when furosemide is added to the regimen. As the blood pressure falls under the potentiating effect of furosemide, a further reduction in dosage or even discontinuation of other antihypertensive drugs may be necessary.

➤*Storage/Stability:*

Furosemide oral solution – Store at controlled room temperature, 15° to 30°C (59° to 86°F). Dispense in original or light-resistant containers as defined in the USP with graduated dropper or graduated spoon (dropper graduated in 5 mg increments at 5, 10, 15, and 20 mg corresponding to 0.5, 1, 1.5, and 2 mL; dispensing spoon graduated in 20 mg increments at 20, 40, 60, and 80 mg corresponding to 2, 4, 6, and 8 mL). Discard opened bottle after 60 days. Protect from light.

Furosemide tablets – Store at controlled room temperature 15° to 30°C (59° to 86°F). Dispense in well-closed, light-resistant containers. Exposure to light might cause a slight discoloration. Discolored tablets should not be dispensed.

FUROSEMIDE — INJECTION

For complete and comparative prescribing information, refer to the Loop Diuretics group monograph.

WARNING

Furosemide is a potent diuretic which, if given in excessive amounts, can lead to a profound diuresis with water and electrolyte depletion. Therefore, careful medical supervision is required and dose and dose schedule must be adjusted to the individual patient's needs (see Administration and Dosage).

Indications

Parenteral therapy should be reserved for patients unable to take oral medication or for patients in emergency clinical situations.

➤*Edema:* For the treatment of edema associated with congestive heart failure, cirrhosis of the liver, and renal disease, including the nephrotic syndrome. Furosemide is particularly useful when an agent with greater diuretic potential is desired.

Furosemide is indicated as adjunctive therapy in acute pulmonary edema. The intravenous (IV) administration of furosemide is indicated when a rapid onset of diuresis is desired (eg, in acute pulmonary edema).

If GI absorption is impaired or oral medication is not practical for any reason, furosemide is indicated by the IV or intramscular (IM) route. Parenteral use should be replaced with oral furosemide as soon as practical.

Administration and Dosage

➤*Approved by the FDA:* May 28, 1982.

➤*Adults:*

Edema – The usual initial dose of furosemide is 20 to 40 mg given as a single dose, injected intramuscularly or intravenously. The IV dose should be given slowly (1 to 2 minutes). Ordinarily a prompt diuresis ensues. If needed, another dose may be administered in the same manner 2 hours later or the dose may be increased. The dose may be raised by 20 mg and given not sooner than 2 hours after the previous dose until the desired

FUROSEMIDE — INJECTION

diuretic effect has been obtained. This individually determined single dose should then be given once or twice daily.

If the physician elects to use high dose parenteral therapy, add the furosemide to either Sodium Chloride Injection, Lactated Ringer's Injection, or Dextrose (5%) Injection after pH has been adjusted to above 5.5, and administer as a controlled IV infusion at a rate not greater than 4 mg/min.

Acute pulmonary edema – The usual initial dose of furosemide is 40 mg injected slowly intravenously (over 1 to 2 minutes). If a satisfactory response does not occur within 1 hour, the dose may be increased to 80 mg injected slowly intravenously (over 1 to 2 minutes).

If necessary, additional therapy (eg, digitalis, oxygen) may be administered concomitantly.

➤*Children:* The usual initial dose of furosemide injection (intravenously or intramuscularly) in pediatric patients is 1 mg/kg body weight and should be given slowly under close medical supervision. If the diuretic response to the initial dose is not satisfactory, dosage may be increased by 1 mg/kg not sooner than 2 hours after the previous dose, until the desired diuretic effect has been obtained. Doses > 6 mg/kg body weight are not recommended.

Literature reports suggest the maximum dose for premature infants should not exceed 1 mg/kg/day (see Warnings, Children).

Incompatibilities – Furosemide injection is a buffered alkaline solution with a pH of about 9 and drug may precipitate at pH values below 7. Care must be taken to ensure that the pH of the prepared infusion solution is in the weakly alkaline to neutral range. Acid solutions, including other parenteral medications (eg, labetalol, ciprofloxacin, amrinone, milrinone) must not be administered concurrently in the same infusion because they may cause precipitation of the furosemide. In addition, furosemide injection should not be added to a running IV line containing any of these acidic products.

➤*Storage/Stability:* Do not use if solution is discolored. Furosemide injection should be inspected visually for particulate matter and discoloration before administration.

Store at controlled room temperature 15° to 30°C (59° to 86°F). Protect from light.

BUMETANIDE

Rx	**Bumex** (Roche)	**Tablets:** 0.5 mg	Lactose. (Roche Bumex 0.5). Green, scored. In 100s, 500s and UD 100s.
		1 mg	Lactose. (Roche Bumex 1). Yellow, scored. In 100s, 500s and UD 100s.
		2 mg	Lactose. (Roche Bumex 2). Peach, scored. In 100s and UD 100s.
Rx	**Bumetanide** (Various, eg, Bedford, Hoffman-LaRoche, Sanofi Winthrop)	**Injection:** 0.25 mg per ml	In 2 ml amps, 2, 4 and 10 ml vials and 4 ml fill in 5 ml vials.

[1] With 0.01% EDTA and 1% benzyl alcohol.

BUMETANIDE — ORAL

For complete and comparative prescribing information, refer to the Loop Diuretics group monograph.

WARNING

Bumetanide is a potent diuretic which, if given in excessive amounts, can lead to a profound diuresis with water and electrolyte depletion. Therefore, careful medical supervision is required and dose and dosage schedule have to be adjusted to the individual patient's needs.

Indications

➤*Edema:* For the treatment of edema associated with congestive heart failure, hepatic and renal disease, including the nephrotic syndrome.

Almost equal diuretic response occurs after oral and parenteral administration of bumetanide. Therefore, if impaired GI absorption is suspected or oral administration is not practical, bumetanide should be given by the IM or IV route.

➤*Unlabeled uses:* Adult nocturia.

Administration and Dosage

➤*Approved by the FDA:* February 28, 1983.

The usual total daily dosage of bumetanide is 0.5 mg to 2 mg and in most patients is given as a single dose.

If the diuretic response to an initial dose of bumetanide is not adequate, in view of its rapid onset and short duration of action, a second or third dose may be given at 4- to 5-hour intervals up to a maximum daily dose of 10 mg. An intermittent dose schedule, whereby bumetanide is given on alternate days or for 3 to 4 days with rest periods of 1 to 2 days in between, is recommended as the safest and most effective method for the continued control of edema. In patients with hepatic failure, the dosage should be kept to a minimum, and if necessary, dosage increased very carefully.

➤*Cross-sensitivity with furosemide:* Because cross-sensitivity with furosemide has rarely been observed, bumetanide can be substituted at approximately a 1:40 ratio of bumetanide to furosemide in patients allergic to furosemide.

Successful treatment with bumetanide following instances of allergic reactions to furosemide suggests a lack of cross-sensitivity.

➤*Storage/Stability:* Store between 15° and 30°C (59° and 86°F). Protect from light.

BUMETANIDE — INJECTION

For complete and comparative prescribing information, refer to the Loop Diuretics group monograph.

WARNING

Bumetanide is a potent diuretic which, if given in excessive amounts, can lead to a profound diuresis with water and electrolyte depletion. Therefore, careful medical supervision is required, and dose and dosage schedule have to be adjusted to the individual patient's needs (see Administration and Dosage).

Indications

➤*Edema:* For the treatment of edema associated with congestive heart failure, and hepatic and renal disease, including the nephrotic syndrome.

Almost equal diuretic response occurs after oral and parenteral administration of bumetanide. Therefore, if impaired GI absorption is suspected or oral administration is not practical, give bumetanide by the IM or IV route.

Administration and Dosage

➤*Approved by the FDA:* February 28, 1983.

➤*Cross-sensitivity with furosemide:* Because cross-sensitivity with furosemide has rarely been observed, bumetanide can be substituted at approximately a 1:40 ratio of bumetanide to furosemide in patients allergic to furosemide.

Successful treatment with bumetanide following instances of allergic reactions to furosemide suggests a lack of cross-sensitivity.

➤*Parenteral administration:* Bumetanide may be administered parenterally (IV or IM) to patients in whom GI absorption may be impaired or in whom oral administration is not practical.

Terminate parenteral treatment and institute oral treatment as soon as possible.

The usual initial dose is 0.5 mg to 1 mg IV or IM. IV administration should be given over a period of 1 to 2 minutes. If the response to an initial dose is deemed insufficient, a second or third dose may be given at intervals of 2 to 3 hours, but should not exceed a daily dosage of 10 mg.

➤*Compatibility:* The compatibility tests of bumetanide injection (0.25 mg/mL, 2 mL ampuls) with 5% Dextrose in Water, 0.9% Sodium Chloride and Lactated Ringer's solution in both glass and plasticized PVC (*Viaflex*) containers have shown no significant absorption effect with either containers, nor a measurable loss of potency due to degradation of the drug. However, solutions should be freshly prepared and used within 24 hours.

➤*Storage/Stability:* Store at controlled room temperature 15° to 30°C (59° to 86°F).

ETHACRYNIC ACID

Rx	**Edecrin** (Merck)	**Tablets:** 25 mg	Lactose. (MSD 65). White, scored. Capsule shape. In 100s.
		50 mg	Lactose. (MSD 90). Green, scored. Capsule shape. In 100s.
Rx	**Edecrin Sodium** (Merck)	**Powder for Injection:** 50 mg (as ethacrynate sodium) per vial	In 50 ml vials for reconstitution.[1]

[1] With 62.5 mg mannitol and 0.1 mg thimerosal.

ETHACRYNIC ACID — ORAL

For complete and comparative prescribing information, refer to the Loop Diuretics group monograph.

WARNING

Ethacrynic acid is a potent diuretic which, if given in excessive amounts, may lead to profound diuresis with water and electrolyte depletion. Therefore, careful medical supervision is required, and dose and dose schedule must be adjusted to the individual patient's needs (see Administration and Dosage).

Indications

For treatment of edema when an agent with greater diuretic potential than those commonly employed is required.

1.) Treatment of the edema associated with congestive heart failure, cirrhosis of the liver, and renal disease, including the nephrotic syndrome.
2.) Short-term management of ascites due to malignancy, idiopathic edema, and lymphedema.
3.) Short-term management of hospitalized pediatric patients, other than infants, with congenital heart disease or the nephrotic syndrome.

Administration and Dosage

➤*Approved by the FDA:* August 23, 1993.

Dosage must be regulated carefully to prevent a more rapid or substantial loss of fluid or electrolyte than is indicated or necessary. The magnitude of diuresis and natriuresis is largely dependent on the degree of fluid accumulation present in the patient. Similarly, the extent of potassium excretion is determined in large measure by the presence and magnitude of aldosteronism.

➤*Dosage:*

To Initiate Diuresis –

In Adults: The smallest dose required to produce gradual weight loss (about 1 to 2 pounds per day) is recommended. Onset of diuresis usually occurs at 50 to 100 mg for adults. After diuresis has been achieved, the minimally effective dose (usually from 50 to 200 mg daily) may be given on a continuous or intermittent dosage schedule. Dosage adjustments are usually in 25 to 50 mg increments to avoid derangement of water and electrolyte excretion.

The patient should be weighed under standard conditions before and during the institution of diuretic therapy with this compound. Small alterations in dose should effectively prevent a massive diuretic response. The following schedule may be helpful in determining the smallest effective dose.

- *Day 1* – 50 mg (single dose) after a meal
- *Day 2* – 50 mg twice daily after meals, if necessary
- *Day 3* – 100 mg in the morning and 50 to 100 mg following the afternoon or evening meal, depending upon response to the morning dose.

A few patients may require initial and maintenance doses as high as 200 mg twice daily. These higher doses, which should be achieved gradually, are most often required in patients with severe, refractory edema.

Children (excluding infants): The initial dose should be 25 mg. Careful stepwise increments in dosage of 25 mg should be made to achieve effective maintenance.

Maintenance Therapy – It is usually possible to reduce the dosage and frequency of administration once dry weight has been achieved.

Ethacrynic Acid may be given intermittently after an effective diuresis is obtained with the regimen outlined above. Dosage may be on an alternate daily schedule or more prolonged periods of diuretic therapy may be interspersed with rest periods. Such an intermittent dosage schedule allows time for correction of any electrolyte imbalance and may provide a more efficient diuretic response.

The chloruretic effect of this agent may give rise to retention of bicarbonate and a metabolic alkalosis. This may be corrected by giving chloride (ammonium chloride or arginine chloride). Ammonium chloride should not be given to cirrhotic patients.

Ethacrynic acid has additive effects when used with other diuretics. For example, a patient who is on maintenance dosage of an oral diuretic may require additional intermittent diuretic therapy, such as an organomercurial, for the maintenance of basal weight. The intermittent use of ethacrynic acid orally may eliminate the need for injections of organomercurials. Small doses of ethacrynic acid may be added to existing diuretic regimens to maintain basal weight. This drug may potentiate the action of carbonic anhydrase inhibitors, with augmentation of natriuresis and kaliuresis. Therefore, when adding ethacrynic acid the initial dose and changes of dose should be in 25 mg increments, to avoid electrolyte depletion. Rarely, patients who failed to respond to ethacrynic acid have responded to older established agents.

While many patients do not require supplemental potassium, the use of potassium chloride or potassium-sparing agents, or both, during treatment with ethacrynic acid is advisable, especially in cirrhotic or nephrotic patients and in patients receiving digitalis.

Salt liberalization usually prevents the development of hyponatremia and hypochloremia. During treatment with ethacrynic acid, salt may be liberalized to a greater extent than with other diuretics. Cirrhotic patients, however, usually require at least moderate salt restriction concomitant with diuretic therapy.

ETHACRYNATE SODIUM — INJECTION

For complete and comparative prescribing information, refer to the Loop Diuretics group monograph.

WARNING

Ethacrynic acid is a potent diuretic which, if given in excessive amounts, may lead to profound diuresis with water and electrolyte depletion. Therefore, careful medical supervision is required, and dose and dose schedule must be adjusted to the individual patient's needs (see Administration and Dosage).

Indications

For treatment of edema when an agent with greater diuretic potential than those commonly employed is required.

1.) Treatment of the edema associated with congestive heart failure, cirrhosis of the liver, and renal disease, including the nephrotic syndrome.
2.) Short-term management of ascites due to malignancy, idiopathic edema, and lymphedema.
3.) Short-term management of hospitalized pediatric patients, other than infants, with congenital heart disease or the nephrotic syndrome.
4.) Intravenous ethacrynic acid is indicated when a rapid onset of diuresis is desired, eg, in acute pulmonary edema, or when gastrointestinal absorption is impaired or oral medication is not practicable.

Administration and Dosage

➤*Approved by the FDA:* August 23, 1993.

➤*Dosage:* Dosage must be regulated carefully to prevent a more rapid or substantial loss of fluid or electrolyte than is indicated or necessary. The magnitude of diuresis and natriuresis is largely dependent on the degree of fluid accumulation present in the patient. Similarly, the extent of potassium excretion is determined in large measure by the presence and magnitude of aldosteronism.

The usual intravenous dose for the average sized adult is 50 mg, or 0.5 to 1 mg/kg of body weight. Usually only one dose has been necessary; occasionally a second dose at a new injection site, to avoid possible thrombophlebitis, may be required. A single intravenous dose not exceeding 100 mg has been used in critical situations.

Intravenous ethacrynic acid is for intravenous use when oral intake is impractical or in urgent conditions, such as acute pulmonary edema.

Insufficient pediatric experience precludes recommendation for this age group.

➤*Reconstitution:* To reconstitute the dry material, add 50 mL of 5% Dextrose Injection, or Sodium Chloride Injection to the vial. Occasionally, some 5% Dextrose Injection solutions may have a low pH (below 5). The resulting solution with such a diluent may be hazy or opalescent. Intravenous use of such a solution is not recommended. Inspect the vial containing intravenous ethacrynic acid for particulate matter and discoloration before use.

➤*Administration:* The solution may be given slowly through the tubing of a running infusion or by direct intravenous injection over a period of several minutes. Do not mix this solution with whole blood or its derivatives. Discard unused reconstituted solution after 24 hours.

Ethacrynic acid should not be given subcutaneously or intramuscularly because of local pain and irritation.

TORSEMIDE

Rx	**Torsemide** (Teva)	**Tablets**: 5 mg	Lactose. In 100s.
Rx	**Demadex** (Roche)		Lactose. (102 5). White, scored. Oval. In UD 100s.
Rx	**Torsemide** (Teva)	10 mg	Lactose. In 100s.
Rx	**Demadex** (Roche)		Lactose. (103 10). White, scored. Oval. In UD 100s.
Rx	**Torsemide** (Teva)	20 mg	Lactose. In 100s.
Rx	**Demadex** (Roche)		Lactose. (104 20). White, scored. Oval. In UD 100s.
Rx	**Torsemide** (Teva)	100 mg	Lactose. In 100s.
Rx	**Demadex** (Roche)		Lactose. (105 100). White, scored. Capsule shape. In UD 100s.
Rx	**Demadex** (Roche)	**Injection**: 10 mg/ml	In 2 and 5 ml amps.

TORSEMIDE — ORAL

For complete and comparative prescribing information, refer to the Loop Diuretics group monograph.

Indications

➤*Edema:* For the treatment of edema associated with congestive heart failure, renal disease, or hepatic disease. Use of torsemide has been found to be effective for the treatment of edema associated with chronic renal failure. Chronic use of any diuretic in hepatic disease has not been studied in adequate and well-controlled trials.

➤*Hypertension:* For the treatment of hypertension alone or in combination with other antihypertensive agents.

Administration and Dosage

➤*Approved by the FDA:* August 23, 1993.

Torsemide tablets may be given at any time in relation to a meal, as convenient. Special dosage adjustment in the elderly is not necessary.

Because of the high bioavailability of torsemide, oral and IV doses are therapeutically equivalent, so patients may be switched to and from the IV form with no change in dose.

➤*Congestive heart failure:* The usual initial dose is 10 mg or 20 mg of once-daily torsemide. If the diuretic response is inadequate, the dose should be titrated upward by approximately doubling until the desired diuretic response is obtained. Single doses higher than 200 mg have not been adequately studied.

➤*Chronic renal failure:* The usual initial dose of torsemide is 20 mg of once-daily torsemide. If the diuretic response is inadequate, the dose should be titrated upward by approximately doubling until the desired diuretic response is obtained. Single doses higher than 200 mg have not been adequately studied.

➤*Hepatic cirrhosis:* The usual initial dose is 5 or 10 mg of once-daily torsemide, administered together with an aldosterone antagonist or a potassium-sparing diuretic. If the diuretic response is inadequate, the dose should be titrated upward by approximately doubling until the desired diuretic response is obtained. Single doses greater than 40 mg have not been adequately studied.

➤*Hypertension:* The usual initial dose is 5 mg once daily. If the 5 mg dose does not provide adequate reduction in blood pressure within 4 to 6 weeks, the dose may be increased to 10 mg once daily. If the response to 10 mg is insufficient, an additional antihypertensive agent should be added to the treatment regimen.

➤*Storage/Stability:* Store all dosage forms at 15° to 30°C (59° to 86°F). Do not freeze.

TORSEMIDE — INJECTION

For complete and comparative prescribing information, refer to the Loop Diuretics group monograph.

Indications

➤*Edema:* For the treatment of edema associated with congestive heart failure, renal disease, or hepatic disease. Use of torsemide has been found to be effective for the treatment of edema associated with chronic renal failure. Chronic use of any diuretic in hepatic disease has not been studied in adequate and well-controlled trials. Torsemide is indicated for the treatment of hypertension alone or in combination with other antihypertensive agents.

Torsemide IV injection is indicated when a rapid onset of diuresis is desired or when oral administration is impractical.

Administration and Dosage

➤*Approved by the FDA:* August 23, 1993.

Because of the high bioavailability of torsemide, oral and IV doses are therapeutically equivalent, so patients may be switched to and from the IV form with no change in dose. Torsemide IV injection should be administered either slowly as a bolus over a period of 2 minutes or administered as a continuous infusion.

If torsemide is administered through an IV line, it is recommended that, as with other injections, the IV line be flushed with normal saline (Sodium Chloride Injection, USP) before and after administration. Torsemide injection is formulated above pH 8.3. Flushing the line is recommended to avoid the potential for incompatibilities caused by differences in pH which could be indicated by color change, haziness or the formation of a precipitate in the solution.

If torsemide is administered as a continuous infusion, stability has been demonstrated through 24 hours at room temperature in plastic containers for the following fluids and concentrations:

Fluids and concentrations	
Demonstrated stability through 24 hours at room temperature in plastic containers	
200 mg torsemide (10 mg/mL) added to:	250 mL Dextrose 5% in water
	250 mL 0.9% Sodium Chloride
	500 mL 0.45% Sodium Chloride

Fluids and concentrations	
Demonstrated stability through 24 hours at room temperature in plastic containers	
50 mg torsemide (10 mg/mL) added to:	500 mL Dextrose 5% in water
	500 mL 0.9% Sodium Chloride
	500 mL 0.45% Sodium Chloride

➤*Congestive heart failure:* The usual initial dose is 10 or 20 mg of once-daily torsemide. If the diuretic response is inadequate, the dose should be titrated upward by approximately doubling until the desired diuretic response is obtained. Single doses greater than 200 mg have not been adequately studied.

➤*Chronic renal failure:* The usual initial dose of torsemide is 20 mg of once-daily torsemide. If the diuretic response is inadequate, the dose should be titrated upward by approximately doubling until the desired diuretic response is obtained. Single doses greater than 200 mg have not been adequately studied.

➤*Hepatic cirrhosis:* The usual initial dose is 5 or 10 mg of once-daily torsemide, administered together with an aldosterone antagonist or a potassium-sparing diuretic. If the diuretic response is inadequate, the dose should be titrated upward by approximately doubling until the desired diuretic response is obtained. Single doses greater than 40 mg have not been adequately studied.

➤*Hypertension:* The usual initial dose is 5 mg once daily. If the 5 mg dose does not provide adequate reduction in blood pressure within 4 to 6 weeks, the dose may be increased to 10 mg once daily. If the response to 10 mg is insufficient, an additional antihypertensive agent should be added to the treatment regimen.

➤*Storage/Stability:* Store all dosage forms at 15° to 30°C (59° to 86°F). Do not freeze.

Actions

➤*Pharmacology:* In the kidney, potassium is filtered at the glomerulus and then absorbed parallel to sodium throughout the proximal tubule and thick ascending limb of the loop of Henle, so that only minor amounts reach the distal convoluted tubule. As a result, potassium appearing in urine is secreted at the distal tubule and collecting duct. The potassium-sparing diuretics interfere with sodium reabsorption at the distal tubule, thus decreasing potassium secretion. They exert a weak diuretic and antihypertensive effect when used alone. Their major use is to enhance the action and counteract the kaliuretic effect of thiazide and loop diuretics.

Spironolactone – Spironolactone, a competitive inhibitor of aldosterone, binds to aldosterone receptors of the distal tubule and prevents the formation of a protein important in sodium transport. The dose of spironolactone required to produce an effect varies according to the amount of aldosterone present. It is effective in primary and secondary hyperaldosteronism. Spironolactone is effective in lowering systolic and diastolic blood pressure in both primary hyperaldosteronism and essential hypertension, although aldosterone secretion may be normal in benign essential hypertension. In addition, spironolactone interferes with testosterone synthesis and may increase peripheral conversion of testosterone to estradiol. This action may be responsible for endocrine abnormalities occasionally noted with therapy.

Amiloride/Triamterene – Amiloride and triamterene not only inhibit sodium reabsorption induced by aldosterone, but they also inhibit basal sodium reabsorption. They are not aldosterone antagonists, but act directly on the renal distal tubule, cortical collecting tubule and collecting duct. They induce a reversal of polarity of the transtubular electrical-potential difference and inhibit active transport of sodium and potassium. Amiloride may inhibit sodium, potassium-ATPase. Amiloride decreases the enhanced urinary excretion of magnesium that occurs when a thiazide or loop diuretic is used alone; it also decreases calcium excretion.

Potassium-Sparing Diuretics: Pharmacological and Pharmacokinetic Properties			
Parameters	Amiloride	Spironolactone	Triamterene
Pharmacology			
Tubular site of action	Proximal = distal	Distal	Distal
Mechanism of action	Na^+, K^+–ATPase inhibition; Na^+/H^+ exchange mechanism inhibition (proximal tubule)	Aldosterone antagonism	Membrane effect
Action:			
Onset (hours)	2	24 to 48	2 to 4
Peak (hours)	6 to 10	48 to 72	6 to 8
Duration (hours)	24	48 to 72	12 to 16
Pharmacokinetics			
Bioavailability	15% to 25%	> 90%	30% to 70%
Protein binding	23%	≥ 98%[1]	50% to 67%
Half-life (hours)	6 to 9	20[2]	3
Active metabolites	none	canrenone	hydroxytriamterene sulfate
Peak plasma levels (hours)	3 to 4	canrenone: 2 to 4[3]	3
Excreted unchanged in urine	≈ 50%[4]	–[4]	≈ 21%
Daily dose (mg)	5 to 20	25 to 400	200 to 300

[1] Canrenone greater than 98%.
[2] 10 to 35 hours for canrenone.
[3] 40% excreted in stool within 72 hours.
[4] Metabolites primarily excreted in urine, but also in bile.

AMILORIDE HYDROCHLORIDE

Rx	**Midamor** (Merck)	**Tablets:** 5 mg	(MSD 92). Yellow. Diamond shape. In 100s.

AMILORIDE — ORAL

Refer to the general discussion of these agents in the Potassium-Sparing Diuretics introduction.

WARNING

Hyperkalemia – Like other potassium-conserving agents, amiloride may cause hyperkalemia (serum potassium levels greater than 5.5 mEq per liter) which, if uncorrected, is potentially fatal. Hyperkalemia occurs commonly (about 10%) when amiloride is used without a kaliuretic diuretic. This incidence is greater in patients with renal impairment, diabetes mellitus (with or without recognized renal insufficiency), and in the elderly. When amiloride is used concomitantly with a thiazide diuretic in patients without these complications, the risk of hyperkalemia is reduced to about 1% to 2%. It is thus essential to monitor serum potassium levels carefully in any patient receiving amiloride, particularly when it is first introduced, at the time of diuretic dosage adjustments, and during any illness that could affect renal function.

Indications

Adjunctive treatment with thiazide diuretics or other kaliuretic-diuretic agents in congestive heart failure or hypertension to:

1.) help restore normal serum potassium levels in patients who develop hypokalemia on the kaliuretic diuretic
2.) prevent development of hypokalemia in patients who would be exposed to particular risk if hypokalemia were to develop (eg, digitalized patients or patients with significant cardiac arrhythmias).

The use of potassium-conserving agents is often unnecessary in patients receiving diuretics for uncomplicated essential hypertension when such patients have a normal diet. Amiloride has little additive diuretic or antihypertensive effect when added to a thiazide diuretic.

Amiloride should rarely be used alone. It has weak (compared with thiazides) diuretic and antihypertensive effects. Used as single agents, potassium sparing diuretics, including amiloride, result in an increased risk of hyperkalemia (approximately 10% with amiloride). Amiloride should be used alone only when persistent hypokalemia has been documented and only with careful titration of the dose and close monitoring of serum electrolytes.

➤*Unlabeled uses:* Reducing lithium-induced polyuria; aerosolized amiloride (drug dissolved in 0.3% saline delivered by nebulizer) appears to slow the progression of pulmonary function reduction in adults with cystic fibrosis.

Administration and Dosage

➤*Approved by the FDA:* January 1986.

Amiloride should be administered with food.

➤*Concomitant therapy:* Amiloride, one 5 mg tablet daily, should be added to the usual antihypertensive or diuretic dosage of a kaliuretic diuretic. The dosage may be increased to 10 mg/day, if necessary. More than two 5 mg tablets of amiloride daily usually are not needed, and there is little controlled experience with such doses. If persistent hypokalemia is documented with 10 mg, the dose can be increased to 15 mg, then 20 mg, with careful monitoring of electrolytes.

In treating patients with congestive heart failure after an initial diuresis has been achieved, potassium loss may also decrease and the need for amiloride should be reevaluated. Dosage adjustment may be necessary. Maintenance therapy may be on an intermittent basis.

➤*Single drug therapy:* If it is necessary to use amiloride alone (see Indications), the starting dosage should be one 5 mg tablet daily. This dosage may be increased to 10 mg per day, if necessary. More than two 5 mg tablets usually are not needed, and there is little controlled experience with such doses. If persistent hypokalemia is documented with 10 mg, the dose can be increased to 15 mg, then 20 mg, with careful monitoring of electrolytes.

➤*Storage/Stability:* Protect from moisture, freezing and excessive heat.

Actions

➤*Pharmacology:* In the kidney, potassium is filtered at the glomerulus and then absorbed parallel to sodium throughout the proximal tubule and thick ascending limb of the loop of Henle, so that only minor amounts reach the distal convoluted tubule. As a result, potassium appearing in urine is secreted at the distal tubule and collecting duct. The potassium-sparing diuretics interfere with sodium reabsorption at the distal tubule, thus decreasing potassium secretion.

Amiloride is a potassium-conserving (antikaliuretic) drug that possesses weak (compared with thiazide diuretics) natriuretic, diuretic, and antihypertensive activity. These effects have been partially additive to the effects of thiazide diuretics in some clinical studies. When administered with a thiazide or loop diuretic, amiloride has been shown to decrease the enhanced urinary excretion of magnesium which occurs when a thiazide or loop diuretic is used alone. Amiloride has potassium-conserving activity in patients receiving kaliuretic-diuretic agents.

Amiloride is not an aldosterone antagonist and its effects are seen even in the absence of aldosterone.

Amiloride exerts its potassium sparing effect through the inhibition of sodium reabsorption at the distal convoluted tubule, cortical collecting tubule and collecting duct; this decreases the net negative potential of the tubular lumen and reduces both potassium and hydrogen secretion and their subsequent excretion. This mechanism accounts in large part for the potassium sparing action of amiloride.

➤*Pharmacokinetics:*

Absorption/Distribution – Approximately 15% to 25% of a dose of amiloride is absorbed from the gastrointestinal tract following oral administration and amiloride is not highly protein bound (23%). Amiloride usually begins to act within 2 hours after an oral dose. Its effect on electrolyte excretion reaches a peak between 6 and 10 hours and lasts about 24 hours. Peak plasma levels are obtained in 3 to 4 hours and the plasma half-life varies from 6 to 9 hours. Effects on electrolytes increase with single doses of amiloride up to approximately 15 mg.

Metabolism/Excretion – Amiloride is not metabolized by the liver but is excreted unchanged by the kidneys. About 50 percent of a 20 mg dose of amiloride is excreted in the urine and 40% in the stool within 72 hours. Amiloride has little effect on glomerular filtration rate or renal blood flow. Because amiloride is not metabolized by the liver, drug accumulation is not anticipated in patients with hepatic dysfunction, but accumulation can occur if the hepatorenal syndrome develops.

AMILORIDE — ORAL

Contraindications

➤*Hyperkalemia:* Amiloride should not be used in the presence of elevated serum potassium levels (greater than 5.5 mEq/L).

➤*Antikaliuretic therapy or potassium supplementation:* Amiloride should not be given to patients receiving other potassium-conserving agents, such as spironolactone or triamterene. Potassium supplementation in the form of medication, potassium-containing salt substitutes or a potassium-rich diet should not be used with amiloride except in severe and/or refractory cases of hypokalemia. Such concomitant therapy can be associated with rapid increases in serum potassium levels. If potassium supplementation is used, careful monitoring of the serum potassium level is necessary.

➤*Renal impairment:* Anuria, acute or chronic renal insufficiency, and evidence of diabetic nephropathy are contraindications to the use of amiloride. Patients with evidence of renal functional impairment (blood urea nitrogen [BUN] levels over 30 mg/100 mL or serum creatinine levels over 1.5 mg/100 mL) or diabetes mellitus should not receive the drug without careful, frequent and continuing monitoring of serum electrolytes, creatinine, and BUN levels. Potassium retention associated with the use of an antikaliuretic agent is accentuated in the presence of renal impairment and may result in the rapid development of hyperkalemia.

➤*Hypersensitivity:* Amiloride is contraindicated in patients who are hypersensitive to this product.

Warnings

➤*Hyperkalemia:* The risk of hyperkalemia may be increased when potassium-conserving agents, including amiloride, are administered concomitantly with an angiotensin-converting enzyme inhibitor (see Drug Interactions). Warning signs or symptoms of hyperkalemia include paresthesias, muscular weakness, fatigue, flaccid paralysis of the extremities, bradycardia, shock, and ECG abnormalities. Monitoring of the serum potassium level is essential because mild hyperkalemia is not usually associated with an abnormal ECG.

When abnormal, the ECG in hyperkalemia is characterized primarily by tall, peaked T waves or elevations from previous tracings. There may also be lowering of the R wave and increased depth of the S wave, widening and even disappearance of the P wave, progressive widening of the QRS complex, prolongation of the PR interval, and ST depression.

➤*Diabetes mellitus:* In diabetic patients, hyperkalemia has been reported with the use of all potassium-conserving diuretics, including amiloride, even in patients without evidence of diabetic nephropathy. Therefore, amiloride should be avoided, if possible, in diabetic patients and, if it is used, serum electrolytes and renal function must be monitored frequently.

Amiloride should be discontinued at least 3 days before glucose tolerance testing.

➤*Metabolic or respiratory acidosis:* Antikaliuretic therapy should be instituted only with caution in severely ill patients in whom respiratory or metabolic acidosis may occur, such as patients with cardiopulmonary disease or poorly controlled diabetes. If amiloride is given to these patients, frequent monitoring of acid-base balance is necessary. Shifts in acid-base balance alter the ratio of extracellular/intracellular potassium, and the development of acidosis may be associated with rapid increases in serum potassium levels.

➤*Hepatic function impairment:* In patients with pre-existing severe liver disease, hepatic encephalopathy manifested by tremors, confusion, and coma, and increased jaundice, have been reported in association with diuretics, including amiloride.

➤*Pregnancy: Category B.* Teratogenicity studies with amiloride in rabbits and mice given 20 and 25 times the maximum human dose, respectively, revealed no evidence of harm to the fetus, although studies showed that the drug crossed the placenta in modest amounts. Reproduction studies in rats at 20 times the expected maximum daily dose for humans showed no evidence of impaired fertility. At approximately 5 or more times the expected maximum daily dose for humans, some toxicity was seen in adult rats and rabbits and a decrease in rat pup growth and survival occurred. There are, however, no adequate and well-controlled studies in pregnant women. Because animal reproduction studies are not always predictive of human response, this drug should be used during pregnancy only if clearly needed.

➤*Lactation:* Studies in rats have shown that amiloride is excreted in milk in concentrations higher than those found in blood, but it is not known whether amiloride is excreted in human milk. Because many drugs are excreted in human milk and because of the potential for serious adverse reactions in nursing infants from amiloride, a decision should be made whether to discontinue nursing or to discontinue the drug, taking into account the importance of the drug to the mother.

➤*Children:* Safety and efficacy have not been established.

Precautions

➤*Electrolyte imbalance and BUN increases:* Hyponatremia and hypochloremia may occur when amiloride is used with other diuretics and increases in BUN levels have been reported. These increases usually have accompanied vigorous fluid elimination, especially when diuretic therapy was used in seriously ill patients, such as those who had hepatic cirrhosis with ascites and metabolic alkalosis, or those with resistant edema. Therefore, when amiloride is given with other diuretics to such patients, careful monitoring of serum electrolytes and BUN levels is important.

Drug Interactions

Amiloride Drug Interactions

Precipitant drug	Object drug*		Description
Amiloride	Digoxin	⬇	In six healthy subjects, amiloride increased the renal clearance and decreased the nonrenal clearance of digoxin. It also appeared to decrease the inotropic effect of digoxin.
Amiloride	Potassium preparations	⬆	Concurrent administration may result in severe hyperkalemia, possibly with cardiac arrhythmias or cardiac arrest. Avoid concomitant use.
ACE inhibitors	Amiloride	⬆	Use of ACE inhibitors may result in elevated serum potassium concentration. Concurrent use with amiloride may lead to significant hyperkalemia.
NSAIDs	Amiloride	⬇	NSAIDs may reduce the therapeutic effect of amiloride. Also, since indomethocin may be associated with increased potassium levels, consider this effect when amiloride is used concurrently.

* ⬆ = Object drug increased. ⬇ = Object drug decreased.

Lithium generally should not be given with diuretics because they reduce its renal clearance and add a high risk of lithium toxicity. However, amiloride may be given to reduce lithium-induced polyuria (see Unlabeled Uses). Read monographs for lithium preparations before use of such concomitant therapy.

Adverse Reactions

Amiloride is usually well tolerated and, except for hyperkalemia (serum potassium levels greater than 5.5 mEq/L, see Warnings), significant adverse effects have been reported infrequently. Minor adverse reactions were reported relatively frequently (about 20%) but the relationship of many of the reports to amiloride is uncertain and the overall frequency was similar in hydrochlorothiazide treated groups. Nausea/anorexia, abdominal pain, flatulence, and mild skin rash have been reported and probably are related to amiloride. Other adverse experiences that have been reported with amiloride are generally those known to be associated with diuresis, or with the underlying disease being treated.

The incidence for column 1 was determined from clinical studies conducted in the United States (837 patients treated with amiloride). The adverse effects listed in column 2 include reports from the same clinical studies and voluntary reports since marketing. The probability of a causal relationship exists between amiloride and these adverse reactions, some of which have been reported only rarely.

Amiloride Adverse Reactions

Incidence > 1%	Incidence ≤ 1%
Miscellaneous	
Headache**	Back pain
Weakness	Chest pain
Fatigability	Neck/shoulder ache
	Pain, extremities
Cardiovascular	
None	Angina pectoris
	Orthostatic hypotension
	Arrhythmia
	Palpitation
GI	
Nausea/anorexia**	Jaundice
Diarrhea**	GI bleeding
Vomiting**	Abdominal fullness
Abdominal pain	GI disturbance
Gas pain	Thirst
Appetite changes	Heartburn
Constipation	Flatulence
	Dyspepsia
Metabolic	
Elevated serum potassium levels (> 5.5 mEq/L)***	None
Dermatologic	
None	Skin rash
	Itching
	Dryness of mouth
	Pruritus
	Alopecia

AMILORIDE — ORAL

Amiloride Adverse Reactions	
Incidence > 1%	Incidence ≤ 1%
Musculoskeletal Muscle cramps	Joint pain Leg ache
CNS Dizziness Encephalopathy	Paresthesia Tremors Vertigo
Psychiatric None	Nervousness Mental confusion Insomnia Decreased libido Depression Somnolence
Respiratory Cough Dyspnea	Shortness of breath
Special senses None	Visual disturbances Nasal congestion Tinnitus Increased intraocular pressure
GU Impotence	Polyuria Dysuria Urinary frequency Bladder spasms
	Gynecomastia

** Reactions occurring in 3% to 8% of patients treated with amiloride. (Those reactions occurring in less than 3% of the patients are unmarked.)
*** See Warnings.

➤*Causal relationship unknown:* Other reactions have been reported but occurred under circumstances where a causal relationship could not be established. However, in these rarely reported events, that possibility cannot be excluded. Therefore, these observations are listed to serve as alerting information to physicians: activation of probable pre-existing peptic ulcer, aplastic anemia, neutropenia, abnormal liver function.

Overdosage

➤*Symptoms:* No data are available in regard to overdosage in humans.

It is not known whether the drug is dialyzable.

The most likely signs and symptoms to be expected with overdosage are dehydration and electrolyte imbalance. These can be treated by established procedures.

➤*Treatment:* Therapy with amiloride should be discontinued and the patient observed closely. There is no specific antidote. Emesis should be induced or gastric lavage performed. Treatment is symptomatic and supportive. If hyperkalemia occurs, active measures should be taken to reduce the serum potassium levels.

Patient Information

May cause GI upset; take with food.

Notify physician if any of the following occurs: Muscular weakness; fatigue; muscle cramps.

May cause dizziness, headache, or visual disturbances; observe caution while driving or performing other tasks requiring alertness, coordination or physical dexterity.

Avoid large quantities of potassium-rich food.

SPIRONOLACTONE

Rx	**Spironolactone** (Various, eg, Geneva, Mylan, Parmed)	**Tablets:** 25 mg	In 100s, 250s, 500s, and 1,000s.
Rx	**Aldactone** (Searle)		(Searle 1001 Aldactone 25). Lt. yellow. Film coated. In 100s, 500s, 1,000s, 2,500s, and UD 100s.
Rx	**Spironolactone** (Various, eg, Mutual, Mylan)	**Tablets:** 50 mg	In 50s, 100s, 250s, 1,000s, and UD 30s and 60s.
Rx	**Aldactone** (Searle)		(Searle 1041 Aldactone 50). Lt. orange, scored. Oval. Film coated. In 100s and UD 100s.
Rx	**Spironolactone** (Various, eg, Mutual, Mylan)	**Tablets:** 100 mg	In 50s, 100s, 250s, 1,000s, and UD 30s and 60s.
Rx	**Aldactone** (Searle)		(Searle 1031 Aldactone 100). Peach, scored. Film coated. In 100s and UD 100s.

SPIRONOLACTONE — ORAL

Refer to the general discussion of these agents in the Potassium-Sparing Diuretics introduction.

WARNING

Spironolactone has been shown to be a tumorigen in chronic toxicity studies in rats. Spironolactone should be used only in those conditions for which it is indicated. Unnecessary use of this drug should be avoided.

Indications

➤*Primary hyperaldosteronism:* Establishing the diagnosis of primary hyperaldosteronism by therapeutic trial. Short-term preoperative treatment of patients with primary hyperaldosteronism. Long-term maintenance therapy for patients with discrete aldosterone-producing adrenal adenomas who are judged to be poor operative risks or who decline surgery. Long term maintenance therapy for patients with bilateral micro- or macronodular adrenal hyperplasia (idiopathic hyperaldosteronism).

➤*Edematous conditions:*

Congestive heart failure – For the management of edema and sodium retention when the patient is only partially responsive to, or is intolerant of, other therapeutic measures. Spironolactone is also indicated for patients with congestive heart failure taking digitalis when other therapies are considered inappropriate.

Cirrhosis of the liver accompanied by edema and/or ascites – Aldosterone levels may be exceptionally high in this condition. Spironolactone is indicated for maintenance therapy together with bed rest and the restriction of fluid and sodium.

The nephrotic syndrome – For nephrotic patients when treatment of the underlying disease, restriction of fluid and sodium intake, and the use of other diuretics do not provide an adequate response.

➤*Essential hypertension:* Usually in combination with other drugs, spironolactone is indicated for patients who cannot be treated adequately with other agents or for whom other agents are considered inappropriate.

➤*Hypokalemia:* For the treatment of patients with hypokalemia when other measures are considered inappropriate or inadequate. Spironolactone is also indicated for the prophylaxis of hypokalemia in patients taking digitalis when other measures are considered inadequate or inappropriate.

➤*Use in pregnancy:* The routine use of diuretics in an otherwise healthy woman is inappropriate and exposes mother and fetus to unnecessary hazard. Diuretics do not prevent development of toxemia of pregnancy, and there is no satisfactory evidence that they are useful in the treatment of developing toxemia.

Spironolactone is indicated in pregnancy when edema is due to pathologic causes just as it is in the absence of pregnancy. However, there are no adequate and well-controlled studies with spironolactone in pregnant women. Spironolactone has known endocrine effects in animals including progestational and antiandrogenic effects. The antiandrogenic effects can result in apparent estrogenic side effects in humans, such as gynecomastia. Therefore, the use of spironolactone in pregnant women requires that the anticipated benefit be weighed against the possible hazards to the fetus. Dependent edema in pregnancy, resulting from restriction of venous return by the expanded uterus, is properly treated through elevation of the lower extremities and use of support hose; use of diuretics to lower intravascular volume in this case is unsupported and unnecessary. There is hypervolemia during normal pregnancy which is not harmful to either the fetus or the mother (in the absence of cardiovascular disease), but which is associated with edema, including generalized edema, in the majority of pregnant women. If this edema produces discomfort, increased recumbency will often provide relief. In rare instances, this edema may cause extreme discomfort which is not relieved by rest. In these cases, a short course of diuretics may provide relief and may be appropriate.

➤*Unlabeled uses:* Hirsutism; premenstrual syndrome (PMS); short-term treatment of acne vulgaris.

The combination of spironolactone and testolactone for at least 6 months may be effective for short-term treatment of familial male precocious puberty.

SPIRONOLACTONE — ORAL

Administration and Dosage

➤*Approved by the FDA:* October 17, 1985.

➤*Primary hyperaldosteronism:* Spironolactone may be employed as an initial diagnostic measure to provide presumptive evidence of primary hyperaldosteronism while patients are on normal diets.

Long test – Spironolactone is administered at a daily dosage of 400 mg for 3 to 4 weeks. Correction of hypokalemia and of hypertension provides presumptive evidence for the diagnosis of primary hyperaldosteronism.

Short test – Spironolactone is administered at a daily dosage of 400 mg for 4 days. If serum potassium increases during spironolactone administration but drops when spironolactone is discontinued, a presumptive diagnosis of primary hyperaldosteronism should be considered.

After the diagnosis of hyperaldosteronism has been established by more definitive testing procedures, spironolactone may be administered in doses of 100 to 400 mg daily in preparation for surgery. For patients who are considered unsuitable for surgery, spironolactone may be employed for long-term maintenance therapy at the lowest effective dosage determined for the individual patient.

➤*Edema in adults (congestive heart failure, hepatic cirrhosis, or nephrotic syndrome):* An initial daily dosage of 100 mg of spironolactone administered in either single or divided doses is recommended, but may range from 25 to 200 mg daily. When given as the sole agent for diuresis, spironolactone should be continued for at least 5 days at the initial dosage level, after which it may be adjusted to the optimal therapeutic or maintenance level administered in either single or divided daily doses. If, after 5 days, an adequate diuretic response to spironolactone has not occurred, a second diuretic which acts more proximally in the renal tubule may be added to the regimen. Because of the additive effect of spironolactone when administered concurrently with such diuretics, an enhanced diuresis usually begins on the first day of combined treatment; combined therapy is indicated when more rapid diuresis is desired. The dosage of spironolactone should remain unchanged when other diuretic therapy is added.

➤*Essential hypertension:* For adults, an initial daily dosage of 50 to 100 mg of spironolactone administered in either single or divided doses is recommended. Spironolactone may also be given with diuretics which act more proximally in the renal tubule or with other antihypertensive agents. Treatment with spironolactone should be continued for at least 2 weeks, since the maximum response may not occur before this time. Subsequently, dosage should be adjusted according to the response of the patient.

➤*Hypokalemia:* Spironolactone in a dosage ranging from 25 mg to 100 mg daily is useful in treating a diuretic-induced hypokalemia, when oral potassium supplements or other potassium-sparing regimens are considered inappropriate.

➤*Storage/Stability:* Store below 25°C (77°F). Dispense in a tight, light-resistant, child-resistant container.

Actions

➤*Pharmacology:* Spironolactone is a specific pharmacologic antagonist of aldosterone, acting primarily through competitive binding of receptors at the aldosterone-dependent sodium-potassium exchange site in the distal convoluted renal tubule. Spironolactone causes increased amounts of sodium and water to be excreted, while potassium is retained. Spironolactone acts both as a diuretic and as an antihypertensive drug by this mechanism. It may be given alone or with other diuretic agents which act more proximally in the renal tubule.

Aldosterone antagonist activity – Increased levels of the mineralocorticoid, aldosterone, are present in primary and secondary hyperaldosteronism. Edematous states in which secondary aldosteronism is usually involved include congestive heart failure, hepatic cirrhosis, and the nephrotic syndrome. By competing with aldosterone for receptor sites, spironolactone provides effective therapy for the edema and ascites in those conditions. Spironolactone counteracts secondary aldosteronism induced by the volume depletion and associated sodium loss caused by active diuretic therapy.

Spironolactone is effective in lowering the systolic and diastolic blood pressure in patients with primary hyperaldosteronism. It is also effective in most cases of essential hypertension, despite the fact that aldosterone secretion may be within normal limits in benign essential hypertension.

Through its action in antagonizing the effect of aldosterone, spironolactone inhibits the exchange of sodium for potassium in the distal renal tubule and helps to prevent potassium loss.

➤*Pharmacokinetics:* Spironolactone is rapidly and extensively metabolized. Sulfur-containing products are the predominant metabolites and are thought to be primarily responsible, together with spironolactone, for the therapeutic effects of the drug. The following pharmacokinetic data were obtained from 12 healthy volunteers following the administration of 100 mg of spironolactone (as tablets) daily for 15 days. On the 15th day, spironolactone was taken immediately after a low-fat breakfast and blood was drawn thereafter.

Spironolactone Pharmacokinetic Data

	Accumulation factor: AUC (0-24 hrs, day 15)/ AUC (0-24 hrs, day 1)	Mean peak serum concentration	Mean (SD) post-steady-state half-life
7-α-(thiomethyl) spirolactone (TMS)	1.25	391 ng/mL at 3.2 hours	13.8 hours (6.4) (terminal)
6-β-hydroxy-7-α-(thiomethyl) spirolactone (HTMS)	1.5	125 ng/mL at 5.1 hours	15 hours (4) (terminal)
Canrenone (C)	1.41	181 ng/mL at 4.3 hours	16.5 hours (6.3) (terminal)
Spironolactone	1.3	80 ng/mL at 2.6 hours	Approximately 1.4 hours (0.5) (β half-life)

The pharmacological activity of spironolactone metabolites in man is not known. However, in the adrenalectomized rat the antimineralocorticoid activities of the metabolites C, TMS, and HTMS, relative to spironolactone, were 1.1, 1.28, and 0.32, respectively. Relative to spironolactone, their binding affinities to the aldosterone receptors in rat kidney slices were 0.19, 0.86, and 0.06, respectively.

In humans the potencies of TMS and 7-α-thiospirolactone in reversing the effects of the synthetic mineralocorticoid, fludrocortisone, on urinary electrolyte composition were 0.33 and 0.26, respectively, relative to spironolactone. However, since the serum concentrations of these steroids were not determined, their incomplete absorption and/or first-pass metabolism could not be ruled out as a reason for their reduced in vivo activities.

Both spironolactone and its metabolites are more than 90% bound to plasma proteins. The metabolites are excreted primarily in the urine and secondarily in bile.

The effect of food on spironolactone absorption (two 100 mg spironolactone tablets) was assessed in a single dose study of 9 healthy, drug-free volunteers. Food increased the bioavailability of unmetabolized spironolactone by almost 100%. The clinical importance of this finding is not known.

Contraindications

Anuria, acute renal insufficiency, significant impairment of renal excretory function, or hyperkalemia.

Warnings

➤*Hyperkalemia:* Potassium supplementation, either in the form of medication or as a diet rich in potassium, should not ordinarily be given in association with spironolactone therapy. Excessive potassium intake may cause hyperkalemia in patients receiving spironolactone. Spironolactone should not be administered concurrently with other potassium-sparing diuretics. Spironolactone, when used with ACE inhibitors or indomethacin, even in the presence of a diuretic, has been associated with severe hyperkalemia. Extreme caution should be exercised when spironolactone is given concomitantly with these drugs.

If hyperkalemia is suspected (warning signs include paresthesia, muscle weakness, fatigue, flaccid paralysis of the extremities, bradycardia and shock) an electrocardiogram (ECG) should be obtained. However, it is important to monitor serum potassium levels because mild hyperkalemia may not be associated with ECG changes.

If hyperkalemia is present, spironolactone should be discontinued immediately. With severe hyperkalemia, the clinical situation dictates the procedures to be employed. These include the intravenous administration of calcium chloride solution, sodium bicarbonate solution and/or the oral or parenteral administration of glucose with a rapid-acting insulin preparation. These are temporary measures to be repeated as required. Cationic exchange resins such as sodium polystyrene sulfonate may be orally or rectally administered. Persistent hyperkalemia may require dialysis.

➤*Renal function impairment:* Spironolactone therapy may cause a transient elevation of BUN, especially in patients with preexisting renal impairment. Spironolactone may cause mild acidosis.

➤*Hepatic function impairment:* Spironolactone should be used with caution in patients with impaired hepatic function because minor alterations of fluid and electrolyte balance may precipitate hepatic coma.

➤*Carcinogenesis:* Orally administered spironolactone has been shown to be a tumorigen in dietary administration studies performed in rats, with its proliferative effects manifested on endocrine organs and the liver. In an 18-month study using doses of about 50, 150 and 500 mg/kg/day, there were statistically significant increases in benign adenomas of the thyroid and testes and, in male rats, a dose-related increase in proliferative changes in the liver (including hepatocytomegaly and hyperplastic nodules). In a 24-month study in which the same strain of rat was administered doses of about 10, 30, 100 and 150 mg spironolactone/kg/day, the range of proliferative effects included significant increases in hepatocellular adenomas and testicular interstitial cell tumors in males, and significant increases in thyroid follicular cell adenomas and carcinomas in both sexes. There was also a statistically significant, but not dose-related, increase in benign uterine endometrial stromal polyps in females.

SPIRONOLACTONE — ORAL

A dose-related (above 20 mg/kg/day) incidence of myelocytic leukemia was observed in rats fed daily doses of potassium canrenoate (a compound chemically similar to spironolactone and whose primary metabolite, canrenone, is also a major product of spironolactone in man) for a period of 1 year. In 2-year studies in the rat, oral administration of potassium canrenoate was associated with myelocytic leukemia and hepatic, thyroid, testicular and mammary tumors.

➤*Mutagenesis:* In the presence of metabolic activation, spironolactone has been reported to be negative in some mammalian mutagenicity tests in vitro and inconclusive (but slightly positive) for mutagenicity in other mammalian tests in vitro. In the presence of metabolic activation, potassium canrenoate has been reported to test positive for mutagenicity in some mammalian tests in vitro, inconclusive in others, and negative in still others.

➤*Fertility impairment:* In a 3-litter reproduction study in which female rats received dietary doses of 15 and 50 mg spironolactone/kg/day, there were no effects on mating and fertility, but there was a small increase in incidence of stillborn pups at 50 mg/kg/day. When injected into female rats (100 mg/kg/day for 7 days, intraperitoneally), spironolactone was found to increase the length of the estrous cycle by prolonging diestrus during treatment and inducing constant diestrus during a 2-week posttreatment observation period. These effects were associated with retarded ovarian follicle development and a reduction in circulating estrogen levels, which would be expected to impair mating, fertility and fecundity. Spironolactone (100 mg/kg/day), administered intraperitoneally to female mice during a 2-week cohabitation period with untreated males, decreased the number of mated mice that conceived (effect shown to be caused by an inhibition of ovulation) and decreased the number of implanted embryos in those that became pregnant (effect shown to be caused by an inhibition of implantation), and at 200 mg/kg, also increased the latency period to mating.

➤*Pregnancy: Category C.*

Teratology studies with spironolactone have been carried out in mice and rabbits at doses of up to 20 mg/kg/day. On a body surface area basis, this dose in the mouse is substantially below the maximum recommended human dose and, in the rabbit, approximates the maximum recommended human dose. No teratogenic or other embryotoxic effects were observed in mice, but the 20 mg/kg dose caused an increased rate of resorption and a lower number of live fetuses in rabbits. Because of its antiandrogenic activity and the requirement of testosterone for male morphogenesis, spironolactone may have the potential for adversely affecting sex differentiation of the male during embryogenesis. When administered to rats at 200 mg/kg/day between gestation days 13 and 21 (late embryogenesis and fetal development), feminization of male fetuses was observed. Offspring exposed during late pregnancy to 50 and 100 mg/kg/day doses of spironolactone exhibited changes in the reproductive tract including dose-dependent decreases in weights of the ventral prostate and seminal vesicle in males, ovaries and uteri that were enlarged in females, and other indications of endocrine dysfunction, that persisted into adulthood. There are no adequate and well-controlled studies with spironolactone in pregnant women. Spironolactone has known endocrine effects in animals including progestational and antiandrogenic effects. The antiandrogenic effects can result in apparent estrogenic side effects in humans, such as gynecomastia. Therefore, the use of spironolactone in pregnant women requires that the anticipated benefit be weighed against the possible hazards to the fetus.

➤*Lactation:* Canrenone, a major (and active) metabolite of spironolactone, appears in human breast milk. Because spironolactone has been found to be tumorigenic in rats, a decision should be made whether to discontinue the drug, taking into account the importance of the drug to the mother. If the drug is deemed essential, an alternative method of infant feeding should be instituted.

➤*Children:* Safety and efficacy have not been established.

Precautions

➤*Monitoring:* All patients receiving diuretic therapy should be observed for evidence of fluid or electrolyte imbalance (eg, hypomagnesemia, hyponatremia, hypochloremic alkalosis, hyperkalemia).

➤*Fluid and electrolyte imbalance:* Serum and urine electrolyte determinations are particularly important when the patient is vomiting excessively or receiving parenteral fluids. Warning signs or symptoms of fluid and electrolyte imbalance, irrespective of cause, include dryness of the mouth, thirst, weakness, lethargy, drowsiness, restlessness, muscle pains or cramps, muscular fatigue, hypotension, oliguria, tachycardia, and gastrointestinal disturbances such as nausea and vomiting. Hyperkalemia may occur in patients with impaired renal function or excessive potassium intake and can cause cardiac irregularities, which may be fatal. Consequently, no potassium supplement should ordinarily be given with spironolactone.

Periodic determination of serum electrolytes to detect possible electrolyte imbalance should be done at appropriate intervals, particularly in the elderly and those with significant renal or hepatic impairments.

➤*Concomitant medications:* See Drug Interactions for more information.

➤*Hyperchloremic metabolic acidosis:* Reversible hyperchloremic metabolic acidosis, usually in association with hyperkalemia, has been reported to occur in some patients with decompensated hepatic cirrhosis, even in the presence of normal renal function.

➤*Hyponatremia:* Dilutional hyponatremia, manifested by dryness of the mouth, thirst, lethargy, and drowsiness, and confirmed by a low serum sodium level, may be caused or aggravated, especially when spironolactone is administered in combination with other diuretics, and dilutional hyponatremia may occur in edematous patients in hot weather; appropriate therapy is water restriction rather than administration of sodium, except in rare instances when the hyponatremia is life-threatening.

➤*Gynecomastia:* Gynecomastia may develop in association with the use of spironolactone; physicians should be alert to its possible onset. The development of gynecomastia appears to be related to both dosage level and duration of therapy and is normally reversible when spironolactone is discontinued. In rare instances some breast enlargement may persist when spironolactone is discontinued.

Drug Interactions

Spironolactone Drug Interactions

Precipitant drug	Object drug*		Description
Spironolactone	Anticoagulants	⬇	The hypoprothrombinemic effect may be decreased.
Spironolactone	Digitalis glycosides	⟷	The interaction is complex and difficult to predict. Spironolactone increases the half-life of digoxin and can decrease its clearance. This may result in increased serum digoxin levels and subsequent toxicity. In addition, the drug may attenuate the inotropic action of digoxin. Spironolactone decreases and increases digitoxin's elimination half-life.
Spironolactone	Mitotane	⬇	One patient failed to respond to mitotane while receiving concurrent spironolactone. Mitotane toxicity developed when the drug was discontinued.
Spironolactone	Potassium preparations	⬆	Concurrent administration may result in hyperkalemia, possibly with cardiac arrhythmias or cardiac arrest. Avoid concomitant use.
ACE inhibitors	Spironolactone	⬆	Use of ACE inhibitors may elevate serum potassium. Concurrent use with spironolactone may lead to significant hyperkalemia.
Salicylates	Spironolactone	⬇	The diuretic effect of spironolactone may be decreased by concurrent salicylate use, possibly due to reduced tubular secretion of canrenone; this interaction is dose-dependent. The antihypertensive action does not appear altered.

* ⬆ = Object drug increased ⬇ = Object drug decreased ⟷ = Undetermined clinical effect

➤*Alcohol, barbiturates, or narcotics:* Potentiation of orthostatic hypotension may occur.

➤*Corticosteroids, ACTH:* Intensified electrolyte depletion, particularly hypokalemia, may occur.

➤*Pressor amines (eg, norepinephrine):* Spironolactone reduces the vascular responsiveness to norepinephrine. Therefore, caution should be exercised in the management of patients subjected to regional or general anesthesia while they are being treated with spironolactone.

➤*Skeletal muscle relaxants, nondepolarizing (eg, tubocurarine):* Possible increased responsiveness to the muscle relaxant may result.

➤*Lithium:* Lithium generally should not be given with diuretics. Diuretic agents reduce the renal clearance of lithium and add a high risk of lithium toxicity.

➤*Nonsteroidal anti-inflammatory drugs (NSAIDs):* In some patients, the administration of an NSAID can reduce the diuretic, natriuretic, and antihypertensive effect of loop, potassium-sparing and thiazide diuretics. Combination of NSAIDs (eg, indomethacin) with potassium-sparing diuretics has been associated with severe hyperkalemia. Therefore, when spironolactone and NSAIDs are used concomitantly, the patient should be observed closely to determine if the desired effect of the diuretic is obtained.

➤*Drug/Lab test interactions:* Several reports of possible interference with digoxin radioimmunoassays by spironolactone, or its metabolites, have appeared in the literature. Neither the extent nor the potential clinical significance of its interference (which may be assay-specific) has been fully established.

Adverse Reactions

The following adverse reactions have been reported and, within each category (body system), are listed in order of decreasing severity.

➤*CNS:* Mental confusion, ataxia, headache, drowsiness, lethargy.

➤*Endocrine:* Gynecomastia (The development of gynecomastia appears to be related to both dosage level and duration of therapy and is normally reversible when spironolactone is discontinued. In rare instances some breast enlargement may persist when spironolactone is discontinued.), inability to achieve or maintain erection, irregular menses or amenorrhea,

SPIRONOLACTONE — ORAL

postmenopausal bleeding. Carcinoma of the breast has been reported in patients taking spironolactone but a cause and effect relationship has not been established.

➤*GI:* Gastric bleeding, ulceration, gastritis, diarrhea and cramping, nausea, vomiting.

➤*Hematologic:* Agranulocytosis.

➤*Hematologic/Lymphatic:* A very few cases of mixed cholestatic/hepatocellular toxicity, with 1 reported fatality, have been reported with spironolactone administration.

➤*Hypersensitivity:* Fever, urticaria, maculopapular or erythematous cutaneous eruptions, anaphylactic reactions, vasculitis.

➤*Renal:* Renal dysfunction (including renal failure).

Overdosage

➤*Symptoms:* The oral LD_{50} of spironolactone is greater than 1000 mg/kg in mice, rats, and rabbits. Acute overdosage of spironolactone may be manifested by drowsiness, mental confusion, maculopapular or erythematous rash, nausea, vomiting, dizziness, or diarrhea. Rarely, instances of hyponatremia, hyperkalemia, or hepatic coma may occur in patients with severe liver disease, but these are unlikely due to acute overdosage. Hyperkalemia may occur, especially in patients with impaired renal function.

➤*Treatment:* Induce vomiting or evacuate the stomach by lavage. There is no specific antidote. Treatment is supportive to maintain hydration, electrolyte balance, and vital functions.

Patients who have renal impairment may develop spironolactone-induced hyperkalemia. In such cases, spironolactone should be discontinued immediately. With severe hyperkalemia, the clinical situation dictates the procedures to be employed. These include the intravenous administration of calcium chloride solution, sodium bicarbonate solution and/or the oral or parenteral administration of glucose with a rapid-acting insulin preparation. These are temporary measures to be repeated as required. Cationic exchange resins such as sodium polystyrene sulfonate may be orally or rectally administered. Persistent hyperkalemia may require dialysis.

Patient Information

Patients who receive spironolactone should be advised to avoid potassium supplements and foods containing high levels of potassium including salt substitutes.

TRIAMTERENE

Rx	**Dyrenium** (SmithKline Beecham)	**Capsules:** 50 mg	(Dyrenium 50). Red. In 100s and UD 100s.
		100 mg	(Dyrenium 100). Red. In 100s, 1000s and UD 100s.

TRIAMTERENE — ORAL

Refer to the general discussion of these agents in the Potassium-Sparing Diuretics introduction.

Indications

➤*Edema:* For the treatment of edema associated with congestive heart failure, cirrhosis of the liver and the nephrotic syndrome; also in steroid-induced edema, idiopathic edema and edema due to secondary hyperaldosteronism.

Triamterene may be used alone or with other diuretics either for its added diuretic effect or its potassium-sparing potential. It also promotes increased diuresis when patients prove resistant or only partially responsive to thiazides or other diuretics because of secondary hyperaldosteronism.

Administration and Dosage

➤*Adult dosage:* Dosage should be titrated to the needs of the individual patient. When used alone, the usual starting dose is 100 mg twice daily after meals. When combined with another diuretic or antihypertensive agent, the total daily dosage of each agent should usually be lowered initially and then adjusted to the patient's needs. The total daily dosage should not exceed 300 mg (see Precautions). When triamterene is added to other diuretic therapy or when patients are switched to triamterene from other diuretics, all potassium supplementation should be discontinued.

➤*Storage/Stability:* Store between 15° and 30°C (59° and 86°F). Protect from light.

Actions

➤*Pharmacology:* Triamterene has a unique mode of action; it inhibits the reabsorption of sodium ions in exchange for potassium and hydrogen ions at that segment of the distal tubule under the control of adrenal mineralocorticoids (especially aldosterone). This activity is not directly related to aldosterone secretion or antagonism; it is a result of a direct effect on the renal tubule.

The fraction of filtered sodium reaching this distal tubular exchange site is relatively small, and the amount that is exchanged depends on the level of mineralocorticoid activity. Thus, the degree of natriuresis and diuresis produced by inhibition of the exchange mechanism is necessarily limited. Increasing the amount of available sodium and the level of mineralocorticoid activity by the use of more proximally acting diuretics will increase the degree of diuresis and potassium conservation.

Triamterene occasionally causes increases in serum potassium, which can result in hyperkalemia. It does not produce alkalosis because it does not cause excessive excretion of titratable acid and ammonium.

Triamterene has been shown to cross the placental barrier and appear in the cord blood of animals.

➤*Pharmacokinetics:*

Absorption/Distribution – Onset of action is 2 to 4 hours after ingestion. In healthy volunteers the mean peak serum levels were 30 ng/mL at 3 hours. Triamterene is rapidly absorbed, with somewhat less than 50% of the oral dose reaching the urine. Most patients will respond to triamterene during the first day of treatment. Maximum therapeutic effect, however, may not be seen for several days.

Metabolism/Excretion – Triamterene is primarily metabolized to the sulfate conjugate of hydroxytriamterene. Both the plasma and urine levels of this metabolite greatly exceed triamterene levels. The average percent of drug recovered in the urine (0 to 48 hours) was 21%. Duration of diuresis depends on several factors, especially renal function, but it generally tapers off 7 to 9 hours after administration.

Contraindications

Anuria. Severe or progressive kidney disease or dysfunction with the possible exception of nephrosis. Severe hepatic disease. Hypersensitivity to the drug.

Triamterene should not be used in patients with preexisting elevated serum potassium, as is sometimes seen in patients with impaired renal function or azotemia, or in patients who develop hyperkalemia while on the drug. Patients should not be placed on dietary potassium supplements, potassium salts or potassium-containing salt substitutes in conjunction with triamterene.

Triamterene should not be given to patients receiving other potassium-sparing agents such as spironolactone, amiloride hydrochloride or other formulations containing triamterene. Two deaths have been reported in patients receiving concomitant spironolactone and triamterene or formulations containing triamterene. Although dosage recommendations were exceeded in 1 case and in the other serum electrolytes were not properly monitored, these 2 drugs should not be given concomitantly.

Warnings

➤*Hyperkalemia:* Abnormal elevation of serum potassium levels (≥ 5.5 mEq/L) can occur with all potassium-sparing agents, including triamterene. Hyperkalemia is more likely to occur in patients with renal impairment and diabetes (even without evidence of renal impairment), and in the elderly or severely ill. Since uncorrected hyperkalemia may be fatal, serum potassium levels must be monitored at frequent intervals especially in patients receiving triamterene, when dosages are changed or with any illness that may influence renal function.

If hyperkalemia is present or suspected, an electrocardiogram (ECG) should be obtained. If the ECG shows no widening of the QRS or arrhythmia in the presence of hyperkalemia, it is usually sufficient to discontinue triamterene and any potassium supplementation and substitute a thiazide alone. Sodium polystyrene sulfonate may be administered to enhance the excretion of excess potassium. The presence of a widened QRS complex or arrhythmia in association with hyperkalemia requires prompt additional therapy. For tachyarrhythmia, infuse 44 mEq of sodium bicarbonate or 10 mL of 10% calcium gluconate or calcium chloride over several minutes. For asystole, bradycardia or A-V block transvenous pacing is also recommended.

The effect of calcium and sodium bicarbonate is transient and repeated administration may be required. When indicated by the clinical situation, excess K+ may be removed by dialysis or oral or rectal administration of sodium polystyrene sulfonate. Infusion of glucose and insulin has also been used to treat hyperkalemia.

➤*Hypersensitivity reactions:* There have been isolated reports of hypersensitivity reactions; therefore, patients should be observed regularly for the possible occurrence of blood dyscrasias, liver damage or other idiosyncratic reactions.

➤*Carcinogenesis:* In studies conducted under the auspices of the National Toxicology Program, groups of rats were fed diets containing 0, 150, 300, or 600 ppm triamterene, and groups of mice were fed diets containing 0, 100, 200, or 400 ppm triamterene. Male and female rats exposed to the highest tested concentration received triamterene at about 25 and 30 mg/kg/day, respectively. Male and female mice exposed to the highest tested concentration received triamterene at about 45 and 60 mg/kg/day, respectively.

There was an increased incidence of hepatocellular neoplasia (primarily adenomas) in male and female mice at the highest dosage level. These doses represent 7.5 and 10 times the maximum recommended human dose (MRHD) of 300 mg/kg/day (or 6 mg/kg/day based on a 50 kg patient) for male and female mice, respectively, when based on body weight of 0.7 and 0.9 times the MRHD when based on body-surface area.

Although hepatocellular neoplasia (exclusively adenomas) in the rat study was limited to triamterene-exposed males, incidence was not dose-dependent and there was no statistically significant difference from control incidence at any dose level.

➤*Mutagenesis:* Triamterene was not mutagenic in bacteria (*Salmonella typhimurium* strains TA98, TA100, TA1535, or TA1537) with or without metabolic activation. It did not induce chromosomal aberrations in Chinese

TRIAMTERENE — ORAL

hamster ovary (CHO) cells in vitro with or without metabolic activation, but it did induce sister chromatid exchanges in CHO cells in vitro with and without metabolic activation.

➤*Pregnancy: Category C.*

The routine use of diuretics in an otherwise healthy woman is inappropriate and exposes mother and fetus to unnecessary hazard. Diuretics do not prevent development of toxemia of pregnancy, and there is no satisfactory evidence that they are useful in the treatment of developed toxemia.

Edema during pregnancy may arise from pathological causes or from the physiologic and mechanical consequences of pregnancy. Diuretics are indicated in pregnancy when edema is due to pathologic causes, just as they are in the absence of pregnancy (see Precautions). Dependent edema in pregnancy, resulting from restriction of venous return by the expanded uterus, is properly treated through elevation of the lower extremities and use of support hose; use of diuretics to lower intravascular volume in this case is illogical and unnecessary. There is hypervolemia during healthy pregnancy that is harmful to neither the fetus nor the mother (in the absence of cardiovascular disease), but that is associated with edema, including generalized edema, in the majority of pregnant women. If this edema produces discomfort, increased recumbency will often provide relief. In rare instances, this edema may cause extreme discomfort which is not relieved by rest. In these cases, a short course of diuretics may provide relief and may be appropriate.

Reproduction studies have been performed in rats at doses as high as 20 times the MRHD on the basis of body weight, and 6 times the MRHD on the basis of body surface area without evidence of harm to the fetus due to triamterene. Because animal reproduction studies are not always predictive of human response, this drug should be used during pregnancy only if clearly needed.

Triamterene has been shown to cross the placental barrier and appear in the cord blood. The use of triamterene in pregnant women requires that the anticipated benefits be weighed against possible hazards to the fetus. These possible hazards include adverse reactions that have occurred in the adult.

➤*Lactation:* Triamterene has not been studied in nursing mothers. Triamterene appears in animal milk and is likely present in human milk. If use of the drug product is deemed essential, the patient should stop nursing.

➤*Children:* Safety and effectiveness have not been established.

Precautions

➤*Monitoring:* Periodic BUN and serum potassium determinations should be made to check kidney function, especially in patients with suspected or confirmed renal insufficiency. It is particularly important to make serum potassium determinations in elderly or diabetic patients receiving the drug; these patients should be observed carefully for possible serum potassium increases.

➤*Electrolyte imbalance:* Electrolyte imbalance often encountered in such diseases as congestive heart failure, renal disease or cirrhosis may be aggravated or caused independently by any effective diuretic agent including triamterene. The use of full doses of a diuretic when salt intake is restricted can result in a low-salt syndrome.

➤*Nitrogen retention:* Triamterene can cause mild nitrogen retention, which is reversible upon withdrawal of the drug and is seldom observed with intermittent (every-other-day) therapy.

➤*Metabolic acidosis:* Triamterene may cause a decreasing alkali reserve with the possibility of metabolic acidosis.

➤*Hematologic effects:* By the very nature of their illness, cirrhotics with splenomegaly sometimes have marked variations in their blood pictures. Since triamterene is a weak folic acid antagonist, it may contribute to the appearance of megaloblastosis in cases where folic acid stores have been depleted. Therefore, periodic blood studies in these patients are recommended. They should also be observed for exacerbations of underlying liver disease.

➤*Uric acid:* Triamterene has elevated uric acid, especially in persons predisposed to gouty arthritis.

➤*Renal stones:* Triamterene has been reported in renal stones in association with other calculus components. Triamterene should be used with caution in patients with histories of renal stones.

➤*Special risk:* Triamterene tends to conserve potassium rather than to promote the excretion as do many diuretics and, occasionally, can cause increases in serum potassium which, in some instances, can result in hyperkalemia. In rare instances, hyperkalemia has been associated with cardiac irregularities.

➤*Lab test abnormalities:* Hyperkalemia will rarely occur in patients with adequate urinary output, but it is a possibility if large doses are used for considerable periods of time. If hyperkalemia is observed, triamterene should be withdrawn. The healthy adult range of serum potassium is 3.5 to 5 mEq/L with 4.5 mEq often being used for a reference point. Potassium levels persistently above 6 mEq/L require careful observation and treatment. Normal potassium levels tend to be higher in neonates (7.7 mEq/L) than in adults.

Serum potassium levels do not necessarily indicate true body potassium concentration. A rise in plasma pH may cause a decrease in plasma potassium concentration and an increase in the intracellular potassium concentration. Because triamterene conserves potassium, it has been theorized that in patients who have received intensive therapy or been given the drug for prolonged periods, a rebound kaliuresis could occur upon abrupt withdrawal. In such patients, withdrawal of triamterene should be gradual.

Drug Interactions

Triamterene Drug Interactions

Precipitant drug	Object drug*		Description
Triamterene	Amantadine	↑	Amantadine plasma levels may increase and urinary excretion may decrease, possibly increasing the risk for developing adverse effects.
Triamterene	Potassium preparations	↑	Concurrent administration may result in severe hyperkalemia, possibly with cardiac arrhythmias or cardiac arrest. Avoid concomitant use.
ACE inhibitors	Triamterene	↑	Use of ACE inhibitors may elevate serum potassium. Concurrent use with triamterene may lead to significant hyperkalemia.
Cimetidine	Triamterene	↑	Cimetidine may increase the bioavailability and decrease the renal clearance and hydroxylation of triamterene.
Indomethacin	Triamterene	↑	Rapid progress into acute renal failure has occurred with concurrent use. Use this combination only when clearly needed.

* ↑ = Object drug increased

Caution should be used when lithium and diuretics are used concomitantly because diuretic-induced sodium loss may reduce the renal clearance of lithium and increase serum lithium levels with risk of lithium toxicity. Patients receiving such combined therapy should have serum lithium levels monitored closely and the lithium dosage adjusted if necessary.

The effects of the following drugs may be potentiated when given together with triamterene: Antihypertensive medication, other diuretics, preanesthetic and anesthetic agents, skeletal muscle relaxants (nondepolarizing).

Triamterene may raise blood glucose levels; for adult-onset diabetes, dosage adjustments of hypoglycemic agents may be necessary during and after therapy; concurrent use with chlorpropamide may increase the risk of severe hyponatremia.

➤*Drug/Lab test interactions:* Triamterene and quinidine have similar fluorescence spectra; thus, triamterene will interfere with the fluorescent measurement of quinidine.

Adverse Reactions

Adverse reactions are listed below. All adverse reactions occur rarely (that is, 1 in 1000, or less).

➤*CNS:* Weakness, fatigue, dizziness, headache, dry mouth.

➤*GI:* Jaundice or liver enzyme abnormalities, nausea and vomiting, diarrhea.

➤*Hematologic:* Thrombocytopenia, megaloblastic anemia.

➤*Hypersensitivity:* Anaphylaxis, rash, photosensitivity.

➤*Metabolic:* Hyperkalemia, hypokalemia.

➤*Renal:* Azotemia, elevated BUN and creatinine, renal stones, acute interstitial nephritis (rare), acute renal failure (1 case of irreversible renal failure has been reported).

Overdosage

➤*Symptoms:* In the event of overdosage it can be theorized that electrolyte imbalance would be the major concern, with particular attention to possible hyperkalemia. Other symptoms that might be seen would be nausea and vomiting, other GI disturbances and weakness. It is conceivable that some hypotension could occur.

➤*Treatment:* Immediate evacuation of the stomach should be induced through emesis and gastric lavage. Careful evaluation of the electrolyte pattern and fluid balance should be made. There is no specific antidote.

Reversible acute renal failure following ingestion of 50 tablets of a product containing a combination of 50 mg triamterene and 25 mg hydrochlorothiazide has been reported. The oral LD_{50} in mice is 380 mg/kg. The amount of drug in a single dose ordinarily associated with symptoms of overdose or likely to be life-threatening is not known. Although triamterene is 67% protein-bound, there may be some benefit to dialysis in cases of overdosage.

Patient Information

To help avoid stomach upset, it is recommended that the drug be taken after meals. If a single daily dose is prescribed, it may be preferable to take it in the morning to minimize the effect of increased frequency of urination on nighttime sleep.

If a dose is missed, the patient should not take more than the prescribed dose at the next dosing interval.

Indications

➤*Glaucoma:* For adjunctive treatment of chronic simple (open-angle) glaucoma and secondary glaucoma; preoperatively in acute angle-closure glaucoma when delay of surgery is desired to lower intraocular pressure (IOP).

➤*Acetazolamide:*

Tablets, sustained release (SR) capsules and injection – For the prevention or amelioration of symptoms associated with acute mountain sickness in climbers attempting rapid ascent and in those who are susceptible to acute mountain sickness despite gradual ascent.

Tablets and injection only – For adjunctive treatment of edema due to chronic heart failure (CHF), drug-induced edema and centrencephalic epilepsy (petit mal, unlocalized seizures).

Actions

➤*Pharmacology:* These agents are nonbacteriostatic sulfonamides that inhibit the enzyme carbonic anhydrase. This action reduces the rate of aqueous humor formation, resulting in decreased IOP. This action is independent of systemic acid-base balance.

By inhibiting hydrogen ion secretion by the renal tubule, these agents cause increased excretion of sodium, potassium, bicarbonate and water, thus producing an alkaline diuresis. Carbonic anhydrase inhibitors (CAIs) cause a decrease in renal blood flow and glomerular filtration rate. Redistribution of flow to the renal cortex occurs. These changes are mild and unrelated to diuretic activity.

Evidence seems to indicate that **acetazolamide** has utility as an adjuvant in the treatment of certain dysfunctions of the CNS (eg, epilepsy). Inhibition of carbonic anhydrase in this area appears to retard abnormal, paroxysmal, excessive discharge from CNS neurons.

➤*Pharmacokinetics:*

Pharmacokinetics of Carbonic Anhydrase Inhibitors

CAI	IOP Lowering Effects			Relative inhibitor potency
	Onset (h)	Peak effect (h)	Duration (h)	
Acetazolamide				
Tablets	1 to 1.5	1 to 4	8 to 12	1
SR capsules	2	3 to 6	18 to 24	
Injection (IV)	2 min	15 min	4 to 5	
Methazolamide	2 to 4	6 to 8	10 to 18	–[a]

[a] Quantitative data not available; reported to be more active than acetazolamide.

Methazolamide – Peak plasma concentrations for the 25, 50 and 100 mg twice daily regimens were 2.5, 5.1 and 10.7 mcg/mL, respectively. Approximately 55% is bound to plasma proteins. The mean steady-state plasma elimination half-life is approximately 14 hours. At steady state approximately 25% of the dose is recovered unchanged in the urine. Renal clearance accounts for 20% to 25% of the total clearance of drug. After repeated dosing, methazolamide accumulates to steady-state concentrations in 7 days.

Contraindications

Hypersensitivity to these agents; depressed sodium or potassium serum levels; marked kidney and liver disease or dysfunction; suprarenal gland failure; hyperchloremic acidosis; adrenocortical insufficiency; cirrhosis (**acetazolamide, methazolamide**); long-term use in chronic noncongestive angle-closure glaucoma, because organic closure of the angle may occur while worsening glaucoma is masked by lowered IOP.

Warnings

➤*Hepatic function impairment:* Use of **methazolamide** in this condition may precipitate hepatic coma.

➤*Pregnancy: Category C.* Animal studies with some of these drugs have demonstrated teratogenicity (skeletal anomalies). Do not use during pregnancy, especially during the first trimester, unless the potential benefits outweigh the potential hazards.

➤*Lactation:* Safety for use in the nursing mother has not been established. It is not known whether all carbonic anhydrase inhibitors are excreted in breast milk. **Acetazolamide** appeared in breast milk of a patient taking 500 mg twice daily. However, the infant ingested only 0.06% of the dose, an amount unlikely to cause adverse reactions.

➤*Children:* Safety and efficacy for use in children have not been established.

Precautions

➤*Monitoring:* Monitor for hematologic reactions common to sulfonamides. Obtain baseline complete blood count and platelet counts before therapy and at regular intervals during therapy.

➤*Hypokalemia:* Hypokalemia may develop when severe cirrhosis is present, during concomitant use of steroids or adrenocorticotropic hormone, and with interference with adequate oral electrolyte intake. Hypokalemia can sensitize or exaggerate the response of the heart to the toxic effects of digitalis (eg, increased ventricular irritability). Hypokalemia may be avoided or treated with potassium supplements or foods with high potassium content.

➤*Dose increases:* Increasing the dose of **acetazolamide** does not increase diuresis and may increase drowsiness or paresthesia; it often results in decreased diuresis. However, very large doses have been given with other diuretics to promote diuresis in complete refractory failure.

➤*Pulmonary conditions:* These drugs may precipitate or aggravate acidosis. Use with caution in patients with pulmonary obstruction or emphysema when alveolar ventilation may be impaired.

➤*Cross-sensitivity:* Cross-sensitivity between antibacterial sulfonamides and sulfonamide derivative diuretics, including **acetazolamide** and various thiazides, has been reported.

Drug Interactions

CAI Drug Interactions

Precipitant drug	Object drug[a]		Description
Acetazolamide	Cyclosporine	↑	Increased trough cyclosporine levels with possible nephrotoxicity and neurotoxicity may occur.
Acetazolamide	Primidone	↓	Primidone serum and urine concentrations may be decreased.
CAIs	Salicylates	↑	Concurrent use may result in accumulation and toxicity of the CAI, including CNS depression and metabolic acidosis. Also, CAI-induced acidosis may allow increased CNS penetration by salicylates.
Salicylates	CAIs	↑	
Diflunisal	CAIs	↑	Concurrent use may result in a significant decrease in intraocular pressure; the effect may be less pronounced with methazolamide. Increased side effects may also occur.

[a] ↑ = Object drug increased. ↓ = Object drug decreased.

Adverse Reactions

Sulfonamide-type adverse reactions may occur (see Systemic Sulfonamides monograph in the Anti-Infectives chapter).

➤*CNS:* Ataxia, confusion, convulsions, depression, disorientation, dizziness, drowsiness, fatigue, flaccid paralysis, headache, lassitude, malaise, nervousness, paresthesias of the extremities, tinnitus, tremor, weakness.

➤*Dermatologic:* Photosensitivity, pruritus, rash (including erythema multiforme, Stevens-Johnson syndrome, toxic epidermal necrolysis), skin eruptions, urticaria.

➤*GI:* Anorexia, constipation, diarrhea, melena, nausea, taste alteration, vomiting.

➤*Hematologic:* Agranulocytosis, bone marrow depression, hemolytic anemia, leukopenia, pancytopenia, thrombocytopenia, thrombocytopenic purpura.

➤*Renal:* Crystalluria, glycosuria, hematuria, phosphaturia, polyuria, renal calculi, renal colic, urinary frequency.

➤*Miscellaneous:* Acidosis (usually corrected with bicarbonate), decreased/absent libido, electrolyte imbalance, fever, hepatic insufficiency, impotence, transient myopia, weight loss.

Overdosage

➤*Symptoms:* Symptoms of overdosage or toxicity may include anorexia, ataxia, dizziness, drowsiness, nausea, paresthesias, tinnitus, tremor, and vomiting.

➤*Treatment:* In the event of overdosage, induce emesis or perform gastric lavage. The electrolyte disturbance most likely to be encountered from overdosage is hyperchloremic acidosis that may respond to bicarbonate administration. Potassium supplementation may be required. Observe carefully; give supportive treatment.

Patient Information

Advise patient that if GI upset occurs, to take with food.

Instruct patient to avoid prolonged exposure to sunlight or sunlamps; this medicine may cause photosensitivity.

This medicine may cause drowsiness; advise patients to observe caution while driving or performing other tasks requiring alertness, coordination, or physical dexterity.

Instruct patient to notify health care provider if sore throat, fever, unusual bleeding or bruising, tingling or tremors in the hands or feet, flank or loin pain, or skin rash occurs.

ACETAZOLAMIDE

Rx	**Acetazolamide** (Various, eg, Mutual, URL)	**Tablets**: 125 mg	In 50s, 100s, and 250s.
Rx	**Acetazolamide** (Various, eg, Qualitest, Schein, URL)	**Tablets**: 250 mg	In 100s, 500s, 1000s and UD 100s.
Rx	**Diamox Sequels** (Barr)	**Capsules, sustained-release**: 500 mg	(Diamox D3). Orange. In 30s and 100s.
Rx	**Acetazolamide** (Various, eg, Bedford Labs)	**Powder for Injection, lyophilized**: 500 mg	In vials.

ACETAZOLAMIDE — ORAL

For complete and comparative prescribing information, see Carbonic Anhydrase Inhibitor monograph.

Indications

For adjunctive treatment of the following: Chronic simple (open-angle) glaucoma, secondary glaucoma, and preoperatively in acute angle-closure glaucoma where delay of surgery is desired in order to lower intraocular pressure. Acetazolamide is also indicated for the prevention or amelioration of symptoms associated with acute mountain sickness in climbers attempting rapid ascent and in those who are very susceptible to acute mountain sickness despite gradual ascent.

➤*Tablets:* Also for adjunctive treatment of the following: Edema due to congestive heart failure; drug-induced edema; centrencephalic epilepsies (petit mal, unlocalized seizures).

Administration and Dosage

➤*Approved by the FDA:* April 25, 1995.

➤*Glaucoma:*

Tablets – Acetazolamide should be used as an adjunct to the usual therapy. The dosage employed in the treatment of chronic simple (open-angle) glaucoma ranges from 250 mg to 1 g of acetazolamide per 24 hours, usually in divided doses for amounts over 250 mg. It has usually been found that a dosage in excess of 1 g per 24 hours does not produce an increased effect. In all cases, the dosage should be adjusted with careful individual attention both to symptomatology and ocular tension. Continuous supervision by a physician is advisable.

In treatment of secondary glaucoma and in the preoperative treatment of some cases of acute congestive (closed-angle) glaucoma, the preferred dosage is 250 mg every 4 hours, although some cases have responded to 250 mg twice daily on short-term therapy. In some acute cases, it may be more satisfactory to administer an initial dose of 500 mg followed by 125 or 250 mg every 4 hours depending on the individual case. IV therapy may be used for rapid relief of ocular tension in acute cases. A complementary effect has been noted when acetazolamide has been used in conjunction with miotics or mydriatics as the case demanded.

Sustained-release capsules – The recommended dosage is 1 capsule (500 mg) 2 times a day. Usually 1 capsule is administered in the morning and 1 capsule in the evening. It may be necessary to adjust the dose, but it has usually been found that dosage in excess of 2 capsules (1 g) does not produce an increased effect. The dosage should be adjusted with careful individual attention both to symptomatology and intraocular tension. In all cases, continuous supervision by a physician is advisable.

In those unusual instances where adequate control is not obtained by the twice-a-day administration of acetazolamide sustained-release capsules the desired control may be established by means of tablets or parenteral. Use tablets or parenteral in accordance with the more frequent dosage schedules recommended for these dosage forms, such as 250 mg every 4 hours, or an initial dose of 500 mg followed by 250 mg or 125 mg every 4 hours, depending on the case in question.

➤*Epilepsy:*

Tablets – It is not clearly known whether the beneficial effects observed in epilepsy are due to direct inhibition of carbonic anhydrase in the CNS or whether they are due to the slight degree of acidosis produced by the divided dosage. The best results to date have been seen in petit mal in children. Good results, however, have been seen in patients, both children and adult, in other types of seizures (eg, grand mal, mixed seizure patterns, myoclonic jerk patterns). The suggested total daily dose is 8 to 30 mg/kg in divided doses. Although some patients respond to a low dose, the optimum range appears to be from 375 to 1000 mg daily. However, some investigators feel that daily doses in excess of 1 g do not produce any better results than a 1 g dose. When acetazolamide is given in combination with other anticonvulsants, it is suggested that the starting dose should be 250 mg once daily in addition to the existing medications. This can be increased to levels as indicated above. The change from other medications to acetazolamide should be gradual and in accordance with usual practice in epilepsy therapy.

➤*Congestive heart failure:*

Tablets – For diuresis in congestive heart failure, the starting dose is usually 250 to 375 mg once daily in the morning (5 mg/kg). If, after an initial response, the patient fails to continue to lose edema fluid, do not increase the dose but allow for kidney recovery by skipping medication for a day. Acetazolamide yields best diuretic results when given on alternate days, or for 2 days alternating with a day of rest.

Failures in therapy may be due to overdosage or too frequent dosage. The use of acetazolamide does not eliminate the need for other therapy such as digitalis, bed rest, and salt restriction.

➤*Drug-induced edema:*

Tablets – Recommended dosage is 250 to 375 mg of acetazolamide once a day for 1 or 2 days, alternating with a day of rest.

➤*Acute mountain sickness:* Dosage is 500 mg to 1000 mg daily, in divided doses using tablets or sustained-release capsules as appropriate. In circumstances of rapid ascent, such as in rescue or military operations, the higher dose level of 1000 mg is recommended. It is preferable to initiate dosing 24 to 48 hours before ascent and to continue for 48 hours while at high altitude, or longer as necessary to control symptoms.

➤*Note:* The dosage recommendations for glaucoma and epilepsy differ considerably from those for congestive heart failure, since the first 2 conditions are not dependent upon carbonic anhydrase inhibition in the kidney which requires intermittent dosage if it is to recover from the inhibitory effect of the therapeutic agent.

➤*Storage/Stability:* Store at controlled room temperature 15° to 30°C (59° to 86°F). Dispense in tight, light-resistant container.

ACETAZOLAMIDE SODIUM — INJECTION

Indications

For adjunctive treatment of the following: Edema due to congestive heart failure; drug-induced edema; centrencephalic epilepsies (petit mal, unlocalized seizures); chronic simple (open-angle) glaucoma, secondary glaucoma, and preoperatively in acute angle-closure glaucoma where delay of surgery is desired in order to lower intraocular pressure.

Administration and Dosage

➤*Approved by the FDA:* December 5, 1990.

➤*Preparation and storage of parenteral solution:* Each 500 mg vial containing sterile acetazolamide sodium should be reconstituted with at least 5 mL of Sterile Water for Injection prior to use. Reconstituted solutions retain their physical and chemical properties for 3 days under refrigeration at 2° to 8°C (36° to 46°F), or 12 hours at room temperature 15° to 30°C (59° to 86°F). Contains no preservative. The direct IV route of administration is preferred. IM administration is not recommended.

➤*Glaucoma:* Acetazolamide should be used as an adjunct to the usual therapy. The dosage employed in the treatment of chronic simple (open-angle) glaucoma ranges from 250 mg to 1 g of acetazolamide per 24 hours, usually in divided doses for amounts greater than 250 mg. It has usually been found that a dosage in excess of 1 g/24 hours does not produce an increased effect. In all cases, the dosage should be adjusted with careful individual attention both to symptomatology and ocular tension. Continuous supervision by a physician is advisable.

In treatment of secondary glaucoma and in the preoperative treatment of some cases of acute congestive (closed-angle) glaucoma, the preferred dosage is 250 mg every 4 hours, although some cases have responded to 250 mg twice daily on short-term therapy. In some acute cases, it may be more satisfactory to administer an initial dose of 500 mg followed by 125 or 250 mg every 4 hours depending on the individual case. IV therapy may be used for rapid relief of ocular tension in acute cases. A complementary effect has been noted when acetazolamide has been used in conjunction with miotics or mydriatics as the case demanded.

➤*Epilepsy:* It is not clearly known whether the beneficial effects observed in epilepsy are due to direct inhibition of carbonic anhydrase in the CNS or whether they are due to the slight degree of acidosis produced by the divided dosage. The best results to date have been seen in petit mal in children. Good results, however, have been seen in patients, both children and adult, in other types of seizures such as grand mal, mixed seizure patterns, and myoclonic jerk patterns. The suggested total daily dose is 8 to 30 mg per kg in divided doses. Although some patients respond to a low dose, the optimum range appears to be from 375 to 1000 mg daily. However, some investigators feel that daily doses in excess of 1 g do not produce any better results than a 1 g dose. When acetazolamide is given in combination with other anticonvulsants, it is suggested that the starting dose should be 250 mg once daily in addition to the existing medications. This can be increased to levels as indicated above.

The change from other medications to acetazolamide should be gradual and in accordance with usual practice in epilepsy therapy.

➤*Congestive heart failure:* For diuresis in congestive heart failure, the starting dose is usually 250 to 375 mg once daily in the morning (5 mg/kg). If, after an initial response, the patient fails to continue to lose edema fluid, do not increase the dose but allow for kidney recovery by skipping medication for a day.

Carbonic Anhydrase Inhibitors

ACETAZOLAMIDE SODIUM — INJECTION

Acetazolamide yields best diuretic results when given on alternate days, or for 2 days alternating with a day of rest. Failures in therapy may be due to overdosage or too frequent dosage. The use of acetazolamide does not eliminate the need for other therapy such as digitalis, bed rest, and salt restriction.

➤*Drug-induced edema:* Recommended dosage is 250 to 375 mg of acetazolamide once a day for 1 or 2 days, alternating with a day of rest.

➤*Note:* The dosage recommendations for glaucoma and epilepsy differ considerably from those for congestive heart failure, since the first two conditions are not dependent upon carbonic anhydrase inhibition in the kidney which requires intermittent dosage if it is to recover from inhibitory effect of the therapeutic agent.

➤*Storage/Stability:* Store drug product at controlled room temperature 15° to 30°C (59° to 86°F). Discard unused portion.

METHAZOLAMIDE

Rx	**Methazolamide** (Various, eg, Mikart)	**Tablets:** 25 mg	In 100s.
		50 mg	In 100s.

METHAZOLAMIDE — ORAL

For complete and comparative prescribing information, refer to the Carbonic Anhydrase Inhibitor group monograph.

Indications

➤*Glaucoma:* Methazolamide is indicated in the treatment of ocular conditions where lowering intraocular pressure is likely to be of therapeutic benefit, such as chronic open-angle glaucoma, secondary glaucoma, and preoperatively in acute angle-closure glaucoma where lowering the intraocular pressure is desired before surgery.

Administration and Dosage

➤*Dosage:* The effective therapeutic dose administered varies from 50 mg to 100 mg 2 to 3 times daily. The drug may be used concomitantly with miotic and osmotic agents.

➤*Storage/Stability:* Store at controlled room temperature 15° to 30°C (59° to 86°F).

Diuretic Combinations

DIURETIC COMBINATIONS

Rx	**Amiloride/ Hydrochlorothiazide** (Various, eg, Goldline, Warner Chilcott)	**Tablets:** 5 mg amiloride HCl and 50 mg hydrochlorothiazide	In 100s, 500s and 1000s.
Rx	**Moduretic** (Merck)		Lactose. (917). Peach, scored. Diamond shape. In 100s and UD 100s.
Rx	**Spironolactone/ Hydrochlorothiazide** (Various, eg, Danbury, Goldline, Mylan)	**Tablets:** 25 mg spironolactone and 25 mg hydrochlorothiazide	In 100s, 250s, 500s and 1000s.
Rx	**Aldactazide** (Searle)		(Searle 1011 Aldactazide 25). Tan. Film coated. In 100s, 500s, 1000s and UD 100s.
Rx	**Aldactazide** (Searle)	**Tablets:** 50 mg spironolactone and 50 mg hydrochlorothiazide	(Searle 1021 Aldactazide 50). Tan, scored. In 100s and UD 100s.
Rx	**Triamterene/ Hydrochlorothiazide** (Various, eg, Geneva)	**Tablets:** 37.5 mg triamterene and 25 mg hydrochlorothiazide	In 100s, 500s and 1000s.
Rx	**Maxzide-25MG** (Bertek)		(Maxzide LL M9). Lt. green, scored. Bow-tie shape. In 100s, UD 100s.
Rx	**Triamterene/Hydrochlorothiazide** (Duramed)	**Capsules:** 37.5 mg triamterene and 25 mg hydrochlorothiazide	Lactose. (DPI/488). White. In 1000s.
Rx	**Dyazide** (SmithKline Beecham)		Lactose. (Dyazide). Red and white. In 1000s, unit-of-use 100s and UD 100s.
Rx	**Triamterene/Hydrochlorothiazide** (Various, eg, Geneva, Goldline, Zenith)	**Capsules:** 50 mg triamterene and 25 mg hydrochlorothiazide	In 100s and 1000s.
Rx	**Triamterene/Hydrochlorothiazide** (Various, eg, Barr, Danbury, Geneva, Goldline, Major, Schein, UDL, Warner Chilcott)	**Tablets:** 75 mg triamterene and 50 mg hydrochlorothiazide	In 100s, 250s, 500s, 1000s, and UD 100s.
Rx	**Maxzide** (Bertek)		(Maxzide LL M8). Lt. yellow, scored. Bow-tie shape. In 100s, 500s, UD 100s.

DIURETIC COMBINATIONS — ORAL

For complete information concerning the components of the combined diuretic products, consult the appropriate drug monographs in the Diuretics section.

Administration and Dosage

Fixed-dose combination drugs are not indicated for initial therapy of edema or hypertension; they require therapy titrated to the individual patient. If the fixed combination represents the determined dosage, its use may be more convenient in patient management. The treatment of hypertension and edema is not static; reevaluate as conditions in each patient warrant.

Dosage for each combination/strength varies. Refer to labeling for specific guidelines.

➤*Amiloride/Hydrochlorothiazide:* 1 to 2 tablets daily with meals.

➤*Spironolactone/Hydrochlorothiazide:*

25 mg/25 mg – 1 to 8 tablets daily.

50 mg/50 mg – 1 to 4 tablets daily.

➤*Triamterene/Hydrochlorothiazide:*

37.5 mg/25 mg – 1 or 2 tablets/capsules daily.

50 mg/25 mg – 1 or 2 capsules twice daily after meals.

75 mg/50 mg – 1 tablet daily.

Actions

➤*Pharmacology:* The combination of a thiazide and a potassium-sparing diuretic provides additive diuretic activity and antihypertensive effects through different mechanisms of action and also minimizes the potassium depletion characteristics of thiazides.

Precautions

➤*Triamterene/Hydrochlorothiazide:*

Bioavailability – Use caution when changing to another triamterene/hydrochlorothiazide combination product. Combination products are not equivalent.

Osmotic Diuretics

Actions

➤*Pharmacology:* Osmotic agents induce diuresis by elevating the osmolarity of the glomerular filtrate, thereby hindering the tubular reabsorption of water. Excretion of sodium and chloride is increased. These agents are freely filtered at the glomerulus; poorly reabsorbed by the renal tubule; not secreted by the tubule; relatively pharmacologically inert; usually resistant to metabolic alteration (except glycerin). Activity in the kidneys depends on the concentration of osmotically active particles in solution.

The main indication for osmotic diuretics (primarily mannitol) is prophylaxis of acute renal failure in conditions in which glomerular filtration is greatly reduced (ie, severe trauma, cardiovascular operations). By maintaining a flow of dilute urine, damage to the nephron by high concentrations of toxic solute does not occur. They are also employed to reduce intracranial pressure and elevated intraocular pressure. In the eyes, these agents act by creating an osmotic gradient between the plasma and ocular fluids.

Mannitol is the most widely used osmotic diuretic. The other agents include urea, glycerin and isosorbide. For specific approved indications, refer to individual drug monographs.

➤*Pharmacokinetics:* **Mannitol** is only slightly metabolized, while the rest is freely filtered by the glomeruli and excreted intact in urine. About 7% is reabsorbed by the renal tubules. Approximately 90% of an injected dose is recovered in urine after 24 hours. In severe renal insufficiency, the rate of mannitol excretion is greatly reduced; retained mannitol may increase extracellular tonicity, expand the extracellular fluid and induce an apparent hyponatremia with increased serum osmolality.

Osmotic Diuretics Pharmacokinetics

Diuretic	Route	Onset (min)	Peak (hrs)	Duration (hrs)	Half-life	Metabolized (%)	Ocular penetration	Distribution
Glycerin	PO	10-30	1-1.5	4-5	30-45 minutes	80	poor	E[1]
Isosorbide	PO	10-30	1-1.5	5-6	5-9.5 hrs	0	good	TBW[2]
Mannitol	IV	30-60	1	6-8	15-100 minutes	7-10	very poor	E[1]
Urea	IV	30-45	1	5-6			good	TBW[2]

[1] E = extracellular water
[2] TBW = total body water

MANNITOL

Rx	**Osmitrol** (Baxter)	**Injection:** 5%	In 1000 ml.
		10%	In 500 and 1000 ml.
		15%	In 500 ml.
		20%	In 250 and 500 ml.
Rx	**Mannitol** (Various, eg, Abbott, American Regent, IMS, Kendall McGaw, Pasadena)	**Injection:** 10%	In 1000 ml.
		Injection: 15%	In 150 and 500 ml.
		Injection: 20%	In 250 and 500 ml.
		Injection: 25%	In 50 ml vials and syringes.
Rx	**Resectisol** (Kendall McGaw)	**Solution:** 5 g/100 ml in distilled water (275 mOsm/L)	In 2000 ml.

MANNITOL — INJECTION

Refer to the general discussion of these agents in the Osmotic Diuretics Introduction.

Indications

Promotion of diuresis, in the prevention or treatment of the oliguric phase of acute renal failure before irreversible renal failure becomes established.

Reduction of intracranial pressure and treatment of cerebral edema by reducing brain mass.

Reduction of elevated intraocular pressure when the pressure cannot be lowered by other means.

Promotion of urinary excretion of toxins.

➤*Urologic irrigation:* Mannitol solution, 25% is indicated as an irrigation solution in transurethral prostatic resection or other transurethral surgical procedures.

Administration and Dosage

The total dosage, concentration, and rate of administration should be governed by the nature and severity of the condition being treated and the patient's fluid requirement and urinary output. The adult dosage ranges from 50 to 200 g in a 24-hour period, but in most cases an adequate response will be achieved at a usual dosage of approximately 100 g/24 hours. The rate of administration is usually adjusted to maintain a urine flow of at least 30 to 50 mL/hr. Lower mannitol concentrations and solutions containing sodium chloride are useful in preventing dehydration and electrolyte depletion. This outline of administration and dosage is only a general guide to therapy.

Dosage requirements for patients 12 years of age and under have not been established. As with adults, dose is dependent on weight, clinical condition, and laboratory results. Follow recommendations of appropriate pediatric reference text.

➤*Test dose:* A test dose of mannitol should be given prior to instituting therapy for patients with marked oliguria or those believed to have inadequate renal function. Such test doses may be approximately 0.2 g/kg (about 75 mL of a 20% solution or 50 mL of a 25% solution) infused in a period of 3 to 5 minutes to produce a urine flow of at least 30 to 50 mL/hr. If urine flow does not increase within 2 or 3 hours, a second test dose may be given. If response is inadequate, the patient should be reevaluated.

➤*Prevention of acute renal failure (oliguria):* When used during cardiovascular and other types of surgery, immediately postoperatively or following trauma, 50 to 100 g of mannitol as a 5% to 25% solution may be given. The concentration and amount will depend upon the fluid requirements of the patient. Following suspected or actual hemolytic transfusion reactions, 20 g of mannitol may be given IV over a 5-minute period to provoke diuresis. If diuresis does not occur, the 20 g dose may be repeated. If there is an adequate urine flow (30 to 50 mL/hr) then IV fluids containing not more than 50 to 75 mEq of sodium per liter should be given in sufficient volume to match the desired urine flow (100 mL/hr) until fluids can be taken orally.

➤*Treatment of oliguria:* The usual dose for treatment of oliguria is 50 to 100 g administered as a 15% to 25% solution.

➤*Reduction of intracranial pressure, cerebral edema, or intraocular pressure:* A 25% solution of mannitol is recommended since its effectiveness depends on establishing intravascular hyperosmolarity. When used before or after surgery, a total dose of 1.5 to 2 g/kg can be given over a period of 30 to 60 minutes. Careful evaluation must be made of the circulatory and renal reserve prior to and during use of mannitol at this relatively high dose and rapid infusion rate. Careful attention must be paid to fluid and electrolyte balance, body weight, and total input and output before and after infusion of mannitol. Evidence of reduced cerebral spinal fluid pressure may be observed within 15 minutes after starting infusion.

Maximal reduction of intraocular pressure occurs 30 to 60 minutes after injection.

➤*10% or 20% mannitol:*

Adjunctive therapy for intoxications – As an agent to promote diuresis in intoxications, 10% or 20% mannitol is indicated. The concentration will depend upon the fluid requirement and urinary output of the patient. Generally, a bolus dose of 20% mannitol is given, followed by a slower infusion of 10% mannitol (with electrolytes) to maintain urine output at the desired level.

It is recommended that 20% mannitol injection be administered through a blood filter set to ensure against infusion of mannitol crystals.

When a hypertonic solution is to be administered peripherally, it should be slowly infused through a small bore needle, placed well within the lumen of a large vein to minimize venous irritation. Carefully avoid infiltration.

➤*25% mannitol:*

Urinary excretion of toxic substances – Mannitol in 5% to 25% solutions is used as an infusion as long as indicated if the level of urinary output remains high. The concentration will depend upon the fluid requirement and urinary output. IV water and electrolytes must be given to replace the loss of these substances in the urine, sweat and expired air. If benefits are not observed after 200 g of mannitol are given, discontinue it.

➤*Directions for use of Excel* container: Do not admix with other drugs.

Caution – Do not use plastic container in series connection.

To open – Tear overwrap down at notch and remove solution container. Check for minute leaks by squeezing solution container firmly. If leaks are found, discard solution as sterility may be impaired.

Before use, perform the following checks: Inspect each container. Read the label. Ensure solution is the one ordered and is within the expiration date. Invert container and carefully inspect the solution in good light for cloudiness, haze, or particulate matter. Any container which is suspect should not be used. Use only if solution is clear and container and seals are intact.

Preparation for administration –
1.) Remove plastic protector from sterile set port at bottom of container.
2.) Attach administration set. Refer to complete directions accompanying set.

➤*Instructions for proper use of vials with flip-tear top seals:* Read instructions carefully. Use proper aseptic technique.

Caution – If it is necessary to introduce filtered air into the vial, this must be done slowly and with caution. If the vial has been warmed, allow vial to cool to room temperature before use.

➤*Storage/Stability:* Exposure of pharmaceutical products to heat should be minimized. Avoid excessive heat. Protect from freezing. Use only if solution is clear and seal intact and undamaged.

10% and 20% solutions – It is recommended that the product be stored at room temperature (25°C; 77°F).

MANNITOL — INJECTION

25% solution – Store at controlled room temperature 15° to 30°C (59° to 86°F). Preservative free. Discard unused portion.

Actions

➤*Pharmacology:* Mannitol is an obligatory osmotic diuretic.

Mannitol occurs naturally in fruits and vegetables and is metabolically inert in humans.

➤*Pharmacokinetics:*

Absorption – Mannitol is poorly absorbed from the GI tract.

Metabolism/Excretion – After IV injection, mannitol is confined to the extracellular space, only slightly metabolized, and rapidly excreted by the kidneys. Approximately 80% of a typical dose appears in the urine within 3 hours. Mannitol is freely filtered by the glomeruli with less than 10% tubular reabsorption; it is not secreted by tubular cells. It induces diuresis by elevating the osmolarity of the glomerular filtrate and thereby hinders tubular reabsorption of water. Urinary output of water and excretion of sodium and chloride are enhanced.

Mannitol injection is free of electrolytes and is used in urology as a nonhemolytic irrigant. The amount of mannitol absorbed intravascularly during transurethral prostatic surgery is variable and depends primarily on the extent of the surgery. Such mannitol is excreted by the kidneys and produces osmotic diuresis.

Contraindications

Well-established anuria due to severe renal disease; severe pulmonary congestion or frank pulmonary edema; active intracranial bleeding except during craniotomy; severe dehydration; progressive renal damage or dysfunction after institution of mannitol therapy, including increasing oliguria and azotemia; progressive heart failure or pulmonary congestion after institution of mannitol therapy.

Warnings

➤*Fluid and electrolyte imbalance:* Excessive loss of water and electrolytes may lead to serious imbalances. Serum sodium and potassium should be carefully monitored during mannitol therapy.

The diuresis after rapid infusion of mannitol may increase preexisting hemoconcentration. With continued use of mannitol, a loss of water in excess of electrolytes can cause hypernatremia.

Shift of sodium-free intracellular fluid into the extracellular compartment after mannitol infusion may lower serum sodium concentration and aggravate preexisting hyponatremia.

➤*Transurethral prostatectomy:* Irrigating solutions used in transurethral prostatectomy have been shown to enter the systemic circulation in relatively large volumes, exert a systemic effect and may significantly alter cardiopulmonary and renal dynamics.

➤*Renal function impairment:* A test dose should be utilized in patients with severe impairment of renal function. A second test dose may be tried if there is an inadequate response, but no more than 2 test doses should be attempted.

➤*Carcinogenesis:* In an early study of 1%, 5% or 10% mannitol, given for 94 weeks in the diet of Wistar rats, a low incidence of benign thymomas occurred in females which was apparently treatment related. A subsequent lifetime study at similar dose levels in Spraque-Dawley, Fischer and Wistar rats revealed no carcinogenic effect in the thymus.

➤*Pregnancy:* *Category B.*

This drug should be used during pregnancy only if clearly needed.

➤*Lactation:* It is not known whether this drug is excreted in human milk. Because many drugs are excreted in human milk, caution should be exercised when mannitol injection is administered to a nursing mother.

➤*Children:* Dosage requirements in children below 12 years of age have not been established.

Precautions

➤*Monitoring:* Clinical evaluation and periodic laboratory determinations are necessary to monitor changes in fluid balance, electrolyte concentrations, and acid-base balance during parenteral therapy with mannitol solutions.

Excessive loss of water and electrolytes may lead to serious imbalances. Serum sodium and potassium should be carefully monitored during mannitol therapy.

Closely monitor the urine output and discontinue mannitol infusion promptly if output is low. Inadequate urine output results in accumulation of mannitol, expansion of extracellular fluid volume and could result in water intoxication or congestive heart failure. Renal function must be closely monitored during mannitol infusion.

➤*Cardiovascular:* The cardiovascular status of the patient should be carefully evaluated before mannitol is administered by rapid IV injection or before and during transurethral resection since expansion of the extracellular fluid may lead to fulminating congestive heart failure.

➤*Hypovolemia:* By sustaining diuresis, mannitol administration may obscure and intensify inadequate hydration or hypovolemia.

➤*Pseudoagglutination:* Electrolyte-free mannitol solutions should not be given conjointly with blood.

Unless it is essential, electrolyte-free mannitol solutions should not be combined with blood. When it is essential to give the combination, at least 20 mEq of sodium chloride should be added per L of mannitol solution to avoid agglomeration of erythrocytes. The contents of opened containers should be used promptly, and unused contents should be discarded.

➤*Crystallization (25% mannitol):* Crystals, if present in mannitol injection, 25% may be dissolved by placing the vial in a hot water bath maintained at 60° to 80°C (140° to 176°F), with occasional shaking. The resulting solution should be allowed to cool to body temperature before injection.

An administration set with a filter should be used for IV infusions of solutions containing 20% or more of mannitol.

A white flocculant mannitol precipitate may result from contact with PVC surfaces which act as nuclei for rapid rate crystallization of small crystals. This condition has also been reported to occur when mannitol has come in contact with other plastic and rough glass surfaces. Attempting to resolubilize the white flocculant precipitate with the aid of heat is not useful because crystallization may recur in a short period of time.

Solutions of mannitol may crystallize when exposed to low temperatures. Concentrations greater than 15% have a greater tendency to crystallization. If crystals are observed, the container should be warmed by appropriate means to not greater than 60°C (140°F), shaken, then cooled to body temperature before administering. If all crystals cannot be completely redissolved, the container must be rejected.

Note – Use of any other method to heat the vial may result in its explosion.

➤*Administration:* Do not use plastic container in series connection.

If administration is controlled by a pumping device, care must be taken to discontinue pumping action before the container runs dry or air embolism may result.

These solutions are intended for IV administration using sterile equipment. It is recommended that IV administration apparatus be replaced at least once every 24 hours.

➤*Special risk:* Mannitol solution must be used with caution in patients with significantly cardiopulmonary or renal dysfunction.

Mannitol solutions should be used with care in patients with hypervolemia, renal insufficiency, urinary tract obstruction, or impending or frank cardiac decompensation.

Adverse Reactions

Reactions which may occur because of the solution or the technique of administration include febrile response, infection at the site of injection, venous thrombosis or phlebitis extending from the site of injection, extravasation and hypervolemia.

Isolated cases of adverse reactions, such as pulmonary congestion, fluid and electrolyte imbalance, acidosis, electrolyte loss, dryness of the mouth, thirst, marked diuresis, urinary retention, edema, headache, blurred vision, convulsions, nausea, vomiting, rhinitis, arm pain, skin necrosis, thrombophlebitis, chills, dizziness, urticaria, dehydration, hypotension, hypertension, tachycardia, fever, and angina-like chest pains have been reported during or following mannitol infusion.

Too rapid infusion of hypertonic solutions may cause local pain and venous irritation. Rate of administration should be adjusted according to tolerance. Use of the largest peripheral vein and a small bore needle is recommended.

If an adverse reaction does occur, discontinue the infusion, evaluate the patient, institute appropriate therapeutic countermeasures and save the remainder of the fluid for examination if deemed necessary.

➤*25% mannitol:* Reactions are infrequent and may include:

Cardiovascular – Pulmonary edema, edema, hypotension, hypertension, tachycardia, angina-like chest pain.

CNS – Headache, convulsions, dizziness.

Dermatologic – Skin necrosis, thrombophlebitis.

GI – Dryness of mouth, nausea, vomiting, diarrhea.

GU – Osmotic nephrosis, urinary retention.

Hypersensitivity – Urticaria.

Metabolic – Fluid and electrolyte imbalance, acidosis, dehydration.

Special senses – Blurred vision, rhinitis.

Miscellaneous – Thirst, arm pain, chills, fever.

Overdosage

➤*Symptoms:* Larger doses than recommended may result in increased electrolyte excretion, particularly sodium, chloride, and potassium. Sodium depletion can result in orthostatic tachycardia or hypotension and decreased central venous pressure. Chloride metabolism closely follows that of sodium. Potassium deficit can impair neuromuscular function and cause intestinal dilatation and ileus.

Mannitol may cause pulmonary edema or water intoxication if urine flow is inadequate.

➤*Treatment:* In the event of a fluid or solute overload during parenteral therapy, reevaluate the patient's condition, and institute appropriate corrective treatment.

UREA

Rx	**Ureaphil** (Abbott)	**Injection:** 40 g per 150 ml	In single-dose containers.

STERILE UREA — INJECTION

Refer to the general discussion of these agents in the Osmotic Diuretics Introduction.

Indications

When administered as a 30% solution, this preparation is indicated for the reduction of intracranial pressure (in the control of cerebral edema) and of intraocular pressure.

➤*Unlabeled uses:* Intra-amniotic injection has been used to induce abortion.

Administration and Dosage

➤*Adults:* For the reduction of increased intracranial or intraocular pressure the adult dose ranges from 1 to 1.5 g (3.3 to 5 mL) per kilogram of body weight; or 0.45 to 0.68 g (1.5 to 2.3 mL) per pound of body weight.

➤*Children:* In pediatric patients the dosage ranges from 0.5 to 1.5 g/kg of body weight. In infants up to 2 years of age as little as 0.1 g/kg may be adequate.

➤*Administration:* The amount to be administered is generally estimated on the basis of g of urea per kilogram of body weight. Dosage also must take into account the clinical condition of the patient, especially the state of hydration, electrolyte balance and integrity of renal function. The total daily dose should not exceed 120 g of urea.

Sterile urea is administered as a 30% solution by slow intravenous infusion. The rate of injection should not exceed 4 mL min.

➤*Preparation of solution:* Sterile urea is prepared by adding an appropriate volume of 5% or 10% Dextrose Injection. The desired diluent can be added directly to the urea container.

To prepare 135 mL of a 30% solution of sterile urea, the contents of one 40 g container are mixed with 105 mL of the diluent, or 2 such containers are mixed with 210 mL of diluent to prepare 270 mL of a 30% solution. Each milliliter of a 30% solution provides 300 mg of urea.

Urea should be freshly prepared in each case. Discard any unused portion.

➤*Storage/Stability:* Store at controlled room temperature 15° to 30°C (59° to 86°F). Discard solution if not used within 24 hours after reconstitution.

Parenteral drug products (reconstituted) should be inspected visually for particulate matter and discoloration prior to administration, whenever solution and container permit.

Actions

➤*Pharmacology:* The reduction of intracranial edema and abnormally elevated cerebrospinal fluid pressure which occurs following intravenous administration of hypertonic urea solutions, depends upon osmotic pressure gradients between the blood, extracellular and intracellular fluid compartments. Thus, the primary mechanism of action appears to be physical. Hypertonic urea rapidly increases blood tonicity thus effecting a greater urea concentration gradient in the blood than in the extravascular fluid. This results in transudation of fluid from the tissues, including the brain and cerebrospinal fluid into the blood.

As the concentration of urea in the glomerular filtrate increases, reabsorption of a proportional amount of water is prevented. Such retardation of proximal tubular reabsorption increases the rate and volume of urine flow.

Contraindications

Severely impaired renal function; active intracranial bleeding; marked dehydration; frank liver failure.

Urea should not be infused in veins of the lower extremities of elderly patients because phlebitis and thrombosis of superficial and deep veins may occur.

Do not administer unless seal of urea container is intact and reconstituted solution is clear. Discard unused portion.

Warnings

➤*Electrolyte imbalance:* Urea may cause depletion of electrolytes which can result in hyponatremia and hypokalemia. Early signs of such depletion may indicate the need for supplementation before serum levels are reduced.

➤*Extravasation:* Extreme care is essential to prevent accidental extravasation of the solution at the site of injection since this may cause local reactions ranging from mild irritation to tissue necrosis.

➤*Renal function impairment:* In the presence of kidney disease, urea should be administered with caution. Mild elevation of blood urea nitrogen does not preclude its use or continued use, but frequent laboratory studies should be made to determine if kidney function is adequate to eliminate the infused urea as well as that produced endogenously.

Patients exhibiting a temporary reduction in urine volume are generally able to maintain a satisfactory elimination of urea. However, if diuresis does not follow the injection of urea to such patients within 6 to 12 hours, the drug should be withdrawn pending further evaluation of renal function.

➤*Hepatic function impairment:* If used in patients with some liver impairment, urea should be administered with great caution since there may be a significant rise in blood ammonia levels.

➤*Pregnancy: Category C.* Animal reproduction studies have not been conducted with sterile urea. It is also not known whether sterile urea can cause fetal harm when given to a pregnant woman or can affect reproduction capacity. Sterile urea should be given to a pregnant woman only if clearly needed.

➤*Lactation:* It is not known whether this drug is excreted in human milk. Because many drugs are excreted in human milk, caution should be exercised when sterile urea is administered to a nursing mother.

Precautions

➤*Comatose patients:* An indwelling urethral catheter should be used in comatose patients receiving urea for injection to insure bladder emptying.

➤*Rapid IV administration:* Rapid intravenous (IV) administration of hypertonic solutions of urea may be associated with hemolysis as well as a direct effect on the cerebral vasomotor centers which may result in increased capillary bleeding. These effects usually can be avoided by not exceeding an infusion rate of 4 mL min. Solutions of urea should not be administered through the same administration set through which blood is being infused.

➤*Intracranial bleeding:* Although arterial oozing has been reported as a nuisance when intracranial surgery is performed on patients following treatment with urea, it has not been a significant problem. However, sterile urea should not be used in the presence of active intracranial bleeding unless such use is preliminary to prompt surgical intervention to control hemorrhage. It should be kept in mind that reduction of brain edema induced by urea may result in reactivation of intracranial bleeding.

➤*Blood loss:* As with other infused solutions, urea may temporarily maintain circulatory volume and blood pressure in spite of considerable blood loss. Consequently, when excessive blood loss occurs within a short period of time, blood replacement should be adequate and simultaneous with the infusion of urea.

➤*Hypothermia:* Hypothermia when used with urea infusion may increase the risk of venous thrombosis and hemoglobinuria.

Adverse Reactions

Headaches (reported to be similar to those which occur in some patients following lumbar puncture), nausea and vomiting, occasionally syncope and disorientation have been known to occur following intravenous administration. Less often reported is a transient agitated confusional state. No serious reactions have been noted when solutions have been infused slowly provided renal function is not seriously impaired or there is no evidence of active intracranial bleeding. Chemical phlebitis and thrombosis near the site of injection have been reported infrequently.

Reactions which may occur because of the solution (reconstituted) or the technique of administration include febrile response, infection at the site of injection, venous thrombosis or phlebitis extending from the site of injection, extravasation and hypervolemia.

If an adverse reaction does occur, discontinue the infusion, evaluate the patient, institute appropriate therapeutic countermeasures and save the remainder of the fluid for examination if deemed necessary.

Overdosage

In the event of overdosage as reflected by unusually elevated blood urea nitrogen (BUN) levels, discontinue the drug, evaluate the patient and institute corrective measures as indicated. (See Warnings and Administration and Dosage.)

GLYCERIN (Glycerol)

Rx	**Osmoglyn** (Alcon)	**Solution**: 50% (0.6 g glycerin/ml)	Lime flavor. In 220 ml.

GLYCERIN — ORAL

Refer to the general discussion of these agents in the Osmotic Diuretics Introduction.

Indications

For the short-term reduction of intraocular pressure. May be used prior to and after intraocular surgery. May be used to interrupt an acute attack of glaucoma.

May be employed in acute angle-closure glaucoma and is also of value in treatment of secondary glaucomas intractable to conventional management.

Administration and Dosage

➤*Dosage:* Usual dosage is 2 to 3 mL of glycerin per kg of body weight (approximately 4 to 6 oz per individual), given 1 to 1½ hours prior to surgery.

➤*Storage / Stability:* Store at room temperature.

Actions

➤*Pharmacology:* An oral osmotic agent for reducing intraocular pressure. It adds to the tonicity of the blood until metabolized and eliminated by the kidneys.

Contraindications

Anuria; severe dehydration; frank or impending acute pulmonary edema; severe cardiac decompensation; and in those with hypersensitivity to any component of this preparation.

Warnings

➤*Pregnancy:* *Category C.*

Animal reproduction studies have not been conducted with glycerin. It is also not known whether glycerin can cause fetal harm when administered to a pregnant woman or can affect reproduction capacity. This drug should be given to a pregnant woman only if clearly needed.

➤*Children:* Safety and efficacy have not been established.

Precautions

➤*Special risk:* When administered prior to surgery, ensure that the patient's bladder is emptied. Prolonged use may cause excess weight gain. Glycerin should be administered with caution to patients with cardiac, renal or hepatic disease. Altered hydration may lead to pulmonary edema or congestive heart failure.

Caution should be exercised in hypervolemia, confused mental states, and congestive heart disease; and in the dehydrated patient (eg, certain diabetics).

Adverse Reactions

➤*Miscellaneous:* Nausea, vomiting, headache, confusion, and disorientation may occur. Severe dehydration, cardiac arrhythmia, or hyperosmolar nonketolic coma which can result in death have been reported.

ISOSORBIDE

Rx	**Ismotic** (Alcon)	**Solution**: 45% (100 g per 220 ml)	With 4.6 mEq sodium and 0.9 mEq potassium per 220 ml. Alcohol, saccharin, sorbitol. Vanilla-mint flavor. In 220 ml.

ISOSORBIDE — ORAL

Refer to the general discussion of these agents in the Osmotic Diuretics Introduction.

Indications

For the short-term reduction of intraocular pressure prior to and after intraocular surgery.

May be used to interrupt an acute attack of glaucoma. Use where less risk of nausea and vomiting than that posed by other oral hyperosmotic agents is needed.

Administration and Dosage

➤*Initial dose:* 1.5 g/kg (equivalent to 1.5 ml/lb).

➤*Dose range:* 1 to 3 g/kg 2 to 4 times a day as indicated.

Palatability may be improved if the medication is poured over cracked ice and sipped.

Contraindications

Well established anuria; severe dehydration; frank or impending acute pulmonary edema; severe cardiac decompensation; hypersensitivity to any component of this preparation.

Warnings

➤*Fluid / Electrolyte balance:* With repeated doses, maintain adequate fluid and electrolyte balance.

➤*Urinary output:* If urinary output continues to decrease, closely review the patient's clinical status. Accumulation may result in overexpansion of the extracellular fluid.

➤*Pregnancy:* *Category B.* There is no adequate information on whether this drug affects fertility in humans or has a teratogenic potential or other adverse fetal effect. Use during pregnancy only if clearly needed.

Precautions

➤*Repetitive doses:* Use repetitive doses with caution, particularly in patients with diseases associated with salt retention. Ensure that the patient's bladder has been emptied prior to surgery.

Adverse Reactions

Nausea; vomiting; headache; confusion; disorientation; gastric discomfort; thirst; hiccoughs; hypernatremia; hyperosmolarity; rash; irritability; syncope; lethargy; vertigo; dizziness; lightheadedness.

NONPRESCRIPTION DIURETICS

otc	**Maximum Strength Aqua•Ban** (Thompson Medical)	**Tablets**: 50 mg pamabrom	Lactose. In 30s.

NONPRESCRIPTION DIURETICS — ORAL

Indications

For the relief of temporary water weight gain, bloating, swelling, or full feeling associated with the premenstrual and menstrual periods.

Administration and Dosage

Take 1 tablet 4 times/day. Do not take more than 4 tablets in a 24-hour period.

Nonprescription diuretic products are promoted for the alleviation of menstrual discomfort. When taken 5 to 6 days before onset of menses, *otc* diuretics may help relieve symptoms related to water retention. These include excess water weight, bloating, swelling, painful breasts, cramps, and tension.

The most frequently used *otc* diuretic agents are ammonium chloride and caffeine. These agents are classified as Category I (generally recognized as safe and effective and not misbranded).

Indications

➤*Bronchodilation:* Relief of reversible bronchospasm associated with acute and chronic bronchial asthma, exercise-induced bronchospasm (EIB), bronchitis, emphysema, bronchiectasis, or other obstructive pulmonary diseases.

According to the National Asthma Education and Prevention Program's Expert Panel Report II, long-acting β_2 agonists (eg, **salmeterol**) are used concomitantly with anti-inflammatory medications for long-term control of symptoms, especially nocturnal symptoms. They also prevent EIB. Short-acting $\beta_2$agonists (eg, **albuterol**, **bitolterol**, **pirbuterol**, **terbutaline**) are the therapy of choice for relief of acute symptoms and prevention of EIB.

Refer to individual monographs for indications of specific agents.

Actions

➤*Pharmacology:* Sympathomimetic agents are used to produce bronchodilation. They relieve reversible bronchospasm by relaxing the smooth muscles of the bronchioles in conditions associated with asthma, bronchitis, emphysema, or bronchiectasis. Bronchodilation may additionally facilitate expectoration. Some agents are also used for other purposes. See monographs for Vasopressors Used in Shock, Nasal Decongestants, and Ophthalmic Decongestants.

The pharmacologic actions of these agents include: Alpha-adrenergic stimulation (vasoconstriction, nasal decongestion, pressor effects); β_1-adrenergic stimulation (increased myocardial contractility and conduction); and β_2-adrenergic stimulation (bronchial dilation and vasodilation, enhancement of mucociliary clearance, inhibition of cholinergic neurotransmission). Beta-adrenergic drugs stimulate adenyl cyclase, the enzyme that catalyzes the formation of cyclic-3'5' adenosine monophosphate (cyclic AMP) from adenosine triphosphate (ATP). Cyclic AMP that is formed inhibits the release of mediators of immediate hypersensitivity from inflammatory cells, especially from mast cells and basophils. This increase of cyclic AMP leads to activation of protein kinase A, which inhibits the phosphorylation of myosin and lowers intracellular ionic calcium concentrations, resulting in relaxation.

Other adrenergic actions include alpha receptor-mediated contraction of GI and urinary sphincters; α and β receptor-mediated lipolysis; α and β receptor-mediated decrease in GI tone; and changes in renin secretion, uterine relaxation, hepatic glycogenolysis/gluconeogenesis, and pancreatic beta cell secretion.

The relative selectivity of action of sympathomimetic agents is the primary determinant of clinical usefulness; it can predict the most likely side effects. β_2 selective agents provide the greatest benefit with minimal side effects. Direct administration via inhalation provides prompt effects and minimizes systemic activity. These drugs also inhibit histamine release from mast cells, produce vasodilation, and increase ciliary motility. Bitolterol functions as a prodrug that must first be hydrolyzed by esterases in tissue and blood to its active moiety, colterol. Isoproterenol is one of the most potent bronchodilators available.

Sympathomimetic Bronchodilators: Pharmacologic Effects and Pharmacokinetic Properties

Sympathomimetic	Adrenergic receptor activity	β_2 potency[1]	Route	Onset (minutes)	Duration (hrs)
Salmeterol[2]	$\beta_1 < \beta_2$	0.5	Inh	within 20	12
Albuterol[2]	$\beta_1 < \beta_2$	2	PO	within 30	4-8
			Inh[3]	within 5	3-6
Bitolterol[2]	$\beta_1 < \beta_2$	5	Inh	2-4	5 ≥ 8
Isoetharine[2]	$\beta_1 < \beta_2$	6	Inh[3]	within 5	2-3
Metaproterenol[2]	$\beta_1 < \beta_2$	15	PO	≈ 30	4
			Inh[3]	5-30	1- ≥ 6
Pirbuterol[2]	$\beta_1 < \beta_2$	5	Inh	within 5	5
Terbutaline[2]	$\beta_1 < \beta_2$	4	PO	30	4-8
			SC	5-15	1.5-4
			Inh	5-30	3-6
Isoproterenol	β_1 β_2	1	IV	immediate	< 1
			Inh[3]	2-5	1-3
Ephedrine	α β_1 β_2	—	PO	15-60	3-5
			SC	> 20	≤ 1
			IM	10-20	≤ 1
			IV	immediate	—
Epinephrine	α β_1 β_2	—	SC	5-10	4-6
			IM	—	1-4
			Inh[3]	1-5	1-3

[1] Relative molar potency: 1 = most potent.
[2] These agents all have minor β_1 activity.
[3] May be administered via aerosol or bulb nebulizer or IPPB administration.

Contraindications

Hypersensitivity to any component (allergic reactions are rare); cardiac arrhythmias associated with tachycardia; angina, preexisting cardiac arrhythmias associated with tachycardia, known hypersensitivity to sympathomimetic amines, and ventricular arrhythmias requiring inotropic therapy, tachycardia or heart block caused by digitalis intoxication (**isoproterenol**); patients with organic brain damage, local anesthesia of certain areas (eg, fingers, toes) because of the risk of tissue sloughing, labor, cardiac dilatation, coronary insufficiency, cerebral arteriosclerosis, organic heart disease (**epinephrine**); in those cases where vasopressors may be contraindicated; narrow-angle glaucoma, nonanaphylactic shock during general anesthesia with halogenated hydrocarbons or cyclopropane (**epinephrine**, **ephedrine**).

Warnings

➤*Special risk patients:* Administer with caution to patients with diabetes mellitus, hyperthyroidism, prostatic hypertrophy (**ephedrine**) or history of seizures; elderly; psychoneurotic individuals, patients with long-standing bronchial asthma and emphysema who have developed degenerative heart disease (**epinephrine**).

In patients with status asthmaticus and abnormal blood gas tensions, improvement in vital capacity and blood gas tensions may not accompany apparent relief of bronchospasm following isoproterenol. Facilities for administering oxygen and ventilatory assistance are necessary.

Diabetes – Large doses of IV **albuterol** and IV **terbutaline** may aggravate preexisting diabetes mellitus and ketoacidosis. Relevance to the use of oral or inhaled albuterol and oral terbutaline is unknown. Diabetic patients receiving any of these agents may require an increase in dosage of insulin or oral hypoglycemic agents.

➤*Cardiovascular effects:* Use with caution in patients with cardiovascular disorders including coronary insufficiency, ischemic heart disease, coronary artery disease, cardiac arrhythmias, CHF, and hypertension.

Beta-adrenergic agonists can produce significant cardiovascular effects measured by pulse rate, blood pressure, symptoms, or ECG changes (eg, flattening of T-waves, prolongation of the QTc interval, and ST-segment depression).

Isoproterenol doses sufficient to increase the heart rate more than 130 bpm may increase the likelihood of inducing ventricular arrhythmias.

These agents may cause toxic symptoms through idiosyncratic response or overdosage. If cardiac rate increases sharply, angina patients may experience anginal pain until the cardiac rate decreases.

Patients who were administered **bitolterol** did not reveal a preferential β-$_2$adrenergic effect. At doses that produced long duration of bronchodilator activity with a mean maximum bronchodilating effect of approximately 40% increase in FEV_1 (forced expiratory volume in 1 second), a less than 10 beat/minute mean maximum increase in heart rate was seen. The effect on the heart rate was transient and similar to the increases seen in the isoproterenol-treated patients in these studies.

Closely monitor patients receiving **epinephrine**. Inadvertently induced high arterial blood pressure may result in angina pectoris, aortic rupture, or cerebral hemorrhage. Cardiac arrhythmias develop in some individuals even after therapeutic doses. Epinephrine causes changes in the ECG even in healthy people, including a decrease in amplitude of the T-wave.

Ephedrine may cause hypertension resulting in intracranial hemorrhage. It may induce anginal pain in patients with coronary insufficiency or ischemic heart disease.

Large doses of inhaled or oral **salmeterol** (12 to 20 times the recommended dose) have been associated with clinically significant prolongation of the QTc interval, which has the potential for producing ventricular arrhythmias.

Significant changes in systolic and diastolic blood pressure can occur in some patients after use of any beta-adrenergic aerosol bronchodilator.

➤*Paradoxical bronchospasm:* Occasional patients have developed severe paradoxical airway resistance with repeated, excessive use of inhalation preparations; the cause is unknown. Discontinue the drug immediately and institute alternative therapy because patients may not respond to other therapy until the drug is withdrawn.

➤*Usual dose response:* Advise patients to contact a physician if they do not respond to their usual dose of a sympathomimetic amine.

Close supervision is recommended in patients requiring more than 3 **isoproterenol** aerosolized treatments. Further therapy with the bronchodilator aerosol alone is inadvisable when 3 to 5 treatments within 6 to 12 hours produce minimal or no relief. Reduce **epinephrine** dose if bronchial irritation, nervousness, restlessness, or sleeplessness occurs. Do not continue to use epinephrine, but seek medical assistance immediately if symptoms are not relieved within 20 minutes or become worse.

➤*CNS effects:* Sympathomimetics may produce CNS stimulation.

IV **albuterol** sulfate in animals has demonstrated that it crosses the blood-brain barrier and reaches brain concentrations of approximately 5% of the plasma concentrations.

➤*Long-term use:* Prolonged use of **ephedrine** may produce a syndrome resembling an anxiety state. Many patients develop nervousness and a sedative may be needed. After prolonged use or overdosage, elevated serum lactic acid levels with severe metabolic acidosis have occurred, as have transient blood glucose elevations.

➤*Acute symptoms:* Do not use **salmeterol** to treat acute asthma symptoms. If the patient's short-acting, inhaled β_2-agonist becomes less effective (eg, the patient needs more inhalations than usual), obtain medical evaluation immediately. Increasing its use in this situation is inappropriate. Do not use salmeterol more frequently than twice daily (morning and evening) at the recommended dose. When prescribing salmeterol, provide patients with a short-acting, inhaled β_2-agonist (eg, albuterol) for treatment of symptoms that occur despite regular twice-daily (morning and evening) use of salmeterol.

Asthma may deteriorate acutely over a period of hours or chronically over several days. In this setting, increased use of inhaled, short-acting β_2-agonists is a marker of destabilization of asthma and requires re-evaluation of the patient. Consider alternative treatment regimens, especially inhaled or systemic corticosteroids. If the patient uses at least 4 inhalations/day of a short-acting β_2-agonist on a regular basis, or if more than 1 canister (200 inhalations per canister) is used in an 8-week period, have the patient see the physician for re-evaluation of treatment.

Use with short-acting β_2-agonists – When patients begin treatment with **salmeterol**, advise those who have been taking short-acting, inhaled β_2-agonists on a regular daily basis to discontinue their regular daily dosing regimen, and clearly instruct them to use short-acting, inhaled β_2-agonists only for symptomatic relief if they develop asthma symptoms while taking salmeterol.

➤*Morbidity/Mortality:* It was previously suggested that an increased risk of death or near death from asthma may be associated with the regular use of inhaled beta agonists. Another study demonstrated that patients with mild intermittent asthma were neither harmed nor did they benefit from regularly scheduled daily use of short-acting inhaled beta agonists. However, regularly scheduled, daily use of beta agonists is not recommended.

Excessive use of inhalants – Deaths from excessive use of inhaled sympathomimetics have been reported; the exact cause is unknown, but cardiac arrest following an unexpected severe acute asthmatic crisis and subsequent hypoxia is suspected.

➤*Overdosage/IV injection:* Overdosage or inadvertent IV injection of conventional SC **epinephrine** doses may cause extremely elevated arterial pressure, which may result in cerebrovascular hemorrhage, particularly in elderly patients; severe peripheral constriction and cardiac stimulation resulting in pulmonary arterial hypertension and potentially fatal pulmonary edema; and ventricular hyperirritability, which may result in death from ventricular fibrillation. Epinephrine is rapidly inactivated in the body, and treatment is primarily supportive. If necessary, pressor effects may be counteracted by rapidly acting vasodilators or alpha-adrenergic blocking drugs. If prolonged hypotension follows such measures, it may be necessary to administer another pressor drug, such as norepinephrine. If an epinephrine overdose induces pulmonary edema that interferes with respiration, treatment consists of a rapidly acting alpha-adrenergic blocking drug (eg, phentolamine) or intermittent positive-pressure respiration. Transient bradycardia followed by tachycardia may also result, and these may be accompanied by potentially fatal cardiac arrhythmias. Ventricular, premature contractions may appear within 1 minute after injection and may be followed by multifocal, ventricular tachycardia (prefibrillation rhythm). Subsidence of the ventricular effects may be followed by atrial tachycardia and occasionally by AV block. Treatment of arrhythmias consists of administration of a beta-adrenergic blocking drug, such as propranolol. Overdosage sometimes also results in extreme pallor and coldness of skin, metabolic acidosis, and kidney failure. Take suitable corrective measures.

➤*Respiratory depression:* When compressed oxygen is used as the aerosol propellant, determine the percentage of oxygen by the patient's individual requirements to avoid depression of respiratory drive.

➤*Hypersensitivity reactions:* Hypersensitivity (allergic) reactions can occur after administration of **bitolterol**, **albuterol**, **metaproterenol**, **terbutaline**, **ephedrine**, **salmeterol**, and possibly other bronchodilators. See Management of Acute Hypersensitivity Reactions.

➤*Carcinogenesis:* A significant increase in the incidence of leiomyomas of the mesovarium and ovarian cysts has been demonstrated with **albuterol** and **terbutaline** in animal studies. **Salmeterol** caused a dose-related increase in the incidence of smooth muscle hyperplasia and cystic glandular hyperplasia of the uterus in mice.

➤*Elderly:* Lower doses may be required because of increased sympathomimetic sensitivity. Observe special caution when using in elderly patients who have concomitant cardiovascular disease that could be adversely affected by this class of drug. Based on available data, no adjustment of **salmeterol** dosage in geriatric patients is warranted.

➤*Pregnancy: Category B* (**terbutaline**). *Category C* (**albuterol**, **bitolterol**, **ephedrine**, **epinephrine**, **isoetharine**, **isoproterenol**, **metaproterenol**, **salmeterol**, **pirbuterol**). Several of these agents are teratogenic and embryocidal in animal studies. There is no evidence that these class effects in animals are relevant to use in humans. There are no adequate and well-controlled studies in pregnant women. Use only when clearly needed and when potential benefits outweigh potential hazards to the fetus.

Labor and delivery – Use of β_2-active sympathomimetics inhibits uterine contractions. Adverse reactions include increased heart rate, transient hyperglycemia, hypokalemia, cardiac arrhythmias, pulmonary edema, cerebral and myocardial ischemia, and increased fetal heart rate and hypoglycemia in the neonate. Although these effects are unlikely with aerosol use, consider the potential for untoward effects.

Oral **albuterol** has the potential to delay preterm labor. There are no well-controlled studies that demonstrate that they stop preterm labor or prevent labor at term. Therefore, use cautiously in pregnant patients when given for relief of bronchospasm to avoid interference with uterine contractility. **Terbutaline** is not indicated for and is not used for the management of preterm labor. Maternal death has occurred with terbutaline and other drugs in this class.

Parenteral administration of **ephedrine** to maintain blood pressure during low or other spinal anesthesia for delivery can cause acceleration of fetal heart rate; do not use in obstetrics when maternal blood pressure exceeds 130/80.

➤*Lactation:* **Terbutaline**, **ephedrine**, and **epinephrine** are excreted in breast milk. It is not known whether other agents are excreted in breast milk. Decide whether to discontinue nursing or to discontinue the drug, taking into account the importance of the drug to the mother.

➤*Children:*

Inhalation – Safety and efficacy for use of **bitolterol**, **pirbuterol**, **isoetharine**, **salmeterol**, and **terbutaline** in children 12 years of age or younger have not been established. **Albuterol** aerosol and inhalation powder in children younger than 4 years of age and **albuterol** solution for inhalation in children younger than 2 years of age have not been established. **Metaproterenol** may be used in children 6 years of age or older.

Injection – Parenteral **terbutaline** is not recommended for use in children younger than 12 years of age. Administer **epinephrine** with caution to infants and children. Syncope has occurred following administration to asthmatic children.

Oral – **Metaproterenol** is not recommended for use in children younger than 6 years of age. **Terbutaline** is not recommended for use in children younger than 12 years of age. Safety and efficacy have not been established for **albuterol** in children younger than 2 years of age (syrup) and younger than 6 years of age (tablets and extended-release tablets). In children, **ephedrine** is effective in the oral therapy of asthma. Because of its CNS-stimulating effect, it is rarely used alone. This effect is usually countered by an appropriate sedative; however, its rationale has been questioned.

Precautions

➤*Tolerance:* Tolerance may occur with prolonged use of sympathomimetic agents, but temporary cessation of the drug restores its original effectiveness.

➤*Hypokalemia:* Decreases in serum potassium levels have occurred, possibly through intracellular shunting, which can produce adverse cardiovascular effects. The decrease is usually transient, not requiring supplementation.

➤*Hyperglycemia:* **Isoproterenol** causes less hyperglycemia than does **epinephrine**. Isoproterenol and epinephrine are equally effective in stimulating the release of free fatty acids and energy production.

Glycogenolysis in the liver is increased by **ephedrine** but not as much as by **epinephrine**; usual doses of ephedrine are unlikely to produce hyperglycemia.

➤*Parkinson's disease:* **Epinephrine** may temporarily increase rigidity and tremor.

➤*Parenteral use:* Administer **epinephrine** with great caution and in carefully circumscribed quantities in areas of the body served by end arteries or with otherwise limited blood supply (eg, fingers, toes, nose, ears, genitals) or if peripheral vascular disease is present to avoid vasoconstriction-induced tissue sloughing.

➤*Combined therapy:* Concomitant use with other sympathomimetic agents is not recommended, as it may lead to deleterious cardiovascular effects. This does not preclude the judicious use of an adrenergic stimulant aerosol bronchodilator in patients receiving tablets. Do not give on a routine basis. If regular coadministration is required, consider alternative therapy.

Do not use greater than or equal to 2 beta-adrenergic aerosol bronchodilators simultaneously because of the potential of additive effects.

Patients must be warned not to stop or reduce corticosteroid therapy without medical advice, even if they feel better when they are being treated with β_2 agonists. These agents are not to be used as a substitute for oral or inhaled corticosteroids.

➤*Sulfites:* Some of these products contain sulfites that may cause allergic-type reactions (including anaphylactic symptoms and life-threatening or less severe asthmatic episodes) in certain susceptible persons. The overall prevalence of sulfite sensitivity in the general population is unknown and probably low. It is seen more frequently in asthmatic or atopic nonasthmatic persons.

➤*Benzyl alcohol:* Benzyl alcohol, contained in some of these products as a preservative, has been associated with a fatal "gasping syndrome" in premature infants.

➤*Drug abuse and dependence:* Prolonged abuse of **ephedrine** can lead to symptoms of paranoid schizophrenia. Patients exhibit such signs as tachycardia, poor nutrition and hygiene, fever, cold sweat, and dilated pupils. Some measure of tolerance develops, but addiction does not occur. With all sympathomimetic aerosols, cardiac arrest and even death may be associated with abuse.

Drug Interactions

Most interactions listed apply to sympathomimetics when used as vasopressors; however, consider the interaction when using the bronchodilator sympathomimetics.

Sympathomimetic Bronchodilator Drug Interactions			
Precipitant drug	Object drug*		Description
Beta blockers	Sympathomimetics	↓	Concomitant use may inhibit cardiac, bronchodilating, and vasodilating effects. Severe bronchospasms may be produced in asthmatic patients taking **albuterol** or **salmeterol**. Consider cardioselective beta blockers, and use with caution if there are no alternatives to beta blocker therapy. With **epinephrine**, an initial hypertensive episode followed by bradycardia may occur.
Furazolidone	Sympathomimetics	↑	The pressor sensitivity to mixed-acting sympathomimetics (eg, **ephedrine**) may be increased. Direct-acting agents (eg, **epinephrine**) are not affected.
Guanethidine	Sympathomimetics Direct Mixed	 ↑ ↓	Guanethidine potentiates the effects of the direct-acting sympathomimetics (eg, **epinephrine**) and inhibits the effects of the mixed-acting agents (eg, **ephedrine**). Guanethidine hypotensive action may also be reversed, requiring increased guanethidine dosage.
Sympathomimetics	Guanethidine	↓	
Methyldopa	Sympathomimetics	↑	Concurrent administration may result in an increased pressor response.
MAO inhibitors	Sympathomimetics	↑	Coadministration of MAO inhibitors and mixed-acting sympathomimetics (eg, **ephedrine**) may result in severe headache, hypertension, and hyperpyrexia, resulting in hypertensive crisis. MAO inhibitors also potentiate the actions of beta-adrenergic agonists on the vascular system. Direct-acting agents (eg, **epinephrine**) interact minimally. Avoid coadministration with sympathomimetics or within 2 weeks.
Oxytocic drugs (eg, ergonovine)	Sympathomimetics	↓	Concurrent administration may result in severe hypotension.
Rauwolfia alkaloids	Sympathomimetics Direct Mixed	 ↑ ↓	Reserpine potentiates the pressor response of the direct-acting sympathomimetics (eg, **epinephrine**), which may result in hypertension. The pressor response of the mixed-acting agents (eg, **ephedrine**) is decreased.

Sympathomimetic Bronchodilator Drug Interactions			
Precipitant drug	Object drug*		Description
Tricyclic antidepressants (TCAs)	Sympathomimetics Direct Mixed	 ↑ ↓	TCAs potentiate the pressor response of direct-acting sympathomimetics (eg, **epinephrine**); dysrhythmias have occurred. The pressor response of mixed-acting agents (eg, **ephedrine**) is decreased. TCAs also potentiate the actions of beta-adrenergic agonists on the vascular system.
Sympathomimetics	Theophylline	↔	Enhanced toxicity, particularly cardiotoxicity, has been noted. Decreased theophylline levels may occur. **Ephedrine** may cause theophylline toxicity.
General anesthetics (eg, halothane, cyclopropane)	Isoproterenol Epinephrine Ephedrine	↑	The potential for the myocardium to be sensitized to the effects of sympathomimetic amines is increased. Arrhythmias may result with coadministration and may respond to beta blockers.
Cardiac glycosides			
Alpha-adrenergic blockers (eg, phentolamine)	Ephedrine Epinephrine	↓	Vasoconstricting and hypertensive effects are antagonized.
Diuretics	Ephedrine Epinephrine	↓	Vascular response may be decreased.
Antihistamines	Epinephrine	↑	**Epinephrine** effects may be potentiated.
Ergot alkaloids Phenothiazines Nitrites	Epinephrine	↓	Pressor effects of epinephrine may be reversed.
Levothyroxine	Epinephrine	↑	**Epinephrine** effects may be potentiated.
Epinephrine	Insulin or oral hypoglycemic agents	↓	Diabetics may require an increased dose of the hypoglycemic agent.
Ergot alkaloids	Isoproterenol	↑	Coadministration may result in additive peripheral vasoconstriction.
Isoproterenol	Ergot alkaloids		
Albuterol Salmeterol	Diuretics	↑	ECG changes and hypokalemia associated with these diuretics may worsen with coadministration.
Albuterol	Digoxin	↓	Digoxin serum levels may be decreased.

* ↑ = Object drug increased. ↓ = Object drug decreased.
↔ = Undetermined clinical effect.

➤*Drug/Lab test interactions:* **Isoproterenol** causes false elevations of bilirubin as measured in vitro by a sequential multiple analyzer. Isoproterenol inhalation may result in enough absorption of the drug to produce elevated urinary **epinephrine** values. Although small with standard doses, the effect is likely to increase with larger doses.

Adverse Reactions

Sympathomimetic Bronchodilator Adverse Reactions (%)[1]

	Adverse reaction	Salmeterol	Albuterol	Bitolterol	Isoetharine	Metaproterenol	Pirbuterol	Terbutaline	Isoproterenol	Ephedrine	Epinephrine
Cardiovascular	Palpitations	1-3	< 1-10	1.5-3	✓[2]	0.3-4	1.3-1.7	≤ 23	< 5-22	✓	7.8-30
	Tachycardia	1-3	1-10	< 3.7	✓	< 17	1.2-1.3	1.3-3	2-12	✓	≤ 2.6
	Blood pressure changes/ hypertension		1-5	< 1	✓	0.3		< 1	2-5		✓
	Chest tightness/pain/discomfort, angina		< 3	≤ 1.5		0.2	< 1.3	1.3-1.5	✓		≤ 2.6
	PVCs, arrhythmias, skipped beats			0.5			< 1	≈ 4	< 1-3	✓	✓
CNS	Tremor	4	< 1-24.2	9-26.6	✓	1-33	1.3-6	< 5-38	< 15		16-18
	Dizziness/vertigo	≥ 3	< 1-7	1-4	✓	1-4	0.6-1.2	1.3-10	1.5-5	✓	3.3-7.8
	Shakiness/ nervousness/ tension	1-3	1-20	1.5-11.1	✓	2.6-14	4.5-7	< 5-31	< 15	✓	8.5-31
	Weakness		< 2		✓	1.3	< 1	≤ 1.3	✓		1.6-2.6
	Drowsiness		< 1			0.7		< 5-11.7	< 5		8.2-14
	Restlessness		< 1		✓						✓
	Hyperactivity/ Hyperkinesia, excitement		1-20	< 1	✓		< 1		✓		
	Headache	28	2-22	≤ 8.4	✓	≤ 4	1.3-2	7.8-10	1.5-10	✓	3.3-10
	Insomnia		1-11	< 1	✓	1.8	< 1	✓	1.5	✓	✓
GI	Nausea/Vomiting	1-3	2-15	≤ 3	✓	< 14	≤ 1.7	1.3-10	< 15	✓	1-11.5
	Heartburn/GI distress/ disorder	1-3	≤ 5			≤ 4		< 10	≤ 5-10		
	Diarrhea	1-3	1			0.7	< 1.3				
	Dry mouth		< 3			1.3	< 1.3				
Respiratory	Cough	7	< 1-5	≤ 4.1		≤ 4	1.2		1-5		
	Wheezing		≤ 1.5					✓	1.5		
	Dyspnea		1.5	≤ 1				≤ 2	≤ 1.5		≤ 2
	Bronchospasm		1-15.4	≤ 1.5					≤ 18		
	Throat dryness/irritation, pharyngitis	≥ 3	≤ 6	2.5-5		≤ 4	< 1	✓	3.1		
Miscellaneous	Flushing		< 1	< 1			< 1	≤ 2.4	✓		≤ 1.3
	Sweating		< 1					≤ 2.4	✓	✓	✓
	Anorexia/ Appetite loss		1				< 1			✓	✓
	Unusual/bad taste or taste/ smell change		< 1			≤ 0.3	< 1	✓			

[1] Data pooled for all routes of administration, all age groups, from separate studies, and are not necessarily comparable.

[2] ✓ = Reported; no incidence given.

Adverse reactions are generally transient, and no cumulative effects have been reported. It is usually not necessary to discontinue treatment; however, in selected cases temporarily reduce dosage. After the reaction has subsided, increase dosage in small increments to optimal dosage. In addition to the table, other adverse reactions are as follows:

➤*Albuterol:*

CNS – CNS stimulation, malaise (1.5%); emotional lability, fatigue, nightmares, aggressive behavior (1%); lightheadedness, disturbed sleep, irritability (less than 1%).

Respiratory – Bronchitis (1.5% to 4%); nasal congestion (1% to 2%); sputum increase (1.5%); epistaxis (1% to 3%); hoarseness (rare in adults; 2% in children 4 to 12 years old).

Miscellaneous – Increased appetite, stomachache (3%); muscle cramps (1% to 3%); pallor, conjunctivitis, anorexia, teeth discoloration, dyspepsia (1%); dilated pupils, epigastric pain, micturition difficulty, muscle spasm, voice changes (less than 1%); urticaria, angioedema, rash, bronchospasm, oropharyngeal edema (rare with oral and inhaled albuterol). Rarely, erythema multiforme and Stevens-Johnson syndrome have been associated with the administration of albuterol sulfate syrup in children. There have been rare reports of GI obstruction in such patients in association with ingestion of products containing delivery systems similar to that contained in albuterol sulfate extended-release tablets.

➤*Bitolterol:*

Miscellaneous – Lightheadedness (6.8%). Elevations of AST, decrease in platelets and WBC counts and proteinuria (rare); clinical relevance or relationship is unknown. The overall incidence of cardiovascular effects was approximately 5%.

➤*Ephedrine:* Precordial pain; contact dermatitis after topical application.

Parenteral: Vesical sphincter spasm from repeated injections resulting in difficult and painful urination; urinary retention in males with prostatism. Confusion, delirium, and hallucinations; cerebral hemorrhage.

➤*Epinephrine:* Anxiety; fear; pallor.

Parenteral: Cerebral hemorrhage; induce or aggravate psychomotor agitation; disorientation; impairment of memory; assaultive behavior; panic; hallucinations; suicidal or homicidal tendencies; schizophrenic-type thought disorders or paranoid delusions; hemiplegia; and subarachnoid and cerebral hemorrhage; direct vasoconstrictive effect on the renal circulation; syncope in children; temporary rigidity and tremor in Parkinson's disease patients; fatal ventricular fibrillation; occlusion of the central retinal artery, shock, and angina in coronary-artery disease; urticaria, wheal, and hemorrhage at injection site; pain at injection site (1.6% to 2.6%); local tissue necrosis from vascular constriction due to repeated injections at the same site.

➤*Isoetharine:*

Miscellaneous – Anxiety.

➤*Isoproterenol:*

Cardiovascular – Adams-Stokes attacks; cardiac arrest; hypotension; precordial ache/distress. In a few patients, presumably with organic disease of the AV node and its branches, isoproterenol has precipitated Adams-Stokes seizures during normal sinus rhythm or transient heart block.

Respiratory – Bronchitis (5%); sputum increase (1.5%); rebound bronchospasm; coronary insufficiency; paradoxical airway resistance; pulmonary edema.

➤*Metaproterenol:*

Respiratory – Asthma exacerbation (1% to 4%); hoarseness, nasal congestion (0.7%).

Miscellaneous – Rash (1.3%); backache, fatigue, skin reaction (0.7%).

➤*Pirbuterol:*

CNS – Anxiety, confusion, depression, fatigue, syncope (less than 1%).

Dermatologic – Alopecia, edema, pruritus, rash, bruising (less than 1%).

GI – Abdominal pain/cramps, glossitis, stomatitis (less than 1%).

Miscellaneous – Hypotension, numbness in extremities, weight gain (less than 1%).

➤*Salmeterol:*

Respiratory – Upper respiratory tract infection, nasopharyngitis (14%); nasal cavity/sinus disease (6%); sinus headache, lower respiratory tract infection (4%); allergic rhinitis (≥ 3%); rhinitis, laryngitis, tracheitis/bronchitis (1% to 3%).

Musculoskeletal – Joint/back pain, muscle cramp/contraction, myalgia/myositis, muscular soreness (1% to 3%).

Miscellaneous – Giddiness, influenza (≥ 3%); viral gastroenteritis, urticaria, dental pain, malaise/fatigue, rash/skin eruption, dysmenorrhea (1% to 3%).

➤*Terbutaline:*

Miscellaneous – ECG changes, such as sinus pause, atrial premature beats, AV block, ventricular premature beats, ST-T-wave depression, T-wave inversion, sinus bradycardia, and atrial escape beat with aberrant conduction; increased heart rate; muscle cramps; central stimulation; pain at injection site (0.5% to 2.6%); elevations in liver enzymes, seizures, and hypersensitivity vasculitis (rare).

Overdosage

➤*Inhalation:*

Symptoms – Exaggeration of the effects listed under Adverse Reactions can occur. Seizures, hypokalemia, anginal pain, hyperglycemia, hypotension, or hypertension may result. Clinically significant prolongation with QTc interval and cardiac arrest have been reported with use.

Treatment – Discontinue medication with general supportive measures. Monitor blood pressure and ECG. The judicious use of a cardioselective β-receptor blocker (ic, mctoprolol, atenolol) is suggested, bearing in mind the danger of inducing an asthmatic attack. Dialysis is not appropriate.

➤*Systemic:*

Symptoms – Palpitations; tachycardia; transient arrhythmias; bradycardia; extrasystoles; heart block; angina; hyperglycemia and increased insulin levels followed by rebound hypoglycemia; hypokalemia; hypo- or hypertension; significant drop in blood pressure caused by peripheral vasodilation; fever; chills; cold perspiration; blanching of the skin; nausea; vomiting; mydriasis. Central actions produce insomnia, anxiety, nervousness, drowsiness, muscle cramps, headache, sweating, and tremor. Delirium, convulsions, collapse, and coma may occur.

The principal manifestation of **ephedrine** sulfate poisoning is convulsions. The following signs and symptoms may also occur: Initially, the patient may have hypertension, followed later by hypotension accompanied by anuria. Nausea, vomiting, chills, cyanosis, irritability, nervousness, fever, suicidal behavior, tachycardia, dilated pupils, blurred vision, opisthotonos, spasms, convulsions, pulmonary edema, gasping respirations, coma, and respiratory failure.

Treatment – Discontinue medication or reduce dosage. Emesis, gastric lavage, or charcoal may be useful following overdosage with oral agents. If pronounced, a β-adrenergic blocker (propranolol) may be used, but consider the possibility of aggravation of airway obstruction; phentolamine may be used to block strong α-adrenergic actions. Treatment includes usual supportive measures. Monitor blood pressure, pulse, respiration, and ECG. If respirations are shallow or cyanosis is present, administer artificial respiration. Vasopressors are contraindicated. In cardiovascular collapse, maintain blood pressure. For hypertension, 5 mg phentolamine mesylate diluted in saline may be administered slowly IV, or 100 mg may be given orally. Convulsions may be controlled by diazepam or paraldehyde. Cool applications and dexamethasone 1 mg/kg administered slowly IV may control pyrexia. Refer to General Management of Acute Overdosage.

Patient Information

➤*Inhalation:* Patient instructions are available with products. Many patients do not use metered-dose inhalers correctly, even after repeated instructions. Do not assume the patient understands the use of inhaled drugs and the proper administration technique. Use verbal instructions as well as an actual demonstration if possible. Repeat instructions at follow-up visits.

Thoroughly shake the inhaler with canister in place for 5 to 10 seconds; breathe out to the end of a normal breath. Hold the inhaler system upright; place the mouthpiece into the mouth, close the lips tightly or position mouthpiece 2 to 3 finger widths from open mouth, and tilt head back slightly. While activating the inhaler, take a slow, deep breath for 3 to 5 seconds; hold the breath for approximately 10 seconds, and exhale slowly. Allow at least 1 minute between inhalations (puffs) if necessary. Allow at least 2 minutes between inhalations for **metaproterenol**. Rinse mouth with water after each use.

Do not exceed recommended dosage; excessive use may lead to adverse effects or loss of effectiveness. Do not stop or adjust the dose.

Do not change brands without consulting the physician or pharmacist.

Notify physician if treatment is less effective, symptoms worsen, or the need to use this product increases in frequency. Usual adverse events include palpitations, chest pain, rapid heart rate, and tremor or nervousness.

Isoproterenol – May cause the patient's saliva to turn pinkish red.

Salmeterol – Shake well before using. Salmeterol is not meant to relieve acute asthmatic symptoms, which should be treated with an inhaled, short-acting bronchodilator. The bronchodilator action usually lasts for greater than or equal to 12 hours; therefore, do not use more often than every 12 hours. While using salmeterol, seek medical attention immediately if the short-acting bronchodilator treatment becomes less effective for symptom relief, if more inhalations than usual are needed, or if more than the maximum number of inhalations of short-acting bronchodilator treatment prescribed for a 24-hour period are needed. If the patient uses greater than or equal to 4 inhalations/day of a short-acting β_2-agonist on a regular basis or if more than 1 canister (200 inhalations/canister) is used in an 8-week period, have the patient see the physician for re-evaluation of treatment. When using salmeterol to prevent exercise-induced bronchospasm, administer the dose greater than or equal to 30 to 60 minutes before exercise.

➤*Metered dose inhalers:* The contents of metered dose inhalers are under pressure. Do not puncture. Do not use or store near heat or open flame. Exposure to temperatures more than 120°F may cause bursting. Never throw container into fire or incinerator. Keep out of reach of children. If unusual smell or taste is noted with use, discontinue use in consultation with physician.

Warn patients that adverse cardiovascular effects may occur (eg, palpitations, chest pain, rapid heart rate, tremor, nervousness).

➤*Proper nebulizer use:* Find a location where the patient can sit comfortably for 10 to 15 minutes. Plug in the compressor. Mix the medication as directed, or empty the prepared unit dose vials (UDVs) into the nebulizer. Do not mix different types of medications without permission from the physician or pharmacist. Assemble the mask or mouthpiece and connect the tubing from this to the port on the compressor. Sit in a comfortable, upright position. Put the mask over nose and mouth (make sure it fits properly so the mist does not flow up into eyes); or if using a mouthpiece, put it into mouth. Turn on the compressor. Take slow, deep breaths. If possible, hold breath for 10 seconds before slowly exhaling. Continue until medication chamber is empty. Wash mask with hot, soapy water. Rinse well and allow to air dry before reuse.

➤*Oral:* Do not exceed prescribed dosage. If GI upset occurs, take with food.

May cause nervousness, restlessness, insomnia (especially **ephedrine**); if these effects continue after reducing dosage, notify physician.

Notify physician if palpitations, tachycardia, chest pain, muscle tremors, dizziness, headache, flushing, or difficult urination (ephedrine) occurs or if breathing difficulty persists.

➤*Epinephrine injection:* In the event of a life-threatening situation, follow these steps immediately to administer epinephrine:

1.) Remove blue plastic needle cover. Hold syringe upright and push plunger to expel air and excess epinephrine (plunger will stop).
2.) Rotate rectangular plunger ¼ turn to the right. Plunger will align with slot in barrel of syringe. Wipe injection site with alcohol swab, if available.
3.) Insert needle straight into arm or thigh.
4.) Push plunger until it stops. Syringe will inject a 0.3 mL dose for adults and children older than 12 years of age. *Children:* Syringe barrel has 0.1 mL graduations so that smaller doses can be measured. *Administer to infants to 2 years of age:* 0.05 to 0.1 mL; *2 to 6 years of age:* 0.15 mL; and *6 to 12 years of age:* 0.2 mL. Once initial injection has been administered, follow these additional steps.
5.) Contact physician, if possible.
6.) Prepare syringe for a possible second injection. Turn the rectangular plunger ¼ turn to the right to line up with rectangular slot in the syringe (a slight wiggling may aid the turning and alignment of the plunger).
7.) *The second injection:* If, after 10 minutes from the first injection, symptoms are not noticeably improved, a second injection is required. Dispose of syringe and remaining contents.
8.) Keep patient warm and avoid exertion.

ISOPROTERENOL HCl

See the Isoproterenol monograph in the Vasopressors Used in Shock section and the group monograph in the Cardiovascular Agents chapter.

EPHEDRINE SULFATE

See the Ephedrine monograph in the Vasopressors Used in Shock section and the group group monograph in the Cardiovascular Agents chapter.

EPINEPHRINE

See the Epinephrine monograph in the Vasopressors Used in Shock section and the group group monograph in the Cardiovascular Agents chapter.

LEVALBUTEROL HYDROCHLORIDE

Rx	**Xopenex** (Sepracor)	**Solution for inhalation**: 0.31 mg per 3 mL (as base)	Preservative-free. Sulfuric acid. In UD 3 mL vials.
		0.63 mg per 3 mL (as base)	Preservative-free. Sulfuric acid. In UD 3 mL vials.
		1.25 mg per 3 mL (as base)	Preservative-free. Sulfuric acid. In UD 3 mL vials.
		Solution for inhalation, concentrate: 1.25 mg per 0.5 mL	Preservative-free. In 0.5 mL UD vials.

LEVALBUTEROL HYDROCHLORIDE — INHALATION

For complete and comparative prescribing information, refer to the Sympathomimetic Bronchodilator group monograph.

Indications

➤*Bronchospasm:* For the treatment or prevention of bronchospasm in adults, adolescents, and children 6 years of age and older with reversible obstructive airway disease.

Administration and Dosage

➤*Approved by the FDA:* March 25, 1999.

➤*Children 6 to 11 years of age:* 0.31 mg administered 3 times/day by nebulization. Do not exceed routine dosing of 0.63 mg 3 times/day.

➤*Adults and adolescents 12 years of age and older:* 0.63 mg administered 3 times/day (every 6 to 8 hours) by nebulization.

Patients 12 years of age and older with more severe asthma or patients who do not respond adequately to a dose of 0.63 mg levalbuterol may benefit from a dosage of 1.25 mg 3 times/day. Closely monitor patients receiving the higher dose for adverse systemic effects and balance the risks of such effects against the potential for improved efficacy.

The use of levalbuterol can be continued as medically indicated to control recurring bouts of bronchospasm. During this time, most patients gain optimal benefit from regular use of the inhalation solution.

If a previously effective dosage regimen fails to provide the expected relief, seek immediate medical advice because this is often a sign of seriously worsening asthma that requires reassessment of therapy.

➤*Administration:* Dilute the concentrated solution (1.25 mg per 0.5 mL) with sterile normal saline before administration by nebulization.

The safety and efficacy of levalbuterol inhalation solution have been established in clinical trials when administered using the *PARI LC Jet* and the *PARI LC Plus* nebulizers, and the *PARI Master Dura-Neb 2000* and *Dura-Neb 3000* compressors. The safety and efficacy of levalbuterol inhalation solution when administered using other nebulizer systems have not been established.

Drug compatibility (physical and chemical), efficacy, and safety of levalbuterol solution for inhalation when mixed with other drugs in a nebulizer have not been established.

➤*Storage/Stability:* Store in the protective foil pouch between 20° and 25°C (68° and 77°F). Protect from light and excessive heat. Keep unopened vials in the foil pouch. Once the foil pouch is opened, use the vials within 2 weeks. If the individual vial is removed from the foil pouch and is not used immediately, protect from light and use within 1 week. Discard the vial if the solution is not colorless.

SALMETEROL XINAFOATE

Rx	**Serevent Diskus** (GlaxoSmithKline)	**Powder for inhalation** : 50 mcg (as base)	Lactose. In 60 blisters and institutional pack containing 28 blisters.

SALMETEROL XINAFOATE — INHALATION

For complete and comparative prescribing information, refer to the Sympathomimetic Bronchodilator group monograph.

WARNING

Long-acting beta$_2$-adrenergic agonists, such as salmeterol, may increase the risk of asthma-related death. Therefore, when treating patients with asthma, salmeterol should only be used as additional therapy for patients not adequately controlled on other asthma-controller medications (e.g., low- to medium-dose inhaled corticosteroids) or whose disease severity clearly warrants initiation of treatment with 2 maintenance therapies, including salmeterol. Data from a large placebo-controlled US study that compared the safety of salmeterol or placebo added to the usual asthma therapy showed an increase in asthma-related deaths in patients receiving salmeterol (13 deaths out of 13,176 patients treated for 28 weeks on salmeterol versus 3 deaths out of 13,179 patients on placebo).

Indications

➤*Asthma/Bronchospasm:* For long-term, twice daily (morning and evening) administration in the maintenance treatment of asthma and in the prevention of bronchospasm in patients 4 years of age and older with reversible obstructive airway disease, including patients with symptoms of nocturnal asthma.

Long-acting beta$_2$-adrenergic agonists, such as salmeterol, may increase the risk of asthma-related death. Therefore, when treating patients with asthma, salmeterol should only be used as additional therapy for patients not adequately controlled on other asthma-controller medications (e.g., low- to medium-dose inhaled corticosteroids) or whose disease severity clearly warrants initiation of treatment with 2 maintenance therapies, including salmeterol. Do not use in patients whose asthma can be managed by occasional use of short-acting, inhaled β_2-agonists or whose asthma can be successfully managed by inhaled corticosteroids or other controller medications along with occasional use of inhaled, short-acting β_2-agonists.

➤*Chronic obstructive pulmonary disease (COPD):* Long-term, twice daily (morning and evening) administration in the maintenance treatment of bronchospasm associated with COPD (including emphysema and chronic bronchitis).

➤*Exercise-induced bronchospasm (EIB):* For the prevention of EIB in patients 4 years of age and older.

Administration and Dosage

➤*Approved by the FDA:* February 4, 1994.

➤*Asthma/Bronchospasm:* Long-acting beta$_2$-adrenergic agonists, such as salmeterol, may increase the risk of asthma-related death. Therefore, when treating patients with asthma, salmeterol should only be used as additional therapy for patients not adequately controlled on other asthma-controller medications (e.g., low- to medium-dose inhaled corticosteroids) or whose disease severity clearly warrants initiation of treatment with 2 maintenance therapies, including salmeterol. Do not use in patients whose asthma can be managed by occasional use of short-acting, inhaled β_2-agonists or whose asthma can be successfully managed by inhaled corticosteroids or other controller medications along with occasional use of inhaled, short-acting β_2-agonists.

The usual dosage for adults and children 4 years of age and older is 1 inhalation (50 mcg) twice daily (morning and evening, approximately 12 hours apart).

If a previously effective dosage regimen fails to provide the usual response, immediately seek medical advice because this is often a sign of destabilization of asthma. Under these circumstances, reevaluate the therapeutic regimen and consider additional therapeutic options, such as inhaled or systemic corticosteroids. If symptoms arise in the period between doses, use a short-acting, inhaled β_2-agonist for immediate relief.

To gain full therapeutic benefit, administer twice daily (morning and evening) in the treatment of reversible airway obstruction.

➤*COPD:* The usual dosage for adults is 1 inhalation (50 mcg) twice daily (morning and evening), approximately 12 hours apart.

➤*Prevention of EIB:* One inhalation at least 30 minutes before exercise protects patients against EIB. When used intermittently as needed for prevention of EIB, this protection may last up to 9 hours in adolescents and adults and up to 12 hours in patients 4 to 11 years of age. Do not use additional doses of salmeterol for 12 hours after the administration of this drug. In patients who are receiving salmeterol twice daily (morning and evening), do not use additional salmeterol for prevention of EIB. If this dose is not effective, consider other appropriate therapy for EIB.

➤*Administration:* Do not exhale into the inhalation device; only activate and use the inhalation device in a level, horizontal position. Do not use a spacer.

➤*Storage/Stability:* Store at controlled room temperature, 20° to 25°C (68° to 77°F), in a dry place away from direct heat or sunlight. Keep out of reach of children. Keep the device dry and never wash the mouthpiece or any part of the device. The inhalation device is not reusable; discard after every blister has been used (when the dose indicator reads "0") or 6 weeks after removal from the moisture-protective foil overwrap pouch, whichever comes first. Do not attempt to take the device apart.

ALBUTEROL

Rx	**Albuterol** (Various, eg, Mylan)	**Tablets**: 2 mg[a]	May contain lactose. In 100s, 500s, and 600s.
Rx	**Proventil** (Schering)		Lactose. (Proventil 2 252). White, scored. In 100s and 500s.
Rx	**Albuterol** (Various, eg, Mylan, UDL)	**Tablets**: 4 mg[a]	May contain lactose. In 100s, 500s, and 600s.
Rx	**Proventil** (Schering)		Lactose. (Proventil 4 573). White, scored. In 100s and 500s.
Rx	**VoSpire ER** (Odyssey)	**Tablets, extended release**: 4 mg[a]	(V 4). Green. In 100s.
Rx	**VoSpire ER** (Odyssey)	**Tablets, extended release**: 8 mg[a]	(V 8). White. In 100s.
Rx	**Albuterol** (Various, eg, Alpharma, Mylan, Teva)	**Syrup**: 2 mg[a] per 5 mL	May contain sorbitol. In 473 mL.
Rx	**Proventil** (Schering)		Saccharin. Strawberry flavor. In 480 mL.
Rx	**Albuterol** (Various, eg, Andrx, Apothecon, Major, Sidmak, Warrick)	**Aerosol**: Delivers 90 mcg/actuation	In 6.8 g (≥ 80 inhalations) and 17 g (≥ 200 inhalations).
Rx	**Albuterol HFA**[a] (Ivax)		In 8.5 g (200 inhalations). Contains no chlorofluorocarbons (CFCs).
Rx	**ProAir HFA**[a] (Ivax)		In 8.5 g (200 inhalations). Contains no chlorofluorocarbons (CFCs).
Rx	**Proventil** (Schering)		In 17 g (200 inhalations).
Rx	**Proventil HFA**[a] (Key)		In 6.7 g (200 inhalations). Contains no CFCs.
Rx	**Ventolin HFA**[a] (GlaxoSmithKline)		In 18 g (200 inhalations). Contains no CFCs.
Rx	**Albuterol** (Various, eg, Alpharma, Dey, Ivax, Nephron)	**Solution for inhalation**: 0.083% (2.5 mg[a] per 3 mL)	In 3 mL UD vials.
Rx	**Proventil** (Schering)		In 3 mL UD vials.
Rx	**Albuterol** (Various, eg, Ivax, Nephron)	**Solution for inhalation**: 0.5% (5 mg[a]/mL)	In 0.5 mL vials and 20 mL with dropper.
Rx	**Proventil** (Schering)		In 20 mL with dropper.
Rx	**AccuNeb** (Dey)	**Solution for inhalation**: 0.021% (0.63 mg[a] per 3 mL)	Preservative-free. In 3 mL UD vials.
Rx	**Albuterol** (Nephron)	**Solution for inhalation**: 0.042% (1.25 mg[a] per 3 mL)	Preservative-free. In 3 mL UD vials.
Rx	**AccuNeb** (Dey)		Preservative-free. In 3 mL UD vials.

[a] As sulfate.

ALBUTEROL SULFATE — ORAL

For complete and comparative prescribing information, refer to the Sympathomimetic Bronchodilator group monograph.

Indications

➤*Tablets and extended-release tablets:* For the relief of bronchospasm in adults and children 6 years of age and older with reversible obstructive airway disease.

➤*Syrup:* For the relief of bronchospasm in adults and children 2 years of age and older with reversible obstructive airway disease.

➤*Unlabeled uses:* Albuterol has been shown to be effective for treating hyperkalemia in patients with renal failure.

Administration and Dosage

➤*Approved by the FDA:* May 7, 1982.

The following dosages are expressed in terms of albuterol base.

➤*Tablets:*

Usual dosage –

Adults and children over 12 years of age: The usual starting dosage is 2 or 4 mg, 3 or 4 times a day.

Children 6 to 12 years of age: The usual starting dosage is 2 mg, 3 or 4 times a day.

Dosage adjustment –

Adults and children over 12 years of age: A dosage above 4 mg 4 times a day should be used only when the patient fails to respond. If a favorable response does not occur with the 4 mg initial dosage, it should be cautiously increased stepwise up to a maximum of 8 mg 4 times a day as tolerated.

Children 6 to 12 years of age: For children from 6 to 12 years of age who fail to respond to the initial starting dosage of 2 mg 4 times a day, the dosage may be cautiously increased stepwise, but not to exceed 24 mg/day (given in divided doses).

Elderly patients and those sensitive to beta-adrenergic stimulators: An initial dosage of 2 mg 3 or 4 times a day is recommended for elderly patients and for those with a history of unusual sensitivity to beta-adrenergic stimulators. If adequate bronchodilation is not obtained, dosage may be increased gradually to as much as 8 mg 3 or 4 times a day. The total daily dose should not exceed 32 mg in adults and children 12 years and older.

➤*Extended-release tablets:*

Usual dosage –

Adults and children over 12 years of age: 8 mg every 12 hours. In some patients, 4 mg every 12 hours may be sufficient.

Children 6 to 12 years of age: 4 mg every 12 hours.

Dosage adjustment in adults and children over 12 years of age – In unusual circumstances, such as adults of low body weight, it may be desirable to use a starting dosage of 4 mg every 12 hours and progress to 8 mg every 12 hours according to response.

If control of reversible airway obstruction is not achieved with the recommended doses in patients on otherwise optimized asthma therapy, the doses may be cautiously increased stepwise under the control of the supervising physician to a maximum dose of 32 mg/day in divided doses (ie, every 12 hours).

Dosage adjustment in children 6 to 12 years of age – If control of reversible airway obstruction is not achieved with the recommended doses in patients on otherwise optimized asthma therapy, the doses may be cautiously increased stepwise under the control of the supervising physician to a maximum dose of 24 mg per day in divided doses (ie, every 12 hours).

Switching from oral albuterol products – Patients currently maintained on albuterol sulfate tablets or albuterol sulfate syrup can be switched to albuterol sulfate extended-release tablets. For example, the administration of one 4 mg albuterol sulfate extended-release tablet every 12 hours is comparable to one 2 mg albuterol sulfate tablet every 6 hours. Multiples of this regimen up to the maximum recommended daily dose also apply. Albuterol sulfate extended-release tablets must be swallowed whole with the aid of liquids. Do not chew or crush these tablets.

➤*Syrup:*

Adults and children over 14 years of age – The usual starting dose is 2 or 4 mg 3 or 4 times a day.

Children over 6 to 14 years of age – The usual starting dose is 2 mg 3 or 4 times a day.

Children 2 to 6 years of age – Initiate at 0.1 mg/kg of body weight 3 times a day. This starting dose should not exceed 2 mg 3 times a day.

Dosage adjustment –

Adults and children over 14 years of age: A dosage above 4 mg 4 times a day should be used only when the patient fails to respond. If a favorable response does not occur with the 4 mg initial dose, it should be cautiously increased stepwise up to a maximum of 8 mg 4 times a day as tolerated.

Children over 6 to 14 years of age who fail to respond to the initial starting dosage of 2 mg 4 times a day: The dosage may be cautiously increased stepwise, but not to exceed 24 mg/day (given in divided doses).

Children 2 to 6 years of age who do not respond satisfactorily to the initial dosage: The dosage may be increased stepwise to 0.2 mg/kg of body weight 3 times a day, but not to exceed a maximum of 4 mg (2 teaspoonfuls) given 3 times a day.

Elderly patients and those sensitive to beta-adrenergic stimulators: The initial dosage should be restricted to 2 mg 3 or 4 times a day and individually adjusted thereafter.

➤*Storage/Stability:* Store at controlled room temperature 15° to 30°C (59° to 86°F). Protect from light. Dispense in a well-closed, light-resistant container using a child-resistant closure. Replace cap securely after each opening.

ALBUTEROL — INHALATION

For complete and comparative prescribing information, refer to the Sympathomimetic Bronchodilator group monograph.

Indications

➤*Asthma/Bronchospasm:* For the relief and prevention of bronchospasm in patients with reversible obstructive airway disease; acute attacks of bronchospasm (inhalation solution); prevention of exercise-induced bronchospasm. Aerosol and inhalation powder are indicated for children 4 years of age and older (12 years of age and older for *Proventil*); solution for inhalation is indicated for children 2 years of age and older.

Administration and Dosage

➤*Inhalation aerosol:*

Adults and children 4 years of age and older (12 years of age and older for Proventil) – 2 inhalations every 4 to 6 hours. In some patients, 1 inhalation every 4 hours may be sufficient. More frequent administration or a larger number of inhalations is not recommended. If previously effective dosage fails to provide relief, this may be a marker of destabilization of asthma and requires reevaluation of the patient and treatment regimen.

Maintenance therapy (Proventil only*)* – For maintenance therapy or to prevent exacerbation of bronchospasm, 2 inhalations 4 times/day should be sufficient.

Continue the use of albuterol inhalation aerosol as medically indicated to control recurring bouts of bronchospasm. During this time most patients gain optimal benefit from regular use of the inhaler. Safe usage for periods extending over several years has been documented.

If a previously effective dosage regimen fails to provide the usual response, this may be a marker of destabilization of asthma and requires reevaluation of the patient and treatment regimen, giving special consideration to the possible need for anti-inflammatory treatment (eg, corticosteroids).

Prevention of exercise-induced bronchospasm –

Adults and children 4 years of age and older (12 years of age and older for Proventil): 2 inhalations 15 minutes prior to exercise.

➤*Inhalation solution:*

Adults and children 12 years of age and older – 2.5 mg 3 to 4 times/day by nebulization. Dilute 0.5 mL of the 0.5% solution with 2.5 mL sterile normal saline. Deliver over approximately 5 to 15 minutes.

Children 2 to 12 years of age (greater than or equal to 15 kg) – 2.5 mg (1 unit dose [UD] vial) 3 to 4 times/day by nebulization. Children weighing less than 15 kg who require less than 2.5 mg/dose (ie, less than a full UD vial) should use the 0.5% inhalation solution. Deliver over approximately 5 to 15 minutes.

AccuNeb: The usual starting dosage for patients 2 to 12 years of age is 1.25 mg or 0.63 mg administered 3 or 4 times/day, as needed, by nebulization. More frequent administration is not recommended. Deliver over 5 to 15 minutes. *AccuNeb* has not been studied in the setting of acute attacks of bronchospasm.

➤*Storage/Stability:* Store between 15° and 30°C (59° and 86°F). Failure to use this product within this temperature range may result in improper dosing. For optimal results, the canister should be at room temperature before use. Shake well before using.

Use the albuterol inhalation aerosol canister only with the actuator provided. Do not use the actuator with other aerosol medication canisters.

ALBUTEROL SULFATE — INHALATION

For complete and comparative prescribing information, refer to the Sympathomimetic Bronchodilator group monograph.

Indications

For the relief of bronchospasm in patients 2 years of age and older with reversible obstructive airway disease and acute attacks of bronchospasm.

For the treatment or prevention of bronchospasm in adults and children 4 years of age and older with reversible obstructive airway disease and for the prevention of exercise-induced bronchospasm in patients 4 years of age and older.

Administration and Dosage

➤*Approved by the FDA:* January 14, 1987.

➤*Inhalation solution 0.5%:* To avoid microbial contamination, proper aseptic techniques should be used each time the bottle is opened. Precautions should be taken to prevent contact of the dropper tip of the bottle with any surface, including the nebulizer reservoir and associated ventilatory equipment. In addition, if the solution changes color or becomes cloudy, it should not be used.

Children 2 to 12 years of age – Initial dosing should be based upon body weight (0.1 to 0.15 mg/kg/dose), with subsequent dosing titrated to achieve the desired clinical response. Dosing should not exceed 2.5 mg 3 to 4 times daily by nebulization.

Approximate Dosing According to Body Weight

Approximate weight (kg)	Approximate weight (lb)	Dose (mg)	Volume of inhalation solution
10 to 15 kg	22 to 33 lb	1.25 mg	0.25 mL
> 15 kg	> 33 lb	2.5 mg	0.5 mL

The appropriate volume of the 0.5% inhalation solution should be diluted in sterile normal saline solution to a total volume of 3 mL prior to administration via nebulization.

Adults and children over 12 years of age – The usual dosage is 2.5 mg of albuterol administered 3 to 4 times daily by nebulization. More frequent administration or higher doses are not recommended. To administer 2.5 mg of albuterol, dilute 0.5 mL of the 0.5% inhalation solution with 2.5 mL of sterile normal saline solution. The flow rate is regulated to suit the particular nebulizer so that albuterol sulfate inhalation solution will be delivered over approximately 5 to 15 minutes.

The use of albuterol sulfate inhalation solution can be continued as medically indicated to control recurring bouts of bronchospasm. During this time most patients gain optimal benefit from regular use of the inhalation solution.

If a previously effective dosage regimen fails to provide the usual relief, medical advice should be sought immediately as this is often a sign of seriously worsening asthma that would require reassessment of therapy.

Drug compatibility (physical and chemical), efficacy, and safety of albuterol sulfate inhalation solution when mixed with other drugs in a nebulizer have not been established.

➤*Inhalation solution 0.083%:* The usual dosage for adults and children weighing at least 15 kg is 2.5 mg of albuterol administered 3 to 4 times daily by nebulization. Children weighing less than 15 kg who require less than 2.5 mg/dose (ie, less than a full nebule) should use albuterol sulfate inhalation solution 0.5% instead of inhalation solution 0.083%. More frequent or higher doses are not recommended. To administer 2.5 mg of albuterol, administer the entire contents of 1 sterile unit dose nebule (3 mL of 0.083% inhalation solution by nebulization). The flow rate is regulated to suit the particular nebulizer so that albuterol sulfate inhalation solution 0.083% will be delivered over approximately 5 to 15 minutes.

The use of albuterol sulfate inhalation solution 0.083% can be continued as medically indicated to control recurring bouts of bronchospasm. During this time, most patients gain optimal benefit from regular use of the inhalation solution 0.083%.

If a previously effective dosage regimen fails to provide the usual relief, medical advice should be sought immediately, as this is often a sign of seriously worsening asthma that would require reassessment of therapy.

Albuterol inhalation solution 0.083% requires no dilution before administration by nebulization.

Drug compatibility (physical and chemical), efficacy, and safety of albuterol sulfate inhalation solution 0.083% when mixed with other drugs in a nebulizer have not been established.

➤*HFA inhalation aerosol:*

Adult and pediatric asthma – For treatment of acute episodes of bronchospasm or prevention of asthmatic symptoms, the usual dosage for adults and children 4 years of age and older is 2 inhalations repeated every 4 to 6 hours; in some patients, 1 inhalation every 4 hours may be sufficient. More frequent administration or a larger number of inhalations is not recommended. It is recommended to prime the inhaler before using for the first time, and in cases where the inhaler has not been used for more than 2 weeks, by releasing 4 test sprays into the air, away from the face.

Albuterol sulfate inhalation aerosol can also be used to relieve acute symptoms of asthma. The use of albuterol sulfate inhalation aerosol can be continued as medically indicated to control recurring bouts of bronchospasm. If a previously effective dosage regimen fails to provide the usual response, this may be a marker of destabilization of asthma and requires reevaluation of the patient and the treatment regimen, giving special consideration to the possible need for anti-inflammatory treatment (eg, corticosteroids).

Safe use of albuterol for periods extending over several years has been documented.

Exercise-induced bronchospasm prevention – The usual dosage for adults and children 4 years and older is 2 inhalations 15 to 30 minutes before exercise. For treatment, see above.

Cleaning – To maintain proper use of this product, it is important that the actuator be washed and dried thoroughly at least once a week. The inhaler may cease to deliver medication if not properly cleaned and dried thoroughly. Keeping the plastic actuator clean is very important to prevent medication build-up and blockage. If the actuator becomes blocked with drug, washing the actuator will remove the blockage.

➤*Storage/Stability:*

Inhalation solution 0.5% – Store between 2° to 25°C (36° to 77°F).

Inhalation solution 0.083% – Protect from light. Store in refrigerator between 2° and 8°C (36° and 46°F). Albuterol sulfate inhalation solution 0.083% may be held at room temperature for up to 2 weeks before use. (Nebules must be used within 2 weeks of removal from refrigerator.) Discard if solution becomes discolored.

HFA inhalation aerosol – The blue actuator supplied with albuterol inhalation aerosol should not be used with any other product canisters, and actuators from other products should not be used with the supplied canister. The correct amount of medication in each canister cannot be ensured after 200 actuations, even though the canister is not completely empty. The canister should be discarded when 200 actuations have been used or 3 months after removal from the moisture-protective foil pouch, whichever comes first.

ALBUTEROL SULFATE — INHALATION

Never immerse the canister into water to determine how full the canister is ("float test").

Contents under pressure: Do not puncture. Do not use or store near heat or open flame. Exposure to temperatures above 48.8°C (120°F) may cause bursting. Never throw container into fire or incinerator. Avoid spraying in eyes.

Store between 15° and 25°C (59° and 77°F). Store canister with mouthpiece down. For best results, the canister should be at room temperature before use. Shake well before using.

BITOLTEROL MESYLATE

Rx	**Tornalate** (Elan)	**Solution for inhalation:** 0.2%	In 10, 30, and 60 mL w/dropper.[a]

[a] With 25% alcohol and propylene glycol.

BITOLTEROL MESYLATE — INHALATION

For complete and comparative prescribing information, refer to the Sympathomimetic Bronchodilator group monograph.

Indications

➤*Asthma/Bronchospasm:* For prophylaxis and treatment of bronchial asthma and reversible bronchospasm. May be used with concurrent theophylline or steroid therapy.

Administration and Dosage

➤*Solution for inhalation:* For adults and children older than 12 years of age, administer during a 10- to 15-minute period. The treatment period can be adjusted by varying the amount of diluent (normal saline solution) placed in the nebulizer with the medication. The total volume (medication plus diluent) is usually adjusted to 2 to 4 mL.

Dosing Regimens for Bitolterol Solution for Inhalation 0.2%

	Continuous flow nebulization		Intermittent flow nebulization	
Doses	Volume (mL)	Bitolterol (mg)	Volume (mL)	Bitolterol (mg)
Usual dose	1.25	2.5	0.5	1
Decreased dose	0.75	1.5	0.25	0.5
Increased dose	1.75	3.5	0.75	1.5

Up to 1 mL of solution for inhalation, 0.2% (2 mg) can be administered with the intermittent flow system to severely obstructed patients.

The usual frequency of treatments is 3 times/day. Treatments may be increased up to 4 times/day; however, the interval between treatments should be greater than or equal to 4 hours. For some patients, 2 treatments a day may be adequate. Seek medical advice immediately if the previously effective dosage regimen fails to provide the usual relief as this is often a sign of seriously worsening asthma that would require reassessment of therapy.

Do not exceed the maximum daily dose of 8 mg with an intermittent flow nebulization system or 14 mg with a continuous flow nebulization system.

ISOETHARINE HYDROCHLORIDE

Rx	**Isoetharine** (Roxane)	**Solution for inhalation:** 1%	EDTA, parabens, sulfites. In 10 and 30 mL w/dropper.

ISOETHARINE HYDROCHLORIDE — INHALATION

For complete and comparative prescribing information, refer to the Sympathomimetic Bronchodilator group monograph.

Indications

➤*Asthma/Bronchospasm:* For bronchial asthma and reversible bronchospasm that occurs with bronchitis and emphysema.

Administration and Dosage

Isoetharine Doses

Method of administration	Usual dose	Range of dose of 1:3 dilution[a]
Hand bulb nebulizer	4 inhalations	3 to 7 inhalations undiluted
Oxygen aerosolization[b]	0.5 mL	1 to 2 mL
IPPB[c]	0.5 mL	1 to 4 mL

[a] Dilution of 1 part isoetharine plus 3 parts of normal saline solution.
[b] Administered with oxygen flow adjusted to 4 to 6 L/min over 15 to 20 minutes.
[c] IPPB = intermittent positive pressure breathing. Usually an inspiratory flow rate of 15 L/min at a cycling pressure of 15 cm H_2O is recommended. It may be necessary, according to patient and type of IPPB apparatus, to adjust flow rate to 6 to 30 L/min, cycling pressure to 10 to 15 cm H_2O, and further dilution according to the needs of the patient.

Usually, treatment does not need to be repeated more often than every 4 hours; although in severe cases, more frequent administration may be necessary.

➤*Storage/Stability:* Do not use if discolored or contains a precipitate. Protect from light.

METAPROTERENOL SULFATE

Rx	**Metaproterenol Sulfate** (Various, eg, Par)	**Tablets:** 10 mg	In 100s and 1000s.
		20 mg	In 100s and 1000s.
Rx	**Metaproterenol Sulfate** (Silarx)	**Syrup:** 10 mg per 5 mL	Saccharin, sorbitol, EDTA. Black cherry flavor. In 473 mL.
Rx	**Alupent** (Boehringer Ingelheim)	**Aerosol:** Delivers 0.65 mg/actuation	In 7 g (100 inhalations) and 14 g canisters and refills (200 inhalations).
Rx	**Metaproterenol Sulfate** (Various, eg, Dey)	**Solution for inhalation:** 0.4%	May contain EDTA. In 2.5 mL UD vials.
Rx	**Alupent** (Boehringer Ingelheim)		EDTA. In 2.5 mL UD vials.[1]
Rx	**Metaproterenol Sulfate** (Various, eg, Dey)	**Solution for inhalation:** 0.6%	May contain EDTA. In 2.5 mL UD vials.
Rx	**Alupent** (Boehringer Ingelheim)		EDTA. In 2.5 mL UD vials.[1]
Rx	**Metaproterenol Sulfate** (Various)	**Solution for inhalation:** 5%	May contain EDTA, benzalkonium chloride. In 10 and 30 mL w/dropper.
Rx	**Alupent** (Boehringer Ingelheim)		EDTA, benzalkonium chloride. In 10 or 30 mL w/dropper.

[1] For use with an IPPB device.

METAPROTERENOL SULFATE — ORAL

For complete and comparative prescribing information, refer to the Sympathomimetic Bronchodilator group monograph.

Indications

➤*Asthma/Bronchospasm:* Bronchial asthma and for reversible bronchospasm which may occur in association with bronchitis and emphysema.

Administration and Dosage

➤*Approved by the FDA:* June 28, 1988.

➤*Syrup:*

Adults – 10 mL (20 mg) 3 or 4 times a day.

Children older than 9 years of age or weight over 60 lbs – 10 mL (20 mg) 3 or 4 times a day.

Children 6 to 9 years of age or weight under 60 lbs – 5 mL (10 mg) 3 or 4 times a day.

Children younger than 6 years of age – Clinical trial experience in children under the age of 6 years is limited. Of 40 children treated with metaproterenol syrup for at least 1 month, daily doses of approximately 1.3 to 2.6 mg/kg were well tolerated.

➤*Tablets:*

Adults – The usual dose is 20 mg 3 to 4 times daily.

Children –

Aged 6 to 9 years or weight under 60 lbs: 10 mg 3 or 4 times a day.
Older than 9 years or weight over 60 lbs: 20 mg 3 or 4 times a day.
Younger than 6 years of age: Metaproterenol tablets are not recommended for use in children under 6 years at this time.

It is recommended that the physician titrate dosage according to each individual patient's response to therapy.

➤*Storage/Stability:* Store between 15° and 30°C (59° and 86°F). Protect from light.

Syrup – Dispense in tight, light-resistant containers.

Tablets – Protect from moisture.

METAPROTERENOL SULFATE — INHALATION

For complete and comparative prescribing information, refer to the Sympathomimetic Bronchodilator group monograph.

Indications

➤*Asthma/Bronchospasm:* In the treatment of asthma and bronchitis or emphysema when a reversible component is present in adults and for the treatment of acute asthmatic attacks in children 6 years of age or older.

Administration and Dosage

➤*Approved by the FDA:* June 30, 1983.

➤*Metaproterenol sulfate inhalation solution:* The dosage and administration data are summarized in the following table:

Population	Method of administration	Usual single dose	Range	Dilution
Adult 12 years and older	Hand-bulb nebulizer	10 inhalations	5 to 15 inhalations	No dilution
	IPPB or nebulizer	0.3 mL	0.2 to 0.3 mL	Diluted in approximately 2.5 mL saline solution or other diluent
Pediatric 6 to 12 years	Nebulizer	0.1 mL	0.1 to 0.2 mL	Diluted in saline solution to a total volume of 3 mL

Metaproterenol sulfate inhalation solution is administered by oral inhalation via IPPB or nebulizer. Usually, treatment need not be repeated more often than every 4 hours to relieve acute attacks of bronchospasm. Metaproterenol sulfate inhalation solution is administered 3 to 4 times a day for the treatment of reversible airways disease in adults. A single dose of nebulized metaproterenol sulfate in the treatment of an acute attack of asthma may not completely abort an attack.

As with all medications, the physician should begin therapy with the lowest effective dose and then titrate the dosage according to the individual patient's requirements.

➤*Metaproterenol sulfate inhalation aerosol:* The usual single dose is 2 to 3 inhalations. With repetitive dosing, inhalation should usually not be repeated more often than about every 3 to 4 hours. Total dosage per day should not exceed 12 inhalations.

Metaproterenol sulfate inhalation aerosol is not recommended for children younger than 12 years of age.

It is recommended that the physician titrate dosage according to each individual patient's response to therapy.

➤*Storage/Stability:* Store between 15° to 25°C (59° to 77°F). Protect from light and excess humidity. Do not use the solution if it is pinkish or darker than slightly yellow or contains a precipitate.

PIRBUTEROL ACETATE

Rx	**Maxair Autohaler** (3M Pharm.)	**Aerosol:** Delivers 0.2 mg (as acetate)/actuation	In 2.8 g (80 inhalations) and 14 g (400 inhalations).

PIRBUTEROL ACETATE — INHALATION

For complete and comparative prescribing information, refer to the Sympathomimetic Bronchodilator group monograph.

Indications

➤*Asthma/Bronchospasm:* For the prevention and reversal of bronchospasm in patients 12 years of age and older with reversible bronchospasm including asthma. It may be used with or without concurrent theophylline and/or corticosteroid therapy.

Administration and Dosage

➤*Approved by the FDA:* December 30, 1986.

The usual dose for adults and children 12 years and older is 2 inhalations (400 mcg) repeated every 4 to 6 hours. One inhalation (200 mcg) repeated every 4 to 6 hours may be sufficient for some patients.

A total daily dose of 12 inhalations should not be exceeded.

If a previously effective dosage regimen fails to provide the usual relief, medical advice should be sought immediately as this is often a sign of seriously worsening asthma which would require reassessment of therapy.

It is recommended to "test spray" pirbuterol acetate inhaler into the air before using for the first time and in cases where the aerosol has not been used for a prolonged period of time.

➤*Storage/Stability:* Store between 15° and 30°C (59° to 86°F). Failure to use this product within this temperature range may result in improper dosing. For optimal results, the canister should be at room temperature before use. Shake well before using.

The contents of pirbuterol acetate inhalation aerosol are under pressure. Do not puncture. Do not use or store near heat or open flame. Exposure to temperature above 120°F may cause bursting. Never throw container into fire or incinerator. Keep out of reach of children. Avoid spraying in eyes.

The light blue plastic actuator supplied with pirbuterol acetate inhalation aerosol should not be used with any other product canisters, and actuators from other product should not be used with pirbuterol acetate inhalation aerosol canister.

TERBUTALINE SULFATE

Rx	**Terbutaline Sulfate** (Global)	**Tablets:** 2.5 mg	Oval. In 100s.
Rx	**Brethine** (aaiPharma)		Lactose. (Geigy 72). White, oval, scored. In 100s, 1000s, and UD 100s.
Rx	**Terbutaline Sulfate** (Global)	**Tablets:** 5 mg	In 100s.
Rx	**Brethine** (aaiPharma)		Lactose. (Geigy 105). White, scored. In 100s, 1000s, and UD 100s.
Rx	**Terbutaline Sulfate** (Various, eg, American Pharmaceutical Partners, Sicor)	**Injection:** 1 mg/mL	In 1 mL single-use vials.
Rx	**Brethine** (aaiPharma)		In 2 mL amp with 1 mL fill.

Sympathomimetics

TERBUTALINE SULFATE — ORAL

For complete and comparative prescribing information, refer to the Sympathomimetic Bronchodilator group monograph.

Indications

➤*Asthma/Bronchospasm:* Prevention and reversal of bronchospasm in patients 12 years of age and older with asthma and reversible bronchospasm associated with bronchitis and emphysema.

➤*Unlabeled uses:* As a tocolytic agent to treat preterm labor.

Administration and Dosage

➤*Adults:* 5 mg administered at approximately 6-hour intervals, 3 times daily, during the hours the patient is usually awake. If side effects are particularly disturbing, the dose may be reduced to 2.5 mg 3 times daily, and still provide a clinically significant improvement in pulmonary function. The total dose within 24 hours should not exceed 15 mg.

➤*Children:* Terbutaline sulfate is not recommended for use in children below the age of 12 years. A dosage of 2.5 mg 3 times daily is recommended for children 12 to 15 years of age. The total dose within 24 hours should not exceed 7.5 mg.

If a previously effective dosage regimen fails to provide the usual relief, medical advice should be sought immediately as this is often a sign of seriously worsening asthma that would require reassessment of therapy.

➤*Storage/Stability:* Store at controlled room temperature 15° to 30°C (59° to 86°F). Dispense in tight, light-resistant container.

TERBUTALINE SULFATE — INJECTION

For complete and comparative prescribing information, refer to the Sympathomimetic Bronchodilator group monograph.

Indications

➤*Asthma/Bronchospasm:* Prevention and reversal of bronchospasm in patients 12 years of age and older with asthma and reversible bronchospasm associated with bronchitis and emphysema.

➤*Unlabeled uses:* As a tocolytic agent to treat preterm labor.

Administration and Dosage

Ampuls should be used only for SC administration and not IV infusion. Sterility and accurate dosing cannot be ensured if the ampuls are not used in accordance with Administration and Dosage.

Discard unused portion after single patient use.

The usual SC dose of terbutaline sulfate injection is 0.25 mg injected into the lateral deltoid area. If significant clinical improvement does not occur within 15 to 30 minutes, a second dose of 0.25 mg may be administered. If the patient then fails to respond within another 15 to 30 minutes, other therapeutic measures should be considered. The total dose within 4 hours should not exceed 0.5 mg.

➤*Storage/Stability:* Keep at controlled room temperature, 15° to 30°C (59° to 86°F). Protect from light by storing ampuls in original carton until dispensed. Do not use if the solution is discolored.

FORMOTEROL FUMARATE

Rx	**Foradil Aerolizer** (Schering)	**Inhalation powder in capsules:** 12 mcg	(CG FXF). In blister pack 18s and 60s with *Aerolizer Inhaler.*[a]

[a] With 25 mg lactose as carrier.

FORMOTEROL FUMARATE — INHALATION

For complete and comparative prescribing information, refer to the Sympathomimetic Bronchodilator group monograph.

Indications

➤*Asthma/Bronchospasm:* For long-term, twice-daily (morning and evening) administration in the maintenance treatment of asthma and in the prevention of bronchospasm in adults and children 5 years of age or older with reversible obstructive airways disease, including patients with symptoms of nocturnal asthma, who require regular treatment with inhaled, short-acting, $beta_2$ agonists. It is not indicated for patients whose asthma can be managed by occasional use of inhaled, short-acting, $beta_2$agonists.

Exercise-induced bronchospasm – For the acute prevention of exercise-induced bronchospasm (EIB) in adults and children 12 years of age or older, when administered on an occasional, as needed basis.

➤*Chronic obstructive pulmonary disease (COPD):* For the long-term, twice-daily (morning and evening) administration in the maintenance treatment of bronchoconstriction in patients with COPD, including chronic bronchitis and emphysema.

Administration and Dosage

➤*Approved by the FDA:* February 16, 2001.

Formoterol fumarate capsules should be administered only by the oral inhalation route and only using the inhaler supplied. Formoterol fumarate capsules should not be ingested (ie, swallowed) orally. Formoterol fumarate capsules should always be stored in the blister, and only removed immediately before use.

➤*For maintenance treatment of asthma:* For adults and children 5 years of age or older, the usual dosage is the inhalation of the contents of one 12 mcg formoterol fumarate capsule every 12 hours using the inhaler supplied. The patient must not exhale into the device. The total daily dose of formoterol fumarate should not exceed 1 capsule twice daily (24 mcg total daily dose). More frequent administration or administration of a larger number of inhalations is not recommended. If symptoms arise between doses, an inhaled short-acting $beta_2$ agonist should be taken for immediate relief.

If a previously effective dosage regimen fails to provide the usual response, medical advice should be sought immediately as this is often a sign of destabilization of asthma. Under these circumstances, the therapeutic regimen should be reevaluated and additional therapeutic options, such as inhaled or systemic corticosteroids, should be considered.

➤*For prevention of exercise-induced bronchospasm (EIB):* For adults and adolescents 12 years of age or older, the usual dosage is the inhalation of the contents of one 12 mcg formoterol fumarate capsule at least 15 minutes before exercise administered on an occasional as needed basis.

Additional doses of formoterol fumarate should not be used for 12 hours after the administration of this drug. Regular, twice-daily dosing has not been studied in preventing EIB. Patients who are receiving formoterol fumarate twice daily for maintenance of their asthma should not use additional doses for prevention of EIB and may require a short-acting bronchodilator.

➤*For maintenance treatment of COPD:* The usual dosage is the inhalation of the contents of one 12 mcg capsule every 12 hours using the inhaler supplied.

A total daily dose of greater than 24 mcg is not recommended.

If a previously effective dosage regimen fails to provide the usual response, medical advice should be sought immediately as this is often a sign of destabilization of COPD. Under these circumstances, the therapeutic regimen should be reevaluated and additional therapeutic options should be considered.

➤*Storage/Stability:*

Prior to dispensing – Store in a refrigerator, 2° to 8°C (36° to 46°F).

After dispensing to patient – Store at 20° to 25°C (68° to 77°F). Protect from heat and moisture. Capsules should always be stored in the blister and only removed from the blister immediately before use.

Diluents

SODIUM CHLORIDE

For Sodium Chloride prescribing information, see the Electrolytes group monograph and the Sodium Chloride monograph in the Nutrients and Nutritional Agents chapter.

Xanthine Derivatives

Indications

Symptomatic relief or prevention of bronchial asthma and reversible bronchospasm associated with chronic bronchitis and emphysema.

➤*Unlabeled uses:* Treatment of apnea and bradycardia of prematurity. Doses of 2 mg/kg/day have been used to maintain serum concentrations between 3 and 5 mcg/mL.

Theophylline 300 mg/day was effective in reducing essential tremor in one study of 20 patients.

Theophylline 10 mg/kg/day may significantly improve pulmonary function and dyspnea in patients with chronic obstructive pulmonary disease.

Administration and Dosage

➤*Parenteral administration:* See theophylline and dextrose and aminophylline.

Individualize dosage. Base dosage adjustments on clinical response and improvement in pulmonary function with careful monitoring of serum levels. If possible, monitor serum levels to maintain levels in the therapeutic range of 10 to 20 mcg/mL. Levels more than 20 mcg/mL may produce toxicity, and it may even occur with levels between 15 to 20 mcg/mL, particularly when factors known to reduce theophylline clearance are present (see Warnings). Once stabilized on a dosage, serum levels tend to remain constant. Data are available that indicate that the serum theophylline concentrations required to produce maximum physiologic benefit may fluctuate with the degree of bronchospasm present and are variable.

Calculate dosages on the basis of lean body weight, since theophylline does not distribute into fatty tissue. Regardless of salt used, dosages should be equivalent based on anhydrous theophylline content.

➤*Individualize frequency of dosing:* With immediate-release products, dosing every 6 hours generally is required, especially in children; intervals up to 8 hours may be satisfactory in adults. Some children and adults requiring higher than average doses (those having rapid rates of clearance; eg, half-lives less than 6 hours) may be more effectively controlled during chronic therapy with sustained-release products. Determine dosage intervals to produce minimal fluctuations between peak and trough serum theophylline concentrations. Consider the absorption profile and the elimination rate. When converting from an immediate-release to a sustained-release product, the total daily dose should remain the same, and only the dosing interval adjusted.

➤*Acute symptoms requiring rapid theophyllinization in patients not receiving theophylline:* To achieve a rapid effect, an initial loading dose is required. Dosage recommendations are for theophylline anhydrous.

Dosage Guidelines for Rapid Theophyllinization[a]

Patient group	Oral loading	Maintenance
Children 1 to 9 years of age	5 mg/kg	4 mg/kg q 6 hr
Children 9 to 16 years of age and young adult smokers	5 mg/kg	3 mg/kg q 6 hr
Otherwise healthy non-smoking adults	5 mg/kg	3 mg/kg q 8 hr
Older patients, patients with cor pulmonale	5 mg/kg	2 mg/kg q 8 hr
Patients with CHF	5 mg/kg	1 to 2 mg/kg q 12 hr

[a] In patients not receiving theophylline.

➤*Infants (preterm to younger than 1 year):*

Theophylline Dosage Guidelines for Infants

Age	Initial maintenance dose
Premature infants	
≤ 24 days postnatal	1 mg/kg q 12 hr
> 24 days postnatal	1.5 mg/kg q 12 hr
Infants (6 to 52 weeks)	([0.2 × age in weeks] + 5) × kg = 24 hr dose in mg
≤ 26 weeks	Divide into q 8 hr dosing
26 to 52 weeks	Divide into q 6 hr dosing

Guide final dosage by serum concentration after a steady state has been achieved.

➤*Acute symptoms requiring rapid theophyllinization in patients receiving theophylline:* Each 0.5 mg/kg theophylline administered as a loading dose will increase the serum theophylline concentration by approximately 1 mcg/mL. Ideally, defer the loading dose if a serum theophylline concentration can be obtained rapidly.

If this is not possible, exercise clinical judgment. When there is sufficient respiratory distress to warrant a small risk, then 2.5 mg/kg of theophylline administered in rapidly absorbed form is likely to increase serum concentration by approximately 5 mcg/mL. If the patient is not experiencing theophylline toxicity, this is unlikely to result in dangerous adverse effects. Maintenance doses are in the Dosage Guidelines table.

➤*Chronic therapy:* Slow clinical titration is generally preferred.

Initial dose – 16 mg/kg/24 hours or 400 mg/24 hours, whichever is less, of anhydrous theophylline in divided doses at 6 or 8 hour intervals.

Increasing dose – The above dosage may be increased in approximately 25% increments at 3-day intervals so long as the drug is tolerated or until the maximum dose (indicated below) is reached.

➤*Maximum dose (where the serum concentration is not measured):* Do not attempt to maintain any dose that is not tolerated.

Maximum Daily Theophylline Dose Based on Age

Age	Maximum daily dose[a]
1 to 9 years	24 mg/kg/day
9 to 12 years	20 mg/kg/day
12 to 16 years	18 mg/kg/day
> 16 years	13 mg/kg/day

[a] Not to exceed listed dose or 900 mg, whichever is less.

Exercise caution in younger children who cannot complain of minor side effects. Older adults and those with cor pulmonale, CHF, or liver disease may have unusually low dosage requirements; they may experience toxicity at the maximal dosages recommended.

➤*Measurement of serum theophylline concentrations during chronic therapy:* Measurement of serum theophylline concentrations during chronic therapy is recommended. Obtain the serum sample at the time of peak absorption, 1 to 2 hours after administration for immediate-release products and 5 to 9 hours after the morning dose for most sustained-release formulations. The patient must not miss doses during the previous 48 hours, and dosing intervals must have been reasonably typical during that period of time. The table below provides guidance to dosage adjustments based on serum theophylline level determinations:

Dosage Adjustment After Serum Theophylline Measurement

If serum theophylline is:		Directions
Too low	5 to 10 mcg/mL	Increase dose by ≈ 25% at 3-day intervals until either the desired clinical response or serum concentration is achieved.[a]
Within desired range	10 to 20 mcg/mL	Maintain dosage if tolerated. Recheck serum theophylline concentration at 6 to 12 month intervals.[b]
Too high	20 to 25 mcg/mL	Decrease doses by ≈ 10%. Recheck serum theophylline concentration after 3 days.[b]
	25 to 30 mcg/mL	Skip next dose and decrease subsequent doses by about 25%. Recheck serum theophylline after 3 days.
	> 30 mcg/mL	Skip next 2 doses and decrease subsequent doses by 50%. Recheck serum theophylline after 3 days.

[a] The total daily dose may need to be administered at more frequent intervals if asthma symptoms occur repeatedly at the end of a dosing interval.

[b] Finer adjustments in dosage may be needed for some patients.

➤*Timed-release capsules:* These dosage forms gradually release the active medication so that the total daily dosage may be administered in 1 to 3 doses divided by 8 to 24 hours, depending on the patient's pharmacokinetic profile, thus reducing the number of daily doses required. In the following timed-release capsule product listings, the manufacturer's recommended average dosing intervals are presented in parentheses. Nevertheless, frequency of dosing must be individualized based on the absorption profile of the drug and the rate of elimination of the drug from the patient. These products are not necessarily interchangeable. If patients are switched from one brand to another, closely monitor their theophylline serum levels; serum concentrations may vary greatly following brand interchange.

Actions

➤*Pharmacology:* The methylxanthines (theophylline, its soluble salts and derivatives) directly relax the smooth muscle of the bronchi and pulmonary blood vessels, stimulate the CNS, induce diuresis, increase gastric acid secretion, reduce lower esophageal sphincter pressure, and inhibit uterine contractions. Theophylline is also a central respiratory stimulant. Aminophylline has a potent effect on diaphragmatic contractility in healthy people and may then be capable of reducing fatigability and thereby improve contractility in patients with chronic obstructive airway disease. The exact mode of action is unclear.

For many years, the proposed main mechanism of action of the xanthines was inhibition of phosphodiesterase, which results in an increase in cyclic adenosine monophosphate (cAMP). However, this effect is negligible at therapeutic concentrations. Other effects that appear to occur at therapeutic concentrations and may collectively play a role in the mechanism of the xanthines include the following: Inhibition of extracellular adenosine (which causes bronchoconstriction), although it is unlikely that this is a main mechanism; stimulation of endogenous catecholamines, although this also does not appear to be a major mechanism; antagonism of prostaglandins PGE_2 and $PGF_{2}\alpha$; direct effect on mobilization of intracellular calcium resulting in smooth muscle relaxation; beta-adrenergic agonist activity on the airways. None of these mechanisms have been proven.

➤*Pharmacokinetics:*

Absorption – Theophylline is well absorbed from oral liquids and uncoated plain tablets; maximal plasma concentrations are reached in 2 hours. Rectal absorption from suppositories is slow and erratic, the oral route is generally preferred. Enteric coated tablets and some sustained release dosage forms may be unreliably absorbed. Food may alter bioavailability and absorption pattern of some sustained release preparations; close monitoring is advised (see Drug Interactions).

Distribution – Average volume of distribution is 0.45 L/kg (range, 0.3 to 0.7 L/kg). Theophylline does not distribute into fatty tissue, but readily crosses the placenta and is excreted into breast milk. Approximately 40% is bound to plasma protein. Therapeutic serum levels generally range from 10 to 20 mcg/mL. Although some bronchodilatory effect occurs at lower concentrations, stabilization of hyperreactive airways is most evident at levels more than 10 mcg/mL, and adverse effects are uncommon at levels less than 20 mcg/mL. Once a patient is stabilized, serum levels tend to remain constant with the same dosage.

Metabolism/Excretion – Xanthines are biotransformed in the liver (85% to 90%) to 1, 3–dimethyluric acid, 3–methylxanthine and 1–methyluric acid; 3–methylxanthine accumulates in concentrations approximately 25% of those of theophylline.

Excretion is by the kidneys; less than 15% of the drug is excreted unchanged. Elimination kinetics vary greatly. Plasma elimination half-life averages about 3 to 15 hours in adult nonsmokers, 4 to 5 hours in adult smokers (1 to 2 packs per day), 1 to 9 hours in children and 20 to 30 hours for premature neonates. In the neonate, theophylline is metabolized partially to caffeine. The premature neonate excretes about 50% unchanged theophylline and may accumulate the caffeine metabolite.

A prolonged half-life may occur in congestive heart failure, liver dysfunction, alcoholism, respiratory infections and patients receiving certain other drugs (see Drug Interactions). Total clearance appears relatively unaffected by renal failure.

Equivalent dose – Because of differing theophylline content, the various salts and derivatives are not equivalent on a weight basis. The table below indicates percentage of anhydrous theophylline and approximate equivalent dose of each compound. Product listings include anhydrous theophylline dosage equivalents.

Theophylline Content and Equivalent Dose of Various Theophylline Salts

Theophylline salts	Theophylline %	Equivalent dose
Theophylline anhydrous	100	100 mg
Theophylline monohydrate	91	110 mg
Aminophylline anhydrous	86	116 mg
Aminophylline dihydrate	79	127 mg
Oxtriphylline	64	156 mg

Dyphylline – A chemical derivative of theophylline, it is not a theophylline salt as are the other agents. It is about one-tenth as potent as theophylline. Following oral administration, dyphylline is 68% to 82% bioavailable. Peak plasma concentrations are reached within 1 hour, and its half-life is 2 hours. The minimal effective therapeutic concentration is 12 mcg/mL. It is not metabolized to theophylline and 83% ± 5% is excreted unchanged in the urine.

Contraindications

Hypersensitivity to any xanthine; peptic ulcer; underlying seizure disorders (unless receiving appropriate anticonvulsant medication).

➤*Aminophylline:* Hypersensitivity to ethylenediamine.

➤*Aminophylline rectal suppositories:* Irritation or infection of rectum or lower colon.

Warnings

➤*Status asthmaticus:* This is a medical emergency and is not rapidly responsive to usual doses of conventional bronchodilators. Optimal therapy frequently requires both parenteral medication and close monitoring, preferably in an intensive care setting. Oral theophylline products alone are not appropriate for status asthmaticus.

➤*Toxicity:* Excessive doses may cause severe toxicity; monitor serum levels to assure maximum benefit with minimum risk. Incidence of toxicity increases significantly at serum levels more than 20 mcg/mL (75% of patients with levels more than 25 mcg/mL). Serum levels more than 20 mcg/mL are rare after appropriate use of recommended doses. However, if theophylline plasma clearance is reduced for any reason (eg, hepatic impairment; patients older than 55 years of age, particularly males and those with chronic lung disease; cardiac failure; sustained high fever; infants younger than 1 year old), even conventional doses may result in increased serum levels and potential toxicity. Frequently, such patients have markedly prolonged levels following drug discontinuation.

Serious side effects such as ventricular arrhythmias, convulsions or even death may appear as the first sign of toxicity without any previous warning. Less serious signs of toxicity (eg, nausea, restlessness) may occur frequently when initiating therapy, but are usually transient; when such signs are persistent during maintenance therapy, they are often associated with serum concentrations greater than 20 mcg/mL. Serious toxicity is not reliably preceded by less severe side effects.

➤*Cardiac effects:* Theophylline may cause dysrhythmias or worsen preexisting arrhythmias. Any significant change in cardiac rate or rhythm warrants monitoring and further investigation. Many patients who require theophylline may exhibit tachycardia due to underlying disease; the relationship to elevated serum theophylline concentrations may not be appreciated. Ventricular arrhythmias respond to lidocaine.

➤*Pregnancy:* *Category C.* It is not known whether theophylline can cause fetal harm when administered to a pregnant woman or can affect reproduction capacity. Give only if clearly needed. Theophylline has been found in cord serum and crosses the placenta; newborns may have therapeutic serum levels. Apnea has been associated with theophylline withdrawal in a neonate. Theophylline-related human congenital defects or malformations have not been reported.

➤*Lactation:* Theophylline distributes readily into breast milk with a milk:plasma ratio of 0.7 and may cause irritability or other signs of toxicity in nursing infants. Decide whether to discontinue nursing or to discontinue the drug, taking into account the importance of the drug to the mother.

➤*Children:* Sufficient numbers of infants younger than 1 year of age have not been studied in clinical trials to support use in this age group; however, there is evidence that the use of dosage recommendations for older infants and young children may result in the development of toxic serum levels. Carefully consider associated benefits and risks in this age group. (See Administration and Dosage and Unlabeled uses.)

Precautions

➤*Use with caution:* Cardiac disease; hypoxemia; hepatic disease; hypertension; congestive heart failure (CHF); alcoholism; elderly (particularly males); and neonates.

➤*GI effects:* Use cautiously in peptic ulcer. Local irritation may occur; centrally mediated GI effects may occur with serum levels more than 20 mcg/mL. Reduced lower esophageal pressure may cause reflux, aspiration and worsening of airway obstruction.

➤*Alcohol:* The addition of alcohol in liquid formulations is not necessary for absorption and may be potentially harmful.

Drug Interactions

Agents that Decrease Theophylline Levels

Aminoglutethimide	Rifampin	Carbamazepine[a]
Barbiturates	Smoking (cigarettes and marijuana)	Isoniazid[a]
Charcoal	Sulfinpyrazone	Loop diuretics[a]
Hydantoins[b]	Sympathomimetics (β-agonists)	
Ketoconazole	Thioamines[c]	

Agents that Increase Theophylline Levels

Allopurinol	Disulfiram	Quinolones
Beta blockers (non-selective)	Ephedrine	Thiabendazole
Calcium channel blockers	Influenza virus vaccine	Thyroid hormones[d]
Cimetidine	Interferon	Carbamazepine[a]
Contraceptives, oral	Macrolides	Isoniazid[a]
Corticosteroids	Mexiletine	Loop diuretics[a]

[a] May increase or decrease theophylline levels.
[b] Decreased hydantoin levels may also occur.
[c] Increased theophylline clearance in hyperthyroid patients.
[d] Decreased theophylline clearance in hypothyroid patients.

➤*Benzodiazepines:* The sedative effects of benzodiazepines may be antagonized by theophyllines, although their pharmacokinetics do not appear to be altered. Coadministration may be beneficial in reversing sedation produced by benzodiazepines.

➤*Beta-agonists:* Acts synergistically with theophylline in vitro; an additive effect has also been demonstrated in vivo.

➤*Halothane:* Coadministration with theophylline has resulted in catecholamine-induced arrhythmias.

➤*Ketamine:* Coadministration with theophylline has resulted in extensor-type seizures.

➤*Lithium:* Plasma levels may be reduced by theophyllines.

➤*Nondepolarizing muscle relaxants:* A dose-dependent reversal of neuromuscular blockade by theophyllines may occur.

➤*Probenecid:* May increase the pharmacologic effects of dyphylline due to decreased dyphylline renal excretion.

➤*Propofol:* Theophyllines may antagonize the sedative effects of propofol.

➤*Ranitidine:* Case reports suggest that theophylline plasma levels may be increased by ranitidine, possibly increasing pharmacologic and toxic effects. However, several controlled studies indicate that an interaction does not occur. It appears that if this interaction occurs, it is rare.

➤*Tetracyclines:* The incidence of theophylline adverse reactions may possibly be enhanced by concurrent tetracyclines.

➤*Drug/Lab test interactions:* Currently available analytical methods for measuring serum theophylline levels are specific, and metabolites and other drugs generally do not affect the results. However, be aware of the specific laboratory method used and whether other factors will interfere with the assay for theophylline.

➤*Drug/Food interactions:* Theophylline elimination is increased (half-life shortened) by a low carbohydrate, high protein diet and charcoal broiled beef (due to a high polycyclic carbon content). Conversely, elimination is decreased (prolonged half-life) by a high carbohydrate low protein diet. Food may alter the bioavailability and absorption pattern of certain sustained release preparations. Some sustained release preparations may be subject to rapid release of their contents when taken with food, resulting in toxicity. It appears that consistent administration in the fasting state allows predictability of effects.

Adverse Reactions

Adverse reactions/toxicity are uncommon at serum theophylline levels less than 20 mcg/mL.

Levels more than 20 mcg/mL – 75% of patients experience adverse reactions (eg, nausea, vomiting, diarrhea, headache, insomnia, irritability).

Levels more than 35 mcg/mL – Hyperglycemia; hypotension; cardiac arrhythmias; tachycardia (more than 10 mcg/mL in premature newborns); seizures; brain damage; death.

➤*Cardiovascular:* Palpitations; tachycardia; extrasystoles; hypotension; circulatory failure; life-threatening ventricular arrhythmias.

➤*CNS:* Irritability; restlessness; headache; insomnia; reflex hyperexcitability; muscle twitching; convulsions.

➤*GI:* Nausea; vomiting; epigastric pain; hematemesis; diarrhea; rectal irritation or bleeding (aminophylline suppositories). Therapeutic doses of theophylline may induce gastroesophageal reflux during sleep or while recumbent, increasing the potential for aspiration which can aggravate bronchospasm.

➤*Renal:* Proteinuria; potentiation of diuresis.

➤*Respiratory:* Tachypnea; respiratory arrest.

➤*Miscellaneous:* Fever; flushing; hyperglycemia; inappropriate antidiuretic hormone syndrome; rash; alopecia. Ethylenediamine in aminophylline can cause sensitivity reactions, including exfoliative dermatitis and urticaria.

Overdosage

➤*Symptoms:* Anorexia; nausea; vomiting; nervousness; insomnia; agitation; irritability; headache; tachycardia; extrasystoles; tachypnea; fasciculation; tonic/clonic convulsions. Convulsions or ventricular arrhythmias may be the first signs of toxicity. Hyperamylasemia, simulating pancreatitis, has also been noted. Other symptoms of intoxication are listed under Adverse Reactions.

Serious adverse effects are rare at serum theophylline concentrations less than 20 mcg/mL. Between 20 and 40 mcg/mL, sinus tachycardia and cardiac arrhythmias occur. Above 40 mcg/mL, seizures and cardiorespiratory arrest can occur. However, convulsions and death have been reported at concentrations as low as 25 mcg/mL.

Acute overdosage appears to be better tolerated with the more serious reactions (eg, seizures) occurring with chronic overdosage (levels more than 40 mcg/mL), but rarely in the acute situation unless levels exceed 100 mcg/mL. Also, symptoms such as hypokalemia, hypercalcemia, hyperglycemia and decreased serum bicarbonate concentrations occur more frequently with acute overdosage.

Overdosage with sustained release preparations may cause a dramatic increase in serum theophylline concentrations much later (at least 12 hours) than the increases that occur with other preparations. Early treatment will help but not prevent these delayed elevated levels.

➤*Treatment:*

Treatment if seizure has not occurred – Induce vomiting, even if emesis has occurred spontaneously; ipecac syrup is preferred. However, do not induce emesis in patients with impaired consciousness. Take precautions against aspiration, especially in infants and children. If vomiting is unsuccessful or contraindicated, perform gastric lavage (of no value at least 1 hour post-ingestion). Administer a cathartic (particularly for sustained-release preparations; sorbitol may be useful) and activated charcoal. Prophylactic phenobarbital may increase the seizure threshold.

If seizure occurs – Establish an airway and administer oxygen. Administer IV diazepam 0.1 to 0.3 mg/kg, up to 10 mg. Monitor vital signs, maintain blood pressure and provide adequate hydration.

Post-seizure coma – Maintain airway and oxygenation. Perform intubation and lavage instead of inducing emesis. Introduce the cathartic and activated charcoal via a large bore gastric lavage tube. Provide full supportive care and adequate hydration while the drug is metabolized. If repeated oral activated charcoal is ineffective, charcoal hemoperfusion may be indicated.

Supportive care – Employ usual supportive measures. Refer to General Management of Acute Overdosage. Do not use stimulants (analeptic agents). Continuously monitor cardiac function. Verapamil has been used to treat atrial arrhythmias; lidocaine or procainamide may be used for ventricular arrhythmias. May need IV fluids to treat dehydration, acid-base imbalance and hypotension; the latter may also be treated with vasopressors. Apnea will require ventilatory support. Treat hyperpyrexia, especially in children, with tepid water sponge baths or a hypothermic blanket.

Monitor theophylline serum level until it falls below 20 mcg/mL because secondary rises of plasma theophylline may occur from redistribution, delayed absorption, etc.; this has been reported with sustained release products.

Dialysis – Charcoal hemoperfusion rapidly removes theophylline and may be indicated when the serum concentration is more than 60 mcg/mL, even in the absence of obvious toxicity. Forced diuresis, peritoneal dialysis and extracorporeal methods are inadequate. However, hemodialysis appears capable of removing approximately 36% to 40% of serum theophylline.

"Gastric dialysis": With oral activated charcoal, 20 to 40 g every 4 hours until serum level is less than 20 mcg/mL, may shorten half-life and speed removal, regardless of route. Mechanism may include enhancing drug concentration gradient into the GI lumen, a disruption of an enterohepatic recycling process or binding unabsorbed drug.

Patient Information

If GI upset occurs with liquid or non-sustained release forms, take with food.

Do NOT chew or crush enteric coated or sustained release tablets or capsules.

Take at the same time, with or without food, each day.

Notify physician if nausea, vomiting, insomnia, jitteriness, headache, rash, severe GI pain, restlessness, convulsions or irregular heartbeat occurs.

Avoid large amounts of caffeine-containing beverages, such as tea, coffee, cocoa and cola drinks or large amounts of chocolate; these products may increase side effects.

➤*Brand interchange:* Do not change from one brand to another without consulting your pharmacist or physician. Products manufactured by different companies may not be equally effective.

Individual doses are determined by response (decrease in symptoms). Blood levels must be checked regularly to avoid underdosing and overdosing. Do not change the dose of your medication without consulting your physician.

THEOPHYLLINE

Rx	**Theophylline** (Various)	**Tablets**: 300 mg	In 100s, 500s and 1000s.
Rx	**Bronkodyl** (Winthrop)	**Capsules**: 100 mg	Brown and white. In 100s.
Rx	**Elixophyllin** (Forest)		Dye free. (Forest 642). In 100s.
Rx	**Bronkodyl** (Winthrop)	**Capsules**: 200 mg	Green and white. In 100s.
Rx	**Elixophyllin** (Forest)		Dye free. (Forest 643). In 100s and 500s.
Rx	**Theophylline** (Various, eg, Balan, Barre-National, Bioline, Geneva, Moore, Rugby, Schein, URL)	**Elixir**: 80 mg per 15 mL (26.7 mg per 5 mL)	In pt and gal and UD 15 and 30 mL.
Rx	**Asmalix** (Century)		20% alcohol. In gal.
Rx	**Elixomin** (Cenci)		20% alcohol. Orange raspberry flavor. In pt.
Rx	**Elixophyllin** (Forest)		20% alcohol. Saccharin. Mixed fruit flavor. In pt, qt and gal.
Rx sf	**Lanophyllin** (Lannett)		20% alcohol. In pt and gal.
Rx	**Theophylline Extended-Release** (Dey)	**Tablets, extended-release**: 100 mg	In 100s, 500s and 1000s.
		200 mg	In 100s, 500s and 1000s.
		300 mg	In 100s, 500s and 1000s.
Rx	**Theo-24** (UCB Pharma)	**Capsules, timed release (24 hours)**: 100 mg	(Theo-24 100 mg Searle 2832). Gold and clear. In 100s and UD 100s.
		200 mg	(Theo-24 200 mg Searle 2842). Orange and clear. In 100s, 500s and UD 100s.
		300 mg	(Theo-24 300 mg Searle 2852). Red and clear. In 100s, 500s and UD100s.
		Note: Patients receiving once daily doses ≥ 13 mg/kg or ≥ 900 mg (whichever is less) should avoid eating a high-fat-content morning meal or should take medication at least 1 hour before eating. If patient cannot comply with this regimen, place on alternative therapy.	
Rx	**Theophylline** (Various, eg, Mason, Parmed)	**Capsules, extended release**: 100 mg	In 100s.
		125 mg	In 100s.
		200 mg	In 100s.
		300 mg	In 100s.

THEOPHYLLINE

Rx	**Theophylline SR** (Various, eg, Balan, Bioline, Geneva, Goldline, Major, Moore, Rugby, Sidmak)	**Tablets, timed release (12 to 24 hours):** 100 mg	In 100s and 500s.
		200 mg	In 100s, 500s, 1000s, UD 100s.
		300 mg	In 100s, 500s, 1000s, UD 100s.
Rx	**Theophylline** (Able)	**Tablets, extended release:** 300 mg	(A379). White to off-white, scored, capsule shape. In 30s, 100s, 500s, and 1,000s.
		400 mg	(A380). White to off-white, scored. In 30s, 100s, 500s, and 1,000s.
		450 mg	(A381). White to off-white, scored, capsule shape. In 30s, 100s, 500s, and 1,000s.
		600 mg	(A382). White to off-white, oval. In 30s, 100s, 500s, and 1,000s.
Rx	**Theochron** (Various, eg, Inwood, Lemmon)	**Tablets, extended release:** 100 mg	In 100s, 500s, 1000s.
		200 mg	In 100s, 500s, 1000s.
		300 mg	In 100s, 500s, 1000s.
Rx	**Theochron** (Forest)	**Tablets, extended release (12 to 24 hours):** 450 mg	(IL3614/450). Off-white, capsule shape, scored. In 100s, 500s, and 1000s.
Rx	**Theocron** (Inwood)	**Tablets, timed release (12 to 24 hours):** 100 mg	Dye free. (IL/3584). White, scored. Convex. In 100s, 500s, 1000s.
		200 mg	Dye free. (IL/3583). White, scored. Oval. In 100s, 500s, 1000s.
		300 mg	Dye free. (IL/3581). White, scored. Capsule shape. In 100s, 500s, 1000s.
Rx	**Uniphyl** (Purdue Frederick)	**Tablets, timed release (24 hours):** 400 mg	(PF U400). White, scored. In 100s, 500s, UD 100s.
		600 mg	(PF U600). White, scored. In 100s.

THEOPHYLLINE — ORAL

For complete and comparative prescribing information, refer to the Xanthine Derivatives group monograph.

Indications

For the treatment of the symptoms and reversible airflow obstruction associated with chronic asthma and other chronic lung diseases (eg, emphysema, chronic bronchitis).

Administration and Dosage

The steady-state peak serum theophylline concentration is a function of the dose, the dosing interval, and the rate of theophylline absorption and clearance in the individual patient. Because of marked individual differences in the rate of theophylline clearance, the dose required to achieve a peak serum theophylline concentration in the 10 to 20 mcg/mL range varies 4-fold among otherwise similar patients in the absence of factors known to alter theophylline clearance (eg, 400 to 1600 mg/day in adults less than 60 years old and 10 to 36 mg/kg/day in children 1 to 9 years old). For a given population there is no single theophylline dose that will provide both safe and effective serum concentrations for all patients. Administration of the median theophylline dose required to achieve a therapeutic serum theophylline concentration in a given population may result in either subtherapeutic or potentially toxic serum theophylline concentrations in individual patients. For example, at a dose of 900 mg/day in adults less than 60 years or 22 mg/kg/day in children 1 to 9 years, the steady-state peak serum theophylline concentration will be less than 10 mcg/mL in about 30% of patients, 10 to 20 mcg/mL in about 50% and 20 to 30 mcg/mL in about 20% of patients. The dose of theophylline must be individualized on the basis of peak serum theophylline concentration measurements in order to achieve a dose that will provide maximum potential benefit with minimal risk of adverse effects.

➤*Dosage adjustment:* Transient caffeine-like adverse effects and excessive serum concentrations in slow metabolizers can be avoided in most patients by starting with a sufficiently low dose and slowly increasing the dose, if judged to be clinically indicated, in small increments. Dose increases should only be made if the previous dosage is well tolerated and at intervals of no less than 3 days to allow serum theophylline concentrations to reach the new steady state. Dosage adjustment should be guided by serum theophylline concentration measurement. Health care providers should instruct patients and care givers to discontinue any dosage that causes adverse effects, to withhold the medication until these symptoms are gone and to then resume therapy at a lower, previously tolerated dosage.

➤*Monitoring:* If the patient's symptoms are well controlled, there are no apparent adverse effects, and no intervening factors that might alter dosage requirements, serum theophylline concentrations should be monitored at 6 month intervals for rapidly growing children and at yearly intervals for all others. In acutely ill patients, serum theophylline concentrations should be monitored at frequent intervals (eg, every 24 hours).

➤*Dosage calculation:* Theophylline distributes poorly into body fat; therefore, mg/kg dose should be calculated on the basis of ideal body weight.

➤*Dosage recommendations:* Application of these general dosing recommendations to individual patients must take into account the unique clinical characteristics of each patient. In general, these recommendations should serve as the upper limit for dosage adjustments in order to decrease the risk of potentially serious adverse events associated with unexpected large increases in serum theophylline concentration.

Dosing initiation and titration (as anhydrous theophylline)*		
Children (12 to 15 years) and adults (16 to 60 years) without risk factors for impaired clearance		
Titration step	Children < 45 kg	Children > 45 kg and adults
Starting dosage	12 to 14 mg/kg/day up to a maximum of 300 mg/day divided every 24 hours[a]	300 to 400 mg/day[1] divided every 24 hours[a]
After 3 days, if tolerated, increase dose to:	16 mg/kg/day up to a maximum of 400 mg/day divided every 24 hours[a]	400 to 600 mg/day[b] divided every 24 hours[a]
After 3 more days, if tolerated and if needed, increase dose to:	20 mg/kg/day up to a maximum of 600 mg/day divided every 24 hours[a]	As with all theophylline products, doses greater than 600 mg should be titrated according to blood level (see table below)
Patients with risk factors for impaired clearance, the elderly (> 60 years), and those in whom it is not feasible to monitor serum theophylline concentrations:		
In children 6 to 15 years of age, the final theophylline dose should not exceed 16 mg/kg/day up to a maximum of 400 mg/day in the presence of risk factors for reduced theophylline clearance or if it is not feasible to monitor serum theophylline concentrations.		
In adolescents ≥ 16 years and adults, including the elderly, the final theophylline dose should not exceed 400 mg/day in the presence of risk factors for reduced theophylline clearance or if it is not feasible to monitor serum theophylline concentrations.		

[a] Patients with more rapid metabolism, clinically identified by higher than average dose requirements, should receive a smaller dose more frequently to prevent breakthrough symptoms resulting from low trough concentrations before the next dose. A reliably absorbed slow-release formulation will decrease fluctuations and permit longer dosing intervals.

[b] If caffeine-like adverse effects occur, then consideration should be given to a lower dose and titrating the dose more slowly.

THEOPHYLLINE — ORAL

Dosage adjustment guided by serum theophylline concentrations	
Peak serum concentration	Dosage adjustment
< 9.9 mcg/mL	If symptoms are not controlled and current dosage is tolerated, increase dose about 25%. Recheck serum concentration after 3 days for further dosage adjustment.
10 to 14.9 mcg/mL	If symptoms are controlled and current dosage is tolerated, maintain dose and recheck serum concentration at 6- to 12-month intervals.[a] If symptoms are not controlled and current dosage is tolerated, consider adding additional medication(s) to treatment regimen.
15 to 19.9 mcg/mL	Consider 10% decrease in dose to provide greater margin of safety even if current dosage is tolerated[a].
20 to 24.9 mcg/mL	Decrease dose by 25% even if no adverse effects are present. Recheck serum concentration after 3 days to guide further dosage adjustment.
25 to 30 mcg/mL	Skip next dose and decrease subsequent doses at least 25% even if no adverse effects are present. Recheck serum concentration after 3 days to guide further dosage adjustment. If symptomatic, consider whether overdose treatment is indicated (see recommendations for chronic overdosage).
> 30 mcg/mL	Treat overdose as indicated (see recommendations for chronic overdosage). If theophylline is subsequently resumed, decrease dose by at least 50% and recheck serum concentration after 3 days to guide further dosage adjustment.

[a] Dose reduction or serum theophylline concentration measurement is indicated whenever adverse effects are present, physiologic abnormalities that can reduce theophylline clearance occur (eg, sustained fever), or a drug that interacts with theophylline is added or discontinued.

Extended-release tablets – Theophylline extended-release tablets can be taken once a day in the morning or evening. It is recommended that theophylline extended-release tablets be taken with meals. Patients should be advised that if they choose to take theophylline extended-release tablets with food it should be taken consistently with food and if they take it in a fasted condition it should routinely be taken fasted. It is important that the product, whenever dosed, be dosed consistently with or without food.

Theophylline extended-release tablets are not to be chewed or crushed. The scored tablet may be split. Infrequently patients receiving theophylline extended-release 400 or 600 mg tablets may pass an intact matrix tablet in the stool or via colostomy. These matrix tablets usually contain little or no residual theophylline. Stabilized patients, 12 years of age or older, who are taking an immediate-release or extended-release theophylline product may be transferred to once-daily administration of 400 or 600 mg theophylline extended-release tablets on a mg-for-mg basis.

It must be recognized that the peak and trough serum theophylline levels produced by the once-daily dosing may vary from those produced by the previous product or regimen.

Extended-release capsules – Theophylline extended-release capsules, like other extended-release theophylline products, is intended for patients with relatively continuous or recurring symptoms who have a need to maintain therapeutic serum levels of theophylline. It is not intended for patients experiencing an acute episode of bronchospasm (associated with asthma, chronic bronchitis, or emphysema). Such patients require rapid relief of symptoms and should be treated with an immediate-release or IV theophylline preparation (or other bronchodilators) and not with extended-release products.

Taking theophylline extended-release capsules immediately after a high-fat meal may alter its rate of absorption. However, the differences are usually small and theophylline extended-release capsules may normally be administered without regard to meals.

Patients who metabolize theophylline at a normal or slow rate are reasonable candidates for once-daily dosing with theophylline extended-release capsules. Patients who metabolize theophylline rapidly (eg, younger patients, smokers, and some nonsmoking adults) and who have symptoms repeatedly at the end of a dosing interval, will require increased doses given once a day or preferably, are likely to be better controlled by a schedule of twice-daily dosing. Those patients who require increased daily doses are more likely to experience relatively wide peak-trough differences and may be candidates for twice-a-day dosing with theophylline extended-release capsules.

Patients should be instructed to take this medicine each morning at approximately the same time and not to exceed the prescribed dose.

Recent studies suggest that dosing of extended-release theophylline products at night (after the evening meal) results in serum concentrations of theophylline which are not identical to those recorded during waking hours and my be characterized by early trough and delayed peak levels. This appears to occur whether the drug is given as an immediate-release, extended-release, or IV product. To avoid this phenomenon when 2 doses per day are prescribed, it is recommended that the second dose be given 10 to 12 hours after the morning dose and before the evening meal.

Food and posture, along with changes associated with circadian rhythm, may influence the rate of absorption or clearance rates of theophylline from extended-release dosage forms administered at night. The exact relationship of these and other factors to nighttime serum concentrations and the clinical significance of such findings require additional study. Therefore, it is not recommended that theophylline extended-release capsules (when used as a once-a-day product) be administered at night.

Patients who require a relatively high dose of theophylline (ie, a dose equal to or greater than 900 mg or 13 mg/kg, whichever is less) should not take theophylline extended-release capsules less than 1 hour before a high-fat-content meal since this may result in significant increase in peak serum level and in the extent of absorption of theophylline as compared to administration in the fasted state.

Once-daily dosing: The slow absorption rate of some preparations may allow once-daily administration in adult nonsmokers with appropriate total body clearance and other patients with low dosage requirements. Once-daily dosing should be considered only after the patient has been gradually and satisfactorily treated to therapeutic levels with every-12-hour dosing. Once-daily dosing should be based on the dosing guidelines in the tables above and should be initiated at the end of the last every 12 hours dosing interval. The trough concentration (C_{min}) obtained following conversion to once-daily dosing may be lower (especially in high clearance patients) and the peak concentration (C_{max}) may be higher (especially in low clearance patients) and the peak concentration (C_{max}) may be higher (especially in low clearance patients) than that obtained with every-12-hour dosing. If symptoms recur, or signs of toxicity appear during the once-daily dosing interval, dosing on the every-12-hour basis should be reinstituted.

It is essential that serum theophylline concentrations be monitored before and after transfer to once-daily dosing. Food and posture, along with changes associated with circadian rhythm, may influence the rate of absorption or clearance rates of theophylline from extended-release dosage forms administered at night. The exact relationship of these and other factors to nighttime serum concentrations and the clinical significance of such findings require additional study. Therefore, it is not recommended that theophylline extended-release capsules, when used as a once-daily product, be administered at night.

Patients with risk factors for impaired clearance, the elderly (greater than 60 years), and those in whom it is not feasible to monitor serum theophylline concentrations: In children 1 to 15 years of age, the final theophylline dose should not exceed 16 mg/kg/day up to a maximum of 400 mg/day in the presence of risk factors for reduced theophylline clearance, or if it is not feasible to monitor serum theophylline concentrations.

In adolescents greater than or equal to 16 years of age and adults, including the elderly, the final theophylline dose should not exceed 400 mg/day in the presence of risk factors for reduced theophylline clearance or if it is not feasible to monitor serum theophylline concentrations.

Patients with more rapid metabolism, clinically identified by higher than average dose requirements, should receive a smaller dose more frequently to prevent breakthrough symptoms resulting from low trough concentrations before the next dose. A reliably absorbed slow-release formulation will decrease fluctuations and permit longer dosing intervals.

Extended-release tablets – Theophylline extended-release tablets are recommended for chronic or long-term management and prevention of symptoms, and not for use in treating acute symptoms of asthma and reversible bronchospasm.

➤*Storage/Stability:*

Elixir and extended-release tablets – Store at controlled room temperature 15° to 30°C (59° to 86°F).

Dispense in tight container.

Extended-release capsules – Store below 25°C (77°F).

Sustained-release tablets – Store between 15° to 25°C (59° to 77°F).

Tablets – Store below 30°C (86°F).

THEOPHYLLINE AND DEXTROSE

Rx	**Theophylline and 5% Dextrose** (Abbott and Baxter)	**Injection**: 200 mg/container	In 50 mL (4 mg/mL) and 100 mL (2 mg/mL).
		400 mg/container	In 100 mL (4 mg/mL), 250 mL (1.6 mg/mL), 500 mL (0.8 mg/mL) and 1000 mL (0.4 mg/mL).
		800 mg/container	In 250 mL (3.2 mg/mL), 500 mL (1.6 mg/mL) and 1000 mL (0.8 mg/mL).

THEOPHYLLINE AND DEXTROSE — INJECTION

For complete and comparative prescribing information, refer to the Xanthine Derivative group monograph.

Administration and Dosage

Substitute oral therapy for IV theophylline as soon as adequate improvement is achieved.

See also aminophylline for parenteral administration guidelines, noting the difference of theophylline content.

➤*The following may be incompatible when mixed with theophylline in IV fluids:* Anileridine; ascorbic acid; chlorpromazine; codeine phosphate; corticotropin; dimenhydrinate; epinephrine HCl; erythromycin gluceptate; hydralazine; hydroxyzine HCl; insulin; levorphanol tartrate; meperidine; methadone; methicillin sodium; morphine sulfate; norepinephrine bitartrate; oxytetracycline; papaverine; penicillin G potassium; phenobarbital sodium; phenytoin sodium; procaine; prochlorperazine maleate; promazine; promethazine; tetracycline; vancomycin; vitamin B complex with C.

➤*Children:* Due to marked variation in theophylline metabolism, use this drug only if clearly needed in infants younger than 6 months of age.

AMINOPHYLLINE (Theophylline Ethylenediamine) – 79% theophylline

Rx	**Aminophylline** (Various, eg, Balan, Bioline, Geneva-Marsam, Goldline, Major, Roxane, Rugby, Searle, URL)	**Tablets**: 100 mg (equiv. to 79 mg theophylline)	Plain or enteric coated. In 100s, 1000s and UD 100s.
Rx	**Aminophylline** (Various, eg, Balan, Bioline, Geneva-Marsam, Goldline, Major, Moore, Roxane, Rugby, Searle, URL)	**Tablets**: 200 mg (equiv. to 158 mg theophylline)	Plain or enteric coated. In 100s, 1000s and UD 100s.
Rx	**Aminophylline** (Various, eg, Abbott, American Regent, Elkins-Sinn, Moore, Solopak)	**Injection**: 250 mg (equiv. to 197 mg theophylline) per 10 mL For IV use.	In 10 and 20 mL amps & vials & syringes.

AMINOPHYLLINE (Theophylline Ethylenediamine) – 79% theophylline — ORAL

For complete and comparative prescribing information, refer to the Xanthine Derivative group monograph. For oral dosage, refer to the Equivalent Dosage table in Actions and to the Administration section in the Xanthine Derivatives group monograph.

AMINOPHYLLINE — INJECTION

For complete and comparative prescribing information, refer to the Xanthine Derivative group monograph.

Indications

➤*Bronchial asthma/reversible bronchospasm:* For the relief of acute bronchial asthma and for reversible bronchospasm associated with chronic bronchitis and emphysema.

Administration and Dosage

➤*Approved by the FDA:* February 1, 1982.

➤*Individual dosage:* Effective use of theophylline (ie, the concentration of drug in the serum associated with optimal benefit and minimal risk of toxicity) is considered to occur when the theophylline concentration is maintained from 10 to 20 mcg/mL. The early studies from which these levels were derived were carried out in patients immediately or shortly after recovery from acute exacerbations of their disease (some hospitalized with status asthmaticus).

Although the 20 mcg/mL level remains appropriate as a critical value (above which toxicity is more likely to occur) for safety purposes, additional data are now available which indicate that the serum theophylline concentrations required to produce maximum physiologic benefit may, in fact, fluctuate with the degree of bronchospasm present and are variable. Therefore, the physician should individualize the range appropriate to the patient's requirements, based on both symptomatic response and improvement in pulmonary function. It should be stressed that serum theophylline concentrations maintained at the upper level of the 10 to 20 mcg/mL range may be associated with potential toxicity when factors known to reduce theophylline clearance are operative.

➤*Dosage guidelines:* Acute symptoms of bronchospasm requiring rapid attainment of theophylline serum levels for bronchodilation.

Theophylline does not distribute into fatty tissue. Dosage should be calculated on the basis of lean (ideal) body weight where mg/kg doses are presented.

Note – Status asthmaticus should be considered a medical emergency and is defined as that degree of bronchospasm which is not rapidly responsive to usual doses of conventional bronchodilators. Optimal therapy for such patients frequently requires both additional medication, parenterally administered, and close monitoring, preferably in an intensive care setting.

Patients not currently receiving theophylline products:

Aminophylline dosage		
	Loading	Maintenance
Children age: 1 to under 9 years	6.3 mg/kg [a] (5)	1 mg/kg/h[a] (0.79)
Children age: 9 to under 16 years and smokers	6.3 mg/kg [a] (5)	0.8 mg/kg/h[a] (0.63)

Aminophylline dosage		
	Loading	Maintenance
Otherwise healthy nonsmoking adults	6.3 mg/kg[a] (5)	0.5 mg/kg/h[a] (0.4)
Older patients and patients with cor pulmonale	6.3 mg/kg[a] (5)	0.3 mg/kg/h[a] (0.24)
Patients with congestive heart failure	6.3 mg/kg[a] (5)	0.1 to 0.2 mg/kg/h[a] (0.08 to 0.16)

[a] Equivalent dosage of theophylline.

Patients currently receiving theophylline products: Determine, where possible, the time, amount, dosage form, and route of administration of the last dose the patient received.

The loading dose for theophylline is based on the principle that each 0.5 mg/kg of theophylline administered as a loading dose will result in a 1 mcg/mL increase in serum theophylline concentration. Ideally, the loading dose should be deferred if a serum theophylline concentration can be obtained rapidly.

If this is not possible, the clinician must exercise his judgement in selecting a dose based on the potential for benefit and risk. When there is sufficient respiratory distress to warrant a small risk, then 2.5 mg/kg of theophylline administered in rapidly absorbed form is likely to increase the serum concentration by approximately 5 mcg/mL. If the patient is not experiencing theophylline toxicity, this is unlikely to result in dangerous adverse effects.

Subsequent to the decision regarding modification of the loading dose for this group of patients, the maintenance dosage recommendations are the same as those described above.

➤*Administration:* The loading dose of aminophylline can be given by very slow IV push or, more conveniently, may be infused in a small quantity (usually 100 to 200 mL) of 5% Dextrose Injection or 0.9% Sodium Chloride Injection. Do not exceed the rate of 25 mg/min.

Thereafter, maintenance therapy can be administered by a large volume infusion to deliver the desired amount of drug each hour. Aminophylline is compatible with most commonly used IV solutions.

Oral therapy should be substituted for intravenous aminophylline as soon as adequate improvement is achieved.

➤*Intravenous admixture incompatibility:* Although there have been reports of aminophylline precipitating in acidic media, these reports do not apply to the dilute solutions found in intravenous infusions. Aminophylline injection should not be mixed in a syringe with other drugs but should be added separately to the intravenous solution.

Xanthine Derivatives

AMINOPHYLLINE — INJECTION

When an intravenous solution containing aminophylline is given "piggy-back", the intravenous system already in place should be turned off while the aminophylline is infused if there is a potential problem with admixture incompatibility.

Because of the alkalinity of aminophylline containing solutions, drugs known to be alkali labile should be avoided in admixtures. These include epinephrine HCl, norepinephrine bitartrate, isoproterenol HCl and penicillin G potassium. It is suggested that specialized literature be consulted before preparing admixtures with aminophylline and other drugs.

Parenteral drug products should be inspected visually for particulate matter and discoloration prior to administration, whenever solution and container permit. Do not administer unless solution is clear and container is undamaged. Discard unused portion. Do not use if crystals have separated from solution.

➤*Special risk patients:* Caution should be exercised for younger children who cannot complain of minor side effects. Older adults, those with cor pulmonale, congestive heart failure, and/or liver disease may have unusually low dosage requirements and thus may experience toxicity at the maximal dosage recommended below.

➤*Storage/Stability:* Store at controlled room temperature, 15° to 30°C (59° to 86°F). Protect from light. Store in carton until time of use. Single dose container. Discard unused portion.

DYPHYLLINE (Dihydroxypropyl Theophylline)

Rx	**Dyphylline** (Various, eg, Balan, Major)	**Tablets:** 200 mg	In 100s and 1000s.
Rx	**Lufyllin** (Medpointe)		(Wallace 521). White, scored. Rectangular. In 100s, 1000s, 5000s and UD 100s.
Rx	**Dyphylline** (Various, eg, Balan, Major, URL)	**Tablets:** 400 mg	In 100s and 1000s.
Rx	**Lufyllin-400** (Medpointe)		(Wallace 731). White, scored. Capsule shape. In 100s, 1000s, 2500s and UD 100s.
Rx	**Dylix** (Lunsco)	**Elixir:** 100 mg per 15 mL	20% alcohol. In 437 mL.

DYPHYLLINE — ORAL

For complete and comparative prescribing information, refer to the Xanthine Derivatives group monograph.

Indications

➤*Bronchial asthma/reversible bronchospasm:* For relief of acute bronchial asthma and for reversible bronchospasm associated with chronic bronchitis and emphysema.

Administration and Dosage

Dosage should be individually titrated according to the severity of the condition and the response of the patient.

➤*Tablets:*

Usual adult dose – Up to 15 mg/kg every 6 hours.

➤*Elixir:*

Usual adult dose – 30 mL to 60 mL (2 to 4 tablespoons) every 6 hours.

➤*Dosage adjustment:* Base dosage adjustments on clinical response and improvement in pulmonary function with careful monitoring of serum levels. This allows an objective assessment of whether therapy should be continued in patients with chronic bronchitis and emphysema.

Appropriate dosage adjustments should be made in patients with impaired renal function.

➤*Storage/Stability:*

Tablets – Store at controlled room temperature 15° to 30°C (59° to 86°F).

Elixir – Store at controlled room temperature 20° to 25°C (68° to 77°F). Dispense in a tight container.

Anticholinergics

IPRATROPIUM BROMIDE

Rx	**Ipratropium Bromide** (Dey)	**Solution for Inhalation:** 0.02% (500 mcg per vial)	Preservative free. In 25 and 60 unit-dose vials (2.5 ml each).
Rx	**Atrovent HFA** (Boehringer Ingelheim)	**Aerosol:** Each actuation delivers 17 mcg	In 12.9 g metered dose inhaler w/mouthpiece (200 inhalations).
Rx	**Atrovent** (Boehringer Ingelheim)	**Aerosol:** Each actuation delivers 18 mcg	In 14.7 g metered dose inhaler w/mouthpiece (200 inhalations).
Rx	**Ipratropium Bromide** (Various, eg, Bausch & Lomb, Roxane)	**Nasal spray:** 0.03%. Each spray delivers 21 mcg	In 30 mL with spray pump (345 sprays).
Rx	**Atrovent** (Boehringer Ingelheim)		In 30 mL bottles with spray pump (345 sprays).
Rx	**Ipratropium Bromide** (Various, eg, Bausch & Lamb, Roxane)	**Nasal spray:** 0.06%. Each spray delivers 42 mcg	In 15 mL with spray pump (165 sprays).
Rx	**Atrovent** (Boehringer Ingelheim)		In 15 mL bottles with spray pump (165 sprays).

IPRATROPIUM BROMIDE — INHALATION

Indications

➤*Chronic obstructive pulmonary disease (COPD):* Alone or with other bronchodilators, especially beta adrenergics, as a bronchodilator for maintenance treatment of bronchospasm associated with COPD, including chronic bronchitis and emphysema.

Administration and Dosage

➤*Approved by the FDA:* December 29, 1986.

➤*HFA aerosol:*

Dose – The usual starting dose is 2 inhalations 4 times a day. Patients may take additional inhalations as required; however, the total number of inhalations should not exceed 12 in 24 hours. Each actuation of ipratropium HFA inhalation aerosol delivers ipratropium 17 mcg from the mouthpiece.

Priming – "Prime" or actuate ipratropium HFA inhalation aerosol before using for the first time by releasing 2 test sprays into the air away from the face. In cases where the inhaler has not been used for more than 3 days, prime the inhaler again by releasing 2 test sprays into the air away from the face.

➤*Solution:*

Dose – The usual dosage is 500 mcg (1 unit-dose vial) administered 3 to 4 times a day by oral nebulization, with doses 6 to 8 hours apart. The unit dose vials contain 500 mcg of ipratropium anhydrous in 2.5 mL normal saline. Ipratropium inhalation solution can be mixed in the nebulizer with albuterol or metaproterenol if used within 1 hour.

Administration – Use of a nebulizer with mouthpiece rather than face mask may be preferable to reduce the likelihood of the nebulizer solution reaching the eyes. Advise patients that ipratropium inhalation solution can be mixed in the nebulizer with albuterol or metaproterenol if used within 1 hour. Drug stability and safety of ipratropium inhalation solution when mixed with other drugs in a nebulizer have not been established. Remind patients that ipratropium inhalation solution should be used consistently as prescribed throughout the course of therapy.

Solution incompatibility – Drug stability and safety of ipratropium inhalation solution when mixed with other drugs in a nebulizer have not been established. Advise patients that ipratropium inhalation solution can be mixed in the nebulizer with albuterol or metaproterenol if used within 1 hour.

➤*Storage/Stability:*

HFA aerosol –

Store at 25°C (77°F). Excursions permitted to 15° to 30°C (59° to 86°F). For optimal results, store the canister at room temperature before use.

Contents under pressure: Do not puncture. Do not use or store near heat or open flame. Exposure to temperatures above 49°C (120°F) may cause bursting. Never throw the inhaler into a fire or incinerator.

Solution – Store between 15° and 30°C (59° and 86°F). Protect from light. Retain in foil pouch until time of use.

Actions

➤*Pharmacology:* Ipratropium bromide is an anticholinergic (parasympathetic) agent that, based on animal studies, appears to inhibit vagally medi-

IPRATROPIUM BROMIDE — INHALATION

ated reflexes by antagonizing the action of acetylcholine, the transmitter agent released at neuromuscular junctions in the lung. Anticholinergics prevent the increase in intracellular concentration of cyclic guanosine monophosphate (cyclic GMP), which are caused by interaction of acetylcholine with the muscarinic receptor on bronchial smooth muscle.

➤*Pharmacokinetics:*

Absorption – The bronchodilation following inhalation of ipratropium is primarily a local, site-specific effect, not a systemic one. Much of an administered dose is swallowed but not absorbed, as shown by fecal excretion studies. Ipratropium is a quaternary amine. Following nebulization of a 2 mg dose, a mean 7% of the dose was absorbed into the systemic circulation either from the surface of the lung or from the GI tract.

Distribution – Ipratropium is minimally bound (0% to 9% in vitro) to plasma albumin and α_1-acid glycoprotein. Its blood/plasma concentration ratio was estimated to be about 0.89. Autoradiographic studies in rats have shown that ipratropium does not penetrate the blood-brain barrier.

Metabolism / Excretion – Ipratropium is partially metabolized to inactive ester hydrolysis products. Following intravenous (IV) administration, approximately one half of the dose is excreted unchanged in the urine.

The half-life of elimination is about 2 hours after inhalation or IV administration. The total body clearance and renal clearance were estimated to be 2,505 and 1,019 mL/min, respectively. The amount of the total dose excreted unchanged in the urine (Ae) within 24 hours was approximately one half of the administered dose.

A pharmacokinetic study with 29 COPD patients (48 to 79 years of age) demonstrated that mean peak plasma ipratropium concentrations of 59 ± 20 pg/mL were obtained following a single administration of 4 inhalations of ipratropium HFA inhalation aerosol (84 mcg). Plasma ipratropium concentrations rapidly declined to 24 ± 15 pg/mL by 6 hours. When these patients were administered 4 inhalations 4 times daily (16 inhalations/day – 336 mcg) for 1 week, the mean peak plasma ipratropium concentration increased to 82 ± 39 pg/mL with a trough (6 hour) concentration of 28 ± 12 pg/mL at steady state.

Contraindications

Hypersensitivity to ipratropium or its components, or atropine or its derivatives.

Warnings

➤*Acute bronchospasm:*

HFA aerosol – Ipratropium HFA inhalation aerosol is a bronchodilator for the maintenance treatment of bronchospasm associated with COPD and is not indicated for the initial treatment of acute episodes of bronchospasm where rescue therapy is required for rapid response.

Inhaled medicines, including ipratropium HFA inhalation aerosol, may cause paradoxical bronchospasm. If this occurs, stop treatment with ipratropium HFA inhalation aerosol and consider other treatments.

Solution – The use of ipratropium inhalation solution as a single agent for the relief of bronchospasm in acute COPD exacerbation has not been adequately studied. Drugs with faster onset of action may be preferable as initial therapy in this situation. Combination of ipratropium and beta agonists has not been shown to be more effective than either drug alone in reversing the bronchospasm associated with acute COPD exacerbation.

➤*Hypersensitivity reactions:* Immediate hypersensitivity reactions may occur after administration of ipratropium as demonstrated by rare cases of urticaria, angioedema, rash, bronchospasm, anaphylaxis, and oropharyngeal edema.

➤*Fertility impairment:* Fertility of male or female rats at oral dosages up to 50 mg/kg/day (approximately 2,000 times the maximum recommended human daily inhalation dosage on a mg/m^2 basis for HFA aerosol) was unaffected by ipratropium administration. At an oral dose of 500 mg/kg (approximately 20,000 times the maximum recommended daily inhalation dose in adults on a mg/m^2 basis), ipratropium inhalation HFA aerosol formulation produced a decrease in the conception rate.

➤*Pregnancy: Category B.*

At oral doses of 90 mg/kg and above in rats in the aerosol HFA formulation (approximately 3,600 times the maximum recommended daily inhalation dose in adults on a mg/m^2 basis) embryotoxicity was observed as increased resorption. This effect is not considered relevant to human use due to the large doses at which it was observed and the difference in route of administration. There are, however, no adequate or well-controlled studies have been conducted in pregnant women. Because animal reproduction studies are not always predictive of human response, use ipratropium during pregnancy only if clearly needed.

➤*Lactation:* It is not known whether ipratropium inhalation solution or aerosol are excreted in human milk. Although lipid-soluble quaternary cations pass into breast milk, it is unlikely that the active component, ipratropium, would reach the infant to an important extent, especially when taken by inhalation. Ipratropium is not well absorbed systemically after inhalation or oral administration. However, because many drugs are excreted in human milk, exercise caution when ipratropium is administered to a breastfeeding woman.

➤*Children:*

HFA aerosol – Safety and efficacy in children have not been established.

Solution – Safety and efficacy in children younger than 12 years of age have not been established.

Precautions

➤*Special risk:* Use ipratropium with caution in patients with narrow-angle glaucoma, prostatic hyperplasia, or bladder-neck obstruction, particularly if they are receiving an anticholinergic by another route. Cases of precipitation or worsening of narrow-angle glaucoma and acute eye pain have been reported with direct eye contact of ipratropium administered by oral inhalation.

Drug Interactions

➤*Anticholinergic agents:* Although ipratropium is minimally absorbed into the systemic circulation, there is some potential for an additive interaction with concomitantly used anticholinergic medications. Caution is therefore advised in the coadministration of ipratropium inhalation with other anticholinergic-containing drugs.

Adverse Reactions

➤*HFA aerosol:*

Adverse Reactions Reported in ≥ 3% of Patients in any Ipratropium Bromide Group

	Placebo-controlled 12-week study 244.1405 and active-controlled 12-week study 244.1408			Active-controlled 1-year study 244.2453	
	Ipratropium HFA aerosol (n = 243)	Ipratropium CFC (n = 183)	Placebo (n = 128)	Ipratropium HFA aerosol (n = 305)	Ipratropium CFC (n = 151)
Adverse reaction	%	%	%	%	%
Total with any adverse reaction	63	68	72	91	87
CNS					
Dizziness	3	3	2	3	1
Headache	6	9	8	7	5
GI					
Dry mouth	4	2	2	2	3
Dyspepsia	1	3	1	5	3
Nausea	4	1	2	4	4
GU					
Urinary tract infection	2	3	1	10	8
Respiratory					
Bronchitis	10	11	6	23	19
COPD exacerbation	8	14	13	23	23
Coughing	3	4	6	5	5
Dyspnea	8	8	4	7	4
Rhinitis	4	2	4	6	2
Sinusitis	1	4	3	11	14
Upper respiratory tract infection	9	10	16	34	34
Miscellaneous					
Back pain	2	3	2	7	3
Influenza-like symptoms	4	2	2	8	5

Overall, in the above mentioned studies, 9.3% of the patients taking ipratropium 42 mcg HFA inhalation aerosol and 8.7% of the patients taking ipratropium 42 mcg inhalation aerosol CFC reported at least 1 adverse reaction that was considered by the investigator to be related to the study drug. The most common drug-related adverse reactions were dry mouth (1.6% of ipratropium HFA inhalation aerosol and 0.9% of ipratropium inhalation aerosol CFC patients) and taste perversion (bitter taste) (0.9% of ipratropium HFA inhalation aerosol and 0.3% of ipratropium inhalation aerosol CFC patients).

As an anticholinergic drug, cases of precipitation or worsening of narrow-angle glaucoma, mydriasis, acute eye pain, hypotension, urinary retention, tachycardia, constipation, and bronchospasm, including paradoxical bronchospasm, have been reported.

Allergic-type reactions such as skin rash; angioedema of tongue, lips, and face; urticaria (including giant urticaria); laryngospasm; and anaphylactic reaction have been reported.

Postmarketing experience –

HFA aerosol: Allergic-type reactions such as skin rash; angioedema of tongue, lips, and face; urticaria (including giant urticaria); laryngospasm; and anaphylactic reactions have been reported, with positive rechallenge in some cases. Many of the patients had a history of allergies to other drugs and/or foods, including soybean.

IPRATROPIUM BROMIDE — INHALATION

Additionally, urinary retention, mydriasis, and bronchospasm, including paradoxical bronchospasm, have been reported during the postmarketing period with use of ipratropium inhalation aerosol CFC.

➤*Solution:*

All Adverse Reactions from a Double-Blind, Parallel, 12-week Study of Patients With COPD[a]

Adverse reaction	Ipratropium (500 mcg 3 times daily) (n = 219)	Metaproterenol (15 mg 3 times daily) (n = 212)	Ipratropium/ Metaproterenol (500 mcg 3 times daily/ 15 mg 3 times daily) (n = 108)	Albuterol (2.5 mg 3 times daily) (n = 205)	Ipratropium/ Albuterol (500 mcg 3 times daily/ 2.5 mg 3 times daily) (n = 100)
Cardiovascular					
Chest pain	3.2%	4.2%	5.6%	2%	1%
Hypertension/ hypertension aggravated	0.9%	1.9%	0.9%	1.5%	4%
CNS					
Dizziness	2.3%	3.3%	1.9%	3.9%	4%
Headache	6.4%	5.2%	6.5%	6.3%	9%
Insomnia	0.9%	0.5%	4.6%	1%	1%
Nervousness	0.5%	4.7%	6.5%	1%	1%
Tremor	0.9%	7.1%	8.3%	1%	0%
GI					
Constipation	0.9%	0%	3.7%	1%	1%
Dry mouth	3.2%	0%	1.9%	2%	3%
Nausea	4.1%	3.8%	1.9%	2.9%	2%
Musculoskeletal					
Arthritis	0.9%	1.4%	0.9%	0.5%	3%
Respiratory					
Bronchitis	14.6%	24.5%	15.7%	16.6%	20%
Bronchospasm	2.3%	2.8%	4.6%	5.4%	5%
Coughing	4.6%	8%	6.5%	5.4%	6%
Dyspnea	9.6%	13.2%	16.7%	12.7%	9%
Pharyngitis	3.7%	4.2%	5.6%	2.9%	4%
Respiratory tract disorder	0%	6.1%	6.5%	2%	4%
Rhinitis	2.3%	4.2%	1.9%	2.4%	0%
Sinusitis	2.3%	2.8%	0.9%	5.4%	4%
Sputum increased	1.4%	1.4%	4.6%	3.4%	0%
Upper respiratory tract infection	13.2%	11.3%	9.3%	12.2%	16%
Miscellaneous					
Back pain	3.2%	1.9%	1.9%	2.4%	0%
Influenza-like symptoms	3.7%	4.7%	8.5%	0.5%	1%
Pain	4.1%	3.3%	0.9%	2.9%	5%

[a] All adverse reactions, regardless of drug relationship, reported by greater than or equal to 3% of patients in the 12-week controlled clinical trials.

Additional adverse reactions reported in less than 3% of the patients treated with ipratropium include tachycardia, palpitations, eye pain, urinary retention, urinary tract infection, and urticaria. Cases of precipitation or worsening of narrow-angle glaucoma and acute eye pain have been reported.

Lower respiratory tract adverse reactions (bronchitis, dyspnea, and bronchospasm) were the most common reactions leading to discontinuation of ipratropium therapy in the 12-week trials. Headache, mouth dryness, and aggravation of COPD symptoms are more common when the total daily dose of ipratropium equals or exceeds 2,000 mcg.

Hypersensitivity – Allergic-type reactions such as skin rash; angioedema of tongue, lips, and face; urticaria; laryngospasm; and anaphylactic reaction have been reported. Many of the patients had a history of allergies to other drugs and/or foods.

Overdosage

Acute overdose by inhalation is unlikely because ipratropium is not well absorbed systemically after inhalation or oral administration.

Patient Information

Advise patients that ipratropium inhalation is for the maintenance treatment of bronchospasm associated with COPD and is not indicated for the initial treatment of acute episodes of bronchospasm where rescue therapy is required for rapid response.

Do not use ipratropium inhalation more frequently than recommended. The dose or frequency of ipratropium inhalation aerosol should not be increased without patients consulting their doctors. If treatment with ipratropium inhalation aerosol becomes less effective for symptomatic relief, their symptoms become worse, and/or patients need to use the product more frequently than usual, seek medical attention immediately. Advise patients who are pregnant or breast-feeding to contact their doctors about the use of ipratropium inhalation. Appropriate use of ipratropium inhalation includes an understanding of the way it should be administered.

Instruct patients to avoid spraying ipratropium in or around the eyes. Caution patients to avoid spraying the aerosol into their eyes and advise them that this may result in precipitation or worsening of narrow-angle glaucoma, mydriasis, eye pain or discomfort, temporary blurring of vision, visual halos, or colored images in association with red eyes from conjunctival and corneal congestion. Advise patients that should any combination of these symptoms develop, they should consult their doctors immediately.

While taking ipratropium inhalation aerosol, other inhaled drugs should not be used unless prescribed.

Remind patients that ipratropium inhalation should be used consistently as prescribed throughout the course of therapy.

➤*HFA aerosol:* The action of ipratropium inhalation aerosol should last 2 to 4 hours. Advise patients that although the taste and inhalation sensation of ipratropium HFA inhalation aerosol may be slightly different from that of the CFC (chlorofluorocarbon) formulation of ipratropium inhalation aerosol, they are comparable in terms of safety and efficacy.

Do not shake the ipratropium HFA inhalation aerosol canister before using it.

"Prime" ipratropium HFA inhalation aerosol 2 times before taking the first dose from a new inhaler or when the inhaler has not been used for more than 3 days. To prime, push the canister against the mouthpiece, allowing the medicine to spray into the air. Avoid spraying the medicine into your eyes while priming ipratropium HFA inhalation aerosol.

Use ipratropium HFA inhalation aerosol exactly as prescribed by your doctor. Do not change your dose or how often you use ipratropium HFA inhalation aerosol without talking with your doctor. Talk to you doctor if you have questions about your medical condition or your treatment.

IPRATROPIUM BROMIDE — INTRANASAL

Indications

➤*Perennial rhinitis 0.03%:* For the symptomatic relief of rhinorrhea associated with allergic and nonallergic perennial rhinitis in adults and children 6 years of age and older. Ipratropium bromide nasal spray 0.03% does not relieve nasal congestion, sneezing, or postnasal drip associated with allergic or nonallergic perennial rhinitis.

➤*Common cold or seasonal allergic rhinitis 0.06%:* For the symptomatic relief of rhinorrhea associated with the common cold or seasonal allergic rhinitis for adults and children 5 years of age and older. Ipratropium bromide 0.06% nasal spray does not relieve nasal congestion or sneezing associated with the common cold or seasonal allergic rhinitis.

Administration and Dosage

➤*Approved by the FDA:* October 20, 1995.

Initial pump priming requires 7 sprays of the pump. If used regularly as recommended, no further priming is required. If not used for more than 24 hours, the pump will require 2 sprays, or if not used for more than 7 days, the pump will require 7 sprays to reprime.

➤*0.03%:* 2 sprays (42 mcg) per nostril 2 or 3 times daily (total dose 168 to 252 mcg/day) for the symptomatic relief of rhinorrhea associated with allergic and nonallergic perennial rhinitis in adults and children 6 years of age and older. Optimum dosage varies with the response of the individual patient.

➤*0.06%:*

For symptomatic relief of rhinorrhea associated with the common cold – 2 sprays (84 mcg) per nostril 3 or 4 times daily (total dose 504 to 672 mcg/day) in adults and children 12 years of age and older. Optimum dosage varies with the response of the individual patient. The recommended dose of ipratropium bromide 0.06% nasal spray for children age 5 to 11 years is 2 sprays (84 mcg) per nostril 3 times daily (total dose of 504 mcg/day).

The safety and effectiveness of the use of ipratropium bromide 0.06% nasal spray beyond 4 days in patients with the common cold have not been established.

For symptomatic relief of rhinorrhea associated with seasonal allergic rhinitis – 2 sprays (84 mcg) per nostril 4 times daily (total dose 672 mcg/day) in adults and children 5 years of age and older.

The safety and efficacy of the use of ipratropium bromide 0.06% nasal spray beyond 3 weeks in patients with seasonal allergic rhinitis have not been established.

➤*Storage/Stability:* Store tightly closed between 15° and 30°C (59° and 86°F). Avoid freezing. Keep out of reach of children. Do not spray in the eyes.

Actions

➤*Pharmacology:* Ipratropium bromide is an anticholinergic agent that inhibits vagally mediated reflexes by antagonizing the action of acetylcholine at the cholinergic receptor. In humans, ipratropium bromide has antisecretory properties and, when applied locally, inhibits secretions from the serous and seromucous glands lining the nasal mucosa. Ipratropium bromide is a quaternary amine that minimally crosses the nasal and GI membranes and the blood-brain barrier, resulting in a reduction of the systemic anticholinergic effects (eg, neurologic, ophthalmic, cardiovascular, GI effects) that are seen with tertiary anticholinergic amines.

➤*Pharmacokinetics:*

Absorption – Ipratropium bromide is poorly absorbed into the systemic circulation following oral administration (2% to 3%). Less than 20% of an 84 mcg per nostril dose was absorbed from the nasal mucosa of healthy volunteers, induced-cold adult volunteers, naturally acquired common cold pediatric patients, or perennial rhinitis adult patients.

Distribution – Ipratropium bromide is minimally bound (0% to 9% in vitro) to plasma albumin and alpha-1-acid glycoprotein. Its blood/plasma concentration ratio was estimated to be approximately 0.89. Studies in rats have shown that ipratropium bromide does not penetrate the blood-brain barrier.

Metabolism – Ipratropium bromide is partially metabolized to ester hydrolysis products, tropic acid, and tropane. These metabolites appear to be inactive based on in vitro receptor affinity studies using rat brain tissue homogenates.

Excretion – After IV administration of 2 mg ipratropium bromide to 10 healthy volunteers, the terminal half-life of ipratropium was approximately 1.6 hours. The total body clearance and renal clearance were estimated to be 2,505 and 1,019 mL/min, respectively. The amount of the total dose excreted unchanged in the urine (Ae) within 24 hours was approximately one-half of the administered dose.

Special populations –

Children:

• *0.03%* – Following administration of 42 mcg of ipratropium bromide 0.03% nasal spray per nostril 2 or 3 times a day in perennial rhinitis patients 6 to 18 years old, the mean amounts of the total dose excreted unchanged in the urine (8.6% to 11.1%) were higher than those reported in adult volunteers or adult perennial rhinitis patients (3.7% to 5.6%). Plasma ipratropium concentrations were relatively low (ranging from undetectable up to 0.49 ng/mL). No correlation of the amount of the total dose excreted unchanged in the urine (Ae) with age or gender was observed in the pediatric population.

• *0.06%* – Following administration of 84 mcg of ipratropium bromide per nostril 3 times a day in patients 5 to 18 years old (n = 42) with a naturally acquired common cold, the mean amount of the total dose excreted unchanged in the urine of 7.8% was comparable to 84 mcg per nostril 4 times a day in an adult induced common cold population (n = 22) of 7.3% to 8.1%. Plasma ipratropium concentrations were relatively low (ranging from undetectable up to 0.62 ng/mL). No correlation of the amount of the total dose excreted unchanged in the urine (Ae) with age or gender was observed in the pediatric population.

Contraindications

History of hypersensitivity to atropine or its derivatives, or to any of the other ingredients.

Warnings

➤*Hypersensitivity reactions:* Immediate hypersensitivity reactions may occur after administration of ipratropium bromide, as demonstrated by rare cases of urticaria, angioedema, rash, bronchospasm, and oropharyngeal edema.

➤*Fertility impairment:* Fertility of male or female rats was unaffected by ipratropium bromide at oral doses up to 50 mg/kg (approximately 1,600 times the maximum recommended daily intranasal dose in adults on a mg/m^2 basis). At an oral dose of 500 mg/kg (approximately 16,000 times the maximum recommended daily intranasal dose in adults on a mg/m^2 basis), ipratropium bromide produced a decrease in the conception rate.

➤*Pregnancy: Category B.* At oral doses greater than 90 mg/kg in rats (approximately 2,900 times for 0.03% ipratropium bromide and approximately 1,100 times for 0.06% ipratropium bromide the maximum recommended daily intranasal dose in adults on a mg/m^2 basis) embryotoxicity was observed as increased resorption. This effect is not considered relevant to human use due to the large doses at which it was observed and the difference in route of administration. However, no adequate or well-controlled studies have been conducted in pregnant women. Because animal reproduction studies are not always predictive of human response, ipratropium bromide nasal spray should be used during pregnancy only if clearly needed.

➤*Lactation:* It is known that some ipratropium bromide is systemically absorbed following nasal administration; however the portion that may be excreted in human milk is unknown. Although lipid-insoluble quaternary bases pass into breast milk, the minimal systemic absorption makes it unlikely that ipratropium bromide would reach the infant in an amount sufficient to cause a clinical effect. However, because many drugs are excreted in human milk, exercise caution when ipratropium bromide nasal spray is administered to a nursing woman.

➤*Children:*

0.03% – Safety and efficacy in patients younger than 6 years of age have not been established.

0.06% – Safety and efficacy in patients younger than 5 years of age have not been established.

Precautions

➤*Special risk:* Ipratropium bromide nasal spray should be used with caution in patients with narrow-angle glaucoma, prostatic hypertrophy, or bladder neck obstruction, particularly if they are receiving an anticholinergic by another route. Cases of precipitation or worsening of narrow-angle glaucoma and acute eye pain have been reported with direct eye contact of ipratropium bromide administered by oral inhalation.

Drug Interactions

No controlled clinical trials were conducted to investigate drug-drug interactions. Ipratropium bromide nasal spray is minimally absorbed into the systemic circulation; nonetheless, there is some potential for an additive interaction with other coadministered anticholinergic medications, including ipratropium bromide for oral inhalation.

Adverse Reactions

➤*0.03%:*

Percentage of Patients Reporting Events[a]				
	Ipratropium bromide nasal spray 0.03% (n = 356)		Vehicle control (n = 347)	
	Incidence (%)	Discontinued (%)	Incidence (%)	Discontinued (%)
Headache	9.8%	0.6%	9.2%	0%
Upper respiratory tract infection	9.8%	1.4%	7.2%	1.4%
Epistaxis[b]	9%	0.3%	4.6%	0.3%
Rhinitis[a]				
Nasal dryness	5.1%	0%	0.9%	0.3%
Nasal irritation[c]	2%	0%	1.7%	0.6%
Other nasal symptoms[d]	3.1%	1.1%	1.7%	0.3%

IPRATROPIUM BROMIDE — INTRANASAL

Percentage of Patients Reporting Events[a]				
	Ipratropium bromide nasal spray 0.03% (n = 356)		Vehicle control (n = 347)	
	Incidence (%)	Discontinued (%)	Incidence (%)	Discontinued (%)
Pharyngitis	8.1%	0.3%	4.6%	0%
Nausea	2.2%	0.3%	0.9%	0%

[a] This table includes adverse events that occurred at an incidence rate of at least 2% in the ipratropium bromide group and more frequently in the ipratropium bromide group than in the vehicle group.All events are listed by their WHO term; rhinitis has been presented by descriptive terms for clarification.
[b] Epistaxis reported by 7% of ipratropium bromide patients and 2.3% of vehicle patients, blood-tinged mucus by 2% of ipratropium bromide patients and 2.3% of vehicle patients.
[c] Nasal irritation includes reports of nasal itching, nasal burning, nasal irritation, and ulcerative rhinitis.
[d] Other nasal symptoms include reports of nasal congestion, increased rhinorrhea, increased rhinitis, posterior nasal drip, sneezing, nasal polyps, and nasal edema.

Ipratropium bromide 0.03% nasal spray was well tolerated by most patients. The most frequently reported nasal adverse events were transient episodes of nasal dryness or epistaxis. These adverse events were mild or moderate in nature, none was considered serious, none resulted in hospitalization and most resolved spontaneously or following a dose reduction. Treatment for nasal dryness and epistaxis was required infrequently (less than or equal to 2%) and consisted of local application of pressure or a moisturizing agent (eg, petroleum jelly, saline nasal spray). Patient discontinuation for epistaxis or nasal dryness was infrequent in both the controlled (less than or equal to 0.3%) and 1-year, open-label (less than or equal to 2%) trials. There was no evidence of nasal rebound (ie, a clinically significant increase in rhinorrhea, posterior nasal drip, sneezing, or nasal congestion severity compared to baseline) upon discontinuation of double-blind therapy in these trials.

Adverse events reported by less than 2% of the patients receiving ipratropium bromide nasal spray 0.03% during the controlled clinical trials or during the open-label follow-up trial, which are potentially related to ipratropium bromide's local effects or systemic anticholinergic effects include the following: Dry mouth/throat, dizziness, ocular irritation, blurred vision, conjunctivitis, hoarseness, cough, and taste perversion.

Additional anticholinergic effects noted with other ipratropium bromide dosage forms (ipratropium bromide inhalation solution, ipratropium bromide inhalation aerosol, and ipratropium bromide 0.06% nasal spray) include the following: Precipitation or worsening of narrow-angle glaucoma, urinary retention, prostatic disorders, tachycardia, constipation, and bowel obstruction.

There were infrequent reports of skin rash in both the controlled and uncontrolled clinical studies. Allergic-type reactions such as skin rash, angioedema of the throat, tongue, lips and face, generalized urticaria, laryngospasm, and anaphylactic reactions have been reported with ipratropium bromide 0.03% nasal spray and other ipratropium bromide products.

➤*0.06%:*

Percentage of Patients with Common Cold Reporting Events[a]		
	Ipratropium bromide 0.06% nasal spray	Vehicle control (n = 351)
Number of patients	352	351
Epistaxis[b]	8.2%	2.3%
Dry mouth/throat	1.4%	0.3%
Nasal congestion	1.1%	0%
Nasal dryness	4.8%	2.8%

[a] This table includes adverse events for which the incidence was greater than or equal to 1% in the ipratropium bromide group and higher in the ipratropium bromide group than in the vehicle group.
[b] Epistaxis was reported by 5.4% of ipratropium bromide patients and 1.4% of vehicle patients, blood-tinged nasal mucus by 2.8% of ipratropium bromide patients, and 0.9% of vehicle patients.

Ipratropium bromide 0.06% nasal spray was well tolerated by most patients. The most frequently reported adverse events were transient episodes of nasal dryness or epistaxis. The majority of these adverse events (96%) were mild or moderate in nature, none was considered serious, and none resulted in hospitalization. No patient required treatment for nasal dryness, and only 3 patients (less than 1%) required treatment for epistaxis, which consisted of local application of pressure or a moisturizing agent (eg, petroleum jelly). No patient receiving ipratropium bromide 0.06% nasal spray was discontinued from the trial due to either nasal dryness or bleeding.

Adverse events reported by less than 1% of patients receiving ipratropium bromide 0.06% nasal spray during the controlled clinical trials, which are potentially related to local effects or systemic anticholinergic effects of ipratropium bromide include taste perversion, nasal burning, conjunctivitis, coughing, dizziness, hoarseness, palpitation, pharyngitis, tachycardia, thirst, tinnitus, and blurred vision. No controlled trial was conducted to address the relative incidence of adverse events for 3-times-daily versus 4-times-daily therapy.

Percent of Patients with SAR Reporting Events[a]		
	Ipratropium bromide 0.06% nasal spray	Vehicle control
Number of patients	218	211
Epistaxis[b]	6%	3.3%
Pharyngitis	5%	3.8%
URI	5%	3.3%
Nasal dryness	4.6%	0.9%
Headache	4.1%	0.5%
Dry mouth/throat	4.1%	0%
Taste perversion	3.7%	1.4%
Sinusitis	2.8%	2.8%
Pain	1.8%	0.9%
Diarrhea	1.8%	0.5%

[a] This table includes adverse events for which the incidence was 1% or greater in the ipratropium bromide group and higher in the ipratropium bromide group than in the vehicle group.
[b] Epistaxis reported by 3.7% of ipratropium bromide and 2.4% of vehicle patients, blood-tinged nasal mucus by 2.3% of ipratropium bromide patients and 1.9% of vehicle patients.

Additional anticholinergic effects noted with other ipratropium bromide dosage forms (ipratropium bromide inhalation solution, ipratropium inhalation aerosol, and ipratropium bromide 0.03% nasal spray) include precipitation or worsening of narrow-angle glaucoma, urinary retention, prostate disorders, constipation, and bowel obstruction.

There were no reports of allergic-type reactions in the controlled clinical trials. Allergic-type reactions such as skin rash, angioedema of the throat, tongue, lips and face, generalized urticaria, laryngospasm, and anaphylactic reactions have been reported with ipratropium bromide 0.06% nasal spray and other ipratropium bromide products.

Overdosage

Acute overdosage by intranasal administration is unlikely since ipratropium bromide is not well absorbed systemically after intranasal or oral administration. Following administration of a 20 mg oral dose (equivalent to ingesting more than 4 bottles of ipratropium bromide 0.03% nasal spray or 2 bottles of ipratropium bromide 0.06% nasal spray) to 10 male volunteers, no change in heart rate or blood pressure was noted. Following a 2 mg IV infusion over 15 minutes to the same 10 male volunteers, plasma ipratropium concentrations of 22 to 45 ng/mL were observed (greater than 100 times the concentrations observed following intranasal administration). Following IV infusion these 10 volunteers had a mean increase of heart rate of 50 bpm and less than 20 mm Hg change in systolic or diastolic blood pressure at the time of peak ipratropium levels.

Patient Information

Advise patients that temporary blurring of vision, precipitation or worsening of narrow-angle glaucoma, or eye pain may result if ipratropium bromide nasal spray comes into direct contact with the eyes. Instruct patients to avoid spraying ipratropium bromide nasal spray in or around their eyes. Instruct patients who experience eye pain, to carefully read and follow the accompanying Patient's instructions for use.

TIOTROPIUM BROMIDE

Rx	**Spiriva** (Boehringer Ingelheim)	**Powder for inhalation:** 18 mcg (as base)	In blister packs containing 6 capsules with inhaler.

TIOTROPIUM BROMIDE — INHALATION

Indications

➤*Chronic obstructive pulmonary disease (COPD):* Long-term, once-daily, maintenance treatment of bronchospasm associated with COPD, including chronic bronchitis and emphysema.

Administration and Dosage

➤*Approved by the FDA:* January 30, 2004.

The recommended dosage of tiotropium bromide is the inhalation of the contents of 1 tiotropium bromide capsule, once-daily, with the tiotropium bromide inhalation device.

Tiotropium bromide capsules are for inhalation only and must not be swallowed.

➤*Storage/Stability:* Store at 25°C (77°F); excursions permitted to 15° to 30°C (59° to 86°F).

The capsules should not be exposed to extreme temperature or moisture. Do not store capsules in the tiotropium bromide inhalation device.

Actions

➤*Pharmacology:* Tiotropium is a long-acting, antimuscarinic agent, which is often referred to as an anticholinergic. It has similar affinity to the sub-

TIOTROPIUM BROMIDE — INHALATION

types of muscarinic receptors, M_1 to M_5. In the airways, it exhibits pharmacological effects through inhibition of M_3-receptors at the smooth muscle leading to bronchodilation. The competitive and reversible nature of antagonism was shown with human and animal origin receptors and isolated organ preparations. In preclinical in vitro as well as in vivo studies prevention of methacholine-induced bronchoconstriction effects were dose-dependent and lasted longer than 24 hours. The bronchodilation following inhalation of tiotropium is predominantly a site-specific effect.

➤*Pharmacokinetics:*

Absorption – Following dry powder inhalation by young healthy volunteers, the absolute bioavailability of 19.5% suggests that the fraction reaching the lung is highly bioavailable. It is expected from the chemical structure of the compound (quaternary ammonium compound) that tiotropium is poorly absorbed from the gastrointestinal tract. Food is not expected to influence the absorption of tiotropium for the same reason. Oral solutions of tiotropium have an absolute bioavailability of 2% to 3%. Maximum tiotropium plasma concentrations were observed 5 minutes after inhalation.

Distribution – Tiotropium shows a volume of distribution of 32 L/kg indicating that the drug binds extensively to tissues. The drug is bound by 72% to plasma proteins. At steady state, peak tiotropium plasma levels in COPD patients were 17 to 19 pg/mL when measured 5 minutes after dry powder inhalation of an 18 mcg dose and decreased rapidly in a multi-compartmental manner. Steady-state trough plasma concentrations were 3 to 4 pg/mL. Local concentrations in the lung are not known, but the mode of administration suggests substantially higher concentrations in the lung. Studies in rats have shown that tiotropium does not readily penetrate the blood-brain barrier.

Metabolism – The extent of biotransformation appears to be small. This is evident from a urinary excretion of 74% of unchanged substance after an intravenous dose to young healthy volunteers. Tiotropium, an ester, is nonenzymatically cleaved to the alcohol N-methylscopine and dithienylglycolic acid, neither of which bind to muscarinic receptors.

In vitro experiments with human liver microsomes and human hepatocytes suggest that a fraction of the administered dose (74% of an intravenous dose is excreted unchanged in the urine, leaving 25% for metabolism) is metabolized by cytochrome P450-dependent oxidation and subsequent glutathione conjugation to a variety of Phase II metabolites. This enzymatic pathway can be inhibited by P450 2D6 and 3A4 inhibitors, such as quinidine, ketoconazole, and gestodene. Thus, P450 2D6 and 3A4 are involved in the metabolic pathway that is responsible for the elimination of a small part of the administered dose. In vitro studies using human liver microsomes showed that tiotropium in supra-therapeutic concentrations does not inhibit P450 1A1, 1A2, 2B6, 2C9, 2C19, 2D6, 2E1, or 3A4.

Excretion – The terminal elimination half-life of tiotropium is between 5 and 6 days following inhalation. Total clearance was 880 mL/min after an intravenous dose in young healthy volunteers with an inter-individual variability of 22%. Intravenously administered tiotropium is mainly excreted unchanged in urine (74%). After dry powder inhalation, urinary excretion is 14% of the dose, the remainder being mainly nonabsorbed drug in the gut which is eliminated via the feces. The renal clearance of tiotropium exceeds the creatinine clearance, indicating active secretion into the urine. After chronic once-daily inhalation by COPD patients, pharmacokinetic steady state was reached after 2 to 3 weeks with no accumulation thereafter.

Special populations –

Renal function impairment: Since tiotropium is predominantly renally excreted, renal impairment was associated with increased plasma drug concentrations and reduced drug clearance after both intravenous infusion and dry powder inhalation. Mild renal impairment (Ccr 50 to 80 mL/min), which is often seen in elderly patients, increased tiotropium plasma concentrations (39% increase in AUC_{0-4} after intravenous infusion). In COPD patients with moderate to severe renal impairment (Ccr less than 50 mL/min), the intravenous administration of tiotropium resulted in doubling of the plasma concentrations (82% increase in AUC_{0-4}), which was confirmed by plasma concentrations after dry powder inhalation.

Elderly: As expected for drugs predominantly excreted renally, advanced age was associated with a decrease of tiotropium renal clearance (326 mL/min in COPD patients less than 58 years to 163 mL/min in COPD patients greater than 70 years), which may be explained by decreased renal function. Tiotropium excretion in urine after inhalation decreased from 14% (young healthy volunteers) to about 7% (COPD patients). Plasma concentrations were numerically increased with advancing age within COPD patients (43% increase in AUC_{0-4} after dry powder inhalation), which was not significant when considered in relation to inter- and intra-individual variability. Tiotropium is administered by dry powder inhalation. In common with other inhaled drugs, the majority of the delivered dose is deposited in the gastrointestinal tract and, to a lesser extent, in the lung, the intended organ. Many of the pharmacokinetic data described below were obtained with higher doses than recommended for therapy.

Contraindications

Hypersensitivity to atropine or its derivatives, including ipratropium, or to any component of this product.

Warnings

➤*QT interval prolongation:* In a multicenter, randomized, double-blind trial that enrolled 198 patients with COPD, the number of subjects with changes from baseline-corrected QT interval of 30 to 60 msec was higher in the tiotropium bromide group as compared with placebo. This difference was apparent using both the Bazett (QTcB) [20 (20%) patients vs 12 (12%) patients] and Fredericia (QTcF) [16 (16%) patients vs 1 (1%) patient] corrections of QT for heart rate. No patients in either group had either QTcB or QTcF of greater than 500 msec. Other clinical studies with tiotropium bromide did not detect an effect of the drug on QTc intervals.

➤*Acute bronchospasm:* Tiotropium bromide is intended as a once-daily maintenance treatment for COPD and is not indicated for the initial treatment of acute episodes of bronchospasm (ie, rescue therapy).

➤*Hypersensitivity reactions:* Immediate hypersensitivity reactions, including angioedema, may occur after administration of tiotropium bromide. If such a reaction occurs, therapy with tiotropium bromide should be stopped at once and alternative treatments should be considered.

Inhaled medicines, including tiotropium bromide, may cause paradoxical bronchospasm. If this occurs, treatment with tiotropium bromide should be stopped and other treatments considered.

➤*Renal function impairment:* As a predominantly renally excreted drug, patients with moderate to severe renal impairment (creatinine clearance of less than or equal to 50 mL/min) treated with tiotropium bromide should be monitored closely.

➤*Fertility impairment:* In rats, decreases in the number of corpora lutea and the percentage of implants were noted at inhalation tiotropium doses of 0.078 mg/kg/day or greater (approximately 35 times the RHDD on a mg/m^2 basis). No such effects were observed at 0.009 mg/kg/day (approximately 4 times than the RHDD on a mg/m^2 basis). The fertility index, however, was not affected at inhalation doses up to 1.689 mg/kg/day (approximately 760 times the RHDD on a mg/m^2 basis). These dose multiples may be overestimated due to difficulties in measuring deposited doses in animal inhalation studies.

➤*Elderly:* Of the total number of patients who received tiotropium bromide in the 1-year clinical trials, 426 were less than 65 years, 375 were 65 to 74 years and 105 were greater than or equal to 75 years of age. Within each age subgroup, there were no differences between the proportion of patients with adverse events in the tiotropium bromide and the comparator groups for most events. Dry mouth increased with age in the tiotropium bromide group (differences from placebo were 9%, 17.1%, and 16.2% in the aforementioned age subgroups). A higher frequency of constipation and urinary tract infections with increasing age was observed in the tiotropium bromide group in the placebo-controlled studies. The differences from placebo for constipation were 0%, 1.8%, and 7.8% for each of the age groups. The differences from placebo for urinary tract infections were −0.6%, 4.6% and 4.5%. No overall differences in effectiveness were observed among these groups. Based on available data, no adjustment of tiotropium bromide dosage in geriatric patients is warranted.

➤*Pregnancy: Category C.* In rats, fetal resorption, litter loss, decreases in the number of live pups at birth and the mean pup weights, and a delay in pup sexual maturation were observed at inhalation tiotropium doses of greater than or equal to 0.078 mg/kg (approximately 35 times the RHDD on a mg/m^2 basis). In rabbits, an increase in post-implantation loss was observed at an inhalation dose of 0.4 mg/kg/day (approximately 360 times the RHDD on a mg/m^2 basis). Such effects were not observed at inhalation doses of 0.009 and up to 0.088 mg/kg/day in rats and rabbits, respectively. These doses correspond to approximately 4 and 80 times the RHDD on a mg/m^2 basis, respectively. These dose multiples may be overestimated due to difficulties in measuring deposited doses in animal inhalation studies.

There are no adequate and well-controlled studies in pregnant women. Tiotropium bromide should be used during pregnancy only if the potential benefit justifies the potential risk to the fetus.

➤*Lactation:* Clinical data from nursing women exposed to tiotropium are not available. Based on lactating rodent studies, tiotropium is excreted into breast milk. It is not known whether tiotropium is excreted in human milk, but because many drugs are excreted in human milk and given these findings in rats, caution should be exercised if tiotropium bromide is administered to a nursing woman.

➤*Children:* Safety and efficacy in pediatric patients have not been established.

Precautions

➤*Special risk:* As an anticholinergic drug, tiotropium bromide may potentially worsen symptoms and signs associated with narrow-angle glaucoma, prostatic hyperplasia or bladder-neck obstruction and should be used with caution in patients with any of these conditions.

Drug Interactions

Tiotropium bromide has been used concomitantly with other drugs commonly used in COPD without increases in adverse drug reactions. These include sympathomimetic bronchodilators, methylxanthines, and oral and inhaled steroids. However, the coadministration of tiotropium bromide with other anticholinergic-containing drugs (eg, ipratropium) has not been studied and is therefore not recommended.

Adverse Reactions

The most commonly reported adverse drug reaction was dry mouth. Dry mouth was usually mild and often resolved during continued treatment. Other reactions reported in individual patients and consistent with possible anticholinergic effects included constipation, increased heart rate, blurred vision, glaucoma, urinary difficulty, and urinary retention.

Four multicenter, 1-year, controlled studies evaluated tiotropium bromide in patients with COPD. The table below shows all adverse events that occurred with a frequency of greater than or equal to 3% in the tiotropium bromide group in the 1-year placebo-controlled trials where the rates in the tiotropium bromide group exceeded placebo by greater than or equal to 1%. The frequency of corresponding events in the ipratropium-controlled trials is included for comparison.

TIOTROPIUM BROMIDE — INHALATION

Adverse experience incidence (% patients) in 1-year COPD clinical trials				
	Placebo-controlled trials		Ipratropium-controlled trials	
Body system (event)	Tiotropium bromide (n = 550)	Placebo (n = 371)	Tiotropium bromide (n = 356)	Ipratropium (n = 179)
Body as a whole				
Accidents	13%	11%	5%	8%
Chest pain (nonspecific)	7%	5%	5%	2%
Dependent edema	5%	4%	3%	5%
GI				
Abdominal pain	5%	3%	6%	6%
Constipation	4%	2%	1%	1%
Dry mouth	16%	3%	12%	6%
Dyspepsia	6%	5%	1%	1%
Vomiting	4%	2%	1%	2%
Musculoskeletal				
Myalgia	4%	3%	4%	3%
Resistance mechanism disorders				
Infection	4%	3%	1%	3%
Moniliasis	4%	2%	3%	2%
Respiratory system (upper)				
Epistaxis	4%	2%	1%	1%
Pharyngitis	9%	7%	7%	3%
Rhinitis	6%	5%	3%	2%
Sinusitis	11%	9%	3%	2%
Upper respiratory tract infection	41%	37%	43%	35%
Skin and appendage disorders				
Rash	4%	2%	2%	2%
Urinary system				
Urinary tract infection	7%	5%	4%	2%

Arthritis, coughing, and influenza-like symptoms occurred at a rate of greater than or equal to 3% in the tiotropium bromide treatment group, but were less than 1% in excess of the placebo group.

Other events that occurred in the tiotropium bromide group at a frequency of 1% to 3% in the placebo-controlled trials where the rates exceeded that in the placebo group include the following:

➤*Cardiovascular:* Angina pectoris (including aggravated angina pectoris).

➤*CNS:* Dysphonia and paresthesia.

➤*GI:* Gastrointestinal disorder not otherwise specified (NOS), gastroesophageal reflux, and stomatitis (including ulcerative stomatitis).

➤*Immunologic:* Herpes zoster.

➤*Metabolic/Nutritional:* Hypercholesterolemia and hyperglycemia.

➤*Musculoskeletal:* Skeletal pain.

➤*Psychiatric:* Depression.

➤*Respiratory:* Laryngitis.

➤*Special senses:* Cataract.

➤*Miscellaneous:* Allergic reaction and leg pain. In addition, among the adverse events observed in the clinical trials with an incidence of less than 1% were atrial fibrillation, supraventricular tachycardia, angioedema, and urinary retention.

In the 1-year trials, the incidence of dry mouth, constipation, and urinary tract infection increased with age.

Two multicenter, 6-month, controlled studies evaluated tiotropium bromide in patients with COPD. The adverse events and the incidence rates were similar to those seen in the 1-year controlled trials.

In addition to adverse events identified during clinical trials, the following adverse reactions have been reported in the worldwide postmarketing experience: Epistaxis, palpitations, pruritus, and urticaria.

Overdosage

➤*Symptoms:* High doses of tiotropium may lead to anticholinergic signs and symptoms. However, there were no systemic anticholinergic adverse effects following a single inhaled dose of up to 282 mcg tiotropium in 6 healthy volunteers. In a study of 12 healthy volunteers, bilateral conjunctivitis and dry mouth were seen following repeated once-daily inhalation of 141 mcg of tiotropium.

Acute intoxication by inadvertent oral ingestion of tiotropium bromide capsules is unlikely since it is not well absorbed systemically.

➤*Treatment:* A case of overdose has been reported from postmarketing experience. A female patient was reported to have inhaled 30 capsules over a 2.5 day period, and developed altered mental status, tremors, abdominal pain, and severe constipation. The patient was hospitalized, tiotropium bromide was discontinued, and the constipation was treated with an enema. The patient recovered and was discharged on the same day.

Patient Information

It is important for patients to understand how to correctly administer tiotropium bromide capsules using the tiotropium bromide inhalation device. Tiotropium bromide capsules should only be administered via the tiotropium bromide inhalation device and the tiotropium bromide inhalation device should not be used for administering other medications.

Capsules should always be stored in sealed blisters and only removed immediately before use. The blister strip should be carefully opened to expose only 1 capsule at a time. Open the blister foil as far as the stop line to remove only 1 capsule at a time. The drug should be used immediately after the packaging over an individual capsule is opened, or else its effectiveness may be reduced. Capsules that are inadvertently exposed to air (ie, not intended for immediate use) should be discarded.

Eye pain or discomfort, blurred vision, visual halos or colored images in association with red eyes from conjunctival congestion and corneal edema may be signs of acute narrow-angle glaucoma. Should any of these signs and symptoms develop, consult a physician immediately. Miotic eye drops alone are not considered to be effective treatment.

Care must be taken not to allow the powder to enter into the eyes as this may cause blurring of vision and pupil dilation.

Tiotropium bromide inhalation device is a once-daily maintenance bronchodilator and should not be used for immediate relief of breathing problems (ie, as a rescue medication).

IPRATROPIUM BROMIDE AND ALBUTEROL SULFATE

Rx	**Combivent** (Boehringer Ingelheim)	**Aerosol**: Each actuation delivers 18 mcg ipratropium bromide and 103 mcg albuterol sulfate (equiv. to 90 mcg albuterol base)	In 14.7 g metered dose inhaler w/mouthpiece (200 inhalations).
Rx	**DuoNeb** (Dey)	**Inhalation solution**: 0.5 mg ipratropium bromide and 3 mg albuterol sulfate (equiv. to 2.5 mg albuterol base)	In 3 mL unit-dose vials. In 30s and 60s.

IPRATROPIUM BROMIDE AND ALBUTEROL SULFATE — INHALATION

For complete and comparative prescribing information, refer to the individual Ipratropium Bromide and Albuterol monographs.

Indications

➤*Bronchospasm:* For use in patients with chronic obstructive pulmonary disease (COPD) on a regular aerosol bronchodilator who continue to have evidence of bronchospasm and require a second bronchodilator.

Administration and Dosage

➤*Approved by the FDA:* October 24, 1996.

➤*Combivent:* Shake well before using.

The recommended dose is 2 inhalations 4 times a day. Patients may take additional inhalations as required; however, advise the patient not to exceed 12 in 24 hours. It is recommended to "test spray" 3 times before using for the first time and in cases where the aerosol has not be used for more than 24 hours.

➤*DuoNeb:* The recommended dose is one 3 mL vial administered 4 times/day via nebulization with up to 2 additional 3 mL doses allowed per day, if needed. Administer via jet nebulizer connected to an air compressor with an adequate air flow, equipped with mouthpiece or suitable face mask.

The use of these agents can be continued as medically indicated to control recurring bouts of bronchospasm. If a previously effective regimen fails to provide the usual relief, medical advice should be sought immediately, as this is often a sign of worsening COPD, which would require reassessment of therapy.

➤*Storage/Stability:* Store *Combivent* between 15° and 30°C (59° and 86°F). Avoid excessive humidity. For optimal results, the canister should be at room temperature before use. Store *DuoNeb* between 2° and 25°C (36° and 77°F). Protect from light.

ZAFIRLUKAST

Rx	**Accolate** (AstraZeneca)	**Tablets:** 10 mg	Lactose, povidone. (ACCOLATE 10 ZENECA). White. Film-coated. In 60s and UD 100s.
		20 mg	Lactose, povidone. (ACCOLATE 20 ZENECA). White. Film-coated. In 60s and UD 100s.

ZAFIRLUKAST — ORAL

Indications

➤*Asthma:* Prophylaxis and chronic treatment of asthma in adults and children 5 years of age and older.

➤*Unlabeled uses:* Treatment of chronic urticaria.

Administration and Dosage

➤*Approved by the FDA:* September 26, 1996.

Because food can reduce the bioavailability of zafirlukast, take at least 1 hour before or 2 hours after meals.

➤*Adults and children 12 years of age and older:* The recommended dose is 20 mg twice daily.

➤*Pediatric patients 5 through 11 years of age:* The recommended dose is 10 mg twice daily.

➤*Hepatic function impairment:* The clearance of zafirlukast is reduced in patients with stable alcoholic cirrhosis such that the C_{max} and AUC are approximately 50% to 60% greater than those of healthy adults. Zafirlukast has not been evaluated in patients with hepatitis or in long-term studies of patients with cirrhosis.

➤*Storage/Stability:* Store at controlled room temperature, 20° to 25°C (68° to 77°F). Protect from light and moisture. Dispense in the original airtight container.

Actions

➤*Pharmacology:* Zafirlukast is a selective and competitive receptor antagonist of leukotriene D_4 and E_4 (LTD_4 and LTE_4), components of slow-reacting substance of anaphylaxis (SRSA). Cysteinyl leukotriene production and receptor occupation have been correlated with the pathophysiology of asthma, including airway edema, smooth muscle constriction, and altered cellular activity associated with the inflammatory process, which contribute to the signs and symptoms of asthma. Patients with asthma were found in 1 study to be 25 to 100 times more sensitive to the bronchoconstricting activity of inhaled LTD_4 than nonasthmatic subjects.

In vitro studies demonstrated that zafirlukast antagonized the contractile activity of 3 leukotrienes (LTC_4, LTD_4, and LTE_4) in conducting airway smooth muscle from laboratory animals and humans. Zafirlukast prevented intradermal LTD_4-induced increases in cutaneous vascular permeability and inhibited inhaled LTD_4-induced influx of eosinophils into animal lungs. Inhalational challenge studies in sensitized sheep showed that zafirlukast suppressed the airway responses to antigen; this included both the early- and late-phase response and the nonspecific hyperresponsiveness.

In humans, zafirlukast inhibited bronchoconstriction caused by several kinds of inhalational challenges. Pretreatment with single oral doses of zafirlukast inhibited the bronchoconstriction caused by sulfur dioxide and cold air in patients with asthma. Pretreatment with single doses of zafirlukast attenuated the early- and late-phase reaction caused by inhalation of various antigens such as grass, cat dander, ragweed, and mixed antigens in patients with asthma. Zafirlukast also attenuated the increase in bronchial hyperresponsiveness to inhaled histamine that followed inhaled allergen challenge.

➤*Pharmacokinetics:*

Absorption – Zafirlukast is rapidly absorbed following oral administration. Peak plasma concentrations are generally achieved 3 hours after oral administration. The absolute bioavailability of zafirlukast is unknown. In 2 separate studies, 1 using a high-fat and the other a high-protein meal, administration of zafirlukast with food reduced the mean bioavailability by approximately 40%.

Distribution – Zafirlukast is more than 99% bound to plasma proteins, predominantly albumin. The degree of binding was independent of concentration in the clinically relevant range. The apparent steady-state volume of distribution (Vss/F) is approximately 70 L, suggesting moderate distribution into tissues. Studies in rats using radiolabeled zafirlukast indicate minimal distribution across the blood-brain barrier.

Metabolism – Zafirlukast is extensively metabolized. The most common metabolic products are hydroxylated metabolites, which are excreted in the feces. The metabolites of zafirlukast identified in plasma are at least 90 times less potent as LTD_4 receptor antagonists than zafirlukast in a standard in vitro test of activity. In vitro studies using human liver microsomes showed that the hydroxylated metabolites of zafirlukast excreted in the feces are formed through the cytochrome P450 2C9 (CYP2C9) pathway. Additional in vitro studies utilizing human liver microsomes show that zafirlukast inhibits the cytochrome P450 CYP3A4 and CYP2C9 isoenzymes at concentrations close to the clinically achieved total plasma concentrations.

Excretion – The apparent oral clearance (CL/f) of zafirlukast is approximately 20 L/h. Studies in the rat and dog suggest that biliary excretion is the primary route of excretion. Following oral administration of radiolabeled zafirlukast to volunteers, urinary excretion accounts for approximately 10% of the dose and the remainder is excreted in feces. Zafirlukast is not detected in urine.

In the pivotal bioequivalence study, the mean terminal half-life of zafirlukast is approximately 10 hours in both healthy adult subjects and patients with asthma. In other studies, the mean plasma half-life of zafirlukast ranged from approximately 8 to 16 hours in both healthy subjects and patients with asthma. The pharmacokinetics of zafirlukast are approximately linear over the range from 5 to 80 mg. Steady-state plasma concentrations of zafirlukast are proportional to the dose and predictable from single-dose pharmacokinetic data. Accumulation of zafirlukast in the plasma following twice-daily dosing is approximately 45%.

Special populations –

Hepatic function impairment: In a study of patients with hepatic impairment (biopsy-proven cirrhosis), there was a reduced clearance of zafirlukast resulting in a 50% to 60% greater C_{max} and AUC compared with healthy subjects.

Elderly: The apparent oral clearance of zafirlukast decreases with age. In patients older than 65 years of age, there is an approximately 2- to 3-fold greater C_{max} and AUC compared with young adult patients.

Children: Following administration of 20 mg zafirlukast to 20 boys and girls between 7 and 11 years of age, and in a second study, to 29 boys and girls between 5 and 6 years of age, the following pharmacokinetic parameters were obtained:

Parameter	Children 5 to 6 years of age Mean (% coefficient of variation)	Children 7 to 11 years of age Mean (% coefficient of variation)
C_{max} (ng/mL)	756 (39%)	601 (45%)
AUC (ng•h/mL)	2,458 (34%)	2,027 (38%)
T_{max} (h)	2.1 (61%)	2.5 (55%)
CL/f (L/h)	9.2 (37%)	11.4 (42%)

Weight unadjusted apparent clearance was 11.4 L/h (42%) in the 7- to 11-year-old children and 9.2 L/h (37%) in the 5- to 6-year-old children, which resulted in greater systemic drug exposures than that obtained in adults for an identical dose. To maintain similar exposure levels in children compared with adults, a dose of 10 mg twice daily is recommended in children 5 to 11 years of age.

Pharmacokinetic parameters –

Mean (% Coefficient of Variation) Pharmacokinetic Parameters of Zafirlukast Following Single 20 mg Oral Dose Administration to Male Volunteers (n = 36)				
C_{max} (ng/mL)	T_{max}[a] (h)	AUC (ng•h/mL)	$t_{½}$ (h)	CL/f (L/h)
326 (31)	2 (0.5 to 5)	1,137 (34)	13.3 (75.6)	19.4 (32)

[a] Median and range.

Contraindications

Hypersensitivity to zafirlukast or any of its inactive ingredients.

Warnings

➤*Acute asthma attacks:* Zafirlukast is not indicated for use in the reversal of bronchospasm in acute asthma attacks, including status asthmaticus. Therapy with zafirlukast can be continued during acute exacerbations of asthma.

➤*Hepatic function impairment:*

See Pharmacokinetics for more information.

➤*Carcinogenesis:* In 2-year carcinogenicity studies, zafirlukast was administered at dietary doses of 10, 100, and 300 mg/kg to mice and 40, 400, and 2,000 mg/kg to rats. Male mice given 300 mg/kg/day (approximately 30 times the maximum recommended daily oral dosage in adults and in children [on a mg/m^2 basis] showed an increased incidence of hepatocellular adenomas; female mice at this dose showed a greater incidence of whole body histocytic sarcomas. Male and female rats given a dietary dose of 2,000 mg/kg/day (approximately 160 times the exposure to drug plus metabolites from the maximum recommended daily oral dosage in adults and in children based on a comparison of the plasma AUC values) of zafirlukast showed an increased incidence of urinary bladder transitional cell papillomas.

The clinical significance of these findings for the long-term use of zafirlukast is unknown.

➤*Elderly:* See Actions for more information.

A total of 8,094 patients were exposed to zafirlukast in North American and European short-term placebo-controlled clinical trials. Of these, 243 patients were elderly (65 years of age and older). No overall difference in adverse reactions was seen in the elderly patients, except for an increase in the frequency of infections among zafirlukast-treated elderly patients compared with placebo-treated elderly patients (7% vs 2.9%). The infections

ZAFIRLUKAST — ORAL

were not severe, occurred mostly in the lower respiratory tract, and did not necessitate withdrawal of therapy.

An open-label, uncontrolled, 4-week trial of 3,759 asthma patients compared the safety and efficacy of 20 mg zafirlukast given twice daily in 3 patient age groups, adolescents (12 to 17 years of age), adults (18 to 65 years of age), and elderly (older than 65 years of age). A higher percentage of elderly patients (n = 384) reported adverse reactions when compared with adults and adolescents. These elderly patients showed less improvement in efficacy measures. In the elderly patients, adverse reactions occurring in greater than 1% of the population included headache (4.7%), diarrhea and nausea (1.8%), and pharyngitis (1.3%). The elderly reported the lowest percentage of infections of all 3 age groups in this study.

➤*Pregnancy: Category B.* At an oral dosage of 2,000 mg/kg/day (approximately 410 times the maximum recommended daily oral dose in adults [on a mg/m^2 basis]) in rats, maternal toxicity and deaths were seen with increased incidence of early fetal resorption. Spontaneous abortions occurred in cynomolgus monkeys at a maternally toxic oral dosage of 2,000 mg/kg/day. There are no adequate and well-controlled trials in pregnant women. Because animal reproduction studies are not always predictive of human response, use zafirlukast during pregnancy only if clearly needed.

➤*Lactation:* Zafirlukast is excreted in breast milk. Following repeated 40 mg twice-a-day dosing in healthy women, average steady-state concentrations of zafirlukast in breast milk were 50 ng/mL compared with 255 ng/mL in plasma. Because of the potential for tumorigenicity shown for zafirlukast in mouse and rat studies and the enhanced sensitivity of neonatal rats and dogs to the adverse effects of zafirlukast, do not administer zafirlukast to mothers who are breastfeeding.

Precautions

➤*Hepatic effects:* Cases of life-threatening hepatic failure have been reported in patients treated with zafirlukast. Cases of liver injury without other attributable cause have been reported from postmarketing adverse reaction surveillance of patients who have received the recommended dosage of zafirlukast (40 mg/day). In most, but not all postmarketing reports, the patient's symptoms abated and the liver enzymes returned to normal or near normal after stopping zafirlukast. In rare cases, patients have either presented with fulminant hepatitis or progressed to hepatic failure, liver transplantation, and death.

Consider the value of liver function testing. Periodic serum transaminase testing has not proven to prevent serious injury but it is generally believed that early detection of drug-induced hepatic injury along with immediate withdrawal of the suspect drug enhances the likelihood for recovery.

Advise patients to be alert for signs and symptoms of liver dysfunction (eg, right upper quadrant abdominal pain, nausea, fatigue, lethargy, pruritus, jaundice, flu-like symptoms, anorexia) and to contact their health care provider immediately if they occur, Ongoing clinical assessment of patients should govern health care provider interventions, including diagnostic evaluations and treatment.

If liver dysfunction is suspected based upon clinical signs or symptoms (eg, right upper quadrant abdominal pain, nausea, fatigue, lethargy, pruritus, jaundice, and flu-like symptoms, anorexia, enlarged liver), discontinue zafirlukast. Liver function tests, in particular serum ALT, should be measured immediately and the patient managed accordingly. If liver function tests are consistent with hepatic dysfunction, do not resume zafirlukast therapy. Patients in whom zafirlukast was withdrawn because of hepatic dysfunction where no other attributable cause is identified should not be re-exposed to zafirlukast.

➤ *Eosinophilic conditions:* In rare cases, patients on zafirlukast therapy may present with systemic eosinophilia, sometimes presenting with clinical features of vasculitis consistent with Churg-Strauss syndrome, a condition that is often treated with systemic steroid therapy. These events usually, but not always, have been associated with the reduction of oral steroid therapy. Be alert to eosinophilia, vasculitic rash, worsening pulmonary symptoms, cardiac complications, or neuropathy presenting in their patients. A causal association between zafirlukast and these underlying conditions has not been established.

Drug Interactions

Because of zafirlukast's inhibition of cytochrome P450 2C9 and 3A4 isoenzymes, use caution with coadministration of drugs known to be metabolized by these isoenzymes.

Zafirlukast Drug Interactions

Precipitant drug	Object drug*		Description
Aspirin	Zafirlukast	↑	Coadministration of zafirlukast with aspirin results in mean increased plasma levels of zafirlukast by ≈ 45%.
Erythromycin	Zafirlukast	↓	Coadministration of a single dose of zafirlukast with erythromycin to steady state results in decreased mean plasma levels of zafirlukast by ≈ 40% because of decreased zafirlukast bioavailability.
Theophylline	Zafirlukast	↓	Coadministration of zafirlukast at steady state with a single dose of a liquid theophylline preparation results in decreased mean plasma levels of zafirlukast by ≈ 30%, but no effects on plasma theophylline levels were observed.
Zafirlukast	Warfarin	↑	Coadministration of zafirlukast with warfarin results in a clinically significant increase in prothrombin time (PT). Closely monitor PT and adjust anticoagulant dose accordingly.

* ↑ = Object drug increased. ↓ = Object drug decreased.

➤*Warfarin:* In a drug interaction study in 16 healthy male volunteers, coadministration of multiple doses of zafirlukast (160 mg/day) to steady state with a single 25 mg dose of warfarin resulted in a significant increase in the mean AUC (+63%) and half-life (+36%) of S-warfarin. The mean PT increased by approximately 35%. This interaction is probably due to an inhibition by zafirlukast of the cytochrome P450 2C9 isoenzyme system. Patients on oral warfarin anticoagulant therapy and zafirlukast should have their prothrombin times monitored closely and anticoagulant dose adjusted accordingly.

➤*Theophylline:* Rare cases of patients experiencing increased theophylline levels with or without clinical signs or symptoms of theophylline toxicity after the addition of zafirlukast to an existing theophylline regimen have been reported. The mechanism of the interaction between zafirlukast and theophylline in these patients is unknown.

Adverse Reactions

➤*Adults and children 12 years of age and older:* A comparison of adverse reactions reported by greater than or equal to 1% of zafirlukast-treated patients, and at rates numerically greater than in placebo-treated patients, is shown for all trials in the following table.

Adverse Reaction	Zafirlukast (n = 4,058)	Placebo (n = 2,032)
Abdominal pain	1.8%	1.1%
Accidental injury	1.6%	1.5%
ALT elevation	1.5%	1.1%
Asthenia	1.8%	1.6%
Back pain	1.5%	1.2%
Diarrhea	2.8%	2.1%
Dizziness	1.6%	1.5%
Dyspepsia	1.3%	1.2%
Fever	1.6%	1.1%
Headache	12.9%	11.7%
Infection	3.5%	3.4%
Myalgia	1.6%	1.5%
Nausea	3.1%	2%
Pain (generalized)	1.9%	1.7%
Vomiting	1.5%	1.1%

The frequency of less common adverse reactions was comparable between zafirlukast and placebo.

➤*Miscellaneous:* Rarely, elevations of 1 or more liver enzymes have occurred in patients receiving zafirlukast in controlled clinical trials. In clinical trials, most of these have been observed in asymptomatic patients at doses 4 times higher than the recommended dose. The following hepatic events (which have occurred predominantly in females) have been reported from postmarketing adverse reaction surveillance of patients who have received the recommended dose of zafirlukast (40 mg/day): cases of symptomatic hepatitis (with or without hyperbilirubinemia) without other attributable cause; and rarely, hyperbilirubinemia without other elevated liver function tests. In most, but not all postmarketing reports, the patient's symptoms abated and the liver enzymes returned to normal or near normal after stopping zafirlukast. In rare cases, patients have presented with fulminant hepatitis or progressed to hepatic failure, liver transplantation, and death.

In clinical trials, an increased proportion of zafirlukast patients older than 55 years of age reported infections as compared with placebo-treated patients. A similar finding was not observed in other age groups studied. These infections were mostly mild or moderate in intensity and predominantly affected the respiratory tract. Infections occurred equally in both sexes, were dose-proportional to total milligrams of zafirlukast exposure, and were associated with coadministration of inhaled corticosteroids. The clinical significance of this finding is unknown.

See Precautions for more information.

Hypersensitivity reactions, including urticaria, angioedema, and rashes, with or without blistering, have been reported in association with zafirlukast therapy. Additionally, there have been reports of patients experiencing agranulocytosis, bleeding, bruising, or edema, arthralgia, and myalgia in association with zafirlukast therapy.

➤*Pediatric patients 5 through 11 years of age:* In pediatric patients receiving zafirlukast in multidose clinical trials, the following reactions occurred with a frequency of greater than or equal to 2% and more frequently than in pediatric patients who received placebo, regardless of causality assessment: headache (4.5% vs 4.2%) and abdominal pain (2.8% vs 2.3%).

Overdosage

➤*Symptoms:* Overdosage with zafirlukast has been reported in 4 patients surviving reported doses as high as 200 mg. The predominant symptoms reported following zafirlukast overdose were rash and upset stomach. There

ZAFIRLUKAST — ORAL

were no acute toxic effects in humans that could be consistently ascribed to the administration of zafirlukast.

➤*Treatment:* It is reasonable to employ the usual supportive measures in the event of an overdose (eg, remove unabsorbed material from the GI, employ clinical monitoring, and institute supportive therapy) if required.

Patient Information

Zafirlukast is indicated for the chronic treatment of asthma; regularly as prescribed, even during symptom-free periods. Zafirlukast is not a bronchodilator; do not use to treat acute episodes of asthma. Do not decrease the dose or stop taking any other antiasthma medications unless instructed by your doctor. Women who are breastfeeding should not take zafirlukast. Alternative antiasthma medication should be considered in such patients.

The bioavailability of zafirlukast may be decreased when taken with food. Take zafirlukast at least 1 hour before or 2 hours after meals.

A rare side effect of zafirlukast is hepatic dysfunction; contact your doctor immediately if you experience signs or symptoms of hepatic dysfunction (eg, right upper quadrant abdominal pain, nausea, fatigue, lethargy, pruritus, jaundice, flu-like symptoms, anorexia). Liver failure resulting in liver transplantation and death has occurred in patients taking zafirlukast.

MONTELUKAST SODIUM

Rx	**Singulair** (Merck)	**Tablets:** 10 mg (as base)	Lactose. (MRK 117 SINGULAIR). Beige, rounded square. Film coated. In unit-of-use 30s and 90s and UD 100s.
		Tablets, chewable: 4 mg (as base)	Mannitol, aspartame, 0.674 mg phenylalanine. (MRK 711 SINGULAIR). Pink, oval. Cherry flavor. In unit-of-use 30s and 90s and UD 100s.
		5 mg (as base)	Mannitol, aspartame, 0.842 mg phenylalanine. (MRK 275 SINGULAIR). Pink. Cherry flavor. In unit-of-use 30s and 90s and UD 100s.
		Granules: 4 mg (as base)/packet	Mannitol. In 30 packets.

MONTELUKAST SODIUM — ORAL

Indications

➤*Asthma:* Prophylaxis and chronic treatment of asthma in adults and children 12 months of age and older.

➤*Allergic rhinitis:* Relief of symptoms of allergic rhinitis (seasonal allergic rhinitis in adults and children 2 years of age and older), and perennial allergic rhinitis in adults and children 6 months of age and older.

➤*Unlabeled uses:* Chronic urticaria, atopic dermatitis.

Administration and Dosage

➤*Approved by the FDA:* February 20, 1998.

Montelukast should be taken once daily. For asthma, the dose should be taken in the evening. For allergic rhinitis, the time of administration may be individualized to suit patient needs.

Patients with both asthma and allergic rhinitis should take only 1 tablet daily in the evening.

➤*Adults and adolescents 15 years of age and older:* One 10 mg tablet daily.

➤*Children 6 to 14 years of age:* One 5 mg chewable tablet daily. No dosage adjustment within this age group is necessary.

➤*Children 2 to 5 years of age:* One 4 mg chewable tablet or 1 packet of 4 mg oral granules daily.

➤*Children 12 to 23 months of age with asthma:* 1 packet of 4 mg oral granules daily to be taken in the evening.

➤*Children 6 to 23 months of age with perennial allergic rhinitis:* 1 packet of 4 mg oral granules daily.

➤*Administration of oral granules:* Montelukast 4 mg oral granules can be administered either directly in the mouth, dissolved in 1 teaspoonful (5 mL) of cold or room temperature baby formula or breast milk, or mixed with a spoonful of cold or room temperature soft foods; based on stability studies, only applesauce, carrots, rice, or ice cream should be used. The packet should not be opened until ready to use. After opening the packet, the full dose (with or without mixing with baby formula, breast milk, or food) must be administered within 15 minutes. If mixed with baby formula, breast milk, or food, montelukast oral granules must not be stored for future use. Discard any unused portion. Montelukast oral granules are not intended to be dissolved in any liquid other than baby formula or breast milk for administration. However, liquids may be taken subsequent to administration. Montelukast oral granules can be administered without regard to time of meals.

➤*Storage/Stability:* Store at 25°C (77°F); excursions permitted to 15° to 30°C (59° to 86°F). Protect from moisture and light. Store in original package. When bulk bottle product container is subdivided, repackage into a well-closed, light-resistant container.

Actions

➤*Pharmacology:* The cysteinyl leukotrienes (LTC_4, LTD_4, LTE_4) are products of arachidonic acid metabolism and are released from various cells, including mast cells and eosinophils. These eicosanoids bind to CysLT receptors. The CysLT type-1 ($CysLT_1$) receptor is found in the human airway (including airway smooth muscle cells and airway macrophages) and on other proinflammatory cells (including eosinophils and certain myeloid stem cells). CysLTs have been correlated with the pathophysiology of asthma and allergic rhinitis.

Asthma – In asthma, leukotriene-mediated effects include airway edema, smooth muscle contraction, and altered cellular activity associated with the inflammatory process.

Allergic rhinitis – In allergic rhinitis, CysLTs are released from the nasal mucosa after allergen exposure during both early- and late-phase reactions and are associated with symptoms of allergic rhinitis. Intranasal challenge with CysLTs has been shown to increase nasal airway resistance and symptoms of nasal obstruction. Montelukast has not been assessed in intranasal challenge studies. The clinical relevance of intranasal challenge studies is unknown.

Montelukast is an orally active compound that binds with high affinity and selectivity to the $CysLT_1$ receptor (in preference to other pharmacologically important airway receptors, such as the prostanoid, cholinergic, or β-adrenergic receptor). Montelukast inhibits physiologic actions of LTD_4 at the $CysLT_1$ receptor without any agonist activity.

➤*Pharmacokinetics:*

Absorption – Montelukast is absorbed rapidly following oral administration. After administration of the 10 mg film-coated tablet to fasted adults, the mean peak montelukast plasma concentration (C_{max}) is achieved in 3 to 4 hours (T_{max}). The mean oral bioavailability is 64%. The oral bioavailability and C_{max} are not influenced by a standard meal in the morning.

For the 5 mg chewable tablet, the mean C_{max} is achieved in 2 to 2.5 hours after administration to adults in the fasted state. The mean oral bioavailability is 73% in the fasted state versus 63% when administered with a standard meal in the morning.

For the 4 mg chewable tablet, the mean C_{max} is achieved 2 hours after administration in children 2 to 5 years of age in the fasted state.

The 4 mg oral granule formulation is bioequivalent to the 4 mg chewable tablet when administered to adults in the fasted state. The coadministration of the oral granule formulation with applesauce did not have a clinically significant effect on the pharmacokinetics of montelukast. A high-fat meal in the morning did not affect the area under the curve (AUC) of montelukast oral granules; however, the meal decreased C_{max} by 35% and prolonged T_{max} from 2.3 ± 1 hours to 6.4 ± 2.9 hours.

Distribution – Montelukast is more than 99% bound to plasma proteins. The steady-state volume of distribution of montelukast averages 8 to 11 L. Studies in rats with radiolabeled montelukast indicate minimal distribution across the blood-brain barrier. In addition, concentrations of radiolabeled material at 24 hours postdose were minimal in all other tissues.

Metabolism – Montelukast is metabolized extensively. In studies with therapeutic doses, plasma concentrations of metabolites of montelukast are undetectable at steady state in adults and children.

In vitro studies using human liver microsomes indicate that cytochromes P-450 3A4 and 2C9 are involved in the metabolism of montelukast. Clinical studies investigating the effect of known inhibitors of cytochromes P-450 3A4 (eg, erythromycin, ketoconazole) or 2C9 (eg, fluconazole) on montelukast pharmacokinetics have not been conducted. Based on further in vitro results in human liver microsomes, therapeutic plasma concentrations of montelukast do not inhibit cytochromes P-450 3A4, 2C9, 1A2, 2A6, 2C19, or 2D6. However, in vitro studies have shown that montelukast is a potent inhibitor of cytochrome P-450 2C8.

Excretion – The plasma clearance of montelukast averages 45 mL/min in healthy adults. Following an oral dose of radiolabeled montelukast, 86% of the radioactivity was recovered in 5-day fecal collections, and less than 0.2% was recovered in urine. Coupled with estimates of montelukast oral bioavailability, this indicates that montelukast and its metabolites are excreted almost exclusively via the bile.

In several studies, the mean plasma half-life of montelukast ranged from 2.7 to 5.5 hours in healthy young adults. The pharmacokinetics of montelukast are nearly linear for oral doses up to 50 mg. During once-daily dosing with montelukast 10 mg, there is little accumulation of the parent drug in plasma (14%).

Special populations –

Hepatic function impairment: Patients with mild to moderate hepatic function impairment and clinical evidence of cirrhosis had evidence of decreased metabolism of montelukast resulting in 41% (90% confidence interval [CI], 7%, 85%) higher mean montelukast AUC following a single 10 mg dose. The elimination of montelukast was slightly prolonged compared with that in healthy subjects (mean half-life, 7.4 hours). No dosage adjustment is required in patients with mild to moderate hepatic function impairment. The pharmacokinetics of montelukast in patients with more severe hepatic function impairment or with hepatitis have not been evaluated.

Elderly: The pharmacokinetic profile and the oral bioavailability of a single 10 mg oral dose of montelukast are similar in elderly and younger adults. The plasma half-life of montelukast is slightly longer in the elderly. No dosage adjustment in the elderly is required.

Children: In children 6 to 11 months of age, the systemic exposure to montelukast and the variability of plasma montelukast concentrations were higher than those observed in adults. Based on population analyses, the mean

MONTELUKAST SODIUM — ORAL

AUC (4,296 ng•h/mL [range, 1,200 to 7,153]) was 60% higher, and the mean C_{max} (667 ng/mL [range, 201 to 1,058]) was 89% higher than those observed in adults (mean AUC, 2,689 ng•h/mL [range, 1,521 to 4,595]); mean C_{max} (353 ng/mL [range, 180 to 548]). The systemic exposure in children 12 to 23 months of age was less variable, but it was still higher than that observed in adults. The mean AUC (3,574 ng•h/mL [range, 2,229 to 5,408]) was 33% higher, and the mean C_{max} (562 ng/mL [range, 296 to 814]) was 60% higher than those observed in adults. Safety and tolerability of montelukast in a single-dose pharmacokinetic study in 26 children 6 to 23 months of age were similar to that of patients 2 years of age and older. Use the 4 mg oral granule formulation for children 12 to 23 months of age for the treatment of asthma, or for children 6 to 23 months of age for the treatment of perennial allergic rhinitis. Because the 4 mg oral granule formulation is bioequivalent to the 4 mg chewable tablet, it can also be used as an alternative formulation to the 4 mg chewable tablet in children 2 to 5 years of age.

Contraindications

Hypersensitivity to any component of this product.

Warnings

➤*Acute asthma attacks:* Montelukast is not indicated for use in the reversal of bronchospasm in acute asthma attacks, including status asthmaticus.

Advise patients to have appropriate rescue medication available. Therapy with montelukast can be continued during acute exacerbations of asthma.

➤*Fertility impairment:* In fertility studies in female rats, montelukast produced reductions in fertility and fecundity indices at an oral dose of 200 mg/kg (estimated exposure was approximately 70 times the AUC for adults at the maximum recommended daily oral dose).

➤*Pregnancy: Category B.* Montelukast crosses the placenta following oral dosing in rats and rabbits. There are, however, no adequate and well-controlled studies in pregnant women. Because animal reproduction studies are not always predictive of human response, use montelukast during pregnancy only if clearly needed.

The manufacturer maintains a registry to monitor the pregnancy outcomes of women exposed to montelukast while pregnant. Health care providers are encouraged to report any prenatal exposure by calling the pregnancy registry at 1-800- 986-8999.

➤*Lactation:* Studies in rats have shown that montelukast is excreted in milk. It is not known if montelukast is excreted in human milk. Because many drugs are excreted in human milk, exercise caution when montelukast is given to a breast-feeding mother.

➤*Children:* Safety and efficacy of montelukast have been established in adequate and well-controlled studies in children with asthma 6 to 14 years of age. Safety and efficacy profiles in this age group are similar to those seen in adults.

The safety and efficacy in children younger than 12 months of age with asthma and 6 months with perennial allergic rhinitis have not been established. Long-term trials evaluating the effect of chronic administration of montelukast on linear growth in children have not been conducted.

Precautions

➤*Exercise-induced bronchoconstriction:* Do not use montelukast as monotherapy for the treatment and management of exercise-induced bronchospasm. Patients who have exacerbations of asthma after exercise should continue to use their usual regimen of inhaled beta-agonists as prophylaxis and have available for rescue a short-acting inhaled beta-agonist.

➤*Concurrent corticosteroids:* While the dose of inhaled corticosteroid may be reduced gradually under medical supervision, do not abruptly substitute montelukast for inhaled or oral corticosteroids.

➤*Aspirin sensitivity:* Patients with known aspirin sensitivity should continue avoidance of aspirin or NSAIDs while taking montelukast. Although montelukast is effective in improving airway function in asthmatic patients with documented aspirin sensitivity, it has not been shown to truncate bronchoconstrictor response to aspirin and other NSAIDs in aspirin-sensitive asthmatic patients.

➤*Eosinophilia:* In rare cases, patients with asthma on therapy with montelukast may present with systemic eosinophilia, sometimes presenting with clinical features of vasculitis consistent with Churg Strauss syndrome, a condition that is often treated with systemic corticosteroid therapy. These events usually, but not always, have been associated with the reduction of oral corticosteroid therapy. Be alert to the presentation of eosinophilia, vasculitic rash, worsening pulmonary symptoms, cardiac complications, and/or neuropathy in patients. A causal association between montelukast and these underlying conditions has not been established.

➤*Phenylketonurics:* Inform phenylketonuric patients that the 4 and 5 mg chewable tablets contain phenylalanine (a component of aspartame) 0.674 and 0.842 mg, respectively.

Drug Interactions

Montelukast Drug Interactions

Precipitant drug	Object drug[a]		Description
Phenobarbital	Montelukast	⬇	Montelukast plasma concentrations may be reduced, decreasing the pharmacologic effect.
Montelukast	Prednisone	⬆	Adverse effects of prednisone (eg, edema) may be increased.

[a] ⬆ = Object drug increased. ⬇ = Object drug decreased.

Adverse Reactions

➤*Asthma:*

Adults and adolescents 15 years of age and older –

Montelukast Adverse Reactions Occurring in ≥ 1% of Patients

	Montelukast 10 mg/day (n = 1,955)	Placebo (n = 1,180)
CNS		
Asthenia/ fatigue	1.8%	1.2%
Dizziness	1.9%	1.4%
Headache	18.4%	18.1%
Dermatologic		
Rash	1.6%	1.2%
GI		
Abdominal pain	2.9%	2.5%
Dyspepsia	2.1%	1.1%
Gastroenteritis, infectious	1.5%	0.5%
Pain, dental	1.7%	1%
Laboratory test abnormalities[a]		
ALT increased	2.1%	2%
AST increased	1.6%	1.2%
Pyuria	1%	0.9%
Respiratory		
Congestion, nasal	1.6%	1.3%
Cough	2.7%	2.4%
Miscellaneous		
Fever	1.5%	0.9%
Influenza	4.2%	3.9%
Trauma	1%	0.8%

[a] Number of patients tested (montelukast and placebo, respectively): ALT and AST, 1,935, 1,170; pyuria, 1,924, 1,159.

➤*Children 6 to 14 years of age with asthma:* In children 6 to 14 years of age receiving montelukast, the following reactions occurred with a frequency greater than or equal to 2% and more frequently than in children who received placebo, regardless of causality assessment:

GI – Diarrhea, dyspepsia, nausea.

Respiratory – Laryngitis, pharyngitis, sinusitis.

Special senses – Otitis.

Miscellaneous – Fever, influenza, viral infection.

➤*Children 2 to 5 years of age with asthma:* In children 2 to 5 years of age receiving montelukast, the following reactions occurred with a frequency greater than or equal to 2% and more frequently than in children who received placebo, regardless of causality assessment:

CNS – Headache.

Dermatologic – Dermatitis, eczema, rash, urticaria, varicella.

GI – Abdominal pain, diarrhea, gastroenteritis.

Respiratory – Cough, pneumonia, rhinorrhea, sinusitis.

Special senses – Conjunctivitis, ear pain, otitis.

Miscellaneous – Fever, influenza.

➤*Children 6 to 23 months of age with asthma:* In children 6 to 23 months of age receiving montelukast, the following reactions occurred with a frequency of greater than or equal to 2% and more frequently than in children who received placebo, regardless of causality assessment:

Respiratory – Cough, pharyngitis, rhinitis, tonsillitis, upper respiratory tract infection, wheezing.

Special senses – Otitis media.

➤*Adults and adolescents 15 years of age and older with seasonal allergic rhinitis:* Montelukast has been evaluated for safety in 2,199 adult and adolescent patients 15 years of age and older in clinical trials. Montelukast administered once daily in the morning or in the evening was generally well tolerated with a safety profile similar to that of placebo. In placebo-controlled clinical trials, the following event was reported with montelukast with a frequency greater than or equal to 1% and at an incidence greater than placebo, regardless of causality assessment: upper respiratory tract infection (1.9% of patients receiving montelukast versus 1.5% of patients receiving placebo). In a 4-week placebo-controlled clinical study, the safety profile was consistent with that observed in 2-week studies. The incidence of somnolence was similar to that of placebo in all studies.

➤*Children 2 to 14 years of age with seasonal allergic rhinitis:* Montelukast has been evaluated in 280 children 2 to 14 years of age in a 2-week multicenter, double-blind, placebo-controlled, parallel-group safety study. Montelukast administered once daily in the evening was generally well tolerated with a safety profile similar to that of placebo. In this study, the following events occurred with a frequency of 2% or more and at an incidence greater than placebo, regardless of causality assessment:

MONTELUKAST SODIUM — ORAL

CNS – Headache.

Respiratory – Pharyngitis, upper respiratory tract infection.

Special senses – Otitis media.

➤*Adults and adolescents 15 years of age and older with perennial allergic rhinitis:* Montelukast has been evaluated for safety in 3,357 adult and adolescent patients 15 years of age and older with perennial allergic rhinitis, of whom 1,632 received montelukast in two 6-week clinical studies. Montelukast administered once daily was generally well tolerated, with a safety profile consistent with that observed in patients with seasonal allergic rhinitis and similar to that of placebo. In these 2 studies, the following events were reported with montelukast with a frequency of 1% or more and at an incidence greater than placebo, regardless of causality assessment:

CNS – Somnolence (incidence was similar to that of placebo).

Lab test abnormalities – Increased ALT.

Respiratory – Cough, epistaxis, sinus headache, sinusitis, upper respiratory tract infection.

➤*Children 6 months to 14 years of age with perennial allergic rhinitis:* The safety in patients 2 to 14 years of age with perennial allergic rhinitis is supported by the established safety in patients 2 to 14 years of age with seasonal allergic rhinitis. The safety in patients 6 to 23 months of age is supported by data from pharmacokinetic and safety and efficacy studies in asthma in this pediatric population and from adult pharmacokinetic studies.

➤*Postmarketing:*

Cardiovascular – Palpitations.

CNS – Agitation (including aggressive behavior), dream abnormalities, drowsiness, hallucinations, hypesthesia, insomnia, irritability, paresthesia, restlessness; seizures (very rarely).

GI – Diarrhea, dyspepsia, nausea, vomiting; pancreatitis (very rarely).

Hematologic – Increased bleeding tendency.

In rare cases, patients with asthma on therapy with montelukast may present with systemic eosinophilia, sometimes presenting with clinical features of vasculitis consistent with Churg-Strauss syndrome, a condition that is often treated with systemic corticosteroid therapy. These events usually, but not always, have been associated with the reduction of oral corticosteroid therapy. Be alert to the presentation of eosinophilia, vasculitic rash, worsening pulmonary symptoms, cardiac complications, and/or neuropathy in patients. A causal association between montelukast and these underlying conditions has not been established.

Hepatic – Rare cases of cholestatic hepatitis, hepatocellular liver injury, and mixed-pattern liver injury have been reported in patients treated with montelukast. Most of these occurred in combination with other confounding factors, such as use of other medications, or when montelukast was administered to patients who had underlying potential for liver disease such as alcohol use or other forms of hepatitis.

Hypersensitivity – Hypersensitivity reactions (including anaphylaxis, angioedema, pruritus, urticaria, and, very rarely, hepatic eosinophilic infiltration).

Musculoskeletal – Arthralgia, myalgia (including muscle cramps).

Miscellaneous – Bruising, edema.

Overdosage

➤*Symptoms:* No mortality occurred following single oral doses of montelukast up to 5,000 mg/kg in mice (estimated exposure was approximately 335 and 210 times the AUC for adults and children, respectively, at the maximum recommended daily oral dose) and rats (estimated exposure was approximately 230 and 145 times the AUC for adults and children, respectively, at the maximum recommended daily oral dose).

➤*Treatment:* No specific information is available on the treatment of overdosage with montelukast. In chronic asthma studies, montelukast has been administered at dosages up to 200 mg/day to adult patients for 22 weeks and, in short-term studies, up to 900 mg/day to patients for approximately a week without clinically important adverse experiences. In the event of overdose, it is reasonable to employ the usual supportive measures (eg, remove unabsorbed material from the GI tract, employ clinical monitoring, institute supportive therapy, if required).

There have been reports of acute overdosage with montelukast in children in postmarketing experience and clinical studies of up to at least 150 mg/day. The clinical and laboratory findings observed were consistent with the safety profile in adults and older children. There were no adverse experiences reported in the majority of overdosage reports. The most frequent adverse experiences observed were thirst, somnolence, mydriasis, hyperkinesia, and abdominal pain.

It is not known whether montelukast is removed by peritoneal dialysis or hemodialysis.

Patient Information

Advise patients to take montelukast daily as prescribed, even when they are asymptomatic, as well as during periods of worsening asthma, and to contact their health care provider if their asthma is not well controlled.

Advise patients that oral montelukast is not for the treatment of acute asthma attacks. They should have appropriate short-acting inhaled beta-agonist medication available to treat asthma exacerbations.

Advise patients that, while using montelukast, medical attention should be sought if short-acting inhaled bronchodilators are needed more often than usual, or if more than the maximum number of inhalations of short-acting bronchodilator treatment prescribed for a 24-hour period are needed.

Instruct patients receiving montelukast not to decrease the dose or stop taking any other asthma medications unless instructed by a health care provider.

Instruct patients who have exacerbations of asthma after exercise to continue to use their usual regimen of inhaled beta-agonists as prophylaxis unless otherwise instructed by their health care provider. All patients should have available for rescue a short-acting inhaled beta agonist.

Advise patients with known aspirin sensitivity to continue avoidance of aspirin or NSAIDs while taking montelukast.

➤*Chewable tablets:*

Phenylketonurics – Inform phenylketonuric patients that the 4 and 5 mg chewable tablets contain phenylalanine (a component of aspartame) 0.674 and 0.842 mg, respectively.

LEUKOTRIENE FORMATION INHIBITORS

ZILEUTON

Rx	**Zyflo** (Abbott)	**Tablets:** 600 mg	(ZL 600). White. Oval. Film coated. In 120s.

ZILEUTON — ORAL

Indications

Prophylaxis and chronic treatment of asthma in adults and children at least 12 years of age.

Administration and Dosage

➤*Approved by the FDA:* December 9, 1996.

The recommended dosage of zileuton for the symptomatic treatment of patients with asthma is one 600 mg tablet 4 times a day for a total daily dose of 2400 mg. For ease of administration, zileuton may be taken with meals and at bedtime.

Hepatic transaminases should be evaluated prior to initiation of zileuton and periodically during treatment.

➤*Storage/Stability:* Store tablets at controlled room temperature between 20° to 25°C (68° to 77°F). Protect from light.

Actions

➤*Pharmacology:* Zileuton is a specific inhibitor of 5-lipoxygenase and thus inhibits leukotriene (LTB_4, LTC_4, LTD_4, and LTE_4) formation. Both the R(+) and S(−) enantiomers are pharmacologically active as 5-lipoxygenase inhibitors in in vitro systems. Leukotrienes are substances that induce numerous biological effects including augmentation of neutrophil and eosinophil migration, neutrophil and monocyte aggregation, leukocyte adhesion, increased capillary permeability, and smooth muscle contraction. These effects contribute to inflammation, edema, mucus secretion, and bronchoconstriction in the airways of asthmatic patients. Sulfido-peptide leukotrienes (LTC_4, LTD_4, LTE_4, also known as the slow-releasing substances of anaphylaxis) and LTB_4, a chemo-attractant for neutrophils and eosinophils, can be measured in a number of biological fluids including bronchoalveolar lavage fluid (BALF) from asthmatic patients.

➤*Pharmacokinetics:*

Absorption – Zileuton is rapidly absorbed upon oral administration with a mean time to peak plasma concentration (t_{max}) of 1.7 hours and a mean peak level (C_{max}) of 4.98 mcg/mL. The absolute bioavailability of zileuton is unknown. Systemic exposure (mean AUC) following 600 mg zileuton administration is 19.2 mcg•hr/mL. Plasma concentrations of zileuton are proportional to dose, and steady-state levels are predictable from single-dose pharmacokinetic data. Administration of zileuton with food resulted in a small but statistically significant increase (27%) in zileuton C_{max} without significant changes in the extent of absorption (AUC) or t_{max}. Therefore, zileuton can be administered with or without food.

Distribution – The apparent volume of distribution (V/F) of zileuton is approximately 1.2 L/kg. Zileuton is 93% bound to plasma proteins, primarily to albumin, with minor binding to α1-acid glycoprotein.

Metabolism/Excretion – Elimination of zileuton is predominantly via metabolism with a mean terminal half-life of 2.5 hours. Apparent oral clearance of zileuton is 7 mL/min/kg. Zileuton activity is primarily due to the parent drug. Studies with radiolabeled drug demonstrated that orally administered zileuton is well absorbed into the systemic circulation with 94.5% and 2.2% of the radiolabeled dose recovered in urine and feces, respectively. Several zileuton metabolites have been identified in human plasma and urine. These include 2 diastereomeric O-glucuronide conjugates (major metabolites) and an N-dehydroxylated metabolite of zileuton. The urinary excretion of the inactive N-dehydroxylated metabolite and unchanged zileuton each accounted for less than 0.5% of the dose. In vitro studies utilizing human liver microsomes have shown that zileuton and its N-dehydroxylated metabolite can be oxidatively metabolized by the cytochrome P450 isoenzymes 1A2, 2C9 and 3A4 (CYP1A2, CYP2C9 and CYP3A4).

Special populations –

Hepatic function impairment: Zileuton is contraindicated in patients with active liver disease.

ZILEUTON — ORAL

Contraindications

Active liver disease or transaminase elevations at least 3 times the upper limit of normal (at least 3 × ULN); hypersensitivity to zileuton or any of its inactive ingredients.

Warnings

➤*Acute asthma attacks:* Zileuton is not indicated for use in the reversal of bronchospasm in acute asthma attacks, including status asthmaticus. Therapy with zileuton can be continued during acute exacerbations of asthma.

➤*Hepatic function impairment:* Zileuton is contraindicated in patients with active liver disease.

Since treatment with zileuton may result in increased hepatic transaminases, zileuton should be used with caution in patients who consume substantial quantities of alcohol or have a history of liver disease.

➤*Carcinogenesis:* In 2-year carcinogenicity studies, increases in the incidence of liver, kidney, and vascular tumors in female mice and a trend towards an increase in the incidence of liver tumors in male mice were observed at 450 mg/kg/day (providing approximately 4 times [females] or 7 times [males] the systemic exposure [AUC] achieved at the maximum recommended human daily oral dose).

In rats, an increase in the incidence of kidney tumors was observed in both sexes at 170 mg/kg/day (providing approximately 6 times [males] or 14 times [females] the systemic exposure [AUC] achieved at the maximum recommended human daily oral dose).

Although a dose-related increased incidence of benign Leydig cell tumors was observed, Leydig cell tumori-genesis was prevented by supplementing male rats with testosterone.

➤*Mutagenesis:* A dose-related increase in DNA adduct formation was reported in kidneys and livers of female mice treated with zileuton. Although some evidence of DNA damage was observed in a UDS assay in hepatocytes isolated from Aroclor-1254 treated rats, no such finding was noticed in hepatocytes isolated from monkeys, where the metabolic profile of zileuton is more similar to that of humans.

➤*Fertility impairment:* In reproductive performance/fertility studies, zileuton produced no effects on fertility in rats at oral doses up to 300 mg/kg/day (providing approximately 8 times [male rats] and 18 times [female rats] the systemic exposure [AUC] achieved at the maximum recommended human daily oral dose). Comparative systemic exposure (AUC) is based on measurements in male rats or nonpregnant female rats at similar dosages. However, reduction in fetal implants was observed at oral doses of 150 mg/kg/day and higher (providing approximately 9 times the systemic exposure [AUC] achieved at the maximum recommended human daily oral dose). Increases in gestation length, prolongation of estrous cycle, and increases in stillbirths were observed at oral doses of 70 mg/kg/day and higher (providing approximately 4 times the systemic exposure [AUC] achieved at the maximum recommended human daily oral dose). In a perinatal/postnatal study in rats, reduced pup survival and growth were noted at an oral dose of 300 mg/kg/day (providing approximately 18 times the systemic exposure [AUC] achieved at the maximum recommended human daily oral dose).

➤*Pregnancy: Category C.* Developmental studies indicated adverse effects (reduced body weight and increased skeletal variations) in rats at an oral dose of 300 mg/kg/day (providing approximately 18 times the systemic exposure [AUC] achieved at the maximum recommended human daily oral dose). Comparative systemic exposure [AUC] is based on measurements in nonpregnant female rats at a similar dosage. Zileuton or its metabolites cross the placental barrier of rats. Three of 118 (2.5%) rabbit fetuses had cleft palates at an oral dose of 150 mg/kg/day (equivalent to the maximum recommended human daily oral dose on a mg/m^2 basis). There are no adequate and well-controlled studies in pregnant women. Zileuton should be used during pregnancy only if the potential benefit justifies the potential risk to the fetus.

➤*Lactation:* Zileuton and its metabolites are excreted in rat milk. It is not known if zileuton is excreted in human milk. Because many drugs are excreted in human milk, and because of the potential for tumorigenicity shown for zileuton in animal studies, a decision should be made whether to discontinue nursing or to discontinue the drug, taking into account the importance of the drug to the mother.

➤*Children:* The safety and effectiveness of zileuton in pediatric patients younger than 12 years of age have not been established.

Precautions

➤*Monitoring:* It is recommended that hepatic transaminases be evaluated at initiation of, and during therapy with, zileuton. Serum ALT should be monitored before treatment begins, once-a-month for the first 3 months, every 2 to 3 months for the remainder of the first year, and periodically thereafter for patients receiving long-term zileuton therapy. If clinical signs or symptoms of liver dysfunction (eg, right upper quadrant pain, nausea, fatigue, lethargy, pruritus, jaundice, or "flu-like" symptoms) develop or transaminase elevations greater than 5 times the ULN occur, zileuton should be discontinued and transaminase levels followed until normal.

➤*Hepatic effects:* Elevations of 1 or more liver function tests may occur during zileuton therapy. These laboratory abnormalities may progress, remain unchanged, or resolve with continued therapy. In a few cases, initial transaminase elevations were first noted after discontinuing treatment, usually within 2 weeks. The ALT test is considered the most sensitive indicator of liver injury. In placebo-controlled clinical trials, the frequency of ALT elevations greater than or equal to 3 times the upper limit of normal (3 × ULN) was 1.9% for zileuton-treated patients, compared with 0.2% for placebo-treated patients.

In a long-term safety surveillance study, 2458 patients received zileuton in addition to their usual asthma care and 489 received their usual asthma care. In patients treated for up to 12 months with zileuton in addition to their usual asthma care, 4.6% developed an ALT of at least 3 × ULN, compared with 1.1% of patients receiving only their usual asthma care. Sixty-one percent of these elevations occurred during the first 2 months of zileuton therapy. After 2 months of treatment, the rate of new ALT elevations greater than or equal to 3 × ULN stabilized at a mean of 0.3% per month for patients receiving zileuton-plus-usual-asthma care compared with 0.11% per month for patients receiving usual asthma care alone. Of the 61 zileuton-plus-usual-asthma-care patients with ALT elevations between 3 to 5 × ULN, 32 patients (52%) had ALT values decrease to below 2 × ULN while continuing zileuton therapy. Twenty-one of the 61 patients (34%) had further increases in ALT levels to greater than or equal to 5 × ULN and were withdrawn from the study in accordance with the study protocol. In patients who discontinued zileuton, elevated ALT levels returned to less than 2 × ULN in an average of 32 days (range, 1 to 111 days).

In controlled and uncontrolled clinical trials involving greater than 5000 patients treated with zileuton, the overall rate of ALT elevation greater than or equal to 3 × ULN was 3.2%. In these trials, 1 patient developed symptomatic hepatitis with jaundice, which resolved upon discontinuation of therapy. An additional 3 patients with transaminase elevations developed mild hyperbilirubinemia that was less than 3 times the upper limit of normal. There was no evidence of hypersensitivity or other alternative etiologies for these findings. In subset analyses, females over the age of 65 appeared to be at an increased risk for ALT elevations. Patients with preexisting transaminase elevations may also be at an increased risk for ALT elevations.

Since treatment with zileuton may result in increased hepatic transaminases, zileuton should be used with caution in patients who consume substantial quantities of alcohol or have a history of liver disease.

➤*Lab test abnormalities:* Elevations of 1 or more liver function tests may occur during zileuton therapy. These laboratory abnormalities may progress, remain unchanged, or resolve with continued therapy. In a few cases, initial transaminase elevations were first noted after discontinuing treatment, usually within 2 weeks. The ALT test is considered the most sensitive indicator of liver injury.

Drug Interactions

➤*Theophylline:* In a drug-interaction study in 16 healthy volunteers, coadministration of multiple doses of zileuton (800 mg every 12 hours) and theophylline (200 mg every 6 hours) for 5 days resulted in a significant decrease (approximately 50%) in steady-state clearance of theophylline, an approximate doubling of theophylline AUC, and an increase in theophylline C_{max} (by 73%). The elimination half-life of theophylline was increased by 24%. Also, during coadministration, theophylline-related adverse events were observed more frequently than after theophylline alone. Upon initiation of zileuton in patients receiving theophylline, the theophylline dosage should be reduced by approximately one-half and plasma theophylline concentrations monitored. Similarly, when initiating therapy with theophylline in a patient receiving zileuton, the maintenance dose or dosing interval of theophylline should be adjusted accordingly and guided by serum theophylline determinations.

➤*Warfarin:* Concomitant administration of multiple doses of zileuton (600 mg every 6 hours) and warfarin (fixed daily dose obtained by titration in each subject) to 30 healthy male volunteers resulted in a 15% decrease in R-warfarin clearance and an increase in AUC of 22%. The pharmacokinetics of S-warfarin were not affected. These pharmacokinetic changes were accompanied by a clinically significant increase in prothrombin times. Monitoring of prothrombin time, or other suitable coagulation tests, with the appropriate dose titration of warfarin is recommended in patients receiving concomitant zileuton and warfarin therapy.

➤*Propranolol:* Coadministration of zileuton and propranolol results in a significant increase in propranolol concentrations. Administration of a single 80 mg dose of propranolol in 16 healthy male volunteers who received zileuton 600 mg every 6 hours for 5 days resulted in a 42% decrease in propranolol clearance. This resulted in an increase in propranolol C_{max}, AUC, and elimination half-life by 52%, 104%, and 25% respectively. There was an increase in β-blockade and decrease in heart rate associated with the coadministration of these drugs. Patients on zileuton and propranolol should be closely monitored and the dose of propranolol reduced as necessary. No formal drug-drug interaction studies between zileuton and other beta-adrenergic blocking agents (ie, β-blockers) have been conducted. It is reasonable to employ appropriate clinical monitoring when these drugs are coadministered with zileuton.

➤*Terfenadine:* In a drug interaction study in 16 healthy volunteers, coadministration of multiple doses of terfenadine (60 mg every 12 hours) and zileuton (600 mg every 6 hours) for 7 days resulted in a decrease in clearance of terfenadine by 22% leading to a statistically significant increase in mean AUC and C_{max} of terfenadine of approximately 35%. This increase in terfenadine plasma concentration in the presence of zileuton was not associated with a significant prolongation of the QTc interval. Although there was no cardiac effect in this small number of healthy volunteers, given the high inter-individual pharmacokinetic variability of terfenadine, coadministration of zileuton and terfenadine is not recommended.

ZILEUTON — ORAL

Adverse Reactions

Proportion of patients experiencing adverse reactions in placebo-controlled studies in asthma		
Body system/reaction	Zileuton 600 mg 4 times daily Percent (%) occurrence (n = 475)	Placebo Percent (%) occurrence (n = 491)
Miscellaneous		
Headache	24.6%	24%
Pain (unspecified)	7.8%	5.3%
Abdominal pain	4.6%	2.4%
Asthenia	3.8%	2.4%
Accidental injury	3.4%	2%
GI		
Dyspepsia	8.2%[a]	2.9%
Nausea	5.5%	3.7%
Musculoskeletal		
Myalgia	3.2%	2.9%

[a] $P \leq 0.05$ vs placebo.

➤*Less common adverse reactions:* Less common adverse reactions occurring at a frequency of greater than 1% and more commonly in zileuton-treated patients included: Arthralgia, chest pain, conjunctivitis, constipation, dizziness, fever, flatulence, hypertonia, insomnia, lymphadenopathy, malaise, neck pain/rigidity, nervousness, pruritus, somnolence, urinary tract infection, vaginitis, and vomiting.

➤*Frequency of discontinuation due to adverse reactions:* The frequency of discontinuation from the asthma clinical studies due to any adverse reaction was comparable between zileuton (9.7%) and placebo-treated (8.4%) groups.

In placebo-controlled clinical trials, the frequency of ALT elevations greater than or equal to 3 × ULN was 1.9% for zileuton-treated patients, compared with 0.2% for placebo-treated patients. In controlled and uncontrolled trials, 1 patient developed symptomatic hepatitis with jaundice, which resolved upon discontinuation of therapy. An additional 3 patients with transaminase elevations developed mild hyperbilirubinemia that was less than 3 times the upper limit of normal. There was no evidence of hypersensitivity or other alternative etiologies for these findings. Zileuton is contraindicated in patients with active liver disease or transaminase elevations greater than or equal to 3 × ULN. It is recommended that hepatic transaminases be evaluated at initiation of and during therapy with zileuton.

Occurrences of low white blood cell count (less than or equal to 2.8×10^9/L) were observed in 1% of 1678 patients taking zileuton and 0.6% of 1056 patients taking placebo in placebo-controlled studies. These findings were transient and the majority of cases returned toward normal or baseline with continued zileuton dosing. All remaining cases returned toward normal or baseline after discontinuation of zileuton. Similar findings were also noted in a long-term safety surveillance study of 2458 patients treated with zileuton plus usual asthma care versus 489 patients treated only with usual asthma care for up to 1 year. The clinical significance of these observations is not known.

In the long-term safety surveillance trial of zileuton plus usual asthma care versus usual asthma care alone, a similar adverse reaction profile was seen as in other clinical trials.

➤*Postmarketing experience:* Rash and urticaria have been reported with zileuton.

Overdosage

➤*Symptoms:* Human experience of acute overdose with zileuton is limited. A patient in a clinical trial took between 6.6 and 9 g of zileuton in a single dose.

➤*Treatment:* Vomiting was induced and the patient recovered without sequelae. Zileuton is not removed by dialysis. Should an overdose occur, the patient should be treated symptomatically and supportive measures instituted as required. If indicated, elimination of unabsorbed drug should be achieved by emesis or gastric lavage; usual precautions should be observed to maintain the airway. A Certified Poison Control Center should be consulted for up-to-date information on management of overdose with zileuton.

Patient Information

- Zileuton is not a bronchodilator and should not be used to treat acute episodes of asthma.
- When taking zileuton, they should not decrease the dose or stop taking any other asthma medications unless instructed by a physician.
- While using zileuton, medical attention should be sought if short-acting bronchodilators are needed more often than usual, or if more than the maximum number of inhalations of short-acting bronchodilator treatment prescribed for a 24-hour period are needed.
- The most serious side effect of zileuton is elevation of liver enzyme tests and that, while taking zileuton, they must return for liver enzyme test monitoring on a regular basis.
- If they experience signs or symptoms of liver dysfunction (eg, right upper quadrant pain, nausea, fatigue, lethargy, pruritus, jaundice, or "flu-like" symptoms), they should contact their physician immediately.

MONOCLONAL ANTIBODIES

OMALIZUMAB

Rx	**Xolair** (Genentech)	**Powder for injection, lyophilized:** 129.6 mg (75 mg per 0.6 mL after reconstitution)	Preservative free. 93.1 mg sucrose. In single-use 5 mL vials.
		202.5 mg (150 mg per 1.2 mL after reconstitution)	Preservative free. 145.5 mg sucrose. In single-use 5 mL vials.

OMALIZUMAB — INJECTION

Indications

➤*Moderate to severe persistent asthma:* For adults and adolescents 12 years of age and older with moderate to severe persistent asthma who have a positive skin test or in vitro reactivity to a perennial aeroallergen and those symptoms are inadequately controlled with inhaled corticosteroids.

➤*Unlabeled uses:* Omalizumab may be beneficial in treating seasonal allergic rhinitis.

Administration and Dosage

➤*Approved by the FDA:* June 20, 2003.

Omalizumab 150 to 375 mg is administered SC every 2 or 4 weeks. Because the solution is slightly viscous, the injection may take 5 to 10 seconds to administer. Doses (mg) and dosing frequency are determined by serum total immunoglobulin E (IgE) level (units/mL), measured before the start of treatment, and body weight (kg). See the dose determination chart below for appropriate dose assignment. Doses of more than 150 mg are divided among more than 1 injection site to limit injections to not more than 150 mg per site.

Omalizumab Doses Administered by SC Injection Every 4 Weeks (mg)				
Pretreatment serum IgE (units/mL)	Body weight (kg)			
	30 to 60	> 60 to 70	> 70 to 90	> 90 to 150
≥ 30 to 100	150	150	150	300
> 100 to 200	300	300	300	See next table
> 200 to 300	300	See next table	See next table	See next table

Omalizumab Doses Administered by SC Injection Every 2 Weeks (mg)				
Pretreatment serum IgE (units/mL)	Body weight (kg)			
	30 to 60	> 60 to 70	> 70 to 90	> 90 to 150
> 100 to 200	See previous table	See previous table	See previous table	225
> 200 to 300	See previous table	225	225	300
> 300 to 400	225	225	300	Do not dose
> 400 to 500	300	300	375	Do not dose
> 500 to 600	300	375	Do not dose	Do not dose
> 600 to 700	375	Do not dose	Do not dose	Do not dose

➤*Dosage adjustment:* Total IgE levels are elevated during treatment and remain elevated for up to 1 year after the discontinuation of treatment. Therefore, retesting of IgE levels during omalizumab treatment cannot be used as a guide for dose determination. Base dose determination after treatment interruptions lasting less than 1 year on serum IgE levels obtained at the initial dose determination. Total serum IgE levels may be retested for dose determination if treatment with omalizumab has been interrupted for 1 year or more.

Adjust doses for significant changes in body weight.

➤*Preparation:* Prepare omalizumab for SC administration by using sterile water for injection only.

The lyophilized product takes 15 to 20 minutes to dissolve. The fully reconstituted product will appear clear or slightly opalescent and may have a few small bubbles or foam around the edge of the vial. The reconstituted product

OMALIZUMAB — INJECTION

is somewhat viscous; in order to obtain the full 0.6 or 1.2 mL dose, all of the product must be withdrawn from the vial before expelling any air or excess solution from the syringe.

1.) Draw 0.9 (75 mg vial) or 1.4 mL (150 mg vial) sterile water for injection into a 3 mL syringe equipped with a 1 inch 18-gauge needle.
2.) Inject the sterile water for injection directly into the product.
3.) Keeping the vial upright, gently swirl the vial for approximately 1 minute to evenly wet the powder. Do not shake.
4.) Gently swirl the vial for 5 to 10 seconds approximately every 5 minutes in order to dissolve any remaining solids. There should be no visible gel-like particles in the solution. Some vials may take longer than 20 minutes to dissolve completely. Do not use if the contents do not dissolve completely by 40 minutes.
5.) Invert the vial for 15 seconds in order to allow the solution to drain toward the stopper. Using a new 3 mL syringe equipped with a 1 inch 18-gauge needle, insert the needle into the inverted vial. Before removing the needle from the vial, pull the plunger all the way back to the end of the syringe barrel in order to remove all of the solution from the inverted vial.
6.) Replace the 18-gauge needle with a 25-gauge needle for SC injection.
7.) Expel air, large bubbles, and any excess solution in order to obtain the required 0.6 or 1.2 mL dose.

Number of Injections and Total Injection Volumes for Asthma

Dose (mg)	Number of vials: 75 mg[a]	Number of vials: 150 mg[b]	Number of injections	Total volume injected (mL)
150	0	1	1	1.2
225	1	1	2	1.8
300	0	2	2	2.4
375	1	2	3	3

[a] 0.6 mL maximum delivered volume per vial.
[b] 1.2 mL maximum delivered volume per vial.

➤*Storage/Stability:* Ship omalizumab at controlled ambient temperature (30°C or lower 86°F or lower). Store omalizumab under refrigerated conditions (2° to 8°C; 36° to 46°F). Do not use beyond the expiration date stamped on carton.

Omalizumab is for single use only and contains no preservatives. The solution may be used for SC administration within 8 hours following reconstitution when stored in the vial at 2° to 8°C (36° to 46°F), or within 4 hours of reconstitution when stored at room temperature.

Protect reconstituted omalizumab vials from direct sunlight.

Actions

➤*Pharmacology:* Omalizumab inhibits the binding of IgE to the high-affinity IgE receptor (FcεRI) on the surface of mast cells and basophils. Reduction in surface-bound IgE on FcεRI-bearing cells limits the degree of release of mediators of the allergic response. Treatment with omalizumab also reduces the number of FcεRI receptors on basophils in atopic patients.

Pharmacodynamics – In clinical studies, serum free IgE levels were reduced in a dose dependent manner within 1 hour following the first dose and maintained between doses. Mean serum free IgE decrease was greater than 96% using recommended doses. Serum total IgE levels (ie, bound and unbound) increased after the first dose due to the formation of omalizumab:IgE complexes, which have a slower elimination rate compared with free IgE. At 16 weeks after the first dose, average serum total IgE levels were 5-fold higher compared with pre-treatment when using standard assays. After discontinuation of omalizumab dosing, the omalizumab-induced increase in total IgE and decrease in free IgE were reversible, with no observed rebound in IgE levels after drug washout. Total IgE levels did not return to pre-treatment levels for up to 1 year after discontinuation of omalizumab.

➤*Pharmacokinetics:*

Absorption/Distribution – After SC administration, omalizumab is absorbed with an average absolute bioavailability of 62%. Following a single SC dose in adult and adolescent patients with asthma, omalizumab was absorbed slowly, reaching peak serum concentrations after an average of 7 to 8 days. The pharmacokinetics of omalizumab are linear at doses greater than 0.5 mg/kg. Following multiple doses of omalizumab, areas under the serum concentration-time curve from day 0 to day 14 at steady state were up to 6-fold of those after the first dose.

In vitro, omalizumab forms complexes of limited size with IgE. Precipitating complexes and complexes larger than 1 million daltons in molecular weight are not observed in vitro or in vivo. Tissue distribution studies in cynomolgus monkeys showed no specific uptake of ^{125}I-omalizumab by any organ or tissue. The apparent volume of distribution in patients following SC administration was 78 ± 32 mL/kg.

Metabolism/Excretion – Clearance of omalizumab involves IgG clearance processes as well as clearance via specific binding and complex formation with its target ligand, IgE. Liver elimination of IgG includes degradation in the liver reticuloendothelial system (RES) and endothelial cells. Intact IgG is also excreted in bile. In studies with mice and monkeys, omalizumab:IgE complexes were eliminated by interactions with Fcγ receptors within the RES at rates that were generally faster than IgG clearance. In asthma patients omalizumab serum elimination half-life averaged 26 days, with apparent clearance averaging 2.4 ± 1.1 mL/kg/day. In addition, doubling body weight approximately doubled apparent clearance.

Contraindications

Severe hypersensitivity reaction to omalizumab.

Warnings

➤*Hypersensitivity reactions:* Anaphylaxis has occurred within 2 hours of the first or subsequent administration of omalizumab in 3 (less than 0.1%) patients without other identifiable allergic triggers. These events included urticaria and throat and/or tongue edema. Patients should be observed after injection of omalizumab, and medications for the treatment of severe hypersensitivity reactions including anaphylaxis should be available. If a severe hypersensitivity reaction to omalizumab occurs, therapy should be discontinued. Omalizumab should not be administered to patients who have experienced a severe hypersensitivity reaction to omalizumab.

➤*Carcinogenesis:* Malignant neoplasms were observed in 20 of 4127 (0.5%) omalizumab-treated patients compared with 5 of 2236 (0.2%) control patients in clinical studies of asthma and other allergic disorders. The observed malignancies in omalizumab-treated patients were a variety of types, with breast, non-melanoma skin, prostate, melanoma, and parotid occurring more than once, and 5 other types occurring once each. The majority of patients were observed for less than 1 year. The impact of longer exposure to omalizumab or use in patients at higher risk for malignancy (eg, elderly, current smokers) is not known.

➤*Pregnancy: Category B.* IgG molecules are known to cross the placental barrier. There are no adequate and well-controlled studies of omalizumab in pregnant women. Because animal reproduction studies are not always predictive of human response, omalizumab should be used during pregnancy only if clearly needed.

➤*Lactation:* The excretion of omalizumab in milk was evaluated in female cynomolgus monkeys receiving SC doses of 75 mg/kg/week. Neonatal plasma levels of omalizumab after in utero exposure and 28 days of nursing were between 11% and 94% of the maternal plasma level. Milk levels of omalizumab were 1.5% of maternal blood concentration. While omalizumab presence in human milk has not been studied, IgG is excreted in human milk and therefore it is expected that omalizumab will be present in human milk. The potential for omalizumab absorption or harm to the infant are unknown; caution should be exercised when administering omalizumab to a nursing woman.

➤*Children:* Safety and effectiveness in pediatric patients below the age of 12 years have not been established.

Precautions

➤*Acute asthma exacerbations:* Omalizumab has not been shown to alleviate asthma exacerbations acutely and should not be used for the treatment of acute bronchospasm or status asthmaticus.

➤*Corticosteroid reduction:* Systemic or inhaled corticosteroids should not be abruptly discontinued upon initiation of omalizumab therapy. Decreases in corticosteroids should be performed under the direct supervision of a physician and may need to be performed gradually.

➤*Lab test abnormalities:* Serum total IgE levels increase following administration of omalizumab due to formation of omalizumab:IgE complexes. Elevated serum total IgE levels may persist for up to 1 year following discontinuation of omalizumab. Serum total IgE levels obtained less than 1 year following discontinuation may not reflect steady state free IgE levels and should not be used to reassess the dosing regimen.

Drug Interactions

None known.

Adverse Reactions

The most serious adverse reactions occurring in clinical studies with omalizumab are malignancies and anaphylaxis. Malignant neoplasms were observed in 20 of 4127 (0.5%) omalizumab-treated patients compared with 5 of 2236 (0.2%) control patients in clinical studies of asthma and other allergic disorders. The observed malignancies in omalizumab-treated patients were a variety of types, with breast, non-melanoma skin, prostate, melanoma, and parotid occurring more than once, and 5 other types occurring once each. Anaphylactic reactions were rare but temporally associated with omalizumab administration. These events included urticaria and throat and/or tongue edema.

The adverse reactions most commonly observed among patients treated with omalizumab included injection site reaction (45%), viral infections (23%), upper respiratory tract infection (20%), sinusitis (16%), headache (15%), and pharyngitis (11%). These events were observed at similar rates in omalizumab-treated patients and control patients. These were also the most frequently reported adverse reactions resulting in clinical intervention (eg, discontinuation of omalizumab, or the need for concomitant medication to treat an adverse reaction).

Adverse events ≥ 1% more frequent in omalizumab-treated patients

Adverse event	Omalizumab (n = 738) (%)	Placebo (n = 717) (%)
Body as a whole		
Pain	7%	5%
Fatigue	3%	2%
Musculoskeletal system		
Arthralgia	8%	6%
Fracture	2%	1%
Leg pain	4%	2%
Arm pain	2%	1%
Nervous system		
Dizziness	3%	2%

OMALIZUMAB — INJECTION

Adverse events ≥ 1% more frequent in omalizumab-treated patients		
Adverse event	Omalizumab (n = 738) (%)	Placebo (n = 717) (%)
Skin and appendages		
Pruritus	2%	1%
Dermatitis	2%	1%
Special senses		
Earache	2%	1%

➤*Injection site reactions:* Injection site reactions of any severity occurred at a rate of 45% in omalizumab-treated patients compared with 43% in placebo-treated patients. The types of injection site reactions included: bruising, redness, warmth, burning, stinging, itching, hive formation, pain, indurations, mass, and inflammation.

Severe injection-site reactions occurred more frequently in omalizumab-treated patients compared with patients in the placebo group (12% versus 9%).

The majority of injection site reactions occurred within 1 hour-post injection, lasted less than 8 days, and generally decreased in frequency at subsequent dosing visits.

➤*Immunogenicity:* Low titers of antibodies to omalizumab were detected in approximately 1/1723 (less than 0.1%) of patients treated with omalizumab. The data reflect the percentage of patients whose test results were considered positive for antibodies to omalizumab in an ELISA assay and are highly dependent on the sensitivity and specificity of the assay. Additionally, the observed incidence of antibody positivity in the assay may be influenced by several factors including sample handling, timing of sample collection, concomitant medications, and underlying disease. Therefore, comparison of the incidence of antibodies to omalizumab with the incidence of antibodies to other products may be misleading.

Allergic – Allergic symptoms, including urticaria, dermatitis, and pruritus were observed in patients treated with omalizumab. There were also 3 cases of anaphylaxis observed within 2 hours of omalizumab administration in which there were no other identifiable allergic triggers.

Overdosage

The maximum tolerated dose of omalizumab has not been determined. Single intravenous doses of up to 4000 mg have been administered to patients without evidence of dose-limiting toxicities. The highest cumulative dose administered to patients was 44,000 mg over a 20-week period, which was not associated with toxicities.

Patient Information

Patients receiving omalizumab should be told not to decrease the dose of, or stop taking any other asthma medications unless otherwise instructed by their physician. Patients should be told that they may not see immediate improvement in their asthma after beginning omalizumab therapy.

RESPIRATORY INHALANT PRODUCTS

Corticosteroids

For additional information, refer to the general discussion of Systemic Glucocorticoids in the Endocrine and Metabolic Agents chapter.

WARNING

Adrenal insufficiency – Deaths caused by adrenal insufficiency have occurred in asthmatic patients during and after transfer from systemic corticosteroids to inhaled corticosteroids. After withdrawal from systemic corticosteroids, several months are required for recovery of hypothalamic-pituitary-adrenal (HPA) function. During this period of HPA suppression, patients may exhibit symptoms of adrenal insufficiency when exposed to trauma, surgery, or infections, particularly gastroenteritis or other conditions with acute electrolyte loss. Although inhaled glucocorticoids may control asthmatic symptoms during these episodes, they do not provide the necessary mineralocorticoid for the treatment of these emergencies. Patients previously maintained on at least 20 mg/day of prednisone (or equivalent) may be most susceptible, especially when their systemic corticosteroids have been almost completely withdrawn.

Stress / Severe asthma attack – During periods of stress or a severe asthmatic attack, have patients withdrawn from systemic corticosteroids resume them (in large doses) immediately and contact a physician. Have patients carry a warning card indicating that they may need supplementary systemic corticosteroids during such periods. To assess the risk of adrenal insufficiency in emergency situations, periodically perform routine adrenal cortical function tests, including measurement of early morning resting cortisol levels in all patients. An early morning resting cortisol level may be accepted as normal only if it falls at or near the normal mean level.

Indications

➤*Asthma, chronic:* Maintenance and prophylactic treatment of asthma; includes patients who require systemic corticosteroids and may benefit from systemic dose reduction/elimination.

For specific labeled indications, refer to individual drug monographs.

Administration and Dosage

➤*Comparative efficacy:* Specific dosage guidelines for individual agents are included in the product listings. The relative anti-inflammatory potency of inhaled corticosteroids are in the following order: Flunisolide = triamcinolone acetonide < beclomethasone dipropionate = budesonide < fluticasone. Current data only supports a difference in potency, not efficacy, among the inhaled corticosteroids. The principle advantage of more potent inhaled corticosteroids may be in improved patient compliance and acceptance.

Estimated Comparative Daily Dosages for Inhaled Corticosteroids (Adults)[a]

Drug	Low dose	Medium dose	High dose
Beclomethasone dipropionate	168 to 504 mcg	504 to 840 mcg	> 840 mcg
42 mcg/puff	4 to 12 puffs	12 to 20 puffs	> 20 puffs
84 mcg/puff	2 to 6 puffs	6 to 10 puffs	> 10 puffs
Budesonide *Turbuhaler*	200 to 400 mcg	400 to 600 mcg	> 600 mcg
200 mcg/dose	1 to 2 inhalations	2 to 3 inhalations	> 3 inhalations
Flunisolide	500 to 1000 mcg	1000 to 2000 mcg	> 2000 mcg
250 mcg/puff	2 to 4 puffs	4 to 8 puffs	> 8 puffs
Fluticasone	88 to 264 mcg	264 to 660 mcg	> 660 mcg
MDI:[b] 44, 110, 220 mcg/puff	2 to 6 puffs (44 mcg) or 2 puffs (110 mcg)	2 to 6 puffs (110 mcg)	> 6 puffs (110 mcg) or > 3 puffs (220 mcg)
DPI:[c] 50, 100, 250 mcg/puff	2 to 6 inhalations (50 mcg)	3 to 6 inhalations (100 mcg)	> 6 inhalations (100 mcg) or > 2 inhalations (250 mcg)
Triamcinolone acetonide	400 to 1000 mcg	1000 to 2000 mcg	> 2000 mcg
100 mcg/puff	4 to 10 puffs	10 to 20 puffs	> 20 puffs

[a] *Guidelines for the Diagnosis and Management of Asthma*. Expert Panel Report 2. National Institutes of Health. National Heart, Lung, and Blood Institute. February 1997. http://www.lungusa.org/asthma/astnhlbi.html

[b] MDI = Metered dose inhaler.

[c] DPI = Dry powder inhaler.

Estimated Comparative Daily Dosages for Inhaled Corticosteroids (Children)[a]			
Drug	Low dose	Medium dose	High dose
Beclomethasone dipropionate (6 to 12 years of age)	84 to 336 mcg	336 to 672 mcg	> 672 mcg
42 mcg/puff	2 to 8 puffs	8 to 16 puffs	> 16 puffs
84 mcg/puff	1 to 4 puffs	4 to 8 puffs	> 8 puffs
Budesonide *Turbuhaler* (≥ 6 years of age)	100 to 200 mcg	200 to 400 mcg	> 400 mcg
200 mcg/dose		1 to 2 inhalations	> 2 inhalations
Flunisolide (6 to 15 years of age)	500 to 750 mcg	1000 to 1250 mcg	> 1250 mcg
250 mcg/puff	2 to 3 puffs	4 to 5 puffs	> 5 puffs
Fluticasone (≥ 12 years of age)	88 to 176 mcg	176 to 440 mcg	> 440 mcg
MDI:[b] 44, 110 mcg/puff	2 to 4 puffs (44 mcg)	4 to 10 puffs (44 mcg) or 2 to 4 puffs (110 mcg)	> 4 puffs (110 mcg)
DPI:[c] 50, 100, 250 mcg/dose	2 to 4 inhalations (50 mcg)	2 to 4 inhalations (100 mcg)	> 4 inhalations (100 mcg) or > 2 inhalations (250 mcg)
Triamcinolone acetonide (6 to 12 years of age)	400 to 800 mcg	800 to 1200 mcg	> 1200 mcg
100 mcg/puff	4 to 8 puffs	8 to 12 puffs	> 12 puffs

[a] *Guidelines for the Diagnosis and Management of Asthma.* Expert Panel Report 2. National Institutes of Health. National Heart, Lung, and Blood Institute. February 1997. http://www.lungusa.org/asthma/astnhlbi.html

[b] MDI = Metered dose inhaler.

[c] DPI = Dry powder inhaler.

➤*Patients receiving concomitant systemic steroids:* Stabilize the patient's asthma before treatment is started. Initially, use inhaled corticosteroids concurrently with usual maintenance dose of systemic steroid. After ≈ 1 week, start gradual withdrawal of the systemic steroid by reducing the daily or alternate daily dose. Make the next reduction after 1 to 2 weeks, depending on response. These decrements should not exceed 2.5 mg prednisone or equivalent. A slow rate of withdrawal cannot be overemphasized.

During withdrawal, some patients may experience symptoms of steroid withdrawal (eg, joint or muscular pain, lassitude, depression) despite maintenance or even improvement of respiratory function. Encourage continuance with the inhaler, but observe for objective signs of adrenal insufficiency. If adrenal insufficiency occurs, increase the systemic steroid dose temporarily and continue further withdrawal more slowly.

During periods of stress or severe asthma attack, transfer patients may require supplementary systemic steroids (see Warning box).

Actions

➤*Pharmacology:* Corticosteroids may have direct inhibitory effects on many cells involved in airway inflammation in asthma (eg, macrophages, T-lymphocytes, eosinophils, airway epithelial cells). In vitro, corticosteroids decrease cytokine-mediated survival of eosinophils, reducing the number of eosinophils in the circulation and airways of patients with asthma during corticosteroid therapy. While corticosteroids may not inhibit the release of mast cells in an allergic reaction, they do reduce the number of mast cells within the airway. Corticosteroids may also inhibit plasma exudation and the secretion of mucous in inflamed airways.

Inhaled corticosteroids have anti-inflammatory effects of the bronchial mucosa of asthma patients. Treatment with inhaled corticosteroids for 1 to 3 months results in a reduction in mast cells, macrophages, T-lymphocytes, and eosinophils in the epithelium and submucosa in the bronchioles. By reducing airway inflammation, inhaled corticosteroids lessen airway hyperresponsiveness in asthmatic adults and children. Long-term therapy reduces airway responsiveness to histamine cholinergic agonists, and allergens. Treatment also lowers responsiveness to exercise, fog, cold air, bradykinin, adenosine, and irritants. Inhaled corticosteroids make the airways less sensitive to these spasmogens and limits the maximal narrowing of the airway. Maximal effects of inhaled corticosteroid treatment may not be seen for several months.

➤*Pharmacokinetics:*

Pharmacokinetics of Inhaled Corticosteroids					
	Corticosteroids				
Parameters	Beclomethasone	Budesonide	Flunisolide	Fluticasone	Triamcinolone
Absorption					
Systemic bioavailability from lungs	≈ 20%	25%	40%	20	21.5%
Distribution					
Vd (L/kg)	NA	4.3	1.8	3.5	1.4
Protein binding	87%	85% to 90%	NA	91%	≈ 68%
Metabolism					
Site	liver (CYP3A)	liver (CYP3A)	liver	liver (CYP3A4)	mostly from liver, less extensively from the kidneys
Metabolites (Activity)	beclomethasone 17-mono-propionate (active), free beclomethasone (very weak anti-inflammatory effects)	16α-hydroxy-prednisolone and 6β-hydroxy-budesonide (< 1% of parent)	6β-OH (low corticosteroid potency)	17β-carboxylic acid (negligible in animal studies)	6β-hydroxy-triamcinolone acetonide, 21-carboxy-triamcinolone acetonide, and 21-carboxy 6β hy droxytriamcinolone acetonide (less active than parent)
Excretion					
Site	feces, urine (less than 10%)	urine (≈ 60%), feces	renal (50%), feces (40%)	feces, urine (less than 0.02%)	urine (≈ 40%), feces (≈ 60%)
$T_{½}$	2.8 hr	2.8 hr	≈ 1.8 hr	3.1 hr	1.5 hr

Contraindications

Relief of acute bronchospasm; primary treatment of status asthmaticus or other acute episodes of asthma when intensive measures are required; hypersensitivity to any ingredients.

➤*Vanceril:* Relief of asthma that can be controlled by bronchodilators and other nonsteroid medications; in patients who require systemic corticosteroid treatment infrequently; treatment of nonasthmatic bronchitis.

Warnings

➤*Infections:* Localized fungal infections with *Candida albicans* or *Aspergillus niger* have occurred in the mouth, pharynx, and occasionally the larynx. Positive cultures for oral *Candida* may be present in up to 34% to 75% of patients. Incidence of clinically apparent infection is low and may require treatment with appropriate antifungal therapy or discontinuance of inhaled steroid treatment. Actions that may minimize the problem include dose reduction, decreasing dose frequency, rinsing mouth after use, and use of an add-on spacer device.

Use inhaled corticosteroids with caution, if at all, in patients with active or quiescent tuberculous infection of the respiratory tract; untreated systemic fungal, bacterial, parasitic, or viral infection; or ocular herpes simplex.

➤*Compromised immune systems:* People who are on drugs that suppress the immune system are more susceptible to infections than healthy individuals. For example, chickenpox and measles can have a more serious or even fatal course in nonimmune children or adults on corticosteroids. In such children or adults who have not had these diseases, take particular care to avoid exposure. How the dose, route, and duration of corticosteroid administration affect the risk of disseminated infection is unknown. The contribution of the underlying disease or prior corticosteroid treatment to the risk is also unknown. If exposed to chickenpox, prophylaxis with varicella-zoster immune globulin (VZIG) may be indicated. If exposed to measles, prophylaxis with pooled IM immunoglobulin (IG) may be indicated. If chickenpox develops, consider treatment with antiviral agents.

➤*Acute asthma:* These products are not bronchodilators and are not for rapid relief of bronchospasm. Contact a physician immediately when asthmatic episodes do not respond to bronchodilators. Patients may require systemic corticosteroids.

There is no evidence that control of asthma can be achieved by inhaled corticosteroids in amounts greater than recommended doses.

➤*Bronchospasm:* This may occur with an immediate increase in wheezing following dosing. If bronchospasm occurs following corticosteroid inhalation, treat immediately with a short-acting inhaled bronchodilator. Discontinue inhalation treatment, and institute an alternative treatment.

Instruct patients to contact their health care provider immediately when episodes of asthma do not respond to bronchodilators during treatment with corticosteroid inhalation. During such episodes, patients may require treatment with systemic corticosteroids.

➤*Combination with prednisone:* Combination therapy of inhaled corticosteroids with systemic corticosteroids may increase the risk of HPA suppression compared to a therapeutic dose of either one alone. Use inhaled corticosteroids with caution in patients already receiving prednisone.

➤*Replacement therapy:* Transfer from systemic steroid therapy may unmask allergic conditions previously suppressed (eg, rhinitis, conjunctivitis, eczema).

➤*Pregnancy: Category C; Category B* (**budesonide** only). Glucocorticoids are teratogenic in rodents. Findings include cleft palate, internal hydrocephaly, and axial skeletal defects; CNS and cranial malformations were observed in monkeys. There are no adequate and well-controlled studies in pregnant women. Use these agents during pregnancy only if the benefit clearly justifies the potential risk to the fetus. Infants born of mothers who received substantial doses during pregnancy should be observed for adrenal insufficiency.

Budesonide – Studies of pregnant women have not shown that *Pulmicort Turbuhaler* increases the risk of abnormalities when administered during pregnancy. The results from a large population-based prospective cohort epidemiological study indicate no increased risk for congenital malformations from the use of inhaled budesonide during early pregnancy. Congenital malformations were studied in 2014 infants born to mothers reporting the use of inhaled budesonide for asthma in early pregnancy (usually 10 to 12 weeks after the last menstrual period), the period when most major organ malformations occur. The rate of recorded congenital malformations was similar compared with the general population rate (3.8% vs 3.5%, respectively). In addition, after exposure to inhaled budesonide, the number of infants born with orofacial clefts was similar to the expected number in the normal population (4 children vs 3.3, respectively).

➤*Lactation:* Glucocorticoids are excreted in breast milk. It is unknown whether inhaled corticosteroids are excreted in breast milk. Decide whether to discontinue nursing or to discontinue the drug.

➤*Children:* Insufficient information is available to warrant use in children younger than 6 years of age or younger than 12 with **fluticasone** and **beclomethasone**. Monitor growth in children and adolescents because there is evidence that oral corticosteroids may suppress growth in a dose-related fashion, particularly in higher doses for extended periods.

Precautions

➤*Steroid withdrawal:* During withdrawal from oral steroids, some patients may experience symptoms of systemically active steroid withdrawal (eg, joint or muscular pain, lassitude, depression), despite maintenance or even improvement of respiratory function. Although steroid withdrawal effects are usually transient and not severe, severe and even fatal exacerbation of asthma can occur if the previous daily oral corticosteroid requirement had significantly exceeded 10 mg/day of prednisone or equivalent.

➤*HPA suppression:* In responsive patients, inhaled corticosteroids may permit control of asthmatic symptoms with less HPA suppression. Because these agents are absorbed and can be systemically active, the beneficial effects in minimizing or preventing HPA dysfunction may be expected only when recommended dosages are not exceeded. When administered in excessive doses or at recommended doses in a minority of susceptible patients, systemic corticosteroid effects (eg, hypercorticoidism, adrenal suppression) may occur. Slowly reduce or discontinue corticosteroid therapy when these events occur. Titrate patients to the lowest effective dose because of individual sensitivity to cortisol product effects. Carefully observe patients for evidence of systemic corticosteroid effects. Take particular care in observing patients postoperatively or during periods of stress for evidence of a decrease in adrenal function.

Flunisolide – Because of the possibility of higher systemic absorption, monitor patients using **flunisolide** for any evidence of systemic corticosteroid effect. If such changes occur, discontinue slowly, consistent with accepted procedures for discontinuing oral corticosteroids. When flunisolide is used chronically at 2 mg/day, monitor patients periodically for effects on the HPA axis.

➤*Glaucoma:* Rare instances of glaucoma, increased intraocular pressure, and cataracts have been reported following the inhaled administration of corticosteroids.

➤*Long-term effects:* The effects of long-term glucocorticoid inhalation are unknown. Although there is no clinical evidence of adverse effects, the local and systemic effects on developmental or immunologic processes in the mouth, pharynx, trachea, and lung are unknown.

There is no information about effects on acute, recurrent, or chronic pulmonary infection (including active or quiescent tuberculosis) or effects of long-term use on lung or other tissues. Use with caution (see Warnings).

➤*Pulmonary infiltrates:* Pulmonary infiltrates with eosinophilia may occur with **beclomethasone** or **flunisolide**. This may manifest because of systemic steroid withdrawal when inhalational agents are used, but a causative role for either agent or vehicle cannot be ruled out.

➤*Reduction in growth velocity:* A reduction in growth velocity in children may occur as a result of inadequate control of chronic diseases such as asthma or from corticosteroid use. Closely follow the growth of adolescents taking corticosteroids by any route, and weigh the benefits of corticosteroid therapy and asthma control against the possibility of growth suppression if an adolescent's growth appears slowed.

Drug Interactions

➤*Ketoconazole:* A potent inhibitor of cytochrome P450 3A4 may increase plasma levels of **budesonide** and **fluticasone** during concomitant dosing. The clinical significance is unknown. Use caution.

Adverse Reactions

Suppression of HPA function (see Warning Box; Warnings).

Inhaled Corticosteroids Adverse Reactions (%)

	Beclomethasone dipropionate	Budesonide inhalation powder	Budesonide inhalation suspension	Flunisolide	Fluticasone propionate aerosol	Fluticasone propionate inhalation powder	Triamcinolone acetonide
Cardiovascular							
Tachycardia	< 2	—	—	1 to 3	—	—	—
Chest pain	< 2	—	1 to 3	3 to 9	—	—	—
CNS							
Headache	12[a] 22 to 27[b]	13 to 14	—	25	17 to 22	9 to 15	7 to 21
Migraine	< 2	1 to 3	—	—	—	1 to 3	—
Insomnia	< 2	1 to 3	—	1 to 3	—	—	—
Dermatological							
Eczema	< 2[b]	—	1 to 3	3 to 9	—	—	—
Pruritus	< 2[b]	—	1 to 3	3 to 9	—	—	—
Rash	Rare[a] < 2	—	< 1 to 4	3 to 9	1 to 3	—	1 to 3
GI							
Nausea	1[a] < 2	1 to 3	—	25	1 to 3		—
Dyspepsia	3 to 6[b]	1 to 4	—	1 to 3	1 to 3	—	—
Dry mouth	—	1 to 3	—	1 to 3	—	—	1 to 3
Oral candidiasis	—	2 to 4	—	3 to 9	2 to 5	3 to 11	1 to 3
Gastroenteritis	—	1 to 3	5	—	—	1 to 3	—
Vomiting	—	1 to 3	2 to 4	25	1 to 3		1 to 3

Inhaled Corticosteroids Adverse Reactions (%)							
	Beclomethasone dipropionate	Budesonide inhalation powder	Budesonide inhalation suspension	Flunisolide	Fluticasone propionate aerosol	Fluticasone propionate inhalation powder	Triamcinolone acetonide
Diarrhea	< 2	—	2 to 4	10	1 to 3	< 4	1 to 3
Abdominal pain	—	1 to 3	2 to 3	3 to 9	—	1 to 3	1 to 3
Anorexia	—	—	1 to 3	3 to 9	—	—	—
GU							
Dysmenorrhea	1 to 3[a] < 4[b]	—	—	—	1 to 3	1 to 3	—
Menstrual disturbance				3 to 9		1 to 3	
Hypersensitivity							
Urticaria	Rare[a] < 2	—	—	1 to 3	Rare	1 to 3	Rare
Angioedema	Rare[a]	—	—	—	Rare	Rare	—
Respiratory							
Upper respiratory tract infections	9[a] < 2	19 to 24	34 to 38	25	15 to 22	16 to 22	—
Pharyngitis	8[a] 11 to 14[b]	5 to 10	—	1 to 3	10 to 14	6 to 13	7 to 25
Rhinitis	6[a]	—	7 to 12	3 to 9	1 to 3	2 to 9	—
Sinusitis	3[a] 3 to 4[b]	2 to 11	—	3 to 9	3 to 6	4 to 6	2 to 9
Nasal congestion	5 to 6[b]	—	—	15	8 to 16	4 to 7	—
Coughing	1 to 3[a] 7 to 9[b]	—	5 to 9	3 to 9	—	—	—
Dysphonia	1 to 3[a] < 2[b]	—	1 to 3	—	3 to 8	< 1 to 6	—
Bronchospasm	Rare[a] < 2	—	—	—	Rare	—	—
Sneezing	2 to 3[b]	—	—	3 to 9	—	1 to 3	—
Epistaxis	—	—	2 to 4	1 to 3	—	1 to 3	—
Chest congestion	< 2	—	—	3 to 9	1 to 3	1 to 3	1 to 3
Bronchitis	< 2	—	—	1 to 3	1 to 3	1 to 4	—
Special senses							
Taste alteration	< 2	1 to 3	—	10	—	—	—
Otitis media	—	—	9 to 12	—	—	1 to 3	—
Ear infection	—	—	2 to 5	3 to 9	—	—	—
Conjunctivitis	—	—	< 1 to 4	—	—	1 to 3	—
Earache	< 2	—	1 to 3	1 to 3	—	1 to 3	—
Miscellaneous							
Infection, viral	5 to 8[b]	—	3 to 5	—	—	—	—
Weight changes	—	1 to 3	—	1 to 3	—	—	1 to 3
Back pain	1[a]	2 to 6	—	—	—	—	2 to 4
Influenza-like syndrome	< 1 to 3[b]	6 to 14	1 to 3	10	3 to 8	3 to 4	2 to 5
Pain	2[a] < 2	5	—	—	—	1 to 3	1 to 3
Fever	< 2	< 4	—	3 to 9	1 to 3	2 to 4	—
Infection	—	1 to 3	1 to 3	—	—	—	—

[a] *QVAR*.

[b] *Vanceril* (both strengths).

➤*Beclomethasone:*

Miscellaneous – Fatigue (2% to 3%); increased asthma symptoms (less than 2% to 3%); rigors, rectal hemorrhage, lacrimation, arthralgia, depression, skin discoloration, UTI, lymphadenopathy, respiratory disorder (less than 2%).

➤*Budesonide inhalation powder:*

Musculoskeletal – Fracture, myalgia, neck pain (1% to 3%).

Miscellaneous – Voice alteration (1% to 6%); ecchymosis, syncope, hypertonia (1% to 3%).

➤*Budesonide inhalation suspension:*

CNS – Hyperkinesias, emotional lability (1% to 3%).

Dermatologic – Pustular rash, contact dermatitis (1% to 3%).

Musculoskeletal – Fracture, myalgia (1% to 3%).

Special senses – Eye infection, otitis externa (1% to 3%).

Miscellaneous – Moniliasis (3% to 4%); allergic reaction, fatigue, stridor, cervical lymphadenopathy, purpura, herpes simplex (1% to 3%).

Postmarketing: Hypersensitivity reactions, symptoms of hypocorticism/hypercorticism, psychiatric symptoms including depression, aggressive reactions, irritability, anxiety and psychosis, bone disorders including avascular necrosis of the femoral head and osteoporosis (less than 1%).

➤*Flunisolide:*

CNS – Dizziness, irritability, nervousness, shakiness (3% to 9%); anxiety, depression, faintness, fatigue, hyperactivity, hypoactivity, moodiness, numbness, vertigo (1% to 3%).

Dermatologic – Acne, hives (1% to 3%).

GI – Upset stomach (10%); heartburn (3% to 9%); constipation, gas, increased appetite (1% to 3%); abdominal fullness (less than 1%).

Hematologic – Capillary fragility, enlarged lymph nodes (1% to 3%).

Respiratory – Sore throat (20%); cold symptoms (15%); runny nose, sinus congestion, sinus drainage, sinus infection, hoarseness, sputum, wheezing (3% to 9%); glossitis, mouth/throat irritation, phlegm, chest tightness, dyspnea, head stuffiness, laryngitis, nasal irritation, pleurisy, pneumonia, sinus discomfort (1% to 3%); shortness of breath (less than 1%).

Special senses – Loss of smell (3% to 9%); blurred vision, eye discomfort, eye infection (1% to 3%).

Miscellaneous – Edema, palpitations (3% to 9%); chills, malaise, peripheral edema, sweating, weakness (1% to 3%).

➤*Fluticasone:*

CNS – Giddiness, nervousness (1% to 3%).

Respiratory – Nasal discharge (4% to 5%); allergic rhinitis (3% to 5%); pain in nasal sinus(es), laryngitis, acute nasopharyngitis, dyspnea, irritation caused by inhalant, tonsillitis (1% to 3%).

GI – Stomach disorder, gastroenteritis/colitis, abdominal discomfort, mouth/throat irritation (1% to 3%).

GU – Moniliasis, candidiasis of vagina, pelvic inflammatory disease, vaginitis/vulvovaginitis (1% to 3%).

Musculoskeletal – Back problems (less than 1% to 4%); joint pain, sprain/strain, aches and pains, limb pain, muscular soreness, disorder/symptoms of neck (1% to 3%).

Special senses – Eye irritation, dental disorder, conjunctivitis (1% to 3%).

Miscellaneous – Dermatitis, rash/skin eruption, injury (1% to 3%).

Postmarketing: Throat soreness and irritation; hoarseness; aphonia; Cushingoid features; growth velocity reduction in children/adolescents; weight gain; hyperglycemia; restlessness; agitation; aggression; depression; immediate bronchospasm; asthma exacerbation; dyspnea; wheezing; chest tightness; cough; pruritus; contusions; ecchymosis; laryngitis; bronchospasm.

➤*Triamcinolone:*

GU – Cystitis, urinary tract infection, vaginal monilia (1% to 3%).

Musculoskeletal – Bursitis, myalgia, tenosynovitis (1% to 3%).

Respiratory – Hoarseness; cough; increased wheezing; irritated throat; dry throat; dry mouth; oral candidiasis.

Miscellaneous – Facial edema, photosensitivity, toothache, easy bruisability, steroid withdrawal symptoms, voice alteration (1% to 3%).

Overdosage

The potential for acute toxic effects following overdose of inhaled corticosteroids is low. Chronic overdosage may result in signs/symptoms of hypercorticoidism.

Patient Information

Patient instructions are available with each product.

Rinse mouth with water without swallowing after each dose to reduce the risk of oral candidiasis. If the infection develops, treat with appropriate therapy. Corticosteroid therapy may need to be interrupted.

Instruct patients whose systemic corticosteroids have been reduced or withdrawn to carry a warning card indicating the need for supplemental systemic steroids in the event of stress or severe asthmatic attack that is unresponsive to bronchodilators.

Advise patients not to stop therapy abruptly. If discontinuation is necessary, contact the physician.

This medication is intended for treatment of asthma. It does not contain medication intended to provide rapid relief of breathing difficulties during an asthma attack. It is very important that the medication is used regularly at the intervals recommended by doctor, and not as an emergency measure.

Warn people who are on immunosuppressant doses of corticosteroids to avoid exposure to chickenpox or measles. Advise patients to seek medical advice without delay if they are exposed.

Advise patients receiving bronchodilators (eg, albuterol) by inhalation to use the bronchodilator several minutes before the corticosteroid inhalant to enhance penetration of the steroid into the bronchial tree and reduce potential toxicity from the inhaled fluorocarbon propellants in the 2 aerosols.

Notify physician if sore throat or sore mouth occurs.

➤*Administration technique:* The success of these agents is a function of proper administration technique. The following guidelines may be useful:

Aerosol – Thoroughly shake the inhaler with canister in place; breathe out to the end of a normal breath. Hold the inhaler system upright; place the mouthpiece into the mouth and close the lips tightly. While activating the inhaler, take a slow, deep breath for 3 to 5 seconds, hold the breath for approximately 10 seconds, and exhale slowly. Allow at least 1 minute between inhalations (puffs). Rinse the mouth with water after each use to help reduce dry mouth and hoarseness.

Inhaled powder – Hold inhaler upright, and twist the cover off. Twist the grip fully to the right as far as it will go, then twist it back. You will hear a click. Exhale; then place the mouthpiece between lips, slightly tilt head back, and inhale deeply and forcefully. Remove inhaler from mouth, and hold breath for approximately 10 seconds. Allow at least 1 minute between inhalations (puffs). Rinse the mouth with water after each use to help reduce dry mouth and hoarseness.

BECLOMETHASONE DIPROPIONATE

Rx	**QVAR** (IVAX)	**Aerosol:** 40 mcg/actuation	In 7.3 g canisters (100 actuations) with actuator.
		80 mcg/actuation	In 7.3 g canisters (100 actuations) with actuator.

BECLOMETHASONE DIPROPIONATE — INHALATION

For complete and comparative prescribing information, refer to the Corticosteroids Respiratory Inhalant group monograph.

Indications

➤*Asthma, chronic:* Maintenance treatment of asthma as prophylactic therapy in patients 5 years of age and older.

For asthma patients who require systemic corticosteroid administration, where adding beclomethasone dipropionate inhalation aerosol may reduce or eliminate the need for the systemic corticosteroids.

Beclomethasone dipropionate HFA inhalation aerosol is not indicated for the relief of acute bronchospasm.

Administration and Dosage

➤*Approved by the FDA:* May 1976.

Patients should prime beclomethasone dipropionate HFA inhalation aerosol by actuating into the air twice before using for the first time or if beclomethasone dipropionate HFA inhalation aerosol has not been used for over 10 days. Avoid spraying in the eyes or face when priming beclomethasone dipropionate HFA inhalation aerosol. Beclomethasone dipropionate HFA inhalation aerosol is a solution aerosol, which does not require shaking. Consistent dose delivery is achieved, whether using the 40 or 80 mcg strengths, due to proportionality of the 2 products (ie, 2 actuations of 40 mcg strength should provide a dose comparable to 1 actuation of the 80 mcg strength).

Beclomethasone dipropionate HFA inhalation aerosol should be administered by the oral inhaled route in patients 5 years of age and older. The onset and degree of symptom relief will vary in individual patients. Improvement in asthma symptoms should be expected within the first or second week of starting treatment, but maximum benefit should not be expected until 3 to 4 weeks of therapy. For patients who do not respond adequately to the starting dose after 3 to 4 weeks of therapy, higher doses may provide additional asthma control. The safety and efficacy of beclomethasone dipropionate when administered in excess of recommended doses has not been established.

Beclomethasone Dipropionate Recommended Dosages

Previous therapy	Recommended starting dose	Highest recommended dose
Adults and adolescents		
Bronchodilators alone	40 to 80 mcg twice daily	320 mcg twice daily
Inhaled corticosteroids	40 to 160 mcg twice daily	320 mcg twice daily
Children 5 to 11 years		
Bronchodilators alone	40 mcg twice daily	80 mcg twice daily
Inhaled corticosteroids	40 mcg twice daily	80 mcg twice daily

The recommended dosage of beclomethasone dipropionate HFA inhalation aerosol relative to chlorofluorocarbon (CFC)-based beclomethasone dipropionate (CFC-BDP) inhalation aerosol is lower due to differences in delivery characteristics between the products. Recognizing that a definitive comparative therapeutic ratio between beclomethasone dipropionate HFA inhalation aerosol and CFC-BDP has not been demonstrated, any patient who is switched from CFC-BDP to beclomethasone dipropionate HFA inhalation aerosol should be dosed appropriately, taking into account the dosing recommendations above, and should be monitored to ensure that the dose of beclomethasone dipropionate HFA inhalation aerosol selected is safe and efficacious. As with any inhaled corticosteroid, physicians are advised to titrate the dose of beclomethasone dipropionate HFA inhalation aerosol downward over time to the lowest level that maintains proper asthma control. This is particularly important in children since a controlled study has shown that beclomethasone dipropionate HFA inhalation aerosol has the potential to affect growth in children.

➤*Patients not receiving systemic corticosteroids:* Patients who require maintenance therapy of their asthma may benefit from treatment with beclomethasone dipropionate HFA inhalation aerosol at the doses recommended above. In patients who respond to beclomethasone dipropionate HFA inhalation aerosol, improvement in pulmonary function is usually apparent within 1 to 4 weeks after the start of therapy. Once the desired effect is achieved, consideration should be given to tapering to the lowest effective dose.

➤*Patients maintained on systemic corticosteroids:* Beclomethasone dipropionate HFA inhalation aerosol may be effective in the management of asthmatics maintained on systemic corticosteroids and may permit replacement or significant reduction in the dosage of systemic corticosteroids.

The patient's asthma should be reasonably stable before treatment with beclomethasone dipropionate HFA inhalation aerosol is started. Initially, beclomethasone dipropionate HFA inhalation aerosol should be used concurrently with the patient's usual maintenance dose of systemic corticosteroid. After approximately 1 week, gradual withdrawal of the systemic corticosteroid is started by reducing the daily or alternate daily dose. Reductions may be made after an interval of 1 or 2 weeks, depending on the response of the patient. A slow rate of withdrawal is strongly recommended. Generally, these decrements should not exceed 2.5 mg of prednisone or its equivalent. During withdrawal, some patients may experience symptoms of systemic corticosteroid withdrawal (eg, joint or muscular pain, lassitude, depression) despite maintenance or even improvement in pulmonary function. Such patients should be encouraged to continue with the inhaler but should be monitored for objective signs of adrenal insufficiency. If evidence of adrenal insufficiency occurs, the systemic corticosteroid doses should be increased temporarily, and, thereafter, withdrawal should continue more slowly.

During periods of stress or a severe asthma attack, transfer patients may require supplementary treatment with systemic corticosteroids.

BECLOMETHASONE DIPROPIONATE — INHALATION

➤*Storage / Stability:* Store beclomethasone dipropionate HFA inhalation aerosol when not being used so that the product rests on the concave end of the canister with the plastic actuator on top. Store at 25°C (77°F). Excursions between 15° and 30°C (59° and 86°F) are permitted. For optimal results, the canister should be at room temperature when used. Beclomethasone dipropionate HFA inhalation aerosol canister should only be used with the beclomethasone dipropionate HFA inhalation aerosol actuator, and the actuator should not be used with any other inhalation drug product.

Contents under pressure – Do not puncture. Do not use or store near heat or open flame. Exposure to temperatures above 49°C (120°F) may cause bursting. Never throw container into fire or incinerator.

BUDESONIDE

Rx	**Pulmicort Turbuhaler** (AstraZeneca)	**Powder:** 200 mcg (each actuation delivers ≈ 160 mcg)/metered dose	(Pulmicort™ 200 mcg). In 200 dose *Turbuhaler.*
Rx	**Pulmicort Respules** (AstraZeneca)	**Inhalation suspension:** 0.25 mg/2 mL	EDTA. In single-dose envelopes. In 30s.
		0.5 mg/2 mL	EDTA. In single-dose envelopes. In 30s.

BUDESONIDE — INHALATION

For complete and comparative prescribing information, refer to the Corticosteroids Respiratory Inhalant group monograph.

WARNING

Particular care is needed for patients who are transferred from systemically active corticosteroids to inhaled corticosteroids (eg, budesonide) because deaths due to adrenal insufficiency have occurred in asthmatic patients during and after transfer from systemic corticosteroids to less systemically available inhaled corticosteroids. After withdrawal from systemic corticosteroids, a number of months are required for recovery of HPA-axis function.

Patients who have been previously maintained on greater than or equal to 20 mg/day of prednisone (or its equivalent) may be most susceptible, particularly when their systemic corticosteroids have been almost completely withdrawn.

During this period of HPA-axis suppression, patients may exhibit signs and symptoms of adrenal insufficiency when exposed to trauma, surgery, or infection (particularly gastroenteritis) or other conditions associated with severe electrolyte loss. Although budesonide may provide control of asthma symptoms during these episodes, in recommended doses it supplies less than normal physiological amounts of corticosteroid systemically and does not provide the mineralocorticoid activity that is necessary for coping with these emergencies.

During periods of stress or a severe asthma attack, patients who have been withdrawn from systemic corticosteroids should be instructed to resume oral corticosteroids (in large doses) immediately and to contact their physicians for further instruction. These patients should also be instructed to carry a medical identification card indicating that they may need supplementary systemic corticosteroids during periods of stress or a severe asthma attack.

Indications

➤*Powder for inhalation:* For the maintenance treatment of asthma as prophylactic therapy in adult and pediatric patients 6 years of age or older. It is also indicated for patients requiring oral corticosteroid therapy for asthma. Many of those patients may be able to reduce or eliminate their requirement for oral corticosteroids over time.

➤*Inhalation suspension:* For the maintenance treatment of asthma and as prophylactic therapy in children 12 months to 8 years of age.

Budesonide is not indicated for the relief of acute bronchospasm.

Administration and Dosage

➤*Approved by the FDA:* June 24, 1997.

➤*Patients maintained on chronic oral corticosteroids:* Initially, budesonide should be used concurrently with the patient's usual maintenance dose of systemic corticosteroid. After approximately 1 week, gradual withdrawal of the systemic corticosteroid is started by reducing the daily or alternate daily dose. The next reduction is made after an interval of 1 or 2 weeks, depending on the response of the patient. Generally, these decrements should not exceed 25% of the prednisone dose or its equivalent. A slow rate of withdrawal is strongly recommended. During reduction of oral corticosteroids, patients should be carefully monitored for asthma instability, including objective measures of airway function, and for adrenal insufficiency. During withdrawal, some patients may experience symptoms of systemic corticosteroid withdrawal (eg, joint or muscular pain, lassitude, depression) despite maintenance or even improvement in pulmonary function. Such patients should be encouraged to continue with budesonide but should be monitored for objective signs of adrenal insufficiency. If evidence of adrenal insufficiency occurs, the systemic corticosteroid doses should be increased temporarily, and thereafter withdrawal should continue more slowly. During periods of stress or a severe asthma attack, transfer patients may require supplementary treatment with systemic corticosteroids.

➤*Powder for inhalation:* Budesonide should be administered by the orally inhaled route in asthmatic patients greater than or equal to 6 years of age. Individual patients will experience a variable onset and degree of symptom relief. Generally, budesonide has a relatively rapid onset of action for an inhaled corticosteroid. Improvement in asthma control following inhaled administration of budesonide can occur within 24 hours of initiation of treatment, although maximum benefit may not be achieved for 1 to 2 weeks or longer. The safety and efficacy of budesonide when administered in excess of recommended doses have not been established.

Budesonide Powder for Inhalation Recommended Dosages

	Previous therapy	Recommended starting dose	Highest recommended dose
Adults	Bronchodilators alone	200 to 400 mcg twice daily	400 mcg twice daily
	Inhaled corticosteroids*	200 to 400 mcg twice daily	800 mcg twice daily
	Oral corticosteroids	400 to 800 mcg twice daily	800 mcg twice daily
Children	Bronchodilators alone	200 mcg twice daily	400 mcg twice daily
	Inhaled corticosteroids*	200 mcg twice daily	400 mcg twice daily
	Oral corticosteroids	The highest recommended dose in children is 400 mcg twice daily.	

* In patients with mild-to-moderate asthma who are well-controlled on inhaled corticosteroids, dosing with budesonide 200 mcg or 400 mcg once daily may be considered. Budesonide can be administered once daily either in the morning or in the evening.

If the once-daily treatment with budesonide does not provide adequate control of asthma symptoms, the total daily dose should be increased or administered as a divided dose.

Note – In all patients, it is desirable to titrate to the lowest effective dose once asthma stability is achieved.

Patients should be instructed to prime budesonide prior to its initial use, and instructed to inhale deeply and forcefully each time the unit is used. Rinsing the mouth after inhalation is also recommended.

➤*Inhalation suspension:* For inhalation use via compressed air driven jet nebulizers only (not for use with ultrasonic devices). Not for injection. Read patient instructions before using.

Budesonide inhalation suspension is indicated for use in asthmatic patients 12 months to 8 years of age. Budesonide inhalation suspension should be administered by the inhaled route via jet nebulizer connected to an air compressor. Individual patients will experience a variable onset and degree of symptom relief. Improvement in asthma control following inhaled administration of budesonide inhalation suspension can occur within 2 to 8 days of initiation of treatment, although maximum benefit may not be achieved for 4 to 6 weeks. The safety and efficacy of budesonide inhalation suspension when administered in excess of recommended doses have not been established. In all patients, it is desirable to downward-titrate to the lowest effective dose once asthma stability is achieved.

Budesonide Inhalation Suspension Recommended Dosages

Previous therapy	Recommended starting dose	Highest recommended dose
Bronchodilators alone	0.5 mg total daily dose administered either once daily or twice daily in divided doses	0.5 mg total daily dose
Inhaled corticosteroids	0.5 mg total daily dose administered either once daily or twice daily in divided doses	1 mg total daily dose
Oral corticosteroids	1 mg total daily dose administered either as 0.5 mg twice daily or 1 mg once daily	1 mg total daily dose

In symptomatic children not responding to nonsteroidal therapy, a starting dose of 0.25 mg once daily of budesonide inhalation suspension may also be considered.

If once-daily treatment with budesonide inhalation suspension does not provide adequate control of asthma symptoms, the total daily dose should be increased or administered as a divided dose.

Patients not receiving systemic (oral) corticosteroids – Patients who require maintenance therapy of their asthma may benefit from treatment

BUDESONIDE — INHALATION

with budesonide inhalation suspension at the doses recommended above. Once the desired clinical effect is achieved, consideration should be given to tapering to the lowest effective dose. For the patients who do not respond adequately to the starting dose, consideration should be given to administering the total daily dose as a divided dose, if a once-daily dosing schedule was followed. If necessary, higher doses, up to the maximum recommended doses, may provide additional asthma control.

Administration – A *Pari-LC-Jet Plus Nebulizer* (with face mask or mouthpiece) connected to a *Pari Master* compressor was used to deliver budesonide inhalation suspension to each patient in 3 US controlled clinical studies. The safety and efficacy of budesonide inhalation suspension delivered by other nebulizers and compressors have not been established.

Budesonide inhalation suspension should be administered via jet nebulizer connected to an air compressor with an adequate air flow, equipped with a mouthpiece or suitable face mask. Ultrasonic nebulizers are not suitable for the adequate administration of budesonide inhalation suspension and, therefore, are not recommended.

The effects of mixing budesonide inhalation suspension with other nebulizable medications have not been adequately assessed. Budesonide inhalation suspension should be administered separately in the nebulizer.

➤*Storage / Stability:*

Powder for inhalation – Store with the cover tightened in a dry place at controlled room temperature 20° to 25°C (68° to 77°F). Keep out of the reach of children.

Inhalation suspension – Budesonide inhalation suspension should be stored upright at controlled room temperature 20° to 25°C (68° to 77°F), and protected from light. When an envelope has been opened, the shelf life of the unused inhalation suspension is 2 weeks when protected. After opening the aluminum foil envelope, the unused inhalation suspension should be returned to the aluminum foil envelope to protect them from light. Any opened inhalation suspension must be used promptly. Gently shake the inhalation suspension using a circular motion before use. Keep out of reach of children. Do not freeze.

FLUNISOLIDE

Rx	**AeroSpan** (Forest)	**Aerosol:** ≈ 80 mcg flunisolide hemihydrate (78 mcg flunisolide)/ actuation	In 5.1 and 8.9 g cannisters (60 and 120 metered actuations, respectively).
Rx	**AeroBid** (Forest)	**Aerosol:** ≈ 250 mcg/actuation	In canisters (100 metered doses).
Rx	**AeroBid-M** (Forest)		Menthol flavor. In canisters (100 metered doses).

FLUNISOLIDE HEMIHYDRATE — INHALATION

Indications

➤*Asthma, chronic:* For the maintenance treatment of asthma as prophylactic therapy in adult and pediatric patients 6 years of age and older. It is also indicated for asthma patients requiring oral corticosteroid therapy, where adding flunisolide HFA inhalation aerosol may reduce or eliminate the need for oral corticosteroids.

Administration and Dosage

Flunisolide should be administered by the orally inhaled route in asthmatic patients 6 years of age and older. The onset and degree of symptom relief with orally inhaled corticosteroids is usually apparent within 2 to 4 weeks after the start of treatment, and varies with individual patients. The time to improvement in asthma control was not evaluated in clinical studies with flunisolide inhalation aerosol. For patients who do not respond adequately to the starting dose after 3 to 4 weeks of therapy, higher doses may provide additional asthma control. The safety and efficacy of flunisolide inhalation aerosol when administered in excess of recommended doses have not been established.

➤*Dosing:* In all patients, it is desirable to titrate to the lowest effective dose once asthma stability is achieved.

Adults (12 years of age and older) – The recommended starting dose is 160 mcg twice daily. The maximum dose should not exceed 320 mcg twice daily. Higher doses have not been studied.

Children (6 to 11 years of age) – The recommended starting dose is 80 mcg twice daily. The maximum dose should not exceed 160 mcg twice daily. Higher doses have not been studied. Pediatric patients should administer this product under adult supervision.

➤*Therapeutic ratio between flunisolide HFA and flunisolide CFC inhalation:* The recommended dosage of flunisolide HFA inhalation aerosol relative to flunisolide CFC inhalation aerosol is lower due to differences in delivery characteristics between the products. Recognizing that a definitive comparative therapeutic ratio between flunisolide HFA inhalation aerosol and flunisolide CFC inhalation aerosol has not been demonstrated, any patient who is switched from flunisolide CFC inhalation aerosol to flunisolide HFA inhalation aerosol should be dosed appropriately, taking into account the dosing recommendations above, and should be monitored to ensure that the dose of flunisolide HFA inhalation aerosol selected is safe and efficacious. As with any inhaled corticosteroid, physicians are advised to select the dose that would be appropriate based upon the patient's disease severity and titrate the dose of flunisolide HFA inhalation aerosol downward over time to the lowest level that maintains proper asthma control.

➤*Concomitant systemic corticosteroid therapy:* Clinical studies with flunisolide hemihydrate HFA inhalation aerosol did not evaluate patients on oral corticosteroids. However, clinical studies with therapeutic doses of flunisolide CFC inhalation aerosol did show efficacy in the management of asthmatics dependent or maintained on systemic corticosteroids.

If a patient is already on a systemic corticosteroid for asthma control, flunisolide HFA inhalation aerosol should be used concurrently with the patient's usual maintenance dose of oral corticosteroid before an attempt is made to withdraw systemic corticosteroid. The patient's asthma should be reasonably stable before withdrawal of oral corticosteroid is initiated. After approximately one week, gradual withdrawal of the systemic corticosteroid may be started by reducing the daily or alternate daily dose. The next reduction may be made after an interval of one or two weeks, depending on the response of the patients. In general, these decrements should not exceed 2.5 mg of prednisone or its equivalent. A slow rate of withdrawal is strongly recommended. During reduction of oral corticosteroids, patients should be carefully monitored for asthma instability, including objective measures of airway function, and for adrenal insufficiency. During their withdrawal from a systemic corticosteroid, some patients may experience symptoms of systemic corticosteroid withdrawal, e.g., joint and/or musculoskeletal pain, lassitude and depression, despite maintenance or even improvements in pulmonary function. Such patients should be encouraged to continue with flunisolide HFA inhalation aerosol and should be monitored for objective signs of adrenal insufficiency. If evidence of adrenal insufficiency occurs, the systemic corticosteroid doses should be increased temporarily and thereafter withdrawal should continue more slowly. During periods of stress or a severe asthma attack, patients being transferred may require supplementary treatment with a systemic corticosteroid.

➤*Storage / Stability:* Store at 25°C (77°F); excursions permitted to 15° to 30°C (59° to 86°F). For best results, the canister should be at room temperature before use.

FLUNISOLIDE — INHALATION

For complete and comparative prescribing information, refer to the Corticosteroids Respiratory Inhalant group monograph.

WARNING

Particular care is needed in patients who are transferred from systemically active corticosteroids to flunisolide inhaler because deaths due to adrenal insufficiency have occurred in asthmatic patients during and after transfer from systemic corticosteroids to aerosol corticosteroids. After withdrawal from systemic corticosteroids, a number of months are required for recovery of hypothalamic-pituitary-adrenal (HPA) function. During this period of HPA suppression, patients may exhibit signs and symptoms of adrenal insufficiency when exposed to trauma, surgery or infections, particularly gastroenteritis. Although flunisolide inhaler may provide control of asthmatic symptoms during these episodes, it does not provide the systemic steroid that is necessary for coping with these emergencies. During periods of stress or a severe asthmatic attack, patients who have been withdrawn from systemic corticosteroids should be instructed to resume systemic steroids (in large doses) immediately and to contact their physician for further instruction. These patients should also be instructed to carry a warning card indicating that they may need supplementary systemic steroids during periods of stress or a severe asthma attack. To assess the risk of adrenal insufficiency in emergency situations, routine tests of adrenal cortical function, including measurement of early morning resting cortisol levels, should be performed periodically in all patients. An early morning resting cortisol level may be accepted as normal if it falls at or near the normal mean level.

Indications

➤*Asthma, chronic:* Maintenance treatment of asthma as prophylactic therapy. Flunisolide is also indicated for asthma patients who require systemic corticosteroid administration, where adding flunisolide may reduce or eliminate the need for the systemic corticosteroids.

Administration and Dosage

➤*Approved by the FDA:* August 17, 1984.

Flunisolide inhaler is for oral inhalation only. Rinsing the mouth after inhalation is advised.

➤*Adults:* The recommended starting dose is 2 inhalations twice daily, morning and evening, for a total daily dose of 1 mg. The maximum daily dose should not exceed 4 inhalations twice a day for a total daily dose of 2 mg. When the drug is used chronically at 2 mg/day, patients should be monitored periodically for effects on the hypothalamic-pituitary-adrenal (HPA) axis.

➤*Pediatric patients:* For children and adolescents 6 to 15 years of age, 2 inhalations may be administered twice daily for a total daily dose of 1 mg. Higher doses have not been studied. Insufficient information is available to warrant use in children under age 6. With chronic use, pediatric patients should be monitored for growth as well as for effects on the HPA axis.

➤*Patients not receiving systemic corticosteroids:* Patients who require maintenance therapy of their asthma may benefit from treatment with flunisolide at the doses recommended above. In patients who respond to flunisolide, improvement in pulmonary function is usually apparent within 1 to 4 weeks after the start of therapy. Once the desired effect is achieved, consideration should be given to tapering to the lowest effective dose.

➤*Patients maintained on systemic corticosteroids:* Clinical studies have shown that flunisolide may be effective in the management of asthmatics dependent or maintained on systemic corticosteroids and may permit replacement or significant reduction in the dosage of systemic corticosteroids. The patient's asthma should be reasonably stable before treatment with flunisolide is started. Initially, flunisolide should be used concurrently with the patient's usual maintenance dose of systemic corticosteroid. After approximately 1 week, gradual withdrawal of the systemic corticosteroid is started by reducing the daily or alternate daily dose. Reductions may be made after an interval of 1 or 2 weeks, depending on the response of the patient. A slow rate of withdrawal is strongly recommended. Generally, these decrements should not exceed 2.5 mg of prednisone or its equivalent. During withdrawal, some patients may experience symptoms of systemic corticosteroid withdrawal (eg, joint or muscular pain, lassitude and depression, despite maintenance or even improvement of pulmonary function). Such patients should be encouraged to continue with the inhaler but should be monitored for objective signs of adrenal insufficiency. If evidence of adrenal insufficiency occurs, the systemic corticosteroid doses should be increased temporarily and thereafter withdrawal should continue more slowly.

During periods of stress or a severe asthma attack, transfer patients may require supplementary treatment with systemic corticosteroids.

FLUTICASONE PROPIONATE

Rx	**Flovent HFA** (GlaxoSmithKline)	**Aerosol:** 44 mcg/actuation	In 10.6 g canister containing 120 metered inhalations. With actuator.
		110 mcg/actuation	In 12 g canister containing 120 metered inhalations. With actuator.
		220 mcg/actuation	In 12 g canister containing 120 metered inhalations. With actuator.
Rx	**Flovent Rotadisk** (GlaxoSmithKline)	**Powder for inhalation:** 50 mcg/actuation	Lactose. In 4 blisters containing 15 *Rotadisks* with inhalation device.
		100 mcg/actuation	Lactose. In 4 blisters containing 15 *Rotadisks* with inhalation device.
		250 mcg/actuation	Lactose. In 4 blisters containing 15 *Rotadisks* with inhalation device.
Rx	**Flovent Diskus** (GlaxoSmithKline)	**Powder for inhalation:** 50 mcg/actuation	In inhalation device containing 28 or 60 blisters.
		100 mcg/actuation	In inhalation device containing 28 or 60 blisters.
		250 mcg/actuation	In inhalation device containing 28 or 60 blisters.

FLUTICASONE PROPIONATE — INHALATION

For complete and comparative prescribing information, refer to the Corticosteroids Respiratory Inhalant group monograph.

WARNING

Particular care is needed for patients who are transferred from systematically active corticosteroids to fluticasone propionate because deaths because of adrenal insufficiency have occurred in patients with asthma during and after transfer from systemic corticosteroids to less systemically available inhaled corticosteroids. After withdrawal from systemic corticosteroids, a number of months are required for recovery of hypothalamic-pituitary-adrenal (HPA) function.

Patients who have been previously maintained on 20 mg/day or more of prednisone (or its equivalent) may be most susceptible, particularly when their systemic corticosteroids have been almost completely withdrawn. During this period of HPA suppression, patients may exhibit signs and symptoms of adrenal insufficiency when exposed to trauma, surgery, or infection (particularly gastroenteritis) or other conditions associated with severe electrolyte loss. Although fluticasone propionate inhalation may provide control of asthma symptoms during these episodes, in recommended doses it supplies less than normal physiological amounts of glucocorticoid systemically and does not provide the mineralocorticoid activity that is necessary for coping with these emergencies.

During periods of stress or a severe asthma attack, patients who have been withdrawn from systemic corticosteroids should be instructed to resume oral corticosteroids (in large doses) immediately and to contact their physicians for further instruction. These patients should also be instructed to carry a warning card indicating that they may need supplementary systemic corticosteroids during periods of stress or a severe asthma attack.

Indications

➤*Asthma, chronic:* For the maintenance treatment of asthma as prophylactic therapy in patients 4 years of age and older. Also indicated for patients requiring oral corticosteroid therapy for asthma. Many of these patients may be able to reduce or eliminate their requirement for oral corticosteroids over time.

Fluticasone is not indicated for relief of acute bronchospasm.

Administration and Dosage

➤*Approved by the FDA:* March 27, 1996.

Advise patients to rinse mouth after inhalation.

Fluticasone should be administered by the orally inhaled route only in patients 4 years of age and older. Individual patients will experience a variable time to onset and degree of symptom relief. Maximum benefit may not be achieved for 1 to 2 weeks or longer after starting treatment.

After asthma stability has been achieved, titrate to the lowest effective dose to reduce side effect possibility. For patients not responding adequately to the starting dose after 2 weeks, higher doses may provide additional asthma control. The safety and efficacy of fluticasone when administered in excess of recommended dosages have not been established.

➤*Fluticasone aerosol:*

Recommended Doses for Fluticasone Aerosol

Previous therapy	Recommended starting dose	Highest recommended dose
Adolescent and adult patients (≥ 12 years)		
Bronchodilators alone	88 mcg twice daily	440 mcg twice daily
Inhaled corticosteroids	88 to 220 mcg twice daily[a]	440 mcg twice daily
Oral corticosteroids[b]	440 mcg twice daily	880 mcg twice daily

FLUTICASONE PROPIONATE — INHALATION

Recommended Doses for Fluticasone Aerosol		
Previous therapy	Recommended starting dose	Highest recommended dose
Pediatric patients (4 to 11 years)[c]		
	88 mcg twice daily	88 mcg twice daily

[a] For patients currently receiving inhaled corticosteroid therapy: Starting doses more than 88 mcg twice daily may be considered for patients with poorer asthma control or those who have previously required doses of inhaled corticosteroids that are in the higher range for that specific agent.
[b] For patients currently receiving chronic oral corticosteroid therapy: Prednisone should be reduced no faster than 2.5 to 5 mg/day on a weekly basis, beginning after at least 1 week of therapy with fluticasone. Patients should be carefully monitored for signs of asthma instability, including serial objective measures of airflow, and for signs of adrenal insufficiency. Once prednisone reduction is complete, the dosage of fluticasone should be reduced to the lowest effective dosage.
[c] Recommended pediatric dosage is 88 mcg twice daily regardless of prior therapy.

Priming – Fluticasone aerosol should be primed before using for the first time by releasing 4 test sprays into the air away from the face, shaking well before each spray. In cases where the inhaler has not been used for more than 7 days or when it has been dropped, prime the inhaler again by shaking well and releasing 1 test spray into the air away from the face.

Elderly – In studies where elderly patients (65 years of age or older) have been treated with fluticasone propionate inhalation aerosol, efficacy and safety did not differ from that in younger patients. Based on available data for fluticasone, no dosage adjustment is recommended.

➤*Fluticasone powder:*

Recommended Doses for Fluticasone Powder		
Previous therapy	Recommended starting dose	Highest recommended dose
Adults and adolescents		
Bronchodilators alone	100 mcg twice daily	500 mcg twice daily
Inhaled corticosteroids	100-250 mcg twice daily[a]	500 mcg twice daily
Oral corticosteroids	500[b]-1000 mcg twice daily	1,000 mcg twice daily
Children 4 to 11 years of age		
Bronchodilators alone	50 mcg twice daily	100 mcg twice daily
Inhaled corticosteroids	50 mcg twice daily	100 mcg twice daily

[a] Starting doses more than 100 mcg twice daily for adults and adolescents and 50 mcg twice daily for children 4 to 11 years of age may be considered for patients with poorer asthma control or those who have previously required doses of inhaled corticosteroids that are in the higher range for that specific agent.
[b] Designated with the *Diskus*.

Concomitant systemic corticosteroid therapy – For patients currently receiving chronic oral corticosteroids, reduce prednisone no faster than 2.5 mg/day on a weekly basis, beginning after at least 1 week of aerosol therapy. Monitor patients for signs of asthma instability, including serial objective measures of airflow, and for signs of adrenal insufficiency. Decrease fluticasone dosage to the lowest effective dose once prednisone reduction is complete (see Administration in group monograph).

➤*Children:* Because individual responses may vary, children previously maintained on fluticasone propionate *Rotadisk* 50 or 100 mcg twice daily may require dosage adjustments upon transfer to the fluticasone propionate *Diskus*.

➤*Storage/Stability:* Shake well before using. Store aerosol at 25°C (77°F); excursions permitted to 15° to 30°C (59° to 86°F). Store powder at 20° to 25°C (68° to 77°F) in a dry place. Store aerosol canister with mouthpiece down. Do not spray in eyes. Do not puncture or incinerate aerosol canister. For best results, the aerosol canister should be at room temperature before use. Protect from freezing and direct heat or sunlight. Use *Rotadisk* blisters within 2 months after opening the moisture-protective foil. The *Diskus* device is not reusable. Discard the *Diskus* device after 6 weeks (50 mcg strength) or 2 months (100 and 250 mcg strengths) after removal from the moisture-protective foil overwrap pouch or after all blisters have been used (when the dose indicator reads "0"), whichever comes first.

TRIAMCINOLONE ACETONIDE

Rx	**Azmacort** (Kos)	**Aerosol:** 100 mcg/actuation from spacer mouthpiece	In 20 g inhaler (60 mg triamcinolone acetonide) with actuator (≥ 240 metered doses).

TRIAMCINOLONE ACETONIDE — INHALATION

For complete and comparative prescribing information, refer to the Corticosteroids Respiratory Inhalant group monograph.

Indications

➤*Asthma, chronic:* In the maintenance treatment of asthma as prophylactic therapy; for asthma patients who require systemic corticosteroids, where adding an inhaled corticosteroid may reduce or eliminate the need for the systemic corticosteroids.

Administration and Dosage

➤*Approved by the FDA:* April 23, 1982.

Rinsing the mouth after inhalation is advised. Different considerations must be given to the following groups of patients in order to obtain the full therapeutic benefit of triamcinolone inhalation aerosol.

Note: In all patients, it is desirable to titrate to the lowest effective dose once asthma stability had been achieved.

➤*Adults:* The usual dosage is 2 inhalations (200 mcg) 3 to 4 times a day or 4 inhalations (400 mcg) twice daily. Do not exceed a maximum daily intake of 16 inhalations (1600 mcg). Higher initial doses (12 to 16 inhalations/day) may be considered in patients with more severe asthma.

➤*Children 6 to 12 years of age:* The usual dosage is 1 or 2 inhalations (100 to 200 mcg) 3 to 4 times a day or 2 to 4 inhalations (200 to 400 mcg) twice daily. Do not exceed a maximum daily intake of 12 inhalations (1200 mcg). There is insufficient information to warrant use in children less than 6 years of age.

In patients who respond to triamcinolone, improvement in pulmonary function is usually apparent within 1 to 2 weeks after the initiation of therapy. Do not increase the prescribed dosage; contact physician if symptoms do not improve or if condition worsens.

➤*Patients not receiving systemic corticosteroids:* Follow above directions. In responsive patients, an improvement in pulmonary function is usually apparent within 1 to 2 weeks.

➤*Concomitant systemic corticosteroid therapy:* See Administration in group monograph.

➤*Storage/Stability:* For best results, keep the canister at room temperature before use. Shake well before using. Do not puncture. Do not use or store near heat or open flame; exposure to greater than 48.8°C (120°F) may cause bursting. Never throw canister into fire or incinerator.

MOMETASONE FUROATE

Rx	**Asmanex Twisthaler** (Schering)	**Powder for inhalation:** 220 mcg (delivers mometasone furoate 200 mcg)/actuation	Lactose. In inhalation device of 14, 30, 60, and 120 units.

MOMETASONE FUROATE — INHALATION

Indications

➤*Asthma, chronic:* For the maintenance treatment of asthma as prophylactic therapy in patients 12 years of age and older. Mometasone also is indicated for asthma patients who require oral corticosteroid therapy, where adding mometasone therapy may reduce or eliminate the need for oral corticosteroids.

Mometasone is not indicated for the relief of acute bronchospasm.

Administration and Dosage

➤*Approved by the FDA:* March 30, 2005.

Administer mometasone by the orally inhaled route in patients 12 years of age and older. Individual patients will experience a variable time to onset and degree of symptom relief. Maximum benefit may not be achieved for 1 to 2 weeks or longer. The safety and efficacy of mometasone when administered in excess of recommended doses have not been established.

In all patients, it is desirable to titrate to the lowest effective dose once asthma stability is achieved.

Mometasone Recommended Dosages		
Previous therapy	Recommended starting dosage	Highest recommended daily dose
Bronchodilators alone	220 mcg once daily in the evening[a]	440 mcg[b]
Inhaled corticosteroids	220 mcg once daily in the evening[a]	440 mcg[b]
Oral corticosteroids[c]	440 mcg twice daily	880 mcg

[a] When administered once daily, mometasone should only be taken in the evening.
[b] The 440 mcg daily dose may be administered in divided doses of 220 mcg twice daily or as 440 mcg once daily.
[c] For patients currently receiving chronic oral corticosteroid therapy, reduce prednisone no faster than 2.5 mg/day on a weekly basis, beginning after at least 1 week of mometasone therapy. Carefully monitor patients for signs of asthma instability, including serial objective measures of airflow, and for signs of adrenal insufficiency. Once prednisone reduction is complete, reduce the dosage of mometasone to the lowest effective dosage.

MOMETASONE FUROATE — INHALATION

➤*Administration:* Instruct patients to inhale rapidly and deeply. Rinsing the mouth after inhalation is advised.

➤*Storage/Stability:* Store in a dry place at 25°C (77°F); excursions permitted to 15° to 30°C (59° to 86°F). Discard the inhaler 45 days after opening the foil pouch or when dose counter reads "00," whichever comes first.

Intranasal Steroids

For information on the systemic use of corticosteroids, refer to the Adrenal Cortical Steroids (glucocorticoids) monograph in the Endocrine and Metabolic Agents chapter.

Indications

See individual product listings for specific labeled indications.

Intranasal Steroids Indications

	Beclomethasone	Budesonide	Flunisolide	Fluticasone	Mometasone	Triamcinolone
Nasal polyps	✓[a]	X[b]		X		
Nonallergic (vasomotor) rhinitis	✓			✓		
Perennial allergic rhinitis	✓	✓	✓	✓	✓	✓
Seasonal allergic rhinitis	✓	✓	✓	✓	✓[c]	✓
Recurrent chronic sinusitis[d]		X		X	X	

[a] ✓ = Approved uses.
[b] X = Unlabeled uses.
[c] Treatment and prophylaxis.
[d] As adjunctive therapy with an antibiotic and/or decongestant.

Administration and Dosage

Please refer to the individual monographs for specific dosing information.

Use intranasal steroids at regular intervals for optimal effect.

➤*Duration of therapy:* Although some symptomatic relief may be achieved sooner, maximum benefit may not be reached until at least 2 weeks of therapy. Generally do not continue use beyond 3 weeks in the absence of significant symptomatic improvement.

Actions

➤*Pharmacology:* These drugs have potent glucocorticoid and weak mineralocorticoid activity. The mechanisms responsible for the anti-inflammatory action of corticosteroids on the nasal mucosa are unknown. However, glucocorticoids have a wide range of inhibitory activities against multiple cell types (eg, mast cells, eosinophils, neutrophils, macrophages, lymphocytes) and mediators (eg, histamine, eicosanoids, leukotrienes, cytokines) involved in allergic and nonallergic/irritant-mediated inflammation. These agents, when administered topically in recommended doses, exert direct local anti-inflammatory effects with minimal systemic effects. Exceeding the recommended dose may result in systemic effects, including hypothalamic-pituitary-adrenal (HPA) function suppression.

➤*Pharmacokinetics:*

Pharmacokinetics of Intranasal Steroids

	Corticosteroids					
Parameters	Beclomethasone	Budesonide	Flunisolide	Fluticasone	Mometasone	Triamcinolone
Bioavailability	44%	≈ 34%	50%	< 2%	Virtually undetectable	Minimal
Vd	20 L, 424 L[a]	2 to 3 L/kg	NA[b]	4.2 L/kg[c]	NA	99.5 L[c]
Protein binding	87%	85% to 90%[d]	NA	91%[c]	98% to 99%[e]	NA
Site of metabolism		Liver (CYP3A)	Liver	Liver (CYP3A4)	Liver (CYP3A4)	Liver
Metabolites (activity)	17-monopropionate (active), free beclomethasone (very weak; prodrug)	16α-hydroxyprednisolone and 6β-hydroxybudesonide (< 1% of parent)	NA	17β-carboxylic acid (inactive)	6β-hydroxymometasone furoate	6β-hydroxytriamcinolone acetonide, 21-carboxytriamcinolone acetonide, and 21-carboxy-6β-hydroxytriamcinolone acetonide (substantially < parent)
Excretion site	Feces (≈ 60%), urine (≈ 12%)[f]	Feces, urine (≈ 66%)	Feces (≈ 50%), urine (≈ 50%)	Feces (> 95%), urine (< 5%)[c]	Feces, urine	Feces (≈ 60%), urine (≈ 40%)
t½	0.5 h, 2.7 h[a,c]	2 to 3 h[c]	1 to 2 h	7.8 h[c]	5.8 h[c]	3.1 h

[a] Value for metabolite.
[b] Not available.
[c] Data from IV administration.
[d] Over a concentration range of 1 to 100 nmol/L.
[e] Over a concentration range of 5 to 500 ng/mL.
[f] Data from oral administration.

Special populations –

Hepatic function impairment: Reduced liver function may affect the elimination of corticosteroids. The systemic availability of oral **budesonide** was doubled by compromised liver function. The relevance of this finding to intranasal budesonide has not been established.

Children: Children had **budesonide** plasma concentrations approximately twice that observed in adults after intranasal administration primarily because of differences in weight.

Contraindications

Untreated localized infections involving the nasal mucosa (**flunisolide**); hypersensitivity to the drug or any component of the product.

Warnings

➤*Special senses:* Rare instances of wheezing, nasal septum perforation, cataracts, glaucoma, and increased intraocular pressure have been reported. Temporary or permanent loss of the sense of smell and taste has been reported with **flunisolide** use (see Adverse Reactions).

➤*Systemic corticosteroids:* The combined administration of alternate-day systemic prednisone with these products may increase the likelihood of HPA suppression. Therefore, use with caution in patients already on alternate-day prednisone.

Replacement of a systemic corticosteroid with intranasal corticosteroids can be accompanied by signs of adrenal insufficiency.

During withdrawal from oral corticosteroids, some patients may experience withdrawal symptoms (eg, joint or muscular pain, lassitude, depression). Carefully monitor patients previously treated with systemic corticosteroids for prolonged periods and then transferred to intranasal steroids to avoid acute adrenal insufficiency in response to stress. This is particularly important in patients who have asthma or other conditions where too rapid a decrease in systemic corticosteroids may cause a severe exacerbation of their symptoms.

➤*Excessive doses/sensitivity:* If recommended doses of intranasal **beclomethasone** are exceeded or if individuals are particularly sensitive or predisposed by virtue of recent systemic steroid therapy, symptoms of hypercorticism may occur, including, very rarely, menstrual irregularities, acneiform lesions, cataracts, and cushingoid features. If such changes occur, discontinue slowly, consistent with accepted procedures for discontinuing oral steroids. Avoid doses greater than recommended.

➤*Hypersensitivity reactions:* Rare cases of immediate and delayed hypersensitivity reactions, including angioedema, bronchospasm, rash, and urticaria have been reported after intranasal administration of corticosteroids. Refer to Management of Acute Hypersensitivity Reactions.

➤*Hepatic function impairment:* Reduced liver function may affect the elimination of corticosteroids. The systemic availability of oral **budesonide** was doubled by compromised liver function. The relevance of this finding to intranasal budesonide has not been established.

➤*Carcinogenesis:*

Flunisolide: Flunisolide was administered to mice at doses of 5, 50, and 500 mcg/kg/day and to rats at doses of 0.5, 1, and 2.5 mcg/kg/day. There was an increased incidence of benign pulmonary adenomas in mice but not rats. Female rats receiving the highest oral dose had an increased incidence of mammary adenocarcinoma compared with control rats.

Budesonide: Budesonide caused a significant increase in the incidence of gliomas and hepatocellular tumors in the male rats receiving an oral dose of 50 mcg/kg (approximately twice the maximum recommended daily intranasal dose in adults and children on a mcg/m^2 basis, respectively).

➤*Fertility impairment:*
Beclomethasone: In rats, beclomethasone caused decreased conception rates at an oral dose of 16 mg/kg (approximately 390 times the intranasal maximum recommended daily dose [MRDD] in adults on a mg/m^2 basis). There was no significant effect of beclomethasone on fertility in rats at oral doses of 1.6 mg/kg (approximately 40 times the intranasal MRDD in adults on a mg/m^2 basis). Inhibition of the estrous cycle in dogs was observed following oral dosing at 0.5 mg/kg (approximately 40 times the intranasal MRDD in adults on a mg/m^2 basis). No inhibition of the estrous cycle in dogs was seen following 12 months exposure at an estimated inhalation dose of 0.33 mg/kg (approximately 25 times the intranasal MRDD in adults on a mg/m^2 basis).
Budesonide: In rats at SC doses of 20 mcg/kg and above (less than the intranasal MRDD in adults on a mcg/m^2 basis), budesonide caused a decrease in prenatal viability and viability of the pups at birth and during lactation, along with a decrease in maternal body-weight gain. No such effects were noted at 5 mcg/kg (less than the intranasal MRDD in adults on a mcg/m^2 basis).
Flunisolide: Female rats receiving high doses of flunisolide (200 mcg/kg/day or 1180 mcg/m^2 body surface area) showed some evidence of impaired fertility.
Triamcinolone: Triamcinolone acetonide caused increased fetal resorptions and stillbirths and decreases in pup weight and survival at doses of 5 mcg/kg and above (approximately one fifth the intranasal MRDD in adults on a mcg/m^2 basis). Doses of 1 mcg/kg did not include the above mentioned effects.

➤*Elderly:* In general, use caution in dose selection for an elderly patient, starting at the low end of the dosing range, reflecting greater frequency of decreased hepatic, renal, or cardiac function, and concomitant disease or other drug therapy.

➤*Pregnancy: Category C.* There are no adequately controlled trials in pregnant women. However, animal studies have demonstrated teratogenic, fetotoxic, and embryocidal effects. Topical administration of recommended doses is unlikely to achieve significant systemic levels; however, use these agents during pregnancy only if the potential benefits outweigh the potential hazards to the fetus.

Carefully observe infants born of mothers who have received substantial doses of corticosteroids during pregnancy for signs of adrenal insufficiency.

➤*Lactation:* It is not known whether these drugs are excreted in breast milk. Because other corticosteroids are excreted in human milk, use caution when administering to nursing women.

➤*Children:*

Beclomethasone, budesonide, flunisolide, triamcinolone – Safety and efficacy for use in children younger than 6 years of age have not been established.

Fluticasone – Safety and efficacy for use in children younger than 4 years of age have not been established.

Mometasone – Safety and efficacy for use in children younger than 2 years of age have not been established. Controlled clinical studies have shown that intranasal corticosteroids may cause a reduction in growth velocity in pediatric patients. This effect has been observed in the absence of laboratory evidence of HPA axis suppression, suggesting that growth velocity is a more sensitive indicator of systemic corticosteroid exposure in pediatric patients than some commonly used tests of HPA-axis function. The long-term effects of this reduction in growth velocity associated with intranasal corticosteroids, including the impact on final adult height, are unknown. The potential for "catch-up" growth following discontinuation of treatment with intranasal corticosteroids has not been adequately studied. Routinely monitor the growth of pediatric patients receiving intranasal corticosteroids (eg, via stadiometry). Weigh the potential growth effects of prolonged treatment against the clinical benefits obtained and the risks/benefits of treatment alternatives. To minimize the systemic effects of intranasal corticosteroids, titrate each patient to the lowest dose that effectively controls his/her symptoms.

Precautions

➤*Monitoring:* Routinely monitor the growth of pediatric patients receiving intranasal corticosteriods (eg, via stadiometry). Carefully monitor patients previously treated for prolonged periods with systemic corticosteroids and then transferred to topical corticosteroids for acute adrenal insufficiency in response to stress. Examine periodically for evidence of *Candida* infection or other signs of adverse effects on the nasal mucosa.

➤*Nasopharyngeal irritation:* If persistent nasopharyngeal irritation occurs, it may be an indication to stop therapy.

➤*Infections:* Localized infections of the nose and pharynx with *Candida albicans* have developed only rarely. When such an infection occurs, it may require treatment with appropriate local or systemic therapy and/or discontinuation of steroid treatment.

Use with caution, if at all, in patients with active or quiescent tuberculosis infections of the respiratory tract, or in untreated fungal, bacterial, or systemic viral infections, or ocular herpes simplex.

Individuals receiving immunosuppressant agents are more susceptible to infections than healthy individuals. For example, chickenpox and measles can have a more serious or fatal course in susceptible children or adults receiving immunosuppressant doses of corticosteroids. Take particular care to avoid exposure in children or adults who have not had these diseases or who have not been properly immunized. Prophylaxis with varicella-zoster immune globulin (VZIG) may be indicated if exposed to chickenpox. If an individual is exposed to measles, prophylaxis with pooled immunoglobulin may be indicated. Consider treatment with antiviral agents if chickenpox develops.

➤*Wound healing:* Because of the inhibitory effect of corticosteroids on wound healing, do not use nasal steroids in patients who have experienced recent nasal septal ulcers, recurrent epistaxis, or nasal surgery or trauma until healing has occurred.

➤*Vasoconstrictors:* In the presence of excessive nasal mucosa secretion or edema of the nasal mucosa, the drug may fail to reach the site of intended action. In such cases, use a nasal vasoconstrictor during the first 2 to 3 days of therapy.

➤*Systemic effects:* Although systemic effects are low when used in recommended dosage, HPA suppression and other systemic effects may occur, especially with excessive doses.

➤*Long-term treatment:* Examine patients periodically over several months or longer for possible changes in the nasal mucosa.

Drug Interactions

Intranasal Corticosteroid Drug Interactions

Precipitant drug	Object drug[a]		Description
Cimetidine	Budesonide	⬆	Coadministration caused a slight decrease in budesonide clearance and a corresponding increase in its oral bioavailability.
Inhibitors of CYP3A4 (eg, ketoconazole, itraconazole, clarithromycin, erythromycin, cimetidine, ritonavir)	Budesonide Fluticasone	⬆	Concomitant administration may inhibit metabolism and increase systemic exposure of the intranasal steroid. After oral administration of ketoconazole, the mean plasma concentration of oral budesonide increased by more than 7-fold. Coadministration of oral ritonavir and intranasal fluticasone resulted in a significant increase in fluticasone plasma concentrations resulting in possible Cushing syndrome and adrenal suppression. Use with caution.

[a] ⬆ = Object drug increased.

Adverse Reactions

Intranasal Corticosteroid Adverse Reactions (%)[a]

Adverse reaction	Beclomethasone	Budesonide	Flunisolide (nasal solution)	Flunisolide (nasal spray)	Fluticasone	Mometasome	Triamcinolone
CNS							
Dizziness					1 to 3		
Headache	< 5		≤ 5		7 to 16	17 to 26	≥ 2
Lightheadedness	< 5						
GI							
Abdominal pain					1 to 3		
Diarrhea					1 to 3	2 to < 5	
Dyspepsia						2 to < 5	
Nausea	< 5		≤ 5	> 1	3 to 5	2 to < 5	
Vomiting			≤ 5		3 to 5	1 to 5	≥ 2

Intranasal Corticosteroid Adverse Reactions (%)[a]							
Adverse reaction	Beclomethasone	Budesonide	Flunisolide (nasal solution)	Flunisolide (nasal spray)	Fluticasone	Mometasome	Triamcinolone
Hypersensitivity reactions							
Anaphylaxis					Rare[b]	✓[b,c]	
Angioedema	Rare	Rare[b]			Rare[b]	✓[b]	
Bronchospasm	Rare				Rare[b]		
Dyspnea					Rare[b]		
Edema of face/tongue					Rare[b]		
Pruritus					Rare[b]		
Rash	Rare				Rare[b]		
Wheezing	Rare	Rare			Rare[b]	2 to < 5	
Urticaria	Rare				Rare[b]		
Respiratory							
Asthma symptoms					3 to 7	2 to < 5	≥ 2
Bronchitis					1 to 3	2 to < 5	
Bronchospasm		2					
Cough		2		> 1	4	7 to 13	2
Epistaxis	< 3	8	≤ 5[d]	3 to 9	6 to 7[d]	8 to 11[d]	3
Mild nasopharyngeal irritation	24						
Nasal burning/stinging			45	13	2 to 3	✓[b]	
Nasal dryness	✓			> 1			
Nasal irritation	✓	2	≤ 5		2 to 3	2 to < 5	
Nasal mucosal ulceration	Rare				Rare[b]	Rare	
Nasal septal perforation	Rare	Rare[b]	Rare	Rare	Rare[b]	Rare[b]	Rare
Nasal stuffiness/ congestion	< 3		≤ 5				
Rhinitis						2 to < 5	≥ 2
Pharyngitis		4		> 1	6 to 8	10 to 12	5
Rhinorrhea	< 3				1 to 3		
Sinusitis				≤ 1		4 to 5	≥ 2
Sneezing	4		≤ 5				
Throat discomfort (burning, itching, swelling, pain)		Rare[b]	≤ 5		Rare[b]		
Throat dryness/irritation	✓	Rare[b]			Rare[b]		
Upper respiratory tract infection						5 to 7	
Special senses							
Aftertaste				17			
Blurred vision					✓[b]		
Cataracts	Rare				Rare[b]		
Conjunctivitis					✓[b]	2 to < 5	
Dry/irritated eyes					✓[b]		
Earache						2 to < 5	
Glaucoma	Rare				Rare[b]		
Hoarseness				≤ 1	Rare[b]		
Increased intraocular pressure	Rare	Rare			Rare[b]	Rare	
Loss of taste/smell	Rare	Rare[b]	≤ 5	≤ 1	✓[b]	Rare[b]	
Otitis media						2 to < 5	≥ 2
Unpleasant taste/smell	✓						
Watery eyes	< 3		≤ 5				
Miscellaneous							
Aches and pains					1 to 3		
Arthralgia						2 to < 5	
Chest pain						2 to < 5	
Dysmenorrhea						1 to 5	
Fever					1 to 3		
Flu-like symptoms					1 to 3	2 to < 5	
Growth suppression	✓	✓			✓[b]		
Infection	Rare[e]	Rare[e]	Rare[e]	Rare[e]	Rare[e]	Rare[e]	Rare[e]
Myalgia						2 to < 5	
Palpitations		Rare[b]					

Intranasal Corticosteroid Adverse Reactions (%)[a]							
Adverse reaction	Beclomethasone	Budesonide	Flunisolide (nasal solution)	Flunisolide (nasal spray)	Fluticasone	Mometasome	Triamcinolone
Viral infection						8 to 14	
Voice changes					Rare[b]		

[a] Data pooled from all age groups and from separate studies and are not necessarily comparable.
[b] Occurred during postmarketing.
[c] ✓ = Reported; no incidence given.
[d] Including bloody mucus.
[e] Localized infections of the nose and pharynx with *Candida albicans*.

Overdosage

Acute overdosage is unlikely with intranasal corticosteroids. However, chronic overdosage may occur and result in hypercorticism and adrenal suppression. If such symptoms occur, slowly discontinue intranasal corticosteroids consistent with accepted procedures for discontinuing oral steroid therapy.

Patient Information

Instruct patients to read the patient instructions provided with the product.

Advise patients that effects may not be immediate and not to exceed the recommended dosage. Benefit requires regular use and usually occurs within a few days. One to 2 weeks may pass before full effect is achieved.

Advise patients to contact their health care provider if symptoms worsen or do not improve by 3 weeks of treatment.

Instruct patients to clear nasal passages before use. If nasal passages are blocked, use of a topical nasal decongestant 5 to 10 minutes prior to administering the intranasal steroid may be beneficial.

Instruct patients to shake bottle gently before each use. Patients will also need to prime the pump the first time it is used and if it has not been used for more than a week.

Instruct patients to close the other nostril with a finger and tilt head slightly forward while using.

Advise patients to avoid blowing nose for at least 10 to 15 minutes after use.

Advise patients to avoid spraying into eyes or directly into nasal septum.

Advise patients not to use the bottle for more than the labeled number of sprays, even if the bottle is not completely empty.

Advise patients on immunosuppressant doses of corticosteroids to avoid exposure to chicken pox or measles and to seek medical advice if exposed.

Advise patients to contact their health care provider if they experience recurrent episodes of epistaxis or nasal septum discomfort.

FLUNISOLIDE

Rx	**Flunisolide** (Bausch & Lomb)	**Solution:** 0.025% (25 mcg/actuation)[a]	In 25 mL nasal pump dispenser (200 sprays/bottle).
Rx	**Nasarel** (Ivax Laboratories)	**Spray:** 0.025% (29 mcg/actuation)[b]	In 25 mL spray bottles (200 sprays/bottle) with meter pump and nasal adapter.

[a] With propylene glycol, polyethylene glycol 3350, benzalkonium chloride, EDTA.
[b] With 0.01% benzalkonium chloride, butylated hydroxytoluene, EDTA, polyethylene glycol 400, sorbitol.

FLUNISOLIDE — INTRANASAL

For complete and comparative prescribing information, refer to the Intranasal Steroids group monograph.

Indications

➤*Allergic rhinitis:* For the relief and management of nasal symptoms of seasonal and perennial allergic rhinitis.

Administration and Dosage

➤*Approved by the FDA:* March 8, 1995.

Encourage patients with blocked nasal passages to use a decongestant just before administration to ensure adequate penetration of the spray. Advise patients to clear their nasal passages of secretions prior to use.

➤*Adults:* 2 sprays in each nostril 2 times/day. The dose may be increased to 2 sprays in each nostril 3 times/day.

➤*Children 6 to 14 years of age:* 1 spray in each nostril 3 times/day or 2 sprays in each nostril 2 times/day.

➤*Maximum dose:*

Adults – 8 sprays in each nostril per day.

Children 6 to 14 years of age – 4 sprays in each nostril per day.

➤*Maintenance dose:* After the desired clinical effect is obtained, reduce the maintenance dose to the smallest amount necessary to control symptoms. Some patients with perennial allergic rhinitis may be maintained on 1 spray in each nostril per day.

➤*Duration:* Improvement in symptoms usually becomes apparent within a few days. However, relief may not occur in some patients for as long as 2 weeks. Do not use for more than 3 weeks in absence of significant symptomatic improvement.

➤*Priming:* Before use, prime the nasal spray by pushing down on the pump 5 or 6 times until a fine mist appears. If the pump has not been used for 5 days or more, the spray must be primed again.

➤*Storage/Stability:* Store between 15° and 30°C (59° and 86°F).

BECLOMETHASONE DIPROPIONATE

Rx	**Beconase AQ** (GlaxoSmithKline)	**Spray:** 0.042% (42 mcg/actuation)[a]	In 25 g bottles (180 metered doses per bottle) with metering atomizing pump and nasal adapter.

[a] With dextrose, polysorbate 80, benzalkonium chloride, 0.25% v/w phenylethyl alcohol.

BECLOMETHASONE DIPROPIONATE — INTRANASAL

For complete and comparative prescribing information, refer to the Intranasal Steroids group monograph.

Indications

➤*Rhinitis:* For the relief of symptoms of seasonal or perennial allergic and nonallergic (vasomotor) rhinitis.

Results from 2 clinical trials have shown that significant symptom relief was obtained within 3 days. However, symptom relief may not occur in some patients for as long as 2 weeks.

➤*Nasal polyps:* For the prevention of recurrence of nasal polyps following surgical removal.

Administration and Dosage

➤*Approved by the FDA:* July 27, 1987.

➤*Adults and children greater than or equal to 12 years of age:* 1 or 2 nasal inhalations (42 to 84 mcg) in each nostril twice a day (total dose, 168 to 336 mcg/day).

➤*Children 6 to 12 years of age:* Patients should be started with 1 nasal inhalation in each nostril twice daily; patients not adequately responding to 168 mcg or those with more severe symptoms may use 336 mcg (2 inhalations in each nostril). Once adequate control is achieved, the dosage should be decreased to 84 mcg (1 spray in each nostril) twice daily. Beclomethasone dipropionate intranasal is not recommended for children below 6 years of age.

The maximum total daily dosage should not exceed 2 sprays in each nostril twice daily (336 mcg/day).

In the presence of excessive nasal mucus secretion or edema of the nasal mucosa, the drug may fail to reach the sites of intended action. In such cases it is advisable to use a topical or oral nasal vasoconstrictor/decongestant during the first 2 to 3 days of beclomethasone dipropionate intranasal therapy.

➤*Directions for use:* Illustrated patient's instructions for proper use accompany each package of beclomethasone dipropionate intranasal.

➤*Storage/Stability:* Store between 15° and 30°C (59° and 86°F).

TRIAMCINOLONE ACETONIDE

Rx	**Nasacort AQ** (Aventis)	**Spray:** 55 mcg/actuation[a]	In 6.5 and 16.5 g bottles (providing 30 and 120 actuations, respectively) with metered-dose pump unit and nasal adapter.
Rx	**Nasacort HFA** (Aventis)	**Aerosol:** 55 mcg/actuation[b]	In 9.3 g metered dose canister (providing 100 actuations) with nasal actuator.

[a] With polysorbate 80, dextrose, benzalkonium chloride, and EDTA.
[b] In tetrafluoroethane (HFA-134a) and dehydrated alcohol 0.7%.

TRIAMCINOLONE ACETONIDE — INTRANASAL

For complete and comparative prescribing information, refer to the Intranasal Steroids group monograph.

Indications

➤*Allergic rhinitis:* For the treatment of the symptoms of seasonal and perennial allergic rhinitis in adults and children 6 years of age and older.

Administration and Dosage

➤*Approved by the FDA:* July 11, 1991.

➤*Adults and children 12 years of age or older:*

Nasal spray – The recommended starting and maximum dose is 220 mcg/day as 2 sprays in each nostril once daily.

Nasal inhaler – The recommended starting dose of triamcinolone acetonide nasal inhaler is 220 mcg/day given as 2 sprays (55 mcg/spray) in each nostril once a day. If needed, the dose may be increased to 440 mcg/day (55 mcg/spray) either as once-a-day dosage or divided up to 4 times a day (ie, twice a day, 2 sprays/nostril), or 4 times a day (1 spray/nostril). After the desired effect is obtained, some patients may be maintained on a dose of as little as 1 spray (55 mcg) in each nostril once a day (total daily dose 110 mcg/day).

➤*Children 6 to 11 years of age:*

Nasal spray – The recommended starting dose is 110 mcg/day given as 1 spray in each nostril once daily. The maximum recommended dose is 220 mcg/day as 2 sprays/nostril once daily.

Nasal inhaler – The recommended starting dose of triamcinolone acetonide nasal inhaler is 220 mcg/day given as 2 sprays (55 mcg/spray) in each nostril once a day. Once the maximal effect has been achieved, it is always desirable to titrate the patient to the minimum effective dose.

➤*Children less than 6 years of age:* Triamcinolone acetonide is not recommended for children less than 6 years of age since adequate numbers of patients have not been studied in this age group.

➤*Individualization of dosage:*

Nasal spray – It is always desirable to titrate an individual patient to the minimum effective dose to reduce the possibility of side effects. In adults, when the maximum benefit has been achieved and symptoms have been controlled, reducing the dose to 110 mcg/day (1 spray in each nostril once a day) has been shown to be effective in maintaining control of the allergic rhinitis symptoms in patients who were initially controlled at 220 mcg/day.

In children 6 to 11 years of age, the recommended starting dose is 110 mcg/day given as 1 spray in each nostril once daily. The maximum recommended daily dose in children 6 to 11 years of age is 220 mcg/day (2 sprays in each nostril once daily). Some patients who do not achieve maximum symptom control at a dose of 110 mcg/day may benefit from a dose of 220 mcg given as 2 sprays in each nostril once daily. The minimum effective dose should be used to ensure continued control of symptoms. Once symptoms are controlled, pediatric patients may be able to be maintained on 110 mcg/day (1 spray in each nostril once daily).

An improvement in some patient symptoms may be seen within the first day of treatment, and generally, it takes 1 week of treatment to reach maximum benefit. Initial assessment for response should be made during this time frame and periodically until the patient's symptoms are stabilized. If adequate relief of symptoms has not been obtained after 3 weeks of treatment, triamcinolone acetonide should be discontinued.

Nasal inhaler – A decrease in symptoms may occur as soon as 12 hours after starting steroid therapy and generally can be expected to occur within a few days of initiating therapy in allergic rhinitis. If improvement is not evident after 2 to 3 weeks, the patients should be reevaluated.

➤*Storage/Stability:* Store at controlled room temperature, 20° to 25°C (68° to 77°F).

Nasal inhaler, pressurized canister, and aerosol – Avoid spraying in eyes. Do not puncture. Do not store or use near heat or open flame. Exposure to temperatures above 49°C (120°F) may cause bursting. Never throw container into fire or incinerator. Keep out of the reach of children.

BUDESONIDE

Rx	**Rhinocort Aqua** (AstraZeneca)	**Spray:** 32 mcg/actuation[a]	In 8.6 g bottles (120 metered sprays) with metered-dose pump.

[a] Dextrose, polysorbate 80, EDTA.

BUDESONIDE — INTRANASAL

For complete and comparative prescribing information, refer to the Intranasal Steroids group monograph.

Indications

For the management of nasal symptoms of seasonal or perennial allergic rhinitis in adults and children 6 years of age and older.

Administration and Dosage

➤*Approved by the FDA:* October 1, 1999.

The recommended starting dose for adults and children 6 years of age and older is 64 mcg/day administered as 1 spray per nostril of 32 mcg budesonide nasal spray once daily. The maximum recommended dose for adults (12 years of age and older) is 256 mcg/day administered as 4 sprays per nostril once daily of 32 mcg budesonide nasal spray, and the maximum recommended dose for children (younger than 12 years of age) is 128 mcg/day administered as 2 sprays per nostril once daily of 32 mcg budesonide nasal spray.

Prior to initial use, shake the container gently and prime the pump by actuating 8 times. If used daily, the pump does not need to be reprimed. If not used for 2 consecutive days, reprime with 1 spray or until a fine spray appears. If not used for greater than 14 days, rinse the applicator and reprime with 2 sprays or until a fine spray appears.

➤*Individualization of dosage:* It is always desirable to titrate an individual patient to the minimum effective dose to reduce the possibility of side effects. In adults and children 6 years of age and older, the recommended starting dose is 64 mcg daily administered as 1 spray per nostril of 32 mcg budesonide nasal spray, once daily. Some patients who do not achieve symptom control at the recommended starting dose may benefit from an increased dose. The maximum daily dose is 256 mcg for adults and 128 mcg for children (younger than 12 years of age). When the maximum benefit has been achieved and symptoms have been controlled, reducing the dose may be effective in maintaining control of the allergic rhinitis symptoms in patients who were initially controlled on higher doses.

➤*Storage/Stability:* Store at controlled room temperature 20° to 25°C (68° to 77°F) with the valve up. Do not freeze. Protect from light. Shake gently before use. Do not spray in eyes.

FLUTICASONE PROPIONATE

Rx	**Fluticasone Propionate** (Par)	**Spray:** 50 mcg/actuation[a]	In 16 g (120 actuations) amber glass bottles with metering atomizing pump and nasal adapter.
Rx	**Flonase** (GlaxoSmithKline)		In 16 g (120 actuations) amber glass bottles with metering atomizing pump and nasal adapter.

[a] With dextrose, polysorbate 80, 0.02% w/w benzalkonium chloride, 0.25% w/w phenylethyl alcohol.

FLUTICASONE PROPIONATE — INTRANASAL

For complete and comparative prescribing information, refer to the Intranasal Steroids group monograph.

Indications

For the management of the nasal symptoms of seasonal and perennial allergic and nonallergic rhinitis in adults and pediatric patients 4 years of age and older.

Administration and Dosage

➤*Approved by the FDA:* October 19, 1994.

➤*Adults:* The recommended starting dosage in adults is 2 sprays (50 mcg of fluticasone propionate each) in each nostril once daily (total daily dose, 200 mcg). The same dosage divided into 100 mcg given twice daily (eg, 8 am and 8 pm) is also effective. After the first few days, patients may be able to reduce their dosage to 100 mcg (1 spray in each nostril) once daily for maintenance therapy. Some patients (12 years of age and older) with seasonal allergic rhinitis may find as-needed use of fluticasone propionate nasal spray (not to exceed 200 mcg daily) effective for symptom control. Greater symptom control may be achieved with scheduled regular use.

➤*Adolescents and children (4 years of age and older):* Patients should be started with 100 mcg (1 spray in each nostril once daily). Patients not adequately responding to 100 mcg may use 200 mcg (2 sprays in each nostril). Once adequate control is achieved, the dosage should be decreased to 100 mcg (1 spray in each nostril) daily.

The maximum total daily dosage should not exceed 2 sprays in each nostril (200 mcg/day).

Fluticasone propionate nasal spray is not recommended for children less than 4 years of age.

➤*Individualization of dosage:* Adult patients may be started on a 200 mcg once-daily regimen (two 50 mcg sprays in each nostril once daily). An alternative 200 mcg/day dosage regimen can be given as 100 mcg twice daily (one 50 mcg spray in each nostril twice daily).

Maximum total daily doses should not exceed 2 sprays in each nostril (total dose, 200 mcg/day). There is no evidence that exceeding the recommended dose is more effective.

➤*Storage/Stability:* Store between 4° and 30°C (39° and 86°F).

Intranasal Steroids

MOMETASONE FUROATE MONOHYDRATE

Rx	**Nasonex** (Schering)	**Spray:** 0.05% (50 mcg/actuation)[a]	In 17 g bottles (120 sprays) with metered-dose manual pump spray unit.

[a] Glycerin, 0.25% w/w phenylethyl alcohol, citric acid, benzalkonium chloride, polysorbate 80.

MOMETASONE FUROATE MONOHYDRATE — INTRANASAL

For complete and comparative prescribing information, refer to the Intranasal Steroids group monograph.

Indications

➤*Allergic rhinitis:* For the treatment of the nasal symptoms of seasonal allergic and perennial allergic rhinitis in adults and pediatric patients 2 years of age and older. Mometasone is indicated for the prophylaxis of the nasal symptoms of seasonal allergic rhinitis in adult and adolescent patients 12 years of age and older. In patients with a known seasonal allergen that precipitates nasal symptoms of seasonal allergic rhinitis, initiation of prophylaxis with mometasone is recommended 2 to 4 weeks prior to the anticipated start of the pollen season. Safety and efficacy of mometasone in pediatric patients younger than 2 years of age have not been established.

➤*Nasal polyps:* For the treatment of nasal polyps in patients 18 years of age and older.

Administration and Dosage

➤*Approved by the FDA:* October 1, 1997.

➤*Allergic rhinitis:*

Adults and children 12 years of age and older – The recommended dose for prophylaxis and treatment of the nasal symptoms of seasonal allergic rhinitis and treatment of the nasal symptoms of perennial allergic rhinitis is 2 sprays (50 mcg of mometasone in each spray) in each nostril once daily (total daily dose of 200 mcg).

In patients with a known seasonal allergen that precipitates nasal symptoms of seasonal allergic rhinitis, prophylaxis with mometasone (200 mcg/day) is recommended 2 to 4 weeks prior to the anticipated start of the pollen season.

Children 2 to 11 years of age – The recommended dose for treatment of the nasal symptoms of seasonal allergic and perennial allergic rhinitis is 1 spray (50 mcg of mometasone in each spray) in each nostril once daily (total daily dose of 100 mcg).

➤*Nasal polyps:*

Adults 18 years of age and older – The recommended dose for nasal polyps is 2 sprays (50 mcg of mometasone in each spray) in each nostril twice daily (total daily dose of 400 mcg). A dose of 2 sprays (50 mcg of mometasone in each spray) in each nostril once daily (total daily dose of 200 mcg) is also effective in some patients.

➤*Storage/Stability:* Store at 25°C (77°F); excursions permitted to 15° to 30°C (59° to 86°F). Protect from light.

When mometasone is removed from its cardboard container, avoid prolonged exposure of the product to direct light. Brief exposure to light, as with normal use, is acceptable.

Mucolytics

ACETYLCYSTEINE (N-Acetylcysteine)

Rx	**Acetylcysteine** (Various, Cetus, DuPont)	**Solution:** 10% (as sodium)	In 4, 10 and 30 ml vials.[a]
Rx	**Mucomyst** (Apothecon)		In 4, 10 and 30 ml vials.[a]
Rx	**Acetylcysteine** (Various, Cetus, Dey, DuPont)	**Solution:** 20% (as sodium)	In 4, 10, 30 and 100 ml vials.[a]
Rx	**Mucomyst** (Apothecon)		In 4, 10 and 30 ml vials.[a]

[a] May contain EDTA.

ACETYLCYSTEINE — INHALATION

WARNING

Not for injection.

Indications

As adjuvant therapy for patients with abnormal, viscid, or inspissated mucous secretions in such conditions as:

- Chronic bronchopulmonary disease (chronic emphysema, emphysema with bronchitis, chronic asthmatic bronchitis, tuberculosis, bronchiectasis and primary amyloidosis of the lung).
- Acute bronchopulmonary disease (pneumonia, bronchitis, tracheobronchitis).
- Pulmonary complications of cystic fibrosis.
- Tracheostomy care.
- Pulmonary complications associated with surgery.
- Use during anesthesia.
- Posttraumatic chest conditions.
- Atelectasis due to mucous obstruction.
- Diagnostic bronchial studies (bronchograms, bronchospirometry, and bronchial wedge catheterization).

➤*Unlabeled uses:* As an ophthalmic solution to treat keratoconjunctivitis sicca (dry eye). It has been used as an enema to treat bowel obstruction due to meconium ileus or its equivalent.

Administration and Dosage

➤*Approved by the FDA:* August 30, 1994.

Acetylcysteine solution 10% and 20% is available in glass vials containing 4 mL, 10 mL or 30 mL. The 20% solution may be diluted to a lesser concentration with either Sodium Chloride Inhalation Solution; Sodium Chloride Injection; or Sterile Water for Injection, or Sterile Water for Inhalation. The 10% solution may be used undiluted.

➤*Nebulization (face mask, mouth piece, tracheostomy):* 1 to 10 mL of the 20% solution or 2 to 20 mL of the 10% solution may be given every 2 to 6 hours; the recommended dose for most patients is 3 to 5 mL of the 20% solution or 6 to 10 mL of the 10% solution 3 to 4 times a day.

➤*Nebulization (tent, croupette):* In special circumstances it may be necessary to nebulize into a tent or croupette, and this method of use must be individualized to take into account the available equipment and the patient's particular needs. This form of administration requires very large volumes of the solution, occasionally as much as 300 mL during a single treatment period.

If a tent or croupette must be used, the recommended dose is the volume of acetylcysteine (using 10% or 20%) that will maintain a very heavy mist in the tent or croupette for the desired period. Administration for intermittent or continuous prolonged periods, including overnight, may be desirable.

➤*Direct instillation:* 1 to 2 mL of a 10% or 20% solution may be given as often as every hour.

When used for the routine nursing care of patients with tracheostomy, 1 to 2 mL of a 10% or 20% solution may be given every 1 to 4 hours by instillation into the tracheostomy.

Acetylcysteine may be introduced directly into a particular segment of the bronchopulmonary tree by inserting (under local anesthesia and direct vision) a small plastic catheter into the trachea. Two to 5 mL of the 20% solution may then be instilled by means of a syringe connected to the catheter.

Acetylcysteine may also be given through a percutaneous intratracheal catheter. One to 2 mL of the 20% or 2 to 4 mL of the 10% solution every 1 to 4 hours may then be given by a syringe attached to the catheter.

➤*Diagnostic bronchograms:* 2 or 3 administrations of 1 to 2 mL of the 20% solution or 2 to 4 mL of the 10% solution should be given by nebulization or by instillation intratracheally, prior to the procedure.

➤*Administration of aerosol:*

Materials – Acetylcysteine may be administered using conventional nebulizers made of plastic or glass. Certain materials used in nebulization equipment react with acetylcysteine. The most reactive of these are certain metals (notably iron and copper) and rubber. Where material may come into contact with acetylcysteine solution, parts made of the following acceptable materials should be used: Glass, plastic, aluminum, anodized aluminum, chromed metal, tantalum, sterling silver, or stainless steel. Silver may become tarnished after exposure, but this is not harmful to the drug action or to the patient.

Nebulizing gases – Compressed tank gas (air) or an air compressor should be used to provide pressure for nebulizing the solution. Oxygen may also be used but should be used with usual precautions in patients with severe respiratory disease and CO_2 retention.

Apparatus – Acetylcysteine is usually administered as fine nebulae, and the nebulizer used should be capable of providing optimal quantities of a suitable range of particle sizes.

Commercially available nebulizers will produce nebulae of acetylcysteine satisfactory for retention in the respiratory tract. Most of the nebulizers tested will supply a high proportion of the drug solution as particles of less than 10 microns in diameter. One study has shown that particles less than 10 microns should be retained in the respiratory tract satisfactorily.

Various intermittent positive pressure breathing devices nebulized acetylcysteine with a satisfactory efficiency including: *No. 40 De Vilbiss* and the *Bennett Twin-Jet Nebulizer*.

The nebulized solution may be inhaled directly from the nebulizer. Nebulizers may also be attached to plastic face masks or plastic mouthpieces. Suitable nebulizers may also be fitted for use with the various intermittent positive pressure breathing (IPPB) machines. The nebulizing equipment should be cleaned immediately after use because the residues may clog the smaller orifices or corrode metal parts.

ACETYLCYSTEINE — INHALATION

Hand bulbs are not recommended for routine use for nebulizing acetylcysteine because their output is generally too small. Also, some hand-operated nebulizers deliver particles that are larger than optimum for inhalation therapy.

Acetylcysteine should not be placed directly into the chamber of a heated (hot pot) nebulizer. A heated nebulizer may be part of the nebulization assembly to provide a warm saturated atmosphere if the acetylcysteine aerosol is introduced by means of a separate unheated nebulizer. Usual precautions for administration of warm saturated nebulae should be observed.

The nebulized solution may be breathed directly from the nebulizer. Nebulizers may also be attached to plastic face masks, plastic face tents, plastic mouth pieces, conventional plastic oxygen tents, or head tents. Suitable nebulizers may also be fitted for use with the various IPPB machines.

The nebulizing equipment should be cleaned immediately after use, otherwise the residues may occlude the fine orifices or corrode metal parts.

Prolonged nebulization – When three-fourths of the initial volume of acetylcysteine solution has been nebulized, a quantity of Sterile Water for Injection (approximately equal to the volume of solution remaining), should be added to the nebulizer. This obviates any concentration of the agent in the residual solvent remaining after prolonged nebulization.

➤*Compatibility:* The physical and chemical compatibility of acetylcysteine with certain other drugs that might be concomitantly administered by nebulization, direct instillation, or topical application, has been studied.

Acetylcysteine should not be mixed with certain antibiotics. For example, the antibiotics tetracycline hydrochloride, oxytetracycline hydrochloride, and erythromycin lactobionate were found to be incompatible when mixed in the same solution. These agents may be administered from separate solutions if administration of these agents is desirable.

The supplying of these data should not be interpreted as a recommendation for combining acetylcysteine with other drugs. The data below are not presented as positive assurance that no incompatibility will be present, since these data are based only on short-term compatibility studies done in the Mead Johnson Research Center. Manufacturers may change their formulations, and this could alter compatibilities. These data are intended to serve only as a guide for predicting compounding problems.

If it is deemed advisable to prepare an admixture, it should be administered as soon as possible after preparation. Do not store unused mixtures.

In Vitro Compatibility[a] Tests of Aacetylcysteine

Product or agent	Compatibility rate	Ratio tested[b]	
		Acetyl-cysteine	Product or agent
Anesthetic, gas			
Halothane	Compatible	20%	Infinite
Nitrous oxide	Compatible	20%	Infinite
Anesthetic, local			
Cocaine HCl	Compatible	10%	5%
Lidocaine HCl	Compatible	10%	2%
Tetracaine HCl	Compatible	10%	1%
Antibacterials (a parenteral form of each antibiotic was used)			
Bacitracin[c,d] (mix and use at once)	Compatible	10%	5000 U/mL
Chloramphenicol sodium succinate	Compatible	20%	20 mg/mL
Carbenicillin disodium[c] (mix and use at once)	Compatible	10%	125 mg/mL
Gentamicin sulfate [c]	Compatible	10%	20 mg/mL
Kanamycin sulfate[c] (mix and use at once)	Compatible	10%	167 mg/mL
	Compatible	17%	85 mg/mL
Lincomycin HCl[c]	Compatible	10%	150 mg/mL
Neomycin sulfate[c]	Compatible	10%	100 mg/mL
Novobiocin sodium[c]	Compatible	10%	25 mg/mL
Penicillin G potassium[c] (mix and use at once)	Compatible	10%	25,000 U/mL
Polymyxin B sulfate[c]	Compatible	10%	50,000 U/mL
Cephalothin sodium	Compatible	10%	110 mg/mL
Colistimethate sodium[c] (mix and use at once)	Compatible	10%	37.5 mg/mL
Vancomycin HCl[c]	Compatible	10%	25 mg/mL
Amphotericin B	Incompatible	4% to 15%	1 to 4 mg/mL
Chlortetracycline HCl[c]	Incompatible	10%	12.5 mg/mL
Erythromycin lactobionate	Incompatible	10%	15 mg/mL
Oxytetracycline HCl	Incompatible	10%	12.5 mg/mL
Ampicillin sodium	Incompatible	10%	50 mg/mL
Tetracycline HCl	Incompatible	10%	12.5 mg/mL

In Vitro Compatibility[a] Tests of Aacetylcysteine

Product or agent	Compatibility rate	Ratio tested[b]	
		Acetyl-cysteine	Product or agent
Bronchodilators			
Isoproterenol HCl[c]	Compatible	3%	0.5%
Isoproterenol HCl[c]	Compatible	10%	0.05%
Isoproterenol HCl[c]	Compatible	20%	0.05%
Isoproterenol HCl	Compatible	13.3% (2 parts)	0.33% (1 part)
Isoetharine HCl	Compatible	13.3% (2 parts)	(1 part)
Epinephrine HCl	Compatible	13.3% (2 parts)	0.33% (1 part)
Contrast media			
Iodized oil	Incompatible	20%/ 20 mL	40%/10 mL
Decongestants			
Phenylephrine HCl[c]	Compatible	3%	0.25%
Phenylephrine HCl	Compatible	13.3% (2 parts)	0.17% (1 part)
Enzymes			
Chymotrypsin	Incompatible	5%	400 γ/mL
Trypsin	Incompatible	5%	400 γ/mL
Solvents			
Alcohol	Compatible	12%	10% to 20%
Propylene glycol	Compatible	3%	10%
Steroids			
Dexamethasone sodium phosphate	Compatible	16%	0.8 mg/mL
Prednisolone sodium phosphate[e]	Compatible	16.7%	3.3 mg/mL
Other agents			
Hydrogen peroxide	Incompatible	(All ratios)	
Sodium bicarbonate	Compatible	20% (1 part)	4.2% (1 part)

[a] The rating, incompatible, is based on the formation of a precipitate, a change in clarity, immiscibility or a rapid loss of potency of acetylcysteine or the active ingredient of the product or agent in the admixture. The rating, compatible, means that there was no significant physical change in the admixture when compared with a control solution of the product or agent, and that there was no predicted chemical incompatibility. All of the admixtures have been tested for short-term chemical compatibility by assaying for the concentration of acetylcysteine after mixing.

[b] Entries are final corrections. Values in parentheses relate volumes of acetylcysteine solution to volume of test solutions.

[c] The active ingredient in the product or agent was also assayed after mixing. Some of the admixtures developed minor physical changes which were considered to be insufficient to rate the admixture incompatible. These are listed in footnotes d, e, and f.

[d] A strong odor developed after storage for 24 hours at room temperature.

[e] A light tan color developed after storage for 24 hours at room temperature.

➤*Storage/Stability:* This product does not contain an antimicrobial agent, and care must be taken to minimize contamination of the sterile solution. If only a portion of the solution in a vial is used, store the remainder in a refrigerator and use for inhalation only within 96 hours.

Actions

➤*Pharmacology:* The viscosity of pulmonary mucous secretions depends on the concentrations of mucoprotein and to a lesser extent deoxyribonucleic acid (DNA). The latter increases with increasing purulence owing to the presence of cellular debris. The mucolytic action of acetylcysteine is related to the sulfhydryl group in the molecule. This group probably "opens" disulfide linkages in mucous thereby lowering the viscosity. The mucolytic activity of acetylcysteine is unaltered by the presence of DNA, and increases with increasing pH. Significant mucolysis occurs between pH 7 and 9.

Acetylcysteine undergoes rapid deacetylation in vivo to yield cysteine or oxidation to yield diacetylcystine.

Occasionally, patients exposed to the inhalation of an acetylcysteine aerosol respond with the development of increased airways obstruction of varying and unpredictable severity. Those patients who are reactors cannot be identified a priori from a random patient population. Even when patients are known to have reacted previously to the inhalation of an acetylcysteine aerosol, they may not react during a subsequent treatment. The converse is also true; patients who have had inhalation treatments of acetylcysteine without incident may still react to a subsequent inhalation with increased airways obstruction. Most patients with bronchospasm are quickly relieved by the use of a bronchodilator given by nebulization. If bronchospasm progresses, the medication should be discontinued immediately.

ACETYLCYSTEINE — INHALATION

Contraindications

Sensitivity to acetylcysteine.

Warnings

➤*Bronchial secretions:* After proper administration of acetylcysteine, an increased volume of liquified bronchial secretions may occur. When cough is inadequate, the open airway must be maintained by mechanical suction if necessary. When there is a mechanical block due to foreign body or local accumulation, the airway should be cleared by endotracheal aspiration, with or without bronchoscopy. Asthmatics under treatment with acetylcysteine should be watched carefully. Most patients with bronchospasm are quickly relieved by the use of a bronchodilator given by nebulization. If bronchospasm progresses, this medication should be discontinued immediately.

➤*Fertility impairment:* Reproductive toxicity studies of acetylcysteine in the rat given oral doses of acetylcysteine up to 1000 mg/kg (5.2 times the human mucolytic dose) have been reported in the literature. The only adverse effect observed was a slight non-dose-related reduction in fertility at dose levels of 500 or 1000 mg/kg/day (2.6 or 5.2 times the human dose) in the segment 1 study.

➤*Pregnancy:* *Category B.* There are no adequate and well-controlled studies in pregnant women. Because animal reproduction studies may not always be predictive of human responses, this drug should be used during pregnancy only if clearly needed.

➤*Lactation:* It is not known whether this drug is excreted in human milk. Because many drugs are excreted in human milk, caution should be exercised when acetylcysteine is administered to a nursing woman.

Precautions

➤*Odor:* With the administration of acetylcysteine, the patient may initially notice a slight disagreeable odor that is soon noticeable. With a face mask there may be a stickiness on the face after nebulization. This is easily removed by washing with water.

➤*Solution color:* Under certain conditions, a color change may occur in the solution of acetylcysteine in the opened bottle. The light purple color is the result of a chemical reaction which does not significantly affect the safety or mucolytic effectiveness of acetylcysteine.

➤*Continued nebulization:* Continued nebulization of an acetylcysteine solution with a dry gas will result in an increased concentration of the drug in the nebulizer because of evaporation of the solvent. Extreme concentration may impede nebulization and efficient delivery of the drug. Dilution of the nebulizing solution with appropriate amounts of Sterile Water for Injection, as a concentration occurs, will obviate this problem.

Drug Interactions

None known.

Adverse Reactions

➤*Hypersensitivity:* Acquired sensitization to acetylcysteine have been reported rarely. Reports of sensitization in patients have not been confirmed by patch testing. Sensitization has been confirmed in several inhalation therapists who reported a history of dermal eruptions after frequent and extended exposure to acetylcysteine.

➤*Local:* Reports of irritation to the tracheal and bronchial tracts have been received and although hemoptysis has occurred in patients receiving acetylcysteine such findings are not uncommon in patients with bronchopulmonary disease and a causal relationship has not been established.

➤*Miscellaneous:* Adverse effects have included stomatitis, nausea, vomiting, fever, rhinorrhea, drowsiness, clamminess, chest tightness, and bronchoconstriction. Clinically overt acetylcysteine induced bronchospasm occurs infrequently and unpredictably even in patients with asthmatic bronchitis or bronchitis complicating bronchial asthma.

DORNASE ALFA (Recombinant human deoxyribonuclease; DNase)

Rx	**Pulmozyme** (Genentech)	**Solution for inhalation:** 1 mg/ml	Preservative free. With 0.15 mg/ml calcium chloride dihydrate and 8.77 mg/ml sodium chloride. In 2.5 ml amps.

DORNASE ALFA — INHALATION

Indications

➤*Cystic fibrosis:* Daily administration of dornase alfa in conjunction with standard therapies is indicated in the management of cystic fibrosis patients to improve pulmonary function. In patients with an FVC greater than or equal to 40% of predicted, daily administration of dornase alfa has also been shown to reduce the risk of respiratory tract infections requiring parenteral antibiotics.

Safety and efficacy of daily administration have not been demonstrated in patients for longer than 12 months.

Administration and Dosage

➤*Approved by the FDA:* December 30, 1993.

The recommended dose for use in most cystic fibrosis patients is one 2.5 mg single-use ampule inhaled once daily using a recommended nebulizer. Some patients may benefit from twice daily administration. Clinical trial results and laboratory information are only available to support use of the following nebulizer/compressor systems.

- *Hudson T Up-draft II* nebulizer with *Pulmo-Aide* compressor
- *Marquest Acorn II* nebulizer with *Pulmo-Aide* compressor
- *Pari LC Jet+* nebulizer with *Pari Proneb* compressor
- *Pari Baby* nebulizer with *Pari Proneb* compressor
- *Durable Sidestream* nebulizer with *Mobilaire* compressor
- *Durable Sidestream* nebulizer with *Porta-Neb* compressor

Note: Patients who are unable to inhale or exhale orally throughout the entire nebulization period may use the *Pari Baby* nebulizer.

Patients who use the *Sidestream* nebulizer with the *Mobilaire* compressor should turn the compressor control knob fully to the right and then turn on the compressor. At this setting, the needle on the pressure gauge should vibrate between 35 and 45 pounds per square inch (highest pressure output).

No data are currently available that support the administration of dornase alfa with other nebulizer systems. The patient should follow the manufacturer's instructions on the use and maintenance of the equipment.

Dornase alfa should not be diluted or mixed with other drugs in the nebulizer. Mixing of dornase alfa with other drugs could lead to adverse physicochemical or functional changes in dornase alfa or the admixed compound. Patients should be advised to squeeze each ampule prior to use in order to check for leaks.

➤*Storage / Stability:* Store under refrigeration (2° to 8°C/36° to 46°F). Ampules should be protected from strong light. Unused ampules should be stored in their protective foil pouch under refrigeration.

Actions

➤*Pharmacology:* In cystic fibrosis patients, retention of viscous purulent secretions in the airways contributes both to reduced pulmonary function and to exacerbations of infection.

Purulent pulmonary secretions contain very high concentrations of extracellular DNA released by degenerating leukocytes that accumulate in response to infection. In vitro, dornase alfa hydrolyzes the DNA in sputum of cystic fibrosis patients and reduces sputum viscoelasticity.

➤*Pharmacokinetics:* When 2.5 mg dornase alfa was administered by inhalation to 18 cystic fibrosis patients, mean sputum concentrations of 3 mcg/mL DNase were measurable within 15 minutes. Mean sputum concentrations declined to an average of 0.6 mcg/mL 2 hours following inhalation. Inhalation of up to 10 mg three times a day of dornase alfa by 4 cystic fibrosis patients for 6 consecutive days, did not result in a significant elevation of serum concentrations of DNase above normal endogenous levels. After administration of up to 2.5 mg of dornase alfa twice daily for 6 months to 321 cystic fibrosis patients, no accumulation of serum DNase was noted.

Dornase alfa, 2.5 mg by inhalation, was administered daily to 98 patients aged 3 months to less than or equal to 10 years, and bronchoalveolar lavage (BAL) fluid was obtained within 90 minutes of the first dose. BAL DNase concentrations were detectable in all patients but showed a broad range, from 0.007 to 1.8 mcg/mL. Over an average of 14 days of exposure, serum DNase concentrations (mean ± SD) increased by 1.3 ± 1.3 ng/mL for the 3 months to less than 5 year age group and by 0.8 ± 1.2 ng/mL for the 5 to less than or equal to 10 year age group. The relationship between BAL or serum DNase concentration and adverse experiences and clinical outcomes is unknown.

Contraindications

Known hypersensitivity to dornase alfa, Chinese hamster ovary cell products, or any component of the product.

Warnings

➤*Pregnancy:* *Category B.* There are no adequate and well-controlled studies in pregnant women. Because animal reproductive studies are not always predictive of the human response, this drug should be used during pregnancy only if clearly needed.

➤*Lactation:* It is not known whether dornase alfa is excreted in human milk. Small amounts of dornase alfa were detected in maternal milk of cynomolgus monkeys when administered a bolus dose (100 mcg/kg) of dornase alfa followed by a 6 hour intravenous infusion (80 mcg/kg/hr). Little or no measurable dornase alfa would be expected in human milk after chronic aerosol administration of recommended doses. Because many drugs are excreted in human milk, caution should still be exercised when dornase alfa is administered to a nursing woman.

➤*Children:* Because of the limited experience with the administration of dornase alfa to patients younger than 5 years of age, its use should be considered only for those patients in whom there is a potential for benefit in pulmonary function or in risk of respiratory tract infection.

Precautions

➤*Administration:* Dornase alfa should be used in conjunction with standard therapies for cystic fibrosis.

Drug Interactions

None known.

DORNASE ALFA — INHALATION

Adverse Reactions

In a randomized, placebo-controlled clinical trial in patients with FVC greater than or equal to 40% of predicted, over 600 patients received dornase alfa once or twice daily for 6 months; most adverse events were not more common on dornase alfa than on placebo and probably reflected the sequelae of the underlying lung disease. In most cases events that were increased were mild, transient in nature, and did not require alterations in dosing. Few patients experienced adverse events resulting in permanent discontinuation from dornase alfa, and the discontinuation rate was similar for placebo (2%) and dornase alfa (3%). Events that were more frequent (greater than 3%) in dornase alfa-treated patients than in placebo-treated patients are listed in the table below.

In a randomized, placebo-controlled trial of patients with advanced disease (FVC less than 40% of predicted) the safety profile for most adverse events was similar to that reported for the trial in patients with mild to moderate disease.

Adverse events increased 3% or more in dornase alfa-treated patients over placebo in cystic fibrosis clinical trials

	Trial in mild to moderate cystic fibrosis patients (FVC greater than or equal to 40% of predicted) treated for 24 weeks			Trial in advanced cystic fibrosis patients (FVC less than 40% of predicted) treated for 12 weeks	
Adverse event (of any severity or seriousness)	Placebo (n = 325)	Dornase alfa every day (n = 322)	Dornase alfa twice a day (n = 321)	Placebo (n = 159)	Dornase alfa every day (n = 161)
Voice alteration	7%	12%	16%	6%	18%
Pharyngitis	33%	36%	40%	28%	32%
Rash	7%	10%	12%	1%	3%
Laryngitis	1%	3%	4%	1%	3%
Chest pain	16%	18%	21%	23%	25%
Conjunctivitis	2%	4%	5%	0%	1%
Rhinitis	< 3%[a]	< 3%[a]	< 3%[a]	24%	30%
FVC decrease of ≥ 10% of predicted[b]	< 3%[a]	< 3%[a]	< 3%[a]	17%	22%
Fever	< 3%[a]	< 3%[a]	< 3%[a]	28%	32%
Dyspepsia	< 3%[a]	< 3%[a]	< 3%[a]	0%	3%
Dyspnea (when reported as serious)	< 3%[c]	< 3%[c]	< 3%[c]	12%[d]	17%[d]

[a] Differences were less than 3% for these adverse events in the trial in mild to moderate cystic fibrosis patients.
[b] Single measurement only, does not reflect overall FVC changes.
[c] Difference was less than 3% for this adverse event in the trial in mild to moderate cystic fibrosis patients.
[d] Total reports of dyspnea (regardless of severity or seriousness) had a difference of less than 3% for the trial in advanced cystic fibrosis patients.

➤*Events observed at similar rates in dornase alfa inhalation solution and placebo-treated patients with FVC greater than or equal to 40% of predicted:*

Allergic – There have been no reports of anaphylaxis attributed to the administration of dornase alfa to date. Urticaria, mild to moderate, and mild skin rash have been observed and have been transient. Within all of the studies, a small percentage (average of 2% to 4%) of patients treated with dornase alfa developed serum antibodies to dornase alfa. None of these patients developed anaphylaxis, and the clinical significance of serum antibodies to dornase alfa is unknown.

GI – Intestinal obstruction, gall bladder disease, liver disease, pancreatic disease.

Metabolic/Nutritional – Diabetes mellitus, hypoxia, weight loss.

Respiratory – Apnea, bronchiectasis, bronchitis, change in sputum, increased cough, dyspnea, hemoptysis, decreased lung function, nasal polyps, pneumonia, pneumothorax, rhinitis, sinusitis, increased sputum, wheeze.

Miscellaneous – Abdominal pain, asthenia, fever, flu syndrome, malaise, sepsis.

Mortality rates observed in controlled trials were similar for the placebo- and dornase alfa-treated patients. Causes of death were consistent with progression of cystic fibrosis and included apnea, cardiac arrest, cardiopulmonary arrest, cor pulmonale, heart failure, massive hemoptysis, pneumonia, pneumothorax, and respiratory failure.

The safety of dornase alfa, 2.5 mg by inhalation, was studied with 2 weeks of daily administration in 98 patients with cystic fibrosis (65 patients aged 3 months to less than 5 years, 33 patients aged 5 to less than or equal to 10 years). The *Pari Baby* reusable nebulizer (which uses a facemask instead of a mouthpiece) was utilized in patients unable to demonstrate the ability to inhale or exhale orally throughout the entire treatment period (54/65, 83% of the younger and 2/33, 6% of the older patients). The number of patients reporting cough was higher in the younger age group as compared to the older age group (29/65, 45% compared to 10/33, 30%) as was the number reporting moderate to severe cough (24/65, 37% as compared to 6/33, 18%). Other events tended to be of mild to moderate severity. The number of patients reporting rhinitis was higher in the younger age group as compared to the older age group (23/65, 35% compared to 9/33, 27%) as was the number reporting rash (4/65, 6% as compared to 0/33, 0%). The nature of adverse events was similar to that seen in the larger trials of dornase alfa inhalation solution.

Overdosage

Cystic fibrosis patients have received up to 20 mg twice daily for up to 6 days and 10 mg twice daily intermittently (2 weeks on/2 weeks off drug) for 168 days. These doses were well tolerated.

Patient Information

Store in the refrigerator at 2° to 8°C (36° to 46°F) and protect from strong light. It should be kept refrigerated during transport and should not be exposed to room temperatures for a total time of 24 hours. The solution should be discarded if it is cloudy or discolored. Dornase alfa contains no preservative and, once opened, the entire contents of the ampule must be used or discarded. Patients should be instructed in the proper use and maintenance of the nebulizer and compressor system used in its delivery.

Dornase alfa should not be diluted or mixed with other drugs in the nebulizer. Mixing of dornase alfa with other drugs could lead to adverse physicochemical and/or functional changes in dornase alfa or the admixed compound.

CROMOLYN SODIUM (Disodium Cromoglycate)

Rx	**Cromolyn Sodium** (Various, eg, Alpharma, Dey)	**Solution for inhalation**: 20 mg/2 mL	In 60 and 120 UD vials or amps.
Rx	**Intal** (Aventis)	**Solution for inhalation**: 20 mg/2 mL	In 60 and 120 UD amps.
		Aerosol: 800 mcg/actuation	In 8.1 g (≥ 112 metered sprays) and 14.2 g (≥ 200 metered sprays).
otc	**Nasalcrom** (Pharmacia)	**Nasal solution**: 40 mg/mL[a] (Each actuation delivers 5.2 mg)	In 13 mL or 26 mL metered spray device.
Rx	**Gastrocrom** (Celltech)	**Oral concentrate**: 100 mg/5 mL	In 8 UD amps/foil pouch.

[a] With benzalkonium chloride and EDTA.

CROMOLYN SODIUM (Disodium Cromoglycate)

Indications

➤*Bronchial asthma (inhalation solution, aerosol):* As prophylactic management of bronchial asthma. Cromolyn is given on a regular, daily basis in patients with frequent symptomatology requiring a continuous medication regimen.

➤*Prevention of bronchospasm (inhalation solution, aerosol):* To prevent acute bronchospasm induced by exercise, toluene diisocyanate, environmental pollutants, and known antigens.

➤*Allergic rhinitis (nasal solution):* To prevent and treat allergic rhinitis caused by airborne pollens from trees, grasses, or ragweed, and by mold, animals, and dust. To prevent and relieve the following nasal symptoms: Runny/itchy nose, sneezing, and allergic stuffy nose.

➤*Mastocytosis (oral):* Improves diarrhea, flushing, headaches, vomiting, urticaria, abdominal pain, nausea, and itching in some patients.

➤*Unlabeled uses:* Cromolyn has been used as an alternative therapy in refractory forms of chronic urticaria/angioedema. Oral cromolyn has been used for the treatment of food allergies and mucosal and serosal eosinophilic gastroenteritis.

Administration and Dosage

➤*Approved by the FDA:* May 28, 1982.

➤*Inhalation solution (adults and children at least 2 years of age):* Initially, 20 mg (1 amp/vial) administered by nebulization 4 times/day at regular intervals. The effectiveness of therapy depends upon administration at regular intervals.

CROMOLYN SODIUM (Disodium Cromoglycate)

Administer solution from a power-operated nebulizer having an adequate flow rate and equipped with a suitable face mask or mouthpiece. Hand operated nebulizers are not suitable.

Introduce cromolyn into the patient's therapeutic regimen when the acute episode has been controlled, the airway has been cleared, and the patient is able to inhale adequately.

Improvement ordinarily occurs within the first 4 weeks of administration, although some patients may demonstrate an immediate response. Efficacy is manifested by a decrease in the severity of clinical symptoms, or the need for concomitant therapy, or both.

Prevention of acute bronchospasm – Inhale 20 mg (1 amp/vial) administered by nebulization shortly before exposure to the precipitating factor.

➤*Aerosol (adults and children at least 5 years of age):* For management of bronchial asthma, the usual starting dose is 2 metered sprays inhaled 4 times/day at regular intervals. Do not exceed this dose. Not all patients will respond to the recommended dose, and a lower dose may provide efficacy in younger patients.

Advise patients with chronic asthma that the effect of therapy is dependent upon its administration at regular intervals, as directed. Introduce therapy into the patient's therapeutic regimen when the acute episode has been controlled, the airway has been cleared, and the patient is able to inhale adequately.

Improvement ordinarily occurs within the first 4 weeks of administration, although some patients may demonstrate an immediate response. Efficacy is manifested by a decrease in the severity of clinical symptoms, or the need for concomitant therapy, or both.

Prevention of acute bronchospasm – The usual dose is inhalation of 2 metered dose sprays shortly (ie, 10 to 15 minutes but not more than 60 minutes) before exposure to the precipitating factor.

➤*Nasal solution:*

Adults and children at least 2 years of age – 1 spray in each nostril 3 to 6 times daily at regular intervals every 4 to 6 hours. Maximum effects may not be seen for 1 to 2 weeks. Clear the nasal passages before administering the spray and inhale through the nose during administration (see Patient Information).

➤*Oral:*

Adults (13 years of age or older) – 2 ampules 4 times/day 30 minutes before meals and at bedtime.

Children 2 to 12 years of age – 1 ampule 4 times/day 30 minutes before meals and at bedtime.

If satisfactory control of symptoms is not achieved within 2 to 3 weeks, the dosage may be increased; do not exceed 40 mg/kg/day.

The effect of therapy is dependent upon its administration at regular intervals as directed. Not for inhalation or injection.

Maintenance – Once a therapeutic response has been achieved, the dose may be reduced to the minimum required to maintain the patient with a lower degree of symptomatology. To prevent relapses, maintain the dosage.

Administer as a solution at least 30 minutes before meals and at bedtime after preparation according to the following directions.

1.) Break open and squeeze liquid contents of ampule(s) into a glass of water.
2.) Stir solution.
3.) Drink all of the liquid.

➤*Nonsteroidal agents:* Add cromolyn (inhalation solution and aerosol) to the patient's existing treatment regimen (eg, bronchodilators). Concomitant medications may be decreased gradually when a clinical response to cromolyn is evident (approximately 2 to 4 weeks) and asthma is under good control. Titrate the frequency of cromolyn administration downward to the lowest effective level if concomitant medications are discontinued or required on no more than an as-needed basis. The usual decrease is from 4 to 3 ampules/vials per day for the nebulizer solution, or from 2 metered inhalations 4 times/day to 3 times/day to twice daily for the inhalation aerosol. Gradually reduce dosage to avoid asthma exacerbations. Clinical deterioration in these patients whose dosage has been decreased to less than 4 ampules/vials or 4 inhalations per day may require an increase in cromolyn dosage and the introduction of, or increase in, symptomatic medications.

➤*Corticosteroids:* Continue concomitant corticosteroid treatment following the introduction of cromolyn (inhalation solution and aerosol). If the patient improves, attempt to decrease corticosteroid dosage. Even if the corticosteroid-dependent patient fails to improve following cromolyn use, attempt gradual tapering of steroid dosage while maintaining close patient supervision. Consider reinstituting steroid therapy for a patient subjected to significant stress (eg, a severe asthmatic attack, surgery, trauma, severe illness) while being treated or within 1 year (occasionally up to 2 years) after corticosteroid treatment has been terminated, in case of adrenocortical insufficiency. When respiratory function is impaired, as may occur in severe exacerbation of asthma, a temporary increase in the amount of corticosteroids or other agents may be required to regain control of the patient's asthma.

It is particularly important to exercise great care if for any reason cromolyn is withdrawn in cases where its use has permitted a reduction in the corticosteroid maintenance dose. In such cases, continued close supervision of the patient is essential because there may be a sudden reappearance of severe manifestations of asthma that will require immediate therapy and possible reintroduction of corticosteroids.

➤*Compatibility:* Cromolyn nebulizer solution has demonstrated compatibility with 5% metaproterenol sulfate, 0.5% isoproterenol HCl, 1% isoetharine HCl, 2.25% epinephrine, 0.1% terbutaline sulfate, 0.02% ipratropium bromide, and 20% acetylcysteine solution for at least 1 hour after their admixture. It also was compatible with 0.6% and 5% metaproterenol sulfate, 0.2% atropine sulfate, 0.5% albuterol sulfate, and 0.9% sodium chloride solution for at least 90 minutes after their admixture. It is important to note that the stated medications may not be identical to the formulations currently marketed in the US.

➤*Storage/Stability:*

Inhalation solution – Store at controlled room temperature 20° to 25°C (68° to 77°F). Protect from light. Do not use if the solution contains a precipitate or becomes discolored. Store ampules in foil pouch until ready to use.

Aerosol and nasal solution – Store at controlled room temperature 20° to 25°C (68° to 77°F). Do not puncture, incinerate, or place the aerosol near sources of heat. Protect nasal solution from light.

Oral concentrate – Store between 15° to 30°C (59° to 86°F). Protect from light. Do not use the concentrate if it contains a precipitate or becomes discolored. Store ampules in foil pouch until ready to use.

Actions

➤*Pharmacology:* Cromolyn is an anti-inflammatory agent. It has no intrinsic bronchodilator, antihistaminic, vasoconstrictor, or glucocorticoid activity. In animal studies, cromolyn inhibits sensitized and mast cells degranulation that occurs after exposure to specific antigens. The drug inhibits the release of mediators, histamine, and SRS-A (the slow-reacting substance of anaphylaxis, a leukotriene) from the mast cell. Studies have demonstrated that cromolyn indirectly inhibits calcium ions from entering the mast cell, resulting in the prevention of mediator release. Immediate and nonimmediate bronchoconstrictive reactions induced by the inhalation of antigens can be inhibited by cromolyn. Cromolyn also attenuates bronchospasms caused by exercise, toluene diisocyanate, aspirin, cold air, sulfur dioxide, and environmental pollutants. Cromolyn acts locally on the lung to which it is directly applied.

➤*Pharmacokinetics:* After inhalation, approximately 8% is absorbed from the lung and rapidly excreted unchanged in bile and urine. The remainder is either exhaled or deposited in the oropharynx, swallowed, and excreted via the alimentary tract.

Cromolyn is poorly absorbed from the GI tract. No more than 1% of an administered dose is absorbed after oral administration, the remainder being excreted in the feces. Very little absorption of cromolyn was seen after oral administration of 500 mg to each of 12 volunteers. From 0.28% to 0.5% of the administered dose was recovered in the first 24 hours of urinary excretion in 3 subjects. The mean urinary excretion over 24 hours in the remaining 9 subjects was 0.45%.

Contraindications

Hypersensitivity to cromolyn or to any ingredient contained in these products.

Warnings

➤*Acute asthma:* Cromolyn has no role in the treatment of acute asthma, especially status asthmaticus; it is a prophylactic drug with no benefit for acute situations.

➤*Hypersensitivity reactions:* Severe anaphylactic reactions may occur rarely with cromolyn. Refer to General Management of Acute Hypersensitivity Reactions.

➤*Renal/Hepatic function impairment:* In view of the biliary and renal routes of excretion, decrease the dose or discontinue the drug in these patients.

➤*Pregnancy: Category B.* There are no adequate and well-controlled studies in pregnant women. Use only when clearly needed. Animal studies have demonstrated adverse fetal effects (increased resorptions, decreased fetal weight) only at very high parenteral doses.

➤*Lactation:* It is not known whether this drug is excreted in human milk. Exercise caution when the drug is administered to a nursing woman.

➤*Children:*

Aerosol – Safety and efficacy in children less than 5 years of age have not been established.

Inhalation solution – Safety and efficacy in children less than 2 years of age have not been established.

Nasal – Do not use in children under 2 years of age unless directed by a physician.

Oral – In neonatal rats, cromolyn increased mortality at oral doses of 1000 mg/kg or greater. In term infants up to 6 months of age, data suggest the dose not exceed 20 mg/kg/day. Reserve use in children less than 2 years of age for patients with severe disease in which potential benefits clearly outweigh risks.

Precautions

➤*Bronchospasm/Cough:* Occasionally, patients experience cough or bronchospasm following inhalation and, at times, may not be able to continue treatment despite prior bronchodilator administration. Rarely, very severe bronchospasm has occurred.

➤*Asthma:* Symptoms may recur if drug is reduced below recommended dosage or discontinued.

CROMOLYN SODIUM (Disodium Cromoglycate)

➤*Eosinophilic pneumonia (pulmonary infiltrates with eosinophilia):* If this occurs during the course of therapy, discontinue the drug.

➤*Aerosol:* Because of the propellants in this preparation, use with caution in patients with coronary artery disease or cardiac arrhythmias.

Adverse Reactions

The most frequently reported adverse reactions attributed to cromolyn sodium (on the basis of recurrence following readministration) involve the respiratory tract and include bronchospasm (sometimes severe, associated with a precipitous fall in pulmonary function [FEV_1]), cough, laryngeal edema (rare), nasal congestion (sometimes severe), pharyngeal irritation, and wheezing.

➤*Aerosol:*

Frequent – Throat irritation or dryness; bad taste; cough; wheeze; nausea.

Infrequent –
CNS: Dizziness; headache.
GU: Dysuria; urinary frequency.
Hypersensitivity: Anaphylaxis; rash; urticaria; angioedema.
Special senses: Lacrimation; swollen parotid gland.
Miscellaneous: Joint swelling and pain; substernal burning; myopathy; pulmonary infiltrates with eosinophilia.

Rare (unclear if attributable to drug) –
CNS: Vertigo; drowsiness.
Dermatologic: Exfoliative dermatitis; photodermatitis.
Musculoskeletal: Myalgia; polymyositis.
Respiratory: Hemoptysis; sneezing; nasal itching; nasal bleeding; nasal burning.
Miscellaneous: Stomachache; anemia; hoarseness; nephrosis; liver disease; serum sickness; periarteritic vasculitis; pericarditis; peripheral neuritis.

➤*Inhalation solution:*

Miscellaneous – Cough; nasal congestion; wheezing; sneezing; nausea; drowsiness; nasal itching; epistaxis; nose burning; serum sickness; stomachache.

➤*Nasal solution:*

Miscellaneous – Sneezing; nasal stinging; nasal irritation.

➤*Oral concentrate:* Most of the adverse events reported in mastocytosis patients have been transient and could represent symptoms of the disease. The most frequently reported adverse events in mastocytosis patients who have received cromolyn during clinical studies were headache and diarrhea. Each occurred in 4 of 87 patients. Pruritus, nausea, and myalgia were each reported in 3 patients and abdominal pain, rash, and irritability in 2 patients. There was also one report of malaise.

Adverse events have been reported during studies in other clinical conditions and during foreign postmarketing surveillances. In most cases, these reports were incomplete and attribution to cromolyn was not determined.

Cardiovascular – Tachycardia; premature ventricular contractions (PVCs); palpitations.

CNS – Dizziness; headache; paresthesia; migraine; hypesthesia; convulsions; psychosis; anxiety; depression; hallucinations; behavior change; insomnia; nervousness.

Dermatologic – Pruritus, rash; flushing; urticaria/angioedema; erythema and burning; photosensitivity.

GI – Diarrhea; nausea; abdominal pain; constipation; dyspepsia; flatulence; glossitis; stomatitis; vomiting; dysphagia; esophagospasm.

Hematologic – Polycythemia; neutropenia; pancytopenia.

Musculoskeletal – Arthralgia; myalgia; leg stiffness/weakness.

Miscellaneous – Pharyngitis; dyspnea; fatigue; edema; unpleasant taste; chest pain; postprandial lightheadedness and lethargy; dysuria; urinary frequency; purpura; hepatic function test abnormal; tinnitus; lupus erythematosus syndrome.

Overdosage

There is no clinical syndrome associated with an overdosage of cromolyn. In several animal species, acute toxicity with cromolyn occurs only with very high exposure levels. No deaths occurred at the highest oral doses tested in mice, 8000 mg/kg (approximately 5100 and 2700 times the maximum recommended daily inhalation doses in adults and children, respectively, on a mg/m^2 basis) or in rats, 8000 mg/kg (approximately 10,000 and 5400 times the maximum recommended daily inhalation doses in adults and children, respectively, on a mg/m^2 basis).

Patient Information

➤*Nasal solution:* Stop using the nasal spray and consult the physician if any of the following occurs: Shortness of breath, wheezing, or chest tightness; hives or swelling of the mouth or throat; symptoms worsen; new symptoms emerge; there is no improvement within 2 weeks; product needed for more than 12 weeks. Other medications (eg, allergy medications) may be used safely with cromolyn nasal solution. Do not use to treat sinus infection, asthma, or cold symptoms.

Directions for use – Blow nose before administering spray. Hold pump with thumb at bottom and nozzle between fingers. If this is the first time using the pump, or if you have not used the pump for several days, spray in the air until you get a fine mist. Insert nozzle into nostril, spray upward while breathing in through the nose. Repeat in other nostril. Brief stinging or sneezing may occur right after use. Keep clean by wiping nozzle. If used more than 12 weeks, consult a physician.

➤*Aerosol:*

Directions for use – Take the cover off the mouthpiece. Shake the inhaler gently. Hold inhaler and breathe out slowly and fully, expelling as much air as possible. Do not breathe into the inhaler; it could clog the inhaler valve. Place the mouthpiece into your mouth, close your lips around it, and tilt your head back. Keep your tongue below the opening of the inhaler. While breathing in deeply and slowly through the mouth, fully depress the top of the metal canister with your index finger. Remove the inhaler from your mouth. Hold your breath for several seconds, then breathe out slowly. Keep track of the number of actuations used from each canister of cromolyn inhaler and discard the canister after 112 actuations from the 8.1 g canister or 200 actuations from the 14.2 g canister.

➤*Inhalation solution:* Do not swallow solution because it is poorly absorbed orally. Empty the ampule into a power-driven nebulizer as directed. Do not mix different types of medications without permission from your health care provider.

Directions for use – Squeeze the contents of the ampule into the solution container of your nebulizer. Once the nebulizer has been assembled and contains cromolyn inhalation solution, hold the mask close to the face and switch on the device. Breathe through the mouth and out through the nose in a normal, relaxed manner. Nebulization should take approximately 5 to 10 minutes.

➤*Oral:* The effect of therapy depends upon administration at regular intervals as directed.

Take at least 30 minutes before meals and at bedtime. Break open ampule(s) and squeeze liquid contents into a glass of water. Stir solution and drink all of the liquid.

NEDOCROMIL SODIUM

Rx	**Tilade** (Monarch)	**Aerosol:** 1.75 mg/actuation	In 16.2 g canisters providing at least 104 metered inhalations. With mouthpiece.

NEDOCROMIL SODIUM — INHALATION

Indications

➤*Asthma, chronic:* For maintenance therapy in the management of adult and pediatric patients 6 years and older with mild to moderate asthma.

Nedocromil sodium is not indicated for the reversal of acute bronchospasm.

Administration and Dosage

➤*Approved by the FDA:* December 30, 1992.

The recommended dosage for adult and pediatric patients 6 years of age and older is 2 inhalations 4 times a day at regular intervals, which provides a dose of 14 mg per day. In patients whose asthma is well controlled on this dosage (eg, patients who only need occasional inhaled or oral beta$_2$-agonists and who are not experiencing serious exacerbations), less frequent administration may be effective. Dosing may be initially reduced to 3 times a day (10.5 mg/day), then after several weeks, to twice a day (7 mg/day) if asthma remains well controlled.

Each nedocromil sodium inhalation canister must be primed with 3 actuations prior to the first use. If a canister remains unused for more than 7 days, then it should be reprimed with 3 actuations.

Nedocromil sodium may be added to the patient's existing treatment regimen (eg, bronchodilators). When a clinical response to nedocromil sodium is evident and if the patient's asthma is under good control, an attempt may be made to decrease concomitant medication usage gradually.

➤*Storage/Stability:* Store between 2° to 30°C (36° to 86°F). Do not freeze. Avoid spraying in eyes. Contents under pressure. Do not puncture, incinerate, place near sources of heat, or use with other mouthpieces. Exposure to temperatures above 49°C (120°F) may cause bursting. Never throw canister into fire or incinerator. Keep out of the reach of children. For best results, the canister should be at room temperature before use.

Shake well before using.

Actions

➤*Pharmacology:* Nedocromil sodium has been shown to inhibit the in vitro activation of, and mediator release from, a variety of inflammatory cell types associated with asthma, including eosinophils, neutrophils, macrophages, mast cells, monocytes, and platelets. In vitro studies on cells obtained by bronchoalveolar lavage from antigen-sensitized macaque monkeys show that nedocromil sodium inhibits the release of mediators including histamine, leukotriene C_4, and prostaglandin D_2. Similar studies with human bronchoalveolar cells showed inhibition of histamine release from mast cells and beta-glucuronidase release from macrophages.

Nedocromil sodium has been tested in experimental models of asthma using allergic animals and shown to inhibit the development of early and late bronchoconstriction responses to inhaled antigen. The development of air-

NEDOCROMIL SODIUM — INHALATION

way hyper-responsiveness to nonspecific bronchoconstrictors was also inhibited. Nedocromil sodium reduced antigen-induced increases in airway microvasculature leakage when administered intravenously in a model system.

In humans, nedocromil sodium has been shown to inhibit acutely the bronchoconstrictor response to several kinds of challenge. Pretreatment with single doses of nedocromil sodium inhibited the bronchoconstriction caused by sulfur dioxide, inhaled neurokinin A, various antigens, exercise, cold air, fog, and adenosine monophosphate.

➤*Pharmacokinetics:*

Absorption – Systemic bioavailability of nedocromil sodium administered as an inhaled aerosol is low. In a single dose study involving 20 healthy adult subjects who were administered a 3.5 mg dose of nedocromil sodium (2 actuations of 1.75 mg each), the mean AUC was 5 ng•hr/mL and the mean C_{max} was 1.6 ng/mL attained about 28 minutes after dosing. The mean half-life was 3.3 hours. Urinary excretion over 12 hours averaged 3.4% of the administered dose, of which approximately 75% was excreted in the first 6 hours of dosing.

In a multiple dose study, 6 healthy adult volunteers (3 males and 3 females) received a 3.5 mg single dose followed by 3.5 mg 4 times a day for 7 consecutive days. Accumulation of the drug was not observed. Following single and multiple dose inhalations, urinary excretion of nedocromil accounted for 5.6% and 12% of the drug administered, respectively. After intravenous administration to healthy adults, urinary excretion of nedocromil was approximately 70%. The absolute bioavailability of nedocromil was thus 8% (5.6/70) for single and 17% (12/70) for multiple inhaled doses.

Similarly, in a multiple dose study of 12 asthmatic adult patients, each given a 3.5 mg single dose followed by 3.5 mg 4 times a day for 1 month, both single dose and multiple dose inhalations gave a mean high plasma concentration of 2.8 ng/mL between 5 and 90 minutes, mean AUC of 5.6 ng•hr/mL, and a mean terminal half-life of 1.5 hours. The mean 24-hour urinary excretion after either single or multiple dose administration represented approximately 5% of the administered dose.

Studies involving very high oral doses of nedocromil (600 mg single dose, and subsequently 200 mg 3 times a day for 7 days) showed an absolute bioavailability of less than 2%. In a radiolabeled (^{14}C) nedocromil intravenous study involving 2 healthy adult males, urinary excretion accounted for 64% of the dose, fecal excretion for 36%.

Although minimal pharmacokinetic data are available in children between the ages of 6 and 11 years, the nedocromil sodium levels obtained at 1 hour after chronic dosing in this age group appear to be similar to those observed in adults.

Distribution –

Protein binding: Nedocromil is approximately 89% protein bound in human plasma over a concentration range of 0.5 to 50 mcg/mL. This binding is reversible.

Metabolism/Excretion – Nedocromil is not metabolized after IV administration and is excreted unchanged.

Contraindications

Hypersensitivity to nedocromil sodium or other ingredients in this preparation.

Warnings

➤*Acute asthma:* Nedocromil sodium inhalation aerosol is not a bronchodilator and, therefore, should not be used for the reversal of acute bronchospasm, particularly status asthmaticus. Nedocromil sodium should ordinarily be continued during acute exacerbations, unless the patient becomes intolerant to the use of inhaled dosage forms.

➤*Bronchospasm:* As with other inhaled asthma medications, bronchospasm, which can be life-threatening, may occur immediately after administration. If this occurs, nedocromil sodium should be discontinued and alternative therapy instituted.

➤*Pregnancy: Category B.* There are no adequate and well-controlled studies in pregnant women. Because animal reproduction studies are not always predictive of human response, this drug should be used during pregnancy only if clearly needed.

➤*Lactation:* It is not known whether this drug is excreted in human milk. Because many drugs are excreted in human milk, caution should be exercised when nedocromil sodium is administered to a nursing woman.

➤*Children:* The safety and effectiveness of nedocromil sodium in patients below the age of 6 years have not been established.

Precautions

➤*Monitoring:* The role of nedocromil sodium as a corticosteroid-sparing agent in patients receiving oral or inhaled corticosteroids remains to be defined. If systemic or inhaled corticosteroid therapy is reduced in patients receiving nedocromil sodium, careful monitoring is necessary.

Drug Interactions

None known.

Adverse Reactions

The reasons for withdrawal were generally similar in the nedocromil sodium and placebo-treated groups, except that patients withdrew due to bad taste statistically more frequently on nedocromil sodium than on placebo. Headache reported as severe or very severe, some with nausea and ill feeling, was experienced by 1% of nedocromil sodium patients and 0.7% of placebo patients.

The events reported with a frequency of 1% or greater across all placebo-controlled studies are displayed for all patients ages 6 years and older who received nedocromil sodium or placebo at 2 inhalations 4 times daily.

The adverse event profile observed in children ages 6 through 11 years was similar to that observed in adults.

Adverse event	% Experiencing adverse event		% Withdrawing	
	Nedocromil (n = 2632)	Placebo (n = 2402)	Nedocromil	Placebo
Special senses				
Unpleasant taste	11.6%	3.1%	1.6%	0%
Respiratory				
Coughing	8.9%	10.2%	1.1%	1.2%
Pharyngitis	7.6%	7.5%	0.5%	0.4%
Rhinitis*	7.3%	6%	0.1%	0.1%
Upper respiratory tract infection	6.7%	6.3%	0.1%	0.2%
Sputum increased	1.5%	1.4%	0.1%	0.2%
Bronchitis	1.1%	1.5%	0.1%	0.1%
Dyspnea	2.5%	3.3%	0.8%	1%
Bronchospasm**	8.4%	11.8%	1.4%	2%
Sinusitis	3.3%	4.1%	1.1%	0%
Respiratory disorder	0.8%	1.1%	0%	0%
GI				
Nausea*	3.9%	2.3%	1.1%	0.5%
Vomiting*	2.5%	1.6%	0.2%	0.3%
Dyspepsia	1.5%	1.1%	0.1%	0.1%
Diarrhea	1.3%	1.2%	0.1%	0%
Abdominal pain*	1.9%	1.3%	0.2%	0.1%
CNS				
Dizziness	0.8%	1.3%	0.1%	0.2%
Miscellaneous				
Headache	8.1%	7.5%	0.4%	0.2%
Chest pain	3.6%	3.8%	0.7%	0.5%
Fatigue	1%	0.8%	0.2%	0%
Fever	3.1%	3.7%	0.1%	0.1%
Resistance mechanism disorders				
Viral infection	2.4%	3.2%	0.1%	0.1%
Ophthalmic				
Conjunctivitis	1.1%	0.7%	0%	0.1%
Dermatologic				
Rash**	0.5%	1.2%	0.1%	0%

* Statistically significant higher frequency on nedocromil sodium, $P < 0.05$.
** Statistically significant higher frequency on placebo, $P < 0.05$.

Other adverse events present at less than the 1% level of occurrence, but that might be related to nedocromil sodium administration, include arthritis, dizziness, rash, tremor, and a sensation of warmth.

In clinical trials with 2632 patients receiving nedocromil sodium, 2 patients (0.08%) developed neutropenia and 3 patients (0.11%) developed leukopenia. Although it is unclear if these reactions were caused by nedocromil sodium, in several cases these abnormal laboratory tests returned to normal when nedocromil sodium was discontinued.

There have been reports of clinically significant elevation of hepatic transaminases (ALT and AST greater than 10 times the upper limit of the normal reference range in 1 patient) associated with the administration of nedocromil sodium. It is unclear if these abnormal laboratory tests in asymptomatic patients were caused by nedocromil sodium.

Cases of bronchospasm immediately following dosing with nedocromil sodium have been reported from postmarketing experience. Isolated cases of pneumonitis with eosinophilia (PIE syndrome) and anaphylaxis have also been reported in which a relationship to drug is undetermined.

Overdosage

There is no experience to date with overdose of nedocromil sodium in humans. There were no deaths in rodents at an oral dose of 4000 mg/kg (approximately 690 times [for mice] and 1370 times [for rats] the maximum recommended human daily inhalation dose on a mg/m^2 basis). The subcutaneous or intravenous lethal dose in rats was between 2000 and 4000 mg/kg (approximately 690 and 1370 times, respectively, the maximum recommended human daily inhalation dose on a mg/m^2 basis). No deaths occurred in mice at a subcutaneous dose of 4000 mg/kg (approximately 690 times the maximum recommended human daily inhalation dose on a mg/m^2 basis), and the intravenous lethal dose in mice was between 2000 and 4000 mg/kg (approximately 345 and 690 times, respectively, the maximum recommended human daily inhalation dose on a mg/m^2 basis). An intravenous dose of 240 mg/kg (approximately 110 times the maximum recommended human daily inhalation dose on a mg/m^2 basis) did not produce any deaths in cats. Head shaking/tremor and

NEDOCROMIL SODIUM — INHALATION

salivation were observed in beagle dogs following daily inhalation doses of 5 mg/kg (approximately 6 times the maximum recommended human daily inhalation dose on a mg/m^2 basis) and transient hypotension was detected following daily subcutaneous doses of 8 mg/kg (approximately 9 times the maximum recommended human daily inhalation dose on a mg/m^2 basis). In addition, clonic convulsions were observed in dogs following daily inhalation doses of 20 mg/kg plus subcutaneous doses of 20 mg/kg giving peak plasma nedocromil levels of 7.6 mcg/mL, some 3 orders of magnitude greater than peak plasma levels (2.5 ng/mL) of the maximum recommended human daily inhalation dose. Specific tests designed to evaluate CNS activity demonstrated no effects due to nedocromil sodium, and nedocromil sodium does not pass the blood brain barrier. Therefore, overdosage is unlikely to result in clinical manifestations requiring more than observation and discontinuation of the drug where appropriate.

Patient Information

- Nedocromil sodium must be taken regularly to achieve benefit, even during symptom-free periods.
- Nedocromil sodium is not meant to relieve acute asthma symptoms. If symptoms do not improve or the patient's condition worsens, the patient should not increase the dosage but should notify the physician immediately.
- They should not decrease the dose without the physician's knowledge. The recommended dose should not be exceeded.
- The full therapeutic effect of nedocromil sodium may not be obtained for 1 week or longer after initiating treatment.
- Because the therapeutic effect depends upon local delivery to the lungs, it is essential that patients be properly instructed in the correct method of use.
- An illustrated leaflet for the patient is included in each nedocromil sodium inhaler pack.

NITRIC OXIDE

Rx	**INOmax** (INO Therapeutics, Inc.)	**Gas:** 100 ppm	In 353 (delivered volume 344 L) and 1963 L (delivered volume 1918 L).
		800 ppm	In 353 (delivered volume 344 L) and 1963 L (delivered volume 1918 L).

NITRIC OXIDE — INHALATION

Indications

➤*Neonates with hypoxic respiratory failure:* Nitric oxide, in conjunction with ventilatory support and other appropriate agents, is indicated for the treatment of term and near-term (greater than 34 weeks) neonates with hypoxic respiratory failure associated with clinical or echocardiographic (ECG) evidence of pulmonary hypertension, where it improves oxygenation and reduces the need for extracorporeal membrane oxygenation.

➤*Unlabeled uses:* Reduce pulmonary artery pressure (PAP) and pulmonary vascular resistance during neonatal cardiac operations; symptomatic treatment of hypoxemia or pulmonary hypertension due to allograft dysfunction subsequent to lung transplantation.

Administration and Dosage

➤*Approved by the FDA:* December 23, 1999.

➤*Dosage:* The recommended dose of nitric oxide is 20 ppm. Treatment should be maintained up to 14 days or until the underlying oxygen desaturation has resolved and the neonate is ready to be weaned from nitric oxide therapy.

An initial dose of 20 ppm was used in the Neonatal Inhaled Nitric Oxide Study (NINOS) and CINRGI trials. In CINRGI, patients whose oxygenation improved with 20 ppm were dose-reduced to 5 ppm as tolerated at the end of 4 hours of treatment. In the NINOS trial, patients whose oxygenation failed to improve on 20 ppm could be increased to 80 ppm, but those patients did not then improve on the higher dose. As the risk of methemoglobinemia and elevated NO_2 levels increases significantly when nitric oxide is administered at doses greater than 20 ppm, doses above this level ordinarily should not be used.

➤*Administration:* Additional therapies should be used to maximize oxygen delivery. In patients with collapsed alveoli, additional therapies might include surfactant and high-frequency oscillatory ventilation.

The safety and effectiveness of inhaled nitric oxide have been established in a population receiving other therapies for hypoxic respiratory failure, including vasodilators, intravenous fluids, bicarbonate therapy, and mechanical ventilation. Different dose regimens for nitric oxide were used in the clinical studies.

Nitric oxide should be administered with monitoring for PaO_2, methemoglobin, and NO_2.

The nitric oxide delivery systems used in the clinical trials provided operator-determined concentrations of nitric oxide in the breathing gas, and the concentration was constant throughout the respiratory cycle. Nitric oxide must be delivered through a system with these characteristics and which does not cause generation of excessive inhaled nitrogen dioxide. The *INOvent* system and other systems meeting these criteria were used in the clinical trials. In the ventilated neonate, precise monitoring of inspired nitric oxide and NO_2 should be instituted, using a properly calibrated analysis device with alarms. The system should be calibrated using a precisely defined calibration mixture of nitric oxide and nitrogen dioxide, such as *INOcal*. Sample gas for analysis should be drawn before the Y-piece, proximal to the patient. Oxygen levels should also be measured.

In the event of a system failure or a wall-outlet power failure, a backup battery power supply and reserve nitric oxide delivery system should be available.

The nitric oxide dose should not be discontinued abruptly as it may result in an increase in pulmonary artery pressure (PAP) or worsening of blood oxygenation (PaO_2). Deterioration in oxygenation and elevation in PAP may also occur in children with no apparent response to nitric oxide. Discontinue/wean cautiously.

➤*Storage/Stability:* Store at 25°C (77°F) with excursions permitted between 15° to 30°C (59° to 86°F).

Occupational exposure – The exposure limit set by the Occupational Safety and Health Administration (OSHA) for nitric oxide is 25 ppm, and for NO_2 the limit is 5 ppm.

Actions

➤*Pharmacology:* Nitric oxide is a compound produced by many cells of the body. It relaxes vascular smooth muscle by binding to the heme moiety of cytosolic guanylate cyclase, activating guanylate cyclase and increasing intracellular levels of cyclic guanosine 3',5'-monophosphate, which then leads to vasodilation. When inhaled, nitric oxide produces pulmonary vasodilation.

Nitric oxide appears to increase the partial pressure of arterial oxygen (PaO_2) by dilating pulmonary vessels in better ventilated areas of the lung, redistributing pulmonary blood flow away from lung regions with low ventilation/perfusion (V/Q) ratios toward regions with normal ratios.

Effects on pulmonary vascular tone in PPHN – Persistent pulmonary hypertension of the newborn (PPHN) occurs as a primary developmental defect or as a condition secondary to other diseases such as meconium aspiration syndrome (MAS), pneumonia, sepsis, hyaline membrane disease, congenital diaphragmatic hernia (CDH), and pulmonary hypoplasia. In these states, pulmonary vascular resistance (PVR) is high, which results in hypoxemia secondary to right-to-left shunting of blood through the patent ductus arteriosus and foramen ovale. In neonates with PPHN, nitric oxide improves oxygenation (as indicated by significant increases in PaO_2).

➤*Pharmacokinetics:*

Metabolism – Methemoglobin disposition has been investigated as a function of time and nitric oxide exposure concentration in neonates with respiratory failure.

Methemoglobin concentrations increased during the first 8 hours of nitric oxide exposure. The mean methemoglobin level remained below 1% in the placebo group and in the 5 ppm and 20 ppm nitric oxide groups, but reached approximately 5% in the 80 ppm nitric oxide group. Methemoglobin levels greater than 7% were attained only in patients receiving 80 ppm, where they comprised 35% of the group. The average time to reach peak methemoglobin was 10 ± 9 (SD) hours (median, 8 hours) in these 13 patients; but 1 patient did not exceed 7% until 40 hours.

Excretion – Nitrate has been identified as the predominant nitric oxide metabolite excreted in the urine, accounting for greater than 70% of the nitric oxide dose inhaled. Nitrate is cleared from the plasma by the kidney at rates approaching the rate of glomerular filtration.

Contraindications

Nitric oxide should not be used in the treatment of neonates known to be dependent on right-to-left shunting of blood.

Warnings

➤*Mutagenesis:* Nitric oxide has demonstrated genotoxicity in *Salmonella* (Ames test), human lymphocytes, and after in vivo exposure in rats.

➤*Pregnancy: Category C.* Animal reproduction studies have not been conducted with nitric oxide. It is not known if nitric oxide can cause fetal harm when administered to a pregnant woman or can affect reproductive capacity. Nitric oxide is not intended for adults.

➤*Lactation:* Nitric oxide is not indicated for use in the adult population, including nursing mothers. It is not known whether nitric oxide is excreted in human milk.

➤*Children:* Nitric oxide for inhalation has been studied in a neonatal population (up to 14 days of age).

Precautions

➤*Rebound:* Abrupt discontinuation of nitric oxide may lead to worsening oxygenation and increasing pulmonary artery pressure.

➤*Methemoglobinemia:* Methemoglobinemia increases with the dose of nitric oxide. In the clinical trials, maximum methemoglobin levels usually were reached approximately 8 hours after initiation of inhalation, although methemoglobin levels have peaked as late as 40 hours following initiation of nitric oxide therapy. In 1 study, 13 of 37 (35%) of neonates treated with nitric

NITRIC OXIDE — INHALATION

oxide 80 ppm had methemoglobin levels exceeding 7%. Following discontinuation or reduction of nitric oxide the methemoglobin levels returned to baseline over a period of hours.

➤*Elevated NO_2 levels:* In 1 study, NO_2 levels were less than 0.5 ppm when neonates were treated with placebo, 5 ppm, and 20 ppm nitric oxide over the first 48 hours. The 80 ppm group had a mean peak NO_2 level of 2.6 ppm.

Drug Interactions

No formal drug-interaction studies have been performed, and a clinically significant interaction with other medications used in the treatment of hypoxic respiratory failure cannot be excluded based on the available data. In particular, although there are no data to evaluate the possibility nitric oxide donor compounds, including sodium nitroprusside and nitroglycerin, may have an additive effect with nitric oxide on the risk of developing methemoglobinemia. Nitric oxide has been administered with tolazoline, dopamine, dobutamine, steroids, surfactant, and high-frequency ventilation.

Adverse Reactions

Controlled studies have included 325 patients on nitric oxide doses of 5 to 80 ppm and 251 patients on placebo. Total mortality in the pooled trials was 11% on placebo and 9% on nitric oxide, a result adequate to exclude nitric oxide mortality being more than 40% worse than placebo.

➤*Adverse reactions with an incidence of at least 5%:*

Adverse reaction in the CINRGI trial		
Adverse reaction	Placebo (n = 89)	Inhaled NO (n = 97)
Hypotension	9 (10%)	13 (13%)
Withdrawal	9 (10%)	12 (12%)
Atelectasis	8 (9%)	9 (9%)
Hematuria	5 (6%)	8 (8%)
Hyperglycemia	6 (7%)	8 (8%)
Sepsis	2 (2%)	7 (7%)
Infection	3 (3%)	6 (6%)
Stridor	3 (3%)	5 (5%)
Cellulitis	0 (0%)	5 (5%)

Overdosage

➤*Symptoms:* Overdosage with nitric oxide will be manifest by elevations in methemoglobin and NO_2. Elevated NO_2 may cause acute lung injury. Elevations in methemoglobinemia reduce the oxygen delivery capacity of the circulation. In clinical studies, NO_2 levels greater than 3 ppm or methemoglobin levels greater than 7% were treated by reducing the dose of, or discontinuing, nitric oxide.

➤*Treatment:* Methemoglobinemia that does not resolve after reduction or discontinuation of therapy can be treated with intravenous vitamin C, intravenous methylene blue, or blood transfusion, based upon the clinical situation.

FLUTICASONE PROPIONATE/SALMETEROL

Rx	Advair Diskus (GlaxoSmithKline)	Powder for inhalation: 100 mcg fluticasone propionate, 50 mcg salmeterol[a]	Lactose. In 28 and 60 blisters in a disposable, purple-colored device.
		250 mcg fluticasone propionate, 50 mcg salmeterol[a]	Lactose. In 28 and 60 blisters in a disposable, purple-colored device.
		500 mcg fluticasone propionate, 50 mcg salmeterol[a]	Lactose. In 28 and 60 blisters in a disposable, purple-colored device.

[a] Supplied as 72.5 mcg salmeterol xinaforte, equivalent to 50 mcg base.

FLUTICASONE PROPIONATE/SALMETEROL — INHALATION

For complete and comparative prescribing information, please refer to the Corticosteroids and Sympathomimetics group monographs.

WARNING

Long-acting β_2-adrenergic agonists, such as salmeterol, one of the active ingredients in fluticasone propionate/salmeterol, may increase the risk of asthma-related death. Therefore, when treating patients with asthma, physicians should only prescribe fluticasone propionate/salmeterol for patients not adequately controlled on other asthma-controller medications (eg, low- to medium-dose inhaled corticosteroids) or whose disease severity clearly warrants initiation of treatment with 2 maintenance therapies. Data from a large placebo-controlled US study that compared the safety of salmeterol or placebo added to usual asthma therapy showed an increase in asthma-related deaths in patients receiving salmeterol (13 deaths out of 13,176 patients treated for 28 weeks on salmeterol versus 3 deaths out of 13,179 on placebo).

Indications

➤*Asthma, chronic:* For the long-term, twice-daily maintenance treatment of asthma in patients 4 years of age and older. Not indicated for the relief of acute bronchospasm.

Long-acting β_2 adrenergic agonists, such as salmeterol, may increase the risk of asthma-related death. When treating patients with asthma, physicians should only prescribe fluticasone propionate/salmeterol for patients not adequately controlled on other asthma-controller medications (eg, low- to medium-dose inhaled corticosteroids) or whose disease severity clearly warrants initiation of treatment with 2 maintenance therapies. It is not indicated in patients whose asthma can be successfully managed by inhaled corticosteroids along with occasional use of inhaled, short-acting β_2- agonists.

➤*Chronic obstructive pulmonary disease (COPD) associated with chronic bronchitis:* For the twice-daily maintenance treatment of airflow obstruction in patients with COPD associated with chronic bronchitis. Fluticasone propionate/salmeterol 250 mcg/50 mcg twice daily is the only approved dosage for the treatment of COPD associated with chronic bronchitis. Higher doses, including fluticasone propionate/salmeterol 500 mcg/50 mcg, are not recommended.

Administration and Dosage

➤*Approved by the FDA:* August 24, 2000.

Administer by the orally inhaled route only. The maximum recommended dose of fluticasone propionate/salmeterol is 500 mcg/50 mcg twice daily.

➤*Asthma, chronic:*

Adults and children 12 years of age and older – One inhalation twice daily (morning and evening, approximately 12 hours apart). More frequent administration or a higher number of inhalations of the prescribed strength is not recommended because some patients are more likely to experience adverse effects with higher doses of salmeterol. The safety and efficacy of fluticasone propionate/salmeterol when administered in excess of recommended doses have not been established.

For all patients, titrate to the lowest effective strength after adequate asthma stability is achieved.

If symptoms arise in the period between doses, administer an inhaled, short-acting β_2-agonist for immediate relief.

Patients receiving fluticasone propionate/salmeterol twice daily should not use additional salmeterol or other inhaled, long-acting β_2-agonists (eg, formoterol) for prevention of exercise-induced bronchospasm or for any other reason.

Improvement in asthma control following inhaled administration of fluticasone propionate/salmeterol can occur within 30 minutes of beginning treatment, although maximum benefit may not be achieved for 1 week or longer after starting treatment. Individual patients will experience a variable time to onset and degree of symptom relief.

Replacing the current strength of fluticasone propionate/salmeterol with a higher strength may provide additional asthma control for patients who do not respond adequately to the starting dose after 2 weeks of therapy.

If a previously effective dosage regimen fails to provide adequate improvement in asthma control, reevaluate the therapeutic regimen and consider additional therapeutic options, such as replacing the current strength of fluticasone propionate/salmeterol with a higher strength, adding an additional inhaled corticosteroid, or initiating oral corticosteroids.

Advise patients to rinse mouth with water after inhalation without swallowing.

Patients not currently on an inhaled corticosteroid – A starting dose of fluticasone propionate/salmeterol 100 mcg/50 mcg or 250 mcg/50 mcg twice daily is recommended for patients who are not currently on an inhaled corticosteroid and whose disease severity warrants treatment with 2 maintenance therapies, including patients on noncorticosteroid maintenance therapy.

Patients currently on an inhaled corticosteroid – The following table provides the recommended starting dose for patients currently on an inhaled corticosteroid.

Recommended Starting Doses of Fluticasone Propionate/Salmeterol for Asthma Patients (Age ≥ 12) Not Adequately Controlled on Inhaled Corticosteroids

Current daily dose of inhaled corticosteroid		Recommended strength and dosing schedule of fluticasone propionate/salmeterol
Beclomethasone dipropionate HFA inhalation aerosol	≤ 160 mcg 320 mcg 640 mcg	100 mcg/50 mcg twice daily 250 mcg/50 mcg twice daily 500 mcg/50 mcg twice daily
Budesonide inhalation aerosol	≤ 400 mcg 800 to 1200 mcg 1600 mcg[a]	100 mcg/50 mcg twice daily 250 mcg/50 mcg twice daily 500 mcg/50 mcg twice daily
Flunisolide inhalation aerosol	≤ 1000 mcg 1250 to 2000 mcg	100 mcg/50 mcg twice daily 250 mcg/50 mcg twice daily
Flunisolide HFA inhalation aerosol	≤ 320 mcg 640 mcg	100 mcg/50 mcg twice daily 250 mcg/50 mcg twice daily
Fluticasone propionate HFA inhalation aerosol	≤ 176 mcg 440 mcg 660 to 880 mcg[a]	100 mcg/50 mcg twice daily 250 mcg/50 mcg twice daily 500 mcg/50 mcg twice daily
Fluticasone propionate inhalation powder	≤ 200 mcg 500 mcg 1000 mcg[a]	100 mcg/50 mcg twice daily 250 mcg/50 mcg twice daily 500 mcg/50 mcg twice daily
Mometasone furoate inhalation powder	220 mcg 440 mcg 880 mcg	100 mcg/50 mcg twice daily 250 mcg/50 mcg twice daily 500 mcg/50 mcg twice daily
Triamcinolone acetonide inhalation aerosol	≤ 1000 mcg 1100 to 1600 mcg	100 mcg/50 mcg twice daily 250 mcg/50 mcg twice daily

[a] Do not use fluticasone propionate/salmeterol for transferring patients from systemic corticosteroid therapy.

Children 4 to 11 years of age – For patients 4 to 11 years of age who are symptomatic on an inhaled corticosteroid, the dosage is 1 inhalation of fluticasone propionate/salmeterol 100 mcg/50 mcg twice daily (morning and evening, approximately 12 hours apart).

➤*COPD associated with chronic bronchitis:* The dosage for adults is 1 inhalation (250 mcg/50 mcg) twice daily (morning and evening, approximately 12 hours apart).

Fluticasone propionate/salmeterol 250 mcg/50 mcg twice daily is the only approved dosage for the treatment of COPD associated with chronic bronchitis. Higher doses, including fluticasone propionate/salmeterol 500 mcg/50 mcg, are not recommended because no additional improvement in lung function was observed in clinical trials and higher doses of corticosteroids increase the risk of systemic effects. The benefit of treating patients with COPD associated with chronic bronchitis with fluticasone propionate/salmeterol 250 mcg/50 mcg for periods longer than 6 months has not been evaluated. Periodically reevaluate patients treated with fluticasone propionate/salmeterol 250 mcg/50 mcg for COPD associated with chronic bronchitis for periods longer than 6 months to assess the continuing benefits and potential risks of treatment.

If shortness of breath occurs in the period between doses, an inhaled, short-acting β_2-agonist should be taken for immediate relief.

Patients who are receiving fluticasone propionate/salmeterol twice daily should not use additional salmeterol or other inhaled, long-acting β_2-agonists (eg, formoterol) for the maintenance treatment of COPD or for any other reason.

➤*Storage/Stability:* Store at 20° to 25°C (68° to 77°F) in a dry place away from direct heat or sunlight. Keep out of the reach of children. The inhalation device is not reusable; therefore, discard 1 month after removal from the moisture-protective, foil overwrap pouch or after every blister has been used (when the dose indicator reads "0"), whichever comes first. Do not attempt to take the device apart.

Indications

➤*Oral:* For temporary relief of nasal congestion due to the common cold, hay fever or other upper respiratory allergies, and nasal congestion associated with sinusitis; to promote nasal or sinus drainage.

➤*Topical:* Symptomatic relief of nasal and nasopharyngeal mucosal congestion due to the common cold, sinusitis, hay fever or other upper respiratory allergies.

Administration and Dosage

Recommended Dosage Guidelines for Oral and Topical Nasal Decongestants (Dosage Maximum/24 h)[a]

Drug and route	Adults ≥ 12 years of age	Children 6 to < 12 years of age	Children 2 to < 6 years of age
Ephedrine sulfate			
Topical			
Sprays	0.25%: 2 or 3 sprays in each nostril no more than q 4 h (6 doses/24 h)	0.25%: 1 or 2 sprays in each nostril no more than q 4 h (6 doses/24 h)	not recommended
Epinephrine HCl			
Topical	0.1%: Apply as drops or spray or with sterile swab as required	same as adults	not recommended
Naphazoline			
Topical			
Sprays	0.05%: 1 or 2 sprays in each nostril no more than q 6 h (4 doses/24 h)	not recommended	not recommended
Drops	0.05%: 1 or 2 drops in each nostril no more than q 6 h (4 doses/24 h)	not recommended	not recommended
Oxymetazoline HCl			
Topical			
Sprays	0.05%: 2 or 3 sprays in each nostril q 10 to 12 h (2 doses/24 h)	same as adults	not recommended
Phenylephrine HCl			
Oral	10-20 mg q 4 h (120 mg/24 h)	10 mg q 4 h (60 mg/24 h)	0.25% drops: 1 mL q 4 h (6 doses/24 h); (15 mg/24 h)
Topical			
Sprays	0.25%, 0.5%, 1%: 2 to 3 sprays in each nostril no more than q 4 h (6 doses/24 h)	0.25%: 2 to 3 sprays in each nostril no more than q 4 h (6 doses/24 h)	not recommended
Drops	0.25%, 0.5%, 1%: 2 to 3 drops in each nostril no more than q 4 h (6 doses/24 h)		0.125%: 2 to 3 drops in each nostril no more than q 4 h (6 doses/24 h)
Pseudoephedrine HCl			
Oral	60 mg q 4 to 6 h (240 mg/24 h)	30 mg q 4 to 6 h (120 mg/24 h)	15 mg q 4 to 6 h (60 mg/24 h)
Oral SR, CR	120 mg SR q 12 h or 240 mg CR q 24 h (240 mg/24 h)	not recommended	not recommended
Pseudoephedrine sulfate			
Oral ER	120 mg ER q 12 h (240 mg/24 h)	not recommended	not recommended
Tetrahydrozoline HCl			
Topical			
Sprays	0.1%: 3 to 4 sprays in each nostril prn, no more than q 3 h (8 doses/24 h)	same as adults	not recommended
Drops	0.1%: 2 to 4 drops in each nostril prn, no more than q 3 h (8 doses/24 h)	same as adults	0.05%: 2 to 3 drops in each nostril prn no more than q 3 h (8 doses/24 h)
Xylometazoline HCl			
Topical			
Sprays	0.1%: 1 to 3 sprays in each nostril q 8 to 10 h (3 doses/24 h)	0.05%: 1 spray in each nostril q 8 to 10 h (3 doses/24 h)	same dose for 2 to 12 years of age
Drops	0.1%: 2 to 3 drops in each nostril q 8 to 10 h (3 doses/24 h)	0.05%: 2 to 3 drops in each nostril q 8 to 10 h (3 doses/24 h)	same dose for 2 to 12 years of age

[a] Refer to manufacturer's directions.
SR = sustained release; CR = controlled release; ER = extended release

Actions

➤*Pharmacology:* Drugs that cause vasoconstriction, such as decongestants, act on the adrenergic receptors in the nasal mucosa by affecting the blood vessels' sympathetic tone and provoking vasoconstriction. Available decongestants include noradrenaline releasers (eg, amphetamines, **pseudoephedrine**), alpha$_1$-adrenergic agonists (eg, **phenylephrine**), and alpha$_2$-adrenergic agonists (eg, **naphazoline**, **oxymetazoline**). Decongestants improve nasal ventilation by shrinking swollen nasal mucosa. Constriction in the mucous membranes results in their shrinkage; this promotes drainage, thus improving ventilation and the stuffy feeling.

Decongestants are sympathomimetic amines administered directly to swollen membranes (eg, via spray, drops) or systemically via the oral route. They are used in acute conditions such as hay fever, allergic rhinitis, vasomotor rhinitis, sinusitis, and the common cold to relieve membrane congestion.

Oral agents are not as effective as topical products, especially on an immediate basis, but generally have a longer duration of action, cause less local irritation, and are not associated with rebound congestion (rhinitis medicamentosa).

Contraindications

Monoamine oxidase inhibitor (MAOI) therapy; hypersensitivity.

➤*Oral:*

Sustained-release pseudoephedrine – Children younger than 12 years of age.

➤*Topical:*

Tetrahydrozoline – 0.1% solution in children younger than 6 years of age; 0.05% solution in infants younger than 2 years of age. Systemic effects are less likely from topical use, but use caution in the conditions listed for oral agents. Adverse reactions are more likely with excessive use, in the elderly, and in children.

Warnings

➤*Special risk patients:* Administer with caution to patients with thyroid disease, diabetes, cardiovascular disease, coronary artery disease, hypertension, intraocular pressure, peripheral vascular disease, heart disease, or difficulty in urination due to enlargement of the prostate gland, unless directed by a physician. Rarely, some tablets may cause bowel obstruction or blockage, usually in people with severe narrowing of the bowel, esophagus, stomach, or intestine. If a patient has had obstruction or narrowing of the bowel, have him or her consult a physician before taking oral tablet products. Advise patients to contact their physician if they experience persistent abdominal pain or vomiting. As with any drug, if a patient is pregnant or nursing a baby, she should seek the advice of a health professional before using these products.

➤*Hypertension:* Hypertensive patients should use these products only with medical advice, as they may experience a change in blood pressure because of the added vasoconstriction. Studies suggest pseudoephedrine is the drug of choice. Sustained-action preparations may affect the cardiovascular system to a lesser degree.

➤*Excessive use:* Do not exceed recommended dosage. If nervousness, dizziness, or sleeplessness occur, discontinue use and have the patient consult a physician. Do not take topical products for greater than 3 days or oral products for greater than 7 days. If symptoms do not improve or are accompanied by a fever, the patient should consult a physician.

➤*Rebound congestion (rhinitis medicamentosa):* Following topical application, this may occur after the vasoconstriction subsides. Patients who increase the amount of drug and frequency of use may produce toxicity and perpetuate the rebound congestion.

Treatment – A simple but uncomfortable solution is to completely withdraw the topical medication. A more acceptable method is to gradually withdraw therapy by initially discontinuing the medication in one nostril, followed by total withdrawal. Substituting an oral decongestant for a topical one also may be useful.

➤*Elderly:* Patients 60 years of age or older are more likely to experience adverse reactions to sympathomimetics. Overdosage may cause hallucinations, convulsions, CNS depression, and death. Demonstrate safe use of a short-acting sympathomimetic before use of a sustained-action formulation in elderly patients.

➤*Pregnancy:* (*Category C* – **tetrahydrozoline**, **pseudoephedrine**, **phenylephrine**, **epinephrine**, **ephedrine**, **oxymetazoline**). It is not known whether these agents can cause fetal harm or affect reproduction capacity. Give only when clearly needed.

➤*Lactation:*

Oral preparations – Consult a physician before using.

Topical – It is not known if these agents are excreted in breast milk. Exercise caution when administering to a nursing woman.

➤*Children:* Use in children is product-specific. Refer to individual product listings.

Precautions

➤*Acute use:* Use topical decongestants only in acute states and not longer than 3 days. Use sparingly (especially the imidazolines) in all patients, particularly infants, children, and patients with cardiovascular disease.

➤*Stinging sensation:* Some individuals may experience a mild, transient stinging sensation after topical application.

➤*Sulfite sensitivity:* Some of the nasal decongestant products contain sulfites that may cause allergic-type reactions including anaphylactic symptoms and life-threatening or less severe asthmatic episodes in certain susceptible people. The overall prevalence of sulfite sensitivity in the general population is unknown but is probably low. Sulfite sensitivity is seen more frequently in asthmatic than in nonasthmatic people. Products containing sulfites are identified in the product listings.

Drug Interactions

Most interactions listed apply to sympathomimetics when used as vasopressors; however, consider the interaction when using the nasal decongestants.

Nasal Decongestant Drug Interactions			
Precipitant drug	Object drug[a]		Description
Beta blockers	Epinephrine	↑	An initial hypertensive episode followed by bradycardia may occur.
Furazolidone	Nasal decongestants	↑	The pressor sensitivity to mixed-acting agents (eg, ephedrine) may be increased. Direct-acting agents (eg, epinephrine) are not affected.
Guanethidine	Nasal decongestants Direct Mixed	 ↑ ↓	Guanethidine potentiates the effects of the direct-acting agents (eg, epinephrine) and inhibits the effects of the mixed-acting agents (eg, ephedrine). Guanethidine's hypotensive action also may be reversed.
Nasal decongestants	Guanethidine	↓	
Methyldopa	Nasal decongestants	↑	Coadministration may result in an increased pressor response.
MAO inhibitors	Nasal decongestants	↑	Concurrent use of MAOIs and mixed-acting agents (eg, ephedrine) may result in severe headache, hypertension, and hyperpyrexia, possibly resulting in hypertensive crisis. Direct-acting agents (eg, epinephrine) interact minimally, if at all.
Rauwolfia alkaloids	Nasal decongestants Direct Mixed	 ↑ ↓	Reserpine potentiates the pressor response of direct-acting agents (eg, epinephrine), which may result in hypotension. The pressor response of mixed-acting agents (eg, ephedrine) is decreased.
Tricyclic antidepressants (TCAs)	Nasal decongestants Direct Mixed	 ↑ ↓	TCAs potentiate the pressor response of direct-acting agents (eg, epinephrine); dysrhythmias have occurred. The pressor response of mixed-acting agents (eg, ephedrine) is decreased.
Urinary acidifiers	Nasal decongestants	↓	Acidification of the urine may increase the elimination of the nasal decongestant; therapeutic effects may be decreased. Conversely, urinary alkalinization may decrease the elimination of these agents, possibly increasing therapeutic or toxic effects.
Urinary alkalinizers		↑	

[a] ↑ = Object drug increased. ↓ = Object drug decreased.

Adverse Reactions

➤*Cardiovascular:* Arrhythmias; palpitations; tachycardia; transient hypertension; bradycardia.

➤*CNS:* Headache; lightheadedness; dizziness; drowsiness; tremor; insomnia; nervousness; restlessness; giddiness; psychological disturbances; prolonged psychosis (eg, paranoia, terror, delusions); weakness.

➤*GI:* Nausea; gastric irritation.

➤*Hypersensitivity:* Hypersensitivity reactions such as rash, urticaria, leukopenia, agranulocytosis, and thrombocytopenia may occur.

➤*Miscellaneous:* Orofacial dystonia; sweating; blepharospasm (eg, ocular irritation, tearing, photophobia); urinary retention may occur in patients with prostatic hypertrophy.

Topical use – Burning; stinging; sneezing; dryness; local irritation, rebound congestion.

Overdosage

➤*Symptoms:* Overdoses have caused hypertension, bradycardia, drowsiness, and rebound hypotension in adults; a shock-like syndrome with hypotension and bradycardia also may occur. In either case, the treatment of overdosage is usually that of watchful expectancy and general supportive measures. If possible, keep the patient warm and maintain fluid balance orally or parenterally, if necessary. Overdosage of **tetrahydrozoline** nasal solution may result in oversedation in young children.

➤*Treatment:* Treatment is supportive; in severe cases, IV phentolamine may be used. See General Management of Acute Overdosage.

Tetrahydrozoline – There is no known antidote. The use of stimulants is contraindicated. If respiratory rate drops to less than or equal to 10, administer oxygen and assist respiration. Monitor blood pressure to prevent hypotensive crisis.

Patient Information

Patients with hypertension, heart disease, or other cardiovascular diseases, thyroid disease, diabetes, or difficulty urinating due to an enlarged prostate should use these products only with medical advice.

➤*Topical:* Notify physician of insomnia, dizziness, weakness, tremor, or irregular heart beat.

Do not exceed recommended dosage and do not use longer than 3 days. If symptoms persist, contact the doctor. Frequent or prolonged use may cause nasal congestion to recur or worsen.

Stinging, burning, sneezing, increased nasal discharge, or drying of the nasal mucosa may occur.

Do not share container with other patients. Do not allow tip of container to touch the nasal passage. Discard after medication is no longer required.

Proper use – Spray – Keep head upright. Sniff hard for a few minutes after use.

Drops – Recline on a bed and hang your head over the edge; remain in this position for several minutes after using the drops, turning the head from side to side.

Inhalers – Warm in the hand before use. Wipe the inhaler after each use.

➤*Oral:* Do not exceed recommended dosage; higher doses may cause nervousness, dizziness, or sleeplessness.

If symptoms do not improve within 7 days or are accompanied by a high fever, consult physician before continuing use.

Arylalkylamines

PSEUDOEPHEDRINE SULFATE

otc	**Drixoral 12 Hour Non-Drowsy Formula** (Schering-Plough Healthcare)	**Tablets, extended-release:** 120 mg	Sugar, lactose, butylparabens. (DRIXORAL NDF). In 10s.

PSEUDOEPHEDRINE SULFATE — ORAL

For complete and comparative prescribing information, refer to the Nasal Decongestants group monograph.

Indications

➤*Nasal congestion:* For temporary relief of nasal congestion due to the common cold, hay fever, or other upper respiratory allergies, and associated with sinusitis.

Administration and Dosage

➤*Adults and children (12 years of age or older).* 120 mg every 12 hours. Do not exceed 240 mg in 24 hours.

Do not crush or chew sustained release preparations.

PSEUDOEPHEDRINE HYDROCHLORIDE (d-Isoephedrine Hydrochloride)

otc	**Pseudoephedrine HCl** (Various, eg, Geneva, Roxane, Rugby)	**Tablets:** 30 mg	In 24s, 100s, 1,000s, blister pack 100s.
otc	**Congestaid** (Zee Medical)		In 24s.
otc	**Genaphed** (Goldline)		In 24s.[1]
otc	**Medi-First Sinus Decongestant** (Textilease Medique[2])		In 100s and 250s.
otc	**Sudodrin** (Textilease Medique[2])		(FR4). In 250s, 250s, and 1000s.
otc	**Simply Stuffy** (McNeil Consumer)		In 24s.[1]
otc	**Sudafed Non-Drowsy, Maximum Strength** (Warner-Lambert Consumer)		(SU). In 24s, and 96s.[3]

Arylalkylamines

PSEUDOEPHEDRINE HYDROCHLORIDE (d-Isoephedrine Hydrochloride)

otc	**Pseudoephedrine HCl** (Various, eg, Geneva, Roxane)	**Tablets**: 60 mg	In 100s, 1,000s, and blister pack 100s.
otc	**Cenafed** (Century)		In 100s.
otc	**Sudafed, Children's Non-Drowsy** (Warner-Lambert Consumer)	**Tablets, chewable**: 15 mg	Orange flavor. In 24s.[4]
otc	**Triaminic Allergy Congestion Softchews** (Novartis Consumer)		Orange flavor. In 18s.[5]
otc	**Sudafed Non-Drowsy 12 Hour Long-Acting** (Warner-Lambert Consumer)	**Tablets, extended-release**: 120 mg	Capsule shape. (SUDAFED 12 HOUR). In 10s.
otc	**Dimetapp, Maximum Strength 12-Hour Non-Drowsy Extentabs** (Whitehall-Robins)		Capsule shape. In 10s.
otc	**Efidac 24 Pseudoephedrine** (Hogil)	**Tablets, controlled-release**: 240 mg (immediate-release 60 mg, controlled-release 180 mg).	In 6s, 12s, and UD 1s.
otc	**Sudafed Non-Drowsy 24 Hour Long-Acting** (Warner-Lambert Consumer)		(SU-24). In 10s.
otc	**Sinustop** (Nature's Way)	**Capsules**: 60 mg	In 20s.[6]
otc	**AllergyCare** (Nature's Way)		In 20s.[7]
otc	**Dimetapp, Maximum Strength, Non-Drowsy Liqui-Gels** (Whitehall-Robins)	**Capsules, softgel**: 30 mg	In 12s.[8]
otc	**Nasal Decongestant, Children's Non-Drowsy** (Various, eg, AmerisourceBergen[9])	**Liquid**: 15 mg/5 mL	In 118 mL.
otc	**Simply Stuffy** (McNeil-PPC)		Corn syrup, sucralose. Alcohol-free. Cherry berry flavor. In 120 mL.
otc	**Triaminic Allergy Congestion** (Novartis Consumer)		In 118 mL.[10]
otc sf	**Sudafed, Children's Non-Drowsy** (Warner-Lambert Consumer)		Alcohol free. Grape flavor. In 118 mL.[11]
otc	**Pseudoephedrine HCl** (Various, eg, Rugby)	**Liquid**: 30 mg/5 mL	In 120 and 473 mL.
otc	**Decofed Syrup** (Various)		In 118 and 473 mL.
otc	**Cenafed Syrup** (Century)		In 120 and 480 mL, and 3.8 L.[12]
otc	**Silfedrine, Children's** (Silarx)		In 118 and 237 mL.[13]
otc	**Unifed** (Altaire)		Methylparaben, glycerin, sorbitol, sucrose. In 118 mL.
otc	**ElixSure Children's Congestion** (Taro Consumer)	**Syrup**: 15 mg/5 mL	Glycerin, propylparaben. Grape and bubble gum flavors. In 118 mL.
otc	**Nasal Decongestant Oral** (Various, eg, ProMetic)	**Drops**: 7.5 mg/0.8 mL	In 15 and 30 mL w/dropper.
otc	**Dimetapp Decongestant Pediatric** (Whitehall-Robins)		In 15 mL.[14]
otc	**Kid Kare** (Rugby)		Alcohol free. Cherry flavor. In 30 mL w/dropper.[15]
otc	**PediaCare Decongestant, Infants'** (Pharmacia Consumer)		Alcohol free. Fruit flavor. In 15 mL w/dropper.[16]

[1] With lactose.
[2] Textilease Medique Products, 900 Lively Blvd., Wood Dale, IL 60191; (630) 694-4100.
[3] With lactose, sucrose.
[4] With aspartame, mannitol, 0.78 mg phenylalanine.
[5] With aspartame, mannitol, sorbitol, sucrose, 17.5 mg phenylalanine.
[6] With echinacea purpura, ginger, goldenseal root.
[7] With brigham tea herb, elder flowers, eyebright, ginger, golden rod herb, licorice root.
[8] With mannitol, sorbitol.
[9] AmerisourceBergen, 1300 Morris Dr., Chesterbrook, PA 19087; (888)276-6034.
[10] With EDTA, sucrose, sorbitol.
[11] With EDTA, saccharin, sorbitol.
[12] With methylparaben.
[13] With methylparaben, saccharin, sucrose.
[14] With corn syrup, menthol, sorbitol, sucrose.
[15] With sorbitol, sugar.
[16] With sorbitol, sucrose.

PSEUDOEPHEDRINE HYDROCHLORIDE — ORAL

For complete and comparative prescribing information, refer to the Nasal Decongestants group monograph.

Indications

➤*Nasal congestion:* Temporary relieves nasal congestion due to the common cold, hay fever, or other upper respiratory allergies, and nasal congestion associated with sinusitis; reduces swelling of nasal passages; relieves sinus pressure; promotes nasal or sinus drainage; restores freer breathing through the nose.

Administration and Dosage

➤*Adults (12 years of age or older):* 60 mg every 4 to 6 hours (120 mg sustained-release every 12 hours, 240 mg controlled-release every 24 hours). Do not exceed 240 mg in 24 hours.

➤*Children (6 to 12 years of age):* 30 mg every 4 to 6 hours. Do not exceed 120 mg in 24 hours.

Children (2 to 5 years of age) – 15 mg every 4 to 6 hours. Do not exceed 60 mg in 24 hours.

Children (younger than 2 years of age) – Consult a physician.

➤*Storage/Stability:* Store at room temperature (15° to 25°C [59° to 77°F]).

PHENYLEPHRINE HYDROCHLORIDE

otc	**Sudafed PE** (Pfizer)	**Tablets**: 10 mg	Acesulfame K. In 18s.
otc	**Sudogest PE** (Major)		Dextrose. In 36s.
Rx	**AH-chew D** (WE Pharm)	**Tablets, chewable**: 10 mg	(WE 07). Scored. Bubble gum flavor. In 100s.
Rx	**Nasop** (Hawthorn)	**Tablets, orally disintegrating** : 10 mg	(HAW 260). Pink. Bubble gum flavor. In 100s.[a]
Rx	**Lusonal** (WraSer)	**Oral liquid**: 7.5 mg per 5 mL	Strawberry flavor. In 473 mL.[b]
otc	**Little Colds Decongestant for Infants and Children** (Vetco)	**Oral drops**: 2.5 mg/mL	Alcohol free. Grape flavor. Glycerin, sorbitol and sucralose. In 30 mL.
otc	**Little Noses Gentle Formula, Infants & Children** (Vetco[c])	**Nasal solution**: 0.125%	**Drops**: Alcohol free. In 15 mL w/dropper.[e]

PHENYLEPHRINE HYDROCHLORIDE

otc	**Afrin Children's Pump Mist** (Schering-Plough Healthcare)	**Nasal solution:** 0.25%	**Spray:** In 15 mL.[e]
otc	**Neo-Synephrine 4-Hour Mild Formula** (Bayer Corp.)		**Spray:** In 15 mL.[f]
otc	**Rhinall** (Scherer)		**Spray:** In 40 mL.[g]
			Drops: In 30 mL.[g]
otc	**Neo-Synephrine 4-Hour Regular Strength** (Bayer Corp.)	**Nasal solution:** 0.5%	**Drops:** In 15 mL.[f]
			Spray: In 15 mL.[f]
otc	**Vicks Sinex Ultra Fine Mist** (Procter & Gamble)		**Spray:** In 14.7 mL.[h]
otc	**Phenylephrine hydrochloride** (Various, cg, Rugby)	**Nasal solution:** 1%	In 480 mL.
otc	**4-Way Fast Acting** (Bristol-Myers)		**Spray:** In 30 mL.[i]
otc	**Neo-Synephrine 4-Hour Extra Strength** (Bayer Corp.)		**Drops:** In 15 mL.[f]
			Spray: In 15 mL.[f]
otc	**Sudafed PE Quick-dissolve** (Pfizer Consumer Healthcare)	**Strips:** 10 mg	1 mg phenylalanine, acesulfame K, aspartame, EDTA, glycerin. Cherry menthol flavor. In 10s.

[a] With phenylalanine 4 mg, aspartame, sorbitol.
[b] With aspartame, phenylalanine, parabens.
[c] Vetco, 105 Baylis Road, Melville, NY 11747; (631)755-1155.
[d] With sorbitol, sucralose.
[e] With EDTA, benzalkonium chloride.
[f] With benzalkonium chloride, thimerosal.
[g] With chlorobutanol, sodium bisulfite, benzalkonium chloride.
[h] With benzalkonium chloride, camphor, EDTA, eucalyptol, menthol, tyloxapol.
[i] With benzalkonium chloride, boric acid, sodium borate.

PHENYLEPHRINE HYDROCHLORIDE — ORAL

For complete and comparative prescribing information, refer to the Nasal Decongestants group monograph.

Indications

➤*Nasal congestion:* Phenylephrine is recommended for the temporary relief of nasal congestion due to the common cold, sinusitis, hay fever, or upper respiratory allergies.

➤*Lusonal:* For temporarily relief of symptoms of upper respiratory tract disorders such as sinusitis, vasomotor rhinitis, and hay fever, as well as for the temporary relief of coughs associated with respiratory tract infections and related conditions such as sinusitis, bronchitis, and asthma, when these conditions are complicated by tenacious mucus and/or mucus plugs and congestion.

Administration and Dosage

➤*Adults (12 years of age or older):*

Tablets – 1 or 2 tablets every 4 hours.

Oral liquid – 10 mL every 6 hours up to 40 mL/day.

➤*Children (6 through 11 years of age):*

Tablets – 1 tablet every 4 hours.

Oral liquid – 5 mL every 6 hours up to 20 mL/day.

➤*Children (2 through 5 years of age):*

0.25% oral drops – 1 dropperful (1 mL) by mouth every 4 hours not to exceed 6 doses in a 24-hour period.

Orally disintegrating tablets – ½ tablet every 4 hours.

Oral liquid – 2.5 mL every 6 hours up to 10 mL/day.

➤*Children (younger than 2 years of age):* Consult a physician.

➤*Chewable tablets:*

Adults and children 12 years of age and older – Chew 1 or 2 tablets every 4 hours.

Children 6 to 12 years of age – Chew 1 tablet every 4 hours.

Children under 6 years of age – Take as recommended by a physician. Tablets may be broken in half for ease of administration.

➤*Oral drops:* See the table below. For accurate dosing, only use the enclosed dropper and follow all dosing instructions.

Age (years)	Dose
Under 2 years of age	Consult physician.
2 to under 6 years of age	2.5 mg

All doses should be taken by mouth only and may be repeated every 4 hours, not to exceed 6 doses in a 24-hour period.

➤*Strips:*

Adults – 1 strip every 4 hour, do not take more than 6 in 24 hours. Place 1 film strip on tongue and allow it to dissolve.

Children younger than 12 years of age – Consult a physician.

➤*Storage/Stability:* Store at controlled room temperature 15° to 30°C (59° to 86°F).

Store strips in a dry place.

PHENYLEPHRINE HYDROCHLORIDE — INTRANASAL

For complete and comparative prescribing information, refer to the Nasal Decongestants group monograph.

Indications

➤*Nasal congestion:* For prompt, temporary relief of nasal congestion due to the common cold, sinusitis, hay fever, or other upper respiratory allergies, or associated with sinusitis.

Administration and Dosage

➤*Adults (12 years of age or older):* Two to 3 sprays or drops in each nostril. Repeat every 3 to 4 hours (0.25% and 0.5%). The 1% solution should be repeated no more often than every 4 hours. Do not give to children younger than 12 years of age unless directed by a physician.

➤*Children (6 through 11 years of age):*

0.25% – 2 to 3 sprays or drops in each nostril not more often than every 4 hours.

➤*Children (2 through 5 years of age):*

0.125% – 2 or 3 drops into each nostril not more often than every 4 hours.

➤*Children (younger than 2 years of age):* Consult a physician.

PHENYLEPHRINE TANNATE

Rx	**AH-chew D** (WE Pharm)	**Oral suspension:** 10 mg (as phenylephrine hydrochloride) per 5 mL	Saccharin, parabens. Grape flavor. In 20 and 118 mL unit-of-use bottles.

PHENYLEPHRINE TANNATE — ORAL

For complete and comparative prescribing information, refer to the Nasal Decongestants group monograph.

Indications

➤*Nasal congestion:* For the temporary relief of nasal congestion caused by the common cold, sinusitis, and hay fever (allergic rhinitis).

Administration and Dosage

➤*Adults and adolescents 12 years of age or older:* 5 to 10 mL every 12 hours.

➤*Children 6 to 12 years of age:* 2.5 to 5 mL every 12 hours.

Consult a health care provider for children younger than 6 years of age.

➤*Storage/Stability:* Store oral suspension at 25°C (77°). Excursions permitted to 15° to 30°C (50° to 86°F).

Imidazolines

NAPHAZOLINE HYDROCHLORIDE

otc	**Privine** (Insight[a])	**Solution:** 0.05%	**Drops:** In 25 mL w/dropper.[b]
			Spray: In 20 mL.[b]

[a] Insight Pharmaceuticals Corp., 1170 Wheeler Way, Suite 150, Langhorne, PA 19047-1749; 1-(267) 852-0505; fax 1-(267) 852-0515.

[b] With benzalkonium chloride, EDTA.

NAPHAZOLINE HYDROCHLORIDE — INTRANASAL

For complete and comparative prescribing information, refer to the Nasal Decongestants group monograph.

Indications

➤*Nasal congestion:* Temporary relief of nasal congestion due to the common cold, hay fever or other upper respiratory tract allergies, or associated with sinusitis.

Administration and Dosage

➤*Approved by the FDA:* March 24, 1972.

➤*Adults and children 12 years of age and over:* 1 or 2 drops or sprays in each nostril not more often than every 6 hours. Do not give to children under 12 years of age unless directed by a doctor.

➤*Storage/Stability:* Store between 15° to 30°C (59° to 86°F).

In case of accidental ingestion, seek professional assistance or contact a poison control center immediately.

OXYMETAZOLINE HYDROCHLORIDE

otc	**Oxymetazoline HCl** (Various, eg, Alpharma, Clay Park, Thames)	**Solution:** 0.05%	**Spray:** In 15 and 30 mL.
otc	**12 Hour Nasal** (Various, eg, URL)		**Spray:** In 15 mL.
otc	**Twice-A-Day 12-Hour Nasal** (Major)		**Spray:** In 15 and 30 mL.[1]
otc	**Neo-Synephrine 12-Hour Extra Moisturizing** (Bayer Corp.)		**Spray:** In 15 mL.[2]
otc	**Neo-Synephrine 12-Hour** (Bayer Corp.)		**Spray:** In 15 mL.[2]
otc	**Duration** (Schering-Plough Healthcare)		**Spray:** In 30 mL.[3]
otc	**Afrin 12-Hour Original Pump Mist** (Schering-Plough Healthcare)		**Spray:** In 15 mL.[3]
otc	**Afrin 12-Hour Original** (Schering-Plough Healthcare)		**Spray:** In 15 mL. [3]
otc	**Afrin Severe Congestion with Menthol** (Schering-Plough Healthcare)		**Spray:** In 15 mL.[4]
otc	**Afrin Sinus with Vapornase** (Schering-Plough Healthcare)		**Spray:** In 15 mL. [4]
otc	**Afrin No-Drip 12-Hour** (Schering-Plough Healthcare)		**Spray:** In 15 mL.[5]
otc	**Afrin No-Drip 12-Hour Extra Moisturizing** (Schering-Plough Healthcare)		**Spray:** In 15 mL.[6]
otc	**Afrin No-Drip 12-Hour Severe Congestion with Menthol** (Schering-Plough Healthcare)		**Spray:** In 15 mL.[7]
otc	**Afrin No-Drip Sinus with Vapornase** (Schering-Plough Healthcare)		**Spray:** In 15 mL.[7]
otc	**Dristan 12-Hr Nasal** (Whitehall-Robins)		**Spray:** In 15 mL.[8]
otc	**Duramist Plus 12-Hr Decongestant** (Pfeiffer)		**Spray:** In 15 mL.[9]
otc	**Genasal** (Goldline)		**Spray:** In 15 and 30 mL.[10]
otc	**Nasal Decongestant, Maximum Strength** (Taro)		**Spray:** In 15 and 30 mL.
otc	**Nasal Relief** (Rugby)		**Spray:** In 15 mL.[11]
otc	**Nōstrilla 12-Hour** (Heritage)		**Spray:** In 15 mL metered pump spray.[12]
otc	**Vicks Sinex 12-Hour Long-Acting** (Procter & Gamble)		**Spray:** In 15 mL.[13]
otc	**Vicks Sinex 12-Hour Ultra Fine Mist for Sinus Relief** (Procter & Gamble)		**Spray:** In 15 mL.[14]

[1] With EDTA, benzalkonium chloride, benzyl alcohol.
[2] With benzalkonium chloride, phenylmercuric acetate, glycine, sorbitol, sodium chloride.
[3] With benzalkonium chloride, EDTA.
[4] With benzalkonium chloride, benzyl alcohol, camphor, EDTA, eucalyptol, menthol.
[5] With carboxymethylcellulose sodium, microcrystalline cellulose, benzalkonium chloride, benzyl alcohol, EDTA.
[6] With carboxymethylcellulose sodium, microcrystalline cellulose, benzalkonium chloride, benzyl alcohol, EDTA, glycerin.
[7] With carboxymethylcellulose sodium, microcrystalline cellulose, benzalkonium chloride, benzyl alcohol, camphor, EDTA, eucalyptol, menthol.
[8] With benzalkonium chloride, hydroxypropylmethylcellulose, thimerosal, sodium chloride.
[9] With benzalkonium chloride, EDTA, sodium chloride.
[10] With benzalkonium chloride, phenylmercuric acetate, sorbitol.
[11] With EDTA, phenylmercuric acetate, sodium chloride.
[12] With benzalkonium chloride, glycine, sorbitol.
[13] With benzalkonium chloride, camphor, chlorhexidine gluconate, EDTA, eucalyptol, menthol, sodium chloride, tyloxapol.
[14] With aromatic vapors (camphor, eucalyptus, menthol), tyloxapol, EDTA, benzalkonium chloride, sodium chloride.

OXYMETAZOLINE HYDROCHLORIDE — INTRANASAL

For complete and comparative prescribing information, refer to the Nasal Decongestants group monograph.

Indications

➤*Nasal congestion:* For the temporary relief of nasal congestion due to a cold, hay fever, or other upper respiratory allergies, or associated with sinusitis. Reduces swelling of nasal passages; shrinks swollen membranes. Temporarily restores freer breathing through the nose; temporarily relieves sinus congestion and pressure.

Administration and Dosage

➤*Adults and children (6 years or older):* 2 or 3 sprays of 0.05% solution in each nostril twice daily, morning and evening, or every 10 to 12 hours. Do not exceed 2 doses in any 24-hour period.

TETRAHYDROZOLINE HYDROCHLORIDE

Rx	**Tyzine Pediatric** (Kenwood)	**Solution:** 0.05%	**Drops:** In 15 mL with dropper.[1]
Rx	**Tyzine** (Kenwood)	**Solution:** 0.1%	**Drops:** In 30 mL with dropper.[1]
			Spray: In 15 mL.[1]

[1] With benzalkonium chloride, EDTA.

TETRAHYDROZOLINE HYDROCHLORIDE — INTRANASAL

For complete and comparative prescribing information, refer to the Nasal Decongestants group monograph.

Indications

➤*Nasal congestion:* Decongestion of nasal and nasopharyngeal mucosa.

Administration and Dosage

➤*Adults and children 6 years and over:* 2 to 4 drops or 3 to 4 sprays of 0.1% solution instilled in each nostril as needed, never more often than every 3 hours. Less frequent administration is usually sufficient since relief is maintained for 4 hours or longer in most cases, and often for as long as 8 hours. Bedtime instillation usually ensures sleep undisturbed by the need for remedication before morning, or by insomnia from central stimulation.

➤*Children 2 to 6 years of age:*

Pediatric nasal drops 0.05% – Do not use tetrahydrozoline HCl 0.1% nasal solution or tetrahydrozoline HCl 0.1% nasal spray. It is recommended that 2 to 3 drops be instilled in each nostril as needed, and never more often than every 3 hours. Relief usually lasts for several hours, so that instillation is usually needed only every 4 to 6 hours. Instillation of nose drops can be most conveniently accomplished with the patient in the lateral head-low position.

➤*Storage/Stability:* Store below 30°C (86°F).

XYLOMETAZOLINE HYDROCHLORIDE

otc	**Otrivin Pediatric Nasal** (Novartis Consumer)	**Solution:** 0.05%	**Drops:** In 25 mL dropper bottle.[1]
otc	**Natru-Vent** (Boehringer Ingelheim Consumer Health)		**Spray:** Preservative free. In metered-dose pump spray bottles (100 sprays).[2]
otc	**Otrivin** (Novartis Consumer)	**Solution:** 0.1%	**Drops:** In 25 mL dropper bottle.[3]
			Spray: In 20 mL.[3]
otc	**Natru-Vent** (Boehringer Ingelheim Consumer Health)		**Spray:** Preservative free. In two 10 mL bottles.[2]

[1] With benzalkonium chloride, EDTA.
[2] With sorbitol.
[3] With benzalkonium chloride, sodium chloride, EDTA.

XYLOMETAZOLINE HYDROCHLORIDE — INTRANASAL

For complete and comparative prescribing information, refer to the Nasal Decongestants group monograph.

Indications

➤*Spray/Drops:* For the temporary relief of nasal congestion due to the common cold, hay fever, or other respiratory allergies.

➤*Pediatric drops:* For temporary relief of nasal and sinus congestion and pressure due to a cold.

Administration and Dosage

➤*Adults (12 years of age or older):* 2 to 3 drops or 1 to 3 sprays (0.1%) in each nostril every 8 to 10 hours. Do not give 0.1% solution to children younger than 12 years of age.

➤*Children (2 to 12 years of age):* 2 to 3 drops or 1 spray (0.05%) in each nostril every 8 to 10 hours. Do not exceed 3 doses in any 24-hour period.

NASAL DECONGESTANT COMBINATIONS

otc	**Dristan Fast Acting Formula** (Whitehall-Robins)	**Solution:** 0.5% phenylephrine HCl and 0.2% pheniramine maleate	**Spray:** In 15 mL.[1]

[1] With mannitol, sorbitol, benzalkonium chloride, benzyl alcohol.

NASAL DECONGESTANT COMBINATIONS — INTRANASAL

For complete and comparative prescribing information, refer to the Nasal Decongestants group monograph.

Indications

➤*Nasal congestion:* Relieves nasal congestion due to colds and sinusitis.

In this combination: **PHENYLEPHRINE HCl** is a decongestant.

PHENIRAMINE MALEATE is an antihistamine.

NASAL DECONGESTANT INHALERS

otc	**Benzedrex** (B.F. Ascher)	**Inhaler:** 250 mg propylhexedrine	In single plastic inhalers.[1]
otc	**Vicks Vapor Inhaler** (Procter & Gamble Consumer)	**Inhaler:** 50 mg levmetamfetamine	In single plastic inhalers.[2]

[1] With menthol, lavender oil.
[2] With camphor, lavender oil, menthol.

NASAL DECONGESTANT INHALERS — INHALATION

For complete and comparative prescribing information, refer to the Nasal Decongestants group monograph.

Indications

➤*Nasal congestion:* For the temporary relief of nasal congestion due to the common cold, hay fever, upper respiratory allergies, or sinusitis.

Administration and Dosage

➤*Adults and children (6 years of age or older):* 1 to 2 inhalations in each nostril (while blocking the other nostril) not more than every 2 hours. Do not exceed recommended dosage. Do not use these products for greater than 3 days. If symptoms persist beyond this time, consult physician.

NASAL PRODUCTS

otc	**Nasal Spray** (Various, eg, Ivax)	**Solution:** Sodium chloride	**Spray:** In 45 mL.
otc	**Pretz Moisturizing** (Parnell)		**Spray:** In 50 mL.[a]
otc	**Afrin Saline, Extra Moisturizing** (Schering-Plough HealthCare)		**Spray:** In 45 mL.[b]
otc	**Simply Saline** (Blairex)		**Spray:** In 44 mL.
otc	**Pretz Irrigation** (Parnell)		**Spray:** In 237 mL.[c]
otc	**SalineX** (Muro)	**Solution:** 0.4% sodium chloride	**Drops:** In 15 mL.[d]
			Mist: In 50 mL.[d]

NASAL PRODUCTS

otc	**Ayr Saline** (B.F. Ascher)	**Solution**: 0.65% sodium chloride	**Drops**: In 50 mL.[b]
			Mist: In 50 mL.[b]
			Gel: In 14 g.[e]
otc	**Breathe Free** (Thompson Medical)		**Spray**: In 45 mL.[f]
otc	**HuMist Moisturizing Mist** (Scherer)		**Spray**: In 45 mL.[g]
otc	**NaSal** (Bayer Corp.)		**Drops**: Alcohol free. In 15 mL.[h]
			Spray: Alcohol free. In 30 mL.[h]
otc	**Nasal Moist** (Blairex)		**Spray**: Alcohol free, dye free. In 45 mL.
			Mist pump: Alcohol free, dye free. In 15 mL.
			Gel: Alcohol free, dye free. In 28.5 g and unit-of-use 2 mL.[i]
otc	**Ocean** (Fleming)		**Spray**: In 45 and 473 mL.[f]
otc	**Ocean for Kids** (Fleming)		**Spray**: Alcohol free. In 37.5 mL.[j]
otc	**Mycinaire Saline Mist** (Pfieffer)		**Spray**: In 45 mL.[f]
otc	**Rhinaris Lubricating Mist** (Pharmascience)	**Solution**: 15% polyethylene glycol, 5% propylene glycol	**Spray**: In 30 mL.[k]
		Solution: 15% polyethylene glycol, 20% propylene glycol	**Gel**: In 28.35 g.[k]
otc	**Nasal•Ease with Zinc** (Health Care Products)	**Solution**: Zinc acetate	**Gel**: In 14.1 g.[l]
otc	**Nasal•Ease with Zinc Gluconate** (Health Care Products)	**Solution**: Zinc gluconate	**Spray**: In 30 mL.[m]
otc	**Ayr Saline** (B.F. Ascher)	**Gel**: methyl gluceth-10, propylene glycol, glycerin	**Swabs**: In 20s.[n]

[a] With glycerin, yerba santa.
[b] With benzalkonium chloride, EDTA.
[c] With yerba santa.
[d] With benzalkonium chloride, propylene glycol, polyethylene glycol, EDTA.
[e] With aloe vera gel, glycerin, parabens.
[f] With benzalkonium chloride.
[g] With chlorobutanol.
[h] With benzalkonium chloride, thimerosal.
[i] With aloe vera.
[j] With benzalkonium chloride, EDTA, glycerin.
[k] With benzalkonium chloride, sodium chloride.
[l] With aloe vera, calendula extract, parabens, glycerin, tocopherol acetate, EDTA.
[m] With sodium chloride, benzalkonium chloride, glycerin.
[n] With glyceryl polymethacrylate, triethanolamine, aloe vera, PEG/PPG-18/18 dimethicone, carbomer, poloxamer 184, sodium chloride, xanthan gum, diazolidinyl urea, parabens, soybean oil, geranium maculatum oil, tocopheryl acetate, blue 1.

NASAL PRODUCTS — INTRANASAL

For complete and comparative prescribing information, refer to the Nasal Decongestants group monograph.

Indications

Can be used as a nasal wash for sinuses and to restore moisture, thin nasal secretions, and relieve dry, crusted, and inflamed nasal membranes due to colds, low humidity, nasal decongestant overuse, allergies, minor nose bleeds, winter dryness, air travel, pregnancy, oxygen therapy, chronic sinusitis, asthma, intranasal and endoscopic sinus surgery, and other irritations.

Administration and Dosage

➤*Spray/Drops:* 2 to 6 sprays/drops in each nostril every 2 hours, as often as needed, or as directed by a doctor. To spray, hold head in upright position and give short, firm squeezes in each nostril. For drops, tilt head back and hold bottle upside down.

➤*HuMist:* Use is suggested for adults 12 years of age or older.

➤*Rhinaris:*

Adults and children (older than 2 years of age) – 1 or 2 sprays into each nostril every 4 hours as needed.

Nasal•Ease with Zinc Gluconate –

Adults and children (4 years of age or older): 1 to 2 sprays/drops in each nostril 2 to 4 times/day. Discontinue use after 5 days.

➤*Gel:* Apply around nostrils, under nose, or in nostrils as needed to help relieve discomfort. Use at bedtime to prevent drying and crusting.

Rhinaris – Apply a small amount of gel into each nostril every 4 hours as needed.

ALPHA$_1$-PROTEINASE INHIBITOR (HUMAN)

Rx	**Aralast** (Baxter)	**Powder for injection, lyophilized:** 400 mg (≥ 16 mg alpha$_1$-PI/mL when reconstituted)	Preservative free. In single-dose vial[1] with 25 mL diluent.
		Powder for injection, lyophilized: 800 mg (≥ 16 mg alpha$_1$-PI/mL when reconstituted)	Preservative free. In single-dose vial[1] with 50 mL diluent.
Rx	**Prolastin** (Bayer)	**Powder for injection, lyophilized:** 500 mg (≥ 20 mg alpha$_1$-PI/mL when reconstituted)	Preservative free. In single-dose vial[2] with 20 mL diluent.
		Powder for injection, lyophilized: 1000 mg (≥ 20 mg alpha$_1$-PI/mL when reconstituted)	Preservative free. In single-dose vial[2] with 40 mL diluent.
Rx	**Zemaira** (Aventis)	**Powder for injection, lyophilized:** 1000 mg	Preservative free. In single-dose vial[3] with 20 mL diluent.

[1] With polyethylene glycol, sodium, and albumin. With total alpha$_1$-PI functional activity in mg stated on the label of each vial.
[2] With polyethylene glycol, sucrose, sodium, and small amounts of other plasma proteins. With total alpha$_1$-PI functional activity in mg as stated on the label of each vial.
[3] With sodium and mannitol. The specific activity is ≥ 0.7 mg of functional alpha$_1$-PI/mg of total protein. The total alpha$_1$-PI functional activity in mg is stated on the label of each vial.

ALPHA$_1$-PROTEINASE INHIBITOR (HUMAN) — INJECTION

Indications

➤*Congenital alpha$_1$-proteinase inhibitor (alpha$_1$-PI; alpha$_1$-antitrypsin) deficiency:* For chronic augmentation therapy in patients having congenital deficiency of alpha$_1$-PI with clinically evident emphysema.

Clinical data demonstrating the long-term effects of chronic augmentation or replacement therapy of individuals with alpha$_1$-PI are not available.

Aralast and *Zemaira* are not indicated as therapy for lung disease patients in whom congenital alpha$_1$-PI deficiency has not been established.

Prolastin is not indicated for use in patients other than those with PiZZ, PiZ(null), or Pi(null)(null) phenotypes.

Administration and Dosage

➤*Approved by the FDA:* December 2, 1987.

➤*Dosage:* The recommended dosage is 60 mg/kg/body weight administered once weekly by IV infusion.

➤*Administration:* For IV use only. Give at a rate of approximately 0.08 mL/kg/min as determined by the response and comfort of the patient. Administer *Zemaira* reconstituted solution through a filter. The infusion should take approximately 15 to 30 minutes to complete. If adverse events occur, reduce the rate or interrupt the infusion until the symptoms subside. The infusion may then be resumed at a rate tolerated by the subject.

➤*Functional activity:* Each vial of *Aralast* and *Prolastin* has the functional activity, as determined by inhibition of porcine pancreatic elastase, stated on the label of the bottle. *Zemaira*'s functional activity is determined by the capacity to neutralize human neutrophil elastase.

➤*Storage / Stability:* Give within 3 hours after reconstitution. Do not refrigerate after reconstitution. Give alone without mixing other agents or diluting solutions. Refrigerate at 2° to 8°C (35° to 46°F) or at temperatures not to exceed 25°C (77°F). Avoid freezing. Do not use after expiration date printed on the label. *Aralast* must be used within 1 month once removed from refrigeration. Discard partially used vials; do not save for future use.

Actions

➤*Pharmacology:* Alpha$_1$-PI functions in the lungs to inhibit serine proteases such as neutrophil elastase (NE), which is capable of degrading protein components of the alveolar walls and is chronically present in the lung. In the healthy lung, alpha$_1$-PI is thought to provide more than 90% of the anti-NE protection in the lower respiratory tract.

Alpha$_1$-PI deficiency is an autosomal, codominant, hereditary disorder characterized by low serum and lung levels of alpha$_1$-PI. Severe forms of the deficiency are frequently associated with slowly progressive, moderate to severe panacinar emphysema that most often manifests in the third to fourth decades of life, resulting in a significantly lower life expectancy. Individuals with alpha$_1$-PI deficiency have little protection against NE released by a chronic, low-level of neutrophils in their lower respiratory tract, resulting in a protease:protease inhibitor imbalance in the lung. The emphysema associated with alpha$_1$-PI deficiency is typically worse in the lower lung zones. It is believed to develop because there are insufficient amounts of alpha$_1$-PI in the lower respiratory tract to inhibit NE. This imbalance allows unopposed destruction of the connective tissue framework of the lung parenchyma.

➤*Pharmacokinetics:* In clinical studies of alpha$_1$-PI in 23 subjects with the PiZZ variant of congenital deficiency of alpha$_1$-antitrypsin deficiency and documented destructive lung disease, the mean in vivo recovery of alpha$_1$-PI was 4.2 mg (immunologic)/dL/mg (functional)/kg administered. Half-life of alpha$_1$-PI in vivo was approximately 4.5 days. Nineteen of the subjects received alpha$_1$-PI replacement therapy, 60 mg/kg/week for up to 26 weeks (average, 24 weeks). Blood levels of alpha$_1$-PI were maintained above 80 mg/dL. Within a few weeks, bronchoalveolar lavage studies demonstrated significantly increased levels of alpha$_1$-PI and functional antineutrophil elastase capacity in the epithelial lining fluid of the lower respiratory tract of the lungs.

In 18 subjects treated with a single dose (60 mg/kg) of *Zemaira*, the AUC and standard deviation (SD) were 144 mcM × day (SD 27), maximum serum concentration was 44.1 mcM (SD 10.8), clearance was 603 mL/day (SD 129), and terminal half-life was 5.1 days (SD 2.4).

Contraindications

In individuals with selective IgA deficiencies (IgA level less than 15 mg/dL) who have known antibody against IgA, because they may experience severe reactions, including anaphylaxis, to IgA that may be present.

➤*Zemaira*: Hypersensitivity to any of its components or a history of anaphylaxis or severe systemic response to alpha$_1$-PI products

Warnings

➤*Infectious transmission:* Because alpha$_1$-PI is derived from pooled human plasma, it may carry a risk of transmitting infectious agents (eg, viruses and, theoretically, the Creutzfeldt-Jakob disease [CJD] agent).

There is also the possibility that unknown infectious agents may be present in such products. Individuals who receive infusions of blood or plasma products may develop signs and/or symptoms of some viral infections, particularly hepatitis C. All infections thought by a physician possibly to have been transmitted by these products should be reported by the physician or other health care provider to Bayer Corporation for *Prolastin* (1-800-228-8371), to Baxter Healthcare Corporation for *Aralast* (1-888-675-2762 [US] or 1-323-225-9735 [international]), or to Aventis Behring for *Zemaira* (1-800-504-5434). Weigh the risks and benefits of the use of this product and discuss with the patient.

Prolastin has been heat-treated in solution at 60°C for 10 hours in order to reduce the potential for transmission of infectious disease. No cases of hepatitis B or hepatitis C have been recorded in individuals receiving *Prolastin*. However, as all individuals receive prophylaxis against hepatitis B, no conclusion can be drawn at this time regarding potential transmission of hepatitis B virus.

During clinical studies, no cases of hepatitis A, B, C, or HIV viral infections were reported with the use of *Zemaira*.

➤*Hypersensitivity reactions:* If anaphylactic or severe anaphylactoid reactions occur, discontinue infusion immediately. Epinephrine and other appropriate supportive therapy should be available for the treatment of any acute anaphylactic or anaphylactoid reaction.

➤*Pregnancy: Category C.* It is not known whether this drug can cause fetal harm when administered to a pregnant woman or can affect reproduction capacity. Use only when clearly needed and when the potential benefits outweigh the potential hazards to the fetus.

➤*Lactation:* It is not known whether alpha$_1$-PI is excreted in human milk. Because many drugs are excreted in human milk, exercise caution when administering alpha$_1$-PI to a nursing woman.

➤*Children:* Safety and efficacy in children have not been established.

Precautions

➤*Monitoring:* The "threshold" level of *Prolastin* in the serum believed to provide adequate antielastase activity in the lung of individuals with alpha$_1$-antitrypsin deficiency is 80 mg/mL (based on commercial standards for alpha$_1$-PI immunologic assay). However, assays of alpha$_1$-PI based on commercial standards measure antigenic activity of alpha$_1$-PI is expressed as actual functional activity (ie, actual capacity to neutralize porcine pancreatic elastase). As functional activity may be less than antigenic activity, serum levels of alpha$_1$-PI determined using commercial immunologic assays may not accurately reflect actual functional alpha$_1$-PI levels. Therefore, although it may be helpful to monitor serum levels of alpha$_1$-PI in individuals receiving *Prolastin* using currently available commercial assays of antigenic activity, do not use results of these assays to determine the required therapeutic dosage.

➤*Circulatory overload:* There will be an increase in plasma volume following IV administration of *Prolastin* and *Zemaira*. Use caution in patients at risk for circulatory overload.

➤*Hepatitis B immunization:* It is recommended that in preparation for receiving *Prolastin*, recipients be immunized against hepatitis B using a licensed hepatitis B vaccine. If it becomes necessary to treat an individual with *Prolastin*, and time is insufficient for adequate antibody response to vaccination, administer a single dose of hepatitis B immune globulin (human), 0.06 mL/kg/body weight, IM, at the time of administration of the initial dose of hepatitis B vaccine.

ALPHA$_1$-PROTEINASE INHIBITOR (HUMAN) — INJECTION

Adverse Reactions

➤*Prolastin:* Delayed fever (maximum temperature rise was 38.9°C, resolving spontaneously over 24 hours) occurring up to 12 hours following treatment (0.77%); lightheadedness, dizziness (0.19%). Mild transient leukocytosis and dilutional anemia several hours after infusion have also been noted.

Postmarketing – Occasional reports of other flu-like symptoms, allergic-like reactions, chills, dyspnea, rash, tachycardia, and rarely, hypotension.

➤*Aralast:* Upper and lower respiratory tract infections (96.3%); COPD exacerbations, headache, somnolence (0.3%); chills, fever, vasodilation, dizziness, pruritus, rash, abnormal vision, chest pain, increased cough, dyspnea (0.1%).

ALT or AST elevations of at least 2 times the upper limit of normal (up to 3.7 times) were noted in 11.1% of subjects. Elevations were transient lasting 3 months or less.

➤*Zemaira:* Asthenia, injection site pain, dizziness, headache, paresthesia, pruritus (1%).

Summary of Adverse Reactions

	Zemaira	*Prolastin*
Subject treated	89	32
Subjects with adverse events regardless of causality (%)	78	63
Subjects with related adverse events (%)	6	13
Subjects with related serious adverse events	0	0
Number of infusions	1296	160
Adverse events regardless of causality (rates per infusion)	298 (0.230)	83 (0.519)
Related adverse events (rates per infusion)	6 (0.005)	5 (0.03)

The frequencies of adverse events per infusion that were at least 0.4% in *Zemaira*-treated subjects, regardless of causality, were: Headache (2.5%); upper respiratory tract infection (1.6%); sinusitis (1.5%); injection site hemorrhage, sore throat (0.9%); bronchitis (0.8%); asthenia, fever (0.6%); pain, rhinitis, bronchospasm, chest pain (0.5%); increased cough, rash, infection (0.4%).

The following adverse events, regardless of causality, occurred at a rate of 0.2% to less than 0.4% per infusion: Abnormal pain; diarrhea; dizziness; ecchymosis; myalgia; pruritus; vasodilation; accidental injury; back pain; dyspepsia; dyspnea; hemorrhage; injection site reaction; lung disorder; migraine; nausea; paresthesia.

Diffuse interstitial lung disease was noted on a routine chest x-ray of 1 subject at week 24. Causality could not be determined.

In a retrospective analysis, during the 10-week blinded portion of the 24-week clinical study, 6 subjects (20%) of the 30 treated with *Zemaira* had a total of 7 exacerbations of their COPD. Nine subjects (64%) of the 14 treated with *Prolastin* had a total of 11 exacerbations of their COPD. The observed difference between groups was 44% (95% confidence interval from 8% to 70%). Over the entire 24-week treatment period of the 30 subjects in the *Zemaira* treatment group, 7 subjects (23%) had a total of 11 exacerbations of their COPD.

Patient Information

Inform patients of the early signs of hypersensitivity reactions including hives, generalized urticaria, tightness of the chest, dyspnea, wheezing, faintness, hypotension, and anaphylaxis. Advise patients to discontinue use of the product and contact their physician and/or seek immediate emergency care, depending on the severity of the reaction, if these symptoms occur.

As with all plasma-derived products, some viruses, such as parvovirus B19, are particularly difficult to remove or inactivate at this time. Parvovirus B19 may most seriously affect pregnant women and immune-compromised individuals. Symptoms of parvovirus B19 include fever, drowsiness, chills, and runny nose followed 2 weeks later by a rash and joint pain. Encourage patients to consult their physician if such symptoms occur.

LUNG SURFACTANTS

BERACTANT (Natural Lung Surfactant)

Rx	**Survanta** (Ross Laboratories)	**Suspension**: 25 mg phospholipids per ml suspended in 0.9% sodium chloride solution.[1]	In single use vials containing 8 ml suspension.

[1] With 0.5 to 1.75 mg triglycerides, 1.4 to 3.5 mg free fatty acids and less than 1 mg protein per ml.

BERACTANT — INTRATRACHEAL

Indications

➤*Respiratory distress syndrome:* Beractant is indicated for prevention and treatment ("rescue") of respiratory distress syndrome (RDS) (hyaline membrane disease) in premature infants. Beractant significantly reduces the incidence of RDS, mortality due to RDS and air-leak complications.

In premature infants less than 1250 g birth weight or with evidence of surfactant deficiency, give beractant as soon as possible, preferably within 15 minutes of birth.

To treat infants with RDS confirmed by x-ray and requiring mechanical ventilation, give beractant as soon as possible, preferably by 8 hours of age.

Administration and Dosage

➤*Approved by the FDA:* July 1, 1991.

For intratracheal administration only.

Marked improvements in oxygenation may occur within minutes of administration of beractant. Therefore, frequent and careful clinical observation and monitoring of systemic oxygenation are essential to avoid hyperoxia.

➤*Dosage:* Each dose of beractant is 100 mg of phospholipids/kg birth weight (4 mL/kg). The beractant information below shows the total dosage for a range of birth weights.

Beractant dosing chart

Weight (grams)	Total dose (mL)
600 to 650	2.6
651 to 700	2.8
701 to 750	3
751 to 800	3.2
801 to 850	3.4
851 to 900	3.6
901 to 950	3.8
951 to 1000	4
1001 to 1050	4.2
1051 to 1100	4.4
1101 to 1150	4.6
1151 to 1200	4.8
1201 to 1250	5
1251 to 1300	5.2
1301 to 1350	5.4
1351 to 1400	5.6
1401 to 1450	5.8

Beractant dosing chart

Weight (grams)	Total dose (mL)
1451 to 1500	6
1501 to 1550	6.2
1551 to 1600	6.4
1601 to 1650	6.6
1651 to 1700	6.8
1701 to 1750	7
1751 to 1800	7.2
1801 to 1850	7.4
1851 to 1900	7.6
1901 to 1950	7.8
1951 to 2000	8

Four doses of beractant can be administered in the first 48 hours of life. Doses should be given no more frequently than every 6 hours.

➤*Directions for use:* Beractant should be inspected visually for discoloration prior to administration. The color of beractant is off-white to light brown. If settling occurs during storage, swirl the vial gently (do not shake) to redisperse. Some foaming at the surface may occur during handling and is inherent in the nature of the product.

Beractant is stored refrigerated (2° to 8°C; 35.6° to 46.4°F). Date and time need to be recorded in the box on front of the carton or vial, whenever beractant is removed from the refrigerator. Before administration, beractant should be warmed by standing at room temperature for at least 20 minutes or warmed in the hand for at least 8 minutes. Artificial warming methods should not be used. If a prevention dose is to be given, preparation of beractant should begin before the infant's birth.

Unopened, unused vials of beractant that have been warmed to room temperature may be returned to the refrigerator within 24 hours of warming, and stored for future use. Beractant should not be removed from the refrigerator for greater than 24 hours. Beractant should not be warmed and returned to the refrigerator more than once. Each single-use vial of beractant should be entered only once. Used vials with residual drug should be discarded.

Beractant does not require reconstitution or sonication before use.

➤*Dosing procedure:* Beractant is administered intratracheally by instillation through a 5 French end-hole catheter. The catheter can be inserted into the infant's endotracheal tube without interrupting ventilation by passing the catheter through a neonatal suction valve attached to the endotracheal tube. Alternatively, beractant can be instilled through the catheter by briefly disconnecting the endotracheal tube from the ventilator.

BERACTANT — INTRATRACHEAL

The neonatal suction valve used for administering beractant should be a type that allows entry of the catheter into the endotracheal tube without interrupting ventilation and also maintains a closed airway circuit system by sealing the valve around the catheter.

If the neonatal suction valve is used, the catheter should be rigid enough to pass easily into the endotracheal tube. A very soft and pliable catheter may twist or curl within the neonatal suction valve. The length of the catheter should be shortened so that the tip of the catheter protrudes just beyond the end of the endotracheal tube above the infant's carina. Beractant should not be instilled into a mainstem bronchus.

To ensure homogenous distribution of beractant throughout the lungs, each dose is divided into 4 quarter doses.

Each quarter dose is administered with the infant in a different position. The recommended positions are as follows:

- Head and body inclined 5° to 10° down, head turned to the right.
- Head and body inclined 5° to 10° down, head turned to the left.
- Head and body inclined 5° to 10° up, head turned to the right.
- Head and body inclined 5° to 10° up, head turned to the left.

The dosing procedure is facilitated if 1 person administers the dose while another person positions and monitors the infant.

First dose – Determine the total dose of beractant from the beractant dosing information, based on the infant's birth weight. Slowly withdraw the entire contents of the vial into a plastic syringe through a large-gauge needle (eg, at least 20 gauge). Do not filter beractant and avoid shaking.

Attach the premeasured 5 French end-hole catheter to the syringe. Fill the catheter with beractant. Discard excess beractant through the catheter so that only the total dose to be given remains in the syringe.

Before administering beractant, ensure proper placement and patency of the endotracheal tube. At the discretion of the clinician, the endotracheal tube may be suctioned before administering beractant. The infant should be allowed to stabilize before proceeding with dosing.

In the prevention strategy, weigh, intubate and stabilize the infant. Administer the dose as soon as possible after birth, preferably within 15 minutes. Position the infant appropriately and gently inject the first quarter dose through the catheter over 2 to 3 seconds.

After administration of the first quarter dose, remove the catheter from the endotracheal tube. Manually ventilate with a handbag with sufficient oxygen to prevent cyanosis, at a rate of 60 breaths/minute, and sufficient positive pressure to provide adequate air exchange and chest wall excursion.

In the rescue strategy, the first dose should be given as soon as possible after the infant is placed on a ventilator for management of RDS. In the clinical trials, immediately before instilling the first quarter dose, the infant's ventilator settings were changed to rate 60/minute, inspiratory time 0.5 second, and $FiO_2 1$.

Position the infant appropriately and gently inject the first quarter dose through the catheter over 2 to 3 seconds. After administration of the first quarter dose, remove the catheter from the endotracheal tube and continue mechanical ventilation.

In both strategies, ventilate the infant for at least 30 seconds or until stable. Reposition the infant for instillation of the next quarter dose.

Instill the remaining quarter doses using the same procedures. After instillation of each quarter dose, remove the catheter and ventilate for at least 30 seconds or until the infant is stabilized. After instillation of the final quarter dose, remove the catheter without flushing it. Do not suction the infant for 1 hour after dosing unless signs of significant airway obstruction occur.

After completion of the dosing procedure, resume usual ventilator management and clinical care.

Repeat doses – The dosage of beractant for repeat doses is also 100 mg phospholipids/kg and is based on the infant's birth weight. The infant should not be reweighed for determination of the beractant dosage. Use the beractant dosing information to determine the total dosage.

The need for additional doses of beractant is determined by evidence of continuing respiratory distress. Using the following criteria for redosing, significant reductions in mortality due to RDS were observed in the multiple-dose clinical trials with beractant.

Dose no sooner than 6 hours after the preceding dose if the infant remains intubated and requires at least 30% inspired oxygen to maintain a PaO_2 less than or equal to 80 torr.

Radiographic confirmation of RDS should be obtained before administering additional doses to those who received a prevention dose.

Prepare beractant and position the infant for administration of each quarter dose as previously described. After instillation of each quarter dose, remove the dosing catheter from the endotracheal tube and ventilate the infant for at least 30 seconds or until stable.

In the clinical studies, ventilator settings used to administer repeat doses were different than those used for the first dose. For repeat doses, the FiO_2 was increased by 0.2 or an amount sufficient to prevent cyanosis. The ventilator delivered a rate of 30/minute with an inspiratory time less than 1 second. If the infant's pretreatment rate was greater than or equal to 30, it was left unchanged during beractant instillation.

Manual handbag ventilation should not be used to administer repeat doses. During the dosing procedure, ventilator settings may be adjusted at the discretion of the clinician to maintain appropriate oxygenation and ventilation.

After completion of the dosing procedure, resume usual ventilator management and clinical care.

➤*Dosing precautions:* If an infant experiences bradycardia or oxygen desaturation during the dosing procedure, stop the dosing procedure and initiate appropriate measures to alleviate the condition. After the infant has stabilized, resume the dosing procedure.

Rales and moist breath sounds can occur transiently after administration of beractant. Endotracheal suctioning or other remedial action is unnecessary unless clear-cut signs of airway obstruction are present.

➤*Storage/Stability:* Store unopened vials at refrigeration temperature (2° to 8°C; 35.6° to 46.4°F). Protect from light. Store vials in carton until ready for use. Vials are for single use only. Upon opening, discard unused drug.

Actions

➤*Pharmacology:* Endogenous pulmonary surfactant lowers surface tension on alveolar surfaces during respiration and stabilizes the alveoli against collapse at resting transpulmonary pressures. Deficiency of pulmonary surfactant causes RDS in premature infants. Beractant replenishes surfactant and restores surface activity to the lungs of these infants.

In vitro, beractant reproducibly lowers minimum surface tension to less than 8 dynes/cm as measured by the pulsating bubble surfactometer and Wilhelmy Surface Balance. In situ, beractant restores pulmonary compliance to excised rat lungs artificially made surfactant-deficient. In vivo, single beractant doses improve lung pressure-volume measurements, lung compliance, and oxygenation in premature rabbits and sheep.

Animal pharmacology – Beractant is administered directly to the target organ, the lungs, where biophysical effects occur at the alveolar surface. In surfactant-deficient premature rabbits and lambs, alveolar clearance of radiolabeled lipid components of beractant is rapid. Most of the dose becomes lung associated within hours of administration, and the lipids enter endogenous surfactant pathways of reutilization and recycling. In surfactant-sufficient adult animals, beractant clearance is more rapid than in premature and young animals. There is less reutilization and recycling of surfactant in adult animals.

Contraindications

None known.

Warnings

➤*Administration:* Beractant is intended for intratracheal use only.

➤*Oxygenation/Lung compliance:* Beractant can rapidly affect oxygenation and lung compliance. Therefore, its use should be restricted to a highly supervised clinical setting with immediate availability of clinicians experienced with intubation, ventilator management, and general care of premature infants. Infants receiving beractant should be frequently monitored with arterial or transcutaneous measurement of systemic oxygen and carbon dioxide.

➤*Transient effects:* During the dosing procedure, transient episodes of bradycardia and decreased oxygen saturation have been reported. If these occur, stop the dosing procedure and initiate appropriate measures to alleviate the condition. After stabilization, resume the dosing procedure.

Precautions

➤*Rales and moist breath sounds:* Rales and moist breath sounds can occur transiently after administration. Endotracheal suctioning or other remedial action is not necessary unless clear-cut signs of airway obstruction are present.

➤*Nosocomial sepsis:* Increased probability of posttreatment nosocomial sepsis in beractant-treated infants was observed in the controlled clinical trials (see information below). The increased risk for sepsis among beractant-treated infants was not associated with increased mortality among these infants. The causative organisms were similar in treated and control infants. There was no significant difference between groups in the rate of posttreatment infections other than sepsis.

➤*Usage:* Use of beractant in infants less than 600 g birth weight or greater than 1750 g birth weight has not been evaluated in controlled trials. There is no controlled experience with use of beractant in conjunction with experimental therapies for RDS (eg, high-frequency ventilation, extracorporeal membrane oxygenation).

No information is available on the effects of doses other than 100 mg phospholipids/kg, greater than 4 doses, dosing more frequently than every 6 hours, or administration after 48 hours of age.

Adverse Reactions

The most commonly reported adverse reactions were associated with the dosing procedure. In the multiple-dose, controlled clinical trials, each dose of beractant was divided into 4 quarter doses which were instilled through a catheter inserted into the endotracheal tube by briefly disconnecting the endotracheal tube from the ventilator. Transient bradycardia occurred with 11.9% of doses. Oxygen desaturation occurred with 9.8% of doses.

Other reactions during the dosing procedure occurred with less than 1% of doses, and included endotracheal tube reflux, pallor, vasoconstriction, hypotension, endotracheal tube blockage, hypertension, hypocarbia, hypercarbia, and apnea. No deaths occurred during the dosing procedure, and all reactions resolved with symptomatic treatment.

The occurrence of concurrent illnesses common in premature infants was evaluated in the controlled trials. The rates in all controlled studies are in the following table:

BERACTANT — INTRATRACHEAL

	All controlled studies		
Concurrent event	Beractant (%)	Control (%)	P-value [a]
Patent ductus arteriosus	46.9%	47.1%	0.814
Intracranial hemorrhage	48.1%	45.2%	0.241
Severe intracranial hemorrhage	24.1%	23.3%	0.693
Pulmonary air leaks	10.9%	24.7%	< 0.001
Pulmonary interstitial emphysema	20.2%	38.4%	< 0.001
Necrotizing enterocolitis	6.1%	5.3%	0.427
Apnea	65.4%	59.6%	0.283
Severe apnea	46.1%	42.5%	0.114
Posttreatment sepsis	20.7%	16.1%	0.019
Posttreatment infection	10.2%	9.1%	0.345
Pulmonary hemorrhage	7.2%	5.3%	0.166

[a] P-value comparing groups in controlled studies.

When all controlled studies were pooled, there was no difference in intracranial hemorrhage. However, in 1 of the single-dose rescue studies and 1 of the multiple-dose prevention studies, the rate of intracranial hemorrhage was significantly higher in beractant patients than control patients (63.3% vs 30.8%, P = 0.001; and 48.8% vs 34.2%, P = 0.047, respectively). The rate in a treatment IND involving approximately 8100 infants was lower than in the controlled trials.

➤*Complications reported in controlled clinical studies in premature infants:*

Cardiovascular – Hypotension, hypertension, tachycardia, ventricular tachycardia, aortic thrombosis, cardiac failure, cardiorespiratory arrest, increased apical pulse, persistent fetal circulation, air embolism, total anomalous pulmonary venous return.

CNS – Seizures.

Endocrine – Adrenal hemorrhage, inappropriate antidiuretic hormone (ADH) secretion, hyperphosphatemia.

GI – Abdominal distention, hemorrhage, intestinal perforations, volvulus, bowel infarct, feeding intolerance, hepatic failure, stress ulcer.

Hematologic – Coagulopathy, thrombocytopenia, disseminated intravascular coagulation.

Musculoskeletal – Inguinal hernia.

Renal – Renal failure, hematuria.

Respiratory – Lung consolidation, blood from the endotracheal tube, deterioration after weaning, respiratory decompensation, subglottic stenosis, paralyzed diaphragm, respiratory failure.

Systemic – Fever, deterioration.

➤*Follow-up evaluations:*

Multiple-dose studies: Six-month, age-adjusted, follow-up evaluations have been completed in 631 (345 treated) of 916 surviving infants. There were significantly less cerebral palsy and need for supplemental oxygen in beractant infants than controls. Wheezing at the time of examination was significantly more frequent among beractant infants, although there was no difference in bronchodilator therapy.

Final, 12-month, follow-up data from the multiple-dose studies are available from 521 (272 treated) of 909 surviving infants. There was significantly less wheezing in beractant infants than controls, in contrast to the 6-month results. There was no difference in the incidence of cerebral palsy at 12 months.

Twenty-four-month, age-adjusted evaluations were completed in 429 (226 treated) of 906 surviving infants. There were significantly fewer beractant infants with rhonchi, wheezing, and tachypnea at the time of examination. No other differences were found.

Overdosage

Rales and moist breath sounds can transiently occur after beractant is given, and do not indicate overdosage. Endotracheal suctioning or other remedial action is not required unless clear-cut signs of airway obstruction are present.

➤*Symptoms:* Overdosage with beractant has not been reported. Based on animal data, overdosage might result in acute airway obstruction.

➤*Treatment:* Treatment should be symptomatic and supportive.

CALFACTANT

Rx	**Infasurf** (Forest Pharmaceuticals)	**Suspension, intratracheal:** 35 mg phospholipids per ml suspended in 0.9% sodium chloride solution[1] and 0.65 mg proteins[2]	In single-use vials, containing 6 ml suspension.

[1] Including 26 mg phosphatidylcholine of which 16 mg is desaturated phosphatidylcholine.

[2] Including 0.26 mg of SP-B.

CALFACTANT — INTRATRACHEAL

Indications

➤*Respiratory distress syndrome:* Calfactant is indicated for the prevention of respiratory distress syndrome (RDS) in premature infants at high risk for RDS and for the treatment ("rescue") of premature infants who develop RDS. Calfactant decreases the incidence of RDS, mortality due to RDS, and air leaks associated with RDS.

Prophylaxis therapy at birth with calfactant is indicated for premature infants younger than 29 weeks of gestational age at significant risk for RDS. Calfactant prophylaxis should be administered as soon as possible, preferably within 30 minutes after birth.

Calfactant therapy is indicated for infants 72 hours of age or younger with RDS (confirmed by clinical and radiologic findings) and requiring endotracheal intubation.

Administration and Dosage

➤*Approved by the FDA:* July 1, 1998.

For intratracheal administration only.

Rapid and substantial increases in blood oxygenation and improved lung compliance often follow calfactant instillation. Close clinical monitoring and surveillance following administration may be needed to adjust oxygen therapy and ventilator pressures appropriately.

➤*Dosage:* Each dose of calfactant is 3 mL/kg body weight at birth. Calfactant has been administered every 12 hours for a total of up to 3 doses.

➤*Directions for use:* Calfactant is a suspension which settles during storage. Gentle swirling or agitation of the vial is often necessary for redispersion. Do not shake. Visible flecks in the suspension and foaming at the surface are normal for calfactant.

Unopened, unused vials of calfactant that have warmed to room temperature can be returned to refrigerated storage within 24 hours for future use. Repeated warming to room temperature should be avoided. Each single-use vial should be entered only once and the vial with any unused material should be discarded after the initial entry.

Calfactant does not require reconstitution. Do not dilute or sonicate.

➤*Dosing procedures:*

General – Calfactant should only be administered intratracheally through an endotracheal tube. The dose of calfactant is 3 mL/kg birth weight. The dose is drawn into a syringe from the single-use vial using a 20 gauge or larger needle with care taken to avoid excessive foaming. Administration is made by instillation of the calfactant suspension into the endotracheal tube.

Administration for treatment of RDS –

Initial dose: Calfactant should be administered intratracheally through a side-port adapter into the endotracheal tube. Two attendants, one to instill the calfactant, the other to monitor the patient and assist in positioning, facilitate the dosing. The dose (3 mL/kg) should be administered in 2 aliquots of 1.5 mL/kg each. After each aliquot is instilled, the infant should be positioned with either the right or the left side dependent. Administration is made while ventilation is continued over 20 to 30 breaths for each aliquot, with small bursts timed only during the inspiratory cycles. A pause followed by evaluation of the respiratory status and repositioning should separate the 2 aliquots.

Repeat doses: Repeat doses of 3 mL/kg of birth weight, up to a total of 3 doses 12 hours apart, have been given in the calfactant controlled clinical trials if the patient was still intubated.

In the calfactant vs beractant trials, calfactant was administered through a 5 French feeding catheter inserted into the endotracheal tube. The total dose was instilled in 4 equal aliquots with the catheter removed between each of the instillations and mechanical ventilation resumed for 0.5 to 2 minutes. Each of the aliquots was administered with the patient in 1 of 4 different positions (prone, supine, right, and left lateral) to facilitate even distribution of the surfactant. Repeat doses were administered as early as 6 hours after the previous dose for a total of up to 4 doses if the infant was still intubated and required at least 30% inspired oxygen to maintain a $P_aO_2 \leq$ BO torr.

Administration for prophylaxis of RDS at birth – The amount of a prophylaxis dose of calfactant should be based on the infant's birth weight. Administration of calfactant should be given as soon as possible after birth. Usually the immediate care and stabilization of the premature infant born with hypoxemia or bradycardia should precede calfactant prophylaxis.

The dosing procedures are described under Administration for Treatment of RDS.

Dosing precautions – During administration of calfactant liquid suspension into the airway, infants often experience bradycardia, reflux of calfactant into the endotracheal tube, airway obstruction, cyanosis, dislodgment of the endotracheal tube, or hypoventilation. If any of these events occur, the administration should be interrupted and the infant's condition should be stabilized using appropriate interventions before the administration of calfactant is resumed. Endotracheal suctioning or reintubation is sometimes needed when there are signs of airway obstruction during the administration of the surfactant.

➤*Storage/Stability:* Store calfactant intratracheal suspension at refrigerated temperature 2° to 8°C (36° to 46°F) and protect from light. Vials are for single use only. After opening, discard unused drug.

Calfactant should be stored at refrigerated temperature 2° to 8°C (36° to 46°F). Warming of calfactant before administration is not necessary.

CALFACTANT — INTRATRACHEAL

Unopened, unused vials of calfactant that have warmed to room temperature can be returned to refrigerated storage within 24 hours for future use. Repeated warming to room temperature should be avoided. Each single-use vial should be entered only once and the vial with any unused material should be discarded after the initial entry.

Actions

➤*Pharmacology:* Endogenous lung surfactant is essential for effective ventilation because it modifies alveolar surface tension thereby stabilizing the alveoli. Lung surfactant deficiency is the cause of respiratory distress syndrome (RDS) in premature infants. Calfactant restores surface activity to the lungs of these infants.

Calfactant absorbs rapidly to the surface of the air:liquid interface and modifies surface tension similarly to natural lung surfactant. A minimum surface tension of less than or equal to 3 mN/m is produced in vitro by calfactant as measured on a pulsating bubble surfactometer. Ex vivo, calfactant restores the pressure volume mechanics and compliance of surfactant-deficient rat lungs. In vivo, calfactant improves lung compliance, respiratory gas exchange, and survival in preterm lambs with profound surfactant deficiency.

➤*Pharmacokinetics:* Calfactant is administered directly to the lung lumen surface, its site of action. No human studies of absorption, biotransformation or excretion of calfactant have been performed. The administration of calfactant with radiolabeled phospholipids into the lungs of adult rabbits results in the persistence of 50% of radioactivity in the lung alveolar lining and 25% of radioactivity in the lung tissue 24 hours later. Less than 5% of the radioactivity is found in other organs. In premature lambs with lethal surfactant deficiency, less than 30% of instilled calfactant is present in the lung lining after 24 hours.

Warnings

➤*Administration:* Calfactant is intended for intratracheal use only.

➤*Oxygenation / Lung compliance:* The administration of exogenous surfactants, including calfactant, often rapidly improves oxygenation and lung compliance. Following administration of calfactant, patients should be carefully monitored so that oxygen therapy and ventilatory support can be modified in response to changes in respiratory status.

➤*Transient effects:* Transient episodes of reflux of calfactant into the endotracheal tube, cyanosis, bradycardia, or airway obstruction have occurred during the dosing procedures. These events require stopping calfactant administration and taking appropriate measures to alleviate the condition. After the patient is stable, dosing can proceed with appropriate monitoring.

➤*Intensive care:* Calfactant therapy is not a substitute for neonatal intensive care. Optimal care of premature infants at risk for RDS and newborn infants with RDS who need endotracheal intubation requires an acute care unit organized, staffed, equipped, and experienced with intubation, ventilator management, and general care of these patients.

Precautions

➤*Usage:* No data are available on the use of calfactant in conjunction with experimental therapies of RDS, eg, high-frequency ventilation.

Data from controlled trials on the efficacy of calfactant are limited to doses of approximately 100 mg phospholipid/kg body weight and up to a total of 4 doses.

➤*Special risk:* When repeat dosing was given at fixed 12-hour intervals in the calfactant vs colfosceril palmitate trials, transient episodes of cyanosis, bradycardia, reflux of surfactant into the endotracheal tube, and airway obstruction were observed more frequently among infants in the calfactant-treated group.

An increased proportion of patients with both intraventricular hemorrhage (IVH) and periventricular leukomalacia (PVL) was observed in calfactant-treated infants in the calfactant-colfosceril palmitate controlled trials. These observations were not associated with increased mortality.

Adverse Reactions

The most common adverse reactions associated with calfactant dosing procedures in the controlled trials were cyanosis (65%), airway obstruction (39%), bradycardia (34%), reflux of surfactant into the endotracheal tube (21%), requirement for manual ventilation (16%), and reintubation (3%). These events were generally transient and not associated with serious complications or death.

➤*Follow-up evaluations:* Two-year follow-up data of neurodevelopmental outcomes in 415 infants enrolled in 5 centers that participated in the calfactant vs colfosceril palmitate controlled trials demonstrated significant developmental delays in equal percentages of calfactant and colfosceril palmitate patients.

➤*Common complications:* The incidence of common complications of prematurity and RDS in the 4 controlled calfactant trials are presented below. Prophylaxis and treatment study results for each surfactant are combined.

Common complications of prematurity and RDS in controlled trials

Complication	Calfactant (n = 1001), %	Colfosceril palmitate (n = 978), %	Calfactant (n = 553), %	Colfosceril palmitate (n = 566), %
Apnea	61	61	76	76
Patient ductus arteriosus	47	48	45	48
Intracranial hemorrhage	29	31	36	36
Severe intracranial hemorrhage[a]	12	10	9	7
IVH and PVL	7	3	5	5
Sepsis	20	22	28	27
Pulmonary air leaks	12	22	15	15
Pulmonary interstitial emphysema	7	17	10	10
Pulmonary hemorrhage	7	7	7	6
Necrotizing enterocolitis	5	5	17	18

[a] Grade III and IV by the method of Papile.

Overdosage

There have been no reports of overdosage with calfactant. While there are no known adverse effects of excess lung surfactant, overdosage would result in overloading the lungs with an isotonic solution. Ventilation should be supported until clearance of the liquid is accomplished.

PORACTANT ALFA (PORCINE ORIGIN)

Rx	**Curosurf** (Dey)	**Suspension, intratracheal:** 80 mg phospholipids/mL[a]	Preservative free. In 1.5 or 3 mL single-use vials.

[a] Includes 54 mg of phosphatidylcholine, of which 30.5 mg is dipalmitoyl phosphatidylcholine and 1 mg of protein, including 0.3 mg of SP-B.

PORACTANT ALFA — INTRATRACHEAL

Indications

➤*Respiratory distress syndrome (RDS):* Poractant alfa is indicated for the treatment (rescue) of respiratory distress syndrome (RDS) in premature infants. Poractant alfa reduces mortality and pneumothoraces associated with RDS.

➤*Unlabeled uses:* Severe meconium aspiration syndrome in term infants; respiratory failure caused by group B streptococcal infection in neonates.

Administration and Dosage

➤*Approved by the FDA:* November 18, 1999.

➤*Initial dose:* The initial recommended dose of poractant alfa is 2.5 mL/kg birth weight. This dose may be determined from the poractant alfa dosing section (see below).

Poractant Alfa Dosing

Weight (g)	Initial dose 2.5 mL/kg	Repeat dose 1.25 mL/kg	Weight (g)	Initial dose 2.5 mL/kg	Repeat dose 1.25 mL/kg
	Each dose (mL)			Each dose (mL)	
600 to 650	1.6	0.8	1,301 to 1,350	3.3	1.65
651 to 700	1.7	0.85	1,351 to 1,400	3.5	1.75
701 to 750	1.8	0.9	1,401 to 1,450	3.6	1.8
751 to 800	2	1	1,451 to 1,500	3.7	1.85
801 to 850	2.1	1.05	1,501 to 1,550	3.8	1.9
851 to 900	2.2	1.1	1,551 to 1,600	4	2

Poractant Alfa Dosing

Weight (g)	Initial dose 2.5 mL/kg	Repeat dose 1.25 mL/kg	Weight (g)	Initial dose 2.5 mL/kg	Repeat dose 1.25 mL/kg
	Each dose (mL)			Each dose (mL)	
901 to 950	2.3	1.15	1,601 to 1,650	4.1	2.05
951 to 1,000	2.5	1.25	1,651 to 1,700	4.2	2.1
1,001 to 1,050	2.6	1.3	1,701 to 1,750	4.3	2.15
1,051 to 1,100	2.7	1.35	1,751 to 1,800	4.5	2.25
1,101 to 1,150	2.8	1.4	1,801 to 1,850	4.6	2.3
1,151 to 1,200	3	1.5	1,851 to 1,900	4.7	2.35
1,201 to 1,250	3.1	1.55	1,901 to 1,950	4.8	2.4
1,251 to 1,300	3.2	1.6	1,951 to 2,000	5	2.5

Repeat doses – Up to 2 repeat doses of 1.25 mL/kg birth weight each may be administered, using the same technique described for the initial dose. Administer repeat doses at approximately 12-hour intervals in infants who remain intubated and in whom RDS is considered responsible for their persisting or deteriorating respiratory status. The maximum recommended total dose (sum of the initial and up to 2 repeat doses) is 5 mL/kg.

PORACTANT ALFA — INTRATRACHEAL

Sufficient information is not available on the effects of administering initial doses of poractant alfa other than 2.5 mL/kg (200 mg/kg), subsequent doses other than 1.25 mL/kg (100 mg/kg), administration of greater than 3 total doses, dosing more frequently than every 12 hours, or initiating therapy with poractant alfa more than 15 hours after diagnosing RDS. Adequate data are not available on the use of poractant alfa in conjunction with experimental therapies of RDS (eg, high-frequency ventilation).

Administration for intratracheal administration only – Poractant alfa is administered intratracheally by instillation through a 5 French end-hole catheter, and briefly disconnecting the endotracheal tube from the ventilator. Alternatively, poractant alfa may be administered through the secondary lumen of a dual lumen endotracheal tube without interrupting mechanical ventilation.

Before administering, ensure proper placement and patency of the endotracheal tube. At the discretion of the clinician, the endotracheal tube may be suctioned before administering poractant alfa. Allow the infant to stabilize before proceeding with dosing.

For endotracheal tube instillation using a 5 French end-hole catheter – Slowly withdraw the entire contents of the vial of poractant alfa into a 3 or 5 mL plastic syringe through a large-gauge needle (eg, at least 20 gauge). Attach the precut 8-centimeter 5 French end-hole catheter to the syringe. Fill the catheter with poractant alfa. Discard excess poractant alfa through the catheter so that only the total dose to be given remains in the syringe.

Immediately before poractant alfa administration, change the infant's ventilator settings to a rate of 40 to 60 breaths/minute, inspiratory time 0.5 second, and supplemental oxygen sufficient to maintain SaO_2 greater than 92%. Keep the infant in a neutral position (head and body in alignment without inclination). Briefly disconnect the endotracheal tube from the ventilator. Insert the precut 5 French catheter into the endotracheal tube and instill the first aliquot (1.25 mL/kg birth weight) of poractant alfa. Position the infant so that either the right or left side is dependent for this aliquot. After the first aliquot is instilled, remove the catheter from the endotracheal tube and manually ventilate the infant with 100% oxygen at a rate of 40 to 60 breaths/minute for 1 minute. When the infant is stable, reposition the infant so that the other side is dependent and administer the remaining aliquot using the same procedures. Do not suction airways for 1 hour after surfactant instillation unless signs of significant airway obstruction occur.

After completion of the dosing procedure, resume usual ventilator management and clinical care. In the clinical trials, ventilator management was modified to maintain a PaO_2 of approximately 55 mm Hg, $PaCO_2$ of 35 to 45, and pH greater than 7.3.

For endotracheal instillation using the secondary lumen of a dual lumen endotracheal tube – Slowly withdraw the entire contents of the vial of poractant alfa into a 3 or 5 mL plastic syringe through a large-gauge needle (eg, at least 20 gauge). Do not attach 5 French end-hole catheter. Keep the infant in a neutral position (head and body in alignment without inclination). Administer poractant alfa through the proximal end of the secondary lumen of the endotracheal tube as a single dose, given over 1 minute, and without interrupting mechanical ventilation. After completion of this dosing procedure, ventilatory management may require transient increases in FiO_2 ventilatory rate or peak inspiratory pressure.

➤*Dosing precautions:* Transient episodes of bradycardia, decreased oxygen saturation, reflux of the surfactant into the endotracheal tube, and airway obstruction have occurred during the dosing procedure of poractant alfa. These events require interrupting the administration of poractant alfa and taking the appropriate measures to alleviate the condition. After stabilization, dosing may resume with appropriate monitoring.

➤*Directions for use:* Visually inspect poractant alfa for discoloration prior to administration. The color of poractant alfa is white to creamy white. Before use, slowly warm the vial to room temperature and gently turn upside-down in order to obtain a uniform suspension. Do not shake.

Unopened, unused vials of poractant alfa that have warmed to room temperature may be returned to refrigerated storage within 24 hours for future use. Do not warm to room temperature and return to refrigerated storage more than once. Protect from light. Enter each single-use vial only once and discard the vial with any unused material after the initial entry.

➤*Storage/Stability:* Store poractant alfa intratracheal suspension in a refrigerator at 2° to 8°C (36° to 46°F). Unopened vials of poractant alfa may be warmed to room temperature for up to 24 hours prior to use. Do not warm poractant alfa to room temperature or return it to the refrigerator more than once. Protect from light. Do not shake. Vials are for single-use only. After opening the vial, discard the unused portion of the drug.

Actions

➤*Pharmacology:* Endogenous pulmonary surfactant reduces surface tension at the air-liquid interface of the alveoli during ventilation and stabilizes the alveoli against collapse at resting transpulmonary pressures. A deficiency of pulmonary surfactant in preterm infants results in RDS, characterized by poor lung expansion, inadequate gas exchange, and a gradual collapse of the lungs (atelectasia). Poractant alfa compensates for the deficiency of surfactant and restores surface activity to the lungs of these infants.

In vitro, poractant alfa lowers minimum surface tension to less than or equal to 4 mN/m as measured by the Wilhelmy Balance System.

In vivo, in several pharmacodynamic studies, poractant alfa improved lung compliance, pulmonary gas exchange, or survival in premature rabbits.

➤*Pharmacokinetics:*

Absorption/Distribution – Poractant alfa is administered directly to the target organ, the lung, where biophysical effects occur at the alveolar surface. No human pharmacokinetic studies to characterize the absorption, biotransformation, or excretion of poractant alfa have been performed. Nonclinical studies have been performed to evaluate the disposition of phospholipids present in poractant alfa.

The concentration of ^{14}C-DPPC in alveolar macrophages was less than or equal to 2% of that in the lung in newborn and adult rabbits. Of the total ^{14}C-DPPC recovered in newborn rabbits, less than 0.6% was found in the serum, liver, kidneys, and brain, respectively, at 48 hours.

Metabolism/Excretion – In both adult and newborn rabbits, approximately 50% of the radiolabeled component rapidly was removed from the alveoli in the first 3 hours after single intratracheal administration of poractant alfa-^{14}C-DPPC (dipalmitoylphosphatidylcholine). Over a 24-hour period, approximately 45% of the labeled DPPC was cleared from the lungs of adult rabbits compared to approximately 20% in newborn rabbits. In newborn rabbits, poractant alfa-^{14}C-DPPC passed from the alveolar space into the lung parenchyma and then was secreted again into the alveoli, whereas in adult rabbits, most of the DPPC was not recycled. The $t_{½}$ in the lung appeared to be approximately 25 hours in adult rabbits and 67 hours in newborn rabbits.

Contraindications

None known.

Warnings

➤*Administration:* Poractant alfa is intended for intratracheal use only. Administer poractant alfa only by those trained and experienced in the care, resuscitation, and stabilization of preterm infants.

➤*Dosing precautions:* Transient adverse effects seen with the administration of poractant alfa include bradycardia, hypotension, endotracheal tube blockage, and oxygen desaturation. These events require stopping poractant alfa administration and taking appropriate measures to alleviate the condition. After the patient is stable, dosing may proceed with appropriate monitoring.

Precautions

➤*Monitoring:* The administration of exogenous surfactants, including poractant alfa, rapidly can affect oxygenation and lung compliance. Therefore, give infants receiving poractant alfa frequent clinical and laboratory assessments so oxygen and ventilatory support can be modified to respond to respiratory changes.

➤*Prior to administration:* Correction of acidosis, hypotension, anemia, hypoglycemia, and hypothermia is recommended prior to poractant alfa administration.

➤*Complications of prematurity:* Surfactant administration can be expected to reduce the severity of RDS, but will not eliminate the mortality and morbidity associated with other complications of prematurity.

Adverse Reactions

Transient adverse effects seen with the administration of poractant alfa include bradycardia, hypotension, endotracheal tube blockage, and oxygen desaturation.

The rates of common complications of prematurity observed in study 1 are shown below.

Complications of Prematurity: Poractant Alfa vs Control (%)		
	Poractant alfa 2.5 mL/kg (200 mg/kg) (n = 78)	Control[a] (n = 66)
Acquired pneumonia	17%	21%
Acquired septicemia	14%	18%
Bronchopulmonary dysplasia	18%	22%
Intracranial hemorrhage	51%	64%
Patent ductus arteriosus	60%	48%
Pneumothorax	21%	36%
Pulmonary interstitial emphysema	21%	38%

[a] Controlled patients were disconnected from the ventilator and manually ventilated for 2 minutes. No surfactant was instilled.

➤*Follow-up:* Seventy-six infants (45 treated with poractant alfa) were evaluated at 1 year of age and 73 infants (44 treated with poractant alfa) at 2 years of age. Data from follow-up evaluations for weight and length, persistent respiratory symptoms, incidence of cerebral palsy, visual impairment, or auditory impairment were similar between treatment groups. In 16 patients (10 treated with poractant alfa and 6 controls) evaluated at 5.5 years of age, the developmental quotient, derived using the Griffiths Mental Developmental Scales, was similar between groups.

Overdosage

➤*Symptoms:* There have been no reports of overdosage following the administration of poractant alfa.

➤*Treatment:* In the event of accidental overdosage, and only if there are clear clinical effects on the infant's respiration, ventilation, or oxygenation, aspirate as much of the suspension as possible and manage the infant with supportive treatment, with particular attention to fluid and electrolyte balance.

Indications

As a group, these agents are used for the relief of manifestations of immediate-type hypersensitivity reactions. The varying degrees of anticholinergic, antihistaminic, and antimuscarinic activity make many antihistamines useful as sedatives, antiemetics, antitussives, antiparkinson agents, adjuncts to pre- or postoperative analgesic therapy, and agents to combat motion sickness. Refer to individual monographs on the following pages for specific indications.

Actions

➤*Pharmacology:*

Antihistamines: Dosage and Effects						
Antihistamine	Dose[a] (mg)	Dosing interval[b] (hrs)	Sedative effects	Antihistaminic activity	Anticholinergic activity	Antiemetic effects
First-Generation (nonselective)						
Alkylamines						
Brompheniramine	4	4 to 6	+	+++	++	—
Chlorpheniramine	4	4 to 6	+	++	++	—
Dexchlorpheniramine	2	4 to 6	+	+++	++	—
Pheniramine	15 to 30	8 to 12	++	—	—	—
Triprolidine	2.5	4 to 6	+	—	—	—
Ethanolamines						
Carbinoxamine	4	6	+++	—	+++	—
Clemastine	1	12	++	+ to ++	+++	++ to +++
Diphenhydramine	25 to 50	6 to 8	+++	+ to ++	+++	++ to +++
Ethylenediamine						
Pyrilamine	25 to 50	6 to 8	+	—	±	—
Phenothiazines						
Promethazine	12.5 to 25	6 to 24	+++	+++	+++	++++
Piperazines						
Hydroxyzine	25 to 100	4 to 8	+++	++ to +++	++	+++
Piperidines						
Azatadine	1 to 2	12	++	++	++	—
Cyproheptadine	4	8	+	++	++	—
Phenindamine	25	4 to 6	±	++	++	—
Second-Generation (peripherally selective)						
Phthalazinone						
Azelastine[c]	0.5	12	±	++ to +++	±	—
Piperazine						
Cetirizine	5 to 10	24	+	++ to +++	±	—
Piperidines						
Desloratadine	5	24	±	—	±	—
Fexofenadine	60	12	±	—	±	—
Loratadine	10	24	±	++ to +++	±	—

* ++++ = very high, +++ = high, ++ = moderate, + = low, ± = low to none.
[a] Usual single adult dose.
[b] For conventional dosage forms.
[c] Some effects may be enhanced or reduced as a result of administration via the nasal route.

Antihistamines are reversible, competitive H_1 receptor antagonists that reduce or prevent most of the physiologic effects that histamine normally induces at the H_1 receptor site. They do not prevent histamine release nor bind with histamine that already has been released. Antihistaminic effects include inhibition of respiratory, vascular, and GI smooth muscle constriction; decreased capillary permeability, which reduces the wheal, flare, and itch response; and decreased histamine-activated exocrine secretions (eg, salivary, lacrimal). Antihistamines with strong anticholinergic (atropine-like) properties also may potentiate the drying effect by suppressing cholinergically innervated exocrine glands. **First-generation antihistamines** bind nonselectively to central and peripheral H_1 receptors and may result in CNS stimulation or depression. CNS depression, which usually occurs with higher therapeutic doses, allows some of these agents to be used clinically for sedation. However, **second-generation antihistamines** are selective for peripheral H_1 receptors and, as a group, are less sedating. Several first-generation agents (eg, diphenhydramine, some piperazines, promethazine) with strong anticholinergic properties bind to central muscarinic receptors and produce antiemetic effects, decreasing nausea, vomiting, and motion sickness (see Antiemetic/Antivertigo agents). At doses much higher than that needed to antagonize histamine, a few agents (especially promethazine) exhibit local anesthetic effects. Some agents (eg, cyproheptadine, azatadine) also have antiserotonergic effects.

Switching from one class of antihistamines to another may restore responsiveness when a patient becomes refractory to the effects of a particular agent.

➤*Pharmacokinetics:*

First-generation agents – Pharmacokinetics of first-generation agents have not been studied extensively. With a few exceptions, these agents are well absorbed following oral administration, have an onset of action within 15 to 30 minutes, are maximal within 1 to 2 hours, and have a duration of action of approximately 4 to 6 hours, although some are much longer acting (see Pharmacology table). Most are metabolized by the liver. Antihistamine metabolites and small amounts of unchanged drug are excreted in urine. Small amounts may be excreted in breast milk.

Second-generation agents – Intranasal administration of **azelastine** yields peak levels in 2 to 3 hours, with an elimination half-life of 22 hours. Metabolism by the P450 system results in steady-state peak levels of a major active metabolite (desmethylazelastine), which are 20% to 50% of azelastine levels. The elimination half-life of the metabolite is predicted to be 54 hours. The major route of excretion is via feces.

Cetirizine is a metabolite of **hydroxyzine**. **Desloratadine** is a metabolite of **loratadine**. The pharmacokinetics of the second-generation agents have been studied more thoroughly and are provided in the table below.

Pharmacokinetics of Peripherally Selective H_1 Antagonists						
	Onset of action	T_{max} (h)	Elimination t½ (h)	Protein binding (%)	CYP450 metabolism	Food effect on absorption
Cetirizine	rapid	1	8.3	93	↓; 50% excreted unchanged	delayed 1.7 h
Desloratadine	≤ 1 h	3	27	82 to 87	—	None
Fexofenadine	rapid	2.6	14.4	60 to 70	↓↓; 95% excreted unchanged	—
Loratadine	rapid	1.3 to 2.5[a]	8.4 to 28[a]	97 (75)[b]	↑; 3A4, 2D6	delayed 1 h

↑ = High, ↓ = Low, ↓↓ = Very low.
[a] All active constituents (parent drug and active metabolites).
[b] Active metabolite.

Contraindications

➤*First-generation antihistamines:* Hypersensitivity to specific or structurally related antihistamines; newborns or premature infants (see Warnings); nursing mothers (see Warnings); monoamine oxidase (MAO) therapy (see Drug Interactions); pregnancy (**hydroxyzine**); angle-closure glaucoma, stenosing peptic ulcer, symptomatic prostatic hypertrophy, bladder neck obstruction, pyloroduodenal obstruction, elderly, debilitated patients (**cyproheptadine**).

➤*Second-generation antihistamines:* Hypersensitivity to specific or structurally related antihistamines. **Desloratadine** is contraindicated in those who are hypersensitive to **loratadine**. **Cetirizine** is contraindicated in those who are hypersensitive to **hydroxyzine**.

Warnings

➤*Neuroleptic malignant syndrome (NMS):* A potentially fatal symptom complex sometimes referred to as NMS has been reported in association with **promethazine** alone or in combination with antipsychotic drugs. Clinical manifestations of NMS are hyperpyrexia, muscle rigidity, altered mental status, and evidence of autonomic instability (eg, irregular pulse or blood pressure, tachycardia, diaphoresis, cardiac dysrhythmias).

➤*CNS depression:* Antihistamines may impair the mental and/or physical abilities required for the performance of potentially hazardous tasks, such as driving a vehicle or operating machinery. The impairment may be amplified by concomitant use of other CNS depressants such as alcohol, sedatives/hypnotics (including barbiturates), narcotics, narcotic analgesics, general anesthetics, tricyclic antidepressants, and tranquilizers. Therefore, such agents either should be eliminated or given in reduced dosage in the presence of certain antihistamines with strong CNS depressant effects.

When given concomitantly with **promethazine**, reduce the dose of barbiturates by at least one half, and reduce the dose of the narcotics by one quarter to one half. Individualize dosage. Excessive amounts of promethazine relative to a narcotic may lead to restlessness and motor hyperactivity in the patient with pain.

➤*Special risk patients:* Use antihistamines with caution in patients with narrow-angle glaucoma, stenosing peptic ulcer, pyloroduodenal obstruction, symptomatic prostatic hypertrophy, bladder neck obstruction, bronchial asthma, increased intraocular pressure, hyperthyroidism, cardiovascular disease, and hypertension.

➤*Carcinogenesis:* Mice and rats given **loratadine** had a higher incidence in hepatocellular tumors (combined adenomas and carcinomas) than controls.

➤*Respiratory disease:* In general, antihistamines are not recommended to treat lower respiratory tract symptoms (eg, emphysema, chronic bronchitis, asthma) because their anticholinergic (drying) effects may thicken secretions and impair expectoration. However, several reports indicate antihistamines may be used safely in asthmatic patients with severe perennial allergic rhinitis without exacerbating the asthma.

➤*Seizure threshold:* **Promethazine** may lower the seizure threshold; consider this when giving to people with known seizure disorders or when giving in combination with narcotics or local anesthetics that also may affect seizure threshold.

➤*Respiratory depression:* Avoid sedatives and CNS depressants in patients with compromised respiratory function (eg, chronic obstructive pulmonary disease [COPD], sleep apnea).

➤*Hypersensitivity reactions:* Hypersensitivity reactions may occur, and any of the usual manifestations of drug allergy may develop. Have epinephrine 1:1000 immediately available. Refer to Management of Acute Hypersensitivity Reactions.

➤*Renal/Hepatic function impairment:* Use a lower initial dose of **loratadine**, **desloratadine**, and **cetirizine** in patients with renal or hepatic impairment.

➤*Elderly:* Antihistamines are more likely to cause dizziness, excessive sedation, syncope, toxic confusional states, and hypotension in elderly patients and also may cause paradoxical stimulation. Dosage reduction may be required.

The phenothiazine side effects (extrapyramidal signs, especially parkinsonism, akathisia, and persistent dyskinesia) are more prone to develop in the elderly.

➤*Pregnancy:* (*Category B* – **Azatadine**, **cetirizine**, **chlorpheniramine**, **clemastine**, **cyproheptadine**, **dexchlorpheniramine**, **diphenhydramine**, **loratadine**; *Category C* – **brompheniramine**, **carbinoxamine**, **desloratadine**, **fexofenadine**, **hydroxyzine**, **pheniramine**, **phenytoloxamine**, **promethazine**, **pyrilamine**, **triprolidine**). Safety for use during pregnancy has not been established. Several possible associations with malformations have been found, but significance is unknown. Use only when clearly needed and when the potential benefits outweigh the potential hazards to the fetus. Do not use during the third trimester; newborn and premature infants may have severe reactions (eg, convulsions) to some antihistamines.

Reports of jaundice, hyperreflexia, and prolonged extrapyramidal symptoms occurred in infants whose mothers received phenothiazines during pregnancy. Promethazine, taken within 2 weeks of delivery, may inhibit newborn platelet aggregation.

➤*Lactation:* The following antihistamines have been reported to be excreted in breast milk: **Cetirizine**, **clemastine**, **desloratadine**, **diphenhydramine**, **loratadine**, **triprolidine**. The use of cetirizine in nursing mothers is not recommended. The American Academy of Pediatrics considers triprolidine to be compatible with breastfeeding. Loratadine and its metabolite pass easily into breast milk and achieve concentrations that are equivalent to plasma levels with an AUC milk/AUC plasma ratio of 1.17 and 0.85, respectively. Because of the higher risk of adverse effects for infants generally, and for newborns and prematures in particular, antihistamine therapy is contraindicated in nursing mothers.

Although there are no quantitative measures, the molecular weight for **fexofenadine**, **hydroxyzine**, and **promethazine** is low enough that excretion into breast milk should be expected.

➤*Children:* Antihistamines may diminish mental alertness; conversely, they may produce excitation occasionally, particularly in the young child.

Promethazine is not recommended in children younger than 2 years of age. Exercise caution when administering promethazine to children because of the potential for fatal respiratory depression. Limit antiemetics to prolonged vomiting of known etiology. The extrapyramidal symptoms that may occur secondary to promethazine may be confused with the CNS signs of undiagnosed primary disease (eg, encephalopathy, Reye syndrome). Avoid use in children whose signs and symptoms may suggest Reye syndrome or other hepatic diseases. In children who are acutely ill associated with dehydration, there is an increased susceptibility to dystonias with the use of promethazine.

Precautions

➤*Hematologic:* Use **promethazine** with caution in bone marrow depression. Leukopenia and agranulocytosis have been reported, usually when used with other marrow-toxic agents.

➤*Anticholinergic effects:* Antihistamines have varying degrees of atropine-like actions; use with caution in patients with a predisposition to urinary retention, history of bronchial asthma, increased intraocular pressure, hyperthyroidism, cardiovascular disease, or hypertension. Antihistamines may thicken bronchial secretions caused by anticholinergic properties and may inhibit expectoration and sinus drainage.

➤*Phenothiazines:* Use phenothiazines with caution in patients with cardiovascular disease, liver dysfunction, or ulcer disease.**Promethazine** has been associated with cholestatic jaundice.

Use cautiously in patients with acute or chronic respiratory impairment, particularly children, because phenothiazines may suppress the cough reflex. If hypotension occurs, epinephrine is not recommended because phenothiazines may reverse its usual pressor effect and cause a paradoxical further lowering of blood pressure. Because these drugs have an antiemetic action, they may obscure signs of intestinal obstruction, brain tumor, or overdosage of toxic drugs.

Phenothiazines elevate prolactin levels, which persist through chronic administration. Approximately ⅓ of breast cancers are prolactin-dependent in vitro, an important factor if these drugs are prescribed for a patient with a history of breast cancer. Although galactorrhea, amenorrhea, gynecomastia, and impotence have been reported, the clinical significance of elevated serum prolactin levels is unknown.

➤*Phenylketonurics:* Inform phenylketonuric patients that some of these products contain phenylalanine.

➤*Tartrazine sensitivity:* Some of these products contain tartrazine (FD&C yellow #5), which may cause allergic-type reactions (including bronchial asthma) in susceptible individuals. Although the incidence of sensitivity is low, it is frequently seen in patients who also have aspirin hypersensitivity. Specific products containing tartrazine are identified in the product listings.

➤*Hazardous tasks:* Antihistamines have varying degrees of sedative effects and may cause drowsiness and reduce mental alertness; instruct patients not to drive or perform other tasks requiring alertness, coordination, or physical dexterity. Supervise children who are taking antihistamines when they engage in potentially hazardous activities (eg, bicycle riding).

➤*Photosensitivity:* Photosensitization may occur; therefore, caution patients to take protective measures (eg, sunscreens, protective clothing) against exposure to ultraviolet light or sunlight until tolerance is determined.

Drug Interactions

Antihistamine Drug Interactions			
Precipitant drug	Object drug*		Description
Antacids, aluminum/ magnesium containing	Antihistamines Fexofenadine	↓	Administration of fexofenadine within 15 minutes of an aluminum- and magnesium-containing antacid decreased fexofenadine AUC by 41% and C_{max} by 43%. Fexofenadine should not be taken closely in time to these antacids.
Cimetidine	Antihistamines Azelastine Desloratadine Loratadine	↑	Concomitant use resulted in substantially increased plasma levels of loratadine and desloratadine and an increase of ≈ 65% in levels of orally administered azelastine.
Erythromycin	Antihistamines Desloratadine Fexofenadine Loratadine	↑	Plasma levels (including metabolites) may be increased. No clinically relevant changes in safety profile.
Ketoconazole	Antihistamines Desloratadine Fexofenadine Loratadine	↑	Plasma levels (including metabolites) may be increased. No clinically relevant changes in safety profile.
MAO inhibitors	Antihistamines	↑	MAOIs may prolong and intensify the anticholinergic and sedative effects of antihistamines; may cause hypotension and extrapyramidal reactions with phenothiazines and severe hypotension with dexchlorpheniramine.
Antihistamines	MAOIs		
Rifamycins (eg, rifampin)	Antihistamines Fexofenadine	↓	Rifampin may reduce the absorption of fexofenadine, thereby decreasing the pharmacologic effect.
Antihistamines	Alcohol, CNS depressants	↑	Additive CNS depressant effects may occur (see Warnings). This may be less likely with second-generation agents.
Antihistamines Cyproheptadine	Metyrapone	↓	Cyproheptadine may diminish the expected pituitary adrenal response to metyrapone. Avoid concurrent use or discontinue cyproheptadine before metyrapone is used.
Antihistamines Cyproheptadine	Selective serotonin reuptake inhibitors (SSRIs) Nefazodone Venlafaxine	↓	SSRIs have serotonergic activity and cyproheptadine is a serotonin antagonist. If a loss of the antidepressant effectiveness occurs, consider discontinuing cyproheptadine.
Antihistamine Diphenhydramine	Beta-blockers	↑	Diphenhydramine may inhibit the CYP2D6 mediated metabolism of certain beta-blockers (eg, metoprolol), producing increased plasma concentrations and cardiovascular effects. Monitor closely.

* ↑ = Object drug increased, ↓ = Object drug decreased.

See the Antipsychotic Agents monograph for a complete discussion of the drug interactions that relate to the phenothiazine antihistamine, promethazine.

➤*Drug/Lab test interactions:* Diagnostic pregnancy tests based on human chorionic gonadotropin (hCG) and anti-hCG may result in false-negative or false-positive interpretations in patients on **promethazine**. Increased blood glucose has occurred in promethazine patients.

Phenothiazines may increase serum cholesterol, spinal fluid protein, and urinary urobilinogen levels; decrease protein bound iodine; yield false-positive urine bilirubin tests; and interfere with urinary ketone and steroid determinations.

Discontinue antihistamines approximately 4 days prior to **skin testing procedures**; these drugs may prevent or diminish otherwise positive reactions to dermal reactivity indicators.

➤*Drug/Food interactions:* Food increased the AUC of **loratadine** by approximately 40% and the metabolite by approximately 15%; absorption was delayed by 1 hour; peak levels were unaffected. Although not expected to be clinically important, take on an empty stomach. The AUC of loratadine rapidly disintegrating tablets was increased by 26% when administered without water compared with water; peak levels were not affected significantly. Bioavailability was unaffected; dissolved remnants may be swallowed with or without water.

Systemic absorption of **cetirizine** was delayed by 1.7 hours, and peak plasma levels were decreased by 23%. However, cetirizine may be taken with or without food.

In one study of **desloratadine** orally disintegrating tablets, administration with food shifted the median T_{max} from 2.5 to 4 hours.

Certain fruit juices (ie, apple, orange, grapefruit) administered with **fexofenadine** significantly reduced the AUC and C_{max} of fexofenadine. Therefore, fexofenadine's clinical effect may be decreased. It would be prudent for patients to take fexofenadine with a liquid other than these juices.

Adverse Reactions

➤*Allergic:* Anaphylactic shock; angioneurotic, laryngeal, and peripheral edema; asthma; dermatitis; drug rash; lupus erythematosus-like syndrome; urticaria.

➤*Cardiovascular:* Bradycardia; cardiac arrest; ECG changes, including blunting of T-waves and prolongation of the QT interval; extrasystoles; faintness; hypertension; hypotension; palpitations; postural hypotension; reflex tachycardia; tachycardia; venous thrombosis at injection site (IV **promethazine**).

➤*CNS:* Disturbed coordination; dizziness; drowsiness (often transient); faintness; sedation; (most frequent). Acute labyrinthitis; blurred vision; catatonic-like states; confusion; convulsions; diplopia; disorientation; disturbing dreams/nightmares; euphoria; excitation; fatigue; grand mal seizures; hallucinations; headache; hysteria; insomnia; lassitude; neuritis; oculogyric crisis; paresthesias; pseudoschizophrenia; restlessness; tinnitus; tongue protrusion (usually in association with IV administration or excessive dosage); torticollis; tremor; vertigo; weakness. Extrapyramidal reactions may occur with high doses; these reactions usually respond to dose reduction.

➤*GI:* Epigastric distress (most frequent, especially ethylenediamines); anorexia; constipation; diarrhea; increased appetite; nausea; stomatitis; vomiting; weight gain.

Nasal spray – Glossitis; increased ALT; ulcerative and aphthous stomatitis.

➤*GU:* Dysuria; early menses; gynecomastia; induced lactation; inhibition of ejaculation; urinary frequency; urinary retention.

➤*Hematologic:* Agranulocytosis; aplastic anemia; hemolytic anemia; hypoplastic anemia; leukopenia; pancytopenia; thrombocytopenia.

➤*Respiratory:* Thickening of bronchial secretions (most frequent); chest tightness; dry mouth, nose, and throat; nasal stuffiness; respiratory depression; sore throat; wheezing.

Nasal spray – Epistaxis; paroxysmal sneezing; rhinitis.

➤*Special senses:*

Nasal spray – Bitter taste (most frequent); conjunctivitis; eye abnormality; eye pain; nasal burning; taste loss; watery eyes.

➤*Miscellaneous:* Chills; elevated spinal fluid proteins; elevation of plasma cholesterol levels; erythema; excessive perspiration; glycosuria; heaviness, tingling, and weakness of the hands; high or prolonged glucose tolerance curves; obstructive jaundice (usually reversible upon drug discontinuation); photosensitivity; thrombocytopenic purpura; tissue necrosis following subcutaneous administration of IV **promethazine**.

Nasal spray – Temporomandibular dislocation.

Adverse Events Greater Than Placebo for Peripherally Selective H_1 Antagonists[a]					
Adverse reaction	Azelastine (n = 391)	Cetirizine (n = 2,034)	Fexofenadine (n = 679)	Loratadine (n = 1,926)	Desloratadine (n = 1,866)
CNS					
Dizziness	2%	2%	—	—	4%
Drowsiness/ Somnolence	11.5%	13.7%	1.3%	8%	2.1%
Fatigue	2.3%	5.9%	1.3%	4%	2.1% to 5%
Headache	14.8%	> 2%	> 1%	12%	14%
Weight gain	2%	—	—	—	—
Ear, nose, throat					
Dry mouth, nose, throat	2.8%	5%	—	3%	3%
Epistaxis	2%	—	—	—	—
Pharyngitis	3.8%	2%	> 1%	—	3% to 4.1%
GI					
Nausea, vomiting, abdominal distress, bowel changes	2.8%	> 2%	1.3% to 1.6%	—	3% to 4%
Miscellaneous					
Dysmenorrhea	—	—	1.5%	—	2.1%
Myalgia	—	—	—	—	2.1% to 3%

[a] Data pooled from several studies and are not necessarily comparable.

➤*Phenothiazines:* These antihistamines infrequently cause typical phenothiazine adverse effects. See the Antipsychotic Agents monograph for a complete discussion.

Overdosage

➤*Symptoms:* Effects may vary from CNS depression (eg, sedation, apnea, diminished mental alertness) and cardiovascular collapse to stimulation (eg, insomnia, hallucinations, tremors, convulsions), especially in children and elderly patients. Profound hypotension, respiratory depression, unconsciousness, coma, and death may occur, particularly in infants and children. Convulsions occur rarely and indicate a poor prognosis. The convulsant dose lies near the lethal dose.

Toxic effects are seen within 30 minutes to 2 hours and result in drowsiness, dizziness, ataxia, tinnitus, blurred vision, and hypotension. Anticholinergic effects result in fixed dilated pupils, flushing, dry mouth, hyperthermia (especially in children), and fever. GI symptoms also may occur. Hyperpyrexia to 41.8°C (107°F) and acute oral and facial dystonic reactions have been reported.

Children often manifest CNS stimulation and may have hallucinations, toxic psychosis, delirium tremens, excitement, ataxia, incoordination, muscle twitching, athetosis, hyperthermia, cyanosis, convulsions, and hyperreflexia followed by postictal depression and cardiorespiratory arrest. Seizures resistant to therapy may follow and may be preceded by mild depression. A paradoxical reaction has been reported in children receiving single doses of 75 to 125 mg oral **promethazine,** characterized by hyperexcitability and nightmares. CNS stimulation in adults usually manifests as seizures. Marked cerebral irritation, resulting in jerking of muscles and possible convulsions, may be followed by deep stupor. Occasionally, respiratory depression, cardiovascular collapse, and death follows a latent period.

Less common findings include ECG changes, such as wandering pacemaker, prolonged QT interval, and nonspecific ST-T wave changes that disappear quickly. The EEG may show general cerebral dysrhythmia and diffuse delta wave activity that may persist after clinical recovery.

➤*Treatment:* Take adequate precautions to protect against aspiration, especially in infants and children. Administer activated charcoal as a slurry with water and a cathartic to minimize absorption. Correct acidosis and electrolyte imbalances. Do not induce emesis in unconscious patients. Gastric lavage is indicated within 3 hours after ingestion and even later if large amounts were taken. Continue therapy directed at reversing the effects of timed-release medication and at supporting the patient. Hemoperfusion may be used in severe cases. **Cetirizine, fexofenadine,** and **loratadine** do not appear to be dialyzable. Refer to General Management of Acute Overdosage.

Hypotension is an early sign of impending cardiovascular collapse; treat vigorously using general supportive measures or specific vasopressor treatment (eg, norepinephrine, phenylephrine, dopamine). Avoid epinephrine; it may worsen hypotension. Propranolol may be used for refractory ventricular arrhythmias.

Administer 0.1 mg/kg IV diazepam slowly for convulsions; repeat as needed. IV physostigmine may reverse central anticholinergic effects. Use with caution. Avoid analeptics; they may cause convulsions. Depressant effects of **promethazine** are not reversed by naloxone.

Ice packs and cooling sponge baths, not alcohol, may help reduce a child's fever.

Patient Information

Instruct patients to inform a physician of a history of glaucoma, peptic ulcer, urinary retention, or pregnancy before starting antihistamine therapy.

Some antihistamines may cause nervousness, insomnia, and dry mouth.

Some antihistamines may cause drowsiness or dizziness; advise patients to observe caution while driving or performing other tasks requiring alertness, coordination, or physical dexterity and to avoid alcohol and other CNS depressants (eg, sedatives, hypnotics, tranquilizers, antianxiety agents).

Some antihistamines may cause GI upset; instruct patients to take with food.

Advise patients to avoid prolonged exposure to sunlight; some agents may cause photosensitivity.

Instruct patients not to crush or chew sustained-release preparations.

➤*Phenothiazines:* Advise patients to report any involuntary muscle movements or unusual sensitivity to sunlight.

Alkylamines, Nonselective

BROMPHENIRAMINE

Rx	**Brompheniramine Tannate** (Brighton)	**Tablets, chewable**: 12 mg brompheniramine tannate	Sucrose. (BP-940). Purple, oval, scored. Grape flavor. In 60s.
Rx	**BrōveX CT** (Athlon)		Sucrose. (273). Yellow, oval, scored. Banana flavor. In 60s.
Rx	**LoHist 12 Hour** (Larken)	**Tablets, extended release**: 6 mg brompheniramine tannate	(LH 12). White, oval, scored. In 100s.
Rx	**Bidhist** (Cypress)	**Tablets, extended release**: 6 mg brompheniramine maleate	(CYP 471). White, oval. In 100s.
Rx	**Lodrane 24** (ECR Pharmaceuticals)	**Capsules, extended release**: 12 mg brompheniramine maleate	(Lodrane 24). White. In 100s.
Rx	**VaZol** (WraSer)	**Liquid**: 2 mg/5 mL brompheniramine tannate	Bubble gum flavor. In 472 mL.
Rx (sf)	**Lodrane XR** (ECR Pharmaceuticals)	**Oral suspension**: 8 mg/5 mL brompheniramine tannate	Alcohol free. Strawberry flavor. In pints and 10 mL.
Rx	**BrōveX** (Athlon)	**Oral suspension**: 12 mg/5 mL brompheniramine tannate	Methylparaben, saccharin, sucrose, tartrazine. Banana flavor. In 20 and 118 mL.

BROMPHENIRAMINE TANNATE — ORAL

For complete and comparative prescribing information, refer to the Antihistamines group monograph.

Indications

➤*Allergies:* For the temporary relief of sneezing, itchy, watery eyes, itchy nose or throat, and runny nose caused by hay fever (allergic rhinitis), or other respiratory allergies.

VaZol also is indicated for the temporary relief of runny nose and sneezing caused by the common cold; treatment of allergic and nonallergic pruritic symptoms; temporary relief of mild, uncomplicated urticaria and angioedema; amelioration of allergic reactions to blood or plasma; adjunctive therapy in anaphylactic reactions.

Administration and Dosage

➤*Tablets, extended release:* Take with food, water, or milk to minimize gastric irritation. Swallow whole; do not crush tablets.

Adults and children older than 12 years of age – 1 or 2 tablets (6 to 12 mg) every 12 hours.

Children 6 to 12 years of age – 1 tablet (6 mg) every 12 hours.

➤*Tablets, chewable:*

Adults and children 12 years of age and older – 1 or 2 tablets (12 to 24 mg) every 12 hours, up to 4 tablets (48 mg) in 24 hours.

Children 6 to younger than 12 years of age – ½ to 1 tablet (6 to 12 mg) every 12 hours, up to 2 tablets (24 mg) in 24 hours.

Children 2 to younger than 6 years of age – ½ tablet (6 mg) every 12 hours, up to 1 tablet (12 mg) in 24 hours.

➤*Capsules, extended release:* Take with food, water or milk to minimize gastric irritation. Swallow whole; do not crush capsules.

Adults and children 12 years of age and older – 1 or 2 capsules (12 to 24 mg) once daily.

Children 6 to younger than 12 years of age – 1 capsule (12 mg) once daily.

➤*Oral suspension:* Shake well before use.

Adults and children 12 years of age and older – 5 to 10 mL (12 to 24 mg) every 12 hours, up to 20 mL (48 mg) in 24 hours.

Children 6 to younger than 12 years of age – 5 mL (12 mg) every 12 hours, up to 10 mL (24 mg) in 24 hours.

Children 2 to younger than 6 years of age – 2.5 mL (6 mg) every 12 hours, up to 5 mL (12 mg) in 24 hours.

Children 12 months to 2 years of age – 1.25 mL (3 mg) every 12 hours, up to 2.5 mL (6 mg) in 24 hours.

➤*Oral liquid:*

Adults and children older than 12 years of age – 10 mL (4 mg) 4 times daily.

Children 6 to 12 years of age – 5 mL (2 mg) 4 times daily.

Children 2 to 6 years of age – 2.5 mL (1 mg) 4 times daily

Children younger than 2 years of age – Titrate dosage individually based on 0.5 mg/kg/day in equally divided doses, 4 times daily.

➤*Lodrane XR:*

Adults and children older than 12 years of age – 5 mL every 12 hours, not to exceed 2 doses in 24 hours.

Children 6 to 12 years of age – 2.5 mL every 12 hours, not to exceed 2 doses in 24 hours.

Children 2 to 6 years of age – 1.25 mL every 12 hours, not to exceed 2 doses in 24 hours.

Children younger than 2 years of age – As recommended by a physician.

➤*Storage/Stability:* Store extended-release tablets, liquid, and oral suspension between 15° and 30°C (59° to 86°F). Dispense in a tight, light-resistant container.

CHLORPHENIRAMINE

otc	**Chlorpheniramine Maleate** (Various, eg, Contract Pharmacal, URL)	**Tablets**: 4 mg (as maleate)	In 24s, 100s, and 1,000s.
otc	**Aller-Chlor** (Rugby)		In 24s, 100s, and 1,000s.
otc	**Allergy** (Major)		Lactose. In 24s and 100s.
otc	**Allergy Relief** (Zee Medical)		In 12s.
otc	**Chlo-Amine** (Hollister-Stier)	**Tablets, chewable**: 2 mg (as maleate)	Sugar. Orange flavor. In 96s.
otc	**Chlor-Trimeton Allergy 8 Hour** (Schering-Plough Healthcare)	**Tablets, extended-release**: 8 mg (as maleate)	(374). In 15s.
otc	**Chlor-Trimeton Allergy 12 Hour** (Schering-Plough Healthcare)	**Tablets, extended-release**: 12 mg (as maleate)	(009). In 10s.
otc	**Efidac 24**[a] (Hogil)	**Tablets, extended-release**: 16 mg (as maleate)	Mannitol. In 6s.
Rx	**QDALL AR**[b] (Atley)	**Capsules, extended-release**: 12 mg (as maleate)	Sucrose. (QD 111). Blue/White. In 100s.
Rx	**Chlorpheniramine Maleate** (Various, eg, Qualitest)	**Capsules, sustained-release**: 8 mg (as maleate)	In 100s and 1,000s.
Rx	**Chlorpheniramine Maleate** (Various, eg, Qualitest)	**Capsules, sustained-release**: 12 mg (as maleate)	In 100s and 1,000s.
Rx	**ED-CHLOR-TAN** (Edwards Pharmaceuticals)	**Caplets**: 8 mg (as tannate)	In 100s.
otc	**Aller-Chlor** (Rugby)	**Syrup**: 2 mg/5 mL (as maleate)	5% alcohol, parabens, sugar. In 118 mL.

[a] 4 mg immediate release, 12 mg controlled release.

[b] 2 mg immediate release, 10 mg sustained release.

CHLORPHENIRAMINE MALEATE — ORAL

For complete and comparative prescribing information, refer to the Antihistamines group monograph.

Indications

➤*Allergic rhinitis:* For the temporary relief of sneezing, itchy, watery eyes, itchy throat, and runny nose caused by hay fever, other upper respiratory allergies, and the common cold.

Administration and Dosage

Individualize dosage.

➤*Tablets or syrup:*

Adults and children 12 years of age and older – 4 mg every 4 to 6 hours. Do not exceed 24 mg in 24 hours.

Children 6 to 12 years of age – 2 mg (break 4 mg tablets in half) every 4 to 6 hours. Do not exceed 12 mg in 24 hours.

Children younger than 6 years of age: Consult a physician.

➤*Tablets, extended-release:*

Adults and children 12 years of age and older – 8 mg every 8 to 12 hours or 12 mg every 12 hours. Do not exceed 24 mg in 24 hours.

Efidac 24 –

Adults and children 12 years of age and older: 16 mg with liquid every 24 hours. Do not exceed 16 mg in 24 hours. Swallow each tablet whole; do not divide, crush, chew, or dissolve.

➤*Capsules, extended-release:*

Adults and children 12 years of age and older – 12 mg once daily, not to exceed 24 mg in 24 hours.

➤*Capsules, sustained-release:*

Adults and children 12 years of age and older – 8 or 12 mg every 12 hours, up to 16 to 24 mg/day.

Children 6 to 12 years of age – 8 mg at bedtime or during the day as indicated.

➤*Caplets:*

Adults and children 12 years of age and older – 8 mg every 12 hours, up to 16 to 24 mg/day.

Children 6 to 12 years of age – Consult a physician.

➤*Storage/Stability:* Store between 15° and 30°C (59° and 86°F).

DEXCHLORPHENIRAMINE MALEATE

Rx	**Dexchlorpheniramine Maleate** (Various, eg, Amide, Breckenridge, URL)	**Tablets, extended-release**: 4 mg	In 100s and 1,000s.
Rx	**Dexchlorpheniramine Maleate** (Various, eg, Amide, Breckenridge, URL)	**Tablets, extended-release**: 6 mg	In 100s and 1,000s.
Rx	**Dexchlorpheniramine Maleate** (Morton Grove)	**Syrup**: 2 mg/5 mL	Alcohol, orange flavor. In 473 mL.

DEXCHLORPHENIRAMINE MALEATE — ORAL

For complete and comparative prescribing information, refer to the Antihistamines group monograph.

Indications

➤*Hypersensitivity reactions, type I:* For the treatment of perennial and seasonal allergic rhinitis; vasomotor rhinitis; allergic conjunctivitis; mild, uncomplicated allergic skin manifestations of urticaria and angioedema; amelioration of allergic reactions to blood or plasma; dermatographism; and adjunctive anaphylactic therapy.

Administration and Dosage

Individualize dosage.

➤*Adults and children 12 years of age and older:* 4 or 6 mg at bedtime or every 8 to 10 hours.

➤*Children 6 to 12 years of age:* 4 mg/day, preferably taken at bedtime.

➤*Storage/Stability:* Store between 2° and 30°C (36° and 86°F).

TRIPROLIDINE

Rx *(sf)*	**Zymine** (Vindex Pharmaceuticals)	**Liquid**: 1.25 mg/5 mL	Alcohol free. Apple flavor. In 15 and 473 mL.

TRIPROLIDINE — ORAL

For complete and comparative prescribing information, refer to the Antihistamines group monograph.

Indications

➤*Allergies:* For the symptomatic relief of perennial and seasonal allergic rhinitis, vasomotor rhinitis, allergic conjunctivitis caused by inhalant allergens and foods, and mild, uncomplicated allergic skin manifestations of urticaria and angioedema.

Administration and Dosage

➤*Adults and children 12 years of age and older:* 10 mL every 4 to 6 hours; do not exceed 40 mL in 24 hours.

➤*Children:*

6 to 12 years of age – 5 mL every 4 to 6 hours; do not exceed 20 mL in 24 hours.

4 to 6 years of age – 3.75 mL every 4 to 6 hours; do not exceed 15 mL in 24 hours.

2 to 4 years of age – 2.5 mL every 4 to 6 hours; do not exceed 10 mL in 24 hours.

4 months to 2 years of age – 1.25 mL every 4 to 6 hours; do not exceed 5 mL in 24 hours.

➤*Storage/Stability:* Store between 15° to 30°C (59° to 86°F). Dispense in tight, light- and child-resistant containers.

Ethanolamines, Nonselective

CARBINOXAMINE

Rx	**Palgic** (Pamlab)	**Tablets:** 4 mg carbinoxamine maleate	Lactose. (PAL 4). White, scored. In 100s and 500s.
Rx	**Histex CT** (Teamm Pharm[a])	**Tablets, timed release:** 8 mg carbinoxamine maleate	(258). Blue, scored. Film-coated. In 30s and 100s.
Rx	**Histex I/E** (Teamm Pharm[a])	**Capsules, extended release:** 10 mg carbinoxamine maleate[b]	(050 HISTEX I/E). Green and white. In 60s.
Rx sf	**Pediatex** (Zyber)	**Liquid:** 1.67 mg per 5 mL carbinoxamine maleate	Saccharin, sorbitol. Alcohol and dye-free. Cotton candy flavor. In 15 and 473 mL.
Rx sf	**Histex Pd** (Teamm Pharm[a])	**Liquid:** 4 mg per 5 mL carbinoxamine maleate	Saccharin, sorbitol. Alcohol and dye free. Gum fruit flavor. In 473 mL.
Rx sf	**Palgic** (Pamlab)		Parabens. Clear. Bubble gum flavor. In 118 and 473 mL.
Rx	**Pediatex 12** (Zyber)	**Oral suspension:** 3.2 mg per 5 mL carbinoxamine tannate	Methylparaben, saccharin, sucrose. Candy apple flavor. In 20 and 473 mL.

[a] Teamm Pharmaceuticals, 3000 Aerial Center Parkway, Suite 110, Morrisville, NC 27560; 919-481-9020, 866-481-9020, fax 919-481-9311.

[b] 2 mg immediate-release and 8 mg extended-release.

CARBINOXAMINE MALEATE — ORAL

For complete and comparative prescribing information, refer to the Antihistamines group monograph.

Indications

➤*Allergies:* For relief of nasal and nonnasal symptoms of seasonal and perennial allergic rhinitis. *Palgic* tablets also are indicated for the symptomatic treatment of vasomotor rhinitis; allergic conjunctivitis caused by inhalant allergens and foods; mild, uncomplicated allergic skin manifestations of urticaria and angioedema; dermatographism; as therapy for anaphylactic reactions adjunctive to epinephrine and other standard measures after the acute manifestations have been controlled; amelioration of the severity of allergic reactions to blood or plasma.

Administration and Dosage

➤*Palgic* tablets:

Adults – 1 or 2 tablets (4 to 8 mg) 3 to 4 times daily.

Children 6 years of age and older – 1 to 1½ tablets (4 to 6 mg) 3 or 4 times daily.

Children 3 to 6 years of age – ½ to 1 tablet (2 to 4 mg) 3 or 4 times daily.

Children 1 to 3 years of age – ½ tablet (2 mg) 3 or 4 times daily.

➤*Tablets:*

Adults and children 12 years of age and older – 1 tablet (8 mg) twice daily (every 12 hours).

Children 6 to 12 years of age – ½ tablet twice daily (every 12 hours). The tablets are not recommended for children younger 6 years of age. Tablets may be broken in half for ease of administration without affecting release of the medication, but should not be crushed or chewed prior to swallowing.

➤*Capsules:*

Adults and children 12 years of age and older – 1 capsule every 12 hours, up to 2 per day.

➤*Liquids:*

Histex Pd –

Adults and children 6 years of age and older: 5 mL 4 times/day.

Children:
- *18 months to 6 years of age* – 2.5 mL 4 times/day.
- *9 to 18 months of age* – 1.25 to 2.5 mL 4 times/day.

Palgic –

Adults: 5 or 10 mL 3 to 4 times/day.

Children:
- *Older than 6 years of age* – 5 to 7.5 mL 3 or 4 times/day.
- *3 to 6 years of age* – 2.5 to 5 mL 3 or 4 times/day.
- *1 to 3 years of age* – 2.5 mL 3 or 4 times/day.

Pediatex –

Adults and children 6 years of age and older: 10 mL 4 times/day.

Children:
- *18 months to 6 years of age* – 5 mL 4 times/day.
- *9 to 18 months of age* – 3.75 to 5 mL 4 times/day.
- *6 to 9 months of age* – 3.75 mL 4 times/day.
- *3 to 6 months of age* – 2.5 mL 4 times/day.
- *1 to 3 months of age* – 1.25 mL 4 times/day.

➤*Oral suspension:* Shake well.

Adults and children 12 years of age and older – 10 to 20 mL every 12 hours.

Children 6 to 12 years of age – 5 to 10 mL every 12 hours.

Children 2 to 6 years of age – 2.5 to 5 mL every 12 hours.

➤*Storage/Stability:* Store between 15° and 30°C (59° to 86°F). Dispense in tight, light-resistant containers.

CLEMASTINE FUMARATE

otc	**Clemastine Fumarate** (Various, eg, Geneva)	**Tablets:** 1.34 mg as fumarate (equivalent to 1 mg clemastine)	In 100s.
otc	**Dayhist-1** (Major)		Lactose. In 8s.
otc	**Tavist Allergy** (Novartis Consumer Health)		Lactose. (TAVIST ALLERGY). In 8s.
Rx	**Clemastine Fumarate** (Various, eg, Teva)	**Tablets:** 2.68 mg (equivalent to 2 mg clemastine)	In 100s.
Rx	**Clemastine Fumarate** (Various, eg, Apotex, Teva)	**Syrup:** 0.67 mg /5 mL (equivalent to 0.5 mg clemastine)	May contain alcohol. In 118 and 120.

CLEMASTINE FUMARATE — ORAL

For complete and comparative prescribing information, refer to the Antihistamines group monograph.

Indications

➤*Allergic rhinitis:* For the relief of symptoms associated with allergic rhinitis or other upper respiratory allergies, such as sneezing, rhinorrhea, pruritus, and lacrimation, in adults (tablets and syrup) and in children 6 to 12 years of age (syrup only).

➤*Urticaria/Angioedema:* For the relief of mild, uncomplicated allergic skin manifestations of urticaria and angioedema in adults (tablets and syrup) and in children 6 to 12 years of age (syrup only).

Administration and Dosage

Individualize dosage.

➤*Allergic rhinitis:*

Adults – 1.34 mg every 12 hours or twice daily. Dosage may be increased as needed. Do not exceed 8.04 mg/day for the syrup or 2.68 mg in 24 hours for the tablets.

Children 6 to 12 years of age (syrup only) – 0.67 mg twice daily. Dosage may be increased as needed. Single doses of up to 2.25 mg clemastine have been well tolerated. Do not exceed 4.02 mg/day.

➤*Urticaria/Angioedema:*

Adults – 2.68 mg twice daily, not to exceed 8.04 mg/day.

Children 6 to 12 years of age (syrup only) – 1.34 mg twice daily, not to exceed 4.02 mg/day.

➤*Storage/Stability:* Store between 15° and 30°C (59° to 86°F).

DIPHENHYDRAMINE

otc	**Diphenhydramine** (Various, eg, Eon, Marlex)	**Tablets:** 25 mg (as hydrochloride)	In 24s and 100s.
otc	**Banophen** (Major)		In 24s and 100s.
otc	**Genahist** (Goldline)		In 24s.
otc	**Benadryl Allergy Ultratabs** (Pfizer)		In 24s, 48s, and 100s.
otc	**Diphenhist Captabs** (Rugby)		Capsule shape. In 100s.

Ethanolamines, Nonselective

DIPHENHYDRAMINE

otc	**AllerMax Caplets, Maximum Strength** (Pfeiffer)	**Tablets**: 50 mg (as hydrochloride)	Lactose. In 24s.
otc	**Benadryl Allergy** (Pfizer)	**Tablets, chewable**: 12.5 mg (as hydrochloride)	Aspartame, 4.2 mg phenylalanine. Grape flavor. In 24s.
Rx	**Dytan** (Hawthorn)	**Tablets, chewable**: 25 mg (as tannate)	Phenylalanine. (HAW 571). Oval-shape, scored. Strawberry flavor. In 60s.
otc	**Children's Benadryl Allergy Fastmelt** (Pfizer)	**Tablets, orally disintegrating**: 12.5 mg (equivalent to 19 mg citrate)	Aspartame, mannitol, 4.5 mg phenylalanine. In 20s.
otc/ Rx[a]	**Diphenhydramine HCl** (Various, eg, Eon, Marlex, Major)	**Capsules**: 25 mg (as hydrochloride)	In 24s, 100s, and 1,000s.
otc	**Banophen** (Major)		In 24s and 100s
otc	**Benadryl Allergy Kapseals** (Pfizer)		Lactose. In 24s and 48s.
otc	**Benadryl Dye-Free Allergy Liqui Gels** (Pfizer)		Sorbitol. In 24s.
otc	**Diphenhist** (Rugby)		Benzyl alcohol, butylparaben, EDTA, lactose, parabens. In 100s.
otc	**Genahist** (Goldline)		Lactose, parabens. In 100s.
otc/ Rx[a]	**Diphenhydramine HCl** (Various, eg, Eon, Major)	**Capsules**: 50 mg (as hydrochloride)	In 100s and 1,000s.
otc	**Triaminic Cough & Runny Nose** (Novartis Consumer Health)	**Strips, orally disintegrating**: 12.5 mg (as hydrochloride)	Alcohol less than 5%, sorbitol, sucralose. Grape flavor. In 16s.
otc	**Triaminic MultiSymptom** (Novartis Consumer Health)	**Strips, orally disintegrating**: 25 mg (as hydrochloride)	Alcohol less than 5%, sorbitol, sucralose. Cherry flavor. In 12s.
otc sf	**Genahist** (Goldline)	**Liquid**: 12.5 mg per 5 mL (as hydrochloride)	Alcohol free. Cherry flavor. In 118 mL.
otc sf	**Scot-Tussin Allergy Relief Formula Clear** (Scot-Tussin)		Menthol, parabens. Alcohol and dye free. Cherry-strawberry flavor. In 118 mL.
otc	**AllerMax** (Pfeiffer)		0.5% alcohol, glucose, saccharin, sorbitol, sucrose, menthol. Raspberry flavor. In 118 mL.
otc	**Benadryl Children's Allergy** (Pfizer)		Sugar. Alcohol free. Cherry flavor. In 118 and 236 mL.
otc sf	**Benadryl Children's Dye-Free Allergy** (Pfizer)		Saccharin, sorbitol. Alcohol free. Bubble gum flavor. In 118 mL.
otc	**Diphen AF** (Morton Grove)		Saccharin, sugar. Alcohol free. Cherry flavor. In 118, 237, and 473 mL.
otc	**Altaryl Children's Allergy** (Altaire)		Alcohol free. Glycerin, saccharin, sugar, 9 mg sodium. Cherry flavor. In 118 mL.
otc	**Diphenhist** (Rugby)	**Oral solution**: 12.5 mg per 5 mL (as hydrochloride)	Glycerin, saccharin, sucrose. Alcohol free. In 473 mL.
otc	**Banophen Allergy** (Major)	**Elixir**: 12.5 mg per 5 mL (as hydrochloride)	Sugar. In 118 mL.
otc	**Siladryl** (Silarx)		5.6% alcohol. Cherry flavor. In 118 mL.
otc/ Rx[a]	**Hydramine Cough** (Various, eg, Alpharma)	**Syrup**: 12.5 mg/5 mL	May contain alcohol. In 473 mL.
otc	**Silphen Cough** (Silarx)		Menthol, parabens, sucrose, 5% alcohol. Strawberry flavor. In 118 mL.
Rx	**Tusstat** (Century)	**Syrup**: 12.5 mg per 5 mL (as hydrochloride)	5% alcohol. In 30, 118, and 473 mL, and 3.8 L.
Rx	**Ben-Tann** (Midlothian)	**Suspension**: 25 mg per 5 mL (as tannate)	Sucrose, saccharin. Strawberry flavor. In 118 mL.
Rx	**Dytan** (Hawthorn)		Phenylalanine. Strawberry flavor. In 118 mL.
Rx	**Diphenhydramine** (Various, eg, Abbott)	**Injection**: 50 mg/mL (as hydrochloride)	In 1 mL fill in 2 mL cartridges.
Rx	**Benadryl** (Parke-Davis)		In 1 mL amps, 1 and 10 mL *Steri-vials*,[b] and 1 mL *Steri-dose* syringe.

[a] Products are available OTC or *Rx*, depending on product labeling.

[b] With benzethonium chloride.

DIPHENHYDRAMINE HYDROCHLORIDE — ORAL

For complete and comparative prescribing information, refer to the Antihistamines group monograph. Also refer to the general discussion in the Antiparkinson Agents introduction and the Anticholinergics group monograph in the CNS chapter. For a complete listing of diphenhydramine sleep aids, see Nonprescription Sleep Aids in the CNS Agents chapter.

Indications

➤*Hypersensitivity reactions, type I:* Perennial and seasonal allergic rhinitis; vasomotor rhinitis and sneezing caused by the common cold; allergic conjunctivitis caused by inhalant allergens and foods; mild, uncomplicated allergic skin manifestations of urticaria and angioedema; amelioration of allergic reactions to blood or plasma in patients with a known history of such reactions; dermatographism; as adjunctive anaphylactic therapy; for uncomplicated allergic conditions of the immediate type. Parenteral therapy also is indicated when oral therapy is impossible or contraindicated.

➤*Antiparkinsonism:* Parkinsonism in the elderly who are unable to tolerate more potent agents; mild cases of parkinsonism in other age groups; in other cases of parkinsonism in combination with centrally acting anticholinergic agents. Parenteral therapy also is indicated when oral therapy is impossible or contraindicated.

➤*Antitussive (syrup and liquid only):* For control of coughs caused by colds or allergy.

➤*Unlabeled uses:* Diphenhydramine also has been used as an antianxiety agent in doses of 25 to 200 mg/day.

Treatment or prophylaxis of chemotherapy-induced emesis; drug-induced extrapyramidal reactions; treatment of mucositis in combination with other drugs.

Administration and Dosage

Individualize dosage.

➤*Hypersensitivity reactions, type I/Antiparkinsonism/Motion sickness:*

Oral –

Adults: 25 to 50 mg, every 4 to 6 hours. Maximum daily dosage is 300 mg. For diphenhydramine tannate, 50 to 100 mg every 12 hours.

Children 6 to younger than 12 years of age: 12.5 to 25 mg, every 4 to 6 hours. Maximum daily dosage is 150 mg. For diphenhydramine tannate, 25 to 50 mg every 12 hours.

Children 2 to younger than 6 years of age: For diphenhydramine tannate oral suspension, 12.5 to 25 mg every 12 hours.

Ethanolamines, Nonselective

DIPHENHYDRAMINE HYDROCHLORIDE — ORAL

➤*Antitussive (syrup and liquid only):*

Syrup –

Adults: 25 mg every 4 hours; do not exceed 150 mg in 24 hours.

Children:

- *6 to 12 years of age* – 12.5 mg every 4 hours; do not exceed 75 mg in 24 hours.
- *2 to 6 years of age* – 6.25 mg every 4 hours; do not exceed 25 mg in 24 hours.

Liquid –

Adults and children 12 years of age and older: 25 to 50 mg every 4 hours; do not exceed 300 mg in 24 hours.

Children:

- *6 to 12 years of age* – 12.5 to 25 mg every 4 hours; do not exceed 150 mg in 24 hours.
- *Younger than 6 years of age* – Consult a physician.

➤*Storage/Stability:* Store at controlled room temperature, 15° to 30°C (59° to 86°F). Protect injection from freezing and light.

DIPHENHYDRAMINE CITRATE — ORAL

For complete and comparative prescribing information, refer to the Antihistamines group monograph. Also refer to the general discussion in the Antiparkinson Agents introduction and the Anticholinergics group monograph in the CNS chapter. For a complete listing of diphenhydramine sleep aids, see Nonprescription Sleep Aids in the CNS Agents chapter.

Indications

➤*Antihistamine:* Temporarily relieves symptoms due to hay fever or other upper respiratory allergies, including runny nose; sneezing; itchy, watery eyes; itching of the nose or throat.

Temporarily relieves runny nose and sneezing symptoms due to the common cold.

➤*Nonprescription sleep aid:* Aid in the relief of insomnia.

➤*Unlabeled uses:* Treatment or prophylaxis of chemotherapy-induced emesis; drug-induced extrapyramidal reactions; treatment of mucositis in combination with other drugs.

Administration and Dosage

➤*Antihistamine:* Take every 4 to 6 hours. Do not take more than 6 doses in 24 hours.

Adults and children 12 years of age and older – 2 to 4 tablets (38 to 76 mg).

Children 6 to less than 12 years of age – 1 to 2 tablets (19 mg to 38 mg).

Children less than 6 years of age – Ask a doctor.

➤*Nonprescription sleep aid:* Administer 38 mg to 76 mg diphenhydramine citrate (2 to 4 tablets) before bedtime.

Do not use in children younger than 12 years of age.

➤*Storage/Stability:* Store at 15° to 25°C (59° to 77°F) in a dry place. Protect from heat, humidity, and light.

DIPHENHYDRAMINE TANNATE — ORAL

For complete and comparative prescribing information, refer to the Antihistamines group monograph. For a complete listing of diphenhydramine sleep aids, see Nonprescription Sleep Aids in the CNS Agents chapter.

Indications

➤*Allergic conditions:* For amelioration of allergic reactions in the absence of acute symptoms or after acute symptoms have been controlled, and for other uncomplicated allergic conditions when oral therapy is indicated.

➤*Unlabeled uses:* Treatment or prophylaxis of chemotherapy-induced emesis; drug-induced extrapyramidal reactions; treatment of mucositis in combination with other drugs.

Administration and Dosage

Administer the recommended dose every 12 hours.

➤*Adults to children 12 years of age and over:* 25 to 50 mg.

➤*Children 6 to under 12 years of age:* 12.5 to 25 mg.

➤*Children under 6 years of age:* Consult a physician.

Oral suspension –

Children 2 to 6 years of age: 6.25 to 12.5 mg (1.25 to 2.5 mL).

Children under 2 years of age: Consult a physician.

➤*Storage/Stability:* Store at controlled room temperature, 15° to 30°C (59° to 86°F).

DIPHENHYDRAMINE HYDROCHLORIDE — INJECTION

For complete and comparative prescribing information, refer to the Antihistamines group monograph. For a complete listing of diphenhydramine sleep aids, see Nonprescription Sleep Aids in the CNS Agents chapter.

Indications

Diphenhydramine in the injectable form is effective in adults and pediatric patients, other than premature infants and neonates, for the following conditions when diphenhydramine in the oral form is impractical.

➤*Allergic conditions:* For amelioration of allergic reactions to blood or plasma, in anaphylaxis as an adjunct to epinephrine and other standard measures after the acute symptoms have been controlled, and for other uncomplicated allergic conditions of the immediate type when oral therapy is impossible or contraindicated.

➤*Motion sickness:* For active treatment of motion sickness.

➤*Antiparkinsonism:* For use in parkinsonism, when oral therapy is impossible or contraindicated, as follows: parkinsonism in the elderly who are unable to tolerate more potent agents; mild cases of parkinsonism in other age groups, and in other cases of parkinsonism in combination with centrally acting anticholinergic agents.

➤*Unlabeled uses:* For antipsychotic-induced dystonia, diphenhydramine 50 mg IM or IV has been shown to be effective. Treatment or prophylaxis of chemotherapy-induced emesis; drug-induced extrapyramidal reactions; treatment of mucositis in combination with other drugs.

Administration and Dosage

This product is for IV or IM administration only.

Diphenhydramine in the injectable form is indicated when the oral form is impractical.

Individualize the dosage according to the needs and the response of the patient.

➤*Pediatric patients, other than premature infants and neonates:* 5 mg/kg per 24 hr or 150 mg/m^2 per 24 hr. Maximum daily dosage is 300 mg. Divide into 4 doses, administered intravenously (IV) at a rate generally not exceeding 25 mg/min, or deep intramuscularly (IM).

➤*Adults:* 10 to 50 mg IV at a rate generally not exceeding 25 mg/min, or deep IM, 100 mg if required; maximum daily dosage is 400 mg.

➤*Storage/Stability:* Store at controlled room temperature 15° to 30°C (59° to 86°F). Protect from light and freezing. Retain in carton until time of use.

Phenothiazines, Nonselective

PROMETHAZINE HYDROCHLORIDE

Rx	**Promethazine Hydrochloride** (Able Labs)	**Tablets:** 12.5 mg	May contain lactose. (A405). Lt. peach. In 30s, 100s, 500s, and 1,000s.
Rx	**Promethazine Hydrochloride** (Various, eg, Able Labs, Geneva)	**Tablets:** 25 mg	May contain lactose. In 30s, 100s, 500s, and 1,000s.
Rx	**Promethazine Hydrochloride** (Various, eg, Able Labs, Geneva)	**Tablets:** 50 mg	May contain lactose. In 30s, 100s, 500s, and 1,000s.
Rx	**Promethazine Hydrochloride** (Various, eg, Morton Grove)	**Syrup:** 6.25 mg/5 mL	Alcohol. In 473 mL.
Rx	**Promethazine Hydrochloride** (Ivax)	**Suppositories:** 12.5 mg	May contain hard fat. In 12s.
Rx	**Phenadoz** (Paddock)		Cocoa butter. In 12s.
Rx	**Promethazine Hydrochloride** (Various, eg, Alpharma, Ivax)	**Suppositories:** 25 mg	May contain hard fat. In 12s.
Rx	**Phenadoz** (Paddock)		Cocoa butter. In 12s.
Rx	**Promethazine Hydrochloride** (Various, eg, Ivax, Major)	**Suppositories:** 50 mg	In 12s.
Rx	**Promethazine Hydrochloride** (Various, eg, Abbott)	**Injection:** 25 mg/mL	May contain EDTA. In 1 mL amps.
Rx	**Phenergan** (Wyeth Labs)		EDTA, 0.25 mg/mL sodium metabisulfite. In 1 mL amps.

PROMETHAZINE HYDROCHLORIDE

Rx	**Promethazine Hydrochloride** (Various, eg, Abbott)	**Injection:** 50 mg/mL	May contain EDTA. In 1 mL amps.
Rx	**Phenergan** (Wyeth Labs)		EDTA, 0.25 mg/mL sodium metabisulfite. In 1 mL amps.

PROMETHAZINE HYDROCHLORIDE — ORAL

For complete and comparative prescribing information, refer to the Antihistamines group monograph. For more information on promethazine as an antiemetic/antivertigo agent, see the Antiemetic/Antivertigo monograph in the CNS Agents chapter.

WARNING

Promethazine should not be used in pediatric patients younger than 2 years of age because of the potential for fatal respiratory depression.

Postmarketing cases of respiratory depression including fatalities, have been reported with use of promethazine in pediatric patients less than 2 years of age. A wide range of weight-based doses of promethazine have resulted in respiratory depression in these patients.

Caution should be exercised when administering promethazine to pediatric patients 2 years of age and older. It is recommended that the lowest effective dose of promethazine be used in pediatric patients 2 years of age and older and concomitant administration of other drugs with respiratory depressant effects be avoided.

Indications

➤*Analgesia:* Adjunctive therapy for control of postoperative pain.

➤*Antiemetic:* Prevention and control of nausea and vomiting associated with certain types of anesthesia and surgery and in postoperative patients.

➤*Hypersensitivity reactions, type I:* Perennial and seasonal allergic rhinitis; vasomotor rhinitis; allergic conjunctivitis caused by inhalant allergens and foods; mild, uncomplicated allergic skin manifestations of urticaria and angioedema; amelioration of allergic reactions to blood or plasma; dermatographism; adjunctive anaphylactic therapy. Parenteral therapy is indicated when oral therapy is impossible or contraindicated.

➤*Motion sickness (oral and rectal only):* Active and prophylactic treatment of motion sickness.

➤*Sedation:* Preoperative, postoperative, or obstetric sedation; relief of apprehension and production of light sleep.

Administration and Dosage

Individualize dosage; after initiation, adjust to smallest effective dose.

➤*Antiemetic:*

Oral/Rectal –

Adults: Usual dose is 25 mg; doses of 12.5 to 25 mg may be repeated every 4 to 6 hours as needed for prophylaxis or treatment of active nausea/vomiting.

Children (older than 2 years of age): Usual dose is 25 mg or 0.5 mg/lb; doses of 12.5 to 25 mg may be repeated every 4 to 6 hours as needed for prophylaxis or treatment of active nausea/vomiting. Adjust dose to the age, weight, and severity of condition for the patient being treated. Antiemetics are not recommended for treatment of uncomplicated vomiting in pediatric patients; limit use to prolonged vomiting of known etiology.

➤*Hypersensitivity reactions, type I:*

Oral/Rectal – May be administered rectally or parenterally if the oral route is not feasible; however, resume oral administration as soon as possible if continued therapy is warranted.

Adults and children (older than 2 years of age): Usual dose is 25 mg at bedtime; 12.5 mg before meals and at bedtime may be given, if necessary. Single 25 mg doses at bedtime or 6.25 to 12.5 mg taken 3 times daily will usually suffice. After initiation of treatment in children or adults, adjust dosage to the smallest amount adequate to relieve symptoms. The administration of promethazine in 25 mg doses will control minor transfusion reactions of an allergic nature.

➤*Motion sickness (oral and rectal only):*

Adults – Usual dose is 25 mg twice daily; take first dose 30 to 60 minutes before anticipated travel; repeat 8 to 12 hours later if needed. On successive travel days, take 25 mg on rising and again before the evening meal.

Children (older than 2 years of age) – 12.5 to 25 mg twice daily.

➤*Pre- and postoperative use:*

Oral/Rectal –

Adults: For preoperative use, 50 mg administered with an appropriately reduced dose of narcotic or barbiturate and the required amount of a belladonna alkaloid.

Postoperative sedation and adjunctive use with analgesics may be obtained by the administration of 25 to 50 mg doses in adults.

For the night before surgery to relieve apprehension and produce a quiet sleep,, administer 50 mg doses for adults.

Children (older than 2 years of age): For preoperative use, 0.5 mg/lb in combination with an appropriately reduced dose of narcotic or barbiturate and the appropriate dose of an atropine-like drug.

Postoperative sedation and adjunctive use with analgesics may be obtained by the administration of 12.5 to 25 mg in children.

For the night before surgery to relieve apprehension and produce a quiet sleep administer 12.5 to 25 mg doses for children.

➤*Sedation:*

Oral/Rectal – If used for preoperative sedation, administer the night before surgery to relieve apprehension and produce quiet sleep.

Adults: 25 to 50 mg at bedtime.

Children (older than 2 years of age): 12.5 to 25 mg at bedtime.

➤*Use in children:* Promethazine tablets are contraindicated for children younger than 2 years of age. Exercise caution when administering promethazine to pediatric patients 2 years of age and older because of the potential for fatal respiratory depression. Antiemetics are not recommended for treatment of uncomplicated vomiting in pediatric patients; limit use to prolonged vomiting of known etiology. The extrapyramidal symptoms that can occur secondary to promethazine administration may be confused with the CNS signs of undiagnosed primary disease (eg, encephalopathy, Reye syndrome). Avoid the use of promethazine in pediatric patients whose signs and symptoms may suggest Reye syndrome or other hepatic diseases. In pediatric patients who are acutely ill associated with dehydration, there is an increased susceptibility to dystonias. Excessive large doses of antihistamines, including promethazine, in pediatric patients may cause hallucinations, convulsions, and sudden death.

➤*Storage/Stability:*

Tablets – Store at controlled room temperature 20° to 25°C (68° to 77°F). Keep tightly closed. Protect from light and dispense in a tight, light-resistant container.

Syrup – Store at controlled room temperature 15° to 25°C (59° to 77°F).

PROMETHAZINE HYDROCHLORIDE — RECTAL

For complete and comparative prescribing information, refer to the Antihistamines group monograph. For more information on promethazine as an antiemetic/antivertigo agent, see the Antiemetic/Antivertigo monograph in the CNS Agents chapter.

WARNING

Promethazine should not be used in pediatric patients younger than 2 years of age because of the potential for fatal respiratory depression.

Postmarketing cases of respiratory depression, including fatalities, have been reported with use of promethazine hydrochloride suppositories in pediatric patients younger than 2 years of age. A wide range of weight-based doses of promethazine have resulted in respiratory depression in these patients.

Caution should be exercised when administering promethazine to pediatric patients 2 years of age and older. It is recommended that the lowest effective dose of promethazine be used in pediatric patients 2 years of age and older and concomitant administration of other drugs with respiratory-depressant effects be avoided.

Indications

Promethazine hydrochloride suppositories are useful for the following:

- Perennial and seasonal allergic rhinitis.
- Vasomotor rhinitis.
- Allergic conjunctivitis due to inhalant allergens and foods.
- Mild, uncomplicated allergic skin manifestations of urticaria and angioedema.
- Amelioration of allergic reactions to blood or plasma.
- Dermographism.
- Anaphylactic reactions, as adjunctive therapy to epinephrine and other standard measures, after the acute manifestations have been controlled.
- Preoperative, postoperative, or obstetric sedation.
- Prevention and control of nausea and vomiting associated with certain types of anesthesia and surgery.
- Therapy adjunctive to meperidine or other analgesics for control of postoperative pain.
- Sedation in both children and adults, as well as relief of apprehension and production of light sleep from which the patient can be easily aroused.
- Active and prophylactic treatment of motion sickness.
- Antiemetic therapy in postoperative patients.

Administration and Dosage

Promethazine hydrochloride rectal suppositories are contraindicated for children under 2 years of age because of the potential for fatal respiratory depression.

Promethazine hydrochloride suppositories are for rectal administration only.

➤*Allergy:* The average dose is 25 mg taken before retiring; however, 12.5 mg may be taken before meals and on retiring, if necessary. Single 25 mg doses at bedtime or 6.25 to 12.5 mg taken 3 times daily will usually suffice. After initiation of treatment in children or adults, dosage should be adjusted to the smallest amount adequate to relieve symptoms. The admin-

PROMETHAZINE HYDROCHLORIDE — RECTAL

istration of promethazine hydrochloride in 25 mg doses will control minor transfusion reactions of an allergic nature.

➤*Motion sickness:* The average adult dose is 25 mg taken twice daily. The initial dose should be taken one-half to 1 hour before anticipated travel and be repeated 8 to 12 hours later, if necessary. On succeeding days of travel, it is recommended that 25 mg be given on arising and again before the evening meal. For children, promethazine hydrochloride rectal suppositories, 12.5 to 25 mg, twice daily, may be administered.

➤*Nausea and vomiting:* Antiemetics should not be used in vomiting of unknown etiology in children and adolescents.

The average effective dose of promethazine hydrochloride for the active therapy of nausea and vomiting in children or adults is 25 mg; 12.5 to 25 mg doses may be repeated, as necessary, at 4- to 6-hour intervals.

For nausea and vomiting in children, the usual dose is 0.5 mg per pound of body weight, and the dose should be adjusted to the age and weight of the patient and the severity of the condition being treated.

For prophylaxis of nausea and vomiting, as during surgery and the postoperative period, the average dose is 25 mg repeated at 4- to 6-hour intervals, as necessary.

➤*Sedation:* This product relieves apprehension and induces a quiet sleep from which the patient can be easily aroused. Administration of 12.5 to 25 mg promethazine hydrochloride by rectal suppository at bedtime will provide sedation in children. Adults usually require 25 to 50 mg for nighttime, presurgical, or obstetrical sedation.

➤*Pre- and postoperative use:* Promethazine hydrochloride suppositories in 12.5 to 25 mg doses for children and 50 mg doses for adults the night before surgery relieves apprehension and produces a quiet sleep.

For preoperative medication children require doses of 0.5 mg per pound of body weight in combination with an appropriately reduced dose of narcotic or barbiturate and the appropriate dose of an atropine-like drug.

Usual adult dosage is 50 mg promethazine hydrochloride suppositories with an appropriately reduced dose of narcotic or barbiturate and the required amount of a belladonna alkaloid.

Postoperative sedation and adjunctive use with analgesics may be obtained by the administration of 12.5 to 25 mg in children and 25 to 50 mg doses in adults.

➤*Use in children:* Promethazine is contraindicated for children younger than 2 years of age.

➤*Storage/Stability:* Store refrigerated between 2° to 8°C (36° to 46°F).

Dispense in a well-closed container.

PROMETHAZINE HYDROCHLORIDE — INJECTION

For complete and comparative prescribing information, refer to the Antihistamines group monograph. For more information on promethazine as an antiemetic/antivertigo agent, see the Antiemetic/Antivertigo monograph in the CNS Agents chapter.

WARNING

Do not use promethazine in children younger than 2 years of age because of the potential for fatal respiratory depression.

Postmarketing cases of respiratory depression, including fatalities, have been reported with use of promethazine in children younger than 2 years of age. A wide range of weight-based doses of promethazine have resulted in respiratory depression in these patients.

Exercise caution when administering promethazine to children 2 years of age and older. It is recommended that the lowest effective dose of promethazine be used in children 2 years of age and older, and that concomitant administration of other drugs with respiratory depressant effects be avoided.

Indications

➤*Analgesia:* Adjunctive therapy for control of postoperative pain.

➤*Antiemetic:* Prevention and control of nausea and vomiting associated with certain types of anesthesia and surgery and in postoperative patients.

➤*Hypersensitivity reactions, type I:* Perennial and seasonal allergic rhinitis; vasomotor rhinitis; allergic conjunctivitis caused by inhalant allergens and foods; mild, uncomplicated allergic skin manifestations of urticaria and angioedema; amelioration of allergic reactions to blood or plasma; dermatographism; adjunctive anaphylactic therapy. Parenteral therapy is indicated when oral therapy is impossible or contraindicated.

➤*Sedation:* Preoperative, postoperative, or obstetric sedation; relief of apprehension and production of light sleep.

Administration and Dosage

Individualize dosage; after initiation, adjust to smallest effective dose.

➤*Antiemetic:*

Parenteral –

Adults: Usual dose is 12.5 to 25 mg; may repeat every 4 hours as needed. If used postoperatively, reduce doses of concomitant analgesics or barbiturates accordingly.

Children (2 to 12 years of age): Do not exceed half the adult dose. Do not use when etiology of vomiting is unknown.

➤*Hypersensitivity reactions, type I:*

Parenteral –

Adults: 25 mg; may repeat dose within 2 hours if needed. Resume oral therapy as soon as patient's circumstances permit.

Children (2 years of age and older): Dose should not exceed half the adult dose.

➤*Pre- and postoperative use:*

Parenteral –

Adults: 25 to 50 mg in combination with appropriately reduced doses of analgesics, hypnotics, and atropine-like drugs as appropriate.

Children (2 to 12 years of age): 0.5 mg/lb in combination with an appropriately reduced dose of narcotic or barbiturate and the appropriate dose of an atropine-like drug.

➤*Sedation:*

Parenteral –

Adults: 25 to 50 mg at bedtime for nighttime sedation. Doses of 50 mg provide sedation and relieve apprehension during early stages of labor. When labor is definitely established, 25 to 75 mg (average dose, 50 mg) promethazine injection may be given IM or IV with an appropriately reduced dose of any desired narcotic. If necessary, promethazine injection with a reduced dose of analgesic may be repeated once or twice at 4-hour intervals. Do not exceed 100 mg/24 hours for patients in labor.

Children (2 to 12 years of age): Do not exceed half the adult dose.

➤*Use in children:* Promethazine is contraindicated for children younger than 2 years of age. Exercise caution when administering promethazine to pediatric patients 2 years of age and older because of the potential for fatal respiratory depression. Antiemetics are not recommended for treatment of uncomplicated vomiting in pediatric patients; limit use to prolonged vomiting of known etiology. The extrapyramidal symptoms that can occur secondary to promethazine administration may be confused with the CNS signs of undiagnosed primary disease (eg, encephalopathy, Reye syndrome). Avoid the use of promethazine in pediatric patients whose signs and symptoms may suggest Reye syndrome or other hepatic diseases. In pediatric patients who are acutely ill associated with dehydration, there is an increased susceptibility to dystonias. Excessive large doses of antihistamines, including promethazine, in pediatric patients may cause hallucinations, convulsions, and sudden death.

➤*Administration for injection:* The preferred parenteral route of administration is deep IM injection; properly administered IV doses are well tolerated, but this method is associated with increased hazard. IV administration should be at a concentration not to exceed 25 mg/mL at a rate no greater than 25 mg/min. Avoid subcutaneous and intra-arterial injection because tissue necrosis and gangrene can result.

➤*Storage/Stability:*

Injection – Store at controlled room temperature 20° to 25°C (68° to 77°F). Protect from light. Keep covered in carton until time of use. Do not use if solution has developed color or contains a precipitate.

HYDROXYZINE

Rx	**Hydroxyzine** (Various, eg, Sidmak, URL)	**Tablets:** 10 mg	In 100s, 500s, and 1,000s.
Rx	**Hydroxyzine** (Various, eg, Sidmak, URL)	**Tablets:** 25 mg	In 100s, 500s, and 1,000s.
Rx	**Hydroxyzine** (Various, eg, Sidmak, URL)	**Tablets:** 50 mg	In 100s, 500s, and 1,000s.
Rx	**Hydroxyzine Pamoate** (Various, eg, Barr, IVAX, URL)	**Capsules:** 25 mg (as pamoate)[a]	In 100s, 500s, 1,000s, and UD 100s.
Rx	**Vistaril** (Pfizer)		Sucrose. Two-tone green. In 100s.
Rx	**Hydroxyzine Pamoate** (Various, eg, Barr, IVAX, URL)	**Capsules:** 50 mg (as pamoate)[a]	In 100s, 500s, 1,000s, and UD 100s.
Rx	**Vistaril** (Pfizer)		Sucrose. Green/white. In 100s.
Rx	**Hydroxyzine Pamoate** (Various, eg, Barr)	**Capsules:** 100 mg (as pamoate)[a]	In 100s, 500s, and 1,000s.
Rx	**Vistaril** (Pfizer)		Sucrose. Green/gray. In 100s.

HYDROXYZINE

Rx	**Hydroxyzine** (Various, eg, Alpharma, Hi-Tech Pharmacal, Morton Grove, URL)	**Syrup**: 10 mg/5 mL	May contain alcohol. In 118 and 473 mL.
Rx	**Vistaril** (Pfizer)	**Oral suspension**: 25 mg/5 mL (as pamoate)[a]	Sorbitol. Lemon flavor. In 120 and 473 mL.
Rx	**Hydroxyzine HCl** (Various, eg, Abbott, American Pharmaceutical Partners, American Regent)	**Injection**: 25 mg/mL	May contain benzyl alcohol. In 1 and 2 mL vials.
Rx	**Hydroxyzine HCl** (Various, eg, Abbott, American Pharmaceutical Partners, American Regent)	**Injection**: 50 mg/mL	May contain benzyl alcohol. In 1, 2, and 10 mL vials.

[a] Hydroxyzine pamoate is equivalent to hydroxyzine.

HYDROXYZINE — ORAL

For complete and comparative prescribing information, refer to the Antihistamines group monograph.

Indications

➤*Pruritus:* Caused by allergic conditions such as chronic urticaria and atopic or contact dermatoses and in histamine-mediated pruritus.

➤*Sedation:* When used as premedication and following general anesthesia.

➤*Anxiety and tension:* Associated with psychoneurosis and as an adjunct in organic disease states in which anxiety is manifested.

Administration and Dosage

➤*Approved by the FDA:* April 1956.

Individualize dosage.

➤*Pruritus:*

Adults – 25 mg 3 or 4 times/day.

Children –

Older than 6 years of age: 50 to 100 mg/day in divided doses.
Younger than 6 years of age: 50 mg/day in divided doses.

➤*Sedation:*

Adults – 50 to 100 mg as premedication or following general anesthesia. Hydroxyzine may potentiate concomitant narcotics (eg, meperidine), non-narcotic analgesics, and barbiturates; reduce dosages accordingly. Atropine and other belladonna alkaloids may be given as appropriate.

Children – 0.6 mg/kg.

➤*Anxiety and tension:*

Adults – 50 to 100 mg 4 times daily.

Children greater than 6 years of age – 50 to 100 mg daily in divided doses.

Children less than 6 years of age – 50 mg daily in divided doses.

➤*Storage/Stability:* Store oral dosage forms at controlled room temperature 15° to 30°C (59° to 86°F). Dispense in a tight, light-resistant container.

Actions

➤*Pharmacology:* Hydroxyzine hydrochloride is unrelated chemically to phenothiazines, reserpine, meprobamate or the benzodiazepines. Hydroxyzine is not a cortical depressant, but its action may be due to a suppression of activity in certain key regions of the subcortical area of the central nervous system (CNS).

Primary skeletal muscle relaxation has been demonstrated experimentally. Bronchodilator activity, and antihistaminic and analgesic effects have been demonstrated experimentally and confirmed clinically. An antiemetic effect, both by the apomorphine test and the veriloid test, has been demonstrated.

Pharmacological and clinical studies indicate that hydroxyzine in therapeutic dosage does not increase gastric secretion or acidity and in most cases has mild antisecretory activity.

➤*Pharmacokinetics:* Hydroxyzine is rapidly absorbed in the gastrointestinal tract and its clinical effects are usually noted within 15 to 30 minutes after oral administration.

Contraindications

Hydroxyzine, when administered to the pregnant mouse, rat and rabbit, induced fetal abnormalities in the rat and mouse at doses substantially above the human therapeutic range. Clinical data in human beings are inadequate to establish safety in early pregnancy. Until such data are available, hydroxyzine is contraindicated in early pregnancy.

Hydroxyzine is contraindicated for patients who have shown a previous hypersensitivity to it.

Warnings

➤*Elderly:* A determination has not been made whether controlled clinical studies of hydroxyzine included sufficient numbers of subjects aged 65 years and over to define a difference in response from younger subjects. Other reported clinical experience has not identified differences in responses between the elderly and younger patients. In general, dose selection for an elderly patient should be cautious, usually starting at the low end of the dosing range, reflecting the greater frequency of decreased hepatic, renal or cardiac function, and of concomitant disease or other drug therapy.

The extent of renal excretion of hydroxyzine has not been determined. Because elderly patients are more likely to have decreased renal function, care should be taken in dose selections.

Sedating drugs may cause confusion and over sedation in the elderly; elderly patients generally should be started on low doses of hydroxyzine and observed closely.

➤*Pregnancy: Category C.* Hydroxyzine, when administered to the pregnant mouse, rat and rabbit, induced fetal abnormalities in the rat and mouse at doses substantially above the human therapeutic range. Clinical data in human beings are inadequate to establish safety in early pregnancy. Until such data are available, hydroxyzine is contraindicated in early pregnancy.

➤*Lactation:* It is not known whether this drug is excreted in human milk. Since many drugs are so excreted, hydroxyzine should not be given to nursing mothers.

Precautions

➤*Hazardous tasks:* Since drowsiness may occur with use of this drug, patients should be warned of this possibility and cautioned against driving a car or operating dangerous machinery while taking hydroxyzine. Patients should also be advised against the simultaneous use of other CNS depressant drugs, and cautioned that the effects of alcohol may be increased.

Adverse Reactions

Side effects reported with the administration of hydroxyzine hydrochloride are usually mild and transitory in nature.

➤*CNS:* Drowsiness is usually transitory and may disappear in a few days of continued therapy or upon reduction of the dose. Involuntary motor activity including rare instances of tremor and convulsions have been reported, usually with doses considerably higher than those recommended. Clinically significant respiratory depression has not been reported at recommended doses.

➤*Miscellaneous:* Dry mouth.

Overdosage

➤*Symptoms:* The most common manifestation of hydroxyzine overdosage is hypersedation. As in the management of overdosage with any drug, it should be borne in mind that multiple agents may have been taken.

➤*Treatment:* Immediate gastric lavage is recommended. General supportive care, including frequent monitoring of the vital signs and close observation of the patient, is indicated. Hypotension, though unlikely, may be controlled with intravenous fluids and levarterenol, norepinephrine, or metaraminol. Do not use epinephrine as hydroxyzine counteracts its pressor action.

There is no specific antidote. It is doubtful that hemodialysis would be of any value in the treatment of overdosage with hydroxyzine. However, if other agents such as barbiturates have been ingested concomitantly, hemodialysis may be indicated. There is no practical method to quantitate hydroxyzine in body fluids or tissue after its ingestion or administration.

HYDROXYZINE HYDROCHLORIDE — INJECTION

For complete and comparative prescribing information, refer to the Antihistamines group monograph.

Indications

➤*Pruritus:* Caused by allergic conditions such as chronic urticaria and atopic or contact dermatoses and in histamine-mediated pruritus.

➤*Sedation:* When used as premedication and following general anesthesia.

➤*Anxiety and tension:* Associated with psychoneurosis and as an adjunct in organic disease states in which anxiety is manifested.

Administration and Dosage

➤*Approved by the FDA:* April 1956.

Individualize dosage. Start patients on IM therapy only when indicated; maintain on oral therapy whenever possible.

Hydroxyzine injection is for deep IM administration only and may be given without further dilution. Avoid IV, subcutaneous, or intra-arterial administration. The preferred site of administration for adults is the upper, outer quadrant of the buttock or the mid-lateral thigh. For children, it is preferable to administer in the mid-lateral thigh; for infants and small children, use the periphery of the upper, outer quadrant of the gluteal region only

Piperazines, Nonselective

HYDROXYZINE HYDROCHLORIDE — INJECTION

when necessary, such as in burn patients, to minimize the possibility of damage to the sciatic nerve. The deltoid area should be used only if well developed such as in certain adults and older children, and then only with caution to avoid radial nerve injury. Do not make IM injections into the lower and mid-third of the upper arm.

➤*Pruritus:*

Adults only – 25 mg 3 to 4 times/day.

➤*Sedation:*

Adults – 50 to 100 mg as premedication or following general anesthesia. Hydroxyzine may potentiate concomitant narcotics (eg, meperidine), non-narcotic analgesics, and barbiturates; reduce dosages accordingly. Atropine and other belladonna alkaloids may be given as appropriate.

Children – 0.6 mg/kg.

➤*Anxiety and tension:* For symptomatic relief of anxiety and tension associated with psychoneurosis and as an adjunct in organic disease states in which anxiety is manifested.

Adults – 50 to 100 mg 4 times daily.

➤*Storage/Stability:* Store injection below 30°C (86°F).

Piperidines, Nonselective

CYPROHEPTADINE

Rx	**Cyproheptadine** (Various, eg, IVAX, Par, Pliva)	**Tablets:** 4 mg	In 100s, 1,000s, and UD 100s.
Rx	**Cyproheptadine** (Various, eg, Alpharma)	**Syrup:** 2 mg/5 mL	May contain alcohol. In 473 mL.

CYPROHEPTADINE HYDROCHLORIDE — ORAL

For complete and comparative prescribing information, refer to the Antihistamines group monograph.

Indications

➤*Hypersensitivity reactions:* Perennial and seasonal allergic rhinitis; vasomotor rhinitis; allergic conjunctivitis caused by inhalant allergens and foods; mild, uncomplicated allergic skin manifestations of urticaria and angioedema; amelioration of allergic reactions to blood or plasma; cold urticaria; dermatographism; adjunctive anaphylactic therapy.

➤*Unlabeled uses:* Prophylactic treatment of pediatric migraines; suppression of vascular headaches; appetite stimulation; treatment of nightmares associated with post-traumatic stress disorder.

Administration and Dosage

➤*Approved by the FDA:* August 1961.

Individualize dosage.

➤*Adults:* 4 to 20 mg/day. Initiate therapy with 4 mg 3 times/day. Most patients require 12 to 16 mg/day and occasionally as much as 32 mg/day. Do not exceed 0.5 mg/kg/day.

➤*Children:* Calculate total daily dosage as approximately 0.25 mg/kg/day or 8 mg/m^2/day.

7 to 14 years of age – 4 mg 2 or 3 times/day. Do not exceed 16 mg/day.

2 to 6 years of age – 2 mg 2 or 3 times/day. Do not exceed 12 mg/day.

➤*Storage/Stability:* Store at controlled room temperature, 15° to 30°C (59° to 86°F), in a well-closed container.

PHENINDAMINE TARTRATE

otc	**Nolahist** (Amarin)	**Tablets:** 25 mg	Alcohol and dye free. In 24s and 100s.

PHENINDAMINE TARTRATE — ORAL

For complete and comparative prescribing information, refer to the Antihistamines group monograph.

Indications

➤*Allergic rhinitis:* Temporarily relieves runny nose, sneezing, itching of the nose or throat, and itchy, watery eyes due to hay fever or other upper respiratory allergic rhinitis.

Administration and Dosage

➤*Adults and children 12 years of age or older:* Oral dosage is 1 tablet every 4 to 6 hours, not to exceed 6 tablets in 24 hours, or as directed by a doctor.

➤*Children 6 to younger than 12 years of age:* Oral dosage is one-half tablet every 4 to 6 hours, not to exceed 3 tablets in 24 hours, or as directed by a doctor.

Children younger than 6 years of age – Consult a doctor.

➤*Storage/Stability:* Store at 15° to 30°C (59° to 86° F) and keep tightly closed away from light.

Phthalazinones, Peripherally selective

AZELASTINE

Rx	**Astelin** (Medpointe)	**Nasal spray:** 137 mcg/spray	Benzalkonium chloride, EDTA. 17 mg (100 metered sprays) per bottle. In 2s.

AZELASTINE HYDROCHLORIDE — INTRANASAL

For complete and comparative prescribing information, refer to the Antihistamines group monograph.

Indications

➤*Seasonal allergic rhinitis:* Such as rhinorrhea, sneezing, and nasal pruritus in adults and children 5 years of age and older.

➤*Vasomotor rhinitis:* Such as rhinorrhea, nasal congestion, and postnasal drip in adults and children 12 years of age and older.

Administration and Dosage

➤*Approved by the FDA:* October 1996.

➤*Seasonal allergic rhinitis:*

Adults and children 12 years of age and older – 2 sprays per nostril twice daily.

Children 5 to 11 years of age – 1 spray per nostril twice daily.

➤*Vasomotor rhinitis:*

Adults and children 12 years of age and older – 2 sprays per nostril twice daily.

➤*Priming:* Before initial use, replace the screw cap on the bottle with the pump unit and prime the delivery system with 4 sprays or until a fine mist appears. When 3 days or more have elapsed since last use, reprime the pump with 2 sprays or until a fine mist appears.

➤*Storage/Stability:* Store at controlled room temperature 20° to 25°C (68° to 77°F). Protect from freezing.

Piperazine, Peripherally Selective

CETIRIZINE

Rx	**Zyrtec** (Pfizer)	**Tablets:** 5 mg	Lactose. (ZYRTEC 5). White, rectangular. Film-coated. In 100s.
		10 mg	Lactose. (ZYRTEC 10). White, rectangular. Film-coated. In 100s.
		Tablets, chewable: 5 mg	Lactose. (ZYRTEC C5). Purple, grape flavor. In 30s.
		10 mg	Lactose. (ZYRTEC C10). Purple, grape flavor. In 30s.
		Syrup: 5 mg/5 mL	Parabens, sugar. Banana-grape flavor. In 120 and 480 mL.

Piperazine, Peripherally Selective

CETIRIZINE HYDROCHLORIDE — ORAL

For complete and comparative prescribing information, refer to the Antihistamines group monograph.

Indications

➤*Chronic urticaria:* For the treatment of the uncomplicated skin manifestations of chronic idiopathic urticaria in adults and children 6 months of age and older. It significantly reduces the occurrence, severity, and duration of hives and significantly reduces pruritus.

➤*Perennial allergic rhinitis:* Caused by allergens such as dust mites, animal dander, and molds in adults and children 6 months of age and older. Symptoms treated effectively include sneezing, rhinorrhea, postnasal discharge, nasal pruritus, ocular pruritus, and tearing.

➤*Seasonal allergic rhinitis:* Caused by allergens such as ragweed, grass, and tree pollens in adults and children 2 years of age and older. Symptoms treated effectively include sneezing, rhinorrhea, nasal pruritus, ocular pruritus, tearing, and redness of the eyes.

➤*Unlabeled uses:* To decrease the initial wheal response and pruritus associated with mosquito bites, and has been shown to improve asthma symptom scores in patients with allergic asthma.

Administration and Dosage

➤*Approved by the FDA:* December 12, 1995.

May be given with or without food.

➤*Adults and children 12 years of age and older:* 5 or 10 mg once daily depending on symptom severity.

➤*Children:*

6 to 11 years of age – 5 or 10 mg once daily depending on symptom severity.

2 to 5 years of age – 2.5 mg once daily. The dosage in this age group can be increased to a maximum dose of 5 mg/day given as 5 mg once daily or as 2.5 mg given every 12 hours.

6 months up to 2 years of age 2.5 mg once daily. The dose in children 12 to 23 months of age can be increased to a maximum dose of 5 mg/day given as 2.5 mg every 12 hours. Syrup is recommended for this age group.

➤*Renal / Hepatic function impairment:* In patients 12 years of age and older with decreased renal function (Ccr 11 to 31 mL/min), hemodialysis patients (Ccr less than 7 mL/min), and in hepatically impaired patients, 5 mg once daily is recommended. Similarly, pediatric patients 6 to 11 years of age with impaired renal or hepatic function should use the lower recommended dose. Because of the difficulty in reliably administering doses of less than cetirizine 2.5 mg in a syrup doseform, and in the absence of pharmacokinetic and safety information in children younger than 6 years of age with impaired renal or hepatic function, its use in this impaired patient population is not recommended.

➤*Elderly (77 years of age and older):* 5 mg once daily as recommended.

➤*Storage / Stability:* Store at 20° to 25°C (68° to 77°F); excursions permitted to 15° to 30°C (59° to 86°F). Syrup also can be refrigerated at 2° to 8°C (36° to 46°F).

Piperidines, Peripherally Selective

DESLORATADINE

Rx	**Clarinex** (Schering)	**Tablets:** 5 mg	Lactose. (C5). Lt. blue. Film-coated. In 100s, 500s, unit-of-use 30s, and UD hospital pack 100s.
Rx	**Clarinex RediTabs** (Schering)	**Tablets, rapidly disintegrating:** 2.5 mg	Mannitol, aspartame, 1.4 mg phenylalanine. (K). Speckled, light red. Tutti frutti flavor. In blister packages of 30.
		5 mg	Mannitol, aspartame, 2.9 mg phenylalanine. (A). Speckled, light red. Tutti frutti flavor. In blister packages of 30.
Rx	**Clarinex** (Schering)	**Syrup:** 2.5 mg per 5 mL	Sugar, EDTA. Bubble gum flavor. In 480 mL.

DESLORATADINE — ORAL

For complete and comparative prescribing information, refer to the Antihistamines group monograph.

Indications

➤*Chronic idiopathic urticaria:* Symptomatic relief of pruritus and reduction in the number and size of hives in patients 6 months of age and older.

➤*Perennial allergic rhinitis:* For the relief of the nasal and nonnasal symptoms of perennial allergic rhinitis in patients 6 months of age and older.

➤*Seasonal allergic rhinitis:* For the relief of the nasal and nonnasal symptoms of seasonal allergic rhinitis in patients 2 years of age and older.

Administration and Dosage

➤*Approved by the FDA:* December 21, 2001.

➤*Adults and children 12 years of age and older:* 5 mg once daily.

➤*Children 6 to 11 years of age:* 2.5 mg once daily.

➤*Children 12 months to 5 years of age:* 1.25 mg once daily.

➤*Children 6 to 11 months of age:* 1 mg once daily.

➤*Rapidly disintegrating tablets:* Place rapidly disintegrating tablets on the tongue immediately after opening the blister; tablet disintegration occurs rapidly. Administer with or without water.

➤*Renal / Hepatic function impairment:* In adults, a starting dose of one 5 mg tablet every other day is recommended.

➤*Storage / Stability:* Protect tablet unit-of-use packaging and UD hospital packs from excessive moisture. Store at 15° to 30°C (59° to 86°F). Heat-sensitive; avoid exposure at or above 30°C (86°F).

Store syrup and disintegrating tablets at 25°C (77°F); excursions permitted between 15° to 30°C (59° to 86°F). Protect syrup from light.

FEXOFENADINE

Rx	**Allegra** (Aventis)	**Tablets:** 30 mg	(03 0088 or 03 E). Peach. Film-coated. In 100s and 500s.
		60 mg	(06 0088 or 06 E). Peach. Film-coated. In 100s, 500s, and blister pack 100s.
		180 mg	(018 0088 or 018 E). Peach. Film-coated. In 100s and 500s.
		Capsules: 60 mg	Lactose. (ALLEGRA 60 mg). White/pink. In 60s, 100s, 500s, and blister pack 100s.

FEXOFENADINE — ORAL

For complete and comparative prescribing information, refer to the Antihistamines group monograph.

Indications

➤*Chronic idiopathic urticaria:* For the treatment of uncomplicated skin manifestations of chronic idiopathic urticaria in adults and children 6 years of age and older. It significantly reduces pruritus and the number of wheals.

➤*Seasonal allergic rhinitis:* For the relief of symptoms associated with seasonal allergic rhinitis in adults and children 6 years of age and older. Symptoms include sneezing; rhinorrhea; itchy nose, palate, and throat; and itchy, watery, and red eyes.

Administration and Dosage

➤*Approved by the FDA:* July 25, 1995.

Fexofenadine should not be taken closely in time with aluminum- and magnesium-containing antacids.

➤*Chronic idiopathic urticaria:*

Adults and children 12 years of age and older – 60 mg twice daily.

Children 6 to 11 years of age – 30 mg twice daily.

➤*Seasonal allergic rhinitis:*

Adults and children 12 years of age and older – 60 mg twice daily or 180 mg once daily.

Children 6 to 11 years of age – 30 mg twice daily.

➤*Renal function impairment:*

Adults and children 12 years of age and older – 60 mg once daily as a starting dose.

Children 6 to 11 years of age – 30 mg once daily as a starting dose.

➤*Storage / Stability:* Store capsules and tablets at controlled room temperature 20° to 25°C (68° to 77°F). Protect from excessive moisture.

LORATADINE

otc	**Loratadine** (Various, Geneva)	**Tablets**: 10 mg	In 100s.
otc	**Claritin 24-Hour Allergy** (Schering-Plough)		Lactose. (Claritin 10 458). 1s, 2s, 5s, 10s, 20s, 30s, and 40s.
otc	**Tavist ND** (Novartis)		Lactose. In 30s.
otc	**Claritin Hives Relief** (Schering)		Lactose. In 10s.
otc	**Clear-Atadine** (Major)		Lactose. In 10s.
otc	**Non-drowsy Allergy Relief** (Major)	**Tablets, orally disintegrating**: 10 mg	0.9 mg phenylalanine. Aspartame, lactose, mannitol. Cherry flavor. In 10s.
otc	**Triaminic Allerchews** (Novartis)		Mannitol. In 8s.
otc	**Dimetapp Children's ND Non-Drowsy Allergy** (Wyeth)		Aspartame, corn syrup, mannitol, 8.4 mg phenylalanine. In 6s and 12s.
otc	**Alavert** (Wyeth Consumer)		Lactose. In 6s, 12s, 15s, 30s, and 48s.
otc	**Claritin Reditabs** (Schering)	**Tablets, rapidly disintegrating**: 10 mg	Mannitol. (C). White to off-white. Mint flavor. In 4s, 10s, 20s, and 30s.
otc	**Claritin** (Schering)	**Syrup**: 5 mg/5 mL	Sucrose, sugar, EDTA. Fruit flavor. In 120 mL.
otc	**Dimetapp Children's ND Non-Drowsy Allergy** (Wyeth)		Sucrose. In 118 mL.
otc	**Alavert Children's** (Wyeth)		
otc	**Non-Drowsy Allergy Relief for Kids** (Major)		Sucrose, glycerin. Fruit flavor. In 120 mL.
otc	**Children's Loratadine Syrup** (Taro)		Fruit flavor. In 120 mL.

LORATADINE — ORAL

For complete prescribing information, refer to the Antihistamines group monograph.

Indications

➤*Allergic rhinitis:* For the relief of nasal and nonnasal symptoms of seasonal allergic rhinitis.

➤*Unlabeled uses:* For the treatment of chronic idiopathic urticaria in patients 2 years of age and older.

Administration and Dosage

➤*Approved by the FDA:* April 12, 1993.

➤*Adults and children 6 years of age and older:* 10 mg once daily.

➤*Children 2 to 5 years of age:* 5 mg (5 mL) syrup once daily.

➤*Hepatic/Renal function impairment (glomerular filtration rate less than 30 mL/min):*

Adults and children 6 years of age and older – 10 mg every other day as starting dose.

Children 2 to 5 years of age – 5 mg every other day as starting dose.

➤*Rapidly disintegrating tablets:* Place tablets on the tongue. Tablet disintegration occurs rapidly. Administer with or without water.

Use within 6 months of opening laminated foil pouch and immediately upon opening individual tablet blister.

➤*Storage/Stability:* Protect unit dose packs, unit-of-use packs, and rapidly disintegrating tablets from excessive moisture. Store tablets between 2° and 30°C (36° and 86°F). Store syrup and rapidly disintegrating tablets between 2° and 25°C (36° and 77°F).

ANTIHISTAMINE COMBINATIONS

Content given per 5 mL.

	Product & Distributor	Antihistamine	Average Dose	Excipients & How Supplied
Rx sf	**Carbinoxamine Maleate and Carbinoxamine Tannate Oral Suspension** (Brighton)	2 mg carbinoxamine maleate, 6 mg carbinoxamine tannate	**6 yr of age or older** - 5 mL q 12 h **18 mo to 6 yr of age** - 2.5 mL q 12 h **9 to 18 mo of age** - 1.25 mL q 12 h **younger than 9 mo of age** - only as directed by physician	Alcohol free, dye free. Saccharin, sorbitol, parabens. Bubble-gum flavor. In 118 and 473 mL.
Rx	**Poly-Histine Elixir** (Sanofi-Synthelabo)	4 mg phenyltoloxamine citrate, 4 mg pyrilamine maleate, 4 mg pheniramine maleate	**12 yr of age or older** - 10 mL q 4 h **6 to 12 yr of age** - 5 mL q 4 h **2 to 6 yr of age** - 2.5 mL q 4 h	4% alcohol. Lemon-lime flavor. In 473 mL.

For complete prescribing information, refer to the Antihistamine group monograph.

BENZONATATE

Rx	**Benzonatate Softgels** (Various, eg, Inwood, Sidmak)	**Capsules**: 100 mg	In 100s and 500s.
Rx	**Tessalon Perles** (Forest)		Parabens. (T). Yellow. In 100s and 500s.
Rx	**Benzonatate Softgels** (Various, eg, Inwood)	**Capsules**: 200 mg	In 100s and 500s.
Rx	**Tessalon** (Forest)		Parabens. (0698). Yellow. In 100s and 500s.

BENZONATATE — ORAL

Indications

➤*Cough:* Benzonatate is indicated for the symptomatic relief of cough.

Administration and Dosage

➤*Approved by the FDA:* February 10, 1958.

➤*Adults and children greater than 10 years of age:* Usual dose is one 100 mg capsule or softgel capsule or 200 mg capsule 3 times daily as required. If necessary, up to 600 mg daily may be given.

➤*Storage/Stability:*

Capsules – Store at controlled room temperature 15° to 30°C (59° to 86°F).

Softgel capsules – The softgels should be protected from light, moisture and humidity, and stored at controlled room temperature 15° to 30°C (59° to 86°F). Dispense in a tight, light-resistant container.

Actions

➤*Pharmacology:* Benzonatate acts peripherally by anesthetizing the stretch receptors located in the respiratory passages, lungs, and pleura by dampening their activity and thereby reducing the cough reflex at its source. It begins to act within 15 to 20 minutes and its effect lasts for 3 to 8 hours. Benzonatate has no inhibitory effect on the respiratory center in recommended dosage.

Contraindications

Hypersensitivity to benzonatate or related compounds.

Warnings

➤*Hypersensitivity reactions:* Severe hypersensitivity reactions (including bronchospasm, laryngospasm, and cardiovascular collapse) have been reported, which are possibly related to local anesthesia from sucking or chewing the capsule or softgel capsule instead of swallowing it. Severe reactions have required intervention with vasopressor agents and supportive measures.

➤*Pregnancy: Category C.* Animal reproduction studies have not been conducted with benzonatate. It is also not known whether benzonatate can cause fetal harm when administered to a pregnant woman or can affect reproduction capacity. Benzonatate should be given to a pregnant woman only if clearly needed.

➤*Lactation:* It is not known whether this drug is excreted in human milk. Because many drugs are excreted in human milk caution should be exercised when benzonatate is administered to a nursing woman.

➤*Children:* Safety and efficacy in children younger than 10 years of age have not been established.

Precautions

➤*CNS effects:* Benzonatate is chemically related to anesthetic agents of the paraaminobenzoic acid class (eg, procaine, tetracaine) and has been associated with adverse CNS effects possibly related to a prior sensitivity to related agents or interaction with concomitant medication.

Drug Interactions

Isolated instances of bizarre behavior, including mental confusion and visual hallucinations, have also been reported in patients taking benzonatate in combination with other prescribed drugs.

Adverse Reactions

Potential adverse reactions to benzonatate may include the following:

➤*CNS:* Sedation, headache, dizziness, mental confusion, and visual hallucinations.

➤*Dermatologic:* Pruritus and skin eruptions.

➤*GI:* Constipation, nausea, and GI upset.

➤*Hypersensitivity:* Hypersensitivity reactions including bronchospasm, laryngospasm, cardiovascular collapse possibly related to local anesthesia from chewing or sucking the capsule or softgel capsules.

➤*Miscellaneous:* Nasal congestion; sensation of burning in the eyes; vague "chilly" sensation; numbness of the chest. Rare instances of deliberate or accidental overdose have resulted in death.

Overdosage

➤*Symptoms:* If capsules or softgel capsules are chewed or dissolved in the mouth, oropharyngeal anesthesia will develop rapidly. CNS stimulation may cause restlessness and tremors, which may proceed to clonic convulsions followed by profound CNS depression.

Overdose may result in death. The drug is chemically related to tetracaine and other topical anesthetics and shares various aspects of their pharmacology and toxicology. Drugs of this type are generally well absorbed after ingestion.

➤*Treatment:* Evacuate gastric contents and administer copious amounts of activated charcoal slurry. Even in the conscious patient, cough and gag reflexes may be so depressed as to necessitate special attention to protection against aspiration of gastric contents and orally administered materials. Convulsions should be treated with a short-acting barbiturate given intravenously and carefully titrated for the smallest effective dosage. Intensive support of respiration and cardiovascular-renal function is an essential feature of the treatment of severe intoxication from overdosage.

Do not use CNS stimulants.

Patient Information

Release of benzonatate from the capsule in the mouth can produce a temporary local anesthesia of the oral mucosa and choking could occur. Therefore, the capsules and softgel capsules should be swallowed without chewing.

DEXTROMETHORPHAN HBr

otc	**Robitussin CoughGels** (Wyeth)	**Gelcaps**: 15 mg	Liquid filled. Sorbitol. In 20s.
otc	**DexAlone** (DexGen)	**Gelcaps**: 30 mg	Liquid filled. Sorbitol. In 30s.
otc	**Hold DM** (B. F. Ascher)	**Lozenges**: 5 mg	Sucrose, corn syrup. Original and cherry flavor. In 10s.
otc sf	**Scot-Tussin DM Cough Chasers** (Scot-tussin)		Peppermint oil, sorbitol. Dye-free. In 20s.
otc	**Trocal** (Textilease)	**Lozenges**: 7.5 mg	Cherry flavor. In 10s, 50s, and 500s.
otc	**Triaminic Thin Strips Long Acting Cough** (Novartis Consumer Health)	**Strips, orally disintegrating**: 7.5 mg	Alcohol (less than 5%), sorbitol, sucralose. Cherry flavor. In 16s.
otc	**Theraflu Thin Strips Long Acting Cough** (Novartis Consumer Health)	**Strips, orally disintegrating**: 15 mg	Alcohol (less than 5%), sorbitol, sucralose. Cherry flavor. In 12s.
otc	**Simply Cough** (McNeil-PPC)	**Liquid**: 5 mg/5 mL	Corn syrup, sucralose. Alcohol free. Cherry berry flavor. In 120 mL.
otc	**Creo-Terpin** (Lee)	**Liquid**: 10 mg/15 mL (3.33 mg/5 mL)	Tartrazine, 25% alcohol, corn syrup, saccharin. In 120 mL.
otc	**Robitussin Maximum Strength Cough** (Whitehall-Robins)	**Liquid**: 15 mg/5 mL	1.4% alcohol, glucose, corn syrup, saccharin. Cherry flavor. In 118 and 237 mL.
otc	**Vicks 44 Cough Relief** (Procter and Gamble)	**Liquid**: 10 mg/5 mL	31 mg sodium/15 mL, alcohol, corn syrup, saccharin. In 118 mL.
otc	**Creomulsion for Children** (Summit)	**Syrup**: 5 mg/5 mL	Alcohol free. Sucrose. Cherry flavor. In 118 mL.
otc sf	**Robitussin Pediatric Cough** (Whitehall-Robins)	**Syrup**: 7.5 mg/5 mL	Alcohol free. Saccharin, sorbitol. Cherry flavor. In 118 mL.
otc	**ElixSure Children's Cough** (Taro Consumer)		Propylparaben, sorbitol. Cherry and bubble gum flavors. In 118 mL.

DEXTROMETHORPHAN HBr

otc	**Silphen DM** (Silarx)	**Syrup:** 10 mg/5 mL	5% alcohol, menthol, methylparaben, sucrose. In 118 mL.
otc	**Creomulsion Adult Formula** (Summit)	**Syrup:** 20 mg/15 mL	Alcohol free. Sucrose. In 118 mL.
otc	**Delsym** (Celltech)	**Oral suspension, extended-release:** Dextromethorphan polistirex equivalent to 30 mg dextromethorphan HBr/5mL.	0.26% alcohol and 5 mg sodium/5 mL, corn syrup, sucrose, parabens. Orange flavor. In 89 mL.
otc	**PediaCare Infants' Long-Acting Cough** (Pfizer Consumer Health)	**Drops:** 3.75 mg/0.8 mL	Alcohol free. Glycerin, sorbitol. Grape flavor. In 15 mL.
otc	**Little Colds Cough Formula** (Vetco)	**Drops:** 7.5 mg/mL	Glycerin, corn syrup. Natural grape flavor. In 30 mL.
otc	**PediaCare Infants' Long-Acting Cough** (Pfizer Consumer Health)	**Freezer pops:** 7.5 mg/25 mL (per pop)	Benzyl alcohol, corn syrup, ethyl maltol, sucralose. Berry flavor. In 8s.

DEXTROMETHORPHAN HYDROBROMIDE — ORAL

Indications

➤*Cough:* Temporarily relieves cough caused by minor throat and bronchial irritation as may occur with the common cold or inhaled irritants.

Administration and Dosage

➤*Gelcaps:*

Adults and children 12 years of age and older – 30 mg every 6 to 8 hours. Do not exceed 120 mg in 24 hours. Do not use in children less than 12 years of age.

➤*Lozenges:*

Adults and children 12 years of age and older – 5 to 15 mg every 1 to 4 hours up to 120 mg/day.

Children 6 to younger than 12 years of age – 5 to 10 mg every 1 to 4 hours up to 60 mg/day. Do not give to children under 6 years of age unless directed by a physician.

➤*Liquid and syrup:*

Adults and children 12 years of age and older – 10 to 20 mg every 4 hours or 30 mg every 6 to 8 hours up to 120 mg/day.

Children –

6 to younger than 12 years of age: 15 mg every 6 to 8 hours up to 60 mg/day.
2 to younger than 6 years of age: 7.5 mg every 6 to 8 hours up to 30 mg/day.

➤*Extended-release suspension:*

Adults and children 12 years of age and older – 60 mg every 12 hours up to 120 mg/day.

Children –

6 to younger than 12 years of age: 30 mg every 12 hours up to 60 mg/day.
2 to younger than 6 years of age: 15 mg every 12 hours up to 30 mg/day.

➤*Strips:* Allow the strip to dissolve on the tongue.

Adults and children 12 years of age and older – 30 mg every 6 to 8 hours, up to 120 mg/day.

Children 6 to younger than 12 years of age – 15 mg every 6 to 8 hours, up to 60 mg/day.

➤*Freezer pops:*

Children 6 to younger than 12 years of age – Two freezer pops (50 mL as liquid). If needed, repeat dose every 6 to 8 hour; do not exceed 4 doses in 24 hours.

Children 2 to younger than 6 years of age – One freezer pop (25 mL as liquid). If needed, repeat dose every 6 to 8 hour; do not exceed 4 doses in 24 hours.

➤*Drops:*

Children 2 to 3 years of age – One dropperful (2 dropperfuls *PediaCare*) for a total of 7.5 mg. If needed, repeat every 6 to 8 hours, up to 30 mg/day.

➤*Storage/Stability:* Store at controlled room temperature (15° to 30°C; 59° to 86°F).

Actions

➤*Pharmacology:* Dextromethorphan is the d-isomer of the codeine analog of levorphanol; it lacks analgesic and addictive properties. Its cough suppressant action is due to a central action on the cough center in the medulla. Dextromethorphan 15 to 30 mg equals codeine 8 to 15 mg as an antitussive.

➤*Pharmacokinetics:*

Absorption – Dextromethorphan is rapidly absorbed in the GI tract.

Metabolism/Excretion – It undergoes metabolism in the liver and is then excreted in the urine as unchanged drug and demethylated metabolites.

Contraindications

Hypersensitivity to any component.

Warnings

➤*Persistent cough:* Do not take this product for persistent or chronic cough such as occurs with smoking, asthma or emphysema, or if cough is accompanied by excessive phlegm (mucus) unless directed by a health care provider. A persistent cough may be a sign of a serious condition. If cough persists for more than 1 week, tends to recur, or if it is accompanied by fever, rash, or persistent headache, consult a health care provider. These could be signs of a serious condition.

➤*Pregnancy: Category C.* It is not known if dextromethorphan can cause fetal harm or affect reproduction capacity when administered to a pregnant woman. Give to a pregnant woman only if clearly needed.

➤*Lactation:* It is not known if dextromethorphan is excreted in breast milk.

➤*Children:*

Gelcaps – Do not give to children younger than 12 years of age.

Lozenges – Do not give to children younger than 6 years of age unless directed by a health care provider.

Liquid, syrup, and pediatric liquid – Do not give to children younger than 2 years of age unless directed by a health care provider.

Precautions

➤*Special risk:*

Asthma, chronic bronchitis, emphysema, or mucus with cough – Because dextromethorphan decreases coughing, it makes it difficult to get rid of the mucus that collects in the lungs and airways with some diseases.

Diabetes – Some products contain sugar and may affect control of blood glucose monitoring.

Slowed breathing – Dextromethorphan may slow the rate or breathing even further.

➤*Drug abuse and dependence:* Anecdotal reports of abuse of dextromethorphan-containing cough/cold products have increased, especially among teenagers. Additional data are needed before determining the abuse and dependency potential of dextromethorphan.

➤*Tartrazine sensitivity:* Some dextromethorphan-containing products contain tartrazine, which may cause allergic-type reactions (including bronchial asthma) in certain susceptible people. Although the overall incidence of tartrazine sensitivity in the general population is low, it is frequently seen in patients who also have aspirin hypersensitivity.

Drug Interactions

Dextromethorphan Drug Interactions

Precipitant drug	Object drug *		Description
MAOIs	Dextromethorphan	↑	Hyperpyrexia, abnormal muscle movement, hypotension, coma, and death have been associated with concurrent use. Avoid coadministration and avoid use for 2 weeks after stopping the MAOI.
Quinidine	Dextromethorphan	↑	Plasma dextromethorphan levels may be elevated because of quinidine inhibiting the metabolism of dextromethorphan (via CYP 2D6). Increased toxic effects may develop. Reduce dose if needed.
Sibutramine	Dextromethorphan	↑	A "serotonin syndrome," including CNS irritability, motor weakness, shivering, myoclonus, and altered consciousness, may occur because of additive serotonergic effects. Coadministration is not recommended.

Adverse Reactions

Adverse reactions may include dizziness, drowsiness, and GI disturbances.

Overdosage

➤*Symptoms:*

Adults – Altered sensory perception, ataxia, dysphoria, slurred speech.

Children – Ataxia, convulsions, respiratory depression.

Patient Information

Do not use if you are currently taking a prescription monoamine oxidase (MAO) inhibitor (certain drugs for depression, psychiatric, or emotional conditions, or Parkinson disease), or for 2 weeks after stopping the MAO inhibitor drug. If you are uncertain whether your prescription drug contains an MAO inhibitor, consult your doctor before taking this product.

DEXTROMETHORPHAN HYDROBROMIDE — ORAL

Do not use dextromethorphan for persistent or chronic cough, such as with smoking, asthma, or emphysema, or if cough is accompanied by excessive phlegm (mucus), unless directed by your doctor. Contact your doctor if cough lasts for more than 1 week, comes back, or is accompanied by fever, rash, or persistent headache. These could be signs of a serious condition.

If you are pregnant or breastfeeding, seek the advice of your doctor before using this product.

DEXTROMETHORPHAN POLISTIREX — ORAL

Indications

➤*Cough:* Temporary relief of cough due to minor throat and bronchial irritation that may occur with the common cold or inhaled irritants.

Administration and Dosage

Shake bottle well before using.

➤*Adults and children 12 years of age and over:* 2 teaspoonfuls every 12 hours, not to exceed 4 teaspoonfuls in 24 hours.

➤*Children 6 to under 12 years of age:* 1 teaspoonful every 12 hours, not to exceed 2 teaspoonfuls in 24 hours.

➤*Children 2 to under 6 years of age:* ½ teaspoonful every 12 hours, not to exceed 1 teaspoonful in 24 hours.

➤*Children under 2 years of age:* Consult a physician.

➤*Storage/Stability:* Store at 15° to 30°C (59° to 86°F).

Warnings

➤*Persistent cough:* Do not take this product for persistent or chronic cough such as occurs with smoking, asthma, or emphysema, or if cough is accompanied by excessive phlegm (mucus) unless directed by a physician. A persistent cough may be a sign of a serious condition. If cough persists for more than 1 week, tends to recur, or is accompanied by fever, rash, or persistent headache, consult a physician.

➤*Pregnancy: Category C.* As with any drug, if you are pregnant or nursing a baby, seek the advice of a health professional before using this product.

Drug Interactions

➤*Monoamine oxidase inhibitor (MAOI):* Do not use this product if you are now taking a prescription MAOI (certain drugs for depression, psychiatric or emotional conditions, or Parkinson's disease), or for 2 weeks after stopping the MAOI drug. If you are uncertain whether your prescription drug contains an MAOI, consult a health professional before taking this product.

Overdosage

In case of accidental overdose, seek professional assistance or contact a poison control center immediately.

DIPHENHYDRAMINE HYDROCHLORIDE

For complete and comparative prescribing information, refer to the Antihistamines group monograph. For a complete listing of diphenhydramine sleep aids, see Nonprescription Sleep Aids in the CNS Agents chapter. For more information on diphenhydramine, refer to diphenhydramine in the ethanolamines.

DEXTROMETHORPHAN HBr/BENZOCAINE

otc	**Cough-X** (B.F. Ascher)	**Lozenges**: 5 mg dextromethorphan and 2 mg benzocaine	Dye free. Menthol-eucalyptus flavor. In 9s.
otc	**Cēpacol Ultra Sore Throat Plus Cough** (Combe)	**Lozenges**: 7.5 mg benzocaine, 5 mg dextromethorphan hydrobromide	Glucose, sucrose. Mixed berry flavor. In 18s.
otc	**Tetra-Formula** (Reese Pharm.)	**Lozenges**: 10 mg dextromethorphan HBr and 15 mg benzocaine	Sucrose, glucose, dextrose. In 10s.

DEXTROMETHORPHAN HBr/BENZOCAINE — ORAL

For complete and comparative prescribing information, refer to the Dextromethorphan HBr and Benzocaine individual monographs.

Indications

Temporarily suppresses cough caused by minor throat and bronchial irritants as may occur with the common cold. Also for the temporary relief of occasional minor irritation and sore throat.

Administration and Dosage

Do not exceed recommended dosage. Do not use for more than 2 days for sore throat or for more than 7 days for cough unless directed by a doctor. Do not use for persistent or chronic cough such as occurs with smoking, asthma, emphysema, or if cough is accompanied by excessive phlegm unless directed by a doctor. Allow lozenge to dissolve slowly in the mouth.

➤*Cough-X:*

Adults and children 6 years of age and older – One lozenge every 2 hours as needed, not to exceed 12 lozenges in 24 hours or as directed by a physician.

Children 2 to 6 years of age – One lozenge every 4 hours not to exceed 6 lozenges in 24 hours, or as directed by a physician.

In children, take care to prevent choking on lozenge.

➤*Tetra-Formula:*

Adults and children 6 years of age and older – Dissolve 1 lozenge slowly in the mouth; do not chew. May be repeated every 4 hours or as directed by a physician.

Children under 6 years of age – Consult a physician.

➤*Storage/Stability:* Store below 86°F and protect from moisture.

EXPECTORANTS

GUAIFENESIN (Glyceryl Guaiacolate)

otc	**Hytuss** (Hyrex)	**Tablets**: 100 mg	(HY). White, scored. In 100s and 1000s.
Rx	**Guaifenesin** (Various, eg, URL)	**Tablets**: 200 mg	In 100s.
Rx	**Organidin NR** (Medpointe)		Rose, scored. In 100s.
otc	**Guaifenesin** (URL)	**Tablets**: 400 mg	Dye-free. In 50s and 100s.
Rx	**Allfen Jr** (MCR American)		Dye-free. (ALLFEN JR). Scored. In 100s.
Rx	**Liquibid** (Capellon)		In 100s.
otc	**Mucinex** (Adams)	**Tablets, extended-release**: 600 mg	Bi-layered. In 20s, 40s, and 500s.
otc	**Humibid Maximum Strength** (Adams)	**Tablets, extended-release**: 1,200 mg	Bi-layered. In 100s.
otc	**Hytuss 2X** (Hyrex)	**Capsules**: 200 mg	EDTA, benzyl alcohol, FD&C Blue No. 1, parabens. In 100s.
otc	**Guaifenesin** (Various, eg, URL)	**Syrup**: 100 mg per 5 mL	In 473 mL.
otc	**Altarussin** (Altaire)		Alcohol-free. Corn syrup, menthol, saccharin. In 118 mL.
otc	**Guiatuss** (Various, eg, Goldline)		May contain corn syrup, saccharin, and menthol. In 118 mL.

GUAIFENESIN (Glyceryl Guaiacolate)

otc sf	**Diabetic Tussin** (Health Care Products)	**Liquid**: 100 mg per 5 mL	Alcohol- and dye-free. 8.4 mg per 5 mL phenylalanine. Aspartame, menthol, methylparaben. In 118 mL.
Rx	**Ganidin NR** (Cypress)		In 473 mL.
Rx	**Guaifenesin NR** (Silarx)		Raspberry flavor. In 473 mL.
Rx	**Organidin NR** (Medpointe)		Saccharin, sorbitol. Raspberry flavor. In 473 mL.
otc	**Robitussin** (Wyeth)		Alcohol-free. Glucose, corn syrup, saccharin, menthol. In 118 and 237 mL.
otc	**Siltussin DAS** (Silarx)		Strawberry flavor. In 118 mL.
otc sf	**Scot-Tussin Expectorant** (Scot-Tussin)		Alcohol- and dye-free. Contains phenylalanine.[a] Aspartame, parabens, menthol. Grape flavor. In 118 mL.
otc	**Siltussin SA** (Silarx)		Strawberry flavor. In 118, 237, and 473 mL.
otc sf	**Naldecon Senior EX** (Sandoz)	**Liquid**: 200 mg per 5 mL	Alcohol-free. Sorbitol, saccharin. In 120 mL.

[a] Amount not specified.

GUAIFENESIN — ORAL

Indications

➤*100 mg tablets:* Guaifenesin 100 mg tablets relieve bronchial drainage, and dry, nonproductive coughs become more productive and less frequent. This medication relieves irritated membranes in the respiratory tract by preventing dryness through increased mucous flow.

➤*200 mg tablets, 200 mg capsules, and 100 mg per 5 mL syrup and liquid:* Guaifenesin help loosen phlegm (mucus) and thin bronchial secretions to rid the bronchial passageways of bothersome mucus, drain bronchial tubes, and make coughs more productive. This medication helps loosen phlegm and thins bronchial secretions in patients with stable chronic bronchitis.

➤*400 and 600 mg tablets:* For the temporary relief of coughs associated with respiratory tract infections and related conditions such as sinusitis, pharyngitis, bronchitis, and asthma, when these conditions are complicated by tenacious mucus or mucus plugs and congestion.

Administration and Dosage

➤*Adults and children over 12 years of age:*

400 mg tablets – One tablet every 4 hours. Maximum daily dose should not exceed 6 doses (6 tablets or 2400 mg) in any 24-hour period.

600 mg sustained-release tablets – One or 2 tablets every 12 hours, not to exceed 4 tablets (2400 mg) in 24 hours.

➤*Adults and children 12 years of age and older:*

200 mg tablets – One or 2 tablets (200 mg to 400 mg) every 4 hours, not to exceed 12 tablets (2400 mg) in 24 hours..

200 mg capsules – One or 2 capsules every 4 hours, not to exceed 12 capsules (2400 mg) in 24 hours.

100 mg per 5 mL syrup and 100 mg per 5 mL liquid – Take 10 to 20 mL (2 to 4 teaspoonfuls) every 4 hours, but not more than 120 mL (24 teaspoonfuls) in 24 hours, or as directed by a doctor.

➤*Children 6 to 12 years of age:*

400 mg tablets – One-half tablet every 4 hours. Maximum daily dose should not exceed 6 doses (3 tablets) in any 24-hour period. Tablets may be broken in half for ease of administration without affecting release of medication, but not crushed or chewed.

600 mg sustained-release tablets – One tablet every 12 hours, not to exceed 2 tablets (1200 mg) in 24 hours.

➤*Children 6 to under 12 years of age:*

200 mg capsules – One capsule every 4 hours, not to exceed 6 capsules (1200 mg) in 24 hours.

100 mg per 5 mL syrup and 100 mg per 5 mL liquid – Take 1 to 2 teaspoonfuls (5 to 10 mL) every 4 hours, but not more than 12 teaspoonfuls (60 mL) in 24 hours, or as directed by a doctor.

➤*Children 2 to under 6 years of age:*

400 mg tablets – Do not administer unless directed by a physician.

200 mg capsules – Consult a doctor.

100 mg per 5 mL syrup – Take one-half to 1 teaspoonful (2.5 to 5 mL) every 4 hours, but not more than 6 teaspoonfuls (30 mL) in 24 hours, or as directed by a doctor.

➤*Children under 2 years of age:* Consult a doctor.

➤*Storage/Stability:* Store at controlled room temperature, 15° to 30°C (59° to 86°F). Dispense in tight, light-resistant containers. Keep this and all medication out of the reach of children. In case of accidental overdose, seek professional assistance or contact a poison control center immediately.

Actions

➤*Pharmacology:* Guaifenesin is an expectorant which increases respiratory tract fluid secretions and helps to loosen phlegm and bronchial secretions. By reducing the viscosity of secretions and increasing sputum volume, guaifenesin increases the efficiency of the cough reflex and of ciliary action in removing accumulated secretions from the trachea and bronchi. As a result, bronchial drainage is improved and less frequent.

➤*Pharmacokinetics:*

Absorption – Guaifenesin is readily absorbed from the gastrointestinal tract.

Metabolism/Excretion – Guaifenesin is rapidly metabolized and excreted in the urine. Guaifenesin has a plasma half-life of 1 hour. The major urinary metabolite is β-(2-methoxyphenoxy) lactic acid.

Contraindications

These products are contraindicated in patients with hypersensitivity to guaifenesin.

Warnings

➤*Kidney stone formation:* Reports in the literature have suggested that consumption of large quantities of guaifenesin-containing medications may be associated with an increased risk of drug-induced kidney stone formation.

➤*Pregnancy:* Category C. Animal reproduction studies have not been conducted. Safe use in pregnancy has not been established relative to possible adverse effects on fetal development. It is not known whether guaifenesin tablets can cause fetal harm when administered to a pregnant woman or can affect reproduction capacity. Therefore, this product should not be used in pregnant patients, unless in the judgment of the physician, the potential benefits outweigh possible hazards. Guaifenesin tablets should be given to a pregnant woman only if clearly needed.

➤*Lactation:* It is not known whether guaifenesin is excreted in human milk. Because many drugs are excreted in human milk, caution should be exercised when guaifenesin is administered to a nursing woman, and a decision should be made whether to discontinue nursing or to discontinue the drug, taking into account the importance of the drug to the mother.

➤*Children:*

400 mg tablets – Guaifenesin 400 mg tablets are not recommended to children under 6 years of age.

600 mg sustained-release tablets – Safety and efficacy of 600 mg sustained-release tablets in pediatric patients under the age of 12 years have not been established.

Precautions

➤*Evaluation:* Before prescribing medication to suppress or modify cough, it is important to ascertain that the underlying cause of cough is identified, that modification of cough does not increase the risk of clinical or physiological complications, and that appropriate therapy for the primary disease is instituted.

Drug Interactions

➤*Drug/Lab test interactions:* Guaifenesin may increase renal clearance for urate and thereby lower serum uric acid levels. Guaifenesin may produce an increase in urinary 5-hydroxyindoleacetic (5-HIAA) acid and may therefore interfere with the interpretation of this test for the diagnosis of carcinoid syndrome. It may also falsely elevate the vanillylmandelic acid (VMA) test for catechols. Administration of this drug should be discontinued 48 hours prior to the collection of urine specimens for such tests.

Adverse Reactions

Guaifenesin is well tolerated and has a wide margin of safety. Products containing guaifenesin have been associated with nausea, vomiting, GI discomfort, dizziness, headache, skin rash, and urticaria.

Overdosage

➤*Symptoms:* Overdosage with guaifenesin is unlikely to produce toxic effects since its toxicity is low. Guaifenesin, when administered by stomach tube to test animals in doses up to 5 g/kg, produced no signs of toxicity.

➤*Treatment:* In severe cases of overdosage, treatment should be aimed at reducing further absorption of the drug. Gastric emptying (emesis or gastric lavage) is recommended as soon as possible after ingestion. Treatment is symptomatic and supportive.

GUAIFENESIN — ORAL

Patient Information

Do not give this product to children under 2 years of age, unless directed by a physician. Do not take guaifenesin for persistent or chronic cough such as occurs with smoking, asthma, chronic bronchitis, emphysema, or if cough is accompanied by excessive phlegm (mucus), unless directed by a physician. A persistent cough may be a sign of a serious condition. If cough persists for more than 1 week, tends to recur, or is accompanied by fever, rash, or persistent headache, consult a physician.

POTASSIUM IODIDE

Rx	**Potassium Iodide** (Various, eg, Balan, Goldline, Harber)	**Solution:** 1 g potassium iodide per ml. *Dose:* 0.3 ml (300 mg) to 0.6 ml (600 mg) 3 or 4 times a day, diluted in water. Do not take more than 12 times a day.	In 30 and 240 ml and pt.
Rx *sf*	**Potassium Iodide** (Roxane)		In 30 and 240 ml.
Rx	**SSKI** (Upsher-Smith)		In 30 and 240 ml.
Rx	**Pima** (Fleming)	**Syrup:** 325 mg potassium iodide per 5 ml. *Dose:* Adults – 5 to 10 ml 3 times daily. Children – 2.5 to 5 ml 3 times daily.	Sugar. Black raspberry flavor. In pt and gal.

POTASSIUM IODIDE — ORAL

Indications

➤*Expectorant:* As an expectorant in the treatment of chronic pulmonary diseases where tenacious mucus complicates the problem. These include bronchial asthma, chronic bronchitis, bronchiectasis, pulmonary emphysema, and sinus congestion.

➤*Unlabeled uses:* Potassium iodide (60 mg 3 times daily) has been used effectively in a limited number of patients for Sweet's syndrome (acute febrile neutrophilic dermatosis) in combination with a potent topical steroid, as an alternative to systemic corticosteroids.

Administration and Dosage

➤*Adults:* One or two teaspoonsful (5 to 10 g) or as recommended by a physician in 120 to 240 mL of water.

➤*Children 3 to 6 years:* One teaspoonful (5 g) every 4 to 6 hours in 120 to 240 mL of water.

➤*Children under 3 years:* One half teaspoonful (2.5 g) every 4 to 6 hours in 120 to 240 mL of water.

Actions

➤*Pharmacology:* Potassium iodide enhances the secretion of respiratory fluids, thus decreasing mucus viscosity.

Warnings

➤*Hypersensitivity reactions:* Patients who are hyperthyroid or who may be sensitive to iodides may temporarily develop iodine-induced swelling of a lymph or salivary gland. Other adverse events in iodide-sensitive patients may include GI upset, metallic taste, minor skin eruptions, nausea, vomiting.

RESPIRATORY COMBINATION PRODUCTS

Combination products are frequently used in respiratory conditions. These products present two problems: (1) The patient may not need the components of the product; (2) the patient may need the components, but in different strengths or intervals.

➤**Product Selection Guidelines**: When recommending a respiratory combination product, consider the following guidelines.

Patient's data –

Symptoms: Pain, fever, congestion, runny nose, productive/nonproductive cough.

Patient's medical history / health: Age, allergy history, pregnancy, heart disease, hypertension, asthma, bronchitis, glaucoma, hyperthyroidism, diabetes, depression.

Drugs patient is currently taking: Other cold or allergy medications; medications for hypertension, diabetes, etc.

Do not exceed the recommended dosage. Do not take an *otc* product for greater than 7 days. If symptoms do not improve or are accompanied by fever, consult a physician.

Humidification of room air and adequate fluid intake (6 to 8 glasses/day) are important in treating cold symptoms.

Sulfite / Tartrazine sensitivity – Some of these products contain sulfites or tartrazine, which may cause allergic-type reactions (eg, hives, itching, wheezing, anaphylaxis) in certain susceptible persons. Although overall prevalence of sensitivity in general population is probably low, it is seen more frequently in asthmatics or in atopic nonasthmatic persons (sulfites) or in those with aspirin hypersensitivity (tartrazine).

Sugar free liquid products (sf) – The small amount of sugar in usual doses of medication is probably insignificant to the well controlled diabetic. However, consider the effects of alcohol and sympathomimetics in addition to the sugar content.

Sustained release formulations – Products with identical active ingredients are listed together. Due to formulation differences, do not consider them bioequivalent.

Dosage – Usually average adult dose. For children, consult package literature or physician.

➤**Groups**: These combination products are presented in groups based on the components of their formulations. Products with identical or similar ingredients are listed adjacent to each other, regardless of therapeutic claims, which may differ even for identical formulations. Pediatric preparations (those products intended mainly or exclusively for children) are grouped at the end of each respective section.

Antiasthmatic Combinations – These contain xanthine derivatives and sympathomimetics for bronchodilation. Many products also contain expectorants to facilitate mobilization of mucus.
Xanthine Combinations
Xanthine-Sympathomimetic Combinations

Upper Respiratory Combinations – These are used primarily for relief of symptoms associated with colds, upper respiratory tract infections and allergic conditions (eg, acute rhinitis, sinusitis).
Decongestant Combinations
Antihistamine and Analgesic Combinations
Decongestant and Antihistamine Combinations
Decongestant, Antihistamine and Analgesic Combinations
Decongestant, Antihistamine and Anticholinergic Combinations

Cough Preparations – These include an antitussive or expectorant, but may also contain ingredients for relief of associated symptoms.
Antitussive Combinations
Expectorant Combinations
Narcotic Antitussives with Expectorants
Nonnarcotic Antitussives with Expectorants
Antitussive and Expectorant Combinations

➤**Ingredients**: An FDA advisory review panel has proposed monographs for all *otc* cold, cough, allergy, bronchodilator and antihistamine products. In addition, the FDA proposes to classify *otc* drugs as "monograph conditions" (old Category I) and "nonmonograph conditions" (old Categories II and III). When using these combination products, consider the prescribing information for each ingredient.

Antihistamines – (See individual monograph). These are used for symptomatic relief from allergic rhinitis (hay fever) including runny nose, sneezing, itching of the nose or throat, and itchy and watery eyes. The anticholinergic effects of antihistamines may cause a thickening of bronchial secretions; therefore, these agents may be counterproductive in respiratory conditions characterized by congestion. Antihistamines may cause drowsiness.

Xanthines – (See individual monograph). These, primarily theophylline, relieve bronchial spasm by direct action on the bronchial smooth muscle in bronchospastic conditions such as asthma and chronic bronchitis. Product listings include anhydrous theophylline dosage equivalents. Some xanthine-containing combination products are available *otc,* but asthmatic patients should use them only under physician supervision.

Sympathomimetics – These are used for their α-adrenergic (vasoconstrictor/decongestant) or β_2 adrenergic (bronchodilator) effects.

Decongestants: Used for temporary relief of nasal congestion due to colds or allergy. Given orally, they are less effective than topical nasal decongestants, and they have a potential for systemic side effects. Frequent or prolonged topical use may lead to local irritation and rebound congestion.

Bronchodilators: Ephedrine common in these combinations, stimulates cardiac (β_1) receptors. Bronchodilation is weaker than with catecholamines; α-adrenergic effects may decrease congestion of mucous membranes. Other β-active agents are effective bronchodilators, but pseudoephedrine is not.

Narcotic antitussives – The antitussive dose is lower than that required for analgesia. Consider general precautions for the use of narcotics, including the potential for abuse, when using these products. See Narcotic Antitussive monograph for complete prescribing information. See also the Narcotic Agonist Analgesics monograph for complete information on the narcotics.

Codeine: 10 to 20 mg every 4 to 6 hours.
Hydrocodone (dihydrocodeinone): 5 to 10 mg every 6 to 8 hours.
Hydromorphone HCl: 2 mg every 4 hours.

Nonnarcotic antitussives – These decrease the cough reflex without inducing many of the common characteristics of narcotic preparations.
Dextromethorphan: 10 to 30 mg every 4 to 8 hours.
Diphenhydramine: 25 mg every 4 hours.

Carbetapentane: This has atropine-like and local anesthetic actions and suppresses cough reflex through selective depression of the medullary cough center.

- *Dose* – 15 to 30 mg, 3 or 4 times daily.

Caramiphen edisylate: A weak anticholinergic and centrally acting antitussive.

- *Dose* –
  - *Adults:* 10 to 20 mg every 4 to 6 hours.
  - *Children (6 to 12):* 5 to 10 mg q 4 to 6 h;
  - *Children (2 to 6):* 2.5 to 5 mg q 4 to 6 h.

Expectorants – In the FDA's final monograph for *otc* expectorants, guaifenesin (see individual monograph) is the only agent approved for use as an expectorant. Guaifenesin may help loosen phlegm and thin bronchial secretions to rid the bronchial passageways of bothersome mucus, drain bronchial tubes or make coughs more productive. Humidification of room air and adequate fluid intake (6 to 8 glasses/day) are important therapeutic measures as well.

Dose:

- *Adults* – 200 to 400 mg every 4 hours, not to exceed 2400 mg in 24 hours.
- *Children* – Lower dosages are specified on labeling. Consult a physician for children younger than 2 years of age.

Other ingredients not upgraded by the FDA include: Ammonium chloride, beechwood creosote, benzoin preparations, camphor, eucalyptol/eucalyptus oil, iodines, ipecac syrup, menthol/peppermint oil, pine tar preparations, potassium guaiacolsulfonate, sodium citrate, squill preparations, terpin hydrate preparations, tolu preparations and turpentine oil. Products containing these ingredients must be reformulated.

Analgesics – These (eg, acetaminophen, aspirin, ibuprofen, sodium salicylate) are frequently included to treat headache, fever, muscle aches, pain. See individual monographs.

Anticholinergics – (See individual monograph). These are included for their drying effects on mucus secretions. This action may be beneficial in acute rhinorrhea; however, drying of respiratory secretions may lead to thickened mucus and more difficult expectoration. Traditionally, anticholinergics have been avoided in patients with asthma or chronic obstructive pulmonary disease (COPD); however, some patients respond well to these agents. Caution is still advised in this group.

An anticholinergic for oral inhalation is available as a bronchodilator for maintenance of bronchospasm associated with COPD, including chronic bronchitis and emphysema (see Ipratropium monograph).

The FDA has ruled that no anticholinergic product for *otc* use is recognized as safe and effective. Therefore, the products must be reapproved by new drug application (NDA) before November 10, 1986, or be regarded as misbranded (*Federal Register* 1985 Nov 8; 50:46582-87).

Papaverine HCl – (See individual monograph). This relaxes the smooth muscle of the bronchial tree.

Barbiturates – (See individual monograph). These are included for sedative effects as "correctives" with xanthines or sympathomimetics which may cause CNS stimulation. The sedative efficacy of low doses (eg, 8 mg phenobarbital) is questionable.

Caffeine – (See individual monograph). This is included for CNS stimulation to counteract antihistamine depression and to enhance concomitant analgesics.

XANTHINE COMBINATIONS, CAPSULES AND TABLETS

Content given per capsule or tablet.

	Product & Distributor	Xanthine[1]	Expectorant	Other	Average Adult Dose	How Supplied
Rx	**Quibron-300 Capsules** (Roberts)	300 mg theophylline	180 mg guaifenesin		16 mg/kg/day or 400 mg theophylline/day, in divided doses, q 6 to 8 h	(Roberts 068). Yellow and white. In 100s.
Rx	**Bronchial Capsules** (Various, eg, Moore)	150 mg theophylline	90 mg guaifenesin		16 mg/kg/day or 400 mg theophylline/day, in divided doses, q 6 to 8 h	In 100s and 1000s.
Rx	**Glyceryl-T Capsules** (Rugby)[2]				1 or 2 bid or tid	In 100s.
Rx	**Quibron Capsules** (BMS)				16 mg/kg/day or 400 mg theophylline/day, in divided doses, q 6 to 8 h	(M022). Yellow. In 100s, 1000s and UD 100s.
Rx	**Mudrane GG-2 Tablets** (ECR Pharm)	111 mg theophylline	100 mg guaifenesin		1 tid or qid	(GG 9533). Green, mottled. In 100s.
Rx	**Dyphylline & Guaifenesin** (Econolab)	200 mg dyphylline	200 mg guaifenesin		1 qid	In 100s.
Rx	**Dyflex-G Tablets** (Econo Med)				1 or 2 qid	In 100s and 1000s.
Rx	**Dyline G.G. Tablets** (Seatrace)				1 tid or qid	(0551 and 0123) Pink, scored. In 100s and 1000s.
Rx	**Lufyllin-GG Tablets** (Medpointe)				1 qid	(Wallace 521). Lt. yellow, scored. In 100s, 1,000s, and 3,000s.
Rx	**Panfil G** (Pan American Labs)	200 mg dyphylline	100 mg guaifenesin		1 tid or qid after meals	Lactose. Orange/green. (PAL/0305). In 100s

[1] Theophylline content given as anhydrous unless otherwise specified.

[2] Form of theophylline unknown.

Refer to the general discussion of these products in the Respiratory Combinations Introduction.

XANTHINE COMBINATIONS, LIQUIDS

Content given per 15 ml.

	Product & Distributor	Xanthine[1]	Expectorant	Other	Average Adult Dose	How Supplied
Rx	**Theolate Liquid** (Various, eg, Barre-National)	150 mg theophylline	90 mg guaifenesin		15 ml q 6 to 8 h	In 118 mL, pt and gal.
Rx	**Glyceryl-T Liquid** (Rugby)					In 480 ml.
Rx	**Synophylate-GG Syrup** (Central)	150 mg theophylline (300 mg theophylline sodium glycinate)	100 mg guaifenesin	10% alcohol. Saccharin, sorbitol, sucrose	3 mg theophylline/kg q 8 h	In pt and gal.
Rx	**Ed-Bron G Liquid** (Edwards Pharmaceuticals, Inc.)	150 theophylline	100 mg guaifenesin	Parabens, aspartame, phenylalanine.	15 to 30 mL 3 to 4 times daily.	Peach flavor. In 30 and 473 mL.
Rx *sf*	**Elixophyllin GG Liquid** (Forest)	100 mg theophylline	100 mg guaifenesin	Sorbitol	3 mg theophylline/kg q 8 h	Alcohol and dye free. In 237 and 473 ml.
Rx	**Theophylline KI Elixir** (Various, eg, Qualitest)[2]	80 mg theophylline	130 mg potassium iodide		3 mg theophylline/kg q 8 h	In 480 ml and gal.
Rx	**Elixophyllin-KI Elixir** (Forest)			Saccharin, sodium bisulfite, sucrose, anise oil		In 237 ml.
Rx	**Iophylline Elixir** (Various, eg, Major)[2]	120 mg theophylline	30 mg iodinated glycerol		15 to 30 ml tid	In 480 ml.
Rx	**Dilor-G Liquid** (Savage)	300 mg dyphylline	300 mg guaifenesin	Saccharin, sorbitol, sucrose, parabens	5 or 10 ml tid or qid	Alcohol free. Mint flavor. In pint and gal.
Rx	**Panfil G** (Pan American Labs)	300 mg dyphylline	150 mg guaifenesin	Parabens, sorbitol, sucrose.	10 ml tid or qid	Vanilla flavor. In pints.
Rx	**Difil-G Forte Liquid** (Stewart-Jackson Pharmacal, Inc.)	300 mg dyphylline	300 mg guaifenesin	Parabens, saccharin, sucrose, sorbitol.	5 to 10 mL tid or qid	Menthol flavor. In 480 mL.
Rx	**Dilex-G Syrup** (Mikart, Inc.)			Parabens, saccharin, sucrose, sorbitol.	5 to 10 mL tid or qid	Menthol flavor. In 480 mL.
Rx	**Dilor-G Liquid** (Savage Laboratories)			Parabens, saccharin,sorbitol, sucrose.	5 to 10 mL tid or qid.	Alcohol free. Mint flavor. In pints and gal.
Rx	**Dy-G Liquid** (Cypress Pharmaceutical, Inc.)				5 to 10 mL tid or qid.	Alcohol free. Mint flavor. In pints.
Rx	**Dyphylline-GG Elixir** (Various, eg, Barre-National, Goldline, Qualitest, Silarx)	100 mg dyphylline	100 mg guaifenesin	17% alcohol. Saccharin, sucrose	30 ml qid	In 473 ml.
Rx	**Lufyllin-GG Elixir** (Medpointe)					Wine flavor. In pt and gal.

[1] Theophylline content given as anhydrous unless otherwise specified.

[2] May contain alcohol.

Refer to the general discussion of these products in the Respiratory Combinations Introduction.

XANTHINE-SYMPATHOMIMETIC COMBINATIONS, TABLETS

Content given per tablet.

	Product & Distributor	Xanthine[1]	Sympathomimetic	Expectorant	Other	Average Adult Dose	How Supplied
otc	**Theodrine Tablets** (Rugby)	120 mg theophylline[2]	22.5 mg ephedrine HCl			1 to 2 q 4 h up to 3 doses/day	In 1000s.
otc	**Tedrigen Tablets** (Goldline)				7.5 mg phenobarbital	1 to 2 q 4 h	In 100s and 1000s.
Rx	**Hydrophed Tablets** (Rugby)	130 mg theophylline	25 mg ephedrine sulfate		10 mg hydroxyzine HCl	1 bid to qid	In 100s and 1000s.
Rx	**Marax Tablets** (Roerig)						Dye free. Scored. M-shaped. In 100s and 500s.
Rx	**Mudrane GG Tablets** (ECR Pharm)	111 mg theophylline (130 mg aminophylline anhydrous)	16 mg ephedrine HCl	100 mg guaifenesin	8 mg phenobarbital	1 tid or qid	(GG 9551). Yellow, mottled, scored. In 100s.
Rx	**Mudrane Tablets** (ECR Pharm)	111 mg theophylline (130 mg aminophylline anhydrous)	16 mg ephedrine HCl	195 mg potassium iodide	8 mg phenobarbital	1 tid or qid	(9550). Yellow, scored. In 100s.
Rx	**Quadrinal Tablets** (Knoll)	65 mg theophylline (130 mg theophylline calcium salicylate)	24 mg ephedrine HCl	320 mg potassium iodide	24 mg phenobarbital	1 tid or qid	(14). White, scored. Biconvex. In 100s.
otc	**Primatene Dual Action Tablets** (Whitehall)	60 mg theophylline	12.5 mg ephedrine HCl	100 mg guaifenesin		2 q 4 h	In 24s.
Rx	**Lufyllin-EPG Tablets** (Wallace)	100 mg dyphylline	16 mg ephedrine HCl	200 mg guaifenesin	16 mg phenobarbital	1 to 2 q 6 h	In 100s.

[1] Theophylline content given as anhydrous unless otherwise specified.
[2] Form of theophylline unknown.

Refer to the general discussion of these products in the Respiratory Combinations Introduction.

XANTHINE-SYMPATHOMIMETIC COMBINATIONS, LIQUIDS

Content given per 15 ml.

	Product & Distributor	Xanthine[1]	Sympathomimetic	Expectorant	Other	Average Adult Dose	How Supplied
Rx	**Lufyllin-EPG Elixir** (Wallace)	150 mg dyphylline	24 mg ephedrine HCl	300 mg guaifenesin	5.5% alcohol. 24 mg phenobarbital	10 to 20 ml q 6 h	In 480 ml.

[1] Theophylline content given as anhydrous unless otherwise specified.

Refer to the general discussion of these products in the Respiratory Combinations Introduction.

PEDIATRIC XANTHINE-SYMPATHOMIMETIC COMBINATIONS

Content given per 15 ml.

	Product & Distributor	Xanthine[1]	Sympathomimetic	Other	Average Adult Dose	How Supplied
Rx	**Theomax DF Syrup** (Various, eg, Barre-National)	97.5 mg theophylline	18.75 mg ephedrine sulfate	5% alcohol. 7.5 mg hydroxyzine HCl	*Children (> 5 yrs)* - 5 ml tid or qid *(2 to 5 yrs)* - 2.5 to 5 ml tid or qid	In pt and gal.
Rx	**Marax-DF Syrup** (Roerig)			7.5 mg hydroxyzine HCl, sucrose[2]	*Children (> 5 yrs)* - 5 ml tid or qid *(2 to 5 yrs)* - 2.5 to 5 ml tid or qid	In pt and gal.

[1] Theophylline content given as anhydrous unless otherwise specified.
[2] May contain alcohol.

Refer to the general discussion of these products in the Respiratory Combinations Introduction.

DECONGESTANT AND ANALGESIC COMBINATIONS

Content given per capsule, tablet, or 5 mL.

	Product & Distributor	Decongestant	Analgesic	Average Adult Dose	Excipients & How Supplied
otc	**Alka-Seltzer Plus Cold & Sinus Tablets** (Bayer)	5 mg phenylephrine HCl	250 mg acetaminophen	2 q 4 h up to 8/day	4 mg phenylalanine, aspartame, acesulfame K, saccharin, sorbitol. In 20s.
otc	**Cepacol Sore Throat Liquid**[1] (J.B. Williams)	10 mg pseudoephedrine HCl	106.7 mg acetaminophen	30 mL q 4 to 6 h up to 120 mL/day	Alcohol free. Tartrazine, honey, saccharin, sorbitol. Honey flavor. In 237 mL.
otc	**Alka-Seltzer Plus Cold & Sinus Liqui-Gels**[1] (Bayer)	30 mg pseudoephedrine HCl	325 mg acetaminophen	2 q 4 h up to 8/day	Liquid-filled. Sorbitol. (AS+ C&S). In 12s and 20s.
otc	**Allerest Allergy & Sinus Relief Maximum Strength Tablets**[1] (Heritage)			2 q 4 to 6 h up to 8/day	In 24s.
otc	**Ornex No Drowsiness Tablets**[1] (B.F. Ascher)				Capsule shape. In 24s and 48s.
otc	**Phenapap Tablets**[1] (Rugby)				In 100s.
otc	**Sinutab Sinus Without Drowsiness Regular Strength Tablets** (Warner-Lambert)			2 q 4 h up to 8/day	In 24s.
otc	**Sudafed Cold & Sinus Non-Drowsy Liqui-Caps** (Warner-Lambert)			2 q 4 to 6 h up to 8/day	Liquid-filled. Sorbitol. In 10s and 20s.
otc	**Daytime Sinus Relief Non-Drowsy Maximum Strength Tablets** (Akyma)	30 mg pseudoephedrine HCl	500 mg acetaminophen	2 q 4 to 6 h up to 8/day	Capsule shape. In 24s.
otc	**Dilotab Tablets** (Zee Medical)			2 q 6 h up to 8/day	In 24s.
otc	**Dristan Cold Non-Drowsy Maximum Strength Tablets** (Whitehall-Robins)			2 q 6 h up to 8/day	Capsule shape. In 20s.
otc	**Mapap Sinus Maximum Strength Geltabs** (Major)			2 q 4 to 6 h up to 8/day	In 24s.
otc	**Nasal Decongestant Sinus Non-Drowsy Tablets** (Topco)			2 q 6 h up to 8/day	In 24s.
otc	**Ornex No Drowsiness Maximum Strength Tablets** (BF Ascher)				(ORNEX MAX). Capsule shape. In 24s and 48s.
otc	**Sine-Off No-Drowsiness Formula Tablets** (Hogil)				(SINE-OFF). Capsule shape. In 24s.
otc	**Sinus-Relief Maximum Strength Tablets** (Major)				Dextrose. Capsule shape. In 24s.
otc	**Sinutab Sinus Without Drowsiness Maximum Strength Tablets** (Warner-Lambert)				Round (tablet); capsule shape (caplet). In 24s and 48s.
otc	**Sudafed Sinus Headache Non-Drowsy Tablets** (Warner-Lambert)				Round (tablet); capsule shape (caplet). In 24s and 48s.
otc	**SudoGest Sinus Maximum Strength Tablets** (Major)				Dextrose. In 24s.
otc	**Tavist Sinus Maximum Strength Tablets** (Novartis)				Lactose, dextrose, methylparaben. (Tavist Sinus). Capsule shape. In 24s.
otc	**Tylenol Sinus Non-Drowsy Maximum Strength Geltabs, Tablets, and Gelcaps** (McNeil)			2 q 4 to 6 h up to 8/day	**Tablets:** (TYLENOL Sinus). Capsule shape. In 24s. **Geltabs:** Parabens. (TYLENOL SINUS). In 24s, 48s, and 60s. **Gelcaps:** Parabens. (TYLENOL SINUS). In 24s, 48s, and 60s.
otc	**Advil Cold & Sinus Tablets** (Whitehall-Robins)	30 mg pseudoephedrine HCl	200 mg ibuprofen	1 to 2 q 4 to 6 h up to 6/day	Parabens, sucrose. (ADVIL COLD & SINUS). Oval. In 40s.
otc	**Advil Cold & Sinus Liqui-gels** (Whitehall-Robins)				Sorbitol. In 16s and 32s.
otc	**Advil Flu & Body Ache Tablets** (Whitehall-Robins)				Parabens, sucrose. Capsule shape. In 20s.
otc	**Dristan Sinus Tablets** (Whitehall-Robins)				Parabens, sucrose. Oval. In 20s.
otc	**Motrin Sinus Headache Tablets** (McNeil)				(Motrin Sinus Headache). Capsule shape. In 20s.
otc	**Aleve Cold & Sinus Tablets** (Bayer)	120 mg pseudoephedrine HCl	220 mg naproxen sodium (200 mg naproxen)	1 q 12 h up to 2/day	Extended release. Lactose. Capsule shape. In 10s, 20s, and 40s.
otc	**Aleve Sinus & Headache Tablets** (Bayer)				Extended release. Lactose. Capsule shape. In 10s.

[1] This product also may be used in children; refer to package labeling for dosing.

For complete and comparative prescribing information, refer to the Respiratory Combinations Introduction.

PEDIATRIC DECONGESTANT AND ANALGESIC COMBINATIONS

Content given per tablet, 5 mL (liquid), or 1 mL (drops).

	Product & Distributor	Decongestant	Analgesic	Average Dose	Excipients & How Supplied
otc	**Tylenol Infants' Drops Plus Cold** (McNeil)	9.375 mg pseudoephedrine HCl	100 mg acetaminophen	***2 to 3 y*** - 1.6 mL q 4 to 6 h up to 6.4 mL/day	Alcohol free. Corn syrup, sorbitol. Bubble-gum flavor. In 15 mL w/dropper.
otc	**Tylenol Children's Plus Cold Suspension** (McNeil)	15 mg pseudoephedrine HCl	160 mg acetaminophen	***6 to 11 y*** - 10 mL q 4 to 6 h up to 40 mL/day; ***2 to 5 y*** - 5 mL q 4 to 6 h up to 20 mL/day	Acesulfame K, corn syrup, sorbitol. Fruit flavor. In 120 mL.
otc	**Triaminic Softchews Allergy Sinus & Headache Tablets** (Novartis)			***6 to 11 y*** - 2 q 4 to 6 h up to 8/day; ***2 to 5 y*** - 1 q 4 to 6 h up to 4/day	11.2 mg phenylalanine, aspartame, mannitol, sorbitol, sucrose. Fruit-punch flavor. In 18s.
otc	**Children's Ibuprofen Cold Suspension** (Major)	15 mg pseudoephedrine HCl	100 mg ibuprofen/5 mL	***6 to 11 y*** - 10 mL q 6 h up to 40 mL/day; ***2 to 5 y*** - 5 mL q 6 h up to 20 mL/day	Alcohol-free. Corn syrup. Berry flavor. In 120 mL.
otc	**Children's Advil Cold Suspension** (Whitehall-Robins)	15 mg pseudoephedrine HCl	100 mg ibuprofen	***6 to 11 y (48 to 95 lbs)*** - 10 mL q 6 h up to 40 mL/day; ***2 to 5 y (24 to 47 lbs)*** - 5 mL q 6 h up to 20 mL/day	Sorbitol, sucrose. Alcohol free. Grape flavor. In 120 mL.
otc	**Dimetapp Children's Cold & Fever Suspension** (Wyeth Consumer Healthcare)				
otc	**Motrin Children's Cold Suspension** (McNeil)			***6 to 11 y*** - 10 mL q 6 h up to 40 mL/day; ***2 to 5 y*** - 5 mL q 6 h up to 20 mL/day	Acesulfame K, sucrose. Berry, dye free berry, or grape flavors. In 118 mL.

Refer to the general discussion of these products in the Respiratory Combinations Introduction. Some of the products in the previous Decongestant and Analgesic Combinations table also may be used in children.

DECONGESTANT AND EXPECTORANT COMBINATIONS

Content given per capsule, tablet, or 5 mL.

	Product & Distributor	Decongestant	Expectorant	Other	Average Adult Dose	Excipients & How Supplied
Rx	**Broncholate Syrup** (Sanofi-Synthelabo)	6.25 mg ephedrine HCl	100 mg guaifenesin		10 to 20 mL every 4 h up to 120 mL/day	Orange flavor. In 473 mL.
Rx	**KIE Syrup**[1] (Laser)	8 mg ephedrine HCl	150 mg potassium iodide		10 to 15 mL every 4 to 6 h up to 60 mL/day	Saccharin, sorbitol, sucrose. Cherry flavor. In 473 mL.
otc	**Mini Two-Way Action Tablets** (BDI Pharm)	12.5 mg ephedrine HCl	200 mg guaifenesin		1 to 2 every 4 h up to 12/day	In 6s, 24s, and 60s.
otc	**Primatene Tablets** (Whitehall-Robins)				2 every 4 h up to 12/day	In 24s and 60s.
otc	**Dynafed Asthma Relief Tablets** (BDI Pharm)	25 mg ephedrine HCl	200 mg guaifenesin		½ to 1 every 4 h up to 6/day	In 60s.
otc	**Mini Two-Way Action Tablets** (BDI Pharm)					In 6s, 48s and 60s.
otc	**Bronkaid Dual Action Tablets** (Bayer)	25 mg ephedrine sulfate	400 mg guaifenesin		1 every 4 h up to 6/day	Capsule shape. In 24s.
Rx sf	**Despec Liquid**[1] (International Ethical)	5 mg phenylephrine HCl	100 mg guaifenesin		10 mL 4 times daily (every 6 h)	Alcohol and dye free. Maltitol, saccharin, sorbitol. Grape flavor. In 15, 120, and 240 mL.
otc	**Rescon-GG Liquid**[1] (Capellon)				10 mL every 4 to 6 h up to 40 mL/day	Alcohol and dye free. Parabens, sorbitol, sugar. Cherry flavor. In 118 and 473 mL.
Rx sf	**Entex Liquid**[1] (Andrx)	7.5 mg phenylephrine HCl	100 mg guaifenesin		5 to 10 mL every 4 to 6 h up to 40 mL/day	Alcohol and dye free. Punch flavor. In 15 and 473 mL.
Rx	**Guaifed-PD Capsules**[1] (Victory)	7.5 mg phenylephrine HCl	200 mg guaifenesin		1 to 2 every 12 h	Extended release. Maltodextrin, parabens, sucrose. (GUAIFED 200-7.5 VERUM). Purple/White. In 30s and 100s.
Rx	**Crantex ER Capsules** (Breckenridge)	10 mg phenylephrine HCl	300 mg guaifenesin		1 or 2 every 12 h	Extended release. Sugar. (B232). Green/white. In 100s.
Rx	**Entex ER Capsules**[1] (Andrx)					Extended release. Maltodextrin, sucrose, parabens. (ENTEX ER 334). White. In 30s and 100s.
Rx	**ExeFen-PD Tablets**[1] (Larken[2])	10 mg phenylephrine HCl	600 mg guaifenesin		1 or 2 every 12 h	Extended release. (LL50). Blue, capsule shape, scored. In 100s.
Rx	**Guaifed Capsules**[1] (Victory)	15 mg phenylephrine HCl	400 mg guaifenesin		1 every 12 h	Extended release. Maltodextrin, parabens, sucrose. (GUAIFED 400-15 VERUM). Purple/White. In 30s and 100s.
Rx	**SINUvent PE Tablets**[1] (WE Pharm)	15 mg phenylephrine HCl	600 mg guaifenesin		2 bid every 12 h	Extended release. (WE). Lt. green, capsule shape, scored. In 100s.
Rx	**Deconsal II Capsules**[1] (Cornerstone Biopharma)	20 mg phenylephrine HCl	375 mg guaifenesin		1 to 2 every 12 h up to 3/day	Extended-release. Sucrose. (Cornerstone Biopharma Deconsal II). Blue, yellow opaque. In 20s and 100s.

DECONGESTANT AND EXPECTORANT COMBINATIONS

	Product & Distributor	Decongestant	Expectorant	Other	Average Adult Dose	Excipients & How Supplied
Rx	**GFN 600/Phenylephrine 20 Tablets**[1] (Cypress)	20 mg phenylephrine HCl	600 mg guaifenesin		1 to 2 every 12 h up to 2/day	Dye free. (CYP 269). White, oval, scored. In 100s.
Rx	**Liquibid-PD Tablets**[1] (Capellon)	25 mg phenylephrine HCl	275 mg guaifenesin		1 or 2 every 12 h up to 4/day	Sustained release. White/Blue bilayered, triangular, scored. In 100s.
Rx	**Duraphen II Tablets**[1] (ProEthic)	25 mg phenylephrine HCl	800 mg guaifenesin		1 every 12 h up to 2 per day	Extended release. Maltodextrin, talc. (PE/822). White, oval shape, scored. In 100s.
Rx	**Duratuss Tablets**[1] (Victory Pharma[3])	25 mg phenylephrine HCl	900 mg guaifenesin		1 every 12 h	Extended release. Maltodextrin, talc. (900/25). White. In 100s.
Rt	**Duratuss GP Tablets** (Victory Pharma[3])	25 mg phenylephrine HCl	1,200 mg guaifenesin		1 every 12 h up to 2 per day	Extended release. Maltodextrin, talc. (1200/25). White. In 100s.
Rx	**Entex LA Capsules**[1] (Andrx)	30 mg phenylephrine HCl	400 mg guaifenesin		1 every 12 h up to 2 per day	Extended release. Maltodextrin, sucrose. (ANDRX 333). Yellow and blue. In 100s.
Rx	**PhenaVent LA Capsules** (Ethex)					Extended release. Sucrose. (ETHEX 095). Opaque blue/opaque light blue. In 30s.
Rx	**Entex LA Tablets**[1] (Andrx)	30 mg phenylephrine HCl	600 mg guaifenesin		1 every 12 h up to 2/day	Sustained release. Dye free. (ENTEX LA 330/330). White, oval, scored. In 100s.
Rx	**PhenaVent LA Tablets** (Ethex)					(ETHEX 443). White to off-white, capsule shape. Film-coated. In 100s.
Rx	**Liquibid-D Tablets**[1] (Capellon)	40 mg phenylephrine HCl	600 mg guaifenesin		1 every 12 h	(LIQUIBID-D). White, oval, scored. In 100s.
Rx	**Liquibid-D 1200 Tablets**[1] (Capellon)	40 mg phenylephrine HCl	1200 mg guaifenesin		1 every 12 h	Sustained release. (1200). Lt. green, capsule shape, scored. Film coated. In 100s.
Rx	**PhenaVent D Tablets** (Ethex)					(ETHEX 444). White to off-white, capsule shape. Film-coated. In 100s.
Rx	**Sina-12X Tablets**[1] (MedPointe)	25 mg phenylephrine tannate	200 mg guaifenesin		1 or 2 q 12 h	(SINA 6301). Purple, capsule shape, scored. In 30s.
otc	**Robafen PE Liquid**[1] (Major)	30 mg pseudoephedrine HCl	100 mg guaifenesin		10 mL every 4 h up to 40 mL/day	Alcohol free. Glucose, corn syrup, saccharin. In 118 mL.
otc	**Robitussin PE Liquid**[1] (Whitehall-Robins)					Corn syrup, glucose, saccharin. In 118 and 237 mL.
otc	**Sudafed Non-Drowsy Non-Drying Sinus Liquid Caps** (Warner-Lambert)	30 mg pseudoephedrine HCl	120 mg guaifenesin		2 every 4 h up to 8/day	Liquid filled. Sorbitol. In 24s.
otc	**Guaifed Syrup**[1] (Muro)	30 mg pseudoephedrine HCl	200 mg guaifenesin		10 mL every 4 to 6 h up to 40 mL/day	Alcohol free. EDTA, menthol, saccharin, sorbitol, sucrose. Cherry flavor. In 473 mL.
otc	**Robitussin Severe Congestion Liqui-Gels**[1] (Whitehall-Robins)				2 every 4 h up to 8/day	Liquid filled. Mannitol, sorbitol. (AHR 8601). In 24s.
otc	**Severe Congestion Tussin Softgels**[1] (AmerisourceBergen)					Sorbitol. In 12s.
otc	**Sinutab Non-Drying Liquid Caps** (Warner-Lambert)					Liquid filled. Sorbitol. In 24s.
otc	**Robitussin Cold Sinus & Congestion Tablets**[1] (Whitehall-Robins)	30 mg pseudoephedrine HCl	200 mg guaifenesin	325 mg acetaminophen	2 every 4 h up to 8/day	Lactose. Capsule shape. In 20s.
otc	**Tylenol Sinus Severe Congestion Tablets** (McNeil)				2 every 4 to 6 h up to 8/day	Capsule shape. In 24s.
Rx	**PanMist-S Syrup**[1] (Pan American)	40 mg pseudoephedrine HCl	200 mg guaifenesin		≤ 10 mL qid	Alcohol free. Grape flavor. In 15 and 473 mL.
Rx	**Stamoist E Tablets**[1] (Magna)	45 mg pseudoephedrine HCl	600 mg guaifenesin		1 tablet bid	(17). White, capsule shape, scored. In 100s.
Rx	**Profen II Tablets**[1] (IVAX)	45 mg pseudoephedrine HCl	800 mg guaifenesin		1 to 1½ every 12 h up to 3/day	Extended release. (PROFEN-II 307). White, scored. In 100s.
Rx	**Pseudoephedrine HCl/Guaifenesin SR Tablets**[1] (URL)	48 mg pseudoephedrine HCl	595 mg guaifenesin		1 or 2 every 12 h up to 4/day	Extended release. (α 1891). White, capsule shape. In 100s.
Rx	**PanMist JR Tablets**[1] (Pan American)					Extended release. (PAL 0768). White, capsule shape. Dye-free. In 100s.
Rx	**Coldmist JR Tablets**[1] (Breckenridge)					Extended release. (B 368). White, scored. In 100s.
Rx	**Respa-1st Tablets**[1] (Respa)	58 mg pseudoephedrine HCl	600 mg guaifenesin		1 or 2 every 12 h	Sustained release. (RESPA 87). White, scored. In 100s.
Rx	**Respaire-60 SR Capsules**[1] (Laser)	60 mg pseudoephedrine HCl	200 mg guaifenesin		2 every 12 h up to 4/day	Extended release. (LASER 0174). Green/clear. In 100s.
Rx	**Versacaps Capsules**[1] (Seatrace)	60 mg pseudoephedrine HCl	300 mg guaifenesin		1 every 12 h	Sustained release. Benzyl alcohol, EDTA, parabens, sucrose. In 100s.

DECONGESTANT AND EXPECTORANT COMBINATIONS

	Product & Distributor	Decongestant	Expectorant	Other	Average Adult Dose	Excipients & How Supplied
otc	**Congestac Tablets**[1] (B.F. Ascher)	60 mg pseudoephedrine HCl	400 mg guaifenesin		1 every 4 to 6 h up to 4/day	(C). Capsule shape. In 12s and 24s.
otc	**Refenesen Plus Severe Strength Cough & Cold Medicine Tablets** (Reese)					Capsule shape. In 16s.
Rx	**Zephrex Tablets**[1] (Sanofi-Synthelabo)				1 every 4 to 6 h	(Sanofi 460). Oval. Film coated. In 100s.
Rx	**AMBI 60/580 Tablets**[1] (AMBI)	60 mg pseudoephedrine HCl	580 mg guaifenesin		1 or 2 every 12 h up to 4/day	(AMBI 121). White, capsule shape. In 100s.
Rx	**Maxifed-G Tablets**[1] (MCR American)				1 or 2 every 12 h	(MAXIFED G 514). White, capsule shape. In 100s.
Rx	**Guaifenesin/Pseudoephedrine HCl Tablets**[1] (Major)	60 mg pseudoephedrine HCl	600 mg guaifenesin		1 or 2 every 12 h up to 4/day	Sustained release. In 100s.
Rx	**AquatabD Dose Pack Tablets**[1] (Adams)					Sustained release. (Adams 044). White, scored. In 56s.
Rx	**Durasal II Tablets**[1] (Prasco)					Sustained release. (300). Mottled blue, capsule shape, scored. In 100s.
Rx	**Guaifenex PSE 60 Tablets**[1] (Ethex)					Extended release. Lactose. (ETHEX/214). Blue, scored. Capsule shape. In 100s.
Rx	**Iosal II Tablets**[1] (Iopharm)					Sustained release. In 100s.
Rx	**G/P 1200/60 Tablets**[1] (Cypress)	60 mg pseudoephedrine HCl	1200 mg guaifenesin		1 every 12 h up to 2/day	Sustained release. (CYP 272). White. In 100s.
Rx	**AquatabD Tablets** (Adams)	75 mg pseudoephedrine HCl	1200 mg guaifenesin		1 every 12 h up to 2/day	Extended release. (Adams 068). Lt. green, oval, scored. In 100s.
Rx	**Maxifed Tablets**[1] (MCR American)	80 mg pseudoephedrine HCl	780 mg guaifenesin		1 to 1½ every 12 h	(MAXIFED/MCR 620). Green, capsule shape, scored. In 100s.
Rx	**Pseudoephedrine HCl/Guaifenesin LA Tablets**[1] (URL)	85 mg pseudoephedrine HCl	795 mg guaifenesin		1 every 12 h up to 3/day	Timed release. (NL 734). White, capsule shape. In 100s.
Rx	**Coldmist LA Tablets**[1] (Breckenridge)				1 every 12 h up to 2/day	Extended release. (B-367). White, scored. In 100s.
Rx	**PanMist LA Tablets**[1] (Pan American)				1 every 12 h up to 3/day	Extended release. (PAL 07/92). Pink with red specks, capsule shape. In 100s.
Rx	**H 9600 SR Tablets**[1] (Hawthorn)	90 mg pseudoephedrine HCl	600 mg guaifenesin		1 every 12 h	Sustained release. Dye-free. (HAW 301). Scored, capsule shape. In 100s.
Rx	**Profen Forte Tablets**[1] (IVAX)	90 mg pseudoephedrine HCl	800 mg guaifenesin		1 every 12 h up to 2/day	Extended release. (PROFEN FORTE 315). White, scored. In 100s.
Rx	**Dynex Tablets**[1] (Athlon)	90 mg pseudoephedrine HCl	1200 mg guaifenesin		1 every 12 h	Dye free. Sustained release. (DG 033). Scored. Capsule shape. In 30s and 100s.
Rx	**Pseudovent Capsules** (Ethex)	120 mg pseudoephedrine HCl	250 mg guaifenesin		1 every 12 h	Sustained release. EDTA, methylparaben, sucrose. (ETHEX 016). White/clear. In 100s.
Rx	**Respaire-120 SR Capsules** (Laser)				1 every 12 h up to 2/day	Extended release. (LASER 0169). Orange/clear. In 100s.
Rx	**Entex PSE Capsules**[1] (Andrx)	120 mg pseudoephedrine HCl	400 mg guaifenesin		1 every 12 h up to 2/day	Extended-release. Maltodextrin, sucrose. (ANDRX 132). (B 366). White and blue. In 100s.
Rx sf	**GP-500 Tablets**[1] (Marnel)	120 mg pseudoephedrine HCl	500 mg guaifenesin		1 bid	Dye free. Sustained release. (GP-500). White, scored, capsule shape. In 100s.
Rx	**Nasatab LA Tablets**[1] (ECR Pharm)					Sustained release. (MX/225). White, scored, capsule shape. Film-coated. In 100s.
Rx	**V-Dec-M Tablets**[1] (Seatrace)					Sustained release. (AM/PM). White, scored. In 12s and 100s.
Rx	**Touro LA Tablets** (Dartmouth)	120 mg pseudoephedrine HCl	525 mg guaifenesin		1 every 12 h	Sustained release. (DP636 TOURO LA). Capsule shape. In 100s.
Rx	**Entex PSE Tablets**[1] (Andrx)	120 mg pseudoephedrine HCl	600 mg guaifenesin		1 every 12 h	Sustained release. Sugar. (Entex PSE 032 032). Yellow, scored. In 100s.
Rx	**Guaifenex PSE 120 Tablets**[1] (Ethex)					Extended release. Dye free. (Ethex 208). White, capsule shape, scored. In 100s.
Rx	**GuaiMAX-D Tablets**[1] (Schwarz)					Extended release. (GUAIMAX-D SP 2055). White to off-white, capsule shape, scored. In 100s.
Rx	**Guaipax PSE Tablets**[1] (Eon)					Sustained release. (E784). White, scored, oval. In 100s, 250s, and 500s.
Rx	**Miraphen PSE Tablets**[1] (Major)					Extended release. In 500s.
Rx	**Zephrex LA Tablets**[1] (Sanofi-Synthelabo)					Extended release. (Sanofi LA). Orange, oval. In 100s.

DECONGESTANT AND EXPECTORANT COMBINATIONS

	Product & Distributor	Decongestant	Expectorant	Other	Average Adult Dose	Excipients & How Supplied
Rx	**GFN/PSE Tablets**[1] (Cypress)	120 mg pseudoephedrine HCl	1200 mg guaifenesin		1 every 12 h up to 2/day.	Sustained release. (CYP 266). White. In 100s.
Rx	**Guaifenex GP Tablets** (Ethex)					Extended release. Dye free. Lactose. (ETHEX 373). White, scored, oval. Film-coated. In 100s.
Rx	**Lusonal Liquid**[1] (Wraser)	7.5 mg pseudoephedrine HCl			10 mL every 6 h up to 40 mL/day	Phenylalanine, parabens, aspartame. In 473 mL.

[1] This product also may be used in children; refer to package labeling for dosing.
[2] Larken Laboratories, 148 Weisenberger Road, Madison, MS 39110; (601) 605-5275.
[3] Victory Pharma, 12707 High Bluff Dr., Suite 200, San Diego, CA 92130; (858) 350-4217, fax (858) 350-4218.

Refer to the general discussion of these products in the Respiratory Combinations Introduction. Some of the products in the following Pediatric Decongestant Expectorant Combinations table also may be used in adults.

PEDIATRIC DECONGESTANT AND EXPECTORANT COMBINATIONS

Content given per capsule or 5 mL.

	Product & Distributor	Decongestant	Expectorant	Average Dose	Excipients & How Supplied
Rx	**Donatussin Drops** (Great Southern)	1.5 mg phenylephrine HCl	20 mg guaifenesin	***1 to 2 yrs*** - 1 to 2 mL q 4 to 6 h up to 4 doses/day; ***6 mo to 1 yr*** - 0.6 to 1 mL q 4 to 6 h up to 4 doses/day; ***3 to 6 mo*** - 0.3 to 0.6 mL q 4 to 6 h up to 4 doses/day; ***1 to 3 mo*** - 2 to 3 drops per month of age q 4 to 6 h up to 4 doses/day	Raspberry flavor. In 30 mL with dropper.
Rx	**PhenaVent PED Capsules**[1] (Ethex Corporation)	7.5 mg phenylephrine HCl	200 mg guaifenesin	**6 to < 12 yrs** - 1 q 12 h	(ETHEX/079) Blue/white capsule. In 100s.
Rx	**Sina-12 X Oral Suspension** (MedPointe)	5 mg phenylephrine tannate	100 mg guaifenesin	***> 6 yrs*** — 5 to 10 mL q 12 h; ***2 to 6 yrs*** — 2.5 to 5 mL q 12 h; ***< 2 yrs*** — titrate dose individually	Methylparaben, saccharin, sucrose. Grape flavor. In 120 mL.
otc	**Thera-Hist Expectorant Chest Congestion Liquid** (Major)	15 mg pseudoephedrine HCl	50 mg guaifenesin	***6 to < 12 yrs*** - 10 mL q 4 to 6 h up to 40 mL/day; ***2 to < 6 yrs*** - 5 mL q 4 to 6 h up to 20 mL/day	EDTA, sorbitol, sucrose. Citrus flavor. In 118 mL.
otc	**Triacting Liquid** (Various, eg, AmerisourceBergen, Topco)				May contain EDTA, sorbitol, or sucrose. In 118 mL.
otc	**Triaminic Chest & Nasal Congestion Liquid** (Novartis)				Alcohol-free. EDTA, sorbitol, sucrose. Citrus flavor. In 118 mL.
Rx	**Pseudovent-PED Capsules**[1] (Ethex)	60 mg pseudoephedrine HCl	300 mg guaifenesin	***6 to 12 yrs*** - 1 q 12 h	Sustained release. EDTA, parabens, sucrose. (ETHEX/015). Blue/clear. In 100s.

[1] This product also may be used in adults; refer to package labeling for dosing.

Refer to the general discussion of these products in the Respiratory Combinations Introduction. Some of the products in the previous Decongestant and Expectorant Combinations table also may be used in children.

ANTIHISTAMINE AND ANALGESIC COMBINATIONS

Content given per capsule or tablet.

	Product & Distributor	Antihistamine	Analgesic	Average Adult Dose	Excipients & How Supplied
otc	**Coricidin HBP Cold & Flu Tablets**[a] (Schering-Plough)	2 mg chlorpheniramine maleate	325 mg acetaminophen	2 q 4 to 6 h up to 12/day	Sugar, lactose, butylparaben. In 24s.
otc	**Tylenol Sore Throat Nighttime Liquid** (McNeil Consumer)	8 mg per 5 mL diphenhydramine hydrochloride	166.6 mg per 5 mL acetaminophen	30 mL q 4 to 6 h up to 120 mL/day	Sucralose, sucrose, sorbitol. Cool burst flavor. In 240 mL.
otc	**Percogesic Extra Strength Tablets** (Medtech)	12.5 mg diphenhydramine HCl	500 mg acetaminophen	2 q 6 h up to 8/day	Dextrose. Capsule shape. In 40s.
otc	**Tylenol Severe Allergy Tablets** (McNeil)			2 q 4 to 6 h up to 8/day	Capsule shape. (TYLENOL Severe Allergy). In 24s.
otc	**Tylenol PM Extra Strength Tablets, Gelcaps, and Geltabs** (McNeil)	25 mg diphenhydramine HCl	500 mg acetaminophen	2 hs	**Tablets**: (TYLENOL PM). Capsule shape. In 24s, 50s, 100s, and 150s. **Gelcaps**: Parabens. (TYLENOL PM). In 50s. **Geltabs**: Parabens. (TYLENOL PM). In 50s and 100s.
Rx	**Ed-Flex Capsules**[1] (Edwards)	20 mg phenyltoloxamine citrate	300 mg acetaminophen 200 mg salicylamide	1 or 2 q 4 h up to 8/day	(ED-FLEX). Red. In 30s and 100s.

ANTIHISTAMINE AND ANALGESIC COMBINATIONS

	Product & Distributor	Antihistamine	Analgesic	Average Adult Dose	Excipients & How Supplied
Rx	**Ed-Flex Capsules**[1] (Edwards)	20 mg phenyltoloxamine citrate	500 mg acetaminophen 500 mg magnesium salicylate		
Rx	**Duraxin Capsules**[1] (Portal)	25 mg phenyltoloxamine citrate	325 mg acetaminophen 200 mg salicylamide	1 or 2 q 4 to 6 h up to 8/day	In 30s.
otc	**Aceta-Gesic Tablets**[1] (Rugby)	30 mg phenyltoloxamine citrate	325 mg acetaminophen	1 or 2 q 4 h up to 8/day	In 24s and 1000s.
otc	**Major-gesic Tablets**[1] (Major)				In 100s and 1000s.
otc	**Percogesic Tablets**[1] (Medtech)				Sucrose. (PERCOGESIC). In 24s, 50s, and 90s.
otc	**Phenylgesic Tablets**[1] (Ivax)				Orange. In 100s and 1000s.
Rx	**Relagesic Tablets**[1] (International Ethical)	50 mg phenyltoloxamine citrate	650 mg acetaminophen	½ or 1 every 4 to 6 h up to 5/day	(RELAGESIC IEL/650). White, scored. In 100s.

[a] This product also may be used in children; refer to package labeling for dosing.

For complete and comparative prescribing information, refer to the Respiratory Combinations Introduction.

DECONGESTANT, ANTIHISTAMINE, AND EXPECTORANT COMBINATIONS

Content given per tablet or 5 mL.

	Product & Distributor	Decongestant	Antihistamine	Expectorant	Average Adult Dose	Excipients & How Supplied
Rx	**Decolate Tablets** (Wesley)	5 mg phenylephrine HCl	4 mg chlorpheniramine maleate	100 mg guaifenesin	1 tid or qid	In 1000s.
Rx	**Ryna-12X Tablets** (MedPointe)[1]	25 mg phenylephrine tannate	60 mg pyrilamine tannate	200 mg guaifenesin	1 to 2 q 12 h	In 30s and 100s.
Rx	**Ryna-12X Suspension** (MedPointe)[1]	5 mg phenylephrine tannate	30 mg pyrilamine tannate	100 mg guaifenesin	5 to 10 mL q 12 h	Methylparaben, saccharin, sucrose. Grape flavor. In 120 mL.
Rx	**Polaramine Expectorant Liquid**[1] (Schering)	20 mg pseudoephedrine sulfate	2 mg dexchlorpheniramine maleate	100 mg guaifenesin	5 to 10 mL tid or qid	7.2% alcohol, menthol, sorbitol, sugar. In 473 mL.

[1] This product also may be used in children; refer to package labeling for dosing instructions.

Refer to the general discussion of these products in the Respiratory Combinations Introduction.

DECONGESTANTS AND ANTIHISTAMINES

Content given per capsule, tablet, or 5 mL.

	Product & Distributor	Decongestant	Antihistamine	Average Adult Dose	Excipients & How Supplied
Rx *sf*	**Alacol Syrup**[a] (Ballay Pharmaceuticals)	5 mg phenylephrine hydrochloride	2 mg brompheniramine maleate	10 mL q 4 h up to 60 mL/day	Alcohol free. Saccharin, sorbitol. Black raspberry flavor. In 473 mL bottles.
Rx	**Bromfed Capsules** (Verum Pharm)	15 mg phenylephrine hydrochloride	12 mg brompheniramine maleate	1 q 12 h	Extended release. Parabens, sucrose. (BROMFED 12-15 VERUM). Purple/Clear. In 100s.
Rx	**Rhinabid Capsules**[a] (Breckenridge)				Extended release. Sugar. (B092). In 100s.
Rx	**Norel LA Tablets** (US Pharmaceutical)	40 mg phenylephrine hydrochloride	8 mg carbinoxamine maleate	1 q 12 h up to 2/day	Extended release. (4 35 US). Maroon and white, bi-layer, triangle shape. In 100s.
otc	**Histatab Plus Tablets**[a] (Century)	5 mg phenylephrine hydrochloride	2 mg chlorpheniramine maleate	2 q 4 h up to 12/day	In 30s, 100s, and 1000s.
Rx	**Ed A-Hist Liquid**[a] (Edwards)	10 mg phenylephrine hydrochloride	4 mg chlorpheniramine maleate	5 mL tid or qid	5% alcohol. Grape flavor. In 473 mL.
Rx *sf*	**Rondec Syrup**[a] (Alliant)	12.5 mg phenylephrine hydrochloride	4 mg chlorpheniramine maleate	5 mL q 4 to 6 h up to 30 mL/day	Alcohol free. Saccharin, sorbitol. Bubble gum flavor. In 20, 118, and 473 mL.
Rx	**Ed A-Hist Tablets** (Edwards)	20 mg phenylephrine hydrochloride	8 mg chlorpheniramine maleate	1 q 12 h	Sustained release. (MAR-CPM). Light brown. In 100s.
Rx	**NoHist Tablets**[a] (Sovereign Pharmaceuticals)				(LL 60). White, capsule shape, scored. In 100s.
Rx *sf*	**Nalex-A Liquid**[a] (Blansett Pharmacal)	5 mg phenylephrine hydrochloride	2.5 mg chlorpheniramine maleate, 7.5 mg phenyltoloxamine citrate	10 mL q 4 h	Alcohol free. Cotton candy flavor. In 437 mL.
Rx	**Nalex-A Tablets**[a] (Blansett Pharmacal)	20 mg phenylephrine hydrochloride	4 mg chlorpheniramine maleate, 40 mg phenyltoloxamine citrate	1 bid or tid	Lactose. (Blansett 3/08). Beige, capsule shape. In 100s.
Rx	**Promethazine Hydrochloride and Phenylephrine Hydrochloride Syrup**[a] (Various, eg, Alpharma)	5 mg phenylephrine hydrochloride	6.25 mg promethazine hydrochloride	5 mL q 4 to 6 h up to 30 mL/day	7% alcohol. May contain sorbitol, sugar, parabens. In 118 and 473 mL and 3.8 L.
Rx	**Phenergan VC Syrup**[a] (Wyeth-Ayerst)				7% alcohol, saccharin. In 118 and 473 mL.
Rx	**Prometh VC Plain Syrup**[a] (Alpharma)				7% alcohol. In 3.8 L.

DECONGESTANTS AND ANTIHISTAMINES

	Product & Distributor	Decongestant	Antihistamine	Average Adult Dose	Excipients & How Supplied
Rx	**J-Tand Suspension**[a] (Jaymac Pharmaceuticals)	5 mg phenylephrine tannate	4 mg brompheniramine tannate	5 to 10 mL q 12 h up to 20 mL/day	Aspartame, parabens. Strawberry cream flavor. In 473 mL.
Rx	**BroveX-D Suspension**[a] (Pharmakon Labs)	20 mg phenylephrine tannate	12 mg brompheniramine tannate	5 to 10 mL q 12 h	Aspartame, parabens. Bubble gum flavor. In 473 mL.
Rx	**R-Tanna Tablets** (Prasco)	25 mg phenylephrine tannate	9 mg chlorpheniramine tannate	1 or 2 q 12 h	(KL142). Mottled tan, capsule shape. In 100s.
Rx	**Nalex-A 12 Suspension**[a] (Blansett Pharmacal)	5 mg phenylephrine tannate	2 mg chlorpheniramine tannate, 12.5 mg pyrilamine tannate	30 mL q 12 h	Sucrose, saccharin, methylparaben. Raspberry flavor. In 118 mL.
Rx	**Tana Cof A12 Suspension**[1] (Larken Laboratories)				Methylparaben saccharin, sucrose. Raspberry flavor. In 118 mL.
Rx	**AllerTan Suspension**[a] (ProEthic)	15 mg phenylephrine tannate	8 mg chlorpheniramine tannate, 12.5 mg pyrilamine tannate	5 to 10 mL every 12 h up to 20 mL/day	Saccharin, sorbitol, methylparaben. Grape flavor. In 473 mL.
Rx	**Dytan-D Chewable Tablets**[a] (Hawthorn)	5 mg phenylephrine tannate	25 mg diphenhydramine tannate	1 to 2 q 12 h	Aspartame, sorbitol, 1.5 mg phenylalanine. (HAW 577). Blue, triangular, scored. Berry flavor. In 60s.
Rx	**D-Tann Suspension**[a] (Midlothian Laboratories)	7.5 mg phenylephrine tannate	25 mg diphenhydramine tannate	5 to 10 mL q 12 h	Methylparaben, saccharin, sucrose. Bubble gum flavor. In 118 mL.
Rx	**AlleRx Suspension**[1] (Cornerstone Biopharma)	7.5 mg phenylephrine tannate	3 mg chlorpheniramine tannate	15 mL q 12 h	Methylparaben, saccharin, sucrose. Raspberry flavor. In 473 mL.
Rx	**K-Tan 4 Suspension**[a] (Prasco Laboratories)	5 mg phenylephrine tannate	30 mg pyrilamine tannate	5 to 10 mL q 12 h	Methylparaben, saccharin, sucrose. Strawberry flavor. In 118 mL unit of use containers.
Rx	**Tanavan Suspension**[a] (Scientific Laboratories)	12.5 mg phenylephrine tannate	30 mg pyrilamine tannate	5 to 10 mL q 12 h	Grape flavor. In 118 and 473 mL.
Rx	**Viravan-S Suspension** (PediaMed)				In 118 and 473 mL.
Rx	**Viravan-T Chewable Tablets**[a] (PediaMed)	25 mg phenylephrine tannate	30 mg pyrilamine tannate	1 q 12 h	Dye free. Sugar, saccharin. (VIRAVAN). Mottled brown, scored. Grape flavor. In 100s.
Rx	**K-Tan**[a] **Tablets** (Prasco Laboratories)	25 mg phenylephrine tannate	60 mg pyrilamine tannate	1 or 2 q 12 h	(PRASCO 525). Buff, capsule shape, scored. In 100s.
Rx	**Ryna-12 Tablets**[a] (Wallace)				(WALLACE 673). Buff, capsule shape, scored. In 100s.
Rx	**Semprex-D Capsules** (Celltech)	60 mg pseudoephedrine hydrochloride	8 mg acrivastine	1 q 4 to 6 h up to 4/day	Lactose. (MEDEVA SEMPREX-D). Dark green opaque/white opaque. In 100s.
otc	**Bromfed Syrup** (Muro)	30 mg pseudoephedrine hydrochloride	2 mg brompheniramine maleate	10 mL q 4 to 6 h up to 40 mL/day	Saccharin, sorbitol, sucrose, methylparaben. Orange-lemon flavor. In 480 mL.
Rx	**Brofed Liquid**[a] (Marnel)	30 mg pseudoephedrine hydrochloride	4 mg brompheniramine maleate	10 mL tid	Parabens, saccharin, sorbitol, sucrose, corn syrup, menthol. Mint flavor. In 473 mL.
Rx	**BPM Pseudo 6/45 mg Tablets**[a] (Boca Pharmacal)	45 mg pseudoephedrine hydrochloride	6 mg brompheniramine maleate	1 or 2 q 12 h	Extended release. (BP 544). White, oval. In 100s.
Rx	**Bidhist-D Tablets**[a] (Cypress Pharmaceutical)				Extended release. (CYP 470). White, oval. In 100s.
Rx	**Lodrane 12 D Tablets**[a] (ECR)				Extended release. Dye free. (ECR 645). White, oval, scored. In 100s.
Rx	**LoHist 12D Tablets**[a] (Pharmakon Labs)				Extended release. Dye free. (LH 12D). White, scored. In 100s.
Rx	**Brompheniramine Maleate/Pseudoephedrine Hydrochloride Syrup**[a] (Cypress)	60 mg pseudoephedrine hydrochloride	4 mg brompheniramine maleate	5 mL qid	Saccharin, sorbitol. Raspberry flavor. In 473 mL.
Rx	**Bromfed Tablets**[a] (Muro)			1 q 4 h up to 6/day	Lactose. (MURO 4060). White, scored. In 100s.
Rx sf	**Lodrane Liquid**[a] (ECR)			5 mL q 4 to 6 h up to 20 mL/day	Alcohol and dye free. Cherry flavor. In 473 mL.
Rx	**Touro Allergy Capsules**[1] (Dartmouth)	60 mg pseudoephedrine hydrochloride	5.75 mg brompheniramine maleate	1 or 2 q 12 h	Sustained release. Sucrose. (TOURO ALLERGY). Orange/clear. In 100s.
Rx	**Lodrane LD Capsules**[a] (ECR)	60 mg pseudoephedrine hydrochloride	6 mg brompheniramine maleate	1 or 2 q 12 h	Dye free. (ECR 6006). Clear. In 100s.
Rx	**Respahist Capsules**[a] (Respa)			1 or 2 q 12 h up to 4/day	Sustained release. In 100s.
Rx	**Brovex SR Capsules**[1] (Athlon Pharmaceuticals)	90 mg pseudoephedrine hydrochloride	9 mg brompheniramine maleate	1 q 12 h up to 2/day	Extended release. Sucrose. (271 9/90). Blue and yellow. In 100s.

DECONGESTANTS AND ANTIHISTAMINES

	Product & Distributor	Decongestant	Antihistamine	Average Adult Dose	Excipients & How Supplied
Rx	**Histex SR Capsules** (Teamm Pharm)	120 mg pseudoephedrine hydrochloride	10 mg brompheniramine maleate	1 q 12 h	Extended release. (SR 089). Peach/clear. In 30s and 100s.
Rx	**Uni-Tex 120/10 ER Capsules**[a] (URL)				Extended release. In 30s and 100s.
Rx	**Bromfenex Capsules** (Ethex)	120 mg pseudoephedrine hydrochloride	12 mg brompheniramine maleate	1 q 12 h	Extended release. Sucrose. (Ethex/019). Lt green/clear. In 100s.
Rx	**ULTRAbrom Capsules** (WE Pharm)				Extended release. In 100s and dispenser pack 10s.
Rx	**Rondec Tablets**[a] (Biovail)	60 mg pseudoephedrine hydrochloride	4 mg carbinoxamine maleate	1 qid	Lactose. (D 22). Orange. In 100s and 500s.
Rx	**Palgic-D Tablets**[a] (Pan American)	80 mg pseudoephedrine hydrochloride	8 mg carbinoxamine maleate	1 q 12 h	Extended release. Dye-free. (PAL 61/31). White, capsule shape, scored. In 100s.
Rx	**Coldec D Tablets**[a] (Breckenridge)				White, capsule shape. In 100s.
Rx	**Rondec-TR Tablets** (Biovail)	120 mg pseudoephedrine hydrochloride	8 mg carbinoxamine maleate	1 bid	Timed release. Dextrose, lactose. (D 25). Blue. In 100s.
Rx	**Zyrtec-D 12 Hour Tablets** (Pfizer)	120 mg pseudoephedrine hydrochloride	5 mg cetirizine hydrochloride	1 bid	Extended release. Lactose. (ZYRTEC-D). White, bilayered. In 100s.
Rx	**PSE CPM**[a] **Tablets** (Boca)	15 mg pseudoephedrine hydrochloride	2 mg chlorpheniramine maleate	2 q 4 to 6 h	Aspartame, sugar. (BOCA 133). Purple, capsule shape, scored. Grape flavor. In 100s.
otc	**Allerest Maximum Strength Tablets** (Heritage Consumer Products)	30 mg pseudoephedrine hydrochloride	2 mg chlorpheniramine maleate	2 q 4 to 6 h up to 8/day	In 24s.
Rx	**Deconamine Syrup**[1] (Kenwood)			5 to 10 mL tid or qid	Alcohol and dye free. Sorbitol, sucrose. Grape flavor. In 473 mL.
Rx	**RE2+30 Syrup**[a] (River's Edge Pharmaceuticals)			5 to 10 mL tid or qid	Saccharin, sorbitol. Grape flavor. In 118 mL.
otc *sf*	**Scot-Tussin Hayfebrol Liquid**[a] (Scot-Tussin)			10 mL q 6 h up to 40 mL/day	Alcohol and dye free. Parabens, menthol. In 120 mL.
Rx	**Histex Liquid**[a] (Teamm Pharm)			10 mL q 4 to 6 h	Peach flavor. In 15, 29.6, and 473 mL.
Rx	**Deconamine Tablets** (Kenwood)	60 mg pseudoephedrine hydrochloride	4 mg chlorpheniramine maleate	1 tid or qid	Lactose. (KENWOOD 184). White, scored. In 100s.
Rx	**Kronofed-A Jr. Capsules** (Ferndale)			1 q 12 h	Sustained release. (FL). In 100s and 500s.
otc	**Sudafed Cold & Allergy Maximum Strength Tablets**[a] (Warner-Lambert)			1 q 4 to 6 h up to 4/day	Lactose. In 24s.
Rx	**Clorfed Tablets**[a] (Stewart-Jackson)			1 to 2 q 12 h	Extended release. (CLORFED). White, scored. In 100s.
Rx *sf*	**Amerifed Liquid**[a] (AMBI Pharm)	80 mg pseudoephedrine hydrochloride	4 mg chlorpheniramine maleate	5 mL q 8 h up to 15 mL/day	Alcohol free. Parabens, aspartame, phenylalanine. Raspberry flavor. In 30 and 473 mL.
Rx	**QDALL** (Atley)	100 mg pseudoephedrine hydrochloride	12 mg chlorpheniramine maleate	1 qd up to 2/day	Sucrose. (QD 112). Blue/yellow. In 100s.
Rx	**Chlorpheniramine Maleate/Pseudoephedrine Hydrochloride ER Capsules** (Various, eg, Eon, Kremers Urban)	120 mg pseudoephedrine hydrochloride	8 mg chlorpheniramine maleate	1 q 12 h	Extended release. May contain parabens and sucrose. In 100s, 250s, 500s, and 1,000s.
Rx	**Deconamine SR Capsules** (Kenwood)				Sustained release. Sugar. (KENWOOD 181). Blue/yellow. In 100s, 500s, and 1,000s.
Rx	**Deconomed SR Capsules** (Iopharm)				Sustained release. Sucrose, parabens. Blue/clear. In 100s and 500s.
Rx	**Kronofed-A Capsules** (Ferndale)				Sustained release. (FL). In 100s and 500s.
Rx	**N D Clear Capsules** (Seatrace)				Sustained release. Clear. In 100s and 1,000s.
Rx	**Time-Hist Capsules** (MCR American)				Sustained release. (PT/026). Clear. In 100s.
Rx	**Biohist-LA Tablets**[a] (IVAX)	120 mg pseudoephedrine hydrochloride	12 mg chlorpheniramine maleate	½ to 1 q 12 h	Sustained release. In 100s.
Rx	**Histade Capsules** (Breckenridge)			1 q 12 h	Sustained release. Sucrose. (B170). Red. In 100s.
Rx *sf*	**Hexafed Tablets** (Alaven Pharmaceutical)	60 mg pseudoephedrine hydrochloride	4 mg dexchlorpheniramine maleate	1 bid up to 3/day	Extended release. (AP 27). White. Film coated. In 100s.
otc	**Benadryl Allergy & Sinus Fastmelt Dissolving Tablets** (Warner-Lambert)	30 mg pseudoephedrine hydrochloride	19 mg diphenhydramine citrate (12.5 mg diphenhydramine hydrochloride)	2 q 4 to 6 h up to 8/day	4.6 mg phenylalanine, aspartame, mannitol. In 20s.
otc	**Benadryl Allergy & Sinus Liquid**[1] (Warner-Lambert)	30 mg pseudoephedrine hydrochloride	12.5 mg diphenhydramine hydrochloride	10 mL q 4 to 6 h up to 40 mL/day	Saccharin, sorbitol. Grape flavor. In 118 mL.

DECONGESTANTS AND ANTIHISTAMINES

	Product & Distributor	Decongestant	Antihistamine	Average Adult Dose	Excipients & How Supplied
otc	**Benadryl Allergy & Sinus Tablets** (Warner-Lambert)	60 mg pseudoephedrine hydrochloride	25 mg diphenhydramine hydrochloride	1 q 4 to 6 h up to 4/day	In 24s.
Rx	**Allegra-D 12 Hour Tablets** (Aventis)	120 mg pseudoephedrine hydrochloride	60 mg fexofenadine hydrochloride	1 bid	Extended release. (06/012D). White, tan. Layered. Film coated. In 100s, 500s, and blister pack 100s.
Rx	**Allegra-D 24 Hour Tablets** (Aventis)	240 mg pseudoephedrine hydrochloride	180 mg fexofenadine hydrochloride	1 q 24 h	Extended release. Alcohols, talc. (308AV). White. Film coated. In 30s, 100s, and 500s.
Rx	**Quadra-Hist D Capsules** (Ethex)	80 mg pseudoephedrine hydrochloride	16 mg pheniramine maleate, 16 mg phenyltoloxamine citrate, 16 mg pyrilamine maleate	1 q 8 to 12 h	Extended release. Sucrose. (ETHEX/056). Opaque pink/white. In 100s.
otc	**Triprolidine Hydrochloride w/Pseudoephedrine Hydrochloride Syrup**[a] (Various, eg, Ivax)	30 mg pseudoephedrine hydrochloride	1.25 mg triprolidine hydrochloride	10 mL q 4 to 6 h up to 40 mL/day	In 118 mL.
otc	**Allerfrim Syrup**[a] (Rugby)				Sucrose, methylparaben, sorbitol, corn syrup. In 118 and 473 mL.
otc	**Aprodine Syrup**[a] (Major)				In 118 mL.
otc	**Silafed Syrup**[a] (Silarx)			10 mL q 4 h up to 40 mL/day	Methylparaben, sucrose, saccharin. In 118 and 237 mL.
otc	**Actifed Cold & Allergy Tablets**[a] (Warner-Lambert)	60 mg pseudoephedrine hydrochloride	2.5 mg triprolidine hydrochloride	1 q 4 to 6 h up to 4/day	Sucrose, lactose. In 12s and 24s.
otc	**Allerfrim Tablets**[a] (Rugby)				Lactose. (Rugby). Scored. Film-coated. In 24s, 100s, and 1,000s.
otc	**Aprodine Tablets**[a] (Major)				Lactose. In 24s.
otc	**Cenafed Plus Tablets**[a] (Century)				In 30s and 1,000s.
otc	**Genac Tablets**[a] (Ivax)				Lactose. White. In 48s.
otc	**Sudafed Sinus Nighttime Maximum Strength Tablets**[a] (Warner-Lambert)				Lactose, sucrose. In 12s.
Rx	**Sudal-12 Chewable Tablets**[a] (Atley Pharmaceuticals)	pseudoephedrine polistirex equivalent to 30 mg pseudoephedrine hydrochloride	chlorpheniramine polistirex equivalent to 4 mg chlorpheniramine maleate	1 to 2 q 12 h	Aspartame, 25 mg phenylalanine. (A/P 30/4). Purple. Grape flavor. In 100s.
Rx	**Sudal-12 Suspension**[a] (Atley Pharmaceuticals)	pseudoephedrine polistirex equivalent to 30 mg pseudoephedrine hydrochloride	chlorpheniramine polistirex equivalent to 6 mg chlorpheniramine maleate	5 to 10 mL q 12 h	Extended release Corn syrup, parabens. Strawberry flavor. In 473 mL.
otc	**Chlor-Trimeton Allergy-D 4 Hour Tablets**[a] (Schering-Plough)	60 mg pseudoephedrine sulfate	4 mg chlorpheniramine maleate	1 q 4 to 6 h up to 4/day	Lactose. In 24s.
otc	**Chlor-Trimeton Allergy-D 12 Hour Tablets** (Schering-Plough)	120 mg pseudoephedrine sulfate	8 mg chlorpheniramine maleate	1 q 12 h up to 2/day	Butylparaben, sugar, lactose. (LA CTM D). In 24s.
Rx	**Clarinex-D 12 Hour Tablets** (Schering)	120 mg pseudoephedrine sulfate	2.5 mg desloratadine	1 bid approximately 12 hours apart	Extended release. EDTA. (D12). Blue and white bilayered, oval. In 100s.
Rx	**Clarinex-D 24 Hour Tablets** (Schering)	240 mg pseudoephedrine sulfate	5 mg desloratadine	1 q 24 h	Extended release. EDTA. (D 24). Light blue, oval. In 100s.
Rx	**Drixomed Tablets** (Iopharm)	120 mg pseudoephedrine sulfate	6 mg dexbrompheniramine maleate	1 q 12 h up to 2/day	Sustained release Green. In 100s and 500s.
otc	**Drixoral Cold & Allergy Tablets** (Schering-Plough)				Sugar, lactose, butylparaben. (DRIXORAL). In 10s.
otc	**Claritin-D 12 Hour Tablets** (Schering-Plough)	120 mg pseudoephedrine sulfate	5 mg loratadine	1 q 12 h	Extended release. Lactose, sugar, butylparaben. (CLARITIN-D). White. In 100s, unit of use 30s, and UD 100s.
otc	**Alavert Allergy & Sinus D-12 Hour Tablets** (Wyeth Consumer)			1 q 12 h up to 2/day	Extended release. Lactose. In 12s.
otc	**Claritin-D 24 Hour Tablets** (Schering-Plough)	240 mg pseudoephedrine sulfate	10 mg loratadine	1 q 24 h	Extended release. Sugar. (CLARITIN-D 24 HOUR). White, oval. In 100s and UD 100s.
otc	**Clear-Atadine D Tablets** (Major)				Extended release. Lactose. In 10s and 15s.

DECONGESTANTS AND ANTIHISTAMINES

	Product & Distributor	Decongestant	Antihistamine	Average Adult Dose	Excipients & How Supplied
Rx sf	**Lodrane D Suspension**[a] (ECR)	90 mg pseudoephedrine tannate	8 mg brompheniramine tannate	5 mL q 12 h up to 10 mL/day	Alcohol free. Strawberry flavor. In 473 mL.
Rx	**C-PHED Tannate Suspension**[a] (Morton Grove)	75 mg pseudoephedrine tannate	4.5 mg chlorpheniramine tannate	10 to 20 mL q 12 h up to 40 mL/day	Strawberry/banana flavor. In 118 mL.
Rx	**CP-TANNIC Suspension**[a] (Cypress)				Strawberry/banana flavor. In 473 mL.
Rx	**Tanafed DP Suspension**[a] (First Horizon)				Methylparaben, saccharin, sucrose. Strawberry-banana flavor. In 20, 118, and 473 mL.

[a] This product also may be used in children; refer to package labeling for dosing.

Refer to the general discussion of these products in the Respiratory Combinations Introduction. Some of the products in the following Pediatric Decongestants and Antihistamines table also may be used in adults.

PEDIATRIC DECONGESTANTS AND ANTIHISTAMINES

Content given per tablet, capsule, 5 mL (liquid), or 1 mL (drops).

	Product & Distributor	Decongestant	Antihistamine	Average Dose	Excipients & How Supplied
Rx	**Bromfed-PD Capsules**[1] (Verum Pharm)	7.5 mg phenylephrine HCl	6 mg brompheniramine maleate	***6 to under 12 yrs*** - 1 q 12 h	Extended release. Parabens, sucrose. (BROMFED-PD 6-7.5 VERUM). Purple. In 100s.
Rx	**Rhinabid PD Capsules**[1] (Breckenridge Pharmaceutical, Inc.)				Extended release. Sugar. (B093). White to off-white beads. In 100s.
Rx	**Dallergy Oral Drops** (Laser)	2 mg phenylephrine HCl	1 mg chlorpheniramine maleate	***12 to 24 mo*** — 1 to 2 mL q 4 to 6 h up to 4 doses/day; ***6 to 12 mo*** — 0.6 to 1 mL q 4 to 6 h up to 4 doses/day; ***3 to 5 mo*** — 0.3 to 0.6 mL q 4 to 6 h up to 4 doses/day; ***1 to 3 mo*** — 2 to 3 drops per month of age q 4 to 6 h up to 4 doses/day	Peach/Tangerine flavor. In 30 mL.
Rx sf	**Rondec Oral Drops** (Alliant)	3.5 mg phenylephrine HCl	1 mg chlorpheniramine maleate	***12 to 24 mos*** - 1 mL qid; ***6 to 12 mos*** - 0.75 mL qid	Alcohol free. Saccharin, sorbitol. Bubble gum flavor. In 30 mL with calibrated dropper.
Rx	**Dallergy-JR Capsules**[1] (Laser)	20 mg phenylephrine HCl	4 mg chlorpheniramine maleate	***6 to 12 yrs*** - 1 q 12 h up to 2/day	Extended release. Sucrose. (DALLERGY JR Laser 176). Maize/Clear. In 100s.
Rx	**Rescon-Jr. Tablets**[1] (Capellon)			***> 12 yrs*** - 1 or 2 q 12 h; ***6 to 12 yrs*** - 1 q 12 h	Extended-release. (RESCON JR). Yellow and white, capsule shape, scored. In 100s.
Rx sf	**Polyhist PD Suspension**[1] (Great Southern Laboratories)	7.5 mg phenylephrine HCl	2 mg chlorpheniramine maleate, 12.5 mg pyrilamine maleate	***6 to 12 yrs*** - 5 mL q 4 to 6 h; ***2 to 6 yrs*** - 2.5 mL q 4 to 6 h; ***< 2 yrs*** - consult physician	Alcohol and dye free. Saccharin, sorbitol. Bubble gum flavor. In 473 mL.
Rx	**Nuhist Suspension** (Dayton)	5 mg phenylephrine tannate	4.5 mg chlorpheniramine tannate	***> 6 yrs*** - 5 to 10 mL q 12 h; ***2 to 6 yrs*** - 2.5 to 5 mL q 12 h; ***< 2 yrs*** - titrate dose	Methylparaben, saccharin, sucrose. In 473 mL.
Rx	**Phenyl Chlor-Tan Suspension** (Hi-Tech)			***> 6 yrs*** - 5 to 10 mL q 12 h; ***2 to 6 yrs*** - 2.5 to 5 mL q 12 h; ***< 2 yrs*** - titrate dose individually	Methylparaben, saccharin, sucrose. Raspberry flavor. In 473 mL.
Rx	**Rhinatate-NF Pediatric Suspension** (Major)				Methylparaben, saccharin, sucrose. In 473 mL.
Rx	**R-Tanna S Pediatric Suspension** (Prasco)				Methylparaben, saccharin, sucrose. Grape flavor. In 118 mL.
Rx	**Rynatan Pediatric Suspension** (Wallace)				Tartrazine, methylparaben, saccharin, sucrose. Strawberry-currant flavor. In 473 mL.
Rx	**Rynatan Chewable Tablets** (MedPointe)			***> 6 yrs*** - 1 or 2 q 12 h; ***2 to 6 yrs*** - 1/2 to 1 q 12 h	Maltodextrin, saccharin, sucrose. (RYNATAN 712). Purple, capsule shape, scored. Grape flavor. In 30s.
Rx	**Dallergy-JR Suspension**[1] (Laser)	20 mg phenylephrine tannate	4 mg chlorpheniramine tannate	***6 to < 12 yrs*** - 5 mL q 12 h up to 10 mL/day, ***2 to < 6 yrs*** - 2.5 mL q 12 h up to 5 mL/day	In 473 mL.

PEDIATRIC DECONGESTANTS AND ANTIHISTAMINES

	Product & Distributor	Decongestant	Antihistamine	Average Dose	Excipients & How Supplied
Rx	**Phenylephrine Tannate/Chlorpheniramine Tannate/Pyrilamine Tannate Pediatric Suspension** (Duramed)	5 mg phenylephrine tannate	2 mg chlorpheniramine tannate, 12.5 mg pyrilamine tannate	***> 6 yrs*** - 5 to 10 mL q 12 h; ***2 to 6 yrs*** - 2.5 to 5 mL q 12 h; ***< 2 yrs*** - titrate dose individually	Methylparaben, saccharin, sucrose. Strawberry-blackberry-currant flavor. In 118 mL unit of use and 473 mL.
Rx	**Rhinatate Pediatric Suspension** (Major)				Methylparaben, saccharin, sucrose. Strawberry-blackberry-currant flavor. In 473 mL.
Rx	**Triotann Pediatric Suspension** (Prasco)				Methylparaben, saccharin, sucrose. Strawberry-blackberry-currant flavor. In 473 mL.
Rx	**Triotann-S Pediatric Suspension** (Duramed)				Methylparaben, saccharin, sucrose. Strawberry-blackberry-currant flavor. In 118 mL unit of use.
Rx	**Duonate-12 Suspension** (URL)	5 mg phenylephrine tannate	30 mg pyrilamine tannate	***> 6 yrs*** - 5 to 10 mL q 12 h; ***2 to 6 yrs*** - 2.5 to 5 mL q 12 h; ***< 2 yrs*** - titrate dose individually	In 118 mL unit of use with oral syringe.
Rx	**R-Tanna 12 Suspension** (Duramed)				Saccharin, sucrose, methylparaben. Strawberry-currant flavor. In 118 mL unit of use with oral syringe.
Rx	**Ryna-12 S Suspension** (Wallace)				Methylparaben, saccharin, sucrose. Strawberry-currant flavor. In 118 mL unit of use with oral syringe.
Rx	**AccuHist Drops** (PediaMed)	12.5 mg pseudoephedrine HCl	1 mg brompheniramine maleate	***12 to 24 mos*** - 1 mL qid up to 4 mL/day; ***6 to 12 mos*** - 0.75 mL qid up to 3 mL/day; ***3 to 6 mos*** - 0.5 mL qid up to 2 mL/day; ***1 to 3 mos*** - 0.25 mL qid up to 1 mL/day.	Saccharin, sorbitol. Cherry flavor. In 30 mL w/dropper.
Rx	**Bromhist-NR Drops** (Cypress)				Saccharin, sorbitol. Alcohol free. Cherry flavor. In 30 mL w/calibrated dropper.
Rx sf	**LoHist-PD Pediatric Drops**				Saccharin, sorbitol. Cherry flavor. In 30 mL bottle with dropper.
otc	**Bromanate Elixir** (Alpharma)	15 mg pseudoephedrine HCl	1 mg brompheniramine maleate	***6 to < 12 yrs*** - 10 mL q 4 h up to 40 mL/day	Alcohol free. Grape flavor. In 118, 237, and 473 mL.
otc	**Dimaphen Elixir**[1] (Major)			***6 to < 12 yrs*** - 10 mL q 4 to 6 h up to 40 mL/day	Alcohol free. Saccharin, sorbitol. Grape flavor. In 118 and 237 mL.
otc	**Dimetapp Cold & Allergy Elixir**[1] (Whitehall-Robins)			***6 to < 12 yrs*** - 10 mL q 4 h up to 40 mL/day	Alcohol free. Corn syrup, saccharin, sorbitol. Grape flavor. In 118 and 237 mL.
Rx	**Brompheniramine Maleate/ Pseudoephedrine HCl Syrup** (Cypress)	30 mg pseudoephedrine HCl	4 mg brompheniramine maleate	***> 6 yrs*** - 5 mL qid; ***2 to 6 yrs*** - 2.5 mL qid	Saccharin, sorbitol. Raspberry flavor. In 473 mL.
Rx	**Bromfenex PD Capsules**[1] (Ethex)	60 mg pseudoephedrine HCl	6 mg brompheniramine maleate	***6 to 12 yrs*** - 1 q 12 h	Extended release. Opaque green/clear. Sucrose. (Ethex/020). In 100s.
Rx	**ULTRAbrom PD Capsules**[1] (WE Pharm)				Extended release. (WE 04). Purple/clear. In 100s.
Rx sf	**AccuHist Drops** (PediaMed)	12.5 mg pseudoephedrine HCl	1 mg brompheniramine maleate	***12 to 24 mos*** - 1 mL qid up to 4 mL/day; ***6 to 12 mos*** - 0.75 mL qid up to 3 mL/day; ***3 to 6 mos*** - 0.5 mL qid up to 2 mL/day; ***1 to 3 mos*** - 0.25 mL qid up to 2 mL/day	Saccharin, sorbitol. Cherry flavor. In 30 mL bottle with dropper.
Rx sf	**Pediatex-D Liquid** (Zyber)	12.5 mg pseudoephedrine HCl	1.67 mg carbinoxamine maleate	≥ ***6 yrs*** - 10 mL qid; ***18 mos to 6 yrs*** - 5 mL qid; ***9 to 18 mos*** - 3.75 to 5 mL qid; ***6 to 9 mos*** - 3.75 mL qid; ***3 to 6 mos*** - 2.5 mL qid; ***1 to 3 mos*** - 1.25 mL qid	Alcohol and dye free. Cotton candy flavor. In 20 and 473 mL.
Rx sf	**Andehist NR Drops** (Silarx)	15 mg pseudoephedrine HCl	1 mg carbinoxamine maleate	***12 to 24 mos*** - 1 mL qid; ***6 to 12 mos*** - 0.75 mL qid; ***3 to 6 mos*** - 0.5 mL qid; ***1 to 3 mos*** - 0.25 mL qid	Alcohol free. Saccharin, sorbitol. In 30 mL bottle with dropper.
Rx sf	**Carbaxefed RF Oral Drops** (Morton Grove)				Alcohol free. Saccharin, sorbitol. Cherry flavor. In 30 mL bottle with dropper.
Rx sf	**Cordron-D Liquid**[1] (Cypress Pharmaceutical, Inc.)	7.5 mg pseudoephedrine HCl	2 mg carbinoxamine maleate	***> 6 yrs*** - 10 mL qid; ***18 mos to 6 yrs*** - 5 mL qid; ***9 to 18 mos*** - 3.75 to 5 mL qid; ***6 to 9 mos*** - 3.75 mL qid; ***3 to 6 mos*** - 2.5 mL qid; ***1 to 3 mos*** - 1.25 mL qid	Alcohol and dye free. Saccharin, sorbitol. Cotton candy flavor. In 473 mL.

PEDIATRIC DECONGESTANTS AND ANTIHISTAMINES

	Product & Distributor	Decongestant	Antihistamine	Average Dose	Excipients & How Supplied
Rx	**Palgic DS Syrup** (Pan American)	25 mg pseudoephedrine HCl	2 mg carbinoxamine maleate	≥ ***6 yrs*** - 10 mL qid; ***18 mos to 6 yrs*** - 5 mL qid; ***10 to 18 mos*** - 5 mL qid; ***7 to 9 mos*** - 3.75 mL qid; ***4 to 6 mos*** - 2.5 mL qid; ***1 to 3 mos*** - 1.25 mL qid	Strawberry/pineapple flavor. In 15 and 473 mL.
Rx sf	**Carbic DS Syrup**[1] (Scientific Laboratories, Inc.)			***18 mos to 6 yrs*** - 5 mL qid; ***9 to 18 mos*** - 3.75 to 5 mL qid; ***6 to 9 mos*** - 3.75 mL qid; ***3 to 6 mos*** - 2.5 mL qid; ***1 to 3 mos*** - 1.25 mL qid	Alcohol and dye free. Strawberry-pineapple fruit flavor. In 473 mL.
Rx sf	**Carbinoxamine Oral Drops** (Morton Grove)			***9 to 18 mos*** - 1 mL qid; ***6 to 9 mos*** - 0.75 mL qid; ***3 to 6 mos*** - 0.5 mL qid; ***1 to 3 mos*** - 0.25 mL qid	Alcohol free. Parabens, sorbitol. Raspberry or fruit flavors. In 30 mL w/dropper.
Rx	**Cydec Oral Drops** (Cypress)				Raspberry flavor. In 30 mL.
Rx sf	**Carbinoxamine Syrup**[1] (Morton Grove)	60 mg pseudoephedrine HCl	4 mg carbinoxamine maleate	***< 6 yrs*** - 5 mL qid; ***18 mos to 6 yrs*** - 2.5 mL qid	Alcohol free. Parabens, sorbitol. Raspberry or fruit flavors. In 118, 237, and 473 mL.
otc	**PediaCare Children's Cold & Allergy Liquid** (Pfizer Consumer Healthcare)	15 mg pseudoephedrine HCl	1 mg chlorpheniramine maleate	***6 to 11 yrs*** - 10 mL q 4 to 6 h up to 40 mL/day	Alcohol free. Corn syrup, sorbitol. Bubble-gum flavor. In 120 mL.
otc	**Thera-Hist Cold & Allergy Syrup** (Major)			***6 to < 12 yrs*** - 10 mL q 4 to 6 h up to 40 mL/day	Sorbitol, sucrose. In 118 mL.
otc	**Tri-Acting Cold & Allergy Syrup** (Topco)				Alcohol free. Sorbitol, sucrose. Orange flavor. In 118 mL.
otc	**Triacting Cold & Allergy Liquid** (AmerisourceBergen)				Alcohol free. Sorbitol, sucrose. Orange flavor. In 118 mL.
otc	**Triaminic Cold & Allergy Liquid** (Novartis)				Alcohol free. Sorbitol, sucrose. Orange flavor. In 118 and 147 mL.
otc	**Triaminic Softchews Tablets** (Novartis)			***6 to < 12 yrs*** - 2 q 4 to 6 h up to 8/day	17.5 mg phenylalanine, aspartame, mannitol, sucrose. Orange flavor. In 18s.
Rx	**Pediox Tablets**[1] (Atley)	15 mg pseudoephedrine HCl	2 mg chlorpheniramine maleate	***6 to < 12 yrs*** - 1 q 4 to 6 h	Chewable. Aspartame, phenylalanine, mannitol, sorbitol, xylitol. Grape flavor. (15 2 P). Purple, scored. In 100s.
otc	**Benadryl Children's Allergy & Cold Fastmelt Tablets**[1] (Warner-Lambert)	30 mg pseudoephedrine HCl	19 mg diphenhydramine citrate (12.5 mg diphenhydramine HCl)	***6 to < 12 yrs*** - 1 q 4 h up to 4/day	4.6 mg phenylalanine, aspartame, mannitol. In 20s.
otc sf	**Benadryl Children's Allergy & Sinus Liquid**[1] (Warner-Lambert)	30 mg pseudoephedrine HCl	12.5 mg diphenhydramine HCl	***6 to < 12 yrs*** - 5 mL q 4 to 6 h up to 20 mL/day	Alcohol free. Saccharin, sorbitol. Grape flavor. In 118 mL.
Rx	**Quadra-Hist D PED Capsules** (Ethex)	40 mg pseudoephedrine HCl	8 mg phenyltoloxamine citrate, 8 mg pyrilamine maleate, 8 mg pheniramine maleate	***6 to 12 yrs*** - 1 q 8 to 12 h	Extended release. Sucrose. (ETHEX/057). White opaque. In 100s.
Rx	**Pediatex 12 D Suspension**[1] (Zyber)	45.2 mg pseudoephedrine tannate	3.6 mg carbinoxamine tannate	***6 to 12 yrs*** - 5 to 10 mL q 12 h; ***2 to 6*** - 2.5 to 5 mL q 12 h	Red. Magnasweet, methylparaben, saccharin, sucrose. Candy apple flavor. In 20 and 473 mL bottles.
Rx sf	**Chlorpheniramine Tannate/Pseudoephedrine Tannate Suspension** (Various, eg, URL)	75 mg pseudoephedrine tannate	4.5 mg chlorpheniramine tannate	***6 to 12 yrs*** - 5 to 10 mL q 12 h up to 20 mL/day; ***2 to 6*** - 2.5 to 5 mL q 12 h up to 10 mL/day	Alcohol free. Strawberry/banana flavor. In 118 and 473 mL.
Rx	**Duotan PD Suspension**[1] (Scientific Laboratories, Inc.)	75 mg pseudoephedrine tannate	2.5 mg dexchlorpheniramine tannate	***6 to 12 yrs*** - 5 to 10 mL q 12 h up to 20 mL/day; ***2 to 6*** - 2.5 to 5 mL q 12 h up to 10 mL/day	Methylparaben, saccharin, sucrose. Strawberry-banana flavor. In 118 and 473 mL.

[1] This product also may be used in adults; refer to package labeling for dosing.

Refer to the general discussion of these products in the Respiratory Combinations Introduction. Some of the products in the previous Decongestants and Antihistamines table also may be used in children.

DECONGESTANT, ANTIHISTAMINE, AND ANALGESIC COMBINATIONS

Content given per capsule, tablet, packet, or 5 mL.

	Product & Distributor	Decongestant	Antihistamine	Analgesic/Other	Average Adult Dose	Excipients & How Supplied
otc	**Onset Forte Micro-Coated Tablets** (Medique Products)	5 mg phenylephrine HCl	2 mg chlorpheniramine maleate	162.5 mg acetaminophen	2 q 4 h, up to 12/day	In 500s.
otc	**Alka-Seltzer Plus Cold Medicine Effervescent Tablets** (Bayer)	5 mg phenylephrine HCl	2 mg chlorpheniramine maleate	250 mg acetaminophen	2 tablets dissolved in 118 mL water q 4 h up to 8/day	Acesulfame K, aspartame, phenylalanine, saccharin, sorbitol. Original, orange, and cherry flavors. In 12s, 20s, 36s, and 48s.
otc	**Decodult Tablets** (Wesley Pharmacal)	5 mg phenylephrine HCl	2 mg chlorpheniramine maleate	300 mg acetaminophen	2 q 4 to 6 h up to 12/day	In 1,000s.
otc	**Dristan Cold Multi-Symptom Formula Tablets** (Whitehall Robins)	5 mg phenylephrine HCl	2 mg chlorpheniramine maleate	325 mg acetaminophen	2 q 4 h up to 12/day	In 20s, 40s, and 75s.
otc	**Dryphen, Multi-Symptom Formula Tablets** (Major)					In 40s.
otc	**Medicidin-D Tablets** (Medique Products)					In 12s, 100s, 200s, and 500s.
otc	**Pyrroxate Extra-Strength Tablets** (Lee Pharmaceuticals)	10 mg phenylephrine HCl	4 mg chlorpheniramine maleate	650 mg acetaminophen	1 q 4 to 6 hours up to 6/day	Capsule-shaped. In 24s.
otc	**Benadryl Allergy & Sinus Headache Tablets**[a] (Pfizer)	5 mg phenylephrine HCl	12.5 mg diphenhydramine HCl	325 mg acetaminophen	2 q 4 h up to 12/day	Capsule shape. In 24s and 48s.
otc	**Benadryl Allergy & Cold Tablets**[a] (Pfizer)					Capsule shape. In 24s.
otc	**Sudafed PE Multi-Symptom Severe Cold Tablets**[a] (Pfizer)					Capsule shape. In 12s and 24s.
Rx	**Norel SR Tablets** (US Pharmaceuticals Corp.)	40 mg phenylephrine HCl	8 mg chlorpheniramine maleate 50 mg phenyltoloxamine citrate	325 mg acetaminophen	1 q 12 h up to 2/day	Extended-release. Yellow/white, triangle-shaped. (04,20/US) In 100s.
otc	**Theraflu Cold & Sore Throat Powder** (Novartis)	10 mg phenylephrine HCl	20 mg pheniramine maleate	325 mg acetaminophen	1 packet dissolved in 240 mL hot water q 4 h up to 6/day	Acesulfame K, maltodextrin, sucrose, 43 mg sodium. Lemon flavor. In 6s.
otc	**Theraflu Flu & Sore Throat Powder** (Novartis)	10 mg phenylephrine HCl	20 mg pheniramine maleate	650 mg acetaminophen	1 packet dissolved in 240 mL hot water q 4 h up to 6/day	Acesulfame K, maltodextrin, sucrose, 44 mg sodium, 7 mg potassium. Apple cinnamon flavor. In 6s.
otc sf	**Scot-Tussin Original Clear 5-Action Cold and Allergy Formula Liquid**[a] (Scot-Tussin)	4.2 mg phenylephrine HCl	13.3 mg pheniramine maleate	83.3 mg Na citrate, 83.3 mg Na salicylate, 25 mg caffeine citrate	5 mL q 3 to 4 h up to qid	Alcohol and dye free. Saccharin, parabens. Cherry-strawberry flavor. In 118 and 473 mL and 3.8 L.
otc	**Scot-Tussin Original 5-Action Cold and Allergy Formula Syrup**[a] (Scot-Tussin)					Alcohol free. Sugar, parabens, sorbitol. Grape flavor. In 118 and 473 mL and 3.8 L.
otc	**Comtrex Nighttime Acute Head Cold Maximum Strength Liquid** (Bristol-Myers Squibb Co.)	10 mg pseudoephedrine HCl	0.67 mg brompheniramine maleate	166.7 mg acetaminophen	30 mL q 6 h up to 120 mL/day	Alcohol 10%, saccharin, sucrose. Strawberry flavor. In 240 mL.
otc	**Comtrex Acute Head Cold Maximum Strength Tablets** (Bristol-Myers Squibb)	30 mg pseudoephedrine HCl	2 mg brompheniramine maleate	500 mg acetaminophen	2 q 6 h up to 8/day	Parabens. Capsule shape. In 20s.
otc	**Comtrex Nighttime Flu Therapy Maximum Strength Liquid** (Bristol-Myers Squibb)	10 mg pseudoephedrine HCl	0.67 mg chlorpheniramine maleate	166.7 mg acetaminophen	30 mL q 6 h up to 12 mL/day	Alcohol 10%, saccharin, sucrose. Cherry flavor. In 240 mL.
otc	**Alka-Seltzer Plus Cold Medicine Liqui-Gels**[a] (Bayer)	30 mg pseudoephedrine HCl	2 mg chlorpheniramine maleate	325 mg acetaminophen	2 q 4 h up to 8/day	Liquid filled. Sorbitol. (AS+ COLD). In 12s and 20s.
otc	**Kolephrin Tablets**[a] (Pfeiffer)				2 q 4 to 6 h up to 8/day	Capsule shape. In 24s and 36s.

DECONGESTANT, ANTIHISTAMINE, AND ANALGESIC COMBINATIONS

	Product & Distributor	Decongestant	Antihistamine	Analgesic/Other	Average Adult Dose	Excipients & How Supplied
otc	**Actifed Cold & Sinus Maximum Strength Tablets** (Warner-Lambert)	30 mg pseudoephedrine HCl	2 mg chlorpheniramine maleate	500 mg acetaminophen	2 q 6 h up to 8/day	Capsule shape. In 20s.
otc	**Comtrex Sinus & Nasal Decongestant Maximum Strength Tablets** (Bristol-Myers Squibb)					Parabens. Capsule shape. In 20s.
otc	**Good Sense Maximum Strength Dose Sinus Tablets** (Perrigo)					Capsule shape. In 24s.
otc	**Good Sense Maximum Strength Pain Relief Allergy Sinus Gelcaps** (Perrigo)					In 24s.
otc	**Sine-Off Sinus Medicine Tablets** (Hogil Pharm.)					Capsule shape. In 24s and 96s.
otc	**Sinutab Sinus Allergy, Maximum Strength Tablets** (Warner-Lambert)					Capsule shape. In 24s.
otc	**Tylenol Allergy Complete Multi-Symptom Tablets, Gelcaps, and Geltabs** (McNeil Consumer Health)				2 q 4 to 6 h up to 8/day	**Tablets**: Mannitol. Capsule shape. In 24s and 48s. **Gelcaps**: Parabens, EDTA. In 24s and 48s. **Geltabs**: Parabens, EDTA. In 24s and 48s.
otc	**Comtrex Day/Night Flu Therapy Maximum Strength Caplets** (Bristol-Myers Squibb)	*Day:* 30 mg pseudoephedrine HCl		500 mg acetaminophen	*Day:* 2 caplets q 6 h up to 4/day *Night:* 2 caplets no sooner than 6 h after last daytime dose	*Day:* Mineral oil. Orange, caplet shape. *Night:* Mineral oil, parabens. Green. In 20s (10 day; 10 night).
		Night: 30 mg pseudoephedrine HCl	2 mg chlorpheniramine maleate	500 mg acetaminophen		
Rx	**Simplet Tablets** (Major)	60 mg pseudoephedrine HCl	4 mg chlorpheniramine maleate	650 mg acetaminophen	1 tid or qid	In 100s.
otc	**Singlet for Adults Tablets** (SmithKline Beecham Consumer)				1 q 4 to 6 h up to 4/day	Sucrose. Capsule shape. In 100s.
otc	**Triaminicin Cold, Allergy, Sinus Medicine Tablets** (Novartis Consumer Health)					Lactose, methylparaben. In 24s.
otc	**TheraFlu Flu & Cold Medicine for Sore Throat, Maximum Strength Powder** (Novartis Consumer Health)	60 mg pseudoephedrine HCl	4 mg chlorpheniramine maleate	1,000 mg acetaminophen	1 packet dissolved in 177 mL hot water q 6 h up to 4/day	Sucrose, aspartame, 20 mg phenylalanine. Apple cinnamon flavor. In 6s.
otc	**Advil Allergy Sinus Tablets** (Wyeth)	30 mg pseudoephedrine HCl	2 mg chlorpheniramine maleate	200 mg ibuprofen	1 q 4 to 6 h up to 6/day	Oval. In 10s and 20s.
otc	**Tavist Allergy/Sinus/Headache Tablets** (Novartis Consumer Health)	30 mg pseudoephedrine HCl	0.335 mg clemastine fumarate	500 mg acetaminophen	2 q 6 h up to 8/day	Methylparaben. Capsule shape. In 24s and 48s.
otc	**Tylenol Allergy Complete Multi-Symptom Day & Night Tablets** (McNeil Consumer)	*Day:* 30 mg pseudoephedrine HCl	2 mg chlorpheniramine maleate	500 mg acetaminophen	2 q 4 to 6 h up to 8/day	Swallow whole. Capsule shape. In 12s.
		Night: 30 mg pseudoephedrine HCl	25 mg diphenhydramine HCl	500 mg acetaminophen	2 q 4 to 6 h up to 8/day	Capsule shape. In 12s.
otc	**Benadryl Allergy & Sinus Headache Gelcaps** (Warner-Lambert)	30 mg pseudoephedrine HCl	12.5 mg diphenhydramine HCl	500 mg acetaminophen	2 q 6 h up to 8/day	(Benadryl). Capsule shape. In 24s and 48s.

DECONGESTANT, ANTIHISTAMINE, AND ANALGESIC COMBINATIONS

	Product & Distributor	Decongestant	Antihistamine	Analgesic/Other	Average Adult Dose	Excipients & How Supplied
otc	**Benadryl Maximum Strength Severe Allergy & Sinus Headache Tablets** (Warner-Lambert)	30 mg pseudoephedrine HCl	25 mg diphenhydramine HCl	500 mg acetaminophen	2 q 6 h up to 8/day	Capsule shape. In 20s.
otc	**Sine-Off Night Time Formula Sinus, Cold, & Flu Medicine Geltabs** (Hogil Pharm.)					Capsule shape. In 10s.
otc	**Sudafed Maximum Strength Sinus Nighttime Plus Pain Relief Tablets** (Warner-Lambert)					(SU NT). Capsule shape. In 20s.
otc	**Tylenol Allergy Complete NightTime Tablets** (McNeil Consumer Health)				2 q 4 to 6 h up to 8/day	Capsule shape. In 24s.
otc	**Tylenol Flu NightTime, Maximum Strength Gelcaps** (McNeil Consumer Healthcare)				2 q 6 h up to 8/day	Parabens. In 24s.
otc	**Tylenol Flu, Maximum Strength Gelcaps** (McNeil Consumer Healthcare)				2 at bedtime; may repeat q 6 h up to 8/day.	Benzyl alcoho , castor oil, parabens. Capsule shape. In 12s.
otc	**Contac Day & Night Allergy/Sinus Relief Tablets** (SmithKline Beecham)	*Day:* 60 mg pseudoephedrine HCl		650 mg acetaminophen	*Day:* 1 q 6 h *Night:* 1 q 6 h (≤ 4/day in any combination)	*Day:* Capsule shape. White. *Night:* Capsule shape. Green. In 20s (15 day; 5 night).
		Night: 60 mg pseudoephedrine HCl	50 mg diphenhydramine HCl	650 mg acetaminophen		
otc	**Tylenol Sinus NightTime, Maximum Strength Tablets** (McNeil Consumer Healthcare)	30 mg pseudoephedrine HCl	6.25 mg doxylamine succinate	500 mg acetaminophen	2 q 4 to 6 h up to 8/day	Capsule shape. In 24s.
otc	**Coricidin 'D' Cold, Flu, & Sinus Tablets**[a] (Schering-Plough Healthcare Products)	30 mg pseudoephedrine sulfate	2 mg chlorpheniramine maleate	325 mg acetaminophen	2 q 4 to 6 h up to 8/day	Lactose. (Coricidin D). In 24s.
otc	**Drixoral Allergy Sinus Tablets** (Schering-Plough Healthcare Products)	60 mg pseudoephedrine sulfate	3 mg dexbrompheniramine maleate	500 mg acetaminophen	2 q 12 h up to 4/day	Extended release. Parabens. (DRIXORAL C + F). In 12s.

[a] This product also may be used in children; refer to package labeling for dosing.

Refer to the general discussion of these products in the Respiratory Combinations Introduction.

PEDIATRIC DECONGESTANT, ANTIHISTAMINE, AND ANALGESIC COMBINATIONS

Content given per tablet or 5 mL.

	Product & Distributor	Decongestant	Antihistamine	Analgesic	Average Dose	Excipients & How Supplied
otc	**Tylenol Children's Cold Chewable Tablets** (McNeil Consumer Healthcare)	7.5 mg pseudoephedrine hydrochloride	0.5 mg chlorpheniramine maleate	80 mg acetaminophen	***6 to 11 y*** - 4 q 4 to 6 h up to 16/day	Aspartame, mannitol, 6 mg phenylalanine. Grape flavor. In 24s.
otc	**Tylenol Children's Cold Liquid** (McNeil Consumer Healthcare)	15 mg pseudoephedrine hydrochloride	1 mg chlorpheniramine maleate	160 mg acetaminophen	***6 to 11 y*** - 10 mL q 4 to 6 h up to 40 mL/day	Sorbitol, sucrose. Alcohol free. Grape flavor. In 120 mL.
otc	**Tylenol Children's Plus Cold Nighttime Oral Suspension** (McNeil Consumer)					Sorbitol. Grape flavor. In 120 mL.

Refer to the general discussion of these products in the Respiratory Combinations Introduction. Some of the products in the previous Decongestant, Antihistamine, and Analgesic Combinations table also may be used in children.

DECONGESTANT, ANTIHISTAMINE, AND ANTICHOLINERGIC COMBINATIONS

Content given per tablet, capsule, or 5 mL.

	Product & Distributor	Decongestant	Antihistamine	Anticholinergic	Average Adult Dosage	Excipients & How Supplied
Rx	**NoHist EXT Tablets**[a] (Larken)		8 mg chlorpheniramine maleate	2.5 mg methscopolamine nitrate	1 every 12 h up to 2/day	Extended release. (LL 61). Blue, capsule shape, scored. In 100s.
Rx	**Ryneze Tablets**[a] (Stewart-Jackson)					Extended release. (SJP 655). Yellow, triangular, bisected. In 100s.
Rx	**Dallergy Syrup**[a] (Laser)	10 mg phenylephrine hydrochloride	2 mg chlorpheniramine maleate	0.625 mg methscopolamine nitrate	10 mL every 4 to 6 h up to 40 mL/day	In 473 mL.
Rx	**QV-Allergy Syrup**[a] (Pharmaceutical Associates)					Sucrose. Grape flavor. In 473 mL.
Rx	**AH-chew Tablets**[a] (WE Pharm.)	10 mg phenylephrine hydrochloride	2 mg chlorpheniramine maleate	1.25 mg methscopolamine nitrate		Chewable. (WE 03). Scored. Grape flavor. In 100s.
Rx	**Dehistine Syrup**[a] (Cypress)				10 mL every 4 to 6 h up to 40 mL/day	Alcohol free. Root beer flavor. In 473 mL.
Rx	**Duradryl Syrup**[a] (Breckenridge)				5 or 10 mL every 3 or 4 h	Corn syrup. In 473 mL.
Rx	**Ex-Histine Syrup**[a] (WE Pharm.)				10 mL every 4 to 6 h up to 40 mL/day	Root beer flavor. In 473 mL.
Rx	**Extendryl Chewable Tablets**[a] (Cornerstone BioPharma[b])				2 every 4 h up to 12/day	Tan, scored. Root beer flavor. In 100s and 1,000s.
Rx	**Extendryl Syrup**[a] (Cornerstone BioPharma[b])				10 mL every 4 to 6 h up to 40 mL/day	Root beer flavor. In 473 mL.
Rx	**AH-chew Suspension**[a] (WE Pharm.)	10 mg phenylephrine hydrochloride	2 mg chlorpheniramine maleate	1.5 mg methscopolamine nitrate	5 to 10 mL every 12 h	Parabens. Grape flavor. In 20 and 118 mL.
Rx	**DuraTan PE Suspension**[a] (ProEthic)				5 to 10 mL every 12 h up to 20 mL/day	Sucralose, parabens. Grape flavor. In 118 mL.
Rx	**Dallergy Tablets**[a] (Laser)	10 mg phenylephrine hydrochloride	4 mg chlorpheniramine maleate	1.25 mg methscopolamine nitrate	1 every 4 to 6 h up to 4/day	(Laser Dallergy). Scored. In 100s.
Rx sf	**Denaze Liquid**[a] (Cypress)				5 to 10 mL every 3 or 4 h	Saccharin, sorbitol. Alcohol and dye free. Blue raspberry flavor. In 473 mL.
Rx	**CPM 8/PE 20/MSC 1.25 Tablets**[a] (Cypress)	20 mg phenylephrine hydrochloride	8 mg chlorpheniramine maleate	1.25 mg methscopolamine nitrate	1 every 12 h up to 2/day	Lactose. (CYP 250). White, capsule shape, scored. In 100s.
Rx	**AeroHist Plus Tablets**[a] (Aero)	20 mg phenylephrine hydrochloride	8 mg chlorpheniramine maleate	2.5 mg methscopolamine nitrate	1 every 12 h up to 2/day	Extended release. (2376 aero). White, capsule shape, scored. In 100s.
Rx	**DriHist SR Tablets**[a] (Prasco)					Sustained release. (110). White, capsule shape, scored. In 100s.
Rx	**Drysec Tablets**[a] (A.G. Marin)					Extended release. (CPM M/D). White, scored. In 100s.
Rx	**Extendryl SR Capsules** (Fleming)					Sustained release. (F SR). Green/Red. In 100s and 1000s.
Rx	**Hista-Vent DA Tablets**[a] (Ethex)					Sustained release. (ETH 227). Brown, capsule shape. In 100s.
Rx	**Pre-Hist-D Tablets**[a] (Marnel)					Sustained release. (MD CPM). White, scored. In 100s.
Rx	**OMNIhist II LA Tablets**[a] (WE Pharm.)	25 mg phenylephrine hydrochloride	8 mg chlorpheniramine maleate	2.5 mg methscopolamine nitrate	1 every 12 h up to 2/day	Dye free. (WE 32). Capsule shape, scored. In 100s.
Rx	**Dallergy Tablets**[a] (Propst)	20 mg phenylephrine hydrochloride	12 mg chlorpheniramine maleate	2.5 mg methscopolamine nitrate	1 every 12 h up to 2/day	Extended release. (DALLERGY 12H). White, capsule shape, scored. In 100s.
Rx	**AccuHist LA Tablets** (PediaMed)	20 mg phenylephrine hydrochloride	8 mg chlorpheniramine maleate	0.19 mg hyoscyamine sulfate, 0.04 mg atropine sulfate, 0.01 mg scopolamine hydrobromide	1 every 12 h up to 2/day	Sustained release. Lactose. (PROPST 010). White, capsule shape. In 100s and 500s.
Rx	**Bellahist-D LA Tablets** (Cypress)					Extended release. Alcohol and dye free. (CYP 449). Capsule shape, scored. In 100s.

DECONGESTANT, ANTIHISTAMINE, AND ANTICHOLINERGIC COMBINATIONS

	Product & Distributor	Decongestant	Antihistamine	Anticholinergic	Average Adult Dosage	Excipients & How Supplied
Rx	**Phenylephrine CM Tablets**[a] (Boca Pharmacal)	40 mg phenylephrine hydrochloride	8 mg chlorpheniramine maleate	2.5 mg methscopolamine nitrate	1 every 12 h	Extended release. (BP 546). Green/White, capsule shape, scored. In 30s and 100s.
Rx	**Ralix Tablets**[a] (Cypress)					Extended release. (CYP 232). White. In 100s.
Rx	**Rescon-MX Tablets** (Capellon)					Extended release. (PHE). Green/White, capsule shape, scored. In 100s.
Rx	**AlleRx-D Tablets** (Adams Labs)	120 mg pseudoephedrine hydrochloride		2.5 mg methscopolamine nitrate	1 every 12 h up to 2/day	Controlled release. (Adams 006). Yellow, elongated, scored. In 60s.
Rx	**PSE 120/MSC 2.5 Tablets** (Cypress)					Sustained release. (CYP 281). White, scored. In 60s.
Rx	**Pannaz S Syrup**[a] (Pan American Labs)	15 mg pseudoephedrine hydrochloride	2 mg carbinoxamine maleate	1.25 mg methscopolamine nitrate	5 to 10 mL 4 times a day	Blueberry flavor. In 15 and 473 mL.
Rx	**Pannaz Tablets** (Pan American Labs)	90 mg pseudoephedrine hydrochloride	8 mg carbinoxamine maleate	2.5 mg methscopolamine nitrate	1 every 12 h up to 2/day	Extended release. (PAL 88). Lt. green, speckled, scored. In 100s.
Rx	**Durahist Tablets**[a] (ProEthic)	60 mg pseudoephedrine hydrochloride	8 mg chlorpheniramine maleate	1.25 mg methscopolamine nitrate	1 every 12 h up to 2/day	Sustained release. Talc. (PE 424). White, scored. In 100s.
Rx	**Stahist Tablets** (Magna)	90 mg pseudoephedrine HCl	8 mg chlorpheniramine maleate	0.19 mg hyoscyamine sulfate, 0.04 mg atropine sulfate, 0.01 mg scopolamine hydrobromide	1 every 12 h up to 2/day	Extended release. Dye free. (27). White, scored. In 100s.
Rx *sf*	**Respa A.R. Tablets** (Respa Pharm.)	90 mg pseudoephedrine hydrochloride	8 mg chlorpheniramine maleate	0.024 mg belladonna alkaloids (atropine, hyoscyamine, scopolamine)	1 every 12 h	Dye free. In 100s.
Rx	**CPM 8/PSE 90/MSC 2.5 Tablets**[a] (Cypress)	90 mg pseudoephedrine hydrochloride	8 mg chlorpheniramine maleate	2.5 mg methscopolamine nitrate	1 every 12 h up to 2/day	Sustained release. (CYP282). White, scored. In 100s.
Rx	**Pannaz Tablets**[a] (Pan American Lab)					Sustained release. (PAL 88). Lt. green, scored. In 100s.
Rx	**Pseudo CM TR Tablets**[a] (Boca Pharmacal)	120 mg pseudoephedrine hydrochloride	8 mg chlorpheniramine maleate	2.5 mg methscopolamine nitrate	1 every 12 h up to 2/day	Extended release. (BOCA123). White, scored. In 100s.
Rx	**Rescon-MX Tablets**[a] (Capellon)					Sustained release. (RES CON). Mottled green, scored. In 100s.
Rx	**Xiral Tablets**[a] (Hawthorn)					Sustained release. Dye free. (HAW 500). White, capsule shape, scored. In 100s.
Rx	**AlleRx Dose Pack Tablets** (Adams Labs)	*Day:* 120 mg pseudoephedrine hydrochloride		2.5 mg methscopolamine nitrate	1 am	*Day:* Controlled release. (Adams/006). Yellow, elongated, scored. *Night:* Controlled release. (Adams/007). Blue, elongated, scored. In 20s (10 day; 10 night).
		Night:	8 mg chlorpheniramine maleate	2.5 mg methscopolamine nitrate	1 pm	
Rx	**Durahist D Tablets**[a] (ProEthic)	45 mg pseudoephedrine hydrochloride	3.5 mg dexchlorpheniramine maleate	1 mg methscopolamine nitrate	1 every 12 h up to 2/day	Extended release. (PE/426). White, capsule shape, scored. In 100s.

[a] This product also may be used in children; refer to package labeling for dosing.

[b] Cornerstone BioPharma, Inc., 2000 Regency Parkway, Cary, NC 27511; 1-888-466-6505.

Refer to the general discussion of these products in the Respiratory Combinations Introduction.

PEDIATRIC DECONGESTANT, ANTIHISTAMINE, AND ANTICHOLINERGIC COMBINATIONS

Content given per capsule.

	Product & Distributor	Decongestant	Antihistamine	Anticholinergic	Average Dose	Excipients & How Supplied
Rx	**Extendryl JR Capsules** (Cornerstone)	10 mg phenylephrine HCl	4 mg chlorpheniramine maleate	1.25 mg methscopolamine nitrate	***6 to 12 yrs*** - 1 q 12 h up to 3/day	Extended release. Sucrose, talc. (CBP JR). Green/Red. In 100s.
Rx	**AeroKid Syrup** (Aero)					Glycerin, sorbitol, saccharin. Raspberry flavor. In 20, 120, and 480 mL.

Refer to the general discussion of these products in the Respiratory Combinations Introduction. Some of the products in the previous Decongestant, Antihistamine, and Anticholinergic Combinations monograph also may be used in children.

ANTITUSSIVE COMBINATIONS

Content given per tablet, capsule, packet, pouch, or 5 mL.

	Product & Distributor	Antitussive	Antihistamine	Decongestant	Other	Average Adult Dose	Excipients & How Supplied
Rx	**Re-Tann Suspension**[a] (Midlothian Labs)	25 mg carbetapentane tannate		75 mg pseudoephedrine tannate		10 mL every 12 hours up to 40 mL/day	Parabens, aspartame, phenylalanine. Cherry flavor. In 473 mL.
Rx	**Levall 12 Suspension**[a] (Athlon)	30 mg carbetapentane tannate		30 mg phenylephrine tannate		5 to 10 mL every 12 hours up to 40 mL/day	Parabens, aspartame, phenylalanine. Strawberry flavor. In 20 and 118 mL.
Rx	**BetaTan Suspension**[a] (Wraser)	30 mg carbetapentane tannate	4 mg brompheniramine tannate	7.5 mg phenylephrine tannate		5 to 10 mL every 12 hours	Parabens, aspartame, phenylalanine. Cotton candy flavor. In 118 mL.
Rx	**Tussizone-12 RF Suspension**[a] (Mallinckrodt)	30 mg carbetapentane tannate	4 mg chlorpheniramine tannate			5 to 10 mL every 12 hours up to 20 mL/day	Tartrazine, methylparaben, saccharin, sucrose. Strawberry currant flavor. In 118 mL.
Rx	**Tannic-12 Tablets** (Cypress)	60 mg carbetapentane tannate	5 mg chlorpheniramine tannate			1 to 2 tablets every 12 hours up to 4 tablets/day	Dye free. (CYP 303). Capsule shape, tan, scored. In 100s.
Rx	**Trionate Tablets** (Breckenridge)						(B072). Capsule shape, off-white. In 100s.
Rx	**Tussi-12 Tablets** (Wallace)						(Wallace 0681). Capsule shape, mauve, scored. In 100s.
Rx	**Tussizone-12 RF Tablets** (Mallinckrodt)						(0037 0681). Capsule shape, mauve, scored. In 100s.
Rx	**Exratuss Suspension**[a] (Midlothian)	30 mg carbetapentane tannate	4 mg chlorpheniramine tannate	12.5 mg phenylephrine tannate		5 to 10 mL every 12 hours up to 20 mL/day	Saccharin, sucrose, methylparaben. Strawberry flavor. In 118 mL.
Rx	**Quad Tann Tablets** (Breckenridge)	60 mg carbetapentane tannate	5 mg chlorpheniramine tannate	10 mg phenylephrine tannate, 10 mg ephedrine tannate		1 to 2 tablets every 12 hours up to 4 tablets/day	(B-816). Capsule shape, beige. In 100s.
Rx	**Rynatuss Tablets** (Medpointe)						(Wallace 717). Capsule shape, mauve, scored. In 100s, 500s, and 2,000s.
Rx	**D-Tann CT Suspension**[a] (Midlothian)	30 mg carbetapentane tannate	25 mg diphenhydramine tannate	7.5 mg phenylephrine tannate		5 to 10 mL every 12 hours	Methylparaben, saccharin, sucrose. Banana and strawberry flavors. In 118 mL.
Rx	**Dytan-CS Suspension**[a] (Hawthorn)						
Rx	**Dytan-CS Tablets**[a] (Hawthorn)	30 mg carbetapentane tannate	25 mg diphenhydramine tannate	10 mg phenylephrine tannate		1 to 2 tablets every 12 hours up to 4 tablets/day	(HAW 581). Triangular, tan. In 60s.
Rx	**C-Tanna 12D Suspension**[a] (Prasco)	30 mg carbetapentane tannate	30 mg pyrilamine tannate	5 mg phenylephrine tannate		5 to 10 mL every 12 hours up to 20 mL/day	Methylparaben, sucrose. Strawberry flavor. In 118 mL.
Rx	**Tannate-12D S Suspension**[a] (Hi-Tech)						Methylparaben, saccharin, sucrose. 118 mL.
Rx	**Tussi-12D S Suspension**[a] (Wallace)						Tartrazine, methylparaben, saccharin, sucrose. Strawberry-currant flavor. In 120 mL with oral syringe.
Rx	**Tussi-12D Tablets**[a] (Medpointe)	60 mg carbetapentane tannate	40 mg pyrilamine tannate	10 mg phenylephrine tannate		1 to 2 tablets every 12 hours	(WALLACE 0692). Capsule shape, pink, scored. In 100s.
c-iii	**Cycofed Syrup**[a] (Cypress)	20 mg codeine phosphate		60 mg pseudoephedrine HCl		5 mL every 6 hours up to 20 mL/day	Spearmint flavor. In 473 mL.
c-iii	**Nucofed Syrup**[a] (Monarch)						Alcohol free. Sorbitol, sucrose. Mint flavor. In 473 mL.
c-iii	**Nucofed Capsules** (Monarch)					1 capsule every 6 hours up to 4 capsules/day	Lactose. (M 018). Green/clear. In 60s.

ANTITUSSIVE COMBINATIONS

	Product & Distributor	Antitussive	Antihistamine	Decongestant	Other	Average Adult Dose	Excipients & How Supplied
c-v	**Dihistine DH Elixir**[a] (Alpharma)	10 mg codeine phosphate	2 mg chlorpheniramine maleate	30 mg pseudoephedrine HCl		10 mL every 4 to 6 hours up to 40 mL/day	5% alcohol. In 118 and 473 mL and 3.8 L.
c-v	**Decohistine DH Liquid** (Morton Grove)					5 to 10 mL every 4 to 6 hours up to 40 mL/day	5.8% alcohol, sugar, menthol, parabens, sorbitol. Grape/honey flavor. In 118 and 473 mL and 3.8 L.
c-v	**Prometh w/Codeine Cough Syrup**[a] (Alpharma)	10 mg codeine phosphate	6.25 mg promethazine HCl			5 mL every 4 to 6 hours up to 30 mL/day	7% alcohol, corn syrup, parabens, saccharin. In 118 mL.
c-v	**Promethazine HCl w/Codeine Syrup**[a] (Various, eg, Major, Morton Grove, URL)						In 118 and 473 mL.
c-v	**Promethazine Hydrochloride, Phenylephrine Hydrochloride and Codeine Phosphate Syrup**[a] (Alpharma)	10 mg codeine phosphate	6.25 mg promethazine HCl	5 mg phenylephrine HCl		5 mL every 4 to 6 hours up to 30 mL/day	7% alcohol. Parabens, saccharin, sucrose, sugar. Strawberry flavor. In 118 mL, 237 mL and 473 mL.
c-v	**Promethazine VC w/Codeine Cough Syrup**[a] (URL)						7.1% alcohol, EDTA, sugar, methylparaben. Cherry/raspberry flavor. In 473 mL.
c-v	**Prometh VC w/Codeine Cough Syrup**[a] (Alpharma)						7% alcohol, parabens, sugar, saccharin. In 118, 237, and 473 mL and 3.8 L.
c-v	**Tricodene Cough & Cold Liquid**[a] (Pfeiffer)	8.2 mg codeine phosphate	12.5 mg pyrilamine maleate			10 mL every 6 to 8 hours up to 60 mL/day	In 120 mL.
c-v	**Codimal PH Syrup**[a] (Schwarz)	10 mg codeine phosphate	8.33 mg pyrilamine maleate	5 mg phenylephrine HCl		10 mL every 4 to 6 hours up to 60 mL/day	Alcohol free. Sucrose. In 118 and 473 mL.
c-v	**Triacin-C Cough Syrup**[a] (Alpharma)	10 mg codeine phosphate	1.25 mg triprolidine HCl	30 mg pseudoephedrine HCl		10 mL every 4 to 6 hours up to 40 mL/day	4.3% alcohol, methylparaben. Caramel flavor. In 118 and 473 mL and 3.8 L.
c-iii	**Codeprex Suspension**[a] (Celltech Pharmaceuticals)	20 mg codeine polistirex		4 mg chlorpheniramine polistirex		10 mL every 12 hours up to 20 mL/day	Extended release. EDTA, parabens, sucrose, vegetable oil. Cherry-cream flavor. In 473 mL.
otc	**Tylenol Cough & Sore Throat Daytime Liquid** (McNeil Consumer)	5 mg dextromethorphan HBr			166.7 mg acetaminophen	30 mL every 6 hours up to 120 mL/day	Sorbitol, sucrose. In 240 mL.
Rx	**Promethazine HCl and Dextromethorphan HBr Syrup**[a] (Various, eg, Hi-Tech)	15 mg dextromethorphan HBr	6.25 mg promethazine HCl			5 mL every 4 to 6 hours up to 30 mL/day	May contain alcohol. In 118 and 437 mL.
otc	**Dimetapp Long Acting Cough Plus Cold Syrup** (Wyeth)	7.5 mg dextromethorphan HBr		15 mg pseudoephedrine HCl		20 mL every 6 hours up to 80 mL/day	Corn syrup, saccharin. Fruit punch flavor. In 118 mL.
otc	**Robitussin Honey Cough & Cold Liquid** (Whitehall-Robins)	10 mg dextromethorphan HBr		20 mg pseudoephedrine HCl		15 mL every 6 hours up to 60 mL/day	Saccharin. In 118 mL.
otc	**Top Care Maximum Strength Soothing Cough & Head Congestion Relief D Liquid**[a] (Topco Assoc.)						5% alcohol, corn syrup, saccharin. Cherry flavor. In 118 mL.
otc	**Vicks 44D Cough & Head Congestion Relief Liquid**[a] (Procter & Gamble)						5% alcohol, saccharin, corn syrup. In 118 and 236 mL.
otc	**Robitussin Maximum Strength Cough & Cold Syrup** (Whitehall-Robins)	15 mg dextromethorphan HBr		30 mg pseudoephedrine HCl		10 mL every 6 hours up to 40 mL/day	1.4% alcohol, corn syrup, saccharin, glucose. In 237 mL.

ANTITUSSIVE COMBINATIONS

	Product & Distributor	Antitussive	Antihistamine	Decongestant	Other	Average Adult Dose	Excipients & How Supplied
otc	**666 Cold Preparation, Maximum Strength Liquid**[a] (Monticello Drug Co.)	3.3 mg dextromethorphan HBr		10 mg pseudoephedrine HCl	108.3 mg acetaminophen	30 mL every 4 hours up to 120 mL/day	Saccharin, sucrose. In 177 mL.
otc	**Vicks DayQuil Multi-Symptom Cold/Flu Relief Liquid**[a] (Procter & Gamble)						Saccharin, sucrose. In 177 mL.
otc	**Tylenol Cold & Flu Severe Daytime Liquid** (McNeil Consumer)	5 mg dextromethorphan HBr		10 mg pseudoephedrine HCl	166.7 mg acetaminophen	30 mL every 6 hours up to 120 mL/day	Sorbitol, sucrose. In 240 mL.
otc	**Robitussin Honey Flu Multi-Symptom Liquid** (Whitehall-Robins)	6.6 mg dextromethorphan HBr		20 mg pseudoephedrine HCl	166.7 mg acetaminophen	15 mL every 4 hours up to 60 mL/day	Saccharin, corn syrup, menthol. In 118 mL.
otc	**Vicks DayQuil Multi-Symptom Cold/Flu Relief LiquiCaps** (Procter & Gamble)	15 mg dextromethorphan HBr		30 mg pseudoephedrine HCl	325 mg acetaminophen	2 liquicaps every 6 hours up to 8 liquicaps/day	Sorbitol. In 12s, 20s, 40s, and 60s.
otc	**Alka-Seltzer Plus Cold & Flu Liqui-Gels**[a] (Bayer)	10 mg dextromethorphan HBr		30 mg pseudoephedrine HCl	325 mg acetaminophen	2 liqui-gels every 4 hours up to 8 liqui-gels/day	Liquid filled. Sorbitol. In 12s.
otc	**Alka-Seltzer Plus Flu Medicine Liqui-Gels** [a] (Bayer)						Liquid filled. Sorbitol. In 12s.
otc	**Histenol-Forte Tablets** (Zee Medical)						In 24s.
otc	**Tylenol Cold Non-Drowsy Formula Gel-caps and Tablets**[a] (McNeil Consumer)	15 mg dextromethorphan HBr		30 mg pseudoephedrine HCl	325 mg acetaminophen	2 gelcaps or tab-lets every 6 hours up to 8 gelcaps or tablets/day	**Gelcaps**: Parabens. (TYLENOL COLD). In 24s. **Tablets**: (TYLENOL Cold). Capsule shape. In 24s.
otc	**Top Care Multi-Symptom Pain Relief Cold Tablets**[a] (Topco Assoc.)						Capsule shape. In 24s.
otc	**Comtrex Multi-Symptom Maximum Strength Non-Drowsy Cold & Cough Relief Tablets** (Bristol-Myers)	15 mg dextromethorphan HBr		30 mg pseudoephedrine HCl	500 mg acetaminophen	2 tablets every 6 hours up to 8 tablets/day	Parabens. Capsule shape. In 24s.
otc	**Theraflu Severe Cold Non-Drowsy Tab-lets** (Novartis Consumer)						Lactose, methylparaben, polydex-trose. Capsule shape. In 12s and 24s.
otc	**Tylenol Flu Maximum Strength Non-Drowsy Gelcaps** (McNeil Consumer)						Parabens. (TYLENOL FLU). In 24s.
otc	**Sudafed Non-Drowsy Severe Cold Formula Maximum Strength Tablets** (Warner-Lambert)						(Sudafed SCF). In 24s.
otc	**Robitussin Honey Flu Non-Drowsy Syrup** (Whitehall-Robins)	20 mg dextromethorphan HBr		60 mg pseudoephedrine HCl	500 mg acetaminophen	1 pouch every 4 hours in 4 to 177 mL of hot beverage (eg, tea)	Corn syrup, saccharin. In 6s.
otc	**TheraFlu Non-Drowsy Flu, Cold & Cough Maximum Strength Powder** (Novartis Consumer)	30 mg dextromethorphan HBr		60 mg pseudoephedrine HCl	1000 mg acetaminophen	1 packet dis-solved in 177 mL hot water every 6 hours up to 4 packets/day	Sucrose. Lemon flavor. In 6s and 12s.
otc	**Theraflu Severe Cold Non-Drowsy Packet** (Novartis Consumer)						17 mg phenylalanine, aspartame, sucrose. Lemon flavor. In 6s.
otc	**TheraFlu Severe Cold & Congestion Non-Drowsy, Maximum Strength Powder** (Novartis Consumer)						Acesulfame K, aspartame, 17 mg phenylalanine, sucrose. Lemon flavor. In 6s.
Rx sf	**Alacol DM Syrup**[a] (Ballay)	10 mg dextromethorphan HBr	2 mg brompheniramine maleate	5 mg phenylephrine HCl		10 mL every 4 hours up to 60 mL/day	Alcohol free. Saccharin, sorbitol. Black raspberry flavor. In 473 mL.

ANTITUSSIVE COMBINATIONS

	Product & Distributor	Antitussive	Antihistamine	Decongestant	Other	Average Adult Dose	Excipients & How Supplied
Rx sf	**Tusdec-DM Liquid**[a] (Cypress)	15 mg dextromethorphan HBr	2 mg brompheniramine maleate	7.5 mg phenylephrine HCl		10 mL every 6 hours up to 40 mL/day	Alcohol and dye and free. Saccharin, sorbitol. Strawberry flavor. In 473 mL.
Rx sf	**Bromatane DX Syrup**[a] (Ivax)	10 mg dextromethorphan HBr	2 mg brompheniramine maleate	30 mg pseudoephedrine HCl		10 mL every 4 to 6 hours up to 40 mL/day	0.95% alcohol. In 473 mL.
Rx	**Bromfed DM Cough Syrup**[a] (Verum Pharm)					10 mL every 4 hours up to 60 mL/day	Saccharin, sorbitol, sucrose, methylparaben. Cherry flavor. In 473 mL.
Rx	**Genebrom-DM Liquid**[a] (PGD)					10 mL every 6 hours up to 40 mL/day	Alcohol free. Parabens, sugar, saccharin. Cherry flavor. In 473 mL.
otc	**Robitussin Allergy & Cough Liquid**[a] (Whitehall-Robins)					10 mL every 4 hours up to 40 mL/day	Alcohol and dye free. Saccharin, sorbitol. In 118 mL.
Rx	**Carbodex DM Syrup**[a] (Tri-Med)	15 mg dextromethorphan HBr	4 mg brompheniramine maleate	45 mg pseudoephedrine HCl		5 mL qid	Menthol, sorbitol. In 473 mL.
Rx	**Carbofed DM Syrup**[a] (Hi-Tech Pharmacal)						Sorbitol. Grape flavor. In 473 mL.
Rx	**Sildec-DM Syrup**[a] (Silarx)						Alcohol free. Saccharin, sorbitol. Grape flavor. In 473 mL.
Rx sf	**Coldec DM**[a] (Silarx)	15 mg dextromethorphan HBr	4 mg brompheniramine maleate	60 mg pseudoephedrine HCl		5 mL qid	Alcohol free. Saccharin, sorbitol. Grape flavor. In 480 mL.
Rx	**Rondamine DM Syrup**[a] (Major)						< 0.2% alcohol. Grape flavor. In 120 and 473 mL and 3.8 L.
Rx sf	**Anaplex-DM Liquid**[a] (ECR)	30 mg dextromethorphan HBr	4 mg brompheniramine maleate	60 mg pseudoephedrine HCl		5 mL every 4 to 6 hours up to 20 mL/day	Alcohol and dye free. Fruit flavor. In 473 mL.
Rx sf	**Bromphenex DM Liquid**[a] (Breckenridge)						Alcohol and dye free. Fruit flavor. Sorbitol, saccharin. In 473 mL.
Rx sf	**Cordron-DM Liquid**[a] (Cypress)	15 mg dextromethorphan HBr	3 mg carbinoxamine maleate	15 mg pseudoephedrine HCl		10 mL 4 times daily	Alcohol and dye free. Cotton candy flavor. Saccharin, sorbitol. In 473 mL
Rx	**DMax Syrup**[a] (Great Southern)	15 mg dextromethorphan HBr	4 mg carbinoxamine maleate	8 mg phenylephrine HCl		10 mL every 6 hours up to 40 mL/day	Berry flavor. In 30 and 473 mL.
Rx	**Balamine DM Syrup**[a] (Ballay)	12.5 mg dextromethorphan HBr	4 mg carbinoxamine maleate	60 mg pseudoephedrine HCl		5 mL qid	Menthol. Grape flavor. In 473 mL.
Rx	**Cydec-DM Syrup**[a] (Cypress)	15 mg dextromethorphan HBr	4 mg carbinoxamine maleate	60 mg pseudoephedrine HCl		5 mL qid	Grape flavor. In 118 and 437 mL and 3.8 L.
Rx sf	**Tussafed Syrup**[a] (Everett)						Alcohol free. Menthol. Grape flavor. In 120 and 480 mL.
otc sf	**Tricodene Sugar Free Liquid**[a] (Pfeiffer)	10 mg dextromethorphan HBr	2 mg chlorpheniramine maleate			10 mL every 4 to 6 hours up to 60 mL/day	Alcohol free. Sorbitol, mannitol, menthol, saccharin. In 120 mL.
otc sf	**Scot-Tussin DM Liquid**[a] (Scot-Tussin)	15 mg dextromethorphan HBr	2 mg chlorpheniramine maleate			10 mL every 6 to 8 hours up to 40 mL/day	Alcohol and dye free. Parabens. In 118, 237, and 473 mL and 3.8 L.
otc	**Coricidin HBP Cough & Cold Tablets** (Schering-Plough)	30 mg dextromethorphan HBr	4 mg chlorpheniramine maleate			1 tablet every 6 hours up to 4 tablets/day	Sugar. (C C + C). In 16s.
otc	**Coricidin HBP Maximum Strength Flu Tablets** (Schering-Plough)	15 mg dextromethorphan HBr	2 mg chlorpheniramine maleate		500 mg acetaminophen	2 tablets every 6 hours up to 8 tablets/day	Lactose. In 20s.

ANTITUSSIVE COMBINATIONS

	Product & Distributor	Antitussive	Antihistamine	Decongestant	Other	Average Adult Dose	Excipients & How Supplied
otc	**Alka-Seltzer Plus Flu Medicine Effervescent Tablets** (Bayer)	15 mg dextromethorphan HBr	2 mg chlorpheniramine maleate		500 mg aspirin	2 tablets dissolved in 118 mL water every 6 hours up to 8 tablets/day	Acesulfame K, aspartame, 6.7 mg phenylalanine, mannitol, saccharin. Honey/orange flavor. In 20s.
Rx	**Extendryl DM Tablets**[a] (Auriga[b])	30 mg dextromethorphan HBr	8 mg chlorpheniramine maleate		2.5 methscopolamine nitrate	1 tablet twice daily up to 2/day	Extended-release. (AP 202). Scored, bisected. In 100s.
otc	**Father John's Medicine Plus Liquid** (Oakhurst Co.)	1.66 mg dextromethorphan HBr	0.66 mg chlorpheniramine maleate	1.66 mg phenylephrine HCl		30 mL every 4 hours up to 180 mL/day	Alcohol free. In 118 mL.
otc	**Alka-Seltzer Plus Cold & Cough Medicine Effervescent Tablets** (Bayer)	10 mg dextromethorphan HBr	2 mg chlorpheniramine maleate	5 mg phenylephrine HCl		2 tablets dissolved in 118 mL water every 4 hours up to 8 tablets/day	Aspartame, 11 mg phenylalanine, sorbitol. In 20s.
Rx sf	**Ameritussa AD Liquid**[a] (AMBI)	15 mg dextromethorphan HBr	3 mg chlorpheniramine maleate	10 mg phenylephrine HCl		10 mL every 6 hours up to 40 mL/day	Alcohol free. Phenylalanine, aspartame. In 473 mL.
Rx sf	**Rondec-DM Syrup**[a] (Alliant)	15 mg dextromethorphan HBr	4 mg chlorpheniramine maleate	12.5 mg phenylephrine HCl		5 mL every 4 to 6 hours up to 30 mL/day	Alcohol free. Saccharin, sorbitol. Grape flavor. In 20, 118, and 437 mL.
Rx sf	**Norel DM Liquid**[a] (US Pharm)	15 mg dextromethorphan HBr	4 mg chlorpheniramine maleate	10 mg phenylephrine HCl		5 mL every 4 hours up to 30 mL/day	Alcohol and dye free. Sorbitol. In 473 mL.
otc	**Alka-Seltzer Plus Nose & Throat Effervescent Tablets** (Bayer)	10 mg dextromethorphan HBr	2 mg chlorpheniramine maleate	5 mg phenylephrine HCl	250 mg acetaminophen	2 tablets fully dissolved in 120 mL water every 4 hours up to 8 tablets/day	Acesulfame K, aspartame, maltodextrin, saccharin, sorbitol, 5.6 mg phenylalanine. Citrus blend flavor. In 20s.
otc	**Robitussin PM Cough & Cold Liquid**[a] (Wyeth Consumer)	7.5 mg dextromethorphan HBr	1 mg chlorpheniramine maleate	15 mg pseudoephedrine HCl		20 mL every 6 hours up to 80 mL/day	Alcohol free. Corn syrup, saccharin. In 118 mL.
otc sf	**Rescon-DM Liquid**[a] (Capellon Pharm.)	10 mg dextromethorphan HBr	2 mg chlorpheniramine maleate	30 mg pseudoephedrine HCl		10 mL every 4 to 6 hours up to 40 mL/day	Alcohol and dye free. In 118 and 473 mL.
otc	**Comtrex Maximum Strength Nighttime Cold & Cough Liquid** (Bristol-Myers)	5 mg dextromethorphan HBr	0.67 mg chlorpheniramine maleate	10 mg pseudoephedrine	166.7 mg acetaminophen	30 mL every 6 hours, not to exceed 120 mL/day	10% alcohol, saccharin, sucrose. In 240 mL.
otc	**Robitussin Flu Liquid**[a] (Whitehall-Robins)	5 mg dextromethorphan HBr	1 mg chlorpheniramine maleate	15 mg pseudoephedrine HCl	160 mg acetaminophen	20 mL every 4 hours up to 80 mL/day	Alcohol free. In 118 mL.
otc	**Vicks 44M Cough, Cold, & Flu Relief Liquid** (Procter & Gamble)	7.5 mg dextromethorphan HBr	1 mg chlorpheniramine maleate	15 mg pseudoephedrine HCl	162.5 mg acetaminophen	20 mL every 6 hours up to 80 mL/day	10% alcohol, corn syrup, saccharin. In 236 mL.

ANTITUSSIVE COMBINATIONS

	Product & Distributor	Antitussive	Antihistamine	Decongestant	Other	Average Adult Dose	Excipients & How Supplied
otc	**Alka-Seltzer Plus Cold & Cough Liqui-Gels**[a] (Bayer)	10 mg dextromethorphan HBr	2 mg chlorpheniramine maleate	30 mg pseudoephedrine HCl	325 mg acetaminophen	2 liqui-gels every 4 hours up to 8 liqui-gels/day	Liquid filled. Sorbitol. (AS+ C&C). In 12s and 20s.
otc	**Kolephrin/DM Tablets**[a] (Pfeiffer)					2 tablets every 4 to 6 hours up to 8 tablets/day	Capsule shape. In 30s.
otc	**Top Care Multi-Symptom Pain Relief Cold Tablets**[a] (Topco Assoc.)	15 mg dextromethorphan HBr	2 mg chlorpheniramine maleate	30 mg pseudoephedrine HCl	325 mg acetaminophen	2 tablets every 6 hours up to 8 tablets/day	Capsule shape. In 24s.
otc	**Tylenol Cold Complete Formula Tablets**[a] (McNeil Consumer)						Capsule shape. In 24s.
otc	**Mapap Cold Formula Tablets**[a] (Major)						In 24s.
otc	**Contac Severe Cold & Flu Maximum Strength Tablets** (SmithKline Beecham)	15 mg dextromethorphan HBr	2 mg chlorpheniramine maleate	30 mg pseudoephedrine HCl	500 mg acetaminophen	2 tablets every 6 hours up to 8 tablets/day	Capsule shape. In 30s.
otc	**Genacol Maximum Strength Cold & Flu Relief Tablets** (Ivax)						In 50s.
otc	**Comtrex Maximum Strength Nighttime Cold & Cough Tablet** (Bristol-Myers Squibb)						Parabens, mineral oil. Capsule shape. In 20s.
otc	**Comtrex Cough and Cold Relief, Multi-Symptom Maximum Strength Tablets**[a] (Bristol-Myers Squibb)						Parabens. Capsule shape. In 24s.
otc	**Cold Symptoms Relief Maximum Strength Tablets** (Major)						In 24s.
otc	**Theraflu Severe Cold Tablets** (Novartis Consumer)						Lactose, methylparaben. Capsule shape. In 24s.
otc	**Comtrex Day & Night Cold & Cough Relief, Multi-Symptom Maximum Strength Tablets** (Bristol-Myers Squibb)	*Day:* 15 mg dextromethorphan HBr		30 mg pseudoephedrine HCl	500 mg acetaminophen	2 caplets every 6 hours up to 4 caplets/day	Parabens, mineral oil. *Day:* Orange. In 10s. *Night:* Blue. In 10s.
		Night:	2 mg chlorpheniramine maleate	30 mg pseudoephedrine HCl	500 mg acetaminophen	2 caplets no sooner than every 6 hours after last daytime caplet up to 2 caplets/day	
otc	**Robitussin Honey Flu Nighttime Syrup** (Whitehall-Robins)	20 mg dextromethorphan HBr	4 mg chlorpheniramine maleate	60 mg pseudoephedrine HCl	500 mg acetaminophen	1 pouch every 4 hours in 4 to 177 mL of hot beverage (eg, tea) up to 4 pouches/day	Corn syrup, saccharin. In 6s.
otc	**Theraflu Cold & Cough Powder** (Novartis Consumer)	20 mg dextromethorphan HBr	4 mg chlorpheniramine maleate	60 mg pseudoephedrine HCl	650 mg acetaminophen	1 packet dissolved in 180 mL (16 oz) hot water every 4 to 6 hours up to 4 doses/day	Aspartame, 13 mg phenylalanine, 19 mg sodium, sucrose. Lemon flavor. In 6s and 12s.

ANTITUSSIVE COMBINATIONS

	Product & Distributor	Antitussive	Antihistamine	Decongestant	Other	Average Adult Dose	Excipients & How Supplied
otc	**TheraFlu Flu, Cold, & Cough and Sore Throat, Maximum Strength Powder** (Novartis Consumer)	30 mg dextromethorphan HBr	4 mg chlorpheniramine maleate	60 mg pseudoephedrine HCl	1000 mg acetaminophen	1 pack dissolved in 6 oz water every 4 to 6 hours up to 4 doses/day	Aspartame, acesulfame K, phenylalanine, sucrose. Cherry flavor. In 6s.
otc	**Theraflu Severe Cold & Cough Powder** (Novartis Consumer)					1 packet dissolved in 180 mL (16 oz) hot water every 6 hours up to 4 doses/day	14 mg sodium, 27 mg phenylalanine, aspartame, sucrose. Cherry flavor. In 6s.
otc	**TheraFlu Flu, Cold, & Cough NightTime, Maximum Strength Powder** (Novartis Consumer)						Sucrose. Lemon flavor. In 6 and 12 packs.
otc	**TheraFlu Severe Cold & Congestion Night Time, Maximum Strength Powder** (Novartis Consumer)						Sucrose. Lemon flavor. In 6s.
otc	**Top Care Maximum Strength Flu, Cold, & Cough Medicine Night Time Powder** (Topco Assoc.)						Sucrose. Lemon flavor. In 6s.
Rx sf	**Tussall Syrup** (Everett)	20 mg dextromethorphan HBr	2 mg dexbrompheniramine maleate	10 mg phenylephrine HCl		5 mL every 4 to 6 hours up to 30 mL/day	Alcohol free. EDTA, saccharin, sorbitol. Strawberry flavor. In 473 mL.
Rx	**Tussall-ER Tablet**[a] (Everett)	30 mg dextromethorphan HBr	6 mg dexbrompheniramine maleate	20 mg phenylephrine HCl		1 tablet every 12 hours up to 2 tablets/day	Extended release. (EV 0471). Capsule shape, white, scored. In 100s.
otc	**Co ntac Day & Night Cold & Flu Tablets** (SmithKline Beecham)	*Day:* 30 mg dextromethorphan HBr		60 mg pseudoephedrine HCl	650 mg acetaminophen	*Day:* 1 tablet every 6 hours *Night:* 1 tablet every 6 hours ≤ 4 in any combination per day	*Day:* Capsule shape, yellow. *Night:* Capsule shape, blue. In 20s (15 day; 5 night).
		Night:	50 mg diphenhydramine HCl	60 mg pseudoephedrine HCl	650 mg acetaminophen		
otc	**Vicks NyQuil Cough Syrup**[a] (Procter & Gamble)	5 mg dextromethorphan HBr	2.1 mg doxylamine succinate			30 mL every 6 to 8 hours up to 120 mL/day	Alcohol, corn syrup, saccharin. Cherry flavor. In 177 mL.
otc	**Alka-Seltzer Plus Night-Time Cold Medicine Effervescent Tablets** (Bayer)	10 mg dextromethorphan HBr	6.25 mg doxylamine succinate	5 mg phenylephrine HCl		2 dissolved in 118 mL water hs or every 4 hours up to 8 tablets/day	Acesulfame K, aspartame, 7.8 mg phenylalanine, sorbitol. In 20s.
otc	**All-Nite Liquid** (Major)	5 mg dextromethorphan HBr	2.1 mg doxylamine succinate	10 mg pseudoephedrine HCl	167 mg acetaminophen	30 mL every 6 hours up to 120 mL/day	10% alcohol, saccharin, corn syrup. Original and cherry flavors. In 177 mL.
otc	**Nite Time Cold Formula for Adults Liquid** (Alpharma)					30 mL hs or every 6 hours up to 120 mL/day	10% alcohol, saccharin, sucrose. In 296 mL.
otc	**Tylenol Flu NightTime, Maximum Strength Liquid**[a] (McNeil Consumer)					30 mL every 6 hours up to 120 mL/day	Corn syrup, saccharin, sorbitol. In 237 mL.
otc	**Vicks NyQuil Multi-Symptom Cold/Flu Relief Liquid** (Procter & Gamble)						10% alcohol, corn syrup, saccharin. Regular and cherry flavors. In 180, 300, and 420 mL.

ANTITUSSIVE COMBINATIONS

	Product & Distributor	Antitussive	Antihistamine	Decongestant	Other	Average Adult Dose	Excipients & How Supplied
otc	**Tylenol Cold & Flu Severe Liquid** (McNeil Consumer)	*Day:* 5 mg dextromethorphan HBr		10 mg pseudoephedrine HCl	166.7 mg acetaminophen	*Day:* 30 mL every 6 hours up to 120 mL/day.	Sorbitol, sucrose. *Day:* In 240 mL. *Night:* In 240 mL.
		Night: 5 mg dextromethorphan HBr	2.1 mg doxylamine succinate	10 mg pseudoephedrine HCl	166.7 mg acetaminophen	*Night:* 30 mL every 6 hours up to 120 mL/day	
otc	**Nighttime Cold Softgels** (Goldline)	10 mg dextromethorphan HBr	6.25 mg doxylamine succinate	30 mg pseudoephedrine HCl	250 mg acetaminophen	2 capsules every 4 hours up to 8 capsules/day	Alcohol free. Sorbitol. In 12s.
otc	**Top Care LiquiCaps Nite Time Multi-Symptom Cold/Flu Relief Capsules** (Topco Assoc.)						Sorbitol. In 20s.
otc	**Alka-Seltzer Plus NightTime Cold Liqui-Gels** (Bayer)	10 mg dextromethorphan HBr	6.25 mg doxylamine succinate	30 mg pseudoephedrine HCl	325 mg acetaminophen	2 capsules hs	Liquid filled. Alcohol free. Sorbitol. In 12s, 20s, and 36s.
otc	**Vicks NyQuil Multi-Symptom Cold & Flu Relief LiquiCaps** (Procter & Gamble)	15 mg dextromethorphan HBr	6.25 mg doxylamine succinate	30 mg pseudoephedrine HCl	325 mg acetaminophen	2 liquicaps every 6 hours up to 8 liquicaps/day	Sorbitol. In 12s, 20s, and 40s.
otc	**Night Time Multi-Symptom Cold/Flu Relief Liquid Caps** (Major)	15 mg dextromethorphan HBr	6.25 mg doxylamine succinate	30 mg pseudoephedrine HCl	325 mg acetaminophen	2 liquid caps every 6 hours up to 8 liquid caps/day	Sorbitol. In 12s.
Rx	**Prometh w/Dextromethorphan Syrup**[a] (Alpharma)	15 mg dextromethorphan HBr	6.25 mg promethazine HCl			5 mL every 4 to 6 hours up to 30 mL/day	7% alcohol, parabens, saccharin. Lemon/mint flavor. In 118, 237, and 473 mL and 3.8 L.
Rx	**Promethazine w/Dextromethorphan Cough Syrup** (Morton Grove)						7.1% alcohol, saccharin. Pineapple flavor. In 118 and 473 mL.
otc sf	**Codal-DM Syrup**[a] (Cypress)	10 mg dextromethorphan HBr	8.33 mg pyrilamine maleate	5 mg phenylephrine HCl		10 mL every 4 hours up to 60 mL/day	Alcohol and dye free. In 473 mL.
otc sf	**Codimal DM Syrup**[a] (Schwarz)						Alcohol and dye free. Menthol, saccharin, sorbitol. In 120 and 473 mL and 3.8 L.
otc sf	**Dicomal-DM Syrup**[a] (Econolab)						Alcohol and dye free. Menthol, saccharin, sorbitol. In 473 mL.
Rx sf	**Poly Hist DM Liquid**[a] (Poly Pharmaceuticals)	15 mg dextromethorphan HBr	12.5 pyrilamine maleate	7.5 mg phenylephrine HCl		5 to 10 mL every 4 to 6 hours up to 40 mL/day	Alcohol and dye free. Saccharin, sorbitol. Grape flavor. In 20 mL and 473 mL.
otc	**Robitussin Night Relief Liquid** (Whitehall-Robins)	5 mg dextromethorphan HBr	8.3 mg pyrilamine maleate	10 mg pseudoephedrine HCl	108.3 mg acetaminophen	30 mL hs or every 6 hours up to 120 mL/day	Alcohol free. Saccharin, sorbitol. Cherry flavor. In 177 mL.
Rx	**Bromatan-DM Suspension**[a] (Cypress)	20 mg dextromethorphan tannate	8 mg brompheniramine tannate	20 mg phenylephrine tannate		10 mL every 12 hours up to 20 mL/day	Alcohol free. Aspartame, phenylalanine, parabens. Bubble gum favor. In 473 mL.
Rx	**DuraTan DM Suspension**[a] (ProEthic)						Alcohol free. Parabens, aspartame, phenylalanine. Bubble gum flavor. In 473 mL.

ANTITUSSIVE COMBINATIONS

	Product & Distributor	Antitussive	Antihistamine	Decongestant	Other	Average Adult Dose	Excipients & How Supplied
Rx	**TanaCof-DM Suspension**[a] (Larken)	25 mg dextromethorphan tannate	2.5 mg dexchlorpheniramine tannate	75 mg pseudoephedrine tannate		10 to 20 mL every 12 hours up to 40 mL/day	Parabens, aspartame, phenylalanine. Cotton candy flavor. In 118 and 473 mL.
Rx	**Tanafed DMX Suspension**[a] (First Horizon)						Methylparaben, saccharin, sucrose. Cotton candy flavor. In 20, 118, and 473 mL.
Rx	**Tannate DMP-DEX Liquid**[a] (Hi-Tech)						Methylparaben, saccharin, sucrose. Cotton candy flavor. In 118 and 473 mL.
Rx *sf*	**Anaplex DMX Syrup**[a] (ECR)	60 mg dextromethorphan tannate	8 mg brompheniramine tannate	90 mg pseudoephedrine tannate		5 mL every 12 hours up to 10 mL/day	Alcohol free. Grape flavor. In 473 mL.
c-v	**Pancof PD Syrup**[a] (Pan American)	3 mg dihydrocodeine bitartrate	2 mg chlorpheniramine maleate	7.5 mg phenylephrine HCl		5 to 10 mL every 4 to 6 hours up to 40 mL/day	In 120 mL.
c-v	**Tricof PD Syrup**[a] (Scientific Laboratories)						Grape flavor. In 473 mL.
c-iii *sf*	**Pancof Syrup**[a] (Pan American)	7.5 mg dihydrocodeine bitartrate	2 mg chlorpheniramine maleate	15 mg pseudoephedrine HCl		5 to 10 mL every 4 to 6 hours	Alcohol and dye free. Saccharin, sorbitol. In 473 mL.
c-iii *sf*	**Tricof Syrup**[a] (Scientific Laboratories)					5 to 10 mL every 4 hours up to 40 mL/every day	Alcohol and dye free. Grape flavor. In 473 mL.
c-iii	**Hycodan Tablets**[a] (Endo)	5 mg hydrocodone bitartrate			1.5 mg homatropine MBr	1 tablet every 4 to 6 hours up to 6 tablets/day	Lactose. (Hycodan). White, scored. In 100s.
c-iii	**Hycodan Syrup**[a] (Endo)					5 mL every 4 to 6 hours up to 30 mL/day	Sorbitol, sugar, parabens. Cherry flavor. In 473 mL.
c-iii	**Hydrocodone Bitartrate and Homatropine Methylbromide Syrup**[a] (Alpharma)						Methylparaben, saccharin, sucrose. Cherry flavor. In 473 and 3,785 mL.
c-iii	**Hydromet Syrup**[a] (Alpharma)						Saccharin, sucrose, methylparaben. Cherry flavor. In 473 mL and 3.8 L.
c-iii	**Hydromide Syrup**[a] (Major)					5 mL every 4 hours up to 30 mL/day	< 0.1% alcohol. Cherry flavor. In 473 mL.
c-iii	**Hydropane Syrup**[a] (Watson)					5 mL every 4 to 6 hours up to 30 mL/day	Parabens, sucrose. Cherry flavor. In 473 mL and 3.8 L.
c-iii	**Tussigon Tablets**[a] (Daniels)					1 tablet every 4 to 6 hours up to 6 tablets/day	(dp 082). Blue, scored. In 100s and 500s.
c-iii *sf*	**Nalex DH Liquid**[a] (Blansett Pharmacal)	2.5 mg hydrocodone bitartrate		5 mg phenylephrine hydrochloride		10 mL every 4 to 6 hours up to 40 mL/day	Alcohol free. Cherry flavor. In 15 and 437 mL.
c-iii *sf*	**Tusdec-HC Liquid**[a] (Cypress)	3.75 mg hydrocodone bitartrate		7.5 mg phenylephrine HCl		5 mL every 4 hours up to 30 mL/day	Alcohol and dye free. Sorbitol. Grape flavor. In 473 mL.
c-iii	**Pancof-HC Syrup** (Pam Laboratories)	3 mg hydrocodone bitartrate		15 mg pseudoephedrine HCl		5 to 10 mL 4 times daily	Saccharin, sorbitol. Grape flavor. In 3,700 mL.

ANTITUSSIVE COMBINATIONS

	Product & Distributor	Antitussive	Antihistamine	Decongestant	Other	Average Adult Dose	Excipients & How Supplied
c-iii	**Detussin Liquid**[a] (Alpharma)	5 mg hydrocodone bitartrate		60 mg pseudoephedrine HCl		5 mL qid	5% alcohol, corn syrup, saccharin, methylparaben. Cherry flavor. In 473 mL.
c-iii	**Histussin D Liquid**[a] (Sanofi-Synthelabo)						In 473 mL.
c-iii	**P-V-Tussin Tablets** (Numark)					1 tablet every 4 to 6 hours up to 4 hours/day	Lactose. (NUMARK 10/91). Capsule shape, orange, scored. In 100s.
c-iii sf	**Anaplex HD Liquid**[a] (ECR Pharmaceuticals)	1.7 mg hydrocodone bitartrate	2 mg brompheniramine maleate	30 mg pseudoephedrine HCl		10 mL every 6 to 8 hours up to 40 mL/day	Alcohol and dye free. Strawberry flavor. In 118 and 473 mL.
c-iii sf	**Bromphenex HD Liquid**[a] (Breckenridge)						Alcohol and dye free. Sorbitol, saccharin. Strawberry flavor. In 473 mL.
c-iii	**Bromplex HD Liquid** (Prasco)						Saccharin, sorbitol. Strawberry flavor. In 473 mL.
c-iii	**M-End Liquid**[a] (R.A. McNeil)	2.5 mg hydrocodone bitartrate	2 mg brompheniramine maleate	15 mg pseudoephedrine HCl		10 mL every 4 to 6 hours	Saccharin, sorbitol. Cherry flavor. In 473 mL.
c-iii sf	**Brompheniramine/Hydrocodone/PSE Liquid**[a] (Varsity Laboratories)	2.5 mg hydrocodone bitartrate	3 mg brompheniramine maleate	30 mg pseudoephedrine HCl		5 to 10 mL every 4 to 6 hours up to 40 mL/day	Alcohol free. Saccharin, sorbitol. Bubble gum flavor. In 473 mL.
c-iii sf	**FluTuss HC Liquid**[a] (Wraser)	2.5 mg hydrocodone bitartrate	2 mg brompheniramine maleate	7.5 mg phenylephrine HCl		5 to 10 mL every 4 to 6 hours up to 30 mL/day	Alcohol free. Tartrazine, saccharin, sorbitol. Peach flavor. In 15 mL and 473 mL.
c-iii	**M-End Max Liquid**[a] (R.A. McNeil)	5 mg hydrocodone bitartrate	2 mg brompheniramine maleate	7.5 mg phenylephrine HCl		5 to 10 mL every 4 to 6 hours up to 30 mL/day	Methylparaben, sucrose. Grape flavor. In 473 mL.
c-iii	**Hydrocodone Bitartrate 5 mg/ Pseudoephedrine HCl 30 mg/ Carbinoxamine Maleate 2 mg Liquid**[a] (URL)	5 mg hydrocodone bitartrate	2 mg carbinoxamine maleate	30 mg pseudoephedrine HCl		5 to 10 mL every 4 to 6 hours up to 30 mL/day	Alcohol free. In 473 mL.
c-iii sf	**Histex HC Liquid**[a] (Teamm Pharm)						Saccharin, sorbitol. Alcohol free. Peach flavor. In 473 mL.
c-iii sf	**S-T Forte 2 Liquid**[a] (Scot-Tussin)	2.5 mg hydrocodone bitartrate	2 mg chlorpheniramine maleate			5 mL tid or qid up to 20 mL/day	Alcohol and dye free. Menthol, parabens. In 473 mL and 3.8 L.
c-iii	**ED-TLC Liquid**[a] (Edwards)	1.67 mg hydrocodone bitartrate	2 mg chlorpheniramine maleate	5 mg phenylephrine HCl		10 mL tid or qid	In 473 mL.
c-iii	**Hydrocodone HD Liquid**[a] (Morton Grove)					10 mL every 4 hours up to 40 mL/day	Alcohol free. Sugar, menthol, parabens. Cherry flavor. In 236 and 473 mL.
c-iii sf	**Triant-HC Liquid**[a] (Hawthorn)					10 mL every 4 to 6 hours up to 40 mL/day	Alcohol free. Strawberry flavor. In 473 mL.
c-iii sf	**Tridal HD Syrup**[a] (Scientific Laboratories)	2 mg hydrocodone bitartrate	2 mg chlorpheniramine maleate	7.5 mg phenylephrine hydrochloride		10 mL every 4 hours up to 40 mL/day	Alcohol free. Cherry flavor. In 473 mL.
c-iii	**Baltussin HC Liquid**[a] (Ballay Pharmaceuticals)	2.5 mg hydrocodone bitartrate	2 mg chlorpheniramine maleate	5 mg phenylephrine hydrochloride		10 mL every 4 hours up to 40 mL/day	Alcohol free. Saccharin, sorbitol. Fruit flavor. In 473 mL.
c-iii sf	**Cotuss HD Syrup**[a] (Scientific Laboratories)	2.5 mg hydrocodone bitartrate	4 mg chlorpheniramine maleate	10 mg phenylephrine hydrochloride		10 mL every 4 to 6 hours up to 40 mL/day	Alcohol free. Cherry flavor. In 473 mL.

ANTITUSSIVE COMBINATIONS

	Product & Distributor	Antitussive	Antihistamine	Decongestant	Other	Average Adult Dose	Excipients & How Supplied
c-iii sf	**Rindal HD Plus Syrup**[a] (Breckenridge)	3.5 mg hydrocodone bitartrate	2 mg chlorpheniramine maleate	7.5 mg phenylephrine hydrochloride		10 mL every 4 hours up to 40 mL/day	Alcohol free. Saccharin, sorbitol. Black raspberry flavor. In 473 mL.
c-iii sf	**Tridal HD Plus Syrup**[a] (Scientific Laboratories)						Black raspberry flavor. In 473 mL.
c-iii (sf)	**Z-Cof HC Liquid**[a] (Zyber)	3.5 mg hydrocodone bitartrate	2.5 mg chlorpheniramine maleate	8 mg phenylephrine hydrochloride		10 mL every 4 to 6 hours up to 40 mL/day	Alcohol free. Saccharin, sorbitol. Raspberry flavor. In 473 mL.
c-iii (sf)	**Coughtuss Liquid**[a] (Breckenridge)	5 mg hydrocodone bitartrate	2 mg chlorpheniramine maleate	5 mg phenylephrine hydrochloride		10 mL every 4 to 6 hours up to 40 mL/day	Alcohol free. Saccharin, sorbitol. Candy apple flavor. In 473 mL.
c-iii (sf)	**Tritussin Syrup**[a] (Scientific Laboratories)						Alcohol free. Candy apple flavor. In 473 mL.
c-iii (sf)	**Cotuss MS Syrup**[a] (Scientific Laboratories)	5 mg hydrocodone bitartrate	2 mg chlorpheniramine maleate	10 mg phenylephrine hydrochloride		10 mL every 4 to 6 hours up to 40 mL/day	Alcohol free. Pineapple-orange flavor. In 473 mL.
c-iii sf	**Endal HD** (PediaMed)	2 mg hydrocodone bitartrate	12.5 mg diphenhydramine HCl	7.5 mg phenylephrine		10 mL every 4 hours up to 40 mL/day	Alcohol free. Cherry flavor. In 473 mL
c-iii sf	**Lortuss HC Liquid**[a] (ProEthic)	3.75 mg hydrocodone bitartrate		7.5 mg phenylephrine		5 mL every 4 hours up to 30 mL/day	Saccharin, sorbitol. Grape flavor. In 20 and 473 mL.
c-iii	**Endagen-HD Liquid**[a] (Jones Pharma)	1.7 mg hydrocodone bitartrate	2 mg chlorpheniramine maleate	5 mg phenylephrine HCl		10 mL tid or qid	Cherry flavor. In 473 mL.
c-iii	**Vanex HD Liquid** (Abana)						Dye free. Cherry flavor. In 480 mL.
c-iii	**Hydro-PC Liquid**[a] (Cypress)	2 mg hydrocodone bitartrate	2 mg chlorpheniramine maleate	5 mg phenylephrine HCl		10 mL every 4 hours up to 40 mL/day	Strawberry flavor. In 473 mL.
c-iii	**Hydro-PC II Liquid**[a] (Cypress)	2 mg hydrocodone bitartrate	2 mg chlorpheniramine maleate	7.5 mg phenylephrine HCl		10 mL every 4 hours up to 40 mL/day	Strawberry flavor. In 473 mL.
c-iii sf	**Comtussin HC Syrup**[a] (Econolab)	2.5 mg hydrocodone bitartrate	2 mg chlorpheniramine maleate	5 mg phenylephrine HCl		10 mL every 4 hours up to 40 mL/day	Sorbitol, saccharin. In 473 mL
c-iii	**Cytuss HC Liquid**[a] (Cypress)						In 473 mL.
c-iii sf	**Histussin HC Syrup** (Sanofi-Synthelabo)					5 mL up to qid	Alcohol free. Orange/pineapple flavor. In 473 mL.
c-iii sf	**Hydrocodone CP Syrup**[a] (Morton Grove)					5 mL qid	Alcohol free. Saccharin, sorbitol. Fruit flavor. In 237 and 473 mL.
c-iii sf	**Histinex HC Syrup**[a] (Ethex)					10 mL every 4 hours up to 40 mL/day	Alcohol free. Saccharin, sorbitol. Fruit flavor. In 473 and 946 mL.
c-iii	**Atuss HC Liquid**[a] (Atley)	2.5 mg hydrocodone bitartrate	2 mg chlorpheniramine maleate	10 mg phenylephrine HCl		10 mL every 4 hours up to 40 mL/day	Menthol, sucrose. Cherry flavor. In 473 mL.
c-iii	**ED Tuss HC Syrup**[a] (Edwards)	2.5 mg hydrocodone bitartrate	4 mg chlorpheniramine maleate	10 mg phenylephrine HCl		5 mL every 4 hours up to 20 mL/day	5% alcohol, saccharin, sorbitol. Grape flavor. In 473 mL.
c-iii	**Maxi-Tuss HC Liquid**[a] (MCR American)					5 mL every 4 hours up to 30 mL/day	In 473 mL.
c-iii sf	**Endal HD Plus Syrup**[a] (PediaMed)	3.5 mg hydrocodone bitartrate	2 mg chlorpheniramine maleate	7.5 mg phenylephrine HCl		10 mL every 4 hours up to 40 mL/day	Alcohol free. Saccharin, sorbitol. Black raspberry flavor. In 473 mL.

ANTITUSSIVE COMBINATIONS

	Product & Distributor	Antitussive	Antihistamine	Decongestant	Other	Average Adult Dose	Excipients & How Supplied
c-iii sf	**Z-Cof HC Syrup**[a] (Zyber)	3.5 mg hydrocodone bitartrate	2.5 mg chlorpheniramine maleate	10 mg phenylephrine HCl		10 mL every 4 to 6 hours up to 40 mL/day	Alcohol free. Saccharin, sorbitol. Raspberry flavor. In 473 mL.
c-iii sf	**Poly-Tussin Syrup**[a] (Pharmakon)	5 mg hydrocodone bitartrate	2 mg chlorpheniramine maleate	5 mg phenylephrine HCl		5 to 10 mL every 4 hours up to 40 mL/day	Alcohol free. Phenylalanine. In 473 mL.
c-iii	**Atuss MS Liquid**[a] (Atley)	5 mg hydrocodone bitartrate	2 mg chlorpheniramine maleate	10 mg phenylephrine HCl		10 mL every 4 hours up to 40 mL/day	Menthol, sucrose. Pineapple/orange flavor. In 473 mL.
c-iii sf	**Hydron CP Liquid**[a] (Cypress)						Saccharin, sorbitol. Pineapple-orange flavor. Alcohol-free. In 473 mL.
c-iii sf	**Maxi-Tuss HCX Liquid**[a] (MCR American Pharmaceuticals)	6 mg hydrocodone bitartrate	2 mg chlorpheniramine maleate	12 mg phenylephrine HCl		5 mL every 4 hours up to 30 mL/day	Alcohol-free. In 480 mL.
c-iii sf	**Cordron-HC Liquid**[a] (Cypress)	1.67 mg hydrocodone bitartrate	2.5 mg chlorpheniramine maleate	20 mg pseudoephedrine hydrochloride		10 mL every 4 to 6 hours	Alcohol free. Saccharin, sorbitol. Vanilla flavor. In 473 mL.
c-iii sf	**Hydrocof-HC Liquid**[a] (Morton Grove)	3 mg hydrocodone bitartrate	2 mg chlorpheniramine maleate	15 mg pseudoephedrine hydrochloride		5 to 10 mL 4 times daily	Alcohol and dye free. Saccharin, sorbitol. Grape flavor. In 473 mL.
c-iii sf	**WellTuss HC Liquid**[a] (Prasco)						Alcohol and dye free. Saccharin, sorbitol. Grape flavor. In 473 mL.
c-iii sf	**Histinex PV Syrup**[a] (Ethex)	2.5 mg hydrocodone bitartrate	2 mg chlorpheniramine maleate	30 mg pseudoephedrine HCl		10 mL every 4 to 6 hours up to 40 mL/day	Alcohol free. Parabens, saccharin, sorbitol. Fruit flavor. In 473 mL.
c-iii	**Hyphed Liquid**[a] (Cypress)						5% alcohol. Raspberry flavor. In 473 mL.
c-iii	**P-V-Tussin Syrup**[a] (Numark)						5% alcohol, glucose, parabens, saccharin, sorbitol, sucrose. Banana flavor. In 473 mL and 3.8 L.
c-iii	**Tussend Syrup**[a] (Monarch)						5% alcohol, corn syrup, parabens, saccharin, sucrose. Banana flavor. In 473 mL.
c-iii sf	**Hydro-Tussin HC Syrup**[a] (Ethex)	3 mg hydrocodone bitartrate	2 mg chlorpheniramine maleate	15 mg pseudoephedrine HCl		5 to 10 mL qid	Alcohol and dye free. In 473 mL.
c-iii sf	**Pancof-HC Liquid**[a] (Pan American Labs)						Alcohol and dye free. In 480 mL.
c-iii sf	**Hydron PSC Liquid**[a] (Cypress)	5 mg hydrocodone bitartrate	2 mg chlorpheniramine maleate	30 mg pseudoephedrine HCl		5 mL tid or qid	Menthol, saccharin, sorbitol. Alcohol free. Vanilla flavor. In 473 mL.
c-iii	**Tussend Tablets**[a] (Monarch)	5 mg hydrocodone bitartrate	4 mg chlorpheniramine maleate	60 mg pseudoephedrine HCl		1 tablets every 4 to 6 hours up to 4 tablets/day	Lactose. (MPC100). Capsule shape, yellow, scored. In 100s.
c-iii sf	**Statuss Green Liquid**[a] (Huckaby)	2.5 mg hydrocodone bitartrate	2 mg chlorpheniramine maleate, 3.3 mg pyrilamine maleate	5 mg phenylephrine HCl, 3.3 mg pseudoephedrine HCl		10 mL every 4 to 6 hours up to 40 mL/day	Alcohol free. In 473 mL.
c-iii	**Tussionex Pennkinetic Suspension**[a] (CellTech)	10 mg hydrocodone (as polistirex)	8 mg chlorpheniramine (as polistirex)			5 mL every 12 hours up to 10 mL/day	Extended release. Alcohol free. Parabens, sucrose, corn syrup. In 473 mL.
c-iii	**Hydex PD Liquid**[a] (Cypress)	4 mg hydrocodone bitartrate	2 mg dexchlorpheniramine maleate	5 mg phenylephrine HCl		5 mL 3 or 4 times daily	Saccharin, sorbitol. Grape flavor. In 473 mL.
c-iii	**Notuss PD Liquid** (Stewart-Jackson)					5 mL tid or qid up to 20 mg/day	Menthol, sorbitol, sugar. Grape flavor. In 473 mL.

ANTITUSSIVE COMBINATIONS

	Product & Distributor	Antitussive	Antihistamine	Decongestant	Other	Average Adult Dose	Excipients & How Supplied
c-iii *sf*	**Hydro-DP Syrup**[a] (Cypress)	2 mg hydrocodone bitartrate	12.5 mg diphenhydramine HCl	7.5 mg phenylephrine HCl		10 mL every 4 hours up to 40 mL/day	Alcohol free. Saccharin, sorbitol. Cherry flavor. In 118 and 473 mL.
c-iii *sf*	**Rindal HPD Syrup**[a] (Breckenridge)						Alcohol free. Saccharin, sorbitol. Cherry flavor. In 473 mL
c-iii	**TussiNATE Syrup**[a] (Pediamed)	3.5 mg hydrocodone bitartrate	12.5 mg diphenhydramine HCl	5 mg phenylephrine HCl		10 mL every 4 to 6 hours up to 40 mL/day	Alcohol free. Saccharin, sucrose. Black raspberry flavor. In 473 mL
c-iii	**Codal-DH Syrup**[a] (Cypress)	1.66 mg hydrocodone bitartrate	8.33 mg pyrilamine maleate	5 mg phenylephrine HCl		5 to 10 mL every 4 hours up to 40 mL/day	In 473 mL.
c-iii	**Codimal DH Syrup**[a] (Schwarz)						Alcohol free. Menthol, sucrose. In 118 and 473 mL.
c-iii	**Dicomal-DH Syrup**[a] (Econolab)						In 473 mL.
c-iii *sf*	**Mintuss MR Syrup**[a] (Breckenridge)	5 mg hydrocodone bitartrate	5 mg pyrilamine maleate	5 mg phenylephrine HCl		10 mL every 4 hours up to 40 mL/day	Alcohol free. Menthol, sucrose. Pineapple-orange flavor. In 473 mL.
c-iii *sf*	**Zymine HC Liquid**[a] (Vindex)	2.5 mg hydrocodone bitartrate	1.25 mg triprolidine HCl	30 mg pseudoephedrine HCl		10 mL every 4 to 6 hours	Alcohol free and dye free. Strawberry bubble gum flavor. In 15 and 473 mL.
c-iii	**HyTan Suspension**[a] (Prasco Labs))	5 mg hydrocodone tannate	4 mg chlorpheniramine tannate			10 mL every 12 hours up to 20 mL in 24 hours	Aspartame, parabens. Tropical fruit flavor. In 118 mL.

[a] This product also may be used in children; refer to package labeling for dosing.

[b] Auriga Pharmaceuticals, 5555 Triangle Parkway, Norcross, GA 30092; (678) 282-1600

For complete and comparative prescribing information, refer to the Respiratory Combinations introduction. Some of the products in the following Pediatric Antitussive Combinations table also may be used in adults.

PEDIATRIC ANTITUSSIVE COMBINATIONS

Content given per tablet, 5 mL (liquid), or 1 mL (drops).

	Product & Distributor	Decongestant	Antihistamine	Antitussive	Other	Average Dose	Excipients & How Supplied
Rx	**Tussi-12 S Suspension** (Wallace)		4 mg chlorpheniramine tannate	30 mg carbetapentane tannate		***> 6 y*** - 5 to 10 mL q 12 h; ***2 to 6 y*** - 2.5 to 5 mL q 12 h	Methylparaben, saccharin, sucrose, tartrazine. Strawberry-currant flavor. In 118 mL with syringe.
Rx *sf*	**DACEX-A Oral Drops** (Cypress)	2 mg phenylephrine HCl	1 mg carbinoxamine maleate	2 mg dextromethorphan HBr		***3 to 6 mo*** - 0.3 to 0.6 mL q 4 to 6 h up to 2.4 mL/day ***6 to 12 mo*** - 0.6 to 1 mL q 4 to 6 h up to 4 mL/day ***12 to 24 mo*** - 1 to 2 mL q 4 to 6 h up to 8 mL/day	Alcohol-free. Saccharin, sorbitol. Cherry flavor. In 30 mL bottle with calibrated dropper.
Rx	**TRITUSS-A Oral Drops** (Everett Laboratories)						Parabens, saccharin, sorbitol. Cherry flavor. In 30 mL bottle with calibrated dropper.
Rx	**DMax Pediatric Drops** (Great Southern)	2 mg phenylephrine HCl	2 mg carbinoxamine maleate	4 mg dextromethorphan HBr		***1 to 3 mo*** - 2 to 3 drops/mo of age qid ***3 to 6 mo*** - 0.5 mL qid ***6 to 12 mo*** - 0.75 mL qid ***12 to 24 mo*** - 1 mL qid	Purple. Berry flavor. In 30 mL bottle with 1 mL dropper.
Rx	**Tannic-12 Suspension** (Cypress)	5 mg phenylephrine tannate	4 mg chlorpheniramine tannate	30 mg carbetapentane tannate		***> 6 y*** - 5 to 10 mL q 12 h; ***2 to 6 y*** - 2.5 to 5 mL q 12 h	Methylparaben, saccharin, sucrose. Strawberry flavor. In 473 mL.
Rx	**Rynatuss Pediatric Suspension** (Wallace)	5 mg phenylephrine tannate, 5 mg ephedrine tannate	4 mg chlorpheniramine tannate	30 mg carbetapentane tannate		***> 6 y*** - 5 to 10 mL q 12 h; ***2 to 6 y*** - 2.5 to 5 mL q 12 h	Tartrazine, methylparaben, saccharin, sucrose. Strawberry-currant flavor. In 237 and 473 mL.
Rx *sf*	**Lortuss DM Liquid**[a] (ProEthic)	7.5 mg phenylephrine HCl	2 mg brompheniramine maleate	15 mg dextromethorphan HBr		***≥ 12 y*** - 10 mL q 6 h up to 40 mL/day ***6 to 12 y*** - 5 mL q 6 h up to 20 mL/day ***< 6 y*** - consult a physician	Alcohol-free. Saccharin, sorbitol. Tutti-fruiti flavor. In 20 and 473 mL.

PEDIATRIC ANTITUSSIVE COMBINATIONS

	Product & Distributor	Decongestant	Antihistamine	Antitussive	Other	Average Dose	Excipients & How Supplied
Rx	**Tannate-V-DM Suspension**[a] (Hi-Tech)	12.5 mg phenylephrine tannate	30 mg pyrilamine tannate	25 mg dextromethorphan tannate		***6 to 12 y*** - 5 mL q 12 h ***2 to 6 y*** - 2.5 mL q 12 h	Methylparaben, sucralose, sucrose. Grape flavor. In 473 mL.
Rx	**Viravan-DM Suspension**[a] (PediaMed)					***6 to 12 y*** - 5 mL q 12 h; ***2 to 6 y*** - 2.5 mL q 12 h	Methylparaben, sucralose, sucrose. Grape flavor. In 473 mL.
Rx	**Viravan-DM Chewable Tablets** (PediaMed)	25 mg phenylephrine tannate	30 mg pyrilamine tannate	25 mg dextromethorphan tannate		***6 to 12 y*** - ½ to 1 q 12 h; ***2 to 6 y*** - ½ q 12 h	Sugar, sucralose. Dye free. (VIRAVAN-DM). Mottled brown, scored. Grape flavor. In 100s
otc	**Dimetapp Decongestant Plus Cough Infant Drops** (Whitehall-Robins)	9.375 mg pseudoephedrine HCl		3.125 mg dextromethorphan HBr		***2 to 3 y*** - 1.6 mL q 4 to 6 h up to 6.4 mL/day	Alcohol free. Corn syrup, menthol, sucrose. Grape flavor. In 15 mL with dropper.
otc	**Pedia Care Infants' Decongestant & Cough Drops** (Pharmacia)						Alcohol free. Sorbitol. Cherry flavor. In 15 mL with dropper.
otc	**Pedia Relief Decongestant Plus Cough Infants' Drops** (Major)						Alcohol free. Sorbitol. Cherry flavor. In 15 mL with dropper.
otc	**Tylenol Plus Cold & Cough Infants' Concentrated Drops** (McNeil)	9.375 mg pseudoephedrine HCl		3.125 mg dextromethorphan HBr	100 mg acetaminophen	***2 to 3 y*** - 1.6 mL q 4 to 6 h up to 6.4 mL/day	Alcohol free. Corn syrup, sorbitol. Cherry flavor. In 15 mL with dropper.
otc sf	**Sudafed Children's Non-Drowsy Cold & Cough Liquid**[a] (Warner-Lambert)	15 mg pseudoephedrine HCl		5 mg dextromethorphan HBr		***6 to < 12 y*** - 10 mL q 4 h up to 40 mL/day; ***2 to < 6 y*** - 5 mL q 4 h up to 20 mL/day	Alcohol free. Saccharin, sorbitol. Cherry-berry flavor. In 118 mL.
otc	**Dimetapp Children's Non-Drowsy Flu Syrup**[a] (Whitehall-Robins)	15 mg pseudoephedrine HCl		5 mg dextromethorphan HBr	160 mg acetaminophen	***6 to < 12 y*** - 10 mL q 4 h up to 40 mL/day; ***2 to < 6 y*** - 5 mL q 4 h up to 20 mL/day	Alcohol free. Corn syrup, saccharin, sorbitol. Fruit flavor. In 118 mL.
otc	**Triaminic Throat Pain & Cough Softchews Tablets**[a] (Novartis)					***6 to < 12 y*** - 2 q 4 to 6 h up to qid; ***2 to < 6 y*** - 1 q 4 to 6 h up qid	Aspartame, mannitol, 28.1 mg phenylalanine. Grape flavor. In 18s.
otc	**PediaCare Children's Long-Acting Cough Plus Cold Liquid** (Pfizer Consumer Health)	15 mg pseudoephedrine HCl		7.5 mg dextromethorphan HBr		***6 to 11 y*** - 10 mL q 6 h up to 40 mL/day; ***2 to 5 y*** - 5 mL q 6 h up to 20 mL/day	Alcohol free. Corn syrup, sorbitol. Grape flavor. In 120 mL.
otc	**Robitussin Pediatric Cough & Cold Formula Liquid**[a] (Whitehall-Robins)					***6 to < 12 y*** - 10 mL q 6 h up to 40 mL/day; ***2 to < 6 y*** - 5 mL q 6 h up to 20 mL/day	Alcohol free. Corn syrup, saccharin. Fruit punch flavor. In 118 mL.
otc	**Triaminic AM Non-Drowsy Cough & Decongestant Liquid**[a] (Novartis)						EDTA, sorbitol, sucrose. Orange/Strawberry flavor. In 118 mL.
otc	**Triaminic Cough Liquid** (Novartis)					***6 to < 12 y*** - 10 mL q 4 to 6 h up to 40 mL/day; ***2 to < 6 y*** - 5 mL q 4 to 6 h up to 20 mL/day	Alcohol free. Sorbitol, sucrose. Cherry flavor. In 118 mL.
otc	**Triaminic Cold & Sore Throat Softchews Tablets** (Novartis)	15 mg pseudoephedrine HCl		5 mg dextromethorphan HBr	160 mg acetaminophen	***6 to < 12 y*** - 2 q 4 to 6 h up to 8/day; ***2 to < 6 y*** - 1 q 4 to 6 h up to 4/day	Aspartame, 28.1 mg phenylalanine, sorbitol, mannitol, sucrose. Grape flavor. In 18s.
otc	**Triaminic Cough & Sore Throat Liquid** (Novartis)					***6 to < 12 y*** - 10 mL q 6 h up to 40 mL/day; ***2 to < 6 y*** - 5 mL q 6 h up to 20 mL/day	Alcohol free. EDTA, sucrose. Grape flavor. In 118 and 237 mL.
Rx sf	**EndaCof-PD Oral Drops** (Larken)	12.5 mg pseudoephedrine HCl	1 mg brompheniramine maleate	3 mg dextromethorphan HBr		***12 to 24 mo*** - 1 mL qid up to 4 mL/day ***6 to 12 mo*** - 0.75 mL qid up to 3 mL/day ***3 to 6 mo*** - 0.5 mL qid up to 2 mL/day ***1 to 3 mo*** - 0.25 mL qid up to 1 mL/day	Alcohol free. Parabens, saccharin. Grape flavor. In 30 mL bottle with 1 mL dropper.

PEDIATRIC ANTITUSSIVE COMBINATIONS

	Product & Distributor	Decongestant	Antihistamine	Antitussive	Other	Average Dose	Excipients & How Supplied
Rx *sf*	**Histacol DM Pediatric Oral Drops** (Breckenridge)	15 mg pseudoephedrine HCl	1 mg brompheniramine maleate	4 mg dextromethorphan HBr		***9 to 18 mo*** - 1 mL qid; ***6 to 9 mo*** - 0.75 mL qid; ***3 to 6 mo*** - 0.5 mL qid; ***1 to 3 mo*** - 0.25 mL qid	Alcohol free. Sorbitol. Grape flavor. In 30 mL with 1 mL dropper.
Rx	**Pediahist DM Drops** (Boca Pharmacal)					***9 to 18 mo*** - 1 mL qid up to 4 mL/day; ***6 to 9 mo*** - 0.75 mL qid up to 3 mL/day; ***3 to 6 mo*** - 0.5 mL qid up to 2 mL/day; ***1 to 3 mo*** - 0.25 mL qid up to 1 mL/day	Sorbitol. Grape flavor. In 30 mL with calibrated dropper.
Rx	**AccuHist PDX Drops** (PediaMed)	12.5 mg pseudoephedrine HCl	1 mg brompheniramine maleate	3 mg dextromethorphan HBr		***12 to 24 mo*** - 1 mL qid, up to 4 mL/day; ***6 to 12 mo*** - 0.75 mL qid, up to 3 mL/day; ***3 to 6 mo*** - 0.5 mL qid, up to 2 mL/day; ***1 to 3 mo*** - 0.25 qid, up to 1 mL/day.	Saccharin, sorbitol. Grape flavor. In 30 mL w/ dropper.
Rx	**Bromhist PDX Drops** (Cypress)	12.5 mg pseudoephedrine HCl	1 mg brompheniramine maleate	3 mg dextromethorphan HBr		***12 to 24 mo*** - 1 mL qid, up to 4 mL/day; ***6 to 12 mo*** - 0.75 mL qid, up to 3 mL/day; ***3 to 6 mo*** - 0.5 mL qid, up to 2 mL/day; ***1 to 3 mo*** - 0.25 qid, up to 1 mL/day.	Sorbitol, saccharin. Alcohol free. Grape flavor. In 30 mL w/ calibrated dropper.
otc	**Bromanate DM Cold & Cough Elixir**[a] (Alpharma)	15 mg pseudoephedrine HCl	1 mg brompheniramine maleate	5 mg dextromethorphan HBr		***6 to < 12 y*** - 5 mL q 4 h up to 30 mL/day	Alcohol free. Grape flavor. In 118 mL.
otc	**Children's Elixir DM Cough & Cold Elixir**[a] (AmerisourceBergen)					***6 to < 12 y*** - 10 mL q 4 to 6 h up to 40 mL/day	Alcohol free. Saccharin, sorbitol. Grape flavor. In 118 mL.
otc	**Dimaphen DM Cold & Cough Elixir**[a] (Major)						Alcohol free. Saccharin, sorbitol. Grape flavor. In 118 mL.
otc	**Dimetapp DM Children's Cold & Cough Elixir**[a] (Whitehall-Robins)					***6 to < 12 y*** - 10 mL q 4 h up to 40 mL/day	Alcohol free. Sorbitol, saccharin, corn syrup. Grape flavor. In 118 and 237 mL.
otc	**Dimetapp Children's Night-time Flu Syrup**[a] (Whitehall-Robins)	15 mg pseudoephedrine HCl	1 mg brompheniramine maleate	5 mg dextromethorphan HBr	160 mg acetaminophen	***6 to < 12 y*** - 10 mL q 4 h up to 40 mL/day	Alcohol free. Corn syrup, saccharin, sorbitol. Bubble gum flavor. In 118 mL.
Rx	**C.P.-DM Drops** (Hi-Tech)	15 mg pseudoephedrine HCl	1 mg carbinoxamine maleate	4 mg dextromethorphan HBr		***12 to 24 mo*** - 1 mL qid; ***6 to 12 mo*** - 0.75 mL qid; ***3 to 6 mo*** - 0.5 mL qid; ***1 to 3 mo*** - 0.25 mL qid.	Saccharin, sorbitol. Grape flavor. In 30 mL with dropper.
Rx *sf*	**Carbofed DM Oral Drops** (Hi-Tech)						Alcohol free. In 30 mL with dropper.
Rx	**Rondec-DM Oral Drops** (Biovail)						Saccharin, sorbitol. Grape flavor. In 30 mL with dropper.
Rx	**Andehist DM NR Oral Drops** (Silarx)						Saccharin, sorbitol. Grape flavor. In 30 mL with dropper.
Rx	**Carbodex DM Drops** (Tri-Med)	15 mg pseudoephedrine HCl	1 mg carbinoxamine maleate	4 mg dextromethorphan HBr		***9 to 18 mo*** - 1 mL qid; ***6 to 9 mo*** - 0.75 mL qid; ***3 to 6 mo*** - 0.5 mL qid; ***1 to 3 mo*** - 0.25 mL qid	In 30 mL.
Rx *sf*	**Sildec-DM Oral Drops** (Silarx)					***12 to 24 mo*** - 1 mL qid; ***6 to 12 mo*** - 0.75 mL qid; ***3 to 6 mo*** - 0.5 mL qid; ***1 to 3 mo*** - 0.25 mL qid	Saccharin, sorbitol. Grape flavor. In 30 mL with dropper.
Rx	**Pediatex-DM Liquid**[a] (Zyber Pharm)	15 mg pseudoephedrine HCl	2 mg carbinoxamine maleate	15 mg dextromethorphan HBr		***6 to 12 y*** - 5 mL qid; ***18 mo to 6 y*** - 2.5 mL qid	Saccharin, sorbitol. Cotton candy flavor. In 20 and 473 mL.
Rx	**Balamine DM Oral Drops** (Ballay)	25 mg pseudoephedrine HCl	2 mg carbinoxamine maleate	3.5 mg dextromethorphan HBr		***9 to 18 mo*** - 1 mL qid; ***6 to 9 mo*** - 0.75 mL qid; ***3 to 6 mo*** - 0.5 mL qid; ***1 to 3 mo*** - 0.25 mL qid	Menthol. Grape flavor. In 30 mL with dropper.
Rx	**Cydec-DM Drops** (Cypress)	25 mg pseudoephedrine HCl	2 mg carbinoxamine maleate	4 mg dextromethorphan HBr			Grape flavor. In 30 mL with dropper.

PEDIATRIC ANTITUSSIVE COMBINATIONS

	Product & Distributor	Decongestant	Antihistamine	Antitussive	Other	Average Dose	Excipients & How Supplied
Rx	**Balamine DM Syrup**[a] (Ballay)	60 mg pseudoephedrine HCl	4 mg carbinoxamine maleate	12.5 mg dextromethorphan HBr		**≥ *6 y*** - 5 mL qid; ***18 mo to 6 y*** - 2.5 mL qid	Menthol. Grape flavor. In 473 mL.
Rx	**Cydec-DM Syrup**[a] (Cypress)	60 mg pseudoephedrine HCl	4 mg carbinoxamine maleate	15 mg dextromethorphan HBr		**≥ *6 y*** - 5 mL qid; ***18 mo to 6 y*** - 2.5 mL qid	Grape flavor. In 118 and 473 mL and 3.8 L.
otc	**Tylenol Children's Cold Plus Cough Chewable Tablets** (McNeil)	7.5 mg pseudoephedrine HCl	0.5 mg chlorpheniramine maleate	2.5 mg dextromethorphan HBr	80 mg acetaminophen	***6 to 11 y*** - 4 q 4 to 6 h up to 16/day	Aspartame, mannitol, 4 mg phenylalanine. (TYLENOL C/C TC/C). Cherry flavor. In 24s.
otc	**All-Nite Children's Cold/Cough Relief Liquid**[a] (Major)	10 mg pseudoephedrine HCl	0.67 mg chlorpheniramine maleate	5 mg dextromethorphan HBr		***6 to 11 y*** – 15 mL q 6 h up to 60 mL/day	Alcohol free. Sucrose. Cherry flavor. In 118 mL.
otc	**Nite Time Children's Liquid**[a] (Topco)						Alcohol free. Sucrose. Cherry flavor. In 118 mL.
otc	**Vicks Children's NyQuil Cold/Cough Relief Liquid**[a] (Procter & Gamble)						Alcohol free. Sucrose. Cherry flavor. In 118 mL.
otc	**Vicks Pediatric 44M Cough & Cold Relief Liquid**[a] (Procter & Gamble)						Alcohol free. Corn syrup, saccharin. Cherry flavor. In 115 mL.
otc	**Kid Kare Children's Cough/Cold Liquid** (Rugby)	15 mg pseudoephedrine HCl	1 mg chlorpheniramine maleate	5 mg dextromethorphan HBr		***6 to 11 y*** - 10 mL q 4 to 6 h up to 40 mL/day	Alcohol free. Sorbitol, corn syrup. Cherry flavor. In 118 mL.
otc	**Pedia Care Cough-Cold Liquid** (Pharmacia)						Alcohol free. Corn syrup, sorbitol. Cherry flavor. In 118 mL.
otc	**Pedia Care Multi-Symptom Cold Liquid** (Pharmacia)						Alcohol free. Corn syrup, sorbitol. Cherry flavor. In 120 mL.
otc	**Thera-Hist Cold & Cough Syrup**[a] (Major)						Sorbitol, sucrose. Cherry flavor. In 118 mL.
otc	**Tri-Acting Cold & Cough Syrup** (Topco)						Alcohol free. Sorbitol, sucrose. Cherry flavor. In 118 mL.
otc	**Triaminic Cold & Cough Liquid** (Novartis)						Alcohol free. Sorbitol, sucrose. Cherry flavor. In 118 mL.
otc	**PediaCare Children's Multi-Symptom Cold Chewable Tablets** (Pfizer Consumer Health)					***6 to < 12 y*** - 2 q 4 h up to 8/day	Aspartame, 8.4 mg phenylalanine, sucrose. Cherry Flavor. In 18s.
otc	**Triaminic Cold & Cough Softchews Tablets**[a] (Novartis)					***6 to < 12 y*** - 2 q 4 to 6 h up to 8/day	Aspartame, mannitol, 17.7 mg phenylalanine, sucrose. (T2). Cherry flavor. In 18s.
otc	**Tylenol Children's Cold Plus Cough Suspension** (McNeil)	15 mg pseudoephedrine HCl	1 mg chlorpheniramine maleate	5 mg dextromethorphan HBr	160 mg acetaminophen	***6 to 11 y*** - 10 mL q 4 to 6 h up to 40 mL/day	Alcohol free. Acesulfame K, butylparaben, corn syrup, sorbitol. Cherry flavor. In 120 mL.
otc	**Pedia Care NightRest Cough & Cold Liquid** (Pharmacia)	15 mg pseudoephedrine HCl	1 mg chlorpheniramine maleate	7.5 mg dextromethorphan HBr		***6 to 11 y*** - 10 mL q 6 to 8 h up to 40 mL/day	Alcohol free. Corn syrup, sorbitol. Cherry flavor. In 120 mL.
otc	**Robitussin Pediatric Night Relief Cough & Cold Liquid** (Whitehall-Robins)					***6 to < 12 y*** - 10 mL q 6 h up to 40 mL/day	Alcohol free. Corn syrup, saccharin. Fruit punch flavor. In 118 mL
otc	**Triaminic Night Time Cough & Cold Liquid** (Novartis)						Alcohol free. Sorbitol, sucrose, EDTA. Grape flavor. In 118 mL.

PEDIATRIC ANTITUSSIVE COMBINATIONS

	Product & Distributor	Decongestant	Antihistamine	Antitussive	Other	Average Dose	Excipients & How Supplied
otc	**Triaminic Flu, Cough & Fever Liquid** (Novartis)	15 mg pseudoephedrine HCl	1 mg chlorpheniramine maleate	7.5 mg dextromethorphan HBr	160 mg acetaminophen	***6 to < 12 y*** - 10 mL q 6 h up to 40 mL/day	Acesulfame K, EDTA, sucrose. Bubble gum flavor. In 118 mL.
otc	**Tylenol Children's Flu Suspension** (McNeil)					***6 to 11 y*** - 10 mL q 6 to 8 h up to 40 mL/day	Alcohol free. Acesulfame K, butylparaben, corn syrup, sorbitol. Bubble gum flavor. In 118 mL.
Rx	**Atuss-12 DM Suspension, extended-release**[a] (Atley)	30 mg pseudoephedrine HCl (as polistirex)	6 mg chlorpheniramine maleate (as polistirex)	30 mg/5 mL dextromethorphan HBr (as polistirex)		***6 to 12 y*** - 2.5 to 5 mL q 12 h; ***2 to 6 y*** - 2.5 mL q 12 h	Corn syrup, parabens. In 20 and 473 mL.
c-iii sf	**Pediatex HC Syrup**[a] (Zyber)	17.5 mg pseudoephedrine HCl	2.5 mg chlorpheniramine maleate	1.67 mg hydrocodone bitartrate		***6 to 12 y*** - 5 mL q 4 to 6 h up to 20 mL/day ***2 to 6 y*** - 2.5 mL q 4 to 6 h up to 10 mL/day	Saccharin, sorbitol. Cotton candy flavor. In 20 and 480 mL.

[a] This product also may be used in adults; refer to package labeling for dosing.

Refer to the general discussion of these products in the Respiratory Combinations Introduction. Some of the products in the previous Antitussive Combinations table also may be used in children.

ANTITUSSIVE AND EXPECTORANT COMBINATIONS

Content given per tablet, 5 mL, or packet.

	Product & Distributor	Antitussive	Expectorant	Decongestant	Antihistamine/ Other	Average Adult Dose	Excipients & How Supplied
Rx	**Levall Liquid**[a] (Athlon Pharmaceuticals)	20 mg carbetapentane citrate	100 mg guaifenesin	15 mg phenylephrine HCl		5 mL q 4 to 6 h up to 20 mL/day	Alcohol free. Strawberry flavor. In 15 and 473 mL.
c-v	**Dihistine Expectorant Liquid** (Alpharma)	10 mg codeine phosphate	100 mg guaifenesin	30 mg pseudoephedrine HCl		10 mL q 4 h up to 40 mL/day	7.5% alcohol, saccharin, sorbitol, sucrose. In 473 mL.
c-v	**Guiatuss DAC Liquid**[a] (Various, eg, Ivax)						May contain alcohol. In 473 mL.
c-v sf	**Mytussin DAC Liquid**[a] (Morton Grove Pharmaceuticals)						1.7% alcohol, menthol, saccharin, sorbitol. Strawberry-raspberry flavor. In 118 and 473 mL.
c-v	**Novagest Expectorant with Codeine Liquid**[a] (Major)						8.2% alcohol, sugar, menthol, parabens. In 118 and 473 mL.
c-iii	**Nucofed Expectorant Syrup**[a] (Monarch)	20 mg codeine phosphate	200 mg guaifenesin	60 mg pseudoephedrine HCl		5 mL q 6 h up to 20 mL/day	12.5% alcohol, saccharin, sucrose. Cherry flavor. In 473 mL.
c-iii	**Nucotuss Expectorant Syrup**[a] (Alpharma)						12.5% alcohol. In 473 mL.
c-v	**Tussirex Syrup** (Scot-Tussin)	10 mg codeine phosphate	83.3 mg sodium citrate	4.17 mg phenylephrine HCl	13.33 mg pheniramine maleate, 83.33 mg sodium salicylate, 25 mg caffeine citrate	5 mL tid	Alcohol and dye free. 0.17 mg menthol. In 473 mL and 3.8 L.
c-v sf	**Tussirex Sugar Free Liquid** (Scot-Tussin)						Alcohol and dye free. 0.17 mg menthol. In 30 and 473 mL and 3.8 L.
Rx	**Donatussin Syrup**[a] (Laser)	15 mg dextromethorphan HBr	100 mg guaifenesin	10 mg phenylephrine HCl	2 mg/5 mL chlorpheniramine maleate	10 mL q 6 h up to 40 mL/day	In 30, 115, and 473 mL.
Rx	**TUSSI-PRES Liquid**[a] (Kramer-Novis[b])	15 mg dextromethorphan HBr	200 mg guaifenesin	5 mg phenylephrine HCl		10 mL q 6 h up to 40 mL/day	14 mg phenylalanine, aspartame, parabens. Cherry flavor. In 237 mL.
Rx	**Tussafed Ex Syrup**[a] (Everett Laboratories)	30 mg dextromethorphan HBr	200 mg guaifenesin	10 mg phenylephrine HCl		5 mL qid	Alcohol free. EDTA, saccharin, sorbitol. Cherry-vanilla flavor. In 473 mL.
Rx	**SINUtuss DM Tablets**[a] (WE Pharm)	30 mg dextromethorphan HBr	600 mg guaifenesin	15 mg phenylephrine HCl		2 tablets bid	Dye-free. (WE 45). Capsule shape, scored. In 100s.
Rx sf	**Lemotussin-DM Liquid**[a] (Seneca)	7.5 mg dextromethorphan HBr	50 mg guaifenesin, 50 mg potassium guaiacolsulfonate	10 mg pseudoephedrine HCl	2 mg chlorpheniramine maleate	5 to 10 mL q 6 to 8 h	Parabens, saccharin, sorbitol. Alcohol free. In 473 mL.

ANTITUSSIVE AND EXPECTORANT COMBINATIONS

	Product & Distributor	Antitussive	Expectorant	Decongestant	Antihistamine/ Other	Average Adult Dose	Excipients & How Supplied
otc	**Robafen CF Syrup**[a] (Major)	10 mg dextromethorphan HBr	100 mg guaifenesin	30 mg pseudoephedrine HCl		10 mL q 4 h up to 40 mL/day	Alcohol free. Saccharin, sorbitol. In 118 and 237 mL.
otc	**Robitussin CF Syrup**[a] (Whitehall-Robins)						Alcohol free. Saccharin, sorbitol. In 355 mL.
otc	**Comtrex Multi-Symptom Deep Chest Cold Softgels** (Bristol-Myers Squibb)	10 mg dextromethorphan HBr	100 mg guaifenesin	30 mg pseudoephedrine HCl	250 mg acetaminophen	2 q 4 h up to 8/day	Sorbitol. In 20s.
otc	**Robitussin Cold, Multi-Symptom Cold & Flu Softgels** (Whitehall-Robins)					2 q 4 h up to 8/day	Sorbitol. (AHR 8602). In 12s.
otc	**Sudafed Multi-Symptom Cold & Cough Liquid Caps** (Warner-Lambert)						Sorbitol. (SMS). In 20s.
otc	**Cold & Cough Tussin Softgels**[a] (AmerisourceBergen)	10 mg dextromethorphan HBr	200 mg guaifenesin	30 mg pseudoephedrine HCl		2 q 4 h up to 8/day	Sorbitol. In 12s.
otc	**Robitussin Cold, Cold & Cough Softgels**[a] (Whitehall-Robins)						Sorbitol. (AHR 8600). In 12s and 20s.
otc	**Robitussin Cold, Cold & Congestion Softgels and Tablets**[a] (Whitehall-Robins)						Capsule shape. In 20s.
otc	**Robitussin Cold, Multi-Symptom Cold & Flu Tablets**[a] (Whitehall-Robins)	10 mg dextromethorphan HBr	200 mg guaifenesin	30 mg pseudoephedrine HCl	325 mg acetaminophen	2 q 4 h up to 8/day	Capsule shape. In 20s.
Rx	**DEKA Liquid**[a] (Dayton)	15 mg dextromethorphan HBr	100 mg guaifenesin	15 mg pseudoephedrine HCl	0.5 mg dexbrompheniramine maleate	10 mL every 4 to 6 h.	Sucrose, saccharin, parabens. Grape flavor. In 120 mL.
Rx sf	**PanMist-DM Syrup**[a] (Pan American Laboratories)	15 mg dextromethorphan HBr	100 mg guaifenesin	40 mg pseudoephedrine HCl		Up to 10 mL tid or qid	Alcohol and dye free. Strawberry flavor. In 15 and 473 mL.
otc	**Tylenol Cold Severe Congestion Tablets** (McNeil Consumer)	15 mg dextromethorphan HBr	200 mg guaifenesin	30 mg pseudoephedrine HCl	325 mg acetaminophen	2 q 6 to 8 h up to 8/day	Mannitol. Capsule shape. In 48s.
Rx sf	**Z-Cof DM Syrup**[a] (Zyber Pharmaceuticals)	15 mg dextromethorphan HBr	200 mg guaifenesin	40 mg pseudoephedrine HCl		10 mL bid or tid up to 30 mL/day	Alcohol free. Grape flavor. In 473 mL.
Rx	**Duraflu Tablets**[a] (ProEthic)	20 mg dextromethorphan HBr	200 mg guaifenesin	60 mg pseudoephedrine HCl	500 mg acetaminophen	1 qid up to 4/day	Dye-free. (PE 723). Scored. In 100s.
otc	**TheraFlu Flu & Chest Congestion Non-Drowsy Powder** (Novartis Consumer Health)	30 mg dextromethorphan HBr	400 mg guaifenesin	60 mg pseudoephedrine HCl	1,000 mg acetaminophen	1 packet dissolved in 6 oz. hot water every 6 h up to 4/day	Aspartame, 24 mg phenylalanine, sucrose. Natural citrus flavor. In 6s.
otc	**TheraFlu Maximum Strength Flu, Cold, & Cough Powder** (Novartis)						Alcohol free. Aspartame, phenylalanine, sucrose. Honey lemon flavor. In 6s.
Rx	**GFN 550/PSE 60/DM 30 Tablets**[a] (Cypress)	30 mg dextromethorphan HBr	550 mg guaifenesin	60 mg pseudoephedrine HCl		1 to 2 q 12 h up to 4/day	Extended release. Dye-free. (CYP 28 7). In 100s.
Rx	**Touro CC Tablets**[a] (Dartmouth Pharmaceuticals)	30 mg dextromethorphan HBr	575 mg guaifenesin	60 mg pseudoephedrine HCl		1 or 2 q 12 h up to 4/day	Sustained release. Dye-free. (TOURO CC/DP). Capsule shape, scored. In 100s.
Rx	**Maxifed DM Tablets**[a] (MCR American Pharmaceutical)	30 mg dextromethorphan HBr	580 mg guaifenesin	60 mg pseudoephedrine HCl		1 to 2 q 12 h up to 4/day.	Extended release. Dye free. (MAXIFED DM). Capsule shape, scored. In 100s.
Rx	**AMBI 60/580/30 Tablets**[a] (AMBI)					1 to 2 q 12 h up to 4/day.	Extended release. Dye free. (AMBI/122). Capsule shape, scored. In 100s.

ANTITUSSIVE AND EXPECTORANT COMBINATIONS

	Product & Distributor	Antitussive	Expectorant	Decongestant	Antihistamine/ Other	Average Adult Dose	Excipients & How Supplied
Rx	**GFN 600/PSE 60/DM 30 Tablets**[a] (Cypress)	30 mg dextromethorphan HBr	600 mg guaifenesin	60 mg pseudoephedrine HCl		1 to 2 q 12 h up to 4/day	Sustained release. Dye-free. White, capsule shape, scored. In 100s.
Rx	**Tussafed-LA Tablets**[a] (Everett)						Sustained release. Dye free. Capsule shape, scored. In 100s.
Rx	**Profen II DM Tablets**[a] (Ivax)	30 mg dextromethorphan HBr	800 mg guaifenesin	45 mg pseudoephedrine HCl		1 or 1½ q 12 h up to 3/day	Extended release. (PROFEN II DM). White, capsule shape, scored. In 100s.
Rx	**Medent-DM Tablets**[a] (Stewart-Jackson Pharmacal)	30 mg dextromethorphan HBr	800 mg guaifenesin	60 mg pseudoephedrine HCl		1 to 1½ q 12 h or 1 q 8 h up to 3/day	Sustained release. Dye free. (SJ/641). Oval, scored. In 100s.
Rx	**PanMist-DM Tablets**[a] (Pan American Laboratories)	32 mg dextromethorphan HBr	595 mg guaifenesin	48 mg pseudoephedrine HCl		1 or 2 q 12 h up to 4/day	Extended release. (PAL 07/59). Green, capsule shape, scored. In 100s.
Rx	**Maxifed DMX Tablets**[a] (MCR American Pharmaceutical)	40 mg dextromethorphan HBr	780 mg guaifenesin	80 mg pseudoephedrine HCl		1 to 1½ q 12 h up to 2/day	Sustained release. Dye free. (MAXIFED DMX). White, oval, scored. In 100s.
Rx	**Humibid DM Capsules**[a] (Carolina Pharmaceuticals)[c]	50 mg dextromethorphan HBr	400 mg guaifenesin	200 mg potassium guaiacol-sulfonate		1 q 12 h up to 2/day	Extended release. Sucrose. (HUMABID DM CAROLINA PHARMA). Lt. blue, white opaque. In 30s and 100s.
Rx	**Profen Forte DM Tablets**[a] (Ivax)	60 mg dextromethorphan HBr	800 mg guaifenesin	90 mg pseudoephedrine HCl		1 q 12 h up to 2/day	Sustained release. (PROFEN FORTE DM/316). White, capsule shape, scored. In 100s.
Rx	**MAXIPHEN DM Tablets**[a] (AMBI)	60 mg dextromethorphan HBr	1000 mg guaifenesin	40 mg phenylephrine HCl		1 q 12 h up to 2/day.	Extended-release. Dye-free. (Maxiphen DM). Capsule shape, scored. In 100s.
Rx	**Aquatab C Tablets** (Adams)	60 mg dextromethorphan HBr	1,200 mg guaifenesin	60 mg pseudoephedrine HCl		1 q 12 h up to 2/day	Extended release. (Adams 063). Lt. yellow, oval, scored. In 100s.
Rx	**GFN 1200/DM 60/PSE 120 Tablets** (Cypress)	60 mg dextromethorphan HBr	1,200 mg guaifenesin	120 mg pseudoephedrine HCl		1 q 12 h up to 2/day	Sustained release. Dye free. (CYP 273). White, capsule shape, scored. In 100s.
Rx	**Pancof-EXP Syrup**[a] (Pan American)	7.5 mg dihydrocodeine bitar-trate	100 mg guaifenesin	15 mg pseudoephedrine		5 to 10 mL q 4 to 6 h	Saccharin, sorbitol, menthol. Alcohol- and dye-free. In 25 and 473 mL.
c-iii	**Atuss-G Syrup**[a] (Atley)	2 mg hydrocodone bitartrate	100 mg guaifenesin	10 mg phenylephrine HCl		10 mL q 4 h up to 40 mL/day	Menthol, saccharin, sucrose. Grape flavor. In 473 mL.
c-iii	**Donatussin DC Syrup**[a] (Laser)	2.5 mg hydrocodone bitartrate	50 mg guaifenesin	7.5 mg phenylephrine HCl		10 mL q 4 to 6 h up to 40 mL/day	Alcohol free. In 118 and 473 mL.
c-iii	**Tussafed HC Syrup**[a] (Everett Laboratories)					10 mL q 4 to 6 h up to 60 mL/day	Alcohol free. In 473 mL.
c-iii	**Duratuss HD Elixir**[a] (Victory Pharma)	2.5 mg hydrocodone bitartrate	225 mg guaifenesin	10 mg phenylephrine HCl		10 mL q 4 to 6 h	Saccharin, sorbitol, sodium ben-zoate. Wild cherry flavor. In 473 mL.
c-iii sf	**Entex HC Liquid**[a] (Andrx Laboratories)	5 mg hydrocodone bitartrate	100 mg guaifenesin	7.5 mg phenylephrine HCl		5 to 10 mL q 4 to 6 h up to 40 mL/day	Alcohol and dye free. Cherry fla-vor. In 15 and 473 mL.
c-iii sf	**Levall 5.0 Liquid**[a] (Athlon Pharmaceuticals)	5 mg hydrocodone bitartrate	100 mg guaifenesin	15 mg phenylephrine HCl		5 mL q 4 to 6 h up to 20 mL/day	Alcohol free. Grape flavor. In 15 and 473 mL.
c-iii	**ZTuss Expectorant Liquid**[a] (Huckaby Pharmacal)	2.5 mg hydrocodone bitartrate	100 mg guaifenesin	15 mg pseudoephedrine HCl	2 mg chlorpheniramine maleate	10 mL q 4 to 6 h	Phenylalanine. In 473 mL.

ANTITUSSIVE AND EXPECTORANT COMBINATIONS

	Product & Distributor	Antitussive	Expectorant	Decongestant	Antihistamine/ Other	Average Adult Dose	Excipients & How Supplied
c-iii	**Hydro-Tussin HD Liquid**[a] (Ethex)	2.5 mg hydrocodone bitartrate	100 mg guaifenesin	30 mg pseudoephedrine HCl		10 mL q 4 to 6 h	Alcohol free. Saccharin, sorbitol. In 473 mL.
c-iii	**Su-Tuss HD Elixir**[a] (Cypress)						5% alcohol. Fruit punch flavor. In 473 mL.
c-iii *sf*	**Pancof-XP Liquid**[a] (Pan American Labs)	3 mg hydrocodone bitartrate	100 mg guaifenesin	15 mg pseudoephedrine HCl		5 to 10 mL qid	Alcohol and dye free. In 473 mL.
c-iii	**Nalex Expectorant Liquid**[a] (Blansett Pharmacal)	5 mg hydrocodone bitartrate	200 mg guaifenesin	60 mg pseudoephedrine HCl		12.5% alcohol. 5 mL qid up to 20 mL/day	In 25 and 473 mL.

[a] This product may also be used in children; refer to package labeling for dosing.
[b] Kramer-Novis, P.O. Box 191775, San Juan, PR 00919-1775; (787) 767-2072, fax (787) 767-7281.
[c] Carolina Pharmaceutical, Inc., 2500 Regency Parkway, Cary, NC 27511.

Refer to the general discussion of these products in the Respiratory Combinations Introduction. Some of the products in the following Pediatric Antitussive and Expectorant Combinations table also may be used in adults.

PEDIATRIC ANTITUSSIVE AND EXPECTORANT COMBINATIONS

Content given per 5 mL or 1 mL (drops).

	Product & Distributor	Decongestant	Antihistamine/Other	Antitussive	Expectorant	Dose	Excipients & How Supplied
Rx *sf*	**Zotex Pediatric Drops** (Vertical Pharmaceuticals, Inc.)	2.5 mg/mL phenylephrine hydrochloride		3 mg/mL dextromethorphan HBr	35 mg/mL guaifenesin	***9 to 18 mo***- 1 mL qid; ***6 to 9 mo***- 0.75 mL qid	Alcohol-free. Parabens, saccharin. Grape flavor. In 30 mL. with dropper.
Rx *sf*	**Tussi-Pres Pediatric**[a] **Liquid** (Kramer-Novis)	2.5 mg phenylephrine hydrochloride		5 mg dextromethorphan hydrobromide	75 mg guaifenesin	***6 to 12 yr (45 to 95 lbs) -*** 10 mL q 6 h. up to 40 mL/day; ***2 to 6 yr (25 to 45 lbs) -*** 5 mL q 6 h, up to 20 mL/day	Alcohol, dye, and saccharin free. Parabens, aspartame, 14 mg per 5 mL phenylalanine. In 473 mL.
Rx	**Phenydex Pediatric Liquid** (Roxmar Laboratories)	2.5 mg phenylephrine hydrochloride		5 mg dextromethorphan hydrobromide	50 mg guaifenesin	***6 to 12 yr*** - 10 mL q 4 h up to 60 mL/day; ***2 to 6 yr*** - 5 mL q 4 h up to 30 mL/day	Phenylalanine. Tutti fruit flavor. In 118 mL.
Rx	**AccuHist PDX Syrup**[a] (PediaMed)	5 mg phenylephrine hydrochloride	2 mg/5 mL brompheniramine maleate	5 mg dextromethorphan hydrobromide	50 mg guaifenesin	***6 to < 12 yr -*** 5 mL q 4 to 6 h, up to 30 mL/day; ***2 to < 6 yr -*** 2.5 mL q 4 to 6 h, up to 15 mL/day.	Sucrose. Grape flavor. In 473 mL.
c-v	**Nucofed Pediatric Expectorant Syrup**[a] (Monarch)	30 mg pseudoephedrine hydrochloride		10 mg codeine phosphate	100 mg guaifenesin	***6 to < 12 yr*** - 5 mL q 6 h up to 20 mL/day; ***2 to < 6 yr*** - 2.5 mL q 6 h up to 10 mL/day	6% alcohol, EDTA, saccharin, sucrose. Strawberry flavor. In 473 mL.
c-v	**Nucotuss Pediatric Expectorant Syrup**[a] (Alpharma)						6% alcohol. Strawberry flavor. In 473 mL.
Rx	**DEKA Pediatric Drops** (Dayton)	12.5 mg pseudoephedrine hydrochloride	0.5 mg dexbrompheniramine maleate	4 mg dextromethorphan hydrobromide	40 mg guaifenesin	***12 to 24 mo*** - 1 mL every 4 to 6 h up to 4 mL daily; ***6 to 12 mo*** - 0.75 mL every 4 to 6 h up to 3 mL daily ***3 to 6 mo*** - 0.5 mL every 4 to 6 h up to 2 mL daily ***1 to 3 mo*** - 0.25 mL every 4 to 6 h up to 1 mL daily	Alcohol free. Sucrose, saccharin, parabens, EDTA. Grape flavor. In 30 mL with calibrated dropper.
Rx *sf*	**Despec Drops** (International Ethical Laboratories, Inc.)	10 mg pseudoephedrine hydrochloride		4 mg dextromethorpan hydrobromide	20 mg guaifenesin	***12 to 23 mo*** - 1 mL q 4 to 6 h up to 4 mL/day; ***6 to 12 mo*** - 0.75 mL q 4 to 6 h up to 3 mL/day; ***3 to 6 mo*** - 0.5 mL q 4 to 6 h up to 2 mL/day; ***1 to 3 mo*** - 0.25 mL q 4 to 6 h up to 1 mL/day	Alcohol and dye free. Grape flavor. In 15 and 30 mL bottles with calibrated dropper.

PEDIATRIC ANTITUSSIVE AND EXPECTORANT COMBINATIONS

	Product & Distributor	Decongestant	Antihistamine/Other	Antitussive	Expectorant	Dose	Excipients & How Supplied
otc	**Robitussin Cough & Cold Infant Drops**[a] (Whitehall-Robins)	6 mg/mL pseudoephedrine hydrochloride		2 mg/mL dextromethorphan hydrobromide	40 mg/mL guaifenesin	***2 to < 6 yr*** - 2.5 mL q 4 h up to 10 mL/day	Corn syrup, menthol, saccharin, sorbitol. In 30 mL.
Rx	**AccuHist DM Pediatric Syrup**[a] (PediaMed)	30 mg pseudoephedrine hydrochloride	2 mg brompheniramine maleate	5 mg dextromethorphan hydrobromide	50 mg guaifenesin	***6 to < 12 yr*** - 5 mL q 6 h up to 20 mL/day; ***2 to < 6 yr*** - 2.5 mL q 6 h up to 10 mL/day	Corn syrup, sucrose. Alcohol free. Grape flavor. In 473 mL.
Rx	**Bromhist-DM Pediatric Syrup**[a] (Cypress)						Alcohol and dye free. Saccharin, sorbitol. Grape flavor.In 473 mL.
Rx	**Histacol DM Pediatric Syrup**[a] (Breckenridge)						Alcohol free. Corn syrup, sorbitol. Grape flavor. In 473 mL.
Rx	**Pediahist DM Syrup**[a] (Boca Pharmacal)						Alcohol free. Corn syrup. Grape flavor. In 473 mL.

[a] This product also may be used in adults; refer to package labeling for dosing.

Refer to the general discussion of these products in the Respiratory Combinations Introduction. Some of the products in the previous Antitussive and Expectorant Combinations table also may be used in children.

ANTITUSSIVES WITH EXPECTORANTS

Content given per tablet or 5 mL.

	Product & Distributor	Antitussive	Expectorant	Average Adult Dose	Excipients & How Supplied
c-v	**Cheracol Cough Syrup**[1] (Lee Pharmaceuticals)	10 mg codeine phosphate	100 mg guaifenesin	10 mL q 4 to 6 h up to 60 mL/day	4.75% alcohol, fructose, sucrose. In 60, 120, and 480 mL.
c-v sf	**Gani-Tuss NR Liquid**[1] (Various, eg, Cypress)			10 mL q 4 h up to 60 mL/day	Alcohol free. Raspberry flavor. In 120 and 473 mL.
c-v sf	**Guiatuss AC Syrup**[1] (Various, eg, Alpharma, Ivax)				3.5% alcohol. In 118 and 473 mL.
c-v sf	**Mytussin AC Cough Syrup**[1] (Morton Grove Pharmaceuticals)			5 to 10 mL q 4 to 6 h up to 60 mL/day	3.5% alcohol, menthol, saccharin, sorbitol. Fruit flavor. In 118, 237, and 473 mL.
c-v sf	**Romilar AC Liquid**[1] (Scot-Tussin)			10 mL q 4 h up to 60 mL/day	Alcohol and dye free. Menthol, aspartame, phenylalanine, parabens. In 473 mL.
c-v	**Tussi-Organidin NR Liquid**[1] (Wallace)				Saccharin, sorbitol. Raspberry flavor. In 473 mL.
c-iii	**Codeine Phosphate and Guaifenesin Tablets** (Ethex)	10 mg codeine phosphate	300 mg guaifenesin	1 q 4 h up to 6/day	Sugar. (ETHEX 223). Red, oval. In 100s.
otc sf	**Benylin Expectorant Liquid**[1] (Warner Lambert)	5 mg dextromethorphan HBr	100 mg guaifenesin	20 mL q 6 to 8 h up to 80 mL/day	Alcohol free. Saccharin, sorbitol. Raspberry flavor. In 118 mL.
otc	**Vicks 44E Cough & Chest Congestion Relief Liquid**[1] (Procter & Gamble)	6.67 mg dextromethorphan HBr	66.7 mg guaifenesin	15 mL q 4 h up to 90 mL/day	5% alcohol, corn syrup, saccharin. In 118 and 236 mL.

ANTITUSSIVES WITH EXPECTORANTS

	Product & Distributor	Antitussive	Expectorant	Average Adult Dose	Excipients & How Supplied
otc	**Cheracol D Cough Formula Syrup**[1] (Lee Pharmaceuticals)	10 mg dextromethorphan HBr	100 mg guaifenesin	10 mL q 4 h up to 60 mL/day	4.75% alcohol, fructose, sucrose. In 118 and 177 mL.
otc	**Cheracol Plus Liquid**[1] (Lee Pharmaceuticals)				4.75% alcohol, fructose, sucrose. In 118 mL.
otc sf	**Diabetic Tussin DM Liquid**[1] (Health Care Products)				Alcohol and dye free. Aspartame, 8.4 mg phenylalanine, methylparaben, menthol. In 118 mL.
otc	**Extra Action Cough Syrup**[1] (Rugby)				Corn syrup, glucose, saccharin. In 118 mL.
Rx sf	**Gani-Tuss-DM NR Liquid**[1] (Cypress)				Alcohol free. Raspberry flavor. In 118 and 473 mL.
otc	**Genatuss DM Syrup**[1] (Ivax)				Alcohol free. Corn syrup, menthol, saccharin. In 118 mL.
otc	**Guaifenesin DM Syrup**[1] (UDL)				Alcohol free. Saccharin, sorbitol. In UD 5 and 10 mL.
Rx sf	**Guaifenesin-DM NR Liquid**[1] (Silarx)				Alcohol free. Methylparaben, saccharin, sorbitol. Raspberry flavor. In 118 and 473 mL and 3.8 L.
otc	**Guiatuss-DM Syrup**[1] (Various, eg, Alpharma, Ivax)				Alcohol free. May contain sucrose. In 118 and 237 mL.
otc	**Mytussin DM Syrup**[1] (Morton Grove Pharmaceuticals)			5 to 10 mL q 4 h up to 60 mL/day	Alcohol free. Sugar, menthol, saccharin. Cherry flavor. In 118 mL and 3.8 L.
otc sf	**Phanatuss DM Cough Syrup**[1] (Pharmakon Labs)			10 mL q 3 to 4 h up to 60 mL/day	Alcohol free. Parabens, saccharin, menthol. In 118 mL.
otc	**Robitussin-DM Liquid**[1] (Whitehall-Robins)			10 mL q 4 h up to 60 mL/day	Glucose, corn syrup, saccharin. In 118, 237, 360, and 473 mL.
otc sf	**Robitussin Sugar Free Cough Liquid**[1] (Whitehall-Robins)				Alcohol and dye free. Methylparaben, saccharin. In 118 mL.
otc	**Siltussin DM Cough Syrup**[1] (Silarx)				Alcohol free. Sucrose, saccharin, methylparaben. In 118 mL.
otc sf	**Tolu-Sed DM Liquid**[1] (Scherer)			5 to 10 mL q 4 h or 15 mL q 6 to 8 h up to 60 mL/day	10% alcohol. In 118 mL.
Rx	**Tussi-Organidin-DM NR Liquid**[1] (Wallace)			10 mL q 4 h up to 60 mL/day	Saccharin, sorbitol. Raspberry flavor. In 473 mL.
otc	**Kolephrin GG/DM Liquid**[1] (Pfeiffer)	10 mg dextromethorphan HBr	150 mg guaifenesin	10 mL q 4 h up to 60 mL/day	Alcohol free. Glucose, saccharin, sucrose. Cherry flavor. In 118 mL.
Rx	**Aquatab DMSyrup**[1] (Adams)	10 mg dextromethorphan HBr	200 mg guaifenesin	5 to 10 mL q 4 h up to 60 mL/day	Acesulfame K, aspartame, menthol, methylparaben, phenylalanine. In 473 mL.
otc	**Coricidin HBP Chest Congestion & Cough-Softgel Capsules** (Schering-Plough)			1 or 2 q 4 h up to 12/day	Sorbitol. In 20s.
otc sf	**Diabetic Tussin Maximum Strength DM Liquid** (Health Care Products)			10 mL q 4 h up to 60 mL/day	Alcohol and dye free. Aspartame, 8.4 mg phenylalanine, menthol, methylparaben. In 118 and 237 mL.
otc	**Robitussin Cough & Congestion Formula Liquid**[1] (Wyeth)				Alcohol free. Corn syrup, menthol, saccharin, sorbitol. In 118 mL.
otc	**Tuss-DM Tablets**[1] (Hyrex)			1 or 2 q 4 h up to 12/day	In 100s, 1000s, and UD 50s.
otc sf	**Safe Tussin Liquid**[1] (Kramer)	15 mg dextromethorphan HBr	100 mg guaifenesin	10 mL q 6 h up to 40 mL/day	Alcohol and dye free. Sorbitol, menthol. Mint flavor. In 120 mL.
otc sf	**Scot-Tussin Senior Clear Liquid** (Scot-tussin)	15 mg dextromethorphan HBr	200 mg guaifenesin	5 mL q 4 h up to 30 mL/day	Parabens, phenylalanine, menthol, aspartame. Alcohol free. In 118 mL.

ANTITUSSIVES WITH EXPECTORANTS

	Product & Distributor	Antitussive	Expectorant	Average Adult Dose	Excipients & How Supplied
Rx	**Hydro-Tussin DM Liquid**[1] (Ethex)	20 mg dextromethorphan HBr	200 mg guaifenesin	5 mL q 4 h up to 30 mL/day	Saccharin, sorbitol. In 473 mL.
Rx	**Maxi-tuss DM Liquid**[1] (MCR American Pharmaceuticals)				Glucose, menthol, parabens, saccharin. Black cherry flavor. In 473 mL.
Rx	**SU-TUSS DM Liquid**[1] (Cypress)				5% alcohol. Fruit flavor. In 473 mL.
Rx	**Duratuss DM Elixir**[1] (Victory Pharma)	25 mg dextromethorphan HBr	225 mg guaifenesin	5 mL every 4 h up to 30 mL in 24 h	Saccharin, sorbitol, sodium benzoate. Grape flavor. in 473 mL.
Rx	**Respa-DM Tablets**[1] (Respa)	28 mg dextromethorphan HBr	600 mg guaifenesin	1 or 2 q 12 h up to 4/day	Sustained release. Dye free. (RESPA 78). Scored. In 100s.
Rx	**Atuss-12 DX Suspension**[1] (Atley)	Dextromethorphan polistirex (equivalent to 30 mg dextromethorphan HBr)	200 mg guaifenesin/ 5 mL	5 to 10 mL q 12 h	Extended release. Parabens, honey. Honey-lemon flavor. In 20 and 473 mL.
Rx	**Dextromethorphan HBr/Guaifenesin Tablets**[1] (URL)	30 mg dextromethorphan HBr	500 mg guaifenesin	1 or 2 q 12 h up to 4/day	Extended release. Dye-free. (NL 736). Capsule shape, scored. In 100s.
Rx	**Sudal-DM Tablets**[1] (Atley Pharmaceuticals)	30 mg dextromethorphan HBr	500 mg guaifenesin	1 or 2 q 12 h up to 4/day	Sustained release. Dye-free. (SUDAL DM/P). Scored. In 100s.
Rx	**Touro DM Tablets**[1] (Dartmouth)	30 mg dextromethorphan HBr	575 mg guaifenesin	1 or 2 q 12 h up to 4/day	Sustained release. (TOURO DM/DP311). Lt. blue, scored. In 100s.
Rx	**Guaifenesin DM Tablets**[1] (Prasco)	30 mg dextromethorphan HBr	600 mg guaifenesin	1 or 2 q 12 h up to 4/day	Extended release. (310). Green, capsule shape. In 100s.
Rx	**Guaifenex DM Tablets**[1] (Ethex)				Extended release. (Ethex/213). Green, capsule shape, scored. In 100s.
Rx	**Guiadrine DM Tablets**[1] (Breckenridge Pharmaceutical)				Sustained release. In 100s and 250s.
Rx	**Iobid DM Tablets**[1] (Iopharm)				Sustained release. In 100s.
otc	**Mucinex DM Tablets** (Adams)	30 dextromethorphan HBr	600 mg guaifenesin	1 or 2 every 12 h up to 4 per day	Extended release. In 20s and 40s.
Rx	**Z-Cof LA Tablets**[1] (Zyber)	30 mg dextromethorphan HBr	650 mg guaifenesin	1 or 2 q 12 h up to 4/day	Sustained release. (ZYBER 105). White, scored. In 100s.
Rx	**GFN 1000/DM 50 Tablets**[1] (Cypress)	50 mg dextromethorphan HBr	1000 mg guaifenesin	1 q 12 h up to 2/day	Extended release. (CYP 288). Capsule shape, scored. In 100s.
Rx	**Allfen-DM Tablets**[1] (MCR American Pharmaceuticals)	55 mg dextromethorphan HBr	1000 mg guaifenesin	1 q 12 h up to 2/day	Extended release. Dye free. (ALLFEN DM). Scored. In 100s.
Rx	**AMBI 1000/55 Tablets**[1] (AMBI)			1 to 1.5 q 12 h or 1 q 8 h up to 3/day	Extended release. Dye Free (AMBI 120). Capsule shape, scored. In 100s.
Rx	**Dex GG TR Tablets**[1] (Boca Pharmacal)	60 mg dextromethorphan HBr	1,000 mg guaifenesin	1 q 12 h up to 2/day	Extended release. (BOCA 122). White. In 100s.
Rx	**GFN 1000/DM 60 Tablets**[1] (Cypress)				Sustained release. (CYP 267). White, capsule shape, scored. In 100s.
Rx	**Guaifenesin 1000 mg and Dextromethorphan HBr 60 mg LA Tablets**[1] (URL Laboratories)				In 100s.
Rx	**Muco-Fen DM Tablets**[1] (Ivax)				Long-acting. Dye-free. (MUCOFEN DM). Scored. In 100s.
Rx	**Aquatab DM Tablets** (Adams)	60 mg dextromethorphan HBr	1,200 mg guaifenesin	1 q 12 h up to 2/day	(Adams 002). Lt. blue, oval, scored. In 100s.
Rx	**GFN 1200/DM 60 Tablets**[1] (Cypress)				Sustained release. (CYP263). White, scored. In 100s.
otc	**Mucinex DM Tablets** (Adams)				Extended release. Bilayered. In 100s and 500s.
Rx	**TUSSI-bid Tablets**[1] (Capellon Pharmaceuticals)				Sustained release. (L/DM). Mottled pink, capsule shape, scored. In 100s.

ANTITUSSIVES WITH EXPECTORANTS

	Product & Distributor	Antitussive	Expectorant	Average Adult Dose	Excipients & How Supplied
c-iii sf	**Maxi-Tuss HCG Liquid**[1] (MCR American Pharmaceutical)	6 mg hydrocodone bitartrate	200 mg/5 mL guaifenesin	5 to 10 mL pc and hs (not less than 4 h apart) up to 50 mL/day	Alcohol free. Aspartame, phenylalanine, parabens. In 480 mL.
c-iii sf	**Pneumotussin 2.5 Cough Syrup**[1] (ECR Pharmaceuticals)	2.5 mg hydrocodone bitartrate	200 mg guaifenesin	10 mL q 4 to 6 h	Alcohol and dye free. Cherry punch flavor. In 473 mL.
c-iii	**Pneumotussin Tablets**[1] (ECR Pharmaceuticals)	2.5 mg hydrocodone bitartrate	300 mg guaifenesin	1 or 2 q 4 to 6 h up to 8/day	Dye free. (ECR 2.5). White, capsule shape, scored. In 100s.
c-iii sf	**Codiclear DH Syrup**[1] (Victory)	3.5 mg hydrocodone bitartrate	100 mg guaifenesin	5 mL q at least 4 h apart pc and hs up to 30 mL/day	Alcohol and dye free. Saccharin, sorbitol. Grape flavor. In 118 and 473 mL.
c-iii sf	**Hydrocodone Bitartrate and Guaifenesin Liquid**[1] (Various, eg, Ethex, Ivax, Kremers Urban, Watson)	5 mg hydrocodone bitartrate	100 mg guaifenesin	5 mL q 4 h pc and hs up to 30 mL/day	Alcohol and dye free. May contain menthol, parabens, sorbitol, saccharin. In 473 and 946 mL.
c-iii	**Hycosin Expectorant Syrup**[1] (Alpharma)				10% alcohol, parabens, saccharin, sorbitol, sucrose. Butterscotch flavor. In 473 mL.
c-iii	**Hycotuss Expectorant Syrup**[1] (Endo)				10% alcohol, saccharin, sorbitol, sugar, parabens. Butterscotch flavor. In 473 mL.
c-iii sf	**Hydrocodone GF Syrup**[1] (Morton Grove Pharmaceuticals)				Alcohol and dye free. Saccharin, sorbitol. Fruit flavor. In 237 and 473 mL.
c-iii sf	**Kwelcof Liquid** [1] (B.F. Ascher & Company)				Alcohol and dye free. Menthol, saccharin, sorbitol. Fruit flavor. In 473 mL.
c-iii sf	**Vitussin Syrup**[1] (Cypress)				Alcohol and dye free. Cherry flavor. In 473 mL.
c-iii sf	**Hydron EX Liquid**[1] (Cypress)	2.5 mg hydrocodone bitartrate	120 mg potassium guaiacolsulfonate	10 to 15 mL q 4 to 6 h up to 60 mL/day	Saccharin, sorbitol. Alcohol-free. Cherry flavor. In 473 mL.
c-iii sf	**Prolex DH Liquid**[1] (Blansett Pharmacal)	4.5 mg hydrocodone bitartrate	300 mg potassium guaiacolsulfonate	5 to 7.5 mL qid	Alcohol free. Saccharin, sorbitol, menthol. Tropical fruit punch flavor. In 25, 118, and 473 mL.
c-iii sf	**Hydron KGS Liquid**[1] (Cypress)	5 mg hydrocodone bitartrate	300 mg potassium guaiacolsulfonate	5 to 7.5 mL qid	Alcohol free. Saccharin, sorbitol. Wild cherry flavor. In 473 mL.
c-iii sf	**Marcof Expectorant Syrup**[1] (Marnel)	5 mg hydrocodone bitartrate	350 mg potassium guaiacolsulfonate	5 mL q 4 h pc and hs up to 30 mL/day	Alcohol and dye free. Menthol, saccharin, sorbitol. In 473 mL.
c-ii	**Dilaudid Cough Syrup** (Knoll)	1 mg hydromorphone HCl	100 mg guaifenesin	5 mL q 3 to 4 h	5% alcohol. Peach flavor. In 473 mL.

[1] This product also may be used in children; refer to package labeling for dosing.

[2] Victory Pharma, 12707 High Bluff Dr., Suite 200, San Diego, CA 92130; (858) 350-4217, fax (858) 350-4218.

Refer to the general discussion of these products in the Respiratory Combinations Introduction. Some of the products in the following Pediatric Antitussives with Expectorant table also may be used in adults.

PEDIATRIC ANTITUSSIVES WITH EXPECTORANTS

Content given per 5 mL (liquid) or 1 mL (drops).

	Product & Distributor	Antitussive	Expectorant	Average Dose	Excipients & How Supplied
otc	**Robitussin DM Infant Drops** (Whitehall-Robins)	2 mg/mL dextromethorphan HBr	40 mg/mL guaifenesin	***2 to < 6 yrs*** - 2.5 mL q 4 h up to 15 mL/day	Alcohol free. Corn syrup, saccharin. Fruit punch flavor. In 30 mL with oral syringe.
otc	**Vicks Pediatric 44e Cough & Chest Congestion Relief Liquid**[1] (Procter & Gamble)	3.3 mg dextromethorphan HBr	33.3 mg guaifenesin	***6 to 11 yrs*** - 15 mL q 4 h up to 90 mL/day; ***2 to 5 yrs*** - 7.5 mL q 4 h up to 45 mL/day	Corn syrup, saccharin. Cherry flavor. In 118 mL.

[1] This product also may be used in adults; refer to package labeling for dosing.

Refer to the general discussion of these products in the Respiratory Combinations Introduction. Some of the products in the previous Antitussives with Expectorants table also may be used in children.

TOPICAL COMBINATIONS

	Product & Distributor	Ingredients	Excipients & How Supplied
otc	**Nose Better Gel** (Lee Pharm)	0.5% allantoin, 0.75% camphor, 0.5% menthol	Lanolin, methylparaben. In 12.9 g.
otc	**TheraPatch Vapor Patch for Kids Cough Suppressant** (LecTec Corp.)	4.7% camphor, 2.6% menthol	Glycerin. Cherry scent. In 7s.
otc	**Triaminic Vapor Patch for Cough** (Novartis Consumer Health)		Glycerin. Cherry and menthol scents. In 6s.
otc	**Mentholatum Cherry Chest Rub for Kids** (Mentholatum Co.)	4.7% camphor, 2.6% menthol, 1.2% eucalyptus oil	Petrolatum. In 28 g.
otc	**TheraFlu Vapor Stick** (Novartis)	4.8% camphor, 2.6% menthol	Cetyl alcohol, eucalyptus oil, parabens. In herbal and menthol scents. In 51 g.
otc	**TheraFlu Vapor Stick Cough & Muscle Aches** (Novartis)		Cetyl alcohol, eucalyptus oil, parabens. In 51 g.
otc	**Tom's of Maine Natural Cough & Cold Rub Cough Suppressant** (Tom's of Maine)		In 92.4 g.
otc	**Vicks VapoRub Cream** (Procter & Gamble)	5.2% camphor, 2.8% menthol, 1.2% eucalyptus oil	Cetyl and stearyl alcohol, EDTA, glycerin, parabens. In 56 g.
otc	**Mentholatum Ointment** (Mentholatum Co.)	9% camphor, 1.3% menthol	Petrolatum. In 28 g.
otc	**Breathe Right Children's Colds Nasal Strips** (CNS Inc.)	Menthol	In 10s.
otc	**Breathe Right Colds Nasal Strips** (CNS Inc.)		In 10s.
otc	**Ayr Mentholated Vapor Inhaler** (B.F. Ascher)	0.5 mL mixture of eucalyptus oil, menthol, lavender oil	In 1s.

CAFFEINE

otc	**Caffedrine** (Various, eg, Blairex)	**Tablets:** 200 mg	In 16s.
otc	**Maximum Strength NoDoz** (Bristol-Myers)		Sucrose. Caplet shape. Coated. In 36s.
otc	**Vivarin** (GlaxoSmithKline)		Dextrose. (V). Coated. In 16s, 24s, 40s, and 80s.
otc	**Keep Alert** (Magno-Humphries Labs.)		Caplet shape. In 60s.
otc	**357 HR Magnum** (BDI)		In 36s, 100s, and 500s.
otc	**Overtime** (BDI)		In 100s and 500s.
otc	**20-20** (BDI)		In 100s and 500s.
otc	**Valentine** (BDI)		In 100s and 500s.
otc	**Keep Going** (Block Drug Co.)		Caplet shape. In 4s.
otc	**44 Magnum** (BDI)	**Capsules:** 200 mg	In 100s and 500s.
otc	**Molie** (BDI)		In 100s and 500s.
otc	**Fastlene** (BDI)		In 100s and 500s.
otc	**Enerjets** (Chilton Labs)	**Lozenges:** 75 mg	Sugar. Coffee, mocha mint, and "bitterscotch" flavors. In 10s.
Rx	**Cafcit** (Mead Johnson)	**Oral solution:** 20 mg/mL (caffeine citrate)[1]	Preservative free. In 3 mL vials.
		Injection: 20 mg/mL (caffeine citrate)[1]	Preservative free. In 3 mL vials.
Rx	**Caffeine and Sodium Benzoate** (Bedford)	**Injection:** 250 mg/mL (121 mg caffeine, 129 mg sodium benzoate)	In 2 mL single-use vials.
Rx	**Caffeine and Sodium Benzoate** (American Regent)	**Injection:** 250 mg/mL (125 mg caffeine, 125 mg sodium benzoate)	In 2 mL single-dose vials.

[1] 2 mg of caffeine citrate is equivalent to 1 mg caffeine base.

[2] Xanodyne Pharmacal, Inc., 7310 Turfway Rd., Suite 490, Florence, KY 41042; 877-XANODYNE, fax 859-371-6391; http://www.xanodyne.com.

CAFFEINE — ORAL

Indications

➤*Fatigue/drowsiness:* Helps restore mental alertness or wakefulness when experiencing fatigue or drowsiness.

➤*Analgesia:* As an adjuvant in analgesic formulations.

➤*Unlabeled uses:*

Obesity – In combination with ephedrine, caffeine causes a modest, but significant, weight loss in obese individuals when energy intake is restricted over an extended period. This reflects a synergistic interaction as it not seen with either agent alone.

Headache – Caffeine enhances the effect of ergotamine and may have direct actions on the extracranial vasculature or on trigeminal afferents in the treatment of migraine. Caffeine has been shown to effectively relieve headache resulting from lumbar puncture, and appears to produce an intrinsic analgesic effect in headaches of nonvascular origin.

Alcohol intoxication – For the treatment of excited or comatose alcoholic patients.

Postprandial hypotension – Postprandial decreases in blood pressure occur in elderly individuals, particularly after meals high in carbohydrates. Caffeine 250 mg, attenuated postprandial hypotension in a small number of patients. Analeptic use of caffeine is strongly discouraged by clinicians.

Administration and Dosage

➤*Fatigue/drowsiness:* 100 to 200 mg by mouth not more often than every 3 to 4 hours, as needed. Not recommended for children younger than 12 years of age.

➤*Storage/Stability:* Store at room temperature.

Avoid excessive heat (greater than 37.7°C [100°F]) or humidity.

Keep this and all drugs out of the reach of children.

Actions

➤*Pharmacology:* Caffeine, a methylxanthine, exerts its pharmacological effects by increasing calcium permeability in sarcoplasmic reticulum, inhibiting phosphodiesterase promoting accumulation of cyclic AMP, and is a competitive, nonselective antagonist at adenosine A_1 and A_{2A} receptors. Evidence suggests that adenosine receptor antagonism is the most important factor responsible for most pharmacological effects of methylxanthines in doses that are administered therapeutically or consumed in xanthine-containing beverages.

Caffeine is a potent stimulant of the CNS. Its cortical effects are milder and of shorter duration than those of the amphetamines. In slightly larger doses, it stimulates medullary, vagal, vasomotor, and respiratory centers, promoting bradycardia, vasoconstriction, and increased respiratory rate. Caffeine produces a positive inotropic effect on the myocardium and a positive chronotropic effect at the sinoatrial node, causing transient increases in heart rate, force of contraction, cardiac output, and heart work. In doses greater than 250 mg, the centrally mediated vagal effects of caffeine may be masked by increased sinus rates, tachycardia, extrasystoles, or other major ventricular arrhythmias. Caffeine constricts cerebral vasculature, but directly peripheral blood vessels, decreasing peripheral vascular resistance. The latter effect (and possibly vagal cardiac stimulation) on blood pressure is offset by increased cardiac output (and possibly stimulation of the medullary vasomotor area). The overall effect of caffeine on heart rate and blood pressure depends on whether CNS or peripheral effects predominate.

Caffeine stimulates voluntary skeletal muscle, increasing the force of contraction and decreasing muscular fatigue. It also stimulates gastric acid secretion from parietal cells. Caffeine increases renal blood flow and glomerular filtration rate and decreases proximal tubular reabsorption of sodium and water, resulting in mild diuresis. It also stimulates glycogenolysis and lipolysis.

Long-term administration of caffeine results in an upregulation of A_1 receptors in the brain, as well as an enhanced sensitivity to adenosine analogs that have an affinity for A_1 receptors. Tolerance to the cardiovascular, CNS, and diuretic effects may develop. Differences in effects of caffeine on various organ systems may be observed in nonusers of caffeine vs habitual consumers. Acute ingestion of caffeine produces increases in systolic blood pressure, plasma catecholamines, plasma renin activity, and heart rate; chronic ingestion has little or no effect on these hemodynamic variables.

➤*Pharmacokinetics:*

Absorption/Distribution – Caffeine is well absorbed orally (99%) and is widely distributed throughout the body. Peak plasma levels of 5 to 25 mcg/mL are achieved 15 to 120 minutes after 250 mg. Protein binding is approximately 17%. Caffeine readily crosses the blood-brain barrier and placenta; low concentrations are also present in breast milk. Therapeutic plasma concentrations are approximately 6 to 13 mcg/mL; those greater than 20 mcg/mL may produce adverse effects. The lethal concentration is greater than 100 mcg/mL.

Metabolism/Excretion – Caffeine is metabolized in the liver and is excreted in the urine as methyluric acid, methylxanthine, and other metabolites with only approximately 1% excreted unchanged. In the adult, plasma half-life ranges from 3 to 7 hours. Half-life is increased with smoking and is prolonged in pregnancy (less than or equal to 18 hours), cirrhosis, and with concomitant use of some drugs.

Contraindications

Hypersensitivity to any components.

Warnings

➤*Pregnancy: Category C.* Safety for use in pregnancy has not been established. Caffeine crosses the placenta and achieves fetal blood and tissue levels similar to maternal concentrations. Excessive caffeine intake (greater than 600 mg/day) has been weakly associated with increased fetal loss, low birth weight, premature deliveries, an increase in the incidence of fetal breathing activity, and a significant fall in baseline fetal heart rate. Three cases of fetal arrhythmia have also been reported. However, when used in moderation, there is no association with these effects or congential manifestations. Caffeine causes birth defects in animals when administered at doses toxic to the mother.

➤*Lactation:* Caffeine appears in the breast milk of nursing mothers. Milk:plasma rations of 0.5 and 0.76 have been reported. Approximately 1.3 to 3.1 mg of caffeine would be ingested by a nursing infant whose mother had 35 to 336 mg of oral caffeine.

➤*Children:* Do not use in children under 12 years old.

Precautions

➤*GI effects:* Theophylline derivatives tend to relax the lower esophageal sphincter and increase gastric acid secretion. Caffeine-containing products may exacerbate duodenal ulcers. Caffeine may also considerably aggravate diarrhea in patients with irritable colon.

CAFFEINE — ORAL

➤*Seizure disorder:* Caffeine is a CNS stimulant and in cases of caffeine overdose, seizures have been reported.

➤*Cardiovascular disease:* Although no cases of cardiac toxicity were reported in the placebo-controlled trial, caffeine has been shown to increase heart rate, left ventricular output, and stroke volume in published studies.

➤*Metabolic effects:* Caffeine stimulates glycogenolysis and lipolysis which increases free fatty acids and produces hyperglycemia. Caffeine also causes a release of catecholamines and increased metabolic activity.

➤*Bone mineral density:* Lifetime caffeinated coffee intake equivalent to 2 cups/day is associated with decreased bone density in older women (mean age, 72.7 years) who do not drink milk on a daily basis. In elderly women whose calcium balance was impaired (less than 800 mg of calcium/day), high caffeine intake predisposed them to bone loss of the hip. However, caffeine or coffee-induced calcium loss and bone loss are insignificant in the face of adequate calcium intake.

➤*Withdrawal:* Symptoms occur within 12 to 24 hours following cessation of chronic caffeine ingestion (as little as 100 mg of caffeine/day) and may endure up to 7 days. The most common symptom is headache, but other frequently reported reactions include fatigue, depression, anxiety, and insomnia.

Drug Interactions

Caffeine Drug Interactions			
Precipitant drug	Object drug*		Description
Allopurinol	Caffeine	↔	Allopurinol inhibits the conversion of caffeine metabolite methylxanthine to methyluric acid.
Cimetidine Contraceptives, oral Disulfiram Fluoroquinolones	Caffeine	↑	Caffeine hepatic metabolism may be impaired, resulting in decreased clearance and increased half-life. Consider avoiding caffeine consumption if excessive CNS or cardiovascular effects occur.
Mexiletine	Caffeine	↑	Concomitant administration reduced the elimination of caffeine by 30% to 50%.
Phenytoin	Caffeine	↓	Phenytoin decreases the half-life of caffeine and increases clearance. Concomitant administration results in lower caffeine levels.
Smoking	Caffeine	↓	Smoking induces hepatic metabolism and increases caffeine clearance.
Caffeine	Aspirin	↑	Caffeine appears to increase the GI absorption of aspirin, but does not appear to affect salicylate elimination.
Caffeine	Clozapine	↑	Caffeine may inhibit clozapine metabolism (P450 1A2), resulting in elevation of clozapine levels; possible increase in side effects may occur.
Caffeine	Lithium	↓	Caffeine may reduce serum lithium concentrations and may enhance renal clearance. Monitoring of serum lithium concentrations and adjustments in lithium dose may be necessary.
Caffeine	Theophylline	↑	Ingestion of caffeine (120 to 630 mg daily) can reduce theophylline clearance 23% and increase the elimination half-life. Serum theophylline levels may be increased. Advise patients to avoid drastic changes in daily caffeine intake.

* ↑ = Object drug increased. ↓ = Object drug decreased.
↔ = Undetermined clinical effect.

➤*Drug/Lab test interactions:* Caffeine produces false-positive elevations of serum urate as measured by the Bittner method. Caffeine also produces slight increases in urine levels of vanillylmandelic acid (VMA), catecholamines, and 5-hydroxyindoleacetic acid. Because high urine levels of VMA or catecholamines may result in false-positive diagnosis of pheochromocytoma or neuroblastoma, avoid caffeine intake during tests for these disorders.

➤*Drug/Food interactions:* Coffee and tea consumed with a meal or 1 hour after meal significantly inhibits the absorption of dietary iron. Clinical significance has not been determined.

Adverse Reactions

➤*Cardiovascular:* Tachycardia, extrasystoles, palpitations, other cardiac arrhythmias.

➤*CNS:* Insomnia, restlessness, excitement, nervousness, tinnitus, scintillating scotoma, muscular tremor, headache, lightheadedness.

Large doses of caffeine also may produce agitation, a condition resembling anxiety neurosis, hyperesthesia, and muscle twitches.

➤*GI:* Nausea, vomiting, diarrhea, stomach pain.

➤*Miscellaneous:* Hypersensitivity (eg, dermatitis, rhinitis, bronchial asthma), urticaria, hyperglycemia, diuresis.

Overdosage

➤*Symptoms:* Ingestion of 15 to 30 mg/kg results in significant toxicity (vomiting, myoclonus, myocardial irritability, hematemesis). Oral doses of 5 to 50 g (mean, 10 g) have produced fatalities; the lethal dose is estimated to be 100 to 200 mg/kg. In adults, IV doses of 57 mg/kg have been fatal. Toxicity correlates to serum caffeine levels. Several cups of coffee may produce caffeine concentrations of 5 to 10 mcg/mL. Symptoms of agitation and myoclonus develop at levels of 5 to 10 mcg/mL; cardiac arrythmias and seizures may develop at 50 to 100 mcg/mL. Caffeine concentrations as low as 80 mcg/mL to up to 1560 mcg/mL have been associated with death, although patients with concentrations up to 200 mcg/mL have survived. Fatalities have also been observed after the use of coffee enemas as a homeopathic therapy. Other symptoms of caffeine overdose that may develop include opisthotonus, decerebrate posturing, generalized muscular hypertonicity, rhabdomyolysis with resultant renal failure, pulmonary edema, hyperglycemia, hypokalemia, leukocytosis, ketosis, and metabolic acidosis.

Infants and children – In one 5-year-old patient, death occurred following oral ingestion of approximately 3 g. Signs and symptoms reported in the literature after caffeine overdose in preterm infants include fever, tachypnea, jitteriness, fine tremor of the extremities, hypertonia, opisthotonos, tonic-clonic movements, nonpurposeful jaw and lip movements, vomiting, hyperglycemia, elevated blood urea nitrogen, and elevated total leukocyte concentration. Seizures have also been reported. One case of caffeine overdose complicated by development of intraventricular hemorrhage and long-term neurological sequelae has been reported. No deaths associated with caffeine overdose have been reported in preterm infants.

➤*Treatment:* Primarily symptomatic and supportive. GI decontamination should include gastric lavage followed by activated charcoal. Control seizures with IV diazepam and phenobarbital. Caffeine levels have been shown to decrease after exchange transfusions. Even though not clearly established, indications for hemodialysis should include a caffeine serum concentration greater than 100 mcg/mL and life-threatening seizures or cardiac arrhythmias, regardless of serum concentration.

Patient Information

Limit the use of caffeine-containing medications, foods, or beverages while taking caffeine products because too much caffeine may cause nervousness, irritability, sleeplessness, and occasionally, rapid heart beat. Discontinue use if increased or abnormal heart rate, dizziness, or palpitations occur.

For occasional use only. Not intended for use as a substitute for sleep. If fatigue or drowsiness persists or continues to recur, consult a doctor.

Do not give to children under 12 years of age. Keep this and all drugs out of the reach of children.

As with any drug, if you are pregnant or nursing a baby, seek the advice of a health professional before using this product. Pregnant women should limit their intake of caffeine and caffeine-containing beverages.

In case of accidental overdose, seek professional assistance or contact a poison control center immediately.

Do not exceed recommended dosage.

CAFFEINE CITRATE — ORAL

Indications

For the short term treatment of apnea of prematurity in infants between 28 and younger than 33 weeks gestational age.

Administration and Dosage

➤*Approved by the FDA:* September 21, 1999.

Prior to initiation of caffeine citrate, baseline serum levels of caffeine should be measured in infants previously treated with theophylline, since preterm infants metabolize theophylline to caffeine. Likewise, baseline serum levels of caffeine should be measured in infants born to mothers who consumed caffeine prior to delivery, since caffeine readily crosses the placenta.

➤*Oral solution:* Caffeine citrate oral solution is available as a clear, colorless, sterile, non-pyrogenic, preservative-free aqueous solution adjusted to pH 4.7 Each mL contains 20 mg caffeine citrate (equivalent to 10 mg of caffeine base).

CAFFEINE CITRATE — ORAL

The recommended loading dose and maintenance doses of caffeine citrate follow:

	Dose of caffeine citrate volume	Dose of caffeine citrate mg/kg	Route	Frequency
Loading dose	1 mL/kg	20 g/kg	IV[a] (over 30 minutes)	One time
Maintenance dose	0.25 mL/kg	5 mg/kg	IV[a] (over 10 minutes) or orally	Every 24 hours[b]

[a] Using a syringe infusion pump.
[b] Beginning 24 hours after the loading dose.

Note that the dose of caffeine base is one-half the dose when expressed as caffeine citrate (eg, 20 mg of caffeine citrate is equivalent to 10 mg of caffeine base).

Serum concentrations of caffeine may need to be monitored periodically throughout treatment to avoid toxicity. Serious toxicity has been associated with serum levels greater than 50 mg/L.

Caffeine citrate should be inspected visually for particulate matter and discoloration prior to administration. Vials containing discolored solution or visible particulate matter should be discarded.

➤*Storage / Stability:* Store at 15° to 30°C (59° to 86°F).

This product is preservative free and is therefore for single use only. Discard unused portion.

Actions

➤*Pharmacology:*

Mechanism of action – Caffeine is structurally related to other methylxanthines, theophylline and theobromine. It is a bronchial smooth muscle relaxant, a CNS stimulant, a cardiac muscle stimulant and a diuretic.

Although the mechanism of action of caffeine in apnea of prematurity is not known, several mechanisms have been hypothesized. These include the following: Stimulation of the respiratory center; increased minute ventilation; decreased threshold to hypercapnia; increased response to hypercapnia; increased skeletal muscle tone; decreased diaphragmatic fatigue; increased metabolic rate; increased oxygen consumption.

Most of these effects have been attributed to antagonism of adenosine receptors, both A_1 and A_2 subtypes, by caffeine, which has been demonstrated in receptor binding assays and observed at concentrations approximating those achieved therapeutically.

➤*Pharmacokinetics:*

Absorption – Caffeine is well absorbed orally and is widely distributed throughout the body. After oral administration of 10 mg caffeine base/kg to preterm neonates, the peak plasma level (C_{max}) for caffeine ranged from 6 to 10 mg/L and the mean time to reach peak concentration (T_{max}) ranged from 30 minutes to 2 hours. The T_{max} was not affected by formula feeding. The absolute bioavailability, however, was not fully examined in preterm neonates.

Distribution – Caffeine is rapidly distributed into the brain across the blood-brain barrier. Caffeine levels in the cerebrospinal fluid of preterm neonates approximate their plasma levels. The mean volume of distribution of caffeine in infants (0.8 to 0.9 L/kg) is slightly higher than that in adults (0.6 L/kg). Plasma protein binding data are not available for neonates or infants. In adults, the mean plasma protein binding in vitro is reported to be approximately 36%.

Metabolism – Hepatic cytochrome P450 1A2 (CYP1A2) is involved in caffeine biotransformation. Caffeine metabolism in preterm neonates is limited due to their immature hepatic enzyme systems.

Interconversion between caffeine and theophylline has been reported in preterm neonates; caffeine levels are approximately 25% of theophylline levels after theophylline administration and approximately 3% to 8% of caffeine administered would be expected to convert to theophylline.

Excretion – In young infants, the elimination of caffeine is much slower than that in adults due to immature hepatic or renal function. Mean half-life ($T_{½}$) and fraction excreted unchanged in urine (A_e) of caffeine in infants have been shown to be inversely related to gestational/postconceptual age. In neonates, the $T_{½}$ is approximately 3 to 4 days and the A_e is approximately 86% (within 6 days). By 9 months of age, the metabolism of caffeine approximates that seen in adults ($T_{½}$ = 5 hours and A_e = 1%).

Contraindications

Hypersensitivity to any of its components.

Warnings

➤*Necrotizing enterocolitis:* During the double-blind, placebo-controlled clinical trial, 6 cases of necrotizing enterocolitis developed among the 85 infants studied (caffeine = 46, placebo = 39), with 3 cases resulting in death. Five of the 6 patients with necrotizing enterocolitis were randomized to or had been exposed to caffeine citrate.

Reports in the published literature have raised a question regarding the possible association between the use of methylxanthines and development of necrotizing enterocolitis, although a causal relationship between methylxanthine use and necrotizing enterocolitis has not been established. Therefore, as with all preterm infants, patients being treated with caffeine citrate should be carefully monitored for the development of necrotizing enterocolitis.

➤*Renal / Hepatic function impairment:* Caffeine citrate should be administered with caution in infants with impaired renal or hepatic function.

➤*Mutagenesis:* Caffeine (as caffeine base) increased the sister chromatid exchange (SCE) SCE/cell metaphase (exposure time dependent) in an in vivo mouse metaphase analysis. Caffeine also potentiated the genotoxicity of known mutagens and enhanced the micronuclei formation (5-fold) in folate-deficient mice.

➤*Fertility impairment:* Caffeine (as caffeine base) administered to male rats at 50 mg/kg/day subcutaneously (approximately equal to the maximum recommended intravenous loading dose for infants on a mg/m^2 basis) for 4 days prior to mating with untreated females, caused decreased male reproductive performance in addition to causing embryotoxicity. In addition, long-term exposure to high oral doses of caffeine (3 g over 7 weeks) was toxic to rat testes as manifested by spermatogenic cell degeneration.

➤*Pregnancy: Category C.* Concern for the teratogenicity of caffeine is not relevant when administered to infants. In studies performed in adult animals, caffeine (as caffeine base) administered to pregnant mice as sustained release pellets at 50 mg/kg (less than the maximum recommended intravenous loading dose for infants on a mg/m^2 basis), during the period of organogenesis, caused a low incidence of cleft palate and exencephaly in the fetuses. There are no adequate and well-controlled studies in pregnant women.

Precautions

➤*Monitoring:* Prior to initiation of caffeine citrate, baseline serum levels of caffeine should be measured in infants previously treated with theophylline, since preterm infants metabolize theophylline to caffeine. Likewise, baseline serum levels of caffeine should be measured in infants born to mothers who consumed caffeine prior to delivery, since caffeine readily crosses the placenta.

In the placebo-controlled clinical trial, caffeine levels ranged from 8 to 40 mg/L. A therapeutic plasma concentration range of caffeine could not be determined from the placebo-controlled clinical trial. Serious toxicity has been reported in the literature when serum caffeine levels exceed 50 mg/L.

In clinical studies reported in the literature, cases of hypoglycemia and hyperglycemia have been observed. Therefore, serum glucose may need to be periodically monitored in infants receiving caffeine citrate.

➤*Apnea:* Apnea of prematurity is a diagnosis of exclusion. Other causes of apnea (eg, central nervous system disorders, primary lung disease, anemia, sepsis, metabolic disturbances, cardiovascular abnormalities, or obstructive apnea) should be ruled out or properly treated prior to initiation of caffeine citrate.

➤*Seizures:* Caffeine is a central nervous system stimulant and in cases of caffeine overdose, seizures have been reported. Caffeine citrate should be used with caution in infants with seizure disorders.

➤*Duration of use:* The duration of treatment of apnea of prematurity in the placebo-controlled trial was limited to 10 to 12 days. The safety and efficacy of caffeine citrate for longer periods of treatment have not been established. Safety and efficacy of caffeine citrate for use in the prophylaxis treatment of sudden infant death syndrome (SIDS) or prior to extubation in mechanically ventilated infants have also not been established.

➤*Cardiovascular effects:* Although no cases of cardiac toxicity were reported in the placebo-controlled trial, caffeine has been shown to increase heart rate, left ventricular output, and stroke volume in published studies. Therefore, caffeine citrate should be used with caution in infants with cardiovascular disease.

Drug Interactions

Few data exist on drug interactions with caffeine in preterm neonates. Based on adult data, lower doses of caffeine may be needed following coadministration of drugs which are reported to decrease caffeine elimination (eg, cimetidine and ketoconazole) and higher caffeine doses may be needed following coadministration of drugs that increase caffeine elimination (eg, phenobarbital and phenytoin).

➤*CYP450 system:* Cytochrome P450 1A2 (CYP1A2) is known to be the major enzyme involved in the metabolism of caffeine. Therefore, caffeine has the potential to interact with drugs that are substrates for CYP1A2, inhibit CYP1A2, or induce CYP1A2.

➤*Ketoprofen:* Caffeine administered concurrently with ketoprofen reduced the urine volume in 4 healthy volunteers. The clinical significance of this interaction in preterm neonates is not known.

➤*Theophylline:* Interconversion between caffeine and theophylline has been reported in preterm neonates. The concurrent use of these drugs is not recommended.

Adverse Reactions

➤*Adverse events that occurred more frequently in caffeine citrate treated patients than placebo during double-blind therapy:*

Caffeine Citrate Oral Adverse Reactions

Adverse reaction	Caffeine citrate (n = 46); n (%)	Placebo (n = 39); n (%)
Cardiovascular		
Hemorrhage	1 (2.2%)	0 (0%)
CNS		
Cerebral hemorrhage	1 (2.2%)	0 (0%)

CAFFEINE CITRATE — ORAL

Caffeine Citrate Oral Adverse Reactions		
Adverse reaction	Caffeine citrate (n = 46); n (%)	Placebo (n = 39); n (%)
Dermatologic		
Dry skin	1 (2.2%)	0 (0%)
Rash	4 (8.7%)	3 (7.7%)
Skin breakdown	1 (2.2%)	0 (0%)
GI		
Necrotizing enterocolitis	2 (4.3%)	1 (2.6%)
Gastritis	1 (2.2%)	0 (0%)
Gastrointestinal hemorrhage	1 (2.2%)	0 (0%)
GU		
Kidney failure	1 (2.2%)	0 (0%)
Hemic/Lymphatic		
Disseminated intravascular coagulation	1 (2.2%)	0 (0%)
Metabolic/Nutritional		
Acidosis	1 (2.2%)	0 (0%)
Healing abnormal	1 (2.2%)	0 (0%)
Respiratory		
Dyspnea	1 (2.2%)	0 (0%)
Lung edema	1 (2.2%)	0 (0%)
Special senses		
Retinopathy of prematurity	1 (2.2%)	0 (0%)
Miscellaneous		
Accidental injury	1 (2.2%)	0 (0%)
Feeding intolerance	4 (8.7%)	2 (5.1%)
Sepsis	2 (4.3%)	0 (0%)

In addition to the cases above, three cases of necrotizing enterocolitis were diagnosed in patients receiving caffeine citrate during the open-label phase of the study.

Three of the infants who developed necrotizing enterocolitis during the trial died. All had been exposed to caffeine. Two were randomized to caffeine, and 1 placebo patient was "rescued" with open-label caffeine for uncontrolled apnea.

Adverse events described in the published literature include: central nervous system stimulation (ie, irritability, restlessness, jitteriness), cardiovascular effects (ie, tachycardia, increased left ventricular output, and increased stroke volume), gastrointestinal effects (ie, increased gastric aspirate, gastrointestinal intolerance), alterations in serum glucose (hypoglycemia and hyperglycemia) and renal effects (increased urine flow rate, increased creatinine clearance, and increased sodium and calcium excretion). Published long-term follow-up studies have not shown caffeine to adversely affect neurological development or growth parameters.

Overdosage

➤*Symptoms:* Following overdose, serum caffeine levels have ranged from approximately 50 mg/L to 350 mg/L. Signs and symptoms reported in the literature after caffeine overdose in preterm infants include fever, tachypnea, jitteriness, fine tremor of the extremities, hypertonia, opisthotonos, tonic-clonic movements, nonpurposeful jaw and lip movements, vomiting, hyperglycemia, elevated blood urea nitrogen, and elevated total leukocyte concentration. Seizures have also been reported in cases of overdose. One case of caffeine overdose complicated by development of intraventricular hemorrhage and long-term neurological sequelae has been reported. No deaths associated with caffeine overdose have been reported in preterm infants.

➤*Treatment:* Treatment of caffeine overdose is primarily symptomatic and supportive. Caffeine levels have been shown to decrease after exchange transfusions. Convulsions may be treated with intravenous administration of diazepam or a barbiturate such as pentobarbital sodium.

Patient Information

Caffeine citrate does not contain any preservatives and each vial is for single use only. Any unused portion of the medication should be discarded. It is important that the dose of caffeine citrate be measured accurately, ie, with a 1 cc or other appropriate syringe.

Consult your physician if the baby continues to have apnea events; do not increase the dose of caffeine citrate without medical consultation. Consult your physician if the baby begins to demonstrate signs of gastrointestinal intolerance, such as abdominal distention, vomiting, or bloody stools, or seems lethargic.

Caffeine citrate should be inspected visually for particulate matter and discoloration prior to its administration. Vials containing discolored solution or visible particulate matter should be discarded.

CAFFEINE CITRATE — INJECTION

Indications

For the short term treatment of apnea of prematurity in infants between 28 and younger than 33 weeks gestational age.

Administration and Dosage

➤*Approved by the FDA:* September 21, 1999.

Prior to initiation of caffeine citrate, baseline serum levels of caffeine should be measured in infants previously treated with theophylline, since preterm infants metabolize theophylline to caffeine. Likewise, baseline serum levels of caffeine should be measured in infants born to mothers who consumed caffeine prior to delivery, since caffeine readily crosses the placenta.

➤*Citrated caffeine parenteral solution:* Caffeine citrate injection for IV administration is available as a clear, colorless, sterile, non-pyrogenic, preservative-free, aqueous solution adjusted to pH 4.7. Each mL contains 20 mg caffeine citrate (equivalent to 10 mg of caffeine base).

Dissolve 10 g caffeine citrate powder (5 g caffeine) in 250 mL Sterile Water for Injection, qs to 500 mL, filter, and autoclave. Final concentration is 10 mg/mL caffeine base (20 mg/mL caffeine citrate). Stable in glass vials for up to 342 days when refrigerated (22°C; 73.4°F) or frozen (4°C; 39.2°F) and protected from light.

The recommended loading dose and maintenance doses of caffeine citrate follow.

	Dose of caffeine citrate volume	Dose of caffeine citrate mg/kg	Route	Frequency
Loading dose	1 mL/kg	20 g/kg	IV[a] (over 30 minutes)	One time
Maintenance dose	0.25 mL/kg	5 mg/kg	IV[a] (over 10 minutes) or orally	Every 24 hours[b]

[a] Using a syringe infusion pump.
[b] Beginning 24 hours after the loading dose.

Note that the dose of caffeine base is one-half the dose when expressed as caffeine citrate (eg, 20 mg of caffeine citrate is equivalent to 10 mg of caffeine base).

Serum concentrations of caffeine may need to be monitored periodically throughout treatment to avoid toxicity. Serious toxicity has been associated with serum levels greater than 50 mg/L.

➤*Drug compatibility:* To test for drug compatibility with common intravenous solutions or medications, 20 mL of caffeine citrate injection were combined with 20 mL of a solution or medication, with the exception of an *Intralipid* admixture, which was combined as 80 mL/80 mL. The physical appearance of the combined solutions was evaluated for precipitation. The admixtures were mixed for 10 minutes and then assayed for caffeine. The admixtures were then continually mixed for 24 hours, with further sampling for caffeine assays at 2, 4, 8, and 24 hours.

Based on this testing, caffeine citrate injection, 60 mg/3 mL is chemically stable for 24 hours at room temperature when combined with the following test products. Dextrose Injection, USP 5%; 50% Dextrose Injection, USP *Intralipid* 20% IV Fat Emulsion; *Aminosyn* 8.5% Crystalline Amino Acid Solution; Dopamine Hydrochloride Injection, USP 40 mg/mL diluted to 0.6 mg/mL with Dextrose Injection, USP 5%; Calcium Gluconate Injection, USP 10% (0.465 mEq/Ca^{+2}/mL); Heparin Sodium Injection, USP 1000 units/mL diluted to 1 unit/mL with Dextrose Injection, USP 5%; Fentanyl Citrate Injection, USP 50 mcg/mL diluted to 10 mcg/mL with Dextrose Injection, USP 5%.

➤*Storage/Stability:* Store at 15° to 30°C (59° to 86°F).

Preservative free. For single use only. Discard unused portion.

Actions

➤*Pharmacology:* Caffeine is structurally related to other methylxanthines, theophylline and theobromine. It is a bronchial smooth muscle relaxant, a CNS stimulant, a cardiac muscle stimulant and a diuretic.

Although the mechanism of action of caffeine in apnea of prematurity is not known, several mechanisms have been hypothesized. These include: Stimulation of the respiratory center; increased minute ventilation; decreased threshold to hypercapnia; increased response to hypercapnia; increased skeletal muscle tone; decreased diaphragmatic fatigue; increased metabolic rate; increased oxygen consumption.

Most of these effects have been attributed to antagonism of adenosine receptors, both A_1 and A_2 subtypes, by caffeine, which has been demonstrated in receptor binding assays and observed at concentrations approximating those achieved therapeutically.

➤*Pharmacokinetics:*

Distribution – Caffeine is rapidly distributed into the brain. Caffeine levels in the cerebrospinal fluid of preterm neonates approximate their plasma levels. The mean volume of distribution of caffeine in infants (0.8 to 0.9 L/kg) is slightly higher than that in adults (0.6 L/kg). Plasma protein binding data are not available for neonates or infants. In adults, the mean plasma protein binding in vitro is reported to be approximately 36%.

CAFFEINE CITRATE — INJECTION

Metabolism – Hepatic cytochrome P450 1A2 (CYP1A2) is involved in caffeine biotransformation. Caffeine metabolism in preterm neonates is limited due to their immature hepatic enzyme systems.

Interconversion between caffeine and theophylline has been reported in preterm neonates; caffeine levels are approximately 25% of theophylline levels after theophylline administration and approximately 3% to 8% of caffeine administered would be expected to convert to theophylline.

Excretion – In young infants, the elimination of caffeine is much slower than that in adults due to immature hepatic or renal function. Mean half-life ($T_{½}$) and fraction excreted unchanged in urine (A_e) of caffeine in infants have been shown to be inversely related to gestational/postconceptual age. In neonates, the $T_{½}$ is approximately 3 to 4 days and the A_e is approximately 86% (within 6 days). By 9 months of age, the metabolism of caffeine approximates that seen in adults ($T_{½}$ = 5 hours and A_e = 1%).

Contraindications

Hypersensitivity to any of its components.

Warnings

➤*Necrotizing enterocolitis:* During the double-blind, placebo-controlled clinical trial, 6 cases of necrotizing enterocolitis developed among the 85 infants studied (caffeine = 46, placebo = 39), with 3 cases resulting in death. Five of the 6 patients with necrotizing enterocolitis were randomized to or had been exposed to caffeine citrate.

Reports in the published literature have raised a question regarding the possible association between the use of methylxanthines and development of necrotizing enterocolitis, although a causal relationship between methylxanthine use and necrotizing enterocolitis has not been established. Therefore, as with all preterm infants, patients being treated with caffeine citrate should be carefully monitored for the development of necrotizing enterocolitis.

➤*Renal/Hepatic function impairment:* Caffeine citrate should be administered with caution in infants with impaired renal or hepatic function.

➤*Mutagenesis:* Caffeine (as caffeine base) increased the sister chromatid exchange (SCE) SCE/cell metaphase (exposure time dependent) in an in vivo mouse metaphase analysis. Caffeine also potentiated the genotoxicity of known mutagens and enhanced the micronuclei formation (5-fold) in folate-deficient mice.

➤*Fertility impairment:* Caffeine (as caffeine base) administered to male rats at 50 mg/kg/day subcutaneously (approximately equal to the maximum recommended intravenous loading dose for infants on a mg/m^2 basis) for 4 days prior to mating with untreated females, caused decreased male reproductive performance in addition to causing embryotoxicity. In addition, long-term exposure to high oral doses of caffeine (3 g over 7 weeks) was toxic to rat testes as manifested by spermatogenic cell degeneration.

➤*Pregnancy: Category C.* Concern for the teratogenicity of caffeine is not relevant when administered to infants. In studies performed in adult animals, caffeine (as caffeine base) administered to pregnant mice as sustained release pellets at 50 mg/kg (less than the maximum recommended intravenous loading dose for infants on a mg/m^2 basis), during the period of organogenesis, caused a low incidence of cleft palate and exencephaly in the fetuses. There are no adequate and well-controlled studies in pregnant women.

Precautions

➤*Monitoring:* Prior to initiation of caffeine citrate, baseline serum levels of caffeine should be measured in infants previously treated with theophylline, since preterm infants metabolize theophylline to caffeine. Likewise, baseline serum levels of caffeine should be measured in infants born to mothers who consumed caffeine prior to delivery, since caffeine readily crosses the placenta.

In the placebo-controlled clinical trial, caffeine levels ranged from 8 to 40 mg/L. A therapeutic plasma concentration range of caffeine could not be determined from the placebo-controlled clinical trial. Serious toxicity has been reported in the literature when serum caffeine levels exceed 50 mg/L.

In clinical studies reported in the literature, cases of hypoglycemia and hyperglycemia have been observed. Therefore, serum glucose may need to be periodically monitored in infants receiving caffeine citrate.

➤*Apnea:* Apnea of prematurity is a diagnosis of exclusion. Other causes of apnea (eg, central nervous system disorders, primary lung disease, anemia, sepsis, metabolic disturbances, cardiovascular abnormalities, or obstructive apnea) should be ruled out or properly treated prior to initiation of caffeine citrate.

➤*Seizures:* Caffeine is a central nervous system stimulant and in cases of caffeine overdose, seizures have been reported. Caffeine citrate should be used with caution in infants with seizure disorders.

➤*Use:* The duration of treatment of apnea of prematurity in the placebo-controlled trial was limited to 10 to 12 days. The safety and efficacy of caffeine citrate for longer periods of treatment have not been established. Safety and efficacy of caffeine citrate for use in the prophylaxis treatment of sudden infant death syndrome (SIDS) or prior to extubation in mechanically ventilated infants have also not been established.

➤*Cardiovascular:* Although no cases of cardiac toxicity were reported in the placebo-controlled trial, caffeine has been shown to increase heart rate, left ventricular output, and stroke volume in published studies. Therefore, caffeine citrate should be used with caution in infants with cardiovascular disease.

Drug Interactions

Few data exist on drug interactions with caffeine in preterm neonates. Based on adult data, lower doses of caffeine may be needed following coadministration of drugs which are reported to decrease caffeine elimination (eg, cimetidine and ketoconazole) and higher caffeine doses may be needed following coadministration of drugs that increase caffeine elimination (eg, phenobarbital and phenytoin).

➤*CYP450 system:* Cytochrome P450 1A2 (CYP1A2) is known to be the major enzyme involved in the metabolism of caffeine. Therefore, caffeine has the potential to interact with drugs that are substrates for CYP1A2, inhibit CYP1A2, or induce CYP1A2.

➤*Ketoprofen:* Caffeine administered concurrently with ketoprofen reduced the urine volume in 4 healthy volunteers. The clinical significance of this interaction in preterm neonates is not known.

➤*Theophylline:* Interconversion between caffeine and theophylline has been reported in preterm neonates. The concurrent use of these drugs is not recommended.

Adverse Reactions

➤*Adverse events that occurred more frequently in caffeine citrate treated patients than placebo during double-blind therapy:*

Caffeine Citrate Injection Adverse Reactions

Adverse reaction	Caffeine citrate (n = 46); n (%)	Placebo (n = 39); n (%)
Cardiovascular		
Hemorrhage	1 (2.2%)	0 (0%)
CNS		
Cerebral hemorrhage	1 (2.2%)	0 (0%)
Dermatologic		
Dry skin	1 (2.2%)	0 (0%)
Rash	4 (8.7%)	3 (7.7%)
Skin breakdown	1 (2.2%)	0 (0%)
GI		
Necrotizing enterocolitis	2 (4.3%)	1 (2.6%)
Gastritis	1 (2.2%)	0 (0%)
Gastrointestinal hemorrhage	1 (2.2%)	0 (0%)
GU		
Kidney failure	1 (2.2%)	0 (0%)
Hemic/Lymphatic		
Disseminated intravascular coagulation	1 (2.2%)	0 (0%)
Metabolic/Nutritional		
Acidosis	1 (2.2%)	0 (0%)
Healing abnormal	1 (2.2%)	0 (0%)
Respiratory		
Dyspnea	1 (2.2%)	0 (0%)
Lung edema	1 (2.2%)	0 (0%)
Special senses		
Retinopathy of prematurity	1 (2.2%)	0 (0%)
Miscellaneous		
Accidental injury	1 (2.2%)	0 (0%)
Feeding intolerance	4 (8.7%)	2 (5.1%)
Sepsis	2 (4.3%)	0 (0%)

In addition to the cases above, 3 cases of necrotizing enterocolitis were diagnosed in patients receiving caffeine citrate during the open-label phase of the study.

Three of the infants who developed necrotizing enterocolitis during the trial died. All had been exposed to caffeine. Two were randomized to caffeine, and 1 placebo patient was "rescued" with open-label caffeine for uncontrolled apnea.

Adverse events described in the published literature include: Central nervous system stimulation (ie, irritability, restlessness, jitteriness), cardiovascular effects (ie, tachycardia, increased left ventricular output, and increased stroke volume), gastrointestinal effects (ie, increased gastric aspirate, gastrointestinal intolerance), alterations in serum glucose (hypoglycemia and hyperglycemia) and renal effects (increased urine flow rate, increased creatinine clearance, and increased sodium and calcium excretion). Published long-term follow-up studies have not shown caffeine to adversely affect neurological development or growth parameters.

CAFFEINE CITRATE — INJECTION

Overdosage

➤*Symptoms:* Following overdose, serum caffeine levels have ranged from approximately 50 mg/L to 350 mg/L. Signs and symptoms reported in the literature after caffeine overdose in preterm infants include fever, tachypnea, jitteriness, fine tremor of the extremities, hypertonia, opisthotonos, tonic-clonic movements, nonpurposeful jaw and lip movements, vomiting, hyperglycemia, elevated blood urea nitrogen, and elevated total leukocyte concentration. Seizures have also been reported in cases of overdose. One case of caffeine overdose complicated by development of intraventricular hemorrhage and long-term neurological sequelae has been reported. No deaths associated with caffeine overdose have been reported in preterm infants.

➤*Treatment:* Treatment of caffeine overdose is primarily symptomatic and supportive. Caffeine levels have been shown to decrease after exchange transfusions. Convulsions may be treated with intravenous administration of diazepam or a barbiturate such as pentobarbital sodium.

Patient Information

➤*What are the possible side effects of caffeine citrate?* Your baby may or may not develop side effects from taking caffeine citrate. Each baby is different. If your baby develops 1 or more of the following symptoms, speak with your baby's doctor right away:

- Restlessness, jitteriness or shakiness.
- Faster heart beat.
- Increased urination (increased diaper wetting).The following symptoms may be caused by serious bowel or stomach problems. Call your baby's doctor right away if your baby develops:
- Bloated abdomen (stomach area).
- Vomiting.
- Bloody stools (bloody bowel movements).
- Loss of energy, lethargy (acting sluggish).

CAFFEINE AND SODIUM BENZOATE — INJECTION

Indications

➤*Respiratory depression:* Caffeine and sodium benzoate injection has been used in conjunction with supportive measure to treat respiratory depression associated with overdosage with CNS-depressant drugs (eg, narcotic analgesics, alcohol). However, because of questionable benefit and transient action, most authorities believe caffeine and other analeptics should not be used in these conditions and recommend other supportive therapy.

➤*Unlabeled uses:*

Postprandial hypotension – Postprandial decreases in blood pressure occur in elderly individuals, particularly after meals high in carbohydrates. Caffeine 250 mg attenuated postprandial hypotension in a small number of patients. Analeptic use of caffeine is strongly discouraged by most clinicians.

Administration and Dosage

Caffeine and sodium benzoate injection may be administered by IM or slow IV injection.

Analeptic use of caffeine is strongly discouraged by most clinicians. However, the manufacturer of caffeine and sodium benzoate injection recommends IM, or in emergency respiratory failure, IV injection of 500 mg of the drug (about 250 mg of anhydrous caffeine) or a maximum single dose of 1 g (about 500 mg of anhydrous caffeine) for the treatment of respiratory depression associated with overdosage of CNS depressants, including narcotic analgesics and alcohol, and with electric shock.

The usual dose is 0.5 g (7½ grains) as frequently directed by the physician. The maximum safe dose is 0.5 g and the total dose in 24 hours should rarely exceed 2.5 g.

➤*Storage/Stability:* Store at controlled room temperature between 15° to 30°C (59° to 86°F).

Actions

➤*Pharmacology:* Caffeine is pharmacologically similar to the other xanthine drugs, such as theobromine and theophylline; however, these 3 agents differ in the intensity of their actions on various structures. Caffeine's CNS and skeletal muscle effects are greater than those of other xanthines. In all other areas, theophylline has greater activity than caffeine, although some studies report that caffeine has greater diuretic effect than theobromine. The increased levels of intracellular cyclic-AMP mediate most of caffeine's pharmacologic actions. Caffeine competitively inhibits phosphodiesterase, the enzyme that degrades cyclic 3'-5' adenosine monophosphate. Caffeine stimulates all levels of the CNS. Caffeine's cortical effects are milder and of shorter duration than those of amphetamines. In slightly larger doses, caffeine stimulates medullary vagal, vasomotor and respiratory centers, promoting bradycardia, vasoconstriction, and increased respiratory rate.

Caffeine produces a positive inotropic effect on the myocardium and a positive chronotropic effect at the sinoatrial node, causing transient increases in heart rate, force of contraction, cardiac output and heart work. In doses greater than 250 mg, the centrally mediated vagal effects of caffeine may be masked by increased sinus rates, tachycardia, extrasystoles, or other major ventricular arrhythmias may result.

Caffeine constricts cerebral vasculature. In contrast, the drug directly dilates peripheral blood vessels, decreasing peripheral vascular resistance. The effect of this decrease in peripheral vascular resistance (and possibly that of vagal cardiac stimulation) on blood pressure is offset by increased cardiac output (and possibly stimulation of the medullary vasomotor area). The overall effect of caffeine on heart rate and blood pressure depends on whether CNS or peripheral effects predominate. Therapeutic doses of caffeine increase blood pressure only slightly.

Caffeine stimulates voluntary skeletal muscle, increasing the force of contraction and decreasing muscular fatigue. The drug also stimulates gastric acid secretion from parietal cells. Caffeine increases renal blood flow and glomerular filtration rate and decreases proximal tubular reabsorption of sodium and water, resulting in mild diuresis.

Caffeine stimulates glycogenolysis and lipolysis, but increase in blood glucose and in plasma lipids are insignificant in healthy patients. Tolerance may develop to the diuretic, cardiovascular, and CNS effects of caffeine.

➤*Pharmacokinetics:*

Distribution – Caffeine is rapidly distributed throughout the body tissues, readily crossing the placenta and blood-brain barrier. Approximately 17% of the drug is bound to plasma proteins. Caffeine has approximately a half-life ($t_{1/2}$) of 3 to 4 hours in adults.

Metabolism/Excretion – In adults, the drug is rapidly metabolized in the liver to 1-methyluric acid, 1-methylxanthine and 7-methylxanthine. Caffeine and its metabolites are excreted primarily by the kidneys.

Precautions

➤*Toxicities:* Large doses of caffeine may produce headache, excitement, agitation, a condition resembling anxiety neurosis, scintillating scotoma, hyperesthia, tinnitus, muscle tremors or twitches, diuresis, tachycardia, extrasystoles, and other cardiac arrhythmias. Further CNS depression may occur when already depressed patients are too vigorously treated with caffeine and sodium benzoate injection.

Drug Interactions

Caffeine and other xanthines may enhance the cardiac inotropic effects of beta-adrenergic-stimulating agents. Caffeine has also been reported to increase its own metabolism and that of other drugs, including phenobarbital and aspirin.

➤*Drug/Lab test interactions:* Caffeine produces false-positive elevations of serum urate as measured by the Bittner method. The drug also produces slight increases in urine levels of vanilamandelic acid (VMA), catecholamines, and 5-hydrocyindoleacetic acid. Because high urine levels of VMA or catecholamines may result in false-positive diagnosis of pheochromocytoma or neuroblastoma, caffeine intake should be avoided during tests for these disorders.

Overdosage

➤*Symptoms:* Acute toxicity involving caffeine has been reported rarely. Mild delirium, insomnia, diuresis, dehydration, and fever commonly occur with overdosage. More serious symptoms of overdosage include cardiac arrhythmias and clonic-tonic convulsions. In adults, IV doses of 57 mg/kg of body weight and oral doses of 18.5 g have been fatal. In one 5-year-old patient, death occurred following oral ingestion of ≈ 3 g of caffeine.

➤*Treatment:* Convulsions may be treated with IV administration of diazepam or a barbiturate such as phenobarbital sodium.

DOXAPRAM HYDROCHLORIDE

Rx	**Doxapram Hydrochloride** (Bedford)	**Injection:** 20 mg/mL	0.9% benzyl alcohol. In 20 mL multiple-dose vials.
Rx	**Dopram** (Baxter Healthcare Corp.)		0.9% benzyl alcohol. In 20 mL multiple-dose vials.

DOXAPRAM HYDROCHLORIDE — INJECTION

Indications

➤*Postanesthesia:* When the possibility of airway obstruction and/or hypoxia have been eliminated, doxapram may be used to stimulate respiration in patients with drug-induced postanesthesia respiratory depression or apnea other than that caused by muscle relaxants.

To pharmacologically stimulate deep breathing in the postoperative patient, a quantitative method of assessing oxygenation, such as pulse oximetry is recommended.

➤*Drug-induced CNS depression:* To stimulate respiration, hasten arousal, and encourage return of laryngopharyngeal reflexes in patients with mild to moderate respiratory and CNS depression caused by overdosage. Exercise care to prevent vomiting and aspiration.

Controlled ventilation and standard supportive care for respiratory depression caused by CNS overdose is safer, more reliable, and more effective than doxapram therapy.

➤*Chronic obstructive pulmonary disease associated with acute hypercapnia:* As a temporary measure in hospitalized patients with acute respiratory insufficiency superimposed on chronic obstructive pulmonary

DOXAPRAM HYDROCHLORIDE — INJECTION

disease (COPD). Use for a short period of time (approximately 2 hours) to prevent elevation of arterial CO_2 tension during the administration of oxygen. Do not use in conjunction with mechanical ventilation.

➤*Unlabeled uses:*

Neonatal apnea (apnea of prematurity) – Doxapram has been used when methylxanthines have failed.

Administration and Dosage

➤*Postanesthetic use (IV):* By IV injection (see table below); slow administration of the drug and careful observation of the patient during administration and for some time subsequently are advisable.

By infusion – Prepare the solution by adding doxapram 250 mg (12.5 mL) to 250 mL of dextrose 5% or 10% in water or normal saline solution. Initiate infusion at a rate of approximately 5 mg/min until a satisfactory respiratory response is observed, and maintained at a rate of 1 to 3 mg/min. Adjust the rate of infusion to sustain the desired level of respiratory stimulation with a minimum of side effects. The maximum total dosage by infusion is 4 mg/kg, or approximately 300 mg for the average adult.

Doxapram Dosage for Postanesthetic Use (IV)

IV administration	Recommended dosage mg/kg	Maximum dose per single injection mg/kg	Maximum total dose[a] mg/kg
Single injection	0.5 to 1	1.5	1.5
Repeat injections (5 min intervals)	0.5 to 1	1.5	2
Infusion	0.5 to 1	-	4

[a] Dose not to exceed 3 g per 24 hours.

➤*Drug-induced CNS depression:*

Doxapram Dosage for Drug-induced CNS Depression

Level of depression	Method 1 Priming dose single/ repeat IV injection mg/kg	Method 2 Rate of intermittent IV infusion mg/kg/hr
Mild[a]	1	1 to 2
Moderate[b]	2	2 to 3

[a] Class 0: Asleep, but can be aroused and can answer questions. Class 1: Comatose, will withdraw from painful stimuli, reflexes intact.

[b] Class 2: Comatose, will not withdraw from painful stimuli, reflexes intact. Class 3: Comatose, reflexes absent, no depression of circulation or respiration.

Using single and/or repeat single IV injections (Method 1) – Give priming IV dose and repeat in 5 minutes. The priming dose for moderate depression is 2 mg/kg and the priming dose for mild depression is 1 mg/kg. Repeat every 1 to 2 hours until patient awakens. Watch for relapse into unconsciousness or development of respiratory depression, because doxapram does not affect the metabolism of CNS depressant drugs.

If relapse occurs, resume every 1 to 2 hours until arousal is sustained, or total maximum daily dose (3 g) is given. After maximum dose has been given, allow patient to sleep until 24 hours has elapsed from first injection, using assisted or automatic respiration if necessary.

Repeat procedure the following day until patient breathes spontaneously and sustains desired level of consciousness, or until maximum dosage (3 g) is given. After maximum dose has been given, administer repetitive doses only to patients who have shown response to the initial dose. Failure to respond appropriately indicates the need for neurologic evaluation for a possible CNS source of sustained coma.

Intermittent IV infusion (method 2) – Give priming dose as in Method 1. If patient awakens, watch for relapse; if no response, continue general supportive treatment for 1 to 2 hours and repeat priming dose of doxapram. If some respiratory stimulation occurs, prepare IV infusion of doxapram 250 mg (12.5 mL) in 250 mL of saline or dextrose solution. Deliver at a rate of 1 to 3 mg/min (60 to 180 mL/h) according to size of patient and depth of coma. Discontinue use at end of 2 hours or if patient begins to awaken.

Continue supportive treatment for 0.5 to 2 hours and repeat the steps following the priming dose as above. Do not exceed 3 g/day.

➤*COPD associated with acute hypercapnia:* Mix doxapram 400 mg in 180 mL of dextrose 5% or 10% or normal saline solution (concentration of 2 mg/mL). Start infusion at 1 to 2 mg/min (0.5 to 1 mL/min); if indicated, increase to maximum of 3 mg/min. Determine arterial blood gases prior to administration and at least every 30 minutes during the 2 hours of infusion to ensure against development of CO_2 retention and acidosis. Altering oxygen concentration or flow rate may necessitate adjustment in doxapram infusion rate.

Predictable blood gas patterns are more readily established with continuous infusion. If the blood gases deteriorate, discontinue infusion. Additional infusions beyond the maximum 2 hour administration period are not recommended.

➤*Admixture compatibility/incompatibility:* Doxapram is compatible with 5% and 10% dextrose in water or normal saline.

Admixture of doxapram with alkaline solutions such as 2.5% thiopental, sodium bicarbonate, furosemide, or aminophylline will result in precipitation or gas formation.

Doxapram is also not compatible with ascorbic acid, cefoperazone, cefotaxime, cefotetan, cefuroxime, folic acid, dexamethasone disodium phosphate, diazepam, hydrocortisone sodium phosphate, methylprednisolone, or hydrocortisone sodium succinate.

Admixture of doxapram and ticarcillin results in an 18% loss of doxapram in 3 hours. When doxapram is mixed with minocycline, there is a loss of 8% of doxapram in 3 hours and a 13% loss of doxapram in 6 hours.

Actions

➤*Pharmacology:* Doxapram produces respiratory stimulation mediated through the peripheral carotid chemoreceptors. The respiratory stimulant action is manifested by an increase in tidal volume associated with a slight increase in respiratory rate. As the dosage is increased, the central respiratory centers in the medulla are stimulated with progressive stimulation of other parts of the brain and spinal cord.

A pressor response caused by improved cardiac output rather than peripheral vasoconstriction may occur. If there is no cardiac impairment, the pressor effect is greater in hypovolemic than in normovolemic states. Following administration, an increased release of catecholamines has occurred.

Although opiate-induced respiratory depression is antagonized by doxapram, the analgesic effect is not affected.

➤*Pharmacokinetics:* The onset of respiratory stimulation following the recommended single IV injection usually occurs in 20 to 40 seconds, with peak effect at 1 to 2 minutes. The duration of effect varies from 5 to 12 minutes.

Contraindications

Hypersensitivity to the drug or any of the injection components; epilepsy or other convulsive states; mechanical disorders of ventilation such as mechanical obstruction, muscle paresis (including neuromuscular blockage), flail chest, pneumothorax, acute bronchial asthma, pulmonary fibrosis, or other conditions resulting in restriction of chest wall, muscles of respiration or alveolar expansion; head injury; cerebrovascular accident; cerebral edema; significant cardiovascular impairment; uncompensated heart failure; severe coronary artery disease; severe hypertension, including that associated with hyperthyroidism or pheochromocytoma; proven or suspected pulmonary embolism.

Warnings

➤*CNS effects:* There is a risk that doxapram will produce adverse effects, including seizures, caused by general CNS stimulation. Muscle involvement may range from fasciculation to spasticity.

➤*Postanesthetic use:* Exercise the same consideration to preexisting disease states as in non-anesthetized individuals. Doxapram is neither an antagonist to muscle relaxant drugs nor a specific narcotic antagonist. More specific tests (eg, peripheral nerve stimulation, airway pressures, head lift, pulse oximetry, end-tidal carbon dioxide) to assess adequacy of ventilation are recommended before administering doxapram. Ensure adequacy of airway and oxygenation prior to use. Administer carefully and only under careful supervision to patients with hypermetabolic states such as hyperthyroidism or pheochromocytoma. Narcosis may recur after stimulation with doxapram, take care to maintain close observation until the patient has been fully alert for 0.5 to 1 hour.

➤*General anesthesia:* In patients who have received general anesthesia utilizing a volatile agent known to sensitize the myocardium to catecholamines, delay administration of doxapram until the volatile agent has been excreted in order to lessen the potential for arrhythmias, including ventricular tachycardia and ventricular fibrillation.

➤*Drug-induced CNS and respiratory depression:* Doxapram alone may not stimulate adequate spontaneous breathing or provide sufficient arousal in patients who are severely depressed either due to respiratory failure or to CNS depressant drugs. May be used as an adjunct to established supportive measures and resuscitative techniques.

➤*COPD:* In an attempt to lower pCO_2, do not increase rate of infusion in severely ill patients because of the associated increased work in breathing. Do not use in conjunction with mechanical ventilation.

In some patients, arrhythmias in acute respiratory failure secondary to COPD are probably the result of hypoxia. Use with caution in these patients.

Obtain arterial blood gases prior to the initiation of doxapram infusion and oxygen administration, then at least every 30 minutes during the infusion period to prevent development of CO_2 retention and acidosis in patients with COPD with acute hypercapnia. Doxapram administration does not diminish the need for careful patient monitoring or the need for supplemental oxygen in acute respiratory failure. Discontinue use if the arterial blood gases deteriorate and initiate mechanical ventilation.

➤*Renal/Hepatic function impairment:* Administer with caution to patients with significant renal or hepatic impairment, as a reduction in the rate of metabolism or excretion of metabolites may alter the response.

➤*Pregnancy:* *Category B.* There are no adequate and well-controlled studies in pregnant women. Use during pregnancy only when clearly needed.

➤*Lactation:* It is not known whether this drug is excreted in breast milk. Exercise caution when administering to a nursing mother.

➤*Children:* Safety and effectiveness in pediatric patients younger than 12 years of age have not been established. This product contains benzyl alcohol as a preservative. Benzyl alcohol, a component of this product, has been associated with serious adverse events and death, particularly in pediatric

DOXAPRAM HYDROCHLORIDE — INJECTION

patients. The "gasping syndrome," (characterized by central nervous system depression, metabolic acidosis, gasping respirations, and high levels of benzyl alcohol and its metabolites found in the blood and urine) has been associated with benzyl alcohol dosages higher than 99 mg/kg/day in neonates and low birth weight neonates. Additional symptoms may include gradual neurological deterioration, seizures, intracranial hemorrhage, hematological abnormalities, skin breakdown, hepatic and renal failure, hypotension, bradycardia, and cardiovascular collapse. Premature and low-birthweight infants, as well as patients receiving high dosages, may be more likely to develop toxicity.

Premature neonates – Premature neonates given doxapram have developed hypertension, irritability, jitteriness, hyperglycemia, glucosuria, abdominal distension, increased gastric residuals, vomiting, bloody stools, necrotizing enterocolitis, erratic limb movements, excessive crying, disturbed sleep, premature eruption of teeth, and QT prologizing that has resulted in heart block. In premature neonates with risk factors such as a previous seizure, perinatal asphyxia, or intracerebral hemorrhage, seizures have occurred. In many instances, doxapram was administered following administration of xanthine derivatives such as caffeine, aminophylline, or theophylline.

Precautions

➤*Monitoring:* Monitor blood pressure, pulse rate, and deep tendon reflexes to prevent overdosage. Monitor for disturbance in cardiac rhythm.

➤*Administration:* Avoid vascular extravasation or use of a single injection site over an extended period; thrombophlebitis or local skin irritation may occur. Rapid infusion may result in hemolysis.

Do not use doxapram in conjunction with mechanical ventilation.

IV short-acting barbiturates, oxygen, and resuscitative equipment should be readily available to manage overdosage manifested by excessive CNS stimulation. Slow administration and careful observation of the patient during and following administration are advisable to ensure that the protective reflexes have been restored and to prevent possible posthyperventilation or hypoventilation. Administer cautiously to patients receiving sympathomimetics or monoamine oxidase inhibitors (MAOIs), as an additive pressor effect may occur. An adequate airway is essential and airway protection should be considered, as doxapram may stimulate vomiting. Employ recommended dosages; do not exceed maximum total dosages. Use the minimum effective dosage to avoid side effects.

➤*Cardiovascular/Respiratory effects:* Blood pressure increases are generally modest, but significant increases have occurred. Not recommended for use in severe hypertension. If sudden hypotension or dyspnea develop, discontinue use. Cardiovascular effects may include various dysrhythmias. Monitor patients receiving doxapram for disturbance of their cardiac rhythm. Monitor blood pressure, pulse rate, and deep tendon reflexes to prevent overdosage.

➤*Lowered pCO_2:* Lowered pCO_2 induced by hyperventilation produces cerebral vasoconstriction and slowing of the cerebral circulation. In certain patients, a pressor effect of doxapram on the pulmonary circulation may result in a fall of the arterial pO_2 probably caused by a worsening of ventilation perfusion-matching in the lungs despite an overall improvement in alveolar ventilation and a fall in pCO_2. Carefully supervise patients, taking into account available blood gas measurements.

➤*Benzyl alcohol:* Doxapram products may contain benzyl alcohol, which has been associated with a fatal "gasping syndrome" in premature infants. Exposure to excessive amounts of benzyl alcohol has been associated with toxicity (hypotension, metabolic acidosis), particularly in neonates, and an increased incidence of kernicterus, particularly in small preterm infants. There have been rare reports of deaths, primarily in preterm infants, associated with exposure to excessive amounts of benzyl alcohol. Administration of high dosages of medications containing this preservative must take into account the total amount of benzyl alcohol administered. The amount of benzyl alcohol at which toxicity may occur is not known. If the patient requires more than the recommended dosages or other medications containing this preservative, consider the daily metabolic load of benzyl alcohol from these combined sources (see Warnings).

Drug Interactions

Doxapram Drug Interactions

Precipitant drug	Object drug[a]		Description
Doxapram	Anesthetics	↑	In patients who have received general anesthesia utilizing a volatile agent known to sensitize the myocardium to catecholamines, delay administration of doxapram until the volatile agent has been excreted in order to lessen the potential for arrhythmias, including ventricular tachycardia and ventricular fibrillation.
Doxapram	MAOIs	↑	Administer cautiously to patients receiving these drugs because an additive pressor effect may occur.
Doxapram	Neuromuscular blocking agents	↓	Doxapram may temporarily mask residual effects of neuromuscular blocking agents.
Doxapram	Sympathomimetics	↑	Administer cautiously to patients receiving these drugs because an additive pressor effect may occur.
Aminophylline Theophylline	Doxapram	↑	Administer cautiously, as increased skeletal muscle activity, agitation, and hyperactivity may occur.

[a] ↑ = Object drug increased. ↓ = Object drug decreased.

Adverse Reactions

➤*Cardiovascular:* Arrhythmias (including ventricular tachycardia and ventricular fibrillation); chest pain; lowered T-waves; phlebitis; tightness in chest; variations in heart rate. A mild to moderate increase in blood pressure is commonly noted and may be of concern in patients with severe cardiovascular diseases (see Precautions).

➤*CNS:* Apprehension; bilateral Babinski; clonus; convulsions; disorientation; dizziness; hallucinations; headache; hyperactivity; involuntary movements; paresthesia (eg, feeling of warmth, burning or hot sensation), especially in the area of the genitalia and perineum.

➤*GI:* Desire to defecate; diarrhea; nausea; vomiting.

➤*GU:* Albuminuria; elevation of BUN; stimulation of urinary bladder with spontaneous voiding; urinary retention.

➤*Hematologic/Lymphatic:* A decrease in hemoglobin, hematocrit, or red blood cell count has occurred in postoperative patients. In the presence of preexisting leukopenia, a further decrease in WBC has occurred following anesthesia and treatment with doxapram; hemolysis with rapid infusion.

➤*Respiratory:* Bronchospasm; cough; dyspnea; hiccoughs; hyperventilation; laryngospasm; rebound hypoventilation; tachypnea.

➤*Miscellaneous:* Flushing; increased deep tendon reflexes; muscle fistulization; muscle spasticity; pruritus; pupillary dilatation; pyrexia; sweating.

Overdosage

➤*Symptoms:* Excessive pressor effect, hypertension, tachycardia, skeletal muscle hyperactivity, and enhanced deep tendon reflexes may be early signs of overdosage. Other effects may include agitation, confusion, sweating, cough, and dyspnea. Evaluate blood pressure, pulse rate, and deep tendon reflexes periodically and adjust dosage or infusion rate accordingly.

➤*Treatment:* There is no specific antidote. Management should be symptomatic. Refer to General Management of Acute Overdosage. Convulsive seizures are unlikely at recommended dosages, but anticonvulsants, oxygen, and resuscitative equipment should be available. There is no evidence that doxapram is dialyzable. Because of the half-life of doxapram, it is unlikely that dialysis would be appropriate treatment for overdosage.

MODAFINIL

c-iv	**Provigil** (Cephalon)	**Tablets:** 100 mg	Lactose, talc. (PROVIGIL 100 MG). White, capsule shape. In 100s.
		200 mg	Lactose, talc. (PROVIGIL 200 MG). White, capsule shape, scored. In 100s.

MODAFINIL — ORAL

Indications

To improve wakefulness in patients with excessive sleepiness associated with narcolepsy, obstructive sleep apnea/hypopnea syndrome (OSAHS), and shift work sleep disorder (SWSD).

In OSAHS, as an adjunct to standard treatment(s) for the underlying obstruction. If continuous positive airway pressure (CPAP) is the treatment of choice for a patient, make a maximal effort to treat with CPAP for an adequate period of time prior to initiating modafinil. If modafinil is used adjunctively with CPAP, the encouragement of and periodic assessment of CPAP compliance is necessary.

➤*Unlabeled uses:* Treatment of fatigue associated with multiple sclerosis.

Administration and Dosage

➤*Approved by the FDA:* December 24, 1998.

The recommended dose of modafinil is 200 mg given once a day.

For patients with narcolepsy and OSAHS, take modafinil as a single dose in the morning.

For patients with SWSD, take modafinil approximately 1 hour prior to the start of their work shift.

Doses up to 400 mg/day, given as a single dose, have been well tolerated, but there is no consistent evidence that this dose confers additional benefit beyond that of the 200 mg dose.

MODAFINIL — ORAL

➤*Concomitant medications:* Consider dosage adjustment for concomitant medications that are substrates for CYP3A4, such as triazolam and cyclosporine.

Drugs that are largely eliminated via CYP2C19 metabolism, such as diazepam, propranolol, phenytoin (also via CYP2C9), or S-mephenytoin may have prolonged elimination upon coadministration with modafinil and may require dosage reduction and monitoring for toxicity.

➤*Hepatic function impairment:* In patients with severe hepatic impairment, reduce the dose of modafinil to one-half of that recommended for patients with normal hepatic function.

See Actions for more information.

➤*Renal function impairment:* There is inadequate information to determine safety and efficacy of dosing in patients with severe renal impairment.

See Warnings for more information.

➤*Elderly:* In elderly patients, elimination of modafinil and its metabolites may be reduced as a consequence of aging. Therefore, give consideration to the use of lower doses in this population. A slight decrease (approximately 20%) in the oral clearance (CL/F) of modafinil was observed in a single dose study at 200 mg in 12 subjects with a mean age of 63 years (range 53 to 72 years), but the change was considered unlikely to be clinically significant. In a multiple-dose study (300 mg/day) in 12 patients with a mean age of 82 years (range 67 to 87 years), the mean levels of modafinil in plasma were approximately 2 times those historically obtained in matched younger subjects. Due to potential effects from the multiple concomitant medications with which most of the patients were being treated, the apparent difference in modafinil pharmacokinetics may not be attributable solely to the effects of aging. However, the results suggest that the clearance of modafinil may be reduced in the elderly. Therefore, give consideration to the use of lower doses in this population.

➤*Storage/Stability:* Store at 20° to 25°C (68° to 77°F).

Actions

➤*Pharmacology:* The precise mechanism(s) through which modafinil promotes wakefulness is unknown. Modafinil has wake-promoting actions like sympathomimetic agents including amphetamine and methylphenidate, although the pharmacologic profile is not identical to that of sympathomimetic amines.

In addition to its wakefulness-promoting effects and increased locomotor activity in animals, in humans, modafinil produces psychoactive and euphoric effects, alterations in mood, perception, thinking, and feelings typical of other CNS stimulants. Modafinil is reinforcing, as evidenced by its self-administration in monkeys previously trained to self-administer cocaine; modafinil was also partially discriminated as stimulant-like.

The optical enantiomers of modafinil have similar pharmacological actions in animals. Two major metabolites of modafinil, modafinil acid and modafinil sulfone, do not appear to contribute to the CNS-activating properties of modafinil.

➤*Pharmacokinetics:*

Absorption – Modafinil is a racemic compound, whose enantiomers have different pharmacokinetics (eg, the half-life of the l-isomer is approximately 3 times that of the d-isomer in humans). The enantiomers do not interconvert. At steady state, total exposure to the L-isomer is approximately 3 times that for the d-isomer. The trough concentration ($C_{min, ss}$) of circulating modafinil after once-daily dosing consists of 90% of the l-isomer and 10% of the d-isomer.

Absorption of modafinil tablets is rapid, with peak plasma concentrations occurring at 2 to 4 hours. The bioavailability of modafinil tablets is approximately equal to that of an aqueous suspension. The absolute oral bioavailability was not determined due to the aqueous insolubility (less than 1 mg/mL) of modafinil, which precluded IV administration. Food has no effect on overall modafinil bioavailability; however, its absorption (T_{max}) may be delayed by approximately 1 hour if taken with food.

Distribution – Modafinil is well distributed in body tissue with an apparent volume of distribution (approximately 0.9 L/kg) larger than the volume of total body water (0.6 L/kg). In human plasma, in vitro, modafinil is moderately bound to plasma protein (approximately 60%, mainly to albumin). At serum concentrations obtained at steady state after doses of 200 mg/day, modafinil exhibits no displacement of protein binding of warfarin, diazepam, or propranolol. Even at much larger concentrations (1,000 mcM; greater than 25 times the C_{max} of 40 mcM at steady state at 400 mg/day), modafinil has no effect on warfarin binding. Modafinil acid at concentrations greater than 500 mcM decreases the extent of warfarin binding, but these concentrations are greater than 35 times those achieved therapeutically.

Metabolism/Excretion – The effective elimination half-life of modafinil after multiple doses is about 15 hours. The enantiomers of modafinil exhibit linear kinetics upon multiple dosing of 200 to 600 mg/day once daily in healthy volunteers. Apparent steady states of total modafinil and l-(-)-modafinil are reached after 2 to 4 days of dosing. The major route of elimination (approximately 90%) is metabolism, primarily by the liver, with subsequent renal elimination of the metabolites. Urine alkalinization has no effect on the elimination of modafinil.

Metabolism occurs through hydrolytic deamidation, S-oxidation, aromatic ring hydroxylation, and glucuronide conjugation. Less than 10% of an administered dose is excreted as the parent compound. In a clinical study using radiolabeled modafinil, a total of 81% of the administered radioactivity was recovered in 11 days postdose, predominantly in the urine (80% vs 1% in the feces). The largest fraction of the drug in urine was modafinil acid, but at least 6 other metabolites were present in lower concentrations. Only 2 metabolites reach appreciable concentrations in plasma (ie, modafinil acid, modafinil sulfone). In preclinical models, modafinil acid, modafinil sulfone, 2-]acetic acid and 4-hydroxy modafinil, were inactive or did not appear to mediate the arousal effects of modafinil.

In humans, decreases in trough levels of modafinil have sometimes been observed after multiple weeks of dosing, suggesting auto-induction, but the magnitude of the decreases and the inconsistency of their occurrence suggest that their clinical significance is minimal. Significant accumulation of modafinil sulfone has been observed after multiple doses due to its long elimination half-life of 40 hours. Induction of metabolizing enzymes, most importantly cytochrome P450 (CYP) 3A4, has also been observed in vitro after incubation of primary cultures of human hepatocytes with modafinil and in vivo after extended administration of modafinil at 400 mg/day.

Special populations –

Renal function impairment: In a single-dose 200 mg modafinil study, severe chronic renal failure (creatinine clearance less than or equal to 20 mL/min) did not significantly influence the pharmacokinetics of modafinil, but exposure to modafinil acid (an inactive metabolite) was increased 9-fold.

Hepatic function impairment: Pharmacokinetics and metabolism were examined in patients with cirrhosis of the liver (6 M and 3 F). Three patients had stage B or B+ cirrhosis (per the child criteria), and 6 patients had stage C or C+ cirrhosis. Clinically 8 of 9 patients were icteric and all had ascites. In these patients, the oral clearance of modafinil was decreased by about 60%, and the steady-state concentration was doubled compared to healthy patients. Reduce the dose of modafinil in patients with severe hepatic impairment.

Contraindications

Known hypersensitivities to modafinil.

Warnings

➤*Excessive sleepiness:* Advise patients with abnormal levels of sleepiness who take modafinil that their level of wakefulness may not return to normal. Frequently reassess patients with excessive sleepiness, including those taking modafinil, for their degrees of sleepiness and, if appropriate, advise them to avoid driving or any other potentially dangerous activity. Prescribers should also be aware that patients may not acknowledge sleepiness or drowsiness until directly questioned about drowsiness or sleepiness during specific activities.

➤*Renal function impairment:* In patients with severe renal impairment (mean creatinine clearance equals 16.6 mL/min), a 200 mg single dose of modafinil did not lead to increased exposure to modafinil but resulted in much higher exposure to the inactive metabolite, modafinil acid, than is seen in subjects with normal renal function. There is little information available about the safety of such levels of this metabolite.

➤*Hepatic function impairment:* In patients with severe hepatic impairment, with or without cirrhosis, modafinil should be administered at a reduced dose as the clearance of modafinil was decreased compared to that in healthy subjects.

➤*Pregnancy:* *Category C.* Modafinil administered orally to pregnant rats throughout the period of organogenesis caused, in the absence of maternal toxicity, an increase in resorptions and an increased incidence of hydronephrosis and skeletal variations in the offspring at a dose of 200 mg/kg/day (10 times the recommended human dose of 200 mg/day on a mg/m^2 basis) but not at 100 mg/kg/day.

However, in a subsequent study in pregnant rabbits, increased resorptions, and increased alterations in fetuses from a single litter (open eyelids, fused digits, rotated limbs), were observed at 180 mg/kg/day (17 times the recommended human dose on a mg/m^2 basis), a dose that was also maternally toxic.

There are no adequate and well-controlled studies in pregnant women. Use modafinil during pregnancy only if the potential benefit justifies the potential risk to the fetus.

Labor and delivery – The effect of modafinil on labor and delivery in humans has not been systematically investigated. Seven healthy births occurred in patients who had received modafinil during pregnancy. One patient gave birth 3 weeks earlier than the expected range of delivery dates (estimated using ultrasound) to a healthy male infant. One woman with a history of spontaneous abortions suffered a spontaneous abortion while being treated with modafinil.

➤*Lactation:* It is not known whether modafinil or its metabolites are excreted in human milk. Because many drugs are excreted in human milk, exercise caution when modafinil tablets are administered to a nursing woman.

➤*Children:* Safety and effectiveness in individuals below 16 years of age have not been established. Leukopenia has been reported in pediatric patients taking modafinil.

Precautions

➤*Diagnosis of sleep disorders:* Use modafinil only in patients who have had complete evaluations of their excessive sleepiness, and in whom a diagnosis of either narcolepsy, OSAHS, or SWSD has been made in accordance with ICSD or DSM diagnostic criteria. Such an evaluation usually consists of a complete history and physical examination, and it may be supplemented with testing in a laboratory setting. Some patients may have more than 1 sleep disorder contributing to their excessive sleepiness (eg, OSAHS and SWSD coincident in the same patient).

MODAFINIL — ORAL

➤*CPAP use in patients with OSAHS:* In OSAHS, modafinil is indicated as an adjunct to standard treatment(s) for the underlying obstruction. If CPAP is the treatment of choice for a patient, make a maximal effort to treat with CPAP for an adequate period of time prior to initiating modafinil. If modafinil is used adjunctively with CPAP, the encouragement of and periodic assessment of CPAP compliance is necessary.

➤*Cardiovascular system:* In clinical studies of modafinil, signs and symptoms, including chest pain, palpitations, dyspnea, and transient ischemic T-wave changes on ECG, were observed in 3 subjects in association with mitral valve prolapse or left ventricular hypertrophy. It is recommended that modafinil tablets not be used in patients with histories of left ventricular hypertrophy or in patients with mitral valve prolapse who have experienced the mitral valve prolapse syndrome when previously receiving CNS stimulants. Such signs may include, but are not limited to, ischemic ECG changes, chest pain, or arrhythmia.

Modafinil has not been evaluated or used to any appreciable extent in patients with recent histories of myocardial infarction or unstable angina. Treat such patients with caution.

Blood pressure monitoring in short-term (less than 3 months) controlled trials showed no clinically significant changes in mean systolic and diastolic blood pressure in patients receiving modafinil as compared to placebo. However, a retrospective analysis of the use of antihypertensive medication in these studies showed that a greater proportion of patients on modafinil required new or increased use of antihypertensive medications (2.4%) compared to patients on placebo (0.7%). The differential use was slightly larger when only studies in OSAHS were included, with 3.4% of patients on modafinil and 1.1% of patients on placebo requiring such alterations in the use of antihypertensive medication. Increased monitoring of blood pressure may be appropriate in patients on modafinil.

➤*CNS effects:* There have been reports of psychotic episodes associated with modafinil. One healthy male volunteer developed ideas of reference, paranoid delusions, and auditory hallucinations in association with multiple daily 600 mg doses of modafinil and sleep deprivation. There was no evidence of psychosis 36 hours after drug discontinuation. Exercise caution when modafinil is given to patients with histories of psychosis.

➤*Drug abuse and dependence:*

Controlled substance class – Modafinil is listed in Schedule IV of the Controlled Substances Act.

Abuse potential and dependence – In addition to its wakefulness-promoting effect and increased locomotor activity in animals, in humans, modafinil produces psychoactive and euphoric effects, alterations in mood, perception, thinking, and feelings typical of other CNS stimulants. In in vitro binding studies, modafinil binds to the dopamine reuptake site and causes an increase in extracellular dopamine, but no increase in dopamine release. Modafinil is reinforcing, as evidenced by its self-administration in monkeys previously trained to self-administer cocaine. In some studies, modafinil was also partially discriminated as stimulant-like. Physicians should follow patients closely, especially those with a history of drug or stimulant (eg, methylphenidate, amphetamine, cocaine) abuse. Observe patients for signs of misuse or abuse (eg, incrementation of doses, drug-seeking behavior).

The abuse potential of modafinil (200, 400, and 800 mg) was assessed relative to methylphenidate (45 and 90 mg) in an inpatient study in individuals experienced with drugs of abuse. Results from this clinical study demonstrated that modafinil produced psychoactive and euphoric effects and feelings consistent with other scheduled CNS stimulants (methylphenidate).

Withdrawal – The effects of modafinil withdrawal were monitored following 9 weeks of modafinil use in 1 US phase 3 controlled clinical trial. No specific symptoms of withdrawal were observed during 14 days of observation, although sleepiness returned in narcoleptic patients.

➤*Hazardous tasks:* Frequently assess patients with excessive sleepiness, including those taking modafinil, and, if appropriate, advise them to avoid driving or any other potentially dangerous activity.

Although modafinil has not been shown to produce functional impairment, any drug affecting the CNS may alter judgment, thinking, or motor skills. Caution patients about operating an automobile or other hazardous machinery until they are reasonably certain that modafinil therapy will not adversely affect their abilities to engage in such activities.

Drug Interactions

➤*CYP450 system:* In in vitro studies using primary human hepatocyte cultures, modafinil was shown to slightly induce CYP1A2, CYP2B6 and CYP3A4 in a concentration-dependent manner. Although induction results based on in vitro experiments are not necessarily predictive of response in vivo, exercise caution when modafinil is coadministered with drugs that depend on these 3 enzymes for their clearance. Specifically, lower blood levels of such drugs could result. In the case of CYP1A2 and CYP2B6, no other evidence of enzyme induction has been observed. A modest induction of CYP3A4 by modafinil has been indicated by other results; hence, the clearance of CYP3A4 substrates such as cyclosporine, steroidal contraceptives and, to a lesser degree, theophylline, may be increased.

The exposure of human hepatocytes to modafinil in vitro produced an apparent concentration-related suppression of expression of CYP2C9 activity suggesting that there is a potential for a metabolic interaction between modafinil and the substrates of this enzyme (eg, S-warfarin, phenytoin). In a subsequent clinical study in healthy volunteers, chronic modafinil treatment did not show a significant effect on the single-dose pharmacokinetics of warfarin when compared to placebo.

In vitro studies using human liver microsomes showed that modafinil reversibly inhibited CYP2C19 at pharmacologically relevant concentrations of modafinil. CYP2C19 is also reversibly inhibited, with similar potency, by a circulating metabolite, modafinil sulfone. Although the maximum plasma concentrations of modafinil sulfone are much lower than those of parent modafinil, the combined effect of both compounds could produce sustained partial inhibition of the enzyme. Drugs that are largely eliminated via CYP2C19 metabolism, such as diazepam, propranolol, phenytoin (also via CYP2C9) or S-mephenytoin may have prolonged elimination upon coadministration with modafinil and may require dosage reduction and monitoring for toxicity.

Tricyclic antidepressants – Due to the partial involvement of CYP3A4 in the metabolic elimination of modafinil, coadministration of potent inducers of CYP3A4 (eg, carbamazepine, phenobarbital, rifampin) or inhibitors of CYP3A4 (eg, ketoconazole, itraconazole) could alter the plasma levels of modafinil.

Modafinil Drug Interactions

Precipitant drug	Object drug[a]		Description
MAO inhibitors	Modafinil	↔	Use caution when administering MAO inhibitors and modafinil.
Methylphenidate Dextroamphetamine	Modafinil	↔	Modafinil absorption may be delayed approximately 1 hour.
Modafinil	Cyclosporine	↓	After 1 month of 200 mg/day modafinil, cyclosporine blood levels were decreased 50% in 1 patient. Cyclosporine dosage adjustment may be needed.
Modafinil	Contraceptives, oral Estrogens	↓	The effectiveness of oral contraceptives and estrogens may be reduced when used with modafinil. Alternative or concomitant methods of contraception are recommended for patients treated with modafinil and for 1 month after discontinuation of modafinil.
Modafinil	Triazolam	↓	Triazolam Cmax, AUC, and half-life may be decreased.
Modafinil	Tricyclic antidepressants	↑	In tricyclic-treated patients deficient in CYP2D6 (ie, poor debrisoquine metabolizers [7% to 10% of the white population; similar or lower in other populations]), the amount of metabolism by CYP2C19 may be substantially increased. Modafinil may cause plasma elevations of certain tricyclics (eg, clomipramine, desipramine) in these patients. A reduction in the dose of tricyclic agents might be needed.

[a] ↑ = Object drug increased. ↓ = Object drug decreased.
↔ = Undetermined clinical effect.

➤*Drug/Food interactions:* Although food has no effect on overall modafinil bioavailability, absorption may be delayed approximately 1 hour.

Adverse Reactions

The most commonly observed adverse events (greater than or equal to 5%) associated with the use of modafinil more frequently than placebo-treated patients in the placebo-controlled clinical studies in primary disorders of sleep and wakefulness were headache, nausea, nervousness, rhinitis, diarrhea, back pain, anxiety, insomnia, dizziness, and dyspepsia. The adverse event profile was similar across these studies.

In the placebo-controlled clinical trials, 74 of the 934 patients (8%) who received modafinil discontinued due to an adverse experience compared to 3% of patients that received placebo. The most frequent reasons for discontinuation that occurred at a higher rate for modafinil than placebo patients were headache (2%), nausea, anxiety, dizziness, insomnia, chest pain, and nervousness (each less than 1%). In a Canadian clinical trial, a 35-year-old obese narcoleptic male with a history of syncopal episodes experienced a 9-second episode of asystole after 27 days of modafinil treatment (300 mg/day in divided doses).

Incidence in controlled trials – The following table presents the adverse reactions that occurred at a rate of 1% or more and were more frequent in patients treated with modafinil than in placebo patients in US placebo-controlled clinical trials.

MODAFINIL — ORAL

Incidence of Treatment-Emergent Adverse Experiences in Parallel-group, Placebo-controlled Clinical Trials[a] in Narcolepsy, OSAHS, and SWSD with Modafinil (200 mg, 300 mg, and 400 mg)[b]

Body system	Preferred term	Modafinil (n = 934)	Placebo (n = 567)
Cardiovascular	Hypertension	3%	1%
	Palpitation	2%	1%
	Tachycardia	2%	1%
	Vasodilatation	2%	0%
CNS	Anxiety	5%	1%
	Agitation	1%	0%
	Confusion	1%	0%
	Depression	2%	1%
	Dizziness	5%	4%
	Dyskinesia[d]	1%	0%
	Emotional lability	1%	0%
	Hyperkinesia	1%	0%
	Hypertonia	1%	0%
	Insomnia	5%	1%
	Nervousness	7%	3%
	Paresthesia	2%	0%
	Somnolence	2%	1%
	Tremor	1%	0%
	Vertigo	1%	0%
Dermatologic	Herpes simplex	1%	0%
	Sweating	1%	0%
GI	Anorexia	4%	1%
	Abnormal liver function[c]	2%	1%
	Constipation	2%	1%
	Diarrhea	6%	5%
	Dry mouth	4%	2%
	Dyspepsia	5%	4%
	Flatulence	1%	0%
	Mouth ulceration	1%	0%
	Nausea	11%	3%
	Thirst	1%	0%
GU	Hematuria	1%	0%
	Pyuria	1%	0%
	Urine abnormality	1%	0%
Hematologic/lymphatic	Eosinophilia	1%	0%
Metabolic-nutritional	Edema	1%	0%
Respiratory	Asthma	1%	0%
	Epistaxis	1%	0%
	Lung disorder	2%	1%
	Pharyngitis	4%	2%
	Rhinitis	7%	6%
Special senses	Abnormal vision	1%	0%
	Amblyopia	1%	0%
	Eye pain	1%	0%
	Taste perversion	1%	0%
Miscellaneous	Back pain	6%	5%
	Chest pain	3%	1%
	Chills	1%	0%
	Flu syndrome	4%	3%
	Headache	34%	23%
	Neck rigidity	1%	0%

[a] Six double-blind placebo-controlled clinical studies in narcolepsy, OSAHS, and SWSD.
[b] Events reported by at least 1% of patients treated with modafinil that were more frequent than in the placebo group are included; incidence is rounded to the nearest 1%. The adverse experience terminology is coded using a standard modified COSTART Dictionary.Events for which the modafinil incidence was at least 1%, but equal to or less than placebo are not listed in the table. These events included the following: infection, pain, accidental injury, abdominal pain, hypothermia, allergic reaction, asthenia, fever, viral infection, neck pain, migraine, abnormal electrocardiogram, hypotension, tooth disorder, vomiting, periodontal abscess, increased appetite, ecchymosis, hyperglycemia, peripheral edema, weight loss, weight gain, myalgia, leg cramps, arthritis, cataplexy, thinking abnormality, sleep disorder, increased cough, sinusitis, dyspnea, bronchitis, rash, conjunctivitis, ear pain, dysmenorrhea (incidence adjusted for gender), urinary tract infection.
[c] Elevated liver enzymes.
[d] Oro-facial dyskinesias.

Dose dependency of adverse reactions – In the placebo-controlled clinical trials which compared doses of 200, 300, and 400 mg/day of modafinil and placebo, the only adverse events that were clearly dose related were headache and anxiety.

Vital sign changes – While there was no consistent change in mean values of heart rate or systolic and diastolic blood pressure, the requirement for antihypertensive medication was slightly greater in patients on modafinil compared to placebo.

➤*Lab test abnormalities:* Clinical chemistry, hematology, and urinalysis parameters were monitored in phase 1, 2 and 3 studies. In these studies, mean plasma levels of gamma-glutamyl transferase (GGT) and alkaline phosphatase (AP) were found to be higher following administration of modafinil, but not placebo. Few subjects, however, had GGT or AP elevations outside of the normal range. Shifts to higher, but not clinically significantly abnormal, GGT and AP values appeared to increase with time in the population treated with modafinil in the phase 3 clinical trials.

➤*Postmarketing:* In addition to the adverse reactions observed during clinical trials, the following adverse reactions have been identified during postapproval use of modafinil in clinical practice: Symptoms of psychosis, symptoms of mania, granulocytosis, urticaria (hives), angioedema.

Because these adverse reactions are reported voluntarily from a population of uncertain size, reliable estimates of their frequency cannot be made.

Overdosage

➤*Symptoms:* In clinical trials, a total of 151 protocol-specified doses of 1,000 to 1,600 mg/day (5 to 8 times the recommended daily dose of 200 mg), have been administered to 32 subjects, including 13 subjects who received doses of 1,000 or 1,200 mg/day for 7 to 21 consecutive days. In addition, several intentional acute overdoses occurred; the 2 largest being 4,500 mg and 4,000 mg taken by 2 subjects participating in foreign depression studies. None of these study subjects experienced any unexpected or life-threatening effects. Adverse experiences that were reported at these doses included excitation or agitation, insomnia, and slight or moderate elevations in hemodynamic parameters. Other observed high-dose effects in clinical studies have included anxiety, irritability, aggressiveness, confusion, nervousness, tremor, palpitations, sleep disturbances, nausea, diarrhea, and decreased prothrombin time.

From postmarketing experience, there have been no reports of fatal overdoses involving modafinil alone (doses up to 12 g). Overdoses involving multiple drugs, including modafinil, have resulted in fatal outcomes. Symptoms most often accompanying modafinil overdose, alone or in combination with other drugs have included the following: insomnia; CNS symptoms such as restlessness, disorientation, confusion, excitation and hallucination; digestive changes such as nausea and diarrhea; and cardiovascular changes such as tachycardia, bradycardia, hypertension, and chest pain.

Cases of accidental ingestion/overdose have been reported in children as young as 11 months of age. The highest reported accidental ingestion on a mg/kg basis occurred in a 3-year-old boy who ingested 800 to 1,000 mg (50 to 63 mg/kg) of modafinil. The child remained stable. The symptoms associated with overdose in children were similar to those observed in adults.

➤*Treatment:* No specific antidote to the toxic effects of modafinil overdose has been identified to date. Manage such overdoses with primarily supportive care, including cardiovascular monitoring. If there are no contraindications, consider induced emesis or gastric lavage. There are no data to suggest the utility of dialysis or urinary acidification or alkalinization in enhancing drug elimination. The physician should consider contacting a poison control center on the treatment of any overdose.

MODAFINIL — ORAL

Patient Information

Physicians are advised to discuss the following issues with patients for whom they prescribe modafinil tablets:

Modafinil is indicated for patients who have abnormal levels of sleepiness. Modafinil has been shown to improve, but not eliminate this abnormal tendency to fall asleep. Therefore, patients should not alter their previous behavior with regard to potentially dangerous activities (eg, driving, operating machinery) or other activities requiring appropriate levels of wakefulness, until and unless treatment with modafinil has been shown to produce levels of wakefulness that permit such activities. Advise patients that modafinil is not a replacement for sleep.

Inform patients that it may be critical that they continue to take their previously prescribed treatments (eg, patients with OSAHS receiving CPAP should continue to do so).

Inform patients of the availability of a patient information leaflet, and instruct them to read the leaflet prior to taking modafinil. See Patient Information at the end of this labeling for the text of the leaflet provided for patients.

➤*Pregnancy:* Advise patients to notify their physicians if they become pregnant or intend to become pregnant during therapy. Caution patients regarding the potentially increased risk of pregnancy when using steroidal contraceptives (including depot or implantable contraceptives) with modafinil tablets and for 1 month after discontinuation of therapy.

➤*Concomitant medication:* Advise patients to inform their physicians if they are taking, or plan to take, any prescription or over-the-counter drugs, because of the potential for interactions between modafinil tablets and other drugs.

➤*Alcohol:* Advise patients that the use of modafinil in combination with alcohol has not been studied. Advise patients that it is prudent to avoid alcohol while taking modafinil tablets.

Amphetamines

WARNING

Amphetamines have a high potential for abuse. Use in weight reduction programs only when alternative therapy has been ineffective. Administration for prolonged periods may lead to drug dependence and must be avoided. Pay particular attention to the possibility of subjects obtaining amphetamines for nontherapeutic use or distribution to others. Prescribe or dispense sparingly.

Indications

➤*Narcolepsy:* To improve wakefulness in patients with excessive day-time sleepiness associated with narcolepsy.

➤*Attention deficit disorder with hyperactivity:* Indicated as an integral part of a total treatment program that includes other remedial measures (psychological, educational, social) for a stabilizing effect in children 3 to 16 years of age with a behavioral syndrome characterized by moderate to severe distractibility, short attention span, hyperactivity, emotional lability, and impulsivity. Do not diagnose this syndrome with finality when these symptoms are only of comparatively recent origin. Nonlocalizing (soft) neurological signs, learning disability, and abnormal EEG may be present and a diagnosis of CNS dysfunction may be warranted.

➤*Exogenous obesity:* As a short-term adjunct in a regimen of weight reduction based on caloric restriction, for patients refractory to alternative therapy (eg, repeated diets, group programs, other drugs). Weigh the limited usefulness against the possible risks inherent in use.

➤*Unlabeled uses:* Cocaine dependence treatment (**dextroamphetamine**), autism (**dextroamphetamine**).

Administration and Dosage

Administer at the lowest effective dosage and adjust individually. Avoid late evening doses, particularly with the long-acting form, because of the resulting insomnia.

When treating attention deficit disorder in children, occasionally interrupt drug administration to determine if there is a recurrence of behavioral symptoms sufficient to require continued therapy.

Actions

➤*Pharmacology:* Amphetamines are sympathomimetic amines with CNS stimulant activity. CNS effects are mediated by release of norepinephrine from central noradrenergic neurons. At higher doses, dopamine may be released in the mesolimbic system.

Peripheral alpha and beta activity includes elevation of systolic and diastolic blood pressures and weak bronchodilator and respiratory stimulant action. At therapeutic doses, the heart rate may be reflexly slowed; large doses may produce cardiac arrhythmias.

There is neither specific evidence that clearly establishes the mechanism whereby amphetamines produce mental and behavioral effects in children, nor conclusive evidence regarding how these effects relate to the condition of the CNS.

The site of action for appetite suppression is thought to be the lateral hypothalamic feeding center.

➤*Pharmacokinetics:*

Special populations –

Children: Children eliminated amphetamine faster than adults.

Gender: Systemic exposure to amphetamine was 20% to 30% higher in women than in men because of the higher dose administered to women on a mg/kg body weight basis. Amphetamine is metabolized in the liver by aromatic hydroxylation, N-dealkylation, and deamination.

Amphetamines are effective after oral administration and effects last for several hours.

Dextroamphetamine – Following administration of three 5 mg tablets, average maximal dextroamphetamine plasma concentrations (C_{max}) of 36.6 ng/mL were achieved at ≈ 3 hours. Following administration of one 15 mg sustained-release capsule, maximal dextroamphetamine plasma concentrations were obtained ≈ 8 hours after dosing. The average C_{max} was 23.5 ng/mL. The average plasma $t_{½}$ was similar for the tablet and sustained-release capsule and was ≈ 12 hours.

Methamphetamine – Methamphetamine is rapidly absorbed from the GI tract. The biological half-life has been reported in the range of 4 to 5 hours. Excretion occurs primarily in the urine and is dependent on urine pH. Alkaline urine will increase the drug half-life significantly. Approximately 62% of an oral dose is eliminated in the urine within the first 24 hours with ≈ 33% as intact drug and the remainder as metabolites.

Amphetamine mixture – Following administration of immediate-release amphetamine mixture tablets, the peak plasma concentrations occurred in ≈ 3 hours for d-amphetamine and l-amphetamine.

The time to reach maximum plasma concentration (T_{max}) for extended-release amphetamine mixture capsules is ≈ 7 hours, which is ≈ 4 hours longer compared with the immediate-release formulation.

A single dose of 20 mg extended-release amphetamine mixture capsules provided comparable plasma concentration profiles of d-amphetamine and l-amphetamine with 10 mg immediate-release amphetamine mixture tablets twice daily administered 4 hours apart.

The mean elimination half-life is 1 hour shorter for d-amphetamine and 2 hours shorter for l-amphetamine in children 6 to 12 years of age compared with that of adults ($t_{½}$ is 10 hours for d-amphetamine and 13 hours for l-amphetamine in adults and 9 and 11 hours, respectively, for children). Extended-release amphetamine mixture capsules demonstrate linear pharmacokinetics over the dose range of 10 to 30 mg. There is no unexpected accumulation at steady state.

Food does not affect the extent of absorption of extended-release amphetamine mixture capsules, but prolongs T_{max} by 2.5 hours (from 5.2 hours at fasted state to 7.7 hours after a high-fat meal). Opening the capsule and sprinkling the contents on applesauce results in comparable absorption to the intact capsule taken in the fasted state.

Contraindications

Advanced arteriosclerosis; symptomatic cardiovascular disease; moderate to severe hypertension; hyperthyroidism; known hypersensitivity or idiosyncrasy to the sympathomimetic amines; glaucoma; agitated states; history of drug abuse; during or within 14 days following administration of MAO inhibitors (hypertensive crises may result).

Warnings

➤*Tolerance:* When tolerance to the anorectic effect develops, do not exceed recommended dose in an attempt to increase the effect; rather, discontinue the drug.

➤*Drug dependence:* Amphetamines have been extensively abused. Tolerance, extreme psychological dependence, and severe social disability have occurred. Patients may increase the dosage to many times that recommended. Abrupt cessation following prolonged high dosage results in extreme fatigue, mental depression, and changes on the sleep EEG.

Manifestations of chronic intoxication – Severe dermatoses, marked insomnia, irritability, hyperactivity, and personality changes have occurred. Disorganization of thoughts, poor concentration, visual hallucinations, and compulsive behavior often occur. The most severe manifestation of chronic intoxication is psychosis, often clinically indistinguishable from paranoid schizophrenia. This is rare with oral amphetamines.

➤*Growth inhibition:* Decrements in the predicted growth (ie, weight gain or height) rate have been reported with the long-term use of stimulants in children. Therefore, carefully monitor patients requiring long-term therapy.

➤*Pregnancy: Category C.* Safety for use during pregnancy has not been established. Reproduction studies in mammals at many times the human dose have suggested an embryotoxic and teratogenic potential. Congenital defects associated with amphetamine use include cardiac abnormalities, bifidexencephaly, and biliary atresia. **Methamphetamine** has been shown to have teratogenic and embryocidal effects in mammals given high multiples of the human dose. There are no adequate and well-controlled studies in pregnant women. Use in women who are or who may become pregnant (especially those in the first trimester) only when clearly needed and when the potential benefits outweigh the potential hazards to the fetus.

Infants born to mothers dependent on amphetamines have an increased risk of premature delivery and low birth weight. Also, these infants may experience symptoms of withdrawal as demonstrated by dysphoria, including agitation and significant lassitude.

➤*Lactation:* Amphetamines are excreted in breast milk. Advise patients to discontinue nursing while taking amphetamines.

➤*Children:* Safety and efficacy have not been established for the use of amphetamines as anorectic agents in children less than 12 years of age.

Amphetamine and **dextroamphetamine** are not recommended in children less than 3 years of age for attention deficit disorder with hyperactivity. In psychotic children, amphetamines may exacerbate symptoms of behavior disturbance and thought disorder. Amphetamines may exacerbate motor and phonic tics and Tourette's syndrome. Therefore, clinical evaluation for tics and Tourette's syndrome in children and their families should precede use of stimulants.

Data are inadequate to determine whether chronic administration of amphetamines may be associated with growth inhibition; therefore, monitor growth during treatment and interrupt treatment in patients who are not growing or gaining weight as expected.

Long-term effects in children have not been well established.

Extended-release amphetamine mixture – Extended-release amphetamine mixture capsules are indicated for children ≥ 6 years of age. Effects in children 3 to 5 years of age have not been studied.

Precautions

➤*Hypertension:* Exercise caution in prescribing amphetamines for patients with even mild hypertension.

➤*Prescribe or dispense:* Prescribe or dispense the least amount feasible at one time to minimize the possibility of overdosage.

➤*Potentially hazardous tasks:* Amphetamines may impair the ability of the patient to engage in potentially hazardous activities such as operating machinery or vehicles; caution the patient accordingly.

➤*Attention deficit disorders:* Drug treatment is not indicated in all cases and should be considered only in light of the complete history and evaluation of the child. Amphetamine use should depend on the chronicity and severity of the child's symptoms and appropriateness for his/her age. Use should not depend solely on the presence of ≥ 1 of the behavioral characteristics.

When these symptoms are associated with acute stress reactions, amphetamine treatment is usually not indicated.

➤*Fatigue:* Do not use **methamphetamine** to combat fatigue or replace rest in normal people.

➤*Tartrazine sensitivity:* Some of these products contain tartrazine, which may cause allergic-type reactions (including bronchial asthma) in susceptible individuals. Although the incidence of tartrazine sensitivity in the general population is low, it is frequently seen in patients who also have aspirin hypersensitivity. Specific products containing tartrazine are identified in the product listings.

Drug Interactions

Insulin requirements in diabetes mellitus may be altered in association with the use of **methamphetamine** and the concomitant dietary regimen.

Amphetamine Drug Interactions

Precipitant drug	Object drug[a]		Description
Furazolidone	Amphetamines	↑	Increased sensitivity to amphetamines may occur. If an interaction is suspected, monitor patient for signs and symptoms of amphetamine toxicity and reduce the amphetamine dose accordingly.
MAO inhibitors	Amphetamines	↑	Exaggerated pharmacologic effects from the amphetamines may occur. Avoid coadministration. The hypertensive reaction may occur for up to several weeks after discontinuing the MAO inhibitor.
SSRIs	Amphetamines	↑	Increased sensitivity to effect of sympathomimetics and increased risk of "serotonin syndrome" may occur. If these agents must be given concurrently, monitor the patient for increased signs and symptoms of CNS effects. Adjust therapy as needed.
Urinary acidifiers	Amphetamines	↓	The elimination of amphetamines is hastened with a concomitant reduction in their duration of action. No special precautions appear necessary. This interaction has been exploited therapeutically in the management of amphetamine overdose.
Urinary alkalinizers	Amphetamines	↑	Alkalinized urine may prolong the effects of amphetamines. Avoid agents that may alkalinize urine, particularly in overdose situations.
Amphetamines	Guanethidine	↓	Amphetamines may reverse the hypotensive effects of guanethidine. Monitor patients. If there is a loss of blood pressure control, stop the amphetamine or switch to alternative hypotensive therapy.

[a] ↑ = Object drug increased. ↓ = Object drug decreased.

➤*Drug/Lab test interactions:* Plasma **corticosteroid** levels may be increased. This increase is greatest in the evening. This should be considered if determination of plasma corticosteroid levels is desired in a person receiving amphetamines. **Urinary steroid** determinations may be altered by amphetamines.

Adverse Reactions

➤*Cardiovascular:* Palpitations; tachycardia; elevation of blood pressure; reflex decrease in heart rate; arrhythmias (at larger doses). There have been isolated reports of cardiomyopathy associated with chronic amphetamine use.

➤*CNS:* Overstimulation; restlessness; dizziness; insomnia; dyskinesia; euphoria; dysphoria; tremor; headache; changes in libido; psychotic episodes at recommended doses (rare). CNS stimulants have exacerbated Tourette's disorder and have exacerbated motor and phonic tics.

➤*GI:* Dry mouth; unpleasant taste; diarrhea; constipation; other GI disturbances. Anorexia and weight loss may occur as undesirable effects when amphetamines are used other than for their anorectic effect.

➤*Miscellaneous:* Urticaria; impotence; changes in libido; suppression of growth in children with long-term stimulant use.

Overdosage

➤*Symptoms:* Individual patient response to amphetamines varies widely. Manifestations of acute overdosage with amphetamines include the following: Restlessness; irritability; insomnia; tremor; hyperreflexia; rhabdomyolysis; rapid respiration; hyperpyrexia; assaultiveness; hallucinations; panic states; diaphoresis; mydriasis; flushing; hyperactivity; confusion; hypertension or hypotension; extrasystoles; tachypnea; fever; delirium; self-injury; marked hypertension; arrhythmias. Fatigue and depression usually follow the central stimulation. Cardiovascular effects include arrhythmias, hypertension or hypotension, and circulatory collapse. GI symptoms include nausea, vomiting, diarrhea, and abdominal cramps. Fatal poisoning usually is preceded by convulsions and coma.

➤*Treatment:* Consult with a certified poison control center for up-to-date guidance and advice. Treatment is largely symptomatic and includes gastric evacuation, although this is usually ineffective more than 4 hours after ingestion. After emptying the stomach, administer activated charcoal and a cathartic. Acidification of the urine increases amphetamine excretion. Experience with hemodialysis and peritoneal dialysis is inadequate to permit recommendations.

If acute, severe hypertension complicates amphetamine overdosage, administration of IV phentolamine has been suggested. However, a gradual drop in blood pressure usually results from sufficient sedation. Chlorpromazine antagonizes the central stimulant effects of amphetamines and can be used to treat amphetamine intoxication.

Because much of the long-acting form of medication is coated for gradual release, direct therapy at reversing the effects of the ingested drug and at supporting the patient; continue until overdosage symptoms subside. Use saline cathartics to hasten the evacuation of pellets that have not released medication.

Amphetamine mixture – Consider the prolonged release of mixed amphetamine salts from extended-release amphetamine mixture capsules when treating patients with overdose.

Patient Information

Regardless of indication, administer amphetamines at the lowest effective dosage and individually adjust dosage. Avoid late evening doses because of the resulting insomnia.

Do not chew or crush sustained-release or long-acting tablets.

Do not increase dosage, except on physician's advice.

Amphetamines may impair the ability of the patient to engage in potentially hazardous activities such as operating machinery or vehicles; caution the patient accordingly.

May cause nervousness, restlessness, insomnia, dizziness, anorexia, dry mouth, and GI disturbances. Notify physician if these effects become pronounced.

DEXTROAMPHETAMINE SULFATE

c-ii	**Dextroamphetamine Sulfate** (Various, eg, Barr)	**Tablets**: 5 mg	In 100s.
c-ii	**Dexedrine** (GlaxoSmithKline)		Tartrazine, lactose, sucrose. (SKF E19). Orange, triangular, scored. In 100s.
c-ii	**DextroStat** (Shire Richwood)		Tartrazine, lactose, sucrose. (RP 51). Yellow, scored. In 100s, 500s, and 1000s.
c-ii	**Dextroamphetamine Sulfate** (Various, eg, Barr)	**Tablets**: 10 mg	In 100s.
c-ii	**DextroStat** (Shire Richwood)		Tartrazine, lactose, sucrose. (RP 52). Yellow, scored. In 100s and 500s.
c-ii	**Dextroamphetamine Sulfate** (Various, eg, Barr)	**Capsules, sustained-release**: 5 mg	In 100s.
c-ii	**Dexedrine Spansules** (GlaxoSmithKline)		Sugar spheres. (5 mg 3512/5 mg SB). Clear and brown. In 100s.
c-ii	**Dextroamphetamine Sulfate** (Various, eg, Barr)	**Capsules, sustained-release**: 10 mg	In 100s.
c-ii	**Dexedrine Spansules** (GlaxoSmithKline)		Sugar spheres. (10 mg 3513/10 mg SB). Clear and brown. In 100s.
c-ii	**Dextroamphetamine Sulfate** (Various, eg, Barr)	**Capsules, sustained-release**: 15 mg	In 100s.
c-ii	**Dexedrine Spansules** (GlaxoSmithKline)		Sugar spheres. (15 mg 3514/15 mg SB). Clear/Brown. In 100s.

DEXTROAMPHETAMINE SULFATE — ORAL

Complete and comparative prescribing information for these products begins in the Amphetamines group monograph.

WARNING

Amphetamines have a high potential for abuse. Administration of amphetamines for prolonged periods of time may lead to drug dependence and must be avoided. Particular attention should be paid to the possibility of subjects obtaining amphetamines for nontherapeutic use or distribution to others, and the drugs should be prescribed or dispensed sparingly.

Indications

In narcolepsy; in attention deficit disorder with hyperactivity, as an integral part of a total treatment program which typically includes other remedial measures (psychological, educational, social) for a stabilizing effect in children (ages 3 years to 16 years) with a behavioral syndrome characterized by the following group of developmentally inappropriate symptoms: Moderate-to-severe distractibility, short attention span, hyperactivity, emotional lability, and impulsivity. The diagnosis of this syndrome should not be made with finality when these symptoms are only of comparatively recent origin. Nonlocalizing (soft) neurological signs, learning disability, and abnormal EEG may or may not be present, and a diagnosis of central nervous system dysfunction may or may not be warranted.

Administration and Dosage

Amphetamines should be administered at the lowest effective dosage and dosage should be individually adjusted. Late evening doses, particularly with the sustained-release or extended-release capsule forms, should be avoided because of the resulting insomnia.

➤*Narcolepsy:* Usual dose 5 to 60 mg per day in divided doses, depending on the individual patient response.

Narcolepsy seldom occurs in children younger than 12 years of age; however, when it does, dextroamphetamine sulfate may be used. The suggested initial dose for patients aged 6 to 12 is 5 mg daily; daily dose may be raised in increments of 5 mg at weekly intervals until optimal response is obtained. In patients greater than or equal to 12 years of age, start with 10 mg daily; daily dosage may be raised in increments of 10 mg at weekly intervals until optimal response is obtained. If bothersome adverse reactions appear (eg, insomnia or anorexia), dosage should be reduced. Sustained- or extended-release capsules may be used for once-a-day dosage wherever appropriate. With tablets, give first dose on awakening; give additional doses (1 or 2) at intervals of 4 to 6 hours.

➤*Attention deficit disorder with hyperactivity:* Not recommended for pediatric patients younger than 3 years of age.

In pediatric patients from 3 to 5 years of age – Start with 2.5 mg daily, by tablet; daily dosage may be raised in increments of 2.5 mg at weekly intervals until optimal response is obtained.

In pediatric patients 6 years of age and older – Start with 5 mg once or twice daily; daily dosage may be raised in increments of 5 mg at weekly intervals until optimal response is obtained. Only in rare cases will it be necessary to exceed a total of 40 mg per day.

Sustained-release or extended-release capsules may be used for once-a-day dosage wherever appropriate.

With tablets, give first dose on awakening; give additional doses (1 or 2) at intervals of 4 to 6 hours.

Where possible, drug administration should be interrupted occasionally to determine if there is a recurrence of behavioral symptoms sufficient to require continued therapy.

➤*Storage/Stability:* Store at controlled room temperature 15° to 30°C (59° to 86°F). Dispense in a tight, light- and child-resistant container.

METHAMPHETAMINE HYDROCHLORIDE (Desoxyephedrine Hydrochloride)

c-ii	**Methamphetamine Hydrochloride** (Able)	**Tablets**: 5 mg	Corn starch, lactose. (A 396). In 30s, 100s, 500s, and 1000s.
c-ii	**Desoxyn** (Abbott)		Lactose. (TE). White. In 100s.

METHAMPHETAMINE HYDROCHLORIDE — ORAL

For complete and comparative prescribing information for these products, refer to the Amphetamines general monograph.

WARNING

Methamphetamine has a high potential for abuse. It should thus be tried only in weight reduction programs for patients in whom alternative therapy has been ineffective. Administration of methamphetamine for prolonged periods of time in obesity may lead to drug dependence and must be avoided. Particular attention should be paid to the possibility of subjects obtaining methamphetamine for nontherapeutic use or distribution to others, and the drug should be prescribed or dispensed sparingly.

Indications

➤*Attention deficit disorder with hyperactivity:* As an integral part of a total treatment program that typically includes other remedial measures (psychological, educational, social) for a stabilizing effect in children greater than 6 years of age with a behavioral syndrome characterized by the following group of developmentally inappropriate symptoms: Moderate to severe distractibility, short attention span, hyperactivity, emotional lability, and impulsivity. The diagnosis of this syndrome should not be made with finality when these symptoms are only of comparatively recent origin. Nonlocalizing (soft) neurological signs, learning disability, and abnormal EEG may or may not be present, and a diagnosis of CNS dysfunction may or may not be warranted.

➤*Exogenous obesity:* As a short-term (ie, a few weeks) adjunct in a regimen of weight reduction based on caloric restriction, for patients in whom obesity is refractory to alternative therapy (eg, repeated diets, group programs, other drugs). The limited usefulness of methamphetamine hydrochloride tablets should be weighed against possible risks inherent in use.

Administration and Dosage

Methamphetamine should be administered at the lowest effective dosage, and dosage should be individually adjusted. Late evening medication should be avoided because of the resulting insomnia.

➤*Attention deficit disorder with hyperactivity:* For treatment of children greater than or equal to 6 years of age with a behavioral syndrome characterized by moderate to severe distractibility, short attention span, hyperactivity, emotional lability, and impulsivity, an initial dose of 5 mg methamphetamine hydrochloride once or twice a day is recommended. Daily dosage may be raised in increments of 5 mg at weekly intervals until an optimum clinical response is achieved. The usual effective dose is 20 to 25 mg daily. The total daily dose may be given in 2 divided doses daily.

Where possible, drug administration should be interrupted occasionally to determine if there is a recurrence of behavioral symptoms sufficient to require continued therapy.

➤*Obesity:* One 5 mg tablet should be taken 30 minutes before each meal. Total daily dose may be given as conventional tablets in 2 divided doses or once daily using the long-acting form. Do not use the long-acting form for

METHAMPHETAMINE HYDROCHLORIDE — ORAL

initiation of dosage or until the titrated daily dose is equal to or greater than the dosage provided in a long-acting tablet. Treatment should not exceed a few weeks in duration. Intermittent or interrupted courses of therapy may be useful. A 3- to 6-week course of therapy followed by a discontinuation period of half the original treatment length has been suggested. Methamphetamine is not recommended for use as an anorectic agent in children less than 12 years of age.

➤*Storage / Stability:* Store below 30°C (86°F).

AMPHETAMINE MIXTURES

c-ii	**Amphetamine Salt Combo** (Barr)	**Tablets:** 5 mg (1.25 mg dextroamphetamine sulfate, 1.25 mg dextroamphetamine saccharate, 1.25 mg amphetamine aspartate, 1.25 mg amphetamine sulfate)	(b 971 5). Blue, oval, scored. In 50s, 100s, and 500s.
c-ii	**Adderall** (Shire Richwood)		Lactose, sucrose. (AD 5). Blue, scored. In 100s.
c-ii	**Adderall** (Shire Richwood)	7.5 mg (1.875 mg dextroamphetamine sulfate, 1.875 mg dextroamphetamine saccharate, 1.875 mg amphetamine aspartate, 1.875 mg amphetamine sulfate)	Lactose, sucrose. (AD 7.5). Blue, scored. In 100s.
c-ii	**Amphetamine Salt Combo** (Barr)	10 mg (2.5 mg dextroamphetamine sulfate, 2.5 mg dextroamphetamine saccharate, 2.5 mg amphetamine aspartate, 2.5 mg amphetamine sulfate)	(b 972 1/0). Blue, oval, scored. In 50s, 100s, and 500s.
c-ii	**Adderall** (Shire Richwood)		Lactose, sucrose. (AD 10). Blue, scored. In 100s.
c-ii	**Adderall** (Shire Richwood)	12.5 mg (3.125 mg dextroamphetamine sulfate, 3.125 mg dextroamphetamine saccharate, 3.125 mg amphetamine aspartate, 3.125 mg amphetamine sulfate)	Lactose, sucrose. (AD 12.5). Orange, scored. In 100s.
c-ii	**Adderall** (Shire Richwood)	15 mg (3.75 mg dextroamphetamine sulfate, 3.75 mg dextroamphetamine saccharate, 3.75 mg amphetamine aspartate, 3.75 mg amphetamine sulfate)	Lactose, sucrose. (AD 15). Orange, scored. In 100s.
c-ii	**Amphetamine Salt Combo** (Barr)	20 mg (5 mg dextroamphetamine sulfate, 5 mg dextroamphetamine saccharate, 5 mg amphetamine aspartate, 5 mg amphetamine sulfate)	(b 973 2/0). Peach, oval, scored. In 50s, 100s, and 500s.
c-ii	**Adderall** (Shire Richwood)		Lactose, sucrose. (AD 20). Orange, scored. In 100s.
c-ii	**Amphetamine Salt Combo** (Barr)	30 mg (7.5 mg dextroamphetamine sulfate, 7.5 mg dextroamphetamine saccharate, 7.5 mg amphetamine aspartate, 7.5 mg amphetamine sulfate)	(b 974 3/0). Peach, oval, scored. In 50s, 100s, and 500s.
c-ii	**Adderall** (Shire Richwood)		Lactose, sucrose. (AD 30). Orange, scored. In 100s.
c-ii	**Adderall XR** (Shire)	**Capsules:** 5 mg (1.25 mg dextroamphetamine saccharate, 1.25 mg amphetamine aspartate monohydrate, 1.25 mg dextroamphetamine sulfate, 1.25 mg amphetamine sulfate)	Sugar spheres, talc. (ADDERALL XR 5 mg). Clear/Blue. In 100s.
		10 mg (2.5 mg dextroamphetamine saccharate, 2.5 mg amphetamine aspartate monohydrate, 2.5 mg dextroamphetamine sulfate, 2.5 mg amphetamine sulfate)	Sugar spheres. (SHIRE 381 10 mg). Blue. In 100s.
		15 mg (3.75 mg dextroamphetamine saccharate, 3.75 mg amphetamine aspartate monohydrate, 3.75 mg dextroamphetamine sulfate, 3.75 mg amphetamine sulfate)	Sugar spheres, talc. (ADDERALL XR 15 mg). Blue/White. In 100s.
		20 mg (5 mg dextroamphetamine saccharate, 5 mg amphetamine aspartate monohydrate, 5 mg dextroamphetamine sulfate, 5 mg amphetamine sulfate)	Sugar spheres. (SHIRE 381 20 mg). Orange. In 100s.
		25 mg (6.25 mg dextroamphetamine saccharate, 6.25 mg amphetamine aspartate monohydrate, 6.25 mg dextroamphetamine sulfate, 6.25 mg amphetamine sulfate)	Sugar spheres, talc. (ADDERALL XR 25 mg). Orange/White. In 100s.
		30 mg (7.5 mg dextroamphetamine saccharate, 7.5 mg amphetamine aspartate monohydrate, 7.5 mg dextroamphetamine sulfate, 7.5 mg amphetamine sulfate)	Sugar spheres. (SHIRE 381 30 mg). Natural/Orange. In 100s.

AMPHETAMINE MIXTURES — ORAL

For complete and comparative prescribing information for these products, refer to the Amphetamines group monograph.

WARNING

Amphetamines have a high potential for abuse. Administration of amphetamines for prolonged periods of time may lead to drug dependence and must be avoided. Particular attention should be paid to the possibility of subjects obtaining amphetamines for non-therapeutic use or distribution to others, and the drugs should be prescribed or dispensed sparingly.

Indications

➤*Attention deficit disorder with hyperactivity:* As an integral part of a total treatment program that typically includes other remedial measures (psychological, educational, social) for a stabilizing effect in children with behavioral syndrome characterized by the following group of developmentally inappropriate symptoms: Moderate to severe distractibility, short attention span, hyperactivity, emotional lability, and impulsivity. The diagnosis of this syndrome should not be made with finality when these symptoms are only of comparatively recent origin. Nonlocalizing (soft) neurological signs, learning disability and abnormal EEG may or may not be present, and a diagnosis of central nervous system dysfunction may or may not be warranted.

➤*Narcolepsy:* Amphetamines tablets are also indicated in narcolepsy.

Administration and Dosage

➤*Approved by the FDA:* February 13, 1996.

➤*Tablets:* Regardless of indication, amphetamines should be administered at the lowest effective dosage and dosage should be individually adjusted. Late evening doses should be avoided because of the resulting insomnia.

Attention deficit disorder with hyperactivity – Not recommended for children less than 3 years of age. In children from 3 to 5 years of age, start with 2.5 mg daily; daily dosage may be raised in increments of 2.5 mg at weekly intervals until optimal response is obtained.

In children 6 years of age and older, start with 5 mg once or twice daily; daily dosage may be raised in increments of 5 mg at weekly intervals until optimal response is obtained. Only in rare cases will it be necessary to exceed a total of 40 mg/day. Give first dose on awakening; additional doses (1 or 2) at intervals of 4 to 6 hours.

Where possible, drug administration should be interrupted occasionally to determine if there is a recurrence of behavioral symptoms sufficient to require continued therapy.

Narcolepsy – Usual dose 5 mg to 60 mg/day in divided doses, depending on the individual patient response.

Narcolepsy seldom occurs in children less than 12 years of age; however, when it does, dextroamphetamine sulfate may be used. The suggested initial dose for patients aged 6 to 12 is 5 mg daily; daily dose may be raised in increments of 5 mg at weekly intervals until optimal response is obtained. In patients 12 years of age and older, start with 10 mg daily; daily dosage may be raised in increments of 10 mg at weekly intervals until optimal response is obtained. If bothersome adverse reactions appear (eg, insomnia or anorexia), dosage should be reduced. Give first dose on awakening; additional doses (1 or 2) at intervals of 4 to 6 hours.

AMPHETAMINE MIXTURES — ORAL

➤*Extended-release capsules:* In children with ADHD who are 6 years of age and older and are either starting treatment for the first time or switching from another medication, start with 10 mg once daily in the morning; daily dosage may be raised in increments of 10 mg at weekly intervals. Dosage should be individualized according to the needs and response of the patient. Amphetamines should be administered at the lowest effective dosage. The maximum recommended dose is 30 mg/day; doses more than 30 mg/day of amphetamine extended-release have not been studied.

Amphetamines are not recommended for children less than 3 years of age. Amphetamine extended-release has not been studied in children less than 6 years of age.

Patients currently using amphetamine immediate-release – Based on bioequivalence data, patients taking divided doses of immediate-release amphetamine, for example twice a day, may be switched to amphetamine extended-release at the same total daily dose taken once daily. Titrate at weekly intervals to appropriate efficacy and tolerability as indicated.

Amphetamine extended-release capsules may be taken whole, or the capsule may be opened and the entire contents sprinkled on applesauce. If the patient is using the sprinkle administration method, the sprinkled applesauce should be consumed immediately; it should not be stored. Patients should take the applesauce with sprinkled beads in its entirety without chewing. The dose of a single capsule should not be divided. The contents of the entire capsule should be taken, and patients should not take anything less than 1 capsule per day.

Amphetamine extended-release capsules should be given upon awakening. Afternoon doses should be avoided because of the potential for insomnia.

Where possible, drug administration should be interrupted occasionally to determine whether there is a recurrence of behavioral symptoms sufficient to require continued therapy.

➤*Storage/Stability:* Dispense in a tight, light-resistant container as defined in the USP.

Store at controlled room temperature 15° to 30°C (59° to 86°F).

DEXMETHYLPHENIDATE HYDROCHLORIDE

c-ii	**Focalin** (Novartis)	**Tablets:** 2.5 mg	Lactose. (D 2.5). Blue. In 100s.
		5 mg	Lactose. (D 5). Yellow. In 100s.
		10 mg	Lactose. (D 10). White. In 100s.
c-ii	**Focalin XR** (Novartis)	**Capsules, extended-release:** 5 mg	Sugar spheres. (NVR D5). Lt. blue. In 100s.
		10 mg	Sugar spheres. (NVR D10). Lt. caramel. In 100s.
		20 mg	Sugar spheres. (NVR D20). White. In 100s.

DEXMETHYLPHENIDATE HYDROCHLORIDE — ORAL

WARNING

Drug dependence – Give dexmethylphenidate cautiously to patients with a history of drug dependence or alcoholism. Chronic, abusive use can lead to marked tolerance and psychological dependence with varying degrees of abnormal behavior. Frank psychotic episodes can occur, especially with parenteral abuse. Careful supervision is required during drug withdrawal from abusive use because severe depression may occur. Withdrawal following chronic therapeutic use may unmask symptoms of the underlying disorder that may require follow-up.

Indications

➤*Attention deficit hyperactivity disorder (ADHD):* For the treatment of ADHD in patients 6 years of age and older. Dexmethylphenidate is indicated as an integral part of a total treatment program for ADHD that may include other measures (eg, psychological, educational, social) for patients with this syndrome. Drug treatment may not be indicated for all patients with this syndrome. Stimulants are not intended for use in the patient who exhibits symptoms secondary to environmental factors or other primary psychiatric disorders, including psychosis.

Administration and Dosage

➤*Approved by the FDA:* November 13, 2001.

Administer dexmethylphenidate immediate-release twice daily, at least 4 hours apart, with or without food. Dexmethylphenidate extended-release capsules are for oral administration once daily in the morning. Capsules may be swallowed whole or alternatively may be administered by sprinkling the capsule contents on a small amount of applesauce (see specific instructions below). Dexmethylphenidate capsules and/or their contents should not be crushed, chewed, or divided.

The capsules may be carefully opened and the beads sprinkled over a spoonful of applesauce. The mixture of drug and applesauce should be consumed immediately in its entirety. The drug and applesauce mixture should not be stored for future use.

Individualize dosage according to the needs and responses of the patient.

➤*Patients new to methylphenidate:* The recommended starting dose of dexmethylphenidate for patients who are not currently taking racemic methylphenidate, or for patients who are on stimulants other than methylphenidate is the following:

Immediate-release – 5 mg/day (2.5 mg twice daily). Dosage may be adjusted in 2.5 to 5 mg increments to a maximum of 20 mg/day (10 mg twice daily). In general, dosage adjustments may proceed at approximately weekly intervals.

Extended-release – 5 mg/day for pediatric patients and 10 mg/day for adult patients. Dosage may be adjusted in 5 mg increments to a maximum of 20 mg/day for pediatric patients and in 10 mg/day increments to a maximum of 20 mg/day for adult patients. In general, dosage adjustments may proceed at approximately weekly intervals.

➤*Patients currently using methylphenidate:* For patients currently using methylphenidate, the recommended starting dose of dexmethylphenidate is half the dose of racemic methylphenidate. The maximum recommended dose is 20 mg/day (10 mg twice daily immediate-release).

➤*Maintenance / Extended treatment:* It is generally agreed that pharmacological treatment of ADHD may be needed for extended periods. The physician who elects to use dexmethylphenidate for extended periods in patients with ADHD should periodically reevaluate the long-term usefulness of the drug for the individual patient with periods off medication to assess the patient's functioning without pharmacotherapy. Improvement may be sustained when the drug is either temporarily or permanently discontinued.

➤*Dose reduction and discontinuation:* If paradoxical aggravation of symptoms or other adverse events occur, reduce the dosage, or, if necessary, discontinue the drug.

If improvement is not observed after appropriate dosage adjustment over a 1-month period, discontinue the drug.

➤*Storage / Stability:* Store at 25°C (77°F); excursions permitted 15° to 30°C (59° to 86°F). Protect from light and moisture.

Actions

➤*Pharmacology:* Dexmethylphenidate hydrochloride is a central nervous system stimulant. Dexmethylphenidate hydrochloride, the more pharmacologically active enantiomer of the d- and l-enantiomers, is thought to block the reuptake of norepinephrine and dopamine into the presynaptic neuron and increase the release of these monoamines into the extraneuronal space. The mode of therapeutic action in ADHD is not known.

➤*Pharmacokinetics:*

Absorption – Dexmethylphenidate hydrochloride is readily absorbed following oral administration. In patients with ADHD, plasma dexmethylphenidate concentrations increase rapidly, reaching a maximum in the fasted state at about 1 to 1½ hours post-dose. No differences in the pharmacokinetics of dexmethylphenidate hydrochloride were noted following single and repeated twice-daily dosing, thus indicating no significant drug accumulation in children with ADHD.

When given to children as capsules in single doses of 2.5 mg, 5 mg, and 10 mg, C_{max} and $AUC_{0\text{-}inf}$ of dexmethylphenidate were proportional to dose. In the same study, plasma dexmethylphenidate levels were comparable to those achieved following single dl-threo-methylphenidate hydrochloride doses given as capsules in twice the total mg amount (equimolar with respect to dexmethylphenidate hydrochloride).

Food effects: In a single-dose study conducted in adults, coadministration of 2 times 10 mg dexmethylphenidate hydrochloride with a high fat breakfast resulted in a dexmethylphenidate t_{max} of 2.9 hours postdose as compared to 1.5 hours postdose when given in a fasting state. C_{max} and $AUC_{0\text{-}inf}$ were comparable in both the fasted and non-fasted states.

Distribution – Plasma dexmethylphenidate concentrations in children decline exponentially following oral administration of dexmethylphenidate hydrochloride.

Metabolism / Excretion – In humans, dexmethylphenidate is metabolized primarily to d-α-phenyl-piperidine acetic acid (also known as d-ritalinic acid) by de-esterification. This metabolite has little or no pharmacological activity. There is little or no in vivo interconversion to the l-threo-enantiomer, based on a finding of minute levels of l-threo-methylphenidate being detectable in a few samples in only 2 of 58 children and adults. After oral dosing of radiolabeled racemic methylphenidate in humans, about 90% of the radioactivity was recovered in urine. The main urinary metabolite was ritalinic acid, accountable for approximately 80% of the dose.

In vitro studies showed that dexmethylphenidate did not inhibit cytochrome P450 isoenzymes.

The mean plasma elimination half-life of dexmethylphenidate is approximately 2.2 hours.

Special populations –

Gender: In a single-dose study conducted in adults, the mean dexmethylphenidate $AUC_{0\text{-}inf}$ values (adjusted for body weight) following single 2 times 10 mg doses of dexmethylphenidate hydrochloride were 25% to 35% higher in adult female volunteers (n = 6) compared to male volunteers (n = 9). Both t_{max} and $t_{½}$ were comparable for males and females.

Contraindications

Marked anxiety, tension, and agitation, since the drug may aggravate these symptoms; hypersensitivity to methylphenidate or other components of the product; glaucoma; motor tics or with a family history or diagnosis of Tourette syndrome; during treatment with monoamine oxidase inhibitors, and also within a minimum of 14 days following discontinuation of a monoamine oxidase inhibitor (hypertensive crises may result).

Warnings

➤*Depression:* Do not use to treat severe depression.

➤*Fatigue:* Do not use for the prevention or treatment of normal fatigue states.

➤*Long-term suppression of growth:* Sufficient data on safety of long-term use of dexmethylphenidate hydrochloride in children are not yet available. Although a causal relationship has not been established, suppression of growth (ie, weight gain or height) has been reported with the long-term use of stimulants in children. Therefore, patients requiring long-term therapy should be carefully monitored. Patients who are not growing or gaining weight as expected should have their treatment interrupted.

➤*Psychosis:* Clinical experience suggests that in psychotic children, administration of methylphenidate may exacerbate symptoms of behavior disturbance and thought disorder.

➤*Seizures:* There is some clinical evidence that methylphenidate may lower the convulsive threshold in patients with a history of seizures, in patients with prior EEG abnormalities in the absence of a history of seizures, and, very rarely, in the absence of a history of seizures and no prior EEG evidence of seizures. In the presence of seizures, the drug should be discontinued.

➤*Visual disturbance:* Symptoms of visual disturbances have been encountered in rare cases following use of methylphenidate. Difficulties with accommodation and blurring of vision have been reported.

➤*Carcinogenesis:* Lifetime carcinogenicity studies have not been carried out with dexmethylphenidate. In a lifetime carcinogenicity study carried out in B6C3F1 mice, racemic methylphenidate caused an increase in hepatocellular adenomas, and in males only, an increase in hepatoblastomas at a

DEXMETHYLPHENIDATE HYDROCHLORIDE — ORAL

daily dose of approximately 60 mg/kg/day. Hepatoblastoma is a relativity rare rodent malignant tumor type. There was no increase in total malignant hepatic tumors. The mouse strain used is sensitive to the development of hepatic tumors, and the significance of these results to humans is unknown.

➤*Mutagenesis:* Sister chromatid exchanges and chromosome aberrations were increased, indicative of a weak clastogenic response, in an in vitro assay of racemic methylphenidate in cultured Chinese hamster ovary (CHO) cells.

➤*Pregnancy: Category C.* Racemic methylphenidate has been shown to have teratogenic effects in rabbits when given in doses of 200 mg/kg/day throughout organogenesis.

Adequate and well-controlled studies in pregnant women have not been conducted. Use during pregnancy only if the potential benefit justifies the potential risk to the fetus.

➤*Lactation:* It is not known whether dexmethylphenidate is excreted in human milk. Because many drugs are excreted in human milk, caution should be exercised if dexmethylphenidate hydrochloride is administered to a nursing woman.

➤*Children:* The safety and efficacy of dexmethylphenidate hydrochloride in children under 6 years old have not been established. Long-term effects of dexmethylphenidate hydrochloride in children have not been well established.

Precautions

➤*Monitoring:* Periodic CBC, differential, and platelet counts are advised during prolonged therapy.

➤*Special risk:*

Hypertension and other cardiovascular conditions – Use cautiously in patients with hypertension. Blood pressure should be monitored at appropriate intervals in all patients taking dexmethylphenidate hydrochloride, especially those with hypertension. In the placebo controlled studies, the mean pulse increase was 2 to 5 bpm for both dexmethylphenidate hydrochloride and racemic methylphenidate compared to placebo, with mean increases of systolic and diastolic blood pressure of 2 to 3 mm Hg, compared to placebo. Therefore, caution is indicated in treating patients whose underlying medical conditions might be compromised by increases in blood pressure or heart rate (eg, those with preexisting hypertension, heart failure, recent myocardial infarction, or hyperthyroidism).

➤*Drug abuse and dependence:*

Controlled substance class – Dexmethylphenidate hydrochloride, like other methylphenidate products, is classified as a schedule II controlled substance by federal regulation.

Abuse, dependence, and tolerance – Dexmethylphenidate hydrochloride should be given cautiously to patients with a history of drug dependence or alcoholism. Chronic, abusive use can lead to marked tolerance and psychological dependence with varying degrees of abnormal behavior. Frank psychotic episodes can occur, especially with parenteral abuse. Careful supervision is required during drug withdrawal from abusive use since severe depression may occur. Withdrawal following chronic therapeutic use may unmask symptoms of the underlying disorder that may require follow-up.

Drug Interactions

Dexmethylphenidate Drug Interactions

Precipitant drug	Object drug*		Description
Methylphenidate (racemic)	Antihypertensive agents	⬇	Methylphenidate may decrease the effectiveness of drugs used to treat hypertension.
Dexmethylphenidate hydrochloride	Pressor agents (eg, dopamine, epinephrine, phenylephrine)	⬇	Because of possible effects on blood pressure, use dexmethylphenidate cautiously with pressor agents.
Methylphenidate (racemic)	Coumarin anticoagulants (eg, warfarin)	⬆	Dexmethylphenidate hydrochloride may inhibit the metabolism of warfarin-like drugs. It may be necessary to adjust the dosage or monitor coagulation times when starting or stopping therapy.
Methylphenidate (racemic)	Anticonvulsants (eg, phenobarbital, phenytoin, primidone)	⬆	Downward dose adjustments of anticonvulsant therapy may be required when given concomitantly with methylphenidate.
Methylphenidate (racemic)	Tricyclic antidepressants (eg, amitriptyline)	⬆	It may be necessary to adjust the dosage of antidepressant therapy when giving these agents concurrently.
Methylphenidate (racemic)	Selective serotonin reuptake inhibitors (SSRIs)	⬆	Methylphenidate may inhibit the metabolism of SSRI antidepressants. It may be necessary to adjust the SSRI dose when given concomitantly with methylphenidate.
Methylphenidate (racemic)	Clonidine	⟷	Serious adverse events have been reported in concomitant use with clonidine; however, no causality for the combination has been established.

* ⬆ = Object drug increased. ⬇ = Object drug decreased. ⟷ = Undetermined clinical effect.

Adverse Reactions

➤*Discontinuation of treatment:* No dexmethylphenidate hydrochloride-treated patients discontinued due to adverse reactions in 2 placebo-controlled trials. Overall, 50 of 684 children treated with dexmethylphenidate hydrochloride (7.3%) experienced an adverse event that resulted in discontinuation. The most common reasons for discontinuation were twitching (described as motor or vocal tics), anorexia, insomnia, and tachycardia (approximately 1% each).

➤*Adverse reactions (≥ 5%):* The table below enumerates treatment-emergent adverse reactions for 2, placebo-controlled, parallel group trials in children with ADHD at dexmethylphenidate hydrochloride doses of 5, 10, and 20 mg/day.

Treatment-Emergent Adverse Reactions[a] Occurring During Double-blind Treatment in Clinical Trials of Dexmethylphenidate Hydrochloride

Body system	Preferred term	Dexmethylphenidate hydrochloride (n = 79)	Placebo (n = 82)
Miscellaneous	Abdominal pain	15%	6%
	Fever	5%	1%
GI	Anorexia	6%	1%
	Nausea	9%	1%

[a] Events, regardless of causality, for which the incidence for patients treated with dexmethylphenidate hydrochloride was at least 5% and twice the incidence among placebo-treated patients. Incidence has been rounded to the nearest whole number.

➤*Adverse reactions with other methylphenidate hydrochloride products:* Nervousness and insomnia are the most common adverse reactions reported with other methylphenidate products. In children, loss of appetite, abdominal pain, weight loss during prolonged therapy, insomnia, and tachycardia may occur more frequently; however, any of the other adverse reactions listed below may also occur.

➤*Other adverse reactions:*

Cardiovascular – Angina, arrhythmia, palpitations, pulse increased or decreased.

Blood pressure increased or decreased, cerebral arteritis or occlusion.

CNS – Dizziness, drowsiness, dyskinesia, headache, rare reports of Tourette's syndrome, toxic psychosis.

GI – Nausea.

Hypersensitivity – Hypersensitivity reactions including skin rash, urticaria, fever, arthralgia, exfoliative dermatitis, erythema multiforme with histopathological findings of necrotizing vasculitis, and thrombocytopenic purpura.

➤*Adverse reactions reported in patients taking methylphenidate:* Although a definite causal relationship has not been established, the following have been reported in patients taking methylphenidate:

Dermatologic – Scalp hair loss.

Hepatic – Abnormal liver function, ranging from transaminase elevation to hepatic coma.

Lymphatic – Leukopenia or anemia.

Psychiatric – Transient depressed mood.

Neuroleptic malignant syndrome (NMS) – Very rare reports of NMS have been received, and, in most of these, patients were concurrently receiving therapies associated with NMS. In a single report, a 10-year-old boy who had been taking methylphenidate for approximately 18 months experienced an NMS-like event within 45 minutes of ingesting his first dose of venlafaxine. It is uncertain whether this case represented a drug-drug interaction, a response to either drug alone or some other cause.

Children – In children, loss of appetite, abdominal pain, weight loss during prolonged therapy, insomnia, and tachycardia may occur more frequently; however, any of the other adverse reactions listed above may also occur.

Overdosage

➤*Symptoms:* Signs and symptoms of acute methylphenidate overdosage, resulting principally from overstimulation of the CNS and from excessive sympathomimetic effects, may include the following: Vomiting, agitation, tremors, hyperreflexia, muscle twitching, convulsions (may be followed by coma), euphoria, confusion, hallucinations, delirium, sweating, flushing, headache, hyperpyrexia, tachycardia, palpitations, cardiac arrhythmias, hypertension, mydriasis, and dryness of mucous membranes.

➤*Treatment:* Treatment consists of appropriate supportive measures. The patient must be protected against self-injury and against external stimuli that would aggravate overstimulation already present. Gastric contents may be evacuated by gastric lavage as indicated. Before performing gastric lavage, control agitation and seizures if present and protect the airway. Other measures to detoxify the gut include administration of activated char-

DEXMETHYLPHENIDATE HYDROCHLORIDE — ORAL

coal and a cathartic. Intensive care must be provided to maintain adequate circulation and respiratory exchange; external cooling procedures may be required for hyperpyrexia.

Efficacy of peritoneal dialysis for dexmethylphenidate hydrochloride overdosage has not been established.

Poison control center – As with the management of all overdosage, the possibility of multiple drug ingestion should be considered. The physician may wish to consider contacting a poison control center for up-to-date information on the management of overdosage with methylphenidate.

Patient Information

Your doctor should be made aware of any current or past physical or mental problems. Tell your doctor if there is a history of drug or alcohol abuse, depression, psychosis, epilepsy or seizure disorders, high blood pressure, glaucoma, facial tics (involuntary movements), or a family history of Tourette's syndrome.

Both your doctor and your pharmacist should also be informed of all medicines that you are taking, even if these drugs are not taken on a regular basis and are available without prescription. Your doctor will decide whether you can take dexmethylphenidate hydrochloride with other medicines. Methylphenidate is known to interact with a number of other drugs. These include medicines to treat depression, such as monoamine oxidase inhibitors (MAOIs); to control seizures; and to thin blood. Sometimes these interactions may require a change in dosage, or occasionally stopping one of the drugs involved.

Tell your doctor if you are pregnant or nursing a baby.

➤*Who should not take dexmethylphenidate hydrochloride?:* You should not take dexmethylphenidate hydrochloride if:
- You have significant anxiety, tension, or agitation since dexmethylphenidate hydrochloride may make these conditions worse.
- You are allergic to methylphenidate or any of the other ingredients in dexmethylphenidate hydrochloride.
- You have glaucoma, an eye disease.
- You have tics or Tourette's syndrome, or a family history of Tourette's syndrome.
- You are taking a monoamine oxidase inhibitor, a type of drug, or have discontinued a monoamine oxidase inhibitor in the last 14 days.

➤*Other important safety information:* Tell your doctor if you have blurred vision when taking dexmethylphenidate hydrochloride.

Slower growth (weight gain or height) has been reported with long-term use of methylphenidate in children. Your doctor will be carefully watching your height and weight. If you are not growing or gaining weight as your doctor expects, your doctor may stop your dexmethylphenidate hydrochloride treatment.

METHYLPHENIDATE HYDROCHLORIDE

c-ii	**Methylphenidate Hydrochloride** (Various, eg, Able, Sandoz, Watson)	**Tablets**: 5 mg	In 100s and 1,000s.
c-ii	**Methylin** (Mallinckrodt)		Lactose, talc. (5 M). White. In 100s and 1,000s.
c-ii	**Ritalin** (Novartis)		Lactose. (CIBA 7). Yellow. In 100s.
c-ii	**Methylphenidate Hydrochloride** (Various, eg, Able, Sandoz, Watson)	**Tablets**: 10 mg	In 100s and 1,000s.
c-ii	**Methylin** (Mallinckrodt)		Lactose, talc. (10 M). White, scored. In 100s and 1,000s.
c-ii	**Ritalin** (Novartis)		Lactose. (CIBA 3). Pale green, scored. In 100s.
c-ii	**Methylphenidate Hydrochloride** (Various, eg, Able, Sandoz, Watson)	**Tablets**: 20 mg	In 100s and 1,000s.
c-ii	**Methylin** (Mallinckrodt)		Lactose, talc. (20 M). White, scored. In 100s and 1,000s.
c-ii	**Ritalin** (Novartis)		Sucrose, talc. (CIBA 34). Pale yellow, scored. In 100s.
c-ii	**Methylin** (Alliant)	**Tablets, chewable**: 2.5 mg	Aspartame, 0.42 mg phenylalanine. (2.5 CHEW). White to cream color, rounded square. Grape flavor. In 100s.
		5 mg	Aspartame, 0.84 mg phenylalanine. (5 CHEW). White to cream color, rounded square. Grape flavor. In 100s.
		10 mg	Aspartame, 1.68 mg phenylalanine. (10 CHEW). White to cream color, rounded square. Grape flavor. In 100s.
c-ii	**Metadate ER** (Celltech)	**Tablets, extended-release**: 10 mg	Cetyl alcohol, lactose. Color-additive free. (561 MD). White, oval. In 100s.
c-ii	**Methylin ER** (Mallinckrodt)		Talc. Color-additive free. (1423 M). White to off-white. In 100s.
c-ii	**Concerta** (McNeil)[a]	**Tablets, extended-release**: 18 mg	Lactose. (alza 18). Yellow. In 100s.
c-ii	**Methylphenidate Hydrochloride** (Various, eg, Able, Sandoz, Watson)	**Tablets, extended-release**: 20 mg	In 30s and 100s.
c-ii	**Metadate ER** (Celltech)		Cetyl alcohol, lactose. Color-additive free. (562 MD). White. In 100s.
c-ii	**Methylin ER** (Mallinckrodt)		Talc. Color-additive free. (1451 M). White to off-white. In 100s.
c-ii	**Concerta** (McNeil)[a]	**Tablets, extended-release**: 27 mg	Lactose. (alza 27). Gray. In 100s.
c-ii	**Concerta** (McNeil)[a]	**Tablets, extended-release**: 36 mg	Lactose. (alza 36). White. In 100s.
c-ii	**Concerta** (McNeil)[a]	**Tablets, extended-release**: 54 mg	Lactose. (alza 54). Brownish-red. In 100s.
c-ii	**Ritalin-SR** (Novartis)	**Tablets, sustained-release**: 20 mg	Cetostearyl alcohol, lactose, mineral oil. Color-additive free. (CIBA 16). White, coated. In 100s.
c-ii	**Metadate CD** (Celltech)[b]	**Capsules, extended-release**: 10 mg	Sugar spheres. (CELLTECH 574 10 mg). Green/White. In 100s and UD 100s.
c-ii	**Ritalin LA** (Novartis)[c]		Sugar spheres, talc. (NVR R10). White/Lt. brown. In 100s.
c-ii	**Metadate CD** (Celltech)[b]	**Capsules, extended-release**: 20 mg	Sugar spheres. (CELLTECH 575 20 mg). Blue/White. In 100s, UD 100s, and dosepack 30s.
c-ii	**Ritalin LA** (Novartis)[c]		Sugar spheres, talc. (NVR R20). White. In 100s.
c-ii	**Metadate CD** (Celltech)[b]	**Capsules, extended-release**: 30 mg	Sugar spheres. (CELLTECH 576 30 mg). Reddish-brown/White. In 100s and UD 100s.
c-ii	**Ritalin LA** (Novartis)[c]		Sugar spheres, talc. (NVR R30). Yellow. In 100s.
c-ii	**Ritalin LA** (Novartis)[c]	**Capsules, extended-release**: 40 mg	Sugar spheres, talc. (NVR R40). Lt. brown. In 100s.
c-ii	**Methylin** (Alliant)	**Oral solution**: 5 mg per 5 mL	Glycerin. Grape flavor. In 500 mL.
		10 mg per 5 mL	Glycerin. Grape flavor. In 500 mL.
c-ii	**Daytrana** (Shire)	**Patch, transdermal**: 10mg	In 10s and 30s.
		15 mg	In 10s and 30s.
		20 mg	In 10s and 30s.
		30 mg	In 10s and 30s.

[a] The initial dose of *Concerta* is released from the outer coating within 1 hour, and the remainder is released at a controlled rate over 5 to 9 hours. Therefore, the total methylphenidate dose is released over 6 to 10 hours.

[b] The immediate-release beads comprise 30% of the total methylphenidate dose (ie, 6 mg of a 20 mg capsule) and provide the initial phase, rapid release of methylphenidate. The second set of beads provides the second, extended-release phase of methylphenidate, and comprise 70% of the total methylphenidate dose (ie, 14 mg from a 20 mg capsule).

[c] Extended-release formulation using Spheroidal Oral Drug Absorption System (*SODAS*) technology, a bimodal release delivery system. Fifty percent of the contents are immediate-release beads to provide rapid onset. The second half of the contents consists of delayed-release beads that are released approximately 4 hours after administration. This delivery system mimics twice-daily administration of immediate-release methylphenidate.

METHYLPHENIDATE HYDROCHLORIDE — ORAL

WARNING

Drug dependence – Give methylphenidate cautiously to emotionally unstable patients (eg, those with a history of drug dependence or alcoholism) because such patients may increase dosage on their own initiative.

Chronically abusive use can lead to marked tolerance and psychic dependence with varying degrees of abnormal behavior. Frank psychotic episodes can occur, especially with parenteral abuse. Careful supervision is required during drug withdrawal because severe depression as well as the effects of chronic overactivity can be unmasked. Long-term follow-up may be required because of the patient's basic personality disturbances.

Indications

➤*Attention deficit disorders/Attention deficit hyperactivity disorder (ADHD):* Attention deficit disorders (previously known as minimal brain dysfunction in children). Other terms being used to describe the behavioral syndrome below include the following: hyperkinetic child syndrome, minimal brain damage, minimal cerebral dysfunction, and minor cerebral dysfunction.

➤*Long-term use:* The effectiveness of methylphenidate extended-release (ER) products (*Concerta, Metadate CD, Ritalin LA*) for long-term use (ie, for more than 4 weeks [*Concerta*], 3 weeks [*Metadate CD*], or 2 weeks [*Ritalin LA*]) has not been systematically evaluated in controlled trials. Therefore, the physician who elects to use methylphenidate for extended periods should periodically reevaluate the long-term usefulness of the drug for the individual patient.

➤*Narcolepsy (except Concerta, Metadate CD,* and *Ritalin LA):* For the treatment of narcolepsy.

➤*Unlabeled uses:* Depression in medically ill (including stroke) elderly persons; alleviation of neurobehavioral symptoms after traumatic brain injury (mixed efficacy); improvement in pain control, sedation, or both in patients receiving opiates.

Administration and Dosage

➤*Approved by the FDA:* December 5, 1955.

Individualize dosage according to the needs and responses of the patient.

➤*Adults:*

Immediate-release (IR) tablets, chewable tablets, and oral solution – Administer in divided doses 2 or 3 times daily, preferably 30 to 45 minutes before meals. The average dosage is 20 to 30 mg daily. Some patients may require 40 to 60 mg daily. In others, 10 to 15 mg daily will be adequate. Patients who are unable to sleep if medication is taken late in the day should take the last dose before 6 pm.

➤*Children (6 years of age and older):* Initiate methylphenidate in small doses, with gradual weekly increments. Daily dosage above 60 mg is not recommended.

If improvement is not observed after appropriate dosage adjustment over a 1-month period, discontinue the drug.

IR tablets and chewable tablets – Start with 5 mg twice daily (before breakfast and lunch), with gradual increments of 5 to 10 mg weekly.

➤*All patients:*

Chewable tablets – Instruct patients to take methylphenidate chewable tablets with at least 240 mL (8 ounces) of water or other fluid. Taking this product without enough liquid may cause choking.

ER and sustained-release (SR) tablets (Metadate ER, Methylin ER, and *Ritalin SR)* – Methylphenidate ER and SR tablets have a duration of action of approximately 8 hours. Therefore, methylphenidate ER and SR tablets may be used in place of methylphenidate tablets when the 8-hour dosage of methylphenidate ER and SR tablets corresponds to the titrated 8-hour dosage of methylphenidate.

Methylphenidate ER and SR tablets must be swallowed whole with the aid of liquids and never crushed, chewed, or divided.

➤*Maintenance/Extended treatment:* There is no body of evidence available from controlled trials to indicate how long the patient with ADHD should be treated with methylphenidate. It is generally agreed, however, that pharmacological treatment of ADHD may be needed for extended periods. Nevertheless, the health care provider who elects to use methylphenidate for extended periods in patients with ADHD should periodically reevaluate the long-term usefulness of the drug for the individual patient with trials off the medication to assess the patient's functioning without pharmacotherapy. Improvement may be sustained when the drug is either temporarily or permanently discontinued.

➤*Dose reduction and discontinuation:* If paradoxical aggravation of symptoms or other adverse reactions occur, reduce the dosage or, if necessary, discontinue the drug.

If improvement is not observed after appropriate dosage adjustment over a 1-month period, discontinue the drug.

Drug treatment should not and need not be indefinite, and usually may be discontinued after puberty.

➤*Concerta:* Administer orally once daily in the morning with or without food because it has been shown to improve attention and behavior for 12 hours after dosing.

Concerta must be swallowed whole with the aid of liquids and must not be chewed, divided, or crushed.

Based on an assessment of clinical benefit and tolerability, doses may be increased at weekly intervals for patients who have not achieved an optimal response at a lower dose.

Patients new to methylphenidate – The recommended starting dosage of *Concerta* for patients who are not currently taking methylphenidate or for patients who are on stimulants other than methylphenidate is 18 mg once daily.

Initial Dosing Recommendations for *Concerta*		
Patient age	Recommended starting dosage	Maximum dosage
Children 6 to 12 years of age	18 mg/day	54 mg/day
Adolescents 13 to 17 years of age	18 mg/day	72 mg/day, not to exceed 2 mg/kg/day

Patients currently using methylphenidate – The recommended dosage of *Concerta* for patients who are currently taking methylphenidate 2 or 3 times daily at dosages of 10 to 45 mg/day is provided in the following table. Dosing recommendations are based on current dose regimen and clinical judgment. Initial conversion dosage should not exceed 54 mg/day. After conversion, dosages may be adjusted to a maximum of 72 mg/day taken once daily in the morning.

In general, dosage adjustment may proceed at approximately weekly intervals.

Recommended Dosage Conversion from Methylphenidate Regimens to *Concerta*	
Previous methylphenidate daily dosage	Recommended *Concerta* starting dosage
Methylphenidate 5 mg 2 or 3 times daily	18 mg every morning
Methylphenidate 10 mg 2 or 3 times daily	36 mg every morning
Methylphenidate 15 mg 2 or 3 times daily	54 mg every morning

For other methylphenidate regimens, use clinical judgment when selecting the starting dose.

A 27 mg strength is available for health care providers who wish to prescribe between the 18 and 36 mg doses.

➤*ER capsules (Metadate CD* and *Ritalin LA):* Methylphenidate ER capsules are administered once daily in the morning before breakfast.

Methylphenidate ER capsules may be swallowed whole with the aid of liquids or, alternatively, may be administered by opening the capsule and sprinkling the capsule contents onto a small amount (tablespoon) of applesauce. Methylphenidate ER capsules and/or their contents should not be crushed or chewed.

The capsules may be carefully opened and the beads sprinkled over a spoonful of applesauce. The applesauce should not be warm because it could affect the modified release properties of *Ritalin LA*. The mixture of drug and applesauce should be consumed immediately in its entirety. Drinking some fluids (eg, water) should follow the intake of the sprinkles with applesauce. The drug and applesauce mixture should not be stored for future use.

The recommended starting dosage of methylphenidate ER capsules is 20 mg once daily. Dosage may be adjusted in weekly 10 to 20 mg increments (10 mg increments for *Ritalin LA*) to a maximum of 60 mg/day taken once daily in the morning before breakfast, depending upon tolerability and degree of efficacy observed. Daily dose above 60 mg is not recommended.

Ritalin LA – When in the judgement of the clinician a lower initial dose is appropriate, patients may begin treatment with *Ritalin LA* 10 mg.

Patients currently receiving methylphenidate: The recommended dosage of *Ritalin LA* for patients currently taking methylphenidate twice daily or SR is provided in the following table.

Previous Methylphenidate Dosage	Recommended *Ritalin LA* Dosage
Methylphenidate 5 mg twice daily	10 mg once daily
Methylphenidate 10 mg twice daily or methylphenidate SR 20 mg	20 mg once daily
Methylphenidate 15 mg twice daily	30 mg once daily
Methylphenidate 20 mg twice daily or methylphenidate SR 40 mg	40 mg once daily
Methylphenidate 30 mg twice daily or methylphenidate SR 60 mg	60 mg once daily

For other methylphenidate regimens, use clinical judgment when selecting a starting dosage. *Ritalin LA* dosage may be adjusted at weekly intervals in 10 mg increments.

➤*Storage/Stability:* Dispense in a tight container with a child-resistant closure.

Keep out of the reach of children.

IR, ER, and SR tablets – Do not store above 30°C (86°F). Protect from light and moisture.

Chewable tablets and oral solution – Store at 20° to 25°C (68° to 77°F). Protect chewable tablets from moisture.

ER capsules – Store at 25°C (77°F); excursions permitted to 15° to 30°C (59° to 86°F). Protect from humidity.

METHYLPHENIDATE HYDROCHLORIDE — ORAL

Actions

➤*Pharmacology:* Methylphenidate is a CNS stimulant. The mode of therapeutic action is not known, but methylphenidate presumably activates the brain stem arousal system and cortex to produce its stimulant effect. Methylphenidate is thought to block the reuptake of norepinephrine and dopamine into the presynaptic neuron and increase the release of these monoamines into the extraneuronal space.

There is neither specific evidence that clearly establishes the mechanism whereby methylphenidate produces its mental and behavioral effects in children, nor conclusive evidence regarding how these effects relate to the condition of the CNS.

Methylphenidate is a racemic mixture comprised of the d- and l-threo enantiomers. The d-threo enantiomer is more pharmacologically active than the l-threo enantiomer.

➤*Pharmacokinetics:*

Absorption –
IR, ER, and SR tablets: Methylphenidate in the ER and SR tablets is more slowly but as extensively absorbed as in the IR tablets. Relative bioavailability of the SR tablet compared with the IR tablet, measured by the urinary excretion of methylphenidate major metabolite (α-phenyl-2-piperidine acetic acid) was 105% (49% to 168%) in children and 101% (85% to 152%) in adults.

The time to peak rate in children was 4.7 hours (1.3 to 8.2 hours) for the ER and SR tablets and 1.9 hours (0.3 to 4.4 hours) for the IR tablets.

• *Concerta* – Methylphenidate is readily absorbed. Following oral administration of *Concerta*, plasma methylphenidate concentrations increase rapidly, reaching an initial maximum at approximately 1 hour, followed by gradual ascending concentrations over the next 5 to 9 hours, after which a gradual decrease begins. Mean times to reach peak plasma concentrations across all doses of *Concerta* occurred between 6 and 10 hours.

Concerta once daily minimizes the fluctuations between peak and trough concentrations associated with IR methylphenidate 3 times daily. The relative bioavailability of *Concerta* once daily and methylphenidate 3 times daily in adults is comparable.

• *Metadate ER* – Pharmacokinetic and statistical analyses for a multiple-dose study demonstrated that 3 times daily administration of 2 *Metadate ER* 10 mg tablets met the requirements for bioequivalence to 1 methylphenidate SR 20 mg tablet when administered every 8 hours. Pharmacokinetic parameters (ie, $AUC_{0-\infty}$, T_{max}, C_{max}, C_{min}, and C_{av}) demonstrated achievement of steady state following 3 times daily administration of 2 *Metadate ER* 10 mg tablets was confirmed.

Bioavailability of *Metadate ER* 20 mg tablets was compared with an SR reference product and an IR product. The extent of absorption for the 3 products was similar, and the rate of absorption of the 2 SR products was not statistically different.

Chewable tablets and oral solution: Methylphenidate chewable tablets and oral solution are readily absorbed. Following oral administration of methylphenidate chewable tablets and oral solution, peak plasma concentrations are achieved at approximately 1 to 2 hours. Methylphenidate chewable tablets and oral solution have been shown to be bioequivalent to methylphenidate IR tablets. The mean C_{max} following a methylphenidate 20 mg chewable tablet dose and 20 mg oral solution dose is approximately 10 and 9 ng/mL, respectively.

ER capsules:
• *Metadate CD* – Methylphenidate is readily absorbed. *Metadate CD* capsules have a plasma/time concentration profile showing 2 phases of drug release with a sharp, initial slope similar to a methylphenidate IR tablet, and a second rising portion approximately 3 hours later, followed by a gradual decline.

• *Ritalin LA* – *Ritalin LA* produces a bimodal plasma concentration-time profile (ie, 2 distinct peaks approximately 4 hours apart) when orally administered to children diagnosed with ADHD and to healthy adults. The initial rate of absorption for *Ritalin LA* is similar to that of *Ritalin* tablets as shown by the similar rate parameters between the 2 formulations (ie, initial lag time [T_{lag}], first peak concentration [C_{max1}], and time to the first peak [T_{max1}], which is reached in 1 to 3 hours). The mean time to the interpeak minimum (T_{minip}) and time to the second peak (T_{max2}) are also similar for *Ritalin LA* given once daily and *Ritalin* tablets given in 2 doses 4 hours apart (see the following table), although the ranges observed are greater for *Ritalin LA*.

Ritalin LA given once daily exhibits a lower second peak concentration (C_{max2}), higher interpeak minimum concentrations (C_{minip}), and less peak and trough fluctuations than *Ritalin* tablets given in 2 doses given 4 hours apart. This is due to an earlier onset and more prolonged absorption from the delayed-release beads.

Distribution – Binding to plasma proteins is low (10% to 33%), and the apparent distribution volume at steady state with intravenous (IV) administration has been reported to be approximately 6 L/kg.

Concerta: Plasma methylphenidate concentrations in adults and adolescents decline bioexponentially following oral administration. The half-life of methylphenidate in adults and adolescents following oral administration of *Concerta* was approximately 3.5 hours.

Metabolism – In humans, methylphenidate is metabolized rapidly primarily via deesterification to alpha-phenyl-piperidine acetic acid (PPA or ritalinic acid). The metabolite has little or no pharmacologic activity.

Concerta: In adults, the metabolism of *Concerta* once daily as evaluated by metabolism to PPA is similar to that of methylphenidate 3 times daily. The metabolism of single and repeated once-daily doses of *Concerta* is similar.

Ritalin LA: The absolute bioavailability of methylphenidate in children has been reported to be approximately 30% (range, 10% to 52%), suggesting pronounced presystemic metabolism. Only small amounts of hydroxylated metabolites (eg, hydroxymethylphenidate and hydroxyritalinic acid) are detectable in plasma.

Excretion –
Chewable tablets and oral solution: After oral dosing of radiolabeled methylphenidate in humans, approximately 90% of the radioactivity was recovered in urine. The main urinary metabolite was PPA, accounting for approximately 80% of the dose. The pharmacokinetics of methylphenidate chewable tablets and oral solution have been studied in healthy adult volunteers. The mean terminal half-life of methylphenidate following administration of methylphenidate 20 mg chewable tablets ($t_{1/2}$ = 3 hours) or 20 mg oral solution ($t_{1/2}$ = 2.7 hours) is comparable to the mean terminal half-life following administration of methylphenidate IR tablets ($t_{1/2}$ = 2.8 hours) in healthy adult volunteers.

ER and SR tablets: After oral dosing of radiolabeled methylphenidate in humans, approximately 90% of the radioactivity was recovered in urine. The main urinary metabolite was PPA, accounting for approximately 80% of the dose. An average of 67% of ER and SR tablet dose was excreted in children as compared with 86% in adults.

ER capsules:
• *Metadate CD* – The mean terminal half-life ($t_{1/2}$) of methylphenidate following administration of methylphenidate ER capsules ($t_{1/2}$ = 6.8 hours) is longer than the mean terminal $t_{1/2}$ following administration of methylphenidate IR tablets ($t_{1/2}$ = 2.9 hours) and methylphenidate SR tablets ($t_{1/2}$ = 3.4 hours) in healthy adult volunteers. This suggests that the elimination process observed for methylphenidate ER capsules is controlled by the release rate of methylphenidate from the ER formulation, and that the drug absorption is the rate-limiting process.

• *Ritalin LA* – In studies with *Ritalin LA* and *Ritalin* tablets in adults, methylphenidate from *Ritalin* tablets is eliminated from plasma with an average half-life of approximately 3.5 hours (range, 1.3 to 7.7 hours). In children, the average half-life is approximately 2.5 hours, with a range of approximately 1.5 to 5 hours. The rapid half-life in both children and adults may result in unmeasurable concentrations between the morning and midday doses with *Ritalin* tablets. No accumulation of methylphenidate is expected following multiple once-a-day dosing with *Ritalin LA*. The half-life of ritalinic acid is approximately 3 to 4 hours.

After oral administration of an IR formulation of methylphenidate, 78% to 97% of the dose is excreted in the urine and 1% to 3% in the feces in the form of metabolites within 48 to 96 hours. Only small quantities (less than 1%) of unchanged methylphenidate appear in the urine. Most of the dose is excreted in the urine as ritalinic acid (60% to 86%), the remainder being accounted for by minor metabolites.

Special populations –
Renal function impairment: There is no experience with the use of methylphenidate in patients with renal insufficiency. After oral administration of radiolabeled methylphenidate in humans, methylphenidate was extensively metabolized and approximately 80% of the radioactivity was excreted in the urine in the form of ritalinic acid. Because renal clearance is not an important route of methylphenidate clearance (less than 1% of a radiolabeled dose is excreted in the urine as unchanged compound), renal insufficiency is expected to have little effect on the pharmacokinetics of methylphenidate.

Hepatic function impairment: There is no experience with the use of methylphenidate in patients with hepatic insufficiency. Hepatic insufficiency is expected to have minimal effect on the pharmacokinetics of methylphenidate because it is metabolized primarily to ritalinic acid by nonmicrosomal hydrolytic esterases that are widely distributed throughout the body.

Children: The pharmacokinetics of methylphenidate after administration have not been studied in children younger than 6 years of age.

• *Concerta* – Increase in age resulted in increased apparent oral clearance (58% increase in adolescents compared with children). Some of these differences could be explained by body weight differences among these populations. This suggests that subjects with higher body weights may have lower exposures of total methylphenidate at similar doses.

• *Ritalin LA* – The pharmacokinetics of *Ritalin LA* was examined in 18 children with ADHD between 7 and 12 years of age. Fifteen of these children were between 10 and 12 years of age. The time until the between-peak minimum and the time until the second peak were delayed and more variable in children compared with adults. After a *Ritalin LA* 20 mg dose, concentrations in children were approximately twice the concentrations observed in adults 18 to 35 years of age. This higher exposure is almost completely due to the smaller body size and total volume of distribution in children, because apparent clearance normalized to body weight is independent of age.

Food effects –
Chewable tablets and oral solution: See Drug Interactions for more information.

Contraindications

➤*Agitation:* Methylphenidate is contraindicated in patients with marked anxiety, tension, and agitation because the drug may aggravate these symptoms.

➤*Hypersensitivity:* Methylphenidate is contraindicated in patients known to be hypersensitive to methylphenidate or other components of the product.

➤*Glaucoma:* Methylphenidate is contraindicated in patients with glaucoma.

➤*Tics:* Methylphenidate is contraindicated in patients with motor tics or with a family history or diagnosis of Tourette syndrome.

➤*Monoamine oxidase inhibitors (MAOIs):* Methylphenidate is contraindicated during treatment with MAOIs and within a minimum of 14 days following discontinuation of an MAOI (hypertensive crises may result).

METHYLPHENIDATE HYDROCHLORIDE — ORAL

Warnings

➤*Depression:* Do not use methylphenidate to treat severe depression of either exogenous or endogenous origin.

➤*Fatigue:* Do not use methylphenidate for the prevention or treatment of normal fatigue states.

➤*Hypertension:* Use cautiously in patients with hypertension. Monitor blood pressure at appropriate intervals in all patients taking methylphenidate, especially those with hypertension. Studies of methylphenidate have shown modest increases of resting pulse and systolic and diastolic blood pressure. Therefore, caution is indicated in treating patients whose underlying medical conditions might be compromised by increases in blood pressure or heart rate (eg, those with preexisting hypertension, heart failure, recent myocardial infarction, or hyperthyroidism).

➤*Long-term suppression of growth:* Sufficient data on safety and efficacy of long-term use of methylphenidate in children are not yet available. Although a causal relationship has not been established, suppression of growth (ie, weight gain and/or height) has been reported with the long-term use of stimulants in children. Therefore, carefully monitor patients requiring long-term therapy. Interrupt treatment in patients who are not growing or gaining weight as expected. In the double-blind, placebo-controlled study of *Ritalin LA*, the mean weight gain was greater for patients receiving placebo (+1 kg) than for patients receiving *Ritalin LA* (+0.1 kg).

➤*Psychosis:* Clinical experience suggests that in psychotic patients, administration of methylphenidate may exacerbate symptoms of behavior disturbance and thought disorder.

➤*Seizures:* There is some clinical evidence that methylphenidate may lower the convulsive threshold in patients with a history of seizures, with prior EEG abnormalities in absence of seizures, and, very rarely, in absence of a history of seizures and no prior EEG evidence of seizures. Safe concomitant use of anticonvulsants and methylphenidate has not been established. In the presence of seizures, discontinue the drug.

➤*Visual disturbances:* Symptoms of visual disturbances have been encountered in rare cases. Difficulties with accommodation and blurring of vision have been reported.

➤*GI obstruction (Concerta only):* Because the *Concerta* tablet is nondeformable and does not appreciably change in shape in the GI tract, it should not be ordinarily administered to patients with preexisting severe GI narrowing (pathologic or iatrogenic) (eg, esophageal motility disorders, small bowel inflammatory disease, "short gut" syndrome caused by adhesions or decreased transit time, history of peritonitis, cystic fibrosis, chronic intestinal pseudo-obstruction, Meckel diverticulum). There have been rare reports of obstructive symptoms in patients with known strictures in association with the ingestion of drugs in nondeformable controlled-release formulations. Because of the controlled-release design of the tablet, only use *Concerta* in patients who are able to swallow the tablet whole.

➤*Carcinogenesis:* In a lifetime carcinogenicity study carried out in B6C3F1 mice, methylphenidate caused an increase in hepatocellular adenomas and, in males only, an increase in hepatoblastomas, at a daily dosage of approximately 60 mg/kg/day. This dose is approximately 30 times and 2.5 (*Methylin* [IR, ER, and chewable tablets, and oral solution], *Metadate ER*) or 4 (*Ritalin, Ritalin-SR, Ritalin LA, Metadate CD*, and *Concerta*) times the maximum recommended human dose (MRHD) on a mg/kg and mg/m^2 basis, respectively. Hepatoblastoma is a relatively rare rodent malignant tumor type. There was no increase in total malignant hepatic tumors. The mouse strain used is sensitive to the development of hepatic tumors, and the significance of these results to humans is unknown.

➤*Mutagenesis:* Methylphenidate was not mutagenic in the in vitro Ames reverse mutation assay or in the in vitro mouse lymphoma cell forward mutation assay. Sister chromatid exchanges and chromosome aberrations were increased, indicative of a weak clastogenic response, in an in vitro assay in cultured Chinese hamster ovary cells. The genotoxic potential of methylphenidate has not been evaluated in an in vivo assay. Methylphenidate was negative in vivo in males and females in the mouse bone marrow micronucleus assay.

➤*Pregnancy: Category C.* Methylphenidate has been shown to have teratogenic effects in rabbits when given in dosages of 200 mg/kg/day, which is approximately 167 and 78 times (100 and 40 times in *Metadate CD*) the MRHD on a mg/kg and mg/m^2 basis, respectively.

In studies conducted in rats and rabbits, methylphenidate was administered orally at dosages of up to 75 and 200 mg/kg/day, respectively, during the period of organogenesis. Teratogenic effects (increased incidence of fetal spina bifida) were observed in rabbits at the highest dose, which is approximately 40 times the MRHD on a mg/m^2 basis. The no-effect level for embryo-fetal development in rabbits was 60 mg/kg/day (11 times the MRHD on a mg/m^2 basis). There was no evidence of specific teratogenic activity in rats, although increased incidences of fetal skeletal variations were seen at the highest dose level (7 times the MRHD on a mg/m^2 basis), which was also maternally toxic. The no-effect level for embryo-fetal development in rats was 25 mg/kg/day (2 times the MRHD on a mg/m^2 basis). When methylphenidate was administered to rats throughout pregnancy and lactation at dosages of up to 45 mg/kg/day, offspring body weight gain was decreased at the highest dosage (4 times the MRHD on a mg/m^2 basis), but no other effects on postnatal development were observed. The no-effect level for pre- and postnatal development in rats was 15 mg/kg/day (equal to the MRHD on a mg/m^2 basis).

A reproduction study in rats revealed no evidence of teratogenicity at oral doses of up to 30 mg/kg/day (15-fold and 3-fold the MRHD of *Concerta* on a mg/kg and mg/m^2 basis, respectively), 58 mg/kg/day, or 75 mg/kg/day (which is 62.5 and 13.5 times the MRHD on a mg/kg and mg/m^2 basis, respectively). However, this dose, which caused some maternal toxicity, resulted in decreased postnatal pup weights and survival when given to the dams from day 1 of gestation through the lactation period. This dose is approximately 30- and 6-fold the MRHD of methylphenidate on a mg/kg and mg/m^2 basis, respectively. The approximate plasma exposure to methylphenidate plus its main metabolite PPA in pregnant rats was 2 times that seen in trials in volunteers and patients with the maximum recommended dose of *Concerta* based on the AUC.

There are no adequate and well-controlled studies in pregnant women. Use methylphenidate during pregnancy only if the potential benefit justifies the potential risk to the fetus.

➤*Lactation:* It is not known whether methylphenidate is excreted in human milk. Because many drugs are excreted in human milk, exercise caution if methylphenidate is administered to a breast-feeding woman.

➤*Children:* Do not use methylphenidate in children younger than 6 years of age because safety and efficacy in this age group have not been established. Long-term effects of methylphenidate in children have not been well established.

Precautions

➤*Monitoring:* Periodic complete blood cell, differential, and platelet counts are advised during prolonged therapy.

Monitor blood pressure at appropriate intervals in all patients taking methylphenidate, especially those with hypertension.

➤*Prescribing:* Drug treatment is not indicated in all cases of this behavioral syndrome and should be considered only in light of the complete history and evaluation of the child. The decision to prescribe methylphenidate should depend on the physician's assessment of the chronicity and severity of the child's symptoms and the appropriateness for the child's age. Prescription should not depend solely on the presence of 1 or more of the behavioral characteristics.

The physician who elects to use methylphenidate for extended periods in patients with ADHD should periodically reevaluate the long-term usefulness of the drug for the individual patient with trials off the medication to assess the patient's functioning without pharmacotherapy.

➤*Acute stress:* When these symptoms are associated with acute stress reactions, treatment with methylphenidate is usually not indicated.

➤*Phenylketonurics:* Phenylalanine is a component of aspartame. Each methylphenidate 2.5 mg chewable tablet contains phenylalanine 0.42 mg, each 5 mg chewable tablet contains phenylalanine 0.84 mg, and each 10 mg chewable tablet contains phenylalanine 1.68 mg.

➤*Special risk:*

Agitation – Patients with an element of agitation may react adversely; discontinue therapy if necessary.

➤*Drug abuse and dependence:* Methylphenidate, like other methylphenidate products, is classified as a schedule II controlled substance by federal regulation.

Give methylphenidate cautiously to emotionally unstable patients (eg, history of drug dependence or alcoholism) because such patients may increase dosage on their own initiative.

Chronically abusive use can lead to marked tolerance and psychic dependence with varying degrees of abnormal behavior. Frank psychotic episodes can occur, especially with parenteral abuse. Careful supervision is required during drug withdrawal because severe depression as well as the effects of chronic overactivity can be unmasked. Long-term follow-up may be required because of the patient's basic personality disturbances.

Drug Interactions

➤*Antacids/Acid suppressants (Ritalin LA):* The effects of GI pH alterations on the absorption of methylphenidate from ER capsules have not been studied. Because the modified release characteristics of methylphenidate ER capsules are pH dependent, the coadministration of antacids or acid suppressants could alter the release of methylphenidate.

➤*Vasopressor agents:* Methylphenidate may decrease the hypotensive effect of guanethidine. Because of possible effects on blood pressure, use cautiously with vasopressor agents.

➤*Drugs requiring dosage adjustments:* Human pharmacologic studies have shown that methylphenidate may inhibit the metabolism of coumarin anticoagulants, anticonvulsants (eg, phenobarbital, phenytoin, diphenylhydantoin, primidone), phenylbutazone, and tricyclic drugs (eg, imipramine, clomipramine, desipramine, selective serotonin reuptake inhibitors [SSRIs]). Downward dosage adjustments of these drugs may be required when given concomitantly with methylphenidate. It may be necessary to adjust the dosage and monitor plasma drug concentrations (or, in the case of coumarin, coagulation times) when initiating or discontinuing concomitant methylphenidate.

➤*Clonidine:* Serious adverse reactions have been reported in concomitant use with clonidine, although no causality for the combination has been established. The safety of using methylphenidate in combination with clonidine or other centrally acting alpha-2 agonists has not been systematically evaluated.

➤*MAOIs:* Do not use methylphenidate in patients being treated (currently or within the proceeding 2 weeks) with MAOIs.

METHYLPHENIDATE HYDROCHLORIDE — ORAL

Methylphenidate Drug Interactions			
Precipitant drug	Object drug[a]		Description
MAOIs	Methylphenidate	↑	Hypertensive crisis may result with coadministration. Monitor blood pressure during combined MAOI and methylphenidate use. This combination is contraindicated.
Methylphenidate	Anticonvulsants (eg, phenytoin, phenobarbital, primidone)	↑	Anticonvulsant levels may be increased, resulting in increased pharmacologic and toxic effects of the anticonvulsant.
Methylphenidate	Coumarin anticoagulants	↑	Human pharmacologic studies have shown that methylphenidate may inhibit the metabolism of coumarin anticoagulants.
Methylphenidate	Guanethidine	↓	Antihypertensive effect of guanethidine may be decreased by concurrent methylphenidate. Arrhythmias were reported in 1 case. Antiarrhythmics may be needed.
Methylphenidate	SSRIs	↑	Coadministration may cause an increased serum concentration of the SSRIs.
Methylphenidate	Tricyclic antidepressants	↑	Coadministration may cause increased serum concentration of tricyclic antidepressants.

[a] ↑ = Object drug increased. ↓ = Object drug decreased.

➤*Drug/Food interactions:*

Chewable tablets and oral solution – In a study in adult volunteers investigating the effects of a high-fat meal on the bioavailability of methylphenidate chewable tablets and oral solution at a dose of 20 mg, the presence of food delayed the peak concentrations by approximately 1 hour (chewable tablets: 1.5 hours fasted, 2.4 hours fed; oral solution: 1.7 hours fasted, 2.7 hours fed). Overall, a high-fat meal increased the C_{max} of methylphenidate oral solution by approximately 13%, and increased the AUC of methylphenidate chewable tablets and oral solution by approximately 20% and 25% on average, respectively. Through a cross-study comparison, the magnitude of food effect is found to be comparable between methylphenidate chewable tablets, oral solution, and IR tablets.

Metadate CD – In a study in adult volunteers to investigate the effects of a high-fat meal on the bioavailability of a dose of *Metadate CD* 40 mg, the presence of food delayed the early peak by approximately 1 hour (range, −2 to 5 hours delay). The plasma levels rose rapidly following the food-induced delay in absorption. Overall, a high-fat meal increased the C_{max} of *Metadate CD* capsules by approximately 30% and AUC by approximately 17%, on average.

Metadate ER – Based on rate of bioavailability ($AUC_{(0-\infty)}$, T_{max}, and C_{max}), no significant difference was found following single-dose administration, in fasting and fed adults, of 2 *Metadate ER* 10 mg tablets, or 1 methylphenidate SR 20 mg tablet. The administration of the ER methylphenidate tablets with food resulted in a greater C_{max} and $AUC_{(0-\infty)}$ than when administered in a fasting condition.

Ritalin LA – Administration times relative to meal and meal composition may need to be individually titrated.

When *Ritalin LA* was administered with a high-fat breakfast to adults, *Ritalin LA* had a longer lag time until absorption began and variable delays in the time until the first peak concentration, the time until interpeak minimum, and the time until the second peak. The first peak concentration and the extent of absorption were unchanged after food relative to the fasting state, although the second peak was approximately 25% lower. The effect of a high-fat lunch was not examined.

Adverse Reactions

➤*Adverse findings in clinical trials with methylphenidate ER:*

Treatment-emergent adverse reactions –

Concerta: The following table enumerates, for a 4-week, placebo-controlled, parallel-group trial in children with ADHD at methylphenidate ER tablet doses of 18, 36, or 54 mg/day, the incidence of treatment-emergent adverse reactions. The table includes only those reactions that occurred in 1% or more of patients treated with methylphenidate ER tablets where the incidence in patients treated with methylphenidate ER tablets was greater than the incidence in placebo-treated patients.

Concerta Adverse Reactions[a] in Children		
Adverse reaction	Methylphenidate ER tablets (n = 106)	Placebo (n = 99)
CNS		
Dizziness	2%	0%
Headache	14%	10%
Insomnia	4%	1%
GI		
Abdominal pain (stomachache)	7%	1%
Anorexia (loss of appetite)	4%	0%
Vomiting	4%	3%
Respiratory		
Cough increased	4%	2%
Pharyngitis	4%	3%
Sinusitis	3%	0%
Upper respiratory tract infection	8%	5%

[a] Events, regardless of causality, for which the incidence for patients treated with methylphenidate ER tablets was at least 1% and greater than the incidence among placebo-treated patients. Incidence has been rounded to the nearest whole number.

The following table lists the incidence of treatment-emergent adverse reactions for a 2-week, placebo-controlled trial (study 4) in adolescents with ADHD at methylphenidate ER tablet doses of 18, 36, 54, or 72 mg/day.

Concerta Adverse Reactions[a] in a 2-Week Clinical Trial in Adolescents		
Adverse reaction	Methylphenidate ER tablets (n = 87)	Placebo (n = 90)
CNS		
Headache	9%	8%
Insomnia	5%	0%
GI		
Anorexia	2%	0%
Diarrhea	2%	0%
Vomiting	3%	0%
GU		
Dysmenorrhea	2%	0%
Respiratory		
Pharyngitis	2%	1%
Rhinitis	3%	2%
Miscellaneous		
Accidental injury	6%	3%
Fever	3%	0%

[a] Events, regardless of causality, for which the incidence for patients treated with methylphenidate ER tablets was at least 2% and greater than the incidence among placebo-treated patients. Incidence has been rounded to the nearest whole number.

• *Tics* – In a long-term uncontrolled study (n = 432 children), the cumulative incidence of new onset tics was 9% after 27 months of treatment with methylphenidate ER tablets.

In a second uncontrolled study (n = 682 children), the cumulative incidence of new onset tics was 1% (9 of 682 children). The treatment period was up to 9 months with mean treatment duration of 7.2 months.

Metadate CD: The following table enumerates, for a pool of the 3 studies in pediatric patients with ADHD, at methylphenidate ER capsule doses of 20, 40, or 60 mg/day, the incidence of treatment-emergent adverse reactions. One study was a 3-week, placebo-controlled, parallel-group trial, 1 study was a controlled, crossover trial, and the third study was an open titration trial. The following table includes only those events that occurred in 5% or more of patients treated with methylphenidate ER capsules where the incidence in patients treated with methylphenidate ER capsules was greater than the incidence in placebo-treated patients.

Metadate CD Adverse Reactions[a]		
Adverse reaction	Methylphenidate (n = 188)	Placebo (n = 190)
CNS		
Headache	12%	8%
Insomnia	5%	2%
GI		
Abdominal pain (stomachache)	7%	4%
Anorexia (loss of appetite)	9%	2%

[a] Events, regardless of causality, for which the incidence for patients treated with methylphenidate was at least 5% and greater than the incidence among placebo-treated patients. Incidence has been rounded to the nearest whole number.

Ritalin LA: Adverse reactions with an incidence of more than 5% during the initial 4-week, single-blind methylphenidate ER capsules titration period of this study were anorexia, decreased appetite, headache, insomnia, and upper abdominal pain.

METHYLPHENIDATE HYDROCHLORIDE — ORAL

Treatment-emergent adverse reactions with an incidence of more than 2% among methylphenidate ER capsule-treated subjects, during the 2-week, double-blind phase of the clinical study were as follows:

Ritalin LA Adverse Reactions		
	Methylphenidate ER capsules (n = 65)	Placebo (n = 71)
Adverse reaction	n (%)	n (%)
Anorexia	2 (3.1%)	0 (0%)
Insomnia	2 (3.1%)	0 (0%)

Adverse reactions associated with discontinuation of treatment –

Concerta: In the 4-week, placebo-controlled, parallel-group trial in children (study 3), 1 methylphenidate ER tablet-treated patient (0.9%; 1 of 106) and 1 placebo-treated patient (1%; 1 of 99) discontinued because of an adverse reaction (sadness and increase in tics, respectively).

In the 2-week, placebo-controlled phase of a trial in adolescents (study 4), no methylphenidate ER tablets-treated patients (0%; 0 of 87) and 1 placebo-treated patient (1.1%; 1 of 90) discontinued because of an adverse reaction (increased mood irritability).

In the 2 open-label, long-term safety trials (studies 5 and 6; one 24-month study in children 6 to 13 years of age and one 9-month study in child, adolescent, and adult patients treated with methylphenidate ER tablets), 6.7% (101 of 1,514) of patients discontinued because of adverse reactions. These reactions with an incidence of more than 0.5% included the following: insomnia (1.5%), twitching (1%), and abdominal pain, anorexia, emotional lability, nervousness (0.7%).

Metadate CD: In the 3-week placebo-controlled, parallel-group trial, 2 *Metadate CD*–treated patients (1%) and no placebo-treated patients discontinued because of an adverse reaction (rash and pruritus; and headache, abdominal pain, and dizziness, respectively).

Ritalin LA: In the 2-week, double-blind treatment phase of a placebo-controlled, parallel-group study in children with ADHD, only 1 *Ritalin LA*–treated subject (1 of 65; 1.5%) discontinued because of an adverse reaction (depression).

In the single-blind titration period of this study, subjects received methylphenidate ER capsules for up to 4 weeks. During this period a total of 6 subjects (6 of 161; 3.7%) discontinued because of adverse reactions. The adverse reactions leading to discontinuation were anger (in 2 patients), anxiety, depressed mood, fatigue, hypomania, lethargy, and migraine.

Postmarketing (Concerta) – Additional very rare undesirable effects reported during the marketing experience include the following: abnormal liver function tests (eg, transaminase elevation), arrhythmia, blurred vision, difficulties in visual accommodation, leukopenia, palpitations, thrombocytopenia.

➤*Adverse reactions with other methylphenidate products:*

Most common – Nervousness and insomnia are the most common adverse reactions but are usually controlled by reducing dosage and omitting the drug in the afternoon or evening.

Other reactions include the following:

Cardiovascular – Angina, blood pressure increased/decreased, cardiac arrhythmia, palpitations, pulse increased/decreased, tachycardia.

CNS – Dizziness, drowsiness, dyskinesia, headache, Tourette syndrome (rare), toxic psychosis.

GI – Abdominal pain, anorexia, nausea.

Hypersensitivity – Hypersensitivity (including skin rash, urticaria, fever, arthralgia, exfoliative dermatitis, erythema multiforme with histopathological findings of necrotizing vasculitis, and thrombocytopenic purpura).

Miscellaneous – Weight loss during prolonged therapy.

Children: In children, loss of appetite, abdominal pain, weight loss during prolonged therapy, insomnia, and tachycardia may occur more frequently; however, any of the other adverse reactions listed above may also occur.

Other (causal relationship not established) – The following adverse reactions have been reported (causal relationship not established): isolated cases of cerebral arteritis or occlusion, anemia and/or leukopenia, or transient depressed mood; a few instances of scalp hair loss; instances of abnormal liver function (ranging from transaminase elevation to hepatic coma).

Neuroleptic malignant syndrome (NMS) (very rare): Very rare reports NMS of have been received, and, in most of these, patients were concurrently receiving therapies associated with NMS. In a single report, a boy 10 years of age who had been taking methylphenidate for approximately 18 months experienced an NMS-like event within 45 minutes of ingesting his first dose of venlafaxine. It is uncertain whether this case represented a drug-drug interaction, a response to either drug alone, or some other cause.

Overdosage

➤*Symptoms:* Signs and symptoms of acute overdosage, resulting principally from overstimulation of the CNS and from excessive sympathomimetic effects, may include the following: agitation, cardiac arrhythmias, confusion, convulsions (may be followed by coma), delirium, dryness of mucous membranes, euphoria, flushing, hallucinations, headache, hyperpyrexia, hyperreflexia, hypertension, muscle twitching, mydriasis, palpitations, sweating, tachycardia, tremors, vomiting.

➤*Treatment:* Consult with a certified poison control center for up-to-date guidance and advice regarding treatment.

As with the management of all overdosage, consider the possibility of multiple drug ingestion.

Treatment consists of appropriate supportive measures. The patient must be protected against self-injury and against external stimuli that would aggravate overstimulation already present. Gastric contents may be evacuated by gastric lavage. In the presence of severe intoxication, use a carefully titrated dosage of a short-acting barbiturate before performing gastric lavage. Before performing gastric lavage, control agitation and seizures if present and protect the airway. Other measures to detoxify the gut include administration of activated charcoal and a cathartic.

Intensive care must be provided to maintain adequate circulation and respiratory exchange; external cooling procedures may be required for hyperpyrexia.

Efficacy of peritoneal dialysis or extracorporeal hemodialysis for methylphenidate overdosage has not been established; also, dialysis is considered unlikely to be of benefit because of the large volume of distribution of methylphenidate.

Consider the prolonged release of methylphenidate from *Concerta*, *Metadate CD*, and *Ritalin LA* when treating patients with overdose.

Patient Information

➤*Chewable tablets:* Taking methylphenidate chewable tablets without adequate fluid may cause them to swell and block the throat or esophagus and may cause choking. Advise patients not to take this product if they have difficulty in swallowing. Instruct patients to seek immediate medical attention if they experience chest pain, vomiting, or difficulty in swallowing or breathing after taking this product.

Instruct patients to take methylphenidate chewable tablets (child or adult dose) with at least 8 ounces (a full glass) of water or other fluid. Taking this product without enough liquid may cause choking.

Phenylalanine is a component of aspartame. Each methylphenidate 2.5 mg chewable tablet contains phenylalanine 0.42 mg, each 5 mg chewable tablet contains phenylalanine 0.84 mg, and each 10 mg chewable tablet contains phenylalanine 1.68 mg.

➤*Concerta*: Instruct patients to swallow methylphenidate ER tablets (*Concerta*) whole with the aid of liquids. Tablets should not be chewed, divided, or crushed. The medication is contained within a nonabsorbable shell designed to release the drug at a controlled rate. The tablet shell, along with insoluble core components, is eliminated from the body; instruct patients not be concerned if they occasionally notice something that looks like a tablet in their stool.

➤*Metadate CD*: Instruct patients using methylphenidate ER capsules (*Metadate CD*) to take 1 dose in the morning before breakfast. Instruct them that the capsule may be swallowed whole, or, alternatively, the capsule may be opened and the capsule contents sprinkled onto a small amount (1 tablespoon) of applesauce and given immediately, and not stored for future use. The capsules and the capsule contents must not be crushed or chewed.

➤*Ritalin LA*: Administer once daily in the morning. Capsules may be swallowed whole or opened and the contents sprinkled onto a spoonful of cool applesauce and consumed immediately in its entirety. Capsules or contents should not be crushed, chewed, or divided.

➤*Methylin, Ritalin*: Take last daily dose early in the evening (prior to 6 pm) to avoid insomnia. It is often recommended that methylphenidate be taken 30 to 45 minutes before meals.

➤*Patient information:*

Concerta, *Metadate CD*, and *Ritalin LA* –

Who should not take methylphenidate?: Do not take methylphenidate if:

- you have significant anxiety, tension, or agitation because methylphenidate may make these conditions worse
- you are allergic to methylphenidate or any other ingredient in the product
- you have glaucoma, an eye disease
- you have tics or Tourette syndrome, or a family history of Tourette syndrome
- you are taking an MAOI, a type of antidepressant, or have discontinued an MAOI in the last 14 days

Can I take methylphenidate with other medicines?: You should not take methylphenidate with MAOIs or within 14 days of stopping an MAOI.

Other important safety information: Before taking methylphenidate, tell your doctor if you are pregnant or plan on becoming pregnant. If you take methylphenidate, it may be in your breast milk. Tell your doctor if you are breast-feeding a baby.

Tell your doctor if you have blurred vision when taking methylphenidate.

Slower growth (weight gain and/or height) has been reported with long-term use of methylphenidate in children. Your doctor will be carefully watching your height and weight. If you are not growing or gaining weight as your doctor expects, your doctor may stop your methylphenidate treatment.

METHYLPHENIDATE HYDROCHLORIDE — TRANSDERMAL

WARNING

Drug dependence – Give methylphenidate cautiously to emotionally unstable patients (eg, those with a history of drug dependence or alcoholism) because such patients may increase dosage on their own initiative.

Chronically abusive use can lead to marked tolerance and psychic dependence with varying degrees of abnormal behavior. Frank psychotic episodes can occur, especially with parenteral abuse. Careful supervision is required during drug withdrawal because severe depression as well as the effects of chronic overactivity can be unmasked. Long-term follow-up may be required because of the patient's basic personality disturbances.

Indications

➤*Attention Deficit Hyperactivity Disorder (ADHD):* For the treatment of ADHD.

Administration and Dosage

➤*Approved by the FDA:* April 6, 2006.

➤*Recommended dose:* It is recommended that methylphenidate be applied to the hip area 2 hours before an effect is needed and should be removed 9 hours after application. Dosage should be titrated to effect. The recommended dose titration schedule is shown in the table below. Dose titration, final dosage, and wear time should be individualized according to the needs and response of the patient.

Methyphenidate Transdermal Recommended Titration Schedule (Patients New to Methylphenidate)

	Upward Titration, If Response is not Maximized			
	Week 1	Week 2	Week 3	Week 4
Patch Size	12.5 cm^2	18.75 cm^2	25 cm^2	37.5[2]
Nominal Delivered Dose* (mg/9 hrs)	10 mg	15 mg	20 mg	30 mg
Delivery Rate*	(1.1 mg/hr)*	(1.6 mg/hr)*	(2.2 mg/hr)*	(3.3 mg/hr)*

* Nominal in vivo delivery rate in pediatric subjects aged 6-12 when applied to the hip, based on a 9-hour wear period.

➤*Conversion:* Patients converting from another formulation of methylphenidate should follow the above titration schedule due to differences in bioavailability of methylphenidate transdermal compared to other products.

➤*Application:* The parent or caregiver should be encouraged to use the administration chart included with each carton of methylphenidate to monitor application and removal time, and method of disposal. The patient information included at the end of the insert also includes a timetable to calculate when to remove methylphenidate, based on the 9-hour application time.

The adhesive side of the patch should be placed on a clean, dry area of the hip. The area selected should not be oily, damaged, or irritated. Apply patch to the hip area. Avoid the waistline, since clothing may cause the patch to rub off. When applying the patch the next morning, place on the opposite hip at a new site if possible.

The patch should be applied immediately after opening the pouch and removing the protective liner. Do not use if the pouch seal is broken. The patch should then be pressed firmly in place with the palm of the hand for approximately 30 seconds, making sure that there is good contact of the patch with the skin, especially around the edges. After proper application, bathing, swimming, or showering have not been shown to affect patch adherence. In the unlikely event that a patch should fall off, a new patch may be applied at a different site, but the total recommended wear time for that day should remain 9 hours.

➤*Disposal:* Upon removal, used patches should be folded so that the adhesive side of the patch adheres to itself and should be flushed down the toilet or disposed of in an appropriate lidded container. If the patient stops using the prescription, each unused patch should be removed from its pouch, separated from the protective liner, folded onto itself, and flushed down the toilet or disposed of in an appropriate lidded container.

The parent should be encouraged to record on the administration chart included with each carton the time that each patch was applied and removed. If a patch was removed without the parent or caregiver's knowledge, or if a patch is missing from the tray, the parent or caregiver should be encouraged to ask the child when and how the patch was removed.

➤*Long-term use:* There is no body of evidence available from controlled clinical trials to indicate how long the patient with ADHD should be treated with methylphenidate. It is generally agreed, however, that pharmacological treatment of ADHD may be needed for extended periods. Nevertheless, the physician who elects to use methylphenidate for extended periods in patients with ADHD should periodically re-evaluate the long-term usefulness of the drug for the individual patient with periods off medication to assess the patient's functioning without pharmacotherapy. Improvement may be sustained when the drug is either temporarily or permanently discontinued.

➤*Dose / Wear Time Reduction and Discontinuation:* The patch may be removed earlier than 9 hours if a shorter duration of effect is desired or late day side effects appear. Plasma concentrations of d-methylphenidate generally begin declining when the patch is removed, although absorption may continue for several hours. Individualization of wear time may help manage some of the side effects caused by methylphenidate. If aggravation of symptoms or other adverse reactions occur, the dosage or wear time should be reduced, or, if necessary, the drug should be discontinued. Residual methylphenidate remains in used patches when worn as recommended.

➤*Storage / Stability:* Do not store patches unpouched. Store at 25°C (77°F); excursions permitted to 15-30°C (59-86°F).

Once the tray is opened, use contents within 2 months. Apply the patch immediately upon removal from the protective pouch. Do not store patches unpouched. For transdermal use only.

Anorexiants

Indications

In addition to the nonamphetamine anorexiants included in this section, amphetamines are also used for short-term obesity therapy.

➤*Exogenous obesity:* As a short-term adjunct in a regimen of weight reduction based on caloric restriction. Measure the limited usefulness of these agents against their inherent risks. Refer to individual monographs for extended indications.

Actions

➤*Pharmacology:* Adrenergic agents (eg, **diethylpropion**, **benzphetamine**, **phendimetrazine**, **phentermine**) act by modulating central norepinephrine and dopamine receptors through the promotion of catecholamine release. Aside from phentermine, other adrenergic agents are infrequently used, perhaps because of the lack of long-term, well-controlled data or the fear of their potential abuse. Older adrenergic weight-loss drugs (eg, amphetamine, methamphetamine, phenmetrazine), which strongly engage in dopamine pathways, are no longer recommended because of the risk of their abuse.

➤*Pharmacokinetics:*

Distribution – **Diethylpropion** is rapidly absorbed from the GI tract after oral administration and is extensively metabolized through a complex pathway of biotransformation involving N-dealkylation and reduction. Many of these metabolites are biologically active and may participate in the therapeutic action of diethylpropion. Diethylpropion and its active metabolites are believed to cross the blood-brain barrier and the placenta, and are excreted mainly by the kidneys with 75% to 106% of the dose recovered in the urine within 48 hours after dosing. The plasma half-life of the aminoketone metabolites is ≈ 4 to 6 hours.

Excretion – Most of the drugs and their metabolites are excreted via the kidneys. The average half-lives for **phendimetrazine** are ≈ 1.9 hours for *Bontril PDM*, 9.8 hours for *Bontril*, and 3.7 hours for *Prelu-2*.

Contraindications

Advanced arteriosclerosis; symptomatic cardiovascular disease; moderate-to-severe hypertension; hyperthyroidism; known hypersensitivity or idiosyncrasy to sympathomimetic amines; glaucoma; highly nervous or agitated states; history of drug abuse; during or within 14 days following the administration of MAO inhibitors (hypertensive crises may result); coadministration with other CNS stimulants.

➤*Pregnancy:* *Category X*. **Benzphetamine hydrochloride** is contraindicated during pregnancy (see Warnings).

Warnings

➤*Tolerance:* Tolerance to the anorectic effects may develop within a few weeks. If tolerance to the anorectic effect develops, do not exceed the recommended dose in an attempt to increase the effect; rather, discontinue the drug.

➤*Other drugs:* These agents should not be used in combination with other anorectic agents, including prescribed drugs (eg, SSRIs [eg, fluoxetine, sertraline, fluvoxamine, paroxetine]), *otc* preparations, and herbal products. When using CNS-active agents, consider the possibility of adverse interactions with alcohol.

➤*Primary pulmonary hypertension (PPH):* PPH, a rare, frequently fatal disease of the lungs, has been reported to occur in patients receiving certain anorectic agents. The initial symptom of PPH is usually dyspnea. Other initial symptoms include the following: Angina pectoris, syncope, or lower extremity edema. Advise patients to report immediately any deterioration in exercise tolerance. Discontinue treatment in patients who develop new, unexplained symptoms of dyspnea, angina pectoris, syncope, or lower extremity edema.

➤*Valvular heart disease:* Serious regurgitant cardiac valvular disease, primarily affecting the mitral, aortic, or tricuspid valves, has been reported in otherwise healthy people who had taken certain anorectic agents in combination for weight loss. The etiology of these valvulopathies has not been established and their course in individuals after the drugs are stopped is not known.

➤*Pregnancy:* (*Category X* - Benzphetamine hydrochloride. *Category B* - Diethylpropion. *Category C* - Phentermine, phendimetrazine). Safety for use during pregnancy has not been established. Use in women who are or who may become pregnant (especially those in the first trimester) only when clearly needed and when the potential benefits outweigh the potential hazards to the fetus.

In animal studies with **phendimetrazine**, conception rate was adversely affected, as well as survival and body weight of pups. Congenital malformations are associated with phendimetrazine use, but a causal relationship has not been proven. Animal and clinical studies have not shown a teratogenic potential for **diethylpropion**. Abuse of diethylpropion during pregnancy may result in withdrawal symptoms in the human neonate.

➤*Lactation:* Safety for use in the nursing mother has not been established. Amphetamines are excreted in human milk. Advise mothers taking amphetamines to refrain from nursing.

Diethylpropion and its metabolites are excreted in breast milk. Exercise caution when administering to a nursing woman.

➤*Children:* **Phendimetrazine** and **benzphetamine** are not recommended for use in children less than 12 years of age. **Diethylpropion** is not recommended for use in pediatric patients less than 16 years of age.

Phentermine – Safety and efficacy have not been established for *Adipex-P*. *Pro-Fast SA*, *ProFast HS*, and *Pro-Fast SR* are not recommended in patients less than 12 years of age. *Ionamin* is not recommended in children less than 16 years of age.

Precautions

➤*Psychological disturbances:* Psychological disturbances occurred in patients who received an anorectic agent together with a restrictive diet.

➤*Cardiovascular disease:* Exercise caution in prescribing amphetamines for patients with even mild hypertension.

➤*Dispensing:* The least amount feasible should be prescribed or dispensed at one time in order to minimize the possibility of overdosage.

➤*Convulsions:* Convulsions may increase in some epileptics receiving **diethylpropion**. Dose titration or drug discontinuance may be necessary.

➤*Diabetes:* Insulin requirements in diabetes mellitus may be altered in association with the use of anorexigenic drugs and the concomitant dietary restrictions.

➤*Drug abuse and dependence:* These drugs are chemically and pharmacologically related to the amphetamines, and have abuse potential. Intense psychological dependence and severe social dysfunction may occur. If this occurs, gradually reduce the dosage to avoid withdrawal symptoms (eg, extreme fatigue, sleep EEG changes, mental depression). Chronic intoxication is manifested by severe dermatoses, marked insomnia, irritability, hyperactivity, and personality changes. Psychosis, often clinically indistinguishable from schizophrenia, is the most severe manifestation.

➤*Hazardous tasks:* May produce dizziness, extreme fatigue, and depression after abrupt cessation of prolonged high-dosage therapy; patients should observe caution while driving or performing other tasks requiring alertness.

➤*Tartrazine sensitivity:* Some of these products contain tartrazine, which may cause allergic-type reactions (including bronchial asthma) in susceptible individuals. Although the incidence of tartrazine sensitivity in the general population is low, it is frequently seen in patients who also have aspirin hypersensitivity. Specific products containing tartrazine are identified in the product listings.

Drug Interactions

Phentermine may decrease the hypotensive effect of adrenergic neuron blocking drugs.

Anorexiant Drug Interactions

Precipitant drug	Object drug[a]		Description
Furazolidone MAO inhibitors	Anorexiants	↑	MAO inhibitors may increase the pressor response to the anorexiants. Possible hypertensive crisis and intracranial hemorrhage may occur. This interaction may also occur with **furazolidone**, an antimicrobial with MAO inhibitor activity. Avoid this combination.
Selective serotonin reuptake inhibitors (SSRIs)	Anorexiants	↑	Increased sensitivity to effect of sympathomimetics and increased risk of "serotonin syndrome" may occur. Monitor patient for increased signs/symptoms of CNS effects.
Anorexiants	Guanethidine	↓	Anorexiants may decrease the hypotensive effect of guanethidine.
Anorexiants	Tricyclic antidepressants	↑	Amphetamines may enhance the effects of tricyclic antidepressants.

[a] ↑ = Object drug increased. ↓ = Object drug decreased.

Adverse Reactions

➤*Cardiovascular:* Palpitations; tachycardia; arrhythmias (including ventricular); precordial pain; primary pulmonary hypertension or regurgitant cardiac valvular disease; elevation of blood pressure. ECG changes have been reported with **diethylpropion**; valvulopathy has been reported with diethylpropion very rarely, but the causal relationship is unknown. Isolated reports of cardiomyopathy have been associated with chronic amphetamine use.

➤*CNS:* Overstimulation; cerebrovascular accident; nervousness; restlessness; dizziness; insomnia; malaise; anxiety; euphoria; drowsiness; depression; agitation; dysphoria; dyskinesia; tremor; headache; psychotic episodes (rare); agitation; jitteriness; depression following withdrawal of the drug. An increase in convulsive episodes occurred in a few epileptics.

➤*GI:* Dry mouth; unpleasant taste; nausea; vomiting; abdominal discomfort; diarrhea; GI disturbances; constipation; stomach pain.

➤*GU:* Dysuria; polyuria; urinary frequency; impotence; menstrual upset; gynecomastia; changes in libido.

➤*Hematologic:* Bone marrow depression; agranulocytosis; leukopenia.

➤*Hypersensitivity:* Urticaria; rash; erythema.

➤*Ophthalmic:* Mydriasis; blurred vision.

➤*Miscellaneous:* Hair loss; muscle pain; excessive sweating; ecchymosis; flushing; dyspnea.

Overdosage

➤*Symptoms:*

CNS – Restlessness; tremor; tachypnea; hyperreflexia; hyperpyrexia; rhabdomyolysis; confusion; belligerence; assaultiveness; hallucinations; panic states. Depression and fatigue usually follow central stimulation.

Convulsions, coma, and death may result.

Cardiovascular – Arrhythmias (tachycardia); hypertension or hypotension; circulatory collapse.

GI – Nausea; vomiting; diarrhea; abdominal cramps.

➤*Treatment:* Includes symptomatic and supportive therapy. Refer to Management of Acute Overdosage.

Sedate patient with a barbiturate or another sedative, and employ gastric lavage. Give activated charcoal if ingestion was recent.

Experience with hemodialysis or peritoneal dialysis is inadequate to permit recommendations.

Patient Information

May cause insomnia; avoid taking medication late in the day.

Caution patients about concomitant use of alcohol or other CNS-active drugs and anorectic agents.

Weight reduction requires strict adherence to dietary restriction.

Do not take more frequently than prescribed.

Notify physician if palpitations, nervousness, or dizziness occurs.

Medication may cause dry mouth and constipation; notify physician if these become pronounced.

May produce dizziness or blurred vision; observe caution while driving or performing other tasks requiring alertness.

These drugs should generally be taken on an empty stomach.

Do not crush or chew sustained-release products.

BENZPHETAMINE HYDROCHLORIDE

c-iii	**Didrex** (Pharmacia)	**Tablets:** 50 mg	Lactose, sorbitol. (DIDREX 50). Peach, scored. In 100s and 500s.

BENZPHETAMINE HYDROCHLORIDE — ORAL

Complete and comparative prescribing information begins in the Anorexiants group monograph.

Indications

➤*Obesity:* Management of exogenous obesity as a short-term adjunct (a few weeks) in a regimen of weight reduction based on caloric restriction. The limited usefulness of agents of this class should be weighed against possible risks inherent in their use.

Administration and Dosage

Dosage should be individualized according to the response of the patient. The suggested dosage ranges from 25 to 50 mg 1 to 3 times daily. Treatment should begin with 25 to 50 mg once daily with subsequent increase in individual dose or frequency according to response. A single daily dose is preferably given midmorning or midafternoon, according to the patient's eating habits. In an occasional patient, it may be desirable to avoid late afternoon administration. Use of benzphetamine hydrochloride is not recommended in individuals under 12 years of age.

➤*Storage/Stability:* Store at controlled room temperature (20° to 25°C; 68° to 77°F).

DIETHYLPROPION HYDROCHLORIDE

c-iv	**Diethylpropion Hydrochloride** (Various, eg, Schein, Watson)	**Tablets:** 25 mg	In 100s.
c-iv	**Tenuate** (Aventis)		Lactose. (TENUATE 25 or MERRELL 697). White. In 100s.
c-iv	**Diethylpropion Hydrochloride** (Various, eg, Watson)	**Tablets, controlled release:** 75 mg	In 100s.
c-iv	**Tenuate Dospan** (Aventis)		Mannitol. (TENUATE 75 or MERRELL 698). White. In 100s and 250s.

DIETHYLPROPION HYDROCHLORIDE — ORAL

Complete and comparative prescribing information begins in the Anorexiants group monograph.

Indications

➤*Obesity:* Management of exogenous obesity as a short-term adjunct (a few weeks) in a regimen of weight reduction based on caloric restriction in patients with an initial body mass index (BMI) of 30 kg/m^2 or higher and who have not responded to appropriate weight reducing regimen (diet and/or exercise) alone.

Administration and Dosage

➤*Approved by the FDA:* November 7, 1960.

➤*Diethylpropion hydrochloride immediate-release:* One 25 mg tablet 3 times daily, 1 hour before meals, and in midevening if desired to overcome night hunger.

➤*Diethylpropion hydrochloride controlled-release:* One 75 mg tablet daily, swallowed whole, in mid-morning.

➤*Storage/Stability:* Keep tightly closed. Store at room temperature, below 30°C (86°F).

PHENDIMETRAZINE TARTRATE

c-iii	**Phendimetrazine** (Various, eg, Camall, Eon, Major, Schein)	**Tablets:** 35 mg	In 100s, 1000s, and 5000s.
c-iii	**Bontril PDM** (Valeant)		Sugar, isopropyl alcohol, lactose. (B 35 V). Green, white, and yellow layered; scored. In 100s and 1,000s.
c-iii	**Bontril Slow-Release** (Valeant)	**Capsules, sustained-release:** 105 mg	(A 047). Green/Yellow. In 100s.
c-iii	**Melfiat-105 Unicelles** (Numark)		Sucrose. (NUMARK 1082). Orange/Clear. In 100s.
c-iii	**Prelu-2** (Roxane)		Sucrose. Celery/Green. In 100s.

PHENDIMETRAZINE TARTRATE — ORAL

Complete and comparative prescribing information begins in the Anorexiants group monograph.

Indications

➤*Obesity:* Management of exogenous obesity as a short-term adjunct (a few weeks) in a regimen of weight reduction based on caloric restriction.

Administration and Dosage

➤*Approved by the FDA:* September 1, 1982.

➤*Tablets:* 35 mg 2 or 3 times a day, 1 hour before meals.

Dosage should be individualized to obtain an adequate response with the lowest effective dosage. In some cases ½ tablet (17.5 mg) per dose may be adequate. Dosage should not exceed 2 tablets 3 times a day.

➤*Sustained-release capsules:* One capsule (105 mg) in the morning, taken 30 to 60 minutes before the morning meal.

Phendimetrazine tartrate is not recommended for use in children under 12 years of age.

➤*Storage/Stability:* Store at controlled room temperature 15° to 30°C (59° to 86°F). Protect from moisture.

Dispense in a tight, light-resistant container as defined in the USP, with a child-resistant closure (as required).

PHENTERMINE HYDROCHLORIDE

c-iv	**Phentermine Hydrochloride** (Various, eg, Camall)	**Tablets:** 8 mg	In 1000s.
c-iv	**Pro-Fast SA** (American Pharmaceuticals)		Lactose, tartrazine. In 100s.
c-iv	**Phentermine Hydrochloride** (Various, eg, Eon)	**Capsules:** 15 mg phentermine resin	In 100s and 1000s.
c-iv	**Ionamin** (Celltech)		Lactose. (Ionamin 15). Yellow/gray. In 100s and 400s.
c-iv	**Phentermine Hydrochloride** (Various, eg, Camall)	**Capsules:** 18.75 mg (equivalent to 15 mg phentermine base)	In 1000s.
c-iv	**Pro-Fast HS** (American Pharmaceuticals)		EDTA, benzyl alcohol, parabens. Gray/Yellow. In 100s.
c-iv	**Phentermine Hydrochloride** (Various, eg, Amide, Camall, Eon)	**Capsules:** 30 mg (equivalent to 24 mg phentermine base)	In 100s and 1000s.
c-iv	**Ionamin** (Celltech)	**Capsules:** 30 mg phentermine resin	Lactose. (Ionamin 30). Yellow. In 100s.
c-iv	**Phentermine Hydrochloride** (Various, eg, Amide, Camall, Purepac)	**Tablets:** 37.5 mg (equivalent to 30 mg phentermine base)	In 100s and 1000s.
c-iv	**Adipex-P** (Gate)		Lactose, sucrose. (ADIPEX-P 9 9). Blue/White, oblong, scored. In 30s, 100s, and 1000s.
c-iv	**Phentermine Hydrochloride** (Various, eg, Amide, Geneva, Ivax, Rugby, URL)	**Capsules:** 37.5 mg (equivalent to 30 mg phentermine base)	In 100s and 1000s.
c-iv	**Adipex-P** (Gate)		Lactose. (ADIPEX-P 37.5). Blue/White. In 100s.
c-iv	**Pro-Fast SR** (American Pharmaceuticals)		Sugar, tartrazine, EDTA, benzyl alcohol, parabens. Black/Yellow. In 100s.

PHENTERMINE HYDROCHLORIDE — ORAL

Complete and comparative prescribing information begins in the Anorexiants group monograph.

Indications

➤*Obesity:* Short-term (a few weeks) adjunct in a regimen of weight reduction based on exercise, behavioral modification and caloric restriction in the management of exogenous obesity for patients with an initial body mass index greater than or equal to 30 kg/m^2, or greater than or equal to 27 kg/m^2 in the presence of other risk factors (eg, hypertension, diabetes, hyperlipidemia).

Administration and Dosage

Dosage should be individualized to obtain an adequate response with the lowest effective dose.

Phentermine hydrochloride is not recommended for use in patients 16 years of age and younger.

Late evening medication should be avoided because of the possibility of resulting insomnia.

➤*Obesity:*

Capsules – The usual dosage is 15 to 30 mg at approximately 2 hours after breakfast for appetite control.

Administration of 1 capsule daily has been found to be adequate in suppression of the appetite for 12 to 14 hours.

Tablets – The usual adult dose is 1 tablet daily, administered before breakfast or 1 to 2 hours after breakfast. The dosage may be adjusted to the

PHENTERMINE HYDROCHLORIDE — ORAL

patient's need. For some patients ½ tablet (18.75 mg) daily may be adequate, while in some cases it may be desirable to give ½ tablet (18.75 mg) 2 times a day.

➤*Storage/Stability:* Dispense in a tight container with a child-resistant closure. Store at controlled room temperature 15° to 30°C (59° to 86°F). Protect from moisture. Keep tightly closed.

PHENTERMINE RESIN — ORAL

Complete and comparative prescribing information begins in the Anorexiants group monograph.

Indications

➤*Obesity:* Short-term (a few weeks) adjunct in a regimen of weight reduction based on exercise, behavioral modification, and caloric restriction in the management of exogenous obesity for patients with an initial body mass index greater than or equal to 30 kg/m^2, or greater than or equal to 27 kg/m^2 in the presence of other risk factors (eg, hypertension, diabetes, hyperlipidemia).

Administration and Dosage

➤*Approved by the FDA:* May 4, 1959.

One capsule daily, before breakfast or 10 to 14 hours before retiring. For individuals exhibiting greater drug responsiveness, phentermine resin 15 mg capsules will usually suffice. Phentermine resin 30 mg capsules are recommended for less responsive patients.

Phentermine resin capsules are not recommended for use in pediatric patients under 16 years of age.

Phentermine resin capsules should be swallowed whole.

➤*Storage/Stability:* Store at 25°C (77°F); excursions permitted to 15° to 30°C (59° to 86°F). Keep out of the reach of children.

SIBUTRAMINE HYDROCHLORIDE

c-iv	**Meridia** (Abbott)	**Capsules:** 5 mg	Lactose. (MERIDIA -5-). Blue/yellow. In 100s.
		10 mg	Lactose. (MERIDIA -10-). Blue/white. In 100s.
		15 mg	Lactose. (MERIDIA -15-). Yellow/white. In 100s.

SIBUTRAMINE HYDROCHLORIDE MONOHYDRATE — ORAL

Indications

➤*Obesity:* Sibutramine is indicated for the management of obesity, including weight loss and maintenance of weight loss, and should be used in conjunction with a reduced calorie diet. Sibutramine is recommended for obese patients with an initial body mass index greater than or equal to 30 kg/m^2, or greater than or equal to 27 kg/m^2 in the presence of other risk factors (eg, hypertension, diabetes, dyslipidemia).

Administration and Dosage

The recommended starting dose of sibutramine is 10 mg administered once daily with or without food. If there is inadequate weight loss, the dose may be titrated after 4 weeks to a total of 15 mg once daily. The 5 mg dose should be reserved for patients who do not tolerate the 10 mg dose. Blood pressure and heart rate changes should be taken into account when making decisions regarding dose titration.

Doses above 15 mg daily are not recommended. In most clinical trials, sibutramine was given in the morning.

➤*Storage/Stability:* Store at 25°C (77°F); excursions permitted to 15° to 30°C (59° to 86°F). Protect from heat and moisture. Dispense in a tight, light-resistant container.

Actions

➤*Pharmacology:* Sibutramine produces its therapeutic effects by norepinephrine, serotonin, and dopamine reuptake inhibition. Sibutramine and its major pharmacologically active metabolites (M_1 and M_2) do not act via release of monoamines.

Sibutramine exerts its pharmacological actions predominantly via its secondary (M_1) and primary (M_2) amine metabolites. The parent compound, sibutramine, is a potent inhibitor of serotonin (5-hydroxytryptamine, 5-HT) and norepinephrine reuptake in vivo, but not in vitro. However, metabolites M_1 and M_2 inhibit the reuptake of these neurotransmitters both in vitro and in vivo.

In human brain tissue, M_1 and M_2 also inhibit dopamine reuptake in vitro, but with approximately 3-fold lower potency than for the reuptake inhibition of serotonin or norepinephrine.

Potencies of sibutramine, M_1 and M_2 as in vitro inhibitors of monoamine reuptake in human brain

	Potency to inhibit monoamine reuptake (Ki;nM)		
	Serotonin	Norepinephrine	Dopamine
Sibutramine	298	5,451	943
M_1	15	20	49
M_2	20	15	45

A study using plasma samples taken from sibutramine-treated volunteers showed monoamine reuptake inhibition of norepinephrine greater than serotonin greater than dopamine; maximum inhibitions were norepinephrine = (73%), serotonin = (54%) and dopamine = (16%).

Sibutramine and its metabolites (M_1 and M_2) are not serotonin, norepinephrine- or dopamine-releasing agents. Following chronic administration of sibutramine to rats, no depletion of brain monoamines has been observed.

Sibutramine, M_1 and M_2 exhibit no evidence of anticholinergic or antihistaminergic actions. In addition, receptor binding profiles show that sibutramine, M_1 and M_2 have low affinity for serotonin (5-HT_1, 5-HT_{1A}, 5-HT_{1B}, 5-HT_{2A}, 5-HT_{2C}), norepinephrine (β, β_1, β_3, α_1 and α_2), dopamine (D_1 and D_2), benzodiazepine, and glutamate (NMDA) receptors. These compounds also lack monoamine oxidase inhibitory activity in vitro and in vivo.

➤*Pharmacokinetics:*

Absorption – Sibutramine is rapidly absorbed from the GI tract (t_{max} of 1.2 hours) following oral administration and undergoes extensive first-pass metabolism in the liver (oral clearance of 1,750 L/hr and half-life of 1.1 hour) to form the pharmacologically active mono- and di- desmethyl metabolites M_1 and M_2. Peak plasma concentrations of M_1 and M_2 are reached within 3 to 4 hours. On the basis of mass balance studies, on average, at least 77% of a single oral dose of sibutramine is absorbed. The absolute bioavailability of sibutramine has not been determined.

Effect of food: Administration of a single 20 mg dose of sibutramine with a standard breakfast resulted in reduced peak M_1 and M_2 concentrations (by 27% and 32%, respectively) and delayed the time to peak by approximately 3 hours. However, the AUCs of M_1 and M_2 were not significantly altered.

Distribution – Radiolabeled studies in animals indicated rapid and extensive distribution into tissues: Highest concentrations of radiolabeled material were found in the eliminating organs, liver and kidney. In vitro, sibutramine, M_1 and M_2 are extensively bound (97%, 94% and 94%, respectively) to human plasma proteins at plasma concentrations seen following therapeutic doses.

Metabolism – Sibutramine is metabolized in the liver principally by the cytochrome P4503A4 isoenzyme, to desmethyl metabolites, M_1 and M_2. These active metabolites are further metabolized by hydroxylation and conjugation to pharmacologically inactive metabolites, M_5 and M_6. Following oral administration of radiolabeled sibutramine, essentially all of the peak radiolabeled material in plasma was accounted for by unchanged sibutramine (3%), M_1 (6%), M_2 (12%), M_5 (52%), and M_6 (27%).

M_1 and M_2 plasma concentrations reached steady-state within 4 days of dosing and were approximately 2-fold higher than following a single dose. The elimination half-lives of M_1 and M_2, 14 and 16 hours, respectively, were unchanged following repeated dosing.

Excretion – Approximately 85% (range, 68% to 95%) of a single orally administered radiolabeled dose was excreted in urine and feces over a 15-day collection period with the majority of the dose (77%) excreted in the urine. Major metabolites in urine were M_5 and M_6; unchanged sibutramine, M_1, and M_2 were not detected. The primary route of excretion for M_1 and M_2 is hepatic metabolism and for M_5 and M_6 is renal excretion.

Special populations –

Renal function impairment: The effect of renal disease has not been studied. However, since sibutramine and its active metabolites M_1 and M_2 are eliminated by hepatic metabolism, renal disease is unlikely to have a significant effect on their disposition. Elimination of the inactive metabolites M_5 and M_6, which are renally excreted, may be affected in this population. Sibutramine, should not be used in patients with severe renal impairment.

Hepatic function impairment: In 12 patients with moderate hepatic impairment receiving a single 15 mg oral dose of sibutramine, the combined AUCs of M_1 and M_2 were increased by 24% compared to healthy subjects while M_5 and M_6 plasma concentrations were unchanged. The observed differences in M_1 and M_2 concentrations do not warrant dosage adjustment in patients with mild to moderate hepatic impairment. Sibutramine should not be used in patients with severe hepatic dysfunction.

Summary of pharmacokinetic parameters –

Mean (% CV) and 95% confidence intervals of pharmacokinetic parameters (dose = 15 mg)

Study population	C_{max} (ng/mL)	t_{max} (hr)	AUC[a] (ng•hr/mL)	t½ (hr)
Metabolite M_1				
Target population:				
Obese subjects	4 (42)	3.6 (28)	25.5 (63)	-
(n = 18)	3.2 to 4.8	3.1 to 4.1	18.1 to 32.9	

SIBUTRAMINE HYDROCHLORIDE MONOHYDRATE — ORAL

Mean (% CV) and 95% confidence intervals of pharmacokinetic parameters (dose = 15 mg)				
Study population	C_{max} (ng/mL)	t_{max} (hr)	AUC[a] (ng•hr/mL)	$t_{½}$ (hr)
Special population:				
Moderate hepatic impairment	2.2 (36)	3.3 (33)	18.7 (65)	-
(n = 12)	1.8 to 2.7	2.7 to 3.9	11.9 to 25.5	
Metabolite M_2				
Target population:				
Obese subjects	6.4 (28)	3.5 (17)	92.1 (26)	17.2 (58)
(n = 18)	5.6 to 7.2	3.2 to 3.8	81.2 to 103	12.5 to 21.8
Special population:				
Moderate hepatic impairment	4.3 (37)	3.8 (34)	90.5 (27)	22.7 (30)
(n = 12)	3.4 to 5.2	3.1 to 4.5	76.9 to 104	18.9 to 26.5

[a] Calculated only up to 24 hours for M_1.

Contraindications

Sibutramine is contraindicated in patients receiving monoamine oxidase inhibitors (MAOIs).

Sibutramine is contraindicated in patients with hypersensitivity to sibutramine or any of the inactive ingredients of sibutramine.

Sibutramine is contraindicated in patients who have a major eating disorder (anorexia nervosa or bulimia nervosa).

Sibutramine is contraindicated in patients taking other centrally acting appetite suppressant drugs.

Warnings

➤*Blood pressure and pulse:* Sibutramine substantially increases blood pressure in some patients. Regular monitoring of blood pressure is required when prescribing sibutramine.

In placebo-controlled obesity studies, sibutramine 5 to 20 mg once daily was associated with mean increases in systolic and diastolic blood pressure of approximately 1 to 3 mm Hg relative to placebo, and with mean increases in pulse rate relative to placebo of approximately 4 to 5 beats per minute. Larger increases were seen in some patients, particularly when therapy with sibutramine was initiated at the higher doses. In premarketing placebo-controlled obesity studies, 0.4% of patients treated with sibutramine were discontinued for hypertension (SBP greater than or equal to 160 mm Hg or DBP greater than or equal to 95 mm Hg), compared with 0.4% in the placebo group, and 0.4% of patients with sibutramine hydrochloride monohydrate were discontinued for tachycardia (pulse rate greater than or equal to 100 bpm), compared with 0.1% in the placebo group. Blood pressure and pulse should be measured prior to starting therapy with sibutramine and should be monitored at regular intervals thereafter. For patients who experience a sustained increase in blood pressure or pulse rate while receiving sibutramine, either dose reduction or discontinuation should be considered. sibutramine should be given with caution to those patients with a history of hypertension, and should not be given to patients with uncontrolled or poorly controlled hypertension.

Percent outliers in studies 1 and 2			
	% Outliers*		
Dose (mg)	SBP	DBP	Pulse
Placebo	9	7	12
5 mg	8	20	16
10 mg	12	15	28
15 mg	13	17	24
20 mg	14	22	37

* Outlier defined as increase from baseline of greater than or equal to 15 mm Hg for 3 consecutive visits (SBP), greater than or equal to 10 mm Hg for 3 consecutive visits (DBP), or pulse greater than or equal to 10 bpm for 3 consecutive visits.

➤*Potential interaction with monoamine oxidase inhibitors:* Sibutramine is a norepinephrine, serotonin and dopamine reuptake inhibitor and should not be used concomitantly with MAOIs. There should be at least a 2-week interval after stopping MAOIs before commencing treatment with sibutramine. Similarly, there should be at least a 2-week interval after stopping sibutramine before starting treatment with MAOIs.

➤*Concomitant cardiovascular disease:* Treatment with sibutramine has been associated with increases in heart rate or blood pressure. Therefore, sibutramine should not be used in patients with a history of coronary artery disease, congestive heart failure, arrhythmias, or stroke.

➤*Glaucoma:* Because sibutramine can cause mydriasis, it should be used with caution in patients with narrow angle glaucoma.

➤*Miscellaneous:* Organic causes of obesity (eg, untreated hypothyroidism) should be excluded before prescribing sibutramine.

➤*Renal/Hepatic function impairment:* Patients with severe renal impairment or severe hepatic dysfunction have not been systematically studied; sibutramine should therefore not be used in such patients.

➤*Carcinogenesis:* Sibutramine was administered in the diet to mice (1.25, 5, or 20 mg/kg/day) and rats (1, 3, or 9 mg/kg/day) for 2 years generating combined maximum plasma AUC's of the 2 major active metabolites equivalent to 0.4 and 16 times, respectively, those following a daily human dose of 15 mg. There was no evidence of carcinogenicity in mice or in female rats. In male rats there was a higher incidence of benign tumors of the testicular interstitial cells; such tumors are commonly seen in rats and are hormonally mediated. The relevance of these tumors to humans is not known.

➤*Fertility impairment:* In rats, there were no effects on fertility at doses generating combined plasma AUCs of the 2 major active metabolites up to 32 times those following a human dose of 15 mg. At 13 times the human combined AUC, there was maternal toxicity, and the dam's nest-building behavior was impaired, leading to a higher incidence of perinatal mortality; there was no effect at approximately 4 times the human combined AUC.

➤*Elderly:* Clinical studies of sibutramine did not include sufficient numbers of patients aged 65 years and over to determine whether they respond differently from younger patients. In general, dose selection for an elderly patient should be cautious, reflecting the greater frequency of decreased hepatic, renal, or cardiac function, and of concomitant disease or other drug therapy.

➤*Pregnancy: Category C.*

Teratogenic – Radiolabeled studies in animals indicated that tissue distribution was unaffected by pregnancy, with relatively low transfer to the fetus. In rats, there was no evidence of teratogenicity at doses of 1, 3, or 10 mg/kg/day generating combined plasma AUCs of the 2 major active metabolites up to approximately 32 times those following the human dose of 15 mg. In rabbits dosed at 3, 15, or 75 mg/kg/day, plasma AUCs greater than approximately 5 times those following the human dose of 15 mg caused maternal toxicity. At markedly toxic doses, Dutch Belted rabbits had a slightly higher than control incidence of pups with a broad short snout, short rounded pinnae, short tail and, in some, shorter thickened long bones in the limbs; at comparably high doses in New Zealand white rabbits, 1 study showed a slightly higher than control incidence of pups with cardiovascular anomalies while a second study showed a lower incidence than in the control group.

No adequate and well-controlled studies with sibutramine have been conducted in pregnant women. The use of sibutramine during pregnancy is not recommended. Women of childbearing potential should employ adequate contraception while taking sibutramine. Patients should be advised to notify their physician if they become pregnant or intend to become pregnant during therapy.

➤*Lactation:* It is not known whether sibutramine or its metabolites are excreted in human milk. Sibutramine is not recommended for use in nursing mothers. Patients should be advised to notify their physician if they are breastfeeding.

➤*Children:* The safety and effectiveness of sibutramine in pediatric patients under 16 years of age have not been established.

Precautions

➤*Pulmonary hypertension:* Certain centrally acting weight loss agents that cause release of serotonin from nerve terminals have been associated with pulmonary hypertension (PPH), a rare but lethal disease. In premarketing clinical studies, no cases of PPH have been reported with sibutramine. Because of the low incidence of this disease in the underlying population, however, it is not known whether or not sibutramine may cause this disease.

➤*Special risk:*

Seizures – During premarketing testing, seizures were reported in less than 0.1% of sibutramine-treated patients. Sibutramine should be used cautiously in patients with a history of seizures. It should be discontinued in any patient who develops seizures.

Bleeding – There have been reports of bleeding in patients taking sibutramine. While a causal relationship is unclear, caution is advised in patients predisposed to bleeding events and those taking concomitant medications known to affect hemostasis or platelet function.

Gallstones – Weight loss can precipitate or exacerbate gallstone formation.

➤*Drug abuse and dependence:*

Controlled substance – Sibutramine is a controlled substance in Schedule IV of the Controlled Substances Act (CSA).

Abuse and physical and psychological dependence – Physicians should carefully evaluate patients for history of drug abuse and follow such patients closely, observing them for signs of misuse or abuse (eg, development of tolerance, incrementation of doses, drug seeking behavior).

➤*Hazardous tasks:*

Interference with cognitive and motor performance – Although sibutramine did not affect psychomotor or cognitive performance in healthy volunteers, any CNS active drug has the potential to impair judgment, thinking or motor skills.

SIBUTRAMINE HYDROCHLORIDE MONOHYDRATE — ORAL

Drug Interactions

➤*CYP450 system:* In vitro studies indicated that the cytochrome P4503A4-mediated metabolism of sibutramine was inhibited by ketoconazole and to a lesser extent by erythromycin. Clinical interaction trials were conducted on these substrates. The potential for such interactions is described below.

Sibutramine Drug Interactions

Precipitant drug	Object drug*		Description
Alcohol	Sibutramine	↑	Concomitant use of sibutramine and excess alcohol is not recommended.
Cimetidine	Sibutramine	↔	Concomitant administration resulted in small increases in combined sibutramine metabolites (M_1 and M_2), plasma C_{max} (3.4%), and AUC (7.3%); these differences are unlikely to be of clinical significance.
Erythromycin	Sibutramine	↔	Concomitant erythromycin resulted in small increases in sibutramine metabolites' AUC (less than 14%) for M_1 and M_2. A small reduction in C_{max} for M_1 (11%) and a slight increase in C_{max} for M_2 (10%) were observed.
Ketoconazole	Sibutramine	↔	Concomitant administration resulted in moderate increases in sibutramine metabolites' AUC and C_{max} of 58% and 36% for M_1 and of 20% and 19% for M_2, respectively.
Sibutramine	Agents that may raise blood pressure or increase heart rate (see Description)	↑	These agents include decongestants, cough, cold, and allergy products that contain agents such as ephedrine or pseudoephedrine. Use caution when using concurrently with sibutramine. See Warnings.
Sibutramine	CNS-active drugs	↑	Caution is advised if the concomitant administration of sibutramine with other centrally acting drugs is indicated. See Warnings.
Sibutramine	MAOIs (eg, phenelzine, selegiline, tranylcypromine)	↑	In patients receiving MAOIs in combination with serotonergic agents (eg, fluoxetine, fluvoxamine, paroxetine, sertraline, venlafaxine), there have been reports of serious, sometimes fatal, reactions ("serotonin syndrome"; see Warnings). Because sibutramine inhibits serotonin reuptake, it should not be used concomitantly with an MAOI. At least 2 weeks should elapse between discontinuation of an MAOI and initiation of treatment with sibutramine. Similarly, ≥ 2 weeks should elapse between discontinuation of therapy and initiation of treatment with an MAOI.
Sibutramine	SSRIs, ergot alkaloids (eg, dihydroergotamine), lithium, certain opioids (eg, dextromethorphan, meperidine, pentazocine, fentanyl), 5-HT_1 receptor agonists (eg, sumatriptan, zolmitriptan), tryptophan	↑	The serotonergic effects of these agents may be additive. A "serotonin syndrome" may occur (see Warnings). Concomitant administration of these agents is not recommended. Carefully monitor patients if concurrent use cannot be avoided.

* ↑ = Object drug increased. ↔ = Undetermined clinical effect.

➤*Drug/Food interactions:* Administration of a single 20 mg dose of sibutramine with a standard breakfast resulted in reduced peak M_1 and M_2 concentrations (by 27% and 32%, respectively) and delayed the time to peak by ≈ 3 hours. However, the AUCs of M_1 and M_2 were not significantly altered.

Adverse Reactions

In placebo-controlled studies, the most common reactions were dry mouth, anorexia, insomnia, constipation, and headache. Adverse reactions in these studies occurring in greater than or equal to 1% of sibutramine treated patients and more frequently than in the placebo group are shown in the following data.

Obese patients in placebo-controlled studies

Body system/adverse reaction	Sibutramine (n = 2,068) % incidence	Placebo (n = 884) % incidence
Miscellaneous		
Headache	30.3%	18.6%
Back pain	8.2%	5.5%
Flu syndrome	8.2%	5.8%
Injury accident	5.9%	4.1%
Asthenia	5.9%	5.3%
Abdominal pain	4.5%	3.6%
Chest pain	1.8%	1.2%
Neck pain	1.6%	1.1%
Allergic reaction	1.5%	0.8%
Cardiovascular		
Tachycardia	2.6%	0.6%
Vasodilation	2.4%	0.9%
Migraine	2.4%	2%
Hypertension/Increased blood pressure	2.1%	0.9%
Palpitation	2%	0.8%
GI		
Anorexia	13%	3.5%
Constipation	11.5%	6%
Increased appetite	8.7%	2.7%
Nausea	5.9%	2.8%
Dyspepsia	5%	2.6%
Gastritis	1.7%	1.2%
Vomiting	1.5%	1.4%
Rectal disorder	1.2%	0.5%
Metabolic/Nutritional		
Thirst	1.7%	0.9%
Generalized edema	1.2%	0.8%
Musculoskeletal		
Arthralgia	5.9%	5%
Myalgia	1.9%	1.1%
Tenosynovitis	1.2%	0.5%
Joint disorder	1.1%	0.6%
CNS		
Dry mouth	17.2%	4.2%
Insomnia	10.7%	4.5%
Dizziness	7%	3.4%
Nervousness	5.2%	2.9%
Anxiety	4.5%	3.4%
Depression	4.3%	2.5%
Paresthesia	2%	0.5%
Somnolence	1.7%	0.9%
CNS stimulation	1.5%	0.5%
Emotional lability	1.3%	0.6%
Respiratory		
Rhinitis	10.2%	7.1%
Pharyngitis	10%	8.4%
Sinusitis	5%	2.6%
Cough increased	3.8%	3.3%
Laryngitis	1.3%	0.9%

SIBUTRAMINE HYDROCHLORIDE MONOHYDRATE — ORAL

Obese patients in placebo-controlled studies		
Body system/adverse reaction	Sibutramine (n = 2,068) % incidence	Placebo (n = 884) % incidence
Dermatologic		
Rash	3.8%	2.5%
Sweating	2.5%	0.9%
Herpes simplex	1.3%	1%
Acne	1%	0.8%
Special senses		
Taste perversion	2.2%	0.8%
Ear disorder	1.7%	0.9%
Ear pain	1.1%	0.7%
GU		
Dysmenorrhea	3.5%	1.4%
Urinary tract infection	2.3%	2%
Vaginal monilia	1.2%	0.5%
Metrorrhagia	1%	0.8%

➤*Premarketing studies:* The following adverse events were reported in greater than or equal to 1% of all patients who received sibutramine in controlled and uncontrolled premarketing studies.

CNS – Agitation, leg cramps, hypertonia, abnormal thinking.

Dermatologic – Pruritus.

GI – Diarrhea, flatulence, gastroenteritis, tooth disorder.

GU – Menstrual disorder.

Metabolic/Nutritional – Peripheral edema.

Musculoskeletal – Arthritis.

Respiratory – Bronchitis, dyspnea.

Special senses – Amblyopia.

Miscellaneous – Fever.

➤*Other adverse events (clinical studies):*

Seizures – Convulsions were reported as an adverse event in 3 of 2,068 (0.1%) sibutramine-treated patients and in none of 884 placebo-treated patients in placebo-controlled premarketing obesity studies. Two of the 3 patients with seizures had potentially predisposing factors (1 had a history of epilepsy; 1 had a subsequent diagnosis of brain tumor). The incidence in all subjects who received sibutramine (3 of 4,588 subjects) was less than 0.1%.

Ecchymosis/bleeding disorders – Ecchymosis (bruising) was observed in 0.7% of sibutramine-treated patients and in 0.2% of placebo-treated patients in premarketing placebo-controlled obesity studies. One patient had prolonged bleeding of a small amount which occurred during minor facial surgery. Sibutramine may have an effect on platelet function due to its effect on serotonin uptake.

Interstitial nephritis – Acute interstitial nephritis (confirmed by biopsy) was reported in 1 obese patient receiving sibutramine during premarketing studies. After discontinuation of the medication, dialysis and oral corticosteroids were administered; renal function normalized. The patient made a full recovery.

Altered laboratory findings – Abnormal liver function tests, including increases in AST, ALT, GGT, LDH, alkaline phosphatase and bilirubin, were reported as adverse events in 1.6% of sibutramine-treated obese patients in placebo-controlled trials compared with 0.8% of placebo patients. In these studies, potentially clinically significant values (total bilirubin greater than or equal to 2 mg/dL; ALT, AST, GGT, LDH, or alkaline phosphatase greater than or equal to 3 times the upper limit of normal) occurred in 0% (alkaline phosphatase) to 0.6% (ALT) of the sibutramine-treated patients and in none of the placebo-treated patients. Abnormal values tended to be sporadic, often diminished with continued treatment, and did not show a clear dose-response relationship.

➤*Postmarketing reports:* Voluntary reports of adverse events temporally associated with the use of sibutramine are listed below. It is important to emphasize that although these events occurred during treatment with sibutramine, they may have no causal relationship with the drug. Obesity itself, concurrent disease states/risk factors, or weight reduction may be associated with an increased risk for some of these events.

Hypersensitivity – Allergic hypersensitivity reactions ranging from mild skin eruptions and urticaria to angioedema and anaphylaxis have been reported.

Psychiatric – Cases of depression, suicidal ideation, and suicide have been reported rarely in patients on sibutramine treatment. However, a relationship has not been established between the occurrence of depression or suicidal ideation and the use of sibutramine. If depression occurs during treatment with sibutramine, further evaluation may be necessary.

Miscellaneous – Abnormal dreams, abnormal ejaculation, abnormal gait, abnormal vision, alopecia, amnesia, anaphylactic shock, anaphylactoid reaction, anemia, anger, angina pectoris, arthrosis, atrial fibrillation, blurred vision, bursitis, cerebrovascular accident, chest pressure, chest tightness, cholecystitis, cholelithiasis, concentration impaired, confusion, congestive heart failure, depression aggravated, dermatitis, dry eye, duodenal ulcer, epistaxis, eructation, eye pain, facial edema, gastrointestinal hemorrhage, Gilles de la Tourette's syndrome, goiter, heart arrest, heart rate decreased, hematuria, hyperglycemia, hyperthyroidism, hypesthesia, hypoglycemia, hypothyroidism, impotence, increased intraocular pressure, increased salivation, increased urinary frequency, intestinal obstruction, leukopenia, libido decreased, libido increased, limb pain, lymphadenopathy, manic reaction, micturition difficulty, mood changes, mouth ulcer, myocardial infarction, nasal congestion, nightmares, otitis externa, otitis media, petechiae, photosensitivity (eyes), photosensitivity (skin), respiratory disorder, serotonin syndrome, short-term memory loss, speech disorder, stomach ulcer, sudden unexplained death, supraventricular tachycardia, syncope, thrombocytopenia, tinnitus, tongue edema, torsade de pointes, transient ischemic attack, tremor, twitch, urinary retention, urticaria, vascular headache, ventricular tachycardia, ventricular extrasystoles, ventricular fibrillation, vertigo, yawn.

Overdosage

➤*Symptoms:* There is very limited experience of overdose with sibutramine. Three cases of overdose have been reported with sibutramine. The first was in a 2-year-old child of 1 patient who ingested up to eight 10 mg capsules. No complications were observed during the overnight hospitalization, and the child was discharged the following day with no sequelae. The second report was in a 30-year-old male in a depression study who ingested approximately 100 mg of sibutramine in an attempt to commit suicide. The patient suffered no adverse effects or ECG abnormalities postingestion. The third report was in the 45-year-old husband of a patient in an obese dyslipidemic study. He ingested 400 mg of his wife's drug supply and was hospitalized for observation; a heart rate of 120 bpm was noted. He was discharged the next day with no apparent sequelae.

➤*Treatment:* There is no specific antidote to sibutramine. Treatment should consist of general measures employed in the management of overdosage: An airway should be established; cardiac and vital sign monitoring is recommended; general symptomatic and supportive measures should be instituted. Cautious use of beta blockers may be indicated to control elevated blood pressure or tachycardia. The benefits of forced diuresis and hemodialysis are unknown.

Patient Information

Patients should be advised to notify their physicians if they develop a rash, hives, or other allergic reactions.

Patients should be advised to inform their physicians if they are taking, or plan to take, any prescription or over-the-counter drugs, especially weight-reducing agents, decongestants, antidepressants, cough suppressants, lithium, dihydroergotamine, sumatriptan, or tryptophan, since there is a potential for interactions.

Patients should be reminded of the importance of having their blood pressure and pulse monitored at regular intervals.

WARNING

Fentanyl transmucosal – Oral transmucosal fentanyl is indicated only for the management of breakthrough cancer pain in patients with malignancies already receiving and tolerant of opioid therapy for their underlying persistent cancer pain. Patients considered opioid tolerant are those who are taking morphine 60 mg/day or more, transdermal fentanyl 50 mcg/h, or an equianalgesic dose of another opioid for a week or longer. It is contraindicated in the management of acute or postoperative pain. Because life-threatening hypoventilation could occur at any dose in patients not taking chronic opiates, do not use in opioid nontolerant patients. Use only in the care of cancer patients and only by oncologists and pain specialists who are knowledgeable of and skilled in the use of schedule II opioids to treat cancer pain. Instruct patients and their caregivers that this drug contains a medicine in an amount that can be fatal to a child. Keep all units out of reach of children, and discard opened units properly.

Fentanyl transdermal system – Fentanyl transdermal systems contain a high concentration of the potent schedule II opioid agonist, fentanyl. Schedule II opioid substances have the highest potential for abuse and associated risk of fatal overdose due to respiratory depression. Fentanyl can be abused and is subject to criminal diversion. The high content of fentanyl in the patches may be a particular target for abuse and diversion.

Fentanyl transdermal system is indicated for management of persistent, moderate to severe chronic pain that:

- requires continuous, around-the-clock opioid administration for an extended period of time, and
- cannot be managed by other means such as nonsteroidal analgesics, opioid combination products, or immediate-release (IR) opioids.

Fentanyl transdermal system should only be used in patients who are already receiving opioid therapy, who have demonstrated opioid tolerance, and who require a total daily dose at least equivalent to fentanyl transdermal system 25 mcg/h. Patients who are considered opioid-tolerant are those who have been taking, for a week or longer, morphine 60 mg/day or more, or oral oxycodone 30 mg/day or more, or oral hydromorphone 8 mg/day or more, or an equianalgesic dose of another opioid.

Because serious or life-threatening hypoventilation could occur, fentanyl transdermal is contraindicated:

- in patients who are not opioid tolerant
- in the management of acute pain or in patients who require opioid analgesia for a short period of time
- in the management of postoperative pain, including use after outpatient or day surgeries (eg, tonsillectomies)
- in the management of mild pain.
- in the management of intermittent pain (eg, use on an as-needed basis).

Because the peak fentanyl levels occur between 24 and 72 hours of treatment, prescribers should be aware that serious or life-threatening hypoventilation may occur, even in opioid-tolerant patients, during the initial application period. The concomitant use of fentanyl transdermal system with potent cytochrome P450 3A4 inhibitors (ritonavir, ketoconazole, itraconazole, troleandomycin, clarithromycin, nelfinavir, and nefazodone) may result in an increase in fentanyl plasma concentrations, which could increase or prolong adverse drug effects and may cause potentially fatal respiratory depression. Carefully monitor patients receiving fentanyl transdermal system and potent CYP3A4 inhibitors for an extended period of time and make dosage adjustments if warranted.

Do not administer fentanyl transdermal system to children younger than 2 years of age. Administer to children only if they are opioid tolerant and 2 years of age or older.

Fentanyl transdermal system is only for use in patients who are already tolerant to opioid therapy of comparable potency. Use in nonopioid-tolerant patients may lead to fatal respiratory depression. Overestimating the fentanyl transdermal system dose when converting patients from another opioid medication can result in fatal overdose with the first dose. Due to the mean elimination half-life of 17 hours of fentanyl transdermal system, patients who are thought to have had a serious adverse event, including overdose, will require monitoring and treatment for at least 24 hours.

Fentanyl transdermal system can be abused in a manner similar to other opioid agonists, legal or illicit. Consider this risk when administering, prescribing, or dispensing in situations where there is concern about increased risk of misuse, abuse, or diversion.

Fentanyl transdermal patches are intended for transdermal use (on intact skin) only. Using damaged or cut fentanyl transdermal patches can lead to the rapid release of the contents of the fentanyl transdermal patch and absorption of a potentially fatal dose of fentanyl.

Hydromorphone –

High potency (HP) injection: HP injection is a highly concentrated solution of hydromorphone intended for use in opioid-tolerant patients. Do not confuse HP injection with standard parenteral formulations of injection or other opioids. Overdose and death could result.

WARNING (cont.)

Extended-release (ER) capsules: Hydromorphone ER capsules are indicated for the management of persistent moderate to severe pain in patients requiring continuous, around-the-clock analgesia with a high potency opioid for an extended period of time (weeks to months) or longer. Use ER capsules only in patients who are already receiving opioid therapy, have demonstrated opioid tolerance, and require a minimum total daily dose of opiate medication equivalent to oral hydromorphone 12 mg. Patients considered opioid tolerant are those taking oral morphine 60 mg/day or more, oral oxycodone 30 mg/day or more, oral hydromorphone 8 mg/day or more, or an equianalgesic dose of another opioid, for a week or longer. Administer ER capsules once every 24 hours.

Appropriate patients for treatment with ER capsules include patients who require high doses of potent opioids on an around-the-clock basis to improve pain control and patients who have difficulty attaining adequate analgesia with IR opioid formulations. ER capsules are contraindicated for use on an as-needed basis.

ER capsules are not intended to be used as the first opioid product prescribed for a patient or in patients who require opioid analgesia for a short period of time.

ER capsules are for opioid-tolerant patients only. Use in nonopioid-tolerant patients may lead to fatal respiratory depression. Overestimating the ER capsule dose when converting patients from another opioid medication can result in fatal overdose with the first dose. Because of the mean apparent 18-hour elimination half-life of ER capsules, patients who receive an overdose will require an extended period of monitoring and treatment that may go beyond 18 hours. Even in the face of improvement, continued medical monitoring is required because of the possibility of extended effects.

Schedule II opioid agonists (eg, hydromorphone, fentanyl, methadone, morphine, oxycodone, oxymorphone) have the highest risk of fatal overdoses because of respiratory depression, as well as the highest potential for abuse. ER capsules can be abused in a manner similar to other opioid agonists, legal or illicit. Consider these risks when administering, prescribing, or dispensing ER capsules in situations where there is concern about increased risk of misuse, abuse, or diversion.

People at increased risk for opioid abuse include those with a personal or family history of substance abuse (including drug or alcohol abuse or addiction) or mental illness (eg, major depression). Assess patients for clinical risks for opioid abuse or addiction prior to prescribing opioids. Routinely monitor all patients receiving opioids for signs of misuse, abuse, and addiction. Patients at increased risk of opioid abuse may still be appropriately treated with modified-release opioid formulations; however, these patients will require intensive monitoring for signs of misuse, abuse, or addiction.

ER capsules are to be swallowed whole, not broken, chewed, opened, dissolved, or crushed. Taking broken, chewed, dissolved, or crushed ER capsules or capsule contents can lead to the rapid release and absorption of a potentially fatal dose of hydromorphone. Overestimating the ER capsule dose when converting the patient from another opioid medication can result in fatal overdose with the first dose. With the long half-life of ER capsules (18 hours), patients who receive the wrong dose will require an extended period of monitoring and treatment that may go beyond 18 hours. Even in the face of improvement, continued medical monitoring is required because of the possibility of extended effects.

Methadone – To treat narcotic addiction in detoxification or maintenance programs, methadone should be dispensed only by hospitals, community pharmacies, and maintenance programs approved by the FDA and designated state authorities. Approved maintenance programs shall dispense and use methadone in oral form only and according to treatment requirements stipulated in *Federal Methadone Regulations*. Failure to abide by the requirements in these regulations may result in criminal prosecution, seizure of drug supply, revocation of program approval, and injunction precluding program operation.

Methadone, used as an analgesic, may be dispensed in any licensed pharmacy.

Methadone dispersible tablets are for oral administration only. This preparation contains insoluble excipients and therefore must not be injected. It is recommended that methadone dispersible tablets, if dispensed, be packaged in child-resistant containers and kept out of the reach of children to prevent accidental ingestion.

Cardiac conduction effects: Laboratory studies, in vivo and in vitro, have demonstrated that methadone inhibits cardiac potassium channels and prolongs the QT interval. Cases of QT interval prolongation and serious arrhythmia (torsades de pointes) have been observed during treatment with methadone. These cases appear to be more commonly associated with, but not limited to, higher dose treatment (greater than 200 mg/day). Most cases involve patients being treated for pain with large, multiple daily doses of methadone, although cases have been reported in patients receiving doses commonly used for maintenance treatment of opioid addiction.

WARNING (cont.)

Morphine –

Avinza: Avinza capsules are a modified-release formulation of morphine sulfate indicated for once-daily administration for the relief of moderate to severe pain requiring continuous, around-the-clock opioid therapy for an extended period of time. *Avinza* capsules are to be swallowed whole or the contents of the capsules sprinkled on applesauce. The capsule beads are not to be chewed, crushed, or dissolved due to the risk of rapid release and absorption of a potentially fatal dose of morphine.

Astromorph PF, Duramorph, Infumorph: Because of the risk of severe adverse effects when the epidural or intrathecal route of administration is employed, patients must be observed in a fully equipped and staffed environment for at least 24 hours after the initial dose.

Infumorph: Infumorph is not recommended for single-dose intravenous (IV), intramuscular (IM), or subcutaneous administration because of the very large amount of morphine in the ampul and the associated risk of overdosage.

Oxycodone – Controlled-release (CR) oxycodone is an opioid agonist and a schedule II controlled substance with an abuse liability similar to morphine.

Oxycodone can be abused in a manner similar to other opioid agonists, legal or illicit. Consider this when prescribing or dispensing oxycodone CR tablets in situations where there is concern about an increased risk of misuse, abuse, or diversion.

Oxycodone CR tablets are indicated for the management of moderate to severe pain when a continuous, around-the-clock analgesic is needed for an extended period of time.

Oxycodone CR tablets are not intended for use as an as-needed analgesic.

Oxycodone 80 and 160 mg CR tablets are for use in opioid-tolerant patients only. These tablet strengths may cause fatal respiratory depression when administered to patients not previously exposed to opioids.

Oxycodone CR tablets are to be swallowed whole and are not to be broken, chewed, or crushed. Taking broken, chewed, or crushed oxycodone CR tablets leads to rapid release and absorption of a potentially fatal dose of oxycodone.

Propoxyphene –

Fatalities:

- Do not prescribe propoxyphene for patients who are suicidal or addiction-prone.
- Prescribe propoxyphene with caution for patients taking tranquilizers or antidepressant drugs and patients who use alcohol in excess.
- Tell patients not to exceed the recommended dose and to limit alcohol intake.

Propoxyphene products in excessive doses, either alone or in combination with other CNS depressants (including alcohol), are a major cause of drug-related deaths. Fatalities within the first hour of overdosage are not uncommon. In a survey of deaths due to overdosage conducted in 1975, in approximately 20% of fatal cases, death occurred within the first hour (5% within 15 minutes). Propoxyphene should not be taken in higher doses than those recommended by the health care provider. Judicious prescribing of propoxyphene is essential for safety. Consider nonnarcotic analgesics for depressed or suicidal patients. Do not prescribe propoxyphene for suicidal or addiction-prone patients. Caution patients about the concomitant use of propoxyphene products and alcohol because of potentially serious CNS-additive effects of these agents. Because of added CNS depressant effects, cautiously prescribe with concomitant sedatives, tranquilizers, muscle relaxants, antidepressants, or other CNS-depressant drugs. Advise patients of the additive depressant effects of these combinations.

Many propoxyphene-related deaths have occurred in patients with histories of emotional disturbances, suicidal ideation or attempts, or misuse of tranquilizers, alcohol, and other CNS-active drugs. Deaths have occurred as a consequence of the accidental ingestion of excessive quantities of propoxyphene alone or in combination with other drugs. Do not exceed the recommended dosage.

Indications

Opioid Analgesic Indications

Drug	Analgesia	Anesthesia	Cough	Diarrhea	Detoxification
Alfentanil	✓	✓			
Codeine	✓		✓[a]		
Fentanyl injection	✓	✓			
Fentanyl transdermal	✓				
Fentanyl transmucosal	✓				
Hydrocodone	✓[a]		✓[a]		
Hydromorphone	✓				
Levorphanol	✓				
Meperidine	✓	✓			
Methadone	✓				✓
Morphine sulfate	✓	✓			
Opium				✓	
Oxycodone	✓				
Oxymorphone	✓	✓			
Propoxyphene	✓				
Remifentanil	✓	✓			
Sufentanil	✓	✓			
Tramadol	✓				

[a] Currently only available for this indication when part of a multi-ingredient product.

➤*Oxymorphone:* Oxymorphone is also indicated for relief of anxiety in patients with dyspnea associated with pulmonary edema secondary to acute left ventricular dysfunction.

Refer to individual product listings for specific indications.

Administration and Dosage

With any potent opioid drug product, it is critical to adjust the dosing regimen for each patient individually, taking into account the patient's prior analgesic treatment experience. Although it is clearly impossible to enumerate every consideration that is important to the selection of initial dose and dosing interval, consider the following:

- the daily dose, potency, and precise characteristics of the opioid the patient has been taking previously (eg, whether it is a pure agonist or mixed agonist/antagonist, elimination half-life);
- the reliability of the relative potency estimate used to calculate the dose of morphine needed (potency estimates may vary with the route of administration);
- the degree of opioid tolerance, if any; and
- the general condition and medical status of the patient.

The following equianalgesic dosing table is based on parenteral **morphine** 10 mg. Dosage adjustments may be needed if the elimination half-life of the new opioid differs from the current opioid (see Pharmacokinetics).

Approximate Equianalgesic Dosing of Opioid Analgesics in Adults[a,b]

Opioid	Equianalgesic dose: Oral	Parenteral (IM, subcutaneous, IV)	Rectal
Codeine	200 mg	120 to 130 mg	NA[c]
Fentanyl[d]	NA	0.1 mg	NA
Hydrocodone	30 mg	NA	NA
Hydromorphone	7.5 mg	1.5 mg	3 mg
Levorphanol	4 mg	2 mg	NA
Meperidine	300 mg	75 mg	NA
Methadone	10 to 20 mg	5 to 10 mg	NA
Morphine	60 mg single dose, 30 mg repeated doses	10 mg	ND[e]
Oxycodone	20 to 30 mg	NA	NA
Oxymorphone	NA	1 mg	10 mg

[a] Table is to be used for estimation only. Data are compiled from multiple references and may be based on single-dose studies.
[b] Caution: Recommended doses do not apply for adult patients with body weight less than 50 kg. Recommended doses do not apply to patients with renal or hepatic insufficiency or other conditions affecting drug metabolism and kinetics. Starting doses should be lower for elderly patients.
[c] NA = Not available commercially for this route of administration.
[d] Refer to Fentanyl Transdermal monograph for dosing conversion.
[e] ND = No data.

Actions

➤*Pharmacology:* The precise mechanism of analgesic action of narcotic or opioid analgesics is unknown. They have affinity for the opioid μ-receptor located in the brain, spinal cord, and smooth muscle.

Narcotic analgesics are classified as full agonists, mixed agonist-antagonists, or partial agonists by their activity at opioid receptors. There are 3 major classes of opioid receptors in the CNS, designated mu (μ), kappa (κ), and delta (δ). Opiate receptors in the CNS mediate analgesic activity. Narcotic agonists occupy the same receptors as endogenous opioid peptides (enkephalins or endorphins), and both may alter the central release of neurotransmitters from afferent nerves sensitive to noxious stimuli.

Consequences of the μ-receptor activation include analgesia, respiratory depression, miosis, reduced GI motility, and euphoria. κ receptors act primarily in the spinal cord and cause analgesia, dysphoria, and psychotomimetic effects. They also cause less intense miosis and respiratory depression than μ-receptor activation. The consequence of δ-receptor stimulation in human beings is unclear. Morphine-like narcotic agonists have activity at the μ, κ, and δ receptors. Opioid agonists include natural opium alkaloids (eg, **morphine, codeine**), semisynthetic analogs (eg, **hydromorphone, oxymorphone, oxycodone**), and synthetic compounds (eg, **methadone, sufentanil, fentanyl, levorphanol, tramadol**).

Tramadol and its active metabolite (M1) appear to bind to μ-opioid receptors and weakly inhibit reuptake of norepinephrine and serotonin.

Mixed *agonist-antagonist* drugs (eg, nalbuphine, pentazocine) have agonist activity at some receptors and antagonist activity at other receptors; also included are the *partial agonists* (eg, butorphanol, buprenorphine) (see the Narcotic Agonist-Antagonist Analgesics group monograph).

Narcotic antagonists – Narcotic antagonists (eg, naloxone) do not have agonist activity at any of the opioid receptor sites (see individual monographs). Antagonists block the opiate receptor, inhibit pharmacological activity of the agonist, and precipitate withdrawal in dependent patients.

Secondary pharmacological effects – The narcotics have a variety of secondary pharmacological effects, including the following:

Cardiovascular: Peripheral vasodilation, reduced peripheral resistance, and inhibition of baroreceptors. Orthostatic hypotension and fainting may occur when the patient sits up.

CNS: Euphoria, drowsiness, apathy, mental confusion, alterations in mood, reduction in body temperature, feelings of relaxation, dysphoria, pupillary constriction. Nausea and vomiting are caused by direct stimulation of the emetic chemoreceptors located in the medulla. **Hydromorphone** increases cerebrospinal (CSF) pressure.

Dermatologic: Histamine release, pruritus, flushing, and red eyes.

Endocrine: Opioid agonists have been shown to have a variety of effects on the secretion of hormones. Opioids inhibit the secretion of adrenocorticotropic hormone, cortisol, and luteinizing hormone in humans. They also stimulate prolactin, growth hormone secretion, and pancreatic secretion of insulin and glucagon in humans and other species, rats, and dogs. Thyroid-stimulating hormone has been shown to be both inhibited and stimulated by opioids.

GI:

- *Stomach* – Decreases gastric motility, thus prolonging gastric emptying time. This may lead to esophageal reflux.
- *Small intestine* – Decreases biliary, pancreatic, and intestinal secretions and delays digestion of food in the small intestine. Resting tone increases and periodic spasms occur.
- *Large intestine* – Propulsive peristaltic waves in the colon are diminished and tone increases until it spasms. This, along with the inattention to the normal stimuli for defecation reflex, contribute to constipation.
- *Biliary tract* – The sphincter of Oddi constricts leading to epigastric distress or biliary colic.

GU: Increases smooth muscle tone in the urinary tract and can induce spasms. Urinary urgency and difficulty with urination may result.

Respiratory: Depressant effects first diminish tidal volume, then respiratory rate, because of reduced sensitivity of the respiratory center to carbon dioxide.

- *Cough* – Suppresses cough reflex by direct effect on cough center in the medulla.

Miscellaneous: **Hydromorphone** causes transient hyperglycemia; **codeine** causes release of antidiuretic hormone.

Comparative pharmacology is summarized below. Consider these comparisons as approximations that may vary widely among patients.

Opioid Analgesics Comparative Pharmacology[a]

Drug	Analgesic	Antitussive	Constipation	Respiratory depression	Sedation	Emesis	Physical dependence
Phenanthrenes							
Codeine	+*	+++	+	+	+	+	+
Hydrocodone	++	+++	nd[b]	nd	nd	nd	++
Hydromorphone	++	++	+	++	+	+	++
Levorphanol	++	++	nd	++	++	+	++
Morphine	++	++	++	++	++	++	++
Oxycodone	++	+++	++	++	++	++	++
Oxymorphone	++	+	+++	+++	nd	+++	+++
Phenylpiperidines							
Fentanyl	++	nd	nd	+	nd	+	nd
Meperidine	++	nd	+	++	+	nd	++
Diphenylheptanes							
Methadone	++	++	+	++	+	+	+
Propoxyphene	+	nd	nd	+	+	+	+

* + = degree of activity from the least (+) to the greatest (+++).
[a] Table adapted from Catalano RB. The medical approach to management of pain caused by cancer. *Semin Oncol.* 1975;2:379-392.
[b] nd – No data available.

➤*Pharmacokinetics:* Administration IV is most reliable and rapid; IM or subcutaneous use may delay absorption and peak effect. Many agents undergo a significant first-pass effect.

Opioid Analgesic Pharmacokinetics

Drug	Onset of effect	Peak effect	Duration of effect	Elimination $t_{½}$	Vd (L/kg)	Protein binding (%)	Metabolism pathway	Active metabolites	Major excretion pathway
Alfentanil	immediate	1.5 to 2 min	< 10 min	1.5 to 1.85 h	0.4 to 1	92%	liver	—	urine
Codeine	Oral: 10 to 30 min, IV: 15 min	0.5 to 1 h	Oral: 4 to 6 h, IV: 5 h	2.5 to 3 h	—	—	liver	Morphine	urine
Fentanyl injection	IV: immediate, IM: 7 to 8 min	—	IV: 0.5 to 1 h, IM: 1 to 2 h	3.65 h	4	Alters with increasing ionization	liver	—	urine
Fentanyl transdermal	—	24 to 72 h	72 h	≈ 17 h	6	Decreases with increasing ionization	liver: CYP3A4	—	urine
Fentanyl transmucosal	—	—	—	7 h	4	80% to 85%	liver: CYP3A4	—	urine
Hydromorphone	IM/Subcutaneous: 15 min, Oral: 30 min	0.5 to 1 h	IR: 4 to 5 h, ER: 24 h, IM/Subcutaneous: 4 to 5 h	IR: 2.3 h, ER: 18.6 h, IM/Subcutaneous: 2.6 h	≈ 4	8% to 20%	liver: glucuronidation	—	urine
Levorphanol	IM: 15 to 30 min	Oral: 1 h	—	IV: 11 to 16 h	IV: 10 to 13	40%	—	—	—
Meperidine	—	—	2 to 4 h	3 to 6 (parent), < 20 h (normeperidine)		60% to 80%	liver	normeperidine	—
Methadone	Parenteral: 10 to 20 min, Oral: 30 to 60 min	—	4 h	8 to 59 h	2 to 6	85% to 90%	liver: primarily CYP3A4 and to lesser extent CYP2D6	—	urine and fecal
Morphine sulfate	IM/Subcutaneous: 10 to 30 min	Epidural: 10 to 15 min, Oral: 1 h	Subcutaneous/IM: 4 to 5 h	1.5 to 2 h	1 to 6	20% to 35%	liver: glucuronidation	morphine-6-glucuronide	urine
Oxycodone	within 60 min	—	IR: 3 to 4 h, CR[a]: 12 h	IR: 3.2 h, CR: 4.5 h	2.6	45%	liver: somewhat involves CYP2D6	noroxycodone and oxymorphone	urine

Opioid Analgesic Pharmacokinetics									
Drug	Onset of effect	Peak effect	Duration of effect	Elimination t½	Vd (L/kg)	Protein binding (%)	Metabolism pathway	Active metabolites	Major excretion pathway
Oxymorphone	Parenteral: 5 to 10 min	—	Parenteral: 3 to 6 h	1.3 h	≈ 3	—	liver	—	urine
Propoxyphene	—	2 to 2.5 h	—	6 to 12 h (parent), 30 to 36 h (norpropoxyphene)	—	80%	liver	norpropoxyphene	urine
Remifentanil	rapid	—	—	10 to 20 min	0.35	70%	hydrolysis by esterases	—	urine
Sufentanil	IV: immediate, Epidural: 10 min[b]	—	Epidural: 1.7 h[b]	2.7 h	—	91% to 93%, 79% in neonates	liver and small intestine	—	—
Tramadol	—	—	2 h (tramadol), 3 h (M1, active metabolite)	6.3 h (tramadol), 7.4 h (M1, active metabolite)	2.6 to 2.9	20%	liver: CYP2D6 and CYP3A4	O-desmethyltramadol (M1) via CYP2D6	urine

[a] CR = controlled-release

[b] With bupivacaine.

Special populations –

Elderly:

• *Alfentanil* – Patients older than 65 years of age have reduced plasma clearance and increased elimination half-life, which may prolong postoperative recovery.

• *Fentanyl* – Clearance may be greatly decreased.

• *Hydromorphone* – Age related increases in exposure have been observed. Greater sensitivity of older individuals cannot be excluded. Adjust dosages according to clinical situation.

• *Meperidine* – Elderly patients have a slower elimination rate compared with younger patients.

• *Morphine* – Elderly patients may have reduced clearance.

• *Oxycodone* – Plasma levels are approximately 15% greater in elderly patients versus young patients.

• *Remifentanil* – The clearance of remifentanil is reduced (approximately 25%) in the elderly (older than 65 years of age) compared with young adults (average 25 years of age). However, remifentanil blood concentrations fall as rapidly after termination of administration in the elderly as in young adults.

• *Tramadol* – In subjects older than 75 years of age, maximum serum concentrations are elevated (208 vs 162 ng/mL) and the elimination half-life is prolonged (7 vs 6 hours) compared with subjects 65 to 75 years of age. Adjustment of the daily dose is recommended for patients older than 75 years of age.

Gender:

• *Oxycodone* – Females exhibit plasma levels up to 25% higher than males on a body weight adjusted basis. The cause of this difference is unknown.

• *Tramadol* – The absolute bioavailability of tramadol was 73% in males and 79% in females. The plasma clearance was 6.4 mL/min/kg in males and 5.7 mL/min/kg in females following an IV dose of tramadol 100 mg. Following a single oral dose, and after adjusting for body weight, females had a 12% higher peak tramadol concentration and a 35% higher AUC compared with males. The clinical significance of this difference is unknown.

Renal function impairment:

• *Hydromorphone* – Possible accumulation with severe impairment. Use with caution.

• *Meperidine* – Accumulation of meperidine and/or normeperidine may occur in patients with renal impairment.

• *Methadone* – Methadone pharmacokinetics have not been extensively evaluated in patients with renal insufficiency. Unchanged methadone and its metabolites are excreted in urine to a variable degree. Methadone is a basic (pKa = 9.2) compound and the luminal pH of the urinary tract can affect its extraction from plasma. Urine acidification has been shown to increase renal elimination of methadone. Forced diuresis, peritoneal dialysis, hemodialysis, or charcoal hemoperfusion have not been established as beneficial for increasing methadone or metabolite elimination.

• *Morphine* – Clearance is decreased and plasma levels increased in patients with renal failure.

• *Oxycodone* – Patients with mild to severe renal impairment (creatinine clearance [Ccr] less than 60 mL/min) show peak plasma oxycodone and noroxycodone concentrations 50% and 20% higher, respectively, and AUC values for oxycodone, noroxycodone, and oxymorphone 60%, 50%, and 40% higher than normal subjects, respectively. This is accompanied by increased sedation but not by differences in respiratory rate, pupillary constriction, or several other measures of drug effect. There was an increase in the elimination half-life for oxycodone of 1 hour.

• *Remifentanil* – In anephric patients, the half-life of the carboxylic acid metabolite increases from 90 minutes to 30 hours. The metabolite is removed by hemodialysis with a dialysis extraction ratio of approximately 30%.

• *Tramadol* – Impaired renal function results in a decreased rate and extent of excretion of tramadol and its active metabolite, M1. In patients with Ccr less than 30 mL/min, adjustment of the dosing regimen is recommended. The total amount of tramadol and M1 removed during a 4-hour dialysis period is less than 7% of the administered dose.

Hepatic function impairment:

• *Alfentanil* – Patients with compromised liver function have reduced plasma clearance and an extended elimination half-life, which may prolong postoperative recovery.

• *Hydromorphone* – Possible accumulation with severe impairment; use with caution.

• *Meperidine* – Accumulation of meperidine and/or normeperidine may occur in patients with hepatic impairment.

• *Methadone* – Methadone is metabolized in the liver and patients with liver impairment may be at risk of accumulating methadone after multiple dosing.

• *Morphine* – Clearance is decreased and half-life is increased in patients with cirrhosis. The 3- and 6-glucuronide metabolites to morphine plasma AUC ratios are also decreased, indicating diminished metabolic activity.

• *Oxycodone* – Patients with mild to moderate hepatic dysfunction show peak plasma oxycodone and noroxycodone concentrations 50% and 20% higher, respectively, and AUC values are 95% and 65% higher, respectively, than normal subjects. Oxymorphone peak plasma levels and AUC values are lower by 30% and 40%. The elimination half-life for oxycodone increased by 2.3 hours.

• *Tramadol* – Metabolism of tramadol and M1 is reduced in patients with advanced cirrhosis of the liver, resulting in both a larger AUC for tramadol and longer tramadol and M1 elimination half-lives (13 hours for tramadol and 19 hours for M1). In cirrhotic patients, adjustment of the dosing regimen is recommended.

Children:

• *Meperidine* – Meperidine has a slower elimination rate in neonates and young children compared with older children and adults.

• *Morphine* – Infants younger than 1 month of age have a prolonged elimination half-life and decreased clearance relative to older infants and pediatric patients. The clearance and half-life begin to approach adult values by the second month of life. Children old enough to take capsules should have pharmacokinetic parameters similar to adults, dosed on a per kilogram basis.

• *Remifentanil* – Clearance and volume of distribution of remifentanil were increased in younger children and declined to young healthy adult values by 17 years of age. The average clearance of remifentanil in neonates (younger than 2 months of age) was approximately 90.5 mL/min/kg while in adolescents (13 to 16 years of age) this value was approximately 57.2 mL/min/kg. The total (steady state) volume of distribution in neonates was approximately 452 mL/kg vs 223 mL/kg in adolescents. The half-life of remifentanil was the same in neonates and adolescents.

Cardiopulmonary bypass (CPB):

• *Remifentanil* – Remifentanil clearance is reduced by approximately 20% during hypothermic CPB.

Race:

• *Morphine* – In 1 study, Chinese subjects given IV morphine had a higher clearance compared with whites (1,852 mL/min compared with 1,495 mL/min).

Contraindications

Hypersensitivity to the drug or known intolerance to other opioids or any components of the products.

➤*Fentanyl:*

Transmucosal – Management of acute or postoperative pain; opioid non-tolerant patients.

Transdermal – Nonopioid-tolerant patients; management of acute pain or in patients who require opioid analgesia for a short period of time; management of postoperative pain, including use after outpatient day surgeries; management of mild or intermittent pain (eg, use on an as-needed basis); respiratory depression; acute or severe bronchial asthma; paralytic ileus; doses exceeding 25 mcg/h at initiation of opioid therapy.

➤*Hydromorphone:*

Oral / Suppositories – Use on as-needed basis; respiratory depression; acute or severe bronchial asthma; paralytic ileus; obstetrical analgesia (8 mg tablets, oral solution, and suppositories only); intracranial lesion associated with increased intracranial pressure (2 and 4 mg tablets only).

Injection – Patients not already receiving large amounts of parenteral narcotics (HP injection only); respiratory depression; status asthmaticus; obstetrical analgesia (hydromorphone injection).

➤*Meperidine:* In patients taking monoamine oxidase inhibitors (MAOIs) or in those who have received such agents within 14 days.

➤*Methadone:*

Injection – Respiratory depression; acute bronchial asthma; hypercarbia.

➤*Morphine:*

IR concentrated oral solution and tablets / suppositories – Respiratory insufficiency or depression; severe CNS depression; attack of bronchial asthma; heart failure secondary to chronic lung disease; cardiac arrhythmias; increased intracranial or CSF pressure; head injuries; brain tumor; acute alcoholism; delirium tremens; convulsive disorders; after biliary tract surgery; suspected surgical abdomen; surgical anastomosis; concomitantly with MAOIs or within 14 days of such treatment; paralytic ileus.

Injection – Heart failure secondary to chronic lung disease; cardiac arrhythmias; brain tumor; acute alcoholism; delirium tremens; idiosyncrasy to the drug; increased intracranial or CSF pressure; head injuries; acute bronchial asthma; upper airway obstruction. Because of its stimulating effect on the spinal cord, morphine should not be used in convulsive states (eg, status epilepticus, tetanus, strychnine poisoning); concomitantly with MAOIs or in those who have received such agents within 14 days.

Epidural/Intrathecal – Presence of infection at the injection microinfusion site; concomitant anticoagulant therapy; uncontrolled bleeding diathesis; parenterally administered corticosteroids within a 2-week period, other concomitant drug therapy or medical condition that would contraindicate the technique of epidural or intrathecal analgesia; acute bronchial asthma; upper airway obstruction.

Soluble tablets for injection – Convulsive states such as those occurring in status epilepticus, tetanus, and strychnine poisoning.

DepoDur – Respiratory depression; acute or severe bronchial asthma; upper airway obstruction; paralytic ileus; head injury; increased intracranial pressure; circulatory shock.

Sustained-release (SR)/ER/CR – Respiratory depression; acute or severe bronchial asthma; paralytic ileus.

➤*Opium:* Diarrhea caused by poisoning until the toxic material is eliminated from the GI tract; use in children (opium tincture only); convulsive states such as those occurring in status epilepticus, tetanus, and strychnine poisoning (*Paregoric* only).

➤*Oxycodone:*

CR/IR tablets (15 and 30 mg)/IR capsules (5 mg)/ER/Concentrated solution – Significant respiratory depression; acute or severe bronchial asthma; hypercarbia; paralytic ileus.

➤*Oxymorphone:* Hypersensitivity to morphine analogs; acute asthma attack; severe respiratory depression or upper airway obstruction; paralytic ileus; pulmonary edema secondary to a chemical respiratory irritant.

➤*Remifentanil:* For epidural or intrathecal administration; hypersensitivity to fentanyl analogs.

➤*Tramadol:* Acute intoxication with alcohol, hypnotics, narcotics, centrally acting analgesics, opioids, or psychotropic drugs.

Warnings

For important warnings associated with **transmucosal** and **transdermal fentanyl**, **hydromorphone**, **methadone**, **morphine**, **oxycodone**, and **propoxyphene**, refer to individual monographs.

➤*Suicide:* Do not prescribe **propoxyphene** for patients who are suicidal or addiction prone. Many of the propoxyphene-related deaths have occurred in patients with histories of emotional disturbances, suicidal ideation, or suicide attempts as well as misuse of tranquilizers, alcohol, and other CNS-active drugs. Some deaths were a consequence of accidental ingestion of excessive quantities of propoxyphene alone or in combination with other drugs. Warn patients not to exceed dosage recommended by health care provider (see Black Box Warning).

➤*Respiratory depression:* Narcotics may be expected to produce serious or potentially fatal respiratory depression if given in an excessive dose, too frequently, or in full dosage to compromised or vulnerable patients because the doses required to produce analgesia in the general clinical population may cause serious respiratory depression in vulnerable patients. Safe use of opioids requires that the dose and dosage interval be individualized to each patient based on the severity of the pain, weight, age, diagnosis, and physical status of the patient, and the type and dose of concurrently administered medication.

Respiratory depression caused by opioid analgesics can be reversed by opioid antagonists, such as naloxone. Because the duration of respiratory depression may last longer than the duration of the opioid antagonist action, maintain appropriate surveillance.

Certain forms of conduction anesthesia, such as spinal anesthesia and some peridural anesthetics, can alter respiration by blocking intercostal nerves. Through other mechanisms, **fentanyl** injection can also alter respiration. Therefore, when fentanyl injection is used to supplement these forms of anesthesia, the anesthetist needs to be aware of the physiological alterations involved and manage them appropriately. Profound analgesia is accompanied by respiratory depression and diminished sensitivity to CO_2 stimulation, which may persist or recur in the postoperative period. Respiratory depression secondary to chest wall rigidity has been reported in the postoperative period. Intraoperative hyperventilation may further alter postoperative response to CO_2. Employ appropriate postoperative monitoring to ensure that adequate spontaneous breathing is established and maintained in the absence of stimulation prior to discharging the patient from the recovery area.

Fentanyl transdermal – Because significant amounts of fentanyl are absorbed from the skin for 17 hours or more after the system is removed, hypoventilation may persist beyond the removal. Consequently, observe patients with hypoventilation carefully for degree of sedation, and monitor their respiratory rate until respiration has stabilized.

Levorphanol – Reduce the initial levorphanol dose by 50% or more when the drug is given to patients with any condition affecting respiratory reserve or in conjunction with other drugs affecting the respiratory center. Then, individually titrate subsequent doses according to patient response. Respiratory depression produced by levorphanol can be reversed by naloxone, a specific antagonist.

Remifentanil – Respiratory depression in spontaneously breathing patients is generally managed by decreasing the rate of infusion of remifentanil by 50% or by temporarily discontinuing the infusion.

➤*CNS depressants:* Use with caution and in reduced dosage in patients concurrently receiving other opioid narcotic analgesics, general anesthetics, phenothiazines, other tranquilizers, sedative-hypnotics (including barbiturates), tricyclic antidepressants, and/or other CNS depressants (including alcohol). Respiratory depression, hypotension, and profound sedation or coma may result.

If **fentanyl** is administered with a tranquilizer such as droperidol, pulmonary arterial pressure may be decreased. Be familiar with the special properties of each drug, particularly the widely differing durations of action, and have available fluids and other countermeasures to manage hypotension when such a combination is used.

➤*Head injury and increased intracranial pressure:* Narcotics may obscure the clinical course of patients with head injuries. The respiratory-depressant effects and the capacity to elevate CSF pressure may be markedly exaggerated in the presence of head injury, brain tumor, other intracranial lesions, impaired consciousness, or preexisting elevated intracranial pressure. Use with extreme caution, and use only if deemed essential. Pupillary changes (miosis) from narcotics may obscure the existence, extent, and course or intracranial pathology. High doses of neuraxial **morphine** may produce myoclonic events.

➤*QT prolongation:* Administer **methadone** with particular caution to patients already at risk for development of prolonged QT interval (eg, cardiac hypertrophy, concomitant diuretic use, hypokalemia, hypomagnesemia). Careful monitoring is recommended when using methadone in patients with a history of cardiac conduction abnormalities, those taking medications affecting cardiac conduction, and in other cases where history or physical exam suggest an increased risk of dysrhythmia. QT prolongation also has been reported in patients with no prior cardiac history who have received high doses of methadone. Evaluate patients developing QT prolongation while on methadone treatment for the presence of modifiable risk factors, such as concomitant medications with cardiac effects, drugs that might cause electrolyte abnormalities, and drugs that might act as inhibitors of methadone metabolism. For use of methadone to treat pain, weigh the risk of QT prolongation and development of dysrhythmias against the benefit of adequate pain management and the availability of alternative therapies. In using methadone, carry out an individualized benefit-to-risk assessment and include evaluation of patient presentation and complete medical history. For patients judged to be at risk, perform careful monitoring of cardiovascular status, including QT prolongation and dysrhythmias and those described previously.

➤*Seizures:* Seizures may be aggravated or may occur in individuals with or without a history of convulsive disorders if dosage is substantially increased above recommended levels because of tolerance. Observe patients with known seizure disorders closely for **meperidine**- or **morphine**-induced seizure activity. Reports of mild to severe seizures and myoclonus have been reported in severely compromised patients administered high doses of parenteral **hydromorphone** for cancer and severe pain. Opioid administration at very high doses is associated with seizures and myoclonus in a variety of diseases where pain control is the primary focus.

Seizures have been reported in patients receiving **tramadol** within the recommended dosage range. Spontaneous postmarketing reports indicate the seizure risk is increased with doses above the recommended range. Concomitant use with selective serotonin reuptake inhibitors (SSRIs or anorectics), tricyclic compounds (eg, TCAs, cyclobenzaprine, promethazine), or other opioids also increases the risk of seizures. Administration of tramadol with neuroleptics, MAOIs (see Warnings), or other drugs that reduce the seizure threshold may also enhance the seizure risk. Risk of convulsions may also increase in patients with epilepsy, those with a history of seizures, or in patients with a recognized risk for seizure (eg, head trauma, metabolic disorders, alcohol and drug withdrawal, CNS infections). In a tramadol overdose, naloxone administration may also increase the risk of seizure (see Overdosage).

➤*Administration:* **Sufentanil**, **fentanyl**, **remifentanil**, **alfentanil**, and **morphine** should be administered only by personnel specifically trained in the use of IV and epidural anesthetics and the management of potent opioid respiratory effects.

An opioid antagonist, resuscitative and intubation equipment, and oxygen should be readily available.

Administer continuous infusions only by an infusion device. Use IV bolus administration of remifentanil only during the maintenance of general anesthesia. In nonintubated patients, administer remifentanil doses over 30 to 60 seconds.

Interruption of infusion – Interruption of an infusion of **remifentanil** will result in rapid offset of effect. Rapid clearance and lack of drug accumulation will result in rapid dissipation of respiratory-depressant and analgesic effects upon discontinuation of remifentanil at recommended doses. Precede discontinuation of an infusion of remifentanil with the establishment of adequate postoperative analgesia.

IV tubing – Make injections of **remifentanil** into IV tubing at or close to the venous cannula. Upon discontinuation of remifentanil, clear the IV tubing to prevent the inadvertent administration of remifentanil at a later point in time. Failure to adequately clear the IV tubing to remove residual remifentanil has been associated with respiratory depression, apnea, and muscle rigidity upon the administration of additional fluids or medications through the same IV tubing.

Do not administer remifentanil into the same IV tubing with blood because of potential inactivation by nonspecific esterases in blood products.

➤*ER, SR, CR products:* These dosage forms must not be chewed, crushed, or dissolved due to the risk of rapid release and absorption of a potentially fatal dose.

➤*Parenteral therapy:* Give by very slow IV injection, preferably as a diluted solution. The patient should be lying down. Rapid IV injection increases the incidence of adverse reactions; respiratory depression, hypotension, apnea, circulatory collapse, cardiac arrest, and anaphylactoid reactions have occurred. Do not administer IV unless a narcotic antagonist and facilities for assisted or controlled respiration are available.

Smooth muscle hypertonicity may result in biliary colic, difficulty in urination, and possible urinary retention requiring catheterization. Give consideration to inherent risks in urethral catheterization (eg, sepsis) when epidural or intrathecal administration is considered, especially in the perioperative period.

➤*Epidural / Intrathecal administration:* Limit epidural or intrathecal administration of preservative-free **morphine** and **sufentanil** to the lumbar area. Intrathecal use has been associated with a higher incidence of respiratory depression than epidural use. Prior to any epidural or intrathecal drug administration, the health care provider should be familiar with patient conditions (eg, infection at the injection site, bleeding diathesis, anticoagulant therapy) that call for special evaluation of the benefit-vs-risk potential.

Thoracic administration has been shown to dramatically increase the incidence of early and late respiratory depression even with morphine 1 to 2 mg. Narcotics should be administered by or under the direction of a health care provider experienced in the technique of epidural administration and who is thoroughly familiar with the drug labeling. Administer only in settings where adequate patient monitoring is possible. Have resuscitative equipment and a specific antagonist (naloxone injection) immediately available for the management of respiratory depression as well as complications that might result from inadvertent intrathecal or intravascular injection (note: intrathecal morphine dosage is usually one-tenth that of epidural dosage). Continue patient monitoring for at least 24 hours after each dose, because delayed respiratory depression may occur.

Verify proper placement of the needle or catheter in the epidural space before injection of sufentanil or preservative-free morphine to ensure that unintentional intravascular or intrathecal administration does not occur. Unintentional intravascular injection of sufentanil could result in a potentially serious overdose, including acute truncal muscular rigidity and apnea. Unintentional intrathecal injection of the full sufentanil/bupivacaine epidural doses and volume could produce effects of high spinal anesthesia, including prolonged paralysis and delayed recovery. If analgesia is inadequate, verify the placement and integrity of the catheter prior to the administration of any additional epidural medications. Administer sufentanil epidurally by slow injection.

➤*Asthma and other respiratory conditions:* The use of bisulfites is contraindicated in asthmatic patients. Bisulfites and **morphine** may potentiate each other, preventing use by causing severe adverse reactions. Use with extreme caution in patients having an acute asthmatic attack, bronchial asthma, chronic obstructive pulmonary disease or cor pulmonale, a substantially decreased respiratory reserve, and preexisting respiratory depression, hypoxia, or hypercapnia. Even usual therapeutic doses of narcotics may decrease respiratory drive while simultaneously increasing airway resistance to the point of apnea. Reserve use for those whose conditions require endotracheal intubation and respiratory support or control of ventilation. In these patients, consider alternative nonopioid analgesics, and employ only under careful medical supervision at the lowest effective dose.

➤*Hypotensive effect:* Opioid analgesics may cause severe hypotension in the postoperative patient or in individuals whose ability to maintain blood pressure has been compromised by a depleted blood volume or coadministration of drugs such as phenothiazines or general anesthetics. In ambulatory patients, orthostatic hypotension may occur.

Carefully observe patients with reduced circulating blood volume, impaired myocardial function, or those on sympatholytic drugs for orthostatic hypotension, particularly in transport.

➤*Renal toxicity: Avinza* doses over 1,600 mg/day contain a quantity of fumaric acid that has not been demonstrated to be safe, which may result in serious renal toxicity. Daily dose of *Avinza* must be limited to a maximum of 1,600 mg/day.

➤*Hypersensitivity reactions:* Although extremely rare, cases of anaphylaxis have been reported.

Serious and rarely fatal anaphylactoid reactions have been reported in patients receiving therapy with **tramadol**. When these events do occur it is often following the first dose. Other reported allergic reactions include pruritus, hives, bronchospasm, angioedema, toxic epidermal necrolysis, and Stevens-Johnson syndrome. Patients with a history of anaphylactoid reactions to **codeine** and other opioids may be at increased risk and therefore should not receive tramadol (see Contraindications).

➤*Renal / Hepatic function impairment:* Renal and hepatic dysfunction may cause a prolonged duration and cumulative effect. Administer with caution; smaller doses may be necessary (see Pharmacokinetics).

Meperidine – In patients with renal or hepatic dysfunction, normeperidine (an active metabolite of meperidine) may accumulate, resulting in increased CNS adverse reactions.

➤*Carcinogenesis:* In **methadone**, studies indicate that there was a significant increase in pituitary adenomas in female mice consuming 15 mg/kg/day for 2 years. This dose was approximately 0.6 times a human daily oral dose of 120 mg/day.

In **tramadol**, a slight, but statistically significant, increase in 2 common murine tumors, pulmonary and hepatic, was observed in a mouse carcinogenicity study, particularly in aged mice. Mice were dosed orally up to 30 mg/kg (90 mg/m^2 or 0.36 times the maximum daily human dosage of 246 mg/m^2) for approximately 2 years.

➤*Mutagenesis:* **Methadone** treatment of male mice increased sex chromosome and autosome univalent chromosomes and translocations in multivalent chromosomes. Methadone tested positive in the *Escherichia coli* DNA repair system and *Neurospora crassa* and mouse lymphoma forward mutation assays.

Morphine was found to increase DNA fragmentation when incubated in vitro with a human lymphoma cell line. In vivo, morphine has been reported to produce an increase in the frequency of micronuclei in bone marrow cells and immature red blood cells in the mouse micronucleus test and to induce chromosomal aberrations in murine lymphocytes and spermatids. Some of the in vivo clastogenic effects reported with morphine in mice may be directly related to increases in glucocorticoid levels produced by morphine in this species.

In the in vitro mouse lymphoma assay with **remifentanil** and **hydromorphone**, mutagenicity was seen only with metabolic activation.

Oxycodone was clastogenic in the human lymphocyte chromosomal assay in the presence of metabolic activation in the human chromosomal aberration test (1,250 mcg/mL or more) at 24 but not 48 hours of exposure and in the mouse lymphoma assay at doses of 50 mcg/mL or more with metabolic activation and at 400 mcg/mL or more without metabolic activation.

With **tramadol**, weakly mutagenic results occurred in the presence of metabolic activation in the mouse lymphoma assay and micronucleus test in rats.

➤*Fertility impairment:* A single daily bolus dose of **fentanyl** has been shown to impair fertility and to have an embryocidal effect in rats at doses 0.3 times the upper human dose for 12 days.

Remifentanil has been shown to reduce fertility in male rats when tested after 70 or more days of daily IV administration of 0.5 mg/kg, or approximately 40 times the maximum recommended human dose.

➤*Elderly:* Appropriately reduce the initial dose in elderly and debilitated patients. Consider the effect of the initial dose in determining supplemental doses. Use caution because opioids have the ability to depress respiration and reduce ventilatory drive to a clinically significant event.

In 1 clinical trial, **alfentanil** doses required to produce anesthesia, as determined by appearance of delta waves in electroencephalogram, were 40% lower in elderly patients than that needed in healthy young patients.

Because elderly, cachectic, or debilitated patients may have altered pharmacokinetics due to poor fat stores, muscle wasting, or altered clearance, do not start them on **transdermal fentanyl** doses more than 25 mcg/h unless they are already taking oral **morphine** 135 mg/day or more or an equivalent dose of another opioid.

In studies with **transmucosal fentanyl**, patients older than 65 years of age were titrated to a mean dose that was about 200 mcg less than the mean dose titrated to by younger patients. Studies with **IV fentanyl** showed that elderly patients are twice as sensitive to the effects of fentanyl as the younger population. The clearance of IV fentanyl may be greatly decreased in patients older than 60 years of age.

Elderly patients have a slower elimination rate compared with young patients and they may be more susceptible to the effects of **meperidine**; a reduction in total daily dose may be required.

The pharmacodynamic effects of neuraxial **morphine** in the elderly are more variable than in the younger population. Base initial doses on careful clinical observation following "test doses," after making due allowances for the effects of the patient's age and infirmity on his/her ability to clear the drug, particularly in patients receiving epidural morphine. Elderly patients may be more susceptible to respiratory depression and/or respiratory arrest following administration of morphine.

In elderly patients, the clearance of **oxycodone** appears to be slightly reduced. Compared with young adults, the plasma concentrations of oxycodone were increased approximately 15%.

The rate of **propoxyphene** metabolism may be reduced in some patients. Consider increased dosing intervals.

After termination of **remifentanil** administration, blood concentrations fell as rapidly in the elderly as in young adults. While the effective biological half-life of remifentanil is unchanged, elderly patients have been shown to be twice as sensitive to the pharmacodynamic effects as younger patients. Decrease the recommended starting dose by 50% in patients older than 65 years of age.

Daily doses greater than **tramadol** 300 mg are not recommended in patients older than 75 years of age (see Administration and Dosage). Patients older than 75 years of age had slightly elevated serum concentrations and a slightly prolonged elimination half-life (see Actions). Patients older than 75 years of age also experienced more treatment-limiting adverse events during clinical trials, as compared with those younger than 65 years of age. Constipation resulted in the discontinuation of treatment in 10% of those older than 75 years of age.

➤*Pregnancy: Category C; Category B* (**oxycodone**). Safety for use during pregnancy has not been established. There are no adequate and well-controlled studies in pregnant women. Use in pregnant women only if the potential benefits outweigh the possible risks.

The placental transfer of narcotics is rapid. Maternal addiction and neonatal withdrawal occurs following use. Withdrawal symptoms include irritability, excessive crying, yawning, sneezing, increased respiratory rate, tremors, convulsions, hyperreflexia, fever, vomiting, increased stools, diarrhea, hyperactivity, abnormal sleep patterns, high-pitched crying, weight loss, and failure to gain weight. Symptoms usually appear during the first days of life, but may be delayed for 2 to 4 weeks.

Alfentanil and **sufentanil** have an embryocidal effect in rats and rabbits when given in doses 2.5 times the upper human dose for 10 days to more than 30 days.

Fentanyl reproduction studies in rats revealed a significant decrease in the pregnancy rate. This decrease was most pronounced in the high-dose group (1.25 mg/kg) in which 1 in 20 animals became pregnant. Female rats were treated with fentanyl 0, 0.025, 0.1, or 0.4 mg/kg/day via IV infusion from day 6 of pregnancy through 3 weeks of lactation. Fentanyl treatment (0.4 mg/kg/day) significantly decreased body weight in male and female pups and also decreased survival in pups at day 4.

In a rat pre- and postnatal study, an increase in pup mortality and a decrease in pup body weight that was associated with maternal toxicity was observed at doses of **hydromorphone** 2 and 5 mg/kg/day. Hydromorphone administration to pregnant hamsters and mice during major organ development revealed teratogenicity likely the result of maternal toxicity associated with sedation and hypoxia. In hamsters given single subcutaneous doses from 14 to 278 mg/kg during organogenesis (gestation days 8 to 10), doses 19 mg/kg or more of hydromorphone produced skull malformations (exencephaly and cranioschisis). Continuous infusion of hydromorphone (5 mg/kg, subcutaneously) via implanted osmotic mini pumps during organogenesis (gestation days 7 to 10) produced soft tissue malformations (cryptochidism, cleft palate, malformed ventricals and retina), and skeletal variations (supraoccipital, checkerboard and split sternebrae, delayed ossification of the paws and ectopic ossification sites). The malformations and variations observed in the hamsters and mice were at doses approximately 3-fold higher and less than 1-fold lower, respectively, than a 32 mg human daily oral dose on a body surface area basis.

Levorphanol has been shown to be teratogenic in mice when given as a single oral dose of 25 mg/kg. The tested dose caused a near 50% mortality of the mouse embryos.

Meperidine should not be used in pregnant women prior to the labor period, because safe use in pregnancy prior to labor has not been established relative to possible adverse effects on fetal development. Meperidine is known to cross the placental barrier.

In humans, the frequency of congenital anomalies has been reported to be no greater than expected among the children of 70 women who were treated with **morphine** during the first 4 months of pregnancy or in 448 women treated with this drug anytime during pregnancy. Furthermore, no malformations were observed in the infant of a woman who attempted suicide by taking an overdose of morphine and other medication during the first trimester of pregnancy. In animals, several reports indicate that morphine administered subcutaneously during the early gestational period in mice and hamsters produced neurological, soft tissue, and skeletal abnormalities. With one exception, the effects that have been reported were following doses that were maternally toxic and the abnormalities noted were characteristic of those observed when maternal toxicity is present. In 1 study, following subcutaneous infusion of doses 0.15 mg/kg or more to mice, exencephaly, hydronephrosis, intestinal hemorrhage, split supraoccipital, malformed sternebrae, and malformed xiphoid were noted in the absence of maternal toxicity. In the hamster, morphine given subcutaneously on gestation day 8 produced exencephaly and cranioschisis.

Oxymorphone was reported to produce malformations in offspring of hamsters that received 1,500 times the recommended human dose on day 8 of gestation.

Tramadol is embryotoxic and fetotoxic in mice (360 mg/m^2), rats (150 mg/m^2), and rabbits (900 mg/m^2) at maternally toxic doses. Embryo and fetal toxicity consisted primarily of decreased fetal weights, skeletal ossification, and increased supernumerary ribs at maternally toxic dose levels. Transient delays in developmental or behavioral parameters were also seen in pups from rat dams allowed to deliver. Embryo and fetal lethality were reported in only 1 rabbit study at 300 mg/kg (3,600 mg/m^2). In peri- and postnatal studies in rats, progeny of dams receiving oral (gavage) dose levels of 50 mg/kg or more had decreased weights, and pup survival was decreased early in lactation at 80 mg/kg.

Methadone – An expert review of published data on experiences with methadone use during pregnancy by Teratogen Information System (TERIS) concluded that maternal use of methadone during pregnancy as part of a supervised, therapeutic regimen is unlikely to pose a substantial teratogenic risk (quantity and quality of data assessed as "limited to fair"); however, the data are insufficient to state that there is no risk (TERIS, last reviewed October 2002). Pregnant women involved in methadone maintenance programs have been reported to have significantly improved prenatal care, improved fetal outcomes, and reduced mortality when compared with pregnant women using illicit drugs. Several factors complicate the interpretation of investigations of the children of women who took methadone during pregnancy. These include: the maternal use of illicit drugs, other maternal factors such as nutrition, infection, and psychosocial circumstances, limited information regarding dose and duration of methadone use during pregnancy, and the fact that most maternal exposure appears to occur after the first trimester of pregnancy. In addition, reported studies generally compare the benefit of methadone to the risk of untreated addiction to illicit drugs; the relevance of these findings to pain patients prescribed methadone during pregnancy is unclear.

Methadone has been detected in amniotic fluid and cord plasma at concentrations proportional to maternal plasma and in newborn urine at lower concentrations than corresponding maternal urine. Several studies suggested that infants born to narcotic-addicted women treated with methadone during all or part of pregnancy have been found to have decreased fetal growth with reduced birth weight, length, and/or head circumference compared with controls. The growth deficit does not appear to persist into later childhood. However, children born to women treated with methadone during pregnancy have been shown to demonstrate mild but persistent deficits in performance on psychometric and behavioral tests.

Following large doses, methadone produced teratogenic effects in the guinea pig, hamster, and mouse. One published study found that in hamster fetuses, subcutaneous methadone doses of 31 mg/kg or more (estimated exposure was approximately 2 times a human daily oral dose of 120 mg/day on a mg/m^2 basis, or equivalent to a human daily IV dose of 120 mg/day) on day 8 of gestation produced exencephaly and neurological effects. Some of the reported effects were observed at doses that were maternally toxic. In another study, a single subcutaneous dose of methadone 22 to 24 mg/kg (estimated exposure was approximately equivalent to a human daily oral dose of 120 mg/day on a mg/m^2 basis; or half a human daily IV dose of 120 mg/day) on day 9 of gestation in mice also produced exencephaly in 11% of the embryos.

There are conflicting reports on whether the risk of sudden infant death syndrome (SIDS) is increased in infants born to women treated with methadone during pregnancy.

Labor – Narcotics cross the placenta and can produce respiratory depression and psychophysiologic effects in the neonate. Resuscitation may be required; have naloxone available. The use of epidurally administered **sufentanil** in combination with bupivacaine 0.125% with or without epinephrine is indicated for labor and delivery. Sufentanil is not recommended for IV use or in larger epidural doses during labor and delivery because of potential risks to the newborn after delivery. In a human clinical trial, the average maternal **remifentanil** concentrations were approximately twice those seen in the fetus. However, in some cases, fetal concentrations were similar to those in the mother. The umbilical arteriovenous ratio of remifentanil concentrations was approximately 30%, suggesting metabolism of remifentanil in the neonate. The use of **alfentanil**, **levorphanol**, **meperidine**, **morphine**, **oxycodone**, and **fentanyl** is not recommended. Do not use **methadone** for obstetrical analgesia. Its long duration of action increases the probability of neonatal respiratory depression. It has also been associated with low infant birthweight.

Opioid analgesics in therapeutic doses may prolong labor. Generally, the effect of opioids on the pregnant uterus appears to depend on the time of administration; administration of the drugs during the latent phase of the first stage of labor, or before cervical dilation of 4 to 5 cm has occurred, may hamper the progress of labor.

Narcotics with mixed agonist-antagonist properties should not be used for pain control during labor in patients chronically treated with methadone because they may precipitate acute withdrawal.

Oral hydromorphone is not recommended to be initiated prior to or during labor or in the immediate postpartum period. Hydromorphone injection is contraindicated in labor and delivery.

Use **oxymorphone** with caution during labor. Sinusoidal fetal heart rate patterns may occur with the use of opioid analgesics.

Tramadol has been shown to cross the placenta; do not use prior to or during labor unless the potential benefits outweigh the risks. The mean ratio of serum tramadol in the umbilical veins compared with maternal veins was 0.83 for 40 women given tramadol during labor.

➤*Lactation:* Most of these agents appear in breast milk, but effects on the infant may not be significant. Some recommend waiting 4 to 6 hours after use before breast-feeding. Withdrawal symptoms can occur in breast-feeding infants when maternal administration of an opioid-analgesic is stopped. Decide whether to discontinue breast-feeding or to discontinue the drug, taking into account the importance of the drug to the mother.

Alfentanil – Significant levels of alfentanil were found in breast milk 4 hours after administration of 60 mcg/kg. No detectable levels were found after 28 hours.

Codeine – Codeine passes into breast milk in very small amounts that are probably insignificant. The American Academy of Pediatrics considers codeine to be compatible with breastfeeding.

Fentanyl – Fentanyl (transmucosal, transdermal) is excreted in human milk; therefore, it is not recommended for use in breast-feeding women because of the possibility of the effects in infants. It is not known whether fentanyl injection is excreted in breast milk; use with caution.

Hydromorphone, oxymorphone – It is not known whether oxymorphone and hydromorphone are excreted in human milk.

Levorphanol – Levorphanol is not recommended for use in breast-feeding mothers, because it is not known if levorphanol is secreted in pharmacologically active amounts in human milk.

Meperidine, oxycodone – Concentrations of these drugs have been detected in breast milk. Meperidine achieves an average milk:plasma ratio of greater than 1 (peak milk levels of 0.13 mcg/mL occur 2 hours after a 50 mg IM dose). Breast-feeding should not be undertaken while receiving these drugs because of the possibility of sedation and/or respiratory depression in the infant.

Methadone – Methadone is secreted into human milk. There is no information on use of parenteral methadone in breast-feeding, or on the safety of the high doses of methadone typically used in chronic pain treatment. The safety of breast-feeding while taking oral methadone is also controversial. At maternal oral doses of 10 to 80 mg/day, methadone concentrations from 50 to 570 mcg/L in milk have been reported, which, in the majority of samples, were lower than maternal serum drug concentrations at steady state. Peak methadone levels in milk occur approximately 4 to 5 hours after an oral dose. Based on an average milk consumption of 150 mL/kg/day, an infant would consume approximately 17.4 mcg/kg/day, which is approximately 2% to 3% of the oral maternal dose. Methadone has been detected in very low plasma concentrations in some infants whose mothers were taking methadone. Women on high-dose methadone maintenance, who are already breast-feeding, should be counseled to wean breast-feeding gradually in order to prevent neonatal abstinence syndrome. Inform methadone-treated mothers considering breast-feeding an opioid-naïve infant of the presence of methadone in breast milk.

Morphine – Low levels of morphine have been detected in maternal milk. The milk:plasma morphine AUC ratio is about 2.5:1.

Propoxyphene – Low levels of propoxyphene have been detected in human milk. In postpartum studies, no adverse effects were seen in infants receiving breast milk from mothers who were given propoxyphene.

Remifentanil, sufentanil – It is not known whether these drugs are excreted in human milk. Because fentanyl analogs are excreted in human milk, use with caution.

Tramadol – Following a single IV 100 mg dose, the cumulative excretion in breast milk within 16 hours postdose was 100 mcg of tramadol (0.1% of the maternal dose) and 27 mcg of M1.

➤*Children:*

Alfentanil – There are no adequate data to support the use of alfentanil in children younger than 12 years of age. Hypotension has occurred in neonates with respiratory distress syndrome receiving alfentanil 20 mcg/kg.

Codeine – Safe dosage of codeine has not been established for children younger than 3 years of age.

Fentanyl – Safety and efficacy of fentanyl (transdermal and injection) in children younger than 2 years of age are not established. Administer transdermal fentanyl only to children 2 years of age or older if they are opioid tolerant. Safety and efficacy of fentanyl transmucosal have not been established in patients younger than 16 years of age. Methemoglobinemia has occurred rarely in premature neonates undergoing emergency anesthesia and surgery including combined use of fentanyl injection, pancuronium, and atropine; a cause-and-effect relationship has not been established.

Meperidine – Meperidine has a slower elimination rate in neonates and young infants compared with older children and adults. Neonates and young infants may also be more susceptible to the effects, especially the respiratory depressant effects. Use with caution in neonates and young infants, and weigh any potential benefits against the relative risk.

Oxycodone – Do not use oxycodone in children; safety and efficacy have not been established.

Remifentanil – Safety and efficacy have been established in patients from birth to 12 years of age for use in the maintenance of general anesthesia in outpatient and inpatient pediatric surgery. Remifentanil has not been studied in children for use as a postoperative analgesic or as an analgesic component of monitored anesthesia care.

Sufentanil – Safety and efficacy of IV sufentanil in children younger than 2 years of age undergoing cardiovascular surgery have been documented in a limited number of cases.

Tramadol – Safety and efficacy in patients younger than 16 years of age have not been established.

Hydromorphone / Levorphanol / Methadone / Morphine / Opium / Oxymorphone / Propoxyphene – Safety and efficacy are not established in children.

Precautions

➤*Monitoring:* Because of the possibility of delayed respiratory depression, continue monitoring patients well after surgery. Monitor vital signs routinely.

Patients receiving monitored anesthesia care (MAC) should be continuously monitored by people not involved in the conduct of the surgical or diagnostic procedure. Oxygen supplementation should be immediately available and provided where clinically indicated. Continuously monitor oxygen saturation. Observe the patient for early signs of hypotension, apnea, upper airway obstruction, or oxygen desaturation.

➤*Acute abdominal conditions:* Narcotics may obscure diagnosis or clinical course. Do not give SR **morphine** to patients with GI obstruction, particularly paralytic ileus, as there is a risk of the product remaining in the stomach for an extended period and the subsequent release of a bolus of morphine when normal gut motility is restored. As with other solid morphine formulations, diarrhea may reduce morphine absorption. Opioids have been shown to decrease bowel motility. Ileus is a common postoperative complication, especially after intra-abdominal surgery with opioid analgesia. Use with caution and monitor for decreased bowel motility in postoperative patients receiving opioids. Implement standard supportive therapy.

➤*Special risk patients:* Use caution and reduce initial dose in elderly or debilitated patients and in those suffering from conditions accompanied by hypoxia or hypercapnia when even moderate therapeutic doses may dangerously decrease pulmonary ventilation. Also exercise caution in patients sensitive to CNS depressants, including those with cardiovascular, pulmonary, renal, or hepatic disease; myxedema; convulsive disorders; increased intracranial or ocular pressure; acute alcoholism; delirium tremens; cerebral arteriosclerosis; fever; decreased respiratory reserve (eg, emphysema, severe obesity, asthma, chronic obstructive pulmonary disease or cor pulmonale, sleep apnea syndrome); inflammatory bowel disease; diarrhea secondary to poisoning until the toxin is eliminated; diarrhea secondary to pseudomembranous colitis; GI hemorrhage; bronchial asthma; hypothyroidism; kyphoscoliosis; Addison disease; prostatic hypertrophy; urethral stricture; gallbladder disease or gallstones; recent GI or GU tract surgery; toxic psychosis; alcohol or drug abuse; sickle cell anemia; bradyarrhythmias; paralysis of the phrenic nerve; inability to swallow.

In obese patients (more than 20% above ideal body weight), determine the **alfentanil**, **remifentanil**, and **sufentanil** dosage on the basis of ideal body weight.

Use **fentanyl transmucosal** with caution in patients with diabetes because it contains approximately 2 g of sugar per unit.

In patients with pheochromocytoma, **meperidine** has been reported to provoke hypertension.

Bradycardia – **Fentanyl**, **sufentanil**, **remifentanil**, and **alfentanil** may produce bradycardia, which may be treated with ephedrine or anticholinergic drugs, such as atropine or glycopyrrolate. Use caution when administering to patients with bradyarrhythmias.

➤*Skeletal muscle rigidity:* **Alfentanil**, **fentanyl**, and **sufentanil** may cause skeletal muscle rigidity, particularly of the truncal muscles. The incidence and severity of muscle rigidity is usually dose related. Alfentanil, fentanyl, and sufentanil may produce muscular rigidity that involves all skeletal muscles, including those of the neck, external eye, and extremities. The incidence may be reduced by the following:

1.) routine methods of administration of neuromuscular-blocking agents for balanced opioid anesthesia;
2.) administration of up to ¼ of the full paralyzing dose of a nondepolarizing neuromuscular-blocking agent just prior to administration of alfentanil, fentanyl, or sufentanil; following loss of consciousness or eyelash reflex, administer a full paralyzing dose of a neuromuscular-blocking agent; or
3.) simultaneous administration of alfentanil, fentanyl, or sufentanil and a full paralyzing dose of a neuromuscular-blocking agent when alfentanil, fentanyl, or sufentanil is used in rapidly administered anesthetic dosages. The neuromuscular-blocking agent should be compatible with the patient's cardiovascular status.

Alfentanil administration at anesthetic dosages (more than 130 mcg/kg) will consistently produce muscular rigidity with an immediate onset.

Skeletal muscle rigidity can be caused by **remifentanil** and is related to the dose and speed of administration. Remifentanil may cause chest wall rigidity (inability to ventilate) after single doses of greater than 1 mcg/kg administered over 30 to 60 seconds, or after infusion rates 0.1 mcg/kg/min or greater. Single doses of less than 1 mcg/kg may cause chest wall rigidity when given concurrently with a continuous infusion of remifentanil.

Muscle rigidity seen during the use of remifentanil in spontaneously breathing patients may be treated by stopping or decreasing the rate of administration of remifentanil. Resolution of muscle rigidity after discontinuing the infusion of remifentanil occurs within minutes. In the case of life-threatening muscle rigidity, a rapid-onset neuromuscular blocker or naloxone may be administered.

➤*Fever / External heat:* Serum **fentanyl** concentrations may increase by approximately one third for patients with a body temperature of 40°C (104°F) because of temperature-dependent increases in fentanyl release from the transdermal system and increased skin permeability. Therefore, monitor patients wearing fentanyl transdermal systems who develop fever for opioid side effects and adjust the dose as necessary. Similar increases also may be observed if the fentanyl transdermal system is exposed to external heat (eg, heating pads, electric blankets, saunas, hot tubs). Therefore, advise patients to avoid exposing the patch application site to direct external heat.

➤*Supraventricular tachycardias:* Use **meperidine** with caution in atrial flutter and other supraventricular tachycardias; vagolytic action may increase the ventricular response rate.

➤*Cardiovascular effects:* Limit use of **levorphanol** in acute MI or in cardiac patients with myocardial dysfunction or coronary insufficiency because the effects of levorphanol on the heart are unknown.

Administer opioids with caution to patients in circulatory shock, because vasodilation produced by the drug may further reduce cardiac output and blood pressure.

➤*Pancreatitis / Biliary tract disease:* Use opioids with caution in patients with biliary tract disease, including acute pancreatitis and in those about to undergo surgery of the biliary tract because it may cause spasm of the sphincter of Oddi and diminish biliary and pancreatic secretions. **Levorphanol** has been shown to cause moderate to marked rises in pressure in the common bile duct when given in analgesic doses; it is not recommended for use in biliary surgery. Opioids may cause increases in serum amylase concentration.

➤*Urinary system disorders:* Initiation of neuraxial opiate analgesia is frequently associated with disturbances of micturition, especially in males with prostatic enlargement. Early recognition of difficulty in urination and prompt intervention in cases of urinary retention is indicated.

➤*Cough reflex:* Cough reflex is suppressed. Exercise caution when using opioid analgesics postoperatively and in patients with pulmonary disease.

➤*Intraoperative awareness:* Intraoperative awareness has been reported in patients younger than 55 years of age when **remifentanil** has been administered with propofol infusion rates of 75 mcg/kg/min or less.

➤*Tolerance:* Tolerance, in which increasingly large doses are required in order to produce the same degree of analgesia, is manifested initially by a shortened duration of analgesic effect, and subsequently by decreases in the intensity of analgesia. The rate of development of tolerance varies among patients. In chronic pain patients, and in opioid-tolerant cancer patients, guide the dose of opioids by the degree of tolerance manifested.

➤*Drug abuse and dependence:* Psychological dependence, physical dependence, and tolerance may develop upon repeated administration of opioids; therefore, prescribe and administer opioids with caution. However, psychological dependence is unlikely to develop when opioids are used for a short time for the treatment of pain. Physical dependence, the condition in which continued administration of the drug is required to prevent the appearance of a withdrawal syndrome, usually assumes clinically significant proportions only after several weeks of continued opioid use, although some mild degree of physical dependence may develop after a few days of opioid therapy. Withdrawal symptoms also may be precipitated in the patient with physical dependence by the administration of a drug with opioid-antagonist activity (eg, naloxone).

Use opioids with caution in patients with alcoholism or other drug dependencies because of the increased frequency of opioid tolerance, dependence, and the risk of addiction observed in these patient populations. Abuse of opioids in combination with other CNS depressants can result in serious risk to the patient.

Abuse of ER dose forms by crushing, chewing, snorting, or injecting the dissolved product will result in the immediate release of the entire daily dose of the opioid and pose a significant risk to the abuser that could result in overdose and death.

Acute abstinence syndrome (withdrawal) – In chronic pain patients in whom opioid analgesics are abruptly discontinued, anticipate a severe abstinence syndrome. This may be similar to the abstinence syndrome noted in patients who withdraw from heroin. Severity is related to the degree of dependence, the abruptness of withdrawal, and the drug used. Generally, withdrawal symptoms develop at the time the next dose would ordinarily be given.

Symptoms of withdrawal – The opioid agonist abstinence syndrome is characterized by some or all of the following: restlessness, lacrimation, rhinorrhea, yawning, perspiration, gooseflesh, restless sleep or "yen", and mydriasis during the first 24 hours. These symptoms often increase in severity and over the next 72 hours may be accompanied by increasing irritability, anxiety, weakness, twitching, and spasms of muscles; kicking movements; severe backache, abdominal and leg pains; abdominal and muscle cramps; hot and cold flashes, insomnia; nausea, anorexia, vomiting, intestinal spasm, diarrhea; coryza and repetitive sneezing; increase in body temperature, blood pressure, respiratory rate and heart rate. Because of excessive loss of fluids through sweating, vomiting, and diarrhea, there is usually marked weight loss, dehydration, ketosis, and disturbances in acid-base balance. Cardiovascular collapse can occur. Without treatment most observable symptoms disappear in 5 to 14 days; however, there appears to be a phase of secondary or chronic abstinence which may last for 2 to 6 months characterized by insomnia, irritability, and muscular aches.

Treatment – Primarily symptomatic and supportive; maintain proper fluid and electrolyte balance and administer a tranquilizer to suppress anxiety. Severe withdrawal symptoms may require narcotic replacement. Gradual withdrawal using successively smaller doses will minimize symptoms.

Methadone is not a tranquilizer; patients may react to problems and stresses with the same anxiety symptoms as others do. Do not confuse such symptoms with narcotic abstinence; do not treat anxiety by increasing the methadone dose.

➤*Hazardous tasks:* May produce drowsiness or dizziness. Patients should use caution while driving or performing other tasks requiring alertness, coordination, or physical dexterity.

➤*Sulfite sensitivity:* May cause allergic-type reactions (eg, hives, itching, wheezing, anaphylaxis) in certain susceptible patients. Although the overall prevalence of sulfite sensitivity in the general population is probably low, it is seen more frequently in asthmatic patients or in atopic nonasthmatic patients. Specific products containing sulfites are identified in the product listings.

Drug Interactions

➤*CYP450 system:* **Fentanyl** is metabolized mainly via CYP3A4; therefore, potential interactions may occur when fentanyl is given concurrently with agents that affect CYP3A4 activity. Coadministration with CYP3A4 inducers may reduce the efficacy of fentanyl while coadministration with CYP3A4 inhibitors may increase fentanyl plasma concentration. Carefully monitor patients receiving fentanyl and potent CYP3A4 inhibitors (eg, ritonavir, ketoconazole, clarithromycin) for an extended period of time and adjust dosage as needed.

Oxycodone is metabolized in part by CYP2D6 to **oxymorphone**. The interaction between oxycodone and CYP2D6 inhibitors (eg, quinidine, amiodarone, paroxetine, fluoxetine, amitriptyline) has not yet been shown to be of clinical significance.

Tramadol is extensively metabolized by a number of pathways including CYP2D6 and CYP3A4. The formation of M1 (active metabolite) is dependent upon CYP2D6 and as such is subject to inhibition, which may affect the therapeutic response. Therefore, coadministration of tramadol with a CYP2D6 inhibitor (eg, fluoxetine, paroxetine, quinidine) may increase concentrations of tramadol and reduce concentrations of M1. Coadministration of tramadol with CYP3A4 inhibitors (eg, macrolide antibiotics, azole antifungals, protease inhibitors) may decrease tramadol clearance and CYP3A4 inducers (eg, rifampin, carbamazepine, phenytoin) may increase tramadol clearance.

Opioid Analgesics Drug Interactions

Precipitant drug	Object drug*		Description
Acyclovir	Opioid analgesics	↑	Plasma concentrations of meperidine and normeperidine may be increased; use with caution.
Amiodarone	Opioid analgesics Fentanyl	↑	Profound bradycardia, sinus arrest, and hypotension have occurred with concomitant administration. Monitor hemodynamic function and administer inotropic, chronotropic, and pressor support as necessary. The bradycardia is usually unresponsive to atropine; large doses of vasopressors have been used.
Anticholinergics	Opioid analgesics	↑	Coadministration may result in increased risk of urinary retention and/or severe constipation which may lead to paralytic ileus.
Azole antifungals	Opioid analgesics Alfentanil Fentanyl Methadone	↑	Coadministration may lead to increased pharmacological and adverse effects of the narcotic. Use with caution, and monitor for prolonged or recurrent respiratory depression. A lower dose of the narcotic may be necessary.
Barbiturate anesthetics	Opioid analgesics	↑	Barbiturate anesthetics may increase the respiratory and CNS-depressant effects of the narcotics because of additive pharmacologic activity.
Opioid analgesics	Barbiturate anesthetics		
Barbiturates	Opioid analgesics Methadone	↓	Coadministration may reduce methadone actions. Patients receiving chronic methadone treatment may experience withdrawal symptoms. A higher dose of methadone may be required during coadministration of barbiturates.
Benzodiazepines	Opioid analgesics Sufentanil	↑	Coadministration may result in decreased mean arterial pressure and systemic vascular resistance (also see CNS depressant interaction).
Benzodiazepines Diazepam	Opioid analgesics Alfentanil Fentanyl	↑	Diazepam may produce cardiovascular depression when given with high doses of fentanyl and alfentanil. Administration prior to or following high doses of alfentanil decreases blood pressure secondary to vasodilation; recovery may be prolonged.
Beta-blockers Calcium channel blockers	Opioid analgesics Sufentanil	↑	Increased incidence and degree of bradycardia and hypotension during induction of sufentanil in patients on chronic calcium channel or beta blocker therapy.
Opioid analgesics Sufentanil	Beta-blockers Calcium channel blockers		
Carbamazepine	Opioid analgesics Tramadol	↓	Because carbamazepine increases tramadol metabolism and because of the seizure risk associated with tramadol, concomitant administration is not recommended.
Cigarette smoking	Opioid analgesics Propoxyphene	↓	Cigarette smoking may induce liver enzymes responsible for the metabolism of propoxyphene; efficacy is reportedly decreased in smokers. Patients may increase the dosage to obtain adequate pain relief.
Cimetidine	Opioid analgesics	↑	The actions of opioid analgesics may be enhanced, resulting in toxicity. Alfentanil clearance may be reduced; therefore, smaller alfentanil doses may be needed.
CNS depressants (eg, barbiturates, tranquilizers, inhalation anesthetics, ethanol)	Opioid analgesics	↑	Both the magnitude and duration of CNS and cardiovascular effects may be enhanced. Reduce the dose of one or both agents during concomitant use.
CYP2D6 inhibitors (eg, fluoxetine, paroxetine, quinidine, amitriptyline)	Opioid analgesics Oxycodone Tramadol	↑	Inhibition of the metabolism of tramadol or oxycodone may occur.

Opioid Analgesics Drug Interactions

Precipitant drug	Object drug*		Description
CYP3A4 inducers (eg, rifampin, phenytoin)	Opioid analgesics Fentanyl Tramadol	⬇	May produce increased clearance of fentanyl and tramadol; use with caution.
CYP3A4 inhibitors (eg, erythromycin, ketoconazole, certain protease inhibitors)	Opioid analgesics Fentanyl Tramadol	⬆	Coadministration may produce increased fentanyl and tramadol concentrations. Carefully monitor patients receiving fentanyl and potent CYP3A4 inhibitors (eg, ritonavir, ketoconazole, clarithromycin) for an extended period of time and adjust the dosage as needed.
Droperidol	Opioid analgesics Fentanyl	⬆	Pulmonary arterial pressure may be depressed and hypotension may occur.
Erythromycin	Opioid analgesics Alfentanil Fentanyl Methadone	⬆	Erythromycin may inhibit the metabolism of the narcotic. Coadministration may result in increased pharmacologic effects of the narcotic. Monitor for prolonged or recurrent respiratory depression and sedation. Consider a lower dose of the narcotic or an alternate narcotic.
Ethanol	Opioid analgesics Alfentanil	⬇	Chronic ethanol consumption may produce a pharmacodynamic tolerance to alfentanil. Chronic ethanol consumers may need higher doses of alfentanil (see also CNS depressants interaction).
Hydantoins (eg, phenytoin)	Opioid analgesics Meperidine Methadone	⬇	Hydantoins may decrease the pharmacologic effects of meperidine and methadone, possibly because of increased hepatic metabolism of the narcotic.
Lidocaine	Opioid analgesics Morphine	⬆	Respiratory depression and loss of consciousness may occur.
Opioid analgesics Morphine	Lidocaine		
MAOIs	Opioid analgesics	⬆	Severe and unpredictable potentiation by MAOIs has been reported with certain opioid analgesics. Opioids are not recommended for use in patients who have received MAOIs within 14 days. Meperidine is contraindicated in patients who have recently received an MAOI. Coadministration could result in adverse reactions that may include agitation, seizures, diaphoresis, and fever, which may progress to coma, apnea, and death. Reactions may occur several weeks following withdrawal of MAOIs.
Opioid analgesics	MAOIs		
Neostigmine	Opioid analgesics Morphine	⬆	Increases the intensity and duration of the analgesic action.
Nitrous oxide	Opioid analgesics Fentanyl Sufentanil	⬆	Nitrous oxide may cause cardiovascular depression with high-dose sufentanil and fentanyl.
Nonnucleoside reverse transcriptase inhibitors (NNRTIs) (eg, nevirapine, efavirenz)	Opioid analgesics Methadone	⬇	Concomitant administration may result in reduced methadone action and opiate withdrawal symptoms. Anticipate an increase in the methadone dose when starting an NNRTI and monitor for withdrawal symptoms. Monitor for methadone overdose signs when an NNRTI is discontinued and adjust the methadone dose accordingly.
Nucleoside reverse transcriptase inhibitors Abacavir	Opioid analgesics Methadone	⬇	When coadministered with abacavir, methadone clearance increased by 22%. Methadone dose adjustment may be needed in a small number of patients. Coadministration may decrease AUC and C_{max} of didanosine and stavudine; however, coadministation may increase zidovudine concentration. Monitor zidovudine effects closely; a lower dose may be needed.
Opioid analgesics Methadone	Nucleoside reverse transcriptase inhibitors Didanosine Stavudine Zidovudine	⬆⬇	
Opioid agonist/antagonist analgesics, opioid partial agonist analgesics	Opioid analgesics	⬇	Do not administer opioid agonist/antagonist analgesics (eg, pentazocine, nalbuphine, butorphanol) or partial agonists (eg, buprenorphine) to a patient who has received or is receiving a course of therapy with a pure agonist opioid analgesic. In opioid-dependent patients, mixed agonist/antagonist analgesics and partial agonists may precipitate withdrawal symptoms.
Phenothiazines	Opioid analgesics	⬆	Although the analgesic effect of narcotics may be potentiated, a higher incidence of toxic effects may occur. Reduce the dose of meperidine.
Propofol	Opioid analgesics Oxycodone	⬆	Increased risk of bradycardia with concomitant use.
Protease inhibitors (eg, ritonavir, saquinavir, nelfinavir)	Opioid analgesics Fentanyl Meperidine Methadone Propoxyphene	⬆⬇	Plasma concentrations of propoxyphene and fentanyl may be increased, possibly causing toxicity. The pharmacologic effects of methadone may be decreased. Meperidine levels may decrease and normeperidine levels may increase, possibly decreasing efficacy but increasing neurologic toxicity. Concurrent use of propoxyphene or meperidine with a protease inhibitor is contraindicated.
Quinidine	Opioid analgesics Codeine	⬇	The analgesic effects of codeine may be decreased. It may be necessary to use an alternative analgesic.
Reserpine	Opioid analgesics Morphine	⬇	Inhibits analgesic action.
Rifamycins (eg, rifampin)	Opioid analgesics Methadone Morphine	⬇	Rifampin appears to stimulate methadone metabolism. Coadministration may result in reduced methadone action and opiate withdrawal symptoms. A higher dose of methadone may be required during coadministration of rifampin. The analgesic effects of morphine may be decreased with concurrent administration. May be necessary to administer an alternative analgesic.
Sibutramine	Opioid analgesics Meperidine	⬆	Serotonergic effects of these agents may be additive, resulting in a serotonin syndrome. Concomitant administration is not recommended.
Opioid analgesics Meperidine	Sibutramine		
SSRIs Nefazodone Venlafaxine	Opioid analgesics Methadone Tramadol	⬆	Fluvoxamine may inhibit methadone metabolism and therefore increase toxicity. Use with caution. The serotonergic effects of tramadol and serotonin reuptake effects of tramadol and serotonin reuptake inhibitors may be additive, increasing the risk for adverse effects such as seizures and serotonin syndrome.
Opioid analgesics Tramadol	SSRIs Nefazodone Venlafaxine		

Opioid Analgesics Drug Interactions

Precipitant drug	Object drug*		Description
Tricyclic antidepressants Amitriptyline Clomipramine Nortriptyline	Opioid analgesics Morphine	↑	Monitor for increased CNS and respiratory depression when administered with morphine.
Urinary acidifiers	Opioid analgesics Methadone	↓	Urinary acidifiers increase the renal clearance of methadone.
Opioid analgesics Methadone	Desipramine	↑	Desipramine blood levels have increased with concurrent methadone therapy.
Opioid analgesics Propoxyphene	Carbamazepine	↑	Propoxyphene may inhibit the metabolism of carbamazepine, thereby increasing carbamazepine serum concentrations and toxicity.
Opioid analgesics Remifentanil	Opioid analgesics Morphine	↓	The analgesic effect of morphine may be decreased with coadministration. May be necessary to titrate morphine to higher levels than expected.
Opioid analgesics Tramadol	Digoxin	↑	Rare reports of digoxin toxicity have been reported in postmarketing surveillance.
Opioid analgesics Morphine	Diuretics	↓	Reduces efficacy by inducing the release of antidiuretic hormone.
Opioid analgesics Morphine Propoxyphene Tramadol	Warfarin	↑	The oral anticoagulant effect of warfarin may be increased. Monitor coagulation tests and adjust dose as needed.
Opioid analgesics	Skeletal muscle relaxants	↑	Coadministration may enhance the neuromuscular blocking action and produce an increased degree of respiratory depression.

* ↑ = Object drug increased. ↓ = Object drug decreased.

➤*Drug/Food interactions:* Grapefruit juice may increase **methadone** serum concentrations, thereby increasing the pharmacologic and adverse effects.

Adverse Reactions

Opioid Analgesic Adverse Reactions[a]

System	Adverse reactions	Alfentanil	Codeine	Fentanyl injection	Fentanyl transdermal: Adults	Fentanyl transdermal: Children (2 to 18 years of age)	Fentanyl transmucosal	Hydromorphone IR*	Hydromorphone ER*	Levorphanol	Meperidine	Methadone	Morphine	Oxycodone IR*	Oxycodone CR*	Oxymorphone	Propoxyphene	Remifentanil: Adults	Remifentanil: Children (≤ 12 years of age)	Sufentanil	Tramadol
Cardiovascular	Abnormal ECG								< 1			✓									PM
	Angina pectoris						< 1		< 1												
	Arrhythmia	14			≥ 1				< 1	✓		✓								0.3-1	
	Atrial fibrillation								< 1				✓					< 1			
	Bradycardia	14	✓	✓	< 1			✓	< 1	✓	✓	✓	✓			✓		1-7		3-9	
	Cardiac arrest		✓	✓				✓		✓	✓	✓	✓	✓							PM
	Cardiomegaly								< 1												
	Chest pain				≥ 1		≥ 1		≥ 1				✓		< 1			< 1			
	Circulatory depression/collapse		✓	✓				✓			✓	✓	✓	✓	✓						
	CHF/heart failure								< 1			✓		< 3							
	Deep thrombophlebitis						≥ 1		< 1					< 3							
	Extrasystoles									✓											
	Faintness		✓					✓				✓	✓								
	Flushing		✓			≥ 1		✓		✓	✓	✓	✓			✓		1			
	Hemorrhage						< 1		< 1					< 3							
	Hypertension	18		✓		≥ 1	0-1	✓	< 1				✓					1-2		3-9	PM
	Hypotension	10	✓ (orthostatic)	✓			< 1	✓	< 1	✓	✓	✓	✓	< 3	1-5	✓		4-19		3-9	< 1
	Migraine						≥ 1		≥ 1					< 3	< 1						PM
	MI								< 1												
	Myocardial ischemia																				PM
	Palpitation		✓				≥ 1	✓	< 1	✓	✓	✓	✓	< 3		✓					PM
	Pallor								< 1				✓								
	Peripheral vascular disorder						< 1														
	Phlebitis										✓	✓	✓ (IV)								
	QT interval prolongation								< 1			✓									
	ST depression														< 1						
	Supraventricular tachycardia								< 1												
	Syncope		✓		≥ 1	≥ 1		✓	< 1		✓	✓	✓		< 1			< 1			< 1
	Tachycardia	12	✓		PM	≥ 1	< 1	✓	≥ 1	✓	✓	✓	✓	< 3		✓		< 1		0.3-1	< 1
	Thrombosis								< 1												
	Vascular disorder						≥ 1														
	Vasodilation						0-4		≥ 1				✓	< 3	< 1						1-5

Opioid Analgesic Adverse Reactions[a]

System	Adverse reactions	Alfentanil	Codeine	Fentanyl injection	Fentanyl transdermal		Fentanyl transmucosal	Hydromorphone IR*	Hydromorphone ER*	Levorphanol	Meperidine	Methadone	Morphine	Oxycodone IR*	Oxycodone CR*	Oxymorphone	Propoxyphene	Remifentanil		Sufentanil	Tramadol
					Adults	Children (2 to 18 years of age)												Adults	Children (≤ 12 years of age)		
CNS	Abnormal coordination				≥1																
	Abnormal dreams				≥ 1		0-1		< 1	✓			✓		1-5						
	Abnormal gait				≥1		0-5		≥ 1				✓		< 1						< 1
	Abnormal thinking				≥ 1		0-2		≥ 1	✓			✓		1-5						< 1
	Acute brain syndrome						< 1														
	Addiction								< 1												
	Agitation		✓		≥ 1	≥ 1	< 1		≥ 1		✓	✓	✓	< 1				< 1			
	Amnesia				≥1		< 1		≥ 1	✓			✓		< 1			< 1			< 1
	Anxiety		✓		3-10	≥ 1	0-15	✓	≥ 1				✓	< 3	1-5			< 1			1-5
	Aphasia				< 1				< 1												
	Apathy								< 1												
	Asthenia				≥ 10	3-10	0-38		3.2				✓		6						6-12
	Ataxia								< 1				✓								
	Cerebral ischemia						< 1														
	Cerebrovascular accident								< 1												
	CNS stimulation									✓						✓					7-14
	Coma									✓			✓					< 1			
	Confusion				≥ 10	≥ 1	0-13		≥ 1	✓		✓	✓	< 3	1-5	✓		< 1			1-5
	Convulsion/ Seizure		✓			≥ 1	0-2		< 1	✓	✓, severe	✓	✓		< 1						< 1
	Delirium								< 1				✓								
	Dementia								< 1												
	Depersonalization				< 1				< 1						< 1						
	Depression				3-10	≥ 1	2-9		≥ 1	✓			✓		< 1	✓					< 1
	Disorientation		✓					✓			✓	✓	✓					< 1			
	Dizziness	3-9	✓	✓	3-10	≥ 1	0-17	✓	≥ 1	✓		✓	✓	✓	13		< 1	< 5			26-33
	Drowsiness							✓	< 1				✓			✓					
	Dyskinesia									✓											
	Dysphoria		✓					✓	< 1		✓	✓		✓		✓	< 1	< 1			
	Emotional lability						< 1		< 1						< 1						
	Euphoria	0.3-1	✓		3-10		< 1	✓	< 1		✓	✓	✓	✓	1-5	✓	< 1				1-5
	Facial paralysis						< 1														
	Fear		✓					✓													
	Foot drop						< 1														
	Hallucinations				3-10	≥ 1	≤ 2	✓	≥ 1		✓		✓		< 1	✓	< 1	< 1			< 1
	Headache	0.3-1	✓		3-10	3-10	3-20	✓	4.7		✓	✓	✓		7	✓	< 1	≤ 18			18-32
	Hemiplegia						< 1														
	Hostility				< 1				< 1												
	Hyperkinesia									✓					< 1						
	Hypertonia				< 1				≥ 1					< 3							1-5

Opioid Analgesic Adverse Reactions[a]

System	Adverse reactions	Alfentanil	Codeine	Fentanyl injection	Fentanyl transdermal		Fentanyl transmucosal	Hydromorphone IR*	Hydromorphone ER*	Levorphanol	Meperidine	Methadone	Morphine	Oxycodone IR*	Oxycodone CR*	Oxymorphone	Propoxyphene	Remifentanil		Sufentanil	Tramadol
					Adults	Children (2 to 18 years of age)												Adults	Children (≤ 12 years of age)		
CNS (cont.)	Hypesthesia						≥ 1		≥ 1						< 1						
	Hypokinesia						≥ 1		< 1	✓											
	Hypotonia				< 1										< 1						
	Impairment of mental and physical performance		✓					✓													
	Incoordination						< 1	✓	< 1		✓		✓								1-5
	Increased intracranial pressure							✓					✓								
	Insomnia		✓		≥ 1	3-10	≤ 8	✓	≥ 1	✓		✓	✓		1-5	✓					
	Lethargy		✓					✓		✓			✓								
	Light-headedness		✓					✓			✓	✓	✓	✓		✓	< 1				
	Mental clouding		✓					✓					✓			✓					
	Mood changes		✓					✓					✓								
	Myoclonic movements	PM					0-4		< 1		✓										
	Nervousness				3-10	3-10	0-4		≥ 1	✓			✓	< 3	1-5	✓					1-5
	Neuralgia								< 1					< 3							
	Neuropathy						≥ 1														
	Paranoid reaction				≥ 1	≥ 1			< 1												
	Paresthesia				≥ 1		≥ 1	✓	≥ 1				✓		< 1			< 1			< 1
	Personality disorder									✓				< 3							
	Postoperative confusion	0.3-1																			
	Psychosis								< 1												
	Restlessness															✓					
	Serotonin syndrome																				< 1
	Shivering	0.3-1			≥ 1													1-5	3		
	Sleep disorder euphoria								< 1												
	Sleepiness/sedation/somnolence	1-3	✓		≥ 10	3-10	7-20	✓	4.7		✓	✓	✓	✓	23	✓	< 1			3-9	16-25
	Speech disorder				≥ 1	≥ 1	≥ 1		≥ 1						< 1			< 1			PM
	Stupor				< 1	≥ 1	0-4		< 1						< 1						
	Subdural hematoma						< 1														
	Suicide attempt/tendency									✓											< 1
	Tremor				≥ 1	≥ 1	0-2	✓	≥ 1		✓		✓	< 3	< 1			< 1			< 1
	Twitching								< 1		✓				1-5			< 1			
	Vertigo				< 1		0-4		< 1				✓		< 1						26-33
	Weakness		✓					✓			✓	✓	✓			✓	< 1				
	Withdrawal syndrome								< 1	✓			✓		< 1						
Dermatological	Alopecia						≥ 1		< 1												
	Application-site reactions				> 1	3-10															
	Dry skin												✓		< 1						
	Erythema																			0.3-1	
	Erythematous rash					≥ 1															
	Exfoliative dermatitis				< 1		< 1								< 1						
	Herpes simplex													< 3							
	Herpes zoster						< 1														
	Itching/pruritus	0.3-1	✓		3-10	3-10	0-5	✓	2.6	✓		✓	✓	✓	13	✓		≤ 18		25	8-11
	Localized skin reaction					≥ 1												< 1			
	Maculopapular rash						< 1		< 1												
	Photosensitivity reaction								< 1					< 3							
	Pustules				< 1																
	Rash				≥ 1	≥ 1	0-8	✓	≥ 1	✓		✓	✓	< 3	1-5		< 1	< 1			1-5
	Skin discoloration						< 1														
	Skin ulcer						≥ 1														
	Stevens-Johnson syndrome/Toxic epidermal necrolysis																				< 1
	Sweating		✓	✓	≥ 10	≥ 1	0-4	✓	≥ 1	✓	✓	✓	✓	< 3	5	✓		6			6-9
	Urticaria	0.3-1					< 1	✓	< 1	✓		✓	✓	< 3	< 1			< 1			< 1
	Vesicles																				< 1
	Vesiculobullous						< 1														

Opioid Analgesic Adverse Reactions[a]

System	Adverse reactions	Alfentanil	Codeine	Fentanyl injection	Fentanyl transdermal		Fentanyl transmucosal	Hydromorphone IR*	Hydromorphone ER*	Levorphanol	Meperidine	Methadone	Morphine	Oxycodone IR*	Oxycodone CR*	Oxymorphone	Propoxyphene	Remifentanil		Sufentanil	Tramadol
					Adults	Children (2 to 18 years of age)												Adults	Children (≤ 12 years of age)		
GI	Abdominal distention				< 1		≥ 1														
	Abdominal pain				3-10	≥ 1	≥ 1		≥ 1	✓		✓		< 3	1-5	✓	< 1				1-5
	Abnormal LFTs								< 1				✓				< 1				PM
	Abnormal stools								< 1												
	Anorexia		✓		3-10	≥ 1		✓	≥ 1			✓	✓	< 3	1-5	✓					1-5
	Appetite increased								< 1						< 1						
	Biliary tract spasm		✓					✓	< 1	✓	✓	✓	✓	✓		✓					
	Cheilitis						< 1														
	Cholangitis								< 1												
	Cholecystitis								< 1												
	Colitis								< 1												
	Colon hemorrhage						< 1														
	Colonic motility increased												✓								
	Constipation		✓		≥ 10	3-10	0-20	✓	15.8		✓	✓	✓	✓	23	✓	< 1	< 1			24-46
	Cramps							✓				✓			✓						
	Dry mouth		✓		≥ 10	≥ 1	0-4	✓	≥ 1	✓	✓	✓	✓	< 3	6	✓					5-10
	Diarrhea				3-10	≥ 1	≥ 1	✓	≥ 1				✓	< 3	1-5			< 1			5-10
	Dyspepsia				3-10		≥ 1		≥ 1	✓			✓	< 3	1-5						5-13
	Dysphagia						≥ 1		≥ 1				✓	< 3	< 1			< 1			
	Enterocolitis								< 1												
	Eructation						≥ 1		< 1						< 1						
	Esophageal stenosis						< 1														
	Esophagitis						< 1		< 1												
	Fecal impaction						< 1		< 1												
	Fecal incontinence						< 1		< 1												
	Flatulence				≥ 1		≥ 1		≥ 1						< 1						1-5
	Gastritis														1-5						
	Gastroenteritis						< 1						✓								
	GI disorder						< 1								< 1						
	GI hemorrhage						≥ 1		< 1												PM
	Gingivitis						≥ 1							< 3							
	Glossitis						≥ 1		< 1			✓		< 3							
	Gum hemorrhage						< 1														
	Gum line erosion						PM														
	Hepatic failure								< 1												PM
	Hepatitis																				PM
	Hepatomegaly								< 1												
	Hepatorenal syndrome						< 1														
	Ileus							✓	< 1				✓		< 1	✓		< 1			

Opioid Analgesic Adverse Reactions[a]

System	Adverse reactions	Alfentanil	Codeine	Fentanyl injection	Fentanyl transdermal		Fentanyl transmucosal	Hydromorphone IR*	Hydromorphone ER*	Levorphanol	Meperidine	Methadone	Morphine	Oxycodone IR*	Oxycodone CR*	Oxymorphone	Propoxyphene	Remifentanil		Sufentanil	Tramadol
					Adults	Children (2 to 18 years of age)												Adults	Children (≤ 12 years of age)		
GI (cont.)	Increased pressure in the biliary tract		✓																		
	Intestinal obstruction						0-4		< 1				✓								
	Jaundice						≥ 1		< 1								< 1				
	Liver tenderness						< 1														
	Melena								< 1												
	Mouth ulceration						≥ 1		< 1												
	Nausea	28	✓	✓	≥ 10	≥ 10	11-45	✓	10.5	✓	✓	✓	✓	< 3	23	✓	< 1	1-4.4	6-8	3-9	24-40
	Oral moniliasis						≥ 1														
	Periodontal abscess						≥ 1														
	Rectal disorder						≥ 1						✓								
	Rectal hemorrhage						≥ 1		< 1												
	Salivation increased								< 1												
	Stomatitis						≥ 1								< 1						PM
	Thirst						< 1		< 1				✓		< 1						
	Tongue edema								< 1												
	Tooth caries						< 1														
	Tooth disorder						< 1														
	Tooth loss						PM														
	Toxic megacolon															✓[b]					
	Vomiting	18	✓	✓	≥ 10	≥ 10	6-31	✓	3.2	✓	✓	✓	✓	< 3	12	✓	< 1	≤ 22	12-16	3-9	9-17
	Weight loss				PM		≥ 1		≥ 1				✓								< 1
GU	Abnormal ejaculation				PM								✓								
	Amenorrhea											✓			< 1						
	Antidiuretic effect		✓					✓			✓	✓	✓		< 1	✓					
	Bladder pain				< 1																
	Breast neoplasm						≥ 1														
	Breast pain						≥ 1														
	Creatinine increased								< 1												PM
	Decreased libido/potency		✓		PM		< 1					✓	✓		< 1						
	Dysmenorrhea								< 1												
	Dysuria						≥ 1		≥ 1				✓		< 1			< 1			< 1
	Hematuria						≥ 1		< 1						< 1						
	Hydronephrosis						≥ 1														
	Impotence								< 1				✓	✓							
	Kidney failure						≥ 1			✓											
	Kidney pain						< 1														
	Menopausal symptoms																				1-5
	Menstrual disorder																				< 1
	Nocturia						< 1														
	Oliguria				< 1		< 1						✓					< 1			
	Polyuria						< 1								< 1						
	Proteinuria																				PM
	Pyelonephritis						< 1														
	Scrotal edema						> 1														
	Spasm of vesical sphincters		✓					✓					✓								
	Ureteral spasm		✓					✓					✓			✓					
	Urinary frequency				< 1				< 1												1-5
	Urinary hesitancy		✓					✓				✓	✓			✓					
	Urinary incontinence						≥ 1		≥ 1									< 1			
	Urinary retention		✓		3-10	≥ 1	0-2	✓	< 1	✓	✓	✓	✓		< 1	✓		< 1		✓	1-5
	Urinary urgency						≥ 1		< 1												
	UTI						≥ 1						✓	< 3							
	Urination impaired						≥ 1		< 1	✓					< 1						
	Vaginal hemorrhage						≥ 1														
	Vaginitis						≥ 1														

Opioid Analgesic Adverse Reactions[a]

System	Adverse reactions	Alfentanil	Codeine	Fentanyl injection	Fentanyl transdermal: Adults	Fentanyl transdermal: Children (2 to 18 years of age)	Fentanyl transmucosal	Hydromorphone IR*	Hydromorphone ER*	Levorphanol	Meperidine	Methadone	Morphine	Oxycodone IR*	Oxycodone CR*	Oxymorphone	Propoxyphene	Remifentanil: Adults	Remifentanil: Children (≤ 12 years of age)	Sufentanil	Tramadol
Hematologic/Lymphatic	Agranulocytosis								< 1												
	Anemia						≥ 1		≥ 1				✓	< 3							
	Bleeding time increased						< 1														
	Ecchymosis						≥ 1		< 1												
	Hemoglobin decrease																				PM
	Leukopenia						≥ 1		≥ 1					< 3							
	Leukocytosis								< 1												
	Lymphadenopathy						≥ 1		< 1						< 1						
	Lymphedema						≥ 1														
	Lymphoma-like reaction								< 1												
	Pancytopenia						≥ 1		< 1												
	Petechia								< 1												
	Thrombocytopenia						≥ 1		< 1			✓	✓								
Hypersensitivity	Allergic reaction		✓			≥ 1	< 1	✓	< 1					< 3		✓[c]					< 1
	Allergic bronchospastic reaction															✓					
	Allergic laryngeal edema															✓					
	Allergic laryngospasm															✓					
	Anaphylaxis/Anaphylactoid	PM		✓								✓	✓		< 1			< 1		PM	< 1
	Edema											✓	✓								
	Hemorrhagic urticaria		Rare									✓	✓								
	Pruritus		✓								✓	✓	✓			✓					
	Skin rash		✓								✓	✓	✓			✓					
	Urticaria		✓								✓	✓	✓			✓					
	Wheal and flare over vein with IV injection							✓			✓	✓	✓								
Metabolic	Acidosis						< 1		< 1												
	Adrenal cortex insufficiency								< 1												
	Cachexia								< 1												
	Cyanosis								< 1		✓										
	Diabetes mellitus								< 1												
	Gout								< 1					< 3							
	Hypercalcemia						≥ 1														
	Hyperglycemia						≥ 1		< 1					< 3				< 1			
	Hypocalcemia						< 1			< 1											
	Hypoglycemia						< 1														
	Hypokalemia						≥ 1		≥ 1			✓									
	Hypomagnesemia						≥ 1		< 1			✓									
	Hyponatremia						< 1		< 1						< 1						
	Hypoproteinemia						< 1														
Musculoskeletal	Arthralgia						≥ 1		≥ 1					< 3							
	Arthritis						< 1							< 3							
	Bone disorder						≥ 1														
	Chest wall rigidity	17		✓																3-9	
	Joint disorder						≥ 1														
	Leg cramps						≥ 1		≥ 1												
	Muscle atrophy						< 1														
	Muscle rigidity			✓				✓					✓					2-11		✓	
	Muscle tremor							✓													
	Myalgia						≥ 1		≥ 1					< 3							
	Myasthenia						< 1		< 1												
	Myopathy						< 1														
	Neck and extremity rigidity	PM																		PM	
	Pathological fracture						≥ 1							< 3							
	Skeletal muscle movement	3-9																			
	Synovitis						< 1														
	Tendon disorder						< 1														

Opioid Analgesic Adverse Reactions[a]																					
System	Adverse reactions	Alfentanil	Codeine	Fentanyl injection	Fentanyl transdermal		Fentanyl transmucosal	Hydromorphone IR*	Hydromorphone ER*	Levorphanol	Meperidine	Methadone	Morphine	Oxycodone IR*	Oxycodone CR*	Oxymorphone	Propoxyphene	Remifentanil		Sufentanil	Tramadol
					Adults	Children (2 to 18 years of age)												Adults	Children (≤ 12 years of age)		
Respiratory	Apnea	1-3		✓	3-10			✓	< 1	✓			✓		✓			≤ 30		0.3-1	
	Asthma				< 1		≥ 1		< 1												
	Atelectasis								< 1							✓					
	Bronchitis				≥ 1		≥ 1							< 3				< 1			
	Bronchospasm	< 1						✓										< 1		0.3-1	
	Cough					≥ 1	≥ 1		≥ 1					< 3	< 1			< 1	1		
	Dyspnea				3-10	≥ 1	2-22		≥ 1				✓	< 3	1-5			< 1			< 1
	Epistaxis						≥ 1		≥ 1					< 3							
	Hemoptysis				≥ 1		≥ 1		< 1												
	Hiccoughs				≥ 1		< 1		≥ 1				✓		1-5			< 1			
	Hypercarbia	0.3-1																			
	Hyperventilation						< 1		< 1												
	Hypoventilation				3-10				< 1	✓			✓								
	Hypoxia								≥ 1									< 1			
	Laryngismus								< 1					< 3							
	Laryngospasm	0.3-1		✓				✓					✓					< 1			
	Lung disorder						< 1							< 3							
	Pharyngitis				3-10		≥ 1		≥ 1					< 3	< 1			< 1			
	Pleural effusion						< 1		≥ 1									< 1			
	Pneumonia						≥ 1		≥ 1												
	Pneumothorax						< 1														
	Pulmonary edema											✓						< 1			PM
	Pulmonary embolus								< 1												PM
	Respiratory arrest		✓	✓			✓	✓			✓	✓	✓	✓	✓						
	Respiratory depression	3-9 (post-op)	✓	✓		≥ 1		✓			✓	✓	✓	✓	✓	✓		< 1		0.3-1	
	Respiratory disorder				< 1																
	Respiratory insufficiency						< 1														
	Rhinitis					≥ 1	≥ 1		≥ 1					< 3							
	Sinusitis						≥ 1							< 3							
	Sputum increased						≥ 1														
	Stertorous breathing				< 1																
	Suppressed cough reflex		✓																		
	Voice alteration						< 1						✓		< 1						
Special senses	Abnormal vision						0-3		< 1	✓					< 1						
	Amblyopia				< 1				≥ 1					< 3							
	Blurred vision	1-3		✓	PM			✓	< 1							✓					
	Cataracts																				PM
	Conjunctivitis						≥ 1														
	Diplopia							✓	< 1	✓			✓			✓					
	Dry eyes								< 1												
	Dysgeusia																				< 1
	Ear disorder						≥ 1														
	Ear pain						< 1														
	Eye hemorrhage						< 1														
	Hyperacusis								< 1												
	Lacrimation disorder						< 1		< 1												
	Miosis		✓				< 1	✓					✓			✓					
	Nystagmus							✓	< 1				✓								
	Partial permanent/transitory deafness						< 1														PM
	Taste perversion						≥ 1	✓	≥ 1				✓		< 1						
	Tinnitus						≥ 1		≥ 1						< 1						PM
	Visual disturbances		✓					✓			✓	✓	✓				✓				1-5

Opioid Analgesic Adverse Reactions[a]

System	Adverse reactions	Alfentanil	Codeine	Fentanyl injection	Fentanyl transdermal Adults	Fentanyl transdermal Children (2 to 18 years of age)	Fentanyl transmucosal	Hydromorphone IR*	Hydromorphone ER*	Levorphanol	Meperidine	Methadone	Morphine	Oxycodone IR*	Oxycodone CR*	Oxymorphone	Propoxyphene	Remifentanil Adults	Remifentanil Children (≤ 12 years of age)	Sufentanil	Tramadol
Miscellaneous	Abscess						< 1														
	Accidental injury				≥ 1		0-9		≥ 1				✓	< 3	< 1						< 1
	Ascites						≥ 1		< 1												
	Back pain				≥ 1		≥ 1							< 3							
	Bone pain						≥ 1		≥ 1					< 3							
	Carcinoma								≥ 1												
	Cellulitis						≥ 1		< 1												
	Chills						≥ 1	✓	≥ 1				✓	< 3	1-5			1			
	Dehydration						≥ 1		≥ 1				✓		< 1						
	Edema				PM		≥ 1		≥ 1			✓	✓	< 3	< 1						
	Face edema								< 1						< 1						
	Fever				≥ 1	≥ 1	≥ 1		≥ 1				✓	< 3	< 1						
	Flank pain								< 1									< 10			
	Flu syndrome				3-10		≥ 1						✓	< 3							
	Fungal infection						≥ 1														
	Hypothermia								< 1												
	Infection				3-10		≥ 1		5.3				✓								
	Injection-site pain/reaction	0.3-1						✓		✓								1			
	Intraoperative muscle movement																			0.3-1	
	Malaise						≥ 1		≥ 1				✓		< 1						1-5
	Neck pain						≥ 1		≥ 1					< 3	< 1						
	Neoplasm								< 1												
	Pain					3-10	≥ 1		≥ 1					< 3	< 1						
	Pelvic pain						≥ 1														
	Sepsis						≥ 1		< 1				✓	< 3							
	Shock		✓					✓		✓	✓	✓	✓	✓	✓						
	Viral infection						≥ 1														

[a] Data polled from separate studies and are not necessarily comparable.
[b] In patients with inflammatory bowel disease.
[c] Including erythema, papules, itching, and edema.
* IR = immediate release, ER = extended release, CR = controlled release, PM = postmarketing.

Management of adverse reactions – Most patients receiving opioids, especially those who are opioid naïve, will experience side effects. Frequently the side effects from opioids are transient but may require evaluation and management. Anticipate adverse events, such as constipation, and treat aggressively and prophylactically with a stimulant laxative and/or stool softener. Patients do not usually become tolerant to the constipating effects of opioids.

Other opioid-related side effects such as sedation and nausea are usually self-limited and often do not persist beyond the first few days. If nausea persists and is unacceptable to the patient, consider treatment with antiemetics or other modalities as they may relieve these symptoms.

Patients receiving some opioids may pass an intact matrix "ghost" in the stool or via colostomy. These ghosts contain little or no residual drug and are of no clinical consequence.

Overdosage

In general, the shorter the onset and duration of action of the opiate, the greater the intensity and rapidity of symptom onset. Infants and children may be relatively more sensitive on a body weight basis. Elderly patients are comparatively intolerant.

➤*Symptoms:* In severe overdosage, mainly by the IV route, apnea, circulatory collapse, convulsions, cardiac arrest, pulmonary edema, and death may occur. The less severely poisoned patient often has a triad of CNS depression, miosis, and respiratory depression. Serious overdosage is characterized by respiratory depression, extreme somnolence progressing to stupor or coma, constricted pupils, skeletal muscle flaccidity, and cold and clammy skin. Hypotension, bradycardia, hypothermia, pulmonary edema, pneumonia, or shock occurs in 40% or less of patients.

➤*Treatment:* Employ supportive measures as indicated. Refer to General Management of Acute Overdosage. Give primary attention to reestablishment of adequate respiratory exchange; provide a patent airway and institute assisted or controlled ventilation.

Administer a narcotic antagonist (eg, naloxone). The duration of respiratory depression following overdosage may be longer than the duration of the opioid antagonist, so repeated administration of the antagonist may be necessary; keep the patient under surveillance. Do not give an antagonist in the absence of clinically significant respiratory or cardiovascular depression. Naloxone is the antagonist of choice (see individual monograph). If necessary to give an antagonist to an opioid-tolerant patient, administer with extreme caution and by titration with smaller than usual doses.

While naloxone will reverse some, but not all, symptoms caused by **tramadol** overdose, the risk of seizures is also increased with naloxone administration. In animals, convulsions following the administration of toxic doses of tramadol were suppressed with barbiturates or benzodiazepines but were increased with naloxone. Hemodialysis is not expected to be helpful in a tramadol overdose because it removed less than 7% of the administered dose in a 4-hour dialysis period.

IV fluids and vasopressors for the treatment of hypotension and other supportive measures may be employed.

In painful conditions, reversal of narcotic effect may result in acute onset of pain and release of catecholamines. Careful administration of naloxone may permit reversal of side effects without affecting analgesia. Parenteral administration of narcotics in patients receiving epidural or intrathecal **morphine** may result in overdosage.

In cases of overdose from the **fentanyl transdermal** patch, remove the patch immediately.

In cases of oral overdose, evacuate the stomach by emesis or gastric lavage if treatment can be instituted within 2 hours following ingestion. Do not induce emesis. Absorption of drugs from the GI tract may be decreased by giving activated charcoal which, in many cases, is more effective than lavage. Observe the patient for a rise in temperature or pulmonary complications that may require antibiotic therapy.

Forced diuresis, peritoneal dialysis, hemodialysis, or charcoal hemoperfusion have not been established as beneficial for a **codeine** or **methadone** overdosage. Dialysis is of little value in poisoning due to **propoxyphene**.

Patient Information

Advise patients to swallow SR, CR, and ER products whole and not to break, crush, chew, open, or dissolve them because doing so may lead to rapid release and absorption of a potentially fatal dose. ER and SR **morphine** capsules may be opened and the beads sprinkled on a small amount of applesauce immediately prior to ingestion; advise patients not to chew, crush, or dissolve the beads.

Instruct patients and caregivers to keep used and unused **fentanyl transdermal** systems out of the reach of children. Used systems should be folded so that the adhesive side of the system adheres to itself and should be flushed down the toilet immediately upon removal. Advise patients to dispose of any systems remaining from a prescription as soon as they are no longer needed. Unused systems should be removed from their pouches and flushed down the toilet.

Keep **fentanyl** lozenges out of the reach of children. Dispose of properly (see individual monograph). Advise diabetic patients that each lozenge contains 2 g of sugar. Consumption of sugar-containing products may increase dental caries. Consult a dentist to ensure proper oral hygiene.

Advise patients that narcotics may cause drowsiness, dizziness, or blurring of vision and to use caution while driving or performing other tasks requiring alertness, coordination, or physical dexterity.

Orthostatic hypotension may occur with the use of this medication, especially in ambulatory patients. Patients should get up slowly from a sitting or lying position.

Instruct patients to avoid alcohol and other CNS depressants.

Instruct patients to notify health care provider if nausea, vomiting, or constipation become prominent.

If GI upset occurs, these agents may be taken with food.

Instruct patients to notify a health care provider if shortness of breath or difficulty in breathing occurs.

Advise patients not to adjust the dose without consulting their health care provider.

Instruct patients to inform a health care provider if pregnant or planning to become pregnant.

Because of the potential for these drugs to be abused, advise patients to protect them from theft and to not give them to anyone else.

Advise the patient to not discontinue the drug abruptly if therapy has lasted more than a few weeks. Instruct them to consult their health care provider.

Instruct patients to avoid exposing the **fentanyl transdermal** system application site to a direct external heat source. There is a potential for temperature-dependent increases in fentanyl release from the system.

ALFENTANIL HYDROCHLORIDE

c-ii	**Alfentanil hydrochloride** (Abbott)	**Injection:** 500 mcg (as base)/mL	Preservative free. In 2, 5, and 10 mL amps.
c-ii	**Alfenta** (Akorn)		Preservative free. In 2, 5, 10, and 20 mL amps.

ALFENTANIL HYDROCHLORIDE — INJECTION

For complete and comparative prescribing information, refer to the Narcotic Agonist Analgesics group monograph.

Indications

➤*Analgesia:* Analgesic adjunct given in incremental doses in the maintenance of anesthesia with barbiturate/nitrous oxide/oxygen.

As an analgesic administered by continuous infusion with nitrous oxide/oxygen in the maintenance of general anesthesia.

➤*Anesthetic:* Primary anesthetic for induction of anesthesia in general surgery when endotracheal intubation and mechanical ventilation are required.

➤*Monitored anesthesia care (MAC):* Analgesic component for MAC.

Administration and Dosage

➤*Approved by the FDA:* December 29, 1986.

Individualize dosage and titrate to desired effect in each patient according to body weight, physical status, underlying pathological conditions, use of other drugs, and type and duration of surgical procedure and anesthesia. In obese patients (more than 20% above ideal total body weight), determine dosage on the basis of lean body weight. Reduce dose in elderly or debilitated patients.

Monitor vital signs routinely.

In patients administered anesthetic (induction) dosages, qualified personnel and adequate facilities are essential for the management of intraoperative and postoperative respiratory depression.

Use a tuberculin syringe or equivalent for accuracy in administering small volumes.

➤*Children (younger than 12 years of age):* Use is not recommended.

➤*Premedication:* Individualize the selection of preanesthetic medications.

➤*Neuromuscular-blocking agents:* Neuromuscular-blocking agents should be compatible with the patient's condition.

➤*General anesthesia:* See table below for the use of alfentanil, such as by the following:

1.) by incremental injection as an analgesic adjunct to anesthesia with barbiturate/nitrous oxide/oxygen for short surgical procedures (expected duration of less than 1 hour);
2.) by continuous infusion as a maintenance analgesic with nitrous oxide/oxygen for general surgical procedures; and
3.) by intravenous (IV) injection in anesthetic doses for the induction of anesthesia for general surgical procedures with a minimum expected duration of 45 minutes; and
4.) by IV injection as the analgesic component for MAC.

Alfentanil Dosage Range for Use During General Anesthesia

Clinical status	Induction[a]	Maintenance	Total dose
Spontaneously breathing/Assisted ventilation	8 to 20 mcg/kg	3 to 5 mcg/kg every 5 to 20 min or 0.5 to 1 mcg/kg/min	8 to 40 mcg/kg
Assisted or controlled ventilation			
Incremental injection (to attenuate response to laryngoscopy and intubation)	20 to 50 mcg/kg	5 to 15 mcg/kg every 5 to 20 min	up to 75 mcg/kg
Continuous infusion[b] (to provide attenuation of response to intubation and incision)	50 to 75 mcg/kg	0.5 to 3 mcg/kg/min. Average infusion rate 1 to 1.5 mcg/kg/min	dependent on duration of procedure
Anesthetic induction (give slowly [over 3 min]).[c] Reduce concentration of inhalation agents by 30% to 50% for initial hour)	130 to 245 mcg/kg	0.5 to 1.5 mcg/kg/min or general anesthetic	dependent on duration of procedure
MAC[d] (for sedated and responsive spontaneously breathing patients)	3 to 8 mcg/kg	3 to 5 mcg/kg every 5 to 20 min or 0.25 to 1 mcg/kg/min	3 to 40 mcg/kg

[a] Administer induction doses of alfentanil slowly (over 3 minutes). Administration may produce loss of vascular tone and hypotension. Consider fluid replacement prior to induction.

[b] 0.5 to 3 mcg/kg/min with nitrous oxide/oxygen in general surgery. Following anesthetic induction dose, reduce infusion rate requirements by 30% to 50% for the first hour of maintenance.
Vital sign changes that indicate response to surgical stress or lightening of anesthesia may be controlled by increasing rate to a max of 4 mcg/kg/min or administering bolus doses of 7 mcg/kg. If changes are not controlled after 3 bolus doses given over 5 minutes, use a barbiturate, vasodilator, and/or inhalation agent. Always adjust infusion rates downward in the absence of these signs until there is some response to surgical stimulation.
Rather than an increase in infusion rate, administer 7 mcg/kg bolus doses of alfentanil or a potent inhalation agent in response to signs of lightening of anesthesia within the last 15 minutes of surgery. Discontinue infusion at least 10 to 15 minutes prior to the end of surgery.

[c] At these doses, expect truncal rigidity and use a muscle relaxant.

[d] During administration of alfentanil for MAC, infusions may be continued to the end of the procedure.

➤*Admixture compatibility:* Physical and chemical compatibilities of alfentanil have been demonstrated in solution with normal saline, 5% dextrose in normal saline, 5% dextrose in water, and lactated Ringers.

➤*Storage/Stability:* Protect from light. Store at room temperature (15° to 25°C, 59° to 77°F).

CODEINE

c-ii	**Codeine Sulfate** (Various, eg, Roxane)	**Tablets:** 15 mg (as sulfate)	In UD 100s.
		30 mg (as sulfate)	In 100s and UD 100s.
		60 mg (as sulfate)	In 100s
c-ii	**Codeine Phosphate** (Roxane)	**Solution, oral:** 15 mg/5 mL (as phosphate)	Parabens. In 500 mL and UD 5 mL.
c-ii	**Codeine Phosphate** (Various, eg, Hospira)	**Injection:** 15 mg/mL (as phosphate)	May contain sulfites. In 2 mL *Carpuject* syringe system.
		30 mg/mL (as phosphate)	May contain sulfites. In 2 mL *Carpuject* syringe system.

CODEINE SULFATE — ORAL

For complete and comparative prescribing information, refer to the Opioid Analgesics group monograph.

Indications

➤*Antitussive:* In combination with other respiratory agents for the treatment of cough (see Upper Respiratory Combinations in the Respiratory chapter).

➤*Pain:* For the relief of mild to moderate pain.

Administration and Dosage

Adjust dosage according to the severity of the pain and the response of the patient. It may occasionally be necessary to exceed the usual dosage recommended in cases of more severe pain or in those patients who have become tolerant to the analgesic effect of narcotics.

➤*Analgesic:*

Adults – 15 to 60 mg every 4 to 6 hours.

➤*Storage/Stability:* Store tablets at 25°C (77°F); excursions permitted to 15° to 30°C (59° to 86°F) and protect from moisture. Dispense in a well-closed container.

CODEINE PHOSPHATE — ORAL

For complete and comparative prescribing information, refer to the Opioid Analgesics group monograph.

Indications

➤*Antitussive:* In combination with other respiratory agents for the treatment of cough (see Upper Respiratory Combinations in the Respiratory chapter).

➤*Pain:* For the relief of mild to moderate pain.

Administration and Dosage

Adjust dosage according to the severity of the pain and the response of the patient. It may occasionally be necessary to exceed the usual dosage recommended in cases of more severe pain or in those patients who have become tolerant to the analgesic effect of narcotics.

➤*Analgesic:*

Adults – 15 to 60 mg every 4 to 6 hours.

➤*Storage/Stability:* Store oral solution at 25°C (77°F); excursions permitted to 15° to 30°C (59° to 86°F) and protect from moisture. Dispense in a well-closed container.

CODEINE PHOSPHATE — INJECTION

For complete and comparative prescribing information, refer to the Opioid Analgesics group monograph.

Indications

➤*Antitussive:* In combination with other respiratory agents for the treatment of cough (see Upper Respiratory Combinations in the Respiratory chapter).

➤*Pain:* For the relief of mild to moderate pain.

Administration and Dosage

Adjust dosage according to the severity of the pain and the response of the patient. It may occasionally be necessary to exceed the usual dosage recommended in cases of more severe pain or in those patients who have become tolerant to the analgesic effect of narcotics.

➤*Analgesic:*

Adults – 30 mg subcutaneously or intramuscularly (IM) every 4 hours as needed. The usual dose range is 15 to 60 mg.

Children – 500 mcg/kg or 15 mg/m^2 subcutaneously or IM every 4 hours as necessary.

➤*Admixture incompatibility:* Codeine is incompatible with soluble barbiturates.

➤*Storage/Stability:* Store injection below 40°C (104°F) and protect from light and freezing.

FENTANYL

c-ii	**Fentanyl** (Various, eg, Baxter)	**Injection:** 50 mcg (as base)/mL	In 2, 5, 10, and 20 mL amps; 30 and 50 mL single-dose vials.
c-ii	**Sublimaze** (Akorn)		Preservative free. In 2, 5, 10, and 20 mL amps.

FENTANYL CITRATE — INJECTION

For complete prescribing information, refer to the Opioid Analgesics group monograph.

Indications

➤*Pain:* For analgesic action of short duration during anesthesia (premedication, induction, maintenance), and in the immediate postoperative period (recovery room) as needed.

For use as an opioid analgesic supplement in general or regional anesthesia.

For administration with a neuroleptic such as droperidol (see monograph in the General Anesthetics section) as an anesthetic premedication, for induction of anesthesia, and as an adjunct in maintenance of general and regional anesthesia.

For use as an anesthetic agent with oxygen in selected high-risk patients (open heart surgery or certain complicated neurological or orthopedic procedures).

Administration and Dosage

➤*Approved by the FDA:* February 19, 1968.

Individualize dosage. Monitor vital signs routinely.

➤*Concomitant anesthesia:* Certain forms of conduction anesthesia, such as spinal anesthesia and some peridural anesthetics, can alter respiration by blocking intercostal nerves. Fentanyl can also alter respiration through other mechanisms.

➤*Concomitant narcotic administration:* The respiratory depressant effect of fentanyl may persist longer than the analgesic effect. Consider the total dose of all opioid analgesics used before ordering narcotic analgesics during recovery from anesthesia. Use opioids in reduced doses initially, ¼ to ⅓ those usually recommended.

➤*Premedication:* 50 to 100 mcg intramuscularly (IM), 30 to 60 minutes prior to surgery.

➤*Adjunct to general anesthesia:*

Total low dose – 2 mcg/kg in small doses for minor, painful surgical procedures and postoperative pain relief.

Maintenance low dose – 2 mcg/kg. Additional doses are needed infrequently in minor procedures.

Total moderate dose – 2 to 20 mcg/kg. In addition to adequate analgesia, some abolition of the stress response should occur. Respiratory depression necessitates artificial ventilation and careful observation of postoperative ventilation.

Maintenance moderate dose – 2 to 20 mcg/kg. Use 25 to 100 mcg intravenously (IV) or IM when movement and/or changes in vital signs indicate surgical stress or lightening of analgesia.

Total high dose – 20 to 50 mcg/kg for "stress free" anesthesia. Use during open heart surgery and complicated neurosurgical and orthopedic procedures where surgery is prolonged and the stress response is detrimental. Inject with nitrous oxide/oxygen to attenuate the stress response. Postoperative ventilation and observation are required.

Maintenance high dose – 20 to 50 mcg/kg, ranging from 25 mcg to half the initial loading dose. Individualize dosage. Administer when vital signs indicate surgical stress and lightening of analgesia.

➤*Adjunct to regional anesthesia:* 50 to 100 mcg IM or slowly IV over 1 to 2 minutes as required.

➤*Postoperatively (recovery room):* 50 to 100 mcg IM for the control of pain, tachypnea, and emergence delirium; repeat dose in 1 to 2 hours as needed.

➤*Children (2 to 12 years of age):* For induction and maintenance, a reduced dose as low as 2 to 3 mcg/kg is recommended.

➤*Elderly/Debilitated patients:* Reduce initial dose in elderly and debilitated patients and patients with renal or hepatic dysfunction.

➤*General anesthetic:* 50 to 100 mcg/kg with oxygen and a muscle relaxant when attenuation of the responses to surgical stress is especially important. Up to 150 mcg/kg may be necessary. It has been used for open heart surgery and other major surgical procedures to protect the myocardium from excess oxygen demand and for complicated neurological and orthopedic procedures.

➤*Storage/Stability:* Protect from light. Store at controlled room temperature (15° to 25°C; 59° to 77°F).

FENTANYL TRANSMUCOSAL SYSTEM

c-ii	**Actiq** (Cephalon)	**Lozenge on a stick:**[a] 200 mcg (as base)	Sugar. Berry flavor. In 30s with gray carton blister packs.
		400 mcg (as base)	Sugar. Berry flavor. In 30s with blue carton blister packs.
		600 mcg (as base)	Sugar. Berry flavor. In 30s with orange carton blister packs.
		800 mcg (as base)	Sugar. Berry flavor. In 30s with purple carton blister packs.
		1,200 mcg (as base)	Sugar. Berry flavor. In 30s with green carton blister packs.
		1,600 mcg (as base)	Sugar. Berry flavor. In 30s with burgundy carton blister packs.

[a] Each unit contains approximately 2 g of sugar.

FENTANYL CITRATE — TRANSMUCOSAL

For complete and comparative prescribing information, refer to the Opioid Analgesics group monograph.

WARNING

Oral transmucosal fentanyl is indicated only for the management of breakthrough cancer pain in patients with malignancies already receiving and tolerant to opioid therapy for their underlying persistent cancer pain. Patients considered opioid tolerant are those who are taking morphine 60 mg/day or more, transdermal fentanyl 50 mcg/h, or an equianalgesic dose of another opioid for a week or longer. Because life-threatening hypoventilation could occur at any dose in patients not taking chronic opiates, it is contraindicated in the management of acute or postoperative pain. Do not use in opioid-nontolerant patients. Use only in the care of cancer patients and only by oncologists and pain specialists who are knowledgeable of and skilled in the use of schedule II opioids to treat cancer pain. Instruct patients and their caregivers that this drug contains a medicine in an amount that can be fatal to a child. Keep all units out of reach of children, and discard opened units properly.

Indications

➤*Breakthrough cancer pain:* Only indicated for the management of breakthrough cancer pain in patients with malignancies who are already receiving and are tolerant of opioid therapy for their underlying persistent cancer pain. Patients considered opioid tolerant are those who are taking morphine 60 mg/day or more, transdermal fentanyl 50 mcg/h, or an equianalgesic dose of another opioid for 1 week or longer.

Administration and Dosage

➤*Approved by the FDA:* November 4, 1998.

Use has not been established with opioid-tolerant children younger than 16 years of age. Keep out of the reach of children.

➤*Administration:* Open the foil package immediately prior to product use. Place the unit in the patient's mouth between the cheek and lower gum, moving it from one side to the other using the handle. Instruct the patient to suck, not chew, the lozenge. A unit dose, if chewed and swallowed, might result in lower peak concentrations and lower bioavailability.

Instruct the patient to consume the lozenge over a 15-minute period. Longer or shorter consumption times may produce less efficacy than reported in clinical trials. If signs of excessive opioid effects appear before the unit is consumed, remove the drug matrix from the patient's mouth immediately and decrease future doses.

➤*Dose titration:* Initial dose to treat episodes of breakthrough cancer pain should be 200 mcg. Prescribe patients an initial titration supply of six 200 mcg units. Advise patients to use all units before increasing to a higher dose.

Redosing within a single episode – Until the appropriate dose is reached, it may be necessary to use an additional unit during a single episode. Redosing may start 15 minutes after the previous unit has been completed (30 minutes after the start of the previous unit). Do not give more than 2 units for each individual breakthrough cancer pain episode while patients are in the titration phase and consuming units that individually may be subtherapeutic.

Increasing the dose – If treatment of several consecutive breakthrough cancer pain episodes requires more than 1 fentanyl lozenge per episode, consider an increase in dose to the next higher available strength. At each new dose during titration, prescribe 6 units of the titration dose. Evaluate each new dose used in the titration period over several episodes of breakthrough cancer pain (generally 1 to 2 days) to determine whether it provides adequate efficacy with acceptable side effects. The incidence of side effects is likely to be greater during this initial titration period compared with later, after the effective dose is determined.

Daily limit – Once a successful dose has been found (ie, an average episode is treated with a single unit), instruct patients to limit consumption to 4 units/day or less. If consumption increases to more than 4 units/day, reevaluate the dose of the long-acting opioid for persistent cancer pain.

➤*Discontinuation:* A gradual downward titration is recommended for discontinuation because it is not known at what dose level the opioid may be discontinued without producing the signs and symptoms of abrupt withdrawal.

➤*Safety and handling:* Fentanyl lozenge is supplied in individually sealed child-resistant foil pouches. The amount of fentanyl contained in the lozenge can be lethal to a child. Keep out of the reach of children.

Health care providers and dispensing pharmacists must specifically question patients and caregivers about the presence of children in the home on a full-time or visiting basis and counsel accordingly regarding the dangers to children of inadvertent exposure to the fentanyl transmucosal system.

➤*Disposal:* Dispose of units remaining from a prescription as soon as they are no longer needed. Dispose of all units immediately after use. Partially consumed units represent a special risk because they are no longer protected by the child-resistant pouch, yet may contain enough medicine to be fatal to a child.

A temporary storage bottle is provided to be used in the event that a partially consumed unit cannot be disposed of promptly.

➤*Storage/Stability:* Store at 20° to 25°C (68° to 77°F) with excursions permitted between 15° and 30°C (59° to 86°F) until ready to use. Protect from freezing and moisture.

FENTANYL TRANSDERMAL SYSTEM

	Product/Distributor	Dose (mcg/h)	System size (cm^2)	Fentanyl content (mg)	How supplied
c-ii	**Duragesic-12** (Janssen)	12.5	5	1.25	In cartons containing 5 individually packaged systems.[a]
c-ii	**Fentanyl Transdermal System** (Various, eg, Mylan, Sandoz)	25	6.25 to 10	2.5 to 2.75	In cartons containing 5 individually packaged systems.
c-ii	**Duragesic-25** (Janssen)	25	10	2.5	In cartons containing 5 individually packaged systems.[a]
c-ii	**Fentanyl Transdermal System** (Various, eg, Mylan, Sandoz)	50	12.5 to 20	5 to 5.5	In cartons containing 5 individually packaged systems.
c-ii	**Duragesic-50** (Janssen)	50	20	5	In cartons containing 5 individually packaged systems.[a]
c-ii	**Fentanyl Transdermal System** (Various, eg, Mylan, Sandoz)	75	18.75 to 30	7.5 to 8.25	In cartons containing 5 individually packaged systems.
c-ii	**Duragesic-75** (Janssen)	75	30	7.5	In cartons containing 5 individually packaged systems.[a]
c-ii	**Fentanyl Transdermal System** (Various, eg, Mylan, Sandoz)	100	25 to 40	10 to 11	In cartons containing 5 individually packaged systems.
c-ii	**Duragesic-100** (Janssen)	100	40	10	In cartons containing 5 individually packaged systems.[a]

[a] < 0.2 mL alcohol is released during use.

FENTANYL — TRANSDERMAL

For complete prescribing information, refer to the Opioid Analgesics group monograph.

WARNING

Fentanyl transdermal systems contain a high concentration of the potent schedule II opioid agonist, fentanyl. Schedule II opioid substances have the highest potential for abuse and associated risk of fatal overdose caused by respiratory depression. Fentanyl can be abused and is subject to criminal diversion. The high content of fentanyl in the patches may be a particular target for abuse and diversion.

Fentanyl transdermal system is indicated for management of persistent, moderate to severe chronic pain that:

- requires continuous, around-the-clock opioid administration for an extended period of time, and
- cannot be managed by other means such as nonsteroidal analgesics, opioid combination products, or immediate-release (IR) opioids.

Fentanyl transdermal system should only be used in patients who are already receiving opioid therapy, who have demonstrated opioid tolerance, and who require a total daily dose at least equivalent to fentanyl transdermal system 25 mcg/h. Patients who are considered opioid tolerant are those who have been taking, for a week or longer, morphine 60 mg/day or more, or oral oxycodone 30 mg/day or more, or oral hydromorphone 8 mg/day or more, or an equianalgesic dose of another opioid.

Because serious or life-threatening hypoventilation could occur, fentanyl transdermal is contraindicated:

- in patients who are not opioid tolerant
- in the management of acute pain or in patients who require opioid analgesia for a short period of time
- in the management of postoperative pain, including use after outpatient or day surgeries (eg, tonsillectomies)
- in the management of mild pain
- in the management of intermittent pain (eg, use on an as-needed basis).

Because the peak fentanyl levels occur between 24 and 72 hours of treatment, prescribers should be aware that serious or life-threatening hypoventilation may occur, even in opioid-tolerant patients, during the initial application period. The concomitant use of fentanyl transdermal system with potent CYP450 3A4 inhibitors (ie, ritonavir, ketoconazole, itraconazole, troleandomycin, clarithromycin, nelfinavir, nefazodone) may result in an increase in fentanyl plasma concentrations, which could increase or prolong adverse drug effects and may cause potentially fatal respiratory depression. Carefully monitor patients receiving fentanyl transdermal system and potent CYP3A4 inhibitors for an extended period of time and adjust dosage if warranted.

Do not administer fentanyl transdermal system to children younger than 2 years of age. Administer to children only if they are opioid tolerant and 2 years of age or older.

Fentanyl transdermal system is only for use in patients who are already tolerant to opioid therapy of comparable potency. Use in nonopioid-tolerant patients may lead to fatal respiratory depression. Overestimating the fentanyl transdermal system dose when converting patients from another opioid medication can result in fatal overdose with the first dose. Because of the 17-hour mean elimination half-life of fentanyl transdermal system, patients who are thought to have had a serious adverse event, including overdose, will require monitoring and treatment for at least 24 hours.

Fentanyl transdermal system can be abused in a manner similar to other opioid agonists, legal or illicit. Consider this risk when administering, prescribing, or dispensing in situations where there is concern about increased risk of misuse, abuse, or diversion.

Fentanyl transdermal patches are intended for transdermal use (on intact skin) only. Using damaged or cut fentanyl transdermal patches can lead to the rapid release of the contents of the fentanyl transdermal patch and absorption of a potentially fatal dose of fentanyl.

Indications

➤*Pain:* Management of persistent moderate to severe chronic pain in patients requiring continuous opioid analgesia for pain that cannot be managed by lesser means such as opioid combinations, nonsteroidal analgesics, or IR opioids.

Fentanyl transdermal systems should only be used in patients who are already receiving opioid therapy, who have demonstrated opioid tolerance, and who require a total daily dose at least equivalent to fentanyl transdermal system 25 mcg/h. Patients who are considered opioid tolerant are those who have been taking, for a week or longer, morphine 60 mg/day or more, oral oxycodone 30 mg/day or more, oral hydromorphone 8 mg/day or more, or an equianalgesic dose of another opioid.

Administration and Dosage

➤*Approved by the FDA:* August 7, 1990.

Individualize dosage. The most important factor to consider in determining the appropriate dose is the extent of preexisting opioid tolerance. Reduce initial doses in elderly or debilitated patients.

➤*Application:* Apply to intact, nonirritated, and nonirradiated skin on a flat surface, such as chest, back, flank, or upper arm. In young children and people with cognitive impairment, adhesion should be monitored. The upper back is the preferred location to minimize the potential of inappropriate patch removal. Clip (do not shave) hair at the application site prior to system application. If the site of application must be cleansed prior to application of the system, do so with clear water. Do not use soaps, oils, lotions, alcohol, or any other agents that might irritate the skin or alter its characteristics. Allow the skin to dry completely prior to system application.

Apply immediately upon removal from the sealed package. Do not alter the system (eg, cut) in any way prior to application. Firmly press the transdermal system in place with the palm of the hand for 30 seconds, making sure the contact is complete, especially around the edges.

Each system may be worn continuously for 72 hours. If analgesia for longer than 72 hours is required, apply a new system to a different skin site after removal of the previous transdermal system.

Keep out of the reach of children. Fold used systems so that the adhesive side of the system adheres to itself, then flush the system down the toilet immediately upon removal. Dispose of any systems remaining from a prescription as soon as they are no longer needed. Remove unused systems from their pouch (fold so that the adhesive side of the patch adheres to itself) and flush down the toilet.

If the gel from the drug reservoir accidentally contacts the skin, the area should be washed with copious amounts of water. Do not use soap, alcohol, or other solvents to remove the gel because they may enhance the drug's ability to penetrate the skin.

➤*Dose selection:* In selecting an initial dose, give attention to the following:

1.) the daily dose, potency, and characteristics of the opioid the patient has been taking previously (eg, whether it is a pure agonist or mixed agonist-antagonist);
2.) the reliability of the relative potency estimates used to calculate the dose needed (potency estimates may vary with the route of administration);
3.) the degree of opioid tolerance;
4.) the general condition and medical status of the patient. Maintain each patient at the lowest dose providing acceptable pain control.

Pediatric patients converting to fentanyl transdermal system therapy with a 25 mcg/h patch should be opioid tolerant and receiving oral morphine equivalents 60 mg/day or more. The dose conversion schedule and method of titration described in the table below were used safely in opioid-tolerant pediatric patients older than 2 years of age with chronic pain.

To convert patients from oral or parenteral opioids to the transdermal system, use the following table:

Dose Conversion Guidelines[a]				
Current analgesic	Daily dose (mg/d)			
Oral morphine	60 to 134	135 to 224	225 to 314	315 to 404
IM/IV morphine	10 to 22	23 to 37	38 to 52	53 to 67
Oral oxycodone	30 to 67	67.5 to 112	112.5 to 157	157.5 to 202
IM/IV oxycodone	15 to 33	33.1 to 56	56.1 to 78	78.1 to 101
Oral codeine	150 to 447	448 to 747	748 to 1047	1,048 to 1,347
Oral hydromorphone	8 to 17	17.1 to 28	28.1 to 39	39.1 to 51
IV hydromorphone	1.5 to 3.4	3.5 to 5.6	5.7 to 7.9	8 to 10
IM meperidine	75 to 165	166 to 278	279 to 390	391 to 503
Oral methadone	20 to 44	45 to 74	75 to 104	105 to 134
IM methadone	10 to 22	23 to 37	38 to 52	53 to 67
Recommended fentanyl transdermal system dose				
Fentanyl transdermal system	25 mcg/h	50 mcg/h	75 mcg/h	100 mcg/h

[a] This table should not be used to convert fentanyl transdermal system to other therapies because this conversion to fentanyl transdermal system is conservative. Use of this table for conversion to other analgesic therapies can overestimate the dose of the new agent. Overdosage of the new analgesic agent is possible.

Alternatively, for adult and pediatric patients taking opioids or doses not listed in the table above, use the following methodology:

1.) Calculate the previous 24-hour analgesic requirement.
2.) Convert this amount to the equianalgesic oral morphine dose using the table in the Actions section of the Opioids Analgesics group monograph.
3.) The following table displays the range of 24-hour oral morphine doses that are recommended for conversion to each transdermal system dose. Use this table to find the calculated 24-hour morphine dose and the corresponding transdermal fentanyl dose. Initiate treatment using the recommended dose and titrate patients upwards until analgesic efficacy is attained. Upward titration may be done no more frequently than 3 days after the initial dose; thereafter, it may be done no more frequently than every 6 days. For delivery rates in excess of 100 mcg/h, multiple systems may be used.

Initial Fentanyl Transdermal Dose Based on Daily Oral Morphine Dose[a]	
Oral 24-hour morphine (mg/day)	Fentanyl transdermal (mcg/h)
60 to 134[b]	25
135 to 224	50
225 to 314	75
315 to 404	100
405 to 494	125

FENTANYL — TRANSDERMAL

Initial Fentanyl Transdermal Dose Based on Daily Oral Morphine Dose[a]	
Oral 24-hour morphine (mg/day)	Fentanyl transdermal (mcg/h)
495 to 584	150
585 to 674	175
675 to 764	200
765 to 854	225
855 to 944	250
945 to 1034	275
1,035 to 1,124	300

[a] Do not use this table to convert from fentanyl transdermal system to other therapies because this conversion to fentanyl is conservative. Use of this table for conversion to other analgesic therapies can overestimate the dose of the new agent. Overdosage of the new analgesic agent is possible.
[b] Pediatric patients initiating therapy on a fentanyl transdermal system 25 mcg/h should be opioid-tolerant and receiving oral morphine equivalents 60 mg/day or more.

The majority of patients are adequately maintained with transdermal fentanyl administered every 72 hours. Some patients may require systems to be applied every 48 hours. Because of the increase in serum fentanyl concentration over the first 24 hours following initial system application, the initial evaluation of the maximum analgesic effect cannot be made before 24 hours of wearing. The initial dosage may be increased after 3 days.

An increase in the fentanyl transdermal dose should be evaluated before changing dosing intervals in order to maintain patients on a 72-hour regimen. Dosing intervals less than every 72 hours were not studied in children and adolescents and are not recommended.

During the initial application, patients should use short-acting analgesics as needed until analgesic efficacy with the transdermal system is attained. Thereafter, some patients may still require periodic supplemental doses of other short-acting analgesics for breakthrough pain.

➤*Dose titration:* The recommended initial fentanyl transdermal dose based upon the daily oral morphine dose is conservative, and 50% of patients are likely to require a dose increase after initial application. The initial dosage may be increased after 3 days, based on the daily dose of supplemental opioid analgesics required by the patient in the second or third day of the initial application.

It may take up to 6 days after increasing the dose for the patient to reach equilibrium on the new dose. Therefore, patients should wear a higher dose through 2 applications before any further increase in dosage is made on the basis of the average daily use of a supplemental analgesic.

Base appropriate dosage increments on the daily dose of supplementary opioids, using the ratio of 45 mg/24 h of oral morphine to a 12.5 mcg/h increase in transdermal fentanyl dose.

➤*Special populations:* Elderly, cachetic, or debilitated patients should not be started on fentanyl transdermal system doses higher than 25 mcg/h unless they are already tolerating an around-the-clock opioid at a dose and potency comparable with fentanyl transdermal system 25 mcg/h.

➤*Discontinuation:* Upon system removal, it takes 17 hours or more for the fentanyl serum concentration to fall by 50%. Titrate the dose of the new analgesic based on the patient's report of pain until adequate analgesia has been attained. For patients requiring discontinuation of opioids, a gradual downward titration is recommended because it is not known at what dose level the opioid may be discontinued without producing the signs and symptoms of abrupt withdrawal.

➤*Storage / Stability:* Do not store above 25°C (77°F). Apply immediately after removal from individually sealed package. Do not use if the seal is broken. For transdermal use only.

HYDROCODONE

Hydrocodone is only available in combination with other ingredients for the treatment of pain and cough. See Upper Respiratory Combinations in the Respiratory chapter or the Opioid Analgesic Combinations.

HYDROMORPHONE HYDROCHLORIDE

c-ii	**Hydromorphone Hydrochloride** (Various, eg, Endo, Ethex, Roxane)	**Tablets:** 2 mg	In 100s, and UD 25s and 100s.
c-ii	**Dilaudid** (Abbott)		Lactose. (2). Orange. In 100s, 500s, and UD 100s.
c-ii	**Hydromorphone Hydrochloride** (Various, eg, Endo, Ethex, Roxane)	**Tablets:** 4 mg	In 100s, and UD 25s and 100s.
c-ii	**Dilaudid** (Abbott)		Lactose. (4). Yellow. In 100s, 500s, and UD 100s.
c-ii	**Hydromorphone Hydrochloride** (Various, eg, Mallinckrodt, Roxane)	**Tablets:** 8 mg	In 100s.
c-ii	**Dilaudid** (Abbott)		Lactose, sodium metabisulfite. (8). White, scored, triangular. In 100s.
c-ii	**Palladone** (Purdue Pharma)	**Capsules, extended-release:** 12 mg	Pellet filled. (P-XL 12 mg). Cinnamon-colored. In 60s and UD 20s.
		16 mg	Pellet filled. (P-XL 16 mg). Pink. In 60s and UD 20s.
		24 mg	Pellet filled. (P-XL 24 mg). Blue. In 60s and UD 20s.
		32 mg	Pellet filled. (P-XL 32 mg). White. In 60s and UD 20s.
c-ii	**Hydromorphone Hydrochloride** (Various, eg, Roxane)	**Oral solution:** 1 mg per 1 mL	In 4 and 8 mL UD patient cups and 250 mL bottles.
c-ii	**Dilaudid** (Abbott)		Parabens, sucrose, glycerin. May contain sodium metabisulfite. In 473 mL.
c-ii	**Hydromorphone Hydrochloride** (Various, eg, Hospira, Baxter)	**Injection:** 1 mg/mL	In 1 mL prefilled syringes.
c-ii	**Dilaudid** (Abbott)		In 1 mL amps.
c-ii	**Hydromorphone Hydrochloride** (Various, eg, Hospira, Baxter)	**Injection:** 2 mg/mL	In 1 and 20 mL vials and 1 mL prefilled syringes.
c-ii	**Dilaudid** (Abbott)		In 1 mL amps and 20 mL multidose vials.[a]
c-ii	**Hydromorphone Hydrochloride** (Various, eg, Hospira, Baxter)	**Injection:** 4 mg/mL	In 1 mL prefilled syringes.
c-ii	**Dilaudid** (Abbott)		In 1 mL amps.
c-ii	**Hydromorphone Hydrochloride** (Various, eg, Faulding, Hospira)	**Injection:** 10 mg/mL	In 1, 5, and 50 mL single-dose vials.
c-ii	**Dilaudid-HP** (Abbott)		In 1 and 5[b] mL amps and 50 mL single-dose vials.[b]
c-ii	**Dilaudid-HP** (Abbott)	**Powder for injection, lyophilized:** 250 mg (10 mg/mL after reconstitution)	In single-dose vials.[b]
c-ii	**Hydromorphone Hydrochloride** (Paddock)	**Suppositories:** 3 mg	In 6s.
c-ii	**Dilaudid** (Abbott)		Cocoa butter. In 6s.

[a] With EDTA and methyl- and propylparabens. Vial stopper contains latex.
[b] For use in the preparation of large volume parenteral solutions.

HYDROMORPHONE HYDROCHLORIDE — INJECTION

For complete prescribing information, refer to the Opioid Analgesics group monograph.

WARNING

HP injection is a highly concentrated solution of hydromorphone intended for use in opioid-tolerant patients. Do not confuse HP injection with standard parenteral formulations of injection or other opioids. Overdose and death could result.

Indications

➤*Pain:* Relief of moderate to severe pain such as that caused by surgery, cancer, trauma (soft tissue and bone), biliary colic, myocardial infarction (MI), burns, and renal colic.

Administration and Dosage

➤*Approved by the FDA:* January 11, 1984.

➤*Parenteral:* The starting dosage is 1 to 2 mg subcutaneously or intramuscularly (IM) every 4 to 6 hours as needed. For opioid-naive patients, a lower dose should be considered to prevent oversedation. May be given by slow intravenous (IV) injection over at least 2 to 3 minutes.

HP – Only give the HP strength (10 mg/mL) to patients tolerant of other narcotics. If converting from regular strength hydromorphone to HP strength hydromorphone, use similar doses, depending on the patient's clinical response to the drug. If HP hydromorphone is substituted for a different opioid analgesic, use the following equivalency table as a guide to determine the appropriate dose of HP hydromorphone.

Because of its high concentration, the delivery of precise doses of HP hydromorphone may be difficult if low doses of hydromorphone are required. Therefore, use HP hydromorphone only if the amount of hydromorphone required can be delivered accurately with this formulation.

Approximate Equianalgesic Doses[a] (IM or Subcutaneous Administration)

Drug	Dose (mg)	Duration compared with morphine
Butorphanol	1.5 to 2.5	Same
Hydromorphone	1.3	Slightly shorter
Levorphanol	2.3	Same
Meperidine	80	Shorter
Methadone	10	Same
Morphine	10	Same
Nalbuphine	12	Same
Oxymorphone	1.1	Slightly shorter
Pentazocine	60	Shorter

[a] Equianalgesic to IM morphine 10 mg in terms of the area under the analgesic time effect curve.

In open clinical trials with HP hydromorphone in patients with terminal cancer, doses ranged from 1 to 14 mg subcutaneously or IM; 1 patient received 30 mg subcutaneously on 2 occasions.

Experience with administration of HP hydromorphone by the IV route is limited. If IV administration is necessary, slowly give the injection over at least 2 to 3 minutes. The IV route is usually painless.

500 mg per 50 mL vial: To use this single-dose presentation, do not penetrate the stopper with a syringe. Instead, remove both the aluminum flipseal and rubber stopper in a suitable work area, such as under a laminar flow hood (or equivalent clean air compounding area). The contents may then be withdrawn for preparation of a single, large volume parenteral solution. Discard any unused portion in an appropriate manner.

Reconstitution of sterile lyophilized powder for injection – Reconstitute immediately prior to use with 25 mL of sterile water for injection to provide a sterile solution containing 10 mg/mL.

➤*Storage / Stability:* Store at 25°C (77°F); excursions permitted to 15° to 30°C (59° to 86°F). Protect from light.

HYDROMORPHONE HYDROCHLORIDE — ORAL

For complete prescribing information, refer to the Opioid Analgesics group monograph.

WARNING

Extended-release (ER) capsules – Hydromorphone ER capsules are indicated for the management of persistent moderate to severe pain in patients requiring continuous, around-the-clock analgesia with a HP opioid for an extended period of time (weeks to months) or longer. Use ER capsules only in patients who are already receiving opioid therapy, have demonstrated opioid tolerance, and require a minimum total daily dose of opiate medication equivalent to oral hydromorphone 12 mg. Patients considered opioid tolerant are those taking oral morphine 60 mg/day or more, oral oxycodone 30 mg/day or more, oral hydromorphone 8 mg/day or more, or an equianalgesic dose of another opioid, for a week or longer. Administer ER capsules once every 24 hours.

Appropriate patients for treatment with ER capsules include patients who require high doses of potent opioids on an around-the-clock basis to improve pain control and patients who have difficulty attaining adequate analgesia with immediate-release (IR) opioid formulations. ER capsules are contraindicated for use on an as-needed basis.

ER capsules are not intended to be used as the first opioid product prescribed for a patient or in patients who require opioid analgesia for a short period of time.

ER capsules are for opioid-tolerant patients only. Use in nonopioid-tolerant patients may lead to fatal respiratory depression. Overestimating the ER capsule dose when converting patients from another opioid medication can result in fatal overdose with the first dose. Because of the mean apparent 18-hour elimination half-life of ER capsules, patients who receive an overdose will require an extended period of monitoring and treatment that may go beyond 18 hours. Even in the face of improvement, continued medical monitoring is required because of the possibility of extended effects.

Schedule II opioid agonists (eg, hydromorphone, fentanyl, methadone, morphine, oxycodone, oxymorphone) have the highest risk of fatal overdoses because of respiratory depression, as well as the highest potential for abuse. ER capsules can be abused in a manner similar to other opioid agonists, legal or illicit. Consider these risks when administering, prescribing, or dispensing ER capsules in situations where there is concern about increased risk of misuse, abuse, or diversion.

People at increased risk for opioid abuse include those with a personal or family history of substance abuse (including drug or alcohol abuse or addiction) or mental illness (eg, major depression). Assess patients for clinical risks for opioid abuse or addiction prior to prescribing opioids. Routinely monitor all patients receiving opioids for signs of misuse, abuse, and addiction. Patients at increased risk of opioid abuse may still be appropriately treated with modified-release opioid formulations; however, these patients will require intensive monitoring for signs of misuse, abuse, or addiction.

WARNING (cont.)

ER capsules are to be swallowed whole, not broken, chewed, opened, dissolved, or crushed. Taking broken, chewed, dissolved, or crushed ER capsules or capsule contents can lead to the rapid release and absorption of a potentially fatal dose of hydromorphone. Overestimating the ER capsule dose when converting the patient from another opioid medication can result in fatal overdose with the first dose. With the long half-life of ER capsules (18 hours), patients who receive the wrong dose will require an extended period of monitoring and treatment that may go beyond 18 hours. Even in the face of improvement, continued medical monitoring is required because of the possibility of extended effects.

Indications

➤*Pain:* Relief of moderate to severe pain such as that caused by surgery, cancer, trauma (soft tissue and bone), biliary colic, myocardial infarction (MI), burns, and renal colic.

ER capsules – For the management of persistent moderate to severe pain in patients requiring continuous, around-the-clock analgesia with a HP opioid for an extended period of time, generally weeks to months or longer, and for patients who have difficulty attaining adequate analgesia with IR opioid formulations (see Warning box).

Administration and Dosage

➤*Approved by the FDA:* January 11, 1984.

➤*Tablets:* The starting dosage is 2 to 4 mg every 4 to 6 hours; 4 mg or more every 4 to 6 hours for more severe pain. If the pain increases in severity, analgesia is not adequate, or tolerance occurs, a gradual increase in dosage may be required. If pain is exceedingly severe, or if prompt response is desired, use parenteral hydromorphone initially in adequate amounts to control the pain.

➤*ER capsules:* Individualize dosage. The extended-release nature of the formulation allows it to be administered once every 24 hours. Capsules are swallowed whole and not broken, chewed, opened, dissolved, or crushed. Taking broken, chewed, dissolved, or crushed capsules or capsule contents can lead to the rapid release and absorption of a potentially fatal dose of hydromorphone.

Capsules are for opioid-tolerant patients only. Use in nonopioid-tolerant patients may lead to fatal respiratory depression. They are not intended to be used on an as-needed basis, as the first opioid product prescribed for a patient, or in patients who require opioid analgesia for a short period of time.

Overestimating the dose when converting patients from another opioid medication can result in fatal overdose with the first dose. Because of the mean apparent 18-hour elimination half-life of the capsule, patients who receive an overdose will require an extended period of monitoring and treatment that may go beyond 18 hours. Even in the face of improvement, continued medical monitoring is required because of the possibility of extended effects.

Use the capsules only in patients who are already receiving opioid therapy, have demonstrated opioid tolerance, and require a minimum total daily dose of opiate medication equivalent to oral hydromorphone 12 mg. Patients con-

HYDROMORPHONE HYDROCHLORIDE — ORAL

sidered opioid tolerant are those who are taking oral morphine 60 mg/day or more, oral oxycodone 30 mg/day or more, oral hydromorphone 8 mg/day or more, or an equianalgesic dose of another opioid, for a week or longer.

Determine the total daily (24-hour) dose of the patient's previous opioid.

1.) Using standard conversion ratio estimates (see the following table), multiply the milligrams per day of the previous opioids by the appropriate conversion factors to obtain the equivalent total daily dose of oral hydromorphone. The conversion ratios represent a reasonable starting point, although they have not been verified in well-controlled, multidose trials.
2.) Modify the dose if indicated.
3.) Round off to a dose that is appropriate for the capsule strengths available (12, 16, 24, and 32 mg capsules).
4.) Discontinue all other around-the-clock opioid analgesics when the ER capsules are initiated.

No fixed conversion ratio is likely to be satisfactory in all patients, especially patients receiving large opioid doses. The recommended doses are only a starting point, and close observation and frequent titration is indicated until a satisfactory dose is obtained on the new therapy.

Multiplication Factors for Converting the Daily Dose of Prior Opioids to the Daily Dose of Oral Hydromorphone[a]

Calculation: mg/day prior opioid × factor = mg/day oral hydromorphone

Prior opioid	Oral factor	Parenteral factor
Codeine	0.04	—
Hydrocodone	0.22	—
Hydromorphone	1	5
Levorphanol	1.88	3.75
Meperidine	0.02	0.1
Methadone	0.38	0.75
Morphine	0.12	0.75
Oxycodone	0.25	—

[a] To be used only for conversion to oral hydromorphone. For patients receiving high-dose parenteral opioids, a more conservative conversion is warranted. For example, for high dose parenteral **morphine**, use 0.38 instead of 0.75 as a multiplication factor (ie, halve the multiplication factor).

Conversion from transdermal fentanyl to ER capsules – ER capsule treatment can be initiated 18 hours following the removal of the transdermal fentanyl patch. Initially, substitute a conservative hydromorphone dosage, approximately 12 mg once a day of ER capsules, for each 50 mcg/h of transdermal fentanyl. Closely observe the patient for early titration, as there is very limited clinical experience with this conversion.

Conversion from opioid combination drugs – Patients currently receiving around-the-clock fixed-combination opioid analgesics, and a daily dose of 45 mg or more oxycodone or hydrocodone equivalents, or 300 mg/day dose of codeine equivalents, may be started on 12 mg of ER capsules once daily. The nonopioid component of the combination product may be continued as a separate drug. Alternatively, a different nonopioid analgesic may be selected.

Supplemental (rescue) analgesics – Most patients given around-the-clock therapy with controlled-release opioids may need to have immediate-release medication available for exacerbations of pain or to treat or prevent pain that occurs predictably during certain patient activities (incident pain). ER capsules can be safely used concomitantly with usual doses of nonopioid analgesics and analgesic adjuvants, provided care is taken to select a proper initial dose.

Individualization of dosage – Once therapy is initiated, frequently assess pain relief and other opioid effects. Titrate the capsules to adequate effect (generally mild or less pain with the regular use of no more than 2 doses of supplemental analgesics per 24 hours). Have rescue medication available. Because steady-state plasma concentrations are achieved within approximately 2 to 3 days of therapy with hydromorphone, dosage adjustment can be carried out as frequently as every 2 days when clinically necessary. If more than 2 doses of rescue medication are needed within a 24-hour period for 2 consecutive days, usually titrate the dose of ER capsules upward. Administer this formulation once every 24 hours. As a guideline, the total daily hydromorphone dose (including rescue) usually can be increased 25% to 50% of the current dose at each upward titration.

If signs of excessive opioid-related adverse reactions are observed, the dose may be reduced. If this adjustment leads to inadequate analgesia, a supplemental dose of IR opioid analgesic may be given. Alternatively, nonopioid analgesic adjuvants may be administered. Make dose adjustments to obtain an appropriate balance between pain relief and opioid-related adverse reactions.

If common opioid-related adverse reactions occur before the therapeutic goal of pain relief is achieved, effectively treat the reactions prior to continuing upward titration of ER capsules. Once adverse reactions are under control, continue upward titration to an acceptable level of pain control.

During periods of changing analgesic requirements, including initial titration, frequent contact is recommended between the health care provider, other members of the health care team, the patient, and the caregiver/family.

Continuation of therapy – The intent of the titration period is to establish a patient-specific daily dose that will provide adequate analgesia with acceptable adverse reactions and minimal rescue doses (2 or less) for as long as pain relief is necessary. If pain recurs, the dose can be increased to reestablish pain control. Employ the method of therapy adjustment outlined to regain pain control.

During chronic around-the-clock opioid therapy, closely follow patients and reassess their pain as clinically indicated. Continue to assess patients for their clinical risks for opioid abuse or addiction, particularly with high dose formulations.

Cessation of therapy – When the patient no longer requires therapy with hydromorphone capsules, gradually taper doses to prevent signs and symptoms of withdrawal in the physically dependent patient. Ensure proper disposal of unused capsules by flushing them down the toilet.

Conversion from capsules to parenteral opioids – To avoid overdose, follow conservative dose conversion ratios.

➤*Oral liquid:* The starting dosage is 2.5 to 10 mg every 3 to 6 hours.

➤*Storage/Stability:* Store oral dosage forms at 25°C (77°F); excursions permitted to 15° to 30°C (59° to 86°F). Protect from light.

HYDROMORPHONE HYDROCHLORIDE — RECTAL

For complete prescribing information, refer to the Opioid Analgesics group monograph.

Indications

➤*Pain:* Relief of moderate to severe pain such as that caused by surgery, cancer, trauma (soft tissue and bone), biliary colic, myocardial infarction (MI), burns, and renal colic.

Administration and Dosage

➤*Approved by the FDA:* January 11, 1984.

➤*Dosage:* 3 mg every 6 to 8 hours or as directed by the health care provider.

➤*Storage/Stability:* Refrigerate suppositories between 2° to 8°C (36° to 46°F).

LEVORPHANOL TARTRATE

c-ii	**Levorphanol Tartrate** (Roxane)	**Tablets:** 2 mg	(54 410). Lactose. White, scored. In 100s.
c-ii	**Levo-Dromoran** (Valeant)		Lactose. (Levo-Dromoran ICN). Scored. In 100s.
c-ii	**Levo-Dromoran** (Valeant)	**Injection:** 2 mg/mL	In 1 mL amps[a] and 10 mL multidose vials.[b]

[a] Contains parabens.

[b] Contains phenol 14.5 mg/mL.

LEVORPHANOL TARTRATE — ORAL

For complete prescribing information, refer to the Opioid Analgesics group monograph.

Indications

➤*Pain:* Management of moderate to severe pain where an opioid analgesic is appropriate.

➤*Preoperative medication (Levo-Dromoran* only): As a preoperative medication where an opioid analgesic is appropriate.

Administration and Dosage

➤*Approved by the FDA:* January 8, 1953.

➤*Dosage:* Recommended starting dose is 2 mg. Repeat in 6 to 8 hours (*Levo-Dromoran*) or 3 to 6 hours (*Levorphanol Tartrate*) as needed, provided the patient is assessed for signs of hypoventilation and excessive sedation.

Levo-Dromoran – If necessary, increase the dose to up to 3 mg every 6 to 8 hours, after adequate evaluation of the patient's response. Higher doses may be appropriate in opioid-tolerant patients. Adjust dosage according to the severity of the pain; the patient's age, weight, physical status, and underlying diseases; use of concomitant medications; and other factors.

Total oral daily doses of more than 6 to 12 mg in 24 hours are generally not recommended as starting doses in nonopioid-tolerant patients; lower total daily doses may be appropriate.

Levorphanol Tartrate – The effective daily dosage range, depending on the severity of the pain, is 8 to 16 mg in 24 hours in the nontolerant patient. Total oral daily doses of more than 16 mg in 24 hours are generally not recommended as starting doses in nonopioid-tolerant patients.

➤*Chronic pain:* Individualize dosage. Levorphanol is 4 to 8 times as potent as morphine and has a longer half-life. Because there is incomplete cross-tolerance among opioids, when converting a patient from morphine to levorphanol, begin the total daily dose of oral levorphanol at approximately 1/15 to 1/12 of the total daily dose of oral morphine that such patients had previously required, and then adjust the dose to the patient's clinical response. If a patient is to be placed on fixed-schedule dosing (round-the-clock) with this drug, take care to allow adequate time after each dose

LEVORPHANOL TARTRATE — ORAL

change (approximately 72 hours) for the patient to reach a new steady state before a subsequent dose adjustment to avoid excessive sedation because of drug accumulation.

➤*Perioperative period (Levo-Dromoran)*: Levorphanol has been used for analgesic action during premedication and the postoperative period. Factors to be considered in determining the dosage include age, body weight, physical status, underlying pathological condition, use of other drugs, type of anesthesia used, the surgical procedure involved, and the severity of pain.

➤*Special populations:* The initial doses of levorphanol should be reduced by 50% or more when the drug is given to elderly or to patients with any condition affecting respiratory reserve or in conjunction with other drugs affecting the respiratory center. Subsequent doses should then be individually titrated according to the patient's response. Respiratory depression produced by levorphanol can be reversed by naloxone, a specific antagonist.

➤*Storage / Stability:* Tablets should be stored at 59° to 86°F (15° to 30°C). Dispense in tight containers as defined in USP/NF.

LEVORPHANOL TARTRATE — INJECTION

For complete prescribing information, refer to the Opioid Analgesics group monograph.

Indications

➤*Pain:* Management of moderate to severe pain where an opioid analgesic is appropriate.

➤*Preoperative medication (Levo-Dromoran* only): As a preoperative medication where an opioid analgesic is appropriate.

Administration and Dosage

➤*Approved by the FDA:* January 8, 1953.

➤*Intravenous (IV):* The usual recommended starting dose for IV administration is up to 1 mg given in divided doses by slow injection. This may be repeated in 3 to 6 hours as needed, provided the patient is assessed for signs of hypoventilation or excessive sedation. Dosage should be adjusted according to the severity of the pain; age, weight and physical status of the patient; the patient's underlying diseases; use of concomitant medications; and other factors (see Warnings, Precautions). Total daily doses of more than 4 to 8 mg IV in 24 hours are generally not recommended as starting doses in nonopioid tolerant patients; lower total daily doses may be appropriate.

➤*Intramuscular (IM) or subcutaneous:* The usual recommended starting dose for IM or subcutaneous administration is 1 to 2 mg. This may be repeated in 6 to 8 hours as needed, provided the patient is assessed for signs of hypoventilation or excessive sedation. Dosage should be adjusted according to the severity of the pain; age, weight, and physical status of the patient; the patient's underlying diseases; use of concomitant medications; and other factors (see Warnings, Precautions). Total daily doses of more then 3 to 8 mg IM in 24 hours are generally not recommended as starting doses in nonopioid-tolerant patients; lower total daily doses may be appropriate.

➤*Chronic pain:* Individualize dosage. Levorphanol is 4 to 8 times as potent as morphine and has a longer half-life. Because there is incomplete cross-tolerance among opioids, when converting a patient from morphine to levorphanol, begin the total daily dose of oral levorphanol at approximately 1⁄15 to 1⁄12 of the total daily dose of oral morphine that such patients had previously required, and then adjust the dose to the patient's clinical response. If a patient is to be placed on fixed-schedule dosing (round-the-clock) with this drug, take care to allow adequate time after each dose change (approximately 72 hours) for the patient to reach a new steady state before a subsequent dose adjustment to avoid excessive sedation because of drug accumulation.

➤*Perioperative period (Levo-Dromoran)*: Levorphanol has been used for analgesic action during premedication and the postoperative period. Factors to be considered in determining the dosage include age, body weight, physical status, underlying pathological condition, use of other drugs, type of anesthesia used, the surgical procedure involved, and the severity of pain.

➤*Premedication (Levo-Dromoran)*: Individualize the preoperative medication dose. The usual dose for healthy young adults is 1 to 2 mg IM or subcutaneously, administered 60 to 90 minutes before surgery. Older or debilitated patients usually require less drug. Levorphanol 2 mg is approximately equivalent to morphine 10 to 15 mg or meperidine 100 mg.

➤*Special populations:* The initial doses of levorphanol should be reduced by 50% or more when the drug is given to elderly or to patients with any condition affecting respiratory reserve or in conjunction with other drugs affecting the respiratory center. Subsequent doses should then be individually titrated according to the patient's response. Respiratory depression produced by levorphanol can be reversed by naloxone, a specific antagonist.

➤*Incompatibilities:* Levorphanol injection has been reported to be physically incompatible with solutions containing aminophylline, ammonium chloride, amobarbital sodium, chlorothiazide sodium, heparin sodium, methicillin sodium, nitrofurantoin sodium, novobiocin sodium, pentobarbital sodium, perphenazine, phenobarbital sodium, phenytoin sodium, secobarbital sodium, sodium bicarbonate, sodium iodide, sulfadiazine sodium, sulfisoxazole diethanolamine, and thiopental sodium.

➤*Safety and handling:* Levorphanol injection is packaged in sealed systems that have a low risk of accidental exposure to health care workers. Ordinary care should be taken to avoid aerosol generation while preparing a syringe for use. Significant absorption from accidental dermal exposure is unlikely, and spilled levorphanol should be washed from the skin by rinsing with cool water. As with all controlled substances, abuse by health care personnel is possible and the drug should be handled accordingly.

➤*Storage / Stability:* Store at 15° to 30°C (59° to 86°F).

MEPERIDINE HYDROCHLORIDE

c-ii	**Meperidine Hydrochloride** (Various, eg, Amide, Barr, Roxane, Watson)	**Tablets**: 50 mg	In 100s, 500s, 1,000s, and UD 25s.
c-ii	**Demerol** (Sanofi-Synthelabo)		White, scored, convex. In 100s, 500s, and UD 25s.
c-ii	**Meperidine Hydrochloride** (Various, eg, Amide, Barr, Roxane, Watson)	**Tablets**: 100 mg	In 100s, 500s, and 1,000s, and UD 25s.
c-ii	**Demerol** (Sanofi-Synthelabo)		White, convex. In 100s.
c-ii	**Demerol** (Sanofi-Synthelabo)	**Syrup**: 50 mg per 5 mL	Glucose, saccharin. Alcohol free. Banana flavor. In 473 mL.
c-ii	**Meperidine Hydrochloride** (Roxane)	**Oral solution**: 50 mg per 5 mL	Sorbitol. In 500 mL.
c-ii	**Meperidine Hydrochloride** (Various, eg, Baxter)	**Injection**: 25 mg/mL	In 1 mL amps and 1 mL vials.
c-ii	**Demerol** (Abbott)		In 1 mL *Carpuject* syringes.[a]
c-ii	**Meperidine Hydrochloride** (Various, eg, Baxter)	**Injection**: 50 mg/mL	In 1 mL amps and 1 mL vials.
c-ii	**Demerol** (Abbott)		In 0.5, 1, 1.5, and 2 mL amps[b], 30 mL multidose vials,[b] and 1 mL *Carpuject*[a] syringes.
c-ii	**Meperidine Hydrochloride** (Various, eg, Baxter)	**Injection**: 75 mg/mL	In 1 mL vials and 1 mL amps
c-ii	**Demerol** (Abbott)		In 1 mL *Carpuject* syringes.[a]
c-ii	**Meperidine Hydrochloride** (Various, eg, Baxter)	**Injection**: 100 mg/mL	In 1 mL vials and 1 mL amps.
c-ii	**Demerol** (Abbott)		In 1 mL amp,[b] 20 mL multidose vials,[b] and 1 mL *Carpuject* syringes.[a]

[a] Ampuls and *Carpuject* syringes are preservative free.
[b] Multidose vials contain metocresol as preservative.

MEPERIDINE HYDROCHLORIDE — ORAL

For complete prescribing information, refer to the Opioid Analgesics group monograph.

Indications

Relief of moderate to severe pain.

Administration and Dosage

➤*Approved by the FDA:* November 10, 1942.

Meperidine is less effective orally than parenterally.

➤*Pain:* Adjust dosage according to the severity of the pain and the response of the patient.

Adults – Usual dosage is 50 to 150 mg every 3 to 4 hours as necessary.

Children – Usual dosage is 1.1 to 1.75 mg/kg (0.5 to 0.8 mg/lb) up to the adult dose, every 3 to 4 hours, as necessary.

➤*Concomitant therapy:* The dose should be proportionately reduced (usually by 25% to 50%) when administered concomitantly with phenothiazines and many other tranquilizers because they potentiate the action of meperidine.

➤*Storage / Stability:* Store at 25°C (77°F); excursions permitted to 15° to 30°C (59° to 86°F) [See USP Controlled Room Temperature].

MEPERIDINE HYDROCHLORIDE — INJECTION

For complete prescribing information, refer to the Opioid Analgesics group monograph.

Indications

Relief of moderate to severe pain.

For preoperative medication, support of anesthesia, and obstetrical analgesia.

Administration and Dosage

➤*Approved by the FDA:* November 10, 1942.

Meperidine is less effective orally than parenterally.

➤*Pain:* Adjust dosage according to the severity of the pain and the response of the patient.

While subcutaneous administration is suitable for occasional use, intramuscular (IM) administration is preferred when repeated doses are required. If intravenous (IV) administration is required, dosage should be decreased and the injection made very slowly, preferably utilizing a diluted solution.

Adults – Usual dosage is 50 to 150 mg IM or subcutaneously every 3 to 4 hours as necessary. Elderly patients should usually be given meperidine at the lower end of the dosage range and observed closely.

Children – Usual dosage is 1.1 to 1.75 mg/kg (0.5 to 0.8 mg/lb) IM or subcutaneously up to the adult dose, every 3 to 4 hours, as necessary.

Concomitant therapy – The dose should be proportionately reduced (usually by 25% to 50%) when administered concomitantly with phenothiazines and many other tranquilizers because they potentiate the action of meperidine.

➤*Preoperative medication:*

Adults – 50 to 100 mg IM or subcutaneously, 30 to 90 minutes before beginning anesthesia.

Elderly: Give elderly patients meperidine at the lower end of the dose range and observe closely.

Children – 1.1 to 2.2 mg/kg (0.5 to 1 mg/lb) IM or subcutaneously, up to adult dose, 30 to 90 minutes before beginning anesthesia.

➤*Support of anesthesia:* Meperidine may be administered by repeated slow IV injections of fractional doses (eg, 10 mg/mL) or by a continuous IV infusion of a more dilute solution (eg, 1 mg/mL). Individualize dosage.

➤*Obstetrical analgesia:* When pain becomes regular, administer 50 to 100 mg IM or subcutaneously; may repeat at 1- to 3-hour intervals.

➤*Storage / Stability:* Store at room temperature up to 25°C (77°F).

METHADONE HYDROCHLORIDE

c-ii	**Methadone Hydrochloride** (Various, eg, Mallinckrodt, Roxane, Vista Pharm)	**Tablets:** 5 mg	In 100s and UD 100s.
c-ii	**Dolophine Hydrochloride** (Roxane)		(54 162). White, scored. In 100s.
c-ii	**Methadose** (Mallinckrodt)		(Methadose 5). White, scored. In 100s.
c-ii	**Methadone Hydrochloride** (Various, eg, Mallinckrodt, Roxane, Vista Pharm)	**Tablets:** 10 mg	In 100s and UD 100s.
c-ii	**Dolophine Hydrochloride** (Roxane)		(54 549). White, scored. In 100s.
c-ii	**Methadose** (Mallinckrodt)		(Methadose 10). White, scored. In 100s.
c-ii	**Methadone Hydrochloride**[a] (Various, eg, Cebert, Vista Pharm)	**Tablets, dispersible:** 40 mg	In 100s.
c-ii	**Methadose**[a] (Mallinckrodt)		(Methadose 40). White, quadrisected. In 100s.
c-ii	**Methadone Hydrochloride** (Roxane)	**Solution, oral:** 5 mg per 5 mL	8% alcohol, sorbitol. Citrus flavor. In 500 mL.
		10 mg per 5 mL	8% alcohol, sorbitol. Citrus flavor. In 500 mL.
c-ii	**Methadone Hydrochloride**[a] (Various, eg, Cebert, VistaPharm)	**Concentrate, oral:** 10 mg/mL	In 946 mL and 1 L.
c-ii	**Methadone Hydrochloride Intensol** (Roxane)		In 30 mL with calibrated dropper.
c-ii	**Methadose**[a] (Mallinckrodt)		Sucrose. Cherry flavor. In 1 L. Also available as sugar free, dye free, unflavored.
c-ii	**Methadone Hydrochloride** (aaiPharma)	**Injection:** 10 mg/mL	In 20 mL multidose vials.[b]

[a] For detoxification and maintenance only.
[b] With 0.5% chlorobutanol.

METHADONE HYDROCHLORIDE — ORAL

For complete prescribing information, refer to the Opioid Analgesics group monograph.

WARNING

To treat narcotic addiction in detoxification or maintenance programs, methadone should be dispensed only by hospitals, community pharmacies, and maintenance programs approved by the FDA and designated state authorities. Approved maintenance programs shall dispense and use methadone in oral form only and according to treatment requirements stipulated in *Federal Methadone Regulations*. Failure to abide by the requirements in these regulations may result in criminal prosecution, seizure of drug supply, revocation of program approval, and injunction precluding program operation.

Methadone, used as an analgesic, may be dispensed in any licensed pharmacy.

Methadone dispersible tablets are for oral administration only. This preparation contains insoluble excipients and therefore must not be injected. It is recommended that methadone dispersible tablets, if dispensed, be packaged in child-resistant containers and kept out of the reach of children to prevent accidental ingestion.

Cardiac conduction effects – Laboratory studies, in vivo and in vitro, have demonstrated that methadone inhibits cardiac potassium channels and prolongs the QT interval. Cases of QT interval prolongation and serious arrhythmia (torsades de pointes) have been observed during treatment with methadone. These cases appear to be more commonly associated with, but not limited to, higher dose treatment (greater than 200 mg/day). Most cases involve patients being treated for pain with large, multiple daily doses of methadone, although cases have been reported in patients receiving doses commonly used for maintenance treatment of opioid addiction.

Indications

➤*Pain / Detoxification:* For relief of severe pain; detoxification and temporary maintenance treatment of narcotic addiction (except dispersible tablets and certain oral concentrates; see product table).

Note – If used to treat heroin dependence for longer than 3 weeks, the procedure passes from treatment of acute withdrawal syndrome (detoxification) to maintenance therapy. Maintenance may be undertaken only by approved methadone programs. This does not preclude maintenance treatment of addicts hospitalized for other conditions and who require temporary maintenance during the critical period of their stays or whose enrollment has been verified in a program approved for maintenance treatment with methadone.

Administration and Dosage

➤*Approved by the FDA:* August 13, 1947.

Oral methadone is about one half as potent as parenteral. Oral administration results in a delay of onset, a lower peak, and an increased duration of analgesic effect. Duration of effect increases with repeated use because of cumulative effects.

➤*Pain:* 2.5 to 10 mg orally every 3 or 4 hours as necessary. Adjust dosage according to the severity of pain and patient response. For exceptionally severe pain, or in those tolerant of opioid analgesia, it may be necessary to exceed the usual recommended dosage.

➤*Dosage adjustment during pregnancy:* Methadone clearance may be increased during pregnancy. Several small studies have demonstrated significantly lower trough methadone plasma concentrations and shorter methadone half-lives in women during their pregnancy compared with after their delivery. During pregnancy, a woman's methadone dose may need to be increased, or their dosing interval decreased. Keep dosage as low as possible. Methadone should be used in pregnancy only if the potential benefit justifies the potential risk to the fetus.

➤*Detoxification treatment:* Detoxification treatment should not exceed 21 days and may not be repeated earlier than 4 weeks after completion of the preceding course. If methadone is administered longer than 3 weeks, the procedure is considered to have progressed from detoxification or treatment of the acute withdrawal syndrome to maintenance treatment, even though the goal and intent may be eventual total withdrawal.

Oral administration is preferred. However, if the patient is unable to ingest oral methadone, the parenteral form may be used. Injectable methadone products are not approved for the outpatient treatment of opioid dependence. Parenteral methadone should be used only for patients who are unable to take oral medication, such as during hospitalization. The patient's oral methadone dose should be converted to an equivalent parenteral dose using the considerations above.

METHADONE HYDROCHLORIDE — ORAL

Initially, a single dose of 15 to 20 mg will often suppress withdrawal symptoms. Provide additional methadone if withdrawal symptoms are not suppressed or if symptoms reappear. When patients are physically dependent on high doses, 40 mg/day in single or divided doses is usually an adequate stabilizing dose. Continue stabilization for 2 to 3 days, then gradually decrease the dose on a daily basis or at 2-day intervals. The rate at which methadone is decreased will be determined separately for each patient. Provide a sufficient amount to keep withdrawal symptoms at a tolerable level. In hospitalized patients, a daily reduction of 20% of total daily dose may be tolerated and may cause little discomfort. In ambulatory patients, a somewhat slower schedule may be needed.

➤*Detoxification maintenance:* Individualize dosage. Initial dosage should control abstinence symptoms following narcotic withdrawal, but should not cause sedation, respiratory depression, or other effects of acute intoxication. If patients have been heavy heroin users up to admission day, they may be given methadone 20 mg 4 to 8 hours after heroin is stopped or 40 mg in a single oral dose. If they enter treatment with little or no narcotic tolerance, initial dosage may be halved. When in doubt, use a smaller dose. Keep the patient under observation. If abstinence symptoms are distressing, give additional 10 mg doses as needed. Adjust dosage as tolerated and required, up to 120 mg/day.

For a complete description of detoxification and maintenance regulations and dosage protocols, consult a local approved methadone program.

➤*Acute pain:* Maintenance patients on a stable methadone dose who experience physical trauma, postoperative pain, or other causes of acute pain cannot be expected to derive analgesia from their stable dose of methadone regimens. Such patients should be given analgesics, including opioids, that would be indicated in other patients experiencing similar nociceptive stimulation. Because of the opioid tolerance induced by methadone, when opioids are required for management of acute pain in methadone patients, somewhat higher and/or more frequent doses will often be required than would be the case for other, nontolerant patients.

➤*Dispersible tablets:* Methadone dispersible tablets have been formulated with insoluble excipients to deter the use of this drug by injection. Dissolve each tablet in approximately 1 ounce of liquid (other than grapefruit juice) and swallow. Do not swallow tablets whole or chew tablets.

➤*Storage/Stability:* Store at controlled room temperature 15° to 30°C (59°to 86°F). Protect from light.

METHADONE HYDROCHLORIDE — INJECTION

For complete prescribing information, refer to the Opioid Analgesics group monograph.

WARNING

To treat narcotic addiction in detoxification or maintenance programs, methadone should be dispensed only by hospitals, community pharmacies, and maintenance programs approved by the FDA and designated state authorities. Approved maintenance programs shall dispense and use methadone in oral form only and according to treatment requirements stipulated in *Federal Methadone Regulations*. Failure to abide by the requirements in these regulations may result in criminal prosecution, seizure of drug supply, revocation of program approval, and injunction precluding program operation.

Methadone, used as an analgesic, may be dispensed in any licensed pharmacy.

Cardiac conduction effects – Laboratory studies, in vivo and in vitro, have demonstrated that methadone inhibits cardiac potassium channels and prolongs the QT interval. Cases of QT interval prolongation and serious arrhythmia (torsades de pointes) have been observed during treatment with methadone. These cases appear to be more commonly associated with, but not limited to, higher dose treatment (greater than 200 mg/day). Most cases involve patients being treated for pain with large, multiple daily doses of methadone, although cases have been reported in patients receiving doses commonly used for maintenance treatment of opioid addiction.

Indications

➤*Pain/Detoxification:* For relief of severe pain; detoxification and temporary maintenance treatment of narcotic addiction.

Note – If used to treat heroin dependence for longer than 3 weeks, the procedure passes from treatment of acute withdrawal syndrome (detoxification) to maintenance therapy. Maintenance may be undertaken only by approved methadone programs. This does not preclude maintenance treatment of addicts hospitalized for other conditions and who require temporary maintenance during the critical period of their stays or whose enrollment has been verified in a program approved for maintenance treatment with methadone.

Administration and Dosage

➤*Approved by the FDA:* August 13, 1947.

Oral methadone is about one half as potent as parenteral. Oral administration results in a delay of onset, a lower peak, and an increased duration of analgesic effect. Duration of effect increases with repeated use because of cumulative effects.

➤*Pain:* As with all opioid drugs, it is necessary to adjust the dosing regimen for each patient individually, taking into account the patient's prior analgesic treatment experience. The following dosing recommendations should only be considered as suggested approaches to what is actually a series of clinical decisions over time in the management of the pain of each individual patient. Prescribers should always follow appropriate pain management principles of careful assessment and ongoing monitoring.

In the selection of an initial dose of methadone injection, attention should be given to the following:

1.) The total daily dose, potency and specific characteristics of the opioid the patient had been taking previously, if any;
2.) The relative potency estimate used to calculate an equianalgesic starting methadone dose, in particular, whether it is intended for use in acute or chronic methadone dosing;
3.) The patient's degree of opioid tolerance;
4.) The age, general condition, and medical status of the patient;
5.) Concurrent medications, particularly other CNS and respiratory depressants;
6.) The type, severity, and expected duration of the patient's pain;
7.) The acceptable balance between pain control and adverse side effects.

Methadone injection may be administered intravenously (IV), subcutaneously, or intramuscularly (IM). The absorption of subcutaneous and IM methadone has not been well characterized and appears to be unpredictable. Local tissue reactions may occur.

Initiation of therapy in opioid-nontolerant patients – Starting dose is 2.5 to 10 mg every 8 to 12 hours, slowly titrated to effect. More frequent administration may be required during methadone initiation in order to maintain adequate analgesia, and extreme caution is necessary to avoid overdosage, taking into account methadone's long elimination half life.

Conversion from oral to parenteral methadone – Initially use a 2:1 dose ratio (eg, oral methadone 10 mg to parenteral methadone 5 mg).

Switching patients to parenteral methadone from other chronic opioids – Switching a patient from another chronically administered opioid to methadone requires caution due to the uncertainty of dose conversion ratios and incomplete cross-tolerance. Deaths have occurred in opioid-tolerant patients during conversion to methadone.

Conversion ratios in many commonly used equianalgesic dosing tables do not apply in the setting of repeated methadone dosing. Although with single-dose administration the onset and duration of analgesic action, as well as the analgesic potency of methadone and morphine, are similar, methadone's potency increases over time with repeated dosing. Furthermore, the conversion ratio between methadone and other opiates varies dramatically depending on baseline opiate (morphine equivalent) use as shown in the table below.

Oral Morphine to IV Methadone Conversion for Chronic Administration

Total daily baseline oral morphine dose	Estimated daily oral methadone requirement as percent of total daily morphine dose	Estimated daily IV methadone as percent of total daily oral morphine dose[a]
< 100 mg	20% to 30%	10% to 15%
100 to 300 mg	10% to 20%	5% to 10%
300 to 600 mg	8% to 12%	4% to 6%
600 to 1,000 mg	5% to 10%	3% to 5%
> 1,000 mg	< 5%	< 3%

[a] The total daily methadone dose derived from the table above may then be divided to reflect the intended dosing schedule (ie, for administration every 8 hours, divide total daily methadone dose by 3).

Parenteral Morphine to IV Methadone Conversion for Chronic Administration[a]

Total daily baseline parenteral morphine dose	Estimated daily parenteral methadone requirement as percent of total daily morphine dose[b]
10 to 30 mg	40% to 66%
30 to 50 mg	27% 66%
50 to 100 mg	22% to 50%
100 to 200 mg	15% to 34%
200 to 500 mg	10% to 20%

[a] Derived from previous table assuming a 3:1 oral:parenteral morphine ratio.
[b] The total daily methadone dose derived from the table above may then be divided to reflect the intended dosing schedule (ie, for administration every 8 hours, divide total daily methadone dose by 3).

Note: Equianalgesic methadone dosing varies not only between patients, but also within the same patient, depending on baseline morphine (or other opioid) dose. The above tables have been included in order to illustrate this concept and to provide a safe starting point for opioid conversion. Methadone dosing should not be based solely on these tables. Methadone conversion and dose titration methods should always be individualized to account for the patient's prior opioid exposure, general medical condition, concomitant medication, and anticipated breakthrough medication use.

➤*Dosage adjustment during pregnancy:* Methadone clearance may be increased during pregnancy. Several small studies have demonstrated significantly lower trough methadone plasma concentrations and shorter methadone half-lives in women during their pregnancy compared with after their delivery. During pregnancy, a woman's methadone dose may need to be increased, or their dosing interval decreased. Keep dosage as low as pos-

METHADONE HYDROCHLORIDE — INJECTION

sible. Methadone should be used in pregnancy only if the potential benefit justifies the potential risk to the fetus.

➤*Detoxification treatment:* Detoxification treatment should not exceed 21 days and may not be repeated earlier than 4 weeks after completion of the preceding course. If methadone is administered longer than 3 weeks, the procedure is considered to have progressed from detoxification or treatment of the acute withdrawal syndrome to maintenance treatment, even though the goal and intent may be eventual total withdrawal.

Oral administration is preferred. However, if the patient is unable to ingest oral methadone, the parenteral form may be used. Injectable methadone products are not approved for the outpatient treatment of opioid dependence. Parenteral methadone should be used only for patients who are unable to take oral medication, such as during hospitalization. The patient's oral methadone dose should be converted to an equivalent parenteral dose using the considerations above.

For a complete description of detoxification and maintenance regulations and dosage protocols, consult a local approved methadone program.

➤*Acute pain:* Maintenance patients on a stable methadone dose who experience physical trauma, postoperative pain, or other causes of acute pain cannot be expected to derive analgesia from their stable dose of methadone regimens. Such patients should be given analgesics, including opioids, that would be indicated in other patients experiencing similar nociceptive stimulation. Because of the opioid tolerance induced by methadone, when opioids are required for management of acute pain in methadone patients, somewhat higher and/or more frequent doses will often be required than would be the case for other, nontolerant patients.

➤*Storage/Stability:* Store at controlled room temperature, 15° to 30°C (59° to 86°F). Protect from light.

MORPHINE SULFATE

c-ii	**Morphine Sulfate** (Various, eg, Ethex, Roxane)	**Tablets**: 15 mg	In 100s and UD 100s.
c-ii	**Morphine Sulfate** (Various, eg, Ethex, Roxane)	**Tablets**: 30 mg	In 100s and UD 100s.
c-ii	**Morphine Sulfate** (Watson)	**Tablets, controlled-release**: 15 mg	Lactose. (ABG 15). Blue. Film-coated. In 100s.
c-ii	**MS Contin** (Purdue Frederick)		Lactose. (PF M15). Blue. In 100s, 500s, and UD 25s.
c-ii	**Oramorph SR** (aaiPharma)		Lactose. (15). White. In 100s and 500s, and UD 100s.
c-ii	**Morphine Sulfate** (Watson)	**Tablets, controlled-release**: 30 mg	Lactose. (ABG 30). Lavender. Film-coated. In 100s.
c-ii	**MS Contin** (Purdue Frederick)		Lactose. (PF M30). Lavender. In 100s, 500s, and UD 25s.
c-ii	**Oramorph SR** (aaiPharma)		Lactose. (30). White. In 50s, 100s, and 250s, and UD 100s.
c-ii	**Morphine Sulfate** (Watson)	**Tablets, controlled-release**: 60 mg	Lactose. (ABG 60). Orange. Film-coated. In 100s.
c-ii	**MS Contin** (Purdue Frederick)		Lactose. (PF M 60). Orange. In 100s, 500s, and UD 25s.
c-ii	**Oramorph SR** (aaiPharma)		Lactose. (60). White. In 100s and UD 25s.
c-ii	**Morphine Sulfate** (Watson)	**Tablets, controlled-release**: 100 mg[a]	(ABG 100). Gray. Film-coated. In 100s.
c-ii	**MS Contin** (Purdue Frederick)		(PF 100). Gray. In 100s, 500s, and UD 25s.
c-ii	**Oramorph SR** (aaiPharma)		Lactose. (100). White. In 100s and UD 25s.
c-ii	**Morphine Sulfate** (Watson)	**Tablets, controlled-release**: 200 mg[a]	(ABG 200). Green, capsule shape. Film-coated. In 100s.
c-ii	**MS Contin** (Purdue Frederick)		(PFM 200). Green. Capsule shape. In 100s.
c-ii	**Morphine Sulfate** (Various, eg, Endo, Mallinckrodt)	**Tablets, extended-release**: 15 mg	In 100s and 500s, UD 100s, and 150 punch cards.
		30 mg	In 50s, 100s, and 500s, UD 100s, and 150 punch cards.
		60 mg	In 100s and 500s, UD 100s, and 150 punch cards.
c-ii	**Morphine Sulfate** (Various, eg, Endo, Mallinckrodt, Watson)	**Tablets, extended-release**: 100 mg	In 100s, 500s, and UD 100s.
c-ii	**Morphine Sulfate** (Various, eg, Endo, Mallinckrodt)	**Tablets, extended-release**: 200 mg[a]	In 100s.
c-ii	**Morphine Sulfate** (Ranbaxy)	**Tablets for injection, soluble**: 10 mg	Lactose and sucrose. In 100s.
		15 mg	Lactose and sucrose. In 100s.
		30 mg	Lactose and sucrose. In 100s.
c-ii	**Avinza** (Ligand)	**Capsules, extended-release pellets**: 30 mg	Sugar starch spheres, fumaric acid. Yellow/White. (e 30 mg 505). In 100s.
		60 mg[a]	Sugar starch spheres, fumaric acid. Bluish-green/White. (e 60 mg 506). In 100s.
		90 mg[a]	Sugar starch spheres, fumaric acid. Red/White. (e 90 mg 507). In 100s.
		120 mg[a]	Sugar starch spheres, fumaric acid. Blue-violet/white. (e 120 mg 508). In 100s.
c-ii	**Kadian** (Alpharma)	**Capsules, sustained-release pellets**: 20 mg	Sucrose. (KADIAN 20 mg). Yellow opaque. In 30s, 60s, and 100s.
		30 mg	Sucrose. (KADIAN 30 mg). Blue violet opaque. In 30s, 60s, and 100s.
		50 mg	Sucrose. (KADIAN 50 mg). Blue opaque. In 30s, 60s, and 100s.
		60 mg	Sucrose. (KADIAN 60 mg). Pink opaque. In 30s, 60s, and 100s.
		100 mg	Sucrose. (KADIAN 100 mg). Green opaque. In 30s, 60s, and 100s.
c-ii	**Morphine Sulfate** (Roxane)	**Oral solution**: 10 mg per 5 mL	In 100 and 500 mL and UD 5 and 10 mL.
c-ii	**MSIR** (Purdue Frederick)		Sugar, sucrose, EDTA. In 120 mL.
c-ii	**Morphine Sulfate** (Roxane)	**Oral solution**: 20 mg per 5 mL	In 100 and 500 mL.
c-ii	**MSIR** (Purdue Frederick)		Sugar, sucrose, EDTA. In 120 mL.
c-ii	**Morphine Sulfate** (Various, Ethex, Mallinckrodt)	**Oral solution (concentrate)**: 20 mg/mL	Alcohol free. In 15, 30, 120, and 240 mL with calibrated dropper or spoon.
c-ii	**MSIR** (Purdue Frederick)		EDTA. In 30 mL with calibrated dropper.
c-ii	**Roxanol** (aaiPharma)		In 30 and 120 mL with calibrated dropper.
c-ii	**Roxanol T** (aaiPharma)		Flavored. In 30 and 120 mL with calibrated dropper.
c-ii	**Roxanol 100** (aaiPharma)	**Oral solution (concentrate)**: 100 mg per 5 mL	In 240 mL with calibrated spoon.

MORPHINE SULFATE

c-ii	**Morphine Sulfate** (Abbott[b], Baxter)	**Injection:** 0.5 mg/mL	In 10 mL amps and vials.
c-ii	**Astramorph PF**[b] (AstraZeneca)		In 2 and 10 mL amps and 10 mL single-use vials.
c-ii	**Duramorph**[b] (Baxter)		In single-use 10 mL amps.
c-ii	**Morphine Sulfate** (Various, eg, Abbott[b], Baxter, International Medication Systems)	**Injection:** 1 mg/mL	In 10 mL amps and vials and 30 mL vials.
c-ii	**Astramorph PF**[b] (AstraZeneca)		In 2 and 10 mL amps and 10 mL single-use vials.
c-ii	**Duramorph**[b] (Baxter)		In 10 mL single-use amps.
c-ii	**Morphine Sulfate** (Various, eg, Abbott, Hospira)	**Injection:** 2 mg/mL	In 30 mL vials, and 1 mL syringes, *Carpuject*, and *Tubex*.
c-ii	**Morphine Sulfate** (Various, eg, Abbott, Hospira)	**Injection:** 4 mg/mL	In 1 and 2 mL disposable syringes, and 1 mL *Carpuject* and *Tubex*.
c-ii	**Morphine Sulfate** (Various, eg, Baxter, Faulding)	**Injection:** 5 mg/mL	In 1 mL vials.
c-ii	**Morphine Sulfate** (Various, eg, Baxter, Hospira)	**Injection:** 8 mg/mL	In 1 mL *Carpuject*, vials, and amps.
c-ii	**Morphine Sulfate** (Various, eg, Baxter, Hospira)	**Injection:** 10 mg/mL	In 1 mL *Carpuject*, vials, and amps and 10 mL multidose vials.
c-ii	**Infumorph 200**[b] (Baxter)		In 20 mL (200 mg) amps.
c-ii	**DepoDur**[b] (Endo)	**Injection, extended-release liposomal:** 10 mg/mL	In 1 mL, 1.5 mL, and 2 mL single-use vials in cartons of 5.
c-ii	**Morphine Sulfate** (Various, eg, Baxter, Hospira)	**Injection:** 15 mg/mL	In 1 mL *Carpuject*, amps, and vials and 20 mL multidose vials.
c-ii	**Morphine Sulfate** (Various, eg, Faulding, International Medication Systems)	**Solution for injection:** 25 mg/mL[d]	In 4, 10, 20, and 40 mL syringes[b] and single-use vials.[c]
c-ii	**Infumorph 500**[b] (Baxter)		In 20 mL (500 mg) amps.
c-ii	**Morphine Sulfate** (Various, eg, Faulding, International Medication Systems)	**Solution for injection:** 50 mg/mL[d]	In 10, 20, 40, 50 mL syringes[b] and single-use vials.[c]
c-ii	**Morphine Sulfate in 5% Dextrose** (Hospira)	**Injection:** 1 mg/mL	In 100 and 250 mL.
c-ii	**Morphine Sulfate** (Various, eg, G & W, Paddock)	**Rectal suppositories:** 5 mg	In 12s.
c-ii	**RMS** (Upsher-Smith)		In 12s.
c-ii	**Morphine Sulfate** (Various, eg, G & W, Paddock)	**Rectal suppositories:** 10 mg	In 12s
c-ii	**RMS** (Upsher-Smith)		In 12s.
c-ii	**Morphine Sulfate** (Various, eg, G & W, Paddock)	**Rectal suppositories:** 20 mg	In 12s.
c-ii	**RMS** (Upsher-Smith)		In 12s.
c-ii	**Morphine Sulfate** (Various, eg, G & W, Paddock)	**Rectal suppositories:** 30 mg	In 12s.
c-ii	**RMS** (Upsher-Smith)		In 12s.

[a] For use only in opioid-tolerant patients.
[b] Some preparations are preservative free.
[c] May contain sulfites; for IV use only.
[d] For IV use after dilution. Not for direct injection.

MORPHINE SULFATE — ORAL

For complete prescribing information, refer to the Opioid Analgesics group monograph.

WARNING

Avinza – *Avinza* capsules are a modified-release formulation of morphine indicated for once-daily administration for the relief of moderate to severe pain requiring continuous, around-the-clock opioid therapy for an extended period of time. *Avinza* capsules are to be swallowed whole or the contents of the capsules sprinkled on a small amount of applesauce immediately prior to ingestion. The capsule beads are not to be chewed, crushed, or dissolved because of the risk of rapid release and absorption of a potentially fatal dose of morphine. Patients must not consume alcoholic beverages while on *Avinza* therapy. Additionally, patients must not use prescription or nonprescription medications containing alcohol while on *Avinza* therapy. Consumption of alcohol while taking *Avinza* may result in the rapid release and absorption of a potentially fatal dose of morphine.

Indications

➤*Controlled-release (CR)/Extended-release (ER)/Sustained-release (SR) tablets/capsules:* Relief of moderate to severe pain in patients requiring continuous, around-the-clock opioid therapy for an extended period of time. Not intended for use as an as-needed analgesic.

➤*Immediate-release (IR) tablets/solution:* Relief of moderate to severe pain.

Administration and Dosage

➤*Approved by the FDA:* September 18, 1984.

➤*IR:* 5 to 30 mg (oral solution or tablets) every 4 hours or as directed by health care provider. For control of severe chronic pain in patients with certain terminal diseases, this drug should be administered on a regularly scheduled basis every 4 hours at the lowest dosage level that will achieve adequate analgesia.

➤*CR/ER/SR:*

Initial therapy – There has been no evaluation of CR/ER/SR morphine as an initial opioid analgesic in the management of pain. Because it may be more difficult to titrate a patient to adequate analgesia using a CR/ER/SR morphine, it is ordinarily advisable to begin treatment using an IR morphine formulation.

The *MS Contin* 200 mg tablet is for use only in opioid-tolerant patients requiring daily morphine-equivalent doses of 400 mg or more. Reserve this strength for patients who have already been titrated to a stable analgesic regimen using lower strengths of *MS Contin* or other opioids. If *Kadian* is chosen, start with 20 mg in those who do not have a proven tolerance to opioids. Increase at a rate of up to 20 mg every other day. Individualize dosage.

The daily dose of *Avinza* must be limited to a maximum of 1,600 mg. *Avinza* dosages of over 1,600 mg/day contain a quantity of fumaric acid that has not been demonstrated to be safe, and may result in serious renal toxicity. The 60, 90, and 120 mg capsules are for use only in opioid-tolerant patients. All doses are intended to be administered once daily.

See the following information on dosing recommendations.

Individualization of dosage:

• *Avinza* – As the initial opioid for patients who do not have a proven tolerance to opioids, patients should be treated initially at a dosage of 30 mg once daily (at 24-hour intervals). For opioid-naïve patients, the dose should be increased conservatively. For such patients, it is recommended that the dose of *Avinza* be adjusted in increments not greater than 30 mg every 4 days. Some degree of tolerance may occur, requiring dosage adjustment until the achievement of a balance between analgesia and opioid side effects. When necessary, the total daily dose of *Avinza* should be increased until pain relief is reached or clinically significant opioid-related adverse reactions occur.

The dose may be titrated as frequently as every other day to control analgesia. In the event that breakthrough pain occurs, *Avinza* may be supplemented with a small dose (5% to 15% of the total daily dose of morphine) of a short-acting analgesic.

• *Kadian* – Administer one half of the estimated total daily oral morphine dose every 12 hours (twice a day) or by administering the total daily oral morphine dose every 24 hours (once a day). To avoid accumulation, the dosing interval should not be reduced below 12 hours. The dose should be titrated no more frequently than every other day to allow the patients to stabilize before escalating the dose. If breakthrough pain occurs, the dose may be supplemented with a small dose (less than 20% of the total daily dose) of a short-acting analgesic. Patients who are excessively sedated after a once-daily dose or who regularly experience inadequate analgesia before the next dose should be switched to a twice-daily dosing. Patients who do not have a proven tolerance to opioids should be started only on the 20 mg strength, and usually should be increased at a rate not greater than 20 mg every other day.

Conversion from conventional IR oral morphine formulations to CR/ER/SR oral morphine –

SR: Administer one half of the patient's total daily oral morphine dose as *Kadian* every 12 hours or by administering the total daily oral morphine dose as *Kadian* every 24 hours. *Kadian* should not be given more frequently than every 12 hours. The first dose of *Kadian* may be taken with the last

MORPHINE SULFATE — ORAL

dose of any IR opioid medication because of the long delay until the peak effect after administration of *Kadian*.

ER (tablets and capsules):

• *Tablets* – A patient's daily morphine requirement is established using IR oral morphine (dosing every 4 to 6 hours). The patient is then converted to morphine ER in either of 2 ways:

1.) by administering one half of the patient's 24-hour requirement as morphine ER on an every- 12-hour schedule; or,
2.) by administering one third of the patient's daily requirement as morphine ER on an every-8-hour schedule.

With either method, dose and dosing interval is then adjusted as needed. The 15 mg ER tablet should be used for initial conversion if the patient's total daily requirement is expected to be less than 60 mg. Morphine ER tablets of 30 mg strength are recommended for patients with a daily morphine requirement of 60 to 120 mg. When the total daily dose is expected to be greater than 120 mg, the appropriate tablet strength should be employed.

• *Capsules* – Patients receiving other oral morphine formulations may be converted to *Avinza* by administering the patient's total daily oral morphine dose as *Avinza* once daily. *Avinza* should not be given more frequently than every 24 hours. Supplemental pain medication may be required until the response to the patient's daily *Avinza* dosage has stabilized (up to 4 days).

CR: The patient may convert in 1 of 2 ways:

1.) by administering one half of the patient's 24-hour requirement as *MS Contin* or *Oramorph SR* on an every-12-hour schedule; or
2.) by administering one third of the patient's daily requirement as *MS Contin* on an every 8-hour schedule.

The 15 mg tablet of *MS Contin* should be used for initial conversion, for patients whose total daily requirement is expected to be less than 60 mg. The 30 mg tablet strength is recommended for patients with a daily morphine requirement of 60 to 120 mg. When the total daily dose is expected to be greater than 120 mg, the appropriate combination of tablet strength should be employed. The 30 mg tablet strength of *Oramorph SR* for initial conversion is recommended for patients with a daily morphine requirement of 120 mg or less.

Conversion from parenteral morphine or other opioids (parenteral or oral) to CR/ER/SR oral morphine – Particular care must be exercised in the conversion process. Because of uncertainty about, and intersubject variation in, relative estimates of opioid potency and cross tolerance, initial dosing regimens should be conservative; that is, an underestimation of the 24-hour oral morphine requirement is preferred to an overestimate. To this end, initial individual doses should be estimated conservatively. In patients whose daily morphine requirements are expected to be no more than 120 mg, the 30 mg tablet strength is recommended for the initial titration period. Once a stable dose regimen is reached, the patient can be converted to the 60 or 100 mg tablet strength or appropriate combination of tablet strengths.

The following general points should be considered regarding opioid conversions:

Parenteral to oral morphine ratio: It may take anywhere from 2 to 6 mg of oral morphine to provide analgesia equivalent to 1 mg of parenteral morphine. A dose of oral morphine 3 times the daily parenteral morphine requirement may be sufficient in chronic use settings. A reasonable starting dose of *Avinza* would be approximately 3 times the previous daily parenteral morphine requirement.

Other parenteral or oral nonmorphine opioids to oral morphine: In general, it is safest to administer half of the estimated daily morphine requirement as the initial dose, and to manage inadequate analgesia by supplementation with IR morphine.

➤*Conversion from CR/ER/SR oral morphine to parenteral opioids:* It is best to assume that the parenteral-to-oral potency is high. For example, to estimate the required 24-hour dose of morphine for intramuscular (IM) use, the health care provider could employ a conversion of 1 mg of morphine IM for every 6 mg of morphine as CR tablet. The IM 24-hour dose would have to be divided by 6 and administered on an every-4-hour regimen. This approach is recommended because it is least likely to cause overdose.

Avinza/Kadian – When converting from *Avinza* or *Kadian* to parenteral opioids, it is best to calculate an equivalent parenteral dose and then initiate treatment at half of this calculated value. As an example, an estimated total 24-hour parenteral morphine requirement of a patient receiving *Avinza* or *Kadian* is one third of the dose of *Avinza* or *Kadian*. This estimated dose should then be divided in half, and this last calculated dose is the total daily dose. This value should be further divided by 6 if the desire is to dose with parenteral morphine every 4 hours.

Consider a patient taking 360 mg of *Avinza* or *Kadian* daily. First, divide by 3 to account for differences in bioavailability between oral and parenteral morphine. This new figure, 120 mg, is the estimated total 24-hour requirement of parenteral morphine. Dividing by 2, the result gives the total daily dose of 60 mg. If it is decided to administer the drug at 4-hour intervals, then administer 10 mg (60 divided by 6) every 4 hours.

Although this approach may require a dosage increase in the first 24 hours for many patients, this method is recommended, as it is less likely to result in overdose. Overdose is more likely to occur when administering an equivalent dose of parenteral morphine without titration. Provision for breakthrough pain should be made.

➤*Conversion of ER (Avinza)* or SR (*Kadian*) to other CR oral morphine formulations: *Kadian* is not bioequivalent to other CR morphine preparations. For a given dose, the same total amount of morphine is available from *Avinza* as from oral morphine solution or CR morphine tablets. Conversion from *Kadian* or *Avinza* to the same total daily dose of another CR morphine formulation may lead to either excessive sedation at peak or inadequate analgesia at trough. Close observation and appropriate dosage adjustments are recommended.

➤*Conversion from Avinza* to other pain control therapies: It is important to remember that the persistence of *Avinza*-derived plasma morphine concentrations may be in excess of 36 hours when making a conversion to other pain control therapies.

➤*Dosage reductions/adjustments:*

IR – During the first 2 to 3 days of effective pain relief, the patient may sleep for many hours. This can be misinterpreted as the effect of excessive analgesic dosing rather than the first sign of relief in a pain-exhausted patient. The dose, therefore, should be maintained for at least 3 days before reduction, if respiratory activity and other vital signs are adequate. Following successful relief of severe pain, periodic attempts to reduce the narcotic dose should be made. Smaller doses or complete discontinuation of the narcotic analgesic may become feasible due to a physiologic change or the improved mental state of the patient.

CR/ER/SR – If signs of excessive opioid effects are observed early in a dosing interval, the next dose should be reduced. If this adjustment leads to inadequate analgesia (ie, breakthrough pain occurs late in the dosing interval) the dosing interval may be shortened. Alternatively, a supplemental dose of a short-acting analgesic may be given. In adjusting dosing requirements, it is recommended that the dosing interval never be extended beyond 12 hours, because the administration of a very large dose may lead to acute overdosage.

➤*Discontinuation of therapy:* When the patient no longer requires therapy, doses should be tapered gradually to prevent signs and symptoms of withdrawal in the physically dependent patient.

➤*Administration:*

CR/ER/SR tablets/capsules – Must be swallowed whole (not chewed, crushed, or dissolved) because of the risk of acute overdose. Ingesting chewed or crushed beads or pellets will lead to the rapid release and absorption of a potentially toxic dose of morphine.

Avinza: Avinza beads sprinkled over applesauce were found to be bioequivalent to *Avinza* capsules swallowed whole under fasting conditions in a study of healthy volunteers. Absorption of the beads sprinkled on other foods has not been tested. Capsules may be opened and the entire bead contents sprinkled on a small amount of applesauce immediately prior to ingestion. The applesauce should be at room temperature or cooler. Patients should ingest the mixture immediately. Patients must swallow the mixture without chewing or crushing beads, then rinse their mouths and swallow to ensure all beads have been ingested. Patients should consume the entire portion and not divide applesauce into separate doses.

Kadian: Capsules may be opened and the entire contents sprinkled on a small amount of applesauce immediately prior to ingestion.

Open the capsule and sprinkle the entire contents over approximately 10 mL of water and flush by swirling through a prewetted 16 French gastrostomy tube fitted with funnel at the port end. Additional aliquots of water are used to transfer all pellets and to flush the tube. Do not attempt the administration of pellets through a nasogastric tube.

May be given once or twice daily.

Concentrate oral solution: Administer with caution because the solution is a highly concentrated solution of morphine. Error in dosage or confusion between milligrams of morphine and milliliters of solution may cause significant overdosage. Dosing instructions should be clearly prescribed in milligrams of morphine and milliliters of solution. Verify correct dose and volume before administration to patient.

➤*Special risk patients:* Morphine may suppress respiration in the elderly, patients taking other CNS depressants, the very ill, and patients with respiratory problems; therefore, lower doses may be required.

➤*Storage/Stability:* Store oral solutions, tablets, and capsules at controlled room temperature (15° to 30°C; 59° to 86°F). Protect from light and moisture.

MORPHINE SULFATE — INJECTION

For complete prescribing information, refer to the Opioid Analgesics group monograph.

WARNING

Astromorph PF, Infumorph, Duramorph – Because of the risk of severe adverse effects when the epidural or intrathecal route of administration is employed, patients must be observed in a fully equipped and staffed environment for at least 24 hours after the initial dose.

Infumorph – Infumorph is not recommended for single-dose intravenous (IV), intramuscular (IM), or subcutaneous administration because of the very large amount of morphine in the ampul and the associated risk of overdosage.

Indications

➤*IV:* Relief of severe pain (eg, pain of myocardial infarction [MI], severe injuries, severe chronic pain associated with terminal cancer after all nonnarcotic analgesics have failed); used preoperatively to sedate the patient and allay apprehension, facilitate anesthesia induction, and reduce anesthetic dosage; control postoperative pain; relieve anxiety and reduce left ventricular work by reducing preload pressure; treatment of dyspnea associated with acute left ventricular failure and pulmonary edema; produce anesthesia for open-heart surgery.

➤*Subcutaneous/IM:* Relief of moderate to severe pain; relieve preoperative apprehension; preoperative sedation; control postoperative pain; supplement to anesthesia; analgesia during labor; acute pulmonary edema; allay anxiety.

➤*Epidural/Intrathecal:* Management of pain not responsive to nonnarcotic analgesics. For the treatment of intractable chronic pain (*Infumorph* only).

➤*ER epidural: DepoDur* is an ER liposome injection of morphine intended for single-dose administration by the epidural route, at the lumbar level, for the treatment of pain following major surgery. *DepoDur* is administered prior to surgery or after clamping the umbilical cord during cesarean section.

Administration and Dosage

➤*Approved by the FDA:* September 18, 1984.

➤*Subcutaneous/IM:*

Analgesia during labor – 10 mg is usually administered.

Adults – 10 mg (range, 5 to 20 mg) every 4 hours as needed.

Children – 0.1 to 0.2 mg/kg every 4 hours as needed. Do not exceed 15 mg/dose.

Soluble tablets – Prepare soluble tablets in sterile water and filter through a 0.22 micron membrane filter.

For preanesthetic medication:

- *Adults* – 10 mg per 70 kg of body weight (range, 5 to 20 mg)
- *Children (1 year of age and older)* – 0.1 mg per kg (maximum dose 10 mg).

For analgesia:

- *Adults* – 10 mg per 70 kg of body weight (range, 5 to 20 mg)
- *Children* – 0.1 to 0.2 mg/kg (maximum dose 15 mg).

➤*IV:*

Adults – 2 to 10 mg per 70 kg of body weight. A strength of 2.5 to 15 mg of morphine may be diluted in 4 to 5 mL of sterile water for injection. Administer slowly over 4 to 5 minutes. Rapid IV use increases the incidence of adverse reactions. Do not administer IV unless an opioid antagonist is immediately available.

For relief of pain and as preanesthetic – The usual adult dose is 10 mg every 4 hours, depending on the severity of the condition and the patient's response. The usual individual dose range is 5 to 15 mg. The usual daily dose range is 12 to 120 mg.

Usual pediatric dose (analgesic) – 50 to 100 mcg IV (0.05 to 0.1 mg) per kg of body weight, administered very slowly. Not to exceed 10 mg per dose.

Severe chronic pain associated with terminal cancer – Prior to initiation of the morphine infusion (in concentrations between 0.2 to 1 mg/mL), a loading dose of 15 mg or more of morphine may be administered by IV push to alleviate pain.

The infusion dosage range is 0.8 to 80 mg/h, though doses up to 144 mg/h have been used. Thus, for the 1 mg/mL solution, the infusion may be run from 0.8 to 80 mL/h, and for a 0.5 mg/mL solution, the infusion may be run from 1.6 to 160 mL/h.

A constant infusion rate must be maintained with an infusion pump in order to assure proper dosage control. Take care to avoid overdosage (respiratory depression) or abrupt cessation of therapy, which may give rise to withdrawal symptoms.

Open heart surgery – Administer large doses (0.5 to 3 mg/kg) of morphine IV as the sole anesthetic or with a suitable anesthetic agent. The patients are given oxygen and cardiovascular function is not depressed by morphine, as long as adequate ventilation is maintained.

MI pain – 8 to 15 mg administered parenterally. For very severe pain, additional smaller doses may be given every 3 to 4 hours as needed.

Incompatibility – Morphine has been reported to be physically or chemically incompatible with various drug products. Specialized references should be consulted for specific compatibility information.

➤*Epidural:* Initial injection of 5 mg in the lumbar region may provide satisfactory pain relief for up to 24 hours. If adequate pain relief is not achieved within 1 hour, carefully administer incremental doses of 1 to 2 mg at intervals sufficient to assess effectiveness. Give no more than 10 mg per 24 hours. Thoracic administration has been shown to dramatically increase the incidence of early and late respiratory depression even at doses of 1 to 2 mg. Patient monitoring should be continued for at least 24 hours after each dose since delayed respiratory depression may occur. Note: Intrathecal dosage is usually one-tenth that of epidural dosage.

For continuous infusion, an initial dose of 2 to 4 mg per 24 hours is recommended. Further doses of 1 to 2 mg may be given if pain relief is not achieved initially.

Aged or debilitated patients – Administer with extreme caution. Doses less than 5 mg may provide satisfactory pain relief for up to 24 hours.

Infumorph – The starting dose must be individualized. The recommended initial epidural dose in patients who are not tolerant to opioids range from 3.5 to 7.5 mg/day. The usual starting dose for continuous epidural infusion, based upon limited data in patients who have some degree of opioid tolerance, is 4.5 to 10 mg/day. The dose requirements may increase significantly during treatment, frequently to 20 to 30 mg/day.

➤*ER epidural:* Patient monitoring should be continued for at least 48 hours after dosing, as delayed respiratory depression may occur.

Major orthopedic surgery – Major orthopedic surgery of the lower extremity is dosed at 15 mg.

Lower abdominal or pelvic surgery – 10 to 15 mg. Some patients may benefit from a 20 mg dose of *DepoDur*, but the incidence of serious adverse respiratory events was dose-related in clinical trials.

Cesarean section – 10 mg. *DepoDur* should not be administered to women for vaginal labor and delivery.

Administration – *DepoDur* is not intended for intrathecal, IV, or IM administration. Administration of *DepoDur* into the thoracic epidural space or higher has not been evaluated and therefore is not recommended. *DepoDur* may be administered via needle or catheter at the lumbar level. *DepoDur* may be administered undiluted or may be diluted up to 5 mL total volume with preservative-free 0.9% normal saline. Do not use an in-line filter during administration of *DepoDur*.

Elderly – DepoDur should be administered to elderly patients (older than 65 years of age) after careful evaluation of their underlying medical condition and consideration of the risks associated with *DepoDur*. Vigilant perioperative monitoring should be exercised for elderly patients receiving *DepoDur*. In general, as with all opiates, the dose for elderly or debilitated patients should be at the low end of the dosing range.

➤*Intrathecal:* A single injection of 0.2 to 1 mg may provide satisfactory pain relief for up to 24 hours. (Caution: This is only 0.4 to 2 mL of the 0.5 mg/mL potency or 0.2 to 1 mL of the 1 mg/mL potency.) Do not inject intrathecally more than 2 mL of the 0.5 mg/mL potency or 1 mL of the 1 mg/mL potency. Use in lumbar area only. Repeated intrathecal injections are not recommended. A constant IV infusion of naloxone 0.6 mg/h for 24 hours after intrathecal injection may reduce incidence of potential side effects. Patient monitoring should be continued for at least 24 hours after each dose, because delayed respiratory depression may occur. Note: Intrathecal dosage is usually one-tenth that of epidural dosage.

Infumorph – Familiarization with the continuous microinfusion device is essential. To minimize risk from glass or other particles, the product must be filtered through not more than a 5 micron microfilter before injecting into the microinfusion device. If dilution is required, 0.9% sodium chloride injection is recommended. Individualize the starting dose. The recommended initial lumbar intrathecal dose range in patients with no tolerance to opioids is 0.2 to 1 mg/day. The published range of doses for individuals who have some degree of opioid tolerance varies from 1 to 10 mg/day. Limited experience with continuous intrathecal infusion of morphine has shown that the daily doses have to be increased over time. Employ doses greater than 20 mg/day with caution since they may be associated with a higher likelihood of serious side effects.

Aged or debilitated patients – Use extreme caution. Lower dose is usually satisfactory.

Repeat dosage – If pain recurs, consider alternative administration routes because experience with repeated doses by this route is limited.

➤*Special risk patients:* Morphine may suppress respiration in the elderly, those taking other CNS depressants, the very ill, and those patients with respiratory problems; therefore, lower doses may be required.

➤*Storage/Stability:* Store soluble tablets for injection at controlled room temperature (15° to 30°C; 59° to 86°F). Protect from light and moisture.

Injection – Store injections at controlled room temperature (15° to 30°C; 59° to 86°F). Solutions may darken with age. Do not use if injection is darker than pale yellow, discolored in any way, or contains a precipitate.

Infumorph, Duramorph, Astromorph PF injections – Protect from light. Store at 20° to 25°C (68° to 77°F), excursions permitted to 15° to 30°C (59° to 86°F) until ready to use. Do not freeze. Contains no preservative or antioxidant. Discard any unused portion. Do not heat sterilize.

DepoDur – *DepoDur* should be routinely stored in the refrigerator at 2° to 8°C (36° to 46°F). *DepoDur* may be held at 15° to 30°C (59° to 86°F) for up to 7 days in sealed, intact (unopened) vials. As a convenience to the hospital pharmacist, each carton of *DepoDur* includes pharmacy stickers for noting when each vial has been removed from refrigeration. Although *DepoDur* is a sterile agent, it does not contain any bacteriostatic agents. Therefore, *DepoDur* must be administered within 4 hours after withdrawal from the vial. Do not heat or gas sterilize. Following withdrawal from the vial, *DepoDur* may

MORPHINE SULFATE — INJECTION

be held at 15° to 30°C (59° to 86°F) for up to 4 hours prior to administration. Protect from freezing; do not administer if it is suspected that the vial has been frozen.

Soluble tablets for injection – Solutions may darken with age. Do not use if the solution is darker than pale yellow, is discolored in any other way, or contains a precipitate.

MORPHINE SULFATE — RECTAL

For complete prescribing information, refer to the Opioid Analgesics group monograph.

Indications

➤*Severe pain:* Morphine is indicated for the relief of severe chronic and acute pain.

Administration and Dosage

➤*Approved by the FDA:* September 18, 1984.

➤*Usual adult dosage:* 10 to 20 mg every 4 hours or as directed by a healthcare provider.

Dosage is a patient-dependent variable; therefore, increased dosage may be required to achieve adequate analgesia.

➤*Dosage reduction:* During the first 2 to 3 days of effective pain relief, the patient may sleep for many hours. This can be misinterpreted as the effect of excessive analgesic dosing rather than the first sign of relief of a pain-exhausted patient. The dose, therefore, should be maintained for at least 3 days before reduction, if respiratory activity and other vital signs are adequate.

Following successful relief of severe pain, periodic attempts to reduce the narcotic dose should be made. Smaller doses or complete discontinuation of the narcotic analgesic may become feasible because of a physiologic change or the improved mental state of the patient.

➤*Special populations:* Morphine may suppress respiration in the elderly, the very ill, and those patients with respiratory problems; therefore, lower doses may be required.

OPIUM

c-ii	**Opium Tincture, Deodorized** (Ranbaxy)	**Liquid**: anhydrous morphine equiv. 10 mg per mL	19% alcohol. In 120 and 473 mL.
c-iii	**Paregoric** (Various, eg, Barre-National)	**Liquid**: anhydrous morphine equiv. 2 mg per 5 mL	45% alcohol.[a] In 473 mL.

[a] May also contain benzoic acid.

OPIUM TINCTURE — ORAL

For complete prescribing information, refer to the Opioid Analgesics group monograph.

Indications

➤*Diarrhea:* For treatment of diarrhea. This preparation should not be used in diarrhea caused by poisoning until the toxic material is eliminated from the GI tract.

Administration and Dosage

➤*Caution:* Opium tincture contains 25 times more morphine than paregoric. Do not confuse opium tincture with paregoric; this may lead to a potentially fatal overdose of morphine.

➤*Opium tincture:*

Adults – 0.6 mL 4 times daily.

➤*Paregoric:*

Adults – 5 to 10 mL 1 to 4 times daily.

Children – 0.25 to 0.5 mL/kg 1 to 4 times daily.

➤*Storage/Stability:* Store at controlled room temperature 15° to 30°C (59° to 86°F). Protect from light.

OXYCODONE HYDROCHLORIDE

c-ii	**Oxycodone Hydrochloride** (Various, eg, Amide, Ethex, Mallinckrodt)	**Tablets**: 5 mg	In 100s, 500s, and UD 100s.
c-ii	**M-oxy** (Mallinckrodt)		(M-OXY 5). White, scored. In 100s.
c-ii	**Roxicodone** (aaiPharma)		(54 582). White, scored. In 100s and UD 100s.
c-ii	**Oxycodone Hydrochloride** (Ethex)	**Tablets**: 10 mg	In 100s and UD 100s.
c-ii	**Oxycodone Hydrochloride** (Various, eg, Amide, Ethex)	**Tablets**: 15 mg	In 100s and UD 100s.
c-ii	**Roxicodone** (aaiPharma)		Lactose. (54 710). Green, scored. In 100s and UD 100s.
c-ii	**Oxycodone Hydrochloride** (Ethex)	**Tablets**: 20 mg	In 100s and UD 100s.
c-ii	**Oxycodone Hydrochloride** (Various, eg, Amide, Ethex)	**Tablets**: 30 mg	In 100s and UD 100s.
c-ii	**Roxicodone** (aaiPharma)		Lactose. (54 199). Blue, scored. In 100s and UD 100s.
c-ii	**Oxycodone Hydrochloride** (Endo)	**Tablets, controlled-release**: 10 mg	(E702 10). White. Coated. In 30s and 500s.
c-ii	**OxyContin** (Purdue Pharma LP)		Lactose. (OC 10). White, convex. In 100s and UD 25s.
c-ii	**Oxycodone Hydrochloride** (Endo)	**Tablets, controlled-release**: 20 mg	(E703 20). Pink. Coated. In 30s and 500s.
c-ii	**OxyContin** (Purdue Pharma LP)		Lactose. (OC 20). Pink, convex. In 100s and UD 25s.
c-ii	**Oxycodone Hydrochloride** (Endo)	**Tablets, controlled-release**: 40 mg	(E705 40). Yellow. Coated. In 30s and 500s.
c-ii	**OxyContin** (Purdue Pharma LP)		Lactose. (OC 40). Yellow, convex. In 100s and UD 25s.
c-ii	**Oxycodone Hydrochloride** (Various, Global, Teva)	**Tablets, controlled-release**: 80 mg[a]	Lactose. In 100s, 500s, and 1,000s.
c-ii	**OxyContin** (Purdue Pharma LP)		Lactose. (OC 80). Green, convex. In 100s and UD 25s.
c-ii	**Oxycodone Hydrochloride** (Ethex)	**Capsules**: 5 mg	Lactose. (Ethex 041). Buff/white. In 100s and UD 100s.
c-ii	**OxyIR** (Purdue Pharma)		Sucrose. (O-IR PF5mg). Beige/orange. In 100s.
c-ii	**Oxycodone Hydrochloride** (Various, eg, Mallinckrodt)	**Solution, oral**: 5 mg per 5 mL	In 500 mL.
c-ii	**Roxicodone** (aaiPharma)		Sorbitol. In 500 mL and UD 5 mL.
c-ii	**Oxycodone Hydrochloride** (Various, eg, Mallinckrodt)	**Solution, concentrate**: 20 mg/mL	In 30 mL.
c-ii	**Roxicodone Intensol** (aaiPharma)		In 30 mL with calibrated dropper.
c-ii	**ETH-Oxydose** (Ethex)		Saccharin, sorbitol. Berry flavor. In 30 mL with dropper.
c-ii	**OxyFAST** (Purdue Pharma LP)		Saccharin. In 30 mL with dropper.

[a] For use in opioid-tolerant patients only.

OXYCODONE — ORAL

For complete prescribing information, refer to the Opioid Analgesics group monograph.

WARNING

Controlled-release (CR) oxycodone is an opioid agonist and a schedule II controlled substance with an abuse liability similar to morphine.

Oxycodone can be abused in a manner similar to other opioid agonists, legal or illicit. This should be considered when prescribing or dispensing oxycodone CR tablets in situations where the health care provider or pharmacist is concerned about an increased risk of misuse, abuse, or diversion.

Oxycodone CR tablets are indicated for the management of moderate to severe pain when a continuous, around-the-clock analgesic is needed for an extended period of time. Oxycodone CR tablets are not intended for use as as-needed analgesics.

Oxycodone 80 and 160 mg CR tablets are for use in opioid-tolerant patients only. These tablet strengths may cause fatal respiratory depression when administered to patients not previously exposed to opioids.

Oxycodone CR tablets are to be swallowed whole and are not to be broken, chewed, or crushed. Taking broken, chewed, or crushed oxycodone CR tablets leads to rapid release and absorption of a potentially fatal dose of oxycodone.

Indications

➤*Pain:*

Oral solution and concentrate solution – Relief of moderate to moderately severe pain.

Immediate-release (IR) tablets – Management of moderate to severe pain where use of an opioid analgesic is appropriate.

CR tablets – Management of moderate to severe pain when a continuous, around-the-clock analgesic is needed for an extended period of time. Not intended for use as an as-needed analgesic.

Individualize treatment in every case, initiating therapy at the appropriate point along a progression from nonopioid analgesics, such as nonsteroidal anti-inflammatory drugs (NSAIDs) and acetaminophen to opioids in a plan of pain management such as outlined by the World Health Organization, the Agency for Healthcare Research and Quality (formerly known as the Agency for Health Care Policy and Research), the Federation of State Medical Boards Model Guidelines, or the American Pain Society.

Not indicated for pain in the immediate postoperative period (the first 12 to 24 hours following surgery), or if the pain is mild or not expected to persist for an extended period of time. Oxycodone CR tablets are only indicated for postoperative use if the patient is already receiving the drug prior to surgery or if the postoperative pain is expected to be moderate to severe and persist for an extended period of time. Individualize treatment, moving from parenteral to oral analgesics as appropriate.

Administration and Dosage

➤*Approved by the FDA:* December 12, 1995

➤*IR tablets:* IR tablets are intended for the management of moderate to severe pain in patients who require treatment with an oral opioid analgesic. Individually adjust the dose according to severity of pain, patient response, and patient size. If the pain increases in severity, analgesia is not adequate, or tolerance occurs, a gradual increase in dosage may be required.

Adults – 10 to 30 mg every 4 hours (5 mg every 6 hours for *OxyIR*, oxycodone IR capsules), as needed. Individualize dosage. More severe pain may require 30 mg or more every 4 hours. If the pain increases in severity, analgesia is not adequate, or tolerance occurs, a gradual increase in dosage may be required.

Children – Not recommended for use in children.

Patients not currently on opioid therapy (opioid naïve) – Start patients who have not been receiving opioid analgesics on IR tablets in a dosing range of 5 to 15 mg every 4 to 6 hours as needed for pain. Titrate the dose based upon the individual patient's response to his/her initial dose of IR tablets. Patients with chronic pain should have their dosage given on an around-the-clock basis to prevent the reoccurrence of pain rather than treating the pain after it has occurred. This dose can then be adjusted to an acceptable level of analgesia, taking into account side effects experienced by the patient.

Severe chronic pain – For control of severe chronic pain, administer on a regularly scheduled basis, every 4 to 6 hours, at the lowest dosage level that will achieve adequate analgesia.

Conversion from fixed-ratio opioid/acetaminophen, opioid/aspirin, or opioid/nonsteroidal combination drugs – When converting patients from fixed-ratio opioid/nonopioid drug regimens, a decision should be made whether or not to continue the nonopioid analgesic. If a decision is made to discontinue the use of the nonopioid analgesic, it may be necessary to titrate the dose of the IR tablets in response to the level of analgesia and adverse effects afforded by the dosing regimen. If the nonopioid regimen is continued as a separate single entity agent, base the starting dose upon the most recent dose of opioid as a baseline for further titration of oxycodone. Gauge incremental increases according to side effects to an acceptable level of analgesia.

Patients currently on opioid therapy – If a patient has been receiving opioid-containing medications prior to taking IR tablets, the potency of the prior opioid relative to oxycodone should be factored into the selection of the total daily dose of oxycodone.

In converting patients from other opioids to IR tablets, close observation and adjustment of dosage based upon the patient's response to IR tablets is imperative. Administration of supplemental analgesia for breakthrough or incident pain and titration of the total daily dose of IR tablets may be necessary, especially in patients who have disease states that are changing rapidly.

Maintenance of therapy – Continual reevaluation of the patient receiving IR tablets is important, with special attention to the maintenance of pain control and the relative incidence of side effects associated with therapy. If the level of pain increases, make efforts to identify the source of increased pain while adjusting the dose as described above to decrease the level of pain.

During chronic therapy, especially for noncancer-related pain (or pain associated with other terminal illnesses), the continued need for the use of opioid analgesics should be reassessed as appropriate.

Cessation of therapy – When a patient no longer requires therapy with IR tablets or other opioid analgesics for the treatment of pain, it is important that therapy be gradually discontinued over time to prevent the development of an opioid abstinence syndrome (narcotic withdrawal). In general, therapy can be decreased by 25% to 50% per day with careful monitoring for signs and symptoms of withdrawal. If the patient develops these signs or symptoms, the dose should be raised to the previous level and titrated down more slowly, either by increasing the interval between decreases, decreasing the amount of change in dose, or both. It is not known at what dose of IR tablets that treatment may be discontinued without risk of the opioid abstinence syndrome.

➤*CR tablets:* Swallow tablets whole; do not break, chew, or crush. Taking broken, chewed, or crushed tablets could lead to the rapid release and absorption of a potentially fatal dose of oxycodone. *OxyContin* is not indicated for rectal administration. Data from a study involving 21 normal volunteers show that *OxyContin* tablets administered per rectum resulted in an AUC 39% greater and a C_{max} 9% higher than tablets administered by mouth. Therefore, there is an increased risk of adverse events with rectal administration.

One 160 mg tablet is comparable to two 80 mg tablets when taken on an empty stomach. However, with a high-fat meal there is a 25% greater peak plasma concentration following one 160 mg tablet. Use dietary caution when patients are initially titrated to 160 mg tablets.

In treating pain, it is vital to assess the patient regularly and systematically. Regularly review therapy and adjust based upon the patient's own reports of pain and side effects and the health care professional's clinical judgment.

CR tablets are intended for the management of moderate to severe pain when a continuous, around-the-clock analgesic is needed for an extended period of time. The CR nature of the formulation allows it to be effectively administered every 12 hours. While symmetric (same AM and PM), around-the-clock, every-12-hour dosing is appropriate for the majority of patients, some patients may benefit from asymmetric (different dose given in AM than in PM) dosing, tailored to their pain pattern. It is usually appropriate to treat a patient with only 1 opioid for around-the-clock therapy.

Initiation of therapy – It is critical to initiate the dosing regimen for each patient individually, taking into account the patient's prior opioid and nonopioid analgesic treatment. Give attention to the following:

1.) the general condition and medical status of the patient;
2.) the daily dose, potency, and kind of the analgesic(s) the patient has been taking;
3.) the reliability of the conversion estimate used to calculate the dose of oxycodone;
4.) the patient's opioid exposure and opioid tolerance (if any);
5.) special safety issues associated with conversion to CR tablet doses at or exceeding 160 mg every 12 hours (see Special Instructions for CR 80 and 160 mg Tablets); and
6.) the balance between pain control and adverse experiences.

Take care to use low initial doses of CR tablets in patients who are not already opioid tolerant, especially those who are receiving concurrent treatment with muscle relaxants, sedatives, or other CNS-active medications.

Patients not already taking opioids (opioid naïve) – A reasonable starting dose for most patients who are opioid naïve is 10 mg every 12 hours. If a nonopioid analgesic (eg, aspirin, acetaminophen, NSAID) is being provided, it may be continued.

Patients currently on opioid therapy –

1.) Using standard conversion ratio estimates (see table below), multiply the mg per day of the previous opioids by the appropriate multiplication factors to obtain the equivalent total daily dose of oral oxycodone.
2.) Divide this 24-hour oxycodone dose in half to obtain the twice-daily (every 12 hours) dose of CR tablets.
3.) Round down to a dose that is appropriate for the tablet strengths available.
4.) Discontinue all other around-the-clock opioid drugs when CR tablet therapy is initiated.

No fixed conversion ratio is likely to be satisfactory in all patients, especially patients receiving large opioid doses. The recommended doses shown in the following table are only a starting point. Close observation and frequent titration are indicated until patients are stable in the new therapy.

OXYCODONE — ORAL

Multiplication Factors for Converting the Daily Dose of Prior Opioids to the Daily Dose of Oral Oxycodone[a]		
mg/day prior opioid × factor = mg/day oral oxycodone		
	Oral prior opioid	Parenteral prior opioid
Oxycodone	1	—
Codeine	0.15	—
Fentanyl transdermal therapeutic system	see below	see below
Hydrocodone	0.9	—
Hydromorphone	4	20
Levorphanol	7.5	15
Meperidine	0.1	0.4
Methadone	1.5	3
Morphine	0.5	3

[a] To be used only for conversion to oral oxycodone. For patients receiving high-dose parenteral opioids, a more conservative conversion is warranted. For example, for high-dose parenteral morphine, use 1.5 instead of 3 as a multiplication factor.

In all cases, supplemental analgesia should be made available in the form of IR oral oxycodone or another suitable short-acting analgesic.

CR tablets can be safely used concomitantly with usual doses of nonopioid analgesics and analgesic adjuvants, provided care is taken to select a proper initial dose.

Conversion from transdermal fentanyl to CR tablets – Eighteen hours following the removal of the transdermal fentanyl patch, treatment with CR tablets can be initiated. Although there has been no systematic assessment of such conversion, a conservative oxycodone dose, approximately 10 mg every 12 hours of CR tablets, should be initially substituted for each fentanyl transdermal patch 25 mcg/h. Closely follow the patient for early titration as there is very limited clinical experience with this conversion.

Dosage individualization – Once therapy is initiated, pain relief and other opioid effects should be frequently assessed. Titrate patients to adequate effect (generally mild or no pain with the regular use of no more than 2 doses of supplemental analgesia per 24 hours). Patients who experience breakthrough pain may require dosage adjustment or rescue medication. Because steady-state plasma concentrations are approximated within 24 to 36 hours, dosage adjustment may be carried out every 1 to 2 days. It is most appropriate to increase the every-12-hour dose, not the dosing frequency. There is no clinical information on dosing intervals shorter than every 12 hours. As a guideline, except for the increase from 10 to 20 mg every 12 hours, the total daily oxycodone dose usually can be increased by 25% to 50% of the current dose at each increase.

If signs of excessive opioid-related adverse experiences are observed, the next dose may be reduced. If this adjustment leads to inadequate analgesia, a supplemental dose of IR oxycodone may be given. Alternatively, nonopioid analgesic adjuvants may be employed. Make dose adjustments to obtain an appropriate balance between pain relief and opioid-related adverse experiences.

If significant adverse events occur before the therapeutic goal of mild or no pain is achieved, the events should be treated aggressively. Once adverse events are under control, upward titration should continue to an acceptable level of pain control.

During periods of changing analgesic requirements, including initial titration, frequent contact is recommended between health care provider, other members of the health care team, the patient, and the caregiver/family.

Special instructions for 80 and 160 mg CR tablets – For use in opioid-tolerant patients only.

CR tablets, 80 and 160 mg, are for use only in opioid-tolerant patients requiring daily oxycodone equivalent dosages of at least 160 mg for the 80 mg tablet and at least 320 mg for the 160 mg tablet. Take care in the prescribing of these tablet strengths. Instruct patients against use by individuals other than the patient for whom it was prescribed, as such inappropriate use may have severe medical consequences, including death.

Supplemental analgesia – Most patients given around-the-clock therapy with CR opioids may need to have IR medication available for "rescue" from breakthrough pain or to prevent pain that occurs predictably during certain patient activities (incident pain).

Therapy maintenance – The intent of the titration period is to establish a patient-specific every-12-hour dosing that will maintain adequate analgesia with acceptable side effects for as long as pain relief is necessary. Should pain recur, the dose can be incrementally increased to reestablish pain control. The method of therapy adjustment outlined above should be employed to reestablish pain control.

During chronic therapy, especially for noncancer pain syndromes, the continued need for around-the-clock opioid therapy should be reassessed periodically (eg, every 6 to 12 months) as appropriate.

Therapy cessation – When the patient no longer requires therapy with the CR tablets, taper doses gradually over several days to prevent signs and symptoms of withdrawal in the physically dependent patient.

Conversion from CR tablets to parenteral opioids – To avoid overdose, follow conservative dose conversion ratios. For patients receiving high-dose parenteral opioids, a more conservative conversion is warranted.

➤*Oral concentrate solutions: Roxicodone Intensol*, *OxyFAST*, and *ETH-Oxydose* 20 mg/mL solution are highly concentrated solutions. Take care in prescribing and dispensing this solution strength. Fill dropper to the level of the prescribed dose (1 mL = 20 mg; 0.75 mL = 15 mg; 0.5 mL = 10 mg; 0.25 mL = 5 mg). For ease of administration, add dose to approximately 30 mL (1 fluid oz) or more of juice or other liquid. May also be added to applesauce, pudding, or other semi-solid foods. The drug-food mixture should be used immediately and not stored for future use.

The usual adult dosage is 5 mg every 6 hours as needed for pain.

➤*Oral solutions:* The usual adult oral dose is 10 to 30 mg every 4 hours as needed for pain or as directed by a physician. The dose must be individually adjusted according to severity of pain, patient response, and patient size. More severe pain may require 30 mg or more every 4 hours. If the pain increases in severity, analgesia is not adequate, or tolerance occurs, a gradual increase in dosage may be required.

For control of severe, chronic pain in patients with certain terminal diseases, this drug should be administered on a regularly scheduled basis, every 4 hours, at the lowest dosage level that will achieve adequate analgesia.

➤*Storage/Stability:* Store at 25°C (77°F); excursions permitted between 15° to 30°C (59° to 86°F). Discard open bottles of oral solution after 90 days.

OXYMORPHONE HYDROCHLORIDE

c-ii	**Numorphan** (Endo Laboratories)	**Injection:** 1 mg/mL	In 1 mL amps.
		1.5 mg/mL	Parabens. In 10 mL multidose vials.
		Suppositories: 5 mg	In 6s.

OXYMORPHONE HYDROCHLORIDE — INJECTION

For complete prescribing information, refer to the Opioid Analgesics group monograph.

Indications

➤*Pain:* Relief of moderate to severe pain.

➤*Preoperative medication/anesthesia/anxiety:* For preoperative medication, support of anesthesia, obstetrical analgesia, and for relief of anxiety in patients with dyspnea associated with pulmonary edema secondary to acute left ventricular dysfunction.

Administration and Dosage

➤*Approved by the FDA:* April 2, 1959.

Use smaller doses of oxymorphone than those recommended below for debilitated and elderly patients and those with severe liver disease.

➤*Intravenous:* Initially, 0.5 mg. In nondebilitated patients, the dose can be cautiously increased until satisfactory pain relief is obtained.

➤*Subcutaneous or intramuscular (IM):* Initially, 1 to 1.5 mg every 4 to 6 hours, as needed. For analgesia during labor, give 0.5 to 1 mg IM.

➤*Storage/Stability:* Protect injections from light; store at 15° to 30°C (59° to 86°F).

Protect from light.

OXYMORPHONE HYDROCHLORIDE — RECTAL

For complete prescribing information, refer to the Opioid Analgesics group monograph.

Indications

➤*Pain:* Relief of moderate to severe pain.

Administration and Dosage

➤*Approved by the FDA:* April 2, 1959.

Use smaller doses of oxymorphone than those recommended below for debilitated and elderly patients and those with severe liver disease.

➤*Rectal:* 5 mg every 4 to 6 hours, as needed. In nondebilitated patients, cautiously increase dose until pain relief is satisfactory.

➤*Storage/Stability:* Refrigerate suppositories at 2° to 8°C (36° to 46°F).

PROPOXYPHENE (Dextropropoxyphene)

c-iv	**Darvon-N** (aaiPharma)	**Tablets**: 100 mg (as napsylate)	Lactose. (Lilly Darvon-N 100). Buff, elliptical. Film-coated. In 100s, 500s, and UD 100s.
c-iv	**Propoxyphene Hydrochloride** (Various, eg, Ivax)	**Capsules**: 65 mg (as hydrochloride)	In 100s.
c-iv	**Darvon Pulvules** (aaiPharma)		(Darvon). Opaque pink, parabola shape. In 100s and 500s.

PROPOXYPHENE NAPSYLATE — ORAL

For complete prescribing information, refer to the Opioid Analgesics monograph.

WARNING

Fatalities –
- Do not prescribe propoxyphene for patients who are suicidal or addiction prone.
- Prescribe propoxyphene with caution for patients taking tranquilizers or antidepressant drugs and patients who use alcohol in excess.
- Tell patients not to exceed the recommended dose and to limit alcohol intake.

Propoxyphene products in excessive doses, either alone or in combination with other CNS depressants (including alcohol), are a major cause of drug-related deaths. Fatalities within the first hour of overdosage are not uncommon. In a survey of deaths due to overdosage conducted in 1975, in approximately 20% of fatal cases, death occurred within the first hour (5% within 15 minutes). Propoxyphene should not be taken in higher doses than those recommended by the health care provider. Judicious prescribing of propoxyphene is essential for safety. Consider nonopioid analgesics for depressed or suicidal patients. Caution patients about the concomitant use of propoxyphene products and alcohol because of potentially serious CNS-additive effects of these agents. Because of added CNS depressant effects, cautiously prescribe with concomitant sedatives, tranquilizers, muscle relaxants, antidepressants, or other CNS-depressant drugs. Advise patients of the additive depressant effects of these combinations.

Many propoxyphene-related deaths have occurred in patients with histories of emotional disturbances, suicidal ideation or attempts, or misuse of tranquilizers, alcohol, and other CNS-active drugs. Deaths have occurred as a consequence of the accidental ingestion of excessive quantities of propoxyphene alone or in combination with other drugs. Do not exceed the recommended dosage.

Indications

For the relief of mild to moderate pain.

Administration and Dosage

➤*Approved by the FDA:* August 16, 1957.

Because of differences in molecular weight, 100 mg of propoxyphene napsylate is required to supply propoxyphene equivalent to 65 mg of the hydrochloride.

➤*Usual dose:* 100 mg every 4 hours as needed. Do not exceed 600 mg/day.

➤*Renal or hepatic function impairment:* Consider a reduced total daily dosage in patients with hepatic or renal impairment.

➤*Elderly:* Propoxyphene metabolism rate may be reduced in some patients. Consider increased dosing interval.

➤*Storage/Stability:* Store at controlled room temperature, 15° to 30°C (59° to 86°F).

PROPOXYPHENE HYDROCHLORIDE — ORAL

For complete prescribing information, refer to the Opioid Analgesics monograph.

WARNING

Fatalities –
- Do not prescribe propoxyphene for patients who are suicidal or addiction prone.
- Prescribe propoxyphene with caution for patients taking tranquilizers or antidepressant drugs and patients who use alcohol in excess.
- Tell patients not to exceed the recommended dose and to limit alcohol intake.

Propoxyphene products in excessive doses, either alone or in combination with other CNS depressants (including alcohol), are a major cause of drug-related deaths. Fatalities within the first hour of overdosage are not uncommon. In a survey of deaths due to overdosage conducted in 1975, in approximately 20% of fatal cases, death occurred within the first hour (5% within 15 minutes). Propoxyphene should not be taken in higher doses than those recommended by the health care provider. Judicious prescribing of propoxyphene is essential for safety. Consider nonopioid analgesics for depressed or suicidal patients. Caution patients about the concomitant use of propoxyphene products and alcohol because of potentially serious CNS-additive effects of these agents. Because of added CNS depressant effects, cautiously prescribe with concomitant sedatives, tranquilizers, muscle relaxants, antidepressants, or other CNS-depressant drugs. Advise patients of the additive depressant effects of these combinations.

Many propoxyphene-related deaths have occurred in patients with histories of emotional disturbances, suicidal ideation or attempts, or misuse of tranquilizers, alcohol, and other CNS-active drugs. Deaths have occurred as a consequence of the accidental ingestion of excessive quantities of propoxyphene alone or in combination with other drugs. Do not exceed the recommended dosage.

Indications

➤*Pain:* Relief of mild to moderate pain.

Administration and Dosage

➤*Approved by the FDA:* August 16, 1957.

Because of differences in molecular weight, 100 mg of propoxyphene napsylate is required to supply propoxyphene equivalent to 65 mg of the hydrochloride.

➤*Usual dose:* 65 mg every 4 hours as needed. Do not exceed 390 mg/day.

➤*Renal or hepatic function impairment:* Consider a reduced total daily dosage in patients with hepatic or renal impairment.

➤*Elderly:* Propoxyphene metabolism rate may be reduced in some patients. Consider increased dosing interval.

➤*Storage/Stability:* Store at controlled room temperature 15° to 30°C (59° to 86°F).

REMIFENTANIL HYDROCHLORIDE

c-ii	**Ultiva** (Abbott)	**Powder for injection:** 1 mg (as base)	Preservative free. 15 mg glycine. In 3 mL vials.
		2 mg (as base)	Preservative free. 15 mg glycine. In 5 mL vials.
		5 mg (as base)	Preservative free. 15 mg glycine. In 10 mL vials.

REMIFENTANIL HYDROCHLORIDE — INJECTION

For complete prescribing information, refer to the Opioid Analgesics group monograph.

Indications

➤*Analgesia:* An analgesic agent for use during the induction and maintenance of general anesthesia for inpatient and outpatient procedures and for continuation as an analgesic into the immediate postoperative period under the direct supervision of an anesthesia practitioner in a postoperative anesthesia care unit or intensive care setting. As an analgesic component of monitored anesthesia care.

Administration and Dosage

➤*Approved by the FDA:* July 12, 1996.

For intravenous (IV) use only. Individualize dosage.

Administer continuous infusions of remifentanil only by an infusion device. The injection site should be close to the venous cannula. Clear all IV tubing at the time of discontinuation of infusion. Use IV bolus administration of remifentanil only during the maintenance of general anesthesia.

➤*General anesthesia:*

Adults – Remifentanil is not recommended as the sole agent in general anesthesia because loss of consciousness cannot be assured and because of a high incidence of apnea, muscle rigidity, and tachycardia. Remifentanil is synergistic with other anesthetics, and doses of thiopental, propofol, isoflurane, and midazolam may need to be reduced by up to 75% with the coadministration of remifentanil.

Remifentanil Dosing Guidelines: General Anesthesia and Continuing as an Analgesic into the Postoperative Care Unit or Intensive Care Setting

Phase	Continuous IV infusion (mcg/kg/min)	Infusion dose range (mcg/kg/min)	Supplemental IV bolus dose (mcg/kg)
Induction of anesthesia (through intubation)	0.5 to 1[a]	NA[b]	NA[b]
Maintenance of anesthesia with:			
Nitrous oxide (66%)	0.4	0.1 to 2	1
Isoflurane (0.4 to 1.5 MAC[c])	0.25	0.05 to 2	1
Propofol (100 to 200 mcg/kg/min)	0.25	0.05 to 2	1
Continuation as an analgesic into the immediate postoperative period	0.1	0.025 to 0.2	Not recommended

[a] An initial dose of 1 mcg/kg may be administered over 30 to 60 seconds.
[b] No data available.
[c] MAC = monitored anesthesia care.

Children (1 year of age and older) – The table below summarizes the recommended doses in pediatric patients, predominantly American Society of Anesthesiologists (ASA) physical status I, II, or III. In pediatric patients, remifentanil was administered with nitrous oxide or nitrous oxide in combination with halothane, sevoflurane, or isoflurane.

Dosing Guidelines in Pediatric Patients — Maintenance of Anesthesia

Phase	Continuous IV infusion[a] (mcg/kg/min)	Infusion dose range (mcg/kg/min)	Supplemental IV bolus dose (mcg/kg)
Maintenance of anesthesia with:			
Halothane (0.3 to 1.5 MAC)	0.25	0.05 to 1.3	1
Sevoflurane (0.3 to 1.5 MAC)	0.25	0.05 to 1.3	1
Isoflurane (0.4 to 1.5 MAC)	0.25	0.05 to 1.3	1

[a] An initial dose of 1 mcg/kg may be administered over 30 to 60 seconds.

➤*Induction of anesthesia:* Administer at an infusion rate of 0.5 to 1 mcg/kg/min with a hypnotic or volatile agent for the induction of anesthesia. If endotracheal intubation is to occur less than 8 minutes after the start of infusion of remifentanil, then an initial dose of 1 mcg/kg may be administered over 30 to 60 seconds.

➤*Maintenance of anesthesia:* After endotracheal intubation, decrease the infusion rate of remifentanil in accordance with the dosing guidelines in the tables above. Because of the rapid onset and short duration of action of remifentanil, the rate of administration during anesthesia can be titrated upward in 25% to 100% increments in adults or up to 50% increments in pediatric patients, or downward in 25% to 50% decrements every 2 to 5 minutes to attain the desired level of μ-opioid effect. In response to light anesthesia or transient episodes of intense surgical stress, supplemental bolus doses of 1 mcg/kg may be administered every 2 to 5 minutes. At infusion rates greater than 1 mcg/kg/min, consider increases in the concomitant anesthetic agents to increase the depth of anesthesia.

➤*Continuation as an analgesic into the immediate postoperative period:* Remifentanil infusions may be continued into the immediate postoperative period for select patients for whom later transition to longer-acting analgesics may be desired. The use of bolus injections of remifentanil to treat pain during the postoperative period is not recommended. When used as an IV analgesic in the immediate postoperative period, administer remifentanil initially by continuous infusion at a rate of 0.1 mcg/kg/min. The infusion rate may be adjusted every 5 minutes in 0.025 mcg/kg/min increments to balance the patient's level of analgesia and respiratory rate. Infusion rates more than 0.2 mcg/kg/min are associated with respiratory depression (respiratory rate less than 8 breaths/min).

➤*Guidelines for discontinuation:* Upon discontinuation of remifentanil, clear the IV tubing to prevent inadvertent administration at a later time.

Because of the rapid offset of action, no residual analgesic activity will be present within 5 to 10 minutes after discontinuation. For patients undergoing surgical procedures where postoperative pain is generally anticipated, administer alternative analgesics prior to discontinuation of remifentanil. The choice of analgesic should be appropriate for the patient's surgical procedure and the level of follow-up care.

➤*Analgesic component of MAC (adults only):* It is strongly recommended that supplemental oxygen be supplied whenever remifentanil is administered.

Remifentanil Dosing Guidelines for Adults - Monitored Anesthesia Care

Method	Timing	Remifentanil alone	Remifentanil + midazolam 2 mg
Single IV dose	Given 90 seconds before local anesthetic	1 mcg/kg over 30 to 60 seconds	0.5 mcg/kg over 30 to 60 seconds
Continuous IV infusion	Beginning 5 minutes before local anesthetic	0.1 mcg/kg/min	0.05 mcg/kg/min
	After local anesthetic	0.05 mcg/kg/min (range: 0.025 to 0.2 mcg/kg/min)	0.025 mcg/kg/min (range: 0.025 to 0.2 mcg/kg/min)

Single dose – A single IV dose of 0.5 to 1 mcg/kg over 30 to 60 seconds may be given 90 seconds before the placement of the local or regional anesthetic block.

Continuous infusion – When used alone as an IV analgesic component of MAC, administer initially by continuous infusion at a rate of 0.1 mcg/kg/min beginning 5 minutes before placement of the local or regional anesthetic block.

Because of the risk for hypoventilation, decrease the infusion rate of remifentanil to 0.05 mcg/kg/min following placement of the block. Thereafter, rate adjustments of 0.025 mcg/kg/min at 5-minute intervals may be used to balance the patient's level of analgesia and respiratory rate. Rates greater than 0.2 mcg/kg/min are generally associated with respiratory depression (respiratory rates less than 8 breaths/min).

Bolus doses of remifentanil administered simultaneously with a continuous infusion of remifentanil to spontaneously breathing patients are not recommended.

➤*Coronary artery bypass surgery:* The table below summarizes the recommended doses for induction, maintenance, and continuation as an analgesic into the intensive care unit (ICU) in adult patients, predominantly ASA physical status III or IV. To avoid hypotension during the induction phase, it is important to consider the concomitant medication regimens used.

Dosing Recommendations — Coronary Artery Bypass Surgery

Phase	Continuous IV infusion (mcg/kg/min)	Infusion dose range (mcg/kg/min)	Supplemental IV bolus dose (mcg/kg)
Induction of anesthesia (through intubation)	1	—	—
Maintenance of anesthesia	1	0.125 to 4	0.5 to 1
Continuation as an analgesic into ICU	1	0.05 to 1	—

➤*Individualization of dosage:*

Elderly – Decrease the starting doses of remifentanil by 50% in elderly patients (older than 65 years of age). Cautiously titrate to effect.

Obesity – Base the starting dose of remifentanil on ideal body weight (IBW) in obese patients (more than 30% over their IBW).

➤*Preanesthetic medication:* The need for premedication and the choice of anesthetic agents must be individualized. In clinical studies, patients who received remifentanil frequently received a benzodiazepine premedication.

➤*Preparation for administration:* To reconstitute solution, add 1 mL of diluent per mg of remifentanil. Shake well to dissolve. When reconstituted

REMIFENTANIL HYDROCHLORIDE — INJECTION

as directed, the solution contains approximately 1 mg of remifentanil activity per mL. Remifentanil should be diluted to a recommended final concentration of 20, 25, 50, or 250 mcg/mL prior to administration. Do not administer remifentanil without dilution.

Reconstitution and Dilution of Remifentanil		
Final concentration	Amount of remifentanil in each vial	Final volume after reconstitution and dilution
20 mcg/mL	1 mg 2 mg 5 mg	50 mL 100 mL 250 mL
25 mcg/mL	1 mg 2 mg 5 mg	40 mL 80 mL 200 mL
50 mcg/mL	1 mg 2 mg 5 mg	20 mL 40 mL 100 mL
250 mcg/mL	5 mg	20 mL

➤*Admixture compatibility and stability:* Remifentanil is stable for 24 hours at room temperature after reconstitution and further dilution to concentrations of 20 to 250 mcg/mL with the following IV fluids: sterile water for injection; 5% dextrose injection; 5% dextrose and 0.9% sodium chloride injection; 0.9% sodium chloride injection; 0.45% sodium chloride injection; lactated Ringer's and 5% dextrose injection.

Remifentanil is stable for 4 hours at room temperature after reconstitution and further dilution to concentrations of 20 to 250 mcg/mL with lactated Ringer's injection.

Remifentanil has been shown to be compatible with propofol when coadministered into a running IV administration set.

➤*Incompatibilities:* Nonspecific esterases in blood products may lead to the hydrolysis of remifentanil to its carboxylic acid metabolite. Therefore, administration of remifentanil into the same IV tubing with blood is not recommended.

➤*Storage/Stability:* Store at 2° to 25°C (36° to 77°F).

SUFENTANIL CITRATE

c-ii	**Sufentanil Citrate** (Various, eg, Baxter)	**Injection:** 50 mcg (as base)/mL	In 1, 2, and 5 mL amps and 1, 2, and 5 mL vials.
c-ii	**Sufenta** (Taylor)		Preservative free. In 1, 2, and 5 ml amps.

SUFENTANIL CITRATE — INJECTION

For complete prescribing information, refer to the Opioid Analgesics group monograph.

Indications

➤*Analgesia:* Analgesic adjunct for the maintenance of balanced general anesthesia in patients who are intubated and ventilated.

➤*Anesthetic:* As a primary anesthetic agent for the induction and maintenance of anesthesia with 100% oxygen in patients undergoing major surgical procedures. In patients who are intubated and ventilated, such as cardiovascular surgery or neurosurgical procedures in the sitting position, to provide favorable myocardial and cerebral oxygen balance or when extended postoperative ventilation is anticipated.

➤*Epidural analgesic:* For epidural administration as an analgesic combined with low-dose bupivacaine, usually 12.5 mg per administration, during labor and vaginal delivery.

Administration and Dosage

➤*Approved by the FDA:* May 4, 1984.

Individualize dosage. Monitor vital signs routinely. Administer by slow intravenous (IV) injection or IV infusion.

Adult Dosage Range Chart — Analgesic Component to General Anesthesia (Total Dosage Requirements of 1 mcg/kg/h or Less are Recommended)	
Total dosage	Maintenance dosage
Analgesic dosages	
Incremental or infusion: 1 to 2 mcg/kg (expected duration of anesthesia is 1 to 2 hours). Approximately ≥ 75% of total sufentanil dosage may be administered prior to intubation by either slow injection or infusion titrated to individual patient response. Dosages in this range are generally administered with nitrous oxide/oxygen in patients undergoing general surgery ≤ 8 hours in which endotracheal intubation and mechanical ventilation are required.	*Incremental:* 10 to 25 mcg (0.2 to 0.5 mL) may be administered in increments as needed when movement and/or changes in vital signs indicate surgical stress or lightening of analgesia. *Infusion:* Sufentanil may be administered as an intermittent or continuous infusion as needed in response to signs of lightening of analgesia. In absence of signs of lightening of analgesia, always adjust infusion rates downward until there is some response to surgical stimulation. Individualize supplemental dosages. Adjust maintenance infusion rates based upon the induction dose of sufentanil so that the total dose does not exceed 1 mcg/kg/h of expected surgical time. Individualize dosage and adjust to remaining operative time anticipated.
Analgesic dosages	
Incremental or infusion: 2 to 8 mcg/kg (expected duration of anesthesia is 2 to 8 hours). Approximately ≤ 75% of the total calculated sufentanil dosage may be administered by slow injection or infusion prior to intubation, titrated to individual patient response. Dosages in this range are generally administered with nitrous oxide/oxygen in more complicated major surgical procedures in which endotracheal intubation and mechanical ventilation are required. Provides some attenuation of sympathetic reflex activity in response to surgical stimuli, hemodynamic stability, and relatively rapid recovery.	*Incremental:* 10 to 50 mcg (0.2 to 1 mL) may be administered in increments as needed when movement and/or changes in vital signs indicate stress or lightening of analgesia. Individualize supplemental dosages. *Infusion:* Sufentanil may be administered as an intermittent or continuous infusion as needed in response to signs of lightening of analgesia. In the absence of signs of lightening of analgesia, infusion rates should always be adjusted downward until there is some response to surgical stimulation. Maintenance infusion rates should be adjusted based upon the induction dose of sufentanil so that the total dose does not exceed 1 mcg/kg/h of expected surgical time. Individualize dosage and adjust to remaining operative time anticipated.
Anesthetic dosages	
Incremental or infusion: 8 to 30 mcg/kg (anesthetic doses). At this anesthetic dosage range, sufentanil is generally administered as a slow injection, as an infusion, or as an injection followed by an infusion. Sufentanil with 100% oxygen and a muscle relaxant produces sleep at doses ≥ 8 mcg/kg and maintains a deep level of anesthesia without additional agents. The addition of N_2O to these dosages will reduce systolic blood pressure. At doses of up to 25 mcg/kg, catecholamine release is attenuated; dosages of 25 to 30 mcg/kg block sympathetic responses including catecholamine release. Use high doses in patients undergoing major surgical procedures in which endotracheal intubation and mechanical ventilation are required (eg, cardiovascular surgery and neurosurgery in the sitting position with maintenance of favorable myocardial and cerebral oxygen balance). Postoperative observation is essential and postoperative mechanical ventilation may be required at the higher dosage range because of extended postoperative respiratory depression. Titrate dosage to individual patient response.	*Incremental:* Depending on the initial dose, maintenance doses of 0.5 to 10 mcg/kg may be administered by slow injection in anticipation of surgical stress, such as incision, sternotomy, or cardiopulmonary bypass. *Infusion:* Sufentanil may be administered by continuous or intermittent infusion as needed in response to signs of lightening of anesthesia. In the absence of lightening of anesthesia, infusion rates should always be adjusted downward until there is some response to surgical stimulation. Base the maintenance infusion rate for sufentanil upon the induction dose so that the total dose for the procedure does not exceed 30 mcg/kg.

SUFENTANIL CITRATE — INJECTION

➤*Epidural use in labor and delivery:* 10 to 15 mcg administered with bupivacaine 0.125% 10 mL with or without epinephrine. Mix sufentanil and bupivacaine together before administration. Doses can be repeated twice (for a total of 3 doses) at not less than 1-hour intervals until delivery.

Administer sufentanil by slow injection. Closely monitor respiration following each administration of an epidural injection of sufentanil.

➤*Children (younger than 12 years of age):* For induction and maintenance of anesthesia in children undergoing cardiovascular surgery, a dose of 10 to 25 mcg/kg administered with 100% oxygen is recommended. Supplemental doses of up to 25 to 50 mcg are recommended for maintenance.

➤*Elderly / Debilitated patients:* Dosage should be reduced.

➤*Premedication:* The selection of preanesthetic medications should be based upon the needs of the individualized patient.

➤*Concomitant medication:* If benzodiazepines, barbiturates, inhalation agents, other opioids, or CNS depressants are used concomitantly, the dose of sufentanil and/or these agents should be reduced. In all cases, dosage should be titrated to individual patient response.

➤*Obesity:* In obese patients (more then 20% above ideal body weight), the dosage of sufentanil should be determined on the basis of lean body weight.

➤*Storage / Stability:* Store at 15° to 25°C (59° to 77°F). Protect from light.

TRAMADOL HYDROCHLORIDE

Rx	**Tramadol** (Various, eg, Caraco, Eon, Ivax, Mallinckrodt, Purepac)	**Tablets:** 50 mg	In 100s, 500s, and 1,000s.
Rx	**Ultram** (Ortho-McNeil)		Lactose. (Ultram 0659). White, capsule shape, scored. Film-coated. In 100s, 500s, and UD 100s.
Rx	**Ultram ER** (Ortho-McNeil)	**Tablets, extended-release:** 100 mg	(100ER). White. In 30s and 90s.
		200 mg	(200ER). White. In 30s and 90s.
		300 mg	(300ER). White. In 30s and 90s.

TRAMADOL HYDROCHLORIDE — ORAL

For complete prescribing information, refer to the Opioid Analgesics group monograph.

Indications

➤*Immediate-release:* Management of moderate to moderately severe pain.

➤*Extended-release:* Management of moderate to moderately severe pain in adults who require around-the-clock treatment of their pain for an extended period of time.

Administration and Dosage

➤*Approved by the FDA:* March 3, 1995.

➤*Immediate-release:* Individualize dose based on the lowest effective dose. Starting at the lowest possible dose and titrating upward as needed has resulted in increased tolerability and fewer discontinuations. Can be administered without regard to meals.

For moderate to moderately severe chronic pain not requiring rapid onset of analgesic effect, administer 25 mg/day in the morning and titrate in 25 mg increments as separate doses every 3 days to reach 100 mg/day (25 mg 4 times/day). Thereafter, increase the dose by 50 mg as tolerated every 3 days to reach 200 mg/day (50 mg 4 times/day). After titration, administer 50 to 100 mg every 4 to 6 hours as needed for pain relief. Do not exceed 400 mg/day.

For patients requiring rapid onset of analgesic relief and for whom the benefits outweigh the risk of discontinuation due to adverse effects associated with higher initial doses, administer 50 to 100 mg every 4 to 6 hours as needed, not to exceed 400 mg/day.

Elderly – Use caution when selecting a dose for patients older than 65 years of age; start at the low end of the dosing range. Do not exceed 300 mg/day in patients 75 years of age and older.

Renal function impairment – In patients with a creatinine clearance less than 30 mL/min, increase the dosing interval to 12 hours, with a maximum daily dose of 200 mg. Because hemodialysis only removes 7% of an administered dose, dialysis patients can receive their regular dose on the day of dialysis.

Hepatic function impairment – The recommended dose for patients with cirrhosis is 50 mg every 12 hours.

➤*Extended-release:*

Adults 18 years of age and older – Extended-release tablets should be initiated at a dose of 100 mg once daily and titrated up as necessary by 100 mg increments every 5 days to relieve pain, depending upon tolerability. Extended-release tablets should not be administered at a dose exceeding 300 mg/day.

Good pain management practice dictates that the dose be individualized according to patient need using the lowest beneficial dose. Start at the lowest beneficial dose. Start at the lowest possible dose and titrate upward as tolerated to achieve an adequate effect. Clinical studies of the extended-release tablets have not demonstrated a clinical benefit at a total daily dose exceeding 300 mg.

Elderly – In general, dosing of an elderly patient (older than 65 years of age) should be initiated cautiously, usually starting at the low end of the dosing range, reflecting the greater frequency of decreased hepatic, renal, or cardiac function and of concomitant disease or other drug therapy. Extended-release tablets should be administered with even greater caution in patients over 75 years of age because of the greater frequency of adverse events seen in this population.

Renal / Hepatic function impairment – Extended-release tablets should not be used in patients with creatinine clearance less than 30 mL/min or severe hepatic impairment (Child-Pugh class C).

➤*Storage / Stability:* Dispense in a tight container. Store at 25°C (77°F); excursions permitted to 15° to 30°C (59° to 86°F).

OPIOID ANALGESIC COMBINATIONS

Content given per tablet, capsule, 5 mL oral solution, and mL injection, or suppository.

	Product and Distributor	Narcotic	Acetaminophen	Aspirin	Other Content	Average Adult Dose	How Supplied
c-v	**Acetaminophen w/Codeine Oral Solution**[a] (Various, eg, Morton Grove, Roxane)	12 mg codeine phosphate	120 mg			15 mL q 4 h	In 120 mL, pt and gal.
c-v	**Capital w/Codeine Suspension** (Carnrick)						Fruit punch flavor. In 473 mL.
c-v	**Tylenol w/Codeine Elixir** (McNeil)				7% alcohol, saccharin, sucrose		Cherry flavor. In 480 mL.
c-iii	**Acetaminophen w/Codeine Tablets** (Various, eg, Lemmon)	15 mg codeine phosphate	300 mg			1 to 4 q 4 h	In 100s and 1000s.
c-iii	**Tylenol w/Codeine No. 2 Tablets** (McNeil)				Sodium metabisulfite		(McNeil Tylenol Codeine 2). White. In 100s and UD 500s.
c-iii	**Acetaminophen w/Codeine Tablets** (Various, eg, Lemmon, Moore, Purepac, Roxane)	30 mg codeine phosphate	300 mg			0.5 to 2 q 4 h	In 100s, 1000s and UD 100s.
c-iii	**Aceta w/Codeine Tablets** (Century)					1 tid	In 100s and 1000s.
c-iii	**Tylenol w/Codeine No. 3 Tablets** (McNeil)				Sodium metabisulfite	0.5 to 2 q 4 h	(McNeil Tylenol Codeine 3). White. In 100s, 500s, 1000s and UD 500s.
c-iii	**Butalbital, Acetaminophen, Caffeine, and Codeine Phosphate Capsules** (Breckenridge)	30 mg codeine phosphate	325 mg		40 mg caffeine, 50 mg butalbital	1 or 2 q 4 h up to 6/day	May contain tartrazine and talc. In 100s and 500s.
c-iii	**Fioricet w/Codeine Capsules** (Watson)						(Fioricet codeine). Dark blue/gray. In 100s and *ControlPak* 25s.
c-iii	**Phrenilin w/Caffeine and Codeine Capsules** (Valeant)						(A 061). Opaque lavender/opaque white. In 100s.
c-iii	**Vopac Tablets** (Athlon)	30 mg codeine phosphate	650 mg			½ to 2 q 4 h up to 6/day	(CM 650). White, scored, capsule-shape. In 100s and 500s.
c-iii	**Aspirin and Codeine Phosphate** (Vintage)	15 mg codeine phosphate		325 mg		1 or 2 q 4 h as needed	In 100s, 500s, and 1000s.
c-iii	**Aspirin w/Codeine No. 3 Tablets** (Various, eg, Goldline, Moore, Schein, URL, Zenith)	30 mg codeine phosphate		325 mg		1 or 2 q 4 h	In 100s and 1000s.
c-iii	**Empirin w/Codeine No. 3 Tablets** (GlaxoWellcome)						(Empirin 3). White. In 100s, 500s, 1000s and *Dispenserpak* 25s.
c-iii	**Ascomp with Codeine Capsules** (Breckenridge)	30 mg codeine phosphate		325 mg	40 mg caffeine, 50 mg butalbital	1 or 2 q 4 h up to 6/day	In 100s and 500s.
c-iii	**Fiorinal w/Codeine Capsules** (Novartis)						(F-C Sandoz 78-107). Blue/yellow. In 100s and *ControlPak* 25s.
c-iii	**Acetaminophen w/Codeine Tabs** (Various, eg, Lemmon, Moore, Purepac)	60 mg codeine phosphate	300 mg			1 q 4 h	In 100s, 500s, 1000s.
c-iii	**Tylenol w/Codeine No. 4 Tablets** (McNeil)				Sodium metabisulfite		(McNeil Tylenol Codeine 4). White. In 100s, 500s, and UD 500s.
c-iii	**Aspirin w/Codeine No. 4 Tablets** (Various, eg, Goldline, Major, Moore, Rugby, URL, Zenith)	60 mg codeine phosphate		325 mg		1 q 4 h	In 100s, 500s and 1000s.
c-iii	**Empirin w/Codeine No. 4 Tablets** (GlaxoWellcome)						(Empirin 4). White. In 100s, 500s and *Dispenserpak* 25s.
c-iii	**Hydrocodone Bitartrate and Ibuprofen** (Teva)	7.5 mg hydrocodone bitartrate			200 mg ibuprofen	1 q 4 to 6 h up to 5/day	Lactose. (5161). White. Film-coated. In 100s.
c-iii	**Vicoprofen Tablets** (Abbott)						(VP). White. Convex. Film coated. In 100s, 500s and UD 100s.

OPIOID ANALGESIC COMBINATIONS

	Product and Distributor	Narcotic	Acetaminophen	Aspirin	Other Content	Average Adult Dose	How Supplied
c-iii	**Hycet Oral Solution** (Xanodyne)	2.5 mg hydrocodone bitartrate	108 mg		7% alcohol, glycerin, parabens, saccharin, sorbitol, sucrose.	15 mL q 4 to 6 h up to 120 mL/day.	In 473 mL.
c-iii	**Lortab Elixir** (Whitby)	2.5 mg hydrocodone bitartrate	167 mg		7% alcohol, saccharin, sorbitol, sucrose, parabens	15 mL q 4 to 6 h up to 6/day	Tropical fruit punch flavor. In 473 mL.
c-iii	**Hydrocodone Bitartrate and Acetaminophen Elixir** (Various, eg, Mallinckrodt, Pharmaceutical Associates)				7% alcohol.	15 mL q 4 to 6 h up to 90 mL/day	In 473 mL.
c-iii	**Hydrocodone Bitartrate and Acetaminophen** (Qualitest)	2.5 mg hydrocodone bitartrate	500 mg		Sucrose	1 or 2 q 4 to 6 h up to 8/day	(3591 V). White w/ pink specks. In 100s, 500s, and 1,000s.
c-iii	**Lortab 2.5/500 Tablets** (Whitby)						(Whitby/901). White/pink specks. In 100s and 500s.
c-iii	**Xodol** (Teamm)	5 mg hydrocodone bitartrate	300 mg			1 or 2 q 4 to 6 hr	(5 300 TP). White, capsule shape, bisected. In 100s and 500s.
c-iii	**Hydrocodone Bitartrate and Acetaminophen, 5 mg/325 mg Tablets** (Various, eg, Mallinckrodt, Watson)	5 mg hydrocodone bitartrate	325 mg			1 or 2 q 4 to 6 hr up to 12/day	In 100s, 500s, 1000s, and UD 100s.
c-iii	**Anexsia Tablets** (Andrx)					1 or 2 q 4 to 6 hr as needed up to 12/day	(M365). White, capsule shape, scored. In 100s and 1000s.
c-iii	**Norco 5/325 Tablets** (Watson)				Sucrose	1 to 2 q t to 6 hr	(Watson 913). White with orange specks, scored, capsule shape. In 100s and 500s.
c-iii	**Zydone Tablets** (Endo)	5 mg hydrocodone bitartrate	400 mg			1 or 2 q 4 to 6 h up to 8/day	(E5). Yellow, convex. Octagonal shape. In 100s, 500s, and UD 100s.
c-iii	**Hydrocodone Bitartrate & Acetaminophen Caps** (Various, eg, Goldline, Rugby)	5 mg hydrocodone bitartrate	500 mg			1 or 2 q 4 to 6 h up to 8/day	In 100s and 500s.
c-iii	**Hydrocodone Bitartrate and Acetaminophen Tablets** (Various, eg, Geneva, Goldline, Moore, Rugby, Watson)						In 100s and 500s.
c-iii	**Bancap HC Capsules** (Forest)						(Forest 610A). Yellow/orange. In 100s and 500s.
c-iii	**Ceta-Plus Capsules** (Seatrace)						(Seatrace). White. In 100s.
c-iii	**Co-Gesic Tablets** (Central)						(500-5) White, scored. Oval. In 100s and 500s.
c-iii	**Hydrocet Capsules** (Carnrick)						(C 8657). Blue/white. In 100s.
c-iii	**Hydrogesic Capsules** (Edwards)	5 mg hydrocodone bitartrate	500 mg			1 or 2 q 4 to 6 h up to 8/day	In 100s.
c-iii	**Hy-Phen Tablets** (B.F. Ascher)						(225-450). White, scored. Capsule shape. In 100s.
c-iii	**Margesic H Capsules** (Marnel)						(Margesic H). Gray/lavender. In 100s.
c-iii	**Lorcet-HD Capsules** (UAD)						(1120). Maroon. In 100s.
c-iii	**Lortab 5/500 Tablets** (Whitby)				Sugar		(UCB 902). White w/blue specks, scored. Capsule shape. In 100s, 500s and UD 100s.
c-iii	**Anexsia 5/500 Tablets** (Mallinckrodt)						(BMP 207). White, scored. In 100s.
c-iii	**Panacet 5/500 Tablets** (ECR Pharm)						(ECR 0141). White, scored. Oval. In 100s.

OPIOID ANALGESIC COMBINATIONS

	Product and Distributor	Narcotic	Acetaminophen	Aspirin	Other Content	Average Adult Dose	How Supplied
c-iii	**Stagesic Capsules** (Huckaby)	5 mg hydrocodone bitartrate	500 mg		Parabens	1 to 2 q 4 to 6 h up to 8/day	(Stagesic). White. In 100s.
c-iii	**T-Gesic Capsules** (T.E. Williams)					1 to 2 q 6 to 8 h	(T-Gesic/TEW). White. In 100s.
c-iii	**Vicodin Tablets** (Abbott)					1 to 2 q 4 to 6 h up to 8/day	(Vicodin). White, scored. Capsule shape. In 100s, 500s and UD 100s.
c-iii	**Hydrocodone Bitartrate and Acetaminophen, 7.5 mg/325 mg Tablets** (Various, eg, Mallinckrodt, Watson)	7.5 mg hydrocodone bitartrate	325 mg			1 q 4 to 6 hr as needed up to 8/day	In 100s, 500s, 1000s, and UD 100s.
c-iii	**Anexsia Tablets** (Andrx)						(M366). White, oval. In 100s and 1000s.
c-iii	**Zydone Tablets** (Endo)	7.5 mg hydrocodone bitartrate	400 mg			1 q 4 to 6 h up to 6/day	(E 7.5). Blue, convex. Octagonal shape. In 100s, 500s, and UD 100s.
c-iii	**Lortab 7.5/500 Tablets** (Whitby)	7.5 mg hydrocodone bitartrate	500 mg		Sucrose	1 q 4 to 6 h	(Whitby/903). White w/green specks, scored. Capsule shape. In 100s, 500s and UD 100s.
c-iii	**Hydrocodone with Acetaminophen Tablets** (Various, eg, Watson)						In 100s and 500s.
c-iii	**Anexsia 7.5/650 Tablets** (Mallinckrodt)	7.5 mg hydrocodone bitartrate	650 mg			1 q 4 to 6 h	(BMP 188). Peach, scored. Capsule shape. In 100s.
c-iii	**Lorcet Plus Tablets** (UAD)						(U 201). White, scored. Capsule shape. In 100s, 500s and UD 100s.
c-iii	**Hydrocodone Bitartrate/Acetaminophen Caplets** (Various, eg, King Pharm)						In 100s and 500s.
c-iii	**Vicodin ES Tablets** (Abbott)	7.5 mg hydrocodone bitartrate	750 mg			1 q 4 to 6 h up to 5/day	(Vicodin ES). White, scored. Oval. In 100s and UD 100s.
c-iii	**Hydrocodone with Acetaminophen Tablets** (Various, eg, Barr,Geneva,Mallinckrodt,Royce, URL, Zenith Goldline)					1 q 4 to 6 h up to 6/day	In 1002, 500s, and 1000s.
c-iii	**Xodol Tablets** (Teamm)	10 mg hydrocodone bitartrate	300 mg			1 q 4 to 6 h up to 6/day	(10 300 TP). White, capsule shape. In 100s and 500s.
c-iii	**Hydrocodone Bitartrate and Acetaminophen** (Mallinckrodt)	10 mg hydrocodone bitartrate	325 mg				(M367). White, oval, bisected. In 100s, 500s, and UD 100s.
c-iii	**Norco Tablets** (Watson Labs)					1 q 4 to 6 h up to 6/day	(NORCO 539). Yellow, bisected. Capsule shape. In 100s and 500s.
c-iii	**Zydone Tablets** (Endo)	10 mg hydrocodone bitartrate	400 mg			1 q 4 to 6 h up to 6/day	(E 10). Red, convex. Octagonal shape. In 100s, 500s, and UD 100s.
c-iii	**Lortab 10/500 Tablets** (UCB Pharma)	10 mg hydrocodone bitartrate	500 mg			1 q 4 to 6 h up to 6/day	(UCB/910). Pink. Capsule shape. In 100s and 500s.
c-iii	**Hydrocodone Bitartrate and Acetaminophen Tablets** (Various, eg, Barr, Mallinckrodt, Qualitest, Watson)						
c-iii	**Hydrocodone Bitartrate and Acetaminophen Tablets** (Major)	10 mg hydrocodone bitartrate	650 mg		In 500s.	1 q 4 to 6 h up to 6/day	
c-iii	**Lorcet 10/650 Tablets** (UAD)	10 mg hydrocodone bitartrate	650 mg			1 q 4 to 6 h	(UAD 6350). Light blue, scored. Capsule shape. In 20s, 100s and UD 100s.

OPIOID ANALGESIC COMBINATIONS

	Product and Distributor	Narcotic	Acetaminophen	Aspirin	Other Content	Average Adult Dose	How Supplied
c-iii	**Hydrocodone Bitartrate and Acetaminophen Tablets** (Various, eg, Inwood, Mallinckrodt)	10 mg hydrocodone bitartrate	660 mg			1 q 4 to 6 h up to 6/day	In 100s and 500s.
c-iii	**Anexsia 10/660 Tablets** (Mallinckrodt)					1 q 4 to 6 h	(KPI 3). White, scored. Capsule shape. In 100s and 1000s.
c-iii	**Vicodin HP Tablets** (Abbott)						(Vicodin HP). White, scored. Oval. In 100s.
c-iii	**Hydrocodone Bitartrate and Acetaminophen, 10 mg/750 mg Tablets** (Mallinckrodt, Watson)	10 mg hydrocodone bitartrate	750 mg			1 q 4 to 6 hr, as needed up to 5/day.	In 100s, 5002, and UD 100s.
c-iii	**Maxidone** (Watson)				Lactose.	1 q 4 to 6 hr, up to 5/day.	(Maxidone 634). Yellow, capsule shape, scored. In 100s and 500s.
c-iii	**Alor 5/500 Tablets** (Atley)	5 mg hydrocodone bitartrate		500 mg		1 to 2 q 4 to 6 h up to 8/day	(AP Alor). In 100s.
c-iii	**Lortab ASA Tablets** (Whitby)					1 or 2 q 4 to 6 h	Pink, scored. In 100s.
c-iii	**Panasal 5/500** Tablets (E.C. Robins)					1 or 2 q 4 to 6 h up to 8/day	(ECR 0131). Pink, mottled, scored. In 100s.
c-iii	**Panlor DC** (Pan American Labs)	16 mg dihydrocodeine bitartrate	356.4 mg	30 mg caffeine	2 q 4 h	(PAL/0016). Red. In 100s.	
c-iii	**Synalgos-DC Capsules** (Leitner)	16 mg dihydrocodeine bitartrate		356.4 mg	30 mg caffeine	2 q 4 h	(Wyeth 4191). Blue/gray. In 100s and 500s.
c-iii	**Panlor SS Tablets** (Pan American Labs)	32 mg dihydrocodeine bitartrate	712.8 mg		60 mg caffeine		(PAL 032). Lavender, oval, scored. in 100s.
c-ii	**Acetaminophen with Oxycodone Tablets** (Various, eg, Goldline, Major)	5 mg oxycodone HCl	325 mg			1 q 6 h	In 100s, 500s 1000s and UD 25s.
c-ii	**Endocet Tablets** (Endo Labs.)	5 mg oxycodone HCl	325 mg			1 q 6 h	(Endo 602). White. In 100s and 500s.
c-ii	**Percocet Tablets** (Du Pont)	5 mg oxycodone HCl	325 mg			1 q 6 h	(Percocet 5). In 100s, 500s and UD 100s.
c-ii	**Roxicet Tablets** (Roxane)						(54 543). White, scored. In 100s, 500s and UD 100s.
c-ii	**Roxicet Oral Solution** (Roxane)				0.4% alcohol, EDTA, saccharin, sucrose	5 mL q 6 h	In 500 mL and UD 5 mL.
c-ii	**Oxycodone with Acetaminophen Capsules** (Various, eg, Goldline, Major, Schein)	5 mg oxycodone HCl	500 mg			1 q 6 h	In 100s, 500s, 1000s and UD 25s.
c-ii	**Roxicet 5/500 Caplets** (Roxane)						(54 730). White, scored. In 100s and UD 100s.
c-ii	**Roxilox Capsules** (Roxane)						(HD532). In 100s.
c-ii	**Tylox Capsules** (McNeil)				Sodium metabisulfite		(Tylox McNeil). Red. In 100s and UD 100s.
c-ii	**Oxycodone HCl and Acetaminophen Tablets** (Mallinckrodt)	7.5 mg oxycodone HCl	325 mg			1 q 6 h prn, not to exceed 8 tablets daily	(M522 7.5/325). White to off-white. Caplet shape. In 20s, 100s, 500s, 1,000s, and UD 100s.
c-ii	**Endocet Tablets** (Endo)						(E700 7.5/325). Peach, capsule shape. In 100s and 500s.

OPIOID ANALGESIC COMBINATIONS

	Product and Distributor	Narcotic	Acetaminophen	Aspirin	Other Content	Average Adult Dose	How Supplied
c-ii	**Oxycodone HCl and Acetaminophen Tablets** (Mallinckrodt)	7.5 mg oxycodone HCl	500 mg			1 q 6 h prn, not to exceed 8 tablets daily	(M582). White to off-white, oval. In 20s, 100s, 500s, 1,000s, and UD 100s.
c-ii	**Endocet Tablets** (Endo)						(E796 7.5). Peach, capsule shape. In 100s and 500s.
c-ii	**Percocet** (Endo)					1 q 6 h	(PERCOCET 7.5). Peach, capsule shape. In 100s and 500s.
c-ii	**Oxycodone HCl and Acetaminophen Tablets** (Mallinckrodt)	10 mg oxycodone HCl	325 mg			1 q 6 h prn, not to exceed 6 tablets daily	(M523 10/325). White to off-white. Caplet shape. In 20s, 100s, 500s, 1,000s, and UD 100s.
c-ii	**Endocet Tablets** (Endo)						(E712 10/325). Yellow, oval. In 100s and 500s.
c-ii	**Percocet** (Endo)					1 q 6 h	In 100s, 500s, and UD 100s.
c-ii	**Oxycodone HCl and Acetaminophen Tablets** (Mallinckrodt)	10 mg oxycodone HCl	650 mg			1 q 6 h prn, not to exceed 6 tablets daily	(M562). White to off-white. Capsule shape. In 20s, 100s, 500s, 1,000s, and UD 100s.
c-ii	**Endocet Tablets** (Endo)						(E797 10). Yellow, oval. In 100s and 500s.
c-ii	**Percocet** (Endo)					1 q 6 h	(PERCOCET 10). Yellow, oval. In 100s and 500s.
c-ii	**Percocet** (Endo)	2.5 mg oxycodone HCl	325 mg				(PERCOCET 2.5). Pink, oval. In 500s and UD 100s.
c-ii	**Combunox** (Forest)	5 mg oxycodone HCl			400 mg ibuprofen	1 tablet; up to 4 per 24 h not to exceed 7 days	(F P 5400). White to off-white, capsule shape, bisected. Film-coated. In 100s.
c-ii	**Percodan-Demi Tablets** (Du Pont)	2.25 mg oxycodone HCl, 0.19 mg oxycodone terephthalate		325 mg		1 or 2 q 6 h	White, scored. In 100s.
c-ii	**Oxycodone with Aspirin Tablets** (Various, eg, Goldline)	4.5 mg oxycodone HCl, 0.38 mg oxycodone terephthalate		325 mg		1 q 6 h	In 100s, 500s, 1000s and UD 25s.
c-ii	**Percodan Tablets** (DuPont)						Yellow, scored. In 500s, 1000s, and UD 250s.
c-ii	**Roxiprin Tablets** (Roxane)						(54 902). White, scored. In 100s, 1000s and UD 100s.
c-iv	**Propoxyphene Napsylate and Acetaminophen Tablets** (Various, eg, Moore)	50 mg propoxyphene napsylate	325 mg			2 q 4 h	In 100s, 500s, 550s, 1000s and UD 100s.
c-iv	**Darvocet-N 50 Tablets** (aaiPharma)	50 mg propoxyphene napsylate	325 mg			2 q 4 h	(Lilly Darvocet-N 50). Orange. In *RxPak* 100s, 500s and UD 100s.
c-iv	**Balacet 325 Tablets** (Cornerstone Biopharma)	100 mg propoxyphene napsylate	325 mg		Lactose	1 q 4 h up to 6/day	(P325). Violet, capsule shaped. Film-coated. In 100s.
c-iv	**Trycet Tablets** (Tryon Laboratories[b])						(P325). Violet, capsule shaped. Film-coated. In 100s.
c-iv	**Propoxyphene Napsylate and Acetaminophen Tablets** (Pliva)	100 mg propoxyphene napsylate	500 mg			1 q 4 h up to 6/day	Lactose. (P500). Pink. Film-coated. In 100s.
c-iv	**Darvocet A500** (aaiPharma)						Film-coated. In 100s.
c-iv	**Propoxyphene Napsylate and Acetaminophen Tablets** (Various, eg, Zenith)	100 mg propoxyphene napsylate	650 mg			1 q 4 h	In 30s, 50s, 100s, 500s, 1,000s and UD 100s.
c-iv	**Darvocet-N 100 Tablets** (aaiPharma)						(Darvocet-N 100). Orange. In *RxPak* 100s, 500s, UD 100s, UD 500s and RN 500s.

OPIOID ANALGESIC COMBINATIONS

	Product and Distributor	Narcotic	Acetaminophen	Aspirin	Other Content	Average Adult Dose	How Supplied
c-iv	**Propoxyphene HCl w/Acetaminophen Tablets** (Various, eg, Moore, Mylan)	65 mg propoxyphene HCl	650 mg			1 q 4 h	In 500s.
c-iv	**Darvon Compound-32 Pulvules** (Lilly)	32 mg propoxyphene HCl		389 mg	32.4 mg caffeine	1 q 4 h	(DARVON COMP). Pink. In 100s.
c-iv	**Darvon Compound-65 Pulvules** (Lilly)	65 mg propoxyphene HCl		389 mg	32.4 mg caffeine	1 q 4 h	Red/gray. Lilly 3111 DARVON COMP. 65. In 500s and *RxPak* 100s.
c-ii	**B & O Supprettes No. 15A Suppositories** (PolyMedica)	30 mg powdered opium			16.2 mg powdered belladonna extract. Polyethylene glycol/Polysorbate 60 base	1 or 2/day	Scored. In 12s.
c-ii	**Opium and Belladonna Suppositories** (Wyeth-Ayerst)	60 mg powdered opium			15 mg belladonna extract. Cocoa butter base	1 or 2/day	In 20s.
c-ii	**B & O Supprettes No.16A Suppositories** (PolyMedica)				16.2 mg powdered belladonna extract. Polyethylene glycol/Polysorbate 60 base	1 or 2/day	Scored. In 12s.
c-ii	**Meperidine Hydrochloride and Promethazine Hydrochloride** (Ethex)	50 mg meperidine hydrochloride, 25 mg promethazine hydrochloride			Lactose	1 every 4 to 6 hours	Lactose. (ETHEX 027). Opaque maroon. In 100s.
Rx	**Tramadol and Acetaminophen Tablets** (Par)	37.5 mg tramadol hydrochloride	325 mg			2 every 4 to 6 hours up to 8/day	(083 KALI). Orange, capsule shape. Film coated. In 20s, 100s, and 500s.
Rx	**Ultracet Tablets** (Ortho-McNeil)						(O-M 650). Yellow, capsule shape. Film coated. In 20s, 100s, 500s, and UD 100s.

[a] May contain alcohol.

[b] Tryon Laboratories, 27368 Via Industria, Temecula, CA 92590; (951) 719-1104; fax (951) 719-1139.

OPIOID ANALGESIC COMBINATIONS

Precautions

➤*Sulfite sensitivity:* Some of these products contain sulfites that may cause allergic-type reactions (eg, hives, itching, wheezing, anaphylaxis) in certain susceptible people. Although the overall prevalence of sulfite sensitivity in the general population is probably low, it is seen more frequently in asthmatics or in atopic nonasthmatic people. Specific products containing sulfites are identified in the product listing.

Mixed opioid agonist-antagonists (pentazocine, butorphanol, and nalbuphine) are primarily κ-opioid receptor agonists and μ-opioid receptor antagonists. They produce analgesia in nontolerant patients but may precipitate withdrawal in those dependent on morphine-like drugs.

A partial agonist analgesic (buprenorphine) is an antagonist at the κ-opioid receptor but is a partial agonist at the μ-opioid receptor. It may also precipitate withdrawal effects in those dependent on morphine-like drugs, but to a lesser degree than mixed agonist-antagonists. Partial agonists also produce less psychotomimetic effects that are seen with mixed agonist-antagonists.

Opioid Agonist-Antagonist Pharmacokinetics

Agonist/Antagonist		Onset (min)	Peak (min)	Duration (h)	Equivalent dose[1] (mg)	Relative antagonist activity
Buprenorphine	IM	15	60	≥ 6	0.3	Equipotent with naloxone
	IV[2]	-	-	-		
Butorphanol	IM	≤ 15	30-60	3-4	2	More potent than pentazocine, but less than naloxone
	IV	Few min	30-60	3-4		
	Nasal	≤ 15	60-120	4-5		
Nalbuphine	SC/IM	< 15	60	3-6	10	10 times that of pentazocine
	IV	2-3	nd			
Pentazocine	SC/IM	15-20	15-60	4-6	30	Weak
	IV	2-3	nd	nd		
	Oral	15-30	nd	≥ 3		

[1] Parenteral dose equivalent to 10 mg morphine.
[2] When given IV, the time to onset and peak effect are shortened
* nd – no data

BUPRENORPHINE HYDROCHLORIDE

c-iii	**Subutex** (Reckitt Benckiser)	**Tablets, sublingual:** 2 mg (as base)	Lactose. White, oval. In 30s.
		8 mg (as base)	Lactose. White, oval. In 30s.
c-iii	**Buprenorphine Hydrochloride** (Abbott)	**Injection:** 0.324 mg (equiv. to 0.3 mg buprenorphine)/mL	In 1 mL *Carpuject*.[1]
c-iii	**Buprenex** (Reckitt Benckiser)		In 1 mL amps.[1]

[1] With 50 mg anhydrous dextrose.

BUPRENORPHINE HYDROCHLORIDE — ORAL

Refer to the general discussion in the Opioid Agonist-Antagonist Analgesic introduction.

Indications

For the treatment of opioid dependence.

Administration and Dosage

➤*Approved by the FDA:* December 30, 1985.

Buprenorphine hydrochloride is administered sublingually as a single daily dose in the range of 12 to 16 mg/day. Buprenorphine hydrochloride is preferred for use during induction. Following induction, buprenorphine hydrochloride/naloxone, due to the presence of naloxone, is preferred when clinical use includes unsupervised administration. The use of buprenorphine hydrochloride for unsupervised administration should be limited to those patients who cannot tolerate buprenorphine hydrochloride/naloxone, for example those patients who have been shown to be hypersensitive to naloxone.

➤*Method of administration:* Buprenorphine hydrochloride tablets should be placed under the tongue until they are dissolved. For doses requiring the use of more than 2 tablets, patients are advised to either place all the tablets at once or alternatively (if they cannot fit in more than 2 tablets comfortably) place 2 tablets at a time under the tongue. Either way, the patients should continue to hold the tablets under the tongue until they dissolve; swallowing the tablets reduces the bioavailability of the drug. To ensure consistency in bioavailability, patients should follow the same manner of dosing with continued use of the product.

➤*Induction:* Prior to induction, consideration should be given to the type of opioid dependence (ie, long- or short-acting opioid), the time since last opioid use, and the degree or level of opioid dependence. To avoid precipitating withdrawal, induction with buprenorphine hydrochloride should be undertaken when objective and clear signs of withdrawal are evident.

In a 1-month study of buprenorphine hydrochloride/naloxone tablets, induction was conducted with buprenorphine hydrochloride tablets. Patients received 8 mg of buprenorphine hydrochloride on day 1 and 16 mg buprenorphine hydrochloride on day 2. From day 3 onward, patients received buprenorphine hydrochloride/naloxone tablets at the same buprenorphine dose as day 2. Induction in the studies of buprenorphine solution was accomplished over 3 to 4 days, depending on the target dose. In some studies, gradual induction over several days led to a high rate of drop-out of buprenorphine patients during the induction period. Therefore, it is recommended that an adequate maintenance dose, titrated to clinical effectiveness, should be achieved as rapidly as possible to prevent undue opioid withdrawal symptoms.

➤*Patients taking heroin or other short-acting opioids:* At treatment initiation, the dose of buprenorphine hydrochloride should be administered at least 4 hours after the patient last used opioids or preferably when early signs of opioid withdrawal appear.

➤*Patients on methadone or other long-acting opioids:* There is little controlled experience with the transfer of methadone-maintained patients to buprenorphine. Available evidence suggests that withdrawal symptoms are possible during induction to buprenorphine treatment. Withdrawal appears more likely in patients maintained on higher doses of methadone (greater than 30 mg) and when the first buprenorphine dose is administered shortly after the last methadone dose.

➤*Maintenance:* Buprenorphine hydrochloride/naloxone is the preferred medication for maintenance treatment due to the presence of naloxone in the formulation.

➤*Adjusting the dose until the maintenance dose is achieved:* The recommended target dose of buprenorphine hydrochloride/naloxone is 16 mg/day. Clinical studies have shown that 16 mg of buprenorphine hydrochloride or buprenorphine hydrochloride/naloxone is a clinically effective dose compared with placebo and indicate that doses as low as 12 mg may be effective in some patients. The dosage of buprenorphine hydrochloride/naloxone should be progressively adjusted in increments/decrements of 2 mg or 4 mg to a level that holds the patient in treatment and suppresses opioid withdrawal effects. This is likely to be in the range of 4 mg to 24 mg per day, depending on the individual.

➤*Reducing dosage and stopping treatment:* The decision to discontinue therapy with buprenorphine hydrochloride/naloxone or buprenorphine hydrochloride after a period of maintenance or brief stabilization should be made as part of a comprehensive treatment plan. Both gradual and abrupt discontinuation have been used, but no controlled trials have been undertaken to determine the best method of dose taper at the end of treatment.

➤*Storage/Stability:* Store at 25°C (77°F), excursions permitted from 15° to 30°C (59° to 86°F).

Actions

➤*Pharmacology:*

Subjective effects – Comparisons of buprenorphine with full agonists such as methadone and hydromorphone suggest that sublingual buprenorphine produces typical opioid agonist effects which are limited by a ceiling effect. In nondependent subjects, acute sublingual doses of buprenorphine hydrochloride/naloxone tablets produced opioid agonist effects, which reached a maximum between doses of 8 mg and 16 mg of buprenorphine hydrochloride. The effects of 16 mg buprenorphine hydrochloride/naloxone were similar to those produced by 16 mg buprenorphine hydrochloride (buprenorphine alone).

Opioid agonist ceiling effects were also observed in a double-blind, parallel group, dose ranging comparison of single doses of buprenorphine sublingual solution (1, 2, 4, 8, 16 or 32 mg), placebo, and a full agonist control at various doses. The treatments were given in ascending dose order at intervals of at least 1 week to 16 opioid-experienced, nondependent subjects. Both drugs produced typical opioid agonist effects. For all the measures for which the drugs produced an effect, buprenorphine produced a dose-related response but, in each case, there was a dose that produced no further effect. In contrast, the highest dose of the full agonist control always produced the greatest effects. Agonist objective rating scores remained elevated for the higher doses of buprenorphine (8 to 32 mg) longer than for the lower doses and did not return to baseline until 48 hours after drug administrations. The onset of effects appeared more rapidly with buprenorphine than with the full agonist control, with most doses nearing peak effect after 100 minutes for buprenorphine compared to 150 minutes for the full agonist control.

Physiologic effects – Buprenorphine in intravenous (2 mg, 4 mg, 8 mg, 12 mg and 16 mg) and sublingual (12 mg) doses has been administered to nondependent subjects to examine cardiovascular, respiratory and subjective effects at doses comparable to those used for treatment of opioid dependence. Compared with placebo, there were no statistically significant differences among any of the treatment conditions for blood pressure, heart rate, respiratory rate, O_2 saturation or skin temperature across time. Systolic BP was higher in the 8 mg group than placebo (3 hour AUC values). Minimum and maximum effects were similar across all treatments. Subjects remained responsive to low voice and responded to computer prompts. Some subjects showed irritability, but no other changes were observed.

BUPRENORPHINE HYDROCHLORIDE — ORAL

The respiratory effects of sublingual buprenorphine were compared with the effects of methadone in a double-blind, parallel group, dose ranging comparison of single doses of buprenorphine sublingual solution (1, 2, 4, 8, 16, or 32 mg) and oral methadone (15, 30, 45, or 60 mg) in nondependent, opioid-experienced volunteers. In this study, hypoventilation not requiring medical intervention was reported more frequently after buprenorphine doses of 4 mg and higher than after methadone. Both drugs decreased O_2 saturation to the same degree.

➤*Pharmacokinetics:*

Absorption – Plasma levels of buprenorphine increased with the sublingual dose of buprenorphine hydrochloride. There was a wide inter-patient variability in the sublingual absorption of buprenorphine. Both C_{max} and AUC of buprenorphine increased in a linear fashion with the increase in dose (in the range of 4 to 16 mg), although the increase was not directly dose-proportional.

Buprenorphine pharmacokinetic parameters after a 16 mg dose were as follows (mean (%CV)):

C_{max} (ng/mL) = 5.47 (23) and $AUC_{0\text{-}48}$ (ng•hr/mL) = 32.63 (25).

Distribution – Buprenorphine is approximately 96% protein bound, primarily to alpha and beta globulin.

Metabolism – Buprenorphine undergoes both N-dealkylation to norbuprenorphine and glucuronidation. The N-dealkylation pathway is mediated by cytochrome P450 3A4 isozyme. Norbuprenorphine, an active metabolite, can further undergo glucuronidation.

Excretion – A mass balance study of buprenorphine showed complete recovery of radiolabel in urine (30%) and feces (69%) collected up to 11 days after dosing. Almost all of the dose was accounted for in terms of buprenorphine, norbuprenorphine, and 2 unidentified buprenorphine metabolites. In urine, most of buprenorphine and norbuprenorphine was conjugated (buprenorphine, 1% free and 9.4% conjugated; norbuprenorphine, 2.7% free and 11% conjugated). In feces, almost all of the buprenorphine and norbuprenorphine were free (buprenorphine, 33% free and 5% conjugated; norbuprenorphine, 21% free and 2% conjugated).

Buprenorphine has a mean elimination half-life from plasma of 37 hours.

Special populations –

Hepatic function impairment: The effect of hepatic impairment on the pharmacokinetics of buprenorphine is unknown. Since it is extensively metabolized, the plasma levels will be expected to be higher in patients with moderate and severe hepatic impairment. Therefore, in patients with hepatic impairment dosage should be adjusted and patients should be observed for symptoms of precipitated opioid withdrawal.

Contraindications

Buprenorphine hydrochloride should not be administered to patients who have been shown to be hypersensitive to buprenorphine.

Warnings

➤*Dependence:* Buprenorphine is a partial agonist at the mu-opiate receptor and chronic administration produces dependence of the opioid type, characterized by withdrawal upon abrupt discontinuation or rapid taper. The withdrawal syndrome is milder than seen with full agonists, and may be delayed in onset.

➤*Head injury and increased intracranial pressure:* Buprenorphine hydrochloride, like other potent opioids, may elevate cerebrospinal fluid pressure and should be used with caution in patients with head injury, intracranial lesions and other circumstances where cerebrospinal pressure may be increased. Buprenorphine hydrochloride can produce miosis and changes in the level of consciousness that may interfere with patient evaluation.

➤*Respiratory depression:* Significant respiratory depression has been associated with buprenorphine, particularly by the intravenous route. A number of deaths have occurred when addicts have intravenously misused buprenorphine, usually with benzodiazepines concomitantly. Deaths have also been reported in association with concomitant administration of buprenorphine with other depressants such as alcohol or other opioids. Patients should be warned of the potential danger of the self-administration of benzodiazepines or other depressants while under treatment with buprenorphine hydrochloride.

In the case of overdose, the primary management should be the reestablishment of adequate ventilation with mechanical assistance of respiration, if required. Naloxone may not be effective in reversing any respiratory depression produced by buprenorphine.

Buprenorphine hydrochloride should be used with caution in patients with compromised respiratory function (eg, chronic obstructive pulmonary disease, cor pulmonale, decreased respiratory reserve, hypoxia, hypercapnia, or preexisting respiratory depression).

➤*Hepatic effects:* Cases of cytolytic hepatitis and hepatitis with jaundice have been observed in the addict population receiving buprenorphine both in clinical trials and in postmarketing adverse event reports. The spectrum of abnormalities ranges from transient asymptomatic elevations in hepatic transaminases to case reports of hepatic failure, hepatic necrosis, hepatorenal syndrome, and hepatic encephalopathy. In many cases, the presence of preexisting liver enzyme abnormalities, infection with hepatitis B or hepatitis C virus, concomitant usage of other potentially hepatotoxic drugs, and ongoing injecting drug use may have played a causative or contributory role. In other cases, insufficient data were available to determine the etiology of the abnormality. The possibility exists that buprenorphine had a causative or contributory role in the development of the hepatic abnormality in some cases. Measurements of liver function tests prior to initiation of treatment is recommended to establish a baseline. Periodic monitoring of liver function tests during treatment is also recommended. A biological and etiological evaluation is recommended when a hepatic event is suspected. Depending on the case, the drug should be carefully discontinued to prevent withdrawal symptoms and a return to illicit drug use, and strict monitoring of the patient should be initiated.

➤*Hypersensitivity reactions:* Cases of acute and chronic hypersensitivity to buprenorphine have been reported both in clinical trials and in the post-marketing experience. The most common signs and symptoms include rashes, hives, and pruritus. Cases of bronchospasm, angioneurotic edema, and anaphylactic shock have been reported. A history of hypersensitivity to buprenorphine is a contraindication to buprenorphine hydrochloride or buprenorphine hydrochloride/naloxone use. A history of hypersensitivity to naloxone is a contraindication to buprenorphine hydrochloride/naloxone use.

➤*Hepatic function impairment:* The effect of hepatic impairment on the pharmacokinetics of buprenorphine is unknown. It is extensively metabolized; therefore, the plasma levels will be expected to be higher in patients with moderate and severe hepatic impairment. Dosage should be adjusted and patients should be watched for symptoms of precipitated opioid withdrawal.

➤*Carcinogenesis:* Carcinogenicity studies of buprenorphine were conducted in Sprague-Dawley rats and CD-1 mice. Buprenorphine was administered in the diet to rats at doses of 0.6, 5.5, and 56 mg/kg/day (estimated exposure was approximately 0.4, 3 and 35 times the recommended human daily sublingual dose of 16 mg on a mg/m^2 basis) for 27 months. Statistically significant dose-related increases in testicular interstitial (Leydig's) cell tumors occurred, according to the trend test adjusted for survival. Pair-wise comparison of the high dose against control failed to show statistical significance. In an 86-week study in CD-1 mice, buprenorphine was not carcinogenic at dietary doses up to 100 mg/kg/day (estimated exposure was approximately 30 times the recommended human daily sublingual dose of 16 mg on a mg/m^2 basis).

➤*Mutagenesis:* Buprenorphine was studied in a series of tests utilizing gene, chromosome, and DNA interactions in both prokaryotic and eukaryotic systems. Results were negative in yeast (*Saccharomyces cerevisiae*) for recombinant, gene convertant, or forward mutations; negative in *Bacillus subtilis* "rec" assay, negative for clastogenicity in CHO cells, Chinese hamster bone marrow and spermatogonia cells, and negative in the mouse lymphoma L5178Y assay. Results were equivocal in the Ames test: Negative in studies in 2 laboratories, but positive for frame shift mutation at a high dose (5 mg/plate) in a third study. Results were positive in the Green-Tweets (*E. coli*) survival test, positive in a DNA synthesis inhibition (DSI) test with testicular tissue from mice, for both in vivo and in vitro incorporation of [^{3}H]thymidine, and positive in unscheduled DNA synthesis (UDS) test using testicular cells from mice.

➤*Pregnancy: Category C.*

Neonatal withdrawal – Neonatal withdrawal has been reported in the infants of women treated with buprenorphine during pregnancy. From post-marketing reports, the time to onset of neonatal withdrawal symptoms ranged from day 1 to day 8 of life with most occurring on day 1. Adverse events associated with neonatal withdrawal syndrome included hypertonia, neonatal tremor, neonatal agitation, and myoclonus. There have been rare reports of convulsions and in 1 case, apnea and bradycardia were also reported.

Teratogenic – Buprenorphine was not teratogenic in rats or rabbits after IM or SC doses up to 5 mg/kg/day (estimated exposure was approximately 3 and 6 times, respectively, the recommended human daily sublingual dose of 16 mg on a mg/m^2 basis), after IV doses up to 0.8 mg/kg/day (estimated exposure was approximately 0.5 times and equal to, respectively, the recommended human daily sublingual dose of 16 mg on a mg/m^2 basis), or after oral doses up to 160 mg/kg/day in rats (estimated exposure was approximately 95 times the recommended human daily sublingual dose of 16 mg on a mg/m^2 basis) and 25 mg/kg/day in rabbits (estimated exposure was approximately 30 times the recommended human daily sublingual dose of 16 mg on a mg/m^2 basis). Significant increases in skeletal abnormalities (eg, extra thoracic vertebra or thoraco-lumbar ribs) were noted in rats after SC administration of 1 mg/kg/day and up (estimated exposure was approximately 0.6 times the recommended human daily sublingual dose of 16 mg on a mg/m^2 basis), but were not observed at oral doses up to 160 mg/kg/day. Increases in skeletal abnormalities in rabbits after IM administration of 5 mg/kg/day (estimated exposure was approximately 6 times the recommended human daily sublingual dose of 16 mg on a mg/m^2 basis) or oral administration of 1 mg/kg/day or greater (estimated exposure was approximately equal to the recommended human daily sublingual dose of 16 mg on a mg/m^2 basis) were not statistically significant.

In rabbits, buprenorphine produced statistically significant pre-implantation losses at oral doses of 1 mg/kg/day or greater and post-implantation losses that were statistically significant at IV doses of 0.2 mg/kg/day or greater (estimated exposure was approximately 0.3 times the recommended human daily sublingual dose of 16 mg on a mg/m^2 basis).

There are no adequate and well-controlled studies of buprenorphine hydrochloride in pregnant women. Buprenorphine hydrochloride should only be used during pregnancy if the potential benefit justifies the potential risk to the fetus.

Nonteratogenic – Dystocia was noted in pregnant rats treated IM with buprenorphine 5 mg/kg/day (approximately 3 times the recommended human daily sublingual dose of 16 mg on a mg/m^2 basis). Both fertility and peri- and postnatal development studies with buprenorphine in rats indicated increases in neonatal mortality after oral doses of 0.8 mg/kg/day and up (approximately 0.5 times the recommended human daily sublingual dose of 16 mg on a mg/m^2 basis), after IM doses of 0.5 mg/kg/day and up (approximately 0.3 times the recommended human daily sublingual dose of 16 mg on a mg/m^2 basis), and after SC doses of 0.1 mg/kg/day and up (approximately 0.06 times the recommended human daily sublingual dose of 16 mg on a

BUPRENORPHINE HYDROCHLORIDE — ORAL

mg/m^2 basis). Delays in the occurrence of righting reflex and startle response were noted in rat pups at an oral dose of 80 mg/kg/day (approximately 50 times the recommended human daily sublingual dose of 16 mg on a mg/m^2 basis).

➤*Lactation:* An apparent lack of milk production during general reproduction studies with buprenorphine in rats caused decreased viability and lactation indices. Use of high doses of sublingual buprenorphine in pregnant women showed that buprenorphine passes into the mother's milk. Breastfeeding is therefore not advised in mothers treated with buprenorphine hydrochloride or buprenorphine hydrochloride/naloxone.

➤*Children:* Buprenorphine hydrochloride is not recommended for use in pediatric patients. The safety and effectiveness of buprenorphine hydrochloride in patients below the age of 16 years have not been established.

Precautions

➤*Acute abdominal conditions:* As with other mu-opioid receptor agonists, the administration of buprenorphine hydrochloride/naloxone or buprenorphine hydrochloride may obscure the diagnosis or clinical course of patients with acute abdominal conditions.

➤*Special risk:* Buprenorphine hydrochloride should be administered with caution in elderly or debilitated patients and those with severe impairment of hepatic, pulmonary, or renal function; myxedema or hypothyroidism, adrenal cortical insufficiency (eg, Addison's disease); CNS depression or coma; toxic psychoses; prostatic hypertrophy or urethral stricture; acute alcoholism; delirium tremens; or kyphoscoliosis.

Buprenorphine has been shown to increase intracholedochal pressure, as do other opioids, and thus should be administered with caution to patients with dysfunction of the biliary tract.

➤*Drug abuse and dependence:* Buprenorphine hydrochloride is controlled as a Schedule III narcotic under the Controlled Substances Act.

Buprenorphine is a partial agonist at the mu-opioid receptor and chronic administration produces dependence of the opioid type, characterized by moderate withdrawal upon abrupt discontinuation or rapid taper. The withdrawal syndrome is milder than seen with full agonists, and may be delayed in onset.

Neonatal withdrawal has been reported in the infants of women treated with buprenorphine hydrochloride during pregnancy.

➤*Hazardous tasks:* Buprenorphine hydrochloride may impair the mental or physical abilities required for the performance of potentially dangerous tasks such as driving a car or operating machinery, especially during drug induction and dose adjustment. Patients should be cautioned about operating hazardous machinery, including automobiles, until they are reasonably certain that buprenorphine therapy does not adversely affect their ability to engage in such activities.

Drug Interactions

Buprenorphine Hydrochloride Drug Interactions

Precipitant drug	Object drug*		Description
Barbiturate anesthetics	Buprenorphine	↑	Barbiturate anesthetics may increase the respiratory and CNS depression of buprenorphine because of additive pharmacologic activity.
Benzodiazepines	Buprenorphine	↑	Coma and death have been associated with the concomitant IV misuse of buprenorphine and benzodiazepines by addicts.
CNS depressants (eg, opioid analgesics, general anesthetics, benzodiazepines, phenothiazines, other tranquilizers, sedative/hypnotics, other CNS depressants including alcohol)	Buprenorphine	↑	Patients receiving both agents may exhibit increased CNS depression. When combined therapy is contemplated, consider reduction of the dose of one or both agents.
CYP3A4 inducers (eg, phenobarbital, carbamazepine, phenytoin, rifampin)	Buprenorphine	↓	Although not investigated, it is recommended to closely monitor patients when buprenorphine is coadministered with a CYP3A4 inducer. May cause possible increased clearance.
CYP3A4 inhibitors (ie, azole antifungals, macrolide antibiotics, protease inhibitors)	Buprenorphine	↑	Coadministration may increase buprenorphine plasma concentrations. Buprenorphine dosage adjustment may be required.
MAO inhibitors	Buprenorphine	↔	Exercise caution. Specific information is not available.

* ↑ = Object drug increased. ↓ = Object drug decreased.
↔ = Undetermined clinical effect.

Adverse Reactions

In a comparative study, adverse event profiles were similar for subjects treated with 16 mg buprenorphine hydrochloride/naloxone or 16 mg buprenorphine hydrochloride. The following adverse events were reported to occur by at least 5% of patients in a 4-week study.

Adverse Events (≥ 5%) by Body System and Treatment Group in a 4-week Study

Body system/ adverse event (COSTART terminology)	n (%) Buprenorphine hydrochloride/ naloxone 16 mg/day (n = 107)	n (%) Buprenorphine hydrochloride 16 mg/day (n = 103)	n (%) Placebo (n = 107)
Body as a whole			
Asthenia	7 (6.5%)	5 (4.9%)	7 (6.5%)
Chills	8 (7.5%)	8 (7.8%)	8 (7.5%)
Headache	39 (36.4%)	30 (29.1%)	24 (22.4%)
Infection	6 (5.6%)	12 (11.7%)	7 (6.5%)
Pain	24 (22.4%)	19 (18.4%)	20 (18.7%)
Abdominal pain	12 (11.2%)	12 (11.7%)	7 (6.5%)
Back pain	4 (3.7%)	8 (7.8%)	12 (11.2%)
Withdrawal syndrome	27 (25.2%)	19 (18.4%)	40 (37.4%)
Cardiovascular system			
Vasodilation	10 (9.3%)	4 (3.9%)	7 (6.5%)
Digestive system			
Constipation	13 (12.1%)	8 (7.8%)	3 (2.8%)
Diarrhea	4 (3.7%)	5 (4.9%)	16 (15%)
Nausea	16 (15%)	14 (13.6%)	12 (11.2%)
Vomiting	8 (7.5%)	8 (7.8%)	5 (4.7%)
Nervous system			
Insomnia	15 (14%)	22 (21.4%)	17 (15.9%)
Respiratory system			
Rhinitis	5 (4.7%)	10 (9.7%)	14 (13.1%)
Skin and appendages			
Sweating	15 (14%)	13 (12.6%)	11 (10.3%)

The adverse event profile of buprenorphine was also characterized in the dose-controlled study of buprenorphine solution, over a range of doses in 4 months of treatment. The following table shows adverse events reported by at least 5% of subjects in any dose group in the dose-controlled study.

Adverse Events (≥ 5%) by Body System and Treatment Group in a 16-week Study

Body system/ adverse event (COSTART terminology)	Buprenorphine dose* Very low* (n =184) n (%)	Low* (n = 180) n (%)	Moderate* (n = 186) n (%)	High* (n = 181) n (%)	Total* (n = 731) n (%)
Body as a whole					
Abscess	9 (5%)	2 (1%)	3 (2%)	2 (1%)	16 (2%)
Asthenia	26 (14%)	28 (16%)	26 (14%)	24 (13%)	104 (14%)
Chills	11 (6%)	12 (7%)	9 (5%)	10 (6%)	42 (6%)
Fever	7 (4%)	2 (1%)	2 (1%)	10 (6%)	21 (3%)
Flu syndrome	4 (2%)	13 (7%)	19 (10%)	8 (4%)	44 (6%)
Headache	51 (28%)	62 (34%)	54 (29%)	53 (29%)	220 (30%)
Infection	32 (17%)	39 (22%)	38 (20%)	40 (22%)	149 (20%)
Accidental injury	5 (3%)	10 (6%)	5 (3%)	5 (3%)	25 (3%)
Pain	47 (26%)	37 (21%)	49 (26%)	44 (24%)	177 (24%)
Back pain	18 (10%)	29 (16%)	28 (15%)	27 (15%)	102 (14%)
Withdrawal syndrome	45 (24%)	40 (22%)	41 (22%)	36 (20%)	162 (22%)
Digestive system					
Constipation	10 (5%)	23 (13%)	23 (12%)	26 (14%)	82 (11%)
Diarrhea	19 (10%)	8 (4%)	9 (5%)	4 (2%)	40 (5%)
Dyspepsia	6 (3%)	10 (6%)	4 (2%)	4 (2%)	24 (3%)
Nausea	12 (7%)	22 (12%)	23 (12%)	18 (10%)	75 (10%)
Vomiting	8 (4%)	6 (3%)	10 (5%)	14 (8%)	38 (5%)
Nervous system					
Anxiety	22 (12%)	24 (13%)	20 (11%)	25 (14%)	91 (12%)
Depression	24 (13%)	16 (9%)	25 (13%)	18 (10%)	83 (11%)
Dizziness	4 (2%)	9 (5%)	7 (4%)	11 (6%)	31 (4%)
Insomnia	42 (23%)	50 (28%)	43 (23%)	51 (28%)	186 (25%)
Nervousness	12 (7%)	11 (6%)	10 (5%)	13 (7%)	46 (6%)
Somnolence	5 (3%)	13 (7%)	9 (5%)	11 (6%)	38 (5%)
Respiratory system					
Cough increase	5 (3%)	11 (6%)	6 (3%)	4 (2%)	26 (4%)
Pharyngitis	6 (3%)	7 (4%)	6 (3%)	9 (5%)	28 (4%)
Rhinitis	27 (15%)	16 (9%)	15 (8%)	21 (12%)	79 (11%)
Skin and appendages					
Sweat	23 (13%)	21 (12%)	20 (11%)	23 (13%)	87 (12%)

BUPRENORPHINE HYDROCHLORIDE — ORAL

Adverse Events (≥ 5%) by Body System and Treatment Group in a 16-week Study

Body system/ adverse event (COSTART terminology)	Buprenorphine dose*				
	Very low* (n =184)	Low* (n = 180)	Moderate* (n = 186)	High* (n = 181)	Total* (n = 731)
	n (%)	n (%)	n (%)	n (%)	n (%)
Special senses					
Runny eyes	13 (7%)	9 (5%)	6 (3%)	6 (3%)	34 (5%)

* *Sublingual solution. Doses in this table cannot necessarily be delivered in tablet form, but for comparison purposes: "Very low" dose (1 mg solution) would be less than a tablet dose of 2 mg; "Low" dose (4 mg solution) approximates a 6 mg tablet dose; "Moderate" dose (8 mg solution) approximates a 12 mg tablet dose; "High" dose (16 mg solution) approximates a 24 mg tablet dose.

➤*CNS:* Patients receiving buprenorphine in the presence of other narcotic analgesics, general anesthetics, benzodiazepines, phenothiazines, other tranquilizers, sedative/hypnotics or other CNS depressants (including alcohol) may exhibit increased CNS depression. When such combined therapy is contemplated, reduction of the dose of 1 or both agents should be considered.

Buprenorphine hydrochloride may impair the mental or physical abilities required for the performance of potentially dangerous tasks such as driving a car or operating machinery, especially during drug induction and dose adjustment. Patients should be cautioned about operating hazardous machinery, including automobiles, until they are reasonably certain that buprenorphine therapy does not adversely affect their ability to engage in such activities. Like other opioids, buprenorphine hydrochloride may produce orthostatic hypotension in ambulatory patients.

Overdosage

➤*Symptoms:* Manifestations of acute overdose include pinpoint pupils, sedation, hypotension, respiratory depression and death.

➤*Treatment:* The respiratory and cardiac status of the patient should be monitored carefully. In the event of depression of respiratory or cardiac function, primary attention should be given to the reestablishment of adequate respiratory exchange through provision of a patent airway and institution of assisted or controlled ventilation. Oxygen, intravenous fluids, vasopressors, and other supportive measures should be employed as indicated.

In the case of overdose, the primary management should be the reestablishment of adequate ventilation with mechanical assistance of respiration, if required naloxone may not be effective in reversing any respiratory depression produced by buprenorphine.

High doses of naloxone hydrochloride, 10 to 35 mg/70 kg may be of limited value in the management of buprenorphine overdose. Doxapram (a respiratory stimulant) also has been used.

Patient Information

Patients should inform their family members that, in the event of emergency, the treating physician or emergency room staff should be informed that the patient is physically dependent on opioids and that the patient is being treated with buprenorphine hydrochloride/naloxone or buprenorphine hydrochloride.

Patients should be cautioned that a serious overdose may occur if benzodiazepines, sedatives, tranquilizers, antidepressants, or alcohol are taken at the same time as buprenorphine hydrochloride/naloxone or buprenorphine hydrochloride.

Patients should be cautioned that buprenorphine hydrochloride/naloxone or buprenorphine hydrochloride may impair the mental or physical abilities required for the performance of potentially dangerous tasks such as driving a car or operating machinery. Patients should be cautioned not to drive or operate complex machinery until they know how buprenorphine hydrochloride/naloxone or buprenorphine hydrochloride affects their ability to function in these circumstances, such as driving a car.

Patients should consult their physician if other prescription medications are currently being used or are prescribed for future use.

BUPRENORPHINE HYDROCHLORIDE — INJECTION

Refer to the general discussion in the Opioid Agonist-Antagonist Analgesic introduction.

Indications

For the relief of moderate to severe pain.

Administration and Dosage

➤*Adults and children 13 years of age and older:* The usual dosage for persons 13 years of age and older is 1 mL buprenorphine hydrochloride (0.3 mg buprenorphine) given by deep IM or slow (over at least 2 minutes) IV injection at up to 6-hour intervals, as needed. Repeat once (up to 0.3 mg) if required, 30 to 60 minutes after initial dosage, giving consideration to previous dose pharmacokinetics, and thereafter only as needed. In high-risk patients (eg, elderly, debilitated, presence of respiratory disease) and in patients where other CNS depressants are present, such as in the immediate postoperative period, the dose should be reduced by approximately one-half. Extra caution should be exercised with the IV route of administration, particularly with the initial dose.

Occasionally, it may be necessary to administer single doses of up to 0.6 mg to adults depending on the severity of the pain and the response of the patient. This dose should only be given IM and only to adult patients who are not in a high-risk category. At this time, there are insufficient data to recommend single doses greater than 0.6 mg for long-term use.

➤*Children:* Buprenorphine hydrochloride has been used in children 2 to 12 years of age at doses between 2 to 6 mcg/kg of body weight given every 4 to 6 hours. There is insufficient experience to recommend a dose in infants less than 2 years of age, single doses greater than 6 mcg/kg of body weight, or the use of a repeat or second dose at 30 to 60 minutes (such as is used in adults). Since there is some evidence that not all children clear buprenorphine faster than adults, fixed interval or "round-the-clock" dosing should not be undertaken until the proper interdose interval has been established by clinical observation of the child. Physicians should recognize that, as with adults, some children may not need to be remedicated for 6 to 8 hours.

➤*Storage/Stability:* Avoid excessive heat (over 40°C or 104°F). Protect from prolonged exposure to light.

Actions

➤*Pharmacology:* Buprenorphine hydrochloride is a parenteral opioid analgesic with 0.3 mg buprenorphine hydrochloride being approximately equivalent to 10 mg morphine sulfate in analgesic and respiratory depressant effects in adults.

Mechanism of analgesic action – Buprenorphine hydrochloride exerts its analgesic effect via high affinity binding to μ subclass opiate receptors in the CNS. Although buprenorphine hydrochloride may be classified as a partial agonist, under the conditions of recommended use it behaves very much like classical μ agonists such as morphine. One unusual property of buprenorphine hydrochloride observed in in vitro studies is its very slow rate of dissociation from its receptor. This could account for its longer duration of action than morphine, the unpredictability of its reversal by opioid antagonists, and its low level of manifest physical dependence.

Narcotic antagonist activity – Buprenorphine demonstrates narcotic antagonist activity and has been shown to be equipotent with naloxone as an antagonist of morphine in the mouse tail flick test.

Cardiovascular effects – Buprenorphine hydrochloride may cause a decrease or, rarely, an increase in pulse rate and blood pressure in some patients.

Effects on respiration – Under usual conditions of use in adults, both buprenorphine hydrochloride and morphine show similar dose-related respiratory depressant effects. At adult therapeutic doses, buprenorphine hydrochloride (0.3 mg buprenorphine) can decrease respiratory rate in an equivalent manner to an equianalgesic dose of morphine (10 mg).

➤*Pharmacokinetics:* Pharmacological effects occur as soon as 15 minutes after IM injection and persist for 6 hours or longer. Peak pharmacologic effects usually are observed at 1 hour. When used intravenously, the times to onset and peak effect are shortened.

The limits of sensitivity of available analytical methodology precluded demonstration of bioequivalence between IM and IV routes of administration. In postoperative adults, pharmacokinetic studies have shown elimination half-lives ranging from 1.2 to 7.2 hours (mean 2.2 hours) after IV administration of 0.3 mg of buprenorphine. A single, 10-patient, pharmacokinetic study of doses of 3 mcg/kg in children (age 5 to 7 years) showed a high interpatient variability, but suggests that the clearance of the drug may be higher in children than in adults. This is supported by at least one repeat-dose study in postoperative pain that showed an optimal interdose interval of 4 to 5 hours in children as opposed to the recommended 6 to 8 hours in adults.

Buprenorphine, in common with morphine and other phenolic opioid analgesics, is metabolized by the liver and its clearance is related to hepatic blood flow. Studies in patients anesthetized with 0.5% halothane have shown that this anesthetic decreases hepatic blood flow by approximately 30%.

Contraindications

Buprenorphine hydrochloride should not be administered to patients who have been shown to be hypersensitive to the drug.

Warnings

➤*Respiratory depression:* As with other potent opioids, clinically significant respiratory depression may occur within the recommended dose range in patients receiving therapeutic doses of buprenorphine. Buprenorphine hydrochloride should be used with caution in patients with compromised respiratory function (eg, chronic obstructive pulmonary disease, cor pulmonale, decreased respiratory reserve, hypoxia, hypercapnia, or preexisting respiratory depression). Particular caution is advised if buprenorphine hydrochloride is administered to patients taking or recently receiving drugs with CNS/respiratory depressant effects. In patients with the physical or pharmacological risk factors above, the dose should be reduced by approximately one-half.

Naloxone may not be effective in reversing the respiratory depression produced by buprenorphine hydrochloride. Therefore, as with other potent opioids, the primary management of overdose should be the reestablishment of adequate ventilation with mechanical assistance of respiration, if required.

➤*Head injury and increased intracranial pressure:* Buprenorphine hydrochloride, like other potent analgesics, may itself elevate cerebrospinal fluid pressure and should be used with caution in patients with head injury, intracranial lesions, and other circumstances where cerebrospinal pressure may be increased. Buprenorphine hydrochloride can produce miosis and changes in the level of consciousness, which may interfere with patient evaluation.

➤*Narcotic-dependent patients:* Because of the narcotic antagonist activity of buprenorphine hydrochloride, use in the physically dependent individual may result in withdrawal effects.

➤*Hepatic function impairment:* Because buprenorphine hydrochloride is metabolized by the liver, the activity of buprenorphine hydrochloride may

BUPRENORPHINE HYDROCHLORIDE — INJECTION

be increased or extended in those individuals with impaired hepatic function or those receiving other agents known to decrease hepatic clearance.

Buprenorphine hydrochloride has been shown to increase intracholedochal pressure to a similar degree as other opioid analgesics, and thus should be administered with caution to patients with dysfunction of the biliary tract.

➤*Carcinogenesis:* Carcinogenicity studies were conducted in Sprague-Dawley rats and CD-1 mice. Buprenorphine was administered in the diet at doses of 0.6, 5.5, and 56 mg/kg/day for 27 months in rats. These doses were approximately equivalent to 5.7, 52 and 534 times the recommended human dose (1.2 mg) on a mg/m^2 body surface area basis. Statistically significant dose-related increases in testicular interstitial (Leydig's) cell tumors occurred, according to the trend test adjusted for survival. Pairwise comparison of the high dose against control failed to show statistical significance. In the mouse study, buprenorphine was administered in the diet at doses of 8, 50, and 100 mg/kg/day for 86 weeks.

The high dose was approximately equivalent to 477 times the recommended human dose (1.2 mg) on a mg/m^2 basis. Buprenorphine was not carcinogenic in mice.

➤*Pregnancy: Category C.* There are no adequate and well-controlled studies in pregnant women. Buprenorphine hydrochloride should be used during pregnancy only if the potential benefit justifies the potential risk to the fetus.

Teratogenic – Buprenorphine was not teratogenic in rats or rabbits after IM or SC doses up to 5 mg/kg/day (approximately 48 and 95 times the recommended human daily dose of 1.2 mg on a mg/m^2 basis), IV doses up to 0.8 mg/kg/day (approximately 8 times and 15 times the recommended human daily dose of 1.2 mg on a mg/m^2 basis), or oral doses up to 160 mg/kg/day in rats (approximately 1525 times the recommended human daily dose of 1.2 mg on a mg/m^2 basis) and 25 mg/kg/day in rabbits (approximately 475 times the recommended human daily dose of 1.2 mg on a mg/m^2 basis). Significant increases in skeletal abnormalities (eg, extra thoracic vertebra or thoraco-lumbar ribs) were noted in rats after SC administration of 1 mg/kg/day and up (approximately 9.5 times the recommended human daily dose of 1.2 mg on a mg/m^2 basis) and in rabbits after IM administration of 5 mg/kg/day (approximately 95 times the recommended human daily dose of 1.2 mg on a mg/m^2 basis), but these increases were not statistically significant. Increases in skeletal abnormalities after oral administration were not observed in rats, and increases in rabbits (1 to 25 mg/kg/day) were not statistically significant.

Labor and delivery – The safety of buprenorphine hydrochloride given during labor and delivery has not been established.

➤*Lactation:* An apparent lack of milk production during general reproduction studies with buprenorphine in rats caused decreased viability and lactation indices. Use of high doses of sublingual buprenorphine in pregnant women showed that buprenorphine passes into the mother's milk. Breastfeeding is therefore not advised in nursing mothers treated with buprenorphine hydrochloride.

➤*Children:* The safety and efficacy of buprenorphine hydrochloride have been established for children between 2 and 12 years of age. Use of buprenorphine hydrochloride in children is supported by evidence from adequate and well-controlled trials of buprenorphine hydrochloride in adults, with additional data from studies of 960 children ranging in age from 9 months to 18 years of age. Data is available from a pharmacokinetic study, several controlled clinical trials, and several large postmarketing studies and case series. The available information provides reasonable evidence that buprenorphine hydrochloride may be used safely in children ranging from 2 to 12 years of age, and that it is of similar effectiveness in children as in adults.

Precautions

➤*Special risk:* Buprenorphine hydrochloride should be administered with caution in the elderly, debilitated patients, in children and those with severe impairment of hepatic, pulmonary, or renal function; myxedema or hypothyroidism; adrenal cortical insufficiency (eg, Addison's disease); CNS depression or coma; toxic psychoses; prostatic hypertrophy or urethral stricture; acute alcoholism; delirium tremens; or kyphoscoliosis.

➤*Drug abuse and dependence:* Buprenorphine hydrochloride is a partial agonist of the morphine type (ie, it has certain opioid properties that may lead to psychic dependence of the morphine type due to an opiate-like euphoric component of the drug). Direct dependence studies have shown little physical dependence upon withdrawal of the drug. However, caution should be used in prescribing to individuals who are known to be drug abusers or ex-narcotic addicts. The drug may not substitute in acutely dependent narcotic addicts due to its antagonist component and may induce withdrawal symptoms.

➤*Hazardous tasks:* Buprenorphine hydrochloride may impair the mental or physical abilities required for the performance of potentially dangerous tasks such as driving a car or operating machinery. Therefore, buprenorphine hydrochloride should be administered with caution to ambulatory patients who should be warned to avoid such hazards.

Drug Interactions

➤*Naloxone:* Naloxone may not be effective in reversing the respiratory depression produced by buprenorphine hydrochloride. Therefore, as with other potent opioids, the primary management of overdose should be the reestablishment of adequate ventilation with mechanical assistance of respiration, if required.

Buprenorphine Hydrochloride Drug Interactions

Precipitant drug	Object drug*		Description
Barbiturate anesthetics	Buprenorphine	↑	Barbiturate anesthetics may increase the respiratory and CNS depression of buprenorphine because of additive pharmacologic activity.
Benzodiazepines	Buprenorphine	↑	Coma and death have been associated with the concomitant IV misuse of buprenorphine and benzodiazepines by addicts.
CNS depressants (eg, opioid analgesics, general anesthetics, benzodiazepines, phenothiazines, other tranquilizers, sedative/hypnotics, other CNS depressants including alcohol)	Buprenorphine	↑	Patients receiving both agents may exhibit increased CNS depression. When combined therapy is contemplated, consider reduction of the dose of one or both agents.
CYP3A4 inducers (eg, phenobarbital, carbamazepine, phenytoin, rifampin)	Buprenorphine	↓	Although not investigated, it is recommended to closely monitor patients when buprenorphine is coadministered with a CYP3A4 inducer. May cause possible increased clearance.
CYP3A4 inhibitors (ie, azole antifungals, macrolide antibiotics, protease inhibitors)	Buprenorphine	↑	Coadministration may increase buprenorphine plasma concentrations. Buprenorphine dosage adjustment may be required.
MAO inhibitors	Buprenorphine	↔	Exercise caution. Specific information is not available.

* ↑ = Object drug increased. ↓ = Object drug decreased. ↔ = Undetermined clinical effect.

Adverse Reactions

The most frequent adverse reaction in clinical studies involving 1133 patients was sedation, which occurred in approximately two-thirds of the patients. Although sedated, these patients could easily be aroused to an alert state.

Other less frequent adverse reactions occurring in 5% to 10% of the patients were nausea and dizziness/vertigo.

Adverse reactions occurring in 1% to 5% of the patients were sweating, headache, miosis, hypotension, nausea/vomiting, vomiting, and hypoventilation.

➤*Less than 1%:* The following adverse reactions were reported to have occurred in less than 1% of the patients:

Cardiovascular – Hypertension; tachycardia; bradycardia.

CNS – Confusion; blurred vision; euphoria; weakness/fatigue; dry mouth; nervousness; depression; slurred speech; paresthesia.

Dermatologic – Pruritus.

GI – Constipation.

Ophthalmic – Diplopia; visual abnormalities.

Respiratory – Dyspnea; cyanosis.

Miscellaneous – Injection site reaction; urinary retention; dreaming; flushing/warmth; chills/cold; tinnitus; conjunctivitis; Wenckebach block; psychosis.

Other effects observed infrequently include malaise, hallucinations, depersonalization, coma, dyspepsia, flatulence, apnea, rash, amblyopia, tremor, and pallor.

The following reactions have been reported to occur rarely: Loss of appetite; dyspheria/agitation; diarrhea; urticaria; convulsions/lack of muscle coordination.

In the United Kingdom, buprenorphine hydrochloride was made available under monitored release regulation during the first year of sale, and yielded data from 1736 physicians on 9123 patients (17,120 administrations). Data on 240 children less than 18 years of age were included in this monitored release program. No important new adverse effects attributable to buprenorphine hydrochloride were observed.

Overdosage

➤*Symptoms:* Clinical experience with buprenorphine hydrochloride overdosage has been insufficient to define the signs of this condition at this time. Although the antagonist activity of buprenorphine may become manifest at doses somewhat above the recommended therapeutic range, doses in the recommended therapeutic range may produce clinically significant respiratory depression in certain circumstances.

BUPRENORPHINE HYDROCHLORIDE — INJECTION

➤*Treatment:* The respiratory and cardiac status of the patients should be monitored carefully. Primary attention should be given to the reestablishment of adequate respiratory exchange through provision of a patent airway and institution of assisted or controlled ventilation. Oxygen, IV fluids, vasopressors, and other supportive measures should be employed as indicated. Doxapram, a respiratory stimulant, may be used.

Naloxone may not be effective in reversing the respiratory depression produced by buprenorphine hydrochloride. Therefore, as with other potent opioids, the primary management of overdose should be the reestablishment of adequate ventilation with mechanical assistance of respiration, if required.

Patient Information

The effects of buprenorphine hydrochloride, particularly drowsiness, may be potentiated by other centrally-acting agents such as alcohol or benzodiazepines. It is particularly important that in these circumstances patients must not drive or operate machinery.

Buprenorphine hydrochloride has some pharmacologic effects similar to morphine, which in susceptible patients may lead to self-administration of the drug when pain no longer exists. Patients must not exceed the dosage of buprenorphine hydrochloride prescribed by their physician. Patients should be urged to consult their physician if other prescription medications are currently being used or are prescribed for future use.

BUPRENORPHINE HYDROCHLORIDE COMBINATIONS

c-iii	**Suboxone** (Reckitt Benckiser)	**Tablets, sublingual:** 2 mg buprenorphine base/ 0.5 mg naloxone	Lactose, acesulfame K. Orange, hexagonal. Lemon/Lime flavor. In 30s.
		8 mg buprenorphine base/2 mg naloxone	Lactose, acesulfame K. Orange, hexagonal. Lemon/Lime flavor. In 30s.

BUPRENORPHINE HYDROCHLORIDE COMBINATIONS — ORAL

Refer to the general discussion in the Opioid Agonist-Antagonist Analgesic introduction and the Buprenorphine and Naloxone monographs.

Indications

➤*Opioid dependence:* Treatment of opioid dependence.

Administration and Dosage

➤*Approved by the FDA:* October 8, 2002.

Buprenorphine/naloxone tablets are administered sublingually as a single daily dose in the range of 12 to 16 mg/day. When taken sublingually, buprenorphine and buprenorphine/naloxone have similar clinical effects and are interchangeable. Buprenorphine tablets contain no naloxone and are preferred for use during induction. Following induction, buprenorphine/naloxone, because of the presence of naloxone, is preferred when clinical use includes unsupervised administration. Limit the use of buprenorphine for unsupervised administration to those patients who cannot tolerate buprenorphine/naloxone (eg, those patients who have been shown to be hypersensitive to naloxone).

➤*Administration:* Place tablets under the tongue until they are dissolved. For doses requiring the use of more than 2 tablets, patients are advised to place all the tablets at once or, alternatively (if they cannot fit in more than 2 tablets comfortably), place 2 tablets at a time under the tongue. Either way, the patient should continue to hold the tablets under the tongue until they dissolve; swallowing the tablets reduces the bioavailability of the drug. To ensure consistency in bioavailability, patients should follow the same manner of dosing with continued use of the product.

➤*Induction:* Prior to induction, consider the type of opioid dependence (ie, long- or short-acting opioid), the time since last opioid use, and the degree or level of opioid dependence. To avoid precipitating withdrawal, undertake induction with buprenorphine when objective and clear signs of withdrawal are evident.

In a 1-month study of buprenorphine/naloxone tablets, induction was conducted with buprenorphine tablets. Patients received 8 mg buprenorphine on day 1 and 16 mg on day 2. From day 3 onward, patients received buprenorphine/naloxone tablets at the same buprenorphine dose as day 2. Induction in the studies of buprenorphine solution was accomplished over 3 to 4 days, depending on the target dose. In some studies, gradual induction over several days led to a high rate of drop-out of buprenorphine patients during the induction period. Therefore, it is recommended that an adequate maintenance dose, titrated to clinical effectiveness, should be achieved as rapidly as possible to prevent undue opioid withdrawal symptoms.

Patients taking heroin or other short-acting opioids – At treatment initiation, administer the dose of buprenorphine at least 4 hours after the patient last used opioids or, preferably, when early signs of withdrawal appear.

Patients on methadone or other long-acting narcotics – There is little controlled experience with the transfer of methadone-maintained patients to buprenorphine. Available evidence suggests that withdrawal symptoms are possible during induction of buprenorphine treatment. Withdrawal appears more likely in patients maintained on higher doses of methadone (more than 30 mg) and when the first buprenorphine dose is administered shortly after the last methadone dose.

➤*Maintenance:* Buprenorphine/Naloxone is the preferred medication for maintenance treatment because of the presence of naloxone in the formulation.

Adjusting the dose until the maintenance dose is achieved – The recommended target dose of buprenorphine/naloxone is 16 mg/day. Clinical studies have shown that 16 mg buprenorphine or buprenorphine/naloxone is a clinically effective dose compared with placebo and indicate that doses as low as 12 mg may be effective in some patients. Progressively adjust the dosage of buprenorphine/naloxone in increments/decrements of 2 or 4 mg to a level that holds the patient in treatment and suppresses opioid withdrawal effects. This is likely to be in the range of 4 to 24 mg/day, depending on the individual.

➤*Reducing dosage and stopping treatment:* Make the decision to discontinue therapy with buprenorphine/naloxone after a period of maintenance or brief stabilization as part of a comprehensive treatment plan. Gradual and abrupt discontinuation have been used, but no controlled trials have been undertaken to determine the best method of dose taper at the end of treatment.

➤*Storage/Stability:* Store at 25°C (77°F). Excursions permitted to 15° to 30°C (59° to 86°F).

Contraindications

Do not administer to patients who have been shown to be hypersensitive to buprenorphine or naloxone.

Warnings

➤*Opioid withdrawal effects:* Because it contains naloxone, buprenorphine/naloxone is highly likely to produce marked and intense withdrawal symptoms if misused parenterally by individuals dependent on opioid agonists (eg, heroin, morphine, methadone). Sublingually, buprenorphine/naloxone may cause opioid withdrawal symptoms in these people if administered before the agonist effects of the opioid have subsided.

BUTORPHANOL TARTRATE

c-iv	**Butorphanol Tartrate** (Various, eg, Apotex, Baxter, Bedford, Bertek, Hospira, Novaplus)	**Injection:** 1 mg/mL[1]	In 2 mL vials.
c-iv	**Stadol** (Bristol-Myers Squibb)		In 1 mL vials.
c-iv	**Butorphanol Tartrate** (Various, eg, Apotex, Baxter, Bedford, Bertek, Hospira, Novaplus)	**Injection:** 2 mg/mL[1]	In 1 and 2 mL vials.
c-iv	**Stadol** (Bristol-Myers Squibb)		In 1, 2 and 10[2] mL vials.
c-iv	**Butorphanol Tartrate** (Various, eg, Mylan, Roxane)	**Nasal spray:** 10 mg/mL	In 2.5 mL.

[1] 1 mg of tartrate salt is equal to 0.68 mg base.

[2] With 0.1 mg/mL benzethonium chloride.

BUTORPHANOL TARTRATE — INJECTION

Refer to the general discussion in the Opioid Agonist-Antagonist Analgesic introduction.

Indications

Butorphanol tartrate injectable is indicated for the management of pain when the use of an opioid analgesic is appropriate.

Butorphanol tartrate injectable is also indicated as a preoperative or preanesthetic medication, as a supplement to balanced anesthesia, and for the relief of pain during labor.

Administration and Dosage

Factors to be considered in determining the dose are age, body weight, physical status, underlying pathological condition, use of other drugs, type of anesthesia to be used, and surgical procedure involved. Use in the elderly, patients with hepatic or renal disease or in labor requires extra caution. The following doses are for patients who do not have impaired hepatic or renal function and who are not on CNS active agents.

➤*Use for pain:*

Intravenous – The usual recommended single dose for IV administration is 1 mg repeated every 3 to 4 hours as necessary. The effective dosage range, depending on the severity of pain, is 0.5 to 2 mg repeated every 3 to 4 hours.

Intramuscular – The usual recommended single dose for IM administration is 2 mg in patients who will be able to remain recumbent, in the event drowsiness or dizziness occurs. This may be repeated every 3 to 4 hours, as necessary. The effective dosage range depending on the severity of pain is 1 to 4 mg repeated every 3 to 4 hours. There are insufficient clinical data to recommend single doses above 4 mg.

BUTORPHANOL TARTRATE — INJECTION

➤*Use as preoperative/preanesthetic medication:* The preoperative medication dosage of butorphanol tartrate injectable should be individualized (see Individualization of dosage). The usual adult dose is 2 mg IM, administered 60 to 90 minutes before surgery. This is approximately equivalent in sedative effect to 10 mg morphine or 80 mg meperidine.

➤*Use in balanced anesthesia:* The usual dose of butorphanol tartrate injectable is 2 mg IV shortly before induction and/or 0.5 to 1 mg IV in increments during anesthesia. The increment may be higher, up to 0.06 mg/kg (4 mg per 70 kg), depending on previous sedative, analgesic, and hypnotic drugs administered. The total dose of butorphanol tartrate injectable will vary; however, patients seldom require less than 4 mg or more than 12.5 mg (approximately 0.06 to 0.18 mg/kg).

➤*Labor:* In patients at full term in early labor a 1 to 2 mg dose of butorphanol tartrate injectable IV or IM may be administered and repeated after 4 hours. Alternative analgesia should be used for pain associated with delivery or if delivery is expected to occur within 4 hours.

If concomitant use of butorphanol tartrate with drugs that may potentiate its effects is deemed necessary, the lowest effective dose should be employed.

➤*Individualization of dosage:* Use of butorphanol in geriatric patients, patients with renal impairment, patients with hepatic impairment, and during labor requires extra caution.

As with other opioids of this class, butorphanol tartrate injectable may not provide adequate intraoperative analgesia in every patient or under all conditions. A failure to achieve successful analgesia during balanced anesthesia is commonly reflected by increases in general sympathetic tone. Consequently, if blood pressure or heart rate continue to rise, consideration should be given to adding a potent volatile liquid inhalation anesthetic or another intravenous medication.

In labor, the recommended initial dose of butorphanol tartrate injectable is 1 or 2 mg IM or IV in mothers with fetuses of 37 weeks gestation or beyond and without signs of fetal distress. Dosage adjustments of butorphanol tartrate injectable in labor should be based on initial response with consideration given to concomitant analgesic or sedative drugs and the expected time of delivery. A dose should not be repeated in less than 4 hours nor administered less than four hours prior to the anticipated delivery.

➤*Elderly and renal/hepatic function impairment:* The initial dose in the elderly and in patients with renal or hepatic impairment should generally be half the recommended adult dose (0.5 mg IV and 1 mg IM). Repeat doses in these patients should be determined by the patient's response rather than at fixed intervals but will generally be no less than 6 hours.

➤*Storage/Stability:* Store at 25°C (77°F) (controlled room temperature).

Actions

➤*Pharmacology:* Butorphanol is a mixed agonist-antagonist with low intrinsic activity at receptors of the μ-opioid type (morphine-like). It is also an agonist against at K-opioid receptors.

Its interactions with these receptors in the central nervous system apparently mediate most of its pharmacologic effects, including analgesia.

In addition to analgesia, CNS effects include depression of spontaneous respiratory activity and cough, stimulation of the emetic center, miosis, and sedation. Effects possibly mediate by non-CNS mechanisms include alteration in cardiovascular resistance and capacitance, bronchomotor tone, gastrointestinal secretory and motor activity, and bladder sphincter activity.

In an animal model, the dose of the butorphanol tartrate required to antagonize morphine analgesia by 50% was similar to that for nalorphine, less than that for pentazocine and more than that for naloxone.

In human studies of butorphanol, sedation is commonly noted at doses of 0.5 mg or more. Narcosis is produced by 10 to 12 mg doses of butorphanol administered over 10 to 15 minutes intravenously.

Butorphanol, like other mixed agonist-antagonists with a high affinity for the kappa receptor, may produce unpleasant psychotomimetic effects in some individuals.

Nausea and/or vomiting may be produced by doses of 1 mg or more administered by any route.

In human studies involving individuals without significant respiratory dysfunction, 2 mg of butorphanol IV and 10 mg of morphine sulfate IV depressed respiration to a comparable degree. At higher doses, the magnitude of respiratory depression with butorphanol is not appreciably increased; however, the duration of respiratory depression is longer. Respiratory depression noted after administration of butorphanol to humans by any route is reversed by treatment with naloxone, a specific opioid antagonist.

Butorphanol tartrate demonstrates antitussive effects in animals at doses less than those required for analgesia.

Hemodynamic changes noted during cardiac catheterization in patients receiving single 0.025 mg/kg IV doses of butorphanol have included increases in pulmonary artery pressure, wedge pressure and vascular resistance, increases in left ventricular and diastolic pressure, and in systemic arterial pressure.

Pharmacodynamics – The analgesic effect of butorphanol is influenced by the route of administration. Onset of analgesia is within a few minutes for intravenous administration and within 15 minutes for IM injection.

Peak analgesic activity occurs within 30 to 60 minutes following IV and IM administration.

The duration of analgesia varies depending on the pain model as well as the route of administration, but is generally 3 to 4 hours with IM and IV doses as defined by the time 50% of patients required remedication. In postoperative studies, the duration of analgesia with IV or IM butorphanol was similar to morphine, meperidine, and pentazocine when administered in the same fashion at equipotent doses.

➤*Pharmacokinetics:*

Absorption/Distribution – Butorphanol tartrate injectable is rapidly absorbed after IM injection and peak plasma levels are reached in 20 to 40 minutes.

Following its initial absorption/distribution phase, the single-dose pharmacokinetics of butorphanol by the IV, IM, and nasal routes of administration are similar.

Serum protein binding is independent of concentration over the range achieved in clinical practice (up to 7 ng/mL) with a bound fraction of approximately 80%.

The drug is transported across the blood:brain and placental barriers and into human milk.

Metabolism/Excretion – Butorphanol is extensively metabolized in the liver. Metabolism is qualitatively and quantitatively similar following IV, IM, or nasal administration. Oral bioavailability is only 5% to 17% because of extensive first-pass metabolism of butorphanol.

The major metabolite of butorphanol is hydroxybutorphanol, while norbutorphanol is produced in small amounts. Both have been detected in plasma following administration of butorphanol, with norbutorphanol present at trace levels at most time points. The elimination half-life of hydroxybutorphanol is about 18 hours and, as a consequence, considerable accumulation (approximately 5-fold) occurs when butorphanol is dosed to steady-state (1 mg transnasally every 6 hours for 5 days).

Elimination occurs by urine and fecal excretion. When ^{3}H-labeled butorphanol is administered to healthy subjects, most (70% to 80%) of the dose is recovered in the urine, while approximately 15% is recovered in the feces.

About 5% of the dose is recovered in the urine as butorphanol. Forty-nine percent (49%) is eliminated in the urine as hydroxybutorphanol. Less than 5% is excreted in the urine as norbutorphanol.

Special populations –

Renal function impairment: In renally impaired patients with creatinine clearances less than 30 mL/min the elimination half-life is approximately doubled and the total body clearance is approximately one half (10.5 hours [clearance 150 L/hr] as compared to 5.8 hours [clearance 260 L/hr] in healthy subjects). No effect was observed on C_{max} or t_{max} after a single dose.

Hepatic function impairment: After IV administration to patients with hepatic impairment, the elimination half-life of butorphanol was approximately tripled and total body clearance was approximately one-half (half-life 16.8 hours, clearance 92 L/hr) compared to healthy subjects (half-life 4.8 hours, clearance 175 L/hr). The exposure of hepatically impaired patients to butorphanol was significantly greater (about 2-fold) than that in healthy subjects.

Pharmacokinetic parameters –

Mean Pharmacokinetic Parameters of Butorphanol in Younger and Elderly Subjects[a]

Parameters	IV	
	Younger	Elderly
AUC (inf)[b] (ng•h/mL)	7.24 (1.57) (4.4 to 9.77)	8.71 (2.02) (4.76 to 13.03)
Half-life (h)	4.56 (1.67) (2.06 to 8.7)	5.61 (1.36) (3.25 to 8.79)
Volume of distribution[c] (L)	487 (155) (305 to 901)	552 (124) (305 to 737)
Total body clearance (L/h)	99 (23) (70 to 154)	82 (21) (52 to 143)

[a] Younger subjects (n = 24) are from 20 to 40 years old and elderly (n = 24) are greater than 65 years of age.
[b] Area under the plasma concentration time curve after a 1 mg dose.
[c] Derived from IV data.

Contraindications

Hypersensitivity to butorphanol tartrate or the preservative benzethonium chloride.

Warnings

➤*Patients dependent on narcotics:* Because of its opioid antagonist properties, butorphanol is not recommended for use in patients dependent on narcotics. Such patients should have an adequate period of withdrawal from opioid drugs prior to beginning butorphanol therapy. In patients taking opioid analgesics chronically, butorphanol has precipitated withdrawal symptoms such as anxiety, agitation, mood changes, hallucinations, dysphoria, weakness and diarrhea.

Because of the difficulty in assessing opioid tolerance in patients who have recently received repeated doses of narcotic analgesic medication, caution should be used in the administration of butorphanol to such patients.

➤*Renal/Hepatic function impairment:* See Administration and Dosage for more information.

➤*Fertility impairment:* Rats treated orally with 160 mg/kg/day (944 mg/m^2) had a reduced pregnancy rate. However, a similar effect was not observed with a 2.5 mg/kg/day (14.75 mg/m^2) subcutaneous dose.

➤*Elderly:* See Administration and Dosage for more information.

Due to changes in clearance, the mean half-life of butorphanol is increased by 25% (to over 6 hours) in patients over the age of 65 years. Elderly

BUTORPHANOL TARTRATE — INJECTION

patients may be more sensitive to the side effects of butorphanol. In clinical studies of butorphanol nasal spray, elderly patients had an increased frequency of headache, dizziness, drowsiness, vertigo, constipation, nausea and/or vomiting, and nasal congestion compared with younger patients. There are insufficient efficacy data for patients 65 years to determine whether they respond differently from younger patients.

Butorphanol and its metabolites are known to be substantially excreted by the kidney, and the risk of toxic reactions to this drug may be greater in patients with impaired renal function. Because elderly patients are more likely to have decreased renal function, care should be taken in dose selection.

➤*Pregnancy: Category C.* Pregnant rats treated subcutaneously with butorphanol at 1 mg/kg (5.9 mg/m^2) had a higher frequency of stillbirths than controls. Butorphanol at 30 mg/kg/oral (360 mg/m^2) and 60 mg/kg/oral (720 mg/m^2) also showed higher incidences of post-implantation loss in rabbits.

There are no adequate and well-controlled studies of butorphanol tartrate in pregnant women before 37 weeks of gestation. Butorphanol tartrate should be used during pregnancy only if the potential benefit justifies the potential risk to the infant.

Labor and delivery – There have been rare reports of infant respiratory distress/apnea following the administration of butorphanol tartrate injectable during labor. The reports of respiratory distress/apnea have been associated with administration of a dose within 2 hours of delivery, use of multiple doses, use with additional analgesic or sedative drugs, or use in preterm pregnancies.

In a study of 119 patients, the administration of 1 mg of IV butorphanol tartrate injectable during labor was associated with transient (10 to 90 minutes) sinusoidal fetal heart rate patterns, but was not associated with adverse neonatal outcomes. In the presence of an abnormal fetal heart rate pattern, butorphanol tartrate injectable should be used with caution.

➤*Lactation:* Butorphanol has been detected in milk following administration of butorphanol tartrate injectable to nursing mothers. The amount an infant would receive is probably clinically insignificant (estimated 4 mcg/L of milk in a mother receiving 2 mg IM 4 times a day).

➤*Children:* Butorphanol is not recommended for use in patients below 18 years of age because safety and efficacy have not been established in the population.

Precautions

➤*Head injury and increased intracranial pressure:* As with other opioids, the use of butorphanol in patients with head injury may be associated with carbon dioxide retention and secondary elevation of cerebrospinal fluid pressure, drug-induced miosis, and alterations in mental state that would obscure the interpretation of the clinical course of patients with head injuries. In such patients, butorphanol should be used only if the benefits of use outweigh the potential risks.

➤*Respiratory depression:* Butorphanol may produce respiratory depression, especially in patients receiving other CNS active agents, or patients suffering from CNS diseases or respiratory impairment.

➤*Cardiovascular effects:* Because butorphanol may increase the work of the heart, especially the pulmonary circuit, the use of butorphanol in patients with acute myocardial infarction, ventricular dysfunction, or coronary insufficiency should be limited to those situations where the benefits clearly outweigh the risk.

Severe hypertension has been reported rarely during butorphanol therapy. In such cases, butorphanol should be discontinued and the hypertension treated with antihypertensive drugs. In patients who are not opioid dependent, naloxone has also been reported to be effective.

➤*Drug abuse and dependence:* Butorphanol is one of a class of drugs known to be abused and thus should be handled accordingly.

Butorphanol tartrate, by all routes of administration, has been associated with episodes of abuse. Of the cases received, there were more reports of abuse with the nasal spray formulation than with the injectable formulation.

Physical dependence, tolerance, and withdrawal – Prolonged, continuous use of butorphanol tartrate may result in physical dependence or tolerance (a decrease in response to a given dose). Abrupt cessation of use by patients with physical dependence may result in symptoms of withdrawal.

➤*Hazardous tasks:* Opioid analgesics, including butorphanol, impair the mental and physical abilities required for the performance of potentially dangerous tasks such as driving a car or operating machinery. Effects such as drowsiness or dizziness can appear, usually within the first hour after dosing. These effects may persist for varying periods of time after dosing. Patients who have taken butorphanol should not drive or operate dangerous machinery for at least 1 hour and until the effects of the drug are no longer present.

Drug Interactions

➤*CNS depressants:* Concurrent use of butorphanol with central nervous system depressants (eg, alcohol, barbiturates, tranquilizers, antihistamines) may result in increased central nervous system depressant effects. When used concurrently with such drugs, the dose of butorphanol should be the smallest effective dose and the frequency of dosing reduced as much as possible when administered concomitantly with drugs that potentiate the action of opioids.

Adverse Reactions

The most frequently reported adverse experiences across all clinical trials with butorphanol tartrate were somnolence (43%), dizziness (19%), nausea and/or vomiting (13%).

The following adverse experiences were reported at a frequency of 1% or greater, and were considered to be probably related to the use of butorphanol:

➤*Cardiovascular:* Vasodilation, palpitations.

➤*CNS:* Anxiety, confusion, dizziness, euphoria, floating feeling, insomnia, nervousness, paresthesia, somnolence, tremor.

➤*Dermatologic:* Sweating/clammy, pruritus.

➤*GI:* Anorexia, constipation, dry mouth, nausea or vomiting, stomach pain.

➤*Respiratory:* Bronchitis, cough, dyspnea, epistaxis, nasal congestion, nasal irritation, pharyngitis, rhinitis, sinus congestion, sinusitis, upper respiratory tract infection.

➤*Special senses:* Blurred vision, ear pain, tinnitus, unpleasant taste.

➤*Miscellaneous:* Asthenia/lethargy, headache, sensation of heat.

➤*The following adverse experiences were reported with a frequency of less than 1% in clinical trials and were considered to be probably related to the use of butorphanol:*

Cardiovascular – Hypotension, syncope.

CNS – Abnormal dreams, agitation, dysphoria, hallucinations, hostility, withdrawal symptoms.

Dermatologic – Rash/hives.

GU – Impaired urination.

➤*Postmarketing:* Postmarketing experience with butorphanol tartrate injection and nasal spray has shown an adverse event profile similar to that seen during the premarketing evaluation of butorphanol by all routes of administration. Adverse experiences that were associated with the use of butorphanol tartrate and that are not listed above have been chosen for inclusion below because of their seriousness, frequency of reporting, or probably relationship to butorphanol. Because they are reported voluntarily from a population of unknown size, estimates of frequency cannot be made. These adverse experiences include apnea, convulsion, delusion, drug dependence, excessive drug effect associated with transient difficulty speaking or executing purposeful movements, overdose, and vertigo. Reports of butorphanol overdose with fatal outcomes have usually but not always been associated with ingestion of multiple drugs.

Overdosage

➤*Symptoms:* The clinical manifestations of overdose are those of opioid drugs in general. Consequences of overdose vary with the amount of butorphanol ingested and individual response to the effects of opiates. The most serious symptoms are hypoventilation, cardiovascular insufficiency, coma, and death. Butorphanol overdose may be associated with ingestion of multiple drugs.

Overdose can occur due to accidental or intentional misuse of butorphanol, especially in young children who may gain access to the drug in the home.

➤*Treatment:* The management of suspected butorphanol overdosage includes maintenance of adequate ventilation, peripheral perfusion, normal body temperature, and protection of the airway. Patients should be under continuous observation with adequate serial measures of mental state, responsiveness and vital signs. Oxygen and ventilatory assistance should be available with continual monitoring by pulse oximetry if indicated. In the presence of coma, placement of an artificial airway may be required. An adequate intravenous portal should be maintained to facilitate treatment of hypotension associated with vasodilation.

The use of a specific opioid antagonist such as naloxone should be considered. As the duration of butorphanol action usually exceeds the duration of action of naloxone, repeated dosing with naloxone may be required.

In managing cases of suspected butorphanol overdose, the possibility of multiple drug ingestion should always be considered.

Patient Information

Drowsiness and dizziness related to the use of butorphanol may impair mental and/or physical abilities required for the performance of potentially hazardous tasks (eg, driving, operating machinery).

Alcohol should not be consumed while using butorphanol. Concurrent use of butorphanol with drugs that affect the central nervous system (eg, alcohol, barbiturates, tranquilizers, antihistamines) may result in increased central nervous system depressant effects such as drowsiness, dizziness and impaired mental function.

BUTORPHANOL TARTRATE — INTRANASAL

Refer to the general discussion in the Opioid Agonist-Antagonist Analgesic introduction.

Indications

Management of pain when the use of an opioid analgesic is appropriate.

Administration and Dosage

Factors to be considered in determining the dose are age, body weight, physical status, underlying pathological condition, use of other drugs, type of anesthesia to be used, and surgical procedure involved. Use in the elderly, patients with hepatic or renal disease or in labor requires extra caution. The following doses are for patients who do not have impaired hepatic or renal function and who are not on CNS active agents.

➤*Use for pain:* The usual recommended dose is 1 mg (1 spray in 1 nostril). Adherence to this dose reduces the incidence of drowsiness and dizziness. If adequate pain relief is not achieved within 60 to 90 minutes, an additional 1 mg dose may be given.

The initial 2 dose sequence outlined above may be repeated in 3 to 4 hours as required after the second dose of the sequence.

Depending on the severity of the pain, an initial dose of 2 mg (1 spray in each nostril) may be used in patients who will be able to remain recumbent in the event drowsiness or dizziness occur. In such patients single additional 2 mg doses should not be given for 3 to 4 hours.

➤*Use in balanced anesthesia:* Use is not recommended because it has not been studied in induction or maintenance of anesthesia.

➤*Use in labor:* Use is not recommended as it has not been studied in labor.

➤*Individualization of dosage:* Use of butorphanol in geriatric patients, patients with renal impairment, patients with hepatic impairment, and during labor requires extra caution.

The initial dose sequence in elderly patients and patients with renal or hepatic impairment should be limited to 1 mg followed, if needed, by 1 mg in 90 to 120 minutes. The repeat dose sequence in these patients should be determined by the patient's response rather than at fixed times but will generally be no less than at 6-hour intervals.

➤*Storage/Stability:* Store at 25°C (77°F) controlled room temperature. Parenteral drug products should be inspected visually for particulate matter and discoloration prior to administration, whenever solution and container permit.

Actions

➤*Pharmacology:* Butorphanol is a mixed agonist-antagonist with low intrinsic activity at receptors of the µ-opioid type (morphine-like). It is also an agonist at κ-opioid receptors.

Its interactions with these receptors in the central nervous system apparently mediate most of its pharmacologic effects, including analgesia.

In addition to analgesia, CNS effects include depression of spontaneous respiratory activity and cough, stimulation of the emetic center, miosis and sedation. Effects possibly mediate by non-CNS mechanisms include alteration in cardiovascular resistance and capacitance, bronchomotor tone, gastrointestinal secretory and motor activity and bladder sphincter activity.

In an animal model, the dose of the butorphanol tartrate required to antagonize morphine analgesia by 50% was similar to that for nalorphine, less than that for pentazocine and more than that for naloxone.

In human studies of butorphanol, sedation is commonly noted at doses of 0.5 mg or more. Narcosis is produced by 10 to 12 mg doses of butorphanol administered over 10 to 15 minutes intravenously.

Butorphanol, like other mixed agonist-antagonists with a high affinity for the kappa receptor, may produce unpleasant psychotomimetic effects in some individuals.

Nausea and/or vomiting may be produced by doses of 1 mg or more administered by any route.

In human studies involving individuals without significant respiratory dysfunction, 2 mg of butorphanol IV and 10 mg of morphine sulfate IV depressed respiration to a comparable degree. At higher doses, the magnitude of respiratory depression with butorphanol is not appreciably increased; however, the duration of respiratory depression is longer. Respiratory depression noted after administration of butorphanol to humans by any route is reversed by treatment with naloxone, a specific opioid antagonist. As the duration of butorphanol action usually exceeds the duration of action of naloxone, repeated dosing with naloxone may be required.

Butorphanol tartrate demonstrates antitussive effects in animals at doses less than those required for analgesia.

Hemodynamic changes noted during cardiac catheterization in patients receiving single 0.025 mg/kg intravenous doses of butorphanol have included increases in pulmonary artery pressure, wedge pressure and vascular resistance, increases in left ventricular and diastolic pressure and in systemic arterial pressure.

Pharmacodynamics – The analgesic effect of butorphanol is influenced by the route of administration. Onset of analgesia is within 15 minutes for the nasal spray dose.

Peak analgesic activity occurs within 1 to 2 hours following the nasal spray administration.

The duration of analgesia varies depending on the pain model as well as the route of administration. Compared to the injectable form and other drugs in this class, butorphanol tartrate nasal spray has a longer duration of action (4 to 5 hours).

➤*Pharmacokinetics:*

Absorption/Distribution – After nasal administration, mean peak blood levels of 0.9 to 1.04 ng/mL occur at 30 to 60 minutes after a 1 mg dose (see below). The absolute bioavailability of butorphanol tartrate is 60% to 70% and is unchanged in patients with allergic rhinitis. In patients using a nasal vasoconstrictor (oxymetazoline) the fraction of the dose absorbed was unchanged, but the rate of absorption was slowed. The peak plasma concentrations were approximately half those achieved in the absence of the vasoconstrictor.

Serum protein binding is independent of concentration over the range achieved in clinical practice (up to 7 ng/mL) with a bound fraction of approximately 80%.

Mean Pharmacokinetic Parameters of Butorphanol in Younger and Elderly Subjects[a]

	IV		Nasal	
Parameters	Younger	Elderly	Younger	Elderly
t_{max}[b] (h)			0.62 (0.32)[e] (0.15 to 1.5)[g]	1.03 (0.74) (0.25 to 3)
C_{max}[c] (ng/mL)			1.04 (0.4) (0.35 to 1.97)	0.9 (0.57) (0.1 to 2.68)
AUC (inf)[d] (ng•h/mL)	7.24 (1.57) (4.4 to 9.77)	8.71 (2.02) (4.76 to 13.03)	4.93 (1.24) (2.16 to 7.27)	5.24 (2.27) (0.3 to 10.34)
Half-life (h)	4.56 (1.67) (2.06 to 8.7)	5.61 (1.36) (3.25 to 8.79)	4.74 (1.57) (2.89 to 8.79)	6.56 (1.51) (3.75 to 9.17)
Absolute bioavailability (%)			69 (16) (44 to 113)	61 (25) (3 to 121)
Volume of distribution[f] (L)	487 (155) (305 to 901)	552 (124) (305 to 737)		
Total body clearance (L/h)	99 (23) (70 to 154)	82 (21) (52 to 143)		

[a] Younger subjects (n = 24) are from 20 to 40 years old and elderly (n = 24) are greater than 65 years of age.
[b] Time to peak plasma concentration.
[c] Peak plasma concentration normalized to 1 mg dose.
[d] Area under the plasma concentration time curve after a 1 mg dose.
[e] Mean (1 SD).
[f] Derived from IV data.
[g] (range of observed values)

Dose proportionality for butorphanol tartrate nasal spray has been determined at steady state in doses up to 4 mg at 6-hour intervals. Steady state is achieved within 2 days. The mean peak plasma concentration at steady state was 1.8-fold (maximal 3-fold) following a single dose.

The drug is transported across the blood:brain and placental barriers and into human milk.

Metabolism/Excretion – Butorphanol is extensively metabolized in the liver. Metabolism is qualitatively and quantitatively similar following intravenous, intramuscular, or nasal administration. Oral bioavailability is only 5% to 17% because of extensive first-pass metabolism of butorphanol.

The major metabolite of butorphanol is hydroxybutorphanol, while norbutorphanol is produced in small amounts. Both have been detected in plasma following administration of butorphanol, with norbutorphanol present at trace levels at most time points. The elimination half-life of hydroxybutorphanol is about 18 hours and, as a consequence, considerable accumulation (approximately 5-fold) occurs when butorphanol is dosed to steady state (1 mg transnasally every 6 hours for 5 days).

Elimination occurs by urine and fecal excretion. When 3H labeled butorphanol is administered to healthy subjects, most (70% to 80%) of the dose is recovered in the urine, while approximately 15% is recovered in the feces.

About 5% of the dose is recovered in the urine as butorphanol. Forty-nine percent is eliminated in the urine as hydroxybutorphanol. Less than 5% is excreted in the urine as norbutorphanol.

Special populations –

Renal function impairment: In renally impaired patients with creatinine clearances less than 30 mL/min, the elimination half-life is approximately doubled and the total body clearance is approximately one half (10.5 hours [clearance 150 L/hr] as compared to 5.8 hours [clearance 260 L/hr] in healthy subjects). No effect was observed on C_{max} or t_{max} after a single dose.

Hepatic function impairment: After intravenous administration to patients with hepatic impairment, the elimination half-life of butorphanol was approximately tripled and total body clearance was approximately one-half (half-life 16.8 hours, clearance 92 L/hr) compared to healthy subjects (half-life 4.8 hours, clearance 175 L/hr). The exposure of hepatically impaired patients to butorphanol was significantly greater (about 2-fold) than that in healthy subjects. Similar results were seen after nasal administration. No effect on C_{max} or t_{max} was observed after a single intranasal dose.

Elderly: Butorphanol pharmacokinetics in the elderly differ from younger patients. The mean absolute bioavailability of butorphanol tartrate in elderly women (48%) was less than that in elderly men (75%), younger men (68%) or younger women (70%). Elimination half-life is increased in the elderly (6.6 hours as opposed to 4.7 hours in younger subjects).

Contraindications

Hypersensitivity to butorphanol tartrate or the preservative benzethonium chloride.

BUTORPHANOL TARTRATE — INTRANASAL

Warnings

➤*Patients dependent on narcotics:* Because of its opioid antagonist properties, butorphanol is not recommended for use in patients dependent on narcotics. Such patients should have an adequate period of withdrawal from opioid drugs prior to beginning butorphanol therapy. In patients taking opioid analgesics chronically, butorphanol has precipitated withdrawal symptoms such as anxiety, agitation, mood changes, hallucinations, dysphoria, weakness and diarrhea.

Because of the difficulty in assessing opioid tolerance in patients who have recently received repeated doses of narcotic analgesic medication, caution should be used in the administration of butorphanol to such patients.

➤*Renal/Hepatic function impairment:* In patients with hepatic or renal impairment, the initial dose sequence of butorphanol tartrate nasal spray should be limited to 1 mg followed, if needed, by 1 mg in 90 to 120 minutes. The repeat dose sequence in these patients should be determined by the patient's response rather than at fixed times but will generally be at intervals of no less than 6 hours.

➤*Fertility impairment:* Rats treated orally with 160 mg/kg/day (944 mg/m^2) had a reduced pregnancy rate. However, a similar effect was not observed with a 2.5 mg/kg/day (14.75 mg/m^2) subcutaneous dose.

➤*Elderly:* See Administration and Dosage for more information.

Due to changes in clearance, the mean half-life of butorphanol is increased by 25% (to over 6 hours) in patients over the age of 65 years. Elderly patients may be more sensitive to the side effects of butorphanol. In clinical studies of butorphanol tartrate nasal spray, elderly patients had an increased frequency of headache, dizziness, drowsiness, vertigo, constipation, nausea and/or vomiting, and nasal congestion compared with younger patients. There are insufficient efficacy data for patients greater than or equal to 65 years to determine whether they respond differently from younger patients.

Butorphanol and its metabolites are known to be substantially excreted by the kidney, and the risk of toxic reactions to this drug may be greater in patients with impaired renal function. Because elderly patients are more likely to have decreased renal function, care should be taken in dose selection.

➤*Pregnancy: Category C.* Pregnant rats treated subcutaneously with butorphanol at 1 mg/kg (5.9 mg/m^2) had a higher frequency of stillbirths than controls. Butorphanol at 30 mg/kg/oral (360 mg/m^2) and 60 mg/kg/oral (720 mg/m^2) also showed higher incidences of post-implantation loss in rabbits.

There are no adequate and well controlled studies of butorphanol tartrate in pregnant women before 37 weeks of gestation. Butorphanol tartrate should be used during pregnancy only if the potential benefit justifies the potential risk to the infant.

Labor and delivery – Butorphanol tartrate nasal spray is not recommended during labor or delivery because there is no clinical experience with its use in this setting.

➤*Lactation:* Although there is no clinical experience with the use of butorphanol tartrate nasal spray in nursing mothers, it should be assumed that butorphanol will appear in the milk following the nasal route of administration.

➤*Children:* Butorphanol is not recommended for use in patients below 18 years of age because safety and efficacy have not been established in the population.

Precautions

➤*Head injury and increased intracranial pressure:* As with other opioids, the use of butorphanol in patients with head injury may be associated with carbon dioxide retention and secondary elevation of cerebrospinal fluid pressure, drug-induced miosis, and alterations in mental state that would obscure the interpretation of the clinical course of patients with head injuries. In such patients, butorphanol should be used only if the benefits of use outweigh the potential risks.

➤*Respiratory depression:* Butorphanol may produce respiratory depression, especially in patients receiving other CNS active agents, or patients suffering from CNS diseases or respiratory impairment.

➤*Cardiovascular effects:* Because butorphanol may increase the work of the heart, especially the pulmonary circuit, the use of butorphanol in patients with acute myocardial infarction, ventricular dysfunction, or coronary insufficiency should be limited to those situations where the benefits clearly outweigh the risk.

Hypotension associated with syncope during the first hour of dosing with butorphanol tartrate nasal spray has been reported rarely, particularly in patients with a history of similar reactions to opioid analgesics. Therefore, patients should be advised to avoid activities with potential risks.

Severe hypertension has been reported rarely during butorphanol therapy. In such cases, butorphanol should be discontinued and the hypertension treated with antihypertensive drugs. In patients who are not opioid dependent, naloxone has also been reported to be effective.

➤*Hazardous tasks:* Opioid analgesics, including butorphanol, impair the mental and physical abilities required for the performance of potentially dangerous tasks such as driving a car or operating machinery. Effects such as drowsiness or dizziness can appear, usually within the first hour after dosing. These effects may persist for varying periods of time after dosing. Patients who have taken butorphanol should not drive or operate dangerous machinery for at least 1 hour and until the effects of the drug are no longer present.

Alcohol should not be consumed while using butorphanol. Concurrent use of butorphanol with drugs that effect the central nervous system (eg, alcohol, barbiturates, tranquilizers, antihistamines) may result in increased central nervous system depressant effects such as drowsiness, dizziness, and impaired mental function.

Butorphanol is one of a class of drugs known to be abused and thus should be handled accordingly.

Patients should be instructed on the proper use of butorphanol tartrate.

➤*Drug abuse and dependence:* Butorphanol tartrate, by all routes of administration, has been associated with episodes of abuse. Of the cases received, there were more reports of abuse with the nasal spray formulation than with the injectable formulation.

Physical dependence, tolerance, and withdrawal – Prolonged, continuous use of butorphanol tartrate may result in physical dependence or tolerance (a decrease in response to a given dose). Abrupt cessation of use by patients with physical dependence may result in symptoms of withdrawal.

Clinical trial experience – In all clinical trials, less than 1% of patients using butorphanol tartrate nasal spray had experiences that suggested the development of physical dependence or tolerance. Much of this information is based on experience with patients who did not have prolonged continuous exposure to butorphanol tartrate nasal spray. However, in 1 controlled clinical trial where patients with chronic pain from nonmalignant disease were treated with butorphanol tartrate nasal spray (n = 303) or placebo (n = 99) for up to 6 months, overuse (which may suggest the development of tolerance) was reported in nine (2.9%) patients receiving butorphanol tartrate nasal spray and no patients receiving placebo. Probable withdrawal symptoms were reported in eight (2.6%) patients using butorphanol tartrate nasal spray and no patients receiving placebo in the chronic nonmalignant pain study. Most of these patients abruptly discontinued butorphanol tartrate nasal spray after extended use or high doses. Symptoms suggestive of withdrawal included anxiety, agitation, tremulousness, diarrhea, chills, sweats, insomnia, confusion, incoordination, and hallucinations.

Postmarketing experience – Butorphanol tartrate has been associated with episodes of abuse and dependence. Of the cases received, there were more reports of abuse with the nasal spray formulation than with the injectable formulation.

Drug Interactions

➤*CNS depressants:* Concurrent use of butorphanol with central nervous system depressants (eg, alcohol, barbiturates, tranquilizers, and antihistamines) may result in increased central nervous system depressant effects. When used concurrently with such drugs, the dose of butorphanol should be the smallest effective dose and the frequency of dosing reduced as much as possible when administered concomitantly with drugs that potentiate the action of opioids.

➤*Sumatriptan:* In healthy volunteers, the pharmacokinetics of a 1 mg dose of butorphanol administered as butorphanol tartrate nasal spray were not affected by the coadministration of a single 6 mg subcutaneous dose of sumatriptan. However, in another study in healthy volunteers, the pharmacokinetics of butorphanol were significantly altered (29% decrease in AUC and 38% decrease in C_{max}) when a 1 mg dose of butorphanol tartrate nasal spray was administered 1 minute after a 20 mg dose of sumatriptan nasal spray. (The 2 drugs were administered in opposite nostrils.) When the butorphanol tartrate nasal spray was administered 30 minutes after the sumatriptan nasal spray, the AUC of butorphanol increased 11% and C_{max} decreased 18%.

In neither case were the pharmacokinetics of sumatriptan affected by coadministration with butorphanol tartrate nasal spray. These results suggest that the analgesic effect of butorphanol tartrate nasal spray may be diminished when it is administered shortly after sumatriptan nasal spray, but by 30 minutes any such reduction in effect should be minimal.

The safety of using butorphanol tartrate nasal spray and sumatriptan nasal spray during the same episode of migraine has not been established. However, it should be noted that both products are capable of producing transient increases in blood pressure.

➤*Nasal vasoconstrictors:* The fraction of butorphanol tartrate absorbed is unaffected by the concomitant administration of a nasal vasoconstrictor (oxymetazoline), but the rate of absorption is decreased. Therefore, a slower onset can be anticipated if butorphanol tartrate is administered concomitantly with, or immediately following, a nasal vasoconstrictor.

Adverse Reactions

The most frequently reported adverse experiences across all clinical trials with butorphanol tartrate injection and nasal spray were somnolence (43%), dizziness (19%), nausea and/or vomiting (13%). In long-term trials with butorphanol tartrate nasal spray only, nasal congestion (13%) and insomnia (11%) were frequently reported.

The following adverse experiences were reported at a frequency of 1% or greater, and were considered to be probably related to the use of butorphanol.

➤*Cardiovascular:* Vasodilation, palpitations.

➤*CNS:* Anxiety, confusion, dizziness, euphoria, floating feeling, insomnia, nervousness, paresthesia, somnolence, tremor.

➤*Dermatologic:* Sweating/clammy, pruritus.

➤*GI:* Anorexia, constipation, dry mouth, nausea and/or vomiting, stomach pain.

➤*Respiratory:* Bronchitis, cough, dyspnea, epistaxis, nasal congestion, nasal irritation, pharyngitis, rhinitis, sinus congestion, sinusitis, upper respiratory tract infection.

➤*Special senses:* Blurred vision, ear pain, tinnitus, unpleasant taste.

BUTORPHANOL TARTRATE — INTRANASAL

➤*Miscellaneous:* Asthenia/lethargy, headache, sensation of heat.

➤*Adverse experiences reported with a frequency of less than 1%:* The following adverse experiences were reported with a frequency of less than 1%, in clinical trials or from postmarketing experience, and were considered to be probably related to the use of butorphanol.

Cardiovascular – Hypotension, syncope.

CNS – Abnormal dreams, agitation, dysphoria, hallucinations, hostility, withdrawal symptoms.

Dermatologic – Rash/hives.

GU – Impaired urination.

➤*Adverse reactions (less than 1% frequency and postmarketing experiences):* The following infrequent additional adverse experiences were reported in a frequency of less than 1% of the patients studied in short-term butorphanol tartrate nasal spray trials and under circumstances where the association between these events and butorphanol administration is unknown. They are being listed as altering information for the physician.

Cardiovascular – Chest pain, hypertension, tachycardia.

CNS – Depression.

Respiratory – Shallow breathing.

Miscellaneous – Edema.

➤*Postmarketing experience:* Postmarketing experience with butorphanol tartrate nasal spray and butorphanol tartrate injection has shown an adverse event profile similar to that seen during the premarketing evaluation of butorphanol by all routes of administration. Adverse experiences that were associated with the use of butorphanol tartrate nasal spray or butorphanol tartrate injection and that are not listed above have been chosen for inclusion below because of their seriousness, frequency of reporting, or probable relationship to butorphanol. Because they are reported voluntarily from a population of unknown size, estimates of frequency cannot be made. These adverse experiences include apnea, convulsion, delusion, drug dependence, excessive drug effect associated with transient difficulty speaking and/or executing purposeful movements, overdose, and vertigo. Reports of butorphanol overdose with a fatal outcome have usually but not always been associated with ingestion of multiple drugs.

Overdosage

➤*Symptoms:* The clinical manifestations of overdose are those of opioid drugs, the most serious of which are hypoventilation, cardiovascular insufficiency, coma, and death. Butorphanol overdose may be associated with ingestion of multiple drugs.

Consequences of overdose vary with the amount of butorphanol ingested and individual response to the effects of opiates.

Overdose can occur due to accidental or intentional misuse of butorphanol, especially in young children who may gain access to the drug in the home.

➤*Treatment:* The management of suspected butorphanol overdosage includes maintenance of adequate ventilation, peripheral perfusion, normal body temperature, and protection of the airway. Patients should be under continuous observation with adequate serial measures of mental state, responsiveness and vital signs. Oxygen and ventilatory assistance should be available with continual monitoring by pulse oximetry if indicated. In the presence of coma, placement of an artificial airway may be required. An adequate intravenous portal should be maintained to facilitate treatment of hypotension associated with vasodilation.

The use of a specific opioid antagonist such as naloxone should be considered. As the duration of butorphanol action usually exceeds the duration of action of naloxone, repeated dosing with naloxone may be required.

In managing cases of suspected butorphanol overdosage, the possibility of multiple drug ingestion should always be considered.

Patient Information

Drowsiness and dizziness related to the use of butorphanol may impair mental and/or physical abilities required for the performance of potentially hazardous tasks (eg, driving, operating machinery).

Alcohol should not be consumed while using butorphanol. Concurrent use of butorphanol with drugs that affect the central nervous system (eg, alcohol, barbiturates, tranquilizers, antihistamines) may result in increased central nervous system depressant effects such as drowsiness, dizziness and impaired mental function.

Patients should be instructed on the proper use of butorphanol tartrate.

NALBUPHINE HYDROCHLORIDE

Rx	**Nalbuphine Hydrochloride** (Various, eg, Hospira)	**Injection:** 10 mg/mL	In 1 and 10 mL vials.
Rx	**Nubain** (Endo)		In 1 mL amps[a] and 10 mL vials. Parabens.
Rx	**Nalbuphine Hydrochloride** (Various, eg, Hospira)	**Injection:** 20 mg/mL	In 1 and 10 mL vials.
Rx	**Nubain** (Endo)		In 1 mL amps[a] and 10 mL vials. Parabens.

[a] Available as sulfite/paraben-free.

NALBUPHINE HYDROCHLORIDE — INJECTION

Refer to the general discussion in the Opioid Agonist-Antagonist Analgesic introduction.

Indications

➤*Pain:* For the relief of moderate to severe pain.

➤*Anesthesia:* For use as a supplement to balanced anesthesia, for preoperative and postoperative analgesia, and for obstetrical analgesia during labor and delivery.

➤*Unlabeled uses:* For the prevention and treatment of intrathecal morphine-induced pruritus after cesarean delivery.

Administration and Dosage

➤*Approved by the FDA:* May 15, 1979.

➤*Pain:*

Adult dose – 10 mg for a 70 kg individual administered subcutaneously, intramuscularly, or IV. May repeat the dose every 3 to 6 hours as necessary.

Nontolerant patients – Recommended single maximum dose is 20 mg with a maximum total daily dose of 160 mg.

➤*Supplement to anesthesia:*

Induction doses – 0.3 to 3 mg/kg IV administered over a 10 to 15 minute period.

Maintenance dose – 0.25 to 0.5 mg/kg in a single IV administration.

➤*Patients dependent on opioids:* Patients who have been taking opioids chronically may experience withdrawal symptoms upon the administration of nalbuphine. If unduly troublesome, opioid withdrawal symptoms may be controlled by the slow IV administration of small increments of morphine until relief occurs. If the previous analgesic was morphine, meperidine, codeine, or another opioid with similar duration of activity, 25% of the anticipated dose of nalbuphine may be administered initially and the patient observed for signs of withdrawal (ie, abdominal cramps, nausea and vomiting, lacrimation, rhinorrhea, anxiety, restlessness, elevation of temperature, piloerection). If untoward symptoms do not occur, progressively larger doses may be tried at appropriate intervals until the desired level of analgesia is obtained.

➤*Renal/Hepatic function impairment:* Use nalbuphine with caution in patients with renal or liver dysfunction and administer in reduced amounts.

➤*Incompatibilities:* Nalbuphine is physically incompatible with nafcillin and ketorolac.

➤*Storage/Stability:* Store at 25°C (77°F); excursions permitted to 15° to 30°C (59° to 86°F). Protect from excessive light. Store in carton until contents have been used.

Actions

➤*Pharmacology:* Nalbuphine is a synthetic opioid agonist-antagonist analgesic of the phenanthrene series. It is related chemically to both the widely used opioid antagonist, naloxone, and the potent opioid analgesic, oxymorphone.

Nalbuphine is a potent analgesic. Its analgesic potency is essentially equivalent to that of morphine on a milligram basis. The opioid antagonist activity of nalbuphine is one-fourth as potent as nalorphine and 10 times that of pentazocine. Receptor studies show that nalbuphine binds to mu, kappa, and delta receptors, but not to sigma receptors. Nalbuphine is primarily a kappa agonist/partial mu antagonist analgesic.

Nalbuphine may produce the same degree of respiratory depression as equianalgesic doses of morphine. However, nalbuphine exhibits a ceiling effect such that increases in dose greater than 30 mg do not produce further respiratory depression.

Nalbuphine by itself has potent opioid antagonist activity at doses equal to or lower than its analgesic dose. When administered following or concurrent with mu agonist opioid analgesics (eg, morphine, oxymorphone, fentanyl), nalbuphine may partially reverse or block opioid-induced respiratory depression from the mu agonist analgesic. Nalbuphine may precipitate withdrawal in patients dependent on opioid drugs. Use nalbuphine with caution in patients who have been receiving mu opioid analgesics on a regular basis.

➤*Pharmacokinetics:* The onset of action of nalbuphine occurs within 2 to 3 minutes after IV administration, and in less than 15 minutes following subcutaneous or intramuscular injection. The plasma half-life of nalbuphine is 5 hours, and in clinical studies the duration of analgesic activity has been reported to range from 3 to 6 hours. Nalbuphine is metabolized in the liver and excreted by the kidneys.

Contraindications

Hypersensitivity to nalbuphine, or to any of the other ingredients in the product.

Warnings

➤*Administration:* Nalbuphine should be given as a supplement to general anesthesia only by persons specifically trained in the use of IV anesthetics

NALBUPHINE HYDROCHLORIDE — INJECTION

and management of the respiratory effects of potent opioids. Naloxone, resuscitative and intubation equipment, and oxygen should be readily available.

➤*Head injury and increased intracranial pressure:* The possible respiratory depressant effects and the potential of potent analgesics to elevate cerebrospinal fluid pressure (resulting from vasodilation following CO_2 retention) may be exaggerated markedly in the presence of head injury, intracranial lesions, or a preexisting increase in intracranial pressure. Furthermore, potent analgesics may produce effects that may obscure the clinical course of patients with head injuries. Therefore, use nalbuphine in these circumstances only when essential, and then administer with extreme caution.

➤*Renal/Hepatic function impairment:* Because nalbuphine is metabolized in the liver and excreted by the kidneys, use nalbuphine with caution in patients with renal or liver dysfunction and administer in reduced amounts.

➤*Mutagenesis:* Nalbuphine induced an increased frequency of mutation in mouse lymphoma cells.

➤*Pregnancy: Category B.* (*Category D* in prolonged use or in high doses at term). Safe use of nalbuphine in pregnancy has not been established. Although animal reproductive studies have not revealed teratogenic or embryotoxic effects, administer nalbuphine to pregnant women only if clearly needed, if the potential benefit outweighs the risk to the fetus, and if appropriate measures such as fetal monitoring are taken to detect and manage any potential adverse effect on the fetus.

Neonatal body weight and survival rates were reduced at birth and during lactation when nalbuphine was administered subcutaneously to female and male rats prior to mating and throughout gestation and lactation or to pregnant rats during the last third of the gestation period and throughout lactation at doses approximately 4 times the maximum recommended human dose.

Severe fetal bradycardia has been reported when nalbuphine is administered during labor. Naloxone may reverse these effects. Although there are no reports of fetal bradycardia earlier in pregnancy, it is possible that this may occur.

Labor and delivery – The placental transfer of nalbuphine is high, rapid, and variable with a maternal to fetal ratio ranging from 1:0.37 to 1:6. Fetal and neonatal adverse effects that have been reported following the administration of nalbuphine to the mother during labor include fetal bradycardia, respiratory depression at birth, apnea, cyanosis, and hypotonia. Maternal administration of naloxone during labor has normalized these effects in some cases. Severe and prolonged fetal bradycardia has been reported. Permanent neurological damage attributed to fetal bradycardia has occurred. A sinusoidal fetal heart rate pattern associated with the use of nalbuphine also has been reported. Use nalbuphine during labor and delivery only if clearly indicated and only if the potential benefit outweighs the risk to the infant. Monitor newborns for respiratory depression, apnea, bradycardia, and arrhythmias if nalbuphine has been used.

➤*Lactation:* Limited data suggest that nalbuphine is excreted in maternal milk but only in a small amount (less than 1% of the administered dose) and with a clinically insignificant effect. Exercise caution when nalbuphine is administered to a nursing woman.

➤*Children:* Safety and effectiveness in pediatric patients below the age of 18 years have not been established.

Precautions

➤*Respiratory depression:* At the usual adult dose of 10 mg/70 kg, nalbuphine causes some respiratory depression approximately equal to that produced by equal doses of morphine. However, in contrast to morphine, respiratory depression is not increased appreciably with higher doses of nalbuphine. Respiratory depression induced by nalbuphine may be reversed by naloxone when indicated. Administer nalbuphine with caution at low doses to patients with impaired respiration (eg, from other medication, uremia, bronchial asthma, severe infection, cyanosis, or respiratory obstructions).

➤*Myocardial infarction:* Use with caution in patients with myocardial infarction who have nausea or vomiting.

➤*Biliary tract surgery:* Use with caution in patients about to undergo surgery of the biliary tract since it may cause spasm of the sphincter of Oddi.

➤*Cardiovascular effects:* During evaluation of nalbuphine in anesthesia, a higher incidence of bradycardia has been reported in patients who did not receive atropine preoperatively.

➤*Drug abuse and dependence:* Observe caution in prescribing nalbuphine to emotionally unstable patients or to individuals with a history of opioid abuse. Closely supervise such patients when long-term therapy is contemplated.

There have been reports of abuse and dependence associated with nalbuphine among health care providers, patients, and bodybuilders. There have been reported instances of psychological and physical dependence and tolerance in patients abusing nalbuphine. Individuals with a prior history of opioid or other substance abuse or dependence may be at greater risk in responding to reinforcing properties of nalbuphine.

Opioid withdrawal effects – Abrupt discontinuation of nalbuphine following prolonged use has been followed by symptoms of opioid withdrawal (ie, abdominal cramps, nausea and vomiting, rhinorrhea, lacrimation, restlessness, anxiety, elevated temperature, piloerection).

➤*Hazardous tasks:* Nalbuphine may impair the mental or physical abilities required for the performance of potentially dangerous tasks such as driving a car or operating machinery. Therefore, administer nalbuphine with caution to ambulatory patients who should be warned to avoid such hazards.

Drug Interactions

Nalbuphine Drug Interactions

Precipitant Drug	Object Drug*		Description
Cimetidine	Nalbuphine	↑	The actions of nalbuphine may be enhanced, resulting in toxicity. If significant CNS depression develops, withdraw the drugs.
Nalbuphine	Barbiturate anesthetics (ie, thiopental)	↑	The dose required to induce anesthesia may need to be reduced in the presence of nalbuphine. Monitor for additive pharmacologic effects such as respiratory depression.
Nalbuphine	CNS depressants (ie, opioid analgesics, general anesthetics, phenothiazines, tranquilizers, sedatives, hypnotics, alcohol)	↑	Concomitant use may exhibit additive CNS depression. When such combined therapy is used, reduce the dose of one or both agents.
CNS depressants (ie, opioid analgesics, general anesthetics, phenothiazines, tranquilizers, sedatives)	Nalbuphine		

* ↑ = Object drug increased.

➤*Drug/Lab test interactions:* Nalbuphine may interfere with enzymatic methods for the detection of opioids depending on the specificity/sensitivity of the test. Please consult the test manufacturer for specific details.

Adverse Reactions

➤*Hypersensitivity:* Anaphylactic/anaphylactoid and other serious hypersensitivity reactions have been reported. These reactions may include shock, respiratory distress, respiratory arrest, bradycardia, cardiac arrest, hypotension, or laryngeal edema. Other allergic-type reactions reported include stridor, bronchospasm, wheezing, edema, rash, pruritus, nausea, vomiting, diaphoresis, weakness, and shakiness.

➤*Cardiovascular:* Bradycardia, hypertension, hypotension, tachycardia (1% or less).

➤*CNS:* Sedation (36%); dizziness/vertigo (5%); headache (3%); confusion, crying, depression, dysphoria, euphoria, faintness, feeling of heaviness, floating, hallucinations, hostility, nervousness, numbness, restlessness, tingling, unreality, unusual dreams (1% or less). The incidence of psychotomimetic effects, such as delusions, depersonalization, dysphoria, hallucinations, and unreality, has been shown to be less than that which occurs with pentazocine.

➤*Dermatologic:* Sweaty/clammy (9%); burning, itching, urticaria (1% or less).

➤*GI:* Nausea/vomiting (6%); dry mouth (4%); bitter taste, cramps, dyspepsia (1% or less).

➤*Respiratory:* Asthma, depression, dyspnea (1% or less).

➤*Miscellaneous:* Blurred vision, flushing and warmth, speech difficulty, urinary urgency (1% or less).

Postmarketing – Other reports include agitation; injection-site reactions such as burning, hot sensations, pain, redness, and swelling; pulmonary edema; seizures.

Overdosage

➤*Symptoms:* The administration of single doses of 72 mg nalbuphine subcutaneously to 8 healthy subjects has been reported to have resulted primarily in symptoms of sleepiness and mild dysphoria.

➤*Treatment:* The immediate IV administration of an opiate antagonist such as naloxone or nalmefene is a specific antidote. Use oxygen, IV fluids, vasopressors, and other supportive measures as indicated.

Patient Information

Nalbuphine is associated with sedation and may impair mental and physical abilities required for the performance of potentially dangerous tasks such as driving a car or operating machinery.

Nalbuphine is to be used as prescribed by a physician. Do not increase dose or frequency without first consulting with a physician since nalbuphine may cause psychological or physical dependence.

The use of nalbuphine with other narcotics may cause signs and symptoms of withdrawal.

Abrupt discontinuation of nalbuphine after prolonged usage may cause signs and symptoms of withdrawal.

PENTAZOCINE

c-iv	**Talwin** (Abbott Hospital Products)	**Injection**: 30 mg (as lactate)/ml	In 10 ml vials[1], 1 ml *Uni-Amps*, 1 ml *Uni-Nest* amps and 1 and 2 ml fill in 2 ml *Carpuject*.[2]

[1] With 2 mg acetone sodium bisulfite and 1 mg methylparaben per ml.

[2] With 1 mg acetone sodium bisulfite.

PENTAZOCINE LACTATE — INJECTION

Refer to the general discussion in the Opioid Agonist-Antagonist Analgesic introduction.

Indications

For the relief of moderate to severe pain. Pentazocine lactate may also be used for preoperative or preanesthetic medication and as a supplement to surgical anesthesia.

Administration and Dosage

➤*Adults, excluding patients in labor:* The recommended single parenteral dose is 30 mg by IM, subcutaneous, or IV route. This may be repeated every 3 to 4 hours. Doses in excess of 30 mg IV or 60 mg IM or subcutaneous are not recommended. Total daily dosage should not exceed 360 mg.

The subcutaneous route of administration should be used only when necessary because of possible severe tissue damage at injection sites (see Warnings). When frequent injections are needed, the drug should be administered intramuscularly. In addition, constant rotation of injection sites (eg, the upper outer quadrants of the buttocks, mid-lateral aspects of the thighs, and the deltoid areas) is essential.

➤*Patients in labor:* A single, IM 30 mg dose has been most commonly administered. An IV 20 mg dose has given adequate pain relief to some patients in labor when contractions become regular, and this dose may be given 2 or 3 times at 2- to 3-hour intervals, as needed.

➤*Children under 12 years of age:* See Warnings for more information.

➤*Incompatibilities:* Pentazocine lactate should not be mixed in the same syringe with soluble barbiturates because precipitation will occur.

Actions

➤*Pharmacology:* Pentazocine lactate is a potent analgesic and 30 mg is usually as effective an analgesic as morphine 10 mg or meperidine 75 mg to 100 mg; however, a few studies suggest the pentazocine lactate to morphine ratio may range from 20 mg to 40 mg pentazocine lactate to 10 mg morphine. The duration of analgesia may sometimes be less than that of morphine. Analgesia usually occurs within 15 to 20 minutes after IM or subcutaneous injection and within 2 to 3 minutes after IV injection. Pentazocine lactate weakly antagonizes the analgesic effects of morphine, meperidine, and phenazocine; in addition, it produces incomplete reversal of cardiovascular, respiratory, and behavioral depression induced by morphine and meperidine. Pentazocine lactate has about 1⁄50 the antagonistic activity of nalorphine. It also has sedative activity.

Contraindications

Hypersensitivity to pentazocine lactate.

Warnings

➤*General information:* In prescribing parenteral pentazocine lactate for chronic use, particularly if the drug is to be self-administered, the physician should take precautions to avoid increases in dose and frequency of injection by the patient.

Just as with all medication, the oral form of pentazocine lactate is preferable for chronic administration.

➤*Tissue damage at injection sites:* Severe sclerosis of the skin, subcutaneous tissues, and underlying muscle have occurred at the injection sites of patients who have received multiple doses of pentazocine lactate. Constant rotation of injection sites is, therefore, essential. In addition, animal studies have demonstrated that pentazocine lactate is not tolerated as well subcutaneously as it is intramuscularly (see Administration and Dosage).

➤*Head injury and increased intracranial pressure:* As in the case of other potent analgesics, the potential of pentazocine lactate injection for elevating cerebrospinal fluid pressure may be attributed to CO_2 retention due to the respiratory depressant effects of the drug. These effects may be markedly exaggerated in the presence of head injury, other intracranial lesions, or a preexisting increase in intracranial pressure. Furthermore, pentazocine lactate can produce effects which may obscure the clinical course of patients with head injuries. In such patients, pentazocine lactate must be used with extreme caution and only if its use is deemed essential.

➤*Acute CNS manifestations:* Patients receiving therapeutic doses of pentazocine have experienced hallucinations (usually visual), disorientation, and confusion which have cleared spontaneously within a period of hours. The mechanism of this reaction is not known. Such patients should be closely observed and vital signs checked. If the drug is reinstituted, it should be done with caution since these acute CNS manifestations may recur.

➤*Myocardial infarction:* Caution should be exercised in the IV use of pentazocine for patients with acute myocardial infarction accompanied by hypertension or left ventricular failure. Data suggest that intravenous administration of pentazocine increases systemic and pulmonary arterial pressure and systemic vascular resistance in patients with acute myocardial infarction.

➤*Renal/Hepatic function impairment:* Although laboratory tests have not indicated that pentazocine lactate causes or increases renal or hepatic impairment, the drug should be administered with caution to patients with such impairment. Extensive liver disease appears to predispose to greater side effects (eg, marked apprehension, anxiety, dizziness, sleepiness) from the usual clinical dose, and may be the result of decreased metabolism of the drug by the liver.

➤*Pregnancy: Category C.* Safe use of pentazocine lactate during pregnancy (other than labor) has not been established. Animal reproduction studies have not demonstrated teratogenic or embryotoxic effects. However, pentazocine lactate should be administered to pregnant patients (other than labor) only when, in the judgment of the physician, the potential benefits outweigh the possible hazards. Patients receiving pentazocine lactate during labor have experienced no adverse effects other than those that occur with commonly used analgesics. Pentazocine lactate should be used with caution in women delivering premature infants.

➤*Children:* Because clinical experience in children under 12 years of age is limited, the use of pentazocine lactate in this age group is not recommended.

Precautions

➤*Biliary surgery:* Narcotic drug products are generally considered to elevate biliary tract pressure for varying periods following their administration. Some evidence suggests that pentazocine may differ from other marketed narcotics in this respect (ie, it causes little or no elevation in biliary tract pressures). The clinical significance of these findings, however, is not yet known.

➤*Respiratory depression:* The possibility that pentazocine lactate may cause respiratory depression should be considered in treatment of patients with bronchial asthma. Pentazocine lactate should be administered only with caution and in low dosage to patients with respiratory depression (eg, from other medication, uremia, or severe infection), severely limited respiratory reserve, obstructive respiratory conditions, or cyanosis.

➤*CNS effect:* Caution should be used when pentazocine lactate is administered to patients prone to seizures; seizures have occurred in a few such patients in association with the use of pentazocine lactate although no cause and effect relationship has been established.

➤*Drug abuse and dependence:* Special care should be exercised in prescribing pentazocine for emotionally unstable patients and for those with a history of drug misuse. Such patients should be closely supervised when more than 4 or 5 days of therapy is contemplated. There have been instances of psychological and physical dependence on pentazocine lactate in patients with such a history and, rarely, in patients without such a history. Extended use of parenteral pentazocine lactate may lead to physical or psychological dependence in some patients. When pentazocine lactate is abruptly discontinued, withdrawal symptoms such as abdominal cramps, elevated temperature, rhinorrhea, restlessness, anxiety, and lacrimation may occur. However, even when these have occurred, discontinuance has been accomplished with minimal difficulty. In the rare patient in whom more than minor difficulty has been encountered, reinstitution of parenteral pentazocine lactate with gradual withdrawal has ameliorated the patient's symptoms. Substituting methadone or other narcotics for pentazocine lactate in the treatment of the pentazocine abstinence syndrome should be avoided. There have been rare reports of possible abstinence syndromes in newborns after prolonged use of pentazocine lactate during pregnancy.

➤*Hazardous tasks:* Since sedation, dizziness, and occasional euphoria have been noted, ambulatory patients should be warned not to operate machinery, drive cars, or unnecessarily expose themselves to hazards.

➤*Sulfite sensitivity:* Some of these products may contain acetone sodium bisulfite, a sulfite that may cause allergic-type reactions including anaphylactic symptoms and life-threatening or less severe asthmatic episodes in certain susceptible people. The overall prevalence of sulfite sensitivity in the general population is unknown and probably low. Sulfite sensitivity is seen more frequently in asthmatic than in nonasthmatic people.

Drug Interactions

Pentazocine Drug Interactions

Precipitant drug	Object drug*		Description
Pentazocine	Alcohol	↑	Due to the potential for increased CNS depressant effects, use cautiously in patients currently receiving pentazocine.
Barbiturate anesthetics	Pentazocine	↑	Barbiturate anesthetics may increase the respiratory and CNS depression of pentazocine because of additive pharmacologic activity.

* ↑ = Object drug increased. ↓ = Object drug decreased.

➤*CNS depressants:* Concomitant use of CNS depressants with parenteral pentazocine lactate may produce additive CNS depression. Adequate equipment and facilities should be available to identify and treat systemic emergencies should they occur.

➤*Patients receiving narcotics:* Pentazocine lactate is a mild narcotic antagonist. Some patients previously given narcotics, including methadone for the daily treatment of narcotic dependence, have experienced withdrawal symptoms after receiving pentazocine lactate.

PENTAZOCINE LACTATE — INJECTION

Adverse Reactions

The most commonly occurring reactions are nausea, dizziness or lightheadedness, vomiting, and euphoria.

➤*Dermatologic:* Soft tissue induration, nodules, and cutaneous depression can occur at injection sites. Ulceration (sloughing) and severe sclerosis of the skin and subcutaneous tissues (and, rarely, underlying muscle) have been reported after multiple doses. Other reported dermatologic reactions include diaphoresis, sting on injection, flushed skin including plethora, dermatitis including pruritus.

➤*Infrequent reactions:*

Cardiovascular – Circulatory depression, shock, hypertension.

CNS – Dizziness, lightheadedness, hallucinations, sedation, euphoria, headache, confusion, disorientation; infrequently weakness, disturbed dreams, insomnia, syncope, visual blurring and focusing difficulty, depression; and rarely tremor, irritability, excitement, tinnitus.

GI – Constipation, dry mouth.

Respiratory – Respiratory depression, dyspnea, transient apnea in a small number of newborn infants whose mothers received pentazocine lactate during labor.

Miscellaneous – Urinary retention, headache, paresthesia, alterations in rate or strength of uterine contractions during labor.

➤*Rare reactions:*

CNS – Muscle tremor, insomnia, disorientation, hallucinations.

GI – Taste alteration, diarrhea and cramps.

Hematologic – Depression of white blood cells (especially granulocytes), which is usually reversible, moderate transient eosinophilia.

Ophthalmic – Blurred vision, nystagmus, diplopia, miosis.

Miscellaneous – other: tachycardia, weakness or faintness, chills, allergic reactions including edema of the face, toxic epidermal necrolysis (see Acute CNS manifestations and Drug abuse under Precautions).

Overdosage

➤*Symptoms:* Clinical experience with pentazocine lactate overdosage has been insufficient to define the signs of this condition.

➤*Treatment:* Oxygen, IV fluids, vasopressors, and other supportive measures should be employed as indicated. Assisted or controlled ventilation should also be considered. For respiratory depression due to overdosage or unusual sensitivity to pentazocine lactate, parenteral naloxone is a specific and effective antagonist.

PENTAZOCINE COMBINATIONS

c-iv	**Talwin Compound** (Sanofi Winthrop)	**Tablets**: 12.5 mg (as hydrochloride) and 325 mg aspirin	White. In 100s.
c-iv	**Pentazocine Hydrochloridel and Acetaminophen** (Watson)	**Tablets**: 25 mg (as hydrochloride) and 650 mg acetaminophen	(396 25 650). Aqua, capsule shape. In 100s, 500s, and 1000s.
c-iv	**Talacen** (Sanofi Winthrop)		Sodium metabisulfite. (Winthrop T37). Blue, scored. In 100s and UD 250s.
c-iv	**Pentazocine and Naloxone Hydrochloride** (Royce)	**Tablets**: 50 mg (as hydrochloride) and 0.5 mg naloxone hydrochloride	In 100s, 500s and 1000s.
c-iv	**Talwin NX** (Sanofi Winthrop)		(T51). Yellow, scored. Oblong. In 100s and UD 250s.

PENTAZOCINE COMBINATIONS — ORAL

Refer to the general discussion in the Opioid Agonist-Antagonist Analgesic introduction. For complete prescribing information, refer to the Pentazocine monograph.

WARNING

Talwin Nx – *Talwin Nx* is intended for oral use only. Severe, potentially lethal reactions (eg, pulmonary emboli, vascular occlusion, ulceration and abscesses, withdrawal symptoms in narcotic-dependent individuals) may result from misuse of this drug by injection or in combination with other substances.

Administration and Dosage

➤*Adults:*

Pentazocine and aspirin – 2 tablets 3 or 4 times daily.

Pentazocine and acetaminophen – 1 tablet every 4 hours, up to 6 tablets per day.

Pentazocine and naloxone – Initially, 50 mg every 3 or 4 hours; increase to 100 mg if necessary. Do not exceed a total daily dosage of 600 mg. When anti-inflammatory or antipyretic effects are desired in addition to analgesia, aspirin can be administered concomitantly.

Pentazocine tablets are intended for oral use only. Severe, potentially lethal reactions may result from misuse by injection or when combined with other substances. Oral pentazocine tablets contain 0.5 mg naloxone, an opioid antagonist, to aid in elimination of the abuse potential.

➤*Children:* Clinical experience is limited; not recommended for children younger than 12 years of age.

CENTRAL ANALGESICS

CLONIDINE HYDROCHLORIDE

Rx	**Duraclon** (aaiPharma)	**Injection**: 100 mcg/ml	Preservative-free. In 10 ml vials.
		500 mcg/ml	Preservative-free. In 10 ml vials.

CLONIDINE HYDROCHLORIDE — INJECTION

WARNING

The 500 mcg/mL strength product should be diluted prior to use in an appropriate solution.

Note – Epidural clonidine is not recommended for obstetrical, postpartum, or peri-operative pain management. The risk of hemodynamic instability, especially hypotension and bradycardia, from epidural clonidine may be unacceptable in these patients. However, in a rare obstetrical, postpartum or peri-operative patient, potential benefits may outweigh the possible risks.

Indications

For the treatment of severe pain in cancer patients that is not adequately relieved by opioid analgesics alone. Epidural clonidine is more likely to be effective in patients with neuropathic pain than somatic or visceral pain.

➤*Unlabeled uses:* Prevention of postanesthetic shivering.

Administration and Dosage

➤*Approved by the FDA:* October 2, 1996.

The recommended starting dose for continuous epidural infusion is 30 mcg/h. Although dosage may be titrated up or down depending on pain relief and occurrence of adverse events, experience with dosage rates above 40 mcg/h is limited.

Familiarization with the continuous epidural infusion device is essential. Patients receiving epidural clonidine from a continuous infusion device should be closely monitored for the first few days to assess their response.

➤*Dilution:* The 500 mcg/mL (0.5 mg/mL) strength product must be diluted prior to use in 0.9% sodium chloride for injection, USP, to a final concentration of 100 mcg/mL, as explained below:

To obtain a final clonidine hydrochloride concentration of 100 mcg/mL, the addition of 4, 8, 12, 16, 20, 24, 28, 32, 36, and 40 mL of 0.9% sodium chloride for injection USP to 1, 2, 3, 4, 5, 6, 7, 8, 9, and 10 mL of 500 mcg/mL clonidine hydrochloride for injection results in a final concentration of 100 mcg/mL or 500 mcg/5 mL, 1,000 mcg/10 mL, 1,500 mcg/15 mL, 2,000 mcg/20 mL, 2,500 mcg/25 mL, 3,000 mcg/30 mL, 4,000 mcg/40 mL, 4,500 mcg/45 mL, and 5,000 mcg/50 mL, respectively.

Clonidine hydrochloride must not be used with a preservative.

➤*Renal function impairment:* Dosage should be adjusted according to the degree of renal impairment, and patients should be carefully monitored. Since only a minimal amount of clonidine is removed during routine hemodialysis, there is no need to give supplemental clonidine following dialysis.

➤*Storage/Stability:* Store at 25°C (77°F) controlled room temperature, see USP. Preservative free; discard unused portion.

Actions

➤*Pharmacology:* Epidurally administered clonidine produces dose-dependent analgesia not antagonized by opiate antagonists. The analgesia is limited to the body regions innervated by the spinal segments where anal-

CLONIDINE HYDROCHLORIDE — INJECTION

gesic concentrations of clonidine are present. Clonidine is thought to produce analgesia at presynaptic and postjunctional alpha-2-adrenoceptors in the spinal cord by preventing pain signal transmission to the brain.

➤*Pharmacokinetics:*

Distribution – Clonidine is highly lipid soluble and readily distributes into extravascular sites including the central nervous system. Clonidine's volume of distribution is 2.1 ± 0.4 L/kg. The binding of clonidine to plasma protein is primarily to albumin and varies between 20% and 40% in vitro. Epidurally administered clonidine readily partitions into plasma via the epidural veins and attains systemic concentrations (0.5 to 2 ng/mL) that are associated with a hypotensive effect mediated by the central nervous system.

Metabolism – In humans, clonidine metabolism follows minor pathways with the major metabolite, p-hydroxyclonidine, being present at less than 10% of the concentration of unchanged drug in urine.

Excretion – Following an intravenous dose of ^{14}C-clonidine, 72% of the administered dose was excreted in urine in 96 hours of which 40% to 50% was unchanged clonidine. Renal clearance for clonidine was determined to be 133 ± 66 mL/min. In a study where ^{14}C-clonidine was given to subjects with varying degrees of kidney function, elimination half-lives varied (17.5 to 41 hours) as a function of creatinine clearance. In subjects undergoing hemodialysis only 5% of body clonidine stores was removed.

Special populations –

Renal function impairment: The pharmacokinetics of epidurally administered clonidine has not been studied in patients with renal disease.

Hepatic function impairment: The pharmacokinetics of epidurally administered clonidine has not been studied in patients with hepatic disease.

Children: The pharmacokinetics of epidurally administered clonidine has not been studied in the pediatric population. Following a 10 minute intravenous infusion of 300 mcg clonidine hydrochloride to five male volunteers, plasma clonidine levels showed an initial rapid distribution phase (mean ± SD $t_{½}$ = 11 ± 9 minutes) followed by a slower elimination phase ($t_{½}$ = 9 ± 2 hours) over 24 hours. Clonidine's total body clearance (CL) was 219 ± 92 mL/min.

Following a 700 mcg clonidine hydrochloride epidural dose given over 5 minutes to 4 male and 5 female volunteers, peak clonidine plasma levels (4.4 ± 1.4 ng/mL) were obtained in 19 ± 27 minutes. The plasma elimination half-life was determined to be 22 ± 15 hours following sample collection for 24 hours. CL was 190 ± 70 mL/min. In cerebral spinal fluid (CSF), peak clonidine levels (418 ± 255 ng/mL) were achieved in 26 ± 11 minutes. The clonidine CSF elimination half-life was 1.3 ± 0.5 hours when samples were collected for 6 hours. Compared to men, women had a lower mean plasma clearance, longer mean plasma half-life, and higher mean peak level of clonidine in both plasma and CSF.

In cancer patients who received 14 days of clonidine hydrochloride epidural infusion (rate = 30 mcg/hr) plus morphine by patient-controlled analgesia (PCA), steady state clonidine plasma concentrations of 2.2 ± 1.1 and 2.4 ± 1.4 ng/mL were obtained on dosing days 7 and 14, respectively. CL was 279 ± 184 and 272 ± 163 mL/min on these days. CSF concentrations were not determined in these patients.

Contraindications

History of sensitization or allergic reactions to clonidine. Epidural administration is contraindicated in the presence of an injection site infection, in patients on anticoagulant therapy, and in those with a bleeding diathesis. Administration of clonidine hydrochloride above the C4 dermatome is contraindicated.

Warnings

➤*Use in postoperative or obstetrical analgesia:* Epidural clonidine is not recommended for obstetrical, post-partum, or peri-operative pain management. The risk of hemodynamic instability, especially hypotension and bradycardia, from epidural clonidine may be unacceptable in these patients.

➤*Hypotension:* Because severe hypotension may follow the administration of clonidine, it should be used with caution in all patients. It is not recommended in most patients with severe cardiovascular disease or in those who are otherwise hemodynamically unstable. The benefit of its administration in these patients should be carefully balanced against the potential risks resulting from hypotension.

Vital signs should be monitored frequently, especially during the first few days of epidural clonidine therapy. When clonidine is infused into the upper thoracic spinal segments, more pronounced decreases in the blood pressure may be seen.

Clonidine decreases sympathetic outflow from the central nervous system resulting in decreases in peripheral resistance, renal vascular resistance, heart rate, and blood pressure. However, in the absence of profound hypotension, renal blood flow and glomerular filtration rate remain essentially unchanged.

In the pivotal double-blind, randomized study of cancer patients, where 38 subjects were administered epidural clonidine hydrochloride at 30 mcg/hr in addition to epidural morphine, hypotension occurred in 45% of subjects. Most episodes of hypotension occurred within the first 4 days after beginning epidural clonidine. However, hypotensive episodes occurred throughout the duration of the trial. There was a tendency for these episodes to occur more commonly in women, and in those with higher serum clonidine levels. Patients experiencing hypotension also tended to weigh less than those who did not experience hypotension. The hypotension usually responded to intravenous fluids and, if necessary, parenteral ephedrine.

Published reports on the use of epidural clonidine for intraoperative or postoperative analgesia also show a consistent and marked hypotensive response to clonidine. Severe hypotension may occur even if intravenous fluid pretreatment is given.

➤*Withdrawal:* Sudden cessation of clonidine treatment, regardless of the route of administration, has, in some cases, resulted in symptoms such as nervousness, agitation, headache, and tremor, accompanied or followed by a rapid rise in blood pressure. The likelihood of such reactions appears to be greater after administration of higher doses or with concomitant betablocker treatment. Special caution is therefore advised in these situations. Rare instances of hypertensive encephalopathy, cerebrovascular accidents and death have been reported after abrupt clonidine withdrawal. Patients with a history of hypertension or other underlying cardiovascular conditions may be at particular risk of the consequences of abrupt discontinuation of clonidine. In the pivotal double-blind, randomized cancer pain study, 4 of 38 subjects receiving 720 mcg of clonidine per day experienced rebound hypertension following abrupt withdrawal. One of these patients with rebound hypertension subsequently experienced a cerebrovascular accident.

Careful monitoring of infusion pump function and inspection of catheter tubing for obstruction or dislodgement can help reduce the risk of inadvertent abrupt withdrawal of epidural clonidine. Patients should notify their physician immediately if clonidine administration is inadvertently interrupted for any reason. Patients should also be instructed not to discontinue therapy without consulting their physician.

When discontinuing therapy with epidural clonidine, the physician should reduce the dose gradually over 2 to 4 days to avoid withdrawal symptoms.

An excessive rise in blood pressure following discontinuation of epidural clonidine can be treated by administration of clonidine or by IV phentolamine. If therapy is to be discontinued in patients receiving a betablocker and clonidine concurrently, the betablocker should be withdrawn several days before the gradual discontinuation of epidural clonidine.

➤*Infections:* Infections related to implantable epidural catheters pose a serious risk. Evaluation of fever in a patient receiving epidural clonidine should include the possibility of a catheter-related infection such as meningitis or epidural abscess.

➤*Fertility impairment:* Fertility of male or female rats was unaffected by oral clonidine hydrochloride doses as high as 150 mcg/kg, or about 0.5 times the MRDHD. Fertility of female rats did, however, appear to be affected in another experiment at oral dose levels of 500 to 2000 mcg/kg, or 2 to 7 times the MRDHD.

➤*Pregnancy: Category C.*

Teratogenic – Reproduction studies in rabbits at clonidine hydrochloride doses up to approximately the MRDHD revealed no evidence of teratogenic or embryotoxic potential. In rats, however, doses as low as one-third the MRDHD were associated with increased resorptions in a study in which dams were treated continuously from 2 months prior to mating. Increased resorptions were not associated with treatment with the same or higher doses up to 0.5 times the MRDHD when dams were treated on days 6 to 15 of gestation. Increased resorptions were observed at higher levels (7 times the MRDHD) in rats and mice treated on days 1 to 14 of gestation.

Clonidine readily crosses the placenta and its concentrations are equal in maternal and umbilical cord plasma; amniotic fluid concentrations can be 4 times those found in serum. There are no adequate and well-controlled studies in pregnant women during early gestation when organ formation takes place. Studies using epidural clonidine during labor have demonstrated no apparent adverse effects on the infant at the time of delivery. However, these studies did not monitor the infants for hemodynamic effects in the days following delivery. Clonidine hydrochloride injection should be used during pregnancy only if the potential benefits justify the potential risk to the fetus.

Labor and delivery – There are no adequate controlled clinical trials evaluating the safety, efficacy, and dosing of clonidine hydrochloride in obstetrical settings. Because maternal perfusion of the placenta is critically dependent on blood pressure, use of clonidine hydrochloride as an analgesic during labor and delivery is not indicated.

➤*Lactation:* Concentrations of clonidine in human breast milk are approximately twice those found in maternal plasma. Caution should be exercised when clonidine is administered to a nursing woman. Because of the potential for severe adverse reactions in nursing infants, a decision should be made to either discontinue nursing or to discontinue clonidine.

➤*Children:* The safety and effectiveness of clonidine hydrochloride in this limited indication and clinical population have been established in patients old enough to tolerate placement and management of an epidural catheter, based on evidence from adequate and well controlled studies in adults and experience with the use of clonidine in the pediatric age group for other indications. The use of clonidine hydrochloride should be restricted to pediatric patients with severe intractable pain from malignancy that is unresponsive to epidural or spinal opiates or other more conventional analgesic techniques. The starting dose of clonidine hydrochloride should be selected on per kilogram basis (0.5 mcg/kg/hr) and cautiously adjusted based on the clinical response.

Precautions

➤*Special risk:*

Cardiac effects – Epidural clonidine frequently causes decreases in heart rate. Symptomatic bradycardia can be treated with atropine. Rarely, atrioventricular block greater than first degree has been reported. Clonidine does not alter the hemodynamic response to exercise, but may mask the increase in heart rate associated with hypovolemia.

Respiratory depression and sedation – Clonidine administration may result in sedation through the activation of alpha-adrenoceptors in the brainstem. High doses of clonidine cause sedation and ventilatory abnormalities that are usually mild. Tolerance to these effects can develop with

CLONIDINE HYDROCHLORIDE — INJECTION

chronic administration. These effects have been reported with bolus doses that are significantly larger than the infusion rate recommended for treating cancer pain.

Depression – Depression has been seen in a small percentage of patients treated with oral or transdermal clonidine. Depression commonly occurs in cancer patients and may be exacerbated by treatment with clonidine. Patients, especially those with a known history of affective disorders, should be monitored for the signs and symptoms of depression.

Pain of visceral or somatic origin – In the clinical investigations, at doses tested, clonidine hydrochloride was most effective in well-localized, "neuropathic" pain that was characterized as electrical, burning, or shooting in nature, and which was localized to a dermatomal or peripheral nerve distribution. Clonidine hydrochloride may be less effective, or possibly ineffective in the treatment of pain that is diffuse, poorly localized, or visceral in origin.

Drug Interactions

Clonidine Drug Interactions			
Precipitant drug	Object drug*		Description
Beta blockers	Clonidine	↑	Beta blockers may exacerbate the hypertensive response seen with clonidine withdrawal. Also, because of the potential for additive effects such as bradycardia and AV block, use caution in patients receiving clonidine with agents known to affect sinus node function or AV nodal conduction (eg, digitalis, calcium channel blockers, beta blockers).
Fluphenazine	Clonidine	↑	There is one reported case of a patient with acute delirium associated with the simultaneous use of fluphenazine and oral clonidine. Symptoms resolved when clonidine was withdrawn and recurred when the patient was rechallenged with clonidine.
Narcotic analgesics	Clonidine	↑	Narcotic analgesics may potentiate the hypotensive effects of clonidine.
Tricyclic antidepressants	Clonidine	↓	Tricyclic antidepressants may antagonize the hypotensive effects of clonidine. The effects of tricyclic antidepressants on clonidine's analgesic actions are not known.
Clonidine	Alcohol/ barbiturates	↑	Clonidine may potentiate the CNS-depressive effect of alcohol, barbiturates or other sedating drugs.
Clonidine	Local anesthetics	↑	Epidural clonidine may prolong the duration of pharmacologic effects of epidural local anesthetics, including sensory and motor blockade.

* ↑ = Object drug increased. ↓ = Object drug decreased.

Adverse Reactions

The following adverse events may be related to administration of either clonidine or morphine.

Clonidine Adverse Reactions		
Adverse Events	Clonidine (%)	Placebo (%)
Total number of patients who experienced ≥ 1 adverse event	97.4	80.5
Hypotension	44.8	10.6
Postural hypotension	31.6	0
Dry mouth	13.2	8.5
Nausea	13.2	21.3
Somnolence	13.2	21.3
Dizziness	13.2	4.3
Confusion	13.2	10.6
Vomiting	10.5	14.9
Nausea/Vomiting	7.9	2.1
Sweating	5.3	0
Anxiety	11	2
Chest pain	5.3	0
Hallucination	5.3	2.1
Tinnitus	5.3	0
Constipation	6	4.3
Tachycardia	2.6	4.3
Hypoventilation	2.6	4.3
Urinary tract infection	22	nd[1]
Dyspnea	6	nd
Infection	8	nd
Asthenia	5	nd
Hyperaesthesia	5	nd
Pain	5	nd
Skin ulcer	5	nd
Decreased heart rate	†[2]	nd
Rebound hypertension	11	nd

[1] nd = No data.
[2] † = Occurs, but the incidence is unknown.

Adverse reactions seen during continuous epidural clonidine infusion are dose-dependent and typical for a compound of this pharmacologic class. The adverse events most frequently reported in the pivotal controlled clinical trial of continuous epidural clonidine administration consisted of hypotension, postural hypotension, decreased heart rate, rebound hypertension, dry mouth, nausea, confusion, dizziness, somnolence, and fever. Hypotension is the adverse event that most frequently requires treatment. The hypotension is usually responsive to intravenous fluids and, if necessary, parenterally-administered ephedrine. Hypotension was observed more frequently in women and in lower weight patients, but no dose-related response was established.

The inadvertent intrathecal administration of clonidine has not been associated with a significantly increased risk of adverse events, but there are inadequate safety and efficacy data to support the use of intrathecal clonidine. Epidural clonidine was compared to placebo in a 2 week double-blind study of 85 terminal cancer patients with intractable pain receiving epidural morphine. The following adverse events were reported in 2 or more patients and may be related to administration of either clonidine hydrochloride or morphine.

Incidence of Adverse Events in the 2-week Trial		
Adverse events	Clonidine (n = 38), n (%)	Placebo (n = 47), n (%)
Total number of patients who experienced at least 1 adverse event	37 (97.4)	38 (80.5)
Hypotension	17 (44.8)	5 (10.6)
Postural hypotension	12 (31.6)	0 (0)
Dry mouth	5 (13.2)	4 (8.5)
Nausea	5 (13.2)	10 (21.3)
Somnolence	5 (13.2)	10 (21.3)
Dizziness	5 (13.2)	2 (4.3)
Confusion	5 (13.2)	5 (10.6)
Vomiting	4 (10.5)	7 (14.9)
Nausea/vomiting	3 (7.9)	1 (2.1)
Sweating	2 (5.3)	0 (0)
Chest pain	2 (5.3)	0 (0)
Hallucinations	2 (5.3)	1 (2.1)
Tinnitus	2 (5.3)	0 (0)
Constipation	1 (2.6)	2 (4.3)

CLONIDINE HYDROCHLORIDE — INJECTION

Incidence of Adverse Events in the 2-week Trial		
Adverse events	Clonidine (n = 38), n (%)	Placebo (n = 47), n (%)
Total number of patients who experienced at least 1 adverse event	37 (97.4)	38 (80.5)
Tachycardia	1 (2.6)	2 (4.3)
Hypoventilation	1 (2.6)	2 (4.3)

➤*Long-term extension of the above trial:* An open-label long-term extension of the above trial was performed. Thirty-two subjects received epidural clonidine and morphine for up to 94 weeks a median dosing period of 10 weeks. The following adverse events (and percent incidence) were reported: Hypotension/postural hypotension (47%); nausea (13%); anxiety/confusion (38%); somnolence (25%); urinary tract infection (22%); constipation, dyspnea, fever, infection (6% each); asthenia, hyperaesthesia, pain, skin ulcer, and vomiting (5% each). Eighteen percent of subjects discontinued this study as a result of catheter-related problems (eg, infections, accidental dislodging), and one subject developed meningitis, possibly as a result of a catheter-related infection. In this study, rebound hypertension was not assessed, and ECG and laboratory data were not systematically sought.

The following adverse reactions have also been reported with the use of any dosage form of clonidine. In many cases patients were receiving concomitant medication and a causal relationship has not been established:

Cardiovascular – Palpitations and tachycardia, and bradycardia, each 0.5%. Syncope, Raynaud's phenomenon, congestive heart failure, and electrocardiographic abnormalities (ie, sinus node arrest, functional bradycardia, high degree AV block) have been reported rarely. Rare cases of sinus bradycardia and atrioventricular block have been reported, both with and without the use of concomitant digitalis.

CNS – Nervousness and agitation, 3%; mental depression, 1%; insomnia, 0.5%. Cerebrovascular accidents, other behavioral changes, vivid dreams or nightmares, restlessness, and delirium have been reported rarely.

Dermatologic – Rash, 1%; pruritus, 0.7%; hives, angioneurotic edema and urticaria, 0.5%; alopecia, 0.2%.

GI – Anorexia and malaise, each 1%; mild transient abnormalities in liver function tests, 1%; hepatitis, parotitis, ileus and pseudo obstruction, and abdominal pain, rarely.

GU – Decreased sexual activity, impotence, and libido, 3%; nocturia, about 1%; difficulty in micturition, about 0.2%; urinary retention, about 0.1%.

Hematologic – Thrombocytopenia, rarely.

Metabolic – Weight gain, 0.1%; gynecomastia, 1%; transient elevation of glucose or serum phosphatase, rarely.

Musculoskeletal – Muscle or joint pain, about 0.6%; leg cramps, 0.3%.

Ophthalmic – Dryness of the eyes, burning of the eyes and blurred vision were rarely reported.

Special senses – Dryness of the nasal mucosa was rarely reported.

Miscellaneous – Weakness, 10%; fatigue, 4%; headache and withdrawal syndrome, each 1%. Also reported were pallor, a weakly positive Coomb's test, and increased sensitivity to alcohol.

Overdosage

➤*Symptoms:* Hypertension may develop early and may be followed by hypotension, bradycardia, respiratory depression, hypothermia, drowsiness, decreased or absent reflexes, irritability, and miosis. With large oral overdoses, reversible cardiac conduction defects or arrhythmias, apnea, coma, and seizures have been reported. As little as 100 mcg of oral clonidine has produced signs of toxicity in pediatric patients.

The largest overdose reported to date involved a 28-year old white male who ingested 100 mg of clonidine hydrochloride powder. This patient developed hypertension followed by hypotension, bradycardia, apnea, hallucinations, semicoma, and premature ventricular contractions. The patient fully recovered after intensive treatment. Plasma clonidine levels were 60 ng/mL after 1 hour, 190 ng/mL after 1.5 hours, 370 ng/mL after 2 hours, and 120 ng/mL after 5.5 and 6.5 hours. In mice and rats, the oral LD_{50} of clonidine is 206 and 465 mg/kg, respectively.

➤*Treatment:* There is no specific antidote for clonidine overdosage. Supportive care may include atropine sulfate for bradycardia, intravenous fluids or vasopressor agents for hypotension. Hypertension associated with overdosage has been treated with intravenous furosemide, diazoxide or alpha-blocking agents such as phentolamine. Naloxone may be a useful adjunct in the treatment of clonidine-induced respiratory depression, hypotension, or coma; blood pressure should be monitored since the administration of naloxone has occasionally resulted in paradoxical hypertension. Tolazoline administration has yielded inconsistent results and is not recommended as first-line therapy. Dialysis is not likely to significantly enhance the elimination of clonidine.

Patient Information

Patients should be instructed about the risks of rebound hypertension and warned not to discontinue clonidine except under the supervision of a physician. Patients should notify their physician immediately if clonidine administration is inadvertently interrupted for any reason. Patients who engage in potentially hazardous activities, such as operating machinery or driving, should be advised of the potential sedative and hypotensive effects of epidural clonidine. They should also be informed that sedative effects may be increased by CNS-depressing drugs such as alcohol and barbiturates, and that hypotensive effects may be increased by opiates.

ACETAMINOPHEN

ACETAMINOPHEN (N-Acetyl-P-Aminophenol, APAP)

otc	**Acetaminophen** (Various, eg, Geneva, Moore, Roxane, Rugby, Schein)	**Tablets**: 325 mg	In 50s, 100s, 1,000s and UD 100s.
otc	**Aceta** (Century)		In 100s and 1,000s.
otc	**Genapap** (Goldline)		In 100s.
otc	**Genebs** (Goldline)		In 100s.
otc	**Mapap Regular Strength** (Major)		Scored. In 100s, 1,000s and UD 100s.
otc	**Maranox** (C.S. Dent)		In 8s.
otc	**Meda Tab** (Circle)		In 100s.
otc	**Tapanol Regular Strength** (Circle)		In 100s and 250s.
otc	**Tylenol Caplets** (McNeil-CPC)		In 24s, 50s and 100s.
otc	**Tylenol Regular Strength Tablets** (McNeil-CPC)		(TYLENOL 325). In 24s, 50s, 100s and 200s.
otc	**Acetaminophen** (Various, eg, Geneva, Moore)	**Tablets**: 500 mg	In 100s, 1,000s and UD 100s.
otc	**Aceta** (Century)		In 100s and 1,000s.
otc	**Aspirin Free Anacin Maximum Strength** (Whitehall)		In 60s.
otc	**Extra Strength Dynafed E.X.** (BDI)		In 36s.
otc	**Genebs Extra Strength** (Goldline)		In 100s.
otc	**Mapap Extra Strength** (Major)		In 30s, 60s, 100s, 200s, 1,000s and UD 100s.
otc	**Panadol Extra Strength** (GlaxoSmithKline Consumer Healthcare)		(P 500). In 30s and 60s.
otc	**Redutemp** (Inter. Ethical Labs)		In 60s.
otc	**Tapanol Extra Strength** (Republic)		In 100s.
otc	**Tylenol Extra Strength** (McNeil-CPC)		(TYLENOL 500). In 100s.
otc	**UN-Aspirin Extra Strength** (Zee Medical)		In 24s.
otc	**Acetaminophen** (Roxane)	**Tablets**: 650 mg	In 1,000s and UD 100s.

ACETAMINOPHEN (N-Acetyl-P-Aminophenol, APAP)

otc	**Acetaminophen** (Various, eg, Moore, Rugby, Schein)	**Tablets, chewable**: 80 mg	In 30s, and 100s.
otc	**Apacet** (Parmed)		In 30s.
otc	**Children's Dynafed Jr.** (BDI)		(44 185). Fruit flavor. In 36s.
otc	**Genapap, Children's** (Goldline)		Fruit flavor. Saccharin free. In 30s.
otc	**Children's Māpap** (Major)		3 mg phenylalanine, aspartame, mannitol, sucrose. Grape, fruit splash flavors. In 30s.
otc	**Children's Tylenol Soft Chews** (McNeil-CPC)		Aspartame. Grape and fruit flavors. In 30s.
otc sf	**Panadol, Children's** (SmithKline Beecham)		(P). Scored. Fruit flavor. In 30s.
otc	**Tempra 3** (Mead Johnson Nutritional)		In 30s.
otc	**Tylenol, Children's** (McNeil-CPC)		(Tylenol 80). Scored. Fruit, bubble gum or grape flavor. In 30s, 48s and 96s.
otc	**Tylenol Junior Strength** (McNeil-CPC)	**Tablets, chewable**: 160 mg	Aspartame (6 mg phenylalanine). (TYLENOL 160). Grape and fruit flavors. In 24s.
otc	**Tylenol Arthritis** (McNeil-CPC)	**Tablets, extended release**: 650 mg	(TYLENOL ER). Caplet-shaped. In 100s.
otc	**Tylenol Children's Meltaways** (McNeil Consumer)	**Tablets, dispersible**: 80 mg	Bubblegum burst flavor. In 4s.
otc sf	**Panadol, Junior Strength** (Sterling Health)	**Caplets**: 160 mg	In 30s.
otc	**Aspirin Free Pain Relief** (Hudson)	**Caplets**: 500 mg	In 100s.
otc	**Genapap Extra Strength** (Goldline)		In 50s and 100s.
otc	**Genebs Extra Strength** (Goldline)		In 100s.
otc	**Tapanol Extra Strength** (Republic)		In 50s, 100s and 175s.
otc	**Tylenol Extended Relief** (McNeil-CPC)	**Caplets**: 650 mg	(Tylenol ER). In 100s.
otc	**Tylenol 8 Hour** (McNeil)	**Caplets, extended-release**: 650 mg	Polyvinyl alcohol, povidone. In 24s, 50s, 100s, and 150s.
otc	**Aspirin Free Anacin Maximum Strength** (Whitehall)	**Gelcaps**: 500 mg	(AF Anacin). In 100s.
otc	**Tapanol Extra Strength** (Republic)		In 100s and 175s.
otc	**Tylenol Extra Strength** (McNeil-CPC)		Gelatin coated. (TYLENOL 500). In 24s, 50s and 100s.
otc	**Tylenol 8 Hour** (McNeil)	**Geltabs, extended-release**: 650 mg	Benzyl alcohol, EDTA, parabens, povidone. In 20s, 40s, and 80s.
otc	**Acetaminophen** (Various, eg, Moore)	**Capsules**: 500 mg	In 50s, 100s and 1,000s.
otc	**Meda Cap** (Circle)		In 100s.
otc	**Acetaminophen** (Various, eg, Roxane, UDL Labs)	**Liquid**: 160 mg/5 mL	In 120 and 500 mL and UD 100s.
otc sf	**Panadol, Children's** (SmithKline Beecham)		Alcohol free. Saccharin, sorbitol. Fruit flavor. In 59 and 118 mL.
otc sf	**Silapap Children's** (Silarx)		Alcohol free. Methylparaben, saccharin. In 118 mL.
otc	**Tempra 2 Syrup** (Mead Johnson Nutritional)		In 120 mL.
otc	**Tylenol Sore Throat Maximum Strength** (McNeil Consumer)	**Liquid**: 166.6 mg/5 mL	Corn syrup, saccharin, sorbitol. Honey lemon, wild cherry flavors. In 240 mL.
otc	**Tylenol Sore Throat Daytime** (McNeil Consumer)		Sorbitol, sucralose, sucrose. Cool burst flavor. In 240 mL.
otc	**Comtrex Maximum Strength Sore Throat** (Bristol-Myers Squibb)		Glycerin, saccharin, sorbitol, sucrose. Honey-lemon flavor. In 240 mL.
otc	**Acetaminophen** (Various, eg, Goldline)	**Liquid**: 500 mg/15 mL	In 237 mL.
otc	**Tylenol Extra Strength** (McNeil-CPC)		7% alcohol. Sorbitol, sucrose. Mint flavor. In 240 mL with dosage cup.
otc	**ElixSure Children's Fever/Pain** (Taro Consumer Healthcare)	**Syrup**: 160 mg/5 mL	Butylparaben, glycerin. Cherry flavor. In 122 mL.
otc	**Silapap, Children's** (Silarx)	**Elixir**: 80 mg/2.5 mL	Alcohol-free. In 237 mL.
otc	**Ridenol** (R.I.D.)	**Elixir**: 80 mg/5 mL	In 120 mL.
otc	**Acetaminophen** (Various, eg, Pharm. Assoc. Inc)	**Elixir**: 120 mg/5 mL	In UD 27 mL (100s).
otc	**Aceta** (Century)		In 120 mL and gal.
otc	**Oraphen-PD** (Great Southern)		In 120 mL.
otc	**Acetaminophen** (Various, eg, Goldline, Rugby, Schein)	**Elixir**: 160 mg/5 mL	In 118 and 120 mL, pt and gal.
otc	**Apra Children's** (Altaire)		Alcohol-free. Sorbitol, sucrose, glycerin. Grape flavor. In 118 mL.
otc	**Genapap, Children's** (Goldline)		In 120 mL.
otc	**Mapap, Children's** (Major)		Alcohol free. Cherry flavor. In 120 mL.
otc	**Tylenol, Children's** (McNeil-CPC)		Alcohol free. Sorbitol, sucrose, butylparaben, corn syrup. Cherry flavor. In 60 and 120 mL.
otc	**Dolono** (R.I.D)		Alcohol free. Sorbitol, sucrose. Cherry flavor. In 120 mL.

ACETAMINOPHEN (N-Acetyl-P-Aminophenol, APAP)

otc	**Acetaminophen Drops** (Various, eg, Bioline, Moore, Schein)	**Drops, oral:** 100 mg/mL	In 15 mL.
otc	**Apacet** (Parmed)		In 15 mL.
otc	**Genapap, Infants' Drops** (Goldline)		Alcohol free. Fruit flavor. In 15 mL w/0.8 mL dropper.
otc	**Infantaire Drops** (Altaire)		In 15 mL w/ 0.8 mL dropper.
otc	**Mapap Infant Drops** (Major)		Alcohol free. Fruit flavor. In 15 and 30 mL.
otc sf	**Panadol, Infants' Drops** (SmithKline Beecham)		Alcohol free. Saccharin. Fruit flavor. In 14.8 mL with 0.8 mL dropper.
otc	**Silapap, Infants** (Silarx)		Alcohol free. Fruit flavor. In 15 mL with dropper.
otc	**Tempra 1** (Mead Johnson Nutritional)		In 15 mL.
otc	**Tylenol, Infants' Drops** (McNeil-CPC)		Alcohol free. Saccharin, butylparaben, corn syrup, sorbitol. Fruit flavor. In 7.5 mL and in 30 mL w/0.8 mL dropper.
otc	**FeverAll, Infants** (Alpharma)	**Suppositories:** 80 mg	In 6s.
otc	**Acetaminophen** (Various, eg, Goldline, Moore, Rugby)	**Suppositories:** 120 mg	In 12s.
otc	**FeverAll** (Alpharma)		In 12s.
otc	**Acephen** (G & W Labs)		In 6s, 12s and UD 12s, 50s and 100s.
otc	**FeverAll, Children's** (Alpharma)		In 6s.
otc	**Neopap** (PolyMedica)	**Suppositories:** 125 mg	In 12s.
otc	**Acetaminophen** (Harber)	**Suppositories:** 300 mg	In 12s.
otc	**Acetaminophen** (Various, eg, Rugby)	**Suppositories:** 325 mg	In 12s.
otc	**FeverAll** (Alpharma)		In 12s.
otc	**Acephen** (G & W Labs)		In 6s, 12s, 50s and 100s.
otc	**FeverAll, Junior Strength** (Alpharma)		In 6s.
otc	**Acetaminophen** (Various, eg, Goldline, Moore, Rugby)	**Suppositories:** 650 mg	In 12s.
otc	**FeverAll** (Alpharma)		In 12s.
otc	**Acephen** (G & W Labs)		In 12s, 500s and UD 50s and 100s.

ACETAMINOPHEN — ORAL

Indications

➤*Adults and children greater than or equal to 12 years of age or older:* For the reduction of fever and temporary relief of minor aches and pains associated with sore throat, common cold, toothache, headache, and muscular aches.

Acetaminophen extra-strength and regular-strength tablets and extended-release tablets are also indicated for the temporary relief of the minor pain of arthritis, backache, and for the pain of menstrual cramps.

➤*Children:* For the reduction of fever. For the temporary relief of minor aches and pains associated with a cold, flu, headache, sore throat, immunizations, teething and toothaches in children 2 to 11 years of age.

➤*Unlabeled uses:* Prophylactic acetaminophen use in children receiving DTP vaccination appears to decrease incidence of fever and injection-site pain. A dose immediately following vaccination and every 4 to 6 hours thereafter for 48 to 72 hours is suggested.

Administration and Dosage

➤*General dosing:*

Adults – 325 to 650 mg every 4 to 6 hours, or 1 g 3 to 4 times a day. Do not exceed 4 g/day.

Children – May repeat doses every 4 hours. Do not exceed 5 doses in 24 hours.

0 to 3 months of age: Administer 40 mg every 4 hours.
4 to 11 months of age: Administer 80 mg every 4 hours.
1 to less than 2 years of age: Administer 120 mg every 4 hours.
2 to 3 years of age: Administer 160 mg every 4 hours.
4 to 5 years of age: Administer 240 mg every 4 hours.
6 to 8 years of age: Administer 320 mg every 4 hours.
9 to 10 years of age: Administer 400 mg every 4 hours.
11 years of age: Administer 480 mg every 4 hours.
12 to 14 years of age: Administer 640 mg every 4 hours.
Greater than 14 years of age: Administer 650 mg every 4 hours.

A 10 to 15 mg/kg/dose schedule has also been recommended.

➤*Children less than 12 years of age:* Consult a physician before using these products in children weighing less than 24 pounds or less than 2 years of age.

Chewable tablets – Chew tablets before swallowing.

Acetaminophen chewable tablets are not the same concentration as junior strength acetaminophen tablets.

Concentrated drops – Shake well before using.

Acetaminophen concentrated drops are more concentrated than other acetaminophen liquids.

Elixir and oral suspension liquid – Shake well before using.

Acetaminophen elixir and oral suspension liquid are not the same concentration as acetaminophen drops.

Children:

- For children under 2 years or under 24 lb, consult a doctor for dosing information.
- For children ages 2 to 3 years or 24 to 35 lb, give 5 mL.
- For children ages 4 to 5 years or 36 to 47 lb, give 7.5 mL.
- For children ages 6 to 8 or 48 to 59 lb, give 10 mL.
- For children ages 9 to 10 or 60 to 71 lb, give 12.5 mL.
- For children age 11 or 72 to 95 lb, give 15 mL.
- All dosages may be repeated every 4 hours, but not more than 5 times daily.

Dispersible tablets – Dissolve in mouth or chew before swallowing. If needed, repeat dose every 4 hours. Do not use more than 5 times in 24 hours.

- For children younger than 2 years of age or under 24 lb, consult a doctor for dosing information.
- For children 2 to 3 years of age or 24 to 35 lb, give 160 mg.
- For children 4 to 5 years of age or 36 to 47 lb, give 240 mg.
- For children 6 to 8 years of age or 48 to 59 lb, give 320 mg.
- For children 9 to 10 years of age or 60 to 71 lb, give 400 mg.
- For children 11 years of age or 72 to 95 lb, give 480 mg.

Acetaminophen regular strength tablets –

Adults: 650 mg every 4 to 6 hours as needed. Do not take more than 3,900 mg in 24 hours, or as directed by a doctor.

Children: 325 mg every 4 to 6 hours as needed. Do not take more than 5 tablets in 24 hours. Do not use this regular strength product in children under 6 years of age. This will provide more than the recommended dose (overdose) of acetaminophen and could cause serious health problems.

➤*Storage/Stability:* Store at room temperature (15° to 30°C; 59° to 86°F). Avoid high humidity and excessive heat 40°C (104°F). Keep product away from direct light. Protect from freezing.

Actions

➤*Pharmacology:* Acetaminophen is the active metabolite of phenacetin and acetanilid.

The site and mechanism of the analgesic effect is unclear. Acetaminophen reduces fever by direct action on the hypothalmic heat-regulating center, which increases dissipation of body heat (via vasodilation and sweating). The action of endogenous pyrogen on heat-regulating centers is inhibited. Acetaminophen is almost as potent as aspirin in inhibiting prostaglandin synthetase in the CNS, but its peripheral inhibition of prostaglandin synthesis is minimal, which may account for its lack of clinically significant antirheumatic or anti-inflammatory effects.

Generally, antipyretic and analgesic effects of acetaminophen and aspirin are comparable. Aspirin is clearly superior to acetaminophen for pain of inflammatory origin. Acetaminophen does not inhibit platelet aggregation, affect prothrombin response, or produce GI ulceration.

ACETAMINOPHEN — ORAL

➤*Pharmacokinetics:*

Absorption – Absorption of acetaminophen is rapid and almost complete from the GI tract. Peak plasma concentrations occur within 0.5 to 2 hours, with slightly faster absorption of liquid preparations. With overdosage, absorption is complete in 4 hours.

Distribution – Serum protein binding varies from 20% to 50% at toxic concentrations.

Metabolism / Excretion – The half-life in plasma is approximately 2 hours. Acetaminophen is relatively uniformly distributed throughout most body fluids. Binding of the drug to plasma proteins is variable; only 20% to 50% may be bound at the concentrations encountered during acute intoxication. Ninety percent (90%) to 100% of the drug is recovered in the urine within the first day, primarily after hepatic conjugation with glucuronic acid (approximately 60%), sulfuric acid (approximately 35%) or cysteine (approximately 3%); small amounts of hydroxylated and deacetylated metabolites also have been detected. Acetaminophen is extensively metabolized and excreted in urine primarily as inactive glucuronate and sulfate conjugates (94%). About 4% is metabolized via cytochrome P450 oxidase to a toxic metabolite normally detoxified by preferential conjugation with cellular glutathione and excreted in urine as conjugates of and mercapturic acid. When acetaminophen is used chronically or taken acutely in large doses, glutathione stores are depleted and hepatic necrosis may occur; 2% is excreted unchanged. Half-life is slightly prolonged in neonates and in cirrhotics.

Warnings

➤*Alcohol warning:* Patients who consume 3 or more alcoholic drinks every day should ask their physicians whether they should take acetaminophen or other pain relievers/fever reducers. Acetaminophen may cause liver damage.

Caution chronic alcoholics to limit acetaminophen intake to less than or equal to 2 g/day.

➤*Hepatic effects:* Hepatotoxicity and severe hepatic failure occurred in chronic alcoholics following therapeutic doses. The hepatotoxicity is believed to be caused by induction of hepatic microsomal enzymes resulting in an increase in toxic metabolites or by the reduced amount of glutathione responsible for conjugating toxic metabolites. A safe dose for a chronic alcohol abuser has not been determined.

➤*Pregnancy: Category B.* Acetaminophen crosses the placenta. It is routinely used during all stages of pregnancy; when used in therapeutic doses, it appears to be safe for short-term use. Continuous high daily dosage probably caused severe anemia in a mother, and the neonate had fatal kidney disease. Although there is no evidence of a relationship between acetaminophen ingestion and congenital malformations, 3 cases of congenital hip dislocation may have been associated with acetaminophen.

➤*Lactation:* Acetaminophen is excreted in breast milk in low concentrations with reported milk:plasma ratios of 0.91 to 1.42 at 1 and 12 hours, respectively. No adverse reactions in nursing infants were reported.

➤*Children:* Consult a physician for use greater than 5 days (children), greater than 10 days (adults), or greater than 3 days for fever (children and adults).

Precautions

➤*Severe or recurrent pain or high or continued fever:* Severe or recurrent pain or high or continued fever may indicate serious illness. If pain persists for greater than 5 days or if redness or swelling is present, consult a phsycian.

Drug Interactions

The potential hepatoxicity of acetaminophen may be increased by large doses or long-term administration of the following agents because of hepatic microsomal enzyme induction: Barbiturates, carbamazepine, hydantoins, isoniazid, rifampin, sulfinpyrazone. The therapeutic effects of acetaminophen may also be decreased.

The potential hepatotoxicity of APAP may be increased by large doses or long-term administration of the following agents because of hepatic microsomal enzyme induction. The therapeutic effects of APAP may also be decreased.

- Barbiturates
- Carbamazepine
- Hydantoins
- Isoniazid
- Rifampin
- Sulfinpyrazone

Acetaminophen Drug Interactions

Precipitant drug	Object drug*		Description
Alcohol, ethyl	APAP	⬆	Hepatotoxicity has occurred in chronic alcoholics following various dose levels (moderate to excessive) of acetaminophen.
Anticholinergics	APAP	⬇	The onset of acetaminophen effect may be delayed or decreased slightly, but the ultimate pharmacological effect is not significantly affected by anticholinergics.
Beta blockers, propranolol	APAP	⬆	Propranolol appears to inhibit the enzyme systems responsible for the glucuronidation and oxidation of acetaminophen. Therefore, the pharmacologic effects of acetaminophen may be increased.
Charcoal, activated	APAP	⬇	Reduces acetaminophen absorption when administered as soon as possible after overdose.
Contraceptives, oral	APAP	⬇	Increase in glucuronidation resulting in increased plasma clearance and a decreased half-life of acetaminophen.
Probenecid	APAP	⬆	Probenecid may increase the therapeutic effectiveness of acetaminophen slightly.
APAP	Lamotrigine	⬇	Serum lamotrigine concentrations may be reduced, producing a decrease in therapeutic effects.
APAP	Loop diuretics	⬇	The effects of the loop diuretic may be decreased because APAP may decrease renal prostaglandin excretion and decrease plasma renin activity.
APAP	Zidovudine	⬇	The pharmacologic effects of zidovudine may be decreased because of enhanced nonhepatic or renal clearance of zidovudine.

* ⬆ = Object drug increased. ⬇ = Object drug decreased.

Overdosage

➤*Symptoms:* Acute poisoning may be manifested by nausea, vomiting, drowsiness, confusion, liver tenderness, low blood pressure, cardiac arrhythmias, jaundice, and acute hepatic and renal failure. These occur within the first 24 hours and may persist for greater than or equal to 1 week. Death has occurred because of liver necrosis. Acute renal failure may also occur. However, there are often no specific early symptoms or signs.

The course of acetaminophen poisoning is divided into 4 stages (postingestion time):

Stage 1 –
12 to 24 hours: Nausea, vomiting, diaphoresis, anorexia.

Stage 2 –
24 to 48 hours: Clinically improved; AST, ALT, bilirubin, and prothrombin levels begin to rise.

Stage 3 –
72 to 96 hours: Peak hepatotoxicity; AST of 20,000 not unusual.

Stage 4 –
7 to 8 days: Recovery.

Hepatotoxicity – Hepatotoxicity may result. The minimal toxic dose is 10 g (140 mg/kg), but liver damage has occurred with a single 5.85 g dose; greater than or equal to 20 to 25 g are potentially fatal. Children appear less susceptible to toxicity than adults because they have less capacity for glucuronidation metabolism. Initial signs of toxicity may include nausea, vomiting, anorexia, malaise, diaphoresis, abdominal pain, and diarrhea. Hepatotoxicity usually is not apparent for 48 to 72 hours. If an acute dose of greater than or equal to 150 mg/kg was ingested, or if the dose cannot be determined, obtain a serum acetaminophen assay after 4 hours following ingestion. If in the toxic range, obtain liver function studies and repeat at 24-hour intervals. Hepatic failure may lead to encephalopathy, coma, and death.

Plasma acetaminophen levels greater than 300 mcg/mL at 4 hours postingestion were associated with hepatic damage in 90% of patients; minimal hepatic damage is anticipated if plasma levels at 4 hours are less than 120 mcg/mL or less than 30 mcg/mL at 12 hours after ingestion.

Chronic excessive use (greater than 4 g/day) eventually may lead to transient hepatotoxicity. The kidneys may undergo tubular necrosis; the myocardium may be damaged.

➤*Treatment:* Oral N-acetylcysteine is a specific antidote for acetaminophen toxicity. Administration IV can cause anaphylaxis. If patient vomits within 1 hour of administration of N-acetylcysteine, repeat the dose. Refer to the acetylcysteine monograph for complete prescribing information and for specific nomogram to guide treatment.

Patient Information

➤*Alcohol warning:* If you consume 3 or more alcoholic drinks every day, ask your physician whether you should take acetaminophen or other pain relievers/fever reducers. Acetaminophen may cause liver damage.

➤*Sore throat:* If sore throat is severe, persists for more than 2 days, is accompanied or followed by fever, headache, rash, nausea, or vomiting, consult a doctor promptly.

Do not exceed the recommended dose.

Do not use capsules, extended-release tablets, extra- or regular-strength tablets, or liquid with any other product containing acetaminophen, for

ACETAMINOPHEN — ORAL

greater than 10 days for pain unless directed by a doctor, or for greater than 3 days for fever unless directed by a doctor. Do not use chewable tablets, concentrated drops, elixir, or oral suspension liquid with any other product containing acetaminophen, for greater than 5 days for pain unless directed by a doctor, or for greater than 3 days for fever unless directed by a doctor.

Stop using this medicine and contact your doctor if symptoms do not improve; new symptoms occur; pain or fever persists or gets worse; redness or swelling is present; or if sore throat is severe, persists for more than 2 days, is accompanied or followed by fever, headache, rash, nausea, or vomiting. These could be signs of a serious condition.

In case of accidental overdose, contact a physician or poison control center immediately. Prompt medical attention is critical for adults as well as for children even if you do not notice any signs or symptoms. Keep out of the reach of children.

Do not use with any other product containing acetaminophen. Do not use if carton is opened, or if neck wrap or foil inner seal imprinted "Safety Seal" is broken or missing.

Stop use and ask a doctor if new symptoms occur; pain gets worse or lasts for more than 5 days; or fever gets worse or lasts for more than 3 days.

As with any drug, if you are pregnant or breastfeeding, seek the advice of a doctor before using this product.

ACETAMINOPHEN — RECTAL

Indications

For the temporary reduction of fever and for the temporary relief of occasional aches and pains, and headaches.

➤*Unlabeled uses:* Prophylactic acetaminophen use in children receiving DTP vaccination appears to decrease incidence of fever and injection site pain. A dose immediately following vaccination every 4 to 6 hours thereafter for 48 to 72 hours is suggested.

Administration and Dosage

Find the right dose. Remove the wrapper and carefully insert suppository well up into the rectum.

➤*80 mg:*

Children less than 3 months of age – Consult a doctor.

Children 3 to 11 months of age – Give 1 suppository every 6 hours.

Children 12 to 36 months of age – Give 1 suppository every 4 hours. Do not give more than a total of 6 suppositories in any 24-hour period.

➤*120 mg:*

Children less than 3 years of age – Consult a doctor.

Children 3 to 6 years of age – Give 1 suppository every 4 to 6 hours. Do not give more than a total of 6 suppositories in any 24-hour period.

➤*325 mg:*

Children less than 6 years of age – Consult a doctor.

Children 6 to 12 years of age – Give 1 suppository every 4 to 6 hours. Do not give more than a total of 6 suppositories in any 24-hour period.

Adults – Use 2 suppositories every 4 to 6 hours. Do not use more than a total of 12 suppositories in any 24-hour period.

➤*650 mg:*

Adults and children 12 years of age and older – Use 1 suppository every 4 to 6 hours while symptoms last. Do not exceed 6 suppositories in any 24-hour period.

Children under 12 years of age – Do not use.

➤*Storage/Stability:* Store at 2° to 27°C (36° to 80°F).

Contraindications

Hypersensitivity to acetaminophen or any other ingredient in this medicine.

Warnings

➤*Use:* Do not use this medicine for fever or pain for more than 3 days unless directed by a doctor.

Consult a doctor if fever or pain persists or gets worse, new symptoms occur, or redness or swelling is present in the painful area. These may be signs of a serious condition.

➤*Hepatic effects:* Acetaminophen may cause liver damage.

➤*Pregnancy: Category B.*

If you are pregnant, seek the advice of a medical professional before using this product.

➤*Lactation:* If you are nursing a baby, seek the advice of a medical professional before using this product.

➤*Children:* Do not use 650 mg suppositories in children under 12 years of age.

Drug Interactions

➤*Alcohol:* If you drink 3 or more alcoholic beverages daily, ask your doctor whether you should take acetaminophen or other pain relievers.

Patient Information

➤*Tamper-resistant:* Suppositories are individually wrapped. Do not use if imprinted wrapper is opened or damaged.

Keep this and all drugs out of the reach of children. In case of accidental ingestion, seek professional assistance or contact a poison control center immediately. Prompt medical attention is critical for adults and children even if you do not notice any signs or symptoms.

SALICYLATES

WARNING

Children and teenagers should not use salicylates for chickenpox or flu symptoms before a doctor is consulted about Reye's syndrome, a rare but serious illness.

Indications

Mild to moderate pain; fever; various inflammatory conditions such as rheumatic fever, rheumatoid arthritis and osteoarthritis.

➤*Aspirin:* Aspirin, for reducing the risk of recurrent transient ischemic attacks (TIAs) or stroke in men who have had transient ischemia of the brain due to fibrin platelet emboli. It has not been effective in women and is of no benefit for completed strokes.

➤*Aspirin:* Aspirin, to reduce the risk of death or nonfatal myocardial infarction (MI) in patients with previous infarction or unstable angina pectoris.

➤*Unlabeled uses:* Possible effect of long-term aspirin-like analgesics to prevent cataract formation is being studied. Dipyridamole is often added to aspirin to prevent MI and stroke, but data do not show improved antithrombotic aspirin efficacy during coadministration. Low-dose aspirin may help prevent toxemia of pregnancy and may be beneficial in pregnant women with inadequate uteroplacental blood flow (eg, systemic lupus erythematosus). Further studies are needed. See Warnings.

Actions

➤*Pharmacology:* The salicylates have analgesic, antipyretic and anti-inflammatory effects. **Aspirin** and other salicylic acid derivatives are hydrolyzed to salicylic acid. Salicylamide and **diflunisal** are structurally related, but are not true salicylates because they are not hydrolyzed to salicylic acid.

Salicylates have analgesic, antipyretic, anti-inflammatory and antirheumatic effects. The pharmacological effects of these agents are qualitatively similar. Salicylates lower elevated body temperature through vasodilation of peripheral vessels, thus enhancing dissipation of excess heat. The anti-inflammatory and analgesic activity may be mediated through inhibition of the prostaglandin synthetase enzyme complex.

Aspirin – Aspirin differs from the other agents in this group in that it more potently inhibits prostaglandin synthesis, has greater anti-inflammatory effects and irreversibly inhibits platelet aggregation. The aspirin molecule's acetyl group is believed to account for these differences. Aspirin inhibits prostaglandin production by acetylating cyclo-oxygenase, the initial enzyme in the prostaglandin biosynthesis pathway.

Irreversible inhibition of platelet aggregation (aspirin) – Single analgesic aspirin doses prolong bleeding time. Acetylation of platelet cyclo-oxygenase prevents synthesis of thromboxane A_2, a prostaglandin derivative, which is a potent vasoconstrictor and inducer of platelet aggregation and platelet release reaction. Aspirin (no other salicylates) inhibits platelet aggregation for the life of the platelet (7 to 10 days).

Aspirin has shown some success as an antiplatelet agent in patients with thromboembolic disease. Low doses of aspirin inhibit platelet aggregation and may be more effective than higher doses. Larger doses inhibit cyclo-oxygenase in arterial walls, interfering with prostacyclin production, a potent vasodilator and inhibitor of platelet aggregation. Combinations of dipyridamole or sulfinpyrazone with aspirin have been recommended for antithrombotic action for prophylaxis in various high risk situations (ie, coronary bypass graft patency, total hip replacement).

Myocardial infarction (MI) – **Aspirin** use in MI patients was associated with ≈ 20% reduction in risk of subsequent death and nonfatal reinfarction, a median absolute decrease of 3% from the 12% to 22% event rates with placebo. Daily aspirin dosage in post-MI studies was 300 mg in one and 900 to 1500 mg in five. In aspirin-treated unstable angina patients (325 mg/day), reduction in risk was about 50%, a reduction in event rate of 5% from the 10% rate with placebo over the 12-week study.

In the Aspirin Myocardial Infarction Study (AMIS) trial, 1 g/day was associated with small increases in systolic BP (average, 1.5 to 2.1 mmHg) and diastolic BP (0.5 to 0.6 mmHg). Uric acid levels and BUN increased by < 1 mg/dl.

In the Second International Study of Infarct Survival (ISIS-2) trial, patients who received a combination of aspirin (160 mg/day) and streptokinase after the onset of suspected acute MI had significantly fewer reinfarctions, strokes and deaths than those patients who received placebo. Also, the combination was significantly better than either drug alone; their separate effects on vascular deaths appeared additive.

Other pharmacological actions – Inhibition of prothrombin synthesis and prolonged prothrombin time are clinically significant only after large doses (≥ 6 g/day). Doses > 3 to 5 g/day have a uricosuric effect; low doses (< 2 g/day) decrease uric acid secretion.

➤*Pharmacokinetics:*

Absorption/Distribution – Salicylates are rapidly and completely absorbed after oral use. Bioavailability is dependent on the dosage form, presence of food, gastric emptying time, gastric pH, presence of antacids or buffering agents and particle size. Bioavailability of some enteric coated products may be erratic. Food slows the absorption of salicylates. Absorption from rectal suppositories is slower, resulting in lower salicylate levels. **Aspirin** is partially hydrolyzed to salicylic acid during absorption and is distributed to all body tissues and fluids, including fetal tissues, breast milk and CNS. Highest concentrations are found in plasma, liver, renal cortex, heart and lungs. Protein binding of salicylates is concentration-dependent. At low therapeutic concentrations (100 mcg/ml), ≈ 90% is bound; at higher plasma concentrations (400 mcg/ml), 76% is bound. Signs of salicylism (eg, tinnitus) occur at serum levels > 200 mcg/ml; severe toxic effects may occur at levels > 400 mcg/ml (see Adverse Reactions).

Metabolism/Excretion – Salicylic acid is eliminated by renal excretion and by oxidation and conjugation of metabolites. **Aspirin** has a half-life of ≈ 15 to 20 minutes. Salicylic acid has a half-life of 2 to 3 hours at low doses; at higher doses, it may exceed 20 hours. In therapeutic anti-inflammatory doses, half-life ranges from 6 to 12 hours. Plasma salicylate levels increase disproportionately as dosage is increased. Elimination is determined by zero order kinetics. Renal excretion of unchanged drug depends upon urine pH. As urinary pH changes from 5 to 8, renal clearance of free ionized salicylate increases from 2% to 3% of amount excreted to > 80%.

Contraindications

Hypersensitivity to salicylates or nonsteroidal anti-inflammatory drugs (NSAIDs). Use extreme caution in patients with history of adverse reactions to salicylates. Cross-sensitivity may exist between aspirin and other NSAIDs which inhibit prostaglandin synthesis, and aspirin and tartrazine. Aspirin cross-sensitivity does not appear to occur with sodium salicylate, salicylamide or choline salicylate. Aspirin hypersensitivity is more prevalent in those with asthma, nasal polyposis, chronic urticaria.

In hemophilia, bleeding ulcers and hemorrhagic states.

➤*Magnesium salicylate:* Magnesium salicylate in advanced chronic renal insufficiency due to magnesium retention.

Warnings

➤*Reye's syndrome:*

Salicylate association – Use of salicylates, particularly **aspirin**, in children or teenagers with influenza or chickenpox may be associated with development of Reye's syndrome. This rare, acute, life-threatening condition is characterized by vomiting, lethargy and belligerence that may progress to delirium and coma. Mortality rate is 20% to 30%; permanent brain damage has been reported in survivors.

A causal relationship is controversial, but CDC, FDA, American Academy of Pediatrics' Committee on Infectious Diseases and Surgeon General advise against salicylate use in children and teens with influenza or chickenpox. (See Warning Box.)

➤*Otic effects:* Discontinue use if dizziness, ringing in ears (tinnitus) or impaired hearing occurs. Tinnitus probably represents blood salicylic acid levels reaching or exceeding the upper limit of the therapeutic range. It is a helpful guide to dose titration. Temporary hearing loss disappears gradually upon discontinuation of the drug.

➤*Use in surgical patients:* Avoid **aspirin**, if possible, for 1 week prior to surgery because of the possibility of postoperative bleeding.

➤*Hypersensitivity reactions:* **Aspirin** intolerance, manifested by acute bronchospasm, generalized urticaria/angioedema, severe rhinitis or shock occurs in 4% to 19% of asthmatics. Symptoms occur within 3 hours after ingestion. The aspirin triad consists of the association of asthma, nasal polyps and aspirin intolerance. Have epinephrine 1:1000 immediately available. Refer to Management of Acute Hypersensitivity Reactions.

Foods – Foods may contribute to a reaction. Some foods with 6 mg/100 g salicylate include curry powder, paprika, licorice, Benedictine liqueur, prunes, raisins, tea, gherkins. A typical American diet contains 10 to 200 mg/day salicylate.

Desensitization – Desensitization has been successfully induced and maintained. Perform in hospital; generally maintain with one **aspirin**/day. Any NSAID can maintain desensitization. However, if maintenance is interrupted, sensitivity will reappear (2 to 5 days).

➤*Hepatic function impairment:* Use caution in liver damage, preexisting hypoprothrombinemia and vitamin K deficiency. Reversible hepatic encephalopathy occurred in a chronic alcoholic with cirrhosis who took ASA 5 g/day for osteoarthritis. Aspirin-induced hepatotoxicity occurred after therapeutic doses for rheumatoid arthritis.

➤*Pregnancy: Category D* (aspirin); *Category C* (salsalate, magnesium salicylate). **Aspirin** may produce adverse maternal effects: Anemia, ante- or postpartum hemorrhage, prolonged gestation and labor. Salicylates readily cross the placenta. By inhibiting prostaglandin synthesis, salicylates may cause constriction of ductus arteriosus, and, possibly, other untoward fetal effects. Maternal aspirin use during later stages of pregnancy may cause adverse fetal effects: Low birth weight, increased incidence of intracranial hemorrhage in premature infants, stillbirths, neonatal death. Salicylates may be teratogens. Avoid use during pregnancy, especially in third trimester.

➤*Lactation:* Salicylates are excreted in breast milk in low concentrations, producing peak milk levels ranging from 1.1 to 10 mcg/ml. Adverse effects on platelet function in the nursing infant have not been reported, but are a potential risk.

➤*Children:* Safety and efficacy of **magnesium salicylate** or **salsalate** have not been established. Administration of **aspirin** to children (including teenagers) with acute febrile illness has been associated with the development of Reye's syndrome. Dehydrated febrile children appear more prone to salicylate intoxication.

Precautions

➤*Renal effects:* Use with caution in chronic renal insufficiency; **aspirin** may cause a transient decrease in renal function, and may aggravate chronic kidney diseases (rare).

In patients with renal impairment, take precautions when administering **magnesium salicylate**. Discontinue other drugs containing magnesium and monitor serum magnesium levels if dosage levels of magnesium salicylate are high.

➤*GI effects:* Use caution in those intolerant to salicylate because of GI irritation, and in gastric ulcers, peptic ulcer, mild diabetes, gout, erosive gastritis or bleeding tendencies. **Salsalate** and **choline salicylate** may cause less GI irritation than **aspirin**.

Although fecal blood loss is less with enteric coated aspirin than with uncoated, give enteric coated aspirin with caution to patients with GI distress, ulcer or bleeding problems. Occult GI bleeding occurs in many patients but is not correlated with gastric distress. The amount of blood lost is usually clinically insignificant (average, 2.5 ml), but with prolonged use, it may result in iron deficiency anemia. Patients developing peptic ulcers while taking salicylates for rheumatic disease have healed during treatment with cimetidine and antacids despite continued salicylate use. In addition, although acute aspirin use results in mucosal lesions, only 20% to 25% of those on chronic aspirin for rheumatism develop mucosal injury.

➤*Hematologic effects:* **Aspirin** interferes with hemostasis. Avoid use if patients have severe anemia, history of blood coagulation defects, or take anticoagulants (see Drug Interactions).

➤*Long-term therapy:* To avoid potentially toxic concentrations, warn patients on long-term therapy not to take other salicylates (nonprescription analgesics, etc).

Periodically monitor plasma salicylic acid concentrations during long-term treatment to aid maintenance of therapeutic levels (100 to 300 mcg/ml). Toxic manifestations are not usually seen until concentrations exceed 300 mcg/ml. Monitor urinary pH regularly; sudden acidification, as from pH 6.5 to 5.5, can double the plasma level, resulting in toxicity.

➤*Salicylism:* Salicylism may require dosage adjustment.

➤*Controlled release aspirin:* Controlled release aspirin, because of its relatively long onset of action, is not recommended for antipyresis or short-term analgesia. Not recommended in children > 12; contraindicated in all children with fever accompanied by dehydration.

➤*Benzyl alcohol:* Some of these products contain the preservative benzyl alcohol, which has been associated with a fatal "gasping syndrome" in premature infants.

➤*Tartrazine sensitivity:* Some of these products contain tartrazine, which may cause allergic-type reactions (including bronchial asthma) in susceptible individuals. Although the incidence of tartrazine sensitivity in the general population is low, it is frequently seen in patients who also have aspirin hypersensitivity. Specific products containing tartrazine are identified in the product listings.

Drug Interactions

Salicylate Drug Interactions

Precipitant drug	Object drug*		Description
Alcohol	Salicylates	⬆	The risk of GI ulceration increases when salicylates are given concomitantly. Ingestion of alcohol during salicylate therapy may also prolong bleeding time.
Ammonium chloride	Salicylates	⬆	Urinary acidifiers decrease salicylate excretion.
Ascorbic acid			
Methionine			
Antacids	Salicylates	⬇	Antacids and urinary alkalinizers may decrease the pharmacologic effects of salicylates. Urinary alkalinization increases the renal excretion of salicylic acid due to decreased tubular reabsorption of un-ionized drug. The magnitude of the antacid interaction depends on the agent, dose and pretreatment urine pH.
Urinary alkalinizers			

Salicylate Drug Interactions

Precipitant drug	Object drug*		Description
Carbonic anhydrase inhibitors	Salicylates	↑	Salicylate intoxication has occurred after coadministration of these agents. However, salicylic acid renal elimination may be increased if urine is kept alkaline. Conversely, salicylates may displace acetazolamide from protein binding sites resulting in toxicity. Further study is needed.
Salicylates	Carbonic anhydrase inhibitors		
Charcoal, activated	Aspirin	↓	Coadministration decreases aspirin absorption, depending on charcoal dose and interval between ingestion. May be useful (see Overdosage).
Corticosteroids	Salicylates	↓	Corticosteroids increase salicylate clearance and decrease serum levels.
Nizatidine	Salicylates	↑	Increased serum salicylate levels have occurred in patients receiving high dose aspirin (3.9 g/day) and concurrent nizatidine.
Aspirin	Anticoagulants, oral	↑	Therapeutic aspirin has an additive hypoprothrombinemic effect. Impaired platelet function may prolong bleeding time. Use caution.
Anticoagulants, oral	Aspirin		
Aspirin	Heparin	↑	Aspirin can increase bleeding risk in heparin anticoagulated patients.
Aspirin	Nitroglycerin	↑	Nitroglycerin, when taken with aspirin, may result in unexpected hypotension. Data are limited. If hypotension occurs, reduce the nitroglycerin dose.
Aspirin	NSAIDs	↓	Aspirin may decrease NSAID serum concentrations. Concomitant use offers no advantage and may significantly increase incidence of GI effects.
Aspirin	Valproic acid	↑	Aspirin displaces the drug from its protein-binding sites and may decrease its total body clearance, thus increasing the pharmacologic effects.
Salicylates	Angiotensin-converting enzyme inhibitors	↓	Antihypertensive effectiveness of these agents may be decreased by concurrent salicylate administration, possibly due to prostaglandin inhibition. Consider discontinuing salicylates if problems occur.
Salicylates	Beta-adrenergic blockers	↓	Beta-adrenergic blockers may have their antihypertensive action blunted by concurrent salicylate administration, possibly due to prostaglandin inhibition. Consider discontinuing salicylates if problems occur.
Salicylates	Loop diuretics	↓	Loop diuretics may be less effective when given with salicylates in patients with compromised renal function or with cirrhosis with ascites; however, data conflict.
Salicylates	Methotrexate	↑	Salicylates increase drug levels causing toxicity by interfering with protein binding and renal elimination of the antimetabolite.
Salicylates	Probenecid	↓	Salicylates antagonize the uricosuric effect of probenecid and sulfinpyrazone. While salicylates in large doses (> 3 g/day) have a uricosuric effect, smaller amounts may reduce the uricosuric effect of these agents.
	Sulfinpyrazone		
Salicylates	Spironolactone	↓	Salicylates may inhibit the diuretic effects; antihypertensive action does not appear altered. Effects depend on the dose of spironolactone.
Salicylates	Sulfonylureas	↑	Salicylates in doses > 2 g/day have a hypoglycemic action, perhaps by altering pancreatic beta cell function. They may potentiate the glucose-lowering effect of these drugs.
	Insulin		

* ↑ = Object drug increased. ↓ = Object drug decreased.

➤*Drug/Lab test interactions:* Salicylates compete with thyroid hormone for binding sites on thyroid binding pre-albumin and possibly thyroid-binding globulin resulting in increases in **protein bound iodine (PBI)**. Salicylates probably do not interfere with T_3 resin uptake.

Serum uric acid – Serum uric acid levels are elevated by salicylate levels < 10 mg/dl and decreased by levels > 10 mg/dl. Combined **phenylbutazone** and salicylates decrease uric acid excretion and may increase serum uric acid by an average of 2 mg/dl.

Salicylates in moderate to large (anti-inflammatory) doses cause false-negative readings for **urine glucose** by the glucose oxidase method and false-positive readings by the copper reduction method.

Salicylates in the urine interfere with **5–HIAA** determinations by fluorescent methods, but not by the nitrosonaphthol colorimetric method.

Salicylates in the urine interact with **urinary ketone** determinations by the ferric chloride (Gerhardt) method producing a reddish color.

Large doses may decrease urinary excretion of **PSP (phenolsulfonphthalein)**.

Salicylates in the urine result in falsely elevated **VMA (vanillylmandelic acid)** with most tests, but falsely decrease VMA determinations by the Pisano method.

Adverse Reactions

➤*Dermatologic:* Hives, rashes and angioedema may occur, especially in patients suffering from chronic urticaria.

➤*GI:* Nausea, dyspepsia (5% to 25%), heartburn, epigastric discomfort, anorexia, acute reversible hepatotoxicity, massive GI bleeding and occult blood loss may occur. Aspirin may potentiate peptic ulcer.

Chronic aspirin use may cause persistent iron deficiency anemia.

➤*Hematologic:* Prolongation of bleeding time, leukopenia, thrombocytopenia, purpura, decreased plasma iron concentration, shortened erythrocyte survival time.

➤*Hepatic:* High aspirin doses reportedly produced reversible hepatic dysfunction.

➤*Miscellaneous:* Fever, thirst, dimness of vision.

Allergic reactions – Allergic and anaphylactic reactions were noted when hypersensitive individuals took aspirin. Fatal anaphylactic shock, while not common, has been reported.

Aspirin intolerance – Aspirin intolerance, manifested by exacerbation of bronchospasm and rhinitis, may occur in patients with a history of nasal polyps, asthma or rhinitis. The mechanism of this intolerance may be the result of aspirin-induced shunting of prostaglandin synthesis to the lipoxygenase pathway and liberation of leukotrienes, ie, slow-reacting substance of anaphylaxis.

Salicylism – Mild "salicylism" may occur after repeated use of large doses and consists of dizziness, tinnitus (manifested as musical perceptions in one patient), difficulty hearing, nausea, vomiting, diarrhea, mental confusion, CNS depression, headache, sweating, hyperventilation and lassitude. Salicylate serum concentrations correlate with pharmacological actions and adverse effects observed. See table below:

Serum Salicylate: Clinical Correlations

Serum salicylate concentration (mcg/ml)	Desired effects	Adverse effects/ intoxication
≈ 100	Antiplatelet Antipyresis Analgesia	GI intolerance and bleeding, hypersensitivity, hemostatic defects
150-300	Anti-inflammatory	Mild salicylism
250-400	Treatment of rheumatic fever	Nausea/vomiting, hyperventilation, salicylism, flushing, sweating, thirst, headache, diarrhea, and tachycardia
> 400-500		Respiratory alkalosis, hemorrhage, excitement, confusion, asterixis, pulmonary edema, convulsions, tetany, metabolic acidosis, fever, coma, cardiovascular collapse, renal and respiratory failure

Overdosage

➤*Symptoms:*

Acute lethal dose (approximate) –

Adults: 10 to 30 g.

Children: 4 g. Respiratory alkalosis is seen initially in acute salicylate ingestions. Hyperpnea and tachypnea occur as a result of increased CO_2 production and a direct stimulatory effect of salicylate on the respiratory center. Other symptoms may include nausea, vomiting, hypokalemia, tinnitus, neurologic abnormalities (eg, disorientation, irritability, hallucinations, lethargy, stupor, coma, seizures), dehydration, hyperthermia, hyperventilation, hyperactivity, thrombocytopenia, platelet dysfunction, hypoprothrombinemia, increased capillary fragility and other hematologic abnormalities. Symptoms may progress quickly to depression, coma, respiratory failure and collapse. Although blood glucose is usually normal or slightly elevated, hypoglycemia may occur with chronic toxicity or in late acute toxicity. A mixed respiratory alkalosis and metabolic acidosis may also develop. Chronic salicylate toxicity may occur when > 100 mg/kg/day is ingested for 2 or more days. It is more difficult to recognize and is associated with increased morbidity and mortality. Compared to acute poisoning, hyperventilation, dehydration, systemic acidosis and severe CNS manifestations occur more frequently.

➤*Treatment:* Initial treatment includes induction of emesis or gastric lavage to remove any unabsorbed drug from the stomach. Activated charcoal diminishes salicylate absorption, most effectively if given within 2 hours after ingestion. Monitor salicylate levels, acid-base and fluid and electrolyte balance. Further therapy is largely supportive. Refer to General Management of Acute Overdosage. Reduce hyperthermia; treat severe convulsions with diazepam. Forced alkaline diuresis will enhance renal excretion of salicylates. Hemodialysis is very efficient in eliminating salicylate, but use only in patients who are severely poisoned, and in those with noncardiogenic pulmonary edema, severe CNS symptoms, renal failure, acidosis refractory to conservative therapy or clinical deterioration despite other therapies. Rarely, IV vitamin K may be indicated to correct hypoprothrombinemia.

Patient Information

May cause GI upset; take with food or after meals.

Do not crush or chew sustained release preparations.

Take with a full glass of water (240 ml) to reduce the risk of lodging medication in the esophagus.

Patients allergic to tartrazine dye should avoid **aspirin**.

Notify physician if ringing in ears or persistent GI pain occurs.

Do not use **aspirin** if it has a strong vinegar-like odor.

ASPIRIN (Acetylsalicylic Acid; ASA)

otc	**Bayer Children's Aspirin** (Bayer)	**Tablets, chewable:** 81 mg	Saccharin. (BAYER BAYER BAYER BAYER). Orange flavor. In 36s.
otc	**St. Joseph Adult Chewable Aspirin** (Schering-Plough)		Saccharin. (SJ). Orange flavor. In 36s.
otc	**Aspergum** (Schering-Plough)	**Gum tablets:** 227.5 mg	Chewable. Glucose, saccharin, sugar. Orange and cherry flavors. In 16s and 40s.
otc	**Aspirin** (Various, eg, Moore, Parmed, Rugby, URL, Warner-C)	**Tablets:** 325 mg	In 100s, 200s, 250s, 500s, and 1,000s.
otc	**Genuine Bayer Aspirin Caplets** (Bayer)		**Caplets:** (BAYER BAYER BAYER BAYER). Film coated. In 50s, 100s, and 200s.
otc	**Empirin** (GlaxoWellcome)		(Tabloid brand). White. In 50s, 100s, and 250s.
otc	**Norwich Regular Strength** (Lee)		Coated. In 100s.
otc	**Aspirin** (URL)	**Tablets:** 500 mg	In 100s.
otc	**Arthritis Foundation Pain Reliever** (McNeil-CPC)		In 50s.
otc	**Maximum Bayer Aspirin Tablets and Caplets** (Bayer)		**Tablets:** Film coated. In 30s, 60s, and 100s.
			Caplets: Film coated. In 30s and 60s.
otc	**Norwich Extra-Strength** (Procter & Gamble)		In 150s.
otc	**Ecotrin Adult Low Strength** (GlaxoSmithKline Consumer Healthcare)	**Tablets, enteric coated:** 81 mg	Tartrazine. (ECOTRIN LOW). In 45s.
otc	**Halfprin 81** (Kramer)		In 90s.
otc	**Heartline** (BDI)		In 36s.
otc	**½ Halfprin** (Kramer)	**Tablets, enteric coated:** 165 mg	Red. In 60s and 200s.
otc	**Aspirin** (Various, eg, Geneva, Major, Moore, Parmed, Rugby, URL)	**Tablets, enteric coated:** 325 mg	In 30s, 60s, 90s, 100s, 1,000s, and UD 100s.
otc	**Ecotrin Tablets and Caplets** (SmithKline Beecham)		**Tablets:** (Ecotrin Reg). In 100s, 250s, and 1,000s.
			Caplets: (Ecotrin Reg). In 100s.
otc	**Ecotrin Maximum Strength Caplets** (SmithKline Beecham)	**Tablets, enteric coated:** 500 mg	**Caplets:** (Ecotrin Max). In 60s.
otc	**Extra Strength Bayer Enteric 500 Aspirin** (Bayer)		(Bayer 500). In 60s.
otc	**Aspirin** (Various, eg, Moore, Rugby)	**Tablets, enteric coated:** 650 mg	In 100s and 1,000s.
otc	**Extended Release Bayer 8-Hour Caplets** (Bayer)	**Tablets, extended release:** 650 mg	White, scored. In 50s.
Rx	**ZORprin** (PAR)	**Tablets, controlled release:** 800 mg	(57). White. Elongated. In 100s.
otc	**Bayer Low Adult Strength** (Bayer)	**Tablets, delayed release:** 81 mg	Lactose. (81). In 120s.
otc	**Aspirin** (Various, eg, Goldline, Moore, Rugby, URL)	**Suppositories**[a]: 120 mg	In 12s.
		200 mg	In 12s.
		300 mg	In 12s.
		600 mg	In 12s and 100s.

[a] Refrigerate.

ASPIRIN — ORAL

For complete and comparative prescribing information, refer to the Salicylates group monograph.

Indications

➤*Vascular indication (ischemic stroke, transient ischemic attack, acute myocardial infarction, prevention of recurrent MI, unstable angina pectoris, and chronic stable angina pectoris):* Aspirin is indicated to:

1.) Reduce the combined risk of death and nonfatal stroke in patients who have had ischemic stroke or transient ischemia of the brain due to fibrin platelet emboli.
2.) Reduce the risk of vascular mortality in patients with a suspected acute MI.
3.) Reduce the combined risk of death and nonfatal MI in patients with a previous MI or unstable angina pectoris.
4.) Reduce the combined risk of MI and sudden death in patients with chronic stable angina pectoris.

Revascularization procedures (coronary artery bypass graft [CABG], percutaneous transluminal coronary angioplasty [PTCA], and carotid endarterectomy) – Aspirin is indicated in patients who have undergone revascularization procedures (ie, CABG, PTCA or carotid endarterectomy) when there is a preexisting condition for which aspirin is already indicated.

➤*Rheumatoid disease indications (rheumatoid arthritis, juvenile rheumatoid arthritis, spondyloarthropathies, osteoarthritis, and the arthritis and pleurisy of systemic lupus erythematosus [SLE]):* Aspirin is indicated for the relief of the signs and symptoms of rheumatoid arthritis, juvenile rheumatoid arthritis, osteoarthritis, spondyloarthropathies, and arthritis and pleurisy associated with SLE.

➤*Analgesic/antipyretic:* Temporary relief of:

- Headache.
- Pain and fever of colds.
- Muscle aches and pains.
- Menstrual pain.
- Toothache pain.
- Minor aches and pains of arthritis.

ASPIRIN — ORAL

Administration and Dosage

Take each dose of aspirin with a full glass of water unless the patient is fluid restricted. Individualize anti-inflammatory and analgesic dosages. When aspirin is used in high doses, the development of tinnitus may be used as a clinical sign of elevated plasma salicylate levels except in patients with high frequency hearing loss.

➤*Ischemic stroke and TIA:* 50 to 325 mg once a day. Continue therapy indefinitely.

➤*Suspected acute MI:* Administer the initial dose of 160 to 325 mg as soon as an MI is suspected. Continue the maintenance dose of 160 to 325 mg a day for 30 days post-infarction. After 30 days, consider further therapy based on dosage and administration for prevention of recurrent MI.

➤*Prevention of recurrent MI:* 75 to 325 mg once a day. Continue therapy indefinitely.

➤*Unstable angina pectoris:* 75 to 325 mg once a day. Continue therapy indefinitely.

➤*Chronic stable angina pectoris:* 75 to 325 mg once a day. Continue therapy indefinitely.

➤*CABG:* 325 mg daily starting 6 hours postprocedure. Continue therapy for 1 year postprocedure.

➤*PTCA:* Give the initial dose of 325 mg 2 hours presurgery. Maintenance dose is 160 to 325 mg daily. Continue therapy indefinitely.

➤*Carotid endarterectomy:* Doses of 80 mg once daily to 650 mg twice daily, started presurgery, are recommended. Continue therapy indefinitely.

➤*Rheumatoid arthritis:* The initial dose is 3 g a day in divided doses. Increase as needed for anti-inflammatory efficacy with target plasma salicylate levels of 150 to 300 mcg/mL. At high doses (ie, plasma levels of greater than 200 mcg/mL), the incidence of toxicity increases.

➤*Juvenile rheumatoid arthritis:* Initial dose is 90 to 130 mg/kg/day in divided doses. Increase as needed for anti-inflammatory efficacy with target plasma salicylate levels of 150 to 300 mcg/mL. At high doses (ie, plasma levels greater than 200 mcg/mL), the incidence of toxicity increases.

➤*Spondyloarthropathies:* Up to 4 g/day in divided doses.

➤*Osteoarthritis:* Up to 3 g/day in divided doses.

➤*Arthritis and pleurisy of SLE:* The initial dose is 3 g/day in divided doses. Increase as needed for anti-inflammatory efficacy with target plasma salicylate levels of 150 to 300 mcg/mL. At high doses (ie, plasma levels of greater than 200 mcg/mL), the incidence of toxicity increases.

➤*Analgesic/antipyretic:*

Adults and children 12 years of age or over – Take 324 to 1,000 mg every 4 to 6 hours as needed up to a maximum of 4,000 mg per 24 hours or as directed by a doctor.

Extended-release products: Take 1,300 mg followed by 650 to 1,300 mg every 8 hours, as needed, up to a maximum of 3,900 mg per 24 hours or as directed by a doctor. For maximum nighttime and early morning relief from stiffness upon arising, take 1,300 mg at bedtime.

Aspirin gum: Chew 454 mg every 4 hours, not to exceed 3,632 mg in 24 hours, or as directed by a doctor.

Children under 12 years of age – 10 to 15 mg/kg/dose every 4 hours (see the following table), up to 60 to 80 mg/kg/day. Do not use in children or teenagers with chickenpox or flu symptoms due to the possibility of Reye's syndrome. Dosage recommendations by age and weight are as follows:

Recommended Aspirin Dosage in Children

Age (years)	Weight		Dosage (mg every 4 hours)	No. of 81 mg tablets (every 4 hours)	No. of 325 mg tablets (every 4 hours)
	lbs	kg			
2 to 3	24 to 35	10.6 to 15.9	162	2	0.5
4 to 5	36 to 47	16 to 21.4	243	3	
6 to 8	48 to 59	21.5 to 26.8	324	4	1
9 to 10	60 to 71	26.9 to 32.3	405	5	
11	72 to 95	32.4 to 43.2	486	6	1.5
12 to 14	≥ 96	≥ 43.3	648	8	2

➤*Storage/Stability:* Store oral aspirin products in a cool dry place at controlled room temperature 15° to 30°C (59° to 86°F). Keep container closed after each use.

Aspirin gum is safety sealed. Do not use if foil imprint is torn or missing.

ASPIRIN — RECTAL

For complete and comparative prescribing information, refer to the Salicylates group monograph.

Indications

For the relief of minor aches, pains, and headache and for reduction of fever.

Administration and Dosage

➤*Directions:* Remove suppository from plastic packet and insert into the rectum as far as possible.

Adult – 1 suppository every 4 hours for no more than 10 days or as directed by a physician.

Children under 12 years of age – Consult a physician.

➤*Storage/Stability:* Store in a cool place 8° to 15°C (46° to 59°F) or refrigerate.

ASPIRIN (Acetylsalicylic Acid; ASA), BUFFERED

otc	**Tri-Buffered Bufferin Tablets and Caplets** (Bristol-Myers Squibb)	**Tablets**: 325 mg with calcium carbonate, magnesium oxide and magnesium carbonate	**Tablets**: (B). White. In 12s, 36s, 60s, 100s, 200s, 275s, 1000s. **Caplets**: (B). White, scored. In 36s, 60s and 100s.
otc	**Buffered Aspirin** (Various, eg, Geneva, Goldline, Major, Moore, Rugby, UDL, URL)	**Tablets**: 325 mg with buffers	In 100s, 500s, 1000s and UD 100s and 200s.
otc	**Bayer Buffered Aspirin** (Bayer)		(Bayer Buffered). In 100s.
otc	**Asprimox** (Invamed)	**Caplets**: 325 mg with buffers	In 100s and 500s.
otc	**Asprimox Extra Protection for Arthritis Pain** (Invamed)		In 100s and 500s.
otc	**Adprin-B** (Pfeiffer)	**Tablets, coated**: 325 mg with calcium carbonate, magnesium carbonate and magnesium oxide	In 130s.
otc	**Asprimox** (Invamed)	**Tablets, coated**: 325 mg with 75 mg aluminum hydroxide, 75 mg magnesium hydroxide and calcium carbonate	Capsule shape. In 100s and 500s.
otc	**Magnaprin** (Rugby)	**Tablets, coated**: 325 mg with 50 mg magnesium hydroxide, 50 mg aluminum hydroxide and calcium carbonate	Film coated. In 100s and 500s.
otc	**Ascriptin** (Rhone-Poulenc Rorer)		(Ascriptin). In 60s.
otc	**Ascriptin A/D** (Rhone-Poulenc Rorer)	**Tablets, coated**: 325 mg with 75 mg magnesium hydroxide, 75 mg aluminum hydroxide and calcium carbonate	(AP Ascriptin). Capsule shape. In 225s.
otc	**Magnaprin Arthritis Strength Captabs** (Rugby)		Capsule shape. In 100s and 500s.
otc	**Bufferin** (Bristol-Myers)	**Tablets, coated**: 325 mg with 158 mg calcium carbonate, 63 mg magnesium oxide and 34 mg magnesium carbonate	(B). In 12s, 36s, 60s, 100s, 200s and UD 150s.
otc	**Extra Strength Bayer Plus Caplets** (Bayer)	**Tablets**: 500 mg with calcium carbonate, magnesium carbonate, and magnesium oxide	In 30s and 60s.
otc	**Bufferin Extra Strength** (Bristol-Myers)		In 130s.
otc	**Ascriptin Maximum Strength** (Novartis)	**Tablets**: 500 mg aspirin, 237 mg calcium carbonate, 33 mg magnesium hydroxide, 33 mg aluminum hydroxide.	Capsule shaped. In 85s.

ASPIRIN (Acetylsalicylic Acid; ASA), BUFFERED

otc	**Ascriptin Extra Strength** (Rhone-Poulenc Rorer)	**Tablets, coated**: 500 mg with 80 mg magnesium hydroxide, 80 mg aluminum hydroxide and calcium carbonate	Capsule shape. In 50s.
otc	**Arthritis Pain Formula** (Whitehall)	**Tablets**: 500 mg with 100 mg magnesium hydroxide and 27 mg aluminum hydroxide	Capsule shape. In 40s, 100s, and 175s.
otc	**Alka-Seltzer with Aspirin** (Bayer)	**Tablets, effervescent**: 325 mg with 1.9 g sodium bicarbonate and 1 g citric acid per dry tablet, 567 mg sodium/tablet	In 12s, 24s, 36s, 72s, 96s, and 100s.
otc	**Alka-Seltzer with Aspirin (Flavored)** (Bayer)	**Tablets, effervescent**: 325 mg with 1.7 g sodium bicarbonate and 1.2 g citric acid per dry tablet, 506 mg sodium/tablet	Saccharin and flavoring. In 12s, 24s and 36s.
otc	**Alka-Seltzer Extra Strength with Aspirin** (Bayer)	**Tablet, effervescent**: 500 mg with 1.9 g sodium bicarbonate and 1 g citric acid	In 12s and 24s.
otc	**Asprimox Extra Protection for Arthritis Pain** (Invamed)	**Tablets** : 325 mg with 75 mg aluminum hydroxide, 75 mg magnesium hydroxide and calcium carbonate	Capsule shape. In 100s and 500s.

ASPIRIN (Acetylsalicylic Acid; ASA), BUFFERED — ORAL

Complete prescribing information for these products begins in the Salicylates monograph.

Administration and Dosage

The addition of small amounts of antacids may decrease GI irritation and increase the dissolution and absorption rates of these products.

DIFLUNISAL

Rx	**Diflunisal** (Various, eg, Lemmon, West Point Pharma)	**Tablets**: 250 mg	In 100s, 500s and unit-of-use 60s.
Rx	**Dolobid** (MSD)		(MSD 675). Peach. Film coated. In unit-of-use 60s and UD 100s.
Rx	**Diflunisal** (Various, eg, Lemmon, West Point Pharma)	**Tablets**: 500 mg	In 100s, 500s and unit-of-use 60s.
Rx	**Dolobid** (MSD)		(MSD 697). In UD 100s and unit-of-use 60s.

DIFLUNISAL — ORAL

WARNING

Cardiovascular risk – Nonsteroidal anti-inflammatory agents (NSAIDs) may cause an increased risk of serious cardiovascular thrombotic events, myocardial infarction, and stroke, which can be fatal. This risk may increase with duration of use. Patients with cardiovascular disease or risk factors for cardiovascular disease may be at greater risk.

Diflunisal is contraindicated for the treatment of peri-operative pain in the setting of coronary artery bypass graft (CABG) surgery.

GI risk – NSAIDs cause an increased risk of serious GI adverse events including bleeding, ulceration, and perforation of the stomach or intestines, which can be fatal. These events can occur at any time during use and without warning symptoms. Elderly patients are at greater risk for serious GI events.

Indications

For acute or long-term use for symptomatic treatment of the following: Mild to moderate pain; osteoarthritis (OA); rheumatoid arthritis (RA).

Administration and Dosage

Concentration-dependent pharmacokinetics prevail when diflunisal is administered; a doubling of dosage produces a greater than doubling of drug accumulation. The effect becomes more apparent with repetitive doses.

➤*Administration:* Diflunisal may be administered with water, milk, or meals. Tablets should be swallowed whole, not crushed or chewed.

➤*Mild to moderate pain:* For mild to moderate pain, an initial dose of 1,000 mg followed by 500 mg every 12 hours is recommended for most patients. Following the initial dose, some patients may require 500 mg every 8 hours.

A lower dosage may be appropriate depending on such factors as pain severity, patient response, weight, or advanced age; for example, 500 mg initially, followed by 250 mg every 8 to 12 hours.

➤*OA / RA:* For OA and RA, the suggested dosage range is 500 to 1,000 mg daily in 2 divided doses. The dosage of diflunisal may be increased or decreased according to patient response.

Maintenance dosages higher than 1,500 mg a day are not recommended.

MAGNESIUM SALICYLATE

otc	**Backache Maximum Strength Relief** (B-M Squibb)	**Caplets**: 467 mg (as tetrahydrate)	Film coated. In 24s and 50s.
Rx	**Novasal** (US Pharmaceutical)	**Tablet**: 600 mg (as tetrahydrate)	(0700/US). Light red, oval, scored. Film-coated. In 100s.
otc	**Extra Strength Doan's** (Ciba Consumer)	**Caplets**: 500 mg	(DOAN'S). In 24s and 48s.
otc	**Bayer Select Maximum Strength Backache** (Bayer)	**Caplets**: 580 mg (as tetrahydrate)	In 24s and 50s.
otc	**Momentum Muscular Backache Formula** (Whitehall)	**Caplets**: 580 mg (as tetrahydrate, equivalent to 467 mg magnesium salicylate anhydrous)	(MSM). In 48s.
Rx	**Magan** (Adria)	**Tablets**: 545 mg	(Adria 412). Pink. In 100s and 500s.
Rx	**Mobidin** (Ascher)	**Tablets**: 600 mg	(0310). Yellow, scored. In 100s and 500s.
otc	**Doan's** (Novartis Consumer Health)	**Tablets**: 377 mg (as tetrahydrate, equivalent to 303.7 mg magnesium salicylate anhydrous)	In 24s.

MAGNESIUM SALICYLATE TETRAHYDRATE — ORAL

Complete prescribing information for these products begins in the Salicylates monograph.

Administration and Dosage

➤*Rx:*

Adults – 600 mg 3 or 4 times per day.

Elderly: A reduced dosage, lower than the recommended schedules, should always be considered for patients 65 years of age and older, because of possible salicylate overdose and precautions pertaining to the renal and neurologic organ system. The dosage in elderly patients should always be at the lowest level to minimize and avoid adverse reactions.

➤*OTC:*

Adults – 2 tablets with a full glass of water every 4 to 6 hours while symptoms persist, or as directed by a health care provider. Patients should not take more than 8 to 12 tablets in any 24-hour period. See labeling information for specific dosing information.

Children younger than 12 years of age – Patients should consult a health care provider.

➤*Storage / Stability:* Store at room temperature, between 15° and 30°C (59° and 86°F).

Dispense in a tight, light-resistant container with a child-resistant closure.

SALICYLATE COMBINATIONS

Rx	**Choline Magnesium Trisalicylate** (Various, eg, Sidmak, Zenith Goldline)	**Tablets**: 500 mg salicylate (as 293 mg choline salicylate, 362 mg Mg salicylate)	(SL 528). Yellow, scored. Film coated, capsule shape. In 100s and 500s.
		750 mg salicylate (as 440 mg choline salicylate, 544 mg Mg salicylate)	(SL 529). Blue, scored. Film coated, capsule shape. In 100s and 500s.
		1000 mg salicylate (as 587 mg choline salicylate, 725 mg Mg salicylate)	(SL 530). Pink, scored. Capsule shape, film coated. In 100s and 500s.
Rx	**Choline Magnesium Trisalicylate** (Various, eg, Cypress)	**Liquid**: 500 mg salicylate (as 293 mg choline salicylate, 362 mg Mg salicylate)/5 ml	In 237 ml.

Complete prescribing information for these products begins in the Salicylates monograph.

SALSALATE (Salicylsalicylic Acid)

Rx	**Salsalate** (Various, eg, Geneva, Goldline, Major, Moore, Rugby, URL, Vitarine)	**Tablets**: 500 mg	In 100s, 500s and UD 100s.
Rx	**Amigesic** (Amide)		(A 019). Yellow or blue. Film coated. In 100s and 500s.
Rx	**Argesic-SA** (Econo Med)		In 100s.
Rx	**Salflex** (Carnrick)		Dye free. (C 8671). White. Film coated. In 100s.
Rx	**Salsitab** (Upsher-Smith)		(500). Blue. Film coated. In 100s, 500s and UD 100s.
Rx	**Salsalate** (Various, eg, Copley, Geneva, Goldline, Major, Moore, Rugby, URL, Vitarine)	**Tablets**: 750 mg	In 100s, 500s and UD 100s.
Rx	**Amigesic Caplets** (Amide)		(A0 10). Yellow or blue, scored. Film coated, Capsule shaped. In 100s and 500s.
Rx	**Artha-G** (T.E. Williams)		(Artha-G). Lavender, scored. In 120s.
Rx	**Marthritic** (Marnel)		In 100s.
Rx	**Salsitab** (Upsher-Smith)		(750). Blue, scored. Film coated. In 100s, 500s and UD 100s.
Rx	**Salflex** (Carnrick)		Dye free. (C 8672). White, scored. Film coated. In 100s and 500s.

SALSALATE — ORAL

Complete prescribing information for these products begins in the Salicylates monograph.

Administration and Dosage

Dosage should be adjusted according to the severity of the disease and the response of the patient.

➤*Adults:* The usual dosage is 3000 mg daily, given in divided doses, such as 2 tablets twice daily or 1 tablet 4 times daily. Some patients, eg, the elderly, may require a lower dosage to achieve therapeutic blood concentrations and to avoid the more common side effects such as auditory disturbances.

Alleviation of symptoms is gradual, and full benefit may not be evident for 3 to 4 days, when plasma salicylate levels have achieved steady state. There is no evidence for development of tissue tolerance (tachyphylaxis) but salicylate therapy may induce increased activity of metabolizing liver enzymes, causing a greater rate of salicyluric acid production and excretion, with a resultant increase in dosage requirement for maintenance of therapeutic serum salicylate levels.

➤*Storage/Stability:* Dispense in a tight container as defined in the USP-NF with a child-resistant closure.

Store at controlled room temperature 15° to 30°C (59° to 86°F).

SODIUM THIOSALICYLATE

Rx	**Sodium Thiosalicylate** (Various)	**Injection**: 50 mg/ml	In 30 ml vials and 2 ml amps.
Rx	**Rexolate** (Hyrex)		In 30 ml vials.

SODIUM THIOSALICYLATE — INJECTION

Complete and comparative prescribing information for these products begins in the Salicylates monograph.

Administration and Dosage

It is advisable to administer this product IM in order to obviate the usual problems associated with IV administration.

➤*Rheumatic fever:* In the symptomatic treatment of rheumatic fever, the usual adult IM dosage is 100 to 150 mg every 4 to 8 hours for 3 days, followed by 100 mg twice daily until the patient is asymptomatic.

➤*Gout:* In the symptomatic treatment of acute gout, the usual adult IM dosage is 100 mg every 3 to 4 hours for 2 days, followed by 100 mg once daily until the patient is asymptomatic.

➤*Muscular pain/disorders:* The usual adult dosage for the symptomatic treatment of muscular pain and musculoskeletal disorders is 50 to 100 mg once daily or once every other day.

➤*Storage/Stability:* Store at 15° to 30°C (59° to 86°F).

NONNARCOTIC ANALGESIC COMBINATIONS

Content given per capsule, tablet, or packet.

<table>
<tr><th></th><th>Product and Distributor</th><th>Acetaminophen</th><th>Aspirin</th><th>Other Analgesics</th><th>Caffeine</th><th>Other Content</th><th>How Supplied</th></tr>
<tr><td>otc</td><td>Painaid Tablets
(Zee Medical)</td><td>110 mg</td><td>162 mg</td><td>152 mg salicylamide</td><td>32.4 mg</td><td></td><td>In 24s.</td></tr>
<tr><td>otc</td><td>Saleto Tablets
(Mallard)</td><td>115 mg</td><td>210 mg</td><td>65 mg salicylamide</td><td>16 mg</td><td></td><td>Pink. In 100s, 1000s, and Sani-Pak 1000s.</td></tr>
<tr><td>otc</td><td>FemBack Caplets
(CCA Laboratories)</td><td>150 mg</td><td></td><td>150 mg salicylamide</td><td></td><td>44 mg phenyltoloxamine citrate</td><td>Coated. In 24s.</td></tr>
<tr><td>otc</td><td>Vanquish Caplets
(Bayer)</td><td>194 mg</td><td>227 mg</td><td></td><td>33 mg</td><td>50 mg magnesium hydroxide, 25 mg aluminum hydroxide</td><td>(Vanquish). In 60s and 100s.</td></tr>
<tr><td>otc</td><td>Excedrin Migraine
(Bristol-Myers Squibb)</td><td rowspan="8">250 mg</td><td rowspan="4">250 mg</td><td rowspan="4"></td><td rowspan="4">65 mg</td><td rowspan="4"></td><td>(E). In 50s and 100s.</td></tr>
<tr><td rowspan="3">otc</td><td rowspan="3">Excedrin Extra Strength Caplets, Tablets, and Geltabs
(Bristol-Myers Squibb)</td><td>Caplets: Saccharin. (E). In 24s, 50s, 100s, 175s, and 275s.</td></tr>
<tr><td>Tablets: Saccharin. (E). In 24s, 50s, 100s, 175s, and 275s.</td></tr>
<tr><td>Geltabs: Saccharin. In 24s, 40s, and 80s.</td></tr>
<tr><td>otc</td><td>Painaid BRF Back Relief Formula Tablets (Zee Medical)</td><td></td><td>250 mg magnesium salicylate tetrahydrate</td><td></td><td></td><td>In 24s.</td></tr>
<tr><td>otc</td><td>Painaid ESF Extra-Strength Formula Tablets
(Zee Medical)</td><td>250 mg</td><td></td><td>65 mg</td><td></td><td>In 24s.</td></tr>
<tr><td>otc</td><td>Pamprin Maximum Pain Relief Caplets
(Chattem)</td><td></td><td>250 mg magnesium salicylate</td><td></td><td>25 mg pamabrom</td><td>In 16s and 32s.</td></tr>
<tr><td>otc</td><td>Summit Extra Strength Caplets
(Pfeiffer Pharmaceuticals)</td><td>250 mg</td><td></td><td>65 mg</td><td></td><td>Coated. In 50s.</td></tr>
<tr><td>otc</td><td>Goody's Extra Strength Headache Powder (GlaxoSmithKline Consumer)</td><td>260 mg</td><td>520 mg</td><td></td><td>32.5 mg</td><td></td><td>Lactose. In 2s, 6s, 24s, and 50s.</td></tr>
<tr><td>Rx</td><td>Duraxin Capsules
(Portal)</td><td rowspan="3">325 mg</td><td></td><td>200 mg salicylamide</td><td></td><td>25 mg phenyltoloxamine citrate</td><td>In 30s.</td></tr>
<tr><td>otc</td><td>Goody's Body Pain Powder
(Goody's Pharmaceuticals)</td><td>500 mg</td><td></td><td></td><td></td><td>Lactose. In 6s and 24s.</td></tr>
<tr><td>otc</td><td>Aceta-Gesic
(Rugby)</td><td></td><td></td><td></td><td>30 mg phenyltoloxamine citrate</td><td>In 24s, 100s, and 1000s.</td></tr>
<tr><td>Rx</td><td>Levacet Tablets
(Pharmakon)</td><td>400 mg</td><td>400 mg</td><td>150 mg salicylamide</td><td>40 mg</td><td>50 mg phenyltoloxamine citrate</td><td>(LEVACET). Yellow, capsule shape. In 50s.</td></tr>
</table>

NONNARCOTIC ANALGESIC COMBINATIONS

	Product and Distributor	Acetaminophen	Aspirin	Other Analgesics	Caffeine	Other Content	How Supplied
otc	**Excedrin Tension Headache Geltabs** and **Caplets** (Bristol-Myers Squibb)	500 mg			65 mg		**Geltabs**: Parabens. In 50s and 100s. **Caplets**: Parabens. Capsule shape. In 50s and 100s.
otc	**Excedrin Aspirin Free Geltabs** and **Caplets** (Bristol-Myers Squibb)				65 mg		**Geltabs**: (AF Excedrin). In 24s, 50s, and 100s. **Caplets**: Saccharin, parabens. (AFE). In 24s, 50s, and 100s.
otc	**Excedrin QuickTabs** (Bristol-Myers Squibb)				65 mg		Mannitol, sucralose. Spearmint and peppermint flavors. In 16s and 32s.
otc	**Prēmsyn PMS Caplets** (Chattem)					25 mg pamabrom, 15 mg pyrilamine maleate	In 20s and 40s.
otc	**Vitelle Lurline PMS Tablets** (Fielding)					25 mg pamabrom, 50 mg pyridoxine hydrochloride	In 50s.
otc	**Pamprin Multi-Symptom Maximum Strength Caplets** and **Tablets** (Chattem)					25 mg pamabrom, 15 mg pyrilamine maleate	**Caplets**: (PAMPRIN). In 24s and 48s. **Tablets**: (PAMPRIN). In 12s, 24s, and 48s.
otc	**Midol Maximum Strength Menstrual Caplets** and **Gelcaps** (Bayer)				60 mg	15 mg pyrilamine maleate	**Caplets**: (Midol MENSTRUAL). In 8s and 24s. **Gelcaps**: EDTA. In 24s.
otc	**Midol Maxiumum Strength PMS Caplets** and **Gelcaps** (Bayer)					25 mg pamabrom, 15 mg pyrilamine maleate	**Caplets**: (MIDOL). In 24s. **Gelcaps**: EDTA. In 24s.
otc	**Fem-1 Tablets** (BDI)					25 mg pamabrom	In 16s.
otc	**Painaid PMF Premenstrual Formula Tablets** (Zee Medical)					25 mg pamabrom	In 24s.
Rx	**Flextra-DS Tablets** (Poly Pharm)					50 mg phenyltoloxamine citrate	In 100s.
otc	**Anacin Aspirin Free Maximum Strength Tablets** (Whitehall)						**Tablets**: In 30s, 60s, 100s, and 750s.
otc	**APAP-Plus Tablets** (Textilease Medique Products Co.)				65 mg		In 100s, 200s, and 500s.
otc	**Midol Teen Maximum Strength Caplets** (Bayer)					25 mg pamabrom	(Midol TEEN). In 24s.
otc	**Anacin Aspirin Free Extra Strength Tablets** (Whitehall)						In 60s.
otc	**Women's Tylenol Multi-Symptom Menstrual Relief Caplets** (McNeil Consumer)					25 mg pamabrom	In 24s.
Rx	**Durabac Forte Tablets** (ProEthic)	500 mg		500 mg magnesium salicylate	50 mg	20 mg phenyltoloxamine citrate	(PE 827). Off-white, scored. In 100s.

NONNARCOTIC ANALGESIC COMBINATIONS

	Product and Distributor	Acetaminophen	Aspirin	Other Analgesics	Caffeine	Other Content	How Supplied
Rx	**Hyflex-650 Tablets** (Breckenridge)	650 mg				60 mg phenyltoloxamine citrate	(B/064). Red, scored. In 100s.
c-iv	**Micrainin Tablets** (Wallace)		325 mg			200 mg meprobamate	(Wallace 37-0120). Capsule-shape. White/orange. In 100s.
otc	**Anacin Caplets** and **Tablets** (Whitehall)		400 mg		32 mg		**Caplets**: In 100s. **Tablets**: Coated. In 30s, 50s, 100s, 200s, and 300s.
otc	**P-A-C Analgesic Tablets** (Lee Pharmaceuticals)						In 100s and 1000s.
otc	**Anacin Maximum Strength Tablets** (Whitehall)		500 mg		32 mg		In 20s, 40s, and 75s.
otc	**Bayer Extra Strength Back & Body Pain** (Bayer)				32.5 mg		Capsule shape. In 50s and 100s.
otc	**Bayer PM Extra Strength Aspirin Plus Sleep Aid Caplet** (Bayer)					25 mg diphenhydramine hydrochloride	(BAYER PM). In 24s.
otc	**Bayer Plus Extra Strength** (Bayer)					250 mg calcium carbonate	In 50s.
otc	**BC Powder Original Formula** (Block)		650 mg	195 mg salicylamide	33.3 mg		Lactose. In 50s.
otc	**BC Powder Arthritis Strength** (Block)		742 mg	222 mg salicylamide	38 mg		Lactose. In 50s.
otc	**Mobigesic Tablets** (BF Ascher)			325 mg magnesium salicylate anhydrous		30 mg phenyltoloxamine citrate	In 18s, 50s, and 100s.
Rx	**Magsal Tablets** (U.S. Pharm)			600 mg magnesium salicylate tetrahydrate		25 mg phenyltoloxamine dihydrogen citrate	(0321/US). Green, oval. In 100s.

NONNARCOTIC ANALGESIC COMBINATIONS — ORAL

Indications

Components of these combinations include the following (see individual monographs):

➤*Nonnarcotic analgesics:* Acetaminophen, aspirin, salicylates, salicylamide.

Barbiturates, meprobamate, and antihistamines – (eg, pyrilamine, diphenhydramine, phenyltoloxamine). Used for their sedative effects.

Antacids – (eg, calcium carbonate, magnesium hydroxide, aluminum hydroxide). Used to minimize gastric upset from salicylates.

Caffeine – A traditional component of many analgesic formulations, may be beneficial in certain vascular headaches.

Pamabrom – Used as a diuretic.

Aminobenzoate – Retards the conjugation of salicylic acid and prolongs the action of salicylates.

Another component listed, but not contributing to the analgesic properties of these products includes pyridoxine hydrochloride.

Administration and Dosage

➤*Dose:* The average adult dose is 1 or 2 capsules or tablets or 1 powder packet every 2 to 6 hours as needed for pain. Each product varies; for complete prescribing information, refer to the product label/packaging information.

NONNARCOTIC ANALGESICS WITH BARBITURATES

Rx	**Butalbital, Acetaminophen, and Caffeine Tablets** (Various, eg, Major, Schein, Teva, Zenith Goldline)	**Tablets**: 325 mg acetaminophen, 40 mg caffeine, 50 mg butalbital	In 30s, 50s, 100s, 500s, 1000s, and UD 100s.
Rx	**Americet** (MCR American)		In 100s.
Rx	**Esgic** (Forest)		(535-11). White, scored. Capsule shape. In 100s.
Rx	**Fioricet** (Novartis)		(Fioricet). Light blue. In 100s, 500s, and UD 100s.
Rx	**Repan** (Everett)		(162E305). White. In 100s.
Rx	**Margesic** (Marnel)	**Capsules**: 325 mg acetaminophen, 40 mg caffeine, 50 mg butalbital	(Margesic/Mar). White. In 100s.
Rx	**Triad** (UAD Laboratories)		(TRIAD/UAD 905). White. In 100s.
Rx	**Esgic** (Gilbert Laboratories)		(535-12). White. In 100s.
Rx	**Medigesic** (US Pharm Corp)		(US/US). White. In 100s.
c-iii	**Butalbital, Aspirin, and Caffeine Capsules** (Various, eg, Lannett, Major)	**Capsules**: 325 mg aspirin, 40 mg caffeine, 50 mg butalbital	In 100s and 1000s.
c-iii	**Butalbital Compound** (Various, eg, Qualitest)		In 100s.
c-iii	**Fiorinal** (Novartis)		Benzyl alcohol, EDTA, parabens. (Fiorinal 78-103). Lime green/green. In 100s, 500s, and UD 25s.
Rx	**Phrenilin** (Carnrick)	**Tablets**: 325 mg acetaminophen, 50 mg butalbital	(C 8650). Violet, scored. In 100s and 500s.
Rx	**Marten-Tab** (Marnel)		(MIA/106). White. Capsule shape. In 100s.
Rx	**Butalbital, Acetaminophen, and Caffeine Tablets** (Various, eg, Able, Inwood, Major, Qualitest, URL, West-Ward)	**Tablets**: 500 mg acetaminophen, 40 mg caffeine, 50 mg butalbital	In 100s and 500s.
Rx	**Esgic-Plus** (Forest)		(Forest 678). White, scored. Capsule shape. In 100s and 500s.
Rx	**Esgic-Plus** (Forest)	**Capsules**: 500 mg acetaminophen, 40 mg caffeine, 50 mg butalbital	(Forest 0372/Esgic Plus). Red. In 20s, 100s, and 500s.
Rx	**Axocet** (Savage)	**Tablets**: 650 mg acetaminophen, 50 mg butalbital	(0389). Blue, capsule shape. In 100s.
Rx	**Bupap** (ECR Pharmaceuticals)		(59010/240). Blue, scored. Capsule shape. In 100s.
Rx	**Dolgic** (Athlon[1])		(MIA/112). Blue. Capsule shape. In 100s.
Rx	**Promacet** (MCR American)		In 100s.
Rx	**Repan CF** (Everett Labs)		(EVERETT 166). Blue, scored. Capsule shape. In 100s.
Rx	**Sedapap** (Merz Pharmaceuticals)		(MP 392). White. Capsule shape. In 100s.
Rx	**Tencon** (International Ethical Labs)		(Tencon 029). White, capsule shape. In 100s.
Rx	**Phrenilin Forte** (Carnrick)	**Capsules**: 650 mg acetaminophen, 50 mg butalbital	Benzyl alcohol, parabens, EDTA. (C 8656). Amethyst. In 100s and 500s.
Rx	**Butex Forte** (Athlon[1])		Benzyl alcohol, EDTA, parabens. (Butex Forte/070). White. In 100s.
Rx	**Bucet** (Forest)		Benzyl alcohol, EDTA, parabens. (Bucet/UAD 307). White. In 20s, 100s, and 500s.
c-iii	**Butalbital, Aspirin, and Caffeine Tablets** (Various, eg, Purepac, Schein, Zenith Goldline)	**Tablets**: 325 mg aspirin, 40 mg caffeine, 50 mg butalbital	In 30s, 50s, 100s, 500s, 1000s, and UD 100s.
c-iii	**Butalbital Compound** (Various, eg, Qualitest)		In 100s and 1000s.

[1] Athlon Pharmaceuticals, Inc., P. O. Box 3181, Ridgeland, MS 39158; (601) 899–5714.

NONNARCOTIC ANALGESICS WITH BARBITURATES — ORAL

For complete prescribing information, refer to the individual component drug monographs.

Administration and Dosage

➤*Adults:* 1 or 2 every 4 hours, as needed.

Precautions

➤*Benzyl alcohol:* Some of these products contain the preservative benzyl alcohol, which has been associated with a fatal "gasping syndrome" in premature infants.

DICLOFENAC SODIUM AND MISOPROSTOL

Rx	**Arthrotec** (Pharmacia)	**Tablets:**[a] 50 mg diclofenac sodium/200 mcg misoprostol	Lactose. (AAAA50 SEARLE 1411). White to off-white. Film-coated. In 60s, 90s, and UD 100s.
		75 mg diclofenac sodium/200 mcg misoprostol	Lactose. (AAAA75 SEARLE 1421). White to off-white. Film-coated. In 60s and UD 100s.

[a] Each tablet consists of an enteric-coated core containing diclofenac sodium surrounded by an outer mantle containing misoprostol.

DICLOFENAC SODIUM AND MISOPROSTOL — ORAL

This is an abbreviated monograph. For complete prescribing information, refer to the NSAID and misoprostol monographs.

WARNING

The administration of this product by any route is contraindicated in pregnant women because its misoprostol component can cause abortion.

Reports, primarily from Brazil, of congenital anomalies and fetal death subsequent to use of misoprostol alone, as an abortifacient, have been received.

Patients must be advised of the abortifacient property and warned not to give the drug to others.

Uterine rupture has been reported when misoprostol was administered intravaginally in pregnant women to induce labor or to induce abortion beyond the first trimester of pregnancy.

Uterine perforation has been reported following administration of combined vaginal and oral misoprostol in pregnant women to induce abortion. In each of these reported cases, the gestational age of the pregnancies was unknown.

Do not use in women with childbearing potential unless the patient requires nonsteroidal anti-inflammatory drug (NSAID) therapy and is at high risk of developing gastric or duodenal ulceration or of developing complications from gastric or duodenal ulcers associated with the use of the NSAID. In such patients, this drug may be prescribed if the patient:

- Had a negative serum pregnancy test within 2 weeks prior to beginning therapy;
- is capable of complying with effective contraceptive measures;
- has received both oral and written warnings of the hazards of misoprostol, the risk of possible contraception failure, and the danger to other women of childbearing potential should the drug be taken by mistake;
- will begin using this product only on the second or third day of the next normal menstrual period.

Indications

➤*Arthritis:* Treatment of the signs and symptoms of osteoarthritis or rheumatoid arthritis in patients at high risk of developing NSAID-induced gastric and duodenal ulcers and their complications.

Administration and Dosage

➤*Approved by the FDA:* December 1997.

Swallow tablets whole; do not chew, crush, or dissolve. May be taken with meals to minimize GI effects. This fixed combination product is not appropriate for patients who would not receive the appropriate dose of both ingredients.

➤*Osteoarthritis:* The recommended dose for maximal GI mucosal protection is 50 mg diclofenac/200 mcg misoprostol 3 times daily. For patients who experience intolerance, 50 mg/200 mcg or 75 mg/200 mcg twice daily can be used, but are less effective in preventing ulcers.

➤*Rheumatoid arthritis:* Recommended dose is 50 mg diclofenac/200 mcg misoprostol 3 or 4 times daily. For patients who experience intolerance, 50 mg/200 mcg or 75 mg/200 mcg twice daily can be used, but are less effective in preventing ulcers.

➤*Special dosing considerations:* For gastric ulcer prevention, 200 mcg 3 and 4 times daily are therapeutically equivalent, but more protective than the twice-daily regimen. For duodenal ulcer prevention, 4 times daily is more protective than the 2- or 3-times daily regimens. However, the 4-times daily regimen is less tolerated.

Dosages may be individualized using the separate products (misoprostol and diclofenac), after which the patient may be changed to the appropriate combination diclofenac/misoprostol dose. If clinically indicated, misoprostol cotherapy with diclofenac/misoprostol, or use of the individual components to optimize the misoprostol dose, or frequency of administration may be appropriate. The total dose of misoprostol should not exceed 800 mcg/day, and do not administer more than 200 mcg of misoprostol at any one time. Doses of diclofenac higher than 150 mg/day in osteoarthritis or higher than 225 mg/day in rheumatoid arthritis are not recommended.

➤*Storage/Stability:* Store at or below 25°C (77°F) in a dry area.

Actions

➤*Pharmacology:* This product is a combination containing diclofenac sodium, an NSAID with analgesic properties, and misoprostol, a GI mucosal protective prostaglandin E_1 analog. Diclofenac sodium has anti-inflammatory, analgesic, and antipyretic properties. The mechanism of action of diclofenac, like other NSAIDs, is not completely understood, but may be related to prostaglandin synthetase inhibition. A deficiency of prostaglandins within the gastric and duodenal mucosa may lead to diminishing bicarbonate and mucus secretion and may contribute to the mucosal damage caused by NSAIDs.

Misoprostol is a synthetic prostaglandin E_1 analog with gastric antisecretory and (in animals) mucosal protective properties. It can increase bicarbonate and mucus production, but in humans this has been shown at doses of 200 mcg and above that are also antisecretory. Therefore, it is not possible to tell whether the ability of misoprostol to prevent gastric and duodenal ulcers is the result of its antisecretory effect, its mucosal protective effect, or both.

➤*Pharmacokinetics:* The pharmacokinetics following oral administration of a single dose or multiple doses of diclofenac/misoprostol to healthy subjects under fasted conditions are similar to the pharmacokinetics of the 2 individual components. Food decreases the multiple-dose bioavailability profile of both formulations.

Contraindications

Hypersensitivity to diclofenac, misoprostol, or other prostaglandins; patients who have experienced asthma, urticaria, or other allergic-type reactions after taking aspirin or other NSAIDs; severe, rarely fatal, anaphylactic-like reactions to diclofenac sodium have been reported; pregnancy (see Black Box Warning).

Warnings

➤*Pregnancy: Category X* (see Black Box Warnings). Contraindicated in pregnancy. One case of amniotic fluid embolism, which resulted in maternal and fetal death, has been reported with use of misoprostol during pregnancy. Severe vaginal bleeding, retained placenta, shock, fetal bradycardia, and pelvic pain also have been reported. These women were administered misoprostol vaginally and/or orally over a range of doses.

Misoprostol may endanger pregnancy (may cause miscarriage) and thereby cause harm to the fetus when administered to a pregnant woman. Misoprostol produces uterine contractions, uterine bleeding, and expulsion of the products of conception. Miscarriages caused by misoprostol may be incomplete.

The diclofenac sodium component, like other NSAIDs, which are prostaglandin-inhibiting drugs, may affect the fetal cardiovascular system causing premature closure of the ductus arteriosus. NSAIDs may also inhibit uterine contractions.

Patients should avoid pregnancy during treatment and for 1 month or through 1 menstrual cycle after discontinuation.

➤*Lactation:* Diclofenac sodium is found in the milk of breastfeeding mothers. It is unlikely that misoprostol is excreted into breast milk because the drug is rapidly metabolized by the body. Excretion of the active metabolite (misoprostol acid) into breast milk is possible but has not been studied. Because of the potential for serious adverse reactions in nursing infants, this product is not recommended during breastfeeding.

➤*Children:* Safety and efficacy in pediatric patients have not been established.

Adverse Reactions

➤*GI:* GI disorders had the highest reported incidence in patients receiving diclofenac/misoprostol. These events were generally minor, but led to discontinuation of therapy in 9% of patients on diclofenac/misoprostol and 5% on diclofenac.

GI Adverse Reactions: Diclofenac/Misoprostol vs Diclofenac (%)

GI disorder	Diclofenac/Misoprostol	Diclofenac
Abdominal pain	21	15
Diarrhea	19	11
Dyspepsia	14	11
Nausea	11	6
Flatulence	9	4

Diarrhea and abdominal pain developed early in the course of therapy and were usually self-limited (resolved after 2 to 7 days). Rare instances of profound diarrhea leading to severe dehydration have been reported in patients receiving misoprostol. Monitor patients with an underlying condition (eg, inflammatory bowel disease, dehydration) carefully if this product is prescribed. The incidence of diarrhea can be minimized by administering diclofenac/misoprostol with food and by avoiding coadministration with magnesium-containing antacids.

Patient Information

Advise patients to report any signs or symptoms of GI ulceration or bleeding, skin rash, weight gain, or swelling. Advise patients to stop therapy and seek immediate medical attention if signs of liver toxicity occur (eg, nausea, fatigue, lethargy, itching, jaundice, right upper quadrant tenderness, "flu-like" symptoms).

Do not take this product if pregnant, and avoid becoming pregnant while taking this medicine and for at least 1 month or through 1 menstrual cycle after discontinuation. If pregnancy occurs during diclofenac/misoprostol therapy, stop taking the drug and contact the physician immediately.

Diarrhea, abdominal pain, upset stomach, and nausea may develop during the first few weeks of therapy and stop after about a week with continued treatment. To minimize diarrhea, take with meals and avoid antacids con-

DICLOFENAC SODIUM AND MISOPROSTOL — ORAL

taining magnesium (if needed, use one containing aluminum or calcium instead). If difficulty persists (more than 7 days), or if experiencing severe diarrhea, cramping, or nausea, call the physician.

Swallow tablets whole. Do not chew, crush, or dissolve.

NAPROXEN AND LANSOPRAZOLE

Rx	**Prevacid NapraPAC 375**[1] (TAP Pharmaceuticals)	**Tablets**: 375 mg naproxen	(NPR LE 375). Pink, oval. In blister cards.
		Capsules, delayed release: 15 mg lansoprazole	Sucrose, FD&C Blue No.1. (PREVACID 15). Pink/green. In blister cards.
Rx	**Prevacid NapraPAC 500**[1] (TAP Pharmaceuticals)	**Tablets**: 500 mg naproxen	(NPR LE 500). Yellow, capsule shape. In blister cards.
		Capsules, delayed release: 15 mg lansoprazole	Sucrose, FD&C Blue No.1. (PREVACID 15). Pink/green. In blister cards.

[1] In weekly (7-day) blister cards containing 14 *Naprosyn* tablets and 7 *Prevacid* capsules and in 1-month administration packs containing 4 weekly blister cards.

For complete prescribing information, refer to the Proton Pump Inhibitors and the Nonsteroidal Anti-Inflammatory Agents group monographs.

NAPROXEN AND LANSOPRAZOLE — ORAL

Indications

➤*Nonsteroidal anti-inflammatory drug (NSAID)-associated gastric ulcers:* For reducing the risk of NSAID-associated gastric ulcers in patients with a history of documented gastric ulcer who require the use of an NSAID for treatment of the signs and symptoms of rheumatoid arthritis, osteoarthritis, and ankylosing spondylitis.

Administration and Dosage

Each daily dose consists of one 15 mg lansoprazole capsule and 2 of either 375 or 500 mg naproxen tablets. Take the lansoprazole capsule and 1 of the naproxen tablets before eating in the morning with a glass of water. Take the second naproxen tablet in the evening with a glass of water. The maximum daily naproxen dose of naproxen/lansoprazole is 1000 mg.

Swallow lansoprazole delayed-release capsules whole. Do not chew or crush.

➤*Dosage adjustment:* For naproxen/lansoprazole, no adjustment of the 15 mg lansoprazole component is necessary in patients with renal insufficiency or for the elderly. However, consider dose adjustment for the naproxen component for patients with renal insufficiency, liver disease, or the elderly.

➤*Storage/Stability:* Store at 25°C (77°F); excursion permitted to 15° to 30°C (59° to 86°F). Protect from light and moisture. Store and dispense in original container.

NONSTEROIDAL ANTI-INFLAMMATORY AGENTS

Indications

NSAIDs: Summary of Indications

Indications (✓ -Labeled; X- Unlabeled)	Celecoxib	Diclofenac potassium	Diclofenac sodium/ Diclofenac sodium XR	Etodolac	Fenoprofen	Flurbiprofen	Ibuprofen	Indomethacin	Indomethacin SR	Ketoprofen	Ketoprofen SR	Ketorolac	Meclofenamate	Mefenamic acid	Meloxicam	Nabumetone	Naproxen	Oxaprozin	Piroxicam	Sulindac	Tolmetin
Rheumatoid arthritis (RA)	✓	✓	✓	✓	✓	✓	✓	✓	✓	✓	✓		✓			✓	✓	✓	✓	✓	✓
Osteoarthritis (OA)	✓	✓	✓	✓	✓	✓	✓	✓	✓	✓	✓		✓		✓	✓	✓	✓	✓	✓	✓
Ankylosing spondylitis		✓	✓[a]	X		X		✓	✓								✓			✓	
Mild to moderate pain				✓	✓		✓						✓	✓[b]							
Pain	✓	✓								✓		✓[c]					✓				
Primary dysmenorrhea	✓	✓				X	✓			✓			✓	✓			✓		X		
Juvenile RA		X	X		X					X							✓		X	X	✓
Tendinitis				X				✓	✓								✓			✓	
Bursitis				X				✓	✓								✓			✓	
Acute painful shoulder			X	X				✓	✓											✓	
Acute gout				X		X		✓									✓			✓	
Fever							✓[d]														
Familial adenomatous polyposis (FAP)	✓																				
Sunburn								X[e]													
Migraine																					
Abortive (acute attack)						X	X					X	X	X			X				
Prophylactic					X		X	X		X			X				X				
Menstrual					X			X		X			X	X			X				
Cluster headache								X													
Polyhydramnios								X													
Acne vulgaris, resistant							X														
Menorrhagia													X								
Premenstrual syndrome														X			X				
Cystoid macular edema								X[e]													
Closure of persistent patent ductus arteriosus								✓[f]													

[a] Sodium only, not sodium XR.
[b] Therapy not to exceed 1 week.
[c] Therapy not to exceed 5 days.
[d] In children only.
[e] Topical formulation.
[f] IV formulation only.

➤*Rheumatoid arthritis (RA) (except* **ketorolac, mefenamic acid,** *and* **meloxicam***) and osteoarthritis (OA) (except* **ketorolac** *and* **mefenamic acid***):* Relief of signs and symptoms; treatment of acute flares and exacerbation; long-term management.

Concomitant therapy – Concomitant therapy with other second-line drugs (eg, gold salts) demonstrates additional therapeutic benefit. Whether they can be used with partially effective doses of corticosteroids for a "steroid-sparing" effect and result in greater improvement is not established.

Use with salicylates is not recommended; greater benefit is not achieved, and the potential for adverse reactions is increased. The use of aspirin with nonsteroidal anti-inflammatory agents (NSAIDs) may cause a decrease in blood levels of the nonaspirin drug.

*Juvenile RA (***tolmetin, naproxen***)* – For the treatment of juvenile RA.

➤*Mild to moderate pain (***diclofenac potassium, etodolac, fenoprofen, ibuprofen, ketoprofen, ketorolac, meclofenamate, mefenamic acid, naproxen, naproxen sodium***):* Postextraction dental pain, postsurgical episiotomy pain, and soft tissue athletic injuries.

➤*Primary dysmenorrhea:* **Celecoxib, diclofenac potassium, ibuprofen, ketoprofen, mefenamic acid, naproxen, naproxen sodium**.

➤*Idiopathic heavy menstrual blood loss:* **Meclofenamate**.

➤*Unlabeled uses:* Selected NSAIDs have been used in the treatment of juvenile RA, symptomatic treatment of sunburn, and for various migraine headaches. For other uses, refer to the Summary of Indications table.

Actions

➤*Pharmacology:* Clinically, there are no clear guidelines to assist in selecting the most appropriate agent. Base selection on clinical experience, patient convenience, side effects, and cost.

NSAIDs exhibit antipyretic, analgesic, and anti-inflammatory activities. The major mechanism of therapeutic effects is believed to result from inhibition of prostaglandin synthesis. NSAIDs inhibit cyclooxygenase (COX), the enzyme that catalyzes the synthesis of cyclic endoperoxides from arachidonic acid to form prostaglandins. In the gastric mucosa, prostaglandins decrease gastric acid synthesis, stimulate the production of glutathione that scavenges superoxides, promote the generation of a protective barrier of mucus and bicarbonate, and promote adequate blood flow to the gastric mucosal cells. Prostaglandin in the kidneys modulates intrarenal plasma flow and electrolyte balance.

Two COX isoenzymes have been identified: COX-1 and COX-2. COX-1, expressed constitutively, is synthesized continuously and is present in all tissues and cell types, most notably in platelets, endothelial cells, the GI tract, renal microvasculature, glomerulus, and collecting ducts. COX-1 is important for homeostatic maintenance, such as platelet aggregation, the regulation of blood flow in the kidney and stomach, and the regulation of gastric acid secretion. Inhibition of COX-1 activity is considered a major contributor to NSAID GI toxicity. COX-2 is considered an inducible isoenzyme, although there is some constitutive expression in the kidney, brain, bone, female reproductive system, neoplasias, and GI tract. The function of the COX-2 isoenzyme is induced during pain and inflammatory stimuli.

Many NSAIDs inhibit both COX-1 and COX-2. Most NSAIDs are mainly COX-1 selective (eg, **aspirin, ketoprofen, indomethacin, piroxicam, sulindac**). Others are considered slightly selective for COX-1 (eg, **ibuprofen, naproxen, diclofenac**) and others may be considered slightly selective for COX-2 (eg, **etodolac, nabumetone, meloxicam**). The mechanism of action of **celecoxib** is primarily selective inhibition of COX-2; at therapeutic concentrations, the COX-1 isoenzyme is not inhibited, thus GI toxicity may be decreased.

Other mechanisms that may contribute to NSAID anti-inflammatory activity include the reduction of superoxide radicals, induction of apoptosis, inhibition of adhesion molecule expression, decrease of nitric oxide synthase, decrease of proinflammatory cytokine levels (tumor necrosis factor-α, interleukin-1), modification of lymphocyte activity, and alteration of cellular membrane functions.

Central analgesic activity has been demonstrated in animal pain models by some NSAIDs such as diclofenac, ibuprofen, indomethacin, and ketoprofen. This may be because of the interference of prostaglandin formation or with transmitters or modulators in the nociceptive system. Other proposals include the central action mediated by opioid peptides, inhibition of serotonin release, or inhibition of excitatory amino acids or N-methyl-D-aspartate receptors. Antipyretic activity of NSAIDs is because of the inhibition of prostaglandin E_2 (PGE_2) synthesis in circumventricular organs in and near the preoptic hypothalamic area. Infections, tissue damage, inflammation, graft rejection, malignancies, and other disease states enhance the formation of cytokines that increase PGE_2 production. PGE_2 triggers the hypothalamus to promote increases in heat generation and decreases in heat loss.

RA – No one NSAID has demonstrated a clear advantage for the treatment of RA. Individual patients have demonstrated variability in response to certain NSAIDs. Anti-inflammatory activity is shown by reduced joint swelling, reduced pain, reduced duration of morning stiffness and disease activity, increased mobility, and by enhanced functional capacity (demonstrated by an increase in grip strength, delay in time-to-onset of fatigue, and a decrease in time to walk 50 feet).

OA – Improvement is demonstrated by increased range of motion and a reduction in the following: Tenderness with pressure, pain in motion and at rest, night pain, stiffness and swelling, overall disease activity, and by increased range of motion. There is no data to suggest superiority of one NSAID over another as therapy for OA in terms of efficacy and toxicity. NSAIDs for OA are to be used intermittently if possible during painful episodes and prescribed at the minimum effective dose to reduce the potential of renal and GI toxicities. Do not use **indomethacin** chronically because of its greater toxicity profile and its potential for accelerating progression of OA.

Acute gouty arthritis, ankylosing spondylitis – Relief of pain; reduced fever, swelling, redness, and tenderness; and increased range of motion have occurred with treatment of NSAIDs.

Dysmenorrhea – Excess prostaglandins may produce uterine hyperactivity. These agents reduce elevated prostaglandin levels in menstrual fluid and reduce resting and active intrauterine pressure, as well as frequency of uterine contractions. Probable mechanism of action is to inhibit prostaglandin synthesis rather than provide analgesia.

➤*Pharmacokinetics:*

Absorption/Distribution – NSAIDs are rapidly and almost completely absorbed. **Naproxen sodium** is more rapidly absorbed than the **naproxen** formulation and is used when more prompt relief is desired. **Diclofenac potassium** is formulated to release diclofenac in the stomach. **Diclofenac sodium** resists dissolution in the low pH of gastric fluid but allows a rapid release of the drug in the higher-pH environment in the duodenum. In general, food delays absorption but does not significantly affect total amount absorbed. However, the rate of absorption of **meclofenamic acid** decreased by 26% and C_{max} was delayed by 3 hours when administered 0.5 hours after a meal. In general, administer NSAIDs with meals to minimize GI effects. Some NSAIDs can be given with an aluminum and magnesium hydroxide antacid, which does not affect absorption. All NSAIDs are highly protein bound (more than 90%). Because **diclofenac** is enteric coated, its time to peak levels are delayed despite its relatively short half-life.

Metabolism/Excretion – Most NSAIDs have negligible hepatic metabolism, except for **etodolac, ketorolac, nabumetone, oxaprozin,** and **meloxicam. Celecoxib** and **mefenamic acid** undergo metabolism via cytochrome P450 2C9 isoenzymes. Excretion is via the kidney, primarily as metabolites. **Sulindac** and **nabumetone** are inactive prodrugs converted by the liver to active metabolites.

Pharmacokinetic Parameters/Maximum Dosage Recommendations of NSAIDs

NSAID	Bioavailability (%)	Half-life (hours)	Volume of distribution	Clearance	Peak (hours)	Protein binding (%)	Renal elimination (%)	Fecal elimination (%)
Acetic acids								
Diclofenac	50 to 60	2	0.1 to 0.2 L/kg	350 mL/min	2	> 99	65	-
Indomethacin	98	4.5	0.29 L/kg	0.084 L/hr/kg	2	90	60	33
Sulindac	90	7.8	NS[a]	≈ 2.71 L/hr	2 to 4	> 93	50	25
Tolmetin	NS[a]	2 to 7	NS[a]	NS[a]	0.5 to 1	NS [a]	≈ 100	-
COX 2 inhibitor								
Celecoxib	NS[a]	11	400 L	27.7 L/hr	3	97	27	57
Fenamates								
Meclofenamate	≈ 100	1.3	23 L	206 mL/min	0.5 to 2	> 99	70	30
Mefenamic acid	NS[a]	2	1.06 L/kg	21.23 L/hr	2 to 4	> 90	52	20
Naphthylalkanones								
Nambumetone	> 80	22.5	0.1 to 0.2 L/kg	26.1 mL/min	9 to 12	> 99	80	9
Oxicams								
Piroxicam	NS[a]	50	0.15 L/kg	0.002 to 0.003 L/kg/hr	3 to 5	98.5	NS[a]	NS[a]
Meloxicam	89	15 to 20	10 L	7 to 9 mL/min	4 to 5	99.4	50	50
Propionic acids								
Fenoprofen	NS[a]	3	NS[a]	NS[a]	2	99	90	-
Flurbiprofen	NS[a]	5.7	0.1 to 0.2 L/kg	1.13 L/hr	≈ 1.5	> 99	> 70	-
Ibuprofen	> 80	1.8 to 2	0.15 L/kg	≈ 3 to 3.5 L/hr	1 to 2	99	45 to 79	-
Ketoprofen	90	2.1	0.1 L/kg	6.9 L/hr	0.5 to 2	> 99	80	-

Pharmacokinetic Parameters/Maximum Dosage Recommendations of NSAIDs								
NSAID	Bioavailability (%)	Half-life (hours)	Volume of distribution	Clearance	Peak (hours)	Protein binding (%)	Renal elimination (%)	Fecal elimination (%)
Ketoprofen ER	90	5.4	0.1 L/kg	6.8 L/hr	6 to 7	> 99	80	-
Naproxen	95	12 to 17	0.16 L/kg	0.13 mL/min/kg	2 to 4	> 99	95	-
Oxaprozin	95	42 to 50	10 to 12.5 L	0.25 to 0.34 L/hr	3 to 5	> 99	65	35
Pyranocarboxylic acid								
Etodolac	≥ 80	7.3	0.362 L/kg	47 mL/hr/kg	≈ 1.5	> 99	72	16
Pyrrolizine carboxylic acid								
Ketorolac	100	5 to 6	≈ 0.2 L/kg	≈ 0.025 L/hr/kg	2 to 3	99	91	6

[a] NS = Not studied.

Contraindications

Hypersensitivity to the drug or any components.

➤*NSAID hypersensitivity:* Because of potential cross-sensitivity to other NSAIDs, do not give these agents to patients in whom aspirin or other NSAIDs have induced symptoms of asthma, rhinitis, urticaria, nasal polyps, angioedema, bronchospasm, and other symptoms of allergic or anaphylactoid reactions. Severe, rarely fatal anaphylactic-like and asthmatic reactions have been reported in such patients receiving NSAIDs.

➤*Fenoprofen or mefenamic acid:* Preexisting renal disease.

➤*Mefenamic acid:* Active ulceration or chronic inflammation of either the upper or lower GI tract.

➤*Indomethacin suppositories:* History of proctitis or recent rectal bleeding.

➤*Celecoxib:* Hypersensitivity to sulfonamides.

➤*Ketorolac:* Active peptic ulcer disease; recent GI bleeding or perforation; a history of peptic ulcer disease or GI bleeding; advanced renal impairment or patients at risk for renal failure because of volume depletion; labor and delivery because, through its prostaglandin synthesis inhibitory effect, it may adversely affect fetal circulation and inhibit uterine contractions, thus increasing the risk of uterine hemorrhage; nursing mothers because of the potential adverse effects of prostaglandin-inhibiting drugs on neonates; previously demonstrated hypersensitivity to ketorolac tromethamine, allergic manifestations to aspirin or other NSAIDs; as prophylactic analgesic before any major surgery; intraoperatively when hemostasis is critical because of the increased risk of bleeding; suspected or confirmed cerebrovascular bleeding, hemorrhagic diathesis, incomplete hemostasis and those at high risk of bleeding; patients currently receiving ASA or NSAIDs because of the cumulative risks of inducing serious NSAID-related adverse events; for neuraxial (epidural or intrathecal) administration because of its alcohol content; concomitant use with probenecid.

Warnings

➤*GI effects:* Serious GI toxicity such as inflammation, bleeding, ulceration and perforation of the stomach, small, or large intestine, can occur at any time, with or without warning symptoms, in patients treated chronically with NSAID therapy. Although minor upper GI problems (eg, dyspepsia) are common, usually developing early in therapy, remain alert for ulceration and bleeding in patients treated chronically with NSAIDs even in the absence of previous GI tract symptoms. In patients observed in clinical trials of several months to 2 years duration, symptomatic upper GI ulcers, gross bleeding, or perforation occurred in approximately 1% of patients treated for 3 to 6 months, and in approximately 2% to 4% of patients treated for 1 year. These trends continue, thus increasing the likelihood of developing a serious GI event at some time during the course of therapy. However, even short-term therapy is not without risk. In patients receiving **nabumetone**, the incidence of peptic ulcers was 0.3% at 3 to 6 months, 0.5% at 1 year, and 0.8% at 2 years. Only 1 in 5 patients who develop a serious upper GI adverse event on NSAID therapy is symptomatic. Inform patients about the signs or symptoms of serious GI toxicity and what steps to take if they occur.

Studies have shown that patients with a history of peptic ulcer disease or GI bleeding and who use NSAIDs, have a greater than 10-fold risk for developing a GI bleed than patients with neither of these risk factors. In addition, treatment with oral corticosteroids or anticoagulants, longer duration of NSAID therapy, smoking, alcoholism, older age, and poor general health status contribute to an increased risk for a GI bleed. High-dose NSAIDs probably carry a greater risk of these reactions, although controlled clinical trials generally do not show this. In considering the use of relatively large doses (within the recommended dosage range), sufficient benefit should offset the potential increased risk of GI toxicity. To minimize the potential risk for an adverse GI event, use the lowest effective dose for the shortest possible duration. For high-risk patients, consider alternate therapies that do not involve NSAIDs.

Ketorolac is contraindicated in patients with previously documented peptic ulcers and GI bleeding. In patients with active peptic ulcer and active RA, attempt to treat the arthritis with nonulcerogenic drugs. Fatalities have occurred. GI bleeding is associated with higher morbidity and mortality in patients acutely ill with other conditions, the elderly, and patients with hemorrhagic disorders. In patients with active GI bleeding or an active peptic ulcer, institute an appropriate ulcer regimen, and have the physician weigh the benefits of therapy with the NSAID against possible hazards, and carefully monitor the patient's progress. When the NSAID is given to patients with a history of upper or lower GI tract disease, it should be given under close supervision and only after consulting the Adverse Reactions section.

Do not give **indomethacin** to patients with active GI lesions or a history of recurrent GI lesions unless the high risk is warranted and patients can be monitored closely. To reduce GI effects, give NSAIDs after meals, with food, or with antacids (does not apply to enteric-coated **diclofenac**).

Higher doses of **meloxicam** (eg, chronic daily 30 mg doses) were associated with increased risk of serious GI effects. Do not exceed daily doses of 15 mg.

If diarrhea occurs with **mefenamic acid** or diarrhea, GI irritation, and abdominal pain occur with **meclofenamate**, reduce dosage or temporarily discontinue use. Some patients may be unable to tolerate further therapy with these agents.

➤*CNS effects:* **Indomethacin** may aggravate depression or other psychiatric disturbances, epilepsy, and parkinsonism; use with considerable caution. If severe CNS adverse reactions develop, discontinue the drug. Some of these agents also may cause headaches (highest incidence with **fenoprofen**, **indomethacin**, **ketorolac**, and **celecoxib**). If headache persists despite dosage reduction, discontinue use.

➤*Hypersensitivity reactions:* A potentially fatal apparent hypersensitivity syndrome has occurred with **sulindac**; this syndrome may include constitutional symptoms, cutaneous findings, involvement of major organs, conjunctivitis, or other less specific findings. The clinical picture of hypersensitivity reactions may vary from vasomotor rhinitis, urticaria, and angioedema to serious bronchoconstriction and, in some cases, anaphylactic shock. This may be because of an allergic immunological hypersensitivity reaction or a pseudoallergic reaction characterized by mast-cell degranulation by complement components, histamine liberation by drugs, and interference with endogenous eicosanoid biosynthesis. The former mechanism appears to be responsible for the anaphylactic shock or urticaria that may develop after taking amidopyrine or noramidopyrine, the latter for the bronchoconstriction encountered after ingestion of aspirin, noramidopyrine, or of aminophenazone and other pyrazole drugs.

Rarely, fever and other evidence of hypersensitivity, including abnormalities in 1 or more liver function tests and severe skin reactions, have occurred during therapy with sulindac. Fatalities have occurred in these patients. Hepatitis, jaundice, or both, with or without fever, may occur usually within the first 1 to 3 months of therapy. Consider determination of liver function whenever a patient on therapy with sulindac develops unexplained fever, rash, or other dermatologic reactions or constitutional symptoms. If unexplained fever or other evidence of hypersensitivity occurs, discontinue therapy with sulindac. The elevated temperature and abnormalities in liver function caused by sulindac characteristically have reverted to normal after discontinuation of therapy. Administration of sulindac should not be reinstituted in such patients.

Anaphylactoid reactions – Anaphylactoid reactions have occurred in patients without known exposure to NSAIDs, but they typically occur in asthmatic patients who experience rhinitis with or without nasal polyps, or who exhibit severe, potentially fatal bronchospasm after taking aspirin or other NSAIDs. Anaphylactoid reactions have occurred in patients with aspirin hypersensitivity and in patients who discontinued **tolmetin**, then restarted it. These reactions appear to occur more often with tolmetin than other NSAIDs not structurally related but data conflict. Refer to Management of Acute Hypersensitivity Reactions.

➤*Renal function impairment:* NSAID metabolites are eliminated primarily by kidneys; use with caution in those with renal function impairment. Assess renal function before and during therapy. Monitor serum creatinine or creatinine clearance. Reduce dosage to avoid excessive accumulation.

In cases of advanced kidney disease, treatment with **piroxicam** and **meloxicam** is not recommended. However, if NSAID therapy must be initiated, close monitoring of the patient's kidney function is advisable. **Sulindac** metabolites have been reported rarely as the major or a minor component in renal stones in association with other calculus components. Use sulindac with caution in patients with a history of renal lithiasis and keep patients well hydrated while receiving the drug.

➤*Hepatic function impairment:* **Naproxen** may exhibit an increase in unbound fraction and a reduced clearance of free drug in cirrhotic liver patients, suggesting an increased potential for toxicity in this group; consider reducing the dose. Also, **sulindac** AUC may increase in patients with cirrhosis because of altered sulfide formation/metabolism. Disposition of total and free **etodolac** is not altered in patients with compensated hepatic cirrhosis. Effects of hepatic disease on other NSAIDs is unknown. Use caution in patients with impaired hepatic function or history of liver disease.

In patients treated with a single 15 mg dose of **meloxicam**, there was no marked difference in plasma concentrations in patients with mild and moderate hepatic impairment compared with healthy subjects. Protein binding of meloxicam was not affected by hepatic insufficiency. No dose adjustment is needed in patients with mild to moderate hepatic insufficiency; patients with severe hepatic impairment have not been adequately studied.

➤*Elderly:* Age appears to increase the possibility of adverse reactions to NSAIDs. The risk of serious ulcer disease is increased in elderly patients (> 65 years of age) taking NSAIDs; this risk appears to increase with the dose. Use with greater care and begin with reduced dosages. In **nabumetone**-treated patients, no differences in overall efficacy and safety were observed between older and younger patients. **Ketorolac** is cleared more slowly by the elderly; use caution and reduce dosage.

➤*Pregnancy: Category B* (**ketoprofen, naproxen, naproxen sodium, flurbiprofen, diclofenac, fenoprofen, ibuprofen, indomethacin, meclofenamate, sulindac**). *Category C* (**etodolac, ketorolac, mefenamic acid, meloxicam, nabumetone, oxaprozin, tolmetin, piroxicam, celecoxib**). All NSAIDs are *Category D* if used in the third trimester or near delivery.

Safety for use during pregnancy has not been established; use is not recommended. There are no adequate and well-controlled studies in pregnant women. An increased incidence of dystocia, increased postimplantation loss, decreased pup survival, increased length of delivery time, embryolethality, septal heart defects, stillbirth, and delayed parturition occurred in animals. Agents that inhibit prostaglandin synthesis may cause closure of the ductus arteriosus and other untoward effects to the fetus. GI tract toxicity increased in pregnant women in the last trimester. Some NSAIDs may prolong pregnancy if given before onset of labor.

The known effects of drugs of this class on the human fetus during the third trimester of pregnancy include: Constriction of the ductus arteriosus prenatally, tricuspid incompetence, and pulmonary hypertension; nonclosure of the ductus arteriosus postnatally, which may be resistant to medical management; myocardial degenerative changes, platelet dysfunction with resultant bleeding, intracranial bleeding, renal dysfunction or failure, renal injury/dysgenesis that may result in prolonged or permanent renal failure, oligohydramnios, GI bleeding or perforation, and increased risk of necrotizing enterocolitis. Avoid during pregnancy, especially in the third trimester.

➤*Lactation:* Most NSAIDs are excreted in breast milk. **Naproxen** appears at ≈ 1% of maternal serum concentration. In 10 healthy women, recovery of **flurbiprofen** in breast milk accounted for 0.05% (range, 0.03% to 0.07%) of a 100 mg dose; average peak concentration in milk was 0.09 mcg/mL. **Ibuprofen** was not detected in breast milk of 12 women who had ingested 400 mg every 6 hours over 24 hours. **Ketorolac** was detected in breast milk at a maximum milk-to-plasma ratio of 0.037. In general, do not use in nursing mothers because of effects on the infant's cardiovascular system.

➤*Children:* **Mefenamic acid** and **meclofenamate** are not recommended in children < 14 years of age. Safety and efficacy of **meloxicam** use has not been established in children < 18 years of age. **Indomethacin's** safety is not established in children; not recommended in children ≤ 14 years of age, except in circumstances that warrant the risk. When using indomethacin in children ≥ 2 years of age, closely monitor liver function. Hepatotoxicity, including fatalities, has occurred in children with juvenile RA. Suggested starting dose is 2 mg/kg/day in divided doses. Do not exceed 4 mg/kg/day or 150 to 200 mg/day, whichever is less. As symptoms subside, reduce dosage or discontinue drug. For use of IV indomethacin in premature infants, see Agents for Patent Ductus Arteriosus. **Tolmetin** and **naproxen** are the only agents labeled for juvenile RA, although studies are being conducted with other agents. Safety and efficacy of tolmetin and naproxen in infants < 2 years of age are not established. Safety and efficacy of other NSAIDs in children are not established.

Precautions

➤*Monitoring:* Serious GI tract ulceration and bleeding can occur without warning. Follow chronically treated patients for signs and symptoms of ulceration and bleeding; inform them of the importance of this follow-up (see Warnings).

Monitor transaminases and other hepatic enzymes in patients treated with NSAIDs. For patients on **diclofenac** therapy, it is recommended that a determination from lab results be made within 4 weeks of initiating therapy and at intervals thereafter. If clinical signs and symptoms consistent with liver disease develop, or if systemic manifestations occur (eg, eosinophilia, rash) and abnormal liver tests are detected, persist, or worsen, discontinue diclofenac immediately.

➤*Corticosteroid use:* NSAIDs cannot be expected to be a substitute for corticosteroids or to treat corticosteroid insufficiency. Abrupt discontinuation of corticosteroids may lead to disease exacerbation.

➤*Functional class IV RA patients (incapacitated, largely or wholly bedridden, confined to wheelchair):* Safety and efficacy are not established.

➤*Steroid dosage:* If corticosteroid dosage is reduced or eliminated during NSAID therapy, reduce dosage slowly and observe patient closely for evidence of adverse effects, including adrenal insufficiency and exacerbation of symptoms (see Adrenalcortical Steroids, Glucocorticoids monograph).

➤*Porphyria:* Avoid the use of NSAIDs in patients with hepatic porphyria. To date, 1 patient has been described in whom **diclofenac** probably triggered a clinical attack of porphyria. The postulated mechanism demonstrated in rats for causing such attacks by diclofenac, as well as some other NSAIDs, is through stimulation of the porphyria precursor delta-aminolevulinic acid (ALA).

➤*Aseptic meningitis:* Aseptic meningitis with fever and coma has been observed on rare occasions in patients on NSAIDs therapy. Although it is probably more likely to occur in patients with systemic lupus erythematosus (SLE) and related connective tissue diseases, it has been reported in patients who do not have an underlying chronic disease. If signs or symptoms of meningitis develop in a patient on NSAID therapy, consider the possibility of it being related to the NSAID.

➤*Platelet aggregation:* NSAIDs can inhibit platelet aggregation; the effect is reversible, quantitatively less, and of shorter duration than that seen with aspirin. These agents prolong bleeding time (within normal range) in healthy subjects. This may be exaggerated in patients with underlying hemostatic defects; use with caution and carefully monitor in people with intrinsic coagulation defects and in those on anticoagulant therapy.

➤*Preexisting asthma:* About 10% of patients with asthma may have aspirin-sensitive asthma. The use of aspirin in patients with aspirin-sensitive asthma has been associated with severe bronchospasm, which can be fatal. Because cross reactivity, including bronchospasm, between aspirin and other NSAIDs has been reported in such aspirin-sensitive patients, do not administer NSAIDs to patients with this form of aspirin sensitivity, and use the drug with caution in patients with preexisting asthma.

➤*Hematologic effects:* Decreased hemoglobin or hematocrit levels have rarely required discontinuation. Anemia may be because of fluid retention, GI blood loss, or an incompletely described effect upon erythropoiesis. If anemia is suspected in patients on long-term therapy, determine hemoglobin and hematocrit values. Frequently determine hemoglobin values in patients with initial values ≤ 10 g/dL who are to receive long-term therapy.

Patients on long-term treatments should have their CBC and a chemistry profile checked periodically. Low white blood cell counts occur rarely, are transient, and usually return to normal while therapy continues. Persistent leukopenia, granulocytopenia, or thrombocytopenia warrants further evaluation and may require discontinuing the drug.

Postoperative hematomas and other signs of wound bleeding have occurred with perioperative IM use of **ketorolac**. Exercise caution when administering pre- or intraoperatively and when administering perioperatively if strict hemostasis is critical.

➤*Cardiovascular effects:* May cause fluid retention and peripheral edema. Use caution in compromised cardiac function, hypertension, in patients on chronic diuretic therapy, or other conditions predisposing to fluid retention. Agents may be associated with significant deterioration of circulatory hemodynamics in severe heart failure and hyponatremia, presumably because of inhibition of prostaglandin-dependent compensatory mechanisms.

➤*Ophthalmologic effects:* Perform ophthalmological studies in patients who develop eye complaints during therapy. Effects include blurred or diminished vision, scotomata, changes in color vision, corneal deposits, and retinal disturbances, including maculas. Discontinue therapy if ocular changes are noted. Blurred vision may be significant and warrants thorough examination, including central visual fields and color vision testing. These changes may be asymptomatic; perform periodic examinations in patients on prolonged therapy.

➤*Infection:* NSAIDs may mask the usual signs of infection. Use with extra care in the presence of existing controlled infection. The pharmacologic activity of NSAIDs in reducing inflammation and possibly fever may diminish the utility of these diagnostic signs in detecting complications of presumed noninfectious, painful conditions.

➤*Renal effects:* Acute renal insufficiency, interstitial nephritis with hematuria, nephrotic syndrome, proteinuria, hyperkalemia, hyponatremia, renal papillary necrosis, and other renal medullary changes may occur.

Long-term administration of NSAIDs has resulted in renal papillary necrosis and other renal medullary changes. Renal toxicity also has been seen in patients in whom renal prostaglandins have a compensatory role in the maintenance of renal perfusion. In these patients, administration of NSAIDs may cause dose-dependent reduction in prostaglandin formation and, secondarily, in renal blood flow, which may precipitate overt renal decompensation. Patients at greatest risk of this reaction are those with impaired renal function, heart failure, liver dysfunction, those taking diuretics and ACE inhibitors, and the elderly. Discontinuation of NSAID therapy is usually followed by recovery to the pretreatment state.

Exercise caution when initiating treatment with NSAIDs in patients with considerable dehydration. It is advisable to rehydrate patients first and then start therapy with NSAIDs. Correct hypovolemia before treatment with **ketorolac** is initiated. They are not recommended in patients with preexisting kidney disease.

Acute renal insufficiency – Patients with pre-existing renal disease or compromised renal perfusion are at greatest risk for acute renal insufficiency. A form of renal toxicity seen in patients with prerenal conditions leads to reduced renal blood flow or blood volume. NSAID use may cause a dose-dependent reduction in prostaglandin formation and precipitate overt renal decompensation. Patients at greatest risk are the elderly; premature infants; those with heart failure, renal or hepatic dysfunction, SLE, chronic glomerulonephritis, dehydration, diabetes mellitus, or impaired renal function; those taking ACE inhibitors; septicemia; pyelonephritis; concomitant use of any nephrotoxic drug; extracellular volume depletion from any cause; and those on diuretics. Recovery usually follows discontinuation.

Those patients at high risk who chronically take NSAIDs should have renal function monitored if they have signs or symptoms that may be consistent with mild azotemia (eg, malaise, fatigue, loss of appetite). Patients occasionally may develop some elevation of serum creatinine and BUN levels without any signs and symptoms. There may also be substantial proteinuria and, on renal biopsy, electron microscopy has shown foot process fusion and T-lymphocyte infiltration in the renal interstitium.

Interstitial nephritis – Interstitial nephritis has occurred with increased frequency in patients receiving NSAIDs and may be due to altered prostaglandin metabolism.

GU tract problems have occurred in patients taking **fenoprofen**, most frequently, dysuria, cystitis, hematuria, interstitial nephritis, and nephrotic syndrome. This may be preceded by fever, rash, arthralgia, oliguria, and azotemia, and may progress to anuria. Rapid recovery followed early recognition and drug withdrawal.

Hyperkalemia – Another potentially serious NSAID-induced renal electrolyte abnormality is hyperkalemia. NSAIDs tend to blunt prostaglandin-mediated renin release, leading to diminished aldosterone formation and, hence, decreased potassium excretion. NSAIDs can augment sodium and chloride reabsorption within the renal tubule in the setting of diminished glomerular filtration rate by opposing natriuretic and diuretic prostaglandins. This decreases the delivery of intraluminal sodium for sodium-potassium exchange at the distal nephron.

Papillary necrosis – Papillary necrosis may present as an acute or chronic form of NSAID nephropathy in the setting of massive NSAID overdose in a dehydrated patient with preexisting normal renal function. The chronic form is associated with analgesic-abuse nephropathy.

➤*Hepatic effects:* Borderline liver function test elevations may occur in ≈ 15% of patients and may progress, remain essentially unchanged, or become transient with continued therapy. The ALT test is probably the most sensitive indicator of liver dysfunction. Meaningful (≥ 3 times upper limit of normal) AST or ALT elevations occurred in ≈ 1% of patients. If symptoms or signs suggesting liver dysfunction, or an abnormal test occurs, evaluate for more severe hepatic reactions. Severe reactions, including jaundice and fatal fulminant hepatitis, liver necrosis, and hepatic failure have occurred rarely, some with fatal outcomes. Evaluate a patient with symptoms and signs suggesting liver dysfunction, or in whom an abnormal liver test has occurred, for evidence of the development of more severe hepatic reactions while on therapy with NSAIDs. If an NSAID is to be used in the presence of impaired liver function, it must be done under strict observation. Discontinue treatment if abnormal tests persist or worsen, if clinical signs and symptoms consistent with liver disease develop, or if systemic manifestations occur (eg, eosinophilia, rash).

➤*Pancreatitis:* Pancreatitis has occurred in patients receiving **sulindac**. If pancreatitis is suspected, discontinue the drug, start supportive therapy, and monitor closely (eg, serum and urine amylase, amylase/creatinine clearance ratio, electrolytes, serum calcium, glucose, lipase). Check for other causes of pancreatitis as well as for conditions that mimic pancreatitis.

➤*Auditory effects:* Perform periodic auditory function tests during chronic **fenoprofen** therapy in patients with impaired hearing.

➤*Heavy menstrual blood loss evaluation:* Prior to prescribing **meclofenamate** for heavy blood flow and primary dysmenorrhea, make a thorough risk/benefit assessment that takes into account the results described in the clinical pharmacology section. It is recommended that meclofenamate treatment not be prescribed for heavy menstrual flow without establishing its idiopathic nature. Fully evaluate spotting or bleeding between cycles and do not treat with meclofenamate. Worsening of menstrual blood loss or excessive blood loss failing to respond to meclofenamate should also be evaluated by an appropriate work-up and not treated with meclofenamate.

➤*Dermatologic effects:* A combination of dermatologic and allergic signs and symptoms suggestive of serum sickness have occasionally occurred in conjunction with the use of **piroxicam**. These include arthralgias, pruritus, fever, fatigue, and rash including vesiculobullous reactions and exfoliative dermatitis.

➤*Concomitant NSAID therapy:* Do not use **naproxen sodium** and **naproxen** concomitantly; both drugs circulate as naproxen anion.

Do not use **diclofenac** immediate-release, delayed-release, and extended-release tablets concomitantly with other diclofenac-containing products because they also circulate in plasma as diclofenac anion.

➤*Photosensitivity:* Photosensitivity may occur; caution patients to take protective measures (ie, sunscreens, protective clothing) against UV or sunlight until tolerance is determined.

Drug Interactions

➤*Cytochrome P450:* Exercise caution when coadministering **celecoxib** and **mefenamic acid** with drugs known to inhibit the isoenzyme 2C9.

NSAID Drug Interactions

Precipitant drug	Object drug*		Description
Bisphosphonates	NSAIDs	↑	Risk of gastric ulceration may be increased. Use cautiously.
Cholestyramine	NSAIDs	↓	The effects of NSAIDs may be decreased. Cholestyramine has enhanced piroxicam and meloxicam plasma clearance and decreased the GI absorption of NSAIDs.
Cimetidine	NSAIDs	↔	NSAID plasma concentrations may be increased or decreased by cimetidine; some studies report no effect. Also, indomethacin and sulindac have increased ranitidine and cimetidine bioavailability.
Colestipol	NSAIDs	↓	The effects of diclofenac may be decreased because colestipol may interfere with the absorption of diclofenac, thereby reducing bioavailability.
Diflunisal	NSAIDs Indomethacin	↑	Diflunisal may decrease the renal clearance and significantly increase indomethacin plasma concentrations that may produce toxicity.
Dimethyl sulfoxide (DMSO)	NSAIDs Sulindac	↓	DMSO may decrease the formation of the active metabolite of sulindac, possibly resulting in a decreased therapeutic effect. Also, topical DMSO with sulindac has resulted in severe peripheral neuropathy.
Fluconazole	NSAIDs Celecoxib	↑	Increase in celecoxib plasma concentration may occur because of inhibition of celecoxib metabolism.
Phenobarbital	NSAIDs Fenoprofen	↓	Phenobarbital, an enzyme inducer, may decrease fenoprofen half-life. Dosage adjustments of fenoprofen may be required if phenobarbital is added or withdrawn.
Phenylbutazone	NSAIDs Etodolac	↑	Phenylbutazone can increase by approximately 80% the free fraction of etodolac. Coadministration is not recommended.
Probenecid	NSAIDs	↑	Probenecid may increase the concentrations and possibly the toxicity of NSAIDs. Do not use ketorolac and probenecid concomitantly.
Ritonavir	NSAIDs Piroxicam	↑	Ritonavir may increase the concentrations and possibly the toxicity of piroxicam by inhibiting its metabolism.
Salicylates	NSAIDs	↓	Plasma concentrations of NSAIDs may be decreased by salicylates. Avoid concurrent use because it offers no therapeutic advantage and may significantly increase the incidence of GI effects.
Salicylates	NSAIDs Ketorolac	↑	Increased risk of serious ketorolac-related side effects may occur. Salicylates may displace ketorolac from protein binding sites and may produce possible synergistic side effects. Ketorolac is contraindicated in patients receiving aspirin.
Sucralfate	NSAIDs	↓	The effects of diclofenac may be decreased, possibly because of decreased absorption. Sucralfate does not appear to alter ketoprofen or naproxen bioavailability.
NSAIDs	ACE inhibitors	↓	Antihypertensive effects of captopril may be blunted or completely abolished by indomethacin. Other reports suggest that NSAIDs may diminish the antihypertensive effect of ACE inhibitors.
NSAIDs	Aminoglycosides	↑	Aminoglycoside plasma concentrations may be elevated in premature infants because of NSAIDs reducing the glomerular filtration rate. Reduce aminoglycoside dose prior to NSAID initiation and monitor serum aminoglycoside levels and renal function.
NSAIDs	Anticoagulants	↑	Coadministration may prolong prothrombin time (PT). Also consider the effects NSAIDs have on platelet function and gastric mucosa. Monitor PT and patients closely, especially the first few days, and instruct patients to watch for signs and symptoms of bleeding.
NSAIDs	Beta blockers	↓	The antihypertensive effect of beta blockers may be impaired, possibly because of NSAID inhibition of renal prostaglandin synthesis, thereby allowing unopposed pressor systems to produce hypertension. Avoid using this combination if possible. Monitor blood pressure and adjust beta blocker dose as needed. Consider using a non-interacting NSAID (eg, sulindac).
NSAIDs	Cyclosporine	↑	Nephrotoxicity of both agents may be increased.
Cyclosporine	NSAIDs		
NSAIDs Ibuprofen Indomethacin	Digoxin	↑	Ibuprofen and indomethacin may increase digoxin serum levels.
NSAIDs Indomethacin	Dipyridamole	↑	Indomethacin and dipyridamole coadministration may augment water retention.
NSAIDs	Diuretics	↓	Effects of diuretics may be decreased.

NSAID Drug Interactions

Precipitant drug	Object drug*		Description
NSAIDs	Hydantoins	↑	Serum phenytoin levels may be increased, resulting in an increase in pharmacologic and toxic effects of phenytoin.
NSAIDs	Lithium	↑	Serum lithium levels may be increased; however, sulindac has no effect or may decrease lithium levels. Monitor for signs of lithium toxicity.
NSAIDs	Methotrexate	↑	The risks of methotrexate toxicity (eg, stomatitis, bone marrow suppression, nephrotoxicity) may be increased. Celecoxib and meloxicam did not have a significant effect on methotrexate pharmacokinetics.
NSAIDs Indomethacin	Penicillamine	↑	Indomethacin may increase the bioavailability of penicillamine.
NSAIDs Indomethacin Diclofenac	Potassium-sparing diuretics	↓	Effects of potassium-diuretics may be decreased. Coadministration may increase serum potassium levels.
NSAIDs	Thiazide diuretics	↔	Decreased antihypertensive and diuretic action of thiazides may occur with concurrent indomethacin. Naproxen also has been implicated. Sulindac may enhance the effects of thiazides.

* ↑ = Object drug increased. ↓ = Object drug decreased. ↔ = Undetermined clinical effect.

➤*Drug/Lab test interactions:* **Naproxen** use may result in increased urinary values for 17-ketogenic steroids because of an interaction between naproxen or its metabolites with m-dinitro-benzene used in this assay. Although 17-hydroxycorticosteroid measurements (Porter-Silber test) do not appear to be artificially altered, temporarily discontinue naproxen therapy 72 hours before adrenal function tests are performed. Naproxen may interfere with some urinary assays of 5-hydroxy indoleacetic acid.

Tolmetin – Tolmetin metabolites in urine give positive tests for proteinuria using acid precipitation tests (eg, sulfosalicylic acid). Use commercially available dye-impregnated reagent strips.

Mefenamic acid – A false-positive reaction for urinary bile, using the diazo tablet test, may result. If biliuria is suspected, use other procedures (ie, the Harrison spot test).

Fenoprofen – *Amerlex-M* kit assay values of total and free triiodothyronine in patients on fenoprofen have been reported as falsely elevated on the basis of a chemical cross-reaction that directly interferes with the assay. Thyroid-stimulating hormone, total thyroxine, and thyrotropin-releasing hormone response are not affected.

Oxaprozin – False-positive urine immunoassay screening tests for benzodiazepines have been reported in patients taking oxaprozin. This is because of the lack of specificity of the screening tests. False-positive test results may be expected for several days following discontinuation of oxaprozin therapy. Confirmatory tests, such as gas chromatography/mass spectrometry, will distinguish oxaprozin from benzodiazepines.

NSAIDs, by decreasing platelet adhesion and aggregation, can prolong bleeding time ≈ 3 to 4 minutes.

➤*Drug/Food interactions:* Administration of **tolmetin** with milk had no effect on peak-plasma tolmetin concentration, but decreased total tolmetin bioavailability by 16%. When tolmetin was taken immediately after a meal, peak plasma concentrations were reduced by 50%, while total bioavailability was again decreased by 16%. Peak concentration of **etodolac** is reduced by approximately 50% and the time to peak is increased by 1.4 to 3.8 hours following administration with food; however, the extent of absorption is not affected. Food may reduce the rate of absorption of **oxaprozin**, but the extent is unchanged.

Adverse Reactions

NSAIDs Adverse Reactions (%)[a]

	Adverse reaction	Celecoxib	Diclofenac	Etodolac	Fenoprofen	Flurbiprofen	Ibuprofen	Indomethacin	Ketoprofen	Ketorolac	Meclofenamate	Mefenamic acid	Meloxicam	Nabumetone	Naproxen	Oxaprozin	Piroxicam	Sulindac	Tolmetin
Cardiovascular	Palpitations	< 2	< 1	< 1	2.5		< 1	< 1	< 1	< 1	< 1	< 1	< 2	< 1	1-3	< 1	< 1	< 1	
	Hypertension		< 1	< 1		< 1	< 1	< 1	< 1	1-3		< 1	< 2	< 1			< 1	< 1	3-9
	MI	< 2	< 1	< 1		< 1			< 1			< 1	< 2	< 1			< 1		
	Tachycardia	< 2	< 1		< 1			< 1	< 1			< 1	< 2				< 1		
	CHF	< 0.1	< 1	< 1			< 1	< 1	< 1			< 1			< 1		< 1	< 1	< 1
	Arrhythmia			< 1		< 1	< 1[b]	< 1	< 1			< 1	< 2	< 1			< 1	< 1	
	Angina/Angina pectoris	< 2				< 1							< 2	< 1					
	CVA	< 0.1		< 1		< 1													
	Pulmonary embolism	< 0.1				< 1													
	Syncope	< 0.1		< 1				< 1		< 1		< 1	< 2	< 1			< 1	< 1	
	Vasculitis	< 0.1		< 1[c]								< 1	< 2	< 1	< 1				
	Flushing		< 1	< 1				< 1											
	Hypotension		< 1					< 1				< 1	< 2				< 1		

NSAIDs Adverse Reactions (%)[a]

	Adverse reaction	Celecoxib	Diclofenac	Etodolac	Fenoprofen	Flurbiprofen	Ibuprofen	Indomethacin	Ketoprofen	Ketorolac	Meclofenamate	Mefenamic acid	Meloxicam	Nabumetone	Naproxen	Oxaprozin	Piroxicam	Sulindac	Tolmetin
CNS	Headache	15.8	3-9	< 1	8.7	3-9	1-3	11.7	3-9	17	3-9	1-10	2.4-8.3	3-9	3-9		1-10	3-9	3-9
	Dizziness	2	1-3	3-9	6.5	1-3	3-9	3-9	1-3	7	3-9	1-10	1.1-3.8	3-9	3-9		1-10	3-9	3-9
	Asthenia/malaise	< 2	< 1	3-9	1-5.4					< 1	< 1	< 1	< 2	< 1	< 1	< 1	< 1		3-9
	Depression	< 2	< 1	1-3	< 1		< 1	1-3		< 1	< 1	< 1	< 2	< 1	< 1		< 1	< 1	1-3
	Nervousness	< 2		1-3	5.7	1-3	1-3	< 1		< 1		< 1	< 2	1-3			< 1	1-3	
	Somnolence	< 2		< 1	8.5		< 1	1-3				< 1	< 2	1-3			< 1	< 1	
	Tremor		< 1		2.2					< 1		< 1	< 2	< 1			< 1		
	Confusion			< 1	1.4	< 1	< 1	< 1	< 1			< 1	< 2	< 1			< 1		
	Fatigue	< 2			1.7			1-3			< 1		< 2	1-3					
	Drowsiness		< 1					< 1		6		< 1			3-9		< 1		1-3
	Insomnia	2.3	< 1	< 1	< 1		< 1	< 1		< 1	< 1	< 1	≤ 3.6	1-3	< 1		< 1	< 1	
	Lightheadedness							< 1							1-3				
	Vertigo	< 2						1-3	< 1	< 1		< 1	2	< 1	1-3		< 1	< 1	
	CNS inhibition[d]															1-3			
	CNS inhibition or excitation					1-3[e]			3-9[f]										
	Paresthesia	< 2	< 1	< 1		< 1	< 1	< 1	< 1	< 1	< 1	< 1	< 2	< 1			< 1	< 1	
	Anxiety	< 2	< 1					< 1				< 1	< 2	< 1			< 1		
	Hypesthesia	< 2																	
	Migraine	< 2							< 1										
	Aseptic meningitis		< 1				< 1[g]		< 1						< 1			< 1	
	Convulsions		< 1			< 1		< 1				< 1	< 2				< 1	< 1	
	Hypertonia	< 2				< 1													
	Hallucinations						< 1		< 1	< 1		< 1					< 1		
	Abnormal dreams/dream abnormalities						< 1			< 1		< 1	< 2		< 1		< 1		
Dermatologic	Rash	2.2	1-3	1-3	3.7	1-3	3-9	< 1	1-3	1-3	3-9	1-10	0.3-3	3-9	< 1	3-9	1-10	3-9	
	Pruritus	< 2	1-3	1-3	4.2	< 1	1-3	< 1	< 1	1-3	1-3	1-10	≤ 2.4	3-9	3-9	< 1	1-10	1-3	
	Increased sweating	< 2	< 1	< 1	4.6	< 1		< 1	< 1	1-3		< 1	< 2	1-3	1-3		< 1		
	Skin eruptions														3-9				
	Urticaria	< 2	< 1	< 1	< 1	< 1	< 1	< 1	< 1	< 1	1-3	< 1	< 2	< 1	< 1	< 1	< 1		< 1
	Skin irritation																		1-3
	Alopecia/Loss of hair	< 2	< 1	< 1	< 1	< 1	< 1	< 1	< 1		< 1	< 1	< 2	< 1	< 1	< 1	< 1	< 1	
	Photosensitivity/Photosensitivity reaction	< 2	< 1	< 1		< 1			< 1			< 1	< 2	< 1	< 1[h]	< 1	< 1	< 1	
	Erythema multiforme	< 0.1	< 1[i]	< 1			< 1	< 1	< 1		< 1	< 1	< 0.1	< 1	< 1	< 1	< 1	< 1	< 1
	Stevens-Johnson syndrome	< 0.1	< 1	< 1	< 1		< 1	< 1	< 1		< 1	< 1	< 0.1	< 1	< 1	< 1	< 1	< 1	
	Toxic epidermal necrolysis/Lyell's syndrome	< 0.1			< 1	< 1	< 1	< 1	< 1				< 0.1	< 1		< 1		< 1	< 1
	Exfoliative dermatitis	< 0.1	< 1		< 1	< 1		< 1	< 1		< 1	< 1				< 1	< 1	< 1	
	Bullous eruption/rash		< 1						< 1				< 2	< 1					
	Eczema		< 1			< 1			< 1										

NSAIDs Adverse Reactions (%)[a]

	Adverse reaction	Celecoxib	Diclofenac	Etodolac	Fenoprofen	Flurbiprofen	Ibuprofen	Indomethacin	Ketoprofen	Ketorolac	Meclofenamate	Mefenamic acid	Meloxicam	Nabumetone	Naproxen	Oxaprozin	Piroxicam	Sulindac	Tolmetin
GI	Abdominal pain or cramps	4.1	3-9	3-9	2	3-9	1-3	1-3	3-9		3-9	1-10	1.9-4.7	12	3-9	1-3	1-10	10 (pain) 1-3 (cramps)	3-9
	Abdominal distension		1-3					< 1											
	Diarrhea	5.6	3-9	3-9	1.8	3-9	1-3	1-3	3-9	7	10-33	1-10	1.9-7.8	14	1-3	3-9	1-10	3-9	3-9
	Nausea	3.5	3-9	3-9	7.7	3-9	3-9	3-9	3-9	12	11	1-10	2.4-7.2	3-9	3-9	3-9	1-10	3-9	11
	Vomiting	< 2	< 1	1-3	2.6	1-3			1-3	1-3		1-10	0.6-2.6	1-3	< 1	1-3	1-10		3-9
	Nausea and vomiting						1-3	1-3			11							1-3	
	Constipation	< 2	3-9	1-3	7	1-3	1-3	1-3	3-9	1-3	1-3	1-10	0.8-2.6	3-9	3-9	3-9	1-10	3-9	1-3
	Flatulence	2.2	1-3	3-9	< 1	1-3	1-3	< 1	3-9	1-3	3-9	1-10	0.4-3.2	3-9		1-3	1-10	1-3	3-9
	Peptic ulcer bleed		1-3	< 1			< 1						< 2			< 1			
	Dyspepsia/Indigestion	8.8	3-9	10	10.3	3-9	1-3	3-9	11	12		1-10	3.8-9.5	13	1-3	3-9	1-10	3-9	3-9
	Gastritis	< 2		1-3	< 1	< 1	< 1		< 1	< 1		< 1	< 2	1-3			< 1	< 1	1-3
	Melena	< 2	< 1	1-3			< 1		< 1			< 1	< 2	< 1	< 1		< 1		
	GI bleeding	< 0.1	0.6		< 1	1-3	< 1					< 1	< 2	< 1	< 1	< 1		< 1	< 1
	Epigastric/GI pain						3-9			13									
	Heartburn						3-9				3-9	1-10			3-9		1-10		
	Abdominal/GI distress						1-3	1-3								1-3			3-9
	Bloating						1-3	< 1											
	GI fullness						1-3			1-3									
	Stomatitis	< 2				< 1			1-3	1-3	1-3	< 1		1-3	1-3	< 1	< 1	< 1	< 1
	Anorexia/Decreased appetite	< 2		< 1	< 1		1-3	< 1	1-3	< 1	1-3			< 1		1-3	1-10	1-3	
	Positive stool guaiac				< 1									3-9					
	Dry mouth	< 2	< 1	< 1	< 1	< 1	< 1		< 1	< 1		< 1	< 2	1-3			< 1		
	Gross bleeding/perforation											1-10					1-10		
	Epigastric discomfort																		
	Peptic ulcer		0.6	< 1	< 1	< 1		< 1	< 1		1-3	1-10	< 2	< 1		< 1	1-10	< 1	1-3
	Hepatitis	< 0.1	< 1	< 1		< 1	< 1		< 1			< 1	< 2			< 1	< 1	< 1	< 1
	Jaundice	< 0.1	< 1	< 1	< 1		< 1		< 1			< 1	< 0.1	< 1	< 1		< 1	< 1[j]	
	Pancreatitis	< 0.1	< 1[k]	< 1	< 1		< 1		< 1			< 1	< 2	< 1	< 1	< 1	< 1	< 1	
	Colitis		< 1	< 1		< 1					< 1		< 2		< 1			< 1	
	Hematemesis					< 1			< 1			< 1	< 2		< 1		< 1		
	Appetite increase	< 2							< 1	< 1			< 2	< 1					
	Eructation	< 2		< 1					< 1	< 1		< 1	< 2	< 1			< 1		
	Esophagitis	< 2		< 1[l]								< 1	< 2				< 1		
	Gastroenteritis	< 2						< 1						< 1				< 1	
	Liver failure	< 0.1		< 1								< 1	< 0.1	< 1			< 1	< 1	
	Appetite change		< 1			< 1						< 1					< 1		
	Rectal bleeding/hemorrhage							< 1	< 1	< 1		< 1		< 1		< 1	< 1		
	Glossitis											< 1		< 1			< 1	< 1	< 1

NSAIDs Adverse Reactions (%)[a]

	Adverse reaction	Celecoxib	Diclofenac	Etodolac	Fenoprofen	Flurbiprofen	Ibuprofen	Indomethacin	Ketoprofen	Ketorolac	Meclofenamate	Mefenamic acid	Meloxicam	Nabumetone	Naproxen	Oxaprozin	Piroxicam	Sulindac	Tolmetin
GU	Dysuria	< 2		1-3	< 1							< 1		< 1		1-3	< 1	< 1	< 1
	Urinary frequency/Polyuria	< 2	< 1	1-3			< 1	< 1		< 1		< 1	0.1-2.4			1-3	< 1		
	Urinary tract infection/symptoms	< 2				3-9			1-3				0.3-6.9						1-3
	Renal function impairment/insufficiency/ abnormal			< 1				< 1	3-9			1-10				< 1	1-10	< 1	
	Hematuria	< 2	< 1	< 1	< 1	< 1	< 1	< 1	< 1	< 1		< 1	< 2	< 1	< 1	< 1	< 1	< 1	< 1
	Interstitial nephritis/acute interstitial nephritis	< 0.1	< 1	< 1	< 1	< 1		< 1	< 1			< 1	< 0.1	< 1	< 1	< 1	< 1	< 1	
	Renal failure			< 1	< 1	< 1		< 1	< 1		< 1	< 1	< 2	< 1	< 1		< 1	< 1	< 1
	Albuminuria	< 2											< 2	< 1					
	Cystitis	< 2		< 1	< 1		< 1					< 1					< 1		
	Menstrual disorder/disturbance	< 2				< 1									< 1				
	Renal calculi/stones	< 2		< 1										< 1				< 1	
	Acute renal failure	< 0.1	< 1				< 1									< 1			
	Azotemia		< 1		< 1		< 1							< 1					
	Impotence		< 1						< 1					< 1					
	Nephrotic syndrome		< 1					< 1	< 1					< 1	< 1	< 1	< 1	< 1	
	Oliguria		< 1		< 1					< 1		< 1					< 1		
	Papillary necrosis/renal papillary necrosis		< 1	< 1	< 1		< 1								< 1				
	Proteinuria		< 1					< 1		< 1		< 1					< 1	< 1	< 1
	Vaginal bleeding/hemorrhage	< 2	< 1			< 1		< 1						< 1				< 1	
	Gynecomastia						< 1	< 1	< 1									< 1	
Hematologic/Lymphatic	Purpura		< 1		< 1				< 1	1-3		< 1	< 2		1-3		< 1	< 1	< 1
	Ecchymoses	< 2		< 1		< 1		< 1				< 1			3-9	< 1	< 1	< 1	
	Anemia	< 2		< 1					< 1	< 1		1-10	≤ 4.1	< 1		< 1	1-10		
	Agranulocytosis	< 0.1	< 1	< 1	< 1		< 1	< 1	< 1		< 1	< 1	< 0.1		< 1	< 1	< 1	< 1	< 1
	Leukopenia	< 0.1	< 1	< 1		< 1		< 1			< 1	< 1	< 2	< 1	< 1	< 1	< 1	< 1	
	Thrombocytopenia	< 0.1	< 1	< 1	< 1	< 1	< 1[m]		< 1			< 1	< 2	< 1	< 1	< 1	< 1	< 1	< 1
	Hemolytic anemia		< 1	< 1	< 1	< 1	< 1	< 1			< 1	< 1			< 1		< 1	< 1	< 1
	Aplastic anemia	< 0.1	< 1		< 1	< 1	< 1	< 1				< 1			< 1		< 1	< 1	
	Pancytopenia	< 0.1		< 1	< 1							< 1				< 1	< 1		
	Eosinophilia		< 1			< 1	< 1			< 1	< 1	< 1			< 1		< 1		
	Neutropenia			< 1			< 1				< 1							< 1	
	Lymphadenopathy				< 1	< 1						< 1					< 1		< 1
Hypersensitivity	Anaphylaxis or anaphylactic/ anaphylactoid reaction	< 0.1	< 1	< 1[n]	< 1	< 1	< 1	< 1	< 1			< 1	< 0.1[o]	< 1	< 1	< 1	< 1	< 1	< 1
	Angioedema/Angioneurotic edema	< 0.1	< 1	< 1	< 1	< 1	< 1	< 1				< 1	< 2	< 1	< 1		< 1	< 1	
	Allergy/Allergic reaction	< 2		< 1					< 1				< 2						
	Serum sickness						< 1									< 1	< 1		< 1
Lab test abnormalities	ALT or AST elevations	< 2	2		< 1								< 2						
	Liver test abnormalities/elevations		3-9	< 1		1-3	< 1				< 1	1-10		< 1	< 1	< 1	1-10	< 1	< 1
	BUN increased	< 2		< 1				< 1	3-9				< 2						1-3
	Bleeding time increased			< 1								1-10					1-10		
	Hemoglobin and hematocrit decreases		< 1			< 1	< 1				< 1								1-3
	Creatinine increase	< 2		< 1									< 2						
Metabolic/Nutritional	Fluid retention		1-3				1-3	< 1											
	Peripheral edema	2.1			5														
	Edema	< 2		< 1		3-9	1-3	< 1	3-9	4	1-3	1-10	0.5-4.5[p]	3-9	3-9	< 1	1-10	1-3	3-9
	Body weight changes			< 1		1-3			< 1			< 1	< 2			< 1	< 1		3-9
	Thirst			< 1					< 1						1-3				
	Lower extremity edema																		
	Hyperglycemia	< 2		< 1[q]				< 1				< 1		< 1	< 1		< 1	< 1	
	Hyperkalemia					< 1		< 1							< 1		< 1	< 1	
	Hypokalemia	< 2												< 1					
	Weight gain	< 2						< 1		< 1				< 1					

NSAIDs Adverse Reactions (%)[a]

	Adverse reaction	Celecoxib	Diclofenac	Etodolac	Fenoprofen	Flurbiprofen	Ibuprofen	Indomethacin	Ketoprofen	Ketorolac	Meclofenamate	Mefenamic acid	Meloxicam	Nabumetone	Naproxen	Oxaprozin	Piroxicam	Sulindac	Tolmetin
Musculoskeletal	Arthralgia	< 2											≤ 5.3						
	Myalgia	< 2							< 1						< 1				
	Muscle weakness							< 1							< 1			< 1	
Respiratory	Dyspnea	< 2	< 1	< 1	2.8	< 1		< 1	< 1	< 1		< 1	< 2	< 1	3-9		< 1	< 1	
	Upper respiratory infection	8.1			1.5								≤ 8.3			< 1			
	Rhinitis	2		< 1		1-3	< 1		< 1	< 1									
	Pharyngitis	2.3		< 1					< 1				0.6-3.2						
	Sinusitis	5		< 1												< 1			
	Bronchitis	< 2		< 1		< 1													
	Coughing	< 2								< 1			0.2-2.4	< 1					
	Epistaxis	< 2	< 1			< 1		< 1	< 1	< 1							< 1	< 1	< 1
	Asthma		< 1	< 1		< 1		< 1				< 1	< 2	< 1			< 1		
	Pneumonia	< 2										< 1					< 1		
	Bronchospasm	< 2					< 1		< 1				< 2					< 1	
	Pulmonary edema				< 1			< 1		< 1									
Special senses	Tinnitus	< 2	1-3	1-3	4.5	1-3	1-3	1-3	1-3	< 1	1-3	1-10	< 2	3-9	3-9	1-3	1-10	1-3	1-3
	Hearing disturbances							< 1							1-3				
	Blurred vision	< 2	< 1	1-3	2.2			< 1		< 1	< 1	< 1				< 1	< 1	< 1	
	Visual disturbances/changes			< 1		1-3			1-3					< 1	1-3			< 1	1-3
	Conjunctivitis	< 2		< 1		< 1	< 1		< 1		< 1	< 1	< 2			< 1	< 1		
	Hearing loss/impairment		< 1[r]		1.6		< 1		< 1	< 1		< 1			< 1	< 1	< 1	< 1	
	Diplopia		< 1		< 1		< 1	< 1											
	Taste disorder/perversion/disturbance/alteration/changes	< 2	< 1	< 1		< 1			< 1		< 1		< 2	< 1		< 1			
Miscellaneous	Chills			1-3		< 1			< 1					< 1	< 1				
	Fever	< 2		1-3	< 1	< 1		< 1		< 1		< 1	< 2	< 1	< 1		< 1		< 1
	Back pain	2.8											0.4-3						
	Injury, accidental	2.9																	
	Influenza-like disease/symptoms	< 2											4.5-5.8				< 1		
	Pain	< 2							< 1				0.9-5.2						
	Accident, household												3.2-4.5						
	Fall												≤ 2.6						
	Chest pain	< 2	< 1					< 1											1-3
	Infection			< 1					< 1	< 1		< 1					< 1		
	Face edema	< 2							< 1				< 2						

[a] Data are pooled from separate studies and are not necessarily comparable.
[b] Sinus tachycardia, sinus bradycardia.
[c] Including necrotizing and allergic.
[d] CNS inhibition (depression, sedation, somnolence, or confusion).
[e] CNS stimulation (eg, anxiety, insomnia, reflexes increased, tremor) or CNS inhibition (eg, amnesia, asthenia, somnolence, malaise, depression).
[f] CNS inhibition (eg, somnolence, malaise, depression) or CNS excitation (eg, insomnia, nervousness, dreams).
[g] With fever and coma.
[h] Resembling porphyria cutanea tarda.
[i] Erythema multiforme major.
[j] Sometimes with fever.
[k] With or without concomitant hepatitis.
[l] With or without stricture or cardiospasm.
[m] With or without purpura.
[n] Anaphylactic/Anaphylactoid reaction (including shock).
[o] Including shock.
[p] Edema, dependent edema, peripheral edema, and leg edema combined.
[q] In previously uncontrolled diabetes.
[r] Reversible and irreversible.

➤*Cardiovascular:*
Celecoxib – Aggravated hypertension, coronary artery disorder (less than 2%); peripheral gangrene, thrombophlebitis, ventricular fibrillation (less than 0.1%).

Diclofenac – Premature ventricular contractions (less than 1%).

Fenoprofen – Atrial fibrillation, ECG changes, supraventricular tachycardia (less than 1%).

Flurbiprofen – Cerebrovascular ischemia, heart failure, vascular diseases, vasodilation (less than 1%).

Indomethacin – Thrombophlebitis (less than 1%).

Ketoprofen – Peripheral vascular disease, vasodilation (less than 1%).

Meloxicam – Cardiac failure (less than 2%).

Nabumetone – Thrombophlebitis (less than 1%).

Oxaprozin – Blood pressure changes (less than 1%).

Piroxicam – Exacerbation of angina (less than 1%).

➤*CNS:*
Celecoxib – Leg cramps, neuralgia, neuropathy (less than 2%); ataxia (less than 0.1%).

Diclofenac – Abnormal coordination, disorientation, irritability, memory disturbance, nightmares, psychotic reaction, tic (less than 1%).

Fenoprofen – Disorientation, personality change, seizures, trigeminal neuralgia (less than 1%).

Flurbiprofen – Ataxia, emotional lability, meningitis, subarachnoid hemorrhage, twitching (less than 1%).

Ibuprofen – Emotional lability, pseudotumor cerebri (less than 1%).

Indomethacin – Aggravation of epilepsy and parkinsonism, coma, depersonalization, dysarthria, peripheral neuropathy, psychic disturbances (including psychotic episodes) (less than 1%).

Ketoprofen – Amnesia, dysphoria, libido disturbances, nightmares, personality disorder (less than 1%).

Ketorolac – Abnormal thinking, euphoria, excessive thirst, extrapyramidal symptoms, hyperkinesis, inability to concentrate, stupor (less than 1%).

Mefenamic acid – Coma, meningitis (less than 1%).

Nabumetone – Agitation, nightmares (less than 1%).

Naproxen – Cognitive dysfunction, inability to concentrate (less than 1%).

Oxaprozin – Sleep disturbance (1% to 3%); weakness (less than 1%).

Piroxicam – Akathisia, coma, meningitis, mood alterations (less than 1%).

Sulindac – Neuritis, psychic disturbances (including acute psychosis) (less than 1%).

➤*Dermatologic:*

Celecoxib – Cellulitis, contact dermatitis, dermatitis, dry skin, herpes simplex, herpes zoster, injection site reaction, nail disorder, rash erythematous, rash maculopapular, skin disorder, skin nodule (less than 2%).

Diclofenac – Dermatitis (less than 1%).

Etodolac – Cutaneous vasculitis with purpura, hyperpigmentation, maculopapular rash, skin peeling, vesiculobullous rash (less than 1%).

Flurbiprofen – Dry skin, herpes simplex zoster, nail disorder (less than 1%).

Ibuprofen – Photoallergic skin reactions, vesiculobullous eruptions (less than 1%).

Indomethacin – Erythema nodosum, petechiae (less than 1%).

Ketoprofen – Onycholysis, purpuric rash, skin discoloration (less than 1%).

Ketorolac – Pallor (less than 1%).

Meclofenamate – Erythema nodosum (less than 1%).

Mefenamic acid – Toxic epidermal necrosis (less than 1%).

Nabumetone – Acne, pseudoporphyria cutanea tarda (less than 1%).

Naproxen – Epidermal necrolysis, epidermolysis bullosa, photosensitive dermatitis (less than 1%).

Oxaprozin – Pseudoporphyria (less than 1%).

Piroxicam – Bruising, desquamation, erythema, onycholysis, petechial rash, toxic epidermal necrosis, vesiculobullous reaction (less than 1%).

Sulindac – Sore or dry mucous membranes (less than 1%).

➤*GI:*

Celecoxib – Diverticulitis, dysphagia, gastroesophageal reflux, hemorrhoids, hepatic function abnormal, hiatal hernia, tenesmus (less than 2%); cholelithiasis, colitis with bleeding, esophageal perforation, ileus, intestinal obstruction, intestinal perforation (less than 0.1%).

Diclofenac – Aphthous stomatitis, bloody diarrhea, cirrhosis, esophageal lesions, hepatic necrosis, hepatorenal syndrome, intestinal perforation (less than 1%).

Etodolac – Cholestatic hepatitis, cholestatic jaundice, duodenitis, intestinal ulceration, liver necrosis, peptic ulcer with or without bleeding and/or perforation, ulcerative stomatitis (less than 1%).

Fenoprofen – Aphthous ulceration of the buccal mucosa, cholestatic hepatitis, metallic taste, peptic ulcer without perforation (less than 1%).

Flurbiprofen – Bloody diarrhea, cholecystitis, cholestatic and noncholestatic jaundice, esophageal disease, exacerbation of inflammatory bowel disease, periodontal abscess, small intestine inflammation with loss of blood and protein (less than 1%).

Ibuprofen – Gastric or duodenal ulcer with bleeding and/or perforation, gingival ulcer (less than 1%).

Indomethacin – Development of ulcerative colitis and regional ileitis, ulcerative stomatitis, toxic hepatitis and jaundice (some fatal cases have been reported), intestinal strictures (diaphragms), GI bleeding without obvious ulcer formation and perforation of pre-existing sigmoid lesions (diverticulum, carcinoma, etc), intestinal ulceration associated with stenosis and obstruction, proctitis, single or multiple ulcerations (including perforation and hemorrhage of the esophagus, stomach, duodenum, or small and large intestines) (less than 1%).

Ketoprofen – Buccal necrosis, cholestatic hepatitis, fecal occult blood, hepatic dysfunction, intestinal ulceration, microvesicular steatosis, GI perforation, salivation, ulcerative colitis (less than 1%).

Meclofenamate – Bleeding and/or perforation with or without obvious ulcer formation, cholestatic jaundice, paralytic ileus (less than 1%).

Meloxicam – Gastroesophageal reflux, intestinal perforation, perforated duodenal ulcer, perforated gastric ulcer, stomatitis ulcerative (less than 2%).

Nabumetone – Duodenitis, dysphagia, gallstones, gingivitis (less than 1%).

Naproxen – GI perforation, nonpeptic GI ulceration, ulcerative stomatitis (less than 1%).

Oxaprozin – Hemorrhoidal bleeding (less than 1%).

Piroxicam – Pain (colic) (less than 1%).

Sulindac – Ageusia, bile duct sludging, biliary calculi, cholestasis, GI perforation, intestinal strictures (diaphragm) (less than 1%).

Tolmetin – GI bleeding without evidence of peptic ulcer, perforation (less than 1%).

➤*GU:*

Celecoxib – Breast fibroadenosis, breast neoplasm, breast pain, dysmenorrhea, moniliasis genital, prostatic disorder, urinary incontinence, vaginitis (less than 2%).

Diclofenac – Nocturia (less than 1%).

Etodolac – Leukorrhea, uterine bleeding irregularities (less than 1%).

Fenoprofen – Anuria, mastodynia, nephrosis (less than 1%).

Flurbiprofen – Prostate disease, uterine hemorrhage, vulvovaginitis (less than 1%).

Indomethacin – Breast changes (including enlargement and tenderness, or gynecomastia) (less than 1%).

Ketoprofen – Menometrorrhagia (less than 1%).

Ketorolac – Urinary retention (less than 1%).

Meclofenamate – Nocturia (less than 1%).

Nabumetone – Bilirubinuria, hyperuricemia (less than 1%).

Naproxen – Glomerular nephritis, renal disease (less than 1%).

Oxaprozin – Decreased menstrual flow, increased menstrual flow (less than 1%).

Sulindac – Crystalluria, urine discoloration (less than 1%).

➤*Hematologic/Lymphatic:*

Celecoxib – Thrombocythemia (less than 2%).

Diclofenac – Allergic purpura, bruising (less than 1%).

Fenoprofen – Bruising, hemorrhage (less than 1%).

Flurbiprofen – Iron deficiency anemia (less than 1%).

Ibuprofen – Bleeding episodes (less than 1%).

Indomethacin – Anemia secondary to obvious or occult GI bleeding, bone marrow depression, disseminated intravascular coagulation, leukemia, thrombocytopenic purpura (less than 1%).

Ketoprofen – Hemolysis, hypocoagulability (less than 1%).

Meclofenamate – Thrombocytopenic purpura (less than 1%).

Meloxicam – Bilirubinemia (less than 2%).

Nabumetone – Granulocytopenia (less than 1%).

Naproxen – Granulocytopenia (less than 1%).

Sulindac – Bone marrow depression (including aplastic anemia) (less than 1%).

Tolmetin – Granulocytopenia (less than 1%).

➤*Hypersensitivity:*

Ibuprofen – Henoch-Schonlein vasculitis, lupus erythematosus syndrome, syndrome of abdominal pain, fever, chills, nausea and vomiting (less than 1%).

Indomethacin – Acute respiratory distress, angiitis, purpura, rapid fall in blood pressure resembling a shock-like state (less than 1%).

Meclofenamate – Lupus, serum sickness-like syndrome (less than 1%).

Piroxicam – Positive ANA (less than 1%).

Sulindac – Hypersensitivity vasculitis, potentially fatal hypersensitivity syndrome (less than 1%).

➤*Metabolic/Nutritional:*

Celecoxib – Diabetes mellitus, hypercholesterolemia, NPN increase (less than 2%); hypoglycemia (less than 0.1%).

Diclofenac – Hypoglycemia, weight loss (less than 1%).

Flurbiprofen – Hyperuricemia (less than 1%).

Ibuprofen – Acidosis, hypoglycemic reactions (less than 1%).

Indomethacin – Glycosuria (less than 1%).

Ketoprofen – Diabetes mellitus (aggravated), hyponatremia (less than 1%).

Meloxicam – Dehydration (less than 2%).

Naproxen – Hypoglycemia (less than 1%).

Piroxicam – Hypoglycemia (less than 1%).

➤*Lab test abnormalities:*

Celecoxib – Alkaline phosphatase increased, CPK increased (less than 2%).

Fenoprofen – Increase in alkaline phosphatase and LDH (less than 1%).

Ibuprofen – Decreased creatinine clearance (less than 1%).

Meloxicam – GGT increased (less than 2%).

Sulindac – Increased prothrombin time (patients taking oral anticoagulants) (less than 1%).

➤*Musculoskeletal:*

Celecoxib – Arthrosis, bone disorder, fracture accidental, neck stiffness, synovitis, tendinitis (less than 2%).

Flurbiprofen – Myasthenia (less than 1%).

Indomethacin – Involuntary muscle movement (less than 1%).

➤*Respiratory:*

Celecoxib – Bronchospasm aggravated, laryngitis (less than 2%).

Diclofenac – Edema of the pharynx, hyperventilation, laryngeal edema (less than 1%).

Etodolac – Pulmonary infiltration with eosinophilia (less than 1%).

Fenoprofen – Nasopharyngitis (1.2%).

Flurbiprofen – Hyperventilation, laryngitis, pulmonary infarct (less than 1%).

Ketoprofen – Hemoptysis, laryngeal edema (less than 1%).

Mefenamic acid – Respiratory depression (less than 1%).

Nabumetone – Eosinophilic pneumonia, hypersensitivity pneumonitis, idiopathic interstitial pneumonitis (less than 1%).

Naproxen – Eosinophilic pneumonitis (less than 1%).

Oxaprozin – Pulmonary infections (less than 1%).

Piroxicam – Respiratory depression (less than 1%).

➤*Special senses:*

Celecoxib – Cataract, deafness, ear abnormality, earache, eye pain, glaucoma, otitis media (less than 2%).

Diclofenac – Amblyopia, night blindness, scotoma, vitreous floaters (less than 1%).

Etodolac – Deafness, photophobia (less than 1%).

Fenoprofen – Burning tongue, optic neuritis (less than 1%).

Flurbiprofen – Corneal opacity, ear disease, glaucoma, parosmia, retinal hemorrhage, retrobulbar neuritis, transient hearing loss (less than 1%).

Ibuprofen – Amblyopia, cataracts, dry eyes, optic neuritis (less than 1%).

Indomethacin – Corneal deposits and retinal disturbances (including those of the macula), deafness (less than 1%).

Ketoprofen – Conjunctivitis sicca, eye pain, retinal hemorrhage and pigmentation change (less than 1%).

Ketorolac – Abnormal taste, abnormal vision (less than 1%).

Meclofenamate – Decreased visual acuity, iritis, macular and perimacular edema, retinal changes including macular fibrosis, reversible loss of color vision, temporary loss of vision (less than 1%).

Meloxicam – Abnormal vision (less than 2%).

Piroxicam – Swollen eyes (less than 1%).

Sulindac – Bitter taste, disturbances of retina and vasculature of retina, metallic taste (less than 1%).

Tolmetin – Optic neuropathy, retinal and macular changes (less than 1%).

➤*Miscellaneous:*

Celecoxib – Allergy aggravated, cyst NOS, hot flushes, infection bacterial/fungal/viral, infection soft tissue, moniliasis, peripheral pain, tooth disorder (less than 2%); sepsis, suicide, sudden death (less than 0.1%).

Diclofenac – Dry mucous membranes, swelling of the lip and tongue (less than 1%).

Ketoprofen – Septicemia, shock (less than 1%).

Ketorolac – Injection site pain (2%).

Mefenamic acid – Death, sepsis (less than 1%).

Meloxicam – Hot flushes (less than 2%).

Piroxicam – Death, sepsis (less than 1%).

Sulindac – Fulminant necrotizing fasciitis (less than 1%).

Overdosage

➤*Symptoms:* The incidence of acute NSAID overdoses result in minimal or no toxicity. Most reports of toxic signs and symptoms are mild to moderate and include GI distress, nausea, vomiting, lethargy, tinnitus, confusion, headache, and blurred vision. More severe symptoms may include seizures, metabolic acidosis, hypotension, hypothermia, hepatic and renal injury, coma, anaphylactoid reactions, and respiratory depression. Severe poisoning may result in hypertension, acute renal failure, hepatic dysfunction, cardiovascular collapse, and cardiac arrest. Anaphylactoid reactions have been reported with therapeutic ingestion of NSAIDs and may occur following an overdose. Acute overdose studies of **ibuprofen** report approximately 60% of adults remaining asymptomatic, 30% to 40% suffer mild to moderate symptoms, and less than 3% experience severe symptoms. Those at risk for toxicity associated with chronic use include the elderly and those with pre-existing renal, cardiovascular, or hepatic disease. Most organ systems are involved; however, the majority of deaths from chronic use are related to GI effects.

Symptoms may include the following: Drowsiness; dizziness; mental confusion; disorientation; lethargy; paresthesia; numbness; vomiting; gastric irritation; nausea; abdominal pain; intense headache; tinnitus; convulsions; blurred vision; respiratory depression; GI bleeding; hypertension; dyspepsia; ataxia; tremor; hyperpyrexia; epigastric pain; metabolic acidosis; anaphylactoid reactions; heartburn; indigestion; elevations in serum creatinine and BUN; renal impairment, coma, seizures, status epilepticus (**mefenamic acid**); hypotension and tachycardia (acute ingestion of **fenoprofen**); stupor, coma, diminished urine output and hypotension (**sulindac**; deaths have occurred); metabolic acidosis (acute **ibuprofen** overdosage); acute renal failure (**diclofenac** 2 g; **fenoprofen**, **oxaprozin** [rare]).

➤*Treatment:* Treatment of NSAID toxicity is primarily supportive and symptomatic. In addition to supportive measures, the use of oral activated charcoal may help to reduce the absorption and reabsorption of the NSAID. Refer to General Management of Acute Overdosage. Syrup of ipecac and gastric lavage have been recommended, but effectiveness has not been studied in NSAID overdose. Gastric lavage performed more than 1 hour after overdosage has little benefit. Take care in administering syrup of ipecac to child ingestions of 100 to 400 mg/kg of **ibuprofen** because ibuprofen at this dose range mimic the symptoms produced by ipecac. Because NSAIDs are rapidly absorbed, decontamination may not benefit more than 2- to 4-hour postingestion. Do not give syrup of ipecac to overdose patients at high risk of seizures, especially those who have ingested **mefenamic acid** or high amounts of other NSAIDs.

Because most NSAIDs are highly protein bound, extensively metabolized, and essentially excreted unchanged, elimination enhancement (hemodialysis, forced diuresis, alkalinization of urine, hemoperfusion, and peritoneal dialysis) may be of little value. However, hemodialysis may be necessary in cases of NSAID-induced prolonged or severe renal failure. Multiple doses of activated charcoal for elimination enhancement have been reported in **indomethacin** and **piroxicam** ingestions and therefore, may be applied to **sulindac**, **diclofenac**, **meloxicam**, and **ibuprofen** to interrupt enterohepatic or enteroenteric recirculation. Use this therapy only in severely symptomatic overdoses.

Meclofenamate – Dialysis may be required to correct serious azotemia or electrolyte imbalance.

Meloxicam – In a clinical trial, 4 g oral cholestyramine 3 times daily accelerated meloxicam clearance.

Patient Information

Side effects of NSAIDs can cause discomfort and, rarely, more serious side effects, such as GI bleeding may occur, which may result in hospitalization and even fatalities. NSAIDs are often essential in the management of arthritis and have a major role in treating pain, but they also may be commonly employed for less serious conditions. Apprise patients of potential risks.

Photosensitivity may occur; caution patients to take protective measures (ie, sunscreens, protective clothing) against UV or sunlight until tolerance is determined.

Avoid **aspirin** and alcoholic beverages while taking medication.

Although serious GI tract ulcerations and bleeding can occur without warning symptoms, alert patients for the signs and symptoms of ulcerations and bleeding, and have patients ask for medical advice when observing any indicative sign or symptoms. Apprise patients of the importance of this follow-up.

Inform patients of the warning signs and symptoms of hepatotoxicity (eg, nausea, fatigue, lethargy, pruritus, jaundice, right upper quadrant tenderness, flu-like symptoms). If these occur, instruct patients to stop therapy and seek immediate medical therapy.

Instruct patients to seek immediate emergency help in the case of an anaphylactoid reaction.

Avoid NSAIDs in late pregnancy because it may cause premature closure of the ductus arteriosus.

If GI upset occurs, take with food, milk, or antacids. For GI upset with **tolmetin**, use antacids other than sodium bicarbonate; bioavailability is affected by food and milk. If GI symptoms persist, notify physician.

Advise women who are taking **meclofenamate** for heavy menstrual flow to consult their doctor if they have spotting or bleeding between cycles or worsening of their menstrual blood flow. These symptoms may be signs of the development of a more serious condition that is not appropriately treated with meclofenamate.

Physicians may wish to discuss the potential risks and likely benefits of NSAID treatment with their patients, particularly when the drugs are used for less serious conditions where treatment without NSAIDs may represent an acceptable alternative to both the patient and physician.

Physicians may want to make specific recommendations to patients about when they should take NSAIDs in relation to food and what patients should do if they experience minor GI symptoms associated with them.

May cause drowsiness, vertigo, depression, dizziness, or blurred vision; patients should observe caution while driving or performing other tasks requiring alertness.

Notify physician if skin rash, GI ulceration, bleeding, visual disturbances, weight gain, edema, black stools, or persistent headache occurs.

➤*Mefenamic acid and meclofenamate:* If rash, diarrhea, or other digestive problems occur, discontinue use and consult a physician.

➤*Ibuprofen (otc use):* Do not take for more than 3 days for fever, or more than 10 days for pain. If symptoms persist, worsen, or if new symptoms develop, contact a physician.

DICLOFENAC

Rx	**Cataflam** (Novartis)	**Tablets:** 50 mg (as potassium)	Sucrose. (CATAFLAM 50). Lt brown. In 100s and UD 100s.
Rx	**Diclofenac Potassium** (Various, eg, Geneva, Mylan, Teva)		In 100s and 500s.
Rx	**Diclofenac Sodium** (Various, eg, Geneva, Roxane, Watson)	**Tablets, delayed-release:** 25 mg (as sodium)	May be enteric-coated. In 60s and 100s.
Rx	**Voltaren** (Novartis)		Enteric-coated. Lactose. (VOLTAREN 25). Yellow, triangular. In 60s, 100s, and UD 100s.
Rx	**Diclofenac Sodium** (Various, eg, Geneva, Martec, Purepac, Roxane, Teva, Watson)	**Tablets, delayed-release:** 50 mg (as sodium)	May be enteric-coated. In 42s, 60s, 100s, 500s, 1000s, and UD 100s.
Rx	**Voltaren** (Novartis)		Enteric-coated. Lactose. (VOLTAREN 50). Lt brown, triangular. In 60s, 100s, 1000s, and UD 100s.
Rx	**Diclofenac Sodium** (Various, eg, Geneva, Martec, Purepac, Roxane, Teva, Watson)	**Tablets, delayed-release:** 75 mg (as sodium)	May be enteric-coated. In 42s, 60s, 100s, 500s, 1000s.
Rx	**Voltaren** (Novartis)		Enteric-coated. Lactose. (VOLTAREN 75). Lt pink, triangular. In 60s, 100s, 1000s, and UD 100s.
Rx	**Diclofenac Sodium** (Various, eg, Geneva, Purepac, Teva)	**Tablets, extended-release:** 100 mg (as sodium)	In 100s.
Rx	**Voltaren-XR** (Novartis)		Sucrose, cetyl alcohol. (Voltaren-XR 100). Lt pink. In 100s and UD 100s.

DICLOFENAC POTASSIUM — ORAL

For complete and comparative prescribing information, refer to the NSAIDs group monograph.

WARNING

Cardiovascular risk – NSAIDs may cause an increased risk of serious cardiovascular thrombotic events, myocardial infarction, and stroke, which can be fatal. This risk may increase with duration of use. Patients with cardiovascular disease or risk factors for cardiovascular disease may be at greater risk.

Diclofenac potassium is contraindicated for treatment of perioperative pain in the setting of coronary artery bypass graft (CABG) surgery.

GI risk – NSAIDs cause an increased risk of serious GI adverse events including inflammation, bleeding, ulceration, and perforation of the stomach or intestines, which can be fatal. These events can occur at any time during use and without warning symptoms. Elderly patients are at greater risk for serious GI events.

Indications

For the acute and chronic treatment of signs and symptoms of osteoarthritis and rheumatoid arthritis; for the treatment of ankylosing spondylitis; for the management of mild to moderate pain and primary dysmenorrhea, when prompt pain relief is desired, because it is formulated to provide earlier plasma concentrations of diclofenac.

Administration and Dosage

➤*Approved by the FDA:* July 1988.

The dose of diclofenac should be individualized to the lowest effective dose to minimize adverse reactions.

In patients weighing less than 60 kg (132 lbs), or where the severity of the disease, concomitant medication, or other diseases warrant, the maximum recommended total daily dose of diclofenac potassium should be reduced. Experience with other NSAIDs has shown that starting therapy with maximum doses in patients at increased risk due to renal or hepatic disease, low body weight (less than 60 kg), advanced age, a known ulcer diathesis, or known sensitivity to NSAID effects, is likely to increase frequency of adverse reactions and is not recommended.

➤*Osteoarthritis:* 100 to 150 mg/day of diclofenac potassium, 50 mg 2 or 3 times daily. Dosages greater than 200 mg/day have not been studied in patients with osteoarthritis.

➤*Rheumatoid arthritis:* 150 to 200 mg/day of diclofenac potassium, 50 mg twice daily or 3 times daily. Doses greater than 225 mg/day are not recommended in patients with rheumatoid arthritis.

➤*Ankylosing spondylitis:* 50 mg twice daily. Stay in the range of 100 to 125 mg/day. Doses greater than 125 mg/day have not been studied in patients with ankylosing spondylitis.

➤*Analgesia and primary dysmenorrhea:* The recommended starting dose is 50 mg 3 times daily. With experience, physicians may find that in some patients, an initial dose of 100 mg of diclofenac potassium, followed by 50 mg doses, will provide better relief. After the first day, when the maximum recommended dose may be 200 mg, the total daily dose should generally not exceed 150 mg.

➤*Storage/Stability:* Do not store above 30°C (86°F). Protect from moisture. Dispense in tight container (USP).

DICLOFENAC SODIUM — ORAL

For complete and comparative prescribing information, refer to the NSAIDs group monograph.

WARNING

Cardiovascular risk – NSAIDs may cause an increased risk of serious cardiovascular thrombotic events, myocardial infarction, and stroke, which can be fatal. This risk may increase with duration of use. Patients with cardiovascular disease or risk factors for cardiovascular disease may be at greater risk.

Diclofenac sodium is contraindicated for treatment of perioperative pain in the setting of coronary artery bypass graft (CABG) surgery.

GI risk – NSAIDs cause an increased risk of serious GI adverse events including inflammation, bleeding, ulceration, and perforation of the stomach or intestines, which can be fatal. These events can occur at any time during use and without warning symptoms. Elderly patients are at greater risk for serious GI events.

Indications

For relief of signs and symptoms of osteoarthritis and rheumatoid arthritis.

➤*Delayed-release tablets:* For acute or long-term use in the relief of ankylosing spondylitis.

Administration and Dosage

➤*Approved by the FDA:* July 28, 1988.

As with other NSAIDs, the lowest dose should be sought for each patient. Therefore, after observing the response to initial therapy with diclofenac sodium, the dose and frequency should be adjusted to suit an individual patient's needs.

Different formulations of diclofenac (diclofenac sodium delayed-release tablets; diclofenac sodium extended-release tablets; diclofenac potassium immediate-release tablets) are not necessarily bioequivalent even if the milligram strength is the same.

➤*Osteoarthritis:*

Delayed-release tablets – 100 to 150 mg/day (50 mg twice daily or 3 times daily, or 75 mg twice daily).

Extended-release tablets – 100 mg/day.

➤*Rheumatoid arthritis:*

Delayed-release tablets – 150 to 200 mg/day in divided doses (50 mg 3 times daily or 4 times daily, or 75 mg twice daily).

Extended-release tablets – 100 mg/day. In the rare patient where diclofenac sodium extended-release tablets 100 mg/day is unsatisfactory, the dose may be increased to 100 mg twice daily if the benefits outweigh the clinical risks of increased side effects.

➤*Ankylosing spondylitis:*

Delayed-release tablets – 100 to 125 mg/day, administered as 25 mg 4 times daily, with an extra 25 mg dose at bedtime if necessary.

➤*Storage/Stability:* Do not store above 30°C (86°F). Protect from moisture. Dispense in a tight container.

ETODOLAC

Rx	**Etodolac** (Various, eg, Eon, Par, Purepac, Ranbaxy, Taro, Teva, Watson, Zenith Goldline)	**Tablets**: 400 mg	In 100s and 500s.
Rx	**Etodolac** (Various, eg, Eon, Par, Purepac, Ranbaxy, Taro, Teva, Watson, Zenith Goldline)	**Tablets**: 500 mg	In 100s, 500s, and 1000s.
Rx	**Etodolac** (Various, eg, ESI Lederle, Purepac, Teva)	**Tablets, extended-release**: 400 mg	In 100s and 500s.
Rx	**Etodolac** (Various, eg, ESI Lederle, Teva)	**Tablets, extended-release**: 500 mg	In 100s.
Rx	**Etodolac** (Various, eg, ESI Lederle, Teva)	**Tablets, extended-release**: 600 mg	In 100s.
Rx	**Etodolac** (Various, eg, Mylan, Par, Taro, Teva, Watson)	**Capsules**: 200 mg	In 100s, 500s, and 1000s.
Rx	**Etodolac** (Various, eg, Mylan, Par, Taro, Teva, Watson)	**Capsules**: 300 mg	In 100s, 500s, and 1000s.

ETODOLAC — ORAL

For complete and comparative prescribing information, refer to the NSAIDs group monograph.

Indications

For the relief of the signs and symptoms of osteoarthritis, rheumatoid arthritis, and juvenile rheumatoid arthritis; for the management of other types of pain.

Administration and Dosage

➤*Approved by the FDA:* January 1991.

As with other nonsteroidal anti-inflammatory drugs (NSAIDs), the lowest dose and longest dosing interval should be sought for each patient. Therefore, after observing the response to initial therapy with etodolac, the dose and frequency should be adjusted to suit an individual patient's needs.

➤*Capsules and tablets:* Dosage adjustment of etodolac is generally not required in patients with mild-to-moderate renal impairment. Etodolac should be used with caution in such patients, because, as with other NSAIDs, it may further decrease renal function in some patients with impaired renal function.

Analgesia – The recommended total daily dose of etodolac for acute pain is up to 1000 mg, given as 200 to 400 mg every 6 to 8 hours. In some patients, if the potential benefits outweigh the risks; the dose may be increased to 1200 mg/day in order to achieve a therapeutic benefit that might not have been achieved with 1000 mg/day. Doses of etodolac greater than 1000 mg/day have not been evaluated adequately in well-controlled clinical trials.

Osteoarthritis and rheumatoid arthritis – The recommended starting dose of etodolac for the management of the signs and symptoms of osteoarthritis is 300 mg 2 times a day or 3 times a day, 400 mg 2 times a day, or 500 mg 2 times a day. During long-term administration, the dose of etodolac may be adjusted up or down, depending on the clinical response of the patient. A lower dose of 600 mg/day may suffice for long-term administration. In patients who tolerate 1000 mg/day, the dose may be increased to 1200 mg/day when a higher level of therapeutic activity is required. When treating patients with higher doses, the physician should observe sufficient increased clinical benefit to justify the higher dose. Physicians should be aware that doses above 1000 mg/day have not been evaluated adequately in well-controlled clinical trials.

In chronic conditions, a therapeutic response to therapy with etodolac is sometimes seen within 1 week of therapy, but most often is observed by 2 weeks. After a satisfactory response has been achieved, the patient's dose should be reviewed and adjusted as required.

➤*Extended-release tablets:*

Juvenile rheumatoid arthritis – For relief of signs and symptoms of juvenile rheumatoid arthritis in patients 6 to 16 years of age, the recommended dose given orally once per day should be based on body weight, according to the following information:

Body weight range (kg)	Dose
20 to 30 kg	400 mg tablet × 1
31 to 45 kg	600 mg tablet × 1
46 to 60 kg	400 mg tablet × 2
> 60 kg	500 mg tablet × 2

Rheumatoid arthritis and osteoarthritis – 400 to 1000 mg, given once daily. During long-term administration, the dose of etodolac extended-release tablets may be adjusted up or down, depending on the patient's clinical response, up to a maximum dose of 1200 mg/day. Doses above 1200 mg/day have not been studied, and thus a dose-efficacy relationship at doses beyond 1200 mg/day has not been established. In chronic conditions, a therapeutic response to therapy with etodolac extended-release tablets is sometimes seen within 1 week of therapy, but most often is observed by 2 weeks.

➤*Storage/Stability:*

Capsules and tablets – Store at controlled room temperature from 15° to 30°C (59° to 86°F). Keep tightly closed. Preserve in tight, light-resistant container. Dispense contents with a child-resistant closure as required.

Extended-release tablets – Store at controlled room temperature from 20° to 25°C (68° to 77°F). Protect from excessive heat and humidity.

FENOPROFEN CALCIUM

Rx	**Fenoprofen** (Various, eg, Geneva, Par, Watson)	**Capsules**: 200 mg	In 100s.
Rx	**Nalfon** (Pedinol)		(RX681). Yellow/White opaque. In 100s.
Rx	**Fenoprofen** (Various, eg, Geneva, Par, Watson)	**Capsules**: 300 mg	In 100s.
Rx	**Nalfon** (Pedinol)		(RX682). Yellow/Yellow opaque. In 100s.
Rx	**Fenoprofen** (Various, eg, Watson, Zenith Goldline)	**Tablets**: 600 mg	In 100s, 500s, and 1000s, UD 100s, unit-of-use 30s, 60s, 90s, and 120s.

FENOPROFEN CALCIUM — ORAL

For complete and comparative prescribing information, refer to the NSAIDs group monograph.

WARNING

Cardiovascular risk – NSAIDs may cause an increased risk of serious cardiovascular thrombotic events, myocardial infarction, and stroke, which can be fatal. This risk may increase with duration of use. Patients with cardiovascular disease or risk factors for cardiovascular disease may be at greater risk.

Fenoprofen is contraindicated for treatment of perioperative pain in the setting of coronary artery bypass graft (CABG) surgery.

GI risk – NSAIDs cause an increased risk of serious GI adverse events including bleeding, ulceration, and perforation of the stomach or intestines, which can be fatal. These events can occur at any time during use and without warning symptoms. Elderly patients are at greater risk for serious GI events.

Indications

For relief of the signs and symptoms of rheumatoid arthritis (RA) and osteoarthritis (OA). It is recommended for the treatment of acute flare-ups and exacerbations and for the long-term management of these diseases.

Fenoprofen calcium is also indicated for the relief of mild-to-moderate pain.

➤*Unlabeled uses:* Selected NSAIDs have been used in the treatment of juvenile RA, symptomatic treatment of sunburn, and for various migraine headaches.

Administration and Dosage

➤*Approved by the FDA:* May 2, 1988.

➤*Analgesia:* For the treatment of mild to moderate pain, the recommended dosage is 200 mg every 4 to 6 hours, as needed.

➤*Rheumatoid arthritis and osteoarthritis:* 300 to 600 mg, 3 or 4 times a day. The dose should be tailored to the needs of the patient and may be increased or decreased depending on the severity of the symptoms. Dosage adjustments may be made after initiation of drug therapy or during exacerbations of the disease. Total daily dosage should not exceed 3200 mg.

If GI complaints occur, fenoprofen calcium may be administered with meals or with milk. Although the total amount absorbed is not affected, peak blood levels are delayed and diminished.

Patients with rheumatoid arthritis generally seem to require larger doses of fenoprofen calcium than do those with osteoarthritis. The smallest dose that yields acceptable control should be employed.

Although improvement may be seen in a few days in many patients, an additional 2 to 3 weeks may be required to gauge the full benefits of therapy.

➤*Storage/Stability:* Store at controlled room temperature, 15° to 30°C (59° to 86°F).

FLURBIPROFEN

Rx	**Flurbiprofen** (Various, eg, Zenith Goldline)	**Tablets**: 50 mg	In 100s.
Rx	**Ansaid** (Pharmacia & Upjohn)		Lactose. (Ansaid 50 mg). White, oval. Film-coated. In 2000s.
Rx	**Flurbiprofen** (Various, eg, Teva, Zenith Goldine)	**Tablets**: 100 mg	In 100s and 500s.
Rx	**Ansaid** (Pharmacia & Upjohn)		Lactose. (Ansaid 100 mg). Blue, oval. Film-coated. In 100s and 2000s.

FLURBIPROFEN — ORAL

For complete and comparative prescribing information, refer to the NSAIDs group monograph.

WARNING

Cardiovascular risk – NSAIDs may cause an increased risk of serious cardiovascular thrombotic events, myocardial infarction, and stroke, which can be fatal. This risk may increase with duration of use. Patients with cardiovascular disease or risk factors for cardiovascular disease may be at greater risk.

Flurbiprofen is contraindicated for treatment of perioperative pain in the setting of coronary artery bypass graft (CABG) surgery.

GI risk – NSAIDs cause an increased risk of serious GI adverse events including bleeding, ulceration, and perforation of the stomach or intestines, which can be fatal. These events can occur at any time during use and without warning symptoms. Elderly patients are at greater risk for serious GI events.

Indications

For the relief of the signs and symptoms of rheumatoid arthritis and osteoarthritis.

Administration and Dosage

➤*Approved by the FDA:* November 1998.

➤*Rheumatoid arthritis and osteoarthritis:* As with other nonsteroidal anti-inflammatory drugs, the lowest dose should be sought for each patient. Therefore, after observing the response to initial therapy with flurbiprofen tablets, adjust the dose and frequency to suit an individual patient's needs.

The recommended starting dose is 200 to 300 mg total daily dose administered 2, 3, or 4 times a day (most experience in rheumatoid arthritis has been with 3 or 4 times daily dosage). The largest recommended single dose in a multiple-dose daily regimen is 100 mg. The dose should be tailored to each patient according to the severity of the symptoms and the response to therapy.

Although a few patients have received higher doses, doses greater than 300 mg/day are not recommended until more clinical experience with flurbiprofen is obtained.

➤*Storage/Stability:* Store at controlled room temperature 20° to 25°C (68° to 77°F).

IBUPROFEN

otc	**Junior Strength Motrin** (McNeil)	**Tablets**: 100 mg	(M 100). Yellow. In 24s.
otc	**Ibuprofen** (Various, eg, Geneva, Goldline, Major, Rugby, Schein, UDL, URL)	**Tablets**: 200 mg	In 24s, 50s, 100s, 250s, 1000s, and UD 100s.
otc	**Advil** (Whitehall-Robins)		Sucrose. (Advil). In 8s, 24s, 50s, 72s, 100s, 165s, and 250s.
otc	**Motrin IB** (McNeil)		**Tablets**: (Motrin IB). In 100s. **Gelcaps**: (Motrin IB). In 8s.
otc	**Ibutab** (Zee Medical)		In 24s.
otc	**Midol Maximum Strength Cramp Formula** (Bayer)		(BAYER BAYER BAYER BAYER). In 24s.
otc	**Menadol** (Rugby)		**Captabs**: In 100s.
otc	**Motrin Migraine Pain** (McNeil Consumer)		**Caplets**: (IB). White. In 24s, 50s, and 100s.
Rx	**Ibuprofen** (Various, eg, Geneva, Greenstone Ltd., Major, Schein, UDL, URL, Zenith Goldline)	**Tablets**: 400 mg	In 100s, 360s, 500s, UD 100s, UD 300s, unit-of-use 100s, *Robot ready* 25s, and *Emergi-script* 60s.
Rx	**Motrin** (Pharmacia & Upjohn)		Lactose. (Motrin 400). White. In 100s, 500s, and UD 100s.
Rx	**Ibuprofen** (Various, eg, Geneva, Greenstone Ltd., Major, Schein, UDL, URL, Zenith Goldline)	**Tablets**: 600 mg	In 100s, 270s, 500s, UD 100s, UD 300s, unit-of-use 100s, *Robot* ready 25s, and *Emergi-script* 60s.
Rx	**Motrin** (Pharmacia & Upjohn)		Lactose. (Motrin 600). White, elliptical. In 90s, 100s, 270s, 500s, and UD 100s.
Rx	**Ibuprofen** (Various, eg, Geneva, Greenstone Ltd., Major, Schein, UDL, URL, Zenith Goldline)	**Tablets**: 800 mg	In 100s, 270s, 500s, UD 100s, UD 300s, unit-of-use 100s, *Robot* ready 25s, and *Emergi-script* 60s.
Rx	**Motrin** (Pharmacia & Upjohn)		Lactose. (Motrin 800). White, elliptical. In 100s, 270s, 500s, and UD 100s.
otc	**Children's Advil** (Whitehall-Robins)	**Tablets, chewable**: 50 mg	Aspartame, 2.1 mg phenylalanine. (Advil 50). Fruit and grape flavor. In 24s and 50s.
otc	**Children's Motrin** (McNeil)		Aspartame, 3 mg phenylalanine. Orange flavor. In 24s.
otc	**Motrin, Junior Strength** (McNeil)	**Tablets, chewable**: 100 mg	Aspartame, 6 mg phenylalanine. (MOTRIN 100). Orange flavor. In 24s.
otc	**Junior Strength Advil** (Whitehall-Robins)		Aspartame, 4.2 mg phenylalanine. Grape and fruit flavor. In 24s.
otc	**Advil Liqui-Gels** (Whitehall-Robins)	**Capsules**: 200 mg	Sorbitol. (Advil). Green. In 4s, 20s, 40s, and 80s.
otc	**Advil Migraine** (Whitehall-Robins)		Sorbitol. (Advil). Brown, oval. In 20s.
otc	**Children's Advil** (Wyeth-Ayerst)	**Suspension**: 100 mg/5 ml	Sorbitol, sucrose, EDTA. Fruit flavor. In 119 and 473 ml.
otc	**Children's Motrin** (McNeil-CPC)		Sucrose. Grape, and bubble gum flavor. In 60 and 120 ml.
otc	**Ibuprofen** (Various, eg, Alpharma, Major, Perrigo)		In 118 ml.
otc	**PediaCare Fever** (Pharmacia & Upjohn)		Sucrose. Berry flavor. In 120 ml.
otc	**Pediatric Advil Drops** (Whitehall-Robins)	**Suspension**: 100 mg/2.5 ml	Sorbitol, sucrose, EDTA, glycerin. Grape flavor. In 7.5 ml.

IBUPROFEN

otc	**Ibuprofen** (Perrigo)	**Oral Drops:** 40 mg/ml	In 15 ml.
otc	**Infants' Motrin** (McNeil)		Sorbitol, sucrose. Berry flavor. In 15 ml with dropper.
otc	**PediaCare Fever** (Pharmacia & Upjohn)		Sorbitol, sucrose. Berry flavor. In 15 ml.

IBUPROFEN — ORAL

For complete and comparative prescribing information, refer to the NSAIDs group monograph.

WARNING

Cardiovascular risk – NSAIDs may cause an increased risk of serious cardiovascular thrombotic events, myocardial infarction, and stroke, which can be fatal. This risk may increase with duration of use. Patients with cardiovascular disease or risk factors for cardiovascular disease may be at greater risk.

Ibuprofen is contraindicated for treatment of perioperative pain in the setting of coronary artery bypass graft (CABG) surgery.

GI risk – NSAIDs cause an increased risk of serious GI adverse events including bleeding, ulceration, and perforation of the stomach or intestines, which can be fatal. These events can occur at any time during use and without warning symptoms. Elderly patients are at greater risk for serious GI events.

Indications

➤*OTC:*

Adults –

Liquid-filled capsules: Treats migraine.

Gelcaps and tablets: Temporarily relieves minor aches and pains due to the common cold, headache, toothache, muscular aches, backache, minor pain of arthritis, menstrual cramps.

Temporarily reduces fever.

Children –

Chewable tablets, junior strength tablets, oral suspension, and oral drops: For the temporary reduction of fever and relief of minor aches and pains due to colds, flu, sore throat, headaches, and toothaches. One dose lasts 6 to 8 hours. Ibuprofen children's chewable tablets are recommended for children 4 to 11 years of age. Ibuprofen junior strength tablets are recommended for children 6 to 11 years of age. Ibuprofen oral suspension is recommended for children 2 to 11 years of age. Ibuprofen oral drops are recommended for children 6 months to 3 years of age (varies by manufacturer).

➤*Rx:* Prescription strength ibuprofen tablets are indicated for relief of mild-to-moderate pain, for relief of the signs and symptoms of rheumatoid arthritis and osteoarthritis, and in the treatment of primary dysmenorrhea.

Administration and Dosage

➤*Approved by the FDA:* 1974.

➤*OTC:*

Adults –

Capsules: Take 2 capsules with a glass of water. If migraine symptoms persist or worsen, ask your doctor. Do not take greater than 2 capsules in 24 hours, unless directed by a doctor.

Gelcaps and tablets: Take 1 gelcap or tablet every 4 to 6 hours while symptoms persist. If pain or fever does not respond to 1 gelcap or tablet, 2 gelcaps or tablets may be used, but do not exceed 6 gelcaps or tablets in 24 hours, unless directed by a doctor. The smallest effective dose should be used. Take with food or milk if occasional and mild heartburn, upset stomach, or stomach pain occurs with use. Consult a doctor if these symptoms are more than mild or if they persist.

Children –

Chewable tablets, junior strength chewable tablets: Find the correct dose. If possible, use weight to dose; otherwise, use age. If needed, repeat dose every 6 to 8 hours. Do not take greater than 4 times a day. If stomach upset occurs while taking this product, give with food or milk.

• *50 mg chewable tablets* – Consult a doctor before giving this medicine to children who are less than 4 years of age or weigh less than 36 pounds.

Children 36 to 47 pounds or 4 to 5 years of age take 3 tablets (150 mg).
Children 48 to 59 pounds or 6 to 8 years of age take 4 tablets (200 mg).
Children 60 to 71 pounds or 9 to 10 years of age take 5 tablets (250 mg).
Children 72 to 95 pounds or 11 years of age take 6 tablets (300 mg).

• *Junior strength 100 mg chewable tablets* – Consult a doctor before giving this medicine to children who are less than 6 years of age or weigh less than 48 pounds.

Children 48 to 59 pounds or 6 to 8 years of age take 2 tablets (200 mg).
Children 60 to 71 pounds or 9 to 10 years of age take 2.5 tablets (250 mg).
Children 72 to 95 pounds or 11 years of age take 3 tablets (300 mg).

• *Oral suspension* – 7.5 mg/kg of body weight. Consult a doctor before giving this medicine to children who are less than 2 years of age or weigh less than 24 pounds.

Children 24 to 35 pounds or 2 to 3 years of age take 1 teaspoonful (100 mg).
Children 36 to 47 pounds or 4 to 5 years of age take 1.5 teaspoonfuls (150 mg).
Children 48 to 59 pounds or 6 to 8 years of age take 2 teaspoonfuls (200 mg).
Children 60 to 71 pounds or 9 to 10 years of age take 2.5 teaspoonfuls (250 mg).
Children 72 to 95 pounds or 11 years of age take 3 teaspoonfuls (300 mg).

• *Oral suspension and oral drops* – Shake well before using.

• *Oral drops* – Consult a doctor before giving this medicine to children who are less than 6 months of age or weigh less than 24 pounds.

Children 12 to 17 pounds or 6 to 11 months of age, give 1.25 mL (50 mg).

Children 18 to 23 pounds or 12 to 23 months of age, give 1.875 mL (75 mg).

➤*Rx:* Do not exceed a 3200 mg total daily dose. If GI complaints occur, administer ibuprofen tablets with meals or milk.

Rheumatoid arthritis and osteoarthritis, including flareups of chronic disease –

Suggested dosage: 1200 mg to 3200 mg daily (300 mg 4 times daily; 400, 600, or 800 mg 3 or 4 times daily). Individual patients may show a better response to 3200 mg daily, as compared with 2400 mg, although in well-controlled clinical trials patients on 3200 mg did not show a better mean response in terms of efficacy. Therefore, when treating patients with 3200 mg/day, the physician should observe sufficient increased clinical benefits to offset potential increased risk.

The dose should be tailored to each patient, and may be lowered or raised depending on the severity of symptoms either at time of initiating drug therapy or as the patient responds or fails to respond.

In general, patients with rheumatoid arthritis seem to require higher doses of ibuprofen than do patients with osteoarthritis.

The smallest dose of ibuprofen that yields acceptable control should be employed. A linear blood-level, dose-response relationship exists with single doses up to 800 mg.

Chronic conditions: In chronic conditions, a therapeutic response to therapy with ibuprofen is sometimes seen in a few days to a week but most often is observed by 2 weeks. After a satisfactory response has been achieved, the patient's dose should be reviewed and adjusted as required.

• *Mild-to-moderate pain* – 400 mg every 4 to 6 hours as necessary for relief of pain.

In controlled analgesic clinical trials, doses of ibuprofen greater than 400 mg were no more effective than the 400 mg dose.

• *Dysmenorrhea* – For the treatment of dysmenorrhea, beginning with the earliest onset of such pain, ibuprofen should be given in a dose of 400 mg every 4 hours as necessary for the relief of pain.

➤*Storage / Stability:* Keep these and all drugs out of the reach of children.

Capsules, gelcaps, and tablets – Store at room temperature 20° to 25°C (68° to 77°F). Avoid excessive heat greater than 40°C (104°F).

Oral suspension and oral drops – Store at 15° to 30°C (59° to 86°F).

INDOMETHACIN

Rx	**Indomethacin** (Various, eg, UDL, URL, Zenith Goldline)	**Capsules:** 25 mg	In 50s, 100s, 500s, 1000s, UD 100s, and *Robot* ready 25s.
Rx	**Indocin** (Merck)		Lactose, lecithin. (Indocin/MSD 25). Blue and white. In 100s and 1000s.
Rx	**Indomethacin** (Various, eg, Lederle, UDL, URL, Zenith Goldline)	**Capsules:** 50 mg	In 100s, 500s, 1000s, UD 100s, and *Robot* ready 25s.
Rx	**Indocin** (Merck)		Lactose, lecithin. (Indocin/MSD 50). Blue/white. In 100s.
Rx	**Indomethacin Extended-Release** (Inwood)	**Capsules, sustained-release:** 75 mg	Sucrose, parabens. (IL-3607). Lavender/clear. In 60s and 100s.
Rx	**Indomethacin SR** (Various, eg, Endo, Eon, Inwood, Zenith Goldline)		In 60s, 100s, and 500s.
Rx	**Indocin SR** (Forte Pharma)		(Indocin SR/695). Blue and clear. In unit-of-use 60s.
Rx	**Indocin** (Merck)	**Oral suspension:** 25 mg/5 ml	1% alcohol, sorbitol. Pineapple coconut mint flavor. In 237 ml.
Rx	**Indocin** (Merck)	**Suppositories:** 50 mg	White. In 30s.

INDOMETHACIN — ORAL

For complete and comparative prescribing information, refer to the NSAIDs group monograph. For information on parenteral indomethacin, see Agents for Patent Ductus Arteriosus.

WARNING

Cardiovascular risk – NSAIDs may cause an increased risk of serious cardiovascular thrombotic events, myocardial infarction, and stroke, which can be fatal. This risk may increase with duration of use. Patients with cardiovascular disease or risk factors for cardiovascular disease may be at greater risk.

Indomethacin is contraindicated for treatment of perioperative pain in the setting of coronary artery bypass graft (CABG) surgery.

GI risk – NSAIDs cause an increased risk of serious GI adverse events including bleeding, ulceration, and perforation of the stomach or intestines, which can be fatal. These events can occur at any time during use and without warning symptoms. Elderly patients are at greater risk for serious GI events.

Indications

Indomethacin has been found effective in active stages of the following:

1.) Moderate-to-severe rheumatoid arthritis, including acute flares of chronic disease.
2.) Moderate-to-severe ankylosing spondylitis.
3.) Moderate-to-severe osteoarthritis.
4.) Acute painful shoulder (bursitis or tendinitis).

➤*Capsules and oral suspension:*

1.) Acute gouty arthritis.

Extended-release capsules – Indomethacin extended-release capsules are not recommended for the treatment of acute gouty arthritis.

Indomethacin may enable the reduction of steroid dosage in patients receiving steroids for the more severe forms of rheumatoid arthritis. In such instances, the steroid dosage should be reduced slowly and the patients followed very closely for any possible adverse reactions.

The use of indomethacin in conjunction with aspirin or other salicylates is not recommended. Controlled clinical studies have shown that the combined use of indomethacin and aspirin does not produce any greater therapeutic effect than the use of indomethacin alone. Furthermore, in one of these clinical studies, the incidence of GI side effects was significantly increased with combined therapy.

➤*Unlabeled uses:* Indomethacin suppresses uterine activity by inhibiting prostaglandin synthesis and has been used to prevent premature labor. Prolonged maternal administration of indomethacin for this purpose could result in prenatal ductus arteriosus closure and increased neonatal morbidity; avoid this use.

Administration and Dosage

The lowest possible effective dose for the individual patient should be prescribed. Increased dosage tends to increase adverse reactions, particularly in doses over 150 to 200 mg/day, without a corresponding increase in clinical benefits.

➤*Extended-release capsules:* Indomethacin extended-release capsules are available for oral use. Indomethacin extended-release capsules can be administered once a day and can be substituted for indomethacin 25 mg capsules 3 times a day. In multiple-dose comparisons, the mean daily steady state plasma level of indomethacin attained with daily administration of indomethacin extended-release capsules 75 mg was indistinguishable from that following indomethacin 25 mg capsules given at 0, 6, and 12 hours daily. However, there will be significant differences between the 2 dosage regimens in indomethacin blood levels, especially after 12 hours. In addition, indomethacin extended-release capsules 75 mg twice a day can be substituted for indomethacin 50 mg capsules 3 times a day. Indomethacin extended-release capsules may be substituted for all the indications of indomethacin capsules except acute gouty arthritis.

Adverse reactions appear to correlate with the size of the dose of indomethacin in most patients but not all. Therefore, every effort should be made to determine the smallest effective dosage for the individual patient.

Always give indomethacin capsules, oral suspension, and extended-release capsules with food, immediately after meals, or with antacids to reduce gastric irritation.

➤*Pediatric use:* Effectiveness in pediatric patients 14 years of age and younger has not been established. Indomethacin should not be prescribed for pediatric patients 14 years of age and younger unless toxicity or lack of efficacy associated with other drugs warrants the risk.

If a decision is made to use indomethacin for pediatric patients 2 years of age or older, such patients should be monitored closely, and periodic assessment of liver function is recommended. There have been cases of hepatotoxicity reported in pediatric patients with juvenile rheumatoid arthritis, including fatalities. If indomethacin treatment is instituted, a suggested starting dose is 2 mg/kg/day given in divided doses. Maximum daily dosage should not exceed 4 mg/kg/day or 150 to 200 mg/day, whichever is less. As symptoms subside, the total daily dosage should be reduced to the lowest level required to control symptoms, or the drug should be discontinued.

In experience with more than 900 pediatric patients reported in the literature or to the manufacturer who were treated with indomethacin capsules, side effects in pediatric patients were comparable to those reported in adults. Experience in pediatric patients has been confined to the use of indomethacin capsules.

➤*Adult use:* The information below are dosage recommendations for active stages of the following conditions:

Moderate-to-severe rheumatoid arthritis (including acute flares of chronic disease), moderate-to-severe ankylosing spondylitis, moderate-to-severe osteoarthritis –

Suggested dosage: Indomethacin capsules 25 mg 2 or 3 times a day. If this is well tolerated, increase the daily dosage by 25 or by 50 mg, if required by continuing symptoms, at weekly intervals until a satisfactory response is obtained or until a total daily dose of 150 to 200 mg is reached. Doses above this amount generally do not increase the effectiveness of the drug.

In patients who have persistent night pain or morning stiffness, the giving of a large portion, up to a maximum of 100 mg, of the total daily dose at bedtime, either orally or by rectal suppositories, may be helpful in affording relief. The total daily dose should not exceed 200 mg. In acute flares of chronic rheumatoid arthritis, it may be necessary to increase the dosage by 25 mg or, if required, by 50 mg daily.

If minor adverse reactions develop as the dosage is increased, reduce the dosage rapidly to a tolerated dose, and observe the patient closely.

If severe adverse reactions occur, stop the drug. After the acute phase of the disease is under control, an attempt to reduce the daily dose should be made repeatedly until the patient is receiving the smallest effective dose or the drug is discontinued.

Careful instructions to, and observations of, the individual patient are essential to the prevention of serious, irreversible (including fatal) adverse reactions.

As advancing years appear to increase the possibility of adverse reactions, indomethacin should be used with greater care in the elderly.

Elderly patients seem to tolerate ulceration or bleeding less well than other individuals, and many spontaneous reports of fatal GI events are in this population.

Indomethacin may cause confusion or, rarely, psychosis; physicians should remain alert to the possibility of such adverse reactions in the elderly.

This drug is known to be substantially excreted by the kidney, and the risk of toxic reactions to this drug may be greater in patients with impaired renal function. Because elderly patients are more likely to have decreased renal function, care should be taken in dose selection, and it may be useful to monitor renal function.

➤*Extended-release capsules:* If indomethacin extended-release capsules are used for initiating indomethacin treatment, 1 capsule daily should be the usual starting dose in order to observe patient tolerance since 75 mg/day

INDOMETHACIN — ORAL

is the maximum recommended starting dose for indomethacin. If indomethacin extended-release capsules are used to increase the daily dose, patients should be observed for possible signs and symptoms of tolerance since the daily increment will exceed the daily increment recommended for other dosage forms. For patients who require 150 mg of indomethacin per day and have demonstrated acceptable tolerance, indomethacin extended-release capsules 75 mg may be prescribed as 1 capsule twice daily.

➤*Acute painful shoulder (bursitis or tendinitis):*

Initial dose – 75 to 150 mg daily in 3 or 4 divided doses. (For extended-release, when 150 mg is prescribed, give as 1 capsule twice daily.)

The drug should be discontinued after the signs and symptoms of inflammation have been controlled for several days. The usual course of therapy is 7 to 14 days.

➤*Capsules and oral suspension:*

Acute gouty arthritis –

Suggested dosage: Indomethacin capsules 50 mg 3 times a day until pain is tolerable. The dose should then be rapidly reduced to complete cessation of the drug. Definite relief of pain has been reported within 2 to 4 hours. Tenderness and heat usually subside in 24 to 36 hours, and swelling gradually disappears in 3 to 5 days.

If a decision is made to use indomethacin for pediatric patients 2 years of age or older, such patients should be monitored closely, and periodic assessment of liver function is recommended. There have been cases of hepatotoxicity reported in pediatric patients with juvenile rheumatoid arthritis, including fatalities. If indomethacin treatment is instituted, a suggested starting dose is 2 mg/kg/day, given in divided doses. Maximum daily dosage should not exceed 4 mg/kg/day or 150 to 200 mg/day, whichever is less. As symptoms subside, the total daily dosage should be reduced to the lowest level required to control symptoms, or the drug should be discontinued.

➤*Storage/Stability:*

Capsules and oral suspension –

Capsules: Store at controlled room temperature 15° to 30°C (59° to 86°F). Protect from light. Dispense in a tight, light-resistant container using a child-resistant closure.

Oral suspension: Store indomethacin oral suspension below 30°C (86°F). Avoid temperatures above 50°C (122°F). Protect from freezing.

Extended-release capsules – Store at controlled room temperature 15° to 30°C (59° to 86°F). Protect from moisture.

INDOMETHACIN — RECTAL

For complete and comparative prescribing information, refer to the NSAIDs group monograph. For information on parenteral indomethacin, see Agents for Patent Ductus Arteriosus.

WARNING

Cardiovascular risk – NSAIDs may cause an increased risk of serious cardiovascular thrombotic events, myocardial infarction, and stroke, which can be fatal. This risk may increase with duration of use. Patients with cardiovascular disease or risk factors for cardiovascular disease may be at greater risk.

Indomethacin is contraindicated for treatment of perioperative pain in the setting of coronary artery bypass graft (CABG) surgery.

GI risk – NSAIDs cause an increased risk of serious GI adverse events including bleeding, ulceration, and perforation of the stomach or intestines, which can be fatal. These events can occur at any time during use and without warning symptoms. Elderly patients are at greater risk for serious GI events.

Indications

Indomethacin has been found effective in active stages of the following:

1.) Moderate to severe rheumatoid arthritis including acute flares of chronic disease.
2.) Moderate to severe ankylosing spondylitis.
3.) Moderate to severe osteoarthritis.
4.) Acute painful shoulder (bursitis or tendinitis).
5.) Acute gouty arthritis.

Indomethacin may enable the reduction of steroid dosage in patients receiving steroids for the more severe forms of rheumatoid arthritis. In such instances the steroid dosage should be reduced slowly and the patients followed very closely for any possible adverse effects.

The use of indomethacin in conjunction with aspirin or other salicylates is not recommended. Controlled clinical studies have shown that the combined use of indomethacin and aspirin does not produce any greater therapeutic effect than the use of indomethacin alone. Furthermore, in one of these clinical studies, the incidence of gastrointestinal side effects was significantly increased with combined therapy.

➤*Unlabeled uses:* Indomethacin suppresses uterine activity by inhibiting prostaglandin synthesis and has been used to prevent premature labor. Prolonged maternal administration of indomethacin for this purpose could result in prenatal ductus arteriosus closure and increased neonatal morbidity; avoid this use.

Administration and Dosage

Indomethacin is available as 25 and 50 mg indomethacin capsules, indomethacin oral suspension, containing 25 mg of indomethacin per 5 mL, and 50 mg indomethacin suppositories for rectal use.

Adverse reactions appear to correlate with the size of the dose of indomethacin in most patients but not all. Therefore, every effort should be made to determine the smallest effective dosage for the individual patient.

➤*Pediatric use:* Indomethacin ordinarily should not be prescribed for pediatric patients 14 years of age and under. Effectiveness in pediatric patients 14 years of age and younger has not been established.

➤*Adult use:*

Dosage recommendations for active stages of the following –

Moderate to severe rheumatoid arthritis including acute flares of chronic disease; moderate to severe ankylosing spondylitis; and moderate to severe osteoarthritis:

• *Suggested dosage* – Indomethacin capsules 25 mg 2 or 3 times a day. If this is well tolerated, increase the daily dosage by 25 or by 50 mg, if required by continuing symptoms, at weekly intervals until a satisfactory response is obtained or until a total daily dose of 150 to 200 mg is reached. Doses above this amount generally do not increase the effectiveness of the drug.

In patients who have persistent night pain or morning stiffness, the giving of a large portion, up to a maximum of 100 mg, of the total daily dose at bedtime, either orally or by rectal suppositories, may be helpful in affording relief. The total daily dose should not exceed 200 mg. In acute flares of chronic rheumatoid arthritis, it may be necessary to increase the dosage by 25 mg or, if required, by 50 mg daily.

If minor adverse effects develop as the dosage is increased, reduce the dosage rapidly to a tolerated dose and observe the patient closely.

If severe adverse reactions occur, stop the drug. After the acute phase of the disease is under control, an attempt to reduce the daily dose should be made repeatedly until the patient is receiving the smallest effective dose or the drug is discontinued.

Careful instructions to, and observations of, the individual patient are essential to the prevention of serious, irreversible, including fatal, adverse reactions.

As advancing years appear to increase the possibility of adverse reactions, indomethacin should be used with greater care in the elderly.

Acute painful shoulder (bursitis or tendinitis) –

Initial dose: 75 to 150 mg daily in 3 or 4 divided doses.

The drug should be discontinued after the signs and symptoms of inflammation have been controlled for several days. The usual course of therapy is 7 to 14 days.

Acute gouty arthritis –

Suggested dosage: Indomethacin 50 mg 3 times a day until pain is tolerable. The dose should then be rapidly reduced to complete cessation of the drug. Definite relief of pain has been reported within 2 to 4 hours. Tenderness and heat usually subside in 24 to 36 hours, and swelling gradually disappears in 3 to 5 days.

➤*Storage/Stability:* Store indomethacin suppositories below 30°C (86°F). Avoid transient temperatures above 40°C (104°F).

KETOPROFEN

Rx	**Ketoprofen** (Various, eg, Teva)	**Capsules:** 50 mg	In 100s.
Rx	**Ketoprofen** (Various, eg, Qualitest, Teva)	**Capsules:** 75 mg	In 100s and 500s.
Rx	**Ketoprofen** (Andrx)	**Capsules, extended-release:** 100 mg	In 100s and 1000s.
Rx	**Ketoprofen** (Andrx)	**Capsules, extended-release:** 150 mg	In 100s and 1000s.
Rx	**Ketoprofen** (Andrx)	**Capsules, extended-release:** 200 mg	In 100s and 1000s.

KETOPROFEN — ORAL

For complete and comparative prescribing information, refer to the NSAIDs group monograph.

Indications

For the management of the signs and symptoms of rheumatoid arthritis and osteoarthritis. Ketoprofen extended-release is not recommended for treatment of acute pain because of its sustained-release characteristics.

Immediate-release ketoprofen is indicated for the management of pain, and the treatment of primary dysmenorrhea.

➤*OTC:* Temporary relief of minor aches and pains associated with common cold, headache, toothache, muscular aches, backache, minor arthritis pain, menstrual cramps, and reduction of fever.

KETOPROFEN — ORAL

Administration and Dosage

➤*Rheumatoid arthritis and osteoarthritis:* The recommended starting dose in otherwise healthy patients is the following:

For immediate-release, 75 mg 3 times or 50 mg 4 times a day, or for sustained-release, 200 mg administered once a day. Smaller doses of ketoprofen should be used initially in small individuals or in debilitated or elderly patients. The recommended maximum daily dose of ketoprofen is 300 mg/day for the immediate-release product or 200 mg/day for the sustained-release product.

Dosages greater than 300 mg/day of immediate-release or 200 mg/day of sustained-release are not recommended because they have not been studied.

➤*Management of pain and dysmenorrhea:*

Immediate-release capsules – 25 to 50 mg every 6 to 8 hours as necessary. A larger dose may be tried if the patient's response to a previous dose was less than satisfactory, but doses greater than 75 mg have not been shown to give added analgesia. Daily doses greater than 300 mg are not recommended because they have not been adequately studied. Because of its typical nonsteroidal anti-inflammatory drug side-effect profile, including as its principal adverse effect GI side effects, higher doses of immediate-release ketoprofen should be used with caution and patients receiving them observed carefully (see Individualization of dosage).

Extended-release capsules – The sustained-release product is not recommended for use in treating acute pain because of its extended-release characteristics.

➤*Individualization of dosage:* The recommended starting dose of ketoprofen in otherwise healthy patients is immediate-release, 75 mg 3 times or 50 mg 4 times a day, or sustained-release, 200 mg administered once a day. Smaller doses should be used initially in small individuals or in debilitated or elderly patients. The recommended maximum daily dose of ketoprofen is 300 mg/day for immediate-release or 200 mg/day for sustained-release. Concomitant use of immediate-release capsules and sustained-release capsules is not recommended.

If minor side effects appear, they may disappear at a lower dose which may still have an adequate therapeutic effect. If well tolerated but not optimally effective, the dosage may be increased. Individual patients may show a better response to 300 mg of immediate-release daily as compared to 200 mg, although, in well-controlled clinical trials, patients on 300 mg did not show greater mean effectiveness. They did, however, show an increased frequency of upper- and lower-GI distress and headaches. It is of interest that women also had an increased frequency of these adverse effects compared to men. When treating patients with 300 mg/day, the physician should observe sufficient increased clinical benefit to offset potential increased risk.

Renal function impairment – In patients with mildly impaired renal function, the maximum recommended total daily dose of ketoprofen is 150 mg. In patients with a more severe renal impairment (GFR less than 25 mL/min/1.73 m^2 or end-stage renal impairment), the maximum total daily dose should not exceed 100 mg.

Elderly patients – In elderly patients, renal function may be reduced with apparently normal serum creatinine or blood urea nitrogen (BUN) levels. Therefore, it is recommended that the initial dosage of immediate-release or sustained-release should be reduced for patients greater than 75 years of age.

Liver function impairment – It is recommended that for patients with impaired liver function and serum albumin concentration less than 3.5 g/dL, the maximum initial total daily dose of ketoprofen should be 100 mg. All patients with metabolic impairment, particularly those with both hypoalbuminemia and reduced renal function, may have increased levels of free (biologically active) ketoprofen and should be closely monitored. The dosage may be increased to the range recommended for the general population, if necessary, only after good individual tolerance has been ascertained.

Hypoalbuminemia and reduced renal function – Because hypoalbuminemia and reduced renal function both increase the fraction of free drug (biologically active form), patients who have both conditions may be at greater risk of adverse effects. Therefore, it is recommended that such patients also be started on lower doses of this medicine and closely monitored.

GI effects – As with other nonsteroidal antiinflammatory drugs, the predominant adverse effects of ketoprofen are GI effects. To attempt to minimize these effects, physicians may wish to prescribe that this agent be taken with antacids, food, or milk. Although food delays the absorption of both formulations, in most of the clinical trials ketoprofen was taken with food or milk.

➤*OTC:*

Adults – 12.5 mg with a full glass of liquid every 4 to 6 hours. If pain or fever persists after 1 hour, follow with 12.5 mg. With experience, some patients may find an initial dose of 25 mg will give better relief. Do not exceed 25 mg in a 4- to 6-hour period or 75 mg in a 24-hour period. Use the smallest effective dose.

Children – Do not give to those < 16 years of age unless directed by a physician.

➤*Storage/Stability:* Store at room temperature 15° to 30°C (59° to 86°F). Dispense in a tight, light-resistant container using a child-resistant closure. Protect from direct light and excessive heat and humidity.

KETOROLAC TROMETHAMINE

Rx	**Ketorolac Tromethamine** (Various, eg, Ethex, Teva)	**Tablets:** 10 mg	In 100s and 500s.
Rx	**Ketorolac Tromethamine** (Bedford)	**Injection:** 15 mg/ml	In 1 ml vials.
		30 mg/mL	In 1 and 2 mL single-dose vials and 10 mL multiple-dose vials.

KETOROLAC TROMETHAMINE — INJECTION

For complete and comparative prescribing information, refer to the NSAIDs group monograph.

WARNING

Ketorolac tromethamine is indicated for the short-term (up to 5 days) management of moderately severe acute pain that requires analgesia at the opioid level in adults. It is not indicated for minor or chronic painful conditions. Ketorolac tromethamine is a potent NSAID analgesic, and its administration carries many risks. The resulting NSAID-related adverse reactions can be serious in certain patients for whom ketorolac tromethamine is indicated, especially when the drug is used inappropriately. Increasing the dose of ketorolac tromethamine beyond the label recommendations will not provide better efficacy but will result in increasing the risk of developing serious adverse reactions.

GI effects – Ketorolac tromethamine can cause peptic ulcers, GI bleeding or perforation. Therefore, it is contraindicated in patients with active peptic ulcer disease, in patients with recent GI bleeding or perforation, and in patients with a history of peptic ulcer disease or GI bleeding.

Renal effects – Ketorolac tromethamine is contraindicated in patients with advanced renal impairment and in patients at risk for renal failure due to volume depletion.

Risk of bleeding – Ketorolac tromethamine inhibits platelet function and is, therefore, contraindicated in patients with suspected or confirmed cerebrovascular bleeding, hemorrhagic diathesis, incomplete hemostasis, and those at high risk of bleeding.

Ketorolac tromethamine is contraindicated as prophylactic analgesic before any major surgery and is contraindicated intraoperatively when hemostasis is critical because of the increased risk of bleeding.

Hypersensitivity – Hypersensitivity reactions ranging from bronchospasm to anaphylactic shock, have occurred and appropriate counteractive measures must be available when administering the first dose of ketorolac tromethamine IV/IM. Ketorolac tromethamine is contraindicated in patients who have previously demonstrated hypersensitivity to ketorolac tromethamine or allergic manifestations to aspirin or other NSAIDs.

WARNING (cont.)

Intrathecal or epidural administration – Ketorolac tromethamine is contraindicated for neuraxial (epidural or intrathecal) administration due to its alcohol content.

Labor, delivery, and nursing – Ketorolac tromethamine is contraindicated in labor and delivery because it may adversely affect fetal circulation and inhibit uterine contractions.

The use of ketorolac tromethamine is contraindicated in nursing mothers because of the potential adverse effects of prostaglandin-inhibiting drugs on neonates.

Concomitant use with NSAIDs – Ketorolac tromethamine is contraindicated in patients currently receiving aspirin or NSAIDs because of the cumulative risks of inducing serious NSAID-related adverse reactions.

Special populations – Dosage should be adjusted for patients greater than or equal to 65 years of age, for patients less than 50 kg (110 lbs) of body weight and for patients with moderately elevated serum creatine. Doses of ketorolac tromethamine IV/IM are not to exceed 60 mg (total dose per day) in these patients. Ketorolac tromethamine is indicated as a single dose therapy in pediatric patients; not to exceed 30 mg for IM administration and 15 mg for IV administration.

Indications

➤*Adult patients:* For the short-term (less than or equal to 5 days) management of moderately severe acute pain that requires analgesia at the opioid level, usually in a postoperative setting.

See Administration and Dosage for more information.

➤*Pediatric patients:* The safety and effectiveness of single doses of ketorolac tromethamine IV/IM have been established in pediatric patients between the ages of 2 and 16 years. Ketorolac tromethamine, as a single injectable dose, has been shown to be effective in the management of moderately severe acute pain that requires analgesia at the opioid level, usually in the postoperative setting. There is limited data available to support the use of multiple doses of ketorolac tromethamine in pediatric patients. Safety and effectiveness have not been established in pediatric patients below the age of 2 years. Use of ketorolac tromethamine in pediatric patients is supported by evidence from adequate and well-controlled studies of ketorolac

KETOROLAC TROMETHAMINE — INJECTION

tromethamine in adults with additional pharmacokinetic, efficacy and safety data on its use in pediatric patients available in the published literature.

Ketorolac tromethamine IV/IM have been used concomitantly with morphine and meperidine and has shown an opioid-sparing effect. For breakthrough pain, it is recommended to supplement the lower end of the ketorolac tromethamine IV/IM dosage range with low doses of narcotics as needed, unless otherwise contraindicated. Ketorolac tromethamine IV/IM and narcotics should not be administered in the same syringe; this will result in precipitation of ketorolac from solution.

Administration and Dosage

➤*Approved by the FDA:* November 1989.

➤*Adult patients:* In adults, the combined duration of use of ketorolac tromethamine IV/IM and ketorolac tromethamine oral is not to exceed 5 days. In adults, the use of ketorolac tromethamine oral is only indicated as continuation therapy to ketorolac tromethamine IV/IM.

Ketorolac tromethamine IV/IM – Ketorolac tromethamine IV/IM may be used as a single or multiple dose on a regular or as needed schedule for the management of moderately severe acute pain that requires analgesia at the opioid level, usually in a postoperative setting. Hypovolemia should be corrected prior to the administration of ketorolac tromethamine. Patients should be switched to alternative analgesics as soon as possible, but ketorolac tromethamine therapy is not to exceed 5 days.

When administering ketorolac tromethamine IV/IM, the IV bolus must be given over no less than 15 seconds. The IM administration should be given slowly and deeply into the muscle. The analgesic effect begins in approximately 30 minutes with maximum effect in 1 to 2 hours after dosing IV or IM. Duration of analgesic effect is usually 4 to 6 hours.

Single-dose treatment – The following regimen should be limited to single administration use only:

IM dosing: Patients less than 65 years of age should be administered 1 dose of 60 mg. Patients greater than or equal to 65 years of age, renally impaired, or less than 50 kg (110 lbs) of body weight should be administered 1 dose of 30 mg.

IV dosing: Patients less than 65 years of age should be administered 1 dose of 30 mg. Patients greater than or equal to 65 years of age, renally impaired, or less than 50 kg (110 lbs) of body weight should be administered 1 dose of 15 mg.

➤*Pediatric patients (2 to 16 years of age):* The pediatric population should receive only a single dose of ketorolac tromethamine injection, as follows:

IM dosing – One dose of 1 mg/kg up to a maximum of 30 mg.

IV dosing – One dose of 0.5 mg/kg up to a maximum of 15 mg.

➤*Multiple-dose treatment (IV or IM) in adults:*

Patients less than 65 years of age – The recommended dose is 30 mg ketorolac tromethamine IV/IM every 6 hours. The maximum daily dose should not exceed 120 mg.

Patients greater than or equal to 65 years of age, renally impaired patients, and patients less than 50 kg (110 lbs) – The recommended dose is 15 mg ketorolac tromethamine IV/IM every 6 hours. The maximum daily dose for these populations should not exceed 60 mg. Because ketorolac tromethamine may be cleared more slowly by the elderly who are also more sensitive to the adverse reactions of NSAIDs, extra caution and reduced dosages must be used when treating the elderly with ketorolac tromethamine IV/IM. Because patients with underlying renal insufficiency are at increased risk of developing acute renal failure, the risks and benefits should be assessed prior to giving ketorolac tromethamine to these patients. For breakthrough pain, do not increase the dose or the frequency of ketorolac tromethamine. Consideration should be given to supplementing these regimens with low doses of opioids as needed unless otherwise contraindicated.

➤*Transition from ketorolac tromethamine IV/IM to ketorolac tromethamine oral in adults:* Ketorolac tromethamine oral is indicated only as continuation therapy to ketorolac tromethamine IV/IM for the management of moderately severe acute pain that requires analgesia at the opioid level. The recommended ketorolac tromethamine oral dose is as follows:

Adult patients less than 65 years of age – Two tablets as a first oral dose for patients who received 60 mg IM single dose, 30 mg IV single dose, or 30 mg multiple dose. Ketorolac tromethamine IV/IM followed by 1 ketorolac tromethamine tablet every 4 to 6 hours, not to exceed 40 mg in 24 hours of ketorolac tromethamine oral.

Patients greater than or equal to 65 years of age, renally impaired, or less than 50 kg (110 lbs) of body weight – One tablet as a first oral dose for patients who received 30 mg IM single dose, 15 IV single dose, or 15 mg multiple dose. Ketorolac tromethamine IV/IM followed by 1 ketorolac tromethamine tablet every 4 to 6 hours, not to exceed 40 mg in 24 hours of ketorolac tromethamine oral.

Shortening the recommended dosing intervals may result in increased frequency and severity of adverse reactions.

In adults, the maximum combined duration of use (parenteral and oral ketorolac tromethamine) is limited to 5 days.

➤*Storage/Stability:* Store at 15° to 30°C (59° to 86°F). Protect from light.

KETOROLAC TROMETHAMINE — ORAL

For complete prescribing information, refer to the NSAIDs group monograph.

WARNING

Ketorolac tromethamine is indicated for the short-term (up to 5 days in adults) management of moderately severe acute pain that requires analgesia at the opioid level. It is not indicated for minor or chronic painful conditions. Ketorolac tromethamine is a potent NSAID analgesic, and its administration carries many risks. The resulting NSAID-related adverse events can be serious in certain patients for whom ketorolac tromethamine is indicated, especially when the drug is used inappropriately. Increasing the dose of ketorolac tromethamine beyond the label recommendations will not provide better efficacy but will result in increasing the risk of developing serious adverse events.

GI effects – Ketorolac tromethamine is contraindicated in patients with active peptic ulcer disease, in patients with recent GI bleeding or perforation, and in patients with a history of peptic ulcer disease or GI bleeding.

Renal effects – Ketorolac tromethamine is contraindicated in patients with advanced renal impairment or in patients at risk for renal failure due to volume depletion.

Risk of bleeding – Ketorolac tromethamine inhibits platelet function and is, therefore, contraindicated in patients with suspected or confirmed cerebrovascular bleeding, hemorrhagic diathesis, incomplete hemostasis, and those at high risk of bleeding.

Ketorolac tromethamine is contraindicated as prophylactic analgesic before any major surgery and is contraindicated intraoperatively when hemostasis is critical because of the increased risk of bleeding.

Hypersensitivity – Ketorolac tromethamine is contraindicated in patients with previously demonstrated hypersensitivity to ketorolac tromethamine or allergic manifestations to aspirin or other NSAIDs.

Labor, delivery, and nursing – Ketorolac tromethamine is contraindicated in labor and delivery because, through its prostaglandin synthesis inhibitory effect, it may adversely affect fetal circulation and inhibit uterine contractions.

The use of ketorolac tromethamine is contraindicated in nursing mothers because of the potential adverse effects of prostaglandin-inhibiting drugs on neonates.

Concomitant use with NSAIDs – Ketorolac tromethamine is contraindicated in patients currently receiving aspirin or NSAIDs because of the cumulative risks of inducing serious NSAID-related adverse events.

Dosage and administration – Ketorolac tromethamine oral is indicated only as continuation therapy to ketorolac tromethamine IV/IM, and the combined duration of use of ketorolac tromethamine IV/IM and ketorolac tromethamine oral is not to exceed 5 days because the increased risk of serious adverse events.

WARNING (cont.)

The recommended total daily dose of ketorolac tromethamine oral (maximum 40 mg) is significantly lower than that for ketorolac tromethamine IV/IM (maximum 120 mg).

Special populations – Dosage should be adjusted for patients 65 years of age and older, for patients less than 50 kg (110 lbs) of body weight, and for patients with moderately elevated serum creatine.

Indications

➤*Adult patients:* For the short-term (less than or equal to 5 days) management of moderately severe acute pain that requires analgesia at the opioid level, usually in a postoperative setting. Therapy should always be initiated with ketorolac tromethamine IV/IM, and ketorolac tromethamine oral is to be used only as continuation treatment, if necessary. Combined use of ketorolac tromethamine IV/IM and ketorolac tromethamine oral is not to exceed 5 days of use because of the potential of increasing the frequency and severity of adverse reactions associated with the recommended doses. Patients should be switched to alternative analgesics as soon as possible, but ketorolac tromethamine therapy is not to exceed 5 days.

Administration and Dosage

➤*Approved by the FDA:* December 20, 1991.

In adults, the combined duration of use of ketorolac tromethamine IV/IM and ketorolac tromethamine oral is not to exceed 5 days. In adults, the use of ketorolac tromethamine oral is only indicated as continuation therapy to ketorolac tromethamine IV/IM.

➤*Transition from ketorolac tromethamine IV/IM to ketorolac tromethamine oral in adults:* The recommended ketorolac tromethamine oral dose is as follows:

Adult patients younger than 65 years of age – Take 2 tablets as a first oral dose for patients who received 60 mg IM single dose, 30 mg IV single dose, or 30 mg multiple dose. Ketorolac tromethamine IV/IM followed by 1 tablet ketorolac tromethamine oral every 4 to 6 hours, not to exceed 40 mg in 24 hours of ketorolac tromethamine oral.

Patients 65 years of age and older, renally impaired, or less than 50 kg (110 lbs) of body weight – Take 1 tablet as a first oral dose for patients who received 30 mg IM single dose, 15 mg IV single dose, or 15 mg multiple dose. Ketorolac tromethamine IV/IM followed by 1 tablet ketorolac tromethamine oral every 4 to 6 hours, not to exceed 40 mg in 24 hours of ketorolac tromethamine oral.

Shortening the recommended dosing intervals may result in increased frequency and severity of adverse reactions.

➤*Storage/Stability:* Store bottles at 15° to 30°C (59° to 86°F).

MECLOFENAMATE SODIUM

Rx	**Meclofenamate Sodium** (Various, eg, Mylan, Schein)	**Capsules:** 50 mg[a]	In 100s, 500s, and 1000s.
Rx	**Meclofenamate Sodium** (Various, eg, Mylan, Schein)	**Capsules:** 100 mg[a]	In 100s, 500s, and 100s.

[a] Meclofenamic acid equivalent, as meclofenamate sodium.

MECLOFENAMATE SODIUM — ORAL

For complete and comparative prescribing information, refer to the NSAIDs group monograph.

Indications

For the relief of mild to moderate pain; for the treatment of primary dysmenorrhea and idiopathic heavy menstrual blood loss; for relief of the signs and symptoms of acute and chronic rheumatoid arthritis and osteoarthritis. As with all nonsteroidal anti-inflammatory drugs, selection of meclofenamate sodium requires a careful assessment of the benefit/risk ratio.

Meclofenamate sodium is not recommended in children because adequate studies to demonstrate safety and efficacy have not been carried out.

Administration and Dosage

➤*Usual dosage:*

Mild to moderate pain – 50 mg every 4 to 6 hours. Doses of 100 mg may be needed in some patients for optimal pain relief. However, the daily dose should not exceed 400 mg.

Excessive menstrual blood loss and primary dysmenorrhea – 100 mg 3 times a day, for up to 6 days, starting at the onset of menstrual flow.

Rheumatoid arthritis and osteoarthritis – For rheumatoid arthritis and osteoarthritis, including acute exacerbations of chronic disease, the dosage is 200 to 400 mg per day, administered in 3 or 4 equal doses.

Therapy should be initiated at the lower dosage, then increased as necessary to improve clinical response. The dosage should be individually adjusted for each patient, depending on the severity of the symptoms and the clinical response. The daily dosage should not exceed 400 mg per day. The smallest dosage of meclofenamate sodium that yields clinical control should be employed.

Although improvement may be seen in some patients in a few days, 2 to 3 weeks of treatment may be required to obtain the optimum therapeutic benefit.

After a satisfactory response has been achieved, the dosage should be adjusted as required. A lower dosage may suffice for long-term administration.

If gastrointestinal complaints occur, meclofenamate sodium may be administered with meals or with milk. It has been reported that following the administration of meclofenamate sodium capsules one-half hour after a meal, the average extent of bioavailability decreased by 26%, the average peak concentration (C_{max}) decreased 4-fold and the time to C_{max} was delayed by 3 hours. If intolerance occurs, the dosage may need to be reduced. Therapy should be terminated if any severe adverse reactions occur.

➤*Storage/Stability:* Store at controlled room temperature 15° to 30°C (59° to 86°F). Protect from light and moisture. Dispense in a tight, light-resistant container using a child-resistant closure.

MEFENAMIC ACID

Rx	**Ponstel** (Parke-Davis)	**Capsules:** 250 mg	Lactose. (FHPC 400). Ivory. In 100s.

MEFENAMIC ACID — ORAL

For complete and comparative prescribing information, refer to the NSAIDs group monograph.

WARNING

Cardiovascular risk – NSAIDs may cause an increased risk of serious cardiovascular thrombotic events, myocardial infarction, and stroke, which can be fatal. This risk may increase with duration of use. Patients with cardiovascular disease or risk factors for cardiovascular disease may be at greater risk.

Mefenamic acid is contraindicated for treatment of perioperative pain in the setting of coronary artery bypass graft (CABG) surgery.

GI risk – NSAIDs cause an increased risk of serious GI adverse events including bleeding, ulceration, and perforation of the stomach or intestines, which can be fatal. These events can occur at any time during use and without warning symptoms. Elderly patients are at greater risk for serious GI events.

Indications

For relief of mild to moderate pain in patients greater than or equal to 14 years of age, when therapy will not exceed one week (7 days); for treatment of primary dysmenorrhea.

Administration and Dosage

As with other NSAIDs, the lowest dose should be sought for each patient. Therefore, after observing the response to initial therapy with mefenamic acid, the dose and frequency should be adjusted to suit an individual patient's needs.

Administration is by the oral route, preferably with food.

For relief of acute pain in adults and adolescents 14 years of age and older, the recommended dose is 500 mg as an initial dose followed by 250 mg every 6 hours as needed, usually not to exceed 1 week.

For the treatment of primary dysmenorrhea, the recommended dose is 500 mg as an initial dose followed by 250 mg every 6 hours, starting with the onset of bleeding and associated symptoms. Clinical studies indicate that effective treatment can be initiated with the start of menses and should not be necessary for more than 2 to 3 days.

➤*Storage/Stability:* Store at controlled room temperature 15° to 30°C (59° to 86°F). Protect from moisture.

MELOXICAM

Rx	**Mobic** (Boehringer Ingelheim/Abbott)	**Tablets:** 7.5 mg	Lactose. (M). Pastel, yellow, biconvex. In 100s.
		15 mg	Lactose. (15 M). Pastel, yellow, oblong. In 100s.
		Oral suspension: 7.5 mg per 5 mL	Sorbitol, saccharin. Raspberry flavor. In 100 mL.

MELOXICAM — ORAL

For complete and comparative prescribing information, refer to the nonsteroidal anti-inflammatory drugs (NSAIDs) group monograph.

WARNING

Cardiovascular risk – Nonsteroidal anti-inflammatory drugs (NSAIDs) may cause an increased risk of serious cardiovascular thrombotic events, myocardial infarction (MI), and stroke, which can be fatal. This risk may increase with duration of use. Patients with cardiovascular disease or risk factors for cardiovascular disease may be at higher risk.

Meloxicam is contraindicated for the treatment of perioperative pain in the setting of coronary artery bypass graft (CABG) surgery.

GI risk – NSAIDs cause an increased risk of serious GI adverse reactions, including bleeding, ulceration, and perforation of the stomach or intestines, which can be fatal. These reactions can occur at any time during use and without warning symptoms. Elderly patients are at highest risk for serious GI reactions.

Indications

Carefully consider the potential benefits and risks of meloxicam and other treatment options before deciding to use meloxicam. Use the lowest effective dose for the shortest duration consistent with individual patient treatment goals.

➤*Osteoarthritis (OA)/Rheumatoid arthritis (RA):* For relief of the signs and symptoms of OA and RA.

➤*Pauciarticular/Polyarticular course juvenile rheumatoid arthritis (JRA):* For relief of the signs and symptoms of pauciarticular or polyarticular course JRA in patients 2 years of age and older.

➤*Unlabeled uses:* For the treatment of ankylosing spondylitis and acute shoulder pain.

Administration and Dosage

➤*Approved by the FDA:* April 14, 2000.

Carefully consider the potential benefits and risks of meloxicam and other treatment options before deciding to use meloxicam. Use the lowest dose for the shortest duration consistent with individual patient treatment goals. After observing the response to initial therapy with meloxicam, the dose should be adjusted to suit the individual patient's needs.

Meloxicam may be taken without regard to meals.

➤*OA/RA:* The recommended starting and maintenance oral dosage of meloxicam is 7.5 mg once daily. Some patients may receive additional benefit by increasing the dosage to 15 mg once daily.

➤*Pauciarticular/Polyarticular course JRA:* To improve dosing accuracy in lesser-weight children, the use of meloxicam oral suspension is recommended. For the treatment of JRA, the recommended oral dosage of

MELOXICAM — ORAL

meloxicam is 0.125 mg/kg once daily, up to a maximum of 7.5 mg. There was no additional benefit demonstrated by increasing the dosage more than 0.125 mg/kg once daily in these clinical trials. Individualize dosage based on the weight of the child.

JRA Dosing with Meloxicam Oral Suspension		
	0.125 mg/kg	
Weight	Dose (1.5 mg/mL)	Delivered dose
12 kg (26 lbs)	1 mL	1.5 mg
24 kg (54 lbs)	2 mL	3 mg
36 kg (80 lbs)	3 mL	4.5 mg
48 kg (106 lbs)	4 mL	6 mg
≥ 60 kg (132 lbs)	5 mL	7.5 mg

➤*Oral suspension:* Meloxicam 7.5 mg per 5 mL or 15 mg per 10 mL oral suspension may be substituted for meloxicam 7.5 or 15 mg tablets, respectively.

Shake the oral suspension gently before using.

➤*Maximum dose:* The maximum recommended daily oral dose of meloxicam is 15 mg, regardless of formulation.

➤*Storage / Stability:* Store at 25°C (77°F); excursions are permitted to 15° to 30°C (59° to 86°F). Keep tablets in a dry place.

Dispense tablets in a tight container. Keep oral suspension container tightly closed.

NABUMETONE

Rx	**Nabumetone** (Various, eg, Eon, Geneva, Teva, UDL)	**Tablets**: 500 mg	In 100s, 500s, and UD 100s.
Rx	**Relafen** (SmithKline Beecham)		(Relafen 500). White. Film-coated. Oval. In 100s and UD 100s.
Rx	**Nabumetone** (Various, eg, Eon, Geneva, Teva)	**Tablets**: 750 mg	In 100s and 500s.
Rx	**Relafen** (SmithKline Beecham)		(Relafen 750). Beige. Film-coated. Oval. In 100s and UD 100s.

NABUMETONE — ORAL

For complete prescribing information, refer to the NSAIDs group monograph.

WARNING

Cardiovascular risk – NSAIDs may cause an increased risk of serious cardiovascular thrombotic events, myocardial infarction, and stroke, which can be fatal. This risk may increase with duration of use. Patients with cardiovascular disease or risk factors for cardiovascular disease may be at greater risk.

Nabumetone is contraindicated for treatment of perioperative pain in the setting of coronary artery bypass graft (CABG) surgery.

GI risk – NSAIDs cause an increased risk of serious GI adverse events including bleeding, ulceration, and perforation of the stomach or intestines, which can be fatal. These events can occur at any time during use and without warning symptoms. Elderly patients are at greater risk for serious GI events.

Indications

Nabumetone is indicated for acute and chronic treatment of signs and symptoms of osteoarthritis and rheumatoid arthritis.

Administration and Dosage

➤*Approved by the FDA:* December 24, 1991.

➤*Osteoarthritis (OA) and rheumatoid arthritis (RA):* The recommended starting dose is 1,000 mg taken as a single dose with or without food. Some patients may obtain more symptomatic relief from 1,500 mg to 2,000 mg per day. Nabumetone can be given in either a single or twice-daily dose. Dosages over 2,000 mg per day have not been studied. The lowest effective dose should be used for chronic treatment.

➤*Storage / Stability:* Store at 25°C (77°F) (excursions permitted to 15° to 30°C [59° to 86°F]) in well-closed container; dispense in light-resistant container.

NAPROXEN

otc	**Naproxen Sodium** (Various, eg, Goldline)	**Tablets**: 200 mg (220 mg naproxen sodium)	In 24s and 50s.
otc	**Aleve** (Bayer)		**Tablets**: (ALEVE). In 24s, 50s, 100s, and 150s. **Capsules**: In 24s, 50s, 100s, 150s, and 200s. **Gelcaps**: (ALEVE). In 20s, 40s, and 80s.
otc	**Midol Extended Relief** (Bayer)		Sodium 20 mg. Capsule shape. In 24s.
Rx	**Naproxen Sodium** (Various, eg, Sidmak)	**Tablets**: 250 mg (275 mg naproxen sodium)	In 100s, 500s, 1,000s, and UD 100s.
Rx	**Anaprox** (Roche)		(Roche 274). Lt. blue, biconvex, oval. In 100s.
Rx	**Naproxen Sodium** (Various, eg, Sidmak)	**Tablets**: 500 mg (550 mg naproxen sodium)	In 100s, 500s, 1,000s, and UD 100s.
Rx	**Anaprox DS** (Roche)		(Roche/Anaprox DS). Dark blue, capsule shape. Film-coated. In 100s and 500s.
Rx	**Naproxen** (Various, eg, Lederle, Qualitest, Sidmak, UDL)	**Tablets**: 250 mg	In 30s, 100s, 500s, 1,000s, UD 100s, unit-of-use 30s, 60s, 90s, and 120s, and *Robot ready* 25s.
Rx	**Naprosyn** (Roche)		(Roche/Naprosyn 250). Yellow. In 100s and 500s.
Rx	**Naproxen** (Various, eg, Lederle, Qualitest, Sidmak, UDL)	**Tablets**: 375 mg	In 30s, 100s, 500s, 1,000s, UD 100s, and unit-of-use 30s, 60s, 90s, and 120s.
Rx	**Naprosyn** (Roche)		(Naprosyn 375). Peach. In 100s and 500s.
Rx	**Naproxen** (Various, eg, Lederle, Qualitest, Sidmak, UDL)	**Tablets**: 500 mg	In 30s, 100s, 500s, 1,000s, UD 100s, UD 300s, unit-of-use 30s, 60s, 90s, and 120s, and *Robot ready* 25s.
Rx	**Naprosyn** (Roche)		(Naprosyn 500). Yellow. In 100s and 500s.
Rx	**Naproxen** (Various, eg, Apothecon, Purepac, Roxane, Teva)	**Tablets, delayed-release**: 375 mg	In 100s and 500s.
Rx	**EC-Naprosyn** (Roche)		(EC-Naprosyn 375). White, capsule shape. Enteric-coated. In 100s.
	Naproxen (Various, eg, Apothecon, Purepac, Roxane, Teva)	**Tablets, delayed-release**: 500 mg	In 100s and 500s.
Rx	**EC-Naprosyn** (Roche)		(EC-Naprosyn 500). White, capsule shape. Enteric-coated. In 100s.
Rx	**Naprelan** (Blansett Pharmacal)	**Tablets, controlled-release**: 375 mg (412.5 mg naproxen sodium)	(N375). White, capsule shape. In 100s.
		500 mg (550 mg naproxen sodium)	(N500). White, capsule shape. In 75s.
Rx	**Naprosyn** (Roche)	**Suspension**: 125 mg/5 mL	Sorbitol, sucrose, parabens. Orange-pineapple flavor. In 473 mL.
Rx	**Naproxen** (Various, eg, Roxane)		Methylparaben, sorbitol, sucrose. Pineapple-orange flavor. In 15, 20, and 500 mL.

NAPROXEN — ORAL

For complete and comparative prescribing information, refer to the NSAIDs group monograph.

WARNING

Cardiovascular risk – NSAIDs may cause an increased risk of serious cardiovascular thrombotic events, myocardial infarction, and stroke, which can be fatal. This risk may increase with duration of use. Patients with cardiovascular disease or risk factors for cardiovascular disease may be at greater risk.

Naproxen (except controlled-release tablets) is contraindicated for the treatment of perioperative pain in the setting of coronary artery bypass graft (CABG) surgery.

Gastrointestinal risk – NSAIDs cause an increased risk of serious gastrointestinal adverse events including bleeding, ulceration, and perforation of the stomach or intestines, which can be fatal. These events can occur at any time during use and without warning symptoms. Elderly patients are at greater risk for serious gastrointestinal events.

Indications

Naproxen tablets, naproxen delayed-release tablets, naproxen sodium tablets and naproxen suspension are indicated for the treatment of rheumatoid arthritis, osteoarthritis, ankylosing spondylitis and juvenile arthritis.

Naproxen suspension is recommended for juvenile rheumatoid arthritis in order to obtain the maximum dosage flexibility based on the patient's weight.

Naproxen tablets, naproxen sodium tablets and naproxen suspension are also indicated for the treatment of tendonitis, bursitis, acute gout, and for the management of pain and primary dysmenorrhea. Naproxen delayed-release tablets is not recommended for initial treatment of acute pain because the absorption of naproxen is delayed compared to absorption from other naproxen-containing products.

Administration and Dosage

➤*Approved by the FDA:* March 11, 1976.

➤*Rheumatoid arthritis, osteoarthritis, and ankylosing spondylitis:*

Rheumatoid Arthritis, Osteoarthritis, and Ankylosing Spondylitis		
Naproxen tablets	250 mg	twice daily
	or 375 mg	twice daily
	or 500 mg	twice daily
Naproxen sodium tablets	275 mg (naproxen 250 mg with 25 mg sodium)	twice daily
Naproxen sodium tablets	550 mg (naproxen 500 mg with 50 mg sodium)	twice daily
Naproxen suspension	250 mg (10 mL/2 tsp)	twice daily
	or 375 mg (15 mL/3 tsp)	twice daily
	or 500 mg (20 mL/4 tsp)	twice daily
Naproxen delayed-release tablets	375 mg	twice daily
	or 500 mg	twice daily

During long-term administration the dose of naproxen may be adjusted up or down depending on the clinical response of the patient. A lower daily dose may suffice for long-term administration. In patients who tolerate lower doses well, the dose may be increased to 1500 mg/day when a higher level of anti-inflammatory/analgesic activity is required. When treating patients with naproxen 1500 mg/day (as naproxen tablets or 1650 mg of naproxen sodium tablets), the physician should observe sufficient increased clinical benefit to offset the potential increased risk. The morning and evening doses do not have to be equal in size and administration of the drug more frequently than twice daily does not generally make a difference in response.

To maintain the integrity of the enteric coating, the naproxen delayed-release tablets should not be broken, crushed or chewed during ingestion.

➤*Juvenile arthritis:* The use of naproxen suspension allows for more flexible dose titration.

The recommended total daily dose of naproxen is approximately 10 mg/kg given in 2 divided doses (ie, 5 mg/kg given twice a day).

Dosing of Naproxen Suspension		
Patient's Weight	Dose	Administered As
13 kg (29 lb)	62.5 mg twice daily	2.5 mL (0.5 tsp) twice daily
25 kg (55 lb)	125 mg twice daily	5 mL (1 tsp) twice daily
38 kg (84 lb)	187.5 mg twice daily	7.5 mL (1.5 tsp) twice daily

➤*Management of pain, primary dysmenorrhea and acute tendinitis and bursitis:* The recommended starting dose is 550 mg of naproxen sodium tablets followed by 550 mg every 12 hours or 275 mg every 6 to 8 hours as required. The initial total daily dose should not exceed 1375 mg of naproxen sodium. Thereafter, the total daily dose should not exceed 1100 mg of naproxen sodium. Naproxen tablets may also be used but naproxen delayed-release tablets are not recommended for initial treatment of acute pain because absorption of naproxen is delayed compared to other naproxen-containing products (see Pharmacokinetics, Indications, and Individualization of dosage).

➤*Acute gout:* The recommended starting dose is 750 mg of naproxen tablets followed by 250 mg every 8 hours until the attack has subsided. Naproxen sodium tablets may also be used at a starting dose of 825 mg followed by 275 mg every 8 hours. Naproxen delayed-release tablets are not recommended because of the delay in absorption.

➤*Individualization of dosage:* Although naproxen tablets, naproxen suspension, naproxen delayed-release tablets and naproxen sodium tablets all circulate in the plasma as naproxen, they have pharmacokinetic differences that may affect onset of action. Onset of pain relief can begin within 30 minutes in patients taking naproxen sodium and within 1 hour in patients taking naproxen. Because naproxen delayed-release tablets dissolve in the small intestine rather than in the stomach, the absorption of the drug is delayed compared to the other naproxen formulations.

The recommended strategy for initiating therapy is to choose a formulation and a starting dose likely to be effective for the patient and then adjust the dosage based on observation of benefit and/or adverse events. A lower dose should be considered in patients with renal or hepatic impairment or in elderly patients.

➤*Storage/Stability:* Store at 15° to 30°C (59° to 86°F) in well-closed containers; dispense in light-resistant containers. Avoid excessive heat (more than 40°C; 104°F).

OXAPROZIN

Rx	**Oxaprozin** (Eon Labs)	**Tablets:** 600 mg	(141). White, capsule shape. Film-coated. In 100s, 500s, 1000s, and blister 100s.
Rx	**Daypro** (Searle)	**Caplets:** 600 mg	(Daypro 1381). White, capsule shape. Scored. Film-coated. In 100s, 500s, and UD 100s.
Rx	**Daypro ALTA** (Pharmacia)	**Tablets:** 678 oxaprozin potassium (equivalent to 600 mg oxaprozin)	(Searle 1391). Blue, capsule shape. Film-coated. In 100s, 500s, and UD 100s.

OXAPROZIN — ORAL

For complete and comparative prescribing information, refer to the NSAIDs group monograph.

WARNING

Cardiovascular risk – NSAIDs may cause an increased risk of serious cardiovascular thrombotic events, myocardial infarction, and stroke, which can be fatal. This risk may increase with duration of use. Patients with cardiovascular disease or risk factors for cardiovascular disease may be at greater risk.

Oxaprozin is contraindicated for treatment of perioperative pain in the setting of coronary artery bypass graft (CABG) surgery.

GI risk – NSAIDs cause an increased risk of serious GI adverse events including bleeding, ulceration, and perforation of the stomach or intestines, which can be fatal. These events can occur at any time during use and without warning symptoms. Elderly patients are at greater risk for serious GI events.

Indications

For acute and long-term use in the management of the signs and symptoms of osteoarthritis and rheumatoid arthritis.

Administration and Dosage

➤*Approved by the FDA:* October 29, 1992.

➤*Rheumatoid arthritis:* 1200 mg (two 600 mg tablets) once a day. Both smaller and larger doses may be required in individual patients.

➤*Osteoarthritis:* The usual starting dose for healthy weight patients with mild to moderate osteoarthritis is 600 mg once a day.

The usual daily dose of oxaprozin for the management of the signs and symptoms of moderate to severe osteoarthritis is 1200 mg (two 600 mg tablets) once a day. For patients of low body weight or with milder disease, an initial dosage of one 600 mg caplet once a day may be appropriate.

Regardless of the indication, the dosage should be individualized to the lowest effective dose of oxaprozin to minimize adverse effects, and the maximum recommended total daily dose is 1800 mg (or 26 mg/kg, whichever is lower) in divided doses.

➤*Individualization of dosage:* Oxaprozin, like other NSAIDs, shows considerable interindividual differences in both pharmacokinetics and clinical response (pharmacodynamics). Therefore, the dosage for each patient should be individualized according to the patient's response to therapy. The

OXAPROZIN — ORAL

usual starting dose for most healthy weight patients with rheumatoid arthritis is 1200 mg, once a day.

In cases where a quick onset of action is important, the pharmacokinetics of oxaprozin allow therapy to be started with a one-time loading dose of 1200 to 1800 mg (not to exceed 26 mg/kg).

Doses greater than 1200 mg/day should be reserved for patients who weigh more than 50 kg, have normal renal and hepatic function, are at low risk of peptic ulcer, and whose severity of disease justifies maximal therapy. Physicians should ensure that patients are tolerating doses in the 600 to 1200 mg/day range without gastroenterologic, renal, hepatic, or dermatologic adverse effects before advancing to the larger doses.

The maximum recommended total daily dosage is 1800 mg in divided doses.

Most patients will tolerate once-a-day dosing with oxaprozin, although divided doses may be tried in patients unable to tolerate single doses. As with all drugs of this class, the frequency and severity of adverse events will depend on the dose of the drug, the age and physical condition of the patient, any concurrent medical diagnoses, individual vulnerability, and the duration of therapy. In clinical trials of oxaprozin, no clear dose-response relationship was seen for serious adverse effects, but physicians are cautioned that the reported safety data were developed in patients who had successfully taken lower doses of oxaprozin before being advanced above 1200 mg/day.

Experience with other NSAIDs has shown that starting therapy with maximal doses in patients at increased risk due to renal or hepatic disease, low body weight, advanced age, a known ulcer diathesis, or known sensitivity to NSAID effects is likely to increase the frequency of adverse events and is not recommended.

➤*Storage/Stability:* Keep bottles tightly closed and store below 25°C (77°F) . Dispense in a tight, light-resistant container with a child-resistant closure. Protect the unit dose from light.

PIROXICAM

Rx	**Piroxicam** (Various, eg, SCS Pharmaceuticals, Teva, UDL, URL, Watson, Zenith Goldline)	**Capsules:** 10 mg	In 100s, 500s, 1000s, and UD 100s.
Rx	**Feldene** (Pfizer)		Lactose. (Feldene Pfizer 322). Blue/maroon. In 100s.
Rx	**Piroxicam** (Various, eg, SCS Pharmaceuticals, Teva, UDL, URL, Watson, Zenith Goldline)	**Capsules:** 20 mg	In 100s.
Rx	**Feldene** (Pfizer)		Lactose. (Feldene Pfizer 323). Maroon. In 100s.

PIROXICAM — ORAL

For complete and comparative prescribing information, refer to the NSAIDs group monograph.

WARNING

Cardiovascular risk – NSAIDs may cause an increased risk of serious cardiovascular thrombotic events, myocardial infarction, and stroke, which can be fatal. This risk may increase with duration of use. Patients with cardiovascular disease or risk factors for cardiovascular disease may be at greater risk.

Piroxicam is contraindicated for treatment of perioperative pain in the setting of coronary artery bypass graft (CABG) surgery.

GI risk – NSAIDs cause an increased risk of serious GI adverse events including bleeding, ulceration, and perforation of the stomach or intestines, which can be fatal. These events can occur at any time during use and without warning symptoms. Elderly patients are at greater risk for serious GI events.

Indications

For use in the relief of signs and symptoms of osteoarthritis and rheumatoid arthritis.

Administration and Dosage

➤*Approved by the FDA:* April, 1982.

As with other NSAIDs, the lowest dose should be sought for each patient. Therefore, after observing the response to initial therapy with piroxicam, the dose and frequency should be adjusted to suit an individual patient's needs.

The recommended dose is 20 mg given orally once per day. If desired, the daily dose may be divided. Because of the long half-life of piroxicam, steady-state blood levels are not reached for 7 to 12 days. Therefore, although the therapeutic effects of piroxicam are evident early in treatment, there is a progressive increase in response over several weeks and the effect of therapy should not be assessed for 2 weeks.

SULINDAC

Rx	**Sulindac** (Various, eg, Allscripts, Major, Mutual, Mylan, UDL, URL, Warner Chilcott, Watson)	**Tablets:** 150 mg	In 100s, 500s, 1000s, UD 100s.
Rx	**Clinoril** (Merck)		(MSD 941/Clinoril). Yellow, hexagonal. In 100s.
Rx	**Sulindac** (Various, eg, Allscripts, Major, Mutual, Mylan, UDL, URL, Warner Chilcott, Watson)	**Tablets:** 200 mg	In 100s, 500s, 1000s, UD 100s.
Rx	**Clinoril** (Merck)		(MSD 942). Yellow, hexagonal, scored. In 100s.

SULINDAC — ORAL

For complete and comparative prescribing information, refer to the NSAIDs group monograph.

WARNING

Cardiovascular risk – Nonsteroidal anti-inflammatory agents (NSAIDs) may cause an increased risk of serious cardiovascular thrombotic events, myocardial infarction, and stroke, which can be fatal. This risk may increase with duration of use. Patients with cardiovascular disease or risk factors for cardiovascular disease may be at greater risk.

Sulindac is contraindicated for the treatment of perioperative pain in the setting of coronary artery bypass graft (CABG) surgery.

GI risk – NSAIDs cause an increased risk of serious GI adverse events including bleeding, ulceration, and perforation of the stomach or intestines, which can be fatal. These events can occur at any time during use and without warning symptoms. Elderly patients are at greater risk for serious GI events.

Indications

Sulindac is indicated for acute or long-term use in the relief of signs and symptoms of the following:

- Osteoarthritis (OA).
- Rheumatoid arthritis (RA) (the safety and efficacy of sulindac have not been established in RA patients who are designated in the American Rheumatism Association classification as Functional Class IV: Incapacitated, largely or wholly bedridden, or confined to wheelchair; little or no self-care).
- Ankylosing spondylitis.
- Acute painful shoulder (acute subacromial bursitis/supraspinatus tendinitis).
- Acute gouty arthritis.

Administration and Dosage

Sulindac should be administered orally twice a day with food. The maximum dosage is 400 mg/day. Dosages above 400 mg/day are not recommended.

➤*OA/RA/ankylosing spondylitis:* In OA, RA, and ankylosing spondylitis, the recommended starting dosage is 150 mg twice a day. The dosage may be lowered or raised depending on response.

A prompt response (within 1 week) can be expected in about one half of patients with OA, ankylosing spondylitis, and RA. Others may require longer to respond.

➤*Acute shoulder pain/acute gouty arthritis:* In acute painful shoulder (acute subacromial bursitis/supraspinatus tendinitis) and acute gouty arthritis, the recommended dosage is 200 mg twice a day. After a satisfactory response has been achieved, the dosage may be reduced according to response. In acute painful shoulder, therapy for 7 to 14 days is usually adequate. In acute gouty arthritis, therapy for 7 days is usually adequate.

TOLMETIN SODIUM

Rx	**Tolmetin Sodium** (Various, eg, Mutual, URL)	**Tablets:** 200 mg tolmetin (as sodium)	In 100s.
Rx	**Tolmetin Sodium** (Various, eg, Mylan, Purepac)	**Tablets:** 600 mg tolmetin (as sodium)	In 100s, 500s, and UD 100s.
Rx	**Tolmetin Sodium** (Various, eg, Allscripts, Mylan, Purepac, Teva)	**Capsules:** 400 mg tolmetin (as sodium)	In 100s, 500s, 1000s, and UD 100s.

TOLMETIN SODIUM — ORAL

For complete and comparative prescribing information, refer to the NSAIDs group monograph.

WARNING

Cardiovascular risk – Nonsteroidal anti-inflammatory agents (NSAIDs) may cause an increased risk of serious cardiovascular thrombotic events, myocardial infarction, and stroke, which can be fatal. This risk may increase with duration of use. Patients with cardiovascular disease or risk factors for cardiovascular disease may be at greater risk.

Tolmetin sodium is contraindicated for the treatment of perioperative pain in the setting of coronary artery bypass graft (CABG) surgery.

GI risk – NSAIDs cause an increased risk of serious GI adverse events including bleeding, ulceration, and perforation of the stomach or intestines, which can be fatal. These events can occur at any time during use and without warning symptoms. Elderly patients are at greater risk for serious GI events.

Indications

For the relief of signs and symptoms of rheumatoid arthritis and osteoarthritis; in the treatment of acute flares and the long-term management of the chronic disease; for treatment of juvenile rheumatoid arthritis. The safety and efficacy of tolmetin sodium have not been established in children under 2 years of age.

Administration and Dosage

➤*Approved by the FDA:* March, 1989.

In adults with rheumatoid arthritis or osteoarthritis, the recommended starting dose is 400 mg 3 times daily (1200 mg daily), preferably including a dose on arising and a dose at bedtime. To achieve optimal therapeutic effect, the dose should be adjusted according to the patient's response after 1 to 2 weeks. Control is usually achieved at doses of 600 to 1800 mg daily in divided doses (generally 3 times daily). Doses larger than 1800 mg/day have not been studied and are not recommended.

The recommended starting dose for children (2 years and older) is 20 mg/kg/day in divided doses (3 times daily or 4 times daily). When control has been achieved, the usual dose ranges from 15 to 30 mg/kg/day. Doses higher than 30 mg/kg/day have not been studied and, therefore, are not recommended.

A therapeutic response to tolmetin sodium can be expected in a few days to a week. Progressive improvement can be anticipated during succeeding weeks of therapy. If GI symptoms occur, tolmetin sodium can be administered with antacids other than sodium bicarbonate. Tolmetin sodium bioavailability and pharmacokinetics are not significantly affected by acute or chronic administration of magnesium and aluminum hydroxides; however, bioavailability is affected by food or milk.

➤*Storage/Stability:* Store at controlled room temperature (15° to 30°C; 59° to 86°F). Protect from light.

Selective COX-2 Inhibitors

CELECOXIB

Rx	**Celebrex** (Searle)	**Capsules:** 100 mg	Lactose. (7767 100). White. In 100s, 500s, and UD 100s.
		200 mg	Lactose. (7767 200). White. In 100s, 500s, and UD 100s.
		400 mg	Lactose. (7767 400). White. In 60s and UD 100s.

CELECOXIB — ORAL

WARNING

Cardiovascular (CV) risk – Celecoxib may cause an increased risk of serious CV thrombotic events, myocardial infarction (MI), and stroke, which can be fatal. All nonsteroidal anti-inflammatory drugs (NSAIDs) may have a similar risk. This risk may increase with duration of use. Patients with CV disease or risk factors for CV disease may be at higher risk.

Celecoxib is contraindicated for the treatment of perioperative pain in the setting of coronary artery bypass graft (CABG) surgery.

GI risk – NSAIDs, including celecoxib, cause an increased risk of serious GI adverse reactions, including bleeding, ulceration, and perforation of the stomach or intestines, which can be fatal. These reactions can occur at any time during use and without warning symptoms. Elderly patients are at higher risk for serious GI events.

Indications

➤*Osteoarthritis (OA):* For relief of the signs and symptoms of OA.

➤*Rheumatoid arthritis (RA):* For relief of the signs and symptoms of RA in adults.

➤*Ankylosing spondylitis (AS):* For the relief of signs and symptoms of AS.

➤*Acute pain:* For the management of acute pain in adults.

➤*Primary dysmenorrhea:* For the treatment of primary dysmenorrhea.

➤*Familial adenomatous polyposis (FAP):* To reduce the number of adenomatous colorectal polyps in FAP, as an adjunct to usual care (eg, endoscopic surveillance, surgery). It is not known whether there is a clinical benefit from a reduction in the number of colorectal polyps in FAP patients. It also is not known whether the effects of celecoxib treatment will persist after celecoxib is discontinued. The safety and efficacy of celecoxib treatment in patients with FAP beyond 6 months have not been studied.

➤*Unlabeled uses:* Used as adjunctive therapy in the treatment of schizophrenia (inconclusive data); treatment of colorectal polyps and prevention of colorectal cancer.

Administration and Dosage

➤*Approved by the FDA:* December 31, 1998.

➤*OA:* 200 mg daily, administered as a single dosage or as 100 mg twice/day.

➤*RA:* 100 to 200 mg twice daily.

➤*AS:* 200 mg daily, single (once daily) or divided (twice daily) doses. If no effect is observed after 6 weeks, a trial of 400 mg daily may be worthwhile. If no effect is observed after 6 weeks on 400 mg daily, a response is not likely, and consideration should be given to alternate treatment options.

➤*Acute pain and primary dysmenorrhea:* 400 mg initially, followed by an additional 200 mg dose if needed on the first day. On subsequent days, the recommended dosage is 200 mg twice daily as needed.

➤*FAP:* Usual medical care for FAP patients should be continued while on celecoxib. To reduce the number of adenomatous colorectal polyps in patients with FAP, the recommended oral dosage is 400 mg twice daily to be taken with food.

➤*Hepatic function impairment:* The daily recommended dose of celecoxib in patients with moderate hepatic function impairment (Child-Pugh class B) should be reduced by approximately 50%. The use of celecoxib in patients with severe hepatic function impairment is not recommended.

➤*Storage/Stability:* Store at 25°C (77°F); excursions permitted to 15° to 30°C (59° to 86°F).

ZICONOTIDE

Rx	**Prialt** (Elan)	**Solution:** 25 mcg/mL[a]	In 20 mL single-use vials.
		100 mcg/mL	In 1, 2, and 5 mL single-use vials.

[a] Only use the diluted 25 mcg/mL formulation for the ziconotide-naive pump priming.

ZICONOTIDE — INTRATHECAL

WARNING

Severe psychiatric symptoms and neurological impairment may occur during treatment with ziconotide. Do not treat patients with a preexisting history of psychosis with ziconotide. Monitor all patients frequently for evidence of cognitive impairment, hallucinations, or changes in mood or consciousness. Ziconotide therapy can be interrupted or discontinued abruptly without evidence of withdrawal effects in the event of serious neurological or psychiatric signs or symptoms.

Indications

➤*Analgesia:* For the management of severe chronic pain in patients for whom intrathecal (IT) therapy is warranted, and who are intolerant of or refractory to other treatment, such as systemic analgesics, adjunctive therapies, or IT morphine.

Administration and Dosage

➤*Approved by the FDA:* December 23, 2004.

Initiate ziconotide IT at no more than 2.4 mcg/day (0.1 mcg/h) and titrate to patient response. Doses may be titrated upward by up to 2.4 mcg/day (0.1 mcg/h) at intervals of no more than 2 to 3 times per week, up to a recommended maximum of 19.2 mcg/day (0.8 mcg/h) by day 21. Dose increases in increments of less than 2.4 mcg/day (0.1 mcg/h) and increases in dose less frequently than 2 to 3 times per week may be used. For each dose titration, assess the dosing requirements and adjust the pump infusion flow rate as required to achieve the new dosing. Although 977 patients have been treated with ziconotide IT in long-term, open-label trials, controlled studies of pain relief have not been conducted for longer than 3 weeks duration.

Adjust the dose of ziconotide IT according to the patient's severity of pain, their response to therapy, and the occurrence of adverse reactions. The effective dose of ziconotide for analgesia is variable. The average dose level at the end of the 21-day titration used in the slow titration clinical trial was 6.9 mcg/day (0.29 mcg/h) and the maximum dose was 19.2 mcg/day (0.8 mcg/h) on day 21. Because of the frequency of adverse reactions, 19.2 mcg/day (0.8 mcg/h) is the maximum recommended dose.

Because of the lower incidence of serious adverse reactions and discontinuation for adverse reactions associated with the slower titration, use a faster titration schedule only if there is an urgent need for analgesia that outweighs the risk to the patient's safety.

In clinical trials, no rebound or other adverse reactions related to discontinuation of ziconotide were noted, although treatment was almost always discontinued abruptly.

➤*Administration:* Administer ziconotide IT under the direction of a physician who is experienced in the technique of IT administration and familiar with the drug and device labeling. Ziconotide is not intended for intravenous (IV) administration.

Ziconotide is intended for IT delivery using a programmable implanted variable-rate microinfusion device or an external microinfusion device and catheter. Refer to the manufacturer's manual for specific instructions and precautions for programming the microinfusion device and/or refilling the reservoir.

Ziconotide is used for therapy, undiluted (25 mcg/mL in 20 mL vial) or diluted (100 mcg/mL in 1, 2, or 5 mL vials). Diluted ziconotide is prepared with 0.9% sodium chloride injection using aseptic procedures to the desired concentration prior to placement in the microinfusion pump. The 100 mcg/mL formulation may be administered undiluted once an appropriate dose has been established. Saline solutions containing preservatives are not appropriate for IT drug administration and should not be used. Refrigerate, but do not freeze, all ziconotide solutions after preparation and begin infusion within 24 hours.

➤*Storage/Stability:* Refrigerate ziconotide during transit. Store ziconotide at 2° to 8°C (36° to 46°F). Ziconotide, once diluted aseptically with saline, may be stored at 2° to 8°C for 24 hours. Do not freeze ziconotide. Protect from light. Discard any ziconotide solution with observed particulate matter or discoloration and any unused portion left in the vial.

Actions

➤*Pharmacology:* Ziconotide binds to N-type calcium channels located on the primary nociceptive (A-δ and C) afferent nerves in the superficial layers (Rexed laminae I and II) of the dorsal horn in the spinal cord. Although the mechanism of action of ziconotide has not been established in humans, results in animals suggest that its binding blocks N-type calcium channels, which leads to a blockade of excitatory neurotransmitter release in the primary afferent nerve terminals and antinociception.

➤*Pharmacokinetics:*

Absorption – The cerebrospinal fluid (CSF) pharmacokinetics (PK) of ziconotide have been studied after 1-hour IT infusions of ziconotide 1 to 10 mcg to patients with chronic pain. The plasma PK following IV infusion (0.3 to 10 mcg/kg/day) have also been studied. Both IT and IV data are shown in the following table.

Ziconotide PK Parameters (Mean ± SD)

Route	Fluid	N	CL (mL/min)	Vd (mL)	t½ (h)
IT	CSF	23	0.38 ± 0.56	155 ± 263	4.6 ± 0.9
IV	Plasma	21	270 ± 44	30,460 ± 6,366	1.3 ± 0.3

Following 1-hour IT administration of ziconotide 1 to 10 mcg, both total exposure (AUC; range: 83.6 to 608 ng•h/mL) and peak exposure (C_{max}; range: 16.4 to 132 ng/mL) values in the CSF were variable and dose-dependent, but appeared approximately dose-proportional. During 5 or 6 days of continuous IT infusions of ziconotide at infusion rates ranging from 0.1 to 7 mcg/h in patients with chronic pain, plasma ziconotide levels could not be quantified in 56% of patients using an assay with a lower limit of detection of approximately 0.04 ng/mL. Predictably, patients requiring higher IT infusion dose rates were more likely to have quantifiable ziconotide levels in plasma. Plasma ziconotide levels, when detectable, remain constant after many months of ziconotide IT infusion in patients followed for up to 9 months.

Distribution – Ziconotide is about 50% bound to human plasma proteins. The mean CSF volume of distribution (Vd) of ziconotide following IT administration approximates the estimated total CSF volume (140 mL).

Metabolism – Ziconotide is cleaved by endopeptidases and exopeptidases at multiple sites on the peptide. Following passage from the CSF into the systemic circulation during continuous IT administration, ziconotide is expected to be susceptible to proteolytic cleavage by various ubiquitous peptidases/proteases present in most organs (eg, kidney, liver, lung muscle), and thus readily degraded to peptide fragments and their individual constituent free amino acids. Human and animal CSF and blood exhibit minimal hydrolytic activity toward ziconotide in vitro. The biological activity of the various expected proteolytic degradation products of ziconotide has not been assessed.

Excretion – Minimal amounts of ziconotide (less than 1%) were recovered in human urine following IV infusion. The terminal half-life of ziconotide in CSF after an IT administration was around 4.6 hours (range, 2.9 to 6.5 hours). Mean CSF clearance (CL) of ziconotide approximates adult human CSF turnover rate (0.3 to 0.4 mL/min).

Contraindications

Hypersensitivity to ziconotide or any of its formulation components and in patients with any other concomitant treatment or medical condition that would render IT administration hazardous; preexisting history of psychosis with ziconotide; presence of infection at the microinfusion injection site; uncontrolled bleeding diathesis; spinal canal obstruction that impairs circulation of CSF.

Warnings

➤*Psychiatric symptoms:* Severe psychiatric symptoms and neurological impairment may occur during treatment with ziconotide. Do not treat patients with a preexisting history of psychosis with ziconotide. Monitor all patients frequently for evidence of cognitive impairment, hallucinations, or changes in mood or consciousness. Ziconotide therapy can be interrupted or discontinued abruptly without evidence of withdrawal effects in the event of serious neurological or psychiatric signs or symptoms.

➤*Opiate withdrawal:* Ziconotide is not an opiate and cannot prevent or relieve the symptoms associated with the withdrawal of opiates. To avoid withdrawal syndrome when opiate withdrawal is necessary, patients must not be abruptly withdrawn from opiates. For patients being withdrawn from IT opiates, gradually taper the IT opiate infusion over a few weeks and replace with a pharmacologically equivalent dose of oral opiates. Ziconotide does not interact with opiate receptors and does not potentiate opiate-induced respiratory depression.

➤*Fertility impairment:* Female fertility in rats was significantly affected following continuous IV infusion at a dose of 10 mg/kg/day. Significant reductions in corpora lutea, implantation sites, and number of live fetuses were observed.

➤*Elderly:* Of the total number of subjects in clinical studies of ziconotide, 22% were 65 years of age and older, while 7% were 75 years of age and older. In all trials, there was a higher incidence of confusion in older patients (42% of patients 65 years of age and older vs 29% of patients younger than 65 years of age). Other reported clinical experience has not identified differences in responses between the elderly and younger patients. In general, the dose selection for an elderly patient should be cautious, usually starting at the low end of the dosing range, reflecting the greater frequency of decreased hepatic, renal, or cardiac function, and of concomitant disease or other drug therapy.

➤*Pregnancy: Category C.* Ziconotide was embryolethal in rats when given as a continuous IV infusion during the major period of organogenesis as evidenced by significant increases in postimplantation loss caused by an absence or a reduced number of live fetuses. Estimated exposure for embryolethality in the rat was approximately 700-fold above the expected exposure resulting from the maximum recommended human daily IT dose of 0.8 mcg/h (19.2 mcg/day). Ziconotide was not teratogenic in female rats when given as a continuous IV infusion at doses up to 30 mg/kg/day or in female rabbits up to 5 mg/kg/day during the major period of organ development. Estimated exposures in the female rat and rabbit were approximately

ZICONOTIDE — INTRATHECAL

26,000- and 940-fold higher than the expected exposure resulting from the maximum recommended human daily IT dose of 0.8 mcg/h (19.2 mcg/day) based on plasma exposure. Maternal toxicity in the rat and rabbit, as evidenced by decreased body weight gain and food consumption, was present at all dose levels. Maternal toxicity in the rat led to reduced fetal weights and transient, delayed ossification of the pubic bones at doses 15 mg/kg/day or higher, which is approximately 8,900-fold higher than the expected exposure resulting from the maximum recommended human daily IT dose of 0.8 mcg/h (19.2 mcg/day) based on plasma exposure. The no observable adverse effect level (NOAEL) for embryo-fetal development in rats was 0.5 mg/kg/day and in rabbits was 5 mg/kg/day. Estimated NOAEL exposures in the rat and rabbit were approximately 400- and 940-fold higher, respectively, than the expected exposure resulting from the maximum recommended human daily IT dose of 0.8 mcg/h (19.2 mcg/day) based on plasma exposure.

In a prenatal and postnatal study in rats, ziconotide given as a continuous IV infusion did not affect pup development or reproductive performance up to a dose of 10 mg/kg/day, which is approximately 3,800-fold higher than the expected exposure resulting from the maximum recommended human daily IT dose of 0.8 mcg/h (19.2 mcg/day) based on plasma exposure. Maternal toxicity as evidenced by clinical observations, and decreases in body weight gain and food consumption were observed at all doses.

No adequate and well-controlled studies have been conducted in pregnant women. Because animal studies are not always predictive of human response, use ziconotide during pregnancy only if the potential benefit justifies the risk to the fetus.

➤*Lactation:* It is not known whether ziconotide is excreted in human breast milk. Because many drugs are excreted in human milk, and because of the potential for serious adverse reactions in breast-feeding infants from ziconotide, decide whether to discontinue breast-feeding or to discontinue the drug, taking into account the importance of the drug to the mother.

➤*Children:* Safety and effectiveness in children have not been established.

Precautions

➤*Meningitis and other infections:* Meningitis can occur because of inadvertent contamination of the microinfusion device and other means, such as CSF seeding caused by hematogenous or direct spread from an infected pump pocket or catheter tract. While meningitis is rare with an internal microinfusion device and surgically implanted catheter, the incidence increases substantially with external devices. In the 1,254 patients in ziconotide clinical trials with an exposure of 662 patient years, meningitis occurred in 3% (40 cases) of the ziconotide group using either internal or external microinfusion devices and 1% (1 case) in the placebo group with an exposure of only 5 patient-years. The risk of meningitis with external microinfusion devices and catheters was higher, with 93% cases (38/41) occurring with external infusion systems (37 ziconotide, 1 placebo).

Patients, caregivers, and health care providers must be particularly vigilant for the signs and symptoms of meningitis, including but not limited to fever, headache, stiff neck, altered mental status (eg, lethargy, confusion, disorientation), nausea or vomiting, and occasionally seizures. Serious infection or meningitis can occur within 24 hours of a breach in sterility such as a disconnected catheter, the most common cause of meningitis with external microinfusion devices. The patient and health care provider should be familiar with the handling of the external microinfusion device and care of the catheter skin exit site at risk of infection. Strict aseptic procedures must be used during the preparation of the ziconotide solution or refilling of the microinfusion device to prevent accidental introduction of any contaminants or other environmental pathogens into the reservoir. In suspected cases (especially in immunocompromised patients) or in confirmed cases of meningitis, CSF cultures must be obtained and appropriate antibiotic therapy must be promptly instituted. Treatment of meningitis usually requires removal of the microinfusion system, catheter, and any other foreign body materials within the IT space and, therefore, discontinuation of ziconotide therapy.

➤*Cognitive and neuropsychiatric effects:* Use of ziconotide has been associated with CNS-related adverse reactions, including psychiatric symptoms, cognitive impairment, and decreased alertness/unresponsiveness. For the 1,254 patients treated, the following cognitive adverse event rates were reported: confusion (33%), memory impairment (22%), speech disorder (14%), aphasia (12%), thinking abnormal (8%), and amnesia (1%). Cognitive impairment may appear gradually after several weeks of treatment. Reduce or discontinue the ziconotide dose if signs or symptoms of cognitive impairment develop, but also consider other contributing causes. The various cognitive effects of ziconotide are generally reversible within 2 weeks after drug discontinuation. The medians for time to reversal of the individual cognitive effects ranged from 3 to 15 days. The elderly (65 years of age and older) are at higher risk for confusion.

Reactions of acute psychiatric disturbances such as hallucinations (12%), paranoid reactions (3%), hostility (2%), delirium (2%), psychosis (1%), and manic reactions (0.4%) have been reported in patients treated with ziconotide. Patients with pretreatment psychiatric disorders may be at an increased risk. Ziconotide may cause or worsen depression with the risk of suicide in susceptible patients. If appropriate, management of psychiatric complications should include discontinuation of ziconotide, treatment with psychotherapeutic agents if appropriate, and/or short-term hospitalization. Before drug is reinitiated, careful evaluation must be performed on an individual basis.

➤*Suicide:* In placebo-controlled trials, there was a higher incidence of suicide, suicide attempts, and suicide ideations in ziconotide-treated patients (N = 3) than in the placebo group (N = 1). The incidence was 0.1/patient-year for placebo patients and 0.27/patient-year for ziconotide patients.

➤*Reduced level of consciousness:* Patients have become unresponsive or stuporous while receiving ziconotide. The incidence of unresponsiveness or stupor in clinical trials was 2%. During these episodes, the patient sometimes appears to be conscious and breathing is not depressed. If reduced levels of consciousness occur, discontinue ziconotide until the event resolves, and consider other etiologies (eg, meningitis). There is no known pharmacologic antagonist for this effect. Patients taking concomitant antiepileptics, neuroleptics, sedatives, or diuretics may be at higher risk of depressed levels of consciousness. If altered consciousness occurs, discontinue other CNS-depressant drugs as clinically appropriate.

➤*Serum CK-muscle isoenzyme (CK-MM) elevation:* In clinical studies (mostly open label), 40% of patients had serum CK levels above the upper limit of normal (ULN), and 11% had CK levels that were at least 3 times the ULN. In cases where CK was fractionated, only the muscle isoenzyme (MM) was elevated. The time to occurrence was sporadic, but the greatest incidence of CK elevation was during the first 2 months of treatment. Elevated CKs were more often seen in men, in patients who were being treated with antidepressants or antiepileptics, and in patients treated with IT morphine. Most patients who experienced elevations in CK, even for prolonged periods of time, did not have limiting side effects. However, 1 case of symptomatic myopathy with EMG findings, and 2 cases of acute renal failure associated with rhabdomyolysis and extreme CK elevations (17,000 to 27,000 units/L) have been reported.

Therefore, it is recommended that physicians monitor serum CK in patients undergoing treatment with ziconotide periodically (eg, every other week for the first month and monthly as appropriate thereafter). Clinically evaluate patients and obtain CK measurements in the setting of new neuromuscular symptoms (eg, myalgias, myasthenia, muscle cramps, asthenia) or a reduction in physical activity. If these symptoms continue and CK levels remain elevated or continue to rise, it is recommended that the physician consider ziconotide dose reduction or discontinuation.

➤*Lab test abnormalities:* In clinical studies (mostly open label), up to 40% of patients had serum CK levels above the ULN, and 11% had CK levels that were at least 3 times the ULN. Most cases of CK elevation were not associated with muscle weakness, however 1 case of myopathy with EMG findings and 2 cases of acute renal failure associated with rhabdomyolysis and extreme CK elevations (17,000 to 27,000 units/L) were reported.

➤*Hazardous tasks:* Caution patients against engaging in hazardous activity requiring complete mental alertness or motor coordination, such as operating machinery or driving a motor vehicle, during treatment with ziconotide. Also caution patients about possible combined effects with other CNS-depressant drugs. Dosage adjustments may be necessary when ziconotide is administered with such agents because of the potentially additive effects.

Drug Interactions

Formal PK drug-drug interaction studies have not been performed with ziconotide. As ziconotide is a peptide, it is expected to be completely degraded by endopeptidases and exopeptidases (Phase I hydrolytic enzymes) widely located throughout the body, and not by other Phase I biotransformation processes (including the cytochrome P450 system) or by Phase II conjugation reactions. Thus, IT administration, low plasma ziconotide concentrations, and metabolism by ubiquitous peptidases make metabolic interactions of other drugs with ziconotide unlikely. Further, as ziconotide is not highly bound in plasma (approximately 50%) and has low plasma exposure following IT administration, clinically relevant plasma protein displacement reactions involving ziconotide and coadministered medications are unlikely.

➤*CNS depressants:* Almost all patients in the ziconotide clinical trials received concomitant non-IT medication. Of the 1,254 patients treated, most received several concomitant drugs, including antidepressants (66%), anxiolytics (52%), antiepileptics (47%), neuroleptics (46%), and sedatives (34%). The use of drugs with CNS-depressant activities may be associated with an increased incidence of CNS adverse reactions such as dizziness and confusion.

➤*Opioids:* Ziconotide does not bind to opioid receptors and its pharmacological effects are not blocked by opioid antagonists. In animal models, ziconotide IT potentiated opioid-induced reduction in GI motility, but did not potentiate morphine-induced respiratory depression. In rats receiving ziconotide IT, additive analgesic effects were observed with concurrent administration of morphine, baclofen, or clonidine. Concurrent administration of ziconotide IT and morphine did not prevent the development of morphine tolerance in rats.

More than 90% of patients treated with ziconotide IT used systemic opiates and in the slow titration study, 98% of patients received opioids.

Combination of ziconotide with IT opiates has not been studied in placebo-controlled clinical trials and is not recommended.

Adverse Reactions

The most frequently reported adverse reactions (25% or more) in the 1,254 patients (662 patient years) in clinical trials were dizziness, nausea, confusion, headache, somnolence, nystagmus, asthenia, and pain. Serious adverse reactions and discontinuation of ziconotide for adverse reactions are less frequent when the drug is slowly titrated over 21 days, than with a faster titration schedule.

The following table summarizes the treatment-emergent adverse reactions with a frequency of 5% or greater in the ziconotide-treated group from the 1 placebo-controlled trial using the slow titration schedule in patients with severe chronic pain. All reactions reported during the initial placebo-controlled period of the studies (21 days in the slow titration schedule) are tabulated, regardless of relationship to ziconotide.

ZICONOTIDE — INTRATHECAL

Ziconotide Adverse Reactions in Slow Titration Placebo-Controlled Trial (Reactions that Occurred in ≥ 5% of Patients)		
Adverse reaction	Ziconotide (n = 112)	Placebo (n = 108)
CNS	81%	51%
Abnormal gait	15%	2%
Anxiety	9%	5%
Aphasia	8%	1%
Ataxia	16%	2%
Confusion	18%	5%
Dizziness	47%	13%
Dysesthesia	7%	2%
Hallucinations	7%	0%
Headache	15%	12%
Hypertonia	11%	5%
Memory impairment	12%	1%
Nervousness	7%	4%
Nystagmus	8%	0%
Paresthesia	7%	3%
Somnolence	22%	15%
Speech disorder	9%	2%
Vertigo	7%	0%
GI	60%	51%
Anorexia	10%	5%
Diarrhea	19%	17%
Nausea	41%	31%
Vomiting	15%	13%
GU	22%	12%
Urinary retention	9%	0%
Special senses	20%	11%
Abnormal vision	10%	4%
Miscellaneous	57%	42%
Asthenia	22%	12%
Fever	7%	3%
Pain	11%	7%

The following adverse reactions assessed as related to ziconotide have been reported in 2% or greater of patients participating in the clinical studies (COSTART terms, by body system):

➤*Cardiovascular:* Hypertension, hypotension, postural hypotension, syncope, tachycardia, vasodilation.

➤*CNS:* Abnormal dreams, abnormal gait, agitation, anxiety, aphasia, ataxia, CSF abnormal, confusion, depression, difficulty concentrating, dizziness, dry mouth, dysesthesia, emotional lability, headache, hostility, hyperesthesia, hypertonia, incoordination, insomnia, memory impairment, mental slowing, meningitis, nervousness, neuralgia, nystagmus, paranoid reaction, paresthesia, reflexes decreased, somnolence, speech disorder, stupor, thinking abnormal, tremor, twitching, vertigo.

➤*Dermatologic:* Cutaneous surgical complication, dry skin, pruritus, rash, skin disorder, sweating.

➤*GI:* Anorexia, constipation, diarrhea, dyspepsia, gastrointestinal disorder, nausea, nausea and vomiting, vomiting.

➤*GU:* Dysuria, urinary incontinence, urinary retention, urinary tract infection, urination impaired.

➤*Hematologic:* Anemia, ecchymosis.

➤*Metabolic/Nutritional:* Creatinine phosphokinase increased, dehydration, edema, hypokalemia, peripheral edema, weight loss.

➤*Musculoskeletal:* Arthralgia, arthritis, leg cramps, myalgia, myasthenia.

➤*Respiratory:* Bronchitis, cough increased, dyspnea, lung disorder, pharyngitis, pneumonia, rhinitis, sinusitis.

➤*Special senses:* Abnormal vision, diplopia, photophobia, taste perversion, tinnitus.

➤*Miscellaneous:* Abdominal pain, accidental injury, asthenia, back pain, catheter complication, catheter-site pain, cellulitis, chest pain, chills, fever, flu syndrome, infection, malaise, neck pain, neck rigidity, pain, pump-site complication, pump-site mass, pump-site pain, viral infection.

At less than 2%, the following reactions were assessed by the clinical investigators as related to ziconotide: acute kidney failure, atrial fibrillation, cerebrovascular accident, electrocardiogram abnormal, grand mal convulsion, meningitis, myoclonus, psychosis, respiratory distress, rhabdomyolysis, sepsis, and suicidal ideations. Rare instances of fatal aspiration pneumonia and suicide were reported (less than 1%).

Overdosage

➤*Symptoms:* The maximum recommended ziconotide IT dose is 19.2 mcg/day. The maximum IT dose of ziconotide in clinical trials was 912 mcg/day. In some patients who received IT doses greater than the maximum recommended dose, exaggerated pharmacological effects (eg, ataxia, nystagmus, dizziness, stupor, unresponsiveness, spinal myoclonus, confusion, sedation, hypotension, word-finding difficulties, garbled speech, nausea, vomiting) were observed. There was no indication of respiratory depression. Overdoses may occur because of pump programming errors or incorrect drug concentration preparations. In these cases, patients were observed and ziconotide was either temporarily discontinued or permanently withdrawn. Most patients recovered within 24 hours after withdrawal of drug.

➤*Treatment:* In the event of an IT overdose, elimination of ziconotide from CSF is expected to remain constant (CSF $t_{1/2}$ = 4.6 hours). Therefore, within 24 hours of stopping therapy, the ziconotide CSF concentration should be less than 5% of peak levels.

There is no known antidote to ziconotide. Administer general medical supportive measures to patients who receive an overdose until the exaggerated pharmacological effects of the drug have resolved. Treatment for an overdose is hospitalization, when needed, and symptom-related supportive care. Ziconotide does not bind to opiate receptors, and its pharmacological effects are not blocked by opioid antagonists.

In the event of an inadvertent IV or epidural administration, adverse reactions could include hypotension, which can be treated with a recumbent posture and blood pressure support as required. The half-life of ziconotide in serum is 1.3 hours.

Patient Information

Caution patients against engaging in hazardous activity requiring complete mental alertness or motor coordination such as operating machinery or driving a motor vehicle during treatment with ziconotide.

Caution patients about possible combined effects with other CNS-depressant drugs. Dosage adjustments may be necessary when ziconotide is administered with such agents because of the potentially additive effects.

Advise patients to contact their physician if they experience new or worsening muscle pain, soreness, or weakness with or without darkened urine.

Advise patients to contact their physician immediately if they experience:
- A change in mental status (eg, lethargy, confusion, disorientation, decreased alertness)
- A change in mood or perception (eg, hallucinations, including unusual tactile sensations in the oral cavity)
- Symptoms of depression or suicidal ideation
- Nausea, vomiting, seizures, fever, headache, and/or stiff neck, as these may be symptoms of developing meningitis.

AGENTS FOR MIGRAINE

In addition to the agents on the following pages, propranolol and timolol are indicated for migraine prophylaxis (see Beta-Adrenergic Blocking Agents monograph).

Serotonin 5-HT_1 Receptor Agonists

Indications

➤*Migraine treatment:* For the acute treatment of migraine with or without aura in adults.

➤*Cluster headache (sumatriptan injection only):* For the acute treatment of cluster headache episodes.

Actions

➤*Pharmacology:* **Sumatriptan**, **naratriptan**, **zolmitriptan**, **rizatriptan**, **frovatriptan**, **eletriptan**, and **almotriptan** are selective 5-hydroxytryptamine$_1$ (5-HT_1 or serotonin) receptor agonists.

Serotonin 5-HT_1 Receptor Agonists Receptor Site Affinity			
Drug	High	Weak	None
Almotriptan	5-HT_{1D}, 5-HT_{1B}, 5-HT_{1F}	5-HT_{1A}, 5-HT_7	5-HT_{2-4}, 5-HT_6, α-adrenergic, β-adrenergic, adenosine (A_1, A_2), angiotensin (AT_1, AT_2), dopaminergic D_1 or D_2, endothelin (ET_A, ET_B), tachykinin receptor sites
Eletriptan	5-HT_{1B}, 5-HT_{1D}, 5-HT_{1F}	5-HT_{1A}, 5-HT_{1E}, 5-HT_{2B}, 5-HT_7	5-HT_{2A}, 5-HT_{2C}, 5-HT_3, 5-HT_4, 5-HT_{5A}, 5-HT_6, α-adrenergic, and β-adrenergic, dopaminergic D_1 or D_2, muscarinic, or opioid receptors
Frovatriptan	5-HT_{1B}, 5-HT_{1D}	none	Benzodiazepine receptor sites
Naratriptan	5-HT_{1D}	none	5-HT_{2-4}, α-adrenergic, β-adrenergic, dopaminergic, muscarinic, benzodiazepine receptor sites

Serotonin 5-HT$_1$ Receptor Agonists Receptor Site Affinity			
Drug	High	Weak	None
Rizatriptan	5-HT$_{1B}$, 5-HT$_{1D}$	5-HT$_{1A}$, 5-HT$_{1E}$, 5-HT$_{1F}$, 5-HT$_7$	5-HT$_2$, 5-HT$_3$, α-adrenergic, β-adrenergic, dopaminergic, muscarinic, benzodiazepine receptor sites
Sumatriptan	5-HT$_1$	5-HT$_{1A}$, 5-HT$_{5A}$, 5-HT$_7$	5-HT$_{2-4}$, α-adrenergic, β-adrenergic, dopaminergic, muscarinic, benzodiazepine receptor sites
Zolmitriptan	5-HT$_{1D}$, 5-HT$_{1B}$	5-HT$_{1A}$	5-HT$_{2-4}$, α-adrenergic, β-adrenergic, dopaminergic, muscarinic, histaminic receptor sites

The vascular 5-HT$_1$ receptor subtype is present on the human basilar artery and in the vasculature of isolated human dura mater. Current theories on the etiology of migraine headaches suggest that symptoms are caused by local cranial vasodilation or the release of vasoactive and proinflammatory peptides from sensory nerve endings in an activated trigeminal system. The therapeutic activity of the serotonin 5-HT$_1$ receptor agonists in migraine most likely can be attributed to agonist effects at 5-HT$_{1B/1D}$ receptors on the extracerebral, intracranial blood vessels that become dilated during a migraine attack and on nerve terminals in the trigeminal system. Activation of these receptors results in cranial vessel constriction, inhibition of neuropeptide release, and reduced transmission in trigeminal pain pathways.

➤*Pharmacokinetics:*

Pharmacokinetic Parameters of Triptans in Healthy Volunteers and in Patients with Migraine							
Drug	Dose and route of administration	T_{max} (h)	C_{max} (mcg/L)	Bioavailability (%)	t½ (h)	AUC (mcg/L•h)	Plasma protein binding (%)
Almotriptan	12.5 mg PO	2.5	49.5	80	3.1	266	≈ 35
	25 mg PO	2.7	64	69	3.6	443	
Eletriptan	20 mg PO	2	–	≈ 50	≈ 4	–	≈ 85
Frovatriptan	2.5 mg PO	3	4.2/7[a]	29.6	25.7	94	≈ 15
	40 mg PO	5	24.7/53.4[a]	17.5	29.7	881	
Naratriptan	2.5 mg PO	2	12.6	74	5.5	98	≈ 28
Rizatriptan	10 mg PO	1, 1.6 to 2.5[b]	19.8	40	2	50	14
Sumatriptan	6 mg SC	0.17	72	96	2	90	14 to 21
	100 mg PO	1.5	54	14	2	158	
	20 mg NAS	1.5	13	15.8	1.8	48	
	25 mg PR	1.5	27	19.2	1.8	78	
Zolmitriptan	2.5 mg PO	1.5, 3[b]	3.3/3.8[a]	39	2.3/2.6[a]	18/21[a]	≈ 25
	5 mg PO	1.5, 3[b]	10	46	3	42	
	5 mg NAS	3	3.93[c]	102[d]	≈ 3	22.4[c]	

[a] Value for men and women, respectively.
[b] Orally-disintegrating tablets.
[c] Values based on 2.5 mg dose.
[d] Compared with oral tablet.

Renal function impairment – Clearance of **zolmitriptan** was reduced by 25% in patients with severe renal impairment (Ccr approximately 5 to 25 mL/min); no significant change was observed in those with moderate renal impairment.

Clearance of **naratriptan** was reduced by 50% in patients with moderate renal impairment (Ccr 18 to 39 mL/min), resulting in an increase in mean half life from 6 hours (healthy) to 11 hours (range, 7 to 20 hours). The mean C_{max} increased by approximately 40%. The effects of severe renal impairment have not been assessed (see Contraindications and Administration and Dosage).

In hemodialysis patients (Ccr less than 2 mL/min/1.73 m^2), the AUC for **rizatriptan** was approximately 44% greater than that in patients with normal renal function.

The clearance of **almotriptan** was approximately 65% lower in patients with severe renal impairment (Ccr between 10 and 30 mL/min) and approximately 40% lower in patients with moderate renal impairment (Ccr between 31 and 71 mL/min).

Because less than 10% of **frovatriptan** is excreted in urine after an oral dose, it is unlikely that the exposure to frovatriptan will be affected by renal impairment. The pharmacokinetics of frovatriptan following a single oral dose of 2.5 mg was not different in patients with renal impairment (5 males and 6 females, Ccr 16 to 73 mL/min) vs subjects with normal renal function.

Hepatic function impairment – The liver plays an important role in the presystemic clearance of oral 5-HT$_1$ agonists. Accordingly, the bioavailability may be markedly increased in patients with liver disease.

Oral: In a small study of hepatically impaired patients, **sumatriptan** AUC and C_{max} increased by approximately 70%, and T_{max} decreased by 40 minutes.

In severely hepatically impaired patients, the mean C_{max}, T_{max}, and AUC of **zolmitriptan** were increased 1.5-, 2-, and 3-fold, respectively. Seven of 27 patients experienced 20 to 80 mm Hg elevations in systolic or diastolic blood pressure after a 10 mg dose. Administer zolmitriptan with caution in patients with liver disease, generally using doses less than 2.5 mg.

Clearance of **naratriptan** was decreased by 30% in patients with moderate hepatic impairment (Child-Pugh grade A or B). This resulted in an approximately 40% increase in the half life (range, 8 to 16 hours). The effects of severe hepatic impairment (Child-Pugh grade C) have not been assessed (see Contraindications).

Following oral administration in patients with hepatic impairment caused by mild to moderate alcoholic cirrhosis of the liver, plasma concentrations of **rizatriptan** were similar in patients with mild hepatic insufficiency compared with a control group of healthy subjects; plasma concentrations of rizatriptan were approximately 30% greater in patients with moderate hepatic insufficiency.

The pharmacokinetics of **almotriptan** have not been assessed in this population. Based on the mechanisms of almotriptan clearance, the maximum decrease expected because of hepatic impairment would be 60%.

The effects of severe hepatic impairment on **eletriptan** metabolism have not been evaluated. Subjects with mild or moderate hepatic impairment demonstrated an increase in AUC (34%) and half life. C_{max} was increased by 18% (see Contraindications).

Elderly – There is a statistically significant increase in **eletriptan** half life (from approximately 4.4 to 5.7 hours) between elderly (65 to 93 years of age) and younger adult subjects (18 to 45 years of age).

Contraindications

Injectable preparations used IV, because of the potential to cause coronary vasospasm; patients with ischemic heart disease (angina pectoris, history of MI, strokes, transient ischemic attacks [TIAs], or documented silent ischemia); Prinzmetal variant angina or other significant underlying cardiovascular disease (see Warnings); patients with signs or symptoms consistent with ischemic heart disease or coronary artery vasospasm; patients with uncontrolled hypertension; concurrent use of (or use within 24 hours of) ergotamine-containing preparations or ergot-type medications such as dihydroergotamine or methysergide; concurrent monoamine oxidase inhibitor (MAOI) therapy (or within 2 weeks of discontinuing an MAOI [except for **eletriptan**]; see Drug Interactions); within 24 hours of another 5-HT$_1$ agonist; hypersensitivity to the product or any of its ingredients; management of hemiplegic or basilar migraine; ischemic bowel disease.

➤*Naratriptan and sumatriptan:* Cerebrovascular or peripheral vascular syndromes, severe hepatic impairment (Child-Pugh grade C); severe renal impairment (Ccr less than 15 mL/min) (naratriptan only).

➤*Frovatriptan and eletriptan:* Peripheral vascular disease.

➤*Eletriptan:* Severe hepatic impairment.

Warnings

Use 5-HT$_1$ agonists only when a clear diagnosis of migraine has been established.

➤*Risk of myocardial ischemia or MI and other adverse cardiac events:* Because of the potential of this class of compounds to cause coronary vasospasm, do not give these agents to patients with documented ischemic or vasospastic coronary artery disease (see Contraindications). It is strongly recommended that 5-HT$_1$ agonists not be given to patients in whom unrecognized coronary artery disease (CAD) is predicted by the presence of risk factors (eg, hypertension, hypercholesterolemia, smoking, obesity, diabetes, strong family history of CAD, female with surgical or physiological menopause, or male older than 40 years of age) unless a cardiovascular evaluation provides satisfactory clinical evidence that the patient is reasonably free of coronary artery and ischemic myocardial disease or other significant underlying cardiovascular disease. The sensitivity of cardiac diagnostic procedures to detect cardiovascular diseases or predisposition to coronary artery vasospasm is modest at best. If, during the cardiovascular evaluation, the patient's medical history, electrocardiogram (ECG), or other investigations reveal findings indicative of, or consistent with, coronary artery vasospasm or myocardial ischemia, do not administer 5-HT$_1$ agonists (see Contraindications). For patients with risk factors predictive of CAD who are determined to have a satisfactory cardiovascular evaluation, it is strongly recommended that administration of the first dose take place in the setting of a physician's office or similar medically staffed and equipped facility, unless the patient has previously received 5-HT$_1$ agonists. Because cardiac ischemia can occur in the absence of clinical symptoms, consider obtaining an ECG during the interval immediately following the first use in a patient with risk factors.

It is recommended that patients who are intermittent long-term users of 5-HT$_1$ agonists who have or acquire risk factors predictive of CAD, as described above, undergo periodic interval cardiovascular evaluation as they continue use.

The systematic approach described above is intended to reduce the likelihood that patients with unrecognized cardiovascular disease will be inadvertently exposed to 5-HT$_1$ agonists.

Zolmitriptan – There is a report of at least 1 patient experiencing coronary vasospasm without history of cardiac disease and with documented absence of CAD.

Patients with symptomatic Wolff-Parkinson-White syndrome or arrhythmias associated with other cardiac accessory conduction pathway disorders should not receive zolmitriptan.

➤*Cardiac events and fatalities associated with 5-HT$_1$ agonists:* Serious adverse cardiac events, including acute MI, life-threatening disturbances of cardiac rhythm, and death have been reported within a few hours following the administration of 5-HT$_1$ agonists. Considering the extent of use of 5-HT$_1$ agonists in patients with migraine, the incidence of these events is extremely low.

➤*Cerebrovascular events and fatalities with 5-HT$_1$ agonists:* Cerebral hemorrhage, subarachnoid hemorrhage, stroke, and other cerebrovascular events have been reported in patients treated with 5-HT$_1$ agonists, and some have resulted in fatalities. In a number of cases, it appears possible that the cerebrovascular events were primary, the agonist having been administered in the incorrect belief that the symptoms experienced were a consequence of migraine, when they were not. It should be noted that patients with migraine may be at increased risk of certain cerebrovascular events (eg, stroke, hemorrhage, TIA).

➤*Other vasospasm-related events:* 5-HT$_1$ agonists may cause vasospastic reactions other than coronary artery vasospasm. Peripheral vascular ischemia and colonic ischemia with abdominal pain and bloody diarrhea have been reported with 5-HT$_1$ agonists.

➤*Increases in blood pressure:* Significant elevations in systemic blood pressure, including hypertensive crisis, have been reported on rare occasions in patients with and without a history of hypertension treated with 5-HT$_1$ agonists. 5-HT$_1$ agonists are contraindicated in patients with uncontrolled hypertension.

➤*Local irritation:* Approximately 5% of patients noted irritation in the nose and throat after using **sumatriptan** nasal spray. Irritative symptoms such as burning, numbness, paresthesia, discharge, and pain or soreness were noted to be severe in approximately 1% of patients treated. The symptoms were transient and, in approximately 60% of the cases, resolved in less than 2 hours. Limited examinations of the nose and throat did not reveal any clinically noticeable injury in these patients. Adverse events of any kind perceived in the nasopharynx were severe in approximately 1% of patients, and approximately 60% resolved in 1 hour. Nasopharyngeal examinations failed to demonstrate any clinically significant changes with repeated use of sumatriptan nasal spray.

➤*CYP3A4 inhibitors:* In vitro studies have shown that **eletriptan** is metabolized by the CYP3A4 enzyme. A clinical study has shown that coadministration of eletriptan with ketoconazole, erythromycin, verapamil, and fluconazole increased the C_{max} and AUC of eletriptan 3- and 6-fold, 2- and 4-fold, 2- and 3-fold, and 1.4- and 2-fold, respectively. Do not use eletriptan within 72 hours of taking drugs that have demonstrated potent CYP3A4 inhibition.

➤*Hypersensitivity reactions:* Hypersensitivity reactions have occurred on rare occasions, and severe anaphylaxis/anaphylactoid reactions have occurred. Such reactions can be life-threatening or fatal. Refer to Management of Acute Hypersensitivity Reactions.

➤*Renal function impairment:* Use **rizatriptan** and **sumatriptan** with caution in dialysis patients because of a decrease in the clearance (see Pharmacokinetics). After **eletriptan** administration, there was no significant change in clearance observed in subjects with mild, moderate, or severe renal impairment, although blood pressure elevations were observed in this population.

➤*Hepatic function impairment:* Administer with caution to patients with diseases that may alter the absorption, metabolism, or excretion of drugs. The liver plays an important role in the presystemic clearance of oral 5-HT$_1$ agonists. Accordingly, the bioavailability may be markedly increased in patients with liver disease (see Pharmacokinetics). No dosage adjustment is necessary when **frovatriptan** or **eletriptan** is given to patients with mild to moderate hepatic impairment. Do not use eletriptan in severe hepatic impairment.

➤*Carcinogenesis:* Thyroid follicular cell hyperplasia and thyroid follicular cell adenomas have been observed in rats receiving no more than 400 mg/kg/day **zolmitriptan** for approximately 104 weeks and 90 mg/kg/day **naratriptan** for 13 weeks. An increased incidence of benign c-cell adenomas in the thyroid also was observed in naratriptan animal studies. The lifetime carcinogenic potential of **rizatriptan** was evaluated in a 100-week study in mice and a 106-week study in rats at oral gavage doses up to 125 mg/kg/day. Exposure data were not obtained, but plasma AUCs of parent drug measured in other studies after 5 and 21 weeks of oral dosing in mice and rats, respectively, indicate that the exposures to parent drug at the highest dose level would have been approximately 150 times (mice) and 240 times (rats) the average AUCs measured in humans after three 10 mg doses, the maximum recommended daily dose (MRDD). There was no evidence of an increase in tumor incidence related to rizatriptan in either species.

In a rat study, there was a statistically significant increase in the incidence of pituitary adenomas in males only at 85 mg/kg/day **frovatriptan**, a dose that produced 250 times the exposure achieved at the maximum recommended human dose (MRHD) based on AUC comparisons. In the 26-week transgenic mouse study, there was an increased incidence of subcutaneous sarcomas in females dosed at 200 and 400 mg/kg/day, or 390 and 630 times the human exposure based on AUC comparisons.

In rats, the incidence of testicular interstitial cell adenomas was increased at the high dose of 75 mg/kg/day **eletriptan**. The estimated exposure (AUC) to parent drug at that dose was approximately 6 times that achieved in humans receiving the MRDD of 80 mg. In mice, the incidence of hepatocellular adenomas was increased at the high dose of 400 mg/kg/day eletriptan. The exposure to parent drug (AUC) at that dose was approximately 18 times that achieved in humans receiving the MRDD of 80 mg.

➤*Fertility impairment:* A treatment-related decrease in fertility secondary to a decrease in mating in animals treated with 50 and 500 mg/kg/day **sumatriptan** was observed. A treatment-related decrease in the number of females exhibiting normal estrous cycles at doses of **naratriptan** 170 mg/kg/day or greater and an increase in preimplantation loss at 60 mg/kg/day or greater was observed. Testicular/epididymal atrophy in high-dose male rats accompanied by spermatozoa depletion reduced mating success and may have contributed to the observed preimplantation loss. In a fertility study in rats, altered estrous cyclicity and delays in time to mating were observed in females treated orally with 100 mg/kg/day **rizatriptan**. Plasma drug exposure (AUC) at this dose was approximately 225 times the exposure in humans receiving the MRDD of 30 mg. The no-effect dose was 10 mg/kg/day (approximately 15 times the human exposure at the MRDD). Male and female rats were dosed with **frovatriptan** prior to and during mating and up to implantation at doses of 100, 500, and 1000 mg/kg/day (equivalent to approximately 130, 650, and 1300 times the MRHD on a mg/m^2 basis). At all dose levels there was an increase in the number of females that mated on the first day of pairing compared with control animals. This occurred in conjunction with a prolongation of the estrous cycle. In addition, females had a decreased mean number of corpora lutea and consequently a lower number of live fetuses per litter, which suggested a partial impairment of ovulation. There were no other fertility-related effects. In a rat fertility and early embryonic development study, there was a prolongation of the estrous cycle at the 200 mg/kg/day **eletriptan** dose because of an increase in duration of estrus. There also were dose-related, statistically significant decreases in mean numbers of corpora lutea per dam at all 3 doses, resulting in decreases in mean numbers of implants and viable fetuses per dam. This suggests a partial inhibition of ovulation by eletriptan. Prolongation of the estrous cycle was observed at a dose of 100 mg/kg/day for **almotriptan**.

➤*Elderly:* Pharmacokinetic disposition of 5-HT$_1$ agonists in the elderly is similar to that seen in younger adults.

The risk of adverse reactions to **naratriptan** and **sumatriptan** may be greater in elderly patients who have reduced renal function and who are more likely to have decreased hepatic function; they are at higher risk for CAD, and blood pressure increases may be more pronounced. Therefore, the use of naratriptan and sumatriptan in elderly patients is not recommended.

Dose selection of **almotriptan** for an elderly patient should be cautious, usually starting at the low end of the dosing range, reflecting the greater frequency of decreased hepatic, renal, or cardiac function, and of concomitant disease or other drug therapy. The recommended dose for elderly patients with normal renal function for their age is the same as that recommended for younger adults.

Mean blood concentrations of **frovatriptan** in elderly subjects were 1.5 to 2 times higher than those seen in younger adults. Because migraine occurs infrequently in the elderly, clinical experience with frovatriptan is limited to such patients.

Eletriptan has been given to only 50 patients older than 65 years of age. Blood pressure was increased to a greater extent in elderly subjects than in younger subjects. There is no information about the safety and efficacy of zolmitriptan in this population because patients older than 65 years of age were excluded from the controlled clinical trials.

➤*Pregnancy:* *Category C.* In rats and rabbits, 5-HT$_1$ agonist administration is associated with embryolethality, fetal abnormalities, and pup mortality. There are no adequate and well-controlled studies in pregnant women. Use during pregnancy only if the potential benefit justifies the potential risk to the fetus.

In reproductive toxicity studies in rats and rabbits, oral administration of **eletriptan** was associated with developmental toxicity (decreased fetal and pup weights and an increased incidence of fetal structural abnormalities). Effects on fetal and pup weights were observed at doses that were 6 to 12 times greater than the clinical MRDD of 80 mg.

When pregnant rats were administered **frovatriptan** during the period of organogenesis at oral doses of 100, 500, and 1000 mg/kg/day (equivalent to

130, 650, and 1300 times the MRHD on a mg/m^2 basis), there were dose-related increases in incidences of both litters and total numbers of fetuses with dilated ureters, unilateral and bilateral pelvic cavitation, hydronephrosis, and hydroureters.

The manufacturer maintains a **sumatriptan** and **naratriptan** pregnancy registry. Register patients by calling (800) 336-2176.

➤*Lactation:* **Sumatriptan** and **eletriptan** are excreted in human breast milk. In one study of 8 women given a single 80 mg dose of eletriptan, the mean total amount in breast milk over 24 hours was approximately 0.02% of the administered dose. The resulting eletriptan concentration-time profile was similar to that seen in the plasma over 24 hours, with very low concentrations of drug (mean, 1.7 ng/mL) still present in the milk 18 to 24 hours postdose. Lactating rats dosed with **zolmitriptan** had milk levels equivalent to maternal plasma levels at 1 hour and 4 times higher than plasma levels at 4 hours. **Naratriptan**-related material is excreted in the milk of rats. **Rizatriptan** is extensively excreted in rat milk, at a level of 5-fold or greater than maternal plasma levels. Lactating rats dosed with **almotriptan** had milk levels equivalent to maternal plasma levels at 0.5 hours and 7 times higher than plasma levels at 6 hours after dosing. **Frovatriptan** and its metabolites are excreted in the milk of lactating rats with the maximum concentration being 4-fold higher than that seen in blood. Exercise caution when administering to a nursing woman.

➤*Children:* Safety and efficacy have not been established.

Clinical trials have evaluated 25 to 100 mg oral **sumatriptan** in 701 pediatric patients, 0.25 to 2.5 mg **naratriptan** in 300 adolescents 12 to 17 years of age, and 40 mg **eletriptan** in 274 adolescents 11 to 17 years of age. These studies did not establish efficacy. Adverse events observed in these clinical trials were similar in nature to those reported in clinical trials in adults. The frequency of all adverse events in sumatriptan patients appeared to be dose- and age-dependent, with younger patients reporting events more commonly than older adolescents.

The use of 5-HT_1 receptor agonists is not recommended in patients younger than 18 years of age.

Precautions

➤*Chest, jaw, or neck tightness:* Chest, jaw, or neck tightness have occurred after 5-HT_1 agonist administration, and atypical sensations over the precordium (pain, tightness, pressure, heaviness) have occurred, but these rarely have been associated with arrhythmias or ischemic ECG changes. Evaluate patients who experience signs or symptoms suggestive of angina for the presence of CAD or a predisposition to Prinzmetal variant angina before receiving additional doses. Monitor ECG if dosing is resumed and similar symptoms recur.

Similarly, patients who experience other symptoms or signs suggestive of decreased arterial flow, such as ischemic bowel syndrome or Raynaud syndrome, following the use of any 5-HT_1 agonist are candidates for further evaluation.

➤*Seizures:* There have been rare reports of seizures following **sumatriptan** use.

➤*Ophthalmic effects:*

Binding to melanin-containing tissues – Because 5-HT_1 agonists bind to melanin, accumulation in melanin-rich tissues (eg, the eye) could occur over time, raising the possibility of toxicity in these tissues after extended use. Be aware of the possibility of long-term ophthalmologic effects.

Corneal effects – **Sumatriptan**, **naratriptan**, and **almotriptan** cause corneal opacities and defects in dogs; naratriptan also caused transient changes in precorneal tear film. These changes may occur in humans. **Eletriptan** caused transient corneal opacities in dogs receiving 5 mg/kg and above.

➤*Phenylketonurics:* Inform phenylketonuric patients that **rizatriptan** and **zolmitriptan** orally-disintegrating tablets contain phenylalanine (a component of aspartame). Each 5 mg rizatriptan orally-disintegrating tablet contains 1.05 mg phenylalanine, and each 10 mg orally-disintegrating tablet contains 2.1 mg phenylalanine. Each 2.5 mg zolmitriptan orally-disintegrating tablet contains 2.81 mg phenylalanine.

➤*Photosensitivity:* Photosensitization (photoallergy or phototoxicity) may occur; therefore, caution patients to take protective measures (ie, sunscreens, protective clothing) against exposure to sunlight or ultraviolet light (eg, tanning beds) until tolerance is determined.

Drug Interactions

Serotonin 5-HT_1 Receptor Agonist Drug Interactions

Precipitant drug	Object drug*		Description
Cimetidine	Zolmitriptan	↑	Following coadministration with cimetidine, the half life and AUC of a 5 mg dose of zolmitriptan and its active metabolite were approximately doubled.
Ergot alkaloids (dihydroergotamine, methysergide)	5-HT_1 agonists	↑↓	The risk of vasospastic reactions may be increased. Use of 5-HT_1 agonists within 24 hours of treatment with an ergot-containing medication is contraindicated. The AUC and C_{max} of frovatriptan (2 × 2.5 mg dose) were reduced by ≈ 25% when coadministered with ergotamine tartrate.
Potent CYP3A4 inhibitors (eg, ketoconazole, itraconazole, nefazodone, troleandomycin, clarithromycin, ritonavir, nelfinavir)	Almotriptan Eletriptan	↑	Coadministration of almotriptan and ketoconazole (400 mg/day for 3 days) resulted in an ≈ 60% increase in AUC and maximal plasma concentration of almotriptan. The AUC and C_{max} of eletriptan are increased with coadministration. Do not use eletriptan within 72 hours of treatment with a potent CYP3A4 inhibitor (see Warnings).
5-HT_1 agonists	5-HT_1 agonists	↑	The risk of vasospastic reactions may be increased. Coadministration of two 5-HT_1 agonists within 24 hours of each other is contraindicated.
MAOIs	Almotriptan Rizatriptan Sumatriptan Zolmitriptan	↑	Use of certain 5-HT_1 agonists concomitantly with or within 2 weeks following the discontinuation of an MAOI is contraindicated. If it is necessary to use such agents together, naratriptan, eletriptan, and frovatriptan appear to be less likely to interact with MAOIs.
Oral contraceptives	Frovatriptan	↑	Mean C_{max} and AUC of frovatriptan are 30% higher in those subjects taking oral contraceptives compared with those not taking oral contraceptives.
Propranolol	Zolmitriptan	↔	C_{max} and AUC of zolmitriptan increased 1.5-fold but decreased for the N-desmethyl metabolite by 30% and 15%, respectively. No effects on blood pressure or pulse rate were observed.
	Rizatriptan	↑	In a study of coadministration of 240 mg/day propranolol and a single dose of 10 mg rizatriptan in healthy subjects, mean plasma AUC for rizatriptan was increased by 70% during propranolol administration, and a 4-fold increase was observed in 1 subject.
	Frovatriptan	↑	Propranolol increased the AUC of 2.5 mg frovatriptan in males by 60% and in females by 29%. The C_{max} of frovatriptan was increased 23% in males and 16% in females in the presence of propranolol.
	Eletriptan	↑	C_{max} and AUC of eletriptan were increased by 10% and 33%, respectively, in the presence of propranolol. No interactive increases in blood pressure were observed.
Sibutramine	Naratriptan Rizatriptan Sumatriptan Zolmitriptan	↑	A "serotonin syndrome," including CNS irritability, motor weakness, shivering, myoclonus, and altered consciousness may occur. Coadministration is not recommended. Monitor the patient for adverse effects if concurrent use cannot be avoided.
Almotriptan Frovatriptan Naratriptan Rizatriptan Sumatriptan Zolmitriptan	SSRIs Fluoxetine Fluvoxamine Paroxetine Sertraline	↑	There have been rare reports of weakness, hyperreflexia, and incoordination with combined use of SSRIs. If concomitant treatment is clinically warranted, observe the patient carefully. No interaction was observed when rizatriptan was administered with paroxetine. Fluoxetine had no effect on almotriptan clearance, but C_{max} increased 18%.

* ↑ = Object drug increased. ↓ = Object drug decreased. ↔ = Undetermined clinical effect.

➤*Drug/Food interactions:* Food has no significant effect on oral 5-HT$_1$ agonist bioavailability, but delays **sumatriptan's** T_{max} by approximately 30 minutes and **rizatriptan's** time to reach peak concentration by 1 hour. AUC and C_{max} of **eletriptan** are increased approximately 20% to 30% following oral administration with a high-fat meal.

Adverse Reactions

Serious coronary artery vasospasm, transient myocardial ischemia, ventricular fibrillation/tachycardia, and MI have been associated with 5-HT$_1$ agonists.

Oral – These agents are generally well tolerated. Across all doses, most adverse reactions were mild and transient and did not lead to long-lasting effects. In patients being treated for multiple migraine attacks for 1 year or less with **naratriptan**, **zolmitriptan**, **eletriptan**, or **frovatriptan**, 3.6%, 8%, 8.3%, and 5% withdrew from the trial because of adverse experiences, respectively. The most common events were asthenia, dizziness, nausea, paresthesia, fatigue, pain, chest or neck tightness or heaviness, somnolence, warm sensation, dry mouth, headache, flushing, hot or cold sensation, and chest pain.

Frovatriptan: Frovatriptan is generally well tolerated. The incidence of adverse events in clinical trials did not increase when up to 3 doses were used within 24 hours. The majority of adverse events were mild or moderate and transient. The incidence of adverse events in 4 placebo-controlled clinical trials was not affected by gender, age, or concomitant medications commonly used by migraine patients. There were insufficient data to assess the impact of race on the incidence of adverse events.

Oral 5-HT$_1$ Agonist Adverse Reactions (%)[a]

	Almotriptan		Eletriptan			Frovatriptan	Naratriptan		Rizatriptan		Sumatriptan			Zolmitriptan		
Adverse reaction	6.25 mg (n = 527)	12.5 mg (n = 1313)	20 mg (n = 431)	40 mg (n = 1774)	80 mg (n = 1932)	2.5 mg (n = 1554)	1 mg (n = 627)	2.5 mg (n = 627)	5 mg (n = 977)	10 mg (n = 1167)	25 mg (n = 417)	50 mg (n = 771)	100 mg (n = 437)	1 mg (n = 163)	2.5 mg (n = 498)	5 mg (n = 1012)
Atypical sensations																
Hot/Cold sensation	—	—	—	—	—	3	—	—	—	—	—	—	—	—	—	—
Hypesthesia	—	—	—	—	—	—	—	—	—	—	—	—	—	1	1	2
Miscellaneous sensations	—	—	—	—	—	—	2	4	4	5	—	—	—	—	—	—
Paresthesia	1	1	3	3	4	4	1	2	3	4	3	5	3	5	7	9
Warm/Cold sensation	—	—	—	—	—	—	—	—	—	—	3	2	3	—	—	—
Warm/Hot sensation	—	—	2	2	2	—	—	—	—	—	—	—	—	6	5	7
CNS																
Asthenia	—	—	4	5	10	—	—	—	—	—	—	—	—	5	3	9
Dizziness	—	—	3	6	7	8	1	2	4	9	> 1	> 1	> 1	6	8	10
Drowsiness	—	—	—	—	—	—	1	2	—	—	> 1	> 1	> 1	—	—	—
Fatigue	—	—	—	—	—	5	2	2	4	7	2	2	3	—	—	—
Headache	—	—	4	3	4	4	—	—	< 2	2	> 1	> 1	> 1	—	—	—
Myasthenia	—	—	—	—	—	—	—	—	—	—	—	—	—	0	1	2
Somnolence	—	—	3	6	7	—	—	—	4	8	—	—	—	5	6	8
Vertigo	—	—	—	—	—	—	—	—	—	—	< 1	< 1	2	0	0	2
Miscellaneous CNS effects	—	—	—	—	—	—	4	7	—	—	—	—	—	—	—	—
GI																
Abdominal pain/discomfort/stomach pain/cramps/pressure	—	—	1	2	2	—	—	—	—	—	—	—	—	—	—	—
Dry mouth	1	1	2	3	4	3	—	—	3	3	> 1	> 1	> 1	5	3	3
Dyspepsia	—	—	1	2	2	2	—	—	—	—	—	—	—	3	2	1
Dysphagia (including throat tightness/difficulty swallowing)	—	—	1	2	2	—	—	—	—	—	—	—	—	0	0	2
Nausea	4	5	4	6	—	—	—	4	9	6	1	2	—	4	5	8
Pain/Pressure sensations																
Chest tightness pressure, and/or heaviness	—	—	1	2	4	2	—	—	< 2	3	1	2	2	2	3	4
Heaviness	—	—	—	—	—	—	—	—	—	—	< 1	< 1	2	1	2	5
Neck/Throat/Jaw	—	—	—	—	—	—	1	2	< 2	2	< 1	2	3	4	7	10
Pain, location specified/unspecified	—	—	—	—	—	—	—	—	6	9	2	1	1	2	2	3
Pressure	—	—	—	—	—	—	—	—	—	—	< 1	2	2	—	—	—
Regional pain	—	—	—	—	—	—	—	—	< 1	2	—	—	—	—	—	—
Tightness	—	—	—	—	—	—	—	—	—	—	< 1	2	2	—	—	—
Skeletal		—	—	—	—	3	—	—	—	—	—	—	—	—	—	—
Other	2	4	3	3	1	1	3	2	2	3	—	—	—	—	—	—
Miscellaneous																
Flushing	—	—	2	2	2	4	—	—	—	—	—	—	—	—	—	—
Myalgia	—	—	—	—	—	—	—	—	—	—	—	—	—	1	1	2
Other	—	—	—	—	—	—	6	7	—	—	—	—	—	—	—	—
Palpitations	—	—	—	—	—	—	—	—	—	—	> 1	> 1	> 1	0	< 1	2
Sweating	—	—	—	—	—	—	—	—	—	—	—	—	—	0	2	3

[a] Data are pooled from separate studies and are not necessarily comparable.

Other adverse reactions include the following:

➤*Almotriptan:*

Cardiovascular – Palpitations, tachycardia, vasodilation (0.1% to 1%); hypertension, syncope (less than 0.1%).

CNS – Dizziness, somnolence (1% or more); anxiety, CNS stimulation, hypesthesia, insomnia, restlessness, shakiness, tremor, vertigo (0.1% to 1%); abnormal coordination, change in dreams, depressive symptoms, euphoria, hyperreflexia, hypertonia, impaired concentration, nervousness, neuropathy, nightmares (less than 0.1%).

Dermatologic – Dermatitis, diaphoresis, erythema, pruritus, rash (0.1% to 1%); photosensitivity reaction (less than 0.1%).

GI – Diarrhea, dyspepsia, vomiting (0.1% to 1%); abdominal cramp or pain, colitis, esophageal reflux, gastritis, gastroenteritis, increased salivation, increased thirst (less than 0.1%).

Metabolic – Hyperglycemia, increased serum CPK (0.1% to 1%); hypercholesterolemia, increased GGT (less than 0.1%).

Musculoskeletal – Muscular weakness, myalgia (0.1% to 1%); arthralgia, arthritis, myopathy (less than 0.1%).

Respiratory – Bronchitis, dyspnea, epistaxis, laryngismus, pharyngitis, rhinitis, sinusitis (0.1% to 1%); hyperventilation, laryngitis, sneezing (less than 0.1%).

Special senses – Conjunctivitis, ear pain, eye irritation, hyperacusis, taste alteration (0.1% to 1%); diplopia, dry eyes, eye pain, nystagmus, otitis media, parosmia, scotoma, tinnitus (less than 0.1%).

Miscellaneous – Headache (1% or more); asthenia, back pain, chest pain, chills, dysmenorrhea, fatigue, neck pain, rigid neck (0.1% to 1%); fever (less than 0.1%).

➤*Eletriptan:*

Cardiovascular – Palpitation (1% or more); hypertension, migraine, peripheral vascular disorder, tachycardia (0.1% to 1%); angina pectoris, arrhythmia, atrial fibrillation, AV block, bradycardia, cerebrovascular disorder, hypotension, syncope, thrombophlebitis, vasospasm, ventricular arrhythmia (less than 0.1%).

CNS – Hypertonia, hypesthesia, vertigo (1% or more); abnormal dreams, agitation, anxiety, apathy, ataxia, confusion, depersonalization, depression, emotional lability, euphoria, hyperesthesia, hyperkinesia, incoordination, insomnia, nervousness, speech disorder, stupor, thinking abnormal, tremor (0.1% to 1%); abnormal gait, amnesia, aphasia, catatonic reaction, dementia, diplopia, dystonia, hallucinations, hemiplegia, hyperalgesia, hypokinesia, hysteria, manic reaction, neuropathy, neurosis, oculogyric crisis, paralysis, psychotic depression, sleep disorder, twitching (less than 0.1%).

Dermatologic – Sweating (1% or more); pruritus, rash, skin disorder (0.1% to 1%); alopecia, dry skin, eczema, exfoliative dermatitis, maculopapular rash, psoriasis, skin discoloration, skin hypertrophy, urticaria (less than 0.1%).

Endocrine – Goiter, thyroid adenoma, thyroiditis (less than 0.1%).

GI – Anorexia, constipation, diarrhea, eructation, esophagitis, flatulence, gastritis, GI disorder, glossitis, increased salivation, liver function tests abnormal (0.1% to 1%); gingivitis, hematemesis, increased appetite, rectal disorder, stomatitis, tongue disorder, tongue edema, tooth disorder (less than 0.1%).

GU – Impotence, polyuria, urinary frequency, urinary tract disorder (0.1% to 1%); breast pain, kidney pain, leukorrhea, menorrhagia, menstrual disorder, vaginitis (less than 0.1%).

Hematologic/Lymphatic – Anemia, cyanosis, leukopenia, lymphadenopathy, monocytosis, purpura (less than 0.1%).

Metabolic – CPK increased, edema, peripheral edema, thirst (0.1% to 1%); alkaline phosphatase increased, bilirubinemia, hyperglycemia, weight gain, weight loss (less than 0.1%).

Musculoskeletal – Arthralgia, arthritis, arthrosis, bone pain, myalgia, myasthenia (0.1% to 1%); bone neoplasm, joint disorder, myopathy, tenosynovitis (less than 0.1%).

Respiratory – Pharyngitis (1% or more); asthma, dyspnea, respiratory disorder, respiratory tract infection, rhinitis, voice alteration, yawn (0.1% to 1%); bronchitis, choking sensation, cough increased, epistaxis, hiccough, hyperventilation, laryngitis, sinusitis, sputum increased (less than 0.1%).

Special senses – Abnormal vision, conjunctivitis, ear pain, eye pain, lacrimation disorder, photophobia, taste perversion, tinnitus (0.1% to 1%); abnormality of accommodation, dry eyes, ear disorder, eye hemorrhage, otitis media, parosmia, ptosis (less than 0.1%).

Miscellaneous – Back pain, chills, pain (1% or more); face edema, malaise (0.1% to 1%); abdomen enlarged, abscess, accidental injury, allergic reaction, fever, flu syndrome, halitosis, hernia, hypothermia, lab test abnormal, moniliasis, rheumatoid arthritis, shock (less than 0.1%).

➤*Frovatriptan:*

Cardiovascular – Palpitation (1% or more); abnormal ECG, tachycardia (0.1% to 1%); bradycardia (less than 0.1%).

CNS – Anxiety, dysesthesia, hypesthesia, insomnia (1% or more); abnormal gait, agitation, amnesia, asthenia, ataxia, confusion, depersonalization, depression, emotional lability, euphoria, hyperesthesia, impaired concentration, involuntary muscle contractions, migraine aggravated, nervousness, rigors, speech disorder, thinking abnormal, tremor, vertigo (0.1% to 1%); abnormal dreaming, abnormal reflexes, depression aggravated, hypertonia, hypotonia, personality disorder, tongue paralysis (less than 0.1%).

Dermatologic – Sweating increased (1% or more); bullous eruption, pruritus (0.1% to 1%).

GI – Abdominal pain, diarrhea, vomiting (1% or more); anorexia, constipation, dysphagia, esophagospasm, flatulence, saliva increased (0.1% to 1%); change in bowel habits, cheilitis, eructation, gastroesophageal reflux, hiccough, peptic ulcer, salivary gland pain, stomatitis, toothache (less than 0.1%).

GU – Micturition frequency, polyuria (0.1% to 1%); abnormal urine, nocturia, renal pain (less than 0.1%).

Hematologic – Epistaxis (0.1% to 1%); purpura (less than 0.1%).

Metabolic/Nutritional – Dehydration, thirst (0.1% to 1%); hypocalcemia, hypoglycemia (less than 0.1%).

Musculoskeletal – Arthralgia, arthrosis, back pain, leg cramps, muscle weakness, myalgia (0.1% to 1%).

Respiratory – Rhinitis, sinusitis (1% or more); pharyngitis, dyspnea, hyperventilation, laryngitis (0.1% to 1%).

Special senses – Tinnitus, vision abnormal (1% or more); abnormal lacrimation, conjunctivitis, earache, eye pain, hyperacusis, taste perversion (0.1% to 1%).

Miscellaneous – Pain (1% or more); fever, hot flushes, malaise, (0.1% to 1%); feeling of relaxation, leg pain, mouth edema, syncope (less than 0.1%).

➤*Naratriptan:*

Atypical sensations – Warm/cold temperature sensations (1% or more); strange feeling and burning/stinging sensation (0.1% to 1%).

Cardiovascular – Abnormal ECG (PR prolongation, QT prolongation, ST/T wave abnormalities, premature ventricular contractions, atrial flutter/fibrillation), increased blood pressure, palpitations, syncope, tachyarrhythmias (0.1% to 1%); bradycardia, heart murmurs, hypotension, varicosities (less than 0.1%).

CNS – Vertigo (1% or more); anxiety, cognitive function disorders, depressive disorders, detachment, equilibrium disorders, sleep disorders, tremors (0.1% to 1%); aggression, agitation, compressed nerve syndromes, confusion, convulsions, coordination disorders, decreased consciousness, dreams, hallucinations, hostility, hyperactivity, hyperesthesia, hypesthesia, motor retardation, muscle twitching/fasciculation, neuralgia, neuritis, panic, paralysis of cranial nerves, psychomotor restlessness, sedation (less than 0.1%).

Dermatologic – Pruritus, skin rashes, sweating, urticaria (0.1% to 1%); acne, allergic skin reactions, dermatitis/dermatosis, folliculitis, hair loss, macular skin/rashes, photodermatitis, photosensitivity, pruritic skin rashes, skin erythema, skin flakiness/dryness (less than 0.1%).

GI – Hyposalivation, vomiting (1% or more); constipation, diarrhea, discomfort/pain, dyspeptic symptoms, gastroenteritis (0.1% to 1%); abnormal bilirubin levels, abnormal liver function tests, altered sense of taste, esophagitis, gastric ulcers, gastritis, hemorrhoids, oral itching and irritation, regurgitation and reflux, salivary gland inflammation (less than 0.1%).

GU – Bladder inflammation, diuresis, polyuria (0.1% to 1%); breast discharge, breast inflammation, decreased libido, endometrium disorders, fallopian tube inflammation, lumps in breast, lumps in female reproductive tract, pyelitis, urinary incontinence, urinary tract hemorrhage, urinary urgency, vaginal inflammation (less than 0.1%).

Hematologic – Increased white cells (0.1% to 1%); anemia, purpura, quantitative red cell or hemoglobin defects, thrombocytopenia (less than 0.1%).

Metabolic/Nutritional – Dehydration, fluid retention, polydipsia, thirst (0.1% to 1%); glycosuria, hypercholesterolemia, hyperglycemia, hyperlipidemia, hypothyroidism, ketonuria, parathyroid neoplasm (less than 0.1%).

Musculoskeletal – Pressure/tightness/heaviness sensations (1% or more); arthralgia, articular rheumatism, joint/muscle stiffness, muscle cramps/spasms, muscle pain, rigidity, tightness (0.1% to 1%); bone/skeletal pain (less than 0.1%).

Respiratory – Bronchitis, cough, pneumonia (0.1% to 1%); airway obstruction/constriction, asthma, pleuritis, tracheitis (less than 0.1%).

Special senses – Photophobia (1% or more); blurred vision (0.1% to 1%); aphasia, difficulty focusing, dry eyes, eye hemorrhage, eye pain/discomfort, scotoma, sensation of eye pressure, (less than 0.1%).

Ear, nose, and throat: Ear, nose, and throat infections (1% or more); phonophobia, sinusitis, tinnitus, upper respiratory tract inflammation (0.1% to 1%); allergic rhinitis, ear/nose/throat hemorrhage, hearing difficulty, labyrinthitis (less than 0.1%).

Miscellaneous – Allergic reactions, allergies, chills, descriptions of odor or taste, edema, fever, swelling (0.1% to 1%); mobility disorders, spasms (less than 0.1%).

Postmarketing reports: These events do not include those already listed in the adverse reactions section above. Because the reports cite events reported spontaneously from worldwide postmarketing experience, frequency of events and the role of naratriptan in their causation cannot be reliably determined.

- *Cardiovascular* – Angina, MI.
- *CNS* – Cerebral vascular accident, including transient ischemic attack, subarachnoid hemorrhage, and cerebral infarction.
- *Miscellaneous* – Dyspnea, hypersensitivity including anaphylaxis/anaphylactoid reactions, in some cases severe (eg, circulatory collapse).

➤*Rizatriptan:*

Cardiovascular – Palpitation (1% or more); arrhythmia, bradycardia, cold extremities, hypertension, tachycardia (0.1% to 1%); angina pectoris (less than 0.1%).

CNS – Euphoria, hypesthesia, mental acuity decreased, tremor (1% or more); agitation, anxiety, ataxia, confusion, depression, disorientation, dream abnormality, dysarthria, gait abnormality, hyperesthesia, insomnia, irritability, memory impairment, nervousness, vertigo (0.1% to 1%); akinesia/bradykinesia, apprehension, depersonalization, dysesthesia, hyperkinesia, hypersomnia, hyporeflexia (less than 0.1%).

Dermatologic – Flushing (1% or more); pruritus, rash, sweating, urticaria (0.1% to 1%); acne, erythema, photosensitivity (less than 0.1%).

GI – Diarrhea, vomiting (1% or more); acid regurgitation, constipation, dyspepsia, dysphagia, flatulence, thirst, tongue edema (0.1% to 1%); anorexia, appetite increased, eructation, gastritis, paralysis (tongue) (less than 0.1%).

GU – Hot flashes (1% or more); menstruation disorder, polyuria, urinary frequency (0.1% to 1%); dysuria (less than 0.1%).

Musculoskeletal – Arthralgia, muscle cramp, muscle spasm, muscle weakness, musculoskeletal pain, myalgia, stiffness (0.1% to 1%).

Respiratory – Dyspnea (1% or more); congestion (nasal), dry nose, dry throat, epistaxis, irritation (nasal), pharyngitis, respiratory congestion (nasal), sinus disorder, upper respiratory tract infection, yawning (0.1% to 1%); cough, hiccough, hoarseness, pharyngeal edema, rhinorrhea, sneezing, tachypnea (less than 0.1%).

Special senses – Blurred vision, burning eye, dry eyes, ear pain, eye irritation, eye pain, tearing, tinnitus (0.1% to 1%); eye swelling, hyperacusis, itching eye, photophobia, photopsia, smell perversion (less than 0.1%).

Miscellaneous – Warm/cold sensations (1% or more); abdominal distention, chills, dehydration, facial edema, hangover effect, heat sensitivity (0.1% to 1%); edema/swelling, fever, orthostatic effects, syncope (less than 0.1%).

Postmarketing reports: The following additional adverse reactions have been reported very rarely and most have been reported in patients with risk factors predictive of CAD: Cerebrovascular accident; MI; myocardial ischemia. The following also have been reported: Dysgeusia; toxic epidermal necrolysis.

➤*Sumatriptan:*

Sumatriptan Adverse Reactions (%)			
Adverse reaction	Tablets	Nasal	Injection
Atypical sensations			
Burning sensation	> 1	0.1 to 1	—
Cold sensation	—	0.1 to 1	—
Dysesthesia	< 0.1	< 0.1	< 0.1
Feeling of heaviness	—	0.1 to 1	—
Feeling strange	—	0.1 to 1	—
Numbness	> 1	0.1 to 1	—
Paresthesia	—	0.1 to 1	0.1 to 1
Pressure sensation	—	0.1 to 1	—
Prickling sensation	—	< 0.1	0.1 to 1
Simultaneous hot/cold sensation	—	—	< 0.1
Stinging sensations	—	—	0.1 to 1
Tickling sensations	—	—	< 0.1
Tight feeling in head	0.1 to 1	0.1 to 1	—
Tingling	—	0.1 to 1	—
Cardiovascular			
Abdominal aortic aneurysm	—	< 0.1	—
Abnormal pulse	—	—	< 0.1
Angina	< 0.1	—	—
Arrhythmia	0.1 to 1	0.1 to 1	0.1 to 1
Atherosclerosis	< 0.1	—	—
Bradycardia	< 0.1	< 0.1	0.1 to 1
Cerebral ischemia	< 0.1	—	—
Cerebrovascular lesion	< 0.1	—	—
ECG changes	0.1 to 1	0.1 to 1	0.1 to 1
Flushing	—	0.1 to 1	—
Heart block	< 0.1	—	—
Hypertension	> 1	0.1 to 1	0.1 to 1
Hypotension	> 1	< 0.1	0.1 to 1
Pallor	0.1 to 1	< 0.1	< 0.1
Palpitations	> 1	0.1 to 1	0.1 to 1
Peripheral cyanosis	< 0.1	—	—
Phlebitis	—	< 0.1	—
Pulsating sensations	0.1 to 1	—	0.1 to 1
Raynaud syndrome	—	—	< 0.1
Syncope	> 1	—	0.1 to 1
Tachycardia	0.1 to 1	0.1 to 1	0.1 to 1
Thrombosis	< 0.1	—	—
Transient myocardial ischemia	< 0.1	—	—
Vasodilation	< 0.1	—	< 0.1
CNS			
Aggressiveness	< 0.1	—	—
Agitation	< 0.1	0.1 to 1	0.1 to 1
Anxiety	< 0.1	0.1 to 1	—
Apathy	< 0.1	< 0.1	—
Bradylogia	< 0.1	—	—
Chills	—	0.1 to 1	0.1 to 1
Cluster headache	< 0.1	—	—
Confusion	0.1 to 1	0.1 to 1	0.1 to 1
Convulsions	< 0.1	—	—
Depression	0.1 to 1	0.1 to 1	< 0.1
Depressive disorders	< 0.1	—	—
Detachment	< 0.1	—	—
Difficulty concentrating	0.1 to 1	< 0.1	< 0.1
Disturbances of emotion	—	< 0.1	—
Drowsiness/Sedation	—	0.1 to 1	—
Dysarthria	0.1 to 1	< 0.1	< 0.1
Dystonic reaction	< 0.1	—	< 0.1
Euphoria	0.1 to 1	< 0.1	0.1 to 1

Sumatriptan Adverse Reactions (%)			
Adverse reaction	Tablets	Nasal	Injection
Facial pain	0.1 to 1	< 0.1	< 0.1
Facial paralysis	< 0.1	—	—
Globus hystericus	—	—	< 0.1
Hallucinations	< 0.1	—	—
Heat sensitivity	0.1 to 1	—	—
Hunger	< 0.1	< 0.1	—
Hyperesthesia	< 0.1	—	< 0.1
Hysteria	< 0.1	—	< 0.1
Incoordination	0.1 to 1	< 0.1	—
Increased alertness	< 0.1	—	—
Intoxication	—	< 0.1	< 0.1
Memory disturbance	< 0.1	< 0.1	—
Monoplegia	0.1 to 1	< 0.1	< 0.1
Motor dysfunction	< 0.1	—	—
Myoclonia	—	—	< 0.1
Neoplasm of pituitary	—	< 0.1	—
Neuralgia	< 0.1	—	—
Neurotic disorders	< 0.1	—	—
Paralysis	< 0.1	—	—
Personality change	< 0.1	—	—
Phobia	< 0.1	—	—
Phonophobia	> 1	—	—
Photophobia	> 1	—	0.1 to 1
Psychomotor disorders	< 0.1	—	—
Radiculopathy	< 0.1	—	—
Raised intracranial pressure	< 0.1	—	—
Relaxation	—	—	0.1 to 1
Rigidity	< 0.1	—	—
Sensation of lightness	—	0.1 to 1	0.1 to 1
Shivering	0.1 to 1	0.1 to 1	0.1 to 1
Sleep disturbance	0.1 to 1	0.1 to 1	< 0.1
Stress	—	< 0.1	—
Suicide	< 0.1	—	—
Syncope	0.1 to 1	0.1 to 1	—
Transient hemiplegia	—	—	< 0.1
Tremor	0.1 to 1	0.1 to 1	0.1 to 1
Twitching	< 0.1	—	—
Yawning	—	—	< 0.1
Dermatologic			
Dry/Scaly skin	< 0.1	—	—
Eczema	< 0.1	—	—
Erythema	0.1 to 1	0.1 to 1	0.1 to 1
Herpes	—	—	< 0.1
Peeling of skin	—	—	< 0.1
Pruritus	0.1 to 1	0.1 to 1	0.1 to 1
Rash	0.1 to 1	0.1 to 1	0.1 to 1
Seborrheic dermatitis	< 0.1	—	—
Skin nodules	< 0.1	—	—
Skin tenderness	0.1 to 1	—	< 0.1
Sweating	> 1	< 0.1	—
Swelling of face	—	—	< 0.1
Tightness of the skin	< 0.1	—	—
Wrinkling of the skin	< 0.1	—	—
Endocrine/Metabolic			
Dehydration	—	—	< 0.1
Elevated TSH levels	< 0.1	—	—
Endocrine cysts	< 0.1	—	—
Fluid disturbances	< 0.1	—	—
Galactorrhea	< 0.1	< 0.1	—
Hyperglycemia	< 0.1	—	—
Hypoglycemia	< 0.1	< 0.1	—
Hypothyroidism	< 0.1	—	—
Polydipsia	< 0.1	—	< 0.1
Thirst	0.1 to 1	0.1 to 1	0.1 to 1
Weight gain	< 0.1	—	—
Weight loss	< 0.1	< 0.1	—
GI			
Abdominal discomfort	—	0.1 to 1	—
Abdominal distention	< 0.1	—	—
Colitis	—	< 0.1	—
Constipation	0.1 to 1	< 0.1	—
Decreased appetite	< 0.1	< 0.1	< 0.1
Diarrhea	> 1	0.1 to 1	0.1 to 1
Dry mouth	—	< 0.1	—
Dyspeptic symptoms	< 0.1	—	—
Dysphagia	0.1 to 1	0.1 to 1	—

Sumatriptan Adverse Reactions (%)			
Adverse reaction	Tablets	Nasal	Injection
Feelings of GI pressure	< 0.1	—	—
Flatulence/Eructation	—	< 0.1	< 0.1
Gallstones	—	—	< 0.1
Gastritis	< 0.1	—	—
Gastroenteritis	< 0.1	< 0.1	—
GERD	0.1 to 1	0.1 to 1	0.1 to 1
GI bleeding	< 0.1	—	—
GI pain	< 0.1	—	—
GI tract hemorrhage	—	< 0.1	—
Hematemesis	< 0.1	< 0.1	—
Hypersalivation	< 0.1	—	—
Intestinal obstruction	—	< 0.1	—
Melena	< 0.1	< 0.1	—
Oral itching/irritation	< 0.1	—	—
Pancreatitis	—	< 0.1	—
Peptic ulcer	< 0.1	—	< 0.1
Retching	—	—	< 0.1
Salivary gland swelling	< 0.1	—	—
Swallowing disorders	< 0.1	—	—
Taste disturbances	< 0.1	0.1 to 1	0.1 to 1
GU			
Breast cysts	< 0.1	—	—
Breast lumps	< 0.1	—	—
Breast masses	< 0.1	—	—
Breast swelling	< 0.1	—	—
Breast tenderness	0.1 to 1	—	—
Dysuria	—	—	< 0.1
Dysmenorrhea	—	—	< 0.1
Nipple discharge	< 0.1	—	—
Primary malignant breast neoplasm	< 0.1	—	—
Renal calculus	—	—	< 0.1
Urinary frequency	—	—	< 0.1
Musculoskeletal			
Acquired musculoskeletal deformity	< 0.1	—	—
Arthralgia	< 0.1	—	—
Arthritis	—	< 0.1	—
Articular rheumatitis	< 0.1	—	—
Backache	—	< 0.1	< 0.1
Intervertebral disc disorder	—	< 0.1	—
Joint symptoms	—	< 0.1	0.1 to 1
Muscle atrophy	< 0.1	—	—
Muscle cramps	0.1 to 1	< 0.1	—
Muscle stiffness	< 0.1	< 0.1	< 0.1
Muscle tightness	< 0.1	—	—
Muscle tiredness	< 0.1	—	< 0.1
Muscle weakness	< 0.1	0.1 to 1	—
Musculoskeletal inflammation	< 0.1	—	—
Myalgia	> 1	0.1 to 1	—
Neck pain/stiffness	—	< 0.1	—
Need to flex calf muscles	—	—	< 0.1
Tetany	< 0.1	< 0.1	—
Respiratory			
Allergic rhinitis	> 1	—	—
Asthma	0.1 to 1	< 0.1	—
Breathing disorders	< 0.1	—	—
Bronchitis	< 0.1	—	—
Coughing	< 0.1	—	—
Dyspnea	> 1	0.1 to 1	0.1 to 1
Hiccoughs	< 0.1	—	< 0.1
Lower respiratory tract infections	—	0.1 to 1	< 0.1
Sinusitis	> 1	—	—
Upper respiratory tract inflammation	> 1	—	—
Special senses			
Accommodation disorders	< 0.1	—	—
Blindness/Low vision	< 0.1	—	—
Burning/Numbness of tongue	—	< 0.1	—
Conjunctivitis	< 0.1	—	—
Disturbance of smell	0.1 to 1	< 0.1	< 0.1
Ear infection	—	0.1 to 1	—
Ear, nose, throat hemorrhage	> 1	—	—
External ocular disorders	< 0.1	—	—
External otitis	> 1	—	—

Sumatriptan Adverse Reactions (%)			
Adverse reaction	Tablets	Nasal	Injection
Eye edema	< 0.1	—	—
Eye hemorrhage	< 0.1	—	—
Eye irritation	< 0.1	0.1 to 1	0.1 to 1
Eye pain	< 0.1	—	—
Feeling of fullness in ears	< 0.1	—	—
Hearing loss	> 1	0.1 to 1	—
Keratitis	< 0.1	—	—
Lacrimation	0.1 to 1	< 0.1	0.1 to 1
Meniere disease	—	< 0.1	—
Mydriasis	< 0.1	—	—
Nasal inflammation	> 1	—	—
Noise sensitivity	> 1	—	—
Otalgia	0.1 to 1	< 0.1	—
Sclera disorders	< 0.1	—	—
Tinnitus	> 1	—	—
Visual disturbances	< 0.1	< 0.1	—
Miscellaneous			
Anemia	< 0.1	—	—
Chest tightness/discomfort/ pressure/heaviness	—	0.1 to 1	—
Dental pain	< 0.1	—	—
Drug abuse	< 0.1	—	—
Fever	—	—	< 0.1
Hypersensitivity	—	—	0.1 to 1
Liver function test disturbance	—	—	0.1 to 1
Serotonin agonist effect	—	—	0.1 to 1

Postmarketing reports (oral, injection): The events enumerated include all except those already listed in the adverse reactions section above or those too general to be informative. Because the reports cite events reported spontaneously from worldwide postmarketing experience, frequency of events and the role of sumatriptan injection in their causation cannot be reliably determined. Systemic reactions following sumatriptan use are likely to be similar regardless of route of administration.

• *Cardiovascular* – Atrial fibrillation, cardiomyopathy, colonic ischemia, Prinzmetal variant angina, pulmonary embolism, shock, thrombophlebitis.

• *CNS* – Cerebrovascular accident, CNS vasculitis, dysphasia, panic disorder, subarachnoid hemorrhage.

• *Dermatologic* – Exacerbation of sunburn, hypersensitivity reactions (allergic vasculitis, erythema, pruritus, rash, shortness of breath, urticaria; in addition, severe anaphylaxis/anaphylactoid reactions have been reported), photosensitivity.

Injection only: Following SC administration of sumatriptan, contusion, induration, pain, redness, SC bleeding, stinging, swelling, and on rare occasions, lipoatrophy (depression in the skin) or lipohypertrophy (enlargement or thickening of tissue) have been reported.

• *GI* – Ischemic colitis with rectal bleeding, xerostomia.

• *Hematologic* – Hemolytic anemia, pancytopenia, thrombocytopenia.

• *Special senses* – Deafness, ischemic optic neuropathy, loss of vision, retinal artery occlusion, retinal vein thrombosis.

• *Miscellaneous* – Acute renal failure, angioneurotic edema, bronchospasm in patients with and without a history of asthma, cyanosis, death, elevated liver function tests, temporal arteritis.

➤*Zolmitriptan:*

Cardiovascular – Arrhythmias, hypertension, syncope (0.1% to 1%); bradycardia, extrasystoles, postural hypotension, QT prolongation, tachycardia, thrombophlebitis (less than 0.1%).

CNS – Agitation, anxiety, depression, emotional lability, hyperesthesia, insomnia (0.1% to 1%); akathisia, amnesia, apathy, ataxia, cerebral ischemia, dystonia, euphoria, hallucinations, hyperkinesia, hypertonia, hypotonia, irritability (less than 0.1%).

Dermatologic – Pruritus, rash, urticaria (0.1% to 1%).

GI – Esophagitis, gastroenteritis, increased appetite, liver function abnormality, thirst, tongue edema (0.1% to 1%); anorexia, constipation, gastritis, hematemesis, melena, pancreatitis, ulcer (less than 0.1%).

GU – Cystitis, hematuria, polyuria, urinary frequency/urgency (0.1% to 1%); dysmenorrhea, miscarriage (less than 0.1%).

Hematologic – Ecchymosis (0.1% to 1%); cyanosis, eosinophilia, leukopenia, thrombocytopenia (less than 0.1%).

Metabolic – Edema (0.1% to 1%); alkaline phosphatase increased, hyperglycemia (less than 0.1%).

Musculoskeletal – Back pain, leg cramps, tenosynovitis (0.1% to 1%); arthritis, tetany, twitching (less than 0.1%).

Respiratory – Bronchitis, bronchospasm, epistaxis, hiccough, laryngitis, yawn (0.1% to 1%); apnea, voice alteration (less than 0.1%).

Special senses – Dry eye, ear pain, eye pain, hyperacusis, parosmia, tinnitus (0.1% to 1%); diplopia, lacrimation (less than 0.1%).

Miscellaneous – Allergic reaction, chills, facial edema, fever, malaise, photosensitivity (0.1% to 1%).

Postmarketing reports: The events enumerated include all except those already listed in the adverse reactions section above or those too general to be informative. Because the reports cite events reported spontaneously from worldwide postmarketing experience, frequency of events and the role of zolmitriptan in their causation cannot be reliably determined: Anaphylaxis/anaphylactoid reactions; angina pectoris; coronary artery vasospasm; headache; hypersensitivity reactions including angioedema, ischemic colitis, GI infarction, GI necrosis; MI; transient myocardial ischemia.

➤*Zolmitraptan nasal spray:*

Zolmitriptan Nasal Spray Adverse Reactions (%)		
Adverse reaction	Zolmitriptan nasal spray 5 mg (n = 236)	Placebo (n = 228)
Atypical sensations		
Hyperesthesia	5	0
Paresthesia	10	6
CNS		
Dizziness	3	4
Somnolence	4	2
GI		
Dry mouth	2	0
Nausea	4	1
Unusual taste	21	3
Pain and pressure sensations		
Pain, location specified	4	1
Pain, throat	4	1
Tightness, throat	2	1
Miscellaneous		
Asthenia	3	1
Disorder/discomfort of nasal cavity	3	2

➤*Other adverse events:*

Cardiovascular – Palpitation (1% or more to less than 2%); arrhythmias, hypertension, syncope, tachycardia, thrombophlebitis (0.01%); angina pectoris, atrial fibrillation, bradycardia, MI, vascular disorder, vasodilation (0.001%).

CNS – Headache, insomnia (1% or more to less than 2%); abnormal coordination, abnormal thinking, agitation, amnesia, anxiety, ataxia, circumoral paresthesia, confusion, depersonalization, depression, hypertonia, insomnia, nervousness, speech disorder, tremor, vertigo (0.01%); abnormal dreams, apathy, convulsions, euphoria, hypertonia, irritability, manic reaction, neuropathy, psychosis, tardive dyskinesia (0.001%).

Dermatologic – Pruritus, rash, skin disorder, sweating (0.01%); eczema, erythema, erythema multiforme, hair disorder, neoplasm.

Endocrine – Hyperthyroidism, thyroid edema (0.001%).

GI – Abdominal pain, dysphagia, vomiting (1% or more to less than 2%); diarrhea, dyspepsia, GI disorder, increased saliva, tongue edema, thirst (0.01%); colitis, constipation, eructation, gastritis, GI carcinoma, gingivitis, hepatic neoplasia, increased appetite, intestinal obstruction, jaundice, sialadenitis, stomatitis (0.001%).

GU – Menorrhagia, polyuria (0.01%); breast carcinoma, breast neoplasm, cystitis, dysmenorrhea, enlarged uterine fibroids, fibrocytic breast, kidney pain, metrorrhagia, pyelonephritis, suspicious PAP smear, unintended pregnancy, urinary frequency, urinary tract disorder, urinary tract infection, urine impaired, urogenital neoplasm, uterine disorder, vaginitis (0.001%).

Hematologic – Cyanosis (0.01%); ecchymosis, leukopenia, lymphadenopathy (0.001%).

Metabolic/Nutritional – Dehydration, increased weight, peripheral edema (0.001%).

Musculoskeletal – Arthralgia, joint disorder, myalgia (0.01%); bone pain, osteoporosis, tenosynovitis, twitching (0.001%).

Respiratory – Bronchitis, dyspnea, epistaxis, increased cough, laryngeal edema, pharyngitis, rhinitis, sinusitis, throat discomfort, voice alteration (0.01%); hiccough, hyperventilation, increased sputum, laryngitis, yawning (0.001%).

Special senses – Amblyopia, disorder of lacrimation, ear pain, eye pain, parosmia, tinnitus (0.01%); conjunctivitis, dry eye, photophobia, pneumonia, visual field defect (0.001%).

Miscellaneous – Chest tightness, reaction aggravation (1% or more to less than 2%); abnormal laboratory test, allergic reaction, back pain, chest heaviness, chest pain, chest pressure, chills, cyst, edema of the face, flu syndrome, infection, jaw pain, jaw tightening, neck pain, neck tightness, neoplasm, pressure other (0.01%); cellulitis, fever, jaw pressure, neck heaviness (0.001%).

Overdosage

➤*Symptoms:* Based on the pharmacology of serotonin agonists, hypertension and other more serious cardiovascular symptoms can occur. Overdosage in animals has been fatal; possible symptoms include seizure, tremor, inactivity, extremity erythema, reduced respiratory rate, cyanosis, ataxia, mydriasis, injection-site reaction, and paralysis.

➤*Treatment:* There is no specific antidote. Consider GI decontamination (ie, gastric lavage followed by activated charcoal) in patients with suspected overdose. Institute standard supportive care. If chest pain or other symptoms of angina are present, perform ECG monitoring for evidence of ischemia. Based on the elimination half life, continue monitoring patients after overdose for at least 10 hours (**sumatriptan**), 12 hours (**rizatriptan**), 15 hours (**zolmitriptan**), 20 hours (**almotriptan**), 24 hours (**naratriptan**), 48 hours (**frovatriptan**), or 20 hours or more (**eletriptan**).

It is unknown what effect hemodialysis or peritoneal dialysis has on the serum concentrations of these agents.

Patient Information

A patient information leaflet is provided for patients.

➤*Injection (sumatriptan):* Instruct patients who are advised to self-administer sumatriptan in medically unsupervised situations on the proper use of the product prior to doing so for the first time, including loading the auto-injector and discarding the empty syringes.

For adults, the usual dose is a single injection given just below the skin. Administer as soon as migraine symptoms appear, but it may be given at any time during an attack. A second injection may be given if symptoms of migraine return. Do not use more than 2 injections/24 hours, and allow at least 1 hour between each dose.

The patient may experience pain or redness at the site of injection, but this usually lasts less than 1 hour.

➤*Intranasal:* For adults, the usual dose is a single nasal spray into 1 nostril. If headache returns, a second nasal spray may be given 2 hours after the first spray. For any attack where the patient has no response to the first nasal spray, do not use a second nasal spray without first consulting a physician. Do not administer more than 40 mg **sumatriptan** or 10 mg **zolmitriptan** nasal spray in any 24-hour period.

➤*Oral:* Take a single dose with fluids as soon as symptoms of migraine appear; a second dose may be taken if symptoms return, but no sooner than 2 hours (**sumatriptan**, **zolmitriptan**, **eletriptan**) or 4 hours (**naratriptan**) following the first dose. For a given attack, if there is no response to the first dose, do not take a second dose without first consulting a physician. Do not take more than 200 mg sumatriptan, more than 5 mg naratriptan, more than 10 mg zolmitriptan, or more than 80 mg eletriptan in any 24-hour period.

Tell a physician if the patient has risk factors for heart disease (eg, high blood pressure, high cholesterol, obesity, diabetes, smoking, strong family history of heart disease or stroke, a male over 40 years of age, postmenopausal woman).

These agents are intended to relieve migraine but not to prevent or reduce the number of attacks. Use only to treat an actual migraine attack or cluster headache (sumatriptan injection only).

Instruct patients not to use these agents if they are pregnant, think they might be pregnant, are trying to become pregnant, or are not using adequate contraception, unless they have discussed this with a physician. The manufacturer maintains a sumatriptan and naratriptan pregnancy registry. Register patients by calling (800) 336-2176.

If pain, tightness, pressure, or heaviness in the chest, throat, neck, or jaw occurs when using these agents, instruct patients to discuss it with a physician before using more. If the chest pain is severe or does not go away, instruct patients to immediately call a physician.

If sudden or severe abdominal pain occurs following naratriptan or sumatriptan administration, instruct patients to immediately call a physician.

If shortness of breath, wheezing, heart throbbing, swelling of eyelids, face, or lips, skin rash, skin lumps, or hives occur, advise patients to immediately tell a physician. Instruct patients not to take additional doses unless directed by the physician.

If feelings of tingling, heat, flushing (redness of face lasting a short time), heaviness, pressure, drowsiness, dizziness, tiredness, or sickness develop, instruct patients to tell a physician.

Migraine or treatment with **rizatriptan** may cause somnolence in some patients; dizziness also has been reported. Evaluate ability to perform complex tasks during migraine attacks and after administration of rizatriptan.

Instruct patients not to remove the blister from the outer pouch until just prior to dosing zolmitriptan or rizatriptan orally-disintegrating tablets. Instruct patients to peel blister packs open with dry hands and to place the orally-disintegrating tablet on the tongue, where it will dissolve and be swallowed with the saliva.

Inform phenylketonuric patients that rizatriptan and zolmitriptan orally-disintegrating tablets contain phenylalanine (a component of aspartame). Each 5 mg rizatriptan orally-disintegrating tablet contains 1.05 mg phenylalanine and each 10 mg orally-disintegrating tablet contains 2.1 mg phenylalanine. Each 2.5 mg zolmitriptan orally-disintegrating tablet contains 2.81 mg phenylalanine.

Photosensitization (photoallergy or phototoxicity) may occur; therefore, caution patients to take protective measures (ie, sunscreens, protective clothing) against exposure to sunlight or ultraviolet light (eg, tanning beds) until tolerance is determined.

FROVATRIPTAN SUCCINATE

Rx	Frova (Elan)	Tablets: 2.5 mg (as base)	Lactose. (77). Film-coated. In blister card 9s.

FROVATRIPTAN SUCCINATE — ORAL

For complete and comparative prescribing information, refer to the Serotonin 5-HT$_1$ Receptor Agonists group monograph.

Indications

➤*Migraines:* For the acute treatment of migraine attacks with or without aura in adults.

Frovatriptan succinate is not intended for the prophylactic therapy of migraine or for use in the management of hemiplegic or basilar migraine. The safety and effectiveness of frovatriptan succinate have not been established for cluster headache, which is present in an older, predominately male population.

Administration and Dosage

The recommended dose is a single tablet taken orally with fluids.

If the headache recurs after initial relief, a second tablet may be taken, providing there is an interval of at least 2 hours between doses. The total daily dose of frovatriptan succinate should not exceed 3 tablets (3 × 2.5 mg/day).

There is no evidence that a second dose of frovatriptan succinate is effective in patients who do not respond to a first dose of the drug for the same headache.

The safety of treating an average of more than 4 migraine attacks in a 30-day period has not been established.

➤*Storage/Stability:* Store at controlled room temperature, 25°C (77°F) excursions permitted to 15° to 30°C (59° to 86°F) (see USP controlled room temperature). Protect from moisture and light.

ELETRIPTAN HBr

Rx	Relpax (Pfizer)	Tablets: 24.2 mg eletriptan HBr (equivalent to 20 mg base)	Lactose. (REP20 Pfizer). Orange. Film-coated. In blister card 12s.
		48.5 mg eletriptan HBr (equivalent to 40 mg base)	Lactose. (REP40 Pfizer). Orange. Film-coated. In blister card 12s.

ELETRIPTAN HYDROBROMIDE — ORAL

For complete prescribing information, refer to the Serotonin 5-HT$_1$ Receptor Agonists group monograph.

Indications

➤*Migraines:* For the acute treatment of migraine with or without aura in adults.

Eletriptan hydrobromide is not intended for the prophylactic therapy of migraine or for use in the management of hemiplegic or basilar migraine. Safety and efficacy of eletriptan hydrobromide tablets have not been established for cluster headache, which is present in an older, predominantly male population.

Administration and Dosage

➤*Approved by the FDA:* December 26, 2002.

In controlled clinical trials, single doses of 20 and 40 mg were effective for the acute treatment of migraine in adults. A greater proportion of patients had a response following a 40 mg dose than following a 20 mg dose. Individuals may vary in response to doses of eletriptan tablets. The choice of dose should, therefore, be made on an individual basis. An 80 mg dose, although also effective, was associated with an increased incidence of adverse reactions. Therefore, the maximum recommended single dose is 40 mg.

If after the initial dose, headache improves but then returns, a repeat dose may be beneficial. If a second dose is required, it should be taken at least 2 hours after the initial dose. If the initial dose is ineffective, controlled clinical trials have not shown a benefit of a second dose to treat the same attack. The maximum daily dose should not exceed 80 mg.

The safety of treating an average of more than 3 headaches in a 30-day period has not been established.

➤*CYP3A4 inhibitors:* Eletriptan is metabolized by the CYP3A4 enzyme. Eletriptan should not be used within at least 72 hours of treatment with the following potent CYP3A4 inhibitors: ketoconazole, itraconazole, nefazodone, troleandomycin, clarithromycin, ritonavir and nelfinavir. Eletriptan should not be used within 72 hours with drugs that have demonstrated potent CYP3A4 inhibition and have this potent effect described in the contraindications, warnings, or precautions sections of their labeling (ie, ketoconazole, itraconazole, nefazodone, troleandomycin, clarithromycin, ritonavir, nelfinavir).

➤*Hepatic function impairment:* The drug should not be given to patients with severe hepatic impairment because the effect of severe hepatic impairment on eletriptan metabolism was not evaluated. No dose adjustment is necessary in mild to moderate impairment. Subjects with mild or moderate hepatic impairment demonstrated an increase in both area under the curve (AUC) (34%) and half-life.

➤*Storage/Stability:* Store at 25°C (77°F); excursions permitted to 15° to 30°C (59° to 86°F).

RIZATRIPTAN BENZOATE

Rx	Maxalt (Merck)	Tablets: 5 mg (as base)	Lactose. (MRK 266). Pale pink, capsule shape. In unit-of-use carrying case of 6 tablets.
		10 mg (as base)	Lactose. (MAXALT MRK 267). Pale pink, capsule shape. In unit-of-use carrying case of 6 tablets.
Rx	Maxalt-MLT (Merck)	Tablets, orally disintegrating: 5 mg (as base)	Lyophilized. 1.05 mg phenylalanine, mannitol, aspartame. White to off-white. Peppermint flavor. In 2 unit-of-use carrying case of 3 tablets (6 tablets total).
		10 mg (as base)	Lyophilized. 2.1 mg phenylalanine, mannitol, aspartame. White to off-white. Peppermint flavor. In 2 unit-of-use carrying case of 3 tablets (6 tablets total).

RIZATRIPTAN BENZOATE — ORAL

For complete and comparative prescribing information, refer to the Serotonin 5-HT$_1$ Receptor Agonists group monograph.

Indications

➤*Migraines:* For the acute treatment of migraine attacks with or without aura in adults.

Rizatriptan benzoate is not intended for the prophylactic therapy of migraine or for use in the management of hemiplegic or basilar migraine (such use is contraindicated). Safety and efficacy of rizatriptan benzoate has not been established for cluster headache, which is present in an older, predominantly male population.

Administration and Dosage

➤*Approved by the FDA:* June 29, 1998.

In controlled clinical trials, single doses of 5 and 10 mg of rizatriptan benzoate tablets or rizatriptan benzoate orally disintegrating tablets were effective for the acute treatment of migraines in adults. There is evidence that the 10 mg dose may provide a greater effect than the 5 mg dose. Individuals may vary in response to doses of rizatriptan benzoate tablets. The choice of dose should therefore be made on an individual basis, weighing the possible benefit of the 10 mg dose with the potential risk for increased adverse events.

➤*Redosing:* Doses should be separated by at least 2 hours; no more than 30 mg should be taken in any 24-hour period.

The safety of treating, on average, greater than 4 headaches in a 30-day period has not been established.

➤*Patients receiving propranolol:* In patients receiving propranolol, the 5 mg dose of rizatriptan benzoate should be used, up to a maximum of 3 doses in any 24-hour period. In a study of concurrent administration of propranolol 240 mg/day and a single dose of rizatriptan 10 mg in healthy subjects (n = 11), mean plasma AUC for rizatriptan was increased by 70% during propranolol administration, and a 4-fold increase was observed in 1 subject. The AUC of the active N-monodesmethyl metabolite of rizatriptan was not affected by propranolol.

➤*Administration of orally disintegrating tablets:* For rizatriptan benzoate orally disintegrating tablets, administration with liquid is not necessary. The orally disintegrating tablet is packaged in a blister within an outer aluminum pouch. Patients should be instructed not to remove the blister from the outer pouch until just prior to dosing. The blister pack should then be peeled open with dry hands and the orally disintegrating tablet placed on the tongue, where it will dissolve and be swallowed with the saliva.

➤*Storage/Stability:* Store rizatriptan benzoate tablets at room temperature, 15° to 30°C (59° to 86°F). Dispense in a tight container, if product is subdivided.

Store rizatriptan benzoate orally disintegrating tablets at room temperature, 15° to 30°C (59° to 86°F). The patient should be instructed not to remove the blister from the outer aluminum pouch until the patient is ready to consume the orally disintegrating tablet inside.

NARATRIPTAN HYDROCHLORIDE

Rx	**Amerge** (GlaxoSmithKline)	**Tablets:** 1 mg (as base)	Lactose. (GX CE3). White, D-shaped. Film-coated. In blister pack 9s.
		2.5 mg (as base)	Lactose. (GX CE5). Green, D-shaped. Film-coated. In blister pack 9s.

NARATRIPTAN HYDROCHLORIDE — ORAL

For complete and comparative prescribing information, refer to the Serotonin 5-HT$_1$ Receptor Agonists group monograph.

Indications

➤*Migraines:* For the acute treatment of migraine attacks with or without aura in adults.

Naratriptan hydrochloride tablets are not intended for the prophylactic therapy of migraine or for use in the management of hemiplegic or basilar migraine. Safety and effectiveness of naratriptan hydrochloride tablets have not been established for cluster headache, which is present in an older, predominantly male population.

Administration and Dosage

➤*Approved by the FDA:* February 10, 1998.

In controlled clinical trials, single doses of 1 and 2.5 mg of naratriptan hydrochloride tablets taken with fluid were effective for the acute treatment of migraines in adults. A greater proportion of patients had headache response following a 2.5 mg dose than following a 1 mg dose. Individuals may vary in response to doses of naratriptan hydrochloride tablets. The choice of dose should therefore be made on an individual basis, weighing the possible benefit of the 2.5 mg dose with the potential for a greater risk of adverse events. If the headache returns or if the patient has only partial response, the dose may be repeated once after 4 hours, for a maximum dose of 5 mg in a 24-hour period. There is evidence that doses of 5 mg do not provide a greater effect than 2.5 mg.

The safety of treating, on average, more than 4 headaches in a 30-day period has not been established.

➤*Renal function impairment:* The use of naratriptan hydrochloride is contraindicated in patients with severe renal impairment (creatinine clearance less than 15 mL/min) because of decreased clearance of the drug. In patients with mild to moderate renal impairment, the maximum daily dose should not exceed 2.5 mg over a 24-hour period and a lower starting dose should be considered.

➤*Hepatic function impairment:* The use of naratriptan hydrochloride is contraindicated in patients with severe hepatic impairment (Child-Pugh grade C) because of decreased clearance. In patients with mild or moderate hepatic impairment, the maximum daily dose should not exceed 2.5 mg over a 24-hour period and a lower starting dose should be considered.

➤*Storage/Stability:* Store at controlled room temperature, 20° to 25°C (68° to 77°F).

SUMATRIPTAN

Rx	**Imitrex** (GlaxoSmithKline)	**Tablets:** 25 mg (as succinate)	(I 25). White, triangular shape. Film-coated. In blister pack 9s.
		50 mg (as succinate)	(IMITREX 50). White, triangular shape. Film-coated. In blister pack 9s.
		100 mg (as succinate)	(IMITREX 100). Pink, triangular shape. Film-coated. In blister pack 9s.
		Injection: 4 mg per 0.5 mL (as succinate)	Sodium chloride 7.6 mg/mL. In 4 mg *STATdose System* (2 prefilled single-dose syringe cartridges, 1 *STATdose Pen*, and instructions for use), injection cartridge pack.[1]
		6 mg per 0.5 mL (as succinate)	Sodium chloride 7 mg/mL. In 6 mg single-dose vials (6 mg/0.5 mL) and *STATdose System* (2 prefilled single-dose syringe cartridges, 1 *STATdose Pen*, and instructions for use) injection cartridge pack.[1]
		Spray, nasal: 5 mg	In 100 mcL unit-dose spray device. In 6s.
		20 mg	In 100 mcL unit-dose spray device. In 6s.

[1] Contains 2 prefilled syringe cartridges for refill of *STATdose System* only.

SUMATRIPTAN SUCCINATE — ORAL

For complete and comparative prescribing information, refer to the Serotonin 5-HT$_1$ Receptor Agonists group monograph.

Indications

➤*Migraines:* For the acute treatment of migraine attacks, with or without aura, in adults.

Sumatriptan tablets are not intended for the prophylactic therapy of migraine or for use in the management of hemiplegic or basilar migraine. Safety and efficacy of sumatriptan tablets have not been established for cluster headache, which is present in an older, predominantly male population.

Administration and Dosage

➤*Approved by the FDA:* December 28, 1992.

In controlled clinical trials, single doses of 25, 50, or 100 mg of sumatriptan tablets were effective for the acute treatment of migraine in adults. There is evidence that doses of 50 and 100 mg may provide a greater effect than 25 mg. There is also evidence that doses of 100 mg do not provide a greater effect than 50 mg. Individuals may vary in response to doses of sumatriptan tablets. The choice of dose should therefore be made on an individual basis, weighing the possible benefit of a higher dose with the potential for a greater risk of adverse reactions.

If the headache returns or the patient has a partial response to the initial dose, the dose may be repeated after 2 hours, not to exceed a total daily dose of 200 mg. If a headache returns following an initial treatment with sumatriptan injection, additional single sumatriptan tablets (up to 100 mg/day) may be given with an interval of at least 2 hours between tablet doses. The safety of treating an average of more than 4 headaches in a 30-day period has not been established.

➤*Hepatic function impairment:* Hepatic disease/functional impairment may also cause unpredictable elevations in the bioavailability of orally administered sumatriptan. The liver plays an important role in the presystemic clearance of orally administered sumatriptan. Accordingly, the bioavailability of sumatriptan following oral administration may be markedly increased in patients with liver disease. Consequently, if treatment is deemed advisable in the presence of liver disease, the maximum single dose should, in general, not exceed 50 mg.

➤*Storage/Stability:* Store between 2° and 30°C (36° and 86°F).

SUMATRIPTAN SUCCINATE — INJECTION

For complete and comparative prescribing information, refer to the Serotonin 5-HT$_1$ Receptor Agonists group monograph.

Indications

➤*Migraines:* For the acute treatment of migraine attacks with or without aura and cluster headache episodes.

Sumatriptan succinate injection is not for use in the management of hemiplegic or basilar migraine.

Administration and Dosage

➤*Approved by the FDA:* December 28, 1992.

The maximum single recommended adult dose of sumatriptan succinate injection is 6 mg injected subcutaneously. Controlled clinical trials have failed to show that clear benefit is associated with the administration of a second 6 mg dose in patients who have failed to respond to a first injection.

The maximum recommended dose that may be given in 24 hours is two 6 mg injections separated by at least 1 hour. Although the recommended dose is 6 mg, if side effects are dose limiting, then lower doses may be used. In vitro studies with human microsomes suggest that sumatriptan is metabolized by monoamine oxidase (MAO), predominantly the A isoenzyme. In a study of 14 healthy females, pretreatment with MAO-A inhibitor decreased the clearance of sumatriptan. Under the conditions of this experiment, the result was a 2-fold increase in the area under the sumatriptan plasma concentration times time curve (AUC), corresponding to a 40% increase in elimination half-life. No significant effect was seen with an MAO-B inhibitor. Accordingly, the coadministration of sumatriptan and an MAO-A inhibitor is not generally recommended. If such therapy is clinically warranted, however, suitable dose adjustment and appropriate observation of the patient is advised.

➤*Administration:* In patients receiving doses less than 6 mg, only the single-dose vial dosage form should be used. An autoinjection device is available for use with 6 mg prefilled syringe cartridges to facilitate self-administration in patients in whom this dose is deemed necessary. With this device, the needle penetrates approximately ¼ inch (5 to 6 mm). Since the injection is intended to be given subcutaneously, intramuscular or intravascular delivery should be avoided. Patients should be directed to use injection sites with an adequate skin and subcutaneous thickness to accommodate the length of the needle.

➤*Storage/Stability:* Store between 2° and 30°C (36° and 86°F). Protect from light.

SUMATRIPTAN — INTRANASAL

For complete and comparative prescribing information, refer to the Serotonin 5-HT$_1$ Receptor Agonists group monograph.

Indications

➤*Migraines:* For the acute treatment of migraine attacks with or without aura in adults.

Sumatriptan nasal spray is not intended for the prophylactic therapy of migraine or for use in the management of hemiplegic or basilar migraine. Safety and effectiveness of sumatriptan nasal spray have not been established for cluster headache, which is present in an older, predominantly male population.

Administration and Dosage

➤*Approved by the FDA:* August 26, 1997.

In controlled clinical trials, single doses of 5, 10, or 20 mg of sumatriptan nasal spray administered into 1 nostril were effective for the acute treatment of migraine in adults. A greater proportion of patients had headache response following a 20 mg dose than following a 5 or 10 mg dose. Individuals may vary in response to doses of sumatriptan nasal spray. The choice of dose should therefore be made on an individual basis, weighing the possible benefit of the 20 mg dose with the potential for a greater risk of adverse events. A 10 mg dose may be achieved by the administration of a single 5 mg dose in each nostril. There is evidence that doses above 20 mg do not provide a greater effect than 20 mg.

If the headache returns, the dose may be repeated once after 2 hours, not to exceed a total daily dose of 40 mg. The safety of treating an average of greater than 4 headaches in a 30-day period has not been established.

➤*Storage/Stability:* Store between 2° and 30°C (36° and 86°F). Protect from light.

ZOLMITRIPTAN

Rx	**Zomig** (MedPointe)	**Tablets:** 2.5 mg	Lactose. (Zomig 2.5). Yellow, scored. Film-coated. In blister pack 6s.
		5 mg	Lactose. (Zomig 5). Pink. Film-coated. In blister pack 3s.
		Spray, nasal: 5 mg	In 100 mcL unit-dose spray device. In 6s.
Rx	**Zomig ZMT** (MedPointe)	**Tablets, orally disintegrating:** 2.5 mg	2.81 mg phenylalanine, mannitol, aspartame. (Z). White, bevelled. Orange flavor. In blister pack 6s.

ZOLMITRIPTAN — ORAL

For complete prescribing information, refer to the Serotonin 5-HT$_1$ Receptor Agonists group monograph.

Indications

➤*Migraines:* For the acute treatment of migraine with or without aura in adults.

Zolmitriptan is not intended for the prophylactic therapy of migraine or for use in the management of hemiplegic or basilar migraine. Safety and efficacy of zolmitriptan have not been established for cluster headache, which is present in an older, predominantly male population.

Administration and Dosage

➤*Approved by the FDA:* November 25, 1997.

➤*Tablets:* In controlled clinical trials, single doses of 1, 2.5, and 5 mg of zolmitriptan were effective for the acute treatment of migraines in adults. A greater proportion of patients had headache response following a 2.5 or 5 mg dose than following a 1 mg dose. In the only direct comparison of 2.5 and 5 mg, there was little added benefit from the larger dose, but side effects are generally increased at 5 mg. Patients should, therefore, be started on 2.5 mg or lower. A dose lower than 2.5 mg can be achieved by manually breaking a scored 2.5 mg tablet in half.

If the headache returns, the dose may be repeated after 2 hours, not to exceed 10 mg within a 24-hour period. Controlled trials have not adequately established the effectiveness of a second dose if the initial dose is ineffective.

The safety of treating an average of more than 3 headaches in a 30-day period has not been established.

➤*Orally disintegrating tablets:* In a controlled clinical trial, a single dose of 2.5 mg of zolmitriptan orally disintegrating tablets was effective for the acute treatment of migraines in adults.

If the headache returns, the dose may be repeated after 2 hours, not to exceed 10 mg within a 24-hour period. Controlled trials have not adequately established the effectiveness of a second dose if the initial dose is ineffective.

The safety of treating an average of more than 3 headaches in a 30-day period has not been established.

Administration with liquid is not necessary. The orally disintegrating tablet is packaged in a blister. Patients should be instructed not to remove the tablet from the blister until just prior to dosing. The blister pack should then be peeled open, and the orally disintegrating tablet placed on the tongue, where it will dissolve and be swallowed with the saliva. It is not recommended to break the orally disintegrating tablet.

➤*Hepatic function impairment:* Patients with moderate to severe hepatic impairment have decreased clearance of zolmitriptan and significant elevation in blood pressure was observed in some patients. Use of a low dose with blood pressure monitoring is recommended. In severely hepatically impaired patients, the mean C_{max}, t_{max}, and $AUC_{0-\infty}$ of zolmitriptan were increased 1.5, 2 (2 vs 4 hours), and 3-fold, respectively, compared to healthy patients. Seven out of 27 patients experienced 20 to 80 mm Hg elevations in systolic and/or diastolic blood pressure after a 10 mg dose. Zolmitriptan should be administered with caution in subjects with liver disease, generally using doses less than 2.5 mg.

➤*Storage/Stability:* Store at controlled room temperature, 20° to 25°C (68° to 77°F). Protect from light and moisture.

ZOLMITRIPTAN — INTRANASAL

For complete and comparative prescribing information, refer to the Serotonin 5-HT$_1$ Receptor Agonists group monograph.

Indications

➤*Migraines:* For the acute treatment of migraine with or without aura in adults.

Zolmitriptan is not intended for the prophylactic therapy of migraine or for use in the management of hemiplegic or basilar migraine. Safety and effectiveness of zolmitriptan have not been established for cluster headache, which is present in an older, predominantly male population.

Administration and Dosage

➤*Approved by the FDA:* September 30, 2003.

Administer 1 dose of zolmitriptan nasal spray 5 mg for the treatment of acute migraine. If the headache returns the dose may be repeated after 2 hours. The maximum daily dose should not exceed 10 mg in any 24-hour period.

The safety of treating an average of more than 4 headaches in a 30-day period has not been established.

➤*Hepatic function impairment:* Patients with moderate to severe hepatic impairment have decreased clearance of zolmitriptan and significant elevation in blood pressure was observed in some patients. Use of a lower dose of an alternate formulation with blood pressure monitoring is recommended.

➤*Storage/Stability:* Store at controlled room temperature, 20° to 25°C (68° to 77°F).

ALMOTRIPTAN MALATE

Rx	**Axert** (Ortho-McNeil)	**Tablets:** 6.25 mg	Mannitol. (2080). White. In UD 6s.
		12.5 mg	Mannitol. (A). White. In UD 6s.

ALMOTRIPTAN MALATE — ORAL

For complete and comparative prescribing information, refer to the Serotonin 5-HT$_1$ Receptor Agonists group monograph.

Indications

➤*Migraines:* For the acute treatment of migraine with or without aura in adults.

Almotriptan malate is not intended for the prophylactic therapy of migraine or for use in the management of hemiplegic or basilar migraine. Safety and effectiveness of almotriptan malate tablets have not been established for cluster headache, which is present in an older, predominantly male population.

Administration and Dosage

➤*Approved by the FDA:* May 7, 2001.

In controlled clinical trials, single doses of 6.25 mg and 12.5 mg of almotriptan malate tablets were effective for the acute treatment of migraines in adults, with the 12.5 mg dose tending to be a more effective dose. Individuals may vary in response to doses of almotriptan malate. The choice of dose should therefore be made on an individual basis.

ALMOTRIPTAN MALATE — ORAL

If the headache returns, the dose may be repeated after 2 hours, but no more than 2 doses should be given within a 24-hour period. Controlled trials have not adequately established the effectiveness of a second dose if the initial dose is ineffective.

The safety of treating an average of greater than 4 headaches in a 30-day period has not been established.

➤*Hepatic function impairment:* The pharmacokinetics of almotriptan have not been assessed in this population. The maximum decrease expected in the clearance of almotriptan due to hepatic impairment is 60%. Therefore, the maximum daily dose should not exceed 12.5 mg over a 24-hour period, and a starting dose of 6.25 mg should be used.

➤*Renal function impairment:* In patients with severe renal impairment, the clearance of almotriptan was decreased. Therefore, the maximum daily dose should not exceed 12.5 mg over a 24-hour period, and a starting dose of 6.25 mg should be used.

➤*Storage/Stability:* Store at 25°C (77°F); excursions permitted to 15° to 30°C (59° to 86°F).

Ergotamine Derivatives

WARNING

Serious and/or life-threatening peripheral ischemia has been associated with the coadministration of dihydroergotamine with potent CYP3A4 inhibitors, including protease inhibitors and macrolide antibiotics. Because CYP3A4 inhibition elevates the serum levels of dihydroergotamine, the risk for vasospasm leading to cerebral ischemia and/or ischemia of the extremities is increased. Hence, concomitant use of these medications is contraindicated.

Indications

➤*Ergotamine:* To abort or prevent vascular headaches such as migraine, migraine variant, and histaminic cephalalgia.

➤*Dihydroergotamine:* For the acute treatment of migraine headaches with or without aura and the acute treatment of cluster headache episodes (injection only). Dihydroergotamine nasal spray is not intended for the prophylactic therapy of migraine or for the management of hemiplegic or basilar migraine.

Administration and Dosage

➤*Ergotamine sublingual:* Initiate therapy as soon as possible after the first symptoms of an attack. Place one 2 mg tablet under the tongue; take another tablet at 30-minute intervals thereafter, if necessary. Do not exceed 3 tablets in any 24-hour period. Do not exceed 5 tablets (10 mg) in any 1 week.

➤*Dihydroergotamine nasal spray:* Start with 1 spray (0.5 mg) in each nostril; repeat in 15 minutes for a total dosage of 4 sprays (2 mg). Studies have shown no additional benefit from acute doses greater than 2 mg for a single migraine administration. The safety of doses greater than 3 mg in a 24-hour period and 4 mg in a 7-day period has not been established. Do not use for chronic daily administration.

➤*Dihydroergotamine injection:* Administer in a dose of 1 mL IV, IM, or SC; may be repeated as needed at 1-hour intervals to a total dose of 3 mL for IM or SC delivery or 2 mL for IV delivery in a 24-hour period. Do not exceed a total weekly dosage of 6 mL. Do not use for chronic daily administration.

Actions

➤*Pharmacology:* Ergotamine has partial agonist or antagonist activity against tryptaminergic, dopaminergic, and alpha-adrenergic receptors, depending upon their site; it is a highly active uterine stimulant. It constricts peripheral and cranial blood vessels and depresses central vasomotor centers.

Ergotamine reduces extracranial blood flow, causes a decline in the amplitude of pulsation in the cranial arteries, and decreases hyperperfusion of the basilar artery territory. It does not reduce cerebral hemispheric blood flow. Small doses increase force and frequency of uterine contractions; larger doses increase resting uterine tone. The gravid uterus is more sensitive to these effects.

Ergotamine is hydrogenated in the 9, 10 position as the mesylate salt. Dihydroergotamine binds with high affinity to 5-$HT_{1D\alpha}$ and 5-$HT_{1D\beta}$ receptors. It also binds with high affinity to serotonin 5-HT_{1A}, 5-HT_{2A}, and 5-HT_{2C} receptors; noradrenaline α_{2A}, α_{2B}, and α_1 receptors; and dopamine D_{2L} and D_3 receptors. The therapeutic activity of dihydroergotamine in migraine generally is attributed to the agonist effect at 5-HT_{1D} receptors. Activation of 5-HT_{1D} receptors located on intracranial blood vessels, including those on arteriovenous anastomoses, leads to vasoconstriction, which correlates with the relief of migraine headache. Dihydroergotamine also possesses oxytocic properties.

➤*Pharmacokinetics:*

Absorption/Distribution – GI and sublingual absorption of ergotamine is poor. Following intranasal administration, however, the mean bioavailability of dihydroergotamine mesylate is 32% relative to the injectable administration. Absorption is variable, probably reflecting intersubject differences of absorption and the technique used for self-administration.

Dihydroergotamine mesylate is 93% plasma protein bound. The apparent steady-state volume of distribution is approximately 800 L.

Metabolism/Excretion – Ergotamine is metabolized by the liver; 90% of the metabolites are excreted in the bile. Unmetabolized drug is erratically secreted in saliva, and only trace amounts of unmetabolized drug are excreted in the feces and urine. Although plasma half-life is about 2 hours, ergotamine has long-lasting effects that may be caused by tissue storage.

Following nasal administration, total metabolites represent only 20% to 30% of plasma AUC. The major metabolite, 8′-β-hydroxydihydroergotamine, exhibits affinity equivalent to its parent for adrenergic and 5-HT receptors and demonstrates equivalent potency in several venoconstrictor activity models. The systemic clearance of dihydroergotamine mesylate following IV and IM administration is 1.5 L/min, which mainly reflects hepatic clearance. After intranasal administration, the urinary recovery of parent drug amounts to about 2% of the administered dose compared with 6% after IM administration. The renal clearance (0.1 L/min) is unaffected by the route of dihydroergotamine administration. The decline of plasma dihydroergotamine is biphasic with a terminal half-life of about 9 to 10 hours.

Contraindications

Pregnancy, women who may become pregnant (powerful uterine stimulant actions of ergotamine and dihydroergotamine may cause fetal harm; see Warnings); hypersensitivity to ergot alkaloids or any component of the formulation; peripheral vascular disease (eg, thromboangiitis obliterans, luetic arteritis, severe arteriosclerosis, thrombophlebitis, Raynaud's disease); hepatic or renal impairment; severe pruritus; coronary artery disease (CAD); hypertension; sepsis.

There have been reports of serious adverse events associated with the coadministration of dihydroergotamine and potent CYP3A4 inhibitors (eg, protease inhibitors, macrolide antibiotics), resulting in vasospasm that led to cerebral ischemia and/or ischemia of the extremities. The use of potent CYP3A4 inhibitors (ritonavir, nelfinavir, indinavir, erythromycin, clarithromycin, troleandomycin, ketoconazole, itraconazole) with dihydroergotamine is, therefore, contraindicated.

Do not give dihydroergotamine to patients with ischemic heart disease (angina pectoris, history of MI, documented silent ischemia) or to patients who have clinical symptoms or findings consistent with coronary artery vasospasm, including Prinzmetal variant angina.

Dihydroergotamine may increase blood pressure; do not give to patients with uncontrolled hypertension.

Do not use dihydroergotamine, 5-HT_1 agonists (eg, sumatriptan), ergotamine-containing or ergot-type medications, or methysergide within 24 hours of each other.

Do not administer dihydroergotamine to patients with hemiplegic or basilar migraine.

Dihydroergotamine should not be used by nursing mothers.

Do not use dihydroergotamine with peripheral and central vasoconstrictors because the combination may result in additive or synergistic elevation of blood pressure.

Warnings

➤*CYP3A4 inhibitors (eg, macrolide antibiotics, protease inhibitors):* There have been rare reports of serious adverse events in connection with the coadministration of dihydroergotamine and potent CYP3A4 inhibitors, such as protease inhibitors and macrolide antibiotics, resulting in vasospasm that led to cerebral ischemia and/or ischemia of the extremities. Avoid the use of potent CYP3A4 inhibitors with dihydroergotamine. Examples of some of the more potent CYP3A4 inhibitors include: Antifungals ketoconazole and itraconazole, protease inhibitors ritonavir, nelfinavir, and indinavir, and macrolide antibiotics erythromycin, clarithromycin, and troleandomycin. Administer other less potent CYP3A4 inhibitors with caution. Less potent inhibitors include the following: Saquinavir, nefazodone, fluconazole, grapefruit juice, fluoxetine, fluvoxamine, zileuton, clotrimazole. These lists are not exhaustive; consider the effects on CYP3A4 of other agents being considered for concomitant use with dihydroergotamine.

➤*Fibrotic complications:* There have been reports of pleural and retroperitoneal fibrosis in patients following prolonged daily use of injectable dihydroergotamine. Rarely, prolonged daily use of other ergot alkaloid drugs has been associated with cardiac valvular fibrosis. Rare cases also have been reported in association with the use of injectable dihydroergotamine; however, in those cases, patients also received drugs known to be associated with cardiac valvular fibrosis.

➤*Risk of myocardial ischemia and/or MI and other adverse cardiac events:* Do not use dihydroergotamine in patients with documented ischemic or vasospastic coronary artery disease. It is strongly recommended that dihydroergotamine not be given to patients in whom unrecognized CAD is predicted by the presence of risk factors (eg, hypertension, hypercholesterolemia, smoking, obesity, diabetes, strong family history of CAD, females who are surgically or physiologically postmenopausal, or males who are over 40 years of age) unless a cardiovascular evaluation provides satisfactory clinical evidence that the patient is reasonably free of coronary artery and ischemic myocardial disease or other significant underlying cardiovascular disease. The sensitivity of cardiac diagnostic procedures to detect cardiovascular disease or predisposition to coronary artery vasospasm is modest, at best. If during the cardiovascular evaluation, the patient's medical history or electrocardiographic investigations reveal findings indicative of or consistent with coronary artery vasospasm or myocardial ischemia, do not administer dihydroergotamine.

For patients with risk factors predictive of CAD who are shown to have a satisfactory cardiovascular evaluation, it is strongly recommended that administration of the first dose of dihydroergotamine take place in the setting of a physician's office or similar medically staffed and equipped facility unless the patient has previously received dihydroergotamine. Because cardiac ischemia can occur in the absence of clinical symptoms, consider obtaining, on the first occasion of use, an electrocardiogram during the interval immediately following dihydroergotamine in these patients with risk factors.

It is recommended that patients who are intermittent long-term users of dihydroergotamine and who have or acquire risk factors predictive of CAD, as described above, undergo periodic interval cardiovascular evaluation as they continue to use dihydroergotamine.

The systematic approach described above is currently recommended as a method to identify patients in whom dihydroergotamine may be used to treat migraine headaches with an acceptable margin of cardiovascular safety.

➤*Cardiac events and fatalities:* No deaths have been reported in patients using dihydroergotamine. The potential for adverse cardiac events exists. Serious adverse cardiac events, including acute MI, life-threatening disturbances of cardiac rhythm, and death have been reported following the administration of dihydroergotamine. Considering the extent of use of dihydroergotamine in patients with migraine, the incidence of these events is extremely low.

➤*Drug-associated cerebrovascular events and fatalities:* Cerebral hemorrhage, subarachnoid hemorrhage, stroke, and other cerebrovascular events have been reported in patients treated with dihydroergotamine; some have resulted in fatalities. It should be noted that patients with migraine may be at increased risk of certain cerebrovascular events (eg, stroke, hemorrhage, transient ischemic attack).

➤*Other vasospasm-related events:* Dihydroergotamine, like other ergot alkaloids, may cause vasospastic reactions other than coronary artery vasospasm. Myocardial and peripheral vascular ischemia have been reported with dihydroergotamine.

Dihydroergotamine associated vasospastic phenomena may also cause muscle pains, numbness, coldness, pallor, and cyanosis of the digits. In patients with compromised circulation, persistent vasospasm may result in gangrene or death. Immediately discontinue dihydroergotamine if signs or symptoms of vasoconstriction develop.

➤*Increase in blood pressure:* Significant elevation in blood pressure has been reported on rare occasions in patients with and without a history of hypertension treated with dihydroergotamine. Dihydroergotamine is contraindicated in patients with uncontrolled hypertension.

➤*Local irritation:* Approximately 30% of patients using dihydroergotamine nasal spray (compared with 9% of placebo patients) have reported irritation in the nose or throat and/or disturbance in taste. Irritative symptoms include congestion, burning sensation, dryness, paresthesia, discharge, epistaxis, pain, or soreness. The symptoms were predominantly mild to moderate in severity and transient. In approximately 70% of the above mentioned cases, the symptoms resolved within 4 hours after dosing with dihydroergotamine.

➤*Pregnancy: Category X.* Although no specific teratogenic effects have been found, the fetus suffers if ergotamine is given to the mother. Retarded fetal growth, increased intrauterine death, and resorption occurred in animals, possibly resulting from drug-induced uterine motility and increased vasoconstriction in the placental vascular bed.

Dihydroergotamine possesses oxytocic properties and, therefore, should not be administered during pregnancy. If this drug is used during pregnancy or if the patient becomes pregnant while taking this drug, apprise the patient of the potential hazard to the fetus. There are no adequate studies of dihydroergotamine in human pregnancy, but developmental toxicity has been demonstrated in experimental animals.

➤*Lactation:* Ergotamine is secreted into breast milk and has caused symptoms of ergotism (eg, vomiting, diarrhea) in the infant. Exercise caution when administering to a nursing woman. Excessive dosing or prolonged administration may inhibit lactation. It is likely that dihydroergotamine is excreted in human milk, but there are no data on the drug concentration excreted. Because of the potential for these serious adverse events in nursing infants exposed to dihydroergotamine, nursing should not be undertaken while on this medication.

➤*Children:* Safety and efficacy for use in children have not been established.

Precautions

➤*Coronary artery vasospasm:* Dihydroergotamine may cause coronary artery vasospasm; patients who experience signs or symptoms suggestive of angina following its administration should, therefore, be evaluated for the presence of CAD or a predisposition to variant angina before receiving additional doses. Similarly, patients who experience other symptoms or signs suggestive of decreased arterial flow, such as ischemic bowel syndrome or Raynaud's syndrome following the use of any 5-HT agonist are candidates for further evaluation.

➤*Ergotism:* Although signs and symptoms of ergotism rarely develop even after long-term intermittent use of ergotamine, exercise care to remain within the limits of recommended dosage.

➤*Drug abuse and dependence:* Patients who take ergotamine for extended periods of time may become dependent upon it and require progressively increasing doses for relief of vascular headaches and for prevention of dysphoric effects that follow withdrawal.

Drug Interactions

Ergot Alkaloid Drug Interactions

Precipitant drug	Object drug*		Description
Beta-blockers	Ergot alkaloids	⬆	Peripheral ischemia manifested by cold extremities, possible peripheral gangrene may occur.
CYP3A4 inhibitors (eg, protease inhibitors, macrolide antibiotics, ketoconazole, itraconazole, nefazodone, fluconazole, fluoxetine, fluvoxamine, delavirdine, efavirenz)	Ergot alkaloids	⬆	The risk of ergot toxicity (ie, peripheral vasospasm/ischemia) may be increased. Coadministration with a potent CYP3A4 inhibitor is contraindicated. Use with caution with less potent CYP3A4 inhibitors (see Warnings and Contraindications).
Nicotine	Ergot alkaloids	⬆	Nicotine may provoke vasoconstriction in some patients, predisposing them to a greater ischemic response to ergot therapy.
Sibutramine	Ergot alkaloids	⬆	A serotonin syndrome may occur. Coadministration is not recommended. Carefully monitor patients if concurrent use cannot be avoided.
Dihydroergotamine	Nitrates	⬇	Functional antagonism between these agents, decreasing the antianginal effects may occur.
Ergot alkaloids	$5\text{-}HT_1$ receptor agonists (eg, sumatriptan, frovatriptan, naratriptan, rizatriptan, zolmitriptan)	⬆	Risk of vasospastic reactions may be increased. Administration of a $5\text{-}HT_1$ receptor agonist or ergot alkaloid within 24 hours of each other is contraindicated.
Ergot alkaloids	Vasoconstrictors	⬆	The pressor effects of concurrent use can combine to cause dangerous hypertension.

* ⬆ = Object drug increased. ⬇ = Object drug decreased.

➤*Drug/Food interactions:* Administration with grapefruit juice may increase the serum levels of the ergotamine derivative. Use with caution.

Adverse Reactions

➤*Ergotamine tartrate:* Nausea and vomiting occur in up to 10% of patients. Numbness and tingling of fingers and toes; muscle pain in the extremities; pulselessness; weakness in the legs; precordial pain; transient tachycardia or bradycardia; localized edema; itching.

➤*Dihydroergotamine injection:* Serious cardiac events, including some that have been fatal, have occurred following use of dihydroergotamine injection but are extremely rare. Events reported have included coronary artery vasospasm, transient myocardial ischemia, MI, ventricular tachycardia, and ventricular fibrillation. Fibrotic complications have been reported in association with long-term use of injectable dihydroergotamine.

➤*Dihydroergotamine nasal spray:* During clinical studies and the foreign postmarketing experience with dihydroergotamine nasal spray, there have been no fatalities caused by cardiac events.

Dihydroergotamine Nasal Spray Adverse Reactions (%)

Adverse reaction	Dihydroergotamine (N = 597)	Placebo (N = 631)
CNS		
Dizziness	4	2
Somnolence	3	2
Paresthesia	2	2
GI		
Nausea	10	4
Altered sense of taste	8	1
Vomiting	4	1
Diarrhea	2	< 1
Respiratory		
Rhinitis	26	7
Pharyngitis	3	1
Sinusitis	1	1
Miscellaneous		
Application site reaction	6	2
Dry mouth	1	1
Fatigue	1	1

Dihydroergotamine Nasal Spray Adverse Reactions (%)		
Adverse reaction	Dihydroergotamine (N = 597)	Placebo (N = 631)
Asthenia	1	0
Hot flushes	1	< 1
Stiffness	1	< 1

Overdosage

➤*Symptoms:* Some cases of ergotamine poisoning have occurred in patients who have taken less than 5 mg. Usually, however, toxicity is seen at doses in excess of about 15 mg in 24 hours or 40 mg in a few days. Overdosage causes nausea, vomiting, weakness of the legs, pain in limb muscles, numbness and tingling of fingers and toes, precordial pain, tachycardia or bradycardia, hypertension or hypotension, and localized edema and itching with signs and symptoms of ischemia caused by vasoconstriction of peripheral arteries and arterioles. The feet and hands become cold, pale, and numb. Muscle pain occurs while walking and also later at rest. Gangrene may ensue. Confusion, depression, drowsiness, and convulsions are occasional signs of ergotamine toxicity. Overdosage is particularly likely to occur in patients with sepsis or impaired renal or hepatic function. Patients with peripheral vascular disease are especially at risk of developing peripheral ischemia following treatment with ergotamine.

➤*Treatment:* Treatment consists of the withdrawal of the drug followed by symptomatic measures, including attempts to maintain adequate circulation in the affected parts. Anticoagulant drugs, low molecular weight dextran, and potent vasodilators all may be beneficial. IV infusion of sodium nitroprusside has been successful. Vasodilators must be used with special care in the presence of hypotension. Ergotamine is dialyzable.

Patient Information

Once the nasal spray applicator has been prepared, discard it (with any remaining drug) after 8 hours.

Dosage is individualized. Take exactly as prescribed.

Do not exceed the dosing guidelines. Do not use for chronic daily administration.

Do not stop taking or change the dose unless directed by your physician.

Take at the first sign or hint of a migraine attack.

Stop taking the drug and notify your physician if you experience the following: Numbness, tingling, coldness, or paleness in fingers or toes; muscle pain in arms or legs; weakness in legs; chest pain; heart rate changes; sudden worsening of headache; swelling; itching.

DIHYDROERGOTAMINE MESYLATE

Rx	**Migranal** (Valeant)	**Spray, nasal:** 4 mg/mL (0.5 mg per spray)[a]	In 3.5 mL vials with nasal sprayer.
Rx	**D.H.E. 45** (Xcel[b])	**Injection:** 1 mg/mL[c]	In 1 mL amps.
Rx	**Dihydroergotamine Mesylate** (Various, eg, Bedford, Paddock)		6% alcohol. In 1 mL vials.

[a] With 10 mg caffeine and 50 mg dextrose.
[b] Xcel Pharmaceuticals, 6363 Greenwich Drive, Suite 100, San Diego, CA 92122; (858) 202-2700, fax (858) 202-2799.
[c] With 6.2% alcohol and 15% glycerin.

DIHYDROERGOTAMINE MESYLATE — INTRANASAL

For complete and comparative prescribing information, refer to the Ergotamine Derivatives group monograph.

WARNING

Serious or life-threatening peripheral ischemia has been associated with the coadministration of dihydroergotamine with potent CYP3A4 inhibitors, including protease inhibitors and macrolide antibiotics. Because CYP3A4 inhibition elevates the serum levels of dihydroergotamine, the risk for vasospasm leading to cerebral ischemia or ischemia of the extremities is increased. Hence, concomitant use of these medications is contraindicated.

Indications

➤*Migraines:* For the acute treatment of migraine headaches with or without aura.

Dihydroergotamine mesylate is not intended for the prophylactic therapy of migraine or for the management of hemiplegic or basilar migraine.

Administration and Dosage

➤*Approved by the FDA:* December 8, 1997.

In clinical trials, dihydroergotamine mesylate nasal spray has been effective for the acute treatment of migraine headaches with or without aura. One spray (0.5 mg) of dihydroergotamine mesylate should be administered in each nostril. Fifteen minutes later, an additional 1 spray (0.5 mg) of dihydroergotamine mesylate should be administered in each nostril, for a total dosage of 4 sprays (2 mg) of dihydroergotamine mesylate nasal spray. Studies have shown no additional benefit from acute doses greater than 2 mg for a single migraine administration. The safety of doses greater than 3 mg in a 24-hour period and 4 mg in a 7-day period has not been established.

Dihydroergotamine mesylate nasal spray should not be used for chronic daily administration.

Prior to administration, the pump must be primed (ie, squeeze 4 times) before use.

Once the nasal spray applicator has been prepared, it should be discarded (with any remaining drug in opened ampul) after 8 hours.

➤*Storage/Stability:* Store below 25°C (77°F). Do not refrigerate or freeze.

DIHYDROERGOTAMINE MESYLATE — INJECTION

For complete and comparative prescribing information, refer to the Ergotamine Derivatives group monograph.

WARNING

Serious and life-threatening peripheral ischemia have been associated with the coadministration of dihydroergotamine with potent CYP3A4 inhibitors including protease inhibitors and macrolide antibiotics. Because CYP3A4 inhibition elevates the serum levels of dihydroergotamine, the risk for vasospasm leading to cerebral ischemia and ischemia of the extremities is increased. Hence, concomitant use of these medications is contraindicated.

Indications

➤*Migraines:* For the acute treatment of migraine headaches with or without aura and cluster headache episodes.

Administration and Dosage

Administer in a dose of 1 mL IV, IM or SC. The dose can be repeated, as needed, at 1-hour intervals to a total dose of 3 mL for IM or SC delivery or 2 mL for IV delivery in a 24-hour period. The total weekly dosage should not exceed 6 mL. Dihydroergotamine mesylate injection should not be used for chronic daily administration.

➤*Storage/Stability:* Store at 20° to 25°C (68° to 77°F), in light-resistant containers. Do not refrigerate or freeze.

To ensure constant potency, protect the vials and ampules from light and heat. Administer only if clear and colorless.

ERGOTAMINE TARTRATE

Rx	**Ergomar** (Lotus Biochemical)	**Tablets, sublingual:** 2 mg	Lactose, saccharin. (LB 2). Green. In 20s.

ERGOTAMINE TARTRATE — ORAL

For complete and comparative prescribing information, refer to the Ergotamine Derivatives group monograph.

Indications

As therapy to abort or prevent vascular headache, (eg, migraine, migraine variants, or so called "histaminic cephalalgia").

Administration and Dosage

➤*Approved by the FDA:* February 24, 1983.

All efforts should be made to initiate therapy as soon as possible after the first symptoms of the attacks are noted, since success is proportional to rapidity of treatment, and lower dosages will be effective. At the first sign of an attack or to relieve symptoms after onset of an attack one 2 mg tablet is placed under the tongue. Another tablet should be taken at half-hour intervals thereafter, if necessary, but dosage must not exceed 3 tablets in any 24-hour period. Dosage should be limited to not more that 5 tablets (10 mg) in any one week.

➤*Storage/Stability:* Protect from light and heat. Keep out of the reach of children.

ISOMETHEPTENE MUCATE/DICHLORALPHENAZONE/ACETAMINOPHEN

c-iv	**Isometheptene/Dichloralphenazone/ Acetaminophen** (Various, eg, URL)	**Capsules:** 65 mg isometheptene mucate, 100 mg dichloralphenazone, 325 mg acetaminophen	In 50s, 100s, 250s, and 500s.
c-iv	**Duradrin** (Barr)		(DPI 364). Scarlet/White. In 100s, 250s, and 1000s.
c-iv	**Midrin** (Women First HealthCare)		(MIDRIN). Red. In 50s, 100s, and 250s.
c-iv	**Migratine** (Major)		Red/White. In 100s and 250s.

ISOMETHEPTENE MUCATE/DICHLORALPHENAZONE/ACETAMINOPHEN

Indications

For relief of tension and vascular headaches.

Based on a review of isometheptene mucate by the National Academy of Sciences-National Research Council and/or other information, FDA has classified it as "possibly" effective in the treatment of migraine headache. Final classification of the less-than-effective indication requires further investigation.

Administration and Dosage

➤*Migraine headache:* Usual adult dosage is 2 capsules at once followed by 1 capsule every hour until headache is relieved, up to 5 capsules within a 12-hour period.

➤*Tension headache:* Usual adult dosage is 1 or 2 capsules every 4 hours, up to 8 capsules per day.

➤*Storage/Stability:* Store at controlled room temperature 15° to 30°C (59° to 86°F) in a dry place.

Actions

➤*Pharmacology:* Isometheptene mucate is an unsaturated aliphatic amine with sympathomimetic properties. It acts by constricting dilated cranial and cerebral arterioles, thus reducing the stimuli that lead to vascular headaches.

Dichloralphenazone, a mild sedative, reduces the patient's emotional reaction to the pain of both vascular and tension headaches.

Acetaminophen raises the threshold to painful stimuli, thus exerting an analgesic effect against all types of headaches. Refer to individual monograph.

Contraindications

Glaucoma; severe cases of renal disease; hypertension; organic heart disease; hepatic disease; monoamine oxidase inhibitor (MAOI) therapy (see Drug Interactions).

Warnings

➤*CNS effects:* The capsules contain 100 mg dichloralphenazone. Because of its structural similarity to chloral hydrate, there is a potential for CNS depressant effects. For this reason, caution patients against engaging in hazardous activitoccupations requiring complete mental alertness (eg, operating machinery, driving a motor vehicle) after ingesting the drug. Also, caution patients about possible combined effects with alcohol and other CNS depressant drugs.

➤*Controlled substance:* The capsules are a controlled substance within Schedule IV because of the dichloralphenazone content.

➤*Drug abuse and dependence:* There have been no published reports of withdrawal signs or other signs of abuse associated with the active ingredients contained in the capsules. Because abuse and withdrawal symptoms are possible with chloral hydrate use, they should therefore also be considered possible in those patients taking the capsules in higher doses or for prolonged use. The risk of dependence is increased in patients with a history of alcoholism, drug abuse, or in patients with marked personality disorders. Such dependence-prone individuals should be under careful surveillance when receiving these capsules.

Precautions

➤*Caution:* Observe caution in hypertension and peripheral vascular disease and after recent cardiovascular attacks.

Drug Interactions

➤*MAOIs:* Because isometheptene has sympathomimetic properties, concurrent use may result in severe headache, hypertension, and hyperpyrexia, possibly resulting in hypertensive crisis. Avoid coadministration. If these are used together and hypertension develops, administer phentolamine.

Adverse Reactions

Transient dizziness and skin rash may appear in hypersensitive patients; this usually can be eliminated by reducing the dose.

MIGRAINE COMBINATIONS

	Product & Distributor	Ergotamine tartrate	Caffeine	Other Content	Dosage	How Supplied
Rx	**Ergotamine Tartrate and Caffeine Tablets** (West-ward)	1 mg	100 mg		2 tablets at first sign of an attack; follow with 1 tablet every ½ hour, if needed. Maximum dose is 6 tablets/attack. Do not exceed 10 tablets/week.	Sugar. (WW 120). Buff. Film-coated. In 30s, 100s, and 500s.
Rx	**Cafergot Supps** (Novartis)	2 mg	100 mg	Cocoa butter		(Cafergot Suppository 78-33 Sandoz). In 12s.

MIGRAINE COMBINATIONS

For complete information on these ingredients, refer to the individual monographs.

Indications

Class	Drug	Indications: Nausea and Vomiting	Motion Sickness	Vertigo
ANTIDOPAMINERGICS				
Other	Chlorpromazine[1]	✓		
	Perphenazine[1]	✓		
	Prochlorperazine	✓		
	Promethazine	✓	✓	
	Thiethylperazine	✓		
Other	Metoclopramide	✓		
ANTICHOLINERGICS				
Antihistamines	Buclizine	✓	✓	
	Cyclizine	✓	✓	
	Dimenhydrinate	✓	✓	✓
	Diphenhydramine		✓	
	Meclizine	✓	✓	✓[2]
Other	Scopolamine		✓	
	Trimethobenzamide	✓		
MISCELLANEOUS				
Miscellaneous	Benzquinamide	✓		
	Cannabinoids	✓		
	Corticosteroids	✓[3]		
	Hydroxyzine HCl	✓[3]		
	Diphenidol	✓		✓
	Phosphorated Carbohydrate Solution	✓		

[1] Also indicated for relief of intractable hiccoughs.
[2] Classified "possibly effective" by the FDA.
[3] This is an *unlabeled* use.

Actions

➤*Pharmacology:* Drug-induced vomiting (eg, drugs, radiation, metabolic disorders) is generally stimulated through the chemoreceptor trigger zone (CTZ), which in turn stimulates the vomiting center (VC) in the brain. Nausea of motion sickness is initiated by stimulation of labyrinthine mechanism of the ear, which sends impulses to CTZ. VC may also be stimulated directly (by GI irritation, motion sickness, vestibular neuritis, etc). Increased activity of central neurotransmitters, dopamine in CTZ or acetylcholine in VC appears to be a major mediator for inducing vomiting.

Patients undergoing cancer chemotherapy often experience nausea and vomiting so intolerable that they may refuse further treatment. Some antineoplastic agents are more emetogenic than others. Prophylaxis with an antiemetic drug before the patient receives chemotherapy and treatment afterward may enable the patient to overcome this unpleasant side effect and continue a potentially curative protocol.

Vertigo is a feeling of whirling or rotation accompanied by involuntary swaying, weakness and lightheadedness. Motion sickness, a functional disorder, is caused by repetitive angular, linear or vertical motion. Both of these conditions are characterized by pallor, sweating, hyperventilation, nausea and vomiting.

The drugs that are effective as antiemetics are the **antidopaminergic** agents (phenothiazines, metoclopramide) which are especially effective for drug-induced emesis. **Anticholinergic agents** (antihistamines, trimethobenzamide, scopolamine) may be more appropriate in motion sickness, labyrinthine disorders, etc. Other agents, whose mechanisms are not known or that may act differently (eg, hydroxyzine, corticosteroids, cannabinoids), are effective in various types of emesis.

The preceding table indicates manufacturers' recommended uses for agents in this group. Several of these are indicated for uses other than as antiemetic/antivertigo agents. For a full discussion, see individual drug monographs.

Warnings

➤*Children:* Not recommended for uncomplicated vomiting in children; limit use to prolonged vomiting of known etiology for three principal reasons:

1.) Although there is no confirmatory evidence, centrally-acting antiemetics may contribute, in combination with viral illnesses (a possible cause of vomiting in children), to the development of Reye's syndrome, a potentially fatal acute childhood encephalopathy. This syndrome follows a nonspecific febrile illness, and is characterized by an abrupt onset of persistent, severe vomiting, lethargy, irrational behavior, visceral fatty degeneration (especially involving the liver), progressive encephalopathy leading to coma, convulsions and death.

2.) The extrapyramidal symptoms that can occur secondary to some drugs may be confused with the CNS signs of an undiagnosed primary disease responsible for the vomiting, eg, Reye's syndrome or other encephalopathy.

3.) Drugs with hepatotoxic potential may unfavorably alter the course of Reye's syndrome. Avoid such drugs in children whose signs and symptoms (vomiting) could represent Reye's syndrome. It should also be noted that salicylates and acetaminophen are hepatotoxic at large doses. Although it is not known whether at usual doses they would represent a hazard in patients with the underlying hepatic disorder of Reye's syndrome, these drugs, too, should be avoided in children whose signs and symptoms could represent Reye's syndrome, unless alternative methods of controlling fever are not successful.

Children with acute illnesses (eg, chickenpox, CNS infections, measles, gastroenteritis) or dehydration seem to be much more susceptible to neuromuscular reactions, particularly dystonias, than are adults. In such patients, use antiemetics only under close supervision. Do not use dimenhydrinate in children less than 2 years of age unless directed by a doctor.

Severe emesis – Severe emesis should not be treated with an antiemetic drug alone; where possible, establish cause of vomiting. Direct primary emphasis toward restoration of body fluids and electrolyte balance, and relief of fever and causative disease process. Avoid overhydration which may result in cerebral edema. Antiemetic effects may impede diagnosis of such conditions as brain tumors, intestinal obstruction and appendicitis, and may obscure signs of toxicity from overdosage of other drugs.

Precautions

➤*Benzyl alcohol:* Some of these products contain benzyl alcohol, which has been associated with a fatal "gasping syndrome" in premature infants.

➤*Tartrazine sensitivity:* Some of these products contain tartrazine, which may cause allergic-type reactions (including bronchial asthma) in susceptible individuals. Although the incidence of sensitivity is low, it is frequently seen in patients who also have aspirin hypersensitivity. Specific products containing tartrazine are identified in the product listings.

➤*Sulfite sensitivity:* Some of these products contain sulfites which may cause allergic-type reactions (eg, hives, itching, wheezing, anaphylaxis) in certain susceptible people. Although the overall prevalence of sulfite sensitivity in the general population is probably low, it is seen more frequently in asthmatics or in atopic nonasthmatic people. Specific products containing sulfites are identified in the product listings.

Patient Information

These agents may cause drowsiness; patients should observe caution while driving or performing other tasks requiring alertness.

Avoid alcohol and other CNS depressants.

Antidopaminergics

CHLORPROMAZINE HYDROCHLORIDE

Refer to the general discussion of these products in the Antiemetic/Antivertigo Agents group monograph. For complete prescribing information, refer to the chlorpromazine HCl oral and injection monographs in the Antipsychotic Agents.

METOCLOPRAMIDE

Refer to the general discussion of these products beginning in the Antiemetic/Antivertigo monograph. For complete prescribing information, refer to the Metoclopramide monographs in the GI Stimulants.

PERPHENAZINE

Refer to the general discussion of these products in the Antiemetic/Antivertigo Agents group monograph.For complete prescribing information, refer to the perphenazine monograph in the Antipsychotic Agents..

PROCHLORPERAZINE

Refer to the general discussion of these products in the Antiemetic/Antivertigo Agents group monograph. For complete prescribing information, refer to the prochlorperazine monographs in the Antipsychotic Agents.

PROMETHAZINE

Refer to the general discussion of these products beginning in the Antiemetic/Antivertigo group monograph. For complete information, refer to the promethazine monographs in the Antihistamines section of the Respiratory Agents.

CYCLIZINE

otc	**Marezine** (Himmel)	**Tablets:** 50 mg (as HCl)	(Marezine T4A). Scored. In 12s and 100s.

CYCLIZINE — ORAL

For complete prescribing information, refer to the Antiemetic/Antivertigo Agents group monograph.

Indications

For the prevention and treatment of the nausea, vomiting or dizziness associated with motion sickness.

Administration and Dosage

➤*Adults and children 12 years of age and over:* 1 tablet every 4 to 6 hours, not to exceed 4 tablets in 24 hours, or as directed by a doctor.

➤*Children 6 to under 12 years of age:* ½ tablet every 6 to 8 hours, not to exceed 1½ tablets in 24 hours, or as directed by a doctor.

Do not give to children under 6 years of age unless directed by a doctor.

For prevention, take the first dose one half-hour before departure.

➤*Storage/Stability:* Store at 15° to 25° C (59° to 77° F) in a dry place and protect from light.

Actions

➤*Pharmacology:* Cyclizine has antiemetic, anticholinergic, and antihistaminic properties. It reduces the sensitivity of the labyrinthine apparatus. The action may be mediated through nerve pathways to the vomiting center (VC) from the chemoreceptor trigger zone (CTZ), peripheral nerve pathways, the VC, or other CNS centers.

Cyclizine has an onset of action of 30 to 60 minutes, depending on dosage; the duration of action is 4 to 6 hours.

Contraindications

Contraindicated in patients with a hypersensitivity to cyclizine.

Do not use in patients with asthma, glaucoma, emphysema, chronic pulmonary disease, shortness of breath, difficulty in breathing or difficulty in urination due to enlargement of the prostate gland unless directed by a doctor. Cyclizine should not be used concurrently with sedatives, tranquilizers or anticholinergic medications.

Warnings

➤*Special risk:* Do not take this product if you have asthma, glaucoma, emphysema, chronic pulmonary disease, shortness of breath, difficulty in breathing or difficulty in urination due to enlargement of the prostate gland unless directed by a doctor.

➤*Pregnancy: Category B.* Cyclizine has been teratogenic in rodents, but large scale human studies have not demonstrated adverse fetal effects. Use only when clearly needed and when the potential benefits outweigh the potential hazards to the fetus.

➤*Lactation:* Safety for use in the nursing mother has not been established.

Precautions

➤*Hypotension:* This drug may have a hypotensive action, which may be confusing or dangerous in postoperative patients.

➤*Hazardous tasks:* May produce drowsiness; patients should observe caution while driving or performing other tasks requiring alertness.

Drug Interactions

➤*CNS depressants:* May have additive effects with alcohol and other CNS depressants (eg, hypnotics, sedatives, tranquilizers, antianxiety agents); use with caution.

Overdosage

➤*Symptoms:* Moderate overdosage may cause hyperexcitability alternating with drowsiness. Massive overdosage may cause convulsions, hallucinations, and respiratory paralysis.

➤*Treatment:* Includes appropriate supportive and symptomatic treatment. Dialysis may be considered.

Caution – Do not use morphine or other respiratory depressants.

Patient Information

Do not take this product if you are taking sedatives, tranquilizers or anticholinergic drugs without first consulting with your doctor.

May cause drowsiness; alcohol, sedatives and tranquilizers may increase the drowsiness effect. Avoid alcoholic beverages while taking this product. Use caution when driving a motor vehicle or operating machinery.

As with any drug, if you are pregnant or nursing a baby, seek the advice of a health professional before using this product.

Not for frequent or prolonged use except on the advice of a doctor.

DIMENHYDRINATE

otc	**Dimenhydrinate** (Various)	**Tablets:** 50 mg	In 12s, 100s, 300s, 500s, 1000s and UD 100s.
otc	**Calm-X** (Republic Drug)		In 16s.
Rx	**Dimetabs** (Jones Medical)		In 1000s.
otc	**Dramamine** (Upjohn)		(DRAMAMINE). White, scored. In UD 100s.
otc	**Triptone** (Del Pharmaceuticals)		Scored. In 12s.
otc	**Dramamine** (Upjohn)	**Tablets, chewable:** 50 mg	(DRAMAMINE).Tartrazine. Aspartame, sorbitol. Orange, scored. Orange flavor. In 8s and 24s.
Rx	**Dimenhydrinate** (Various)	**Injection:** 50 mg/ml	In 1 and 10 ml vials and 1 ml amps.
Rx	**Dinate** (Seatrace)		In 10 ml vials.[1]
Rx	**Dramanate** (Pasadena)		In 10 ml vials.[1]
Rx	**Dymenate** (Keene)		In 10 ml vials.[1]
Rx	**Hydrate** (Hyrex)		In 10 ml vials.[1]
Rx	**Dramamine** (Upjohn)	**Liquid:** 15.62 mg/5 ml	In 480 ml.
otc	**Dimenhydrinate** (Various)	**Liquid:** 12.5 m/4 ml	In pt and gal.
otc	**Dramamine** (Upjohn)		5% alcohol. Cherry flavor. In 90 ml.
otc	**Children's Dramamine** (Upjohn)	**Liquid:** 12.5 mg per/5 ml	5% alcohol, sucrose. Cherry flavor. In 120 ml.

[1] In benzyl alcohol and propylene glycol.

DIMENHYDRINATE — ORAL

Refer to the general discussion of these products beginning in the Antiemetic/Antivertigo group monograph.

Indications

For the prevention and treatment of nausea, vomiting, and dizziness associated with motion sickness.

Administration and Dosage

To prevent motion sickness, the first dose should be taken one-half to 1 hour before starting activity. This medication should not be given to children under 2 years of age unless directed by a doctor.

➤*Adults and children 12 years of age and older:* Patients should take 1 to 2 chewable tablets or tablets (50 to 100 mg) every 4 to 6 hours, not to exceed 8 chewable tablets or tablets (400 mg) in 24 hours, or as directed by a doctor.

➤*Children 6 to under 12 years of age:* Patients should take ½ to 1 chewable tablet or tablet (25 to 50 mg) every 6 to 8 hours, not to exceed 3 tablets in 24 hours or as directed by a doctor.

➤*Children 2 to under 6 years of age:* Patients should take ¼ to ½ chewable tablet or tablet (12.5 to 25 mg) every 6 to 8 hours, not to exceed 1 ½ tablets in 24 hours or as directed by a doctor.

➤*Storage/Stability:* This medication should be stored at room temperature. Patients should not use if the blister card is broken. Patients should see bottom of vial for expiration date.

Actions

➤*Pharmacology:* Dimenhydrinate consists of equimolar proportions of diphenhydramine and chlorotheophylline.

➤*Pharmacokinetics:* Dimenhydrinate has a depressant action of hyperstimulated labyrinthine function. The precise mode of action is not known.

DIMENHYDRINATE — ORAL

The antiemetic effects are believed to be due to the diphenhydramine, an antihistamine also used as an antiemetic agent.

Warnings

➤*Special risk:* Patients or parents of patients should ask a doctor before use if they or their children have breathing problems such as emphysema or chronic bronchitis, glaucoma, or difficulty in urination due to enlargement of the prostate gland.

➤*Use:* This medication is not for frequent or prolonged use except on advice of a doctor. Do not exceed recommended dosage.

➤*Pregnancy: Category B.*

If pregnant, the patient should ask a health professional before use.

Safety for use during pregnancy has not been established. Patients should use only when clearly needed and when the potential benefits outweigh the potential hazards to the fetus.

➤*Lactation:* If breastfeeding, the patient should ask a health professional before use.

Small amounts of dimenhydrinate are excreted in breast milk. Because of the potential for adverse reactions in nursing infants, it should be decided whether to discontinue nursing or to discontinue the drug, taking into account the importance of the drug to the mother.

➤*Children:* This medication should not be given to children under 2 years of age unless directed by a doctor.

Precautions

➤*Benzyl alcohol:* Some of these products contain the preservative benzyl alcohol, which has been associated with a fatal "gasping syndrome" in premature infants.

➤*Hazardous tasks:* Patients should use caution when driving a motor vehicle or operating machinery.

➤*Tartrazine sensitivity:*

Chewable tablets – Dimenhydramine chewable tablets contain FD&C Yellow No. 5 (tartrazine) as a color additive.

Drug Interactions

Dimenhydrinate Drug Interactions			
Precipitant drug	Object drug*		Description
Dimenhydrinate	Alcohol, CNS depressants	↑	Concomitant use of alcohol or other CNS depressants with dimenhydrinate may have an additive effect.
Dimenhydrinate	Antibiotics	↑	Use caution when given in conjunction with certain antibiotics that may cause ototoxicity; dimenhydrinate is capable of masking ototoxic symptoms, and irreversible damage may result.

* ↑ = Object drug increased.

Patients should ask a doctor or pharmacist before use if they are taking sedatives or tranquilizers.

Overdosage

➤*Symptoms:* Drowsiness is the usual side effect. Convulsions, coma, and respiratory depression may occur with massive overdosage.

➤*Treatment:* No specific antidote is known. If respiratory depression occurs, initiate mechanically assisted respiration and administer oxygen. Treat convulsions with appropriate doses of diazepam. Give phenobarbital (5 to 6 mg/kg) to control convulsions in children.

Patient Information

Do not use in children under 2 years of age unless directed by a doctor.

Ask a doctor before use if you have:
- A breathing problem such as emphysema or chronic bronchitis.
- Glaucoma.
- Difficulty in urination due to enlargement of the prostate gland.

Ask a doctor or pharmacist before use if you are taking sedatives or tranquilizers.

When using this product:
- Marked drowsiness may occur.
- Avoid alcoholic drinks.
- Alcohol, sedatives, and tranquilizers may increase drowsiness.
- Be careful when driving a motor vehicle or operating machinery.

DIMENHYDRINATE — INJECTION

Refer to the general discussion of these products beginning in the Antiemetic/Antivertigo group monograph.

Indications

For the prevention and treatment of nausea, vomiting, or vertigo of motion sickness.

Administration and Dosage

Dimenhydrinate in the injectable form is indicated when the oral form is impractical.

➤*Adults:* Nausea or vomiting may be expected to be controlled for approximately 4 hours with 50 mg, and prevented by a similar dose every 4 hours. Its administration may be attended by some degree of drowsiness in some patients, and 100 mg every 4 hours may be given in conditions in which drowsiness is not objectionable or even desirable.

For intramuscular (IM) administration, each milliliter (50 mg) of solution is injected as needed, but for intravenous (IV) administration, each milliliter (50 mg) of solution must be diluted in 10 mL of 0.9% sodium chloride injection and injected over a period of 2 minutes.

➤*Pediatric:* For IM administration, 1.25 mg/kg of body weight or 37.5 mg/m^2 of body surface area is administered 4 times daily. The maximum dose should not exceed 300 mg daily. Do not treat neonates with dimenhydrinate.

Note – Some of these products contain benzyl alcohol. Benzyl alcohol has been associated with a fatal "gasping syndrome" in premature infants and infants of low birth weight.

➤*Storage/Stability:* Store at 20° to 25°C (68° to 77°F). Protect from light.

Actions

➤*Pharmacology:* While the precise mode of action of dimenhydrinate is not known, it has a depressant action on hyperstimulated labyrinthine function.

Contraindications

Do not treat neonates or patients with a history of hypersensitivity to dimenhydrinate or its components (diphenhydramine or 8-chlorotheophylline) with dimenhydrinate.

Warnings

➤*Pregnancy: Category B.* Reproduction studies have been performed in rats at doses up to 20 times the human dose, and in rabbits at doses up to 25 times the human dose (on a mg/kg basis), and have revealed no evidence of impaired fertility or harm to the fetus due to dimenhydrinate.

There are no adequate and well-controlled studies in pregnant women. However, clinical studies in pregnant women have not indicated that dimenhydrinate increases the risk of abnormalities when administered in any trimester of pregnancy. It would appear that the possibility of fetal harm is remote when the drug is used during pregnancy. Nevertheless, because the studies in humans cannot rule out the possibility of harm, use dimenhydrinate during pregnancy only if clearly needed.

Labor and delivery – The safety of dimenhydrinate given during labor and delivery has not been established. Reports have indicated dimenhydrinate may have an oxytocic effect. Caution is advised when this effect is unwanted or in situations where it may prove detrimental.

➤*Lactation:* Small amounts of dimenhydrinate are excreted in breast milk. Because of the potential for adverse reactions in breast-feeding infants from dimenhydrinate, decide whether to discontinue breast-feeding or discontinue the drug, taking into account the importance of the drug to the mother.

➤*Children:* As in adults, antihistamines may diminish mental alertness in pediatric patients. Particularly in the young child, they may produce excitation, hallucinations, convulsions, or death in overdose situations. Do not treat neonates with dimenhydrinate.

Note – Some of these products contain benzyl alcohol. Benzyl alcohol has been associated with a fatal "gasping syndrome" in premature infants and infants of low birth weight.

Precautions

➤*Drowsiness:* Drowsiness may be experienced by some patients, especially with high dosage. This effect frequently is not undesirable in conditions for which the drug is used.

➤*Administration:* Do not inject the preparation intra-arterially.

➤*Special risk:* Use caution when dimenhydrinate is given in conjunction with certain antibiotics that may cause ototoxicity because dimenhydrinate is capable of masking ototoxic symptoms, and an irreversible state may be reached.

Use dimenhydrinate with caution in patients with conditions that might be aggravated by anticholinergic therapy (eg, prostatic hypertrophy, stenosing peptic ulcer, pyloroduodenal obstruction, bladder neck obstruction, narrow-angle glaucoma, bronchial asthma, cardiac arrhythmias).

DIMENHYDRINATE — INJECTION

➤*Hazardous tasks:* This drug may impair the mental and/or physical abilities required for the performance of potentially hazardous tasks, such as driving a vehicle or operating machinery. The concomitant use of alcohol or other CNS depressants may have an additive effect. Warn patients accordingly.

Adverse Reactions

The most frequent adverse reaction to dimenhydrinate is drowsiness. Dizziness may also occur. Symptoms of dry mouth, nose, and throat; blurred vision; difficult or painful urination; headache; anorexia; nervousness, restlessness, or insomnia (especially in pediatric patients); skin rash; thickening of bronchial secretions; tachycardia; epigastric distress; lassitude; excitation; and nausea have been reported.

Overdosage

➤*Symptoms:* Drowsiness is the usual clinical side effect. Convulsions, coma, and respiratory depression may occur with massive overdosage.

➤*Treatment:* No specific antidote is known. If respiratory depression occurs, initiate mechanically assisted respiration and administer oxygen. Treat convulsions with appropriate doses of diazepam. Phenobarbital (5 to 6 mg/kg) may be given to control convulsions in pediatric patients.

Patient Information

Because of the potential for drowsiness, caution patients taking dimenhydrinate against operating automobiles or dangerous machinery.

DIPHENHYDRAMINE

Refer to the general discussion of these products beginning in the Antiemetic/Antivertigo group monograph.

MECLIZINE

Rx	**Meclizine HCl** (Various)	**Tablets:** 12.5 mg	In 30s, 60s, 100s, 500s, 1000s, and UD 100s.
Rx	**Antivert** (Pfizer US)		(Antivert 210). In 100s, 1000s, and UD 100s.
Rx	**Antrizine** (Major)		In 100s, 500s, and 1000s.
otc/ Rx[1]	**Meclizine HCl** (Various)	**Tablets:** 25 mg	In 12s, 20s, 30s, 60s, 100s, 500s, 1000s, and UD 32s and 100s.
Rx	**Antivert/25** (Pfizer US)		(Antivert 211). In 100s, 1000s, and UD 100s.
otc	**Dramamine Less Drowsy Formula** (Pharmacia and Upjohn)		Lactose. In 8s.
otc/ Rx[1]	**Meclizine HCl** (Various, eg, Rugby, Goldline)	**Tablets, chewable:** 25 mg	In 20s, 30s, 60s, 100s, 1000s, and UD 100s.
Rx	**Meclizine HCl** (Various)	**Tablets:** 50 mg	In 100s.
Rx	**Antivert/50** (Pfizer US)		(Antivert 214). Scored. In100s.
Rx	**Meni-D** (Seatrace)	**Capsules:** 25 mg	(Meni-D 1-4X Day). Light blue/clear. In 100s.

[1] Products are available *otc* or *Rx*, depending on product labeling.

MECLIZINE — ORAL

For complete prescribing information, refer to the Antiemetic/Antivertigo Agents group monograph.

Indications

For the prevention and treatment of nausea, vomiting, or dizziness associated with motion sickness.

Meclizine is "possibly effective" for the management of vertigo associated with diseases affecting the vestibular system.

Administration and Dosage

➤*Motion sickness:*

Adults and children 12 years of age and older – The initial dose of 25 to 50 mg meclizine HCl should be taken 1 hour prior to travel for protection against motion sickness. Thereafter, the dose may be repeated every 24 hours for the duration of the journey. No more than 2 tablets in 24 hours should be taken.

Children under 12 years of age – Ask a doctor.

➤*Vertigo:* The patient should take 25 to 100 mg daily in divided doses.

➤*Chewable tablets:*

Directions – Do not exceed recommended daily dose. Tablets may be chewed or swallowed with water.

➤*Storage / Stability:*

Tablets – Store at controlled room temperature 15° to 30°C (59° to 86°F). Dispense in tight, light-resistant containers.

Chewable tablets – Store below 30°C (86°F).

Actions

➤*Pharmacology:* Meclizine HCl is an antihistamine which shows marked protective activity against nebulized histamine and lethal doses of IV injected histamine in guinea pigs. It has a marked effect in blocking the vasopressor response to histamine but only a slight blocking action against acetylcholine. Its activity is relatively weak in inhibiting the spasmogenic action of histamine on isolated guinea pig ileum.

➤*Pharmacokinetics:* Meclizine tablets have an onset of action of 30 to 60 minutes, depending on dosage; their duration of action is 4 to 6 hours and 12 to 24 hours, respectively.

Contraindications

Hypersensitivity to meclizine.

Warnings

➤*Pregnancy: Category B.* Reproduction studies in rats have shown cleft palates at 25 to 50 times the human dose. Epidemiological studies in pregnant women, however, do not indicate that meclizine HCl increases the risk of abnormalities when administered during pregnancy. Despite the animal findings, it would appear that the possibility of fetal harm is remote. Nevertheless, meclizine HCl, or any other medication, should be used during pregnancy only if clearly necessary.

Patients should contact a health professional before using this medication if they are pregnant.

➤*Lactation:* Patients should contact a health professional before using this medication if they are breastfeeding.

➤*Children:* Clinical studies establishing safety and effectiveness in children have not been done; therefore, use is not recommended in children under 12 years of age.

Precautions

➤*Special risk:* Due to its potential anticholinergic action, this drug should be used with caution in patients with asthma, emphysema, chronic bronchitis, glaucoma, or enlargement of the prostate gland.

➤*Hazardous tasks:* Since drowsiness may, on occasion, occur with use of this drug, patients should be warned of this possibility and cautioned against driving a car or operating dangerous machinery.

➤*Tartrazine sensitivity:* The meclizine HCl 25 mg and 50 mg tablets may contain FD&C Yellow No. 5 (tartrazine), which may cause allergic-type reactions (including bronchial asthma) in certain susceptible individuals. Although the overall incidence of FD&C Yellow No. 5 (tartrazine) sensitivity in the general population is low, it is frequently seen in patients who also have aspirin hypersensitivity.

Drug Interactions

Patients should avoid alcoholic beverages while taking this drug. Alcohol, sedatives, and tranquilizers may increase drowsiness.

Adverse Reactions

➤*Cardiovascular:* Hypotension; palpitations; tachycardia.

➤*CNS:* Drowsiness; restlessness; excitation; nervousness; insomnia; euphoria; blurred vision; diplopia; vertigo; tinnitus; auditory and visual hallucinations (particularly when dosage recommendations are exceeded).

➤*Dermatologic:* Urticaria; rash.

➤*GI:* Dry mouth; anorexia; nausea; vomiting; diarrhea; constipation; cholestatic jaundice (cyclizine).

➤*GU:* Urinary frequency; difficult urination; urinary retention.

➤*Miscellaneous:* Dry nose and throat.

Overdosage

➤*Symptoms:* Moderate overdosage may cause hyperexcitability alternating with drowsiness. Massive overdosage may cause convulsions, hallucinations and respiratory paralysis.

➤*Treatment:* Includes appropriate supportive and symptomatic treatment. In case of accidental overdose, seek professional assistance or contact a poison control center immediately.

Do not use morphine or other respiratory depressants.

MECLIZINE — ORAL

Patient Information

➤*Chewable tablets:* Do not give this medication to children under 12 years of age unless directed by a doctor. Keep this medication out of the reach of children.

Ask a doctor before use if you have:
- Glaucoma.
- Breathing problems such as emphysema or chronic bronchitis.
- Trouble in urination due to enlargement of the prostate gland.

Ask a doctor or pharmacist before use if you are taking tranquilizers or sedatives.

When using this product:
- You may get drowsy.
- Avoid alcoholic beverages.
- Alcohol, sedatives, and tranquilizers may increase drowsiness.
- Do not drive or operate dangerous machinery.

If you are pregnant or breastfeeding, ask a health professional before use.

In case of overdose, get medical help or contact a poison control center right away.

SCOPOLAMINE — ORAL

Refer to the general discussion of these products beginning in the Antiemetic/Antivertigo group monograph. For complete prescribing information for Oral Scopolamine, see the monograph in the GI Anticholinergics section.

SCOPOLAMINE — TRANSDERMAL

Rx	**Transderm-Scōp** (Baxter)	**Transdermal patch:** 1.5 mg scopolamine (delivers approximately 1 mg scopolamine over 3 days)	In 10s and 24s.

SCOPOLAMINE — TRANSDERMAL

Refer to the general discussion of these products beginning in the Antiemetic/Antivertigo group monograph.

Indications

Prevention of nausea and vomiting associated with motion sickness and recovery from anesthesia and surgery in adults.

➤*Unlabeled uses:* Used transdermally in the treatment of sialorrhea (excessive salivation).

Administration and Dosage

➤*Initiation of therapy:* Apply one system to the postauricular skin (ie, behind the ear) at least 4 hours before the antiemetic effect is required. To prevent postoperative nausea and vomiting, apply the patch the evening before scheduled surgery. To minimize exposure of the newborn baby to the drug, apply the patch 1 hour prior to cesarean section. Scopolamine approximately 1 mg will be delivered over 3 days. Wear only one disc at a time. Do not cut the patch.

For perioperative use, keep patch in place for 24 hours following surgery, then remove and discard.

➤*Handling:* After applying the disc on dry skin behind the ear, wash hands thoroughly with soap and water, then dry them. Discard the removed disc and wash the hands and application site thoroughly with soap and water to prevent any traces of scopolamine from coming into direct contact with the eyes.

➤*Continuation of therapy:* If the disc is displaced, discard it and place a fresh one on the hairless area behind the other ear. For motion sickness, if therapy is required for more than 3 days, discard the first disc and place a fresh one on the hairless area behind the other ear.

➤*Storage/Stability:* Store at controlled room temperature 20° to 25°C (68° to 77°F).

Actions

➤*Pharmacology:* The sole active agent is scopolamine, a belladonna alkaloid with well-known pharmacological properties. It is an anticholinergic agent which acts as a competitive inhibitor at postganglionic muscarinic receptor sites of the parasympathetic nervous system, and on smooth muscles that respond to acetylcholine but lack cholinergic innervation. It has been suggested that scopolamine acts in the CNS by blocking cholinergic transmission from the vestibular nuclei to higher centers in the CNS and from the reticular formation to the vomiting center. Scopolamine can inhibit the secretion of saliva and sweat, decrease GI secretions and motility, cause drowsiness, dilate the pupils, increase heart rate, and depress motor function.

➤*Pharmacokinetics:*

Absorption – Scopolamine's activity is due to the parent drug. The pharmacokinetics of scopolamine delivered via the system are due to the characteristics of both the drug and dosage form. The system is programmed to deliver in vivo ≈ 1 mg of scopolamine at an approximately constant rate to the systemic circulation over 3 days. Upon application to the postauricular skin, an initial priming dose of scopolamine is released from the adhesive layer to saturate skin binding sites. The subsequent delivery of scopolamine to the blood is determined by the rate-controlling membrane and is designed to produce stable plasma levels in a therapeutic range. Following removal of the used system, there is some degree of continued systemic absorption of scopolamine bound in the skin layers.

Scopolamine is well absorbed percutaneously. Following application to the skin behind the ear, circulating plasma levels are detected within 4 hours with peak levels being obtained, on average, within 24 hours. The average plasma concentration produced is 87 pg/mL for free scopolamine and 354 pg/mL for total scopolamine (free + conjugates).

Distribution – The distribution of scopolamine is not well characterized. It crosses the placenta and the blood-brain barrier and may be reversibly bound to plasma proteins.

Metabolism – Although not well characterized, scopolamine is extensively metabolized and conjugated with less than 5% of the total dose appearing unchanged in the urine.

Excretion – The exact elimination pattern of scopolamine has not been determined. Following patch removal, plasma levels decline in a log linear fashion with an observed half-life of 9.5 hours; less than 10% of the total dose is excreted in the urine as parent and metabolites over 108 hours.

Contraindications

Hypersensitivity to scopolamine or other belladonna alkaloids, or any ingredient or component in the formulation or delivery system, or in patients with angle-closure (narrow angle) glaucoma.

Warnings

➤*Ophthalmic effects:* Glaucoma therapy in patients with chronic open-angle (wide-angle) glaucoma should be monitored and may need to be adjusted during scopolamine use, as the mydriatic effect of scopolamine may cause an increase in intraocular pressure.

➤*Idiosyncratic reactions:* Rarely, idiosyncratic reactions may occur with ordinary therapeutic doses of scopolamine. The most serious of these that have been reported are acute toxic psychosis, including confusion, agitation, rambling speech, hallucinations, paranoid behaviors, and delusions.

➤*Elderly:* Scopolamine should be used with caution in the elderly.

➤*Pregnancy: Category C.* Scopolamine hydrobromide has been shown to have a marginal embryotoxic effect in rabbits when administered by daily IV injection at doses producing plasma levels ≈ 100 times the level achieved in humans using a transdermal system. During a clinical study among women undergoing cesarean section treated with scopolamine in conjunction with epidural anesthesia and opiate analgesia, no evidence of CNS depression was found in the newborns. There are no other adequate and well-controlled studies in pregnant women. Other than in the adjunctive use for delivery by cesarean section, scopolamine should be used in pregnancy only if the potential benefit justifies the potential risk to the fetus.

Teratogenic – Teratogenic studies were performed in pregnant rats and rabbits with scopolamine hydrobromide administered by daily IV injection. No adverse effects were recorded in rats.

➤*Lactation:* Because scopolamine is excreted in human milk, caution should be exercised when scopolamine is administered to a nursing woman.

➤*Children:* The safety and effectiveness of scopolamine in children has not been established. Children are particularly susceptible to the side effects of belladonna alkaloids. Scopolamine should not be used in children because it is not known whether this system will release an amount of scopolamine that could produce serious adverse effects in children.

Precautions

➤*Special risk:* Scopolamine should be used with caution in patients with pyloric obstruction or urinary bladder neck obstruction. Caution should be exercised when administering an antiemetic or antimuscarinic drug to patients suspected of having intestinal obstruction.

Scopolamine should be used with caution in the elderly or in individuals with impaired liver or kidney functions because of the increased likelihood of CNS effects.

Caution should be exercised in patients with a history of seizures or psychosis, since scopolamine can potentially aggravate both disorders.

➤*Hazardous tasks:* Since drowsiness, disorientation, and confusion may occur with the use of scopolamine, patients should be warned of the possibility and cautioned against engaging in activities that require mental alertness, such as driving a motor vehicle or operating dangerous machinery.

Drug Interactions

The absorption of oral medications may be decreased during the concurrent use of scopolamine because of decreased gastric motility and delayed gastric emptying.

Scopolamine should be used with care in patients taking other drugs that are capable of causing CNS effects such as sedatives, tranquilizers, or alcohol. Special attention should be paid to potential interactions with drugs having anticholinergic properties (eg, other belladonna alkaloids, antihistamines, (including meclizine) tricyclic antidepressants, and muscle relaxants).

SCOPOLAMINE — TRANSDERMAL

➤*Drug/Lab test interactions:* Scopolamine will interfere with the gastric secretion test.

Adverse Reactions

➤*Motion sickness:* In motion sickness clinical studies of scopolamine, the most frequent adverse reaction was dryness of the mouth. This occurred in about two-thirds of patients on the drug. A less frequent adverse drug reaction was drowsiness, which occurred in less than one-sixth of patients on the drug. Transient impairment of eye accommodation, including blurred vision and dilation of the pupils, was also observed.

➤*Postoperative nausea and vomiting:* In a total of 5 clinical studies in which scopolamine was administered perioperatively to a total of 461 patients and safety was assessed, dry mouth was the most frequently reported adverse drug experience, which occurred in ≈ 29% of patients on the drug. Dizziness was reported by ≈ 12% of patients on the drug.

➤*Postmarketing:* In addition to the adverse experiences reported during clinical testing of scopolamine, the following are spontaneously reported adverse events from postmarketing experience. Because the reports cite events reported spontaneously from worldwide postmarketing experience, frequency of events and the role of scopolamine in their causation cannot be reliably determined: Acute angle-closure (narrow-angle) glaucoma; confusion; difficulty urinating; dry, itchy, or conjunctival injection of eyes; restlessness; hallucinations; memory disturbances; rashes and erythema; and transient changes in heart rate.

➤*Drug withdrawal/postremoval symptoms:* Symptoms such as dizziness, nausea, vomiting, and headache occur following abrupt discontinuation of antimuscarinics. Similar symptoms, including disturbances of equilibrium, have been reported in some patients following discontinuation of use of the scopolamine system. These symptoms usually do not appear until 24 hours or more after the patch has been removed. Some symptoms may be related to adaptation from a motion environment to a motion-free environment. More serious symptoms including muscle weakness, bradycardia and hypotension may occur following discontinuation of scopolamine.

Overdosage

➤*Symptoms:* The signs and symptoms of anticholinergic toxicity include lethargy, somnolence, coma, confusion, agitation, hallucinations, convulsion, visual disturbance, dry flushed skin, dry mouth, decreased bowel sounds, urinary retention, tachycardia, hypertension, and supraventricular arrhythmias.

The symptoms of overdose/toxicity due to scopolamine should be carefully distinguished from the occasionally observed syndrome of withdrawal (see Adverse Reactions). Although mental confusion and dizziness may be observed with both acute toxicity and withdrawal, other characteristic findings differ: Tachyarrhythmias, dry skin, and decreased bowel sounds suggest anticholinergic toxicity, while bradycardia, headache, nausea and abdominal cramps, and sweating suggest post-removal withdrawal. Obtaining a careful history is crucial to making the correct diagnosis.

➤*Treatment:* Because strategies for the management of drug overdose continually evolve, it is strongly recommended that a poison control center be contacted to obtain up-to-date information regarding the management of scopolamine patch overdose. The prescriber should be mindful that antidotes used routinely in the past may no longer be considered optimal treatment. For example, physostigmine, used more or less routinely in the past, is seldom recommended for the routine management of anticholinergic syndromes.

Until up-to-date authoritative advice is obtained, routine supportive measures should be directed to maintaining adequate respiratory and cardiac function.

Most cases of toxicity involving the use of the product will resolve with simple removal of the patch. Serious symptomatic cases of overdosage involving multiple patch applications or ingestion may be managed by initially ensuring the patient has an adequate airway, and supporting respiration and circulation. This should be rapidly followed by removal of all patches from the skin and the mouth. If there is evidence of patch ingestion, gastric lavage, endoscopic removal of swallowed patches, or administration of activated charcoal should be considered, as indicated by the clinical situation. In any case where there is serious overdosage or signs of evolving acute toxicity, continuous monitoring of vital signs and ECG, establishment of IV access, and administration of oxygen are all recommended.

Patient Information

Since scopolamine can cause temporary dilation of the pupils and blurred vision if it comes in contact with the eyes, patients should be strongly advised to wash their hands thoroughly with soap and water immediately after handling the patch. In addition, it is important that used patches be disposed of properly to avoid contact with children or pets.

Patients should be advised to remove the patch immediately and promptly and to contact a physician in the unlikely event that they experience symptoms of acute narrow-angle glaucoma (pain and reddening of the eyes, accompanied by dilated pupils). Patients should also be instructed to remove the patch if they develop any difficulties in urinating.

Patients who expect to participate in underwater sports should be cautioned regarding the potentially disorienting effects of scopolamine. A patient brochure is available.

TRIMETHOBENZAMIDE HYDROCHLORIDE

Rx	**Trimethobenzamide** (Various, eg, Amide, Mutual)	**Capsules:** 300 mg	In 100, 250s, 500s, 1000s, UD 30s, and UD 60s.
Rx	**Tigan** (Monarch)		(Tigan MO79). Purple. In 100s.
Rx	**Trimethobenzamide** (Various)	**Pediatric suppositories:** 100 mg	In 10s.
Rx	**Pediatric Triban** (Great Southern)		In 10s.[1]
Rx	**Tebamide** (G & W Labs)		In 10s.[1]
Rx	**T-Gen** (Goldline)		In 10s.[1]
Rx	**Tigan** (Monarch)		In 10s.[1]
Rx	**Trimazide** (Major)		In 10s.
Rx	**Trimethobenzamide** (Various)	**Adult suppositories:** 200 mg	In 10s and 50s.
Rx	**Tebamide** (G & W Labs)		In 10s[1] and 50s.[1]
Rx	**T-Gen** (Goldline)		In 10s[1] and 50s.[1]
Rx	**Tigan** (Monarch)		In 10s[1] and 50s.[1]
Rx	**Triban** (Great Southern)		In 10s[1] and 50s.[1]
Rx	**Trimazide** (Major)		In 10s.
Rx	**Trimethobenzamide HCl** (Various)	**Injection:** 100 mg/ml	In 2 ml amps and 20 ml vials.
Rx	**Tigan** (Monarch)		In 2 ml amps[3], 20 ml vials,[2] and 2 ml syringe.[4]

[1] With 2% benzocaine.
[2] With phenol.
[3] With methyl- and propylparabens.
[4] With phenol and EDTA.

TRIMETHOBENZAMIDE HYDROCHLORIDE — ORAL

Refer to the general discussion of these products beginning in the Antiemetic/Antivertigo monograph.

Indications

For the treatment of postoperative nausea and vomiting and for nausea associated with gastroenteritis.

Administration and Dosage

Adjust dosage adjusted according to the indication for therapy, severity of symptoms, and the response of the patient.

➤*Usual adult dosage:* One 300 mg capsule 3 or 4 times daily.

➤*Storage/Stability:* Store at 20° to 25°C (68° to 77°F). Dispense in a tight, light-resistant container.

Actions

➤*Pharmacology:* The mechanism of action of trimethobenzamide as determined in animals is obscure, but may involve the chemoreceptor trigger zone (CTZ), an area in the medulla oblongata through which emetic impulses are conveyed to the vomiting center; direct impulses to the vomiting center apparently are not similarly inhibited. In dogs pretreated with trimethobenzamide, the emetic response to apomorphine is inhibited, while little or no protection is afforded against emesis induced by intragastric copper sulfate.

➤*Pharmacokinetics:*

Absorption – The pharmacokinetics of trimethobenzamide have been studied in healthy adult subjects. Following administration of 200 mg (100 mg/mL) trimethobenzamide IM injection, the time to reach maximum plasma concentration (t_{max}) was about 30 minutes, about 15 minutes longer for 300 mg trimethobenzamide oral capsule than an IM injection. A single dose of 300 mg trimethobenzamide oral capsule provided a plasma concentration profile of trimethobenzamide similar to 200 mg trimethobenzamide IM. The relative bioavailability of the capsule formulation compared to the solution is 100%.

Excretion – The mean elimination half-life of trimethobenzamide is 7 to 9 hours.

TRIMETHOBENZAMIDE HYDROCHLORIDE — ORAL

Contraindications

Hypersensitivity to trimethobenzamide.

Warnings

➤*Pregnancy:* Category C. Trimethobenzamide was studied in reproduction experiments in rats and rabbits and no teratogenicity was suggested. The only effects observed were an increased percentage of embryonic resorptions or stillborn pups in rats administered 20 mg and 100 mg/kg and increased resorptions in rabbits receiving 100 mg/kg. In each study these adverse effects were attributed to 1 or 2 dams. The relevance to humans is not known. Since there is no adequate experience in pregnant women who have received this drug, safety in pregnancy has not been established.

➤*Lactation:* Since there is no adequate experience in lactating women who have received this drug, safety in nursing mothers has not been established.

➤*Children:* Exercise caution when administering trimethobenzamide to children for the treatment of vomiting. Antiemetics are not recommended for treatment of uncomplicated vomiting in children. Limit their use to prolonged vomiting of known etiology. There are 2 principal reasons for caution:

1.) The extrapyramidal symptoms which can occur secondary to trimethobenzamide may be confused with the central nervous system signs of an undiagnosed primary disease responsible for the vomiting (eg, Reye's syndrome or other encephalopathy).
2.) It has been suspected that drugs with hepatotoxic potential, such as trimethobenzamide, may unfavorably alter the course of Reye's syndrome. Therefore, avoid such drugs in children whose signs and symptoms (vomiting) could represent Reye's syndrome.

Precautions

➤*Special risk:* During the course of acute febrile illness, encephalitides, gastroenteritis, dehydration and electrolyte imbalance, especially in children and the elderly or debilitated, CNS reactions such as opisthotonos, convulsions, coma and extrapyramidal symptoms have been reported with and without use of trimethobenzamide or other antiemetic agents. In such disorders, exercise caution in administering trimethobenzamide, particularly to patients who recently received other CNS-acting agents (phenothiazines, barbiturates, belladonna derivatives). It is recommended that severe emesis not be treated with an antiemetic drug alone; where possible the cause of vomiting should be established. Direct primary emphasis toward the restoration of body fluids and electrolyte balance, the relief of fever and relief of the causative disease process. Avoid overhydration because it may result in cerebral edema.

The antiemetic effects of trimethobenzamide may render diagnosis more difficult in such conditions as appendicitis and obscure signs of toxicity due to overdosage of other drugs.

Reye's syndrome – Reye's syndrome has been associated with the use of trimethobenzamide and other drugs, including antiemetics, although their contribution, if any, to the cause and course of the disease has not been established. This syndrome is characterized by an abrupt onset shortly following a non-specific febrile illness, with persistent, severe vomiting, lethargy, irrational behavior, progressive encephalopathy leading to coma, convulsions, and death.

➤*Hazardous tasks:* Trimethobenzamide may produce drowsiness. Patients should not operate motor vehicles or other dangerous machinery until their individual responses have been determined.

Drug Interactions

➤*Use with alcohol:* Concomitant use of alcohol with trimethobenzamide may result in an adverse drug interaction.

Adverse Reactions

There have been reports of hypersensitivity reactions and Parkinson-like symptoms. There have been instances of hypotension reported following parenteral administration to surgical patients. There have been reports of blood dyscrasias, blurring of vision, coma, convulsions, depression of mood, diarrhea, disorientation, dizziness, drowsiness, headache, jaundice, muscle cramps and opisthotonos. If these occur, discontinue the administration of the drug. Allergic-type skin reactions have been observed; therefore, discontinue the drug at the first sign of sensitization. While these symptoms will usually disappear spontaneously, symptomatic treatment may be indicated in some cases.

Patient Information

Trimethobenzamide may produce drowsiness. Do not operate motor vehicles or other dangerous machinery until their individual responses have been determined.

TRIMETHOBENZAMIDE HYDROCHLORIDE — RECTAL

Refer to the general discussion of these products beginning in the Antiemetic/Antivertigo monograph.

Indications

For the control of nausea and vomiting.

Administration and Dosage

Adjust the dosage according to the indication for therapy, severity of symptoms, and the response of the patient.

➤*200 mg suppositories (not to be used in premature or newborn infants):*

Usual adult dosage – 1 suppository (200 mg) 3 times daily or 4 times daily.

Usual children's dosage –

Under 30 lbs: ½ suppository (100 mg) 3 times daily or 4 times daily.
30 to 90 lbs: ½ to 1 suppository (100 to 200 mg) 3 times daily or 4 times daily.

➤*Pediatric 100 mg suppositories (not to be used in premature or newborn infants):*

Usual children's dosage –

Under 30 lbs: 1 suppository (100 mg) 3 times daily or 4 times daily.
30 to 90 lbs: 1 to 2 suppositories (100 to 200 mg) 3 times daily or 4 times daily.

➤*Storage/Stability:* Store at 25°C (77°F); excursions permitted to 15° to 30°C (59° to 86°F).

Actions

➤*Pharmacology:* The mechanism of action of trimethobenzamide as determined in animals is obscure, but may be the chemoreceptor trigger zone (CTZ), an area in the medulla oblongata through which emetic impulses are conveyed to the vomiting center; direct impulses to the vomiting center apparently are not similarly inhibited. In dogs pretreated with trimethobenzamide, the emetic response to apomorphine is inhibited, while little or no protection is afforded against emesis induced by intragastric copper sulfate.

➤*Pharmacokinetics:*

Absorption/Distribution – The pharmacokinetics of trimethobenzamide have been studied in healthy adult subjects. Following administration of 200 mg (100 mg/mL) trimethobenzamide IM injection, the time to reach maximum plasma concentration (T_{max}) was about half an hour, about 15 minutes longer for trimethobenzamide 300 mg oral capsule than an IM injection. A single dose of trimethobenzamide 300 mg oral capsule provided a plasma concentration profile of trimethobenzamide similar to trimethobenzamide 200 mg IM. The relative bioavailability of the capsule formulation compared to the solution is 100%.

Excretion – The mean elimination half-life of trimethobenzamide is 7 to 9 hours.

Contraindications

Premature or newborn infants; hypersensitivity to trimethobenzamide. Since the suppositories contain benzocaine, do not use them in patients known to be sensitive to this or similar local anesthetics.

Warnings

➤*Pregnancy:* Category C. Trimethobenzamide was studied in reproduction experiments in rats and rabbits and no teratogenicity was suggested. The only effects observed were an increased percentage of embryonic resorptions or stillborn pups in rats administered 20 mg and 100 mg/kg and increased resorptions in rabbits receiving 100 mg/kg. In each study these adverse effects were attributed to 1 or 2 dams. The relevance to humans is not known. Since there is no adequate experience in pregnant women who have received this drug, safety in pregnancy has not been established.

➤*Lactation:* Safety in nursing mothers has not been established.

➤*Children:* Exercise caution when administering trimethobenzamide to children for the treatment of vomiting. Antiemetics are not recommended for treatment of uncomplicated vomiting in children; limit their use to prolonged vomiting of known etiology. There are 3 principal reasons for caution:

1.) There has been some suspicion that centrally acting antiemetics may contribute, in combination with viral illnesses (a possible cause of vomiting in children), to development of Reye's syndrome, a potentially fatal acute childhood encephalopathy with visceral fatty degeneration, especially involving the liver. Although there is no confirmation of this suspicion, caution is nevertheless recommended.
2.) The extrapyramidal symptoms which can occur secondary to trimethobenzamide may be confused with the central nervous system signs of an undiagnosed primary disease responsible for the vomiting (eg, Reye's syndrome or other encephalopathy).
3.) It has been suspected that drugs with hepatotoxic potential, such as trimethobenzamide, may unfavorably alter the course of Reye's syndrome. Therefore, avoid such drugs in children whose signs and symptoms (vomiting) could represent Reye's syndrome. It should also be noted that salicylates and acetaminophen are hepatotoxic at large doses. Although it is not known that at usual doses they would represent a hazard in patients with the underlying hepatic disorder of Reye's syndrome, also avoid these drugs in children whose signs and symptoms could represent Reye's syndrome, unless alternative methods of controlling fever are not successful.

Precautions

➤*Reye's syndrome:* Reye's syndrome has been associated with the use of trimethobenzamide and other drugs, including antiemetics, although their contribution, if any, to the cause and course of the disease has not been established. This syndrome is characterized by an abrupt onset shortly following a non-specific febrile illness, with persistent, severe vomiting, lethargy, irrational behavior, progressive encephalopathy leading to coma, convulsions, and death.

➤*Special risk:* During the course of acute febrile illness, encephalitides, gastroenteritis, dehydration and electrolyte imbalance, especially in chil-

TRIMETHOBENZAMIDE HYDROCHLORIDE — RECTAL

dren and the elderly or debilitated, CNS reactions such as opisthotonos, convulsions, coma and extrapyramidal symptoms have been reported with and without use of trimethobenzamide or other antiemetic agents. In such disorders, exercise caution in administering trimethobenzamide, particularly in patients who recently received other CNS-acting agents (phenothiazines, barbiturates, belladonna derivatives). Do not treat severe emesis with an antiemetic drug alone; where possible, establish the cause of vomiting. Direct primary emphasis toward the restoration of body fluids and electrolyte balance, relief of fever, and relief of the causative disease process. Avoid overhydration because it may result in cerebral edema.

The antiemetic effects of trimethobenzamide may render diagnosis more difficult in such conditions as appendicitis and obscure signs of toxicity due to overdosage of other drugs.

➤*Hazardous tasks:* Trimethobenzamide may produce drowsiness. Patients should not operate motor vehicles or other dangerous machinery until their individual responses have been determined.

Drug Interactions

➤*Use with alcohol:* Concomitant use of alcohol with trimethobenzamide may result in an adverse drug interaction.

Adverse Reactions

There have been reports of hypersensitivity reactions and Parkinson-like symptoms. There have been instances of hypotension and hypertension reported following parenteral administration to surgical patients. There have been reports of blood dyscrasias, blurring of vision, coma, convulsions, depression of mood, diarrhea, disorientation, dizziness, drowsiness, headache, jaundice, muscle cramps, and opisthotonos. If these occur, discontinue the administration of the drug. Allergic-type skin reactions have been observed; therefore, discontinue the drug at the first sign of sensitization. While these symptoms will usually disappear spontaneously, symptomatic treatment may be indicated in some cases.

Patient Information

Trimethobenzamide may produce drowsiness. Do not operate motor vehicles or other dangerous machinery until individual response has been determined.

Concomitant use of alcohol with trimethobenzamide may result in an adverse drug interaction.

TRIMETHOBENZAMIDE HYDROCHLORIDE — INJECTION

Refer to the general discussion of these products beginning in the Antiemetic/Antivertigo monograph.

Indications

For the treatment of postoperative nausea and vomiting and for nausea associated with gastroenteritis.

Administration and Dosage

Intramuscular administration may cause pain, stinging, burning, redness and swelling at the site of injection. Such effects may be minimized by deep injection into the upper outer quadrant of the gluteal region, and by avoiding the escape of solution along the route.

➤*Note:* The injectable form is intended for intramuscular administration only; it is not recommended for intravenous use.

Dosage should be adjusted according to the indication for therapy, severity of symptoms, and the response of the patient.

➤*Injectable, 100 mg/mL (not recommended for use in pediatric patients):*

Usual adult dosage –

For the treatment of nausea secondary to gastroenteritis: 200 mg IM.

For the treatment of nausea and vomiting postoperatively: 200 mg IM injection, followed in 1 hour by a second 200 mg IM injection.

➤*Storage/Stability:* Store at room temperature up to 30°C (86°F).

Actions

➤*Pharmacology:* The mechanism of action of trimethobenzamide hydrochloride as determined in animals is obscure, but may be the chemoreceptor trigger zone (CTZ), an area in the medulla oblongata through which emetic impulses are conveyed to the vomiting center; direct impulses to the vomiting center apparently are not similarly inhibited. In dogs pretreated with trimethobenzamide hydrochloride, the emetic response to apomorphine is inhibited, while little or no protection is afforded against emesis induced by intragastric copper sulfate.

➤*Pharmacokinetics:*

Absorption – Oral and parenteral trimethobenzamide are not bioequivalent. An oral dose of 400 mg of trimethobenzamide yields plasma levels approximately equivalent to a 200 mg intramuscular dose.

The pharmacokinetics of trimethobenzamide have been studied in healthy adult subjects. Following administration of 200 mg (100 mg/mL) trimethobenzamide hydrochloride IM injection, the time to reach maximum plasma concentration (t_{max}) was about half an hour, about 15 minutes longer for trimethobenzamide hydrochloride 300 mg oral capsule than an IM injection. A single dose of trimethobenzamide hydrochloride 300 mg oral capsule provided a plasma concentration profile of trimethobenzamide similar to trimethobenzamide hydrochloride 200 mg IM. The relative bioavailability of the capsule formulation compared to the solution is 100%. The mean elimination half-life of trimethobenzamide is 7 to 9 hours.

Contraindications

Pediatric patients; hypersensitivity to trimethobenzamide.

Warnings

➤*Reye's syndrome:* Reye's syndrome has been associated with the use of trimethobenzamide hydrochloride and other drugs, including antiemetics, although their contribution, if any, to the cause and course of the disease has not been established. This syndrome is characterized by an abrupt onset shortly following a nonspecific febrile illness, with persistent, severe vomiting, lethargy, irrational behavior, progressive encephalopathy leading to coma, convulsions, and death.

➤*Pregnancy: Category C.* Trimethobenzamide hydrochloride was studied in reproduction experiments in rats and rabbits and no teratogenicity was suggested. The only effects observed were an increased percentage of embryonic resorptions or stillborn pups in rats administered 20 mg and 100 mg/kg and increased resorptions in rabbits receiving 100 mg/kg. In each study these adverse effects were attributed to 1 or 2 dams. The relevance to humans is not known. Since there is no adequate experience in pregnant women who have received this drug, safety in pregnancy has not been established.

➤*Lactation:* Since there is no adequate experience in lactating women who have received this drug, safety in nursing mothers has not been established.

➤*Children:* Caution should be exercised when administering trimethobenzamide hydrochloride to children for the treatment of vomiting. Antiemetics are not recommended for treatment of uncomplicated vomiting in children and their use should be limited to prolonged vomiting of known etiology. There are 3 principal reasons for caution:

1.) There has been some suspicion that centrally acting antiemetics may contribute, in combination with viral illnesses (a possible cause of vomiting in pediatric patients), to development of Reye's syndrome, a potentially fatal acute childhood encephalopathy with visceral fatty degeneration, especially involving the liver. Although there is no confirmation of this suspicion, caution is nevertheless recommended.
2.) The extrapyramidal symptoms which can occur secondary to trimethobenzamide hydrochloride may be confused with the central nervous system signs of an undiagnosed primary disease responsible for the vomiting (eg, Reye's syndrome or other encephalopathy).
3.) It has been suspected that drugs with hepatotoxic potential, such as trimethobenzamide hydrochloride, may unfavorably alter the course of Reye's syndrome. Such drugs should therefore be avoided in pediatric patients whose signs and symptoms (vomiting) could represent Reye's syndrome. It should also be noted that salicylates and acetaminophen are hepatotoxic at large doses. Although it is not known that at usual doses they would represent a hazard in patients with the underlying hepatic disorder of Reye's syndrome, these drugs, too, should be avoided in pediatric patients whose signs and symptoms could represent Reye's syndrome, unless alternative methods of controlling fever are not successful.

Precautions

➤*Special risk:* The antiemetic effects of trimethobenzamide hydrochloride may render diagnosis more difficult in such conditions as appendicitis and obscure signs of toxicity due to overdosage of other drugs.

During the course of acute febrile illness, encephalitides, gastroenteritis, dehydration and electrolyte imbalance, especially in children and the elderly or debilitated, CNS reactions such as opisthotonos, convulsions, coma and extrapyramidal symptoms have been reported with and without use of trimethobenzamide hydrochloride or other antiemetic agents. In such disorders, caution should be exercised in administering trimethobenzamide hydrochloride, particularly to patients who recently received other CNS-acting agents (phenothiazines, barbiturates, belladonna derivatives). It is recommended that severe emesis should not be treated with an antiemetic drug alone; where possible the cause of vomiting should be established. Primary emphasis should be directed toward the restoration of body fluids and electrolyte balance, the relief of fever and relief of the causative disease process. Overhydration should be avoided since it may result in cerebral edema.

➤*Hazardous tasks:* Trimethobenzamide hydrochloride may produce drowsiness. Patients should not operate motor vehicles or other dangerous machinery until their individual responses have been determined.

Drug Interactions

➤*Use with alcohol:* Concomitant use of alcohol with trimethobenzamide hydrochloride may result in an adverse drug interaction.

Adverse Reactions

There have been reports of hypersensitivity reactions and Parkinson-like symptoms. There have been instances of hypotension reported following parenteral administration to surgical patients. There have been reports of blood dyscrasias, blurring of vision, coma, convulsions, depression of mood, diarrhea, disorientation, dizziness, drowsiness, headache, jaundice, muscle cramps and opisthotonos. If these occur, the administration of the drug should be discontinued. Allergic-type skin reactions have been observed; therefore, the drug should be discontinued at the first sign of sensitization. While these symptoms will usually disappear spontaneously, symptomatic treatment may be indicated in some cases.

Indications

➤*Antiemetic:* Prevention of nausea and vomiting associated with initial and repeat courses of emetogenic cancer therapy, including high-dose cisplatin; prevention of postoperative nausea or vomiting (**ondansetron** and **dolasetron**); prevention of nausea and vomiting associated with radiotherapy in patients receiving either total body irradiation, single high-dose fraction, or daily fractions to the abdomen (oral **ondansetron** and **granisetron**); treatment of postoperative nausea or vomiting (IV **dolasetron**).

➤*Unlabeled uses:*

Granisetron – Acute nausea and vomiting following surgery (1 to 3 mg IV).

Dolasetron – Radiotherapy-induced nausea and vomiting (40 mg IV or 0.3 mg/kg IV).

Actions

➤*Pharmacology:* Selective 5-hydroxytryptamine$_3$ (5-HT_3) receptor antagonists are antinauseant and antiemetic agents with little or no affinity for other serotonin receptors, alpha- or beta-adrenergic, dopamine-D_2, histamine-H_1, benzodiazepine, picrotoxin, or opioid receptors.

Serotonin receptors of the 5-HT_3 type are located peripherally on vagal nerve terminals, enteric neurons in the GI tract, and centrally in the chemoreceptor trigger zone. During chemotherapy, mucosal enterochromaffin cells from the small intestine release serotonin, which stimulates the 5-HT_3 receptors. This evokes vagal afferent discharge, inducing vomiting. In IBS, it is presumed the pain, distension, and exaggerated motor response are at least in part caused by stimulation of the 5-HT_3 receptors.

5-HT_3 antagonists have little effect on blood pressure. **Ondansetron** and **granisetron** have little effect on heart rate or ECG. No evidence of an effect on plasma prolactin or aldosterone concentrations has been found. Ondansetron has no effect on esophageal and gastric motility, lower esophageal sphincter pressure or small intestinal transit time, cardiac output, and stroke volume. Multi day administration of ondansetron and oral granisetron have been shown to slow colonic transit.

➤*Pharmacokinetics:*

Distribution – Plasma protein binding is 65% for **granisetron** and 70% to 76% for **ondansetron**. Both drugs distribute into erythrocytes.

5-HT_3 Antagonist Pharmacokinetics

	Mean C_{max} (ng/ml)	Mean t½ (hr)	Mean Cl (L/hr/kg)	Mean V_d (L/kg)
IV				
Dolasetron				
Adults (100 mg)	320	7.3	0.564	5.8
Elderly[a] (2 to 4 mg/kg)	620	6.9	0.498	4.69
Cancer patients				
Adults	505	7.5	0.612	
Adolescents	562	5.5	0.75	
Children	505	4.4	1.152	≈ 5.2
Pediatric surgery	255	4.8	0.786	
Renal function impairment[b]	867	10.9	0.3	
Granisetron (single 40 mcg/kg dose)				
Adults	64	5	0.79	3
Elderly[c]	57	7.5	0.44	4
Cancer patients	84	9	0.38	3
Ondansetron (single 0.15 mg/kg dose)				
Adults	104	4.1	0.35	NA[e]
Elderly[d]	170	5.5	0.262	NA[e]
Cancer/Surgery	NA[e]	3.5	NA[e]	NA[e]
Oral				
Dolasetron				
Adults	556	8.1	0.804	5.8
Elderly[a]	662	7.2	0.57	5.63
Cancer patients				
Adults	NA[e]	7.9	0.774	
Adolescents	374	6.4	1.59	
Children	217	5.5	2.652	
Pediatric surgery	159	5.9	1.248	
Renal function impairment[b]	701	10.7	0.432	
Hepatic function impairment	410	11	0.528	
Granisetron				
Adults (single 1 mg dose)	3.6	6	0.41	4
Cancer patients (1 mg BID × 7 days)	6	NA[e]	0.52	NA[e]
Ondansetron (single 8 mg dose)				
Adults, male (female)	25 (47)	3.6 (4.2)	0.3935 (0.3045)	NA[e]
Elderly,[d] male (female)	37 (46)	4.5 (6)	0.277 (0.249)	NA[e]

[a] 65 to 75 years of age.
[b] Creatinine clearance ≤ 10 ml/min.
[c] ≥ 65 years of age.
[d] ≥ 75 years of age.
[e] NA = not available.

Special populations –
Gender: Plasma concentrations are 30% to 50% lower and less variable in men compared with women given the same oral dose.

Contraindications

Hypersensitivity to the drug or components of the product; markedly prolonged QTc or atrioventricular block II to III (**dolasetron**) (see Warnings); patients receiving class I or III antiarrhythmic agents (**dolasetron**) (see Warnings).

Warnings

➤*Postoperatively:* Routine prophylaxis is not recommended for patients in whom there is little expectation that nausea or vomiting will occur postoperatively. In patients in when nausea or vomiting must be avoided postoperatively, IV **ondansetron** is recommended even when the incidence of postoperative nausea or vomiting is low. For patients who have postoperative nausea or vomiting, ondansetron may be given to prevent further episodes.

➤*Cardiac effects:* Acute, usually reversible, ECG changes (PR and QTc prolongation; QRS widening) caused by **dolasetron** have been observed in healthy volunteers and controlled clinical trials. The active metabolites of dolasetron may block sodium channels, a property unrelated to its ability to block 5-HT_3 receptors. QTc prolongation is primarily caused by QRS widening. Dolasetron appears to prolong both depolarization and, to a lesser extent, repolarization time. The magnitude and frequency of the ECG changes increased with dose (related to peak plasma concentrations of hydrodolasetron but not the parent compound). These ECG interval prolongations usually returned to baseline within 6 to 8 hours, but in some patients were present at 24-hour follow up.

Administer dolasetron with caution in patients who have or may develop prolongation of cardiac conduction intervals, particularly QTc. These include patients with hypokalemia or hypomagnesemia, patients taking diuretics with the potential for inducing electrolyte abnormalities, patients with congenital QT syndrome, patients taking antiarrhythmic drugs or other drugs that lead to QT prolongation, and cumulative high-dose anthracycline therapy.

➤*Peristalsis:* **Ondansetron** does not stimulate gastric or intestinal peristalsis. Do not use instead of nasogastric suction. Use in abdominal surgery may mask a progressive ileus or gastric distension.

➤*Hypersensitivity reactions:* Rare cases of hypersensitivity reactions, sometimes severe (eg, anaphylaxis, bronchospasm, shortness of breath, hypotension, shock, angioedema, urticaria, facial edema) have occurred. Refer to Management of Acute Hypersensitivity Reactions.

➤*Carcinogenesis:* Rats were treated orally with **granisetron** 1, 5, or 50 mg/kg/day (16, 81, and 405 times the recommended human clinical dose). There was a statistically significant increase in the incidence of hepatocellular carcinomas and adenomas. Treatment with granisetron 100 mg/kg/day (1622 times the recommended human dose) produced hepatocellular adenomas in male and female rats.

In a 24-month carcinogenicity study, there was a statistically significant increase in the incidence of combined hepatocellular adenomas and carcinomas in male mice treated with ≥ 150 mg/kg/day (≥ 6.8 times the recommended dose).

Granisetron produced a significant increase in UDS in HeLa cells in vitro and a significantly increased incidence of cells with polyploidy in an in vitro human lymphocyte chromosomal aberration test.

➤*Elderly:* Dosage adjustment is not needed in patients > 65 years of age. Prevention of nausea and vomiting in elderly patients was no different than in younger age groups.

➤*Pregnancy: Category B.* There are no adequate and well-controlled studies in pregnant women. Use during pregnancy only if the potential benefit justifies the potential risk to the fetus.

➤*Lactation:* **Ondansetron** is excreted in the breast milk of rats. It is not known whether 5-HT_3 antagonists are excreted in human breast milk. Exercise caution when 5-HT_3 antagonists are administered to a nursing woman.

➤*Children:*

Granisetron – Safety and efficacy of the injection in children < 2 years of age have not been established. See Administration and Dosage for use in children ≥ 2 years of age.Safety and efficacy of the oral doseform in children have not been established.

Ondansetron – Little information is available about dosage in children ≤ 3 years of age. See Administration and Dosage for use in children 4 to 18 years of age.

Dolasetron – Safety and efficacy in children < 2 years of age have not been established. See Administration and Dosage for use in children ≥ 2 years of age.

Precautions

➤*Benzyl alcohol:* Some of these products contain benzyl alcohol, which has been associated with a fatal "gasping syndrome" in premature infants.

Drug Interactions

Because 5-HT_3 antagonists are metabolized by hepatic cytochrome P450 enzymes, inducers or inhibitors of these enzymes may change the clearance and, hence, the half-life of 5-HT_3 antagonists. However, on the basis of available data, no dosage adjustment is recommended for patients on these drugs.

5-HT_3 Receptor Antagonist Drug Interactions			
Precipitant drug	Object drug*		Description
Atenolol	Dolasetron	↑	Clearance of hydrodolasetron decreased by ≈ 27% when dolasetron was administered IV concomitantly with atenolol.
Cimetidine	Dolasetron	↑	Blood levels of hydrodolasetron increased 24% when dolasetron was coadministered with cimetidine for 7 days.
Rifampin	Dolasetron	↓	Blood levels of hydrodolasetron decreased 28% with coadministration of rifampin for 7 days.
Rifampin	Ondansetron	↓	Plasma concentrations of ondansetron may be reduced, decreasing its antiemetic effect.

* ↑ = Object drug increased. ↓ = Object drug decreased.

➤*Drug/Food interactions:*

Granisetron – When a single dose of oral granisetron 10 mg was administered with food, AUC was decreased by 5% and C_{max} increased by 30% in non-fasting healthy volunteers.

Ondansetron – The extent of absorption of oral ondansetron is significantly increased (≈ 17%) by food but is not believed to be clinically relevant. C_{max} and T_{max} are not significantly affected.

Adverse Reactions

5-HT_3 Receptor Antagonist Adverse Reactions[a] (%)			
Adverse event	Dolasetron	Granisetron	Ondansetron
Cardiovascular			
Hypertension	2.2 to 2.9	2	2.5
Bradycardia	4 to 5.1	-	-
Tachycardia	2.2 to 3	-	-
Hypotension	5.3	-	3 to 5
CNS			
Anxiety/Agitation	-	-	6
Dizziness	2.2 to 4.4	-	7
Drowsiness/Sedation	1.3 to 2.4[b]	-	8
Headache	7 to 24.3[b]	14 to 21	9 to 27[c,d]
Malaise/Fatigue	2.6 to 5.7	-	9 to 13
Chills/Shivering	1.3 to 2.2	5	7
GI			
Abdominal pain	3.2	6	3[c]
Constipation	-	18	6 to 9
Diarrhea	2.1 to 12.4	8	6
Xerostomia	-	-	2
Dyspepsia	2.2 to 3	-	-
Miscellaneous			
Asthenia	-	14	-
Cold sensation	-	-	2
Fever/Pyrexia	3.5 to 4.3	-	2 to 8
Gynecological disorder	-	-	7
Hypoxia	-	-	9
Injection site reaction	-	-	4
Paresthesia	-	-	2
Pruritus	3.1	-	2 to 5
Urinary retention	2[b]	-	5
Weakness	-	-	2[c]
Increase in AST and ALT	3.6	3.4	3.4
Pain	0 to 3.1	2	2
Oliguria	2.6	-	-

[a] Greater than placebo or comparator regardless of route of administration or indication. Data from separate studies; not necessarily comparable.
[b] More common in placebo.
[c] More common with PO tid vs bid dosing.
[d] More common with single high dose IV.

➤*Cardiovascular:*

Ondansetron – Arrhythmias (6%); hypotension (3% to 5%); chest pain (2%); angina, syncope (rare).

Granisetron – Hypertension (2%); angina, arrhythmias, syncope (rare).

Dolasetron – Hypotension; edema, peripheral edema, mobitz I AV block, chest pain, orthostatic hypotension, myocardial ischemia, syncope, severe bradycardia, palpitations, peripheral ischemia, thrombophlebitis/phlebitis (rare); bradycardia; tachycardia; T-wave change; ST-T wave change; sinus arrhythmia; extrasystole (APCs or VPCs); poor R-wave progression; bundle branch block (left and right); nodal arrhythmia; U wave change; atrial flutter/fibrillation. (See Warnings).

➤*CNS:*

Ondansetron – Extrapyramidal syndrome (6%); grand mal seizures (rare).

Granisetron – CNS stimulation; somnolence (3% to 5%); insomnia (< 2% to 3%); extrapyramidal syndrome (rare).

Dolasetron – Flushing; vertigo; paresthesia; tremor; agitation; sleep disorder; depersonalization; ataxia, twitching, confusion, anxiety, abnormal dreaming (rare).

➤*Dermatologic:*

Dolasetron – Rash; increased sweating.

➤*GI:*

Granisetron – Nausea (15%); vomiting (9%); decreased appetite (5%); taste disorder (2%).

Dolasetron – Constipation; dyspepsia; abdominal pain; anorexia; pancreatitis (rare).

➤*GU:*

Dolasetron – Dysuria, polyuria, acute renal failure (rare).

➤*Hematologic:*

Granisetron – Leukopenia (11%); anemia (4%); thrombocytopenia (3%).

Dolasetron – Hematuria, epistaxis, prolonged prothrombin time, PTT increased, anemia, purpura/hematoma, thrombocytopenia (rare).

Ondansetron – Hypokalemia (rare).

➤*Hepatic:*

Dolasetron – Transient increases in AST and ALT (< 1%); hyperbilirubinemia, increased GGT (rare).

➤*Hypersensitivity:*

Dolasetron – Anaphylactic reaction, facial edema, urticaria (rare).

➤*Lab test abnormalities:*

Dolasetron – Transient increases in AST or ALT values have been reported as adverse events in < 1% of adult patients receiving dolasetron in clinical trials. The increases did not appear to be related to dose or duration of therapy nor associated with symptomatic hepatic disease.

➤*Metabolic/Nutritional:*

Dolasetron – Increased alkaline phosphatase (rare).

➤*Musculoskeletal:*

Ondansetron – Musculoskeletal pain (10%).

Dolasetron – Myalgia, arthralgia (rare).

➤*Respiratory:*

Ondansetron – Bronchospasm (rare).

Dolasetron – Dyspnea, bronchospasm (rare).

➤*Special senses:*

Ondansetron – Transient blurred vision (rare).

Dolasetron – Taste perversion; abnormal vision; tinnitus, photophobia (rare).

➤*Miscellaneous:*

Ondansetron – Wound problem (28%); shivers (7%); postoperative CO_2-related pain (2%); hypersensitivity (rare).

Granisetron – Shivers (5%); alopecia (3%); hypersensitivity (rare).

Overdosage

➤*Symptoms:* A 59-year-old man with metastatic melanoma developed severe hypotension and dizziness 40 minutes after receiving a 15-minute IV infusion of 1000 mg (13 mg/kg) of **dolasetron**.

"Sudden blindness" (amaurosis) of a 2- to 3-minute duration plus severe constipation occurred in one patient who was given a single 72 mg IV dose of **ondansetron**. Hypotension and faintness occurred in a patient who took 48 mg ondansetron orally. Following the infusion of a 32 mg dose of ondansetron over only a 4-minute period, a vasovagal episode with transient second-degree heart block was observed. In all instances, the events completely resolved. Individual doses as large as 145 mg and total daily dosages (3 doses) as large as 252 mg have been administered IV without significant adverse events. Overdosage of up to 38.5 mg **granisetron** injection has been reported without symptoms or with only the occurrence of a slight headache.

➤*Treatment:* Manage patients with appropriate supportive therapy. Following a suspected overdose of **dolasetron** injection, a patient found to have second-degree or higher AV conduction block should undergo cardiac telemetry monitoring. Refer to General Management of Acute Overdosage.

PALONOSETRON HYDROCHLORIDE

Rx	**Aloxi** (MGI Pharma)	**Injection:** 0.25 mg/5 mL (as base)	207.5 mg mannitol. In single-use vials.

PALONOSETRON HYDROCHLORIDE — INJECTION

For complete and comparative prescribing information, refer to the 5-HT_3 Receptor Antagonists group monograph.

Indications

Palonosetron HCl injection is indicated for the prevention of acute nausea and vomiting associated with initial and repeat courses of moderately and highly emetogenic cancer chemotherapy, and for the prevention of delayed nausea and vomiting associated with initial and repeat courses of moderately emetogenic cancer chemotherapy.

Administration and Dosage

➤*Approved by the FDA:* July 25, 2003.

➤*Dosage for adults:* The recommended dosage of palonosetron HCl injection is 0.25 mg administered as a single dose approximately 30 minutes before the start of chemotherapy. Repeated dosing of palonosetron HCl injection within a 7-day interval is not recommended because the safety and efficacy of frequent (consecutive or alternate day) dosing in patients has not been evaluated.

➤*Use in geriatric patients and in patients with impaired renal or hepatic function:* No dosage adjustment is recommended.

➤*Dosage for pediatric patients:* A recommended intravenous dosage has not been established for pediatric patients.

➤*Administration:* Palonosetron HCl is to be infused intravenously over 30 seconds. Palonosetron HCl should not be mixed with other drugs. Flush the infusion line with normal saline before and after administration of palonosetron HCl injection.

➤*Storage/Stability:* Store at controlled room temperature 20° to 25°C (68° to 77°F). Excursions permitted to 15° to 30°C (59° to 86°F). Protect from freezing and light.

Stability – Parenteral drug products should be inspected visually for particulate matter and discoloration before administration, whenever solution and container permit.

DOLASETRON MESYLATE

Rx	**Anzemet** (Aventis)	**Tablets:** 50 mg	Lactose. (A 50). Pink. Film-coated. In 5s, blister-pack 5s, and UD 10s.
		100 mg	Lactose. (ANZEMET 100). Pink, oval. Film-coated. In 5s, blister-pack 5s, and UD 10s.
		Injection: 20 mg/mL	38.2 mg/mL mannitol. In single-use 0.625 mL amps, 0.625 mL fill in 2 mL *Carpuject*, single-use 5 mL vials, and 25 mL multi-dose vial.

DOLASETRON MESYLATE— ORAL

For complete and comparative prescribing information, refer to the 5-HT_3 Receptor Antagonists group monograph.

Indications

Dolasetron mesylate tablets are indicated for the prevention of nausea and vomiting associated with moderately emetogenic cancer chemotherapy, including initial and repeat courses, and for the prevention of postoperative nausea and vomiting.

➤*Unlabeled uses:* Radiotherapy-induced nausea and vomiting (40 mg IV or 0.3 mg/kg IV).

Administration and Dosage

➤*Approved by the FDA:* September 11, 1997.

The recommended doses of dolasetron mesylate tablets should not be exceeded.

➤*Prevention of cancer chemotherapy-induced nausea and vomiting:*

Adults – The recommended oral dose of dolasetron mesylate is 100 mg given within 1 hour before chemotherapy.

Children – The recommended oral dose in pediatric patients 2 to 16 years of age is 1.8 mg/kg given within 1 hour before chemotherapy, up to a maximum of 100 mg. Safety and efficacy in pediatric patients under 2 years of age have not been established.

Use in the elderly, in renal failure patients, or in hepatically impaired patients – No dosage adjustment is recommended.

➤*Prevention of postoperative nausea and vomiting:*

Adults – The recommended oral dosage of dolasetron mesylate is 100 mg within 2 hours before surgery.

Children – The recommended oral dosage in pediatric patients 2 to 16 years of age is 1.2 mg/kg given within 2 hours before surgery, up to a maximum of 100 mg. Safety and efficacy in pediatric patients under 2 years of age have not been established.

Use in the elderly, renal failure patients, or hepatically impaired patients – No dosage adjustment is recommended (see Pharmacokinetics).

➤*Storage/Stability:* Store at controlled room temperature 20° to 25°C (68° to 77°F). Protect from light.

DOLASETRON MESYLATE — INJECTION

For complete and comparative prescribing information, refer to the 5-HT_3 Receptor Antagonists group monograph.

Indications

Dolasetron mesylate injection is indicated for the following:

1.) The prevention of nausea and vomiting associated with initial and repeat courses of emetogenic cancer chemotherapy, including high dose cisplatin.
2.) The prevention of postoperative nausea and vomiting. As with other antiemetics, routine prophylaxis is not recommended for patients in whom there is little expectation that nausea or vomiting will occur postoperatively. In patients where nausea or vomiting must be avoided postoperatively, dolasetron mesylate injection is recommended even where the incidence of postoperative nausea or vomiting is low.
3.) The treatment of postoperative nausea or vomiting.

Administration and Dosage

➤*Approved by the FDA:* September 11, 1997.

The recommended dose of dolasetron mesylate injection should not be exceeded.

➤*Prevention of cancer chemotherapy-induced nausea and vomiting:*

Adults – The recommended IV dosage of dolasetron mesylate injection from clinical trial results is 1.8 mg/kg given as a single dose approximately 30 minutes before chemotherapy (see Administration). Alternatively, for most patients, a fixed dose of 100 mg can be administered over 30 seconds.

Children – The recommended IV dosage in pediatric patients 2 to 16 years of age is 1.8 mg/kg given as a single dose approximately 30 minutes before chemotherapy, up to a maximum of 100 mg (see Administration). Safety and effectiveness in pediatric patients under 2 years of age have not been established.

Dolasetron mesylate injection mixed in apple or apple-grape juice may be used for oral dosing of pediatric patients. When dolasetron mesylate injection is administered orally, the recommended dosage in pediatric patients 2 to 16 years of age is 1.8 mg/kg up to a maximum 100 mg dose given within 1 hour before chemotherapy.

The diluted product may be kept up to 2 hours at room temperature before use.

➤*Prevention or treatment of postoperative nausea or vomiting:*

Adults – The recommended IV dosage of dolasetron mesylate injection is 12.5 mg given as a single dose approximately 15 minutes before the cessation of anesthesia (prevention) or as soon as nausea or vomiting presents (treatment).

Children – The recommended IV dosage in pediatric patients 2 to 16 years of age is 0.35 mg/kg, with a maximum dose of 12.5 mg, given as a single dose approximately 15 minutes before the cessation of anesthesia or as soon as nausea or vomiting presents.

Safety and effectiveness in pediatric patients under 2 years of age have not been established.

Dolasetron mesylate injection mixed in apple or apple-grape juice may be used for oral dosing of pediatric patients. When dolasetron mesylate injection is administered orally, the recommended oral dosage in pediatric patients 2 to 16 years of age is 1.2 mg/kg up to a maximum 100 mg dose given within 2 hours before surgery. The diluted product may be kept up to 2 hours at room temperature before use.

➤*Use in the elderly, in renal failure patients, or in hepatically impaired patients:* No dosage adjustment is recommended.

➤*Administration:* Dolasetron mesylate injection can be safely infused intravenously as rapidly as 100 mg/30 seconds or diluted in a compatible IV solution to 50 mL and infused over a period of up to 15 minutes. Dolasetron mesylate injection should not be mixed with other drugs. Flush the infusion line before and after administration of dolasetron mesylate injection.

Parenteral drug products should be inspected visually for particulate matter and discoloration before administration whenever solution and container permit.

DOLASETRON MESYLATE — INJECTION

➤*Storage / Stability:*

Storage – Store at 20° to 25°C (68° to 77°F) with excursions permitted to 15° to 30°C (59° to 86°F). Protect from light.

Stability – After dilution, dolasetron mesylate injection is stable under normal lighting conditions at room temperature for 24 hours or under refrigeration for 48 hours with the following compatible IV fluids: 0.9% sodium chloride injection, 5% dextrose injection, 5% dextrose, and 0.45% sodium chloride injection, 5% dextrose and Lactated Ringer's injection, Lactated Ringer's injection, and 10% mannitol injection. Although dolasetron mesylate injection is chemically and physically stable when diluted as recommended, sterile precautions should be observed because diluents generally do not contain preservative. After dilution, do not use beyond 24 hours, or 48 hours if refrigerated.

Parenteral drug products should be inspected visually for particulate matter and discoloration before administration whenever solution and container permit.

GRANISETRON HYDROCHLORIDE

Rx	**Kytril** (Roche)	**Tablets**: 1 mg (1.12 mg as hydrochloride)	Lactose. (K1). White, triangular. Film-coated. In SUP 20s and unit-of-use 2s.
		Oral solution: 1 mg/5 mL (1.12 mg per 5 mL as hydrochloride)	Sorbitol. Orange flavor. In 30 mL.
		Injection: 1 mg/mL (1.12 mg/mL as hydrochloride)	10 mg benzyl alcohol and 9 mg sodium chloride per mL. In 1 mL single-dose and 4 mL multi-dose vials.

GRANISETRON HYDROCHLORIDE — ORAL

For complete and comparative prescribing information, refer to the 5-HT_3 Receptor Antagonists group monograph.

Indications

➤*Antiemetic:* Prevention of nausea and/or vomiting associated with initial and repeat courses of emetogenic cancer therapy, including high-dose cisplatin.

Nausea and vomiting associated with radiation, including total body irradiation and fractionated abdominal radiation.

Administration and Dosage

➤*Approved by the FDA:* March 16, 1995.

➤*Emetogenic chemotherapy:* Adult dosage of 2 mg once daily or 1 mg twice daily. In the 2 mg once-daily regimen, two 1 mg tablets or 10 mL of oral solution are given up to 1 hour before chemotherapy. In the 1 mg twice-daily regimen, give the first 1 mg tablet or 1 teaspoonful (5 mL) of oral solution up to 1 hour before chemotherapy and the second tablet or second teaspoonful (5 mL) oral solution 12 hours after the first. Either regimen is administered only on the day(s) chemotherapy is given. Continued treatment while not on chemotherapy has not been found to be useful.

➤*Radiation (total body irradiation or fractionated abdominal radiation):* Adult dose of 2 mg once daily. Two 1 mg tablets or 10 mL of oral solution are taken within 1 hour of radiation.

➤*Storage / Stability:* Keep tightly closed. Protect from light.

Tablets – Store between 15° to 30°C (59° to 86°F).

Oral solution – Store at 25°C (77°F); excursions permitted to 15° to 30°C (59° to 86°F). Store bottle in an upright position.

GRANISETRON HYDROCHLORIDE — INJECTION

Indications

➤*Antiemetic:* For the prevention of nausea and vomiting associated with initial and repeat courses of emetogenic cancer therapy, including high-dose cisplatin.

➤*Postoperative nausea and vomiting:* For the prevention and treatment of postoperative nausea and vomiting. As with other antiemetics, routine prophylaxis is not recommended in patients in whom there is little expectation that nausea or vomiting will occur postoperatively. In patients where nausea or vomiting must be avoided during the postoperative period, granisetron injection is recommended even where the incidence of postoperative nausea or vomiting is low.

Administration and Dosage

➤*Approved by the FDA:* March 11, 1994.

➤*Note:* Granisetron injection 1 mg/mL contains benzyl alcohol.

➤*Prevention of chemotherapy-induced nausea and vomiting:* The recommended dosage for granisetron injection is 10 mcg/kg administered intravenously (IV) within 30 minutes before initiation of chemotherapy, and only on the day(s) chemotherapy is given.

Infusion preparation – Granisetron injection may be administered IV undiluted over 30 seconds, or diluted with 0.9% sodium chloride or 5% dextrose and infused over 5 minutes.

Children – The recommended dose in children 2 to 16 years of age is 10 mcg/kg. Children younger than 2 years of age have not been studied.

Elderly, renal / hepatic function impairment – No dosage adjustment is recommended.

➤*Prevention and treatment of postoperative nausea and vomiting:* The recommended dosage for prevention of postoperative nausea and vomiting is granisetron 1 mg, undiluted, administered IV over 30 seconds, before induction of anesthesia or immediately before reversal of anesthesia.

The recommended dosage for the treatment of nausea or vomiting after surgery is granisetron 1 mg, undiluted, administered IV over 30 seconds.

Children – Safety and efficacy of granisetron injection have not been established in children for the prevention or treatment of postoperative nausea or vomiting.

Elderly, renal / hepatic function impairment – No dosage adjustment is recommended.

Incompatibilities – As a general precaution, do not mix granisetron injection in a solution with other drugs.

➤*Storage / Stability:* Prepare IV infusion of granisetron injection at the time of administration. However, granisetron injection has been shown to be stable for at least 24 hours when diluted in 0.9% sodium chloride or 5% dextrose and stored at room temperature under normal lighting conditions.

Visually inspect parenteral drug products for particulate matter and discoloration before administration whenever solution and container permit.

Store single- and multi-use vials at 25°C (77°F); excursions permitted to 15° to 30°C (59° to 86°F).

Once the multi-use vial is penetrated, use its contents within 30 days.

Do not freeze. Protect from light.

ONDANSETRON HYDROCHLORIDE

Rx	**Zofran** (GlaxoSmithKline)	**Tablets**: 4 mg (as HCl dihydrate)	Lactose. (Zofran 4). White, oval. Film-coated. In 30s, UD 100s, and 1 × 3 daily UD packs.
		8 mg (as HCl dihydrate)	Lactose. (Zofran 8). Yellow, oval. Film-coated. In 30s, UD 100s, and 1 × 3 daily UD packs.
		24 mg (as HCl dihydrate)	Lactose. (GX CF7/24). Pink, oval. Film-coated. In 1 × 1 daily UD packs.
		Solution, oral: 4 mg/5 mL (5 mg as HCl dihydrate)	Sorbitol. Strawberry flavor. In 50 mL bottles.
		Injection: 2 mg/mL (as HCl dihydrate)	Parabens. In 2 mL single-dose vials and 20 mL multidose vials (singles).
		32 mg/50 mL (as HCl dihydrate) (premixed)	Preservative-free. 2500 mg dextrose, 26 mg citric acid, and 11.5 mg sodium citrate/50 mL. In 50 mL single-dose containers.
Rx	**Zofran ODT** (GlaxoSmithKline)	**Tablets, orally disintegrating**: 4 mg (as base)	< 0.03 mg phenylalanine, aspartame, mannitol, parabens. (Z4). White. Strawberry flavor. In UD 30s.
		8 mg (as base)	< 0.03 mg phenylalanine, aspartame, mannitol, parabens. (Z8). White. Strawberry flavor. In UD 10s and 30s.

ONDANSETRON — ORAL

For complete and comparative prescribing information, refer to the 5-HT_3 Receptor Antagonists group monograph.

Indications

Prevention of nausea and vomiting associated with highly emetogenic cancer chemotherapy, including cisplatin ≥ 50 mg/m².

Prevention of nausea and vomiting associated with initial and repeat courses of moderately emetogenic cancer chemotherapy.

Prevention of nausea and vomiting associated with radiotherapy in patients receiving either total body irradiation, single high-dose fraction to the abdomen, or daily fractions to the abdomen.

Prevention of postoperative nausea or vomiting. As with other antiemetics, routine prophylaxis is not recommended for patients in whom there is little expectation that nausea or vomiting will occur postoperatively. In patients where nausea or vomiting must be avoided postoperatively, ondansetron tablets, ondansetron orally disintegrating tablets, and ondansetron oral solution are recommended even where the incidence of postoperative nausea or vomiting is low.

Administration and Dosage

➤*Approved by the FDA:* December 31, 1992.

➤*Instructions for use / handling of ondansetron orally disintegrating tablets:* Do not attempt to push ondansetron orally disintegrating tablets through the foil backing. With dry hands, peel back the foil backing of 1 blister and gently remove the tablet. Immediately place the ondansetron orally disintegrating tablet on top of the tongue where it will dissolve in seconds, then swallow with saliva. Administration with liquid is not necessary.

➤*Prevention of nausea and vomiting associated with highly emetogenic cancer chemotherapy:* The recommended adult oral dosage of ondansetron is a single 24 mg tablet administered 30 minutes before the start of single-day highly emetogenic chemotherapy, including cisplatin ≥ 50 mg/m². Multiday, single-dose administration of ondansetron 24 mg tablets has not been studied.

Pediatric use – There is no experience with the use of 24 mg ondansetron tablets in children.

Geriatric use – The dosage recommendation is the same as for the general population.

➤*Prevention of nausea and vomiting associated with moderately emetogenic cancer chemotherapy:* The recommended adult oral dosage is one 8 mg ondansetron tablet or one 8 mg ondansetron orally disintegrating tablet or 10 mL (2 teaspoonfuls equivalent to 8 mg of ondansetron) of ondansetron oral solution given twice a day. The first dose should be administered 30 minutes before the start of emetogenic chemotherapy, with a subsequent dose 8 hours after the first dose. One 8 mg ondansetron tablet or one 8 mg ondansetron orally disintegrating tablet or 10 mL (2 teaspoonfuls equivalent to 8 mg of ondansetron) of ondansetron oral solution should be administered twice a day (every 12 hours) for 1 to 2 days after completion of chemotherapy.

Pediatric use – For patients ≥ 12 years of age, the dosage is the same as for adults. For patients 4 through 11 years of age, the dosage is one 4 mg ondansetron tablet or one 4 mg ondansetron orally disintegrating tablet or 5 mL (1 teaspoonful equivalent to 4 mg of ondansetron) of ondansetron oral solution given 3 times a day. The first dose should be administered 30 minutes before the start of emetogenic chemotherapy, with subsequent doses 4 and 8 hours after the first dose. One 4 mg ondansetron tablet or one 4 mg ondansetron orally disintegrating tablet or 5 mL (1 teaspoonful equivalent to 4 mg of ondansetron) of ondansetron oral solution should be administered 3 times a day (every 8 hours) for 1 to 2 days after completion of chemotherapy.

Geriatric use – The dosage is the same as for the general population.

➤*Prevention of nausea and vomiting associated with radiotherapy, either total body irradiation, or single high-dose fraction or daily fractions to the abdomen:* The recommended oral dosage is one 8 mg ondansetron tablet or one 8 mg ondansetron orally disintegrating tablet or 10 mL (2 teaspoonfuls equivalent to 8 mg of ondansetron) of ondansetron oral solution given 3 times a day.

For total body irradiation, one 8 mg ondansetron tablet or one 8 mg ondansetron orally disintegrating tablet or 10 mL (2 teaspoonfuls equivalent to 8 mg of ondansetron) of ondansetron oral solution should be administered 1 to 2 hours before each fraction of radiotherapy administered each day.

For single high-dose fraction radiotherapy to the abdomen, one 8 mg ondansetron tablet or one 8 mg ondansetron orally disintegrating tablet or 10 mL (2 teaspoonfuls equivalent to 8 mg of ondansetron) of ondansetron oral solution should be administered 1 to 2 hours before radiotherapy, with subsequent doses every 8 hours after the first dose for 1 to 2 days after completion of radiotherapy.

For daily fractionated radiotherapy to the abdomen, one 8 mg ondansetron tablet or one 8 mg ondansetron orally disintegrating tablet or 10 mL (2 teaspoonfuls equivalent to 8 mg of ondansetron) of ondansetron oral solution should be administered 1 to 2 hours before radiotherapy, with subsequent doses every 8 hours after the first dose for each day radiotherapy is given.

Pediatric use – There is no experience with the use of ondansetron tablets, ondansetron orally disintegrating tablets, or ondansetron oral solution in the prevention of radiation-induced nausea and vomiting in children.

Geriatric use – The dosage recommendation is the same as for the general population.

➤*Postoperative nausea and vomiting:* The recommended dosage is 16 mg given as two 8 mg ondansetron tablets or two 8 mg ondansetron orally disintegrating tablets or 20 mL (4 teaspoonfuls equivalent to 16 mg of ondansetron) of ondansetron oral solution 1 hour before induction of anesthesia.

Pediatric use – There is no experience with the use of ondansetron tablets, ondansetron orally disintegrating tablets, or ondansetron oral solution in the prevention of postoperative nausea and vomiting in children.

Geriatric use – The dosage is the same as for the general population.

➤*Dosage adjustment for patients with impaired renal function:* The dosage recommendation is the same as for the general population. There is no experience beyond first-day administration of ondansetron.

➤*Dosage adjustment for patients with impaired hepatic function:* In patients with severe hepatic impairment according to Child-Pugh criteria, clearance is reduced, apparent volume of distribution is increased with a resultant increase in plasma half-life, and bioavailability approaches 100%. In such patients, a total daily dose of 8 mg should not be exceeded.

➤*Storage / Stability:*

Tablets – Store between 2° and 30°C (36° and 86°F). Protect from light. Store blisters and bottles in cartons.

Orally disintegrating tablets – Store between 2° and 30°C (36° and 86°F).

Oral solution – Store upright between 15° and 30°C (59° and 86°F). Protect from light. Store bottles upright in cartons.

ONDANSETRON — INJECTION

For complete and comparative prescribing information, refer to the 5-HT_3 Receptor Antagonists group monograph.

Indications

Prevention of nausea and vomiting associated with initial and repeat courses of emetogenic cancer chemotherapy, including high-dose cisplatin. Efficacy of the 32 mg single dose beyond 24 hours in these patients has not been established.

Prevention of postoperative nausea or vomiting. As with other antiemetics, routine prophylaxis is not recommended for patients in whom there is little expectation that nausea or vomiting will occur postoperatively. In patients where nausea or vomiting must be avoided postoperatively, ondansetron injection is recommended even where the incidence of postoperative nausea or vomiting is low. For patients who do not receive prophylactic ondansetron injection and experience nausea or vomiting postoperatively, ondansetron injection may be given to prevent further episodes.

Administration and Dosage

➤*Approved by the FDA:* January 4, 1991.

➤*Prevention of chemotherapy-induced nausea and vomiting:* The recommended IV dosage of ondansetron is a single 32 mg dose or three 0.15 mg/kg doses. A single 32 mg dose is infused over 15 minutes beginning 30 minutes before the start of emetogenic chemotherapy. The recommended infusion rate should not be exceeded. With the 3-dose (0.15 mg/kg) regimen, the first dose is infused over 15 minutes beginning 30 minutes before the start of emetogenic chemotherapy. Subsequent doses (0.15 mg/kg) are administered 4 and 8 hours after the first dose of ondansetron.

Ondansetron injection should not be mixed with solutions for which physical and chemical compatibility have not been established. In particular, this applies to alkaline solutions as a precipitate may form.

Vial – Dilute before use. Ondansetron injection should be diluted in 50 mL of 5% Dextrose Injection or 0.9% Sodium Chloride Injection before administration.

Flexible plastic container – Ondansetron injection premixed, 32 mg in 5% Dextrose, 50 mL, requires no dilution.

Children – On the basis of the limited available information, the dosage in children 4 to 18 years of age should be three 0.15 mg/kg doses (see above). Little information is available about dosage in children ≤ 3 years of age.

Elderly – The dosage recommendation is the same as for the general population.

➤*Prevention of postoperative nausea and vomiting:* The recommended IV dosage of ondansetron for adults is 4 mg undiluted administered intravenously in not less than 30 seconds, preferably over 2 to 5 minutes, immediately before induction of anesthesia, or postoperatively if the patient experiences nausea or vomiting occurring shortly after surgery. Alternatively, 4 mg undiluted may be administered IM as a single injection for adults. While recommended as a fixed dose for patients weighing > 40 kg, few patients above 80 kg have been studied. In patients who do not achieve adequate control of postoperative nausea and vomiting following a single, prophylactic, preinduction, IV dose of ondansetron 4 mg, administration of a second IV dose of 4 mg ondansetron postoperatively does not provide additional control of nausea and vomiting.

Vial – Ondansetron injection requires no dilution for administration for postoperative nausea and vomiting.

Children – The recommended IV dosage of ondansetron for children (2 to 12 years of age) is a single 0.1 mg/kg dose for children weighing < 40 kg, or a single 4 mg dose for children weighing > 40 kg. The rate of administration

ONDANSETRON — INJECTION

should not be less than 30 seconds, preferably over 2 to 5 minutes. Little information is available about dosage in children < 2 years of age.

Elderly – The dosage recommendation is the same as for the general population.

➤*Dosage adjustment for patients with impaired renal function:* The dosage recommendation is the same as for the general population. There is no experience beyond first-day administration of ondansetron.

➤*Dosage adjustment for patients with impaired hepatic function:* In patients with severe hepatic impairment according to Child-Pugh criteria, a single maximal daily dose of 8 mg to be infused over 15 minutes beginning 30 minutes before the start of the emetogenic chemotherapy is recommended. There is no experience beyond first-day administration of ondansetron.

➤*Ondansetron injection premixed in flexible plastic containers:*

Instructions for use – To open, tear outer wrap at notch and remove solution container. Check for minute leaks by squeezing container firmly. If leaks are found, discard unit as sterility may be impaired.

Preparation for administration – Use aseptic technique.

1.) Close flow control clamp of administration set.
2.) Remove cover from outlet port at bottom of container.
3.) Insert piercing pin of administration set into port with a twisting motion until the pin is firmly seated. See full directions on administration set carton.
4.) Suspend container from hanger.
5.) Squeeze and release drip chamber to establish proper fluid level in chamber during infusion of ondansetron injection premixed.
6.) Open flow control clamp to expel air from set. Close clamp.
7.) Attach set to venipuncture device. If device is not indwelling, prime and make venipuncture.
8.) Perform venipuncture.
9.) Regulate rate of administration with flow control clamp.

Caution – Ondansetron injection premixed in flexible plastic containers is to be administered by IV drip infusion only. Ondansetron injection premixed should not be mixed with solutions for which physical and chemical compatibility have not been established. In particular, this applies to alkaline solutions as a precipitate may form. If used with a primary IV fluid system, the primary solution should be discontinued during ondansetron injection premixed infusion.

Do not administer unless solution is clear and container is undamaged.

Warning – Do not use flexible plastic container in series connections.

➤*Precaution:* Occasionally, ondansetron precipitates at the stopper/vial interface in vials stored upright. Potency and safety are not affected. If a precipitate is observed, resolubilize by shaking the vial vigorously.

➤*Storage/Stability:*

Injection – Store between 2° and 30°C (36° and 86°F). Protect from light.

Premixed injection – Store between 2° and 30°C (36° and 86°F). Protect from light. Avoid excessive heat. Protect from freezing. Ondansetron injection is stable at room temperature under normal lighting conditions for 48 hours after dilution with the following IV fluids: 0.9% Sodium Chloride Injection, 5% Dextrose Injection, 5% Dextrose and Injection in 5% Dextrose and 0.9% Sodium Chloride Injection, 5% Dextrose and 0.45% Sodium Chloride Injection, and 3% Sodium Chloride Injection.

Although ondansetron injection is chemically and physically stable when diluted as recommended, sterile precautions should be observed because diluents generally do not contain preservative. After dilution, do not use beyond 24 hours.

Parenteral drug products should be inspected visually for particulate matter and discoloration before administration whenever solution and container permit.

ALOSETRON HYDROCHLORIDE

Rx	**Lotronex** (GlaxoSmithKline)	**Tablets:** 0.5 mg (as base)	Lactose (GX EX1). White, oval. Film-coated. In 30s.
		1 mg (as base)	Lactose. (GX CT1). Blue, oval. Film-coated. In 30s.

ALOSETRON HYDROCHLORIDE — ORAL

For complete prescribing information refer to the 5-HT_3 Receptor Antagonists group monograph.

WARNING

Infrequent but serious GI adverse reactions have been reported with the use of alosetron. These events, including ischemic colitis and serious complications of constipation, have resulted in hospitalization, and rarely, blood transfusion, surgery, and death.

- The prescribing program for alosetron was implemented to help reduce risks of serious GI adverse reactions. Only health care providers who have enrolled in GlaxoSmithKline's prescribing program for alosetron, based on their understanding of the benefits and risks, should prescribe alosetron.
- Alosetron is indicated only for women with severe diarrhea-predominant irritable bowel syndrome (IBS) who have failed to respond to conventional therapy. Before receiving the initial prescription for alosetron, the patient must read and sign the patient-physician agreement for alosetron.
- Discontinue alosetron immediately in patients who develop constipation or symptoms of ischemic colitis. Patients should immediately report constipation or symptoms of ischemic colitis to their health care provider. Do not resume alosetron in patients who develop ischemic colitis. Patients who have constipation should immediately contact their health care provider if the constipation does not resolve after alosetron is discontinued. Patients with resolved constipation should resume alosetron only on the advice of their treating health care provider.

Indications

➤*IBS:* Alosetron is indicated only for women with severe diarrhea-predominant IBS who have chronic IBS symptoms (generally lasting 6 months or longer), have had anatomic or biochemical abnormalities of the GI tract excluded, and have not responded adequately to conventional therapy.

Diarrhea-predominant IBS is severe if it includes diarrhea and 1 or more of the following: frequent and severe abdominal pain/discomfort, frequent bowel urgency or fecal incontinence, and/or disability or restriction of daily activities due to IBS.

Because of infrequent but serious GI adverse reactions associated with alosetron, the indication is restricted to those patients for whom the benefit-to-risk balance is most favorable.

Clinical studies have not been performed to adequately confirm the benefits of alosetron in men.

Administration and Dosage

➤*Approved by the FDA:* February 9, 2000.

➤*Prescribing program:* For safety reasons, only health care providers who enroll in the GlaxoSmithKline prescribing program for alosetron should prescribe alosetron.

➤*Adult dosage:* To lower the risk of constipation, alosetron should be started at a dosage of 0.5 mg twice a day. Patients well controlled on 0.5 mg twice a day may be maintained on this regimen. If, after 4 weeks, the 0.5 mg twice daily dosage is well tolerated but does not adequately control IBS symptoms, the dosage can be increased to up to 1 mg twice a day, the dosage used in controlled clinical trials.

Alosetron may be taken with or without food.

Discontinue therapy – Alosetron should be discontinued in patients who have not had adequate control of IBS symptoms after 4 weeks of treatment with 1 mg twice a day.

Alosetron should be discontinued immediately in patients who develop constipation or signs of ischemic colitis. Alosetron should not be restarted in patients who develop ischemic colitis.

➤*Special populations:* Clinical trial and postmarketing experience suggest that debilitated patients or patients taking additional medications that decrease GI motility may be at greater risk of serious complications of constipation. Therefore, appropriate caution and follow-up should be exercised if alosetron is prescribed for these patients.

➤*Pharmacists information:* Alosetron may be dispensed only on presentation of a prescription for alosetron with a sticker for the prescribing program for alosetron attached. A *MedGuide* for alosetron must be given to the patient each time alosetron is dispensed, as required by law. No telephone, facsimile, or computerized prescriptions are permitted with this program. Refills are permitted to be written on prescriptions.

➤*Storage/Stability:* Store at 25°C (77°F); excursions permitted to 15° to 30°C (59° to 86°F). Protect from light and moisture.

Miscellaneous

APREPITANT

Rx	**Emend** (Merck)	**Capsules:** 80 mg	Sucrose. (461 80 mg). White. In 30s and UD[1] 5s.
		125 mg	Sucrose. (462 125 mg). White/Pink. In 30s and UD[1] 5s.

[1] Unit of use tri-fold pack containing one 125 mg capsule and two 80 mg capsules.

APREPITANT — ORAL

Indications

➤*Prevention of nausea/vomiting associated with highly emetogenic cancer chemotherapy:* Aprepitant, in combination with other antiemetic agents, is indicated for the prevention of acute and delayed nausea and vomiting associated with initial and repeat courses of highly emetogenic cancer chemotherapy, including high-dose cisplatin.

➤*Prevention of nausea/vomiting associated with moderately emetogenic cancer chemotherapy:* Aprepitant, in combination with other antiemetic agents, is indicated for the prevention of nausea and vomiting associated with initial and repeat courses of moderately emetogenic cancer chemotherapy.

Administration and Dosage

➤*Approved by the FDA:* March 26, 2003.

➤*Dosage regimen:* Aprepitant is given for 3 days as part of a regimen that includes a corticosteroid and a 5-HT_3 antagonist. The recommended dose of aprepitant is 125 mg orally 1 hour prior to chemotherapy treatment (day 1) and 80 mg once daily in the morning on days 2 and 3.

Aprepitant may be taken with or without food.

Highly emetogenic cancer chemotherapy – In clinical studies, the following regimen was used for the prevention of nausea and vomiting associated with highly emetogenic cancer chemotherapy:

Aprepitant Dosage Regimen for Highly Emetogenic Cancer Chemotherapy				
Treatment	Day 1	Day 2	Day 3	Day 4
Aprepitant[a]	125 mg	80 mg	80 mg	none
Dexamethasone[b]	12 mg orally	8 mg orally	8 mg orally	8 mg orally
Ondansetron[c]	32 mg intravenous (IV)	none	none	none

[a] Aprepitant was administered orally 1 hour prior to chemotherapy treatment on day 1 and in the morning on days 2 and 3.
[b] Dexamethasone was administered 30 minutes prior to chemotherapy treatment on day 1 and in the morning on days 2 through 4. The dose of dexamethasone was chosen to account for drug interactions.
[c] Ondansetron was administered 30 minutes prior to chemotherapy treatment on day 1.

Moderately emetogenic cancer chemotherapy – In a clinical study, the following regimen was used for the prevention of nausea and vomiting associated with moderately emetogenic cancer chemotherapy:

Aprepitant Dosage Regimen for Moderately Emetogenic Cancer Chemotherapy			
Treatment	Day 1	Day 2	Day 3
Aprepitant[a]	125 mg	80 mg	80 mg
Dexamethasone[b]	12 mg orally	none	none
Ondansetron[c]	8 mg orally × 2	none	none

[a] Aprepitant was administered orally 1 hour prior to chemotherapy treatment on day 1 and in the morning on days 2 and 3.
[b] Dexamethasone was administered 30 minutes prior to chemotherapy treatment on day 1. The dexamethasone dose was chosen to account for drug interactions.
[c] One ondansetron 8 mg capsule was administered 30 to 60 minutes prior to chemotherapy treatment, and a second 8 mg capsule was administered 8 hours after the first dose on day 1.

➤*Concomitant corticosteroid therapy:*

Dexamethasone – The oral dexamethasone doses should be reduced approximately 50% when coadministered with aprepitant.

Methylprednisolone – The IV methylprednisolone dose should be reduced approximately 25%, and the oral methylprednisolone dose should be reduced approximately 50% when coadministered with aprepitant.

➤*Storage/Stability:* Store bottles and blisters at 20° to 25°C (68° to 77°F). The desiccant should remain in the original bottle.

Actions

➤*Pharmacology:* Aprepitant is a selective high-affinity antagonist of human substance P/neurokinin 1 (NK_1) receptors. Aprepitant has little or no affinity for serotonin (5-HT_3), dopamine, and corticosteroid receptors, the targets of existing therapies for chemotherapy-induced nausea and vomiting (CINV).

Aprepitant has been shown in animal models to inhibit emesis induced by cytotoxic chemotherapeutic agents, such as cisplatin, via central actions. Animal and human Positron Emission Tomography (PET) studies with aprepitant have shown that it crosses the blood brain barrier and occupies brain NK_1 receptors. Animal and human studies show that aprepitant augments the antiemetic activity of the 5-HT_3-receptor antagonist ondansetron and the corticosteroid dexamethasone and inhibits the acute and delayed phases of cisplatin-induced emesis.

➤*Pharmacokinetics:*

Absorption – The mean absolute oral bioavailability of aprepitant is approximately 60% to 65% and the mean peak plasma concentration (C_{max}) of aprepitant occurred at approximately 4 hours (T_{max}). Oral administration of the capsule with a standard breakfast had no clinically meaningful effect on the bioavailability of aprepitant.

The pharmacokinetics of aprepitant are nonlinear across the clinical dose range. In healthy young adults, the increase in area under the curve ($AUC_{0-\infty}$) was 26% greater than dose proportional between 80 and 125 mg single doses administered in the fed state.

Following oral administration of a single aprepitant 125 mg dose on day 1 and 80 mg once daily on days 2 and 3, the AUC_{0-24h} was approximately 19.6 mcg•h/mL and 21.2 mcg•h/mL on day 1 and day 3, respectively. The C_{max} of 1.6 mcg/mL and 1.4 mcg/mL were reached in approximately 4 hours (T_{max}) on day 1 and day 3, respectively.

Distribution – Aprepitant is more than 95% bound to plasma proteins. The mean apparent volume of distribution at steady state (Vd_{ss}) is approximately 70 L in humans.

Aprepitant crosses the placenta in rats and rabbits and crosses the blood-brain barrier in humans. Animal and human PET studies with aprepitant have shown that it crosses the blood-brain barrier and occupies brain NK_1 receptors.

Metabolism – Aprepitant undergoes extensive metabolism. In vitro studies using human liver microsomes indicate that aprepitant is metabolized primarily by CYP3A4 with minor metabolism by CYP1A2 and CYP2C19. Metabolism is largely via oxidation at the morpholine ring and its side chains. No metabolism by CYP2D6, CYP2C9, or CYP2E1 was detected. In healthy young adults, aprepitant accounts for approximately 24% of the radioactivity in plasma over 72 hours following a single oral dose of [^{14}C]-aprepitant 300 mg, indicating a substantial presence of metabolites in the plasma. Seven metabolites of aprepitant, which are only weakly active, have been identified in human plasma.

Excretion – Following administration of a single IV dose of [^{14}C]-aprepitant 100 mg prodrug to healthy subjects, 57% of the radioactivity was recovered in urine and 45% in feces. A study was not conducted with radiolabeled capsule formulation. The results after oral administration may differ.

Aprepitant is eliminated primarily by metabolism; aprepitant is not renally excreted. The apparent plasma clearance of aprepitant ranged from approximately 62 to 90 mL/min. The apparent terminal half-life ranged from approximately 9 to 13 hours.

Special populations –

Renal function impairment: A single dose of aprepitant 240 mg was administered to patients with severe renal insufficiency (creatinine clearance [Ccr] less than 30 mL/min) and to patients with ESRD requiring hemodialysis.

In patients with severe renal insufficiency, the $AUC_{0-\infty}$ of total aprepitant (unbound and protein bound) decreased 21% and C_{max} decreased 32%, relative to healthy subjects. In patients with ESRD undergoing hemodialysis, the area under the curve ($AUC_{0-\infty}$) of total aprepitant decreased 42% and C_{max} decreased 32%. Because of modest decreases in protein binding of aprepitant in patients with renal disease, the AUC of pharmacologically active unbound drug was not significantly affected in patients with renal insufficiency compared with healthy subjects. Hemodialysis conducted 4 or 48 hours after dosing had no significant effect on the pharmacokinetics of aprepitant; less than 0.2% of the dose was recovered in the dialysate.

No dosage adjustment for aprepitant is necessary for patients with renal insufficiency or for patients with ESRD undergoing hemodialysis.

Hepatic function impairment: Aprepitant was well tolerated in patients with mild to moderate hepatic insufficiency. Following administration of a single dose of aprepitant 125 mg on day 1 and 80 mg once daily on days 2 and 3 to patients with mild hepatic insufficiency (Child-Pugh score 5 to 6), the AUC_{0-24h} of aprepitant was 11% lower on day 1 and 36% lower on day 3, compared with healthy subjects given the same regimen. In patients with moderate hepatic insufficiency (Child-Pugh score 7 to 9), the AUC_{0-24h} of aprepitant was 10% higher on day 1 and 18% higher on day 3, as compared with healthy subjects given the same regimen. These differences in AUC_{0-24h} are not considered clinically meaningful; therefore, no dosage adjustment for aprepitant is necessary in patients with mild to moderate hepatic insufficiency.

There are no clinical or pharmacokinetic data in patients with severe hepatic insufficiency (Child-Pugh score higher than 9).

Elderly: Following oral administration of a single dose of aprepitant 125 mg on day 1 and 80 mg once daily on days 2 through 5, the AUC_{0-24h} of aprepitant was 21% higher on day 1 and 36% higher on day 5 in elderly (65 years of age and older) relative to younger adults. The C_{max} was 10% higher on day 1 and 24% higher on day 5 in elderly relative to younger adults. These differences are not considered clinically meaningful. No dosage adjustment for aprepitant is necessary in elderly patients.

Gender: Following oral administration of a single dose of aprepitant 125 mg, no difference in AUC_{0-24h} was observed between men and women. The C_{max} for aprepitant is 16% higher in women compared with men. The half-life of aprepitant is 25% lower in women compared with men, and T_{max} occurs at approximately the same time. These differences are not considered clinically meaningful. No dosage adjustment for aprepitant is necessary based on gender.

Race: Following oral administration of a single dose of aprepitant 125 mg, the AUC_{0-24h} is approximately 25% and 29% higher in Hispanic subjects compared with white and black subjects, respectively. The C_{max} is 22% and 31% higher in Hispanic subjects compared with white and black subjects, respectively. These differences are not considered clinically meaningful. There was no difference in AUC_{0-24h} or C_{max} between white and black subjects. No dosage adjustment for aprepitant is necessary based on race.

Contraindications

Aprepitant is a moderate CYP3A4 inhibitor. Do not use aprepitant concurrently with pimozide, terfenadine, astemizole, or cisapride. Inhibition of

APREPITANT — ORAL

cytochrome P-450 isoenzyme 3A4 (CYP3A4) by aprepitant could result in elevated plasma concentrations of these drugs, potentially causing serious or life-threatening reactions.

Aprepitant is contraindicated in patients who are hypersensitive to any component of the product.

Warnings

➤*Hepatic function impairment:* There are no clinical or pharmacokinetic data in patients with severe hepatic insufficiency (Child-Pugh score higher than 9). Therefore, exercise caution when aprepitant is administered in these patients.

➤*Carcinogenesis:* Three 2-year carcinogenicity studies of aprepitant (2 in Sprague-Dawley rats and 1 in CD-1 mice) were conducted with aprepitant. Dose selection for the studies was based on saturation of absorption in both species. In the rat carcinogenicity studies, animals were treated with oral dosages of 0.05, 0.25, 1, 5, 25, 125 mg/kg twice daily. The highest dosage tested produced a systemic exposure to aprepitant (plasma $AUC_{0\text{-}24h}$) of 0.4 to 1.4 times the human exposure ($AUC_{0\text{-}24h}$ equal to 19.6 mcg•h/mL) at the recommended dosage of 125 mg/day. Treatment with aprepitant at dosages of 5 to 125 mg/kg twice daily produced thyroid follicular cell adenomas and carcinomas in male rats. In female rats, it produced increased incidences of hepatocellular adenoma at 25 and 125 mg/kg twice daily, and thyroid follicular adenoma at the 125 mg/kg twice-daily dosage. In the mouse carcinogenicity study, animals were treated with oral dosages of 2.5, 25, 125, and 500 mg/kg/day. The highest tested dosage produced a systemic exposure of about 2.2 to 2.7 times the human exposure at the recommended dosage. Treatment with aprepitant produced skin fibrosarcomas in male mice of 125 and 500 mg/kg/day groups.

➤*Pregnancy: Category B.*

There are no adequate and well-controlled studies in pregnant women. Because animal reproduction studies are not always predictive of human response, use this drug during pregnancy only if clearly needed.

➤*Lactation:* Aprepitant is excreted in the milk of rats. It is not known whether this drug is excreted in human milk. Because many drugs are excreted in human milk, because of the potential for possible serious adverse reactions in breast-feeding infants from aprepitant, and because of the potential for tumorigenicity shown for aprepitant in rodent carcinogenicity studies, decide whether to discontinue breast-feeding or the drug, taking into account the importance of the drug to the mother.

➤*Children:* Safety and efficacy of aprepitant in children have not been established.

Precautions

➤*Chronic therapy:* Chronic continuous use of aprepitant for prevention of nausea and vomiting is not recommended because it has not been studied and because the drug interaction profile may change during chronic continuous use.

Drug Interactions

➤*CYP450 system:* Aprepitant is a substrate, a moderate inhibitor, and an inducer of CYP3A4. Aprepitant also is an inducer of CYP2C9.

Aprepitant Drug Interactions

Precipitant drug	Object drug[a]		Description
CYP 3A4 inhibitors (eg, clarithromycin, diltiazem, itraconazole, ketoconazole, nefazodone, nelfinavir, ritonavir, troleandomycin)	Aprepitant	↑	Concurrent use of CYP3A4 inhibitors with aprepitant may increase aprepitant plasma concentrations. Use with caution.
CYP3A4 inducers (eg, carbamazepine, phenytoin, rifampin)	Aprepitant	↓	Coadministration may decrease aprepitant plasma concentrations and delay efficacy.
Paroxetine	Aprepitant	↓	Concurrent use decreased the AUC ≈ 25% and C_{max} ≈ 20% of both aprepitant and paroxetine.
Aprepitant	Paroxetine		
Aprepitant	Contraceptives, oral	↓	The efficacy of oral contraceptives may be reduced during and for 28 days after administration of the last dose of aprepitant. Alternative or backup methods of contraception are recommended during treatment and for 1 month following the last dose of aprepitant.
Aprepitant	CYP2C9 substrates (eg, phenytoin, tolbutamide, warfarin)	↓	Aprepitant is a CYP2C9 inducer and has been shown to induce the metabolism of warfarin and tolbutamide, resulting in lower plasma levels. In patients on chronic warfarin therapy, closely monitor the INR in the 2-week period, particularly at 7 to 10 days, following the initiation of aprepitant.
Aprepitant	CYP3A4 substrates (eg, pimozide, cisapride[b], astemizole[c], terfenadine[c], dexamethasone, methylprednisolone, midazolam, alprazolam, triazolam, docetaxel, paclitaxel, etoposide, irinotecan, ifosfamide, imatinib, vinorelbine, vinblastine, vincristine)	↑	Aprepitant is a moderate inhibitor of CYP3A4 and can increase plasma concentration of coadministered products that are metabolized through CYP3A4. Aprepitant is contraindicated with astemizole, terfenadine, pimozide, or cisapride. Reduce the dexamethasone dose ≈ 50% when given with aprepitant. Reduce the dose of methylprednisolone IV ≈ 25% and the oral dose ≈ 50% when given with aprepitant.

[a] ↓ = Object drug decreased. ↑= Object drug increased.
[b] Available on a limited access basis only.
[c] No longer available in the United States.

Adverse Reactions

The overall safety of aprepitant was evaluated in approximately 3,800 individuals.

➤*Highly emetogenic chemotherapy:* In 2 well-controlled clinical trials in patients receiving highly emetogenic cancer chemotherapy, 544 patients were treated with aprepitant during cycle 1 of chemotherapy, and 413 of these patients continued into the multiple-cycle extension for up to 6 cycles of chemotherapy. Aprepitant was given in combination with ondansetron and dexamethasone and was generally well tolerated. Most adverse reactions reported in these clinical studies were described as mild to moderate in intensity.

In cycle 1, clinical adverse reactions were reported in approximately 69% of patients treated with the aprepitant regimen compared with approximately 68% of patients treated with standard therapy. The following table shows the percent of patients with clinical adverse reactions reported at an incidence greater than or equal to 3%.

Aprepitant Adverse Reactions in Patients Receiving Highly Emetogenic Chemotherapy (Incidence ≥ 3%) (Cycle 1)

Adverse reaction	Aprepitant regimen (n = 544)	Standard therapy (n = 550)
CNS		
Asthenia/Fatigue	17.8%	11.8%
Dizziness	6.6%	4.4%
Headache	8.5%	8.7%
Insomnia	2.9%	3.1%
GI		
Abdominal pain	4.6%	3.3%
Anorexia	10.1%	9.5%
Constipation	10.3%	12.2%
Diarrhea	10.3%	7.5%
Epigastric discomfort	4%	3.1%
Gastritis	4.2%	3.1%
Heartburn	5.3%	4.9%
Nausea	12.7%	11.8%
Vomiting	7.5%	7.6%
Hematologic/Lymphatic		
Neutropenia	3.1%	2.9%
Respiratory		
Hiccups	10.8%	5.6%
Special senses		
Tinnitus	3.7%	3.8%
Miscellaneous		
Dehydration	5.9%	5.1%
Fever	2.9%	3.5%
Mucous membrane disorder	2.6%	3.1%

In addition, isolated cases of serious adverse reactions (regardless of causality) of bradycardia, disorientation, and perforating duodenal ulcer were reported in highly emetogenic CINV clinical studies.

APREPITANT — ORAL

➤*Moderately emetogenic chemotherapy:* During cycle 1 of a moderately emetogenic chemotherapy study, 438 patients were treated with the aprepitant regimen, and 385 of these patients continued into the multiple-cycle extension for up to 4 cycles of chemotherapy. In cycle 1, clinical adverse reactions were reported in approximately 73% of patients treated with the aprepitant regimen compared with approximately 75% of patients treated with standard therapy.

The adverse reaction profile in the moderately emetogenic chemotherapy study was generally comparable with the highly emetogenic chemotherapy studies. The following table shows the percentage of patients with clinical adverse reactions reported at an incidence of greater than or equal to 3%.

Aprepitant Adverse Reactions in Patients Receiving Moderately Emetogenic Chemotherapy (Incidence ≥ 3%) (Cycle 1)		
Adverse reaction	Aprepitant regimen (n = 438)	Standard therapy (n = 428)
Cardiovascular		
Hot flush	3%	1.4%
CNS		
Dizziness	3.4%	4.2%
Fatigue	21.9%	21.5%
Headache	16.4%	16.4%
Insomnia	4.1%	5.6%
Dermatologic		
Alopecia	24%	22.2%
GI		
Anorexia	4.3%	5.8%
Constipation	12.3%	18%
Diarrhea	5.5%	6.3%
Dyspepsia	8.4%	4.9%
Nausea	7.1%	7.5%
Stomatitis	53%	4.4%
Hematologic/Lymphatic		
Neutropenia	8.9%	8.4%
Respiratory		
Pharynolaryngeal pain	3%	2.3%
Miscellaneous		
Asthenia	3.4%	3.7%
Mucosal inflammation	2.5%	3.5%

Isolated cases of serious adverse reactions (regardless of causality) of dehydration, enterocolitis, febrile neutropenia, hypertension, hypesthesia, neutropenic sepsis, pneumonia, and sinus tachycardia were reported in the moderately emetogenic CINV clinical study.

➤*Highly and moderately emetogenic chemotherapy:* The following additional clinical adverse reactions (incidence more than 0.5% and more than standard therapy), regardless of causality, were reported in patients treated with aprepitant regimen:

Cardiovascular – Deep venous thrombosis, flushing, hypertension, hypotension, myocardial infarction, palpitations, pulmonary embolism, tachycardia.

CNS – Anxiety disorder, confusion, depression, peripheral neuropathy, rigors, sensory neuropathy, taste disturbance, tremor.

Dermatologic – Acne, diaphoresis, rash.

GI – Acid reflux, deglutition disorder, dry mouth, dysgeusia, dysphagia, eructation, flatulence, increased salivation, obstipation.

GU – Dysuria, pelvic pain, urinary tract infection.

Hematologic / Lymphatic – Anemia, febrile neutropenia, thrombocytopenia.

Metabolic / Nutritional – Decreased appetite, diabetes mellitus, edema, hypokalemia, weight loss.

Musculoskeletal – Arthralgia, back pain, muscular weakness, musculoskeletal pain, myalgia.

Ophthalmic – Conjunctivitis.

Renal – Renal insufficiency.

Respiratory – Cough, dyspnea, lower respiratory tract infection, nasal secretion, pharyngitis, pneumonitis, respiratory insufficiency, upper respiratory tract infection, vocal disturbance.

Miscellaneous – Candidiasis, herpes simplex, malaise, neoplasm (benign, malignant, and unspecified [including cysts and polyps]), non-small cell lung carcinoma, septic shock.

➤*Lab test abnormalities:* The following table shows the percent of patients with laboratory adverse experiences reported at an incidence greater than or equal to 3% in patients receiving highly emetogenic chemotherapy.

Aprepitant Lab Test Abnormalities in Patients Receiving Highly Emetogenic Chemotherapy (Incidence ≥ 3%) (Cycle 1)		
	Aprepitant regimen (n = 544)	Standard therapy (n = 550)
ALT increased	6%	4.3%
AST increased	3%	1.3%
Serum urea nitrogen (BUN) increased	4.7%	3.5%
Serum creatinine increased	3.7%	4.3%
Proteinuria	6.8%	5.3%

The following additional laboratory adverse reactions (incidence more than 0.5% and more than standard therapy), regardless of causality, were reported in patients treated with aprepitant regimen: alkaline phosphatase increased, erythrocyturia, hyperglycemia, hyponatremia, leukocytes increased, leukocyturia.

The adverse reactions of increased AST and ALT were generally mild and transient.

The following laboratory adverse reactions were reported at an incidence of 3% or more during cycle 1 of the moderately emetogenic chemotherapy study in patients treated with the aprepitant regimen or standard therapy, respectively: decreased hemoglobin (2.3%, 4.7%) and decreased white blood cell count (9.3%, 9%).

The adverse reaction profiles in the multiple-cycle extensions for up to 6 cycles of chemotherapy were generally similar to those observed in cycle 1.

Other adverse reactions – Stevens-Johnson syndrome was reported in a patient receiving aprepitant with cancer chemotherapy in another CINV study. Angioedema and urticaria were reported in a patient receiving aprepitant in a non-CINV study.

Overdosage

➤*Symptoms:* Single doses up to 600 mg of aprepitant were generally well tolerated in healthy subjects. Aprepitant was generally well tolerated when administered as 375 mg once daily for up to 42 days to patients in non-CINV studies. In 33 cancer patients, administration of a single dose of aprepitant 375 mg on day 1 and 250 mg once daily on days 2 to 5 was generally well tolerated.

Drowsiness and headache were reported in 1 patient who ingested 1,440 mg of aprepitant.

➤*Treatment:* No specific information is available on the treatment of overdosage with aprepitant. In the event of overdose, discontinue aprepitant and provide general supportive treatment and monitoring. Because of the antiemetic activity of aprepitant, drug-induced emesis may not be effective.

Aprepitant cannot be removed by hemodialysis.

Patient Information

Instruct patients to read the patient package insert before starting therapy with aprepitant and to reread it each time the prescription is renewed.

Instruct patients to take aprepitant only as prescribed. Advise patients to take their first dose (125 mg) of aprepitant 1 hour prior to chemotherapy treatment.

Aprepitant may interact with some drugs including chemotherapy; therefore, advise patients to report to their health care providers the use of any other prescription or nonprescription medicines, vitamins, or herbal products.

Instruct patients on chronic warfarin therapy to have their clotting status closely monitored in the 2-week period, particularly at 7 to 10 days, following initiation of the 3 day regimen of aprepitant with each chemotherapy cycle.

Administration of aprepitant may reduce the efficacy of oral contraceptives. Advise patients to use alternative or backup methods of contraception during treatment with aprepitant and for 1 month following the last dose of aprepitant.

NABILONE

c-ii	**Cesamet** (Valeant Pharmaceuticals International)	**Capsules:** 1 mg	Corn starch. (Valeant 0247). Purple and white. In 20s.

NABILONE — ORAL

Indications

➤*Antiemetic:* For the treatment of the nausea and vomiting associated with cancer chemotherapy in patients who have failed to respond adequately to conventional antiemetic treatments. This restriction is required because a substantial proportion of any group of patients treated with nabilone can be expected to experience disturbing psychotomimetic reactions not observed with other antiemetic agents.

Because of its potential to alter the mental state, nabilone is intended for use under circumstances that permit close supervision of the patient by a responsible individual, particularly during the initial use of nabilone and during dose adjustments.

Nabilone is not intended for use on an as-needed basis or as the first antiemetic product prescribed for a patient.

Administration and Dosage

➤*Approved by the FDA:* May 15, 2006.

NABILONE — ORAL

➤*Adults:* 1 or 2 mg twice a day. On the day of chemotherapy, the initial dose should be given 1 to 3 hours before the chemotherapeutic agent is administered. To minimize adverse reactions, it is recommended that the lower starting dose be used and that the dose be increased as necessary. A dose of 1 or 2 mg the night before may be useful. The maximum recommended daily dose is 6 mg given in divided doses 3 times a day.

Nabilone may be administered 2 or 3 times daily during the entire course of each cycle of chemotherapy and, if needed, for 48 hours after the last dose of each cycle of chemotherapy.

➤*Storage/Stability:* Store at controlled room temperature, 25°C (77°F); excursions permitted from 15 to 30°C (59° to 86°F).

Actions

➤*Pharmacology:* Nabilone is an orally active synthetic cannabinoid that, like other cannabinoids, has complex effects on the CNS. It has been suggested that the antiemetic effect of nabilone is caused by interaction with the cannabinoid receptor system (the CB 1 receptor), which has been discovered in neural tissues.

Nontherapeutic effects – Nabilone, a synthetic cannabinoid, has the potential to be abused and to produce psychological dependence. Nabilone has complex effects on the CNS. Its effects on the mental state ("inner mental life") are similar to those of cannabis. Subjects given nabilone may experience changes in mood (eg, anxiety, depression, detachment, euphoria, panic, paranoia), decrements in cognitive performance and memory, a decreased ability to control drives and impulses, and alterations in the experience of reality (eg, distortions in the perception of objects and the sense of time, hallucinations). These phenomena appear to be more common when larger doses of nabilone are administered; however, a full-blown picture of psychosis (psychotic organic brain syndrome) may occur in patients receiving doses within the lower portion of the therapeutic range. Tolerance to these effects develops rapidly and is readily reversible.

Data on the chronic use of nabilone are not available; experience with cannabis suggests that chronic use of cannabinoids may be associated with a variety of untoward effects on motivation, cognition, and judgment, as well as other mental status changes. Whether these phenomena reflect the underlying character of individuals chronically abusing cannabis or are a result of the use of cannabis is not known.

The simultaneous use of nabilone and alcohol or barbiturates may produce additive depressive effects on CNS function. Possible changes in mood and other adverse behavioral effects may occur in patients receiving nabilone. Patients should remain under the supervision of a responsible adult while using nabilone.

Nabilone has CNS activity. It produces relaxation, drowsiness, and euphoria in the recommended dosage range. Tolerance to these effects develops rapidly and is readily reversible.

In addition to effects on the mental state, nabilone has several systemic actions; the most prominent are dry mouth and hypotension. Nabilone has been observed to elevate supine and standing heart rates and to cause supine and orthostatic hypotension. In clinical studies, oral administration of nabilone 2 mg did produce some decrease in airway resistance in healthy controls but had no effect in patients with asthma. No other nontherapeutic effects of clinical significance due to nabilone have been reported.

➤*Pharmacokinetics:*

Absorption/Distribution – Nabilone appears to be completely absorbed from the human GI tract when administered orally. Following oral administration of a dose of radiolabeled nabilone 2 mg, peak plasma concentrations of approximately 2 ng/mL of nabilone and 10 ng equivalents/mL of total radioactivity are achieved within 2 hours. The initial rapid disappearance of radioactivity represents uptake and distribution of nabilone into tissue and the slower-phase elimination by metabolism and excretion. The apparent volume of distribution of nabilone is approximately 12.5 L/kg.

Nabilone exhibits dose linearity within its therapeutic range.

Metabolism – Metabolism of nabilone is extensive, and several metabolites have been identified. Precise information concerning the metabolites that may accumulate is not available. The relative activities of the metabolites and the parent drug have not been established. There are at least 2 metabolic pathways involved in the biotransformation of nabilone. A minor pathway is initiated by the stereospecific enzymatic reduction of the 9-keto moiety of nabilone to produce the isomeric carbinol metabolite. The peak concentrations of nabilone and its carbinol metabolites are comparable, but their combined exposures in plasma do not account for more than 20% of that of total radioactivity. Secondly, a metabolite of nabilone in feces has been identified as a diol formed by reduction of the 9-keto group plus oxidation at the penultimate carbon of the dimethylheptyl side chain. In addition, there is evidence of extensive metabolism of nabilone by multiple P-450 enzyme isoforms. However, in clinical use, the very low nabilone plasma concentration is unlikely to interfere with the P-450–mediated degradation of coadministered drugs. Chronic oral administration of 1 mg 3 times daily for 14 days to 3 subjects gave no indication there was any significant accumulation of nabilone. Available evidence suggests that 1 or more of the metabolites has a terminal elimination half-life that exceeds that of nabilone. Consequently, in repeated use, the metabolites may accumulate at concentrations in excess of the parent drug.

Excretion – The plasma half-life ($t_{1/2}$) values for nabilone and total radioactivity of identified and unidentified metabolites are approximately 2 and 35 hours, respectively. The route and rate of the elimination of nabilone and its metabolites are similar to those observed with other cannabinoids, including delta-9-THC (dronabinol). When nabilone is administered intravenously, the drug and its metabolites are eliminated mainly in the feces (approximately 67%) and, to a lesser extent, in the urine (approximately 22%) within 7 days. Of the 67% recovered from the feces, 5% corresponded to the parent compound and 16% to its carbinol metabolite. Following oral administration, approximately 60% of nabilone and its metabolites were recovered in the feces and approximately 24% in urine. Therefore, it appears that the major excretory pathway is the biliary system.

Contraindications

History of hypersensitivity to any cannabinoid.

Warnings

➤*Duration of effects:* The effects of nabilone may persist for a variable and unpredictable period of time following its oral administration. Adverse psychiatric reactions can persist for 48 to 72 hours following cessation of treatment.

➤*CNS effects:* Nabilone has the potential to affect the CNS and might manifest itself in dizziness, drowsiness, euphoria ("high"), ataxia, anxiety, disorientation, depression, hallucinations, and psychosis.

➤*Cardiovascular effects:* Nabilone can cause tachycardia and orthostatic hypotension.

➤*Close supervision:* Because of individual variation in response and tolerance to the effects of nabilone, patients should remain under the supervision of a responsible adult, especially during initial use of nabilone and during dose adjustments.

➤*Elderly:* Clinical studies of nabilone did not include sufficient numbers of subjects 65 years of age and older to determine whether they respond differently than younger subjects. In general, be cautious in dose selection for an elderly patient, usually starting at the low end of the dosing range, reflecting the greater frequency of decreased hepatic, renal, or cardiac function, and of concomitant disease or other drug therapy. Use nabilone with caution in elderly patients 65 years of age and older because they are generally more sensitive to the psychoactive effects of drugs and nabilone can elevate supine and standing heart rates and cause postural hypotension.

➤*Pregnancy: Category C.* Teratology studies conducted in pregnant rats at dosages up to 12 mg/kg/day (about 16 times the human dose on a body surface area basis [BSA]) and pregnant rabbits at dosages up to 3.3 mg/kg/day (about 9 times the human dose on a BSA basis) did not disclose any evidence for a teratogenic potential of nabilone. However, there was dose-related developmental toxicity in both species which was displayed by increases in embryolethality, fetal resorptions, decreased fetal weights, and pregnancy disruptions. In rats, postnatal developmental toxicity was also observed. There are no adequate and well-controlled studies in pregnant women. Because animal studies cannot rule out the possibility of harm, only use nabilone during pregnancy if the potential benefit justifies the potential risk to the fetus.

➤*Lactation:* It is not known whether this drug is excreted in breast milk. Because many drugs, including some cannabinoids, are excreted in breast milk, it is not recommended that nabilone be given to breast-feeding mothers.

➤*Children:* Safety and efficacy have not been established in patients younger than 18 years of age. Caution is recommended in prescribing nabilone to children because of psychoactive effects.

Precautions

➤*Monitoring:* As with all controlled drugs, monitor patients receiving nabilone for signs of excessive use, abuse, and misuse. Patients who may be at increased risk for substance abuse include those with a personal or family history of substance abuse (eg, drug, alcohol abuse) or mental illness.

➤*Special risk:* Carefully evaluate the benefit/risk ratio of nabilone use in patients with the following medical conditions because of individual variation in response and tolerance to the effects of nabilone.

- Because nabilone can elevate supine and standing heart rates and cause postural hypotension, use it with caution in the elderly and in patients with hypertension or heart disease.
- Use nabilone with caution in patients with current or previous psychiatric disorders (eg, bipolar disorder, depression, schizophrenia) because the symptoms of these disease states may be unmasked by the use of cannabinoids.
- Use nabilone with caution in patients with a history of substance abuse, including alcohol abuse or dependence and marijuana use, because nabilone contains a similar active compound to marijuana.

➤*Drug abuse and dependence:* Nabilone, a synthetic cannabinoid pharmacologically related to *Cannabis sativa L*(Marijuana; delta-9-THC) is a highly abusable substance. Nabilone is controlled under schedule II of the Controlled Substances Act. Limit prescriptions for nabilone to the amount necessary for a single cycle of chemotherapy (ie, a few days). Nabilone may produce subjective adverse reactions that may be interpreted as a euphoria or marijuana-like "high" at therapeutic doses.

It is not known what proportion of individuals exposed chronically to nabilone or other cannabinoids will develop either psychological or physical dependence. Long-term use of these compounds has been associated with disorders of motivation, judgment, and cognition. However, it is not clear if these are a manifestation of the underlying personalities of chronic users of this class of drugs or if cannabinoids are directly responsible for these effects. An abstinence syndrome has been reported following discontinuation of delta-9-THC at high doses of 200 mg per day for 12 to 16 consecutive days. The acute phase was characterized by psychic distress, insomnia, and signs of autonomic hyperactivity (hiccups, loose stools, rhinorrhea, sweating). A

NABILONE — ORAL

protracted abstinence phase may have occurred in subjects who reported sleep disturbances for several weeks after delta-9-THC discontinuation.

Abuse – Nabilone was qualitatively and quantitatively similar to approved oral delta-9-THC in the production of cannabis-like effects, demonstrating its potential for abuse.

Preclinical studies performed in dogs and monkeys demonstrated that nabilone was cannabinoid-like. As with delta-9-THC, tolerance develops rapidly to the pharmacological effects in the dog and monkey. Cross-tolerance between nabilone and delta-9-THC was demonstrated in the monkey.

Dependence – The physical dependence capacity of nabilone is unknown at this time. Patients who participated in clinical trials of up to 5 days' duration evidenced no withdrawal symptoms upon cessation of dosing.

➤*Hazardous tasks:* Specifically warn patients receiving nabilone treatment not to drive, operate machinery, or engage in any hazardous activity while receiving nabilone.

Drug Interactions

➤*CYP-450 system:* In vitro P-450 inhibition studies using human liver microsomes showed that nabilone did not significantly inhibit CYP1A2, 2A6, 2C19, 2D6, and 3A4 (using midazolam and nifedipine as substrates). Nabilone had a weak inhibitory effect on CYP2E1 and 3A4 (using testosterone; IC_{50} greater than 50 mcM) and had a moderate inhibitory effect on CYP2C8 and 2C9 (IC_{50} greater than 10 mcM).

Cannabinoid Drug Interactions

Precipitant drug	Object drug[a]		Description
Amphetamines Cocaine Other sympathomimetic agents	Cannabinoids	↑	Additive hypertension, tachycardia, and possibly cardiotoxicity may occur.
Cannabinoids	Amphetamines Cocaine Other sympathomimetic agents		
Antihistamines Atropine Scopolamine Other anticholinergic agents	Cannabinoids	↑	Additive or super-additive tachycardia, or drowsiness may occur.
Cannabinoids	Antihistamines Atropine Scopolamine Other anticholinergic agents		
Barbiturates Benzodiazepines Buspirone Ethanol Lithium Muscle relaxants Opioids Other CNS depressants	Cannabinoids	↑	Additive drowsiness and CNS-depressant effects. Psychomotor function was particularly impaired with concurrent use of nabilone and diazepam. Based on smoked marijuana, an increase in the positive subjective mood effects may occur when used with alcohol.
Cannabinoids	Barbiturates Benzodiazepines Buspirone Ethanol Lithium Muscle relaxants Opioids Other CNS depressants		
Naltrexone	Cannabinoids	↑	Oral THC effects were enhanced by opioid receptor blockade.
Opioids	Cannabinoids	↓	Cross-tolerance and mutual potentiation may occur.
Cannabinoids	Opioids		
Tricyclic antidepressants (eg, amitriptyline, amoxapine)	Cannabinoids	↑	Additive tachycardia, hypertension, or drowsiness may occur.
Cannabinoids	Tricyclic antidepressants (eg, amitriptyline, amoxapine)		
Cannabinoids	Antipyrine Barbiturates	↑	Decreased clearance of antipyrine and barbiturates, presumably via competitive inhibition of metabolism.

Cannabinoid Drug Interactions

Precipitant drug	Object drug[a]		Description
Cannabinoids	Disulfiram	↓	A reversible hypomanic reaction was reported in a 28-year-old man who smoked marijuana; confirmed by dechallenge and rechallenge.
Cannabinoids	Fluoxetine	↓	A 21-year-old woman with depression and bulimia receiving fluoxetine 20 mg/day for 4 weeks became hypomanic after smoking marijuana; symptoms resolved after 4 days.
Cannabinoids	Theophylline	↓	Increased theophylline metabolism reported with smoking marijuana; effect similar to that following smoking tobacco.

[a] ↑ = Object drug increased. ↓ = Object drug decreased.

Adverse Reactions

During controlled clinical trials of nabilone, virtually all patients experienced at least 1 adverse reaction. The most commonly encountered reactions were ataxia, concentration difficulties, dry mouth, drowsiness, euphoria (feeling "high"), headache, and vertigo.

➤*Comparative incidence of reactions:* The following tables list the adverse reactions encountered by a substantial proportion of patients treated with nabilone participating in representative controlled clinical trials.

Incidence of Nabilone Adverse Reactions in Placebo-Controlled Studies

Adverse reaction	Nabilone (n = 132)		Placebo (n = 119)	
	Patients	Percent	Patients	Percent
CNS				
Ataxia	19	14%	0	0%
Depersonalization	2	2%	1	1%
Disorientation	3	2%	0	0%
Drowsiness	69	52%	6	5%
Dysphoria	12	9%	0	0%
Euphoria	14	11%	1	1%
Headache	8	6%	0	0%
Sleep disturbance	14	11%	1	1%
Vertigo	69	52%	3	3%
GI				
Dry mouth	47	36%	2	2%
Nausea	5	4%	0	0%

Incidence of Nabilone Adverse Reactions in Active-Controlled Studies

Adverse reaction	Nabilone (n = 250)		Prochlorperazine (n = 232)	
	Patients	Percent	Patients	Percent
Cardiovascular				
Hypotension	20	8%	3	1%
CNS				
Asthenia	19	8%	10	4%
Ataxia	32	13%	4	2%
Concentration difficulties	31	12%	3	1%
Depression	35	14%	37	16%
Drowsiness	165	66%	108	47%
Euphoria	95	38%	12	5%
Headache	18	7%	14	6%
Sedation	7	3%	2	1%
Vertigo/Dizziness	147	59%	53	23%
Visual disturbance	32	13%	9	4%
GI				
Anorexia	19	8%	22	9%
Dry mouth	54	22%	11	5%
Increased appetite	6	2%	2	1%

➤*Adverse reactions by body system:* The following list of adverse reactions is organized within body systems for patients treated with nabilone in controlled clinical trials. All reactions are listed regardless of causality assessment.

Cardiovascular – Arrhythmia, cerebral vascular accident, flushing, hypertension, hypotension, orthostatic hypotension, palpitation, syncope, tachycardia.

NABILONE — ORAL

CNS – Abnormal dreams, akathisia, anxiety, apathy, asthenia, ataxia, confusion, convulsions, coordination disturbance, decreased concentration, depersonalization syndrome, depression, disorientation, dizziness, drowsiness, dysphoria, dystonia, emotional disorder, euphoria (feeling "high"), fatigue, hallucinations, headache, hyperactivity, inebriated feeling, inhibited walking, insomnia, irritability, light-headedness, malaise, memory disturbance, mood swings, nervousness, numbness, panic disorder, paranoia, paresthesia, perception disturbance, phobic neurosis, postural dizziness, sedation, sleep disturbance, speech disorder, thought disorder, toxic psychosis, tremor, twitch, unconsciousness, vertigo, withdrawal.

Dermatologic – Allergic reactions, anhidrosis, photosensitivity, pruritus, rash.

GI – Abdominal pain, anorexia, aphthous ulcer, constipation, diarrhea, dry mouth, dyspepsia, excessive appetite, gastritis, mouth irritation, nausea, taste change, vomiting.

GU – Decreased urination, frequency of micturition, hot flashes, impaired urination, increased urination, urinary retention.

Hematologic – Anemia.

Metabolic – Thirst.

Musculoskeletal – Back pain, joint pain, muscle pain, neck pain, unspecified pain.

Respiratory – Chest pain, cough, dry nose, dry throat, dyspnea, nasal congestion, nosebleed, pharyngitis, sinus headache, thick tongue, voice change, wheezing.

Special senses – Amblyopia, ear tightness, equilibrium dysfunction, eye disorder, eye dryness, eye irritation, eye swelling, eyelid diseases, photophobia, pupil dilation, tinnitus, vision disturbance, visual field defect.

Miscellaneous – Bacterial infection, chills, excessive sweating, fever, hypotonia.

➤*Postmarketing:* Nabilone has been marketed internationally since 1982. The following adverse reactions listed by body system have been reported since nabilone has been marketed. All reactions are listed regardless of causality assessment.

Cardiovascular – Hypotension, tachycardia.

CNS – Abnormal thinking, anxiety, ataxia, circumoral paresthesia, CNS depression, CNS stimulation, confusion, convulsion, depersonalization, depression, dizziness, dysphoria, emotional lability, euphoria, hallucinations, headache, insomnia, psychosis, somnolence, stupor, vertigo.

GI – Constipation, dry mouth, nausea, vomiting.

Hematologic – Leukopenia.

Special senses – Visual disturbances.

Miscellaneous – Chest pain, face edema, lack of effect.

Overdosage

➤*Symptoms:* Signs and symptoms of overdosage are an extension of the psychotomimetic and physiologic effects of nabilone. In overdose settings, pay attention to vital signs because hypertension and hypotension have been known to occur; tachycardia and orthostatic hypotension were most commonly reported. No cases of overdosage with more than 10 mg/day of nabilone were reported during clinical trials. Signs and symptoms that would be expected to occur in large overdose situations are psychotic episodes (eg, anxiety reactions, coma, hallucinations, respiratory depression).

➤*Treatment:* To obtain up-to-date information about the treatment of overdose, a good resource is your certified regional poison control center. In managing overdosage, consider the possibility of multiple drug overdoses, interaction among drugs, and unusual drug kinetics in the patient.

Overdosage may be considered to have occurred, even at prescribed dosages, if disturbing psychiatric symptoms are present. In these cases, observe the patient in a quiet environment and use supportive measures, including reassurance. Withhold subsequent doses until the patient has returned to baseline mental status; routine dosing may then be resumed if clinically indicated. In such instances, a lower initiating dose is suggested. In controlled clinical trials, alterations in mental status related to the use of nabilone resolved within 72 hours without specific medical therapy.

If psychotic episodes occur, manage the patient conservatively, if possible. For moderate psychotic episodes and anxiety reactions, verbal support and comforting may be sufficient. In more severe cases, antipsychotic drugs may be useful; however, the utility of antipsychotic drugs in cannabinoid psychosis has not been systematically evaluated. Support for their use is drawn from limited experience using antipsychotic agents to manage cannabis overdoses. Because of the potential for drug interactions (eg, additive CNS depressant effects due to nabilone and chlorpromazine), monitor such patients closely.

Protect the patient's airway and support ventilation and perfusion. Meticulously monitor and maintain, within acceptable limits, the patient's vital signs, blood gases, and serum electrolytes, as well as other laboratory values and physical assessments. Absorption of drugs from the GI tract may be decreased by giving activated charcoal, which, in many cases, is more effective than emesis or lavage; consider charcoal instead of or in addition to gastric emptying. Repeated doses of charcoal over time may hasten elimination of some drugs that have been absorbed. Safeguard the patient's airway when employing gastric emptying or charcoal.

The use of forced diuresis, peritoneal dialysis, hemodialysis, charcoal hemoperfusion, or cholestyramine has not been reported. In the presence of normal renal function, most of a dose of nabilone is eliminated through the biliary system.

Treatment for respiratory depression and comatose state consists of symptomatic and supportive therapy. Pay particular attention to the occurrence of hypothermia. If the patient becomes hypotensive, consider fluids, inotropes, and/or vasopressors.

The estimated oral median lethal dose in female mice is between 1,000 and 2,000 mg/kg; in the female rat, it is greater than 2,000 mg/kg.

Patient Information

Alert patients taking nabilone to the potential for additive CNS depression resulting from simultaneous use of nabilone and alcohol or other CNS depressants such as benzodiazepines and barbiturates. Avoid this combination. Specifically warn patients receiving treatment with nabilone not to drive, operate machinery, or engage in any hazardous activity. Make patients using nabilone aware of possible changes in mood and other adverse behavioral effects of the drug so as to avoid panic in the event of such manifestations. Tell patients to remain under the supervision of a responsible adult while using nabilone.

DRONABINOL

c-iii	**Marinol** (Solvay)	**Capsules, gelatin:**[1] 2.5 mg	Parabens. (RL). White. In 25s, 60s, and 100s.
		5 mg	Parabens. (RL). Brown. In 25s and 100s.
		10 mg	Parabens. (RL). Orange. In 25s and 60s.

[1] In sesame oil.

DRONABINOL — ORAL

Refer to the general discussion of these products beginning in the Antiemetic/Antivertigo Agents monograph.

Indications

For the treatment of anorexia associated with weight loss in patients with acquired immune deficiency syndrome (AIDS); and nausea and vomiting associated with cancer chemotherapy in patients who have failed to respond adequately to conventional antiemetic treatments.

Administration and Dosage

➤*Approved by the FDA:* May 31, 1985.

➤*Appetite stimulation:* Initially, 2.5 mg dronabinol should be administered orally twice daily, before lunch and supper. For patients unable to tolerate this 5 mg/day dosage of dronabinol, the dosage can be reduced to 2.5 mg/day, administered as a single dose in the evening or at bedtime. If clinically indicated and in the absence of significant adverse effects, the dosage may be gradually increased to a maximum of 20 mg/day dronabinol, administered in divided oral doses. Caution should be exercised in escalating the dosage of dronabinol because of the increased frequency of dose-related adverse experiences at higher dosages. The dosage may be increased to 2.5 mg before lunch and 5 mg before supper (or 5 mg at lunch and 5 mg after supper). Although most patients respond to 2.5 mg twice daily, 10 mg twice daily has been tolerated in approximately 50% of patients.

➤*Antiemetic:* Dronabinol is best administered at an initial dose of 5 mg/m^2, given 1 to 3 hours prior to the administration of chemotherapy, then every 2 to 4 hours after chemotherapy is given, for a total of 4 to 6 doses/day. Should the 5 mg/m^2 dose prove to be ineffective, and in the absence of significant side effects, the dose may be escalated by 2.5 mg/m^2 increments to a maximum of 15 mg/m^2 per dose. Caution should be exercised in dose escalation, however, as the incidence of disturbing psychiatric symptoms increases significantly at maximum dose. Dronabinol should be used with caution and careful psychiatric monitoring in patients with mania, depression, or schizophrenia because dronabinol may exacerbate these illnesses.

➤*Individualization of dosages:* The pharmacologic effects of dronabinol are dose-related and subject to considerable interpatient variability. Therefore, dosage individualization is critical in achieving the maximum benefit of dronabinol treatment.

Appetite stimulation – In the clinical trials, the majority of patients were treated with 5 mg/day dronabinol, although the dosages ranged from 2.5 to 20 mg/day.

Adults:

1.) Begin with 2.5 mg before lunch and 2.5 mg before supper. If CNS symptoms (feeling high, dizziness, confusion, somnolence) do occur, they usually resolve in 1 to 3 days with continued dosage.
2.) If CNS symptoms are severe or persistent, reduce the dose to 2.5 mg before supper. If symptoms continue to be a problem, taking the single dose in the evening or at bedtime may reduce their severity.
3.) When adverse effects are absent or minimal and further therapeutic effect is desired, increase the dose to 2.5 mg before lunch and 5 mg before supper or 5 and 5 mg. Although most patients respond to 2.5 mg twice daily, 10 mg twice daily has been tolerated in about half of the patients in appetite stimulation studies. The pharmacologic effects of dronabinol are reversible upon treatment cessation.

DRONABINOL — ORAL

➤*Antiemetic:* Most patients respond to 5 mg 3 or 4 times daily. Dosage may be escalated during a chemotherapy cycle or at subsequent cycles, based upon initial results. Therapy should be initiated at the lowest recommended dosage and titrated to clinical response. Administration of dronabinol with phenothiazines, such as prochlorperazine, has resulted in improved efficacy as compared to either drug alone, without additional toxicity.

➤*Pediatrics:* Dronabinol is not recommended for AIDS-related anorexia in pediatric patients because it has not been studied in this population. The pediatric dosage for the treatment of chemotherapy-induced emesis is the same as in adults. Caution is recommended in prescribing dronabinol for children because of the psychoactive effects.

➤*Storage / Stability:* Dronabinol should be packaged in a well-closed container and stored in a cool environment between 8° and 15°C (46° and 59°F) and alternatively could be stored in a refrigerator. Protect from freezing.

Actions

➤*Pharmacology:* Dronabinol is an orally active cannabinoid which, like other cannabinoids, has complex effects on the CNS, including central sympathomimetic activity. Cannabinoid receptors have been discovered in neural tissues. These receptors may play a role in mediating the effects of dronabinol and other cannabinoids. Dronabinol is the principal psychoactive substance present in *Cannabis sativa* L. (marijuana). Nontherapeutic effects of dronabinol are identical to those of marijuana and other centrally active cannabinoids. The mechanism of action is unknown.

Pharmacodynamics – Dronabinol-induced sympathomimetic activity may result in tachycardia or conjunctival injection. Its effects on blood pressure are inconsistent, but occasional subjects have experienced orthostatic hypotension and/or syncope upon abrupt standing.

Dronabinol also demonstrates reversible effects on appetite, mood, cognition, memory, and perception. These phenomena appear to be dose-related, increasing in frequency with higher dosages, and subject to great interpatient variability.

Patients may experience mood changes (eg, euphoria, detachment, depression, anxiety, panic, paranoia), decrements in cognitive performance and memory, a decreased ability to control drives and impulses, and alterations of reality (eg, distortions in perception of objects and sense of time, hallucinations). These latter phenomena are more common with larger doses; however, a full-blown picture of psychosis (psychotic organic brain syndrome) may occur in patients receiving doses in the lower portion of the therapeutic range.

After oral administration, dronabinol has an onset of action of approximately 0.5 to 1 hours and peak effect at 2 to 4 hours. Duration of action for psychoactive effects is 4 to 6 hours, but the appetite stimulant effect of dronabinol may continue for 24 hours or longer after administration.

Tachyphylaxis and tolerance develop to some of the pharmacologic effects of dronabinol and other cannabinoids with chronic use, suggesting an indirect effect on sympathetic neurons. In a study of the pharmacodynamics of chronic dronabinol exposure, healthy male volunteers (n = 12) received 210 mg/day dronabinol, administered orally in divided doses, for 16 days. An initial tachycardia induced by dronabinol was replaced successively by normal sinus rhythm and then bradycardia. A decrease in supine blood pressure, made worse by standing, was also observed initially. These volunteers developed tolerance to the cardiovascular and subjective adverse CNS effects of dronabinol within 12 days of treatment initiation. In 1 study, a slight but consistent decrease in oral temperature was recorded.

Tachyphylaxis and tolerance do not, however, appear to develop to the appetite stimulant effect of dronabinol. In studies involving patients with acquired immune deficiency syndrome (AIDS), the appetite stimulant effect of dronabinol has been sustained for up to 5 months in clinical trials, at dosages ranging from 2.5 mg/day to 20 mg/day.

➤*Pharmacokinetics:*

Absorption / Distribution – Dronabinol is almost completely absorbed (90% to 95%) after single oral doses. Due to the combined effects of first-pass hepatic metabolism and high lipid solubility, only 10% to 20% of the administered dose reaches the systemic circulation. Dronabinol has a large apparent volume of distribution, approximately 10 L/kg, because of its lipid solubility. The plasma protein binding of dronabinol and its metabolites is approximately 97%.

The elimination phase of dronabinol can be described using a 2 compartment model with an initial (alpha) half-life of about 4 hours and a terminal (beta) half-life of 25 to 36 hours. Because of its large volume of distribution, dronabinol and its metabolites may be excreted at low levels for prolonged periods of time.

Metabolism – Dronabinol undergoes extensive first-pass hepatic metabolism, primarily by microsomal hydroxylation, yielding both active and inactive metabolites. Dronabinol and its principal active metabolite, 11-OH-delta-9-THC, are present in approximately equal concentrations in plasma. Concentrations of both parent drug and metabolite peak at approximately 2 to 4 hours after oral dosing and decline over several days. Values for clearance average about 0.2 L/kg/hr, but are highly variable due to the complexity of cannabinoid distribution.

Excretion – Dronabinol and its biotransformation products are excreted in both feces and urine. Biliary excretion is the major route of elimination with about half of a radiolabeled oral dose being recovered from the feces within 72 hours as contrasted with 10% to 15% recovered from urine. Less than 5% of an oral dose is recovered unchanged in the feces.

Following single dose administration, low levels of dronabinol metabolites have been detected for more than 5 weeks in the urine and feces.

In a study of dronabinol involving AIDS patients, urinary cannabinoid/creatinine concentration ratios were studied biweekly over a 6-week period. The urinary cannabinoid/creatinine ratio was closely correlated with dose. No increase in the cannabinoid/creatinine ratio was observed after the first 2 weeks of treatment, indicating that steady-state cannabinoid levels had been reached. This conclusion is consistent with predictions based on the observed terminal half-life of dronabinol. Extended use at recommended doses may cause accumulation of toxic amounts of dronabinol and metabolites.

Contraindications

Hypersensitivity to any cannabinoid or sesame oil.

Warnings

➤*Fertility impairment:* In a long-term study (77 days) in rats, oral administration of dronabinol at doses of 30 to 150 mg/m^2, equivalent to 0.3 to 1.5 times maximum recommended human dose (MRHD) of 90 mg/m^2/day in cancer patients or 2 to 10 times MRHD of 15 mg/m^2/day in AIDS patients, reduced ventral prostate, seminal vesicle and epididymal weights and caused a decrease in seminal fluid volume. Decreases in spermatogenesis, number of developing germ cells, and number of Leydig cells in the testis were also observed. However, sperm count, mating success, and testosterone levels were not affected. The significance of these animal findings in humans is not known.

➤*Elderly:* Caution is advised in prescribing dronabinol capsules in elderly patients because they are generally more sensitive to the psychoactive effects of drugs. In antiemetic studies, no difference in tolerance or efficacy was apparent in patients greater than 55 years of age.

➤*Pregnancy: Category C.* Reproduction studies with dronabinol have been performed in mice at 15 to 450 mg/m^2, equivalent to 0.2 to 5 times maximum recommended human MRHD of 90 mg/m^2/day in cancer patients or 1 to 30 times MRHD of 15 mg/m^2/day in AIDS patients, and in rats at 74 to 295 mg/m^2 (equivalent to 0.8 to 3 times MRHD of 90 mg/m^2 in cancer patients or 5 to 20 times MRHD of 15 mg/m^2/day in AIDS patients). These studies have revealed no evidence of teratogenicity due to dronabinol. At these dosages in mice and rats, dronabinol decreased maternal weight gain and number of viable pups and increased fetal mortality and early resorptions. Such effects were dose dependent and less apparent at lower doses which produced less maternal toxicity. There are no adequate and well-controlled studies in pregnant women. Dronabinol should be used only if the potential benefit justifies the potential risk to the fetus.

➤*Lactation:* Use of dronabinol is not recommended in nursing mothers since, in addition to the secretion of HIV virus in breast milk, dronabinol is concentrated in and secreted in human breast milk and is absorbed by the nursing baby. The effects of chronic exposure to the drug and its metabolites on the infant are unknown.

➤*Children:* Dronabinol capsules are not recommended for AIDS-related anorexia in pediatric patients because it has not been studied in this population. The pediatric dosage for the treatment of chemotherapy-induced emesis is the same as in adults. Caution is recommended in prescribing dronabinol capsules for children because of the psychoactive effects.

Precautions

➤*Monitoring:* Because of individual variation, clinically determine the period of time the patient needs to be supervised. Closely observe patients within an inpatient setting, if possible. This is especially important during treatment of patients with no prior experience with *Cannabis* or dronabinol. However, even patients experienced with these agents may have serious untoward responses not predicted by prior uneventful exposures. Closely observe any patient who has a psychotic experience with dronabinol until the mental state returns to normal. Do not give additional doses until the patient has been examined and the circumstances evaluated. If the situation warrants, give a lower dose under very close supervision.

➤*Special risk:*

Dronabinol use should be carefully evaluated in patients with the following medical condition – The risk/benefit ratio of dronabinol use should be carefully evaluated in patients with the following medical conditions because of individual variation in response and tolerance to the effects of dronabinol:

Dronabinol should be used with caution in patients with cardiac disorders because of occasional hypotension, possible hypertension, syncope, or tachycardia.

Dronabinol should be used with caution in patients with a history of substance abuse, including alcohol abuse or dependence, because they may be more prone to abuse dronabinol as well. Multiple substance abuse is common and marijuana, which contains the same active compound, is a frequently abused substance.

Dronabinol should be used with caution and careful psychiatric monitoring in patients with mania, depression, or schizophrenia because dronabinol may exacerbate these illnesses.

Dronabinol should be used with caution in patients receiving concomitant therapy with sedatives, hypnotics, or other psychoactive drugs because of the potential for additive or synergistic CNS effects.

Dronabinol should be used with caution in pregnant patients, nursing mothers, or pediatric patients because it has not been studied in these patient populations.

➤*Drug abuse and dependence:* Dronabinol is one of the psychoactive compounds present in cannabis, and is abusable and controlled [Schedule III (CIII)] under the Controlled Substances Act. Both psychological and physiological dependence have been noted in healthy individuals receiving dronabinol, but addiction is uncommon and has only been seen after prolonged

DRONABINOL — ORAL

high dose administration. Limit prescriptions to the amount necessary for a single cycle of chemotherapy.

Chronic abuse of cannabis has been associated with decrements in motivation, cognition, judgement, and perception. The etiology of these impairments is unknown, but may be associated with the complex process of addiction rather than an isolated effect of the drug. No such decrements in psychological, social or neurological status have been associated with the administration of dronabinol for therapeutic purposes.

An abstinence syndrome has been reported after the abrupt discontinuation of dronabinol in volunteers receiving dosages of 210 mg/day for 12 to 16 consecutive days. Within 12 hours after discontinuation, these volunteers manifested symptoms such as irritability, insomnia, and restlessness. By approximately 24 hours post-dronabinol discontinuation, withdrawal symptoms intensified to include "hot flashes", sweating, rhinorrhea, loose stools, hiccoughs, and anorexia.

These withdrawal symptoms gradually dissipated over the next 48 hours. The syndrome was essentially complete within 96 hours. Electroencephalographic changes consistent with the effects of drug withdrawal (hyperexcitation) were recorded in patients after abrupt dechallenge. Patients also complained of disturbed sleep for several weeks after discontinuing therapy with high dosages of dronabinol.

➤*Hazardous tasks:* Patients receiving treatment with dronabinol should be specifically warned not to drive, operate machinery, or engage in any hazardous activity until it is established that they are able to tolerate the drug and to perform such tasks safely. Effects may persist for a variable and unpredictable period of time.

Drug Interactions

In studies involving patients with AIDS and/or cancer, dronabinol has been coadministered with a variety of medications (eg, cytotoxic agents, anti-infective agents, sedatives, or opioid analgesics) without resulting in any clinically significant drug/drug interactions. Although no drug/drug interactions were discovered during the clinical trials of dronabinol, cannabinoids may interact with other medications through both metabolic and pharmacodynamic mechanisms. Dronabinol is highly protein bound to plasma proteins, and therefore, might displace other protein-bound drugs. Although this displacement has not been confirmed in vivo, practitioners should monitor patients for a change in dosage requirements when administering dronabinol to patients receiving other highly protein-bound drugs. Published reports of drug/drug interactions involving cannabinoids are summarized in the following table.

Cannabinoid Drug Interactions

Precipitant drug	Object drug*		Description
Dronabinol	Amphetamines Cocaine Sympathomimetics	↑	Additive hypertension, tachycardia, possibly cardiotoxicity, may occur.
Dronabinol	Anticholinergics Antihistamines	↑	Additive or super-additive tachycardia, or drowsiness may occur.
Dronabinol	Antidepressants, tricyclic	↑	Additive tachycardia, hypertension, or drowsiness may occur.
Dronabinol	Alcohol Sedatives Hypnotics Psychomimetics	↑	Additive or synergistic CNS effects may occur. Also, clearance of barbiturates may be decreased, possibly because of inhibition of metabolism.
Cannabinoids	Disulfiram	↑	A reversible hypomanic reaction occurred in a patient who smoked marijuana; confirmed by rechallenge.
Cannabinoids	Fluoxetine	↑	A patient with depression and bulimia became hypomanic after smoking marijuana; symptoms resolved after 4 days.
Cannabinoids	Theophylline	↓	Increased theophylline metabolism was reported with marijuana smoking.

* ↑ = Object drug increased. ↓ = Object drug decreased.

Adverse Reactions

A cannabinoid dose-related "high" (easy laughing, elation, and heightened awareness) has been reported by patients receiving dronabinol in both the antiemetic (24%) and the lower dose appetite stimulant clinical trials (8%).

The most frequently reported adverse experiences in patients with AIDS during placebo-controlled clinical trials involved the CNS and were reported by 33% of patients receiving dronabinol. About 25% of patients reported a minor CNS adverse event during the first 2 weeks and about 4% reported such an event each week for the next 6 weeks thereafter.

➤*Probably causally related: Incidence greater than 1%:* Rates derived from clinical trials in AIDS-related anorexia (n = 157) and chemotherapy-related nausea (n = 317). Rates were generally higher in the antiemetic use (given in parentheses).

Cardiovascular – Palpitations, tachycardia, vasodilation/facial flush.

CNS – (Amnesia), anxiety/nervousness, (hallucination), (ataxia), confusion, depersonalization.
Incidence of events 3% to 10%: Dizziness, euphoria, paranoid reaction, somnolence, abnormal thinking.

GI –
Incidence of events 3% to 10%: Abdominal pain, nausea, vomiting.

Miscellaneous – Asthenia.

➤*Probably causally related: Incidence less than 1%:* Event rates derived from clinical trials in AIDS-related anorexia (n = 157) and chemotherapy-related nausea (n = 317).

Cardiovascular –
Incidence 0.3% to 1%: Hypotension.

CNS – Depression, nightmares, speech difficulties, tinnitus, emotional lability, tremors.

Dermatologic –
Incidence 0.3% to 1%: Flushing.

GI – Fecal incontinence.
Incidence 0.3% to 1%: Diarrhea.

Musculoskeletal – Myalgias.

Special senses –
Incidence 0.3% to 1%: Conjunctivitis. Vision difficulties.

➤*Causal relationship unknown: Incidence less than 1%:* The clinical significance of the association of these events with dronabinol treatment is unknown, but they are reported as alerting information for the clinician.

Dermatologic – Sweating.

GI – Anorexia, hepatic enzyme elevation.

Respiratory – Cough, rhinitis, sinusitis.

Miscellaneous – Chills, headache, malaise.

Overdosage

The estimated lethal human dose of intravenous dronabinol is 30 mg/kg (2100 mg/70 kg). Significant CNS symptoms in antiemetic studies followed oral doses of 0.4 mg/kg (28 mg/70 kg) of dronabinol.

➤*Symptoms:* Signs and symptoms following mild dronabinol intoxication include drowsiness, euphoria, heightened sensory awareness, altered time perception, reddened conjunctiva, dry mouth and tachycardia; following moderate intoxication include memory impairment, depersonalization, mood alteration, urinary retention, and reduced bowel motility; and following severe intoxication include decreased motor coordination, lethargy, slurred speech, and postural hypotension. Apprehensive patients may experience panic reactions, and seizures may occur in patients with existing seizure disorders.

➤*Treatment:* A potentially serious oral ingestion, if recent, should be managed with gut decontamination. In unconscious patients with a secure airway, instill activated charcoal (30 to 100 g in adults, 1 to 2 g/kg in infants) via a nasogastric tube. A saline cathartic or sorbitol may be added to the first dose of activated charcoal. Patients experiencing depressive, hallucinatory or psychotic reactions should be placed in a quiet area and offered reassurance. Benzodiazepines (5 to 10 mg diazepam by mouth) may be used for treatment of extreme agitation. Hypotension usually responds to Trendelenburg position and IV fluids. Pressors are rarely required.

Patient Information

Patients receiving treatment with dronabinol should be alerted to the potential for additive CNS depression if dronabinol is used concomitantly with alcohol or other CNS depressants such as benzodiazepines and barbiturates.

Patients receiving treatment with dronabinol should be specifically warned not to drive, operate machinery, or engage in any hazardous activity until it is established that they are able to tolerate the drug and to perform such tasks safely.

Patients using dronabinol should be advised of possible changes in mood and other adverse behavioral effects of the drug so as to avoid panic in the event of such manifestations. Patients should remain under the supervision of a responsible adult during initial use of dronabinol and following dosage adjustments.

Miscellaneous

PHOSPHORATED CARBOHYDRATE SOLUTION

otc	**Emetrol** (Pharmacia & Upjohn)	**Solution:** 1.87 g dextrose, 1.87 g fructose, 21.5 mg phosphoric acid per 5 mL	Methylparaben. Lemon mint or cherry flavor. In 118, 236, and 473 mL.
otc	**Formula EM** (Major)		Methylparaben. Cherry flavor. In 118 mL.
otc	**Nausea Relief** (Zenith Goldline)		Methylparaben. In 118 mL.
otc	**Nausetrol** (Walsh Dohmen)		Glycerin, methylparaben. Cherry flavor. In 118 mL.

PHOSPHORATED CARBOHYDRATE SOLUTION — ORAL

Refer to the general discussion beginning in the Antiemetic/Antivertigo Agents monograph.

Indications

➤*Antiemetic:* Relief of nausea caused by upset stomach from intestinal flu, stomach flu and food or drink indiscretions.

➤*Unlabeled uses:* Regurgitation in infants; morning sickness; motion sickness; nausea and vomiting caused by drug therapy or inhalation anesthesia.

Administration and Dosage

Do not dilute. Do not take oral fluids immediately before the dose or for at least 15 minutes after the dose.

➤*Nausea:* Dose may be repeated every 15 minutes until distress subsides. Do not take for more than 1 hour or more than 5 doses.

Children 2 to 12 years of age – 5 or 10 ml.

Adults – 15 or 30 ml.

➤*Regurgitation in infants:* 5 or 10 ml, 10 to 15 minutes before each feeding; in refractory cases, 10 or 15 ml, 30 minutes before feeding.

➤*Morning sickness:* 15 to 30 ml on arising; repeat every 3 hours or when nausea threatens.

➤*Motion sickness or nausea and vomiting caused by drug therapy or inhalation anesthesia:*

Children – 5 ml doses.

Adults – 15 ml doses.

Actions

➤*Pharmacology:* Hyperosmolar carbohydrate solutions with phosphoric acid relieve nausea and vomiting by a direct local action on the wall of the GI tract that reduces smooth muscle contraction.

Precautions

➤*Nausea:* Nausea may signal a serious condition. If symptoms are not relieved or recur often, consult a physician.

➤*Diabetic patients:* Diabetic patients should avoid these preparations because they contain significant amounts of sugar.

➤*Hereditary fructose intolerance:* These preparations contain fructose and should be avoided by individuals with hereditary fructose intolerance.

Adverse Reactions

Large doses of fructose can cause abdominal pain and diarrhea.

ANTIANXIETY AGENTS

Benzodiazepines

Indications

➤*Anxiety:* For the management of anxiety disorders or for the short-term relief of the symptoms of anxiety. Anxiety or tension associated with the stress of everyday life usually does not require treatment with an antianxiety agent.

Consult individual drug monographs for specific indications.

In addition to use as antianxiety agents, some benzodiazepines are also useful as hypnotics, anticonvulsants, and muscle relaxants. **Midazolam**, an injectable short-acting benzodiazepine, is used for induction of general anesthesia, preoperative sedation, conscious sedation for diagnostic procedures, and to supplement nitrous oxide and oxygen for short surgical procedures (see individual monograph).

➤*Unlabeled uses:* Management of irritable bowel syndrome (**chlordiazepoxide, diazepam, clorazepate, lorazepam, oxazepam, alprazolam**); panic attacks (alprazolam, diazepam); depression (alprazolam); premenstrual syndrome (alprazolam); status epilepticus, chemotherapy-induced nausea and vomiting, acute alcohol withdrawal syndrome, psychogenic catatonia (lorazepam injection); chronic insomnia (lorazepam).

Actions

➤*Pharmacology:* Benzodiazepines appear to potentiate the effects of gamma-aminobutyrate (GABA) (ie, they facilitate inhibitory GABA neurotransmission) and other inhibitory transmitters by binding to specific benzodiazepine receptor sites. Recent evidence suggest there are at least 2 benzodiazepine receptors, BZ_1 and BZ_2. BZ_1 is thought to be associated with sleep mechanisms; BZ_2 with memory, motor, sensory, and cognitive functions. The activity of the benzodiazepines may involve the following sites: spinal cord (muscle relaxation); brain stem (anticonvulsant properties); cerebellum (ataxia); limbic and cortical areas (emotional behavior). Anxiolytic effects are distinct from nonspecific consequences of CNS depression (ie, sedation and motor impairment). A distinctive feature of the benzodiazepines is the wide margin of safety between therapeutic and toxic doses. Ataxia and sedation occur only at doses beyond those needed for anxiolytic effects.

Clonazepam suppresses the spike and wave discharge in petit mal seizures and decreases frequency, amplitude, duration and spread of discharge in minor motor seizures.

➤*Pharmacokinetics:*

Absorption – The major determinant of the onset and intensity of action of a single oral dose of a benzodiazepine is the rate of absorption from the GI tract. Benzodiazepines are readily absorbed following oral administration.

Intramuscular (IM) administration of **chlordiazepoxide** and **diazepam** results in slow erratic absorption and lower peak plasma levels than oral or intravenous (IV) administration. However, IM administration of diazepam into the deltoid muscle is more likely to be rapid and complete. **Lorazepam** IM is rapidly and completely absorbed.

Distribution – The highly lipid soluble benzodiazepines are widely distributed in the body tissues and highly bound to plasma proteins (70% to 99%). The duration of action is related to their lipid solubility. Highly lipophilic drugs, like **diazepam**, are rapidly taken into the brain and then rapidly redistributed throughout the body.

Metabolism – The effect of lipid solubility on duration of action is complicated by hepatic biotransformation to active metabolites. The benzophenone metabolite of **alprazolam** is inactive, while alpha-hydroxy-alprazolam is approximately 50% as active as the parent compound; both metabolites have the same half-life as alprazolam. Other benzodiazepines have active metabolites with very long half-lives; cumulative effects occur with chronic administration. Desmethyldiazepam is an active metabolite common to many of these agents (eg, **clorazepate, diazepam**); clorazepate is hydrolyzed in the stomach and absorbed as desmethyldiazepam. **Chlordiazepoxide** has several active intermediate metabolites. Five metabolites of clonazepam have been identified. Biotransformation of **clonazepam** is by oxidative hydroxylation and reduction.

Because hepatic biotransformation is the predominant route for benzodiazepine metabolism, the disposition of these drugs may be impaired in patients with chronic liver disease. **Oxazepam** and **lorazepam** are metabolized to inactive compounds and therefore have relatively short half-lives and duration of activity. Because of their simple 1-step inactivation, oxazepam or lorazepam may be preferred in patients with liver disease and in the elderly. Sustained clinical effects require multiple daily doses; significant accumulation does not occur. The other agents with prolonged half-lives may be administered as a single daily dose at bedtime. The elimination half-life of diazepam and desmethyldiazepam is prolonged in obese patients; total metabolic clearance does not change.

BENZODIAZEPINE METABOLIC PATHWAYS

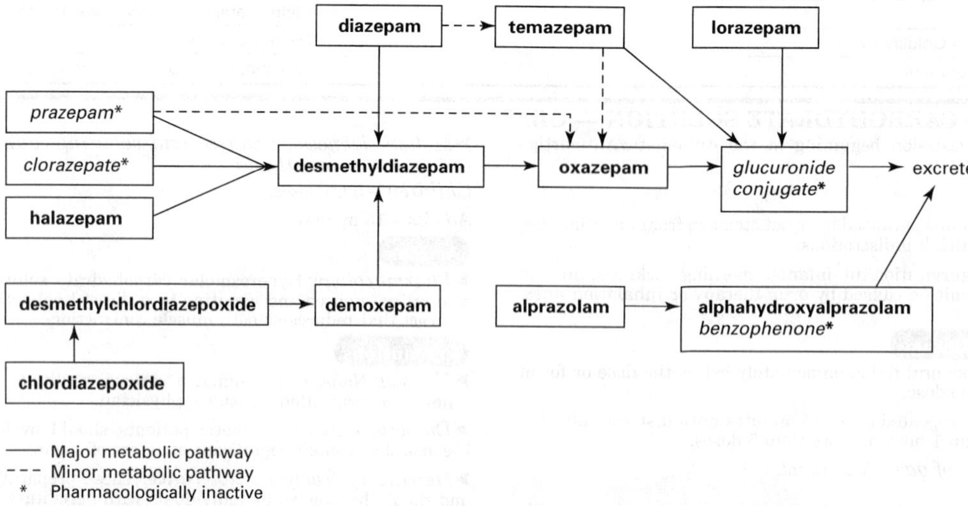

Excretion – Most benzodiazepines are excreted almost entirely in the urine and in the form of oxidized and glucuronide-conjugated metabolites. There is little clinical evidence to suggest that one benzodiazepine is more effective than another. The major differences are reflected in their pharmacokinetic profiles and relative costs. The following table summarizes the major pharmacokinetic variables of these agents:

Benzodiazepine Pharmacokinetics						
Drug	Dosage range (mg/d)[a]	Peak plasma level (h)[a]	Elimination t½ (h)	Metabolites	Speed of onset[a]	Protein binding
Alprazolam	0.75 to 4	1 to 2	6.3 to 26.9	Alpha-hydroxy-alprazolam; Benzophenone	intermediate	80%
Chlordiazepoxide	15 to 100	0.5 to 4	5 to 30	Desmethylchlordiazepoxide[b]; Demoxepam; Desmethyl-diazepam	intermediate	96%
Clonazepam	1.5 to 20	1 to 2	18 to 50	Inactive 7–amino or 7–acetyl-amino derivatives[b]	intermediate	97%
Clorazepate	15 to 60	1 to 2	40 to 50	Desmethyl-diazepam	fast	97% to 98%[c]
Diazepam	4 to 40	0.5 to 2	20 to 80	Desmethyl-diazepam[b]; nordiazepam	very fast	98%
Lorazepam	2 to 4	2 to 4	10 to 20	Inactive glucuronide conjugate	intermediate	85%
Oxazepam	30 to 120	2 to 4	5 to 20	Inactive glucuronide conjugate	slow	87%

[a] Oral administration.
[b] Major metabolite.
[c] Nordiazepam (active metabolite).

Contraindications

Hypersensitivity to benzodiazepines; psychoses; acute narrow-angle glaucoma (may be used in patients with open-angle glaucoma and appropriate therapy); patients with clinical or biochemical evidence of significant liver disease (**clonazepam**); intra-arterial use (**lorazepam** injection); children younger than 6 months of age; lactation (**diazepam**); coadministration with ketoconazole and itraconazole due to inhibition of cytochrome P450 3A (see Warnings).

Warnings

➤*Psychiatric disorders:* These agents are not intended for use in patients with a primary depressive disorder or psychosis, nor in those psychiatric disorders in which anxiety is not a prominent feature.

➤*Long-term use (longer than 4 months):* Effectiveness has not been assessed by systematic clinical studies. Periodically reassess the usefulness of the drug for the individual patient.

➤*Dependence:* Prolonged use of therapeutic doses can lead to dependence. Withdrawal syndrome has occurred after as little as 4 to 6 weeks treatment. It is more likely if the drug is short-acting (eg, **alprazolam**), taken regularly for longer than 3 months and abruptly discontinued.

After rapid decrease of dosage or abrupt discontinuation, withdrawal seizures were reported in alprazolam patients.

Onset is within 1 to 10 days; duration of reaction may be 5 days to 1 month depending on agent, dose, etc. Symptoms generally begin with anxiety-like manifestations; the following may occur in 50% or more of cases: anorexia; concentration difficulties; confusion; dizziness; dysphoria; fatigue; hallucinations; headache; increased anxiety; insomnia; memory impairment; muscle tension/cramps; muscle twitching; paranoid delusions; "psychosis"; seizures (generalized tonic-clonic); sensory disturbances (hypercusis, hypersomnia, metallic taste, paresthesias, photophobia); tremor; vomiting.

Abrupt withdrawal of **clonazepam**, particularly in those patients on long-term, high-dose therapy, may precipitate status epilepticus. While clonazepam is being gradually withdrawn, the simultaneous substitution of another anticonvulsant may be indicated. Other symptoms include diarrhea, sweating, and vomiting.

When discontinuing therapy in patients who have used these agents for prolonged periods, decrease dosage gradually over 4 to 8 weeks to avoid the possibility of withdrawal symptoms, especially in patients with a history of seizures or epilepsy, regardless of their concomitant anticonvulsant drug therapy. Patients on short-acting benzodiazepines may be switched to longer-acting drugs (eg, **diazepam**) which produce a gradual decrease in drug concentration and decrease the chance of withdrawal symptoms. Clonidine, propranolol, and carbamazepine have been used as adjuncts in the treatment of benzodiazepine withdrawal symptoms.

➤*Parenteral administration:* Parenteral (IM or IV) therapy is indicated primarily in acute states. Keep patients under observation, preferably in bed, for up to 3 hours.

Do not inject intra-arterially; this may produce arteriospasm, resulting in gangrene which may require amputation.

Administer parenterally with extreme care (particularly IV) to the elderly, very ill, and those with limited pulmonary reserve. Because of possible apnea or cardiac arrest, resuscitative facilities should be available. Not recommended for obstetric use. Do not administer to patients in shock, coma or in acute alcohol intoxication.

Hypotension or muscular weakness is possible, particularly when benzodiazepines are used with narcotics, barbiturates, or alcohol.

➤*Renal function impairment:* Observe usual precautions in the presence of impaired renal or hepatic function to avoid accumulation of these agents. **Lorazepam** injection is not recommended in these patients. Metabolites of **clonazepam** are excreted by the kidneys; to avoid excess accumulation, exercise caution in patients with renal function impairment. Also, clonazepam is contraindicated in patients with significant liver disease.

➤*Elderly:* The initial dose should be small and dosage increments made gradually, in accordance with the response of the patient, to preclude ataxia or excessive sedation. Hypotension is rare; however, use with caution if cardiac complications may result from a drop in blood pressure.

➤*Pregnancy: Category D* (No category designation for **clonazepam**). Benzodiazepines and their metabolites freely cross the placenta and accumulate in the fetal circulation. An increased risk of congenital malformations associated with the use of minor tranquilizers during the first trimester of pregnancy has been suggested. Malformations reported include cleft lip or palate. Recent studies suggest **diazepam** use in the first trimester does not cause an increased risk of this. Because use of these drugs is rarely a matter of urgency, avoid them during this period. Consider the possibility that a woman of childbearing potential may be pregnant at the time of institution of therapy. Advise patients that if they become pregnant, or plan to become pregnant, they should discuss the desirability of discontinuing the drug.

Labor and delivery – Benzodiazepines have been found in maternal and cord blood, indicating placental transfer of drug. Therefore, benzodiazepines are not recommended for obstetrical use.

Neonatal withdrawal consisting of severe tremulousness and irritability has been attributed to maternal ingestion of benzodiazepines as well as neonatal flaccidity and respiratory problems. Use during labor has resulted in a "floppy infant" syndrome, manifested by hypotonia, lethargy, and sucking difficulties.

Prolonged CNS depression has been observed in neonates, apparently due to inability to biotransform **diazepam** into inactive metabolites.

➤*Lactation:* Benzodiazepines are excreted in breast milk (**lorazepam** excretion is not known). Because neonates metabolize benzodiazepines at a slower rate than adults, accumulation of the drug and its metabolites to toxic levels is possible. Chronic **diazepam** use in breast-feeding mothers reportedly caused infants to become lethargic and to lose weight; do not give to breast-feeding mothers.

➤*Children:* The initial dose should be small and dosage increments made gradually, in accordance with the response of the patient, to preclude ataxia or excessive sedation. Hypotension is rare; however, use with caution if cardiac complications may result from a drop in blood pressure.

Alprazolam – Safety and efficacy for use in patients younger than 18 years of age have not been established.

Chlordiazepoxide – Chlordiazepoxide is not recommended in children younger than 6 years of age (oral) or 12 years of age (injectable).

Clorazepate – Not recommended for use in patients younger than 9 years of age.

Diazepam – Not for use in children younger than 6 months of age (oral); safety and efficacy have not been established in the neonate (30 days or less of age; injectable).

Lorazepam – Do not use in patients younger than 18 years of age (injection); safety and efficacy for use in patients younger than 12 years of age are not established (oral).

Precautions

➤*Monitoring:* Because of isolated reports of neutropenia and jaundice, perform periodic blood counts and liver function tests during long-term therapy. There have been reports of abnormal liver and kidney function tests and of decrease in hematocrit.

➤*Suicide:* In those patients in whom depression accompanies anxiety, suicidal tendencies may be present, and protective measures may be required. Dispense the least amount of drug feasible to the patient.

➤*Paradoxical reactions:* Excitement, stimulation, and acute rage have occurred in psychiatric patients and hyperactive aggressive children. These reactions may be secondary to relief of anxiety and usually appear in the first 2 weeks of therapy. Acute hyperexcited states, anxiety, hallucinations, increased muscle spasticity, insomnia, and sleep disturbances also have occurred. Should these occur, discontinue the drug. Minor EEG changes, usually low voltage fast activity, have been observed during and after therapy and are of no known significance. Anger, hostility and episodes of mania and hypomania have been reported with **alprazolam**.

➤*Multiple seizure type:* When used in patients in whom several different types of seizure disorders coexist, **clonazepam** may increase the incidence or precipitate the onset of generalized tonic-clonic (grand mal) seizures. This may require the addition of other anticonvulsants or an increase in their dosage.

Diazepam – If use in patients with seizure disorders results in an increase in the frequency or severity of grand mal seizures, there may be a need to increase the dosage of standard anticonvulsant medication.

➤*Chronic respiratory disease:* **Clonazepam** may produce an increase in salivation. Use with caution in patients if increased salivation causes respiratory difficulty. Due to the possibility of respiratory depression, use with caution in such patients.

➤*Benzyl alcohol:* Some of these products contain benzyl alcohol, which has been associated with a fatal "gasping syndrome" in premature infants.

➤*Hazardous tasks:* May produce drowsiness or dizziness; observe caution while driving or performing other tasks requiring alertness.

➤*Tartrazine sensitivity:* Some of these products contain tartrazine, which may cause allergic-type reactions (including bronchial asthma) in susceptible individuals. Although the incidence of tartrazine sensitivity in the general population is low, it is frequently seen in patients who also have aspirin hypersensitivity. Specific products containing tartrazine are identified in the product listings.

Drug Interactions

Benzodiazepine Drug Interactions

Precipitant drug	Object drug[a]		Description
Alcohol/CNS depressants (eg, barbiturates, narcotics)	Benzodiazepines	↑	Increased CNS effects (eg, impaired psychomotor function, sedation) may occur.
Benzodiazepines	Alcohol/CNS depressants (eg, barbiturates, narcotics)		
Antacids	Benzodiazepines	↓	Antacids may alter the rate but generally not the extent of GI absorption. Staggering administration times may help avoid possible interaction.
Cimetidine Contraceptives, oral Disulfiram Fluoxetine Isoniazid Ketoconazole Metoprolol Propoxyphene Propranolol Valproic acid	Alprazolam Chlordiazepoxide Clorazepate Diazepam	↑	The elimination of benzodiazepines that undergo oxidative hepatic metabolism (alprazolam, chlordiazepoxide, clorazepate, diazepam) may be decreased by the following drugs due to inhibition of hepatic metabolism. Pharmacologic effects of these benzodiazepines may be increased and excessive sedation/impaired psychomotor function may occur.
Contraceptives, oral	Lorazepam Oxazepam	↓	The clearance rate of benzodiazepines that undergo glucuronidation (lorazepam, oxazepam) may be increased.
Probenecid	Benzodiazepines	↑	Probenecid may interfere with benzodiazepine conjugation in the liver, possibly resulting in a more rapid onset or prolonged effect.
Ranitidine	Diazepam	↓	Ranitidine may reduce the GI absorption of diazepam.
Rifampin	Benzodiazepines	↓	The oxidative metabolism of benzodiazepines may be increased due to microsomal enzyme induction. Pharmacologic effects of some benzodiazepines may be decreased.
Scopolamine	Lorazepam	↑	Scopolamine, used concomitantly with parenteral lorazepam, may increase the incidence of sedation, hallucinations, and irrational behavior.
Theophyllines	Benzodiazepines	↓	Theophyllines may antagonize the sedative effects of the benzodiazepines.
Benzodiazepines	Digoxin	↑	Digoxin's serum concentrations may be increased. Toxicity characterized by GI and neuropsychiatric symptoms and cardiac arrhythmias may occur. Monitor digoxin serum levels.
Benzodiazepines	Levodopa	↓	Levodopa's antiparkinson efficacy may be decreased by coadministration of benzodiazepines.

Benzodiazepines

Benzodiazepine Drug Interactions			
Precipitant drug	Object drug[a]		Description
Benzodiazepines	Neuromuscular blocking agents	↔	Benzodiazepines may potentiate, counteract, or have no effect on the actions of these agents.
Benzodiazepines	Phenytoin	↑	Phenytoin serum concentrations may be increased, resulting in toxicity, but data are conflicting. Phenytoin may increase oxazepam clearance.

[a] ↑ = Object drug increased. ↓ = Object drug decreased. ↔ = Undetermined clinical effect.

Adverse Reactions

Discontinuation of therapy due to undesirable effects is rare. Transient, mild drowsiness is commonly seen in the first few days of therapy. Drowsiness, ataxia and confusion have occurred, especially in elderly and debilitated patients. If these reactions are persistent, reduce dosage. Ataxia is rare with **oxazepam** and does not appear to be specifically related to dose or age. Other adverse reactions less frequently reported include:

➤*Cardiovascular:* Bradycardia; cardiovascular collapse; edema; hypertension; hypotension; palpitations; phlebitis and thrombosis at IV sites; tachycardia. Decrease in systolic blood pressure has been observed.

➤*CNS:* Agitation; akathisia; anterograde amnesia; apathy; aphonia; ataxia; coma; confusion; crying; delirium; depression; difficulty in concentration; disorientation; dizziness; dysarthria; dystonia; euphoria; extrapyramidal symptoms; fatigue; "glassy-eyed" appearance; headache; hemiparesis; hypoactivity; hypotonia; inability to perform complex mental functions; incoordination; irritability; lethargy; light-headedness; memory impairment; nervousness; paradoxical reactions (see Precautions); psychomotor retardation; restlessness; rigidity; sedation and sleepiness; seizures; slurred speech; sobbing; stupor; syncope; tremor; unsteadiness; vertigo; vivid dreams; weakness.

➤*Dermatologic:* Ankle and facial edema; dermatitis; hair loss; hirsutism; pruritus; urticaria; skin rash, including morbilliform, urticarial, and maculopapular.

➤*GI:* Anorexia; change in appetite; coated tongue; constipation; diarrhea; difficulty in swallowing; dry mouth; gastritis; increased salivation; nausea; sore gums; vomiting.

➤*GU:* Changes in libido; incontinence; menstrual irregularities; urinary retention.

➤*Ophthalmic:* Diplopia; nystagmus; visual disturbances.

➤*Psychiatric:* Behavior problems; hysteria; psychosis; suicidal tendencies.

➤*Miscellaneous:* Anemia; auditory disturbances; blood dyscrasias including agranulocytosis; depressed hearing; diaphoresis; dehydration; elevations of LDH, alkaline phosphatase, ALT, and AST; eosinophilia; fever; galactorrhea; gynecomastia; hepatic dysfunction (including hepatitis and jaundice); hiccups; increase or decrease in body weight; joint pain; leukopenia; lymphadenopathy; muscular disturbance; nasal congestion; pain, burning, and redness following IM injection; paresthesias; respiratory disturbances; thrombocytopenia. Partial airway obstruction has occurred and is believed to be due to excessive sedation at time of procedure (**lorazepam** injection).

Overdosage

There are no well-documented fatal overdoses resulting from oral ingestion of benzodiazepines alone. Most overdose-related fatalities implicate benzodiazepines only as a component in multiple drug ingestions.

➤*Symptoms:* Mild symptoms include confusion, diminished reflexes, drowsiness, impaired coordination, lethargy, and somnolence. These agents rarely cause significant respiratory or circulatory depression, particularly when they are the sole agents ingested. Serious symptoms may include ataxia, hypotonia, hypotension, hypnosis, stages 1 to 3 coma, and rarely, death. Consider multiple drug ingestion.

Unlike oral ingestions, IV administration of **diazepam** is associated with a 1.7% incidence of life-threatening reactions, including hypotension and respiratory or cardiac arrest.

➤*Treatment:* Induce vomiting if it has not occurred spontaneously. Employ general supportive measures, along with immediate gastric lavage or ipecac. Follow with activated charcoal administration and a saline cathartic. Monitor respiration, pulse, and blood pressure. Administer IV fluids and maintain an adequate airway. Treat hypotension with norepinephrine or metaraminol. With normal kidney function, forced diuresis with osmotic diuretics, IV fluids, and electrolytes may accelerate the elimination of benzodiazepines. Dialysis is of limited value; however, in more critical situations, renal dialysis and exchange blood transfusions may be indicated. Refer to General Management of Acute Overdosage.

Infusion of physostigmine 0.5 to 4 mg IV at the rate of 1 mg/min may reverse symptoms suggestive of central anticholinergic overdose (eg, confusion, delirium, hallucinations, memory disturbance, visual disturbances); however, weigh the hazards associated with the use of physostigmine (eg, induction of seizures) against its possible clinical benefit.

There have been occasional reports of excitation in patients following overdosage with **chlordiazepoxide**; if this occurs, do not give barbiturates.

Patient Information

Inform patients that these drugs may cause drowsiness and to avoid driving or other tasks requiring alertness.

Advise patients to avoid alcohol or other CNS depressants.

Inform patients that medication may be taken with food or water if stomach upset occurs.

Patients on long-term or high-dosage therapy may experience withdrawal symptoms on abrupt cessation of therapy; advise patients not to discontinue therapy abruptly or change dosage except on advice of the health care provider.

Inform patients that concomitant ingestion with antacids may alter the rate of absorption of these drugs (documented with **diazepam** and **chlordiazepoxide**).

➤*Clonazepam, clorazepate, and diazepam:* Patient should carry identification (*Medic Alert*) indicating medication usage and epilepsy.

ALPRAZOLAM

c-iv	**Alprazolam** (Various, eg, Geneva, Mylan, Purepac)	**Tablets:** 0.25 mg	In 100s, 500s, 1000s, and UD 100s.
c-iv	**Xanax** (Pfizer)		Lactose. (Xanax 0.25). White, oval, scored. In 100s, 500s, 1000s, and UD 100s.
c-iv	**Alprazolam** (Various, eg, Geneva, Mylan, Purepac)	**Tablets:** 0.5 mg	In 100s, 500s, 1000s, and UD 100s.
c-iv	**Xanax** (Pfizer)		Lactose. (Xanax 0.5). Peach, oval, scored. In 100s, 500s, 1000s, and UD 100s.
c-iv	**Alprazolam** (Various, eg, Geneva, Mylan, Purepac)	**Tablets:** 1 mg	In 100s, 500s, 1000s, and UD 100s.
c-iv	**Xanax** (Pfizer)		Lactose, FD & C Blue No. 2. (Xanax 1.0). Blue, oval, scored. In 100s, 500s, and 1000s.
c-iv	**Alprazolam** (Various, eg, Mylan, Purepac)	**Tablets:** 2 mg	In 100s and 500s.
c-iv	**Xanax** (Pfizer)		Lactose. (XANAX 2). White, oblong, multi-scored. In 100s and 500s.
c-iv	**Alprazolam Extended-Release** (Various, eg, Greenstone, Mylan)	**Tablets, extended-release:** 0.5 mg	May contain lactose. In 60s and 500s.
c-iv	**Xanax XR** (Pfizer)		Lactose. (X 0.5). White, pentagonal. In 60s.
c-iv	**Alprazolam Extended-Release** (Various, eg, Greenstone, Mylan)	**Tablets, extended-release:** 1 mg	May contain lactose. In 60s and 500s.
c-iv	**Xanax XR** (Pfizer)		Lactose. (X 1). Yellow, square. In 60s.
c-iv	**Alprazolam Extended-Release** (Various, eg, Greenstone, Mylan)	**Tablets, extended-release:** 2 mg	May contain lactose. In 60s and 500s.
c-iv	**Xanax XR** (Pfizer)		Lactose, FD & C Blue No. 2. (X 2). Blue. In 60s.
c-iv	**Alprazolam Extended-Release** (Various, eg, Greenstone, Mylan)	**Tablets, extended-release:** 3 mg	May contain lactose. In 60s and 500s.
c-iv	**Xanax XR** (Pfizer)		Lactose, FD & C Blue No. 2. (X 3). Green, triangular. In 60s.

ALPRAZOLAM

c-iv	**Niravam** (Schwarz Pharma)	**Tablets, orally disintegrating:** 0.25 mg	Sucralose, sucrose. (SP 321 0.25). Yellow, scored. Orange flavor. In 100s.
		0.5 mg	Sucralose, sucrose. (SP 322 0.5). Yellow, scored. Orange flavor. In 100s.
		1 mg	Sucralose, sucrose. (SP 323 1). White, scored. Orange flavor. In 100s.
		2 mg	Sucralose, sucrose. (SP 324 2). White, scored. Orange flavor. In 100s.
c-iv	**Alprazolam Intensol** (Roxane)	**Oral solution:** 1 mg/mL	Flavorless. In 30 mL with calibrated dropper.

ALPRAZOLAM — ORAL

Complete and comparative prescribing information begins in the Benzodiazepines monograph.

Indications

➤*Panic disorder (Niravam, Xanax, Xanax XR):* Treatment of panic disorder, with or without agoraphobia.

➤*Anxiety disorders (immediate-release tablets and intensol):* For the management of anxiety disorders or for the short-term relief of the symptoms of anxiety. Anxiety associated with depression is also responsive.

Alprazolam given sublingually is absorbed as rapidly as after oral administration; completeness of absorption is comparable.

Administration and Dosage

Individualize dosage. Increase cautiously to avoid adverse effects. Reduce gradually when terminating or decreasing daily dose. Decrease no more than 0.5 mg every 3 days.

➤*Anxiety disorders (immediate-release tablets and intensol):* Initial dose is 0.25 to 0.5 mg 3 times/day. Titrate to a maximum total dose of 4 mg/day in divided doses at intervals of 3 to 4 days. If side effects occur with starting dose, decrease dose.

➤*Panic disorder (Niravam, Xanax, Xanax XR):*

Immediate-release tablets – Initial dose is 0.5 mg 3 times/day. Depending on response, increase dose at intervals of 3 to 4 days in increments of no more than 1 mg/day.

Successful treatment has required doses more than 4 mg/day; in controlled studies, doses in the range of 1 to 10 mg/day were used. The mean dosage employed was approximately 5 to 6 mg/day.

Extended-release tablets – Administer once daily, preferably in the morning. Take the tablets intact; do not chew, crush, or break.

Treatment may be initiated with 0.5 to 1 mg once daily. The suggested total daily dose ranges between 3 and 6 mg/day. The suggested total daily dosages will meet the needs of most patients; however, there will be some who require doses greater than 6 mg/day.

Dose maintenance: In controlled trials, a dose range of 1 to 10 mg/day was used. Most patients showed efficacy in the range of 3 to 6 mg/day. Occasionally as much as 10 mg/day was required to achieve successful response.

Immediate/Extended-release tablets –

Dose titration: Depending on response, the dose may be increased at intervals of 3 to 4 days in increments of no more than 1 mg/day. Slower titration to the dose levels may be advisable to allow full expression of the pharmacodynamic effect. Advance dose until an acceptable therapeutic response (ie, a substantial reduction in or total elimination of panic attacks) is achieved, intolerance occurs, or the maximum recommended dose is attained.

Duration: The necessary duration of treatment for responding patients is unknown. However, periodic reassessment is advised. After a period of extended freedom from attacks, a carefully supervised tapered discontinuation may be attempted, but there is evidence that this may often be difficult to accomplish without recurrence of symptoms and/or the manifestations of withdrawal phenomena.

Dose reduction: Because of the danger of withdrawal, avoid abrupt discontinuation. Gradually reduce dosage in all patients when discontinuing therapy or when decreasing the daily dosage. Although there are no systematically collected data to support a specific discontinuation schedule, it is suggested that the daily dosage be decreased by no more than 0.5 mg every 3 days. Some patients may require an even slower dosage reduction. Some patients may prove resistant to all discontinuation regimens.

In any case, reduction of dose must begin under close supervision and must be gradual. If significant withdrawal symptoms develop, reinstitute the previous dosing schedule and attempt a less rapid schedule of discontinuation only after stabilization. In a controlled postmarketing discontinuation study of panic disorder that compared this recommended taper schedule with a slower taper schedule, no difference was observed between groups in the proportion of patients who tapered to zero dose; however, the slower schedule was associated with a reduction in symptoms associated with a withdrawal syndrome.

Switching from immediate-release to extended-release tablets: Patients currently treated with divided doses of immediate-release tablets (eg, 3 to 4 times/day) may be switched to extended-release tablets at the same total daily dose taken once daily. If the therapeutic response after switching is inadequate, dosage may be titrated as outlined above.

➤*Elderly, advanced hepatic disease, or debilitated patients:*

Immediate-release tablets and intensol – Starting dose is 0.25 mg, given 2 or 3 times/day. Gradually increase if needed and tolerated.

Extended-release tablets – The usual starting dose is 0.5 mg once/day. Gradually increase if needed and tolerated. The elderly may be especially sensitive to the effects of benzodiazepines.

➤*Administration of oral solution:* Alprazolam intensol is a concentrated oral solution. It is recommended that the oral solution be mixed with liquids or semi-solid food such as water, juices, soda or soda-like beverages, applesauce, and puddings. Use only the calibrated dropper provided with this product. Draw into the dropper the amount prescribed for a single dose. Then squeeze the dropper contents into a liquid or semi-solid food. Stir the liquid or food gently for a few seconds. The formulation blends quickly and completely. Consume the entire amount of the mixture of drug and liquid or drug and food immediately. Do not store for future use.

➤*Administration of orally disintegrating tablets:* Just prior to administration, with dry hands, remove the tablet from the bottle. Immediately place the tablet on top of the tongue where it will disintegrate and be swallowed with saliva. Administration with liquid is not necessary. If only one-half of a scored tablet is used for dosing, discard the unused portion of the tablet immediately because it may not remain stable. Discard any cotton that was included in the bottle and reseal the bottle tightly to prevent introducing moisture that might cause the tablets to disintegrate.

➤*Storage/Stability:* Store at controlled room temperature, 15° to 30°C (59° to 86°F). Protect from moisture.

CLORAZEPATE DIPOTASSIUM

c-iv	**Clorazepate Dipotassium** (Various, eg, Able, Mylan, Taro, Watson)	**Tablets:** 3.75 mg	In 100s, 500s, 1000s, and UD 100s.
c-iv	**Tranxene T-tab** (Ovation)		FD & C Blue No. 2. (TL). Blue, scored. In 100s, 500s, and UD 100s.
c-iv	**Clorazepate Dipotassium** (Various, eg, Able, Mylan, Taro, Watson)	**Tablets:** 7.5 mg	In 20s, 100s, 500s, 1000s, and UD 100s and 500s.
c-iv	**Tranxene T-tab** (Ovation)		(TM). Peach, scored. In 100s, 500s, and UD 100s.
c-iv	**Clorazepate Dipotassium** (Various, eg, Able, Mylan, Taro, Watson)	**Tablets:** 15 mg	In 100s, 500s, 1000s, and UD 100s.
c-iv	**Tranxene T-tab** (Ovation)		(TN). Lavender, scored. In 100s, 500s, and UD 100s.
c-iv	**Tranxene-SD Half Strength** (Ovation)	**Tablets, extended-release:** 11.25 mg	Lactose. (TX). Blue. In 100s.
c-iv	**Tranxene-SD** (Ovation)	**Tablets, extended-release:** 22.5 mg	Lactose. (TY). Tan. In 100s.

CLORAZEPATE DIPOTASSIUM — ORAL

Complete prescribing information begins in the Benzodiazepines monograph. Also see the Anticonvulsant monograph section.

Indications

➤*Anxiety:* For the management of anxiety disorders or for the short-term relief of the symptoms of anxiety. Anxiety or tension associated with the stress of everyday life usually does not require treatment with an anxiolytic.

CLORAZEPATE DIPOTASSIUM — ORAL

➤*Seizures:* As adjunctive therapy in the management of partial seizures.

➤*Alcohol withdrawal:* For the symptomatic relief of acute alcohol withdrawal.

Administration and Dosage

➤*Symptomatic relief of anxiety:* Administer orally in divided doses. The usual daily dose is 30 mg. The dose should be adjusted gradually within the range of 15 to 60 mg daily in accordance with the response of the patient. In elderly or debilitated patients it is advisable to initiate treatment at a daily dose of 7.5 to 15 mg.

May also administer in a single dose daily at bedtime; the recommended initial dose is 15 mg. After the initial dose, the response of the patient may require adjustment of subsequent dosage. Lower doses may be indicated in the elderly patient. Drowsiness may occur at the initiation of treatment and with dosage increment.

➤*Symptomatic relief of acute alcohol withdrawal:* The following dosage schedule is recommended:

First 24 hours (day 1) – 30 mg clorazepate dipotassium initially, followed by 30 to 60 mg in divided doses.

Second 24 hours (day 2) – 45 to 90 mg in divided doses.

Third 24 hours (day 3) – 22.5 to 45 mg in divided doses.

Day 4 – 15 to 30 mg in divided doses.

Thereafter, gradually reduce the daily dose to 7.5 to 15 mg. Discontinue drug therapy as soon as patient's condition is stable.

The maximum recommended total daily dose is 90 mg. Avoid excessive reductions in the total amount of drug administered on successive days.

➤*As an adjunct to antiepileptic drugs:* In order to minimize drowsiness, the recommended initial dosages and dosage increments should not be exceeded.

Adults – The maximum recommended initial dose in patients greater than 12 years old is 7.5 mg 3 times a day. Dosage should be increased by no more than 7.5 mg every week and should not exceed 90 mg/day.

Children (9 to 12 years) – The maximum recommended initial dose is 7.5 mg 2 times a day. Dosage should be increased by no more than 7.5 mg every week and should not exceed 60 mg/day.

➤*Storage/Stability:* Store at controlled room temperature 15° to 30°C (59° to 86°F). Protect from moisture and light. Dispense in a tight, light-resistant container using a child-resistant closure.

CHLORDIAZEPOXIDE HYDROCHLORIDE

c-iv	**Chlordiazepoxide HCl** (Various, eg, Barr, Geneva, Major, Watson)	**Capsules**: 5 mg	In 20s, 100s, 500s, 1000s, and UD 100s.
c-iv	**Librium** (ICN Pharmaceuticals)		Lactose, parabens. (LIBRIUM 5). Green and yellow. In 100s.
c-iv	**Chlordiazepoxide HCl** (Various, eg, Barr, Major, UDL, Watson)	**Capsules**: 10 mg	In 20s, 100s, 500s, 1000s, and UD 100s.
c-iv	**Librium** (ICN Pharmaceuticals)		Lactose, parabens. (LIBRIUM 10). Green and black. In 100s.
c-iv	**Chlordiazepoxide HCl** (Various, eg, Barr, Major, UDL, Watson)	**Capsules**: 25 mg	In 20s, 100s, 500s, 1000s, and UD 100s.
c-iv	**Librium** (ICN Pharmaceuticals)		Lactose, parabens. (LIBRIUM 25). Green and white. In 100s.
c-iv	**Librium** (ICN Pharmaceuticals)	**Powder for injection**: 100 mg	In 5 mL amp with 2 mL amp of IM diluent.[a]

[a] With 1.5% benzyl alcohol, polysorbate 80, and 20% propylene glycol.

CHLORDIAZEPOXIDE HYDROCHLORIDE — ORAL

Complete and comparative prescribing information begins in the Benzodiazepines monograph.

Indications

➤*Anxiety disorders:* For the management of anxiety disorders or for short-term relief of anxiety symptoms.

➤*Acute alcohol withdrawal:* For the symptoms of acute alcohol withdrawal.

➤*Preoperative:* For preoperative apprehension and anxiety.

Administration and Dosage

Individualize dosage.

➤*Mild to moderate anxiety:* 5 or 10 mg 3 to 4 times/day.

➤*Severe anxiety:* 20 or 25 mg 3 to 4 times/day.

➤*Elderly patients or patients with debilitating disease:* 5 mg 2 to 4 times/day.

➤*Preoperative apprehension and anxiety:* On days preceding surgery, 5 to 10 mg 3 or 4 times/day.

➤*Acute alcohol withdrawal:* 50 to 100 mg; repeat as needed (up to 300 mg/day). Parenteral form usually used initially. Reduce to maintenance levels.

➤*Children:* Initially, 5 mg 2 to 4 times/day. (May be increased in some children to 10 mg 2 or 3 times/day.) Not recommended in children younger than 6 years of age.

➤*Storage/Stability:* Store at controlled room temperature 15° to 30°C (59° to 86°F). Dispense in a tight, light-resistant container as defined in USP/NF.

CHLORDIAZEPOXIDE HYDROCHLORIDE — INJECTION

Complete and comparative prescribing information begins in the Benzodiazepines monograph.

Indications

➤*Anxiety disorders:* For the management of anxiety disorders or for short-term relief of anxiety symptoms.

➤*Acute alcohol withdrawal:* For the symptoms of acute alcohol withdrawal.

➤*Preoperative:* For preoperative apprehension and anxiety.

Administration and Dosage

Use lower doses (25 to 50 mg) for elderly or debilitated patients and for children 12 years of age or older. Acute symptoms may be rapidly controlled by parenteral administration; subsequent treatment, if necessary, may be given orally. While 300 mg may be given during a 6-hour period, do not exceed this dose in any 24-hour period. Not recommended in children younger than 12 years of age.

➤*Acute alcohol withdrawal:* 50 to 100 mg IM or IV initially; repeat in 2 to 4 hours if necessary.

➤*Acute or severe anxiety:* 50 to 100 mg IM or IV initially; then 25 to 50 mg 3 to 4 times/day if necessary.

➤*Preoperative apprehension and anxiety:* 50 to 100 mg IM 1 hour prior to surgery.

➤*Preparation and administration of injections:* Prepare solution immediately before administration. Discard any unused portion.

IM – Add 2 mL of special IM diluent to contents of 5 mL ampule of chlordiazepoxide sterile powder (100 mg). Avoid excessive pressure when injecting diluent into the ampule containing the powder because bubbles form on the surface of the solution. Agitate gently until completely dissolved. Do not use diluent if it is opalescent or hazy. Do not give solutions made with physiological saline or sterile water for injection IM because of the pain on injection. Give deep IM injection slowly into the upper outer quadrant of the gluteus muscle. Do not give IV solution made with the IM diluent because of the bubbles that form when the IM diluent is added to the chlordiazepoxide powder.

IV – When rapid action is mandatory, administer IV. Add 5 mL of sterile physiological saline or sterile water for injection to contents of amp (100 mg). Agitate gently until thoroughly dissolved. Give injection slowly over 1 minute.

➤*Storage/Stability:* Store at 25°C (77°F); excursions permitted to 15° to 30°C (59° to 86°F).

CLONAZEPAM

c-iv	**Clonazepam** (Various, eg, Mylan, PAR, Teva, TorPharm, UDL, Watson)	**Tablets**: 0.5 mg	May contain lactose. In 100s, 500s, 1000s, and UD 100s.
c-iv	**Klonopin** (Roche)		Lactose, FD&C Blue No. 1 and 2. (1/2 KLONOPIN ROCHE). Orange, scored. In 100s.

CLONAZEPAM

c-iv	**Clonazepam** (Various, eg, Mylan, PAR, Teva, TorPharm, UDL, Watson)	1 mg	May contain lactose. In 100s, 500s, 1000s, and UD 100s.
c-iv	**Klonopin** (Roche)		Lactose, FD&C Blue No. 1 and 2. (1 KLONOPIN ROCHE). Blue. In 100s.
c-iv	**Clonazepam** (Various, eg, Mylan, PAR, Teva, TorPharm, UDL, Watson)	2 mg	May contain lactose. In 100s, 500s, 1000s, and UD 100s.
c-iv	**Klonopin** (Roche)		Lactose, FD&C Blue No. 1 and 2. (2 KLONOPIN ROCHE). White. In 100s.
c-iv	**Clonazepam** (Barr)	**Tablets, orally disintegrating**: 0.125 mg	Aspartamine, xylitol, mannitol, 2.4 mg phenylalanine. (b 94 1/8). Strawberry flavor. White to off-white. In blister packages of 60.
c-iv	**Klonopin Wafers** (Roche)		Mannitol, parabens. (1/8). White. In blister packages of 60.
c-iv	**Clonazepam** (Barr)	**Tablets, orally disintegrating**: 0.25 mg	Aspartamine, xylitol, mannitol, 2.4 mg phenylalanine. (b 95 1/4). Strawberry flavor. White to off-white. In blister packages of 60.
c-iv	**Klonopin Wafers** (Roche)		Mannitol, parabens. (1/4). White. In blister packages of 60.
c-iv	**Clonazepam** (Barr)	**Tablets, orally disintegrating**: 0.5 mg	Aspartamine, xylitol, mannitol, 2.4 mg phenylalanine. (b 96 1/2). Strawberry flavor. White to off-white. In blister packages of 60.
c-iv	**Klonopin Wafers** (Roche)		Mannitol, parabens. (1/2). White. In blister packages of 60.
c-iv	**Clonazepam** (Barr)	**Tablets, orally disintegrating**: 1 mg	Aspartamine, xylitol, mannitol, 2.4 mg phenylalanine. (b 97 1). Strawberry flavor. White to off-white. In blister packages of 60.
c-iv	**Klonopin Wafers** (Roche)		Mannitol, parabens. (1). White. In blister packages of 60.
c-iv	**Clonazepam** (Barr)	**Tablets, orally disintegrating**: 2 mg	Aspartamine, xylitol, mannitol, 2.4 mg phenylalanine. (b 98 2). Strawberry flavor. White to off-white. In blister packages of 60.
c-iv	**Klonopin Wafers** (Roche)		Mannitol, parabens. (2). White. In blister packages of 60.

For additional information, refer to the Benzodiazepines group monograph in the Antianxiety Agents section and to the Anticonvulsants introduction.

CLONAZEPAM — ORAL

Complete and comparative prescribing information begins in the Benzodiazepines monograph.

Indications

➤*Seizure disorders:* Alone or as an adjunct in the treatment of the Lennox-Gastaut syndrome (petit mal variant), akinetic and myoclonic seizures. In patients with absence seizures (petit mal) who have failed to respond to succinimides, clonazepam may be useful.

➤*Panic disorder:* For the treatment of panic disorder, with or without agoraphobia, as defined in DSM-IV.

➤*Unlabeled uses:* Periodic leg movements during sleep. Parkinsonian (hypokinetic) dysarthria. Acute manic episodes of bipolar affective disorder. Multifocal tic disorders. Adjunct in the treatment of schizophrenia. Neuralgias (deafferentation pain syndromes).

Administration and Dosage

The tablets should be administered with water by swallowing the tablet whole. The orally disintegrating tablet should be administered as follows: After opening the pouch, peel back the foil on the blister. Do not push the tablet through foil. Immediately upon opening the blister, using dry hands, remove the tablet and place it in the mouth. Tablet disintegration occurs rapidly in saliva so it can be easily swallowed with or without water.

➤*Seizure disorders:*

Adults – The initial dose should not exceed 1.5 mg/day divided into 3 doses. Dosage may be increased in increments of 0.5 to 1 mg every 3 days until seizures are adequately controlled or until side effects preclude any further increase. Maintenance dosage must be individualized for each patient depending upon response. Maximum recommended daily dose is 20 mg.

The use of multiple anticonvulsants may result in an increase of depressant adverse effects. This should be considered before adding clonazepam to an existing anticonvulsant regimen.

Children – In order to minimize drowsiness, the initial dose for infants and children (less than or equal to 10 years of age or 30 kg of body weight) should be between 0.01 and 0.03 mg/kg/day but not to exceed 0.05 mg/kg/day given in 2 or 3 divided doses. Dosage should be increased by no more than 0.25 to 0.5 mg every third day until a daily maintenance dose of 0.1 to 0.2 mg/kg of body weight has been reached, unless seizures are controlled or side effects preclude further increase. Whenever possible, the daily dose should be divided into 3 equal doses. If doses are not equally divided, the largest dose should be given before retiring.

Therapeutic serum concentrations of clonazepam are 20 to 80 ng/mL.

Elderly – There is no clinical trial experience with clonazepam tablets in seizure disorder patients 65 years of age and older. In general, elderly patients should be started on low doses of clonazepam tablets and observed closely.

➤*Panic disorder:*

Adults – The initial dose is 0.25 mg twice daily. An increase to the target dose for most patients of 1 mg/day may be made after 3 days. The recommended dose of 1 mg/day is based on the results from a fixed dose study in which the optimal effect was seen at 1 mg/day. Higher doses of 2, 3, and 4 mg/day in that study were less effective than the 1 mg/day dose and were associated with more adverse effects. Nevertheless, it is possible that some individual patients may benefit from doses of up to a maximum dose of 4 mg/day, and in those instances, the dose may be increased in increments of 0.125 to 0.25 mg twice daily every 3 days until panic disorder is controlled or until side effects make further increases undesired. To reduce the inconvenience of somnolence, administration of 1 dose at bedtime may be desirable.

Treatment should be discontinued gradually, with a decrease of 0.125 mg twice daily every 3 days, until the drug is completely withdrawn.

There is no body of evidence available to answer the question of how long the patient treated with clonazepam should remain on it. Therefore, the physician who elects to use clonazepam for extended periods should periodically reevaluate the long-term usefulness of the drug for the individual patient.

Children – There is no clinical trial experience with clonazepam in panic disorder patients less than 18 years of age.

➤*Storage / Stability:* Store at 25°C (77°F); excursions permitted to 15° to 30°C (59° to 86°F). Protect from moisture.

DIAZEPAM

c-iv	**Diazepam** (Roxane)	**Oral solution**: 5 mg/5 mL	Sorbitol. Wintergreen-spice flavor. In 500 mL and 5 and 10 mg patient cups.
c-iv	**Diazepam Intensol** (Roxane)	**Oral solution**: 5 mg/mL	19% alcohol. In 30 mL with dropper.
c-iv	**Diazepam** (Various, eg, Barr, Danbury, Ivax, Mylan, Purepac, Zenith)	**Tablets**: 2 mg	May contain lactose. In 100s, 500s, 1000s, and 5000s.
c-iv	**Valium** (Roche)		Lactose. (Roche 2 Valium). White, scored. In 100s and 500s.
c-iv	**Diazepam** (Various, eg, Barr, Danbury, Ivax, Mylan, Purepac, Zenith)	**Tablets**: 5 mg	May contain lactose. In 100s, 500s, 1000s, and 5000s.
c-iv	**Valium** (Roche)		Lactose. (Roche 5 Valium). Yellow, scored. In 100s and 500s.
c-iv	**Diazepam** (Various, eg, Barr, Danbury, Ivax, Mylan, Purepac, Zenith)	**Tablets**: 10 mg	May contain lactose, FD& C Blue No 1. In 100s, 500s, 1000s, and 5000s.
c-iv	**Valium** (Roche)		Lactose, FD& C Blue No 1. (Roche 10 Valium). Blue, scored. In 100s and 500s.
c-iv	**Diazepam** (Various, eg, Hospira)	**Injection**: 5 mg/mL[a]	In 2 mL *Carpuject* cartridges.

Benzodiazepines

DIAZEPAM

c-iv	**Diastat** (Xcel)	**Gel, rectal:** 2.5 mg (pediatric)	1.5% benzyl alcohol, 10% ethyl alcohol. In twin packs. Includes lubricating jelly and plastic applicator with flexible, molded tip in 2 lengths.
		5 mg (pediatric)	1.5% benzyl alcohol, 10% ethyl alcohol. In twin packs. Includes lubricating jelly and plastic applicator with flexible, molded tip in 2 lengths.
		10 mg	1.5% benzyl alcohol, 10% ethyl alcohol. In twin packs. Includes lubricating jelly and plastic applicator with flexible, molded tip in 2 lengths.
		15 mg (adult)	1.5% benzyl alcohol, 10% ethyl alcohol. In twin packs. Includes lubricating jelly and plastic applicator with flexible, molded tip in 2 lengths.
		20 mg (adult)	1.5% benzyl alcohol, 10% ethyl alcohol. In twin packs. Includes lubricating jelly and plastic applicator with flexible, molded tip in 2 lengths.

[a] With 40% propylene glycol, 10% ethyl alcohol, 5% sodium benzoate, benzoic acid, and 1.5% benzyl alcohol.

DIAZEPAM — ORAL

For complete and comparative prescribing information, refer to the Benzodiazepine monograph in the Antianxiety Agents section. Also refer to the general discussion beginning in the Anticonvulsants introduction.

Indications

➤*Anxiety disorders:* For the management of anxiety disorders or for the short-term relief of the symptoms of anxiety.

➤*Acute alcohol withdrawal:* May be useful in symptomatic relief of acute agitation, tremor, impending or acute delirium, tremens, and hallucinosis.

➤*Muscle relaxant:* As an adjunct for the relief of skeletal muscle spasm because of reflex spasm caused by local pathology (eg, inflammation of muscles or joints, secondary to trauma); spasticity caused by upper motor neuron disorders (eg, cerebral palsy, paraplegia); athetosis; stiff-man syndrome. Used parenterally in the treatment of tetanus.

➤*Anticonvulsant:* Oral diazepam may be used adjunctively in convulsive disorders.

Administration and Dosage

Individualize dosage. Increase dosage cautiously to avoid adverse effects.

➤*Management of anxiety disorders and relief of symptoms of anxiety (depending upon severity of symptoms):* 2 to 10 mg 2 to 4 times/day.

➤*Acute alcohol withdrawal:* 10 mg 3 or 4 times during first 24 hours; reduce to 5 mg 3 or 4 times/day, as needed.

➤*Adjunct in skeletal muscle spasm:* 2 to 10 mg 3 or 4 times/day.

➤*Adjunct in convulsive disorders:* 2 to 10 mg 2 to 4 times/day.

➤*Elderly patients or in the presence of debilitating disease:* 2 to 2.5 mg 1 or 2 times/day initially; increase gradually as needed and tolerated.

➤*Children:* 1 to 2.5 mg 3 or 4 times/day initially; increase gradually as needed and tolerated. Not for use in children under 6 months of age. For sedation or muscle relaxation, a dosage of 0.12 to 0.8 mg/kg/24 hours divided 3 to 4 times/day has been recommended.

➤*Intensol:* Diazepam intensol is a concentrated oral solution as compared with standard oral liquid medications. It is recommended that the intensol is mixed with liquid or semisolid food such as water, juices, soda or soda-like beverages, applesauce, and puddings.

Use only the calibrated dropper provided with the product. Draw into the dropper the amount prescribed for a single dose. Then squeeze the dropper contents into a liquid or semi-solid food. Stir the liquid or food gently for a few seconds. Consume the entire amount of the mixture immediately. Do not store for future use.

➤*Storage/Stability:* Store at controlled room temperature, 15° to 30°C (59° to 86°F). Protect from light and moisture.

DIAZEPAM — INJECTION

For complete and comparative prescribing information, refer to the Benzodiazepine monograph in the Antianxiety Agents section. Also refer to the general discussion beginning in the Anticonvulsants introduction.

Indications

➤*Anxiety disorders:* For the management of anxiety disorders or for the short-term relief of the symptoms of anxiety.

➤*Acute alcohol withdrawal:* May be useful in symptomatic relief of acute agitation, tremor, impending or acute delirium, tremens, and hallucinosis.

➤*Muscle relaxant:* As an adjunct for the relief of skeletal muscle spasm because of reflex spasm caused by local pathology (eg, inflammation of muscles or joints, secondary to trauma); spasticity caused by upper motor neuron disorders (eg, cerebral palsy, paraplegia); athetosis; stiff-man syndrome. Used parenterally in the treatment of tetanus.

➤*Anticonvulsant:* Parenteral diazepam is a useful adjunct in status epilepticus and severe recurrent convulsive seizures.

➤*Preoperative:* Used parenterally for the relief of anxiety and tension in patients undergoing surgical procedures; IV prior to cardioversion for the relief of anxiety and tension and to diminish patient's recall; as an adjunct prior to endoscopic procedures for apprehension, anxiety, or acute stress reactions and to diminish patient's recall.

Administration and Dosage

➤*Parenteral:* Individualize dosage.

Older children and adults – 2 to 20 mg IM or IV, depending on the indication and its severity. In some conditions (eg, tetanus) larger doses may be required. In acute conditions, the injection may be repeated within 1 hour; although, an interval of 3 to 4 hours is usually satisfactory. Use lower doses (2 to 5 mg) and more gradual increases in dosage for elderly and debilitated patients and when other sedatives are administered.

IV – When used IV, observe the following procedures to reduce the possibility of venous thrombosis, phlebitis, local irritation, swelling, and rarely, vascular impairment: Inject slowly, take at least 1 minute per 5 mg (1 mL); do not use small veins (ie, dorsum of hand or wrist); avoid intra-arterial administration or extravasation. Do not mix or dilute with other solutions or drugs in syringe or infusion flask. If not feasible to administer directly IV, inject slowly through infusion tubing as close as possible to the vein insertion. Because of the possibility of precipitation of diazepam in IV fluids and the instability of the drug in plastic (PVC) bags and infusion tubing, IV infusion of diazepam is not recommended. Glass, polypropylene, polyethylene, or polyolefin solution bottles and infusion tubing have been used with negligible loss of diazepam. Once acute symptoms are controlled with injectable diazepam, place patient on oral therapy.

Children – To obtain maximum clinical effect with minimum amount of drug and to reduce the risk of hazardous side effects such as apnea or prolonged periods of somnolence, administer slowly over 3 minutes. Do not exceed 0.25 mg/kg. After an interval of 15 to 30 minutes, the initial dose can be repeated. If relief of symptoms is not obtained after a third dose, appropriate adjunctive therapy is recommended. When IV use is indicated, facilities for respiratory assistance should be readily available.

Moderate anxiety disorders and symptoms of anxiety (adults) – 2 to 5 mg IM or IV. Repeat in 3 to 4 hours if necessary.

Severe anxiety disorders and symptoms of anxiety (adults) – 5 to 10 mg IM or IV. Repeat in 3 to 4 hours if necessary.

Acute alcohol withdrawal (adults) – 10 mg IM or IV initially; then 5 to 10 mg in 3 to 4 hours if necessary.

Endoscopic procedures (adults) –

IV: Titrate dosage to desired sedative response, such as slurring of speech. Administer slowly just prior to procedure. Reduce narcotic dosage by at least one third, and in some cases, they may be omitted; 10 mg or less is usually adequate; up to 20 mg may be used, especially when concomitant narcotics are omitted.

IM: 5 to 10 mg 30 minutes prior to procedure if IV route cannot be used.

Muscle spasm (adults) – 5 to 10 mg IM or IV initially; then 5 to 10 mg in 3 to 4 hours if necessary. Tetanus may require larger doses.

Sedation or muscle relaxation (children) – 0.04 to 0.2 mg/kg/dose every 2 to 4 hours, maximum of 0.6 mg/kg within an 8-hour period.

Tetanus –

Infants (older than 30 days of age): 1 to 2 mg IM or IV slowly, repeated every 3 to 4 hours as necessary.

Children (5 years of age or older): 5 to 10 mg repeated every 3 to 4 hours may be required.

Status epilepticus and severe recurrent convulsive seizures – The IV route is preferred; administer slowly. Use the IM route if IV administration is impossible. Administer 5 to 10 mg initially; repeat if necessary at 10- to 15-minute intervals up to a maximum dose of 30 mg in adults. If necessary, repeat therapy in 2 to 4 hours. Exercise extreme caution in patients with chronic lung disease or unstable cardiovascular status. Although seizures

DIAZEPAM — INJECTION

may be controlled promptly, many patients experience a return to seizure activity, presumably because of the short-lived effect of IV diazepam; be prepared to readminister the drug. Diazepam is not recommended for maintenance. Once seizures are controlled, consider other agents for long-term control.

Infants (older than 30 days of age) and children (younger than 5 years of age): Inject 0.2 to 0.5 mg slowly every 2 to 5 minutes up to a maximum of 5 mg.

Children (5 years of age or older): Inject 1 mg every 2 to 5 minutes up to a maximum of 10 mg. Repeat in 2 to 4 hours if necessary. EEG monitoring of seizure may be helpful.

Neonates: 0.3 to 0.75 mg/kg/dose every 15 to 30 minutes for 2 to 3 doses has been suggested.

Preoperative medication (adults) – 10 mg IM before surgery. If atropine, scopolamine, or other premedications are desired, administer in separate syringes.

Cardioversion (adults) – 5 to 15 mg IV, 5 to 10 minutes prior to procedure.

➤*Storage/Stability:* Store at controlled room temperature, 15° to 30°C (59° to 86°F). Protect from light and moisture.

DIAZEPAM — RECTAL

For complete and comparative prescribing information, refer to the Benzodiazepine monograph in the Antianxiety Agents section. Also refer to the general discussion beginning in the Anticonvulsants introduction.

Indications

➤*Anticonvulsant:* For the management of selected, refractory, patients with epilepsy, on stable regimens of antiepileptic drugs (AEDs), who require intermittent use of diazepam to control bouts of increased seizure activity.

Administration and Dosage

➤*Convulsive disorders:* Individualize dosage. Some patients may require higher doses than those given below. In such cases, increase dosage cautiously to avoid adverse effects. Use lower doses and slowly increase the dose in elderly or debilitated patients and when other sedative drugs are administered.

➤*Rectal:* 0.2 to 0.5 mg/kg, depending on age. Calculate the recommended dose by rounding upward to the next available unit dose. A second dose, when required, may be given 4 to 12 hours after the first dose. Do not treat more than 5 episodes/month or more than 1 episode every 5 days.

Children 2 to 5 years of age – 0.5 mg/kg.

Children 6 to 11 years of age – 0.3 mg/kg.

Adults and children older than 12 years of age – 0.2 mg/kg.

Diazepam Rectal Dosing Based on Age and Weight

2 to 5 years of age weight (kg)	6 to 11 years of age weight (kg)	≥ 12 years of age weight (kg)	Dose (mg)
6 to 11	10 to 18	14 to 27	5
12 to 22	19 to 37	28 to 50	10
23 to 33	38 to 55	51 to 75	15
34 to 44	56 to 74	76 to 111	20

A 2.5 mg supplemental dose may be given for patients requiring more precise dose titration or as a partial replacement dose for patients who may expel a portion of the first dose.

Elderly and/or debilitated patients – Adjust dosage downward to reduce ataxia or oversedation.

➤*Storage/Stability:* Store at controlled room temperature 15° to 30°C (59° to 86°F). Protect from moisture.

LORAZEPAM

c-iv	**Lorazepam** (Various, eg, Geneva, Major, Mylan, Squibb Mark, UDL)	**Tablets:** 0.5 mg	In 100s, 500s, and 1000s.
		1 mg	In 100s, 500s, and 1000s.
		2 mg	In 100s, 500s, and 1000s.
c-iv	**Lorazepam Intensol** (Roxane)	**Concentrated oral solution:** 2 mg/mL	Alcohol and dye free. In 10 and 30 mL with dropper.
c-iv	**Lorazepam** (Hospira)	**Injection:** 2 mg/mL	In 1 mL prefilled syringes, and 1 mL single and 10 mL multidose vials.[a]
c-iv	**Ativan** (Baxter)		In single and 10 mL multidose vials[a], in boxes of 10 *TUBEX*.
c-iv	**Lorazepam** (Hospira)	**Injection:** 4 mg/mL	In 1 mL prefilled syringes, and 1 mL single and 10 mL multidose vials.[a]
c-iv	**Ativan** (Baxter)		In single and 10 mL multidose vials[a], in boxes of 10 *TUBEX*.

[a] With PEG 400, propylene glycol, and 2% benzyl alcohol.

LORAZEPAM — ORAL

Complete and comparative prescribing information begins in the Benzodiazepines group monograph. Also see the Anticonvulsant monograph.

Indications

➤*Anxiety:* For the management of anxiety disorders or for the short-term relief of the symptoms of anxiety or of anxiety associated with depressive symptoms.

The efficacy of lorazepam in long-term use (ie, greater than 4 months), has not been assessed by systematic clinical studies. Periodically reassess the usefulness of the drug for the individual patient.

➤*Unlabeled uses:* Short-term improvement of chronic insomnia.

Administration and Dosage

➤*Approved by the FDA:* March 29, 1991.

For optimal results, individualize dose, frequency of administration, and duration of therapy according to patient response.

➤*Usual dose:* 2 to 6 mg/day given in divided doses, the largest dose being taken before bedtime. The daily dosage may vary from 1 to 10 mg/day.

➤*Anxiety:* 2 to 3 mg/day of tablets or solution given 2 or 3 times daily.

➤*Insomnia due to anxiety or transient situational stress:* A single daily dose of 2 to 4 mg of tablet or solution may be given, usually at bedtime.

➤*Elderly or debilitated patients:* An initial dosage of 1 to 2 mg/day of tablet or solution in divided doses is recommended, to be adjusted as needed and tolerated. Gradually increase the dosage of lorazepam when needed to help avoid adverse reactions. When higher dosage is indicated, increase the evening dose before the daytime doses.

➤*Oral solution:*

Proper use – An intensol is a concentrated oral solution as compared with standard oral liquid medications. It is recommended that an intensol be mixed with liquid or semisolid food such as water, juices, soda or soda-like beverages, applesauce, and puddings.

Use only the calibrated dropper provided with this product. Draw into the dropper the amount prescribed for a single dose. Then squeeze the dropper contents into a liquid or semisolid food. Stir the liquid or food gently for a few seconds. The intensol formulation blends quickly and completely. The entire amount of the mixture, of drug and liquid or drug and food, should be consumed immediately. Do not store for future use.

➤*Storage/Stability:*

Tablets – Store at controlled room temperature 15° to 30°C (59° to 86°F). Protect from light. Dispense in a tight, light-resistant container using a child-resistant closure. Keep tightly closed.

Oral solution – Store at cold temperature. Refrigerate 2° to 8°C (36° to 46°F). Protect from light.

LORAZEPAM — INJECTION

Complete and comparative prescribing information begins in the Benzodiazepines group monograph. Also see the Anticonvulsant monograph.

Indications

➤*Status epilepticus:* For the treatment of status epilepticus.

➤*Preanesthetic:* In adult patients for preanesthetic medication, producing sedation (sleepiness or drowsiness), relief of anxiety, and a decreased ability to recall events related to the day of surgery.

Administration and Dosage

➤*Approved by the FDA:* July 25, 1980.

Lorazepam must never be used without individualization of dosage particularly when used with other medications capable of producing CNS depression.

Equipment necessary to maintain a patent airway should be immediately available prior to IV administration of lorazepam.

➤*Status epilepticus:*

IV injection – The usual recommended dose is 4 mg given slowly (2 mg/min) for patients 18 years and older. If seizures cease, no additional lorazepam injection is required. If seizures continue or recur after a 10- to 15-minute observation period, an additional 4 mg IV dose may be slowly administered. Experience with further doses of lorazepam is very limited. Employ the usual precautions in treating status epilepticus. Start an IV

Benzodiazepines

LORAZEPAM — INJECTION

infusion, monitor vital signs, maintain an unobstructed airway, and have artificial ventilation equipment available.

IM injection – IM lorazepam is not preferred in the treatment of status epilepticus because therapeutic lorazepam levels may not be reached as quickly as with IV administration. However, when an IV port is not available, the IM route may prove useful.

➤*Preanesthetic:*

IM injection – For the designated indications as a premedicant, the usual recommended dose of lorazepam for IM injection is 0.05 mg/kg up to a maximum of 4 mg. As with all premedicant drugs, the dose should be individualized. Doses of other CNS-depressant drugs ordinarily should be reduced. For optimum effect, measured as lack of recall, administer IM lorazepam at least 2 hours before the anticipated operative procedure. Administer narcotic analgesics at their usual preoperative time.

IV injection – For the primary purpose of sedation and relief of anxiety, the usual recommended initial dose of lorazepam for IV injection is 2 mg total, or 0.02 mg/lb (0.044 mg/kg), whichever is smaller. This dose will suffice for sedating most adult patients and ordinarily should not be exceeded in patients over 50 years of age. In those patients in whom a greater likelihood of lack of recall for perioperative events would be beneficial, larger doses as high as 0.05 mg/kg up to a total of 4 mg may be administered. Doses of other injectable CNS-depressant drugs ordinarily should be reduced. For optimum effect, measured as lack of recall, administer IV lorazepam 15 to 20 minutes before the anticipated operative procedure.

➤*Dose administration in special populations:*

Renal function impairment – For acute dose administration, adjustment is not needed for patients with renal disease. However, in patients with renal disease, exercise caution if frequent doses are given over relatively short periods of time.

Concomitant medications – The dose of lorazepam should be reduced by 50% when coadministered with probenecid or valproate. It may be necessary to increase the dose of lorazepam in female patients who are concomitantly taking oral contraceptives.

➤*Administration:* When given intramuscularly, lorazepam injection, undiluted, should be injected deep in the muscle mass.

Injectable lorazepam can be used with atropine sulfate, narcotic analgesics, other parenterally used analgesics, commonly used anesthetics, and muscle relaxants.

Immediately prior to IV use, lorazepam injection must be diluted with an equal volume of compatible solution. Contents should be mixed thoroughly by gently inverting the container repeatedly until a homogenous solution results. Do not shake vigorously, as this will result in air entrapment. When properly diluted, the drug may be injected directly into a vein or into the tubing of an existing IV infusion. The rate of injection should not exceed 2 mg per minute.

Lorazepam injection is compatible for dilution purposes with the following solutions: Sterile Water for Injection; Sodium Chloride Injection; 5% Dextrose Injection.

➤*Storage / Stability:* Store in a refrigerator. Protect from light. Use carton to protect contents from light.

OXAZEPAM

c-iv	**Serax** (Alpharma)	**Tablets:** 15 mg	Lactose. (S SERAX 15). Yellow, five-sided. In 100s.
c-iv	**Oxazepam** (Various, eg, Balan, Mark, Moore, Ivax, Squibb)	**Capsules:** 10 mg	In 100s, 500s, and UD 100s.
c-iv	**Serax** (Alpharma)		Lactose. (327 SERAX 10). Pink and white. In 100s.
c-iv	**Oxazepam** (Various, eg, Balan, Mark, Moore, Ivax, Squibb)	**Capsules:** 15 mg	In 100s, 500s, and UD 100s.
c-iv	**Serax** (Alpharma)		Lactose. (328 SERAX 15). Red and white. In 100s.
c-iv	**Oxazepam** (Various, eg, Balan, Mark, Moore, Ivax, Squibb)	**Capsules:** 30 mg	In 100s, 500s, and UD 100s.
c-iv	**Serax** (Alpharma)		Lactose. (329 SERAX 30). Maroon and white. In 100s.

OXAZEPAM — ORAL

Complete prescribing information begins in the Benzodiazepines group monograph.

Indications

➤*Anxiety:* For the management of anxiety disorders or for the short-term relief of the symptoms of anxiety. Anxiety associated with depression is also responsive to oxazepam therapy. This product has been found particularly useful in the management of anxiety, tension, agitation, and irritability in older patients.

➤*Alcohol withdrawal:* Alcoholics with acute tremulousness, inebriation, or with anxiety associated with alcohol withdrawal are responsive to therapy.

The effectiveness of oxazepam in long-term use, that is, more than 4 months, has not been assessed by systematic clinical studies. The physician should reassess periodically the usefulness of the drug for the individual patient.

➤*Unlabeled uses:* Management of irritable bowel syndrome.

Administration and Dosage

➤*Approved by the FDA:* August 3, 1987.

Because of the flexibility of this product and the range of emotional disturbances responsive to it, dosage should be individualized for maximum beneficial effects.

Oxazepam Dosing

Use	Usual dose
Mild-to-moderate anxiety, with associated tension, irritability, agitation, or related symptoms of functional origin or secondary to organic disease.	10 to 15 mg, 3 or 4 times daily.
Severe anxiety syndromes, agitation, or anxiety associated with depression.	15 to 30 mg, 3 or 4 times daily.
Older patients with anxiety, tension, irritability, and agitation.	Initial dosage: 10 mg, 3 times daily. If necessary, increase cautiously to 15 mg, 3 or 4 times daily.
Alcoholics with acute inebriation, tremulousness, or anxiety on withdrawal.	15 to 30 mg, 3 or 4 times daily.

This product is not indicated in children under 6 years of age. Absolute dosage for children 6 to 12 years of age is not established.

➤*Storage / Stability:* Store at controlled room temperature 25°C (77°F). Keep tightly closed and dispense in a tight container.

Miscellaneous Agents

BUSPIRONE HYDROCHLORIDE

Rx	**Buspirone HCl** (Various, eg, Amide, Ethex, PAR, Teva, UDL)	**Tablets:** 5 mg (4.6 mg as base)	May contain lactose. In 100s and 500s.
Rx	**BuSpar** (Bristol-Myers Squibb)		Lactose. (MJ 5 mg BuSpar). White, ovoid-rectangular, scored. In 100s and 500s.
Rx	**Buspirone HCl** (Par)	**Tablets:** 7.5 mg (6.85 as base)	May contain lactose. In 100s and 500s.
Rx	**Buspirone HCl** (Various, eg, Amide, Ethex, PAR, Teva, UDL)	**Tablets:** 10 mg (9.1 mg as base)	May contain lactose. In 100s and 500s.
Rx	**BuSpar** (Bristol-Myers Squibb)		Lactose. (MJ 10 mg BuSpar). White, ovoid-rectangular, scored. In 100s and 500s.
Rx	**Buspirone HCl** (Various, eg, Amide, Ethex, PAR, Teva, UDL)	**Tablets:** 15 mg (13.7 mg as base)	May contain lactose. In 100s and 500s.
Rx	**BuSpar** (Bristol-Myers Squibb)		Lactose. (MJ 822/5 5 5). White, ovoid-rectangular, scored. In DIVIDOSE 60s and 180s.
Rx	**Buspirone HCl** (Mylan)	**Tablets:** 30 mg (27.4 mg as base)	Scored. In 60s, 100s, and 180s.
Rx	**BuSpar** (Bristol-Myers Squibb)		Lactose. (824/10 10 10). Pink, scored. In DIVIDOSE 60s.

BUSPIRONE HYDROCHLORIDE — ORAL

Indications

➤*Anxiety:* For the management of anxiety disorders or the short-term relief of the symptoms of anxiety.

➤*Unlabeled uses:* Decreasing the symptoms (eg, aches, pains, fatigue, cramps, irritability) of premenstrual syndrome.

Administration and Dosage

➤*Approved by the FDA:* April 22, 1996.

➤*Dosage:* The recommended initial dose is 15 mg daily (7.5 mg 2 times a day). To achieve an optimal therapeutic response, at intervals of 2 to 3 days, the dosage may be increased 5 mg/day, as needed. The maximum daily dosage should not exceed 60 mg/day. In clinical trials allowing dose titration, divided doses of 20 to 30 mg/day were commonly employed.

➤*Administration:* Consequently, patients should take buspirone in a consistent manner with regard to the timing of dosing; either always with or always without food.

➤*Concomitant therapy:* When buspirone is to be given with a potent inhibitor of CYP3A4, a low dose of buspirone (eg, 25 mg twice daily) is recommended.

➤*Storage/Stability:* Dispense in a tight, light-resistant container as defined in the USP. Use child-resistant closure. Store at controlled room temperature 15° to 30°C (59° to 86°F). Protect from temperatures greater than 30°C (86°F).

Actions

➤*Pharmacology:* The mechanism of action of buspirone is unknown. Buspirone differs from typical benzodiazepine anxiolytics in that it does not exert anticonvulsant or muscle relaxant effects. It also lacks the prominent sedative effect that is associated with more typical anxiolytics. In vitro preclinical studies have shown that buspirone has a high affinity for serotonin ($5\text{-}HT_{1A}$) receptors. Buspirone has no significant affinity for benzodiazepine receptors and does not affect GABA binding in vitro or in vivo when tested in preclinical models.

Buspirone has moderate affinity for brain D_2-dopamine receptors. Some studies do suggest that buspirone may have indirect effects on other neurotransmitter systems.

➤*Pharmacokinetics:*

Absorption/Distribution – Buspirone is rapidly absorbed in man and undergoes extensive first-pass metabolism. In a radiolabeled study, unchanged buspirone in the plasma accounted for only about 1% of the radioactivity in the plasma. Following oral administration, plasma concentrations of unchanged buspirone are very low and variable between subjects. Peak plasma levels of 1 to 6 ng/mL have been observed 40 to 90 minutes after single oral doses of 20 mg. The single-dose bioavailability of unchanged buspirone when taken as a tablet is on the average about 90% of an equivalent dose of solution, but there is large variability.

The effects of food upon the bioavailability of buspirone have been studied in 8 subjects. They were given a 20 mg dose with and without food; the area under the plasma concentration-time curve (AUC) and peak plasma concentration (C_{max}) of unchanged buspirone increased by 84% and 116%, respectively, but the total amount of buspirone immunoreactive material did not change. This suggests that food may decrease the extent of presystemic clearance of buspirone, but the clinical significance of these findings is unknown.

A multiple-dose study conducted in 15 subjects suggests that buspirone has nonlinear pharmacokinetics. Thus, dose increases and repeated dosing may lead to somewhat higher blood levels of unchanged buspirone than would be predicted from results of single-dose studies.

An in vitro protein binding study indicated that approximately 86% of buspirone is bound to plasma proteins. It was also observed that aspirin increased the plasma levels of free buspirone by 23%, while flurazepam decreased the plasma levels of free buspirone by 20%. However, it is not known whether these drugs cause similar effects on plasma levels of free buspirone in vivo, or whether such changes, if they do occur, cause clinically significant differences in treatment outcome. An in vitro study indicated that buspirone did not displace highly protein-bound drugs such as phenytoin, warfarin, and propranolol from plasma protein, and that buspirone may displace digoxin.

Metabolism/Excretion – Buspirone is metabolized primarily by oxidation, which in vitro has been shown to be mediated by cytochrome P450 3A4 (CYP3A4). Several hydroxylated derivatives and a pharmacologically active metabolite, 1-pyrimidinylpiperazine (1-PP), are produced. In animal models predictive of anxiolytic potential, 1-PP has about one quarter of the activity of buspirone, but is present in up to 20-fold greater amounts. However, this is probably not important in humans: Blood samples from humans chronically exposed to buspirone HCl do not exhibit high levels of 1-PP; mean values are approximately 3 ng/mL and the highest human blood level recorded among 108 chronically dosed patients was 17 ng/mL, less than 1/200th of 1-PP levels found in animals given large doses of buspirone without signs of toxicity.

In a single-dose study using ^{14}C-labeled buspirone, 29% to 63% of the dose was excreted in the urine within 24 hours, primarily as metabolites; fecal excretion accounted for 18% to 38% of the dose. The average elimination half-life of unchanged buspirone after single doses of 10 to 40 mg is about 2 to 3 hours.

Special populations –

Renal function impairment: After multiple-dose administration of buspirone to renally impaired (Ccr = 10 to 70 mL/min/1.73 m^2) patients, steady-state AUC of buspirone increased 4-fold compared with healthy (Ccr greater than or equal to 80 mL/min/1.73 m^2) subjects. Therefore, administration of buspirone to patients with severe renal impairment cannot be recommended.

Hepatic function impairment: After multiple-dose administration of buspirone to patients with hepatic impairment, steady-state AUC of buspirone increased 13-fold compared with healthy subjects. Therefore, administration of buspirone to patients with severe hepatic impairment cannot be recommended.

Contraindications

Hypersensitivity to buspirone.

Warnings

Because buspirone has no established antipsychotic activity, it should not be employed in lieu of appropriate antipsychotic treatment.

➤*Renal/Hepatic function impairment:* See Actions for more information.

➤*Pregnancy: Category B.* In humans, however, adequate and well-controlled studies during pregnancy have not been performed. Because animal reproduction studies are not always predictive of human response, this drug should be used during pregnancy only if clearly needed.

➤*Lactation:* The extent of the excretion in human milk of buspirone or its metabolites is not known. In rats, however, buspirone and its metabolites are excreted in milk. Buspirone administration to nursing women should be avoided if clinically possible.

➤*Children:* The safety and efficacy of buspirone were evaluated in 2 placebo-controlled 6-week trials involving a total of 559 pediatric patients (ranging from 6 to 17 years of age) with GAD. Doses studied were 7.5 to 30 mg twice daily (15 to 60 mg/day). There were no significant differences between buspirone and placebo with regard to the symptoms of GAD following doses recommended for the treatment of GAD in adults. Pharmacokinetic studies have shown that, for identical doses, plasma exposure to buspirone and its active metabolite, 1-PP, are equal to or higher in pediatric patients than adults. No unexpected safety findings were associated with buspirone in these trials. There are no long-term safety or efficacy data in this population.

Precautions

➤*Potential for withdrawal reactions in sedative/hypnotic/anxiolytic drug-dependent patients:* Because buspirone does not exhibit cross-tolerance with benzodiazepines and other common sedative/hypnotic drugs, it will not block the withdrawal syndrome often seen with cessation of therapy with these drugs. Therefore, before starting therapy with buspirone, it is advisable to withdraw patients gradually, especially patients who have been using a CNS-depressant drug chronically, from their prior treatment. Rebound or withdrawal symptoms may occur over varying time periods, depending in part on the type of drug, and its effective half-life of elimination.

The syndrome of withdrawal from sedative/hypnotic/anxiolytic drugs can appear as any combination of irritability, anxiety, agitation, insomnia, tremor, abdominal cramps, muscle cramps, vomiting, sweating, flu-like symptoms without fever, and occasionally, even as seizures.

➤*Possible concerns related to buspirone's binding to dopamine receptors:* Because buspirone can bind to central dopamine receptors, a question has been raised about its potential to cause acute and chronic changes in dopamine-mediated neurological function (eg, dystonia, pseudo-parkinsonism, akathisia, tardive dyskinesia). Clinical experience in controlled trials has failed to identify any significant neuroleptic-like activity; however, a syndrome of restlessness, appearing shortly after initiation of treatment, has been reported in some small fraction of buspirone-treated patients. The syndrome may be explained in several ways. For example, buspirone may increase central noradrenergic activity; alternatively, the effect may be attributable to dopaminergic effects (ie, represent akathisia). Obviously, the question cannot be totally resolved at this point in time. Generally, long-term sequelae of any drug's use can be identified only after several years of marketing.

➤*Drug abuse and dependence:* Although there is no direct evidence that buspirone causes physical dependence or drug-seeking behavior, it is difficult to predict from experiments the extent to which a CNS-active drug will be misused, diverted, or abused once marketed. Consequently, physicians should carefully evaluate patients for a history of drug abuse and follow such patients closely, observing them for signs of buspirone misuse or abuse (eg, development of tolerance, incrementation of dose, drug-seeking behavior).

➤*Hazardous tasks:* Studies indicate that buspirone is less sedating than other anxiolytics and that it does not produce significant functional impairment. However, its CNS effects in any individual patient may not be predictable. Therefore, patients should be cautioned about operating an automobile or using complex machinery until they are reasonably certain that buspirone treatment does not affect them adversely.

BUSPIRONE HYDROCHLORIDE — ORAL

Drug Interactions

Buspirone Drug Interactions			
Precipitant drug	Object drug*		Description
Cimetidine	Buspirone	↑	Coadministration increased buspirone C_{max} (40%) and T_{max} (2-fold), but had minimal effects on AUC.
CYP3A4 inhibitors (eg, itraconazole, ketoconazole, erythromycin, clarithromycin, diltiazem, verapamil, fluvoxamine, ritonavir)	Buspirone	↑	Plasma buspirone concentrations may be elevated because of inhibition of its metabolism (CYP3A4). Adjust buspirone dosage as needed. If given with erythromycin, a low dose of buspirone (eg, 2.5 mg twice/day) is recommended. If given with itraconazole, a low dose of buspirone (eg, 2.5 mg/day) is recommended.
CYP3A4 inducers (eg, rifampin, rifabutin, phenytoin, phenobarbital, carbamazepine, dexamethasone)	Buspirone	↓	Plasma buspirone concentrations may be decreased because of induction of its metabolism (CYP3A4). Adjust the buspirone dose as needed.
Fluoxetine	Buspirone	↓	Effects of buspirone may be decreased. Paradoxical worsening of OCD has occurred.
Nefazodone	Buspirone	↑	Coadministration increased plasma buspirone concentrations (up to 20-fold in C_{max} and up to 50-fold in AUC) and statistically significant decreases (≈ 50%) in plasma concentrations of the buspirone active metabolite. Slight increases (23%) in AUC were observed for nefazodone. If the 2 drugs are to be used in combination, a low dose of buspirone (eg, 2.5 mg/day) is recommended.
Buspirone	Nefazodone		
Buspirone	Diazepam	↑	Although coadministration produced no differences in diazepam kinetic parameters (C_{max}, AUC, and C_{min}), increases (about 15%) in nordiazepam kinetics were seen. Minor effects (dizziness, headache, and nausea) were observed.
Buspirone	Alcohol	↔	Formal studies of the interaction of buspirone with alcohol indicate that buspirone does not increase alcohol-induced impairment in motor and mental performance, but it is prudent to avoid concomitant use.
Buspirone	Haloperidol	↑	Haloperidol and buspirone coadministration may result in increased serum haloperidol concentrations.
Buspirone	MAO inhibitors	↑	There have been reports of elevated blood pressure when buspirone was added to a regimen including an MAOI. Therefore, do not use concomitantly.
Buspirone	Trazodone	↔	One report suggests that concomitant use may have caused 3- to 6-fold elevations of ALT in a few patients. In a similar study attempting to replicate this finding, no interactive effect on hepatic transaminases was identified.

* ↑ = Object drug increased. ↓ = Object drug decreased. ↔ = Undetermined clinical effect.

➤*Drug/Food interactions:*

Grapefruit juice – Coadministration of buspirone (10 mg as a single dose) with grapefruit juice (200 mL double strength 3 times daily for 2 days) increased plasma buspirone concentrations (4.3-fold increase in C_{max}; 9.2-fold increase in AUC). Patients receiving buspirone should be advised to avoid drinking such large amounts of grapefruit juice.

Adverse Reactions

Commonly observed – Dizziness, nausea, headache, nervousness, lightheadedness, and excitement.

Associated with discontinuation of treatment – Approximately 10% of the 2200 anxious patients who participated in the buspirone premarketing clinical efficacy trials in anxiety disorders lasting 3 to 4 weeks discontinued treatment due to an adverse reaction. The more common reactions causing discontinuation included central nervous system disturbances (3.4%), primarily dizziness, insomnia, nervousness, drowsiness, and lightheadedness; gastrointestinal disturbances (1.2%), primarily nausea; and miscellaneous disturbances (1.1%), primarily headache and fatigue. In addition, 3.4% of patients had multiple complaints, none of which could be characterized as primary.

Incidence in controlled clinical trials –

Buspirone Adverse Reactions Incidence in Clinical Trials* (% of Patients Reporting)		
Adverse reaction	Buspirone HCl (n = 477)	Placebo (n = 464)
	Cardiovascular	
Tachycardia/ palpitations	1%	1%
	CNS	
Dizziness	12%	3%
Drowsiness	10%	9%
Nervousness	5%	1%
Insomnia	3%	3%
Lightheadedness	3%	< 1%
Decreased concentration	2%	2%
Excitement	2%	< 1%
Anger/hostility	2%	< 1%
Confusion	2%	< 1%
Depression	2%	2%
	Special senses	
Blurred vision	2%	< 1%
	Gastrointestinal	
Nausea	8%	5%
Dry mouth	3%	4%
Abdominal/gastric distress	2%	2%
Diarrhea	2%	< 1%
Constipation	1%	2%
Vomiting	1%	2%
	Musculoskeletal	
Musculoskeletal aches/pains	1%	< 1%
	Neurological	
Numbness	2%	< 1%
Paresthesia	1%	< 1%
Incoordination	1%	< 1%
Tremor	1%	< 1%
	Dermatologic	
Skin rash	1	< 1%
	Miscellaneous	
Headache	6%	3%
Fatigue	4%	4%
Weakness	2%	< 1%
Sweating/ clamminess	1%	< 1%

* Reactions reported by at least 1% of buspirone patients are included.

➤*Other reactions:* The following definitions of frequency are used: Frequent adverse reactions are defined as those occurring in at least 1/100 patients. Infrequent adverse reactions are those occurring in 1/100 to 1/1000 patients, while rare reactions are those occurring in less than 1/1000 patients.

Cardiovascular – Frequent was nonspecific chest pain; infrequent were syncope, hypotension, and hypertension; rare were cerebrovascular accident, congestive heart failure, myocardial infarction, cardiomyopathy, and bradycardia.

CNS – Frequent were dream disturbances; infrequent were depersonalization, dysphoria, noise intolerance, euphoria, akathisia, fearfulness, loss of interest, dissociative reaction, hallucinations, involuntary movements, slowed reaction time, suicidal ideation, and seizures; rare were feelings of claustrophobia, cold intolerance, stupor, and slurred speech and psychosis.

Dermatologic – Infrequent were edema, pruritus, flushing, easy bruising, hair loss, dry skin, facial edema, and blisters; rare were acne and thinning of nails.

Endocrine – Rare were galactorrhea and thyroid abnormality.

BUSPIRONE HYDROCHLORIDE — ORAL

GI – Infrequent were flatulence, anorexia, increased appetite, salivation, irritable colon, and rectal bleeding; rare was burning of the tongue.

GU – Infrequent were decreased or increased libido, urinary frequency, urinary hesitancy, menstrual irregularity and spotting, and dysuria; rare were amenorrhea, delayed ejaculation, impotence, pelvic inflammatory disease, enuresis, and nocturia.

Lab test abnormalities – Infrequent were increases in hepatic aminotransferases (ALT, AST); rare were eosinophilia, leukopenia, and thrombocytopenia.

Musculoskeletal – Infrequent were muscle cramps, muscle spasms, rigid/stiff muscles, and arthralgias; rare was muscle weakness.

Respiratory – Infrequent were hyperventilation, shortness of breath, and chest congestion; rare was epistaxis.

Special senses – Frequent were tinnitus, sore throat, and nasal congestion; infrequent were redness and itching of the eyes, altered taste, altered smell, and conjunctivitis; rare were inner ear abnormality, eye pain, photophobia, and pressure on eyes.

Miscellaneous – Infrequent were weight gain, fever, roaring sensation in the head, weight loss, and malaise; rare were alcohol abuse, bleeding disturbance, loss of voice, and hiccoughs.

Overdosage

➤*Symptoms:* In clinical pharmacology trials, doses as high as 375 mg/day were administered to healthy male volunteers. As this dose was approached, the following symptoms were observed: Nausea, vomiting, dizziness, drowsiness, miosis, and gastric distress. A few cases of overdosage have been reported, with complete recovery as the usual outcome. No deaths have been reported following overdosage with buspirone alone. Rare cases of intentional overdosage with a fatal outcome were invariably associated with ingestion of multiple drugs or alcohol, and a causal relationship to buspirone could not be determined. Toxicology studies of buspirone yielded the following LD_{50} values: Mice, 655 mg/kg; rats, 196 mg/kg; dogs, 586 mg/kg; and monkeys, 356 mg/kg. These dosages are 160 to 550 times the recommended human daily dose.

➤*Treatment:* General symptomatic and supportive measures should be used along with immediate gastric lavage. Respiration, pulse, and blood pressure should be monitored as in all cases of drug overdosage. No specific antidote is known to buspirone, and dialyzability of buspirone has not been determined.

Patient Information

1.) Inform your physician of any medications, prescription or nonprescription, alcohol, or drugs that you are now taking or plan to take during your treatment with buspirone.
2.) Inform your physician if you are pregnant, or if you are planning to become pregnant, or if you become pregnant while you are taking buspirone.
3.) Inform your physician if you are breastfeeding an infant.
4.) Until you experience how this medication affects you, do not drive a car or operate potentially dangerous machinery.
5.) You should take buspirone consistently, either always with or always without food.
6.) During your treatment with buspirone, avoid drinking large amounts of grapefruit juice.

HYDROXYZINE

For Hydroxyzine prescribing information, refer to the Antihistamine group monograph and the individual monograph in Antihistamines.

MEPROBAMATE

c-iv	**Meprobamate** (Various, eg, Watson)	**Tablets:** 200 mg	In 20s, 100s, and 1000s.
c-iv	**Miltown** (Wallace)		Sugar. (Wallace 37 1101). White. In 100s.
c-iv	**Meprobamate** (Various, eg, Watson)	**Tablets:** 400 mg	In 20s, 100s, 500s, 1000s, and UD 100s.
c-iv	**Miltown** (Wallace)		(Wallace 37 1001). White, scored. In 100s, 500s, and 1000s.

MEPROBAMATE — ORAL

Indications

➤*Anxiety:* For the management of anxiety disorders or for the short-term relief of the symptoms of anxiety. The effectiveness of meprobamate in long-term use, that is, more than 4 months, has not been assessed by systematic clinical studies. The physician should periodically reassess the usefulness of the drug for the individual patient.

Administration and Dosage

➤*Adults:* Doses of meprobamate above 2400 mg daily are not recommended. The usual dosage is 1200 to 1600 mg daily, in 3 or 4 divided doses.

➤*Children:* The usual dosage for children ages 6 to 12 is 100 to 200 mg, 2 or 3 times daily. Meprobamate is not recommended for children under 6.

➤*Storage/Stability:* Store at room temperature 25°C (77°F). Keep tightly closed. Dispense in tight container.

Actions

➤*Pharmacology:* Meprobamate is a carbamate derivative which has been shown (in animal and human studies) to have effects at multiple sites in the central nervous system, including the thalamus and limbic system.

Contraindications

Acute intermittent porphyria as well as allergic or idiosyncratic reactions to meprobamate or related compounds such as carisoprodol, mebutamate, or carbromal.

Warnings

➤*Additive effects:* Since the CNS-suppressant effects of meprobamate and alcohol or meprobamate and other CNS depressants or psychotropic drugs may be additive, appropriate caution should be exercised with patients who take more than 1 of these agents simultaneously.

➤*Renal/Hepatic function impairment:* Meprobamate is metabolized in the liver and excreted by the kidney; to avoid its excess accumulation, caution should be exercised in administration to patients with compromised liver or kidney function.

➤*Pregnancy: Category D.* An increased risk of congenital malformations associated with the use of minor tranquilizers (meprobamate, chlordiazepoxide, and diazepam) during the first trimester of pregnancy has been suggested in several studies. Because use of these drugs is rarely a matter of urgency, their use during this period should almost always be avoided. The possibility that a woman of childbearing potential may be pregnant at the time of institution of therapy should be considered. Patients should be advised that if they become pregnant they should communicate with their physicians about the desirability of discontinuing the drug.

➤*Lactation:* Meprobamate passes the placental barrier. It is present both in umbilical cord blood at or near maternal plasma levels and in breast milk of lactating mothers at concentrations 2 to 4 times that of maternal plasma. When use of meprobamate is contemplated in breastfeeding patients, the drug's higher concentration in breast milk as compared to maternal plasma levels should be considered.

➤*Children:* See Administration and Dosage for more information.

Precautions

➤*Special risk:* The lowest effective dose should be administered, particularly to elderly or debilitated patients, in order to preclude oversedation.

The possibility of suicide attempts should be considered and the least amount of drug feasible should be prescribed at any one time.

Meprobamate occasionally may precipitate seizures in epileptic patients.

➤*Drug abuse and dependence:* Physical dependence, psychological dependence, and abuse have occurred. When chronic intoxication from prolonged use occurs, it usually involves ingestion of greater than recommended doses and is manifested by ataxia, slurred speech, and vertigo. Therefore, careful supervision of dose and amounts prescribed is advised, as well as avoidance of prolonged administration, especially for alcoholics and other patients with a known propensity for taking excessive quantities of drugs.

Sudden withdrawal of the drug after prolonged and excessive use may precipitate recurrence of preexisting symptoms, such as anxiety, anorexia, or insomnia, or withdrawal reactions, such as vomiting, ataxia, tremors, muscle twitching, confusional states, hallucinosis, and, rarely, convulsive seizures. Such seizures are more likely to occur in persons with central nervous system damage or preexistent or latent convulsive disorders. Onset of withdrawal symptoms occurs usually within 12 to 48 hours after discontinuation of meprobamate; symptoms usually cease within the next 12 to 48 hours.

When excessive dosage has continued for weeks or months, dosage should be reduced gradually over a period of 1 or 2 weeks rather than abruptly stopped. Alternatively, a short-acting barbiturate may be substituted, then gradually withdrawn.

➤*Hazardous tasks:* Patients should be warned that meprobamate may impair the mental or physical abilities required for the performance of potentially hazardous tasks such as driving a motor vehicle or operating machinery.

Drug Interactions

Meprobamate Drug Interactions

Precipitant drug	Object drug*		Description
Alcohol	Meprobamate	↑	Acute ingestion may result in a decreased clearance of meprobamate through inhibition of hepatic metabolic systems; enhanced CNS depressant effects may occur. Tolerance may occur with chronic alcohol ingestion, presumably due to enhanced metabolic capacity.
Meprobamate	CNS depressants (eg, barbiturates, narcotics)	↑	Anticipate additive CNS depressant effects.
CNS depressants (eg, barbiturates, narcotics)	Meprobamate		

* ↑ = Object drug increased.

Adverse Reactions

➤*Allergic:* Milder reactions are characterized by an itchy, urticarial, or erythematous maculopapular rash which may be generalized or confined to the groin

Other reactions have included leukopenia, acute nonthrombocytopenic purpura, petechiae, ecchymoses, eosinophilia, peripheral edema, adenopathy, fever, fixed drug eruption with cross reaction to carisoprodol, and cross-sensitivity between meprobamate/mebutamate and meprobamate/carbromal.

More severe hypersensitivity reactions, rarely reported, include hyperpyrexia, chills, angioneurotic edema, bronchospasm, oliguria, and anuria. Also, anaphylaxis, erythema multiforme, exfoliative dermatitis, stomatitis, and proctitis, Stevens-Johnson syndrome, and bullous dermatitis, including 1 fatal case of the latter following administration of meprobamate in combination with prednisolone have occurred.

➤*Cardiovascular:* Palpitations, tachycardia, various forms of arrhythmia, transient ECG changes, syncope, hypotensive crises.

➤*CNS:* Drowsiness, ataxia, dizziness, slurred speech, headache, vertigo, weakness, paresthesias, impairment of visual accommodation, euphoria, overstimulation, paradoxical excitement, fast EEG activity.

➤*GI:* Nausea, vomiting, diarrhea.

➤*Hematologic:* (See also Allergic.) Agranulocytosis and aplastic anemia have been reported, although no causal relationship has been established. These cases rarely were fatal. Rare cases of thrombocytopenic purpura have been reported.

➤*Miscellaneous:* Exacerbation of porphyric symptoms.

Overdosage

➤*Symptoms:* Suicidal attempts with meprobamate have resulted in drowsiness, lethargy, stupor, ataxia, coma, shock, vasomotor and respiratory collapse. Some suicidal attempts have been fatal. The following data on meprobamate tablets have been reported in the literature and from other sources. These data are not expected to correlate with each case (considering factors such as individual susceptibility and length of time from ingestion to treatment), but represent the usual ranges reported.

Acute simple overdose (meprobamate alone) – Death has been reported with ingestion of as little as 12 g meprobamate and survival with as much as 40 g.

Blood levels – Blood levels of 0.5 to 2 mg/dL represents the usual blood level range of meprobamate after therapeutic doses. The level may occasionally be as high as 3 mg%. Blood levels of 3 to 10 mg/dL usually corresponds to findings of mild to moderate symptoms of overdosage, such as stupor or light coma. Blood levels of 10 to 20 mg/dL usually corresponds to deeper coma, requiring more intensive treatment. Some fatalities occur. At levels greater than 20 mg/dL, more fatalities than survivals can be expected.

➤*Treatment:* In cases where excessive doses have been taken, sleep ensues rapidly and blood pressure, pulse, and respiratory rates are reduced to basal levels. Any drug remaining in the stomach should be removed and symptomatic therapy given. Should respiration or blood pressure become compromised, respiratory assistance, central nervous system stimulants and

MEPROBAMATE — ORAL

pressor agents should be administered cautiously as indicated. Meprobamate is metabolized in the liver and excreted by the kidney. Diuresis, osmotic (mannitol) diuresis, peritoneal dialysis, and hemodialysis have been used successfully. Careful monitoring of urinary output is necessary and caution should be taken to avoid overhydration. Relapse and death, after initial recovery, have been attributed to incomplete gastric emptying and delayed absorption.

ANTIDEPRESSANTS

Drugs with clinically useful antidepressant effects include the tricyclic antidepressants (TCAs), tetracyclic antidepressants, trazodone, bupropion, venlafaxine, nefazodone, selective serotonin reuptake inhibitors (SSRIs), and the monoamine oxidase inhibitors (MAOIs). The antidepressant agents all appear effective in the treatment of depression. "Major depressive episode" implies a prominent and relatively persistent (nearly every day for ≥ 2 weeks) depressed or dysphoric mood that usually interferes with daily functioning, and includes ≥ 5 of the following 9 symptoms: Depressed mood; markedly diminished interest or pleasure in all, for almost all activities; significant weight loss or gain when not dieting, or decrease or increase in appetite; insomnia or hypersomnia; psychomotor agitation or retardation; fatigue or loss of energy; feelings of worthlessness, or excessive or inappropriate guilt; diminished ability to think or concentrate, or indecisiveness; recurrent thoughts of death, suicidal ideation, or suicide attempt. These symptoms are not because of the direct physiologic effects of a substance or a general medical condition (eg, hypothyroidism). The symptoms are not better accounted for by bereavement (ie, after the loss of a loved one), persist for > 2 months, or are characterized by marked functional impairment, morbid preoccupation with worthlessness, suicidal ideation, psychotic symptoms, or psychomotor retardation.

➤*Mechanism of action:* Effective antidepressant activity has traditionally been associated with the "biogenic amine hypothesis of depression." The theory is that depression is due to reduced functional activity of ≥ 1 of the endogenous monoamines (norepinephrine, serotonin) in the brain. It was believed that certain types of depression were caused by brain neurotransmitter deficiency and that antidepressants relieved depression by inhibiting the reuptake of serotonin and norepinephrine, thereby correcting this deficiency and facilitating neurotransmission. This explanation is now being questioned for several reasons. First, several antidepressant agents lack any apparent effect on neurotransmitter reuptake. More importantly, the blockade of neurotransmitter reuptake occurs within minutes to hours of antidepressant drug initiation, while the antidepressant effects usually take 1 to 4 weeks to manifest.

The emphasis of research has shifted from acute reuptake effects to the slower adaptive changes in norepinephrine and serotonin receptor systems induced by chronic antidepressant therapy. Postsynaptic receptors participate in nerve impulse neurotransmission while the presynaptic receptors regulate neurotransmitter release and reuptake, an important mechanism of neurotransmitter inactivation. Long-term antidepressant treatment produces complex changes in the sensitivities of both presynaptic and postsynaptic receptor sites. The available antidepressant agents may increase the sensitivity of postsynaptic alpha (α_1) adrenergic and serotonin receptors and may decrease the sensitivity of presynaptic receptor sites. The net effect is the correction (re-regulation) of an abnormal receptor-neurotransmitter relationship. Clinically, this re-regulatory action speeds up the patient's natural recovery process from the depressive episode by normalizing neurotransmission efficacy.

➤*Drug selection:* The non-MAOIs are used more frequently than the MAOIs, mainly because of the perception that MAOIs are less effective than the non-MAOI antidepressants and the risk of hypertensive crisis from ingesting foods containing tyramine or from drug interactions (eg, sympathomimetics) with the MAOIs. However, when MAOIs are used in therapeutic doses, they are probably equally effective to non-MAOIs for the treatment of depression. In general, MAOIs are used for atypical depression.

Base antidepressant drug selection on the patient's history of drug response (if any), the specific drug's side effect profile relative to patient medical conditions and other factors, and clinician familiarity with specific antidepressants. Nortriptyline and desipramine are preferred TCAs in a patient without a history of favorable response to a specific antidepressant because they cause less sedation and have less anticholinergic activity than tertiary TCAs such as amitriptyline and, in the case of nortriptyline, are less likely to cause orthostatic hypotension. Trazodone has less anticholinergic activity than TCAs and causes fewer problems than TCAs when taken in overdose. SSRIs generally lack the adverse reactions (eg, sedation, anticholinergic effects) associated with TCAs, cause few cardiovascular side effects (including orthostasis), are associated with initial weight loss rather than weight gain as is the case with TCAs, and cause fewer problems than TCAs when taken in overdose. Newer information has shown that during long-term use, SSRIs cause similar weight gain as compared with TCAs. However, their use is associated with other side effects such as headache, nervousness, and insomnia. Fluoxetine and paroxetine are recommended to be taken in the morning; sertraline can be taken morning or evening. Use maprotiline, mirtazapine, and bupropion only when other antidepressants have not proven effective. In cases of mild depression, drug therapy and psychotherapy appear to be equally effective.

As a general guideline, continue treatment for 9 months after remission in patients who experience their first episode of depression; following a second episode, continue treatment for 5 years after remission; with a third episode, treat indefinitely.

➤*Actions:* The following table summarizes some of the important pharmacologic and pharmacokinetic data of these agents.

Antidepressant Pharmacologic and Pharmacokinetic Parameters

0 -none + -slight ++ -moderate +++ -high ++++ -very high +++++ -highest	Major side effects			Amine uptake blocking activity		Half-life (hours)	Therapeutic plasma level (ng/ml)	Time to reach steady state (days)	Dose range (mg/day)
	Anticholinergic	Sedation	Orthostatic hypotension	Norepinephrine	Serotonin				
Tricyclics - Tertiary Amines									
Amitriptyline	++++	++++	++	++	++++	31-46	110-250[a]	4-10	50-300
Clomipramine	+++	+++	++	++	+++++	19-37	80-100	7-14	25-250
Doxepin	++	+++	++	+	++	8-24	100-200[a]	2-8	25-300
Imipramine	++	++	+++	++[b]	++++	11-25	200-350[a]	2-5	30-300
Trimipramine	++	+++	++	+	+	7-30	180[a]	2-6	50-300
Tricyclics - Secondary Amines									
Amoxapine[c]	+++	++	+	+++	++	8[d]	200-500	2-7	50-600
Desipramine	+	+	+	++++	++	12-24	125-300	2-11	25-300
Nortriptyline	++	++	+	++	+++	18-44	50-150	4-19	30-100
Protriptyline	+++	+	+	++++	++	67-89	100-200	14-19	15-60
Tetracyclics									
Maprotiline	++	++	+	+++	0/+	21-25	200-300[a]	6-10	50-225
Mirtazapine	++	+++	++	+++	+++	20-40	-	5	15-45
Triazolopyridine									
Trazodone	+	++++	++	0	+++	4-9	800-1600	3-7	150-600
Aminoketone									
Bupropion[5]	++	++	+	0/+	0/+	8-24	-	1.5-8	200-450
Phenethylamine									
Venlafaxine	0	0	0	+++	+++	5-11[a]	-	3-4	75-375
Phenylpiperazine									
Nefazodone	0/+	++	+	0/+	+++++	2-4	-	4-5	200-600

Antidepressant Pharmacologic and Pharmacokinetic Parameters

0 -none + -slight ++ -moderate +++ -high ++++ -very high +++++ -highest	Major side effects			Amine uptake blocking activity					
	Anticholinergic	Sedation	Orthostatic hypotension	Norepinephrine	Serotonin	Half-life (hours)	Therapeutic plasma level (ng/ml)	Time to reach steady state (days)	Dose range (mg/day)
Selective Serotonin Reuptake Inhibitors									
Citalopram	0/+	0/+	0/+	0/+	++++	33	-	7	20-60
Fluoxetine	0/+	0/+	0/+	0/+	+++++	1-16 days[a]	-	2-4 weeks	20-80
Fluvoxamine	0/+	0/+	0	0/+	+++++	15.6	-	≈ 7	50-300
Paroxetine	0	0/+	0	0/+	+++++	10-24	-	7-14	10-50
Sertraline	0	0/+	0	0/+	+++++	1-4 days[a]	-	7	50-200
Monoamine Oxidase Inhibitors									
Phenelzine	+	+	+	-	-	-	-	-	45-90
Tranylcypromine	+	+	0	-	-	2.4-2.8	-	-	30-60

[a] Parent compound plus active metabolite.
[b] Via desipramine, the major metabolite.
[c] Also blocks dopamine receptors.
[d] 30 hours for major metabolite 8-hydroxyamoxapine.
[e] Inhibits dopamine uptake.

Tricyclic Compounds

Refer to the Antidepressants introduction.

Indications

➤*Depression:* Relief of symptoms of depression (except **clomipramine**). The activating properties of **protriptyline** make it particularly suitable for withdrawn and anergic patients.

Agents with significant sedative action may be useful in depression associated with anxiety and sleep disturbances.

➤*Amoxapine:* Relief of depressive symptoms in patients with neurotic or reactive depressive disorders and endogenous and psychotic depression; depression accompanied by anxiety or agitation.

➤*Doxepin:* Treatment of psychoneurotic patients with depression or anxiety; depression or anxiety associated with alcoholism (not to be taken concomitantly with alcohol); depression or anxiety associated with organic disease (the possibility of drug interaction should be considered if the patient is receiving other drugs concomitantly); psychotic depressive disorders with associated anxiety including involutional depression and manic-depressive disorders. The target symptoms of psychoneurosis that respond particularly well to doxepin include anxiety, tension, depression, somatic symptoms and concerns, sleep disturbances, guilt, lack of energy, fear, apprehension, and worry.

➤*Imipramine:* Treatment of enuresis in children ≥ 6 years of age as temporary adjunctive therapy.

➤*Clomipramine:* Only for treatment of obsessive-compulsive disorder (OCD).

➤*Unlabeled uses:* Analgesic adjuncts for phantom limb pain, chronic pain (migraine, chronic tension headache, diabetic neuropathy, tic douloureux, cancer pain, peripheral neuropathy with pain, postherpetic neuralgia, arthritic pain): Amitriptyline 75 to 300 mg/day; doxepin 30 to 300 mg/day; imipramine 75 to 300 mg/day; nortriptyline 50 to 150 mg/day; desipramine 75 to 300 mg/day; amoxapine 100 to 300 mg/day; protriptyline 15 to 60 mg/day.

Pathologic laughing and weeping secondary to forebrain disease – Amitriptyline 30 to 75 mg/day.

Obstructive sleep apnea – Protriptyline.

Peptic ulcer disease – Trimipramine 25 to 50 mg/day; doxepin 50 to 150 mg/day.

Facilitation of cocaine withdrawal – Desipramine 50 to 200 mg/day; imipramine 150 to 300 mg/day.

Panic disorder – Imipramine; clomipramine; desipramine; nortriptyline. Other antidepressants may also be used.

Eating disorders (effective in bulimia nervosa) – Imipramine; desipramine; amitriptyline.

Premenstrual symptoms – Nortriptyline 50 to 125 mg/day; desipramine 100 to 150 mg/day for depression; clomipramine 25 to 75 mg/day for irritability and dysphoria.

Dermatologic disorders (chronic urticaria and angioedema, nocturnal pruritus in atopic eczema) – Doxepin 10 to 30 mg/day; desipramine 100 to 150 mg/day; nortriptyline 20 to 75 mg/day; amitriptyline 10 to 50 mg/day.

Administration and Dosage

If minor side effects develop, reduce dosage. Discontinue treatment promptly if serious adverse effects or allergic manifestations occur.

➤*Plasma levels:* Determination of plasma levels may be useful in identifying patients who appear to have toxic effects and may have excessively high levels of the drug, or those in whom lack of absorption or noncompliance is suspected. Make adjustments in dosage according to patient's clinical response, not based on plasma levels.

➤*Adolescent, elderly, and outpatients:* Lower dosages are recommended. Initiate therapy at a low dosage and increase gradually, noting the clinical response and any evidence of intolerance. Most antidepressant drugs have a lag period of 10 days to 4 weeks before a therapeutic response is noted. Increasing the dose will not shorten this period but rather increase the incidence of adverse reactions. Following remission, maintenance medication may be required for a longer time at the lowest dose that will maintain remission. Continue maintenance therapy ≥ 3 months to decrease the possibility of relapse.

➤*Single daily dose:* A single daily dose may be used for maintenance therapy. A single daily dose at bedtime is convenient, will minimize daytime side effects (sedation and anticholinergic effects), and the sedative effect at bedtime may be beneficial in patients with sleep disorders. Because of increased risk of cardiovascular and other complications, the elderly may not tolerate single daily doses. **Protriptyline** may have a mild stimulant effect; it is generally not given as a single bedtime dose.

➤*Tricyclic / MAOI combined use:* Tricyclic/MAOI combined use is traditionally contraindicated because of the potential serious adverse reactions (see Drug Interactions). Such combinations may offer significant advantages in patients refractory to more conservative therapy. In conservative dosages, with observance of MAOI dietary restrictions, and under close medical observation, combined therapy has been safe. At least 7 to 10 days should elapse between MAOI discontinuation and TCA institution.

Specific dosage guidelines for individual agents are included in the product listings.

Actions

➤*Pharmacology:* The tricyclic antidepressants (TCAs), structurally related to the phenothiazine antipsychotic agents, possess 3 major pharmacologic actions in varying degrees: Blocking of the amine pump, sedation, and peripheral and central anticholinergic action. In contrast to phenothiazines, which act on dopamine receptors, TCAs inhibit reuptake of norepinephrine or serotonin (5-hydroxytryptamine, 5-HT) at the presynaptic neuron. **Amoxapine**, a metabolite of loxapine, retains some of the postsynaptic dopamine receptor-blocking action of neuroleptics.

Amine uptake inhibition – The amine hypothesis of depression proposes a relationship between depression and levels of CNS bioamines at postsynaptic adrenergic receptors in the brain. TCAs can be characterized by their ability to inhibit presynaptic reuptake of norepinephrine and serotonin (see table in Introduction).

Although amine pump blockade may be immediate, antidepressant response can take days to weeks.

Other pharmacologic effects – Inhibition of histamine and acetylcholine activity. Clinical effects, in addition to antidepressant effects, include sedation, anticholinergic effects, mild peripheral vasodilator effects, and possible "quinidine-like" actions.

Contraindications

Prior sensitivity to any tricyclic drug. Not recommended for use during the acute recovery phase following MI. Concomitant use of monoamine oxidase inhibitors (MAOIs) is generally contraindicated (see Warnings, Drug Interactions).

➤*Doxepin:* Patients with glaucoma or a tendency to have urinary retention.

Cross-sensitivity may occur among the dibenzazepines (**clomipramine**, **desipramine**, **imipramine**, **nortriptyline**, and **trimipramine**). In addition, dibenzoxepines (**doxepin**, **amoxapine**) may produce cross-sensitivity. **Amitriptyline** may block the antihypertensive action of guanethidine or similarly active compounds.

Warnings

➤*Tardive dyskinesia:* Tardive dyskinesia, a syndrome consisting of potentially irreversible, involuntary, dyskinetic movements may develop in patients treated with neuroleptics (eg, antipsychotics). **Amoxapine** is not an antipsychotic, but it has substantive neuroleptic activity. Although the syndrome appears most often among the elderly, especially elderly women, it is impossible to determine which patients will develop the syndrome. Whether or not neuroleptic drugs differ in their potential to cause tardive dyskinesia is unknown. For a more complete discussion of tardive dyskinesia, see the Antipsychotic Agents group monograph.

➤*Neuroleptic malignant syndrome (NMS):* NMS is a potentially fatal condition reported in association with antipsychotic drugs and with **amoxapine**. Clinical manifestations of NMS are hyperpyrexia, muscle rigidity, altered mental status, and evidence of autonomic instability (irregular pulse or blood pressure, tachycardia, diaphoresis, and cardiac arrhythmias). The management of NMS should include the following: (1) Immediate discontinuation of antipsychotic drugs, amoxapine, and other drugs not essential to concurrent therapy, (2) intensive symptomatic treatment and medical monitoring, and (3) treatment of any concomitant serious medical problems for which specific treatments are available. There is no general agreement about specific pharmacologic treatment regimens for uncomplicated NMS.

Once the NMS is resolved, use a different antidepressant drug if the patient continues to require antidepressant treatment.

Hyperthermia has occurred with **clomipramine**; most cases occurred when it was used with other drugs (eg, neuroleptics) and may be an example of NMS.

➤*Seizure disorders:* Because TCAs lower the seizure threshold, use with caution in patients with a history of seizures or other predisposing factors (eg, brain damage of varying etiology, alcoholism, concomitant drugs known to lower the seizure threshold). However, seizures have occurred in patients with and without a history of seizure disorders. Seizure was identified as the most significant risk of **clomipramine** use in premarket evaluation.

➤*Anticholinergic effects:* Use with caution in patients with a history of urinary retention, narrow-angle glaucoma, or increased intraocular pressure. In angle-closure glaucoma, even average doses may precipitate an attack. In occasional susceptible patients or in those receiving anticholinergics (including antiparkinson agents), the atropine-like effects may become more pronounced (eg, paralytic ileus). See table in Introduction for relative anticholinergic actions.

➤*Cardiovascular disorders:* Use with extreme caution in patients with cardiovascular disorders because of the possibility of conduction defects, arrhythmias, CHF, sinus tachycardia, MI, strokes, and tachycardia. These patients require cardiac surveillance at all dose levels of the drug. In high doses, TCAs may produce arrhythmias, sinus tachycardia, conduction defects, and prolonged conduction time. Tachycardia and postural hypotension may occur more frequently with **protriptyline**.

➤*Hyperthyroid patients:* Hyperthyroid patients or those receiving thyroid medication require close supervision because of the possibility of cardiovascular toxicity, including arrhythmias.

➤*Psychiatric patients:* Schizophrenic or paranoid patients may exhibit a worsening of psychosis with TCA therapy. In overactive or agitated patients, increased anxiety or agitation may occur. Neuropsychiatric signs and symptoms (eg, delusions, hallucinations, psychotic episodes, confusion, paranoia) have been reported with **clomipramine** use. Paranoid delusions, with or without associated hostility, may be exaggerated. Reduction of TCA dosage and concomitant antipsychotic therapy (eg, perphenazine) may be necessary.

The possibility of suicide in depressed patients remains during treatment and until significant remission occurs. Patients should not have easy access to large quantities of the drug; advise the physician to prescribe small quantities of TCAs.

➤*Mania/Hypomania:* Hypomanic or manic episodes may occur, particularly in patients with cyclic disorders. Such reactions may necessitate discontinuation of the drug. If needed, **imipramine pamoate** may be resumed in lower doses when these episodes are relieved. Administration of a tranquilizer may be useful in controlling such episodes. Manic-depressive patients may experience a shift to a hypomanic or manic phase, which may necessitate discontinuation and possibly resuming at a lower dose when these episodes are relieved.

➤*MAOIs:* Do not give MAOIs with or immediately following TCAs. Such combinations can produce hyperpyretic crises, severe convulsions, sweating, coma, hyperexcitability, hyperthermia, tachycardia, tachypnea, headache, mydriasis, flushing, confusion, hypotension, disseminated intravascular coagulation, and death. Allow at least 14 days to elapse between MAOI discontinuation and TCA institution. Some TCAs have been used safely and successfully with MAOIs. Initiate TCA cautiously with gradual dosage increase until achieving optimum response. **Furazolidone** may interact similarly with TCAs.

➤*Rash:* Antidepressant drugs can cause skin rashes or "drug fever" in susceptible individuals. These allergic reactions may, in rare cases, be severe. They are more likely to occur during the first few days of treatment but may also occur later. Discontinue if rash or fever develop.

➤*Renal/Hepatic function impairment:* Use with caution and in reduced doses in patients with hepatic impairment; metabolism may be impaired, leading to drug accumulation. **Clomipramine** was occasionally associated with AST and ALT elevations (incidence of ≈ 1% and 3%, respectively) of potential clinical importance (values > 3 times the upper limit of normal) but was not associated with other clinical findings suggestive of hepatic injury. Rare reports of more severe liver injury, some fatal, have been reported. Use caution in treating patients with known liver disease, and periodic monitoring of hepatic enzyme levels is recommended in such patients. Use with caution in patients with significantly impaired renal function.

➤*Elderly:* Be cautious in dose selection for an elderly patient, usually starting at the low end of the dosing range. This reflects the greater frequency of decreased hepatic function, concomitant disease, and other drug therapy in elderly patients. Elderly patients may be sensitive to the anticholinergic side effects of TCAs.

Elderly patients taking **amitriptyline** may be at increased risk for falls; start on low doses of amitriptyline and observe closely.

➤*Pregnancy:* (*Category D* - amitriptyline, imipramine, nortriptyline; *Category C* - amoxapine, clomipramine, desipramine, doxepin, protriptyline, trimipramine). Clinical experience is limited. These agents have demonstrated teratogenicity and embryotoxicity in animals at doses greater than maximum human doses. There have been clinical reports of congenital malformations associated with **imipramine**. Limb reduction anomalies have been reported with **amitriptyline** and **nortriptyline**, and neonatal withdrawal symptoms have been seen with **clomipramine**, **desipramine**, and **imipramine**. All are isolated reports.

Safety for use during pregnancy has not been established; use only when clearly needed and when the potential benefits outweigh the potential hazards to the fetus.

➤*Lactation:* These agents are excreted into breast milk in low concentrations (approximate milk:plasma ratio of 0.4 to 1.5). Exercise caution when using in a nursing woman.

➤*Children:* Not recommended for patients < 12 years of age. Safety and efficacy have not been established for **amoxapine** in children < 16 years of age, or **clomipramine** in children < 10 years of age. The safety and efficacy of **imipramine** as temporary adjunctive therapy for nocturnal enuresis in pediatric patients < 6 years of age have not been established. The safety of the drug for long-term, chronic use as adjunctive therapy for nocturnal enuresis in pediatric patients ≥ 6 years of age has not been established. Safety and efficacy are not established in the pediatric age group for **trimipramine**, **nortriptyline**, **protriptyline**, and **desipramine**.

Do not exceed 2.5 mg/kg/day of **imipramine**. ECG changes of unknown significance have occurred in pediatric patients with doses twice this amount. Effectiveness of imipramine in children for conditions other than nocturnal enuresis has not been established.

Precautions

➤*Monitoring:* Perform baseline and periodic leukocyte and differential counts and liver function studies. Fever or sore throat may signal serious neutrophil depression; discontinue therapy if there is evidence of pathological neutropenia.

Monitor ECG prior to initiation of large doses of TCAs and at appropriate intervals thereafter. Patients with cardiovascular disease require cardiac surveillance at all dosage levels. Elderly patients and patients with cardiac disease or a history of cardiac disease are at special risk of developing cardiac abnormalities with TCAs.

➤*Electroconvulsive therapy:* Electroconvulsive therapy with TCAs may increase the hazards of therapy.

➤*Elective surgery:* Discontinue therapy for as long as possible before elective surgery.

➤*Blood sugar levels:* Elevated and lowered blood sugar levels have occurred.

➤*Sexual dysfunction:* Sexual dysfunction was markedly increased in male patients with OCD taking **clomipramine** (42% ejaculatory failure, 20% impotence) compared with placebo.

➤*Weight changes:* Weight gain has been observed in clinical trials involving all TCAs. Weight gain occurred in 18% of patients receiving **clomipramine**. Some patients had weight gain in excess of 25% of their initial body weight.

➤*Serotonin syndrome:* Some TCAs inhibit neuronal reuptake of serotonin and can increase synaptic serotonin levels (eg, **clomipramine**, **amitriptyline**). Either therapeutic or excessive doses of these drugs, in combination with other drugs that also increase synaptic serotonin levels (such as MAOIs), can cause a serotonin syndrome consisting of tremor, agitation, delirium, rigidity, myoclonus, hyperthermia, and obtundation.

➤*Benzyl alcohol:* Some of these products contain benzyl alcohol, which has been associated with a fatal "gasping syndrome" in premature infants.

➤*Hazardous tasks:* May impair mental or physical abilities required for the performance of potentially hazardous tasks; have patients observe caution while driving or performing other tasks requiring alertness, coordination, or physical dexterity.

➤*Photosensitivity:* Photosensitization (photoallergy or phototoxicity) may occur; therefore, caution patients to take protective measures (ie, sunscreens, protective clothing) against exposure to ultraviolet light or sunlight until tolerance is determined.

➤*Sulfite sensitivity:* Some of the injectable antidepressant products contain sulfites that may cause allergic-type reactions including anaphylactic symptoms and life-threatening or less-severe asthmatic episodes in certain susceptible people. The overall prevalence of sulfite sensitivity in the general population is unknown but is probably low. Sulfite sensitivity is seen more frequently in asthmatic than in non-asthmatic people. Products containing sulfites are identified in the product listings.

Drug Interactions

➤*P450 system:* Concomitant use of TCAs with other drugs metabolized by cytochrome P450 2D6 may require lower doses than those usually prescribed for either the TCA or the other drug. Therefore, exercise caution in the coadministration of TCAs with other drugs that are metabolized by this isoenzyme, including other antidepressants, phenothiazines, carbamazepine, and type 1C antiarrhythmics (eg, propafenone, flecainide, encainide), or that inhibit this enzyme (eg, quinidine).

Tricyclic Drug Interactions

Precipitant drug	Object drug*		Description
Barbiturates	TCAs	⬇	Barbiturates may lower serum levels of TCAs; central and respiratory depressant effects may be additive.
Bupropion	TCAs	⬆	Plasma concentrations of TCAs may be elevated, producing an increase in pharmacologic and adverse effects.
Carbamazepine	TCAs	⬇	Carbamazepine may decrease TCA levels. Serum carbamazepine levels may be increased resulting in an increase in pharmacologic and toxic effects.
TCAs	Carbamazepine	⬆	
Charcoal	TCAs	⬇	Charcoal can prevent TCA absorption, thereby reducing their effectiveness or toxicity.
Cimetidine	TCAs	⬆	Cimetidine has increased serum TCA concentrations. Anticholinergic symptoms (eg, severe dry mouth, urinary retention, blurred vision) have been associated with elevated TCA serum levels when cimetidine therapy is initiated. Additionally, higher than expected TCA levels have occurred when they are initiated in patients already taking cimetidine. Other H_2 antagonists may be suitable alternatives.
Haloperidol	TCAs	⬆	Haloperidol may increase serum concentrations of TCAs; a tonic-clonic seizure occurred in 1 patient.
Histamine H_2 antagonists	TCAs	⬆	Increased serum concentrations of the TCAs have occurred; mild symptoms have been noted.
MAO Inhibitors	TCAs	⬆	Such combinations can produce hyperpyretic crisis, severe convulsions, sweating, coma, hyperexcitability, hyperthermia, tachycardia, tachypnea, headache, mydriasis, flushing, confusion, hypotension, disseminated intravascular coagulation, and death. However, some MAOIs have been used safely and successfully with TCAs. See Warnings.
Rifamycins	TCAs	⬇	TCA levels may be decreased, resulting in a decrease in pharmacologic effects.
Smoking	TCAs	⬇	Smoking may increase the metabolic biotransformation of TCAs.
SSRIs	TCAs	⬆	SSRIs may increase the pharmacologic and toxic effects of TCAs; symptoms may persist for several weeks after discontinuation of the SSRI. At least 5 weeks may be necessary when switching from fluoxetine to a TCA.
Valproic acid	TCAs	⬆	Plasma concentrations and side effects of TCAs may be increased.
Venlafaxine	Desipramine	⬆	Desipramine AUC, C_{max}, and C_{min} increased by ≈ 35% in the presence of venlafaxine. The 2-OH-desipramine AUC increased by at least 2.5- to 4.5-fold. The clinical significance of elevated 2-OH-desipramine levels is unknown.
TCAs	Anticholinergics	⬆	The anticholinergic effects may be enhanced by the coadministration of certain TCAs. Paralytic ileus may occur.
TCAs	Clonidine	⬆	Dangerous elevations in blood pressure and hypertensive crisis have occurred in patients receiving concurrent TCAs. Avoid coadministration.
TCAs	Dicumarol	⬆	TCAs may increase the half-life or bioavailability of dicumarol, possibly resulting in increased anticoagulation effects.
TCAs	Guanethidine	⬇	TCAs may antagonize guanethidine's antihypertensive action by inhibiting uptake into adrenergic neurons. Avoid this combination when possible; if concurrent therapy is required, monitor blood pressure. At up to 150 mg/day, doxepin may be given with guanethidine without reducing antihypertensive effect.
TCAs	Levodopa	⬇	Levodopa absorption may be delayed and its bioavailability decreased by TCAs. Hypertensive episodes have also occurred.
TCAs	Quinolones Grepafloxacin Sparfloxacin	⬆	The risk of life-threatening cardiac arrhythmias, including torsades de pointes, may be increased.
TCAs	Sympathomimetics	⬇	TCAs potentiate the pressor response of the direct-acting sympathomimetics; dysrhythmias have occurred. The pressor response to the indirect-acting sympathomimetics is decreased by the TCAs.

* ⬆ = Object drug increased. ⬇ = Object drug decreased.

Adverse Reactions

Sedation and anticholinergic effects are reported most frequently. Tolerance to these effects develops, but side effects may be minimized by starting with a low dose and then gradually increasing the dose or reducing dosage.

Anticholinergic – Dry mouth, and rarely, associated sublingual adenitis or gingivitis; blurred vision; disturbance of accommodation; increased intraocular pressure; mydriasis; constipation; paralytic ileus; urinary retention; delayed micturition; urinary tract dilation; hyperpyrexia.

Withdrawal symptoms – Although not indicative of addiction, abrupt cessation after prolonged therapy may produce dizziness, nausea, headache, vomiting, malaise, sleep disturbances, hyperthermia, irritability, or worsening of psychiatric status. Gradual dosage reduction may produce, within 2 weeks, transient symptoms including irritability, restlessness, and dream and sleep disturbance. Rarely mania or hypomania occurred within 2 to 7 days following cessation of chronic therapy.

Enuretic children – Consider adverse reactions reported with adult use. The most common reactions are nervousness, sleep disorders, tiredness, and mild GI disturbances. These usually disappear with continued therapy or dosage reduction. Other reported reactions include the following: Constipation; convulsions; anxiety; emotional instability; syncope; collapse. Do not exceed 2.5 mg/kg/day of **imipramine**.

➤*Cardiovascular:*

General – Arrhythmias; changes in AV conduction; ECG changes (most frequently with toxic doses); flushing; heart block; hot flushes; hypertension; hypotension; orthostatic hypotension; palpitations; precipitation of CHF; premature ventricular contractions; stroke; sudden death; syncope; tachycardia.

Clomipramine – Aneurysm; atrial flutter; bradycardia; bundle branch block; cardiac arrest/failure; cerebral hemorrhage; extrasystoles; MI; myocardial ischemia; pallor; peripheral ischemia; postural hypotension; thrombophlebitis; vasospasm; ventricular fibrillation; ventricular tachycardia.

Desipramine – Hypertensive episodes during surgery. There has been a report of an "acute collapse" and "sudden death" in an 8-year-old (18 kg) male, treated with desipramine for 2 years for hyperactivity. There have been reports of sudden death in children.

➤*CNS:*

General – Agitation; akathisia; alterations in EEG patterns; anxiety; ataxia; coma; confusion (especially in the elderly); disorientation; disturbed concentration; dizziness; drowsiness; dysarthria; exacerbation of psychosis; excitement; excessive appetite; extrapyramidal symptoms including abnormal involuntary movements and tardive dyskinesia; fatigue; hallucinations; delusions; headache; hyperthermia; hypomania; incoordination; insomnia; mania; nervousness; neuroleptic malignant syndrome; nightmares; numbness; panic; paresthesias of extremities; peripheral neuropathy; restlessness; tremors; seizures; tingling; weakness.

Clomipramine – Abnormal dreaming; abnormal gait; abnormal thinking; aggressive reaction; anticholinergic syndrome; apathy; asthenia; aphasia; apraxia; ataxia; catalepsy; cholinergic syndrome; choreoathetosis; coma; convulsions; decrease in memory; delirium; depersonalization; depression; dyskinesia; dysphonia; emotional lability; encephalopathy; euphoria; extrapyramidal disorder; hostility; hemiparesis; hyperkinesia; hyperreflexia; hypertonia; hypnagogic hallucinations; hypoesthesia; hypokinesia; illusion; impaired impulse control; indecisiveness; irritability; leg cramps; manic reaction; migraine; mutism; myoclonus; neuralgia; neuropathy; nystagmus; oculogyric crisis; oculomotor nerve paralysis; panic reaction; paranoia; paresis; phobic disorder; psychosis; psychosomatic disorder; sensory disturbance; schizophrenic reaction; sleep disorder; somnambulism; somnolence; generalized spasm; speech disorder; stimulation; stupor; suicide; suicide attempt; suicidal ideation; teeth-grinding; twitching; vertigo; yawning.

➤*Dermatologic:* **Clomipramine**, **imipramine** - Acne; alopecia; cellulitis; chloasma; cyst; dermatitis; dry skin; eczema; erythematous rash; folliculitis; genital pruritus; maculopapular rash; photosensitivity reaction; piloerection; psoriasis; pustular rash; seborrhea; skin discoloration; skin hypertrophy; skin ulceration.

➤*GI:*

General – Abdominal pain/cramps; anorexia; aphthous stomatitis; black tongue; constipation; diarrhea; dysphagia; epigastric distress; flatulence; increased pancreatic enzymes; indigestion; GI disorder; nausea and vomiting; parotid swelling; stomatitis; taste disturbance; peculiar taste; ulcerative stomatitis.

Clomipramine – Abnormal hepatic function; blood in stool; cheilitis; chronic enteritis; colitis; discolored feces; duodenitis; dyspepsia; oral/pharyngeal edema; eructation; esophagitis; gastric dilatation; gastric ulcer; gastritis; gastroesophageal reflux; gingival bleeding; gingivitis; glossitis; hemorrhoids; hiccough; increased salivation; intestinal obstruction; irritable bowel syndrome; peptic ulcer; rectal hemorrhage; salivary gland enlargement; tongue ulceration; tooth caries; tooth disorder.

➤*GU:*

General – Gynecomastia and testicular swelling in the male; breast enlargement, menstrual irregularity and galactorrhea in the female; impotence; increased or decreased libido; painful ejaculation; nocturia; testicular swelling; urinary frequency.

Clomipramine – Albuminuria; amenorrhea; anorgasmy; breast engorgement; breast fibroadenosis; breast pain; cervical dysplasia; cystitis; dysmenorrhea; dysuria; endometrial hyperplasia; ejaculation failure; endometriosis; epididymitis; hematuria; lactation (nonpuerperal); leukorrhea; menstrual disorder; micturition disorder/frequency; nocturia; oliguria; ovarian cyst; perineal pain; polyuria; premature ejaculation; prostatic disorder; pyelonephritis; pyuria; renal calculus/cyst/pain; urinary retention; vaginitis; urethral disorder; urinary incontinence; uterine hemorrhage or inflammation; vaginal hemorrhage; vulvar disorder.

➤*Hematologic:*

General – Bone marrow depression including agranulocytosis; aplastic anemia; eosinophilia; leukopenia; purpura; thrombocytopenia.

Clomipramine – Anemia; leukemoid reaction; lymphadenopathy; lymphoma-like disorder.

➤*Hepatic:*

General – Rarely, hepatitis and jaundice (simulating obstructive); elevation in transaminase; changes in alkaline phosphatase; altered liver function.

➤*Hypersensitivity:*

General – Cross-sensitivity with other TCAs; drug fever; edema (general or of face and tongue); itching; petechiae; photosensitization; pruritus; rash; urticaria; vasculitis.

➤*Metabolic / Nutritional:*

General – Change in blood glucose; elevation or depression of blood sugar levels; elevation of prolactin levels; inappropriate ADH secretion.

Clomipramine – Dehydration; diabetes mellitus; fat intolerance; glycosuria; goiter; gout; hypercholesterolemia; hyperglycemia; hyperuricemia; hypokalemia; hypothyroidism; hyperthyroidism.

➤*Musculoskeletal:*

Clomipramine – Arthrosis; bruising; dystonia; exostosis; lupus erythematosus rash; myopathy; myositis; polyarteritis nodosa; torticollis.

➤*Respiratory:*

General – Exacerbation of asthma.

Clomipramine – Bronchitis; bronchospasm; coughing; cyanosis; dyspnea; epistaxis; hemoptysis; hyperventilation; hypoventilation; increased sputum; laryngismus; laryngitis; pharyngitis; pneumonia; rhinitis; sinusitis.

➤*Special senses:*

General – Abnormal lacrimation; tinnitus.

Clomipramine – Abnormal accommodation; abnormal vision; anisocoria; blepharospasm; blepharitis; chromatopsia; conjunctival hemorrhage; conjunctivitis; deafness; diplopia; earache; exophthalmos; eye pain; foreign body sensation; glaucoma; hyperacusis; keratitis; labyrinth disorder; mydriasis; night blindness; ocular allergy; otitis media; parosmia; photophobia; retinal disorder; scleritis; strabismus; taste loss; vestibular disorder; visual field defect.

➤*Miscellaneous:*

General – Alopecia; fever; hyperthermia; hyperpyrexia; local edema; nasal stuffiness; increased perspiration; proneness to falling; weight gain or loss.

Clomipramine – Abnormal skin odor; arthralgia; back pain; chest pain; chills; dependent edema; general edema; fever; halitosis; increased susceptibility to infection; malaise; muscle weakness; myalgia; pain; thirst; withdrawal syndrome.

Overdosage

Children are reportedly more sensitive than adults to acute overdose. Consider any overdose in infants or young children to be serious and potentially fatal. The response of the patient to toxic overdosage of TCAs may vary in severity and is conditioned by factors such as age, amount ingested, amount absorbed, and the interval between ingestion and start of treatment. Deaths may occur from overdosage with this class of drugs. Multiple drug ingestion (including alcohol) is common in deliberate TCA overdose. It is strongly recommended that the physician contact a poison control center for current information on treatment. Signs and symptoms of toxicity develop rapidly after TCA overdose; therefore, hospital monitoring is required as soon as possible.

➤*Symptoms:*

CNS – Early signs include confusion, agitation, hallucinations, drowsiness, and stupor. Seizures are common, especially with **amoxapine**, and may begin within 12 hours after ingestion; status epilepticus may develop. Overdoses with amoxapine are particularly characterized by CNS toxicity, such as coma; acidosis may also occur. Physical examination may reveal clonus, choreoathetosis, hyperactive reflexes, and a positive Babinski's sign.

Anticholinergic – Flushing; dry mouth; mydriasis; dilated pupils; hyperpyrexia; paralytic ileus; urinary retention; decreased GI motility; may not be observed in acute overdose. Anticholinergic effects are not prominent with **amoxapine**.

Cardiovascular – Cardiovascular toxicity is the leading cause of death in overdose. TCAs exert cardiotoxicity because of anticholinergic activity and quinidine-like effect that depresses myocardial contractility, heart rate, and coronary blood flow. Arrhythmias include tachycardia, intraventricular blocks, and complete AV block. Changes in ECG are clinical indicators of TCA toxicity. Any combination of 1) rightward axis of the terminal 40 msec of the QRS complex (a prominent R-wave in lead aVR), 2) QRS duration ≥ 100 msec (≥ 0.1 sec), 3) tachycardia, or 4) QT_c interval ≥ 440 msec suggest serious TCA poisoning. With up to 20 mg/kg, re-entry ventricular arrhythmias, premature ventricular contractions, ventricular tachycardia, or fibrillation may occur. Sudden cardiac arrest has been reported. Pulmonary edema, conduction abnormalities, and hypotension are common. Severe cardiotoxicity usually occurs within 6 hours; however, ECG changes may be noted up to 48 hours postingestion.

Renal – Rhabdomyolysis and renal failure may appear if prolonged seizures or coma occurs. Renal failure may develop 2 to 5 days after toxic overdosage of **amoxapine** in patients who may appear otherwise recovered; acute tubular necrosis with rhabdomyolysis and myoglobinuria is most common. This probably occurs in < 5% of overdose cases, and is typical in those who have experienced multiple seizures.

Other – Respiratory depression, cyanosis, shock, diaphoresis, aspiration, and ARDS may occur in severe overdoses. Hyperthermia and hypothermia have been reported. Polyradiculoneuropathy has been reported with **amitriptyline**. Muscle rigidity, disorders of ocular motility, vomiting, or any other symptoms under adverse events are signs of overdose.

➤*Treatment:* Hospitalize and closely observe with ECG monitoring. Observe for signs of CNS or respiratory depression, hypotension, cardiac dysrhythmias or conduction blocks, and seizures for a minimum of 6 hours even when the amount ingested is thought to be small or the initial degree of intoxication appears slight to moderate. Blood and urine levels are unreliable indicators for clinical management. Closely monitor patients with ECG abnormalities for at least 6 hours and until well after cardiac status returns to normal. A prolonged QRS interval (≥ 100 msec) may indicate the patient is at higher risk for developing seizures, arrhythmias, or hypotension. Relapses may occur after apparent recovery.

Maintain adequate respiratory exchange. Do not use respiratory stimulants. Use normal or half-normal saline to avoid water intoxication, especially in children. Instillation of activated charcoal slurry after large volume gastric lavage may help reduce absorption. Consider gastric lavage in symptomatic patients only after intubation and only if the procedure can be done in the first hour after ingestion. Emesis is contraindicated. Refer to General Management of Acute Overdosage.

Treat cardiovascular effects aggressively. A maximal limb-lead QRS duration of ≥ 0.1 seconds may be an indication of overdose severity. Sodium bicarbonate (hypertonic, 1 M) by IV infusion has effectively treated cardiac dysrhythmias and hypotension. It is usually given 50 mEq (1 mEq/ml) IV bolus, followed by repeated doses to maintain the blood at pH 7.45 to 7.55. If hypotension does not respond to sodium bicarbonate, fluid expansion and vasopressors (eg, norepinephrine 0.1 to 0.2 mcg/kg/min [first choice] or dopamine 10 to 20 mcg/kg/min) may be required. If cardiac dysrhythmias do not respond, lidocaine, bretylium, or phenytoin may be used. Isoproterenol may help control bradyarrhythmias and torsades de pointes ventricular tachycardia while overdrive pacing is being established. Propranolol (0.01 to 0.1 mg/kg/dose over 10 minutes; maximum is 1 mg/dose) is used for life-threatening ventricular arrhythmias in children. The propranolol dose for adults is 1 mg/dose IV administered no faster than 1 mg/min repeated every 2 to 5 minutes until desired response is seen or a maximum of 5 mg has been given. Quinidine, procainamide, and disopyramide are contraindicated for TCA overdose. Serious cardiovascular effects are remarkably rare following **amoxapine** overdosage, and the ECG typically remains within normal limits, except for sinus tachycardia. Hence, prolongation of the QRS interval beyond 100 msec within the first 24 hours is not a useful guide to the severity of overdosage with this drug.

In rare instances, hemoperfusion may be beneficial in acute refractory cardiovascular instability in patients with acute toxicity. Hemodialysis, peritoneal dialysis, exchange transfusions, and forced diuresis have generally been ineffective because of the rapid fixation of TCAs in the tissues.

Treat shock and metabolic acidosis with supportive measures (eg, IV fluids, bicarbonate, oxygen, corticosteroids). Digitalis may increase conduction abnormalities and further irritate an already sensitized myocardium. Exercise care if CHF necessitates rapid digitalization. Closely monitor cardiac function for at least 5 days. Support renal function.

Minimize external stimulation (darken the room) to prevent seizures. Control seizures with benzodiazepines. If these are ineffective, use anticonvulsants (eg, phenytoin, phenobarbital). If phenobarbital and phenytoin are ineffective, consider paralysis or barbiturate coma. Physostigmine is not recommended except to treat life-threatening symptoms that have been unresponsive to other therapies, and then only in consultation with a poison control center. With **amoxapine**, seizures may appear precipitously in otherwise relatively asymptomatic patients. Consider prophylactic anticonvulsants. With other antidepressants, administer diazepam IV bolus (adult: 5 to 10 mg initially that may be repeated every 15 minutes as needed up to 30 mg; child: 0.25 to 0.4 mg/kg dose up to 10 mg/dose) or lorazepam IV bolus (adult: 4 to 8 mg; child: 0.05 to 0.1 mg/kg). Control hyperpyrexia by any available means, including external cooling (ice packs, cooling blankets, sponge baths), benzodiazepines to control agitation and seizures, and paralysis with a neuromuscular blocker, if necessary.

Patient Information

Before using, tell your physician and pharmacist (1) if you have other medical conditions; (2) what other medications you are currently taking (including *otc* and alternative medicines); (3) if you have ever had an unusual or allergic reaction to any TCA; (4) if you are pregnant or may become pregnant; and (5) if you are breastfeeding.

Discontinue drug and get emergency help if any of the following occurs: Seizures; difficult or fast breathing; fever with increased sweating; loss of bladder control; severe muscle stiffness; unusual tiredness or weakness.

Warn patients of the risk of seizure.

Advise patients to complete full course of therapy; may take 4 to 6 weeks to see full benefits.

Warn male patients receiving **clomipramine** of the high incidence of sexual dysfunction.

Given the likelihood that some patients exposed chronically to neuroleptics will develop tardive dyskinesia, it is advised that all patients in whom chronic use is contemplated be given, if possible, full information about this risk. The decision to inform patients or their guardians must obviously take into account the clinical circumstances and the competency of the patient to understand the information provided.

Caution patients against use of alcohol, barbiturates, and other CNS depressants because effects may be exacerbated by TCAs.

Do not discontinue therapy or take other drugs without consent of physician. Abrupt discontinuation of therapy may cause nausea, headache, and malaise.

May cause drowsiness, dizziness, or blurred vision; use caution when driving or performing other tasks requiring alertness, coordination, or physical dexterity. Avoid alcohol and other CNS depressant drugs.

If serious adverse effects occur, dosage should be reduced or treatment should be altered.

Avoid prolonged exposure to sunlight or sunlamps; photosensitivity may occur.

AMITRIPTYLINE HYDROCHLORIDE

Rx	**Amitriptyline HCl** (Various, eg, Geneva, Mutual, Sidmak, URL, Zenith Goldline)	**Tablets:** 10 mg	In 100s, 1,000s, UD 100s, and blister pack 100s and 600s.
Rx	**Amitriptyline HCl** (Various, eg, Geneva, Mutual, Sidmak, UDL, URL, Zenith Goldline)	25 mg	In 100s, 1,000s, UD 100s, and blister pack 25s, 100s, and 600s.
Rx	**Amitriptyline HCl** (Various, eg, Geneva, Mutual, Sidmak)	50 mg	In 100s, 1,000s, UD 100s, and blister pack 25s, 100s, and 600s.
Rx	**Amitriptyline HCl** (Various, eg, Geneva, Mutual, Sidmak, UDL, Zenith Goldline)	75 mg	In 100s, 500s, 1,000s, UD 100s, and blister pack 100s.
Rx	**Amitriptyline HCl** (Various, eg, Geneva, Mutual, Sidmak, UDL, URL, Zenith Goldline)	100 mg	In 100s, 500s, 1,000s, UD 100s, and blister pack 100s.
Rx	**Amitriptyline HCl** (Various, eg, Geneva, Mutual, Sidmak, UDL, Zenith Goldline)	150 mg	In 100s, 1,000s, and UD 100s.

AMITRIPTYLINE HYDROCHLORIDE — ORAL

For complete and comparative prescribing information, refer to the Tricyclic Compounds group monograph.

WARNING

Suicidality in children and adolescents – Antidepressants increased the risk of suicidal thinking and behavior (suicidality) in short-term studies in children and adolescents with major depressive disorder (MDD) and other psychiatric disorders. Anyone considering the use of amitriptyline or any other antidepressant in a child or adolescent must balance this risk with the clinical need. Patients who are started on therapy should be observed closely for clinical worsening, suicidality, or unusual changes in behavior. Families and caregivers should be advised of the need for close observation and communication with the prescriber. Amitriptyline is not approved for use in pediatric patients.

Pooled analyses of short-term (4 to 16 weeks) placebo-controlled trials of 9 antidepressant drugs (SSRIs and others) in children and adolescents with MDD, obsessive-compulsive disorder (OCD), or other psychiatric disorders (a total of 24 trials involving over 4,400 patients) have revealed a greater risk of adverse reactions representing suicidal thinking or behavior (suicidality) during the first few months of treatment in those receiving antidepressants. The average risk of such reactions in patients receiving antidepressants was 4%, twice the placebo risk of 2%. No suicides occurred in these trials.

Indications

➤*Depression:* For the relief of symptoms of depression. Endogenous depression is more likely to be alleviated than are other depressive states.

Administration and Dosage

➤*Approved by the FDA:* May 20, 1983.

➤*Outpatients:* 75 mg/day in divided doses. May gradually increase to 150 mg/day. Make increases preferably in late afternoon or at bedtime. A sedative effect may be apparent before the antidepressant effect is noted. An adequate therapeutic effect may take as long as 30 days to develop.

Alternatively, initiate therapy with 50 to 100 mg at bedtime. Increase by 25 to 50 mg as necessary, to a total of 150 mg/day.

➤*Hospitalized patients:* Hospitalized patients may require 100 mg/day initially. Gradually increase to 200 to 300 mg/day, if necessary.

➤*Adolescent and elderly patients:* 10 mg 3 times/day with 20 mg at bedtime may be satisfactory in adolescent and elderly patients who cannot tolerate higher dosages.

➤*Maintenance:* 40 to 100 mg/day. Total daily dose may be given in a single dose, preferably at bedtime. When patient has satisfactorily improved, reduce dosage to the lowest effective amount. Continue at least 3 months to lessen the possibility of relapse.

➤*IM:* Do not administer IV. Initially, 20 to 30 mg IM 4 times/day. The effects may be more rapid with IM than with oral administration. When used for initial therapy in patients unable or unwilling to take tablets, replace the injection with the tablets as soon as possible.

➤*Children:* Not recommended for children younger than 12 years of age.

➤*Storage / Stability:* Avoid storage at temperatures above 30°C (86°F). Protect from light and store in a well-closed, light-resistant container.

AMOXAPINE

Rx	**Amoxapine** (Various, eg, Geneva, URL, Watson)	**Tablets:** 25 mg	In 30s, 100s, 1,000s, and blister pack 100s.
Rx	**Amoxapine** (Various, eg, Geneva, URL, Watson)	**Tablets:** 50 mg	In 30s, 100s, 500s, 1,000s, and blister pack 100s.
Rx	**Amoxapine** (Various, eg, Geneva, URL, Watson)	**Tablets:** 100 mg	In 30s, 100s, and 1,000s.
Rx	**Amoxapine** (Various, eg, Geneva, URL, Watson)	**Tablets:** 150 mg	In 30s, 100s, and 1,000s.

AMOXAPINE — ORAL

For complete and comparative prescribing information, refer to the Tricyclic Compounds group monograph.

WARNING

Suicidality in children and adolescents – Antidepressants increased the risk of suicidal thinking and behavior (suicidality) in short-term studies in children and adolescents with major depressive disorder (MDD) and other psychiatric disorders. Anyone considering the use of amoxapine or any other antidepressant in a child or adolescent must balance this risk with the clinical need. Patients who are started on therapy should be observed closely for clinical worsening, suicidality, or unusual changes in behavior. Families and caregivers should be advised of the need for close observation and communication with the prescriber. Amoxapine is not approved for use in pediatric patients.

Pooled analyses of short-term (4 to 16 weeks) placebo-controlled trials of 9 antidepressant drugs (SSRIs and others) in children and adolescents with MDD, obsessive-compulsive disorder (OCD), or other psychiatric disorders (a total of 24 trials involving over 4,400 patients) have revealed a greater risk of adverse reactions representing suicidal thinking or behavior (suicidality) during the first few months of treatment in those receiving antidepressants. The average risk of such reactions in patients receiving antidepressants was 4%, twice the placebo risk of 2%. No suicides occurred in these trials.

Indications

➤*Depression:* For the relief of symptoms of depression in patients with neurotic or reactive depressive disorders as well as endogenous and psychotic depressions. It is indicated for depression accompanied by anxiety or agitation.

Administration and Dosage

Usual effective dosage is 200 to 300 mg/day. Three weeks is an adequate trial period providing dosage has reached 300 mg/day (or a lower level of tolerance) for at least 2 weeks. If no response is seen at 300 mg, increase dosage, depending upon tolerance, to 400 mg/day. Hospitalized patients refractory to antidepressant therapy and who have no history of convulsive seizures may have dosage cautiously increased up to 600 mg/day in divided doses.

➤*Adults:* Initially, 50 mg 2 or 3 times daily. Depending upon tolerance, increase dosage to 100 mg 2 or 3 times daily by the end of the first week. Initial dosage of 300 mg/day may cause sedation during the first few days of therapy. Increase above 300 mg/day only if 300 mg/day has been ineffective for at least 2 weeks. Once an effective dosage is established, the drug may be given in a single bedtime dose (not to exceed 300 mg). If the total daily dosage exceeds 300 mg, give in divided doses.

➤*Elderly patients:* Lower dosages are recommended. Initially, 25 mg 2 or 3 times/day. If tolerated, dosage may be increased by the end of the first week to 50 mg 2 or 3 times/day. Although 100 to 150 mg/day may be adequate for many elderly patients, some may require higher dosage; carefully increase up to 300 mg/day. Once an effective dosage is established, give amoxapine in a single bedtime dose, not to exceed 300 mg.

➤*Maintenance:* Maintenance dosage is the lowest dose that will maintain remission. If symptoms reappear, increase dosage to the earlier level until they are controlled. For maintenance therapy at doses of 300 mg or less, a single bedtime dose is recommended.

➤*Storage/Stability:* Store at controlled room temperature, 15° to 30°C (59° to 86°F). Dispense in a tight container as defined in the USP.

CLOMIPRAMINE HYDROCHLORIDE

Rx	**Clomipramine Hydrochloride** (Various, eg, Teva, Watson)	**Capsules:** 25 mg	(Watson 594/25 mg). In 100s and 1,000s.
Rx	**Anafranil** (Novartis)		Parabens. (Anafranil 25 mg). Ivory and melon yellow. In 100s and UD 100s.
Rx	**Clomipramine HCl** (Various, eg, Teva, Watson)	**Capsules:** 50 mg	(Watson 595/50 mg). In 100s and 1,000s.
Rx	**Anafranil** (Novartis)		Parabens. (Anafranil 50 mg). Ivory and aqua blue. In 100s and UD 100s.
Rx	**Clomipramine HCl** (Various, eg, Teva, Watson)	**Capsules:** 75 mg	(Watson 596/75 mg). In 100s and 1,000s.
Rx	**Anafranil** (Novartis)		Parabens. (Anafranil 75 mg). Ivory and yellow. In 100s and UD 100s.

CLOMIPRAMINE HYDROCHLORIDE — ORAL

WARNING

Suicidality in children and adolescents – Antidepressants increased the risk of suicidal thinking and behavior (suicidality) in short-term studies in children and adolescents with major depressive disorder (MDD) and other psychiatric disorders. Anyone considering the use of clomipramine or any other antidepressant in a child or adolescent must balance the risk with the clinical need. Closely observe patients who are started on therapy for clinical worsening, suicidality, or unusual changes in behavior. Advise families and caregivers of the need for close observation and communication with the prescriber. Clomipramine is not approved for use in pediatric patients except for patients with obsessive compulsive disorder (OCD).

Pooled analysis of short-term (4 to 16 weeks) placebo-controlled trials of 9 antidepressant drugs (selective serotonin reuptake inhibitors [SSRIs] and others) in children and adolescence with MDD, OCD, or other psychiatric disorders (a total of 24 trials involving over 4,400 patients) have revealed a greater risk of adverse reactions representing suicidal thinking or behavior (suicidality) during the first few months of treatment in those receiving antidepressants. The average risk of such events in patients receiving antidepressants was 4%, twice the placebo risk of 2%. No suicides occurred in these trials.

Indications

➤*OCD:* Clomipramine is indicated for the treatment of obsessions and compulsions in patients with OCD. The obsessions or compulsions must cause marked distress, be time consuming, or significantly interfere with social or occupational functioning in order to meet the *Diagnostic and Statistical Manual of Mental Disorders, Third Edition, Revised* (*DSM-III-R*) (circa 1989) diagnosis of OCD.

➤*Unlabeled uses:* Panic disorder, premenstrual symptoms.

Administration and Dosage

➤*Approved by the FDA:* December 29, 1989

➤*Adults:* Treatment with clomipramine should be initiated at a dosage of 25 mg/day and gradually increased, as tolerated, to approximately 100 mg during the first 2 weeks. During initial titration, clomipramine should be given in divided doses with meals to reduce GI side effects. Thereafter, the dosage may be increased gradually over the next several weeks, up to a maximum of 250 mg/day. After titration, the total daily dose may be given once daily at bedtime to minimize daytime sedation.

➤*Children and adolescents:* As with adults, the starting dosage is 25 mg daily and should be gradually increased (also given in divided doses with meals to reduce GI side effects) during the first 2 weeks, as tolerated, up to a daily maximum of 3 mg/kg or 100 mg, whichever is smaller. Thereafter, the dosage may be increased gradually over the next several weeks up to a daily maximum of 3 mg/kg or 200 mg, whichever is smaller. As with adults, after titration, the total daily dose may be given once daily at bedtime to minimize daytime sedation.

➤*Maintenance (adults, children, and adolescents):* While there are no systematic studies that answer the question of how long to continue clomipramine, OCD is a chronic condition and it is reasonable to consider continuation for a responding patient. Although the efficacy of clomipramine after 10 weeks has not been documented in controlled trials, patients have been continued in therapy under double-blind conditions for up to 1 year without loss of benefit. However, dosage adjustments should be made to maintain the patient on the lowest effective dosage, and patients should be periodically reassessed to determine the need for treatment. During maintenance, the total daily dose may be given once daily at bedtime.

➤*Dose titration:* The treatment regimens described are based on those used in controlled clinical trials of clomipramine in 520 adults and 91 children and adolescents with OCD. During initial titration, clomipramine should be given in divided doses with meals to reduce GI side effects. The goal of this initial titration phase is to minimize side effects by permitting tolerance to side effects to develop, or allowing the patient time to adapt if tolerance does not develop.

Because both clomipramine and its active metabolite, desmethylclomipramine, have long elimination half-lives, take into consideration the fact that steady-state plasma levels may not be achieved until 2 to 3 weeks after dosage change. Therefore, after initial titration, it may be appropriate to wait 2 to 3 weeks between further dosage adjustments.

➤*Storage/Stability:* Store at 20° to 25°C (68° to 77°F). Dispense in well-closed containers with a child-resistant closure. Protect from moisture.

DESIPRAMINE HYDROCHLORIDE

Rx	**Desipramine HCl** (Various, eg, Eon, Geneva)	**Tablets**: 10 mg	In 100s and 1,000s.
Rx	**Norpramin** (Hoechst Marion Roussel)		(68-7). Blue. Coated. In 100s.[1]
Rx	**Desipramine HCl** (Various, eg, EON, Geneva, Sidmak, URL, Zenith Goldline)	**Tablets**: 25 mg	In 100s, 500s, 1,000s, UD 100s, and blister pack 100s and 600s.
Rx	**Norpramin** (Hoechst Marion Roussel)		(NORPRAMIN 25). Yellow. Coated. In 100s and UD 100s.[a]
Rx	**Desipramine HCl** (Various, eg, Eon, Geneva, Sidmak, UDL, URL, Zenith Goldline)	**Tablets**: 50 mg	In 100s, 500s, 1,000s, UD 100s, and blister pack 100s and 600s.
Rx	**Norpramin** (Hoechst Marion Roussel)		(NORPRAMIN 50). Green. Coated. In 100s and UD 100s.[a]
Rx	**Desipramine HCl** (Various, eg, Eon, Geneva, Sidmak, UDL, URL)	**Tablets**: 75 mg	In 100s, 500s, 1,000s, UD 100s, and blister pack 100s and 600s.
Rx	**Norpramin** (Hoechst Marion Roussel)		(NORPRAMIN 75) Orange. Coated. In 100s.[a]
Rx	**Desipramine HCl** (Various, eg, EON, Geneva, Sidmak)	**Tablets**: 100 mg	In 100s, 500s, and 1,000s.
Rx	**Norpramin** (Hoechst Marion Roussel)		(NORPRAMIN 100). Peach. Coated. In 100s.[a]
Rx	**Desipramine HCl** (Various, eg, EON, Geneva, Sidmak)	**Tablets**: 150 mg	In 50s, 100s, and 1,000s.
Rx	**Norpramin** (Hoechst Marion Roussel)		(NORPRAMIN 150). White. Coated. In 50s.[a]

[a] With mannitol and sucrose.

DESIPRAMINE HYDROCHLORIDE — ORAL

For complete and comparative prescribing information, refer to the Tricyclic Compounds group monograph.

WARNING

Suicidality in children and adolescents – Antidepressants increased the risk of suicidal thinking and behavior (suicidality) in short-term studies in children and adolescents with major depressive disorder (MDD) and other psychiatric disorders. Anyone considering the use of desipramine or any other antidepressant in a child or adolescent must balance this risk with the clinical need. Patients who are started on therapy should be observed closely for clinical worsening, suicidality, or unusual changes in behavior. Families and caregivers should be advised of the need for close observation and communication with the prescriber. Desipramine is not approved for use in pediatric patients.

Pooled analyses of short-term (4 to 16 weeks) placebo-controlled trials of 9 antidepressant drugs (SSRIs and others) in children and adolescents with MDD, obsessive-compulsive disorder (OCD), or other psychiatric disorders (a total of 24 trials involving over 4,400 patients) have revealed a greater risk of adverse reactions representing suicidal thinking or behavior (suicidality) during the first few months of treatment in those receiving antidepressants. The average risk of such reactions in patients receiving antidepressants was 4%, twice the placebo risk of 2%. No suicides occurred in these trials.

Indications

Desipramine HCl is indicated for relief of symptoms in various depressive syndromes, especially endogenous depression.

Administration and Dosage

➤*Approved by the FDA:* February 11, 1982.

This medication is not recommended for use in children.

Lower dosages are recommended for elderly patients and adolescents. Lower dosages are also recommended for outpatients compared to hospitalized patients, who are closely supervised. Dosage should be initiated at a low level and increased according to clinical response and any evidence of intolerance. Following remission, maintenance medication may be required for a period of time and should be at the lowest dose that will maintain remission.

➤*Usual adult dose:* The usual adult dose is 100 to 200 mg/day. In more severely ill patients, dosage may be further increased gradually to 300 mg/day if necessary. Dosages above 300 mg/day are not recommended.

Dosage should be initiated at a lower level and increased according to tolerance and clinical response.

Treatment of patients requiring as much as 300 mg, should generally be initiated in hospitals, where regular visits by the physician, skilled nursing care, and frequent electrocardiograms (ECGs) are available.

The best available evidence of impending toxicity from very high doses of desipramine is prolongation of the QRS or QT intervals on the ECG. Prolongation of the PR interval is also significant, but less closely correlated with plasma levels. Clinical symptoms of intolerance, especially drowsiness, dizziness, and postural hypotension, should also alert the physician to the need for reduction in dosage. Plasma desipramine measurement would constitute the optimal guide to dosage monitoring.

Initial therapy may be administered in divided doses or a single daily dose.

Maintenance therapy may be given on a once-daily schedule for patient convenience and compliance.

➤*Adolescent and geriatric dose:* The usual adolescent and geriatric dose is 25 to 100 mg daily.

Dosage should be initiated at a lower level and increased according to tolerance and clinical response to a usual maximum of 100 mg daily. In more severely ill patients, dosage may be further increased to 150 mg/day. Doses above 150 mg/day are not recommended in these age groups.

Initial therapy may be administered in divided doses or a single daily dose.

Maintenance therapy may be given on a once-daily schedule for patient convenience and compliance.

➤*Storage/Stability:* Store at controlled room temperature 15° to 30°C (59° to 86°F). Protect from moisture.

DOXEPIN HYDROCHLORIDE

Rx	**Doxepin HCl** (Various, eg, Par, UDL, URL, Watson)	**Capsules** : 10 mg	In 100s, 500s, 1,000s, and blister pack 100s.
Rx	**Sinequan** (Roerig)		(Sinequan Roerig 534). In 100s and 1,000s.
Rx	**Doxepin HCl** (Various, eg, Par, UDL, Watson)	**Capsules**: 25 mg	In 100s, 500s, 1,000s, and blister pack 25s and 100s.
Rx	**Sinequan** (Roerig)		(Sinequan Roerig 535). In 100s, 1,000s, and 5000s.
Rx	**Doxepin HCl** (Various, eg, Par, UDL, Watson)	**Capsules**: 50 mg	In 100s, 500s, 1,000s, and blister pack 25s and 100s.
Rx	**Sinequan** (Roerig)		(Sinequan Roerig 536). In 100s, 1,000s, and 5000s.
Rx	**Doxepin HCl** (Various, eg, Par, UDL)	**Capsules**: 75 mg	In 100s, 500s, 1,000s, and blister pack 100s.
Rx	**Sinequan** (Roerig)		(Sinequan Roerig 539). In 100s and 1,000s.
Rx	**Doxepin HCl** (Various, eg, Par, UDL, URL)	**Capsules**: 100 mg	In 100s, 500s, 1,000s, and blister pack 100s.
Rx	**Sinequan** (Roerig)		(Sinequan Roerig 538). In 100s and 1,000s.
Rx	**Doxepin HCl** (Various, eg, Par)	**Capsules**: 150 mg	In 50s, 100s, 500s, and 1,000s.
Rx	**Sinequan** (Roerig)		(Sinequan Roerig 537). In 50s and 500s.
Rx	**Doxepin HCl** (Various, eg, Copley, Morton Grove)	**Oral concentrate**: 10 mg/mL	In 120 mL.
Rx	**Sinequan** (Roerig)		Parabens, peppermint oil, sorbitol. In 118 ml with calibrated dropper.

DOXEPIN HYDROCHLORIDE — ORAL

For complete and comparative prescribing information, refer to the Tricyclic Compounds group monograph.

WARNING

Suicidality in children and adolescents – Antidepressants increased the risk of suicidal thinking and behavior (suicidality) in short-term studies in children and adolescents with major depressive disorder (MDD) and other psychiatric disorders. Anyone considering the use of doxepin or any other antidepressant in a child or adolescent must balance this risk with the clinical need. Patients who are started on therapy should be observed closely for clinical worsening, suicidality, or unusual changes in behavior. Families and caregivers should be advised of the need for close observation and communication with the prescriber. Doxepin is not approved for use in pediatric patients.

Pooled analyses of short-term (4 to 16 weeks) placebo-controlled trials of 9 antidepressant drugs (SSRIs and others) in children and adolescents with MDD, obsessive-compulsive disorder (OCD), or other psychiatric disorders (a total of 24 trials involving over 4,400 patients) have revealed a greater risk of adverse reactions representing suicidal thinking or behavior (suicidality) during the first few months of treatment in those receiving antidepressants. The average risk of such reactions in patients receiving antidepressants was 4%, twice the placebo risk of 2%. No suicides occurred in these trials.

Indications

Doxepin is recommended for the treatment of:

1.) Psychoneurotic patients with depression or anxiety.
2.) Depression or anxiety associated with alcoholism (not to be taken concomitantly with alcohol).
3.) Depression or anxiety associated with organic disease (consider the possibility of drug interaction if the patient is receiving other drugs concomitantly).
4.) Psychotic depressive disorders with associated anxiety including involutional depression and manic-depressive disorders.

The target symptoms of psychoneurosis that respond particularly well to doxepin include anxiety, tension, depression, somatic symptoms and concerns, sleep disturbances, guilt, lack of energy, fear, apprehension, and worry.

Administration and Dosage

➤*Approved by the FDA:* March 11, 1974.

➤*Mild to moderate illness:* Initially, 75 mg/day. Individualize dosage. Usual optimum dosage is 75 to 150 mg/day. Alternatively, the total daily dosage, up to 150 mg, may be given at bedtime. Maximum dose is 150 mg/day.

➤*Mild symptomatology or emotional symptoms accompanying organic disease:* 25 to 50 mg/day is often effective.

➤*More severe anxiety or depression:* Higher doses (eg, 50 mg 3 times/day) may be required; if necessary, gradually increase to 300 mg/day. Additional effectiveness is rarely obtained by exceeding 300 mg/day.

Although optimal antidepressant response may not be evident for 2 to 3 weeks, antianxiety activity is rapidly apparent.

➤*Oral concentrate:* Dilute oral concentrate with approximately 120 mL of water, milk, or fruit juice just prior to administration. The oral concentrate is not physically compatible with a number of carbonated beverages. Do not prepare or store bulk dilutions.

➤*Storage/Stability:* Preparation and storage of doxepin oral concentrate bulk dilutions is not recommended.

IMIPRAMINE HYDROCHLORIDE

Rx	**Imipramine HCl** (Various, eg, Geneva, Mutual, Par, URL)	**Tablets:** 10 mg	In 100s, 250s, 500s, and 1,000s.
Rx	**Tofranil** (Novartis)		(Geigy 32). Coral. Sugar-coated. Triangular. In 100s.
Rx	**Imipramine HCl** (Various, eg, Geneva, Mutual, Par, URL)	**Tablets:** 25 mg	In 100s, 250s, 500s, and 1,000s.
Rx	**Tofranil** (Novartis)		(Geigy 140). Coral, biconvex. Sugar-coated. In 100s.
Rx	**Imipramine HCl** (Various, eg, Geneva, Mutual, Par, URL)	**Tablets:** 50 mg	In 50s, 100s, 250s, 500s, 1,000s, and UD 20s.
Rx	**Tofranil** (Novartis)		(Geigy 136). Coral, biconvex. Sugar-coated. In 100s.

IMIPRAMINE HYDROCHLORIDE — ORAL

For complete and comparative prescribing information, refer to the Tricyclic Compounds group monograph.

WARNING

Suicidality in children and adolescents – Antidepressants increased the risk of suicidal thinking and behavior (suicidality) in short-term studies in children and adolescents with major depressive disorder (MDD) and other psychiatric disorders. Anyone considering the use of imipramine or any other antidepressant in a child or adolescent must balance this risk with the clinical need. Patients who are started on therapy should be observed closely for clinical worsening, suicidality, or unusual changes in behavior. Families and caregivers should be advised of the need for close observation and communication with the prescriber. Imipramine is not approved for use in pediatric patients except for patients with nocturnal enuresis.

Pooled analyses of short-term (4 to 16 weeks) placebo-controlled trials of 9 antidepressant drugs (SSRIs and others) in children and adolescents with MDD, obsessive-compulsive disorder (OCD), or other psychiatric disorders (a total of 24 trials involving over 4,400 patients) have revealed a greater risk of adverse reactions representing suicidal thinking or behavior (suicidality) during the first few months of treatment in those receiving antidepressants. The average risk of such reactions in patients receiving antidepressants was 4%, twice the placebo risk of 2%. No suicides occurred in these trials.

Indications

➤*Depression:* For the relief of symptoms of depression. Endogenous depression is more likely to be alleviated than other depressive states. One to 3 weeks of treatment may be needed before optimal therapeutic effects are evident.

➤*Childhood enuresis:* May be useful as temporary adjunctive therapy in reducing enuresis in children aged 6 years and older, after possible organic causes have been excluded by appropriate tests. In patients having daytime symptoms of frequency and urgency, examination should include voiding cystourethrography and cystoscopy, as necessary. The effectiveness of treatment may decrease with continued drug administration.

Administration and Dosage

➤*Depression:* Lower dosages are recommended for elderly patients and adolescents. Lower dosages are also recommended for outpatients as compared to hospitalized patients who will be under close supervision. Dosage should be initiated at a low level and increased gradually, noting carefully the clinical response and any evidence of intolerance. Following remission, maintenance medication may be required for a longer period of time, at the lowest dose that will maintain remission.

Usual adult dose –

Hospitalized patients: Initially, 100 mg/day in divided doses gradually increased to 200 mg/day as required. If no response after 2 weeks, increase to 250 mg to 300 mg/day.

Outpatients: Initially, 75 mg/day increased to 150 mg/day. Dosages over 200 mg/day are not recommended. Maintenance, 50 mg to 150 mg/day.

Adolescent and geriatric patients: Initially, 30 mg to 40 mg/day; it is generally not necessary to exceed 100 mg/day.

➤*Childhood enuresis:* Initially, an oral dose of 25 mg/day should be tried in children aged 6 and older. Medication should be given 1 hour before bedtime. If a satisfactory response does not occur within 1 week, increase the dose to 50 mg nightly in children under 12 years; children over 12 may receive up to 75 mg nightly. A daily dose greater than 75 mg does not enhance efficacy and tends to increase side effects. Evidence suggests that in early night bedwetters, the drug is more effective given earlier and in divided amounts (ie, 25 mg in midafternoon, repeated at bedtime). Consideration should be given to instituting a drug-free period following an adequate therapeutic trial with a favorable response. Dosage should be tapered off gradually rather than abruptly discontinued; this may reduce the tendency to relapse. Children who relapse when the drug is discontinued do not always respond to a subsequent course of treatment.

A dose of 2.5 mg/kg/day should not be exceeded. ECG changes of unknown significance have been reported in pediatric patients with doses twice this amount.

➤*Storage/Stability:* Store between 15° to 30°C (59° to 86°F). Dispense in tight container (USP).

IMIPRAMINE PAMOATE

Rx	**Tofranil-PM** (Novartis)	**Capsules:**[a] 75 mg	Parabens. (Geigy 20). Coral. In 30s and 100s.
		100 mg	Parabens. (Geigy 40). Dark yellow/coral. In 30s and 100s.
		125 mg	Parabens. (Geigy 45). Ivory/coral. In 30s and 100s.
		150 mg	Parabens. (Geigy 22). Coral. In 30s and 100s.

[a] Strengths are expressed as imipramine HCl equivalent.

IMIPRAMINE PAMOATE — ORAL

For complete and comparative prescribing information, refer to the Tricyclic Compounds group monograph.

WARNING

Suicidality in children and adolescents – Antidepressants increased the risk of suicidal thinking and behavior (suicidality) in short-term studies in children and adolescents with major depressive disorder (MDD) and other psychiatric disorders. Anyone considering the use of imipramine pamoate or any other antidepressant in a child or adolescent must balance this risk with the clinical need. Patients who are started on therapy should be observed closely for clinical worsening, suicidality, or unusual changes in behavior. Families and caregivers should be advised of the need for close observation and communication with the prescriber. Imipramine pamoate is not approved for use in pediatric patients.

Pooled analyses of short-term (4 to 16 weeks) placebo-controlled trials of 9 antidepressant drugs (SSRIs and others) in children and adolescents with MDD, obsessive-compulsive disorder (OCD), or other psychiatric disorders (a total of 24 trials involving over 4,400 patients) have revealed a greater risk of adverse reactions representing suicidal thinking or behavior (suicidality) during the first few months of treatment in those receiving antidepressants. The average risk of such reactions in patients receiving antidepressants was 4%, twice the placebo risk of 2%. No suicides occurred in these trials.

Indications

➤*Depression:* For the relief of symptoms of depression. Endogenous depression is more likely to be alleviated than other depressive states. One to 3 weeks of treatment may be needed before optimal therapeutic effects are evident.

Administration and Dosage

The following recommended dosages for imipramine pamoate should be modified as necessary by the clinical response and any evidence of intolerance.

As with all tricyclics, the antidepressant effect of imipramine may not be evident for 1 to 3 weeks in some patients.

➤*Initial adult dosage:*

Outpatients – Therapy should be initiated at 75 mg/day. Dosage may be increased to 150 mg/day which is the dose level at which optimum response is usually obtained. If necessary, dosage may be increased to 200 mg/day.

Dosage higher than 75 mg/day may also be administered on a once-a-day basis after the optimum dosage and tolerance have been determined. The daily dosage may be given at bedtime. In some patients it may be necessary to employ a divided-dose schedule.

Hospitalized patients – Therapy should be initiated at 100 to 150 mg/day and may be increased to 200 mg/day. If there is no response after 2 weeks, dosage should be increased to 250 to 300 mg/day.

Dosage higher than 150 mg/day may also be administered on a once-a-day basis after the optimum dosage and tolerance have been determined. The daily dosage may be given at bedtime. In some patients it may be necessary to employ a divided-dose schedule.

➤*Adult maintenance dosage:* Following remission, maintenance medication may be required for a longer period of time at the lowest dose that will maintain remission after which the dosage should gradually be decreased.

The usual maintenance dosage is 75 to 150 mg/day. The total daily dosage can be administered on a once-a-day basis, preferably at bedtime. In some patients it may be necessary to employ a divided-dose schedule.

In cases of relapse due to premature withdrawal of the drug, the effective dosage of imipramine should be reinstituted.

➤*Adolescent and geriatric patients:* Therapy in these age groups should be initiated with imipramine hydrochloride tablets at a total daily dosage of 25 to 50 mg, since imipramine pamoate capsules are not available in these strengths. Dosage may be increased according to response and tolerance, but it is generally unnecessary to exceed 100 mg/day in these patients. Imipramine pamoate capsules may be used when total daily dosage is established at 75 mg or higher.

The total daily dosage can be administered on a once-a-day basis, preferably at bedtime. In some patients it may be necessary to employ a divided-dose schedule.

Adolescent and geriatric patients can usually be maintained at lower dosage. Following remission, maintenance medication may be required for a longer period of time at the lowest dose that will maintain remission after which the dosage should gradually be decreased.

In cases of relapse due to premature withdrawal of the drug, the effective dosage of imipramine should be reinstituted.

➤*Storage/Stability:* Do not store above 30°C (86°F). Dispense in tight container (USP).

NORTRIPTYLINE HYDROCHLORIDE

Rx	**Nortriptyline HCl** (Various, eg, Geneva, Teva, UDL)	**Capsules:** 10 mg	In 100s, 500s, 1,000s, blister pack 25s, 100s, and 600s, and UD 100s.
Rx	**Pamelor** (Novartis)		(Sandoz PAMELOR 10 mg). In 100s and UD 100s.[a]
Rx	**Nortriptyline HCl** (Various, eg, Geneva, Teva, UDL)	**Capsules:** 25 mg	In 100s, 500s, 1,000s, blister pack 25s, 100s, and 600s, and UD 100s.
Rx	**Aventyl HCl Pulvules** (Eli Lilly)		(Lilly H19). White/yellow. In 100s and 500s.
Rx	**Pamelor** (Novartis)		(Sandoz PAMELOR 25 mg). In 100s, 500s, and UD 100s.[a]
Rx	**Nortriptyline HCl** (Various, eg, Geneva, Teva, UDL)	**Capsules:** 50 mg	In 100s, 500s, 1,000s, blister pack 25s, 100s, and 600s, and UD 100s.
Rx	**Pamelor** (Novartis)		(Sandoz PAMELOR 50 mg). In 100s and UD 100s.[a]
Rx	**Nortriptyline HCl** (Various, eg, Geneva, Teva)	**Capsules:** 75 mg	In 100s, 500s, 1,000s, and blister pack 100s and 600s.
Rx	**Pamelor** (Novartis)		(Sandoz PAMELOR 75 mg). In 100s.[a]
Rx	**Nortriptyline HCl** (Ranbaxy)	**Solution:** 10 mg base/5 ml	In 480 mL.[b]
Rx	**Pamelor** (Novartis)		In 480 mL.[c]

[a] With benzyl alcohol, EDTA, parabens.
[b] With 4% alcohol, sorbitol.
[c] With 3.4% alcohol.

NORTRIPYLINE HYDROCHLORIDE — ORAL

For complete and comparative prescribing information, refer to the Tricyclic Compounds group monograph.

WARNING

Suicidality in children and adolescents – Antidepressants increased the risk of suicidal thinking and behavior (suicidality) in short-term studies in children and adolescents with major depressive disorder (MDD) and other psychiatric disorders. Anyone considering the use of nortriptyline or any other antidepressant in a child or adolescent must balance this risk with the clinical need. Patients who are started on therapy should be observed closely for clinical worsening, suicidality, or unusual changes in behavior. Families and caregivers should be advised of the need for close observation and communication with the prescriber. Nortriptyline is not approved for use in pediatric patients.

Pooled analyses of short-term (4 to 16 weeks) placebo-controlled trials of 9 antidepressant drugs (SSRIs and others) in children and adolescents with MDD, obsessive-compulsive disorder (OCD), or other psychiatric disorders (a total of 24 trials involving over 4,400 patients) have revealed a greater risk of adverse reactions representing suicidal thinking or behavior (suicidality) during the first few months of treatment in those receiving antidepressants. The average risk of such reactions in patients receiving antidepressants was 4%, twice the placebo risk of 2%. No suicides occurred in these trials.

Indications

➤*Depression:* Nortriptyline HCl is indicated for the relief of symptoms of depression. Endogenous depressions are more likely to be alleviated than are other depressive states.

Administration and Dosage

Not recommended for use in children.

➤*Adults:* 25 mg 3 or 4 times daily; begin at a low level and increase as required. The total daily dose can be given at bedtime. When doses greater than 100 mg/day are given, plasma levels of nortriptyline should be monitored and maintained in the optimum range of 50 to 150 ng/mL. Doses greater than 150 mg/day are not recommended. Higher concentrations may be associated with more adverse experiences. Plasma concentrations are difficult to measure, and physicians should consult with the laboratory professional staff.

➤*Elderly and adolescent patients:* 30 to 50 mg daily in divided doses or total daily dose may be given once/day.

➤*Storage/Stability:* Store nortriptyline HCl capsules, USP below 30°C (86°F) in a tight container.

Store nortriptyline HCl solution, USP at 25°C (77°F); excursions permitted to 15° to 30°C (59° to 86°F) in a tight, light-resistant container. [See USP controlled temperature]

PROTRIPTYLINE HYDROCHLORIDE

Rx	**Protriptyline HCl** (Various, eg, Sidmak)	**Tablets:** 5 mg	In 100s and 1,000s.
Rx	**Vivactil** (Merck)		Lactose. (MSD 26). Orange. Oval. Film coated. In 100s.
Rx	**Protriptyline HCl** (Various, eg, Sidmak)	**Tablets:** 10 mg	In 100s and 1,000s.
Rx	**Vivactil** (Merck)		Lactose. (MSD 47). Yellow. Oval. Film coated. In 100s and UD 100s.

PROTRIPTYLINE HYDROCHLORIDE — ORAL

For complete and comparative prescribing information, refer to the Tricyclic Compounds group monograph.

WARNING

Suicidality in children and adolescents – Antidepressants increased the risk of suicidal thinking and behavior (suicidality) in short-term studies in children and adolescents with major depressive disorder (MDD) and other psychiatric disorders. Anyone considering the use of protriptyline or any other antidepressant in a child or adolescent must balance this risk with the clinical need. Closely observe patients who are started on therapy for clinical worsening, suicidality, or unusual changes in behavior. Advise families and caregivers of the need for close observation and communication with the prescriber. Protriptyline is not approved for use in pediatric patients.

Pooled analyses of short-term (4 to 16 weeks) placebo-controlled trials of 9 antidepressant drugs (selective serotonin reuptake inhibitors [SSRIs] and others) in children and adolescents with MDD, obsessive-compulsive disorder (OCD), or other psychiatric disorders (a total of 24 trials involving over 4,400 patients) have revealed a greater risk of adverse reactions representing suicidal thinking or behavior (suicidality) during the first few months of treatment in those receiving antidepressants. The average risk of such reactions in patients receiving antidepressants was 4%, twice the placebo risk of 2%. No suicides occurred in these trials.

Indications

➤*Depression:* Protriptyline is indicated for the treatment of symptoms of mental depression in patients who are under close medical supervision. Its activating properties make it particularly suitable for withdrawn and anergic patients.

Administration and Dosage

Dosage should be initiated at a low level and increased gradually, noting carefully the clinical response and any evidence of intolerance.

➤*Adults:* 15 to 40 mg/day divided into 3 or 4 doses. If necessary, dosage may be increased to 60 mg/day. Dosages above this amount are not recommended. Increases should be made in the morning dose.

➤*Adolescent and elderly patients:* In general, lower dosages are recommended for these patients. 5 mg 3 times/day may be given initially, and increased gradually if necessary. In elderly patients, the cardiovascular system must be monitored closely if the daily dose exceeds 20 mg.

➤*Maintenance:* When satisfactory improvement has been reached, dosage should be reduced to the smallest amount that will maintain relief of symptoms.

➤*Dosage adjustments for adverse reactions:* Minor adverse reactions require reduction in dosage. Major adverse reactions or evidence of hypersensitivity require prompt discontinuation of the drug.

➤*Children:* The safety and efficacy of protriptyline in pediatric patients have not been established.

➤*Storage/Stability:* Store in a tightly closed container. Store at controlled room temperature 20° to 25°C (68° to 77°F).

TRIMIPRAMINE MALEATE

Rx	**Surmontil** (Wyeth)	**Capsules:** 25 mg	Lactose. (Wyeth 4132). Opaque blue/yellow. In 100s.
		50 mg	Lactose. (Wyeth 4133). Opaque blue/orange. In 100s and UD 100s.
		100 mg	Lactose. (Wyeth 4158). Opaque blue/white. In 100s.

TRIMIPRAMINE MALEATE — ORAL

For complete and comparative prescribing information, refer to the Tricyclic Compounds group monograph.

WARNING

Suicidality in children and adolescents – Antidepressants increased the risk of suicidal thinking and behavior (suicidality) in short-term studies in children and adolescents with major depressive disorder (MDD) and other psychiatric disorders. Anyone considering the use of trimipramine or any other antidepressant in a child or adolescent must balance this risk with the clinical need. Patients who are started on therapy should be observed closely for clinical worsening, suicidality, or unusual changes in behavior. Families and caregivers should be advised of the need for close observation and communication with the prescriber. Trimipramine is not approved for use in pediatric patients.

WARNING (cont.)

Pooled analyses of short-term (4 to 16 weeks) placebo-controlled trials of 9 antidepressant drugs (SSRIs and others) in children and adolescents with MDD, obsessive-compulsive disorder (OCD), or other psychiatric disorders (a total of 24 trials involving over 4,400 patients) have revealed a greater risk of adverse reactions representing suicidal thinking or behavior (suicidality) during the first few months of treatment in those receiving antidepressants. The average risk of such reactions in patients receiving antidepressants was 4%, twice the placebo risk of 2%. No suicides occurred in these trials.

Indications

➤*Depression:* Trimipramine maleate is indicated for the relief of symptoms of depression. Endogenous depression is more likely to be alleviated than other depressive states. In studies with neurotic outpatients, the drug

TRIMIPRAMINE MALEATE — ORAL

appeared to be equivalent to amitriptyline in the less-depressed patients but somewhat less effective than amitriptyline in the more severely depressed patients. In hospitalized depressed patients, trimipramine and imipramine were equally effective in relieving depression.

Administration and Dosage

➤*Approved by the FDA:* September 15, 1982.

Not recommended for use in children.

➤*Adult outpatients:* Initially, 75 mg/day in divided doses; increase to 150 mg/day. Do not exceed 200 mg/day. The total dosage requirement may be given at bedtime.

➤*Adult hospitalized patients:* Initially, 100 mg/day in divided doses, increase gradually in a few days to 200 mg/day depending upon individual response and tolerance. If improvement does not occur in 2 to 3 weeks, increase to a maximum dose of 250 to 300 mg/day.

➤*Adolescent and elderly patients:* Initially, 50 mg/day, with gradual increments up to 100 mg/day.

➤*Maintenance:* Maintenance medication may be required at the lowest dose that will maintain remission (range, 50 to 150 mg/day). Administer as a single bedtime dose. To minimize relapse, continue maintenance therapy for approximately 3 months.

➤*Storage/Stability:* Store at 20° to 25°C (68° to 77°F). Keep bottles tightly closed. Dispense in a tight container.

Tetracyclic Compounds

Refer to the Antidepressants introduction.

Indications

➤*Depression:* Treatment of depression.

➤*Unlabeled uses:* **Maprotiline** is also effective for the relief of anxiety associated with depression.

Actions

➤*Pharmacology:* The mechanism of action is unknown. Tetracyclics enhance central noradrenergic and serotonergic activity. They do not inhibit monoamine oxidase. Although **maprotiline** and **mirtazapine** are in the same chemical class, they each affect different neurotransmitters and thus have different side effect profiles. Maprotiline primarily acts by blocking reuptake of norepinephrine at nerve endings. This pharmacologic action is thought to be responsible for its antidepressant and anxiolytic effects. They act as antagonists at central presynaptic α_2-adrenergic inhibitory autoreceptors and heteroreceptors, an action that is postulated to result in an increase in central noradrenergic and serotonergic activity.

Mirtazapine is a potent antagonist of 5-HT_2 and 5-HT_3 receptors. It does not have significant affinity for the 5-HT_{1A} and 5-HT_{1B} receptors. It is a potent antagonist of histamine (H_1) receptors, a property that may explain its prominent sedative effects. It is also a moderate antagonist at muscarinic receptors, a property that may explain the relatively low incidence of anticholinergic side effects. Mirtazapine is a moderate peripheral α_1-adrenergic antagonist, a property that may explain the occasional orthostatic hypotension associated with its use.

➤*Pharmacokinetics:*

Maprotiline – The mean time to peak is 12 hours. Steady-state levels measured prior to the morning dose on a 1-dosage regimen demonstrated an average minimum concentration of 238 ng/ml and 95% confidence limits of 181 to 295 ng/ml. Binding to serum proteins is approximately 88%. Following a 50 mg oral dose of maprotiline in healthy subjects, the peak plasma level occurred between 9 and 16 hours. Range of apparent volume of distribution is 13 to 24 L/kg, and it is more concentrated in the liver, lung, kidney, brain, and heart than in blood. The average elimination half-life in healthy subjects is 43 hours (range, 27 to 58 hours). Maprotiline is metabolized in the liver. After 21 days of IV maprotiline, 57% was found in the urine and 30% in the feces. Maprotiline is excreted via the bile.

Mirtazapine – Mirtazapine is rapidly and completely absorbed following oral administration and has a half–life of approximately 20 to 40 hours. Peak plasma concentrations are reached within approximately 2 hours following an oral dose. The presence of food in the stomach has a minimal effect on the rate and extent of absorption and does not require a dosage adjustment. Steady-state plasma levels of mirtazapine are attained within 5 days. Mirtazapine is approximately 85% bound to plasma protein.

Metabolism/Excretion: Mirtazapine is extensively metabolized after oral administration. Major pathways of biotransformation are demethylation and hydroxylation followed by glucuronide conjugation. In vitro, cytochrome 2D6 and 1A2 are involved in the formation of the 8-hydroxy metabolite of mirtazapine, whereas cytochrome 3A is considered to be responsible for the formation of the N-desmethyl and N-oxide metabolites. Mirtazapine has an absolute bioavailability of approximately 50%. It is eliminated predominantly via urine (75%) with 15% in feces. Several unconjugated metabolites possess pharmacologic activity but are present in the plasma at very low levels. The (-) enantiomer has an elimination half-life that is approximately twice as long as the (+) enantiomer and, therefore, achieves plasma levels that are approximately 3 times as high.

Plasma levels are linearly related to dose over a dose range of 15 to 80 mg. The mean elimination half-life of mirtazapine after oral administration ranges from approximately 20 to 40 hours, with females of all ages exhibiting significantly longer elimination half-lives than males (37 hours vs 26 hours).

Contraindications

Hypersensitivity to maprotiline or mirtazapine; coadministration with monamine oxidase inhibitors (MAOIs; see Warnings).

➤*Maprotiline:* Known or suspected seizure disorders; during acute phase of MI.

Warnings

➤*Agranulocytosis:* In clinical trials, 2 patients treated with **mirtazapine** developed agranulocytosis (absolute neutrophil count [ANC] less than 500/mm^3 with associated signs and symptoms [eg, fever, infection]) and a third patient developed severe neutropenia (ANC less than 500/mm^3 without any associated symptoms). For these 3 patients, onset of severe neutropenia was detected on days 61, 9, and 14 of treatment, respectively. All 3 patients recovered after mirtazapine was stopped. If a patient develops a sore throat, fever, stomatitis, or other signs of infection, along with a low WBC count, discontinue treatment with the tetracyclic and monitor the patient closely.

➤*Anticholinergic properties:* Administer **maprotiline** with caution in patients with increased intraocular pressure, history of urinary retention, or history of narrow-angle glaucoma because of the drug's anticholinergic properties.

➤*CNS effects:* **Maprotiline** may enhance the response to alcohol, barbiturates, and other CNS depressants, requiring appropriate caution during administration.

➤*Monamine oxidase inhibitors (MAOIs):* Do not give tetracyclics with MAOIs. Allow a minimum of 14 days to elapse after discontinuation of MAOIs before starting a tetracyclic.

➤*Seizures:* Seizures are rare. Most of the seizures have occurred in patients with a history of seizures. In premarketing clinical trials, only 1 seizure was reported among the 2796 patients treated with **mirtazapine**. **Maprotiline** is associated with seizures in overdose and with therapeutic doses. The risk of seizures may be increased when tetracyclics are taken concomitantly with phenothiazines, when the dosage of benzodiazepines is rapidly tapered in patients receiving tetracyclics, or when the recommended dosage of the tetracyclic is exceeded. While a cause-and-effect relationship has not been established, the risk of seizures in patients treated with tetracyclics may be reduced by the following:

- Initiating therapy at a low dosage.
- Maintaining the initial dosage for 2 weeks before raising it gradually in small increments as necessary.
- Keeping the dosage at the minimally effective level during maintenance therapy.

➤*Cardiovascular effects:* Use with caution in patients with a history of MI and angina because of the possibility of conduction defects, arrhythmia, MI, strokes, and tachycardia. Use with caution in patients predisposed to hypotension.

➤*Electroshock therapy:* Avoid concurrent administration of **maprotiline** with electroshock therapy because of the lack of experience in this area.

➤*Renal function impairment:* Following a single 15 mg dose of **mirtazapine**, patients with moderate (glomerular filtration rate [GFR] = 11 to 39 ml/min/1.73 m^2) and severe (GFR < 10 ml/min/1.73 m^2) renal impairment had reductions in mean oral clearance of approximately 30% and 50%, respectively, compared with healthy subjects.

➤*Hepatic function impairment:* Following a single 15 mg dose of **mirtazapine**, the oral clearance decreased by approximately 30% in hepatically impaired patients. Use mirtazapine with caution in patients with impaired hepatic function.

➤*Carcinogenesis:* There was an increased incidence of hepatocellular adenoma and carcinoma in male mice at high doses of **mirtazapine** and an increase in thyroid follicular adenoma/cystadenoma and carcinoma in male rats at high doses. Hepatocellular adenoma increased in female rats with mid and high doses of mirtazapine. **Maprotiline** did not show any drug- or dose-related occurrence of carcinogenesis in rats.

➤*Elderly:* Following administration of 20 mg/day **mirtazapine** for 7 days to subjects 25 to 74 years of age, oral clearance was reduced in the elderly subjects compared with the younger subjects. The differences were most striking in males, with a 40% lower clearance in elderly males compared with younger males, while the clearance in elderly females was only 10% lower compared with younger females. Caution is indicated in administering mirtazapine to elderly patients.

➤*Pregnancy:*

Maprotiline – (*Category B*, maprotiline; *Category C*, mirtazapine). There are no adequate and well-controlled studies in pregnant women. Use during pregnancy only if clearly needed.

➤*Lactation:*

Maprotiline – Maprotiline is excreted in breast milk. At steady state, the concentration in milk corresponds closely to the concentrations in whole blood. Exercise caution when maprotiline is administered to a nursing woman.

Mirtazapine – It is not known if mirtazapine is excreted in breast milk. Use caution when mirtazapine is administered to nursing women.

➤*Children:* Safety and efficacy in children (younger than 18 years of age for **maprotiline**) have not been established.

Precautions

➤*Monitoring:* Discontinue **maprotiline** if there is evidence of pathological neutrophil depression. Perform leukocyte and differential counts in patients who develop fever and sore throat during therapy.

➤*Somnolence:* Somnolence was reported in 54% of patients treated with **mirtazapine**. Somnolence resulted in discontinuation of treatment in 10.4% of patients. It is unclear whether or not tolerance develops to the somnolent effects. Because mirtazapine has potentially significant effects on performance, caution patients about engaging in activities requiring alertness until they have been able to assess the drug's effect on their psychomotor performance.

➤*Dizziness:* Dizziness was reported in 7% of patients treated with **mirtazapine**. It is unclear whether or not tolerance to the dizziness develops.

➤*Increased appetite/weight gain:* Appetite increase was reported in 17% of patients treated with **mirtazapine**. In some trials, weight gain of ≥ 7% of body weight was reported in 7.5% of patients. Of patients receiving mirtazapine, 8% discontinued because of weight gain.

➤*Cholesterol/Triglycerides:* Nonfasting cholesterol increases to ≥ 20% above the upper limits of normal were observed in 15% of **mirtazapine** patients. In some cases, nonfasting triglyceride increases to ≥ 500 mg/dl were observed in 6% of patients treated with mirtazapine compared with 3% for placebo and 3% for amitriptyline.

➤*Mania/Hypomania:* Mania/Hypomania occurred in ≈ 0.2% of patients receiving **mirtazapine**. Hypomanic or manic episodes have occurred in some patients taking tricyclic antidepressant drugs, particularly in patients with cyclic disorders. Such occurrences have also been noted rarely with **maprotiline**. Although the incidence of mania/hypomania is rare during treatment with tetracyclics, use carefully in patients with a history of mania/hypomania.

➤*Suicide:* Suicidal ideation is inherent in depression and may persist until significant remission occurs. As with any patient receiving antidepressants, closely supervise high-risk patients during initial drug therapy. Physicians should write prescriptions for **mirtazapine** and **maprotiline** for the smallest quantity consistent with good patient management in order to reduce the risk of overdose.

➤*Elective surgery:* Prior to elective surgery, discontinue **maprotiline** for as long as possible, because little is known about the interaction between maprotiline and general anesthetics.

➤*Orthostatic hypotension:* **Mirtazapine** was associated with significant orthostatic hypotension in clinical trials with healthy volunteers. Orthostatic hypotension was infrequently observed in clinical trials with depressed patients.

➤*Lab test abnormalities:* Clinically significant ALT elevations (≥ 3 times the upper limit of the normal range) were observed in 2% of patients exposed to **mirtazapine**. Most of these patients did not develop signs or symptoms associated with compromised liver function. While some patients were discontinued for the ALT increases, in other cases, enzyme levels returned to normal despite continued mirtazapine treatment.

➤*Hazardous tasks:* Caution patients about engaging in hazardous activities until they are reasonably certain that tetracyclics do not adversely affect their ability to engage in such activities; because of their prominent sedative effects, tetracyclics may impair judgement, thinking, and particularly, motor skills.

Drug Interactions

➤*Drugs that are metabolized by or inhibit cytochrome P450 enzymes:* Many drugs are metabolized by or inhibit various cytochrome P450 enzymes (eg, 2D6, 1A2, 3A4). In vitro, **mirtazapine** is a substrate for several of these enzymes, including 2D6, 1A2, and 3A4. While in vitro studies have shown that mirtazapine is not a potent inhibitor of any of these enzymes, an indication that mirtazapine is not likely to have a clinically significant inhibitory effect on the metabolism of other drugs that are substrates for these cytochrome P450 enzymes, the concomitant use of mirtazapine with most other drugs metabolized by these enzymes has not been formally studied. Consequently, it is not possible to make any definitive statements about the risks of coadministration of mirtazapine with such drugs.

Because of the pharmacologic similarity of **maprotiline** to the tricyclic antidepressants, the plasma concentration of maprotiline may be increased when the drug is given concomitantly with hepatic enzyme inhibitors (eg, cimetidine, fluoxetine) and decreased by concomitant administration with hepatic enzyme inducers (eg, barbiturates, phenytoin), as has occurred with tricyclic antidepressants. Adjustment of the dosage of maprotiline may therefore be necessary in such cases.

Tetracyclic Drug Interactions

Precipitant drug	Object drug*		Description
Benzodiazepines	Maprotiline	↑	The risk of seizures may be increased when the dosage of benzodiazepines is rapidly tapered in patients receiving maprotiline (see Warnings).
Phenothiazines	Maprotiline	↑	The risk of seizures may be increased with concomitant use (see Warnings).
Thyroid hormones	Maprotiline	↑	Use caution when administering maprotiline to hyperthyroid patients or those on thyroid medication because of the possibility of enhanced potential for cardiovascular toxicity of maprotiline.
Maprotiline	Anticholinergics, Sympathomimetics	↑	Additive atropine-like effects may occur. Closely supervise and carefully adjust dosage when administering concomitantly.
Maprotiline	Guanethidine	↓	Maprotiline may block the pharmacologic effects of guanethidine or similar drugs.
Mirtazapine	Alcohol	↑	Concomitant administration has a minimal effect on plasma levels of mirtazapine. However, the impairment of cognitive and motor skills produced by mirtazapine are additive with those produced by alcohol. Advise patients to avoid alcohol while taking mirtazapine.
Mirtazapine	Diazepam	↑	Concomitant administration has a minimal effect on plasma levels of mirtazapine. However, the impairment of motor skills produced by mirtazapine is additive with those caused by diazepam. Advise patients to avoid diazepam and other similar drugs while taking mirtazapine.

* ↑ = Object drug increased. ↓ = Object drug decreased.

Adverse Reactions

Approximately 16% of the 453 patients who received **mirtazapine** tablets in 6–week controlled US clinical trials discontinued treatment because of an adverse experience, compared with 7% of the 361 placebo-treated patients in those studies. The most common events (≥ 1%) associated with discontinuation and considered to be drug-related (ie, those events associated with dropout at a rate of at least twice that of placebo) included somnolence (10.4%) and nausea (1.5%).

Adverse Reactions: Maprotiline vs Mirtazapine (%)[1]

Adverse reactions	Maprotiline	Mirtazapine
Cardiovascular		
Hypertension	rare	≥ 1
Hypotension	rare	0.1-1
CNS		
Abnormal dreams	-	4
Agitation	2	≥ 1
Anxiety	3	≥ 1
Ataxia	rare	0.1-1
Confusion	rare	2
Dizziness	8	7
Drowsiness	16	-
Extrapyramidal symptoms	rare	0.1-1
Hallucinations	rare	0.1-1
Headache	4	-
Insomnia	2	-
Mania	rare	0.1-1
Nervousness	6	-
Somnolence	-	54
Abnormal thinking	-	3
Tremor	3	2
Weakness and fatigue	4	-
Dermatologic		
Alopecia	rare	< 1
Pruritus	-	≥ 1
Rash	rare	≥ 1
GI		
Dry mouth	22	25
Constipation	6	13
Increased appetite	-	17
Nausea	2	0.1-1
Vomiting	rare	≥ 1
Metabolic/Nutritional		
Edema	rare	1
Peripheral edema	-	2
Weight gain	rare	12
Weight loss	rare	0.1-1

Adverse Reactions: Maprotiline vs Mirtazapine (%)[1]		
Adverse reactions	Maprotiline	Mirtazapine
Miscellaneous		
Altered liver function	rare	0.1-1
Asthenia	-	8
Back pain	-	2
Blurred vision	4	-
Dyspnea	-	1
Flu syndrome	-	5
Myalgia	-	2
Urinary frequency	rare	2

[1] Data are pooled from different studies and are not necessarily comparable.

➤*Maprotiline:*

Cardiovascular – Tachycardia, palpitation, arrhythmia, heart block, syncope (rare).

CNS – Disorientation, delusions, restlessness, nightmares, hypomania, exacerbation of psychosis, decrease in memory, feelings of unreality, numbness, tingling, motor hyperactivity, akathisia, seizures, EEG alterations, tinnitus, dysarthria (rare).

Endocrine – Increased or decreased libido, impotence, elevation or depression of blood sugar levels (rare).

GI – Epigastric distress, diarrhea, bitter taste, abdominal cramps, dysphagia (rare).

Hypersensitivity – Skin rash, petechiae, itching, photosensitization, edema, drug fever (rare).

Miscellaneous – Accommodation disturbances, jaundice, mydriasis, urinary retention and delayed micturition, excessive perspiration, flushing, increased salivation, nasal congestion (rare).

Because of maprotiline's pharmacologic similarity to tricyclic antidepressants and isolated reports of the following adverse reactions, consider each reaction when administering maprotiline: Bone marrow depression (including agranulocytosis, eosinophilia, purpura, and thrombocytopenia), MI, stroke, peripheral neuropathy, sublingual adenitis, black tongue, stomatitis, paralytic ileus, gynecomastia in the male, breast enlargement and galactorrhea in the female, and testicular swelling.

Several voluntary reports of interstitial pneumonitis, which were in some cases associated with eosinophilia and increased liver enzymes, have been received since market introduction. However, there is no clear causal relationship.

➤*Mirtazapine:*

Cardiovascular – Vasodilatation (1% or more); angina pectoris, MI, bradycardia, ventricular extrasystoles, syncope, migraine (0.1% to 1%); atrial arrhythmia, bigeminy, vascular headache, pulmonary embolus, cerebral ischemia, cardiomegaly, phlebitis, left heart failure (less than 0.1%).

CNS – Hypesthesia, apathy, depression, hypokinesia, vertigo, twitching, amnesia, hyperkinesia, paresthesia (1% or more); delirium, delusions, depersonalization, dyskinesia, increased libido, abnormal coordination, dysarthria, neurosis, dystonia, hostility, increased reflexes, emotional lability, euphoria, paranoid reaction (0.1% to 1%); aphasia, nystagmus, akathisia, stupor, dementia, diplopia, drug dependence, paralysis, grand mal convulsion, hypotonia, myoclonus, psychotic depression, withdrawal syndrome (less than 0.1%).

Dermatologic – Acne, exfoliative dermatitis, dry skin, herpes simplex (0.1% to 1%); urticaria, herpes zoster, skin hypertrophy, seborrhea, skin ulcer (less than 0.1%).

Endocrine – Goiter, hypothyroidism (less than 0.1%).

GI – Anorexia (1% or more); eructation, glossitis, cholecystitis, gum hemorrhage, stomatitis, colitis (0.1% to 1%); tongue discoloration, ulcerative stomatitis, salivary gland enlargement, increased salivation, intestinal obstruction, pancreatitis, aphthous stomatitis, cirrhosis of the liver, gastritis, gastroenteritis, oral moniliasis, tongue edema (less than 0.1%).

GU – Urinary tract infection (1% or more); kidney calculus, cystitis, dysuria, urinary incontinence, urinary retention, vaginitis, hematuria, breast pain, amenorrhea, dysmenorrhea, leukorrhea, impotence (0.1% to 1%); polyuria, urethritis, metrorrhagia, menorrhagia, abnormal ejaculation, breast engorgement, breast enlargement, urinary urgency (less than 0.1%).

Hematologic/Lymphatic – Lymphadenopathy, leukopenia, petechiae, anemia, thrombocytopenia, lymphocytosis, pancytopenia (less than 0.1%).

Metabolic/Nutritional – Thirst (1% or more); dehydration (0.1% to 1%); gout, AST increased, healing abnormal, acid phosphatase increased, ALT increased, diabetes mellitus (less than 0.1%).

Musculoskeletal – Myasthenia, arthralgia (1% or more); arthritis, tenosynovitis (0.1% to 1%); pathological fracture, osteoporosis fracture, bone pain, myositis, tendon rupture, arthrosis, bursitis (< 0.1%).

Respiratory – Cough increased, sinusitis (1% or more); epistaxis, bronchitis, asthma, pneumonia (0.1% to 1%); asphyxia, laryngitis, pneumothorax, hiccough (less than 0.1%).

Special senses – Eye pain, abnormality of accommodation, conjunctivitis, deafness, keratoconjunctivitis, lacrimation disorder, glaucoma, hyperacusis, ear pain (0.1% to 1%); blepharitis, partial transitory deafness, otitis media, taste loss, parosmia (less than 0.1%).

Miscellaneous – Malaise, abdominal pain, acute abdominal syndrome (1% or more); chills, fever, face edema, ulcer, photosensitivity reaction, neck rigidity, neck pain, enlarged abdomen (0.1% to 1%); cellulitis, substernal chest pain (less than 0.1%).

Overdosage

➤*Maprotiline:*

Symptoms – Deaths may occur from overdosage with this class of drugs. Signs and symptoms of maprotiline overdose are similar to those seen with tricyclic overdose. Critical manifestations of overdose include cardiac dysrhythmias, severe hypotension, convulsions, and CNS depression, including coma. Changes in the ECG, particularly in QRS axis or width, are clinically significant indicators of toxicity. Other clinical manifestations include drowsiness, tachycardia, ataxia, vomiting, cyanosis, shock, restlessness, agitation, hyperpyrexia, muscle rigidity, athetoid movements, and mydriasis. Because CHF has been seen with overdosage of tricyclic antidepressants, consider CHF with maprotiline overdosage as well.

Management – Obtain an ECG and immediately initiate cardiac monitoring. Protect the patient's airway, establish an IV line, and initiate gastric decontamination. A minimum of 6 hours of observation with cardiac monitoring and observation for signs of CNS or respiratory depression, hypotension, cardiac dysrhythmias or conduction blocks, and seizures is necessary. If signs of toxicity occur at any time during this period, extended monitoring is required. There are case reports of patients succumbing to fatal dysrhythmias late after tricyclic overdose; these patients had clinical evidence of significant poisoning prior to death and most received inadequate GI decontamination. Monitoring of plasma drug levels should not guide management of the patient.

GI decontamination: All patients suspected of overdose should receive GI decontamination. This should include large volume gastric lavage followed by activated charcoal. Emesis is contraindicated.

Cardiovascular: A maximal limb-lead QRS duration of ≥ 0.1 seconds may be the best indication of the severity of the overdose. Use IV sodium bicarbonate to maintain the serum pH of 7.45 to 7.55. A pH greater than 7.6 or a Pco_2 < 20 mmHg is undesirable. Dysrhythmias unresponsive to sodium bicarbonate therapy/hyperventilation may respond to lidocaine, bretylium, or phenytoin. Type 1A and 1C antiarrhythmics are generally contraindicated (eg, quinidine, disopyramide, procainamide).

In rare instances, hemoperfusion may be beneficial in acute refractory cardiovascular instability in patients with acute toxicity. However, hemodialysis, peritoneal dialysis, exchange transfusions, and forced diuresis generally have been ineffective.

CNS: In patients with CNS depression, early intubation is advised because of the potential for abrupt deterioration. Control seizures with benzodiazepines, or if these are ineffective, other anticonvulsants (eg, phenobarbital, phenytoin). Physostigmine is not recommended except to treat life-threatening symptoms that have been unresponsive to other therapies and then only in consultation with a poison control center.

➤*Mirtazapine:*

Symptoms – There is very limited experience with mirtazapine overdose. In premarketing clinical studies, there were 8 reports of mirtazapine overdose alone or in combination with other pharmacologic agents. The only drug-overdose death reported while taking mirtazapine was in combination with amitriptyline and chlorprothixene. All other premarketing overdose cases resulted in full recovery. Signs and symptoms reported in association with overdose included disorientation, drowsiness, impaired memory, and tachycardia. There were no reports of ECG abnormalities, coma, or convulsions following overdose with mirtazapine alone.

Management – Employ general measures to manage overdose with any antidepressant. There are no specific antidotes for mirtazapine. If the patient is unconscious, establish and maintain an airway to ensure adequate oxygenation and ventilation. Consider gastric evacuation either by the induction of emesis or lavage or both. Also consider activated charcoal for overdose treatment. Monitoring of cardiac and vital signs is recommended along with general symptomatic and supportive measures.

Consider the possibility of multiple-drug involvement. Consider contacting a poison control center for additional information on the treatment of any overdose.

Patient Information

Warn patients who are to receive **mirtazapine** about the risk of developing agranulocytosis. Instruct patients to contact their physician if they experience any indication of infection such as fever, chills, sore throat, mucous membrane ulceration, or other possible signs of infection. Pay particular attention to any flu-like complaints or other symptoms that might suggest infection.

Caution patients about engaging in hazardous activities until they are reasonably certain that tetracyclics do not adversely affect their ability to engage in such activities; because of their prominent sedative effects, tetracyclics may impair judgement, thinking, and particularly, motor skills.

Advise patients to inform their physician if they are taking or intend to take any prescription, *otc*, or alternative medicinal drugs because there is a potential for tetracyclics to interact with other drugs.

Advise patients to avoid alcohol while taking tetracyclics because of the additive impairment of cognitive and motor skills.

Advise patients to notify their physician if they become pregnant or intend to become pregnant or are breastfeeding during tetracyclic therapy.

Warn patients of the association between seizures and **maprotiline** use. Inform patients that this association is enhanced in patients with a history of seizures and in those taking certain other drugs.

While patients may notice improvement with therapy in 1 to 4 weeks, advise them to continue therapy as directed.

Advise patients to avoid sunlight or sunlamps or wear protective clothing; photosensitivity may occur.

MAPROTILINE HCl

Rx	**Maprotiline HCl** (Various, eg, Mylan)	**Tablets:** 25 mg	In 30s, 100s, and 500s.
Rx	**Maprotiline HCl** (Various, eg, Mylan)	**Tablets:** 50 mg	In 30s, 100s, and 500s.
Rx	**Maprotiline HCl** (Various, eg, Mylan)	**Tablets:** 75 mg	In 30s, 100s, and 500s.

MAPROTILINE HYDROCHLORIDE — ORAL

For complete and comparative prescribing information, refer to the Tetracyclic Compounds group monograph.

WARNING

Suicidality in children and adolescents – Antidepressants increased the risk of suicidal thinking and behavior (suicidality) in short-term studies in children and adolescents with major depressive disorder (MDD) and other psychiatric disorders. Anyone considering the use of maprotiline or any other antidepressant in a child or adolescent must balance this risk with the clinical need. Patients who are started on therapy should be observed closely for clinical worsening, suicidality, or unusual changes in behavior. Families and caregivers should be advised of the need for close observation and communication with the prescriber. Maprotiline is not approved for use in pediatric patients.

Pooled analyses of short-term (4 to 16 weeks) placebo-controlled trials of 9 antidepressant drugs (SSRIs and others) in children and adolescents with MDD, obsessive-compulsive disorder (OCD), or other psychiatric disorders (a total of 24 trials involving over 4,400 patients) have revealed a greater risk of adverse reactions representing suicidal thinking or behavior (suicidality) during the first few months of treatment in those receiving antidepressants. The average risk of such reactions in patients receiving antidepressants was 4%, twice the placebo risk of 2%. No suicides occurred in these trials.

Indications

Maprotiline HCl is indicated for the treatment of depressive illness in patients with depressive neurosis (dysthymic disorder) and manic-depressive illness, depressed type (major depressive disorder). Maprotiline HCl is also effective for the relief of anxiety associated with depression.

Administration and Dosage

➤*Approved by the FDA:* September 30, 1982.

May be given as a single daily dose or in divided doses. Therapeutic effects are sometimes seen within 3 to 7 days, although 2 to 3 weeks are usually necessary.

➤*Initial adult dosage:* An initial dosage of 75 mg/day is suggested for outpatients with mild to moderate depression. In some patients, especially the elderly, an initial dosage of 25 mg/day may be used. Because of the long half-life of maprotiline, maintain the initial dosage for 2 weeks. The dose may then be increased gradually in 25 mg increments, as required and tolerated. A maximum daily dose of 150 mg/day will result in therapeutic efficacy in most outpatients, but dosages as high as 225 mg/day may be required.

➤*Severe depression:* Give hospitalized patients an initial daily dose of 100 to 150 mg, which may be gradually increased as required and tolerated. Most hospitalized patients with moderate to severe depression respond to a daily dose of 150 mg although daily doses as high as 225 mg may be required. Do not exceed 225 mg/day.

➤*Maintenance:* Keep dosage during prolonged maintenance therapy at the lowest effective level. Dosage may be reduced to 75 to 150 mg/day with adjustment depending on therapeutic response.

➤*Elderly:* In general, lower doses are recommended for patients older than 60 years of age. Doses of 50 to 75 mg/day are satisfactory as maintenance therapy for elderly patients who do not tolerate higher amounts.

➤*Storage/Stability:* Store at controlled room temperature 15° to 30°C (59° to 86°F). Dispense in a tight, light-resistant container.

MIRTAZAPINE

Rx	**Mirtazapine** (Various, eg, Aurobindo Pharma[a], Caraco)	**Tablets:** 7.5 mg	In 30s, 100s, 500s, and 1,000s.
Rx	**Mirtazapine** (Various, eg, Aurobindo Pharma[a], Par, Teva, Watson)	**Tablets:** 15 mg	In 30s, 100s, 500s, and 1,000s.
Rx	**Remeron** (Organon)		Lactose. (Organon TZ3). Yellow, oval, scored. Film-coated. In 30s, 100s, and UD 100s.
Rx	**Mirtazapine** (Various, eg, Aurobindo Pharma, Par, Teva, Watson)	**Tablets:** 30 mg	In 30s, 100s, 500s, and 1,000s.
Rx	**Remeron** (Organon)		Lactose. (Organon TZ5). Red-brown, oval, scored. Film-coated. In 30s and 100s.
Rx	**Mirtazapine** (Various, eg, Aurobindo Pharma, Par, Teva, Watson)	**Tablets:** 45 mg	In 30s, 100s, 500s, and 1,000s.
Rx	**Remeron** (Organon)		Lactose. (Organon TZ7). White, oval. Film-coated. In 30s.
Rx	**Remeron SolTab** (Organon)	**Tablets, orally disintegrating:** 15 mg	Aspartame, mannitol, 2.6 mg phenylalanine. (TZ1). In UD 30s and 90s.
		30 mg	Aspartame, mannitol, 5.2 mg phenylalanine. (TZ2). In UD 30s and 90s.
		45 mg	Aspartame, mannitol, 7.8 mg phenylalanine. (TZ4). In UD 30s and 90s.

[a] Aurobindo Pharma USA, Inc., 2615 Route 130 South, Cranbury, NJ 08512; (866) 850-2876, Fax (716) 916-1142

MIRTAZAPINE — ORAL

For complete and comparative prescribing information, refer to the Tetracyclic Compounds group monograph.

WARNING

Suicidality in children and adolescents – Antidepressants increased the risk of suicidal thinking and behavior (suicidality) in short-term studies in children and adolescents with major depressive disorder (MDD) and other psychiatric disorders. Anyone considering the use of mirtazapine or any other antidepressant in a child or adolescent must balance this risk with the clinical need. Closely observe patients who are started on therapy for clinical worsening, suicidality, or unusual changes in behavior. Advise families and caregivers of the need for close observation and communication with the prescriber. Mirtazapine is not approved for use in pediatric patients.

Pooled analyses of short-term (4 to 16 weeks) placebo-controlled trials of 9 antidepressant drugs (selective serotonin reuptake inhibitors [SSRIs] and others) in children and adolescents with MDD, obsessive compulsive disorder (OCD), or other psychiatric disorders (a total of 24 trials involving over 4,400 patients) have revealed a greater risk of adverse reactions representing suicidal thinking or behavior (suicidality) during the first few months of treatment in those receiving antidepressants. The average risk of such reactions in patients receiving antidepressants was 4%, twice the placebo risk of 2%. No suicides occurred in these trials.

Indications

➤*MDD:* Mirtazapine tablets are indicated for the treatment of MDD.

The efficacy of mirtazapine in the treatment of MDD was established in 6-week controlled trials of outpatients whose diagnoses corresponded most closely to the category of MDD. Overall, these studies demonstrated mirtazapine to be superior to placebo on at least 3 of the following 4 measures: 21-item Hamilton Depression Rating Scale (HDRS) total score, HDRS Depressed Mood Item, Clinical Global Impression (CGI) severity score, and Montgomery and Asberg Depression Rating Scale (MADRS). Superiority of mirtazapine over placebo was also found for certain factors of the HDRS, including anxiety/somatization factor and sleep disturbance factor. The mean mirtazapine dosage for patients who completed these 4 studies ranged from 21 to 32 mg/day. A fifth study of similar design utilized a higher dose (up to 50 mg/day) and also showed efficacy.

A major depressive episode implies a prominent and relatively persistent (nearly every day for at least 2 weeks) depressed or dysphoric mood that usually interferes with daily functioning, and includes at least 5 of the following 9 symptoms: depressed mood, loss of interest in usual activities, significant change in weight or appetite, insomnia or hypersomnia, psychomotor agitation or retardation, increased fatigue, feelings of guilt or worthlessness, slowed thinking or impaired concentration, or a suicide attempt or suicidal ideation.

The efficacy of mirtazapine in hospitalized, depressed patients has not been adequately studied.

The efficacy of mirtazapine in maintaining a response in patients with MDD for up to 40 weeks following 8 to 12 weeks of initial open-label treatment was demonstrated in a placebo-controlled trial. Nevertheless, health care providers who prescribe mirtazapine for extended periods should periodically reevaluate the long-term usefulness of the drug for the individual patient.

Administration and Dosage

➤*Approved by the FDA:* June 14, 1996.

➤*Initial treatment:* The recommended starting dosage for mirtazapine is 15 mg/day, administered in a single dose, preferably in the evening prior to sleep. In the controlled clinical trials establishing the efficacy of mirtazapine in the treatment of major depressive disorder, the effective dosage range was generally 15 to 45 mg/day. While the relationship between dose and satisfactory response in the treatment of MDD for mirtazapine has not been adequately explored, patients not responding to the initial 15 mg dose may benefit from dose increases up to a maximum of 45 mg/day. Mirtazapine has an elimination half-life of approximately 20 to 40 hours; therefore, dose changes should not be made at intervals of less than 1 to 2 weeks in order to allow sufficient time for evaluation of the therapeutic response to a given dose.

➤*Elderly and renal or hepatic function impairment:* The clearance of mirtazapine is reduced in elderly patients and in patients with moderate to severe renal or hepatic impairment. Consequently, be aware that plasma mirtazapine levels may be increased in these patient groups, compared with levels observed in younger adults without renal or hepatic impairment. Mirtazapine clearance is decreased in patients with moderate (glomerular filtration rate [GFR], 11 to 39 mL/min/1.73 m^2) and severe (GFR, less than 10 mL/min/1.73 m^2) renal impairment, and also in patients with hepatic impairment. Caution is indicated when administering mirtazapine to such patients.

Approximately 190 elderly individuals (65 years of age and older) participated in clinical studies with mirtazapine tablets. This drug is known to be substantially excreted by the kidney (75%) and the risk of decreased clearance of this drug is greater in patients with impaired renal function. Because elderly patients are more likely to have decreased renal function, take care in dose selection. Sedating drugs may cause confusion and oversedation in the elderly. No unusual adverse age-related phenomena were identified in this group. Pharmacokinetic studies revealed a decreased clearance in the elderly. Caution is indicated in administering mirtazapine to elderly patients.

➤*Maintenance / Extended treatment:* It is generally agreed that acute episodes of depression require several months or longer of sustained pharmacological therapy beyond responses to the acute episode. Systematic evaluation of mirtazapine has demonstrated that its efficacy in MDD is maintained for periods of up to 40 weeks following 8 to 12 weeks of initial treatment at a dosage of 15 to 45 mg/day. Based on these limited data, it is unknown whether the dose of mirtazapine needed for maintenance treatment is identical to the dose needed to achieve an initial response. Periodically reassess patients to determine the need for maintenance treatment and the appropriate dose for such treatment.

➤*Switching patients to or from a monoamine oxidase (MAO) inhibitor:* Allow at least 14 days to elapse between discontinuation of an MAO inhibitor and initiation of therapy with mirtazapine. In addition, allow at least 14 days after stopping mirtazapine before starting an MAO inhibitor.

➤*Orally disintegrating tablets:* Instruct patients to open the tablet blister pack with dry hands and place the tablet on the tongue. The tablet should be used immediately after removal from its blister; once removed, it cannot be stored. Mirtazapine orally disintegrating tablets will disintegrate rapidly on the tongue and can be swallowed with saliva. No water is needed for taking the tablet. Patients should not attempt to split the tablet.

➤*Storage / Stability:* Store at 25°C (77°F); excursions permitted to 15° to 30°C (59° to 86°F). Protect from light and moisture.

Use the orally disintegrating tablet immediately upon opening individual tablet blister.

TRAZODONE HYDROCHLORIDE

Rx	**Trazodone Hydrochloride** (Various, eg, Barr, Mutual)	**Tablets:** 50 mg	In 100s, 500s, and 1,000s.
Rx	**Desyrel** (Apothecon)		(Desyrel MJ 775). Orange, scored. Film-coated. In 100s, 1,000s, and UD 100s.
Rx	**Trazodone Hydrochloride** (Various, eg, Barr, Mutual)	**Tablets:** 100 mg	In 100s, 500s, and 1,000s.
Rx	**Desyrel** (Apothecon)		(Desyrel MJ 776). White, scored. Film-coated. In 100s, 1,000s, and UD 100s.
Rx	**Trazodone Hydrochloride** (Various, eg, Barr, Mutual)	**Tablets:** 150 mg	In 100s and 500s.
Rx	**Desyrel Dividose** (Apothecon)		(MJ 778 50 50 50). Orange, double-scored. In 100s and 500s.
Rx	**Trazodone Hydrochloride** (Barr)	**Tablets:** 300 mg	(barr 733 100 100 100). White, oval, scored. In 100s.
Rx	**Desyrel Dividose** (Apothecon)		(MJ 796 100 100 100). Yellow, double-scored. In 100s.

TRAZODONE HYDROCHLORIDE — ORAL

WARNING

Suicidality in children and adolescents – Antidepressants increase the risk of suicidal thinking and behavior (suicidality) in short-term studies in children and adolescents with Major Depressive Disorder (MDD) and other psychiatric disorders. Anyone considering the use of trazodone or any other antidepressant in a child or adolescent must balance the risk with the clinical need. Closely observe patients who are started on therapy for clinical worsening, suicidality, or unusual changes in behavior. Advise families and caregivers of the need for close observation and communication with the prescriber. Trazodone is not approved for use in children.

Pooled analyses of short-term (4 to 16 weeks) placebo-controlled trials of 9 antidepressant drugs (selective serotonin reuptake inhibitors [SSRIs] and others) in children and adolescents with MDD, obsessive compulsive disorder (OCD), or other psychiatric disorders (a total of 24 trials involving over 4,400 patients) have revealed a greater risk of adverse reactions representing suicidal thinking or behavior (suicidality) during the first few months of treatment in those receiving antidepressants. The average risk of such reactions in patients receiving antidepressants was 4%; twice the placebo risk of 2%. No suicides occurred in these trials.

Indications

➤*Depression:* Trazodone is indicated for the treatment of depression. The efficacy of trazodone has been demonstrated in both inpatient and outpatient settings and for depressed patients with and without prominent anxiety. The depressive illness of patients studied corresponds to the Major Depressive Episode criteria of the American Psychiatric Association's *Diagnostic and Statistical Manual of Mental Disorders, Third Edition.* Major Depressive Episode implies a prominent and relatively persistent (nearly every day for at least 2 weeks) depressed or dysphoric mood that usually interferes with daily functioning, and includes at least 4 of the following 8 symptoms: change in appetite, change in sleep, psychomotor agitation or retardation, loss of interest in usual activities or decrease in sexual drive, increased fatigability, feelings of guilt or worthlessness, slowed thinking or impaired concentration, and suicidal ideation or attempts.

➤*Unlabeled uses:* Trazodone 50 mg twice daily and tryptophan 500 mg twice daily have been successful in the treatment of aggressive behavior. Dose adjustments were made until therapeutic response was achieved or unacceptable adverse reactions developed. Low dosages (50 to 100 mg daily) decreased cravings for alcohol, depression, and anxious symptoms in patients with alcoholism. A dosage of 300 mg/day may also be useful for treatment of patients with panic disorder or agoraphobia with panic attacks. Low-dose (25 to 75 mg) trazodone is also used to treat insomnia often in conjunction with an SSRI.

Trazodone has been used to treat cocaine withdrawal.

Administration and Dosage

The dosage should be initiated at a low level and increased gradually, noting the clinical response and any evidence of intolerance. Occurrence of drowsiness may require the administration of a major portion of the daily dose at bedtime or a reduction of dosage. Trazodone should be taken shortly after a meal or light snack. Symptomatic relief may be seen during the first week with optimal antidepressant effects typically evident within 2 weeks. Twenty-five percent of those who respond to trazodone require more than 2 weeks (up to 4 weeks) of drug administration.

➤*Adults:* An initial dosage of 150 mg/day in divided doses is suggested. The dosage may be increased by 50 mg/day every 3 to 4 days. The maximum dosage for outpatients usually should not exceed 400 mg/day in divided doses. Inpatients (ie, more severely depressed patients) may be given up to but not in excess of 600 mg/day in divided doses.

➤*Maintenance:* Dosage during prolonged maintenance therapy should be kept at the lowest effective level. Once an adequate response has been achieved, dosage may be gradually reduced, with subsequent adjustment depending on therapeutic response.

Duration – Although there has been no systematic evaluation of the efficacy of trazodone beyond 6 weeks, it is generally recommended that a course of antidepressant drug treatment should be continued for several months.

➤*Storage/Stability:* Store at room temperature, between 15° and 30°C (59° and 86°F). Protect from temperatures above 40°C (104°F).

Dispense in a tight, light-resistant container.

Actions

➤*Pharmacology:* The mechanism of trazodone's antidepressant action in man is not fully understood. In animals, trazodone selectively inhibits serotonin uptake by brain synaptosomes and potentiates the behavioral changes induced by the serotonin precursor, 5-hydroxytryptophan. Cardiac conduction effects of trazodone in the anesthetized dog are qualitatively dissimilar and quantitatively less pronounced than those seen with tricyclic antidepressants. Trazodone is not a monoamine oxidase inhibitor and, unlike amphetamine-type drugs, does not stimulate the CNS.

➤*Pharmacokinetics:*

Absorption – Trazodone is well absorbed after oral administration without selective localization in any tissue. When trazodone is taken shortly after ingestion of food, there may be an increase in the amount of drug absorbed, a decrease in maximum concentration, and a lengthening in the time to maximum concentration.

Distribution – Peak plasma levels occur approximately 1 hour after dosing when trazodone is taken on an empty stomach or 2 hours after dosing when taken with food.

Metabolism – In vitro studies in human liver microsomes show that trazodone is metabolized to an active metabolite, m-chlorophenylpiperazine (mCPP) by cytochrome P-450 3A4 (CYP3A4). Other metabolic pathways that may be involved in metabolism of trazodone have not been well characterized.

Excretion – In some patients, trazodone may accumulate in the plasma.

Contraindications

Trazodone is contraindicated in patients hypersensitive to trazodone.

Warnings

➤*Clinical worsening and suicide risk:* Patients with MDD, both adult and pediatric, may experience worsening of their depression and/or the emergence of suicidal ideation and behavior (suicidality) or unusual changes in behavior, whether or not they are taking antidepressant medications, and this risk may persist until significant remission occurs. There has been a long-standing concern that antidepressants may have a role in inducing worsening of depression and the emergence of suicidality in certain patients. Antidepressants increased the risk of suicidality in short-term studies in children and adolescents with MDD and other psychiatric disorders.

Pooled analyses of short-term, placebo-controlled trials of 9 antidepressant drugs (SSRIs and others) in children and adolescents with MDD, OCD, or other psychiatric disorders (a total of 24 trials involving over 4,400 patients) have revealed a greater risk of adverse reactions representing suicidality during the first few months of treatment in those receiving antidepressants. The average risk of such reactions in patients receiving antidepressants was 4%, twice the placebo risk of 2%. There was considerable variation in risk among drugs but a tendency toward an increase for almost all drugs studied. The risk of suicidality was most consistently observed in the MDD trials, but there were signals of risk arising from some trials in other psychiatric indications (OCD and social anxiety disorder) as well. No suicides occurred in any of these trials. It is unknown whether the suicidality risk in pediatric patients extends to longer-term use, (ie, beyond several months). It is also unknown whether the suicidality risk extends to adults.

Closely observe all pediatric patients being treated with antidepressants for any indication of clinical worsening, suicidality, or unusual changes in behavior, especially during the initial few months of a course of drug therapy, or at times of dose changes (either increases or decreases). Such observation would generally include at least weekly face-to-face contact with patients or their family members or caregivers during the first 4 weeks of treatment, then every other week visits for the next 4 weeks, then at 12 weeks, and, as clinically indicated, beyond 12 weeks. Additional contact by telephone may be appropriate between face-to-face visits.

Similarly observe adults with MDD or comorbid depression in the setting of other psychiatric illness being treated with antidepressants for clinical worsening and suicidality, especially during the initial few months of a course of drug therapy, or at times of dose changes either increases or decreases).

The following symptoms, including anxiety, agitation, panic attacks, insomnia, irritability, hostility, aggressiveness, impulsivity, akathisia (psychomotor restlessness), hypomania, and mania, have been reported in adult and pediatric patients being treated with antidepressants for MDD as well as for other indications, both psychiatric and nonpsychiatric. Although a causal link between the emergence of such symptoms and either the worsening of depression and/or the emergence of suicidal impulses has not been established, there is concern that such symptoms may represent precursors to emerging suicidality.

Give consideration to changing the therapeutic regimen, including possibly discontinuing the medication, in patients whose depression is persistently worse or those who are experiencing emergent suicidality or symptoms that might be precursors to worsening depression or suicidality, especially if these symptoms are severe, abrupt in onset, or were not part of the patient's presenting symptoms.

Alert families and caregivers of pediatric patients being treated with antidepressants for MDD or other indications, both psychiatric and nonpsychiatric, about the need to monitor patients for the emergence of agitation, irritability, unusual changes in behavior, and the other symptoms described previously, as well as the emergence of suicidality, and to report such symptoms immediately to health care providers. Such monitoring should include daily observation by families and caregivers. Write prescriptions for trazodone for the smallest quantity of tablets consistent with good patient management, in order to reduce the risk of overdose. Similarly advise families and caregivers of adults being treated for depression.

➤*Screening patients for bipolar disorder:* A major depressive episode may be the initial presentation of bipolar disorder. It is generally believed (though not established in controlled trials) that treating such an episode with an antidepressant, alone may increase the likelihood of precipitation of a mixed/manic episode in patients at risk for bipolar disorder. Whether any of the symptoms described previously represent such a conversion is unknown. However, prior to initiating treatment with an antidepressant, adequately screen patients with depressive symptoms to determine if they are at risk for bipolar disorder; such screening should include a detailed psychiatric history, including a family history of suicide, bipolar disorder, and depression. Note that trazodone is not approved for use in treating bipolar depression.

TRAZODONE HYDROCHLORIDE — ORAL

➤*Priapism:* Trazodone has been associated with the occurrence of priapism. In many of the cases reported, surgical intervention was required and, in a portion of these cases, permanent impairment of erectile function or impotence resulted. Male patients with prolonged or inappropriate erections should immediately discontinue the drug and consult their health care provider.

The detumescence of priapism and drug-induced penile erections has been accomplished by pharmacologic (eg, the intracavernosal injection of alpha-adrenergic stimulants, such as epinephrine and norepinephrine) and surgical procedures. Perform any pharmacologic or surgical procedure utilized in the treatment of priapism under the supervision of a urologist or a health care provider familiar with the procedure, and do not initiate without urologic consultation if the priapism has persisted for more than 24 hours.

➤*Preexisting cardiac disease:* Trazodone is not recommended for use during the initial recovery phase of myocardial infarction.

Use caution when administering trazodone to patients with cardiac disease and closely monitor such patients, because antidepressant drugs (including trazodone) have been associated with the occurrence of cardiac arrhythmias. Recent clinical studies in patients with preexisting cardiac disease indicate that trazodone may be arrhythmogenic in some patients in that population. Arrhythmias identified included isolated premature ventricular contractions, ventricular couplets, and, in 2 patients, short episodes (3 to 4 beats) of ventricular tachycardia.

➤*Pregnancy: Category C.* Trazodone has been shown to cause increased fetal resorption and other adverse reactions on the fetus in 2 studies using the rat when given at dose levels approximately 30 to 50 times the proposed maximum human dose. There was also an increase in congenital anomalies in 1 of 3 rabbit studies at approximately 15 to 50 times the maximum human dose. There are no adequate and well-controlled studies in pregnant women. Use trazodone during pregnancy only if the potential benefit justifies the potential risk to the fetus.

➤*Lactation:* Trazodone and/or its metabolites have been found in the milk of lactating rats, suggesting that the drug may be secreted in human milk. Exercise caution when trazodone is administered to a breast-feeding woman.

➤*Children:* See Black Box Warning for more information.

Precautions

➤*Hypotension:* Hypotension, including orthostatic hypotension and syncope, has been reported in patients receiving trazodone. Coadministration of antihypertensive therapy with trazodone may require a reduction in the dose of the antihypertensive drug.

➤*Suicide:* The possibility of suicide in seriously depressed patients is inherent in the illness and may persist until significant remission occurs. Therefore, write prescriptions for the smallest number of tablets consistent with good patient management.

➤*Elective surgery:* Little is known about the interaction between trazodone and general anesthetics; therefore, prior to elective surgery, discontinue trazodone for as long as clinically feasible.

➤*Electroconvulsive therapy:* Avoid coadministration with electroshock therapy because of the absence of experience in this area.

➤*Lab test abnormalities:* Occasional low white blood cell and neutrophil counts have been noted in patients receiving trazodone. These were not considered clinically significant and did not necessitate discontinuation of the drug; however, discontinue the drug in any patient whose white blood cell count or absolute neutrophil count falls below normal levels. White blood cell and differential counts are recommended for patients who develop fever and sore throat (or other signs of infection) during therapy.

➤*Hazardous tasks:* Antidepressants may impair the mental or physical abilities required for the performance of potentially hazardous tasks, such as operating an automobile or machinery; caution the patient accordingly.

Drug Interactions

➤*CYP3A4 inhibitors:* In vitro drug metabolism studies suggest there is a potential for drug interactions when trazodone is given with CYP3A4 inhibitors. Ritonavir, a potent CYP3A4 inhibitor, increased the C_{max}, AUC, and elimination half-life, and decreased clearance of trazodone after administration of ritonavir twice daily for 2 days. Adverse reactions, including nausea, hypotension, and syncope, were observed when ritonavir and trazodone were coadministered. It is likely that ketoconazole, indinavir, and other CYP3A4 inhibitors, such as itraconazole or nefazodone, may lead to substantial increases in trazodone plasma concentrations, with the potential for adverse reactions. If trazodone is used with a potent CYP3A4 inhibitor, consider a lower dose of trazodone.

Trazodone Drug Interactions

Precipitant drug	Object drug[a]		Description
Azole antifungals (eg, itraconazole, ketoconazole)	Trazodone	⬆	Coadministration may lead to substantial increases in trazodone plasma concentrations, with the potential for adverse reactions. Monitor patient response and adjust dose of trazodone as needed.
Carbamazepine	Trazodone	⬇	Plasma concentrations of trazodone and its active metabolite may be decreased, producing a decrease in therapeutic effect. Monitor patient when starting or stopping either agent and adjust therapy as needed.
Phenothiazines (eg, chlorpromazine, fluphenazine)	Trazodone	⬆	Elevated trazodone serum concentrations have occurred, increasing the pharmacologic and toxic effects. Monitor patient and adjust dose of trazodone as needed.
Protease inhibitors (eg, indinavir, ritonavir)	Trazodone	⬆	Trazodone plasma concentrations may be elevated, increasing the pharmacologic and adverse reactions. Monitor patient and adjust dose of trazodone as needed.
SSRI antidepressants (eg, fluoxetine, nefazodone, paroxetine, venlafaxine)	Trazodone	⬆	A "serotonin syndrome," including irritability, increased muscle tone, shivering, myoclonus, and altered consciousness, may occur. If coadministration cannot be avoided, start with a low dose of trazodone and closely monitor the patient.
Trazodone	Alcohol, barbiturates, CNS depressants	⬆	Trazodone may enhance the CNS-depressant response to these agents.
Trazodone	Carbamazepine	⬆	Coadministration may increase carbamazepine plasma levels, increasing the therapeutic and adverse reactions. Monitor patient and adjust carbamazepine therapy as needed.
Trazodone	Digoxin	⬆	Increased serum digoxin levels have been reported to occur in patients receiving concurrent trazodone. Monitor digoxin levels regularly.
Trazodone	MAO inhibitors (eg, isocarboxazid, phenelzine)	⟷	It is not known whether interactions will occur between trazodone and MAO inhibitors. If MAO inhibitors are discontinued shortly before, or are to be given concomitantly with trazodone, initiate therapy cautiously with gradual increase in dosage until optimum response is achieved.
Trazodone	Phenytoin	⬆	Phenytoin serum levels were increased with concurrent trazodone therapy. Monitor phenytoin plasma levels regularly.
Trazodone	Warfarin	⬆⬇	There have been reports of increased and decreased prothrombin time occurring in patients taking warfarin and trazodone concurrently. Monitor anticoagulant parameters frequently when starting or stopping trazodone. Avoid as needed use of trazodone in patients receiving warfarin.

[a] ⬆ = Object drug increased. ⬇ = Object drug decreased. ⟷ = Undetermined clinical effect.

➤*Drug/Food interactions:* See Actions for more information.

Adverse Reactions

Trazodone Adverse Reactions

	Inpatients		Outpatients	
Adverse reaction	Trazodone (n = 142)	Placebo (n = 95)	Trazodone (n = 157)	Placebo (n = 158)
Cardiovascular				
Hypertension	2.1%	1.1%	1.3%	< 1%
Hypotension	7%	1.1%	3.8%	0%
Syncope	2.8%	2.1%	4.5%	1.3%

TRAZODONE HYDROCHLORIDE — ORAL

Trazodone Adverse Reactions				
	Inpatients		Outpatients	
Adverse reaction	Trazodone (n = 142)	Placebo (n = 95)	Trazodone (n = 157)	Placebo (n = 158)
Tachycardia/ Palpitations	0%	0%	7%	7%
CNS				
Anger/Hostility	3.5%	6.3%	1.3%	2.5%
Confusion	4.9%	0%	5.7%	7.6%
Decreased concentration	2.8%	2.1%	1.3%	0%
Disorientation	2.1%	0%	< 1%	0%
Dizziness/Lightheadedness	19.7%	5.3%	28%	15.2%
Drowsiness	23.9%	6.3%	40.8%	19.6%
Excitement	1.4%	1.1%	5.1%	5.7%
Fatigue	11.3%	4.2%	5.7%	2.5%
Headache	9.9%	5.3%	19.8%	15.8%
Head full (heavy)	2.8%	0%	0%	0%
Impaired memory	1.4%	0%	< 1%	< 1%
Incoordination	4.9%	0%	1.9%	0%
Insomnia	9.9%	10.5%	6.4%	12%
Malaise	2.8%	0%	0%	0%
Nervousness	14.8%	10.5%	6.4%	8.2%
Nightmares/ Vivid dreams	< 1%	1.1%	5.1%	5.7%
Paresthesia	1.4%	0%	0%	< 1%
Tremors	2.8%	1.1%	5.1%	3.8%
Dermatologic				
Skin condition/ Edema	2.8%	1.1%	7%	1.3%
Sweating/ Clamminess	1.4%	1.1%	< 1%	< 1%
GI				
Abdominal/ Gastric disorder	3.5%	4.2%	5.7%	4.4%
Bad taste in mouth	1.4%	0%	0%	0%
Constipation	7%	4.2%	7.6%	5.7%
Decreased appetite	3.5%	5.3%	0%	< 1%
Diarrhea	0%	1.1%	4.5%	1.9%
Dry mouth	14.8%	8.4%	33.8%	20.3%
Nausea/ Vomiting	9.9%	1.1%	12.7%	9.5%
GU				
Decreased libido	< 1%	1.1%	1.3%	< 1%
Musculoskeletal				
Musculoskeletal aches/pains	5.6%	3.2%	5.1%	2.5%
Respiratory				
Nasal/Sinus congestion	2.8%	0%	5.7%	3.2%
Shortness of breath	< 1%	1.1%	1.3%	0%
Special senses				
Blurred vision	6.3%	4.2%	14.7%	3.8%
Eyes red/tired/ itching	2.8%	0%	0%	0%
Tinnitus	1.4%	0%	0%	< 1%
Miscellaneous				
Weight gain	1.4%	0%	4.5%	1.9%
Weight loss	< 1%	3.2%	5.7%	2.5%

Sinus bradycardia – Occasional sinus bradycardia has occurred in long-term studies.

Other adverse reactions reported – In addition to the relatively common (greater than 1%) adverse reactions enumerated previously, the following adverse reactions have been reported to occur in association with the use of trazodone in the controlled clinical studies:

CNS – Akathisia, hallucinations/delusions, hypomania, impaired speech, increased libido, numbness.

GI – Flatulence, hypersalivation, increased appetite.

GU – Delayed urine flow, early menses, hematuria, impotence, increased urinary frequency, missed periods, retrograde ejaculation.

Miscellaneous – Allergic reaction, anemia, chest pain, muscle twitches.

➤*Postmarketing:*

Cardiovascular – The following cardiovascular system reactions have been reported: arrhythmia, atrial fibrillation, bradycardia, cardiac arrest, cardiospasm, cerebrovascular accident, conduction block, congestive heart failure, myocardial infarction, orthostatic hypotension and syncope, palpitations, vasodilation, and ventricular ectopic activity, including ventricular tachycardia.

CNS – Abnormal dreams, agitation, anxiety, aphasia, ataxia, extrapyramidal symptoms, generalized tonic-clonic seizures, hallucinations, insomnia, paranoid reaction, paresthesia, psychosis, stupor, tardive dyskinesia, vertigo, weakness.

Dermatologic – Alopecia, hirsutism, leukonychia, pruritus, psoriasis, rash, urticaria.

GI – Cholestatis, increased salivation, nausea/vomiting (most frequently).

GU – Breast enlargement or engorgement, clitorism, lactation, priapism (some patients have required surgical intervention), urinary incontinence, urinary retention.

Hematologic/Lymphatic – Hemolytic anemia, leukocytosis, methemoglobinemia.

Hepatic – Hyperbilirubinemia, jaundice, liver enzyme alterations.

Metabolic/Nutritional – Edema, increased amylase.

Miscellaneous – Apnea, chills, diplopia, syndrome of inappropriate secretion of antidiuretic hormone, unexplained death.

Overdosage

➤*Symptoms:* Death from overdosage has occurred in patients ingesting trazodone and other drugs concurrently (namely, alcohol; alcohol, chloral hydrate, and diazepam; amobarbital chlordiazepoxide; or meprobamate).

The most severe reactions reported to have occurred with overdosage of trazodone alone have been priapism, respiratory arrest, seizures, and electrocardiogram changes. The reactions reported most frequently have been drowsiness and vomiting. Overdosage may cause an increase in incidence or severity of any of the reported adverse reactions.

➤*Treatment:* There is no specific antidote for trazodone. Treatment should be symptomatic and supportive in the case of hypotension or excessive sedation. Empty the stomach by gastric lavage of any patient suspected of having taken an overdosage. Forced diuresis may be useful in facilitating elimination of the drug.

Patient Information

Inform patients, their families, and their caregivers about the benefits and risks associated with treatment with trazodone and counsel them in its appropriate use. A patient medication guide about using antidepressants in children and teenagers is available for trazodone. Instruct patients, their families, and their caregivers to read the medication guide and assist them in understanding its contents. Give patients the opportunity to discuss the contents of the medication guide and to obtain answers to any questions they may have. Following is the complete text of the medication guide.

Advise patients of the following issues and ask them to alert their health care provider if these occur while taking trazodone.

➤*Clinical worsening and suicide risk:* Encourage patients, their families, and their caregivers to be alert to the emergence of anxiety, agitation, panic attacks, insomnia, irritability, hostility, aggressiveness, impulsivity, akathisia (psychomotor restlessness), hypomania, mania, other unusual changes in behavior, worsening of depression, and suicidal ideation, especially early during antidepressant treatment and when the dose is adjusted up or down. Advise families and caregivers of patients to observe for the emergence of such symptoms on a day to day-basis, since changes may be abrupt. Advise them to report such symptoms to the patient's health care provider, especially if they are severe, abrupt in onset, or were not part of the patient's presenting symptoms. Symptoms such as these may be associated with an increased risk for suicidal thinking and behavior and indicate a need for very close monitoring and possibly changes in the medication.

Because priapism has been reported to occur in patients receiving trazodone, advise patients with prolonged or inappropriate penile erection to immediately discontinue the drug and consult with the health care provider.

Antidepressants may impair the mental or physical abilities required for the performance of potentially hazardous tasks, such as operating an automobile or machinery; caution the patient accordingly.

Trazodone may enhance the response to alcohol, barbiturates, and other CNS depressants.

Give trazodone shortly after a meal or light snack. Within any individual patient, total drug absorption may be up to 20% higher when the drug is taken with food rather than on an empty stomach. The risk of dizziness/light-headedness may increase under fasting conditions.

BUPROPION HYDROCHLORIDE

Rx	**Bupropion HCl** (Various, eg, Geneva, Teva)	**Tablets:** 75 mg	In 100s.
Rx	**Wellbutrin** (GlaxoSmithKline)		(Wellbutrin 75). Yellow-gold, biconvex. Film-coated. In 100s.
Rx	**Bupropion HCl** (Various, eg, Geneva, Teva)	**Tablets:** 100 mg	In 100s.
Rx	**Wellbutrin** (GlaxoSmithKline)		(Wellbutrin 100). Red, biconvex. Film-coated. In 100s.
Rx	**Bupropion HCl** (Various, eg, Eon, Watson)	**Tablets, sustained release (12 hour):** 100 mg	In 60s, 100s, and 500s.
Rx	**Budeprion SR**[a] (Teva)		(G 2442). Yellow, biconvex. Film-coated. In 100s.
Rx	**Wellbutrin SR**[a] (GlaxoSmithKline)		(Wellbutrin SR 100). Blue, biconvex. Film-coated. In 60s.
Rx	**Bupropion HCl** (Various, eg, Eon, Watson)	**Tablets, sustained release (12 hour):** 150 mg	In 60s and 250s.
Rx	**Budeprion SR**[a] (Teva)		Light-yellow. Film-coated. (G 2444). In 100s.
Rx	**Wellbutrin SR**[a] (GlaxoSmithKline)		(Wellbutrin SR 150). Purple, biconvex. Film-coated. In 60s.
Rx	**Zyban** (GlaxoSmithKline)	**Tablets, sustained release:** 150 mg	(ZYBAN 150). Purple, biconvex. Film-coated. In 60s.
Rx	**Bupropion HCl** (Various, eg, Global, Watson)	**Tablets, sustained release (12 hour):** 200 mg	In 60s, 180s, and 500s.
Rx	**Wellbutrin SR**[a] (GlaxoSmithKline)		(Wellbutrin SR 200). Lt. pink, biconvex. Film-coated. In 60s.
Rx	**Wellbutrin XL**[a] (GlaxoSmithKline)	**Tablets, extended release (24 hour):** 150 mg	(Wellbutrin XL 150). Creamy-white to pale yellow. In 30s.
Rx	**Wellbutrin XL**[a] (GlaxoSmithKline)	**Tablets, extended release (24 hour):** 300 mg	(Wellbutrin XL 300). Creamy-white to pale yellow. In 30s.

[a] Please note that "SR" refers to the 12-hour tablets and "XL" refers to the 24-hour tablets.

BUPROPION — ORAL

For additional information, refer to the Antidepressants introduction. Bupropion also is used as a smoking deterrent. Refer to the Smoking Deterrents section of this chapter for complete prescribing information.

WARNING

Suicidality in children and adolescents – Although *Zyban* is not indicated for treatment of depression, it contains the same active ingredient as the antidepressant bupropion medications *Wellbutrin, Wellbutrin SR*, and *Wellbutrin XL*.

Antidepressants increased the risk of suicidal thinking and behavior (suicidality) in short-term studies in children and adolescents with Major Depressive Disorder (MDD) and other psychiatric disorders. Anyone considering the use of bupropion or any other antidepressant in a child or adolescent must balance this risk with the clinical need. Closely observe patients who are started on therapy for clinical worsening, suicidality, or unusual changes in behavior. Advice families and caregivers of the need for close observation and communication with the prescriber. Bupropion is not approved for use in pediatric patients.

Pooled analyses of short-term (4 to 16 weeks), placebo-controlled trials of 9 antidepressant drugs (selective serotonin reuptake inhibitors [SSRIs] and others) in children and adolescents with MDD, obsessive compulsive disorder (OCD), or other psychiatric disorders (a total of 24 trials involving more than 4,400 patients) have revealed a greater risk of adverse reactions representing suicidal thinking or behavior (suicidality) during the first few months of treatment in those receiving antidepressants. The average risk of such reactions in patients receiving antidepressants was 4%, twice the placebo risk of 2%. No suicides occurred in these trials.

Indications

➤*Depression:* Bupropion (immediate release) IR, *Wellbutrin (sustained release) SR*, and bupropion (extended release) XL are indicated for the treatment of depression.

➤*Smoking cessation (Zyban* only): Indicated as an aid to smoking-cessation treatment.

➤*Unlabeled uses:* Bupropion SR has been effective in the treatment of neuropathic pain and enhancement of weight loss. Bupropion also has been shown to be effective in the treatment of attention deficit hyperactivity disorder.

Administration and Dosage

➤*Approved by the FDA:* December 30, 1985.

➤*General dosing considerations:* It is particularly important to administer bupropion IR, *Wellbutrin SR*, and bupropion XL in a manner most likely to minimize the risk of seizure. Gradual escalation in dosage also is important if agitation, motor restlessness, and insomnia, often seen during the initial days of treatment, are to be minimized. If necessary, these effects may be managed by temporary reduction of the dose or the short-term administration of an intermediate- to long-acting sedative hypnotic. A sedative hypnotic usually is not required beyond the first week of treatment. Insomnia also may be minimized by avoiding bedtime doses. If distressing, untoward effects supervene, dose escalation should be stopped.

➤*Bupropion IR:* No single dose of bupropion IR tablets should exceed 150 mg. Bupropion IR should be administered 3 times daily, preferably with at least 6 hours between successive doses.

Usual dosage for adults – The usual adult dose is 300 mg/day, given 3 times daily. Dosing should begin at 200 mg/day, given as 100 mg twice daily. Based on clinical response, this dose may be increased to 300 mg/day, given as 100 mg 3 times daily, no sooner than 3 days after beginning therapy (see the following table). Increases in dose should not exceed 100 mg/day in a 3-day period.

Bupropion IR Dosing Regimen					
Treatment day	Total daily dose	Tablet strength	Number of tablets		
			Morning	Midday	Evening
1	200 mg	100 mg	1	0	1
4	300 mg	100 mg	1	1	1

Increasing the dosage above 300 mg/day – As with other antidepressants, the full antidepressant effect of bupropion IR may not be evident until 4 weeks of treatment or longer. An increase in dosage, up to a maximum of 450 mg/day, given in divided doses of not more than 150 mg each, may be considered for patients in whom no clinical improvement is noted after several weeks of treatment at 300 mg/day. Dosing above 300 mg/day may be accomplished using the 75 or 100 mg tablets. The 100 mg tablet must be administered 4 times/day with at least 4 hours between successive doses, in order not to exceed the limit of 150 mg in a single dose. Bupropion IR should be discontinued in patients who do not demonstrate an adequate response after an appropriate period of treatment at 450 mg/day.

Maintenance – The lowest dose that maintains remission is recommended. Although it is not known how long the patient should remain on bupropion IR, it is generally recognized that acute episodes of depression require several months or longer of antidepressant drug treatment.

➤*Wellbutrin SR*: *Wellbutrin SR* should be swallowed whole, not crushed, divided, or chewed.

Initial treatment – The usual adult target dose for *Wellbutrin SR* tablets is 300 mg/day, given as 150 mg twice daily. Dosing should begin at 150 mg/day, given as a single daily dose in the morning. If the 150 mg initial dose is adequately tolerated, an increase to the 300 mg/day target dose, given as 150 mg twice daily, may be made as early as day 4 of dosing. There should be an interval of at least 8 hours between successive doses.

Increasing the dosage above 300 mg/day – As with other antidepressants, the full antidepressant effect of *Wellbutrin SR* may not be evident until 4 weeks of treatment or longer. An increase in dosage to the maximum of 400 mg/day, given as 200 mg twice daily, may be considered for patients in whom no clinical improvement is noted after several weeks of treatment at 300 mg/day.

Maintenance – It is generally agreed that acute episodes of depression require several months or longer of sustained pharmacological therapy beyond response to the acute episode.

It is unknown whether or not the dose of *Wellbutrin SR* needed for maintenance treatment is identical to the dose needed to achieve an initial response. Patients should be periodically reassessed to determine the need for maintenance treatment and the appropriate dose for such treatment.

➤*Bupropion XL:* Bupropion XL should be swallowed whole, not crushed, divided, or chewed.

Bupropion XL may be taken without regard to meals.

Initial treatment – The usual adult target dose for bupropion XL tablets is 300 mg/day, given once daily in the morning. Dosing with bupropion XL tablets should begin at 150 mg/day, given as a single daily dose in the morning. If the 150 mg initial dose is adequately tolerated, an increase to the 300 mg/day target dose, given once daily, may be made as early as day 4 of dosing. There should be an interval of at least 24 hours between successive doses.

Increasing the dosage above 300 mg/day – As with other antidepressants, the full antidepressant effect of bupropion XL tablets may not be evident until 4 weeks of treatment or longer. An increase in dosage to the maximum of 450 mg/day, given as a single dose, may be considered for patients in whom no clinical improvement is noted after several weeks of treatment at 300 mg/day.

BUPROPION — ORAL

Maintenance – It is generally agreed that acute episodes of depression require several months or longer of sustained pharmacological therapy beyond response to the acute episode.

It is unknown whether or not the dose of bupropion XL needed for maintenance treatment is identical to the dose needed to achieve an initial response. Patients should be periodically reassessed to determine the need for maintenance treatment and the appropriate dose for such treatment.

Switching to bupropion XL – When switching patients from bupropion IR to bupropion XL or from *Wellbutrin SR* to bupropion XL, give the same total daily dose when possible. Patients who are currently being treated with bupropion IR tablets at 300 mg/day (for example, 100 mg 3 times/day) may be switched to bupropion XL 300 mg once daily. Patients who are currently being treated with *Wellbutrin SR* tablets at 300 mg/day (for example, 150 mg twice daily) may be switched to bupropion XL 300 mg once daily.

➤*Zyban*:

Usual dosage for adults – The recommended and maximum dose of *Zyban* is 300 mg/day, given as 150 mg twice daily. Dosing should begin at 150 mg/day given every day for the first 3 days, followed by a dose increase for most patients to the recommended usual dose of 300 mg/day. There should be an interval of at least 8 hours between successive doses. Doses above 300 mg/day should not be used. *Zyban* should be swallowed whole, not crushed, divided, or chewed.

Treatment with *Zyban* should be initiated while the patient is still smoking, because approximately 1 week of treatment is required to achieve steady-state blood levels of bupropion. Patients should set a "target quit date" within the first 2 weeks of treatment with *Zyban*, generally in the second week. Treatment with *Zyban* should be continued for 7 to 12 weeks; longer treatment should be guided by the relative benefits and risks for individual patients. If a patient has not made significant progress towards abstinence by the seventh week of therapy with *Zyban*, it is unlikely that he or she will quit during that attempt, and treatment should probably be discontinued. Conversely, a patient who successfully quits after 7 to 12 weeks of treatment should be considered for ongoing therapy with *Zyban*. Dose tapering of *Zyban* is not required when discontinuing treatment. It is important that patients continue to receive counseling and support throughout treatment with *Zyban*, and for a period of time thereafter.

Maintenance – Systematic evaluation of *Zyban* 300 mg/day for maintenance therapy demonstrated that treatment for up to 6 months was efficacious. Whether to continue treatment with *Zyban* for periods longer than 12 weeks for smoking cessation must be determined for individual patients.

Combination treatment with Zyban *and a nicotine transdermal system (NTS)* – Combination treatment with *Zyban* and NTS may be prescribed for smoking cessation.

Monitoring for treatment-emergent hypertension in patients treated with the combination of *Zyban* and NTS is recommended.

➤*Hepatic function impairment:* Bupropion should be used with caution in patients with hepatic impairment (including mild-to-moderate hepatic cirrhosis), and a reduced frequency and/or dose (reduced frequency of dosing for *Zyban*) should be considered in patients with mild-to-moderate hepatic cirrhosis.

Bupropion should be used with extreme caution in patients with severe hepatic cirrhosis. The dose should not exceed the following:

Bupropion IR – 75 mg once daily.

Wellbutrin SR – 100 mg every day or 150 mg every other day.

Bupropion XL – 150 mg every other day.

Zyban – 150 mg every other day.

➤*Renal function impairment:* Bupropion should be used with caution in patients with renal function impairment, and a reduced frequency and/or dose (reduced frequency of dosing for *Zyban*) should be considered.

➤*Storage/Stability:*

Bupropion IR – Store at 15° to 25°C (59° to 77°F). Protect from light and moisture.

Wellbutrin SR and *Zyban* – Store at controlled room temperature, 20° to 25°C (68° to 77°F). Dispense in a tight, light resistant container.

Bupropion XL – Store at 25°C (77°F); excursions permitted to 15° to 30°C (59° to 86°F).

Actions

➤*Pharmacology:* Bupropion, an antidepressant of the aminoketone class or a nonnicotine aid to smoking cessation, is chemically unrelated to other known antidepressants. Bupropion is a relatively weak inhibitor of the neuronal uptake of norepinephrine, serotonin, and dopamine, and does not inhibit monoamine oxidase. While the mechanism of action of bupropion as an antidepressant or as a smoking deterrent is unknown, it is presumed that this action is mediated by noradrenergic and/or dopaminergic mechanisms.

Bupropion produces dose-related CNS-stimulant effects in animals, as evidenced by increased locomotor activity, increased rates of responding in various schedule-controlled operant behavior tasks, and, at high doses, induction of mild stereotyped behavior.

Bupropion causes convulsions in rodents and dogs at doses approximately 10-fold the dose recommended as the human antidepressant dose.

➤*Pharmacokinetics:*

Absorption – Bupropion is a racemic mixture. The pharmacologic activity and pharmacokinetics of the individual enantiomers have not been studied. Bupropion follows biphasic pharmacokinetics best described by a 2-compartment model. The steady-state plasma concentrations of bupropion are reached within 8 days.

Plasma bupropion concentrations are dose proportional following single doses of 100 to 250 mg; however, it is not known if the proportionality between dose and plasma level are maintained in chronic use.

Bupropion has not been administered IV to humans; therefore, the absolute bioavailability of bupropion tablets in humans has not been determined. However, it appears likely that only a small proportion of any orally administered dose reaches the systemic circulation intact. In rat and dog studies, the bioavailability of bupropion ranged from 5% to 20%.

In a study comparing chronic dosing with *Wellbutrin SR* tablets 150 mg twice daily to bupropion IR 100 mg 3 times daily, peak plasma concentrations of bupropion at steady state for *Wellbutrin SR* tablets were approximately 85% of those achieved with the IR formulation. There was equivalence for bupropion AUCs, and equivalence for peak plasma concentration and AUCs for all 3 of the detectable bupropion metabolites. Thus, at steady state, *Wellbutrin SR* tablets given twice daily and bupropion IR given 3 times daily are essentially bioequivalent for bupropion and the 3 quantitatively important metabolites.

In a study comparing 14-day dosing with bupropion XL 300 mg once daily to bupropion IR at 100 mg 3 times daily, equivalence was demonstrated for peak plasma concentration and AUC for bupropion and the 3 metabolites (hydroxybupropion, threohydrobupropion, and erythrohydrobupropion).

Additionally, in a study comparing 14-day dosing with bupropion XL 300 mg once daily to *Wellbutrin SR* 150 mg 2 times daily, equivalence was demonstrated for peak plasma concentration and AUC for bupropion and the 3 metabolites.

Bupropion IR: In humans, following oral administration of bupropion IR, peak plasma concentrations are usually achieved within 2 hours, followed by a biphasic decline.

Zyban and *Wellbutrin SR*: Following oral administration of *Zyban* or *Wellbutrin SR* to healthy volunteers, peak plasma concentrations of bupropion are achieved within 3 hours. The mean C_{max} values were 91 and 143 ng/mL from 2 single-dose (150 mg) studies. At steady state, the mean C_{max} following a 150 mg dose every 12 hours is 136 ng/mL.

Bupropion XL: Following oral administration of bupropion XL tablets to healthy volunteers, T_{max} for bupropion was approximately 5 hours, and food did not affect the C_{max} or AUC of bupropion.

Distribution – In vitro tests show that bupropion is 84% bound to human plasma protein at concentrations up to 200 mcg/mL. The extent of protein binding of the hydroxybupropion metabolite is similar to that of bupropion, whereas the extent of protein binding of the threohydrobupropion metabolite is about half that seen with bupropion.

The distribution phase has a mean half-life of 3 to 4 hours.

Zyban: The volume of distribution (Vss/F) estimated from a single 150 mg dose given to 17 subjects is 1950 L (20% CV).

Metabolism/Excretion – Bupropion is extensively metabolized in humans. The following 3 metabolites have been shown to be active: hydroxybupropion, which is formed via hydroxylation of the tert-butyl group of bupropion, and the amino-alcohol isomers threohydrobupropion and erythrohydrobupropion, which are formed via reduction of the carbonyl group. In vitro findings suggest that cytochrome P-450 2B6 (CYP2B6) is the principal isoenzyme involved in the formation of hydroxybupropion, while cytochrome P-450 isoenzymes are not involved in the formation of threohydrobupropion. Oxidation of the bupropion side chain results in the formation of a glycine conjugate of metachlorobenzoic acid, which then is excreted as the major urinary metabolite. The potency and toxicity of the metabolites relative to bupropion have not been fully characterized. However, it has been demonstrated in an antidepressant screening test in mice that hydroxybupropion is one-half as potent as bupropion, while threohydrobupropion and erythrohydrobupropion are 5-fold less potent than bupropion. This may be of clinical importance because their plasma concentrations are as high or higher than those of bupropion.

Bupropion and its metabolites exhibit linear kinetics following chronic administration of 300 to 450 mg/day.

In humans, peak plasma concentrations of hydroxybupropion occur approximately 3 hours after administration of bupropion IR, approximately 6 hours after *Wellbutrin SR* and *Zyban* tablets, and approximately 7 hours after administration of bupropion XL. For the IR tablets and SR tablets, peak plasma concentrations of hydroxybupropion are approximately 10 times the peak level of the parent drug at steady state. Following administration of bupropion XL, peak plasma concentrations of hydroxybupropion are approximately 7 times the peak level of the parent drug at steady state. The elimination half-life of hydroxybupropion is approximately 20 (± 5) hours, and its AUC at steady state is about 17 times that of bupropion for the IR tablets and SR tablets, and about 13 times that of bupropion for bupropion XL tablets. The times to peak concentrations for the erythrohydrobupropion and threohydrobupropion metabolites are similar to that of the hydroxybupropion metabolite. However, their elimination half-lives are longer, approximately 33 (± 10) and 37 (± 13) hours, respectively, and steady-state AUCs are 1.5 (1.4 for bupropion XL) and 7 times that of bupropion, respectively.

Following oral administration of ^{14}C-bupropion 200 mg in humans, 87% and 10% of the radioactive dose were recovered in the urine and feces, respectively. However, the fraction of the oral dose of bupropion excreted unchanged was only 0.5%, a finding consistent with the extensive metabolism of bupropion.

BUPROPION — ORAL

The mean elimination half-life (± SD) of bupropion after chronic dosing is 21 (± 9) hours.

Bupropion IR: The terminal phase has a mean half-life of 14 hours, with a range of 8 to 24 hours.

Zyban: The terminal phase has a mean half-life (± % CV) of 21 hours (± 20%). The mean (± % CV) apparent clearance (Cl/F) estimated from 2 single-dose (150 mg) studies are 135 (± 20%) and 209 L/hr (± 21%). Following chronic dosing of 150 mg of *Zyban* every 12 hours for 14 days (n = 34), the mean Cl/F at steady state was 160 L/hr (± 23%). The mean elimination half-life of *Zyban*, estimated from a series of studies, is approximately 21 hours. Estimates of the half-lives of the metabolites determined from a multiple-dose study were 20 hours (± 25%) for hydroxybupropion, 37 hours (± 35%) for threohydrobupropion, and 33 hours (± 30%) for erythrohydrobupropion. Steady-state plasma concentrations of bupropion and its metabolites are reached within 5 and 8 days, respectively.

Special populations –

Renal function impairment: The effect of renal disease on the pharmacokinetics of bupropion has not been studied. The elimination of the major metabolites of bupropion may be affected by reduced renal function.

Hepatic function impairment: The effect of hepatic function impairment on the pharmacokinetics of bupropion was characterized in 2 single-dose studies, 1 in patients with alcoholic liver disease and 1 in patients with mild-to-severe cirrhosis. The first study showed that the half-life of hydroxybupropion was significantly longer in 8 patients with alcoholic liver disease than in 8 healthy volunteers (32 ± 14 hours vs 21 ± 5 hours, respectively). Although not statistically significant, the AUCs for bupropion and hydroxybupropion were more variable and tended to be greater (by 53% to 57%) in patients with alcoholic liver disease. The differences in half-life for bupropion and the other metabolites in the 2 patient groups were minimal.

The second study showed that there were no statistically significant differences in the pharmacokinetics of bupropion and its active metabolites in 9 patients with mild-to-moderate hepatic cirrhosis compared with 8 healthy volunteers. However, more variability was observed in some of the pharmacokinetic parameters for bupropion (AUC, C_{max}, and t_{max}) and its active metabolites ($t_{1/2}$) in patients with mild-to-moderate hepatic cirrhosis. In addition, in patients with severe hepatic cirrhosis, the bupropion C_{max} and AUC were substantially increased (mean difference: approximately 70% and 3-fold, respectively) and more variable when compared with values in healthy volunteers; the mean bupropion half-life also was longer (29 hours in patients with severe hepatic cirrhosis vs 19 hours in healthy subjects). For the metabolite hydroxybupropion, the mean C_{max} was approximately 69% lower.

For the combined amino-alcohol isomers threohydrobupropion and erythrohydrobupropion, the mean C_{max} was approximately 31% lower.

The mean AUC increased about 1.5-fold (28% for *Zyban*) for hydroxybupropion and about 2.5-fold (50% for *Zyban*) for threo/erythrohydrobupropion.

The median t_{max} was observed 19 hours later for hydroxybupropion and 31 hours (21 hours later with *Zyban*) later for threo/erythrohydrobupropion. The mean half-lives for hydroxybupropion and threo/erythrohydrobupropion were increased 5- and 2-fold (2- and 4-fold respectively with *Zyban*), respectively, in patients with severe hepatic cirrhosis compared with healthy volunteers.

Contraindications

Bupropion is contraindicated in patients with a seizure disorder.

Bupropion is contraindicated in patients treated with any other form of bupropion or any other medications that contain bupropion because the incidence of seizure is dose dependent.

Bupropion is contraindicated in patients with a current or prior diagnosis of bulimia or anorexia nervosa because of a higher incidence of seizures noted in patients treated for bulimia with bupropion IR.

Bupropion is contraindicated in patients undergoing abrupt discontinuation of alcohol or sedatives (including benzodiazepines).

The coadministration of bupropion and a monoamine oxidase (MAO) inhibitor is contraindicated. Allow at least 14 days to elapse between discontinuation of an MAO inhibitor and initiation of treatment with bupropion.

Bupropion is contraindicated in patients who have shown an allergic response to bupropion or the other ingredients that make up any doseform of bupropion.

Warnings

➤*Clinical worsening and suicide risk:* Adults and children with MDD may experience worsening of their depression and/or the emergence of suicidal ideation and behavior (suicidality) or unusual changes in behavior, whether or not they are taking antidepressant medications; this risk may persist until significant remission occurs. There has been a long-standing concern that antidepressants may have a role in inducing worsening of depression and the emergence of suicidality in certain patients. Antidepressants increased the risk of suicidal thinking and behavior (suicidality) in short-term studies in children and adolescents with MDD and other psychiatric disorders. A causal role for antidepressants in inducing suicidality has been established in pediatric patients.

Closely observe all children being treated with antidepressants (for any indication) for clinical worsening, suicidality, and unusual changes in behavior, especially during the initial few months of a course of drug therapy, or at times of dose changes, increases or decreases. Such observation would generally include at least weekly face-to-face contact with patients or their family members or caregivers during the first 4 weeks of treatment, then every other week visits for the next 4 weeks, then at 12 weeks, and as clinically indicated beyond 12 weeks. Additional contact by telephone may be appropriate between face-to-face visits.

Observe adults with MDD or co-morbid depression in the setting of other psychiatric illness being treated with antidepressants similarly for clinical worsening and suicidality, especially during the initial few months of a course of drug therapy, or at times of dose changes, increases or decreases.

The following symptoms, anxiety, agitation, panic attacks, insomnia, irritability, hostility, aggressiveness, impulsivity, akathisia (pyschomotor restlessness), hypomania, and mania, have been reported in adult and pediatric patients being treated with antidepressants for MDD and other indications, psychiatric and nonpsychiatric.

Although a causal link between the emergence of such symptoms and either the worsening of depression and/or emergence of suicidal impulses has not been established, there is concern that such symptoms may represent precursors to emerging suicidality.

Consider changing the therapeutic regimen, including possibly discontinuing the medication, in patients whose depression is persistently worse, or who are experiencing emergent suicidality or symptoms that might be precursors to worsening depression or suicidality, especially if these symptoms are severe, abrupt in onset, or were not part of the patient's presenting symptoms.

Alert families and caregivers of children being treated with antidepressants for MDD or other indications, psychiatric and nonpsychiatric, about the need to monitor patients for the emergence of agitation, irritability, unusual changes in behavior, and the other symptoms described above, as well as the emergence of suicidality, and to report such symptoms immediately to health care providers. Such monitoring should include daily observation by families and caregivers. Write prescriptions for bupropion for the smallest quantity of tablets consistent with good patient management, to reduce the risk of overdose. Similarly advise families and caregivers of adults being treated for depression.

➤*Screening patients for bipolar disorder:* A major depressive episode may be the initial presentation of bipolar disorder. It generally is believed (though not established in controlled trials) that treating such an episode with an antidepressant alone may increase the likelihood of precipitation of a mixed/manic episode in patients at risk for bipolar disorder. Whether any of the symptoms described above represent such a conversion is unknown. However, prior to initiating treatment with an antidepressant, adequately screen patients with depressive symptoms to determine if they are at risk for bipolar disorder; such screening should include a detailed psychiatric history, including a family history of suicide, bipolar disorder, and depression. Note that bupropion is not approved for use in treating bipolar depression.

➤*Other bupropion medications:* Inform patients that bupropion IR, *Wellbutrin SR*, and bupropion XL, for the treatment of MDD, contain the same active ingredient that is found in *Zyban*, used as an aid to smoking-cessation treatment, and that bupropion IR, *Wellbutrin SR*, and bupropion XL should not be used in combination or with *Zyban* or any other medications that contain bupropion.

➤*Anorexia nervosa / bulimia:* Do not give with current or prior diagnosis of bulimia or anorexia nervosa because of a higher incidence of seizures noted in patients treated for bulimia with the bupropion IR.

➤*Seizures:* Bupropion is associated with a dose-related risk of seizures. Discontinue bupropion and do not restart in patients who experience a seizure while on treatment.

➤*Bupropion IR:* Given the wide variability among individuals and their capacity to metabolize and eliminate drugs this disproportionate increase in seizure incidence with dose incrementation calls for caution in dosing.

The risk of seizure appears to be strongly associated with dose. Sudden and large increments in dose may contribute to increased risk. While many seizures occurred early in the course of treatment, some seizures did occur after several weeks at fixed dose.

Dose – Data for bupropion IR revealed a seizure incidence of approximately 0.4% (ie, 13 of 3,200 patients followed prospectively) in depressed patients treated at doses in a range of 300 to 450 mg/day.

This seizure incidence (0.4%) may exceed that of some other marketed antidepressants by as much as 4–fold. This relative risk is only an approximate estimate because no direct comparative studies have been conducted.

Additional data accumulated for bupropion IR suggested that the estimated seizure incidence increases almost 10-fold between 450 and 600 mg/day, which is twice the usually required daily dose (300 mg) and one and one-third the maximum recommended daily dose (450 mg) of bupropion IR (twice the usual adult dose and one and one-half the maximum recommended daily dose [400 mg] of Wellbutrin SR and twice the usual adult dose and one and one-third the maximum recommended daily dose [450 mg] of bupropion XL). This disproportionate increase in seizure incidence with dose incrementation calls for caution in dosing.

➤*Wellbutrin SR*:

Dose – At doses of *Wellbutrin SR* up to a dose of 300 mg/day, the incidence of seizure is approximately 0.1% and increases to approximately 0.4% at the maximum recommended dose of 400 mg/day.

The 450 mg/day upper limit of this dose range is close to the currently recommended maximum dose of 400 mg/day for *Wellbutrin SR* tablets. This seizure incidence (0.4%) may exceed that of other marketed antidepressants and *Wellbutrin SR* tablets up to 300 mg/day by as much as 4-fold. This relative risk is only an approximate estimate because no direct comparative studies have been conducted.

BUPROPION — ORAL

Data for *Wellbutrin SR* tablets revealed a seizure incidence of approximately 0.1% (3 of 3,100 patients followed prospectively) in patients treated at doses in a range of 100 to 300 mg/day. It is not possible to know if the lower seizure incidence observed in this study involving *Wellbutrin SR* resulted from the different formulation or the lower dose used. However, as noted previously, the IR and SR formulations are bioequivalent with regard to rate and extent of absorption during steady state (the most pertinent condition to estimating seizure incidence), because most observed seizures occur under steady-state conditions.

➤*Bupropion XL:* As bupropion XL and *Wellbutrin SR* are bioequivalent to bupropion IR, the seizure incidence with bupropion XL, while not formally evaluated in clinical trials, may be similar to that presented for bupropion IR and *Wellbutrin SR*.

➤*Zyban:* Because the use of bupropion is associated with a dose-dependent risk of seizures, clinicians should not prescribe doses higher than 300 mg/day for smoking cessation.

Dose – For smoking cessation, do not use doses higher than 300 mg/day. The seizure rate associated with doses of sustained-release bupropion up to 300 mg/day is approximately 0.1%. This incidence was prospectively determined during an 8-week treatment exposure in approximately 3,100 depressed patients.

The risk of seizures also is related to patient factors, clinical situations, and concurrent medications, which must be considered in selection of patients for therapy with bupropion.

➤*Patient factors:* Predisposing factors that may increase the risk of seizure with bupropion use include history of head trauma or prior seizure, CNS tumor, the presence of severe hepatic cirrhosis, and concomitant medications that lower seizure threshold.

➤*Clinical situations:* Circumstances associated with an increased seizure risk include, among others, excessive use of alcohol or sedatives (including benzodiazepines); addiction to opiates, cocaine, or stimulants; use of over-the-counter stimulants and anorectics; and diabetes treated with oral hypoglycemics or insulin.

➤*Concomitant medications:* Many medications (eg, antipsychotics, antidepressants, theophylline, systemic steroids) are known to lower seizure threshold.

➤*Recommendations for reducing the risk of seizure:* Use extreme caution when bupropion is administered to patients with a history of seizure, cranial trauma, or other predisposition(s) toward seizure, or prescribed with other agents (eg, antipsychotics, other antidepressants, theophylline, systemic steroids) that lower seizure threshold.

Retrospective analysis of clinical experience gained during the development of bupropion suggests that the risk of seizure may be minimized by the following:

Bupropion IR
- The total daily dose of bupropion IR does not exceed 450 mg.
- The daily dose is administered 3 times daily, with each single dose not to exceed 150 mg to avoid high peak concentrations of bupropion and/or its metabolites.
- The rate of incrementation of dose is very gradual.

Wellbutrin SR
- The total daily dose of *Wellbutrin SR* tablets does not exceed 400 mg.
- The daily dose is administered twice daily.
- The rate of incrementation of dose is gradual.
- No single dose should exceed 200 mg to avoid high peak concentrations of bupropion and/or its metabolites.

Bupropion XL
- The total daily dose of bupropion XL tablets does not exceed 450 mg.
- The rate of incrementation of dose is gradual.

Zyban
- The total daily dose of *Zyban* does not exceed 300 mg (the maximum recommended dose for smoking cessation).
- The recommended daily dose for most patients (300 mg/day) is administered in divided doses (150 mg twice daily).
- No single dose should exceed 150 mg to avoid high peak concentrations of bupropion and/or its metabolites.

➤*Hypersensitivity reactions:* Anaphylactoid/anaphylactic reactions characterized by symptoms such as pruritus, urticaria, angioedema, and dyspnea requiring medical treatment have been reported in clinical trials with bupropion. In clinical trials with *Zyban*, the reported rate was 1 to 3 per thousand. In addition, there have been rare spontaneous postmarketing reports of erythema multiforme, Stevens-Johnson syndrome, and anaphylactic shock associated with bupropion. A patient should stop taking bupropion and consult a doctor if experiencing allergic or anaphylactoid/anaphylactic reactions (eg, skin rash, pruritus, hives, chest pain, edema, shortness of breath) during treatment.

Arthralgia, myalgia, and fever with rash and other symptoms suggestive of delayed hypersensitivity have been reported in association with bupropion. These symptoms may resemble serum sickness.

➤*Renal function impairment:* No studies have been conducted in patients with renal impairment.

Use bupropion with caution in patients with renal impairment, and consider a reduced frequency and/or dose (reduced frequency with *Zyban*) as bupropion and its metabolites may accumulate in such patients to a greater extent than usual. Closely monitor the patient for possible adverse effects that could indicate high drug or metabolite levels.

➤*Hepatic function impairment:* See Administration and Dosage for more information.

Closely monitor all patients with hepatic impairment for possible adverse effects that could indicate high drug and metabolite levels.

Hepatotoxicity – In rats receiving large doses of bupropion chronically, there was an increase in incidence of hepatic hyperplastic nodules and hepatocellular hypertrophy. In dogs receiving large doses of bupropion chronically, various histologic changes were seen in the liver, and laboratory tests suggesting mild hepatocellular injury were noted.

➤*Mutagenesis:* Bupropion produced a positive response (2 to 3 times control mutation rate) in 2 of 5 strains in the Ames bacterial mutagenicity test and an increase in chromosomal aberrations in 1 of 3 in vivo rat bone marrow cytogenetic studies.

Bupropion produced, at a high oral dose (300 mg/kg, but not 100 or 200 mg/kg), a low incidence of chromosomal aberrations in rats. The relevance of these results in estimating the risk of human exposure to therapeutic doses is unknown.

➤*Elderly:* A single-dose, pharmacokinetic study demonstrated that the disposition of bupropion and its metabolites in elderly subjects was similar to that of younger subjects; however, another pharmacokinetic study, single and multiple dose, has suggested that elderly individuals are at increased risk for accumulation of bupropion and its metabolites.

Bupropion is extensively metabolized in the liver to active metabolites, which are further metabolized and excreted by the kidneys. The risk of toxic reaction to this drug may be greater in patients with impaired renal function. Because elderly patients are more likely to have decreased renal function, take care in dose selection; it may be useful to monitor renal function.

➤*Pregnancy: Category C.* There are no adequate and well-controlled studies in pregnant women.

Pregnancy registry – To monitor fetal outcomes of pregnant women exposed to bupropion, GlaxoSmithKline maintains a Bupropion Pregnancy Registry. Health care providers are encouraged to register patients by calling (800) 336-2176.

Labor and delivery – The effect of bupropion on labor and delivery in humans is unknown.

➤*Lactation:* Like many other drugs, bupropion and its metabolites are secreted in human milk. Because of the potential for serious adverse reactions in breast-feeding infants from bupropion, a decision should be made whether to discontinue breast-feeding or to discontinue the drug, taking into account the importance of the drug to the mother.

➤*Children:* The safety and efficacy of bupropion in children have not been established. Anyone considering the use of bupropion in a child or adolescent must balance the potential risks with clinical need.

See the Warning box for more information.

Precautions

➤*Monitoring:* Closely monitor all patients with hepatic function impairment for possible adverse effects that could indicate high drug and metabolite levels. Monitoring of blood pressure is recommended in patients who receive the combination of bupropion and nicotine replacement.

➤*CNS effects:*

Bupropion IR – A substantial proportion of patients treated with bupropion IR experiences some degree of increased restlessness, agitation, anxiety, and insomnia, especially shortly after initiation of treatment. In clinical studies, these symptoms were sometimes of sufficient magnitude to require treatment with sedative/hypnotic drugs. In approximately 2% of patients, symptoms were sufficiently severe to require discontinuation of treatment with bupropion IR.

Wellbutrin SR – Patients in placebo-controlled trials with *Wellbutrin SR* experienced agitation, anxiety, and insomnia as shown in the following table.

Incidence of Agitation, Anxiety, and Insomnia in Placebo-Controlled Trials with *Wellbutrin SR*

Adverse reaction	*Wellbutrin SR* 300 mg/day (n = 376)	*Wellbutrin SR* 400 mg/day (n = 114)	Placebo (n = 385)
Agitation	3%	9%	2%
Anxiety	5%	6%	3%
Insomnia	11%	16%	6%

In clinical studies, these symptoms were sometimes of sufficient magnitude to require treatment with sedative/hypnotic drugs.

Symptoms were sufficiently severe to require discontinuation of treatment in 1% and 2.6% of patients treated with 300 and 400 mg/day, respectively, of *Wellbutrin SR* and 0.8% of patients treated with placebo.

➤*Insomnia:*

Zyban – In the dose-response, smoking-cessation trial, 29% of patients treated with 150 mg/day of *Zyban* and 35% of patients treated with 300 mg/day of *Zyban* experienced insomnia, compared with 21% of placebo-treated patients. Symptoms were sufficiently severe to require discontinuation of treatment in 0.6% of patients treated with *Zyban* and none of the patients treated with placebo.

BUPROPION — ORAL

In the comparative trial, 40% of the patients treated with 300 mg/day of *Zyban*, 28% of the patients treated with 21 mg/day of NTS, and 45% of the patients treated with the combination of *Zyban* and NTS experienced insomnia compared with 18% of placebo-treated patients. Symptoms were sufficiently severe to require discontinuation of treatment in 0.8% of patients treated with *Zyban* and none of the patients in the other 3 treatment groups.

Insomnia may be minimized by avoiding bedtime doses and, if necessary, reduction in dose.

➤*Neuropsychiatric phenomena:* Depressed patients treated with bupropion have been reported to show a variety of neuropsychiatric signs and symptoms, including delusions, hallucinations, psychosis, concentration disturbance, paranoia, and confusion. In some cases, these symptoms abated upon dose reduction and/or withdrawal of treatment.

➤*Psychosis or mania:* Antidepressants can precipitate manic episodes in bipolar disorder (bipolar manic-depressive) patients during the depressed phases of their illnesses and may activate latent psychosis in other susceptible patients.

Bupropion is expected to pose similar risks.

➤*Depression and nicotine withdrawal:* Depressed mood may be a symptom of nicotine withdrawal. Depression, rarely including suicidal ideation, has been reported in patients undergoing a smoking cessation attempt.

➤*Altered appetite and weight:*

Bupropion IR – A weight loss of more than 5 lbs (2.3 kg) occurred in 28% of patients receiving bupropion IR. This incidence is approximately double that seen in comparable patients treated with tricyclics or placebo. Furthermore, while 34.5% of patients receiving tricyclic antidepressants gained weight, only 9.4% of patients treated with bupropion IR did. Consequently, if weight loss is a major presenting sign of a patient's depressive illness, consider the anorectic and/or weight-reducing potential of bupropion IR.

Wellbutrin SR – In placebo-controlled studies using *Wellbutrin SR*, patients experienced weight gain or weight loss as shown in the following table.

Incidence of Weight Gain and Weight Loss in Placebo-Controlled Trials of *Wellbutrin SR*

Weight change	*Wellbutrin SR* 300 mg/day (n = 339)	*Wellbutrin SR* 400 mg/day (n = 112)	Placebo (n = 347)
Gained > 5 lbs	3%	2%	4%
Lost > 5 lbs	14%	19%	6%

In studies conducted with bupropion IR, 35% of patients receiving tricyclic antidepressants gained weight, compared with 9% of patients treated with bupropion IR. If weight loss is a major presenting sign of a patient's depressive illness, consider the anorectic and/or weight-reducing potential of bupropion.

➤*Cardiovascular effects:* In clinical practice, hypertension, in some cases severe, requiring acute treatment, has been reported in patients receiving bupropion alone and in combination with nicotine-replacement therapy. These events have been observed in patients with and without evidence of pre-existing hypertension.

➤*Drug abuse and dependence:*

Controlled substance class – Bupropion is not a controlled substance.

Abuse potential – Controlled clinical studies of bupropion IR conducted in healthy volunteers, in subjects with a history of multiple drug abuse, and in depressed patients showed some increase in motor activity and agitation/excitement.

There have been few reported cases of drug dependence and withdrawal symptoms associated with bupropion IR.

In human studies of abuse liability, individuals experienced with drugs of abuse reported that bupropion produced a feeling of euphoria and desirability. In these subjects, a single dose of bupropion 400 mg (1.33 times the recommended daily dose of *Zyban*) produced mild amphetamine-like activity as compared with placebo on the Morphine-Benzedrine Subscale of the Addiction Research Center Inventories (ARCI), which is indicative of euphorigenic properties, and a score intermediate between placebo and amphetamine on the Liking Scale of the ARCI. These scales measure general feelings of euphoria and drug desirability.

Findings in clinical trials, however, are not known to reliably predict the abuse potential of drugs. Nonetheless, evidence from single-dose studies does suggest that the recommended daily dosage of bupropion when administered in divided doses is not likely to be especially reinforcing to amphetamine or stimulant abusers. However, higher doses that could not be tested because of the risk of seizure might be modestly attractive to those who abuse stimulant drugs.

Zyban: *Zyban* is likely to have a low abuse potential.

When evaluating the desirability of including the drug in smoking cessation programs of individual patients, keep in mind the possibility that bupropion may induce dependence.

➤*Photosensitivity:* Photosensitization may occur; therefore, caution patients to take protective measures (eg, sunscreens, protective clothing) against exposure to ultraviolet light or sunlight until tolerance is determined.

Drug Interactions

Bupropion Drug Interactions

Precipitant drug	Object drug[a]		Description
Amantadine Levodopa	Bupropion	⬆	There is a higher incidence of adverse experiences with concurrent use of these agents. Use small initial doses and small gradual dose increases of bupropion.
Carbamazepine	Bupropion	⬇	Serum concentrations of bupropion may be decreased, decreasing the pharmacologic effects. Adjust therapy as needed.
MAOIs	Bupropion	⬆	Animal data demonstrate bupropion's acute toxicity is enhanced by phenelzine. Coadministration is contraindicated. Allow at least 14 days between discontinuation of an MAOI and initiation of bupropion.
Nicotine replacement	Bupropion	⬆	Coadministration may cause hypertension. Monitor blood pressure.
Ritonavir	Bupropion	⬆	Large increases in serum bupropion concentrations may occur, increasing the risk of bupropion toxicity. Avoid coadministration.
Bupropion	Alcohol	⬆	There have been rare reports of adverse neuropsychiatric reactions or reduced alcohol tolerance. Minimize or avoid consumption of alcohol during treatment with bupropion.
Bupropion	Drugs metabolized by CYP450 2D6 (eg, SSRIs, many TCAs, beta-blockers, type 1C antiarrhythmics, antipsychotics)	⬆	Bupropion and hydroxybupropion are inhibitors of the CYP2D6 isoenzyme. If bupropion is added to the treatment regimen of a patient receiving a drug metabolized by CYP2D6, consider a dose reduction in the original medication.
Bupropion	Warfarin	⬆	Altered PT or INR are infrequently associated with hemorrhagic or thrombotic complications when bupropion is coadministered with warfarin.

[a] ⬆ = Object drug increased. ⬇ = Object drug decreased.

Adverse Reactions

Adverse reactions with bupropion IR – Adverse reactions commonly encountered in patients treated with bupropion hydrochloride IR tablets are agitation, dry mouth, insomnia, headache/migraine, nausea/vomiting, constipation, and tremor.

Discontinuation of treatment: Adverse reactions were sufficiently troublesome to cause discontinuation of treatment with bupropion IR in approximately 10% of the 2,400 patients and volunteers who participated in clinical trials during the product's initial development. The more common reactions causing discontinuation include neuropsychiatric disturbances (3%), primarily agitation and abnormalities in mental status; GI disturbances (2.1%), primarily nausea and vomiting; neurological disturbances (1.7%), primarily seizures, headaches, and sleep disturbances; and dermatologic problems (1.4%), primarily rashes. It is important to note, however, that many of these reactions occurred at doses that exceed the recommended daily dose.

Bupropion IR Adverse Reactions (≥ 1%)[a]

Adverse reaction	Bupropion IR (n = 323)	Placebo patients (n = 185)
Cardiovascular		
Cardiac arrhythmias	5.3%	4.3%
Dizziness	22.3%	16.2%
Hypertension	4.3%	1.6%
Hypotension	2.5%	2.2%
Palpitations	3.7%	2.2%
Syncope	1.2%	0.5%
Tachycardia	10.8%	8.6%
CNS		
Akathisia	1.5%	1.1%
Akinesia/bradykinesia	8%	8.6%

BUPROPION — ORAL

Bupropion IR Adverse Reactions (≥ 1%)[a]

Adverse reaction	Bupropion IR (n = 323)	Placebo patients (n = 185)
Cutaneous temperature disturbance	1.9%	1.6%
Headache/ migraine	25.7%	22.2%
Impaired sleep quality	4%	1.6%
Increased salivary flow	3.4%	3.8%
Insomnia	18.6%	15.7%
Muscle spasms	1.9%	3.2%
Pseudoparkin sonism	1.5%	1.6%
Sedation	19.8%	19.5%
Sensory disturbance	4%	3.2%
Tremor	21.1%	7.6%
Dermatologic		
Excessive sweating	22.3%	14.6%
Pruritus	2.2%	0%
Rash	8%	6.5%
GI		
Anorexia	18.3%	18.4%
Appetite increase	3.7%	2.2%
Constipation	26%	17.3%
Diarrhea	6.8%	8.6%
Dry mouth	27.6%	18.4%
Dyspepsia	3.1%	2.2%
Nausea/ vomiting	22.9%	18.9%
Weight gain	13.6%	22.7%
Weight loss	23.2%	23.2%
GU		
Impotence	3.4%	3.1%
Menstrual complaints	4.7%	1.1%
Urinary frequency	2.5%	2.2%
Urinary retention	1.9%	2.2%
Musculoskeletal		
Arthritis	3.1%	2.7%
Psychiatric		
Agitation	31.9%	22.2%
Anxiety	3.1%	1.1%
Confusion	8.4%	4.9%
Decreased libido	3.1%	1.6%
Delusions	1.2%	1.1%
Disturbed concentration	3.1%	3.8%
Euphoria	1.2%	0.5%
Hostility	5.6%	3.8%
Respiratory		
Upper respiratory complaints	5%	11.4%
Special senses		
Auditory disturbance	5.3%	3.2%
Blurred vision	14.6%	10.3%
Gustatory disturbance	3.1%	1.1%
Miscellaneous		
Fatigue	5%	8.6%
Fever/chills	1.2%	0.5%

[a] Reactions reported by at least 1% of patients receiving bupropion IR are included.

➤*Other reactions observed during the development of bupropion IR:*

Cardiovascular – Edema (at least 1%). Chest pain, electrocardiogram (ECG) abnormalities (premature beats and nonspecific ST-T changes), and shortness of breath/dyspnea (0.1% to 1%). Flushing, pallor, phlebitis, and myocardial infarction (less than 0.1%).

CNS – Ataxia/incoordination, seizure, myoclonus, dyskinesia, dystonia (at least 1%); mydriasis, vertigo, dysarthria (0.1% to 1%); electroencephalogram (EEG) abnormality, abnormal neurological exam, impaired attention, sciatica, aphasia (less than 0.1%).

Seizures: During the initial development, 25 among approximately 2,400 patients treated with bupropion IR experienced seizures. At the time of seizure, 7 patients were receiving daily doses of 450 mg or less for an incidence of 0.33% within the recommended dose range. Twelve patients experienced seizures at 600 mg/day (2.3% incidence); 6 additional patients had seizures at daily doses between 600 and 900 mg (2.8% incidence).

A separate, prospective study was conducted to determine the incidence of seizure during an 8-week treatment exposure in approximately 3,200 additional patients who received daily doses of up to 450 mg. Patients were permitted to continue treatment beyond 8 weeks if clinically indicated. Eight seizures occurred during the initial 8-week treatment period, and 5 seizures were reported in patients continuing treatment beyond 8 weeks, resulting in a total seizure incidence of 0.4%.

The risk of seizure appears to be strongly associated with dose. Sudden and large increments in dose may contribute to increased risk. While many seizures occurred early in the course of treatment, some seizures did occur after several weeks at fixed dose. Discontinue and do not restart bupropion IR in patients who experience a seizure while on treatment.

CNS effects: See Precautions for more information.

Dermatologic – Nonspecific rashes (at least 1%); alopecia, dry skin (0.1% to 1%); change in hair color, hirsutism, acne (less than 0.1%).

Endocrine – Gynecomastia (0.1% to 1%); glycosuria, hormone level change (less than 0.1%).

GI – Stomatitis (at least 1%); bruxism, dysphagia, gum irritation, oral edema, thirst disturbance, toothache (0.1% to 1%); colitis, GI bleeding, glossitis, intestinal perforation, rectal complaints, stomach ulcer (less than 0.1%).

Altered appetite and weight: See Precautions for more information.

GU – Nocturia (at least 1%); vaginal irritation, testicular swelling, urinary tract infection, painful erection, retarded ejaculation (0.1% to 1%); dysuria, enuresis, urinary incontinence, menopause, ovarian disorder, pelvic infection, cystitis, dyspareunia, painful ejaculation (less than 0.1%).

Hematologic/Lymphatic – Lymphadenopathy, anemia, pancytopenia (less than 0.1%).

Hepatic – Liver damage/jaundice (0.1% to 1%).

Hypersensitivity – See Warnings for more information.

Musculoskeletal – Musculoskeletal chest pain (less than 0.1%).

Psychiatric – Mania/hypomania, increased libido, hallucinations, decrease in sexual function, depression (at least 1%); memory impairment, depersonalization, psychosis, dysphoria, mood instability, paranoia, formal thought disorder, frigidity (0.1% to 1%); suicidal ideation (less than 0.1%).

Respiratory – Bronchitis, shortness of breath/dyspnea (0.1% to 1%); epistaxis, rate or rhythm disorder, pneumonia, pulmonary embolism (less than 0.1%).

Special senses – Visual disturbance (0.1% to 1%); diplopia (less than 0.1%).

Miscellaneous – Flu-like symptoms (at least 1%); nonspecific pain (0.1% to 1%); body odor, surgically related pain, infection, medication reaction, overdose (less than 0.1%).

➤*Postmarketing:* Voluntary reports of adverse reactions temporally associated with bupropion that have been received since market introduction and which may have no causal relationship with the drug include the following:

Cardiovascular – Hypertension (in some cases severe), orthostatic hypotension, third-degree heart block.

See Precautions for more information.

CNS – Coma, delirium, dream abnormalities, paresthesia, unmasking of tardive dyskinesia.

Dermatologic – Stevens-Johnson syndrome, angioedema, exfoliative dermatitis, urticaria.

Endocrine – Syndrome of inappropriate antidiuretic hormone secretion, hyperglycemia, hypoglycemia.

GI – Esophagitis.

Hematologic/Lymphatic – Ecchymosis, leukocytosis, leukopenia, thrombocytopenia. Altered PT and/or INR, infrequently associated with hemorrhagic or thrombotic complications, were observed when bupropion was coadministered with warfarin.

Hepatic – Hepatitis, liver damage.

Musculoskeletal – Arthralgia, myalgia, muscle rigidity/fever/ rhabdomyolysis, muscle weakness.

Special senses – Tinnitus.

Miscellaneous – Arthralgia, myalgia, and fever with rash and other symptoms suggestive of delayed hypersensitivity. These symptoms may resemble serum sickness.

➤*Wellbutrin SR:*

Discontinuation of treatment with Wellbutrin SR: In placebo-controlled clinical trials, 9% and 11% of patients treated with 300 and 400 mg/day, respectively, of *Wellbutrin SR* tablets and 4% of patients treated with placebo discontinued treatment because of adverse reactions. The specific adverse reactions in these trials that led to discontinuation in at least 1% of patients treated with 300 or 400 mg/day of *Wellbutrin SR* tablets and at a rate at least twice the placebo rate are listed in the following table.

BUPROPION — ORAL

Treatment Discontinuation of *Wellbutrin SR*			
Adverse reaction	*Wellbutrin SR* 300 mg/day (n = 376)	*Wellbutrin SR* 400 mg/day (n = 114)	Placebo (n = 385)
Rash	2.4%	0.9%	0%
Nausea	0.8%	1.8%	0.3%
Agitation	0.3%	1.8%	0.3%
Migraine	0%	1.8%	0.3%

In clinical trials with bupropion IR, 10% of patients and volunteers discontinued because of an adverse reaction. Events resulting in discontinuation, in addition to those listed above for *Wellbutrin SR*, include vomiting, seizures, and sleep disturbances.

Adverse reactions occurring at an incidence of 1% or more among patients treated with Wellbutrin SR tablets:

Wellbutrin SR Adverse Reactions (≥ 1%)[a]			
Adverse reaction	*Wellbutrin SR* 300 mg/day (n = 376)	*Wellbutrin SR* 400 mg/day (n = 114)	Placebo (n = 385)
Cardiovascular			
Flushing	1%	4%	-
Hot flashes	1%	3%	1%
Migraine	1%	4%	1%
Palpitation	2%	6%	2%
CNS			
Agitation	3%	9%	2%
Anxiety	5%	6%	3%
CNS stimulation	2%	1%	1%
Dizziness	7%	11%	5%
Headache	26%	25%	23%
Insomnia	11%	16%	6%
Irritability	3%	2%	2%
Memory decreased	-	3%	1%
Nervousness	5%	3%	3%
Paresthesia	1%	2%	1%
Somnolence	2%	3%	2%
Tremor	6%	3%	1%
Dermatologic			
Pruritus	2%	4%	2%
Rash	5%	4%	1%
Sweating	6%	5%	2%
Urticaria	2%	1%	0%
GI			
Abdominal pain	3%	9%	2%
Anorexia	5%	3%	2%
Constipation	10%	5%	7%
Diarrhea	5%	7%	6%
Dry mouth	17%	24%	7%
Dysphagia	0%	2%	0%
Nausea	13%	18%	8%
Vomiting	4%	2%	2%
GU			
Arthralgia	1%	4%	1%
Arthritis	0%	2%	0%
Urinary frequency	2%	5%	2%
Urinary tract infection	1%	0%	-
Urinary urgency	-	2%	0%
Vaginal hemorrhage[b]	0%	2%	-
Musculoskeletal			
Myalgia	2%	6%	3%
Twitch	1%	2%	-
Respiratory			
Increased cough	1%	2%	1%
Pharyngitis	3%	11%	2%
Sinusitis	3%	1%	2%
Special senses			
Amblyopia	3%	2%	2%
Taste perversion	2%	4%	-
Tinnitus	6%	6%	2%
Miscellaneous			
Asthenia	2%	4%	2%
Chest pain	3%	4%	1%
Fever	1%	2%	-
Infection	8%	9%	6%
Pain	2%	3%	2%

[a] Adverse reactions that occurred in at least 1% of patients treated with 300 or 400 mg/day of *Wellbutrin SR* tablets, but equally or more frequently in the placebo group, were abnormal dreams, accidental injury, acne, appetite increased, back pain, bronchitis, dysmenorrhea, dyspepsia, flatulence, flu syndrome, hypertension, neck pain, respiratory disorder, rhinitis, and tooth disorder.
[b] Incidence based on the number of women.
- Hyphen denotes adverse reactions occurring in more than 0 but less than 0.5% of patients.

Incidence of commonly observed adverse reactions in controlled clinical trials: Adverse reactions from the previous table occurring in at least 5% of patients treated with *Wellbutrin SR* tablets and at a rate at least twice the placebo rate are listed below for the 300 and 400 mg/day dose groups.

- *Wellbutrin SR* 300 mg/day – Anorexia, dry mouth, rash, sweating, tinnitus, and tremor.
- *Wellbutrin SR* 400 mg/day – Abdominal pain, agitation, anxiety, dizziness, dry mouth, insomnia, myalgia, nausea, palpitation, pharyngitis, sweating, tinnitus, and urinary frequency.

➤*Other adverse reactions:*

Cardiovascular – Flushing, migraine, postural hypotension, stroke, tachycardia, vasodilation (0.1% to 1%); syncope (less than 0.1%).
Also observed: CV disorder, complete atrioventricular block, extrasystoles, hypotension, hypertension (in some cases severe), MI, phlebitis, and pulmonary embolism (PE).

CNS –
Seizures: See Warnings for more information.

See Warnings for more information.
Agitation and insomnia: Symptoms were sufficiently severe to require discontinuation of treatment in 1% and 2.6% of patients treated with 300 and 400 mg/day, respectively, of *Wellbutrin SR* and 0.8% of patients treated with placebo. Agitation, depression, irritability (at least 1%); abnormal coordination, CNS stimulation, confusion, decreased libido, decreased memory, depersonalization, dysphoria, emotional lability, hostility, hyperkinesia, hypertonia, hypesthesia, paresthesia, suicidal ideation, vertigo (0.1% to 1%); amnesia, ataxia, derealization, hypomania (less than 0.1%).
Also observed: Abnormal EEG, akinesia, aphasia, coma, delirium, delusions, dysarthria, dyskinesia, dystonia, euphoria, extrapyramidal syndrome, hallucinations, hypokinesia, increased libido, manic reaction, neuralgia, neuropathy, paranoid reaction, unmasking tardive dyskinesia.

Dermatologic – Sweating (at least 1%); acne, dry skin (0.1% to 1%); maculopapular rash (less than 0.1%).
Also observed: Alopecia, angioedema, exfoliative dermatitis, hirsutism.

Endocrine –
Also observed: Hyperglycemia, hypoglycemia, syndrome of inappropriate antidiuretic hormone.

GI – Dyspepsia, flatulence, vomiting (at least 1%); bruxism, dysphagia, gastric reflux, gingivitis, glossitis, increased salivation, mouth ulcers, stomatitis, thirst (0.1% to 1%); edema of tongue (less than 0.1%).
Also observed: Colitis, esophagitis, gastrointestinal hemorrhage, gum hemorrhage, intestinal perforation, pancreatitis, stomach ulcer, stool abnormality.

GU – Urinary frequency (at least 1%); impotence, polyuria, prostate disorder, urinary urgency (0.1% to 1%).
Also observed: Abnormal ejaculation, cystitis, dyspareunia, dysuria, gynecomastia, menopause, painful erection, salpingitis, urinary incontinence, urinary retention, urinary tract disorder, vaginitis.

Hematologic/Lymphatic – Ecchymosis (0.1% to 1%).
Also observed: Anemia, leukocytosis, leukopenia, lymphadenopathy, pancytopenia, thrombocytopenia; altered PT and/or INR, infrequently associated with hemorrhagic or thrombotic complications, were observed when bupropion was coadministered with warfarin.

Hepatic – Abnormal liver function, jaundice (0.1% to 1%).
Also observed: Hepatitis, liver damage.

Hypersensitivity – Anaphylactoid/anaphylactic reactions characterized by symptoms such as pruritus, urticaria, angioedema, and dyspnea requiring medical treatment have been reported with bupropion. In clinical trials with *Zyban*, the rate 1 to 3 per thousand. In addition, there have been rare spontaneous postmarketing reports of erythema multiforme, Stevens-Johnson syndrome, and anaphylactic shock associated with bupropion.

Metabolic/Nutritional –
Altered appetite and weight: Edema, increased weight, and peripheral edema (0.1% to 1%).

See Precautions for more information.

Incidence of Weight Gain and Weight Loss in Placebo-Controlled Trials			
Weight change	*Wellbutrin SR* 300 mg/day (n = 339)	*Wellbutrin SR* 400 mg/day (n = 112)	Placebo (n = 347)
Gained > 5 lbs	3%	2%	4%
Lost > 5 lbs	14%	19%	6%

BUPROPION — ORAL

Also observed: Glycosuria.

Musculoskeletal – Leg cramps, twitching (0.1% to 1%).
Also observed: Arthritis, muscle rigidity/fever/rhabdomyolysis, muscle weakness.

Respiratory – Bronchospasm (less than 0.1%).
Also observed: Pneumonia.

Special senses – Amblyopia (at least 1%); accommodation abnormality, dry eye (0.1% to 1%).
Also observed: Deafness, diplopia, mydriasis.

Miscellaneous – Asthenia, fever, headache (at least 1%); back pain, chills, facial edema, inguinal hernia, musculoskeletal chest pain, pain, photosensitivity (0.1% to 1%). Malaise (less than 0.1%).
Also observed: Arthralgia, myalgia, fever with rash and other symptoms suggestive of delayed hypersensitivity. These symptoms may resemble serum sickness.

➤*Adverse reactions with Zyban:*
Discontinuation of treatment with Zyban: Adverse reactions were sufficiently troublesome to cause discontinuation of treatment in 8% of the 706 patients treated with *Zyban* and 5% of the 313 patients treated with placebo. The more common reactions leading to discontinuation of treatment with *Zyban* included nervous system disturbances (3.4%), primarily tremors, and skin disorders (2.4%), primarily rashes.
Incidence of commonly observed adverse reactions: The most commonly observed adverse reactions consistently associated with the use of *Zyban* were dry mouth and insomnia. The most commonly observed adverse reactions were defined as those that consistently occurred at a rate of 5 percentage points higher than that for placebo across clinical studies.
Dose dependency of adverse reactions: The incidence of dry mouth and insomnia may be related to the dose of *Zyban*. The occurrence of these adverse reactions may be minimized by reducing the dose of *Zyban*. In addition, insomnia may be minimized by avoiding bedtime doses.
Adverse reactions occurring at an incidence of 1% or more among patients treated with Zyban:

Zyban Adverse Reactions in the Dose-Response Trial (≥ 1%)[a]

Adverse reaction	*Zyban* 100 to 300 mg/day (n = 461)	Placebo (n = 150)
Cardiovascular		
Hot flashes	1%	0%
Hypertension	1%	< 1%
CNS		
Dizziness	8%	7%
Insomnia	31%	21%
Somnolence	2%	1%
Thinking abnormality	1%	0%
Tremor	2%	1%
Dermatologic		
Dry skin	2%	0%
Pruritus	3%	< 1%
Rash	3%	< 1%
Urticaria	1%	0%
GI		
Anorexia	1%	< 1%
Dry mouth	11%	5%
Increased appetite	2%	< 1%
Musculoskeletal		
Arthralgia	4%	3%
Myalgia	2%	1%
Respiratory		
Bronchitis	2%	0%
Special senses		
Taste perversion	2%	< 1%
Miscellaneous		
Allergic reaction	1%	0%
Neck pain	2%	< 1%

[a] Selected adverse reactions with an incidence of at least 1% of patients treated with *Zyban* and more frequent than in the placebo group.

Zyban Adverse Reactions in the Comparative Trial (≥ 1%)[a]

Adverse reaction (COSTART Term)	*Zyban* 300 mg/day (n = 243)	NTS 21 mg/day (n = 243)	*Zyban* and NTS (n = 244)	Placebo (n = 159)
Cardiovascular				
Hypertension	1%	< 1%	2%	0%
Palpitations	2%	0%	1%	0%
CNS				
Anxiety	8%	6%	9%	6%
Disturbed concentration	9%	3%	9%	4%
Dizziness	10%	2%	8%	6%
Dream abnormality	5%	18%	13%	3%
Dysphoria	< 1%	1%	2%	1%
Insomnia	40%	28%	45%	18%
Nervousness	4%	< 1%	2%	2%
Tremor	1%	< 1%	2%	0%
Dermatologic				
Application site reaction[b]	11%	17%	15%	7%
Pruritus	3%	1%	5%	1%
Rash	4%	3%	3%	2%
Urticaria	2%	0%	2%	0%
GI				
Abdominal pain	3%	4%	1%	1%
Anorexia	3%	1%	5%	1%
Constipation	8%	4%	9%	3%
Diarrhea	4%	4%	3%	1%
Dry mouth	10%	4%	9%	4%
Mouth ulcer	2%	1%	1%	1%
Nausea	9%	7%	11%	4%
Thirst	< 1%	< 1%	2%	0%
Musculoskeletal				
Arthralgia	5%	3%	3%	2%
Myalgia	4%	3%	5%	3%
Respiratory				
Dyspnea	1%	0%	2%	1%
Epistaxis	2%	1%	1%	0%
Increased cough	3%	5%	< 1%	1%
Pharyngitis	3%	2%	3%	0%
Rhinitis	12%	11%	9%	8%
Sinusitis	2%	2%	2%	1%
Special senses				
Taste perversion	3%	1%	3%	2%
Tinnitus	1%	0%	< 1%	0%
Miscellaneous				
Accidental injury	2%	2%	1%	1%
Chest pain	< 1%	1%	3%	1%
Facial edema	< 1%	0%	1%	0%
Neck pain	2%	1%	< 1%	0%

[a] Selected adverse reactions with an incidence of at least 1% of patients treated with *Zyban*, NTS, or the combination of *Zyban* and NTS and more frequent than in the placebo group.
[b] Patients randomized to *Zyban* or placebo received placebo patches.

Overdosage

➤*Symptoms:* There has been extensive clinical experience with overdosage of bupropion IR. Thirteen overdoses occurred during clinical trials. Twelve patients ingested 850 to 4,200 mg and recovered without significant sequelae. Another patient who ingested bupropion IR 9,000 mg and tranylcypromine 300 mg experienced a grand mal seizure and recovered without further sequelae.

Since introduction, overdoses of up to bupropion IR 17,500 mg have been reported. Seizure was reported in approximately one third of all cases. Other serious reactions reported with overdoses of bupropion IR alone included hallucinations, loss of consciousness, and sinus tachycardia. Fever, muscle rigidity, rhabdomyolysis, hypotension, stupor, coma, and respiratory failure have been reported when bupropion IR was part of multiple drug overdoses.

Although most patients recovered without sequelae, deaths associated with overdoses of bupropion IR alone have been reported rarely in patients ingesting massive doses of the drug. Multiple uncontrolled seizures, bradycardia, cardiac failure, and cardiac arrest prior to death were reported in these patients.

Wellbutrin SR – There has been very limited experience with overdosage of *Wellbutrin SR* tablets; 3 cases were reported during clinical trials in depressed patients. One patient ingested *Wellbutrin SR* 3,000 mg tablets and vomited quickly after the overdose; the patient experienced blurred vision and lightheadedness. A second patient ingested a "handful" of *Wellbutrin SR* tablets and experienced confusion, lethargy, nausea, jitteriness, and seizure. A third patient ingested *Wellbutrin SR* 3,600 mg and a bottle of wine; the patient experienced nausea, visual hallucinations, and "grogginess." None of the patients experienced further sequelae.

➤*Treatment:* Ensure an adequate airway, oxygenation, and ventilation. Monitor cardiac rhythm and vital signs. EEG monitoring also is recommended for the first 48 hours postingestion. General supportive and symptomatic measures also are recommended. Induction of emesis is not recommended. Gastric lavage with a large-bore orogastric tube with appropriate airway protection, if needed, may be indicated if performed soon after ingestion or in symptomatic patients.

BUPROPION — ORAL

Administer activated charcoal. There is no experience with the use of forced diuresis, dialysis, hemoperfusion, or exchange transfusion in the management of bupropion overdoses. No specific antidotes for bupropion are known.

Because of the dose-related risk of seizures with bupropion, consider hospitalization following suspected overdose. Based on studies in animals, it is recommended that seizures be treated with intravenous (IV) benzodiazepine administration and other supportive measures, as appropriate.

In managing overdosage, consider the possibility of multiple drug involvement. Consider contacting a poison control center for additional information on the treatment of any overdose.

Patient Information

Prescribers or other health professionals should inform patients, their families, and their caregivers about the benefits and risks associated with treatment with bupropion and should counsel them in its appropriate use. A patient Medication Guide About Using Antidepressants in Children and Teenagers is available for bupropion. The prescriber or health professional should instruct patients, their families, and their caregivers to read the Medication Guide and should assist them in understanding its contents. Patients should be given the opportunity to discuss the contents of the Medication Guide and to obtain answers to any questions they may have.

Patients should be advised of the following issues and asked to alert their prescriber if these occur while taking bupropion.

➤*Clinical worsening and suicide risk:* Patients, their families, and their caregivers should be encouraged to be alert to the emergence of anxiety, agitation, panic attacks, insomnia, irritability, hostility, aggressiveness, impulsivity, akathisia (psychomotor restlessness), hypomania, mania, other unusual changes in behavior, worsening of depression, and suicidal ideation, especially early during antidepressant treatment and when the dose is adjusted up or down. Families and caregivers of patients should be advised to observe for the emergence of such symptoms on a day-to-day basis, since changes may be abrupt. Such symptoms should be reported to the patient's prescriber or health professional, especially if they are severe, abrupt in onset, or were not part of the patient's presenting symptoms. Symptoms such as these may be associated with an increased risk for suicidal thinking and behavior and indicate a need for very close monitoring and possibly changes in the medication.

➤*Bupropion IR, Wellbutrin SR,* bupropion XL: Patients should be made aware that bupropion IR, *Wellbutrin SR*, and bupropion XL contain the same active ingredient found in *Zyban*, used as an aid to smoking cessation, and that bupropion IR, *Wellbutrin SR*, and bupropion XL should not be used in combination with *Zyban* or any other medications that contain bupropion.

Physicians are advised to discuss the following issues with patients:

- Bupropion IR and *Wellbutrin SR* should be discontinued and not restarted if they experience a seizure while on treatment.
- Any CNS-active drug like bupropion IR, *Wellbutrin SR*, and bupropion XL may impair their abilities to perform tasks requiring judgment or motor and cognitive skills. Consequently, until they are reasonably certain that bupropion IR, *Wellbutrin SR*, or bupropion XL does not adversely affect their performance, they should refrain from driving an automobile or operating complex, hazardous machinery.
- Excessive use or abrupt discontinuation of alcohol or sedatives (including benzodiazepines) may alter the seizure threshold. Some patients have reported lower alcohol tolerance during treatment with bupropion IR, *Wellbutrin SR*, or *Wellbutrin XL*. Patients should be advised that the consumption of alcohol should be minimized or avoided.
- Patients should be advised to inform their physicians if they are taking or plan to take any prescription or over-the-counter drugs. Concern is warranted because bupropion IR, *Wellbutrin SR*, *Wellbutrin XL* and other drugs may affect each other's metabolism.
- Patients should be advised to notify their physicians if they become pregnant or intend to become pregnant during therapy.

Bupropion IR – Patients should be instructed to take bupropion IR in equally divided doses 3 or 4 times a day to minimize the risk of seizure.

Wellbutrin SR – Patients should be advised to swallow *Wellbutrin SR* tablets whole so that the release rate is not altered. Patients should not chew, divide or crush tablets.

As dose is increased during initial titration to doses above 150 mg/day, patients should be instructed to take *Wellbutrin SR* tablets in 2 divides doses, preferably with at least 8 hours between successive doses, to minimize the risk of seizures.

Bupropion XL – Patients should be advised to swallow bupropion XL tablets whole so that the release rate is not altered. Patients should not chew, divide or crush tablets.

Patients should be advised that they may notice in their stool something that looks like a tablet. This is normal. The medication in bupropion XL is contained in a nonabsorbable shell that has been specially designed to slowly release drug in the body. When this process is completed, the empty shell is eliminated from the body.

NEFAZODONE HYDROCHLORIDE

Rx	**Nefazodone HCl** (Various, eg, Eon, Par, Teva)	**Tablets:** 50 mg	In 60s and 100s.
		100 mg	In 60s.
		150 mg	In 60s.
		200 mg	In 60s.
		250 mg	In 60s.

NEFAZODONE HYDROCHLORIDE — ORAL

For additional information, refer to the Antidepressants introduction.

WARNING

Cases of life-threatening hepatic failure have been reported in patients treated with nefazodone.

The reported rate in the US is approximately 1 case of liver failure resulting in death or transplant per 250,000 to 300,000 patient-years of nefazodone treatment. The total patient-years is a summation of each patient's duration of exposure expressed in years. For example, 1 patient-year is equal to 2 patients each treated for 6 months, 3 patients each treated for 4 months, etc. This represents a rate of about 3 to 4 times the estimated background rate of liver failure. This rate is an underestimate because of underreporting, and the true risk could be considerably greater than this. A large cohort study of antidepressant users found no cases of liver failure leading to death or transplant among nefazodone users in approximately 30,000 patient-years of exposure. The spontaneous report data and the cohort study results provide estimates of the upper and lower limits of the risk of liver failure in nefazodone-treated patients, but are not capable of providing a precise risk estimate.

Ordinarily, treatment with nefazodone should not be initiated in individuals with active liver disease or with elevated baseline serum transaminases. There is no evidence that preexisting liver disease increases the likelihood of developing liver failure; however, baseline abnormalities can complicate patient monitoring.

Advise patients to be alert for signs and symptoms of liver dysfunction (eg, jaundice, anorexia, GI complaints, malaise) and to report them to their health care provider immediately if they occur.

Discontinue nefazodone if clinical signs or symptoms suggest liver failure. If nefazodone-treated patients develop evidence of hepatocellular injury such as increased serum AST or serum ALT levels greater than or equal to 3 times the upper limit of normal, withdraw the drug. These patients should be presumed to be at increased risk for liver injury if nefazodone is reintroduced. Accordingly, do not consider such patients for retreatment.

Indications

➤*Depression:* For the treatment of depression.

Administration and Dosage

➤*Approved by the FDA:* December 22, 1994.

➤*Initial treatment:* The recommended starting dosage for nefazodone is 200 mg/day, administered in 2 divided doses twice a day. In the controlled clinical trials establishing the antidepressant efficacy of nefazodone, the effective dosage range was generally 300 to 600 mg/day. Consequently, most patients, depending on tolerability and the need for further clinical effect, should have their dose increased. Dosage increases should occur in increments of 100 to 200 mg/day, again on a twice-daily schedule, at intervals of no less than 1 week. As with all antidepressants, several weeks on treatment may be required to obtain a full antidepressant response.

➤*Dosage for elderly or debilitated patients:* The recommended initial dosage for elderly or debilitated patients is 100 mg/day, administered in 2 divided doses twice daily. These patients often have reduced nefazodone clearance or increased sensitivity to the side effects of CNS-active drugs. It may also be appropriate to modify the rate of subsequent dose titration. As steady-state plasma levels do not change with age, the final target dose based on a careful assessment of the patient's clinical response may be similar in healthy younger and older patients.

➤*Maintenance/continuation/extended treatment:* There is no body of evidence available from controlled trials to indicate how long the depressed patient should be treated with nefazodone. It is generally agreed, however, that pharmacological treatment for acute episodes of depression should continue for up to 6 months or longer. Whether the dose of antidepressant needed to induce remission is identical to the dose needed to maintain euthymia is unknown. Systematic evaluation of the efficacy of nefazodone has shown that efficacy is maintained for periods of up to 36 weeks following 16 weeks of open-label acute treatment (treated for 52 weeks total) at dosages that averaged 438 mg/day. For most patients, their maintenance dose was that associated with response during acute treatment. The safety of

NEFAZODONE HYDROCHLORIDE — ORAL

nefazodone in long-term use is supported by data from both double-blind and open-label trials involving more than 250 patients treated for at least 1 year.

➤*Switching patients to or from a monoamine oxidase inhibitor (MAOI):* At least 14 days should elapse between discontinuation of an MAOI and initiation of therapy with nefazodone. In addition, allow at least 7 days after stopping nefazodone before starting an MAOI.

➤*Storage/Stability:* Store at controlled room temperature, 15° to 30°C (59° to 86°F) and dispense in a tight, light-resistant container using a child-resistant closure.

Actions

➤*Pharmacology:* The mechanism of action of nefazodone, as with other antidepressants, is unknown.

Preclinical studies have shown that nefazodone inhibits neuronal uptake of serotonin and norepinephrine.

Nefazodone occupies central 5-HT_2 receptors at nanomolar concentrations, and acts as an antagonist at this receptor. Nefazodone was shown to antagonize alpha-1-adrenergic receptors, a property which may be associated with postural hypotension. In vitro binding studies showed that nefazodone had not significant affinity for the following receptors: alpha-2 and beta-adrenergic, 5-HT_{1A}, cholinergic, dopaminergic, or benzodiazepine.

➤*Pharmacokinetics:*

Absorption – Nefazodone is rapidly and completely absorbed but is subject to extensive metabolism, so that its absolute bioavailability is low (about 20%) and variable. Peak plasma concentrations occur at about 1 hour and the half-life of nefazodone is 2 to 4 hours.

Both nefazodone and its pharmacologically similar metabolite, hydroxynefazodone, exhibit nonlinear kinetics for both dose and time, with AUC and C_{max} increasing more than proportionally with dose increases and more than expected upon multiple dosing over time, compared with single dosing. For example, in a multiple-dose study involving twice-daily dosing with 50, 100, and 200 mg, the AUC for nefazodone and hydroxynefazodone increased by about 4-fold with an increase in dosage from 200 to 400 mg/day; C_{max} increased by about 3-fold with the same dose increase. In a multiple-dose study involving twice-daily dosing with 25, 50, 100, and 150 mg, the accumulation ratios for nefazodone and hydroxynefazodone AUC, after 5 days of twice-daily dosing relative to the first dose, ranged from approximately 3 to 4 at the lower dosages (50 to 100 mg/day) and from 5 to 7 at the higher dosages (200 to 300 mg/day); there were also approximately 2- to 4-fold increases in C_{max} after 5 days of twice-daily dosing relative to the first dose, suggesting extensive and greater than predicted accumulation of nefazodone and its hydroxy metabolite with multiple dosing. Steady-state plasma nefazodone and metabolite concentrations are attained within 4 to 5 days of initiation of twice-daily dosing or upon dose increase or decrease.

Effect of food: Food delays the absorption of nefazodone and decreases the bioavailability of nefazodone by approximately 20%.

Distribution – Nefazodone is widely distributed in body tissues, including the CNS. In humans the volume of distribution of nefazodone ranges from 0.22 to 0.87 L/kg.

Metabolism – Nefazodone is extensively metabolized after oral administration by n-dealkylation and aliphatic and aromatic hydroxylation, and less than 1% of administered nefazodone is excreted unchanged in urine. Attempts to characterize 3 metabolites identified in plasma, hydroxynefazodone (HO-NEF), meta-chlorophenylpiperazine (mCPP), and a triazoledione metabolite, have been carried out. The AUC (expressed as a multiple of the AUC for nefazodone dosed at 100 mg twice daily) and elimination half-lives for these 3 metabolites were as follows:

AUC Multiples and t ½ for 3 Metabolites of Nefazodone (100 mg twice a day)		
Metabolite	AUC multiple	t ½
HO-NEF	0.4	1.5 to 4 hours
mCPP	0.07	4 to 8 hours
Triazole-dionemetabolite	4	18 hours

HO-NEF possesses a pharmacological profile qualitatively and quantitatively similar to that of nefazodone. mCPP has some similarities to nefazodone, but also has agonist activity at some serotonergic receptor subtypes. The pharmacological profile of the triazole-dione metabolite has not yet been well characterized. In addition to the above compounds, several other metabolites were present in plasma but have not been tested for pharmacological activity.

Excretion – After oral administration of radiolabeled nefazodone, the mean half-life of total label ranged between 11 and 24 hours. Approximately 55% of the administered radioactivity was detected in urine and about 20% to 30% in feces.

Special populations –

Renal function impairment: In studies involving 29 renally impaired patients, renal impairment (creatinine clearances ranging from 7 to 60 mL/min/1.73 m^2) had no effect on steady-state nefazodone plasma concentrations.

Liver function impairment: In a multidose study of patients with liver cirrhosis, the AUC values for nefazodone and HO-NEF at steady state were approximately 25% greater than those observed in healthy volunteers.

Age/gender effects: After single doses of 300 mg to younger (18 to 45 years of age) and older patients (older than 65 years of age), C_{max} and AUC for nefazodone and hydroxynefazodone were up to twice as high in the older patients. With multiple doses, however, differences were much smaller, 10% to 20%. A similar result was seen for gender, with a higher C_{max} and AUC in women after single doses but no difference after multiple doses.

Initiate treatment with nefazodone initiated at half the usual dose in elderly patients, especially women; however, the therapeutic dose range is similar in younger and older patients.

Contraindications

Coadministration of terfenadine, astemizole, cisapride, pimozide, or carbamazepine with nefazodone is contraindicated.

Nefazodone tablets are contraindicated in patients withdrawn from nefazodone because of evidence of liver injury. Nefazodone tablets are also contraindicated in patients who have demonstrated hypersensitivity to nefazodone, its inactive ingredients, or other phenylpiperazine antidepressants.

The coadministration of triazolam and nefazodone causes a significant increase in the plasma level of triazolam; a 75% reduction in the initial triazolam dosage is recommended if the 2 drugs are to be given together. Because not all commercially available dosage forms of triazolam permit a sufficient dosage reduction, the coadministration of triazolam and nefazodone should be avoided for most patients, including the elderly.

Warnings

➤*Hepatotoxicity:* See the Warning box for more information.

The time to liver injury for the reported liver failure cases resulting in death or transplant generally ranged from 2 weeks to 6 months on nefazodone therapy. Although some reports described dark urine and nonspecific prodromal symptoms (eg, anorexia, malaise, GI symptoms), other reports did not describe the onset of clear prodromal symptoms prior to the onset of jaundice.

Consider the value of liver function testing. Periodic serum transaminase testing has not been proven to prevent serious injury, but it is generally believed that early detection of drug-induced hepatic injury along with immediate withdrawal of the suspect drug enhances the likelihood for recovery.

Advise patients to be alert for signs and symptoms of liver dysfunction (jaundice, anorexia, GI complaints, malaise) and to report them to their health care provider immediately if they occur. Ongoing clinical assessment of patients should govern physician interventions, including diagnostic evaluations and treatment.

➤*Potential for interaction with MAOIs:* In patients receiving antidepressants with pharmacological properties similar to nefazodone in combination with a MAOI, there have been reports of serious, sometimes fatal, reactions. For an SSRI, these reactions have included hyperthermia, rigidity, myoclonus, autonomic instability with possible rapid fluctuations of vital signs, and mental status changes that include extreme agitation progressing to delirium and coma. These reactions have also been reported in patients who have recently discontinued that drug and have been started on an MAOI. Some cases presented with features resembling neuroleptic malignant syndrome. Severe hyperthermia and seizures, sometimes fatal, have been reported in association with the combined use of tricyclic antidepressants and MAOIs. These reactions have also been reported in patients who have recently discontinued these drugs and have been started on an MAOI.

Although the effects of combined use of nefazodone and MAOIs have not been evaluated in humans or animals, because nefazodone is an inhibitor of both serotonin and norepinephrine reuptake, do not use nefazodone in combination with an MAOI, or within 14 days of discontinuing treatment with an MAOI. Allow at least 1 week after stopping nefazodone before starting an MAOI.

➤*Interaction with triazolobenzodiazepines:* Interaction studies of nefazodone with 2 triazolobenzodiazepines (ie, triazolam and alprazolam) metabolized by cytochrome P450 3A4, have revealed substantial and clinically important increases in plasma concentrations of these compounds when administered concomitantly with nefazodone.

Triazolam – See Drug Interactions for more information.

Alprazolam – See Drug Interactions for more information.

➤*Fertility impairment:* A fertility study in rats showed a slight decrease in fertility at 200 mg/kg/day (approximately 3 times the maximum human daily dosage on a mg/m^2 basis) but not at 100 mg/kg/day (approximately 1.5 times the maximum human daily dosage on a mg/m^2 basis).

➤*Elderly:* Of the approximately 7,000 patients in clinical studies who received nefazodone for the treatment of depression, 18% were 65 years of age or older, while 5% were 75 years of age or older. Based on monitoring of adverse reactions, vital signs, electrocardiograms, and results of laboratory tests, no overall differences in safety between elderly and younger patients were observed in clinical studies. Efficacy in the elderly has not been demonstrated in placebo-controlled trials. Other reported clinical experience has not identified differences in responses between elderly and younger patients, but greater sensitivity of some older individuals cannot be ruled out.

Due to the increased systemic exposure to nefazodone seen in single-dose studies in elderly patients, initiate treatment at half the usual dose; titration upward should take place over the same range as in younger patients. Observe the usual precautions in elderly patients who have concomitant medical illnesses or who are receiving concomitant drugs.

➤*Pregnancy: Category C.*

Teratogenic – Reproduction studies have been performed in pregnant rabbits and rats at daily doses up to 200 and 300 mg/kg, respectively (approximately 6 and 5 times, respectively, the maximum human daily dose on a mg/m^2 basis). No malformations were observed in the offspring as a result of nefazodone treatment. However, increased early pup mortality was seen in rats at a dose approximately 5 times the maximum human dose, and

NEFAZODONE HYDROCHLORIDE — ORAL

decreased pup weights were seen at this and lower doses, when dosing began during pregnancy and continued until weaning. The cause of these deaths is not known. The no-effect dose for rat pup mortality was 1.3 times the human dose on a mg/m² basis. There are no adequate and well-controlled studies in pregnant women. Use nefazodone during pregnancy only if the potential benefit justifies the potential risk to the fetus.

Labor and delivery – The effect of nefazodone on labor and delivery in humans is unknown.

➤*Lactation:* It is not known whether nefazodone or its metabolites are excreted in human milk. Because many drugs are excreted in human milk, exercise caution when nefazodone is administered to a nursing woman.

➤*Children:* Safety and efficacy in individuals younger than 18 years of age have not been established.

Precautions

➤*Electroconvulsive therapy (ECT):* There are no clinical studies of the combined use of ECT and nefazodone.

➤*Postural hypotension:* A pooled analysis of the vital signs monitored during placebo-controlled premarketing studies revealed that 5.1% of nefazodone patients compared with 2.5% of placebo patients ($P \le 0.01$) met criteria for a potentially important decrease in blood pressure at some time during treatment (systolic blood pressure less than or equal to 90 mm Hg and a change from baseline of greater than or equal to 20 mm Hg). While there was no difference in the proportion of nefazodone and placebo patients having adverse reactions characterized as "syncope" (nefazodone, 0.2%; placebo, 0.3%), the rates for adverse reactions characterized as "postural hypotension" were as follows: nefazodone (2.8%), tricyclic antidepressants (10.9%), SSRIs (1.1%), and placebo (0.8%). Thus, the prescriber should be aware that there is some risk of postural hypotension in association with nefazodone use. Use nefazodone with caution in patients with known cardiovascular or cerebrovascular disease that could be exacerbated by hypotension (history of myocardial infarction [MI], angina, or ischemic stroke) and conditions that would predispose patients to hypotension (dehydration, hypovolemia, and treatment with antihypertensive medication).

➤*Activation of mania/hypomania:* During premarketing testing, hypomania or mania occurred in 0.3% of nefazodone-treated unipolar patients, compared with 0.3% of tricyclic- and 0.4% of placebo-treated patients. In patients classified as bipolar the rate of manic episodes was 1.6% for nefazodone, 5.1% for the combined tricyclic-treated groups, and 0% for placebo-treated patients. Activation of mania/hypomania is a known risk in a small proportion of patients with major affective disorder treated with other marketed antidepressants. As with all antidepressants, use nefazodone cautiously in patients with a history of mania.

➤*Suicide:* The possibility of a suicide attempt is inherent in depression and may persist until significant remission occurs. Closely supervise high-risk patients during initial drug therapy. Write prescriptions for nefazodone for the smallest quantity of tablets consistent with good patient management in order to reduce the risk of overdose.

➤*Seizures:* During premarketing testing, a recurrence of a petit mal seizure was observed in a patient receiving nefazodone who had a history of such seizures. One nonstudy participant took 2,000 to 3,000 mg nefazodone with methocarbamol and alcohol; this person reportedly experienced a convulsion (type not documented). Neither of these patients died. Rare occurrences of convulsions (including grand mal seizures) following nefazodone administration have been reported since market introduction. A causal relationship to nefazodone has not been established.

➤*Priapism:* While priapism did not occur during premarketing experience with nefazodone, rare reports of priapism have been received since market introduction. A causal relationship to nefazodone has not been established. If patients present with prolonged or inappropriate erections, they should discontinue therapy immediately and consult their health care providers. If the condition persists for more than 24 hours, consult a urologist to determine appropriate management.

➤*Use in patients with concomitant illness:* Nefazodone has not been evaluated or used to any appreciable extent in patients with a history of MI or unstable heart disease. Patients with these diagnoses were systematically excluded from clinical studies during the product's premarketing testing. Evaluation of electrocardiograms of 1,153 patients who received nefazodone in 6- to 8-week, double-blind, placebo-controlled trials did not indicate that nefazodone is associated with the development of clinically important ECG abnormalities. However, sinus bradycardia, defined as heart rate less than or equal to 50 bpm and a decrease of at least 15 bpm from baseline, was observed in 1.5% of nefazodone-treated patients compared with 0.4% of placebo-treated patients ($P \le 0.05$). Because patients with a history of MI or unstable heart disease were excluded from clinical trials, treat such patients with caution.

In patients with cirrhosis of the liver, the AUC values of nefazodone and HO-NEF were increased by approximately 25%.

➤*Hazardous tasks:* Since any psychoactive drug may impair judgment, thinking, or motor skills, caution patients about operating hazardous machinery, including automobiles, until they are reasonably certain that nefazodone therapy does not adversely affect their ability to engage in such activities.

Drug Interactions

➤*CYP450 system:* Terfenadine, astemizole, cisapride, and pimozide are all metabolized by the cytochrome P450 3A4 (CYP3A4) isozyme, and it has been demonstrated that ketoconazole, erythromycin, and other inhibitors of CYP3A4 can block the metabolism of these drugs, which can result in increased plasma concentrations of parent drug. Increased plasma concentrations of terfenadine, astemizole, cisapride, and pimozide are associated with QT prolongation and with rare cases of serious cardiovascular adverse reactions, including death, principally caused by ventricular tachycardia of the torsades de pointes type. Nefazodone has been shown in vitro to be an inhibitor of CYP3A4. Consequently, do not use nefazodone not be used in combination with either terfenadine, astemizole, cisapride, or pimozide.

➤*Drugs highly bound to plasma protein:* Because nefazodone is highly bound to plasma protein, administration of nefazodone to a patient taking another drug that is highly protein bound may cause increased free concentrations of the other drug, potentially resulting in adverse reactions. Conversely, adverse reactions could result from displacement of nefazodone by other highly bound drugs.

➤*CNS-active drugs:*

MAOIs –

Potential for interaction with MAOIs: In patients receiving antidepressants with pharmacological properties similar to nefazodone in combination with an MAOI, there have been reports of serious, sometimes fatal, reactions. For an SSRI, these reactions have included hyperthermia, rigidity, myoclonus, autonomic instability with possible rapid fluctuations of vital signs, and mental status changes that include extreme agitation progressing to delirium and coma. These reactions have also been reported in patients who have recently discontinued that drug and have been started on an MAOI. Some cases presented with features resembling neuroleptic malignant syndrome. Severe hyperthermia and seizures, sometimes fatal, have been reported in association with the combined use of tricyclic antidepressants and MAOIs. These reactions have also been reported in patients who have recently discontinued these drugs and have been started on an MAOI.

Although the effects of combined use of nefazodone and MAOI have not been evaluated in humans or animals, because nefazodone is an inhibitor of both serotonin and norepinephrine reuptake, do not use nefazodone in combination with an MAOI, or within 14 days of discontinuing treatment with an MAOI. Allow at least 1 week after stopping nefazodone before starting an MAOI.

Haloperidol – When a single oral dose of 5 mg haloperidol was coadministered with twice daily 200 mg nefazodone at steady state, haloperidol apparent clearance decreased by 35% with no significant increase in peak haloperidol plasma concentrations or time of peak. This change is of unknown clinical significance. Pharmacodynamic effects of haloperidol were generally not altered significantly. There were no changes in the pharmacokinetic parameters for nefazodone. Dosage adjustment of haloperidol may be necessary when coadministered with nefazodone.

Triazolam/alprazolam –

Triazolam: When a single oral dose of 0.25 mg triazolam was coadministered with twice daily 200 mg nefazodone at steady state, triazolam half-life and AUC increased 4-fold and peak concentrations increased 1.7-fold. Nefazodone plasma concentrations were unaffected by triazolam. Coadministration of nefazodone potentiated the effects of triazolam on psychomotor performance tests. If triazolam is coadministered with nefazodone, a 75% reduction in the initial triazolam dosage is recommended. Because not all commercially available dosage forms of triazolam permit sufficient dosage reduction, avoid coadministration of triazolam with nefazodone for most patients, including the elderly. In the exceptional case where coadministration of triazolam with nefazodone may be considered appropriate, use only the lowest possible dose of triazolam.

Alprazolam: When 1 mg alprazolam and 200 mg nefazodone were coadministered twice daily, steady-state peak concentrations, AUC and half-life values for alprazolam increased by approximately 2-fold. Nefazodone plasma concentrations were unaffected by alprazolam. If alprazolam is coadministered with nefazodone, reduce the initial alprazolam dosage by 50%. No dosage adjustment is required for nefazodone.

Alcohol – Although nefazodone did not potentiate the cognitive and psychomotor effects of alcohol in experiments with healthy subjects, the concomitant use of nefazodone and alcohol in depressed patients is not advised.

Buspirone – In a study of steady-state pharmacokinetics in healthy volunteers, twice daily coadministration of 2.5 or 5 mg buspirone with 250 mg nefazodone resulted in marked increases in plasma buspirone concentrations (increases up to 20-fold in C_{max} and up to 50-fold in AUC) and statistically significant decreases (about 50%) in plasma concentrations of the buspirone metabolite 1-pyrimidinylpiperazine. With twice-daily doses of 5 mg buspirone, slight increases in AUC were observed for nefazodone (23%) and its metabolites hydroxynefazodone (17%) and mCPP (9%). Subjects receiving 250 mg nefazodone twice daily and 5 mg buspirone twice daily experienced light-headedness, asthenia, dizziness, and somnolence, adverse reactions also observed with either drug alone. If the 2 drugs are to be used in combination, a low dose of buspirone (eg, 2.5 mg daily) is recommended. Base subsequent dose adjustment of either drug clinical assessment.

Fluoxetine – When 20 mg fluoxetine once daily and 200 mg nefazodone twice daily were administered at steady state, there were no changes in the pharmacokinetic parameters for fluoxetine or its metabolite, norfluoxetine. Similarly, there were no changes in the pharmacokinetic parameters of nefazodone or HO-NEF; however, the mean AUC levels of the nefazodone metabolites mCPP and triazole-dione increased by 3- to 6-fold and 1.3-fold, respectively. When a 200 mg nefazodone dose was administered to subjects who had been receiving fluoxetine for 1 week, there was an increased incidence of transient adverse events such as headache, light-headedness, nausea, or paresthesia, possibly due to the elevated mCPP levels. Patients who are switched from fluoxetine to nefazodone without an adequate washout period may experience similar transient adverse events. The possibility of this happening can be minimized by allowing a washout period before initiating nefazodone therapy and by reducing the initial dose of nefazodone.

NEFAZODONE HYDROCHLORIDE — ORAL

Because of the long half-life of fluoxetine and its metabolites, this washout period may range from 1 to several weeks depending on the dose of fluoxetine and other individual patient variables.

Desipramine – When 150 mg nefazodone twice daily and 75 mg desipramine once daily were administered together, there were no changes in the pharmacokinetics of desipramine or its metabolite, 2-hydroxy desipramine. There were also no changes in the pharmacokinetics of nefazodone or its triazole-dione metabolite, but the AUC and C_{max} of mCPP increased by 44% and 48%, respectively, while the AUC of HO-NEF decreased by 19%. No changes in doses of either nefazodone or desipramine are necessary when the 2 drugs are given concomitantly. Subsequent dose adjustments should be made on the basis of clinical response.

Carbamazepine – The coadministration of 200 mg nefazodone twice daily for 5 days to 12 healthy subjects on carbamazepine who had achieved steady state (200 mg twice daily) was found to be well-tolerated. Steady-state conditions for carbamazepine, nefazodone, and several of their metabolites were achieved by day 5 of coadministration. With coadministration of the 2 drugs there were significant increases in the steady-state C_{max} and AUC of carbamazepine (23% and 23%, respectively), while the steady-state C_{max} and the AUC of the carbamazepine metabolite, 10,11 epoxycarbamazepine, decreased by 21% and 20%, respectively. The coadministration of the 2 drugs significantly reduced the steady-state C_{max} and AUC of nefazodone by 86% and 93%, respectively. Similar reductions in the C_{max} and AUC of HO-NEF were also observed (85% and 94%), while the reductions in C_{max} and AUC of mCPP and triazole-dione were more modest (13% and 44% for the former and 28% and 57% for the latter). Due to the potential for coadministration of carbamazepine to result in insufficient plasma nefazodone and hydroxynefazodone concentrations for achieving an antidepressant effect for nefazodone, it is recommended that nefazodone not be used in combination with carbamazepine.

General anesthetics – Little is known about the potential for interaction between nefazodone and general anesthetics; therefore, prior to elective surgery, discontinue nefazodone for as long as clinically feasible.

➤*Cardiovascularly active drugs:*

Digoxin – When 200 mg nefazodone twice daily and 0.2 mg digoxin once daily were coadministered for 9 days to healthy male volunteers (n = 18) who were phenotyped as CYP2D6 extensive metabolizers, C_{max}, C_{min}, and AUC of digoxin were increased by 29%, 27%, and 15%, respectively. Digoxin had no effects on the pharmacokinetics of nefazodone and its active metabolites. Because of the narrow therapeutic index of digoxin, exercise caution when nefazodone and digoxin are coadministered; plasma level monitoring for digoxin is recommended.

Propranolol – The coadministration of 200 mg nefazodone twice daily and 40 mg propranolol twice daily for 5.5 days to healthy male volunteers (n = 18), including 3 poor and 15 extensive CYP2D6 metabolizers, resulted in 30% and 14% reductions in C_{max} and AUC of propranolol, respectively, and a 14% reduction in C_{max} for the metabolite, 4-hydroxypropranolol. The kinetics of nefazodone, hydroxynefazodone, and triazole-dione were not affected by coadministration of propranolol. However, C_{max}, C_{min}, and AUC of m-chlorophenylpiperazine were increased by 23%, 54%, and 28%, respectively. No change in initial dose of either drug is necessary; make dose adjustments on the basis of clinical response.

HMG-CoA reductase inhibitors – When single 40 mg doses of simvastatin or atorvastatin, both substrates of CYP3A4, were given to healthy adult volunteers who had received 200 mg nefazodone twice daily for 6 days, approximately 20-fold increases in plasma concentrations of simvastatin and simvastatin acid and 3- to 4-fold increases in plasma concentrations of atorvastatin and atorvastatin lactone were seen. These effects appear to be due to the inhibition of CYP3A4 by nefazodone because, in the same study, nefazodone had no significant effect on the plasma concentrations of pravastatin, which is not metabolized by CYP3A4 to a clinically significant extent.

There have been rare reports of rhabdomyolysis involving patients receiving the combination of nefazodone and either simvastatin or lovastatin, also a substrate of CYP3A4. Rhabdomyolysis has been observed in patients receiving HMG-CoA reductase inhibitors administered alone (at recommended dosages) and in particular, for certain drugs in this class, when given in combination with inhibitors of the CYP3A4 isozyme.

Use caution if nefazodone is administered in combination with HMG-CoA reductase inhibitors that are metabolized by CYP3A4, such as simvastatin, atorvastatin, and lovastatin, and dosage adjustments of these HMG-CoA reductase inhibitors are recommended. Since metabolic interactions are unlikely between nefazodone and HMG-CoA reductase inhibitors that undergo little or no metabolism by the CYP3A4 isozyme, such as pravastatin or fluvastatin, dosage adjustments should not be necessary.

➤*Immunosuppressive agents:* There have been reports of increased blood concentrations of cyclosporine and tacrolimus into toxic ranges when patients received these drugs concomitantly with nefazodone. Both cyclosporine and tacrolimus are substrates of CYP3A4, and nefazodone is known to inhibit this enzyme. If either cyclosporine or tacrolimus is administered with nefazodone, blood concentrations of the immunosuppressive agent should be monitored and dosage adjusted accordingly.

➤*Pharmacokinetics of nefazodone in "poor metabolizers" and potential interaction with drugs that inhibit or are metabolized by cytochrome P450 isozymes:*

CYP3A4 isozyme – Nefazodone has been shown in vitro to be an inhibitor of CYP3A4. This is consistent with the interactions observed between nefazodone and triazolam, alprazolam, buspirone, atorvastatin, and simvastatin, drugs metabolized by this isozyme. Consequently, caution is indicated in the combined use of nefazodone with any drugs known to be metabolized by CYP3A4. In particular, avoid the combined use of nefazodone with triazolam for most patients, including the elderly. The combined use of nefazodone with terfenadine, astemizole, cisapride, or pimozide is contraindicated.

CYP2D6 isozyme – A subset (3% to 10%) of the population has reduced activity of the drug-metabolizing enzyme CYP2D6. Such individuals are referred to commonly as "poor metabolizers" of drugs such as debrisoquin, dextromethorphan, and the tricyclic antidepressants. The pharmacokinetics of nefazodone and its major metabolites are not altered in these "poor metabolizers." Plasma concentrations of 1 minor metabolite (mCPP) are increased in this population; the adjustment of nefazodone dosage is not required when administered to "poor metabolizers." Nefazodone and its metabolites have been shown in vitro to be extremely weak inhibitors of CYP2D6. Thus, it is not likely that nefazodone will decrease the metabolic clearance of drugs metabolized by this isozyme.

CYP1A2 isozyme – Nefazodone and its metabolites have been shown in vitro not to inhibit CYP1A2. Thus, metabolic interactions between nefazodone and drugs metabolized by this isozyme are unlikely.

Adverse Reactions

➤*Associated with discontinuation of treatment:* Approximately 16% of the 3,496 patients who received nefazodone in worldwide premarketing clinical trials discontinued treatment due to an adverse reaction. The more common (greater than or equal to 1%) reactions in clinical trials associated with discontinuation and considered to be drug related (ie, those reactions associated with dropout at a rate approximately twice or greater for nefazodone compared with placebo) included the following: nausea (3.5%), dizziness (1.9%), insomnia (1.5%), asthenia (1.3%), and agitation (1.2%).

➤*Commonly observed adverse reactions in controlled clinical trials:* The most commonly observed adverse reactions associated with the use of nefazodone (incidence of greater than or equal to 5%) and not seen at an equivalent incidence among placebo-treated patients (ie, significantly higher incidence for nefazodone compared with placebo, $P \le 0.05$), derived from the following table, were the following: somnolence, dry mouth, nausea, dizziness, constipation, asthenia, light-headedness, blurred vision, confusion, and abnormal vision.

Adverse reactions occurring at an incidence of 1% or more among nefazodone-treated patients – The table that follows enumerates adverse reactions that occurred at an incidence of greater than or equal to 1%, and were more frequent than in the placebo group, among nefazodone-treated patients who participated in short-term (6- to 8-week) placebo-controlled trials in which patients were dosed with nefazodone to ranges of 300 to 600 mg/day. This table shows the percentage of patients in each group who had at least 1 episode of a reaction at some time during their treatment. Reported adverse reactions were classified using standard Coding Symbols for a Thesaurus of Adverse Reaction Terms (COSTART)-based dictionary terminology.

Treatment-Emergent Adverse Reaction Incidence in 6- to 8-Week Placebo-Controlled Clinical Trials[a] Nefazodone 300 to 600 mg/day Dosage Range

Body system	Preferred term	Percent of patients: Nefazodone (n = 393)	Percent of patients: Placebo (n = 394)
Cardiovascular	Hypotension	2%	1%
	Postural hypotension	4%	1%
CNS	Abnormal dreams	3%	2%
	Ataxia	2%	0%
	Concentration decreased	3%	1%
	Confusion	7%	2%
	Dizziness	17%	5%
	Hypertonia	1%	0%
	Incoordination	2%	1%
	Insomnia	11%	9%
	Libido decreased	1%	< 1%
	Light-headedness	10%	3%
	Memory impairment	4%	2%
	Paresthesia	4%	2%
	Psychomotor retardation	2%	1%
	Somnolence	25%	14%
	Tremor	2%	1%
	Vasodilatation[b]	4%	2%
Dermatologic	Pruritus	2%	1%
	Rash	2%	1%

NEFAZODONE HYDROCHLORIDE — ORAL

Treatment-Emergent Adverse Reaction Incidence in 6- to 8-Week Placebo-Controlled Clinical Trials[a] Nefazodone 300 to 600 mg/day Dosage Range

Body system	Preferred term	Percent of patients	
		Nefazodone (n = 393)	Placebo (n = 394)
GI	Constipation	14%	8%
	Diarrhea	8%	7%
	Dry mouth	25%	13%
	Dyspepsia	9%	7%
	Increased appetite	5%	3%
	Nausea	22%	12%
	Nausea/vomiting	2%	1%
GU	Breast pain[d]	1%	< 1%
	Urinary frequency	2%	1%
	Urinary retention	2%	1%
	Urinary tract infection	2%	1%
	Vaginitis[d]	2%	1%
Metabolic	Peripheral edema	3%	2%
	Thirst	1%	< 1%
Musculoskeletal	Arthralgia	1%	< 1%
Respiratory	Cough increased	3%	1%
	Pharyngitis	6%	5%
Special senses	Abnormal vision[d]	7%	1%
	Blurred vision	9%	3%
	Taste perversion	2%	1%
	Tinnitus	2%	1%
	Visual field defect	2%	0%
Miscellaneous	Asthenia	11%	5%
	Chills	2%	1%
	Fever	2%	1%
	Flu syndrome	3%	2%
	Headache	36%	33%
	Infection	8%	6%
	Neck rigidity	1%	0%

[a] Reactions reported by at least 1% of patients treated with nefazodone and more frequent than the placebo group are included; incidence is rounded to the nearest 1% (< 1% indicates an incidence less than 0.5%). Reactions for which the nefazodone incidence was equal to or less than placebo are not listed in the table, but included the following: abdominal pain, pain, back pain, accidental injury, chest pain, neck pain, palpitation, migraine, sweating, flatulence, vomiting, anorexia, tooth disorder, weight gain, edema, myalgia, cramp, agitation, anxiety, depression, hypesthesia, CNS stimulation, dysphoria, emotional lability, sinusitis, rhinitis, dysmenorrhea, dysuria.
[b] Vasodilatation (flushing, feeling warm).
[c] Abnormal vision (scotoma, visual trails).
[d] Incidence adjusted for gender.

➤*Dose dependency of adverse reactions:* The table that follows enumerates adverse reactions that were more frequent in the nefazodone dosage range of 300 to 600 mg/day than in the nefazodone dosage range of up to 300 mg/day. This table shows only those adverse reactions for which there was a statistically significant difference ($P \le 0.05$) in incidence between the nefazodone dose ranges as well as a difference between the high dose range and placebo.

Dose Dependency of Adverse Reactions in Placebo-Controlled Trials[a]

Body system	Preferred term	Percent of patients		
		Nefazodone 300 to 600 mg/day (n = 209)	Nefazodone ≤ 300 mg/day (n = 211)	Placebo (n = 212)
CNS	Confusion	8%	2%	1%
	Dizziness	22%	11%	4%
	Somnolence	28%	16%	13%
GI	Constipation	17%	10%	9%
	Nausea	23%	14%	12%
Special senses	Abnormal vision	10%	0%	2%
	Blurred vision	9%	3%	2%
	Tinnitus	3%	0%	1%

[a] Reactions for which there was a statistically significant difference ($P \le 0.05$) between the nefazodone dose groups.

➤*Visual disturbances:* In controlled clinical trials, blurred vision occurred in 9% of nefazodone-treated patients compared with 3% of placebo-treated patients. In these same trials, abnormal vision, including scotomata and visual trails, occurred in 7% of nefazodone-treated patients compared with 1% of placebo-treated (see the preceding table). Dose dependency was observed for these reactions in these trials, with none of the scotomata and visual trails at doses below 300 mg/day. However, scotomata and visual trails observed at dosages less than 300 mg/day have been reported in postmarketing experience with nefazodone.

➤*Vital sign changes:*

Postural hypotension – See Precautions for more information.

➤*Weight changes:* In a pooled analysis of placebo-controlled premarketing studies, there were no differences between nefazodone and placebo groups in the proportions of patients meeting criteria for potentially important increases or decreases in body weight (a change of greater than or equal to 7%).

➤*Laboratory changes:* Of the serum chemistry, serum hematology, and urinalysis parameters monitored during placebo-controlled premarketing studies with nefazodone, a pooled analysis revealed a statistical trend between nefazodone and placebo for hematocrit (ie, 2.8% of nefazodone patients met criteria for a potentially important decrease in hematocrit [less than or equal to 37% in men or less than or equal to 32% in women]) compared with 1.5% of placebo patients (0.05 less than $P \le 0.1$). Decreases in hematocrit, presumably dilutional, have been reported with many other drugs that block alpha-1-adrenergic receptors. There was no apparent clinical significance of the observed changes in the few patients meeting these criteria.

➤*ECG changes:* Of the ECG parameters monitored during placebo-controlled premarketing studies with nefazodone, a pooled analysis revealed a statistically significant difference between nefazodone and placebo for sinus bradycardia (ie, 1.5% of nefazodone patients met criteria for a potentially important decrease in heart rate [less than or equal to 50 bpm and a decrease of greater than or equal to 15 bpm]) compared with 0.4% of placebo patients ($P < 0.05$). There was no obvious clinical significance of the observed changes in the few patients meeting these criteria.

➤*Other reactions observed during the premarketing evaluation of nefazodone:* During its premarketing assessment, multiple doses of nefazodone were administered to 3,496 patients in clinical studies, including more than 250 patients treated for at least 1 year. The conditions and duration of exposure to nefazodone varied greatly, and included (in overlapping categories) open and double-blind studies, uncontrolled and controlled studies, inpatient and outpatient studies, fixed-dose and titration studies. Untoward reactions associated with this exposure were recorded by clinical investigators using terminology of their own choosing. Consequently, it is not possible to provide a meaningful estimate of the proportion of individuals experiencing adverse reactions without first grouping similar types of untoward reactions into a smaller number of standardized reaction categories.

Reactions are further categorized by body system and listed in order of decreasing frequency according to the following definitions: frequent adverse reactions are those occurring on 1 or more occasions in at least 1 of 100 patients (only those not already listed in the tabulated results from placebo-controlled trials appear in this listing); infrequent adverse reactions are those occurring in 1 of 100 to 1 of 1,000 patients; rare reactions are those occurring in less than 1 of 1,000 patients.

Cardiovascular –

Infrequent: Tachycardia, hypertension, syncope, ventricular extrasystoles, and angina pectoris.

Rare: AV block, congestive heart failure, hemorrhage, pallor, and varicose vein.

CNS –

Infrequent: Vertigo, twitching, depersonalization, hallucinations, suicide attempt, apathy, euphoria, hostility, suicidal thoughts, abnormal gait, thinking abnormal, attention decreased, derealization, neuralgia, paranoid reaction, dysarthria, increased libido, suicide, and myoclonus.

Rare: Hyperkinesia, increased salivation, cerebrovascular accident, hyperesthesia, hypotonia, ptosis, and neuroleptic malignant syndrome.

Dermatologic –

Infrequent: Dry skin, acne, alopecia, urticaria, maculopapular rash, vesiculobullous rash, and eczema.

GI –

Frequent: Gastroenteritis.

Infrequent: Eructation, periodontal abscess, abnormal liver function tests, gingivitis, colitis, gastritis, mouth ulceration, stomatitis, esophagitis, peptic ulcer, and rectal hemorrhage.

Rare: Glossitis, hepatitis, dysphagia, GI hemorrhage, oral moniliasis, and ulcerative colitis.

GU –

Frequent: Impotence.

Infrequent: Cystitis, urinary urgency, metrorrhagia, amenorrhea, polyuria, vaginal hemorrhage, breast enlargement, menorrhagia, urinary incontinence, abnormal ejaculation, hematuria, nocturia, and kidney calculus.

Rare: Uterine fibroids enlarged, uterine hemorrhage, anorgasmia, and oliguria.

Hematologic/Lymphatic –

Infrequent: Ecchymosis, anemia, leukopenia, and lymphadenopathy.

Metabolic/Nutritional –

Infrequent: Weight loss, gout, dehydration, lactic dehydrogenase increased, AST increased, and ALT increased.

Rare: Hypercholesteremia and hypoglycemia.

Musculoskeletal –

Infrequent: Arthritis, tenosynovitis, muscle stiffness, and bursitis.

Rare: Tendinous contracture.

NEFAZODONE HYDROCHLORIDE — ORAL

Respiratory –

Frequent: Dyspnea and bronchitis.

Infrequent: Asthma, pneumonia, laryngitis, voice alteration, epistaxis, hiccup.

Rare: Hyperventilation and yawn.

Special senses –

Frequent: Eye pain.

Infrequent: Dry eye, ear pain, abnormality of accommodation, diplopia, conjunctivitis, mydriasis, keratoconjunctivitis, hyperacusis, and photophobia.

Rare: Deafness, glaucoma, night blindness, and taste loss.

Miscellaneous –

Infrequent: Allergic reaction, malaise, photosensitivity reaction, face edema, hangover effect, abdomen enlarged, hernia, pelvic pain, and halitosis.

Rare: Cellulitis.

➤*Postmarketing:* Postmarketing experience with nefazodone has shown an adverse reaction profile similar to that seen during the premarketing evaluation of nefazodone. Voluntary reports of adverse reactions temporally associated with nefazodone have been received since market introduction that are not listed above and for which a causal relationship has not been established. These include the following:

Hypersensitivity – Anaphylactic reactions; angioedema; convulsions (including grand mal seizures); galactorrhea; gynecomastia (men); hyponatremia; liver necrosis and liver failure, in some cases leading to liver transplantation or death; priapism; prolactin increased; rhabdomyolysis involving patients receiving the combination of nefazodone and lovastatin or simvastatin; serotonin syndrome; Stevens-Johnson syndrome; and thrombocytopenia.

Overdosage

➤*Symptoms:*

Human experience – In premarketing clinical studies, there were 7 reports of nefazodone overdose alone or in combination with other pharmacological agents. The amount of nefazodone ingested ranged from 1,000 mg to 11,200 mg. Commonly reported symptoms from overdose of nefazodone included nausea, vomiting, and somnolence. One nonstudy participant took 2,000 to 3,000 mg nefazodone with methocarbamol and alcohol; this person reportedly experienced a convulsion (type not documented). None of these patients died. In postmarketing experience, overdose with nefazodone alone and in combination with alcohol or other substances has been reported. Commonly reported symptoms were similar to those reported from overdose in premarketing experience. While there have been rare reports of fatalities in patients taking overdoses of nefazodone, predominantly in combination with alcohol or other substances, no causal relationship to nefazodone has been established.

➤*Treatment:* Treatment should consist of those general measures employed in the management of overdosage with any antidepressant.

Ensure an adequate airway, oxygenation, and ventilation. Monitor cardiac rhythm and vital signs. General supportive and symptomatic measures are also recommended. Induction of emesis is not recommended. Gastric lavage with a large-bore orogastric tube with appropriate airway protection, if needed, may be indicated if performed soon after ingestion, or in symptomatic patients.

Administer activated charcoal. Due to the wide distribution of nefazodone in body tissues, forced diuresis, dialysis, hemoperfusion, and exchange transfusion are unlikely to be of benefit. No specific antidotes for nefazodone are known.

In managing overdosage, consider the possibility of multiple drug involvement. Consider contacting a poison control center for additional information on the treatment of any overdose.

Patient Information

Discuss the following issues with nefazodone-treated patients:

➤*Hepatotoxicity:* Patients should be informed that nefazodone therapy has been associated with liver abnormalities ranging from asymptomatic reversible serum transaminase increases to cases of liver failure resulting in transplant or death. At present, there is no way to predict who is likely to develop liver failure. Ordinarily, patients with active liver disease should not be treated with nefazodone. Advise patients to be alert for signs of liver dysfunction (eg, jaundice, anorexia, GI complaints, malaise) and to report them to their health care provider immediately if they occur.

➤*Time to response/continuation:* As with all antidepressants, several weeks on treatment may be required to obtain the full antidepressant effect. Once improvement is noted, it is important for patients to continue drug treatment as directed by their health care provider.

➤*Interference with cognitive and motor performance:* Since any psychoactive drug may impair judgment, thinking, or motor skills, caution patients about operating hazardous machinery, including automobiles, until they are reasonably certain that nefazodone therapy does not adversely affect their ability to engage in such activities.

➤*Pregnancy:* Advise patients to notify their health care provider if they become pregnant or intend to become pregnant during therapy. Reproduction studies have been performed in pregnant rabbits and rats at daily doses up to 200 and 300 mg/kg, respectively (approximately 6 and 5 times, respectively, the maximum human daily dose on a mg/m^2 basis). No malformations were observed in the offspring as a result of nefazodone treatment. However, increased early pup mortality was seen in rats at a dose approximately 5 times the maximum human dose, and decreased pup weights were seen at this and lower doses, when dosing began during pregnancy and continued until weaning. The cause of these deaths is not known. The no-effect dose for rat pup mortality was 1.3 times the human dose on a mg/m^2 basis. There are no adequate and well-controlled studies in pregnant women. Use nefazodone during pregnancy only if the potential benefit justifies the potential risk to the fetus.

➤*Nursing:* Advise patients to notify their health care provider if they are breastfeeding an infant. It is not known whether nefazodone or its metabolites are excreted in human milk. Because many drugs are excreted in human milk, exercise caution when nefazodone is administered to a nursing woman.

➤*Concomitant medication:* Advise patients to inform their health care providers if they are taking, or plan to take, any prescription or over-the-counter drugs, since there is a potential for interactions. Significant caution is indicated if nefazodone is to be used in combination with alprazolam; concomitant use with triazolam should be avoided for most patients, including the elderly; and concomitant use with terfenadine (not available in the US), astemizole (not available in the US), cisapride, pimozide, or carbamazepine is contraindicated.

➤*Alcohol:* Advise patients to avoid alcohol while taking nefazodone.

➤*Allergic reactions:* Advise patients to notify their health care provider if they develop a rash, hives, or a related allergic phenomenon.

➤*Visual disturbances:* There have been reports of visual disturbances associated with the use of nefazodone, including blurred vision, scotoma, and visual trails. Advise patients to notify their healthcare provider if they develop visual disturbances. In controlled clinical trials, blurred vision occurred in 9% of nefazodone-treated patients compared to 3% of placebo-treated patients. In these same trials, abnormal vision, including scotomata and visual trails, occurred in 7% of nefazodone-treated patients compared with 1% of placebo-treated patients. Dose dependency was observed for these reactions in these trials, with none of the scotomata and visual trails at dosages below 300 mg/day. However, scotomata and visual trails observed at dosages below 300 mg/day have been reported in postmarketing experience with nefazodone.

Serotonin and Norepinephrine Reuptake Inhibitors

DULOXETINE HYDROCHLORIDE

Rx	**Cymbalta** (Eli Lilly)	**Capsules**[a]: 20 mg (as base)	Sucrose, sugar spheres. (20 mg LILLY 3235). Opaque green. In 60s and unit-dose 100s.
		30 mg (as base)	Sucrose, sugar spheres. (30 mg LILLY 3240). Opaque white and opaque blue. In 30s, 90s, and 1,000s; unit-dose 100s.
		60 mg (as base)	Sucrose, sugar spheres. (60 mg LILLY 3237). Opaque green and opaque blue. In 30s, 90s, and 1,000s; unit-dose 100s.

[a] Contains enteric-coated pellets.

DULOXETINE HYDROCHLORIDE — ORAL

WARNING

Suicidality in children and adolescents – Antidepressants increased the risk of suicidal thinking and behavior (suicidality) in short-term studies in children and adolescents with major depressive disorder (MDD) and other psychiatric disorders. Anyone considering the use of duloxetine or any other antidepressant in a child or adolescent must balance this risk with the clinical need. Patients who are started on therapy should be observed closely for clinical worsening, suicidality, or unusual changes in behavior. Families and caregivers should be advised of the need for close observation and communication with the prescriber. Duloxetine is not approved for use in pediatric patients (see Clinical worsening and suicide risk and Children sections in Warnings).

Pooled analyses of short-term (4 to 16 weeks) placebo-controlled trials of 9 antidepressant drugs (SSRIs and others) in children and adolescents with MDD, obsessive-compulsive disorder (OCD), or other psychiatric disorders (a total of 24 trials involving over 4,400 patients) have revealed a greater risk of adverse reactions representing suicidal thinking or behavior (suicidality) during the first few months of treatment in those receiving antidepressants. The average risk of such reactions in patients receiving antidepressants was 4%, twice the placebo risk of 2%. No suicides occurred in these trials.

Indications

➤*Diabetic peripheral neuropathic (DPN) pain:* For the management of neuropathic pain associated with diabetic peripheral neuropathy.

➤*Major depressive disorder (MDD):* For the treatment of MDD as defined in the DSM-IV.

➤*Unlabeled uses:* Fibromyalgia; stress urinary incontinence (SUI).

Administration and Dosage

➤*Approved by the FDA:* August 3, 2004.

Duloxetine should be swallowed whole and should not be chewed or crushed, nor should the contents be sprinkled on food or mixed with liquids.

➤*Diabetic peripheral neuropathic pain:*

Initial treatment – Administer as a total dose of 60 mg/day given once daily without regard to meals. There is no evidence that doses greater than 60 mg/day confer any additional benefit.

Maintenance/Continuation/Extended treatment – Because the progression of diabetic peripheral neuropathy is highly variable and management of pain is empirical, assess the effectiveness of duloxetine individually. Efficacy beyond 12 weeks has not been studied.

➤*MDD:*

Initial treatment – Administer as a total dose of 40 mg/day (given as 20 mg twice daily) to 60 mg/day (given either once a day or as 30 mg twice daily) without regard to meals. There is no evidence that doses greater than 60 mg/day confer any additional benefits.

Maintenance/Continuation/Extended treatment – Acute episodes of major depression require several months or longer of sustained pharmacologic therapy. Periodically reassess patients to determine the need for maintenance treatment and the appropriate dose for such treatment.

➤*Discontinuing treatment:* Symptoms associated with discontinuation of duloxetine and other selective serotonin reuptake inhibitors (SSRIs) and serotonin norepinephrine reuptake inhibitors (SNRIs) have been reported. Monitor patients for symptoms including dizziness, nausea, headache, paresthesia, vomiting, irritability, and nightmares when discontinuing treatment. A gradual reduction in the dose rather than abrupt cessation is recommended whenever possible. If intolerable symptoms occur following a decrease in the dose or upon discontinuation of treatment, then resuming the previously prescribed dose may be considered. Subsequently, the physician may continue decreasing the dose but at a more gradual rate.

➤*Switching patients to or from a monoamine oxidase inhibitor (MAOI):* At least 14 days should elapse between discontinuation of an MAOI and initiation of therapy with duloxetine. In addition, allow at least 5 days after stopping duloxetine before starting an MAOI.

➤*Storage/Stability:* Store at 25°C (77°F); excursions permitted to 15° to 30°C (59° to 86°F).

Actions

➤*Pharmacology:* Although the mechanism of the antidepressant and central pain inhibitory action of duloxetine in humans is unknown, it is believed to be related to its potentiation of serotonergic and noradrenergic activity in the CNS. Preclinical studies have shown that duloxetine is a potent inhibitor of neuronal serotonin and norepinephrine reuptake and a less potent inhibitor of dopamine reuptake. Duloxetine has no significant affinity for dopaminergic, adrenergic, cholinergic, histaminergic, opioid, glutamate, and gamma-aminobutyric acid (GABA) receptors in vitro. Duloxetine does not inhibit monoamine oxidase (MAO).

➤*Pharmacokinetics:*

Absorption/Distribution – Orally administered duloxetine is well absorbed. There is a median 2-hour lag until absorption begins, with maximal plasma concentrations (C_{max}) of duloxetine occurring 6 hours postdose. Food does not affect the C_{max} of duloxetine but delays the time to reach peak concentration from 6 to 10 hours; it marginally decreases the extent of absorption (AUC) by approximately 10%. There is a 3-hour delay in absorption and a one-third increase in apparent clearance of duloxetine after an evening dose as compared with a morning dose.

The apparent volume of distribution averages approximately 1,640 L. Duloxetine is highly bound (greater than 90%) to proteins in human plasma, binding primarily to albumin and α_1-acid glycoprotein. Plasma protein binding of duloxetine is not affected by renal or hepatic impairment. Steady-state plasma concentrations are typically achieved after 3 days of dosing.

Metabolism/Excretion – Duloxetine undergoes extensive metabolism, but the major circulating metabolites have not been shown to contribute significantly to the pharmacologic activity of duloxetine.

Duloxetine has an elimination half-life of approximately 12 hours (range, 8 to 17 hours). Elimination of duloxetine is mainly through hepatic metabolism involving two P-450 isozymes, CYP2D6 and CYP1A2.

Duloxetine comprises approximately 3% of the total radiolabeled material in the plasma, indicating that it undergoes extensive metabolism to numerous metabolites. The major biotransformation pathways for duloxetine involve oxidation of the naphthyl ring followed by conjugation and further oxidation. Both CYP2D6 and CYP1A2 catalyze the oxidation of the naphthyl ring in vitro. Metabolites found in plasma include 4-hydroxy duloxetine glucuronide and 5-hydroxy, 6-methoxy duloxetine sulfate. Many additional metabolites have been identified in urine, some representing only minor pathways of elimination. Only trace (less than 1% of the dose) amounts of unchanged duloxetine are present in the urine. Most (approximately 70%) of the duloxetine dose appears in the urine as metabolites of duloxetine; approximately 20% is excreted in the feces.

Special populations –

Age/Gender effects: A single dose of 40 mg was compared in healthy elderly females (65 to 77 years of age) and healthy middle-age females (32 to 50 years of age). There was no difference in the C_{max}, but the AUC of duloxetine was somewhat (approximately 25%) higher and the half-life approximately 4 hours longer in the elderly females. Dosage adjustment based on the age of the patient is not necessary.

Smoking: Duloxetine bioavailability (AUC) appears to be reduced by approximately one third in smokers. Dosage modifications are not recommended for smokers.

Renal function impairment: After a single dose of duloxetine 60 mg, C_{max} and AUC values were approximately 100% greater in patients with end-stage renal disease (ESRD) receiving chronic intermittent hemodialysis than in subjects with normal renal function. However, the elimination half-life was similar in both groups. The AUCs of the major circulating metabolites, 4-hydroxy duloxetine glucuronide and 5-hydroxy, 6-methoxy duloxetine sulfate, largely excreted in urine, were approximately 7- to 9-fold higher and would be expected to increase further with multiple dosing. For this reason, duloxetine is not recommended for patients with ESRD (requiring dialysis) or severe renal impairment (creatinine clearance less than 30 mL/min).

Hepatic function impairment: Patients with clinically evident hepatic insufficiency have decreased duloxetine metabolism and elimination. After a single dose of duloxetine 20 mg, 6 cirrhotic patients with moderate liver impairment (Child-Pugh class B) had a mean plasma duloxetine clearance approximately 15% that of age- and gender-matched healthy subjects, with a 5-fold increase in mean exposure (AUC). Although C_{max} was similar to healthy patients in the cirrhotic patients, the half-life was approximately 3 times longer. It is recommended that duloxetine not be administered to patients with any hepatic insufficiency.

Contraindications

Known hypersensitivity to duloxetine or any ingredient of the product; concomitant use in patients taking MAOIs; use in patients with uncontrolled narrow-angle glaucoma (see Precautions).

Warnings

➤*Clinical worsening and suicide risk:* Patients with MDD, both adult and pediatric, may experience worsening of their depression and/or the emergence of suicidal ideation and behavior (suicidality) or unusual changes in behavior, whether or not they are taking antidepressant medications, and this risk may persist until significant remission occurs. There has been a long-standing concern that antidepressants may have a role in inducing worsening of depression and the emergence of suicidality in certain patients. Antidepressants increased the risk of suicidal thinking and behavior (suicidality) in short-term studies in children and adolescents with MDD and other psychiatric disorders.

Pooled analyses of short-term, placebo-controlled trials of 9 antidepressant drugs (SSRIs and others) in children and adolescents with MDD, OCD, or other psychiatric disorders (a total of 24 trials involving over 4,400 patients) have revealed a greater risk of adverse reactions representing suicidal behavior or thinking (suicidality) during the first few months of treatment in those receiving antidepressants. The average risk of such reactions in patients receiving antidepressants was 4%, twice the placebo risk of 2%. There was considerable variation in risk among drugs, but a tendency toward an increase for almost all drugs studied. The risk of suicidality was most consistently observed in the MDD trials, but there were signals of risk arising from some trials in other psychiatric indications (OCD and social anxiety disorder) as well. No suicides occurred in any of these trials. It is unknown whether the suicidality risk in pediatric patients extends to longer-term use (ie, beyond several months). It also is unknown whether the suicidality risk extends to adults.

Closely observe all pediatric patients being treated with antidepressants for any indication for clinical worsening, suicidality, and unusual changes in behavior, especially during the initial few months of a course of drug therapy, or at times of dose changes, either increases or decreases. Such

DULOXETINE HYDROCHLORIDE — ORAL

observation would generally include at least weekly face-to-face contact with patients or their family members or caregivers during the first 4 weeks of treatment, then every-other-week visits for the next 4 weeks, then at 12 weeks, and as clinically indicated beyond 12 weeks. Additional contact by telephone may be appropriate between face-to-face visits.

Similarly observe adults with MDD or co-morbid depression in the setting of other psychiatric illness being treated with antidepressants for clinical worsening and suicidality, especially during the initial few months of a course of drug therapy, or at times of dose changes, either increases or decreases.

The following symptoms, anxiety, agitation, panic attacks, insomnia, irritability, hostility, aggressiveness, impulsivity, akathisia (psychomotor restlessness), hypomania, and mania, have been reported in adult and pediatric patients being treated with antidepressants for MDD as well as for other indications, both psychiatric and nonpsychiatric. Although a causal link between the emergence of such symptoms and either the worsening of depression and/or the emergence of suicidal impulses has not been established, there is concern that such symptoms may represent precursors to emerging suicidality.

Give consideration to changing the therapeutic regimen, including possibly discontinuing the medication, in patients whose depression is persistently worse, or who are experiencing emergent suicidality or symptoms that might be precursors to worsening depression or suicidality, especially if these symptoms are severe, abrupt in onset, or were not part of the patient's presenting symptoms.

If the decision has been made to discontinue treatment, taper medication as rapidly as is feasible, but with recognition that abrupt discontinuation can be associated with certain symptoms (see Discontinuation of treatment section in Precautions for a description of the risks of discontinuation of duloxetine).

Alert families and caregivers of pediatric patients being treated with antidepressants for MDD or other indications, both psychiatric and nonpsychiatric, about the need to monitor patients for the emergence of agitation, irritability, unusual changes in behavior, and the other symptoms described above, as well as the emergence of suicidality, and to report such symptoms immediately to health care providers. Such monitoring should include daily observation by families and caregivers. Write prescriptions for duloxetine for the smallest quantity of tablets consistent with good patient management in order to reduce the risk of overdose. Similarly advise families and caregivers of adults being treated for depression.

➤*Screening patients for bipolar disorder:* A major depressive episode may be the initial presentation of bipolar disorder. It is generally believed (though not established in controlled trials) that treating such an episode with an antidepressant alone may increase the likelihood of precipitation of a mixed/manic episode in patients at risk for bipolar disorder. Whether any of the symptoms described above represent such a conversion is unknown. However, prior to initiating treatment with an antidepressant, adequately screen patients with depressive symptoms to determine if they are at risk for bipolar disorder; such screening should include a detailed psychiatric history, including a family history of suicide, bipolar disorder, and depression. It should be noted that duloxetine is not approved for use in treating bipolar depression.

➤*MAOIs:* In patients receiving a serotonin reuptake inhibitor in combination with an MAOI, there have been reports of serious, sometimes fatal, reactions including hyperthermia, rigidity, myoclonus, autonomic instability with possible rapid fluctuations of vital signs, and mental status changes that include extreme agitation progressing to delirium and coma. These reactions also have been reported in patients who have recently discontinued serotonin reuptake inhibitors and are then started on an MAOI. Some cases presented with features resembling neuroleptic malignant syndrome. The effects of combined use of duloxetine and MAOIs have not been evaluated in humans or animals. Therefore, because duloxetine is an inhibitor of serotonin and norepinephrine reuptake, it is recommended that duloxetine not be used in combination with an MAOI, or within at least 14 days of discontinuing treatment with an MAOI. Based on the half-life of duloxetine, allow at least 5 days after stopping duloxetine before starting an MAOI.

➤*Hepatotoxicity:* Duloxetine increases the risk of elevation of serum transaminase levels. Liver transaminase elevations resulted in the discontinuation of 0.4% of duloxetine-treated patients. In these patients, the median time to detection of the transaminase elevation was approximately 2 months. In controlled trials in MDD, elevations of ALT greater than 3 times the upper limit of normal (ULN) occurred in 0.9% of duloxetine-treated patients and in 0.3% of placebo-treated patients. In the full cohort of placebo-controlled trials in any indication, 1% of duloxetine-treated patients had a greater than 3 times the ULN elevation of ALT compared with 0.2% of placebo-treated patients. In placebo-controlled studies using a fixed-dose design, there was evidence of a dose-response relationship for ALT and AST elevation of greater than 3 and 5 times the ULN, respectively.

The combination of transaminase elevations and elevated bilirubin, without evidence of obstruction, is generally recognized as an important predictor of severe liver injury. Three duloxetine patients had elevations of transaminases and bilirubin, but also had elevation of alkaline phosphatase, suggesting an obstructive process; in these patients, there was evidence of heavy alcohol use and this may have contributed to the abnormalities. Two placebo-treated patients also had transaminase elevations with elevated bilirubin. Because it is possible that duloxetine and alcohol may interact to cause liver injury, duloxetine should ordinarily not be prescribed to patients with substantial alcohol use.

➤*Renal function impairment:* Increased plasma concentrations of duloxetine, and especially of its metabolites, occur in patients with ESRD and severe renal impairment (Ccr less than 30 mL/min). For this reason, duloxetine is not recommended for patients with ESRD or severe renal impairment.

➤*Hepatic function impairment:* Do not administer duloxetine to patients with hepatic insufficiency; markedly increased exposure occurs.

➤*Carcinogenesis:* Duloxetine was administered by diet to mice and rats for 2 years. In female mice receiving duloxetine at dietary doses of approximately 140 mg/kg/day (11 times the maximum recommended human dose [MRHD] of 60 mg/day on a mg/m^2 basis), there was an increased incidence of hepatocellular adenomas and carcinomas; the no-effect level was approximately 50 mg/kg (4 times the MRHD on a mg/m^2 basis).

➤*Elderly:* Caution should be exercised in treating elderly patients. When individualizing the dosage, take extra care when increasing the dose.

➤*Pregnancy:* *Category C.* There are no adequate and well-controlled studies in pregnant women; therefore, use during pregnancy only if the potential benefit justifies the potential risk to the fetus.

Neonates exposed to SSRIs or SNRIs late in the third trimester have developed complications requiring prolonged hospitalization, respiratory support, and tube feeding. Such complications can arise immediately upon delivery. Reported clinical findings have included apnea, constant crying, cyanosis, feeding difficulty, hyperreflexia, hypertonia, hypoglycemia, hypotonia, irritability, jitteriness, respiratory distress, seizures, temperature instability, tremor, and vomiting. These features are consistent with either a direct toxic effect of SSRIs and SNRIs or, possibly, a drug discontinuation syndrome. It should be noted that, in some cases, the clinical picture is consistent with serotonin syndrome. When treating a pregnant woman with duloxetine during the third trimester, carefully consider the potential risks and benefits of treatment. The physician may consider tapering duloxetine in the third trimester.

In animal reproduction studies, duloxetine has been shown to have adverse effects on embryo/fetal and postnatal development. When duloxetine was administered orally to pregnant rats and rabbits during the period of organogenesis at doses up to 45 mg/kg/day (7 and 15 times the MRHD on a mg/m^2 basis in rats and rabbits, respectively), fetal weights were decreased. When duloxetine was administered orally to pregnant rats throughout gestation and lactation, the survival of pups to 1-day postpartum and pup body weights at birth and during the lactation period were decreased following maternal exposure to 30 mg/kg/day (5 times the MRHD on a mg/m^2 basis). Furthermore, behaviors consistent with increased reactivity, such as increased startle response to noise and decreased habituation of locomotor activity, were observed in pups following maternal exposure to 30 mg/kg/day.

➤*Lactation:* Duloxetine and/or its metabolites are excreted into the milk of lactating rats. It is unknown whether or not duloxetine and/or its metabolites are excreted into human milk, but nursing while taking duloxetine is not recommended.

➤*Children:* Safety and efficacy in the pediatric population have not been established for duloxetine (see Clinical worsening and suicide risk section in Warnings). Anyone considering the use of duloxetine in a child or adolescent must balance the potential risks with the clinical need.

Precautions

➤*Monitoring:* Monitor patients for the emergence of agitation, irritability, and other symptoms, as well as the emergence of suicidality; monitor blood pressure prior to initiation and periodically during treatment.

➤*Blood pressure effects:* In clinical trials, duloxetine treatment was associated with mean increases in blood pressure, averaging 2 mm Hg systolic and 0.5 mm Hg diastolic and an increase in the incidence of at least 1 measurement of systolic blood pressure over 140 mm Hg compared with placebo. Measure blood pressure prior to initiating treatment and periodically throughout treatment.

➤*Discontinuation of treatment:* Following abrupt discontinuation in placebo-controlled clinical trials of up to 9-weeks' duration, the following symptoms occurred at a rate of 2% or more and at a significantly higher rate in duloxetine-treated patients compared with those discontinuing from placebo: dizziness, headache, irritability, nausea, nightmare, paresthesia, and vomiting.

During marketing of other SSRIs and SNRIs, there have been spontaneous reports of adverse events occurring upon discontinuation of these drugs, particularly when abrupt, including the following: agitation, anxiety, confusion, dizziness, dysphoric mood, emotional lability, headache, hypomania, insomnia, irritability, lethargy, seizures, sensory disturbances (eg, paresthesias such as electric shock sensations), and tinnitus. Although these events are generally self-limiting, some have been reported to be severe.

Monitor patients for these symptoms when discontinuing treatment with duloxetine. A gradual reduction in the dose rather than abrupt cessation is recommended whenever possible. If intolerable symptoms occur following a decrease in the dose or upon discontinuation of treatment, resuming the previously prescribed dose may be considered. Subsequently, the physician may continue decreasing the dose but at a more gradual rate.

➤*Special risk:*

Mania / Hypomania activation – In placebo-controlled trials in patients with MDD, activation of mania or hypomania was reported in 0.1% of duloxetine-treated patients and 0.1% of placebo-treated patients. Activation of mania/hypomania has been reported in a small proportion of patients with mood disorders who were treated with other marketed drugs effective in the treatment of MDD. As with these other agents, cautiously use duloxetine in patients with a history of mania.

DULOXETINE HYDROCHLORIDE — ORAL

Seizures – In placebo-controlled clinical trials in patients with MDD, seizures occurred in 0.1% of patients treated with duloxetine and 0% of patients treated with placebo. Like other drugs effective in the treatment of MDD, prescribe duloxetine with care in patients with a history of a seizure disorder.

Controlled narrow-angle glaucoma – In clinical trials, duloxetine was associated with an increased risk of mydriasis; therefore, use cautiously in patients with controlled narrow-angle glaucoma.

Concomitant illness – Duloxetine is rapidly hydrolyzed in acidic media to naphthol; caution is advised in using duloxetine in patients with conditions that may slow gastric emptying (eg, some forms of diabetes).

Diabetes – In clinical trials, small increases in fasting blood glucose were observed in duloxetine-treated patients; however, overall diabetic control did not worsen as evidenced by stable HbA_{1c} values.

➤*Drug abuse and dependence:* Duloxetine has not been systematically studied in humans for its abuse potential; there was no indication of drug-seeking behavior in the clinical trials. However, it is not possible to predict on the basis of premarketing experience the extent to which a CNS-active drug will be misused, diverted, and/or abused once marketed. Consequently, physicians should carefully evaluate patients for a history of drug abuse and follow such patients closely, observing them for signs of misuse or abuse of duloxetine (eg, development of tolerance, incrementation of dose, drug-seeking behavior).

➤*Hazardous tasks:* Caution patients about operating hazardous machinery, including automobiles, until they are reasonably certain that duloxetine therapy does not adversely affect their ability to engage in such activities.

Drug Interactions

Duloxetine Drug Interactions

Precipitant drug	Object drug*		Description
CYP1A2 inhibitors (eg, fluvoxamine, quinolone antibiotics)	Duloxetine	↑	Concomitant use of duloxetine with fluvoxamine results in approximately 6-fold increase in AUC and approximately 2.5-fold increase in C_{max} of duloxetine. Some quinolone antibiotics would be expected to have similar effects. Avoid these combinations.
CYP2D6 inhibitors (eg, fluoxetine, quinidine, paroxetine)	Duloxetine	↑	Concomitant use of duloxetine with potent inhibitors of CYP2D6 may result in higher concentrations of duloxetine. Paroxetine (20 mg every day) increased the concentration of duloxetine (40 mg every day) by approximately 60%.
Duloxetine	Alcohol	↑	Liver injury, as manifested by ALT and total bilirubin elevations, with evidence of obstruction have occurred from coadministration of alcohol and duloxetine.
Alcohol	Duloxetine	↑	
Duloxetine	CNS-acting drugs	↑	Given the primary CNS effects of duloxetine, it should be used with caution when taken in combination with or substituted for other centrally acting drugs, including those with a similar mechanism of action.
Duloxetine	Drugs extensively metabolized by CYP2D6 (eg, flecainide, phenothiazines, propafenone, tricyclic antidepressants, thioridazine)	↑	Approach coadministration of duloxetine with other drugs extensively metabolized by CYP2D6 and that have a narrow therapeutic index with caution. Because of the risk of serious ventricular arrhythmias and sudden death associated with elevated plasma levels of thioridazine, do not coadminister duloxetine and thioridazine.
Duloxetine	Drugs highly bound to plasma proteins (eg, warfarin)	↑	Because duloxetine is highly protein bound, administration of duloxetine with another highly protein-bound drug may increase free concentrations of the other drug, potentially resulting in adverse effects.
Duloxetine	MAOIs	↑	Coadministration is contraindicated. Do not use duloxetine in combination with an MAOI, or within at least 14 days of discontinuing treatment with an MAOI. Allow at least 5 days after stopping duloxetine before starting an MAOI (see Contraindications and Warnings).

* ↑ = Object drug increased.

➤*Drug/Food interactions:* Food does not affect the C_{max} of duloxetine but delays the time to reach peak concentration from 6 to 10 hours; it marginally decreases the extent of absorption (AUC) by about 10%.

Adverse Reactions

Duloxetine Adverse Reactions (MDD) (%)[a]

Adverse reaction	Duloxetine (N = 1,139)	Placebo (N = 777)
CNS		
Anxiety	3%	2%
Decreased libido	3%	1%
Dizziness	9%	5%
Insomnia[b]	11%	6%
Somnolence	7%	3%
Tremor	3%	1%
Dermatologic		
Increased sweating	6%	2%
GI		
Constipation	11%	4%
Diarrhea	8%	6%
Dry mouth	15%	6%
Nausea	20%	7%
Vomiting	5%	3%
GU		
Ejaculation delayed[c]	3%	1%
Ejaculatory dysfunction[c,d]	3%	1%
Erectile dysfunction[c]	4%	1%
Orgasm abnormal[e]	3%	1%
Metabolic/Nutritional		
Decreased appetite[f]	8%	2%
Decreased weight	2%	1%
Ophthalmic		
Vision blurred	4%	1%
Miscellaneous		
Fatigue	8%	4%
Hot flushes	2%	1%

[a] Events reported by at least 2% of patients treated with duloxetine and more often than placebo. The following events were reported by at least 2% of patients treated with duloxetine and had an incidence equal to or less than placebo: Arthralgia, back pain, cough, dyspepsia, headache, nasopharyngitis, palpitations, pharyngitis, upper abdominal pain, and upper respiratory tract infection.
[b] Term includes middle insomnia.
[c] Male patients only.
[d] Term includes ejaculation disorder and ejaculation failure.
[e] Term includes anorgasmia.
[f] Term includes anorexia.

Duloxetine Adverse Reactions in Diabetic Peripheral Neuropathic Pain (%)[a]

Adverse reaction	Duloxetine 60 mg twice a day (N = 225)	Duloxetine 60 mg every day (N = 228)	Duloxetine 20 mg every day (N = 115)	Placebo (N = 223)
CNS				
Asthenia	8%	4%	2%	1%
Dizziness	17%	14%	6%	6%
Fatigue	12%	10%	2%	5%
Headache	15%	13%	13%	10%
Insomnia	13%	8%	9%	7%
Somnolence	21%	15%	7%	5%
Tremor	5%	1%	0%	0%
Dermatologic				
Hyperhidrosis	8%	6%	6%	2%
GI				
Constipation	15%	11%	5%	3%
Diarrhea	7%	11%	13%	6%
Dry mouth	12%	7%	5%	4%
Dyspepsia	4%	4%	4%	3%
Loose stools	2%	3%	2%	1%

DULOXETINE HYDROCHLORIDE — ORAL

Duloxetine Adverse Reactions in Diabetic Peripheral Neuropathic Pain (%)[a]

Adverse reaction	Duloxetine 60 mg twice a day (N = 225)	Duloxetine 60 mg every day (N = 228)	Duloxetine 20 mg every day (N = 115)	Placebo (N = 223)
Nausea	30%	22%	14%	9%
Vomiting	5%	5%	6%	4%
GU				
Erectile dysfunction[b]	4%	1%	0%	0%
Pollakiuria	5%	1%	3%	2%
Metabolic/ Nutritional				
Anorexia	5%	3%	3%	< 1%
Decreased appetite	11%	4%	3%	< 1%
Musculoskeletal				
Muscle cramp	4%	4%	5%	3%
Myalgia	4%	1%	3%	< 1%
Respiratory				
Cough	5%	3%	6%	4%
Pharyngolaryngeal pain	6%	1%	3%	1%
Miscellaneous				
Nasopharyngitis	9%	7%	9%	5%
Pyrexia	3%	1%	2%	1%

[a] Events reported by at least 2% of patients treated with duloxetine and more often than placebo. The following events were reported by at least 2% of patients treated with duloxetine for DPN and had an incidence equal to or less than placebo: arthralgia, back pain, edema peripheral, influenza, pain in extremity, pruritus, and upper respiratory tract infection.
[b] Male patients only.

➤*Other adverse events reported:*

Cardiovascular – Peripheral edema, phlebitis, hypertensive crisis, atrial fibrillation, bundle branch block right, cardiac failure, CHF, coronary artery disease, myocardial infarction (0.1% to 1%).

Electrocardiograms were obtained from 321 duloxetine-treated patients with MDD and from 528 duloxetine-treated patients with DPN. The rate-corrected QT (QT_c) interval in duloxetine-treated patients did not differ from that seen in placebo-treated patients. No clinically significant differences were observed for QT, PR, and QRS intervals between duloxetine- and placebo-treated patients.

In clinical trials of 40 to 120 mg daily doses, increases in blood pressure averaging 2 mm Hg systolic and 0.5 mm Hg diastolic compared with placebo and an increase in the incidence of at least 1 measurement of systolic blood pressure over 140 mm Hg have occurred.

Duloxetine treatment in placebo-controlled clinical trials caused a small increase in heart rate (approximately 2 beats per minute) compared with placebo.

CNS – Hypoesthesia, initial insomnia, irritability, lethargy, nervousness, nightmare, restlessness, rigors, sleep disorder (at least 1%); ataxia, completed suicide, dysarthria, feeling jittery, mania, mood swings, pressure of speech, sluggishness, suicide attempt (0.1% to 1%).

Dermatologic – Night sweats, pruritus, rash, skin ulcer (at least 1%); acne, alopecia, cold sweat, ecchymosis, eczema, erythema, erythematous rash, exfoliative dermatitis, face edema, hyperkeratosis, increased tendency to bruise, photosensitivity reaction, pruritic rash (0.1% to 1%).

GI – Gastritis (at least 1%); aphthous stomatitis, blood in stool, colitis, dysphagia, diverticulitis, esophageal stenosis acquired, gastric irritation, gastric ulcer, gingivitis, impaired gastric emptying, irritable bowel syndrome, lower abdominal pain, melena (0.1% to 1%).

GU – Dysuria (at least 1%); blood creatinine increased, micturition urgency, nephropathy, urinary hesitation, urinary incontinence, urinary retention, urine flow decreased, urine output decreased (0.1% to 1%).

Duloxetine is in a class of drugs known to affect urethral resistance. If symptoms of urinary hesitation develop during treatment with duloxetine, consider the possibility that they might be drug-related.

Hematologic – Anemia, leukopenia, increased white blood cell count, lymphadenopathy, thrombocytopenia (0.1% to 1%).

➤*Lab test abnormalities:* Small mean increases from baseline to endpoint in ALT, AST, CPK, and alkaline phosphatase. Infrequent, modest, transient, abnormal values were observed for these analytes in duloxetine-treated patients when compared with placebo-treated patients.

➤*Ophthalmic:* Diplopia, glaucoma, keratoconjunctivitis sicca, macular degeneration, maculopathy, photopsia, and retinal detachment (0.1% to 1%).

➤*Metabolic/Nutritional:* Hypoglycemia, increased appetite, weight increased (at least 1%); dehydration, dyslipidemia, edema, hypercholesterolemia, hyperlipidemia, hypertriglyceridemia, thirst (0.1% to 1%).

In MDD placebo-controlled clinical trials, patients treated with duloxetine for up to 9 weeks experienced a mean weight loss of approximately 0.5 kg, compared with a mean weight gain of approximately 0.2 kg in placebo-treated patients.

In DPN pain placebo-controlled clinical trials, patients treated with duloxetine for up to 13 weeks experienced a mean weight loss of approximately 1.1 kg, compared with a mean weight gain of approximately 0.2 kg in placebo-treated patients.

➤*Miscellaneous:* Oropharyngeal swelling, muscular weakness, hepatitis steatosis, influenza-like illness (0.1% to 1%).

Overdosage

➤*Symptoms:* There is limited clinical experience with duloxetine overdose in humans. In premarketing clinical trials as of October 2003, no cases of fatal acute overdose with duloxetine have been reported. Four nonfatal, acute ingestions of duloxetine (300 to 1,400 mg), alone or in combination with other drugs, have been reported.

➤*Treatment:* There is no specific antidote to duloxetine. In case of acute overdose, treatment should consist of those general measures employed in the management of overdose with any drug.

Ensure an adequate airway, oxygenation, and ventilation, and monitor cardiac rhythm and vital signs. Induction of emesis is not recommended. If needed, gastric lavage with a large-bore orogastric tube with appropriate airway protection may be indicated if performed soon after ingestion or in symptomatic patients.

Activated charcoal may be useful in limiting absorption of duloxetine from the GI tract. Administration of activated charcoal has been shown to decrease AUC and C_{max} by an average of one third, although some subjects had a limited effect from activated charcoal. Because of the large volume of distribution of this drug, forced diuresis, dialysis, hemoperfusion, and exchange transfusion are unlikely to be beneficial.

In managing overdose, consider the possibility of multiple-drug involvement.

Patient Information

Inform patients, their families, and their caregivers about the benefits and risks associated with treatment with duloxetine and counsel them in their appropriate use. A patient Medication Guide About Using Antidepressants in Children and Teenagers is available for duloxetine. Instruct patients, their families, and their caregivers to read the Medication Guide and assist them in understanding its contents. Give patients the opportunity to discuss the contents of the Medication Guide and to obtain answers to any questions they may have.

Advise patients of the following issues and ask them to alert their prescriber if these occur while taking duloxetine.

➤*Clinical worsening and suicide risk:* Encourage patients, their families, and their caregivers to be alert to the emergence of anxiety, agitation, panic attacks, insomnia, irritability, hostility, aggressiveness, impulsivity, akathisia (psychomotor restlessness), hypomania, mania, other unusual changes in behavior, worsening of depression, and suicidal ideation, especially early during antidepressant treatment and when the dose is adjusted up or down. Advise families and caregivers of patients to observe for the emergence of such symptoms on a day-to-day basis because changes may be abrupt. Such symptoms should be reported to the patient's prescriber or health professional, especially if they are severe, abrupt in onset, or were not part of the patient's presenting symptoms. Symptoms such as these may be associated with an increased risk for suicidal thinking and behavior and indicate a need for very close monitoring and possibly changes in the medication.

Inform patients that duloxetine should be swallowed whole and should not be chewed or crushed, nor should the contents be sprinkled on food or mixed with liquids. All of these actions might affect the enteric coating.

Caution patients about operating hazardous machinery, including automobiles, until they are reasonably certain that duloxetine therapy does not affect their ability to engage in such activities.

Advise patients that use of duloxetine concomitantly with heavy alcohol intake may be associated with severe liver injury. For this reason, duloxetine should ordinarily not be prescribed for patients with substantial alcohol use.

Advise patients to notify their health care providers if they become pregnant or intend to become pregnant during therapy or if they are breastfeeding.

While patients may notice improvement with duloxetine therapy in 1 to 4 weeks, they should be advised to continue therapy as directed.

VENLAFAXINE HYDROCHLORIDE

Rx	**Effexor** (Wyeth-Ayerst)	**Tablets:** 25 mg	Lactose. (25 W 701). Peach, shield shape, scored. In 100s and *Redipak* 100s.
		37.5 mg	Lactose. (37.5 W 781). Peach, shield shape, scored. In 100s and *Redipak* 100s.
		50 mg	Lactose. (50 W 703). Peach, shield shape, scored. In 100s and *Redipak* 100s.
		75 mg	Lactose. (75 W 704). Peach, shield shape, scored. In 100s and *Redipak* 100s.
		100 mg	Lactose. (100 W 705). Peach, shield shape, scored. In 100s and *Redipak* 100s.

VENLAFAXINE HYDROCHLORIDE

Rx	**Effexor XR** (Wyeth-Ayerst)	**Capsules, extended-release:** 37.5 mg	(W Effexor XR 37.5). Gray/Peach. In 100s and *Redipak* 100s.
		75 mg	(W Effexor XR 75). Peach. In 100s and *Redipak* 100s.
		150 mg	(W Effexor XR 150). Dk orange. In 100s and *Redipak* 100s.

VENLAFAXINE HYDROCHLORIDE — ORAL

For additional information, refer to the Antidepressants introduction.

WARNING

Suicidality in children and adolescents – Antidepressants increased the risk of suicidal thinking and behavior (suicidality) in short-term studies in children and adolescents with major depressive disorder (MDD) and other psychiatric disorders. Anyone considering the use of venlafaxine or any other antidepressant in a child or adolescent must balance this risk with the clinical need. Closely observe patients who are started on therapy for clinical worsening, suicidality, or unusual changes in behavior. Advise families and caregivers of the need for close observation and communication with the prescriber. Venlafaxine is not approved for use in pediatric patients.

Pooled analyses of short-term (4 to 16 weeks) placebo-controlled trials of 9 antidepressant drugs (selective serotonin reuptake inhibitors [SSRIs] and others) in children and adolescents with MDD, obsessive compulsive disorder (OCD), or other psychiatric disorders (a total of 24 trials involving over 4,400 patients) have revealed a greater risk of adverse events representing suicidal thinking or behavior (suicidality) during the first few months of treatment in those receiving antidepressants. The average risk of such events in patients receiving antidepressants was 4%, twice the placebo risk of 2%. No suicides occurred in these trials.

Indications

➤*MDD:* For the treatment of MDD.

➤*Generalized anxiety disorder (extended-release):* For the treatment of generalized anxiety disorder (GAD) as defined in DSM-IV. Anxiety or tension associated with the stress of everyday life usually does not require treatment with an anxiolytic.

➤*Social anxiety disorder (extended-release):* For the treatment of social anxiety disorder, also known as social phobia, as defined in DSM-IV.

➤*Unlabeled uses:* Hot flashes, premenstrual dysphoric disorder (PMDD), posttraumatic stress disorder (PTSD) (not recommended for use after no response with an SSRI for 8 weeks).

Administration and Dosage

➤*Approved by the FDA:* December 28, 1993.

➤*Immediate-release:*

Initial treatment – The recommended starting dose is 75 mg/day, administered in 2 or 3 divided doses, taken with food. Depending on tolerability and the need for further clinical effect, the dose may be increased to 150 mg/day. If needed, further increase the dose up to 225 mg/day. When increasing the dose, make increments of up to 75 mg/day at intervals of no less than 4 days. In outpatient settings there was no evidence of usefulness of doses greater than 225 mg/day for moderately depressed patients, but more severely depressed inpatients responded to a mean dose of 350 mg/day. Certain patients, including more severely depressed patients, may therefore respond more to higher doses, up to a maximum of 375 mg/day, generally in 3 divided doses.

➤*Extended-release:* Administer in a single dose with food either in the morning or in the evening at approximately the same time each day. Each capsule should be swallowed whole with fluid and not divided, crushed, chewed, or placed in water, or it may be administered by carefully opening the capsule and sprinkling the entire contents on a spoonful of applesauce. This drug/food mixture should be swallowed immediately without chewing and followed with a glass of water to ensure complete swallowing of the pellets.

Initial treatment –

MDD: For most patients, the recommended starting dose for venlafaxine extended-release is 75 mg/day, administered in a single dose. In the clinical trials establishing the efficacy of venlafaxine extended-release in moderately depressed outpatients, the initial dose of venlafaxine extended-release was 75 mg/day. For some patients, it may be desirable to start at 37.5 mg/day for 4 to 7 days, to allow new patients to adjust to the medication before increasing to 75 mg/day. While the relationship between dose and antidepressant response for venlafaxine extended-release has not been adequately explored, patients not responding to the initial 75 mg/day dose may benefit from dose increases to a maximum of approximately 225 mg/day. Make dose increases in increments of up to 75 mg/day, as needed, and at intervals of no less than 4 days, since steady-state plasma levels of venlafaxine and its major metabolites are achieved in most patients by day 4. In the clinical trials establishing efficacy, upward titration was permitted at intervals of 2 weeks or more; the average doses were about 140 to 180 mg/day.

It should be noted that, while the maximum recommended dose for moderately depressed outpatients is also 225 mg/day for the immediate-release form of venlafaxine, more severely depressed inpatients in 1 study of the development program for that product responded to a mean dose of 350 mg/day (range of 150 to 375 mg/day). Whether or not higher doses of venlafaxine extended-release are needed for more severely depressed patients is unknown; however, the experience with venlafaxine extended-release doses higher than 225 mg/day is very limited.

GAD: For most patients, the recommended starting dose for venlafaxine extended-release is 75 mg/day, administered in a single dose. In clinical trials establishing the efficacy of venlafaxine extended-release in outpatients with GAD, the initial dose of venlafaxine was 75 mg/day. For some patients, it may be desirable to start at 37.5 mg/day for 4 to 7 days to allow new patients to adjust to the medication before increasing to 75 mg/day. Although a dose-response relationship for effectiveness in GAD was not clearly established in fixed-dose studies, certain patients not responding to the initial 75 mg/day dose may benefit from dose increases to a maximum of approximately 225 mg/day. Make dose increases in increments of up to 75 mg/day, as needed, and at intervals of no less than 4 days.

Social anxiety disorder (social phobia): For most patients, the recommended starting dose for venlafaxine extended-release is 75 mg/day, administered in a single dose. In clinical trials establishing the efficacy of venlafaxine extended-release in outpatients with social anxiety disorder, the initial dose of venlafaxine extended-release was 75 mg/day and the maximum dose was 225 mg/day. For some patients, it may be desirable to start at 37.5 mg/day for 4 to 7 days to allow new patients to adjust to the medication before increasing to 75 mg/day. Although a dose-response relationship for effectiveness in patients with social anxiety disorder was not clearly established in fixed-dose studies, certain patients not responding to the initial 75 mg/day dose may benefit from dose increases to a maximum of approximately 225 mg/day. Make dose increases in increments of up to 75 mg/day, as needed, and at intervals of no less than 4 days.

Switching patients from venlafaxine to venlafaxine extended-release – Depressed patients who are currently being treated at a therapeutic dose with venlafaxine may be switched to venlafaxine extended-release at the nearest equivalent dose (mg/day) (eg, venlafaxine 37.5 mg 2 times daily to venlafaxine extended-release 75 mg once daily). However, individual dosage adjustments may be necessary.

➤*Discontinuing venlafaxine:* When discontinuing venlafaxine after more than 1 week of therapy, it is generally recommended that the dose be tapered to minimize the risk of discontinuation symptoms. Taper the dose gradually over at least a 2-week period in patients who have received venlafaxine for 6 weeks or more.

See Precautions for more information.

Extended-release – In clinical trials with venlafaxine extended-release, tapering was achieved by reducing the daily dose by 75 mg at 1-week intervals. Individualization of tapering may be necessary.

➤*Special populations:*

Pregnant women during the third trimester – Neonates exposed to venlafaxine, other SNRIs (serotonin and norepinephrine reuptake inhibitors), or SSRIs, late in the third trimester have developed complications requiring prolonged hospitalization, respiratory support, and tube feeding. When treating pregnant women with venlafaxine during the third trimester, carefully consider the potential risks and benefits of treatment. Consider tapering venlafaxine in the third trimester.

Hepatic function impairment – In 9 patients with hepatic cirrhosis, the pharmacokinetic disposition of both venlafaxine and O-desmethylvenlafaxine (ODV) was significantly altered after oral administration of venlafaxine. Venlafaxine elimination half-life was prolonged by about 30%, and clearance decreased by about 50% in cirrhotic patients compared to healthy subjects. ODV elimination half-life was prolonged by about 60% and clearance decreased by about 30% in cirrhotic patients compared to healthy subjects. A large degree of intersubject variability was noted. Three patients with more severe cirrhosis had a more substantial decrease in venlafaxine clearance (about 90%) compared to healthy subjects. Given the decrease in clearance and increase in elimination half-life for both venlafaxine and ODV that is observed in patients with hepatic cirrhosis compared with healthy subjects, it is recommended that the starting dose be reduced by 50% in patients with moderate hepatic impairment. Because there was much individual variability in clearance between patients with cirrhosis, individualization of dosage may be desirable in some patients.

Renal function impairment – In a renal impairment study, venlafaxine elimination half-life after oral administration was prolonged by about 50% and clearance was reduced by about 24% in renally impaired patients (GFR = 10 to 70 mL/min), compared to healthy subjects. In dialysis patients, venlafaxine elimination half-life was prolonged by about 180% and clearance was reduced by about 57% compared to healthy subjects. Similarly, ODV elimination half-life was prolonged by about 40%, although clearance was unchanged in patients with renal impairment (GFR = 10 to 70 mL/min) compared with healthy subjects. In dialysis patients, ODV elimination half-life was prolonged by about 142% and clearance was reduced by about 56% compared to healthy subjects. A large degree of intersubject variability was noted. Given the decrease in clearance for venlafaxine and the increase in elimination half-life for both venlafaxine and ODV that is observed in patients with renal impairment (GFR = 10 to 70 mL/min) compared with healthy subjects, it is recommended that the total daily dose be reduced by 25% to 50% for venlafaxine extended-release. For patients with mild to moderate renal impairment, reduce the dose by 25% for venlafaxine. In patients undergoing hemodialysis, it is recommended that the total daily dose be reduced by 50% and that the dose be withheld until the dialysis treatment is completed (4 hours). Because there was much individual variability in clear-

VENLAFAXINE HYDROCHLORIDE — ORAL

ance between patients with renal impairment, individualization of dosage may be desirable in some patients.

Elderly patients – No dose adjustment is recommended for elderly patients solely on the basis of age. As with any drug for the treatment of MDD, GAD, or social anxiety disorder, however, exercise caution in treating the elderly. When individualizing the dosage, take extra care when increasing the dose.

➤*Maintenance treatment:* It is generally agreed that acute episodes of MDD require several months or longer of sustained pharmacological therapy beyond response to the acute episode. In 1 study, in which patients responding during 8 weeks of acute treatment with venlafaxine extended-release were assigned randomly to placebo or to the same dose of venlafaxine extended-release (75, 150, or 225 mg/day, every morning) during 26 weeks of maintenance treatment as they had received during the acute stabilization phase, longer-term efficacy was demonstrated. A second longer-term study has demonstrated the efficacy of venlafaxine in maintaining a response in patients with recurrent MDD who had responded and continued to be improved during an initial 26 weeks of treatment and were then randomly assigned to placebo or venlafaxine for periods of up to 52 weeks on the same dose (100 to 200 mg/day, on a twice-daily schedule). Based on these limited data, it is not known whether the dose of venlafaxine/venlafaxine extended-release needed for maintenance treatment is identical to the dose needed to achieve an initial response. Patients should be periodically reassessed to determine the need for maintenance treatment and the appropriate dose for such treatment.

Extended-release – There is no body of evidence available from controlled trials to indicate how long patients with MDD, GAD, or social anxiety disorder should be treated with venlafaxine extended-release.

In patients with GAD, venlafaxine extended-release has been shown to be effective in 6-month clinical trials. Periodically reassess the need for continuing medication in patients with GAD who improve with venlafaxine extended-release treatment.

In patients with social anxiety disorder, there are no efficacy data beyond 12 weeks of treatment with venlafaxine extended-release. The need for continuing medication in patients with social anxiety disorder who improve with venlafaxine extended-release treatment should be periodically reassessed.

➤*Discontinuing venlafaxine:* Symptoms associated with discontinuation of venlafaxine, other SNRIs, and SSRIs, have been reported. Patients should be monitored for these symptoms when discontinuing treatment. A gradual reduction in the dose rather than abrupt cessation is recommended whenever possible. If intolerable symptoms occur following a decrease in the dose or upon discontinuation of treatment, then resuming the previously prescribed dose may be considered. Subsequently, the physician may continue decreasing the dose but at a more gradual rate. In clinical trials with venlafaxine, tapering was achieved by reducing the daily dose by 75 mg at 1 week intervals. Individualization of tapering may be necessary.

➤*Switching patients to or from a monoamine oxidase inhibitor (MAOI):* Adverse reactions, some of which were serious, have been reported in patients who have recently been discontinued from an MAOI and started on venlafaxine, or who have recently had venlafaxine therapy discontinued prior to initiation of an MAOI. These reactions have included tremor, myoclonus, diaphoresis, nausea, vomiting, flushing, dizziness, hyperthermia with features resembling neuroleptic malignant syndrome, seizures, and death. In patients receiving antidepressants with pharmacological properties similar to venlafaxine in combination with an MAOI, there have also been reports of serious, sometimes fatal, reactions. For a selective serotonin reuptake inhibitor, these reactions have included hyperthermia, rigidity, myoclonus, autonomic instability with possible rapid fluctuations of vital signs, and mental status changes that include extreme agitation progressing to delirium and coma. Some cases presented with features resembling neuroleptic malignant syndrome. Severe hyperthermia and seizures, sometimes fatal, have been reported in association with the combined use of tricyclic antidepressants and MAOIs. These reactions have also been reported in patients who have recently discontinued these drugs and have been started on an MAOI. The effects of combined use of venlafaxine and MAOIs have not been evaluated in humans or animals. At least 14 days should elapse between discontinuation of an MAOI and initiation of therapy with venlafaxine. In addition, allow at least 7 days after stopping venlafaxine before starting an MAOI.

➤*Storage/Stability:* Store at controlled room temperature, 20° to 25°C (68° to 77°F) in a dry place. Dispense in a well-closed container.

Extended-release – Protect from light.

Actions

➤*Pharmacology:* The mechanism of the antidepressant action of venlafaxine in humans is believed to be associated with its potentiation of neurotransmitter activity in the CNS. Preclinical studies have shown that venlafaxine and its active metabolite, ODV, are potent inhibitors of neuronal serotonin and norepinephrine reuptake and weak inhibitors of dopamine reuptake. Venlafaxine and ODV have no significant affinity for muscarinic cholinergic, H_1-histaminergic, or α_1-adrenergic receptors in vitro. Pharmacologic activity at these receptors is hypothesized to be associated with the various anticholinergic, sedative, and cardiovascular effects seen with other psychotropic drugs. Venlafaxine and ODV do not possess monoamine oxidase (MAO) inhibitory activity.

➤*Pharmacokinetics:*

Absorption/Distribution – Venlafaxine is well absorbed and extensively metabolized in the liver. ODV is the only major active metabolite. On the basis of mass balance studies, at least 92% of a single oral dose of venlafaxine is absorbed. The absolute bioavailability of venlafaxine is about 45%.

Steady-state concentrations of venlafaxine and ODV in plasma are attained within 3 days of oral multiple-dose therapy. Venlafaxine and ODV exhibited linear kinetics over the dose range of 75 to 450 mg/day. Mean ± SD steady-state plasma clearance of venlafaxine and ODV is 1.3 ± 0.6 and 0.4 ± 0.2 L/hr/kg, respectively; apparent elimination half-life is 5 ± 2 and 11 ± 2 hours, respectively; and apparent (steady-state) volume of distribution is 7.5 ± 3.7 and 5.7 ± 1.8 L/kg, respectively. Venlafaxine and ODV are minimally bound at therapeutic concentrations to plasma proteins (27% and 30%, respectively). When equal daily doses of venlafaxine immediate-release were administered as either twice-daily or 3-times-daily regimens, the drug exposure (AUC) and fluctuation in plasma levels of venlafaxine and ODV were comparable following both regimens.

Immediate-release: The degree of binding of venlafaxine to human plasma is 27% ± 2% at concentrations ranging from 2.5 to 2,215 ng/mL. The degree of ODV binding to human plasma is 30% ± 12% at concentrations ranging from 100 to 500 ng/dL. Protein-binding-induced drug interactions with venlafaxine are not expected.

The relative bioavailability of venlafaxine from a tablet was 100% when compared to an oral solution. Food has no significant effect on the absorption of venlafaxine or on the formation of ODV.

Extended-release: Administration of venlafaxine extended-release (150 mg every 24 hours) generally resulted in lower C_{max} (150 ng/mL for venlafaxine and 260 ng/mL for ODV) and later T_{max} (5.5 hours for venlafaxine and 9 hours for ODV) than for immediate-release venlafaxine tablets (C_{max} for immediate-release 75 mg every 12 hours was 225 ng/mL for venlafaxine and 290 ng/mL for ODV; T_{max} was 2 hours for venlafaxine and 3 hours for ODV). When equal daily doses of venlafaxine were administered as either an immediate-release tablet or the extended-release capsule, the exposure to both venlafaxine and ODV was similar for the 2 treatments, and the fluctuation in plasma concentrations was slightly lower with the venlafaxine extended-release capsule. Venlafaxine extended-release, therefore, provides a slower rate of absorption, but the same extent of absorption compared with the immediate-release tablet.

Food did not affect the bioavailability of venlafaxine or its active metabolite, ODV. Time of administration (am vs pm) did not affect the pharmacokinetics of venlafaxine and ODV from the venlafaxine extended-release 75 mg capsule.

Metabolism/Excretion – Following absorption, venlafaxine undergoes extensive presystemic metabolism in the liver, primarily to ODV, but also to N-desmethylvenlafaxine, N,O-didesmethylvenlafaxine, and other minor metabolites. In vitro studies indicate that the formation of ODV is catalyzed by CYP2D6; this has been confirmed in a clinical study showing that patients with low CYP2D6 levels ("poor metabolizers") had increased levels of venlafaxine and reduced levels of ODV compared to people with normal CYP2D6 ("extensive metabolizers"). The differences between the CYP2D6 poor and extensive metabolizers, however, are not expected to be clinically important because the sum of venlafaxine and ODV is similar in the 2 groups and venlafaxine and ODV are pharmacologically approximately equiactive and equipotent.

Approximately 87% of a venlafaxine dose is recovered in the urine within 48 hours as unchanged venlafaxine (5%), unconjugated ODV (29%), conjugated ODV (26%), or other minor inactive metabolites (27%). Renal elimination of venlafaxine and its metabolite is thus the primary route of excretion.

Special populations –

Renal function impairment: See Administration and Dosage for more information.

Hepatic function impairment: See Administration and Dosage for more information.

Age and gender: A population pharmacokinetic analysis of 404 venlafaxine-treated patients from 2 studies involving both twice-daily and 3-times-daily regimens showed that dose-normalized trough plasma levels of either venlafaxine or ODV were unaltered by age or gender differences. Dosage adjustment based on the age or gender of a patient is generally not necessary.

Poor/extensive metabolizers (extended-release): Plasma concentrations of venlafaxine were higher in CYP2D6 poor metabolizers than extensive metabolizers. Because the total exposure (AUC) of venlafaxine and ODV was similar in poor and extensive metabolizer groups, however, there is no need for different venlafaxine dosing regimens for these 2 groups.

Contraindications

Hypersensitivity to venlafaxine or to any excipients in the formulation.

Concomitant use in patients taking MAOIs is contraindicated.

Warnings

➤*Clinical worsening and suicide risk:* Patients with MDD, both adult and pediatric, may experience worsening of their depression and/or the emergence of suicidal ideation and behavior (suicidality) or unusual changes in behavior, whether or not they are taking antidepressant medications, and this risk may persist until significant remission occurs. There has been a long-standing concern that antidepressants may have a role in inducing worsening of depression and the emergence of suicidality in certain patients. Antidepressants increased the risk of suicidal thinking and behavior (suicidality) in short-term studies in children and adolescents with MDD and other psychiatric disorders.

Pooled analyses of short-term placebo-controlled trials of 9 antidepressant drugs (SSRIs and others) in children and adolescents with MDD, OCD, or other psychiatric disorders (a total of 24 trials involving over 4,400 patients) have revealed a greater risk of adverse events representing suicidal behavior or thinking (suicidality) during the first few months of treatment in those

VENLAFAXINE HYDROCHLORIDE — ORAL

receiving antidepressants. The average risk of such events in patients receiving antidepressants was 4%, twice the placebo risk of 2%. There was considerable variation in risk among drugs, but a tendency toward an increase for almost all drugs studied. The risk of suicidality was most consistently observed in the MDD trials, but there were signals of risk arising from some trials in other psychiatric indications (OCD and social anxiety disorder) as well. No suicides occurred in any of these trials. It is unknown whether the suicidality risk in pediatric patients extends to longer-term use (beyond several months). It is also unknown whether the suicidality risk extends to adults.

Closely observe all pediatric patients being treated with antidepressants for any indication for clinical worsening, suicidality, and unusual changes in behavior, especially during the initial few months of a course of drug therapy, or at times of dose changes, either increases or decreases. Such observation generally include at least weekly face-to-face contact with patients or their family members or caregivers during the first 4 weeks of treatment, then every-other-week visits for the next 4 weeks, then at 12 weeks, and as clinically indicated beyond 12 weeks. Additional contact by telephone may be appropriate between face-to-face visits.

Similarly observe adults with MDD or comorbid depression in the setting of other psychiatric illness being treated with antidepressants for clinical worsening and suicidality, especially during the initial few months of a course of drug therapy, or at times of dose changes, either increases or decreases.

The following symptoms, anxiety, agitation, panic attacks, insomnia, irritability, hostility, aggressiveness, impulsivity, akathisia (psychomotor restlessness), hypomania, and mania, have been reported in adult and pediatric patients being treated with antidepressants for MDD as well as for other indications, both psychiatric and nonpsychiatric. Although a causal link between the emergence of such symptoms and either the worsening of depression and/or the emergence of suicidal impulses has not been established, there is concern that such symptoms may represent precursors to emerging suicidality.

Consider changing the therapeutic regimen, including possibly discontinuing the medication, in patients whose depression is persistently worse, or who are experiencing emergent suicidality or symptoms that might be precursors to worsening depression or suicidality, especially if these symptoms are severe, abrupt in onset, or were not part of the patient's presenting symptoms.

If the decision has been made to discontinue treatment, taper the medication as rapidly as is feasible, but with recognition that abrupt discontinuation can be associated with certain symptoms.

Alert families and caregivers of pediatric patients being treated with antidepressants for MDD or other indications, both psychiatric and nonpsychiatric, to the need to monitor patients for the emergence of agitation, irritability, unusual changes in behavior, and the other symptoms described above, as well as the emergence of suicidality, and to report such symptoms immediately to health care providers. Such monitoring should include daily observation by families and caregivers. Prescriptions for venlafaxine should be written for the smallest quantity of capsules consistent with good patient management, in order to reduce the risk of overdose. Similarly advise families and caregivers of adults being treated for depression.

➤*Screening patients for bipolar disorder:* A major depressive episode may be the initial presentation of bipolar disorder. It is generally believed (though not established in controlled trials) that treating such an episode with an antidepressant alone may increase the likelihood of precipitation of a mixed/manic episode in patients at risk for bipolar disorder. Whether any of the symptoms described above represent such a conversion is unknown. However, prior to initiating treatment with an antidepressant, adequately screen patients with depressive symptoms to determine if they are at risk for bipolar disorder; such screening should include a detailed psychiatric history, including a family history of suicide, bipolar disorder, and depression. It should be noted that venlafaxine is not approved for use in treating bipolar depression.

➤*Potential for interaction with MAOIs:* Adverse reactions, some of which were serious, have been reported in patients who have recently been discontinued from an MAOI and started on venlafaxine, or who have recently had venlafaxine therapy discontinued prior to initiation of an MAOI. These reactions have included tremor, myoclonus, diaphoresis, nausea, vomiting, flushing, dizziness, hyperthermia with features resembling neuroleptic malignant syndrome, seizures, and death. In patients receiving antidepressants with pharmacological properties similar to venlafaxine in combination with an MAOI, there have also been reports of serious, sometimes fatal, reactions. For a selective serotonin reuptake inhibitor, these reactions have included hyperthermia, rigidity, myoclonus, autonomic instability with possible rapid fluctuations of vital signs, and mental status changes that include extreme agitation progressing to delirium and coma. Some cases presented with features resembling neuroleptic malignant syndrome. Severe hyperthermia and seizures, sometimes fatal, have been reported in association with the combined use of tricyclic antidepressants and MAOIs. These reactions have also been reported in patients who have recently discontinued these drugs and have been started on an MAOI. The effects of combined use of venlafaxine and MAOIs have not been evaluated in humans or animals. Therefore, because venlafaxine is an inhibitor of both norepinephrine and serotonin reuptake, it is recommended that venlafaxine or venlafaxine extended-release not be used in combination with an MAOI, or within at least 14 days of discontinuing treatment with an MAOI. Based on the half-life of venlafaxine, allow at least 7 days after stopping venlafaxine before starting an MAOI.

➤*Immediate-release:*

Sustained hypertension – Venlafaxine treatment is associated with sustained increases in blood pressure in some patients.

In a premarketing study comparing 3 fixed doses of venlafaxine (75, 225, and 375 mg/day) and placebo, a mean increase in supine diastolic blood pressure (SDBP) of 7.2 mm Hg was seen in the 375 mg/day group at week 6 compared to essentially no changes in the 75 and 225 mg/day groups and a mean decrease in SDBP of 2.2 mm Hg in the placebo group.

An analysis for patients meeting criteria for sustained hypertension (defined as treatment-emergent SDBP greater than or equal to 90 mm Hg and greater than or equal to 10 mm Hg above baseline for 3 consecutive visits) revealed a dose-dependent increase in the incidence of sustained hypertension for venlafaxine:

Probability of Sustained Elevation in SDBP (Pool or Premarketing Venlafaxine Studies)	
Treatment group	Incidence of sustained elevation in SDBP
Venlafaxine	
< 100 mg/day	3%
101 to 200 mg/day	5%
201 to 300 mg/day	7%
> 300 mg/day	13%
Placebo	2%

An analysis of the patient with sustained hypertension and the 19 venlafaxine patients who were discontinued from treatment because of hypertension (less than 1% of total venlafaxine-treated group) revealed that most of the blood pressure increases were in a modest range (10 to 15 mm Hg, SDBP). Nevertheless, sustained increases of this magnitude could have adverse consequences. Therefore, it is recommended that patients receiving venlafaxine have regular monitoring of blood pressure. For patients who experience a sustained increase in blood pressure while receiving venlafaxine, consider either dose reduction or discontinuation.

➤*Extended-release:*

Sustained hypertension – Venlafaxine is associated with sustained increases in blood pressure in some patients. Among patients treated with venlafaxine extended-release 75 to 375 mg per day in premarketing studies in patients with MDD, 3% (19 of 705) experienced sustained hypertension [defined as treatment-emergent supine diastolic blood pressure (SDBP) greater than or equal to 90 mm Hg and greater than or equal to 10 mm Hg above baseline for 3 consecutive on-therapy visits]. Among patients treated with venlafaxine extended-release 37.5 to 225 mg per day in premarketing GAD studies, 0.5% (5 of 1,011) experienced sustained hypertension. Among patients treated with venlafaxine extended-release 75 to 225 mg/day in premarketing social anxiety disorder studies, 1.4% (4 of 277) experienced sustained hypertension. Experience with the immediate-release venlafaxine showed that sustained hypertension was dose-related, increasing from 3% to 7% at 100 to 300 mg per day to 13% at doses above 300 mg per day. An insufficient number of patients received mean doses of venlafaxine over 300 mg/day to fully evaluate the incidence of sustained increases in blood pressure at these higher doses.

In placebo-controlled premarketing studies in patients with MDD with venlafaxine extended-release 75 to 225 mg/day, a final on-drug mean increase in supine diastolic blood pressure (SDBP) of 1.2 mm Hg was observed for venlafaxine extended-release-treated patients compared with a mean decrease of 0.2 mm Hg for placebo-treated patients. In placebo-controlled premarketing GAD studies with venlafaxine extended-release 37.5 to 225 mg/day, up to 8 weeks or up to 6 months, a final on-drug mean increase in SDBP of 0.3 mm Hg was observed for venlafaxine extended-release-treated patients compared with a mean decrease of 0.9 and 0.8 mm Hg, respectively, for placebo-treated patients. In placebo-controlled premarketing social anxiety disorder studies with venlafaxine extended-release 75 to 225 mg/day up to 12 weeks, a final on-drug mean increase in SDBP of 1.3 mm Hg was observed for venlafaxine extended-release-treated patients compared with a mean decrease of 1.3 mm Hg for placebo-treated patients.

In premarketing MDD studies, 0.7% (5 of 705) of the venlafaxine extended-release-treated patients, respectively, discontinued treatment because of elevated blood pressure. Among these patients, most of the blood pressure increases were in a modest range (12 to 16 mm Hg, SDBP). In premarketing GAD studies up to 8 weeks and up to 6 months, 0.7% (10 of 1,381) and 1.3% (7 of 535) of the venlafaxine extended-release-treated patients, respectively, discontinued treatment because of elevated blood pressure. Among these patients, most of the blood pressure increases were in a modest range (12 to 25 mm Hg, SDBP up to 8 weeks; 8 to 28 mm Hg up to 6 months). In premarketing social anxiety disorder studies up to 12 weeks, 0.4% (1 of 277) of the venlafaxine extended-release-treated patients discontinued treatment because of elevated blood pressure. In this patient, the blood pressure increase was modest (13 mm Hg, SDBP).

Sustained increases of SDBP could have adverse consequences. Therefore, it is recommended that patients receiving venlafaxine extended-release have regular monitoring of blood pressure. For patients who experience a sustained increase in blood pressure while receiving venlafaxine, consider dose reduction or discontinuation.

➤*Renal/Hepatic function impairment:* In patients with renal impairment (GFR = 10 to 70 mL/min) or cirrhosis of the liver, the clearances of venlafaxine and its active metabolites were decreased, thus prolonging the elimination half-lives of these substances. A lower dose may be necessary. It is recommended that the total daily dose be reduced by 25% to 50% for ven-

VENLAFAXINE HYDROCHLORIDE — ORAL

lafaxine extended-release. For patients with mild to moderate renal impairment, decrease the dose by 25% for venlafaxine immediate-release. In patients undergoing hemodialysis, it is recommended that the total daily dose be reduced by 50% and that the dose be withheld until the dialysis treatment is completed (4 hours). Because there was much individual variability in clearance between patients with renal impairment, individualization of dosage may be desirable in some patients. Like all antidepressants, use venlafaxine with caution in such patients.

➤*Mutagenesis:* There was a clastogenic response in the in vivo chromosomal aberration assay in rat bone marrow in male rats receiving 200 times, on a mg/kg basis, or 50 times, on a mg/m^2 basis, the maximum human daily dose. The no-effect dose was 67 times (mg/kg) or 17 times (mg/m^2) the human dose.

➤*Elderly:* No overall differences in effectiveness or safety were observed between geriatric patients and younger patients, and other reported clinical experience generally has not identified differences in response between the elderly and younger patients. However, greater sensitivity of some older individuals cannot be ruled out. As with other antidepressants, several cases of hyponatremia and syndrome of inappropriate antidiuretic hormone secretion (SIADH) have been reported, usually in the elderly.

➤*Pregnancy: Category C.*

Teratogenic – Venlafaxine did not cause malformations in offspring of rats or rabbits given doses up to 11 times (rat) or 12 times (rabbit) the maximum recommended human daily dose on a mg/kg basis, or 2.5 times (rat) and 4 times (rabbit) the human daily dose on a mg/m^2 basis. However, in rats, there was a decrease in pup weight, an increase in stillborn pups, and an increase in pup deaths during the first 5 days of lactation, when dosing began during pregnancy and continued until weaning. The cause of these deaths is not known. These effects occurred at 10 times (mg/kg) or 2.5 times (mg/m^2) the maximum human daily dose. The no effect dose for rat pup mortality was 1.4 times the human dose on a mg/kg basis or 0.25 times the human dose on a mg/m^2 basis. There are no adequate and well-controlled studies in pregnant women. Because animal reproduction studies are not always predictive of human response, use this drug during pregnancy only if clearly needed.

Nonteratogenic – Neonates exposed to venlafaxine, other SNRIs, or SSRIs late in the third trimester have developed complications requiring prolonged hospitalization, respiratory support, and tube feeding. Such complications can arise immediately upon delivery. Reported clinical findings have included respiratory distress, cyanosis, apnea, seizures, temperature instability, feeding difficulty, vomiting, hypoglycemia, hypotonia, hypertonia, hyperreflexia, tremor, jitteriness, irritability, and constant crying. These features are consistent with either a direct toxic effect of SSRIs and SNRIs or, possibly, a drug discontinuation syndrome. It should be noted that, in some cases, the clinical picture is consistent with serotonin syndrome. When treating a pregnant woman with venlafaxine during the third trimester, carefully consider the potential risks and benefits of treatment.

Labor and delivery – The effect of venlafaxine on labor and delivery in humans is unknown.

➤*Lactation:* Venlafaxine and ODV have been reported to be excreted in human milk. Because of the potential for serious adverse reactions in nursing infants from venlafaxine, decide whether to discontinue breast—feeding or to discontinue the drug, taking into account the importance of the drug to the mother.

➤*Children:* Safety and effectiveness in the pediatric population have not been established. Two placebo-controlled trials in 766 pediatric patients with MDD and 2 placebo-controlled trials in 793 pediatric patients with GAD have been conducted with venlafaxine extended-release, and the data were not sufficient to support a claim for use in pediatric patients.

Anyone considering the use of venlafaxine in a child or adolescent must balance the potential risks with the clinical need.

Although no studies have been designed to primarily assess the impact of venlafaxine's extended-release on the growth, development, and maturation of children and adolescents, the studies that have been done suggest that venlafaxine extended-release may adversely affect weight and height. Should the decision be made to treat a pediatric patient with venlafaxine, regular monitoring of weight and height is recommended during treatment, particularly if it is to be continued long term. The safety of venlafaxine extended-release treatment for pediatric patients has not been systematically assessed for chronic treatment longer than 6 months in duration.

In the studies conducted in pediatric patients (6 to 17 years of age), the occurrence of blood pressure and cholesterol increases considered to be clinically relevant in pediatric patients was similar to that observed in adult patients. Consequently, the precautions for adults apply to pediatric patients.

Precautions

➤*Discontinuation of treatment with venlafaxine:* Discontinuation symptoms have been systematically evaluated in patients taking venlafaxine to include prospective analyses of clinical trials in GAD and retrospective surveys of trials in MDD. Abrupt discontinuation or dose reduction of venlafaxine at various doses has been found to be associated with the appearance of new symptoms, the frequency of which increased with increased dose level and with longer duration of treatment. Reported symptoms include agitation, anorexia, anxiety, confusion, coordination impaired, diarrhea, dizziness, dry mouth, dysphoric mood, fasciculation, fatigue, headaches, hypomania, insomnia, nausea, nervousness, nightmares, sensory disturbances (including shock-like electrical sensations), somnolence, sweating, tremor, vertigo, and vomiting.

During marketing of venlafaxine, other SNRIs, and SSRIs, there have been spontaneous reports of adverse events occurring upon discontinuation of these drugs, particularly when abrupt, including the following: dysphoric mood, irritability, agitation, dizziness, sensory disturbances (eg, paresthesias such as electric shock sensations), anxiety, confusion, headache, lethargy, emotional lability, insomnia, hypomania, tinnitus, and seizures. While these events are generally self-limiting, there have been reports of serious discontinuation symptoms.

Monitor patients for these symptoms when discontinuing treatment with venlafaxine. A gradual reduction in the dose rather than abrupt cessation is recommended whenever possible. If intolerable symptoms occur following a decrease in the dose or upon discontinuation of treatment, then resuming the previously prescribed dose may be considered. Subsequently, the physician may continue decreasing the dose but at a more gradual rate.

➤*Suicide:* The possibility of a suicide attempt is inherent in depression or MDD and may persist until significant remission occurs. Close supervision of high-risk patients should accompany initial drug therapy. Write prescriptions for venlafaxine for the smallest quantity of capsules or tablets consistent with good patient management in order to reduce the risk of overdose.

Observe the same precautions observed when treating patients with depression when treating patients with GAD or social anxiety disorder.

➤*Hyponatremia:* Hyponatremia or the syndrome of inappropriate antidiuretic hormone secretion (SIADH) may occur with venlafaxine. Take this into consideration in patients who are, for example, volume-depleted, elderly, or taking diuretics.

➤*Mydriasis:* Mydriasis has been reported in association with venlafaxine; therefore monitor patients with raised intraocular pressure or at risk of acute narrow-angle glaucoma (angle-closure glaucoma).

➤*Serum cholesterol elevation:* Clinically relevant increases in serum cholesterol were recorded in 5.3% of venlafaxine-treated patients and 0% of placebo-treated patients treated for at least 3 months in placebo-controlled trials. Consider measurement of serum cholesterol levels during long-term treatment.

➤*Abnormal bleeding:* There have been reports of abnormal bleeding (most commonly ecchymosis) associated with venlafaxine treatment. While a causal relationship to venlafaxine is unclear, impaired platelet aggregation may result from platelet serotonin depletion and contribute to such occurrences.

➤*Immediate-release:*

Concomitant illness – Venlafaxine has not been evaluated or used to any appreciable extent in patients with a recent history of myocardial infarction or unstable heart disease. Patients with these diagnoses were systemically excluded from many clinical studies during venlafaxine's premarketing testing. Evaluation of the electrocardiograms for 769 patients who received venlafaxine in 4- to 6-week double-blind, placebo-controlled trials, however, showed that the incidence of trial-emergent conduction abnormalities did not differ from that with placebo. The mean heart rate in venlafaxine-treated patients was increased relative to baseline by about 4 beats per minute.

The electrocardiograms were analyzed for 357 patients who received venlafaxine extended-release and 285 patients who received placebo in 8- to 12-week double-blind, placebo-controlled trials were analyzed. The mean change from baseline in corrected QT interval (QTc) for venlafaxine extended-release-treated patients was increased relative to that for placebo-treated patients (increase of 4.7 msec for venlafaxine extended-release and decrease of 1.9 msec for placebo). In these same trials, the mean change from baseline in heart rate for venlafaxine extended-release-treated patients was significantly higher than that for placebo (a mean increase of 4 beats per minute for venlafaxine extended-release and 1 beat per minute for placebo). In a flexible-dose study, with venlafaxine doses in the range of 200 to 375 mg/day and mean dose greater than 300 mg/day, venlafaxine-treated patients had a mean increase in heart rate of 8.5 beats per minute compared with 1.7 beats per minute in the placebo group.

As increases in heart rate were observed, exercise caution in patients whose underlying medical conditions might be compromised by increases in heart rate (eg, patients with hyperthyroidism, heart failure, or recent myocardial infarction), particularly when using doses of venlafaxine above 200 mg/day.

Anxiety and insomnia – Treatment-emergent anxiety, nervousness, and insomnia were more commonly reported for venlafaxine-treated patients compared with placebo-treated patients in a pooled analysis of short-term, double-blind, placebo-controlled depression studies:

Symptom	Venlafaxine (n = 1,033)	Placebo (n = 609)
Anxiety	6%	3%
Insomnia	18%	10%
Nervousness	13%	6%

Anxiety, nervousness, and insomnia led to drug discontinuation in 2%, 2%, and 3%, respectively, of the patients treated with venlafaxine in the phase 2 and 3 depression studies.

Changes in weight –

Adult patients: A dose-dependent weight loss was noted in patients treated with venlafaxine for several weeks. A loss of 5% or more of body weight occurred in 6% of patients treated with venlafaxine compared with 1% of patients treated with placebo and 3% of patients treated with another antidepressant. However, discontinuation for weight loss associated with venlafaxine was uncommon (0.1% of venlafaxine-treated patients in the phase 2 and phase 3 depression trials).

VENLAFAXINE HYDROCHLORIDE — ORAL

The safety and efficacy of venlafaxine therapy in combination with weight loss agents, including phentermine, have not been established. Coadministration of venlafaxine and weight loss agents is not recommended. Venlafaxine is not indicated for weight loss alone or in combination with other products.

Changes in appetite –

Adult patients: Treatment-emergent anorexia was more commonly reported for venlafaxine-treated (11%) than placebo-treated patients (2%) in the pool of short-term, double-blind, placebo-controlled depression studies.

Activation of mania/hypomania – During phase 2 and 3 trials, hypomania or mania occurred in 0.5% of patients treated with venlafaxine. Activation of mania/hypomania has also been reported in a small proportion of patients with major affective disorder who were treated with other marketed antidepressants. As with all antidepressants, use venlafaxine cautiously in patients with a history of mania.

Seizures – During premarketing testing, seizures were reported in 0.26% (8/3082) of venlafaxine-treated patients. Most seizures (5 of 8) occurred in patients receiving doses of 150 mg/day or less. Use venlafaxine cautiously in patients with a history of seizures. Discontinue the drug in any patient who develops seizures.

➤*Extended-release:*

Insomnia and nervousness – Treatment-emergent insomnia and nervousness were more commonly reported for patients treated with venlafaxine extended-release than with placebo in pooled analyses of short-term MDD, GAD, and social anxiety disorder studies, as shown in the table below:

Incidence of Insomnia and Nervousness in Placebo-Controlled MDD, GAD, and Social Anxiety Disorder Trials

	MDD		GAD		Social anxiety disorder	
Symptom	Venlafaxine ER (n = 357)	Placebo (n = 285)	Venlafaxine ER (n = 1,381)	Placebo (n = 555)	Venlafaxine ER (n = 277)	Placebo (n = 274)
Insomnia	17%	11%	15%	10%	23%	7%
Nervousness	10%	5%	6%	4%	11%	3%

Insomnia and nervousness each led to drug discontinuation in 0.9% of the patients treated with venlafaxine extended-release in MDD studies.

In GAD trials, insomnia and nervousness led to drug discontinuation in 3% and 2%, respectively, of the patients treated with venlafaxine extended-release up to 8 weeks and 2% and 0.7%, respectively, of the patients treated with venlafaxine extended-release up to 6 months.

In social anxiety disorder trials, insomnia and nervousness led to drug discontinuation in 3% and 0%, respectively, of the patients treated with venlafaxine extended-release up to 12 weeks.

Changes in weight –

Adult patients: A loss of 5% or more of body weight occurred in 7% of venlafaxine extended-release-treated and 2% of placebo-treated patients in the short-term placebo-controlled MDD trials. The discontinuation rate for weight loss associated with venlafaxine extended-release was 0.1% in MDD studies. In placebo-controlled GAD studies, a loss of 7% or more of body weight occurred in 3% of venlafaxine extended-release patients and 1% of placebo patients who received treatment for up to 6 months. The discontinuation rate for weight loss was 0.3% for patients receiving venlafaxine extended-release in GAD studies for up to 8 weeks. In placebo-controlled social anxiety disorder trials, 3% of the venlafaxine extended-release-treated and 0.4% of the placebo-treated patients sustained a loss of 7% or more of body weight during up to 12 weeks of treatment. None of the patients receiving venlafaxine in social anxiety disorder studies discontinued for weight loss.

The safety and efficacy of venlafaxine therapy in combination with weight loss agents, including phentermine, have not been established. Coadministration of venlafaxine and weight loss agents is not recommended. Venlafaxine is not indicated for weight loss alone or in combination with other products.

Children: Weight loss has been observed in pediatric patients (6 to 17 years of age) receiving venlafaxine extended-release. In a pooled analysis of four 8-week, double-blind, placebo-controlled, flexible dose outpatient trials for MDD and GAD, venlafaxine extended-release-treated patients lost an average of 0.45 kg (n = 333), while placebo-treated patients gained an average of 0.77 kg (n = 333). More patients treated with venlafaxine extended-release than with placebo experienced a weight loss of at least 3.5% in both the MDD and the GAD studies (18% of venlafaxine extended-release-treated patients vs 3.6% of placebo-treated patients; $P < 0.001$). Weight loss was not limited to patients with treatment-emergent anorexia.

The risks associated with longer-term venlafaxine extended-release use were assessed in an open-label study of children and adolescents who received venlafaxine extended-release for up to 6 months. The children and adolescents in the study had increases in weight that were less than expected based on data from age- and sex-matched peers. The difference between observed weight gain and expected weight gain was larger for children (younger than 12 years of age) than for adolescents (older than 12 years of age).

Changes in height (children) – During the 8-week, placebo-controlled GAD studies, venlafaxine extended-release-treated patients (6 to 17 years of age) grew an average of 0.3 cm (n = 122), while placebo-treated patients grew an average of 1 cm (n = 132); $P = 0.041$. This difference in height increase was most notable in patients younger than 12 years of age. During the 8-week placebo-controlled MDD studies, venlafaxine extended-release-treated patients grew an average of 0.8 cm (n = 146), while placebo-treated patients grew an average of 0.7 cm (n = 147). In the 6-month open-label study, children and adolescents had height increases that were less than expected based on data from age- and sex-matched peers. The difference between observed growth rates and expected growth rates was larger for children (younger than 12 years of age) than for adolescents (older than 12 years of age).

Changes in appetite –

Adult patients: Treatment-emergent anorexia was more commonly reported for venlafaxine extended-release-treated (8%) than placebo-treated patients (4%) in the pool of short-term, double-blind, placebo-controlled MDD studies. The discontinuation rate for anorexia associated with venlafaxine extended-release was 1% in MDD studies. Treatment-emergent anorexia was more commonly reported for venlafaxine extended-release-treated (8%) than placebo-treated patients (2%) in the pool of short-term, double-blind, placebo-controlled GAD studies. The discontinuation rate for anorexia was 0.9% for patients receiving venlafaxine extended-release for up to 8 weeks in GAD studies. Treatment-emergent anorexia was more commonly reported for venlafaxine extended-release-treated (20%) than placebo-treated patients (2%) in the pool of short-term, double-blind, placebo-controlled social anxiety disorder studies. The discontinuation rate for anorexia was 0.4% for patients receiving venlafaxine for up to 12 weeks in social anxiety disorder studies.

Children: Decreased appetite has been observed in pediatric patients receiving venlafaxine extended-release. In the placebo-controlled trials for GAD and MDD, 10% of patients 6 to 17 years of age treated with venlafaxine extended-release for up to 8 weeks and 3% of patients treated with placebo reported treatment-emergent anorexia (decreased appetite). None of the patients receiving venlafaxine extended-release discontinued for anorexia or weight loss.

Activation of mania/hypomania – During premarketing MDD studies, mania or hypomania occurred in 0.3% of venlafaxine extended-release-treated patients and 0% placebo patients. In premarketing GAD studies, 0% of venlafaxine extended-release-treated patients and 0.2% of placebo-treated patients experienced mania or hypomania. In premarketing social anxiety disorder studies, no venlafaxine extended-release-treated patients and no placebo-treated patients experienced mania or hypomania. In all premarketing MDD trials with venlafaxine, mania or hypomania occurred in 0.5% of venlafaxine-treated patients compared with 0% of placebo patients. Mania/hypomania has also been reported in a small proportion of patients with mood disorders who were treated with other marketed drugs to treat MDD. As with all drugs effective in the treatment of MDD, use venlafaxine extended-release cautiously in patients with a history of mania.

Seizures – During premarketing experience, no seizures occurred among 705 venlafaxine extended-release-treated patients in the MDD studies, among 1,381 venlafaxine extended-release-treated patients in GAD studies, or among 277 venlafaxine extended-release-treated patients in social anxiety disorder studies. In all premarketing MDD trials with venlafaxine, seizures were reported at various doses in 0.3% (8 of 3,082) of venlafaxine-treated patients. Like many antidepressants, use venlafaxine extended-release cautiously in patients with a history of seizures and discontinue in any patient who develops seizures.

Concomitant illness – Venlafaxine has not been evaluated or used to any appreciable extent in patients with a recent history of myocardial infarction or unstable heart disease. Patients with these diagnoses were systemically excluded from many clinical studies during venlafaxine's premarketing testing.

The electrocardiograms were analyzed for 275 patients who received venlafaxine extended-release and 220 patients who received placebo in 8- to 12-week double-blind, placebo-controlled trials in MDD, for 610 patients who received venlafaxine extended-release and 298 patients who received placebo in 8-week double-blind, placebo-controlled trials in GAD, and for 195 patients who received venlafaxine extended-release and 228 patients who received placebo in 12-week double-blind, placebo-controlled trials in social anxiety disorder. The mean change from baseline in corrected QT interval (QTc) for venlafaxine extended-release-treated patients in MDD studies was increased relative to that for placebo-treated patients (increase of 4.7 msec for venlafaxine extended-release and decrease of 1.9 msec for placebo). The mean change from baseline in corrected QT interval (QTc) for venlafaxine extended-release-treated patients in the GAD studies did not differ significantly from that with placebo. The mean change from baseline in QTc for venlafaxine extended-release-treated patients in the social anxiety disorder studies was increased relative to that for placebo-treated patients (increase of 2.8 msec for venlafaxine extended-release and decrease of 2 msec for placebo).

In these same trials, the mean change from baseline in heart rate for venlafaxine extended-release-treated patients in the MDD studies was significantly higher than that for placebo (a mean increase of 4 beats per minute for venlafaxine extended-release and 1 beat per minute for placebo). The mean change from baseline in heart rate for venlafaxine extended-release-treated patients in the GAD studies was significantly higher than that for placebo (a mean increase of 3 beats per minute for venlafaxine extended-release and no change for placebo). The mean change from baseline in heart rate for venlafaxine extended-release-treated patients in the GAD studies was significantly higher than that for placebo (a mean increase of 3 beats per minute for venlafaxine extended-release and no change for placebo). The mean change from baseline in heart rate for venlafaxine extended-release-treated patients in the social anxiety disorder studies was significantly higher than that for placebo (a mean increase of 5 beats per minute for venlafaxine extended-release and no change for placebo).

In a flexible-dose study, with venlafaxine doses in the range of 200 to 375 mg/day and mean dose greater than 300 mg/day, venlafaxine-treated patients had a mean increase in heart rate of 8.5 beats per minute compared with 1.7 beats per minute in the placebo group.

VENLAFAXINE HYDROCHLORIDE — ORAL

As increases in heart rate were observed, exercise caution in patients whose underlying medical conditions might be compromised by increases in heart rate (eg, patients with hyperthyroidism, heart failure, or recent myocardial infarction), particularly when using doses of venlafaxine above 200 mg/day.

➤*Electroconvulsive therapy:* There are no clinical data establishing the benefit of electroconvulsive therapy combined with venlafaxine treatment.

Drug Interactions

➤*Drugs metabolized by cytochrome P-450 isoenzymes:*

CYP2D6 – In vitro studies indicate that venlafaxine is a relatively weak inhibitor of CYP2D6. These findings have been confirmed in a clinical drug interaction study comparing the effect of venlafaxine with that of fluoxetine on the CYP2D6-mediated metabolism of dextromethorphan to dextrorphan.

➤*CNS-active drugs:* The risk of using venlafaxine in combination with other CNS-active drugs has not been systematically evaluated (except in the case of those CNS-active drugs noted above). Consequently, caution is advised if the concomitant administration of venlafaxine and such drugs is required. Based on the mechanism of action of venlafaxine and the potential for serotonin syndrome, caution is advised when venlafaxine is coadministered with other drugs that may affect the serotonergic neurotransmitter systems, such as triptans, serotonin reuptake inhibitors, or lithium.

Venlafaxine Drug Interactions

Precipitant drug	Object drug[a]		Description
Cimetidine	Venlafaxine	↑	Concomitant use resulted in inhibition of first-pass metabolism of venlafaxine in 18 healthy subjects. Oral clearance was reduced by ≈ 43%, and AUC and C_{max} were increased by ≈ 60%. However, cimetidine had no apparent effect on ODV. Consequently, the overall pharmacologic activity is expected to increase only slightly.
Cyproheptadine	Venlafaxine	↓	Decreased pharmacologic effects of venlafaxine.
MAO inhibitors	Venlafaxine	↑	Serious, sometimes fatal reactions may occur, including hyperthermia, rigidity, myoclonus, autonomic instability with possible rapid fluctuation of vital signs, and mental status changes that include extreme agitation progressing to delirium and coma (see Warnings). Concomitant use is contraindicated.
Venlafaxine	Clozapine	↑	There have been reports of elevated clozapine levels resulting in adverse events including seizures following the addition of venlafaxine.
Venlafaxine	Desipramine	↑	Desipramine AUC, C_{max}, and C_{min} increased ≈ 35% in the presence of venlafaxine. The 2-OH-desipramine AUC increased at least 2.5- to 4.5-fold. The clinical significance of elevated 2-OH-desipramine levels is unknown.
Venlafaxine	Haloperidol	↑	Venlafaxine decreased total oral-dose clearance of a single dose of haloperidol 42%, which resulted in a 70% increase in haloperidol AUC. In addition, the haloperidol C_{max} increased 88%.
Venlafaxine	Indinavir	↓	Venlafaxine resulted in a 28% decrease in the AUC of a single oral dose of indinavir and a 36% decrease in indinavir C_{max}. The clinical significance of this is unknown.
Venlafaxine	Sibutramine Sumatriptan Tramadol Trazodone	↑	A "serotonin syndrome" including irritability, increased muscle tone, shivering, myoclonus, and altered consciousness may occur.
Venlafaxine	St. John's wort	↑	A "serotonin syndrome," including irritability, increased muscle tone, shivering, myoclonus, and altered consciousness may occur.
Venlafaxine	Warfarin	↑	There have been reports on increases in PT, PTT, or INR when venlafaxine was administered to patients also receiving warfarin.

[a] ↑ = Object drug increased. ↓ = Object drug decreased.

Adverse Reactions

➤*Immediate-release tablets:*

Associated with discontinuation of treatment – Nineteen percent (537 of 2,897) of venlafaxine patients in phase 2 and 3 depression studies discontinued treatment due to an adverse event. The more common events (greater than or equal to 1%) associated with discontinuation and considered to be drug-related (ie, those events associated with dropout at a rate approximately twice or greater for venlafaxine compared to placebo) included the following:

Venlafaxine Adverse Reactions Associated with Discontinuation

Adverse reaction	Venlafaxine	Placebo
CNS		
Anxiety	2%	1%
Dizziness	3%	< 1%
Dry mouth	2%	< 1%
Headache	3%	1%
Insomnia	3%	1%
Nervousness	2%	< 1%
Somnolence	3%	1%
GI		
Nausea	6%	1%
GU		
Abnormal ejaculation[a]	3%	< 1%
Miscellaneous		
Asthenia	2%	< 1%
Sweating	2%	< 1%

[a] Percentages based on the number of men.

Incidence in controlled trials –

Commonly observed adverse events in controlled clinical trials: The most commonly observed adverse events associated with the use of venlafaxine (incidence of 5% or greater) and not seen at an equivalent incidence among placebo-treated patients (ie, incidence for venlafaxine at least twice that for placebo), derived from the 1% incidence table below, were asthenia, sweating, nausea, constipation, anorexia, vomiting, somnolence, dry mouth, dizziness, nervousness, anxiety, tremor, and blurred vision as well as abnormal ejaculation/orgasm and impotence in men.

Adverse events occurring at an incidence of 1% or more among venlafaxine-treated patients:

Treatment-Emergent Adverse Experience Incidence in 4- to 8-Week Placebo-Controlled Clinical Trials[a]

Body system	Preferred term	Venlafaxine (n = 1,033)	Placebo (n = 609)
Cardiovascular	Increased blood pressure/ hypertension	2%	< 1%
	Postural hypotension	1%	< 1%
	Tachycardia	2%	< 1%
	Vasodilation	4%	3%
CNS	Abnormal dreams	4%	3%
	Abnormal thinking	2%	1%
	Agitation	2%	< 1%
	Anxiety	6%	3%
	Confusion	2%	1%
	Decreased libido	2%	< 1%
	Depersonalization	1%	< 1%
	Depression	1%	< 1%
	Dizziness	19%	7%
	Headache	25%	24%
	Insomnia	18%	10%
	Nervousness	13%	6%
	Paresthesia	3%	2%
	Somnolence	23%	9%
	Tremor	5%	1%
	Twitching	1%	< 1%
Dermatological	Pruritus	1%	< 1%
	Rash	3%	2%
	Sweating	12%	3%

VENLAFAXINE HYDROCHLORIDE — ORAL

Treatment-Emergent Adverse Experience Incidence in 4- to 8-Week Placebo-Controlled Clinical Trials[a]			
Body system	Preferred term	Venlafaxine (n = 1,033)	Placebo (n = 609)
GI	Anorexia	11%	2%
	Constipation	15%	7%
	Diarrhea	8%	7%
	Dry mouth	22%	11%
	Dyspepsia	5%	4%
	Flatulence	3%	2%
	Nausea	37%	11%
	Vomiting	6%	2%
GU	Abnormal ejaculation/ orgasm	12%[b]	< 1%[b]
	Impotence	6%[b]	< 1%[b]
	Orgasm disturbance	2%[c]	< 1%[c]
	Urinary frequency	3%	2%
	Urination impaired	2%	< 1%
	Urinary retention	1%	< 1%
Metabolic	Weight loss	1%	< 1%
Respiratory	Yawn	3%	< 1%
Special senses	Blurred vision	6%	2%
	Mydriasis	2%	< 1%
	Taste perversion	2%	< 1%
	Tinnitus	2%	< 1%
Miscellaneous	Asthenia	12%	6%
	Chest pain	2%	1%
	Chills	3%	< 1%
	Hypertonia	3%	2%
	Infection	6%	5%
	Trauma	2%	1%

[a] Events reported by at least 1% of patients treated with venlafaxine are included, and are rounded to the nearest percent. Events for which the venlafaxine incidence was less than or equal to placebo are not listed in the table, but included the following: Abdominal pain, pain, back pain, flu syndrome, fever, palpitation, increased appetite, myalgia, arthralgia, amnesia, hypesthesia, rhinitis, pharyngitis, sinusitis, increased cough, and dysmenorrhea.
[b] Incidence based on number of men.
[c] Incidence based on number of women.

Dose dependency of adverse events: A comparison of adverse event rates in a fixed-dose study comparing venlafaxine 75, 225, and 375 mg/day with placebo revealed a dose dependency for some of the more common adverse events associated with venlafaxine use, as shown in the table that follows. The rule for including events was to enumerate those that occurred at an incidence of 5% or more for at least 1 of the venlafaxine groups and for which the incidence was at least twice the placebo incidence for at least 1 venlafaxine group. Tests for potential dose relationships for these events (Cochran-Armitage test, with a criterion of exact 2-sided $P \leq 0.05$) suggested a dose-dependency for several adverse events in this list, including chills, hypertension, anorexia, nausea, agitation, dizziness, somnolence, tremor, yawning, sweating, and abnormal ejaculation.

Treatment-Emergent Adverse Experience Incidence in a Dose Comparison Trial				
		Venlafaxine (mg/day)		
Body system/ Preferred term	Placebo (n = 92)	75 (n = 89)	225 (n = 89)	375 (n = 88)
Cardiovascular				
Hypertension	1.1%	1.1%	2.2%	4.5%
Vasodilatation	0%	4.5%	5.6%	2.3%
CNS				
Agitation	0%	1.1%	2.2%	4.5%
Anxiety	4.3%	11.2%	4.5%	2.3%
Dizziness	4.3%	19.1%	22.5%	23.9%
Decreased libido	1.1%	2.2%	1.1%	5.7%
Insomnia	9.8%	22.5%	20.2%	13.6%
Nervousness	4.3%	21.3%	13.5%	12.5%
Somnolence	4.3%	16.9%	18%	26.1%
Tremor	0%	1.1%	2.2%	10.2%
Dermatologic				
Sweating	5.4%	6.7%	12.4%	19.3%
GI				
Abdominal pain	3.3%	3.4%	2.2%	8%
Anorexia	2.2%	14.6%	13.5%	17%
Dyspepsia	2.2%	6.7%	6.7%	4.55
Nausea	14.1%	32.6%	38.2%	58%
Vomiting	1.1%	7.9%	3.4%	6.8%
GU				
Abnormal ejaculation/ orgasm	0%	4.5%	2.2%	12.5%

Treatment-Emergent Adverse Experience Incidence in a Dose Comparison Trial				
		Venlafaxine (mg/day)		
Body system/ Preferred term	Placebo (n = 92)	75 (n = 89)	225 (n = 89)	375 (n = 88)
Impotence (number of men)	0% (n = 63)	5.8% (n = 52)	2.1% (n = 48)	3.6% (n = 56)
Respiratory				
Yawn	0%	4.5%	5.6%	8%
Special senses				
Abnormality of accommodation	0%	9.1%	7.9%	5.6%
Miscellaneous				
Asthenia	3.3%	16.9%	14.6%	14.8%
Chills	1.1%	2.2%	5.6%	6.8%
Infection	2.2%	2.2%	5.6%	2.3%

Adaptation to certain adverse events: Over a 6-week period, there was evidence of adaptation to some adverse events with continued therapy (eg, dizziness and nausea), but less to other effects (eg, abnormal ejaculation and dry mouth).

Vital sign changes – Venlafaxine treatment (averaged over all dose groups) in clinical trials was associated with a mean increase in pulse rate of approximately 3 beats per minute, compared to no change for placebo. In a flexible-dose study, with doses in the range of 200 to 375 mg/day and mean dose greater than 300 mg/day, the mean pulse was increased by about 2 beats per minute compared with a decrease of about 1 beat per minute for placebo.

In controlled clinical trials, venlafaxine was associated with mean increases in diastolic blood pressure ranging from 0.7 to 2.5 mm Hg averaged over all dose groups, compared to mean decreases ranging from 0.9 to 3.8 mm Hg for placebo. However, there is a dose dependency for blood pressure increase. Experience with the immediate-release venlafaxine showed that sustained hypertension was dose-related, increasing from 3% to 7% at 100 to 300 mg/day to 13% at doses above 300 mg/day. An insufficient number of patients received mean doses of venlafaxine over 300 mg/day to fully evaluate the incidence of sustained increases in blood pressure at these higher doses.

Lab test abnormalities – Of the serum chemistry and hematology parameters monitored during clinical trials with venlafaxine, a statistically significant difference with placebo was seen only for serum cholesterol. In premarketing trials, treatment with venlafaxine tablets was associated with a mean final on-therapy increase in total cholesterol of 3 mg/dL. Patients treated with venlafaxine tablets for at least 3 months in placebo-controlled 12-month extension trials had a mean final on-therapy increase in total cholesterol of 9.1 mg/dL compared with a decrease of 7.1 mg/dL among placebo-treated patients. This increase was duration dependent over the study period and tended to be greater with higher doses. Clinically relevant increases in serum cholesterol, defined as a final on-therapy increase in serum cholesterol greater than or equal to 50 mg/dL from baseline and to a value greater than or equal to 261 mg/dL or an average on-therapy increase in serum cholesterol greater than or equal to 50 mg/dL from baseline and to a value of greater than or equal to 261 mg/dL, were recorded in 5.3% of venlafaxine-treated patients and 0% of placebo-treated patients.

Electrocardiogram (ECG) changes – In an analysis of ECGs obtained in 769 patients treated with venlafaxine and 450 patients treated with placebo in controlled clinical trials, the only statistically significant difference observed was for heart rate (ie, a mean increase from baseline of 4 beats per minute for venlafaxine). In a flexible-dose study, with doses in the range of 200 to 375 mg/day and mean dose greater than 300 mg/day, the mean change in heart rate was 8.5 beats per minute compared with 1.7 beats per minute for placebo.

Other events observed during premarketing evaluation of venlafaxine – During its premarketing assessment, multiple doses of venlafaxine were administered to 2,897 patients in phase 2 and phase 3 studies. In addition, in premarketing assessment, multiple doses of venlafaxine extended-release were administered to 705 patients in phase 3 MDD studies and venlafaxine was administered to 96 patients. During its premarketing assessment, multiple doses of venlafaxine extended-release were also administered to 1,381 patients in phase 3 GAD studies and 277 patients in phase 3 social anxiety disorder studies. In addition, in premarketing assessment of venlafaxine, multiple doses were administered to 2,897 patients in phase 2 and 3 studies for MDD. The conditions and duration of exposure to venlafaxine in both development programs varied greatly, and included (in overlapping categories) open and double-blind studies, uncontrolled and controlled studies, inpatient (venlafaxine only) and outpatient studies, fixed-dose, and titration studies. Untoward events associated with this exposure were recorded by clinical investigators using terminology of their own choosing. Consequently, it is not possible to provide a meaningful estimate of the proportion of individuals experiencing adverse events without first grouping similar types of untoward events into a smaller number of standardized event categories.

Events are further categorized by body system and listed in order of decreasing frequency using the following definitions: Frequent adverse events are defined as those occurring on 1 or more occasions in at least 1/100 patients; infrequent adverse events are those occurring in 1/100 to 1/1,000 patients; rare events are those occurring in fewer than 1/1,000 patients.

Cardiovascular – Angina pectoris, arrhythmia, extrasystoles, hypotension, peripheral vascular disorder (mainly cold feet or cold hands), syncope, thrombophlebitis (infrequent); aortic aneurysm, arteritis, bigeminy, bradycardia, bundle branch block, capillary fragility, cardiovascular disorder (mitral valve and circulatory disturbances), cerebral ischemia, coronary artery disease, congestive heart failure, first-degree atrioventricular block, heart arrest, mitral valve disorder, mucocutaneous hemorrhage, myocardial infarct, pallor (rare).

CNS – Migraine, trismus, vertigo (frequent); abnormal speech, akathisia, apathy, ataxia, circumoral paresthesia, CNS stimulation, emotion lability, euphoria, hallucinations, hostility, hyperesthesia, hyperkinesia, hypotonia, incoordination, libido increased, manic reaction, myoclonus, neuralgia, neuropathy, psychosis, seizure, stupor (infrequent); abnormal gait, akinesia, alcohol abuse, aphasia, bradykinesia, buccoglossal syndrome, cerebrovascular accident, loss of consciousness, delusions, dementia, dystonia, facial paralysis, feeling drunk, Guillain-Barre syndrome, hyperchlorhydria, hypokinesia, impulse control difficulties, neuritis, nystagmus, paranoid reaction, paresis, psychotic depression, reflexes decreased, reflexes increased, suicidal ideation, torticollis (rare).

Dermatologic – Acne, alopecia, brittle nails, contact dermatitis, dry skin, eczema, skin hypertrophy, maculopapular rash, psoriasis, urticaria (infrequent); erythema nodosum, exfoliative dermatitis, lichenoid dermatitis, hair discoloration, skin discoloration, furunculosis, hirsutism, leukoderma, petechial rash, pustular rash, vesiculobullous rash, seborrhea, skin atrophy, skin striae (rare).

Endocrine – Goiter, hyperthyroidism, hypothyroidism, thyroid nodule, thyroiditis (rare).

GI – Eructation (frequent); bruxism, colitis, dysphagia, tongue edema, esophagitis, gastritis, gastroenteritis, gastrointestinal ulcer, gingivitis, glossitis, hemorrhoids, melena, mouth ulceration, oral moniliasis, rectal hemorrhage, stomatitis (infrequent); cheilitis, cholecystitis, cholelithiasis, duodenitis, esophageal spasm, hematemesis, increased salivation, gastrointestinal hemorrhage, gum hemorrhage, hepatitis, ileitis, jaundice, intestinal obstruction, parotitis, periodontitis, proctitis, soft stools, tongue discoloration (rare).

GU – Metrorrhagia†, prostatic disorder (prostatitis and enlarged prostate†), vaginitis†; (frequent); albuminuria, amenorrhea†, cystitis, dysuria, hematuria, leukorrhea†, menorrhagia†, nocturia, bladder pain, breast pain, polyuria, pyuria, urinary incontinence, urinary urgency, vaginal hemorrhage† (infrequent); abortion†, anuria, balanitis†, breast discharge, breast engorgement, breast enlargement, endometriosis†, female lactation†, fibrocystic breast, calcium crystalluria, cervicitis†, ovarian cyst†, prolonged erection†, gynecomastia (male)†, hypomenorrhea†, kidney calculus, kidney pain, kidney function abnormal, mastitis, menopause†, pyelonephritis, oliguria, orchitis†, salpingitis†, urolithiasis, uterine hemorrhage†, uterine spasm†, vaginal dryness† (rare).

Hematologic/Lymphatic – Ecchymosis (frequent); anemia, leukocytosis, leukopenia, lymphadenopathy, thrombocythemia, thrombocytopenia (infrequent); basophilia, bleeding time increased, cyanosis, eosinophilia, lymphocytosis, multiple myeloma, purpura (rare).

Metabolic/Nutritional – Edema, weight gain (frequent); alkaline phosphatase increased, ALT increased, AST increased, dehydration, hypercholesteremia, hyperglycemia, hyperlipemia, hypokalemia, thirst (infrequent); alcohol intolerance, bilirubinemia, serum urea nitrogen (BUN) increased, creatinine increased, diabetes mellitus, glycosuria, gout, healing abnormal, hemochromatosis, hypercalcinuria, hyperkalemia, hyperphosphatemia, hyperuricemia, hypocholesterolemia, hypoglycemia, hyponatremia, hypophosphatemia, hypoproteinemia, uremia (rare).

Musculoskeletal – Arthritis, arthrosis, bone pain, bone spurs, bursitis, leg cramps, myasthenia, tenosynovitis (infrequent); myopathy, osteoporosis, osteosclerosis, pathological fracture, plantar fasciitis, rheumatoid arthritis, tendon rupture (rare).

Respiratory – Bronchitis, dyspnea (frequent); asthma, chest congestion, epistaxis, hyperventilation, laryngismus, laryngitis, pneumonia, voice alteration (infrequent); atelectasis, hemoptysis, hypoventilation, hypoxia, larynx edema, pleurisy, pulmonary embolus, sleep apnea (rare).

Special senses – Abnormality of accommodation, abnormal vision (frequent); cataract, conjunctivitis, corneal lesion, diplopia, dry eyes, eye pain, hyperacusis, otitis media, parosmia, photophobia, taste loss, visual field defect (infrequent); blepharitis, chromatopsia, conjunctival edema, deafness, decreased pupillary reflex, exophthalmos, glaucoma, retinal hemorrhage, keratitis, labyrinthitis, miosis, papilledema, otitis externa, scleritis, subconjunctival hemorrhage, uveitis (rare).

Miscellaneous – Accidental injury, chest pain substernal, neck pain (frequent); face edema, intentional injury, malaise, moniliasis, neck rigidity, pelvic pain, photosensitivity reaction, suicide attempt, withdrawal syndrome (infrequent); appendicitis, bacteremia, carcinoma, cellulitis, withdrawal syndrome (rare).

Postmarketing – Voluntary reports of other adverse events temporarily associated with the use of the immediate-release form of venlafaxine that have been received since market introduction and that may have no causal relationship with the use of venlafaxine include the following: agranulocytosis, anaphylaxis, aplastic anemia, catatonia, congenital anomalies, creatinine phosphokinase increased, deep vein thrombophlebitis, delirium, ECG abnormalities (such as QT prolongation); cardiac arrhythmias including atrial fibrillation, supraventricular tachycardia, ventricular extrasystoles, and rare reports of ventricular fibrillation and ventricular tachycardia including torsades de pointes, epidermal necrosis/Stevens-Johnson syndrome, erythema multiforme, extrapyramidal symptoms (including tardive dyskinesia), hemorrhage (including eye and gastrointestinal bleeding), hepatic events (including gamma-glutamyltranferase [GGT] elevation; abnormalities of unspecified liver function tests; liver damage, necrosis, or failure; and fatty liver), involuntary movements, lactase dehydrogenase (LDH) increased, neuroleptic malignant syndrome-like events (including a case of a 10-year-old who may have been taking methylphenidate, was treated and recovered), pancreatitis, panic, prolactin increased, renal failure, serotonin syndrome, shock-like electrical sensations or tinnitus (in some cases, subsequent to the discontinuation of venlafaxine or tapering of dose), and syndrome of inappropriate antidiuretic hormone secretion (usually in the elderly); angle-closure glaucoma, neutropenia, night sweats, pancytopenia, pulmonary eosinophilia, rhabdomyolysis.

There have been reports of elevated clozapine levels that were temporally associated with adverse events, including seizures, following the addition of venlafaxine. There have been reports of increases in prothrombin time, partial thromboplastin time, or international normalized ratio (INR) when venlafaxine was given to patients receiving warfarin therapy.

➤*Extended-release:*

Adverse findings observed in short-term, placebo-controlled studies with venlafaxine extended-release –

Adverse events associated with discontinuation of treatment: Approximately 11% of the 357 patients who received venlafaxine extended-release in placebo-controlled clinical trials for depression discontinued treatment due to an adverse experience, compared with 6% of the 285 placebo-treated patients in those studies. Approximately 18% of the 1,381 patients who received venlafaxine extended-release in placebo-controlled clinical trials for GAD discontinued treatment due to an adverse experience, compared with 12% of the 555 placebo-treated patients in those studies. Approximately 17% of the 277 patients who received venlafaxine extended-release capsules in placebo-controlled clinical trials for social anxiety disorder discontinued treatment due to an adverse experience, compared with 5% of the 274 placebo-treated patients in those studies. The most common events leading to discontinuation and considered to be drug-related (ie, leading to discontinuation in at least 1% of the venlafaxine extended-release-treated patients at a rate at least twice that of placebo for either indication) are shown in the table below:

Common Adverse Events Leading to Discontinuation of Treatment in Placebo-Controlled Trials[a]

Adverse event	Percentage of Patients Discontinuing due to Adverse Event					
	MDD indication[b]		GAD indication[c,d]		Social anxiety disorder indication	
	Venlafaxine extended-release (n = 357)	Placebo (n = 285)	Venlafaxine extended-release (n = 1,381)	Placebo (n = 555)	Venlafaxine extended-release (n = 277)	Placebo (n = 274)
CNS						
Anxiety	-	-	-	-	1%	< 1%
Dizziness	2%	1%	-	-	2%	0%
Headache	-	-	-	-	2%	< 1%
Insomnia	1%	< 1%	3%	< 1%	3%	< 1%
Nervousness	-	-	2%	< 1%	-	-
Somnolence	2%	< 1%	3%	< 1%	2%	< 1%
Tremor	-	-	1%	0%	-	-
Dermatologic						
Sweating	-	-	2%	< 1%	1%	0%
GI						
Anorexia	1%	< 1%	-	-	-	-
Dry mouth	1%	0%	2%	< 1%	-	-
Nausea	4%	< 1%	8%	< 1%	4%	0%
Vomiting	-	-	1%	< 1%	-	-
GU						
Impotence[e]	-	-	-	-	3%	0%

† Based on the number of men and women as appropriate.

VENLAFAXINE HYDROCHLORIDE — ORAL

Common Adverse Events Leading to Discontinuation of Treatment in Placebo-Controlled Trials[a]

Adverse event	Percentage of Patients Discontinuing due to Adverse Event					
	MDD indication[b]		GAD indication[c,d]		Social anxiety disorder indication	
	Venlafaxine extended-release (n = 357)	Placebo (n = 285)	Venlafaxine extended-release (n = 1,381)	Placebo (n = 555)	Venlafaxine extended-release (n = 277)	Placebo (n = 274)
Miscellaneous						
Asthenia	-	-	3%	< 1%	1%	< 1%

[a] Two of the MDD studies were flexible dose and 1 was fixed dose. Four of the GAD studies were fixed dose and 1 was flexible dose. Both of the social anxiety disorder studies were flexible dose.
[b] In US placebo-controlled trials for MDD, the following were also common events leading to discontinuation and were considered to be drug-related for venlafaxine extended-release-treated patients (% venlafaxine extended-release [n = 192], % placebo [n = 202]): hypertension (1%, less than 1%); diarrhea (1%, 0%); paresthesia (1%, 0%); tremor (1%, 0%); abnormal vision, mostly blurred vision (1%, 0%); and abnormal, mostly delayed ejaculation (1%, 0%).
[c] In 2 short-term US placebo-controlled trials for GAD, the following were also common events leading to discontinuation and were considered to be drug-related for venlafaxine extended-release-treated patients (% venlafaxine extended-release [n = 476]), % placebo [n = 201]: headache (4%, < 1%); vasodilation (1%, 0%); anorexia (2%, < 1%); dizziness (4%, 1%); thinking abnormal (1%, 0%); and abnormal vision (1%, 0%).
[d] In long-term placebo-controlled trials for GAD, the following was also a common event leading to discontinuation and was considered to be drug-related for venlafaxine extended-release-treated patients (% venlafaxine extended-release [n = 535], % placebo [n = 257]): decreased libido (1%, 0%).
[e] Incidence is based on the number of men (venlafaxine extended-release = 158, placebo = 153).

Commonly observed adverse events –

MDD: Note in particular the following adverse events that occurred in at least 5% of the venlafaxine extended-release patients and at a rate at least twice that of the placebo group for all placebo-controlled trials for MDD: abnormal ejaculation, gastrointestinal complaints (nausea, dry mouth, and anorexia), CNS complaints (dizziness, somnolence, and abnormal dreams), and sweating. In the 2 US placebo-controlled trials, the following additional events occurred in at least 5% of venlafaxine extended-release-treated patients (n = 192) and at a rate at least twice that of the placebo group: Abnormalities of sexual function (impotence in men, anorgasmia in women, and libido decreased), gastrointestinal complaints (constipation and flatulence), CNS complaints (insomnia, nervousness, and tremor), problems of special senses (abnormal vision), cardiovascular effects (hypertension and vasodilation), and yawning.

Treatment-emergent Adverse Event Incidence in Short-Term Placebo-Controlled Venlafaxine Extended-Release Clinical Trials in Patients with MDD [a,b]

Preferred term	Percentage reporting event	
	Venlafaxine extended-release (n = 357)	Placebo (n = 285)
Cardiovascular		
Hypertension	4%	1%
Vasodilation[c]	4%	2%
CNS		
Abnormal dreams[d]	7%	2%
Agitation	3%	1%
Decreased libido	3%	< 1%
Depression	3%	< 1%
Dizziness	20%	9%
Dry mouth	12%	6%
Insomnia	17%	11%
Nervousness	10%	5%
Paresthesia	3%	1%
Somnolence	17%	8%
Tremor	5%	2%
Dermatologic		
Sweating	14%	3%
GI		
Anorexia	8%	4%
Constipation	8%	5%
Flatulence	4%	3%
Nausea	31%	12%
Vomiting	4%	2%
GU		
Abnormal ejaculation (male)[e,f]	16%	< 1%
Anorgasmia (female)[g,h]	3%	< 1%
Impotence[f]	4%	< 1%
Metabolic/Nutritional		
Weight loss	3%	0%
Respiratory		
Pharyngitis	7%	6%
Yawn	3%	0%
Special senses		
Abnormal vision[i]	4%	< 1%
Miscellaneous		
Asthenia	8%	7%

[a] Incidence, rounded to the nearest percent, for events reported by at least 2% of patients treated with venlafaxine extended-release, except the following events which had an incidence less than or equal to placebo: Abdominal pain, accidental injury, anxiety, back pain, bronchitis, diarrhea, dysmenorrhea, dyspepsia, flu syndrome, headache, infection, pain, palpitation, rhinitis, and sinusitis.
[b] Less than 1% indicates an incidence greater than 0 but less than 1%.
[c] Mostly "hot flashes."
[d] Mostly "vivid dreams," "nightmares," and "increased dreaming."
[e] Mostly "delayed ejaculation."
[f] Incidence is based on the number of men.
[g] Mostly "delayed orgasm" or "anorgasmia."
[h] Incidence is based on the number of female patients.
[i] Mostly "blurred vision" and "difficulty focusing eyes."

GAD – Note in particular the following adverse events that occurred in at least 5% of the venlafaxine extended-release patients and at a rate at least twice that of the placebo group for all placebo-controlled trials for the GAD indication: Abnormalities of sexual function (abnormal ejaculation and impotence in men), gastrointestinal complaints (nausea, dry mouth, anorexia, and constipation), problems of special senses (abnormal vision), and sweating.

Treatment-Emergent Adverse Event Incidence in Short-Term Placebo-Controlled Venlafaxine Extended-Release Clinical Trials in GAD Patients[a,b]

Preferred term	Percentage reporting event	
	Venlafaxine extended-release (n = 1,381)	Placebo (n = 555)
Cardiovascular		
Vasodilation[c]	4%	2%
CNS		
Abnormal dreams[d]	3%	2%
Dizziness	16%	11%
Hypertonia	3%	2%
Insomnia	15%	10%
Libido decreased	4%	2%
Nervousness	6%	4%
Paresthesia	2%	1%
Somnolence	14%	8%
Tremor	4%	< 1%
Dermatologic		
Sweating	10%	3%
GI		
Anorexia	8%	2%
Constipation	10%	4%
Dry mouth	16%	6%
Nausea	35%	12%
Vomiting	5%	3%
GU		
Abnormal ejaculation (male)[e,f]	11%	< 1%
Impotence[f]	5%	< 1%
Orgasmic dysfunction (female)[g,h]	2%	0%

VENLAFAXINE HYDROCHLORIDE — ORAL

Treatment-Emergent Adverse Event Incidence in Short-Term Placebo-Controlled Venlafaxine Extended-Release Clinical Trials in GAD Patients[a,b]

Preferred term	Percentage reporting event	
	Venlafaxine extended-release (n = 1,381)	Placebo (n = 555)
Respiratory		
Yawn	3%	< 1%
Special senses		
Abnormal vision[i]	5%	< 1%
Miscellaneous		
Asthenia	12%	8%

[a] Adverse events for which the venlafaxine extended-release reporting rate was less than or equal to the placebo rate are not included. These events are abdominal pain, accidental injury, anxiety, back pain, diarrhea, dysmenorrhea, dyspepsia, flu syndrome, headache, infection, myalgia, pain, palpitation, pharyngitis, rhinitis, tinnitus, and urinary frequency.
[b] Less than 1% means greater than zero but less than 1%.
[c] Mostly "hot flashes."
[d] Mostly "vivid dreams", "nightmares", and "increased dreaming."
[e] Mostly "delayed ejaculation" and "anorgasmia."
[f] Percentages based on the number of males (venlafaxine extended-release = 525, placebo = 220).
[g] Includes "delayed orgasm", "abnormal orgasm", and "anorgasmia."
[h] Percentages based on the number of females (venlafaxine extended-release = 856, placebo = 335).
[i] Mostly "blurred vision," and "difficulty focusing eyes."

Social anxiety disorder – Note in particular the following adverse events that occurred in at least 5% of the venlafaxine extended-release patients and at a rate at least twice that of the placebo group for the 2 placebo-controlled trials for the social anxiety disorder indication: asthenia, gastrointestinal complaints (anorexia, dry mouth, nausea), CNS complaints (anxiety, insomnia, libido decreased, nervousness, somnolence, dizziness), abnormalities of sexual function (abnormal ejaculation, orgasmic dysfunction, impotence), yawn, sweating, and abnormal vision.

Treatment-Emergent Adverse Event Incidence in Short-Term Placebo-Controlled Venlafaxine Extended-Release Clinical Trials in Social Anxiety Disorder Patients[a,b]

Preferred term	Percentage reporting event	
	Venlafaxine extended-release (n = 277)	Placebo (n = 274)
Cardiovascular		
Hypertension	5%	4%
Palpitation	3%	1%
Vasodilation[c]	3%	1%
CNS		
Abnormal dreams[d]	4%	< 1%
Agitation	4%	1%
Anxiety	5%	3%
Dizziness	16%	8%
Headache	34%	33%
Insomnia	23%	7%
Libido decreased	9%	< 1%
Nervousness	11%	3%
Paresthesia	3%	< 1%
Somnolence	16%	8%
Tremor	4%	< 1%
Twitching	2%	0%
Dermatologic		
Sweating	13%	2%
GI		
Abdominal pain	4%	3%
Anorexia[e]	20%	1%
Constipation	8%	4%
Diarrhea	6%	5%
Dry mouth	17%	4%
Eructation	2%	0%
Nausea	29%	9%
Vomiting	3%	2%
GU		
Abnormal ejaculation[f,g]	16%	1%
Impotence[g]	10%	1%
Orgasmic dysfunction[h,i]	8%	0%
Metabolic/Nutritional		
Weight loss	4%	0%
Respiratory		
Sinusitis	2%	1%
Yawn	5%	< 1%
Special senses		
Abnormal vision[j]	6%	3%
Miscellaneous		
Accidental injury	5%	3%
Asthenia	17%	8%
Flu syndrome	6%	5%

[a] Adverse events for which the venlafaxine extended-release reporting rate was less than or equal to the placebo rate are not included. These events are back pain, depression, dysmenorrhea, dyspepsia, infection, myalgia, pain, pharyngitis, rash, rhinitis, and upper respiratory tract infection.
[b] Less than 1% means greater than zero but less than 1%.
[c] Mostly "hot flashes."
[d] Mostly "vivid dreams," "nightmares," and "increased dreaming."
[e] Mostly "decreased appetite" and "loss of appetite."
[f] Includes "delayed ejaculation" and "anorgasmia."
[g] Percentages based on the number of males (venlafaxine extended-release = 158, placebo = 153).
[h] Includes "abnormal orgasm" and "anorgasmia."
[i] Percentages based on the number of females (venlafaxine extended-release = 119, placebo = 121).
[j] Mostly "blurred vision."

Vital sign changes – Venlafaxine extended-release treatment for up to 12 weeks in premarketing placebo-controlled MDD trials was associated with a mean final on-therapy increase in pulse rate of approximately 2 beats per minute, compared with 1 beat per minute for placebo. Venlafaxine extended-release treatment for up to 8 weeks in premarketing placebo-controlled GAD trials was associated with a mean final on-therapy increase in pulse rate of approximately 2 beats per minute, compared with less than 1 beat per minute for placebo. Venlafaxine extended-release treatment for up to 12 weeks in the premarketing placebo-controlled social anxiety disorder trials was associated with mean final on-therapy increase in pulse rate of approximately 4 beats per minute, compared with an increase of about 1 beat per minute for placebo.

In a flexible-dose study, with venlafaxine doses in the range of 200 to 375 mg/day and mean dose greater than 300 mg/day, the mean pulse was increased by about 2 beats per minute compared with a decrease of about 1 beat per minute for placebo.

Lab test abnormalities – Venlafaxine extended-release treatment for up to 12 weeks in premarketing placebo-controlled MDD trials and for up to 8 weeks in premarketing placebo-controlled GAD trials was associated with a mean final on-therapy increases in serum cholesterol concentration of approximately 1.5 mg/dL compared with a mean final decrease of 7.4 mg/dL for placebo. Venlafaxine extended-release treatment for up to 8 weeks and up to 6 months in premarketing placebo-controlled GAD trials was associated with mean final on-therapy increases in serum cholesterol concentration of approximately 1 mg/dL and 2.3 mg/dL, respectively, while placebo subjects experienced mean final decreases of 4.9 mg/dL and 7.7 mg/dL, respectively. Venlafaxine extended-release treatment for up to 12 weeks in premarketing placebo-controlled social anxiety disorder trials was associated with mean final on-therapy increases in serum cholesterol concentration of approximately 11.4 mg/dL compared with a mean final decrease of 2.2 mg/dL for placebo.

Patients treated with venlafaxine for at least 3 months in placebo-controlled 12-month extension trials had a mean final on-therapy increase in total cholesterol of 9.1 mg/dL compared with a decrease of 7.1 mg/dL among placebo-treated patients. This increase was duration dependent over the study period and tended to be greater with higher doses. Clinically relevant increases in serum cholesterol, defined as a final on-therapy increase in serum cholesterol greater than or equal to 50 mg/dL from baseline and to a value greater than or equal to 261 mg/dL, or an average on-therapy increase in serum cholesterol greater than or equal to 50 mg/dL from baseline and to a value greater than or equal to 261 mg/dL, were recorded in 5.3% of venlafaxine-treated patients and 0% of placebo-treated patients.

ECG changes – In a flexible-dose study, with venlafaxine doses in the range of 200 to 375 mg/day and mean dose greater than 300 mg/day, the mean change in heart rate was 8.5 beats per minute compared with 1.7 beats per minute for placebo.

VENLAFAXINE HYDROCHLORIDE — ORAL

Other adverse events observed during premarketing evaluation – Events are further categorized by body system and listed in order of decreasing frequency using the following definitions: Frequent adverse events are defined as those occurring on 1 or more occasions in at least 1/100 patients; infrequent adverse events are those occurring in 1/100 to 1/1,000 patients; rare events are those occurring in fewer than 1/1,000 patients.

Cardiovascular – Migraine, orthostatic hypotension, tachycardia (frequent); angina pectoris, arrhythmia, extrasystoles, hypotension, peripheral vascular disorder (mainly cold feet or cold hands), syncope, thrombophlebitis (infrequent); aortic aneurysm, arteritis, bigeminy, bradycardia, bundle branch block, capillary fragility, cardiovascular disorder (mitral valve disorder and circulatory disturbance), cerebral ischemia, congestive heart failure, coronary artery disease, first-degree atrioventricular block, heart arrest, mucocutaneous hemorrhage, myocardial infarct, pallor (rare).

CNS – Abnormal thinking, amnesia, confusion, depersonalization, hypesthesia, trismus, vertigo (frequent); abnormal speech, akathisia, apathy, ataxia, circumoral paresthesia, CNS stimulation, emotional lability, euphoria, hallucinations, hostility, hyperesthesia, hyperkinesia, hypotonia, incoordination, libido increased, manic reaction, myoclonus, neuralgia, neuropathy, psychosis, seizure, stupor (infrequent); abnormal gait, akinesia, alcohol abuse, aphasia, bradykinesia, buccoglossal syndrome, cerebrovascular accident, feeling drunk, loss of consciousness, delusions, dementia, dystonia, facial paralysis, Guillain-Barre syndrome, hyperchlorhydria, hypokinesia, impulse control difficulties, paranoid reaction, paresis, neuritis, nystagmus, psychotic depression, reflexes decreased, reflexes increased, suicidal ideation, torticollis (rare).

Dermatologic – Pruritus (frequent); acne, alopecia, brittle nails, contact dermatitis, dry skin, eczema, maculopapular rash, psoriasis, skin hypertrophy, urticaria (infrequent); erythema nodosum, exfoliative dermatitis, hair discoloration, furunculosis, hirsutism, leukoderma, lichenoid dermatitis, petechial rash, pustular rash, seborrhea, skin atrophy, skin discoloration, skin striae, vesiculobullous rash (rare).

Endocrine – Goiter, hyperthyroidism, hypothyroidism, thyroid nodule, thyroiditis (rare).

GI – Increased appetite (frequent); bruxism, colitis, dysphagia, esophagitis, gastritis, gastroenteritis, gastrointestinal ulcer, gingivitis, glossitis, rectal hemorrhage, hemorrhoids, melena, mouth ulceration, oral moniliasis, stomatitis, tongue edema (infrequent); cheilitis, cholecystitis, cholelithiasis, esophageal spasms, duodenitis, hematemesis, increased salivation, gastrointestinal hemorrhage, gum hemorrhage, hepatitis, ileitis, jaundice, intestinal obstruction, parotitis, periodontitis, proctitis, soft stools, tongue discoloration (rare).

GU – Metrorrhagia†, prostatic disorder (prostatitis and enlarged prostate)†, urination impaired, vaginitis† (frequent); albuminuria, amenorrhea†, cystitis, dysuria, hematuria, leukorrhea†, menorrhagia†, nocturia, bladder pain, breast pain, polyuria, pyuria, urinary incontinence, urinary retention, urinary urgency, vaginal hemorrhage† (infrequent); abortion†, anuria, breast discharge, breast engorgement, balanitis†, breast enlargement, endometriosis†, female lactation†, fibrocystic breast, calcium crystalluria, cervicitis†, orchitis†, ovarian cyst†, prolonged erection†, gynecomastia (male)†, hypomenorrhea†, kidney calculus, kidney pain, kidney function abnormal, mastitis, menopause†, pyelonephritis, oliguria, salpingitis†, urolithiasis, uterine hemorrhage†, uterine spasm†, vaginal dryness† (rare).

Hematologic/Lymphatic – Ecchymosis (frequent); anemia, leukocytosis, leukopenia, lymphadenopathy, thrombocythemia, thrombocytopenia (infrequent); basophilia, bleeding time increased, cyanosis, eosinophilia, lymphocytosis, multiple myeloma, purpura (rare).

Metabolic/Nutritional – Edema, weight gain (frequent); alkaline phosphatase increased, dehydration, hypercholesteremia, hyperglycemia, hyperlipemia, hypokalemia, AST increased, ALT increased, thirst (infrequent); alcohol intolerance, bilirubinemia, BUN increased, creatinine increased, diabetes mellitus, glycosuria, gout, healing abnormal, hemochromatosis, hypercalcinuria, hyperkalemia, hyperphosphatemia, hyperuricemia, hypocholestermia, hypoglycemia, hyponatremia, hypophosphatemia, hypoproteinemia, uremia (rare).

Musculoskeletal – Arthralgia (frequent); arthritis, arthrosis, bone pain, bone spurs, bursitis, leg cramps, myasthenia, tenosynovitis (infrequent); pathological fracture, myopathy, osteoporosis, osteosclerosis, plantar fasciitis, rheumatoid arthritis, tendon rupture (rare).

Respiratory – Cough increased, dyspnea (frequent); asthma, chest congestion, epistaxis, hyperventilation, laryngismus, laryngitis, pneumonia, voice alteration (infrequent); atelectasis, hemoptysis, hypoventilation, hypoxia, larynx edema, pleurisy, pulmonary embolus, sleep apnea (rare).

Special senses – Abnormality of accommodation, mydriasis, taste perversion (frequent); cataract, conjunctivitis, corneal lesion, diplopia, dry eyes, exophthalmos, eye pain, hyperacusis, otitis media, parosmia, photophobia, taste loss, visual field defect (infrequent); blepharitis, chromatopsia, conjunctival edema, deafness, exophthalmos, glaucoma, retinal hemorrhage, subconjunctival hemorrhage, keratitis, labyrinthitis, miosis, papilledema, decreased pupillary reflex, otitis externa, scleritis, uveitis (rare).

Miscellaneous – Chest pain substernal, chills, fever, neck pain (frequent); face edema, intentional injury, malaise, moniliasis, neck rigidity, pelvic pain, photosensitivity reaction, suicide attempt, withdrawal syndrome (infrequent); appendicitis, bacteremia, carcinoma, cellulitis (rare).

Postmarketing – Voluntary reports of other adverse events temporarily associated with the use of venlafaxine that have been received since market introduction and that may have no causal relationship with the use of venlafaxine include the following: agranulocytosis, anaphylaxis, angle-closure glaucoma, aplastic anemia, catatonia, congenital anomalies, CPK increased, deep vein thrombophlebitis, delirium, ECG abnormalities such as QT prolongation; cardiac arrhythmias including atrial fibrillation, and rare reports of ventricular fibrillation and ventricular tachycardia, including torsade de pointes; epidermal necrosis/Stevens-Johnson syndrome, erythema multiforme, extrapyramidal symptoms (including dyskinesia and tardive dyskinesia), hemorrhage (including eye and gastrointestinal bleeding), hepatic events (including GGT elevation; abnormalities of unspecified liver function tests; liver damage, necrosis, or failure; and fatty liver), involuntary movements, LDH increased, neuroleptic malignant syndrome-like events (including a case of a 10-year-old who may have been taking methylphenidate, was treated and recovered), neutropenia, night sweats, pancreatitis, pancytopenia, panic, prolactin increased, pulmonary eosinophilia, renal failure, rhabdomyolysis, serotonin syndrome, shock-like electrical sensations (in some cases, subsequent to the discontinuation of venlafaxine or tapering of dose), and syndrome of inappropriate antidiuretic hormone secretion (usually in the elderly).

There have been reports of elevated clozapine levels that were temporally associated with adverse events, including seizures, following the addition of venlafaxine. There have been reports of increases in prothrombin time, partial thromboplastin time, or INR when venlafaxine was given to patients receiving warfarin therapy.

Overdosage

➤*Symptoms:* There were 14 reports of acute overdose with venlafaxine, either alone or in combination with other drugs or alcohol, among the patients included in the premarketing evaluation. The majority of the reports involved ingestions in which the total dose of venlafaxine taken was estimated to be no more than several-fold higher than the usual therapeutic dose. The 3 patients who took the highest doses were estimated to have ingested approximately 6.75 g, 2.75 g, and 2.5 g. The resultant peak plasma levels of venlafaxine for the latter 2 patients were 6.24 and 2.35 mcg/mL, respectively, and the peak plasma levels of ODV were 3.37 and 1.3 mcg/mL, respectively. Plasma venlafaxine levels were not obtained for the patient who ingested venlafaxine 6.75 g. All 14 patients recovered without sequelae. Most patients reported no symptoms. Among the remaining patients, somnolence was the most commonly reported symptom. The patient who ingested venlafaxine 2.75 g was observed to have 2 generalized convulsions and a prolongation of QTc to 500 msec, compared with 405 msec at baseline. Mild sinus tachycardia was reported in 2 of the other patients.

Extended-release – Among the patients included in the premarketing evaluation of venlafaxine extended-release, there were 2 reports of acute overdosage with venlafaxine extended-release in depression trials, either alone or in combination with other drugs. One patient took a combination of venlafaxine extended-release 6 g and lorazepam 2.5 mg. This patient was hospitalized, treated symptomatically, and recovered without any untoward effects. The other patient took venlafaxine extended-release 2.85 g. This patient reported paresthesia of all 4 limbs but recovered without sequelae.

There were 2 reports of acute overdose with venlafaxine extended-release in GAD trials. One patient took a combination of venlafaxine extended-release 0.75 g and paroxetine 200 mg and zolpidem 50 mg. This patient was described as being alert, able to communicate, and a little sleepy. This patient was hospitalized, treated with activated charcoal, and recovered without any untoward effects. The other patient took venlafaxine extended-release 1.2 g. This patient recovered and no other specific problems were found. The patient had moderate dizziness, nausea, numb hands and feet, and hot-cold spells 5 days after the overdose. These symptoms resolved over the next week.

There were no reports of acute overdose with venlafaxine extended-release in social anxiety disorder trials.

In postmarketing experience, overdose with venlafaxine has occurred predominantly in combination with alcohol or other drugs. Electrocardiogram changes (eg, prolongation of QT interval, bundle branch block, QRS prolongation), sinus and ventricular tachycardia, bradycardia, hypotension, altered level of consciousness (ranging from somnolence to coma), seizures, vertigo, and death have been reported.

➤*Treatment:* Treatment should consist of those general measures employed in the management of overdosage with any antidepressant.

Ensure an adequate airway, oxygenation, and ventilation. Monitor cardiac rhythm and vital signs. General supportive and symptomatic measures are also recommended. Induction of emesis is not recommended. Gastric lavage with a large bore orogastric tube with appropriate airway protection, if needed, may be indicated if performed soon after ingestion or in symptomatic patients.

Administer activated charcoal. Because of the large volume of distribution of this drug, forced diuresis, dialysis, hemoperfusion, and exchange transfusion are unlikely to be of benefit. No specific antidotes for venlafaxine are known.

In managing overdosage, consider the possibility of multiple drug involvement. Consider contacting a poison control center for additional information on the treatment of any overdose.

Patient Information

➤*Clinical worsening and suicide risk:* Encourage patients, their families, and their caregivers to be alert to the emergence of anxiety, agitation, panic attacks, insomnia, irritability, hostility, aggressiveness, impulsivity, akathisia (psychomotor restlessness), hypomania, mania, other unusual changes in behavior, worsening of depression, and suicidal ideation, especially early during antidepressant treatment and when the dose is adjusted up or down. Advise families and caregivers of patients to observe for the emergence

† Based on the number of men and women as appropriate.

VENLAFAXINE HYDROCHLORIDE — ORAL

of such symptoms on a day-to-day basis, since changes may be abrupt. Such symptoms should be reported to the patients prescriber or health professional, especially if they are severe, abrupt in onset, or were not part of the patients presenting symptoms. Symptoms such as these may be associated with an increased risk for suicidal thinking and behavior and indicate a need for very close monitoring and possibly changes in the medication.

Discuss the following issues with patients for whom venlafaxine is prescribed.

➤*Interference with cognitive and motor performance:* Clinical studies were performed to examine the effects of venlafaxine on behavioral performance of healthy individuals. The results revealed no clinically significant impairment of psychomotor, cognitive, or complex behavior performance. However, since any psychoactive drug may impair judgment, thinking, or motor skills, patients should be cautioned about operating hazardous machinery, including automobiles, until they are reasonably certain that venlafaxine therapy does not adversely affect their ability to engage in such activities.

➤*Alcohol:* Although venlafaxine has not been shown to increase the impairment of mental and motor skills caused by alcohol, advise patients to avoid alcohol while taking venlafaxine.

➤*Allergic reactions:* Advise patients to notify their physician if they develop a rash, hives, or a related allergic phenomenon.

➤*Pregnancy:* Advise patients to notify their physician if they become pregnant or intend to become pregnant during therapy.

➤*Nursing:* Advise patients to notify their physician if they are breast-feeding an infant.

Selective Serotonin Reuptake Inhibitors

Refer to the Antidepressants introduction.

Indications

Refer to individual monographs for further information.

SSRIs — Summary of Indications

Indication ✓ - Labeled X - Unlabeled	Citalopram	Escitalopram	Fluoxetine	Fluvoxamine	Paroxetine	Sertraline
Bulimia nervosa			✓	X		
Depression	✓	✓	✓	X	✓	✓
Generalized anxiety disorder (GAD)	X	✓	X		✓[a]	
Obsessive-compulsive disorder (OCD)	X		✓	✓	✓[a]	✓
Panic disorder	X	X	✓	X	✓	✓
Premenstrual dysphoric disorder (PMDD)	X		✓[b]		✓[c]	✓
Posttraumatic stress disorder (PTSD)	X		X		✓[a]	✓
Social anxiety disorder				X	✓	✓

[a] Immediate-release only.
[b] *Sarafem* only.
[c] Controlled-release only.

➤*Unlabeled uses:* See the above table.

Fluoxetine – Raynaud phenomenon (20 to 60 mg/day); hot flashes (20 mg/day); second-line prophylaxis of migraines (10 to 40 mg/day).

Paroxetine – Hot flashes (20 mg/day or 12.5 to 25 mg/day controlled-release formulation); diabetic neuropathy.

Actions

➤*Pharmacology:* Selective serotonin reuptake inhibitors (SSRIs) are oral antidepressant agents chemically unrelated to the tricyclic, tetracyclic, or other available antidepressants. The antidepressant action of the SSRIs is presumed to be linked to their inhibition of CNS neuronal uptake of serotonin (5HT). Human and in vitro studies have demonstrated that **fluoxetine** (and its active metabolite S-norfluoxetine), **fluvoxamine**, **paroxetine**, **sertraline**, **escitalopram**, and **citalopram** are potent and selective inhibitors of neuronal serotonin reuptake, and they also have a weak effect on norepinephrine and dopamine neuronal reuptake. SSRIs have little affinity for muscarinic, gamma aminobutyric acid (GABA), benzodiazepine, $alpha_1$, $alpha_2$, beta-adrenergic, dopamine (D_2), $5\text{-}HT_1$, $5\text{-}HT_2$, and histamine (H_1) receptors; antagonism of muscarinic, histaminergic, and $alpha_1$-adrenergic receptors has been associated with various anticholinergic, sedative, and cardiovascular effects for other psychotropic drugs. The chronic administration of sertraline in animals was found to down-regulate brain norepinephrine receptors, as has been observed with other clinically effective antidepressants.

➤*Pharmacokinetics:*

SSRI Pharmacokinetics

SSRIs	Time to peak plasma concentration (h)	Peak plasma concentration (ng/mL)	Half-life (h)	Protein binding (%)	Time to reach steady state (days)	Primary route of elimination	Bioavailability (%)
Citalopram	≈ 4	nd*	≈ 35	≈ 80	≈ 7	20% renal, fecal	≈ 80
Escitalopram	5	nd*	27 - 32	≈ 56	≈ 7	7% renal	80[b]
Fluoxetine	6 - 8	15 - 55	24 - 384[a]	≈ 94.5	≈ 28	hepatic	nd*
Fluvoxamine	3 - 8	88 - 546	13.6 - 15.6	≈ 80	≈ 7	≈ 94% renal	53
Paroxetine	5.2	61.7	21	≈ 93-95	≈10	64% renal, 36% fecal	100
Paroxetine CR	6 - 10	30	15 - 20		14		
Sertraline	4.5 - 8.4	nd*	26 - 104[a]	98	≈ 7	40% - 45% renal, 40% - 45% fecal	nd*

[a] t½ includes the active metabolite.
[b] Based on citalopram data.
* nd = No data.

Special populations –
Elderly:
• *Citalopram* – In a single-dose study, citalopram AUC and half-life were increased in the elderly by 30% and 50%, respectively, whereas in a multiple-dose study they were increased by 23% and 30%, respectively.
• *Escitalopram* – Half-life was increased by approximately 50% in elderly subjects, and C_{max} was unchanged.
• *Fluvoxamine* – Mean C_{max} was 40% higher in elderly subjects, and the elimination half-life also increased. The clearance also was reduced by approximately 50%.
• *Paroxetine* – C_{min} concentrations were approximately 70% to 80% higher in elderly patients.
• *Sertraline* – Plasma clearance was approximately 40% lower in elderly patients. Therefore, steady state should be achieved after 2 to 3 weeks in older patients.

Hepatic function impairment:
• *Citalopram* – Oral clearance was reduced by 37% and half-life was doubled in patients with reduced hepatic function.
• *Fluoxetine* – Elimination half-life was prolonged in a study of cirrhotic patients, with a mean of 7.6 days; norfluoxetine elimination also was delayed, with a mean duration of 12 days for cirrhotic patients.
• *Fluvoxamine* – Clearance decreased 30% in patients with hepatic dysfunction.
• *Paroxetine* – Patients with hepatic function impairment had about a 2-fold increase in plasma concentrations (AUC, C_{max}).
• *Sertraline* – In patients with mild liver impairment, clearance was reduced, resulting in approximately 3-fold greater exposure.
Renal function impairment:
• *Citalopram* – In patients with mild to moderate renal function impairment, oral clearance was reduced by 17%.

• *Fluoxetine* – In depressed patients on dialysis (N = 12), fluoxetine administered as 20 mg once daily for 2 months produced steady-state fluoxetine and norfluoxetine plasma concentrations comparable with those seen in patients with normal renal function. The possibility exists that renally excreted metabolites of fluoxetine may accumulate to higher levels in patients with severe renal dysfunction.

• *Paroxetine* – The mean plasma concentrations in patients with Ccr less than 30 mL/min were approximately 4 times greater than normal subjects. Patients with Ccr of 30 to 60 mL/min had about a 2-fold increase in plasma concentrations (AUC, C_{max}).

Contraindications

Hypersensitivity to SSRIs or any inactive ingredients; in combination with a monoamine oxidase inhibitor (MAOI), or within 14 days of discontinuing an MAOI (see Drug Interactions);administration of thioridazine with **fluoxetine** or within a minimum of 5 weeks after fluoxetine has been discontinued; coadministration of **fluvoxamine** with cisapride, thioridazine or pimozide (see Drug Interactions); concomitant use of thioridazine with **paroxetine**; concomitant use of pimozide with **sertraline**; coadministration of sertraline oral concentrate and disulfiram.

Warnings

➤*Long-term use:* The effectiveness of long-term use of SSRIs for OCD, panic disorder, social anxiety disorder, PMDD, PTSD, GAD, and bulimia has not been systematically evaluated. However, the long-term use of SSRIs for depression has been evaluated and demonstrated to maintain antidepressant response for up to 1 year. Periodically reevaluate the SSRI used for extended periods to determine long-term usefulness of the drug for the individual patient.

➤*MAOIs:* In patients receiving an SSRI in combination with an MAOI, serious, sometimes fatal reactions have occurred, including hyperthermia, rigidity, myoclonus, autonomic instability with possible rapid fluctuations of vital signs, and mental status changes that include confusion, irritability, extreme agitation progressing to delirium, and coma. These reactions also have occurred in patients who have recently discontinued an SSRI and have been started on an MAOI. Some cases presented with features resembling neuroleptic malignant syndrome. While no human data show such an interaction with **paroxetine**, limited animal data suggest that the drugs may act synergistically to elevate blood pressure and evoke behavioral excitation. Therefore, it is recommended that SSRIs not be used in combination with an MAOI or within 14 days of discontinuing treatment with an MAOI. Allow at least 2 weeks after stopping the SSRIs before starting an MAOI; allow at least 5 weeks after stopping **fluoxetine** before starting an MAOI (see Drug Interactions).

➤*Suicide risk:* Patients with major depressive disorder, both adult and pediatric, may experience worsening of their depression and/or the emergence of suicidal ideation and behavior (suicidality), whether or not they are taking antidepressant medications, and this risk may persist until significant remission occurs. Although there has been a long-standing concern that antidepressants may have a role in inducing worsening of depression and the emergence of suicidality in certain patients, a causal role for antidepressants in inducing such behaviors has not been established. Nevertheless, closely observe patients being treated with antidepressants for clinical worsening and suicidality, especially at the beginning of a course of drug therapy or at the time of dose changes, either increases or decreases. Consider changing the therapeutic regimen, including possibly discontinuing the medication, in patients whose depression is persistently worse or whose emergent suicidality is severe, abrupt in onset, or was not part of the patient's presenting symptoms. Write prescriptions for the smallest quantity of tablets or capsules in order to reduce the risk of overdose.

➤*Rash and accompanying events:* Seven percent of patients taking **fluoxetine** have developed a rash and/or urticaria; almost one third were withdrawn from treatment. Clinical findings reported in association with rash include: arthralgias, edema, carpal tunnel syndrome, fever, leukocytosis, lymphadenopathy, mild transaminase elevation, proteinuria, and respiratory distress. Most patients improved promptly with discontinuation of fluoxetine and/or adjunctive treatment with antihistamines or steroids; all patients recovered completely. Two patients treated with fluoxetine developed a serious cutaneous systemic illness. Neither had an unequivocal diagnosis, but one had a leukocytoclastic vasculitis; the other had a severe desquamating syndrome that was considered to be vasculitis or erythema multiforme. Other patients have had systemic syndromes suggestive of serum sickness.

Systemic events, possibly related to vasculitis and including lupus-like syndrome, have developed in patients with rash. Although rare, these events may be serious, involving the lung, kidney, or liver. Death has been associated with the events. Anaphylactoid events, including bronchospasm, angioedema, and urticaria, alone and in combination, have occurred with fluoxetine. Pulmonary events, including inflammatory processes of varying histopathology and/or fibrosis, have occurred rarely. These events have occurred with dyspnea as the only preceding symptom. Whether these systemic events and rash have a common underlying cause or are caused by different etiologies or pathogenic processes is not known. Furthermore, a specific underlying immunologic basis for these events has not been identified. Upon the appearance of rash or of other possibly allergic phenomena for which an alternative etiology cannot be identified, discontinue the SSRI.

➤*Renal function impairment:* In depressed patients on dialysis (N = 12), **fluoxetine** administered as 20 mg once daily for 2 months produced steady-state fluoxetine and norfluoxetine plasma concentrations comparable with those seen in patients with normal renal function. The possibility exists that renally excreted metabolites of fluoxetine may accumulate to higher levels in patients with severe renal dysfunction. Use of a lower or less-frequent dose for renally impaired patients is not routinely necessary (see Administration and Dosage).

Increased plasma concentrations of **paroxetine** occur in subjects with severe renal (Ccr less than 30 mL/min). Reduce the initial dosage of paroxetine in patients with severe renal impairment; if necessary, increase upward titration intervals (see Administration and Dosage).

Because **sertraline** and **escitalopram** are extensively metabolized by the liver, excretion of unchanged drug in the urine is a minor route of elimination. However, use with caution in patients with severe renal impairment.

In patients with mild to moderate renal function impairment, oral clearance of **citalopram** was reduced by 17% compared with healthy subjects. No adjustment of dosage for such patients is recommended. No information is available about pharmacokinetics of citalopram in patients with severely reduced renal function (Ccr less than 20 mL/min). Because citalopram is extensively metabolized, excretion of unchanged drug in urine is a minor route of elimination. Until an adequate number of patients with severe renal impairment have been evaluated during chronic treatment with citalopram, use with caution in such patients.

The mean minimum plasma concentrations in renally impaired patients (Ccr 5 to 45 mL/min) after 4 and 6 weeks of treatment (50 mg twice daily, n = 13) were comparable to each other, suggesting no accumulation of **fluvoxamine** in these patients.

➤*Hepatic function impairment:* SSRIs are extensively metabolized by the liver. Use with caution in patients with severe liver impairment. The elimination half-life of **fluoxetine** was prolonged in a study of cirrhotic patients, with a mean of 7.6 days; norfluoxetine elimination also was delayed, with a mean duration of 12 days. **Fluvoxamine** clearance was decreased by 30%; slowly titrate fluvoxamine during initiation of treatment. Increased plasma concentrations of **paroxetine** occur in patients with severe hepatic impairment. Initial dose should be reduced and upward titration, if necessary, should be at increased intervals. The clearance of **sertraline** is decreased in mild, chronic liver impairment. Give a lower or less-frequent dose in patients with liver impairment; if necessary, increase upward titration intervals.

Citalopram oral clearance was reduced by 37% and half-life was doubled in patients with reduced hepatic function compared with healthy subjects. The recommended dose for most hepatically impaired patients is 20 mg.

In subjects with hepatic impairment, clearance of racemic citalopram was decreased and plasma concentrations were increased. The recommended dose of **escitalopram** in hepatically impaired patients is 10 mg/day.

➤*Carcinogenesis:* In mice and rats given **paroxetine** at 2 to 4 times the maximum recommended human dose (MRHD) on a mg/m^2 basis, there was a significantly greater number of male rats with reticulum cell sarcomas and a significantly increased linear trend across dose groups for the occurrence of lymphoreticular tumors in male rats. There was a dose-related increase in the incidence of liver adenomas in male mice receiving **sertraline** at 10 to 40 mg/kg (0.25 to 1 times the MRHD on a mg/m^2 basis). Liver adenomas have a variable rate of spontaneous occurrence in the CD-1 mouse and are of unknown significance to humans. There was an increase in follicular adenomas of the thyroid in female rats receiving sertraline at 40 mg/kg; this was not accompanied by thyroid hyperplasia. While there was an increase in uterine adenocarcinomas in rats receiving sertraline at 10 to 40 mg/kg compared with placebo controls, this effect was not clearly drug-related.

Citalopram was administered in the diet to mice and rats for 18 and 24 months, respectively. There was an increased incidence of small intestine carcinoma in rats receiving 8 or 24 mg/kg/day doses, which are approximately 1.3 and 4 times the MRHD, respectively, on a mg/m^2 basis. A no-effect dose for this finding was not established. The relevance of these findings to humans is unknown.

➤*Mutagenesis:* **Citalopram** was mutagenic in the in vitro bacterial reverse mutation assay (Ames test) in 2 of 5 bacterial strains (*Salmonella* TA98 and TA1537) in the absence of metabolic activation. It was clastogenic in the in vitro Chinese hamster lung cell assay for chromosomal aberrations in the presence and absence of metabolic activation.

➤*Fertility impairment:* A decrease in fertility was seen with **sertraline** in 1 of 2 rat studies at a dose of 80 mg/kg (4 times the MRHD on a mg/m^2 basis).

Two fertility studies conducted in rats at doses of up to 7.5 and 12.5 mg/kg/day (approximately 0.9 and 1.5 times the MRHD on a mg/m^2 basis) indicated that **fluoxetine** had no adverse effects on fertility.

When **citalopram** was administered orally to male and female rats prior to and throughout mating and gestation at doses of 32, 48, and 72 mg/kg/day, mating was decreased at all doses and fertility was decreased at doses of 32 mg/kg/day or more (approximately 5 times the MRHD of 60 mg/day on a body surface area [mg/m^2] basis). Gestation duration was increased at 48 mg/kg/day, approximately 8 times the MRHD.

A reduced pregnancy rate was found in reproduction studies in rats at a dose of 15 mg/kg/day **paroxetine**, which is 2.9 times the MRHD for depression or 2.4 times the MRHD for OCD on a mg/m^2 basis. Irreversible lesions occurred in the reproductive tract of male rats after dosing in toxicity studies for 2 to 52 weeks. These lesions consisted of vacuolation of epididymal tubular epithelium at 50 mg/kg/day and atrophic changes in the seminiferous tubules of the testes with arrested spermatogenesis at 25 mg/kg/day (9.8 and 4.9 times the MRHD for depression; 8.2 and 4.1 times the MRHD for OCD and panic disorder on a mg/m^2 basis).

➤*Elderly:* The disposition of single doses of **fluoxetine** in healthy elderly subjects (older than 65 years of age) did not differ significantly from that in younger healthy subjects. However, data are insufficient to rule out possible age-related differences during chronic use. Clearance of **fluvoxamine** is decreased by approximately 50% in elderly patients, and greater sensitivity of some older individuals cannot be ruled out. Consequently, slowly titrate fluvoxamine during initiation of therapy. **Paroxetine** pharmacokinetic studies revealed a decreased clearance in the elderly, and a lower starting dose is recommended; there was, however, no overall difference in the adverse event profile between elderly and younger patients, and efficacy was similar. For **sertraline**, the pattern of adverse reactions in the elderly was similar to that in younger patients. However, sertraline plasma clearance may be lower (see Pharmacokinetics). In 2 pharmacokinetic studies, **citalopram** AUC was increased by 23% and 30%, respectively, in elderly subjects as compared with younger subjects, and its half-life was increased by 30% and 50%, respectively. In 2 pharmacokinetic studies, **escitalopram** half-life was increased by approximately 50% in elderly subjects as compared with young subjects and C_{max} was unchanged.

➤*Pregnancy: Category C.* There are no adequate and well-controlled studies in pregnant women. Use during pregnancy only if clearly needed. In a study involving 228 women who had received **fluoxetine** during pregnancy, 5.5% of the women who took fluoxetine in the first trimester delivered infants with major structural anomalies. At doses 0.5 to 4 times the MRHD mg/kg, **sertraline** was associated with delayed ossification in fetuses of rats and rabbits, respectively. The decrease in pup survival was most probably caused by in utero exposure to sertraline. In rats, **fluvoxamine** increased pup mortality at birth and decreased postnatal pup weight and survival. **Paroxetine** reproduction studies in rats revealed no evidence of teratogenic effects. However, in rats, there was an increase in pup deaths during the first 4 days of lactation when dosing occurred during the last trimester of gestation and continued throughout lactation. In 2 rat embryo/fetal development studies, oral administration of **citalopram** (32, 56, or 112 mg/kg/day) to pregnant animals during the period of organogenesis resulted in decreased embryo/fetal growth and survival and an increased incidence of fetal abnormalities (including cardiovascular and skeletal defects) at the high dose, which is approximately 18 times the MRHD. Female rats treated with citalopram from late gestation through weaning increased offspring mortality during the first 4 days after birth, and persistent offspring growth retardation was observed at the highest dose (32 mg/kg/day).

Oral administration of **escitalopram** to pregnant animals during the period of organogenesis resulted in decreased fetal body weight and associated delays in ossification. Maternal toxicity (clinical signs and decreased body weight gain and food consumption) was present at all dose levels. When female rats were treated with escitalopram during pregnancy and through weaning, slightly increased offspring mortality and growth retardation were noted at 48 mg/kg/day. Slight maternal toxicity (clinical signs and decreased body weight gain and food consumption) were seen at this dose.

Neonates exposed to SSRIs or serotonin-norepinephrine reuptake inhibitors (SNRIs) late in the third trimester have developed complications requiring prolonged hospitalization, respiratory support, and tube feeding. Such complications can arise immediately upon delivery. Reported clinical findings have included apnea, constant crying; cyanosis, feeding difficulty, hyperreflexia, hypertonia, hypoglycemia, hypotonia, irritability, jitteriness, respiratory distress, seizures, temperature instability, tremor, vomiting. These features are consistent with either a direct toxic effect of SSRIs and SNRIs or, possibly, a drug discontinuation syndrome. It should be noted that, in some cases, the clinical picture is consistent with serotonin syndrome. When treating a pregnant woman with SSRIs during the third trimester, the physician should carefully consider the potential risks and benefits of treatment.

➤*Lactation:* **Fluoxetine**, **fluvoxamine**, **paroxetine**, **citalopram**, and **escitalopram** are excreted in breast milk. It is not known whether **sertraline** or its metabolites are excreted in breast milk. In one breast milk sample, the concentration of fluoxetine plus norfluoxetine was 70.4 ng/mL; the mother's plasma concentration was 295 ng/mL. No adverse effects were noted in the infant. In another case, an infant nursed by a mother on fluoxetine developed crying, sleep disturbance, vomiting, and watery stools. The infant's plasma drug levels were 340 ng/mL of fluoxetine and 208 ng/mL of norfluoxetine on the second day of feeding. There have been 2 reports of infants experiencing excessive somnolence, decreased feeding, and weight loss in association with breastfeeding from a citalopram-treated mother; in one case, the infant was reported to recover completely upon discontinuation of citalopram by its mother. Exercise caution when SSRIs are administered to a nursing woman. Decide whether to discontinue nursing or discontinue the drug taking into account the importance of the drug to the mother.

➤*Children:* Safety and efficacy in children have not been established.

Regular monitoring of weight and growth is recommended if treatment of a child with an SSRI is to be continued long-term.

The safety and efficacy in pediatric patients younger than 8 years of age in major depressive disorder and younger than 7 years of age in OCD have not been established.

The efficacy of **sertraline** for the treatment of OCD was demonstrated in a 12-week, multicenter, placebo-controlled study with 187 outpatients 6 to 17 years of age. The efficacy of sertraline in pediatric patients with depression, panic disorder, PTSD, PMDD, or social anxiety disorder has not been established.

The efficacy of **fluvoxamine** for the treatment of OCD was demonstrated in a 10-week, multicenter, placebo-controlled study with 120 outpatients 8 to 17 years of age. The adverse event profile was similar to that observed in adult studies. The risks, if any, that may be associated with fluvoxamine's extended use in children and adolescents with OCD have not been systematically assessed. Have the prescriber be mindful that the evidence supporting fluvoxamine use in children and adolescents derives from relatively short-term clinical studies and from extrapolation of experience gained with adult patients.

Precautions

➤*Monitoring:* In patients receiving SSRIs and suffering from SIADH, displacement syndromes, edematous states, adrenal disease, or conditions of fluid loss, it is recommended that serum electrolytes, especially sodium, as well as BUN and plasma creatinine be monitored regularly. Monitor patients for the emergence of agitation, irritability, and other symptoms, as well as emergence of suicidality, especially at the beginning of drug therapy or at the time of dose changes. Regular monitoring of weight and growth is recommended, especially if treatment of a child with an SSRI is to be continued long-term.

➤*Abnormal bleeding:* Altered platelet function and/or abnormal results from laboratory studies in patients taking **fluoxetine**, **paroxetine**, or **sertraline** have occurred. There have been reports of abnormal bleeding or purpura in several patients; it is unclear whether the SSRIs had a causative role.

Published case reports have documented the occurrence of bleeding episodes in patients treated with psychotropic drugs that interfere with serotonin reuptake. Subsequent epidemiological studies, both of the case-control and cohort design, have demonstrated an association between the use of psychotropic drugs that interfere with serotonin reuptake and the occurrence of upper GI bleeding. In 2 studies, concurrent use of a nonsteroidal anti-inflammatory drug (NSAID) or aspirin potentiated the risk of bleeding. Although these studies focused on upper GI bleeding, there is reason to believe that bleeding at other sites may be similarly potentiated. Caution patients regarding the risk of bleeding associated with the concomitant use of SSRIs with NSAIDs, aspirin, or other drugs that affect coagulation.

➤*Anxiety, nervousness, and insomnia:* Anxiety, nervousness, and insomnia occurred in 2% to 22% of patients treated with an SSRI. In clinical trials for bulimia nervosa, insomnia occurred in 33% of patients treated with **fluoxetine**.

➤*Altered appetite and weight:* Significant weight loss, especially in underweight depressed or bulimic patients, has occurred. Approximately 3% to 17% of patients treated with an SSRI initially experienced anorexia. Significant weight loss may be an undesirable result of treatment for some patients but on average, patients in controlled trials treated with **paroxetine**, **citalopram**, or **sertraline** had a minimal 1- to 2-pound weight loss vs smaller changes with placebo. Only rarely have the SSRIs been discontinued because of weight loss or anorexia (see Adverse Reactions); however, after prolonged treatments, patients tend to gain weight. Monitor weight change during therapy.

➤*Activation of mania/hypomania:* Activation of mania/hypomania occurred infrequently in approximately 0.1% to 2.6% of patients taking SSRIs. Activation of mania/hypomania also has occurred in a small proportion of patients with major affective disorder treated with other antidepressants. Use cautiously in patients with a history of mania.

➤*Seizures:* Seizures have occurred with **fluoxetine** (0.1%), **fluvoxamine** (0.2%), **paroxetine** (0.1%), **sertraline** (0.2%), and **citalopram** (0.3%). Sertraline, citalopram, and **escitalopram** have not been evaluated in patients with a seizure disorder. These percentages appear similar to the rate associated with other antidepressants and placebo treatment. Use with care in patients with history of seizures; discontinue therapy if seizures occur.

➤*Cardiac effects:* SSRIs have not been systematically evaluated in patients with a recent history of MI or unstable heart disease. Patients with these diagnoses were generally excluded from clinical studies during the product's premarketing testing. However, the ECGs of patients who received SSRIs in clinical trials were evaluated and the data indicate that they are not associated with the development of clinically significant ECG abnormalities.

➤*Fluoxetine dose changes:* The long elimination half-life of **fluoxetine** and norfluoxetine means that changes in dose will not be fully reflected in plasma for several weeks, affecting titration to final dose and withdrawal from treatment.

➤*Concomitant illness:* Clinical experience is limited. Use caution in patients with diseases or conditions that could affect metabolism or hemodynamic responses.

➤*Glaucoma:* Mydriasis has been reported infrequently in premarketing studies with SSRIs. A few cases of acute angle-closure glaucoma associated with **paroxetine** therapy have been reported in the literature. As mydriasis can cause acute angle closure in patients with narrow-angle glaucoma, use caution when SSRIs are prescribed for patients with narrow-angle glaucoma.

➤*Effects of smoking:* Smokers had a 25% increase in the metabolism of **fluvoxamine** compared with nonsmokers.

➤*Electroconvulsive therapy (ECT):* There are no clinical studies establishing the benefit of the combined use of ECT and SSRIs. Rare prolonged seizure in patients on **fluoxetine** has occurred.

➤*Hyponatremia:* Several cases of **fluoxetine**, **fluvoxamine**, **sertraline**, **paroxetine**, **escitalopram**, and **citalopram**-induced hyponatremia (some with serum sodium less than 110 mmol/L) have occurred. The hyponatremia appeared to be reversible when fluoxetine, sertraline, paroxetine, citalopram, escitalopram, and fluvoxamine were discontinued. Although these cases were complex with varying possible etiologies, some were possibly because of the syndrome of inappropriate antidiuretic hormone secretion (SIADH). The majority have been in older patients and in patients taking diuretics or who were otherwise volume-depleted.

➤*Diabetes:* **Fluoxetine** may alter glycemic control. Hypoglycemia has occurred during therapy, and hyperglycemia has developed following discontinuation of the drug. The dosage of insulin and/or oral hypoglycemic agents may need to be adjusted when fluoxetine is started or discontinued.

➤*Uricosuric effect:* **Sertraline** is associated with a mean decrease in serum uric acid of approximately 7%. The clinical significance of this weak uricosuric effect is unknown.

➤*Discontinuation of SSRIs:* During marketing of SSRIs and SNRIs, there have been spontaneous reports of adverse events occurring upon discontinuation of these drugs, particularly when abrupt, including the following: agitation, anxiety, confusion, dizziness, dysphoric mood, emotional lability, headache, hypomania, insomnia, irritability, lethargy, and sensory disturbances (eg, paresthesias such as electric shock sensations). While these events are generally self-limiting, there have been reports of serious discontinuation symptoms.

Monitor patients for these symptoms when discontinuing treatment with SSRIs. A gradual reduction in the dose rather than abrupt cessation is recommended whenever possible. If intolerable symptoms occur following a decrease in the dose or upon discontinuation of treatment, then resuming the previously prescribed dose may be considered. Subsequently, the physician may continue decreasing the dose but at a more gradual rate.

➤*Drug abuse and dependence:* Premarketing clinical experience did not reveal any tendency for a withdrawal syndrome or any drug-seeking behavior. It is not possible to predict on the basis of this limited experience the extent to which a CNS-active drug will be misused, diverted, or abused once marketed. Consequently, before starting an SSRI, carefully evaluate patients for history of drug abuse and follow such patients closely, observing them for signs of misuse or abuse.

➤*Hazardous tasks:* Any psychoactive drug may impair judgment, thinking, or motor skills; caution patients about operating hazardous machinery, including automobiles, until they are reasonably certain that the drug treatment does not affect them adversely.

➤*Photosensitivity:* Photosensitization may occur; therefore, caution patients to take protective measures (eg, sunscreens, protective clothing) against exposure to ultraviolet light or sunlight until tolerance is determined.

Drug Interactions

➤*Drugs highly bound to plasma protein:* Because SSRIs are highly bound to plasma protein, administration to a patient taking another drug that is highly protein-bound (eg, warfarin, digoxin) may cause increased free concentrations of the other drug, potentially resulting in adverse events. Conversely, adverse effects could result from displacement of SSRIs by other highly bound drugs.

➤*CYP450 system:* Concomitant use of SSRIs with drugs metabolized by cytochrome P450 2D6 may require lower doses than usually prescribed for either SSRIs or the other drug because SSRIs may significantly inhibit the activity of this isozyme. In most patients (more than 90%), this isozyme is saturated early during dosing. Therefore, coadministration of **paroxetine** with other drugs that are metabolized by this isozyme (eg, certain antidepressants, phenothiazines, risperidone, type IC antiarrhythmics) or drugs that inhibit this enzyme (eg, quinidine) should be approached with caution. **Fluvoxamine** is a relatively weak inhibitor of this isozyme. However, in vitro the drug inhibits the 1A2, 2C9, and 3A4 isozymes, which are involved in the metabolism of warfarin, theophylline, propranolol, and alprazolam. Therapy with medications that are predominantly metabolized by the CYP2D6 system and that have a relatively narrow therapeutic index (eg, flecainide, vinblastine, TCAs) should be initiated at the low end of the dose range if a patient is receiving **fluoxetine** concurrently or has taken it in the previous 5 weeks.

In vitro studies indicate that cytochrome P450 3A4 and 2C19 are the primary enzymes involved in metabolism of **citalopram** and **escitalopram**. Inhibitors of 3A4 (eg, azole antifungals, macrolide antibiotics) and 2C19 (eg, omeprazole) would be expected to increase plasma citalopram levels. Inducers of 3A4 (eg, carbamazepine) would be expected to decrease citalopram and escitalopram levels.

➤*Serotonin syndrome:* The serotonin syndrome is a complication of therapy with serotonergic drugs. It is most commonly observed when 2 drugs that potentiate serotonergic neurotransmission are used concurrently. When this problem occurs with SSRIs, it is most commonly in the setting of other concurrent medications, such as MAOIs, which increase serotonin by different mechanisms. Other such drugs include tryptophan, amphetamines, or other psychostimulants, other antidepressants that increase 5-HT levels, buspirone, lithium, or dopamine agonists (eg, amantadine, bromocriptine). Serotonin syndrome has been reported in 2 patients who were concomitantly receiving linezolid, an antibiotic that is a reversible non-selective MAOI.

➤*Drugs that interfere with hemostasis (eg, NSAIDs, aspirin, warfarin):* Serotonin release by platelets plays an important role in hemostasis. Epidemiological studies of the case-control and cohort design that have demonstrated an association between use of psychotropic drugs that interfere with serotonin reuptake and the occurrence of upper GI bleeding also have shown that concurrent use of an NSAID or aspirin potentiated the risk of bleeding. Thus, caution patients about the use of such drugs concurrently with an SSRI.

SSRI Drug Interactions

Precipitant drug	Object drug*		Description
Barbiturates	SSRIs Paroxetine	↓	Phenobarbital decreased the AUC and half-life of paroxetine by 25% and 38%, respectively.
Cimetidine	SSRIs	↑	Cimetidine increased steady-state paroxetine concentrations by ≈ 50%. Cimetidine increased sertraline AUC (50%), C_{max} (24%), and half-life (26%). Citalopram and escitalopram AUC (43%) and C_{max} (39%) also increased. Adjust paroxetine dosage as needed.
Cyproheptadine	SSRIs Fluoxetine Paroxetine	↓	The pharmacologic effects of SSRIs may be decreased or reversed.
Linezolid	SSRIs	↑	A serotonin syndrome has been reported to occur after coadministration of linezolid and paroxetine. It may be prudent to allow at least 2 weeks after stopping linezolid before giving an SSRI.
MAO inhibitors	SSRIs	↑	Serious, sometimes fatal, reactions have occurred in patients receiving SSRIs in combination with a MAOI or who have recently discontinued the SSRI and are then started on an MAOI (see Warnings).
Metoclopramide Sibutramine Tramadol	SSRIs	↑	A serotonin syndrome (eg, CNS irritability, shivering, myoclonus, altered consciousness) may occur.
Phenytoin	SSRIs Paroxetine	↓	Phenytoin reduced the AUC and half-life of paroxetine by 50% and 35%, respectively. Also, paroxetine reduced the AUC of phenytoin by 12%, and sertraline, fluoxetine, and fluvoxamine may increase hydantoin levels.
SSRIs Fluoxetine Fluvoxamine Sertraline	Hydantoins	↑↓	
Smoking	SSRIs Fluvoxamine	↓	Smokers had a 25% increase in the metabolism of fluvoxamine.
L-tryptophan	SSRIs	↑	Concurrent use with fluoxetine or paroxetine may produce symptoms related to both central toxicity (eg, headache, sweating, dizziness, agitation, restlessness) and peripheral toxicity (eg, GI distress, nausea, vomiting). Concomitant use is not recommended. Tryptophan may enhance the serotonergic effects of fluvoxamine; use the combination with caution. Severe vomiting has been reported with the coadministration of fluvoxamine and tryptophan.
St. John's wort	SSRIs Paroxetine Sertraline	↑	Increased sedative-hypnotic effects may occur. Avoid concurrent use.
SSRIs	Alcohol	↔	Although potentiation of impairment of mental and motor skills caused by alcohol has not occurred, concurrent use is not recommended in patients.
SSRIs	Antidepressants, tricyclic	↑	Plasma TCA levels may be increased; use caution when coadministering. Monitor TCA levels; may need to reduce TCA dose.

SSRI Drug Interactions			
Precipitant drug	Object drug*		Description
SSRIs Fluoxetine Fluvoxamine Sertraline	Benzodiazepines	↑	Clearance of benzodiazepines metabolized by hepatic oxidation may be decreased; those metabolized by glucuronidation are unlikely to be affected. Coadministration of alprazolam and fluoxetine or fluvoxamine has resulted in increased alprazolam levels and decreased psychomotor performance. Halve the initial alprazolam dose, and titrate to the lowest effective dose. Avoid coadministration of fluvoxamine and diazepam.
SSRIs	Beta blockers	↑	Certain SSRIs may inhibit the metabolism of certain beta blockers. Concurrent use of citalopram or escitalopram and metoprolol produced an increase in metoprolol levels. Fluvoxamine administered with propranolol produced a 5-fold increase in propranolol C_{min}. If propranolol or metoprolol is given with fluvoxamine, reduce the initial beta blocker dose.
SSRIs Fluoxetine Fluvoxamine	Buspirone	↓	Effects of buspirone may be decreased; plasma concentrations may be increased with fluvoxamine but clinical response may be decreased. Paradoxical worsening of OCD or serotonin syndrome has occurred.
SSRIs Fluoxetine Fluvoxamine	Carbamazepine	↑	Serum carbamazepine levels may be increased with fluoxetine or fluvoxamine, possibly resulting in toxicity. The clearance of citalopram and escitalopram may be increased. The therapeutic effect of sertraline may be decreased.
Carbamazepine	SSRIs Citalopram Escitalopram Sertraline	↓	
SSRIs Fluvoxamine Sertraline	Cisapride	↓	Concurrent use of sertraline and cisapride reduced cisapride AUC and C_{max}. Use with fluvoxamine is contraindicated.
SSRIs Citalopram Fluoxetine Fluvoxamine Sertraline	Clozapine	↑	Elevated serum clozapine levels have occurred. Closely monitor patients on concomitant administration.
SSRIs Fluoxetine Fluvoxamine	Cyclosporine	↑	Elevated cyclosporine concentrations were reported in case reports during concomitant administration.
SSRIs Paroxetine	Digoxin	↓	Paroxetine decreased the AUC of digoxin by 15%. The coadministration of paroxetine and digoxin should be undertaken with caution.
SSRIs Fluvoxamine	Diltiazem	↑	Bradycardia has occurred with concurrent use.
SSRIs Fluoxetine Fluvoxamine	Haloperidol	↑	Serum concentrations of haloperidol may be increased. Closely monitor patients on concomitant therapy.
SSRIs Citalopram	Ketoconazole	↓	Coadministration decreased ketoconazole C_{max} (21%) and AUC (10%).
SSRIs Citalopram Escitalopram Fluoxetine Fluvoxamine Sertraline	Lithium	↑↓	Lithium levels may be increased or decreased by fluoxetine with possible neurotoxicity and increased serotonergic effects. In healthy volunteers, sertraline did not affect lithium levels. It is recommended that plasma lithium levels be monitored following initiation of sertraline, fluoxetine, citalopram, and escitalopram with appropriate adjustments to lithium dose. Concurrent use may enhance serotonergic effects of SSRIs. Use caution when coadministering. Lithium may enhance the serotonergic effects of fluvoxamine. Use with caution in combination; seizures have been reported.
Lithium	SSRIs	↑	
SSRIs Fluvoxamine	Methadone	↑	Significantly increased methadone concentrations have occurred. One patient developed opioid intoxication; another had opioid withdrawal symptoms with fluvoxamine discontinuation.
SSRIs Fluvoxamine	Mexiletine	↑	Mexiletine serum levels may be elevated, increasing the risk of side effects.
SSRIs	NSAIDs	↑	The risk of GI adverse effects may be increased. If possible, avoid concurrent use.
SSRIs Fluoxetine Fluvoxamine	Olanzapine	↑	Olanzapine plasma concentrations may be elevated. Observe the patient closely.
SSRIs Fluoxetine Fluvoxamine Paroxetine	Phenothiazines	↑	Plasma phenothiazine concentrations may be elevated, increasing the pharmacologic and adverse effects, including life-threatening cardiac arrhythmias. Thioridazine is contraindicated with fluvoxamine, fluoxetine, and paroxetine (see Contraindications).
SSRIs Fluvoxamine Sertraline	Pimozide	↑	Concurrent use of sertraline and pimozide 2 mg produced a mean increase in pimozide AUC and C_{max} of ≈ 40%, increasing the risk of life-threatening cardiac arrhythmias. Because of pimozide's narrow therapeutic index, administration with sertraline or fluvoxamine is contraindicated.
SSRIs Paroxetine	Procyclidine	↑	Paroxetine increased the AUC, C_{max}, and C_{min} of procyclidine by 35%, 37%, and 67%, respectively. Reduce procyclidine dose if anticholinergic effects occur.
SSRIs Fluoxetine	Propafenone	↑	Coadministration of fluoxetine and propafenone produced elevated propafenone plasma levels. Certain SSRIs may inhibit the metabolism (CYP2D6) of propafenone.
SSRIs Paroxetine	Risperidone	↑	Coadministration may increase risperidone concentrations, increasing the risk of side effects. Serotonin syndrome may occur.
SSRIs Fluoxetine	Ritonavir	↑	The AUC of ritonavir may be increased. Serotonin syndrome may occur.
SSRIs Fluvoxamine	Ropivacaine	↑	Ropivacaine plasma concentrations may be elevated; the pharmacologic effects may be prolonged, increasing the risk of toxicity.
SSRIs Fluvoxamine Sertraline	Sulfonylureas Glimepiride Tolbutamide	↑	Fluvoxamine and sertraline have been shown to decrease the clearance of tolbutamide. Fluvoxamine also has been shown to increase the peak plasma concentration of glimepiride.

SSRI Drug Interactions

Precipitant drug	Object drug*		Description
SSRIs	Sumatriptan	↑	Weakness, hyperreflexia, and incoordination have occurred with coadministration. Observe patient closely.
SSRIs	Sympathomimetics	↑	Increased sensitivity to the effect of sympathomimetics and increased risk of serotonin syndrome may occur.
SSRIs Fluvoxamine	Tacrine	↑	Plasma tacrine concentrations may be elevated, increasing the pharmacologic and cholinergic adverse effects.
SSRIs Fluvoxamine Paroxetine	Theophylline	↑	Clearance of theophylline may be decreased by 3-fold when coadministered with fluvoxamine; reduce dosage. Elevated theophylline levels have occurred with paroxetine. It is recommended that theophylline levels be monitored when these drugs are concurrently administered.
SSRIs Fluoxetine Paroxetine	Trazodone	↑	Plasma trazodone levels may be elevated, resulting in increased pharmacologic and toxic effects. If coadministration cannot be avoided, start with a low dose of the SSRI or trazodone.
SSRIs	Warfarin	↑	A pharmacodynamic interaction of altered anticoagulant effects including increased bleeding diathesis with unaltered prothrombin time (PT) may occur with paroxetine or fluoxetine. Coadministration of sertraline and warfarin and citalopram and warfarin has resulted in an 8% and 5% increase in PT, respectively, and delayed PT normalization. Fluvoxamine increased warfarin plasma levels by 98%; PT was prolonged. Monitor PT. Use caution with coadministration and monitor patient.
SSRIs Sertraline	Zolpidem	↑	Coadministration of sertraline and zolpidem produced a shortened onset of action of zolpidem and an increased effect.

* ↑ = Object drug increased. ↓ = Object drug decreased. ↔ = Undetermined clinical effect.

➤*Drug/Food interactions:* In one study following a single dose of **sertraline** with and without food, sertraline AUC was slightly increased with food and C_{max} was 25% greater. Time to reach peak plasma level decreased from 8 hours post dosing to 5.5 hours. For **paroxetine**, AUC was only slightly increased (6%) when drug was administered with food but the C_{max} was 29% greater, while the time to reach peak plasma concentration decreased from 6.4 hours postdosing to 4.9 hours.

Food does not appear to affect systemic bioavailability of **fluoxetine**, although it may delay absorption by 1 to 2 hours. **Fluvoxamine** and paroxetine CR bioavailability are not affected by food. **Citalopram** and **escitalopram** absorption is not affected by food. Thus, all SSRIs may be given with or without food.

Adverse Reactions

Discontinuation of treatment – In clinical trials, 9.4% to 20% of **paroxetine** patients, 3% to 13% of paroxetine CR patients, 10% to 15% of **sertraline** patients, 22% of **fluvoxamine** patients, 16% of **citalopram** patients, and 6% to 8% of **escitalopram** patients discontinued treatment because of an adverse event.

SSRIs Adverse Reactions (%)[a]

Adverse reaction	Citalopram	Escitalopram	Fluoxetine	Fluvoxamine	Paroxetine IR/CR		Sertraline
Cardiovascular							
Chest pain	—	≥ 1	≥ 1	—	3	1	≥ 1
Hot flushes	0.1 - 1	≥ 1	—	—	—	—	0.1 - 1
Hypertension	0.1 - 1	≥ 1	≥ 1	≥ 1	≥ 1	2	0.1 - 1
Hypotension (postural)	≥ 1	—	0.1 - 1	≥ 1	—	0.1 - 1	0.1 - 1
Palpitations	—	≥ 1	1 - 3	3	2 - 3	0.1 - 1	≥ 1
Syncope	0.1 - 1	0.1 - 1	0.1 - 1	≥ 1	≥ 1	—	0.1 - 1
Tachycardia	≥ 1	0.1 - 1	0.1 - 1	≥ 1	≥ 1	1 - 2	0.1 - 1
Vasodilation	—	—	2 - 3	3	2 - 4	2 - 3	< 0.1
CNS							
Abnormal dreams	—	3	3	—	3 - 4	1	0.1 - 1
Abnormal thinking	—	—	2 - 6	—	0.1 - 1	0.1 - 1	—
Agitation	3	0.1 - 1	≥ 1	2	3 - 6	2 - 3	1 - 6
Amnesia	≥ 1	0.1 - 1	≥ 1	≥ 1	2	0.1 - 1	0.1 - 1
Anxiety	4	—	12 - 13	1 - 5	2 - 6	2 - 5	4
Apathy	≥ 1	0.1 - 1	—	≥ 1	—	—	0.1 - 1
CNS stimulation	—	—	0.1 - 1	2	—	—	—
Concentration, decreased/impaired	≥ 1	≥ 1	—	—	3 - 4	1 - 3	—
Confusion	≥ 1	0.1 - 1	≥ 1	—	1	1	0.1 - 1
Depersonalization	0.1 - 1	0.1 - 1	0.1 - 1	0.1 - 1	3	0.1 - 1	—
Depression	≥ 1	0.1 - 1	—	2	—	2	0.1 - 1
Dizziness	—	4 - 7	2 - 11	2 - 11	6 - 14	6 - 14	6 - 17
Drugged feeling	—	—	—	—	2	—	—
Emotional lability	0.1 - 1	0.1 - 1	≥ 1	0.1 - 1	≥ 1	0.1 - 1	0.1 - 1
Fatigue	5	2-8	—	—	—	—	10 - 16
Headache	—	24	13 - 24	3 - 22	17 - 18	15 - 27	25
Hypertonia	0.1 - 1	—	0.1 - 1	2	0.1 - 1	2 - 3	≥ 1
Hypoesthesia	0.1 - 1	—	0.1 - 1	—	0.1 - 1	0.1 - 1	≥ 1
Hypo-/Hyperkinesia	0.1 - 1	—	—	≥ 1	0.1 - 1	0.1 - 1	0.1 - 1
Insomnia	15	7 - 14	9 - 24	4 - 21	11 - 24	7 - 20	12 - 28
Libido decreased	1 - 4	3 - 7	3 - 9	2	3 - 12	7 - 12	1 - 11
Manic reaction	—	—	—	≥ 1	—	—	—
Myoclonus/twitching	—	0.1 - 1	0.1 - 1	≥ 1	2 - 3	1 - 2	0.1 - 1
Nervousness	—	0.1 - 1	3 - 14	2 - 12	3 - 9	2 - 8	5
Paresthesia	≥ 1	2	—	—	4	1 - 3	2
Psychotic reaction	—	—	—	≥ 1	—	—	—
Sleep disorder	—	—	≥ 1	0.1-1	—	—	—
Somnolence	18	4 - 13	12 - 13	4 - 22	13 - 24	3 - 22	2 - 15
Tremor	8	0.1 - 1	9 - 12	5	4 - 15	4 - 8	< 1 - 11
Vertigo	0.1 - 1	0.1 - 1	—	0.1 - 1	≥ 1	2	0.1 - 1

Selective Serotonin Reuptake Inhibitors

SSRIs Adverse Reactions (%)[a]

Adverse reaction	Citalopram	Escitalopram	Fluoxetine	Fluvoxamine	Paroxetine IR/CR		Sertraline
Dermatologic							
Acne	0.1 - 1	0.1 - 1	0.1 - 1	0.1 - 1	0.1 - 1	0.1 - 1	0.1 - 1
Pruritus	≥ 1	0.1 - 1	3	—	≥ 1	0.1 - 1	0.1 - 1
Rash	≥ 1	≥ 1	4 - 5	—	2 - 3	≥ 1	3
Sweating, excessive/increased	11	3 - 8	7 - 8	7	1 - 14	6 - 14	3 - 11
GI							
Abdominal pain	3	2	6	1	4	3-7	2-7
Anorexia	4	—	10 - 11	1 - 6	—	—	3-11
Constipation	—	3 - 6	5	10	5 - 16	2 - 13	1 - 8
Decreased appetite	—	3	—	—	2 - 9	1 - 12	—
Diarrhea/loose stools	8	6 - 14	2 - 11	1 - 11	9 - 19	6 - 18	13 - 24
Dry mouth	20	4 - 9	9 - 11	1 - 14	9 - 21	2 - 18	6 - 16
Dyspepsia	5	2 - 6	7 - 8	1 - 10	2 - 5	2 - 13	6 - 13
Dysphagia	0.1 - 1	—	0.1 - 1	2	0.1 - 1	—	0.1 - 1
Flatulence	≥ 1	2	3	4	4	6 - 8	—
Gastroenteritis	0.1 - 1	≥ 1	0.1 - 1	0.1 - 1	0.1 - 1	0.1 - 1	0.1 - 1
Increased appetite	≥ 1	≥ 1	≥ 1	—	2 - 4	—	≥ 1
Melena	—	—	0.1 - 1	—	—	—	< 0.1
Nausea	21	15 - 18	9 - 27	9 - 40	15 - 36	17 - 23	13 - 30
Oropharynx disorder	—	—	—	—	2	—	—
Tooth disorder/caries	—	2	—	3	< 0.1	0.1 - 1	0.1 - 1
Vomiting	4	3	1 - 3	2 - 5	2 - 3	2	4
GU							
Abnormal ejaculation	6	9 - 14	—	8	6 - 28	15 - 27	7 - 19
Female genital disorders	—	—	—	—	2 - 9	2 - 10	—
Male genital disorders, others	—	—	—	—	4 - 10	—	—
Menstrual disorder	—	2	—	—	—	1 - 2	0.1 - 1
Sexual dysfunction/impotence/ anorgasmia	1 - 3	2 - 6	0.1 - 1	2	2 - 13	5 - 10	≥ 1
Urinary frequency	—	≥ 1	2	3	2 - 3	2	0.1 - 1
Urinary tract infection	—	≥ 1	—	0.1 - 1	2	3	—
Urination disorder/retention	0.1 - 1	—	0.1- 1	1	3	2	0.1 - 1
Musculoskeletal							
Arthralgia	2	≥ 1	—	0.1 - 1	≥ 1	2	0.1 - 1
Myalgia	2	≥ 1	—	—	2 - 4	5	≥ 1
Myasthenia	—	—	< 0.1	0.1 - 1	1	< 0.1	—
Myopathy	—	—	< 0.1	< 0.1	2	< 0.1	—
Respiratory							
Bronchitis	0.1 - 1	≥ 1	—	0.1 - 1	0.1 - 1	1 - 2	< 0.1
Cough (increased)	≥ 1	≥ 1	—	≥ 1	≥ 1	1 - 2	0.1 - 1
Dyspnea	0.1 - 1	—	—	2	0.1 - 1	—	0.1 - 1
Pharyngitis	—	—	6 - 10	—	4	8	—
Respiratory disorder	—	—	—	—	7	—	—
Rhinitis	5	5	16 - 23	—	3	4	≥ 1
Sinusitis	3	3	—	≥ 1	4	4 - 8	0.1 - 1
Upper respiratory tract infection	5	—	—	9	—	—	0.1 - 1
Yawn	2	2	3 - 5	2	2 - 5	2 - 5	≥ 1
Special senses							
Amblyopia	—	—	—	3	—	—	—
Taste perversion/change	≥ 1	0.1 - 1	≥ 1	3	2	2	—
Tinnitus	0.1 - 1	≥ 1	≥ 1	—	≥ 1	0.1 - 1	≥ 1
Vision disturbances/blurred vision/ abnormal vision	≥ 1	≥ 1	2 - 3	—	2 - 8	1 - 5	3
Miscellaneous							
Accidental injury/trauma	—	—	1 - 8	≥ 1	3 - 6	3 - 8	—
Allergy/allergic reaction	—	≥ 1	—	0.1 - 1	0.1 - 1	2	< 0.1
Asthenia	—	0.1 - 1	8 - 14	2 - 14	3 - 22	14 - 18	≥ 1
Back pain		—	—	—	3	4 - 5	≥ 1
Chills	—	0.1 - 1	≥ 1	2	2	0.1 - 1	—
Edema	0.1 - 1	—	—	≥ 1	0.1 - 1	0.1 - 1	0.1 - 1
Fever	2	≥ 1	2 - 5	—	—	0.1 - 1	0.1 - 1
Flu syndrome	0.1 - 1	5	3 - 12	3	5 - 6	6 - 8	—
Malaise	—	0.1 - 1	0.1 - 1	≥ 1	0.1 - 1	0.1 - 1	< 1 - 10
Pain	—	—	3 - 9			3	1 - 6
Weight gain	≥ 1	≥ 1	≥ 1	≥ 1	≥ 1	1 - 3	≥ 1
Weight loss	≥ 1	0.1 - 1	2 - 3	≥ 1	0.1 - 1	1	0.1 - 1

[a] Data are pooled from different studies and are not necessarily comparable.

Dose dependency of adverse reactions – A comparison of adverse event rates in a fixed-dose study comparing **paroxetine** 10, 20, 30, and 40 mg/day with placebo revealed a clear dose dependency for some of the more common adverse events associated with paroxetine use.

Adverse Reactions by Indications of Fluoxetine								
	Depression		OCD		Bulimia		Panic disorder	
Adverse reaction	Fluoxetine (n = 1728)	Placebo (n = 975)	Fluoxetine (n = 266)	Placebo (n = 89)	Fluoxetine (n = 450)	Placebo (n = 267)	Fluoxetine (n = 425)	Placebo (n = 342
CNS								
Abnormal dreams	1	1	5	2	5	3	1	1
Anxiety	12	7	14	7	15	9	6	2
Insomnia	16	9	28	22	33	13	10	7
Libido decreased	3	< 1	11	2	5	1	1	2
Nervousness	14	9	14	15	11	5	8	6
Somnolence	13	6	17	7	13	5	5	2
Tremor	10	3	9	1	13	1	3	1
Dermatologic								
Rash	4	3	6	3	4	4	2	2
Sweating	8	3	7	< 1	8	3	2	2
GI								
Anorexia	11	2	17	10	8	4	4	1
Diarrhea	12	8	18	13	8	6	9	4
Dry mouth	10	7	12	3	9	6	4	4
Dyspepsia	7	5	10	4	10	6	6	2
Nausea	21	9	26	13	29	11	12	7
GU								
Abnormal ejaculation	< 1	< 1	7	< 1	7	< 1	2	1
Impotence	2	< 1	< 1	< 1	7	< 1	1	< 1
Respiratory								
Pharyngitis	3	3	11	9	10	5	3	3
Sinusitis	1	4	5	2	6	4	2	3
Yawn	< 1	< 1	7	< 1	11	< 1	1	< 1
Miscellaneous								
Asthenia	9	5	15	11	21	9	7	7
Flu syndrome	3	4	10	7	8	3	5	5
Vasodilation	3	2	5	< 1	2	1	1	< 1

Adaptation to certain adverse events – Over a 4- to 6-week period, there was evidence of adaptation to some adverse events with continued therapy (eg, nausea, dizziness), but less to other effects (eg, dry mouth, somnolence, asthenia).

➤*Cardiovascular:*

Citalopram – Angina pectoris, bradycardia, cardiac failure, cerebrovascular accident, extrasystoles, MI, myocardial ischemia (0.1% to 1%); atrial fibrillation, bundle branch block, cardiac arrest, phlebitis, pulmonary embolism, transient ischemic attack (less than 0.1%); chest pain, torsade de pointes, ventricular arrhythmia, QT prolonged (postmarketing).

Escitalopram – Bradycardia, ECG abnormal, varicose vein (0.1% to 1%); atrial fibrillation, hypotension, MI, orthostatic hypotension, pulmonary embolism, QT prolongation, torsade de pointes, ventricular tachycardia (postmarketing).

Fluoxetine – Hemorrhage (at least 1%); angina pectoris, arrhythmia, CHF, hypotension, migraine, myocardial infarct, vascular headache (0.1% to 1%); atrial fibrillation, bradycardia, cerebral embolism, cerebral ischemia, cerebrovascular accident, extrasystoles, heart arrest, heart block, pallor, peripheral vascular disorder, phlebitis, shock, thrombophlebitis, thrombosis, vasospasm, ventricular arrhythmia, ventricular extrasystoles, ventricular fibrillation (less than 0.1%); atrial fibrillation, cerebrovascular accident, heart arrest, pulmonary embolism, pulmonary hypertension, QT prolongation, ventricular tachycardia (including torsade de pointes) (postmarketing).

Fluvoxamine – Angina pectoris, bradycardia, cardiomyopathy, cardiovascular disease, cold extremities, conduction delay, heart failure, MI, pallor, pulse irregular, ST segment changes (0.1% to 1%); AV block, cerebrovascular accident, coronary artery disease, embolus, pericarditis, phlebitis, pulmonary infarction, supraventricular extrasystoles (less than 0.1%); ventricular tachycardia (including torsade de pointes) (postmarketing).

Paroxetine and paroxetine CR – Bradycardia, hematoma, hypotension, supraventricular tachycardia, syncope (0.1% to 1%); angina pectoris, arrhythmia nodal, atrial fibrillation, bundle branch block, cardiospasm, cerebral ischemia, cerebrovascular accident, CHF, heart block, low cardiac output, MI, myocardial ischemia, pallor, phlebitis, pulmonary embolus, supraventricular/ventricular extrasystoles, thrombophlebitis, thrombosis, vascular headache (less than 0.1%); pulmonary hypertension, ventricular fibrillation, ventricular tachycardia (including torsade de pointes) (postmarketing).

Sertraline – Edema (dependent, general, periorbital, peripheral), hypotension, peripheral ischemia, postural dizziness (0.1% to 1%); aggravated hypertension, cerebrovascular disorder, MI, precordial/substernal chest pain (less than 0.1%); atrial arrhythmias, AV block, bradycardia, pulmonary hypertension, QT prolongation, ventricular tachycardia (including torsade de pointes-type arrhythmias) (postmarketing).

➤*CNS:*

Citalopram – Aggravated depression, increased appetite, migraine, suicide attempt (at least 1%); abnormal gait, aggressive reaction, alcohol intolerance, ataxia, delusion, drug dependence, dystonia, euphoria, extrapyramidal disorder, hallucinations, increased libido, involuntary muscle contractions, leg cramps, neuralgia, panic reaction, paranoia, paranoid reaction, psychosis, psychotic depression, rigors (0.1% to 1%); abnormal coordination, catatonic reaction, hyperesthesia, melancholia, ptosis, stupor (less than 0.1%); choreoathetosis; delirium; dyskinesia; neuroleptic malignant syndrome; serotonin syndrome; withdrawal syndrome; grand mal convulsions (postmarketing).

Escitalopram – Irritability, lethargy, lightheaded feeling, migraine (at least 1%); aggravated depression, aggravated restlessness, anxiety attack, auditory hallucination, bruxism, carbohydrate craving, carpal tunnel syndrome, coordination abnormal, crying abnormal, disorientation, dysequilibrium, excitability, faintness, feeling unreal, forgetfulness, hyperreflexia, jitteriness, panic reaction, restless legs, shaking, sluggishness, suicidal tendency, suicide attempt, tics, tremulousness nervous (0.1% to 1%); abnormal gait, aggression, dystonia, extrapyramidal disorders, grand mal seizures (or convulsions), neuroleptic malignant syndrome, seizures, serotonin syndrome, visual hallucinations (postmarketing).

Fluoxetine – Abnormal gait, acute brain syndrome, akathisia, apathy, ataxia, buccoglossal syndrome, CNS depression, euphoria, hallucinations, hostility, hyperkinesia, incoordination, increased libido, neuralgia, neuropathy, neurosis, paranoid reaction, personality disorder, psychosis, vertigo (0.1% to 1%); abnormal EEG, antisocial reaction, circumoral paresthesia, coma, delusions, dysarthria, dystonia, extrapyramidal syndrome, foot drop, hyperesthesia, neuritis, paralysis, reflexes decreased/increased, stupor, (less than 0.1%); confusion, dyskinesia, movement disorders, neuroleptic malignant syndrome-like events, suicidal ideation, violent behaviors, serotonin syndrome (postmarketing).

Fluvoxamine – Agoraphobia, akathisia, ataxia, CNS depression, convulsion, delirium, delusion, drug dependence, dyskinesia, dystonia, euphoria, extrapyramidal syndrome, gait unsteady, hallucinations, hemiplegia, hostility, hypersomnia, hypochondriasis, hypotonia, hysteria, incoordination, increased salivation, increased libido, neuralgia, paralysis, paranoid reaction, phobia, psychosis, stupor, twitching (0.1% to 1%); akinesia, coma, fibrillations, mutism, obsessions, reflexes decreased, slurred speech, tardive dyskinesia, torticollis, trismus, withdrawal syndrome (less than 0.1%); neuropathy, serotonin syndrome (postmarketing).

Paroxetine and paroxetine CR – Alcohol abuse, ataxia, dyskinesia, dystonia, euphoria, hallucinations, hostility, incoordination, increased libido, lack of emotion, manic reaction, migraine, neuralgia, neurosis, neuropathy, paralysis, paranoid reaction (0.1% to 1%); abnormal gait, akinesia, antisocial reaction, aphasia, choreoathetosis, circumoral paresthesias, coma, convulsion, delirium, delusions, diplopia, drug dependence, dysarthria, extrapyramidal syndrome, fasciculations, grand mal convulsion, hostility, hyperalgesia, hysteria, manic-depressive reaction, meningitis, myelitis, nystagmus, peripheral neuritis, psychosis, psychotic depression, reflexes decreased/increased, stupor, torticollis, trismus, withdrawal syndrome (less than 0.1%); akathisia; irritability; meningitis; myelitis; peripheral neuritis; psychosis; psychotic depression; reflexes decreased; reflexes increased; stupor; extrapyramidal symptoms (which have included akathisia, bradykinesia, cogwheel rigidity, dystonia, and hypertonia), Guillain-Barre syndrome, neuroleptic malignant syndrome-like events, serotonin syndrome associated in some cases with concomitant use of serotonergic drugs and with drugs that may have impaired paroxetine metabolism (symptoms included agitation, confusion, diaphoresis, hallucinations, hyperreflexia, myoclonus, shivering, tachycardia, and tremor), status epilepticus, tremor (postmarketing).

Sertraline – Abnormal coordination, abnormal gait, aggravated depression, aggressive reaction, ataxia, delusion, euphoria, hallucination, hyperesthesia, leg cramps, migraine, nystagmus, paranoid reaction, paroniria (0.1% to 1%); choreoarthrosis, coma, dyskinesia, dysphonia, hyporeflexia, hypotonia, illusion, libido increased, ptosis, somnambulism, suicidal ideation, withdrawal syndrome (less than 0.1%); extrapyramidal symptoms, neuroleptic malignant syndrome-like events, psychosis, serotonin syndrome (postmarketing).

➤*Dermatologic:*

Citalopram – Alopecia, dermatitis, dry skin, eczema, photosensitivity reaction, psoriasis, skin discoloration, urticaria (0.1% to 1%); cellulitis, decreased sweating, hypertrichosis, keratitis, melanosis, pruritus ani (less than 0.1%); angioedema, epidermal necrolysis, erythema multiforme (postmarketing).

Escitalopram – Alopecia, dermatitis, dry lips, dry skin, eczema, folliculitis, furunculosis, lipoma, skin nodule (0.1% to 1%); toxic epidermal necrolysis (postmarketing).

Fluoxetine – Alopecia, contact dermatitis, eczema, maculopapular rash, skin discoloration, skin ulcer, vesiculobullous rash (0.1% to 1%); furunculosis, herpes zoster, hirsutism, petechial rash, photosensitivity, psoriasis, purpuric rash, pustular rash, seborrhea (less than 0.1%); epidermal necrolysis, erythema nodosum, exfoliative dermatitis, Stevens-Johnson syndrome (postmarketing).

Fluvoxamine – Alopecia, dry skin, eczema, exfoliative dermatitis, furunculosis, photosensitivity, seborrhea, skin discoloration, urticaria (0.1% to 1%); bullous eruption, Henoch-Schöenlein purpura, Stevens Johnson syndrome, toxic epidermal necrolysis, porphyria (postmarketing).

Paroxetine and paroxetine CR – Acne, alopecia, contact dermatitis, dry skin, ecchymosis, eczema, herpes simplex, photosensitivity, urticaria (0.1% to 1%); angioedema, erythema multiforme, erythema nodosum, exfoliative dermatitis, fungal dermatitis, furunculosis, herpes zoster, hirsutism, maculopapular rash, pustular rash, seborrhea, skin discoloration, skin hypertrophy, skin ulcer, vesiculobullous rash, ecchymosis, skin hypertrophy, sweating decreased (less than 0.1%); toxic epidermal necrolysis (postmarketing).

Sertraline – Alopecia, cold clammy skin, dry skin, erythematous rash, maculopapular rash, photosensitivity, urticaria (0.1% to 1%); bullous eruption, contact dermatitis, dermatitis, eczema, hypertrichosis, follicular rash, pustular rash, skin discoloration (less than 0.1%); severe skin reactions that potentially can be fatal, such as Stevens-Johnson syndrome, vasculitis, photosensitivity, and other severe cutaneous disorders (postmarketing).

➤*GI:*

Citalopram – Increased saliva (at least 1%); eructation, esophagitis, gastritis, gingivitis, hemorrhoids, stomatitis, teeth grinding, thirst (0.1% to 1%); cholecystitis, cholelithiasis, colitis, diverticulitis, duodenal ulcer, gastric ulcer, gastroesophageal reflux, glossitis, hiccoughs, jaundice, rectal hemorrhage (less than 0.1%); GI hemorrhage, pancreatitis (postmarketing).

Escitalopram – Abdominal cramp, heartburn (at least 1%); abdominal discomfort, belching, bloating, gagging, gastritis, gastroesophageal reflux, hemorrhoids, increased stool frequency, polyposis gastric, swallowing difficulty (0.1% to 1%); GI hemorrhage, pancreatitis (postmarketing).

Fluoxetine – Abnormal liver function tests, aphthous stomatitis, cholelithiasis, colitis, eructation, esophagitis, gastritis, glossitis, gum hemorrhage, hyperchlorhydria, increased salivation, melena, mouth ulceration, stomach ulcer/hemorrhage, stomatitis, thirst (0.1% to 1%); biliary pain, bloody diarrhea, cholecystitis, duodenal ulcer, enteritis, esophageal ulcer, fecal incontinence, GI hemorrhage, hematemesis, hemorrhage of colon, hepatitis, intestinal obstruction, liver fatty deposit, pancreatitis, peptic ulcer, rectal hemorrhage, salivary gland enlargement, tongue edema (less than 0.1%).

Fluvoxamine – Colitis, eructation, esophagitis, gastritis, GI hemorrhage, GI ulcer, gingivitis, glossitis, hemorrhoids, melena, rectal hemorrhage, stomatitis (0.1% to 1%); biliary pain, cholecystitis, cholelithiasis, fecal incontinence, hematemesis, intestinal obstruction, jaundice (less than 0.1%).

Paroxetine and paroxetine CR – Abnormal liver function tests, bruxism, colitis, dysphagia, eructation, gastritis, gastroesophageal reflux, gingivitis, glossitis, hemorrhoids, increased salivation, pancreatitis, rectal hemorrhage, ulcerative stomatitis (0.1% to 1%); aphthous stomatitis, bloody diarrhea, bulimia, cholelithiasis, duodenitis, enteritis, esophagitis, fecal impaction/incontinence, gum hemorrhage/hyperplasia, hematemesis, hepatitis, hepatosplenomegaly, ileitis, ileus, intestinal obstruction, jaundice, melena, mouth ulceration, peptic ulcer, salivary gland enlargement, stomach ulcer, stomatitis, throat tightness, tongue discoloration, tongue edema, sialadenitis (less than 0.1%).

Sertraline – Eructation, esophagitis, increased saliva, teeth grinding, (0.1% to 1%); aphthous stomatitis, colitis, diverticulitis, fecal incontinence, gastritis, glossitis, gum hyperplasia, hemorrhagic peptic ulcer, hiccough, melena, proctitis, rectal hemorrhage, stomatitis, tenesmus, tongue edema/ulceration, ulcerative stomatitis (less than 0.1%).

➤*GU:*

Citalopram – Dysmenorrhea (3%); amenorrhea, polyuria (at least 1%); breast enlargement, breast pain, dysuria, galactorrhea, micturition frequency, urinary incontinence, vaginal hemorrhage (0.1% to 1%); facial edema, hematuria, oliguria, pyelonephritis, renal calculus, renal pain (less than 0.1%); priapism, spontaneous abortion, acute renal failure (postmarketing).

Escitalopram – Menstrual cramps (at least 1%); blood in urine, breast neoplasm, dysuria, kidney stone, menorrhagia, pelvic inflammation, premenstrual syndrome, spotting between menses, urinary urgency (0.1% to 1%); acute renal failure (postmarketing).

Fluoxetine – Abortion, albuminuria, amenorrhea, breast enlargement, breast pain, cystitis, dysuria, female lactation, fibrocystic breast, hematuria, leukorrhea, menorrhagia, metrorrhagia, nocturia, polyuria, urinary incontinence/urgency, vaginal hemorrhage (0.1% to 1%); breast engorgement, hypomenorrhea, glycosuria, kidney pain, oliguria, priapism, uterine fibroids enlarged, uterine hemorrhage (less than 0.1%); gynecomastia, kidney failure, priapism, vaginal bleeding after drug withdrawal (postmarketing).

Fluvoxamine – Anuria, breast pain, cystitis, delayed menstruation, dysuria, female lactation, hematuria, menopause, menorrhagia, metrorrhagia, nocturia, polyuria, premenstrual syndrome, urinary incontinence/urgency, urination impaired, vaginal hemorrhage, vaginitis (0.1% to 1%); hematospermia, kidney calculus, oliguria (less than 0.1%); priapism (postmarketing).

Paroxetine and paroxetine CR – Dysmenorrhea (at least 1%); albuminuria, amenorrhea, breast pain, cystitis, dysuria, hematuria, menorrhagia, nocturia, polyuria, prostate disorder, prostatitis, pyuria, urinary incontinence/retention/urgency, vaginitis (0.1% to 1%); abortion, breast atrophy/enlargement/neoplasm, ejaculatory disturbance, endometrial disorder; epididymitis, female lactation, fibrocystic breast, kidney calculus, kidney pain, leukorrhea, mastitis, metrorrhagia, nephritis, oliguria, pregnancy and puerperal disorders, salpingitis, urethritis, urinary casts, urolith, uterine fibroids enlarged, uterine spasm, urethritis, vaginal hemorrhage, vaginal moniliasis (less than 0.1%); acute renal failure, priapism (postmarketing).

Sertraline – Amenorrhea, dysmenorrhea, dysuria, intermenstrual bleeding, leukorrhea, nocturia, polyuria, urinary incontinence, vaginal hemorrhage (0.1% to 1%); acute female mastitis, atrophic vaginitis, balanoposthitis, breast enlargement, cystitis, female breast pain, gynecomastia, hematuria, libido increased, menorrhagia, oliguria, priapism, pyelonephritis, renal pain, strangury (less than 0.1%); acute renal failure (postmarketing).

➤*Musculoskeletal:*

Citalopram – Arthritis, muscle weakness, skeletal pain (0.1% to 1%); bursitis, osteoporosis (less than 0.1%).

Escitalopram – Neck/Shoulder pain (3%); arthritis, arthropathy, back discomfort, jaw pain, jaw stiffness, joint stiffness, muscle contractions involuntary, muscle cramp, muscle stiffness, muscle weakness, muscular tone increased (0.1% to 1%).

Fluoxetine – Arthritis, bone pain, bursitis, leg cramps, tenosynovitis (0.1% to 1%); arthrosis, chondrodystrophy, myositis, osteomyelitis, osteoporosis, rheumatoid arthritis (less than 0.1%).

Fluvoxamine – Arthritis, bursitis, generalized muscle spasm, tendinous contracture, tenosynovitis (0.1% to 1%); arthrosis, pathological fracture (less than 0.1%).

Paroxetine and paroxetine CR – Arthritis, arthrosis, tendonitis (0.1% to 1%); bursitis, generalized spasm, myositis, osteoporosis, tenosynovitis, tetany (less than 0.1%).

Sertraline – Arthrosis, dystonia, muscle cramps/weakness (0.1% to 1%).

➤*Respiratory:*

Citalopram – Pneumonia (0.1% to 1%); asthma, bronchospasm, laryngitis, pneumonitis, sputum increased (less than 0.1%).

Escitalopram – Nasal congestion, sinus congestion, sinus headache (at least 1%); asthma, breath shortness, laryngitis, pneumonia, tracheitis (0.1% to 1%).

Fluoxetine – Asthma, epistaxis, hiccoughs, hyperventilation (0.1% to 1%); apnea, atelectasis, cough decreased, emphysema, hemoptysis, hypoventilation, hypoxia, laryngeal edema, lung edema, pneumothorax, stridor (less than 0.1%); eosinophilic pneumonia (postmarketing).

Fluvoxamine – Asthma, epistaxis, hoarseness, hyperventilation (0.1% to 1%); apnea, congestion of upper airway, hemoptysis, hiccoughs, laryngismus, obstructive pulmonary disease, pneumonia (less than 0.1%).

Paroxetine and paroxetine CR – Asthma, epistaxis, hyperventilation, laryngitis, pneumonia, respiratory flu (0.1% to 1%); dysphonia; emphysema, hemoptysis, hiccoughs, lung fibrosis, pulmonary edema, sputum increased, stridor, voice alterations (less than 0.1%).

Sertraline – Bronchospasm, epistaxis (0.1% to 1%); apnea, bradypnea, hemoptysis, hyperventilation, hypoventilation, laryngismus, laryngitis, stridor (less than 0.1%).

➤*Special senses:*

Citalopram – Conjunctivitis, dry eyes, eye pain (0.1% to 1%); abnormal lacrimation, cataract, diplopia, mydriasis, photophobia, taste loss (less than 0.1%); nystagmus (postmarketing).

Escitalopram – Conjunctivitis, dry eyes, earache, eye infection, eye irritation, metallic taste, pupils dilated, vision abnormal, visual disturbance (0.1% to 1%); diplopia (postmarketing).

Fluoxetine – Ear pain (at least 1%); conjunctivitis, dry eyes, mydriasis, photophobia (0.1% to 1%); blepharitis, deafness, diplopia, exophthalmos, eye hemorrhage, glaucoma, hyperacusis, iritis, parosmia, scleritis, strabismus, taste loss, visual field defect (less than 0.1%); cataract, optic neuritis (postmarketing).

Fluvoxamine – Abnormal accommodation, conjunctivitis, deafness, diplopia, dry eyes, ear pain, eye pain, mydriasis, otitis media, parosmia, photophobia, taste loss, visual field defect (0.1% to 1%); corneal ulcer, retinal detachment (less than 0.1%).

Paroxetine and paroxetine CR – Abnormal accommodation, conjunctivitis, ear ache/pain, eye pain, keratoconjunctivitis, mydriasis, otitis media, (0.1% to 1%); amblyopia, anisocoria, blepharitis, cataract, conjunctival edema, corneal ulcer, deafness, exophthalmos, eye hemorrhage, glaucoma, hyperacusis, night blindness, otitis externa, parosmia, photophobia, ptosis, retinal hemorrhage, taste loss, visual field defect (less than 0.1%).

Sertraline – Abnormal accommodation, conjunctivitis, earache, eye pain, mydriasis (0.1% to 1%); abnormal lacrimation, diplopia, exophthalmos, glaucoma, hyperacusis, labyrinthine disorder, photophobia, scotoma, visual field defect, xerophthalmia (less than 0.1%) blindness, optic neuritis, cataract (postmarketing).

➤*Miscellaneous:*

Citalopram – Abnormal glucose tolerance, anemia, epistaxis, increased alkaline phosphatase, increased hepatic enzymes, leukocytosis, leukopenia, lymphadenopathy, purpura (0.1% to 1%); bilirubinemia, coagulation disorder, dehydration, gingival bleeding, goiter, granulocytopenia, gynecomastia, hayfever; hepatitis, hypochromic anemia, hypoglycemia, hypokalemia, hypothyroidism, lymphocytosis, lymphopenia, obesity (less than 0.1%);akathisia, allergic reaction, anaphylaxis, ecchymosis, hemolytic anemia, hepatic necrosis, myoclonus, prolactinemia, prothrombin decreased, rhabdomyolysis, thrombocytopenia, thrombosis (postmarketing).

Escitalopram – Lethargy (3%); pain in limb (at least 1%); anaphylaxis, anemia, bilirubin increased, bruise, edema of extremities, fall, gout, hematoma, hepatic enzymes increased, hypercholesterolemia, hyperglycemia, leg pain, lymphadenopathy cervical, nosebleed, thirst, tightness of chest (0.1% to 1%); angioedema, hepatitis, rhabdomyolysis, SIADH, thrombocytopenia (postmarketing).

Fluoxetine – Anemia, dehydration, ecchymosis, facial edema, generalized edema, gout, hypercholesterolemia, hyperlipemia, hypokalemia, hypothyroidism, intentional overdose, pelvic pain, peripheral edema; suicide attempt (0.1% to 1%); abdominal syndrome acute, alcohol intolerance, alkaline phosphatase increased, ALT increased, blood dyscrasia, BUN increased, creatine phosphokinase increased, diabetic acidosis, diabetes mellitus, hyperkalemia, hyperuricemia, hypocalcemia, hypochromic anemia, hypothermia, intentional injury, iron deficiency anemia, leukopenia, lymphedema, lymphocytosis, neuroleptic malignant syndrome, petechiae, purpura, thrombocythemia, thrombocytopenia (less than 0.1%); aplastic anemia, cholestatic jaundice, hepatic failure/necrosis, hyperprolactinemia, immune-related hemolytic anemia, misuse/abuse, pancreatitis, pancytopenia, sudden unexpected death, thrombocytopenic purpura, hypoglycemia (postmarketing).

Fluvoxamine – Increased liver transaminase (at least 1%); anemia, dehydration, ecchymosis, hypercholesterolemia, hypothyroidism, leukocytosis, lymphadenopathy, neck pain/rigidity, overdose, suicide attempt, thrombocytopenia (0.1% to 1%); cyst, diabetes mellitus, goiter, hyperglycemia, hyperlipidemia, hypoglycemia, hypokalemia, lactate dehydrogenase increased, leukopenia, pelvic pain, purpura, sudden death (less than 0.1%); acute renal failure, agranulocytosis, anaphylactic reaction, aplastic anemia, hepatitis, hyponatremia, ileus, laryngismus, pancreatitis, vasculitis, angioedema (postmarketing).

Paroxetine and paroxetine CR – Trauma (6%); infection (5% to 6%); pain (at least 1%); anemia, AST/ALT increased, facial edema, flu syndrome, leukopenia, lymphadenopathy, moniliasis, neck pain, purpura, peripheral edema, thirst (0.1% to 1%); abnormal erythrocytes, abnormal lymphocytes, abscess, adrenergic syndrome, anisocytosis, anticholinergic syndrome, basophilia, bilirubinemia, bleeding time increased, BUN increased, cellulitis, creatine phosphokinase increased, dehydration, diabetes mellitus, eosinophilia, goiter, gout, hypercalcemia, hypercholesterolemia, hyperglycemia, hyperkalemia, hyperphosphatemia, hyperthyroidism, hypocalcemia, hypochromic anemia, hypoglycemia, hypokalemia, hyponatremia, hypothermia, hypothyroidism, increased alkaline phosphatase, increased lactic dehydrogenase, increased gamma globulins, iron deficiency anemia, ketosis, leukocytosis, lymphedema, lymphocytosis, lymphopenia, microcytic/normocytic anemia, monocytosis, neck rigidity, non-protein nitrogen increased, obesity, pelvic pain, peritonitis, sepsis, thrombocythemia, thrombocytopenia, thyroiditis, ulcer, varicose vein (less than 0.1%); acute pancreatitis, allergic alveolitis, anaphylaxis, elevated liver function tests (the most severe cases were deaths because of liver necrosis and grossly elevated transaminases associated with severe liver dysfunction), events related to impaired hematopoiesis (including aplastic anemia, pancytopenia, bone marrow aplasia, and agranulocytosis), hemolytic anemia, laryngismus, myopathy, oculogyric crisis which has been associated with concomitant use of pimozide, optic neuritis, porphyria, symptoms suggestive of prolactinemia and galactorrhea, syndrome of inappropriate ADH secretion, vasculitis syndromes (such as Henoch-Schönlein purpura) (postmarketing).

Sertraline – Thirst (0.1% to 1%); abnormal hepatic function, anemia, anterior chamber eye hemorrhage, facial edema, hypoglycemia, pallor, rigors (less than 0.1%); anaphylactoid reaction, angioedema, agranulocytosis, aplastic anemia, galactorrhea, hyperglycemia, hyperprolactinemia, hypothyroidism, increased coagulation time, leukopenia; lupus-like syndrome, oculogyric crisis, pancreatitis, pancytopenia, serum sickness, thrombocytopenia, liver events including elevated enzymes, increased bilirubin, hepatomegaly, hepatitis, jaundice, abdominal pain, vomiting, liver failure, and death (postmarketing).

➤*Lab test abnormalities:*

Sertraline – Asymptomatic elevations in serum transaminases (AST or ALT) have occurred infrequently (approximately 0.8%) in association with sertraline administration. These hepatic enzyme elevations usually occurred within the first 1 to 9 weeks of drug treatment and promptly diminished upon drug discontinuation.

Sertraline therapy was associated with small mean increases in total cholesterol (approximately 3%) and triglycerides (approximately 5%) and a small mean decrease in serum uric acid (approximately 7%) of no apparent clinical importance.

Overdosage

➤*Symptoms:*

Citalopram – Although there were no reports of fatal citalopram overdose in clinical trials involving overdoses of up to 2,000 mg, postmarketing reports of drug overdoses involving citalopram have included 12 fatalities, 10 in combination with other drugs and/or alcohol, and 2 with citalopram alone (2,800 and 3,920 mg), as well as nonfatal overdoses of up to 6,000 mg. Symptoms most often accompanying citalopram overdose, alone or in combination with other drugs or alcohol, included dizziness, nausea, sinus tachycardia, somnolence, sweating, tremor, and vomiting. In more rare cases, observed symptoms included amnesia, coma, confusion, convulsions, cyanosis, hyperventilation, rhabdomyolysis, and ECG changes (including nodal rhythm, QT_c prolongation, ventricular arrhythmia, and 1 possible case of torsade de pointes).

Escitalopram – There have been reports of escitalopram overdose involving doses of up to 600 mg. All patients recovered and no symptoms associated with the overdoses were reported.

Fluoxetine – Of the 1578 cases of overdose involving fluoxetine, alone or with other drugs, there were 195 deaths. Among 633 adult patients who overdosed on fluoxetine alone, 34 resulted in a fatal outcome, 378 completely recovered, and 15 patients experienced sequelae after overdosage, including abnormal accommodation, abnormal gait, confusion, unresponsiveness, nervousness, pulmonary dysfunction, vertigo, tremor, elevated blood pressure, impotence, movement disorder, and hypomania. The remaining 206 patients had an unknown outcome. The most common signs and symptoms associated with nonfatal overdosage were seizures, somnolence, nausea, tachycardia, and vomiting. The largest known ingestion of fluoxetine in adult patients was 8 g in a patient who took fluoxetine alone and who subsequently recovered. However, in an adult patient who took fluoxetine alone, an ingestion as low as 520 mg has been associated with lethal outcome, but causality has not been established.

Among pediatric patients (3 months to 17 years of age), there were 156 cases of overdose involving fluoxetine alone or in combination with other drugs. Six patients died, 127 patients completely recovered, 1 patient experienced renal failure, and 22 patients had an unknown outcome. One of the 6 fatalities was a boy 9 years of age who had a history of OCD, Tourette syndrome with tics, attention deficit disorder, and fetal alcohol syndrome. He had been receiving 100 mg fluoxetine daily for 6 months in addition to clonidine, methylphenidate, and promethazine. Mixed-drug ingestion or other methods of suicide complicated all 6 overdoses in children that resulted in fatalities. The largest ingestion in a pediatric patient was 3 g, which was nonlethal.

Other important adverse events reported with fluoxetine overdose (single or multiple drugs) include coma, delirium, ECG abnormalities (such as QT interval prolongation and ventricular tachycardia, including torsade de pointes-type arrhythmias), hypotension, mania, neuroleptic malignant syndrome-like events, pyrexia, stupor, and syncope.

Fluvoxamine – Of the 462 cases of deliberate or accidental overdose involving fluvoxamine, there were 44 deaths. Of these, 6 were in patients taking fluvoxamine alone and the remaining 38 were in patients taking fluvoxamine along with other drugs. Among nonfatal overdose cases, 373 patients had complete recovery; 4 patients experienced adverse sequelae of overdosage, including persistent mydriasis, unsteady gait, kidney complications (from trauma associated with overdose), and bowel infarction requiring a hemicolectomy. In the remaining 41 patients, the outcome was unknown. The largest known ingestion of fluvoxamine involved 12,000 mg (equivalent of 2 to 3 months' dosage). The patient fully recovered. However, ingestion as low as 1,400 mg have been associated with lethal outcome, indicating considerable prognostic variability.

Commonly (at least 5%) observed adverse events associated with fluvoxamine overdose include coma, hypokalemia, hypotension, nausea, respiratory difficulties, somnolence, tachycardia, and vomiting. Other notable signs and symptoms seen with fluvoxamine overdose (single or multiple drugs) included bradycardia, ECG abnormalities (such as heart arrest, QT interval prolongation, first-degree atrioventricular block, bundle branch block, and junctional rhythm), convulsions, tremor, diarrhea, and increased reflexes.

Paroxetine – Since the introduction of paroxetine in the United States, 342 spontaneous cases of deliberate or accidental overdosage during paroxetine treatment have been reported worldwide. These include overdoses with paroxetine alone and in combination with other substances. Of these, 48 cases were fatal and of the fatalities, 17 appeared to involve paroxetine alone. Eight fatal cases that documented the amount of paroxetine ingested were generally confounded by the ingestion of other drugs or alcohol or the presence of significant comorbid conditions. Of 145 nonfatal cases with known outcome, most recovered without sequelae. The largest known ingestion involved 2,000 mg paroxetine (33 times the maximum recommended daily dose) in a patient who recovered. Commonly reported adverse events associated with paroxetine overdosage include coma, confusion, dizziness, nausea, somnolence, tachycardia, tremor, and vomiting. Other notable signs and symptoms observed with overdoses involving paroxetine (alone or with other substances) include acute renal failure, aggressive reactions, bradycardia, convulsions (including status epilepticus), dystonia, hypertension, hypotension, manic reactions, mydriasis, myoclonus, rhabdomyolysis, serotonin syndrome, stupor, symptoms of hepatic dysfunction (including hepatic failure, hepatic necrosis, jaundice, hepatitis, and hepatic steatosis), syncope, urinary retention, and ventricular dysrhythmias (including torsade de pointes).

Sertraline – Of 1027 cases of overdose involving sertraline worldwide, alone or with other drugs, there were 72 deaths.

Among 634 overdoses in which sertraline was the only drug ingested, 8 resulted in fatal outcome, 75 completely recovered, and 27 patients experienced sequelae after overdosage to include alopecia, decreased libido, diarrhea, ejaculation disorder, fatigue, insomnia, serotonin syndrome, and somnolence. The remaining 524 cases had an unknown outcome. The most common signs and symptoms associated with nonfatal sertraline overdosage were agitation, dizziness, nausea, somnolence, tachycardia, tremor, and vomiting.

The largest known ingestion was 13.5 g in a patient who took sertraline alone and subsequently recovered. However, another patient who took 2.5 g sertraline alone experienced a fatal outcome.

Other important adverse events reported with sertraline overdose (single or multiple drugs) include bradycardia, bundle branch block, coma, convulsions, delirium, hallucinations, hypertension, hypotension, manic reactions, pancreatitis, QT interval prolongation, serotonin syndrome, stupor, and syncope.

➤*Treatment:* There are no specific antidotes. Establish and maintain an airway; ensure adequate oxygenation and ventilation. Activated charcoal, which may be used with sorbitol, may be as or more effective than emesis or lavage.

Monitor cardiac and vital signs along with general symptomatic and supportive measures. SSRI-induced seizures that fail to respond spontaneously may respond to diazepam.

Because of the large volume of distribution of SSRIs, forced diuresis, dialysis, hemoperfusion, and exchange transfusion are unlikely to be of benefit.

Treatment includes usual supportive measures. Refer to General Management of Acute Overdosage.

During overdose management, consider the possibility that multiple medications were ingested. Consider contacting a poison control center for advice.

Patient Information

➤*Hazardous tasks:* Any psychoactive drug may impair judgment, thinking, or motor skills; caution patients about operating hazardous machinery, including automobiles, until they are reasonably certain that the drug treatment does not affect them adversely.

➤*Alcohol:* Although SSRIs have not been shown to increase the impairment of mental and motor skills caused by alcohol, advise patients to avoid alcohol during therapy.

➤*Concomitant medication:* Advise patients to consult their physician or pharmacist before taking concomitant OTC, prescription, or alternative medicinal drugs (see Drug Interactions). Instruct patients to avoid alcohol or other depressant medications.

Caution patients about the concomitant use of SSRIs and NSAIDs, aspirin, or other drugs that affect coagulation because the combined use of psychotropic drugs that interfere with serotonin reuptake and these agents has been associated with an increased risk of bleeding.

➤*Pregnancy or lactation:* Women should notify their physician if they are pregnant, intend to become pregnant, or are breastfeeding.

➤*Rash:* Advise patients to notify their physician if rash, hives, or a related allergic phenomenon develops.

➤*Completing course of therapy:* While patients may notice improvement in 1 to 4 weeks, advise patients to continue therapy as directed.

➤*Photosensitivity:* May cause photosensitivity (sensitivity to sunlight). Instruct patients to avoid prolonged exposure to the sun and other ultraviolet light and to use sunscreens and wear protective clothing until tolerance is determined.

➤*Emergence of adverse reactions:* Encourage patients and their families to be alert to the emergence of akathisia, anxiety, agitation, hostility, hypomania, impulsivity, insomnia, irritability, mania, panic attacks, suicidal ideation, and worsening of depression, especially early during antidepressant treatment. Such symptoms should be reported to the patient's physician, especially if they are severe, abrupt in onset, or were not part of the patient's presenting symptoms.

➤*Controlled-release tablet:* Instruct patients to swallow **paroxetine** CR whole and not to chew or crush.

➤*Citalopram/escitalopram:* Advise patients that **escitalopram** is the active isomer of **citalopram** and that the 2 medications should not be taken concomitantly.

➤*Disulfiram:* Advise patients taking disulfiram not to take concomitant paroxetine oral concentrate because of the alcohol content of the concentrate.

CITALOPRAM HYDROBROMIDE

Rx	**Citalopram Hydrobromide** (Various, eg, Apotex, Caraco, Eon, Ivax, Watson)	**Tablets:** 10 mg (as base)	May contain lactose. In 30s, 100s, 500s, 1,000s, and 5,000s.
Rx	**Celexa** (Forest)		Lactose. (FP 10 mg). Beige, oval. Film-coated. In 100s.
Rx	**Citalopram Hydrobromide** (Various, eg, Apotex, Caraco, Eon, Ivax, Watson)	**Tablets:** 20 mg (as base)	May contain lactose. In 30s, 100s, 500s, 1,000s, 5,000s, and UD 100s.
Rx	**Celexa** (Forest)		Lactose. (F P 20 mg). Pink, oval, scored. Film-coated. In 100s and UD 100s.
Rx	**Citalopram Hydrobromide** (Various, eg, Apotex, Caraco, Eon, Ivax, Watson)	**Tablets:** 40 mg (as base)	May contain lactose. In 30s, 100s, 500s, 1,000s, 5,000s, and UD 100s.
Rx	**Celexa** (Forest)		Lactose. (F P 40 mg). White, oval, scored. Film-coated. In 100s and UD 100s.
Rx	**Citalopram Hydrobromide** (Roxane)	**Solution, oral:** 10 mg (as base) per 5 mL	Sorbitol, parabens. Peppermint flavor. In 240 mL.
Rx	**Celexa** (Forest)		Sorbitol, parabens. Peppermint flavor. In 240 mL.

CITALOPRAM HYDROBROMIDE — ORAL

WARNING

Suicidality in children and adolescents – Antidepressants increased the risk of suicidal thinking and behavior (suicidality) in short-term studies in children and adolescents with major depressive disorder (MDD) and other psychiatric disorders. Anyone considering the use of citalopram or any other antidepressant in a child or adolescent must balance this risk with the clinical need. Closely observe patients who are started on therapy for clinical worsening, suicidality, or unusual changes in behavior. Advise families and caregivers of the need for close observation and communication with the health care provider. Citalopram is not approved for use in pediatric patients.

Pooled analyses of short-term (4- to 16-week), placebo-controlled trials of 9 antidepressant drugs (selective serotonin reuptake inhibitors [SSRIs] and others) in children and adolescents with MDD, obsessive-compulsive disorder (OCD), or other psychiatric disorders (a total of 24 trials involving over 4,400 patients) have revealed a greater risk of adverse reactions representing suicidal thinking or behavior (suicidality) during the first few months of treatment in those receiving antidepressants. The average risk of such reactions in patients receiving antidepressants was 4%, twice the placebo risk of 2%. No suicides occurred in these trials.

Indications

➤*Depression:* For the treatment of depression.

➤*Unlabeled uses:* OCD; panic disorder; premenstrual dysphoric syndrome; generalized anxiety disorder; posttraumatic stress disorder.

Administration and Dosage

➤*Approved by the FDA:* July 24, 1998.

➤*Initial treatment:* 20 mg once daily, in the morning or evening, with or without food, generally with an increase to a dosage of 40 mg/day. Dose increases should usually occur in increments of 20 mg at intervals of no less than 1 week. Although certain patients may require a dosage of 60 mg/day, the only study pertinent to dose response for efficacy did not demonstrate an advantage for the 60 mg/day dosage over the 40 mg/day dosage; doses above 40 mg are therefore not ordinarily recommended.

➤*Maintenance treatment:* Acute episodes of depression require several months or longer of sustained pharmacologic therapy. Systematic evaluation of citalopram in 2 studies has shown that its antidepressant efficacy is maintained for periods of up to 24 weeks following 6 or 8 weeks of initial treatment (32 weeks total). In 1 study, patients were assigned randomly to placebo or to the same dosage of citalopram (20 to 60 mg/day) during maintenance treatment as they had received during the acute stabilization phase, while in the other study, patients were assigned randomly to continuation of citalopram 20 or 40 mg/day or placebo for maintenance treatment. In the latter study, the rates of relapse to depression were similar for the 2 dose groups. Based on these limited data, it is not known whether the dose of citalopram needed to maintain euthymia is identical to the dose needed to induce remission. If adverse reactions are bothersome, a decrease in dosage to 20 mg/day can be considered.

CITALOPRAM HYDROBROMIDE — ORAL

➤*Elderly:* 20 mg/day, with titration to 40 mg/day only for nonresponsive patients.

➤*Hepatic function impairment:* 20 mg/day, with titration to 40 mg/day only for nonresponsive patients.

➤*Renal function impairment:* Use with caution in patients with severe renal impairment.

➤*Treatment discontinuation:* Symptoms associated with discontinuation of citalopram and other SSRIs and serotonin-norepinephrine reuptake inhibitors (SNRIs) such as irritability, agitation, headache, and insomnia have been reported. Monitor patients for these symptoms when discontinuing treatment. A gradual reduction in the dose rather than abrupt cessation is recommended whenever possible. If intolerable symptoms occur following a decrease in the dose or upon discontinuation of treatment, then resuming the previously prescribed dose may be considered. Subsequently, the health care provider may continue decreasing the dose but at a more gradual rate.

➤*Monoamine oxidase inhibitor (MAOI):* At least 14 days should elapse between discontinuation of an MAOI and initiation of citalopram. Allow at least 14 days after stopping citalopram before starting an MAOI.

➤*Storage/Stability:* Store at 25°C (77°F); excursions are permitted to 15° to 30°C (59° to 86°F).

ESCITALOPRAM OXALATE

Rx	**Lexapro** (Forest)	**Tablets:** 5 mg (as base)	Talc. (FL 5). White to off-white. Film-coated. In 100s.
		10 mg (as base)	Talc. (F L 10). White to off-white, scored. Film-coated. In 100s and UD 100s.
		20 mg (as base)	Talc. (F L 20). White to off-white, scored. Film-coated. In 100s and UD 100s.
		Solution, oral: 5 mg (as base) per 5 mL	Sorbitol, parabens. Peppermint flavor. In 240 mL.

ESCITALOPRAM OXALATE — ORAL

For complete prescribing information, refer to the SSRIs group monograph.

WARNING

Suicidality in children and adolescents – Antidepressants increased the risk of suicidal thinking and behavior (suicidality) in short-term studies in children and adolescents with major depressive disorder (MDD) and other psychiatric disorders. Anyone considering the use of escitalopram or any other antidepressant in a child or adolescent must balance this risk with the clinical need. Patients who are started on therapy should be observed closely for clinical worsening, suicidality, or unusual changes in behavior. Families and caregivers should be advised of the need for close observation and communication with the prescriber. Escitalopram is not approved for use in pediatric patients.

Pooled analyses of short-term (4 to 16 weeks) placebo-controlled trials of 9 antidepressant drugs (SSRIs and others) in children and adolescents with MDD, obsessive-compulsive disorder (OCD), or other psychiatric disorders (a total of 24 trials involving over 4,400 patients) have revealed a greater risk of adverse reactions representing suicidal thinking or behavior (suicidality) during the first few months of treatment in those receiving antidepressants. The average risk of such reactions in patients receiving antidepressants was 4%, twice the placebo risk of 2%. No suicides occurred in these trials.

Indications

➤*Generalized anxiety disorder (GAD):* For the treatment of GAD.

➤*Major depressive disorder (MDD):* For the treatment of MDD as defined in the DSM-IV.

➤*Unlabeled uses:* Panic disorder.

Administration and Dosage

➤*Approved by the FDA:* August 14, 2002.

Administer once daily in the morning or evening, with or without food.

➤*GAD:*

Initial therapy – 10 mg once daily. If the dose is increased to 20 mg, this should occur after a minimum of 1 week.

Maintenance therapy – GAD is recognized as a chronic condition. The efficacy of escitalopram in the treatment of GAD beyond 8 weeks has not been systematically studied. The physician who elects to use escitalopram for extended periods should periodically reevaluate the long-term usefulness of the drug for the individual patient.

➤*MDD:*

Initial therapy – 10 mg once daily. A fixed dose trial of escitalopram demonstrated the effectiveness of 10 and 20 mg but failed to demonstrate a greater benefit of 20 mg over 10 mg. If the dose is increased to 20 mg, this should occur after a minimum of 1 week.

Maintenance therapy – Antidepressant efficacy was maintained on 10 or 20 mg/day in clinical trials for periods of up to 36 weeks following 8 weeks of initial treatment. Periodically reassess to determine the need for maintenance treatment.

➤*Elderly/Hepatic function impairment:* 10 mg/day is the recommended dose for most elderly patients and patients with hepatic impairment.

➤*Renal function impairment:* Use with caution in patients with severe renal impairment; no dosage adjustment is necessary for patients with mild or moderate renal impairment.

➤*Pregnancy:* Neonates exposed to escitalopram and other SSRIs or serotonin-norepinephrine reuptake inhibitors (SNRIs) late in the third trimester have developed complications requiring prolonged hospitalization, respiratory support, and tube feeding. When treating pregnant women with escitalopram during the third trimester, the physician should carefully consider the potential risks and benefits of treatment. The physician may consider tapering escitalopram in the third trimester.

➤*Discontinuation of treatment:* Symptoms associated with discontinuation of escitalopram and other SSRIs and SNRIs have been reported. Monitor patients for these symptoms (eg, dysphoric mood, irritability, agitation, dizziness, sensory disturbances, anxiety, confusion, headache, lethargy, emotional lability, hypomania, insomnia) when discontinuing treatment. A gradual reduction in the dose rather than abrupt cessation is recommended whenever possible. If intolerable symptoms occur following a decrease in the dose or upon discontinuation of treatment, consider resuming the previously prescribed dose. Subsequently, the health care provider may continue decreasing the dose at a more gradual rate.

➤*Switching to or from a monoamine oxidase inhibitor (MAOI):* Allow at least 14 days to elapse between discontinuation of an MAOI and initiation of escitalopram therapy. Similarly, allow at least 14 days after stopping escitalopram before starting an MAOI.

➤*Storage/Stability:* Store at 25°C (77°F); excursions permitted to 15° to 30°C (59° to 86°F).

FLUOXETINE HYDROCHLORIDE

Rx	**Fluoxetine HCl** (Various, eg, Geneva, Ivax, Teva)	**Tablets:** 10 mg (as base)	In 30s, 100s, 500s, 1000s, 5000s, and UD 100s.
Rx	**Prozac** (Eli Lilly/Dista)		(PROZAC 10). Green, elliptical, scored. In 30s and 100s.
Rx	**Fluoxetine HCl** (Various, eg, Geneva)	**Tablets:** 20 mg (as base)	In 30s, 100s, and 1000s.
Rx	**Fluoxetine HCl** (Various, eg, Barr, Geneva, Ivax, Mylan, Par, Teva)	**Capsules:** 10 mg (as base)	May contain parabens, EDTA, or lactose. In 100s, 1000s, 2000s, unit of use 30s, and UD 100s.
Rx	**Prozac Pulvules** (Eli Lilly/Dista)		(DISTA 3104 Prozac 10 mg). Green. In 100s, 2000s, and blister card 31s.
Rx	**Sarafem Pulvules** (Warner Chilcott)		(Sarafem 10 mg). Lavender. In blister 28s.
Rx	**Fluoxetine HCl** (Various, eg, Barr, Geneva, Ivax, Par, Teva)	**Capsules:** 20 mg (as base)	May contain parabens, EDTA, or lactose. In 30s, 100s, 1000s, 2000s, and unit of use 30s.
Rx	**Prozac Pulvules** (Eli Lilly/Dista)		(DISTA 3105 Prozac 20 mg). Green/Off-white. In 30s, 100s, 2000s, blister card 31s, and UD 100s.
Rx	**Sarafem Pulvules** (Warner Chilcott)		(Sarafem 20 mg). Pink/Lavender. In blister 28s.
Rx	**Fluoxetine HCl** (Various, eg, Geneva, Teva)	**Capsules:** 40 mg (as base)	In 30s and 100s.
Rx	**Prozac Pulvules** (Eli Lilly/Dista)		(DISTA 3107 Prozac 40 mg). Green/Orange. In 30s.

FLUOXETINE HYDROCHLORIDE

Rx	**Prozac Weekly** (Eli Lilly/Dista)	**Capsules, delayed-release**: 90 mg (as base)	Sucrose, sugar spheres. (Lilly 3004 90 mg). Green/Clear. Enteric-coated pellets. In blister 4s.
Rx	**Fluoxetine HCl** (Various, eg, Alpharma, Apotex, Geneva, Teva)	**Solution, oral**: 20 mg per 5 mL (as base)	May contain alcohol, sucrose. In 120 and 473 mL.
Rx	**Prozac** (Eli Lilly/Dista)		0.23% alcohol, sucrose. Mint flavor. In 120 mL.

FLUOXETINE HYDROCHLORIDE — ORAL

For complete and comparative prescribing information, refer to the SSRIs group monograph.

WARNING

Suicidality in children and adolescents – Antidepressants increased the risk of suicidal thinking and behavior (suicidality) in short-term studies in children and adolescents with major depressive disorder (MDD) and other psychiatric disorders. Anyone considering the use of fluoxetine or any other antidepressant in a child or adolescent must balance this risk with the clinical need. Patients who are started on therapy should be observed closely for clinical worsening, suicidality, or unusual changes in behavior. Families and caregivers should be advised of the need for close observation and communication with the prescriber. Fluoxetine is approved for use in pediatric patients with MDD and obsessive-compulsive disorder (OCD).

Pooled analyses of short-term (4 to 16 weeks) placebo-controlled trials of 9 antidepressant drugs (SSRIs and others) in children and adolescents with MDD, OCD, or other psychiatric disorders (a total of 24 trials involving over 4,400 patients) have revealed a greater risk of adverse reactions representing suicidal thinking or behavior (suicidality) during the first few months of treatment in those receiving antidepressants. The average risk of such reactions in patients receiving antidepressants was 4%, twice the placebo risk of 2%. No suicides occurred in these trials.

Indications

➤*Bulimia nervosa:* For the treatment of binge-eating and vomiting behaviors in patients with moderate to severe bulimia nervosa.

➤*Major depressive disorder:* For the treatment of major depressive disorder as defined in the DSM-IV.

➤*Obsessive-compulsive disorder (OCD):* For the treatment of obsessions and compulsions in patients with OCD, as defined in the DSM-III-R.

➤*Panic disorder:* For the treatment of panic disorder, with or without agoraphobia, as defined in DSM-IV.

➤*Premenstrual dysphoric disorder (PMDD; Sarafem* only): For the treatment of PMDD.

➤*Unlabeled uses:* Posttraumatic stress disorder; Raynaud phenomenon (20 to 60 mg/day); generalized anxiety disorder (20 mg/day); hot flashes (20 mg/day); second-line prophylaxis of migraines (10 to 40 mg/day).

Administration and Dosage

➤*Approved by the FDA:* December 29, 1987.

➤*Bulimia nervosa:*

Initial – 60 mg/day administered in the morning. For some patients, it may be advisable to titrate up to this target dose over several days. Doses above 60 mg/day have not been systematically studied in patients with bulimia.

Maintenance – Patients have been continued on therapy for an additional 52 weeks after an initial 8 weeks of treatment without loss of benefit. Adjust dose to maintain patient on lowest effective dosage. Periodically reassess patients to determine need for continued treatment.

➤*Major depressive disorder:*

Initial –

Adult: 20 mg/day in the morning. Consider a dose increase after several weeks if insufficient clinical improvement is observed. Administer doses above 20 mg/day on a once- (morning) or twice- (eg, morning and noon) daily schedule. Do not exceed a maximum dose of 80 mg/day.

Children (8 to 18 years of age): Initiate treatment with a dose of 10 or 20 mg/day. After 1 week at 10 mg/day, increase the dose to 20 mg/day. However, because of higher plasma levels in lower weight children, the starting and target dose in this group may be 10 mg/day. A dose increase to 20 mg/day may be considered after several weeks if insufficient clinical improvement is observed. The full antidepressant effect may be delayed until 4 weeks of treatment or longer.

Maintenance – Acute episodes of major depression generally require several months or longer of sustained pharmacologic therapy. Whether the dose of antidepressant needed to induce remission is identical to the dose needed to maintain and/or sustain euthymia is unknown.

Weekly dosing – Initiate *Prozac Weekly* 7 days after the last 20 mg daily dose. If satisfactory response is not maintained, consider reestablishing a daily dosing regimen.

➤*OCD:*

Initial –

Adults: 20 mg/day in the morning. Consider a dose increase after several weeks if insufficient clinical improvement is observed. The full therapeutic effect may be delayed until 5 weeks of treatment or longer. Administer doses above 20 mg/day on a once- (morning) or twice- (morning and noon) daily schedule. A dose range of 20 to 60 mg/day is recommended; however, doses of up to 80 mg/day have been well tolerated. Do not exceed 80 mg/day.

Children (8 to 18 years of age): In adolescents and higher weight children, initiate treatment with a dose of 10 mg/day. After 2 weeks, increase the dose to 20 mg/day. Additional dose increases may be considered after several more weeks if insufficient clinical improvement is observed. A dose range of 20 to 60 mg/day is recommended.

In lower weight children, initiate treatment with a dose of 10 mg/day. Additional dose increases may be considered after several more weeks if insufficient clinical improvement is observed. A dose range of 20 to 30 mg/day is recommended. Experience with daily doses greater than 20 mg is very minimal; there is no experience with doses greater than 60 mg.

Maintenance – OCD is a chronic condition, and it is reasonable to consider continuation for a responding patient. Patients have been continued on therapy for an additional 6 months after an initial 13 weeks of treatment without loss of benefit. Adjust dose to maintain patient on lowest effective dosage. Periodically reassess patient to determine need for continued treatment.

➤*Panic disorder:*

Initial – Initiate treatment with a dose of 10 mg/day. After 1 week, increase the dose to 20 mg/day. The most frequently administered dose in the 2 flexible-dose clinical trials was 20 mg/day. A dose increase may be considered after several weeks if no clinical improvement is observed. Fluoxetine doses above 60 mg/day have not been systematically evaluated in patients with panic disorder.

Maintenance – Panic disorder is a chronic condition and it is reasonable to consider continuation for a responding patient. Nevertheless, periodically reassess patients to determine the need for continued treatment.

➤*PMDD (Sarafem* only):

Initial – 20 mg/day given continuously (every day of the menstrual cycle) or intermittently (defined as starting a daily dose 14 days prior to the anticipated onset of menstruation through the first full day of menses and repeating with each new cycle). The dosing regimen should be determined by the physician based on individual patient characteristics. Do not exceed a maximum dose of 80 mg/day.

Maintenance/Continuation treatment – Systematic evaluation has shown that its efficacy is maintained for periods up to 6 months at a dose of 20 mg/day given continuously and up to 3 months at a dose of 20 mg/day given intermittently. Reassess patients periodically to determine the need for continued treatment.

➤*Hepatic function impairment:* Use lower or less frequent dosing.

➤*Special risk patients:* Consider lower or less frequent dosing for elderly patients, patients with concurrent diseases, or those who are taking multiple medications.

➤*Switching to a tricyclic antidepressant (TCA):* Dosage of TCA may need to be reduced, and plasma TCA concentrations may need to be monitored temporarily when fluoxetine is coadministered or has been recently discontinued.

➤*Switching to or from a monoamine oxidase inhibitor (MAOI):* At least 14 days should elapse between discontinuation of an MAOI and initiation of therapy with fluoxetine. In addition, allow at least 5 weeks, perhaps longer, after stopping fluoxetine before starting an MAOI.

➤*Thioridazine:* Do not administer thioridazine with fluoxetine or within a minimum of 5 weeks after fluoxetine has been discontinued.

➤*Storage/Stability:* Store at controlled room temperature, 15° to 30°C (59° to 86°F). Protect from light.

FLUVOXAMINE MALEATE

Rx	**Fluvoxamine Maleate** (Various, eg, Ivax, Mylan)	**Tablets**: 25 mg	In 100s and 500s.
Rx	**Fluvoxamine Maleate** (Various, eg, Ivax, Mylan)	**Tablets**: 50 mg	In 100s, 500s, and 1000s.
Rx	**Fluvoxamine Maleate** (Various, eg, Ivax, Mylan)	**Tablets**: 100 mg	In 100s and 1000s.

FLUVOXAMINE MALEATE — ORAL

For complete and comparative prescribing information, refer to the SSRIs group monograph.

WARNING

Suicidality in children and adolescents – Antidepressants increased the risk of suicidal thinking and behavior (suicidality) in short-term studies in children and adolescents with major depressive disorder (MDD) and other psychiatric disorders. Anyone considering the use of fluvoxamine or any other antidepressant in a child or adolescent must balance this risk with the clinical need. Patients who are started on therapy should be observed closely for clinical worsening, suicidality, or unusual changes in behavior. Families and caregivers should be advised of the need for close observation and communication with the prescriber. Fluvoxamine is not approved for use in pediatric patients except for patients with obsessive-compulsive disorder (OCD).

Pooled analyses of short-term (4 to 16 weeks) placebo-controlled trials of 9 antidepressant drugs (SSRIs and others) in children and adolescents with MDD, OCD, or other psychiatric disorders (a total of 24 trials involving over 4,400 patients) have revealed a greater risk of adverse reactions representing suicidal thinking or behavior (suicidality) during the first few months of treatment in those receiving antidepressants. The average risk of such reactions in patients receiving antidepressants was 4%, twice the placebo risk of 2%. No suicides occurred in these trials.

Indications

➤*Obsessive-compulsive disorder (OCD):* For the treatment of obsessions and compulsions in patients with OCD, as defined in the DSM-III-R.

➤*Unlabeled uses:* Bulimia nervosa; depression; panic disorder; social phobia.

Administration and Dosage

➤*Approved by the FDA:* December 5, 1994.

➤*Adults:*

Initial – 50 mg as a single daily bedtime dose. In trials, patients were titrated within a range of 100 to 300 mg/day. Increase dose in 50 mg increments every 4 to 7 days, as tolerated, until maximum therapeutic benefit is achieved (not to exceed 300 mg/day). It is advisable to give total daily doses greater than 100 mg in 2 divided doses; if doses are unequal, give larger dose at bedtime.

➤*Children (8 to 17 years of age):*

Initial – 25 mg administered as a single daily dose at bedtime. Physicians should consider age and gender differences when dosing pediatric patients. The maximum dose in children up to 11 years of age should not exceed 200 mg/day. Therapeutic effect in female children may be achieved with lower doses. Dose adjustment in adolescents (up to the adult maximum dose of 300 mg) may be indicated to achieve therapeutic benefit. Increase the dose in 25 mg increments every 4 to 7 days as tolerated, until maximum therapeutic benefit is achieved. Divide total daily doses more than 50 mg into 2 doses. If the 2 divided doses are not equal, give the larger dose at bedtime.

➤*Maintenance:* OCD is a chronic condition, although efficacy has not been documented for beyond 10 weeks in controlled trials; it is reasonable to consider continuation for a responding patient. Adjust dose to maintain patient on lowest effective dosage. Periodically reassess patient to determine need for continued treatment.

➤*Elderly / Hepatic function impairment:* Decreased fluvoxamine clearance has been observed in these patients. It may be appropriate to modify initial dose and subsequent dose titration.

➤*Storage / Stability:* Store at controlled room temperature 15° to 30°C (59° to 86°F). Protect from high humidity and dispense in tight, light-resistant containers.

PAROXETINE

Rx	**Paroxetine** (Various, eg, Apotex, Par, Sandoz)	**Tablets**: 10 mg (as hydrochloride)	In 30s, 100s, 1,000s, and UD 100s.
Rx	**Paxil** (GlaxoSmithKline)		(PAXIL 10). Yellow, oval, scored. Film-coated. In 30s.
Rx	**Paroxetine** (Various, eg, Apotex, Par, Sandoz)	**Tablets**: 20 mg (as hydrochloride)	In 30s, 100s, 1,000s, and UD 100s.
Rx	**Paxil** (GlaxoSmithKline)		(PAXIL 20). Pink, oval, scored. Film-coated. In 30s, 100s, and SUP[a] 100s.
Rx	**Paroxetine** (Various, eg, Apotex, Par, Sandoz)	**Tablets**: 30 mg (as hydrochloride)	In 30s, 100s, 1,000s, and UD 100s.
Rx	**Paxil** (GlaxoSmithKline)		(PAXIL 30). Blue, oval. Film-coated. In 30s.
Rx	**Paroxetine** (Various, eg, Apotex, Par, Sandoz)	**Tablets**: 40 mg (as hydrochloride)	In 30s, 100s, 1,000s, and UD 100s.
Rx	**Paxil** (GlaxoSmithKline)		(PAXIL 40). Green, oval. Film-coated. In 30s.
Rx	**Pexeva** (Synthon)	**Tablets**: 10 mg (as mesylate)	(POT 10). White, oval. In 30s.
		20 mg (as mesylate)	(POT 20). Dark orange, oval, scored. In 30s, 100s, and 500s.
		30 mg (as mesylate)	(POT 30). Yellow, oval. In 30s.
		40 mg (as mesylate)	(POT 40). Rose, oval. In 30s.
Rx	**Paxil CR** (GlaxoSmithKline)	**Tablets, controlled-release**: 12.5 mg (as hydrochloride)	Lactose. (Paxil CR 12.5). Yellow. Enteric-coated. In 30s and 100s.
		25 mg (as hydrochloride)	Lactose. (Paxil CR 25). Pink. Enteric-coated. In 30s, 100s, and SUP[a] 100s.
		37.5 mg (as hydrochloride)	Lactose. (Paxil CR 37.5). Blue. Enteric-coated. In 30s.
Rx	**Paxil** (GlaxoSmithKline)	**Suspension, oral**: 10 mg (as hydrochloride) per 5 mL	Parabens, saccharin, sorbitol. Orange flavor. In 250 mL.

[a] SUP = Single unit packages. Intended for institutional use only.

PAROXETINE — ORAL

For complete prescribing information, refer to the SSRIs group monograph.

WARNING

Suicidality in children and adolescents – Antidepressants increased the risk of suicidal thinking and behavior (suicidality) in short-term studies in children and adolescents with major depressive disorder (MDD) and other psychiatric disorders. Anyone considering the use of paroxetine or any other antidepressant in a child or adolescent must balance this risk with the clinical need. Patients who are started on therapy should be observed closely for clinical worsening, suicidality, or unusual changes in behavior. Families and caregivers should be advised of the need for close observation and communication with the prescriber. Paroxetine is not approved for use in pediatric patients.

Pooled analyses of short-term (4 to 16 weeks) placebo-controlled trials of 9 antidepressant drugs (SSRIs and others) in children and adolescents with MDD, obsessive-compulsive disorder (OCD), or other psychiatric disorders (a total of 24 trials involving over 4,400 patients) have revealed a greater risk of adverse reactions representing suicidal thinking or behavior (suicidality) during the first few months of treatment in those receiving antidepressants. The average risk of such reactions in patients receiving antidepressants was 4%, twice the placebo risk of 2%. No suicides occurred in these trials.

Indications

➤*Generalized anxiety disorder (GAD) (immediate-release; except Pexeva)*: For the treatment of generalized anxiety disorder, as defined in the DSM-IV.

➤*Major depressive disorder (immediate- and controlled-release):* For the treatment of major depressive disorder, as defined in the DSM-III or DSM-IV.

➤*Obsessive-compulsive disorder (OCD) (immediate-release):* For the treatment of obsessions and compulsions in patients with OCD, as defined in the DSM-IV.

➤*Panic disorder (immediate- and controlled-release):* For the treatment of panic disorder, with or without agoraphobia, as defined in the DSM-IV.

➤*Posttraumatic stress disorder (PTSD) (immediate-release; except Pexeva)*: For the treatment of PTSD, as defined in the DSM-IV.

➤*Premenstrual dysphoric disorder (PMDD) (controlled-release):* For the treatment of PMDD, as defined in the DSM-IV.

➤*Social anxiety disorder (immediate- and controlled-release; except Pexeva)*: For the treatment of social anxiety disorder, also known as social phobia, as defined in the DSM-IV.

PAROXETINE — ORAL

➤*Unlabeled uses:* Hot flashes (20 mg/day or 12.5 to 25 mg/day controlled release); diabetic neuropathy.

Administration and Dosage

➤*Approved by the FDA:* December 29, 1992.

Swallow controlled-release tablet whole; do not chew or crush.

➤*GAD (immediate-release):*

Initial – 20 mg/day. Administer as a single daily dose with or without food, usually in the morning. Usual range is 20 to 50 mg/day. Change doses in 10 mg/day increments and at intervals of at least 1 week. There is not sufficient evidence to suggest a greater benefit to doses higher than 20 mg/day.

Maintenance – Continued therapy for up to 24 weeks has demonstrated a benefit of such maintenance. GAD is recognized as a chronic condition, and it is reasonable to consider continuation of treatment for a responding patient. Make dosage adjustments to maintain the patient on the lowest effective dosage, and periodically reassess patients to determine the need for continued treatment.

➤*Major depressive disorder:*

Initial –

Immediate-release: 20 mg/day. Administer as a single daily dose with or without food, usually in the morning. Usual range is 20 to 50 mg/day. As with all drugs for the treatment of major depressive disorder, the full effect may be delayed. Some patients not responding to a 20 mg dose may benefit from dose increases in 10 mg/day increments up to a maximum of 50 mg/day. Change doses at intervals of at least 1 week.

Controlled-release: 25 mg/day. Administer as a single daily dose with or without food, usually in the morning. Usual range is 25 to 62.5 mg/day. As with all drugs for the treatment of major depressive disorder, the full effect may be delayed. Some patients not responding to a 25 mg dose may benefit from dose increases in 12.5 mg/day increments up to a maximum of 62.5 mg/day. Change doses at intervals of at least 1 week. Swallow controlled-release tablet whole; do not chew or crush.

Maintenance – There is no body of evidence available concerning the duration of paroxetine therapy. It generally is agreed that acute episodes of major depressive disorder require several months or longer of sustained pharmacologic therapy. Whether the dose needed to induce remission is identical to the dose needed to maintain and/or sustain euthymia is unknown. Efficacy of immediate-release paroxetine has been maintained for periods of up to 1 year with doses that averaged approximately 30 mg, which corresponds to a 37.5 mg dose of controlled-release paroxetine based on relative bioavailability considerations.

➤*OCD (immediate-release):*

Initial – 20 mg/day. Administer as a single daily dose with or without food, usually in the morning. May be increased in 10 mg/day increments. Change doses at intervals of at least 1 week. The recommended dose is 40 mg/day. Usual range is 20 to 60 mg/day. Do not exceed the maximum dosage of 60 mg/day.

Maintenance – Patients have been continued on therapy for 6 months. However, make dosage adjustments to maintain the patient on the lowest effective dosage, and periodically reassess the patient to determine the need for continued treatment. OCD is a chronic condition, and it is reasonable to consider continuation for a responding patient.

➤*Panic disorder:*

Initial –

Immediate-release: 10 mg/day. Administer as a single daily dose with or without food, usually in the morning. May be increased in 10 mg/day increments. The target dose is 40 mg/day. Usual range is 10 to 60 mg/day. Do not exceed the maximum dosage of 60 mg/day. Change doses at intervals of at least 1 week.

Controlled-release: 12.5 mg/day. Administer as a single daily dose with or without food, usually in the morning. Usual range is 12.5 to 75 mg/day. Dose changes should occur in 12.5 mg/day increments. Change doses at intervals of at least 1 week. Do not exceed the maximum dosage of 75 mg/day. Swallow controlled-release tablet whole; do not chew or crush.

Maintenance – Long-term maintenance of efficacy with the immediate-release formulation has been demonstrated in a 3-month relapse prevention trial. In this trial, patients with panic disorder assigned to paroxetine demonstrated a lower relapse rate compared with patients on placebo. Make dosage adjustments to maintain the patient on the lowest effective dosage, and periodically reassess the patient to determine the need for continued treatment. Panic disorder is a chronic condition, and it is reasonable to consider continuation for a responding patient.

➤*PMDD (controlled-release):*

Initial – 12.5 mg/day. Administer as a single daily dose with or without food, usually in the morning. Paroxetine CR may be administered either daily throughout the menstrual cycle or limited to the luteal phase of the menstrual cycle, depending on physician assessment. Usual range is 12.5 to 25 mg/day. Change doses at intervals of at least 1 week. Swallow controlled-release tablet whole; do not chew or crush.

Maintenance – The effectiveness for a period exceeding 3 menstrual cycles has not been systematically evaluated in controlled trials. Women commonly report that symptoms worsen with age until relieved by the onset of menopause. It is reasonable to consider continuation of treatment for a responding patient; periodically reassess patients to determine the need for continued treatment.

➤*PTSD (immediate-release):*

Initial – 20 mg/day. Administer as a single daily dose with or without food, usually in the morning. Usual range is 20 to 50 mg/day. There is not sufficient evidence to suggest a greater benefit for a dose of 40 mg/day compared with 20 mg/day. Change doses, if indicated, in 10 mg/day increments and at intervals of at least 1 week.

Maintenance – Although the efficacy beyond 12 weeks of dosing has not been demonstrated, PTSD is recognized as a chronic condition, and it is reasonable to consider continuation of treatment for a responding patient. Make dosage adjustments to maintain the patient on the lowest effective dosage, and periodically reassess patients to determine the need for continued treatment.

➤*Social anxiety disorder:*

Initial –

Immediate-release: 20 mg/day. Administer as a single daily dose with or without food, usually in the morning. Usual range is 20 to 60 mg/day. Available information does not suggest any additional benefit for doses above 20 mg/day.

Controlled-release: 12.5 mg/day. Administer as a single daily dose with or without food, usually in the morning. Usual range is 12.5 to 37.5 mg/day. If necessary, increase dose at intervals of at least 1 week, in increments of 12.5 mg/day up to a maximum of 37.5 mg/day. Swallow controlled-release tablets whole; do not chew or crush.

Maintenance – Although the efficacy beyond 12 weeks of dosing has not been demonstrated in controlled clinical trials, social anxiety disorder is recognized as a chronic condition, and it is reasonable to consider continuation of treatment for a responding patient. Make dosage adjustments to maintain the patient on the lowest effective dosage, and periodically reassess the patient to determine the need for continued treatment.

➤*Pregnancy:* Neonates exposed to paroxetine and other SSRIs or selective-norepinephrine reuptake inhibitors (SNRIs) late in the third trimester have developed complications requiring prolonged hospitalization, respiratory support, and tube feeding. When treating pregnant women with paroxetine during the third trimester, the physician should carefully consider the potential risks and benefits of treatment. Consider tapering paroxetine in the third trimester.

➤*Elderly or debilitated or patients with severe renal or hepatic impairment:* The recommended initial dose is 10 mg/day (immediate-release) or 12.5 mg/day (controlled-release). Increases may be made if indicated. Do not exceed 40 mg/day (immediate-release) or 50 mg/day (controlled-release).

➤*Switching patients to or from a monoamine oxidase inhibitor (MAOI):* Allow at least 14 days between discontinuation of an MAOI and initiation of paroxetine therapy. Similarly, allow at least 14 days after stopping paroxetine before starting an MAOI.

➤*Discontinuation of treatment:* Symptoms associated with discontinuation of paroxetine have been reported. When discontinuing treatment, monitor for symptoms such as dizziness, sensory disturbances (eg, paresthesias such as electric shock sensations), agitation, anxiety, nausea, and sweating. A gradual reduction in the dose rather than abrupt cessation is recommended whenever possible. If intolerable symptoms occur following a decrease in the dose or upon discontinuation of treatment, then consider resuming the previously prescribed dose. Subsequently, the physician may continue decreasing the dose but at a more gradual rate.

➤*Administration of suspension:* Shake suspension well before using.

➤*Storage / Stability:*

Tablets – Store immediate-release tablets between 15° and 30°C (59° and 86°F) and controlled-release tablets at or below 25°C (77°F).

Suspension – Store at or below 25°C (77°F).

SERTRALINE HYDROCHLORIDE

Rx	**Zoloft** (Pfizer)	**Tablets:** 25 mg (as base)	(ZOLOFT 25 mg). Lt. green, capsule shape, scored. Film-coated. In 50s.
		50 mg (as base)	(ZOLOFT 50 mg). Lt. blue, capsule shape, scored. Film-coated. In 100s, 500s, 5,000s, and UD 100s.
		100 mg (as base)	(ZOLOFT 100 mg). Lt. yellow, capsule shape, scored. Film-coated. In 100s, 500s, 5,000s, and UD 100s.
		Oral concentrate: 20 mg/mL (as base)	12% alcohol, menthol. In 60 mL.[a]

[a] Dropper dispenser contains dry natural rubber.

SERTRALINE HYDROCHLORIDE — ORAL

For complete and comparative prescribing information, refer to the SSRIs group monograph.

WARNING

Suicidality in children and adolescents – Antidepressants increased the risk of suicidal thinking and behavior (suicidality) in short-term studies in children and adolescents with major depressive disorder (MDD) and other psychiatric disorders. Anyone considering the use of sertraline or any other antidepressant in a child or adolescent must balance this risk with the clinical need. Patients who are started on therapy should be observed closely for clinical worsening, suicidality, or unusual changes in behavior. Families and caregivers should be advised of the need for close observation and communication with the prescriber. Sertraline is not approved for use in pediatric patients except for patients with obsessive-compulsive disorder (OCD).

Pooled analyses of short-term (4 to 16 weeks) placebo-controlled trials of 9 antidepressant drugs (SSRIs and others) in children and adolescents with MDD, OCD, or other psychiatric disorders (a total of 24 trials involving over 4,400 patients) have revealed a greater risk of adverse reactions representing suicidal thinking or behavior (suicidality) during the first few months of treatment in those receiving antidepressants. The average risk of such reactions in patients receiving antidepressants was 4%, twice the placebo risk of 2%. No suicides occurred in these trials.

Indications

➤*Major depressive disorder:* For the treatment of major depressive disorder as defined in the DSM-III.

➤*Obsessive-compulsive disorder (OCD):* For the treatment of obsessions and compulsions in patients with OCD, as defined in the DSM-III-R.

➤*Panic disorder:* For the treatment of panic disorder with or without agoraphobia, as defined in the DSM-IV.

➤*Posttraumatic stress disorder (PTSD):* For the treatment of PTSD as defined in the DSM-III-R.

➤*Premenstrual dysphoric disorder (PMDD):* For the treatment of PMDD as defined in the DSM-III-R/IV.

➤*Social anxiety disorder:* For the treatment of social anxiety disorder (social phobia) as defined by DSM-IV.

Administration and Dosage

➤*Approved by the FDA:* December 1991.

Administer sertraline once daily in the morning or evening. Given the 24-hour elimination half-life of sertraline, dose changes should not occur at intervals of less than 1 week.

➤*Major depressive disorder:*

Adults, initial treatment – 50 mg once daily.

Maintenance/Continuation/Extended treatment – It is generally agreed that acute episodes of major depressive disorder require several months or longer of sustained pharmacological therapy. It is not known whether the dose of sertraline needed for maintenance treatment is identical to the dose needed to achieve an initial response. Periodically reassess patients to determine the need for maintenance treatment. Systematic evaluation of sertraline has shown that the antidepressant efficacy is maintained for a period of up to 44 weeks following 8 weeks of initial treatment at doses of 50 to 200 mg/day (mean dose, 70 mg/day).

➤*OCD:*

Adults, initial treatment – 50 mg once daily.

Adults, maintenance/continuation/extended treatment – It is generally agreed that OCD requires several months or longer of sustained pharmacological therapy beyond response to initial treatment. Systematic evaluation of continuing sertraline for periods of up to 28 weeks in patients with OCD and who have responded while taking sertraline during initial treatment phases of 24 to 52 weeks at a dose range of 50 to 200 mg/day has demonstrated a benefit. It is not known whether the dose of sertraline needed for maintenance treatment is identical to the dose needed to achieve an initial response. Nevertheless, periodically reassess patients to determine the need for maintenance treatment.

Children and adolescents – Initiate dosage with 25 mg once daily for children 6 to 12 years of age and 50 mg once daily in adolescents 13 to 17 years of age. While a relationship between dose and effect has not been established for OCD, patients were dosed in a range of 25 to 200 mg/day in trials for children 6 to 17 years of age with OCD. Patients not responding to an initial dose of 25 or 50 mg/day may benefit from dose increases up to a maximum of 200 mg/day. To avoid excess dosing in children with OCD, take into account their generally lower body weights compared with adults when increasing the dose. Given the 24-hour elimination half-life of sertraline, dose changes should not occur at intervals of less than 1 week.

➤*Panic disorder:*

Adults, initial treatment – 25 mg once daily. After 1 week, increase the dose to 50 mg once daily.

Maintenance/Continuation/Extended treatment – It is generally agreed that panic disorder requires several months or longer of sustained pharmacological therapy beyond response to initial treatment. Systematic evaluation of continuing sertraline for periods of up to 28 weeks in patients with panic disorder who have responded while taking sertraline during initial treatment phases of 24 to 52 weeks at a dose range of 50 to 200 mg/day has demonstrated a benefit. It is not known whether the dose of sertraline needed for maintenance treatment is identical to the dose needed to achieve an initial response. Nevertheless, periodically reassess patients to determine the need for maintenance treatment.

➤*PTSD:*

Adults, initial treatment – 25 mg once daily. After 1 week, increase the dose to 50 mg once daily.

Maintenance/Continuation/Extended treatment – It is generally agreed that PTSD requires several months or longer of sustained pharmacological therapy beyond response to initial treatment. Systematic evaluation of sertraline has demonstrated that its efficacy in PTSD is maintained for periods of up to 28 weeks following 24 weeks of treatment at a dose of 50 to 200 mg/day. It is not known whether the dose of sertraline needed for maintenance treatment is identical to the dose needed to achieve an initial response. Periodically reassess patients to determine the need for maintenance treatment.

➤*PMDD:*

Adults, initial treatment – 50 mg/day, either daily throughout the menstrual cycle or limited to the luteal phase of the menstrual cycle, depending on physician assessment.

While a relationship between dose and effect has not been established for PMDD, patients were dosed in the range of 50 to 150 mg/day with dose increases at the onset of each new menstrual cycle. Patients not responding to a 50 mg/day dose may benefit from dose increases (at 50 mg increments per menstrual cycle) up to 150 mg/day when dosing daily throughout the menstrual cycle, or 100 mg/day when dosing during the luteal phase of the menstrual cycle. If a 100 mg/day dose has been established with luteal phase dosing, utilize a 50 mg/day titration step for 3 days at the beginning of each luteal phase dosing period.

Maintenance/Continuation/Extended treatment – The effectiveness of sertraline in long-term use (ie, for more than 3 menstrual cycles) has not been systematically evaluated in controlled trials. However, as women commonly report that symptoms worsen with age until relieved by the onset of menopause, it is reasonable to consider continuation of a responding patient. Dosage adjustments, which may include changes between dosage regimens (eg, daily throughout the menstrual cycle vs during the luteal phase of the menstrual cycle), may be needed to maintain the patient on the lowest effective dosage. Periodically reassess patients to determine the need for continued treatment.

➤*Social anxiety disorder:*

Adults, initial treatment – 25 mg once daily. After 1 week, increase the dose to 50 mg once daily.

Maintenance/Continuation/Extended treatment – Social anxiety disorder is a chronic condition that may require several months or longer of sustained pharmacological therapy beyond response to initial treatment. Systematic evaluation of sertraline has demonstrated that its efficacy in social anxiety disorder is maintained for periods of up to 24 weeks following 20 weeks of treatment at a dose of 50 to 200 mg/day. Make dosage adjustments to maintain patients on the lowest effective dose and periodically reassess patients to determine the need for long-term treatment.

➤*Hepatic function impairment:* Give a lower or less-frequent dosage in patients with hepatic impairment. Use with caution in these patients.

➤*Pregnant women during the third trimester:* Neonates exposed to sertraline and other selective serotonin reuptake inhibitors (SSRIs) or serotonin and norepinephrine reuptake inhibitors (SNRIs) late in the third trimester, have developed complications requiring prolonged hospitalization, respiratory support, and tube feeding. When treating pregnant women with sertraline during the third trimester, carefully consider the potential risks and benefits of treatment. Consider tapering sertraline in the third trimester.

➤*Switching patients to or from a monoamine oxidase inhibitor (MAOI):* At least 14 days should elapse between discontinuation of an MAOI and initiation of therapy with sertraline. In addition, allow at least 14 days after stopping sertraline before starting an MAOI.

➤*Discontinuation of sertraline:* Symptoms associated with discontinuation of sertraline and other SSRIs and SNRIs have been reported. Monitor patients for these symptoms (eg, dysphoric mood, irritability, agitation, dizziness, sensory disturbances, anxiety, confusion, headache, lethargy, emotional lability, insomnia, hypomania) when discontinuing treatment. A gradual reduction in the dose rather than abrupt cessation is recommended whenever possible. If intolerable symptoms occur following a decrease in the dose or upon discontinuation of treatment, then resuming the previously prescribed dose may be considered. Subsequently, the health care provider may continue decreasing the dose but at a more gradual rate.

➤*Oral concentrate:* Dilute prior to use with 4 oz (one-half cup) of water, ginger ale, lemon/lime soda, lemonade, or orange juice only. Do not mix with anything other than the liquids listed. Take the dose immediately after mixing; do not mix in advance. A slight haze may appear after mixing; this is normal. Note: Exercise caution in patients with latex sensitivity as the dropper dispenser contains dry natural rubber.

The oral concentrate is contraindicated with disulfiram because of the alcohol content of the concentrate.

➤*Storage/Stability:* Store at 25°C (77°F); excursions permitted to 15° to 30°C (59° to 86°F).

Indications

➤*Depression:* In general, the MAOIs are indicated in patients with atypical (exogenous) depression and in some patients unresponsive to other antidepressive therapy. They are rarely a drug of first choice.

➤*Unlabeled uses:* MAOIs have shown promise in the treatment of bulimia (having characteristics of atypical depression). Phenelzine has been investigated in the treatment of cocaine addiction; careful supervision is required. Anecdotal cases and small studies indicate beneficial effects of phenelzine in patients with night terrors (30 mg twice daily); posttraumatic stress disorder (60 to 75 mg/day); some migraines resistant to other therapies (15 mg 3 times/day); likewise, with tranylcypromine in Binswanger's encephalopathy (40 mg/day), seasonal affective disorder (≈ 30 mg/day), and subjective symptoms in multiple sclerosis patients (10 to 120 mg/day). MAOIs have also been used in the treatment of panic disorder with associated agoraphobia and globus hystericus syndrome.

Actions

➤*Pharmacology:* Monoamine oxidase is a complex enzyme system, widely distributed throughout the body, which is responsible for the metabolic decomposition of biogenic amines (eg, norepinephrine, epinephrine, dopamine, serotonin). Monoamine oxidase inhibitors (MAOIs) inhibit this enzyme system, causing an increase in the concentration of these endogenous amines.

Two types of MAO enzymes have been identified, MAO-A and MAO-B, which exhibit different preferences for substrates and different sensitivities to inhibitors. MAO-A preferentially de-aminates epinephrine, norepinephrine, and serotonin, while MAO-B metabolizes benzylamine and phenylethylamine. Dopamine and tyramine are metabolized by both isozymes. In neural tissues, this enzyme system regulates the metabolic decomposition of catecholamines and serotonin. Hepatic MAO inactivates circulating monoamines or those that are introduced via the GI tract into portal circulation (eg, tyramine).

Except for selegiline, MAOIs currently in use in the US are nonselective. Selegiline, an MAO-B selective agent, is used therapeutically for the treatment of Parkinson's disease. The nonselective agents are used for their antidepressant effects. All of these agents are irreversible inhibitors of MAO, and therefore, may require up to 2 weeks for normal amine metabolism to be restored following drug discontinuation. Studies have also indicated that chronic therapy with MAOIs causes down-regulation in adrenergic and serotonergic receptors.

Drugs that have MAOI activity cause a wide range of clinical effects and have the potential for serious interactions with other substances. Clinicians and patients should be fully aware of the potential hazards associated with their use.

➤*Pharmacokinetics:*

Absorption/Distribution – Limited information is available on MAOI pharmacokinetics. They appear to be well absorbed following oral administration. Peak levels of tranylcypromine and phenelzine are reached in ≈ 2 and 3 hours, respectively. However, maximal inhibition of MAO occurs within 5 to 10 days.

Metabolism/Excretion – The hydrazine MAOIs (phenelzine, isocarboxazid) are thought to be metabolized with the release of active metabolites. Inactivation is primarily by acetylation. The clinical effects of phenelzine may continue for up to 2 weeks after discontinuation of therapy. Upon withdrawal of tranylcypromine, MAO activity is recovered in 3 to 5 days (possibly up to 10 days). Phenelzine and isocarboxazid are excreted in the urine mostly as metabolites.

Special populations –

"Slow acetylators": Slow acetylation of hydrazine MAOIs may yield exaggerated effects after standard dosing.

Contraindications

Hypersensitivity to these agents; pheochromocytoma; CHF; history of liver disease or abnormal liver function tests; severe impairment of renal function; confirmed or suspected cerebrovascular disorders; cardiovascular disease; hypertension; history of headache; coadministration with other MAOIs; dibenzazepine-related agents including tricyclic antidepressants, carbamazepine, and cyclobenzaprine; bupropion; SSRIs; buspirone; sympathomimetics; meperidine; dextromethorphan; anesthetic agents; CNS depressants; antihypertensives; caffeine; cheese or other foods with high tyramine content (see Warnings and Drug Interactions).

Warnings

➤*Hypertensive crises:* The most serious reactions involve changes in blood pressure; it is inadvisable to use these drugs in elderly or debilitated patients or in the presence of hypertension, cardiovascular or cerebrovascular disease, or coadministered with certain drugs or foods (see Warnings and Drug Interactions).

Hypertensive crises have sometimes been fatal. These crises usually occur within several hours after ingestion of a contraindicated substance and are characterized by some or all of the following symptoms: Occipital headache that may radiate frontally; palpitation; neck stiffness/soreness; nausea; vomiting; sweating (sometimes with fever or cold, clammy skin); dilated pupils; photophobia. Either tachycardia or bradycardia may be present and can be associated with constricting chest pain.

Note – Intracranial bleeding (sometimes fatal) has been reported in association with the paradoxical increase in blood pressure. Monitor blood pressure frequently to detect evidence of any pressor response. Do not rely completely on blood pressure readings, but observe patient frequently.

Discontinue therapy immediately if palpitations or frequent headaches occur. These signs may be prodromal of a hypertensive crisis.

Treatment – If a hypertensive crisis occurs, discontinue these drugs immediately and institute therapy to lower blood pressure. Do not use parenteral reserpine. Headaches tend to abate as blood pressure is lowered. Administer alpha-adrenergic blocking agents such as phentolamine 5 mg IV slowly to avoid producing an excessive hypotensive effect. Manage fever by means of external cooling.

Warning to the patient – Warn all patients against eating foods with high tyramine, dopamine, or tryptophan content (see table) during treatment and for 2 weeks after discontinuing MAOIs. Any high-protein food that is aged or undergoes breakdown by putrefaction process to improve flavor is suspect of being able to produce a hypertensive crisis in patients taking MAOIs. Also warn patients against drinking alcoholic beverages and against self-medication with certain proprietary agents such as cold, hay fever, or weight reduction preparations containing sympathomimetic amines while undergoing therapy. Instruct patients not to consume excessive amounts of caffeine in any form and to report promptly the occurrence of headache or other unusual symptoms.

Tyramine-Containing Foods[a]		
Cheese/Dairy Products		
American	Cheddar[b]	Romano
Blue[b]	Emmenthaler[b]	Roquefort
Boursault[b]	Gruyere	Sour cream
Brie	Mozzarella	Stilton[b]
Camembert[b]	Parmesan	Swiss[b]
		Yogurt
Meat/Fish		
Anchovies	Fermented sausages (bologna, pepperoni, salami, summer sausage)[b]	Meat extracts
Beef or chicken liver,[b] other meats, fish (unrefrigerated, fermented, spoiled, smoked, pickled)	Dried fish (salted herring)	Meats prepared with tenderizer
Caviar	Dry sausage	Herring, pickled, spoiled[b]
	Game meat[b]	Shrimp paste
Alcoholic Beverages (Undistilled)		
Beer (imports, some nonalcoholic)	Red wine (especially Chianti)[b]	Sherry[b]
		Distilled spirits
		Liqueurs
Fruit/Vegetables		
Bananas	Fruit (eg, avocados, especially overripe)	Sauerkraut[b]
Bean curd	Figs, canned (overripe)	Soy sauce
Dried fruits (eg, raisins, prunes)	Miso soup	Yeast extracts (eg, Marmite)[b]
	Raspberries	
Foods Containing Other Vasopressors		
Broad beans (eg, fava beans, overripe) – dopa[b]	Caffeine (eg, coffee, tea, colas)	Chocolate – phenylethylamine
		Ginseng

[a] Tyramine contents are not predictable and may vary. The amounts of tyramine are estimated from low to very high.
[b] Contains high to very high amounts of tyramine.

➤*Suicidal risks:* In patients who may be suicidal, no single form of treatment, such as MAOIs, electroconvulsive, or other therapy, should be relied upon as a sole therapeutic measure. Strict supervision and, preferably, hospitalization are advised.

➤*Concomitant antidepressants:* In patients receiving a selective serotonin reuptake inhibitor (SSRI) in combination with an MAOI, there have been reports of serious, sometimes fatal, reactions including hyperthermia, rigidity, myoclonus, autonomic instability with possible rapid fluctuations of vital signs, and mental status changes that include extreme agitation progressing to delirium and coma. These reactions have also occurred in patients who have recently discontinued an SSRI and have been started on a MAOI. Some cases presented with features resembling neuroleptic malignant syndrome. It is recommended that SSRIs not be used in combination with a MAOI, or within 14 days of a MAOI. Allow at least 2 weeks after stopping the SSRI before starting a MAOI (see Drug Interactions). Allow at least 5 weeks after stopping fluoxetine before starting a MAOI.

Do not administer MAOIs with or immediately following tricyclic antidepressants (TCAs). Such combinations can produce seizures, sweating, coma, hyperexcitability, hyperthermia, tachycardia, tachypnea, headache, mydriasis, flushing, confusion, disseminated intravascular coagulation, and death. Allow at least 14 days to elapse between the discontinuation of the MAOIs and the institution of a TCA. Some TCAs have been used safely and successfully in combination with MAOIs.

➤*Withdrawal:* Withdrawal may be associated with nausea, vomiting, and malaise. An uncommon withdrawal syndrome following abrupt withdrawal of MAOIs has been infrequently reported. Signs and symptoms of this syndrome generally commence 24 to 72 hours after drug discontinuation and may range from vivid nightmares with agitation to frank psychosis and convulsions. This syndrome generally responds to reinstitution of low-dose MAOI therapy followed by cautious downward titration and discontinuation.

➤*Coexisting symptoms:* **Tranylcypromine** and **isocarboxazid** may aggravate coexisting symptoms in depression, such as anxiety and agitation.

➤*Renal function impairment:* Observe caution in patients with impaired renal function because there is a possibility of cumulative effects in such patients.

➤*Carcinogenesis:* **Phenelzine**, like other hydrazine derivatives, has induced pulmonary and vascular tumors in an uncontrolled lifetime study in mice.

➤*Elderly:* Older patients may suffer more morbidity than younger patients during and following an episode of hypertension or malignant hyperthermia with MAOI use. Older patients have less compensatory reserve to cope with any serious adverse reactions. Therefore, use **tranylcypromine** with caution in the elderly.

➤*Pregnancy: Category C.* Safety for use during pregnancy has not been established. Use during pregnancy or in women of childbearing age only when clearly needed and when the potential benefits outweigh the potential hazards to the fetus.

Doses of **phenelzine** in pregnant mice well exceeding the maximum recommended human dose have caused a significant decrease in the number of viable offspring per mouse. The growth of dogs and rats has been retarded by doses exceeding the maximum human dose. **Tranylcypromine** passes through the placental barrier of animals into the fetus.

➤*Lactation:* Safety for use during lactation has not been established. **Tranylcypromine** is excreted in breast milk. Because of the potential for serious adverse effects in the nursing infant, decide whether to discontinue nursing or the drug, taking into account the importance of the drug to the mother.

➤*Children:* Not recommended for patients < 16 years of age.

Precautions

➤*Hypotension:* Observe all patients for symptoms of postural hypotension. Hypotensive side effects have occurred in hypertensive as well as healthy and hypotensive patients. Blood pressure usually returns to pretreatment levels rapidly when the drug is discontinued or the dosage is reduced.

At doses > 30 mg/day, postural hypotension is a major side effect and may result in syncope. Make dosage increases more gradually in patients showing a tendency toward hypotension at the beginning of therapy. Postural hypotension may be relieved by the patient lying down until blood pressure returns to normal.

➤*Hypomania:* Hypomania has been the most common severe psychiatric side effect reported. This has been largely limited to patients in whom disorders characterized by hyperkinetic symptoms coexist with, but are obscured by, depressive affect; hypomania usually appeared as depression improved. If agitation is present, it may be increased with MAOIs. Hypomania and agitation have also occurred at higher than recommended doses or following long-term therapy.

These drugs may cause excessive stimulation in agitated or schizophrenic patients; in manic-depressive states, it may result in a swing from a depressive to a manic phase.

➤*Diabetes:* There is conflicting evidence as to whether MAOIs affect glucose metabolism or potentiate hypoglycemic agents. Consider this if used in diabetics.

➤*Epilepsy:* The effect of MAOIs on the convulsive threshold may vary. Do not use with metrizamide; discontinue MAOI ≥ 48 hours prior to myelography and resume ≥ 24 hours postprocedure.

➤*Hepatotoxicity:* There is a low incidence of altered liver function or jaundice in patients treated with **isocarboxazid**. In the past, it was difficult to differentiate most cases of drug-induced hepatocellular jaundice from viral hepatitis although this is no longer true. Perform periodic liver chemistry tests during therapy. Discontinue the drug at the first sign of hepatic dysfunction or jaundice.

➤*Myocardial ischemia:* MAOIs may suppress anginal pain that would otherwise serve as a warning of myocardial ischemia.

➤*Hyperthyroid patients:* Use **tranylcypromine** and **isocarboxazid** cautiously because of increased sensitivity to pressor amines.

➤*Switching MAOIs:* In several case reports, hypertensive crisis, cerebral hemorrhage, and death have possibly resulted from switching from one MAOI to another without a waiting period. However, in other patients no adverse reactions occurred. Nevertheless, a waiting period of 10 to 14 days is recommended when switching from one MAOI to another or from a dibenzazepine-related agent (eg, amitriptyline, perphenazine).

➤*Drug abuse and dependence:* There have been reports of drug dependency in patients using doses of **tranylcypromine** and **isocarboxazid** significantly in excess of the therapeutic range. Some of these patients had a history of previous substance abuse. The following withdrawal symptoms have been reported: Restlessness; anxiety; depression; confusion; hallucinations; headaches; weakness; diarrhea.

Drug Interactions

MAOI Drug Interactions

Precipitant drug	Object drug*		Description
Methylphenidate	MAOIs	↑	Coadministration may cause a hypertensive crisis.
Metrizamide	MAOIs	↑	Discontinue MAOIs at least 48 hours before myelography and do not resume for at least 24 hours postprocedure because of the decrease of the seizure threshold.
MAOIs	Anesthetics	↑	Patients taking MAOIs should not undergo elective surgery requiring general anesthesia. Do not give cocaine or local anesthesia containing sympathomimetic vasoconstrictors. Keep in mind the possible combined hypotensive effects of MAOIs and spinal anesthesia. Discontinue the MAOI at least 10 days before elective surgery.
MAOIs	Antidepressants	↑	Do not administer MAOIs together with or immediately following these agents (see Warnings). There have been reports of serious, sometimes fatal, reactions (including hyperthermia, rigidity, myoclonus, autonomic instability with possible fluctuations of vital signs, and mental status changes that include extreme agitation and confusion progressing to delirium and coma). Do not administer MAOIs together or in rapid succession with other MAOIs.
MAOIs	Antidiabetic agents	↑	MAOIs may potentiate the hypoglycemic response to insulin or sulfonylureas and delay recovery from hypoglycemia.
MAOIs	Barbiturates	↑	Give barbiturates at a reduced dose with MAOIs.
MAOIs	Beta blockers	↑	Bradycardia may develop during concurrent use of certain MAOIs and beta blockers.
MAOIs	Bupropion	↑	The concurrent use of an MAOI and bupropion HCl is contraindicated. Allow at least 14 days between discontinuation of an MAOI and initiation of bupropion HCl treatment.
MAOIs	Buspirone	↑	Do not take isocarboxazid in combination with buspirone. Several cases of elevated blood pressure have occurred. Allow at least 10 days between discontinuation of isocarboxazid and institution of buspirone.
MAOIs	Carbamazepine	↑	Hypertensive crises, severe convulsive seizures, coma, or circulatory collapse may occur in patients receiving such combinations.
MAOIs	Cyclobenzaprine	↑	Because cyclobenzaprine is structurally related to the tricyclic antidepressants, use with caution with MAOIs (see MAOIs/Antidepressants).
MAOIs	Dextromethorphan	↑	Hyperpyrexia, abnormal muscle movement, psychosis, bizarre behavior, hypotension, coma, and death have been associated with this combination.
MAOIs	Guanethidine	↓	MAOIs may inhibit the hypotensive effects of guanethidine.
MAOIs	Levodopa	↑	Hypertensive reactions occur if levodopa is given to patients receiving MAOIs.
MAOIs	Meperidine	↑	Coadministration or use within 2 to 3 weeks of one another may result in agitation, seizures, diaphoresis, and fever, and progress to coma, apnea, and death. Adverse reactions are possible weeks after MAOI withdrawal. Avoid this combination; administer other narcotic analgesics with caution.
MAOIs	Methyldopa	↑	Coadministration may cause loss of blood pressure control or signs of central stimulation (eg, excitation, hallucinations).

MAOI Drug Interactions			
Precipitant drug	Object drug*		Description
MAOIs	Rauwolfia alkaloids	↑	MAOIs inhibit the destruction of serotonin and norepinephrine, which are believed to be released from tissue stores by rauwolfia alkaloids. Exercise caution when rauwolfia is used concomitantly with MAOIs.
MAOIs	Sulfonamide	↑	Coadministration may cause sulfonamide or MAOI toxicity.
Sulfonamide	MAOIs		
MAOIs	Sumatriptan	↑	Systemic exposure to sumatriptan may be increased, producing toxicity.
MAOIs	Sympathomimetics	↑	The MAOIs' potentiation of indirect- or mixed-acting sympathomimetic substances, including anorexiants, may result in severe headache, hypertension, high fever, and hyperpyrexia, possibly resulting in hypertensive crisis; avoid coadministration.
MAOIs	Thiazide diuretics	↑	Exaggerated hypotensive effects may result from concurrent use.
MAOIs	L-Tryptophan	↑	Coadministration may result in hyperreflexia, confusion, disorientation, shivering, myoclonic jerks, agitation, amnesia, delirium, hypomanic signs, ataxia, ocular oscillations, Babinski signs.

* ↑ = Object drug increased. ↓ = Object drug decreased.

➤*Drug/Food interactions:* Warn all patients against eating foods with a high **tyramine** content. Hypertensive crisis may result (see Warnings).

Adverse Reactions

➤*Common:*

Cardiovascular – Orthostatic and postural hypotension; syncope; palpitations; tachycardia.

CNS – Dizziness; headache; hyperreflexia; tremors; muscle twitching; mania; hypomania (see Precautions); confusion; memory impairment; sleep disturbances including hypersomnia and insomnia; weakness; myoclonic movements; fatigue; drowsiness; restlessness; overstimulation including increased anxiety, agitation, and manic symptoms.

GI – Constipation; GI disturbances; nausea; diarrhea; abdominal pain.

Miscellaneous – Edema; dry mouth; elevated serum transaminases; weight gain; sexual disturbances; anorexia; blurred vision; impotence; chills.

➤*Less common:*

CNS – Jitteriness; euphoria; palilalia; paresthesia; chills; myoclonic jerks; anxiety; hyperactivity; lethargy; sedation.

GU – Urinary retention/frequency; impotence.

Hematologic – Hematologic changes including anemia, agranulocytosis and thrombocytopenia; leukopenia.

Ophthalmic – Glaucoma; nystagmus; blurred vision.

Miscellaneous – Sweating; skin rash; hypernatremia; syncope; heavy feeling; palpitations.

➤*Rare:*

CNS – Convulsions; ataxia; shock-like coma; acute anxiety reaction; precipitation of schizophrenia; toxic delirium; manic reaction; headaches without blood pressure elevation; muscle spasm; myoclonic jerks; numbness; confusion; memory loss.

GU – Impaired water excretion compatible with the syndrome of inappropriate secretion of antidiuretic hormone (SIADH).

Hepatic – Reversible jaundice; hepatitis; fatal progressive necrotizing hepatocellular damage.

Metabolic – Hypermetabolic syndrome that may include, but is not limited to, hyperpyrexia, tachycardia, tachypnea, muscular rigidity, elevated CK levels, metabolic acidosis, hypoxia, and coma and may resemble an overdose.

Miscellaneous – Edema of the glottis; transient respiratory and cardiovascular depression following ECT; leukopenia; lupus-like syndrome; fever associated with increased muscle tone; tinnitus; localized scleroderma, cystic acne flare-up, ataxia, akinesia, disorientation, urinary frequency or incontinence, urticaria, fissuring in corner of mouth (tranylcypromine); skin rash; ejaculation problems; tremors.

Overdosage

➤*Symptoms:* Depending on the amount of overdosage, a mixed clinical picture may develop involving signs and symptoms of the CNS, cardiovascular stimulation or depression. Signs and symptoms may be absent or minimal during the initial 12–hour period following ingestion and may develop slowly thereafter, reaching a maximum in 24 to 48 hours. Some symptoms may persist for 8 to 14 days. Immediate hospitalization, with continuous patient monitoring throughout this period, is essential.

Early symptoms of MAOI toxicity include: Irritability; hyperactivity; anxiety; hypotension; vascular collapse; insomnia; restlessness; dizziness; faintness; weakness; drowsiness; hallucinations; trismus; flushing; sweating; tachypnea; tachycardia; movement disorders including grimacing, opisthotonus, rigidity, clonic movements and muscular fasciculation; severe headache. In serious cases, coma, convulsions, hypertension with severe headache, precordial pain, respiratory depression and failure, pyrexia, hyperpyrexia, diaphoresis, cool and clammy skin, cardiorespiratory arrest, incoherence, agitation, mental confusion, extreme dizziness, shock, and death may occur. Rare instances have been reported in which hypertension was accompanied by twitching or myoclonic fibrillation of skeletal muscles with hyperpyrexia, sometimes progressing to generalized rigidity and coma.

➤*Treatment:* Induce emesis or gastric lavage with instillation of charcoal slurry in early poisoning; protect the airway against aspiration. Support respiration by appropriate measures, including management of the airway, use of supplemental oxygen, and mechanical ventilatory assistance, as required. Refer to General Management of Acute Overdosage.

Cardiovascular – Cardiovascular complications include hypertension and hypotension; hence, any cardiovascular agent must be administered cautiously and blood pressure monitored frequently. Severe hypertension may be treated with an alpha-adrenergic blocker (eg, phentolamine, phenoxybenzamine). Beta blocking agents are not necessarily contraindicated and may be useful for tachycardia, tachypnea, and hyperpyrexia; however, more data are needed. Treat hypotension and vascular collapse with IV fluids and, if necessary, titrate blood pressure with an IV infusion of a dilute pressor agent. Administration of pressor amines such as norepinephrine may be of limited value; their effects may be potentiated. Plasma may be of value, as well. Adrenergic agents may produce a markedly increased pressor response.

CNS – CNS stimulation, including convulsions, may be treated with IV diazepam given slowly. Avoid phenothiazine derivatives and CNS stimulants. Monitor body temperature closely. Intensive management of hyperpyrexia may be required. Maintenance of fluid and electrolyte balance is essential.

Hemodialysis, peritoneal dialysis, and charcoal hemoperfusion may be of value in massive overdosage, but sufficient data are not available to recommend their routine use. External cooling is recommended if hyperpyrexia occurs. Barbiturates have been reported to help relieve myoclonic reactions.

The pathophysiologic effects of massive overdosage may persist for several days; recovery from mild overdosage may be expected within 3 to 4 days. Continue treatment for several days until homeostasis is restored. Liver function studies are recommended during the 4 to 6 weeks after recovery. It is not known if tranylcypromine is dialyzable.

Patient Information

Do not discontinue this medication or adjust dosage except on the advice of a physician. Consult physician before taking any other medication, including *otc* items.

Avoid tyramine-containing foods and certain *otc* drug products (see Warnings).

May cause drowsiness or blurred vision; use with caution when driving or performing other tasks requiring alertness, coordination, or physical dexterity.

Dizziness, weakness, or fainting may occur when arising from a sitting position.

Effects may be delayed a few weeks. Take as directed. Avoid alcohol and tryptophan.

Notify physician if severe headache, palpitation, or tachycardia, a sense of constriction in the throat or chest, sweating, dizziness, neck stiffness, nausea or vomiting, or other unusual symptoms occur.

Inform physician and dentist about the use of MAOIs.

PHENELZINE SULFATE

Rx	**Nardil** (Parke-Davis)	**Tablets:** 15 mg (as base)	Isopropyl alcohol, mannitol. (P-D 270). Orange. Biconvex. Film coated. In 100s.

PHENELZINE SULFATE — ORAL

WARNING

Suicidality in children and adolescents – Antidepressants increased the risk of suicidal thinking and behavior (suicidality) in short-term studies in children and adolescents with Major Depressive Disorder (MDD) and other psychiatric disorders. Anyone considering the use of phenelzine or any other antidepressant in a child or adolescent must balance this risk with the clinical need. Closely observe patients who are started on therapy for clinical worsening, suicidality, or unusual changes in behavior. Advise families and caregivers of the need for close observation and communication with the prescriber. Phenelzine is not approved for use in pediatric patients. Safety and efficacy in the pediatric population have not been established.

Pooled analyses of short-term (4 to 16 weeks) placebo-controlled trials of 9 antidepressant drugs (SSRIs and others) in children and adolescents with major depressive disorder (MDD), obsessive compulsive disorder (OCD), or other psychiatric disorders (a total of 24 trials involving over 4,400 patients) have revealed a greater risk of adverse reactions representing suicidal thinking or behavior (suicidality) during the first few months of treatment in those receiving antidepressants. The average risk of such events in patients receiving antidepressants was 4%, twice the placebo risk of 2%. No suicides occurred in these trials.

Indications

➤*Depression:* Phenelzine has been found to be effective in depressed patients clinically characterized as "atypical," "nonendogenous," or "neurotic." These patients often have mixed anxiety and depression and phobic or hypochondriacal features. There is less conclusive evidence of its usefulness with severely depressed patients with endogenous features.

Phenelzine should rarely be the first antidepressant drug used. Rather, it is more suitable for use with patients who have failed to respond to the drugs more commonly used for these conditions.

➤*Unlabeled uses:* Monoamine oxidase inhibitors (MAOIs) have shown efficacy in the treatment of bulimia; post-traumatic stress disorder (PTSD) (not considered first- or second-line); chronic migraine not responsive to standard agents; and social anxiety disorder (SAD).

Administration and Dosage

➤*Initial dose:* The usual starting dose of phenelzine is 1 tablet (15 mg) 3 times a day.

➤*Early phase treatment:* Dosage should be increased to at least 60 mg per day at a fairly rapid pace consistent with patient tolerance. It may be necessary to increase dosage up to 90 mg per day to obtain sufficient MAO inhibition. Many patients do not show a clinical response until treatment at 60 mg has been continued for at least 4 weeks.

➤*Maintenance dose:* After maximum benefit from phenelzine is achieved, dosage should be reduced slowly over several weeks. Maintenance dosage may be as low as 1 tablet (15 mg) a day or every other day, and should be continued for as long as is required.

➤*Storage/Stability:* Store between 15° and 30°C (59° and 86°F).

TRANYLCYPROMINE SULFATE

Rx	**Parnate** (GlaxoSmithKline)	**Tablets:** 10 mg (as sulfate)	Lactose. (PARNATE SKF). Rose-red. Film coated. In 100s.

TRANYLCYPROMINE SULFATE — ORAL

WARNING

Suicidality in children and adolescents – Antidepressants increased the risk of suicidal thinking and behavior (suicidality) in short-term studies in children and adolescents with major depressive disorder (MDD) and other psychiatric disorders. Anyone considering the use of tranylcypromine or any other antidepressant in a child or adolescent must balance the risk with the clinical need. Closely observe patients who are started on therapy for clinical worsening, suicidality, or unusual changes in behavior. Advise families and caregivers of the need for close observation and communication with the health care provider. Tranylcypromine is not approved for use in pediatric patients.

Pooled analyses of short-term (4- to 16-week) placebo-controlled trials of 9 antidepressant drugs (selective serotonin reuptake inhibitors [SSRIs] and others) in children and adolescents with MDD, obsessive-compulsive disorder (OCD), or other psychiatric disorders (a total of 24 trials involving over 4,400 patients) have revealed a greater risk of adverse reactions representing suicidal thinking or behavior (suicidality) during the first few months of treatment in those receiving antidepressants. The average risk of such reactions in patients receiving antidepressants was 4%, twice the placebo risk of 2%. No suicides occurred in these trials.

Indications

➤*Major depression:* For the treatment of a major depressive episode without melancholia.

Use tranylcypromine in adult patients who can be closely supervised. It should rarely be the first antidepressant drug given. Rather, the drug is suited for patients who have failed to respond to the drugs more commonly administered for depression.

➤*Unlabeled uses:* For migraine prevention; social anxiety disorder; panic disorder; bipolar depression; Alzheimer and Parkinson disease (only in individuals who are unresponsive or unable to take other agents).

Administration and Dosage

➤*Approved by the FDA:* August 16, 1985.

➤*Usual dose:* The usual effective dosage is 30 mg per day, usually given in divided doses. If there are no signs of improvement after a reasonable period (up to 2 weeks), the dosage may be increased in 10 mg per day increments at intervals of 1 to 3 weeks; the dosage range may be extended to a maximum of 60 mg per day from the usual 30 mg per day.

Dosage should be adjusted to the requirements of the individual patient. Improvement should be seen within 48 hours to 3 weeks after starting therapy.

➤*Storage/Stability:* Store between 15° and 30°C (59° and 86°F).

ISOCARBOXAZID

Rx	**Marplan** (Oxford)	**Tablets:** 10 mg	Lactose. Peach. Scored. In 100s.

ISOCARBOXAZID — ORAL

For complete prescribing information, refer to the MAOIs group monograph.

WARNING

Suicidality in children and adolescents – Antidepressants increased the risk of suicidal thinking and behavior (suicidality) in short-term studies in children and adolescents with major depressive disorder (MDD) and other psychiatric disorders. Anyone considering the use of isocarboxazid or any other antidepressant in a child or adolescent must balance this risk with the clinical need. Patients who are started on therapy should be observed closely for clinical worsening, suicidality, or unusual changes in behavior. Families and caregivers should be advised of the need for close observation and communication with the prescriber. Isocarboxazid is not approved for use in pediatric patients.

Pooled analyses of short-term (4 to 16 weeks) placebo-controlled trials of 9 antidepressant drugs (SSRIs and others) in children and adolescents with MDD, obsessive-compulsive disorder (OCD), or other psychiatric disorders (a total of 24 trials involving over 4,400 patients) have revealed a greater risk of adverse reactions representing suicidal thinking or behavior (suicidality) during the first few months of treatment in those receiving antidepressants. The average risk of such reactions in patients receiving antidepressants was 4%, twice the placebo risk of 2%. No suicides occurred in these trials.

Indications

➤*Depression:* Treatment of depression. Because of potentially serious side effects, isocarboxazid is not a first-choice antidepressant in the treatment of newly diagnosed depressed patients.

Administration and Dosage

➤*Approved by the FDA:* August 21, 1998.

➤*Initial dosage:* 10 mg twice daily. If tolerated, increase dosage by 10 mg every 2 to 4 days to achieve a dosage of 40 mg by the end of the first week of treatment. Increase dosage by increments of up to 20 mg/week, if needed and tolerated, to a maximum recommended dosage of 60 mg/day. Daily dosage should be divided into 2 to 4 doses.

➤*Maintenance dosage:* After maximum clinical response is achieved, attempt to reduce the dosage slowly over a period of several weeks without jeopardizing therapeutic response. Beneficial effect may not be seen in some patients for 3 to 6 weeks. If no response is obtained by then, discontinue therapy.

Because of the limited experience with systematically monitored patients receiving isocarboxazid at the higher end of the currently recommended dose range of up to 60 mg/day, caution is indicated in patients for whom a dose of 40 mg/day is exceeded.

WARNING

Atypical antipsychotics –

Increased mortality in elderly patients with dementia-related psychosis: Elderly patients with dementia-related psychosis treated with atypical antipsychotic drugs are at an increased risk of death compared with placebo. Analyses of 17 placebo-controlled trials (modal duration of 10 weeks) in these patients revealed a risk of death in the drug-treated patients of between 1.6 to 1.7 times that seen in placebo-treated patients. Over the course of a typical 10-week controlled trial, the rate of death in drug-treated patients was about 4.5%, compared with a rate of about 2.6% in the placebo group. Although the causes of death were varied, most of the deaths appeared to be either cardiovascular (eg, heart failure, sudden death) or infectious (eg, pneumonia) in nature. Atypical antipsychotics are not approved for the treatment of patients with dementia-related psychosis.

Clozapine –

Agranulocytosis: Because of a significant risk of agranulocytosis, a potentially life-threatening adverse event, reserve **clozapine** use in 1) the treatment of severely ill patients with schizophrenia who fail to show an acceptable response to adequate courses of standard antipsychotic drug treatment, or 2) for reducing the risk of recurrent suicidal behavior in patients with schizophrenia or schizoaffective disorder who are judged to be at risk of re-experiencing suicidal behavior. Patients being treated with clozapine must have a baseline white blood cell (WBC) and differential count before initiation of treatment, as well as regular WBC counts during treatment and for 4 weeks after discontinuation of treatment. Clozapine is available only through a distribution system that ensures monitoring of WBC counts according to the schedule described below, prior to delivery of the next supply of medication (see Warnings).

WARNING (cont.)

Seizures: Seizures have been associated with the use of **clozapine**. Dose appears to be an important seizure predictor, with a greater likelihood at higher clozapine doses. Use caution when administering clozapine to patients with a history of seizures or other predisposing factors. Advise patients not to engage in any activity where sudden loss of consciousness could cause serious risk to themselves or others (see Warnings).

Myocarditis: Analyses of postmarketing safety databases suggest **clozapine** is associated with an increased risk of fatal myocarditis, especially during, but not limited to, the first month of therapy. In patients in whom myocarditis is suspected, discontinue clozapine treatment promptly (see Warnings).

Other adverse cardiovascular and respiratory effects: Orthostatic hypotension, with or without syncope, can occur with **clozapine** treatment. Rarely, collapse can be profound and accompanied by respiratory and/or cardiac arrest. Orthostatic hypotension is more likely to occur during initial titration in association with rapid dose escalation. In patients who have had even a brief interval off clozapine (2 or more days since the last dose), start treatment with 12.5 mg once or twice daily (see Warnings). Because collapse, respiratory arrest, and cardiac arrest during initial treatment have occurred in patients receiving benzodiazepines or other psychotropic drugs, caution is advised when clozapine is initiated in patients taking a benzodiazepine or any other psychotropic drug (see Warnings).

Mesoridazine, thioridazine – Some antipsychotics have been shown to prolong the QTc interval in a dose-related manner, and drugs with this potential, including **mesoridazine** and **thioridazine**, have been associated with torsade-de-pointes-type arrhythmias and sudden death. Because of their potential for significant, possibly life-threatening, proarrhythmic effects, reserve use of mesoridazine and thioridazine in the treatment of schizophrenic patients who fail to show an acceptable response to adequate courses of treatment with other antipsychotic drugs, either because of insufficient effectiveness or the inability to achieve an effective dose because of intolerable adverse effects from those drugs.

Indications

Antipsychotics — Summary of Indications[a]

Indications (✓ = labeled; X = unlabeled)	Aripiprazole	Chlorpromazine	Clozapine	Fluphenazine	Haloperidol	Loxapine	Mesoridazine	Molindone	Olanzapine	Perphenazine	Pimozide	Prochlorperazine	Quetiapine	Risperidone	Thioridazine	Thiothixene	Trifluoperazine	Ziprasidone
Acute agitation associated with bipolar I mania									✓ (IM)[b]									
Acute agitation in schizophrenia									✓ (IM)[b]									✓ (IM)[b]
Acute intermittent porphyria		✓																
Acute manic and/or mixed episodes associated with bipolar disorder	✓	✓	X						✓				✓	✓				✓
Hyperactivity (pediatric patients)		✓			✓													
Intractable hiccoughs		✓			X													
Nausea/Vomiting		✓		X	X					✓		✓						
Nonpsychotic anxiety												✓					✓	
Presurgical apprehension/restlessness		✓																
Psychotic disorders				✓	✓					✓								
Recurrent suicidal behavior			✓															
Schizophrenia	✓	✓	✓	✓		✓	✓	✓	✓	✓	X	✓	✓	✓	✓	✓	✓	✓
Severe behavioral problems (pediatric patients)		✓			✓									X				
Tetanus		✓																
Tourette disorder					✓						✓							
Unlabeled uses																		
Behavioral problems associated with autism														X				
Migraines (acute treatment)		X										X						
Obsessive-compulsive disorder (refractory to SSRIs)									X					X				
PCP-induced psychosis					X													
Psychosis/Agitation in dementia or Alzheimer disease			X		X				X				X	X	X			X
Psychosis in Parkinson disease			X										X	X				

[a] For more detailed information, see the information below and individual drug monographs.

[b] IM = intramuscular

➤*Acute agitation associated with bipolar I mania:* **Olanzapine** IM.

➤*Acute agitation in schizophrenia:* **Ziprasidone** IM is indicated for the treatment of acute agitation in schizophrenic patients for whom treatment with ziprasidone is appropriate and who need IM antipsychotic medication for rapid control of the agitation.

➤*Acute intermittent porphyria:* **Chlorpromazine**.

➤*Acute manic and/or mixed episodes associated with bipolar disorder:* **Chlorpromazine** is indicated to control the manifestations of the manic type of manic-depressive illness. **Olanzapine** is indicated as monotherapy for the acute mixed or manic episodes associated with bipolar I disorder and for the maintenance monotherapy of bipolar disorder or in combination with lithium or valproate for the short-term treatment of acute manic episodes associated with bipolar I disorder. **Quetiapine** is indicated for the short-term treatment of acute manic episodes associated with bipolar I disorder, as either monotherapy or adjunct therapy to lithium or divalproex. **Ziprasidone** IM is indicated for the treatment of acute manic or mixed episodes associated with bipolar disorder, with or without psychotic features. **Aripiprazole** is indicated for the treatment of acute manic and mixed episodes associated with bipolar disorder. **Risperidone** is indicated for the short-term treatment of acute manic or mixed episodes associated with bipolar I disorder.

➤*Behavioral problems (pediatric patients):* **Chlorpromazine** and **haloperidol**. For the treatment of severe behavioral problems in children marked by combativeness and/or explosive hyperexcitable behavior (out of proportion to immediate provocations).

➤*Hyperactivity (pediatric patients):* **Chlorpromazine** and **haloperidol**. For the short-term treatment of hyperactive children who show excessive motor activity with accompanying conduct disorders consisting of some or all of the following symptoms: Aggressiveness, difficulty sustaining attention, impulsiveness, mood lability, poor frustration tolerance.

➤*Intractable hiccoughs:* **Chlorpromazine**.

➤*Nausea/Vomiting:* **Chlorpromazine**, **perphenazine**, and **prochlorperazine**. To control severe nausea and vomiting.

➤*Nonpsychotic anxiety:* **Prochlorperazine** and **trifluoperazine**. For the short-term treatment of generalized nonpsychotic anxiety; however, they are not the first drugs to be used.

➤*Presurgical apprehension/restlessness:* **Chlorpromazine** is indicated for relief of restlessness and apprehension before surgery.

➤*Psychotic disorders:* **Fluphenazine**, **haloperidol**, and **perphenazine**. For use in the management of the manifestations of psychotic disorders.

➤*Recurrent suicidal behavior:* **Clozapine** is indicated for reducing the risk of recurrent suicidal behavior in patients with schizophrenia or schizoaffective disorder who are judged to be at chronic risk for re-experiencing suicidal behavior.

➤*Schizophrenia:* **Aripiprazole**, **chlorpromazine**, **clozapine**, **fluphenazine**, **loxapine**, **mesoridazine**, **molindone**, **olanzapine**, **perphenazine**, **prochlorperazine**, **quetiapine**, **risperidone**, **thioridazine**, **thiothixene**, **trifluoperazine**, and **ziprasidone**. Clozapine, mesoridazine, and thioridazine should only be used in patients who have failed to respond adequately to other antipsychotic drugs.

➤*Tetanus:* **Chlorpromazine** is indicated as an adjunct in the treatment of tetanus.

➤*Tourette disorder:* **Haloperidol** is indicated for the control of tics and vocal utterances of Tourette disorder in children and adults. **Pimozide** is indicated for the suppression of motor and phonic tics in patients with Tourette disorder who have failed to respond satisfactorily to standard treatment.

➤*Unlabeled uses:*

Acute manic episodes associated with bipolar disorder – **Clozapine** also may be an option in the treatment of refractory bipolar mania.

Behavioral problems associated with autism – **Risperidone** was shown to be effective for the treatment of tantrums, aggression, or self-injurious behavior in autistic children.

Behavioral problems (pediatric patients) – **Risperidone** has demonstrated efficacy in reducing aggression in children with a variety of comorbid disorders. Risperidone has also improved severely disruptive behavior in children with subaverage intelligence.

Intractable hiccoughs – **Haloperidol** (2 to 5 mg every 4 to 8 hours) has been used as an alternative agent in the treatment of persistent hiccoughs.

Migraines – **Chlorpromazine** (50 to 100 mg IM) and **prochlorperazine** (10 to 25 mg IM) have been used as abortive treatments of acute migraine attacks in adults.

Nausea/Vomiting – **Haloperidol** and **fluphenazine** also have been used as antiemetics.

Obsessive-compulsive disorder (refractory to SSRIs) – Patients with OCD refractory to SSRIs may respond to the addition of **risperidone** or **olanzapine**.

Phencyclidine (PCP) psychosis – **Haloperidol** has shown to be effective in improving PCP-induced aggression, combativeness, and schizophreniform symptoms (eg, hallucinations, delusions, disorganized thinking.)

Psychosis/Agitation in dementia or Alzheimer disease patient – **Clozapine**, **haloperidol**, **olanzapine**, **quetiapine**, **risperidone**, **thioridazine**, and **ziprasidone** may be useful in the management of agitation and psychotic events in patients with dementia and Alzheimer disease.

Psychosis in Parkinson disease – In the treatment of psychosis in patients with Parkinson disease, **clozapine** has been shown to be beneficial in alleviating psychosis without compromising motor function. Other alternatives include **quetiapine** and **risperidone**.

Tourette disorder – **Risperidone** has shown efficacy in the treatment of tics in patients with Tourette disorder.

Administration and Dosage

See individual product listings for specific dosing.

Individualize dosage. The milligram-for-milligram potency relationship among all dosage forms has not been precisely established. Increase dosage until symptoms are controlled. Increase dosage gradually in elderly, debilitated, or emaciated patients. In continued therapy, gradually reduce dosage to the lowest effective maintenance level after symptoms have been controlled.

Actions

➤*Pharmacology:* The exact mechanism of action of the antipsychotic agents is unknown; however, it is thought to be caused by their antagonistic actions on the receptors of several neurotransmitters. The following table provides information on antipsychotic receptor affinity. All produce antagonist effects on the receptors unless otherwise specified.

Antipsychotic Receptor Affinity	
Antipsychotic agent	Receptor affinity
Conventional agents	
Chlorpromazine	**High** — adrenergic **Weak** — peripheral anticholinergic, histaminergic, serotonergic
Fluphenazine	Dopamine D_2, histamine H_1, alpha-adrenergic, serotonin 5-HT_2
Haloperidol	Dopamine D_2, alpha-adrenergic, serotonin 5-HT_2
Loxapine	Dopamine D_2, histamine H_1, alpha-adrenergic, muscarinic M_1
Mesoridazine	Dopamine D_2, histamine H_1, alpha-adrenergic, muscarinic M_1
Molindone	**Low** — dopamine D_2, alpha-adrenergic, serotonin 5-HT_2
Perphenazine	Dopamine D_2, histamine H_1, alpha-adrenergic
Pimozide	Dopamine D_2, alpha-adrenergic, serotonin 5-HT_2
Prochlorperazine	Dopamine D_2, histamine H_1, alpha-D_2adrenergic, serotonin 5-HT_2
Promethazine[a]	Histamine H_1, muscarinic, some serotonin
Thioridazine	Dopamine D_2, histamine H_1, alpha-adrenergic, muscarinic M_1, serotonin 5-HT_2
Thiothixene	**High** — dopamine D_2 **Low** — histamine H_1, alpha-adrenergic
Trifluoperazine	Dopamine D_2, histamine H_1, alpha-adrenergic, muscarinic M_1, serotonin 5-HT_2
Atypical agents	
Aripiprazole	**High** — dopamine D_2[b], D_3, serotonin 5-HT_{1A}[b], 5-HT_{2A} **Moderate** — dopamine D_4, 5-HT_{2C}, 5-HT_7, $alpha_1$-adrenergic, histamine H_1
Clozapine	**High** — dopamine D_4 Other receptors — dopamine D_1, D_2, D_3, D_5, adrenergic, cholinergic, histaminergic, serotonergic
Olanzapine	**High** — serotonin 5-HT_{2A}, 5-HT_{2C}, dopamine D_1, D_2, D_3, D_4, muscarinic M_1, M_2, M_3, M_4, M_5, histamine H_1, $alpha_1$adrenergic **Weak** — $GABA_A$, benzodiazepine receptor, beta-adrenergic
Quetiapine	Serotonin 5-HT_{1A}, 5-HT_2, dopamine D_1, D_2, $alpha_{1 \text{ and } 2}$-adrenergic, histamine H_1
Risperidone	**High** — dopamine D_2, serotonin 5-HT_2 **Low to moderate** — 5-HT_{1C}, 5-HT_{1D}, 5-HT_{1A}, histamine H_1, alpha-adrenergic **Weak** — D_1, haloperidol-sensitive sigma site
Ziprasidone	**High** — dopamine D_2, D_3, 5-HT_{2A}, 5-HT_{2C}, 5-HT_{1A}[1], 5-HT_{1D}, $alpha_1$adrenergic **Moderate** — histamine H_1

[a] Promethazine is classified as a phenothiazine but not indicated as an antipsychotic.
[b] Partial agonist activity.

Conventional (typical) antipsychotics can be grouped into several classes; the phenothiazines, structurally related thioxanthenes, butyrophenones (phenylbutylpiperadines), diphenylbutylpiperadines, and the indolones.As a group, these agents are dopamine receptor antagonists with a higher affinity for D_2 over D_1 receptors. They exhibit varying degrees of selectivity among the cortical dopamine tracts: Nigrostriatal (movement disorders), mesolimbic (relief of hallucinations and delusions), mesocortical (relief of psychosis, worsening of negative symptoms) or tuberoinfundibular (prolactin release). They also bind with varying affinities to nondopaminergic sites, such as cholinergic, $alpha_1$-adrenergic and histaminic receptors, which can partially explain the varied side effect profiles for each agent. Typical antipsychotics are likely to induce extrapyramidal side effects (EPS) and have similar efficacies when used in equipotent doses. Lower-potency agents tend to be more sedating and high-potency agents usually have a higher incidence of acute EPS.

Novel (atypical) antipsychotics were introduced with the development of **clozapine** and can be structurally classified as dibenzepines, benzisoxazoles, or quinolinone. As a group, they have diverse pharmacodynamic profiles differing considerably from the typical antipsychotics but in general have an increased affinity for serotonin 5-HT_2 receptors compared with D_2 receptors. They act upon several neurotransmitter systems including antagonism at one or more types of dopamine receptors (eg, D_1, D_2, D_4, D_5); selectivity for limbic dopamine receptors; antagonism at 1 or more types of serotonin receptors (eg, 5-HT_1, 5-HT_2); antagonism at $alpha_1$ adrenergic receptors; and activity at muscarinic or histamine H_1 receptors. They are considered atypical because of their decreased ability or inability to induce EPS; newer agents also have a decreased propensity to induce agranulocytosis compared with clozapine. Studies indicate that some atypical agents are effective in patients resistant to conventional antipsychotic therapy and may be more effective in relieving negative symptoms than conventional agents.

Pharmacological Parameters of Antipsychotics

Antipsychotic agent	Approx. equiv. dose (mg)	Usual oral adult daily dose range (mg)	Sedation	EPS	Anticholinergic effects	Orthostatic hypotension	Weight gain
Phenothiazines							
Aliphatic							
Chlorpromazine	100	30-800	+++	++	++	+++	
Piperazine							
Fluphenazine	2	1-40	+	++++	+	+	
Perphenazine	10	12-64	++	++	+	+	
Prochlorperazine		15-150					
Trifluoperazine	5	2-15	+	+++	+	+	
Piperidines							
Mesoridazine	50	100-400	+++	+	+++	++	
Thioridazine	100	150-800	+++	+	+++	+++	
Thioxanthenes							
Thiothixene	4	6-60	+	+++	+	+	
Phenylbutylpiperadines							
Butyrophenone							
Haloperidol	2	1-100	+	++++	+	+	
Diphenylbutylpiperadine							
Pimozide		1-10	+	+++	++	+	
Dihydroindolones							
Molindone	10	15-225	+	++	+	+	
Ziprasidone		40-200	++	++	+	++	+
Dibenzepines							
Dibenzoxazepines							
Loxapine	10	20-250	+	++	+	+	
Dibenzodiazepine							
Clozapine	50	300-900	+++	0	+++	+++	++++
Thienbenzodiazepine							
Olanzapine		5-20	++	+	++	++	++++
Dibenzothiazepine							
Quetiapine		50-800	++	0	0-+	++	+++
Benzisoxazole							
Risperidone		4-16	+	++	0-+	++	+++
Quinolinone							
Aripiprazole		10-30	+	0	0-+	+	+

++++ = Very high incidence of side effects, +++ = High incidence of side effects, ++ = Moderate incidence of side effects, + = Low incidence of side effects

➤*Pharmacokinetics:*

Metabolism – CYP2D6 is the enzyme responsible for metabolism of many antipsychotics. CYP2D6 is subject to genetic polymorphism and to inhibition by a variety of substrates and some nonsubstrates. Extensive CYP2D6 metabolizers convert drugs rapidly, whereas poor metabolizers convert the drugs much more slowly.

Special populations –

Renal function impairment:

• *Aripiprazole* – In patients with severe renal impairment (Ccr less than 30 mL/min), **aripiprazole** and dehydro-aripiprazole C_{max} increased 36% and 53%, respectively. AUC decreased 15% for aripiprazole and increased 7% for dehydro-aripiprazole.

• *Quetiapine* – Patients with severe renal failure (Ccr 10 to 30 mL/min/1.73 m^2) had a 25% lower mean oral clearance than normal subjects (Ccr greater than 80 mL/min/1.73m^2); however, plasma concentrations were within the same range.

• *Ziprasidone* – Intramuscular **ziprasidone** has not been fully evaluated in renal impairment; however, the cyclodextrin excipient is cleared renally. Therefore, administer IM formulation with caution in these patients.

• *Risperidone* – In patients with moderate to severe renal disease, clearance of the sum of **risperidone** and its active metabolite decreased 60%. Reduce dose in renal disease.

Hepatic function impairment:

• *Aripiprazole* – AUC increased 31% in mild, 8% in moderate, and decreased 20% in severe hepatic impairment.

• *Quetiapine* – Mean oral clearance decreased 30% in patients with hepatic impairment and AUC and C_{max} increased by 3 times. Dosage adjustment may be needed.

• *Ziprasidone* – In patients with clinically significant cirrhosis (Child-Pugh Class A and B), an increase in AUC of 13% and 34% occurred, respectively, and half-life was 7.1 hours compared with 4.8 hours in healthy subjects.

• *Risperidone* – The mean free fraction in plasma was increased by about 35% because of the diminished concentration of albumin and alpha acid glycoprotein. Reduce dose in hepatic impairment.

Elderly:

• *Aripiprazole* – Clearance decreased 20% after a single 15 mg dose in patients 65 years of age or older.

• *Quetiapine* – Oral clearance decreased 40% in patients 65 years of age or older. A dosage adjustment may be necessary.

• *Risperidone* – Renal clearance of **risperidone** and its active metabolite were decreased. Modify dose accordingly.

• *Olanzapine* – Mean elimination half-life was about 1.5 times greater in patients 65 years of age or older.

Gender:

• *Aripiprazole* – C_{max} and AUC of **aripiprazole** and dehydro-aripiprazole are 30% to 40% higher in women and correspondingly the oral clearance is lower in women. These differences are largely explained by differences in body weight.

• *Olanzapine* – Clearance is approximately 30% lower in women.

Race:

• *Olanzapine* – Comparisons between study data collected in Japan vs the United States suggest exposure to **olanzapine** could be about 2-fold greater in Japanese patients when equivalent doses are administered.

Smoking:

• *Olanzapine* – Clearance is about 40% higher in smokers.

Antipsychotic Pharmacokinetics

Drug	Bioavailability	Mean C_{max}	T_{max}	Mean Vd	Protein bound (%)	Routes of metabolism	Active metabolite	T½	Routes of excretion
Conventional agents									
Chlorpromazine	20%- 40%	25-150 ng/mL	1-4 h	≈ 21 L/kg	92%-97%			24 h	
Fluphenazine	2.7% (oral); 3.4% (SC/IM)	≈ 2.3 ng/mL (oral); 1.3 ng/mL (SC/IM)	≈ 2.8 h (oral); 24-48 h (SC/IM)	20 L/kg				18 h (oral)	
Haloperidol	60%-65% (oral)	≈ 9.2 ng/mL (oral). ≈ 22 ng/mL (IM)	6 days (decanoate)	≈ 18 L/kg	≈ 92%			≈ 18 h (oral); ≈ 3 wk (decanoate)	Feces, urine (≈ 1%)
Loxapine	≈ 100%							8 h	Urine, feces
Mesoridazine								30 h	
Molindone			1.5 h					12 h	Urine, feces
Perphenazine	20%	984 pg/mL	1-3 h	10-34 L/kg		Sulfoxidation, hydroxylation, dealkylation, and glucuronidation by CYP2D6		9-12 h	
Pimozide	> 50%	≈ 10 ng/mL	4 to 12 h	≈ 28 L/kg[a]	99%	N-dealkylation by CYP3A and CYP1A2 to a lesser extent		≈ 55 h	Urine (main route)
Prochlorperazine				20 L/kg				3-5 h (oral); 6.9 h (IV)	

Antipsychotic Pharmacokinetics

Drug	Bioavailability	Mean C_{max}	T_{max}	Mean Vd	Protein bound (%)	Routes of metabolism	Active metabolite	$T_{½}$	Routes of excretion
Promethazine[b]			2-3 h	13 L/kg	76%-80%	N-demethylation and sulfoxidation		5-14 h	Urine, bile
Thioridazine				18 L/kg	99%		mesoridazine	24 h	
Thiothixene								34 h	
Trifluoperazine								18 h	
Atypical agents									
Aripiprazole	87%		3-5 h	4.9 L/kg[a]	> 99%[c]	Dehydrogenation, hydroxylation, and N-dealkylation by CYP3A4 and CYP2D6	Dehydro-aripiprazole	75[d]-146[e] h	Feces (≈ 55%), urine (≈ 25%)
Clozapine	27%-47%	319 ng/mL[a]	2.5 h	≈ 5.4 L/kg	≈ 97%	Demethylation, hydroxylation, and N-oxidation	Desmethyl metabolite has limited activity	8 h[f]; 12 h[a]	Urine (≈ 50%), feces (≈ 30%)
Olanzapine	≈ 60%	≈ 12.9 ng/mL	≈ 6 h	≈ 1000 L	93% over a concentration range of 7-1100 ng/mL	Glucuronidation and oxidation by CYP1A2 and CYP2D6		21-54 h	Urine (≈ 57%), feces (≈ 30%)
Quetiapine	≥ 73%	778-1080 mcg/L	1.5 h	≈ 10 L/kg	83%[b]	Sulfoxidation and oxidation by CYP3A4	None	≈ 6 h	Urine (≈ 73%), feces (≈20%)
Risperidone	70%	10 ng/mL	≈ 1 h	1-2 L/kg	90%	Hydroxylation by CYP2D6 and N-dealkylation	9-hydroxy-risperidone	3[d]-20[e] h	Urine (≈ 70%), feces (≈ 14%)
Ziprasidone	≈ 60% (oral); 100% (IM)	44.6-139.4 mcg/L	6-8 h (oral); ≈ 60 min (IM)	1.5 L/kg	> 99%	Reduction by aldehyde oxidase, methylation, and oxidation by CYP3A4 and CYP1A2 to a lesser extent		≈ 7 h (oral); 2-5 h (IM)	Feces (≈ 66%), urine (≈ 20%)

[a] At steady-state
[b] Promethazine is classified as a phenothiazine but not indicated as an antipsychotic.
[c] At therapeutic concentrations
[d] Extensive metabolizers
[e] Poor metabolizers
[f] Single dose

Contraindications

Hypersensitivity to drug or any other component of the product (cross-sensitivity between phenothiazines may occur); comatose or greatly depressed states because of CNS depressants or from any other cause (phenothiazines, **clozapine**, **loxapine**, **molindone**, **pimozide**, **haloperidol**); coadministration with other drugs that prolong the QT interval and in patients with congenital long QT syndrome or history of cardiac arrhythmias (**mesoridazine**, **thioridazine**, **pimozide**, **ziprasidone**; see Drug Interactions).

➤*Phenothiazines:* Suspected or established subcortical brain damage (**fluphenazine**); blood dyscrasias (**perphenazine**, **trifluoperazine**, **fluphenazine**); bone marrow depression (**perphenazine**, **trifluoperazine**, **fluphenazine**); preexisting liver damage (**perphenazine**, **trifluoperazine**, **fluphenazine**); pediatric surgery (**prochlorperazine**); hypertensive or hypotensive heart disease of extreme degree (**thioridazine**).

➤*Thiothixene:* Circulatory collapse; blood dyscrasias.

➤*Haloperidol:* Parkinson disease.

➤*Pimozide:* Treatment of simple tics or tics other than those associated with Tourette disorder; in combination with drugs (eg, pemoline, methylphenidate, amphetamines) that may themselves cause motor or phonic tics until it is determined whether or not the drugs, rather than Tourette disorder, are responsible for the tics. See also Drug Interactions.

➤*Clozapine:* Myeloproliferative disorders; uncontrolled epilepsy; history of **clozapine**-induced agranulocytosis or severe granulocytopenia; should not be used with other agents having a well-known potential to cause agranulocytosis or suppress bone marrow function.

➤*Ziprasidone:* Recent acute MI; uncompensated heart failure.

Warnings

➤*Tardive dyskinesia (TD):* TD, a syndrome consisting of potentially irreversible, involuntary dyskinetic movements, may develop in patients treated with antipsychotic drugs. Although prevalence of TD appears highest among the elderly, especially women, it is impossible to rely upon prevalence estimates to predict, at the inception of antipsychotic treatment, which patients are likely to develop the syndrome. Whether antipsychotic drugs differ in their potential to cause TD is unknown. However, atypical antipsychotics appear to have a lower risk of TD. Both the risk of developing TD and the likelihood that it will become irreversible are increased as duration of treatment and total cumulative dose administered increase. However, the syndrome can develop, although much less commonly, after relatively brief treatment periods at low doses.

There is no known treatment for established cases of TD, although it may remit, partially or completely, if antipsychotics are withdrawn. Antipsychotic treatment itself, however, may suppress (or partially suppress) signs and symptoms of TD, possibly masking the underlying disease process. The effect of symptomatic suppression on the long-term course of the syndrome is unknown.

Given these considerations, prescribe antipsychotics in a manner most likely to minimize the occurrence of tardive dyskinesia. In general, reserve chronic antipsychotic treatment for patients who suffer from a chronic illness that responds to antipsychotic drugs and for whom alternative, equally effective, but potentially less harmful treatments are not available or appropriate. In patients who require chronic treatment, use the smallest dose and the shortest duration of treatment producing a satisfactory clinical response. Periodically reassess the need for continued treatment.

If signs and symptoms of TD appear, consider drug discontinuation. However, some patients may require treatment despite the presence of the syndrome.

➤*Extrapyramidal symptoms (EPS):* Dystonic reactions develop primarily with the use of traditional antipsychotics. EPS has occurred during the administration of **haloperidol** and **pimozide** frequently, often during the first few days of treatment. EPS during the administration of haloperidol have been reported frequently, often during the first few days of treatment. EPS can be categorized generally as Parkinson symptoms, akathisia, or dystonia (including opisthotonos and oculogyric crisis). While all can occur at relatively low doses, they occur more frequently and with greater severity at higher doses. The symptoms may be controlled with dose reductions or administration of antiparkinson drugs such as benztropine mesylate or trihexyphenidyl HCl. It should be noted that persistent EPS has been reported; the drug may have to be discontinued in such cases.

➤*Neuroleptic malignant syndrome (NMS):* A potentially fatal symptom complex sometimes referred to as NMS has been reported in association with administration of antipsychotic drugs. Two possible cases of NMS (2/2387 [0.1%]) have been reported in clinical trials with **quetiapine**. Clinical manifestations of NMS are hyperpyrexia, muscle rigidity, altered mental status, and evidence of autonomic instability (irregular pulse or BP, tachycardia, diaphoresis, cardiac dysrhythmia). Additional signs may include elevated creatine phosphokinase, myoglobinuria (rhabdomyolysis), and acute renal failure. The onset may be after hours to months of treatment or may occur after discontinuation of therapy. Once started, NMS proceeds rapidly over 24 to 72 hours.

The risk of NMS is higher in patients receiving high-potency, injectable, or depot antipsychotics. NMS may occur with atypical antipsychotics, but the risk is lower. There have been several reported cases of NMS in patients receiving **clozapine** alone or in combination with lithium or other CNS-active agents. The diagnostic evaluation of patients with this syndrome is complicated. In arriving at a diagnosis, it is important to exclude cases where the clinical presentation includes both serious medical illness (eg, pneumonia, systemic infection) and untreated or inadequately treated EPS. Other important considerations in the differential diagnosis include central anticholinergic toxicity, heat stroke, drug fever, and primary CNS pathology.

Include the following in the management of NMS: 1) Immediate discontinuation of antipsychotic drugs and other drugs not essential to concurrent therapy; 2) intensive symptomatic treatment and medical monitoring; and 3) treatment of any concomitant serious medical problems for which specific treatments are available. There is no general agreement about specific pharmacological treatment regimens for NMS.

If a patient requires antipsychotic drug treatment after recovery from NMS, carefully consider the potential reintroduction of drug therapy. Carefully monitor the patient because recurrences of NMS have been reported.

➤*CNS effects:* These agents may impair mental or physical abilities, especially during the first few days. Drowsiness may occur during the first or second week, after which it generally disappears. If troublesome, lower the dosage. Caution patients against activities requiring alertness (eg, operating vehicles or machinery). Use cautiously in depressed patients. Use caution in agitated states with depression, (particularly if a suicidal tendency is recognized). When **haloperidol** is used for mania in cyclic disorders, a rapid mood swing to depression may occur.

Encephalopathic syndrome – An encephalopathic syndrome (characterized by weakness, lethargy, fever, tremulousness and confusion, extrapyramidal symptoms, leukocytosis, elevated serum enzymes, BUN, fasting blood sugar) has occurred in a few patients treated with lithium plus an antipsychotic (**haloperidol**). In some instances, the syndrome was followed by irreversible brain damage. Because of a possible causal relationship between these events and the coadministration of lithium and antipsychotics, closely monitor patients receiving such combined therapy for early evidence of neurologic toxicity and promptly discontinue treatment if such signs appear. This encephalopathic syndrome may be similar to or the same as NMS.

➤*Cardiovascular effects:* Use with caution in patients with cardiovascular disease (history of MI or ischemic heart disease, heart failure, or conduction abnormalities), cerebrovascular disease, conditions that would predispose patients to hypotension (dehydration, hypovolemia, and treatment with antihypertensive medications), or mitral insufficiency. Increased pulse rates occur in most patients. Large doses and parenteral administration should be avoided in patients with impaired cardiovascular systems. To minimize the occurrence of hypotension after injection, keep patient lying down and observe for at least 30 minutes. One result of therapy may be an increase in mental and physical activity. For example, a few patients with angina pectoris have complained of increased pain while taking **trifluoperazine**. Therefore, withdraw the drug from angina patients if an unfavorable response is noted.

ECG changes – A minority of **clozapine** patients experience ECG repolarization changes similar to those seen with other antipsychotic drugs, including S-T segment depression and flattening or inversion of T waves, all of which normalize after discontinuation of clozapine. The clinical significance is unclear. However, several patients have experienced significant cardiac events, including ischemic changes, MI, arrhythmias, and sudden death. In addition there have been postmarketing reports of CHF, pericarditis, and pericardial effusions. Causality assessment was difficult in many of these cases because of serious preexisting cardiac disease and plausible alternative causes. Rare instances of sudden death have been reported in psychiatric patients, with or without associated antipsychotic drug treatment, and the relationship of these events to antipsychotic drug use is unknown.

Ziprasidone, **pimozide**, **mesoridazine**, and **thioridazine** have been shown to prolong the QT interval, and drugs with this potential have been associated with torsade de pointes-type arrhythmias and sudden death. Certain circumstances may increase the risk of torsade de pointes and/or sudden death in association with the used of drugs that prolong the QT interval, including the following: 1) Bradycardia; 2) hypokalemia or hypomagnesemia; 3) concomitant use of other drugs that prolong the QT interval; and 4) presence of congenital prolongation of the QT interval. Perform a baseline ECG and measure serum potassium and magnesium before initiation of treatment and periodically during treatment, especially during a period of dose adjustment. Patients with QT interval over 450 msec should not receive mesoridazine or thioridazine. Ziprasidone should be avoided in patients with histories of significant cardiovascular illness (eg, QT prolongation, recent acute MI, uncompensated heart failure, cardiac arrhythmia). Replete patients with low potassium and/or magnesium with those electrolytes before proceeding with treatment. Discontinue treatment if the QT interval is over 500 msec. Patients who experience symptoms that may be associated with the occurrence of torsade de pointes (eg, dizziness, palpitations, syncope) may warrant further cardiac evaluation; in particular, consider Holter monitoring. (See Black Box Warning, Contraindications, and Drug Interactions).

Nonspecific ECG changes, usually reversible Q- and T-wave distortions, have been observed in some patients receiving phenothiazines. Nonspecific ECG changes have been observed in some patients receiving **thiothixene**. These changes are usually reversible and frequently disappear on continued thiothixene therapy. The incidence of these changes is lower than that observed with some phenothiazines. The clinical significance of these changes is not known.

Haloperidol has been associated with ECG changes, including QT interval prolongation and ECG pattern changes compatible with the polymorphous configuration of torsade de pointes.

Rare, transient, nonspecific T-wave changes have been reported on ECG in patients taking **molindone**.

Prolongation of the QT interval and torsade de pointes have been reported with risperidone overdoses.

Other drugs that prolong the QT interval have been associated with the occurrence of torsade de pointes. Bradycardia, electrolyte imbalance, concomitant use with other drugs that prolong QT, or the presence of congenital prolongation in QT can increase the risk.

Myocarditis – Postmarketing **clozapine** surveillance data from 4 countries revealed cases of myocarditis, some fatal. The rate of myocarditis in clozapine-treated patients appears to be 17 to 322 times greater than the general population and is associated with an increased risk of fatal myocarditis that is 14 to 161 times greater than the general population. Therefore, consider the possibility of myocarditis in patients receiving clozapine who present with unexplained fatigue, dyspnea, tachypnea, fever, chest pain, palpitations, other signs or symptoms of heart failure, or ECG findings such as ST-T wave abnormalities or arrhythmias. It is not known whether eosinophilia is a reliable predictor of myocarditis. Tachycardia, which has been associated with clozapine treatment, also has been noted as a presenting sign in patients with myocarditis. Therefore, tachycardia during the first month of therapy warrants close monitoring for other signs of myocarditis. Prompt discontinuation of clozapine treatment is warranted upon suspicion of myocarditis. Patients with clozapine-related myocarditis should not be rechallenged with clozapine.

Cardiomyopathy – Cases of cardiomyopathy have been reported in patients treated with **clozapine**. Approximately 80% of clozapine-treated patients in whom cardiomyopathy was reported were younger than 50 years of age; the duration of treatment with clozapine prior to cardiomyopathy diagnosis varied, but was more than 6 months in 65% of the reports. Dilated cardiomyopathy was most frequently reported. Signs and symptoms suggestive of cardiomyopathy, particularly exertional dyspnea, fatigue, orthopnea, paroxysmal nocturnal dyspnea, and peripheral edema should alert the clinician to perform further investigations. If the diagnosis of cardiomyopathy is confirmed, discontinue clozapine unless the benefit to the patient clearly outweighs the risk.

Pulmonary embolism – Consider the possibility of pulmonary embolism in patients receiving **clozapine** who present with deep vein thrombosis, acute dyspnea, chest pain, or with other respiratory signs and symptoms. Deep vein thrombosis also has been observed in association with clozapine therapy. Whether pulmonary embolus can be attributed to clozapine or some characteristics of its users is not clear, but the occurrence of deep vein thrombosis or respiratory symptomatology should suggest its presence.

Hypotension – Orthostatic hypotension with or without syncope can occur, especially during initial titration in association with rapid dose escalation, and may represent a continuing risk in some patients. In 1 report, initial **clozapine** doses as low as 12.5 mg were associated with collapse and respiratory arrest.

Severe, acute hypotension has occurred with the use of phenothiazines and is particularly likely to occur in patients with mitral insufficiency or pheochromocytoma. Rebound hypertension may occur in pheochromocytoma patients.

Carefully watch patients who are undergoing surgery, and who are on large doses of phenothiazines, for hypotensive phenomena. It may be necessary to reduce amounts of anesthetics or CNS depressants. The hypotensive effects may occur after the first injection of the antipsychotic, occasionally after subsequent injections, and rarely after the first oral dose. Recovery is usually spontaneous and symptoms disappear within 0.5 to 2 hours. If hypotension occurs, place the patient in a recumbent position. Females have a greater tendency to experience orthostatic hypotension. Patients with hypovolemia have increased sensitivity to the hypotensive effects of these agents. Volume replacement, when needed, should precede use of vasopressors. If a vasopressor is indicated, use phenylephrine or norepinephrine. Avoid using epinephrine in drug-induced hypotension (see Drug Interactions).

Tachycardia – Tachycardia, which may be sustained, also has been observed in approximately 25% of patients taking **clozapine**, with an average increase in pulse rate of 10 to 15 bpm. The sustained tachycardia is not simply a reflex response to hypotension, and is present in all positions monitored. Either tachycardia or hypotension may pose a serious risk for an individual with compromised cardiovascular function. Pulse rates have increased in most patients receiving antipsychotics.

➤*Cerebrovascular effects:* Cerebrovascular adverse events (eg, stroke, transient ischemic attack), including fatalities, were reported in patients (mean, 85 years of age; range, 73 to 97 years of age) in trials of **risperidone** in elderly patients with dementia-related psychosis. In placebo-controlled trials, there was a significantly higher incidence of cerebrovascular adverse events in patients treated with risperidone compared with patients treated with placebo. **Risperidone** is not approved for the treatment of patients with dementia-related psychosis.

➤*Sudden death:* Sudden, unexpected, and unexplained deaths have been reported in psychotic patients receiving phenothiazines. Previous brain damage or seizures may be predisposing factors; avoid high doses in known seizure patients. Several patients have shown sudden flare-ups of psychotic behavior patterns shortly before death. In some cases, death was apparently caused by cardiac arrest; in others, asphyxia was caused by failure of the cough reflex. Autopsy findings usually reveal acute fulminating pneumonia or pneumonitis, aspiration of gastric contents, or intramyocardial lesions. In some patients, cause could not be determined.

Sudden unexpected deaths have occurred in experimental studies of **pimozide** in conditions other than Tourette disorder. These deaths occurred while patients were receiving pimozide dosages in the range of 1 mg/kg. One possible mechanism for such deaths is prolongation of the QT interval predisposing patients to ventricular arrhythmia.

➤*Priapism:* Rare cases of priapism have been associated with **risperidone**, **ziprasidone**, **quetiapine**, **aripiprazole**, and **olanzapine**. While the relationship of the event to these antipsychotics has not been established, other drugs with alpha-adrenergic blocking effects have been reported to induce priapism. Severe priapism may require surgical intervention.

➤*Hyperprolactinemia:* Antipsychotic drugs elevate prolactin levels; the elevation persists during chronic administration. However, in contrast to more typical antipsychotic drugs, **clozapine** therapy produces little or no prolactin elevation. Drugs that antagonize dopamine D_2 receptors elevate prolactin levels. Experiments indicate that approximately 33% of human breast cancers are prolactin-dependent in vitro, a factor of potential importance if the prescription of these drugs is contemplated in a patient with previously detected breast cancer.

Although disturbances such as galactorrhea, amenorrhea, gynecomastia, and impotence have been reported with prolactin-elevating compounds, the clinical significance of elevated serum prolactin levels is unknown for most patients.

Risperidone, **ziprasidone**, and **olanzapine** elevate prolactin levels. As is common with compounds that increase prolactin release, an increase in pituitary gland, mammary gland, and pancreatic islet cell hyperplasia or neoplasia was observed in risperidone carcinogenicity studies conducted in mice and rats. An increase in mammary gland neoplasia was observed in the olanzapine and ziprasidone carcinogenicity studies conducted in mice and in the olanzapine studies in rats.

Elevated prolactin levels were not demonstrated in clinical trials with **quetiapine**. However, increased prolactin levels were observed in rats studied with this compound.

➤*Hyperglycemia and diabetes mellitus:* Hyperglycemia, in some cases extreme and associated with ketoacidosis or hyperosmolar coma or death, has been reported in patients treated with atypical antipsychotics. Assessment of the relationship between atypical antipsychotic use and glucose abnormalities is complicated by the possibility of an increased background risk of diabetes mellitus in patients with schizophrenia and the increasing incidence of diabetes mellitus in the general population. Given these confounders, the relationship between atypical antipsychotic use and hyperglycemia-related adverse events is not completely understood. However, epidemiological studies suggest an increased risk of treatment-emergent hyperglycemia-related adverse events in patients treated with atypical antipsychotics. Precise risk estimates for hyperglycemia-related adverse events in patients treated with atypical antipsychotics are not available.

Regularly monitor patients with an established diagnosis of diabetes mellitus who are started on atypical antipsychotics for worsening of glucose control. Patients with risk factors for diabetes mellitus (eg, obesity, family history of diabetes) who are starting treatment with atypical antipsychotics should undergo fasting blood glucose testing at baseline and periodically during treatment. Monitor any patient treated with atypical antipsychotics for symptoms of hyperglycemia, including polydipsia, polyuria, polyphagia, and weakness. Patients who develop symptoms of hyperglycemia during treatment with atypical antipsychotics should undergo fasting blood glucose testing. In some cases, hyperglycemia resolved when the atypical antipsychotic was discontinued; however, some patients required continuation of antidiabetic treatment despite discontinuation of the suspect drug.

➤*Antiemetic effects:* Drugs with an antiemetic effect can obscure signs of toxicity of other drugs (eg, cancer chemotherapeutic drugs) or mask symptoms of disease (eg, brain tumor, intestinal obstruction, Reye syndrome). They can suppress the cough reflex; aspiration of vomitus is possible.

Risperidone, **thiothixene**, **loxapine**, and **molindone** have an antiemetic effect in animals that may also occur in humans.

➤*Pulmonary:* Cases of bronchopneumonia (some fatal) have followed the use of antipsychotic agents. Lethargy and decreased sensation of thirst caused by central inhibition may lead to dehydration, hemoconcentration, and reduced pulmonary ventilation. If the above signs appear, especially in the elderly, institute remedial therapy promptly.

Use with caution in respiratory impairment caused by acute pulmonary infections or chronic respiratory disorders, such as severe asthma or emphysema. "Silent pneumonias" may develop in patients treated with **phenothiazines**.

➤*Agranulocytosis:* Agranulocytosis, defined as an absolute neutrophil count (ANC) of less than 500/mm^3, occurs in association with **clozapine** use at a cumulative incidence at 1 year of approximately 1.3%, based on 15 cases out of 1743 patients exposed to clozapine during clinical testing. All of these cases occurred when the need for close monitoring of WBC counts was already recognized. This reaction could prove fatal if not detected early and therapy interrupted. Of the 149 cases of agranulocytosis reported worldwide in association with clozapine use as of December 31, 1989, 32% were fatal. However, few of these deaths occurred since 1977, when knowledge of clozapine-induced agranulocytosis became more widespread, and close monitoring of WBC counts more widely practiced. In the United States, under a weekly WBC monitoring system with clozapine, there have been 585 cases of agranulocytosis as of August 21, 1997; 19 were fatal. During this period 150,409 patients received clozapine. The incidence rates of agranulocytosis based upon a weekly monitoring schedule, rose steeply during the first 2 months of therapy, peaking in the third month. Among clozapine patients who continued the drug beyond the third month, the weekly incidence of agranulocytosis fell to a substantial degree, so that by the sixth month, the weekly incidence of agranulocytosis was reduced to 3 per 1000 person-years. After 6 months, the weekly incidence of agranulocytosis declined still further, however, never reaching zero.

Patients must have a blood sample drawn for a WBC count before initiation of treatment with **clozapine**, and must have subsequent WBC counts done at least weekly for the first 6 months of treatment, as well as for 4 weeks after discontinuation. The distribution of clozapine is contingent upon performance of the required blood tests (see Administration and Dosage of individual monograph).

Except for evidence of significant bone marrow suppression during initial **clozapine** therapy, there are no established risk factors for the development of agranulocytosis. However, a disproportionate number of the US cases of agranulocytosis occurred in patients of Jewish background compared with the overall proportion of such patients exposed during clozapine's domestic development. Most of the US cases occurred within 4 to 10 weeks of exposure, but neither dose nor duration is a reliable predictor. No patient characteristics have been clearly linked to the development of agranulocytosis in association with clozapine use, but agranulocytosis associated with other antipsychotic drugs occurred with a greater frequency in women, the elderly, and in patients who are cachetic or have serious underlying medical illness; such patients may also be at particular risk with clozapine.

To reduce the risk of agranulocytosis developing undetected, **clozapine** will be dispensed only within the clozapine Patient Management System. For more information, call 1-800-448-5938.

➤*Ophthalmic effects:* As with all drugs that exert anticholinergic effect and/or cause mydriasis, use with caution in patients with a history of glaucoma. During prolonged therapy, ocular changes may occur; these include particle deposition in the cornea and lens, progressing in more severe cases to star-shaped lenticular opacities.

Pigmentary retinopathy – Careful observation should be made for pigmentary retinopathy and lenticular pigmentation (fine lenticular pigmentation has been noted in a small number of patients treated for prolonged periods. Pigmentary retinopathy, which has been observed primarily in patients taking larger than recommended thioridazine doses, is characterized by diminution of visual acuity, brownish coloring of vision, and impairment of night vision; examination of the fundus discloses deposits of pigment.

Cataracts – In dogs receiving **quetiapine** for 6 or 12 months, focal triangular cataracts occurred at the junction of the posterior sutures in the outer cortex of the lens at a dose of 4 times the maximum recommended human dose. The finding may be because of inhibition of cholesterol biosynthesis by quetiapine.

Lens changes have also been observed in patients during long-term treatment, but a causal relationship has not been established. Examination of the lens by methods adequate to detect cataract formation, such as slit-lamp exam, is recommended at initiation of treatment or shortly thereafter, and at 6-month intervals.

➤*Seizure disorders:* Some antipsychotics can lower the convulsive threshold and may precipitate seizures. Grand mal seizures have occurred, particularly in patients with EEG abnormalities or a history of such disorders. Use cautiously in patients with a history of epilepsy or those in a state of alcohol withdrawal. These drugs may be used concomitantly with anticonvulsants; maintain an adequate anticonvulsant dosage (see Drug Interactions).

Seizure has been estimated to occur in association with **clozapine** use at a cumulative incidence at 1 year of approximately 5%, based on the occurrence of 1 or more seizures during its clinical testing prior to domestic marketing. Dose appears to be an important predictor of seizure, with a greater likelihood of seizure at the higher clozapine doses used. Exercise caution in administering clozapine to patients having a history of seizures or other predisposing factors. Because of the substantial risk of seizure associated with clozapine use, advise patients not to engage in any activity where sudden loss of consciousness could cause serious risk to themselves or others.

➤*GI dysmotility:* Esophageal dysmotility and aspiration have been associated with antipsychotic drug use. Aspiration pneumonia is a common cause of morbidity and mortality in elderly patients, in particular those with advanced Alzheimer dementia. Use **quetiapine**, **ziprasidone**, **risperidone**, **olanzapine**, **aripiprazole**, and others cautiously in patients at risk for aspiration pneumonia.

➤*Increased mortality in elderly patients with dementia-related psychosis:* Elderly patients with dementia-related psychosis treated with atypical antipsychotic drugs are at an increased risk of death compared with placebo. Atypical antipsychotics are not approved for the treatment of patients with dementia-related psychosis (see Boxed WARNING).

➤*Hypersensitivity reactions:* Patients who have demonstrated a hypersensitivity reaction (eg, blood dyscrasias, jaundice) with a phenothiazine should not be re-exposed to any phenothiazine unless the potential benefits of treatment outweigh the possible hazards.

➤*Renal function impairment:* Administer cautiously to those with diminished renal function. Monitor renal function in long-term therapy; lower the dose or discontinue if BUN becomes abnormal.

➤*Hepatic function impairment:* Jaundice usually occurs between the second and fourth weeks of **phenothiazine** treatment and is regarded as a hypersensitivity reaction. The clinical picture resembles infectious hepatitis with laboratory features of obstructive jaundice. It is usually reversible; however, chronic jaundice has occurred. If fever with flu-like symptoms occurs, perform liver function tests. If tests are abnormal, discontinue treatment. Withhold exploratory laparotomy until extrahepatic obstruction is confirmed. Because of the possibility of liver damage, periodically monitor hepatic function. There is no conclusive evidence that preexisting liver disease makes patients more susceptible to jaundice. Alcoholics with cirrhosis have been successfully treated with **chlorpromazine** without complications. Nevertheless, use cautiously in patients with liver disease. Do not re-expose patients who have experienced jaundice to a **phenothiazine**.

Use with caution in patients with impaired hepatic function. Patients with a history of hepatic encephalopathy caused by cirrhosis have increased sensitivity to the CNS effects of antipsychotic drugs (eg, impaired cerebration and abnormal slowing of the EEG).

Elevations of serum transaminase and alkaline phosphatase, usually transient, have been infrequently observed in some patients. No clinically confirmed cases of jaundice attributable to **thiothixene** have been reported.

Caution is advised in patients using **clozapine** who have concurrent hepatic disease. Hepatitis has been reported in both patients with normal and preexisting liver function abnormalities. Immediately perform liver function tests in patients who develop nausea, vomiting, and/or anorexia during clozapine treatment. If the elevation of these values is clinically relevant or if symptoms of jaundice occur, discontinue clozapine treatment.

Patients with impaired hepatic function may have increases in the free fraction of **risperidone**, possibly resulting in an enhanced effect.

Six percent of **quetiapine** and 2% of **olanzapine** patients had transaminase elevations over 3 times the upper limit of normal. Hepatic enzyme elevations usually occurred within the first 3 weeks of quetiapine treatment and promptly returned to prestudy levels with ongoing treatment. Because quetiapine is extensively metabolized by the liver, higher plasma levels are expected in the hepatically impaired population and dosage adjustment may be needed.

➤*Carcinogenesis:* Antipsychotic drugs elevate prolactin levels, which persist during chronic use. Tissue culture experiments indicate approximately 33% of human breast cancers are prolactin-dependent in vitro, a factor of potential importance if use of these drugs is contemplated in a patient with previously detected breast cancer. Although disturbances such as galactorrhea, amenorrhea, gynecomastia, and impotence have occurred, clinical significance of elevated serum prolactin levels is unknown for most patients. An increase in mammary neoplasia has occurred in rodents after chronic neuroleptic use. Studies, however, have not shown an association between chronic use of these drugs and mammary tumorigenesis.

In mice, **pimozide** causes a dose-related increase in pituitary and mammary tumors.

In female mice at 5 to 20 times the highest initial daily dose of **haloperidol** for chronic or resistant patients, there was a statistically significant increase in mammary gland neoplasia and total tumor incidence; at 20 times the same daily dose there was a statistically significant increase in pituitary gland neoplasia. **Risperidone** administered to rats and mice at doses up to 10 mg/kg for up to 25 months produced statistically significant increases in pituitary gland adenomas, endocrine pancreas adenomas, and mammary gland adenocarcinomas.

The incidence of liver hemangiomas and hemangiosarcomas was significantly increased in 1 mouse study in female mice dosed at 8 mg/kg/day of **olanzapine**. The incidence of mammary gland adenomas and adenocarcinomas also was significantly increased in another study in rodents.

In female mice, the incidences of pituitary gland adenomas and mammary gland adenocarcinomas and adenoacanthomas were increased at dietary doses of 3 to 30 mg/kg/day of **aripiprazole**. The incidence of mammary gland fibroadenomas and adrenocortical carcinomas and combined adrenocortical adenomas/carcinomas also were increased in female rats.

Quetiapine was administered to rats and there were statistically significant increases in thyroid gland follicular adenomas, mammary gland adenomas, and thyroid follicular cell adenomas.

In female mice, there were dose-related increases in the incidences of pituitary gland adenoma and carcinoma, and mammary gland adenocarcinoma at doses of 50, 100, or 200 mg/kg/day of **ziprasidone** tested.

➤*Mutagenesis:* Abnormal sperm and chromosomal aberrations in spermatocytes have occurred in rodents treated with certain fandc-hcp10202.

Aripiprazole and a metabolite were clastogenic in the in vitro chromosomal aberration assay.

Quetiapine produced a reproducible increase in mutations in one *Salmonella typhimurium* tester strain in the presence of metabolic activation.

Ziprasidone produced a reproducible mutagenic response in the Ames assay in 1 strain of *S. typhimurium* in the absence of metabolic activation. Positive results were obtained in both the in vitro mammalian cell gene mutation assay and in the in vitro chromosomal aberration assay in human lymphocytes.

➤*Fertility impairment:* **Quetiapine** decreased mating and fertility in male rats at oral doses of 50 and 150 mg/kg and in female rats at oral doses of 50 mg/kg. An increase in irregular estrus cycles was observed at doses of 10 and 50 mg/kg.

Ziprasidone was shown to increase time to copulation in rats. Fertility rate was reduced at 160 mg/kg/day.

Estrus cycle irregularities and increased corpora lutea were seen at doses of 2, 6, and 20 mg/kg/day of **aripiprazole**. Increased preimplantation loss was seen at 6 and 20 mg/kg, and decreased fetal weight was seen at 20 mg/kg. Male rats had disturbances in spermatogenesis at 60 mg/kg, and prostate atrophy at 40 and 60 mg/kg, but no impairment of fertility was seen.

Risperidone was shown to impair mating, but not fertility, in female rats. In dogs given 0.31 to 5 mg/kg, sperm motility and concentration and serum testosterone were decreased.

Rats treated with **olanzapine** showed impaired male mating performance, but not fertility, at a dose of 22.4 mg/kg/day and female fertility was decreased at a dose of 3 mg/kg/day. Diestrous was prolonged and estrus delayed at 1.1 mg/kg/day; therefore, olanzapine may produce a delay in ovulation.

Female rats administered **pimozide** had prolonged estrus cycles, an effect also produced by other antipsychotics.

➤*Elderly:* Dosages in the lower range are sufficient for most elderly patients. Because these patients appear more susceptible to various cardiovascular, neuromuscular, and anticholinergic reactions, observe patients closely. The prevalence of tardive dyskinesia appears to be highest among the elderly, especially elderly women. Monitor response and adjust dosage accordingly. Increase dosage gradually in elderly patients.

➤*Pregnancy: Category C; Category B* (**clozapine**). Safety for use during pregnancy has not been established. Use only when clearly needed and when potential benefits outweigh potential hazards to the fetus.

There are reported instances of prolonged jaundice, extrapyramidal signs, hyperreflexia or hyporeflexia in newborn infants whose mothers received **phenothiazines**. **Prochlorperazine** is not recommended for use in pregnant patients except in cases of severe nausea and vomiting that are so serious and intractable that drug intervention is required and potential benefits outweigh possible hazards.

Reproductive studies of **chlorpromazine** in rodents have demonstrated potential for embryotoxicity and increased neonatal mortality. Tests in the offspring of the rodent demonstrate decreased performance. The possibility of permanent neurological damage cannot be excluded. It is not recommended that chlorpromazine be given to pregnant patients except when it is essential.

There are reports of cases of limb malformations observed following maternal use of **haloperidol**. Causal relationships were not established in these cases.

Perinatal studies have shown renal papillary abnormalities in offspring of rats treated from mid-pregnancy with **loxapine** doses of 0.6 to 1.8 mg/kg.

In the rat, doses of **pimozide** up to 8 times the maximum human dose resulted in decreased pregnancies and in the retarded development of fetuses. In the rabbit, maternal toxicity, mortality, decreased weight gain, and embryotoxicity including increased resorption were dose-related.

In animal studies, **ziprasidone** and **aripiprazole** demonstrated developmental toxicity, including possible teratogenic effects.

Placental transfer of **risperidone** occurs in rat pups and studies showed a decrease in the number of live pups and an increase in the number of dead pups at birth, and decrease in birth weight in pups. There was one report of a case of agenesis of the corpus callosum in an infant exposed to risperidone in utero. The causal relationship is unknown.

Placental transfer of **olanzapine** occurs in rat pups and studies showed early resorptions and increased numbers of nonviable fetuses.

Animal studies of **quetiapine** showed evidence of embryo/fetal toxicity including delays in skeletal ossification, reduced fetal body weights, increased incidence of a minor soft tissue anomaly, increases in fetal and pup death, and decreases in mean litter weight. Evidence of maternal toxicity was also observed at high doses.

Reproductive studies in animals and clinical experience to date have failed to show a teratogenic effect with **thioridazine**, **thiothixene**, **clozapine**, and **molindone**.

➤*Lactation:* There is evidence that **phenothiazines** are excreted in the breast milk of nursing mothers. Decide whether to discontinue nursing or discontinue the drug, taking into account the importance of the drug to the mother.

Animal studies suggest that **loxapine** (and its metabolites), **risperidone** (and its metabolites), **clozapine**, **olanzapine**, **quetiapine**, and **aripiprazole** may be excreted in breast milk. Risperidone also is excreted in human breast milk. Avoid nursing during loxapine therapy if possible. Women receiving risperidone, clozapine, olanzapine, quetiapine, or aripiprazole should not breastfeed.

Infants should not be nursed during **haloperidol** or **ziprasidone** treatment.

Because of the tumorigenicity and unknown cardiovascular effects in the infant, decide whether to discontinue nursing or discontinue **pimozide**, taking into account the importance of the drug to the mother.

➤*Children:* Children with acute illnesses (eg, chickenpox, CNS infections, measles, gastroenteritis) or dehydration are much more susceptible to neuromuscular reactions, particularly dystonias, than adults. Children seem more prone to develop extrapyramidal reactions, even at moderate doses. Therefore, use the lowest effective dosage.

Extrapyramidal symptoms can occur and be confused with CNS signs of an undiagnosed primary disease responsible for the vomiting (eg, Reye syndrome or other encephalopathy). Avoid antipsychotics and other potential hepatotoxins in children and adolescents whose signs and symptoms suggest Reye syndrome.

Safety and effectiveness of **fluphenazine**, **clozapine**, **haloperidol** (decanoate), **mesoridazine**, **loxapine**, **olanzapine**, **risperidone**, **aripiprazole**, **quetiapine**, and **ziprasidone** in pediatric patients have not been established.

Thiothixene, **perphenazine**, and **molindone** are not recommended in children under 12 years of age. Information on the use and efficacy of **pimozide** in patients less than 12 years of age is limited. **Trifluoperazine** is indicated for the treatment of schizophrenia in children 6 to 12 years of age. When treating children for severe nausea and vomiting, **prochlorperazine** should not to be used in children under 9 kg (20 lb) in weight or 2 years of age. **Chlorpromazine** should not be used in pediatric patients under 6 months of age except where potentially life-saving. Oral **haloperidol** is not intended for children under 3 years of age.

Precautions

➤*Anticholinergic effects:* Use caution in patients with clinically significant prostatic hypertrophy, narrow-angle glaucoma, or a history of paralytic ileus. Anticholinergic effects of **clozapine** are very potent. **Clozapine** use has been associated with varying degrees of impairment of intestinal peristalsis, ranging from constipation to intestinal obstruction, fecal impaction, and paralytic ileus. On rare occasions, these cases have been fatal. Constipation should be initially treated by ensuring adequate hydration, and use of ancillary therapy such as bulk laxatives. **Olanzapine** exhibits in vitro muscarinic receptor affinity and was associated with constipation, dry mouth, and tachycardia. **Thiothixene** and **chlorpromazine** exhibit rather weak anticholinergic properties. **Risperidone**, **aripiprazole**, **ziprasidone**, and **quetiapine** have no affinity for cholinergic muscarinic receptors.

➤*Cholesterol:* **Quetiapine**-treated patients had increases from baseline in cholesterol and triglyceride of 11% and 17%, respectively.

➤*Concomitant conditions:* Use with caution in patients: Exposed to extreme heat or phosphorus insecticides; atropine or related drugs because of additive anticholinergic effects; in a state of alcohol withdrawal; with dermatoses or other allergic reactions to phenothiazine derivatives because of the possibility of cross-sensitivity; who have exhibited idiosyncrasy to other centrally acting drugs. Risperidone has not been evaluated or used to any appreciable extent in patients with a recent history of MI or unstable heart disease; use with caution.

➤*Hematologic:* Various blood dyscrasias have occurred (see Adverse Reactions). In clinical trials, 1% of **clozapine** patients developed eosinophilia, which, in rare cases, can be substantial. If a differential count reveals a total eosinophil count above 4000/mm^3, clozapine therapy should be interrupted until eosinophil count falls below 3000/mm^3. If sore throat or other sign of infection occurs, or if white cell and differential counts indicate cellular depression, stop treatment and institute an antibiotic and other suitable therapy. A single case of transient granulocytopenia has been associated with **mesoridazine**. Patients with bone marrow depression with a phenothiazine should not receive any phenothiazines, unless the potential benefits outweigh the possible hazard.

Routine blood counts are advisable during therapy because blood dyscrasias, including leukopenia, agranulocytosis, thrombocytopenic or nonthrombocytopenic purpura, eosinophilia, and pancytopenia have been observed with phenothiazine derivatives.

➤*Myelography:* Discontinue phenothiazines at least 48 hours before myelography because of the possibility of seizures; do not resume therapy for at least 24 hours postprocedure. Do not use phenothiazines to control nausea and vomiting occurring before or after myelography.

➤*Thrombotic thrombocytopenic purpura (TTP):* A single case of TTP was reported in a 28-year-old female patient receiving **risperidone**. She experienced jaundice, fever, and bruising, but eventually recovered after receiving plasmapheresis. The relationship to therapy is unknown.

➤*Thyroid:* Severe neurotoxicity (rigidity, inability to walk or talk) may occur in patients with thyrotoxicosis who also are receiving antipsychotics.

Hypothyroidism – **Quetiapine** demonstrated a dose-related decrease in total and free thyroxine (T_4) of approximately 20% at the higher end of the therapeutic dose range that was maximal in the first 2 to 4 weeks of treatment and maintained without adaptation or progression during more chronic therapy. Generally, these changes were of no clinical significance and TSH and TBG were unchanged in most patients, but approximately 0.4% of quetiapine patients did experience TSH increases. Six of the patients with TSH increases needed replacement thyroid treatment.

➤*Hyperpyrexia:* A significant, not otherwise explained rise in body temperature may indicate intolerance to antipsychotics. Discontinue in this case. Disruption of the body's ability to reduce core body temperature has been attributed to antipsychotic agents. Appropriate care is advised for patients who will be experiencing conditions that may contribute to an elevation in core body temperature (eg, exercising strenuously, exposure to extreme heat, receiving concomitant medication with anticholinergic activity, being subject to dehydration). Heat stroke has been reported with **haloperidol** use.

During **clozapine** therapy, patients may experience transient temperature elevations above 100.4°F (38°C), with the peak incidence within the first 3 weeks of treatment. While this fever is generally benign and self-limiting, it may necessitate discontinuing patients from treatment. On occasion, there may be an associated increase or decrease in WBC count. Carefully evaluate patients with fever to rule out the possibility of an underlying infectious process or the development of agranulocytosis. In the presence of high fever, the possibility of NMS must be considered.

➤*Abrupt withdrawal:* These drugs are not known to cause psychic dependence. However, following abrupt withdrawal of high-dose therapy, symptoms such as gastritis, nausea, vomiting, dizziness, headache, restlessness, sweating, increased salivation, and insomnia have occurred. To lessen the likelihood of adverse reactions related to cumulative drug effects, periodically determine whether the maintenance dosage could be lowered or drug therapy discontinued. These symptoms can be reduced by gradual reduction of the dosage or by continuing antiparkinson agents for several weeks after the antipsychotic is withdrawn.

Some patients on **pimozide** or **haloperidol** maintenance treatment experience transient dyskinetic signs after abrupt withdrawal. This may be indistinguishable from the syndrome of persistent tardive dyskinesia except for duration. It is not known whether gradual withdrawal of antipsychotic drugs will reduce the rate of occurrence, but it seems reasonable to gradually withdraw use of the drug.

➤*Suicide:* Suicide remains a possibility in psychotic illnesses and bipolar disorder. Do not allow patients of this type to have access to large quantities of the drug.

➤*Cutaneous pigmentation changes:* Rare instances of skin pigmentation have occurred, primarily in females on long-term, high-dose phenothiazine therapy. These changes, restricted to exposed areas of the skin, range from almost imperceptible darkening to a slate gray color, sometimes with a violet hue. Pigmentation may fade following drug discontinuation.

➤*Phenylketonurics:* Inform phenylketonuric patients that some of these products contain phenylalanine.

➤*Benzyl alcohol:* Some of these products contain benzyl alcohol, which has been associated with a fatal "gasping syndrome" in premature infants.

➤*Drug abuse and dependence:* Evaluate patients for history of drug abuse, and observe such patients closely for signs of misuse or abuse (eg, development of tolerance, increases in dose, drug-seeking behavior).

➤*Photosensitivity:* Because photosensitivity has been reported (rarely with **thioridazine**), undue exposure to the sun should be avoided during phenothiazine treatment.

➤*Sulfite sensitivity:* Some of these products contain sulfites that may cause allergic-type reactions, including anaphylactic symptoms and life-threatening or less severe asthmatic episodes in certain susceptible persons. The overall prevalence of sulfite sensitivity in the general population is unknown and probably low. It is seen more frequently in asthmatic or atopic nonasthmatic persons.

Drug Interactions

➤*CYP450:* Several antipsychotics are metabolized by the cytochrome P450 (CYP450) enzyme system. Therefore, several drug interactions may be possible involving drugs that are potent inhibitors or inducers of this enzyme system. Monitor and adjust therapy as needed when these antipsychotics are coadministered with potent inhibitors or inducers of the following isoenzymes.

Antipsychotics and Enzymes Involved with Metabolism

Antipsychotic agent	Enzyme(s)
Aripiprazole	CYP3A4, 2D6
Clozapine	CYP1A2, 2D6, 3A4
Olanzapine	CYP1A2, 2D6
Perphenazine	CYP2D6
Pimozide	CYP3A, 1A2
Quetiapine	CYP3A4
Risperidone	CYP2D6
Thioridazine	CYP2D6
Ziprasidone	Aldehyde oxidase, CYP3A4, 1A2

Antipsychotic Contraindications

Antipsychotic	Contraindicated with
Clozapine	Drugs having a well-known potential to cause agranulocytosis or suppress bone marrow function.
Phenothiazines	Cisapride, sparfloxacin (because of possible additive QT interval prolongation.
Mesoridazine Ziprasidone	Drugs that prolong the QT interval.[a]
Pimozide	Drugs that prolong the QT interval;[a] CYP3A inhibitors (eg, clarithromycin, dirithromycin, erythromycin, itraconazole, ketoconazole, nefazodone, protease inhibitors, sertraline, telithromycin troleandomycin, voriconazole).
Thioridazine	Drugs that prolong the QT interval;[a] CYP2D6 inhibitors (eg, fluoxetine, fluvoxamine, paroxetine, pindolol, propranolol).

[a] The following drugs may prolong the QT interval and increase the risk of life-threatening cardiac arrhythmias, including torsade de pointes: Antiarrhythmic agents (eg, amiodarone, bretylium, disopyramide, dofetilide, procainamide, quinidine, sotalol), arsenic trioxide, chlorpromazine, cisapride, dolasetron mesylate, droperidol, gatifloxacin, halofantrine, levomethadyl acetate, mefloquine, mesoridazine, moxifloxacin, pentamidine, pimozide, probucol, sparfloxacin, tacrolimus, thioridazine, ziprasidone.

Antipsychotic Drug Interactions

Precipitant drug	Object drug*		Description
Anticholinergic agents	Haloperidol	⬇	Decreased serum concentrations of haloperidol, worsening schizophrenic symptoms, and tardive dyskinesia have been reported with coadministration. Coadminister with caution.
Anticholinergic agents	Phenothiazines	⬆⬇	Therapeutic effects of phenothiazines may be decreased by centrally acting anticholinergics. Coadministration may lead to an increase in anticholinergic effects. Coadminister with caution.
Phenothiazines	Anticholinergic agents		
Antipsychotic agents	Alcohol CNS depressants	⬆	Coadministration may lead to enhanced CNS depression, especially impairment of motor skills. Dystonic reactions may be precipitated by alcohol. Avoid concurrent use or use with caution.
Antipsychotic agents	Antihypertensive agents	⬆	May enhance the effects of antihypertensive agents. Antipsychotics produce alpha-adrenergic blockage and may potentiate orthostatic hypotension.
Antipsychotic agents	Dopamine Epinephrine	⬇	For the treatment of antipsychotic-induced hypotension, do not use epinephrine, dopamine, or other sympathomimetics with beta-agonist activity because beta stimulation may worsen the hypotension caused by the antipsychotic-induced alpha blockade.
Azole antifungal agents	Haloperidol	⬆	Haloperidol plasma concentrations may be elevated, increasing risk of side effects with coadministration. Adjust dose of haloperidol as needed.
Beta-blockers (eg, pindolol, propranolol)	Phenothiazines (eg, thioridazine, chlorpromazine)	⬆	Coadministration may lead to increased effects from either or both drugs, including increased risk of life-threatening arrhythmias with thioridazine. Thioridazine is contraindicated in patients taking pindolol or propranolol.
Phenothiazines (eg, thioridazine, chlorpromazine)	Beta-blockers (eg, pindolol, propranolol)		
Caffeine	Clozapine	⬆	Plasma levels of clozapine may be increased, resulting in increased adverse effects. Avoid caffeine if interaction is suspected.
Carbamazepine	Aripiprazole Olanzapine Risperidone Ziprasidone	⬇	The antipsychotic plasma concentrations may be decreased, resulting in decreased therapeutic effect. Adjust antipsychotic dose as needed. When carbamazepine is added to aripiprazole therapy, double the aripiprazole dose.
Carbamazepine	Haloperidol	⬇	Therapeutic effects of haloperidol may be decreased. Adjust dose of therapy as needed.
Haloperidol	Carbamazepine	⬆	
Charcoal	Antipsychotics	⬇	Charcoal can decrease the absorption of antipsychotics, reducing their effectiveness or toxicity.
Cimetidine	Quetiapine	⬆	Cimetidine decreased quetiapine oral clearance 20%.
Citalopram Fluoxetine Fluvoxamine Sertraline	Clozapine	⬆	Plasma levels of clozapine may be increased, resulting in increased pharmacologic and toxic effects. Adjust clozapine dose as needed when starting or stopping certain SSRIs.
Clozapine Loxapine	Benzodiazepines	⬆	Cases of orthostatic hypotension, collapse, respiratory arrest, and cardiac arrest have been reported with concomitant use of certain benzodiazepines. Coadminister with caution.
Clozapine	Risperidone	⬆	Chronic administration of clozapine with risperidone may decrease risperidone clearance.
CYP1A2 inducers (eg, carbamazepine, omeprazole, rifampin)	Clozapine Olanzapine	⬇	May decrease clozapine or olanzapine serum concentrations. May need dosage increase for olanzapine. Carbamazepine increased olanzapine clearance 50%.
CYP1A2 inhibitors (eg, fluvoxamine)	Clozapine Olanzapine	⬆	May increase clozapine or olanzapine serum concentrations. Dose reduction may be needed. Fluvoxamine decreased olanzapine clearance, resulting in a mean increase in C_{max} of 54% in female nonsmokers and 77% in male smokers; AUC increased 52% and 108%, respectively.
CYP3A4 inhibitors (eg, ketoconazole)	Aripiprazole Clozapine Quetiapine Ziprasidone	⬆	The plasma concentrations of the antipsychotic may be increased. Reduce aripiprazole dose 50% with coadministration of ketoconazole, then increase the aripiprazole dose when the CYP3A4 inhibitor is withdrawn.
Famotidine	Aripiprazole	⬇	Coadministration of a single dose of aripiprazole and famotidine resulted in decreased aripiprazole solubility and, therefore, decreased its rate of absorption, C_{max}, and AUC.
Fluoxetine	Haloperidol	⬆	Coadministration has been associated with an increase in haloperidol concentrations. Severe extrapyramidal reactions also have been reported.
Fluoxetine	Olanzapine	⬆	Coadministration resulted in a small (approximately 16%) increase in C_{max} and decrease in olanzapine clearance.
Fluoxetine Paroxetine	Risperidone	⬆	Risperidone concentrations may be elevated, increasing the risk of adverse effects. Fluoxetine increased risperidone plasma levels 2.5- to 2.8-fold. Adjust risperidone dose as needed.
Haloperidol	Lithium	⬆	Alterations in consciousness, encephalopathy, extrapyramidal effects, fever, leukocytosis, and increased serum enzymes have occurred with coadministration. Monitor coadministration closely and discontinue either drug if interaction is suspected.
Lithium	Haloperidol		
Meperidine	Phenothiazines	⬆	Excessive sedation and hypotension may occur with coadministration. Coadministration not recommended.
Phenothiazines	Meperidine		
Olanzapine Quetiapine Risperidone Ziprasidone	Levodopa and dopamine agonists	⬇	May antagonize the effects of levodopa and dopamine agonists.

Antipsychotic Drug Interactions

Precipitant drug	Object drug*		Description
Paroxetine	Phenothiazines	↑	Phenothiazine plasma levels may be increased, increasing the pharmacologic and adverse effects of these agents. Thioridazine is contraindicated. Adjust other phenothiazine doses as needed.
Phenobarbital	Clozapine	↓	Plasma levels of clozapine may be decreased, resulting in decreased pharmacologic effects.
Phenothiazines	Guanethidine	↓	Hypotensive effect of guanethidine is inhibited. Use alternate antihypertensive therapy if blood pressure is uncontrolled.
Phenothiazines	Oral anticoagulants	↓	Phenothiazines may diminish oral anticoagulant effects.
Phenothiazines	Phenytoin	↑↓	Phenothiazines have been reported to increase or decrease phenytoin levels. Monitor phenytoin levels.
Phenothiazines	Thiazide diuretics	↑	Coadministration may potentiate orthostatic hypotension.
Thiazide diuretics	Phenothiazines		
Prochlorperazine	Dofetilide	↑	Elevated dofetilide concentrations may occur with increased risk of ventricular arrhythmia, including torsade de pointes. It is not recommended to use prochlorperazine in patients receiving dofetilide.
Quetiapine	Lorazepam	↑	Lorazepam mean oral clearance was reduced 20% with coadministration.
Quinidine	Aripiprazole	↑	Coadministration increased aripiprazole AUC 112% and decreased the AUC of the active metabolite 35%. Reduce aripiprazole dose 50% with coadministration.
Rifamycins	Haloperidol	↓	Rifamycins may decrease the plasma concentration and therapeutic effects of haloperidol. Adjust haloperidol as needed.
Phenytoin	Quetiapine	↓	Quetiapine plasma levels may be decreased, resulting in decreased pharmacologic effects. Adjust quetiapine dose as needed.
Risperidone	Clozapine	↑	Pharmacologic and adverse effects of clozapine may be increased. Adjust dose as needed.
Risperidone	Valproate	↑	Coadministration resulted in a 20% increase in valproate C_{max}. Adjust therapy as needed.
Ritonavir	Clozapine Perphenazine Risperidone Thioridazine	↑	Increases in serum antipsychotic concentrations may occur, increasing risk of toxicity.
Thioridazine	Quetiapine	↓	Thioridazine increased quetiapine oral clearance 65%.
Valproate	Aripiprazole	↓	Aripiprazole C_{max} and AUC were decreased 25% with coadministration.

↑ = Object drug increased. ↓ = Object drug decreased.

➤*Drug/Lab test interactions:* Phenothiazines may produce false-positive phenylketonuria (PKU) test results. Phenothiazines may cause false-positive pregnancy test results.

➤*Drug/Food interactions:* Grapefruit juice may inhibit the metabolism of **pimozide** via CYP3A. Food slows the absorption of oral **prochlorperazine** and decreases C_{max} 23% and AUC 13%.

Adverse Reactions

Antipsychotic Adverse Reactions[a] (%)

		Conventional Antipsychotics												Atypical Antipsychotics					
	Adverse reactions	Chlorpromazine	Fluphenazine	Haloperidol	Loxapine	Mesoridazine	Molindone	Perphenazine	Pimozide	Prochlorperazine	Thioridazine	Thiothixene	Trifluoperazine	Aripiprazole	Clozapine	Olanzapine	Quetiapine	Risperidone	Ziprasidone, oral (IM)
Cardiovascular	Angina pectoris													0.1-1	1		< 0.1	< 0.1	0.1-1
	Atrial contractions, premature/ atrial fibrillation/flutter													0.1-1	✓	< 0.1	< 0.1	< 0.1	0.1-1
	AV block													0.1-1			< 0.1	0.1-1	< 0.1
	Bradycardia							✓						> 1	✓	0.1-1	0.1-1		0.1-1 (≤ 2)
	Cardiac arrest	✓						✓		✓	Rare	✓	✓	0.1-1		0.1-1			
	Cerebral vascular accident													0.1-1		0.1-1	0.1-1	✓	< 0.1
	CHF													0.1-1	✓	0.1-1	< 0.1		
	ECG changes	✓	✓	✓	✓	✓	✓	✓	✓	✓	✓	✓	✓		1				✓
	Hypertension		✓	✓	✓			✓	✓					2	4	2	✓	0.1-1	> 1 (≤ 2)
	Hypotension	✓	Rare	✓	✓[b]	✓	Rare	✓	✓[b]	✓[c]	✓	✓	✓[c]	> 1	9	3-5[b]	7[b]	0.1-1	1[b] (≤ 5)
	MI													0.1-1	✓			0.1-1	
	Palpitation								✓					0.1-1		0.1-1	> 1	0.1-1	
	Phlebitis													0.1-1	✓			< 0.1	< 0.1
	QTc interval prolongation			✓		✓			✓		✓			0.1-1			0.1-1		✓
	Pulmonary embolus													< 0.1	✓	< 0.1		✓	< 0.1
	Q- and T-wave distortions	✓								✓			✓						
	T-wave flattening					✓			✓		✓				✓		0.1-1		
	T-wave inversion					✓			✓		✓				✓		0.1-1	< 0.1	
	Tachycardia	✓	✓	✓	✓		✓[d]	✓	✓			✓		> 1	25	3	7	3-5	2
	Thrombophlebitis, including deep													< 0.1	✓		0.1-1		< 0.1
	Twitch													0.1-1	✓		0.1-1		
	Vasodilation													0.1-1		0.1-1	0.1-1		(≤ 1)
CNS	Accommodation abnormality															0.1-1	< 0.1	0.1-1	
	Agitation	✓		✓	✓	✓				✓	✓	✓	✓	25	4			22-26	> 1 (≤ 2)
	Akathisia		✓	✓	Freq	✓	✓	✓	40	✓	✓	✓	✓	15-17	3	3			8 (≤ 2)
	Akinesia				✓	✓	✓		40		✓			0.1-1	4	< 0.1			> 1
	Amnesia													0.1-1	✓	0.1-1	0.1-1	0.1-1	> 1
	Anxiety			✓										20	1			12-20	(≤ 2)
	Apathy													0.1-1			0.1-1	0.1-1	
	Asthenia								45					8		10-15	4		5 (≤ 2)
	Ataxia					✓		✓						0.1-1	1	0.1-1	0.1-1		> 1
	Catatonic-like states	Rare	✓	✓				✓		✓			✓				0.1-1	0.1-1	
	Confusion			✓	✓	✓		✓[e]			Rare[e]			> 1	3		0.1-1	0.1-1	> 1
	Convulsions[f]	✓		✓	✓			✓	✓	✓		Infreq	✓		3				
	Delirium													0.1-1	✓	0.1-1	< 0.1	< 0.1	> 1
	Depression			✓			✓		10					> 1	1			0.1-1	
	Dizziness	✓			✓	✓		✓	✓	✓			✓		19	11-18	10	4-7	8 (3-10)
	Dreams, abnormal/ bizarre/increased		✓			✓		✓	3		✓			≥ 1	✓	> 1	0.1-1	≥ 1	
	Drowsiness/sedation/ somnolence	✓	✓	✓	✓	✓	✓	✓	25-70	✓	✓	✓	✓	7.5-15.3	39-46	29-35	18	3-8	14 (8-20)
	Dysarthria													0.1-1	✓	0.1-1	> 1	0.1-1	> 1
	Dyskinesia		✓					✓	✓	✓			✓	0.1-1		≤ 2	0.1-1		> 1
	Dystonia	✓	✓	✓		✓	✓	✓	✓	✓	✓	✓	✓	0.1-1		2-3			4
	Euphoria			✓			✓							< 0.1		> 1	< 0.1	0.1-1	
	Excitement		✓			✓		✓	✓		✓								
	Extrapyramidal symptoms	✓	✓	Freq	Freq	✓	✓	✓	Freq	✓	Infreq	✓	✓	6			✓	17-34	5 (≤ 2)
	Fainting/Faintness	✓			✓	✓		✓	✓										
	Fatigue												✓		2			> 1	
	Gait abnormal													> 1		6	0.1-1		> 1
	Gait, staggering/shuffling	✓			✓					✓			✓						
	Hallucinations			✓										≥ 1	✓		0.1-1		
	Headache		✓	✓	✓			✓	5-22	✓	Rare		✓	31	7		19	12-14	(3-13)
	Hostility													> 1			✓		> 1

Antipsychotic Adverse Reactions[a] (%)																			
		Conventional Antipsychotics												Atypical Antipsychotics					
	Adverse reactions	Chlorpromazine	Fluphenazine	Haloperidol	Loxapine	Mesoridazine	Molindone	Perphenazine	Pimozide	Prochlorperazine	Thioridazine	Thiothixene	Trifluoperazine	Aripiprazole	Clozapine	Olanzapine	Quetiapine	Risperidone	Ziprasidone, oral (IM)
CNS (cont.)	Hyperactivity						✓	✓			Rare			0.1-1					
	Hyperkinesia								6					0.1-1	1		0.1-1		> 1
	Hyperreflexia		✓					✓	✓	✓		✓	✓	0.1-1				< 0.1	< 0.1
	Hypesthesia													0.1-1		0.1-1		< 0.1	> 1
	Hypokinesia													0.1-1	4	0.1-1			> 1
	Incoordination													< 0.1		0.1-1	0.1-1		> 1
	Insomnia	✓		✓	✓			✓	10	✓		✓	✓	20	2	12	✓	23-26	< 3
	Jitteriness	✓								✓			✓						
	Lethargy		✓	✓				✓			Rare				1				
	Libido, increased		✓[g]	✓			✓							0.1-1	✓	0.1-1	0.1-1	0.1-1	
	Libido decreased/loss of							✓	✓					0.1-1	✓		< 0.1	≥ 5	
	Lightheadedness				✓							✓		11					
	Malaise													0.1-1		0.1-1	0.1-1	0.1-1	
	Migraine													0.1-1		0.1-1	0.1-1	< 0.1	
	Motor restlessness (EPS)	✓				✓	✓	✓	✓	✓	✓		✓						
	Nervousness													> 1			✓	≥ 1	
	Neuroleptic malignant syndrome (NMS)	✓	✓	✓	Freq	✓		✓	✓	✓	✓	✓	✓			✓			
	Neuropathy													0.1-1		< 0.1			> 1
	Paresthesia				✓									0.1-1		> 1	✓	0.1-1	> 1 (≤ 2)
	Pseudoparkinsonism	✓	✓	✓	✓	✓	✓	✓	✓	✓	Infreq	✓	✓		< 1	✓		✓	
	Psychosis	Rare	✓	✓		✓		✓		✓	Rare	Infreq	✓	✓	✓		0.1-1		(≤ 1)
	Restlessness		✓	✓		✓		✓			Rare	✓			4				
	Speech slurred				✓	✓		✓							1				
	Suicide attempt/thought													0.1-1/ < 1		> 1	0.1-1		
	Stupor													0.1-1			0.1-1	0.1-1	
	Syncope				✓							✓			6				
	Tardive dyskinesia	✓	✓	✓	✓	✓	✓	✓	✓	✓	✓	✓	✓	0.1-1		0.1-1	0.1-1		> 1
	Tardive dystonia	✓		✓						✓				4-9					
	Tremor	✓			✓	✓	✓		1	✓	✓		✓		6	4-6	✓		> 1
	Trismus	✓				✓		✓		✓	✓		✓						< 0.1
	Vertigo			✓										0.1-1	19	0.1-1	0.1-1	0.1-1	> 1
	Weakness				✓	✓						✓	✓		1				
Dermatologic	Acne			✓										0.1-1		0.1-1	0.1-1	0.1-1	
	Alopecia			✓	✓									0.1-1		0.1-1		0.1-1	0.1-1
	Dermatitis	✓[h,i]	✓[h]		✓	✓[h,i]		✓[h,i]		✓[h]	Infreq[h,i]		✓	< 0.1[h]	✓	0.1-1	0.1-1	0.1-1	0.1-2[h,i,j]
	Ecchymosis													> 1	✓	5	0.1-1		0.1-1
	Eczema		✓					✓		✓			✓	0.1-1	✓	0.1-1	0.1-1	2-4	0.1-1
	Erythema		✓			✓		✓		✓	✓		✓		✓				
	Maculopapular skin reactions			✓										< 0.1		0.1-1	✓		0.1-1
	Pallor							✓			✓			0.1-1		0.1-1		< 0.1	
	Photosensitivity	✓	✓	✓				✓		✓	Rare	✓	✓	0.1-1	✓	0.1-1	0.1-1	> 1	> 1
	Pruritus		✓		✓	✓		✓		✓		✓	✓	0.1-1		0.1-1	0.1-1	0.1-1	
	Psoriasis													0.1-1			< 0.1	< 0.1	
	Purpura, thrombocytopenic	✓	✓					✓		✓			✓						
	Rash				✓	✓	✓		8			✓	✓	✓	2		4	2-5	4
	Rash, vesiculobullous													0.1-1		0.1-1			0.1-1
	Seborrhea		✓		✓									0.1-1		0.1-1	0.1-1	≤ 1	
	Skin pigmentation changes	✓	✓			✓		✓		✓	✓		✓						
	Urticaria		✓					✓		✓	Infreq	✓	✓	< 0.1	✓	< 0.1		< 0.1	0.1-1

Antipsychotic Adverse Reactions[a] (%)																			
		Conventional Antipsychotics												Atypical Antipsychotics					
	Adverse reactions	Chlorpromazine	Fluphenazine	Haloperidol	Loxapine	Mesoridazine	Molindone	Perphenazine	Pimozide	Prochlorperazine	Thioridazine	Thiothixene	Trifluoperazine	Aripiprazole	Clozapine	Olanzapine	Quetiapine	Risperidone	Ziprasidone, oral (IM)
GI	Abdominal discomfort/pain													✓	4		3	1-4	> 1 (≤ 2)
	Abdominal distention/ enlargement													0.1-1		0.1-1	< 0.1	< 0.1	
	Adynamic ileus	✓						✓		✓		✓	✓						
	Anorexia		✓	✓		✓		✓	✓		✓	✓	✓	✓	1		> 1	> 1	2 (≤ 2)
	Appetite increased	✓						✓	5	✓		✓	✓	0.1-1	✓	3-6	0.1-1	0.1-1	
	Atonic colon	✓								✓			✓						
	Constipation	✓	✓	✓	✓	✓	✓	✓	20	✓	✓	Infreq	✓	13	14	9-11	9	7-13	9 (≤ 2)
	Diarrhea			✓				✓	5		✓	✓		✓	2		✓	≥ 5	5 (≤ 3)
	Diverticulitis																	< 0.1	
	Drooling	✓								✓			✓						
	Dry mouth	✓	✓	✓	✓	✓	✓	✓	25	✓	✓	Infreq	✓	✓	6	9-22	7	≥ 5	4 (≤ 1)
	Dyspepsia			✓										15	14	7-11	6	5-10	8 (1-3)
	Dysphagia	✓						✓	3	✓			✓	0.1-1	✓	0.1-1	0.1-1	0.1-1	0.1-1
	Eructation													0.1-1	✓	0.1-1		< 0.1	
	Esophageal ulcer/esophagitis													< 0.1		< 0.1		< 0.1	
	Fecal impaction		✓					✓						0.1-1	✓	0.1-1			< 0.1
	Flatulence													0.1-1		0.1-1	0.1-1	0.1-1	
	Gastritis													0.1-1		0.1-1	0.1-1	0.1-1	
	Gastroenteritis													0.1-1	✓	0.1-1	0.1-1	< 0.1	
	Gastroesophageal reflux													0.1-1	4		0.1-1	< 0.1	
	Gingivitis													0.1-1		0.1-1	0.1-1	< 0.1	
	Glossitis													< 0.1		< 0.1	< 0.1		
	Gum hemorrhage													< 0.1			0.1-1		< 0.1
	Hematemesis													< 0.1	✓		< 0.1	< 0.1	< 0.1
	Hemorrhoids													0.1-1			0.1-1	0.1-1	
	Incontinence, fecal													0.1-1		0.1-1	0.1-1	< 0.1	
	Intestinal obstruction													0.1-1	✓	< 0.1	< 0.1	✓	
	Melena													< 0.1		0.1-1	0.1-1	0.1-1	< 0.1
	Mouth ulceration													0.1-1		0.1-1	0.1-1		
	Nausea	✓	✓	✓	✓	✓	✓	✓	✓	✓	✓	✓	✓	16	5	0.1-1	✓	4-6	10 (4-12)
	Obstipation	✓				✓		✓		✓	✓		✓						
	Paralytic ileus		✓		✓	✓					✓					< 0.1			
	Polydipsia				✓				5			✓	✓	0.1-1		> 1	0.1-1	> 1	0.1-1 (≤ 2)
	Rectal hemorrhage													0.1-1	✓	0.1-1	0.1-1		< 2
	Salivation		✓	✓	✓		✓	✓	14			Infreq		3	31	> 1	0.1-1	≤ 2	✓
	Stomatitis													0.1-1		0.1-1	0.1-1	0.1-1	0.1-1
	Taste altered								5					0.1-1			0.1-1		
	Tongue discoloration															< 0.1		< 0.1	
	Tongue protrusion	✓	✓					✓		✓			✓						
	Tooth caries													0.1-1		0.1-1	0.1-1		
	Vomiting			✓	✓	✓		✓	✓		✓	✓	✓	11	3	4	✓	5-7	> 1 (< 3)
	Weight gain	✓			✓	✓	✓	✓	✓	✓	✓	✓	✓	3 8[k]	4	5-6	2	18	10[k]
	Weight loss				✓		✓		✓					> 1	✓		0.1-1	0.1-1	

Antipsychotic Adverse Reactions[a] (%)

		Conventional Antipsychotics												Atypical Antipsychotics					
	Adverse reactions	Chlorpromazine	Fluphenazine	Haloperidol	Loxapine	Mesoridazine	Molindone	Perphenazine	Pimozide	Prochlorperazine	Thioridazine	Thiothixene	Trifluoperazine	Aripiprazole	Clozapine	Olanzapine	Quetiapine	Risperidone	Ziprasidone, oral (IM)
GU	Albuminuria													0.1-1		< 0.1			0.1-1
	Amenorrhea	✓			Rare		Infreq	✓		✓	✓	✓	✓	0.1-1		> 1	0.1-1	0.1-1	0.1-1
	Breast engorgement	✓		✓				✓			✓								
	Dysmenorrhea													✓	✓		0.1-1	0.1-1	(≤ 2)
	Ejaculation disorders	✓				✓		✓		✓	✓		✓	0.1-1	1	0.1-1	0.1-1	≥ 5	0.1-1
	Galactorrhea	✓	✓	✓	Rare	✓	Infreq	✓		✓	✓	✓	✓			0.1-1	0.1-1	0.1-1	0.1-1
	Glycosuria	✓						✓		✓		✓	✓	< 0.1		0.1-1	< 0.1		0.1-1
	Gynecomastia	✓	✓	✓	Rare	✓	Infreq	✓		✓	✓	✓	✓	0.1-1		< 0.1	< 0.1	< 0.1	< 0.1
	Hematuria													0.1-1		> 1		0.1-1	0.1-1
	Impotence	✓	✓	✓		✓			15	✓		Infreq	✓	0.1-1	✓	0.1-1	0.1-1	≥ 5	0.1-1
	Incontinence, urinary					✓		✓			✓			> 1		2	0.1-1	0.1-1	
	Mastalgia			✓										0.1-1	✓	0.1-1		0.1-1	
	Menorrhagia						✓							< 0.1		0.1-1		≥ 5	0.1-1
	Menstrual irregularities		✓	✓	Rare	✓		✓		✓	✓		✓						
	Metrorrhagia															> 1	0.1-1		0.1-1
	Nocturia								✓					< 0.1			< 0.1		< 0.1
	Polyuria		✓					✓						< 0.1		0.1-1	< 0.1	> 1	0.1-1
	Priapism	✓		✓		✓	✓			✓	✓		✓	< 0.1	✓	0.1-1			(≤ 1)
	Renal failure, acute		✓											0.1-1			< 0.1		
	Urinary frequency/ urgency increased							✓	✓					0.1-1	1	0.1-1	0.1-1		
	Urinary retention	✓		✓	✓	✓	✓	✓		✓	✓		✓	0.1-1	1	0.1-1	0.1-1	> 1	0.1-1
	Vaginal hemorrhage													0.1-1		0.1-1	0.1-1	0.1-1	< 0.1
Hematologic/Lymphatic	Agranulocytosis	✓	✓	Rare	Rare	✓		✓		✓	✓		✓		1				
	Anemia			✓		✓					✓			> 1	✓	0.1-1	0.1-1	0.1-1	0.1-1
	Anemia, aplastic	✓				✓				✓	✓		✓						
	Anemia, hemolytic	✓						✓	✓	✓			✓						
	Anemia, hypochromic													0.1-1			0.1-1	0.1-1	< 0.1
	Blood dyscrasias		✓					✓		✓			✓						
	Eosinophilia	✓	✓			✓		✓		✓	✓		✓	< 0.1	1		0.1-1		0.1-1
	Hemorrhage													0.1-1		0.1-1		< 0.1	
	Hypercholesterolemia													0.1-1		0.1-1	✓		0.1-1
	Hyperglycemia	✓		✓				✓		✓		✓	✓	0.1-1	✓	0.1-1	0.1-1	✓	0.1-1
	Hyperkalemia													0.1-1		< 0.1			< 0.1
	Hyperlipemia													0.1-1		0.1-1	0.1-1		< 0.1
	Hyperuricemia													0.1-1	✓				< 0.1
	Hypoglycemia	✓		✓				✓		✓		✓	✓	0.1-1		0.1-1	0.1-1	< 0.1	< 0.1
	Hypokalemia													0.1-1		0.1-1	< 0.1	< 0.1	0.1-1
	Hyponatremia			✓					✓					0.1-1	✓	0.1-1		0.1-1	< 0.1
	Hypoproteinemia															< 0.1		< 0.1	< 0.1
	Leukocytosis		✓	✓			Rare					✓		0.1-1	✓	0.1-1	0.1-1	< 0.1	0.1-1
	Leukopenia	✓	✓	✓	Rare	✓	Rare	✓		✓	✓	✓	✓	0.1-1	3	> 1	> 1	< 0.1	0.1-1
	Lymphadenopathy													0.1-1		0.1-1	0.1-1		0.1-1
	Pancytopenia	✓	✓					✓		✓	✓		✓						< 0.1
	Thrombocythemia													< 0.1	✓	0.1-1			< 0.1
	Thrombocytopenia				Rare	✓					✓			< 0.1	✓	0.1-1	< 0.1		< 0.1
Hepatic	ALT/AST elevation				✓							Infreq		0.1-1			✓	0.1-1	0.1-1
	Biliary stasis					✓		✓		✓	✓		✓						
	Cholecystitis													0.1-1				< 0.1	
	Cholelithiasis													0.1-1	✓			< 0.1	
	Hepatitis				Rare									< 0.1	✓	0.1-1		< 0.1	< 0.1
	Jaundice	✓	✓[l]	✓	Rare	✓		✓		✓[l]	✓		✓		✓			✓	< 0.1[l]
	Liver function impaired		✓	✓			Rare	✓		✓			✓		1				

Antipsychotic Adverse Reactions[a] (%)

	Adverse reactions	Conventional Antipsychotics												Atypical Antipsychotics					
		Chlorpromazine	Fluphenazine	Haloperidol	Loxapine	Mesoridazine	Molindone	Perphenazine	Pimozide	Prochlorperazine	Thioridazine	Thiothixene	Trifluoperazine	Aripiprazole	Clozapine	Olanzapine	Quetiapine	Risperidone	Ziprasidone, oral (IM)
Hypersensitivity	Allergic reaction	✓								✓			✓	✓	✓	✓		< 0.1	
	Anaphylactoid reactions	✓	✓					✓		✓		Rare	✓			✓		✓	
Lab Test Abn.	Alkaline phosphatase increased											Infreq		0.1-1		0.1-1	0.1-1		0.1-1
	Cerebrospinal fluid proteins abnormality	✓	✓					✓		✓		✓	✓						
	CPK elevated		✓											> 1	✓				0.1-1
	Creatinine increased													0.1-1			0.1-1	0.1-1	< 0.1
Metabolic/Nutritional	Edema, cerebral	✓	✓					Rare		✓		✓	✓						
	Cyanosis													0.1-1	✓	0.1-1	0.1-1		
	Edema					✓					✓			0.1-1	✓			0.1-1	
	Edema, angioneurotic	✓	✓			✓		✓		✓	✓		✓						
	Edema, facial				✓									0.1-1		0.1-1	0.1-1		> 1
	Edema, laryngeal	✓	✓			✓		✓		✓	✓		✓						
	Edema, peripheral	✓	✓					✓		✓	✓	✓	✓	2		3	> 1		0.1-1
	Edema, tongue													0.1-1		0.1-1	0.1-1	< 0.1	0.1-1
Musculoskeletal	Arthralgia/Joint pain													0.1-1	✓	5	0.1-1	2-3	✓
	Arthritis													0.1-1		0.1-1	0.1-1	< 0.1	
	Bone pain													0.1-1		< 0.1	0.1-1		
	Bursitis													0.1-1		0.1-1		< 0.1	
	Muscle rigidity		✓			✓	✓		15	✓	✓				✓				
	Muscle weakness							✓					✓	0.1-1	1		0.1-1		
	Myalgia								3					4	1		✓	0.1-1	1
	Myoclonus				✓									0.1-1	1		0.1-1		< 0.1
	Myopathy													0.1-1		< 0.1			< 0.1
	Opisthotonos	✓	✓	✓		✓		✓	✓	✓	✓		✓						< 0.1
	Rigidity					✓			10						5			0.1-1	
	Spasm, carpopedal	✓								✓	✓		✓						
	Spasm of neck muscles	✓			✓					✓	✓		✓						
	Torticollis	✓				✓		✓	3	✓	✓		✓					< 0.1	< 0.1
Respiratory	Apnea													< 0.1		0.1-1		✓	
	Asphyxia	✓						✓		✓		✓	✓						
	Aspiration														✓			< 0.1	
	Asthma	✓	✓			✓		✓		✓	✓		✓	≥ 1		0.1-1	0.1-1	< 0.1	
	Cough, increased													3	✓	6	> 1	3	3
	Cough reflex failure	✓						✓		✓		✓	✓						
	Dyspnea				✓									> 1	1	> 1	> 1	≤ 1	> 1
	Epistaxis													0.1-1	✓	0.1-1	0.1-1	0.1-1	0.1-1
	Hemoptysis													< 0.1		0.1-1			< 0.1
	Hyperventilation														✓		< 0.1	0.1-1	
	Nasal congestion	✓	✓		✓	✓		✓		✓	✓	Infreq	✓		1				
	Pharyngitis													4		4	> 1	2-3	
	Pneumonia													> 1	✓	0.1-1	0.1-1	0.1-1	0.1-1
	Rhinitis													4		7	3	8-10	4 (≤ 1)

Antipsychotic Adverse Reactions[a] (%)

		Conventional Antipsychotics												Atypical Antipsychotics					
	Adverse reactions	Chlorpromazine	Fluphenazine	Haloperidol	Loxapine	Mesoridazine	Molindone	Perphenazine	Pimozide	Prochlorperazine	Thioridazine	Thiothixene	Trifluoperazine	Aripiprazole	Clozapine	Olanzapine	Quetiapine	Risperidone	Ziprasidone, oral (IM)
Special senses	Blepharitis													0.1-1		0.1-1	0.1-1	< 0.1	0.1-1
	Cataracts			✓					✓					0.1-1		0.1-1			0.1-1
	Conjunctivitis													> 1	✓	> 1	0.1-1		0.1-1
	Diplopia													< 0.1		0.1-1		< 0.1	> 1
	Dry eyes													0.1-1		0.1-1	0.1-1		0.1-1
	Epithelial keratopathy	✓						✓		✓			✓						
	Eye hemorrhage													0.1-1		0.1-1			< 0.1
	Glaucoma		✓					✓							✓[m]	< 0.1	< 0.1		
	Lenticular/corneal opacities	✓	✓			✓		✓		✓	✓		✓						
	Miosis	✓				✓		✓		✓	✓	✓	✓			< 0.1			
	Mydriasis	✓						✓		✓		✓	✓			< 0.1			
	Oculogyric crisis	✓	✓	✓	✓			✓	✓	✓	✓		✓	< 0.1					> 1
	Parotid swelling					p		Rare			Rare				✓				
	Photophobia					✓		✓						< 0.1				< 0.1	0.1-1
	Pigmentary retinopathy	✓						✓		✓			✓						
	Tinnitus													0.1-1		0.1-1	0.1-1		0.1-1
	Vision abnormal																0.1-1	1-2	3
	Vision blurred		✓	✓	✓	✓	✓	✓	✓	✓	✓	Infreq	✓	3					
	Visual disturbances			✓											5				
Miscellaneous	Accidental injury													6		12	✓		4
	Back pain													✓	1	5	2	≤ 2	(≤ 1)
	Chest pain								✓					> 1	1	3	✓	2-3	
	Chills													0.1-1	✓	0.1-1	0.1-1		> 1
	Choreoathetosis																< 0.1	< 0.1	> 1
	Cogwheel rigidity	✓								✓			✓	0.1-1		0.1-1			> 1 (≤ 1)
	Dehydration													≥ 1		0.1-1	0.1-1	< 0.1	0.1-1
	Diaphoresis		✓	✓				✓	✓			Infreq		> 1	6	> 1	> 1	0.1-1	(≤ 2)
	Fever	✓				✓		✓		✓	✓		✓	≥ 1	5	6	2	2-3	> 1
	Flu syndrome													> 1		> 1	> 1	0.1-1	> 1 (≤ 1)
	Gout													< 0.1		< 0.1	< 0.1		< 0.1
	Hyperpyrexia/Hyperthermia	✓	✓	✓	✓	✓		✓	✓	✓	✓	✓	✓						
	Hyperthyroidism													< 0.1			< 0.1		< 0.1
	Hypertonia													✓		3	> 1		3
	Hypothyroidism													0.1-1			0.1-1		< 0.1
	Hypotonia													< 0.1		0.1-1		< 0.1	> 1
	Mask-like faces	✓								✓			✓						
	Moniliasis															0.1-1	0.1-1		
	Neck pain/rigidity													> 1	1	0.1-1	0.1-1		
	Pain, pelvic													≥ 1		0.1-1	0.1-1		
	Pillrolling motion	✓								✓			✓						
	Ptosis				✓														
	Sudden death	✓	✓	✓		✓		Rare	✓	✓	✓	✓	✓		✓	< 0.1		< 0.1	
	Systemic lupus erythematosus-like syndrome	✓	✓			✓		✓		✓	✓		✓						
	Thyroiditis															0.1-1		< 0.1	< 0.1
	Withdrawal syndrome			✓					✓							1		< 0.1	> 1

✓ = Occurs; incidence unknown.
[a] Data are pooled from separate trials and are not necessarily comparable.
[b] Includes orthostatic.
[c] Sometimes fatal.
[d] Especially with sudden marked increase in dosage.
[e] Nocturnal confusion.
[f] Includes petit and grand mal seizures.
[g] In women.
[h] Exfoliative dermatitis included.
[i] Contact dermatitis included.
[j] Fungal dermatitis.
[k] Gained at least 7% body weight.
[l] Includes cholestatic.
[m] Narrow-angle glaucoma.

➤*Other adverse reactions:*

Chlorpromazine: Ocular changes; back muscle rigidity; shock-like reaction.

Fluphenazine: Altered EEG tracings; nonthrombocytopenic purpura; appetite decreased; weight change; local tissue reactions (rare).

Loxapine: Flushed face; numbness; tension.

Mesoridazine: Hypertrophic papillae of tongue; incontinence.

Molindone: Menses resumption; blood glucose alteration; BUN alteration; RBC alteration; thyroid function alteration.

Perphenazine: Pulse-rate change; paranoid reaction; polyphagia; throat tight; ocular changes; inappropriate ADH secretion; limb ache/numbness; shock-like reaction; hypnotic effects; tongue ache; tongue rounding; circulatory collapse (rare).

Pimozide: Adverse behavior effect (5% to 10%); sensitivity of eyes to light (5%); accommodation decrease (4%); speech disorder, stooped posture (2%); gingival hyperplasia, handwriting change (1%); skin irritation; GI distress; tonic spasm; transient dyskinetic signs; periorbital edema; T-wave notching; U-wave appearance.

Thioridazine: Arrhythmias; torsade de pointes-type arrhythmias; autonomic instability; blood glucose alteration; conjunctiva pigmentation; cornea discoloration; altered mental status; paradoxical reaction; irregular pulse; sclera discoloration; altered libido; U-wave appearance; skin eruption (infrequent).

Trifluoperazine: Skin reaction; back muscle rigidity; heat prolongation/intensification.

Haloperidol: BP fluctuations; torsade de pointes-type arrhythmias; hyperammonemia (postmarketing); lymphomonocytosis; RBC count decreased; bronchospasm; laryngospasm; respiration depth increased; retinopathy; heat stroke; local tissue reactions; transient dyskinetic signs.

Atypicals –

Aripiprazole: Ear pain (0.1% to 1%), manic reaction, muscle cramp, dry skin, skin ulcer (at least 1%); deep vein thrombosis, concentration impaired, bloating, periodontal abscess, cystitis, uterine hemorrhage (less than 0.1%), bilirubinemia, increased BUN, increased lactic dehydrogenase (less than 0.1%), jaw pain/tightness, depersonalization, diabetes mellitus, iron deficiency anemia, bradykinesia, chest tightness, colitis, dysphoria, dysuria, extrasystoles, eye pain, hiccough, hypersomnia, GI hemorrhage, kidney calculus, laryngitis, leukorrhea, impaired memory, myocardial ischemia, obesity, otitis media, panic attack, peptic ulcer (less than 0.1%), restless leg, spasm, thinking slowed, vaginal moniliasis; hyperesthesia, arthrosis (0.1% to 1); cardiomegaly, throat tight, anorgasmia, hepatomegaly, amblyopia, increased lacrimation, tenosynovitis, heat stroke, increased sputum, cerebral ischemia, deafness, macrocytic anemia (0.1% to 1%), aspiration pneumonia (0.1% to 1%), increased blinking, blunted affect, cervicitis, cheilitis, decreased consciousness, duodenal ulcer, pulmonary edema, goiter, head heaviness, intracranial hemorrhage, hypernatremia, hypoxia, Mendelson syndrome, dry nasal passages, obsessive thought, otitis externa, pancreatitis, decreased reflexes, respiratory failure, rhabdomyolysis, rheumatoid arthritis, tendonitis, throat pain (0.1% to 1%), urinary burning (0.1% to 1%), urolithiasis, vasovagal reaction buccoglossal syndrome (less than 0.1%); oral moniliasis (0.1% to 1%); upper respiratory infection; dental pain; QT interval shortened; vaginitis.

Clozapine: Arrhythmias, cardiomyopathy, deep vein thrombosis, ST-depression, aphasia, altered EEG tracings, GI distress, hypothermia, periorbital edema, delusions, amentia, bitter taste, bronchitis, mild cataplexy, chills with fever, cholestasis, poor coordination, ear disorder, epileptiform movements, erythema multiforme, increased ESR, eyelid disorder, bloodshot eyes, gastric ulcer, granulocytopenia, elevated hematocrit, elevated hemoglobin, histrionic movements, hot flashes, acute interstitial nephritis, involuntary movements, irritability, ischemic changes, laryngitis, impaired memory, numbness, overdose, acute pancreatitis, pericardial effusions, pericarditis, petechiae, pleural effusion, pneumonia-like symptoms, premature ventricular contraction, rhabdomyolysis, rhinorrhea, sepsis, shakiness, sneezing, status epilepticus, Stevens-Johnson syndrome, stuttering, abnormal stools, dry throat, throat pain/discomfort, tics, tongue numb/sore, vaginal infections/itch, vasculitis, ventricular fibrillation, wheezing, nightmares, sleep disturbance (4%); neutropenia, WBC decreased (3%); urinary abnormalities (2%); incontinence, cardiac abnormality, leg pain (1%).

Olanzapine: Personality disorder (8%); extremity pain (not joint) (5%); amblyopia (3%); articulation impaired, UTI (2%); angioedema, dental pain, intentional injury (at least 1%); antisocial reaction, CNS stimulation, arthrosis, voice alteration, laryngitis, obsessive compulsive symptoms, phobias, tobacco misuse (0.1% to 1%); normocytic anemia, arteritis, fatty liver deposits, keratoconjunctivitis, nystagmus, ketosis, hangover effect, encephalopathy, hiccough, hyperventilation, hypoxia, lung edema, stridor, breast pain, cystitis, uterine fibroids (less than 0.1%); aphthous stomatitis, enteritis, periodontal abscess, acidosis, bilirubinemia, atelectasis, alcohol misuse, coma (rare).

Quetiapine: UTI, infection, pain, ear pain, dry skin, increased triglycerides (1%); bundle branch block, paranoid reaction, cystitis, vulvovaginitis, leg cramps, increased GGT, alcohol intolerance, bruxism, cerebral ischemia, delusions, depersonalization, diabetes mellitus, dysuria, eye pain, hemiplegia, involuntary movements, leukorrhea, manic reaction, orchitis, pathological fracture, irregular pulse, QRS duration, skin ulcer, abnormal thinking, vaginitis (0.1% to 1%); aphasia, emotional lability, deafness, hand edema, hemolysis, hiccough, neuralgia, neutropenia, skin discoloration, ST abnormality, ST elevated, stuttering, subdural hematoma, T-wave abnormality, water intoxication (less than 0.1%).

Risperidone: Lymphedema (8%); upper respiratory infection (3%); angioedema, cerebral vascular disorder, aggressive reaction (1% to 3%); toothache, sinusitis (2% or less); hyperpigmentation (at least 1%); concentration impaired, hyperkeratosis, nonthrombocytopenic purpura, skin exfoliation, bronchospasm, stridor, xerophthalmia (0.1% to 1%); myocarditis, ST-depression, cholinergic syndrome, emotional lability, nightmares, bullous eruption, furunculosis, hypertrichosis, skin ulceration, verruca, feces discoloration, GI hemorrhage, tongue paralysis, genital pruritus, normocytic anemia, ascites, yawning, eye pain, abnormal lacrimation, photopsia, arthrosis, leg cramps, cachexia, coma, increased sputum, sarcoidosis (less than 0.1%).

Ziprasidone: Injection site pain (7% to 9%); respiratory disorder (8%); personality disorder, speech disorder, furunculosis (2% or less); hypotonia, buccoglossal syndrome, accidental fall, hypothermia, motor vehicle accident, flank pain, hypertonia (at least 1%); tooth disorder (less than 1%); cerebral infarct, polycythemia, anorgasmia, male sex dysfunction, tenosynovitis, increased lactic dehydrogenase (0.1% to 1%); bundle branch block, cardiomegaly, myocarditis, keratitis, leukoplakia of the mouth, female sex dysfunction, uterine hemorrhage, basophilia, hypocalcemia, hypochloremia, hypocholesterolemia, lymphedema, lymphocytosis, monocytosis, fatty liver deposits, hepatomegaly, laryngismus, respiratory alkalosis, keratoconjunctivitis, nystagmus, visual field defect, increased BUN, increased GGT, decreased glucose tolerance, ketosis, cerebral infarct, hyperchloremia, oliguria (less than 0.1%).

Overdosage

➤*Symptoms:* CNS depression to the point of somnolence, deep sleep from which patient cannot be aroused, or coma. Hypotension and extrapyramidal symptoms may occur. Other manifestations include: Agitation; restlessness; convulsions; fever; hypothermia; hyperthermia; coma; autonomic reactions; ECG changes; cardiac arrhythmias; tachycardia; hypertension; vomiting; NMS; slurred speech; delirium; respiratory depression or failure; seizures; renal failure (**loxapine**); dry mouth; salivation; ileus; hyperpyrexia; dilated or constricted pupils; cardiac arrest; death.

Other symptoms temporally related to risperidone overdose include torsade de pointes, prolonged QT interval, and cardiopulmonary arrest.

➤*Treatment:* Includes usual supportive measures. Refer to General Management of Acute Overdosage. In case of acute overdosage, establish and maintain an airway and ensure adequate oxygenation and ventilation. Establish IV access and consider gastric lavage (after intubation, if patient is unconscious) and administration of activated charcoal. The possibility of obtundation, seizure, or dystonic reaction of the head and neck following overdose may create a risk of aspiration with induced emesis. Cardiovascular monitoring should commence immediately and include continuous ECG monitoring to detect possible arrhythmias. Treat extrapyramidal symptoms with anticholinergic drugs or diphenhydramine (see Adverse Reactions).

If hypotension occurs, initiate the standard measures for managing circulatory shock, including volume replacement. If a vasoconstrictor is desired, use norepinephrine or phenylephrine. Do not administer epinephrine, dopamine, or other sympathomimetics with beta-agonist activity, because beta stimulation may worsen hypotension of drug-induced alpha blockade (eg, **olanzapine**, **quetiapine**, **risperidone**, **ziprasidone**; see Drug Interactions).

Disopyramide, procainamide, and quinidine carry a theoretical hazard of QT-prolonging effects when administered in patients with acute overdosing. Similarly, it is reasonable to expect that the alpha-adrenergic blocking properties of bretylium might be additive, resulting in problematic hypertension.

Limited experience indicates antipsychotic drugs are not dialyzable.

Because of the long half-life of **pimozide**, patients should be observed for at least 4 days. Additional surveillance after overdosage of **clozapine** and **thioridazine** should be continued for several days because of the risk for delayed effects.

Patient Information

Because some patients exposed chronically to antipsychotics will develop tardive dyskinesia, inform all patients in whom chronic use is contemplated, if possible, about this risk. The decision to inform patients or their guardians must obviously take into account the clinical circumstances and the patient's competence to understand the information (see Warnings).

May cause impaired judgment, thinking, or motor skills; use caution while driving or performing other tasks requiring alertness. Avoid alcohol and other CNS depressants because of possible additive effects and hypotension.

Avoid skin contact with injection and oral concentrates (contact dermatitis may occur). Oral concentrates are most conveniently used when diluted in fruit juices or other liquids. Use immediately after dilution. See individual products for specific guidelines.

Photosensitivity may occur with some antipsychotics. Avoid exposure to ultraviolet light or sunlight. Use sunscreen and protective clothing until tolerance is determined.

Advise patients of the risk of orthostatic hypotension, especially during the period of initial dose titration.

Use caution in hot weather. These drugs may increase susceptibility to heat stroke. Avoid overheating and dehydration.

Notify physician if sore throat, fever, skin rash, impaired vision, tremors, involuntary muscle twitching, muscle stiffness, or jaundice occurs.

Patients should notify their physician if they become pregnant or intend to become pregnant during therapy.

Patients should notify their physician if they are taking, or plan to take, any prescription or over-the-counter drugs or alcohol.

Advise patients not to breastfeed if they are taking **clozapine**, **olanzapine**, **loxapine**, **risperidone**, **aripiprazole**, **ziprasidone**, **haloperidol**, or **quetiapine**. Safety of the typical antipsychotics in the breastfeeding mother has not been established.

False-positive pregnancy tests have occurred with some **phenothiazines** but are less likely to occur when a serum test is used.

Warn patients who are to receive **clozapine** about the significant risk of developing agranulocytosis and that frequent blood tests are required. Patients should report immediately the appearance of lethargy, weakness, fever, sore throat, malaise, mucous membrane ulceration, or other possible signs of infection. Inform patients of the significant risk of seizures during clozapine treatment. Inform patients that if they stop taking clozapine for more than 2 days, they should not restart their medication at the same dosage, but should contact their physician for dosing instructions.

CHLORPROMAZINE HYDROCHLORIDE

Rx	**Chlorpromazine HCl** (Various, eg, Geneva, Major)	**Tablets:** 10 mg	In 100s, 1000s, and UD 100s.
Rx	**Chlorpromazine HCl** (Various, eg, Geneva, Major)	**Tablets:** 25 mg	In 100s, 1000s, and UD 100s.
Rx	**Thorazine** (GlaxoSmithKline)		Lactose, parabens. (SKF T74). Orange. In 100s.
Rx	**Chlorpromazine HCl** (Various, eg, Geneva, Major)	**Tablets:** 50 mg	In 100s, 1000s, and UD 100s.
Rx	**Thorazine** (GlaxoSmithKline)		Lactose, parabens. (SKF T76). Orange. In 100s.
Rx	**Chlorpromazine HCl** (Various, eg, Geneva, Major)	**Tablets:** 100 mg	In 100s, 1000s, and UD 100s.
Rx	**Thorazine** (GlaxoSmithKline)		Lactose, parabens. (SKF T77). Orange. In 100s.
Rx	**Chlorpromazine HCl** (Various, eg, Geneva, Major)	**Tablets:** 200 mg	In 100s, 1000s, and UD 100s.
Rx	**Thorazine** (GlaxoSmithKline)		Lactose, parabens. (SKF T79). Orange. In 100s.
Rx	**Chlorpromazine HCl** (Various, eg, Alpharma)	**Oral concentrate:** 100 mg/mL	May contain parabens, sulfites, sorbitol, and saccharin. In 237 mL with calibrated dropper graduated in 25 mg increments.
Rx	**Thorazine** (GlaxoSmithKline)	**Suppositories (as base):** 100 mg	In 12s.
Rx	**Chlorpromazine HCl** (Various, eg, Elkins-Sinn)	**Injection:** 25 mg/mL	In 1 and 2 mL amps.[a]
Rx	**Thorazine** (GlaxoSmithKline)		In 1 and 2 mL amps.[b]

[a] With sodium metabisulfite and sodium sulfite.
[b] With sodium bisulfite and sodium sulfite.

CHLORPROMAZINE — ORAL

Complete and comparative prescribing information begins in the Antipsychotic Agents group monograph. Also see the Antiemetic/Antivertigo Agents monograph.

Indications

➤*Emesis / Hiccoughs:* For the control of nausea and vomiting and relief of intractable hiccoughs (see Antiemetic/Antivertigo Agents).

➤*Manic-depressive illness:* For the control of manifestations of the manic type of manic-depressive illness.

➤*Porphyria, acute intermittent:* For the treatment of acute intermittent porphyria.

➤*Schizophrenia:* For the treatment of schizophrenia.

➤*Surgery:* For the relief of restlessness and apprehension prior to surgery.

➤*Behavioral problems:* For the treatment of severe behavioral problems in children 1 to 12 years of age marked by combativeness and/or explosive hyperexcitable behavior (out of proportion to immediate provocations).

➤*Hyperactivity:* For the short-term treatment of hyperactive children who show excessive motor activity with accompanying conduct disorders consisting of some or all of the following symptoms: Impulsivity, difficulty sustaining attention, aggressiveness, mood lability, and poor frustration tolerance.

Administration and Dosage

➤*Approved by the FDA:* April 27, 1983.

Individualize dosage based on condition severity. Increase dosage until symptoms are controlled, then gradually reduce dosage to the lowest effective maintenance level. Increase parenteral dosage only if hypotension has not occurred.

➤*Oral concentrate:* Add desired dosage to 60 mL or more of diluent just prior to administration. Suggested vehicles are tomato or fruit juice, milk, simple syrup, orange syrup, carbonated beverages, coffee, tea, or water. Semisolid foods (eg, soups, puddings) may also be used.

➤*Nausea and vomiting:*

Adults –
Oral: 10 to 25 mg every 4 to 6 hours, as needed; increase if necessary.

Children – Do not use in children < 6 months of age except where potentially lifesaving. Do not use in conditions for which specific children's dosages have not been established. The activity following IM use may last 12 hours.

Oral – 0.25 mg/lb (0.55 mg/kg) every 4 to 6 hours, as needed.

➤*Intractable hiccoughs:*

Adults – Orally, 25 to 50 mg 3 or 4 times daily. If symptoms persist for 2 to 3 days, give 25 to 50 mg IM. Should symptoms persist, use slow IV infusion with patient flat in bed. Administer 25 to 50 mg in 500 to 1000 ml of saline. Monitor blood pressure.

➤*Psychotic disorders:* Maximum improvement may not be seen for weeks or even months. Continue optimum dosage for 2 weeks, then gradually reduce to lowest effective maintenance level; 200 mg/day is not unusual. Some patients require higher dosages (eg, 800 mg/day is not uncommon in discharged mental patients).

Hospitalized patients –
Acute schizophrenic or manic states:
• *Less acutely disturbed –*
Oral: 25 mg 3 times/day. Increase gradually until effective dose is reached, usually 400 mg/day.

Outpatients –
Oral: Initial oral dose is 10 mg 3 or 4 times/day or 25 mg 2 or 3 times/day.

More severe cases –
Oral: Give 25 mg 3 times/day. After 1 or 2 days, daily dosage may be increased by 20 to 50 mg at semiweekly intervals until patient becomes calm and cooperative.

➤*Behavioral disorders / Hyperactivity:* Generally, do not use chlorpromazine in children younger than 6 months of age except where potentially lifesaving. It should not be used in conditions for which specific children's dosages have not been established.

Outpatients –
Oral: 0.5 mg/kg (0.25 mg/lb) every 4 to 6 hours, as needed.

Hospitalized patients –
Oral: Start with low doses and increase gradually. In severe behavior disorders, 50 to 100 mg/day, or in older children, 200 mg/day or more may be necessary. There is little evidence that improvement in severely disturbed mentally retarded patients is enhanced by doses beyond 500 mg/day.

➤*Surgery:*

Adults –
Preoperative apprehension: 25 to 50 mg orally 2 to 3 hours before surgery.

Children –
Preoperative apprehension: 0.5 mg/kg (0.25 mg/lb) orally 2 to 3 hours before operation.

➤*Acute intermittent porphyria (adults):* 25 to 50 mg orally 3 or 4 times/day.

➤*Elderly / Debilitated / Emaciated:* Lower initial doses and more gradual adjustments are recommended.

➤*Storage / Stability:* Store between 15° and 30°C (59° to 86°F). The oral concentrate is light sensitive; protect from light and dispense in amber glass bottle. Refrigeration is not required.

CHLORPROMAZINE — RECTAL

Complete and comparative prescribing information begins in the Antipsychotic Agents group monograph. Also see the Antiemetic/Antivertigo Agents monograph.

Indications

➤*Emesis:* For the control of nausea and vomiting (see Antiemetic/Antivertigo Agents).

➤*Manic-depressive illness:* For the control of manifestations of the manic type of manic-depressive illness.

➤*Schizophrenia:* For the treatment of schizophrenia.

➤*Behavioral problems:* For the treatment of severe behavioral problems in children 1 to 12 years of age marked by combativeness and/or explosive hyperexcitable behavior (out of proportion to immediate provocations).

➤*Hyperactivity:* For the short-term treatment of hyperactive children who show excessive motor activity with accompanying conduct disorders consisting of some or all of the following symptoms: Impulsivity, difficulty sustaining attention, aggressiveness, mood lability, and poor frustration tolerance.

Administration and Dosage

Individualize dosage based on condition severity. Increase dosage until symptoms are controlled, then gradually reduce dosage to the lowest effective maintenance level. Increase parenteral dosage only if hypotension has not occurred.

➤*Nausea and vomiting:*

Adults –
Rectal: 50 to 100 mg every 6 to 8 hours, as needed.

CHLORPROMAZINE — RECTAL

Children – Do not use in children < 6 months of age except where potentially lifesaving. Do not use in conditions for which specific children's dosages have not been established. The activity following IM use may last 12 hours.

Rectal: 0.5 mg/lb (1.1 mg/kg) every 6 to 8 hours, as needed.

➤*Behavioral disorders/Hyperactivity:* Generally, do not use chlorpromazine in children younger than 6 months of age except where potentially lifesaving. It should not be used in conditions for which specific children's dosages have not been established.

Outpatients –

Rectal: 1 mg/kg (0.5 mg/lb) every 6 to 8 hours, as needed.

➤*Elderly/Debilitated/Emaciated:* Lower initial doses and more gradual adjustments are recommended.

➤*Storage/Stability:* Store between 15° and 30°C (59° and 86°F).

CHLORPROMAZINE — INJECTION

Complete and comparative prescribing information begins in the Antipsychotic Agents group monograph. Also see the Antiemetic/Antivertigo Agents monograph.

Indications

➤*Emesis/Hiccoughs:* For the control of nausea and vomiting and relief of intractable hiccoughs.

➤*Manic-depressive illness:* For the control of manifestations of the manic type of manic-depressive illness.

➤*Porphyria, acute intermittent:* For the treatment of acute intermittent porphyria.

➤*Schizophrenia:* For the treatment of schizophrenia.

➤*Surgery:* For the relief of restlessness and apprehension prior to surgery.

➤*Tetanus:* An adjunct in treatment of tetanus.

➤*Behavioral problems:* For the treatment of severe behavioral problems in children 1 to 12 years of age marked by combativeness and/or explosive hyperexcitable behavior (out of proportion to immediate provocations).

➤*Hyperactivity:* For the short-term treatment of hyperactive children who show excessive motor activity with accompanying conduct disorders consisting of some or all of the following symptoms: Impulsivity, difficulty sustaining attention, aggressiveness, mood lability, and poor frustration tolerance.

Administration and Dosage

Individualize dosage based on condition severity. Increase dosage until symptoms are controlled, then gradually reduce dosage to the lowest effective maintenance level. Increase parenteral dosage only if hypotension has not occurred.

➤*Injection:* SC is not advised. Inject IM slowly, deep into upper outer quadrant of buttock. Because of possible hypotensive effects, reserve for bedfast patients or for acute ambulatory cases and keep patient recumbent for at least ½ hour after injection. If irritation is a problem, dilute injection with saline or 2% procaine; do not mix with other agents in the syringe. Avoid injecting undiluted into vein. Use the IV route only for severe hiccoughs, surgery, and tetanus. Slight yellowing will not alter potency. Discard if markedly discolored.

Because of the possibility of contact dermatitis, avoid getting solution on hands or clothing.

➤*Nausea and vomiting:*

Adults –

IM: 25 mg. If no hypotension occurs, give 25 to 50 mg every 3 to 4 hours, as needed, until vomiting stops. Then switch to oral dosage.

Children – Do not use in children < 6 months of age except where potentially lifesaving. Do not use in conditions for which specific children's dosages have not been established. The activity following IM use may last 12 hours.

IM: 0.25 mg/lb (0.55 mg/kg) every 6 to 8 hours, as needed.

Maximum IM dosage: Children up to 5 years of age — 40 mg/day.

Children 5 to 12 years of age — 75 mg/day, except in severe cases.

➤*Intractable hiccoughs:*

Adults – Orally, 25 to 50 mg 3 or 4 times daily. If symptoms persist for 2 to 3 days, give 25 to 50 mg IM. Should symptoms persist, use slow IV infusion with patient flat in bed. Administer 25 to 50 mg in 500 to 1000 ml of saline. Monitor blood pressure.

➤*Psychotic disorders:* Maximum improvement may not be seen for weeks or even months. Continue optimum dosage for 2 weeks, then gradually reduce to lowest effective maintenance level; 200 mg/day is not unusual. Some patients require higher dosages (eg, 800 mg/day is not uncommon in discharged mental patients).

Hospitalized patients –

Acute schizophrenic or manic states:

• *IM* – 25 mg initially. If necessary, give an additional 25 to 50 mg injection in 1 hour. Increase gradually over several days (up to 400 mg every 4 to 6 hours in exceptionally severe cases) until patient is controlled. Patient usually becomes quiet and cooperative within 24 to 48 hours. Substitute oral dosage and increase until the patient is calm; 500 mg/day is usually sufficient. While gradual increases to 2000 mg or more/day may be necessary, little therapeutic gain is achieved by exceeding 1000 mg/day for extended periods.

Prompt control of severe symptoms –

IM: 25 mg; if necessary, repeat in 1 hour. Give subsequent doses orally, 25 to 50 mg 3 times/day.

➤*Behavioral disorders/Hyperactivity:* Generally, do not use chlorpromazine in children younger than 6 months of age except where potentially lifesaving. It should not be used in conditions for which specific children's dosages have not been established.

Outpatients –

IM: 0.5 mg/kg (0.25 mg/lb) every 6 to 8 hours, as needed.

Hospitalized patients –

IM:

• *5 years of age or younger or 50 lbs* – Do not exceed 40 mg/day.

• *5 to 12 years of age or 50 to 100 lbs* – Do not exceed 75 mg/day, except in unmanageable cases.

➤*Surgery:*

Adults –

Preoperative apprehension: 12.5 to 25 mg IM 1 to 2 hours before surgery.

Intraoperative (to control acute nausea/vomiting):

• *IM* – 12.5 mg. Repeat in ½ hour if necessary and if no hypotension occurs.

• *IV* – 2 mg per fractional injection at 2-minute intervals. Do not exceed 25 mg (dilute 1 mg/mL with saline).

Children –

Preoperative apprehension: 0.5 mg/kg (0.25 mg/lb) IM 1 to 2 hours before operation.

Intraoperative (to control acute nausea/vomiting):

• *IM* – 0.25 mg/kg (0.125 mg/lb); repeat in ½ hour if needed and if no hypotension occurs.

• *IV* – 1 mg per fractional injection at 2-minute intervals; do not exceed IM dosage. Always dilute to 1 mg/mL with saline.

➤*Tetanus:*

Adults – 25 to 50 mg IM 3 or 4 times/day, usually with barbiturates. For IV use, 25 to 50 mg diluted to at least 1 mg/mL and administered at a rate of 1 mg/min.

Children – 0.5 mg/kg (0.25 mg/lb) IM or IV every 6 to 8 hours. When given IV, dilute to at least 1 mg/mL and administer at a rate of 1 mg per 2 minutes. In children up to 23 kg (50 lbs), do not exceed 40 mg/day; 23 to 45 kg (50 to 100 lbs), do not exceed 75 mg/day, except in severe cases.

➤*Acute intermittent porphyria (adults):* 25 mg IM 3 or 4 times/day until patient can take oral therapy.

➤*Elderly/Debilitated/Emaciated:* Lower initial doses and more gradual adjustments are recommended.

➤*Storage/Stability:* Store between 15° and 30°C (59° and 86°F). Protect the injection solution from light.

FLUPHENAZINE

Rx	**Fluphenazine HCl** (Various, eg, Geneva)	**Tablets:** 1 mg	In 50s, 100s, 500s, 1000s, and UD 100s.
Rx	**Fluphenazine HCl** (Various, eg, Geneva)	**Tablets:** 2.5 mg	In 50s, 100s, 500s, 1000s, and UD 100s.
Rx	**Fluphenazine HCl** (Various, eg, Geneva)	**Tablets:** 5 mg	In 50s, 100s, 500s, 1000s, and UD 100s.
Rx	**Fluphenazine HCl** (Various, eg, Geneva, Par)	**Tablets:** 10 mg	In 50s, 100s, 500s, 1000s, and UD 100s.
Rx	**Fluphenazine HCl** (Various, eg, Pharmaceuticals Associates)	**Elixir:** 2.5 mg/5 mL	May contain 14% alcohol and sucrose. In 60 and 473 mL.
Rx	**Fluphenazine HCl** (Pharmaceuticals Associates)	**Oral solution, concentrate:** 5 mg/mL	14% alcohol. In 120 mL with safety-cap dropper calibrated at 0.1 mL and in 0.2 mL increments.
Rx	**Fluphenazine HCl** (American Pharmaceutical Partners)	**Injection:** 2.5 mg/mL	Parabens. In 10 mL vials.
Rx	**Fluphenazine Decanoate** (Various, eg, Bedford Labs, Geneva)	**Injection:** 25 mg/mL	May contain sesame oil and benzyl alcohol. In 5 mL multidose vials.
Rx	**Prolixin Decanoate** (Apothecon)		In sesame oil with benzyl alcohol. In 5 mL multidose vials.

FLUPHENAZINE HYDROCHLORIDE — ORAL

Complete and comparative prescribing information begins in the Antipsychotic Agents group monograph.

Indications

➤*Psychotic disorders:* For the management of manifestations of psychotic disorders.

Administration and Dosage

Individualize dosage. The oral dose is approximately 2 to 3 times the parenteral dose. Institute treatment with a low initial dosage; increase as necessary. Therapeutic effect is often achieved with doses under 20 mg/day. However, daily doses up to 40 mg may be needed.

➤*Oral:*

Adults – Initially administer 2.5 to 10 mg/day in divided doses at 6 to 8 hour intervals. When symptoms are controlled, reduce dosage gradually to daily maintenance doses of 1 or 5 mg, often given as a single daily dose. Continued treatment is needed to achieve maximum therapeutic benefits; further adjustments in dosage may be necessary during the course of therapy to meet the patient's requirements.

Elderly: Initially, 1 to 2.5 mg/day, adjusted according to response.

For psychotic patients stabilized on a fixed daily dosage of orally administered fluphenazine, conversion from oral therapy to the long-acting injectable fluphenazine decanoate may be indicated.

➤*Oral concentrate:* When the oral concentrate dosage form is to be used, the desired dose (measured by a calibrated device only) should be added to at least 60 mL (2 fluid ounces) of a suitable diluent just prior to administration to ensure palatability and stability. Suggested diluents include tomato or fruit juice, milk, and uncaffeinated soft drinks. The oral concentrate should not be mixed with beverages containing caffeine (coffee, cola), tannics (tea), or pectinates (apple juice) because of the potential incompatibility.

➤*Storage/Stability:* Store at room temperature 15° to 30°C (59° to 86°F); avoid excessive heat. Protect from light and keep tightly closed. Do not freeze elixir or oral concentrate.

FLUPHENAZINE HYDROCHLORIDE — INJECTION

Complete and comparative prescribing information begins in the Antipsychotic Agents group monograph.

Indications

➤*Psychotic disorders:* For the management of manifestations of psychotic disorders.

Administration and Dosage

➤*Approved by the FDA:* April 16, 1987.

Individualize dosage. The oral dose is approximately 2 to 3 times the parenteral dose. Institute treatment with a low initial dosage; increase as necessary. Therapeutic effect is often achieved with doses under 20 mg/day. However, daily doses up to 40 mg may be needed.

➤*Injection:*

Hydrochloride formulation – Administer IM. Average starting dose for adult patients is 1.25 mg (0.5 mL) IM. Initial total daily dose may range from 2.5 to 10 mg and should be divided and given at 6- to 8-hour intervals. Use dosages exceeding 10 mg per day with caution. When symptoms are controlled, oral maintenance therapy can generally be instituted often with single daily doses.

➤*Storage/Stability:* Solutions should be protected from exposure to light. Parenteral solutions may vary in color from essentially colorless to light amber. If a solution has become any darker than light amber or is discolored in any other way, it should not be used.

Store at controlled room temperature 15° to 30°C (59° to 86°F); avoid excessive heat. Protect from light. Do not freeze.

FLUPHENAZINE DECANOATE — INJECTION

Complete and comparative prescribing information begins in the Antipsychotic Agents group monograph.

Indications

➤*Psychotic disorders:* For patients requiring prolonged and parenteral neuroleptic therapy (eg, chronic schizophrenic patients).

Administration and Dosage

➤*Approved by the FDA:* July 14, 1987.

Individualize dosage. The oral dose is approximately 2 to 3 times the parenteral dose. Institute treatment with a low initial dosage; increase as necessary. Therapeutic effect is often achieved with doses under 20 mg/day. However, daily doses up to 40 mg may be needed.

For psychotic patients stabilized on a fixed daily dosage of orally administered fluphenazine, conversion from oral therapy to the long-acting injectable fluphenazine decanoate may be indicated.

Administer IM or SC. Use a dry syringe and needle of at least 21 gauge. A wet needle or syringe may cause the solution to become cloudy. Initiate with 12.5 to 25 mg (0.5 to 1 mL). The onset of action generally appears between 24 and 72 hours after injection, and the effects of the drug on psychotic symptoms become significant within 48 to 96 hours. Determine subsequent injections and dosage interval in accordance with patient response. When administered as maintenance therapy, a single injection may be effective in controlling schizophrenic symptoms up to 4 weeks or longer. The response to a single dose has been found to last as long as 6 weeks in a few patients on maintenance therapy.

Initially, treat patients who have never taken phenothiazines with a shorter-acting form of the drug before administering the decanoate. This helps to determine the response to fluphenazine and to establish appropriate dosage.

No precise formula can be given to convert to fluphenazine decanoate use. However, in a controlled multicenter study, oral 20 mg/day fluphenazine HCl was equivalent to 25 mg fluphenazine decanoate every 3 weeks. This is an approximate conversion ratio of 0.5 mL (12.5 mg) decanoate every 3 weeks for every 10 mg fluphenazine HCl daily. Do not exceed 100 mg. If doses greater than 50 mg are needed, increase succeeding doses cautiously in 12.5 mg increments.

Once conversion to fluphenazine decanoate is made, careful clinical monitoring of the patient and appropriate dosage adjustment should be made at the time of each injection.

➤*Severely agitated patients:* Initially treat with a rapid-acting phenothiazine. When acute symptoms subside, administer 25 mg of the fluphenazine decanoate; adjust subsequent dosage as necessary.

➤*"Poor risk" patients:* In "poor risk" patients (known phenothiazine hypersensitivity or with disorders predisposing to undue reactions), cautiously initiate oral or parenteral fluphenazine. When appropriate dosage is established, give equivalent dose of fluphenazine decanoate.

The optimal amount of the drug and the frequency of administration must be determined for each patient because dosage requirements have been found to vary with clinical circumstances as well as with individual response to the drug.

➤*Storage/Stability:* Store at controlled room temperature 15° to 30°C (59° to 86°F); avoid excessive heat. Do not freeze. Protect from light. Retain vial in carton until ready for use.

PERPHENAZINE

Rx	**Perphenazine** (Various, eg, Geneva, Ivax)	**Tablets:** 2 mg	In 100s, 1000s, and UD 100s.
Rx	**Perphenazine** (Various, eg, Geneva, Ivax)	**Tablets:** 4 mg	In 100s, 500s, 1000s, and UD 100s.
Rx	**Perphenazine** (Various, eg, Geneva, Ivax)	**Tablets:** 8 mg	In 100s, 500s, 1000s, and UD 100s.
Rx	**Perphenazine** (Various, eg, Geneva, Ivax)	**Tablets:** 16 mg	In 100s, 1000s, and UD 100s.
Rx	**Perphenazine** (Pharmaceutical Associates)	**Oral concentrate:** 16 mg/5 mL	Sorbitol, sucrose. Berry flavor. In 118 mL with graduated calibrated dropper.

PERPHENAZINE — ORAL

For complete and comparative prescribing information refer to the Antipsychotic Agents group monograph.

Indications

➤*Psychotic disorders:* For the treatment of schizophrenia (tablets); management of manifestations of psychotic disorders (oral concentrate).

➤*Emesis:* To control severe nausea and vomiting in adults.

Administration and Dosage

Individualize the dosage and adjust according to the severity of the condition and the response obtained.

➤*Moderately disturbed, nonhospitalized patients with schizophrenia:* 4 to 8 mg 3 times/day initially; reduce as soon as possible to minimum effective dosage.

➤*Hospitalized patients with schizophrenia:* 8 to 16 mg 2 to 4 times/day; avoid dosages greater than 64 mg/day.

Reserve prolonged administration of doses exceeding 24 mg/day for hospitalized patients or patients under continued observation for early detection and management of adverse reactions. An antiparkinsonian agent, such as trihexyphenidyl HCl or benztropine mesylate, is valuable in controlling drug-induced extrapyramidal symptoms.

PERPHENAZINE — ORAL

➤*Nausea / Vomiting / Intractable hiccoughs:* 8 to 16 mg daily in divided doses; occasionally, 24 mg may be necessary. Early dosage reduction is desirable.

➤*Oral concentrate:* Dilute perphenazine oral solution (concentrate) only with water, saline, *7-Up*, homogenized milk, carbonated orange drink, and pineapple, apricot, prune, orange, *V-8*, tomato, and grapefruit juices. Do not mix perphenazine oral solution (concentrate) with beverages containing caffeine (eg, coffee, cola), tannics (eg, tea), or pectinates (eg, apple juice) because physical incompatibility may result. Suggested dilution is approximately 2 fluid ounces of diluent for each 5 mL (16 mg) or teaspoonful of perphenazine oral solution (concentrate). A graduated dropper marked to measure 8 mg or 4 mg is supplied with each bottle.

➤*Children:* Not recommended for children younger than 12 years of age.

➤*Elderly:* Geriatric patients are particularly sensitive to the side effects of antipsychotics. Start on lower doses and observe closely.

➤*Storage / Stability:*

Tablets – Store at controlled room temperature 15° to 30°C (59° to 86°F). Dispense in a tight, light-resistant container.

Oral concentrate – Store between 2° and 30°C (36° and 86°F); protect from light. Dispense concentrate in amber bottles; shake well before using.

PROCHLORPERAZINE

Rx	**Prochlorperazine** (Various, eg, Barr, Geneva, Par, UDL, Ivax)	**Tablets**: 5 mg (as maleate)	In 100s, 500s, 1000s, blister pack 25s, and UD 100s.
Rx	**Compazine** (GlaxoSmithKline)		Lactose. (SKF C66). Yellow-green. In 100s and UD 100s.
Rx	**Prochlorperazine** (Various, eg, Barr, Geneva, Par, UDL, Ivax)	**Tablets**: 10 mg (as maleate)	In 100s, 500s, 1000s, blister pack 25s, and UD 100s.
Rx	**Compazine** (GlaxoSmithKline)		Lactose. (SKF C67). Yellow-green. In 100s and UD 100s.
Rx	**Compazine** (GlaxoSmithKline)	**Spansules (sustained-release capsules)**: 10 mg (as maleate)	Sugar spheres. (10 mg 3344 10 mg SB). Black/Natural. In 50s.
		15 mg (as maleate)	Sugar spheres. (15 mg 3346 15 mg SB). Black/Natural. In 50s.
Rx	**Compazine** (GlaxoSmithKline)	**Syrup**: 5 mg/5 mL (as edisylate)	Sucrose. Fruit flavor. In 120 mL.
Rx	**Prochlorperazine** (Various, eg, Abbott)	**Injection**: 5 mg/mL (as edisylate)	In 2 mL vials.
Rx	**Compazine** (GlaxoSmithKline)		In 2 and 10 mL vials.[a]
Rx	**Compazine** (GlaxoSmithKline)	**Suppositories**: 2.5 mg	Glycerin and coconut oil. In 12s.
		5 mg	Glycerin and coconut oil. In 12s.
Rx	**Prochlorperazine** (Various, eg, G & W Labs)	**Suppositories**: 25 mg	In 12s.
Rx	**Compazine** (GlaxoSmithKline)		Glycerin. In 12s.
Rx	**Compro** (Paddock)		Glycerin and coconut oil. In 12s.

[a] With sodium saccharin, benzyl alcohol, sodium biphosphate, and sodium tartrate.

PROCHLORPERAZINE — ORAL

For complete and comparative prescribing information refer to the Antipsychotic Agents group monograph. See also the Antiemetic/Antivertigo Agents monograph.

Indications

➤*Schizophrenia:* For the treatment of schizophrenia.

➤*Nonpsychotic anxiety:* For the short-term treatment of generalized nonpsychotic anxiety; however, prochlorperazine is not the first drug of choice for this indication.

➤*Emesis:* To control severe nausea and vomiting.

Administration and Dosage

➤*Approved by the FDA:* October 1, 1982.

➤*Adults:* Increase dosage more gradually in debilitated or emaciated patients.

Schizophrenia – Adjust dosage in adult psychiatric disorders to the response of the individual and according to the severity of the condition. Begin with the lowest recommended dose. Although response is ordinarily seen within a day or 2, longer treatment is usually required before maximal improvement is seen.

Mild conditions: 5 or 10 mg 3 or 4 times/day.

Moderate to severe conditions: 10 mg 3 or 4 times/day. Gradually Increase dosage until symptoms are controlled or side effects become bothersome. When dosage is increased by small increments over 2 or 3 days, side effects either do not occur or are easily controlled. Some patients respond satisfactorily on 50 to 75 mg/day.

Severe conditions: 100 to 150 mg/day.

Nonpsychotic anxiety in adults – 5 mg 3 to 4 times/day; by spansule capsule, usually one 15 mg capsule on arising or one 10 mg capsule every 12 hours. Do not administer in doses of more than 20 mg/day or for longer than 12 weeks.

Control of severe nausea and vomiting – Usually, 5 to 10 mg, 3 or 4 times daily; 15 mg (sustained release) on arising; 10 mg (sustained release) every 12 hours.

➤*Children:* Do not use in pediatric patients under 20 lb or younger than 2 years of age. Do not use in conditions for which children's dosages have not been established.

Children seem more prone to develop extrapyramidal reactions, even on moderate doses. Use the lowest effective dose. Occasionally the patients may react to the drug with signs of restlessness and excitement. Do not administer additional doses if this occurs. Take particular precaution in administering the drug to children with acute illnesses or dehydration.

Adjust dosage and frequency of administration according to the severity of the symptoms and the response of the patient.

Schizophrenia in children – For children 2 to 12 years of age, starting dosage is $2\frac{1}{2}$ mg 2 or 3 times/day. Do not give more than 10 mg on the first day. Then increase dosage according to the patient's response.

Children (2 to 5 years of age): Usual total daily dose does not exceed 20 mg.

Children (6 to 12 years of age): Usual total daily dose does not exceed 25 mg.

Control of severe nausea and vomiting – More than 1 days' therapy is seldom necessary.

20 to 29 lbs (9.1 to 13.2 kg): 2.5 mg 1 or 2 times/day (not to exceed 7.5 mg/day).

30 to 39 lbs (13.6 to 17.7 kg): 2.5 mg 2 or 3 times/day (not to exceed 10 mg/day).

40 to 85 lbs (18.2 to 38.6 kg): 2.5 mg 3 times/day or 5 mg twice daily (not to exceed 15 mg/day).

➤*Elderly:* Dosages in the lower range are sufficient for most elderly patients. Because they appear to be more susceptible to hypotension and neuromuscular reactions, observe such patients closely. Tailor dosage to the individual, carefully monitor response, and adjust dose accordingly. Increase dosage more gradually in elderly patients.

➤*Storage / Stability:* Store between 15° and 30°C (59° and 86°F). Protect from light.

PROCHLORPERAZINE — INJECTION

For complete and comparative prescribing information refer to the Antipsychotic Agents group monograph. See also the Antiemetic/Antivertigo Agents monograph.

Indications

➤*Schizophrenia:* For the treatment of schizophrenia.

➤*Nonpsychotic anxiety:* For the short-term treatment of generalized nonpsychotic anxiety; however, prochlorperazine is not the first drug of choice for this indication.

➤*Emesis:* To control severe nausea and vomiting.

Administration and Dosage

➤*Approved by the FDA:* October 1, 1982

➤*Adults:* Increase dosage more gradually in debilitated or emaciated patients.

Schizophrenia – Adjust dosage in adult psychiatric disorders to the response of the individual and according to the severity of the condition. Begin with the lowest recommended dose. Although response is ordinarily seen within a day or 2, longer treatment is usually required before maximal improvement is seen.

IM: SC administration is not advisable because of local irritation.

Inject an initial dose of 10 to 20 mg (2 to 4 mL) deeply into the upper outer quadrant of the buttock. Many patients respond shortly after the first injection. Repeat the initial dose every 2 to 4 hours (or, in resistant cases, every hour) to gain control of the patient, if necessary. More than 3 or 4 doses are seldom necessary. After control is achieved, switch patient to an oral form of

PROCHLORPERAZINE — INJECTION

the drug at the same dosage levels or higher. If, in rare cases, parenteral therapy is needed for a prolonged period, give 10 to 20 mg (2 to 4 mL) every 4 to 6 hours.

Control of severe nausea and vomiting –

IM: Initially, 5 to 10 mg. If necessary, repeat every 3 or 4 hours. Do not exceed 40 mg/day.

SC: Do not administer SC because of local irritation.

Adult surgery –

Control of severe nausea and vomiting: Total parenteral dosage should not exceed 40 mg/day. Hypotension may occur if the drug is given IV or by infusion.

IM: 5 to 10 mg, 1 to 2 hours before induction of anesthesia (may repeat once in 30 minutes), or to control acute symptoms during and after surgery (may repeat once).

IV injection: 5 to 10 mg, 15 to 30 minutes before induction of anesthesia, or to control acute symptoms during or after surgery. Repeat once if necessary. Prochlorperazine may be administered either undiluted or diluted in isotonic solution, but do not exceed 10 mg in a single dose of the drug. Do not exceed 5 mg/ml/min. Do not use bolus injection.

IV infusion: 20 mg/L of isotonic solution. Do not dilute in < 1 L of isotonic solution. Add to IV infusion 15 to 30 minutes before induction.

In one study, a dosage of 30 or 40 mg prochlorperazine in 100 ml normal saline was significantly superior to a 10 mg dose in treating cisplatin-induced emesis; toxicity was only moderate.

➤*Children:* Do not use in pediatric patients under 20 lb or younger than 2 years of age. Do not use in conditions for which children's dosages have not been established.

Children seem more prone to develop extrapyramidal reactions, even on moderate doses. Use the lowest effective dose. Occasionally the patients may react to the drug with signs of restlessness and excitement. Do not administer additional doses if this occurs. Take particular precaution in administering the drug to children with acute illnesses or dehydration.

Adjust dosage and frequency of administration according to the severity of the symptoms and the response of the patient. The duration of activity following IM administration may last up to 12 hours. Subsequent doses may be given by the same route if necessary.

Schizophrenia in children –

IM: For ages under 12, calculate the dose on the basis of 0.06 mg/lb of body weight; give by deep IM injection. Control is usually obtained with 1 dose. After control is achieved, switch the patient to an oral form of the drug at the same dosage level or higher.

Control of severe nausea and vomiting –

IM: 0.06 mg/lb (0.132 mg/kg). Give by deep IM injection. Control is usually obtained with one dose. Duration of action may be 12 hours. Subsequent doses may be given if necessary.

➤*Elderly:* Dosages in the lower range are sufficient for most elderly patients. Because they appear to be more susceptible to hypotension and neuromuscular reactions, observe such patients closely. Tailor dosage to the individual, carefully monitor response, and adjust dose accordingly. Increase dosage more gradually in elderly patients.

➤*Compatibility:* Do not mix prochlorperazine injection with other agents in the syringe.

➤*Storage/Stability:* Store at controlled room temperature 15° to 30°C (59° to 86°F). Do not freeze. Protect from light.

PROCHLORPERAZINE — RECTAL

For complete and comparative prescribing information refer to the Antipsychotic Agents group monograph. See also the Antiemetic/Antivertigo Agents monograph.

Indications

➤*Schizophrenia:* For the treatment of schizophrenia.

➤*Nonpsychotic anxiety:* For the short-term treatment of generalized nonpsychotic anxiety; however, prochlorperazine is not the first drug of choice for this indication.

➤*Emesis:* To control severe nausea and vomiting. (*Compro* is only indicated for severe nausea and vomiting in adults.)

Administration and Dosage

➤*Adults:* Dosage should be increased more gradually in debilitated or emaciated patients.

Elderly patients – In general, dosages in the lower range are sufficient for most elderly patients. Since they appear to be more susceptible to hypotension and neuromuscular reactions, such patients should be observed closely. Dosage should be tailored to the individual, response carefully monitored and dosage adjusted accordingly. Dosage should be increased more gradually in elderly patients.

To control severe nausea and vomiting – Adjust dosage to the response of the individual. Begin with the lowest recommended dosage.

Rectal dosage – 25 mg twice daily.

➤*Children:* Do not use in pediatric surgery.

Children seem more prone to develop extrapyramidal reactions, even on moderate doses. Therefore, use lowest effective dosage. Tell parents not to exceed prescribed dosage, since the possibility of adverse reactions increases as dosage rises.

Occasionally the patient may react to the drug with signs of restlessness and excitement; if this occurs, do not administer additional doses. Take particular precaution in administering the drug to children with acute illnesses or dehydration.

Severe nausea and vomiting in children – Prochlorperazine should not be used in pediatric patients under 20 pounds in weight or 2 years of age. It should not be used in conditions for which children's dosages have not been established. Dosage and frequency of administration should be adjusted according to the severity of the symptoms and the response of the patient. Subsequent doses may be given by the same route if necessary.

More than 1 day's therapy is seldom necessary.

Weight	Usual dosage	Not to exceed
Under 20 lbs: not recommended		
20 to 29 lbs	2.5 mg 1 or 2 times/day	7.5 mg/day
30 to 39 lbs	2.5 mg 2 or 3 times/day	10 mg/day
40 to 85 lbs	2.5 mg 3 times/day or 5 mg 2 times/day	15 mg/day

In children with schizophrenia – For children 2 to 12 years, starting dosage is 2.5 mg 2 or 3 times daily. Do not give more than 10 mg the first day. Then increase dosage according to patient's response.

For ages 2 to 5, total daily dosage usually does not exceed 20 mg.

For ages 6 to 12, total daily dosage usually does not exceed 25 mg.

➤*Storage/Stability:* Store between 15° and 30°C (59° and 86°F). Protect from light.

TRIFLUOPERAZINE HYDROCHLORIDE

Rx	**Trifluoperazine** (Various, eg, Sandoz, UDL)	**Tablets:** 1 mg	In 100s, 500s, 1000s, and UD 100s.
		2 mg	In 100s, 500s, 1000s, and UD 100s.
		5 mg	In 100s, 500s, 1000s, and UD 100s.
		10 mg	In 100s, 500s, 1000s, and UD 100s.

TRIFLUOPERAZINE HYDROCHLORIDE — ORAL

For complete and comparative prescribing information refer to the Antipsychotic Agents group monograph.

Indications

➤*Schizophrenia:* For the management of schizophrenia.

➤*Nonpsychotic anxiety:* For the short-term treatment of nonpsychotic anxiety (not the first drug of choice in most patients).

Administration and Dosage

➤*Approved by the FDA:* 1958.

Individualize dosage. Increase dosage more gradually in debilitated or emaciated patients. When maximum response is achieved, reduce dosage gradually to a maintenance level. Use the lowest effective dosage. Patients may be controlled with once- or twice-daily administration.

➤*Schizophrenia:*

Oral –

Adults: 2 to 5 mg orally twice daily. Start small or emaciated patients on the lower dosage. Most patients will show optimum response with 15 or 20 mg/day, although a few may require 40 mg/day or more. Optimum therapeutic dosage levels should be reached within 2 or 3 weeks.

Children (6 to 12 years of age): Adjust dosage to the weight of the child and severity of the symptoms. These dosages are for children 6 to 12 years of age who are hospitalized or under close supervision. Initial dose is 1 mg once or twice daily. Dosage may be increased gradually until symptoms are controlled or until side effects become troublesome. While it is usually not necessary to exceed 15 mg/day, older children with severe symptoms may require higher doses.

➤*Nonpsychotic anxiety:* 1 or 2 mg twice daily. Do not administer more than 6 mg/day or for longer than 12 weeks because trifluoperazine use at higher doses or for longer intervals may cause persistent tardive dyskinesia that may prove irreversible.

Phenothiazine Derivatives

TRIFLUOPERAZINE HYDROCHLORIDE — ORAL

➤*Elderly patients:* Usually, lower dosages are sufficient. The elderly appear more susceptible to hypotension and neuromuscular reactions; observe closely and increase dosage gradually.

➤*Storage/Stability:* Store between 15° and 30°C (59° and 86°F).

THIORIDAZINE HYDROCHLORIDE

Rx	**Thioridazine HCl** (Various, eg, Geneva, Mylan, URL/Mutual)	**Tablets:** 10 mg	In 60s, 100s, 1000s, and UD 100s.
Rx	**Thioridazine HCl** (Various, eg, Geneva)	**Tablets:** 15 mg	In 100s, 1000s, and UD 100s.
Rx	**Thioridazine HCl** (Various, eg, Geneva, Mylan, URL/Mutual)	**Tablets:** 25 mg	In 60s, 100s, 1000s, and UD 100s.
Rx	**Thioridazine HCl** (Various, eg, Geneva, Mylan, URL/Mutual)	**Tablets:** 50 mg	In 60s, 100s, 1000s, and UD 100s.
Rx	**Thioridazine HCl** (Various, eg, Geneva, Mylan, URL/Mutual)	**Tablets:** 100 mg	In 60s, 100s, 1000s, and UD 100s.
Rx	**Thioridazine HCl** (Various, eg, Geneva)	**Tablets:** 150 mg	In 100s and 1000s.
Rx	**Thioridazine HCl** (Various, eg, Geneva)	**Tablets:** 200 mg	In 100s and 1000s.

THIORIDAZINE HYDROCHLORIDE — ORAL

For complete and comparative prescribing information refer to the Antipsychotic Agents group monograph.

WARNING

Thioridazine has been shown to prolong the QTc interval in a dose-related manner. Drugs with this potential, including thioridazine, have been associated with torsade de pointes-type arrhythmias and sudden death. Because of its potential for significant, possibly life-threatening, proarrhythmic effects, reserve thioridazine use in the treatment of schizophrenic patients who fail to show an acceptable response to adequate courses of treatment with other antipsychotic drugs, either because of insufficient effectiveness or the inability to achieve an effective dose because of intolerable adverse effects from those drugs.

Indications

➤*Schizophrenia:* For the management of schizophrenic patients who fail to respond adequately to treatment with other antipsychotic drugs. Before initiating treatment with thioridazine, it is strongly recommended that a patient be given at least 2 trials, each with a different antipsychotic drug product, at an adequate dose and for an adequate duration.

Administration and Dosage

Dosage must be individualized and the smallest effective dosage should be determined for each patient.

➤*Adults:* Starting dose is 50 to 100 mg 3 times/day with a gradual increment to a maximum of 800 mg/day, if necessary. Once effective control of symptoms has been achieved, the dosage may be reduced gradually to determine the minimum maintenance dose. The total daily dosage ranges from 200 to 800 mg, divided into 2 to 4 doses.

➤*Children:* For patients unresponsive to other agents, the recommended initial dose is 0.5 mg/kg/day given in divided doses. Dosage may be increased gradually until optimum therapeutic effect is obtained or the maximum dose of 3 mg/kg/day has been reached.

➤*Storage/Stability:* Store at controlled room temperature 15° to 30°C (59° to 86°F); dispense in a tight, light-resistant container.

Thioxanthene Derivatives

THIOTHIXENE

Rx	**Thiothixene** (Various, eg, Geneva)	**Capsules:** 1 mg	In 100s, and 1000s.
Rx	**Navane** (Roerig)		Lactose. In 100s.
Rx	**Thiothixene** (Various, eg, Geneva)	**Capsules:** 2 mg	In 100s, 1000s, and UD 100s.
Rx	**Navane** (Roerig)		Lactose. In 100s.
Rx	**Thiothixene** (Various, eg, Geneva)	**Capsules:** 5 mg	In 100s, 1000s, and UD 100s.
Rx	**Navane** (Roerig)		Lactose. In 100s.
Rx	**Thiothixene** (Various, eg, Geneva)	**Capsules:** 10 mg	In 100s, 1000s, and UD 100s.
Rx	**Navane** (Roerig)		Lactose. In 100s.
Rx	**Navane** (Roerig)	**Capsules:** 20 mg	Lactose. In 100s.

THIOTHIXENE — ORAL

For complete and comparative prescribing information refer to the Antipsychotic Agents group monograph.

Indications

➤*Schizophrenia:* For the management of schizophrenia.

Administration and Dosage

➤*Approved by the FDA:* June 5, 1987.

Individualize dose depending on the chronicity and severity of the symptoms. Use small doses initially and gradually increase to the optimal effective level based on patient response. Some patients have been successfully maintained on once-a-day therapy.

Not recommended for use in children younger than 12 years of age.

➤*Mild conditions:* Initially, 2 mg 3 times/day. If indicated, an increase to 15 mg/day is often effective.

➤*Severe conditions:* Initially, 5 mg twice daily. Optimal is 20 to 30 mg/day. If indicated, 60 mg/day is often effective. Exceeding 60 mg/day rarely increases the beneficial response.

➤*Storage/Stability:* Store at controlled room temperature up to 30°C (86°F).

Phenylbutylpiperadine Derivatives

HALOPERIDOL

Rx	**Haloperidol** (Various, eg, Geneva, Mylan)	**Tablets:** 0.5 mg	In 100s, 1000s, and UD 100s.
		1 mg	In 100s, 1000s, and UD 100s.
		2 mg	In 100s, 1000s, and UD 100s.
		5 mg	In 100s, 1000s, and UD 100s.
Rx	**Haloperidol** (Various, eg, Geneva)	**Tablets:** 10 mg	In 100s, 1000s, and UD 100s.
		20 mg	In 100s and UD 100s.
Rx	**Haloperidol** (Various, eg, Ivax, Major)	**Oral concentrate:** 2 mg (as lactate)/mL	In 15 and 120 mL, and 5 and 10 mL UD 100s.
Rx	**Haloperidol** (Various, eg, Bedford)	**Injection:** 5 mg (as lactate)/mL	May contain parabens. In 1 mL vials and 10 mL multidose vials.
Rx	**Haldol** (McNeil-CPC)		Parabens. In 1 mL amps and 10 mL multidose vials.

Phenylbutylpiperadine Derivatives

HALOPERIDOL

Rx	**Haloperidol Decanoate** (Various, eg, Apotex, Bedford, Gensia Sicor)	**Injection**: 50 mg (equiv. to 70.5 mg decanoate)/mL	May contain sesame oil and 1.2% benzyl alcohol. In 1 and 5 mL multidose vial.
Rx	**Haldol Decanoate 50** (McNeil, Bedford)		In 1 mL amps[a] and 5 mL vials.
Rx	**Haloperidol Decanoate** (Various, eg, Apotex, Bedford, Gensia Sicor)	**Injection**: 100 mg (equiv. to 141.04 mg decanoate)/mL	May contain sesame oil and 1.2% benzyl alcohol. In 1 mL and 5 mL multidose vial.
Rx	**Haldol Decanoate 100** (McNeil)		In 1 mL amps[a] and 5 mL vials.[a]

[a] In sesame oil with 1.2% benzyl alcohol.

HALOPERIDOL — ORAL

For complete and comparative prescribing information refer to the Antipsychotic Agents group monograph.

Indications

➤*Psychotic disorders:* For the treatment of psychotic disorders (eg, schizophrenia).

➤*Tourette disorder:* For the control of tics and vocal utterances in Tourette disorder.

➤*Behavioral problems:* For the treatment of behavioral problems in children with combative, explosive hyperexcitability that cannot be accounted for by immediate provocation. Reserve for use in these children only after failure to respond to psychotherapy or medications other than antipsychotics.

➤*Hyperactivity:* For short-term treatment of hyperactive children who show excessive motor activity with accompanying conduct disorders consisting of impulsivity, difficulty sustaining attention, aggression, mood lability, or poor frustration tolerance. Reserve for use in these children only after failure to respond to psychotherapy or medications other than antipsychotics.

➤*Unlabeled uses:* Prevention and treatment of chemotherapy-induced nausea or vomiting.

Administration and Dosage

➤*Approved by the FDA:* June 10, 1986.

Individualize dosage. Children, debilitated or geriatric patients, and those with a history of adverse reactions to neuroleptic drugs may require less haloperidol; optimal response is usually obtained with more gradual dosage adjustments and at lower dosage levels. Upon achieving a satisfactory therapeutic response, gradually reduce dosage to the lowest effective maintenance level.

➤*Psychotic disorders:*

Adults: Initial dosage – Moderate symptoms or geriatric or debilitated patients: 0.5 to 2 mg given 2 or 3 times daily; severe symptoms or chronic or resistant patients: 3 to 5 mg 2 or 3 times daily. To achieve prompt control, higher doses may be required.

Patients who remain severely disturbed or inadequately controlled may require dosage adjustment. Daily dosages up to 100 mg may be necessary.

Infrequently, doses greater than 100 mg have been used for severely resistant patients; however, safety of prolonged administration of such doses has not been demonstrated.

Children (3 to 12 years of age; weight range 15 to 40 kg) – Do not use in children younger than 3 years of age. Initial dose is 0.5 mg/day (25 to 50 mcg/kg/day). If required, increase in 0.5 mg increments at 5- to 7-day intervals up to 0.15 mg/kg/day or until therapeutic effect is obtained. Total dose may be divided and given 2 or 3 times daily. The dose in this age group has not been well established.

Conversion from IM to oral – Replace the injectable with the oral form as soon as feasible. For an approximation of the total daily dose required, use the parenteral dose administered in the preceding 24 hours; carefully monitor the patient for the first several days. Give the first oral dose within 12 to 24 hours following the last parenteral dose.

➤*Tourette disorder:*

Adults – A starting dose of 0.5 to 1.5 mg 3 times/day by mouth has been suggested; up to about 10 mg/day may be needed. Requirements vary considerably and the dose must be very carefully adjusted to obtain the optimum response.

Children (3 to 12 years of age; 15 to 40 kg) – 0.05 to 0.075 mg/kg/day. Severely disturbed psychotic children may require higher doses.

➤*Behavioral disorders/hyperactivity:*

Children (3 to 12 years of age; 15 to 40 kg) – 0.05 to 0.075 mg/kg/day. Severely disturbed psychotic children may require higher doses.

In severely disturbed, nonpsychotic children or in hyperactive children with conduct disorders, short-term administration may suffice. There is little evidence that behavior improvement is further enhanced by dosages greater than 6 mg/day.

➤*Elderly/Debilitated:* Lower initial doses and more gradual adjustments are recommended.

➤*Storage/Stability:* Store at controlled room temperature 15° to 30°C (59° to 86°F). Protect from light. Dispense in a tight, light-resistant container using a child-resistant closure.

HALOPERIDOL LACTATE — ORAL

For complete and comparative prescribing information refer to the Antipsychotic Agents group monograph.

Indications

➤*Psychotic disorders:* For the treatment of psychotic disorders (eg, schizophrenia).

➤*Tourette disorder:* For the control of tics and vocal utterances in Tourette disorder.

➤*Behavioral problems:* For the treatment of behavioral problems in children with combative, explosive hyperexcitability that cannot be accounted for by immediate provocation. Reserve for use in these children only after failure to respond to psychotherapy or medications other than antipsychotics.

➤*Hyperactivity:* For short-term treatment of hyperactive children who show excessive motor activity with accompanying conduct disorders consisting of impulsivity, difficulty sustaining attention, aggression, mood lability, or poor frustration tolerance. Reserve for use in these children only after failure to respond to psychotherapy or medications other than antipsychotics.

➤*Unlabeled uses:* Prevention and treatment of chemotherapy-induced nausea or vomiting.

Administration and Dosage

➤*Approved by the FDA:* April 12, 1967.

Individualize dosage. Children, debilitated or geriatric patients, and those with a history of adverse reactions to neuroleptic drugs may require less haloperidol; optimal response is usually obtained with more gradual dosage adjustments and at lower dosage levels. Upon achieving a satisfactory therapeutic response, gradually reduce dosage to the lowest effective maintenance level.

➤*Psychotic disorders:*

Adults: Initial dosage – Moderate symptoms or geriatric or debilitated patients: 0.5 to 2 mg given 2 or 3 times daily; severe symptoms or chronic or resistant patients: 3 to 5 mg 2 or 3 times daily. To achieve prompt control, higher doses may be required.

Patients who remain severely disturbed or inadequately controlled may require dosage adjustment. Daily dosages up to 100 mg may be necessary.

Infrequently, doses greater than 100 mg have been used for severely resistant patients; however, safety of prolonged administration of such doses has not been demonstrated.

Children (3 to 12 years of age; weight range 15 to 40 kg) – Do not use in children younger than 3 years of age. Initial dose is 0.5 mg/day (25 to 50 mcg/kg/day). If required, increase in 0.5 mg increments at 5- to 7-day intervals up to 0.15 mg/kg/day or until therapeutic effect is obtained. Total dose may be divided and given 2 or 3 times daily. The dose in this age group has not been well established.

Conversion from IM to oral – Replace the injectable with the oral form as soon as feasible. For an approximation of the total daily dose required, use the parenteral dose administered in the preceding 24 hours; carefully monitor the patient for the first several days. Give the first oral dose within 12 to 24 hours following the last parenteral dose.

➤*Tourette disorder:*

Adults – A starting dose of 0.5 to 1.5 mg 3 times/day by mouth has been suggested; up to about 10 mg/day may be needed. Requirements vary considerably and the dose must be very carefully adjusted to obtain the optimum response.

Children (3 to 12 years of age; 15 to 40 kg) – 0.05 to 0.075 mg/kg/day. Severely disturbed psychotic children may require higher doses.

➤*Behavioral disorders/hyperactivity:*

Children (3 to 12 years of age; 15 to 40 kg) – 0.05 to 0.075 mg/kg/day. Severely disturbed psychotic children may require higher doses.

In severely disturbed, nonpsychotic children or in hyperactive children with conduct disorders, short-term administration may suffice. There is little evidence that behavior improvement is further enhanced by dosages greater than 6 mg/day.

➤*Elderly/Debilitated:* Lower initial doses and more gradual adjustments are recommended.

➤*Storage/Stability:* Store haloperidol lactate concentrate at controlled room temperature (15° to 30°C; 59° to 86°F). Protect from light. Do not freeze.

Dispense the haloperidol lactate concentrate in a tight, light-resistant container as defined in the official compendium.

HALOPERIDOL LACTATE — ORAL

Store tablets at controlled room temperature 15° to 30°C (59° to 86°F). Dispense in tight, light-resistant container.

HALOPERIDOL LACTATE — INJECTION

For complete and comparative prescribing information refer to the Antipsychotic Agents group monograph.

Indications

➤*Psychotic disorders:* For the treatment of psychotic disorders (eg, schizophrenia).

➤*Tourette disorder:* For the control of tics and vocal utterances in Tourette disorder.

➤*Unlabeled uses:* Prevention and treatment of chemotherapy-induced nausea or vomiting.

Administration and Dosage

➤*Approved by the FDA:* 1971.

Individualize dosage. Children, debilitated or geriatric patients, and those with a history of adverse reactions to neuroleptic drugs may require less haloperidol; optimal response is usually obtained with more gradual dosage adjustments and at lower dosage levels. Upon achieving a satisfactory therapeutic response, gradually reduce dosage to the lowest effective maintenance level.

➤*Psychotic disorders:*

IM administration – 2 to 5 mg haloperidol lactate for prompt control of the acutely agitated schizophrenic patient with moderately severe to very severe symptoms. Depending on response, administer subsequent doses as often as every 60 minutes, although 4- to 8-hour intervals may be satisfactory.

The safety and efficacy of IM administration in children have not been established.

Conversion from IM to oral – Replace the injectable with the oral form as soon as feasible. For an approximation of the total daily dose required, use the parenteral dose administered in the preceding 24 hours; carefully monitor the patient for the first several days. Give the first oral dose within 12 to 24 hours following the last parenteral dose.

➤*Elderly / Debilitated:* Lower initial doses and more gradual adjustments are recommended.

➤*Storage / Stability:* Store at 25°C (77°F); excursions permitted to 15° to 30°C (59° to 86°F [see USP controlled room temperature]). Protect from light; do not freeze.

HALOPERIDOL DECANOATE — INJECTION

For complete and comparative prescribing information refer to the Antipsychotic Agents group monograph.

Indications

➤*Psychotic disorders:* For the treatment of psychotic disorders (eg, schizophrenia). Haloperidol decanoate is for patients who require prolonged parenteral antipsychotic therapy.

Administration and Dosage

➤*Approved by the FDA:* January 14, 1986.

Individualize dosage. Children, debilitated or geriatric patients, and those with a history of adverse reactions to neuroleptic drugs may require less haloperidol; optimal response is usually obtained with more gradual dosage adjustments and at lower dosage levels. Upon achieving a satisfactory therapeutic response, gradually reduce dosage to the lowest effective maintenance level.

➤*Haloperidol decanoate injection:* Individualize dosage and provide close clinical supervision during initiation and stabilization of therapy. The recommended interval between doses is monthly or every 4 weeks. However, variation in patient response may dictate a need for adjustment of the dosing interval as well as the dose. To determine the minimum effective dose, begin with lower initial doses and adjust the dose upward as needed.

Intended for use in chronic psychotic patients who require prolonged parenteral antipsychotic therapy. These patients should be previously stabilized on antipsychotic medication, and should have been treated with, and well tolerated on short-acting haloperidol in order to exclude the possibility of an unexpected adverse sensitivity to haloperidol. Close clinical supervision is required during the initial period of dose adjustment in order to minimize the risk of overdosage or reappearance of psychotic symptoms before the next injection. During dose adjustment or episodes of exacerbation of psychotic symptoms, haloperidol decanoate therapy can be supplemented with short-acting forms of haloperidol.

Haloperidol Decanoate Dosing Recommendations[a]

Patients	1st Month[b]	Monthly maintenance
Stabilized on low daily oral doses (≤ 10 mg/day)	10 to 15 × daily oral dose	10 to 15 × previous daily oral dose
Elderly or debilitated		
Stabilized on higher doses; risk of relapse	20 × daily oral dose	10 to 15 × previous daily oral dose
Tolerant to oral haloperidol		

[a] Clinical experience with doses greater than 450 mg/month has been limited.
[b] Initial dose should not exceed 100 mg. See below.

Initial dosage – The initial dose should not exceed 100 mg regardless of previous antipsychotic dose requirements. If the conversion requires more than 100 mg of haloperidol decanoate as an initial dose, administer that dose in 2 injections (maximum of 100 mg initially followed by the balance in 3 to 7 days).

Maintenance dosage – Individualize with titration upward or downward based on therapeutic response.

Administration – Administer by deep IM injection. A 21-gauge needle is recommended. The maximum volume per injection site should not exceed 3 mL. Do not administer IV.

➤*Elderly / Debilitated:* Lower initial doses and more gradual adjustments are recommended.

➤*Storage / Stability:* Store at controlled room temperature 15° to 30°C (59° to 86°F). Do not refrigerate or freeze. Protect from light. Retain vial in carton until contents are used.

PIMOZIDE

Rx	**Orap** (Teva)	**Tablets:** 1 mg	Lactose. (ORAP 1). White, oval, scored. In 100s.
		2 mg	Lactose. (LEMMON ORAP 2). White, oval, scored. In 100s.

PIMOZIDE — ORAL

For complete and comparative prescribing information, refer to the Antipsychotic Agents group monograph.

Indications

➤*Tourette disorder:* For suppression of motor and phonic tics in patients with Tourette disorder who have failed to respond satisfactorily to standard treatment. Pimozide is not intended as a treatment of first choice, nor is it intended for the treatment of tics that are merely annoying or cosmetically troublesome. Reserve pimozide use for Tourette disorder patients whose development and/or daily life function is severely compromised by the presence of motor and phonic tics.

➤*Unlabeled uses:* Treatment of chronic delusional parasitosis refractory to other treatments.

Administration and Dosage

➤*Approved by the FDA:* July 31, 1984.

The suppression of tics by pimozide requires a slow and gradual introduction of the drug. Carefully adjust the patient's dose to a point where the suppression of tics and the relief afforded is balanced against the untoward side effects of the drug. Perform ECG at baseline and periodically thereafter, especially during dosage adjustment.

➤*Tourette:*

Adults –

Initial dose: 1 to 2 mg/day in divided doses. Thereafter, increase dose every other day.

Maintenance dose: Less than 0.2 mg/kg/day or 10 mg/day, whichever is less. Doses greater than 0.2 mg/kg/day or 10 mg/day are not recommended.

Children –

Initiate at a dose of 0.05 mg/kg preferably taken once at bedtime; dose may be increased every third day to a maximum of 0.2 mg/kg, not to exceed 10 mg/day.

Gradual withdrawal – Periodically attempt to reduce dosage to see if tics persist. Increases of tic intensity and frequency may represent a transient, withdrawal-related phenomenon rather than a return of symptoms. Allow 1 or 2 weeks to elapse before concluding that an increase in tic manifestations is due to the underlying disease rather than drug withdrawal. A gradual withdrawal is recommended in any case.

➤*Storage / Stability:* Store at controlled room temperature 15° to 30°C (59° to 86°F). Dispense in a tight, light-resistant container as defined in the official compendium.

Dihydroindolone Derivatives

MOLINDONE HYDROCHLORIDE

Rx	**Moban** (Endo)	**Tablets:** 5 mg	Lactose. (Moban 5). Orange. In 100s.
		10 mg	Lactose. (Moban 10). Lavender. In 100s.
		25 mg	Lactose. (Moban 25). Green. In 100s.
		50 mg	Lactose. (Moban 50). Blue. In 100s.

MOLINDONE HYDROCHLORIDE — ORAL

For complete and comparative prescribing information refer to the Antipsychotic Agents group monograph.

Indications

➤*Schizophrenia:* For the management of schizophrenia.

Administration and Dosage

Individualize dosage.

➤*Initial dosage:* 50 to 75 mg/day, increase to 100 mg/day in 3 or 4 days. Based on severity of symptomatology, dosage may be titrated up or down depending on individual patient response. An increase to 225 mg/day may be required. Start elderly and debilitated patients on lower dosage.

➤*Maintenance therapy:*

Mild – 5 to 15 mg 3 or 4 times/day.

Moderate – 10 to 25 mg 3 or 4 times/day.

Severe – 225 mg/day may be required.

➤*Storage/Stability:* Store at 25°C (77°F); excursions permitted to 15° to 30°C (59° to 86°F). Dispense in a tight, light-resistant container with child-resistant closure. Keep tightly closed.

Dibenzapine Derivatives

CLOZAPINE

Rx	**Clozapine** (Various, eg, IVAX)	**Tablets:** 12.5 mg	In 30s and 100s.
Rx	**Clozapine** (Various, eg, Mylan, UDL, IVAX)	**Tablets:** 25 mg	In 100s and 500s.
Rx	**Clozaril** (Novartis)		Lactose, talc. (CLOZARIL 25). Pale yellow, scored. In 100s, 500s, and UD 100s.
Rx	**Clozapine** (IVAX)	**Tablets:** 50 mg	In 30s, 100s, 500s, and UD 100s.
Rx	**Clozapine** (Various, eg, Mylan, UDL, IVAX)	**Tablets:** 100 mg	In 100s and 500s.
Rx	**Clozaril** (Novartis)		Lactose, talc. (CLOZARIL 100). Pale yellow, scored. In 100s, 500s, and UD 100s.
Rx	**Clozapine** (IVAX)	**Tablets:** 200 mg	In 30s, 100s, 500s, and UD 100s.
Rx	**FazaClo** (Alamo)	**Tablets, orally disintegrating:** 25 mg	Aspartame, 1.74 mg phenylalanine, mannitol. (A01). Yellow, scored. In 48s.
		100 mg	Aspartame, 6.96 mg phenylalanine, mannitol. (A02). Yellow, scored. In 48s.

CLOZAPINE — ORAL

For complete and comparative prescribing information refer to the Antipsychotic Agents group monograph.

WARNING

Agranulocytosis – Because of a significant risk of agranulocytosis, a potentially life-threatening adverse reaction, reserve clozapine for use in the treatment of severely ill patients with schizophrenia who fail to show an acceptable response to adequate courses of standard antipsychotic drug treatment because of insufficient efficacy or the inability to achieve an effective dose because of intolerable adverse reactions from those drugs, or for reducing the risk of recurrent suicidal behavior in patients with schizophrenia or schizoaffective disorder who are judged to be at risk of reexperiencing suicidal behavior.

Patients being treated with clozapine must have a baseline white blood cell (WBC) count and absolute neutrophil count (ANC) before initiation of treatment as well as regular WBC counts and ANCs during treatment and for at least 4 weeks after discontinuation of treatment.

Clozapine is available only through a distribution system that ensures monitoring of WBC counts and ANCs according to the following schedule prior to delivery of the next supply of medication.

Seizures – Seizures have been associated with the use of clozapine. Dose appears to be an important predictor of seizure, with a greater likelihood at higher clozapine doses. Use caution when administering clozapine to patients who have a history of seizures or other predisposing factors. Advise patients not to engage in any activity in which sudden loss of consciousness could cause serious risk to themselves or others.

Myocarditis – Analyses of postmarketing safety databases suggest that clozapine is associated with an increased risk of fatal myocarditis, especially during, but not limited to, the first month of therapy. In patients in whom myocarditis is suspected, promptly discontinue clozapine treatment.

Other adverse cardiovascular and respiratory reactions – Orthostatic hypotension, with or without syncope, can occur with clozapine treatment. Rarely, collapse can be profound and be accompanied by respiratory and/or cardiac arrest. Orthostatic hypotension is more likely to occur during initial titration in association with rapid dose escalation. In patients who have had even a brief interval off clozapine (2 or more days since the last dose), start treatment with 12.5 mg once or twice daily.

Because collapse, respiratory arrest, and cardiac arrest during initial treatment have occurred in patients who were being administered benzodiazepines or other psychotropic drugs, caution is advised when clozapine is initiated in patients taking a benzodiazepine or any other psychotropic drug.

WARNING (cont.)

Elderly patients with dementia-related psychosis – Elderly patients with dementia-related psychosis treated with atypical antipsychotics drugs are at an increased risk of death compared with placebo. Analyses of 17 placebo-controlled trials (modal duration of 10 weeks) in these patients revealed a risk of death in the drug-treated patients of between 1.6 and 1.7 times that seen in placebo-treated patients. Over the course of a typical 10-week controlled trial, the rate of death in drug-treated patients was about 4.5%, compared with a rate of about 2.6% in the placebo group. Although the causes of death were varied, most of the deaths appeared to be either cardiovascular (eg, heart failure, sudden death) or infectious (eg, pneumonia) in nature. Clozapine is not approved for the treatment of patients with dementia-related psychosis.

Indications

➤*Recurrent suicidal behavior (except orally disintegrating tablets):* For reducing the risk of recurrent suicidal behavior in patients with schizophrenia or schizoaffective disorder who are judged to be at chronic risk for reexperiencing suicidal behavior, based on history and recent clinical state. Suicidal behavior refers to actions by a patient that put himself or herself at risk for death.

The efficacy of clozapine in reducing the risk of recurrent suicidal behavior was demonstrated over a 2-year treatment period in the International Suicide Prevention (InterSePT) trial. Therefore, continue clozapine treatment to reduce the risk of suicidal behavior for at least 2 years.

Be aware that a majority of patients in both treatment groups in InterSePT received other treatments as well as to reduce suicide risk, such as antidepressants and other medications, hospitalization, and/or psychotherapy. The contributions of these additional measures are unknown.

➤*Schizophrenia:* For the management of severely ill schizophrenic patients who fail to respond adequately to standard drug treatment for schizophrenia. Because of the significant risk of agranulocytosis and seizure associated with its use, use clozapine only in patients who have failed to respond adequately to treatment with appropriate courses of standard drug treatments for schizophrenia, either because of insufficient effectiveness or the inability to achieve an effective dose because of intolerable adverse reactions from those drugs.

The efficacy of clozapine in a treatment-resistant schizophrenic population was demonstrated in a 6-week study comparing clozapine and chlorpromazine. Patients meeting *Diagnostic and Statistical Manual of Mental Disorders, Third Edition* criteria for schizophrenia and having a mean Brief Psychiatric Rating scale total score of 61 were demonstrated to be treatment resistant by history and by open, prospective treatment with haloperidol before entering into the double-blind phase of the study. The superiority of clozapine to chlorpromazine was documented in statistical analyses employing both categorical and continuous measures of treatment effect.

CLOZAPINE — ORAL

Because of the significant risk of agranulocytosis and seizure, events which present a continuing risk over time, ordinarily avoid the extended treatment of patients failing to show an acceptable level of clinical response. In addition, periodically reevaluate the need for continuing treatment in patients exhibiting beneficial clinical responses.

Administration and Dosage

➤*Approved by the FDA:* September 26, 1989.

➤*Schizophrenia:* Drug dispensing should not ordinarily exceed a weekly supply. Upon initiation of clozapine therapy, up to a 1-week supply of additional clozapine may be provided to the patient to be held for emergencies (eg, weather, holidays).

If a patient is eligible for WBC count and ANC testing every 2 weeks, then a 2-week supply of clozapine can be dispensed. If a patient is eligible for WBC count and ANC testing every 4 weeks, then a 4-week supply of clozapine can be dispensed. Dispensing is contingent upon the WBC count and ANC test results.

Initial treatment – It is recommended that treatment with clozapine begin with one half of a 25 mg tablet or orally disintegrating tablet (12.5 mg) once or twice daily. The remaining one half of the orally disintegrating tablet should be destroyed. The dosing should be continued with daily dosage increments of 25 to 50 mg/day, if well tolerated, to achieve a target dose of 300 to 450 mg/day by the end of 2 weeks. Subsequent dosage increments should be made no more than once or twice weekly, in increments not to exceed 100 mg. Cautious titration and a divided dosage schedule are necessary to minimize the risks of hypotension, seizure, and sedation.

In the multicenter study that provides primary support for the efficacy of clozapine in patients resistant to standard drug treatment for schizophrenia, patients were titrated during the first 2 weeks up to a maximum dosage of 500 mg/day, on a 3-times-daily basis, and were then dosed in a total daily dosage range of 100 to 900 mg/day, on a 3-times-daily basis thereafter, with clinical response and adverse reactions as guides to correct dosing.

Dosage adjustment – Daily dosing should continue on a divided basis as an effective and tolerable dose level is sought. While many patients may respond adequately at dosages between 300 and 600 mg/day, it may be necessary to raise the dosage to 600 to 900 mg/day range to obtain an acceptable response. (Note: In the multicenter study providing the primary support for the superiority of clozapine in treatment-resistant patients, the mean and median clozapine dosages were both approximately 600 mg/day.

Because of the possibility of increased adverse reactions at higher doses, particularly seizures, patients should ordinarily be given adequate time to respond to a given dose level before escalation to a higher dose is contemplated. Clozapine can cause electroencephalographic (EEG) changes, including the occurrence of spike and wave complexes. It lowers the seizures threshold in a dose-dependent manner and may induce myoclonic jerks or generalized seizures. These symptoms may be likely to occur with rapid dose increase and in patients with preexisting epilepsy. In this case, the dose should be reduced and, if necessary, anticonvulsant treatment initiated.

Maximum dosage: Dosing should not exceed 900 mg/day. Because of the significant risk of agranulocytosis and seizure, events which both present a continuing risk over time, the extended treatment of patients failing to show an acceptable level of clinical response should ordinarily be avoided.

Maintenance – While the maintenance efficacy of clozapine in schizophrenia is still under study, the efficacy of maintenance treatment is well established for many other drugs used to treat schizophrenia. It is recommended that responding patients be continued on clozapine, but at the lowest level needed to maintain remission. Because of the significant risk associated with the use of clozapine, patients should be periodically reassessed to determine the need for maintenance treatment.

Discontinuation – In the event of planned termination of clozapine therapy, gradual reduction in dose is recommended over a 1- to 2-week period. However, if a patient's medical condition requires abrupt discontinuation (eg, leukopenia), the patient should be carefully observed for the recurrence of psychotic symptoms and symptoms related to cholinergic rebound, such as headache, nausea, vomiting, and diarrhea.

Reinitiation of treatment – When restarting patients who have had even a brief interval off clozapine (ie, 2 days or more since the last dose), it is recommended that treatment be reinitiated with one half of a 25 mg tablet (12.5 mg) once or twice daily. If that dose is well tolerated, it may be feasible to titrate patients back to a therapeutic dose more quickly than is recommended for initial treatment. However, any patient who has previously experienced respiratory or cardiac arrest with initial dosing, but was then able to be successfully titrated to a therapeutic dose, should be retitrated with extreme caution even after 24 hours of discontinuation.

Certain additional precautions seem prudent when reinitiating treatment. The mechanisms underlying clozapine-induced adverse reactions are unknown. It is conceivable, however, that reexposure of a patient might enhance the risk of an untoward event's occurrence and increase its severity. Such phenomena, for example, occur when immune-mediated mechanisms are responsible. Consequently, during the reinitiation of treatment, additional caution is advised.

Patients discontinued for WBC counts below 2,000/mm^3 or an ANC below 1,000/mm^3 must not be restarted on clozapine.

➤*Recurrent suicidal behavior (except orally disintegrating tablets):* The dosage and administration recommendations outlined above regarding the use of clozapine in patients with treatment-resistant schizophrenia should also be followed when treating patients with schizophrenia or schizoaffective disorder at risk for recurrent suicidal behavior.

The InterSePT study demonstrated the efficacy of clozapine in treatment of patients with schizophrenia or schizoaffective disorder at risk for recurrent suicidal behavior where the mean daily dose was about 300 mg (range, 12.5 to 900 mg).

Patients previously treated with other antipsychotics were cross-titrated to clozapine over a 1-month interval; the dose of the previous antipsychotic was gradually decreased simultaneously with a gradual increase in clozapine dose over the first month of the study. Patients on depot antipsychotic medication began clozapine after 1 full dosing interval since the last injection.

Duration of therapy – The results of the InterSePT study demonstrated that, for a 2-year treatment period, the probability of a suicide attempt or a hospitalization because of imminent suicide risk is stable at approximately 24% after 1 year of treatment with clozapine. A course of treatment with clozapine of at least 2 years is therefore recommended in order to maintain the reduction of risk for suicidal behavior. After 2 years, it is recommended that the health care provider's risk of suicidal behavior be assessed. If the physician's assessment indicates that a significant risk for suicidal behavior is still present, treatment with clozapine should be continued. Thereafter, the decision to continue treatment with clozapine should be revisited at regular intervals, based on thorough assessments of the patient's risk for suicidal behavior during treatment. If the health care provider determines that the patient is no longer at risk for suicidal behavior, treatment with clozapine may be discontinued (see the recommendations regarding discontinuation of treatment) and treatment of the underlying disorder with an antipsychotic medication to which the patient has previously responded may be resumed.

➤*Orally disintegrating tablets:* Clozapine rapidly disintegrates after placement in the mouth. The clozapine orally disintegrating tablet should be left in the unopened blister until time of use. The orally disintegrating tablet should not be pushed through the foil. Just prior to use, peel the foil from the blister and gently remove the orally disintegrating tablet. Immediately place the tablet in the mouth and allow it to disintegrate and swallow with saliva. No water is needed to take clozapine orally disintegrating tablets.

➤*Storage / Stability:*

Tablets – Storage temperature should not exceed 30°C (86°F).

Orally disintegrating tablets – Store clozapine orally disintegrating tablets at 25°C (77°F); excursions are permitted to 15° to 30°C (59° to 86°F). Protect from moisture. Instruct the patient not to remove the orally disintegrating tablet from the blister until the patient is ready to consume the tablet.

LOXAPINE

Rx	**Loxapine Succinate** (Various, eg, Dixon-Shane, UDL, Watson)	**Capsules:** 5 mg (6.8 mg as loxapine succinate)	In 100s and 1,000s.
Rx	**Loxitane** (Watson)		Lactose. (WATSON LOXITANE 5 mg). Dark green. In 100s and 1,000s.
Rx	**Loxapine Succinate** (Various, eg, Dixon-Shane, UDL, Watson)	**Capsules:** 10 mg (13.6 mg as loxapine succinate)	In 100s.
Rx	**Loxitane** (Watson)		Lactose. (WATSON LOXITANE 10 mg). Dark green/yellow. In 100s and 1,000s.
Rx	**Loxapine Succinate** (Various, eg, Dixon-Shane, UDL, Watson)	**Capsules:** 25 mg (34 mg as loxapine succinate)	In 100s.
Rx	**Loxitane** (Watson)		Lactose. (WATSON LOXITANE 25 mg). Two-tone green. In 100s and 1,000s.
Rx	**Loxapine Succinate** (Various, eg, Dixon-Shane, UDL, Watson)	**Capsules:** 50 mg (68.1 mg loxapine succinate)	In 100s.
Rx	**Loxitane** (Watson)		Lactose. (WATSON LOXITANE 50 mg). Dark green/blue. In 100s and 1,000s.

LOXAPINE — ORAL

For complete and comparative prescribing information, refer to the Antipsychotic Agents group monograph.

Indications

➤*Schizophrenia:* For the treatment of schizophrenia.

Administration and Dosage

Individualize dosage. Administer in divided doses, 2 to 4 times/day.

➤*Initial:* 10 mg twice daily. In severely disturbed patients, up to 50 mg/day may be desirable. Increase dosage fairly rapidly over the first 7 to 10 days until symptoms are controlled.

➤*Maintenance:* Reduce dosage to the lowest level compatible with control of symptoms.

Usual therapeutic and maintenance range is 60 to 100 mg/day. Many patients have been maintained satisfactorily at dosages in the range of 20 to 60 mg/day. Dosages higher than 250 mg/day are not recommended.

➤*Storage/Stability:* Store at controlled room temperature 15° to 30°C (59° to 86°F). Dispense capsules in a tight, child-resistant container.

OLANZAPINE

Rx	**Zyprexa** (Eli Lilly)	**Tablets**: 2.5 mg	Lactose. (LILLY 4112). White. In 60s, 1,000s, and UD 100s.
		5 mg	Lactose. (LILLY 4115). White. In 60s, 1,000s, and UD 100s.
		7.5 mg	Lactose. (LILLY 4116). White. In 60s, 1,000s, and UD 100s.
		10 mg	Lactose. (LILLY 4117). White. In 60s, 1,000s, and UD 100s.
		15 mg	Lactose. (LILLY 4415). Blue, elliptical. In 60s, 1,000s, and UD 100s.
		20 mg	Lactose. (LILLY 4420). Pink, elliptical. In 60s, 1,000s, and UD 100s.
Rx	**Zyprexa Zydis** (Eli Lilly)	**Tablets, orally disintegrating**: 5 mg	(5). Yellow. In dose pack 30s.[a]
		10 mg	(10). Yellow. In dose pack 30s.[b]
		15 mg	(15). Yellow. In dose pack 30s.[c]
		20 mg	(20). Yellow. In dose pack 30s.[d]
Rx	**Zyprexa IntraMuscular** (Eli Lilly)	**Powder for injection**: 10 mg	In vials.

[a] With aspartame, parabens, mannitol, 0.34 mg phenylalanine.
[b] With aspartame, parabens, mannitol, 0.45 mg phenylalanine.
[c] With aspartame, parabens, mannitol, 0.67 mg phenylalanine.
[d] With aspartame, parabens, mannitol, 0.9 mg phenylalanine.

OLANZAPINE — ORAL

For complete and comparative prescribing information, refer to the Antipsychotic Agents group monograph.

Indications

➤*Bipolar disorder:*

Monotherapy – For the treatment of acute mixed or manic episodes associated with bipolar I disorder and for the maintenance monotherapy of bipolar disorder.

Combination therapy – In combination with lithium or valproate for the short-term treatment of acute manic episodes associated with bipolar I disorder.

➤*Schizophrenia:* For the treatment of schizophrenia.

Administration and Dosage

➤*Approved by the FDA:* September 30, 1996 (oral).

➤*Bipolar disorder:*

Monotherapy – Initial dose is 10 to 15 mg orally once daily without regard to meals. Adjust dosage, if indicated, at 5 mg/day increments or decrements in intervals not less than 24 hours.

Short-term (3 to 4 weeks) antimanic efficacy was demonstrated in a dose range of 5 to 20 mg/day in clinical trials. The safety of doses above 20 mg/day has not been evaluated.

Maintenance monotherapy – The benefit of maintaining bipolar patients on monotherapy with olanzapine at a dose of 5 to 20 mg/day, after achieving a responder status for an average duration of 2 weeks, was demonstrated in a controlled trial. Periodically reevaluate olanzapine use in patients taking the drug for extended periods.

Combination therapy – When coadministered with lithium or valproate, generally begin olanzapine dosing with 10 mg orally once daily without regard to meals.

Short-term (6 weeks) antimanic efficacy was demonstrated in a dose range of 5 to 20 mg/day in clinical trials. The safety of doses above 20 mg/day has not been evaluated in clinical trials.

➤*Schizophrenia:* Initial dose is 5 to 10 mg orally once daily without regard to meals, with a target dose of 10 mg/day within several days of initiation. Adjust dosage, if indicated, at 5 mg/day increments or decrements in intervals not less than 1 week.

Efficacy was demonstrated in a dose range of 10 to 15 mg/day in clinical trials. However, increases in efficacy were not demonstrated in doses above 10 mg/day. Doses above 10 mg/day are recommended only after clinical assessment. The safety of doses above 20 mg/day has not been evaluated in clinical trials.

Maintenance treatment – Periodically reassess patients to determine the need for maintenance treatment.

➤*Administration of orally disintegrating tablets:* Peel back foil on blister; do not push tablet through foil. Using dry hands, remove and place the entire tablet in the mouth. The tablet will disintegrate rapidly in saliva so it can be easily swallowed with or without liquid.

➤*Special populations:* The recommended starting dose is 5 mg in patients who are debilitated, who have a predisposition to hypotensive reactions, who otherwise exhibit a combination of factors that may result in slower metabolism of olanzapine (eg, nonsmoking women 65 years of age and older), or who may be more pharmacodynamically sensitive to olanzapine. When indicated, use caution with dose escalation.

➤*Storage/Stability:* Store at controlled room temperature, 20° to 25°C (68° to 77°F). Protect from light and moisture.

OLANZAPINE — INJECTION

For complete and comparative prescribing information, refer to the Antipsychotic Agents group monograph.

WARNING

Increased mortality in elderly patients with dementia-related psychosis – Elderly patients with dementia-related psychosis treated with atypical antipsychotic drugs are at an increased risk of death compared with placebo. Analyses of 17 placebo-controlled trials (modal duration of 10 weeks) in these patients revealed a risk of death in the drug-treated patients between 1.6 to 1.7 times that seen in placebo-treated patients. Over the course of a typical 10-week controlled trial, the rate of death in drug-treated patients was about 4.5%, compared with a rate of about 2.6% in the placebo group. Although the causes of death were varied, most of the deaths appeared to be either cardiovascular (eg, heart failure, sudden death) or infectious (eg, pneumonia) in nature. Olanzapine is not approved for the treatment of patients with dementia-related psychosis.

Indications

➤*Agitation associated with schizophrenia and bipolar I mania:* Olanzapine intramuscular (IM) is indicated for the treatment of agitation associated with schizophrenia and bipolar I mania. Psychomotor agitation is defined in *Diagnostic and Statistical Manual of Mental Disorders-Fourth Edition (DSM-IV)* as excessive motor activity associated with a feeling of inner tension. Patients experiencing agitation often manifest behaviors that interfere with their diagnosis and care (eg, threatening behaviors, escalating or urgently distressing behavior, self-exhausting behavior), leading health care providers to the use of IM antipsychotic medications to achieve immediate control of the agitation.

Administration and Dosage

➤*Approved by the FDA:* September 30, 1996.

The efficacy of olanzapine IM injection in controlling agitation in these disorders was demonstrated in a dose range of 2.5 to 10 mg. The recommended dose in these patients is 10 mg. A lower dose of 5 or 7.5 mg may be considered when clinical factors warrant. If agitation warranting additional IM doses persists following the initial dose, subsequent doses up to 10 mg may be given. However, the efficacy of repeated doses of IM olanzapine for injection in agitated patients has not been systematically evaluated in controlled clinical trials. Also, the safety of total daily doses greater than 30 mg, or 10 mg injections given more frequently than 2 hours after the initial dose and 4 hours after the second dose, have not been evaluated in clinical trials. Maximal dosing of olanzapine IM (eg, 3 doses of 10 mg administered 2 to 4 hours apart) may be associated with a substantial occurrence of significant orthostatic hypotension. Thus, it is recommended that patients requiring

OLANZAPINE — INJECTION

subsequent IM injections be assessed for orthostatic hypotension prior to the administration of any subsequent doses of olanzapine IM injection. The administration of an additional dose to a patient with a clinically significant postural change in systolic blood pressure is not recommended.

If ongoing olanzapine therapy is clinically indicated, olanzapine oral may be initiated in a range of 5 to 20 mg/day as soon as clinically appropriate.

➤*Special populations:*

Elderly – A dose of 5 mg per injection should be considered for geriatric patients or when other clinical factors warrant.

Debilitated patients – A lower dose of 2.5 mg per injection should be considered for patients who otherwise might be debilitated, predisposed to hypotensive reactions, or more pharmacodynamically sensitive to olanzapine.

➤*Administration:* Olanzapine injection is intended for IM use only. Do not administer intravenously (IV) or subcutaneously. Inject slowly, deep into the muscle mass.

Directions for preparation – Dissolve the contents of the vial using 2.1 mL of sterile water for injection to provide a solution containing approximately 5 mg/mL of olanzapine. The resulting solution should appear clear and yellow. Olanzapine reconstituted with sterile water for injection should be used immediately (within 1 hour) after reconstitution. Discard any unused portion.

The following table provides injection volumes for delivering various doses of olanzapine IM for injection reconstituted with sterile water for injection.

Olanzapine IM Injection Volume

Olanzapine dose (mg)	Volume of injection (mL)
10	1.5
7.5	1
5	0.5
2.5	

Admixture incompatibility – Olanzapine injection should be reconstituted only with sterile water for injection. Olanzapine injection should not be combined in a syringe with diazepam injection because precipitation occurs when these products are mixed. Lorazepam injection should not be used to reconstitute olanzapine injection as this combination results in a delayed reconstitution time. Olanzapine injection should not be combined in a syringe with haloperidol injection because the resulting low pH has been shown to degrade olanzapine over time.

➤*Storage/Stability:* Store olanzapine vials (before reconstitution) at controlled room temperature, 20° to 25°C (68° to 77°F). Reconstituted olanzapine may be stored at controlled room temperature, 20° to 25°C (68° to 77°F) for up to 1 hour if necessary. Discard any unused portion of reconstituted olanzapine.

Protect olanzapine injection from light. Do not freeze.

QUETIAPINE FUMARATE

Rx	**Seroquel** (AstraZeneca)	**Tablets:** 25 mg	Lactose. (SEROQUEL 25). Peach. Film-coated. In 100s, 1,000s, and UD 100s.
		50 mg	Lactose. (SEROQUEL 50). White. Film-coated. In 100s, 1,000s, and UD 100s.
		100 mg	Lactose. (SEROQUEL 100). Yellow. Film-coated. In 100s and UD 100s.
		200 mg	Lactose. (SEROQUEL 200). White. Film-coated. In 100s and UD 100s.
		300 mg	Lactose. (SEROQUEL 300). White, capsule shape. Film-coated. In 60s and UD 100s.
		400 mg	Lactose. (SEROQUEL 400). Yellow, capsule shape. Film-coated. In 100s and UD 100s.

QUETIAPINE — ORAL

For complete and comparative prescribing information, refer to the Antipsychotic Agents group monograph.

WARNING

Increased mortality in elderly patients with dementia-related psychosis – Elderly patients with dementia-related psychosis treated with atypical antipsychotic drugs are at an increased risk of death compared with placebo. Analyses of 17 placebo-controlled trials (modal duration of 10 weeks) in these patients revealed a risk of death in the drug-treated patients between 1.6 to 1.7 times of that seen in placebo-treated patients. Over the course of a typical 10-week controlled trial, the rate of death in drug-treated patients was about 4.5%, compared with a rate of about 2.6% in the placebo group. Although the causes of death were varied, most of the deaths appeared to be either cardiovascular (eg, heart failure, sudden death) or infectious (eg, pneumonia) in nature. Quetiapine is not approved for the treatment of patients with dementia-related psychosis.

Indications

➤*Bipolar mania:* For the treatment of acute manic episodes associated with bipolar I disorder, as either monotherapy or adjunct therapy to lithium or divalproex.

➤*Schizophrenia:* For the treatment of schizophrenia.

Administration and Dosage

➤*Approved by the FDA:* September 26, 1997.

➤*Bipolar mania:* When used as monotherapy or adjunct therapy (with lithium or divalproex), initiate quetiapine in twice-daily doses totaling 100 mg/day on day 1, increase to 400 mg/day on day 4 in increments of up to 100 mg/day in twice-daily divided doses. Further dosage adjustments up to 800 mg/day on day 6 should be in increments of no greater than 200 mg/day. Data indicate that the majority of patients responded to dosages between 400 and 800 mg/day. The safety of dosages above 800 mg/day has not been evaluated in clinical trials.

➤*Schizophrenia:*

Usual dose – Generally, administer quetiapine with an initial dosage of 25 mg twice daily, with increases in increments of 25 to 50 mg 2 or 3 times daily on the second and third day, as tolerated, to a target dosage range of 300 to 400 mg/day by the fourth day, given 2 or 3 times daily. Further dosage adjustments, if indicated, should generally occur at intervals of no less than 2 days, as steady state for quetiapine would not be achieved for approximately 1 to 2 days in the typical patient. When dosage adjustments are necessary, increments/decrements of 25 to 50 mg twice daily are recommended. Most efficacy data with quetiapine were obtained using 3-times-daily regimens, but in 1 controlled trial, quetiapine 225 mg twice daily also was effective.

Efficacy in schizophrenia was demonstrated in a dosage range of 150 to 750 mg/day in clinical trials supporting the efficacy of quetiapine. In a dose-response study, dosages greater than 300 mg/day were not demonstrated to be more efficacious than the 300 mg/day dosage. In other studies, however, dosages in the range of 400 to 500 mg/day appeared to be needed. The safety of dosages greater than 800 mg/day has not been evaluated in clinical trials.

➤*Maintenance treatment:* While there is no body of evidence available to answer the question of how long the patient should remain on quetiapine, the efficacy of maintenance treatment is well established for many other drugs used to treat schizophrenia. It is recommended that responding patients be continued on quetiapine, but at the lowest dose needed to maintain remission. Periodically reassess patients to determine the need for maintenance treatment.

➤*Hepatic function impairment:* Start patients with hepatic function impairment on 25 mg/day. Increase the dose daily in increments of 25 to 50 mg/day to an effective dosage, depending on the clinical response and tolerability of the patient.

➤*Special populations:* Consider a slower rate of dose titration and a lower target dose in elderly patients and in patients who are debilitated or who have a predisposition to hypotensive reactions. When indicated, perform dose escalation with caution in these patients.

➤*Reinitiation of treatment in patients previously discontinued:* Although there are no data to specifically address reinitiation of treatment, it is recommended that when restarting patients who have had an interval of less than 1 week off quetiapine, titration of quetiapine is not required and the maintenance dose may be reinitiated. When restarting therapy for patients who have been off quetiapine for longer than 1 week, follow the initial titration schedule.

➤*Switching from other antipsychotics:* There are no systematically collected data to specifically address switching patients with schizophrenia from antipsychotics to quetiapine, or concerning administration with antipsychotics. While immediate discontinuation of the previous antipsychotic treatment may be acceptable for some patients with schizophrenia, more gradual discontinuation may be most appropriate for others. In all cases, minimize the period of overlapping antipsychotic administration. When switching patients with schizophrenia from depot antipsychotics, if medically appropriate, initiate quetiapine therapy in place of the next scheduled injection. Periodically reevaluate the need for continuing existing extrapyramidal symptoms (EPS) medication.

➤*Storage/Stability:* Store at 25°C (77°F); excursions permitted to 15° to 30°C (59° to 86°F).

RISPERIDONE

Rx	**Risperdal** (Janssen)	**Tablets**: 0.25 mg	Lactose. (JANSSEN Ris 0.25). Dark yellow. In 60s and 500s.
		0.5 mg	Lactose. (JANSSEN Ris 0.5). Red-brown. In 60s and 500s.
		1 mg	Lactose. (JANSSEN R 1). White. In 60s, 500s, and blister pack 100s.
		2 mg	Lactose. (JANSSEN R 2). Orange. In 60s, 500s, and blister pack 100s.
		3 mg	Lactose. (JANSSEN R 3). Yellow. In 60s, 500s, and blister pack 100s.
		4 mg	Lactose. (JANSSEN R 4). Green. In 60s and blister pack 100s.
Rx	**Risperdal M-TAB** (Janssen)	**Tablets, orally disintegrating**: 0.5 mg	0.14 mg phenylalanine, mannitol, aspartame, peppermint oil. (R0.5). Light coral. In 7 blister packs of 4 or bingo card of 30.
		1 mg	0.28 mg phenylalanine, mannitol, aspartame, peppermint oil. (R1). Light coral, square. In 7 blister packs of 4 or bingo card of 30.
		2 mg	0.56 mg phenylalanine, mannitol, aspartame, peppermint oil. (R2). Light coral. In 7 blister packs of 4.
Rx	**Risperdal** (Janssen)	**Oral solution**: 1 mg/mL	In 30 mL with calibrated pipette.
Rx	**Risperdal Consta** (Janssen)	**Powder for injection**: 25 mg	In vials. Dose pack contains prefilled syringe and 2 mL of diluent.
		37.5 mg	
		50 mg	

RISPERIDONE — ORAL

WARNING

Increased mortality in elderly patients with dementia-related psychosis – Elderly patients with dementia-related psychosis treated with atypical antipsychotic drugs are at an increased risk of death compared with placebo. Analyses of 17 placebo-controlled trials (modal duration of 10 weeks) in these patients revealed a risk of death in the drug-treated patients of between 1.6 to 1.7 times that seen in placebo-treated patients. Over the course of a typical 10-week controlled trial, the rate of death in drug-treated patients was about 4.5%, compared with a rate of about 2.6% in the placebo group. Although the causes of death were varied, most of the deaths appeared to be either cardiovascular (eg, heart failure, sudden death) or infectious (eg, pneumonia) in nature. Risperidone is not approved for the treatment of patients with dementia-related psychosis.

Indications

➤*Schizophrenia:* For the treatment of schizophrenia.

➤*Bipolar mania:*

Monotherapy – For the short-term treatment of acute manic or mixed episodes associated with bipolar I disorder.

Combination therapy – The combination of risperidone with lithium or valproate is indicated for the short-term treatment of acute manic or mixed episodes associated with bipolar I disorder.

➤*Unlabeled uses:* Treatment of certain behavioral problems in children (with or without autism); improve severely disruptive behavior in children with subaverage intelligence; treatment of patients with obsessive-compulsive disorder refractory to selective serotonin reuptake inhibitors (SSRIs); treatment of psychosis in patients with Parkinson disease; treatment of tics in patients with Tourette disorder.

Administration and Dosage

➤*Approved by the FDA:* December 29, 1993.

➤*Schizophrenia:*

Initial dose – Risperidone can be administered on either a twice daily or once daily schedule. In early clinical trials, risperidone was generally administered at 1 mg twice daily initially, with increases in increments of 1 mg twice daily on the second and third day, as tolerated, to a target dosage of 3 mg twice daily by the third day. Subsequent controlled trials have indicated that total daily risperidone doses of up to 8 mg on an every day regimen are also safe and effective. However, regardless of which regimen is employed, in some patients a slower titration may be medically appropriate. Further dosage adjustments, if indicated, should generally occur at intervals of not less than 1 week, since steady state for the active metabolite would not be achieved for approximately 1 week in the typical patient. When dosage adjustments are necessary, small dose increments/decrements of 1 to 2 mg are recommended.

Efficacy in schizophrenia was demonstrated in a dosage range of 4 to 16 mg/day in the clinical trials supporting effectiveness of risperidone; however, maximal effect was generally seen in a range of 4 to 8 mg/day. Dosages greater than 6 mg/day for twice daily dosing were not demonstrated to be more efficacious than lower dosages, were associated with more extrapyramidal symptoms and other adverse reactions, and are not generally recommended. In a single study supporting once daily dosing, the efficacy results were generally stronger for 8 mg than for 4 mg. The safety of dosages greater than 16 mg/day has not been evaluated in clinical trials.

➤*Maintenance therapy:* While there is no body of evidence available to answer the question of how long the schizophrenic patient treated with risperidone should remain on it, the effectiveness of risperidone 2 to 8 mg/day at delaying relapse was demonstrated in a controlled trial in patients who had been clinically stable for at least 4 weeks and were then followed for a period of 1 to 2 years. In this trial, risperidone was administered on a once-daily schedule, at 1 mg once daily initially, with increases to 2 mg once daily on the second day and to a target dosage of 4 mg once daily on the third day. Nevertheless, patients should be periodically reassessed to determine the need for maintenance treatment with appropriate dose.

➤*Reinitiation of treatment:* Although there are no data to specifically address reinitiation of treatment, it is recommended that when restarting patients who have had an interval off risperidone, the initial titration schedule should be followed.

➤*Switching from other antipsychotics:* There are no systematically collected data to specifically address switching from other antipsychotics to risperidone, or concerning coadministration with other antipsychotics. While immediate discontinuation of the previous antipsychotic treatment may be acceptable for some patients, more gradual discontinuation may be most appropriate for other patients. In all cases, the period of overlapping antipsychotic administration should be minimized. When switching patients from depot antipsychotics, if medically appropriate, initiate risperidone therapy in place of the next scheduled injection. The need for continuing existing extrapyramidal symptom medication should be reevaluated periodically.

➤*Bipolar mania:*

Usual dose – Risperidone should be administered on a once daily schedule, starting with 2 to 3 mg per day. Dosage adjustments, if indicated, should occur at intervals of not less than 24 hours and in dosage increments/decrements of 1 mg per day, as studied in the short-term, placebo-controlled trials. In these trials, short-term (3-week) anti-manic efficacy was demonstrated in a flexible dosage range of 1 to 6 mg per day. Risperidone doses higher than 6 mg per day were not studied.

Maintenance therapy – There is no body of evidence available from controlled trials to guide in the longer-term management of a patient who improves during treatment of an acute manic episode with risperidone. While it is generally agreed that pharmacological treatment beyond an acute response in mania is desirable, both for maintenance of the intitial response and for prevention of new manic episodes, there are not systematically obtained data to support the use of risperidone in such longer-term treatment (ie, beyond 3 weeks).

➤*Concomitant therapy:* Coadministration of carbamazepine and other enzyme inducers (eg, phenytoin, rifampin, phenobarbital) with risperidone would be expected to cause decreases in the plasma concentrations of active moiety (the sum of risperidone and 9-hydroxyrisperidone), which could lead to decreased efficacy of risperidone treatment. The dose of risperidone needs to be titrated accordingly for patients receiving these enzyme inducers, especially during initiation or discontinuation of therapy with these inducers.

Fluoxetine and paroxetine have been shown to increase the plasma concentration of risperidone 2.5- to 2.8-fold and 3.9-fold, respectively. Fluoxetine did not affect the plasma concentration of 9-hydroxyrisperidone an average of 13%. The dose of risperidone needs to be titrated accordingly when fluoxetine or paroxetine is coadministered.

➤*Special populations:* The recommended initial dose is 0.5 mg twice daily in patients who are elderly or debilitated, patients with severe renal or hepatic impairment, and patients either predisposed to hypotension or for whom hypotension would pose a risk. Dosage increases in these patients should be in increments of no more than 0.5 mg twice daily. Increases to dosages greater than 1.5 mg twice daily should generally occur at intervals of at least 1 week. In some patients, slower titration may be medically appropriate.

Elderly or debilitated patients, and patients with renal impairment, may have less ability to eliminate risperidone than healthy adults. Patients with impaired hepatic function may have increases in the free fraction of the risperidone, possibly resulting in an enhanced effect. Risperidone doses should be reduced in patients with liver disease. Patients with a predisposition to hypotensive reactions or for whom such reactions would pose a particular risk likewise need to be titrated cautiously and carefully monitored. A dose reduction should be considered if hypotension occurs. If a once-a-day dosing regimen in the elderly or debilitated patient is being considered, it is recommended that the patient be titrated on a twice-a-day regimen for 2 to 3 days at the target dose. Subsequent switches to a once-a-day dosing regimen can be done thereafter.

RISPERIDONE — ORAL

➤*Orally disintegrating tablets:* Do not open the blister until ready to administer. For single tablet removal, separate 1 of the 4 blister units by tearing apart at the perforations. Bend the corner where indicated. Peel back foil to expose the tablet. Do not push the tablet through the foil because this could damage the tablet.

Using dry hands, remove the tablet from the blister unit and immediately place the entire risperidone orally disintegrating tablet on the tongue. The risperidone orally disintegrating tablet should be consumed immediately, as the tablet cannot be stored once removed from the blister unit. Risperidone orally disintegrating tablets disintegrate in the mouth within seconds and can be swallowed subsequently with or without liquid. Patients should not attempt to split or to chew the tablet.

➤*Storage/Stability:* Keep out of the reach of children.

Risperidone tablets should be stored at controlled room temperature, 15° to 25°C (59° to 77°F), and protect from light and moisture.

Risperidone 1 mg/mL oral solution should be stored at controlled room temperature, 15° to 25°C (59° to 77°F), and protect from light and freezing.

Risperidone orally disintegrating tablets should be stored at controlled room temperature, 15° to 25°C (59° to 77°F).

RISPERIDONE — INJECTION

WARNING

Increased mortality in elderly patients with dementia-related psychosis – Elderly patients with dementia-related psychosis treated with atypical antipsychotic drugs are at an increased risk of death compared with placebo. Analyses of 17 placebo-controlled trials (modal duration of 10 weeks) in these patients revealed a risk of death in the drug-treated patients of between 1.6 and 1.7 times that seen in placebo-treated patients. Over the course of a typical 10-week controlled trial, the rate of death in drug-treated patients was about 4.5%, compared with a rate of about 2.6% in the placebo group. Although the causes of death were varied, most of the deaths appeared to be either cardiovascular (eg, heart failure, sudden death) or infectious (eg, pneumonia) in nature. Risperidone is not approved for the treatment of patients with dementia-related psychosis.

Indications

➤*Schizophrenia:* For the treatment of schizophrenia.

Administration and Dosage

➤*Approved by the FDA:* December 29, 1993 (oral).

For patients who have never taken oral risperidone, it is recommended to establish tolerability with oral risperidone prior to initiating treatment with risperidone injection.

➤*Administration:* Risperidone should be administered every 2 weeks by deep intramuscular (IM) gluteal injection. Each injection should be administered by a healthcare provider using the enclosed safety needle. Injections should alternate between the 2 buttocks. Do not administer intravenously. Do not combine 2 different dosage strengths of risperidone in a single administration.

➤*Dosage:* The recommended dosage is 25 mg IM every 2 weeks. Although dose response for effectiveness has not been established for risperidone, some patients not responding to 25 mg may benefit from a higher dose of 37.5 mg or 50 mg. The maximum dosage should not exceed 50 mg every 2 weeks. No additional benefit was observed with doses greater than 50 mg; however, a higher incidence of adverse reactions was observed.

Oral risperidone (or another antipsychotic medication) should be given with the first injection of risperidone and continued for 3 weeks (and then discontinued) to ensure that adequate therapeutic plasma concentrations are maintained prior to the main release phase of risperidone from the injection site.

➤*Dosage adjustment:* Upward dosage adjustment should not be made more frequently than every 4 weeks. The clinical effects of this dose adjustment should not be anticipated earlier than 3 weeks after the first injection with the higher dose (main release phase begins from 3 weeks onward).

➤*Special populations:*

Elderly – For elderly patients treated with risperidone, the recommended dosage is 25 mg IM every 2 weeks.

Renal/Hepatic function impairment – Patients with renal or hepatic impairment should be treated with titrated doses of oral risperidone prior to initiating treatment with risperidone injection. The recommended starting dosage is oral risperidone 0.5 mg twice daily during the first week, which can be increased to 1 mg twice daily or 2 mg once daily during the second week. If a dose of at least oral risperidone 2 mg is well tolerated, an injection of risperidone 25 mg can be administered every 2 weeks.

Oral supplementation should be continued for 3 weeks after the first injection until the main release of risperidone from the injection site has begun. In some patients, slower titration may be medically appropriate.

See Warnings for more information.

Predisposition to hypotension – Elderly patients and patients with a predisposition to hypotensive reactions or for whom such reactions would pose a particular risk should be instructed in nonpharmacologic interventions that help to reduce the occurrence of orthostatic hypotension (eg, sitting on the edge of the bed for several minutes before attempting to stand in the morning and slowly rising from a seated position). These patients should avoid sodium depletion or dehydration, and circumstances that accentuate hypotension (eg, alcohol intake, high ambient temperature). Monitoring of orthostatic vital signs should be considered.

➤*Maintenance therapy:* Although no controlled studies have been conducted to answer the question of how long patients should be treated with risperidone injection, oral risperidone has been shown to be effective in delaying time to relapse in longer-term use. It is recommended that responding patients be continued on treatment with risperidone injection at the lowest dose needed. Patients should be periodically reassessed to determine the need for continued treatment.

➤*Reinitiation of treatment:* There are no data to specifically address reinitiation of treatment. When restarting patients who have had an interval off treatment with risperidone injection, supplementation with oral risperidone (or another antipsychotic medication) should be administered.

➤*Switching from other antipsychotics:* There are no systematically collected data to specifically address switching schizophrenic patients from other antipsychotics to risperidone, or concerning coadministration with other antipsychotics. Previous antipsychotics should be continued for 3 weeks after the first injection of risperidone to ensure that therapeutic concentrations are maintained until the main release phase of risperidone from the injection site has begun. For schizophrenic patients who have never taken oral risperidone, it is recommended to establish tolerability with oral risperidone prior to initiating treatment with risperidone injection. As recommended with other antipsychotic medications, the need for continuing existing extrapyramidal symptom medication should be reevaluated periodically.

➤*Concomitant therapy:* Coadministration of carbamazepine and other enzyme inducers (eg, phenytoin, rifampin, phenobarbital) with risperidone would be expected to cause decreases in the plasma concentrations of active moiety (the sum of risperidone and 9-hydroxyrisperidone), which could lead to decreased efficacy of risperidone treatment. The dose of risperidone needs to be titrated accordingly for patients receiving these enzyme inducers, especially during initiation or discontinuation of therapy with these inducers. At the initiation of therapy with carbamazepine or other known hepatic enzyme inducers, patients should be closely monitored during the first 4 to 8 weeks, since the dose of risperidone may need to be adjusted. A dose increase, or additional oral risperidone, may need to be considered. On discontinuation of carbamazepine or other hepatic enzyme inducers, the dosage of risperidone should be reevaluated and, if necessary, decreased. Patients may be placed on a lower dose of risperidone between 2 to 4 weeks before the planned discontinuation of carbamazepine therapy to adjust for the expected increase in plasma concentrations of risperidone plus 9-hydroxyrisperidone. For patients treated with the lowest available dose (25 mg) of risperidone, it is recommended to continue treatment with the 25 mg dose unless clinical judgement necessitates interruption of treatment with risperidone.

Fluoxetine and paroxetine have been shown to increase the plasma concentration of risperidone 2.5- to 2.8-fold and 3 to 9-fold, respectively. Fluoxetine did not affect the plasma concentration of 9-hydroxyrisperidone. Paroxetine lowered the concentration of 9-hydroxyrisperidone an average of 13%. The dose of risperidone needs to be titrated acordingly when fluoxetine or paroxetine is coadministered. When either concomitant fluoxetine or paroxetine is initiated or discontinued, the health care provider should reevaluate the dosage of risperidone. When initiation of fluoxetine or paroxetine is considered, patients may be placed on a lower dose of risperidone between 2 to 4 weeks before the planned start of fluoxetine or paroxetine therapy to adjust for the expected increase in plasma concentrations of risperidone. For patients treated with the lowest available dose (25 mg), it is recommended to continue treatment with the 25 mg dose unless clinical judgement necessitates interruption of treatment with risperidone. The effects of discontinuation of concomitant fluoxetine or paroxetine therapy on the pharmacokinetics of risperidone and 9-hydroxyrisperidone have not been studied.

➤*Preparation for use:* Risperidone must be suspended only in the diluent supplied in the dose pack, and must be administered with the needle supplied in the dose pack. All components are required for administration. Do not substitute any components of the dose pack.

Remove the dose pack of risperidone from the refrigerator and allow it to come to room temperature prior to reconstitution.

Upon suspension in the diluent, it is recommended to use risperidone immediately. Risperidone must be used within 6 hours of suspension. Resuspension of risperidone will be necessary prior to administration, as settling will occur over time once the product is in suspension. Keeping the vial upright, shake vigorously back and forth for as long as it takes to resuspend the microspheres.

➤*Storage/Stability:* The entire dose pack should be stored in the refrigerator (2° to 8°C; 36° to 46°F) and protected from light. If refrigeration is unavailable, risperidone can be stored at temperatures not exceeding 25°C (77°F) for no more than 7 days prior to administration. Do not expose unrefrigerated product to temperatures above 25°C (77°F). Once in suspension, the product should not be exposed to temperatures above 25°C (77°F).

Benzisoxazole Derivatives

ZIPRASIDONE

Rx	**Geodon** (Pfizer)	**Capsules**: 20 mg (as hydrochloride)	Lactose. (Pfizer 396). Blue/white. In 60s and UD 80s.
		40 mg (as hydrochloride)	Lactose. (Pfizer 397). Blue/blue. In 60s and UD 80s.
		60 mg (as hydrochloride)	Lactose. (Pfizer 398). White/white. In 60s and UD 80s.
		80 mg (as hydrochloride)	Lactose. (Pfizer 399). Blue/white. In 60s and UD 80s.
		Powder for Injection: 20 mg (as mesylate)	In single-use vials.

ZIPRASIDONE HYDROCHLORIDE — ORAL

For complete and comparative prescribing information, refer to the Antipsychotic Agents group monograph.

WARNING

Increased mortality in elderly patients with dementia-related psychosis – Elderly patients with dementia-related psychosis treated with atypical antipsychotic drugs are at an increased risk of death compared with placebo. Analyses of 17 placebo-controlled trials (modal duration of 10 weeks) in these patients revealed a risk of death in the drug-treated patients between 1.6 to 1.7 times that seen in placebo-treated patients. Over the course of a typical 10-week controlled trial, the rate of death in drug-treated patients was about 4.5%, compared with a rate of about 2.6% in the placebo group. Although the causes of death were varied, most of the deaths appeared to be either cardiovascular (eg, heart failure, sudden death) or infectious (eg, pneumonia) in nature. Ziprasidone is not approved for the treatment of patients with dementia-related psychosis.

Indications

➤*Bipolar mania:* For the treatment of acute manic or mixed episodes associated with bipolar disorder, with or without psychotic features. A manic episode is a distinct period of abnormally and persistently elevated, expansive, or irritable mood. A mixed episode is characterized by the criteria for a manic episode in conjunction with those for a major depressive episode (depressed mood, loss of interest or pleasure in nearly all activities).

➤*Schizophrenia:* For the treatment of schizophrenia. When deciding among the alternative treatments available for this condition, consider the finding of ziprasidone's greater capacity to prolong the QT/QTc interval compared with several other antipsychotic drugs. Prolongation of the QTc interval is associated in some other drugs with the ability to cause torsades de pointes–type arrhythmia, a potentially fatal polymorphic ventricular tachycardia, and sudden death. In many cases, this would lead to the conclusion that other drugs should be tried first. Whether ziprasidone will cause torsades de pointes or increase the rate of sudden death is not yet known.

Administration and Dosage

➤*Approved by the FDA:* February 5, 2001.

➤*Bipolar mania:*

Initial dosage – Administer oral ziprasidone at an initial dosage of 40 mg twice daily with food. Then, increase the dosage to 60 or 80 mg twice/day on the second day of treatment and subsequently adjust on the basis of toleration and efficacy within the range of 40 to 80 mg twice/day. In the flexible-dose clinical trials, the mean daily dose administered was approximately 120 mg.

Maintenance dosage – There is no body of evidence available from controlled trials to guide a clinician in the longer-term management of a patient who improves during treatment of mania with ziprasidone. While it is generally agreed that pharmacological treatment beyond an acute response in mania is desirable, for maintenance of the initial response and prevention of new manic episodes, there are no systematically obtained data to support the use of ziprasidone in such longer-term treatment (eg, beyond 3 weeks).

➤*Schizophrenia:* When deciding among the alternative treatments available for schizophrenia, consider ziprasidone's higher capacity to prolong the QT/QTc interval compared with other antipsychotic drugs.

Initial dosage – Administer ziprasidone at an initial dosage of 20 mg twice daily with food. In some patients, daily dosage subsequently may be adjusted on the basis of individual clinical status up to 80 mg twice daily. If indicated, dosage adjustments generally should occur at intervals of 2 days or more, as steady state is achieved within 1 to 3 days. To ensure use of the lowest effective dose, observe patients for improvement for several weeks before upward dosage adjustment.

Efficacy in schizophrenia was demonstrated in a dosage range of 20 to 100 mg twice daily in short-term, placebo-controlled, clinical trials. There were trends toward dosage response within the range of 20 to 80 mg twice daily, but results were not consistent. Generally, an increase to a dosage more than 80 mg twice daily is not recommended. The safety of dosages above 100 mg twice daily has not been systematically evaluated in clinical trials.

Maintenance dosage – While there is no body of evidence available to answer the question of how long to treat a patient with ziprasidone, systematic evaluation of ziprasidone has shown that its efficacy in schizophrenia is maintained for periods of up to 52 weeks at a dosage of 20 to 80 mg twice daily. No additional benefit was demonstrated for dosages above 20 mg twice daily. Periodically reassess patients to determine the need for maintenance treatment.

➤*Special populations:* Dosage adjustments are generally not required on the basis of age, gender, race, or renal or hepatic impairment.

➤*Storage/Stability:* Store at controlled room temperature, 15° to 30°C (59° to 86°F).

ZIPRASIDONE — INJECTION

For complete and comparative prescribing information, refer to the Antipsychotic Agents group monograph.

Indications

➤*Acute agitation:* For the treatment of acute agitation in schizophrenic patients for whom treatment with ziprasidone is appropriate and who need intramuscular (IM) antipsychotic medication for rapid control of the agitation.

Administration and Dosage

When deciding among the alternative treatments available for schizophrenia, the health care provider should consider the finding of ziprasidone's greater capacity to prolong the QT/QTc interval compared with several other antipsychotic drugs.

➤*Acute agitation:* The recommended dose is 10 to 20 mg administered as required, up to a maximum dosage of 40 mg/day. Doses of 10 mg may be administered every 2 hours; doses of 20 mg may be administered every 4 hours, up to a maximum of 40 mg/day. IM administration of ziprasidone for more than 3 consecutive days has not been studied.

If long-term therapy is indicated, ziprasidone oral should replace the IM administration as soon as possible.

Because there is no experience regarding the safety of administering ziprasidone IM to schizophrenic patients already taking ziprasidone oral, the practice of coadministration is not recommended.

➤*Preparation for administration:* Ziprasidone for injection should only be administered by IM injection. Single-dose vials require reconstitution prior to administration; any unused portion should be discarded.

Add 1.2 mL of sterile water for injection to the vial and shake vigorously until all the drug is dissolved. Each milliliter of reconstituted solution contains ziprasidone 20 mg. To administer a 10 mg dose, draw up 0.5 mL of the reconstituted solution. To administer a 20 mg dose, draw up 1 mL of the reconstituted solution. Because no preservative or bacteriostatic agent is present in this product, aseptic technique must be used in preparation of the final solution. This product must not be mixed with other medicinal products or solvents other than sterile water for injection.

➤*Storage/Stability:* Store at controlled room temperature, 15° to 30°C (59° to 86°F), in dry form. Protect from light. Following reconstitution, ziprasidone can be stored, when protected from light, for up to 24 hours at controlled room temperature or up to 7 days refrigerated, 2° to 8°C (36° to 46°F).

ARIPIPRAZOLE

Rx	**Abilify** (Bristol-Myers Squibb/Otsuka America)	**Tablets**: 2 mg	Lactose. (A-006 2). Green, rectangular. In 30s and blister 100s.
		5 mg	Lactose. (A-007 5). Blue, rectangular. In 30s and blister 100s.
		10 mg	Lactose. (A-008 10). Pink, rectangular. In 30s and blister 100s.
		15 mg	Lactose. (A-009 15). Yellow. In 30s and blister 100s.
		20 mg	Lactose. (A-010 20). White. In 30s and blister 100s.
		30 mg	Lactose. (A-011 30). Pink. In 30s and blister 100s.
		Oral solution: 1 mg/mL	Fructose, sucrose, parabens. Orange cream flavor. In 50, 150, and 480 mL.

ARIPIPRAZOLE — ORAL

WARNING

Increased mortality in elderly patients with dementia-related psychosis – Elderly patients with dementia-related psychosis treated with atypical antipsychotic drugs are at an increased risk of death, compared with placebo. Analyses of 17 placebo-controlled trials (modal duration, 10 weeks) in these patients revealed a risk of death in the drug-treated patients of between 1.6 to 1.7 times that seen in placebo-treated patients. Over the course of a typical 10-week controlled trial, the rate of death in drug-treated patients was about 4.5%, compared with a rate of about 2.6% in the placebo group. Although the causes of death were varied, most of the deaths appeared to be either cardiovascular (eg, heart failure, sudden death) or infections (eg, pneumonia) in nature. Aripiprazole is not approved for the treatment of patients with dementia-related psychosis.

Indications

➤*Bipolar mania:* For the treatment of acute manic and mixed episodes associated with bipolar disorder.

The efficacy of aripiprazole was established in two 3-week placebo-controlled trials of inpatients with *Diagnostic and Statistical Manual of Mental Disorders, Fourth Edition* (*DSM-IV*) criteria for bipolar I disorder who were experiencing an acute manic or mixed episode with or without psychotic features.

The efficacy of aripiprazole in maintaining efficacy in patients with bipolar I disorder with a recent manic or mixed episode who had been stabilized and then maintained for at least 6 weeks was demonstrated in a double-blind, placebo-controlled trial. Prior to entering the double-blind, randomization phase of this trial, patients were clinically stabilized and maintained their stability for 6 consecutive weeks on aripiprazole. Following this 6-week maintenance phase, patients were randomized to either placebo or aripiprazole and monitored for relapse. Health care providers who elect to use aripiprazole for extended periods (ie, longer than 6 weeks) should periodically reevaluate the long-term usefulness of the drug for the individual patients.

➤*Schizophrenia:* For the treatment of schizophrenia.

The efficacy of aripiprazole in the treatment of schizophrenia was established in short-term (4- and 6-week) controlled trials of schizophrenic inpatients.

The efficacy of aripiprazole in maintaining stability in patients with schizophrenia who had been symptomatically stable on other antipsychotic medications for periods of 3 months or longer, were discontinued from those other medications, and were then administered aripiprazole 15 mg/day and observed for relapse during a period of up to 26 weeks was demonstrated in a placebo-controlled trial. Health care providers who elect to use aripiprazole for extended periods should periodically reevaluate the long-term usefulness of the drug for the individual patient.

Administration and Dosage

➤*Approved by the FDA:* November 15, 2002.

➤*Bipolar mania:*

Usual dosage – In clinical trials, the starting dosage was 30 mg/day. A dosage of 30 mg/day was found to be effective when administered as the tablet formulation. Approximately 15% of patients had their dose decreased to 15 mg based on assessment of tolerability. The safety of dosages above 30 mg/day has not been evaluated in clinical trials.

Maintenance treatment – While there is no body of evidence available on how long a patient treated with aripiprazole should remain on the drug, patients with bipolar I disorder who had been symptomatically stable on aripiprazole tablets (15 or 30 mg/day, with a starting dosage of 30 mg/day) for at least 6 consecutive weeks and then randomized to aripiprazole tablets (15 or 30 mg/day) or placebo and monitored for relapse demonstrated a benefit of such maintenance treatment. While it is generally agreed that pharmacological treatment beyond an acute response in mania is desirable, both for maintenance of the initial response and for prevention of new manic episodes, there are no systematically obtained data to support the use of aripiprazole in longer-term treatment (ie, beyond 6 weeks).

➤*Schizophrenia:*

Usual dosage – The recommended starting and target dosage for aripiprazole is 10 or 15 mg/day administered on a once-a-day schedule without regard to meals. Aripiprazole has been systematically evaluated and shown to be effective in a dosage range of 10 to 30 mg/day when administered as the tablet formulation; however, dosages higher than 10 or 15 mg/day, the lowest doses in these trials, were not more effective than 10 or 15 mg/day. Do not make dosage increases before 2 weeks, the time needed to achieve steady state.

Maintenance therapy – While there is no body of evidence available on how long a patient treated with aripiprazole should remain on the drug, systematic evaluation of patients with schizophrenia who had been symptomatically stable on other antipsychotic medications for periods of 3 months or longer, were discontinued from those medications, and were then administered aripiprazole 15 mg/day and observed for relapse during a period of up to 26 weeks demonstrated a benefit of such maintenance treatment. Periodically reassess patients to determine the need for maintenance treatment.

Switching from other antipsychotics – There are no systematically collected data to specifically address switching patients with schizophrenia from other antipsychotics to aripiprazole or concerning coadministration with other antipsychotics. While immediate discontinuation of the previous antipsychotic treatment may be acceptable for some patients with schizophrenia, more gradual discontinuation may be most appropriate for others. In all cases, minimize the period of overlapping antipsychotic administration.

➤*Special populations:* Dosage adjustments are not routinely indicated on the basis of age, gender, race, or renal or hepatic function impairment status.

Concomitant use with potential CYP3A4 inhibitors – When coadministering ketoconazole with aripiprazole, reduce the aripiprazole dose to one half of the usual dose. When the CYP3A4 inhibitor is withdrawn from the combination therapy, increase the aripiprazole dose.

Concomitant use with potential CYP2D6 inhibitors – When coadministering potential CYP2D6 inhibitors such as quinidine, fluoxetine, or paroxetine with aripiprazole, reduce the aripiprazole dose at least to one half of its normal dose. When the CYP2D6 inhibitor is withdrawn from the combination therapy, increase the aripiprazole dose.

Concomitant use with potential CYP3A4 inducers – When a potential CYP3A4 inducer such as carbamazepine is added to aripiprazole therapy, double the aripiprazole dose (to 20 to 30 mg). Base additional dose increases on clinical evaluation. When carbamazepine is withdrawn from the combination therapy, reduce the aripiprazole dose to 10 to 15 mg.

Oral solution – The oral solution can be given on a mg-per-mg basis in place of the 5, 10, 15, or 20 mg tablet strengths. Solution doses can be substituted for the tablet doses on a mg-per-mg basis up to the 25 mg tablet. Patients receiving 30 mg tablets should receive 25 mg of the solution.

➤*Storage / Stability:*

Tablets – Store at 25°C (77°F); excursions are permitted to 15° to 30°C (59° to 86°F).

Oral solution – Store in a refrigerator at 2° to 8°C (36° to 46°F). Open bottles of aripiprazole oral solution should be stored in a refrigerator and can be used for up to 6 months after opening.

LITHIUM

Rx	**Lithium Carbonate** (Various, eg, Harber, International Labs, Roxane)	**Tablets**: 300 mg lithium carbonate (8.12 mEq lithium)	In 100s, 1,000s, and UD 100s.
Rx	**Lithium Carbonate** (Various, eg, Roxane)	**Tablets, extended-release**: 300 mg lithium carbonate (8.12 mEq lithium)	In 100s and 500s.
Rx	**Lithobid** (Solvay)		(Solvay 4492). Peach. Film coated. In 100s, 1,000s, and UD 100s.
Rx	**Lithium Carbonate** (Roxane)	**Tablets, extended-release**: 450 mg lithium carbonate	In 100s.
Rx	**Eskalith CR** (GlaxoSmithKline)	**Tablets, controlled-release**: 450 mg lithium carbonate (12.18 mEq lithium)	(SKF J10). Yellow, scored. In 100s.
Rx	**Lithium Carbonate** (Roxane)	**Capsules**: 150 mg lithium carbonate (4.06 mEq lithium)	(54 213). White. In 100s, 1,000s, and UD 100s.
Rx	**Lithium Carbonate** (Various, eg, Dixon-Shane, Geneva, Goldline, Moore, Roxane)	**Capsules**: 300 mg lithium carbonate (8.12 mEq lithium)	In 100s, 500s, 1,000s, and UD 100s.
Rx	**Eskalith** (GlaxoSmithKline)		(Eskalith SB). Yellow and gray. In 100s.
Rx	**Lithium Carbonate** (Roxane)	**Capsules**: 600 mg lithium carbonate (16.24 mEq lithium)	(54 702). White and flesh. In 100s, 1,000s, and UD 100s.
Rx	**Lithium Citrate** (Various, eg, Geneva, Major, PBI, Roxane, Xactdose)	**Syrup**: 8 mEq lithium (as citrate equivalent to 300 mg lithium carbonate) per 5 mL	In 480 and 500 mL and UD 5 and 10 mL.

LITHIUM CARBONATE — ORAL

Complete prescribing information begins in the Antipsychotic Agents group monograph.

WARNING

Lithium toxicity is closely related to serum lithium levels, and can occur at doses close to therapeutic levels. Facilities for prompt and accurate serum lithium determinations should be available before initiating therapy.

Indications

➤*Bipolar disorder:* Lithium is indicated in the treatment of manic episodes of manic-depressive illness.

Maintenance therapy reduces the frequency of manic episodes and diminishes the intensity of those episodes which may occur.

Typical symptoms of mania include pressure of speech, motor hyperactivity, reduced need for sleep, flight of ideas, grandiosity, elation, poor judgment, aggressiveness, and possibly hostility. When given to a patient experiencing a manic episode, lithium may produce a normalization of symptomatology within 1 to 3 weeks.

➤*Unlabeled uses:* Lithium carbonate (300 to 1000 mg/day) has improved the neutrophil count in patients with cancer chemotherapy-induced neutropenia, in children with chronic neutropenia, and in AIDS patients receiving zidovudine.

Lithium has also been used successfully in the prophylaxis of cluster headache; premenstrual tension; bulimia; alcoholism (especially if patient has a concomitant affective disorder such as depression); syndrome of inappropriate secretion of antidiuretic hormone (ADH); tardive dyskinesia; hyperthyroidism; postpartum affective psychosis; corticosteroid-induced psychosis.

A topical lithium succinate preparation has been studied in the treatment of seborrheic dermatitis and genital herpes.

Administration and Dosage

Individualize dosage according to both serum levels and clinical response. Immediate-release products are usually given 3 or 4 times daily. Extended-release products are usually given twice daily (12-hour intervals). Swallow extended/controlled-release tablets whole; do not chew or crush.

➤*Serum lithium levels:* Draw blood samples immediately prior to the next dose (8 to 12 hours after the previous dose) when lithium concentrations are relatively stable. Do not rely on serum levels alone.

➤*Acute mania:* Optimal patient response is usually established and maintained with 600 mg 3 times daily or 900 mg twice/day for the slow-release form. Such doses normally produce an effective serum lithium level ranging between 1 and 1.5 mEq/L.

Determine serum levels twice weekly during the acute phase and until the serum level and clinical condition of the patient have been stabilized.

➤*Long-term use:* The desirable serum levels are 0.6 to 1.2 mEq/L. Dosage will vary, but 900 to 1,200 mg daily in divided doses will usually maintain this level. Monitor serum levels in uncomplicated cases on maintenance therapy during remission at least every 2 months.

➤*Storage / Stability:* Store at 25°C (77°F); excursions permitted between 15° to 30°C (59° to 86°F). Protect from moisture. Dispense in tight, child-resistant container.

Actions

➤*Pharmacology:* Preclinical studies have shown that lithium alters sodium transport in nerve and muscle cells and effects a shift toward intraneuronal metabolism of catecholamines, but the specific biochemical mechanism of lithium action in mania is unknown.

➤*Pharmacokinetics:* The distribution space of lithium approximates that of total body water. Lithium is primarily excreted in urine with insignificant excretion in feces. Renal excretion of lithium is proportional to its plasma concentration. The half-life of elimination of lithium is approximately 24 hours. Lithium decreases sodium reabsorption by the renal tubules which could lead to sodium depletion. Therefore, it is essential for the patient to maintain a normal diet, including salt, and an adequate fluid intake (2500 to 3000 mL) at least during the initial stabilization period. Decreased tolerance to lithium has been reported to ensue from protracted sweating or diarrhea and, if such occur, supplemental fluid and salt should be administered under careful medical supervision and lithium intake reduced or suspended until the condition is resolved.

Contraindications

Lithium should generally not be given to patients with significant renal or cardiovascular disease, severe debilitation or dehydration, or sodium depletion, and to patients receiving diuretics or angiotensin-converting enzyme (ACE) inhibitors, since the risk of lithium toxicity is very high in such patients. If the psychiatric indication is life-threatening, and if such a patient fails to respond to other measures, lithium treatment may be undertaken with extreme caution, including daily serum lithium determinations and adjustment to the usually low doses ordinarily tolerated by these individuals. In such instances, hospitalization is a necessity.

Warnings

➤*Toxicity:* Lithium toxicity is closely related to serum lithium levels, and can occur at doses close to therapeutic levels. The desirable serum lithium levels are 0.6 to 1.2 mEq/L. Patients abnormally sensitive to lithium may exhibit toxic signs at serum levels of 1 to 1.5 mEq/L.

Outpatients and their families should be warned that the patient must discontinue lithium therapy and contact his physician if such clinical signs of lithium toxicity as diarrhea, vomiting, tremor, mild ataxia, drowsiness, or muscular weakness occur.

➤*Renal function impairment:* Chronic lithium therapy may be associated with diminution of renal concentrating ability, occasionally presenting as nephrogenic diabetes insipidus, with polyuria and polydipsia. Such patients should be carefully managed to avoid dehydration with resulting lithium retention and toxicity. This condition is usually reversible when lithium is discontinued.

Morphologic changes with glomerular and interstitial fibrosis and nephron atrophy have been reported in patients on chronic lithium therapy. Morphologic changes have also been seen in bipolar patients never exposed to lithium. The relationship between renal functional and morphologic changes and their association with lithium therapy has not been established. To date, lithium in therapeutic doses has not been reported to cause end-stage renal disease.

When kidney function is assessed, for baseline data prior to starting lithium therapy or thereafter, routine urinalysis and other tests may be used to evaluate tubular function (eg, urine specific gravity or osmolality following a period of water deprivation, or 24-hour urine volume) and glomerular function (eg, serum creatinine or creatinine clearance). During lithium therapy, progressive or sudden changes in renal function, even within the normal range, indicate the need for reevaluation of treatment.

➤*Elderly:* Elderly patients often require lower lithium dosages to achieve therapeutic serum levels. They may also exhibit adverse reactions at serum levels ordinarily tolerated by younger patients.

In general, dose selection for an elderly patient should be cautious, usually starting at the low end of the dosing range, reflecting the greater frequency of decreased hepatic, renal, or cardiac function, and of concomitant disease or other therapy.

➤*Pregnancy:* *Category D.* In humans, lithium may cause fetal harm when administered to a pregnant woman. There have been reports of lithium having adverse effects on nidations in rats, embryo viability in mice, and metabolism in vitro of rat testis and human spermatozoa have been attributed to lithium, as have teratogenicity in submammalian species, and cleft palate in mice. Studies in rats, rabbits and monkeys have shown no evidence of lithium-induced teratology. Data from lithium birth registries suggest an increase in cardiac and other anomalies, especially Ebstein's anomaly. If the patient becomes pregnant while taking lithium, she should be apprised of

LITHIUM CARBONATE — ORAL

the potential risk to the fetus. If possible, lithium should be withdrawn for at least the first trimester unless it is determined that this would seriously endanger the mother.

➤*Lactation:* Lithium is excreted in human milk. Nursing should not be undertaken during lithium therapy except in rare and unusual circumstances where, in the view of the physician, the potential benefits to the mother outweigh possible hazards to the child. Signs and symptoms of lithium toxicity such as hypertonia, hypothermia, cyanosis and ECG changes have been reported in some infants and neonates.

➤*Children:* Since information regarding the safety and effectiveness of lithium in children under 12 years of age is not available, its use in such patients is not recommended at this time.

There has been a report of a transient syndrome of acute dystonia and hyperreflexia occurring in a 15 kg child who ingested 300 mg of lithium carbonate.

Precautions

➤*Monitoring:* Previously existing underlying thyroid disorders do not necessarily constitute a contraindication to lithium treatment; where hypothyroidism exists, careful monitoring of thyroid function during lithium stabilization and maintenance allows for correction of changing thyroid parameters, if any. Where hypothyroidism occurs during lithium stabilization and maintenance, supplemental thyroid treatment may be used.

Lithium levels should be closely monitored when patients initiate or discontinue NSAID use. In some cases, lithium toxicity has resulted from interactions between an NSAID and lithium.

Kidney function should be assessed prior to and during lithium therapy. Routine urinalysis and other tests may be used to evaluate tubular function (eg, urine specific gravity or osmolality following a period of water deprivation, or 24-hour urine volume) and glomerular function (eg, serum creatinine or creatinine clearance). During lithium therapy, progressive or sudden changes in renal function, even within the normal range, indicate the need for reevaluation of treatment.

The ability to tolerate lithium is greater during the acute manic phase and decreases when manic symptoms subside.

The distribution space of lithium approximates that of total body water. Lithium is primarily excreted in urine with insignificant excretion in feces. Renal excretion of lithium is proportional to its plasma concentration. The half-life of elimination of lithium is approximately 24 hours. Lithium decreases sodium reabsorption by the renal tubules which could lead to sodium depletion. Therefore, it is essential for the patient to maintain a normal diet, including salt, and an adequate fluid intake (2500 to 3000 mL) at least during the initial stabilization period. Decreased tolerance to lithium has been reported to ensue from protracted sweating or diarrhea and, if such occur, supplemental fluid and salt should be administered under careful medical supervision and lithium intake reduced or suspended until the condition is resolved. In addition to sweating and diarrhea, concomitant infection with elevated temperatures may also necessitate a temporary reduction or cessation of medication.

➤*Special risk:* Lithium should generally not be given to patients with significant renal or cardiovascular disease, severe debilitation, dehydration, sodium depletion, and to patients receiving diuretics, or ACE inhibitors, since the risk of lithium toxicity is very high in such patients. If the psychiatric indication is life threatening, and if such a patient fails to respond to other measures, lithium treatment may be undertaken with extreme caution, including daily serum lithium determinations and adjustment to the usually low doses ordinarily tolerated by these individuals. In such instances, hospitalization is a necessity.

➤*Hazardous tasks:* Lithium may impair mental or physical abilities. Caution patients about activities requiring alertness (eg, operating vehicles or machinery).

Drug Interactions

Lithium Drug Interactions

Precipitant drug	Object drug*		Description
Acetazolamide	Lithium	↓	Increased renal excretion of lithium.
Carbamazepine	Lithium	↑	Increased neurotoxic effects despite therapeutic serum levels and normal dosage range.
Fluoxetine	Lithium	↓↑	Increased lithium serum levels; mechanism unknown.
Haloperidol	Lithium	↑	Increased or decreased neurotoxic effects despite therapeutic serum levels and normal dosage range.
Loop diuretics	Lithium	↑	Increased lithium serum levels; mechanism unknown.
Methyldopa	Lithium	↑	Increased neurotoxic effects with or without increased lithium serum levels.
NSAIDs	Lithium	↑	Decreased renal clearance of lithium possibly caused by inhibition of renal prostaglandin synthesis.
Osmotic diuretics (urea)	Lithium	↓	Increased renal excretion of lithium.
Theophyllines	Lithium	↓	Increased renal excretion of lithium.
Thiazide diuretics	Lithium	↑	Increased lithium serum levels caused by decreased renal lithium clearance.
Urinary alkalinizers	Lithium	↓	Enhanced renal lithium clearance.
Verapamil	Lithium	↔	Both a reduction in lithium levels and lithium toxicity have occurred.
Lithium	Iodide salts	↑	Synergistic action to more readily produce hypothyroidism.
Lithium	Neuromuscular blocking agents	↑	Neuromuscular blocking effects may be increased; profound and severe respiratory depression may occur.
Lithium	Phenothiazines	↔	Neurotoxicity, decreased phenothiazine concentrations or increased lithium concentrations may occur.
Lithium	Sympathomimetics	↓	The pressor sensitivity of the sympathomimetic may be decreased.
Lithium	Tricyclic antidepressants	↑	Pharmacologic effects of the tricyclic may be increased.

* ↑ = Object drug increased. ↓ = Object drug decreased.
↔ = Undetermined clinical effect.

The following drugs can lower serum lithium concentrations by increasing urinary lithium excretion: Acetazolamide, urea, xanthine preparations and alkalinizing agents such as sodium bicarbonate.

The following have also been shown to interact with lithium: Methyldopa and phenytoin.

➤*Antipsychotic medication:* The possibility of similar adverse interactions with other antipsychotic medication exists.

➤*Calcium channel blocking agents:* Concurrent use of calcium channel blocking agents with lithium may increase the risk of neurotoxicity in the form of ataxia, tremors, nausea, vomiting, diarrhea or tinnitus. Caution is recommended.

➤*Diuretics or angiotensin-converting enzyme (ACE) inhibitors:* In general, the concomitant use of diuretics or angiotensin-converting enzyme (ACE) inhibitors with lithium carbonate should be avoided. In those cases where concomitant use is necessary, extreme caution is advised since sodium loss from these drugs may reduce the renal clearance of lithium resulting in increased serum lithium concentrations with the risk of lithium toxicity.

There is evidence that ACE inhibitors, such as enalapril and captopril, and angiotensin II receptor antagonists, such as losartan, may substantially increase steady-state plasma lithium levels, sometimes resulting in lithium toxicity. When such combinations are used, the lithium dosage may need to be decreased, and more frequent monitoring of lithium serum concentrations is recommended.

➤*Neuroleptics:* An encephalopathic syndrome (characterized by weakness, lethargy, fever, tremulousness and confusion, extrapyramidal symptoms, leucocytosis, elevated serum enzymes, BUN and FBS) followed by irreversible brain damage has occurred in a few patients treated with lithium plus a neuroleptic, most notably haloperidol. Because of a possible causal relationship between these events and the concomitant administration of lithium and neuroleptic drugs, patients receiving such combined therapy or patients with organic brain syndrome or other CNS impairment should be monitored closely for early evidence of neurological toxicity and treatment discontinued promptly if such signs appear. This encephalopathic syndrome may be similar to or the same as neuroleptic malignant syndrome (NMS).

➤*Metronidazole:* Concurrent use of metronidazole with lithium may provoke lithium toxicity due to reduced renal clearance. Patients receiving such combined therapy should be monitored closely.

➤*Selective serotonin reuptake inhibitors:* The concomitant administration of lithium with selective serotonin reuptake inhibitors (SSRIs) should be undertaken with caution as this combination has been reported to result in symptoms such as diarrhea, confusion, tremor, dizziness, and agitation.

Adverse Reactions

➤*Lithium toxicity:* The likelihood of toxicity increases with increasing serum lithium levels. Serum lithium levels greater than 1.5 mEq/L carry a greater risk than lower levels. However, patients sensitive to lithium may exhibit toxic signs at serum levels below 1.5 mEq/L.

Diarrhea, vomiting, drowsiness, muscular weakness and lack of coordination may be early signs of lithium toxicity, and can occur at lithium levels below 2 mEq/L. At higher levels, giddiness, ataxia, blurred vision, tinnitus and a large output of dilute urine may be seen. Serum lithium levels above 3 mEq/L may produce a complex clinical picture involving multiple organs and organ systems. Serum lithium levels should not be permitted to exceed 2 mEq/L during the acute treatment phase.

LITHIUM CARBONATE — ORAL

Fine hand tremor, polyuria and mild thirst may occur during initial therapy for the acute manic phase, and may persist throughout treatment. Transient and mild nausea and general discomfort may also appear during the first few days of lithium administration.

These side effects are an inconvenience rather than a disabling condition, and usually subside with continued treatment or a temporary reduction or cessation of dosage. If persistent, a cessation of dosage is indicated.

➤*Adverse reactions directly related to serum lithium levels:* The following adverse reactions have been reported and appear to be directly related to serum lithium levels, including concentrations within the therapeutic range.

Cardiovascular – Cardiac arrhythmia, hypotension, peripheral circulatory collapse, bradycardia, sinus node dysfunction with severe bradycardia (which may result in syncope).

EKG changes: Reversible flattening, isoelectricity or inversion of T-waves.

CNS – Blackout spells, epileptiform seizures, slurred speech, dizziness, vertigo, incontinence of urine or feces, somnolence, psychomotor retardation, restlessness, confusion, stupor, coma, acute dystonia, downbeat nystagmus, tongue movements, tics, tinnitus, hallucinations, poor memory, slowed intellectual functioning, startled response, worsening of organic brain syndromes, myasthenia gravis (rarely).

Cases of pseudotumor cerebri (increased intracranial pressure and papilledema) have been reported with lithium use. If undetected, this condition may result in enlargement of the blind spot, constriction of visual fields and eventual blindness due to optic atrophy. Lithium should be discontinued, if clinically possible, if this syndrome occurs.

Autonomic nervous system: Blurred vision, dry mouth, impotence/sexual dysfunction.

EEG changes: Diffuse slowing, widening of frequency spectrum, potentiation and disorganization of background rhythm.

Dermatologic – Drying and thinning of hair, anesthesia of skin, acne, chronic folliculitis, xerosis cutis, alopecia and exacerbation of psoriasis, generalized pruritus with or without rash, angioedema, cutaneous ulcers.

Endocrine – Euthyroid goiter or hypothyroidism (including myxedema) accompanied by lower T_3 and T_4. ^{131}Iodine uptake may be elevated. Paradoxically, rare cases of hyperthyroidism have been reported.

GI – Anorexia, nausea, vomiting, diarrhea, gastritis, salivary gland swelling, abdominal pain, excessive salivation, flatulence, indigestion.

GU – Albuminuria, oliguria, polyuria, glycosuria, decreased creatinine clearance, symptoms of nephrogenic diabetes insipidus including polyuria, thirst and polydipsia.

Musculoskeletal – Tremor, muscle hyperirritability (fasciculations, twitching, clonic movements of whole limbs), ataxia, hypertonicity, choreoathetotic movements, hyperactive deep tendon reflexes, extrapyramidal symptoms including acute dystonia, cogwheel rigidity.

Miscellaneous – Fatigue, lethargy, transient scotomata, dehydration, weight loss, tendency to sleep.

Miscellaneous reactions unrelated to dosage are: Transient electroencephalographic and electrocardiographic changes, leucocytosis, headache, diffuse nontoxic goiter with or without hypothyroidism, transient hyperglycemia, excessive weight gain, edematous swelling of ankles or wrists, and metallic taste.

Exophthalmos, hypercalcemia, hyperparathyroidism, dysgeusia/taste distortion, salty taste, swollen lips, tightness in chest, swollen or painful joints, fever, polyarthralgia, dental caries.

A few reports have been received of the development of painful discoloration of fingers and toes and coldness of the extremities within 1 day of the starting of treatment of lithium. The mechanism through which these symptoms (resembling Raynaud's syndrome) developed is not known. Recovery followed discontinuance.

Some reports of nephrogenic diabetes insipidus, hyperparathyroidism, and hypothyroidism which persist after lithium discontinuation have been received.

Overdosage

➤*Symptoms:* The toxic concentrations for lithium (greater than or equal to 1.5 mEq/L) are close to the therapeutic concentrations (0.6 to 1.2 mEq/L). It is therefore important that patients and their families be cautioned to watch for early symptoms and to discontinue the drug and inform the physician should they occur. Diarrhea, vomiting, drowsiness, muscular weakness, and lack of coordination may be early signs of lithium toxicity, and can occur at lithium levels below 2 mEq/L. At higher levels, giddiness, ataxia, blurred vision, tinnitus, and a large output of dilute urine may be seen. Serum lithium levels above 3 mEq/L may produce a complex clinical picture involving multiple organs and organ systems. Serum lithium levels should not be permitted to exceed 2 mEq/L during the acute treatment phase.

➤*Treatment:* No specific antidote for lithium poisoning is known. Treatment is supportive. Early symptoms of lithium toxicity can usually be treated by reduction of cessation of dosage of the drug and resumption of the treatment at a lower dose after 24 to 48 hours. In severe cases of lithium poisoning, the first and foremost goal of treatment consists of elimination of this ion from the patient.

Treatment is essentially the same as that used in barbiturate poisoning:

1.) Gastric lavage.
2.) Correction of fluid and electrolyte imbalance.
3.) Regulation of kidney functioning.

Urea, mannitol, and aminophylline all produce significant increases in lithium excretion. Hemodialysis is an effective and rapid means of removing the ion from the severely toxic patient. However, patient recovery may be slow. Infection prophylaxis, regular chest x-rays, and preservation of adequate respiration are essential.

Patient Information

Outpatients and their families should be warned that the patient must discontinue lithium therapy and contact his physician if such clinical signs of lithium toxicity as diarrhea, vomiting, tremor, mild ataxia, drowsiness, or muscular weakness occur.

Lithium may impair mental or physical abilities. Caution patients about activities requiring alertness (eg, operating vehicles or machinery).

Take immediately after meals or with food or milk to avoid stomach upset.

Drink 8 to 12 glasses of water or other liquid every day while on this drug. Prolonged exposure to the sun can lead to dehydration. Maintain a regular diet (including salt). Contact a physician if fever or diarrhea develops.

LITHIUM CITRATE — ORAL

Complete prescribing information begins in the Antipsychotic Agents group monograph.

WARNING

Lithium toxicity is closely related to serum lithium levels, and can occur at doses close to therapeutic levels. Facilities for prompt and accurate serum lithium determinations should be available before initiating therapy.

Indications

➤*Bipolar disorder:* Lithium is indicated in the treatment of manic episodes of bipolar disorder.

Maintenance therapy reduces the frequency of manic episodes and diminishes the intensity of those episodes which may occur.

Typical symptoms of mania include pressure of speech, motor hyperactivity, reduced need for sleep, flight of ideas, grandiosity, elation, poor judgment, aggressiveness, and possibly hostility. When given to a patient experiencing a manic episode, lithium may produce a normalization of symptomatology within 1 to 3 weeks.

Administration and Dosage

➤*Acute mania:* Optimal patient response to lithium citrate syrup usually can be established and maintained with 10 mL (2 full teaspoons) (16 mEq of lithium) 3 times daily. Such doses will normally produce an effective serum lithium level ranging between 1 and 1.5 mEq/L. Dosage must be individualized according to serum levels and clinical response. Regular monitoring of the patient's clinical state and of serum lithium levels is necessary. Serum levels should be determined twice per week during the acute phase, and until the serum level and clinical condition of the patient has been stabilized.

➤*Long-term control:* The desirable serum lithium levels are 0.6 to 1.2 mEq/L. Dosage will vary from one individual to another, but usually 5 mL (1 full teaspoon) (8 mEq of lithium) of lithium citrate syrup 3 or 4 times daily will maintain this level. Serum lithium levels in uncomplicated cases receiving maintenance therapy during remission should be monitored at least every 2 months.

Patients abnormally sensitive to lithium may exhibit toxic signs at serum levels of 1 to 1.5 mEq/L. Elderly patients often respond to reduced dosage, and may exhibit signs of toxicity at serum levels ordinarily tolerated by other patients.

➤*Blood samples:* Blood samples for serum lithium determination should be drawn immediately prior to the next dose when lithium concentrations are relatively stable (ie, 8 to 12 hours after the previous dose). Total reliance must not be placed on serum levels alone. Accurate patient evaluation requires both clinical and laboratory analysis.

Actions

➤*Pharmacology:* Preclinical studies have shown that lithium alters sodium transport in nerve and muscle cells and effects a shift toward intraneuronal metabolism of catecholamines, but the specific biochemical mechanism of lithium action in mania is unknown.

➤*Pharmacokinetics:* The distribution space of lithium approximates that of total body water. Lithium is primarily excreted in urine with insignificant excretion in feces. Renal excretion of lithium is proportional to its plasma concentration. The half-life of elimination of lithium is approximately 24 hours. Lithium decreases sodium reabsorption by the renal tubules which could lead to sodium depletion. Therefore, it is essential for the patient to maintain a normal diet, including salt, and an adequate fluid intake (2500 to 3000 mL) at least during the initial stabilization period. Decreased tolerance to lithium has been reported to ensue from protracted sweating or diarrhea and, if such occur, supplemental fluid and salt should be administered.

Contraindications

Lithium should generally not be given to patients with significant renal or cardiovascular disease, severe debilitation or dehydration, or sodium depletion, and to patients receiving diuretics, since the risk of lithium toxicity is very high in such patients. If the psychiatric indication is life-threatening, and if such a patient fails to respond to other measures, lithium treatment

LITHIUM CITRATE — ORAL

may be undertaken with extreme caution, including daily serum lithium determinations and adjustment to the usually low doses ordinarily tolerated by these individuals. In such instances, hospitalization is a necessity.

Warnings

➤*Toxicity:* Lithium toxicity is closely related to serum lithium levels, and can occur at doses close to therapeutic levels. The desirable serum lithium levels are 0.6 to 1.2 mEq/L. Patients abnormally sensitive to lithium may exhibit toxic signs at serum levels of 1 to 1.5 mEq/L.

➤*Renal effects:* Chronic lithium therapy may be associated with diminution of renal concentrating ability, occasionally presenting as nephrogenic diabetes insipidus, with polyuria and polydipsia. Such patients should be carefully managed to avoid dehydration with resulting lithium retention and toxicity. This condition is usually reversible when lithium is discontinued.

Morphologic changes with glomerular and interstitial fibrosis and nephron-atrophy have been reported in patients on chronic lithium therapy. Morphologic changes have also been seen in bipolar patients never exposed to lithium. The relationship between renal functional and morphologic changes and their association with lithium therapy has not been established. To date, lithium in therapeutic doses has not been reported to cause end-stage renal disease.

When kidney function is assessed, for baseline data prior to starting lithium therapy or thereafter, routine urinalysis and other tests may be used to evaluate tubular function (eg, urine specific gravity or osmolality following a period of water deprivation, or 24-hour urine volume) and glomerular function (eg, serum creatinine or creatinine clearance). During lithium therapy, progressive or sudden changes in renal function, even within the normal range, indicate the need for reevaluation of treatment.

➤*Elderly:* Elderly patients often require lower lithium dosages to achieve therapeutic serum concentrations. They may also exhibit adverse reactions at serum concentrations ordinarily tolerated by younger patients. Additionally, patients with renal impairment may also require lower lithium doses.

➤*Pregnancy: Category D.* Lithium may cause fetal harm when administered to a pregnant woman. There have been reports of lithium having adverse effects on nidations in rats, embryo viability in mice, and metabolism in vitro of rat testis and human spermatozoa have been attributed to lithium, as have teratogenicity in submammalian species, and cleft palates in mice. Studies in rats, rabbits and monkeys have shown no evidence of lithium-induced teratology. Data from lithium birth registries suggest an increase in cardiac and other anomalies, especially Ebstein's anomaly. If the patient becomes pregnant while taking lithium, she should be apprised of the potential risk to the fetus. If possible, lithium should be withdrawn for at least the first trimester unless it is determined that this would seriously endanger the mother.

➤*Lactation:* Lithium is excreted in human milk. Nursing should not be undertaken during lithium therapy except in rare and unusual circumstances where, in the view of the physician, the potential benefits to the mother outweigh possible hazards to the child.

➤*Children:* Since information regarding the safety and effectiveness of lithium in children under 12 years of age is not available, its use in such patients is not recommended at this time. There has been a report of a transient syndrome of acute dystonia and hyperreflexia occurring in a 15 kg child who ingested 300 mg of lithium carbonate.

Precautions

➤*Monitoring:* Previously existing underlying thyroid disorders do not necessarily constitute a contraindication to lithium treatment; where hypothyroidism exists, careful monitoring of thyroid function during lithium stabilization and maintenance allows for correction of changing thyroid parameters, if any. Where hypothyroidism occurs during lithium stabilization and maintenance, supplemental thyroid treatment may be used.

The ability to tolerate lithium is greater during the acute manic phase and decreases when manic symptoms subside.

➤*Special risk:* In addition to sweating and diarrhea, concomitant infection with elevated temperatures may also necessitate a temporary reduction or cessation of medication.

➤*Hazardous tasks:* Lithium may impair mental or physical abilities. Caution patients about activities requiring alertness (eg, operating vehicles or machinery).

Drug Interactions

The following drugs can lower serum lithium concentrations by increasing urinary lithium excretion: Acetazolamide, urea, xanthine preparations and alkalinizing agents such as sodium bicarbonate.

The following have also been shown to interact with lithium: Methyldopa and phenytoin.

➤*Antipsychotic medication:* The possibility of similar adverse interactions with other antipsychotic medication exists (see Haloperidol).

➤*Calcium channel blocking agents:* Concurrent use of calcium channel blocking agents with lithium may increase the risk of neurotoxicity in the form of ataxia, tremors, nausea, vomiting, diarrhea or tinnitus.

➤*Carbamazepine:* Concomitant administration of carbamazepine and lithium may increase the risk of neurotoxic side effects.

➤*Diuretics or angiotensin-converting enzyme (ACE) inhibitors:* Caution should be used when lithium and diuretics or angiotensin-converting enzyme (ACE) inhibitors are used concomitantly because sodium loss may reduce the renal clearance of lithium and increase serum lithium levels with risk of lithium toxicity. When such combinations are used, the lithium dosage may need to be decreased, and more frequent monitoring of lithium plasma levels is recommended.

There is evidence that angiotensin-converting enzyme inhibitors (eg, enalapril and captopril) may substantially increase steady-state plasma lithium levels, sometimes resulting in lithium toxicity.

➤*Fluoxetine:* Concurrent use of fluoxetine with lithium has resulted in both increased and decreased serum lithium concentrations. Patients receiving such combined therapy should be monitored closely.

➤*Haloperidol:* An encephalopathic syndrome (characterized by weakness, lethargy, fever, tremulousness and confusion, extrapyramidal symptoms, leucocytosis, elevated serum enzymes, BUN and fasting blood sugar [FBS]) followed by irreversible brain damage has occurred in a few patients treated with lithium plus haloperidol. A causual relationship between these events and the concomitant administration of lithium and haloperidol has not been established; however, patients receiving such combined therapy should be monitored closely for early evidence of neurological toxicity and treatment discontinued promptly if such signs appear.

➤*NSAIDs:* Indomethacin and piroxicam have been reported to increase significantly, steady state plasma lithium levels. In some cases lithium toxicity has resulted from such interactions. There is also evidence that other nonsteroidal, anti-inflammatory agents may have a similar effect. When such combinations are used, increased plasma lithium level monitoring is recommended. Lithium levels should be closely monitored when patients initiate or discontinue NSAID use.

➤*Iodide preparations:* Concomitant extended use of iodide preparations, especially potassium iodide, with lithium may produce hypothyroidism.

➤*Metronidazole:* Concurrent use of metronidazole with lithium may provoke lithium toxicity due to reduced renal clearance. Patients receiving such combined therapy should be monitored closely.

➤*Neuromuscular blocking agents:* Lithium may prolong the effects of neuromuscular blocking agents. Therefore, neuromuscular blocking agents should be given with caution to patients receiving lithium.

➤*Selective serotonin reuptake inhibitors:* The concomitant administration of lithium with selective serotonin reuptake inhibitors should be undertaken with caution as this combination has been reported to result in symptoms such as diarrhea, confusion, tremor, dizziness and agitation.

Adverse Reactions

➤*Lithium toxicity:* The likelihood of toxicity increases with increasing serum lithium levels. Serum lithium levels greater than 1.5 mEq/L carry a greater risk than lower levels. However, patients sensitive to lithium may exhibit toxic signs at serum levels below 1.5 mEq/L.

Diarrhea, vomiting, drowsiness, muscular weakness and lack of coordination may be early signs of lithium toxicity, and can occur at lithium levels below 2 mEq/L. At higher levels, giddiness, ataxia, blurred vision, tinnitus and a large output of dilute urine may be seen. Serum lithium levels above 3 mEq/L may produce a complex clinical picture involving multiple organs and organ systems. Serum lithium levels should not be permitted to exceed 2 mEq/L during the acute treatment phase.

Fine hand tremor, polyuria and mild thirst may occur during initial therapy for the acute manic phase, and may persist throughout treatment. Transient and mild nausea and general discomfort may also appear during the first few days of lithium administration.

These side effects are an inconvenience rather than a disabling condition, and usually subside with continued treatment or a temporary reduction or cessation of dosage. If persistent, a cessation of dosage is indicated.

➤*Adverse reactions not directly related to serum lithium levels:* The following adverse reactions have been reported and do not appear to be directly related to serum lithium levels.

Cardiovascular – Cardiac arrhythmia, hypotension, peripheral circulatory collapse, sinus node dysfunction with severe bradycardia (which may result in syncope).

EKG changes: Reversible flattening, isoelectricity or inversion of T-waves.

CNS – Blackout spells, epileptiform seizures, slurred speech, dizziness, vertigo, incontinence of urine or feces, somnolence, psychomotor retardation, restlessness, confusion, stupor, coma, acute dystonia, downbeat nystagmus.

Autonomic nervous system: Blurred vision, dry mouth.

EEG changes: Diffuse slowing, widening of frequency spectrum, potentiation and disorganization of background rhythm.

Neurological: Cases of pseudotumor cerebri (increased intracranial pressure and papilledema) have been reported with lithium use. If undetected, this condition may result in enlargement of the blind spot, constriction of visual fields and eventual blindness due to optic atrophy. Lithium should be discontinued, if clinically possible, if this syndrome occurs.

Dermatologic – Drying and thinning of hair, anesthesia of skin, chronic folliculitis, xerosis cutis, alopecia and exacerbation of psoriasis.

GI – Anorexia, nausea, vomiting, diarrhea.

GU – Albuminuria, oliguria, polyuria, glycosuria.

Musculoskeletal – Tremor, muscle hyperirritability (fasciculations, twitching, clonic movements of whole limbs), ataxia, choreoathetotic movements, hyperactive deep tendon reflexes.

Endocrine – Euthyroid goiter or hypothyroidism (including myxedema) accompanied by lower T_3 and T_4. Iodine 131 uptake may be elevated. Paradoxically, rare cases of hyperthyroidism have been reported.

Miscellaneous – Fatigue, lethargy, transient scotomata, dehydration, weight loss, tendency to sleep.

LITHIUM CITRATE — ORAL

Miscellaneous reactions unrelated to dosage are the following: Transient electroencephalographic and electrocardiographic changes, leucocytosis, headache, diffuse nontoxic goiter with or without hypothyroidism, transient hyperglycemia, generalized pruritus with or without rash, cutaneous ulcers, albuminuria, worsening of organic brain syndromes, excessive weight gain, edematous swelling of ankles or wrists, and thirst or polyuria, sometimes resembling diabetes insipidus, and metallic taste.

A single report has been received of the development of painful discoloration of fingers and toes and coldness of the extremities within 1 day of the starting of treatment of lithium. The mechanism through which these symptoms (resembling Raynaud's syndrome) developed is not known. Recovery followed discontinuance.

Overdosage

➤*Symptoms:* The toxic levels for lithium are close to the therapeutic levels. It is therefore important that patients and their families be cautioned to watch for early symptoms and to discontinue the drug and inform the physician should they occur. Toxic symptoms include the following: Giddiness; ataxia; blurred vision; tinnitus; vertigo; increasing confusion; slurred speech; blackouts; fasciculations; myoclonic twiching o rmovement of entire limbs; choreoathetoid movements; urinary or fecal incontinence; agitation or manic-like behavior; hyperreflexia; hypertonia; dysarthria; seizures (generalized and focal); arrhythmias; hypotension; peripheral vascular collapse; stupor; muscle group twitching; spasticity; coma.

➤*Treatment:* No specific antidote for lithium poisoning is known. Early symptoms of lithium toxicity can usually be treated by reduction of cessation of dosage of the drug and resumption of the treatment at a lower dose after 24 to 48 hours. In severe cases of lithium poisoning, the first and foremost goal of treatment consists of elimination of this ion from the patient.

Treatment is essentially the same as that used in barbiturate poisoning:
1.) Gastric lavage.
2.) Correction of fluid and electrolyte imbalance.
3.) Regulation of kidney functioning. Urea, mannitol, and aminophylline all produce significant increases in lithium excretion. Hemodialysis is an effective and rapid means of removing the ion from the severely toxic patient. Infection prophylaxis, regular chest x-rays, and preservation of adequate respiration are essential.

Patient Information

Outpatients and their families should be warned that the patient must discontinue lithium therapy and contact his physician if such clinical signs of lithium toxicity as diarrhea, vomiting, tremor, mild ataxia, drowsiness, or muscular weakness occur.

Lithium may impair mental or physical abilities. Caution patients about activities requiring alertness (eg, operating vehicles or machinery).

Take immediately after meals or with food or milk to avoid stomach upset.

Drink 8 to 12 glasses of water or other liquid every day while on this drug. Prolonged exposure to the sun can lead to dehydration. Maintain a regular diet (including salt). Contact a physician if fever or diarrhea develops.

NMDA Receptor Antagonists

MEMANTINE HYDROCHLORIDE

Rx	**Namenda** (Forest Laboratories)	**Tablets:** 5 mg	Lactose. (5 FL). Tan, capsule shape. Film-coated. In 60s, 200s, 2,000s, UD 100s, and titration paks.[a]
		10 mg	Lactose. (10 FL). Gray, capsule shape. Film-coated. In 60s, 200s, 2,000s, UD 100s, and titration paks.[a]
		Oral solution: 2 mg/mL	Sorbitol, parabens. Alcohol free, sugar free. Peppermint flavor. In 360 mL.

[a] Titration paks are blister packages containing 49 tablets (28 × 5 mg and 21 × 10 mg).

MEMANTINE HYDROCHLORIDE — ORAL

Indications

➤*Alzheimer disease:* For the treatment of moderate to severe dementia of the Alzheimer type.

➤*Unlabeled uses:* Treatment of vascular dementia.

Administration and Dosage

➤*Approved by the FDA:* October 16, 2003.

Memantine can be taken with or without food.

➤*Dosage:* The recommended starting dosage of memantine is 5 mg once daily. The recommended target dosage is 20 mg/day. The dosage should be increased in 5 mg increments to 10 mg/day (5 mg twice a day), 15 mg/day (5 and 10 mg as separate doses), and 20 mg/day (10 mg twice a day). The minimum recommended interval between dose increases is 1 week.

➤*Renal function impairment:* Dose reduction in patients with moderate renal function impairment should be considered. In patients with severe renal function impairment, the use of memantine has not been systematically evaluated and is not recommended.

➤*Storage/Stability:* Store at 25°C (77°F); excursions permitted from 15° to 30°C (59° to 86°F).

Actions

➤*Pharmacology:* Persistent activation of CNS N-methyl-D-aspartate (NMDA) receptors by the excitatory amino acid glutamate has been hypothesized to contribute to the symptomatology of Alzheimer disease. Memantine is postulated to exert its therapeutic effect through its action as a low to moderate affinity uncompetitive (open-channel) NMDA receptor antagonist, which binds preferentially to the NMDA receptor-operated cation channels. There is no evidence that memantine prevents or slows neurodegeneration in patients with Alzheimer disease.

Memantine showed low to negligible affinity for gamma-amminobutyric acid, benzodiazepine, dopamine, adrenergic, histamine and glycine receptors and for voltage-dependent Ca^{2+}, Na^+ or K^+ channels. Memantine also showed antagonistic effects at the 5-HT_3 receptor with a potency similar to that for the NMDA receptor and blocked nicotinic acetylcholine receptors with ⅙ to ⅒ the potency.

➤*Pharmacokinetics:*

Absorption/Distribution – Memantine is well-absorbed after oral administration and has linear pharmacokinetics over the therapeutic dose range. Following oral administration, memantine is highly absorbed with peak concentrations reached in about 3 to 7 hours. Food has no effect on the absorption of memantine. The mean volume of distribution of memantine is 9 to 11 L/kg and the plasma protein binding is low (45%).

Metabolism/Excretion – Memantine undergoes little metabolism, with the majority (57% to 82%) of an administered dose excreted unchanged in urine; the remainder is converted primarily to 3 polar metabolites: N-gludantan conjugate, 6-hydroxy memantine, and 1-nitroso-deaminated memantine. These metabolites possess minimal NMDA receptor antagonist activity. The hepatic microsomal P-450 enzyme system does not play a significant role in the metabolism of memantine. Renal clearance involves active tubular secretion moderated by pH-dependent tubular reabsorption. It is excreted predominantly in the urine, unchanged, and has a terminal elimination half-life of about 60 to 80 hours.

Special populations –

Gender: Following multiple-dose administration of memantine 20 mg twice daily, women had about 45- higher exposure than men, but there was no difference in exposure when body weight was taken into account.

Contraindications

Hypersensitivity to memantine or to any excipients used in the formulation.

Warnings

➤*Renal function impairment:* See Administration and Dosage for more information.

➤*Pregnancy: Category B.* Slight maternal toxicity, decreased pup weights, and an increased incidence of nonossified cervical vertebrae were seen at an oral dosage of 18 mg/kg/day in a study in which rats were given oral memantine beginning premating and continuing through the postpartum period. Slight maternal toxicity and decreased pup weights also were seen at this dose in a study in which rats were treated from day 15 of gestation through the postpartum period. The no-effect dose for these effects was 6 mg/kg, which is 3 times the MRHD on a mg/m^2 basis.

There are no adequate and well-controlled studies of memantine in pregnant women. Use memantine during pregnancy only if the potential benefit justifies the potential risk to the fetus.

➤*Lactation:* It is not known whether memantine is excreted in human breast milk. Because many drugs are excreted in human milk, exercise caution when memantine is administered to a breast-feeding mother.

➤*Children:* There are no adequate and well-controlled trials documenting the safety and efficacy of memantine in any illness occurring in children.

Precautions

➤*Genitourinary conditions:* Conditions that raise urine pH may decrease the urinary elimination of memantine resulting in increased plasma levels of memantine.

Drug Interactions

➤*NMDA antagonists:* The combined use of memantine with other NMDA antagonists (amantadine, ketamine, and dextromethorphan) has not been systematically evaluated; approach such use with caution.

➤*Drugs highly bound to plasma proteins:* Because the plasma protein binding of memantine is low (45%), an interaction with drugs that are highly bound to plasma proteins, such as warfarin and digoxin, is unlikely.

➤*Drugs eliminated via renal mechanisms:* Because memantine is eliminated in part by tubular secretion, coadministration of drugs that use the same renal cationic system, including hydrochlorothiazide, triamterene, cimetidine, ranitidine, quinidine, and nicotine, could potentially result in altered plasma levels of both agents. However, coadministration of meman-

MEMANTINE HYDROCHLORIDE — ORAL

tine and hydrochlorothiazide/triamterene did not affect the bioavailability of memantine or triamterene, and the bioavailability of hydrochlorothiazide decreased 20%.

➤*Drugs that make the urine alkaline:* The clearance of memantine was reduced by about 80% under alkaline urine conditions at pH 8. Therefore, alterations of urine pH towards the alkaline condition may lead to an accumulation of the drug with a possible increase in adverse effects. Urine pH is altered by diet, drugs (eg, carbonic anhydrase inhibitors, sodium bicarbonate) and clinical state of the patient (eg, renal tubular acidosis, severe infections of the urinary tract). Hence, use memantine with caution under these conditions.

Adverse Reactions

➤*Adverse reactions reported in controlled trials:*

Memantine Adverse Reactions (≥ 2% and Higher Frequency than Placebo)		
Adverse reaction	Memantine (n = 940)	Placebo (n = 922)
Cardiovascular		
Hypertension	4%	2%
CNS		
Confusion	6%	5%
Dizziness	7%	5%
Hallucination	3%	2%
Headache	6%	3%
Somnolence	3%	2%
GI		
Constipation	5%	3%
Vomiting	3%	2%
Musculoskeletal		
Back pain	3%	2%
Respiratory		
Coughing	4%	3%
Dyspnea	2%	1%
Miscellaneous		
Fatigue	2%	1%
Pain	3%	1%

Other adverse reactions occurring with an incidence of at least 2% in memantine-treated patients but at a greater or equal rate on placebo were agitation, fall, inflicted injury, urinary incontinence, diarrhea, bronchitis, insomnia, urinary tract infection, influenza-like symptoms, gait abnormal, depression, upper respiratory tract infection, anxiety, peripheral edema, nausea, anorexia, and arthralgia.

➤*Vital sign changes:* Memantine and placebo groups were compared with respect to the following: 1) mean change from baseline in vital signs (pulse, systolic blood pressure, diastolic blood pressure, and weight) and 2) the incidence of patients meeting criteria for potentially clinically significant changes from baseline in these variables. There were no clinically important changes in vital signs in patients treated with memantine. A comparison of supine and standing vital sign measures for memantine and placebo in elderly healthy patients indicated that memantine treatment is not associated with orthostatic changes.

➤*Lab test abnormalities:* Memantine and placebo groups were compared with respect to the following: 1) mean change from baseline in various serum chemistry, hematology, and urinalysis variables and 2) the incidence of patients meeting criteria for potentially clinically significant changes from baseline in these variables. These analyses revealed no clinically important changes in laboratory test parameters associated with memantine treatment.

➤*Electrocardiogram (ECG) changes:* Memantine and placebo groups were compared with respect to the following: 1) mean change from baseline in various ECG parameters and 2) the incidence of patients meeting criteria for potentially clinically significant changes from baseline in these variables. These analyses revealed no clinically important changes in ECG parameters associated with memantine treatment.

➤*Other adverse reactions:*

Cardiovascular – Cardiac failure, syncope (at least 1%).

Angina pectoris, atrial fibrillation, bradycardia, cardiac arrest, hypotension, myocardial infarction, postural hypotension, pulmonary edema, pulmonary embolism, thrombophlebitis (0.1% to 1%).

CNS – Aggressive reaction, ataxia, cerebrovascular accident, hypokinesia, transient ischemic attack, vertigo (at least 1%).

Abnormal coordination, abnormal crying, abnormal thinking, amnesia, apathy, aphasia, cerebral hemorrhage, convulsions, delirium, delusion, depersonalization, emotional lability, extrapyramidal disorder, hemiplegia, hyperkinesia, hypertonia, hypesthesia, increased appetite, increased libido, involuntary muscle contractions, nervousness, neuralgia, neuropathy, neurosis, paranoid reaction, paresthesia, paroniria, personality disorder, psychosis, ptosis, sleep disorder, stupor, suicide attempt, tremor (0.1% to 1%).

Dermatologic – Rash (at least 1%). Alopecia, cellulitis, dermatitis, eczema, erythematous rash, pruritus, skin ulceration, urticaria (0.1% to 1%).

GI – Diverticulitis, esophageal ulceration, gastroenteritis, GI hemorrhage, melena (0.1% to 1%).

GU – Frequent micturition (at least 1%). Dysuria, hematuria, urinary retention (0.1% to 1%).

Hematologic/Lymphatic – Anemia (at least 1%).

Leukopenia (0.1% to 1%).

Metabolic/Nutritional – Decreased weight, increased alkaline phosphatase (at least 1%). Aggravated diabetes mellitus, dehydration, hyponatremia (0.1% to 1%).

Respiratory – Pneumonia (at least 1%). Apnea, asthma, hemoptysis (0.1% to 1%).

Special senses – Cataract, conjunctivitis (at least 1%). Abnormal lacrimation, blepharitis, blurred vision, conjunctival hemorrhage, corneal opacity, decreased hearing, decreased visual acuity, diplopia, eye pain, glaucoma, macula lutea degeneration, myopia, retinal detachment, retinal hemorrhage, tinnitus, xerophthalmia (0.1% to 1%).

Miscellaneous – Allergic reaction, hypothermia (0.1% to 1%). Memantine has been commercially available outside the United States since 1982, and has been evaluated in clinical trials including trials in patients with neuropathic pain, Parkinson disease, organic brain syndrome, and spasticity. The following adverse reactions of possible importance for which there is inadequate data to determine the causal relationship have been reported to be temporally associated with memantine treatment in more than 1 patient and are not described elsewhere in labeling: acne, bone fracture, carpal tunnel syndrome, claudication, hyperlipidemia, impotence, otitis media, thrombocytopenia.

Overdosage

➤*Symptoms:* In a documented case of an overdosage with up to 400 mg of memantine, the patient experienced restlessness, psychosis, visual hallucinations, somnolence, stupor, and loss of consciousness. The patient recovered without permanent sequelae.

Animal toxicology – Memantine induced neuronal lesions (vacuolation and necrosis) in the multipolar and pyramidal cells in cortical layers 3 and 4 of the posterior cingulate and retrosplenial neocortices in rats, similar to those which are known to occur in rodents administered other NMDA receptor antagonists. Lesions were seen after a single dose of memantine. In a study in which rats were given daily oral doses of memantine for 14 days, the no-effect dose for neuronal necrosis was 6 times the MRHD on a mg/m^2 basis. The potential for induction of central neuronal vacuolation and necrosis by NMDA receptor antagonists in humans is unknown.

➤*Treatment:* Utilize general supportive measures and symptomatic treatment. Elimination of memantine can be enhanced by acidification of urine.

Patient Information

Instruct caregivers in the recommended administration (twice daily for doses above 5 mg) and dose escalation (minimum interval of 1 week between dose increases)

➤*Patient instructions for memantine oral solution:* Remove oral dosing syringe along with the green cap and plastic tube from its protective plastic bag. Attach the tube to the green cap if it isn't already attached.

The bottle comes with a child-resistant cap. Open it by pushing down on the cap while turning the cap counterclockwise (to the left). Remove the unscrewed cap. Carefully remove the seal from the bottle and discard.

Insert the plastic tube fully into the bottle and screw the green cap tightly onto the bottle by turning the cap clockwise (to the right).

The green cap has an attached lid for sealing the product in between doses. Keeping the bottle upright on the table, remove the lid to uncover the opening on the top of the cap. With the plunger fully depressed, insert the tip of syringe firmly into the opening in the cap.

While holding the syringe, gently pull the plunger of the syringe up to draw medicine into the syringe.

Remove the syringe from the opening of the cap. Invert the syringe (point tip upwards) and slowly press the plunger to a level that pushes out any large air bubbles that may be present. Keep the plunger in this position. Do not worry about a few tiny bubbles. This will not affect your dose in any way.

CHOLINESTERASE INHIBITORS

TACRINE HYDROCHLORIDE (Tetrahydroacridinamine; THA)

Rx	**Cognex** (Parke-Davis)	**Capsules:** 10 mg	Lactose. (Cognex 10). Yellow/dark green. In 120s and UD 100s.
		20 mg	Lactose. (Cognex 20). Yellow/light blue. In 120s and UD 100s.
		30 mg	Lactose. (Cognex 30). Yellow/orange. In 120s and UD 100s.
		40 mg	Lactose. (Cognex 40). Yellow/lavender. In 120s and UD 100s.

TACRINE HYDROCHLORIDE — ORAL

Indications

➤*Alzheimer disease:* For the treatment of mild-to-moderate dementia of the Alzheimer type.

Administration and Dosage

➤*Approved by the FDA:* September 9, 1993.

Following initiation of therapy, or any dosage increase, patients should be observed carefully for adverse effects. Tacrine HCl should be taken between meals whenever possible; however, if minor GI upset occurs, tacrine HCl may be taken with meals to improve tolerability. Taking tacrine HCl with meals can be expected to reduce plasma levels approximately 30% to 40%.

➤*Initiation of treatment:* The initial dose of tacrine HCl is 40 mg/day (10 mg 4 times daily). This dose should be maintained for a minimum of 4 weeks with every other week monitoring of transaminase levels beginning 4 weeks after initiation of treatment. It is important that the dose not be increased during this period because of the potential for delayed onset of transaminase elevations.

➤*Dose titration:* Following 4 weeks of treatment at 40 mg/day (10 mg 4 times daily), the dose of tacrine HCl should then be increased to 80 mg/day (20 mg 4 times daily), providing there are no significant transaminase elevations and the patient is tolerating treatment. Patients should be titrated to higher doses (120 and 160 mg/day, in divided doses on a 4 times daily schedule) at 4-week intervals on the basis of tolerance.

➤*Dose adjustment:* Serum ALT should be monitored every other week from at least week 4 to week 16 following initiation of treatment, after which monitoring may be decreased to every 3 months. For patients who develop ALT elevations greater than 2 times the upper limit of normal, the dose and monitoring regimen should be modified as described below.

A full monitoring and dose titration sequence must be repeated in the event that a patient suspends treatment with tacrine HCl for more than 4 weeks.

Recommended Dose and Monitoring Regimen Modification in Response to ALT Elevations

ALT level	Treatment and monitoring regimen
≤ 2 × ULN	Continue treatment according to recommended titration and monitoring schedule.
> 2 to ≤ 3 × ULN	Continue treatment according to recommended titration. Monitor ALT levels weekly until levels return to normal limits.
> 3 to ≤ 5 × ULN	Reduce the daily dose of tacrine HCl by 40 mg/day. Monitor ALT levels weekly. Resume dose titration and every other week monitoring when the levels of the ALT return to normal limits.
> 5 × ULN	Stop tacrine HCl treatment. Monitor the patient closely for signs and symptoms associated with hepatitis and follow ALT levels until within normal limits. See Rechallenge section below.
	Experience is limited in patients with ALT > 10 × ULN. The risk of rechallenge must be considered against demonstrated clinical benefit.
	Patients with clinical jaundice confirmed by a significant elevation in total bilirubin (> 3 mg/dL) or those exhibiting clinical signs or symptoms of hypersensitivity (eg, rash, fever) in association with ALT elevations should immediately and permanently discontinue tacrine HCl and not be rechallenged.

➤*Rechallenge:* Patients who are required to discontinue tacrine HCl treatment because of ALT elevations may be rechallenged once ALT levels return to healthy limits.

Rechallenge of patients with ALT elevations < 10 times ULN has not resulted in serious liver injury. However, because experience in the rechallenge of patients who had elevations > 10 times ULN is limited, the risks associated with the rechallenge of these patients are not well characterized. Careful, frequent (weekly) monitoring of serum ALT should be undertaken when rechallenging such patients.

If rechallenged, patients should be given an initial dose of 40 mg/day (10 mg 4 times daily) and ALT levels monitored weekly. If, after 6 weeks on 40 mg/day, the patient is tolerating the dosage with no unacceptable elevations in ALT, the recommended dose-titration may be resumed. Weekly monitoring of the ALT levels should continue for a total of 16 weeks after which monitoring may be decreased to monthly for 2 months and every 3 months thereafter.

➤*Storage/Stability:* Store at controlled room temperature 15° to 30°C (59° to 86°F) away from moisture.

Actions

➤*Pharmacology:* Although widespread degeneration of multiple CNS neuronal systems eventually occurs, early pathological changes in Alzheimer disease involve, in a relatively selective manner, cholinergic neuronal pathways that project from the basal forebrain to the cerebral cortex and hippocampus. The resulting deficiency of cortical acetylcholine is believed to account for some of the clinical manifestations of mild-to-moderate dementia. Tacrine HCl, an orally bioavailable, centrally active, reversible cholinesterase inhibitor, presumably acts by elevating acetylcholine concentrations in the cerebral cortex by slowing the degradation of acetylcholine released by still intact cholinergic neurons. If this theoretical mechanism of action is correct, tacrine HCl's effects may lessen as the disease process advances and fewer cholinergic neurons remain functionally intact. There is no evidence that tacrine HCl alters the course of the underlying dementing process.

➤*Pharmacokinetics:*

Absorption – Tacrine HCl is rapidly absorbed after oral administration; maximal plasma concentrations occur within 1 to 2 hours. The rate and extent of tacrine HCl absorption following administration of tacrine HCl capsules and solution are virtually indistinguishable. Absolute bioavailability of tacrine HCl is ≈ 17 (SD ± 13)%. Food reduces tacrine HCl bioavailability by ≈ 30% to 40%; however, there is no food effect if tacrine HCl is administered at least 1 hour before meals. The effect of achlorhydria on the absorption of tacrine HCl is unknown.

Distribution – Mean volume of distribution of tacrine HCl is ≈ 349 (SD ± 193) L. Tacrine HCl is ≈ 55% bound to plasma proteins. The extent and degree of tacrine HCl's distribution within various body compartments has not been systematically studied. However, 336 hours after the administration of a single radiolabeled dose, ≈ 25% of the radiolabel was not recovered in a mass balance study, suggesting the possibility that tacrine HCl or one or more of its metabolites may be retained.

Metabolism – Tacrine HCl is extensively metabolized by the cytochrome P450 system to multiple metabolites, not all of which have been identified. The vast majority of radiolabeled species present in the plasma following a single dose of ^{14}C radiolabeled tacrine HCl are unidentified (ie, only 5% of radioactivity in plasma has been identified [tacrine HCl and 3-hydroxylated metabolites; 1-, 2-, and 4-hydroxytacrine]).

Studies utilizing human liver preparations demonstrated that cytochrome P450 1A2 is the principal isozyme involved in tacrine HCl metabolism. These findings are consistent with the observation that tacrine HCl or one of its metabolites inhibits the metabolism of theophylline in humans (see Drug Interactions). Results from a study utilizing quinidine to inhibit cytochrome P450 2D6 indicate that tacrine HCl is not metabolized extensively by this enzyme system.

Following aromatic ring hydroxylation, tacrine HCl's metabolites undergo glucuronidation. Whether tacrine HCl or its metabolites undergo biliary excretion or enterohepatic circulation is unknown.

Excretion – Tacrine HCl undergoes presystemic clearance (ie, first-pass metabolism). The extent of this first-pass metabolism depends upon the dose of tacrine HCl administered. Because the enzyme system involved can be saturated at relatively low doses, a larger fraction of a high dose of tacrine HCl will escape first-pass elimination than of a smaller dose. Thus, when a 40 mg daily dose is increased by 40 mg, the average plasma concentration will be increased by ≈ 6 ng/mL. However, when a daily dose of 80 or 120 mg is increased by 40 mg, the increment in average plasma concentration is ≈ 10 ng/mL.

Elimination of tacrine HCl from the plasma, however, is not dose dependent (ie, the half-life is independent of dose or plasma concentration). The elimination half-life is ≈ 2 to 4 hours. Following initiation of therapy or a change in daily dose, steady-state tacrine HCl plasma concentration should be attained within 24 to 36 hours.

Special populations –

Gender: Average tacrine HCl plasma concentrations are ≈ 50% higher in females than in males. This is not explained by differences in body surface area or elimination half-life. The difference is probably due to higher systemic availability after oral dosing and may reflect the known lower activity of cytochrome P450 1A2 in women.

Smoking: Mean plasma tacrine HCl concentrations in current smokers are approximately one-third the concentrations in nonsmokers. Cigarette smoking is known to induce cytochrome P450 1A2.

Contraindications

Hypersensitivity to tacrine HCl or acridine derivatives; in patients previously treated with tacrine HCl who developed treatment-associated jaundice; a serum bilirubin ≥ 3 mg/dL; or those exhibiting clinical signs or symptoms of hypersensitivity (eg, rash or fever) in association with ALT elevations.

Warnings

➤*Anesthesia:* Tacrine, as a cholinesterase inhibitor, is likely to exaggerate succinylcholine-type muscle relaxation during anesthesia.

➤*Cardiovascular conditions:* Because of its cholinomimetic action, tacrine HCl may have vagotonic effects on the heart rate (eg, bradycardia). This action may be particularly important to patients with conduction abnormalities, bradyarrhythmia, or a sick sinus syndrome.

➤*GI effects:* Tacrine HCl is an inhibitor of cholinesterase and may be expected to increase gastric acid secretion due to increased cholinergic activity. Therefore, patients are at increased risk for developing ulcers. Those with a history of ulcer disease or those receiving concurrent nonsteroidal anti-inflammatory drugs (NSAIDs) should be monitored closely for symptoms of active or occult GI disease.

Tacrine HCl also as a predictable consequence of its pharmacological properties, can cause nausea, vomiting, and loose stools at recommended doses.

➤*Genitourinary effects:* Cholinomimetics may cause bladder outflow obstruction.

TACRINE HYDROCHLORIDE — ORAL

➤*Neurological conditions:*

Seizures – Cholinomimetics are believed to have some potential to cause generalized convulsions; seizure activity may, however, also be a manifestation of Alzheimer disease.

Sudden worsening of the degree of cognitive impairment – Worsening of cognitive function has been reported following abrupt discontinuation of tacrine HCl or after a large reduction in total daily dose (≥ 80 mg/day).

➤*Pulmonary conditions:* Because of its cholinomimetic action, tacrine HCl should be prescribed with care to patients with a history of asthma.

➤*Hepatic effects:* The use of tacrine HCl in patients without a history of liver disease is commonly associated with serum aminotransferase elevations, some to levels ordinarily considered to indicate clinically important hepatic injury (see above information).

Experience gained in more than 12,000 patients who received tacrine HCl in clinical studies and the treatment IND program indicates that if tacrine HCl is promptly withdrawn following detection of these elevations, clinically evident signs and symptoms of liver injury are rare.

Long-term follow-up of patients who experience transaminase elevations, however, is limited and it is impossible, therefore, to exclude, with certainty, the possibility of chronic sequelae.

➤*Hepatic function impairment:* Tacrine HCl should be prescribed with care in patients with current evidence or history of abnormal liver function indicated by significant abnormalities in serum transaminase (ALT; AST), bilirubin, and gamma-glutamyl transpeptidase (GGT) levels.

Clinically evident liver toxicity – One of more than 12,000 patients exposed to tacrine HCl in clinical studies and the treatment IND program had documented elevated bilirubin (5.3 times upper limit of normal, [ULN]) and jaundice with transaminase levels (AST) nearly 20 times the ULN.

Rare cases of liver toxicity associated with jaundice, raised serum bilirubin, pyrexia, hepatitis and liver failure have been reported in postmarketing experience. Most of these cases have been reversible but some deaths have occurred. Since there was multiple pathology including infection, gallstones and carcinoma it was not possible to clearly establish the relationship to tacrine HCl treatment.

Blood chemistry signs of liver injury – Experience from the 30-week clinical study (described earlier) provides a representative estimate of the frequency of ALT elevations expected for patients whose transaminase levels are monitored weekly and who receive tacrine HCl according to the recommended regimen for dose introduction and titration (see below). A dosing regimen employing a more rapid escalation of the daily dose of tacrine HCl may be associated with more serious clinical events (see below).

Cumulative Incidence of ALT Elevations Based on Maximum Values with Weekly Monitoring During the 30-week Study

Maximum ALT	Males (n = 229)	Females (n = 250)	Total (n = 479)
Within normal limits	121 (53%)	100 (40%)	221 (46%)
> ULN	108 (47%)	150 (60%)	258 (54%)
> 2 times ULN	77 (34%)	104 (42%)	181 (38%)
> 3 times ULN	58 (25%)	81 (32%)	139 (29%)
> 10 times ULN	12 (5%)	19 (8%)	31 (6%)
> 20 times ULN	3 (1%)	6 (2%)	9 (2%)

Experience in 2446 patients who participated in all clinical trials, including the 30-week study, indicates ≈ 50% of patients treated with tacrine HCl can be expected to have at least 1 ALT level above ULN; ≈ 25% of patients are likely to develop elevations > 3 times ULN, and ≈ 7% of patients may develop elevations > 10 times ULN. Data collected from the treatment IND program were consistent with those obtained during clinical studies, and showed 3% of 5665 patients experiencing an ALT elevation > 10 times ULN.

In clinical trials where transaminases were monitored weekly, the median time to onset of the first ALT elevation above ULN was ≈ 6 weeks, with maximum ALT occurring 1 week later, even in instances when tacrine HCl treatment was stopped. Under the conditions of forced slow upwards dose titration (increases of 40 mg/day every 6 weeks) employed in clinical studies, 95% of transaminase elevations > 3 times ULN occurred within the first 18 weeks of tacrine HCl therapy, and 99% of the 10-fold elevations occurred by the 12th week and on not more than 80 mg; note, however, that for most patients ALT was monitored weekly and tacrine HCl was stopped when liver enzymes exceeded 3 times ULN. A total of 276 patients were monitored for ALT levels every other week in 2 double-blind clinical studies, an open-label study, and amended treatment IND. The incidence, severity, time to onset, peak and recovery of ALT levels were similar to weekly monitoring. With less frequent monitoring than every other week or the less stringent discontinuation criteria recommended below, it is possible that marked elevations might be more common. It must also be appreciated that experience with prolonged exposure to the high dose (160 mg/day) is limited. In all cases, transaminase levels returned to within normal limits upon discontinuation of tacrine HCl treatment or following dosage reduction, usually within 4 to 6 weeks.

This relatively benign experience may be the consequence of careful laboratory monitoring that facilitated the discontinuation of patients early on after the onset of their transaminase elevations. Consequently, frequent monitoring of serum transaminase levels is recommended.

Liver biopsy experience – Liver biopsy results in 7 patients who received tacrine HCl (1 in a Parke-Davis sponsored study and 6 in studies reported in the literature) revealed hepatocellular necrosis in 6 patients, and granulomatous changes in the seventh. In all cases, liver function tests returned to normal with no evidence of persisting hepatic dysfunction.

Experience with the rechallenge of patients with transaminase elevations following recovery – Two hundred and twelve patients among the 866 patients assigned to tacrine HCl in the 12- and 30-week studies were withdrawn because they developed transaminase elevations > 3 times ULN. One hundred and forty-five of these patients were subsequently rechallenged with weekly monitoring of ALT. During their initial exposure to tacrine, 20 of these 145 had experienced initial elevations > 10 times ULN, while the remainder had experienced elevations between 3 and 10 times ULN.

Upon rechallenge with an initial dose of 40 mg/day, only 48 (33%) of the 145 patients developed transaminase elevations > 3 times ULN. Of these patients, 44 had elevations that were between 3 and 10 times ULN and 4 had elevations that were > 10 times ULN.

The mean time to onset of elevations occurred earlier on rechallenge than on initial exposure (22 vs 48 days). Of the 145 patients rechallenged, 127 (88%) were able to continue tacrine HCl treatment, and 91 of these 127 patients titrated to doses higher than those associated with the initial transaminase elevation.

Predictors of the risk of transaminase elevations – The incidence of transaminase elevations is higher among females. There are no other known predictors of the risk of hepatocellular injury.

Monitoring of liver function and the management of the patient who develops transaminase elevations –

Blood chemistries: Serum transaminase levels (specifically ALT) should be monitored every other week from at least week 4 to week 16 following initiation of treatment, after which monitoring may be decreased to every 3 months. For patients who develop ALT elevations > 2 times the ULN, the dose and monitoring regimen should be modified.

A full monitoring sequence should be repeated in the event that a patient suspends treatment with tacrine HCl for > 4 weeks.

If ALT elevations occur, the frequency of monitoring and the dose of tacrine HCl should be modified.

Rechallenge: Patients with clinical jaundice confirmed by a significant elevation in total bilirubin (> 3 mg/dL) or those exhibiting clinical signs or symptoms of hypersensitivity (eg, rash, fever) in association with ALT elevations should immediately and permanently discontinue tacrine HCl and not be rechallenged. Other patients who are required to discontinue tacrine HCl treatment because of ALT elevations may be rechallenged once ALT levels return to within healthy limits.

See Administration and Dosage for more information.

Liver biopsy: Liver biopsy is not indicated in cases of uncomplicated transaminase elevation.

➤*Carcinogenesis:* Overall, the results of tests, along with the fact that tacrine HCl belongs to a chemical class (acridines) containing some members which are animal carcinogens, suggest that tacrine HCl may be carcinogenic.

➤*Mutagenesis:* Tacrine HCl was mutagenic to bacteria in the Ames test. Unscheduled DNA synthesis was induced in rat and mouse hepatocytes in vitro. Results of cytogenetic (chromosomal aberration) studies were equivocal. Tacrine HCl was not mutagenic in an in vitro mammalian mutation test.

➤*Pregnancy: Category C.* Animal reproduction studies have not been conducted with tacrine HCl. It is also not known whether tacrine HCl can cause fetal harm when administered to a pregnant woman or can affect reproductive capacity.

➤*Lactation:* It is not known whether this drug is excreted in human milk.

➤*Children:* There are no adequate and well-controlled trials to document the safety and efficacy of tacrine HCl in any dementing illness occurring in pediatric patients.

Precautions

➤*Monitoring:* See Warnings for more information.

➤*Lab test abnormalities:* An absolute neutrophil count (ANC) < 500/mcL occurred in 4 patients who received tacrine HCl during the course of clinical trials. Three of the 4 patients had concurrent medical conditions commonly associated with a low ANC; 2 of these patients remained on tacrine. The fourth patient, who had a history of hypersensitivity (penicillin allergy), withdrew from the study as a result of a rash and also developed an ANC < 500/mcL, which returned to normal; this patient was not rechallenged and, therefore, the role played by tacrine HCl in this reaction is unknown.

Six patients had an absolute neutrophil count ≤ 1500/mcL, associated with an elevation of ALT.

The total clinical experience in > 12,000 patients does not indicate a clear association between tacrine HCl treatment and serious white blood cell abnormalities.

Drug Interactions

➤*CYP450 system:* Tacrine HCl is primarily eliminated by hepatic metabolism via cytochrome P450 drug metabolizing enzymes. Drug interactions may occur when tacrine HCl is given concurrently with agents such as theophylline that undergo extensive metabolism via cytochrome P450 1A2.

TACRINE HYDROCHLORIDE — ORAL

Tacrine Drug Interactions			
Precipitant drug	Object drug*		Description
Cimetidine	Tacrine	↑	Cimetidine increased the C_{max} and AUC of tacrine by ≈ 54% and 64%, respectively.
Tacrine	Anticholinergics	↓	Because of its mechanism of action, tacrine has the potential to interfere with the activity of anticholinergic medications.
Tacrine	Cholinomimetics/ Cholinesterase inhibitors	↑	A synergistic effect is expected when tacrine is given concurrently with succinylcholine, cholinesterase inhibitors or cholinergic agonists (eg, bethanechol).
Tacrine	Theophylline	↑	Coadministration increased theophylline elimination half-life and average plasma levels by ≈ 2-fold; monitor plasma theophylline concentrations and reduce theophylline dose as appropriate.

* ↑ = Object drug increased. ↓ = Object drug decreased.

➤*Fluvoxamine:* In a study of 13 healthy, male volunteers, a single 40 mg dose of tacrine HCl added to fluvoxamine 100 mg/day administered at steady-state was associated with 5- and 8-fold increases in tacrine HCl C_{max} and AUC, respectively, compared to the administration of tacrine HCl alone. Five subjects experienced nausea, vomiting, sweating, and diarrhea following coadministration, consistent with the cholinergic effects of tacrine.

Adverse Reactions

➤*Common adverse events leading to discontinuation:* In clinical trials, ≈ 17% of the 2706 patients who received tacrine and 5% of the 1886 patients who received placebo withdrew permanently because of adverse events. It should be noted that some of the placebo-treated patients were exposed to tacrine HCl prior to receiving placebo due to the variety of study designs used, including crossover studies. Apart from withdrawals due to transaminase elevations, 244 patients (9%) withdrew for adverse events while receiving tacrine HCl.

Hepatic – Transaminase elevations were the most common reason for withdrawals during tacrine treatment (8% of all tacrine-treated patients, or 212 of 456 patients withdrawn). The controlled clinical trial protocols required that any patient with an ALT elevation > 3 times ULN be withdrawn, because of concern about potential hepatotoxicity.

Miscellaneous – Other adverse events that most frequently led to the withdrawal of tacrine-treated patients in clinical trials were nausea or vomiting (1.5%), agitation (0.9%), rash (0.7%), anorexia (0.7%), and confusion (0.5%). These adverse events also most frequently led to the withdrawal of placebo-treated patients, although at lower frequencies (0.1% to 0.2%).

➤*Most frequent:* The events identified here are those that occurred at an absolute incidence of at least 5% of patients treated with tacrine HCl, and at a rate at least 2-fold higher in patients treated with tacrine HCl than placebo. The most common adverse events associated with the use of tacrine HCl were elevated transaminases, nausea or vomiting, diarrhea, dyspepsia, myalgia, anorexia, and ataxia. Of these events, nausea or vomiting, diarrhea, dyspepsia, and anorexia appeared to be dose dependent.

➤*Adverse events reported in controlled trials:*

Adverse Events Occurring in at least 2% of Patients Receiving Tacrine HCl at a Starting Dose of 40 mg/day with Titration in 40 mg/day Increments Every 6 weeks in Controlled Clinical Trials		
Body system/adverse events	Tacrine HCl (n = 634)	Placebo (n = 342)
Laboratory abnormalities		
Elevated transaminase [a]	184 (29%)	5 (2%)
Miscellaneous		
Headache	67 (11%)	52 (15%)
Fatigue	26 (4%)	9 (3%)
Chest pain	24 (4%)	18 (5%)
Weight decrease	21 (3%)	4 (1%)
Back pain	15 (2%)	14 (4%)
Asthenia	15 (2%)	7 (2%)
GI		
Nausea or vomiting	178 (28%)	29 (9%)
Diarrhea	99 (16%)	18 (5%)
Dyspepsia	57 (9%)	22 (6%)
Anorexia	54 (9%)	11 (3%)
Abdominal pain	48 (8%)	24 (7%)
Flatulence	22 (4%)	5 (2%)
Constipation	24 (4%)	8 (2%)
Hematologic-lymphatic system		
Purpura	15 (2%)	8 (2%)
Musculoskeletal system		
Myalgia	54 (9%)	18 (5%)
CNS		
Dizziness	73 (12%)	39 (11%)
Confusion	42 (7%)	24 (7%)
Ataxia	36 (6%)	12 (4%)
Insomnia	37 (6%)	18 (5%)
Somnolence	22 (4%)	11 (3%)
Tremor	14 (2%)	2 (< 1%)
Psychiatric		
Agitation	43 (7%)	30 (9%)
Depression	22 (4%)	14 (4%)
Thinking abnormal	17 (3%)	14 (4%)
Anxiety	16 (3%)	7 (2%)
Hallucination	15 (2%)	12 (4%)
Hostility	15 (2%)	5 (2%)
Respiratory system		
Rhinitis	51 (8%)	22 (6%)
Upper respiratory tract infection	18 (3%)	11 (3%)
Coughing	17 (3%)	18 (5%)
Dermatologic		
Rash [b]	46 (7%)	18 (5%)
Facial flushing, skin flushing	16 (3%)	3 (< 1%)
GU		
Urination frequency	21 (3%)	12 (4%)
Urinary tract infection	21 (3%)	20 (6%)
Urinary incontinence	16 (3%)	9 (3%)

[a] ALT or AST value of ≈ 3 x ULN or greater or that resulted in a change in patient management. Patients were monitored weekly.
[b] Includes COSTART terms: rash, rash-erythematous, rash-maculopapular, urticaria, petechial rash, rash-vesiculobullous, and pruritus.

➤*Other adverse events observed during all clinical trials:* Tacrine HCl has been administered to 2706 individuals during clinical trials. A total of 1471 patients were treated for at least 3 months, 1137 for at least 6 months, and 773 for at least 1 year. Any untoward reactions that occurred during these trials were recorded as adverse events by the clinical investigators using terminology of their own choosing. To provide a meaningful estimate of the proportion of individuals having similar types of events, the events were grouped into a smaller number of standardized categories using a modified dictionary. These categories are used in the listing below. The frequencies represent the proportion of the 2706 individuals exposed to tacrine HCl who experienced that event while receiving tacrine HCl. All adverse events are included except those already listed in the previous paragraphs and those terms too general to be informative. Events are further classified by body system categories and listed using the following definitions: Frequent adverse events are defined as those occurring in at least 1/100 patients; infrequent adverse events are those occurring in 1/100 to 1/1000 patients; and rare adverse events are those occurring in < 1/1000 patients. These adverse events are not necessarily related to tacrine HCl treatment. Only rare adverse events deemed to be potentially important are included.

Cardiovascular –
Frequent: Hypotension, hypertension.
Infrequent: Heart failure, MI, angina pectoris, cerebrovascular accident, transient ischemic attack, phlebitis, venous insufficiency, abdominal aortic aneurysm, atrial fibrillation or flutter, palpitation, tachycardia, bradycardia, pulmonary embolus, migraine, hypercholesterolemia.
Rare: Heart arrest, premature atrial contractions, AV block, bundle branch block.

CNS –
Frequent: Convulsions, vertigo, syncope, hyperkinesia, paresthesia.
Infrequent: Dreaming abnormal, dysarthria, aphasia, amnesia, wandering, twitching, hypesthesia, delirium, paralysis, bradykinesia, movement disorder, cogwheel rigidity, paresis, neuritis, hemiplegia, Parkinson's disease, neuropathy, extrapyramidal syndrome, reflexes decreased/absent.
Rare: Tardive dyskinesia, dysesthesia, dystonia, encephalitis, coma, apraxia, oculogyric crisis, akathisia, oral facial dyskinesia, Bell's palsy, exacerbation of Parkinson's disease.

Dermatologic –
Frequent: Sweating increased.
Infrequent: Acne, alopecia, dermatitis, eczema, skin dry, herpes zoster, psoriasis, cellulitis, cyst, furunculosis, herpes simplex, hyperkeratosis, basal cell carcinoma, skin cancer.
Rare: Desquamation, seborrhea, squamous cell carcinoma, ulcer (skin), skin necrosis, melanoma.

Endocrine –
Infrequent: Diabetes.
Rare: Hyperthyroid, hypothyroid.

GI –
Infrequent: Glossitis, gingivitis, mouth or throat dry, stomatitis, increased salivation, dysphagia, esophagitis, gastritis, gastroenteritis, GI hemorrhage, stomach ulcer, hiatal hernia, hemorrhoids, stools bloody, diverticulitis, fecal impaction, fecal incontinence, hemorrhage (rectum), cholelithiasis, cholecystitis, increased appetite.
Rare: Duodenal ulcer, bowel obstruction.

TACRINE HYDROCHLORIDE — ORAL

GU –

Infrequent: Hematuria, renal stone, kidney infection, glycosuria, dysuria, polyuria, nocturia, pyuria, cystitis, urinary retention, urination urgency, vaginal hemorrhage, pruritus (genital), breast pain, impotence, prostate cancer.

Rare: Bladder tumor, renal tumor, renal failure, urinary obstruction, breast cancer, epididymitis, carcinoma (ovary).

Hematologic / Lymphatic –

Infrequent: Anemia, lymphadenopathy.

Rare: Leukopenia, thrombocytopenia, hemolysis, pancytopenia.

Musculoskeletal –

Frequent: Fracture, arthralgia, arthritis, hypertonia.

Infrequent: Osteoporosis, tendinitis, bursitis, gout.

Rare: Myopathy.

Psychiatric –

Frequent: Nervousness.

Infrequent: Apathy, increased libido, paranoia, neurosis.

Rare: Suicidal ideation, psychosis, hysteria.

Respiratory –

Frequent: Pharyngitis, sinusitis, bronchitis, pneumonia, dyspnea.

Infrequent: Epistaxis, chest congestion, asthma, hyperventilation, lower respiratory tract infection.

Rare: Hemoptysis, lung edema, lung cancer, acute epiglottitis.

Special senses –

Frequent: Conjunctivitis.

Infrequent: Cataract, eyes dry, eye pain, visual field defect, diplopia, amblyopia, glaucoma, hordeolum, deafness, earache, tinnitus, inner ear infection, otitis media, unusual taste.

Rare: Vision loss, ptosis, blepharitis, labyrinthitis, inner ear disturbance.

Miscellaneous –

Frequent: Chill, fever, malaise, peripheral edema.

Infrequent: Face edema, dehydration, weight increase, cachexia, edema (generalized), lipoma.

Rare: Heat exhaustion, sepsis, cholinergic crisis, death.

➤*Postmarketing:* Voluntary reports of adverse events temporally associated with tacrine HCl that have been received since market introduction, that are not listed above, and that may have no causal relationship with the drug include the following: Pancreatitis, perforated peptic ulcer, and falling.

Overdosage

➤*Symptoms:* Overdosage with cholinesterase inhibitors can cause a cholinergic crisis characterized by severe nausea/vomiting, salivation, sweating, bradycardia, hypotension, collapse, and convulsions. Increasing muscle weakness is a possibility and may result in death if respiratory muscles are involved.

➤*Treatment:* As in any case of overdose, general supportive measures should be used. Tertiary anticholinergics such as atropine may be used as an antidote for tacrine HCl overdosage. IV atropine sulfate titrated to effect is recommended.

It is not known whether tacrine HCl or its metabolites can be eliminated by dialysis (hemodialysis, peritoneal dialysis, or hemofiltration).

Patient Information

Patients and caregivers should be advised that the effect of tacrine HCl therapy is thought to depend upon its administration at regular intervals, as directed.

The caregiver should be advised about the possibility of adverse effects. Two types should be distinguished: Those occurring in close temporal association with the initiation of treatment or an increase in dose (eg, nausea, vomiting, loose stools, diarrhea), and those with a delayed onset (eg, rash, jaundice, changes in the color of stool—black, very dark or light [ie, acholic]).

Patients and caregivers should be encouraged to inform the physician about the emergence of new events or any increase in the severity of existing adverse clinical events.

Caregivers should be advised that abrupt discontinuation of tacrine HCl or a large reduction in total daily dose (≥ 80 mg/day) may cause a decline in cognitive function and behavioral disturbances. Unsupervised increases in the dose of tacrine HCl may also have serious consequences. Consequently, changes in dose should not be undertaken in the absence of direct instruction of a physician.

DONEPEZIL HYDROCHLORIDE

Rx	**Aricept** (Eisai/Pfizer)	**Tablets:** 5 mg	White. (ARICEPT 5). In 30s, 90s, and UD blister pack 100s.
		10 mg	Yellow. (ARICEPT 10). In 30s, 90s, and UD blister pack 100s.
Rx	**Aricept ODT** (Eisai/Pfizer)	**Tablets, orally disintegrating:** 5 mg	White. (ARICEPT 5). In UD blister pack 30s.
		10 mg	Yellow. (ARICEPT 10). In UD blister pack 30s.

DONEPEZIL HYDROCHLORIDE — ORAL

Indications

➤*Alzheimer disease:* For treatment of mild to moderate dementia of the Alzheimer type.

➤*Unlabeled uses:* Possible treatment for vascular dementia; improvement of memory in multiple sclerosis patients.

Administration and Dosage

The dosages of donepezil are 5 and 10 mg once daily.

The higher dose of 10 mg did not provide a statistically significant clinical benefit greater than that of 5 mg. There is a suggestion, however, based upon order of group mean scores and dose trend analyses of data, that a daily dose of donepezil 10 mg might provide additional benefit for some patients. Do not increase to 10 mg until patients have been on a daily dose of 5 mg for 4 to 6 weeks.

Take donepezil in the evening, just prior to retiring.

Donepezil may be taken with or without food; allow donepezil orally disintegrating tablets to dissolve on the tongue and follow with water.

Actions

➤*Pharmacology:* Donepezil is postulated to exert its therapeutic effect by enhancing cholinergic function. Deficiency of cholinergic neurotransmission may be the cause of Alzheimer disease. This increase in cholinergic function is accomplished by increasing the concentration of acetylcholine through reversible inhibition of its hydrolysis by acetylcholinesterase (AChE). If this proposed mechanism of action is correct, donepezil's effect may lessen as the disease process advances and fewer cholinergic neurons remain functionally intact. There is no evidence that donepezil alters the course of the underlying dementing process.

➤*Pharmacokinetics:*

Absorption – Donepezil is well absorbed with a relative oral bioavailability of 100% and reaches peak plasma concentrations in 3 to 4 hours. Pharmacokinetics are linear over a dose range of 1 to 10 mg given once daily. Neither food nor time of administration (morning vs evening dose) influences the rate or extent of absorption.

Distribution – Following multiple-dose administration, donepezil accumulates in plasma by 4- to 7-fold and steady state is reached within 15 days. The steady-state volume of distribution is 12 L/kg. Donepezil is approximately 96% bound to human plasma proteins, mainly to albumins (approximately 75%) and alpha$_1$-acid glycoprotein (approximately 21%) over the concentration range of 2 to 1,000 ng/mL.

Metabolism – Donepezil is excreted in the urine intact and extensively metabolized to 4 major metabolites (2 of which are known to be active) and a number of minor metabolites, not all of which have been identified. Donepezil is metabolized by the CYP450 isoenzymes 2D6 and 3A4 and undergoes glucuronidation. Following administration of donepezil, plasma radioactivity was present primarily as intact donepezil (53%) and as 6-O-desmethyl donepezil (11%), which has been reported to inhibit AChE to the same extent as donepezil in vitro and was found in plasma at concentrations equal to approximately 20% of donepezil.

Excretion – The elimination half-life of donepezil is approximately 70 hours, and the mean apparent plasma clearance is 0.13 L/hr/kg. Approximately 57% and 15% of the total dose was recovered in urine and feces, respectively, over a period of 10 days, while 28% remained unrecovered, with approximately 17% of the donepezil dose recovered in the urine as unchanged drug.

Special populations –

Hepatic function impairment: In a study of 10 patients with stable alcoholic cirrhosis, the clearance of donepezil was decreased 20% relative to 10 healthy age- and sex-matched subjects.

Contraindications

Hypersensitivity to donepezil or to piperidine derivatives.

Warnings

➤*Anesthesia:* Donepezil, as a cholinesterase inhibitor, is likely to exaggerate succinylcholine-type muscle relaxation during anesthesia.

➤*Cardiovascular effects:* Because of their pharmacological action, cholinesterase inhibitors may have vagotonic effects on the sinoatrial and atrioventricular nodes. This effect may manifest as bradycardia or heart block in patients with and without known underlying cardiac conduction abnormalities. Syncopal episodes have been reported in association with the use of donepezil.

➤*GI effects:* Through their primary action, cholinesterase inhibitors may be expected to increase gastric acid secretion because of increased cholinergic activity. Therefore, monitor patients closely for symptoms of active or occult GI bleeding, especially those at increased risk for developing ulcers (eg, those with a history of ulcer disease or those receiving concurrent nonsteroidal anti-inflammatory drugs [NSAIDs"). Clinical studies of donepezil have shown no increase relative to placebo in the incidence of peptic ulcer disease or GI bleeding.

Donepezil, as a predictable consequence of its pharmacological properties, has been shown to produce diarrhea, nausea, and vomiting. These effects, when they occur, appear more frequently with the 10 mg/day dose than with the 5 mg/day dose. In most cases, these effects have been mild and transient, sometimes lasting 1 to 3 weeks, and have resolved during continued use of donepezil.

➤*GU effects:* Although not observed in clinical trials, cholinomimetics may cause bladder outflow obstruction.

DONEPEZIL HYDROCHLORIDE — ORAL

➤*Pulmonary effects:* Because of their cholinomimetic actions, prescribe cholinesterase inhibitors with care for patients with a history of asthma or obstructive pulmonary disease.

➤*Seizures:* Cholinomimetics are believed to have some potential to cause generalized convulsions. However, seizure activity also may be a manifestation of Alzheimer disease.

➤*Pregnancy: Category C.* In a study in which pregnant rats were given up to 10 mg/kg/day from day 17 of gestation through day 20 postpartum, there was a slight increase in still births and a slight decrease in pup survival through day 4 postpartum at this dose. There are no adequate or well-controlled studies in pregnant women. Use donepezil during pregnancy only if the potential benefit justifies the potential risk to the fetus.

➤*Lactation:* It is not known whether donepezil is excreted in breast milk.

➤*Children:* There are no adequate and well-controlled trials to document the safety and efficacy of donepezil in any illness occurring in children.

Drug Interactions

Donepezil Drug Interactions

Precipitant drug	Object drug*		Description
Donepezil	Anticholinergics	↓	Because of their mechanism of action, cholinesterase inhibitors have the potential to interfere with the activity of anticholinergic medications.
Donepezil	Cholinomimetics/cholinesterase inhibitors	↑	A synergistic effect may be expected when cholinesterase inhibitors are given concurrently with succinylcholine, similar neuromuscular blocking agents, or cholinergic agonists, such as bethanechol.
Donepezil	NSAIDs	↑	Donepezil increases gastric acid secretions caused by increased cholinergic activity. Therefore, monitor for active or occult GI bleeding (see Warnings).
CYP450 3A4 and 2D6 inhibitors (eg, ketoconazole, quinidine)	Donepezil	↑	Ketoconazole 200 mg daily increased mean donepezil 5 mg daily concentrations (AUC_{0-24} and C_{max}) 36%. The clinical relevance of this increase in concentration is unknown.
CYP450 3A4 and 2D6 inducers (eg, carbamazepine, dexamethasone, phenobarbital, phenytoin, rifampin)	Donepezil	↓	Inducers of CYP3A4 and CYP2D6 could increase the rate of elimination of donepezil.

* ↑ = Object drug increased. ↓ = Object drug decreased.

Adverse Reactions

➤*Adverse events leading to discontinuation:* The rates of discontinuations from controlled clinical trials of donepezil caused by adverse events for donepezil 5 mg/day treatment groups were comparable with those of placebo-treatment groups at approximately 5%. The rate of discontinuation of patients who received 7-day escalations from 5 to 10 mg/day was higher at 13%.

The most common adverse events leading to discontinuation, defined as those occurring in at least 2% of patients and at twice the incidence seen in placebo patients, are shown below.

Adverse Events Leading to Withdrawal from Clinical Trials by Dose Group (%)

Adverse Event	Placebo (n = 355)	Donepezil 5 mg/day (n = 350)	Donepezil 10 mg/day (n = 315)
Diarrhea	0%	< 1%	3%
Nausea	1%	1%	3%
Vomiting	< 1%	< 1%	2%

The most common adverse events, defined as those occurring at a frequency of at least 5% in patients receiving 10 mg/day and twice the placebo rate, are largely predicted by donepezil's cholinomimetic effects. These include anorexia, diarrhea, fatigue, insomnia, muscle cramps, nausea, and vomiting. These adverse events were often of mild intensity and transient, resolving during continued donepezil treatment without the need for dose modification.

Adverse Events in Patients Titrated to 10 mg/day Over 1 and 6 Weeks (%)

	No titration		1-week titration	6-week titration
Adverse Event	Placebo (n = 315)	Donepezil 5 mg/day (n = 311)	Donepezil 10 mg/day (n = 315)	Donepezil 10 mg/day (n = 269)
Anorexia	2%	3%	7%	3%
Diarrhea	5%	8%	15%	9%
Fatigue	3%	4%	8%	3%
Insomnia	6%	6%	14%	6%
Muscle cramps	2%	6%	8%	3%
Nausea	6%	5%	19%	6%
Vomiting	3%	3%	8%	5%

The table below lists treatment emergent signs and symptoms that were reported in at least 2% of patients in placebo-controlled trials who received donepezil and for which the rate of occurrence was greater for donepezil- than placebo-assigned patients. In general, adverse events occurred more frequently in female patients and with advancing age.

Donepezil Adverse Events (≥ 2%)

Adverse Event	Placebo (n = 355)	Donepezil (n = 747)
CNS		
Abnormal dreams	0%	3%
Depression	< 1%	3%
Dizziness	6%	8%
Fatigue	3%	5%
Headache	9%	10%
Insomnia	6%	9%
Somnolence	< 1%	2%
GI		
Anorexia	2%	4%
Diarrhea	5%	10%
Nausea	6%	11%
Vomiting	3%	5%
Musculoskeletal		
Arthritis	1%	2%
Muscle Cramps	2%	6%
Miscellaneous		
Accident	6%	7%
Ecchymosis	3%	4%
Frequent urination	1%	2%
Pain, various locations	8%	9%
Syncope	1%	2%
Weight decrease	1%	3%

➤*Cardiovascular:* Atrial fibrillation, hot flashes, hypertension, hypotension, vasodilation (at least 1%); angina pectoris, arteritis, AV block (first degree), bradycardia, congestive heart failure, deep vein thrombosis, myocardial infarction, peripheral vascular disease, postural hypotension, supraventricular tachycardia (0.1% to 1%).

➤*CNS:* Abnormal crying, aggression, aphasia, ataxia, delusions, increased libido, irritability, nervousness, paresthesia, restlessness, tremor, vertigo (at least 1%); cerebrovascular accident, coldness (localized), decreased libido, dysarthria, dysphasia, dysphoria, emotional lability, emotional withdrawal, gait abnormality, hostility, hypertonia, hypokinesia, intracranial hemorrhage, melancholia, muscle spasm, neuralgia, neurodermatitis, numbness (localized), nystagmus, pacing, paranoia, transient ischemic attack (0.1% to 1%).

➤*Dermatologic:* Diaphoresis, pruritus, urticaria (at least 1%); alopecia, dermatitis, erythema, fungal dermatitis, herpes zoster, hirsutism, hyperkeratosis, night sweats, skin discoloration, skin striae, skin ulcer (0.1% to 1%).

➤*Endocrine:* Diabetes mellitus, goiter (0.1% to 1%).

➤*GI:* Bloating, epigastric pain, fecal incontinence, GI bleeding (at least 1%); cholelithiasis, diverticulitis, drooling, dry mouth, duodenal ulcer, epigastric distress, eructation, fever sore, flatulence, gastritis, gastroenteritis, gingivitis, hemorrhoids, ileus, increased appetite, increased thirst, increased transaminases, irritable colon, jaundice, melena, periodontal abscess, polydipsia, stomach ulcer, tongue edema (0.1% to 1%).

➤*GU:* Nocturia, urinary incontinence (at least 1%); breast fibroadenosis, cystitis, dysuria, enuresis, fibrocystic breast, hematuria, inability to empty bladder, mastitis, metrorrhagia, prostate hypertrophy, pyelonephritis, pyuria, renal failure, urinary urgency, vaginitis (0.1% to 1%).

➤*Hematologic/Lymphatic:* Anemia, eosinophilia, erythrocytopenia, thrombocythemia, thrombocytopenia (0.1% to 1%).

➤*Metabolic/Nutritional:* Dehydration (at least 1%); face edema, gout, hyperglycemia, hypokalemia, increased creatine kinase, increased lactate dehydrogenase, weight increase (0.1% to 1%).

➤*Musculoskeletal:* Bone fracture (at least 1%); muscle fasciculation, muscle weakness (0.1% to 1%).

DONEPEZIL HYDROCHLORIDE — ORAL

➤*Respiratory:* Bronchitis, dyspnea, sore throat (at least 1%); epistaxis, hyperventilation, hypoxia, pharyngitis, pleurisy, pneumonia, postnasal drip, pulmonary collapse, pulmonary congestion, sleep apnea, snoring, wheezing (0.1% to 1%).

➤*Special senses:* Cataract, eye irritation, vision blurred (at least 1%); bad taste, blepharitis, conjunctival hemorrhage, decreased hearing, dry eyes, ear buzzing, earache, glaucoma, motion sickness, otitis externa, otitis media, retinal hemorrhage, spots before eyes, tinnitus (0.1% to 1%).

➤*Miscellaneous:* Chest pain, influenza, toothache (at least 1%); abscess, cellulitis, chills, fever, generalized coldness, head fullness, hiatal hernia, listlessness, periorbital edema (0.1% to 1%).

➤*Postmarketing:* Abdominal pain, agitation, cholecystitis, confusion, convulsions, hallucinations, heart block (all types), hemolytic anemia, hepatitis, hyponatremia, neuroleptic malignant syndrome, pancreatitis, rash.

Overdosage

➤*Symptoms:* Overdosage with cholinesterase inhibitors can result in cholinergic crisis characterized by severe nausea, vomiting, salivation, sweating, bradycardia, hypotension, respiratory depression, collapse, and convulsions. Increasing muscle weakness is a possibility and may result in death if respiratory muscles are involved.

➤*Treatment:* As in any case of overdose, use general supportive measures. Tertiary anticholinergics such as atropine may be used as an antidote for donepezil overdosage. IV atropine sulfate titrated to effect is recommended: An initial dose of 1 to 2 mg IV with subsequent doses based upon clinical response. Atypical responses in blood pressure and heart rate have been reported with other cholinomimetics when coadministered with quarternary anticholinergics such as glycopyrrolate. It is not known whether donepezil or its metabolites can be removed by dialysis (eg, hemodialysis, peritoneal dialysis, hemofiltration).

Patient Information

Take donepezil in the evening, just prior to retiring.

Donepezil may be taken with or without food.

Allow orally disintegrating tablets to dissolve on tongue and follow with water.

RIVASTIGMINE TARTRATE

Rx	**Exelon** (Novartis)	**Capsules**: 1.5 mg (as base)	(Exelon 1.5 mg). Yellow. In 60s, 500s, and UD 100s.
		3 mg (as base)	(Exelon 3 mg). Orange. In 60s, 500s, and UD 100s.
		4.5 mg (as base)	(Exelon 4.5 mg). Red. In 60s, 500s, and UD 100s.
		6 mg (as base)	(Exelon 6 mg). Orange/red. In 60s, 500s, and UD 100s.
		Solution: 2 mg/mL (as base)	In 120 mL bottles.

RIVASTIGMINE TARTRATE — ORAL

Indications

➤*Alzheimer dementia:* Rivastigmine is indicated for the treatment of mild to moderate dementia of the Alzheimer type.

➤*Unlabeled uses:* Treatment of the behavioral symptoms in Lewy-body dementia.

Administration and Dosage

➤*Approved by the FDA:* April 21, 2000.

The dosage of rivastigmine shown to be effective in controlled clinical trials is 6 to 12 mg/day, given as twice-a-day dosing (daily doses of 3 to 6 mg twice daily). There is evidence from the clinical trials that doses at the higher end of this range may be more beneficial.

The starting dose of rivastigmine is 1.5 mg twice a day. If this dose is well tolerated after a minimum of 2 weeks of treatment, the dose may be increased to 3 mg twice daily. Subsequent increases to 4.5 mg twice daily and 6 mg twice daily should be attempted after a minimum of 2 weeks at the previous dose. If adverse reactions (eg, nausea, vomiting, abdominal pain, loss of appetite) cause intolerance during treatment, the patient should be instructed to discontinue treatment for several doses and then restart at the same or next lower dose level. If treatment is interrupted for longer than several days, treatment should be reinitiated with the lowest daily dose and titrated as described above. The maximum dose is 6 mg twice daily (12 mg/day).

Rivastigmine should be taken with food in divided doses in the morning and evening.

Rivastigmine oral solution and rivastigmine capsules may be interchanged at equal doses.

➤*Administration of oral solution:* Patients should be instructed to remove the oral dosing syringe provided from its protective case and, using the provided syringe, withdraw the prescribed amount of rivastigmine oral solution from the container. Each dose of rivastigmine oral solution may be swallowed directly from the syringe or first mixed with a small glass of water, cold fruit juice, or soda. Patients should be instructed to stir and drink the mixture.

➤*Storage/Stability:*

Capsules – Store at 25°C (77°F); excursions permitted to 15° to 30°C (59° to 86°F). Store in a tight container.

Oral Solution – Store at 25°C (77°F); excursions permitted to 15° to 30°C (59° to 86°F). Store in an upright position and protect from freezing.

When rivastigmine oral solution is combined with cold fruit juice or soda, the mixture is stable at room temperature for up to 4 hours.

Actions

➤*Pharmacology:* Pathological changes in dementia of the Alzheimer type involve cholinergic neuronal pathways that project from the basal forebrain to the cerebral cortex and hippocampus. These pathways are thought to be intricately involved in memory, attention, learning, and other cognitive processes. While the precise mechanism of rivastigmine's action is unknown, it is postulated to exert its therapeutic effect by enhancing cholinergic function. This is accomplished by increasing the concentration of acetylcholine through reversible inhibition of its hydrolysis by cholinesterase. If this proposed mechanism is correct, rivastigmine's effect may lessen as the disease process advances and fewer cholinergic neurons remain functionally intact. There is no evidence that rivastigmine alters the course of the underlying dementing process. After a 6 mg dose of rivastigmine, anticholinesterase activity is present in cerebrospinal fluid (CSF) for about 10 hours, with a maximum inhibition of about 60% five hours after dosing.

In vitro and in vivo studies demonstrate that the inhibition of cholinesterase by rivastigmine is not affected by the coadministration of memantine, an N-methyl-D-aspartate receptor antagonist.

➤*Pharmacokinetics:*

Absorption – Rivastigmine is rapidly and completely absorbed, with absolute bioavailability of about 40% (3 mg dose). It shows linear pharmacokinetics up to 3 mg twice daily but is nonlinear at higher doses. Doubling the dose from 3 to 6 mg twice daily results in a 3-fold increase in the area under the curve (AUC). Peak plasma concentrations are reached in approximately 1 hour. Administration of rivastigmine with food delays absorption (T_{max}) by 90 minutes, lowers C_{max} approximately 30% and increases AUC approximately 30%.

Distribution – Rivastigmine is widely distributed throughout the body, with a volume of distribution in the range of 1.8 to 2.7 L/kg. Rivastigmine penetrates the blood-brain barrier, reaching CSF peak concentrations in 1.4 to 2.6 hours. the mean $AUC_{1\text{-}12\ h}$ ratio of CSF/plasma averaged 40 ± 0.5% following 1 to 6 mg twice daily doses.

Rivastigmine is about 40% bound to plasma proteins at concentrations of 1 to 400 ng/mL, which cover the therapeutic concentration range. Rivastigmine distributes equally between blood and plasma, with a blood-to-plasma partition ratio of 0.9 at concentrations ranging from 1 to 400 ng/mL.

Metabolism – Rivastigmine is rapidly and extensively metabolized, primarily via cholinesterase-mediated hydrolysis to the decarbamylated metabolite. Based on evidence from in vitro and animal studies, the major cytochrome P-450 isozymes are minimally involved in rivastigmine metabolism. Consistent with these observations is the finding that no drug interactions related to cytochrome P-450 have been observed in humans.

Excretion – The elimination half-life is about 1.5 hours, with most elimination as metabolites via the urine. The major pathway of elimination is via the kidneys. Following administration of ^{14}C-rivastigmine to 6 healthy volunteers, total recovery of radioactivity over 120 hours was 97% in urine and 0.4% in feces. No parent drug was detected in urine. The sulfate conjugate of the decarbamylated metabolite is the major component excreted in urine and represents 40% of the dose. Mean oral clearance of rivastigmine is 1.8 ± 0.6 L/min after 6 mg twice daily.

Special populations –

Renal function impairment: Following a single 3 mg dose, mean oral clearance of rivastigmine is 64% lower in moderately impaired renal patients (n = 8; glomerular filtration rate [GFR], 10 to 50 mL/min) than in healthy subjects (n = 10; GFR, greater than or equal to 60 mL/min); plasma clearance, 1.7 L/min (coefficient of variation [cv] = 45%) and 4.8 L/min (cv = 80%), respectively. In severely impaired renal patients (n = 8; GFR, less than 10 mL/min), mean oral clearance of rivastigmine is 43% higher than in healthy subjects (n = 10; GFR, greater than or equal to 60 mL/min); plasma clearance, 6.9 and 4.8 L/min, respectively. For unexplained reasons, the severely impaired renal patients had a higher clearance of rivastigmine than moderately impaired patients. However, dosage adjustment may not be necessary in renally impaired patients because the dose of the drug is individually titrated to tolerability.

Hepatic function impairment: Following a single 3 mg dose, mean oral clearance of rivastigmine was 60% lower in hepatically impaired patients (n = 10; biopsy proven) than in healthy subjects (n = 10). After multiple 6 mg twice daily oral dosing, the mean clearance of rivastigmine was 65% lower in mild (n = 7; Child-Pugh score 5 to 6) and moderate (n = 3; Child-Pugh score 7 to 9) hepatically impaired patients (biopsy proven, liver cirrhosis) than in healthy subjects (n = 10). Dosage adjustment is not necessary in hepatically impaired patients because the dose of drug is individually titrated to tolerability.

RIVASTIGMINE TARTRATE — ORAL

Age: Following a single 2.5 mg oral dose to elderly volunteers (older than 60 years of age; n = 24) and younger volunteers (n = 24), mean oral clearance of rivastigmine was 30% lower in elderly (7 L/minutes) than in younger subjects (10 L/minutes).

Gender and race: No specific pharmacokinetic study was conducted to investigate the effect of gender and race on the disposition of rivastigmine, but a population pharmacokinetic analysis indicates that gender (men, n = 277; women, n = 348) and race (white, n = 575; black, n = 34; Asian, n = 4; other, n = 12) did not affect the clearance of rivastigmine.

Nicotine use: Population pharmacokinetic analysis showed that nicotine use increases the oral clearance of rivastigmine 23% (smokers, n = 75; nonsmokers, n = 549).

Drug interactions:

• *Effect of rivastigmine on the metabolism of other drugs* – Rivastigmine is primarily metabolized through hydrolysis by esterases. Minimal metabolism occurs via the major cytochrome P-450 isoenzymes. Based on in vitro studies, no pharmacokinetic drug interactions with drugs metabolized by the following isoenzyme systems are expected: CYP1A2, CYP2D6, CYP3A4/5, CYP2E1, CYP2C9, CYP2C8, or CYP2C19.

No pharmacokinetic interaction was observed between rivastigmine and digoxin, warfarin, diazepam, or fluoxetine in studies in healthy volunteers. The elevation of prothrombin time induced by warfarin is not affected by administration of rivastigmine.

• *Effect of other drugs on the metabolism of rivastigmine* – Drugs that induce or inhibit CYP450 metabolism are not expected to alter the metabolism of rivastigmine. Single-dose pharmacokinetic studies demonstrated that the metabolism of rivastigmine is not significantly affected by coadministration of digoxin, warfarin, diazepam, or fluoxetine.

Population pharmacokinetic analysis with a database of 625 patients showed that the pharmacokinetics of rivastigmine were not influenced by commonly prescribed medications such as antacids (n = 77), antihypertensives (n = 72), beta-blockers (n = 42), calcium channel blockers (n = 75), antidiabetics (n = 21), nonsteroidal anti-inflammatory drugs (NSAIDs) (n = 79), estrogens (n = 70), salicylate analgesics (n = 177), antianginals (n = 35), and antihistamines (n = 15).

Contraindications

Rivastigmine is contraindicated in patients with known hypersensitivity to rivastigmine, other carbamate derivatives, or other components of the formulation.

Warnings

➤*GI adverse reactions:* Rivastigmine use is associated with significant GI adverse reactions, including nausea and vomiting, anorexia, and weight loss. For this reason, always start patients at a dosage of 1.5 mg twice daily and titrate to their maintenance dosage. If treatment is interrupted for longer than several days, reinitiate treatment with the lowest daily dose to reduce the possibility of severe vomiting and its potentially serious sequelae (eg, there has been 1 postmarketing report of severe vomiting with esophageal rupture following inappropriate reinitiation of treatment with a 4.5 mg dose after 8 weeks of treatment interruption).

Nausea and vomiting – In the controlled clinical trials, 47% of the patients treated with a rivastigmine dose in the therapeutic range of 6 to 12 mg/day (n = 1,189) developed nausea (compared with 12% in placebo). A total of 31% of rivastigmine-treated patients developed at least 1 episode of vomiting (compared with 6% for placebo). The rate of vomiting was higher during the titration phase (24% vs 3% for placebo) than in the maintenance phase (14% vs 3% for placebo). The rates were higher in women than men. Five percent of patients discontinued for vomiting, compared with less than 1% for patients on placebo. Vomiting was severe in 2% of rivastigmine-treated patients and was rated as mild or moderate in 14% of patients. The rate of nausea was higher during the titration phase (43% vs 9% for placebo) than in the maintenance phase (17% vs 4% for placebo).

Weight loss – In the controlled trials, approximately 26% of women on high dosages of rivastigmine (greater than 9 mg/day) had weight loss of greater than or equal to 7% of their baseline weight, compared with 6% in the placebo-treated patients. About 18% of the men in the high-dosage group experienced a similar degree of weight loss, compared with 4% in placebo-treated patients. It is not clear how much of the weight loss was caused by anorexia, nausea, vomiting, and diarrhea associated with the drug.

Anorexia – In the controlled trials, of the patients treated with a rivastigmine dosage of 6 to 12 mg/day, 17% developed anorexia, compared with 3% of the placebo patients. Neither the time course or the severity of the anorexia is known.

Peptic ulcers / GI bleeding – Because of their pharmacological action, cholinesterase inhibitors may be expected to increase gastric acid secretion because of increased cholinergic activity. Therefore, monitor patients closely for symptoms of active or occult GI bleeding, especially those at increased risk for developing ulcers (eg, those with a history of ulcer disease or those receiving concurrent NSAIDs). Clinical studies of rivastigmine have shown no significant increase, relative to placebo, in the incidence of peptic ulcer disease or GI bleeding.

➤*Anesthesia:* Rivastigmine, as a cholinesterase inhibitor, is likely to exaggerate succinylcholine-type muscle relaxation during anesthesia.

➤*Cardiovascular effects:* Drugs that increase cholinergic activity may have vagotonic effects on heart rate (eg, bradycardia). The potential for this action may be particularly important to patients with sick sinus syndrome or other supraventricular cardiac conduction conditions. In clinical trials, rivastigmine was not associated with any increased incidence of cardiovascular adverse reactions, heart rate or blood pressure changes, or electrocardiogram (ECG) abnormalities. Syncopal episodes have been reported in 3% of patients receiving rivastigmine 6 to 12 mg/day, compared with 2% of placebo patients.

➤*Urinary obstruction:* Although this was not observed in clinical trials of rivastigmine, drugs that increase cholinergic activity may cause urinary obstruction.

➤*Seizures:* Drugs that increase cholinergic activity are believed to have some potential for causing seizures. However, seizure activity also may be a manifestation of Alzheimer disease.

➤*Pulmonary effects:* Like other drugs that increase cholinergic activity, use rivastigmine with care in patients with a history of asthma or obstructive pulmonary disease.

➤*Carcinogenesis:* In carcinogenicity studies conducted at dosage levels up to 1.1 mg base/kg/day in rats and 1.6 mg base/kg/day in mice, rivastigmine was not carcinogenic. These dosage levels are approximately 0.9 and 0.7 times the maximum recommended human daily dose (MRHD) of 12 mg/day on a mg/m^2 basis.

➤*Mutagenesis:* Rivastigmine was clastogenic in 2 in vitro assays in the presence, but not the absence, of metabolic activation. It caused structural chromosomal aberrations in V79 Chinese hamster lung cells and structural and numerical (polyploidy) chromosomal aberrations in human peripheral blood lymphocytes. Rivastigmine was not genotoxic in 3 in vitro assays: the Ames test, the unscheduled DNA synthesis (UDS) test in rat hepatocytes (a test for induction of DNA repair synthesis), and the hypoxanthine-guanine phosphoribosyl transferase (HGPRT) test in V79 Chinese hamster cells. Rivastigmine was not clastogenic in the in vivo mouse micronucleus test.

➤*Fertility impairment:* Rivastigmine had no effect on fertility or reproductive performance in the rat at dosage levels up to 1.1 mg base/kg/day. This dosage is approximately 0.9 times the MRHD of 12 mg/day on a mg/m^2 basis.

➤*Pregnancy: Category B.* Reproduction studies conducted in pregnant rats at dosages up to 2.3 mg base/kg/day (approximately 2 times the MRHD on a mg/m^2 basis) and in pregnant rabbits at doses up to 2.3 mg base/kg/day (approximately 4 times the MRHD on a mg/m^2 basis) revealed no evidence of teratogenicity. Studies in rats showed slightly decreased fetal/pup weights, usually at doses causing some maternal toxicity; decreased weights were seen at doses that were several fold lower than the MRHD on a mg/m^2 basis. There are no adequate or well-controlled studies in pregnant women. Because animal reproduction studies are not always predictive of human response, use rivastigmine during pregnancy only if the potential benefit justifies the potential risk to the fetus.

➤*Lactation:* It is not known whether rivastigmine is excreted in breast milk. Rivastigmine has no indication for use in breast-feeding mothers.

➤*Children:* There are no adequate and well-controlled trials documenting the safety and efficacy of rivastigmine in any illness occurring in children.

Drug Interactions

➤*Effect of rivastigmine on the metabolism of other drugs:* Rivastigmine is primarily metabolized through hydrolysis by esterases. Minimal metabolism occurs via the major cytochrome P-450 isoenzymes. Based on in vitro studies, no pharmacokinetic drug interactions with drugs metabolized by the following isoenzyme systems are expected: CYP1A2, CYP2D6, CYP3A4/5, CYP2E1, CYP2C9, CYP2C8, or CYP2C19.

No pharmacokinetic interaction was observed between rivastigmine and digoxin, warfarin, diazepam, or fluoxetine in studies in healthy volunteers. The elevation of prothrombin time induced by warfarin is not affected by administration of rivastigmine.

➤*Effect of other drugs on the metabolism of rivastigmine:* Drugs that induce or inhibit CYP450 metabolism are not expected to alter the metabolism of rivastigmine. Single-dose pharmacokinetic studies demonstrated that the metabolism of rivastigmine is not significantly affected by coadministration of digoxin, warfarin, diazepam, or fluoxetine.

Population pharmacokinetic analysis with a database of 625 patients showed that the pharmacokinetics of rivastigmine were not influenced by commonly prescribed medications such as antacids (n = 77), antihypertensives (n = 72), β-blockers (n = 42), calcium channel blockers (n = 75), antidiabetics (n = 21), NSAIDs (n = 79), estrogens (n = 70), salicylate analgesics (n = 177), antianginals (n = 35), and antihistamines (n = 15).

➤*Anticholinergics:* Because of their mechanism of action, cholinesterase inhibitors have the potential to interfere with the activity of anticholinergic medications.

➤*Cholinomimetics and other cholinesterase inhibitors:* A synergistic effect may be expected when cholinesterase inhibitors are given concurrently with succinylcholine, similar neuromuscular blocking agents, or cholinergic agonists such as bethanechol.

➤*Drug / Food interactions:* Administration of rivastigmine with food delays absorption (T_{max}) by 90 minutes, lowers C_{max} approximately 30%, and increases AUC approximately 30%.

Adverse Reactions

The rate of discontinuation because of adverse reactions in controlled clinical trials of rivastigmine was 15% for patients receiving 6 to 12 mg/day, compared with 5% for patients on placebo, during forced weekly-dose titration. While on a maintenance dose, the rates were 6% for patients on rivastigmine, compared with 4% for those on placebo.

The most common adverse reactions leading to discontinuation, defined as those occurring in at least 2% of patients and at twice the incidence seen in placebo patients, are shown in the following table.

RIVASTIGMINE TARTRATE — ORAL

Rivastigmine Adverse Reactions Leading to Withdrawal From Clinical Trials (% Discontinuing)						
	Titration		Maintenance		Overall	
Adverse reaction	Placebo (n = 868)	Rivastigmine ≥ 6 to 12 mg/day (n = 1,189)	Placebo (n = 788)	Rivastigmine ≥ 6 to 12 mg/day (n = 987)	Placebo (n = 868)	Rivastigmine ≥ 6 to 12 mg/day (n = 1,189)
Anorexia	0%	2%	< 1%	1%	< 1%	3%
Dizziness	< 1%	2%	< 1%	1%	< 1%	2%
Nausea	< 1%	8%	< 1%	1%	1%	8%
Vomiting	< 1%	4%	< 1%	1%	< 1%	5%

➤*Most common adverse reactions:* The most common adverse reactions, defined as those occurring at a frequency of at least 5% and twice the placebo rate, are largely predicted by rivastigmine's cholinergic effects. These include anorexia, asthenia, dyspepsia, nausea, and vomiting.

GI – Rivastigmine use is associated with significant nausea, vomiting, and weight loss.

Nausea and vomiting: In the controlled clinical trials, 47% of the patients treated with a rivastigmine dose in the therapeutic range of 6 to 12 mg/day (n = 1,189) developed nausea (compared with 12% in placebo). A total of 31% of rivastigmine-treated patients developed at least 1 episode of vomiting (compared with 6% for placebo). The rate of vomiting was higher during the titration phase (24% vs 3% for placebo) than in the maintenance phase (14% vs 3% for placebo). The rates were higher in women than men. Five percent of patients discontinued for vomiting, compared with less than 1% for patients on placebo. Vomiting was severe in 2% of rivastigmine-treated patients and was rated as mild or moderate in 14% of patients. The rate of nausea was higher during the titration phase (43% vs 9% for placebo) than in the maintenance phase (17% vs 4% for placebo).

Weight loss: In the controlled trials, approximately 26% of women on high dosages of rivastigmine (greater than 9 mg/day) had weight loss of greater than or equal to 7% of their baseline weight, compared with 6% in the placebo-treated patients. About 18% of the men in the high-dose group experienced a similar degree of weight loss, compared with 4% in placebo-treated patients. It is not clear how much of the weight loss was due to anorexia, nausea, vomiting, and diarrhea associated with the drug.

➤*Adverse reactions reported in controlled trials:* The following are treatment-emergent signs and symptoms that were reported in at least 2% of patients in placebo-controlled trials and for which the rate of occurrence was greater for patients treated with rivastigmine dosages of 6 to 12 mg/day than for those treated with placebo (see the following table). Be aware that these figures cannot be used to predict the frequency of adverse reactions in the course of usual medical practice, when patient characteristics and other factors may differ from those prevailing during clinical studies. Similarly, the cited frequencies cannot be directly compared with figures obtained from other clinical investigations involving different treatments, uses, or investigators. An inspection of these frequencies, however, does provide 1 basis by which to estimate the relative contribution of drug and nondrug factors to the adverse reaction incidences in the population studied.

In general, adverse reactions were less frequent later in the course of treatment.

No systematic effect of race or age could be determined on the incidence of adverse reactions in the controlled studies. Nausea, vomiting, and weight loss were more frequent in women than men.

Rivastigmine Adverse Reactions (≥ 2%)		
Adverse reaction	Placebo (n = 868)	Rivastigmine (6 to 12 mg/day) (n = 1,189)
Percent of patients with any adverse reaction	79%	92%
Cardiovascular		
Hypertension	2%	3%
CNS		
Aggressive reaction	2%	3%
Anxiety	3%	5%
Confusion	7%	8%
Depression	4%	6%
Dizziness	11%	21%
Hallucination	3%	4%
Headache	12%	17%
Insomnia	7%	9%
Somnolence	3%	5%
Syncope	2%	3%
Tremor	1%	4%
GI		
Abdominal pain	6%	13%
Anorexia	3%	17%
Constipation	4%	5%
Diarrhea	11%	19%
Dyspepsia	4%	9%
Eructation	1%	2%
Flatulence	2%	4%
Nausea	12%	47%
Vomiting	6%	31%
Respiratory		
Rhinitis	3%	4%
Miscellaneous		
Accidental trauma	9%	10%
Asthenia	2%	6%
Fatigue	5%	9%
Influenza-like symptoms	2%	3%
Malaise	2%	5%
Sweating increased	1%	4%
Urinary tract infection	6%	7%
Weight decrease	< 1%	3%

Other adverse reactions observed at a rate of 2% or more on rivastigmine 6 to 12 mg/day but at a greater or equal rate on placebo were agitation, arthralgia, back pain, bone fracture, bronchitis, chest pain, coughing, delusion, infection (general), nervousness, pain, paranoid reaction, peripheral edema, pharyngitis, rash (general), upper respiratory tract infections, urinary incontinence, vertigo.

➤*Other adverse reactions observed during clinical trials:* Rivastigmine has been administered to over 5,297 patients during clinical trials worldwide. Of these, 4,326 patients have been treated for at least 3 months, 3,407 patients have been treated for at least 6 months, 2,150 patients have been treated for 1 year, 1,250 have been treated for 2 years, and 168 have been treated for over 3 years. With regard to exposure to the highest dose, 2,809 patients were exposed to doses of 10 to 12 mg; 2,615 patients have been treated for 3 months, 2,328 patients have been treated for 6 months, 1,378 patients have been treated for 1 year, 917 patients have been treated for 2 years, and 129 have been treated for over 3 years.

Treatment-emergent signs and symptoms that occurred during 8 controlled clinical trials and 9 open-label trials in North America, Western Europe, Australia, South Africa, and Japan were recorded as adverse reactions by the clinical investigators using terminology of their own choosing. To provide an overall estimate of the proportion of individuals having similar types of events, the reactions were grouped into a smaller number of standardized categories using a modified World Health Organization (WHO) dictionary, and event frequencies were calculated across all studies. These categories are used in the listing below. The frequencies represent the proportion of 5,297 patients from these trials who experienced that event while receiving rivastigmine. All adverse reactions occurring in at least 6 patients (approximately 0.1%) are included, except for those already listed elsewhere in labeling, WHO terms too general to be informative, relatively minor reactions, or reactions unlikely to be drug-caused. Reactions are classified by body system and listed using the following definitions: frequent adverse reactions, those occurring in at least 1/100 patients; infrequent adverse reactions, those occurring in 1/100 to 1/1,000 patients. These adverse reactions are not necessarily related to rivastigmine treatment and in most cases were observed at a similar frequency in placebo-treated patients in the controlled studies.

➤*Cardiovascular:* Angina pectoris, atrial fibrillation, bradycardia, cardiac failure, hypotension, myocardial infarction, palpitation, postural hypotension (1% or more).

Aneurysm, atrioventricular block, bundle-branch block, cardiac arrest, deep thrombophlebitis, extrasystoles, intracranial hemorrhage, peripheral ischemia, pulmonary embolism, sick sinus syndrome, supraventricular tachycardia, tachycardia, thrombosis (0.1% to 1%).

➤*CNS:* Abnormal gait, ataxia, confusion, convulsions, paraesthesia, paranoid reaction (1% or more).

Abnormal dreaming, amnesia, apathy, aphasia, apraxia, decreased libido, delirium, dementia, depersonalization, dysphonia, emotional lability, hyperkinesia, hyperreflexia, hypertonia, hypesthesia, hypokinesia, impaired concentration, increased libido, migraine, neuralgia, neurosis, nystagmus, paresis, peripheral neuropathy, personality disorder, psychosis, suicidal ideation, suicide attempt (0.1% to 1%).

➤*Dermatologic:* Rashes of various kinds (bullous, eczema, erythematous, exfoliative, maculopapular, psoriaform) (1% or more).

Alopecia, cold clammy skin, dermatitis contact, flushing, skin ulceration, urticaria (0.1% to 1%).

➤*Endocrine:* Goiter, hypothyroidism (0.1% to 1%).

➤*GI:* Fecal incontinence, gastritis (1% or more).

Colitis, dry mouth, duodenal ulcer, dysphagia, esophagitis, gastric ulcer, gastritis, gastroenteritis, gastroesophageal reflux, gingivitis, GI hemorrhage, glossitis, hematemesis, hernia, increased saliva, intestinal obstruction, melena, pancreatitis, rectal hemorrhage, tenesmus, ulcerative stomatitis (0.1% to 1%).

➤*GU:* Hematuria (1% or more).

RIVASTIGMINE TARTRATE — ORAL

Acute renal failure, albuminuria, atrophic vaginitis, breast pain, dysuria, impotence, micturition urgency, nocturia, oliguria, polyuria, renal calculus, urinary retention (0.1% to 1%).

➤*Hematologic/Lymphatic:* Anemia, epistaxis (1% or more).

Hematoma, hypochromic anemia, leukocytosis, purpura, thrombocytopenia (0.1% to 1%).

➤*Hepatic:* Abnormal hepatic function, cholecystitis (0.1% to 1%).

➤*Metabolic/Nutritional:* Dehydration, hypokalemia (1% or more).

Cachexia, diabetes mellitus, gout, hypercholesterolemia, hyperglycemia, hyperlipemia, hypoglycemia, hyponatremia, thirst (0.1% to 1%).

➤*Musculoskeletal:* Arthritis, leg cramps, myalgia (1% or more).

Cramps, hernia, muscle weakness (0.1% to 1%).

➤*Ophthalmic:* Cataract (1% ore more).

Blepharitis, conjunctival hemorrhage, diplopia, eye pain, glaucoma (0.1% to 1%).

➤*Respiratory:* Apnea, bronchospasm, laryngitis (0.1% to 1%).

➤*Special senses:* Tinnitus (1% or more).

Loss of taste, perversion of taste (0.1% to 1%).

➤*Miscellaneous:* Accidental trauma, allergy, edema, fever, hot flushes, rigors (1% or more).

Cellulitis, cystitis, edema, feeling cold, halitosis, hemorrhoids, herpes simplex, hypothermia, otitis media, periorbital or facial edema (0.1% to 1%).

➤*Postmarketing:* Voluntary reports of adverse reactions temporally associated with rivastigmine that have been received since market introduction that are not listed above, and that may or may not be causally related to the drug include the following: Stevens-Johnson syndrome.

Overdosage

➤*Symptoms:* Overdosage with cholinesterase inhibitors can result in cholinergic crisis, characterized by severe nausea, vomiting, salivation, sweating, bradycardia, hypotension, respiratory depression, collapse, and convulsions. Increasing muscle weakness is a possibility and may result in death if respiratory muscles are involved. Atypical responses in blood pressure and heart rate have been reported with other drugs that increase cholinergic activity when coadministered with quaternary anticholinergics such as glycopyrrolate.

➤*Treatment:* Because strategies for the management of overdose are continually evolving, it is advisable to contact a poison control center to determine the latest recommendations for the management of an overdose of any drug.

As rivastigmine has a short plasma half-life of about 1 hour and a moderate duration of acetylcholinesterase inhibition of 8 to 10 hours, it is recommended that a further dose of rivastigmine not be administered for the next 24 hours in cases of asymptomatic overdoses.

As in any case of overdose, general supportive measures should be utilized.

Because of the short half-life of rivastigmine, dialysis (hemodialysis, peritoneal dialysis, or hemofiltration) would not be clinically indicated in the event of an overdose.

In overdoses accompanied by severe nausea and vomiting, consider using antiemetics. In a documented case of a rivastigmine 46 mg overdose, the patient experienced vomiting, incontinence, hypertension, psychomotor retardation, and loss of consciousness. The patient fully recovered within 24 hours and conservative management was all that was required for treatment.

Patient Information

Advise caregivers of the high incidence of nausea and vomiting associated with the use of the drug, along with the possibility of anorexia and weight loss. Encourage caregivers to monitor for these adverse reactions and inform their health care provider if they occur. It is critical to inform caregivers that if therapy has been interrupted for more than several days, not to administer the next dose until they have discussed with this with their health care provider.

Instruct caregivers in the correct procedure for administering rivastigmine oral solution. In addition, inform caregivers of the existence of an instruction sheet (included with the product) describing how the solution is to be administered. They should be urged to read this sheet prior to administering rivastigmine oral solution. Tell caregivers to direct questions about the administration of the solution to their doctor or pharmacist.

➤*Rivastigmine oral solution instructions for use:* Remove oral dosing syringe from its protective case. Push down and twist child-resistant closure to open bottle.

Insert tip of syringe into opening of white stopper.

While holding the syringe, pull the plunger up to the level (see markings on side of syringe) that equals the dose prescribed by your doctor.

Before removing syringe containing prescribed dose from bottle, push out large bubbles by moving plunger up and down a few times. After the large bubbles are gone, pull the plunger again to the level that equals the dose prescribed by your doctor. Do not worry about a few tiny bubbles. This will not affect your dose in any way.

Remove the syringe from the bottle.

You may swallow rivastigmine oral solution directly from the syringe or mix with a small glass of water, cold fruit juice, or soda. If mixing with water, juice, or soda, be sure to stir completely and to drink the entire mixture.

Do not mix with other liquids.

After use, wipe outside of syringe with a clean tissue and put it back into its case.

Close bottle using child resistant closure.

GALANTAMINE HBr

Rx	**Razadyne** (Janssen)	**Tablets:** 4 mg (as base)	Lactose. (JANSSEN G 4). Off-white. Film-coated. In 60s.
		8 mg (as base)	Lactose. (JANSSEN G 8). Pink. Film-coated. In 60s.
		12 mg (as base)	Lactose. (JANSSEN G 12). Orange-brown. Film-coated. In 60s.
Rx	**Razadyne ER** (Janssen)	**Capsules, extended-release:** 8 mg (as base)	Sucrose. (GAL 8). White opaque. Pellet-filled. In 30s.
		16 mg (as base)	Sucrose. (GAL 16). Pink opaque. Pellet-filled. In 30s.
		24 mg (as base)	Sucrose. (GAL 24). Caramel opaque. Pellet-filled. In 30s.
Rx	**Razadyne** (Janssen)	**Oral solution:** 4 mg/mL	Saccharin. In 100 mL w/ calibrated pipette.

GALANTAMINE HYDROBROMIDE — ORAL

Indications

➤*Alzheimer disease:* Treatment of mild to moderate dementia of the Alzheimer type.

➤*Unlabeled uses:* Vascular dementia.

Administration and Dosage

➤*Approved by the FDA:* February 28, 2001.

Inform patients and caregivers that if therapy has been interrupted for several days or longer, the patient should be restarted at the lowest dose and the dose escalated to the current dose.

The abrupt withdrawal of galantamine in those patients who had been receiving doses in the effective range was not associated with an increased frequency of adverse events in comparison with those continuing to receive the same doses of that drug. However, the beneficial effects of galantamine are lost when the drug is discontinued.

➤*Immediate-release:* 16 to 32 mg/day given twice daily. The 32 mg/day dose is not as well tolerated as the lower doses and does not provide increased effectiveness; therefore, the recommended dose range is 16 to 24 mg/day given twice daily.

Starting dose is 4 mg twice daily (8 mg/day). After a minimum of 4 weeks of treatment, if well tolerated, increase the dose to 8 mg twice daily (16 mg/day). Attempt a further increase to 12 mg twice daily (24 mg/day) only after a minimum of 4 weeks at the previous dose.

Administer galantamine twice daily, preferably with morning and evening meals.

➤*Extended-release:* The dosage shown to be effective in controlled clinical trials is 16 to 24 mg/day.

The recommended starting dose is 8 mg/day. Increase the dose to the initial maintenance dose of 16 mg/day after a minimum of 4 weeks. A further increase to 24 mg/day should be attempted after a minimum of 4 weeks of 16 mg/day. Base dose increases on assessment of clinical benefit and tolerability of the previous dose.

Administer once daily in the morning, preferably with food. Advise patients and caregivers to be sure to drink adequate amounts of fluid during treatment.

➤*Hepatic impairment:* Galantamine plasma concentrations may be increased in patients with moderate to severe hepatic impairment. In patients with moderately impaired hepatic function (Child-Pugh 7 to 9), the dose generally should not exceed 16 mg/day. The use of galantamine in patients with severe hepatic impairment (Child-Pugh 10 to 15) is not recommended.

➤*Renal impairment:* For patients with moderate renal impairment, the dose generally should not exceed 16 mg/day. In patients with severe renal impairment (Ccr < 9 mL/min), the use of galantamine is not recommended.

➤*Storage/Stability:* Store galantamine at 25°C (77°F); excursions permitted to 15° to 30°C (59° to 86°F).

Actions

➤*Pharmacology:* Galantamine, a tertiary alkaloid, is a competitive and reversible inhibitor of acetylcholinesterase. While the precise mechanism of galantamine's action is unknown, it may exert its therapeutic effect by enhancing cholinergic function. This is accomplished by increasing the concentration of acetylcholine through reversible inhibition of its hydrolysis by cholinesterase. If this mechanism is correct, galantamine's effect may lessen as the disease process advances and fewer cholinergic neurons remain func-

GALANTAMINE HYDROBROMIDE — ORAL

tionally intact. There is no evidence that galantamine alters the course of the underlying dementing process.

➤*Pharmacokinetics:*

Absorption/Distribution – Galantamine is rapidly and completely absorbed with time-to-peak concentration in ≈ 1 hour. Galantamine has an absolute oral bioavailability of ≈ 90%. Bioavailability of the tablet was the same as the bioavailability of an oral solution. Food did not affect the AUC of galantamine but C_{max} decreased by 25% and T_{max} was delayed by 1.5 hours. The mean volume of distribution of galantamine is 175 L.

The plasma protein binding of galantamine is 18% at therapeutically relevant concentrations. In whole blood, galantamine mainly is distributed to blood cells (52.7%). The blood to plasma concentration ratio of galantamine is 1:2.

Metabolism/Excretion – Galantamine is metabolized by hepatic cytochrome P450 enzymes, glucuronidated, and excreted unchanged in the urine. In vitro studies indicated that CYP2D6 and CYP3A4 were the major cytochrome P450 isoenzymes involved in the metabolism of galantamine, and inhibitors of both pathways modestly increase oral bioavailability of galantamine. O-demethylation mediated by CYP2D6 was greater in extensive metabolizers of CYP2D6 than in poor metabolizers. However, in plasma from poor and extensive metabolizers, unchanged galantamine and its glucuronide accounted for much of the sample radioactivity.

Up to 8 hours postdose, unchanged galantamine accounted for 39% to 77% of the total radioactivity in the plasma, and galantamine glucuronide for 14% to 24%. By 7 days, 93% to 99% of the radioactivity had been recovered, with ≈ 95% in urine and ≈ 5% in the feces. Total urinary recovery of unchanged galantamine accounted for ≈ 32% of the dose and that of galantamine glucuronide for ≈ 12%.

After IV or oral administration, ≈ 20% of the dose was excreted as unchanged galantamine in the urine in 24 hours, representing a renal clearance of ≈ 65 mL/min, about 20% to 25% of the total plasma clearance of ≈ 300 mL/min. Galantamine has a terminal elimination half-life of ≈ 7 hours (range, 4.4 to 10) and pharmacokinetics are linear over the range of 8 to 32 mg/day.

The maximum inhibition of anticholinesterase activity of ≈ 40% was achieved in ≈ 1 hour after a single oral dose of 8 mg galantamine in healthy men.

Special populations –

CYP2D6 poor metabolizers: Approximately 7% of the normal population has a genetic variation that leads to reduced levels of activity of the CYP2D6 isozyme. They are referred to as poor metabolizers. After a single oral dose of 4 or 8 mg galantamine, CYP2D6 poor metabolizers demonstrated a similar C_{max} and ≈ 35% AUC increase of unchanged galantamine compared with extensive metabolizers. Dosage adjustment is not necessary in patients identified as poor metabolizers as the dose of drug is individually titrated to tolerability.

Hepatic impairment: Following a single 4 mg dose of galantamine in patients with moderate hepatic impairment, galantamine clearance was decreased by ≈ 25% compared with healthy volunteers. Exposure would be expected to increase further with an increasing degree of hepatic impairment.

Renal impairment: Following a single 8 mg dose of galantamine, AUC increased by 37% and 67% in moderate and severely renal-impaired patients compared with normal volunteers.

Elderly: Data from clinical trials in patients with Alzheimer's disease indicated that galantamine concentrations are 30% to 40% higher than in healthy young subjects.

Gender: No specific pharmacokinetic study was conducted to investigate the effect of gender on the disposition of galantamine, but a population pharmacokinetic analysis indicates that galantamine clearance is ≈ 20% lower in females than in males (explained by lower body weight in females).

Contraindications

Known hypersensitivity to galantamine or to any excipients used in the formulation.

Warnings

➤*Renal function impairment:* In patients with moderately impaired renal function, proceed cautiously with dose titration. In patients with severely impaired renal function (Ccr < 0 mL/min), galantamine is not recommended.

➤*Hepatic function impairment:* In patients with moderately impaired hepatic function, proceed cautiously with dose titration. The use of galantamine in patients with severe hepatic impairment is not recommended.

➤*Pregnancy: Category B.* There are no adequate and well-controlled studies in pregnant women. Use during pregnancy only if the potential benefit justifies the potential risk to the fetus.

➤*Lactation:* It is not known whether galantamine is excreted in breast milk. Galantamine has no indication for use in nursing mothers.

➤*Children:* Safety and efficacy of galantamine in children have not been established. Therefore, the use of galantamine in children is not recommended.

Precautions

➤*Anesthesia:* Galantamine, as a cholinesterase inhibitor, is likely to exaggerate the neuromuscular blockade effects of succinylcholine-type and similar neuromuscular blocking agents during anesthesia.

➤*Cardiovascular conditions:* Because of their pharmacological action, cholinesterase inhibitors have vagotonic effects on the sinoatrial and atrioventricular nodes, leading to bradycardia and AV block. These actions may be particularly important to patients with supraventricular cardiac conduction disorders or to patients taking other drugs concomitantly that significantly slow heart rate. However, postmarketing surveillance of marketed anticholinesterase inhibitors has shown that bradycardia and all types of heart block have been reported in patients with and without known underlying cardiac conduction abnormalities. Therefore, consider all patients to be at risk for adverse effects on cardiac conduction.

In randomized controlled trials, bradycardia was reported more frequently in galantamine-treated patients than in placebo-treated patients, but rarely led to treatment discontinuation. The overall frequency of this event was 2% to 3% for galantamine doses up to 24 mg/day compared with < 1% for placebo. No increased incidence of heart block was observed at the recommended doses.

Patients treated with galantamine ≥ 24 mg/day using the recommended dosing schedule showed a dose-related increase in risk of syncope.

➤*GI conditions:* Cholinomimetics may increase gastric acid secretion because of increased cholinergic activity. Therefore, monitor patients closely for symptoms of active or occult GI bleeding, especially those with an increased risk for developing ulcers (eg, those with a history of ulcer disease or patients using concurrent nonsteroidal anti-inflammatory drugs [NSAIDs]).

Galantamine, as a predictable consequence of its pharmacological properties, has been shown to produce nausea, vomiting, diarrhea, anorexia, and weight loss. In patients who experienced nausea, the median duration was 5 to 7 days.

➤*GU:* Although this was not observed in clinical trials with galantamine, cholinomimetics may cause bladder outflow obstruction.

➤*Neurological conditions:* Cholinesterase inhibitors are believed to have some potential to cause generalized convulsions. However, seizure activity may be a manifestation of Alzheimer's disease.

➤*Pulmonary conditions:* Because of its cholinomimetic action, prescribe galantamine with care to patients with a history of severe asthma or obstructive pulmonary disease.

Drug Interactions

Galantamine Drug Interactions

Precipitant drug	Object drug*		Description
Cholinesterase inhibitors	Succinylcholine, bethanechol	↑	A synergistic effect is expected when combined.
Succinylcholine, bethanechol	Cholinesterase inhibitors		
Cimetidine	Galantamine	↑	Cimetidine increased the bioavailability of galantamine by ≈ 16%. Ranitidine had no effect.
Ketoconazole	Galantamine	↑	Ketoconazole increased the AUC of galantamine by ≈ 30%.
Paroxetine	Galantamine	↑	Paroxetine increased the oral bioavailability of galantamine by ≈ 40%.
Erythromycin	Galantamine	↑	Erythromycin increased the AUC of galantamine by 10%.

* ↑ = Object drug increased.

Adverse Reactions

In a 5-month trial with escalation of the dose by 8 mg/day every 4 weeks, the overall risk of discontinuation because of an adverse event was 7%, 7%, and 10% for the placebo, 16 mg/day galantamine, and 24 mg/day galantamine groups, respectively, with GI adverse effects the principal reason for discontinuing galantamine. The most frequent adverse events leading to discontinuation in this study are listed in the following table.

Most Frequent Galantamine Adverse Events Leading to Discontinuation[1] (%)

Adverse reaction	16 mg/day (n = 279)	24 mg/day (n = 273)	Placebo (n = 286)
Nausea	2	4	< 1
Dizziness	2	1	< 1
Vomiting	1	3	0
Anorexia	1	< 1	< 1
Syncope	0	1	0

[1] Placebo-controlled, double-blind trial with 4-week dose escalation schedule.

Adverse Events Occurring in ≥ 5% Galantamine and ≥ 2 Times Placebo[1]

Adverse event	Galantamine 16 mg/day (n = 279)	Galantamine 24 mg/day (n= 273)	Placebo (n = 286)
Nausea	13	17	5
Diarrhea	12	6	6
Anorexia	7	9	3
Vomiting	6	10	1
Weight decrease	5	5	1

[1] Placebo-controlled trial with 4-week dose escalation schedule.

GALANTAMINE HYDROBROMIDE — ORAL

Galantamine Adverse Events Occurring in ≥ 2% of Patients at a Frequency Greater than Placebo		
Adverse reaction	Galantamine[1] (n = 1040)	Placebo (n = 801)
CNS		
Dizziness	9	6
Headache	8	5
Depression	7	5
Insomnia	5	4
Somnolence	4	3
Tremor	3	2
GI		
Nausea	24	9
Vomiting	13	4
Diarrhea	9	7
Anorexia	9	3
Abdominal pain	5	4
Dyspepsia	5	2
GU		
Urinary tract infection	8	7
Hematuria	3	2
Miscellaneous		
Weight decrease	7	2
Fatigue	5	3
Rhinitis	4	3
Anemia	3	2
Syncope	2	1
Bradycardia	2	1

[1] Adverse events in patients treated with 16 or 24 mg/day of galantamine in 4 placebo-controlled trials are included.

Adverse events occurring with an incidence of ≥ 2% in placebo-treated patients that was either equal to or greater than with galantamine treatment were the following: Constipation, agitation, confusion, anxiety, hallucination, injury, back pain, peripheral edema, asthenia, chest pain, urinary incontinence, upper respiratory tract infection, bronchitis, coughing, hypertension, fall, and purpura.

➤*Other adverse events observed during clinical trials:* These adverse events are not necessarily related to galantamine treatment and in most cases were observed at a similar frequency in placebo-treated patients in the controlled studies.

Cardiovascular – Chest pain (> 1%); postural hypotension, hypotension, dependent edema, cardiac failure, AV block, palpitation, atrial fibrillation, QT prolonged, bundle branch block, supraventricular tachycardia, T-wave inversion, ventricular tachycardia, purpura, epistaxis, thrombocytopenia (0.1% to 1%).

CNS – Vertigo, hypertonia, convulsions, involuntary muscle contractions, paresthesia, ataxia, hypokinesia, hyperkinesia, apraxia, aphasia, apathy, paroniria, paranoid reaction, libido increased, delirium (0.1% to 1%).

GI – Flatulence (> 1%); gastritis, melena, dysphagia, rectal hemorrhage, dry mouth, saliva increased, diverticulitis, gastroenteritis, hiccough (0.1% to 1%); esophageal perforation (< 0.1%).

GU – Incontinence (> 1%); hematuria, micturition frequency, cystitis, urinary retention, nocturia, renal calculi (0.1% to 1%).

Metabolic – Hyperglycemia, alkaline phosphatase increased (0.1% to 1%).

Overdosage

➤*Symptoms:* Signs and symptoms of significant overdosing of galantamine are predicted to be similar to those of overdosing of other cholinomimetics. These effects generally involve the CNS, the parasympathetic nervous system, and the neuromuscular junction. In addition to muscle weakness or fasciculations, some or all of the following signs of cholinergic crisis may develop: Severe nausea, vomiting, GI cramping, salivation, lacrimation, urination, defecation, sweating, bradycardia, hypotension, respiratory depression, collapse, and convulsions. Increasing muscle weakness is a possibility and may result in death if respiratory muscles are involved.

➤*Treatment:* As in any case of overdose, use general supportive measures. Tertiary anticholinergics such as atropine may be used as an antidote for galantamine overdosage. IV atropine sulfate titrated to effect is recommended at an initial dose of 0.5 to 1 mg IV with subsequent doses based on clinical response. Atypical responses in blood pressure and heart rate have been reported with other cholinomimetics when coadministered with quaternary anticholinergics. It is not known whether galantamine or its metabolites can be removed by dialysis (eg, hemodialysis, peritoneal dialysis, hemofiltration).

Patient Information

Instruct caregivers in the recommended administration (twice daily, preferably with morning and evening meal) and dose escalation (dose increases should follow minimum of 4 weeks at prior dose). If therapy has been interrupted for several days or longer, restart the patient at the lowest dose and escalate the dose to the current dose.

Advise patients and caregivers that the most frequent adverse events can be minimized by following the recommended dosage and administration. GI symptoms may be reduced by administering with food or antiemetic medication or ensuring adequate fluid intake.

Instruct caregivers in the correct procedure for administering galantamine oral solution. In addition, inform them of the existence of an instruction sheet (included with the product) describing how the solution is to be administered.

MISCELLANEOUS PSYCHOTHERAPEUTIC AGENTS

ATOMOXETINE HYDROCHLORIDE

Rx	**Strattera** (Eli Lilly)	**Capsules:** 10 mg (as base)	(LILLY 3227 10 mg). White. In 30s.
		18 mg (as base)	(LILLY 3238 18 mg). Gold/White. In 30s.
		25 mg (as base)	(LILLY 3228 25 mg). Blue/White. In 30s.
		40 mg (as base)	(LILLY 3229 40 mg). Blue. In 30s.
		60 mg (as base)	(LILLY 3239 60 mg). Blue/Gold. In 30s.
		80 mg (as base)	(LILLY 3250 80 mg). Opaque brown, opaque white. In 30s and 2,000s.
		100 mg (as base)	(LILLY 3251 100 mg). Opaque brown. In 30s and 1,500s.

ATOMOXETINE HYDROCHLORIDE — ORAL

WARNING

Suicidal ideation in children and adolescents – Atomoxetine increased the risk of suicidal ideation in short-term studies in children or adolescents with Attention-Deficit/Hyperactivity Disorder (ADHD). Anyone considering the use of atomoxetine in a child or adolescent must balance this risk with the clinical need. Patients who are started on therapy should be monitored closely for suicidality (suicidal thinking and behavior), clinical worsening, or unusual changes in behavior. Families and caregivers should be advised of the need for close observation and communication with the prescriber. Atomoxetine is approved for ADHD in pediatric and adult patients. Atomoxetine is not approved for major depressive disorder.

Pooled analysis of short-term (6 to 18 weeks) placebo-controlled trials of atomoxetine in children and adolescents (a total of 12 trials involving over 2200 patients, including 11 trials in ADHD and 1 trial in enuresis) have revealed a greater risk of suicidal ideation early during treatment in those receiving atomoxetine compared to placebo. The average risk of suicidal ideation in patients receiving atomoxetine was 0.4% (5/1357 patients), compared to none in placebo-treated patients (851 patients). No suicides occurred in these trials.

Indications

➤*Attention-deficit/hyperactivity disorder (ADHD):* For the treatment of ADHD.

Administration and Dosage

➤*Approved by the FDA:* January 23, 2003

➤*Initial treatment:*

Children up to 70 kg body weight – Initiate atomoxetine at a total daily dose of approximately 0.5 mg/kg, and increase after a minimum of 3 days to a target total daily dose of approximately 1.2 mg/kg administered either as a single daily dose in the morning or as evenly divided doses in the morning and late afternoon/early evening. No additional benefit has been demonstrated for doses higher than 1.2 mg/kg/day.

The total daily dose in children and adolescents should not exceed 1.4 mg/kg or 100 mg, whichever is less.

Adults and children over 70 kg body weight – Initiate atomoxetine at a total daily dose of 40 mg, and increase after a minimum of 3 days to a target total daily dose of approximately 80 mg administered either as a single daily dose in the morning or as evenly divided doses in the morning and late afternoon/early evening. After 2 to 4 additional weeks, the dose may be increased to a maximum of 100 mg in patients who have not achieved an optimal response. There are no data that support increased effectiveness at higher doses.

The maximum recommended total daily dose in children and adolescents over 70 kg and adults is 100 mg.

➤*Maintenance/extended treatment:* There is no evidence available from controlled trials to indicate how long the patient with ADHD should be

ATOMOXETINE HYDROCHLORIDE — ORAL

treated with atomoxetine. It is generally agreed, however, that pharmacological treatment of ADHD may be needed for extended periods. Nevertheless, the physician who elects to use atomoxetine for extended periods should periodically reevaluate the long-term usefulness of the drug for the individual patient.

➤*General dosing information:* Atomoxetine may be taken with or without food. Atomoxetine capsules are not intended to be opened, they should be taken whole. The safety of single doses over 120 mg and total daily doses above 150 mg have not been systematically evaluated.

➤*Hepatic function impairment:* See Actions for more information.

➤*Dosing adjustment for use with a strong CYP2D6 inhibitor:*

Children up to 70 kg body weight – In children and adolescents up to 70 kg body weight administered strong CYP2D6 inhibitors (eg, paroxetine, fluoxetine, quinidine), initiate atomoxetine at 0.5 mg/kg/day, and only increase to the usual target dose of 1.2 mg/kg/day if symptoms fail to improve after 4 weeks and initial dose is well tolerated.

Adults and children over 70 kg body weight – In children and adolescents over 70 kg body weight and in adults administered strong CYP2D6 inhibitors (eg, paroxetine, fluoxetine, quinidine), initiate atomoxetine at 40 mg/day, and only increase to the usual target dose of 80 mg/day if symptoms fail to improve after 4 weeks and the initial dose is well tolerated.

➤*Discontinuation:* Can be discontinued without being tapered.

➤*Storage/Stability:* Store at 25°C (77°F); excursions permitted to 15° to 30°C (59° to 86°F).

Actions

➤*Pharmacology:* The precise mechanism by which atomoxetine produces its therapeutic effects in ADHD is unknown, but is thought to be related to selective inhibition of the pre-synaptic norepinephrine transporter, as determined in ex vivo uptake and neurotransmitter depletion studies.

➤*Pharmacokinetics:*

Absorption/Distribution – Atomoxetine is rapidly absorbed after oral administration, with absolute bioavailability of about 63% in extensive metabolizers and 94% in poor metabolizers. Maximal plasma concentrations (C_{max}) are reached approximately 1 to 2 hours after dosing.

Atomoxetine can be administered with or without food. Administration of atomoxetine with a standard high-fat meal in adults did not affect the extent of oral absorption of atomoxetine (AUC), but did decrease the rate of absorption, resulting in a 37% lower C_{max}, and delayed T_{max} by 3 hours. In clinical trials with children and adolescents, administration of atomoxetine with food resulted in a 9% lower C_{max}.

The steady-state volume of distribution after intravenous administration is 0.85 L/kg indicating that atomoxetine distributes primarily into total body water. Volume of distribution is similar across the patient weight range after normalizing for body weight.

At therapeutic concentrations, 98% of atomoxetine in plasma is bound to protein, primarily albumin.

Metabolism/Excretion – Atomoxetine is metabolized primarily through the CYP2D6 enzymatic pathway. People with reduced activity in this pathway (poor metabolizers) have higher plasma concentrations of atomoxetine compared with people with normal activity (extensive metabolizers). For poor metabolizers, AUC of atomoxetine is approximately 10-fold and $C_{ss,max}$ is about 5-fold greater than extensive metabolizers. Laboratory tests are available to identify CYP2D6 poor metabolizers. Coadministration of atomoxetine with potent inhibitors of CYP2D6, such as fluoxetine, paroxetine, or quinidine, results in a substantial increase in atomoxetine plasma exposure, and dosing adjustment may be necessary. Atomoxetine did not inhibit or induce the CYP2D6 pathway.

The major oxidative metabolite formed, regardless of CYP2D6 status, is 4-hydroxyatomoxetine, which is glucuronidated. 4-Hydroxyatomoxetine is equipotent to atomoxetine as an inhibitor of the norepinephrine transporter but circulates in plasma at much lower concentrations (1% of atomoxetine concentration in extensive metabolizers and 0.1% of atomoxetine concentration in poor metabolizers). 4-Hydroxyatomoxetine is primarily formed by CYP2D6, but in poor metabolizers, 4-hydroxyatomoxetine is formed at a slower rate by several other cytochrome P450 enzymes. N-desmethylatomoxetine is formed by CYP2C19 and other cytochrome P450 enzymes, but has substantially less pharmacological activity compared with atomoxetine and circulates in plasma at lower concentrations (5% of atomoxetine concentration in extensive metabolizers and 45% of atomoxetine concentration in poor metabolizers).

Mean apparent plasma clearance of atomoxetine after oral administration in adult extensive metabolizers is 0.35 L/h/kg and the mean half-life is 5.2 hours. Following oral administration of atomoxetine to poor metabolizers, mean apparent plasma clearance is 0.03 L/h/kg and mean half-life is 21.6 hours. For poor metabolizers, AUC of atomoxetine is approximately 10-fold and $C_{ss,max}$ is about 5-fold greater than extensive metabolizers. The elimination half-life of 4-hydroxyatomoxetine is similar to that of N-desmethylatomoxetine (6 to 8 hours) in extensive metabolizers subjects, while the half-life of N-desmethylatomoxetine is much longer in poor metabolizer subjects (34 to 40 hours).

Atomoxetine is excreted primarily as 4-hydroxyatomoxetine-O-glucuronide, mainly in the urine (greater than 80% of the dose) and to a lesser extent in the feces (less than 17% of the dose). Only a small fraction of the atomoxetine dose is excreted as unchanged atomoxetine (less than 3% of the dose), indicating extensive biotransformation.

Special populations –

Hepatic function impairment: Atomoxetine exposure (AUC) is increased, compared with healthy subjects, in extensive metabolizer subjects with moderate (Child-Pugh class B) (2-fold increase) and severe (Child-Pugh class C) (4-fold increase) hepatic impairment. Dosage adjustment is recommended for patients with moderate or severe hepatic impairment. For patients with moderate hepatic impairment (Child-Pugh class B), reduce initial and target doses to 50% of the normal dose (for patients without hepatic impairment). For patients with severe hepatic impairment (Child-Pugh Class C), reduce initial dose and target doses to 25% of normal.

Contraindications

In patients known to be hypersensitive to atomoxetine or other constituents of the product.

Atomoxetine should not be taken with an MAOI, or within 2 weeks after discontinuing an MAOI. Treatment with an MAOI should not be initiated within 2 weeks after discontinuing atomoxetine. With other drugs that affect brain monoamine concentrations, there have been reports of serious, sometimes fatal, reactions (including hyperthermia, rigidity, myoclonus, autonomic instability with possible rapid fluctuations of vital signs, and mental status changes that include extreme agitation progressing to delirium and coma) when taken in combination with an MAOI. Some cases presented features resembling neuroleptic malignant syndrome. Such reactions may occur when these drugs are given concurrently or in close proximity.

In clinical trials, atomoxetine use was associated with an increased risk of mydriasis; therefore, its use is not recommended in patients with narrow-angle glaucoma.

Warnings

➤*Hypersensitivity reactions:* Although uncommon, allergic reactions, including angioneurotic edema, urticaria, and rash, have been reported in patients taking atomoxetine.

➤*Growth:* Monitor growth during treatment with atomoxetine. During acute treatment studies (up to 9 weeks), atomoxetine-treated patients lost an average of 0.4 kg, while placebo patients gained an average of 1.5 kg. In a controlled trial that randomized patients to placebo or 1 of 3 atomoxetine doses, 1.3%, 7.1%, 19.3%, and 29.1% of patients lost at least 3.5% of their body weight in the placebo, 0.5, 1.2, and 1.8 mg/kg/day atomoxetine dose groups, respectively. During acute treatment studies, atomoxetine-treated patients grew an average of 0.9 cm, while placebo-treated patients grew an average of 1.1 cm. There are no long-term, placebo-controlled data to evaluate the effect of atomoxetine on growth. Weight and height were assessed during open-label studies of 12 and 18 months, and mean rates of growth were compared to normal growth curves. Patients treated with atomoxetine for at least 18 months gained an average of 6.5 kg while mean weight percentile decreased slightly from 68 to 60. For this same group of patients, the average gain in height was 9.3 cm with a slight decrease in mean height percentile from 54 to 50. Among patients treated for at least 6 months, mean weight gain was lower for poor metabolizer patients compared with extensive metabolizer patients (+0.7 kg compared with +3 kg), while mean growth for poor metabolizer patients was 4.3 cm and mean growth for extensive metabolizer patients was 4.4 cm. Whether final adult height or weight is affected by treatment with atomoxetine is unknown. Monitor patients requiring long-term therapy, and consider interrupting therapy in patients who are not growing or gaining weight satisfactorily.

➤*Mutagenesis:* Atomoxetine was negative in a battery of genotoxicity studies that included a reverse point mutation assay (Ames test), an in vitro mouse lymphoma assay, a chromosomal aberration test in Chinese hamster ovary cells, an unscheduled DNA synthesis test in rat hepatocytes, and an in vivo micronucleus test in mice. However, there was a slight increase in the percentage of Chinese hamster ovary cells with diplochromosomes, suggesting endoreduplication (numerical aberration).

➤*Pregnancy: Category C.* Pregnant rabbits were treated with up to 100 mg/kg/day of atomoxetine by gavage throughout the period of organogenesis. At this dose, in 1 of 3 studies, a decrease in live fetuses and an increase in early resorption was observed. Slight increases in the incidences of atypical origin of carotid artery and absent subclavian artery were observed. These findings were observed at doses that caused slight maternal toxicity. The no-effect dose for these findings was 30 mg/kg/day. The 100 mg/kg dose is approximately 23 times the maximum human dose on a mg/m^2 basis; plasma levels (AUC) of atomoxetine at this dose in rabbits are estimated to be 3.3 times (extensive metabolizers) or 0.4 times (poor metabolizers) those in humans receiving the maximum human dose.

Rats were treated with up to approximately 50 mg/kg/day of atomoxetine (approximately 6 times the maximum human dose on a mg/m^2 basis) in the diet from 2 weeks (females) or 10 weeks (males) prior to mating through the periods of organogenesis and lactation. In 1 of 2 studies, decreases in pup weight and pup survival were observed. The decreased pup survival was also seen at 25 mg/kg (but not at 13 mg/kg). In a study in which rats were treated with atomoxetine in the diet from 2 weeks (females) or 10 weeks (males) prior to mating throughout the period of organogenesis, a decrease in fetal (female only) weight and an increase in the incidence of incomplete ossification of the vertebral arch in fetuses were observed at 40 mg/kg/day (approximately 5 times the maximum human dose on a mg/m^2 basis) but not at 20 mg/kg/day.

No adequate and well-controlled studies have been conducted in pregnant women. Atomoxetine should not be used during pregnancy unless the potential benefit justifies the potential risk to the fetus.

➤*Lactation:* Atomoxetine or its metabolites were excreted in the milk of rats. It is not known if atomoxetine is excreted in human milk. Exercise caution if atomoxetine is administered to a breastfeeding woman.

ATOMOXETINE HYDROCHLORIDE — ORAL

➤*Children:* The safety and efficacy of atomoxetine in pediatric patients less than 6 years of age have not been established. The efficacy of atomoxetine beyond 9 weeks and safety of atomoxetine beyond 1 year of treatment have not been systematically evaluated.

A study was conducted in young rats to evaluate the effects of atomoxetine on growth and neurobehavioral and sexual development. Rats were treated with 1, 10, or 50 mg/kg/day (approximately 0.2, 2, and 8 times, respectively, the maximum human dose on a mg/m^2 basis) of atomoxetine given by gavage from the early postnatal period (day 10 of age) through adulthood. Slight delays in onset of vaginal patency (all doses) and preputial separation (10 and 50 mg/kg), slight decreases in epididymal weight and sperm number (10 and 50 mg/kg), and a slight decrease in corpora lutea (50 mg/kg) were seen, but there were no effects on fertility or reproductive performance. A slight delay in onset of incisor eruption was seen at 50 mg/kg. A slight increase in motor activity was seen on day 15 (males at 10 and 50 and females at 50 mg/kg) and on day 30 (females at 50 mg/kg) but not on day 60 of age. There were no effects on learning and memory tests. The significance of these findings to humans is unknown.

Precautions

➤*Effects on urine outflow from the bladder:* In adult ADHD controlled trials, the rates of urinary retention (3%, 7 out of 269) and urinary hesitation (3%, 7 out of 269) were increased among atomoxetine subjects compared with placebo subjects (0%, 0 out of 263). Two adult atomoxetine subjects and no placebo subjects discontinued from controlled clinical trials because of urinary retention. A complaint of urinary retention or urinary hesitancy should be considered potentially related to atomoxetine.

➤*Special risk:*

Effects on blood pressure and heart rate – Use atomoxetine with caution in patients with hypertension, tachycardia, or cardiovascular or cerebrovascular disease because it can increase blood pressure and heart rate. Measure pulse and blood pressure at baseline, following atomoxetine dose increases, and periodically while on therapy.

In pediatric placebo-controlled trials, atomoxetine-treated subjects experienced a mean increase in heart rate of about 6 beats/minute compared with placebo subjects. At the final study visit before drug discontinuation, 3.6% (12 out of 335) of atomoxetine-treated subjects had heart rate increases of at least 25 beats per minute and a heart rate of at least 110 beats per minute, compared with 0.5% (1 out of 204) of placebo subjects. No pediatric subject had a heart rate increase of at least 25 beats per minute and a heart rate of at least 110 beats per minute on more than one occasion. Tachycardia was identified as an adverse event for 1.5% (5 out of 340) of these pediatric subjects compared with 0.5% (1 out of 207) of placebo subjects. The mean heart rate increase in extensive metabolizer patients was 6.7 beats per minute, and in poor metabolizer patients 10.4 beats per minute.

Atomoxetine-treated pediatric subjects experienced mean increases of about 1.5 mm Hg in systolic and diastolic blood pressures compared with placebo. At the final study visit before drug discontinuation, 6.8% (22 out of 324) of atomoxetine-treated pediatric subjects had high systolic blood pressure measurements compared with 3% (6 out of 197) of placebo subjects. High systolic blood pressures were measured on 2 or more occasions in 8.6% (28 out of 324) of atomoxetine-treated subjects and 3.6% (7 out of 197) of placebo subjects. At the final study visit before drug discontinuation, 2.8% (9 out of 326) of atomoxetine-treated pediatric subjects had high diastolic blood pressure measurements compared with 0.5% (1 out of 200) of placebo subjects. High diastolic blood pressures were measured on 2 or more occasions in 5.2% (17 out of 326) of atomoxetine-treated subjects and 1.5% (3 out of 200) placebo subjects. (High systolic and diastolic blood pressure measurements were defined as those exceeding the 95th percentile, stratified by age, gender, and height percentile - National High Blood Pressure Education Working Group on Hypertension Control in Children and Adolescents.)

In adult placebo-controlled trials, atomoxetine-treated subjects experienced a mean increase in heart rate of 5 beats/minute compared with placebo subjects. Tachycardia was identified as an adverse reaction for 3% (8 out of 269) of these adult atomoxetine subjects compared with 0.8% (2 out of 263) of placebo subjects.

Atomoxetine-treated adult subjects experienced mean increases in systolic (about 3 mm Hg) and diastolic (about 1 mm Hg) blood pressures compared with placebo. At the final study visit before drug discontinuation, 1.9% (5 out of 258) of atomoxetine-treated adult subjects had systolic blood pressure measurements greater than or equal to 150 mm Hg compared with 1.2% (3 out of 256) of placebo subjects. At the final study visit before drug discontinuation, 0.8% (2 out of 257) of atomoxetine-treated adult subjects had diastolic blood pressure measurements greater than or equal to 100 mm Hg compared with 0.4% (1 out of 257) of placebo subjects. No adult subject had a high systolic or diastolic blood pressure detected on more than one occasion.

Orthostatic hypotension has been reported in subjects taking atomoxetine. In short-term child- and adolescent-controlled trials, 1.8% (6 out of 340) of atomoxetine-treated subjects experienced symptoms of postural hypotension compared with 0.5% (1 out of 207) of placebo-treated subjects. Use atomoxetine with caution in any condition that may predispose patients to hypotension.

➤*Hazardous tasks:* Patients should use caution when driving a car or operating hazardous machinery until they are reasonably certain that their performance is not affected by atomoxetine.

Drug Interactions

Atomoxetine Drug Interactions			
Precipitant drug	Object drug*		Description
Atomoxetine	Albuterol	↑	Administer with caution because the cardiovascular action of albuterol can be potentiated.
CYP2D6 inhibitors	Atomoxetine	↑	Coadministration causes an increase in the AUC and C_{max} at steady state. Dosage adjustment may be necessary.
MAOIs	Atomoxetine	↑	Coadministration is contraindicated (see Warnings).
Pressor agents	Atomoxetine	↑	Administer with caution because of possible effects on blood pressure.
Atomoxetine	Pressor agents		

* ↑ = Object drug increased.

Adverse Reactions

➤*Child and adolescent clinical trials:*

Discontinuation: In acute child and adolescent placebo-controlled trials, 3.5% (15 out of 427) of atomoxetine subjects and 1.4% (4 out of 294) placebo subjects discontinued for adverse reactions. For all studies, (including open-label and long-term studies), 5% of extensive metabolizer patients and 7% of poor metabolizer patients discontinued because of an adverse reaction. Among atomoxetine-treated patients, aggression (0.5%, n = 2); irritability (0.5%, n = 2); somnolence (0.5%, n = 2); and vomiting (0.5%, n = 2) were the reasons for discontinuation reported by more than 1 patient.

Commonly observed adverse reactions: The most commonly observed adverse reactions in patients treated with atomoxetine (incidence of 5% or greater and at least twice the incidence in placebo patients, for either twice daily or every day dosing) were dyspepsia, nausea, vomiting, fatigue, appetite decreased, dizziness, and mood swings.

Atomoxetine Adverse Reactions		
	Percentage of patients reporting reactions from twice-daily trials	
Adverse reaction[a]	Atomoxetine (n = 340)	Placebo (n = 207)
	CNS disorders	
Dizziness (excluding vertigo)	6%	3%
Headache	27%	25%
Somnolence	7%	5%
	Dermatologic	
Dermatitis	4%	1%
	GI	
Constipation	3%	1%
Dyspepsia	4%	2%
Upper abdominal pain	20%	16%
Vomiting	11%	9%
	Infections	
Ear infection	3%	1%
Influenza	3%	1%
	Metabolic-nutritional	
Appetite decreased	14%	6%
Weight decreased	2%	0%
	Psychiatric	
Crying	2%	1%
Irritability	8%	5%
Mood swings	2%	0%
	Respiratory	
Cough	11%	7%
Rhinorrhea	4%	3%

[a] Reactions reported by at least 2% of patients treated with atomoxetine, and greater than placebo. The following reactions did not meet this criterion but were reported by more atomoxetine-treated patients than placebo-treated patients and are possibly related to atomoxetine treatment: anorexia, blood pressure increased, early morning awakening, flushing, mydriasis, sinus tachycardia, tearfulness. The following reactions were reported by at least 2% of patients treated with atomoxetine, and equal to or less than placebo: arthralgia, gastroenteritis viral, insomnia, sore throat, nasal congestion, nasopharyngitis, pruritus, sinus congestion, upper respiratory tract infection.

ATOMOXETINE HYDROCHLORIDE — ORAL

Atomoxetine Adverse Reactions

Adverse reaction	Percentage of patients reporting reactions from twice-daily trials		Percentage of patients reporting reactions from once-daily trials	
	Atomoxetine (n = 340)	Placebo (n = 207)	Atomoxetine (n = 85)	Placebo (n = 85)
GI				
Constipation	3%	1%	0%	0%
Diarrhea	3%	6%	4%	1%
Dry mouth	1%	2%	4%	1%
Dyspepsia	4%	2%	8%	0%
Nausea	7%	8%	12%	2%
Upper abdominal pain	20%	16%	16%	9%
Vomiting	11%	9%	15%	1%
Psychiatric				
Mood swings	2%	0%	5%	2%
Miscellaneous				
Fatigue	4%	5%	9%	1%

The following adverse reactions occurred in at least 2% of poor metabolizer patients and were either twice as frequent or statistically significantly more frequent in poor metabolizer patients compared with extensive metabolizers patients: decreased appetite (23% of poor metabolizers, 16% of extensive metabolizers); insomnia (13% of poor metabolizers, 7% of extensive metabolizers); sedation (4% of poor metabolizers, 2% of extensive metabolizers); depression (6% of poor metabolizers, 2% of extensive metabolizers); tremor (4% of poor metabolizers, 1% of extensive metabolizers); early morning awakening (3% of poor metabolizers, 1% of extensive metabolizers); pruritus (2% of poor metabolizers, 1% of extensive metabolizers); mydriasis (2% of poor metabolizers, 1% of extensive metabolizers).

➤*Adult clinical trials:*

Discontinuation: In the acute adult placebo-controlled trials, 8.5% (23 out of 270) atomoxetine subjects and 3.4% (9 out of 266) placebo subjects discontinued for adverse reactions. Among atomoxetine-treated patients, insomnia (1.1%, n = 3); chest pain (0.7%, n = 2); palpitations (0.7%, n = 2); and urinary retention (0.7%, n = 2) were the reasons for discontinuation reported by more than 1 patient.

Commonly observed adverse reactions: Commonly observed adverse reactions associated with the use of atomoxetine (incidence of 2% or greater) and not observed at an equivalent incidence among placebo-treated patients (atomoxetine incidence greater than placebo) are listed in the table above. The most commonly observed adverse reactions in patients treated with atomoxetine (incidence of 5% or greater and at least twice the incidence in placebo patients) were constipation, dry mouth, nausea, appetite decreased, dizziness, insomnia, decreased libido, ejaculatory problems, impotence, urinary hesitation or urinary retention or difficulty in micturition, and dysmenorrhea.

Atomoxetine Adverse Reactions

Adverse reaction[a]	Percentage of patients reporting reaction	
System organ class/ adverse reaction	Atomoxetine (n = 269)	Placebo (n = 263)
Cardiovascular		
Palpitations	4%	1%
CNS		
Dizziness	6%	2%
Headache	17%	17%
Hot flushes	3%	1%
Insomnia or middle insomnia	16%	8%
Paraesthesia	4%	2%
Sinus headache	3%	1%
Dermatologic		
Dermatitis	2%	1%
Increased sweating	4%	1%
GI		
Constipation	10%	4%
Dry mouth	21%	6%
Dyspepsia	6%	4%
Flatulence	2%	1%
Nausea	12%	5%
GU		
Abnormal orgasm	2%	1%
Delayed menses[b]	2%	1%
Dysmenorrhea[b]	7%	3%
Ejaculation failure[c] or ejaculation disorder[c]	5%	2%
Erectile disturbance[c]	7%	1%
Impotence[c]	3%	0%
Irregular menstruation[b]	2%	0%
Menstrual disorder[b]	3%	2%
Prostatitis[c]	3%	0%
Urinary hesitation or urinary retention or difficulty in micturition	8%	0%
Metabolic-nutritional		
Appetite decreased	10%	3%
Decreased weight	2%	1%
Musculoskeletal		
Myalgia	3%	2%
Psychiatric		
Abnormal dreams	4%	3%
Libido decreased	6%	2%
Sleep disorder	4%	2%
Respiratory		
Sinusitis	6%	4%
Miscellaneous		
Fatigue or lethargy	7%	4%
Pyrexia	3%	2%
Rigors	3%	1%

[a] Reactions reported by at least 2% of patients treated with atomoxetine, and greater than placebo. The following reactions did not meet this criterion but were reported by more atomoxetine-treated patients than placebo-treated patients and are possibly related to atomoxetine treatment: Early morning awakening, peripheral coldness, tachycardia. The following reactions were reported by at least 2% of patients treated with atomoxetine, and equal to or less than placebo: Abdominal pain upper, arthralgia, back pain, cough, diarrhea, influenza, irritability, nasopharyngitis, sore throat, upper respiratory tract infection, vomiting.
[b] Based on total number of females (atomoxetine, n = 95; placebo, n = 91).
[c] Based on total number of males (atomoxetine, n = 174; placebo, n = 172).

Male and female sexual dysfunction: Atomoxetine appears to impair sexual function in some patients. Changes in sexual desire, sexual performance, and sexual satisfaction are not well assessed in most clinical trials because they need special attention and because patients and physicians may be reluctant to discuss them. Accordingly, estimates of the incidence of untoward sexual experience and performance cited in product labeling are likely to underestimate the actual incidence. The table below displays the incidence of sexual side effects reported by at least 2% of adult patients taking atomoxetine in placebo-controlled trials.

Atomoxetine Sexual Adverse Reactions (≥ 2%)

	Atomoxetine	Placebo
Erectile disturbance[a]	7%	1%
Impotence[a]	3%	0%
Abnormal orgasm	2%	1%

[a] Males only.

Overdosage

➤*Symptoms:* There is limited clinical trial experience with atomoxetine overdose and no fatalities were observed. During postmarketing, there have been reports of acute and chronic overdoses of atomoxetine. No fatal overdoses of atomoxetine alone have been reported. The most commonly reported symptoms accompanying acute and chronic overdoses were somnolence. agitation, hyperactivity, abnormal behavior, and GI symptoms. Sign and symptoms consistent with sympathetic nervous system activation (eg, mydriasis, tachycardia, dry mouth) have also been observed.

➤*Treatment:* An airway should be established. Monitoring of cardiac and vital signs is recommended, along with appropriate symptomatic and supportive measures. Gastric lavage may be indicated if performed soon after

ATOMOXETINE HYDROCHLORIDE — ORAL

ingestion. Activated charcoal may be useful in limiting absorption. Because atomoxetine is highly protein-bound, dialysis is not likely to be useful in the treatment of overdose.

Patient Information

Patients may take atomoxetine with or without food.

If patients miss a dose, they should take it as soon as possible, but should not take more than the prescribed total daily amount of atomoxetine in any 24-hour period.

Patients should use caution when driving a car or operating hazardous machinery until they are reasonably certain that their performance is not affected by atomoxetine.

Do not take atomoxetine if:
- You took a medicine known as a monoamine oxidase inhibitor (MAOI) in the last 2 weeks. An MAOI is a medicine sometimes used for depression and other mental problems. Some names of MAOI medicines are *Nardil* (phenelzine sulfate) and *Parnate* (tranylcypromine sulfate). Taking atomoxetine with an MAOI could cause serious side effects or be life-threatening.
- You have narrow-angle glaucoma, an eye disease.
- You are allergic to atomoxetine hydrochloride or any of its ingredients. The active ingredient is atomoxetine. The inactive ingredients are listed at the end of this section.

SODIUM OXYBATE

c-iii	**Xyrem**[a] (Orphan Medical)	**Oral solution**: 500 mg/mL[b]	In 180 mL with syringe and dosing cups.

[a] Available only through the *Xyrem* Success Program. Call 1-866-997-3688 for more information.

[b] With ≥ 83 mg/mL sodium.

SODIUM OXYBATE — ORAL

WARNING

Sodium oxybate is a gamma hydroxybutyrate (GHB), a known drug of abuse. Abuse has been associated with some important CNS adverse reactions (including death). Even at recommended doses, use has been associated with confusion, depression, and other neuropsychiatric events. Reports of respiratory depression occurred in clinical trials. Almost all of the patients who received sodium oxybate during clinical trials were receiving CNS stimulants.

Important CNS adverse reactions associated with abuse of sodium oxybate include seizure, respiratory depression, and profound decreases in level of consciousness, with instances of coma and death. For reactions that occurred outside of clinical trials, in people taking GHB for recreational purposes, the circumstances surrounding the reactions often are unclear (eg, dose of GHB taken, the nature and amount of alcohol or any concomitant drugs).

Sodium oxybate is available through the *Xyrem* Success Program, using a centralized pharmacy 1-866-997-3688. The Success Program provides educational materials to the prescriber and the patient explaining the risks and proper use of sodium oxybate and the required prescription form. Once it is documented that the patient has read and/or understands the materials, the drug will be shipped to the patient. The *Xyrem* Success Program also recommends patient follow-up every 3 months. Physicians are expected to report all serious adverse reactions to the manufacturer.

Indications

➤*Excessive daytime sleepiness/cataplexy:* For the treatment of excessive daytime sleepiness and cataplexy in patients with narcolepsy.

➤*Unlabeled uses:* Fibromyalgia pain and fatigue.

Administration and Dosage

➤*Approved by the FDA:* July 17, 2002.

➤*Dosage:* Sodium oxybate is required to be taken at bedtime while in bed and again 2.5 to 4 hours later. The dose of sodium oxybate should be titrated to effect. The recommended starting dosage is 4.5 g/night divided into 2 equal doses of 2.25 g. The starting dosage then can be increased to a maximum of 9 g/night in increments of 1.5 g/night (0.75 g per dose). One to 2 weeks are recommended between dosage increases to evaluate clinical response and minimize adverse reactions. The effective dose range of sodium oxybate is 6 to 9 g/night. The efficacy and safety of sodium oxybate at doses higher than 9 g/night have not been investigated, and doses more than 9 g/night ordinarily should not be administered.

Because food significantly reduces the bioavailability of sodium oxybate, the patient should allow at least 2 hours after eating before taking the first dose of sodium oxybate. Patients should try to minimize variability in time of dosing in relation to meals.

➤*Preparation and administration:* Prepare both doses of sodium oxybate prior to bedtime. Each dose of sodium oxybate must be diluted with 2 ounces (ie, 60 mL, ¼ cup, 4 tablespoons) of water in the child-resistant dosing cups provided prior to ingestion. The first dose is to be taken at bedtime while in bed and the second taken 2.5 to 4 hours later; both doses should be taken while seated in bed. Patients probably will need to set an alarm to awaken for the second dose. The second dose must be prepared prior to ingesting the first dose and should be placed in close proximity to the patient's bed. After ingesting each dose, patients should lie down and remain in bed.

➤*Hepatic function impairment:* Patients with compromised liver function will have increased elimination half-life and systemic exposure along with reduced clearance. As a result, the starting dose should be decreased by one-half and dose increments should be titrated to effect while closely monitoring potential adverse reactions.

➤*Handling and disposal:* Sodium oxybate is a schedule III drug under the Controlled Substances Act. Sodium oxybate should be handled according to state and federal regulations. It is safe to dispose of sodium oxybate oral solution down the sanitary sewer.

➤*Storage/Stability:* Store at 25°C (77°F); excursions permitted up to 15° to 30°C (59° to 86°F). Solutions prepared following dilution should be consumed within 24 hours to minimize bacterial growth and contamination.

Actions

➤*Pharmacology:* The precise mechanism by which sodium oxybate produces an effect on cataplexy is unknown.

➤*Pharmacokinetics:*

Absorption – Sodium oxybate is absorbed rapidly following oral administration, with an absolute bioavailability of about 25%. The average peak plasma concentrations (1st and 2nd peak) following administration of a 9 g daily dose divided into 2 equivalent doses given 4 hours apart were 78 and 142 mcg/mL, respectively. The average time to peak plasma concentration (T_{max}) ranged from 0.5 to 1.25 hours in 8 pharmacokinetic studies. Following oral administration, the plasma levels of sodium oxybate increase more than proportionally with increasing dose. Single doses greater than 4.5 g have not been studied. Administration of sodium oxybate immediately after a high-fat meal resulted in delayed absorption (average T_{max} increased from 0.75 to 2 hours) and a reduction in peak plasma level (C_{max}) by a mean of 58% and systemic exposure (area under the curve [AUC") by 37%.

Sodium oxybate is rapidly but incompletely absorbed after oral administration; absorption is delayed and decreased by a high-fat meal. Pharmacokinetics are nonlinear, with blood levels increasing 3.7-fold as dose is doubled from 4.5 to 9 g. The pharmacokinetics are not altered with repeat dosing.

Distribution – Sodium oxybate is a hydrophilic compound with an apparent volume of distribution averaging 190 to 384 mL/kg. At sodium oxybate concentrations ranging from 3 to 300 mcg/mL, less than 1% is bound to plasma proteins.

Metabolism – Animal studies indicate that metabolism is the major elimination pathway for sodium oxybate, producing carbon dioxide and water via the tricarboxylic acid (Krebs) cycle and secondarily by beta-oxidation. The primary pathway involves a cytosolic $NADP^+$-linked enzyme, sodium oxybate dehydrogenase, that catalyses the conversion of sodium oxybate to succinic semialdehyde, which is then biotransformed to succinic acid by the enzyme succinic semialdehyde dehydrogenase. Succinic acid enters the Krebs cycle where it is metabolized to carbon dioxide and water. A second mitochondrial oxidoreductase enzyme, a transhydrogenase, also catalyses the conversion to succinic semialdehyde in the presence of α-ketoglutarate. An alternate pathway of biotransformation involves β-oxidation via 3,4-dihydroxybutyrate to carbon dioxide and water. No active metabolites have been identified.

Excretion – The clearance of sodium oxybate is almost entirely by biotransformation to carbon dioxide, which is then eliminated by expiration. On average, less than 5% of unchanged drug appears in human urine within 6 to 8 hours after dosing. Fecal excretion is negligible. It is eliminated mainly by metabolism with a half-life of 0.5 to 1 hour.

Special populations –

Hepatic function impairment: Sodium oxybate undergoes significant presystemic (hepatic first-pass) metabolism. The kinetics of sodium oxybate in 16 cirrhotic patients, half without ascites (Child's class A) and half with ascites (Child's class C), were compared with the kinetics in 8 healthy adults after a single oral dose of 25 mg/kg. AUC values were double in the cirrhotic patients, with apparent oral clearance reduced from 9.1 in healthy adults to 4.5 and 4.1 mL/min/kg in class A and class C patients, respectively. Elimination half-life was significantly longer in class C and class A patients than in control subjects (mean $t_{½}$ of 59 and 32 versus 22 minutes). It is prudent to reduce the starting dose of sodium oxybate by half in patients with liver dysfunction.

Contraindications

Patients being treated with sedative hypnotic agents; succinic semialdehyde dehydrogenase deficiency.

Warnings

➤*CNS depression/Respiratory depression:* Sodium oxybate is a CNS depressant with the potential to impair respiratory drive, especially in patients with already compromised respiratory function. In overdoses, life-threatening respiratory depression has been reported. In clinical trials, 2 subjects had profound CNS depression. A healthy 39-year-old female volunteer, received a single dose of sodium oxybate 4.5 g after fasting for 10 hours. An hour later, while asleep, she developed decreased respiration and was treated with an oxygen mask. An hour later, this event recurred. She also vomited and had fecal incontinence. In another case, a 64-year-old narcoleptic man was found unresponsive on the floor on day 170 of treatment with

SODIUM OXYBATE — ORAL

sodium oxybate at a total daily dose of 4.5 g. He was taken to an emergency room where he was intubated. He improved and was able to return home later the same day. Two other patients discontinued sodium oxybate because of severe difficulty breathing and an increase in obstructive sleep apnea.

The respiratory depressant effects of sodium oxybate, at recommended doses, were assessed in 21 patients with narcolepsy, and no dose-related changes in oxygen saturation were demonstrated in the group as a whole. One of these patients had significant concomitant pulmonary illness, and 4 of the 21 had moderate to severe sleep apnea. One of the 4 patients with sleep apnea had significant worsening of the apnea/hypopnea index during treatment, but worsening did not increase at higher doses. Another patient discontinued treatment because of a perceived increase in clinical apnea events. Observe caution if sodium oxybate is prescribed to patients with compromised respiratory function. Be aware that sleep apnea has been reported with a high incidence (even 50%) in some cohorts of narcoleptic patients.

➤*Confusion / Neuropsychiatric adverse reactions:* During clinical trials, 7% of patients treated with sodium oxybate experienced confusion. Fewer than 1% of patients discontinued the drug because of confusion. Confusion was reported at all recommended dosages from 6 to 9 g/day. In a controlled trial in which patients were randomized to fixed total daily doses of 3, 6, and 9 g or placebo, a dose-response relationship for confusion was demonstrated, with 17% of patients at 9 g/day experiencing confusion. In all cases, the confusion resolved soon after termination of treatment. In the majority of cases, confusion resolved with continued treatment. However, fully evaluate patients treated with sodium oxybate who become confused, and consider appropriate intervention on an individual basis.

Other neuropsychiatric events included psychosis, paranoia, hallucinations, and agitation. The emergence of thought disorders and/or behavior abnormalities when patients are treated with sodium oxybate requires careful and immediate evaluation.

➤*Depression:* In clinical trials, 6% of patients treated with sodium oxybate reported depressive symptoms. In the majority of cases, no change in sodium oxybate treatment was required. Three patients (less than 1%) discontinued because of depressive symptoms. In the controlled clinical trial, in which patients were randomized to fixed dosages of 3, 6, and 9 g/day or placebo, there was a single event of depression at the 3 g/day dosage.

Among patients with a previous history of depressive psychiatric disorder, there were 2 suicides and 1 attempted suicide recorded in the 448 patient dataset. Of the 2 suicides, 1 patient used sodium oxybate in conjunction with other drugs. Sodium oxybate was not involved in the second suicide. Sodium oxybate was the only drug involved in the attempted suicide. A fourth patient without a history of depression attempted suicide by taking an overdose of a drug other than sodium oxybate.

The emergence of depression when patients are treated with sodium oxybate requires careful and immediate evaluation. Monitor patients with a history of a depressive illness and/or suicide attempt especially carefully for the emergence of depressive symptoms while taking sodium oxybate.

➤*Hepatic function impairment:* See Administration and Dosage for more information.

➤*Elderly:* There is very limited experience with sodium oxybate in the elderly. Therefore, closely monitor elderly patients for impaired motor and/or cognitive function when taking sodium oxybate.

➤*Pregnancy: Category B.* Reproduction studies conducted in pregnant rats at doses up to 1,000 mg/kg (approximately equal to the maximum recommended human daily dose on a mg/m^2 basis) and in pregnant rabbits at doses up to 1,200 mg/kg (approximately 3 times the maximum recommended human daily dose on a mg/m^2 basis) revealed no evidence of teratogenicity. In a study in which rats were given sodium oxybate from day 6 of gestation through day 21 postpartum, slight decreases in pup and maternal weight gains were seen at 1,000 mg/kg; there were no drug effects on other developmental parameters. There are, however, no adequate and well-controlled studies in pregnant women. Because animal reproduction studies are not always predictive of human response, use this drug during pregnancy only if clearly needed.

Labor and delivery – Sodium oxybate has not been studied in labor or delivery. In obstetric anesthesia using an injectable formulation of sodium oxybate, newborns had stable cardiovascular and respiratory measures but were very sleepy, causing a slight decrease in Apgar scores. There was a fall in the rate of uterine contractions 20 minutes after injection. Placental transfer is rapid, but umbilical vein levels of sodium oxybate were no more than 25% of the maternal concentration. No sodium oxybate was detected in the infant's blood 30 minutes after delivery. Elimination curves of sodium oxybate between a 2-day-old infant and a 15-year-old patient were similar.

➤*Lactation:* It is not known whether sodium oxybate is excreted in human milk. Because many drugs are excreted in human milk, exercise caution when sodium oxybate is administered to a breast-feeding woman.

➤*Children:* Safety and efficacy in patients younger than 16 years of age have not been established.

Precautions

➤*Monitoring:* Monitor patients with a history of a depressive illness and/or suicide attempt especially carefully for the emergence of depressive symptoms while taking sodium oxybate. Monitor elderly patients closely for impaired motor and/or cognitive function when taking sodium oxybate.

➤*Incontinence:* During clinical trials, 9% of narcoleptic patients treated with sodium oxybate experienced either a single episode of, or sporadic, nocturnal urinary incontinence, and less than 1% experienced a single episode of nocturnal fecal incontinence. Less than 1% of patients discontinued as a result of incontinence. Incontinence has been reported at all doses tested. In a controlled trial where patients were randomized to fixed total daily doses of 3, 6, and 9 g or placebo, a dose-response relationship for urinary incontinence was demonstrated, with 14% of patients at 9 g/day experiencing urinary incontinence. In the same trial, 1 patient experienced fecal incontinence at a dosage of 9 g/day and discontinued treatment as a result.

If a patient experiences urinary or fecal incontinence during sodium oxybate therapy, consider pursuing investigations to rule out underlying etiologies, including worsening sleep apnea or nocturnal seizures, although there is no evidence to suggest that incontinence has been associated with seizures in patients being treated with sodium oxybate.

➤*Sleepwalking:* The term "sleepwalking" in this section refers to confused behavior occurring at night and, at times, associated with wandering. It is unclear if some or all of these episodes correspond to true somnambulism, which is a parasomnia occurring during non–rapid eye movement sleep, or to any other specific medical disorder. Sleepwalking was reported in 7% of 448 patients treated in clinical trials with sodium oxybate. In sodium oxybate–treated patients, less than 1% discontinued due to sleepwalking. In controlled trials of up to 4 weeks duration, the incidence of sleepwalking was 1% in both placebo– and sodium oxybate–treated patients. Sleepwalking was reported by 32% of patients treated with sodium oxybate for periods up to 16 years in one independent, uncontrolled trial. Fewer than 1% of the patients discontinued because of sleepwalking. Five instances of significant injury or potential injury were associated with sleepwalking during a clinical trial of sodium oxybate, including a fall, clothing set on fire while attempting to smoke, attempted ingestion of nail polish remover, and overdose of oxybate. Therefore, episodes of sleepwalking should be fully evaluated and appropriate interventions considered.

➤*Sodium intake:* Daily sodium intake in patients taking sodium oxybate ranges from 0.5 g (for a sodium oxybate 3 g dose) to 1.6 g (for a sodium oxybate 9 g dose). Consider this in patients with heart failure, hypertension, or compromised renal function.

➤*Lab test abnormalities:* In an open-label trial of long-term exposure to sodium oxybate, which extended as long as 16 years for some patients, 30% (26/87) of patients tested had at least 1 positive anti-nuclear antibody (ANA) test. Of the 26, 17 patients had multiple positive ANA tests over time. The clinical course of these patients was not always clearly recorded, but 1 patient was clearly diagnosed with rheumatoid arthritis at the time of the first recorded positive ANA test.

➤*Drug abuse and dependence:*

Abuse – Although sodium oxybate has not been systematically studied in clinical trials for its potential for abuse, illicit use and abuse have been reported. Sodium oxybate is a psychoactive drug that produces a wide range of pharmacological effects. It is a sedative-hypnotic that produces dose- and concentration-dependent CNS effects in humans. The onset of effect is rapid, enhancing its desirability as a drug of abuse or misuse.

The rapid onset of sedation, coupled with the amnestic features of sodium oxybate, particularly when combined with alcohol, has proven to be dangerous for the voluntary and involuntary (assault victim) user.

Sodium oxybate is abused in social settings primarily by young adults. Sodium oxybate has some commonalties with ethanol over a limited dose range and some cross tolerance with ethanol has been reported as well. Cases of severe dependence and craving for sodium oxybate have been reported. Dependence is indicated by the use of increasingly large doses, increased frequency of use, and continued use despite adverse consequences. Some of the doses reported abused in the "rave" setting have been similar to the dose range studied for therapeutic treatment of cataplexy.

Hospital emergency department (ED) reports increased 100-fold from 1992 to 1999 (source: Substance Abuse Mental Health Services Administration, Drug Abuse Warning Network [DAWN"). Sixty percent (60%) of the ED reports involved individuals 25 years of age and younger. Numerous deaths have been reported, typically involving sodium oxybate in combination with alcohol and other drugs, including 5 in the DAWN system in which sodium oxybate was the only drug that could be identified.

Dependence – There have been case reports of dependence after illicit use of sodium oxybate at frequent repeated dosages (18 to 250 g/day), in excess of the therapeutic dosage range. In these cases, the signs and symptoms of abrupt discontinuation included an abstinence syndrome consisting of insomnia, restlessness, anxiety, psychosis, lethargy, nausea, tremor, sweating, muscle cramps, and tachycardia. These symptoms generally abated in 3 to 14 days. The discontinuation effects of sodium oxybate have not been systematically evaluated in controlled clinical trials. An abstinence syndrome has not been reported in clinical investigations. Although the clinical trial experience with sodium oxybate in narcolepsy/cataplexy patients at therapeutic doses does not show clear evidence of a withdrawal syndrome, 2 patients reported anxiety and 1 reported insomnia following abrupt discontinuation at the termination of the clinical trial; in the 2 patients with anxiety, the frequency of cataplexy had increased markedly at the same time.

Tolerance – Tolerance to sodium oxybate has not been systematically studied in controlled clinical trials. Open-label, long-term (greater than or equal to 6 months) clinical trials did not demonstrate development of tolerance. There have been some case reports of symptoms of tolerance developing after illicit use at dosages far in excess of the recommended sodium oxybate dosage regimen. Clinical studies of sodium oxybate in the treatment of alcohol withdrawal suggest a potential cross-tolerance with alcohol. Because illicit use and abuse of sodium oxybate have been reported, carefully evaluate patients for a history of drug abuse and follow such patients closely, observing them for signs of misuse or abuse of sodium oxybate (eg, increase in size or frequency of dosing, drug-seeking behavior). Document the diagnosis and indication for sodium oxybate, being alert to drug-seeking behavior and/or feigned cataplexy.

➤*Hazardous tasks:* Because of the rapid onset of its CNS-depressant effects, sodium oxybate should only be ingested at bedtime, and while in bed.

SODIUM OXYBATE — ORAL

For at least 6 hours after ingesting sodium oxybate, patients must not engage in hazardous occupations or activities requiring complete mental alertness or motor coordination, such as operating machinery, driving a motor vehicle, or flying an airplane. When patients first start taking sodium oxybate or any other sleep medicine, until they know whether the medicine will still have some carryover effect on them the next day, they should use extreme care while driving a car, operating heavy machinery, or performing any other task that could be dangerous or requires full mental alertness.

Drug Interactions

➤*CNS agents:* Interactions between sodium oxybate and 3 drugs commonly used in patients with narcolepsy (zolpidem, protriptyline, and modafinil) have been evaluated in formal studies. Sodium oxybate, in combination with these drugs, produced no significant pharmacokinetic changes for either drug. However, pharmacodynamic interactions cannot be ruled out. Nonetheless, do not use sodium oxybate in combination with sedative hypnotics or other CNS depressants.

The combined use of alcohol (ethanol) with sodium oxybate may result in potentiation of the CNS-depressant effects of sodium oxybate and alcohol. Therefore, warn patients strongly against the use of any alcoholic beverages in conjunction with sodium oxybate. Do not use sodium oxybate in combination with sedative hypnotics or other CNS depressants.

In animal models, sodium oxybate and depressant drug combinations generally gave greater CNS depressant effects than did either drug alone. Coadministration to animals of sodium oxybate and benzodiazepines, barbiturates, or ethanol increases sleep duration. In primates, sodium oxybate blood levels were elevated with phenytoin pretreatment and reduced with levodopa, ethosuximide, and trimethadione.

Adverse Reactions

A total of 448 narcoleptic patients were exposed to sodium oxybate in clinical trials. The most commonly observed adverse reactions associated with the use of sodium oxybate were as follows: headache (25%), nausea (21%), dizziness (17%), pain (16%), somnolence (13%), pharyngitis (11%), infection (10%), viral infection (10%), flu syndrome (9%), accidental injury (9%), diarrhea (8%), urinary incontinence (8%), vomiting (8%), rhinitis (8%), asthenia (8%), sinusitis (7%), nervousness (7%), back pain (7%), confusion (7%), sleepwalking (7%), depression (6%), dyspepsia (6%), abdominal pain (6%), abnormal dreams (6%), insomnia (5%).

Two deaths occurred in these clinical trials, both from drug overdoses. Both of these deaths resulted from ingestion of multiple drugs, including sodium oxybate in 1 patient.

In these clinical trials, 13% of patients discontinued because of adverse reactions.

The most frequent (greater than 1%) reasons for discontinuation were nausea (2%) and headache (1.3%).

Approximately 6% of patients receiving sodium oxybate in 3 controlled clinical trials (n = 147) withdrew because of an adverse reaction, compared with 1% receiving placebo (n = 79). The reasons for discontinuation that occurred more frequently in sodium oxybate–treated patients than placebo-treated patients were: nausea (3%), somnolence (2%) and confusion (1%). Amnesia, asthenia, chest pain, dizziness, dyspnea, fecal incontinence, hallucinations, headache, hyperkinesia, paranoid reaction, thinking abnormal, vertigo, and vomiting each caused discontinuation in a single patient.

➤*Most commonly reported adverse reactions:* The most commonly reported adverse reactions associated with the use of sodium oxybate and occurring with at least 5% greater frequency than seen in placebo-treated patients were dizziness (23%), headache (20%), nausea (16%), pain (12%), sleep disorder (9%), confusion (7%), infection (7%), vomiting (6%), and urinary incontinence (5%). These incidences are based on combined data from trial 1 and 2 smaller randomized, double-blind, placebo-controlled, crossover trials (n = 181).

Trial 1, the parallel group, placebo-controlled trial, used 3 fixed doses of sodium oxybate (3, 6, and 9 g). In that trial, dizziness, nausea, urinary incontinence, and vomiting were more common at higher doses, with the majority of reactions occurring in the 6 and 9 g dose groups.

➤*Adverse reactions with an incidence of at least 6% (2 reactions) in 1 or more treatment groups in trial 1:*

Sodium Oxybate Adverse Reactions from Trial 1

Adverse reaction	Placebo (n = 34)	Sodium oxybate dose 3 g (n = 34)	6 g (n = 33)	9 g (n = 35)
Cardiovascular				
Hypertension	1 (3%)	0 (0%)	2 (6%)	0 (0%)
CNS				
Abnormal dream	0 (0%)	0 (0%)	3 (9%)	1 (3%)
Abnormal thinking	0 (0%)	1 (3%)	0 (0%)	2 (6%)
Amnesia	0 (0%)	1 (3%)	0 (0%)	2 (6%)
Anxiety	1 (3%)	1 (3%)	0 (0%)	2 (6%)
Confusion	1 (3%)	3 (9%)	1 (3%)	5 (14%)
Dizziness	2 (6%)	8 (24%)	10 (30%)	12 (34%)
Headache	7 (21%)	3 (9%)	5 (15%)	11 (31%)
Hypesthesia	0 (0%)	2 (6%)	0 (0%)	0 (0%)
Sleep disorder	1 (3%)	2 (6%)	4 (12%)	5 (14%)
Somnolence	4 (12%)	5 (15%)	4 (12%)	5 (14%)

Sodium Oxybate Adverse Reactions from Trial 1

Adverse reaction	Placebo (n = 34)	Sodium oxybate dose 3 g (n = 34)	6 g (n = 33)	9 g (n = 35)
Dermatologic				
Increased sweating	0 (0%)	1 (3%)	1 (3%)	4 (11%)
GI				
Diarrhea	0 (0%)	0 (0%)	2 (6%)	2 (6%)
Dyspepsia	2 (6%)	0 (0%)	3 (9%)	2 (6%)
Nausea	2 (6%)	2 (6%)	5 (15%)	12 (34%)
Nausea/ Vomiting	0 (0%)	0 (0%)	2 (6%)	2 (6%)
Vomiting	0 (0%)	0 (0%)	2 (6%)	4 (11%)
GU				
Dysmenorrhea	1 (3%)	1 (3%)	0 (0%)	2 (6%)
Urinary incontinence	0 (0%)	0 (0%)	2 (6%)	5 (14%)
Musculoskeletal				
Myasthenia	0 (0%)	2 (6%)	1 (3%)	0 (0%)
Special senses				
Amblyopia	1 (3%)	2 (6%)	0 (0%)	0 (0%)
Tinnitus	0 (0%)	2 (6%)	0 (0%)	0 (0%)
Miscellaneous				
Asthenia	1 (3%)	0 (0%)	2 (6%)	0 (0%)
Flu syndrome	0 (0%)	1 (3%)	0 (0%)	2 (6%)
Infection	1 (3%)	3 (9%)	5 (15%)	0 (0%)
Pain	2 (6%)	3 (9%)	4 (12%)	7 (20%)
Viral infection	1 (3%)	1 (3%)	3 (9%)	0 (0%)

➤*Other adverse reactions:* During clinical trials, sodium oxybate was administered to 448 patients with narcolepsy and 125 healthy volunteers. A total of 150 patients received 9 g/day, the maximum recommended dosage. A total of 223 patients received sodium oxybate for at least 1 year. To establish the rate of adverse reactions, data from all subjects receiving any dose of sodium oxybate were pooled. All adverse reactions reported by at least 2 people are included except for those already listed elsewhere in the labeling, terms too general to be informative, or reactions unlikely to be drug induced. These reactions are not necessarily related to sodium oxybate treatment.

Cardiovascular – Syncope (0.1% to 1%).

CNS – Agitation, ataxia, convulsion, stupor, tremor (at least 1%); akathisia, apathy, coma, decreased libido, depersonalization, euphoria, hypertonia, myoclonus, neuralgia, paralysis (0.1% to 1%).

Dermatologic – Acne, alopecia, rash (at least 1%); contact dermatitis, urticaria (0.1% to 1%).

GI – Anorexia, constipation (at least 1%); mouth ulceration, stomatitis (0.1% to 1%).

GU – Albuminuria, cystitis, hematuria, metrorrhagia, urinary frequency (at least 1%); urinary urgency (0.1% to 1%).

Hematologic / Lymphatic – Anemia, ecchymosis, leukocytosis, lymphadenopathy, polycythemia (0.1% to 1%).

Metabolic / Nutritional – Alkaline phosphatase increased, edema, hypercholesteremia, hypocalcemia, weight gain (at least 1%); bilirubinemia, dehydration, hyperglycemia, hypernatremia, hyperuricemia, increased AST, increased ALT, increased creatinine, thirst (0.1% to 1%).

Musculoskeletal – Arthritis, leg cramps, myalgia (at least 1%).

Respiratory – Dyspnea (at least 1%); apnea, epistaxis, hiccup (0.1% to 1%).

Special senses – Taste loss (0.1% to 1%).

Miscellaneous – Allergic reaction, chills (at least 1%); enlarged abdomen, hangover effect, neck rigidity (0.1% to 1%).

Overdosage

➤*Symptoms:* Information regarding overdose with sodium oxybate is derived from reports in the medical literature that describe symptoms and signs in individuals who have ingested the drug illicitly or for medically unapproved purposes. In these circumstances the co-ingestion of other drugs and alcohol is common, and may influence the presentation and severity of clinical manifestations of overdose.

In clinical trials, 2 cases of overdose with sodium oxybate were reported. In the first case, an estimated dose of 150 g, more than 15 times the maximum recommended dose, caused a patient to be unresponsive with brief periods of apnea and to be incontinent of urine and feces. This individual recovered without sequelae. In the second case, death was reported following a multiple-drug overdose consisting of sodium oxybate and numerous other drugs.

Information about signs and symptoms associated with overdosage with sodium oxybate derives from reports of its illicit use. Patient presentation following overdose is influenced by the dose ingested, the time since ingestion, the co-ingestion of other drugs and alcohol, and the fed or fasted state. Patients have exhibited varying degrees of depressed consciousness that may fluctuate rapidly between a confusional, agitated, combative state with ataxia and coma. Emesis (even when obtunded), diaphoresis, headache, and impaired psychomotor skills may be observed. No typical pupillary changes have been described to assist in diagnosis; pupillary reactivity to light is

SODIUM OXYBATE — ORAL

maintained. Blurred vision has been reported. An increasing depth of coma has been observed at higher doses. Myoclonus and tonic-clonic seizures have been reported. Respiration may be unaffected or compromised in rate and depth. Cheyne-Stokes respiration and apnea have been observed. Bradycardia and hypothermia may accompany unconsciousness, as well as muscular hypotonia, but tendon reflexes remain intact.

➤*Treatment:* Immediately institute general symptomatic and supportive care, and consider gastric decontamination if co-ingestants are suspected. Because emesis may occur in the presence of obtundation, appropriate posture (left lateral recumbent position) and protection of the airway by intubation may be warranted. Although the gag reflex may be absent in deeply comatose patients, even unconscious patients may become combative to intubation; consider rapid-sequence induction (without the use of sedative). Closely monitor vital signs and consciousness. The bradycardia reported with sodium oxybate overdose has been responsive to atropine intravenous administration. No reversal of the CNS-depressant effects of sodium oxybate can be expected from naloxone or flumazenil administration. The use of hemodialysis and other forms of extracorporeal drug removal have not been studied in sodium oxybate overdose. However, because of the rapid metabolism of sodium oxybate, these measures are not warranted.

As with the management of all cases of drug overdosage, consider the possibility of multiple drug ingestion. Collect urine and blood samples for routine toxicologic screening, and consult with a regional poison control center for current treatment recommendations.

Patient Information

The *Xyrem* Patient Success Program includes detailed information about the safe and proper use of sodium oxybate, as well as information to help the patient prevent accidental use or abuse of sodium oxybate by others. Patients must confirm that they have read the materials before the first prescription will be filled. Discuss the details of the program and the treatment (including the procedure for preparing the dose to be administered) prior to the initiation of treatment. Inform patients that they must be seen by their health care providers frequently during the course of their treatment, and that a detailed account of the adverse reactions they may have experienced will be taken. Food significantly decreases the bioavailability of sodium oxybate. Administration of sodium oxybate immediately after a high-fat meal resulted in delayed absorption (average T_{max} increased from 0.75 to 2 hours) and a reduction in peak plasma level (C_{max}) by a mean of 58% and of systemic exposure (AUC) by 37%. Whether sodium oxybate is taken in the fed or fasted state may affect both the efficacy and safety of sodium oxybate for a given patient. Patients should be made aware of this and try to take the first dose several hours after a meal. Inform patients that sodium oxybate is associated with urinary and, less frequently, fecal incontinence. Instruct patients to lie down and sleep after each dose of sodium oxybate, and not to take sodium oxybate at any time other than at night, immediately before bedtime and again 2.5 to 4 hours later. Instruct patients that they should not take alcohol or other sedative hypnotics with sodium oxybate.

Psychotherapeutic Combinations

OLANZAPINE AND FLUOXETINE HYDROCHLORIDE

Rx	**Symbyax** (Eli Lilly)	**Capsules:** 6 mg olanzapine/25 mg fluoxetine	Mustard yellow/Lt. yellow. In 30s, 100s, 1,000s, and blister UD 100s.
		6 mg olanzapine/50 mg fluoxetine	Mustard yellow/Lt. grey. In 30s, 100s, 1,000s, and blister UD 100s.
		12 mg olanzapine/25 mg fluoxetine	Red/Lt. yellow. In 30s, 100s, 1,000s, and blister UD 100s.
		12 mg olanzapine/50 mg fluoxetine	Red/Lt. grey. In 30s, 100s, 1,000s, and blister UD 100s.

For additional information, refer to the Selective Serotonin Reuptake Inhibitors and the Antipsychotic Agents group monographs.

OLANZAPINE AND FLUOXETINE HYDROCHLORIDE — ORAL

For additional information, refer to the Selective Serotonin Reuptake Inhibitors and the Antipsychotic Agents group monographs.

WARNING

Suicidality in children and adolescents – Antidepressants increased the risk of suicidal thinking and behavior (suicidality) in short-term studies in children and adolescents with major depressive disorder (MDD) and other psychiatric disorders. Anyone considering the use of olanzapine/fluoxetine or any other antidepressant in a child or adolescent must balance this risk with the clinical need. Patients who are started on therapy should be observed closely for clinical worsening, suicidality, or unusual changes in behavior. Families and caregivers should be advised of the need for close observation and communication with the prescriber. Olanzapine/fluoxetine is not approved for use in pediatric patients.

Pooled analyses of short-term (4 to 16 weeks) placebo-controlled trials of 9 antidepressant drugs (SSRIs and others) in children and adolescents with MDD, obsessive-compulsive disorder (OCD), or other psychiatric disorders (a total of 24 trials involving over 4,400 patients) have revealed a greater risk of adverse reactions representing suicidal thinking or behavior (suicidality) during the first few months of treatment in those receiving antidepressants. The average risk of such reactions in patients receiving antidepressants was 4%, twice the placebo risk of 2%. No suicides occurred in these trials.

Indications

➤*Bipolar disorder:* For the treatment of depressive episodes associated with bipolar disorder.

Administration and Dosage

Administer once daily in the evening, generally beginning with the 6 mg/25 mg capsule. While food has no appreciable effect on the absorption of olanzapine and fluoxetine given individually, the effect of food on the absorption of olanzapine/fluoxetine has not been studied. Dosage adjustments, if indicated, can be made according to efficacy and tolerability. Antidepressant efficacy was demonstrated with olanzapine/fluoxetine in a dose range of olanzapine 6 to 12 mg and fluoxetine 25 to 50 mg. The safety of doses above 18 mg/75 mg has not been evaluated in clinical studies.

➤*Special populations:* Use a starting dose of 6 mg/25 mg for patients with a predisposition to hypotensive reactions, patients with hepatic impairment, or patients who exhibit a combination of factors that may slow the metabolism of olanzapine/fluoxetine (eg, female gender, elderly, nonsmoking status). When indicated, perform dose escalation with caution in these patients. Olanzapine/fluoxetine has not been systemically studied in patients older than 65 years of age or in patients younger than 18 years of age.

➤*Storage / Stability:* Store at 25°C (77°F); excursions permitted to 15° to 30°C (59° to 86°F). Keep tightly closed and protect from moisture.

CHLORDIAZEPOXIDE AND AMITRIPTYLINE

c-iv	**Chlordiazepoxide and Amitriptyline** (Various, eg, Geneva, Lemmon, Par)	**Tablets:** 5 mg chlordiazepoxide and 12.5 mg amitriptyline	In 100s and 500s.
c-iv	**Chlordiazepoxide and Amitriptyline** (Various, eg, Goldline, Lemmon)	**Tablets:** 10 mg chlordiazepoxide and 25 mg amitriptyline	In 100s and 500s.
c-iv	**Limbitrol DS 10-25** (Roche)		(Limbitrol DS). White. Film coated. In 100s, 500s, unit-of-use 50s and UD 100s.

CHLORDIAZEPOXIDE AND AMITRIPTYLINE — ORAL

Consider the prescribing information for chlordiazepoxide in the Antianxiety Agents monograph and amitriptyline in the Antidepressants monograph.

WARNING

Suicidality in children and adolescents – Antidepressants increased the risk of suicidal thinking and behavior (suicidality) in short-term studies in children and adolescents with major depressive disorder (MDD) and other psychiatric disorders. Anyone considering the use of chlordiazepoxide/amitriptyline or any other antidepressant in a child or adolescent must balance this risk with the clinical need. Patients who are started on therapy should be observed closely for clinical worsening, suicidality, or unusual changes in behavior. Families and caregivers should be advised of the need for close observation and communication with the prescriber. Chlordiazepoxide/amitriptyline is not approved for use in pediatric patients.

WARNING (cont.)

Pooled analyses of short-term (4 to 16 weeks) placebo-controlled trials of 9 antidepressant drugs (SSRIs and others) in children and adolescents with MDD, obsessive-compulsive disorder (OCD), or other psychiatric disorders (a total of 24 trials involving over 4,400 patients) have revealed a greater risk of adverse reactions representing suicidal thinking or behavior (suicidality) during the first few months of treatment in those receiving antidepressants. The average risk of such reactions in patients receiving antidepressants was 4%, twice the placebo risk of 2%. No suicides occurred in these trials.

Indications

➤*Severe depression:* Treatment of moderate to severe depression associated with moderate to severe anxiety. The therapeutic response to this combination has occurred earlier and with fewer treatment failures than when either ingredient is used alone. Symptoms likely to respond in the first week

CHLORDIAZEPOXIDE AND AMITRIPTYLINE — ORAL

of treatment include: Insomnia; feelings of guilt or worthlessness; agitation; psychic and somatic anxiety; suicidal ideation; anorexia.

Administration and Dosage

Initially, administer 10 mg chlordiazepoxide with 25 mg amitriptyline 3 or 4 times daily in divided doses; increase to 6 times daily, as required. Some patients respond to smaller doses and can be maintained on 2 tablets daily.

After a satisfactory response is obtained, reduce dosage to smallest amount needed. The larger portion of the total daily dose may be taken at bedtime. In some patients, a single dose at bedtime may be sufficient. In general, lower dosages are recommended for elderly patients.

PERPHENAZINE AND AMITRIPTYLINE HYDROCHLORIDE

Rx	**Perphenazine/Amitriptyline** (Various, eg, Bolar, Geneva, Goldline, Lemmon, Par, Rugby, Zenith)	**Tablets:** 2 mg perphenazine and 10 mg amitriptyline	In 21s, 100s, 500s and 1000s.
Rx	**Etrafon 2-10** (Schering)		(Schering ANA or 287). Yellow. In 500s.
Rx	**Perphenazine/Amitriptyline** (Various, eg, Bolar, Geneva, Goldline, Lemmon, Par, Rugby, Zenith)	**Tablets:** 2 mg perphenazine and 25 mg amitriptyline	In 100s, 500s and 1000s.
Rx	**Etrafon** (Schering)		(Schering ANC or 598). Pink. Sugar coated. In 500s.
Rx	**Perphenazine/Amitriptyline** (Various, eg, Bolar, Geneva, Goldline, Lemmon, Par, Rugby, Zenith)	**Tablets:** 4 mg perphenazine and 10 mg amitriptyline	In 100s, 250s, 500s and 1000s.
Rx	**Etrafon-A** (Schering)		(Schering ANB or 119). Orange. In 100s, 500s, UD 100s.
Rx	**Perphenazine/Amitriptyline** (Various, eg, Bolar, Geneva, Goldline, Lemmon, Par, Rugby, Zenith)	**Tablets:** 4 mg perphenazine and 25 mg amitriptyline	In 100s, 500s, 800s and 1000s.
Rx	**Etrafon-Forte** (Schering)		(Schering ANE or 720). Red. Sugar coated. In 500s.
Rx	**Perphenazine/Amitriptyline** (Various, eg, Bolar, Geneva, Goldline, Lemmon, Par, Rugby, Zenith)	**Tablets:** 4 mg perphenazine and 50 mg amitriptyline	In 100s and 250s.

PERPHENAZINE AND AMITRIPTYLINE HYDROCHLORIDE — ORAL

Consider the prescribing information for perphenazine in the Antipsychotic Agents monograph and amitriptyline in the Antidepressants monograph.

WARNING

Suicidality in children and adolescents – Antidepressants increased the risk of suicidal thinking and behavior (suicidality) in short-term studies in children and adolescents with major depressive disorder (MDD) and other psychiatric disorders. Anyone considering the use of perphenazine/amitriptyline or any other antidepressant in a child or adolescent must balance this risk with the clinical need. Patients who are started on therapy should be observed closely for clinical worsening, suicidality, or unusual changes in behavior. Families and caregivers should be advised of the need for close observation and communication with the prescriber. Perphenazine/amitriptyline is not approved for use in pediatric patients.

Pooled analyses of short-term (4 to 16 weeks) placebo-controlled trials of 9 antidepressant drugs (SSRIs and others) in children and adolescents with MDD, obsessive-compulsive disorder (OCD), or other psychiatric disorders (a total of 24 trials involving over 4,400 patients) have revealed a greater risk of adverse reactions representing suicidal thinking or behavior (suicidality) during the first few months of treatment in those receiving antidepressants. The average risk of such reactions in patients receiving antidepressants was 4%, twice the placebo risk of 2%. No suicides occurred in these trials.

Indications

➤*Anxiety/Agitation/Depression:* Treatment of moderate to severe anxiety or agitation and depressed mood; patients with depression in whom anxiety or agitation are moderate or severe; patients with anxiety and depression associated with chronic physical disease; patients in whom depression and anxiety cannot be clearly differentiated; schizophrenic patients who have associated symptoms of depression.

Many patients presenting symptoms such as agitation, anxiety, insomnia, psychomotor retardation, functional somatic complaints, tiredness, loss of interest and anorexia have responded well to this combination.

Administration and Dosage

Initially, 2 to 4 mg perphenazine with 10 to 50 mg amitriptyline, 3 or 4 times daily. After a satisfactory response is noted, reduce to smallest amount necessary to obtain relief. Not recommended for use in children.

ERGOLOID MESYLATES (Dihydrogenated Ergot Alkaloids, Dihydroergotoxine)

Rx	**Ergoloid Mesylates** (Various, eg, Ivax, Major, Mutual, URL)	**Tablets, sublingual:** 1 mg	In 100s, 500s, 1000s and UD 100s.
Rx	**Ergoloid Mesylates** (Various, eg, Ivax, Major, Mutual, URL)	**Tablets, oral:** 1 mg	In 60s, 100s, 500s, 1000s and UD 32s, 100s and 1000s.

ERGOLOID MESYLATES — ORAL

Indications

➤*Mental capacity decline:* A proportion of individuals older than 60 years of age who manifest signs and symptoms of an idiopathic decline in mental capacity (ie, cognitive and interpersonal skills, mood, self-care, apparent motivation) can experience some symptomatic relief upon treatment with ergoloid mesylates preparations. The identity of the specific trait(s) or condition(s), if any, which would usefully predict a response to ergoloid mesylates therapy is not known. It appears, however, that those individuals who do respond come from groups of patients who would be considered clinically to suffer from some ill-defined process related to aging or to have some underlying dementing condition (ie, primary progressive dementia, Alzheimer's dementia, senile onset, multi-infarct dementia).

Administration and Dosage

The recommended dosage is 1 mg 3 times daily.

Alleviation of symptoms is usually gradual and results may not be observed for 3 to 4 weeks.

➤*Storage/Stability:* Store in a tight, light-resistant container below 25°C (77°F).

Actions

➤*Pharmacology:* There is no specific evidence which clearly establishes the mechanism by which ergoloid mesylates preparations produce mental effects, nor is there conclusive evidence that the drug particularly affects cerebral arteriosclerosis or cerebrovascular insufficiency.

➤*Pharmacokinetics:* Pharmacokinetic studies have been performed in healthy volunteers with the help of radiolabeled drug as well as employing a specific radioimmunoassay technique. From the urinary excretion quotient of orally and intravenously administered tritium-labelled ergoloid mesylates the absorption of ergoloid was calculated to be 25%. Following oral administration, peak levels of 0.5 ng Eq/mL/mg were achieved within 1.5 to 3 hours. Bioavailability studies with the specific radioimmunoassay confirm that ergoloid is rapidly absorbed from the gastrointestinal tract, with mean peak levels of 0.05 to 0.13 ng/mL/mg (with extremes of 0.03 and 0.18 ng/mL/mg) achieved within 0.6 to 1.3 hours (with extremes of 0.4 and 2.8 hours). The finding of lower peak levels of ergoloid compared to the total drug-metabolite composite is consistent with a considerable first pass liver metabolism, with < 50% of the therapeutic moiety reaching the systemic circulation. The elimination of radioactivity, representing ergoloid plus metabolites bearing the radiolabel, was biphasic with half-lives of 4 and 13 hours. The mean half-life of unchanged ergoloid in plasma is about 2.6 to 5.1 hours; after 3 half-lives ergoloid plasma levels are < 10% of radioactivity levels, and by 24 hours no ergoloid is detectable.

Bioequivalence studies were performed comparing ergoloid mesylates oral tablets (administered orally) with ergoloid mesylates sublingual tablets (administered sublingually).

Contraindications

Individuals who have previously shown hypersensitivity to the drug; in patients who have psychosis, acute or chronic, regardless of etiology.

Psychotherapeutic Combinations

ERGOLOID MESYLATES — ORAL

Precautions

Practitioners are advised that because the target symptoms are of unknown etiology, careful diagnosis should be attempted before prescribing ergoloid mesylates preparations.

Adverse Reactions

Ergoloid mesylates preparations have not been found to produce serious side effects. Transient nausea and gastric disturbances have been reported. Ergoloid mesylates preparations do not possess the vasoconstrictor properties of the natural ergot alkaloids.

SEDATIVES AND HYPNOTICS, NONBARBITURATE

The following is a general discussion of nonbarbiturate sedative/hypnotics.

To facilitate comparison, the products are divided into two groups: The miscellaneous nonbarbiturates and the benzodiazepines. Although sedative doses can be given, these agents are primarily intended to be hypnotics (agents that produce drowsiness and facilitate sleep). Agents intended primarily for sedation or tranquilization are discussed in other parts of this chapter.

In the table below, some pharmacokinetic properties of the nonbarbiturate sedative/hypnotics are compared. Do not use this table to predict exact duration of effect, but use as a guide in drug selection.

Nonbarbiturate Sedative/Hypnotics Pharmacokinetic Parameters

Drug	Adult oral dose		Onset (min)	Duration of action (hrs)	Half-life (hrs)	Protein binding (%)	Urinary excretion, unchanged (%)
	Hypnotic	Sedative					
Imidazopyridines							
Zolpidem	10 mg	na*	nd*	nd*	≈ 2.5	92.5	0
Ureides							
Acetylcarbromal	nd*	250-500 mg bid or tid	nd*	nd*	nd*	nd*	nd*
Tertiary Acetylenic Alcohols							
Ethchlorvynol	500 mg	100-200 mg bid or tid	15-60	5	10-20[2]	nd*	40[3]
Piperidine Derivatives							
Glutethimide	250-500 mg	nd*	30	4-8	10-12	50	< 2
Benzodiazepines							
Estazolam	1-2 mg	na*	nd*	nd*	10-24	93	< 5
Flurazepam	15-30 mg	na*	17	7-8	50-100[4]	97	< 1[4]
Quazepam	15 mg	na*	nd*	nd*	25-41	> 95	trace
Temazepam	15-30 mg	na*	nd*	nd*	10-17	98	1.5
Triazolam	0.125-0.5 mg	na*	nd*	nd*	1.5-5.5	90	2
Miscellaneous nonbarbiturates							
Chloral hydrate	0.5-1 g	250 mg tid pc	30	nd*	7-10[1]	35-41	nd*
Paraldehyde	10-30 ml	5-10 ml	10-15	8-12	3.4-9.8	nd*	small
Propiomazine	nd*	10-20 mg	nd*	nd*	nd*	nd*	nd*

* na – Not applicable. nd = No data.
[1] Trichloroethanol, the principal metabolite.
[2] In acute use, half-life of the distribution phase (1 to 3 hours) is more appropriate.
[3] Free and conjugated forms of the major metabolite, secondary alcohol of ethchlorvynol.
[4] Active metabolite, desalkylflurazepam.

Imidazopyridines

ZOLPIDEM TARTRATE

c-iv	**Ambien** (Sanofi-Synthelabo)	**Tablets:** 5 mg	Lactose. (AMB 5 5401). Pink. Film coated. In 100s, 500s, UD 100s, and *Ambien PAK* UD 30s.
		10 mg	Lactose. (AMB 10 5421). White. Film coated. In 100s, 500s, UD 100s, and *Ambien PAK* UD 30s.
c-iv	**Ambien CR** (Sanofi-Synthelabo)	**Tablets, extended-release:** 6.25 mg	Lactose. (A~). Pink, bilayered. In 100s, 500s, and unit-dose 30s.
		12.5 mg	Lactose. (A~). Blue, bilayered. In 100s, 500s, and unit-dose 30s.

ZOLPIDEM TARTRATE — ORAL

Refer to the general discussion beginning in the Sedatives and Hypnotics, Nonbarbiturate introduction.

Indications

➤*Insomnia:*

Immediate-release – For the short-term treatment of insomnia. Hypnotics should generally be limited to 7 to 10 days of use, and reevaluation of the patient is recommended if hypnotics are to be taken for more than 2 to 3 weeks.

Do not prescribe zolpidem in quantities exceeding a 1-month supply.

Extended-release – For the treatment of insomnia, characterized by difficulties with sleep onset and/or sleep maintenance (as measured by wake time after sleep onset).

Administration and Dosage

➤*Approved by the FDA:* December 16, 1992 (immediate-release formulation).

➤*Immediate-release:* The recommended dose for adults is 10 mg immediately before bedtime.

Downward dosage adjustment may be necessary when zolpidem is administered with agents having known CNS-depressant effects because of the potentially additive effects.

The total zolpidem dose should not exceed 10 mg.

➤*Extended-release:* The recommended dose for adults is 12.5 mg immediately before bedtime. Extended-release tablets should be swallowed whole and not be divided, crushed, or chewed.

The effect of zolpidem extended-release tablets may be slowed by ingestion with or immediately after a meal.

➤*Elderly or debilitated patients:* See Warnings for more information.

➤*Hepatic function impairment:* Patients with hepatic insufficiency do not clear the drug as rapidly as healthy patients. The recommended dose is 5 mg of the immediate-release tablet or 6.25 mg of the extended-release tablet taken immediately before bedtime.

➤*Storage/Stability:*

Immediate-release – Store at controlled room temperature, 20° to 25°C (68° to 77°F).

Extended-release – Store between 15° to 25°C (59° to 77°F). Limited excursions are permissible up to 30°C (86°F).

Actions

➤*Pharmacology:* Zolpidem, the active moiety of zolpidem, is a hypnotic agent with a chemical structure unrelated to benzodiazepines, barbiturates, pyrrolopyrazines, pyrazolopyrimidines, or other drugs with known hypnotic properties; interacts with a GABA-benzodiazepine receptor complex; and shares some of the pharmacological properties of the benzodiazepines. In contrast to the benzodiazepines, which nonselectively bind to and activate all benzodiazepine or omega receptor subtypes, zolpidem in vitro binds the benzodiazepine$_1$ receptor preferentially with a high affinity ratio of the alpha$_1$/alpha$_5$ subunits. The benzodiazepine$_1$ receptor is found primarily on the lamina IV of the sensorimotor cortical regions, substantia nigra (pars reticulata), cerebellum molecular layer, olfactory bulb, ventral thalamic complex, pons, inferior colliculus, and globus pallidus. This selective binding of zolpidem on the benzodiazepine$_1$— receptor is not absolute, but it may

ZOLPIDEM TARTRATE — ORAL

explain the relative absence of myorelaxant and anticonvulsant effects in animal studies as well as the preservation of deep sleep (stages 3 and 4) in human studies of zolpidem at hypnotic doses.

➤*Pharmacokinetics:*

Absorption/Distribution – Total protein binding was found to be 92.5 ± 0.1% and remained constant, independent of concentration between 40 and 790 ng/mL.

Immediate-release: The pharmacokinetic profile of zolpidem is characterized by rapid absorption from the GI tract and a short elimination half-life ($t_{½}$) in healthy subjects.

In a single-dose crossover study in 45 healthy subjects administered zolpidem 5 and 10 mg tablets, the mean peak concentrations (C_{max}) were 59 (range, 29 to 113) and 121 (range, 58 to 272) ng/mL, respectively, occurring at a mean time (T_{max}) of 1.6 hours for both. Zolpidem demonstrated linear kinetics in the dose range of 5 to 20 mg.

A food-effect study in 30 healthy male volunteers compared the pharmacokinetics of zolpidem 10 mg when administered while fasting or 20 minutes after a meal. Results demonstrated that with food, mean area under the curve (AUC) and C_{max} were decreased by 15% and 25%, respectively, while mean T_{max} was prolonged by 60% (from 1.4 to 2.2 hours). The half-life remained unchanged. These results suggest that, for faster sleep onset, zolpidem should not be administered with or immediately after a meal.

Extended-release: Zolpidem extended-release exhibits biphasic absorption characteristics, which results in rapid initial absorption from the GI tract similar to zolpidem immediate-release, then provides extended plasma concentrations beyond 3 hours after administration. A study in 24 healthy men was conducted to compare mean zolpidem plasma concentration-time profiles obtained after single oral administration of zolpidem 12.5 mg extended-release and of an immediate-release formulation of zolpidem 10 mg. The $t_{½}$ observed with zolpidem 12.5 mg extended-release was similar to that obtained with zolpidem 10 mg immediate-release.

Following administration of zolpidem extended-release, administered as a single 12.5 mg dose in healthy men, the C_{max} of zolpidem was 134 ng/mL (range, 68.9 to 197 ng/mL) occurring at a median time (T_{max}) of 1.5 hours. The mean AUC of zolpidem was 740 ng•h/mL (range, 295 to 1,359 ng•h/mL).

A food-effect study in 45 healthy volunteers compared the pharmacokinetics of zolpidem 12.5 mg extended-release when administered while fasting or within 30 minutes after a meal. Results demonstrated that with food, mean AUC and C_{max} were decreased by 23% and 30%, respectively, while median T_{max} was increased from 2 hours to 4 hours. The half-life was not changed. These results suggest that, for faster sleep onset, zolpidem extended-release should not be administered with or immediately after a meal.

Metabolism/Excretion – Zolpidem is converted to inactive metabolites that are eliminated primarily by renal excretion.

Immediate-release: The mean zolpidem elimination half-life was 2.6 (range, 1.4 to 4.5) and 2.5 (range, 1.4 to 3.8) hours, for the 5 and 10 mg tablets, respectively. Zolpidem did not accumulate in young adults following nightly dosing with zolpidem 20 mg tablets for 2 weeks.

Extended-release: When zolpidem extended-release was administered as a single 12.5 mg dose in healthy men, the mean zolpidem $t_{½}$ was 2.8 hours (range, 1.62 to 4.05 hours).

Special populations –

Hepatic function impairment:

• *Immediate-release* – The pharmacokinetics of zolpidem in 8 patients with chronic hepatic insufficiency were compared with results in healthy subjects. Following a single 20 mg oral zolpidem dose, mean C_{max} and AUC were found to be 2 times (250 vs 499 ng/mL) and 5 times (788 vs 4203 ng•h/mL) higher, respectively, in hepatically compromised patients, T_{max} did not change. The mean half-life in cirrhotic patients of 9.9 hours (range, 4.1 to 25.8 hours) was greater than that observed in healthy patients of 2.2 hours (range, 1.6 to 2.4 hours). Modify dosing accordingly in patients with hepatic insufficiency.

Elderly:

• *Immediate-release* – In the elderly, the dose for zolpidem should be 5 mg. This recommendation is based on several studies in which the mean C_{max}, $t_{½}$, and AUC were significantly increased when compared with results in young adults. In 1 study of 8 elderly subjects (older than 70 years of age), the means for C_{max}, $t_{½}$, and AUC significantly increased by 50% (255 vs 384 ng/mL), 32% (2.2 vs 2.9 hours), and 64% (955 vs 1,562 ng•h/mL), respectively, as compared with younger adults (20 to 40 years of age) following a single oral zolpidem 20 mg dose. Zolpidem did not accumulate in elderly subjects following nightly oral dosing of 10 mg for 1 week.

• *Extended-release* – In 24 elderly (at least 65 years of age) healthy subjects administered a single 6.25 mg dose of zolpidem extended-release, the mean C_{max} of zolpidem was 70.6 (range, 35 to 161) ng/mL occurring at a T_{max} of 2 hours. The mean AUC of zolpidem was 413 ng•h/mL (range, 124 to 1,190 ng•h/mL) and the mean $t_{½}$ was 2.9 hours (range, 1.59 to 5.5 hours).

Contraindications

There are no known contraindications for zolpidem immediate-release.

Zolpidem extended-release is contraindicated in patients with known hypersensitivity to zolpidem or to any of the inactive ingredients in the formulation.

Warnings

➤*Psychiatric/Physical disorder:* Because sleep disturbances may be the presenting manifestation of a physical and/or psychiatric disorder, initiate symptomatic treatment of insomnia only after a careful evaluation of the patient. The failure of insomnia to remit after 7 to 10 days of treatment may indicate the presence of a primary psychiatric and/or medical illness that should be evaluated. Worsening of insomnia or the emergence of new thinking or behavior abnormalities may be the consequence of an unrecognized psychiatric or physical disorder. Such findings have emerged during the course of treatment with sedative/hypnotic drugs, including zolpidem. Because some of the important adverse effects of zolpidem appear to be dose related, it is important to use the smallest possible effective dose, especially in the elderly.

➤*CNS effects:* A variety of abnormal thinking and behavior changes have been reported to occur in association with the use of sedative/hypnotics. Some of these changes may be characterized by decreased inhibition (eg, aggressiveness and extroversion that seemed out of character), similar to effects produced by alcohol and other CNS depressants. Visual and auditory hallucinations have been reported, as well as behavioral changes such as bizarre behavior, agitation, and depersonalization. Amnesia, anxiety, and other neuropsychiatric symptoms may occur unpredictably. In primarily depressed patients, worsening of depression, including suicidal thinking, has been reported in association with the use of sedative/hypnotics.

It can rarely be determined with certainty whether a particular instance of the abnormal behaviors listed above are drug induced, spontaneous in origin, or a result of an underlying psychiatric or physical disorder. Nonetheless, the emergence of any new behavioral sign or symptom of concern requires careful and immediate evaluation.

➤*Abrupt discontinuation:* See Precautions for more information.

➤*Renal/Hepatic function impairment:* As a general precaution, closely monitor these patients.

➤*Elderly:*

Use in the elderly or debilitated patients – Impaired motor or cognitive performance after repeated exposure or unusual sensitivity to sedative/hypnotic drugs is a concern in the treatment of elderly or debilitated patients. Therefore, the recommended zolpidem extended-release dose is 6.25 mg and the recommended zolpidem immediate-release dose is 5 mg in such patients to decrease the possibility of side effects. Monitor these patients closely.

➤*Pregnancy: Category B* (immediate-release); *Category C* (extended-release).

Immediate-release – In rats, adverse maternal and fetal effects occurred at 20 and 100 mg base/kg and included dose-related maternal lethargy and ataxia and a dose-related trend to incomplete ossification of fetal skull bones. Underossification of various fetal bones indicates a delay in maturation and is often seen in rats treated with sedative/hypnotic drugs. There were no teratogenic effects after zolpidem administration. The no-effect dose for maternal or fetal toxicity was 4 mg base/kg or 5 times the maximum human dose on a mg/m^2 basis.

In rabbits, dose-related maternal sedation and decreased weight gain occurred at all doses tested. At the high dose, 16 mg base/kg, there was an increase in postimplantation fetal loss and underossification of sternebrae in viable fetuses. These fetal findings in rabbits are often secondary to reductions in maternal weight gain. There were no frank teratogenic effects. The no-effect dose for fetal toxicity was 4 mg base/kg or 7 times the maximum human dose on a mg/m^2 basis.

Because animal reproduction studies are not always predictive of human response, use this drug during pregnancy only if clearly needed.

Extended-release – Zolpidem was administered to pregnant Sprague-Dawley rats by oral gavage during the period of organogenesis at dosages of 4, 20, or 100 mg base/kg/day. Adverse maternal and embryo/fetal effects occurred at doses of 20 mg base/kg and higher, manifesting as dose-related lethargy and ataxia in pregnant rats while examination of fetal skull bones revealed a dose-related trend toward incomplete ossification. Teratogenicity was not observed at any dose level. The no-effect dose of zolpidem for maternal and embryo/fetal toxicity was 4 mg base/kg/day (4 times the maximum recommended human dose "MRHD" of zolpidem extended-release on a mg/m^2 basis).

Administration of zolpidem to pregnant Himalayan albino rabbits at dosages of 1, 4, or 16 mg base/kg/day by oral gavage (up to 30 times the MRHD of zolpidem extended-release on a mg/m^2 basis) during the period of organogenesis produced dose-related maternal sedation and decreased maternal body weight gain at all doses. At the high dose of 16 mg base/kg, there was an increase in postimplantation fetal loss and underossification of sternebrae in viable fetuses. Teratogenicity was not observed at any dose level. The no-effect dosage of zolpidem for maternal toxicity was below 1 mg base/kg/day (less than 2 times the MRHD of zolpidem extended-release on a mg/m^2 basis). The no-effect dosage for embryofetal toxicity was 4 mg base/kg/day (8 times the MRHD of zolpidem extended-release on a mg/m^2 basis).

Administration of zolpidem at dosages of 4, 20, or 100 mg base/kg/day to pregnant Sprague-Dawley rats starting on day 15 of gestation and continuing through day 21 of the postnatal lactation period produced dose-dependent lethargy and ataxia in dams at doses of 20 mg base/kg and higher. Decreased maternal body weight gain as well as evidence on nonsecreting mammary glands and a single incidence of maternal death was observed at 100 mg base/kg. Effects observed on rat pups included decreased body weight with maternal doses of 20 mg base/kg and higher and decreased pup survival at maternal doses of 100 mg base/kg. The no-effect dose for maternal and offspring toxicity was 4 mg base/kg (4 times the MRHD of zolpidem extended-release on a mg/m^2 basis).

There are no adequate and well-controlled studies in pregnant women. Use zolpidem extended-release during pregnancy only if the potential benefit justifies the potential risk to the fetus.

Studies to assess the effects on children whose mothers took zolpidem during pregnancy have not been conducted. However, children born of mothers

ZOLPIDEM TARTRATE — ORAL

taking sedative/hypnotic drugs may be at some risk for withdrawal symptoms from the drug during the postnatal period. In addition, neonatal flaccidity has been reported in infants born to mothers who received sedative/hypnotic drugs during pregnancy.

➤*Lactation:* Studies in lactating mothers indicate that the half-life of zolpidem is similar to that in young healthy volunteers (2.6 ± 0.3 hours). Between 0.004% and 0.019% of the total administered dose is excreted into milk, but the effect of zolpidem on the infant is unknown.

In addition, in a rat study, zolpidem inhibited the secretion of milk. The no-effect dose was 4 mg base/kg or 6 times the recommended human dose in mg/m^2.

The use of zolpidem in breast-feeding mothers is not recommended.

➤*Children:* Safety and efficacy in children younger than 18 years of age have not been established.

Precautions

➤*Concomitant illness:* Clinical experience with zolpidem in patients with concomitant systemic illness is limited. Caution is advisable in using zolpidem in patients with diseases or conditions that could effect metabolism or hemodynamic responses. Although studies did not reveal respiratory-depressant effects at hypnotic doses of zolpidem in healthy patients or in patients with mild to moderate chronic obstructive pulmonary disease, a reduction in the Total Arousal Index together with a reduction in lowest oxygen saturation and increase in the times of oxygen desaturation below 80% and 90% was observed in patients with mild to moderate sleep apnea when treated with an immediate-release formulation of zolpidem (10 mg) when compared with placebo. However, observe precautions if zolpidem is prescribed to patients with compromised respiratory function, because sedative/hypnotics have the capacity to depress respiratory drive. Postmarketing reports of respiratory insufficiency in patients receiving immediate-release zolpidem, most of which involved patients with preexisting respiratory impairment, have been received.

➤*Depression:* As with other sedative/hypnotic drugs, administer zolpidem with caution to patients exhibiting signs or symptoms of depression. Suicidal tendencies may be present in such patients and protective measures may be required. Intentional overdosage is more common in this group of patients; therefore, prescribe the least amount of drug that is feasible for the patient at any one time.

➤*History of psychiatric disorders or addiction to drugs/alcohol:* Because persons with a history of psychiatric disorders or addiction to, or abuse of, drugs or alcohol are at increased risk for misuse, abuse and addiction of zolpidem, monitor these patients carefully when administering zolpidem or any other hypnotic.

➤*Drug abuse and dependence:* Sedative/hypnotics have produced withdrawal signs and symptoms following abrupt discontinuation. These reported symptoms range from mild dysphoria and insomnia to a withdrawal syndrome that may include abdominal and muscle cramps, vomiting, sweating, tremors, and convulsions. The US clinical trial experience from zolpidem does not reveal any clear evidence for withdrawal syndrome. Nevertheless, the following adverse reactions included in *DSM-III-R* criteria for uncomplicated sedative/hypnotic withdrawal were reported during US clinical trials following placebo substitution occurring within 48 hours following last zolpidem treatment: fatigue, nausea, flushing, light-headedness, uncontrolled crying, emesis, stomach cramps, panic attack, nervousness, and abdominal discomfort. See Warnings for more information.

➤*Hazardous tasks:* Zolpidem, like other sedative/hypnotic drugs, has CNS-depressant effects. Because of the rapid onset of action, zolpidem should only be ingested immediately prior to going to bed. Caution patients against engaging in hazardous occupations requiring complete mental alertness or motor coordination, such as operating machinery or driving a motor vehicle after ingesting the drug, including potential impairment of the performance of such activities that may occur the day following ingestion of zolpidem. Zolpidem showed additive effects when combined with alcohol and should not be taken with alcohol. Also caution patients about possible combined effects with other CNS-depressant drugs. Dosage adjustments may be necessary when zolpidem is administered with such agents because of the potentially additive effects.

Drug Interactions

Zolpidem Drug Interactions			
Precipitant drug	Object drug[a]		Description
Azole antifungals (eg, fluconazole, itraconazole, ketoconazole)	Zolpidem	↑	Plasma concentrations and therapeutic effects of zolpidem may be increased. Monitor closely and adjust the zolpidem dose as needed.
Chlorpromazine	Zolpidem	↑	Coadministration produced an additive effect of decreased alertness and psychomotor performance.
Zolpidem	Chlorpromazine		
Flumazenil	Zolpidem	↓	Zolpidem's effect may be reversed by flumazenil.
Imipramine	Zolpidem	↑↓	Coadministration produced a 20% decrease in peak levels of imipramine; however, an additive effect of decreased alertness was seen.
Zolpidem	Imipramine		
Rifamycins (eg, rifampin)	Zolpidem	↓	Plasma concentrations and therapeutic effects of zolpidem may be decreased. Monitor closely and adjust the zolpidem dose as needed.
Ritonavir	Zolpidem	↑	Coadministration may cause severe sedation and respiratory depression. Concurrent use is contraindicated.
Selective serotonin reuptake inhibitors (SSRIs; eg, sertraline)	Zolpidem	↑	The onset of action of zolpidem may be shortened and the effect increased. Coadministration with sertraline produced an increase in zolpidem C_{max} (43%) and a decrease in T_{max} (53%). Observe closely.
Zolpidem	CNS depressants (eg, alcohol)	↑	May enhance the CNS depressant effects of zolpidem. An additive effect of psychomotor performance between alcohol and zolpidem has been demonstrated.
CNS depressants (eg, alcohol)	Zolpidem		

[a] ↑ = Object drug increased. ↓ = Object drug decreased.

➤*Drug/Lab test interactions:* Zolpidem is not known to interfere with commonly employed clinical laboratory tests. In addition, clinical data indicate that zolpidem does not cross-react with benzodiazepines, opiates, barbiturates, cocaine, cannabinoids, or amphetamines in 2 standard urine drug screens.

➤*Drug/Food interactions:* See Actions for more information.

Adverse Reactions

➤*Associated with discontinuation of treatment:*

Immediate-release – Approximately 4% of 1,701 patients who received zolpidem at all doses (1.25 to 90 mg) in US premarketing clinical trials discontinued treatment because of an adverse clinical reaction. Reactions most commonly associated with discontinuation from US trials were daytime drowsiness (0.5%), dizziness (0.4%), headache (0.5%), nausea (0.6%), and vomiting (0.5%).

Approximately 4% of 1,959 patients who received zolpidem at all doses (1 to 50 mg) in similar foreign trials discontinued treatment because of an adverse reaction. Reactions most commonly associated with discontinuation from these trials were daytime drowsiness (1.1%), dizziness/vertigo (0.8%), amnesia (0.5%), nausea (0.5%), headache (0.4%), and falls (0.4%).

Data from a clinical study in which SSRI-treated patients were given zolpidem revealed that 4 of the 7 discontinuations during double-blind treatment with zolpidem (n = 95) were associated with impaired concentration, continuing or aggravated depression, and manic reaction; 1 patient treated with placebo (n = 97) was discontinued after an attempted suicide.

Extended-release – In clinical trials with zolpidem extended-release, 3.5% of 201 patients receiving 6.25 or 12.5 mg of zolpidem extended-release discontinued treatment because of an adverse reaction. Reactions most commonly associated with discontinuation were somnolence (1%) and dizziness (1%).

Most commonly observed adverse reactions in controlled trials:

- *Immediate-release* – During short-term treatment (up to 10 nights) with zolpidem at doses up to 10 mg, the most commonly observed adverse reactions associated with the use of zolpidem and seen at statistically significant differences from placebo-treated patients were drowsiness (reported by 2% of zolpidem patients), dizziness (1%), and diarrhea (1%). During longer-term treatment (28 to 35 nights) with zolpidem at doses up to 10 mg, the most commonly observed adverse reactions associated with the use of zolpidem and seen at statistically significant differences from placebo-treated patients were dizziness (5%) and drugged feelings (3%).
- *Extended-release* – During treatment with zolpidem extended-release in adults and elderly at daily doses of 12.5 and 6.25 mg, respectively, each for 3 weeks, the most commonly observed adverse reactions associated with the use of zolpidem extended-release were headache, somnolence, and dizziness.

➤*Adverse reactions observed at an incidence of greater than or equal to 1% in controlled trials:*

Immediate-release –

Short-term placebo controlled trials: The following table was derived from a pool of 11 placebo-controlled short-term US efficacy trials involving zolpidem in doses ranging from 1.25 to 20 mg. The information is limited to data from doses up to and including 10 mg, the highest dose recommended for use.

ZOLPIDEM TARTRATE — ORAL

Zolpidem Immediate-Release Adverse Reactions in Short-Term, Placebo-Controlled, Clinical Trials (%)

Adverse reaction[a]	Zolpidem (≤ 10 mg) (n = 685)	Placebo (n = 473)
CNS		
Dizziness	1%	—
Drowsiness	2%	—
Headache	7%	6%
GI		
Diarrhea	1%	—
Nausea	2%	3%
Musculoskeletal		
Myalgia	1%	2%

[a] Reactions reported by at least 1% of zolpidem patients are included.

Long-term placebo controlled clinical trials – The following table was derived from a pool of 3 placebo-controlled long-term efficacy trials involving zolpidem. These trials involved patients with chronic insomnia who were treated for 28 to 35 nights with zolpidem at doses of 5, 10, or 15 mg. The information is limited to data from doses up to and including 10 mg, the highest dose recommended for use. The table includes only adverse reactions occurring at an incidence of at least 1% for zolpidem patients.

Zolpidem Immediate-Release Adverse Reactions in Long-Term, Placebo-Controlled, Clinical Trials (%)

Adverse reaction[a]	Zolpidem (≤ 10 mg) (n = 152)	Placebo (n = 161)
Cardiovascular		
Palpitation	2%	—
CNS		
Abnormal dreams	1%	—
Amnesia	1%	—
Anxiety	1%	1%
Depression	2%	1%
Dizziness	5%	1%
Drowsiness	8%	5%
Drugged feeling	3%	—
Fatigue	1%	2%
Headache	19%	22%
Lethargy	3%	1%
Light-headedness	2%	1%
Nervousness	1%	3%
Sleep disorder	1%	—
Dermatologic		
Rash	2%	1%
GI		
Abdominal pain	2%	2%
Anorexia	1%	1%
Constipation	2%	1%
Diarrhea	3%	2%
Dry mouth	3%	1%
Dyspepsia	5%	6%
Nausea	6%	6%
Vomiting	1%	1%
GU		
Urinary tract infection	2%	2%
Musculoskeletal		
Arthralgia	4%	4%
Back pain	3%	2%
Myalgia	7%	7%
Respiratory		
Pharyngitis	3%	1%
Rhinitis	1%	3%
Sinusitis	4%	2%
Upper respiratory tract infection	5%	6%
Miscellaneous		
Allergy	4%	1%
Chest pain	1%	—
Infection	1%	1%
Influenza-like symptoms	2%	—

[a] Reactions reported by at least 1% of patients treated with zolpidem.

Extended-release –

Placebo-controlled clinical trials in healthy adults: The following tables were derived from results of 2 placebo-controlled efficacy trials involving zolpidem extended-release. These trials involved patients with primary insomnia who were treated for 3 weeks with zolpidem extended-release at doses of 12.5 or 6.25 mg, respectively. The tables include only adverse reactions occurring at an incidence of at least 1% for zolpidem extended-release patients and with an incidence greater than that seen in the placebo patients.

Zolpidem Extended-Release Adverse Reactions (%)

Adverse reaction[a]	Zolpidem extended-release 12.5 mg (n = 102)	Placebo (n = 110)
Cardiovascular		
Blood pressure increased	1%	—
CNS		
Anxiety	2%	—
Ataxia	1%	—
Balance disorder	2%	—
Binge eating	1%	—
Depersonalization	1%	—
Depression	2%	—
Disinhibition	1%	—
Disorientation	3%	2%
Disturbance in attention	2%	—
Dizziness	12%	5%
Euphoric mood	1%	—
Fatigue	3%	2%
Hallucinations[b]	4%	—
Headache	19%	16%
Hypoesthesia	2%	1%
Memory disorders[c]	3%	—
Mood swings	1%	—
Paresthesia	1%	—
Psychomotor retardation	2%	—
Somnolence	15%	2%
Stress symptoms	1%	—
Dermatologic		
Rash	1%	—
Skin wrinkling	1%	—
Urticaria	1%	—
GI		
Abdominal discomfort	1%	—
Abdominal tenderness	1%	—
Constipation	2%	—
Frequent bowel movements	1%	—
Gastroenteritis	1%	—
Gastroesophageal reflux disease	1%	—
Nausea	7%	4%
Vomiting	1%	—
GU		
Menorrhagia	1%	—
Musculoskeletal		
Back pain	4%	3%
Myalgia	4%	—
Neck pain	1%	—
Respiratory		
Throat irritation	1%	—

ZOLPIDEM TARTRATE — ORAL

Zolpidem Extended-Release Adverse Reactions (%)		
Adverse reaction[a]	Zolpidem extended-release 12.5 mg (n = 102)	Placebo (n = 110)
Special senses		
Altered visual depth perception	1%	—
Asthenopia	1%	—
Eye redness	2%	—
Labyrinthitis	1%	—
Tinnitus	1%	—
Vertigo	2%	—
Vision blurred	2%	1%
Visual disturbance	3%	—
Miscellaneous		
Appetite disorder	1%	—
Asthenia	1%	—
Body temperature increased	1%	—
Chest discomfort	1%	—
Contusion	1%	—
Exposure to poisonous plant	1%	—
Influenza	3%	—

[a] Reactions reported by at least 1% of patients treated with zolpidem extended-release and at greater frequency than in the placebo group.
[b] Hallucinations included hallucinations not otherwise specified as well as visual and hypnogogic hallucinations.
[c] Memory disorders include: amnesia, anterograde amnesia, memory impairment.

Placebo-controlled clinical trials in elderly:

Zolpidem Extended-Release Adverse Reactions (%)		
Adverse reaction[a]	Zolpidem 6.25 mg extended-release (n = 99)	Placebo (n = 106)
Cardiovascular		
Palpitations	2%	—
CNS		
Anxiety	3%	2%
Apathy	1%	—
Burning sensation	1%	—
Depressed mood	1%	—
Dizziness	8%	3%
Dizziness postural	1%	—
Headache	14%	11%
Memory disorders[b]	1%	—
Muscle contractions, involuntary	1%	—
Paresthesia	1%	—
Psychomotor retardation	2%	—
Somnolence	6%	5%
Tremor	1%	—
Dermatologic		
Rash	1%	—
Urticaria	1%	—
GI		
Flatulence	1%	—
Vomiting	1%	—
GU		
Dysuria	1%	—
Vulvovaginal dryness	1%	—
Musculoskeletal		
Arthralgia	2%	—
Muscle cramp	2%	1%
Neck pain	2%	—
Respiratory		
Lower respiratory tract infection	1%	—
Nasopharyngitis	6%	4%
Otitis externa	1%	—
Upper respiratory tract infection	1%	—
Miscellaneous		
Dry throat	1%	—
Influenza like illness	1%	—
Neck injury	1%	—
Pyrexia	1%	—

[a] Reactions reported by at least 1% of patients treated with zolpidem extended-release and at greater frequency than in the placebo group.
[b] Memory disorders include: amnesia, anterograde amnesia, memory impairment.

Dose relationship for adverse reactions: There is evidence from dose comparison trials suggesting a dose relationship for many of the adverse reactions associated with zolpidem use, particularly for certain CNS and GI adverse reactions.

➤*Other adverse reactions observed during the premarketing evaluation of zolpidem extended-release:* Adverse reactions are further classified within body system categories and enumerated in order of decreasing frequency.

Cardiovascular – Palpitation (greater than 1%); cerebrovascular disorder, hypertension, postural hypotension, syncope, tachycardia (0.1% to 1%); angina pectoris, arrhythmia, arteritis, circulatory failure, extrasystoles, hypertension aggravated, hypotension, myocardial infarction, phlebitis, postural hypotension, pulmonary edema, pulmonary embolism, syncope, varicose veins, ventricular tachycardia (greater than 0.1%).

CNS – Ataxia, confusion, depression, dizziness, drowsiness, drugged feeling, dry mouth, euphoria, headache, insomnia, lethargy, light-headedness, vertigo (greater than 1%); abnormal dreams, agitation, amnesia, anxiety, decreased cognition, detached feeling, difficulty concentrating, dysarthria, emotional lability, hallucination, hypoesthesia, illusion, leg cramps, migraine, nervousness, paresthesia, sleep disorder, sleeping (after daytime dosing), speech disorder, stupor, tremor (0.1% to 1%); abnormal gait, abnormal thinking, aggressive reaction, apathy, appetite increased, decreased libido, delusion, dementia, depersonalization, dysphasia, feeling strange, hypokinesia, hypotonia, hysteria, intoxicated feeling, manic reaction, neuralgia, neuritis, neuropathy, neurosis, panic attacks, paresis, personality disorder, somnambulism, suicide attempts, tenesmus, tetany, yawning (greater than 0.1%).

Dermatologic – Rash (greater than 1%); increased sweating, pallor, pruritus (0.1% to 1%); acne, bullous eruption, dermatitis, flushing, furunculosis, injection-site inflammation, photosensitivity reaction, urticaria (greater than 0.1%).

GI – Abdominal pain, diarrhea, dyspepsia, hiccup, nausea (greater than 1%); anorexia, constipation, dysphagia, flatulence, gastroenteritis, vomiting (0.1% to 1%); altered saliva, enteritis, eructation, esophagospasm, gastritis, hemorrhoids, increased saliva, intestinal obstruction, rectal hemorrhage, tooth caries (greater than 0.1%).

GU – Urinary tract infection (greater than 1%); cystitis, menstrual disorder, urinary incontinence, vaginitis (0.1% to 1%); acute renal failure, breast fibroadenosis, breast neoplasm, breast pain, dysuria, impotence, micturition frequency, nocturia, polyuria, pyelonephritis, renal pain, urinary retention (greater than 0.1%).

Hematologic/Lymphatic – Anemia, hyperhemoglobinemia, leukopenia, lymphadenopathy, macrocytic anemia, purpura, thrombosis (greater than 0.1%).

Hepatic – Abnormal hepatic function, increased ALT (0.1% to 1%); bilirubinemia, increased AST (greater than 0.1%).

Metabolic/Nutritional – Edema, hyperglycemia, thirst (0.1% to 1%); gout, hypercholesteremia, hyperlipidemia, increased alkaline phosphatase, increased serum urea nitrogen (BUN), periorbital edema, weight decrease (greater than 0.1%).

Musculoskeletal – Arthralgia, myalgia (greater than 1%); arthritis (0.1% to 1%); arthrosis, muscle weakness, sciatica, tendinitis (greater than 0.1%).

Respiratory – Pharyngitis, sinusitis, upper respiratory infection (greater than 1%); bronchitis, coughing, dyspnea, rhinitis (0.1% to 1%); bronchospasm, epistaxis, hypoxia, laryngitis, pneumonia (greater than 0.1%).

Special senses – Diplopia, vision abnormal (greater than 1%); eye irritation, eye pain, scleritis, taste perversion, tinnitus (0.1% to 1%); abnormal accommodation, conjunctivitis, corneal ulceration, glaucoma, lacrimation abnormal, parosmia, photopsia (greater than 0.1%).

Miscellaneous – Allergy, asthenia, back pain, influenza-like symptoms (greater than 1%); chest pain, falling, fatigue, fever, infection, malaise, trauma (0.1% to 1%); abdominal body sensation, abscess, allergic reaction, allergy aggravated, anaphylactic shock, face edema, herpes simplex, herpes zoster, hot flashes, increased erythrocyte sedimentation rate, otitis externa, otitis media, pain, restless legs, rigors, tolerance increased, (greater than 0.1%).

Overdosage

➤*Symptoms:* In postmarketing reports of overdose with zolpidem immediate-release alone, impairment of consciousness has ranged from somnolence to light coma. There was 1 case each of cardiovascular and res-

Imidazopyridines

ZOLPIDEM TARTRATE — ORAL

piratory compromise. Individuals have fully recovered from zolpidem overdoses up to 400 mg (40 times the maximum recommended dose of the immediate-release product). Overdose cases involving multiple CNS-depressant agents, including zolpidem, have resulted in more severe symptomatology, including fatal outcomes.

➤*Treatment:* As with the management of all overdosage, consider the possibility of multiple drug ingestion. Also consider contacting a poison control center for up-to-date information on the management of hypnotic drug product overdosage. Use general symptomatic and supportive measures along with immediate gastric lavage where appropriate. Administer IV fluids as needed. Flumazenil may be useful. As in all cases of drug overdose, monitor respiration, pulse, blood pressure, and other appropriate signs and general supportive measures employed. Monitor hypotension and CNS depression and treat by appropriate medical intervention. Withhold sedating drugs following zolpidem overdosage, even if excitation occurs. The value of dialysis in the treatment of overdosage has not been determined, although hemodialysis studies in patients with renal failure receiving therapeutic doses have demonstrated that zolpidem is not dialyzable.

Pyrazolopyrimidine

ZALEPLON

c-iv	**Sonata** (King)	**Capsules:** 5 mg	Lactose, tartrazine. (5 mg SONATA). Green/pale green. In 100s.
		10 mg	Lactose, tartrazine. (10 mg SONATA). Green/lt. green. In 100s.

ZALEPLON — ORAL

Indications

➤*Insomnia:* Zaleplon is indicated for the short-term treatment of insomnia. Zaleplon has been shown to decrease the time to sleep onset for up to 30 days in controlled clinical studies. It has not been shown to increase total sleep time or decrease the number of awakenings.

Hypnotics should generally be limited to 7 to 10 days of use, and reevaluation of the patient is recommended if they are to be taken for > 2 to 3 weeks. Zaleplon should not be prescribed in quantities exceeding a 1-month supply.

Administration and Dosage

➤*Approved by the FDA:* August 13, 1999.

The dose of zaleplon should be individualized. The recommended dose of zaleplon for most non-elderly adults is 10 mg. For certain low weight individuals, 5 mg may be a sufficient dose. Although the risk of certain adverse events associated with the use of zaleplon appears to be dose dependent, the 20 mg dose has been shown to be adequately tolerated and may be considered for the occasional patient who does not benefit from a trial of a lower dose. Doses above 20 mg have not been adequately evaluated and are not recommended.

Zaleplon should be taken immediately before bedtime or after the patient has gone to bed and has experienced difficulty falling asleep. Taking zaleplon with or immediately after a heavy, high-fat meal results in slower absorption and would be expected to reduce the effect of zaleplon on sleep latency.

➤*Special populations:*

Elderly and debilitated patients – Elderly patients and debilitated patients appear to be more sensitive to the effects of hypnotics, and respond to 5 mg of zaleplon. The recommended dose for these patients is therefore 5 mg. Doses over 10 mg are not recommended.

Hepatic function impairment – Patients with mild to moderate hepatic impairment should be treated with zaleplon 5 mg because clearance is reduced in this population. Zaleplon is not recommended for use in patients with severe hepatic impairment.

Patients taking cimetidine – An initial dose of 5 mg should be given to patients concomitantly taking cimetidine because zaleplon clearance is reduced in this population (see Drug Interactions).

➤*Storage/Stability:* Store at controlled room temperature, 20° to 25°C (68° to 77°F). Dispense in a light-resistant container.

Actions

➤*Pharmacology:* While zaleplon is a hypnotic agent with a chemical structure unrelated to benzodiazepines, barbiturates, or other drugs with known hypnotic properties, it interacts with the gamma-aminobutyric acid-benzodiazepine (GABA-BZ) receptor complex. Subunit modulation of the GABA-BZ receptor chloride channel macromolecular complex is hypothesized to be responsible for some of the pharmacological properties of benzodiazepines, which include sedative, anxiolytic, muscle relaxant, and anticonvulsive effects in animal models.

Other nonclinical studies have also shown that zaleplon binds selectively to the brain omega-1 receptor situated on the alpha subunit of the $GABA_A$/chloride ion channel receptor complex and potentiates t-butyl-bicyclophosphorothionate (TBPS) binding. Studies of binding of zaleplon to recombinant $GABA_A$ receptors ($\alpha_1\beta_1\gamma_2$ "omega-1" and $\alpha_2\beta_1\gamma_2$ "omega-2") have shown that zaleplon has a low affinity for these receptors, with preferential binding to the omega-1 receptor.

➤*Pharmacokinetics:*

Absorption – The pharmacokinetics of zaleplon have been investigated in more than 500 healthy subjects (young and elderly), nursing mothers, and patients with hepatic disease or renal disease. In healthy subjects, the pharmacokinetic profile has been examined after single doses of up to 60 mg and once-daily administration at 15 mg and 30 mg for 10 days. Zaleplon was rapidly absorbed with a time to peak concentration (t_{max}) of ≈ 1 hour and a terminal-phase elimination half-life ($t_{1/2}$) of ≈ 1 hour. Zaleplon does not accumulate with once-daily administration and its pharmacokinetics are dose proportional in the therapeutic range.

Zaleplon is rapidly and almost completely absorbed following oral administration. Peak plasma concentrations are attained within ≈ 1 hour after oral administration. Although zaleplon is well absorbed, its absolute bioavailability is ≈ 30% because it undergoes significant presystemic metabolism.

Effect of food: In healthy adults a high-fat/heavy meal prolonged the absorption of zaleplon compared to the fasted state, delaying t_{max} by ≈ 2 hours and reducing C_{max} by ≈ 35%. Zaleplon AUC and elimination half-life were not significantly affected. These results suggest that the effects of zaleplon on sleep onset may be reduced if it is taken with or immediately after a high-fat/heavy meal.

Distribution – Zaleplon is a lipophilic compound with a volume of distribution of ≈ 1.4 L/kg following intravenous (IV) administration, indicating substantial distribution into extravascular tissues. The in vitro plasma protein binding is ≈ 60% ± 15% and is independent of zaleplon concentration over the range of 10 ng/mL to 1000 ng/mL. This suggests that zaleplon disposition should not be sensitive to alterations in protein binding. The blood to plasma ratio for zaleplon is ≈ 1, indicating that zaleplon is uniformly distributed throughout the blood with no extensive distribution into red blood cells.

Metabolism – After oral administration, zaleplon is extensively metabolized, with < 1% of the dose excreted unchanged in urine. Zaleplon is primarily metabolized by aldehyde oxidase to form 5-oxo-zaleplon. Zaleplon is metabolized to a lesser extent by cytochrome P450 (CYP) 3A4 to form desethylzaleplon, which is quickly converted, presumably by aldehyde oxidase, to 5-oxo-desethylzaleplon. These oxidative metabolites are then converted to glucuronides and eliminated in urine. All of zaleplon's metabolites are pharmacologically inactive.

Excretion – After either oral or IV administration, zaleplon is rapidly eliminated with a mean $t_{1/2}$ of ≈ 1 hour. The oral-dose plasma clearance of zaleplon is about 3 L/hr/kg and the IV zaleplon plasma clearance is ≈ 1 L/hr/kg. Assuming normal hepatic blood flow and negligible renal clearance of zaleplon, the estimated hepatic extraction ratio of zaleplon is ≈ 0.7, indicating that zaleplon is subject to high first-pass metabolism.

After administration of a radiolabeled dose of zaleplon, 70% of the administered dose is recovered in urine within 48 hours (71% recovered within 6 days), almost all as zaleplon metabolites and their glucuronides. An additional 17% is recovered in feces within 6 days, most as 5-oxo-zaleplon.

Special populations –

Hepatic function impairment: Zaleplon is metabolized primarily by the liver and undergoes significant presystemic metabolism. Consequently, the oral clearance of zaleplon was reduced by 70% and 87% in compensated and decompensated cirrhotic patients, respectively, leading to marked increases in mean C_{max} and AUC (up to 4-fold and 7-fold in compensated and decompensated patients, respectively), in comparison with healthy subjects. The dose of zaleplon should therefore be reduced in patients with mild to moderate hepatic impairment (see Administration and Dosage). Zaleplon is not recommended for use in patients with severe hepatic impairment.

Race: The pharmacokinetics of zaleplon have been studied in Japanese subjects as representative of Asian populations. For this group, C_{max} and AUC were increased 37% and 64%, respectively. This finding can likely be attributed to differences in body weight, or alternatively, may represent differences in enzyme activities resulting from differences in diet, environment, or other factors. The effects of race on pharmacokinetic characteristics in other ethnic groups have not been well characterized.

Contraindications

None known.

Warnings

➤*Psychiatric/Physical disorder:* Because sleep disturbances may be the presenting manifestation of a physical or psychiatric disorder, symptomatic treatment of insomnia should be initiated only after a careful evaluation of the patient. The failure of insomnia to remit after 7 to 10 days of treatment may indicate the presence of a primary psychiatric or medical illness that should be evaluated. Worsening of insomnia or the emergence of new thinking or behavior abnormalities may be the consequence of an unrecognized psychiatric or physical disorder. Such findings have emerged during the course of treatment with sedative/hypnotic drugs, including zaleplon. Because some of the important adverse effects of zaleplon appear to be dose-

ZALEPLON — ORAL

related, it is important to use the lowest possible effective dose, especially in the elderly (see Administration and Dosage).

A variety of abnormal thinking and behavior changes have been reported to occur in association with the use of sedative/hypnotics. Some of these changes may be characterized by decreased inhibition (eg, aggressiveness and extroversion that seem out of character), similar to effects produced by alcohol and other CNS depressants. Other reported behavioral changes have included bizarre behavior, agitation, hallucinations, and depersonalization. Amnesia and other neuropsychiatric symptoms may occur unpredictably. In primarily depressed patients, worsening of depression, including suicidal thinking, has been reported in association with the use of sedative/hypnotics.

It can rarely be determined with certainty whether a particular instance of the abnormal behaviors listed above are drug induced, spontaneous in origin, or a result of an underlying psychiatric or physical disorder. Nonetheless, the emergence of any new behavioral sign or symptom of concern requires careful and immediate evaluation.

Following rapid dose decrease or abrupt discontinuation of the use of sedative/hypnotics, there have been reports of signs and symptoms similar to those associated with withdrawal from other CNS-depressant drugs (see Precautions, Drug abuse and dependence).

➤*Hepatic function impairment:* The dose of zaleplon should be reduced to 5 mg in patients with mild to moderate hepatic impairment. It is not recommended for use in patients with severe hepatic impairment.

➤*Carcinogenesis:* Lifetime carcinogenicity studies of zaleplon were conducted in mice and rats. Mice received doses of 25 mg/kg/day, 50 mg/kg/day, 100 mg/kg/day, and 200 mg/kg/day in the diet for 2 years. These doses are equivalent to 6 to 49 times the maximum recommended human dose (MRHD) of 20 mg on a mg/m^2 basis. There was a significant increase in the incidence of hepatocellular adenomas in female mice in the high dose group. Rats received doses of 1 mg/kg/day, 10 mg/kg/day, and 20 mg/kg/day in the diet for 2 years. These doses are equivalent to 0.5 to 10 times the MRHD of 20 mg on a mg/m^2 basis. Zaleplon was not carcinogenic in rats.

➤*Mutagenesis:* Zaleplon was clastogenic, both in the presence and absence of metabolic activation, causing structural and numerical aberrations (polyploidy and endoreduplication), when tested for chromosomal aberrations in the in vitro Chinese hamster ovary cell assay. In the in vitro human lymphocyte assay, zaleplon caused numerical but not structural aberrations, only in the presence of metabolic activation at the highest concentrations tested. In other in vitro assays, zaleplon was not mutagenic in the Ames bacterial gene mutation assay or the Chinese hamster ovary HGPRT gene mutation assay. Zaleplon was not clastogenic in 2 in vivo assays, the mouse bone marrow micronucleus assay and the rat bone marrow chromosomal aberration assay, and did not cause DNA damage in the rat hepatocyte unscheduled DNA synthesis assay.

➤*Fertility impairment:* In a fertility and reproductive performance study in rats, mortality and decreased fertility were associated with administration of an oral dose of zaleplon of 100 mg/kg/day to males and females prior to and during mating. This dose is equivalent to 49 times the MRHD of 20 mg on a mg/m^2 basis. Follow-up studies indicated that impaired fertility was due to an effect on the female.

➤*Elderly:* A total of 628 patients in double-blind, placebo-controlled, parallel-group clinical trials who received zaleplon were at least 65 years of age; of these, 311 received 5 mg and 317 received 10 mg. In both sleep laboratory and outpatient studies, elderly patients with insomnia responded to a 5 mg dose with a reduced sleep latency, and thus 5 mg is the recommended dose in this population. During short-term treatment (14 night studies) of elderly patients with zaleplon, no adverse event with a frequency of at least 1% occurred at a significantly higher rate with either 5 mg or 10 mg zaleplon than with placebo.

➤*Pregnancy: Category C.* In embryofetal development studies in rats and rabbits, oral administration of up to 100 mg/kg/day and 50 mg/kg/day, respectively, to pregnant animals throughout organogenesis produced no evidence of teratogenicity. These doses are equivalent to 49 (rat) and 48 (rabbit) times the MRHD of 20 mg on a mg/m^2 basis. In rats, pre- and postnatal growth was reduced in the offspring of dams receiving 100 mg/kg/day. This dose was also maternally toxic, as evidenced by clinical signs and decreased maternal body weight gain during gestation. The no-effect dose for rat offspring growth reduction was 10 mg/kg (a dose equivalent to 5 times the MRHD of 20 mg on a mg/m^2 basis). No adverse effects on embryofetal development were observed in rabbits at the doses examined.

In a pre- and postnatal development study in rats, increased stillbirth and postnatal mortality, and decreased growth and physical development, were observed in the offspring of females treated with doses of 7 mg/kg/day or greater during the latter part of gestation and throughout lactation. There was no evidence of maternal toxicity at this dose. The no-effect dose for offspring development was 1 mg/kg/day (a dose equivalent to 0.5 times the MRHD of 20 mg on a mg/m^2 basis). When the adverse effects on offspring viability and growth were examined in a cross-fostering study, they appeared to result from both in utero and lactational exposure to the drug.

There are no studies of zaleplon in pregnant women; therefore, zaleplon is not recommended for use in women during pregnancy.

Labor and delivery – Zaleplon has no established use in labor and delivery.

➤*Lactation:* A study in lactating mothers indicated that the clearance and half-life of zaleplon is similar to that in young healthy subjects. A small amount of zaleplon is excreted in breast milk, with the highest excreted amount occurring during a feeding at ≈ 1 hour after zaleplon administration. Since the small amount of the drug from breast milk may result in potentially important concentrations in infants, and because the effects of zaleplon on a nursing infant are not known, it is recommended that nursing mothers not take zaleplon.

➤*Children:* The safety and effectiveness of zaleplon in pediatric patients have not been established.

Precautions

➤*Timing of drug administration:* Zaleplon should be taken immediately before bedtime or after the patient has gone to bed and has experienced difficulty falling asleep. As with all sedative/hypnotics, taking zaleplon while still up and about may result in short-term memory impairment, hallucinations, impaired coordination, dizziness, and lightheadedness.

➤*Special risk:*

Use in the elderly or debilitated patients – Impaired motor or cognitive performance after repeated exposure or unusual sensitivity to sedative/hypnotic drugs is a concern in the treatment of elderly or debilitated patients. A dose of 5 mg is recommended for elderly patients to decrease the possibility of side effects (see Administration and Dosage). Elderly or debilitated patients should be monitored closely.

Use in patients with concomitant illness – Clinical experience with zaleplon in patients with concomitant systemic illness is limited. Zaleplon should be used with caution in patients with diseases or conditions that could affect metabolism or hemodynamic responses.

Although preliminary studies did not reveal respiratory depressant effects at hypnotic doses of zaleplon in healthy subjects, caution should be observed if zaleplon is prescribed to patients with compromised respiratory function, because sedative/hypnotics have the capacity to depress respiratory drive. Controlled trials of acute administration of zaleplon 10 mg in patients with chronic obstructive pulmonary disease or moderate obstructive sleep apnea showed no evidence of alterations in blood gases or apnea/hypopnea index, respectively. However, patients with compromised respiration due to preexisting illness should be monitored carefully.

Use in patients with depression – As with other sedative/hypnotic drugs, zaleplon should be administered with caution to patients exhibiting signs or symptoms of depression. Suicidal tendencies may be present in such patients and protective measures may be required. Intentional overdosage is more common in this group of patients (see Overdosage); therefore, the least amount of drug that is feasible should be prescribed for the patient at any one time.

➤*Drug abuse and dependence:*

Abuse – Two studies assessed the abuse liability of zaleplon at doses of 25 mg, 50 mg, and 75 mg in subjects with known histories of sedative drug abuse. The results of these studies indicate that zaleplon has an abuse potential similar to benzodiazepine and benzodiazepine-like hypnotics.

Dependence – The potential for developing physical dependence on zaleplon and a subsequent withdrawal syndrome was assessed in controlled studies of 14-, 28-, and 35-night durations and in open-label studies of 6- and 12-month durations by examining for the emergence of rebound insomnia following drug discontinuation. Some patients (mostly those treated with 20 mg) experienced a mild rebound insomnia on the first night following withdrawal that appeared to be resolved by the second night. The use of the Benzodiazepine Withdrawal Symptom Questionnaire and examination of any other withdrawal emergent events did not detect any other evidence for a withdrawal syndrome following abrupt discontinuation of zaleplon therapy in premarketing studies.

However, available data cannot provide a reliable estimate of the incidence of dependence during treatment at recommended doses of zaleplon. Other sedative/hypnotics have been associated with various signs and symptoms following abrupt discontinuation, ranging from mild dysphoria and insomnia to a withdrawal syndrome that may include abdominal and muscle cramps, vomiting, sweating, tremors, and convulsions. Seizures have been observed in 2 patients, one of which had a prior seizure, in clinical trials with zaleplon. Seizures and death have been seen following the withdrawal of zaleplon from animals at doses many times higher than those proposed for human use. Because individuals with a history of addiction to, or abuse of, drugs or alcohol are at risk of habituation and dependence, they should be under careful surveillance when receiving zaleplon or any other hypnotic.

➤*Hazardous tasks.* Zaleplon, like other hypnotics, has CNS depressant effects. Because of the rapid onset of action, zaleplon should only be ingested immediately prior to going to bed or after the patient has gone to bed and has experienced difficulty falling asleep. Patients receiving zaleplon should be cautioned against engaging in hazardous occupations requiring complete mental alertness or motor coordination (eg, operating machinery or driving a motor vehicle) after ingesting the drug, including potential impairment of the performance of such activities that may occur the day following ingestion of zaleplon. Zaleplon, as well as other hypnotics, may produce additive CNS depressant effects when coadministered with other psychotropic medications, anticonvulsants, antihistamines, ethanol, and other drugs that themselves produce CNS depression. Zaleplon should not be taken with alcohol. Dosage adjustment may be necessary when zaleplon is administered with other CNS-depressant agents because of the potentially additive effects.

➤*Tartrazine sensitivity:* This product contains FD&C Yellow No. 5 (tartrazine) which may cause allergic-type reactions (including bronchial asthma) in certain susceptible persons. Although the overall incidence of FD&C Yellow No. 5 (tartrazine) sensitivity in the general population is low, it is frequently seen in patients who also have aspirin hypersensitivity.

ZALEPLON — ORAL

Drug Interactions

➤*CNS-active drugs:*

Ethanol – Zaleplon 10 mg potentiated the CNS-impairing effects of ethanol 0.75 g/kg on balance testing and reaction time for 1 hour after ethanol administration and on the digit symbol substitution test (DSST), symbol copying test, and the variability component of the divided attention test for 2.5 hours after ethanol administration. The potentiation resulted from a CNS pharmacodynamic interaction; zaleplon did not affect the pharmacokinetics of ethanol.

Imipramine – Coadministration of single doses of zaleplon 20 mg and imipramine 75 mg produced additive effects on decreased alertness and impaired psychomotor performance for 2 to 4 hours after administration. The interaction was pharmacodynamic with no alteration of the pharmacokinetics of either drug.

Thioridazine – Coadministration of single doses of zaleplon 20 mg and thioridazine 50 mg produced additive effects on decreased alertness and impaired psychomotor performance for 2 to 4 hours after administration. The interaction was phamacodynamic with no alteration of the pharmacokinetics of either drug.

➤*Drugs that induce CYP3A4:*

Rifampin – CYP3A4 is ordinarily a minor metabolizing enzyme of zaleplon. Multiple-dose administration of the potent CYP3A4 inducer rifampin (600 mg every 24 hours for 14 days), however, reduced zaleplon C_{max} and AUC by ≈ 80%. The coadministration of a potent CYP3A4 enzyme inducer, although not posing a safety concern, thus could lead to ineffectiveness of zaleplon. An alternative non-CYP3A4 substrate hypnotic agent may be considered in patients taking CYP3A4 inducers such as rifampin, phenytoin, carbamazepine, and phenobarbital.

➤*Drugs that inhibit both aldehyde oxidase and CYP3A4:*

Cimetidine – Cimetidine inhibits both aldehyde oxidase (in vitro) and CYP3A4 (in vitro and in vivo), the primary and secondary enzymes, respectively, responsible for zaleplon metabolism. Concomitant administration of zaleplon (10 mg) and cimetidine (800 mg) produced an 85% increase in the mean C_{max} and AUC of zaleplon. An initial dose of 5 mg should be given to patients who are concomitantly being treated with cimetidine.

Adverse Reactions

➤*Adverse findings observed in short-term, placebo-controlled trials:*

Adverse events occurring at an incidence of 1% or more among zaleplon 20 mg-treated patients – The table below enumerates the incidence of treatment-emergent adverse events for a pool of three 28-night and one 35-night placebo-controlled studies of zaleplon at doses of 5 mg or 10 mg and 20 mg. The table includes only those events that occurred in 1% or more of patients treated with zaleplon 20 mg and that had a higher incidence in patients treated with zaleplon 20 mg than in placebo-treated patients.

Incidence (%) of treatment-emergent adverse events in long-term (28 and 35 nights) placebo-controlled clinical trials of zaleplon[1]

Body system/ preferred term	Placebo (n = 344)	Zaleplon 5 mg or 10 mg (n = 569)	Zaleplon 20 mg (n = 297)
Miscellaneous			
Abdominal pain	3%	6%	6%
Asthenia	5%	5%	7%
Headache	35%	30%	42%
Malaise	< 1%	< 1%	2%
Photosensitivity reaction	< 1%	< 1%	1%
GI			
Anorexia	< 1%	< 1%	2%
Colitis	0%	0%	1%
Nausea	7%	6%	8%
Metabolic and nutritional			
Peripheral edema	< 1%	< 1%	1%
CNS			
Amnesia	1%	2%	4%
Confusion	< 1%	< 1%	1%
Depersonalization	< 1%	< 1%	2%
Dizziness	7%	7%	9%
Hallucinations	< 1%	< 1%	1%
Hypertonia	< 1%	1%	1%
Hypesthesia	< 1%	< 1%	2%
Paresthesia	1%	3%	3%
Somnolence	4%	5%	6%
Tremor	1%	2%	2%
Vertigo	< 1%	< 1%	1%
Respiratory			
Epistaxis	< 1%	< 1%	1%
Special senses			
Abnormal vision	< 1%	< 1%	2%
Ear pain	0%	< 1%	1%
Eye pain	2%	4%	3%
Hyperacusis	< 1%	1%	2%
Parosmia	< 1%	< 1%	2%
GU			
Dysmenorrhea	2%	3%	4%

[1] Events for which the incidence for zaleplon 20 mg-treated patients was at least 1% and greater than the incidence among placebo-treated patients. Incidence greater than 1% has been rounded to the nearest whole number.

➤*Other adverse events observed during the premarketing evaluation of zaleplon:* Events are further categorized by body system and listed in order of decreasing frequency according to the following definitions: Frequent adverse events are those occurring on one or more occasions in at least 1/100 patients; infrequent adverse events are those occurring in < 1/100 patients but at least 1/1000 patients; rare events are those occurring in < 1/1000 patients.

Cardiovascular –
Frequent: Migraine.
Infrequent: Angina pectoris, bundle branch block, hypertension, hypotension, palpitation, syncope, tachycardia, vasodilatation, ventricular extrasystoles.
Rare: Bigeminy, cerebral ischemia, cyanosis, pericardial effusion, postural hypotension, pulmonary embolus, sinus bradycardia, thrombophlebitis, ventricular tachycardia.

CNS –
Frequent: Anxiety, depression, nervousness, thinking abnormal (mainly difficulty concentrating).
Infrequent: Abnormal gait, agitation, apathy, ataxia, circumoral paresthesia, emotional lability, euphoria, hyperesthesia, hyperkinesia, hypotonia, incoordination, insomnia, libido decreased, neuralgia, nystagmus.
Rare: CNS stimulation, delusions, dysarthria, dystonia, facial paralysis, hostility, hypokinesia, myoclonus, neuropathy, psychomotor retardation, ptosis, reflexes decreased, reflexes increased, sleep talking, sleep walking, slurred speech, stupor, trismus.

Dermatologic –
Frequent: Pruritus, rash.
Infrequent: Acne, alopecia, contact dermatitis, dry skin, eczema, maculopapular rash, skin hypertrophy, sweating, urticaria, vesiculobullous rash.
Rare: Melanosis, psoriasis, pustular rash, skin discoloration.

Endocrine –
Rare: Diabetes mellitus, goiter, hypothyroidism.

GI –
Frequent: Constipation, dry mouth, dyspepsia.
Infrequent: Eructation, esophagitis, flatulence, gastritis, gastroenteritis, gingivitis, glossitis, increased appetite, melena, mouth ulceration, rectal hemorrhage, stomatitis.
Rare: Aphthous stomatitis, biliary pain, bruxism, cardiospasm, cheilitis, cholelithiasis, duodenal ulcer, dysphagia, enteritis, gum hemorrhage, increased salivation, intestinal obstruction, abnormal liver function tests, peptic ulcer, tongue discoloration, tongue edema, ulcerative stomatitis.

GU –
Infrequent: Bladder pain, breast pain, cystitis, decreased urine stream, dysuria, hematuria, impotence, kidney calculus, kidney pain, menorrhagia, metrorrhagia, urinary frequency, urinary incontinence, urinary urgency, vaginitis.
Rare: Albuminuria, delayed menstrual period, leukorrhea, menopause, urethritis, urinary retention, vaginal hemorrhage.

Hematologic/Lymphatic –
Infrequent: Anemia, ecchymosis, lymphadenopathy.
Rare: Eosinophilia, leukocytosis, lymphocytosis, purpura.

Metabolic/Nutritional –
Infrequent: Edema, gout, hypercholesteremia, thirst, weight gain.
Rare: Bilirubinemia, hyperglycemia, hyperuricemia, hypoglycemia, hypoglycemic reaction, ketosis, lactose intolerance, AST increased, ALT increased, weight loss.

Musculoskeletal –
Frequent: Arthralgia, arthritis, myalgia.
Infrequent: Arthrosis, bursitis, joint disorder (mainly swelling, stiffness, and pain), myasthenia, tenosynovitis.
Rare: Myositis, osteoporosis.

Special senses –
Frequent: Conjunctivitis, taste perversion.
Infrequent: Diplopia, dry eyes, photophobia, tinnitus, watery eyes.
Rare: Abnormality of accommodation, blepharitis, cataract specified, corneal erosion, deafness, eye hemorrhage, glaucoma, labyrinthitis, retinal detachment, taste loss, visual field defect.

Miscellaneous –
Frequent: Back pain, chest pain, fever.
Infrequent: Chest pain substernal, chills, face edema, generalized edema, hangover effect, neck rigidity.

Overdosage

➤*Symptoms:* Signs and symptoms of overdose effects of CNS depressants can be expected to present as exaggerations of the pharmacological effects noted in preclinical testing. Overdose is usually manifested by degrees of central nervous system depression ranging from drowsiness to coma. In mild

Pyrazolopyrimidine

ZALEPLON — ORAL

cases, symptoms include drowsiness, mental confusion, and lethargy; in more serious cases, symptoms may include ataxia, hypotonia, hypotension, respiratory depression, rarely coma, and very rarely death.

There is limited premarketing clinical experience with the effects of an overdosage of zaleplon. Two cases of overdose were reported. One was the accidental ingestion by a 2½-year-old boy of 20 mg to 40 mg of zaleplon. The second was a 20-year-old man who took 100 mg zaleplon plus 2.25 mg of triazolam. Both were treated and recovered uneventfully.

➤*Treatment:* General symptomatic and supportive measures should be used along with immediate gastric lavage where appropriate. Intravenous fluids should be administered as needed. Animal studies suggest that flumazenil is an antagonist to zaleplon. However, there is no premarketing clinical experience with the use of flumazenil as an antidote to a zaleplon overdose. As in all cases of drug overdose, respiration, pulse, blood pressure, and other appropriate signs should be monitored and general supportive measures employed. Hypotension and CNS depression should be monitored and treated by appropriate medical intervention.

Melatonin Receptor Agonist

RAMELTEON

Rx	**Rozerem** (Takeda Pharmaceutical)	**Tablets:** 8 mg	Lactose. (TAK RAM-8). Film coated. In 30s, 100s, and 500s

RAMELTEON — ORAL

Indications

➤*Insomnia:* Ramelteon is indicated for the treatment of insomnia characterized by difficulty with sleep onset.

Administration and Dosage

➤*Approved by the FDA:* July 22, 2005.

➤*Dosage:* The recommended dose of ramelteon is 8 mg taken within 30 minutes of going to bed. It is recommended that ramelteon not be taken with or immediately after a high-fat meal.

➤*Hepatic function impairment:* Ramelteon should not be used in patients with severe hepatic function impairment. Ramelteon should be used with caution in patients with moderate hepatic function impairment.

➤*Concomitant medications:* Ramelteon should not be used in combination with fluvoxamine.

Ramelteon should be used with caution in patients taking other CYP1A2-inhibiting drugs.

➤*Storage/Stability:* Store at 25°C (77°F); excursions permitted to 15° to 30°C (59° to 86°F). Keep container tightly closed; protect from moisture and humidity.

Actions

➤*Pharmacology:*

Pharmacodynamics – Ramelteon is a melatonin receptor agonist with high affinity for melatonin MT_1 and MT_2 receptors and selectivity over the MT_3 receptor. Ramelteon demonstrates full agonist activity in vitro in cells expressing human MT_1 or MT_2 receptors, and high selectivity for human MT_1 and MT_2 receptors compared with the MT_3 receptor.

The activity of ramelteon at the MT_1 and MT_2 receptors is believed to contribute to its sleep-promoting properties, as these receptors, acted upon by endogenous melatonin, are thought to be involved in the maintenance of the circadian rhythm underlying the normal sleep-wake cycle.

The major metabolite of ramelteon, M-II, is active and has approximately one tenth and one fifth the binding affinity of the parent molecule for the human MT_1 and MT_2 receptors, respectively, and is 17- to 25-fold less potent than ramelteon in in vitro functional assays. Although the potency of M-II at MT_1 and MT_2 receptors is lower than the parent drug, M-II circulates at higher concentrations than the parent, producing 20- to 100-fold greater mean systemic exposure when compared with ramelteon. M-II has weak affinity for the serotonin 5-HT_{2B} receptor but no appreciable affinity for other receptors or enzymes. Similar to ramelteon, M-II does not interfere with the activity of a number of endogenous enzymes.

➤*Pharmacokinetics:*

Absorption – The pharmacokinetic profile of ramelteon has been evaluated in healthy subjects as well as in subjects with hepatic or renal impairment.

Ramelteon is absorbed rapidly, with median peak concentrations occurring at approximately 0.75 hours (range, 0.5 to 1.5 hours) after fasted oral administration. Although the total absorption of ramelteon is at least 84%, the absolute oral bioavailability is only 1.8% because of extensive first-pass metabolism.

Food effect: When administered with a high-fat meal, the area under the curve $(AUC)_{0-\infty}$ for a single 16 mg dose of ramelteon was 31% higher, and the maximum serum concentration (C_{max}) was 22% lower, than when given in a fasted state. Median time to maximum serum concentration (T_{max}) was delayed by approximately 45 minutes when ramelteon was administered with food. Effects of food on the AUC values for M-II were similar. It is therefore recommended that ramelteon not be taken with or immediately after a high-fat meal.

Distribution – In vitro protein binding of ramelteon is approximately 82% in human serum, independent of concentration. Binding to albumin accounts for most of that binding because 70% of the drug is bound in human serum albumin.

Ramelteon is not distributed selectively to red blood cells. Ramelteon has a mean volume of distribution after intravenous (IV) administration of 73.6 L, suggesting substantial tissue distribution.

Metabolism – When administered orally to humans in doses ranging from 4 to 64 mg, ramelteon undergoes rapid, high first-pass metabolism, and exhibits linear pharmacokinetics. C_{max} and AUC data show substantial intersubject variability, consistent with the high first-pass effect; the coefficient of variation for these values is approximately 100%. Several metabolites have been identified in human serum and urine.

Metabolism of ramelteon consists primarily of oxidation to hydroxyl and carbonyl derivatives, with secondary metabolism producing glucuronide conjugates. CYP1A2 is the major isozyme involved in the hepatic metabolism of ramelteon; the CYP2C subfamily and CYP3A4 isozymes also are involved to a minor degree.

The rank order of the principal metabolites by prevalence in human serum is M-II, M-IV, M-I, and M-III. These metabolites are formed rapidly and exhibit a monophasic decline and rapid elimination. The overall mean systemic exposure of M-II is approximately 20- to 100-fold higher than the parent drug.

Excretion – Following oral administration of radiolabeled ramelteon, 84% of total radioactivity was excreted in urine and approximately 4% in feces, resulting in a mean recovery of 88%. Less than 0.1% of the dose was excreted in urine and feces as the parent compound. Elimination was essentially complete by 96 hours postdose.

Repeated once-daily dosing with ramelteon does not result in significant accumulation because of the short elimination half-life of ramelteon (on average, approximately 1 to 2.6 hours).

The half-life of M-II is 2 to 5 hours and is independent of dose. Serum concentrations of the parent drug and its metabolites in humans are at or below the lower limits of quantitation within 24 hours.

Special populations –

Hepatic function impairment: Exposure to ramelteon was increased almost 4-fold in subjects with mild hepatic function impairment after 7 days of dosing with 16 mg/day; exposure was further increased (more than 10-fold) in subjects with moderate hepatic function impairment. Exposure to M-II was only marginally increased in mildly and moderately impaired subjects relative to healthy matched controls. The pharmacokinetics of ramelteon have not been evaluated in subjects with severe hepatic function impairment (Child-Pugh class C). Use ramelteon with caution in patients with moderate hepatic function impairment.

Elderly: In a group of 24 elderly subjects 63 to 79 years of age administered a single ramelteon 16 mg dose, the mean C_{max} and $AUC_{0-\infty}$ values were 11.6 ng/mL (standard deviation "SD", 13.8) and 18.7 ng•h/mL (SD, 19.4), respectively. The elimination half-life was 2.6 hours (SD, 1.1). Compared with younger adults, the total exposure ($AUC_{0-\infty}$) and C_{max} of ramelteon were 97% and 86% higher, respectively, in elderly subjects. The $AUC_{0-\infty}$ and C_{max} of M-II were increased by 30% and 13%, respectively, in elderly subjects.

Gender: There are no clinically meaningful gender-related differences in the pharmacokinetics of ramelteon or its metabolites.

Contraindications

Ramelteon is contraindicated in patients with a hypersensitivity to ramelteon or any components of the ramelteon formulation.

Warnings

➤*Psychiatric/Physical disorder:* Because sleep disturbances may be the presenting manifestation of a physical and/or psychiatric disorder, initiate symptomatic treatment of insomnia only after a careful evaluation of the patient. The failure of insomnia to remit after a reasonable period of treatment may indicate the presence of a primary psychiatric and/or medical illness that should be evaluated. Worsening of insomnia, or the emergence of new cognitive or behavioral abnormalities, may be the result of an unrecognized underlying psychiatric or physical disorder and requires further evaluation of the patient. As with other hypnotics, exacerbation of insomnia and emergence of cognitive and behavioral abnormalities were seen with ramelteon during the clinical development program.

A variety of cognitive and behavior changes have been reported to occur in association with the use of hypnotics. Primarily in depressed patients, worsening of depression, including suicidal ideation, has been reported in association with the use of hypnotics.

After taking ramelteon, patients should confine their activities to those necessary to prepare for bed.

➤*Hepatic function impairment:* Do not use ramelteon in patients with severe hepatic function impairment.

➤*Carcinogenesis:* In a 2-year carcinogenicity study, B6C3F1 mice were administered ramelteon at dosages of 0, 30, 100, 300, or 1,000 mg/kg/day by oral gavage. Male mice exhibited a dose-related increase in the incidence of hepatic tumors at dosage levels of 100 mg/kg/day or more, including hepatic adenoma, hepatic carcinoma, and hepatoblastoma. Female mice developed a dose-related increase in the incidence of hepatic adenomas at dosage levels of 300 mg/kg/day or more and hepatic carcinoma at the 1,000 mg/kg/day dosage

RAMELTEON — ORAL

level. The no-effect level for hepatic tumors in male mice was 30 mg/kg/day (103 times and 3 times the therapeutic exposure to ramelteon and the active metabolite M-II, respectively, at the maximum recommended human dosage "MRHD" based on an AUC comparison). The no-effect level for hepatic tumors in female mice was 100 mg/kg/day (827 and 12 times the therapeutic exposure to ramelteon and M-II, respectively, at the MRHD based on AUC).

In a 2-year carcinogenicity study conducted in the Sprague-Dawley rat model, male and female rats were administered ramelteon at dosages of 0, 15, 60, 250, or 1,000 mg/kg/day by oral gavage. Male rats exhibited a dose-related increase in the incidence of hepatic adenoma and benign Leydig cell tumors of the testis at dosage levels greater than or equal to 250 mg/kg/day and hepatic carcinoma at the 1,000 mg/kg/day dosage level. Female rats exhibited a dose-related increase in the incidence of hepatic adenoma at dosage levels greater than or equal to 60 mg/kg/day and hepatic carcinoma at the 1,000 mg/kg/day dosage level. The no-effect level for hepatic tumors and benign Leydig cell tumors in male rats was 60 mg/kg/day (1,429 times and 12 times the therapeutic exposure to ramelteon and M-II, respectively, at the MRHD based on AUC). The no-effect level for hepatic tumors in female rats was 15 mg/kg/day (472 times and 16 times the therapeutic exposure to ramelteon and M-II, respectively, at the MRHD based on AUC).

The development of hepatic tumors in rodents following chronic treatment with nongenotoxic compounds may be secondary to microsomal enzyme induction, a mechanism for tumor generation not thought to occur in humans. Leydig cell tumor development following treatment with nongenotoxic compounds in rodents has been linked to reductions in circulating testosterone levels with compensatory increases in luteinizing hormone release, which is a known proliferative stimulus to Leydig cells in the rat testis. Rat Leydig cells are more sensitive to the stimulatory effects of luteinizing hormone than human Leydig cells. In mechanistic studies conducted in the rat, daily ramelteon administration at 250 and 1,000 mg/kg/day for 4 weeks was associated with a reduction in plasma testosterone levels. In the same study, luteinizing hormone levels were elevated over a 24-hour period after the last ramelteon treatment; however, the durability of this luteinizing hormone finding and its support for the proposed mechanistic explanation was not clearly established.

➤*Mutagenesis:* Ramelteon was not genotoxic in the following: in vitro bacterial reverse mutation (Ames) assay; in vitro mammalian cell gene mutation assay using the mouse lymphoma TK+/- cell line; in vivo/in vitro unscheduled DNA synthesis assay in rat hepatocytes; and in in vivo micronucleus assays conducted in mouse and rat. Ramelteon was positive in the chromosomal aberration assay in Chinese hamster lung cells in the presence of S9 metabolic activation.

Separate studies indicated that the concentration of the M-II metabolite formed by the rat liver S9 fraction used in the in vitro genetic toxicology studies described above, exceeded the concentration of ramelteon; therefore, the genotoxic potential of the M-II metabolite also was assessed in these studies.

➤*Fertility impairment:* Ramelteon was administered to male and female Sprague-Dawley rats in an initial fertility and early embryonic development study at dosage levels of 6, 60, or 600 mg/kg/day. No effects on male or female mating or fertility were observed with a ramelteon dosage up to 600 mg/kg/day (786 times higher than the MRHD on a mg/m^2 basis). Irregular estrus cycles, reduction in the number of implants, and reduction in the number of live embryos were noted with dosing females at greater than or equal to 60 mg/kg/day (79 times higher than the MRHD on a mg/m^2 basis). A reduction in the number of corpora lutea occurred at the 600 mg/kg/day dosage level. Administration of ramelteon up to 600 mg/kg/day to male rats for 7 weeks had no effect on sperm quality, and when the treated male rats were mated with untreated female rats there was no effect on implants or embryos. In a repeat of this study using oral administration of ramelteon at 20, 60, or 200 mg/kg/day for the same study duration, females demonstrated irregular estrus cycles with dosages greater than or equal to 60 mg/kg/day, but no effects were seen on implantation or embryo viability. The no-effect dosage for fertility end points was 20 mg/kg/day in females (26 times the MRHD on a mg/m^2 basis) and 600 mg/kg/day in males (786 times higher than the MRHD on a mg/m^2 basis) when considering all studies.

➤*Pregnancy: Category C.* Ramelteon has been shown to be a developmental teratogen in the rat when given in doses 197 times higher than the MRHD on a mg/m^2 basis. There are no adequate and well-controlled studies in pregnant women. Use ramelteon during pregnancy only if the potential benefit justifies the potential risk to the fetus.

The effects of ramelteon on embryo-fetal development were assessed in both the rat and rabbit. Pregnant rats were administered ramelteon by oral gavage at dosages of 0, 10, 40, 150, or 600 mg/kg/day during gestation days 6 to 17, which is the period of organogenesis in this species. Evidence of maternal toxicity and fetal teratogenicity was observed at dosages of 150 mg/kg/day or more. Maternal toxicity was chiefly characterized by decreased body weight and, at 600 mg/kg/day, ataxia and decreased spontaneous movement. At maternally toxic dosages (150 mg/kg/day or more), the fetuses demonstrated visceral malformations consisting of diaphragmatic hernia and minor anatomical variations of the skeleton (irregularly shaped scapula). At 600 mg/kg/day, reductions in fetal body weights and malformations, including cysts on the external genitalia were additionally observed. The no-effect level for teratogenicity in this study was 40 mg/kg/day (1,892 times and 45 times higher than the therapeutic exposure to ramelteon and the active metabolite M-II, respectively, at the MRHD based on AUC). Pregnant rabbits were administered ramelteon by oral gavage at dosages of 0, 12, 60, or 300 mg/kg/day during gestation days 6 to 18, which is the period of organogenesis in this species. Although maternal toxicity was apparent with a ramelteon dosage of 300 mg/kg/day, no evidence of fetal effects or teratogenicity was associated with any dose level. The no-effect level for teratogenicity was, therefore, 300 mg/kg/day (11,862 times and 99 times higher than the therapeutic exposure to ramelteon and M-II, respectively, at the MRHD based on AUC).

The effects of ramelteon on pre- and postnatal development in rats were studied by administration of ramelteon to the pregnant rats by oral gavage at dosages of 0, 30, 100, or 300 mg/kg/day from day 6 of gestation through parturition to postnatal (lactation) day 21, at which time offspring were weaned. Maternal toxicity was noted at dosages of 100 mg/kg/day or more and consisted of reduced body weight gain and increased adrenal gland weight. Reduced body weight during the postweaning period also was noticed in the offspring of the groups given 100 mg/kg/day or more. Offspring in the 300 mg/kg/day group demonstrated physical and developmental delays including delayed eruption of the lower incisors, delayed acquisition of the righting reflex, and alteration of emotional response. These delays are often observed in the presence of reduced offspring body weight but may still be indicative of developmental delay. An apparent decrease in the viability of offspring in the 300 mg/kg/day group was likely caused by altered maternal behavior and function observed at this dosage level. Offspring of the 300 mg/kg/day group also showed evidence of diaphragmatic hernia, a finding observed in the embryo-fetal development study previously described. There were no effects on the reproductive capacity of offspring and the resulting progeny were not different from those of vehicle-treated offspring. The no-effect level for pre- and postnatal development in this study was 30 mg/kg/day (39 times higher than the MRHD on a mg/m^2 basis).

Labor and delivery – The potential effects of ramelteon on the duration of labor and/or delivery, for either the mother or the fetus, have not been studied. Ramelteon has no established use in labor and delivery.

➤*Lactation:* Ramelteon is secreted into the milk of lactating rats. It is not known whether this drug is excreted in human milk. No clinical studies in breast-feeding mothers have been performed. The use of ramelteon in breast-feeding mothers is not recommended.

➤*Children:* Safety and efficacy of ramelteon in children have not been established. Further study is needed prior to determining that this product may be used safely in prepubescent and pubescent patients.

Use in adolescents and children – Ramelteon has been associated with an effect on reproductive hormones in adults (eg, decreased testosterone levels, increased prolactin levels). It is not known what effect chronic or even chronic, intermittent use of ramelteon may have on the reproductive axis in developing humans.

Precautions

➤*Monitoring:* For patients presenting with unexplained amenorrhea, galactorrhea, decreased libido, or problems with fertility, consider assessment of prolactin levels and testosterone levels as appropriate.

➤*Special risk:* Ramelteon has not been studied in subjects with severe sleep apnea or severe COPD and is not recommended for use in those populations. Advise patients to exercise caution if they consume alcohol in combination with ramelteon.

➤*Hazardous tasks:* Patients should avoid engaging in hazardous activities that require concentration (eg, operating a motor vehicle or heavy machinery) after taking ramelteon.

Drug Interactions

➤*CYP450 enzymes:* Ramelteon has a highly variable intersubject pharmacokinetic profile (approximately 100% coefficient of variation in C_{max} and AUC). As noted above, CYP1A2 is the major isozyme involved in the metabolism of ramelteon; the CYP2C subfamily and CYP3A4 isozymes also are involved to a minor degree.

Ramelteon Drug Interactions

Precipitant drug	Object drug[a]		Description
Alcohol	Ramelteon	⬆	Concomitant use may produce additive CNS effects.
Azole antifungals (ketoconazole, fluconazole)	Ramelteon	⬆	When administered with ketoconazole, the AUC and C_{max} of ramelteon increased by approximately 84% and 36%, respectively. The AUC and C_{max} of ramelteon also was increased by approximately 150% when administered with fluconazole. Similar increases also were seen in M-II exposure.
Fluvoxamine	Ramelteon	⬆	Ramelteon AUC increased approximately 190-fold, and the C_{max} increased approximately 70-fold. Do not use ramelteon in combination with fluvoxamine.
Rifampin	Ramelteon	⬇	Ramelteon and metabolite M-II had a decrease in both AUC and C_{max} by approximately 80% when administered with rifampin.

[a] ⬇ = Object drug decreased. ⬆ = Object drug increased.

➤*Drug/Food interactions:* When administered with a high-fat meal, the $AUC_{0-\infty}$ for a single 16 mg dose of ramelteon was 31% higher, and the C_{max} was 22% lower, than when given in a fasted state. Median T_{max} was delayed

Melatonin Receptor Agonist

RAMELTEON — ORAL

by approximately 45 minutes when ramelteon was administered with food. Effects of food on the AUC values for M-II were similar. It is therefore recommended that ramelteon not be taken with or immediately after a high-fat meal.

Adverse Reactions

➤*Adverse reactions resulting in discontinuation of treatment:* Five percent of the 3,594 individual subjects exposed to ramelteon in clinical trials discontinued treatment because of an adverse reaction, compared with 2% of the 1,370 subjects receiving placebo. The most frequent adverse reactions leading to discontinuation in subjects receiving ramelteon were somnolence (0.8%), dizziness (0.5%), nausea (0.3%), fatigue (0.3%), headache (0.3%), and insomnia (0.3%).

Most commonly observed adverse reactions in phase 1 through 3 trials –

Ramelteon Adverse Reactions (%)		
Adverse reaction	Placebo (n = 1,370)	8 mg (n = 1,250)
CNS		
Depression	1%	2%
Dizziness	3%	5%
Fatigue	2%	4%
Headache	7%	7%
Insomnia exacerbated	2%	3%
Somnolence	3%	5%
GI		
Diarrhea	2%	2%
Dysgeusia	1%	2%
Nausea	2%	3%
Miscellaneous		
Arthralgia	1%	2%
Blood cortisol decreased	0%	1%
Influenza	0%	1%
Myalgia	1%	2%
Upper respiratory tract infection	2%	3%

Overdosage

➤*Symptoms:* No cases of ramelteon overdose have been reported during clinical development.

Ramelteon was administered in single doses up to 160 mg in an abuse liability trial. No safety or tolerability concerns were seen.

➤*Treatment:* Use general symptomatic and supportive measures, along with immediate gastric lavage when appropriate. Administer IV fluids as needed. As in all cases of drug overdose, monitor respiration, pulse, blood pressure, and other appropriate vital signs, and employ general supportive measures.

Hemodialysis does not effectively reduce exposure to ramelteon. Therefore, the use of dialysis in the treatment of overdosage is not appropriate.

Patient Information

Advise patients to take ramelteon within 30 minutes prior to going to bed and to confine their activities to those necessary to prepare for bed.

Advise patients to avoid engaging in hazardous activities (eg, operating a motor vehicle or heavy machinery) after taking ramelteon.

Advise patients not to take ramelteon with or immediately after a high-fat meal.

Advise patients to consult their health care provider if they experience worsening of insomnia or any new behavioral signs or symptoms of concern.

Advise patients to consult their health care provider if they experience 1 of the following: cessation of menses or galactorrhea in women, decreased libido, or problems with fertility.

Advise patients to exercise caution if they consume alcohol in combination with ramelteon.

Benzodiazepines

Refer to the general discussion beginning in the Sedative and Hypnotic, Nonbarbiturate introduction. For information on benzodiazepines used as antianxiety agents, refer to the group monograph in the Antianxiety Agents section.

Indications

➤*Insomnia:* Insomnia characterized by difficulty in falling asleep, frequent nocturnal awakenings or early morning awakening. Can be used for recurring insomnia or poor sleeping habits and in acute or chronic medical situations requiring restful sleep.

Insomnia is often transient and intermittent; therefore, prolonged administration is generally not recommended. Because insomnia may be a symptom of other disorders, consider the possibility that the complaint may be related to a condition for which there is more specific treatment.

Actions

➤*Pharmacology:* Estazolam, flurazepam, quazepam, temazepam and triazolam are benzodiazepine derivatives useful as hypnotics. Benzodiazepines are believed to potentiate gamma aminobutyric acid (GABA) neuronal inhibition. The sedative and anticonvulsant actions involve GABA receptors located in the limbic, neocortical and mesencephalic reticular systems.

At least two benzodiazepine receptor subtypes have been identified in the brain, BZ_1 and BZ_2. BZ_1 is thought to be associated with sleep mechanisms; BZ_2 with memory, motor, sensory and cognitive functions. Quazepam and its active metabolite 2-oxoquazepam have a high affinity for BZ_1 receptors; this selectivity is not seen with estazolam, flurazepam, temazepam and triazolam. It is possible this selectivity of quazepam facilitates GABA transmission; however, further study is needed to determine the clinical significance of this receptor sensitivity.

Benzodiazepines generally decrease sleep latency, the number of awakenings and the time spent in stage 0 (awake stage). Flurazepam, quazepam and temazepam decrease stage 1 (descending drowsiness). Stage 2 (unequivocal sleep) is increased by all benzodiazepines, and most benzodiazepines shorten stages 3 and 4 (slow wave sleep). Temazepam has prolonged stage 3 and shortened stage 4 in neurotic patients or patients with depression. All but flurazepam prolong REM latency. REM sleep is usually shortened, but with temazepam or low-dose flurazepam, this may not be the case. The result of benzodiazepine administration is an increase in total sleep time.

If benzodiazepines are discontinued after 3 or 4 weeks of continued use, the patient may experience REM rebound; however, REM rebound with flurazepam, quazepam and possibly estazolam is slight.

➤*Pharmacokinetics:*

Absorption – These agents are rapidly and completely absorbed within 1 to 3 hours of oral administration. All have high lipid:water distribution coefficients in the non-ionized form. Times to peak plasma concentration range from 0.5 to 2 hours for parent compounds. The major active metabolite of flurazepam reaches peak plasma levels in ≈ 10 hours.

Distribution – Plasma protein binding ranges from 70% to 99% with free-drug concentrations closely approximating CSF levels. IV and rapidly absorbed oral benzodiazepines are rapidly taken into the brain and other highly perfused organs. Redistribution, favoring lipophilic compounds, follows and can greatly influence the duration of CNS effects. They also cross the placenta and are secreted into breast milk.

Metabolism – Benzodiazepines are extensively metabolized in the liver. Biotransformation to active metabolites is an important factor in product selection especially in the elderly or patients with severe liver disease. Flurazepam is biotransformed to an active metabolite, N-desalkylflurazepam, which has a half-life ranging from 47 to 100 hours. Quazepam is extensively metabolized to 2-oxoquazepam, an active metabolite; 2-oxoquazepam is further biotransformed to N-desalkyl-2-oxoquazepam, which is identical to N-desalkylflurazepam and is therefore also active. Temazepam, estazolam and triazolam do not form active long-acting metabolites.

Select Benzodiazepine (Hypnotic) Pharmacokinetic Parameters					
Drug	Usual adult oral dose (mg)	Time to peak plasma levels (hrs)	Half-life (hrs)	Protein binding (%)	Urinary excretion, unchanged (%)
Estazolam	1-2	2	8-28	93	< 5
Flurazepam	15-30	0.5-1 (7.6-13.6)[1]	2-3 (47-100)[1]	97	< 1
Quazepam	7.5-15	2 (1-2)	41 (47-100)[1]	> 95	trace
Temazepam	15-30	1.2-1.6	3.5-18.4 (9-15)	96	0.2
Triazolam	0.125-0.5	1-2	1.5-5.5	78-89	2

[1] N-desalkylflurazepam, active metabolite.

Contraindications

Hypersensitivity to other benzodiazepines; pregnancy (see Warnings); established or suspected sleep apnea (quazepam).

Concurrent use with ketoconazole, itraconazole and nefazodone, medications that significantly impair the oxidative metabolism of **triazolam** mediated by cytochrome P450 3A (CYP3A).

Warnings

➤*Anterograde amnesia:* Anterograde amnesia of varying severity and paradoxical reactions have occurred following therapeutic doses of **triazolam**. Although these effects generally occurred with a 0.5 mg dose, they have also been reported with 0.125 and 0.25 mg doses. These effect may occur with some other benzodiazepines, but data suggest that they may occur at a higher rate with triazolam.

Cases of "traveler's amnesia" have been reported by individuals who have taken **triazolam** to induce sleep while traveling. In some of these cases, insufficient time was allowed for the sleep period prior to awakening and before beginning activity. Also, the concomitant use of alcohol may have been a factor in some cases.

➤*Renal/Hepatic function impairment:* Observe usual precautions under these conditions; the potential for excessive sedation or impaired coordination exists.

Abnormal liver function tests as well as blood dyscrasias have been reported with benzodiazepines.

➤*Elderly:* The risk of developing oversedation, dizziness, confusion or ataxia increases substantially with larger doses of benzodiazepines in elderly and debilitated patients. Initiate with lowest effective dose.

➤*Pregnancy: Category X* (estazolam, quazepam, temazepam, triazolam). Flurazepam is contraindicated in pregnancy.

A neonate whose mother received 30 mg **flurazepam** nightly for insomnia during the 10 days prior to delivery appeared hypotonic and inactive during the first 4 days of life. Serum levels of N–desalkylflurazepam in the infant indicated transplacental circulation.

Teratogenic – Benzodiazepines may cause fetal damage when administered during pregnancy. An increased risk of congenital malformations associated with the use of diazepam and chlordiazepoxide during the first trimester of pregnancy has been suggested. Transplacental distribution results in neonatal CNS depression following ingestion of therapeutic doses of a benzodiazepine hypnotic during the last weeks of pregnancy.

Reproduction studies with **temazepam** in animals demonstrated an increased nursling mortality, increased fetal resorptions and increased occurrence of rudimentary ribs. Exencephaly and fusion or asymmetry of the ribs occurred without dose relationship.

Warn the patient of the potential risk to the fetus if there is a likelihood of the patient becoming pregnant while receiving benzodiazepines. Instruct patients to discontinue the drug prior to becoming pregnant. Consider the possibility that a woman of childbearing potential may be pregnant at the time of therapy institution.

Nonteratogenic – A child born to a mother taking benzodiazepines may be at some risk of withdrawal symptoms during the postnatal period. Neonatal flaccidity has occurred in an infant whose mother had been receiving benzodiazepines.

➤*Lactation:* Safety for use in the nursing mother has not been established. Benzodiazepines are excreted in breast milk. One study showed only 0.11% of quazepam and its metabolites were excreted in breast milk 48 hours after administration. Animal studies indicate that **triazolam, estazolam** and their metabolites are secreted in milk. Therefore, administration to nursing mothers is not recommended.

➤*Children:*

Flurazepam – Not for use in children < 15 years of age.

Estazolam, quazepam, temazepam, triazolam – Not for use in children < 18 years of age.

Precautions

➤*Monitoring:* When triazolam or estazolam treatment is protracted, obtain periodic blood counts, urinalysis and blood chemistry analyses. Minor EEG changes, usually low-voltage fast activity, are of no known significance.

➤*Depression:* Administer with caution in severely depressed patients or in those in whom there is evidence of latent depression or suicidal tendencies. Signs or symptoms of depression may be intensified by hypnotic drugs. Protective measures may be required. Intentional overdosage is more common in these patients, and the least amount of drug that is feasible should be available to the patient at any one time.

➤*Rebound sleep disorder:* Rebound sleep disorder, which is characterized by recurrence of insomnia to levels worse than before treatment began, may occur following abrupt withdrawal of triazolam, usually during the first 1 to 3 nights. Gradual rather than abrupt discontinuation of the drug may help avoid this syndrome. Rebound insomnia appears to be less likely after withdrawal of agents with intermediate or long half-lives (eg, estazolam, flurazepam, quazepam).

➤*Disturbed nocturnal sleep:* Disturbed nocturnal sleep may occur for the first or second night after discontinuing use.

➤*Early morning insomnia:* Early morning insomnia, or early morning awakenings, appears to be more common with the use of short half-life agents (temazepam, triazolam) than agents with intermediate or long half-lives (estazolam, flurazepam, quazepam). However, daytime sleepiness appears to be more prevalent with the long half-life agents.

➤*Respiratory depression and sleep apnea:* Observe caution. In patients with compromised respiratory function, respiratory depression and sleep apnea have occurred. Estazolam may cause dose-related respiratory depression that is ordinarily not clinically relevant at recommended doses in patients with normal respiratory function. However, patients with compromised respiratory function may be at risk; therefore, monitor appropriately. Benzodiazepines have the capacity to depress respiratory drive, although there are insufficient data to characterize the relative potency of these agents in depressing respiratory drive at clinically recommended doses.

➤*Drug abuse and dependence:* Withdrawal symptoms following abrupt discontinuation of benzodiazepines have occurred in patients receiving excessive doses over extended periods of time. Symptoms are similar to those noted with barbiturates and alcohol following abrupt discontinuance and range from mild dysphoria to abdominal and muscle cramps, vomiting, sweating, tremor and convulsions. Milder withdrawal symptoms infrequently occur following abrupt discontinuance of higher therapeutic levels of benzodiazepines taken continuously for several months. Exercise caution in administering to individuals known to be addiction-prone or those who may increase the dosage on their own initiative. Limit repeated prescriptions without adequate medical supervision.

Gradual withdrawal is the preferred course for any patient taking benzodiazepines for a prolonged period. Patients with a history of seizures, regardless of their concomitant anti-seizure therapy, should not be withdrawn abruptly from benzodiazepines.

➤*Hazardous tasks:* Observe caution while driving or performing tasks requiring alertness. Be aware of potential impairment of the performance of such activities the day following ingestion.

Amnesia, paradoxical reactions (eg, excitement, agitation) and other adverse behavioral effects may occur unpredictably.

Drug Interactions

Benzodiazepine (Hypnotic) Drug Interactions

Precipitant drug	Object drug*		Description
Alcohol/CNS depressants	Benzodiazepines	↑	Additive CNS depressant effects. Potential for this interaction continues for several days following flurazepam withdrawal.
Cimetidine Contraceptives, oral Disulfiram Isoniazid	Benzodiazepines (metabolized by oxidation)	↑	The hepatic metabolism of the benzodiazepines may be inhibited, their half-life prolonged and their clearance decreased, possibly resulting in increased pharmacologic and CNS depressant effects. Temazepam, metabolized by glucuronidation, would probably not interact; however, its half-life may be decreased by oral contraceptive agents.
Probenecid	Benzodiazepines	↑	More rapid onset or more prolonged benzodiazepine effect.
Rifampin	Benzodiazepines (metabolized by oxidation)	↓	Increased clearance and decreased half-life of benzodiazepines may occur. Temazepam would probably not interact.
Smoking	Benzodiazepines	↓	Benzodiazepine clearance is increased in cigarette smokers, probably due to enzyme induction.
Theophyllines	Benzodiazepines	↓	Benzodiazepine pharmacologic effects may be antagonized.
Macrolides	Triazolam	↑	Bioavailability of triazolam may be increased.
Benzodiazepines	Digoxin	↑	Digoxin serum levels and toxicity may increase.
Benzodiazepines	Neuromuscular blocking agents (nondepolarizing)	↔	Benzodiazepines may potentiate, counteract or have no effect on these agents.
Benzodiazepines	Phenytoin	↑	Phenytoin serum levels may be increased, resulting in toxicity, but data are conflicting.

* ↑ = Object drug increased. ↓ = Object drug decreased. ↔ = Undetermined clinical effect.

Adverse Reactions

➤*Cardiovascular:* Palpitations; chest pains; tachycardia; hypotension (rare).

➤*CNS:* Headache; nervousness; talkativeness; apprehension; irritability; confusion; euphoria; relaxed feeling; weakness; tremor; lack of concentration; coordination disorders; confusional states/memory impairment; depression; dreaming/nightmares; insomnia; paresthesia; restlessness; tiredness; dysesthesia. Hallucinations, horizontal nystagmus and paradoxical reactions, including excitement, stimulation and hyperactivity were rare. Dizziness, drowsiness, lightheadedness, staggering, ataxia, falling, particularly in elderly or debilitated patients. Severe sedation, lethargy, disorientation and coma are probably indicative of drug intolerance or overdosage.

➤*Dermatologic:* Dermatitis/allergy; sweating, flushes, pruritus, skin rash (rare).

➤*GI:* Heartburn; nausea; vomiting; diarrhea; constipation; GI pain; anorexia; taste alterations; dry mouth; excessive salivation (rare); death from hepatic failure in a patient also receiving diuretics; jaundice; glossitis, stomatitis (triazolam).

➤*Lab test abnormalities:* Elevated AST, ALT, total and direct bilirubin and alkaline phosphatase with **flurazepam**.

➤*Miscellaneous:* Body/joint pain; tinnitus; GU complaints; cramps/pain; congestion. Leukopenia, granulocytopenia, blurred vision, burning eyes, faintness, difficulty in focusing, visual disturbances, shortness of breath, apnea, slurred speech (rare).

➤*Estazolam:* Other adverse reactions reported only for estazolam include the following:

Cardiovascular – Arrhythmia, syncope (< 0.1%).

CNS – Somnolence (42%); asthenia (11%); hypokinesia (8%); hangover (3%); abnormal thinking (2%); anxiety (1%); agitation, amnesia, apathy, emotional lability, hostility, seizure, sleep disorder, stupor, twitch (0.1% to 1%); ataxia, decreased libido, decreased reflexes, neuritis (< 0.1%).

Dermatologic – Urticaria (0.1% to 1%); acne, dry skin, photosensitivity (< 0.1%).

GI – Dyspepsia (2%); decreased/increased appetite, flatulence, gastritis (0.1% to 1%); enterocolitis, melena, mouth ulceration (< 0.1%).

GU – Frequent urination, menstrual cramps, urinary hesitancy/urgency, vaginal discharge/itching (0.1% to 1%); hematuria, nocturia, oliguria, penile discharge, urinary incontinence (< 0.1%).

Respiratory – Cold symptoms (3%); pharyngitis (1%); asthma, cough, dyspnea, rhinitis, sinusitis (0.1% to 1%); epistaxis, hyperventilation, laryngitis (< 0.1%).

Special senses – Ear pain, eye irritation/pain/swelling, photophobia (0.1% to 1%); decreased hearing, diplopia, nystagmus, scotomata (< 0.1%).

Miscellaneous – Lower extremity/back/abdominal pain (1% to 3%); stiffness (1%); allergic reaction, chills, fever, neck/upper extremity pain, thirst, arthritis, muscle spasm, myalgia (0.1% to 1%); edema, jaw pain, swollen breast, thyroid nodule, purpura, swollen lymph nodes, agranulocytosis, increased AST, weight gain/loss, arthralgia (< 0.1%).

Overdosage

➤*Symptoms:* Somnolence; confusion with reduced or absent reflexes; respiratory depression; apnea; hypotension; impaired coordination; slurred speech; seizures; ultimately, coma. Death has occurred with overdoses of benzodiazepines alone and with alcohol.

➤*Treatment:* If excitation occurs, do not use barbiturates. Consider the possibility that multiple agents may have been ingested. Monitor respiration, pulse and blood pressure. Employ general supportive measures. Administer IV fluids and maintain an adequate airway. Perform gastric lavage. Refer to General Management of Acute Overdosage. Hemodialysis and forced diuresis are of little value.

Use of IV pressor agents may be necessary to treat hypotension. Administer IV fluids to encourage diuresis.

Patient Information

Avoid alcohol and other CNS depressants. Do not exceed prescribed dosage.

Do not discontinue medication abruptly after prolonged therapy.

Advise patients that they may experience disturbed nocturnal sleep for the first or second night after discontinuing the drug.

May cause drowsiness or dizziness; observe caution while driving or performing other tasks requiring alertness.

Inform your physician if you are planning to become pregnant, if you are pregnant, or if you become pregnant while taking this medicine.

➤*Triazolam:* Advise patients not to take triazolam in circumstances where a full night's sleep and clearance of the drug from the body are not possible before they would again need to be active and functional.

ESTAZOLAM

Rx	**Estazolam** (Zenith-Goldline)	**Tablets:** 1 mg	In 30s, 100s, 500s and 1000s.
c-iv	**ProSom** (Abbott)		Lactose. (UC). White, scored. In 100s and UD 100s.
Rx	**Estazolam** (Zenith-Goldline)	2 mg	In 30s, 100s, 500s and 1000s.
c-iv	**ProSom** (Abbott)		Lactose. (UD). Coral, scored. In 100s and UD 100s.

ESTAZOLAM — ORAL

For complete and comparative prescribing information, refer to the Benzodiazepines group monograph.

Indications

➤*Insomnia:* Estazolam is indicated for the short-term management of insomnia characterized by difficulty in falling asleep, frequent nocturnal awakenings, and/or early morning awakenings. Both outpatient studies and a sleep laboratory study have shown that estazolam administered at bedtime improved sleep induction and sleep maintenance.

Administration and Dosage

➤*Approved by the FDA:* December 26, 1990.

The recommended initial dose for adults is 1 mg at bedtime; however, some patients may need a 2 mg dose. In healthy elderly patients, 1 mg is also the appropriate starting dose, but increases should be initiated with particular care. In small or debilitated older patients, a starting dose of 0.5 mg, while only marginally effective in the overall elderly population, should be considered.

➤*Storage/Stability:* Store at controlled room temperature 15° to 30°C (59° to 86°F).

FLURAZEPAM HYDROCHLORIDE

c-iv	**Flurazepam** (Various, eg, Goldline, Major, PBI, Warner Chilcott)	**Capsules:** 15 mg	In 100s and 100s.
c-iv	**Dalmane** (Valeant[a])		Orange/ivory. In 100s and 500s.
c-iv	**Flurazepam** (Various, eg, Goldline, Major, PBI, Warner Chilcott)	**Capsules:** 30 mg	In 100s and 100s.
c-iv	**Dalmane** (Valeant[a])		(DALMANE 30 ICN). Red/Ivory. In 100s and 500s.

[a] Valeant Plaza, 3300 Hyland Avenue, Costa Mesa, CA 92626; (800) 548-5100

FLURAZEPAM HYDROCHLORIDE — ORAL

For complete and comparative prescribing information, refer to the Benzodiazepines group monograph.

Indications

➤*Insomnia:* Flurazepam hydrochloride is a hypnotic agent useful for the treatment of insomnia characterized by difficulty in falling asleep, frequent nocturnal awakenings, or early morning awakening. Flurazepam hydrochloride can be used effectively in patients with recurring insomnia or poor sleeping habits, and in acute or chronic medical situations requiring restful sleep. Sleep laboratory studies have objectively determined that flurazepam hydrochloride is effective for at least 28 consecutive nights of drug administration. Since insomnia is often transient and intermittent, short-term use is usually sufficient. Prolonged use of hypnotics is usually not indicated and should only be undertaken concomitantly with appropriate evaluation of the patient.

Administration and Dosage

➤*Approved by the FDA:* November 27, 1985.

Dosage should be individualized for maximal beneficial effects. The usual adult dosage is 30 mg before retiring. In some patients, 15 mg may suffice. In elderly or debilitated patients, 15 mg is usually sufficient for a therapeutic response and it is therefore recommended that therapy be initiated with this dosage.

➤*Storage/Stability:* Store at controlled room temperature 15° to 30°C (59° to 86°F). Protect from light. Dispense in a tight, light-resistant container using a child-resistant closure.

TEMAZEPAM

c-iv	**Restoril** (Mallinckrodt)	**Capsules:** 7.5 mg	Lactose. (FOR SLEEP M RESTORIL 7.5 mg). Blue/pink. In 30s and 100s.
c-iv	**Temazepam** (Various, eg, Goldline, Lederle, Moore, PBI, Warner Chilcott)	**Capsules:** 15 mg	In 100s, 500s and UD 100s.
c-iv	**Restoril** (Mallinckrodt)		Lactose. (FOR SLEEP M RESTORIL 15 mg). Maroon/pink. In 100s and 500s.
c-iv	**Restoril** (Mallinckrodt)	**Capsules:** 22.5 mg	Lactose. (FOR SLEEP M RESTORIL 22.5 mg). Opaque blue. In 30s and 100s.
c-iv	**Temazepam** (Various, eg, Goldline, PBI, Warner-Chilcott)	**Capsules:** 30 mg	In 100s, 500s and UD 100s.
c-iv	**Restoril** (Mallinckrodt)		Lactose. (FOR SLEEP M RESTORIL 30 mg). Maroon/blue. In 100s and 500s.

TEMAZEPAM — ORAL

For complete and comparative prescribing information, refer to the Benzodiazepines group monograph.

Indications

➤*Insomnia:* Temazepam is indicated for the relief of insomnia associated with the complaints of difficulty in falling asleep, frequent nocturnal awakenings, or early morning awakenings. In clinical trials there is a perception by patients that temazepam decreases sleep latency, but sleep laboratory studies have not confirmed such an effect when the drug was administered within 30 minutes of retiring.

Administration and Dosage

The recommended usual adult dose is 30 mg before retiring. In some patients, 15 mg may be sufficient. As with all medications, dosage should be individualized for maximal beneficial effects. In elderly or debilitated patients it is recommended that therapy be initiated with 15 mg until individual responses are determined.

➤*Elderly and debilitated patients:* Since the risk of the development of oversedation, dizziness, confusion or ataxia increases substantially with larger doses of benzodiazepines in elderly and debilitated patients. Fifteen milligrams of temazepam is recommended as the initial dosage for such patients.

➤*Storage/Stability:* Dispense in a tight, light-resistant container. Store at controlled temperature 15° to 30°C (59° to 86°F).

TRIAZOLAM

c-iv	**Triazolam** (Various, eg, Geneva, Goldline, Par, Roxane)	**Tablets:** 0.125 mg	In 10s, 100s, 500s and UD 100s.
c-iv	**Halcion** (Upjohn)		(0.125 Halcion 10). White. In 100s, 500s, UD 100s, *Visipak* 100s.
c-iv	**Triazolam** (Various, eg, Geneva, Goldline, Par, Roxane)	**Tablets:** 0.25 mg	In 10s, 100s, 500s and UD 100s.
c-iv	**Halcion** (Upjohn)		(0.25 Halcion 17). Blue, scored. In 100s, 500s, UD 100s, *Visipak* 100s.

TRIAZOLAM — ORAL

For complete and comparative prescribing information, refer to the Benzodiazepines group monograph.

Indications

➤*Insomnia:* Triazolam is indicated for the short-term treatment of insomnia (generally 7 to 10 days). Use for more than 2 to 3 weeks requires complete reevaluation of the patient.

Administration and Dosage

It is important to individualize the dosage of triazolam tablets for maximum beneficial effect and to help avoid significant adverse effects.

The recommended dose for most adults is 0.25 mg before retiring. A dose of 0.125 mg may be found to be sufficient for some patients (eg, low body weight). A dose of 0.5 mg should be used only for exceptional patients who do not respond adequately to a trial of a lower dose since the risk of several adverse reactions increases with the size of the dose administered. A dose of 0.5 mg should not be exceeded.

➤*Elderly/debilitated patients:* In elderly or debilitated patients the recommended dosage range is 0.125 mg to 0.25 mg to decrease the possibility of development of oversedation, dizziness, or impaired coordination. Therapy should be initiated at 0.125 mg in this group and the 0.25 mg dose should be used only for exceptional patients who do not respond to a trial of the lower dose. A dose of 0.25 mg should not be exceeded in these patients.

As with all medications, the lowest effective dose should be used.

➤*Storage/Stability:* Store at controlled room temperature 20° to 25°C (68° to 77°F).

QUAZEPAM

c-iv	**Doral** (Wallace)	**Tablets:** 7.5 mg	(7.5 Doral). Light orange w/white speckles. Capsule shaped. In 100s, 500s, UD 100s.
		15 mg	(15 Doral). Light orange w/white speckles. Capsule shaped. In 100s, 500s, UD 100s.

QUAZEPAM — ORAL

For complete and comparative prescribing information, refer to the Benzodiazepines group monograph.

Indications

➤*Insomnia:* Quazepam tablets are indicated for the treatment of insomnia characterized by difficulty in falling asleep, frequent nocturnal awakenings, or early morning awakenings. The effectiveness of quazepam has been established in placebo-controlled clinical studies of 5 nights' duration in acute and chronic insomnia. The sustained effectiveness of quazepam has been established in chronic insomnia in a sleep lab (polysomnographic) study of 28 nights duration.

Administration and Dosage

➤*Approved by the FDA:* December 27, 1985.

➤*Adults:* Initiate therapy at 15 mg until individual responses are determined. In some patients, the dose may then be reduced to 7.5 mg.

➤*Elderly and debilitated patients:* Because the elderly and debilitated may be more sensitive to benzodiazepines, attempts to reduce the nightly dosage after the first 1 or 2 nights of therapy are suggested.

A well-controlled sleep laboratory study (n = 30) demonstrated that both quazepam 7.5 mg and quazepam 15 mg were safe and effective treatment for insomnia in geriatric patients (older than 60 years of age). Initiate therapy in geriatric patients at 7.5 mg; if not effective after 1 to 2 nights, dosage may be increased to 15 mg.

➤*Storage/Stability:* Store quazepam at controlled room temperature 20° to 25°C (68° to 77°F). Protect unit doses from excessive moisture.

CHLORAL HYDRATE

c-iv	**Chloral Hydrate** (Various, eg, Balan, Dixon-Shane, Goldline, Lannett, URL)	**Capsules**: 500 mg	In 100s, 500s, 1000s and UD 100s.
c-iv	**Somnote** (Breckenridge		(B-080). In 50s and UD 50s.
c-iv	**Chloral Hydrate** (Various, eg, Pharmaceutical Assoc., Roxane)	**Syrup**: 250 mg/5 ml	In UD 10 ml (40s and 100s).
c-iv	**Chloral Hydrate** (Various, eg, Balan, Dixon-Shane, Geneva, UDL, URL)	**Syrup**: 500 mg/5 ml	In pt, gal and UD 5 ml (100s) and 10 ml (40s and 100s).
c-iv	**Aquachloral Supprettes** (Polymedica)	**Suppositories**: 324 mg	Tartrazine. In 12s.
c-iv	**Aquachloral Supprettes** (Polymedica)	**Suppositories**: 648 mg	In 12s.

CHLORAL HYDRATE

Refer to the general discussion beginning in the Sedative and Hypnotic, Nonbarbiturate introduction.

Indications

Nocturnal sedation; preoperative sedation to lessen anxiety and induce sleep without depressing respiration or cough reflex; in postoperative care and control of pain as an adjunct to opiates and analgesics; preventing or suppressing alcohol withdrawal symptoms (rectal).

Chloral hydrate is effective as a hypnotic only for short-term use; it loses much of its effectiveness for inducing and maintaining sleep after 2 weeks of use.

Administration and Dosage

Take capsules with a full glass of liquid. Administer syrup in ½ glass of water, fruit juice or ginger ale.

➤*Adults:* Single doses or daily dosage should not exceed 2 g.

Hypnotic – 500 mg to 1 g 15 to 30 minutes before bedtime or 30 minutes before surgery.

Sedative – 250 mg 3 times daily after meals.

➤*Children:*

Hypnotic – 50 mg/kg/day, up to 1 g per single dose. May be given in divided doses.

Sedative – 25 mg/kg/day, up to 500 mg per single dose. May be given in divided doses.

Dental sedation – Higher doses than those suggested by the manufacturer are generally used. Doses of 75 mg/kg, supplemented by nitrous oxide may provide better sedation than the lower dose with no change in the vital signs or adverse effects.

Actions

➤*Pharmacology:* The mechanism of action by which the CNS is affected is not known. Hypnotic dosage produces mild cerebral depression and quiet, deep sleep. In therapeutic doses, chloral hydrate has little effect on respiration, blood pressure and reflexes. "Hangover" is less common than with most barbiturates and some benzodiazepines. It has generally been replaced by safer and more effective agents.

➤*Pharmacokinetics:* Chloral hydrate is readily absorbed and metabolized to trichloroethanol, the principal active metabolite. Trichloroethanol has a plasma half-life of 7 to 10 hours; plasma protein binding is 35% to 41%. The drug is converted in the liver and kidney to trichloroacetic acid and excreted in the urine and bile. Although inactive, trichloroacetic acid is 71% to 88% protein bound and can displace other acidic drugs from plasma protein binding sites.

Contraindications

Marked hepatic or renal impairment; severe cardiac disease; gastritis; hypersensitivity or idiosyncrasy to chloral derivatives.

Warnings

➤*Pregnancy: Category C.* Safety for use during pregnancy has not been established. Chloral hydrate crosses the placenta; chronic use during pregnancy may cause withdrawal symptoms in the neonate. Congenital defects have not been reported. Use only when clearly needed and when potential benefits outweigh potential hazards to the fetus.

➤*Lactation:* Chloral hydrate is excreted in breast milk; use by nursing mothers may cause sedation in the infant.

Precautions

➤*Cardiac disease:* Continued use of therapeutic doses does not have a deleterious effect on the heart. However, do not use large doses in patients with severe cardiac disease.

➤*GI conditions:* Avoid use in patients with esophagitis, gastritis or gastric or duodenal ulcers.

➤*Acute intermittent porphyria:* Acute intermittent porphyria attacks may be precipitated by chloral hydrate; use with caution in susceptible patients.

➤*Skin/mucous membrane irritation:* Chloral derivatives irritate the skin and mucous membranes; gastric necrosis has occurred following intoxicating doses.

➤*Drug abuse and dependence:* May be habit forming. Exercise caution in administering to patients prone to addiction. Slurred speech, incoordination, tremulousness and nystagmus should arouse suspicion. Drowsiness, lethargy and hangover are frequently observed from excessive drug intake. Prolonged use of large doses may result in psychic and physical dependence. Tolerance and psychologic dependence may develop by the second week of continued administration. Chloral hydrate addicts may take huge doses of the drug (up to 12 g nightly). Sudden withdrawal may result in CNS excitation with tremor, anxiety, hallucinations or even delirium, which may be fatal. Gastritis, skin eruptions and parenchymatous renal injury may also occur. Undertake withdrawal in a hospital using supportive therapy similar to that used for barbiturate withdrawal.

➤*Hazardous tasks:* May produce drowsiness; patients should observe caution while driving or performing other tasks requiring alertness.

➤*Tartrazine sensitivity:* Some of these products contain tartrazine, which may cause allergic-type reactions (including bronchial asthma) in susceptible individuals. Although the incidence of tartrazine sensitivity in the general population is low, it is frequently seen in patients who also have aspirin hypersensitivity. Specific products containing tartrazine are identified in the product listings.

Drug Interactions

Chloral Hydrate Drug Interactions

Precipitant drug	Object drug*		Description
Alcohol	Chloral hydrate	↑	Alcohol may have synergistic effects with chloral hydrate. With alcohol, there is mutual inhibition of metabolism in addition to the combined depressant effect. Disulfiram-like reactions (eg, increased respiration and pulse rate, flushing), although rare, have occurred. Avoid concomitant use.
Chloral hydrate	Alcohol		
Chloral hydrate	Anticoagulants, oral	↑	Hypoprothrombinemic effects may occur by displacement from protein binding sites. However, this effect is usually small and fleeting. Monitor prothrombin levels and adjust coumarin dose accordingly.
Chloral hydrate	CNS depressants	↑	CNS depressants (eg, barbiturates, narcotics) may have additive CNS effects with chloral hydrate coadministration.
CNS depressants	Chloral hydrate		
Furosemide	Chloral hydrate	↑	Administration of chloral hydrate followed by IV furosemide may result in sweating, hot flashes, tachycardia, hypertension, weakness and nausea.
Chloral hydrate	Hydantoins	↓	The elimination of phenytoin may be increased by concurrent chloral hydrate, possibly reducing its effectiveness.

* ↑ = Object drug increased. ↓ = Object drug decreased.

➤*Drug/Lab test interactions:* Chloral hydrate may interfere with the **copper sulfate test** for glycosuria (confirm suspected glycosuria by a glucose oxidase test), **fluorometric tests** for urine catecholamines (do not administer medication for 48 hours preceding the test) or **urinary 17-hydroxycorticosteroid determinations** (when using the Reddy, Jenkins and Thorn procedure).

Adverse Reactions

➤*CNS:* Somnambulism, disorientation, incoherence, paranoid behavior (occasional); excitement, delirium, drowsiness, staggering gait, ataxia, lightheadedness, vertigo, dizziness, nightmares, malaise, mental confusion, headache, hallucinations (rare).

➤*Dermatologic:* Allergic skin rashes including hives, erythema, eczematoid dermatitis, urticaria, scarlatiniform exanthems (occasional).

➤*GI:* Gastric irritation; nausea and vomiting (occasional); flatulence; diarrhea; unpleasant taste in mouth.

➤*Hematologic:* Leukopenia, eosinophilia (occasional).

➤*Miscellaneous:* Hangover, idiosyncratic syndrome, ketonuria (rare).

CHLORAL HYDRATE

Overdosage

➤*Symptoms:* Stupor; coma; pinpoint pupils; hypotension; slow or rapid and shallow respiration; hypothermia; areflexia; muscle flaccidity.

Corrosive action – Nausea; vomiting; esophagitis; gastritis; hemorrhagic gastritis; gastric necrosis; enteritis.

Organ damage – Hepatic damage (jaundice); renal damage (albuminuria); cardiac damage (ventricular and atrial arrhythmias).

Doses > 2 g may produce symptoms of toxicity. The toxic oral dose of chloral hydrate for adults is approximately 5 to 10 g; however, death has occurred following doses of 1.25 and 3 g; some patients have survived after taking 36 g.

➤*Treatment:* Perform gastric lavage or induce vomiting to empty the stomach. Activated charcoal may prevent drug absorption. Treatment includes usual supportive measures. Refer to General Management of Acute Overdosage. Hemoperfusion and hemodialysis are effective, but peritoneal dialysis is not useful. Hemodialysis is reported to promote the clearance of trichloroethanol.

Patient Information

May cause GI upset. Take capsules with a full glass of water or fruit juice; swallow capsules whole – do not chew. Dilute syrup in a half glass of water or fruit juice.

May cause drowsiness; use caution when performing tasks requiring alertness. Avoid alcohol and other CNS depressants.

May be habit forming; do not discontinue the drug abruptly.

DEXMEDETOMIDINE HYDROCHLORIDE

Rx	**Precedex** (Abbott)	**Injection:** 100 mcg/mL	Preservative-free. 9 mg sodium chloride. In 2 mL vials.

DEXMEDETOMIDINE HYDROCHLORIDE — INJECTION

Indications

➤*Sedation:* Dexmedetomidine is indicated for sedation of initially intubated and mechanically ventilated patients during treatment in an intensive care setting. Dexmedetomidine should be administered by continuous infusion, not to exceed 24 hours.

➤*Unlabeled uses:* To treat shivering; as an adjunct to regional or general anesthesia; as a bridge to ICU sedation and analgesia; as a supplement to regional block in patients undergoing carotid endarterectomy or during awake craniotomy; in selected patients with congestive heart failure; to control agitation while receiving noninvasive ventilatory support such as mask continuous or bilevel positive airway pressure; to minimize withdrawal phenomena in critically ill patients who have received long-term benzodiazepines and opioids during their hospitalization.

Administration and Dosage

➤*Approved by the FDA:* December 24, 1999.

Dexmedetomidine should be administered using a controlled infusion device.

Dexmedetomidine dosing should be individualized and titrated to the desired clinical effect. For adult patients, dexmedetomidine is generally initiated with a loading infusion of 1 mcg/kg over 10 minutes, followed by a maintenance infusion of 0.2 to 0.7 mcg/kg/hr. The rate of the maintenance infusion should be adjusted to achieve the desired level of sedation. Dexmedetomidine is not indicated for infusions lasting longer than 24 hours.

Dexmedetomidine has been continuously infused in mechanically ventilated patients prior to extubation, during extubation, and postextubation. It is not necessary to discontinue dexmedetomidine prior to extubation provided the infusion does not exceed 24 hours.

➤*Dosage adjustment:* Dosage reductions may need to be considered for patients with renal or hepatic impairment.

➤*Dilution prior to administration:* Dexmedetomidine must be diluted in 0.9% sodium chloride solution prior to administration.

Preparation of solutions is the same, whether for the loading dose or for the maintenance infusion.

To prepare the infusion, withdraw 2 mL of dexmedetomidine and add to 48 mL of 0.9% sodium chloride injection to a total of 50 mL. Shake gently to mix well.

➤*Administration with other fluids:* Compatibility of dexmedetomidine with coadministration of blood, serum, or plasma has not been established. Dexmedetomidine has been shown to be compatible when administered with the following IV fluids and drugs: Lactated ringers; 5% dextrose in water; 0.9% sodium chloride in water; 20% mannitol; thiopental sodium; etomidate; vecuronium bromide; pancuronium bromide; succinylcholine; atracurium besylate; mivacurium chloride; glycopyrrolate bromide; phenylephrine HCl; atropine sulfate; midazolam; morphine sulfate; fentanyl citrate; plasma substitute.

➤*Handling procedures:* Compatibility studies have demonstrated the potential for adsorption of dexmedetomidine to some types of natural rubber. Although dexmedetomidine is dosed to effect, it is advisable to use administration components made with synthetic or coated natural rubber gaskets.

➤*Storage/Stability:* Store at controlled room temperature, 25°C (77°F) with excursions allowed from 15° to 30°C (59° to 86°F).

Actions

➤*Pharmacology:* Dexmedetomidine is a relatively selective $alpha_2$-adrenoceptor agonist with sedative properties. $Alpha_2$ selectivity was observed in animals following slow IV infusion of low and medium doses (10 to 300 mcg/kg).

Both $alpha_1$ and $alpha_2$ activity was observed following slow IV infusion of high doses (greater than or equal to 1000 mcg/kg) or with rapid IV administration.

In a study involving healthy volunteers (n = 10), respiratory rate and oxygen saturation remained within normal limits, and there was no evidence of respiratory depression when dexmedetomidine was administered by IV infusion at doses within the recommended dose range (0.2 to 0.7 mcg/kg).

➤*Pharmacokinetics:*

Distribution – Following IV administration, dexmedetomidine exhibits the following pharmacokinetic parameters: A rapid distribution phase with a distribution half-life ($t_{½}$) of approximately 6 minutes; a terminal elimination half-life ($t_{½}$) of approximately 2 hours; and steady-state volume of distribution (V_{ss}) of approximately 118 L. Clearance is estimated to be approximately 39 L/hr. The mean body weight associated with this clearance estimate was 72 kg.

Dexmedetomidine exhibits linear kinetics in the dosage range of 0.2 to 0.7 mg/kg/hr when administered by IV infusion for up to 24 hours. The mean ± SD pharmacokinetic parameters show the main pharmacokinetic parameters when dexmedetomidine was infused (after appropriate loading doses) at maintenance infusion rates of 0.17 mcg/kg/hr (target concentration of 0.3 ng/mL) for 12 and 24 hours, 0.33 mcg/kg/hr (target concentration of 0.6 ng/mL) for 24 hours, and 0.7 mcg/kg/hr (target concentration of 1.25 ng/mL) for 24 hours.

Mean ± SD Pharmacokinetic Parameters

Parameter	Loading infusion (min)/total infusion duration (hours)			
	10 min/12 h	10 min/24 h	10 min/24 h	35 min/24 h
	Dexmedetomidine target concentration (ng/mL) and dose (mcg/kg/hr)			
	0.3/0.17	0.3/0.17	0.6/0.33	1.25/0.7
$t_{½}$*, hour	1.78 ± 0.3	2.22 ± 0.59	2.23 ± 0.21	2.5 ± 0.61
CL liter/hour	46.3 ± 8.3	43.1 ± 6.5	35.3 ± 6.8	36.5 ± 7.5
V_{ss} liter	88.7 ± 22.9	102.4 ± 20.3	93.6 ± 17	99.6 ± 17.8
Avg C_{ss}, ng/mL	0.27 ± 0.05	0.27 ± 0.05	0.67 ± 0.1	1.37 ± 0.2

* Presented as a harmonic mean and pseudo standard deviation.
** Avg C_{ss} = Average steady-state concentration of dexmedetomidine (2.5—9-hour samples for 12-hour infusion and 2.5—18-hour samples for 24-hour infusions).

The steady state volume of distribution of dexmedetomidine is approximately 118 L. Dexmedetomidine protein binding was assessed in the plasma of healthy male and female volunteers. The average protein binding was 94% and was constant across the different concentrations tested. Protein binding was similar in males and females. The fraction of dexmedetomidine that was bound to plasma proteins was statistically significantly decreased in subjects with hepatic impairment compared to healthy subjects.

Metabolism – Dexmedetomidine undergoes almost complete biotransformation with very little unchanged dexmedetomidine excreted in urine and feces. Biotransformation involves both direct glucuronidation as well as cytochrome P450-mediated metabolism. The major metabolic pathways of dexmedetomidine are as follows: Direct N-glucuronidation to inactive metabolites; aliphatic hydroxylation (mediated primarily by CYP2A6) of dexmedetomidine to generate 3-hydroxy dexmedetomidine, the glucuronide of 3-hydroxy dexmedetomidine, and 3-carboxy dexmedetomidine; and N-methylation of dexmedetomidine to generate 3-hydroxy N-methyl dexmedetomidine, 3-carboxy N-methyl dexmedetomidine, and N-methyl O-glucuronide dexmedetomidine.

Excretion – The terminal elimination half-life ($t_{½}$) of dexmedetomidine is approximately 2 hours, and clearance is estimated to be approximately 39 L/hr. A mass-balance study demonstrated that after 9 days an average of 95% of the radioactivity, following IV administration of radiolabeled dexmedetomidine, was recovered in the urine and 4% in the feces. No unchanged dexmedetomidine was detected in the urine. Approximately 85% of the radioactivity recovered in the urine was excreted within 24 hours after the infusion. Fractionation of the radioactivity excreted in urine demonstrated that products of N-glucouronidation accounted for approximately 34% of the cumulative urinary excretion. In addition, aliphatic hydroxylation of parent drug to form 3-hydroxy dexmedetomidine, the glucuronide of 3-hydroxy dexmedetomidine, and 3-carboxylic acid dexmedetomidine together represented approximately 14% of the dose in urine. N-methylation of dexmedetomidine to form 3-hydroxy N-methyl dexmedetomidine, 3-carboxy N-methyl dexmedetomidine, and N-methyl O-glucuronide dexmedetomidine accounted for approximately 18% of the dose in urine. The N-methyl metabolite itself was a minor circulating component and was undetected in urine. Approximately 28% of the urinary metabolites have not been identified.

Warnings

➤*Administration:* Dexmedetomidine should be administered only by persons skilled in the management of patients in the intensive care setting. Due to the known pharmacological effects of dexmedetomidine, patients should be continuously monitored while receiving dexmedetomidine.

DEXMEDETOMIDINE HYDROCHLORIDE — INJECTION

➤*Cardiac effects:* Clinically significant episodes of bradycardia and sinus arrest have been associated with dexmedetomidine administration in young, healthy volunteers with high vagal tone or with different routes of administration, including rapid IV or bolus administration.

Reports of hypotension and bradycardia have been associated with dexmedetomidine infusion. If medical intervention is required, treatment may include decreasing or stopping the infusion of dexmedetomidine, increasing the rate of IV fluid administration, elevation of the lower extremities, and use of pressor agents. Because dexmedetomidine has the potential to augment bradycardia induced by vagal stimuli, clinicians should be prepared to intervene. The IV administration of anticholinergic agents (eg, atropine) should be considered to modify vagal tone. In clinical trials, atropine or glycopyrrolate were effective in the treatment of most episodes of dexmedetomidine-induced bradycardia. However, in some patients with significant cardiovascular dysfunction, more advanced resuscitative measures were required.

Transient hypertension has been observed primarily during the loading dose in association with the initial peripheral vasoconstrictive effects of dexmedetomidine. Treatment of the transient hypertension has generally not been necessary, although reduction of the loading infusion rate may be desirable.

➤*Renal function impairment:* Dexmedetomidine pharmacokinetics (C_{max}, t_{max}, AUC, $t_{½}$, CL, and V_{ss}) were not significantly different in subjects with severe renal impairment (creatinine clearance less than 30 mL/min) compared to healthy subjects. However, the pharmacokinetics of the metabolites of dexmedetomidine have not been evaluated in patients with impaired renal function. Since the majority of metabolites are excreted in the urine, it is possible that the metabolites may accumulate upon long-term infusions in patients with impaired renal function.

➤*Hepatic function impairment:* In subjects with varying degrees of hepatic impairment (Child-Pugh class A, B, or C), clearance values for dexmedetomidine were lower than in healthy subjects. The mean clearance values for subjects with mild, moderate, and severe hepatic impairment were 74%, 64%, and 53% of those observed in healthy subjects, respectively. Mean clearances for free drug were 59%, 51%, and 32% of those observed in healthy subjects, respectively.

Although dexmedetomidine is dosed to effect, it may be necessary to consider dose reduction in patients with hepatic impairment.

➤*Mutagenesis:* Dexmedetomidine was not mutagenic in vitro, in either the bacterial reverse mutation assay (*E. coli* and *Salmonella typhimurium*) or the mammalian cell forward mutation assay (mouse lymphoma). Dexmedetomidine was clastogenic in the in vitro human lymphocyte chromosome aberration test with, but not without, metabolic activation. Dexmedetomidine was also clastogenic in the in vitro mouse micronucleus test.

➤*Elderly:* A total of 531 subjects in the clinical studies were greater than or equal to 65 years of age. A total of 129 subjects in the clinical studies were greater than or equal to 75 years of age. In patients greater than 65 years of age, a higher incidence of bradycardia and hypotension was observed following administration of dexmedetomidine. Therefore a dose reduction may be considered in patients greater than 65 years of age.

Dexmedetomidine is known to be substantially excreted by the kidney, and the risk of adverse reactions to this drug may be greater in patients with impaired renal function. Because elderly patients are more likely to have decreased renal function, care should be taken in dose selection in elderly patients, and it may be useful to monitor renal function.

➤*Pregnancy: Category C.*

Teratogenic – Teratogenic effects were not observed following administration of dexmedetomidine at SC doses up to 200 mcg/kg in rats from day 5 to day 16 of gestation and IV doses up to 96 mcg/kg in rabbits from day 6 to day 18 of gestation. The dose in rats is approximately 2 times the maximum recommended human IV dose on a mcg/m^2 basis. The exposure in rabbits is approximately equal to that in humans at the maximum recommended IV dose based on plasma area-under-the-curve values. However, fetal toxicity, as evidenced by increased postimplantation losses and reduced live pups, was observed in rats at a SC dose of 200 mcg/kg. The no-effect dose was 20 mcg/kg (less than the maximum recommended human IV dose on a mcg/m^2 basis). In another reproductive study when dexmedetomidine was administered SC to pregnant rats from gestation day 16 through nursing, it caused lower pup weights at doses of 8 and 32 mcg/kg as well as fetal and embryocidal toxicity of second generation offspring at a dose of 32 mcg/kg (less than the maximum recommended human IV dose on a mcg/m^2 basis). Dexmedetomidine also produced delayed motor development in pups at a dose of 32 mcg/kg (less than the maximum recommended human IV dose on a mcg/m^2 basis). No such effects were observed at a dose of 2 mcg/kg (less than the maximum recommended human IV dose on a mcg/m^2 basis).

Placental transfer of dexmedetomidine was observed when radiolabeled dexmedetomidine was administered SC to pregnant rats.

There are no adequate and well-controlled studies in pregnant women. Dexmedetomidine should be used during pregnancy only if the potential benefits justify the potential risk to the fetus.

Labor and delivery – The safety of dexmedetomidine during labor and delivery has not been studied. Therefore, dexmedetomidine is not recommended during labor and delivery, including cesarean section deliveries.

➤*Lactation:* It is not known whether dexmedetomidine is excreted in human milk. Radiolabeled dexmedetomidine administered SC to lactating female rats was excreted in milk. Because many drugs are excreted in human milk, caution should be exercised when dexmedetomidine is administered to a nursing woman.

➤*Children:* There have been no clinical studies to establish the safety and efficacy of dexmedetomidine in children less than 18 years of age. Therefore, dexmedetomidine is not recommended for use in this population.

Precautions

➤*Alertness:* Some patients receiving dexmedetomidine have been observed to be arousable and alert when stimulated. This alone should not be considered an evidence of lack of efficacy in the absence of other clinical signs and symptoms.

➤*Administration:* Dexmedetomidine infusion should not be coadministered through the same IV catheter with blood or plasma since physical compatibility has not been established. Safety and efficacy of dexmedetomidine have not been evaluated in infusions over 24 hours. Dexmedetomidine is not indicated for infusions lasting over 24 hours.

➤*Withdrawal:* Although not specifically studied, if dexmedetomidine is administered chronically and stopped abruptly, withdrawal symptoms similar to those reported for another alpha-2-adrenergic agent, clonidine, may result. These symptoms may include nervousness, agitation, and headaches, accompanied or followed by a rapid rise in blood pressure and elevated catecholamine concentrations in the plasma. Dexmedetomidine should not be administered for greater than 24 hours.

➤*Adrenal insufficiency:* Dexmedetomidine had no effect on ACTH-stimulated cortisol release in dogs after a single dose; however, after the SC infusion of dexmedetomidine for 1 week, the cortisol response to ACTH was diminished by approximately 40%.

➤*Special risk:* Caution should be exercised when administering dexmedetomidine HCl injection to patients with advanced heart block or severe ventricular dysfunction. Because dexmedetomidine HCl injection decreases sympathetic nervous system activity, hypotension or bradycardia may be expected to be more pronounced in hypovolemic patients and in those with diabetes mellitus or chronic hypertension and in the elderly.

In situations where other vasodilators or negative chronotropic agents are administered, coadministration of dexmedetomidine HCl injection could have an additive pharmacodynamic affect and should be administered with caution.

➤*Drug abuse and dependence:* Dexmedetomidine is not a controlled substance. The dependence potential of dexmedetomidine has not been studied in humans. However, since studies in rodents and primates have demonstrated that dexmedetomidine exhibits pharmacologic actions similar to those of clonidine, it is possible that dexmedetomidine may produce a clonidine-like withdrawal syndrome upon abrupt discontinuation.

Drug Interactions

➤*Anesthetics, sedatives, hypnotics, and opioids:* Coadministration of dexmedetomidine with anesthetics, sedatives, hypnotics, and opioids is likely to lead to an enhancement of effects. Specific studies have confirmed these effects with sevoflurane, isoflurane, propofol, alfentanil, and midazolam. No pharmacokinetic interactions between dexmedetomidine and isoflurane, propofol, alfentanil, and midazolam have been demonstrated. However, due to possible pharmacodynamic interactions, when coadministered with dexmedetomidine, a reduction in dosage of dexmedetomidine on the concomitant anesthetic, sedative, hypnotic, or opioid may be required.

➤*Neuromuscular blockers:* In one study of 10 healthy volunteers, administration of dexmedetomidine for 45 minutes at a plasma concentration of 1 ng/mL resulted in no clinically meaningful increases in the magnitude or neuromuscular blockade associated with rocuronium administration.

Adverse Reactions

Adverse event information is derived from the placebo-controlled, continuous infusion trials of dexmedetomidine for sedation in the ICU setting in which 387 patients received dexmedetomidine. Overall, the most frequently observed treatment-emergent adverse reactions included hypotension, hypertension, nausea, bradycardia, fever, vomiting hypoxia, tachycardia, and anemia (see the table below).

Treatment-Emergent Adverse Reactions Occurring in > 1% of All Dexmedetomidine-Treated Patients in the Randomized Placebo-Controlled Continuous Infusion ICU Sedation Studies

Adverse reaction	Randomized dexmedetomidine (n = 387)	Placebo (n = 379)
Hypotension	28%	13%
Hypertension	16%	18%
Nausea	11%	9%
Bradycardia	7%	3%
Fever	5%	4%
Vomiting	4%	6%
Atrial fibrillation	4%	3%
Hypoxia	4%	4%
Tachycardia	3%	5%
Hemorrhage	3%	4%
Anemia	3%	2%
Dry mouth	3%	1%
Rigors	2%	3%
Agitation	2%	3%

DEXMEDETOMIDINE HYDROCHLORIDE — INJECTION

Treatment-Emergent Adverse Reactions Occurring in > 1% of All Dexmedetomidine-Treated Patients in the Randomized Placebo-Controlled Continuous Infusion ICU Sedation Studies

Adverse reaction	Randomized dexmedetomidine (n = 387)	Placebo (n = 379)
Hyperpyrexia	2%	3%
Pain	2%	2%
Hyperglycemia	2%	2%
Acidosis	2%	2%
Pleural effusion	2%	1%
Oliguria	2%	< 1%
Thirst	2%	< 1%

The treatment-emergent adverse events below were reported in less than or equal to 1% of all dexmedetomidine-treated patients in the continuous infusion ICU sedation trials and are potentially clinically relevant.

Potentially Clinically Relevant Treatment-Emergent Adverse Reactions to Dexmedetomidine Reported in ≤ 1% of Patients in the Continuous Infusion ICU Sedation Trials

Body system	Preferred term
Miscellaneous	Fever, hyperpyrexia, hypovolemia, light anesthesia, pain, rigors
Cardiovascular, general	Blood pressure fluctuation, heart disorder, aggravated hypertension
Central/peripheral nervous	Dizziness, headache, neuralgia, neuritis, speech disorder
GI	Abdominal pain, diarrhea, vomiting
Heart rate and rhythm	Arrhythmia, ventricular arrhythmia, AV block, cardiac arrest, extrasystoles, atrial fibrillation, heart block, T wave inversion, tachycardia, supraventricular tachycardia, ventricular tachycardia

Potentially Clinically Relevant Treatment-Emergent Adverse Reactions to Dexmedetomidine Reported in ≤ 1% of Patients in the Continuous Infusion ICU Sedation Trials

Body system	Preferred term
Liver and biliary	Increased GGT, increased AST, increased ALT
Metabolic/nutritional	Acidosis, respiratory acidosis, hyperkalemia, increased alkaline phosphatase, thirst
Psychiatric	Agitation, confusion, delirium, hallucination, illusion, somnolence
Hematologic	Anemia
Respiratory	Apnea, bronchospasm, dyspnea, hypercapnia, hypoventilation, hypoxia, pulmonary congestion
Dermatologic and appendages	Increased sweating
Ophthalmic	Photopsia, abnormal vision

Overdosage

The tolerability of dexmedetomidine was noted in 1 study in which healthy subjects were administered doses at and above the recommended dose of 0.2 to 0.7 mcg/kg/hr. The maximum blood concentration achieved in this study was approximately 13 times the upper boundary of the therapeutic range. The most notable effects observed in 2 subjects who achieved the highest doses were first-degree AV block and second-degree heart block. No hemodynamic compromise was noted with the AV block and the heart block resolved spontaneously within 1 minute.

Five patients received an overdose of dexmedetomidine in the ICU sedation studies. Two of these patients had no symptoms reported; 1 patient received a 2 mcg/kg loading dose over 10 minutes (twice the recommended loading dose), and 1 patient received a maintenance infusion of 0.8 mcg/kg/hr. Two other patients who received a 2 mcg/kg loading dose over 10 minutes experienced bradycardia or hypotension. One patient who received a loading bolus dose of undiluted dexmedetomidine (19.4 mcg/kg) had cardiac arrest from which he was successfully resuscitated.

ESZOPICLONE

c-iv	**Lunesta** (Sepracor)	**Tablets:** 1 mg	Lactose. (S190). Lt. blue. Film-coated. In 100s.
		2 mg	Lactose. (S191). White. Film-coated. In 100s; cartons of 90s.
		3 mg	Lactose. (S193). Dk. blue. Film-coated. In 100s; cartons of 90s.

ESZOPICLONE — ORAL

Indications

➤*Insomnia:* Eszopiclone is indicated for the treatment of insomnia. In controlled outpatient and sleep laboratory studies, eszopiclone administered at bedtime decreased sleep latency and improved sleep maintenance.

Administration and Dosage

➤*Approved by the FDA:* December 15, 2004.

➤*Adults:* Individualize the dose of eszopiclone. The recommended starting dose for eszopiclone for most nonelderly adults is 2 mg immediately before bedtime. Dosing can be initiated at or raised to 3 mg if clinically indicated because 3 mg is more effective for sleep maintenance.

➤*Elderly:* The recommended starting dose of eszopiclone for elderly patients whose primary complaint is difficulty falling asleep is 1 mg immediately before bedtime. In these patients, the dose may be increased to 2 mg if clinically indicated. For elderly patients whose primary complaint is difficulty staying asleep, the recommended dose is 2 mg immediately before bedtime.

➤*Administration:* Taking eszopiclone with or immediately after a heavy, high-fat meal results in slower absorption and would be expected to reduce the effect of eszopiclone on sleep latency.

➤*Hepatic function impairment:* The starting dose of eszopiclone should be 1 mg in patients with severe hepatic impairment. Use eszopiclone with caution in these patients.

➤*Coadministration with CYP3A4 inhibitors:* Do not exceed a 1 mg starting dose of eszopiclone in patients coadministered eszopiclone with potent CYP3A4 inhibitors (eg, ketoconazole). If needed, the dose can be raised to 2 mg.

➤*Storage/Stability:* Store at 25°C (77°F); excursions permitted to 15° to 30°C (59° to 86°F).

Actions

➤*Pharmacology:* The precise mechanism of action of eszopiclone as a hypnotic is unknown, but its effect is believed to result from its interaction with gamma aminobutyric acid (GABA)-receptor complexes at binding domains located close to or allosterically coupled to benzodiazepine receptors. Eszopiclone is a nonbenzodiazepine hypnotic, which is a pyrrolopyrazine derivative of the cyclopyrrolone class, with a chemical structure unrelated to pyrazolopyrimidines, imidazopyridines, benzodiazepines, barbiturates, or other drugs with known hypnotic properties.

➤*Pharmacokinetics:*

Absorption/Distribution – The pharmacokinetics of eszopiclone have been investigated in healthy subjects (adult and elderly) and in patients with hepatic disease or renal disease. In healthy subjects, the pharmacokinetic profile was examined after single doses of up to 7.5 mg and after once-daily administration of 1, 3, and 6 mg for 7 days. Eszopiclone is rapidly absorbed, with a time to peak concentration (T_{max}) of approximately 1 hour. In healthy adults, eszopiclone does not accumulate with once-daily administration, and its exposure is dose-proportional over the range of 1 to 6 mg.

Eszopiclone is weakly bound to plasma protein (52% to 59%). The large free fraction suggests that eszopiclone disposition should not be affected by drug-drug interactions caused by protein binding. The blood-to-plasma ratio for eszopiclone is less than 1, indicating no selective uptake by red blood cells.

Metabolism – Following oral administration, eszopiclone is extensively metabolized by oxidation and demethylation. The primary plasma metabolites are (*S*)-zopiclone-N-oxide and (*S*)-N-desmethyl zopiclone; the latter compound binds to GABA receptors with substantially lower potency than eszopiclone, and the former compound shows no significant binding to this receptor. In vitro studies have shown that CYP3A4 and CYP2E1 enzymes are involved in the metabolism of eszopiclone. Eszopiclone did not show any inhibitory potential on CYP450 1A2, 2A6, 2C9, 2C19, 2D6, 2E1, and 3A4 in cryopreserved human hepatocytes.

Excretion – After oral administration, eszopiclone is eliminated with a mean $t_{1/2}$ of approximately 6 hours. Up to 75% of an oral dose of racemic zopiclone is excreted in the urine, primarily as metabolites. A similar excretion profile would be expected for eszopiclone, the S-isomer of racemic zopiclone. Less than 10% of the oral eszopiclone dose is excreted in the urine as parent drug.

Special populations –

Hepatic function impairment: Pharmacokinetics of an eszopiclone 2 mg dose were assessed in 16 healthy volunteers and in 8 subjects with mild, moderate, and severe liver disease. Exposure was increased 2-fold in severely impaired patients compared with healthy volunteers. C_{max} and T_{max} were unchanged. Do not increase the dose of eszopiclone above 2 mg in patients with severe hepatic impairment. No dose adjustment is necessary for patients with mild to moderate hepatic impairment. Use eszopiclone with caution in patients with hepatic impairment.

Elderly: Compared with nonelderly adults, subjects 65 years of age and older had an increase of 41% in total exposure (AUC) and a slightly prolonged elimination of eszopiclone ($t_{1/2}$ approximately 9 hours). C_{max} was

ESZOPICLONE — ORAL

unchanged. Therefore, in elderly patients, decrease the starting dose of eszopiclone to 1 mg. The dose should not exceed 2 mg.

Effect of food – In healthy adults, administration of an eszopiclone 3 mg dose after a high-fat meal resulted in no change in AUC, a reduction in mean maximal drug concentration (C_{max}) of 21%, and delayed T_{max} by approximately 1 hour. The half-life remained unchanged, approximately 6 hours. The effects of eszopiclone on sleep onset may be reduced if it is taken with or immediately after a high-fat/heavy meal.

Contraindications

None known.

Warnings

➤*Psychiatric/physical disorder:* Because sleep disturbances may be the presenting manifestation of a physical and/or psychiatric disorder, initiate symptomatic treatment of insomnia only after a careful evaluation of the patient. The failure of insomnia to remit after 7 to 10 days of treatment may indicate the presence of a primary psychiatric and/or medical illness that should be evaluated. Worsening of insomnia or the emergence of new thinking or behavior abnormalities may be the consequence of an unrecognized psychiatric or physical disorder. Such findings have emerged during the course of treatment with sedative/hypnotic drugs, including eszopiclone. Because some of the important adverse effects of eszopiclone appear to be dose-related, it is important to use the lowest possible effective dose, especially in the elderly.

A variety of abnormal thinking and behavior changes have been reported to occur in association with the use of sedative/hypnotics. Some of these changes may be characterized by decreased inhibition (eg, aggressiveness and extroversion that seem out of character), similar to effects produced by alcohol and other CNS depressants. Other reported behavioral changes have included bizarre behavior, agitation, hallucinations, and depersonalization. Amnesia and other neuropsychiatric symptoms may occur unpredictably. In primarily depressed patients, worsening of depression, including suicidal thinking, has been reported in association with the use of sedative/hypnotics.

It can rarely be determined with certainty whether a particular instance of the abnormal behaviors listed above are drug-induced, spontaneous in origin, or a result of an underlying psychiatric or physical disorder. Nonetheless, the emergence of any new behavioral sign or symptom of concern requires careful and immediate evaluation.

➤*Rapid dose decrease/discontinuation:* Following rapid dose decrease or abrupt discontinuation of the use of sedative/hypnotics, there have been reports of signs and symptoms similar to those associated with withdrawal from other CNS-depressant drugs.

➤*CNS effects:* Eszopiclone, like other hypnotics, has CNS-depressant effects. Because of the rapid onset of action, eszopiclone should only be ingested immediately prior to going to bed or after the patient has gone to bed and has experienced difficulty falling asleep. Eszopiclone, like other hypnotics, may produce additive CNS-depressant effects when coadministered with other psychotropic medications, anticonvulsants, antihistamines, ethanol, and other drugs that produce CNS depression. Eszopiclone should not be taken with alcohol. Dose adjustment may be necessary when eszopiclone is administered with other CNS-depressant agents because of the potentially additive effects.

➤*Hepatic function impairment:* Reduce the dose of eszopiclone to 1 mg in patients with severe hepatic impairment because systemic exposure is doubled in such subjects. No dose adjustment appears necessary for subjects with mild or moderate hepatic impairment.

➤*Carcinogenesis:* In a carcinogenicity study in Sprague-Dawley rats in which eszopiclone was given by oral gavage, no increases in tumors were seen; plasma levels (AUC) of eszopiclone at the highest dosage used in this study (16 mg/kg/day) are estimated to be 80 (females) and 20 (males) times those in humans receiving the maximum recommended human dose (MRHD). However, in a carcinogenicity study in Sprague-Dawley rats in which racemic zopiclone was given in the diet, and in which plasma levels of eszopiclone were reached that were greater than those reached in the above study of eszopiclone, an increase in mammary gland adenocarcinomas in females and an increase in thyroid gland follicular cell adenomas and carcinomas in males were seen at the highest dosage of 100 mg/kg/day. Plasma levels of eszopiclone at this dosage are estimated to be 150 (females) and 70 (males) times those in humans receiving the MRHD. The mechanism for the increase in mammary adenocarcinomas is unknown. The increase in thyroid tumors is thought to be caused by increased levels of thyroid-stimulating hormone (TSH) secondary to increased metabolism of circulating thyroid hormones, a mechanism that is not considered to be relevant to humans.

In a carcinogenicity study in B6C3F1 mice in which racemic zopiclone was given in the diet, an increase in pulmonary carcinomas and carcinomas plus adenomas in females and an increase in skin fibromas and sarcomas in males were seen at the highest dosage of 100 mg/kg/day. Plasma levels of eszopiclone at this dosage are estimated to be 8 (females) and 20 (males) times those in humans receiving the MRHD. The skin tumors were caused by skin lesions induced by aggressive behavior, a mechanism that is not relevant to humans. A carcinogenicity study also was performed in which CD-1 mice were given eszopiclone at dosages up to 100 mg/kg/day by oral gavage; although this study did not reach a maximum tolerated dose, and was thus inadequate for overall assessment of carcinogenic potential, no increases in either pulmonary or skin tumors were seen at doses producing plasma levels of eszopiclone estimated to be 90 times those in humans receiving the MRHD (ie, 12 times the exposure in the racemate study).

➤*Mutagenesis:* Eszopiclone was positive in the mouse lymphoma chromosomal aberration assay and produced an equivocal response in the Chinese hamster ovary cell chromosomal aberration assay. It was not mutagenic or clastogenic in the bacterial Ames gene mutation assay, in an unscheduled DNA synthesis assay, or in an in vivo mouse bone marrow micronucleus assay.

(*S*)-N-desmethyl zopiclone, a metabolite of eszopiclone, was positive in the Chinese hamster ovary cell and human lymphocyte chromosomal aberration assays. It was negative in the bacterial Ames mutation assay, in an in vitro ^{32}P-postlabeling DNA adduct assay, and in an in vivo mouse bone marrow chromosomal aberration and micronucleus assay.

➤*Fertility impairment:* Eszopiclone was given by oral gavage to male rats at doses up to 45 mg/kg/day from 4 weeks premating through mating and to female rats at dosages up to 180 mg/kg/day from 2 weeks premating through day 7 of pregnancy. An additional study was performed in which only females were treated, up to 180 mg/kg/day. Eszopiclone decreased fertility, probably because of effects in both males and females, with no females becoming pregnant when both males and females were treated with the highest dosage; the no-effect dose in both sexes was 5 mg/kg (16 times the MRHD on a mg/m^2 basis). Other effects included increased preimplantation loss (no-effect dose 25 mg/kg), abnormal estrus cycles (no-effect dose 25 mg/kg), and decreases in sperm number and motility and increases in morphologically abnormal sperm (no-effect dose 5 mg/kg).

➤*Elderly:* A total of 287 subjects in double-blind, parallel-group, placebo-controlled clinical trials who received eszopiclone were 65 to 86 years of age. The overall pattern of adverse reactions for elderly subjects (median age, 71 years) in 2-week studies with nighttime dosing of eszopiclone 2 mg was not different from that seen in younger adults. Eszopiclone 2 mg exhibited significant reduction in sleep latency and improvement in sleep maintenance in the elderly population.

➤*Pregnancy: Category C.* Eszopiclone administered by oral gavage to pregnant rats and rabbits during the period of organogenesis showed no evidence of teratogenicity up to the highest doses tested (250 and 16 mg/kg/day in rats and rabbits, respectively; these dosages are 800 and 100 times, respectively, the MRHD on a mg/m^2 basis). In the rat, slight reductions in fetal weight and evidence of developmental delay were seen at maternally toxic dosages of 125 and 150 mg/kg/day, but not at 62.5 mg/kg/day (200 times the MRHD on a mg/m^2 basis).

Eszopiclone also was administered by oral gavage to pregnant rats throughout the pregnancy and lactation periods at dosages of up to 180 mg/kg/day. Increased postimplantation loss, decreased postnatal pup weights and survival, and increased pup startle response were seen at all doses; the lowest dose tested, 60 mg/kg/day, is 200 times the MRHD on a mg/m^2 basis. These doses did not produce significant maternal toxicity. Eszopiclone had no effects on other behavioral measures or reproductive function in the offspring.

There are no adequate and well-controlled studies of eszopiclone in pregnant women. Use eszopiclone during pregnancy only if the potential benefit justifies the potential risk to the fetus.

Labor and delivery – Eszopiclone has no established use in labor and delivery.

➤*Lactation:* It is not known whether eszopiclone is excreted in human milk. Because many drugs are excreted in human milk, exercise caution when eszopiclone is administered to a breast-feeding woman.

➤*Children:* Safety and efficacy of eszopiclone in children younger than 18 years of age have not been established.

Precautions

➤*Timing of drug administration:* Eszopiclone should be taken immediately before bedtime. Taking a sedative/hypnotic while still ambulatory may result in short-term memory impairment, hallucinations, impaired coordination, dizziness, and light-headedness.

➤*Special risk:*

Elderly/Debilitated patients – Impaired motor and/or cognitive performance after repeated exposure or unusual sensitivity to sedative/hypnotic drugs is a concern in the treatment of elderly and/or debilitated patients. The recommended starting dose of eszopiclone for these patients is 1 mg.

Patients with concomitant illness – A study in healthy volunteers did not reveal respiratory-depressant effects at doses 2.5-fold higher (7 mg) than the recommended dose of eszopiclone. Caution is advised, however, if eszopiclone is prescribed to patients with compromised respiratory function.

Depression – Administer sedative/hypnotic drugs with caution to patients exhibiting signs and symptoms of depression. Suicidal tendencies may be present in such patients, and protective measures may be required. Intentional overdose is more common in this group of patients; therefore, prescribe the least amount of drug that is feasible for the patient at any one time.

➤*Drug abuse and dependence:*

Abuse and dependence – In a study of abuse liability conducted in individuals with known histories of benzodiazepine abuse, doses of eszopiclone 6 and 12 mg produced euphoric effects similar to those of diazepam 20 mg. In this study, at doses 2-fold or greater than the maximum recommended doses, a dose-related increase in reports of amnesia and hallucinations was observed for both eszopiclone and diazepam.

The clinical trial experience with eszopiclone revealed no evidence of a serious withdrawal syndrome. Nevertheless, the following adverse reactions included in *Diagnostic and Statistical Manual of Mental Disorders, Fourth Edition* (DSM-IV) criteria for uncomplicated sedative/hypnotic withdrawal were reported during clinical trials following placebo substitution occurring within 48 hours following the last eszopiclone treatment: abnormal dreams, anxiety, nausea, and upset stomach. These reported adverse reactions occurred at an incidence of 2% or less. Use of benzodiazepines and similar

ESZOPICLONE — ORAL

agents may lead to physical and psychological dependence. The risk of abuse and dependence increases with the dose and duration of treatment and concomitant use of other psychoactive drugs. The risk also is greater for patients who have a history of alcohol or drug abuse or history of psychiatric disorders. These patients should be under careful surveillance when receiving eszopiclone or any other hypnotic.

➤*Hazardous tasks:* Caution patients receiving eszopiclone against engaging in hazardous occupations requiring complete mental alertness or motor coordination (eg, operating machinery, driving a motor vehicle) after ingesting the drug, and caution them about potential impairment of the performance of such activities on the day following ingestion of eszopiclone.

Drug Interactions

➤*Olanzapine:* Coadministration of eszopiclone 3 mg and olanzapine 10 mg produced a decrease in DSST scores. The interaction was pharmacodynamic; there was no alteration in the pharmacokinetics of either drug.

Eszopiclone Drug Interactions

Precipitant drug	Object drug[a]		Description
CYP3A4 inducers (eg, rifampin)	Eszopiclone	⬇	Racemic zopiclone exposure was decreased 80% by concomitant use of rifampin. A similar effect would be expected with eszopiclone.
CYP3A4 inhibitors (eg, ketoconazole, clarithromycin, nefazodone, ritonavir)	Eszopiclone	⬆	The AUC, C_{max}, and $t_{½}$ of eszopiclone may be increased when given with a strong CYP3A4 inhibitor. Do not exceed a starting dose of eszopiclone 1 mg when coadministered with potent CYP3A4 inhibitors.
Ethanol	Eszopiclone	⬆	An additive effect on psychomotor performance was seen with coadministration of eszopiclone and ethanol 0.7 g/kg for up to 4 hours after ethanol administration.
Eszopiclone	Ethanol		

[a] ⬆ = Object drug increased. ⬇ = Object drug decreased.

➤*Drug/Food interactions:* See Actions for more information.

Adverse Reactions

➤*Adverse findings observed in placebo-controlled trials:*

Adverse reactions resulting in discontinuation of treatment – In placebo-controlled, parallel-group clinical trials in the elderly, 3.8% of 208 patients who received placebo, 2.3% of 215 patients who received eszopiclone 2 mg, and 1.4% of 72 patients who received eszopiclone 1 mg discontinued treatment because of an adverse reaction. In the 6-week, parallel-group study in adults, no patients in the 3 mg arm discontinued because of an adverse reaction. In the long-term, 6-month study in adult insomnia patients, 7.2% of 195 patients who received placebo and 12.8% of 593 patients who received eszopiclone 3 mg discontinued because of an adverse reaction. No reaction that resulted in discontinuation occurred at a rate of greater than 2%.

Adverse reactions observed at an incidence of at least 2% in controlled trials – The following table shows the incidence of treatment-emergent adverse reactions from a phase 3, placebo-controlled study of eszopiclone at doses of 2 or 3 mg in nonelderly adults. Treatment duration in this trial was 44 days. The table includes only reactions that occurred in 2% or more of patients treated with eszopiclone 2 or 3 mg in which the incidence in patients treated with eszopiclone was greater than the incidence in placebo-treated patients.

Incidence of Treatment-Emergent Adverse Reactions in a 6-Week, Placebo-Controlled Study in Nonelderly Adults with Eszopiclone[a]

Adverse reaction	Placebo (n = 99)	Eszopiclone 2 mg (n = 104)	Eszopiclone 3 mg (n = 105)
CNS			
Anxiety	0%	3%	1%
Confusion	0%	0%	3%
Depression	0%	4%	1%
Dizziness	4%	5%	7%
Hallucinations	0%	1%	3%
Headache	13%	21%	17%
Libido decreased	0%	0%	3%
Nervousness	3%	5%	0%
Somnolence	3%	10%	8%
Dermatologic			
Rash	1%	3%	4%
GI			
Dry mouth	3%	5%	7%
Dyspepsia	4%	4%	5%
Nausea	4%	5%	4%
Vomiting	1%	3%	0%
GU			
Dysmenorrhea[b]	0%	3%	0%
Gynecomastia[c]	0%	3%	0%
Respiratory			
Infection	3%	5%	10%
Special senses			
Unpleasant taste	3%	17%	34%
Miscellaneous			
Viral infection	1%	3%	3%

[a] Reactions for which the eszopiclone incidence was equal to or less than placebo are not listed in the table, but included the following: abnormal dreams, accidental injury, back pain, diarrhea, flu syndrome, myalgia, pain, pharyngitis, and rhinitis.
[b] Gender-specific adverse reactions in women.
[c] Gender-specific adverse reactions in men.

Adverse reactions from the previous table that suggest a dose-response relationship in adults include dizziness, dry mouth, hallucinations, infection, rash, unpleasant taste, and viral infection, with this relationship clearest for unpleasant taste.

The following table shows the incidence of treatment-emergent adverse reactions from combined phase 3, placebo-controlled studies of eszopiclone at doses of 1 or 2 mg in elderly adults (65 to 86 years of age). Treatment duration in these trials was 14 days. The table includes only reactions that occurred in 2% or more of patients treated with eszopiclone 1 or 2 mg in which the incidence in patients treated with eszopiclone was greater than the incidence in placebo-treated patients.

Incidence of Treatment-Emergent Adverse Reactions in Elderly Adults (65 to 86 Years of Age) in 2-Week, Placebo-Controlled Trials with Eszopiclone[a]

Adverse reaction	Placebo (n = 208)	Eszopiclone 1 mg (n = 72)	Eszopiclone 2 mg (n = 215)
CNS			
Abnormal dreams	0%	3%	1%
Dizziness	2%	1%	6%
Headache	14%	15%	13%
Nervousness	1%	0%	2%
Neuralgia	0%	3%	0%
Dermatologic			
Pruritus	1%	4%	1%
GI			
Diarrhea	2%	4%	2%
Dry mouth	2%	3%	7%
Dyspepsia	2%	6%	2%
GU			
Urinary tract infection	0%	3%	0%
Special senses			
Unpleasant taste	0%	8%	12%
Miscellaneous			
Accidental injury	1%	0%	3%
Pain	2%	4%	5%

[a] Reactions for which the eszopiclone incidence was equal to or less than placebo are not listed in the table, but included the following: abdominal pain, asthenia, nausea, rash, and somnolence.

Adverse reactions from the previous table that suggest a dose-response relationship in elderly adults include dry mouth, pain, and unpleasant taste, with this relationship, again, clearest for unpleasant taste.

➤*Other reactions observed during the premarketing evaluation of eszopiclone:*

Cardiovascular – Migraine (1% or more); hypertension (0.1% to less than 1%); thrombophlebitis (less than 0.1%).

CNS – Agitation, apathy, ataxia, emotional lability, hostility, hypertonia, hypesthesia, incoordination, insomnia, memory impairment, neurosis, nystagmus, paresthesia, reflexes decreased, thinking abnormal (mainly difficulty concentrating), vertigo (0.1% to less than 1%); abnormal gait, euphoria, hyperesthesia, hypokinesia, neuritis, neuropathy, stupor, tremor (less than 0.1%).

Dermatologic – Acne, alopecia, contact dermatitis, dry skin, eczema, skin discoloration, sweating, urticaria (0.1% to less than 1%); erythema multiforme, furunculosis, herpes zoster, hirsutism, maculopapular rash, vesiculobullous rash (less than 0.1%).

GI – Anorexia, cholelithiasis, increased appetite, melena, mouth ulceration, thirst, ulcerative stomatitis (0.1% to less than 1%); colitis, dysphagia, gastritis, hepatitis, hepatomegaly, liver damage, rectal hemorrhage, stomach ulcer, stomatitis, tongue edema (less than 0.1%).

GU – Amenorrhea, breast engorgement, breast enlargement, breast neoplasm, breast pain, cystitis, dysuria, female lactation, hematuria, kidney calculus, kidney pain, mastitis, menorrhagia, metrorrhagia, urinary frequency, urinary incontinence, uterine hemorrhage, vaginal hemorrhage, vaginitis (0.1% to less than 1%); oliguria, pyelonephritis, urethritis (less than 0.1%).

Hematologic/Lymphatic – Anemia, lymphadenopathy (0.1% to less than 1%).

Metabolic/Nutritional – Peripheral edema (1% or more); hypercholesteremia, weight gain, weight loss (0.1% to less than 1%); dehydration, gout, hyperlipemia, hypokalemia (less than 0.1%).

ESZOPICLONE — ORAL

Musculoskeletal – Arthritis, bursitis, joint disorder (mainly pain, stiffness, and swelling), leg cramps, myasthenia, twitching (0.1% to less than 1%); arthrosis, myopathy, ptosis (less than 0.1%).

Respiratory – Asthma, bronchitis, dyspnea, epistaxis, hiccup, laryngitis (0.1% to less than 1%).

Special senses – Conjunctivitis, dry eyes, ear pain, otitis externa, otitis media, tinnitus, vestibular disorder (0.1% to less than 1%); hyperacusis, iritis, mydriasis, photophobia (less than 0.1%).

Miscellaneous – Chest pain (1% or more); allergic reaction, cellulitis, face edema, fever, halitosis, heat stroke, hernia, malaise, neck rigidity, photosensitivity (0.1% to less than 1%).

Overdosage

➤*Symptoms:* Signs and symptoms of overdose effects of CNS depressants can be expected to present as exaggerations of the pharmacological effects noted in preclinical testing. Impairment of consciousness ranging from somnolence to coma has been described. Rare individual instances of fatal outcomes following overdose with racemic zopiclone have been reported in European postmarketing reports, most often associated with overdose with other CNS-depressant agents.

➤*Treatment:* Use general symptomatic and supportive measures along with immediate gastric lavage where appropriate. Administer intravenous fluids as needed. Flumazenil may be useful. As in all cases of drug overdose, monitor respiration, pulse, blood pressure, and other appropriate signs and employ general supportive measures. Monitor hypotension and CNS depression and treat by appropriate medical intervention. The value of dialysis in the treatment of overdosage has not been determined.

As with the management of all overdosage, consider the possibility of multiple drug ingestion. The physician may wish to consider contacting a poison control center (1-800-221-2222) for up-to-date information on the management of hypnotic drug product overdosage.

SEDATIVES AND HYPNOTICS, BARBITURATES

The following general discussion of the barbiturates refers to their use as sedative-hypnotic agents and as anticonvulsants. In addition, barbiturates are discussed under General Anesthetics, Barbiturates.

Indications

The following indications apply to most barbiturates. For specific indications, refer to the individual monographs.

➤*Acute convulsive episodes:* Emergency control of certain acute convulsive episodes (eg, those associated with status epilepticus, cholera, eclampsia, meningitis, tetanus, and toxic reactions to strychnine or local anesthetics).

➤*Anticonvulsant (mephobarbital, phenobarbital):* Treatment of partial and generalized tonic-clonic and cortical focal seizures.

➤*Hypnotic:* Short-term treatment of insomnia, since barbiturates appear to lose their effectiveness in sleep induction and maintenance after 2 weeks. If insomnia persists, seek alternative therapy (including nondrug) for chronic insomnia.

➤*Preanesthetic:* Used as preanesthetic sedatives.

➤*Sedation:* Although traditionally used as nonspecific CNS depressants for daytime sedation, the barbiturates generally have been replaced by the benzodiazepines.

Administration and Dosage

Individualize dosage; consider patient's age, weight and condition. Use parenteral routes only when oral administration is impossible or impractical.

➤*Intramuscular (IM) injection:* IM injection of the sodium salts should be made deeply into a large muscle. Do not exceed 5 mL at any one site because of possible tissue irritation. Monitor patient's vital signs.

➤*Intravenous (IV):* Restrict to conditions in which other routes are not feasible, either because the patient is unconscious (as in cerebral hemorrhage, eclampsia or status epilepticus), or because the patient resists (as in delirium), or because prompt action is imperative. Slow IV injection is essential; observe patients carefully during administration. Maintain blood pressure, respiratory and cardiac function, monitor vital signs, and have equipment for resuscitation and artificial ventilation available.

➤*Rectal administration:* Rectally administered barbiturates are absorbed from the colon and are used occasionally in infants for prolonged convulsive states, or when oral or parenteral administration may be undesirable. If the rectal form is not available, the soluble sodium salt may be incorporated in a retention enema.

➤*Elderly/Debilitated:* Reduce dosage because these patients may be more sensitive to barbiturates.

➤*Hepatic/Renal function impairment:* Reduce dosage.

Actions

➤*Pharmacology:* Barbiturates can produce all levels of CNS mood alteration from excitation to mild sedation, hypnosis, and deep coma. In sufficiently high therapeutic doses, barbiturates induce anesthesia. Overdosage can produce death.

These agents depress the sensory cortex, decrease motor activity, alter cerebellar function, and produce drowsiness, sedation, and hypnosis.

Barbiturates have little analgesic action at subanesthetic doses and may increase the reaction to painful stimuli. All barbiturates exhibit anticonvulsant activity in anesthetic doses. However, only phenobarbital and mephobarbital are effective as oral anticonvulsants in subhypnotic doses.

Barbiturates are respiratory depressants; the degree of respiratory depression is dose-dependent. With hypnotic doses, respiratory depression is similar to that which occurs during physiologic sleep and is accompanied by a slight decrease in blood pressure and heart rate.

➤*Pharmacokinetics:*

Absorption – Barbiturates are absorbed in varying degrees following oral, rectal, or parenteral administration. The salts are more rapidly absorbed than the acids. The rate of absorption is increased if the sodium salt is ingested as a dilute solution or taken on an empty stomach.

Onset: Onset of action for oral or rectal administration varies from 20 to 60 minutes. For IM administration, onset is slightly faster than the oral route. Following IV administration, onset ranges from almost immediate for pentobarbital sodium and secobarbital to 5 minutes for phenobarbital sodium. Maximal CNS depression may not occur for at least 15 minutes after IV administration of phenobarbital sodium.

Duration: Duration of action varies and is related to dose and to the rate at which the barbiturates are redistributed throughout the body. In the following table, the barbiturates are classified according to their duration of action. Do not use this classification to predict the exact duration of effect, but use as a guide in drug selection.

Pharmacokinetics of Sedatives and Hypnotic Barbiturates

	Barbiturate	Half-life (h) Range	Half-life (h) Mean	Oral dosage range (mg) Sedative[a]	Oral dosage range (mg) Hypnotic	Onset (min)	Duration (h)
Long-Acting	Mephobarbital	11 to 67	34	32 to 200	—	30 to ≥ 60	10 to 16
	Phenobarbital	53 to 118	79	30 to 120	100 to 320		
Intermediate	Amobarbital[b]	16 to 40	25	—	—	45 to 60	6 to 8
	Butabarbital	66 to 140	100	45 to 120	50 to 100		
Short-Acting	Pentobarbital	15 to 50	†[c]	40 to 120	100	10 to 15	3 to 4
	Secobarbital	15 to 40	28	—	100		

[a] Total daily dose; administered in 2 to 4 divided doses.
[b] Available as injection only.
[c] May follow dose-dependent kinetics. Mean half-life is 50 hours for 50 mg and 22 hours for 100 mg.

Distribution – Barbiturates are weak acids that are rapidly distributed to all tissues and fluids with high concentrations in the brain, liver, and kidneys. Lipid solubility of the barbiturates is the dominant factor in their distribution. The more lipid soluble the barbiturate, the more rapidly it penetrates body tissue. Barbiturates are bound to plasma and tissue proteins; the degree of binding increases directly as a function of lipid solubility.

Phenobarbital has the lowest lipid solubility, plasma binding and brain protein binding, the longest delay in onset of activity, and the longest duration of action. Secobarbital has the highest lipid solubility, plasma protein binding and brain protein binding, the shortest delay in onset of activity, and the shortest duration of action.

Excretion – Barbiturates are metabolized primarily by the hepatic microsomal enzyme system, and the metabolic products are excreted in the urine, and less commonly, in the feces. Approximately 25% to 50% of a phenobarbital dose is eliminated unchanged in the urine, whereas the amount of other barbiturates excreted unchanged in the urine is negligible. The excretion of unmetabolized barbiturate is one feature that distinguishes the long-acting agents. The inactive metabolites of the barbiturates are excreted as conjugates of glucuronic acid.

Contraindications

Barbiturate sensitivity; manifest or latent porphyria; marked liver function impairment; severe respiratory disease when dyspnea or obstruction is evident; nephritic patients; patients with respiratory disease where dyspnea or obstruction is present; intra-arterial administration (consequences vary from transient pain to gangrene); subcutaneous administration (produces tissue irritation ranging from tenderness and redness to necrosis); previous addiction to the sedative/hypnotic group (ordinary doses may be ineffective and may contribute to further addiction).

Warnings

➤*Habit forming:* Tolerance or psychological and physical dependence may occur with continued use (see Drug abuse and dependence in the Precautions section). Administer with caution, if at all, to patients who are mentally depressed, have suicidal tendencies or a history of drug abuse (eg, alcoholics, opiate abusers, other sedative-hypnotic and amphetamine abusers). Limit prescribing and dispensing to the amount required for the interval until the next appointment.

➤*IV administration:* Too rapid administration may cause respiratory depression, apnea, laryngospasm, or vasodilation with fall in blood pressure. Parenteral solutions of barbiturates are highly alkaline. Therefore, use extreme care to avoid perivascular extravasation or intra-arterial injection. Extravascular injection may cause local tissue damage with subsequent necrosis; consequences of intra-arterial injection may vary from transient pain to gangrene of the limb. Any complaint of pain in the limb warrants stopping the injection.

Phenobarbital sodium may be administered IM or IV as an anticonvulsant for emergency use. When administered IV, it may require at least 15 minutes before reaching peak concentrations in the brain. Therefore, injecting phenobarbital sodium until the convulsions stop may cause the brain level to exceed that required to control the convulsions and may lead to severe barbiturate-induced depression.

➤*Pain:* Exercise caution when administering to patients with acute or chronic pain, because paradoxical excitement may be induced or important symptoms may be masked. However, the use of barbiturates as sedatives in postoperative surgery and as adjuncts to cancer chemotherapy is well established.

➤*Seizure disorders:* Status epilepticus may result from abrupt discontinuation, even when administered in small daily doses in the treatment of epilepsy.

➤*Effects on vitamin D:* Barbiturates may increase vitamin D requirements, possibly by increasing the metabolism of vitamin D via enzyme induction. Rickets and osteomalacia have been reported rarely following prolonged use of barbiturates.

➤*Renal function impairment:* Barbiturates are excreted either partially or completely unchanged in the urine and are contraindicated in patients with renal function impairment.

➤*Hepatic function impairment:* Barbiturates are metabolized primarily by hepatic microsomal enzymes. Administer with caution and initially in reduced doses to patients with hepatic function impairment. Do not use in patients showing premonitory signs of hepatic coma.

➤*Elderly:* May produce marked excitement, depression, and confusion in elderly patients. In some people, barbiturates repeatedly produce excitement rather than depression.

➤*Pregnancy: Category D.* Barbiturates may cause fetal damage when administered to a pregnant woman. Studies suggest a connection between maternal consumption of barbiturates and a higher incidence of fetal abnormalities. If this drug is used during pregnancy, or if the patient becomes pregnant while taking this drug, apprise her of the potential hazards to the fetus.

Barbiturates readily cross the placental barrier and are distributed throughout fetal tissues. Fetal blood levels approach maternal blood levels following parenteral use.

Withdrawal symptoms occur in infants born to mothers who receive barbiturates throughout the last trimester of pregnancy. Reports include the acute withdrawal syndrome of seizures and hyperirritability from birth to a delayed onset of up to 14 days.

Anticonvulsant use – Because of the strong possibility of precipitating status epilepticus with attendant hypoxia and the risk to the mother and unborn child, do not discontinue anticonvulsants when used to prevent major seizures. However, consider discontinuing anticonvulsants prior to and during pregnancy when the nature, frequency and severity of the seizures do not pose a serious threat to the patient. It is not known whether even minor seizures constitute some risk to the embryo or fetus.

Maternal ingestion of anticonvulsants, particularly barbiturates, may be associated with a neonatal coagulation defect that may cause bleeding, usually within 24 hours of birth. The defect is characterized by decreased levels of vitamin K-dependent clotting factors, and prolongation of prothrombin time, partial thromboplastin time or both. Give prophylactic vitamin K to the mother 1 month prior to and during delivery, and to the infant immediately after birth.

Labor and delivery – Hypnotic doses do not appear to significantly impair uterine activity during labor. Full anesthetic doses decrease the force and frequency of uterine contractions. Administration to the mother during labor may result in respiratory depression in the newborn; premature infants are particularly susceptible. If barbiturates are used during labor and delivery, have resuscitation equipment available.

➤*Lactation:* Exercise caution when administering to a breast-feeding mother, because small amounts of drug are excreted in breast milk. Drowsiness in the nursing infant has been reported.

➤*Children:* In some patients, especially children, barbiturates repeatedly produce excitement rather than depression. Barbiturates may produce irritability, excitability, inappropriate tearfulness, and aggression in children. Hyperkinetic states also may be induced and are primarily related to a specific drug sensitivity. Cognitive deficits have been associated with phenobarbital use for complicated febrile seizures in children. Safety and efficacy of amobarbital (children < 6 years of age) have not been established.

Precautions

➤*Monitoring:* During prolonged therapy, perform periodic laboratory evaluation of organ systems, including hematopoietic, renal, and hepatic systems.

➤*Special risk:* Untoward reactions may occur in the presence of fever, hyperthyroidism, diabetes mellitus, and severe anemia. Use with caution.

Use **mephobarbital** with caution in patients with myasthenia gravis and myxedema.

➤*Drug abuse and dependence:* Barbiturates may be habit forming. Tolerance, psychological dependence, and physical dependence may occur, especially following prolonged use of high doses. Doses in excess of 400 mg/day **pentobarbital** or **secobarbital** for approximately 90 days are likely to produce some degree of physical dependence. A dose of 600 to 800 mg taken for at least 35 days is sufficient to produce withdrawal seizures. The average daily dose for the barbiturate addict is usually about 1.5 g. As tolerance develops, the amount needed to maintain the same level of intoxication increases; tolerance to a fatal dosage, however, does not increase more than 2-fold. As this occurs, the margin between an intoxicating dosage and fatal dosage becomes smaller.

Intoxication – Symptoms of acute intoxication include unsteady gait, slurred speech, and sustained nystagmus. Mental signs of chronic intoxication include confusion, poor judgment, irritability, insomnia, and somatic complaints. If an individual appears to be intoxicated with alcohol to a degree that is radically disproportionate to the amount of alcohol in his/her blood, suspect the use of barbiturates. The lethal dose of a barbiturate is less if accompanied with alcohol.

Dependence – Symptoms are similar to those of chronic alcoholism and include the following: a strong desire or need to continue taking the drug; tendency to increase the dose; psychological dependence on the effects of the drug related to subjective and individual appreciation of those effects; and physical dependence on the effects of the drug requiring its presence for maintenance of homeostasis resulting in a definite, characteristic, and self-limited abstinence syndrome when the drug is withdrawn.

Withdrawal symptoms – Withdrawal symptoms can be severe and may cause death.

Minor symptoms: These may appear 8 to 12 hours after the last dose of a barbiturate and usually appear in the following order: anxiety, muscle twitching, tremor of hands and fingers, progressive weakness, dizziness, distortion in visual perception, nausea, vomiting, insomnia, and orthostatic hypotension.

Major symptoms: Convulsions and delirium may occur within 16 hours and last up to 5 days after abrupt cessation of these drugs. Intensity of withdrawal symptoms gradually declines within about 15 days.

Treatment of dependence – Treatment of dependence consists of cautious and gradual withdrawal of the drug, which takes an extended period of time.

One method involves substituting 30 mg phenobarbital for each 100 to 200 mg barbiturate dose the patient is taking. The total daily amount of **phenobarbital** is administered in 3 to 4 divided doses, not to exceed 600 mg/day. Should signs of withdrawal occur on the first day of treatment, administer an IM loading dose of phenobarbital 100 to 200 mg in addition to the oral dose. After stabilization on phenobarbital, decrease the total daily dose by 30 mg/day as long as withdrawal is proceeding smoothly. A modification of this regimen involves initiating treatment at the patient's regular dosage level and decreasing the daily dosage by 10%, if tolerated. Severely dependent individuals generally may be withdrawn over 2 to 3 weeks.

Infants physically dependent on barbiturates may be given phenobarbital 3 to 10 mg/kg/day. After withdrawal symptoms (eg, hyperactivity, disturbed sleep, tremors, hyperreflexia) are relieved, gradually decrease the dosage of phenobarbital; completely withdraw over 2 weeks.

➤*Tartrazine sensitivity:* Some of these products contain tartrazine, which may cause allergic-type reactions (including bronchial asthma) in susceptible individuals. Although the incidence of tartrazine sensitivity in the general population is low, it is frequently seen in patients who also have aspirin hypersensitivity. Specific products containing tartrazine are identified in the product listings.

Drug Interactions

Most reports of clinically significant drug interactions occurring with the barbiturates have involved phenobarbital.

Sedative/Hypnotic Barbiturate Drug Interactions

Precipitant drug	Object drug[a]		Description
Alcohol	Barbiturates	↑	Concomitant use may produce additive CNS effects and death.
Charcoal	Barbiturates	↓	Charcoal may reduce the absorption of barbiturates. Depending on the clinical situation, this will reduce their efficacy or toxicity.
Chloramphenicol	Barbiturates	↓	Chloramphenicol may inhibit phenobarbital metabolism. Barbiturates may enhance chloramphenicol metabolism.
Barbiturates	Chloramphenicol	↑	
Monoamine oxidase inhibitors	Barbiturates	↑	MAOIs may enhance the sedative effects of barbiturates.
Rifampin	Barbiturates	↓	Rifampin induces hepatic microsomal enzymes and may decrease the effectiveness of barbiturates.
Valproic acid	Barbiturates	↑	Valproic acid appears to decrease barbiturate metabolism, resulting in an increased effect.
Barbiturates	Anticoagulants	↓	Barbiturates may increase metabolism of anticoagulants, resulting in a decreased response. Patients stabilized on anticoagulants may require dosage adjustments if barbiturates are added to or withdrawn from their regimen.
Barbiturates	Beta blockers	↓	Pharmacokinetic parameters of certain beta-blockers (metoprolol and propranolol) may be altered by barbiturates. Timolol does not appear to be affected.
Barbiturates	Carbamazepine	↓	Decreased serum carbamazepine levels may occur.
Barbiturates	Clonazepam	↓	Increased clonazepam clearance may occur, which may lead to lower steady-state levels and loss of efficacy.
Barbiturates	Contraceptives, oral	↓	Decreased contraceptive effect may occur due to induction of microsomal enzymes. Menstrual irregularities (eg, spotting, breakthrough bleeding) or pregnancy may occur. An alternate form of birth control is suggested.
Barbiturates	Corticosteroids	↓	Barbiturates may enhance corticosteroid metabolism through the induction of hepatic microsomal enzymes.
Barbiturates	Digitoxin	↓	Barbiturates may increase digitoxin metabolism.
Barbiturates	Doxorubicin	↓	Total doxorubicin plasma clearance may be increased.
Barbiturates	Doxycycline	↓	Phenobarbital decreases doxycycline's half-life and serum levels, which may persist for 2 weeks after barbiturate therapy is discontinued.
Barbiturates	Felodipine	↓	Felodipine plasma levels and bioavailability may be reduced.
Barbiturates	Fenoprofen	↓	Fenoprofen bioavailability may be decreased.
Barbiturates	Griseofulvin	↓	Phenobarbital appears to interfere with the absorption of oral griseofulvin, thus decreasing its blood level; however, the effect on therapeutic response has not been established.
Barbiturates	Hydantoins	↔	The effect of barbiturates on metabolism is unpredictable; monitor hydantoin and barbiturate blood levels frequently if these drugs are given concurrently.
Barbiturates	Methoxyflurane	↑	Enhanced renal toxicity may occur.
Barbiturates	Metronidazole	↓	Barbiturates may decrease the antimicrobial effectiveness of metronidazole.
Barbiturates	Narcotics	↔	Methadone actions may be reduced. CNS depressant effects of meperidine may be prolonged.
Barbiturates	Phenylbutazone	↓	The elimination half-life of phenylbutazone may be reduced.
Barbiturates	Quinidine	↓	Phenobarbital may significantly reduce the serum levels and half-life of quinidine.
Barbiturates	Theophylline	↓	Barbiturates decrease theophylline levels, possibly resulting in decreased effects.
Barbiturates	Verapamil	↓	The clearance of verapamil may be increased and its bioavailability decreased.

[a] ↓ = Object drug decreased. ↑ = Object drug increased. ↔ = Undetermined clinical effect.

Adverse Reactions

The following adverse reactions and their incidence were from observations of hospitalized patients. Because such patients may be less aware of milder adverse reactions of barbiturates, the incidence may be higher in fully ambulatory patients.

➤*Cardiovascular:* Bradycardia, hypotension, syncope (less than 1%).

➤*CNS:* Somnolence (1% to 3%); abnormal thinking, agitation, anxiety, ataxia, CNS depression, confusion, dizziness, fever (especially with chronic phenobarbital use), hallucinations, headache, hyperkinesia, insomnia, nervousness, nightmares, psychiatric disturbance (less than 1%); drowsiness; lethargy; residual sedation (hangover effect); vertigo.

Emotional disturbances and phobias may be accentuated with phenobarbital use. In some patients, barbiturates repeatedly produce excitement rather than depression; the patient may appear to be inebriated. Irritability and hyperactivity can occur in children.

Barbiturates, when given in the presence of pain, may cause restlessness, excitement, and even delirium. Rarely, the use of barbiturates results in localized or diffuse myalgic, neuralgic, or arthritic pain, especially in psychoneurotic patients with insomnia. The pain may appear in paroxysms, is most intense in the early morning hours, and is most frequently located in the region of the neck, shoulder girdle, and upper limbs. Symptoms may last for days after the drug is discontinued.

➤*GI:* Constipation, nausea, vomiting (less than 1%); liver damage, particularly with chronic **phenobarbital** use (less than 1%).

➤*Hematologic:* Megaloblastic anemia (rarely, following chronic **phenobarbital** use).

➤*Hypersensitivity:* Skin rashes, angioedema (particularly following chronic phenobarbital use) (less than 1%); exfoliative dermatitis (eg, Stevens-Johnson syndrome and toxic epidermal necrolysis) may be caused by phenobarbital and may be fatal (rare).

Acquired hypersensitivity to barbiturates consists chiefly in allergic reactions that occur especially in persons who tend to have asthma, urticaria, angioedema, and similar conditions. Hypersensitivity reactions in this category include localized swelling, particularly of the eyelids, cheeks or lips, and erythematous dermatitis. The skin eruption may be associated with fever, delirium, and marked degenerative changes in the liver and other parenchymatous organs.

➤*Local:* Inadvertent intra-arterial injection may produce arterial spasm with resultant thrombosis and gangrene of an extremity. Reactions range from transient pain to severe tissue necrosis and neurological deficit. Subcutaneous injection may produce tissue necrosis, pain, tenderness and redness. Injection into or near peripheral nerves may result in permanent neurological deficit. Thrombophlebitis after IV use and pain at IM injection site have been reported.

➤*Respiratory:* Apnea, hypoventilation (less than 1%); circulatory collapse; respiratory depression.

Overdosage

The toxic dose of barbiturates varies considerably. In general, an oral dose of 1 g produces serious poisoning in an adult. Death commonly occurs after 2 to 10 g of ingested barbiturate.

➤*Symptoms:* Onset of symptoms may not occur until several hours after ingestion. Acute barbiturate overdosage is manifested by CNS and respiratory depression which may progress to Cheyne-Stokes respiration, areflexia, constriction of the pupils to a slight degree (though in severe poisoning they may show paralytic dilation), nystagmus, ataxia, oliguria, tachycardia, hypotension, lowered body temperature, and coma. Typical shock syndrome (eg, apnea, circulatory collapse, respiratory arrest, death) may occur.

In extreme overdose, all electrical activity in the brain may cease, in which case a "flat" electroencephalogram normally equated with clinical death cannot be accepted. This effect is fully reversible unless hypoxic damage occurs. Consider the possibility of barbiturate intoxication even in situations that appear to involve trauma.

Complications such as pneumonia, pulmonary edema, cardiac arrhythmias, congestive heart failure and renal failure may occur. Uremia may increase CNS sensitivity to barbiturates if renal function is impaired. Differential diagnosis should include hypoglycemia, head trauma, cerebrovascular accidents, convulsive states and diabetic coma.

➤*Treatment:* Treatment is mainly supportive. Maintain an adequate airway, with assisted respiration and oxygen administration, as necessary. Monitor vital signs and fluid balance. Refer to General Management of Acute Overdosage.

Administer 30 g activated charcoal. Nasogastric administration of multiple doses of activated charcoal has been successful in accelerating the elimination of phenobarbital from the body. Consider gastric lavage with a cuffed endotracheal tube in place with the patient in the face-down position. Activated charcoal may be left in the emptied stomach and a saline cathartic administered.

Administer fluid and other standard treatments for shock, if needed. If renal function is normal, forced diuresis may aid in the elimination of the barbiturate. However, diuresis and peritoneal dialysis are of little value. Alkalinization of the urine increases renal excretion of some barbiturates, especially **phenobarbital** and **mephobarbital** (which is metabolized to phenobarbital).

Hemodialysis and hemoperfusion may be used in severe barbiturate intoxication or if the patient is anuric or in shock. The patient should be rolled from side to side every 30 minutes.

Patient Information

Instruct the patient not to increase the dose of the drug without consulting a health care provider.

Advise patients that barbiturates may impair mental or physical abilities required for the performance of potentially hazardous tasks (eg, driving, operating machinery).

Advise patients not to consume alcohol while taking barbiturates. Concurrent use of barbiturates with other CNS depressants (eg, alcohol, narcotics, tranquilizers, antihistamines) may result in additional CNS depressant effects.

Instruct patient to notify the health care provider if any of the following occur: fever; sore throat; mouth sores; easy bruising or bleeding; tiny broken blood vessels under the skin.

Patients may use these drugs on a limited basis as a sleep aid; advise patients not to use for longer than 2 weeks.

Long-Acting

PHENOBARBITAL

c-iv	**Phenobarbital** (Various, eg, Harber, Lilly, Major, Moore, PBI, Parmed, Roxane, Rugby, Warner Chilcott)	**Tablets**: 15 mg	In 100s, 1000s, 5,000s, and UD 100s.
c-iv	**Solfoton** (ECR Pharm.)	**Tablets**: 16 mg	In 100s and 500s.
c-iv	**Phenobarbital** (Various, eg, Goldline, Harber, Lilly, Major, Moore, PBI, Parmed, Roxane, Rugby)	**Tablets**: 30 mg	In 100s, 1,000s, 5,000s, and UD 100s.
c-iv	**Phenobarbital** (Various, eg, Century, Harber, Lilly, Moore, PBI, Parmed, Roxane)	**Tablets**: 60 mg	In 100s, 1,000s, and UD 100s.
c-iv	**Phenobarbital** (Various, eg, URL)	**Tablets**: 90 mg	In 1,000s.
c-iv	**Phenobarbital** (Various, eg, Century, Harber, Lilly, Roxane)	**Tablets**: 100 mg	In 100s and 1,000s.
c-iv	**Solfoton** (ECR Pharm.)	**Capsules**: 16 mg	In 100s and 500s.
c-iv	**Phenobarbital** (Pharmaceutical Associates)	**Elixir**: 15 mg per 5 mL	13.5% alcohol. Fruit flavor. In pt and UD 5, 10, and 20 mL.
c-iv	**Phenobarbital** (Various, eg, Barre-National, Century, Goldline, Harber, Lilly, Roxane)	**Elixir**: 20 mg per 5 mL	Alcohol. In pt, gal, UD 5 mL and UD 7.5 mL.
c-iv	**Phenobarbital Sodium** (Wyeth-Ayerst)	**Injection**: 30 mg/mL	In 1 mL *Tubex*.
c-iv	**Luminal Sodium** (Hospira)	**Injection**: 60 mg/mL	In 1 mL *Carpuject* with *Luer Lock*.[1]
c-iv	**Phenobarbital Sodium** (Wyeth-Ayerst)		In 1 mL *Tubex*.
c-iv	**Phenobarbital Sodium** (Wyeth-Ayerst)	**Injection**: 65 mg/mL	In 1 mL vials.
c-iv	**Phenobarbital Sodium** (Various, eg, Elkins-Sinn)	**Injection**: 130 mg/mL	In 1 mL *Tubex* and 1 mL vials.
c-iv	**Luminal Sodium** (Hospira)		In 1 mL *Carpuject* with *Luer Lock*.[1]

[1] With 10% alcohol and 67.8% propylene glycol.

PHENOBARBITAL — ORAL

For complete and comparative prescribing information, refer to the Barbiturates group monograph.

Indications

Phenobarbital is indicated for use as a sedative or as an anticonvulsant for the treatment of generalized and partial seizures.

Administration and Dosage

The dose of phenobarbital must be individualized, with full knowledge of its particular characteristics. Factors of consideration are the patient's age, weight, and condition.

➤*Sedation:* For sedation, the drug may be administered in single doses of 30 to 120 mg repeated at intervals; frequency will be determined by the patient's response. It is generally considered that no more than 400 mg of phenobarbital should be administered during a 24-hour period.

Adults –

Daytime sedation: 30 to 120 mg daily in 2 to 3 divided doses.
Oral hypnotic: 100 to 200 mg.

➤*Anticonvulsant use:* Clinical laboratory reference values should be used to determine the therapeutic anticonvulsant level of phenobarbital in the serum. To achieve the blood levels considered therapeutic in children, higher per-kilogram dosages are generally necessary for phenobarbital and most other anticonvulsants. In children and infants, phenobarbital at a loading dose of 15 to 20 mg/kg produces blood levels of about 20 mcg/mL shortly after administration.

Phenobarbital has been used in the treatment and prophylaxis of febrile seizures. However, it has not been established that prevention of febrile seizures influences the subsequent development of epilepsy.

Adults – 60 to 200 mg/day.

Children – 3 to 6 mg/kg/day.

➤*Special patient populations:* Dosage should be reduced in the elderly or debilitated because these patients may be more sensitive to barbiturates.

Dosage should be reduced for patients with impaired renal function or hepatic disease.

➤*Storage/Stability:* Keep tightly closed. Store at controlled room temperature 20° to 25°C (68° to 77°F).

PHENOBARBITAL SODIUM — INJECTION

For complete and comparative prescribing information, refer to the Barbiturates group monograph.

Indications

As a hypnotic, for the short-term management of insomnia.

As a sedative, for the relief of anxiety, tension, and apprehension.

As an anticonvulsant, for the treatment of epilepsy (generalized tonic-clonic and cortical focal seizures).

In the emergency control of certain acute convulsive episodes (eg, those associated with status epilepticus, cholera, eclampsia, meningitis, tetanus, and toxic reactions to strychnine or local anesthetics); phenobarbital sodium may be administered IM or IV as an anticonvulsant for emergency use. When administered IV, it may require 15 or more minutes before reaching peak concentrations in the brain. Therefore, injecting phenobarbital sodium until the convulsions stop may cause the brain level to exceed that required to control the convulsions and lead to severe barbiturate-induced depression.

Administration and Dosage

Intravenous injection should be administered slowly and restricted to conditions in which other administration is not feasible either because the patient is unconscious (as in cerebral hemorrhage, eclampsia, or status epilepticus), or because he resists (as in delirium), or because very prompt action is imperative.

The average dose of phenobarbital sodium injection for adults ranges from 100 mg to 320 mg. Larger doses may occasionally be necessary in persons with status epilepticus, psychoses, and pronounced excitement, and in mental patients with insomnia. However, the total dose should not exceed 600 mg in 24 hours. The effect of large doses must be closely watched. Alkalis should be given and the bowels regulated during prolonged use.

➤*Storage/Stability:* Do not use the solution if more than slightly discolored or contains a precipitate. Protect from light. Store at room temperature up to 30°C (86°F).

Long-Acting

MEPHOBARBITAL

c-iv	**Mebaral** (Ovation)	**Tablets:** 32 mg	(M 31). In 250s.
		50 mg	(M 32). In 250s.
		100 mg	(M 33). In 250s.

MEPHOBARBITAL — ORAL

For complete and comparative prescribing information, refer to the Barbiturates group monograph.

Indications

Mephobarbital is indicated for use as a sedative for the relief of anxiety, tension, and apprehension, and as an anticonvulsant for the treatment of grand mal and petit mal epilepsy.

Administration and Dosage

➤*Epilepsy:*

Average dose for adults – 400 mg to 600 mg (6 grain to 9 grain) daily.

Children < 5 years – 16 mg to 32 mg (¼ grain to ½ grain) 3 or 4 times daily.

Children > 5 years – 32 mg to 64 mg (½ grain to 1 grain) 3 or 4 times daily. Mephobarbital is best taken at bedtime if seizures generally occur at night, and during the day if attacks are diurnal.

Treatment should be started with a small dose which is gradually increased over 4 or 5 days until the optimum dosage is determined. If the patient has been taking some other antiepileptic drug, it should be tapered off as the doses of mephobarbital are increased, to guard against the temporary marked attacks that may occur when any treatment for epilepsy is changed abruptly. Similarly, when the dose is lowered to a maintenance level or to be discontinued, the amount should be reduced gradually over 4 or 5 days.

➤*Special patient populations:* Dosage should be reduced in the elderly or debilitated because these patients may be more sensitive to barbiturates. Dosage should be reduced for patients with impaired renal function or hepatic disease.

➤*Combination with other drugs:* Mephobarbital may be used in combination with phenobarbital, either in the form of alternating courses or concurrently. When the 2 drugs are used at the same time, the dose should be about one-half the amount of each used alone. The average daily dose for an adult is from 50 mg to 100 mg (¾ grain to 1½ grain) of phenobarbital and from 200 mg to 300 mg (3 grain to 4½ grain) of mephobarbital.

Mephobarbital may also be used with phenytoin sodium; in some cases, combined therapy appears to give better results than either agent used alone, since phenytoin sodium is particularly effective for the psychomotor types of seizure but relatively ineffective for petit mal. When the drugs are employed concurrently, a reduced dose of phenytoin sodium is advisable, but the full dose of mephobarbital may be given. Satisfactory results have been obtained with an average daily dose of 230 mg (3½ grain) of phenytoin sodium plus about 600 mg (9 grain) of mephobarbital.

➤*Sedation:*

Adults – 32 mg to 100 mg (½ grain to 1½ grain); optimum dose: 50 mg (¾ grain) 3 to 4 times daily.

Children – 16 mg to 32 mg (¼ grain to ½ grain) 3 to 4 times daily.

➤*Storage/Stability:* Store at room temperature up to 25°C (77°F).

Intermediate-Acting

AMOBARBITAL SODIUM

c-ii	**Amytal Sodium** (Lilly)	**Powder for injection**	In 250 and 500 mg vials.

AMOBARBITAL SODIUM — INJECTION

For complete prescribing information, refer to the Barbiturates group monograph.

Indications

➤*Sedative/hypnotic:* For use as a sedative, hypnotic (short-term treatment of insomnia since it appears to lose its effectiveness after 2 weeks), or preanesthetic.

Administration and Dosage

The dose of amobarbital must be individualized with full knowledge of its particular characteristics and recommended rate of administration. Factors of consideration are the patient's age, weight, and condition.

➤*Adults:* The maximum single dose for an adult is 1 g.

Sedative – 30 to 50 mg given 2 or 3 times daily.

Hypnotic – 65 to 200 mg at bedtime.

➤*Special patient population:*

Elderly – Dosage should be reduced in the elderly or debilitated because these patients may be more sensitive to barbiturates.

Renal/hepatic function impariment – Dosage should be reduced for patients with impaired renal function or hepatic disease.

Children – Ordinarily, an intravenous (IV) dose of 65 mg to 0.5 g may be given to a child 6 to 12 years of age.

➤ *Intramuscular (IM) use:* IM injection of the sodium salts of barbiturates should be made deeply into a large muscle. The average IM dose ranges from 65 mg to 0.5 g. A volume of 5 mL (irrespective of concentration) should not be exceeded at any one site because of possible tissue irritation. Twenty percent solutions may be used so that a small volume can contain a large dose. After IM injection of a hypnotic dose, the patient's vital signs should be monitored. Superficial IM or subcutaneous injections may be painful and may produce sterile abscesses or sloughs.

➤*IV use:* IV injection is restricted to conditions in which other routes are not feasible, either because the patient is unconscious (as in cerebral hemorrhage, eclampsia, or status epilepticus), the patient resists (as in delirium), or prompt action is imperative. Slow IV injection is essential, and patients should be carefully observed during administration. This requires that blood pressure, respiration, and cardiac function be maintained, vital signs be recorded, and equipment for resuscitation and artificial ventilation be available. The rate of IV injection for adults should not exceed 50 mg/min to prevent sleep or sudden respiratory depression. The final dosage is determined to a great extent by the patient's reaction to the slow administration of the drug.

➤*Preparation of solution:* Add sterile water for injection to the vial. The vial should be rotated to facilitate solution of the powder. Do not shake the vial.

Several minutes may be required for the drug to dissolve completely, but under no circumstances should a solution be injected if it has not become absolutely clear within 5 minutes. Also, a solution that forms a precipitate after clearing should not be used. Amobarbital hydrolyzes in solution or on exposure to air. No more than 30 minutes should elapse from the time the vial is opened until its contents are injected. Prior to administration, parenteral drug products should be inspected visually for particulate matter and discoloration whenever solution containers permit.

The following table will aid in preparing solutions of various concentrations. Ordinarily, a 10% solution is used.

Reconstitution of Amobarbital With Sterile Water[a]

Content in weight	1%	2.5%	5%	10%	20%
0.5 g	50 mL	20 mL	10 mL	5 mL	2.5 mL

[a] Quantity of sterile water for injection required to dilute the contents of a given vial of amobarbital sodium to obtain the percentages listed. Solutions derived will be in weight/volume.

➤*Storage/Stability:* Store at 59° to 86°F (15° to 30°C). Do not use a solution that is not absolutely clear after 5 minutes; amobarbital sodium hydrolyzes in solution or upon exposure to air. No more than 30 minutes should elapse from the time the vial is opened until the contents are injected.

BUTABARBITAL SODIUM

c-iii	**Butabarbital Sodium** (Various)	**Tablets:** 15 mg	In 1000s.
c-iii	**Butisol Sodium** (Wallace)		(Butisol Sodium 37 112). Lavender, scored. In 100s and 1000s.
c-iii	**Butabarbital Sodium** (Various)	**Tablets:** 30 mg	In 100s and 1000s.
c-iii	**Butisol Sodium** (Wallace)		Tartrazine. (Butisol Sodium 37 113). Green, scored. In 100s and 1000s.
c-iii	**Butisol Sodium** (Wallace)	**Tablets:** 50 mg	Tartrazine. (Butisol Sodium 37 114). Orange, scored. In 100s.
c-iii	**Butisol Sodium** (Wallace)	**Tablets:** 100 mg	(Butisol Sodium 37 115). Pink, scored. In 100s.

Intermediate-Acting

BUTABARBITAL SODIUM

c-iii	**Butabarbital Sodium** (Various, eg, Harber, Major)	**Elixir:** 30 mg/5 ml	In pt.
c-iii	**Butisol Sodium** (Wallace)		7% alcohol, tartrazine, saccharin. In pt and gal.

BUTABARBITAL SODIUM — ORAL

For complete prescribing information, refer to the Barbiturates group monograph.

Indications

Sedative or hypnotic. Barbiturates appear to lose their effectiveness for sleep induction and maintenance after 2 weeks.

Administration and Dosage

➤*Adults:*

Daytime sedation – 15 to 30 mg, 3 or 4 times daily.

Bedtime hypnotic – 50 to 100 mg.

Preoperative sedation – 50 to 100 mg, 60 to 90 minutes before surgery.

➤*Children:*

Preoperative sedation – 2 to 6 mg/kg; maximum 100 mg.

➤*Elderly/Debilitated:* Reduce dosage; these patients may be more sensitive to the drug.

➤*Hepatic/Renal function impairment:* Reduce dosage.

Short-Acting

SECOBARBITAL SODIUM

c-ii	**Seconal Sodium Pulvules** (Ranbaxy)	**Capsules:** 100 mg	(F40). Orange. In 100s and UD 100s.

SECOBARBITAL SODIUM — ORAL

For complete and comparative prescribing information, refer to the Barbiturates group monograph.

Indications

Hypnotic, for the short-term treatment of insomnia, since it appears to lose its effectiveness for sleep induction and sleep maintenance after 2 weeks.

Preanesthetic.

Administration and Dosage

Dosages of barbiturates must be individualized with full knowledge of their particular characteristics. Factors of consideration are the patient's age, weight, and condition.

➤*Adults:* As a hypnotic, 100 mg at bedtime. Preoperatively, 200 to 300 mg 1 to 2 hours before surgery.

➤*Children:* Preoperatively, 2 to 6 mg/kg, with a maximum dosage of 100 mg.

➤*Special patient population:* Dosage should be reduced in the elderly or debilitated because these patients may be more sensitive to barbiturates. Dosage should be reduced for patients with impaired renal function or hepatic disease.

➤*Storage/Stability:* Store at controlled room temperature, 15° to 30°C (59° to 86°F). Dispense in a tight container.

PENTOBARBITAL SODIUM

c-ii	**Pentobarbital Sodium** (Wyeth-Ayerst)	**Injection:** 50 mg/ml	In 2 ml Tubex.[1]

[1] With propylene glycol and 10% alcohol.

PENTOBARBITAL SODIUM — INJECTION

For complete and comparative prescribing information, refer to the Barbiturates group monograph.

Indications

Hypnotic, for the short-term treatment of insomnia, since barbiturates appear to lose their effectiveness for sleep induction and sleep maintenance after 2 weeks; anticonvulsant, in anesthetic doses, for the emergency control of certain acute convulsive episodes (eg, those associated with status epilepticus, eclampsia, meningitis, tetanus and toxic reactions to strychnine or local anesthetics).

Preanesthetic in pediatric patients.

Administration and Dosage

Dosages of barbiturates must be individualized with full knowledge of their particular characteristics and recommended rate of administration. Factors of consideration are the patient's age, weight, and condition.

➤*Pediatric dosage - Recommended by the American Academy of Pediatrics (intended as a guide):*

Preoperative sedation – 2 to 6 mg/kg - maximum 100 mg IM.

➤*Adult dosage - (intended as a guide):*

Bedtime hypnosis –

IM: 150 to 200 mg - do not exceed a volume of 5 mL at any one site because of possible tissue irritation.

IV: 70 kg adult, 100 mg initially.

➤*Administration:* IM injection of the sodium salts of barbiturates should be made deeply into a large muscle, and a volume of 5 mL should not be exceeded at any one site because of possible tissue irritation. After IM injection of a hypnotic dose, the patient's vital signs should be monitored.

IV injection is restricted to conditions in which other routes are not feasible, either because the patient is unconscious (as in cerebral hemorrhage, eclampsia, or status epilepticus), or because the patient resists (as in delirium), or because prompt action is imperative. Slow IV injection is essential, and patients should be carefully observed during administration. The rate of IV injection should not exceed 50 mg/min. No average IV dose can be relied upon to produce similar effects in different patients. The possibility of overdose and respiratory depression is remote when the drug is injected slowly in fractional doses. The clinical response is the basis for dosage determination, although the patient's weight and age may influence the total amount of the drug required. Watch the physical signs closely to accurately obtain and maintain the desired degree of sedation. This requires that blood pressure, respiration, and cardiac function be maintained, vital signs be recorded, and equipment for resuscitation and artificial ventilation be available.

Initially administer 100 mg in the 70 kg adult. Reduce dosage proportionally for pediatric or debilitated patients. At least 1 minute is necessary to determine the full effect. If needed, small increments of the drug may be given to a total of 200 to 500 mg for healthy adults. The usual dosage is 150 to 200 mg; children's dosage frequently ranges from 2 to 6 mg/kg as a single IM injection, not to exceed 100 mg.

Any vein may be used, but preference should be given to a larger vein (to minimize the risk of irritation with the possibility of resultant thrombosis). Avoid administration into varicose veins, because circulation there is retarded.

The *Tubex Blunt Pointe* sterile cartridge unit is suitable for substances to be administered intravenously only. It is intended for use with injection sets specifically manufactured as "needle-less" injection systems. *Tubex Blunt Pointe* is compatible with Abbott's *LifeShield* prepierced reseal injection site, Baxter's *InterLink* injection site, and B. Braun Medical's *SafSite* reflux valve. Consult manufacturer's recommendations regarding "Directions for Use" of the "needle-less" system. It is also intended for admixture with, and convenient administration of, various medicaments when using Drug Vial Adapters for "needle-less" injection systems.

The *Tubex* sterile cartridge-needle unit is suitable for substances to be administered intravenously or intramuscularly.

➤*Treatment of adverse effects due to inadvertent error in administration:* Extravasation into subcutaneous tissues causes tissue irritation. This may vary from slight tenderness and redness to necrosis. Recommended treatment includes the application of moist heat and the injection of 0.5% procaine solution into the affected area.

Intra-arterial injection of any barbiturate must be avoided. The accidental intra-arterial injection of a small amount of the solution may cause spasm and severe pain along the course of the artery. The injection should be terminated if the patient complains of pain or if other indications of accidental intra-arterial injection occur, such as a white hand with cyanosed skin or patches of discolored skin and delayed onset of hypnosis.

The consequences of intra-arterial injection of pentobarbital can vary from transient pain to gangrene. It is not possible to formulate strict rules for management of such accidents. Although no specific treatment has proved entirely successful, the following procedures have been suggested:

1.) release of the tourniquet or restrictive garments to permit dilution of injected drug,
2.) relief of arterial spasm by injecting 10 mL of a 1% procaine solution into the artery and, if considered necessary, brachial plexus block,
3.) prevention of thrombosis by early anticoagulant therapy, and
4.) supportive treatment.

➤*Anticonvulsant use:* To achieve the blood levels considered therapeutic in children, higher per-kilogram dosages are generally necessary for phenobarbital and most other anticonvulsants. Inject slowly with regard to the time needed for the drug to penetrate the blood-brain barrier.

In status epilepticus, it is imperative to achieve therapeutic blood levels of a barbiturate (or other anticonvulsants) as rapidly as possible.

Short-Acting

PENTOBARBITAL SODIUM — INJECTION

A barbiturate-induced depression may occur along with a postictal depression once the seizures are controlled, therefore, it is important to use the minimal amount required and to wait for the anticonvulsant effect to develop before administering a second dose.

➤*Special patient population:* Dosage should be reduced in the elderly or debilitated because these patients may be more sensitive to barbiturates. Dosage should be reduced for patients with impaired renal function or hepatic disease.

➤*Storage / Stability:* Store at room temperature, approximately 25° C (77° F).

Oral Combinations

ORAL COMBINATIONS

Combined barbiturate products are promoted to provide a more balanced effect through the combination of those with differing rates of action and dissipation.

c-ii	**Tuinal 100 mg Pulvules** (LIlly)	**Capsules:** 50 mg amobarbital sodium and 50 mg secobarbital sodium	Blue and orange. In 100s.
c-ii	**Tuinal 200 mg Pulvules** (Lilly)	**Capsules:** 100 mg amobarbital sodium and 100 mg secobarbital sodium	Blue and orange. In 100s.

NONPRESCRIPTION SLEEP AIDS

otc	**Unisom Nighttime Sleep-Aid** (Pfizer)	**Tablets**: 25 mg doxylamine succinate	(Unisom). Blue, scored. Oval. In 8s, 16s, 32s, 48s.
otc	**Dormin** (Randob)	**Tablets**: 25 mg diphenhydramine hydrochloride	In 32s.
otc	**Miles Nervine** (Miles)		(Nervine). In 12s and 30s.
otc	**Nytol** (Block)		Lactose. (N). In 16s, 32s and 72s.
otc	**Simply Sleep** (McNeil)		In 24s and 48s.
otc	**Sleep-eze 3** (Whitehall)		In 12s and 24s.
otc	**Sleepwell 2-nite** (Rugby)		Sucrose. In 72s.
otc	**Sominex** (SmithKline Beecham)		(S). In 16s, 32s and 72s.
otc	**Extra Strength Tylenol PM** (McNeil-CPC)	**Tablets**: 25 mg diphenhydramine, 500 mg acetaminophen	**Tablets**: (Tylenol PM). In 24s, 50s. **Caplets**: (Tylenol PM). In 24s and 50s.
otc	**Exedrine P.M.** (Bristol-Myers Squibb)		Sorbitol. In 20s and 40s.
otc	**Bayer Select Maximum Strength Night Time Pain Relief** (Bayer)		In 24s and 50s.
otc	**Sominex Pain Relief** (SmithKline-Beecham)		In 16s and 32s.
otc	**Tycolene P.M.** (Pfeiffer Pharmaceuticals)		In 50s.
otc	**Extra Strength Doan's P.M.** (Ciba)	**Tablets**: 25 mg diphenhydramine hydrochloride, 500 mg magnesium salicylate	(DOAN'S PM). In 20s.
otc	**Bufferin AF Nite Time** (B-M Squibb)		Parabens. Light blue. In 24s and 50s.
otc	**Unisom with Pain Relief** (Pfizer)	**Tablets**: 50 mg diphenhydramine hydrochloride, 650 mg acetaminophen	In 16s.
otc	**Diphenhydramine hydrochloride** (Rugby)	**Tablets**: 50 mg diphenhydramine hydrochloride	Blue. In 50s.
otc	**Compoz Nighttime Sleep Aid** (Medtech)		Lactose. In 12s and 24s.
otc	**40 Winks** (Roberts Med)		In 30s.
otc	**Maximum Strength Nytol** (Block)		Lactose. (N). In 8s and 16s.
otc	**Snooze Fast** (BDI)		In 36s.
otc	**Midol PM** (Sterling Health)		In 16s.
otc	**Sominex** (SmithKline-Beecham)		(S). In 8s, 16s and 32s.
otc	**Twilite** (Pfeiffer)		Lactose. In 20s.
otc	**Excedrin PM Liquigels** (Bristol-Myers)	**Capsules**: 25 mg diphenhydramine hydrochloride, 500 mg acetaminophen	Sorbitol. In 20s and 40s.
otc	**Extra Strength Tylenol PM Gelcaps** (McNeil-CPC)		EDTA, propylparaben. In 20s and 40s.
otc	**Legatrin PM** (Columbia)	**Tablets**: 50 mg diphenhydramine hydrochloride, 500 mg acetaminophen	In 30s and 50s.
otc	**Melagesic PM** (B.F. Ascher)	**Tablets**: 500 mg acetaminophen, 1.5 mg melatonin.	In 32s.
otc	**Compoz Gel Caps** (Medtech)	**Capsules**: 25 mg diphenhydramine hydrochloride	In 16s.
otc	**Dormin** (Randob)		Lactose. In 32s and 72s.
otc	**Advil PM** (Wyeth Consumer Health)	**Capsules**: 25 mg diphenhydramine hydrochloride, 200 mg ibuprofen	Sorbitol. In 32s.
otc	**Maximum Strength Sleepinal Capsules and Soft Gels** (Thompson)	**Capsules**: 50 mg diphenhydramine hydrochloride	**Capsules**: Lactose. In 16s. **Soft Gels**: Sorbitol. (Sleepinal). In 16s.
otc	**Maximum Strength Unisom SleepGels** (Pfizer)		Sorbitol. (UNISOM). In 8s.
otc	**Nighttime Pamprin** (Chattem)	**Powder**: 50 mg diphenhydramine hydrochloride, 650 mg acetaminophen	Sugar. Apple cinnamon and hot chocolate flavors. In 4s.
otc	**Excedrin P.M.** (B-M Squibb)	**Liquid**: 167 mg acetaminophen, 8.3 mg diphenhydramine hydrochloride/5 mL	10% alcohol, sucrose. Wild berry flavor. In 180 mL.
		Liquid: 1000 mg acetaminophen 50 mg diphenhydramine hydrochloride/30 mL.	10% alcohol, sucrose. Wild berry flavor. In 180 mL.
otc	**Advil PM** (Wyeth Consumer Health)	**Tablets**: 38 mg diphenhydramine citrate, 200 mg ibuprofen	Lactose. Capsule shape. In 20s and UD 50s.

NONPRESCRIPTION SLEEP AIDS — ORAL

For complete prescribing information for the antihistamines and for a complete listing of diphenhydramine hydrochloride products, refer to the Antihistamines monograph in the Respiratory Drugs section.

Indications

Aid in the relief of insomnia.

Traditionally, products containing analgesics have been used for relief of insomnia due to minor pain.

Administration and Dosage

Administer 25 mg doxylamine or 50 mg diphenhydramine hydrochloride (76 mg diphenhydramine citrate) before bedtime.

Actions

➤*Pharmacology:* These products contain antihistamines which act on the CNS, producing prominent sedative effects.

Contraindications

Asthma, glaucoma or prostate gland enlargement, except under a physician's advice.

Warnings

➤*Prolonged insomnia:* Not for use more than 2 weeks. If insomnia persists for more than 2 weeks, consult a physician; it may be a symptom of a serious underlying illness.

➤*Pregnancy:* Consult a physician before using these products. **Doxylamine** should not be taken by pregnant women.

➤*Lactation:* **Doxylamine** should not be taken by a nursing woman.

➤*Children:* Do not use in children younger than 12 years of age.

Precautions

➤*Hazardous tasks:* May cause drowsiness; observe caution while driving or performing other tasks requiring alertness, coordination or physical dexterity.

Adverse Reactions

Occasional anticholinergic effects may occur with doxylamine.

Overdosage

Antihistamine overdosage reactions may vary from CNS depression to stimulation. See the Antihistamines monograph for a more complete description of reactions.

NONPRESCRIPTION SLEEP AIDS — ORAL

Patient Information

Avoid alcoholic beverages while taking this product. Do not take this product if you are taking sedatives or tranquilizers without first consulting the physician.

May cause drowsiness; observe caution while driving or performing other tasks requiring alertness, coordination or physical dexterity.

Do not use if you have asthma, glaucoma, emphysema, chronic pulmonary disease, shortness of breath, difficulty in breathing or difficulty in urination due to prostate enlargement unless directed by the physician.

GENERAL ANESTHETICS

Barbiturates

Indications

Induction of anesthesia; supplementation of other anesthetic agents; IV anesthesia for short surgical procedures with minimal painful stimuli; induction of a hypnotic state.

➤*Thiopental (IV):* Control of convulsive states and in neurosurgical patients with increased intracranial pressure if adequate ventilation is provided.

➤*Thiopental (rectal suspension):* Used when preanesthetic sedation or basal narcosis by the rectal route is desired. It may be employed as the sole agent in selected brief, minor procedures where muscular relaxation and analgesia are not required.

Actions

➤*Pharmacology:* The ultrashort-acting barbiturates, thiopental and methohexital, depress the CNS to produce hypnosis and anesthesia without analgesia. Methohexital does not possess muscle relaxant properties. These drugs are frequently used to provide hypnosis during balanced anesthesia with other agents for muscle relaxation and analgesia.

Biotransformation products of thiopental are pharmacologically inactive and mostly excreted in the urine.

➤*Pharmacokinetics:* The rapid onset and brief duration of action of these drugs is a function of their high lipid solubility. They quickly cross the blood-brain barrier and are rapidly redistributed from the brain to other body tissues, first to highly perfused visceral organs (liver, kidneys, heart) and muscle, and later to fatty tissues.

Administered IV as the sodium salts, these agents produce anesthesia within 1 minute. Recovery after a small dose is rapid, with somnolence and retrograde amnesia. Muscle relaxation occurs at the onset of anesthesia. The duration of anesthetic activity following a single IV dose is 20 to 30 minutes for thiopental and somewhat shorter for methohexital. Thiopental is readily absorbed by the rectal route when administered as a suspension; onset of action usually occurs within 8 to 10 minutes. Thiopental IV produces hypnosis within 30 to 40 seconds following administration. Repeated doses or continuous infusion of these agents causes accumulation. Slow release of the drug from lipoidal storage sites results in prolonged anesthesia, somnolence, and respiratory and circulatory depression. The plasma half-life is 3 to 8 hours.

Contraindications

➤*Absolute:* Latent or manifest porphyria; hypersensitivity to barbiturates; absence of suitable veins for IV administration.

➤*Relative:* Severe cardiovascular disease; hypotension or shock; conditions in which hypnotic effects may be prolonged or potentiated (excessive premedication, Addison disease, hepatic or renal dysfunction, myxedema, increased blood urea, severe anemia); increased intracranial pressure; asthma; myasthenia gravis; status asthmaticus (thiopental).

If barbiturates are used in conditions involving relative contraindications, reduce dosage and administer slowly.

➤*Rectal suspension:* Patients who are to undergo rectal surgery; presence of inflammatory, ulcerative, bleeding, or neoplastic lesions of the lower bowel; patients with acute asthmatic attacks, and variegate or acute intermittent porphyria.

Warnings

➤*Status asthmaticus:* Use **methohexital** with extreme caution in patients with status asthmaticus.

➤*Repeated or continuous infusion:* Repeated or continuous infusion may cause cumulative effects resulting in prolonged somnolence and respiratory and circulatory depression. Have resuscitative and endotracheal intubation equipment and oxygen immediately available. Maintain patency of the airway at all times.

➤*Pregnancy: Category C* (thiopental); *Category B* (methohexital). Safety for use during pregnancy has not been established. Use only when clearly needed and when the potential benefits outweigh the potential hazards to the fetus.

Thiopental – Thiopental readily crosses the placental barrier.

Methohexital – Methohexital has been used in cesarean section delivery, but because of its solubility and lack of protein binding, it readily and rapidly traverses the placenta.

➤*Lactation:* Small amounts of **thiopental** may appear in breast milk following administration of large doses. Exercise caution when administering barbiturates to a breast-feeding woman.

➤*Children:*

Methohexital – Safety and efficacy in children have not been established.

Precautions

➤*Extravascular injection:* Extravascular injection may cause pain, swelling, ulceration, and necrosis. Intra-arterial injection is dangerous and may produce gangrene on an extremity.

➤*Rectal dose:* If evacuation of the instilled rectal dose occurs, assess the effects of any retained portion before administering a repeat dose.

➤*Special risk:* Respiratory depression, apnea, or hypotension may occur due to individual variations in tolerance or to the physical status of the patient. Exercise caution in debilitated patients, or those with impaired function of respiratory, circulatory, cardiac, renal, hepatic, or endocrine systems.

➤*Drug abuse and dependence:* May be habit-forming.

Drug Interactions

Barbiturate Drug Interactions

Precipitant Drug	Object Drug[a]		Description
Narcotics	Barbiturate anesthetics	↑	The barbiturate dose required to induce anesthesia may be reduced. Apnea may be more common with this combination.
Phenothiazines	Barbiturate anesthetics	↑	Preanesthetic use of phenothiazines may raise the frequency and severity of neuromuscular excitation and hypotension in patients who receive barbiturate anesthesia.
Probenecid	Barbiturate anesthetics	↑	The anesthesia produced by the barbiturate may be extended or achieved at lower doses.
Sulfisoxazole	Barbiturate anesthetics	↑	Sulfisoxazole may enhance the anesthetic effects of the barbiturate.

[a] ↑ = Object drug increased.

➤*Drug/Lab test interactions:* Body segment parameter and liver function studies may be influenced by administration of a single dose of barbiturates.

Adverse Reactions

➤*Cardiovascular:* Circulatory depression; thrombophlebitis; hypotension; peripheral vascular collapse; convulsions in association with cardiorespiratory arrest; myocardial depression; cardiac arrhythmias.

➤*CNS:* Emergence delirium; headache; restlessness; anxiety; seizures; prolonged somnolence and recovery.

➤*GI:* Nausea; emesis; abdominal pain. Rectal irritation; diarrhea; cramping; rectal bleeding (rectal administration).

➤*Hypersensitivity:*

Acute allergic reactions – Erythema; pruritus; urticaria; anaphylactic reaction.

➤*Respiratory:* Respiratory depression including apnea; dyspnea; rhinitis; laryngospasm, bronchospasm, sneezing, coughing.

➤*Miscellaneous:* Salivation; hiccups skin rashes; skeletal muscle hyperactivity; shivering.

Rarely, immune hemolytic anemia with renal failure and radial nerve palsy have occurred.

Overdosage

➤*Symptoms:* Overdosage may occur from too rapid or repeated injections. Too rapid injection may be followed by an alarming fall in blood pressure, even to shock levels. Apnea, occasional laryngospasm, coughing, and other respiratory difficulties with excessive or too rapid injections may occur.

➤*Treatment:* In the event of suspected or apparent overdosage, discontinue the drug, maintain or establish a patent airway (intubate if necessary), and administer oxygen with assisted ventilation if necessary. The lethal dose of barbiturates varies and cannot be stated with certainty. Lethal blood levels may be as low as 1 mg/dL for short-acting barbiturates; less if other depressant drugs or alcohol are also present.

THIOPENTAL SODIUM

c-iii	**Thiopental Sodium** (IMS)	**Powder for Injection**: 2% (20 mg/ml)	In 400 mg *Min-I-Mix* vials with *Min-I-Mix* injector.
c-iii	**Pentothal** (Abbott)		In 1, 2.5 and 5 g kits, 400 mg *Ready-to-Mix* syringes and 400 mg *Ready-to-Mix LifeShield* syringes.
c-iii	**Thiopental Sodium** (Various, eg, Gensia, IMS)	**Powder for Injection**: 2.5% (25 mg/ml)	In 250 and 500 mg *Min-I-Mix* vials with *Min-I-Mix* and 500 mg, 1, 2.5, 5 and 10 g kits.
c-iii	**Pentothal** (Abbott)		In 1, 2.5, 5 g and 500 mg kits, 250 and 500 mg *Ready-to-Mix* syringes and 250 and 500 mg *Ready-to-Mix LifeShield* syringes.

THIOPENTAL SODIUM — INJECTION

For complete and comparative prescribing information refer to the Barbiturate Anesthetics group monograph.

Indications

As the sole anesthetic agent for brief (15 minute) procedures; induction of anesthesia prior to administration of other anesthetic agents; to supplement regional anesthesia; to provide hypnosis during balanced anesthesia with other agents for analgesia or muscle relaxation; for the control of convulsive states during or following inhalation anesthesia, local anesthesia or other causes; in neurosurgical patients with increased intracranial pressure, if adequate ventilation is provided; for narcoanalysis and narcosynthesis in psychiatric disorders.

Administration and Dosage

The volume and choice of diluent for preparing thiopental sodium for injection solutions for clinical use depends on the concentration and vehicle desired. Thiopental sodium for injection Kits provide only Sterile Water for Injection as the diluent for individual or multi-patient use or 0.9% Sodium Chloride Injection as the diluent for individual patient use.

Thiopental sodium for injection is administered by the intravenous route only. Individual response to the drug is so varied that there can be no fixed dosage. The drug should be titrated against patient requirements as governed by age, sex, and body weight. Younger patients require relatively larger doses than middle-aged and elderly patients: The latter metabolize the drug more slowly. Prepuberty requirements are the same for both sexes, but adult females require less than adult males. Dose is usually proportional to body weight, and obese patients require a larger dose than relatively lean persons of the same weight.

➤*Premedication:* Premedication usually consists of atropine or scopolamine to suppress vagal reflexes and inhibit secretions. In addition, a barbiturate or an opiate is often given. Sodium pentobarbital injection is suggested because it provides a preliminary indication of how the patient will react to barbiturate anesthesia. Ideally, the peak effect of these medications should be reached shortly before the time of induction.

➤*Test dose:* It is advisable to inject a small "test" dose of 25 mg to 75 mg (1 mL to 3 mL of a 2.5% solution) of thiopental sodium for injection, USP to assess tolerance or unusual sensitivity to thiopental sodium for injection, USP and pausing to observe patient reaction for at least 60 seconds. If unexpectedly deep anesthesia develops or if respiratory depression occurs consider these possibilities:

1.) the patient may be unusually sensitive to thiopental sodium for injection, USP,
2.) the solution may be more concentrated than had been assumed, or
3.) the patient may have received too much premedication.

➤*Use in anesthesia:* Moderately slow induction can usually be accomplished in the "average" adult by injection of 50 mg to 75 mg (2 mL to 3 mL of a 2.5% solution) at intervals of 20 to 40 seconds, depending on the reaction of the patient. Once anesthesia is established, additional injections of 25 mg to 50 mg can be given whenever the patient moves.

Slow injection is recommended to minimize respiratory depression and the possibility of overdosage. The smallest dose consistent with attaining the surgical objective is the desired goal. Momentary apnea following each injection is typical, and progressive decrease in the amplitude of respiration appears with increasing dosage. Pulse remains normal or increases slightly and returns to normal. Blood pressure usually falls slightly but returns toward normal. Muscles usually relax about 30 seconds after unconsciousness is attained, but this may be masked if a skeletal muscle relaxant is used. The tone of jaw muscles is a fairly reliable index. The pupils may dilate but later contract; sensitivity to light is not usually lost until a level of anesthesia deep enough to permit surgery is attained. Nystagmus and divergent strabismus are characteristic during early stages, but at the level of surgical anesthesia, the eyes are central and fixed. Corneal and conjunctival reflexes disappear during surgical anesthesia.

When thiopental sodium for injection, USP is used for induction in balanced anesthesia with a skeletal muscle relaxant and an inhalation agent, the total dose of thiopental sodium for injection, USP can be estimated and then injected in 2 to 4 fractional doses. With this technique, brief periods of apnea may occur, which may require assisted or controlled pulmonary ventilation. As an initial dose, 210 mg to 280 mg (3 to 4 mg/kg) of thiopental sodium for injection, USP is usually required for rapid induction in the average adult (70 kg).

When thiopental sodium for injection, USP is used as the sole anesthetic agent, the desired level of anesthesia can be maintained by injection of small repeated doses as needed or by using a continuous intravenous drip in a 0.2% or 0.4% concentration. (Sterile water should not be used as the diluent in these concentrations, since hemolysis will occur.) With continuous drip, the depth of anesthesia is controlled by adjusting the rate of infusion.

➤*Use in convulsive states:* For the control of convulsive states following anesthesia (inhalation or local) or other causes 75 mg to 125 mg (3 mL to 5 mL of a 2.5% solution) should be given as soon as possible after the convulsion begins. Convulsions following the use of a local anesthetic may require 125 mg to 250 mg of thiopental sodium for injection, USP given over a 10-minute period. If the convulsion is caused by a local anesthetic, the required dose of thiopental sodium for injection, USP will depend upon the amount of local anesthetic given and its convulsant properties.

➤*Use in neurosurgical patients with increased intracranial pressure:* In neurosurgical patients, intermittent bolus injections of 1.5 to 3.5 mg/kg of body weight may be given to reduce intraoperative elevations of intracranial pressure, if adequate ventilation is provided.

➤*Use in psychiatric disorders:* For narcoanalysis and narcosynthesis in psychiatric disorders, premedication with an anticholinergic agent may precede administration of thiopental sodium for injection, USP. After a test dose, thiopental sodium for injection, USP is injected at a slow rate of 100 mg/min (4 mL/min of a 2.5% solution) with the patient counting backwards from 100. Shortly after counting becomes confused, but before actual sleep is produced, the injection is discontinued. Allow the patient to return to a semidrowsy state where conversation is coherent. Alternatively, thiopental sodium for injection, USP may be administered by rapid IV drip using 0.2% concentration in 5% dextrose and water. At this concentration, the rate of administration should not exceed 50 mL/min.

➤*Preparation of solutions:* Thiopental sodium for injection, USP is supplied as a yellowish, hygroscopic powder in a variety of different containers. Solutions should be prepared aseptically with one of the 3 following diluents: Sterile Water for Injection, USP, 0.9% Sodium Chloride Injection, USP or 5% Dextrose Injection, USP. Clinical concentrations used for intermittent intravenous administration vary between 2% and 5%. A 2% or 2.5% solution is most commonly used. A 3.4% concentration in sterile water for injection is isotonic; concentrations less than 2% in this diluent are not used because they cause hemolysis. For continuous intravenous drip administration, concentrations of 0.2% or 0.4% are used. Solutions may be prepared by adding thiopental sodium for injection, USP to 5% Dextrose Injection, USP, 0.9% Sodium Chloride Injection, USP or a combined electrolyte solution (pH 7.4).

Since thiopental sodium for injection, USP contains no added bacteriostatic agent, extreme care in preparation and handling should be exercised at all times to prevent the introduction of microbial contaminants. Solutions should be freshly prepared and used promptly; when reconstituted for administration to several patients, unused portions should be discarded after 24 hours. Sterilization by heating should not be attempted.

Warning – The 2.5 g and larger sizes contain adequate medication for several patients.

➤*Compatibility:* Any solution of thiopental sodium for injection, USP with a visible precipitate should not be administered. The stability of thiopental sodium for injection, USP solutions depends on several factors, including the diluent, temperature of storage and the amount of carbon dioxide from room air that gains access to the solution. Any factor or condition that tends to lower pH (increase acidity) of thiopental sodium for injection, USP solutions will increase the likelihood of precipitation of thiopental acid. Such factors include the use of diluents that are too acidic and the absorption of carbon dioxide, which can combine with water to form carbonic acid.

Solutions of succinylcholine, tubocurarine, or other drugs that have an acid pH should not be mixed with thiopental sodium for injection, USP solutions. The most stable solutions are those reconstituted in water or isotonic saline, kept under refrigeration, and tightly stoppered. The presence or absence of a visible precipitate offers a practical guide to the physical compatibility of prepared solutions of thiopental sodium for injection, USP.

Calculations for Various Concentrations

Concentration desired		Thiopental sodium for injection	Diluent
Percent	mg/mL	g	mL
0.2	2	1	500
0.4	4	1	250
		2	500
2	20	5	250
		10	500
2.5	25	1	40
		5	200
5	50	1	20
		5	100

THIOPENTAL SODIUM — INJECTION

➤*Storage/Stability:* Store product prior to reconstitution at controlled room temperature 15° to 30°C (59° to 86°F). Store reconstituted solution in a cool place and use within 24 hours of mixing. Administer only clear solution.

METHOHEXITAL SODIUM

c-iv	**Brevital Sodium** (Monarch)	**Powder for Injection:** 2.5 g	In 20 ml vials.

METHOHEXITAL SODIUM — INJECTION

For complete and comparative prescribing information, refer to the Barbiturate Anesthetics group monograph.

WARNING

Use methohexital only in hospital or ambulatory care settings that provide for continuous monitoring of respiratory (eg, pulse oximetry) and cardiac function. Ensure immediate availability of resuscitative drugs and age- and size-appropriate equipment for bag/valve/mask ventilation and intubation and personnel trained in their use and skilled in airway management. For deeply sedated patients, a designated individual other than the practitioner performing the procedure should be present to continuously monitor the patient.

Indications

➤*Adult usage:* Methohexital can be used in adults as follows:
- For IV induction of anesthesia prior to the use of other general anesthetic agents.
- For IV induction of anesthesia and as an adjunct to subpotent inhalational anesthetic agents (such as nitrous oxide in oxygen) for short surgical procedures; give methohexital by infusion or intermittent injection.
- For use along with other parenteral agents, usually narcotic analgesics, to supplement subpotent inhalational anesthetic agents (such as nitrous oxide in oxygen) for longer surgical procedures.
- As IV anesthesia for short surgical, diagnostic, or therapeutic procedures associated with minimal painful stimuli.
- As an agent for inducing a hypnotic state.

➤*Child usage:* Methohexital can be used in children older than 1 month as follows:
- For IM induction of anesthesia prior to the use of other general anesthetic agents.
- For IM induction of anesthesia and as an adjunct to subpotent inhalational anesthetic agents for short surgical procedures.
- As IM anesthesia for short surgical, diagnostic, or therapeutic procedures associated with minimal painful stimuli.

Administration and Dosage

➤*Approved by the FDA:* July 13, 2001.

Methohexital may be administered by direct IV injection or continuous IV drip or IM routes. Reconstituting instructions vary depending on the route of administration.

Facilities for assisting ventilation and administering oxygen are necessary adjuncts for all routes of administration of anesthesia. Since cardiorespiratory arrest may occur, carefully observe patients during and after use of methohexital. Age- and size-appropriate resuscitative equipment (ie, intubation and cardioversion equipment, oxygen, suction, and a secure IV line) and personnel qualified in its use must be immediately available.

Preanesthetic medication is generally advisable. Methohexital may be used with any of the recognized preanesthetic medications.

➤*Preparation of solution:* Freshly prepare and use promptly solutions of methohexital. Reconstituted solutions of methohexital are chemically stable at room temperature for 24 hours.

Diluents – Do not use diluents containing bacteriostatics.
Preferred diluent: Sterile water for injection.
Acceptable diluents: 5% dextrose injection, 0.9% sodium chloride injection.
Incompatible diluents: Lactated Ringer injection.

Dilution instructions – 1% solutions (10 mg/mL) should be prepared for IV use. Contents of vials should be diluted as follows:

Strength	Amount of Diluent to be Added to the Contents of the Vial	For 1% Solution
500 mg	50 mL	No further dilution needed
2.5 g	15 mL	Added to 235 mL for 250 mL total volume

When the first dilution is made with the 2.5 g, the solution in the vial will be yellow. When further diluted to make a 1% solution, it must be clear and colorless or should not be used.

For continuous drip anesthesia, prepare a 0.2% solution by adding 500 mg methohexital to 250 mL of diluent. For this dilution, either 5% glucose solution or isotonic (0.9%) sodium chloride solution is recommended instead of distilled water to avoid extreme hypotonicity.

➤*IM administration:* Contents of the vials should be diluted as follows:

For IM Administration		
Strength	Amount of diluent to be added to the contents of the vial	Concentration after dilution
500 mg vial	10 mL	5% solution (50 mg/mL)
2.5 g vial	50 mL	5% solution (50 mg/mL)

➤*Administration:* Dosage is highly individualized; the drug should be administered only by those completely familiar with its quantitative differences from other barbiturate anesthetics.

Adults – Administer methohexital IV in a concentration no higher than 1%. Higher concentrations markedly increase the incidence of muscular movements and irregularities in respiration and blood pressure.

Induction of anesthesia: For induction of anesthesia, a 1% solution is administered at a rate of about 1 mL per 5 seconds. Gaseous anesthetics and/or skeletal muscle relaxants may be administered concomitantly. The dose required for induction may range from 50 to 120 mg or more but averages about 70 mg. The usual dose in adults ranges from 1 to 1.5 mg/kg. The induction dose usually provides anesthesia for 5 to 7 minutes.

- *Maintenance of anesthesia* – Maintenance of anesthesia may be accomplished by intermittent injections of the 1% solution or, more easily, by continuous IV drip of a 0.2% solution. Give intermittent injections of about 20 to 40 mg (2 to 4 mL of a 1% solution) as required, usually every 4 to 7 minutes. For continuous drip, the average rate of administration is about 3 mL of a 0.2% solution/minute (1 drop/second). Individualize the rate of flow for each patient. For longer surgical procedures, gradual reduction in the rate of administration is recommended. Prolonged administration may result in cumulative effects, including extended somnolence, protracted unconsciousness, and respiratory and cardiovascular depression. Respiratory depression in the presence of an impaired airway may lead to hypoxia, cardiac arrest, and death. Other parenteral agents, usually narcotic analgesics, are ordinarily employed along with methohexital during longer procedures.

Pediatric patients: Administer methohexital IM in a 5% concentration.

- *Induction of anesthesia* – For the induction of anesthesia by the IM route of administration, the usual dose ranges from 6.6 to 10 mg/kg of the 5% concentration.

➤*Compatibility information:* Do not mix solutions of methohexital in the same syringe or administer simultaneously during IV infusion through the same needle with acid solutions, such as atropine sulfate, metocurine iodide, and succinylcholine chloride. Alteration of pH may cause free barbituric acid to be precipitated. Solubility of the soluble sodium salts of barbiturates, including methohexital, is maintained only at a relatively high (basic) pH.

Because of numerous requests from anesthesiologists for information regarding the chemical compatibility of these mixtures, the following chart contains information obtained from compatibility studies in which a 1% solution of methohexital was mixed with therapeutic amounts of agents whose solutions have a low (acid) pH.

Active ingredient	Potency per mL	Volume used	Immediate	15 min	Physical change 30 min	1 h
Methohexital	10 mg	10 mL			control	
Atropine sulfate	1/150 gr	1 mL	none	haze		
Atropine sulfate	1/100 gr	1 mL	none	precipitate	precipitate	
Succinylcholine chloride	0.5 mg	4 mL	none	none	haze	
Succinylcholine chloride	1 mg	4 mL	none	none	haze	
Metocurine iodide	0.5 mg	4 mL	none	none	precipitate	
Metocurine iodide	1 mg	4 mL	none	none	precipitate	
Scopolamine hydrobromide	1/120 g	1 mL	none	none	none	haze
Tubocurarine chloride	3 mg	4 mL	none	haze		

➤*Storage/Stability:* Store at controlled room temperature 20° to 25°C (68° to 77°F).

METHOHEXITAL SODIUM — RECTAL

For complete and comparative prescribing information, refer to the Barbiturate Anesthetics group monograph.

WARNING

Methohexital sodium should be used only in hospital or ambulatory care settings that provide for continuous monitoring of respiratory (eg, pulse oximetry) and cardiac function. Immediate availability of resuscitative drugs and age- and size-appropriate equipment for bag/valve/mask ventilation and intubation and personnel trained in their use and skilled in airway management should be assured. For deeply sedated patients, a designated individual other than the practitioner performing the procedure should be present to continuously monitor the patient.

Indications

➤*Child usage:* Methohexital sodium can be used in children older than 1 month as follows:

- For rectal induction of anesthesia prior to the use of other general anesthetic agents.
- For rectal induction of anesthesia and as an adjunct to subpotent inhalational anesthetic agents for short surgical procedures.
- As rectal anesthesia for short surgical, diagnostic, or therapeutic procedures associated with minimal painful stimuli.

Administration and Dosage

➤*Approved by the FDA:* July 13, 2001.

Methohexital sodium may be administered by the rectal route. Reconstituting instructions vary depending on the route of administration.

Facilities for assisting ventilation and administering oxygen are necessary adjuncts for all routes of administration of anesthesia. Since cardiorespiratory arrest may occur, patients should be observed carefully during and after use of methohexital sodium. Age- and size-appropriate resuscitative equipment (ie, intubation and cardioversion equipment, oxygen, suction, and a secure IV line) and personnel qualified in its use must be immediately available.

Preanesthetic medication is generally advisable. Methohexital sodium may be used with any of the recognized preanesthetic medications.

➤*Rectal administration:*

Strength (vial number)	Amount of diluent to be added to the contents of the vial	Concentration after dilution
500 mg vial (660)	50 mL	1% solution (10 mg/mL)
2.5 g vial (663) (larger vial needed)	250 mL	1% solution (10 mg/mL)

Administration – Dosage is highly individualized; the drug should be administered only by those completely familiar with its quantitative differences from other barbiturate anesthetics.

Pediatric patients: Methohexital sodium is administered rectally as a 1% solution.

• *Induction of anesthesia* – For rectal administration, the usual dose for induction is 25 mg/kg using the 1% solution.

KETAMINE HYDROCHLORIDE

c-iii	**Ketamine HCl** (Various, eg, Bedford)	**Injection:** 10 mg/ml	In 20 ml vials.[1]
		50 mg/ml	In 10 ml vials.[1]
		100 mg/ml	In 5 ml vials.[1]
c-iii	**Ketalar** (Monarch)	**Injection:** Ketamine base (as HCl): 10 mg/ml	In 20 ml vials (10s).[1]
		50 mg/ml	In 10 ml vials (10s).[1]
		100 mg/ml	In 5 ml vials (10s).[1]

[1] With benzethonium chloride.

KETAMINE HYDROCHLORIDE — INJECTION

WARNING

Special note – Emergence reactions have occurred in approximately 12% of patients.

The psychological manifestations vary in severity between pleasant dreamlike states, vivid imagery, hallucinations, and emergence delirium. In some cases, these states have been accompanied by confusion, excitement, and irrational behavior which a few patients recall as an unpleasant experience. The duration ordinarily is no more than a few hours; in a few cases, however, recurrences have taken place up to 24 hours postoperatively. No residual psychological effects are known to have resulted from use of ketamine hydrochloride.

The incidence of these emergence phenomena is least in the young (less than or equal to 15 years of age) and elderly (greater than 65 years of age) patient. Also, they are less frequent when the drug is given IM, and the incidence is reduced as experience with the drug is gained.

The incidence of psychological manifestations during emergence, particularly dreamlike observations and emergence delirium, may be reduced by using lower recommended dosages of ketamine hydrochloride in conjunction with IV diazepam during induction and maintenance of anesthesia (see Administration and Dosage). Also, these reactions may be reduced if verbal, tactile, and visual stimulation of the patient is minimized during the recovery period. This does not preclude the monitoring of vital signs.

In order to terminate a severe emergence reaction, the use of a small hypnotic dose of a short-acting or ultra, short-acting barbiturate may be required.

When ketamine hydrochloride is used on an outpatient basis, the patient should not be released until recovery from anesthesia is complete and then should be accompanied by a responsible adult.

Indications

As the sole anesthetic agent for diagnostic and surgical procedures that do not require skeletal muscle relaxation. Ketamine hydrochloride is best suited for short procedures, but it can be used, with additional doses, for longer procedures.

For the induction of anesthesia prior to the administration of other general anesthetic agents.

To supplement low-potency agents, such as nitrous oxide.

Administration and Dosage

➤*Approved by the FDA:* March 22, 1996.

➤*Note:* Barbiturates and ketamine hydrochloride, being chemically incompatible because of precipitate formation, should not be injected from the same syringe.

If the ketamine hydrochloride dose is augmented with diazepam, the 2 drugs must be given separately. Do not mix ketamine hydrochloride and diazepam in syringe or infusion flask.

➤*Preoperative preparations:* While vomiting has been reported following ketamine hydrochloride administration, some airway protection may be afforded because of active laryngeal-pharyngeal reflexes. However, since aspiration may occur with ketamine hydrochloride, and since protective reflexes may also be diminished by supplementary anesthetics and muscle relaxants, the possibility of aspiration must be considered. Ketamine hydrochloride is recommended for use in the patient whose stomach is not empty when, in the judgment of the practitioner, the benefits of the drug outweigh the possible risks.

Atropine, scopolamine, or another drying agent should be given at an appropriate interval prior to induction.

➤*Onset and duration:* Because of rapid induction following the initial IV injection, the patient should be in a supported position during administration.

The onset of action of ketamine hydrochloride is rapid; an IV dose of 2 mg/kg (1 mg/lb) of body weight usually produces surgical anesthesia within 30 seconds after injection, with the anesthetic effect usually lasting 5 to 10 minutes. If a longer effect is desired, additional increments can be administered IV or IM to maintain anesthesia without producing significant cumulative effects.

IM doses, from experience primarily in pediatric patients, in a range of 9 to 13 mg/kg (4 to 6 mg/lb) usually produce surgical anesthesia within 3 to 4 minutes following injection, with the anesthetic effect usually lasting 12 to 25 minutes.

➤*Dosage:* As with other general anesthetic agents, the individual response to ketamine hydrochloride is somewhat varied depending on the dose, route of administration, and age of patient, so that dosage recommendation cannot be absolutely fixed. The drug should be titrated against the patient's requirements.

➤*Induction:*

IV route – The initial dose of ketamine hydrochloride administered IV may range from 1 to 4.5 mg/kg (0.5 to 2 mg/lb). The average amount required to produce 5 to 10 minutes of surgical anesthesia has been 2 mg/kg (1 mg/lb).

Alternatively, in adult patients, an induction dose of 1 to 2 mg/kg IV ketamine at a rate of 0.5 mg/kg/min may be used for induction of anesthesia. In addition, diazepam in 2 to 5 mg doses, administered in a separate syringe over 60 seconds, may be used. In most cases, less than or equal to 15 mg of IV diazepam will suffice. The incidence of psychological manifestations during emergence, particularly dreamlike observations and emergence delirium, may be reduced by this induction dosage program.

Note: The 100 mg/mL concentration of ketamine hydrochloride should not be injected IV without proper dilution. It is recommended the drug be diluted with an equal volume of either Sterile Water for injection, USP, Normal Saline, or 5% Dextrose in Water.

Rate of administration: It is recommended that ketamine hydrochloride be administered slowly (over a period of 60 seconds). More rapid administration may result in respiratory depression and enhanced pressor response.

IM route – The initial dose of ketamine hydrochloride administered IM may range from 6.5 to 13 mg/kg (3 to 6 mg/lb). A dose of 10 mg/kg (5 mg/lb) will usually produce 12 to 25 minutes of surgical anesthesia.

➤*Maintenance of anesthesia:* The maintenance dose should be adjusted according to the patient's anesthetic needs and whether an additional anesthetic agent is employed.

Increments of one-half to the full induction dose may be repeated as needed for maintenance of anesthesia. However, it should be noted that purposeless and tonic-clonic movements of extremities may occur during the course of anesthesia. These movements do not imply a light plane and are not indicative of the need for additional doses of the anesthetic.

It should be recognized that the larger the total dose of ketamine hydrochloride administered, the longer will be the time to complete recovery.

Adult patients induced with ketamine hydrochloride augmented with IV diazepam may be maintained on ketamine hydrochloride given by slow microdrip infusion technique at a dose of 0.1 to 0.5 mg/min, augmented with diazepam 2 to 5 mg administered IV as needed. In many cases, 20 mg or less of IV diazepam total for combined induction and maintenance will suffice. However, slightly more diazepam may be required depending on the nature and duration of the operation, physical status of the patient, and other factors. The incidence of psychological manifestations during emergence, particularly dreamlike observations and emergence delirium, may be reduced by this maintenance dosage program.

➤*Dilution:* To prepare a dilute solution containing 1 mg of ketamine per mL, aseptically transfer 10 mL (50 mg/mL *Steri-Vial*) or 5 mL (100 mg/mL *Steri-Vial*) to 500 mL of 5% Dextrose Injection, USP or Sodium Chloride (0.9%) Injection, USP (Normal Saline) and mix well. The resultant solution will contain 1 mg of ketamine per mL.

The fluid requirements of the patient and duration of anesthesia must be considered when selecting the appropriate dilution of ketamine hydrochloride. If fluid restriction is required, ketamine hydrochloride can be added to a 250 mL infusion as described above to provide a ketamine hydrochloride concentration of 2 mg/mL.

Ketamine hydrochloride *Steri-Vials* 10 mg/mL are not recommended for dilution.

➤*Supplementary agents:* Ketamine hydrochloride is clinically compatible with the commonly used general and local anesthetic agents when an adequate respiratory exchange is maintained.

The regimen of a reduced dose of ketamine hydrochloride supplemented with diazepam can be used to produce balanced anesthesia by combination with other agents such as nitrous oxide and oxygen.

➤*Storage/Stability:* Store between 15° to 30°C (59° to 86°F). Protect from light.

Actions

➤*Pharmacology:* Ketamine hydrochloride is a rapidly acting general anesthetic producing an anesthetic state characterized by profound analgesia, normal pharyngeal-laryngeal reflexes, normal or slightly enhanced skeletal muscle tone, cardiovascular and respiratory stimulation, and occasionally a transient and minimal respiratory depression.

A patent airway is maintained partly by virtue of unimpaired pharyngeal and laryngeal reflexes.

The anesthetic state produced by ketamine hydrochloride has been termed "dissociative anesthesia" in that it appears to selectively interrupt association pathways of the brain before producing somatesthetic sensory blockade.

KETAMINE HYDROCHLORIDE — INJECTION

It may selectively depress the thalamoneocortical system before significantly obtunding the more ancient cerebral centers and pathways (reticular-activating and limbic systems).

Elevation of blood pressure begins shortly after injection, reaches a maximum within a few minutes, and usually returns to preanesthetic values within 15 minutes after injection. In the majority of cases, the systolic and diastolic blood pressure peaks from 10% to 50% above preanesthetic levels shortly after induction of anesthesia, but the elevation can be higher or longer in individual cases (see Contraindications).

Ketamine has a wide margin of safety; several instances of unintentional administration of overdoses of ketamine hydrochloride (up to 10 times that usually required) have been followed by prolonged but complete recovery.

➤*Pharmacokinetics:*

Absorption/Distribution – Following IV administration, the ketamine concentration has an initial slope (alpha phase) lasting about 45 minutes with a half-life of 10 to 15 minutes. This first phase corresponds clinically to the anesthetic effect of the drug. The anesthetic action is terminated by a combination of redistribution from the CNS to slower equilibrating peripheral tissues and by hepatic biotransformation to metabolite I. This metabolite is about ⅓ as active as ketamine in reducing halothane requirements (MAC) of the rat.

Metabolism/Excretion – The later half-life of ketamine (beta phase) is 2.5 hours.

The biotransformation of ketamine hydrochloride includes N-dealkylation (metabolite 1), hydroxylation of the cyclohexone ring (metabolites 3 and 4), conjugation with glucuronic acid and dehydration of the hydroxylated metabolites to form the cyclohexene derivative (metabolite 2).

Contraindications

Those in whom a significant elevation of blood pressure would constitute a serious hazard; hypersensitivity to the drug.

Warnings

➤*Confusional states:* Postoperative confusional states may occur during the recovery period.

➤*Respiratory depression:* Respiratory depression may occur with overdosage or too rapid a rate of administration of ketamine hydrochloride, in which case supportive ventilation should be employed. Mechanical support of respiration is preferred to administration of analeptics.

➤*Pregnancy:* Since the safe use in pregnancy, including obstetrics (either vaginal or abdominal delivery), has not been established, such use is not recommended.

Animal reproduction – To determine the effect of ketamine hydrochloride on the perinatal and postnatal period, pregnant rats were given twice the average human IM dose during days 18 to 21 of pregnancy. Litter characteristics at birth and through the weaning period were equivalent to those of the control animals. There was a slight increase in incidence of delayed parturition by 1 day in treated dams of this group. Three groups each of mated beagle bitches were given 2.5 times the average human IM dose twice weekly for the 3 weeks of the first, second, and third trimesters of pregnancy, respectively, without the development of adverse reactions in the pups.

➤*Children:* As with other general anesthetic agents, the individual response to ketamine hydrochloride is somewhat varied depending on the dose, route of administration, and age of patient, so that dosage recommendation cannot be absolutely fixed. The drug should be titrated against the patient's requirements.

Precautions

➤*Monitoring:* Cardiac function should be continually monitored during the procedure in patients found to have hypertension or cardiac decompensation.

➤*Administration:* Ketamine hydrochloride should be used by or under the direction of physicians experienced in administering general anesthetics and in maintenance of an airway and in the control of respiration.

Because pharyngeal and laryngeal reflexes are usually active, ketamine hydrochloride should not be used alone in surgery or diagnostic procedures of the pharynx, larynx, or bronchial tree. Mechanical stimulation of the pharynx should be avoided, whenever possible, if ketamine hydrochloride is used alone. Muscle relaxants, with proper attention to respiration, may be required in both of these instances.

Resuscitative equipment should be ready for use.

The incidence of emergence reactions may be reduced if verbal and tactile stimulation of the patient is minimized during the recovery period. This does not preclude the monitoring of vital signs.

The IV dose should be administered over a period of 60 seconds. More rapid administration may result in respiratory depression or apnea and enhanced pressor response.

In surgical procedures involving visceral pain pathways, ketamine hydrochloride should be supplemented with an agent which obtunds visceral pain.

➤*Special risk:* Use with caution in the chronic alcoholic and the acutely alcohol-intoxicated patient.

An increase in CSF pressure has been reported following administration of ketamine hydrochloride. Use with extreme caution in patients with preanesthetic elevated cerebrospinal fluid pressure.

➤*Drug abuse and dependence:* Ketamine has been reported being used as a drug of abuse. Reports suggest that ketamine produces a variety of symptoms including, but not limited to, flashbacks, hallucinations, dysphoria, anxiety, insomnia, or disorientation. Ketamine dependence and tolerance may develop in individuals with a history of drug abuse or dependence. Therefore, ketamine should be prescribed and administered with caution.

➤*Hazardous tasks:* The patients should be cautioned that driving an automobile, operating hazardous machinery or engaging in hazardous activities should not be undertaken for 24 hours or more (depending upon the dosage of ketamine hydrochloride and consideration of other drugs employed) after anesthesia.

Drug Interactions

Ketamine Drug Interactions			
Precipitant drug	Object drug*		Description
Ketamine	Nondepolarizing muscle relaxants	↑	Ketamine may increase the neuromuscular effects resulting in prolonged respiratory depression.
Ketamine	Thiopental	↓	The hypnotic effect of thiopental may be antagonized.
Barbiturates/ Narcotics	Ketamine	↑	Prolonged recovery time may occur if used with ketamine.
Halothane	Ketamine	↓	Cardiac output, blood pressure and pulse rate may be decreased. Halothane blocks the cardiovascular stimulatory effects of ketamine. Closely monitor cardiac function if ketamine and halothane are used together.
Theophyllines	Ketamine	↔	Unpredictable extensor-type seizures have been reported with coadministration.
Thyroid hormones	Ketamine	↑	Concurrent use may produce hypertension and tachycardia.

* ↑ = Object drug increased. ↓ = Object drug decreased. ↔ = Undetermined effect.

Adverse Reactions

➤*Cardiovascular:* Blood pressure and pulse rate are frequently elevated following administration of ketamine hydrochloride alone. However, hypotension and bradycardia have been observed. Arrhythmia has also occurred.

➤*CNS:* In some patients, enhanced skeletal muscle tone may be manifested by tonic and clonic movements sometimes resembling seizures (see Administration and Dosage).

➤*Dermatologic:* Transient erythema or morbilliform rash have also been reported.

➤*GI:* Anorexia, nausea and vomiting have been observed; however, this is not usually severe and allows the great majority of patients to take liquids by mouth shortly after regaining consciousness (see Administration and Dosage).

➤*Hypersensitivity:* Anaphylaxis.

➤*Local:* Local pain and exanthema at the injection site have infrequently been reported.

➤*Ophthalmic:* Diplopia and nystagmus have been noted following ketamine hydrochloride administration. It also may cause a slight elevation in intraocular pressure measurement.

➤*Psychiatric:* See Warning Box.

➤*Respiratory:* Although respiration is frequently stimulated, severe depression of respiration or apnea may occur following rapid IV administration of high doses of ketamine hydrochloride. Laryngospasms and other forms of airway obstruction have occurred during ketamine hydrochloride anesthesia.

Overdosage

➤*Symptoms:* Respiratory depression may occur with overdosage or too rapid a rate of administration of ketamine hydrochloride.

➤*Treatment:* In case of respiratory depression, supportive ventilation should be employed. Mechanical support of respiration is preferred to administration of analeptics.

Patient Information

As appropriate, especially in cases where early discharge is possible, the duration of ketamine hydrochloride and other drugs employed during the conduct of anesthesia should be considered. The patients should be cautioned that driving an automobile, operating hazardous machinery or engaging in hazardous activities should not be undertaken for 24 hours or more (depending upon the dosage of ketamine hydrochloride and consideration of other drugs employed) after anesthesia.

ETOMIDATE

Rx	**Amidate** (Hospira)	**Injection:** 2 mg/mL	In 10, 20 mL amps, 20 mL *Abboject.*

ETOMIDATE — INJECTION

Indications

For the induction of general anesthesia. When considering use of etomidate, the usefulness of its hemodynamic properties should be weighed against the high frequency of transient skeletal muscle movements.

For the supplementation of subpotent anesthetic agents, such as nitrous oxide in oxygen, during maintenance of anesthesia for short operative procedures such as dilation and curettage or cervical conization.

Administration and Dosage

➤*Approved by the FDA:* September 7, 1982.

Etomidate injection is intended for administration only by the intravenous route. The dose for induction of anesthesia in adult patients and in children above the age of 10 years will vary between 0.2 and 0.6 mg/kg of body weight, and it must be individualized in each case. The usual dose for induction in these patients is 0.3 mg/kg, injected over a period of 30 to 60 seconds. There are inadequate data to make dosage recommendations for induction of anesthesia in patients below the age of 10 years; therefore, such use is not recommended.

Smaller increments of intravenous etomidate may be administered to adult patients during short operative procedures to supplement subpotent anesthetic agents, such as nitrous oxide. The dosage employed under these circumstances, although usually smaller than the original induction dose, must be individualized. There are insufficient data to support this use of etomidate for longer adult procedures or for any procedures in children; therefore, such use is not recommended. The use of intravenous fentanyl and other neuroactive drugs employed during the conduct of anesthesia may alter the etomidate dosage requirements. Consult the prescribing information for all other such drugs before using.

➤*Premedication:* Etomidate injection is compatible with commonly administered pre-anesthetic medications, which may be employed as indicated.

➤*Storage / Stability:* Store at controlled room temperature 15° to 30° C (59° to 86° F).

Actions

➤*Pharmacology:* Etomidate is a hypnotic drug without analgesic activity. Intravenous injection of etomidate produces hypnosis characterized by a rapid onset of action, usually within 1 minute. Duration of hypnosis is dose dependent but relatively brief, usually 3 to 5 minutes when an average dose of 0.3 mg/kg is employed. Immediate recovery from anesthesia (as assessed by awakening time, time needed to follow simple commands and time to perform simple tests after anesthesia as well as they were performed before anesthesia), based upon data derived from short operative procedures where intravenous etomidate was used for both induction and maintenance of anesthesia, is about as rapid as, or slightly faster than, immediate recovery after similar use of thiopental. These same data revealed that the immediate recovery period will usually be shortened in adult patients by the intravenous administration of ≈ 0.1 mg of intravenous fentanyl, 1 or 2 minutes before induction of anesthesia, probably because less etomidate is generally required under these circumstances (consult the package insert for fentanyl before using).

The most characteristic effect of intravenous etomidate on the respiratory system is a slight elevation in arterial carbon dioxide tension ($PaCO_2$).

Reduced plasma cortisol and aldosterone levels have been reported following induction doses of etomidate. These results persist for ≈ 6 to 8 hours and appear to be unresponsive to ACTH stimulation. This probably represents blockage of 11 beta-hydroxylation within the adrenal cortex.

The intravenous administration of up to 0.6 mg/kg of etomidate to patients with severe cardiovascular disease has little or no effect on myocardial metabolism, cardiac output, peripheral circulation or pulmonary circulation. The hemodynamic effects of etomidate have in most cases been qualitatively similar to those of thiopental sodium, except that the heart rate tended to increase by a moderate amount following administration of thiopental under conditions where there was little or no change in heart rate following administration of etomidate. There are insufficient data concerning use of etomidate in patients with recent severe trauma or hypovolemia to predict cardiovascular response under such circumstances.

Etomidate induction is associated with a transient 20% to 30% decrease in cerebral blood flow. This reduction in blood flow appears to be uniform in the absence of intracranial space occupying lesions. As with other intravenous induction agents, reduction in cerebral oxygen utilization is roughly proportional to the reduction in cerebral blood flow. In patients with and without intracranial space occupying lesions, etomidate induction is usually followed by a moderate lowering of intracranial pressure, lasting several minutes. All of these studies provided for avoidance of hypercapnia. Information concerning regional cerebral perfusion in patients with intracranial space occupying lesions is too limited to permit definitive conclusions.

Preliminary data suggest that etomidate will usually lower intraocular pressure moderately.

➤*Pharmacokinetics:* Etomidate is rapidly metabolized in the liver. Minimal hypnotic plasma levels of unchanged drug are ≥ 0.23 mcg/mL; they decrease rapidly up to 30 minutes following injection and thereafter more slowly with a half-life value of about 75 minutes. Approximately 75% of the administered dose is excreted in the urine during the first day after injection. The chief metabolite is R-(+)-1-(1-phenylethyl)-1H-imidazole-5-carboxylic acid, resulting from hydrolysis of etomidate, and accounts for about 80% of the urinary excretion. Limited pharmacokinetic data in patients with cirrhosis and esophageal varices suggest that the volume of distribution and elimination half-life of etomidate are approximately double that seen in healthy subjects.

Contraindications

Hypersensitivity to etomidate.

Warnings

➤*Administration:* Intravenous etomidate should be administered only by persons trained in the administration of general anesthetics and in the management of complications encountered during the conduct of general anesthesia.

Because of the hazards of prolonged suppression of endogenous cortisol and aldosterone production, this formulation is not intended for administration by prolonged infusion.

➤*Pregnancy: Category C.* Etomidate has been shown to have an embryocidal effect in rats when given in doses 1 and 4 times the human dose. There are no adequate and well-controlled studies in pregnant women. Etomidate should be used during pregnancy only if the potential benefit justifies the potential risks to the fetus. Etomidate has not been shown to be teratogenic in animals. Reproduction studies with etomidate have been shown to:

1.) Decrease pup survival at 0.3 and 5 mg/kg in rats (≈ 1x and 16x human dosage, respectively) and at 1.5 and 4.5 mg/kg in rabbits (≈ 5x and 15x human dosage, respectively). No clear dose-related pattern was observed.
2.) Increase slightly the number of stillborn fetuses in rats at 0.3 and 1.25 mg/kg (~ 1x and 4x human dosage, respectively).
3.) Cause maternal toxicity with deaths of 6/20 rats at 5 mg/kg (≈ 16x human dosage) and 6/20 rabbits at 4.5 mg/kg (≈ 15x human dosage).

Labor and delivery – There are insufficient data to support use of intravenous etomidate in obstetrics, including Cesarean section deliveries. Therefore, such use is not recommended.

➤*Lactation:* It is not known whether this drug is excreted in human milk. Because many drugs are excreted in human milk, caution should be exercised when etomidate is administered to a nursing mother.

➤*Children:* There are inadequate data to make dosage recommendations for induction of anesthesia in patients below the age of 10 years; therefore, such use is not recommended (see Administration and Dosage).

Precautions

➤*Plasma cortisol levels:* Induction doses of etomidate have been associated with reduction in plasma cortisol and aldosterone concentrations. These have not been associated with changes in vital signs or evidence of increased mortality; however, where concern exists for patients undergoing severe stress, exogenous replacement should be considered.

Adverse Reactions

The most frequent adverse reactions associated with use of intravenous etomidate are transient venous pain on injection and transient skeletal muscle movements, including myoclonus:

1.) Transient venous pain was observed immediately following intravenous injection of etomidate in about 20% of the patients, with considerable difference in the reported incidence (1.2% to 42%). This pain is usually described as mild to moderate in severity but it is occasionally judged disturbing. The observation of venous pain is not associated with a more than usual incidence of thrombosis or thrombophlebitis at the injection site. Pain also appears to be less frequently noted when larger, more proximal arm veins are employed and it appears to be more frequently noted when smaller, more distal, hand or wrist veins are employed.
2.) Transient skeletal muscle movements were noted following use of intravenous etomidate in about 32% of the patients, with considerable difference in the reported incidence (22.7% to 63%). Most of these observations were judged mild to moderate in severity but some were judged disturbing. The incidence of disturbing movements was less when 0.1 mg of fentanyl was given immediately before induction. These movements have been classified as myoclonic in the majority of cases (74%), but averting movements (7%), tonic movements (10%), and eye movements (9%) have also been reported. No exact classification is available, but these movements may also be placed into 3 groups by location:
   a.) Most movements are bilateral. The arms, legs, shoulders, neck, chest wall, trunk, and all 4 extremities have been described in some cases, with 1 or more of these muscle groups predominating in each individual case. Results of electroencephalographic studies suggest that these muscle movements are a manifestation of disinhibition of cortical activity; cortical electroencephalograms, taken during periods when these muscle movements were observed, have failed to reveal seizure activity.
   b.) Other movements are described as either unilateral or having a predominance of activity of 1 side over the other. These movements sometimes resemble a localized response to some stimuli, such as venous pain on injection, in the lightly anesthetized patient (averting movements). Any muscle group or groups may be involved, but a predominance of movement of the arm in which the intravenous infusion is started is frequently noted.

ETOMIDATE — INJECTION

c.) Still other movements probably represent a mixture of the first 2 types.

Skeletal muscle movements appear to be more frequent in patients who also manifest venous pain on injection.

➤*Cardiovascular:* Hypertension, hypotension, tachycardia, bradycardia and other arrhythmias have occasionally been observed during induction and maintenance of anesthesia. One case of severe hypotension and tachycardia, judged to be anaphylactoid in character, has been reported.

➤*GI:* Postoperative nausea or vomiting following induction of anesthesia with etomidate is probably no more frequent than the general incidence. When etomidate was used for both induction and maintenance of anesthesia in short procedures such as dilation and curettage, or when insufficient analgesia was provided, the incidence of postoperative nausea or vomiting was higher than that noted in control patients who received thiopental.

➤*Respiratory:* Hyperventilation, hypoventilation, apnea of short duration (5 to 90 seconds with spontaneous recovery), laryngospasm, hiccup and snoring suggestive of partial upper airway obstruction have been observed in some patients. These conditions were managed by conventional countermeasures.

Overdosage

➤*Symptoms:* Overdosage may occur from too rapid or repeated injections. Too rapid injection may be followed by a fall in blood pressure. No adverse cardiovascular or respiratory effects attributable to etomidate overdose have been reported.

➤*Treatment:* In the event of suspected or apparent overdosage, the drug should be discontinued, a patent airway established (intubate, if necessary) or maintained and oxygen administered with assisted ventilation, if necessary.

MIDAZOLAM HYDROCHLORIDE

c-iv	**Midazolam Hydrochloride** (Roxane)	**Syrup:** 2 mg/mL	EDTA, saccharin, sorbitol. Cherry flavor. In 118 mL.
c-iv	**Midazolam Hydrochloride** (Various, eg, Bedford, Hospira)	**Injection:** 1 mg (as HCl)/mL	In 2 and 5 mL vials and *Carpuject* vials and 10 mL vials.
		5 mg (as HCl)/mL	In 1, 2, and 5 mL vials and *Carpuject* vials, 10 mL vials, and 2 mL syringes.

MIDAZOLAM HYDROCHLORIDE — ORAL

WARNING

Midazolam syrup has been associated with respiratory depression and respiratory arrest, especially when used for sedation in noncritical care settings. Midazolam syrup has been associated with reports of respiratory depression, airway obstruction, desaturation, hypoxia, and apnea, most often when used concomitantly with other CNS depressants (eg, opioids). Midazolam syrup should be used only in hospital or ambulatory care settings, including physicians' and dentists' offices, that can provide for continuous monitoring of respiratory and cardiac function. Immediate availability of resuscitative drugs and age- and size-appropriate equipment for ventilation and intubation, and personnel trained in their use and skilled in airway management should be ensured (see Warnings). For deeply sedated patients, a dedicated individual, other than the practitioner performing the procedure, should monitor the patient throughout the procedure.

Indications

➤*Sedation/Anxiolysis/Amnesia:* For use in children for sedation, anxiolysis and amnesia prior to diagnostic, therapeutic or endoscopic procedures or before induction of anesthesia.

Administration and Dosage

➤*Approved by the FDA:* October 15, 1998.

Indicated for use as a single dose (0.25 to 1 mg/kg with a maximum dose of 20 mg) for preprocedural sedation and anxiolysis in pediatric patients. Midazolam hydrochloride syrup is not intended for chronic administration.

➤*Monitoring:* See Warnings for more information.

Patient response to sedative agents, and resultant respiratory status, is variable. Regardless of the intended level of sedation or route of administration, sedation is a continuum; a patient may move easily from light to deep sedation, with potential loss of protective reflexes, particularly when coadministered with anesthetic agents and other CNS depressants. This is especially true in pediatric patients. The healthcare practitioner who uses this medication in pediatric patients should be aware of and follow accepted professional guidelines for pediatric sedation appropriate to their situation.

➤*Dosage:* Midazolam hydrochloride syrup must never be used without individualization of dosage, particularly when used with other medications capable of producing CNS depression. Younger (< 6 years of age) pediatric patients may require higher dosages (mg/kg) than older pediatric patients, and may require close monitoring.

The recommended dose for pediatric patients is a single dose of 0.25 to 0.5 mg/kg, depending on the status of the patient and desired effect, up to a maximum dose of 20 mg. In general, it is recommended that the dose be individualized and modified based on patient age, level of anxiety, and medical need. The younger (6 months to < 6 years of age) and less cooperative patients may require a higher than usual dose up to 1 mg/kg. A dose of 0.25 mg/kg may suffice for older (6 to < 16 years of age) or cooperative patients, especially if the anticipated intensity and duration of sedation is less critical. For all pediatric patients, a dose of 0.25 mg/kg should be considered when midazolam hydrochloride syrup is administered to patients with cardiac or respiratory compromise, other higher-risk surgical patients, and patients who have received concomitant narcotics or other CNS depressants. As with any potential respiratory depressant, these patients must be monitored for signs of cardiorespiratory depression after receiving midazolam hydrochloride syrup. In obese pediatric patients, the dose should be calculated based on ideal body weight. Midazolam hydrochloride syrup has not been studied, nor is it intended for chronic use.

➤*Concomitant therapy:* When midazolam hydrochloride syrup is given in conjunction with opioids or other sedatives, the potential for respiratory depression, airway obstruction, or hypoventilation is increased. The healthcare practitioner who uses this medication in pediatric patients should be aware of and follow accepted professional guidelines for pediatric sedation appropriate to their situation.

➤*Storage/Stability:* Store at 25°C (77°F); excursions permitted to 15° to 30°C (59° to 86°F).

Actions

➤*Pharmacology:* Midazolam is a short-acting benzodiazepine CNS depressant.

Pharmacodynamic properties of midazolam and its metabolites, which are similar to those of other benzodiazepines, include sedative, anxiolytic, amnesic and hypnotic activities. Benzodiazepine pharmacologic effects appear to result from reversible interactions with the gamma-amino butyric acid (GABA) benzodiazepine receptor, the major inhibitory neurotransmitter in the CNS. The action of midazolam is readily reversed by the benzodiazepine receptor antagonist, flumazenil.

See Warnings for more information.

See Drug Interactions for more information.

➤*Pharmacokinetics:*

Absorption – Midazolam is rapidly absorbed after oral administration and is subject to substantial intestinal and hepatic first-pass metabolism. The pharmacokinetics of midazolam and its major metabolite, alpha-hydroxymidazolam, and the absolute bioavailability of midazolam hydrochloride syrup were studied in pediatric patients of different ages (6 months to < 16 years old) over a 0.25 to 1 mg/kg dose range. Pharmacokinetic parameters from this study are presented in the following paragraphs. The mean t_{max} values across dose groups (0.25, 0.5, and 1 mg/kg) range from 0.17 to 2.65 hours. Midazolam exhibits linear pharmacokinetics between oral doses of 0.25 to 1 mg/kg (up to a maximum dose of 40 mg) across the age groups ranging from 6 months to < 16 years. Linearity was also demonstrated across the doses within the age group of 2 years to < 12 years having 18 patients at each of the 3 doses. The absolute bioavailability of the midazolam syrup in pediatric patients is about 36%, which is not affected by pediatric age or weight. The $AUC_{0-\infty}$ ratio of alpha-hydroxymidazolam to midazolam for the oral dose in pediatric patients is higher than for an IV dose (0.38 to 0.75 vs 0.21 to 0.39 across the age group of 6 months to < 16 years), and the $AUC_{0-\infty}$ ratio of alpha-hydroxymidazolam to midazolam for the oral dose is higher in pediatric patients than in adults (0.38 to 0.75 vs 0.4 to 0.56).

Number of subjects/age	Dose (mg/kg)	t_{max} (hr)	C_{max} (ng/mL)	t½ (hr)	$AUC_{0-\infty}$ (ng•hr/mL)
6 months to < 2 years old					
1	0.25	0.17	28	5.82	67.6
1	0.5	0.35	66	2.22	152
1	1	0.17	61.2	2.97	224
2 to < 12 years old					
18	0.25	0.72 ± 0.44	63 ± 30	3.16 ± 1.5	138 ± 89.5
18	0.5	0.95 ± 0.53	126 ± 75.8	2.71 ± 1.09	306 ± 196
18	1	0.88 ± 0.99	201 ± 101	2.37 ± 0.96	743 ± 642
12 to < 16 years old					
4	0.25	2.09 ± 1.35	29.1 ± 8.2	6.83 ± 3.84	155 ± 84.6
4	0.5	2.65 ± 1.58	118 ± 81.2	4.35 ± 3.31	821 ± 568
2	1	0.55 ± 0.28	191 ± 47.4	2.51 ± 0.18	566 ± 15.7

Distribution – The extent of plasma protein binding of midazolam is moderately high and concentration-independent. In adults and pediatric patients > 1 year of age, midazolam is ≈ 97% bound to plasma protein, principally albumin. In healthy volunteers, alpha-hydroxymidazolam is bound to the extent of 89%. In pediatric patients (6 months to < 16 years) receiving

MIDAZOLAM HYDROCHLORIDE — ORAL

0.15 mg/kg IV midazolam, the mean steady-state volume of distribution ranged from 1.24 to 2.02 L/kg.

Metabolism – Midazolam is primarily metabolized in the liver and gut by human cytochrome P450 3A4 (CYP3A4) to its pharmacologic active metabolite, alpha-hydroxymidazolam, followed by glucuronidation of the alpha-hydroxyl metabolite which is present in unconjugated and conjugated forms in human plasma. The alpha-hydroxymidazolam glucuronide is then excreted in urine. In a study in which adult volunteers were administered IV midazolam (0.1 mg/kg) and alpha-hydroxymidazolam (0.15 mg/kg), the pharmacodynamic parameter values of the maximum effect (E_{max}) and concentration eliciting half-maximal effect (EC_{50}) were similar for both compounds. The effects studied were reaction time and errors in tracing tests. The results indicate that alpha-hydroxymidazolam is equipotent and equally effective as unchanged midazolam on a total plasma concentration basis. After oral or IV administration, 63% to 80% of midazolam is recovered in urine as alpha-hydroxymidazolam glucuronide. No significant amount of parent drug or metabolites is extractable from urine before beta-glucuronidase and sulfatase deconjugation, indicating that the urinary metabolites are excreted mainly as conjugates.

Midazolam is also metabolized to 2 other minor metabolites: 4-hydroxy metabolite (about 3% of the dose) and 1,4-dihydroxy metabolite (about 1% of the dose) are excreted in small amounts in the urine as conjugates.

Excretion – The mean elimination half-life of midazolam ranged from 2.2 to 6.8 hours following single oral doses of 0.25, 0.5, and 1 mg/kg of midazolam (midazolam hydrochloride syrup). Similar results (ranged from 2.9 to 4.5 hours) for the mean elimination half-life were observed following IV administration of 0.15 mg/kg of midazolam to pediatric patients (6 months to < 16 years old). In the same group of patients receiving the 0.15 mg/kg IV dose, the mean total clearance ranged from 9.3 to 11 mL/min/kg.

Special populations –

Hepatic function impairment: Chronic hepatic disease alters the pharmacokinetics of midazolam. Following oral administration of 15 mg of midazolam, C_{max} and bioavailability values were 43% and 100% higher, respectively, in adult patients with hepatic cirrhosis than adult subjects with healthy liver function. In the same patients with hepatic cirrhosis, following IV administration of 7.5 mg of midazolam, the clearance of midazolam was reduced by about 40% and the elimination half-life was increased by about 90% compared with subjects with healthy liver function. Midazolam should be titrated for the desired effect in patients with chronic hepatic disease.

Congestive heart failure: Following oral administration of 7.5 mg of midazolam, elimination half-life values were 43% higher in adult patients with congestive heart failure than in control subjects.

Contraindications

Hypersensitivity to the drug or allergies to cherries or formulation excipients; acute narrow-angle glaucoma. Benzodiazepines may be used in patients with open-angle glaucoma only if they are receiving appropriate therapy. Measurements of intraocular pressure in patients without eye disease show a moderate lowering following induction of general anesthesia with injectable midazolam hydrochloride; patients with glaucoma have not been studied.

Warnings

➤*Respiratory effects:* Serious respiratory adverse reactions have occurred after administration of oral midazolam hydrochloride, most often when midazolam hydrochloride was used in combination with other CNS depressants. These adverse reactions have included respiratory depression, airway obstruction, oxygen desaturation, apnea, and rarely, respiratory or cardiac arrest. When oral midazolam is administered as the sole agent at recommended doses respiratory depression, airway obstruction, oxygen desaturation, and apnea occur infrequently.

Patients should be continuously monitored for early signs of hypoventilation, airway obstruction, or apnea with means for detection readily available (eg, pulse oximetry). Hypoventilation, airway obstruction, and apnea can lead to hypoxia or cardiac arrest unless effective countermeasures are taken immediately. The immediate availability of specific reversal agents (flumazenil) is highly recommended. Vital signs should continue to be monitored during the recovery period. Because midazolam hydrochloride can depress respiration (see Pharmacology), especially when used concomitantly with opioid agonists and other sedatives (see Administration and Dosage), it should be used for sedation/anxiolysis/amnesia only in the presence of personnel skilled in early detection of hypoventilation, maintaining a patent airway, and supporting ventilation.

Episodes of oxygen desaturation, respiratory depression, apnea, and airway obstruction have been occasionally reported following premedication (sedation prior to induction of anesthesia) with oral midazolam; such events are markedly increased when oral midazolam is combined with other CNS-depressing agents and in patients with abnormal airway anatomy, patients with cyanotic congenital heart disease, or patients with sepsis or severe pulmonary disease.

➤*Monitoring:* Prior to the administration of midazolam hydrochloride in any dose, the immediate availability of oxygen, resuscitative drugs, age- and size-appropriate equipment for bag/valve/mask ventilation and intubation, and skilled personnel for the maintenance of a patent airway and support of ventilation should be ensured. Midazolam hydrochloride syrup must never be used without individualization of dosage, particularly when used with other medications capable of producing CNS depression.

Midazolam hydrochloride syrup should be used only in hospital or ambulatory care settings, including physicians' and dentists' offices, that are equipped to provide continuous monitoring of respiratory and cardiac function. Midazolam hydrochloride syrup must only be administered to patients if they will be monitored by direct visual observation by a healthcare professional. If midazolam hydrochloride syrup will be administered in combination with other anesthetic drugs or drugs which depress the CNS, patients must be monitored by persons specifically trained in the use of these drugs and, in particular, in the management of respiratory effects of these drugs, including respiratory and cardiac resuscitation of patients in the age group being treated.

➤*Improper dosing:* Reactions such as agitation, involuntary movements (including tonic/clonic movements and muscle tremor), hyperactivity and combativeness have been reported in both adult and pediatric patients. Consideration should be given to the possibility of paradoxical reaction. Should such reactions occur, the response to each dose of midazolam hydrochloride and all other drugs, including local anesthetics, should be evaluated before proceeding. Reversal of such responses with flumazenil has been reported in pediatric and adult patients.

➤*Special risk:* Higher-risk pediatric surgical patients may require lower doses, whether or not concomitant, sedating medications have been administered. Pediatric patients with cardiac or respiratory compromise may be unusually sensitive to the respiratory-depressant effect of midazolam hydrochloride. Pediatric patients undergoing procedures involving the upper airway such as upper endoscopy or dental care, are particularly vulnerable to episodes of desaturation and hypoventilation due to partial airway obstruction. Patients with chronic renal failure and patients with congestive heart failure eliminate midazolam more slowly.

➤*Carcinogenesis:* Midazolam maleate was administered with diet in mice and rats for 2 years at dosages of 1, 9, and 80 mg/kg/day. In female mice in the highest dose (10 times the highest oral dose of 1 mg/kg for a pediatric patient, on a mg/m^2 basis) group there was a marked increase in the incidence of hepatic tumors. In high-dose (19 times the pediatric dose) male rats there was a small but statistically significant increase in benign thyroid follicular cell tumors. Dosages of 9 mg/kg/day of midazolam maleate (1 to 2 times the pediatric dose) did not increase the incidence of tumors in mice or rats. The pathogenesis of induction of these tumors is not known. These tumors were found after chronic administration, whereas human use will ordinarily be single or intermittent doses.

➤*Pregnancy: Category D.* Although midazolam hydrochloride syrup has not been studied in pregnant patients, an increased risk of congenital malformations associated with the use of benzodiazepine drugs (diazepam and chlordiazepoxide) have been suggested in several studies. If this drug is used during pregnancy, the patient should be apprised of the potential hazard to the fetus.

Labor and delivery – In humans, measurable levels of midazolam were found in maternal venous serum, umbilical venous and arterial serum and amniotic fluid, indicating placental transfer of the drug. The use of midazolam hydrochloride syrup in obstetrics has not been evaluated in clinical trials. Because midazolam is transferred transplacentally and because other benzodiazepines given in the last weeks of pregnancy have resulted in neonatal CNS depression, midazolam hydrochloride syrup is not recommended for obstetrical use.

➤*Lactation:* Midazolam is excreted in human milk. Caution should be exercised when midazolam hydrochloride syrup is administered to a nursing woman.

➤*Children:* Midazolam hydrochloride syrup has not been studied in patients < 6 months of age.

Precautions

➤*Use with other CNS depressants:* The efficacy and safety of midazolam hydrochloride in clinical use are functions of the dose administered, the clinical status of the individual patient, and the use of concomitant medications capable of depressing the CNS. Anticipated effects may range from mild sedation to deep levels of sedation with a potential loss of protective reflexes, particularly when coadministered with anesthetic agents or other CNS depressants. Care must be taken to individualize the dose of midazolam hydrochloride based on the patient's age, underlying medical/surgical conditions, concomitant medications, and to have the personnel, age- and size-appropriate equipment and facilities available for monitoring and intervention. Practitioners administering midazolam hydrochloride must have the skills necessary to manage reasonably foreseeable adverse effects, particularly skills in airway management.

➤*Special risk:* Following oral administration of 7.5 mg of midazolam to adult patients with congestive heart failure, the half-life of midazolam was 43% higher than in control subjects. One study suggests that hypercarbia or hypoxia following premedication with oral midazolam might pose a risk to children with congenital heart disease and pulmonary hypertension, although there are no known reports of pulmonary hypertensive crises that had been triggered by premedication. In the study, 22 children were premedicated with oral midazolam (0.75 mg/kg) or IM morphine plus scopolamine prior to elective repair of congenital cardiac defects. Both premedication regimens increased $PtcCO_2$ and decreased SpO_2 and respiratory rates preferentially in patients with pulmonary hypertension.

➤*Drug abuse and dependence:* Midazolam hydrochloride syrup is a benzodiazepine and is a schedule IV controlled substance that can produce drug dependence of the diazepam-type. Therefore, midazolam hydrochloride syrup may be subject to misuse, abuse and addiction. Benzodiazepines can cause physical dependence. Physical dependence results in withdrawal symptoms in patients who abruptly discontinue the drug. Withdrawal symptoms (ie, convulsions, hallucinations, tremors, abdominal and muscle cramps, vomiting and sweating), similar in characteristics to those noted with barbiturates and alcohol have occurred following abrupt discontinuation of midazolam following chronic administration. Abdominal distention, nausea, vomiting, and tachycardia are prominent symptoms of withdrawal

MIDAZOLAM HYDROCHLORIDE — ORAL

in infants. The handling of midazolam hydrochloride syrup should be managed to minimize the risk of diversion, including restriction of access and accounting procedures as appropriate to the clinical setting and as required by law.

➤*Hazardous tasks:* The decision as to when patients who have received midazolam hydrochloride syrup, particularly on an outpatient basis, may again engage in activities requiring complete mental alertness, operate hazardous machinery or drive a motor vehicle must be individualized. Gross tests of recovery from the effects of midazolam hydrochloride syrup (see Pharmacology) cannot be relied upon to predict reaction time under stress. It is recommended that no patient operate hazardous machinery or a motor vehicle until the effects of the drug, such as drowsiness, have subsided or until one full day after anesthesia and surgery, whichever is longer. Particular care should be taken to assure safe ambulation.

Drug Interactions

➤*CNS agents:* Concomitant use of barbiturates, alcohol or other CNS depressants may increase the risk of hypoventilation, airway obstruction, desaturation, or apnea and may contribute to profound or prolonged drug effect. Narcotic premedication also depresses the ventilatory response to carbon dioxide stimulation.

➤*Inhibitors of CYP3A4 isozymes:*

Interacting drug	Adult doses studied	% Increase in C_{max} of oral midazolam	% Increase in AUC of oral midazolam
Cimetidine	800 to 1200 mg up to 4 times daily in divided doses	6 to 138	10 to 102
Diltiazem	60 mg 3 times daily	105	275
Erythromycin	500 mg 3 times daily	170 to 171	281 to 341
Fluconazole	200 mg once daily	150	250
Grapefruit juice	200 mL	56	52
Itraconazole	100 to 200 mg once daily	80 to 240	240 to 980
Ketoconazole	400 mg once daily	309	1490
Ranitidine	150 mg twice daily or 3 times daily; 300 mg once daily	15 to 67	9 to 66
Roxithromycin	300 mg once daily	37	47
Saquinavir	120 mg 3 times daily	235	514
Verapamil	80 mg 3 times daily	97	192

Other drugs known to inhibit the effects of CYP3A4 would be expected to have similar effects on these midazolam pharmacokinetic parameters.

➤*Inducers of CYP3A4 isozymes:*

Interacting drug	Adult doses studied	% Decrease in C_{max} of oral midazolam	% Decrease in AUC of oral midazolam
Carbamazepine	Therapeutic doses	93	94
Phenytoin	Therapeutic doses	93	94
Rifampin	600 mg/day	94	96

Although not tested, phenobarbital, rifabutin and other drugs known to induce the effects of CYP3A4 would be expected to have similar effects on these midazolam pharmacokinetic parameters.

➤*CNS depressants:* One case was reported of inadequate sedation with chloral hydrate and later with oral midazolam due to a possible interaction with methylphenidate administered chronically in a 2-year-old boy with a history of Williams syndrome. The difficulty in achieving adequate sedation may have been the result of decreased absorption of the sedatives due to both the GI effects and stimulant effects of methylphenidate.

The sedative effect of midazolam hydrochloride syrup is accentuated by any concomitantly administered medication which depresses the CNS, particularly narcotics (eg, morphine, meperidine, fentanyl), propofol, ketamine, nitrous oxide, secobarbital and droperidol. Consequently, the dose of midazolam hydrochloride syrup should be adjusted according to the type and amount of concomitant medications administered and the desired clinical response.

Adverse Reactions

The distribution of adverse reactions occurring in patients evaluated in a randomized, double-blind, parallel-group trial are presented below by body system in order of decreasing frequency. For the premedication period (eg, sedation period prior to induction of anesthesia) alone, see the first table below. For over the entire monitoring period including premedication, anesthesia and recovery, see the second table below.

The distribution of adverse events occurring during the premedication period, before induction of anesthesia, is presented in the first table below. Emesis, which occurred in 31/397 (8%) patients over the entire monitoring period (premedication, anesthesia and recovery), occurred in 3/397 (0.8%) of patients during the premedication period (from midazolam administration to mask induction). Nausea, which occurred in 14/397 (4%) patients over the entire monitoring period, occurred in 2/397 (0.5%) patients during the premedication period.

For the entire monitoring period (premedication, anesthesia and recovery), adverse reactions were reported by 82/397 (21%) patients who received midazolam overall. The most frequently reported adverse reactions were emesis occurring in 31/397 (8%) patients and nausea occurring in 14/397 (4%) patients. Most of these GI events occurred after the administration of other anesthetic agents.

For the respiratory system overall, adverse events (hypoxia, laryngospasm, rhonchi, coughing, respiratory depression, airway obstruction, upper-airway congestion, shallow respirations), occurred during the entire monitoring period in 31/397 (8%) patients and increased in frequency as dosage was increased: 7/132 (5%) patients in the 0.25 mg/kg dose group, 9/132 (7%) patients in the 0.5 mg/kg dose group, and 15/133 (11%) patients in the 1 mg/kg dose group.

Most of the respiratory adverse events occurred during induction, general anesthesia or recovery. One patient (0.25%) experienced a respiratory system adverse event (laryngospasm) during the premedication period. This adverse event occurred precisely at the time of induction. Although many of the respiratory complications occurred in settings of upper airway procedures or concurrently administered opioids, a number of these events occurred outside of these settings as well. In this study, administration of midazolam hydrochloride syrup was generally accompanied by a slight decrease in both systolic and diastolic blood pressures, as well as a slight increase in heart rate.

Midazolam Adverse Reactions

Adverse reaction	0.25 mg/kg (n = 132)	0.5 mg/kg (n = 132)	1 mg/kg (n = 133)	(n = 397)
GI				
Emesis	1 (0.76%)	1 (0.76%)	1 (0.75%)	3 (0.76%)
Nausea			2 (1.5%)	2 (0.5%)
Respiratory				
Laryngospasm			1 *(0.75%)	1 (0.25%)
Sneezing/rhinorrhea			1 (0.75%)	1 (0.25%)
All body systems	1 (0.76%)	1 (0.76%)	5 (3.8%)	1 (1.8%)

* This adverse reaction occurred precisely at the time of induction.

Midazolam Adverse Reactions (≥ 1%)

Adverse reaction	0.25 mg/kg (n = 132)	0.5 mg/kg (n = 132)	1 mg/kg (n = 133)	(n = 397)
GI				
Emesis	11 (8%)	5 (4%)	15 (11%)	31 (8%)
Nausea	6 (5%)	2 (2%)	6 (5%)	14 (4%)
Overall	16 (12%)	8 (6%)	16 (12%)	40 (10%)
Respiratory				
Hypoxia	0	5 (4%)	4 (3%)	9 (2%)
Laryngospasm	0	1 (< 1%)	5 (4%)	6 (2%)
Respiratory depression	2 (2%)	1 (< 1%)	2 (2%)	5 (1%)
Rhonchi	2 (2%)	1 (< 1%)	2 (2%)	5 (1%)
Airway obstruction	2 (2%)	2 (2%)	0	4 (1%)
Upper airway congestion	2 (2%)	0	2 (2%)	4 (1%)
Overall	7 (5%)	9 (7%)	15 (11%)	31 (8%)
Psychiatric				
Agitated	1 (< 1%)	2 (2%)	3 (2%)	6 (2%)
Overall	1 (< 1%)	3 (2%)	4 (3%)	8 (2%)
Heart rate, rhythm disorders				
Bradycardia	1 (< 1%)	3 (2%)	0	4 (1%)
Bigeminy	2 (2%)	0	0	2 (< 1%)
Overall	3 (2%)	3 (2%)	1 (< 1%)	7 (2%)
Central/peripheral nervous system				
Prolonged sedation	0	0	2 (2%)	2 (< 1%)
Overall	2 (2%)	0	3 (2%)	5 (1%)
Dermatologic				
Rash	2 (2%)	0	0	2 (< 1%)
Overall	2 (2%)	2 (2%)	0	4 (1%)
All body systems	26 (20%)	23 (17%)	33 (25%)	82 (21%)

There were no deaths during the study, and no patient withdrew from the study due to adverse events. Serious adverse events (both respiratory disorders) were experienced postoperatively by 2 patients: 1 case of airway obstruction and desaturation (SpO_2 of 33%) in a patient given midazolam hydrochloride syrup 0.25 mg/kg, and 1 case of upper airway obstruction and respiratory depression following 0.5 mg/kg. Both patients had received IV morphine sulfate (1.5 mg total for both patients).

Other adverse reactions that have been reported in the literature with the oral administration of midazolam (not necessarily midazolam hydrochloride syrup), are listed below. The incidence rate for these events was generally < 1%.

MIDAZOLAM HYDROCHLORIDE — ORAL

➤*Cardiovascular:* Decreased systolic and diastolic blood pressure, increased heart rate.

➤*CNS:* Dysphoria, disinhibition, excitation, aggression, mood swings, hallucinations, adverse behavior, agitation, dizziness, confusion, ataxia, vertigo, dysarthria.

➤*GI:* Nausea, vomiting, hiccoughs, gagging, salivation, drooling.

➤*Respiratory:* Apnea, hypercarbia, desaturation, stridor.

➤*Special senses:* Diplopia, strabismus, loss of balance, blurred vision.

Overdosage

➤*Symptoms:* The manifestations of midazolam hydrochloride overdosage reported are similar to those observed with other benzodiazepines, including sedation, somnolence, confusion, impaired coordination, diminished reflexes, coma, and deleterious effects on vital signs. No evidence of specific organ toxicity from midazolam hydrochloride overdosage has been reported.

➤*Treatment:* Treatment of midazolam hydrochloride overdosage is the same as that followed for overdosage with other benzodiazepines. Respiration, pulse rate and blood pressure should be monitored and general supportive measures should be employed. Attention should be given to the maintenance of a patent airway and support of ventilation, including administration of oxygen. Should hypotension develop, treatment may include IV fluid therapy, repositioning, judicious use of vasopressors appropriate to the clinical situation, if indicated, and other appropriate countermeasures. There is no information as to whether peritoneal dialysis, forced diuresis or hemodialysis are of any value in the treatment of midazolam overdosage.

GI decontamination with lavage or activated charcoal once the patient's airway is secure is also recommended.

Flumazenil, a specific benzodiazepine-receptor antagonist, is indicated for the complete or partial reversal of the sedative effects of midazolam hydrochloride and may be used in situations when an overdose with a benzodiazepine is known or suspected. There are anecdotal reports of adverse hemodynamic responses associated with midazolam hydrochloride following administration of flumazenil to pediatric patients. Prior to the administration of flumazenil, necessary measures should be instituted to secure the airway, ensure adequate ventilation, and establish adequate IV access. Flumazenil is intended as an adjunct to, not as a substitute for, proper management of benzodiazepine overdose. Patients treated with flumazenil should be monitored for resedation, respiratory depression and other residual benzodiazepine effects for an appropriate period after treatment. The prescriber should be aware of a risk of seizure in association with flumazenil treatment, particularly in long-term benzodiazepine users and in cyclic antidepressant overdose. The complete flumazenil package insert, including Contraindications, Warnings and Precautions, should be consulted prior to use.

Patient Information

Inform your physician about any alcohol consumption and medicine you are now taking, especially blood pressure medication and antibiotics, including drugs you buy without a prescription. Alcohol has an increased effect when consumed with benzodiazepines; therefore, caution should be exercised regarding simultaneous ingestion of alcohol during benzodiazepine treatment.

Inform your physician if you are pregnant or are planning to become pregnant.

Inform your physician if you are nursing.

Patients should be informed of the pharmacological effects of midazolam hydrochloride syrup, such as sedation and amnesia, which in some patients may be profound. The decision as to when patients who have received midazolam hydrochloride syrup, particularly on an outpatient basis, may again engage in activities requiring complete mental alertness, operate hazardous machinery or drive a motor vehicle must be individualized.

Midazolam hydrochloride syrup should not be taken in conjunction with grapefruit juice.

For pediatric patients, particular care should be taken to ensure safe ambulation.

MIDAZOLAM HYDROCHLORIDE — INJECTION

Benzodiazepine compounds used as antianxiety agents appear under the Antianxiety Agents monograph.

WARNING

Adults and pediatrics – IV midazolam hydrochloride has been associated with respiratory depression and respiratory arrest, especially when used for sedation in noncritical care settings. In some cases, where this was not recognized promptly and treated effectively, death or hypoxic encephalopathy has resulted. IV midazolam hydrochloride should be used only in hospital or ambulatory care settings, including physicians' and dental offices, that provide for continuous monitoring of respiratory and cardiac function (ie, pulse oximetry). Immediate availability of resuscitative drugs and age- and size-appropriate equipment for bag/valve/mask ventilation and intubation, and personnel trained in their use and skilled in airway management should be ensured. Patients should be continuously monitored with some means of detection for early signs of hypoventilation, airway obstruction, or apnea (ie, pulse oximetry). Hypoventilation, airway obstruction, and apnea can lead to hypoxia or cardiac arrest unless effective countermeasures are taken immediately. The immediate availability of specific reversal agents (flumazenil) is highly recommended. Vital signs should continue to be monitored during the recovery period. For deeply sedated pediatric patients, a dedicated individual, other than the practitioner performing the procedure, should monitor the patient throughout the procedure.

The initial dose for sedation in adult patients may be as little as 1 mg, but should not exceed 2.5 mg in a healthy adult. Lower doses are necessary for older (over 60 years) or debilitated patients and in patients receiving concomitant narcotics or other CNS depressants. The initial dose and all subsequent doses should always be titrated slowly; administer over at least 2 minutes and allow an additional 2 or more minutes to fully evaluate the sedative effect. The use of the 1 mg/mL formulation or dilution of the 1 mg/mL or 5 mg/mL formulation is recommended to facilitate slower injection. Doses of sedative medications in pediatric patients must be calculated on a mg/kg basis, and initial doses and all subsequent doses should always be titrated slowly. The initial pediatric dose of midazolam hydrochloride for sedation/anxiolysis/amnesia is age, procedure, and route dependent.

Neonates – Midazolam hydrochloride should not be administered by rapid injection in the neonatal population. Rapid injection should be avoided in the neonatal population. Midazolam hydrochloride administered rapidly as an IV injection (less than 2 minutes) has been associated with severe hypotension in neonates, particularly when the patient has also received fentanyl. Likewise, severe hypotension has been observed in neonates receiving a continuous infusion of midazolam who then receive a rapid IV injection of fentanyl. Seizures have been reported in several neonates following rapid IV administration.

Indications

IM or IV for preoperative sedation/anxiolysis/amnesia; IV as an agent for sedation/anxiolysis/amnesia prior to or during diagnostic, therapeutic, or endoscopic procedures, such as bronchoscopy, gastroscopy, cystoscopy, coronary angiography, cardiac catheterization, oncology procedures, radiologic procedures, suture of lacerations, and other procedures either alone or in combination with other CNS depressants; IV for induction of general anesthesia, before administration of other anesthetic agents. With the use of narcotic premedication, induction of anesthesia can be attained within a relatively narrow dose range and in a short period of time. IV midazolam hydrochloride can also be used as a component of IV supplementation of nitrous oxide and oxygen (balanced anesthesia); continuous IV infusion for sedation of intubated and mechanically ventilated patients as a component of anesthesia or during treatment in a critical care setting.

Administration and Dosage

➤*Approved by the FDA:* December 20, 1985.

Midazolam hydrochloride is a potent sedative agent that requires slow administration and individualization of dosage. Clinical experience has shown midazolam hydrochloride to be 3 to 4 times as potent per mg as diazepam. Because serious and life-threatening cardiorespiratory adverse events have been reported, provision for monitoring, detection and correction of these reactions must be made for every patient to whom midazolam hydrochloride injection is administered, regardless of age or health status. Excessive single doses or rapid IV administration may result in respiratory depression, airway obstruction or arrest. The potential for these latter effects is increased in debilitated patients, those receiving concomitant medications capable of depressing the CNS, and patients without an endotracheal tube but undergoing a procedure involving the upper airway such as endoscopy or dental.

See Warnings for more information.

➤*Administration:* Midazolam hydrochloride should only be administered IM or IV. The safety and efficacy of midazolam hydrochloride following non-IV and non-IM routes of administration have not been established.

Care should be taken to avoid intra-arterial injection or extravasation. Adverse events have included local reactions, as well as isolated reports of seizure activity in which no clear causal relationship was established. Precautions against unintended intra-arterial injection should be taken. Extravasation should also be avoided.

➤*Compatibility:* Midazolam hydrochloride injection may be mixed in the same syringe with the following frequently used premedications: Morphine sulfate, meperidine, atropine sulfate or scopolamine. Midazolam hydrochloride, at a concentration of 0.5 mg/mL, is compatible with 5% dextrose in water and 0.9% sodium chloride for up to 24 hours and with lactated Ringer's solution for up to 4 hours. Both the 1 mg/mL and 5 mg/mL formulations of midazolam hydrochloride may be diluted with 0.9% sodium chloride or 5% dextrose in water.

➤*Monitoring:* Patient response to sedative agents, and resultant respiratory status, is variable. Regardless of the intended level of sedation or route of administration, sedation is a continuum; a patient may move easily from light to deep sedation, with potential loss of protective reflexes. This is especially true in pediatric patients. Sedative doses should be individually titrated, taking into account patient age, clinical status and concomitant use of other CNS depressants. Continuous monitoring of respiratory and cardiac function is required (ie, pulse oximetry).

Adults and pediatrics – Titration to effect with multiple small doses is essential for safe administration. It should be noted that adequate time to achieve peak CNS effect (3 to 5 minutes) for midazolam should be allowed between doses to minimize the potential for oversedation. Sufficient time must elapse between doses of concomitant sedative medications to allow the effect of each dose to be assessed before subsequent drug administration. This is an important consideration for all patients who receive IV midazolam hydrochloride. Immediate availability of resuscitative drugs and age- and size-appropriate equipment and personnel trained in their use and skilled in airway management should be ensured. Patients should be continuously monitored with some means of detection for early signs of

MIDAZOLAM HYDROCHLORIDE — INJECTION

hypoventilation, airway obstruction, or apnea (ie, pulse oximetry). Hypoventilation, airway obstruction, and apnea can lead to hypoxia or cardiac arrest unless effective countermeasures are taken immediately. The immediate availability of specific reversal agents (flumazenil) is highly recommended. Vital signs should continue to be monitored during the recovery period.

➤*Usual adult dose:*

IM – For preoperative sedation/anxiolysis/amnesia (induction of sleepiness or drowsiness and relief of apprehension, impairment of memory of perioperative events) the recommended premedication dose of midazolam for good risk (ASA Physical Status I & II) adult patients below the age of 60 years is 0.07 to 0.08 mg/kg IM (approximately 5 mg IM) administered up to 1 hour before surgery.

For IM use, midazolam should be injected deep in a large muscle mass. The dose must be individualized and reduced when the IM midazolam is administered to patients with chronic obstructive pulmonary disease, other higher risk surgical patients, patients greater than or equal to 60 years of age, and patients who have received concomitant narcotics or other CNS depressants. Administration of IM midazolam hydrochloride to elderly or higher risk surgical patients has been associated with rare reports of death under circumstances compatible with cardiorespiratory depression. In most of these cases, the patients also received other CNS depressants capable of depressing respiration, especially narcotics. In a study of patients 60 years or older, who did not receive concomitant administration of narcotics, 2 to 3 mg (0.02 to 0.05 mg/kg) of midazolam produced adequate sedation during the preoperative period. The dose of 1 mg IM midazolam may suffice for some older patients if the anticipated intensity and duration of sedation is less critical. As with any potential respiratory depressant, these patients require observation for signs of cardiorespiratory depression after receiving IM midazolam.

Onset is within 15 minutes, peaking 30 to 60 minutes. It can be administered concomitantly with atropine sulfate or scopolamine hydrochloride and reduced doses of narcotics.

IV – Midazolam 1 mg/mL formulation is recommended for sedation/anxiolysis/amnesia for procedures to facilitate slower injection. Both the 1 mg/mL and the 5 mg/mL formulations may be diluted with 0.9% sodium chloride or 5% dextrose in water.

Healthy adults below the age of 60: Titrate slowly to the desired effect (eg, the initiation of slurred speech). Some patients may respond to as little as 1 mg. No more than 2.5 mg should be given over a period of at least 2 minutes. Wait an additional 2 or more minutes to fully evaluate the sedative effect. If further titration is necessary, continue to titrate, using small increments, to the appropriate level of sedation. Wait an additional 2 or more minutes after each increment to fully evaluate the sedative effect. A total dose greater than 5 mg is not usually necessary to reach the desired endpoint. If narcotic premedication or other CNS depressants are used, patients will require approximately 30% less midazolam than unpremedicated patients.

Patients age 60 or older, and debilitated or chronically ill patients: Because the danger of hypoventilation, airway obstruction, or apnea is greater in elderly patients and those with chronic disease states or decreased pulmonary reserve, and because the peak effect may take longer in these patients, increments should be smaller and the rate of injection slower. Titrate slowly to the desired effect (eg, the initiation of slurred speech). Some patients may respond to as little as 1 mg. No more than 1.5 mg should be given over a period of no less than 2 minutes. Wait an additional 2 or more minutes to fully evaluate the sedative effect. If additional titration is necessary, it should be given at a rate of no more than 1 mg over a period of 2 minutes, waiting an additional 2 or more minutes each time to fully evaluate the sedative effect. Total doses greater than 3.5 mg are not usually necessary. If concomitant CNS-depressant premedications are used in these patients, they will require at least 50% less midazolam than healthy young unpremedicated patients.

Maintenance dose: Additional doses to maintain the desired level of sedation may be given in increments of 25% of the dose used to first reach the sedative endpoint, but again only by slow titration, especially in the elderly and chronically ill or debilitated patient. These additional doses should be given only after a thorough clinical evaluation clearly indicates the need for additional sedation.

Induction of anesthesia: For induction of general anesthesia, before administration of other anesthetic agents. Individual response to the drug is variable, particularly when a narcotic premedication is not used. The dosage should be titrated to the desired effect according to the patient's age and clinical status. When midazolam is used before other IV agents for induction of anesthesia, the initial dose of each agent may be significantly reduced, at times to as low as 25% of the usual initial dose of the individual agents.

Unpremedicated patients: In the absence of premedication, an average adult under the age of 55 years will usually require an initial dose of 0.3 to 0.35 mg/kg for induction, administered over 20 to 30 seconds and allowing 2 minutes for effect. If needed to complete induction, increments approximately 25% of the patient's initial dose may be used; induction may instead be completed with inhalational anesthetics. In resistant cases, up to 0.6 mg/kg total dose may be used for induction, but such larger doses may prolong recovery. Unpremedicated patients over the age of 55 years usually require less midazolam for induction; an initial dose of 0.3 mg/kg is recommended. Unpremedicated patients with severe systemic disease or other debilitation usually require less midazolam for induction. An initial dose of 0.2 to 0.25 mg/kg will usually suffice; in some cases, as little as 0.15 mg/kg may suffice.

Premedicated patients: When the patient has received sedative or narcotic premedication, particularly narcotic premedication, the range of recommended doses is 0.15 to 0.35 mg/kg. In average adults below the age of 55 years, a dose of 0.25 mg/kg, administered over 20 to 30 seconds and allowing 2 minutes for effect, will usually suffice. The initial dose of 0.2 mg/kg is recommended for good risk (ASA I & II) surgical patients over the age of 55 years. In some patients with severe systemic disease or debilitation, as little as 0.15 mg/kg may suffice. Narcotic premedication frequently used during clinical trials included fentanyl (1.5 to 2 mcg/kg IV, administered 5 minutes before induction), morphine (dosage individualized, up to 0.15 mg/kg IM), and meperidine (dosage individualized, up to 1 mg/kg IM). Sedative premedications were hydroxyzine pamoate (100 mg orally) and sodium secobarbital (200 mg orally). Except for IV fentanyl, administered 5 minutes before induction, all other premedications should be administered approximately 1 hour prior to the time anticipated for midazolam induction.

Injectable midazolam can also be used during maintenance of anesthesia, for surgical procedures, as a component of balanced anesthesia. Effective narcotic premedication is especially recommended in such cases. Incremental injections of approximately 25% of the induction dose should be given in response to signs of lightening of anesthesia and repeated as necessary.

Continuous infusion – For continuous infusion, midazolam 5 mg/mL formulation is recommended diluted to a concentration of 0.5 mg/mL with 0.9% sodium chloride or 5% dextrose in water.

Usual adult dose: If a loading dose is necessary to rapidly initiate sedation, 0.01 to 0.05 mg/kg (approximately 0.5 to 4 mg for a typical adult) may be given slowly or infused over several minutes. This dose may be repeated at 10- to 15-minute intervals until adequate sedation is achieved. For maintenance of sedation, the usual initial infusion rate is 0.02 to 0.1 mg/kg/hr (1 to 7 mg/hr). Higher loading or maintenance infusion rates may occasionally be required in some patients. The lowest recommended doses should be used in patients with residual effects from anesthetic drugs, or in those concurrently receiving other sedatives or opioids. Individual response to midazolam is variable. The infusion rate should be titrated to the desired level of sedation, taking into account the patient's age, clinical status and current medications. In general, midazolam should be infused at the lowest rate that produces the desired level of sedation. Assessment of sedation should be performed at regular intervals and the midazolam infusion rate adjusted up or down by 25% to 50% of the initial infusion rate so as to ensure adequate titration of sedation level. Larger adjustments or even a small incremental dose may be necessary if rapid changes in the level of sedation are indicated. In addition, the infusion rate should be decreased by 10% to 25% every few hours to find the minimum effective infusion rate. Finding the minimum effective infusion rate decreases the potential accumulation of midazolam and provides for the most rapid recovery once the infusion is terminated. Patients who exhibit agitation, hypertension, or tachycardia in response to noxious stimulation, but who are otherwise adequately sedated, may benefit from concurrent administration of an opioid analgesic. Addition of an opioid will generally reduce the minimum effective midazolam infusion rate.

➤*Children:* Unlike adult patients, pediatric patients generally receive increments of midazolam on a mg/kg basis. As a group, pediatric patients generally require higher dosages of midazolam (mg/kg) than do adults. Younger (less than 6 years) pediatric patients may require higher dosages (mg/kg) than older pediatric patients, and may require close monitoring (see tables below). In obese pediatric patients, the dose should be calculated based on ideal body weight. When midazolam is given in conjunction with opioids or other sedatives, the potential for respiratory depression, airway obstruction, or hypoventilation is increased. IV midazolam hydrochloride should be used only in hospital or ambulatory care settings, including physicians' and dental offices, that provide for continuous monitoring of respiratory and cardiac function (ie, pulse oximetry). Immediate availability of resuscitative drugs and age- and size-appropriate equipment for bag/valve/mask ventilation and intubation, and personnel trained in their use and skilled in airway management should be ensured. For deeply sedated pediatric patients, a dedicated individual, other than the practitioner performing the procedure, should monitor the patient throughout the procedure. The healthcare practitioner who uses this medication in pediatric patients should be aware of and follow accepted professional guidelines for pediatric sedation appropriate to their situation.

➤*IM:*

Usual pediatric dose (nonneonatal) – For sedation/anxiolysis/amnesia prior to anesthesia or for procedures, IM midazolam can be used to sedate pediatric patients to facilitate less traumatic insertion of an IV catheter for titration of additional medication. Sedation after IM midazolam is age and dose dependent; higher doses may result in deeper and more prolonged sedation. Doses of 0.1 to 0.15 mg/kg are usually effective and do not prolong emergence from general anesthesia. For more anxious patients, doses up to 0.5 mg/kg have been used. Although not systematically studied, the total dose usually does not exceed 10 mg. If midazolam is given with an opioid, the initial dose of each must be reduced.

➤*IV by intermittent injection:*

Usual pediatric dose (nonneonatal) – For sedation/anxiolysis/amnesia prior to and during procedures or prior to anesthesia. It should be recognized that the depth of sedation/anxiolysis needed for pediatric patients depends on the type of procedure to be performed. For example, simple light sedation/anxiolysis in the preoperative period is quite different from the deep sedation and analgesia required for an endoscopic procedure in a child. For this reason, there is a broad range of dosage. For all pediatric patients, regardless of the indication for sedation/anxiolysis, it is vital to titrate midazolam and other concomitant medications slowly to the desired clinical effect. The initial dose of midazolam should be administered over 2 to 3 minutes. Since midazolam is water soluble, it takes approximately 3 times longer than diazepam to achieve peak EEG effects; therefore, one must wait an additional 2 to 3 minutes to fully evaluate the sedative effect before initiating a procedure or repeating a dose. If further sedation is necessary, continue to titrate with small increments until the appropriate level of sedation is achieved. If other medications capable of depressing the CNS are coadministered, the peak effect of those concomitant medications must be considered and the dose of midazolam adjusted. The importance of drug titration to effect is vital to the safe sedation/anxiolysis of the pediatric

MIDAZOLAM HYDROCHLORIDE — INJECTION

patient. The total dose of midazolam will depend on patient response, the type and duration of the procedure, as well as the type and dose of concomitant medications.

Pediatric patients less than 6 months of age – Limited information is available in nonintubated pediatric patients less than 6 months of age. It is uncertain when the patient transfers from neonatal physiology to pediatric physiology; therefore, the dosing recommendations are unclear. Pediatric patients less than 6 months of age are particularly vulnerable to airway obstruction and hypoventilation; therefore, titration with small increments to clinical effect and careful monitoring are essential.

Pediatric patients 6 months to 5 years of age – Initial dose 0.05 to 0.1 mg/kg; total dose up to 0.6 mg/kg may be necessary to reach the desired endpoint but usually does not exceed 6 mg. Prolonged sedation and risk of hypoventilation may be associated with the higher doses.

Pediatric patients 6 to 12 years of age – Initial dose 0.025 to 0.05 mg/kg; total dose up to 0.4 mg/kg may be needed to reach the desired endpoint but usually does not exceed 10 mg. Prolonged sedation and risk of hypoventilation may be associated with the higher doses.

Pediatric patients 12 to 16 years of age – Should be dosed as adults. Prolonged sedation may be associated with higher doses; some patients in this age range will require higher than recommended adult doses but the total dose usually does not exceed 10 mg. The dose of midazolam must be reduced in patients premedicated with opioid or other sedative agents including midazolam. Higher risk or debilitated patients may require lower dosages whether or not concomitant sedating medications have been administered.

➤*Continuous IV infusion:*

Usual pediatric dose (nonneonatal) – For sedation/anxiolysis/amnesia in critical care settings. To initiate sedation, an IV loading dose of 0.05 to 0.2 mg/kg administered over at least 2 to 3 minutes can be used to establish the desired clinical effect in patients whose trachea is intubated. (Midazolam should not be administered as a rapid IV dose.) This loading dose may be followed by a continuous IV infusion to maintain the effect. An infusion of midazolam has been used in patients whose trachea was intubated but who were allowed to breathe spontaneously. Assisted ventilation is recommended for pediatric patients who are receiving other CNS-depressant medications such as opioids. Based on pharmacokinetic parameters and reported clinical experience, continuous IV infusions of midazolam should be initiated at a rate of 0.06 to 0.12 mg/kg/hr (1 to 2 mcg/kg/min). The rate of infusion can be increased or decreased (generally by 25% of the initial or subsequent infusion rate) as required, or supplemental IV doses of midazolam can be administered to increase or maintain the desired effect. Frequent assessment at regular intervals using standard pain/sedation scales is recommended. Drug elimination may be delayed in patients receiving erythromycin or other P450 3A4 enzyme inhibitors and in patients with liver dysfunction, low cardiac output (especially those requiring inotropic support), and in neonates. Hypotension may be observed in patients who are critically ill, particularly those receiving opioids or when midazolam is rapidly administered.

When initiating an infusion with midazolam in hemodynamically compromised patients, the usual loading dose of midazolam should be titrated in small increments and the patient monitored for hemodynamic instability (eg, hypotension). These patients are also vulnerable to the respiratory depressant effects of midazolam and require careful monitoring of respiratory rate and oxygen saturation.

➤*Continuous IV infusion:*

Usual neonatal dose – For sedation in critical care settings. Based on pharmacokinetic parameters and reported clinical experience in preterm and term neonates whose trachea was intubated, continuous IV infusions of midazolam should be initiated at a rate of 0.03 mg/kg/hr (0.5 mcg/kg/min) in neonates less than 32 weeks and 0.06 mg/kg/hr (0.5 mcg/kg/min) in neonates greater than 32 weeks. IV loading doses should not be used in neonates. Rather, the infusion may be run more rapidly for the first several hours to establish therapeutic plasma levels. The rate of infusion should be carefully and frequently reassessed, particularly after the first 24 hours so as to administer the lowest possible effective dose and reduce the potential for drug accumulation. This is particularly important because of the potential for adverse effects related to metabolism of the benzyl alcohol. Exposure to excessive amounts of benzyl alcohol has been associated with toxicity (hypotension, metabolic acidosis), particularly in neonates, and an increased incidence of kernicterus, particularly in small preterm infants. There have been rare reports of deaths, primarily in preterm infants, associated with exposure to excessive amounts of benzyl alcohol. The amount of benzyl alcohol from medications is usually considered negligible compared to that received in flush solutions containing benzyl alcohol. Administration of high dosages of medications (including midazolam hydrochloride) containing this preservative must take into account the total amount of benzyl alcohol administered. The recommended dosage range of midazolam hydrochloride for preterm and term infants includes amounts of benzyl alcohol well below that associated with toxicity; however, the amount of benzyl alcohol at which toxicity may occur is not known. If the patient requires more than the recommended dosages or other medications containing this preservative, the practitioner must consider the daily metabolic load of benzyl alcohol from these combined sources. Hypotension may be observed in patients who are critically ill and in preterm and term infants, particularly those receiving fentanyl or when midazolam is administered rapidly. Due to an increased risk of apnea, extreme caution is advised when sedating preterm and former preterm patients whose trachea is not intubated.

➤*Storage/Stability:* Store at 15° to 30°C (59° to 86°F).

Actions

➤*Pharmacology:* Midazolam hydrochloride is a short-acting benzodiazepine CNS depressant.

The effects of midazolam hydrochloride on the CNS are dependent on the dose administered, the route of administration, and the presence or absence of other medications. Onset time of sedative effects after IM administration in adults is 15 minutes, with peak sedation occurring 30 to 60 minutes following injection. In 1 adult study, when tested the following day, 73% of the patients who received midazolam hydrochloride IM had no recall of memory cards shown 30 minutes following drug administration; 40% had no recall of the memory cards shown 60 minutes following drug administration. Onset time of sedative effects in the pediatric population begins within 5 minutes and peaks at 15 to 30 minutes depending upon the dose administered. In pediatric patients, up to 85% had no recall of pictures shown after receiving IM midazolam hydrochloride compared with 5% of the placebo controls.

Sedation in adult and pediatric patients is achieved within 3 to 5 minutes after IV injection; the time of onset is affected by total dose administered and the concurrent administration of narcotic premedication. Seventy-one percent (71%) of the adult patients in endoscopy studies had no recall of introduction of the endoscope; 82% of the patients had no recall of withdrawal of the endoscope. In 1 study of pediatric patients undergoing lumbar puncture or bone marrow aspiration, 88% of patients had impaired recall vs 9% of the placebo controls. In another pediatric oncology study, 91% of midazolam hydrochloride treated patients were amnestic compared with 35% of patients who had received fentanyl alone.

When midazolam hydrochloride is given IV as an anesthetic induction agent, induction of anesthesia occurs in approximately 1.5 minutes when narcotic premedication has been administered and in 2 to 2.5 minutes without narcotic premedication or other sedative premedication. Some impairment in a test of memory was noted in 90% of the patients studied. A dose-response study of pediatric patients premedicated with 1 mg/kg IM meperidine found that only 4 out of 6 pediatric patients who received 600 mcg/kg IV midazolam hydrochloride lost consciousness, with eye closing at 108 ± 140 seconds. This group was compared with pediatric patients who were given thiopental 5 mg/kg IV; 6 out of 6 closed their eyes at 20 ± 3.2 seconds. Midazolam hydrochloride did not dependably induce anesthesia at this dose despite concomitant opioid administration in pediatric patients.

Midazolam hydrochloride, used as directed, does not delay awakening from general anesthesia in adults. Gross tests of recovery after awakening (orientation, ability to stand and walk, suitability for discharge from the recovery room, return to baseline Trieger competency) usually indicate recovery within 2 hours, but recovery may take up to 6 hours in some cases. When compared with patients who received thiopental, patients who received midazolam generally recovered at a slightly slower rate. Recovery from anesthesia or sedation for procedures in pediatric patients depends on the dose of midazolam hydrochloride administered, coadministration of other medications causing CNS depression and duration of the procedure.

The usual recommended IM premedicating doses of midazolam hydrochloride do not depress the ventilatory response to carbon dioxide stimulation to a clinically significant extent in adults. IV induction doses of midazolam hydrochloride depress the ventilatory response to carbon dioxide stimulation for 15 minutes or more beyond the duration of ventilatory depression following administration of thiopental in adults. Impairment of ventilatory response to carbon dioxide is more marked in adult patients with chronic obstructive pulmonary disease (COPD). Sedation with IV midazolam hydrochloride does not adversely affect the mechanics of respiration (resistance, static recoil, most lung volume measurements); total lung capacity and peak expiratory flow decrease significantly, but static compliance and maximum expiratory flow at 50% of awake total lung capacity (V_{max}) increase. In 1 study of pediatric patients under general anesthesia, IM midazolam hydrochloride (100 or 200 mcg/kg) was shown to depress the response to carbon dioxide in a dose-related manner.

In cardiac hemodynamic studies in adults, IV induction of general anesthesia with midazolam hydrochloride was associated with a slight-to-moderate decrease in mean arterial pressure, cardiac output, stroke volume and systemic vascular resistance. Slow heart rates (less than 65/minute), particularly in patients taking propranolol for angina, tended to rise slightly; faster heart rates (eg, 85/minute) tended to slow slightly. In pediatric patients, a comparison of IV midazolam hydrochloride (500 mcg/kg) with propofol (2.5 mg/kg) revealed a mean 15% decrease in systolic blood pressure in patients who had received IV midazolam hydrochloride vs a mean 25% decrease in systolic blood pressure following propofol.

➤*Pharmacokinetics:*

Absorption – The absolute bioavailability of the IM route was greater than 90% in a crossover study in which healthy subjects (n = 17) were administered a 7.5 mg IV or IM dose. The mean peak concentration (C_{max}) and time to peak (t_{max}) following the IM dose was 90 ng/mL (20% CV) and 0.5 hour (50% CV). C_{max} for the 1-hydroxy metabolite following the IM dose was 8 ng/mL (t_{max} = 1 hour).

Following IM administration, C_{max} for midazolam and its 1-hydroxy metabolite were approximately one-half of those achieved after IV injection.

Distribution – The volume of distribution (Vd), determined from 6 single-dose pharmacokinetic studies involving healthy adults, ranged from 1 to 3.1 L/kg. Female gender, old age, and obesity are associated with increased values of midazolam Vd. In humans, midazolam has been shown to cross the placenta and enter into fetal circulation and has been detected in human milk and CSF.

In adults and pediatric patients greater than 1 year of age, midazolam is approximately 97% bound to plasma protein, principally albumin.

Metabolism – In vitro studies with human liver microsomes indicate that the biotransformation of midazolam is mediated by cytochrome P450 3A4. This cytochrome also appears to be present in GI tract mucosa as well as liver. Sixty to seventy percent (60% to 70%) of the biotransformation products is 1-hydroxy-midazolam (also termed alpha-hydroxy-midazolam), while 4-hydroxy-midazolam constitutes less than or equal to 5%. Small amounts of

MIDAZOLAM HYDROCHLORIDE — INJECTION

dihydroxy derivative have also been detected but not quantified. The principal urinary excretion products are glucuronide conjugates of the hydroxylated derivatives.

Drugs that inhibit the activity of cytochrome P450 3A4 may inhibit midazolam clearance and elevate steady-state midazolam concentrations.

Studies of the IV administration of 1-hydroxy-midazolam in humans suggest that 1-hydroxy-midazolam is at least as potent as the parent compound and may contribute to the net pharmacologic activity of midazolam. In vitro studies have demonstrated that the affinities of 1- and 4-hydroxy-midazolam for the benzodiazepine receptor are approximately 20% and 7%, respectively, relative to midazolam.

Excretion – Clearance of midazolam is reduced in association with old age, congestive heart failure, liver disease (cirrhosis) or conditions which diminish cardiac output and hepatic blood flow.

The principal urinary excretion product is 1-hydroxy-midazolam in the form of a glucuronide conjugate; smaller amounts of the glucuronide conjugates of 4-hydroxy- and dihydroxy-midazolam are detected as well. The amount of midazolam excreted unchanged in the urine after a single IV dose is less than 0.5% (n = 5). Following a single IV infusion in 5 healthy volunteers, 45% to 57% of the dose was excreted in the urine as 1-hydroxymethyl midazolam conjugate.

Midazolam's activity is primarily due to the parent drug. Elimination of the parent drug takes place via hepatic metabolism of midazolam to hydroxylated metabolites that are conjugated and excreted in the urine. Six (6) single-dose pharmacokinetic studies involving healthy adults yield pharmacokinetic parameters for midazolam in the following ranges: Volume distribution (Vd), 1 to 3.1 L/kg; elimination half-life, 1.8 to 6.4 hours (mean approximately 3 hours); total clearance (Cl), 0.25 to 0.54 L/hr/kg. In a parallel-group study, there was no difference in the clearance, in subjects administered 0.15 mg/kg (n = 4) and 0.3 mg/kg (n = 4) IV doses indicating linear kinetics. The clearance was successively reduced by approximately 30% at doses of 0.45 mg/kg (n = 4) and 0.6 mg/kg (n = 5) indicating nonlinear kinetics in this dose range.

Special populations –

Renal function impairment: Patients with renal impairment may have longer elimination half-lives for midazolam and its metabolites, which may result in slower recovery.

Hepatic function impairment: Midazolam pharmacokinetics were studied after an IV single dose (0.075 mg/kg) was administered to 7 patients with biopsy-proven alcoholic cirrhosis and 8 control patients. The mean half-life of midazolam increased 2.5-fold in the alcoholic patients. Clearance was reduced by 50% and the Vd increased by 20%. In another study in 21 male patients with cirrhosis, without ascites and with healthy kidney function as determined by creatinine clearance, no changes in the pharmacokinetics of midazolam or 1-hydroxy-midazolam were observed when compared to healthy individuals.

Elderly: In 3 parallel-group studies, the pharmacokinetics of midazolam administered IV or IM were compared in young (mean age 29, n = 52) and healthy elderly subjects (mean age 73, n = 53). Plasma half-life was approximately 2-fold higher in the elderly. The mean Vd based on total body weight increased consistently between 15% to 100% in the elderly. The mean Cl decreased approximately 25% in the elderly in 2 studies and was similar to that of the younger patients in the other.

Children: In seriously ill neonates, the terminal elimination half-life of midazolam is substantially prolonged (6.5 to 12 hours) and the clearance reduced (0.07 to 0.12 L/hr/kg) compared to healthy adults or other groups of pediatric patients. It cannot be determined if these differences are due to age, immature organ function or metabolic pathways, underlying illness or debility.

Obese patients: In a study comparing healthy patients (n = 20) and obese patients (n = 20), the mean half-life was greater in the obese group (5.9 vs 2.3 hours). This was due to an increase of approximately 50% in the Vd corrected for total body weight. The clearance was not significantly different between groups.

Congestive heart failure: In patients suffering from congestive heart failure, there appeared to be a 2-fold increase in the elimination half-life, a 25% decrease in the plasma clearance and a 40% increase in the volume of distribution of midazolam.

Continuous infusion – The pharmacokinetic profile of midazolam following continuous infusion, based on 282 adult subjects, has been shown to be similar to that following single-dose administration for subjects of comparable age, gender, body habits and health status. However, midazolam can accumulate in peripheral tissues with continuous infusion. The effects of accumulation are greater after long-term infusions than after short-term infusions. The effects of accumulation can be reduced by maintaining the lowest midazolam infusion rate that produces satisfactory sedation.

Infrequent hypotensive episodes have occurred during continuous infusion; however, neither the time to onset nor the duration of the episode appeared to be related to plasma concentrations of midazolam or alpha-hydroxy-midazolam. Furthermore, there does not appear to be an increased chance of occurrence of a hypotensive episode with increased loading doses.

Contraindications

Hypersensitivity to the drug; acute narrow-angle glaucoma. Benzodiazepines may be used in patients with open-angle glaucoma only if they are receiving appropriate therapy. Measurements of intraocular pressure in patients without eye disease show a moderate lowering following induction with midazolam hydrochloride; patients with glaucoma have not been studied.

Midazolam hydrochloride is not intended for intrathecal or epidural administration due to the presence of the preservative benzyl alcohol in the dosage form.

Warnings

➤*Administration:* See the Warning box for more information.

➤*Respiratory depression effects:* Hypoventilation, airway obstruction, and apnea can lead to hypoxia or cardiac arrest unless effective countermeasures are taken immediately. The immediate availability of specific reversal agents (flumazenil) is highly recommended. Vital signs should continue to be monitored during the recovery period. Because IV midazolam hydrochloride depresses respiration, and because opioid agonists and other sedatives can add to this depression, midazolam hydrochloride should be administered as an induction agent only by a person trained in general anesthesia and should be used for sedation/anxiolysis/amnesia only in the presence of personnel skilled in early detection of hypoventilation, maintaining a patent airway and supporting ventilation. When used for sedation/anxiolysis/amnesia, midazolam hydrochloride should always be titrated slowly in adult or pediatric patients. Adverse hemodynamic events have been reported in pediatric patients with cardiovascular instability; rapid IV administration should also be avoided in this population.

➤*Cardiorespiratory effects:* Serious cardiorespiratory adverse reactions have occurred after administration of midazolam hydrochloride. These have included respiratory depression, airway obstruction, oxygen desaturation, apnea, respiratory arrest or cardiac arrest, sometimes resulting in death or permanent neurologic injury. There have also been rare reports of hypotensive episodes requiring treatment during or after diagnostic or surgical manipulations particularly in adult or pediatric patients with hemodynamic instability. Hypotension occurred more frequently in the sedation studies in patients premedicated with a narcotic.

➤*Improper dosing:* Reactions such as agitation, involuntary movements (including tonic/clonic movements and muscle tremor), hyperactivity and combativeness have been reported in both adult and pediatric patients. These reactions may be due to inadequate or excessive dosing or improper administration of midazolam hydrochloride; however, consideration should be given to the possibility of cerebral hypoxia or true paradoxical reactions. Should such reactions occur, the response to each dose of midazolam hydrochloride and all other drugs, including local anesthetics, should be evaluated before proceeding. Reversal of such responses with flumazenil has been reported in pediatric patients.

➤*Special risk:* Higher risk adult and pediatric surgical patients, elderly patients and debilitated adult and pediatric patients require lower dosages, whether or not concomitant sedating medications have been administered. Adult or pediatric patients with chronic obstructive pulmonary disease (COPD) are unusually sensitive to the respiratory-depressant effect of midazolam hydrochloride. Pediatric and adult patients undergoing procedures involving the upper airway such as upper endoscopy or dental care, are particularly vulnerable to episodes of desaturation and hypoventilation due to partial airway obstruction. Adult and pediatric patients with chronic renal failure and patients with congestive heart failure eliminate midazolam more slowly. Because elderly patients frequently have inefficient function of 1 or more organ systems, and because dosage requirements have been shown to decrease with age, reduced initial dosage of midazolam hydrochloride is recommended, and the possibility of profound or prolonged effect should be considered.

Injectable midazolam hydrochloride should not be administered to adult or pediatric patients in shock or coma, or in acute alcohol intoxication with depression of vital signs. Particular care should be exercised in the use of IV midazolam hydrochloride in adult or pediatric patients with uncompensated acute illnesses, such as severe fluid or electrolyte disturbances.

➤*Intra-arterial injection:* There have been limited reports of intra-arterial injection of midazolam hydrochloride. Adverse events have included local reactions, as well as isolated reports of seizure activity in which no clear causal relationship was established. Precautions against unintended intra-arterial injection should be taken. Extravasation should also be avoided.

➤*Carcinogenesis:* Midazolam maleate was administered with diet in mice and rats for 2 years at dosages of 1, 9 and 80 mg/kg/day. In female mice in the highest dose group, there was a marked increase in the incidence of hepatic tumors. In high-dose male rats, there was a small but statistically significant increase in benign thyroid follicular cell tumors. Dosages of 9 mg/kg/day of midazolam maleate (25 times a human dose of 0.35 mg/kg) do not increase the incidence of tumors. The pathogenesis of induction of these tumors is not known. These tumors were found after chronic administration, whereas human use will ordinarily be of single or several doses.

➤*Elderly:* Because geriatric patients may have altered drug distribution and diminished hepatic or renal function, reduced doses of midazolam hydrochloride are recommended; IV and IM doses of midazolam hydrochloride should be decreased for elderly and for debilitated patients, whether or not concomitant sedating medications have been administered, and subjects over 70 years of age may be particularly sensitive. These patients will also probably take longer to recover completely after midazolam hydrochloride administration for the induction of anesthesia. Administration of IM and IV midazolam hydrochloride to elderly or high-risk surgical patients has been associated with rare reports of death under circumstances compatible with cardiorespiratory depression. In most of these cases, the patients also received other CNS depressants capable of depressing respiration, especially narcotics.

➤*Pregnancy:* *Category D.* An increased risk of congenital malformations associated with the use of benzodiazepine drugs (diazepam and chlordiazepoxide) has been suggested in several studies. If this drug is used during pregnancy, the patient should be apprised of the potential hazard to the fetus.

Labor and delivery – The use of injectable midazolam hydrochloride in obstetrics has not been evaluated in clinical studies. Because midazolam is transferred transplacentally and because other benzodiazepines given in the

MIDAZOLAM HYDROCHLORIDE — INJECTION

last weeks of pregnancy have resulted in neonatal CNS depression, midazolam hydrochloride is not recommended for obstetrical use.

➤*Lactation:* Midazolam is excreted in human milk. Caution should be exercised when midazolam hydrochloride is administered to a nursing woman.

➤*Children:* The safety and efficacy of midazolam hydrochloride for sedation/anxiolysis/amnesia following single-dose IM administration, IV by intermittent injections and continuous infusion have been established in pediatric and neonatal patients. Onset time of sedative effects in the pediatric population begins within 5 minutes and peaks at 15 to 30 minutes depending upon the dose administered. The following adverse reactions related to the use of IV midazolam hydrochloride in pediatric patients were reported in the medical literature: Desaturation (4.6%), apnea (2.8%), hypotension (2.7%), paradoxical reactions (2%), hiccups (1.2%), seizure-like activity (1.1%) and nystagmus (1.1%). The majority of airway-related events occurred in patients receiving other CNS depressing medications and in patients where midazolam hydrochloride was not used as a single sedating agent. Midazolam hydrochloride is a potent sedative agent that requires slow administration and individualization of dosage. Clinical experience has shown midazolam hydrochloride to be 3 to 4 times as potent per mg as diazepam. Because serious and life-threatening cardiorespiratory adverse events have been reported, provision for monitoring, detection and correction of these reactions must be made for every patient to whom midazolam hydrochloride injection is administered, regardless of age or health status. Unlike adult patients, pediatric patients generally receive increments of midazolam hydrochloride on a mg/kg basis. As a group, pediatric patients generally require higher dosages of midazolam hydrochloride (mg/kg) than do adults. Younger (less than 6 years of age) pediatric patients may require higher dosages (mg/kg) than older pediatric patients, and may require closer monitoring. In obese pediatric patients, the dose should be calculated based on ideal body weight. When midazolam hydrochloride is given in conjunction with opioids or other sedatives, the potential for respiratory depression, airway obstruction, or hypoventilation is increased. The healthcare practitioner who uses this medication in pediatric patients should be aware of and follow accepted professional guidelines for pediatric sedation appropriate to their situation.

Preterm infants and neonates – Rapid injection should be avoided in the neonatal population. Midazolam hydrochloride administered rapidly as an IV injection (less than 2 minutes) has been associated with severe hypotension in neonates, particularly when the patient has also received fentanyl. Likewise, severe hypotension has been observed in neonates receiving a continuous infusion of midazolam who then receive a rapid IV injection of fentanyl. Seizures have been reported in several neonates following rapid IV administration.

The neonate also has reduced and immature organ function and is also vulnerable to profound or prolonged respiratory effects of midazolam hydrochloride.

Precautions

➤*Benzyl alcohol:* Exposure to excessive amounts of benzyl alcohol has been associated with toxicity (hypotension, metabolic acidosis), particularly in neonates, and an increased incidence of kernicterus, particularly in small preterm infants. There have been rare reports of deaths, primarily in preterm infants, associated with exposure to excessive amounts of benzyl alcohol. The amount of benzyl alcohol from medications is usually considered negligible compared to that received in flush solutions containing benzyl alcohol. Administration of high dosages of medications (including midazolam hydrochloride) containing this preservative must take into account the total amount of benzyl alcohol administered. The recommended dosage range of midazolam hydrochloride for preterm and term infants includes amounts of benzyl alcohol well below that associated with toxicity; however, the amount of benzyl alcohol at which toxicity may occur is not known. If the patient requires more than the recommended dosages or other medications containing this preservative, the practitioner must consider the daily metabolic load of benzyl alcohol from these combined sources.

➤*Intracranial pressure/cardiac effects:* Midazolam hydrochloride does not protect against the increase in intracranial pressure or against the heart rate rise and blood pressure rise associated with endotracheal intubation under light general anesthesia.

➤*Use with other CNS depressants:* The efficacy and safety of midazolam hydrochloride in clinical use are functions of the dose administered, the clinical status of the individual patient, and the use of concomitant medications capable of depressing the CNS. Anticipated effects range from mild sedation to deep levels of sedation virtually equivalent to a state of general anesthesia where the patient may require external support of vital functions. Care must be taken to individualize and carefully titrate the dose of midazolam hydrochloride to the patient's underlying medical/surgical conditions; administer to the desired effect, being certain to wait an adequate time for peak CNS effects of both midazolam hydrochloride and concomitant medications, and have the personnel and size-appropriate equipment and facilities available for monitoring and intervention. IV midazolam hydrochloride should be used only in hospital or ambulatory care settings, including physicians' and dental offices, that provide for continuous monitoring of respiratory and cardiac function (ie, pulse oximetry). For deeply sedated pediatric patients, a dedicated individual, other than the practitioner performing the procedure, should monitor the patient throughout the procedure. Practitioners administering midazolam hydrochloride must have the skills necessary to manage reasonably foreseeable adverse reactions, particularly skills in airway management.

➤*Drug abuse and dependence:* Midazolam produced physical dependence of a mild-to-moderate intensity in cynomolgus monkeys after 5 to 10 weeks of administration. Available data concerning the drug abuse and dependence potential of midazolam suggest that its abuse potential is at least equivalent to that of diazepam.

Withdrawal symptoms, similar in character to those noted with barbiturates and alcohol (convulsions, hallucinations, tremor, abdominal and muscle cramps, vomiting and sweating), have occurred following abrupt discontinuation of benzodiazepines, including midazolam. Abdominal distention, nausea, vomiting, and tachycardia are prominent symptoms of withdrawal in infants. The more severe withdrawal symptoms have usually been limited to those patients who had received excessive doses over an extended period of time. Generally milder withdrawal symptoms (eg, dysphoria, insomnia) have been reported following abrupt discontinuance of benzodiazepines taken continuously at therapeutic levels for several months. Consequently, after extended therapy, abrupt discontinuation should generally be avoided and a gradual dosage tapering schedule followed. There is no consensus in the medical literature regarding tapering schedules; therefore, practitioners are advised to individualize therapy to meet patient's needs. In some case reports, patients who have had severe withdrawal reactions due to abrupt discontinuation of high-dose, long-term midazolam, have been successfully weaned off of midazolam over a period of several days.

➤*Hazardous tasks:* The decision as to when patients who have received injectable midazolam hydrochloride, particularly on an outpatient basis, may again engage in activities requiring complete mental alertness, operate hazardous machinery or drive a motor vehicle must be individualized. Gross tests of recovery from the effects of midazolam hydrochloride cannot be relied upon to predict reaction time under stress. Gross tests of recovery after awakening (orientation, ability to stand and walk, suitability for discharge from the recovery room, return to baseline Trieger competency) usually indicate recovery within 2 hours, but recovery may take up to 6 hours in some cases. It is recommended that no patient operate hazardous machinery or a motor vehicle until the effects of the drug, such as drowsiness, have subsided, or until 1 full day after anesthesia and surgery, whichever is longer. For pediatric patients, particular care should be taken to ensure safe ambulation.

Drug Interactions

➤*CNS agents:* Concomitant use of barbiturates, alcohol or other CNS depressants may increase the risk of hypoventilation, airway obstruction, desaturation, or apnea and may contribute to profound or prolonged drug effect. Narcotic premedication also depresses the ventilatory response to carbon dioxide stimulation.

The sedative effect of IV midazolam is accentuated by any concomitantly administered medication which depresses the CNS, particularly narcotics (eg, morphine, meperidine, fentanyl) and also secobarbital and droperidol. Consequently, the dosage of midazolam should be adjusted according to the type and amount of concomitant medications administered and the desired clinical response.

➤*CYP450 system:* Caution is advised when midazolam is administered concomitantly with drugs that are known to inhibit the P450 3A4 enzyme system such as cimetidine (not ranitidine), erythromycin, diltiazem, verapamil, ketoconazole and itraconazole. These drug interactions may result in prolonged sedation due to a decrease in plasma clearance of midazolam.

➤*H_2 blockers:* The effect of single oral doses of 800 mg cimetidine and 300 mg ranitidine on steady-state concentrations of midazolam was examined in a randomized crossover study (n = 8). Cimetidine increased the mean steady-state concentration from 57 to 71 ng/mL. Ranitidine increased the mean steady-state concentration to 62 ng/mL. No change in choice reaction time or sedation index was detected after dosing with the H_2 receptor antagonists.

➤*Erythromycin:* In a placebo-controlled study, erythromycin administered as a 500 mg dose 3 times daily for 1 week (n = 6) reduced the clearance of midazolam following a single 0.5 mg/kg IV dose. The half-life was approximately doubled. Caution is advised when midazolam is administered to patients receiving erythromycin since this may result in a decrease in the plasma clearance of midazolam.

➤*Calcium channel blockers:* The effects of diltiazem (60 mg 3 times daily) and verapamil (80 mg 3 times daily) on the pharmacokinetics and pharmacodynamics of midazolam were investigated in a 3-way crossover study (n = 9). The half-life of midazolam increased from 5 to 7 hours when midazolam was taken in conjunction with verapamil or diltiazem. No interaction was observed in healthy subjects between midazolam and nifedipine.

➤*Thiopental:* A moderate reduction in induction dosage requirements of thiopental (about 15%) has been noted following use of IM midazolam hydrochloride for premedication in adults.

➤*Halothane:* The IV administration of midazolam hydrochloride decreases the minimum alveolar concentration (MAC) of halothane required for general anesthesia. This decrease correlates with the dose of midazolam hydrochloride administered; no similar studies have been carried out in pediatric patients, but there is no scientific reason to expect that pediatric patients would respond differently than adults.

➤*Other agents:* In neonates, severe hypotension has been reported with concomitant administration of fentanyl. This effect has been observed in neonates on an infusion of midazolam who received a rapid injection of fentanyl and in patients on an infusion of fentanyl who have received a rapid injection of midazolam.

Adverse Reactions

Fluctuations in vital signs were the most frequently seen findings following parenteral administration of midazolam hydrochloride in adults and included decreased tidal volume or respiratory rate decrease (23.3% of patients following IV and 10.8% of patients following IM administration) and apnea (15.4% of patients following IV administration), as well as variations in blood pressure and pulse rate. The majority of serious adverse reac-

MIDAZOLAM HYDROCHLORIDE — INJECTION

tions, particularly those associated with oxygenation and ventilation, have been reported when midazolam hydrochloride is administered with other medications capable of depressing the CNS. The incidence of such events is higher in patients undergoing procedures involving the airway without the protective effect of an endotracheal tube (eg, upper endoscopy, dental procedures).

➤*Cardiorespiratory effects:* See Warnings for more information.

➤*Improper dosing:* See Warnings for more information.

Adults – The following additional adverse reactions were reported after IM administration: Headache (1.3%) was reported as an adverse reaction. Local adverse effects at the IM injection site reported included pain (3.7%), induration (0.5%), redness (0.5%), and muscle stiffness (0.3%).

Administration of IM midazolam hydrochloride to elderly or higher risk surgical patients has been associated with rare reports of death under circumstances compatible with cardiorespiratory depression. In most of these cases, the patients also received other CNS depressants capable of depressing respiration, especially narcotics.

The following additional adverse reactions were reported subsequent to IV administration as a single sedative/anxiolytic/amnestic agent in adult patients: Hiccups (3.9%), nausea (2.8%), vomiting (2.6%), coughing (1.3%), "oversedation" (1.6%), headache (1.5%), and drowsiness (1.2%). Local adverse effects at the IV site reported included the following: Tenderness (5.6%), pain during injection (5%), redness (2.6%), induration (1.7%), and phlebitis (0.4%).

Children – The following adverse reactions related to the use of IV midazolam hydrochloride in pediatric patients were reported in the medical literature: Desaturation (4.6%), apnea (2.8%), hypotension (2.7%), paradoxical reactions (2%), hiccups (1.2%), seizure-like activity (1.1%) and nystagmus (1.1%). The majority of airway-related events occurred in patients receiving other CNS depressing medications and in patients where midazolam hydrochloride was not used as a single sedating agent.

Neonates – See Warnings for more information.

➤*Occurrence less than 1% in adults and children:* Other adverse reactions, observed mainly following IV injection as a single sedative/anxiolytic/amnesia agent and occurring at an incidence of less than 1% in adult and pediatric patients, are as follows:

Cardiovascular – Bigeminy, premature ventricular contractions, vasovagal episode, bradycardia, tachycardia, nodal rhythm.

CNS – Retrograde amnesia, euphoria, hallucination, confusion, argumentativeness, nervousness, anxiety, grogginess, restlessness, emergence delirium or agitation, prolonged emergence from anesthesia, dreaming during emergence, sleep disturbance, insomnia, nightmares, athetoid movements, seizure-like activity, ataxia, dizziness, dysphoria, slurred speech, dysphonia, paresthesia.

GI – Acid taste, excessive salivation, retching.

Hypersensitivity – Allergic reactions including anaphylactoid reactions, hives, rash, pruritus.

Local – Hive-like elevation at injection site, swelling or feeling of burning, warmth or coldness at injection site.

Respiratory – Laryngospasm, bronchospasm, dyspnea, hyperventilation, wheezing, shallow respirations, airway obstruction, tachypnea.

Special senses – Blurred vision, diplopia, nystagmus, pinpoint pupils, cyclic movements of eyelids, visual disturbance, difficulty focusing eyes, ears blocked, loss of balance, lightheadedness.

Miscellaneous – Yawning, lethargy, chills, weakness, toothache, faint feeling, hematoma.

Overdosage

➤*Symptoms:* The manifestations of midazolam hydrochloride overdosage reported are similar to those observed with other benzodiazepines, including sedation, somnolence, confusion, impaired coordination, diminished reflexes, coma and untoward effects on vital signs. No evidence of specific organ toxicity from midazolam hydrochloride overdosage has been reported.

➤*Treatment:* Treatment of injectable midazolam hydrochloride overdosage is the same as that followed for overdosage with other benzodiazepines. Respiration, pulse rate and blood pressure should be monitored and general supportive measures should be employed. Attention should be given to the maintenance of a patent airway and support of ventilation, including administration of oxygen. An IV infusion should be started. Should hypotension develop, treatment may include IV fluid therapy, repositioning, judicious use of vasopressors appropriate to the clinical situation, if indicated, and other appropriate countermeasures. There is no information as to whether peritoneal dialysis, forced diuresis or hemodialysis are of any value in the treatment of midazolam overdosage.

Flumazenil, a specific benzodiazepine-receptor antagonist, is indicated for the complete or partial reversal of the sedative effects of benzodiazepines and may be used in situations when an overdose with a benzodiazepine is known or suspected. There are anecdotal reports of reversal of adverse hemodynamic responses associated with midazolam hydrochloride following administration of flumazenil to pediatric patients. Prior to the administration of flumazenil, necessary measures should be instituted to secure the airway, ensure adequate ventilation, and establish adequate IV access. Flumazenil is intended as an adjunct to, not as a substitute for, proper management of benzodiazepine overdose. Patients treated with flumazenil should be monitored for resedation, respiratory depression and other residual benzodiazepine effects for an appropriate period after treatment. Flumazenil will only reverse benzodiazepine-induced effects but will not reverse the effects of other concomitant medications. The reversal of benzodiazepine effects may be associated with the onset of seizures in certain high-risk patients. The prescriber should be aware of a risk of seizure in association with flumazenil treatment, particularly in long-term benzodiazepine users and in cyclic antidepressant overdose. The complete flumazenil monograph, including Contraindications, Warnings and Precautions, should be consulted prior to use.

Patient Information

Inform your physician about any alcohol consumption and medicine you are now taking, especially blood pressure medication and antibiotics, including drugs you buy without a prescription. Alcohol has an increased effect when consumed with benzodiazepines; therefore, caution should be exercised regarding simultaneous ingestion of alcohol during benzodiazepine treatment.

Inform your physician if you are pregnant or are planning to become pregnant.

Inform your physician if you are breastfeeding.

Patients should be informed of the pharmacological effects of midazolam hydrochloride, such as sedation and amnesia, which in some patients may be profound. The decision as to when patients who have received injectable midazolam hydrochloride, particularly on an outpatient basis, may again engage in activities requiring complete mental alertness, operate hazardous machinery or drive a motor vehicle must be individualized.

Patients receiving continuous infusion of midazolam in critical care settings over an extended period of time, may experience symptoms of withdrawal following abrupt discontinuation.

PROPOFOL

Rx	**Propofol** (Baxter)	**Injectable emulsion:** 10 mg/mL	In 20 mL single-use vials and 50 and 100 mL single-use infusion vials.[1]
Rx	**Diprivan** (AstraZeneca)		In 20 mL single-use amps, 50 and 100 mL single-use infusion vials, and 50 mL prefilled single-use syringes.[2]

[1] With 100 mg/mL soybean oil, 22.5 mg/mL glycerol, 12 mg/mL egg yolk phospholipid, and 0.25 mg/mL sodium metabisulfite. pH = 4.5 to 6.4.

[2] With 100 mg/mL soybean oil, 22.5 mg/mL glycerol, 12 mg/mL egg lecithin, and 0.005% EDTA. pH = 7 to 8.5.

PROPOFOL — INJECTION

Indications

➤*Anesthesia:* Induction or maintenance of anesthesia as part of a balanced anesthetic technique for inpatient and outpatient surgery in adults and children ≥ 3 years of age. Can also be used for maintenance of anesthesia as part of a balanced anesthetic technique for inpatient and outpatient surgery in adult patients and pediatric patients > 2 months of age. Propofol is not recommended for induction of anesthesia in patients < 3 years of age or for maintenance of anesthesia in patients < 2 months of age because safety and efficacy have not been established in those populations.

➤*Monitored anesthesia care (MAC) sedation:* To initiate and maintain MAC sedation during diagnostic procedures in adults, and it may also be used for MAC sedation in conjunction with local/regional anesthesia in patients undergoing surgical procedures.

➤*Intensive care unit (ICU) sedation:* Continuous sedation and control of stress responses in intubated or respiratory-controlled adult patients in ICUs. Not indicated in pediatric ICU sedation because safety and efficacy have not been established.

Administration and Dosage

➤*Approved by the FDA:* October 1989.

➤*Administration:* Individualize dosage and rate of administration and titrate to the desired effect, according to clinically relevant factors, including preinduction and concomitant medications, age, American Society of Anesthesiologists (ASA) physical classification, and level of debilitation of the patient.

In the elderly, debilitated, and ASA III/IV patients, do not use rapid bolus doses as this will increase cardiorespiratory effects including hypotension, apnea, airway obstruction, or oxygen desaturation.

Propofol blood concentrations at steady state are generally proportional to infusion rates, especially within an individual patient. Undesirable effects such as cardiorespiratory depression are likely to occur at higher blood levels which result from bolus dosing or rapid increase in the infusion rate. An adequate interval (3 to 5 minutes) must be allowed between clinical dosage adjustments in order to assess drug effects.

When administering propofol by infusion, syringe pumps or volumetric pumps are recommended to provide controlled infusion rates. When infusing propofol to patients undergoing magnetic resonance imaging, metered control devices may be used if mechanical pumps are impractical.

Changes in vital signs (increases in pulse rate, blood pressure, sweating, and/or tearing) that indicate a response to surgical stimulation or lightening

PROPOFOL — INJECTION

of anesthesia may be controlled by the administration of 25 to 50 mg (2.5 to 5 mL) incremental boluses and/or by increasing the infusion rate.

For minor surgical procedures (ie, body surface), 60% to 70% nitrous oxide can be combined with a variable rate infusion to provide satisfactory anesthesia. With more stimulating surgical procedures (eg, intra-abdominal), or if supplementation with nitrous oxide is not provided, increase administration rate(s) of propofol or opioids in order to provide adequate anesthesia.

Always titrate infusion rates downward in the absence of clinical signs of light anesthesia until a mild response to surgical stimulation can be perceived in order to avoid the administration of propofol at rates higher than are clinically necessary. Generally, achieve infusion rates of 50 to 100 mcg/kg/min in adults during maintenance in order to optimize recovery times.

Other drugs that cause CNS depression (eg, hypnotics/sedatives, inhalational anesthetics, opioids) can increase CNS depression induced by propofol. Morphine premedication (0.15 mg/kg) with nitrous oxide 67% in oxygen decreases the necessary propofol injection maintenance infusion rate and therapeutic blood concentrations when compared to non-narcotic (eg, lorazepam) premedication.

➤*Induction of general anesthesia:*

Adults – Most adult patients < 55 years of age and classified ASA I/II require 2 to 2.5 mg/kg of propofol for induction when unpremedicated or when premedicated with oral benzodiazepines or IM opioids. For induction, titrate propofol (≈ 40 mg every 10 seconds) against the response of the patient until the clinical signs show the onset of anesthesia.

Elderly, debilitated, or ASA III/IV patients – Because of the reduced clearance and higher blood concentrations, most elderly, debilitated, or ASA III/IV patients require ≈ 1 to 1.5 mg/kg (≈ 20 mg every 10 seconds) of propofol for induction of anesthesia according to their condition and responses. Do not use a rapid bolus, as this will increase the likelihood of undesirable cardiorespiratory depression, including hypotension, apnea, airway obstruction, and/or oxygen desaturation.

Children – Most patients 3 through 16 years of age and classified ASA I/II require 2.5 to 3.5 mg/kg for induction when unpremedicated or when lightly premedicated with oral benzodiazepines or IM opioids. Within this dosage range, younger pediatric patients may require higher induction doses than older pediatric patients. A lower dosage is recommended for pediatric patients classified as ASA III/IV. Attempt to minimize pain on injection when administering propofol to pediatric patients. Boluses of propofol may be administered via small veins if pretreated with lidocaine or via antecubital or larger veins.

Neurosurgical patients – Slower induction is recommended using boluses of 20 mg every 10 seconds. Slower boluses or infusions of propofol for induction of anesthesia, titrated to clinical responses, will generally result in reduced induction dosage requirements (1 to 2 mg/kg).

Cardiac anesthesia – Morphine premedication (0.15 mg/kg) with nitrous oxide 67% in oxygen has been shown to decrease the necessary propofol maintenance infusion rates and therapeutic blood concentrations when compared to nonnarcotic (lorazepam) premedication. Determine the rate of propofol administration based on the patient's premedication and adjust according to clinical responses.

Avoid rapid bolus injection. Use a slow rate of ≈ 20 mg every 10 seconds until induction onset (0.5 to 1.5 mg/kg). In order to assure adequate anesthesia, when propofol is used as the primary agent, maintenance infusion rates should not be < 100 mcg/kg/min and should be supplemented with analgesic levels of continuous opioid administration. When an opioid is used as the primary agent, propofol maintenance rates should be < 50 mcg/kg/min and care should be taken to ensure amnesia with concomitant benzodiazepines. Higher doses of propofol will reduce the opioid requirements (see table below). When propofol is used as the primary anesthetic, it should not be administered with the high-dose opioid technique, as this may increase the likelihood of hypotension.

Propofol Cardiac Anesthesia Techniques

Primary agent	Rate	Secondary agent/rate (following induction with primary agent)
Propofol		Opioid[1] 0.05 to 0.075 mcg/kg/min (no bolus)
Preinduction anxiolysis	25 mcg/kg/min	
Induction	0.5 to 1.5 mcg/kg over 60 sec	
Maintenance (titrated to clinical response)	100 to 150 mcg/kg/min	
Opioid[2]		Propofol 50 to 100 mcg/kg/min (no bolus)
Induction	25 to 50 mcg/kg	
Maintenance	0.2 to 0.3 mcg/kg/min	

[1] Opioid is defined in terms of fentanyl equivalents, ie, 1 mcg fentanyl = 5 mcg alfentanil (for bolus), 10 mcg alfentanil (for maintenance), or 0.1 mcg sufentanil.
[2] Take care to ensure amnesia with concomitant benzodiazepine therapy.

➤*Maintenance of general anesthesia:*

Adults – In adults, anesthesia can be maintained by administering propofol by infusion or intermittent IV bolus injection. The patient's clinical response will determine the infusion rate or the amount and frequency of incremental injections.

Continuous infusion: Propofol 100 to 200 mcg/kg/min administered in a variable rate infusion with 60% to 70% nitrous oxide and oxygen provides anesthesia for patients undergoing general surgery. Maintenance by infusion should immediately follow the induction dose in order to provide satisfactory or continuous anesthesia during the induction phase. During this initial period following the induction dose, higher rates of infusion are generally required (150 to 200 mcg/kg/min) for the first 10 to 15 minutes. Subsequently decrease infusion rates 30% to 50% during the first half hour of maintenance. Generally, rates of 50 to 100 mcg/kg/min in adults should be achieved during maintenance in order to optimize recovery times.

Intermittent bolus: Increments of propofol 25 to 50 mg (2.5 to 5 mL) may be administered with nitrous oxide in adult patients undergoing general surgery. The incremental boluses should be administered when changes in vital signs indicate a response to surgical stimulation or light anesthesia.

Children – Propofol administered as a variable rate infusion supplemented with nitrous oxide 60% to 70% provides satisfactory anesthesia for most children ≥ 2 months of age, ASA class I or II, undergoing general anesthesia.

In general, for the pediatric population, maintenance by infusion of propofol at a rate of 200 to 300 mcg/kg/min should immediately follow the induction dose. Following the first half hour of maintenance, infusion rates of 125 to 150 mcg/kg/min are typically needed. Titrate propofol to achieve the desired clinical effect. Younger children may require higher maintenance infusion rates than older children.

➤*Initiation of MAC sedation:*

Adults – Either an infusion or a slow injection method may be used while closely monitoring cardiorespiratory function. With the infusion method, sedation may be initiated by infusing propofol at 100 to 150 mcg/kg/min (6 to 9 mg/kg/hr) for a period of 3 to 5 minutes and titrating to the desired clinical effect while closely monitoring respiratory function. With the slow injection method for initiation, patients will require ≈ 0.5 mg/kg administered over 3 to 5 minutes and titrated to clinical responses. When propofol is administered slowly over 3 to 5 minutes, most patients will be adequately sedated, and the peak drug effect can be achieved while minimizing undesirable cardiorespiratory effects occurring at high plasma levels.

Elderly, debilitated, or ASA III/IV patients – Do not use rapid (single or repeated) bolus dose administration for MAC sedation. The rate of administration should be over 3 to 5 minutes and the dosage of propofol should be reduced to ≈ 80% of the usual adult dosage in these patients according to their condition, responses, and changes in vital signs. Can be the sole agent for maintenance of MAC sedation during surgical/diagnostic procedures, supplemented with opioids or benzodiazepines, which increase sedative and respiratory effects and may also result in a slower recovery profile.

➤*Maintenance of MAC sedation:* Propofol can be administered as the sole agent for maintenance as MAC sedation during surgical/diagnostic procedures.

Adults – A variable rate infusion method is preferable over an intermittent bolus dose method. With the variable rate infusion method, patients will generally require maintenance rates of 25 to 75 mcg/kg/min (1.5 to 4.5 mg/kg/hr) during the first 10 to 15 minutes of sedation maintenance. Subsequently decrease infusion rates over time to 25 to 50 mcg/kg/min and adjust to clinical response. In titrating to clinical effect, allow ≈ 2 minutes for onset of peak drug effect.

Always titrate downward in the absence of clinical signs of light sedation until mild responses to stimulation are obtained in order to avoid sedative administration at rates higher than are clinically necessary.

If intermittent bolus method is used, 10 or 20 mg (1 or 2 mL) increments can be given and titrated to desired level of sedation. With the intermittent bolus method of sedation maintenance, there is the potential for respiratory depression, transient increases in sedation depth, or prolongation of recovery.

Elderly, debilitated, or ASA III/IV patients – Do not use rapid (single or repeated) bolus dose administration for MAC sedation. Reduce the rate of administration and the dosage to ≈ 80% of the usual adult dosage in these patients according to their condition, responses, and changes in vital signs.

➤*ICU sedation:*

Adults – For intubated, mechanically ventilated adult patients, initiate slowly with a continuous infusion to titrate to desired clinical effect and minimize hypotension.

In clinical studies, the mean infusion maintenance rate for all patients was ≈ 27 mcg/kg/min. The maintenance infusion rates required to maintain adequate sedation ranged from 2.8 to 130 mcg/kg/min. The infusion rate was lower in patients > 55 years of age (≈ 20 mcg/kg/min) compared to patients < 55 years of age (≈ 38 mcg/kg/min). In these studies, morphine or fentanyl was used as needed for analgesia.

Most adult ICU patients recovering from the effects of general anesthesia or deep sedation will require maintenance rates of 5 to 50 mcg/kg/min (0.3 to 3 mg/kg/hr) individualized and titrated to clinical response. With medical ICU patients or patients who have recovered from the effect of general anesthesia or deep sedation, the rate of administration of ≥ 50 mcg/kg/min may be required to achieve adequate sedation. These higher rates may increase the likelihood of hypotension.

Although there are reports of reduced analgesic requirements, most patients received opioids for analgesia during maintenance of ICU sedation. Some patients also received benzodiazepines or neuromuscular blocking agents. During long-term maintenance of sedation, some ICU patients were awakened once or twice every 24 hours for assessment of neurologic or respiratory function.

In post-coronary artery bypass graft (CABG) patients, the maintenance rate of propofol administration was usually low (median, 11 mcg/kg/min) because of the intraoperative administration of high opioid doses. Avoid discontinuation prior to weaning or for daily evaluation of sedation levels. This may

PROPOFOL — INJECTION

result in rapid awakening with associated anxiety, agitation, and resistance to mechanical ventilation. Adjust infusions to maintain light sedation through these processes.

Propofol Dosage Guidelines[1]

Indication	Induction/Initiation	Maintenance
General anesthesia (outpt/inpt):		
Healthy < 55 years	2 to 2.5 mg/kg (40 mg every 10 sec until onset)	100 to 200 mcg/kg/min intermittent bolus; increments of 20 to 50 mg as needed
Elderly, debilitated, ASA III/IV	1 to 1.5 mg/kg (20 mg every 10 sec until onset)	50 to 100 mcg/kg/min
General anesthesia (pediatric): > 3 years	2.5 to 3.5 mg/kg over 20 to 30 sec	200 to 300 mcg/kg/min (1st 30 min) 125 to 150 mcg/kg/min (remainder)
General anesthesia (cardiac):	0.5 to 1.5 mg/kg (a slow rate of ≈ 20 mg every 10 sec until onset); avoid rapid bolus induction	Primary propofol injection with secondary opioid: 100 to 150 mcg/kg/min Low-dose propofol injection w/ primary opioids: 50 to 100 mcg/kg/min (no bolus)
General anesthesia (neuro):	1 to 2 mg/kg (20 mg every 10 sec until onset	100 to 200 mcg/kg/min
MAC sedation:		
Healthy < 55 years:		
Slow infusion/ variable rate	100 to 150 mcg/kg/min for 3 to 5 min	25 to 75 mcg/kg/min for 10 to 15 min; decreased to 25 to 50 mcg/kg/min
Slow injection/ intermittent bolus	0.5 mg/kg over 3 to 5 min	Incremental bolus doses of 10 to 20 mg
Elderly, debilitated, ASA III/IV patients:		
Slow infusion/ variable rate	Usually same as healthy adult, but avoid rapid bolus dose	80% of adult dose; do not use rapid bolus dose
Slow injection/ intermittent bolus	Usually same as healthy adult, but avoid rapid bolus dose	80% of adult dose; do not use rapid bolus dose
ICU sedation:	Initial infusion: 5 mcg/ kg/min for ≥ 5 min Subsequent increments of 5 to 10 mcg/kg/min over 5 to 10 min intervals until desired sedation level is achieved	Infusion rates of 5 to 50 mcg/kg/min or higher may be required

[1] Following the first half hour of maintenance, if clinical signs of light anesthesia are not present, decrease the infusion rate.

➤*Handling:* Always maintain strict aseptic technique during handling. Propofol injectable emulsion is a single-use parenteral product that contains sodium metabisulfite (0.25 mg/mL) or 0.005% EDTA to retard the rate of growth of microorganisms in the event of accidental extrinsic contamination. However, propofol injectable emulsion can still support the growth of microorganisms as it is not an antimicrobially preserved product under USP standards. Do not use if contamination is suspected.

➤*Admixture compatibility and stability:* Although propofol appears to be compatible with other therapeutic agents for a very limited amount of time, the manufacturers do not recommend mixing it with other agents prior to administration.

➤*Dilution prior to administration:* Propofol is provided as a ready-to-use formulation. However, should dilution be necessary, only dilute with 5% Dextrose Injection and do not dilute to a concentration < 2 mg/mL because it is an emulsion. In diluted form it is more stable when in contact with glass than with plastic (95% potency after 2 hours of running infusion in plastic).

➤*Administration with other fluids:* Compatibility of propofol with the coadministration of blood/serum/plasma has not been established (see Warnings). Propofol is compatible with the following IV fluids when administered using a y-type infusion set: 5% Dextrose Injection; Lactated Ringer's Injection; Lactated Ringer's and 5% Dextrose Injection; 5% Dextrose and 0.45% Sodium Chloride Injection; 5% Dextrose and 0.2% Sodium Chloride Injection.

➤*Storage/Stability:* Do not use if there is evidence of separation of the phases of the emulsion. Discard any unused portions of propofol or solutions containing propofol at the end of the anesthetic procedure or at 6 hours, whichever occurs sooner; for ICU sedation, discard after 12 hours (if administered directly from the vial or prefilled syringe) or 6 hours (if transferred to a syringe or other container).

Store at 4° to 22°C (40° to 72°F). Do not freeze. Protect from light. Shake well before use. Propofol undergoes oxidative degradation in the presence of oxygen, and is therefore packaged under nitrogen to eliminate this degradation path.

Actions

➤*Pharmacology:* Propofol is an IV hypnotic/sedative agent for induction and maintenance of anesthesia or sedation. IV injection of a therapeutic dose produces hypnosis rapidly and smoothly with minimal excitation, usually within 40 seconds from the start of an injection. As with other rapidly acting IV anesthetic agents, the half-time of blood-brain equilibration is ≈ 1 to 3 minutes, and this accounts for the rapid induction of anesthesia.

Pharmacodynamic properties of propofol depend on the therapeutic blood propofol concentrations. Steady-state concentrations are generally proportional to infusion rates, especially within an individual patient. Undesirable side effects such as cardiorespiratory depression are likely to occur at higher blood levels that result from bolus dosing or rapid increase in infusion rate. Allow an adequate interval (3 to 5 minutes) between clinical dosage adjustments in order to assess drug effects.

The hemodynamic effects of propofol injection during induction of anesthesia vary. If spontaneous ventilation is maintained, major cardiovascular effects are arterial hypotension (sometimes > 30% decrease) with little or no change in heart rate and no appreciable decrease in cardiac output. If ventilation is assisted or controlled (positive pressure ventilation), degree and incidence of decrease in cardiac output are accentuated. Addition of a potent opioid (eg, fentanyl) as a premedication further decreases cardiac output and respiratory drive.

If anesthesia is continued by infusion of propofol, endotracheal intubation and surgical stimulation may return arterial pressure towards normal. However, cardiac output may remain depressed. In comparative clinical studies, hemodynamic effects of propofol during induction are generally more pronounced than with traditional IV induction agents.

Induction of anesthesia with propofol is frequently associated with apnea. In 1573 adult patients given propofol (2 to 2.5 mg/kg), apnea lasted 0 to 30 sec in 7%, 30 to 60 seconds in 24%, and > 60 seconds in 12% of patients. In 218 children from birth to 16 years of age assessable for apnea who received bolus doses of propofol 1 to 3.6 mg/kg, the values were 12%, 10%, and 5%, respectively. During maintenance, propofol causes a decrease in ventilation usually associated with an increase in carbon dioxide tension which may be marked depending on the rate of administration and other concurrent agents (eg, opioids, sedatives).

In humans and animals, propofol does not suppress the adrenal response to ACTH. Preliminary findings in patients with normal intraocular pressure indicate that propofol anesthesia produces a decrease in intraocular pressure, which may be associated with a concomitant decrease in systemic vascular resistance. Animal studies and limited experience in susceptible patients have not indicated any propensity of propofol to induce malignant hyperthermia. Propofol is rarely associated with elevation of plasma histamine levels and does not cause signs of histamine release.

➤*Pharmacokinetics:*

Distribution – Following an IV bolus dose, plasma levels initially decline rapidly due to both high metabolic clearance and rapid drug distribution into tissues. Distribution accounts for about half of this decline following a bolus of propofol.

However, distribution is not constant over time, but decreases as body tissues equilibrate with plasma and become saturated. The rate at which equilibration occurs is a function of the rate and duration of the infusion. When equilibration occurs, there is no longer a net transfer of propofol between tissues and plasma.

Discontinuation of the recommended doses of propofol after the maintenance of anesthesia for ≈ 1 hour, or for sedation in the ICU for 1 day, results in a prompt decrease in blood propofol concentrations and rapid awakening. Longer infusions (10 days of ICU sedation) result in accumulation of significant tissue stores of propofol, such that the reduction in circulating propofol is slowed and the time to awakening is increased.

By daily titration of propofol dosage to achieve only the minimum effective therapeutic concentration, rapid awakening within 10 to 15 minutes will occur even after long-term administration. However, if higher than necessary infusion levels have been maintained for a long time, propofol will be redistributed from fat and muscle to the plasma, and this return of propofol from peripheral tissues will slow recovery.

The large contribution of distribution (≈ 50%) to the fall of propofol plasma levels following brief infusions means that after very long infusions (at steady state), about half the initial rate will maintain the same plasma levels. Thus, titration to clinical response and daily evaluation of sedation levels are important during use of propofol infusion for ICU sedation, especially infusions of long duration.

Clearance ranges from 23 to 50 mL/kg/min. It is chiefly eliminated by hepatic conjugation to inactive metabolites that are excreted by the kidneys. A glucuronide conjugate accounts for ≈ 50% of dose. Steady-state volume of distribution approaches 60 L/kg. Terminal half-life after a 10-day infusion is 1 to 3 days.

Special populations –

Elderly: With increasing age, the dose needed to achieve a defined anesthetic endpoint (dose requirement) decreases. This does not appear to be an age-related change. With increasing age, higher peak plasma levels occur, which can explain the decreased dose requirement. These higher levels can predispose patients to cardiorespiratory effects, including hypotension, apnea, airway obstruction, or oxygen desaturation. Lower doses are, therefore, recommended in the elderly.

PROPOFOL — INJECTION

Contraindications

When general anesthesia or sedation are contraindicated; hypersensitivity to propofol or components of the product.

Warnings

➤*Administration:* Only people trained in the administration of general anesthesia and not involved in the conduct of the surgical/diagnostic procedure should administer propofol. Continuously monitor patients. Facilities for maintenance of a patent airway, artificial ventilation, and oxygen enrichment and circulatory resuscitation must be immediately available. For sedation of intubated, mechanically ventilated patients in the ICU, administer only by people skilled in the management of critically ill patients and trained in cardiovascular resuscitation and airway management.

See Administration and Dosage for more information.

➤*Blood/Plasma coadministration:* Do not coadminister through the same IV catheter with blood or plasma because compatibility has not been established. In vitro, aggregates of the globular component of the emulsion vehicle have occurred with blood/plasma/serum from humans and animals.

➤*Aseptic technique:* See Administration and Dosage for more information.

➤*Anaphylaxis:* Rarely, features of anaphylaxis, which may include angioedema, bronchospasm, erythema, and hypotension, have occurred after the administration of propofol, although the use of other drugs in most instances makes the relationship to propofol unclear.

➤*Elderly:* See Actions for more information.

➤*Pregnancy: Category B.* Reproduction studies have been performed in rats and rabbits at IV doses of 15 mg/kg/day (approximately equivalent to the recommended human induction dose on a mg/m^2 basis) and have revealed no evidence of impaired fertility or harm to the fetus caused by propofol. However, propofol has been shown to cause maternal deaths in rats and rabbits and decreased pup survival during the lactating period in dams treated with 15 mg/kg/day. The pharmacological activity (anesthesia) of the drug on the mother is probably responsible for the adverse effects seen in the offspring. However, there are no adequate and well-controlled studies in pregnant women. Use during pregnancy only if clearly needed.

Labor and delivery – Not recommended for obstetrics, including cesarean section deliveries. Propofol crosses the placenta and may be associated with neonatal depression.

➤*Lactation:* Not recommended for use in nursing mothers because propofol is excreted in breast milk and the effects of oral absorption of small amounts of propofol are not known.

➤*Children:* Safety and efficacy of propofol have been established for induction of anesthesia in children ≥ 3 years of age and for the maintenance of anesthesia in children ≥ 2 months of age. Not recommended for the induction of anesthesia in children < 3 years of age, in the maintenance of anesthesia in children < 2 months of age, or for ICU or MAC sedation in children because safety and efficacy have not been established. In pediatric patients, administration of fentanyl concomitantly with propofol may result in serious bradycardia. Although no causal relationship has been established, serious adverse events (including fatalities) have been reported in children with respiratory tract infections given propofol for ICU sedation. In pediatric patients, abrupt discontinuation following prolonged infusion may result in flushing of the hands and feet, agitation, tremulousness, and hyperirritability. Increased incidences of bradycardia (5%), agitation (4%), and jitteriness (9%) also have been reported.

Precautions

➤*Monitoring:* MAC sedation patients should be continuously monitored by people not involved in the conduct of the surgical or diagnostic procedure; oxygen supplementation should be immediately available and provided where clinically indicated. Monitor oxygen saturation in all patients. Continuously monitor patients for early signs of hypotension, apnea, airway obstruction, or oxygen desaturation. These cardiorespiratory effects are more likely to occur following rapid initiation (loading) boluses or during supplemental maintenance boluses, especially in the elderly, debilitated, or ASA III/IV patients.

➤*Special risk patients:* Use a lower induction dose and a slower maintenance rate of administration in elderly, debilitated, and ASA III/IV patients. Continuously monitor patients for early signs of significant hypotension or bradycardia. Treatment may include increasing the rate of IV fluid administration, elevation of lower extremities, use of pressor agents, or administration of atropine. Apnea often occurs during induction and may persist for > 60 seconds. Ventilatory support may be required. Because propofol is an emulsion, use caution in patients with lipid metabolism disorders (eg, primary hyperlipoproteinemia, diabetic hyperlipidemia, pancreatitis).

➤*Epilepsy:* When administered to an epileptic patient, there may be a risk of seizure during the recovery phase.

➤*Transient local pain:* Transient local pain may occur during IV injection, which may be reduced if the larger veins of the forearm or antecubital fossa are used or by prior injection of IV lidocaine (1 mL of a 1% solution). Venous sequelae (phlebitis or thrombosis) have occurred rarely (< 1%). In 2 well-controlled clinical studies using dedicated IV catheters, no instances of venous sequelae were reported up to 14 days following induction. Intentional injection into SC or perivascular tissues of animals caused minimal tissue reaction. Intra-arterial injection in animals did not induce local tissue effects. Accidental intra-arterial injections have been reported in patients, and other than pain, there were no major sequelae.

➤*Perioperative myoclonia:* Perioperative myoclonia, rarely including convulsions and opisthotonus, has occurred.

➤*Pulmonary edema:* Pulmonary edema has been reported rarely with propofol use, although a causal relationship is not known.

➤*Cardiovascular effects:* Propofol has no vagolytic activity and has been associated with reports of bradycardia, asystole, and, rarely, cardiac arrest. Consider the IV administration of anticholinergic agents (eg, atropine, glycopyrrolate) to modify potential increases in vagal tone caused by concomitant agents (eg, succinylcholine) or surgical stimuli. There have been rare reports of cardiac arrest. Monitor patients for early signs of significant hypotension or cardiovascular depression, which may be profound. These effects are responsive to discontinuation of propofol, IV fluid administration, or vasopressor therapy.

➤*Hyperlipidemia:* Because propofol is formulated in an oil-in-water emulsion, elevations in serum triglycerides may occur when it is administered for extended periods of time. Monitor patients at risk of hyperlipidemia for increases in serum triglycerides or serum turbidity. Adjust if fat is being inadequately cleared from the body. A reduction in the quantity of concurrently administered lipids is indicated to compensate for the amount of lipid infused as part of the formulation; 1 mL of propofol contains ≈ 0.1 g of fat (1.1 kcal).

➤*Neurosurgical anesthesia:* When propofol is used in patients with increased intracranial pressure (ICP) or impaired cerebral circulation, avoid significant decreases in mean arterial pressure because of the resultant decreases in cerebral perfusion pressure. To avoid significant hypotension and decreases in cerebral perfusion pressure, use an infusion or slow bolus of ≈ 20 mg every 10 seconds instead of rapid, more frequent, and larger boluses. Slower induction titrated to clinical responses generally will result in reduced induction dosage requirements (1 to 2 mg/kg). When increased ICP is suspected, hyperventilation and hypocarbia should accompany use of propofol.

➤*Cardiac anesthesia:* Use slower rates of administration in premedicated patients, geriatric patients, patients with recent fluid shifts, or patients who are hemodynamically unstable. Correct any fluid deficits prior to administration. In those patients where additional fluid therapy may be contraindicated, other measures (eg, elevation of lower extremities, use of pressor agents) may be useful to offset the hypotension that is associated with the induction of anesthesia with propofol.

➤*Additives:*

Sodium metabisulfite – Propofol formulations that contain sodium metabisulfite, a sulfite, may cause allergic-type reactions including anaphylactic symptoms and life-threatening or less severe asthmatic episodes in certain susceptible people. The overall prevalence of sulfite sensitivity in the general population is unknown and probably low. Sulfite sensitivity is seen more frequently in asthmatic than nonasthmatic people.

EDTA – EDTA is a strong chelator of trace metals, including zinc. Although with propofol there are no reports of decreased zinc levels or zinc deficiency-related adverse events, do not infuse propofol for > 5 days without providing a drug holiday to safely replace estimated or measured urine zinc losses.

In clinical trials, mean urinary zinc loss was ≈ 2.5 to 3 mg/day in adult patients and 1.5 to 2 mg/day in pediatric patients. In patients who are predisposed to zinc deficiency, such as those with burns, diarrhea, or major sepsis, consider the need for supplemental zinc during prolonged therapy.

At high doses (2 to 3 g/day) EDTA has been reported, on rare occasions, to be toxic to the renal tubules. Studies to date in patients with normal or impaired renal function, have not shown any alterations in renal function with propofol injectable emulsion containing 0.005% EDTA. In patients at risk for renal impairment, check urinalysis and urine sediment before initiation of sedation and then monitor on alternate days during sedation.

Drug Interactions

➤*CNS depressants:* CNS depressants (eg, hypnotics/sedatives, inhalational anesthetics, opioids) can increase the CNS depression induced by propofol. Morphine premedication with nitrous oxide decreases the necessary propofol maintenance infusion rate and therapeutic blood concentrations when compared to nonnarcotic (eg, lorazepam) premedication (see Administration and Dosage). In addition, the induction dose requirements of propofol may be reduced in patients with IM or IV premedication, particularly with narcotics alone or in combination with sedatives. These agents may increase the anesthetic or sedative effects of propofol and may also result in more pronounced decreases in systolic, diastolic, and mean arterial pressures and cardiac output.

Adverse Reactions

➤*Anesthesia/MAC sedation:*

Cardiovascular – Hypotension (3% to 10%); arrhythmia, tachycardia, bradycardia (1% to 3%); hemorrhage/bleeding, premature atrial contractions, syncope, atrial fibrillation, atrial arrhythmia, AV heartblock, bigeminy, bundle branch block, cardiac arrest, abnormal ECG, edema, extrasystole, heart block, hypertension, MI, myocardial ischemia, PVCs, ST segment depression, supraventricular tachycardia, ventricular fibrillation (< 1%).

CNS – Movement (3% to 10%); hypertonia/dystonia, paresthesia, abnormal dreams, agitation, anxiety, bucking/jerking/thrashing, chills/shivering, clonic/myoclonic movement, combativeness, confusion, delirium, depression, dizziness, emotional lability, euphoria, fatigue, headache, hysteria, insomnia, moaning, rigidity, seizures, somnolence, tremor, twitching, amorous behavior, hypotonia, hallucinations, neuropathy, opisthotonos (< 1%).

Dermatologic – Rash, pruritus (1% to 3%); flushing, diaphoresis, urticaria (< 1%).

PROPOFOL — INJECTION

GI – Hypersalivation, cramping, diarrhea, dry mouth, enlarged parotid, nausea, swallowing, vomiting (< 1%).

GU – Cloudy urine, oliguria, urine retention (< 1%).

Local – Burning/stinging or pain (17.6%); hives/itching, phlebitis, redness/discoloration (< 1%).

Respiratory – Apnea (1% to 3%); bronchospasm, burning in throat, wheezing, cough, dyspnea, hiccough, hypoventilation, hyperventilation, hypoxia, laryngospasm, pharyngitis, sneezing, tachypnea, upper airway obstruction, decreased lung function (< 1%).

Special senses – Amblyopia, diplopia, ear pain, eye pain, taste perversion, tinnitus, conjunctival hyperemia, nystagmus, abnormal vision (< 1%).

Miscellaneous – Awareness, extremity pain, fever, increased drug effect, neck rigidity/stiffness, chest/trunk pain, myalgia, coagulation disorder, leukocytosis, hyperkalemia, asthenia, hyperlipidemia, anaphylaxis/anaphylactoid reaction, perinatal disorder, anticholinergic syndrome, hypomagnesemia (< 1%).

➤*ICU sedation:*

Cardiovascular – Hypotension (26%); bradycardia, decreased cardiac output (1% to 3%); arrhythmia, atrial fibrillation, bigeminy, cardiac arrest, extrasystole, ventricular tachycardia, right heart failure (< 1%).

CNS – Agitation, chills/shivering, intracranial hypertension, seizures, somnolence, abnormal thinking (< 1%).

Metabolic/Nutritional – Hyperlipidemia (3% to 10%); increased BUN, creatinine, and osmolality, dehydration, hyperglycemia, metabolic acidosis (< 1%).

Respiratory – Respiratory acidosis during weaning (3% to 10%); hypoxia (< 1%).

Miscellaneous – Fever, sepsis, trunk pain, weakness, rash, ileus, abnormal liver function, green urine, kidney failure (< 1%).

➤*Children:* Generally, the adverse reaction profile in children 6 days to 16 years of age is similar to adults. The following reactions have occurred: Hypotension, movement (17%); burning/stinging or pain (10%); hypertension (8%); rash (5%); pruritus (2%); nodal tachycardia (1.6%); arrhythmia (1.2%); apnea.

Overdosage

If accidental overdosage occurs, discontinue propofol immediately. Overdosage is likely to cause cardiorespiratory depression. Treat respiratory depression by artificial ventilation with oxygen. Cardiovascular depression may require raising the patient's legs, increasing the flow rate of IV fluids, and administering pressor agents or anticholinergic agents. Refer to General Management of Acute Overdosage.

Patient Information

Performance of activities requiring mental alertness, coordination, or physical dexterity may be impaired for some time after general anesthesia or sedation.

DROPERIDOL

Rx	**Droperidol** (Various, eg, Hospira, American Regent)	**Injection:** 2.5 mg/mL	In 2 mL vials.
Rx	**Inapsine** (Akorn)		In 1 and 2 mL amps or vials.

DROPERIDOL — INJECTION

WARNING

Cases of QT prolongation and/or torsade de pointes have been reported in patients receiving droperidol at doses at or below recommended doses. Some cases have occurred in patients with no known risk factors for QT prolongation, and some cases have been fatal.

Due to its potential for serious proarrhythmic effects and death, reserve droperidol for use in the treatment of patients who fail to show an acceptable response to other adequate treatments, either because of insufficient effectiveness or the inability to achieve an effective dose due to intolerable adverse effects from those drugs.

Cases of QT prolongation and serious arrhythmias (eg, torsade de pointes) have been reported in patients treated with droperidol. Based on these reports, all patients should undergo a 12-lead ECG prior to administration of droperidol to determine if a prolonged QT interval (ie, QTc greater than 440 msec for males or 450 msec for females) is present. If there is a prolonged QT interval, do not administer droperidol. For patients in whom the potential benefit of droperidol treatment is felt to outweigh the risks of potentially serious arrhythmias, perform ECG monitoring prior to treatment and continue for 2 to 3 hours after completing treatment to monitor for arrhythmias.

Droperidol is contraindicated in patients with known or suspected QT prolongation, including patients with congenital long QT syndrome.

Administer droperidol with extreme caution to patients who may be at risk for development of prolonged QT syndrome (eg, congestive heart failure, bradycardia, use of a diuretic, cardiac hypertrophy, hypokalemia, hypomagnesemia, or administration of other drugs known to increase the QT interval). Other risk factors may include age greater than 65 years, alcohol abuse, and use of agents such as benzodiazepines, volatile anesthetics, and IV opiates. Initiate droperidol at a low dose and adjust upward, with caution, as needed to achieve the desired effect.

Indications

➤*Antiemetic:* To reduce the incidence of nausea and vomiting associated with surgical and diagnostic procedures.

➤*Unlabeled uses:* Treatment of breakthrough chemotherapy-induced nausea and vomiting; acute treatment of chemotherapy-induced nausea and vomiting. Prevention of nausea or vomiting associated with chemotherapy.

Administration and Dosage

➤*Approved by the FDA:* February 29, 1988.

Individualize dosage. Some of the factors to be considered in determining the dose are age, body weight, physical status, underlying pathological condition, use of other drugs, type of anesthesia to be used and the surgical procedure involved.

➤*Adult:* The maximum recommended initial dose of droperidol is 2.5 mg IM or slow IV. Additional 1.25 mg doses of droperidol may be administered to achieve the desired effect. However, administer additional doses with caution, and only if the potential benefit outweighs the potential risk.

➤*Children:* For children 2 to 12 years of age, the maximum recommended dose is 0.1 mg/kg, taking into account the patient's age and other clinical factors. However, administer additional doses with caution and only if the potential benefit outweighs the potential risk.

➤*CNS depressant drugs:* Other CNS depressant drugs (eg, barbiturates, tranquilizers, opioids, and general anesthetics) have additive or potentiating effects with droperidol. When patients have received such drugs, the dose of droperidol required will be less than usual. Following the administration of droperidol, reduce the dose of other CNS depressant drugs.

➤*Storage/Stability:* Protect from light. Store at room temperature 15° to 30°C (59° to 86°F).

Actions

➤*Pharmacology:* Droperidol produces marked tranquilization and sedation. It allays apprehension and provides a state of mental detachment and indifference while maintaining a state of reflex alertness.

Droperidol produces an antiemetic effect as evidenced by the antagonism of apomorphine in dogs. It lowers the incidence of nausea and vomiting during surgical procedures and provides antiemetic protection in the postoperative period.

Droperidol potentiates other CNS depressants. It produces mild alpha-adrenergic blockade, peripheral vascular dilatation, and reduction of the pressor effect of epinephrine. It can produce hypotension and decreased peripheral vascular resistance and may decrease pulmonary arterial pressure (particularly if it is abnormally high). It may reduce the incidence of epinephrine-induced arrhythmias, but it does not prevent other cardiac arrhythmias.

The onset of action of single IM and IV doses is from 3 to 10 minutes following administration, although the peak effect may not be apparent for up to 30 minutes. The duration of the tranquilizing and sedative effects generally is 2 to 4 hours, although alteration of alertness may persist for as long as 12 hours.

Contraindications

Known or suspected QT prolongation (ie, QTc interval greater than 440 msec for males or 450 msec for females). This would include patients with congenital long QT syndrome.

Hypersensitivity to the drug.

Warnings

➤*Risks for prolonged QT syndrome:* Administer droperidol with extreme caution in the presence of risk factors for development of prolonged QT syndrome, such as:

1.) clinically significant bradycardia (less than 50 bpm),
2.) any clinically significant cardiac disease,
3.) treatment with Class I and Class III antiarrhythmics,
4.) treatment with monoamine oxidase inhibitors (MAOIs),
5.) concomitant treatment with other drug products known to prolong the QT interval,
6.) electrolyte imbalance, in particular hypokalemia and hypomagnesemia, or concomitant treatment with drugs (eg, diuretics) that may cause electrolyte imbalance.

DROPERIDOL — INJECTION

➤*Effects on cardiac conduction:* See the Warning box for more information.

Hypotension – Keep fluids and other countermeasures to manage hypotension readily available.

Opioids – When required, initially use opioids in reduced doses.

Neuroleptic malignant syndrome – As with other neuroleptic agents, very rare reports of neuroleptic malignant syndrome (altered consciousness, muscle rigidity and autonomic instability) have occurred in patients who have received droperidol.

Since it may be difficult to distinguish neuroleptic malignant syndrome from malignant hyperpyrexia in the perioperative period, consider prompt treatment with dantrolene if increases in temperature, heart rate, or carbon dioxide production occur.

➤*Special risk:* Reduce the initial dose of droperidol appropriately in elderly, debilitated and other poor-risk patients. Consider the effect of the initial dose in determining incremental doses.

➤*Renal/Hepatic function impairment:* Administer droperidol with caution to patients with liver and kidney dysfunction because of the importance of these organs in the metabolism and excretion of drugs.

➤*Pregnancy: Category C.* Droperidol administered intravenously has been shown to cause a slight increase in mortality of the newborn rat at 4.4 times the upper human dose. At 44 times the upper human dose, mortality rate was comparable to that for control animals. Following IM administration, increased mortality of the offspring at 1.8 times the upper human dose is attributed to CNS depression in the dams who neglected to remove placentae from their offspring. Droperidol has not been shown to be teratogenic in animals. There are no adequate and well-controlled studies in pregnant women. Use during pregnancy only if the potential benefit justifies the potential risk to the fetus.

Labor and delivery – There are insufficient data to support the use of droperidol in labor and delivery. Therefore, such use is not recommended.

➤*Lactation:* It is not known whether droperidol is excreted in human milk. Because many drugs are excreted in human milk, exercise caution when droperidol is administered to a nursing mother.

➤*Children:* The safety of droperidol in children less than 2 years of age has not been established.

Precautions

➤*Monitoring:* Monitor vital signs and ECG routinely. When the EEG is used for postoperative monitoring, it may be found that the EEG pattern returns to normal slowly.

As with other CNS depressant drugs, patients who have received droperidol should have appropriate surveillance.

➤*Conduction anesthesia:* Certain forms of conduction anesthesia, such as spinal anesthesia and some peridural anesthetics, can alter respiration by blocking intercostal nerves and can cause peripheral vasodilatation and hypotension because of sympathetic blockade. Through other mechanisms, droperidol can also alter circulation. Therefore, when droperidol is used to supplement these forms of anesthesia, the anesthetist should be familiar with the physiological alterations involved, and be prepared to manage them in the patients elected for these forms of anesthesia.

➤*Hypotension:* If hypotension occurs, consider the possibility of hypovolemia and manage with appropriate parenteral fluid therapy. Consider repositioning the patient to improve venous return to the heart when operative conditions permit. It should be noted that in spinal and peridural anesthesia, tilting the patient into a head-down position may result in a higher level of anesthesia than is desirable, as well as impair venous return to the heart. Exercise care in moving and positioning of patients because of a possibility of orthostatic hypotension. If volume expansion with fluids plus these other countermeasures do not correct the hypotension, then consider the administration of pressor agents other than epinephrine. Epinephrine may paradoxically decrease the blood pressure in patients treated with droperidol due to the alpha-adrenergic blocking action of droperidol.

➤*Pulmonary arterial pressure:* Since droperidol may decrease pulmonary arterial pressure, those who conduct diagnostic or surgical procedures where interpretation of pulmonary arterial pressure measurements might determine final management of the patient should consider this fact.

➤*Pheochromocytoma:* In patients with diagnosed/suspected pheochromocytonia, severe hypertension and tachycardia have been observed after the administration of droperidol.

Drug Interactions

➤*Potentially arrhythmogenic agents:* Do not use any drug known to have the potential to prolong the QT interval together with droperidol. Possible pharmacodynamic interactions can occur between droperidol and potentially arrhythmogenic agents such as Class I or III antiarrhythmics, antihistamines that prolong the QT interval, antimalarials, calcium channel blockers, neuroleptics that prolong the QT interval, and antidepressants.

Use caution when patients are taking concomitant drugs known to induce hypokalemia or hypomagnesemia as they may precipitate QT prolongation and interact with droperidol. These would include diuretics, laxatives, and supraphysiological use of steroid hormones with mineralocorticoid potential.

Droperidol Drug Interactions

Precipitant drug	Object drug*		Description
Droperidol	Anesthesia	↑	Certain forms of conduction anesthesia (eg, spinal anesthesia, some peridural anesthetics) can cause peripheral vasodilation and hypotension because of sympathetic blockade. Droperidol can alter circulation through other mechanisms.
CNS depressants (eg, barbiturates, tranquilizers, opioids, general anesthetics)	Droperidol	↑	CNS depressants have additive or potentiating CNS effects with droperidol; thus, droperidol dose will be less than usual. Likewise, following the droperidol, reduce the dose of other CNS depressants.
Droperidol	CNS depressants (eg, barbiturates, tranquilizers, opioids, general anesthetics)		
Epinephrine	Droperidol	↑	Epinephrine may paradoxically enhance droperidol-induced hypotension because of the alpha-adrenergic blocking action of droperidol. Epinephrine is not recommended as treatment of droperidol-induced hypotension.
Parenteral analgesics (eg, fentanyl)	Droperidol	↑	Hypertension has been reported following coadministration of droperidol and fentanyl or other parenteral analgesics and may be due to unexplained alterations in sympathetic activity following large doses.

* ↑ = Object drug increased.

Adverse Reactions

See the Warning box for more information.

Be alert to palpitations, syncope, or other symptoms suggestive of episodes of irregular cardiac rhythm in patients taking droperidol and promptly evaluate such cases.

The most common somatic adverse reactions reported to occur with droperidol are mild to moderate hypotension and tachycardia, but these effects usually subside without treatment. If hypotension occurs and is severe or persists, consider the possibility of hypovolemia, and manage with appropriate parenteral fluid therapy.

The most common behavioral adverse effects of droperidol include dysphoria, postoperative drowsiness, restlessness, hyperactivity, and anxiety, which can either be the result of an inadequate dosage (lack of adequate treatment effect) or of an adverse drug reaction (part of the symptom complex of akathisia).

Take care to search for extrapyramidal signs and symptoms (dystonia, akathisia, oculogyric crisis) to differentiate these different clinical conditions. When extrapyramidal symptoms are the cause, they can usually be controlled with anticholinergic agents.

Postoperative hallucinatory episodes (sometimes associated with transient periods of mental depression) have also been reported.

Other less common reported adverse reactions include anaphylaxis, dizziness, chills or shivering, laryngospasm, and bronchospasm.

Elevated blood pressure, with or without preexisting hypertension, has been reported following administration of droperidol combined with fentanyl citrate or other parenteral analgesics. This might be due to unexplained alterations in sympathetic activity following large doses; however, it is also frequently attributed to anesthetic or surgical stimulation during light anesthesia.

Overdosage

➤*Symptoms:* The manifestations of droperidol overdosage are an extension of its pharmacologic actions and may include QT prolongation and serious arrhythmias (eg, torsade de pointes).

➤*Treatment:* In the presence of hypoventilation or apnea, administer oxygen, and assist or control respiration as indicated. Maintain a patent airway; an oropharyngeal airway or endotracheal tube might be indicated. Carefully observe the patient for 24 hours; maintain body warmth and adequate fluid intake. If hypotension occurs and is severe or persists, consider the possibility of hypovolemia and manage with appropriate parenteral fluid therapy.

If significant extrapyramidal reactions occur in the context of an overdose, administer an anticholinergic.

HALOTHANE

Rx	**Halothane** (Abbott)	In 250 ml.[1]

[1] With 0.01% thymol. [2] With 0.01% thymol and up to 0.00025% ammonia.

HALOTHANE — INHALATIONAL

Indications

➤*Anesthesia:* For the induction and maintenance of general anesthesia.

Administration and Dosage

Halothane may be administered by the non-rebreathing technique, partial rebreathing, or closed technique. The induction dose varies from patient to patient but is usually within the range of 0.5% to 3%. The maintenance dose varies from 0.5% to 1.5%.

Halothane may be administered with either oxygen or a mixture of oxygen and nitrous oxide.

Halothane should not be kept indefinitely in vaporizer bottles not specifically designed for its use. Thymol does not volatilize along with halothane and, therefore, accumulates in the vaporizer and may, in time, impart a yellow color to the remaining liquid or to wicks in vaporizers. The development of such discolorations may be used as an indicator that the vaporizer should be drained and cleaned, and the discolored halothane discarded. Accumulation of thymol may easily be washed out with a small amount of fresh halothane.

Because of the more rapid uptake of halothane and the increased blood concentration required for anesthesia in younger patients, the minimum alveolar concentration (MAC) values will decrease with age.

Age	MAC percent
Infants	1.08%
3 years	0.91%
10 years	0.87%
15 years	0.92%
24 years	0.84%
42 years	0.76%
81 years	0.64%

➤*Storage/Stability:* Avoid excessive heat. Store in a tight, closed container. Protect from light. Use carton to protect contents from light.

Actions

➤*Pharmacology:* Induction and recovery are rapid, and depth of anesthesia can be rapidly altered. Halothane progressively depresses respiration. There may be tachypnea with reduced tidal volume and alveolar ventilation. Halothane is not an irritant to the respiratory tract, and no increase in salivary or bronchial secretions ordinarily occurs. Pharyngeal and laryngeal reflexes are rapidly obtunded. It causes bronchodilation. Hypoxia, acidosis, or apnea may develop during deep anesthesia.

Halothane reduces the blood pressure and frequently decreases the pulse rate. The greater the concentration of the drug, the more evident these changes become. Atropine may reverse the bradycardia. Halothane does not cause the release of catecholamines from adrenergic stores. Halothane also causes dilation of the vessels of the skin and skeletal muscles. Cardiac arrhythmias may occur, during halothane anesthesia. These include nodal rhythm, AV dissociation, ventricular extrasystoles, and asystole. Halothane sensitizes the myocardial conduction system to the action of epinephrine and norepinephrine, and the combination may cause serious cardiac arrhythmias. Halothane increases cerebrospinal-fluid pressure. Halothane produces moderate muscular relaxation. Muscle relaxants are used as adjuncts in order to maintain lighter levels of anesthesia. Halothane augments the action of nondepolarizing relaxants and ganglionic-blocking agents. Halothane is a potent uterine relaxant.

Contraindications

Obstetrical anesthesia except when uterine relaxation is required.

Warnings

➤*Hepatic effects:* When previous exposure to halothane was followed by unexplained hepatic dysfunction and/or jaundice, consideration should be given to the use of other agents.

➤*Mutagenesis:* Mutagenesis testing of halothane revealed both positive and negative results. In the rat, one-year exposure to trace concentrations of halothane (1 and 10 ppm) and nitrous oxide produced chromosomal damage to spermatogonia cells and bone marrow cells. Negative mutagenesis tests included: Ames bacterial assay, Chinese hamster lung fibroblast assay, sister chromatid exchange in Chinese hamster ovary cells, and human leukocyte culture assay.

➤*Fertility impairment:* Reproduction studies of halothane (10 ppm) and nitrous oxide in the rat caused decreased fertility. This trace concentration corresponds to 1/1000 the human maintenance dose.

➤*Pregnancy: Category C.* Some studies have shown halothane to be teratogenic, embryotoxic, and fetotoxic in the mouse, rat, hamster, and rabbit at subanesthetic and/or anesthetic concentrations. There are no adequate and well-controlled studies in pregnant women. Halothane should be used during pregnancy only if the potential benefit justifies the potential risk to the fetus..

➤*Lactation:* It is not known whether this drug is excreted in human milk. Because many drugs are excreted in human milk, caution should be exercised when halothane is administered to a nursing woman.

➤*Children:* Extensive clinical experience reveals that maintenance concentrations of halothane are generally higher in infants and children, and that maintenance requirements decrease with age. See MAC information, based upon age, in Administration and Dosage.

Precautions

➤*Vaporizers:* Halothane should be used in vaporizers that permit a reasonable approximation of output, and preferably of the calibrated type. The vaporizer should be placed out of circuit in closed-circuit rebreathing systems; otherwise, overdosage is difficult to avoid. The patient should be closely observed for signs of overdosage, ie, depression of blood pressure, pulse rate, and ventilation, particularly during assisted or controlled ventilation.

➤*Cerebrospinal-fluid pressure:* Halothane increases cerebrospinal-fluid pressure. Therefore, in patients with markedly raised intracranial pressure, if halothane is indicated, administration should be preceded by measures ordinarily used to reduce cerebrospinal-fluid pressure. Ventilation should be carefully assessed, and it may be necessary to assist or control ventilation to ensure adequate oxygenation and carbon dioxide removal.

➤*Skeletal-muscle hypermetabolic state:* In susceptible individuals, halothane anesthesia may trigger a skeletal-muscle hypermetabolic state leading to a high oxygen demand and the clinical syndrome known as malignant hyperthermia. The syndrome includes nonspecific features such as muscle rigidity, tachycardia, tachypnea, cyanosis, arrhythmias, and unstable blood pressure. (It should also be noted that many of these nonspecific signs may appear with light anesthesia, acute hypoxia, etc.) An increase in overall metabolism may be reflected in an elevated temperature (which may rise rapidly, early or late in the case, but usually is not the first sign of augmented metabolism) and an increased usage of the CO_2 absorption system (hot canister). PaO_2 and pH may decrease, and hyperkalemia and a base deficit may appear. Treatment includes discontinuance of triggering agents (eg, halothane), administration of intravenous dantrolene, and application of supportive therapy. Such therapy includes vigorous efforts to restore body temperature to normal, respiratory and circulatory support as indicated, and management of electrolyte-fluid-acid-base derangements. Renal failure may appear later, and urine flow should be sustained if possible. It should be noted that the syndrome of malignant hyperthermia secondary to halothane appears to be rare.

Drug Interactions

Epinephrine or norepinephrine should be employed cautiously, if at all, during halothane anesthesia, since their simultaneous use may induce ventricular tachycardia or fibrillation. Nondepolarizing relaxants and ganglionic-blocking agents should be administered cautiously, since their actions are augmented by halothane. Clinical experience and animal experiments suggest that pancuronium should be given with caution to patients receiving chronic tricyclic antidepressant therapy who are anesthetized with halothane, because severe ventricular arrhythmias may result from such usage.

Adverse Reactions

The following adverse reactions have been reported: Mild, moderate, and severe hepatic dysfunction (including hepatic necrosis); cardiac arrest; hypotension; respiratory arrest; cardiac arrhythmias; hyperpyrexia; shivering; nausea; and emesis.

Overdosage

In the event of overdosage, or what may appear to be overdosage, drug administration should be stopped, and assisted or controlled ventilation with pure oxygen initiated.

Patient Information

When appropriate, as in some cases where discharge is anticipated soon after general anesthesia, patients should be cautioned not to drive automobiles, operate hazardous machinery, or engage in hazardous sports for 24 hours or more (depending on the total dose of halothane, condition of the patient, and consideration given to other drugs administered after anesthesia).

ENFLURANE

Rx	**Enflurane** (Abbott)	In 125 and 250 mL.
Rx	**Ethrane** (Ohmeda)	In 125 and 250 mL.
Rx	**Compound 347** (Minrad)	In 250 mL.

ENFLURANE — INHALATION

Indications

➤*Anesthesia:* For induction and maintenance of general anesthesia. Enflurane may be used to provide analgesia for vaginal delivery. Low concentrations of enflurane may also be used to supplement other general anesthetic agents during delivery by Cesarean section. Higher concentrations of enflurane may produce uterine relaxation and an increase in uterine bleeding.

Administration and Dosage

The concentration of enflurane being delivered from a vaporizer during anesthesia should be known. This may be accomplished by using vaporizers calibrated specifically for enflurane or vaporizers from which delivered flows can easily and readily be calculated.

➤*Preanesthetic medication:* Preanesthetic medication should be selected according to the need of the individual patient, taking into account that secretions are weakly stimulated by enflurane and that enflurane does not alter heart rate. The use of anticholinergic drugs is a matter of choice.

➤*Surgical anesthesia:* Induction may be achieved using enflurane alone with oxygen or in combination with oxygen-nitrous oxide mixtures. Under these conditions some excitement may be encountered. If excitement is to be avoided, a hypnotic dose of a short-acting barbiturate should be used to induce unconsciousness, followed by the enflurane mixture. In general, inspired concentrations of 2% to 4.5% enflurane produce surgical anesthesia in 7 to 10 minutes.

➤*Maintenance:* Surgical levels of anesthesia may be maintained with 0.5% to 3% enflurane. Maintenance concentrations should not exceed 3%. If added relaxation is required, supplemental doses of muscle relaxants may be used. Ventilation to maintain the tension of carbon dioxide in arterial blood in the 35 to 45 mmHg range is preferred. Hyperventilation should be avoided in order to minimize possible CNS excitation. The level of blood pressure during maintenance is an inverse function of enflurane concentration in the absence of other complicating problems. Excessive decreases (unless related to hypovolemia) may be due to depth of anesthesia and in such instances should be corrected by lightening the level of anesthesia.

➤*Analgesia:* Enflurane 0.25% to 1% provides analgesia for vaginal delivery equal to that produced by 30% to 60% nitrous oxide. These concentrations normally do not produce amnesia.

➤*Cesarean section:* Enflurane should ordinarily be administered in the concentration range of 0.5% to 1% to supplement other general anesthetics.

➤*Storage/Stability:* Store at room temperature 15° to 30°C (59° to 86°F). Enflurane contains no additives and has been demonstrated to be stable at room temperature for periods in excess of 5 years.

Actions

➤*Pharmacology:* The MAC (minimum alveolar concentration) in man is 1.68% in pure oxygen, 0.57 in 70% nitrous oxide, 30% oxygen, and 1.17 in 30% nitrous oxide, 70% oxygen.

Induction of and recovery from anesthesia with enflurane are rapid. Enflurane has a mild, sweet odor. Enflurane may provide a mild stimulus to salivation or tracheobronchial secretions. Pharyngeal and laryngeal reflexes are readily obtunded. The level of anesthesia can be changed rapidly by changing the inspired enflurane concentration. Enflurane reduces ventilation as depth of anesthesia increases. High $PaCO_2$ levels can be obtained at deeper levels of anesthesia if ventilation is not supported. Enflurane provokes a sigh response reminiscent of that seen with diethyl ether.

There is a decrease in blood pressure with induction of anesthesia, followed by a return to near normal with surgical stimulation. Progressive increases in depth of anesthesia produce corresponding increases in hypotension. Heart rate remains relatively constant without significant bradycardia. Electrocardiographic monitoring or recordings indicate that cardiac rhythm remains stable. Elevation of the carbon dioxide level in arterial blood does not alter cardiac rhythm.

Muscle relaxation may be adequate for intra-abdominal operations at normal levels of anesthesia. Muscle relaxants may be used to achieve greater relaxation and all commonly used muscle relaxants are compatible with enflurane. The nondepolarizing muscle relaxants are potentiated. In the healthy 70 kg adult, 6 to 9 mg of d-tubocurarine or 1 to 1.5 mg of pancuronium will produce a 90% or greater depression of twitch height. Neostigmine does not reverse the direct effect of enflurane.

➤*Pharmacokinetics:* Biotransformation of enflurane in man results in low peak levels of serum fluoride averaging 15 mcmol/L. These levels are well below the 50 mcmol/L threshold level which can produce minimal renal damage in healthy subjects. However, patients chronically ingesting isoniazid or other hydrazine-containing compounds may metabolize greater amounts of enflurane. Although no significant renal dysfunction has been found thus far in such patients, peak serum fluoride levels can exceed 50 mcmol/L, particularly when anesthesia goes beyond 2 MAC hours. Depression of lymphocyte transformation does not follow prolonged enflurane anesthesia in man in the absence of surgery. Thus enflurane does not depress this aspect of the immune response.

Contraindications

Seizure disorders; sensitivity to enflurane or other halogenated anesthetics; known or suspected genetic susceptibility to malignant hyperthermia.

Warnings

➤*EEG changes:* Increasing depth of anesthesia with enflurane may produce a change in the electroencephalogram characterized by high voltage, fast frequency, progressing through spike-dome complexes alternating with periods of electrical silence to frank seizure activity. The latter may or may not be associated with motor movement. Motor activity, when encountered, generally consists of twitching or "jerks" of various muscle groups; it is self-limiting and can be terminated by lowering the anesthetic concentration. This electroencephalographic pattern associated with deep anesthesia is exacerbated by low arterial carbon dioxide tension. A reduction in ventilation and anesthetic concentrations usually suffices to eliminate seizure activity. Cerebral blood flow and metabolism studies in healthy volunteers immediately following seizure activity show no evidence of cerebral hypoxia. Mental function testing does not reveal any impairment of performance following prolonged enflurane anesthesia associated with or not associated with seizure activity.

➤*Depth of anesthesia:* Since levels of anesthesia may be altered easily and rapidly, only vaporizers producing predictable concentrations should be used. Hypotension and respiratory exchange can serve as a guide to depth of anesthesia. Deep levels of anesthesia may produce marked hypotension and respiratory depression.

➤*Hepatic effects:* When previous exposure to a halogenated anesthetic is known to have been followed by evidence of unexplained hepatic dysfunction, consideration should be given to use of an agent other than enflurane.

➤*Malignant hyperthermia:* In susceptible individuals, enflurane anesthesia may trigger a skeletal muscle hypermetabolic state leading to high oxygen demand and the clinical syndrome known as malignant hyperthermia. The syndrome includes nonspecific features such as muscle rigidity, tachycardia, tachypnea, cyanosis, arrhythmias, and unstable blood pressure. (It should also be noted that many of these nonspecific signs may appear with light anesthesia, acute hypoxia, etc. The syndrome of malignant hyperthermia secondary to enflurane appears to be rare; by March 1980, 35 cases had been reported in North America for an approximate incidence of 1:725,000 enflurane anesthetics.) An increase in overall metabolism may be reflected in an elevated temperature (which may rise rapidly early or late in the case, but usually is not the first sign of augmented metabolism) and an increased usage of CO_2 absorption system (hot cannister). PaO_2 and pH may decrease, and hyperkalemia and a base deficit may appear. Treatment includes discontinuance of triggering agents (eg, enflurane), administration of intravenous dantrolene sodium, and application of supportive therapy. Such therapy includes vigorous efforts to restore body temperature to normal, respiratory and circulatory support as indicated, and management of electrolyte-fluid-acid-base derangement. (Consult prescribing information for dantrolene sodium intravenous for additional information on patient management.) Renal failure may appear later or damage may occur in already impaired kidneys due to release of fluoride ion; urine flow should be sustained if possible.

➤*Mutagenesis:* Exposure of mice to 20 hours of 1.2% enflurane causes a small (about 1/2 of 1%) but statistically significant increase in sperm abnormalities. In contrast to these results, in vitro approaches to the study of mutagenesis (Ames test, sister chromatid exchange test, and the 8-azaguanine system) have not shown a mutagenic effect of enflurane.

➤*Pregnancy:* *Category B.* There are no adequate and well-controlled studies in pregnant women. Because animal reproduction studies are not always predictive of human response, this drug should be used during pregnancy only if clearly needed.

➤*Lactation:* It is not known whether this drug is excreted in human milk. Because many drugs are excreted in human milk, caution should be exercised when enflurane is administered to a nursing woman.

Precautions

➤*Monitoring:* Bromsulfalein (BSP) retention is mildly elevated postoperatively in some cases. This may relate to the effect of surgery since prolonged anesthesia (5 to 7 hours) in human volunteers does not result in BSP elevation. There is some elevation of glucose and white blood count intraoperatively. Glucose elevation should be considered in diabetic patients.

➤*Special risk:* Enflurane should be used with caution in patients who by virtue of medical or drug history could be considered more susceptible to cortical stimulation produced by the drug. Enflurane, like some other inhalational anesthetics, can react with desiccated carbon dioxide (CO_2) absorbents to produce carbon monoxide which may result in elevated levels of carboxyhemoglobin in some patients. Case reports suggest that barium hydroxide lime and soda lime become desiccated when fresh gases are passed through the CO_2 absorber cannister at high flow rates over many hours or days. When a clinician suspects that CO_2 absorbent may be desiccated, it should be replaced before the administration of enflurane.

Drug Interactions

The action of nondepolarizing relaxants is augmented by enflurane. Less than the usual amounts of these drugs should be used. If the usual amounts of nondepolarizing relaxants are given, the time for recovery from neuromuscular blockade will be longer in the presence of enflurane than when halothane or nitrous oxide with a balanced technique are used.

Adverse Reactions

➤*Cardiovascular:* Hypotension, arrhythmias.

➤*CNS:* Shivering motor activity exemplified by movements of various muscle groups or seizures may be encountered with deep levels of enflurane, USP, anesthesia, or light levels with hypocapnia.

➤*GI:* Nausea and vomiting have been reported.

➤*Hematologic:* Elevation of the white blood count has been observed.

ENFLURANE — INHALATION

➤*Hepatic:* Unexplained mild, moderate, and severe liver injury may rarely follow anesthesia with enflurane. Serum transaminases may be increased and histologic evidence of injury may be found. The histologic changes are neither unique nor consistent. In several of these cases, it has not been possible to exclude enflurane as the cause or as a contributing cause to liver injury. The incidence of unexplained hepatotoxicity following the administration of enflurane is unknown, but it appears to be rare and not dose related.

➤*Respiratory:* Respiratory depression has been reported.

➤*Miscellaneous:* Malignant hyperthermia (see Warnings).

Overdosage

In the event of overdosage, or what may appear to be overdosage, the following action should be taken: Stop drug administration, establish a clear airway, and initiate assisted or controlled ventilation with pure oxygen.

Patient Information

Enflurane, as well as other general anesthetics, may cause a slight decrease in intellectual function for 2 to 3 days following anesthesia. As with other anesthetics, small changes in moods and symptoms may persist for several days following administration.

ISOFLURANE

Rx	**Isoflurane** (Abbott)	In 100 mL.
Rx	**Forane** (Anaquest)	In 100 mL.
Rx	**Terrell** (Minrad)	In 100 and 250 mL.

ISOFLURANE — INHALATION

Indications

➤*Anesthesia:* For induction and maintenance of general anesthesia. Adequate data have not been developed to establish its application in obstetrical anesthesia.

Administration and Dosage

➤*Premedication:* Premedication should be selected according to the need of the individual patient, taking into account that secretions are weakly stimulated isoflurane, and the heart rate tends to be increased. The use of anticholinergic drugs is a matter of choice.

➤*Induction:* Induction with isoflurane in oxygen or in combination with oxygen-nitrous oxide mixtures may produce coughing, breath holding, or laryngospasm. These difficulties may be avoided by the use of a hypnotic dose of an ultra-short-acting barbiturate. Inspired concentrations of 1.5% to 3% isoflurane usually produce surgical anesthesia in 7 to 10 minutes.

➤*Maintenance:* Surgical levels of anesthesia may be sustained with a 1% to 2.5% concentration when nitrous oxide is used concomitantly. An additional 0.5% to 1% may be required when isoflurane is given using oxygen alone. If added relaxation is required, supplemental doses of muscle relaxants may be used.

The level of blood pressure during maintenance is an inverse function of isoflurane concentration in the absence of other complicating problems. Excessive decreases may be due to depth of anesthesia and in such instances may be corrected by lightening anesthesia.

➤*Storage / Stability:* Store at room temperature 15° to 30°C (59° to 86°F). Isoflurane contains no additives and has been demonstrated to be stable at room temperature for periods in excess of 5 years.

Actions

➤*Pharmacology:* Isoflurane is an inhalation anesthetic. The MAC (minimum alveolar concentration) in man is as follows:

Age	100% oxygen	70% N_2O
26 ± 4	1.28	0.56
44 ± 7	1.15	0.5
64 ± 5	1.05	0.37

Induction of and recovery from isoflurane anesthesia are rapid. Isoflurane has a mild pungency which limits the rate of induction, although excessive salivation or tracheobronchial secretions do not appear to be stimulated. Pharyngeal and laryngeal reflexes are readily obtunded. The level of anesthesia may be changed rapidly with isoflurane. Isoflurane is a profound respiratory depressant. Respiration must be monitored closely and supported when necessary. As anesthetic dose is increased, tidal volume decreases and respiratory rate is unchanged. This depression is partially reversed by surgical stimulation, even at deeper levels of anesthesia. Isoflurane evokes a sigh response reminiscent of that seen with diethyl ether and enflurane, although the frequency is less than with enflurane.

Blood pressure decreases with induction of anesthesia but returns toward normal with surgical stimulation. Progressive increases in depth of anesthesia produce corresponding decreases in blood pressure. Nitrous oxide diminishes the inspiratory concentration of isoflurane required to reach a desired level of anesthesia and may reduce the arterial hypotension seen with isoflurane alone. Heart rhythm is remarkably stable. With controlled ventilation and normal $PaCO_2$, cardiac output is maintained despite increasing depth of anesthesia, primarily through an increase in heart rate which compensates for a reduction in stroke volume. The hypercapnia which attends spontaneous ventilation during isoflurane anesthesia further increases heart rate and raises cardiac output above awake levels. Isoflurane does not sensitize the myocardium to exogenously administered epinephrine in the dog. Limited data indicate that subcutaneous injection of 0.25 mg of epinephrine (50 mL of 1:200,000 solution) does not produce an increase in ventricular arrhythmias in patients anesthetized with isoflurane.

Muscle relaxation is often adequate for intra-abdominal operations at normal levels of anesthesia. Complete muscle paralysis can be attained with small doses of muscle relaxants. All commonly used muscle relaxants are markedly potentiated with isoflurane, the effect being most profound with the nondepolarizing type. Neostigmine reverses the effect of nondepolarizing muscle relaxants in the presence of isoflurane. All commonly used muscle relaxants are compatible with isoflurane.

Isoflurane can produce coronary vasodilation at the arteriolar level in selected animal models; the drug is probably also a coronary dilator in humans. Isoflurane, like some other coronary arteriolar dilators, has been shown to divert blood from collateral dependent myocardium to normally perfused areas in an animal model ("coronary steal"). Clinical studies to date evaluating myocardial ischemia, infarction and death as outcome parameters have not established that the coronary arteriolar dilation property of isoflurane is associated with coronary steal or myocardial ischemia in patients with coronary artery disease.

➤*Pharmacokinetics:* Isoflurane undergoes minimal biotransformation in man. In the postanesthesia period, only 0.17% of the isoflurane taken up can be recovered as urinary metabolites.

Contraindications

Known sensitivity to isoflurane or to other halogenated agents. Known or suspected genetic susceptibility to malignant hyperthermia.

Warnings

➤*Depth of anesthesia:* Since levels of anesthesia may be altered easily and rapidly, only vaporizers producing predictable concentrations should be used. Hypotension and respiratory depression increase as anesthesia is deepened.

➤*Blood loss:* Increased blood loss comparable to that seen with halothane has been observed in patients undergoing abortions.

➤*Cerebral spinal fluid pressure:* Isoflurane markedly increased cerebral blood flow at deeper levels of anesthesia. There may be a transit rise in cerebral spinal fluid pressure which is fully reversible with hyperventilation.

➤*Pregnancy: Category C.* Isoflurane has been shown to have a possible anesthetic-related fetotoxic effect in mice when given in doses 6 times the human dose. There are no adequate and well-controlled studies in pregnant women. Isoflurane should be used during pregnancy only if the potential benefit justifies the potential risk to the fetus.

➤*Lactation:* It is not known whether this drug is excreted in human milk. Because many drugs are excreted in human milk, caution should be exercised when isoflurane is administered to a nursing woman.

Precautions

➤*Maintenance of normal hemodynamics:* Regardless of the anesthetics employed, maintenance of normal hemodynamics is important to the avoidance of myocardial ischemia in patients with coronary artery disease.

➤*Desiccated carbon dioxide:* Isoflurane, like some other inhalational anesthetics, can react with desiccated carbon dioxide (CO_2) absorbents to produce carbon monoxide which may result in elevated levels of carboxyhemoglobin in some patients. Case reports suggest that barium hydroxide lime and soda have become desiccated when fresh gases are passed through the CO_2 absorber cannister at high flow rates over many hours or days. When a clinician suspects that CO_2 absorbent may be desiccated, it should be replaced before the administration of isoflurane.

➤*Hepatic effects:* As with other halogenated anesthetic agents, isoflurane may cause sensitivity hepatitis in patients who have been sensitized by previous exposure to halogenated anesthetics. Known sensitivity to isoflurane or other halogenated agents is a contraindication to the use of this drug.

➤*Malignant hyperthermia:* In susceptible individuals, isoflurane anesthesia may trigger a skeletal muscle hypermetabolic state leading to high oxygen demand and the clinical syndrome known as malignant hyperthermia. The syndrome includes nonspecific features such as muscle rigidity, tachycardia, tachypnea, cyanosis, arrhythmias, and unstable blood pressure. (It should also be noted that many of these nonspecific signs may appear with light anesthesia, acute hypoxia, etc.) An increase in overall metabolism may be reflected in an elevated temperature, (which may rise rapidly early or late in the case, but usually is not the first sign of augmented metabolism) and an increased usage of the CO_2 absorption system (hot cannister). PaO_2 and pH may decrease, and hyperkalemia and a base deficit may appear. Treatment includes discontinuance of triggering agents (eg, isoflurane), administration of IV dantrolene sodium, and application of supportive therapy. Such therapy includes vigorous efforts to restore body temperature to normal, respiratory and circulatory support as indicated,

ISOFLURANE — INHALATION

and management of electrolyte-fluid-acid-base derangements. Renal failure may appear later, and urine flow should be sustained if possible.

If patients judged malignant hyperthermia susceptible are administered IV or oral dantrolene sodium preoperatively, anesthetic preparation must still follow a standard malignant hyperthermia susceptible regimen, including the avoidance of known triggering agents. Monitoring for early clinical and metabolic signs of malignant hyperthermia is indicated because attenuation of malignant hyperthermia, rather than prevention, is possible. These signs usually call for the administration of additional IV dantrolene sodium.

➤*Lab test abnormalities:* Transient increases in BSP retention, blood glucose and serum creatinine with decrease in BUN, serum cholesterol and alkaline phosphatase have been observed.

Drug Interactions

Isoflurane potentiates the muscle relaxant effect of all muscle relaxants, most notably nondepolarizing muscle relaxants, and MAC (minimum alveolar concentration) is reduced by concomitant administration of N_2O. Nitrous oxide diminishes the inspiratory concentration of isoflurane required to reach a desired level of anesthesia and may reduce the arterial hypotension seen with isoflurane alone.

Adverse Reactions

Adverse reactions encountered in the administration of isoflurane are in general dose dependent extensions of pharmacophysiologic effects and include respiratory depression, hypotension and arrhythmias. Shivering, nausea, vomiting and ileus have been observed in the postoperative period. As with all other general anesthetics, transient elevations in white blood count have been observed even in the absence of surgical stress. See Precautions for information regarding malignant hyperthermia. In susceptible individuals, isoflurane anesthesia may trigger a skeletal muscle hypermetabolic state leading to high oxygen demand and the clinical syndrome known as malignant hyperthermia. The syndrome includes nonspecific features such as muscle rigidity, tachycardia, tachypnea, cyanosis, arrhythmias, and unstable blood pressure. (It should also be noted that many of these nonspecific signs may appear with light anesthesia, acute hypoxia, etc.) An increase in overall metabolism may be reflected in an elevated temperature, (which may rise rapidly early or late in the case, but usually is not the first sign of augmented metabolism) and an increased usage of the CO_2 absorption system (hot cannister). PaO_2 and pH may decrease, and hyperkalemia and a base deficit may appear.

During marketing, there have been rare reports of mild, moderate and severe (some fatal) postoperative hepatic dysfunction and hepatitis.

Overdosage

In the event of overdosage, or what may appear to be overdosage, the following action should be taken.

Stop drug administration, establish a clear airway, and initiate assisted or controlled ventilation with pure oxygen.

Patient Information

Isoflurane, as well as other general anesthetics, may cause a slight decrease in intellectual function for 2 or 3 days following anesthesia. As with other anesthetics, small changes in moods and symptoms may persist for up to 6 days after administration.

DESFLURANE

Rx	**Suprane** (Ohmeda)	In 240 ml.

DESFLURANE — INHALATION

Indications

➤*Anesthesia:* For induction or maintenance of anesthesia for inpatient and outpatient surgery in adults.

Desflurane is not recommended for induction of anesthesia in pediatric patients because of a high incidence of moderate-to-severe upper airway adverse events. After induction of anesthesia with agents other than desflurane, and tracheal intubation, desflurane is indicated for maintenance of anesthesia in infants and children.

Administration and Dosage

➤*Approved by the FDA:* September 18, 1992.

Deliver desflurane from a vaporizer specifically designed and designated for use with desflurane.

The administration of general anesthesia must be individualized based on the patient's response. The following table provides mean relative potency based upon age and drug interaction studies in predominantly ASA physical status I or II patients.

Effect of Age on MAC of Desflurane Mean ± SD (% Atmospheres)

Age	n*	O_2 100%	n	N_2O 60%
2 weeks	6	9.2 ± 0	-	-
10 weeks	5	9.4 ± 0.4	-	-
9 months	4	10 ± 0.7	5	7.5 ± 0.8
2 years	3	9.1 ± 0.6	-	-
3 years	-	-	5	6.4 ± 0.4
4 years	4	8.6 ± 0.6	-	-
7 years	5	8.1 ± 0.6.	-	-
25 years	4	7.3 ± 0	4	4 ± 0.3
45 years	4	6 ± 0.3	6	2.8 ± 0.6
70 years	6	5.2 ± 0.6	6	1.7 ± 0.4

* n = number of crossover pairs (using up-and-down method of quantal response).

Desflurane MAC with Fentanyl or Midazolam Mean ± SD (% reduction)

Dose	18 to 30 years of age	31 to 65 years of age
No fentanyl	6.4 ± 0	6.3 ± 0.4
3 mcg/kg fentanyl	3.5 ± 1.9 (46%)	3.1 ± 0.6 (51%)
6 mcg/kg fentanyl	3 ± 1.2 (53%)	2.3 ± 1 (64%)
No midazolam	6.9 ± 0.1	5.9 ± 0.6
25 mcg/kg midazolam	-	4.9 ± 0.9 (16%)
50 mcg/kg midazolam	-	4.9 ± 0.5 (17%)

During the maintenance of anesthesia with inflow rates of greater than or equal to 2 L/min, the alveolar concentration of desflurane will usually be within 10% of the inspired concentration. (F_A/F_I).

➤*Individualization of dose:*

Preanesthetic medication – Issues such as whether or not to premedicate and the choice of premedicant(s) must be individualized. In clinical studies, patients scheduled to be anesthetized with desflurane frequently received IV preanesthetic medication, such as opioid or benzodiazepine.

Induction: In adults, some premedicated with opioid, a frequent starting concentration was 3% desflurane, increased in 0.5% to 1% increments every 2 to 3 breaths. End-tidal concentrations of 4% to 11% desflurane with and without N_2O, produced anesthesia within 2 to 4 minutes. When desflurane was tested as the primary anesthetic induction agent, the incidence of upper airway irritation (apnea, breathholding, laryngospasm, coughing and secretions) was high (see Adverse Reactions). During induction in adults, the overall incidence of oxyhemoglobin desaturation ($SpO_2 < 90\%$) was 6%.

After induction in adults with an IV drug such as thiopental or propofol, desflurane can be started at ≈ 0.5 to 1 MAC, whether the carrier gas is O_2 or N_2O/O_2.

Maintenance: Surgical levels of anesthesia in adults may be maintained with concentrations of 2.5% to 8.5% desflurane with or without the concomitant use of nitrous oxide. In children, surgical levels of anesthesia may be maintained with concentrations of 5.2% to 10% desflurane with or without the concomitant use of nitrous oxide.

During the maintenance of anesthesia, increasing concentrations of desflurane produce dose-dependent decreases in blood pressure. Excessive decreases in blood pressure may be due to depth of anesthesia and in such instances may be corrected by decreasing the inspired concentration of desflurane.

Concentrations of desflurane exceeding 1 MAC may increase heart rate. Thus with this drug, an increased heart rate may not serve reliably as a sign of inadequate anesthesia. Desflurane decreases the doses of neuromuscular-blocking agents required.

➤*Storage/Stability:* Store at room temperature, 15° to 30°C (59° to 86°F). Desflurane has been demonstrated to be stable for the period defined by the expiration dating on the label.

Actions

➤*Pharmacology:* Desflurane is a volatile liquid inhalation anesthetic minimally biotransformed in the liver in humans. Less than 0.02% of the desflurane absorbed can be recovered as urinary metabolites (compared to 0.2% for isoflurane).

Minimum alveolar concentration (MAC) of desflurane in oxygen for a 25-year-old adult is 7.3%. The MAC of desflurane decreases with increasing age and with addition of depressants such as opioids or benzodiazepines (see Administration and Dosage).

➤*Pharmacokinetics:* Due to the volatile nature of desflurane in plasma samples, the washin-washout profile of desflurane was used as a surrogate of plasma pharmacokinetics. Eight healthy male volunteers first breathed 70% N_2O/30% O_2 for 30 minutes and then a mixture of desflurane 2%, isoflurane 0.4%, and halothane 0.2% for another 30 minutes. During this time, inspired and end-tidal concentrations (F_I and F_A) were measured. The F_A/F_I (washin) value at 30 minutes for desflurane was 0.91, compared to 1 for N_2O, 0.74 for isoflurane, and 0.58 for halothane. The washin rates for halothane and isoflurane were similar to literature values. The washin was faster for desflurane than for isoflurane and halothane at all time points. The F_A/F_{AO} (washout) value at 5 minutes was 0.12 for desflurane, 0.22 for

DESFLURANE — INHALATION

isoflurane, and 0.25 for halothane. The washout for desflurane was more rapid than that for isoflurane and halothane at all elimination time points. By 5 days, the F_A/F_{AO} for desflurane is one-twentieth of that for halothane or isoflurane.

Contraindications

Known or suspected genetic susceptibility to malignant hyperthermia; sensitivity to desflurane or to other halogenated agents.

Warnings

➤*Administration:* Desflurane should be administered only by persons trained in the administration of general anesthesia, using a vaporizer specifically designed and designated for use with desflurane. Facilities for maintenance of a patent airway, artificial ventilation, oxygen enrichment, and circulatory resuscitation must be immediately available. Hypotension and respiratory depression increase as anesthesia is deepened.

➤*Fertility impairment:* Fertility was not affected after 1 MAC-hour per day exposure (cumulative 63 and 14 MAC-hours for males and females, respectively). At higher doses, parental toxicity (mortalities and reduced weight gain) was observed, which could affect fertility.

➤*Elderly:* The average MAC for desflurane in a 70–year-old patient is two-thirds the MAC for a 20–year-old patient.

➤*Pregnancy: Category B.* There are no adequate and well-controlled studies in pregnant women. Desflurane should be used during pregnancy only if the potential benefit justifies the potential risk to the fetus.

No teratogenic effect was observed at ≈ 10 and 13 cumulative MAC-hour exposures at 1 MAC-hour/day during organogenesis in rats or rabbits. At higher doses increased incidences of post-implantation loss and maternal toxicity were observed. However, at 10 MAC-hours cumulative exposure in rats, about 6% decrease in the weight of male pups was observed at preterm caesarean delivery.

➤*Lactation:* The concentrations of desflurane in milk are probably of no clinical importance 24 hours after anesthesia. Because of rapid washout, desflurane concentrations in milk are predicted to be below those found with other volatile potent anesthetics.

➤*Children:* Desflurane is not recommended for induction of general anesthesia via mask in infants or children because of the high incidence of moderate to severe laryngospasm in 50% of patients, coughing 72%, breathholding 68%, increase in secretions 21% and oxyhemoglobin desaturation 26%.

Precautions

➤*Cardiovascular effects:* During the maintenance of anesthesia, increasing concentrations of desflurane produce dose-dependent decreases in blood pressure. Excessive decreases in blood pressure may be related to depth of anesthesia and in such instances may be corrected by decreasing the inspired concentration of desflurane.

Concentrations of desflurane exceeding 1 MAC may increase heart rate. Thus an increased heart rate may not be a sign of inadequate anesthesia.

➤*Intracranial space occupying lesions:* In patients with intracranial space occupying lesions, desflurane should be administered at 0.8 MAC or less, in conjunction with a barbiturate induction and hyperventilation (hypocapnia). Appropriate measures should be taken to maintain cerebral perfusion pressure.

➤*Coronary artery disease:* In patients with coronary artery disease, maintenance of normal hemodynamics is important to the avoidance of myocardial ischemia. Desflurane should not be used as the sole agent for anesthetic induction in patients with coronary artery disease or patients where increases in heart rate or blood pressure are undesirable. It should be used with other medications, preferably IV opioids and hypnotics (see Clinical trials).

➤*Concentrations greater than 12%:* Inspired concentrations of desflurane more than 12% have been safely administered to patients, particularly during induction of anesthesia. Such concentrations will proportionately dilute the concentration of oxygen; therefore, maintenance of an adequate concentration of oxygen may require a reduction of nitrous oxide or air if these gases are used concurrently.

➤*Desiccated carbon dioxide:* Desflurane, like some other inhalational anesthetics, can react with desiccated carbon dioxide (CO_2) absorbents to produce carbon monoxide which may result in elevated levels of carboxyhemoglobin in some patients. Case reports suggest that barium hydroxide lime and soda lime become desiccated when fresh gases are passed through the CO_2 absorber cannister at high flow rates over many hours or days. When a clinician suspects that CO_2 absorbent may be desiccated, it should be replaced before the administration of desflurane.

➤*Hepatic effects:* As with other halogenated anesthetic agents, desflurane may cause sensitivity hepatitis in patients who have been sensitized by previous exposure to halogenated anesthetics.

➤*Malignant hyperthermia:* In susceptible individuals, potent inhalation anesthetic agents may trigger a skeletal muscle hypermetabolic state leading to high oxygen demand and the clinical syndrome known as malignant hyperthermia. In genetically susceptible pigs, desflurane-induced malignant hyperthermia. The clinical syndrome is signalled by hypercapnia, and may include muscle rigidity, tachycardia, tachypnea, cyanosis, arrhythmias, or unstable blood pressure. Some of these nonspecific signs may also appear during light anesthesia: Acute hypoxia, hypercapnia, and hypovolemia.

Treatment of malignant hyperthermia includes discontinuation of triggering agents, administration of IV dantrolene sodium, and application of supportive therapy. (Consult prescribing information for dantrolene sodium IV for additional information on patient management.) Renal failure may appear later, and urine flow should be monitored and sustained if possible.

➤*Neurosurgical use:* Desflurane may produce a dose-dependent increase in cerebrospinal fluid pressure (CSFP) when administered to patients with intracranial space occupying lesions. Desflurane should be administered at 0.8 MAC or less, and in conjunction with a barbiturate induction and hyperventilation (hypocapnia) until cerebral decompression in patients with known or suspected increases in CSFP. Appropriate attention must be paid to maintain cerebral perfusion pressure.

➤*Lab test abnormalities:* Transient elevations in glucose and white blood cell count may occur as with use of other anesthetic agents.

Drug Interactions

➤*Benzodiazepines and opioids (MAC reduction):* See Administration and Dosage for more information.

➤*Neuromuscular-blocking agents:* Anesthetic concentrations of desflurane at equilibrium (administered for 15 or more minutes before testing) reduced the ED_{95} of succinylcholine by ≈ 30% and that of atracurium and pancuronium by ≈ 50% compared to N_2O/opioid anesthesia. The effect of desflurane on duration of nondepolarizing neuromuscular blockade has not been studied.

Dosage of Muscle Relaxant Causing 95% Depression in Neuromuscular Blockade			
Desflurane concentration	Mean ED_{95} (mcg/kg)		
	Pancuronium	Atracurium	Succinylcholine
0.65 MAC 60% N_2O/O_2	26	123	—
1.25 MAC 60% N_2O/O_2	18	91	—
1.25 MAC O_2	22	120	362

Dosage reduction of neuromuscular-blocking agents during induction of anesthesia may result in delayed onset of conditions suitable for endotracheal intubation or inadequate muscle relaxation, because potentiation of neuromuscular blocking agents requires equilibration of muscle with the delivered partial pressure of desflurane.

Among nondepolarizing drugs, only pancuronium and atracurium interactions have been studied. In the absence of specific guidelines:

For endotracheal intubation, do not reduce the dose of nondepolarizing muscle relaxants or succinylcholine.

During maintenance of anesthesia, the dose of nondepolarizing muscle relaxants is likely to be reduced compared to that during N_2O/opioid anesthesia. Administration of supplemental doses of muscle relaxants should be guided by the response to nerve stimulation.

Adverse Reactions

➤*Probably causally related:*

Incidence greater than 1% –

Desflurane Induction (Use as a Mask Inhalation Agent)	
Adult patients (n = 370)	
Coughing	34%
Breathholding	30%
Apnea	15%
Increased secretions	*
Laryngospasm	*
Oxyhemoglobin desaturation (SpO_2 < 90%)	*
Pharyngitis	*
Pediatric patients (n = 152)	
Coughing	72%
Breathholding	68%
Laryngospasm	50%
Oxyhemoglobin desaturation (SpO_2 < 90%)	26%
Increased secretions	21%
Bronchospasm	*

* Incidence of events: 3% to 10%

➤*Maintenance and recovery (probably causally related):* The following adverse events occurred in greater than 1% of patients during maintenance and recovery in adult and pediatric patients (n = 687) and are probably causally related:

Cardiovascular – Bradycardia, hypertension, nodal arrhythmia, tachycardia.

CNS – Increased salivation.

GI – Nausea (27%) and vomiting (16%).

Respiratory – Apnea (incidence 3% to 10%), breathholding, increased cough (incidence 3% to 10%), laryngospasm (incidence 3% to 10%), pharyngitis.

DESFLURANE — INHALATION

Special senses – Conjunctivitis (conjunctival hyperemia).

Miscellaneous – Headache.

➤*Probably causally related (incidence < 1%):* Other adverse events that were probably causally related and that were reported in < 1% of patients (3 or more patients, n = 1843) are as follows:

Cardiovascular – Arrhythmia, bigeminy, abnormal electrocardiogram, myocardial ischemia, vasodilation.

CNS – Agitation, dizziness.

Hepatic – Hepatitis was not seen in clinical trials, but has been reported in postmarketing experience or in the literature, and is considered rare.

Respiratory – Asthma, dyspnea, and hypoxia.

➤*Causal relationship unknown (incidence < 1%):* See Warnings for information regarding pediatric use and malignant hyperthermia.

For the following adverse events, which were reported in < 1% of patients, a causal relationship could not be established:

Cardiovascular – Hemorrhage, myocardial infarction (MI).

Dermatologic – Pruritus.

Metabolic/Nutritional – Increased creatine phosphokinase.

Musculoskeletal – Myalgia.

Miscellaneous – Fever.

Overdosage

➤*Treatment:* In the event of overdosage, or suspected overdosage take the following actions: Discontinue administration of desflurane, maintain a patent airway, initiate assisted or controlled ventilation with oxygen, and maintain adequate cardiovascular function.

SEVOFLURANE

Rx	**Ultane** (Abbott)	In 250 mL.

SEVOFLURANE — INHALATION

Indications

➤*Anesthesia:* Induction and maintenance of general anesthesia in adults and children for inpatient and outpatient surgery.

Administration and Dosage

➤*Approved by the FDA:* June 7, 1995.

The concentration of sevoflurane being delivered from a vaporizer should be known. This may be accomplished by using a vaporizer calibrated specifically for sevoflurane. Administration of general anesthesia must be individualized based on patient response.

➤*Replacement of CO_2 absorbents:* Before administration of sevoflurane, replace the CO_2 absorbent if it is desiccated. The exothermic reaction that occurs with sevoflurane and CO_2 absorbents is increased when the CO_2 absorbent becomes desiccated, such as after an extended period of dry gas flow through the CO_2 absorbent canisters. Extremely rare cases of spontaneous fire in the respiratory circuit of the anesthesia machine have been reported during sevoflurane use in conjunction with the use of a desiccated CO_2 absorbent. Rapid changes in the color of some CO_2 absorbents or an unusually delayed rise in the delivered (inspired) gas concentration of sevoflurane compared with the vaporizer setting may indicate excessive heating of the CO_2 absorbent canister and chemical breakdown of sevoflurane.

➤*Preanesthetic medication:* No specific premedication is either indicated or contraindicated. The decision as to whether or not to premedicate and choice of premedication is left to the discretion of the anesthesiologist.

➤*Induction:* Sevoflurane has a nonpungent odor and does not cause respiratory irritability; it is suitable for mask induction in children and adults.

➤*Maintenance:* Surgical levels of anesthesia can usually be obtained with concentrations of 0.5% to 3% with or without the concomitant use of nitrous oxide. Sevoflurane can be administered with any type of anesthesia circuit.

➤*Storage/Stability:* Store at controlled room temperature (15° to 30°C; 59° to 86°F).

Actions

➤*Pharmacology:* Sevoflurane is an inhalational anesthetic. Minimum alveolar concentration (MAC) of sevoflurane in oxygen for an adult 40 years of age is 2.1%. The MAC of sevoflurane decreases with age.

Alveolar concentration/inspired concentration (F_A/F_I) of sevoflurane was compared with F_A/F_I data of other halogenated anesthetics in healthy volunteers. When all data were normalized to isoflurane, the uptake and distribution of sevoflurane was faster than isoflurane and halothane but slower than desflurane. Sevoflurane is a dose-related cardiac depressant. It does not produce increases in heart rate at doses less than 2 MAC.

➤*Pharmacokinetics:*

Metabolism/Excretion – Sevoflurane is metabolized by cytochrome P450 2E1 to hexafluoroisopropanol (HFIP) with release of inorganic fluoride and CO_2. Once formed HFIP is rapidly conjugated with glucuronic acid and eliminated as a urinary metabolite. No other metabolic pathways for sevoflurane have been identified. In vivo metabolism studies suggest that approximately 5% of the sevoflurane dose may be metabolized.

The low solubility of sevoflurane facilitates rapid elimination via the lungs. In healthy volunteers, rate of elimination was similar compared with desflurane, but faster compared with halothane or isoflurane. Up to 3.5% of the sevoflurane dose appears in the urine as inorganic fluoride. Studies on fluoride indicate that up to 50% of fluoride clearance is nonrenal (via fluoride being taken up into bone).

Contraindications

Known sensitivity to sevoflurane or to other halogenated agents nor in patients with known or suspected susceptibility to malignant hyperthermia.

Precautions

➤*Malignant hyperthermia:* Malignant hyperthermia may be triggered by most of the potent inhalational anesthetics. Treatment of malignant hyperthermia includes discontinuation of triggering agents, administration of IV dantrolene sodium and supportive therapy. Sevoflurane may present an increased risk in patients with known sensitivity to volatile halogenated anesthetic agents (see Contraindications).

This information on local anesthetics is not intended to be comprehensive. Consult standard textbooks for further discussion of techniques and applications.

WARNING

Obstetrical anesthesia – The 0.75% concentration of **bupivacaine** is not recommended for obstetrical anesthesia. Cardiac arrest with difficult resuscitation or death has occurred during use for epidural anesthesia in obstetrical patients. Resuscitation has been difficult or impossible despite adequate preparation and appropriate management. Cardiac arrest has occurred after convulsions resulting from systemic toxicity, presumably following unintentional intravascular injection. Reserve the 0.75% concentration for surgical procedures where a high degree of muscle relaxation and prolonged effect are necessary.

Historically, pregnant patients were reported to have a high risk for cardiac arrhythmias, cardiac/circulatory arrest, and death when bupivacaine was inadvertently rapidly injected IV. Avoid 0.75% levobupivacaine in obstetrical patients. The concentration is indicated only for nonobstetrical surgery requiring profound muscle relaxation and long duration. For Cesarean section, the 5 mg/mL (0.5%) levobupivacaine solution in doses up to 150 mg is recommended.

Have resuscitative equipment and drugs immediately available when any local anesthetic is used.

Do not use preparations containing preservatives for caudal epidural anesthesia. When using preparations without preservatives, discard any unused drug remaining in vial.

Indications

Refer to individual product listings.

Administration and Dosage

The dose of local anesthetic administered varies with the procedure, vascularity of the tissues, depth of anesthesia, degree of required muscle relaxation, duration of anesthesia desired, and the physical condition of the patient. Reduce dosages for children, the elderly, debilitated patients, and patients with cardiac or liver disease.

➤*Infiltration or regional block anesthesia:* Always inject slowly, with frequent aspirations, to prevent intravascular injection.

For detailed Administration and Dosage, refer to individual product listings and specific manufacturers' labeling.

Actions

➤*Pharmacology:* These agents prevent generation and conduction of nerve impulses by inhibiting ionic fluxes, increasing electrical excitation threshold, slowing nerve impulse propagation, and reducing rate of rise of action potential. Progression of anesthesia is related to the diameter, myelination, and conduction velocity of affected nerve fibers. The order of loss of nerve function is: Pain, temperature, touch, proprioception, and skeletal muscle tone.

Systemic absorption of local anesthetics affects the cardiovascular system and CNS. At blood concentrations achieved with normal therapeutic doses, changes in cardiac conduction, excitability, refractoriness, contractility, and peripheral vascular resistance are minimal. However, toxic blood concentrations depress cardiac conduction and excitability, which may lead to atrioventricular block and ultimately to cardiac arrest. In addition, with toxic blood concentrations, myocardial contractility may be depressed and peripheral vasodilation may occur, leading to decreased cardiac output and arterial blood pressure.

Following systemic absorption, toxic blood concentrations can produce CNS stimulation, depression, or both. Apparent central stimulation may manifest as restlessness, tremors, and shivering, which may progress to convulsions. Depression and coma may occur, possibly progressing ultimately to respiratory arrest. Local anesthetics have a primary depressant effect on the medulla and on higher centers. The depressed stage may occur without a prior stage of CNS stimulation.

The use of vasoconstrictors (eg, epinephrine) with local anesthetics promotes local hemostasis, decreases systemic absorption and prolongs duration of action.

➤*Pharmacokinetics:* Various pharmacokinetic parameters can be significantly altered by the presence of hepatic or renal disease, addition of epinephrine, factors affecting urinary pH, renal blood flow, administration route and age of patient, and the presence or absence of epinephrine in the anesthetic solution.

Injectable Local Anesthetics Pharmacokinetics

Anesthetic	Onset (minutes)	Duration (hours)	Equivalent anesthetic concentration (%)	pKa	Partition coefficient	Systemic protein binding (%)
Esters						
Procaine[1]	2-5	0.25-1	2	9.1	0.02[3]	5.8[4]
(w/epinephrine)	nd	0.5-1.5				
(Epidural)[2]	15-25	0.5-1.5				
Chloroprocaine[1]	6-12	0.5	2	9	0.14[3]	nd
(w/epinephrine)	nd	0.5-1.5				
(Epidural)[2]	5-15	0.5-1.5				
Tetracaine[1]	≤ 15	2-3	0.25	8.5	4.1[3]	75.6[5]
(Epidural)[2]	20-30	3-5				
(Spinal)	nd	1.25-3				

Injectable Local Anesthetics Pharmacokinetics

Anesthetic	Onset (minutes)	Duration (hours)	Equivalent anesthetic concentration (%)	pKa	Partition coefficient	Systemic protein binding (%)
Amides						
Lidocaine[1]	< 2	0.5-1	1	7.9	2.9[3]	64.3
(w/epinephrine)	< 2	2-6				
(Epidural)[2]	5-15	1-3				
(Spinal)	nd	0.5-1.5				
Prilocaine[1]	< 2	≥ 1	1	7.9	0.9[3]	55
(w/epinephrine)	< 2	2.25				
(Epidural)[2]	5-15	1-3				
Mepivacaine[1]	3-5	0.75-1.5	1	7.8	0.8[3]	77.5[5]
(w/epinephrine)	nd	2-6				
(Epidural)[2]	5-15	1-3				
(Spinal)	nd	0.5-1.5				
Bupivacaine[1]	5	2-4	0.25	8.2	27.5[3]/ 1565[6]	95.6[5]
(w/epinephrine)	nd	3-7				
(Epidural)[2]	10-20	3-5				
(Spinal)	nd	1.25-2.5				
Levobupivacaine	—	—	—	8.09	1624[6]	> 97[5]
(Epidural)[7]	≈ 10	≈ 8	nd			
Articaine	—	—	nd	7.8	17[8]	60-80
(w/epinephrine)	1-6	1				
Ropivacaine	—	—	nd	8.07	2.9[9]	94
(Epidural)	10-30	0.5-6				

[1] Values in this line are for infiltrative anesthesia. nd – No data.
[2] With epinephrine 1:200,000.
[3] n-Heptane/Buffer, pH 7.4.
[4] Nerve homogenate binding.
[5] Plasma protein binding.
[6] Oleyl alcohol/water buffer.
[7] Administration in Cesarean section.
[8] n-octanol/Soerensen buffer, pH 7.35.
[9] n-heptane buffer.

Rate of systemic absorption depends on total dose and concentration of drug, vascularity of administration site, and presence of vasoconstrictors. Depending on route, local anesthetics are distributed to some extent to all body tissues. High concentrations are found in highly perfused organs (eg, liver, lungs, heart, brain). Rate and extent of placental diffusion are determined by plasma protein binding, ionization, and lipid solubility. Fetal/maternal ratios are inversely related to degree of protein binding. Only free, unbound drug is available for placental transfer. Drugs with the highest protein binding capacity may have the lowest fetal/maternal ratios. Lipid soluble, nonionized drugs readily enter fetal blood from maternal circulation.

The onset of local anesthesia is dependent on the dissociation constant (pKa), lipid solubility, pH at the injection site, protein binding and molecular size. In general, local anesthetics with high lipid solubility or low pKa have a faster onset.

Local anesthetics are divided into 2 groups: Esters, which are derivatives of para-aminobenzoic acid, and amides, which are derivatives of aniline. The "ester" local anesthetics are metabolized by hydrolysis of the ester linkage by plasma esterase, probably plasma cholinesterase. The "amide" local anesthetics are metabolized primarily in the liver, then excreted primarily in the urine as metabolites, with a small fraction of unchanged drug.

Contraindications

Hypersensitivity to local anesthetics or any components of the products, para-aminobenzoic acid (esters only) or parabens; congenital or idiopathic methemoglobinemia (**prilocaine**); spinal and caudal anesthesia in septicemia, existing neurologic disease, spinal deformities, and severe hypertension, hemorrhage, shock, or heart block; subarachnoid administration (**chloroprocaine**).

➤*Bupivacaine / Levobupivacaine:* Obstetrical paracervical block anesthesia (such use has resulted in fetal bradycardia and death); IV regional anesthesia (Bier block; cardiac arrest and death have occurred) (see Warnings).

Warnings

➤*Head and neck area:* Small doses of local anesthetics injected into the head and neck area, including retrobulbar, dental, and stellate ganglion blocks, may produce adverse reactions similar to systemic toxicity seen with unintentional intravascular injections of larger doses. The injection procedures require the utmost care. Confusion, convulsions, respiratory depression or arrest, and cardiovascular stimulation or depression have been reported. These reactions may be caused by intra-arterial injection of the local anesthetic with retrograde flow to cerebral circulation. They also may be caused by puncture of the dural sheath of the optic nerve during retrobulbar block with diffusion of any local anesthetic along the subdural space to the midbrain. Observe patient carefully. Monitor respiration and circulation. Do not exceed dosage recommendations.

Ophthalmic surgery – When local anesthetic solutions are used for retrobulbar block, complete corneal anesthesia usually precedes onset of clinically acceptable external ocular muscle akinesia. Therefore, presence of akinesia rather than anesthesia alone should determine readiness of the patient for surgery. Clinicians who perform retrobulbar blocks should be aware that there have been reports of respiratory arrest following local anesthetic injection.

Dentistry – Because of the long duration of anesthesia of **bupivacaine with epinephrine**, caution patients about the possibility of inadvertent trauma to tongue, lips, and buccal mucosa and advise against chewing solid foods or testing anesthetized area by biting or probing.

Cardiovascular reactions – Cardiovascular reactions are depressant. They may be the result of direct drug effect, the result of vasovagal reaction, particularly if the patient is in the sitting position. Failure to recognize premonitory signs such as sweating, feeling of faintness, changes in pulse, or sensorium may result in progressive cerebral hypoxia and seizure, or serious cardiovascular catastrophe. Place patient in recumbent position and administer oxygen.

➤*Intravascular or subarachnoid administration:* It is essential that aspiration for blood or cerebrospinal fluid (where applicable) be done prior to injecting any local anesthetic, both the original dose and all subsequent doses, to avoid intravascular or subarachnoid injection. However, a negative aspiration does not ensure against an intravascular or subarachnoid injection.

In performing **ropivacaine** blocks, unintended intravascular injection is possible and may result in cardiac arrhythmia or cardiac arrest. The potential for successful resuscitation has not been studied in humans. Administer ropivacaine in incremental doses. It is not recommended for emergency situations where a fast onset of surgical anesthesia is necessary. Historically, pregnant patients were reported to have a high risk for cardiac arrhythmias, cardiac/circulatory arrest, and death when 0.75% **bupivacaine** was inadvertently rapidly injected IV.

➤*Spinal anesthesia:* The following conditions may preclude the use of spinal anesthesia, depending upon the physician's evaluation of the situation and ability to deal with the following complications or complaints that may occur:

- Pre-existing diseases of the CNS, such as those attributable to pernicious anemia, poliomyelitis, syphilis, or tumor.
- Hematological disorders predisposing to coagulopathies or patients on anticoagulant therapy. Trauma to a blood vessel during the conduct of spinal anesthesia may, in some instances, result in uncontrollable CNS hemorrhage or soft tissue hemorrhage.
- Chronic backache and preoperative headache.
- Hypotension and hypertension.
- Technical problems (persistent paresthesias, persistent bloody tap).
- Arthritis or spinal deformity.
- Extremes of age.
- Psychosis or other causes of poor cooperation by the patient.

➤*Hypersensitivity reactions:* These include anaphylaxis and may occur in a small segment of the population allergic to para-aminobenzoic acid derivatives (eg, procaine, tetracaine, benzocaine). The amide-type local anesthetics have not shown cross-sensitivity with the esters.

Reactions resulting in fatality have occurred on rare occasions with the use of local anesthetics, even in the absence of a history of hypersensitivity.

Administer ester-type local anesthetics cautiously to patients with abnormal or reduced levels of plasma esterases.

➤*Renal function impairment:* Use **mepivacaine** with caution in patients with renal disease.

➤*Hepatic function impairment:* Because amide-type local anesthetics are metabolized primarily in the liver and ester-type local anesthetics are hydrolyzed by plasma cholinesterase produced by the liver, patients with hepatic disease, especially severe hepatic disease, may be more susceptible to potential toxicity. Use cautiously in such patients.

➤*Elderly:* Repeated doses may cause accumulation of the drug or its metabolites or slow metabolic degradation; give reduced doses.

➤*Pregnancy: Category B* (**levobupivacaine**, **lidocaine**, **prilocaine**, **ropivacaine**). *Category C* (**articaine**, **bupivacaine**, **chloroprocaine**, **mepivacaine**, **procaine**, **tetracaine**). Safety for use in pregnant women, other than those in labor, has not been established. Local anesthetics rapidly cross the placenta. When used for epidural, caudal, paracervical, or pudendal block, they can cause varying degrees of maternal, fetal, and neonatal toxicity involving alterations of the CNS, peripheral vascular tone, and cardiac function. The incidence and degree of toxicity depend upon the procedure, type and amount of drug used, and technique of administration.

Labor, delivery, and abortion – Fetal bradycardia and fetal acidosis may occur in patients receiving anesthetics for paracervical block. Always monitor fetal heart rate prior to and during paracervical anesthesia. Added risk appears to be present in prematurity, toxemia of pregnancy, and fetal distress. Weigh the possible advantages against dangers when considering paracervical block in these conditions. The use of some local anesthetics during labor and delivery may be followed by diminished muscle strength and tone for the infant's first day or 2 of life.

Careful adherence to recommended dosage is extremely important. Failure to achieve adequate analgesia via intended paracervical or pudendal block or both with these doses may indicate intravascular or fetal intracranial injection. Babies so affected present with unexplained neonatal depression at birth and usually manifest seizures within 6 hours. Prompt use of supportive measures and forced urinary excretion of the local anesthetic have been used successfully.

Maternal hypotension – Maternal hypotension has resulted from regional anesthesia. Local anesthetics produce vasodilation by blocking sympathetic nerves. Elevating the patient's legs and positioning her on her left side will help prevent decreases in blood pressure. Continuously monitor fetal heart rate; electronic monitoring is advisable. It is extremely important to avoid aortacaval compression by the gravid uterus during administration of regional block.

Epidural, caudal, paracervical, or pudendal anesthesia – These may alter the forces of parturition through changes in uterine contractility or maternal expulsive efforts. Epidural anesthesia has been reported to prolong the second stage of labor by removing the parturient's reflex urge to bear down or by interfering with motor function. The use of obstetrical anesthesia may increase the need for forceps assistance.

Maternal convulsions and cardiovascular collapse following use of some local anesthetics for paracervical block in early pregnancy (as anesthesia for elective abortion) suggest that systemic absorption may be rapid. Therefore, do not exceed the recommended maximum dose. Inject slowly, with frequent aspirations. Allow a 5-minute interval between sides.

➤*Lactation:* Safety for use in the nursing mother has not been established. **Bupivacaine** has been reported to be excreted in breast milk. However, it is not known whether local anesthetic drugs are excreted in breast milk.

➤*Children:* Because of lack of clinical experience, the administration of **bupivacaine** to children < 12 years of age and bupivacaine 0.75% in dextrose to children < 18 years of age is not recommended.

Safety and efficacy of **tetracaine**, **levobupivacaine**, and **ropivacaine** in children have not been established.

Lidocaine 0.5% to 2% with or without epinephrine (except for dentistry indications) is not indicated in children ≤ 3 years of age. Lidocaine 5% in dextrose is not indicated in children < 16 years of age. Lidocaine 1.5% in dextrose is not indicated in children.

Articaine is not indicated in children < 4 years of age. **Chloroprocaine** is not indicated in children < 3 years of age.

Reduce dosages in children, commensurate with age, body weight, and physical condition.

Precautions

➤*Dosage:* Use the lowest dosage that results in effective anesthesia to avoid high plasma levels and serious adverse effects. Inject slowly, with frequent aspirations before and during the injection, to avoid intravascular injection. Perform syringe aspirations before and during each supplemental injection in continuous (intermittent) catheter techniques. During the administration of epidural anesthesia, it is recommended that a test dose be administered initially and that the patient be monitored for CNS toxicity and cardiovascular toxicity, as well as for signs of unintended intrathecal administration, before proceeding.

➤*Inflammation or sepsis:* Use local anesthetic procedures with caution when there is inflammation or sepsis in the region of proposed injection.

➤*CNS toxicity:* Monitor cardiovascular and respiratory vital signs and state of consciousness after each injection. Restlessness, anxiety, incoherent speech, lightheadedness, numbness, and tingling of the mouth and lips, metallic taste, tinnitus, dizziness, blurred vision, tremors, twitching, depression, or drowsiness may be early signs of CNS toxicity.

➤*Malignant hyperthermia:* Many drugs used during anesthesia are considered potential triggering agents for familial malignant hyperthermia. It is not known whether local anesthetics may trigger this reaction and the need for supplemental general anesthesia cannot be predicted in advance; therefore, have a standard protocol for management available.

➤*Vasoconstrictors:* Use solutions containing a vasoconstrictor with caution and in carefully circumscribed quantities in areas of the body supplied by end arteries or having otherwise compromised blood supply (eg, digits, nose, external ear, penis). Use with extreme caution in patients whose medical history and physical evaluation suggest the existence of hypertension, peripheral vascular disease, arteriosclerotic heart disease, cerebral vascular insufficiency, or heart block; these individuals may exhibit exaggerated vasoconstrictor response.

Serious dose-related cardiac arrhythmias may occur if preparations containing a vasoconstrictor such as epinephrine are employed in patients during or following the administration of potent inhalation agents.

➤*IV regional anesthesia:* Cardiac arrest and death are reported with the use of **bupivacaine** for IV regional anesthesia (Bier block). Bupivacaine is not recommended for this technique.

➤*Special risk:*

Debilitated patients/acutely ill patients/the elderly/children – Repeated doses may cause accumulation of the drug or its metabolites or slow metabolic degradation. Give reduced doses. Use anesthetics with caution in patients with severe disturbances of cardiac rhythm, hypotension, shock, or heart block. Also use local anesthetics with caution in patients with impaired cardiovascular function because they may be less able to compensate for functional changes associated with the prolongation of A-V conduction produced by these drugs.

➤*Sulfite sensitivity:* Some of these products contain sulfites. Sulfites may cause allergic-type reactions (eg, hives, itching, wheezing, anaphylaxis) in certain susceptible people. Although the overall prevalence of sulfite sensitivity in the general population is probably low, it is seen more frequently in asthmatics or in atopic nonasthmatic people.

Drug Interactions

➤*Intercurrent use:* Mixtures of local anesthetics are sometimes employed to compensate for the slower onset of one drug and the shorter duration of action of the second drug. Toxicity is probably additive with mixtures of local anesthetics, but some experiments suggest synergisms. Exercise caution regarding toxic equivalence when mixtures of local anesthetics are employed.

Some preparations contain vasoconstrictors. Keep this in mind when using concurrently with other drugs that may interact with vasoconstrictors (refer to the Vasopressors Used in Shock monographs).

➤*CYP450:* The metabolism of **levobupivacaine** may be affected by the known CYP3A4 inducers (eg, phenytoin, phenobarbital, rifampin), CYP3A4 inhibitors (azole antimycotics, eg, ketoconazole; certain protease inhibitors, eg, ritonavir; macrolide antibiotics, eg, erythromycin; and calcium channel antagonists, eg, verapamil), CYP1A2 inducers (omeprazole), and CYP1A2 inhibitors (furafylline and clarithromycin). Dosage adjustment may be warranted when levobupivacaine is concurrently administered with CYP3A4 inhibitors and CYP1A2 inhibitors as systemic levobupivacaine levels may rise, resulting in toxicity.

The plasma concentration of **ropivacaine** was reduced 70% during coadministration of fluvoxamine (25 mg twice daily for 2 days), a selective and potent CYP1A2 inhibitor. Thus strong inhibitors of cytochrome P4501A2 such as fluvoxamine, given concomitantly during administration of ropivacaine, can interact with ropivacaine, leading to increased ropivacaine plasma levels. Exercise caution when CYP1A2 inhibitors are coadministered. Possible interactions with drugs known to be metabolized by CYP1A2 via competitive inhibition (eg, theophylline, imipramine) may also occur. Coadministration of a selective and potent inhibitor of CYP3A4, ketoconazole (100 mg bid for 2 days with ropivacaine infusion administered 1 hour after ketoconazole) caused a 15% reduction in in vivo plasma clearance of ropivacaine.

Injectable Local Anesthetic Drug Interactions

Precipitant drug	Object drug*		Description
Local anesthetics	Sedatives	⬆	If employed to reduce patient apprehension during dental procedures, use reduced doses, since local anesthetics used in combination with CNS depressants may have additive effects. Give young children minimal doses of each agent.
Local anesthetics	Sulfonamides	⬇	The para-aminobenzoic acid metabolite of procaine, chloroprocaine, and tetracaine inhibits the action of sulfonamides. Therefore, do not use procaine, chloroprocaine, or tetracaine in any condition in which a sulfonamide drug is employed.

* ⬆ = Object drug increased. ⬇ = Object drug decreased.

Adverse Reactions

The most common acute adverse reactions are related to the CNS and cardiovascular systems. These are generally dose-related and may result from overdosage, rapid absorption from the injection site, diminished tolerance, or unintentional intravascular injection.

➤*Cardiovascular:* Myocardial depression, hypotension (with spinal anesthesia caused by vasomotor paralysis and pooling of blood in the venous bed), hypertension, decreased cardiac output, heart block, bradycardia, ventricular arrhythmias (including tachycardia and fibrillation), cardiac arrest, and fetal bradycardia (see Warnings).

➤*CNS:* Restlessness, anxiety, dizziness, tinnitus, blurred vision, chills, pupil constriction or tremors may occur, possibly proceeding to convulsions (≈ 0.1% of local anesthetic epidural administrations). Excitement may be transient or absent, with depression being the first manifestation. This may quickly be followed by drowsiness merging into unconsciousness and respiratory arrest.

Postspinal headache, meningismus, arachnoiditis, palsies, apprehension, double vision, euphoria, sensation of heat, cold, numbness, and spinal nerve paralysis (spinal anesthesia) have also occurred.

➤*GI:* Nausea, vomiting.

➤*Hypersensitivity:* Cutaneous lesions, urticaria, pruritus, erythema, angioneurotic edema (including laryngeal edema), sneezing, syncope, excessive sweating, elevated temperature, and anaphylactoid symptoms (including severe hypotension). Skin testing is of limited value.

➤*Respiratory:* Respiratory impairment or paralysis caused by level of anesthesia (spinal) extending to upper thoracic and cervical segments (see Warnings).

➤*Miscellaneous:* Occasional unintentional penetration of the subarachnoid space by the catheter may occur. Subsequent adverse effects may depend partially on amount of drug administered intrathecally. These may include the following: High or total spinal block; hypotension secondary to spinal block; urinary retention; fecal or urinary incontinence; loss of perineal sensation and sexual function; persistent anesthesia; paresthesia, weakness, and paralysis of the lower extremities and loss of sphincter control; headache and backache; septic meningitis; meningismus; slowing of labor and increased incidence of forceps delivery; cranial nerve palsies caused by traction on nerves from loss of cerebrospinal fluid; arachnoiditis; persistent motor, sensory, or autonomic deficit of some lower spinal segments with slow (several months), incomplete, or no recovery.

Methemoglobinemia – **Prilocaine** may produce dose-dependent methemoglobinemia. While methemoglobin values of < 20% do not generally produce any clinical symptoms, evaluate the appearance of cyanosis at 2 to 4 hours following administration in terms of the patient's status.

➤*Articaine:*

Articaine Adverse Reactions (≥ 1%)

Adverse reaction	Articaine (n = 882)
Pain	13
Headache	4
Face edema	1
Gingivitis	1
Infection	1
Paresthesia	1

The following list includes adverse and intercurrent events that were recorded in ≥ 1 patients, but occurred at an overall rate of < 1% and were considered clinically relevant.

Cardiovascular – Hemorrhage; migraine; syncope; tachycardia.

CNS – Dizziness; dry mouth; facial paralysis; hyperesthesia; increased salivation; nervousness; neuropathy; paresthesia; somnolence.

Dermatologic – Pruritus; skin disorder.

GI – Abdominal pain; constipation; diarrhea; dyspepsia; glossitis; gum hemorrhage; mouth ulceration; nausea; stomatitis; tongue edema; tooth disorder; vomiting.

Hematologic/Lymphatic – Ecchymosis; lymphadenopathy.

Metabolic/Nutritional – Edema; thirst.

Musculoskeletal – Arthralgia; myalgia; osteomyelitis.

Respiratory – Pharyngitis; rhinitis.

Special senses – Ear pain; taste perversion.

Miscellaneous – Accidental injury; asthenia; back pain; dysmenorrhea; injection site pain; malaise; neck pain.

➤*Levobupivacaine:*

Levobupivacaine Adverse Reactions (≥ 1%)

Adverse reaction	Levobupivacaine (n = 509)
Cardiovascular	
Hypotension	19.6
ECG abnormal	3.1
Bradycardia	2.2
Tachycardia	1.8
Hypertension	1
CNS	
Fetal distress	9.6
Delivery delayed	6.3
Dizziness	5.1
Headache	4.5
Hypoesthesia	2.6
Paresthesia	1.8
Somnolence	1.2
Anxiety	1
Dermatologic	
Pruritus	3.7
Purpura	1.4
GI	
Nausea	11.6
Vomiting	8.3
Abdomen enlarged	2.9
Constipation	2.8
Flatulence	2.4
Abdominal pain	2.2
Dyspepsia	2
Diarrhea	1
GU	
Albuminuria	2.9
Hematuria	2
Urine abnormal	1.8
Urinary incontinence	1.2
Breast pain (female)	1
Urine flow decreased	1
Urinary tract infection	1
Miscellaneous	
Anemia	9.6
Postoperative pain	7.3
Fever	6.5
Back pain	5.7
Pain	3.5
Rigors	2.9
Diplopia	2.6
Hypothermia	2.2
Hemorrhage in pregnancy	1.8
Wound drainage increased	1.4
Coughing	1.2

Levobupivacaine Adverse Reactions (≥ 1%)	
Adverse reaction	Levobupivacaine (n = 509)
Leukocytosis	1.2
Anesthesia, local	1

The following adverse events were reported at an overall rate of < 1% and were considered clinically relevant.

Cardiovascular – Postural hypotension; arrhythmia; extrasystoles; atrial fibrillation; cardiac arrest.

CNS – Hypokinesia; involuntary muscle contraction; spasm (generalized); tremor; syncope; confusion.

Dermatologic – Increased sweating; skin discoloration.

Respiratory – Apnea; bronchospasm; dyspnea; pulmonary edema; respiratory insufficiency.

Miscellaneous – Asthenia; edema; elevated bilirubin; ileus.

➤*Ropivacaine:* For the indications of epidural administration in surgery, Cesarean section, postoperative pain management, peripheral nerve block, and local infiltration, the following treatment-emergent adverse events were reported with an incidence of ≥ 5% in all clinical studies (n = 3988): Hypotension (37%); nausea (24.8%); vomiting (11.6%); bradycardia (9.3%); fever (9.2%); pain (8%); postoperative complications (7.1%); anemia (6.1%); paresthesia (5.6%); headache, pruritus (5.1%); back pain (5%).

Urinary retention, dizziness, rigors, hypertension, tachycardia, anxiety, oliguria, hypesthesia, chest pain, hypokalemia, dyspnea, cramps, and urinary tract infection occurred with an incidence of 1% to 5%.

Ropivacaine Adverse Events (≥ 1%) in Adult Patients Receiving Regional or Local Anesthesia[1]		
Adverse reaction	Ropivacaine (n = 1661)	Bupivacaine (n =1433)
Cardiovascular		
Hypotension	32.3	28.5
Bradycardia	5.8	5.1
CNS		
Headache	5.1	4.7
Paresthesia	4.9	4
Dizziness	2.5	1.6
Anxiety	1.3	0.8
GI		
Nausea	17	14.4
Vomiting	7	6.1
GU		
Urinary retention	1.4	1.4
Breast disorder, breast feeding	1.3	0.8
Miscellaneous		
Back pain	4.4	5.2
Pain	4.3	5
Pruritus	3.8	2.8
Fever	3.7	2.6
Rigors (chills)	2.5	1.7
Postoperative complications	2.5	3.1
Hypesthesia	1.6	1.7
Progression of labor poor/failed	1.4	1.5
Rhinitis	1.1	0.9

[1] Surgery, labor, Cesarean section, postoperative pain management, peripheral nerve block, local infiltration.

The following adverse events were reported during the clinical program in > 1 patient (n = 3988), occurred at an overall incidence of < 1%, and were considered relevant.

Cardiovascular – Vasovagal reaction; syncope; postural hypotension; nonspecific ECG abnormalities; extrasystoles; nonspecific arrhythmias; atrial fibrillation; ST segment changes; MI; deep vein thrombosis; phlebitis; pulmonary embolism.

CNS – Tremor; Horner's syndrome; paresis; dyskinesia; neuropathy; vertigo; coma; convulsion; hypokinesia; hypotonia; ptosis; stupor; agitation; confusion; somnolence; nervousness; amnesia; hallucination; emotional lability; insomnia; nightmares.

Dermatologic – Rash; urticaria.

GI – Fecal incontinence; tenesmus; neonatal vomiting.

GU – Poor progression of labor; uterine atony; urinary incontinence; micturition disorder.

Special senses – Tinnitus; hearing abnormalities; vision abnormalities.

Respiratory – Bronchospasm; coughing.

Miscellaneous – Injection site pain; hypothermia; malaise; asthenia; accident or injury; jaundice; hypomagnesemia; myalgia.

For the indication of epidural anesthesia for surgery, the 15 most common adverse events were compared between different concentrations of **ropivacaine** and **bupivacaine**. The following table is based on data from trials in the US and other countries where ropivacaine was administered as an epidural anesthetic for surgery.

Ropivacaine Common Adverse Events (Epidural Administration) (%)					
	Ropivacaine			Bupivacaine	
Adverse reaction	5 mg/mL (n = 256)	7.5 mg/mL (n = 297)	10 mg/mL (n = 207)	5 mg/mL (n = 236)	7.5 mg/mL (n = 174)
Hypotension	38.7	49.2	54.6	38.6	51.1
Nausea	13.3	22.9	—	17.4	20.7
Bradycardia	11.3	19.5	19.3	13.6	14.4
Back pain	7	7.7	16.4	8.9	13.2
Vomiting	7	11.1	11.1	8.1	8
Headache	4.7	6.7	7.7	5.5	5.2
Fever	3.1	1.7	8.7	4.7	—
Chills	2.3	2.4	2.9	1.7	1.7
Urinary retention	2	2.7	4.8	4.2	—
Paresthesia	2	3.4	2.4	3	—
Pruritus	—	4.7	1.4	—	4

Overdosage

Acute emergencies from local anesthetics are generally related to high plasma levels encountered during therapeutic use or to unintended subarachnoid injection.

➤*Management:* The first consideration is prevention.

Convulsions – Convulsions, as well as underventilation or apnea, are caused by unintentional subarachnoid injection; maintain patent airway and assist or control ventilation with oxygen and a delivery system capable of permitting immediate positive airway pressure by mask. Evaluate circulation. If convulsions persist despite respiratory support, and if the status of the circulation permits, give small increments of an ultra short-acting barbiturate (eg, thiopental) or a benzodiazepine (eg, diazepam) IV. Circulatory depression may require administration of IV fluids and a vasopressor.

If not treated immediately, convulsions and cardiovascular depression can result in hypoxia, acidosis, bradycardia, arrhythmias, and cardiac arrest. Underventilation or apnea may produce these same signs and also lead to cardiac arrest if ventilatory support is not instituted. If cardiac arrest occurs, institute standard cardiopulmonary resuscitative measures.

Endotracheal intubation may be indicated.

The supine position is dangerous in pregnant women at term because of aortacaval compression by the gravid uterus. Therefore, during treatment of systemic toxicity, maternal hypotension or fetal bradycardia following regional block, maintain the parturient in the left lateral decubitus position if possible, or accomplish manual displacement of the uterus off the great vessels. Resuscitation of obstetrical patients may take longer than resuscitation of nonpregnant patients and closed-chest cardiac compression may be ineffective. Rapid delivery of the fetus may improve the response to resuscitation efforts.

Patient Information

When appropriate, inform patients in advance that they may experience temporary loss of sensation and motor activity, usually in the lower half of the body, following proper administration of caudal or epidural anesthesia.

Advise the patient to exert caution to avoid inadvertent trauma to the lips, tongue, cheek, mucosae, or soft palate when these structures are anesthetized. The ingestion of food should therefore be postponed until normal function returns.

Advise the patient to consult the dentist if anesthesia persists or a rash develops.

Amide Local Anesthetics

ARTICAINE HYDROCHLORIDE

Rx	**Septocaine** (Septodont)	**Injection**: 4% with 1:100,000 epinephrine	In 1.7 mL cartridges in boxes and cans of 50.[1]

[1] With 1.6 mg/mL sodium chloride and 0.5 mg/mL sodium metabisulfite.

ARTICAINE HYDROCHLORIDE — INJECTION

For complete prescribing information, refer to the Injectable Local Anesthetics group monograph.

Indications

For local, infiltrative, or conductive anesthesia in simple and complex dental and periodontal procedures.

Administration and Dosage

➤*Approved by the FDA:* April 3, 2000.

Articaine HCl Recommended Dosages[1]		
Procedure	Volume (mL)	Total dose of articaine HCl (mg)
Infiltration	0.5 to 2.5	20 to 100
Nerve block	0.5 to 3.4	20 to 136
Oral surgery	1 to 5.1	40 to 204

[1] The above suggested volumes serve only as a guide. Other volumes may be used provided the total maximum recommended dose is not exceeded.

➤*Maximum recommended dosages:*

Adults – For healthy adults, the maximum dose of articaine administered by submucosal infiltration and nerve block should not exceed 7 mg/kg (0.175 mL/kg) or 3.2 mg/lb (0.0795 mL/lb) of body weight.

Children – Use in pediatric patients < 4 years of age is not recommended. Determine the quantity to be injected by the age and weight of the child and the magnitude of the operation. Do not exceed the equivalent of 7 mg/kg (0.175 mL/kg) or 3.2 mg/lb (0.0795 mL/lb) of body weight.

BUPIVACAINE HYDROCHLORIDE

Rx	**Bupivacaine HCl** (Hospira)	**Injection:** 0.25%	In 20, 30, and 50 mL amps, 10 and 30 mL vials, 50 mL multidose vials,[1] and 50 mL *Abboject.*
Rx	**Marcaine** (Abbott)		In 50 mL single-dose amps, 10 and 30 mL single-dose vials, 50 mL multidose vials.[1]
Rx	**Sensorcaine** (AstraZeneca)		In 50[1] mL multidose vials.
Rx	**Sensorcaine MPF** (AstraZeneca)		In 30 mL single-dose amps and 10 and 30 mL single-dose vials.
Rx	**Bupivacaine HCl** (Hospira)	**Injection:** 0.5%	In 10 and 30 mL vials, 20 and 30 mL amps, 30 mL *Abboject,* and 50 mL multidose vials.[1]
Rx	**Marcaine** (Abbott)		In 10 and 30 mL single-dose vials, 30 mL single-dose amps, and 50 mL multidose vials.[1]
Rx	**Sensorcaine** (AstraZeneca)		In 50[1] mL multidose vials.
Rx	**Sensorcaine MPF** (AstraZeneca)		In 10 and 30 mL single-dose vials.
Rx	**Bupivacaine HCl** (Hospira)	**Injection:** 0.75%	In 20 and 30 mL amps and 10 and 30 mL vials.
Rx	**Marcaine** (Abbott)		In 30 mL single-dose amps and 10 and 30 mL single-dose vials.
Rx	**Sensorcaine MPF** (AstraZeneca)		In 30 mL single-dose amps and 10 and 30 mL single-dose vials.
Rx	**Bupivacaine HCl with Epinephrine 1:200,000** (Hospira)	**Injection:** 0.25% with 1:200,000 epinephrine	In 50 mL amps, 10 and 30 mL vials, and 50 mL flip-top multidose vials.[1]
Rx	**Marcaine** (Abbott)		In 50 mL amps[2] and 10,[2] 30,[2] and 50[1,2] mL vials.
Rx	**Sensorcaine** (AstraZeneca)		In 50 mL multidose vials.[1]
Rx	**Sensorcaine MPF** (AstraZeneca)		In 10 and 30 mL single-dose vials.[3]
Rx	**Bupivacaine HCl with Epinephrine 1:200,000** (Hospira)	**Injection:** 0.5% with 1:200,000 epinephrine	In 30 mL amps, 10 and 30 mL vials, and 50 mL flip-top multidose vials.[1]
Rx	**Marcaine** (Abbott)		In 3 and 30 mL single-dose amps[2] and 10 and 30 mL single-dose vials.[2]
Rx	**Sensorcaine** (AstraZeneca)		In 50 mL multidose vials.[1]
Rx	**Sensorcaine MPF** (AstraZeneca)		In 5 mL single-dose amps and 10 and 30 mL single-dose vials.[3]
Rx	**Marcaine** (Eastman-Kodak)		In 1.8 mL dental cartridges.[2]
Rx	**Bupivacaine HCl with Epinephrine 1:200,000** (Hospira)	**Injection:** 0.75% with 1:200,000 epinephrine	In 30 mL amps.
Rx	**Marcaine** (Abbott)		In 30 mL amps.[2]
Rx	**Sensorcaine-MPF Spinal** (AstraZeneca)	**Injection:** 0.75% in 8.25% dextrose	In 2 mL amps.
Rx	**Bupivacaine Spinal** (Abbott)		Preservative-free. In 2 mL amps.

[1] With 1 mg methylparaben per mL.
[2] With 0.5 mg sodium metabisulfite and 0.1 mg EDTA per mL.
[3] With 0.5 mg sodium metabisulfite per mL.

BUPIVACAINE HYDROCHLORIDE — INJECTION

For complete and comparative prescribing information, refer to the Injectable Local Anesthetics group monograph.

WARNING

Injection – The 0.75% concentration of bupivacaine is not recommended for obstetrical anesthesia. There have been reports of cardiac arrest with difficult resuscitation or death during use of bupivacaine for epidural anesthesia in obstetrical patients. In most cases, this has followed use of the 0.75% concentration. Resuscitation has been difficult or impossible despite apparently adequate preparation and appropriate management. Cardiac arrest has occurred after convulsions resulting from systemic toxicity, presumably following unintentional intravascular injection. The 0.75% concentration should be reserved for surgical procedures where a high degree of muscle relaxation and prolonged effect are necessary.

Indications

➤*Injection:* For the production of local or regional anesthesia or analgesic for surgery, dental and oral surgery procedures, diagnostic and therapeutic procedures, and for obstetrical procedures. Only the 0.25% and 0.5% concentrations are indicated for obstetrical anesthesia.

Experience with nonobstetrical surgical procedures in pregnant patients is not sufficient to recommend use of 0.75% concentration of bupivacaine hydrochloride in these patients.

Bupivacaine hydrochloride is not recommended for IV regional anesthesia (Bier Block).

The routes of administration and indicated bupivacaine hydrochloride concentrations are local infiltration (0.25%); peripheral nerve block (0.25% and 0.5%); retrobulbar block (0.75%); sympathetic block (0.25%); lumbar epidural (0.25%, 0.5%, and 0.75%) (0.75% not for obstetrical anesthesia); caudal (0.25% and 0.5%); epidural test dose (0.5% with epinephrine 1:200,000); dental blocks (0.5% with epinephrine 1:200,000).

➤*Dextrose injection for spinal anesthesia:* Bupivacaine hydrochloride spinal is indicated for the production of subarachnoid block (spinal anesthesia). Standard textbooks should be consulted to determine the accepted procedures and techniques for the administration of spinal anesthesia.

BUPIVACAINE HYDROCHLORIDE — INJECTION

Administration and Dosage

➤*Approved by the FDA:* May 4, 1984.

The dose of any local anesthetic administered varies with the anesthetic procedure, the area to be anesthetized, the vascularity of the tissues, the number of neuronal segments to be blocked, the depth of anesthesia and degree of muscle relaxation required, the duration of anesthesia desired, individual tolerance, and the physical condition of the patient. The smallest dose and concentration required to produce the desired result should be administered. Dosages of bupivacaine hydrochloride should be reduced for elderly and debilitated patients and patients with cardiac or liver disease. The rapid injection of a large volume of local anesthetic solution should be avoided and fractional (incremental) doses should be used when feasible.

For specific techniques and procedures, refer to standard textbooks.

➤*Injection:* In recommended doses, bupivacaine hydrochloride produces complete sensory block, but the effect on motor function differs among the three concentrations.

0.25% – When used for caudal, epidural, or peripheral nerve block, produces incomplete motor block. Should be used for operations in which muscle relaxation is not important, or when another means of providing muscle relaxation is used concurrently. Onset of action may be slower than with the 0.5% or 0.75% solutions.

0.5% – Provides motor blockade for caudal, epidural, or nerve block, but muscle relaxation may be inadequate for operations in which complete muscle relaxation is essential.

0.75% – Produces complete motor block. Most useful for epidural block in abdominal operations requiring complete muscle relaxation, and for retrobulbar anesthesia. Not for obstetrical anesthesia.

The duration of anesthesia with bupivacaine hydrochloride is such that for most indications, a single dose is sufficient.

Maximum dosage limit must be individualized in each case after evaluating the size and physical status of the patient, and the usual rate of systemic absorption from a particular injection site. Most experience to date is with single doses of bupivacaine hydrochloride up to 225 mg with epinephrine 1:200,000 and 175 mg without epinephrine; more or less drug may be used depending on individualization of each case.

These doses may be repeated up to once every 3 hours. In clinical studies to date, total daily doses have been up to 400 mg. Until further experience is gained, this dose should not be exceeded in 24 hours. The duration of anesthetic effect may be prolonged by the addition of epinephrine.

The dosages below have generally proved satisfactory and are recommended as a guide for use in the average adult. These dosages should be reduced for elderly or debilitated patients. Until further experience is gained, bupivacaine hydrochloride is not recommended for children < 12 years of age. Bupivacaine hydrochloride is contraindicated for obstetrical paracervical blocks, and is not recommended for IV regional anesthesia (Bier Block).

Use in epidural anesthesia – During epidural administration of bupivacaine hydrochloride, 0.5% and 0.75% solutions should be administered in incremental doses of 3 mL to 5 mL with sufficient time between doses to detect toxic manifestations of unintentional intravascular or intrathecal injection. In obstetrics, only the 0.5% and 0.25% concentrations should be used; incremental doses of 3 mL to 5 mL of the 0.5% solution not exceeding 50 to 100 mg at any dosing interval are recommended. Repeat doses should be preceded by a test dose containing epinephrine if not contraindicated. Use only the single-dose ampuls and single-dose vials for caudal or epidural anesthesia; the multiple-dose vials contain a preservative and therefore should not be used for these procedures.

Test dose for caudal and lumbar epidural blocks – The test dose of bupivacaine hydrochloride (0.5% bupivacaine with 1:200,000 epinephrine in a 3 mL ampul) is recommended for use as a test dose when clinical conditions permit prior to caudal and lumbar epidural blocks. This may serve as a warning of unintended intravascular or subarachnoid injection (see Precautions). The pulse rate and other signs should be monitored carefully immediately following each test dose administration to detect possible intravascular injection, and adequate time for onset of spinal block should be allotted to detect possible intrathecal injection. An intravascular or subarachnoid injection is still possible even if results of the test dose are negative. The test dose itself may produce a systemic toxic reaction, high spinal or cardiovascular effects from the epinephrine.

Dentistry – The 0.5% concentration with epinephrine is recommended for infiltration and block injection in the maxillary and mandibular area when a longer duration of local anesthetic action is desired, such as for oral surgical procedures generally associated with significant postoperative pain. The average dose of 1.8 mL (9 mg) per injection site will usually suffice; an occasional second dose of 1.8 mL (9 mg) may be used if necessary to produce adequate anesthesia after making allowance for 2 to 10 minutes onset time (see Pharmacokinetics). The lowest effective dose should be employed and time should be allowed between injections; it is recommended that the total dose for all injection sites, spread out over a single dental sitting, should not ordinarily exceed 90 mg for a healthy adult patient (ten 1.8 mL injections of 0.5% bupivacaine hydrochloride with epinephrine). Injections should be made slowly and with frequent aspirations. Until further experience is gained, bupivacaine hydrochloride in dentistry is not recommended for children < 12 years of age.

Recommended Concentrations and Doses of Bupivacaine

Type of block	Concentration	Each dose (mL)	Each dose (mg)	Motor block[1]
Local infiltration	0.25%[4]	up to maximum	up to maximum	-
Epidural	0.75%[2,4]	10 to 20	75 to 150	complete
	0.5%[4]	10 to 20	50 to 100	moderate to complete
	0.25%[4]	10 to 20	25 to 50	partial to moderate
Caudal	0.5%[4]	15 to 30	75 to 150	moderate to complete
	0.25%[4]	15 to 30	37.5 to 75	moderate
Peripheral nerves	0.5%[4]	5 to max.	25 to max.	moderate to complete
	0.25%[4]	5 to max.	12.5 to max.	moderate to complete
Retrobulbar[3]	0.75%[4]	2 to 4	15 to 30	complete
Sympathetic	0.25%	20 to 50	50 to 125	-
Dental[3]	0.5% w/epinephrine	1.8 to 3.6 per site	9 to 18 per site	-
Epidural[3] test dose	0.5% w/epinephrine	2 to 3	10 to 15 (10 to 15 mcg epinephrine)	-

[1] With continuous (intermittent) techniques, repeat doses increase the degree of motor block. The first repeat dose of 0.5% may produce complete motor block. Intercostal nerve block with 0.25% may also produce complete motor block for intra-abdominal surgery.
[2] For single-dose use, not for intermittent epidural technique. Not for obstetrical anesthesia.
[3] See Precautions.
[4] Solutions with or without epinephrine.

➤*Dextrose injection for spinal anesthesia:* The extent and degree of spinal anesthesia depend upon several factors including dosage, specific gravity of the anesthetic solution, volume of solution used, force of injection, level of puncture, and position of the patient during and immediately after injection.

7.5 mg or 1 mL bupivacaine hydrochloride spinal has generally proven satisfactory for spinal anesthesia for lower extremity and perineal procedures including TURP and vaginal hysterectomy. 12 mg or 1.6 mL has been used for lower abdominal procedures such as abdominal hysterectomy, tubal ligation, and appendectomy. These doses are recommended as a guide for use in the average adult and may be reduced for the elderly or debilitated patients. Because experience with bupivacaine hydrochloride spinal is limited in patients < 18 years of age, dosage recommendations in this age group cannot be made.

Obstetrical use – Doses as low as 6 mg bupivacaine hydrochloride have been used for vaginal delivery under spinal anesthesia. The dose range of 7.5 to 10.5 mg (1 mL to 1.4 mL) bupivacaine hydrochloride has been used for Cesarean section under spinal anesthesia.

In recommended doses, bupivacaine hydrochloride spinal produces complete motor and sensory block.

➤*Storage/Stability:* Store at controlled room temperature, between 15° and 30°C (59° and 86°F).

Dextrose injection for spinal anesthesia – Bupivacaine hydrochloride spinal solution may be autoclaved once at 15 pound pressure, 121°C (250°F) for 15 minutes. Do not administer any solution that is discolored or contains particulate matter.

LIDOCAINE HYDROCHLORIDE

Rx	**Lidocaine HCl** (Various, eg, Hospira)	**Injection:** 0.5%	In 50 mL single-dose vials and 50 mL multidose vials.[1]
Rx	**Xylocaine** (AstraZeneca)		In 50 mL multidose vials.[2]
Rx	**Xylocaine MPF** (AstraZeneca)		In 50 mL single-dose vials.

LIDOCAINE HYDROCHLORIDE

Rx	**Lidocaine HCl** (Various, eg, Hospira, American Regent, Elkins-Sinn)	**Injection**: 1%	In 2 and 5 mL amps, 5 mL vials,[3] 30 mL single-dose vials, 20,[1] 30,[1] and 50 mL[1] multidose vials, 5 mL syringes, and cartridges.
Rx	**Xylocaine** (AstraZeneca)		In 10, 20, and 50 mL multidose vials.[2]
Rx	**Xylocaine MPF** (AstraZeneca)		In 2, 5 and 30 mL amps, 10 and 20 mL *PolyAmp DuoFit*, and 2, 5, 10, and 30 mL single-dose vials.
Rx	**Lidocaine HCl** (Various, eg, Hospira)	**Injection**: 1.5%	In 20 mL amps.
Rx	**Xylocaine MPF** (AstraZeneca)		In 20 mL amps, 10 and 20 mL *PolyAmp DuoFit*, and 5 and 10 mL single-dose vials.
Rx	**Lidocaine HCl** (Various, eg, Hospira, American Regent, Elkins-Sinn)	**Injection**: 2%	In 2 and 10 mL amps, 5 mL vials,[3] 10 mL single-dose vials, 20[1] and 50 mL[1] multidose vials, and 5 mL syringes.
Rx	**Xylocaine** (AstraZeneca)		In 10, 20, and 50 mL multidose vials[2] and 1.8 mL cartridges.
Rx	**Xylocaine MPF** (AstraZeneca)		In 2 and 10 mL amps, 10 mL *PolyAmp DuoFit*, and 2, 5, and 10 mL single-dose vials.
Rx	**Lidocaine HCl** (Hospira)	**Injection**: 4%	In 5 mL single-dose amps.
Rx	**Xylocaine MPF** (AstraZeneca)		In 5 mL amps and 5 mL syringe with laryngotracheal cannula.
Rx	**Lidocaine and Epinephrine** (Abbott)	**Injection**: 0.5% with 1:200,000 epinephrine	In 50 mL multidose vials.[4]
Rx	**Xylocaine** (AstraZeneca)		In 50 mL multidose vials.[2]
Rx	**Lidocaine and Epinephrine** (Abbott)	**Injection**: 1% with 1:100,000 epinephrine	In 20, 30, and 50 mL multidose vials.[4]
Rx	**Xylocaine** (AstraZeneca)		In 10, 20, and 50 mL multidose vials.[2]
Rx	**Lidocaine and Epinephrine** (Abbott)	**Injection**: 1% with 1:200,000 epinephrine	In 30 mL single-dose amps.[5]
Rx	**Xylocaine MPF** (AstraZeneca)		In 30 mL amps and 5, 10, and 30 mL single-dose vials.[5]
Rx	**Lidocaine HCl** (Abbott)	**Injection**: 1.5% with 1:200,000 epinephrine	In 5 and 30 mL amps and 30 mL single-dose vials.[5]
Rx	**Lidocaine and Epinephrine** (Abbott)		In 5 and 30 mL single-dose amps and 30 mL single-dose vials.[5]
Rx	**Xylocaine MPF** (AstraZeneca)		In 5 and 30 mL amps and 5, 10, and 30 mL single-dose vials.[5]
Rx	**Octocaine** (Septodont)	**Injection**: 2% with 1:50,000 epinephrine	In 1.8 mL cartridges.[6]
Rx	**Xylocaine** (AstraZeneca)		In 1.8 mL dental cartridges.[5]
Rx	**Lidocaine HCl and Epinephrine** (Eastman Kodak)		In 1.8 mL dental cartridges.[5]
Rx	**Lidocaine and Epinephrine** (Various, eg, Abbott, Eastman Kodak)	**Injection**: 2% with 1:100,000 epinephrine	In 1.8 mL cartridges and 20, 30, and 50 mL multidose vials.[7]
Rx	**Octocaine** (Septodont)		In 1.8 mL cartridges.[6]
Rx	**Xylocaine** (AstraZeneca)		In 10[4], 20[4] and 50 mL[4] multidose vials and 1.8 mL cartridges.[5]
Rx	**Lidocaine and Epinephrine** (Abbott)	**Injection**: 2% with 1:200,000 epinephrine	In 20 mL single-dose vials.[5]
Rx	**Xylocaine MPF** (AstraZeneca)		In 20 mL amps and 5, 10, and 20 mL single-dose vials.[5]
Rx	**Lidocaine HCl** (Abbott)	**Injection**: 1.5% with 7.5% dextrose	In 2 mL amps.
Rx	**Xylocaine** (AstraZeneca)		In 2 mL amps.
Rx	**Xylocaine-MPF** (AstraZeneca)		In 2 mL amps.
Rx	**Lidocaine HCl** (Abbott)	**Injection**: 5% with 7.5% dextrose	In 2 mL single-dose amps.
Rx	**Xylocaine MPF** (AstraZeneca)		In 2 mL amps.

[1] May contain methylparaben.
[2] With methylparaben.
[3] Preservative-free.
[4] With methylparaben and sodium metabisulfite.
[5] With sodium metabisulfite.
[6] With sodium bisulfite.
[7] May contain sodium metabisulfite and methylparaben.

LIDOCAINE HYDROCHLORIDE — INJECTION

For complete and comparative prescribing information, refer to the Injectable Local Anesthetics group monograph.

Indications

➤*For infiltration and nerve block:* For production of local or regional anesthesia by infiltration techniques such as percutaneous injection and IV regional anesthesia by peripheral nerve block techniques such as brachial plexus and intercostal and by central neural techniques such as lumbar and caudal epidural blocks, when the accepted procedures for these techniques as described in standard textbooks are observed.

➤*For cardiac arrhythmias:*

IV – In the acute management of:

1.) Ventricular arrhythmias occurring during cardiac manipulation, such as cardiac surgery.
2.) Life-threatening arrhythmias, particularly those which are ventricular in origin, such as those which occur during acute MI.

IM – Single doses are justified in the following exceptional circumstances: When ECG equipment is not available to verify the diagnosis but the potential benefits outweigh the possible risks; when facilities for IV administration are not readily available; by the patient in the prehospital phase of suspected acute MI, directed by qualified medical personnel viewing the transmitted ECG.

➤*Unlabeled uses:* In pediatric patients with cardiac arrest, less than 10% develop ventricular fibrillation, and others develop ventricular tachycardia; the hemodynamically compromised child may develop ventricular couplets or frequent premature ventricular beats. In these cases, lidocaine 1 mg/kg should be administered by the IV, intraosseous, or endotracheal route. A second 1 mg/kg dose may be given in 10 to 15 minutes. Start a lidocaine infusion if the second dose is required; a third bolus may be needed in 10 to 15 minutes to maintain therapeutic levels.

Administration and Dosage

➤*Approved by the FDA:* November 1948.

➤*IM:* 300 mg. The deltoid muscle is preferred. Avoid intravascular injection. Use only the 10% solution for IM injection.

Replacement therapy – As soon as possible, change the patient to IV lidocaine or to an oral antiarrhythmic preparation for maintenance therapy. However, if necessary, an additional IM injection may be administered after 60 to 90 minutes.

➤*Lidocaine HCl injection for infiltration and nerve block:* The table below summarizes the recommended volumes and concentrations of lidocaine HCl injection for various types of anesthetic procedures. The dosages suggested in this information are for healthy adults and refer to the use of

LIDOCAINE HYDROCHLORIDE — INJECTION

epinephrine-free solutions. When larger volumes are required, only solutions containing epinephrine should be used, except in those cases where vasopressor drugs may be contraindicated.

These recommended doses serve only as a guide to the amount of anesthetic required for most routine procedures. The actual volumes and concentrations to be used depend on a number of factors, such as type and extent of surgical procedure, depth of anesthesia, and degree of muscular relaxation required, duration of anesthesia required, and the physical condition of the patient. In all cases, the lowest concentration and smallest dose that will produce the desired result should be given. Dosages should be reduced for children, for elderly and debilitated patients, and for patients with cardiac or liver disease.

The onset of anesthesia, the duration of anesthesia, and the degree of muscular relaxation are proportional to the volume and concentration (ie, total dose) of local anesthetic used. Thus, an increase in volume and concentration of lidocaine HCl injection will decrease the onset of anesthesia, prolong the duration of anesthesia, provide a greater degree of muscular relaxation, and increase the segmental spread of anesthesia. However, increasing the volume and concentration of lidocaine HCl injection may result in a more profound fall in blood pressure when used in epidural anesthesia. Although the incidence of side effects with lidocaine HCl is quite low, caution should be exercised when employing large volumes and concentrations, since the incidence of side effects is directly proportional to the total dose of local anesthetic agent injected.

For IV regional anesthesia, only the 50 mL, single-dose vial containing lidocaine HCl 0.5% injection should be used.

Epidural anesthesia – For epidural anesthesia, only the following dosage forms of lidocaine HCl injection are recommended:

Lidocaine Epidural Anesthesia Dosage Forms	
1% without epinephrine	10 mL *Polyamp DuoFit*
1% without epinephrine	20 mL *Polyamp DuoFit*
1% without epinephrine	30 mL single-dose solutions
1.5% without epinephrine	10 mL *Polyamp DuoFit*
1.5% without epinephrine	20 mL *Polyamp DuoFit*
1.5% without epinephrine	20 mL ampules, 20 mL single-dose solutions
2% without epinephrine	10 mL *Polyamp DuoFit*
2% without epinephrine	10 mL ampules, 10 mL single-dose solutions

Although these solutions are intended specifically for epidural anesthesia, they may also be used for infiltration and peripheral nerve block, provided they are employed as single-dose units. These solutions contain no bacteriostatic agent.

In epidural anesthesia, the dosage varies with the number of dermatomes to be anesthetized (generally 2 to 3 mL of the indicated concentration per dermatome).

Caudal and lumbar epidural block – As a precaution against the adverse reaction sometimes observed following unintentional penetration of the subarachnoid space, a test dose such as 2 to 3 mL of 1.5% lidocaine HCl should be administered at least 5 minutes prior to injecting the total volume required for a lumbar or caudal epidural block. The test dose should be repeated if the patient is moved in a manner that may have displaced the catheter. Epinephrine, if contained in the test dose, (10 to 15 mcg have been suggested), may serve as a warning of unintentional intravascular injection. If injected into a blood vessel, this amount of epinephrine is likely to produce a transient "epinephrine response" within 45 seconds, consisting of an increase in heart rate and systolic blood pressure, circumoral pallor, palpitations, and nervousness in the unsedated patient. The sedated patient may exhibit only a pulse rate increase of 20 or more beats/minute for 15 or more seconds. Patients on beta blockers may not manifest changes in heart rate, but blood pressure monitoring can detect an evanescent rise in systolic blood pressure. Adequate time should be allowed for onset of anesthesia after administration of each test dose. The rapid injection of a large volume of lidocaine HCl injection through the catheter should be avoided, and, when feasible, fractional doses should be administered.

In the event of the known injection of a large volume of local anesthetic solution into the subarachnoid space, after suitable resuscitation and if the catheter is in place, consider attempting the recovery of drug by draining a moderate amount of cerebrospinal fluid (such as 10 mL) through the epidural catheter.

Maximum recommended dosages –

Adult patients: For healthy adults, the maximum individual dose should not exceed 7 mg/kg (3.5 mg/lb) of body weight, and in general it is recommended that the maximum total dose does not exceed 500 mg. When used without epinephrine, the maximum total dose should not exceed 4.5 mg/kg (2 mg/lb) of body weight, and in general, it is recommended that the maximum total dose does not exceed 300 mg. For continuous epidural or caudal anesthesia, the maximum recommended dosage should not be administered at intervals of less than 90 minutes. When continuous lumbar or caudal epidural anesthesia is used for nonobstetrical procedures, more drug may be administered if required to produce adequate anesthesia.

The maximum recommended dose per 90-minute period of lidocaine HCl for paracervical block in obstetrical patients and nonobstetrical patients is 200 mg total. One-half of the total dose is usually administered to each side. Inject slowly, 5 minutes between sides.

For IV regional anesthesia, the dose administered should not exceed 4 mg/kg in adults.

Pediatric patients: It is difficult to recommend a maximum dose of any drug for children, since this varies as a function of age and weight. For children over 3 years of age who have a normal lean body mass and normal body development, the maximum dose is determined by the child's age and weight. For example, in a child of 5 years of age weighing 50 lbs, the dose of lidocaine HCl should not exceed 75 to 100 mg (1.5 to 2 mg/lb). The use of even more dilute solutions (ie, 0.25% to 0.5%) and total dosages not to exceed 3 mg/kg (1.4 mg/lb) are recommended for induction of IV regional anesthesia in children.

In order to guard against systemic toxicity, the lowest effective concentration and lowest effective dose should be used at all times. In some cases, it will be necessary to dilute available concentrations with 0.9% sodium chloride injection in order to obtain the required final concentration.

Recommended Dosages			
	Lidocaine HCl injection (without epinephrine)		
Procedure	Conc (%)	Volume (mL)	Total dose (mg)
Infiltration			
Percutaneous	0.5 or 1	1 to 60	5 to 300
Intravenous regional	0.5	10 to 60	50 to 300
Peripheral nerve blocks			
Brachial	1.5	15 to 20	225 to 300
Dental	2	1 to 5	20 to 100
Intercostal	1	3	30
Paravertebral	1	3 to 5	30 to 50
Pudendal (each side)	1	10	100
Paracervical			
Obstetrical analgesia (each side)	1	10	100
Sympathetic nerve blocks			
Cervical (stellate ganglion)	1	5	50
Lumbar	1	5 to 10	50 to 100
Central neural blocks*			
Thoracic epidural	1	20 to 30	200 to 300
Lumbar epidural (analgesia)	1	25 to 30	250 to 300
Lumbar epidural (anesthesia)	1.5	15 to 20	225 to 300
	2	10 to 15	200 to 300
Caudal			
Obstetrical analgesia	1	20 to 30	200 to 300
Surgical anesthesia	1.5	15 to 20	225 to 300

* Dose determined by number of dermatomes to be anesthetized (2 to 3 mL/dermatome).

The above suggested concentrations and volumes serve only as a guide. Other volumes and concentrations may be used provided the total maximum recommended dose is not exceeded.

➤*Lidocaine HCl injection for cardiac arrhythmias:* This product is for direct infusion only. For continuous infusion protocol, see information for lidocaine HCl for infusion solution.

Adults patients – The usual dose is 50 to 100 mg administered intravenously under ECG monitoring. This dose may be administered at the rate of approximately 25 to 50 mg/min. Sufficient time should be allowed to enable a slow circulation to carry the drug to the site of action. If the initial injection of 50 to 100 mg does not produce a desired response, a second dose may be repeated after 5 minutes.

No more than 200 to 300 mg of lidocaine HCl injection should be administered during a 1 hour period.

Pediatric patients – Although controlled clinical studies to establish pediatric dosing schedules have not been conducted, the American Heart Association's Standards and Guidelines recommends a bolus dose of 1 mg/kg followed by an infusion rate of 30 mcg/kg/min.

➤*Sterilization and technical procedures:* Disinfecting agents containing heavy metals, which cause release of respective ions (eg, mercury, zinc, copper) should not be used for skin or mucous membrane disinfection, as they have been related to incidents of swelling and edema. When chemical disinfection of multidose vials is desired, either isopropyl alcohol (91%) or ethyl alcohol (70%) is recommended. Many commercially available brands of rubbing alcohol, as well as solutions of ethyl alcohol not of USP grade, contain denaturants which are injurious to rubber and therefore are not to be used.

➤*Storage/Stability:* All solutions should be stored at room temperature, approximately 25°C (77°F). Protect from light.

Stable for 24 hours after dilution in 5% Dextrose in Water.

MEPIVACAINE HYDROCHLORIDE

Rx	**Carbocaine** (Hospira)	**Injection**: 1%	In 30 mL single-dose vials and 50 mL[1] multidose vials.
Rx	**Polocaine** (AstraZeneca)		In 50 mL multidose vials.[1]
Rx	**Polocaine MPF** (AstraZeneca)		In 30 mL single-dose vials.[1]
Rx	**Carbocaine** (Hospira)	**Injection**: 1.5%	In 30 mL single-dose vials.
Rx	**Polocaine MPF** (AstraZeneca)		In 30 mL single-dose vials.
Rx	**Carbocaine** (Hospira)	**Injection**: 2%	In 20 mL single-dose vials and 50 mL[1] multidose vials.
Rx	**Polocaine** (AstraZeneca)		In 50 mL multidose vials.[1]
Rx	**Polocaine MPF** (AstraZeneca)		In 20 mL single-dose vials.
Rx	**Mepivacaine HCl** (Septodont)	**Injection**: 3%	In 1.8 mL dental cartridge.
Rx	**Carbocaine** (Eastman-Kodak)		In 1.8 mL dental cartridge.[2]
Rx	**Polocaine** (AstraZeneca)		In 1.8 mL dental cartridge.[3]
Rx	**Carbocaine with Neo-Cobefrin** (Eastman-Kodak)	**Injection**: 2% with 1:20,000 levonordefrin	In 1.8 mL dental cartridge.[2]
Rx	**Mepivacaine HCl and Levonordefrin** (Septodont)		In 1.8 mL dental cartridge.[3]
Rx	**Polocaine with Levonordefrin** (AstraZeneca)		In 1.8 mL dental cartridge.[4]

[1] With methylparaben.
[2] With acetone sodium bisulfite.
[3] With sodium bisulfite.
[4] With sodium metabisulfite.

MEPIVACAINE HYDROCHLORIDE — INJECTION

For complete and comparative prescribing information, refer to the Injectable Local Anesthetics group monograph.

Indications

➤*Peripheral nerve block (eg, cervical, brachial, intercostal, pudendal):* 1% or 2% solution.

➤*Transvaginal block (paracervical plus pudendal):* 1% solution.

➤*Paracervical block in obstetrics:* 1% solution.

➤*Caudal and epidural block:* 1%, 1.5%, or 2% solution.

➤*Infiltration:* 0.5% (via dilution) or 1% solution

➤*Therapeutic block (pain management):* 1% or 2% solution.

➤*Dental procedures (infiltration or nerve block):* 3% solution or 2% solution with levonordefrin.

Administration and Dosage

➤*Approved by the FDA:* August 21, 1984.

Avoid the rapid injection of a large volume of a local anesthetic solution and use fractional (incremental) doses. Administer the smallest dose and concentration required to produce the desired result.

➤*Maximum dosage:* The recommended single adult dose (or the total of a series of doses given in 1 procedure) for unsedated, healthy, normal-sized individuals should not usually exceed 400 mg. The total dose for any 24-hour period should not exceed 1000 mg. Carefully measure the pediatric dose as a percentage of the total adult dose, based on weight, and do not exceed 5 to 6 mg/kg (2.5 to 3 mg/lb) in pediatric patients, especially those weighing < 30 lb. In pediatric patients < 3 years of age or weighing < 30 lb, use concentrations < 2% (eg, 0.5% to 1.5%).

➤*Dental procedures (infiltration or nerve block):* In the upper or lower jaw, the average dose of 1 cartridge usually will suffice. Five cartridges (180 mg of the 2% solution or 270 mg of the 3% solution) usually are adequate to effect anesthesia of the entire oral cavity.

➤*Recommended dosages in various procedures:*

Mepivacaine HCl Recommended Concentrations and Doses

Procedure	Conc. (%)	Total dose mL	Total dose mg	Comments
Cervical, brachial, intercostal, pudendal nerve block	1 2	5 to 40 5 to 20	50 to 400 100 to 400	Pudendal block: one half of total dose injected each side.
Transvaginal block (paracervical plus pudendal)	1	up to 30 (both sides)	up to 300 (both sides)	One-half of total dose injected each side.
Paracervical block	1	up to 20 (both sides)	up to 200 (both sides)	One half of total dose injected each side. This is maximum recommended dose per 90-minute period in obstetrical and nonobstetrical patients. Inject slowly, 5 minutes between sides.
Caudal and epidural block	1 1.5 2	15 to 30 10 to 25 10 to 20	150 to 300 150 to 375 200 to 400	Use only single-dose vials that do not contain a preservative.
Infiltration	1	up to 40	up to 400	An equivalent amount of a 0.5% solution (prepared by diluting the 1% solution with Sodium Chloride Injection) may be used for large areas.
Therapeutic block (pain management)	1 2	1 to 5 1 to 5	10 to 50 20 to 100	—

➤*Storage/Stability:* Store at 15° to 30°C (59° to 86°F).

PRILOCAINE HYDROCHLORIDE

Rx	**Citanest Plain** (AstraZeneca)	**Injection**: 4%	In 1.8 mL cartridge.
Rx	**Citanest Forte** (AstraZeneca)	**Injection**: 4% with 1:200,000 epinephrine	In 1.8 mL cartridge.[1]

[1] With sodium metabisulfite.

PRILOCAINE HYDROCHLORIDE — INJECTION

For complete prescribing information, refer to the Injectable Local Anesthetics group monograph.

Indications

➤*For local anesthesia by nerve block or infiltration in dental procedures:* 4% solution.

Administration and Dosage

Administer the least volume of injection required.

➤*Maximum dosage:* In patients weighing < 150 lbs (70 kg), administer no more than 4 mg/lb (8 mg/kg). In patients weighing ≥ 150 lbs, administer no more than 600 mg (8 cartridges) as a single injection. In children < 10 years of age, it is rarely necessary to administer more than one-half cartridge (40 mg).

➤*Inferior alveolar block:* There are no practical clinical differences between prilocaine with and without epinephrine when used for inferior alveolar blocks.

➤*Maxillary infiltration:* Prilocaine without epinephrine is recommended for use in maxillary infiltration anesthesia for procedures in which the painful aspects can be completed within 15 minutes after the injection. For long procedures, or those involving maxillary posterior teeth where soft tissue numbness is not troublesome to the patient, prilocaine with epinephrine is recommended.

For most routine procedures, initial dosages of 1 to 2 mL of prilocaine with or without epinephrine usually will provide adequate infiltration or major nerve block anesthesia.

➤*Storage/Stability:* Store at ≈ 25°C (77°F).

ROPIVACAINE HYDROCHLORIDE

Rx	**Naropin** (AstraZeneca)	**Injection:** 0.2%	Preservative-free. In 10 and 20 mL *PolyAmp DuoFit Sterile Paks* and 100 and 200 mL single-dose infusion bottles.
		0.5%	Preservative-free. In 20 mL *PolyAmp DuoFit Sterile Paks* and 30 mL single-dose vials.
		0.75%	Preservative-free. In 20 mL *PolyAmp DuoFit Sterile Paks.*
		1%	Preservative free. In 10 and 20 mL *PolyAmp DuoFit Sterile Paks.*

ROPIVACAINE — INJECTION

For complete and comparative prescribing information, refer to the Injectable Local Anesthetics group monograph.

Indications

➤*Acute pain management:* Epidural continuous infusion or intermittent bolus (eg, postoperative or labor); local infiltration.

➤*Surgical anesthesia:* For the production of local or regional anesthesia for surgery. Epidural block for surgery including cesarean section; major nerve block; local infiltration.

Administration and Dosage

➤*Approved by the FDA:* September 24, 1996.

➤*Administration:* Avoid the rapid administration of a large volume of local anesthetic solution and use fractional (incremental) doses. Administer the smallest dose and concentration required to produce the desired result.

➤*Test dose:* Use an adequate test dose (3 to 5 mL of a short-acting local anesthetic containing epinephrine) prior to induction of complete block. Repeat this test dose if patient movement potentiates epidural catheter displacement. Allow adequate time for onset of anesthesia following administration of each test dose.

Ropivacaine Dosage Recommendations

Procedures	Concentration (mg/mL)	Volume (mL)	Dose (mg)	Onset (min)	Duration (hours)
Surgical anesthesia					
Lumbar epidural administration for Surgery	5 (0.5%)	15 to 30	75 to 150	15 to 30	2 to 4
	7.5 (0.75%)	15 to 25	113 to 188	10 to 20	3 to 5
	10 (1%)	15 to 20	150 to 200	10 to 20	4 to 6
Lumbar epidural administration for Cesarean section	5 (0.5%)	20 to 30	100 to 150	15 to 25	2 to 4
	7.5 (0.75%)	15 to 20	113 to 150	10 to 20	3 to 5
Thoracic epidural administration for Surgery	5 (0.5%)	5 to 15	25 to 75	10 to 20	na[d]
	7.5 (0.75%)	5 to 15	38 to 113	10 to 20	na
Major nerve block (eg, brachial plexus block)[a]	5 (0.5%)	35 to 50	175 to 250	15 to 30	5 to 8
	7.5 (0.75%)	10 to 40	75 to 300	10 to 25	6 to 10
Field block (eg, minor nerve blocks and infiltration)	5 (0.5%)	1 to 40	5 to 200	1 to 15	2 to 6
Labor pain management					
Lumbar epidural administration Initial dose	2 (0.2%)	10 to 20	20 to 40	10 to 15	0.5 to 1.5
Continuous infusion[b]	2 (0.2%)	6 to 14 mL/hr	12 to 28 mg/hr	na	na
Incremental injections (top-up)[b]	2 (0.2%)	10 to 15 mL/hr	20 to 30 mg/hr	na	na
Postoperative pain management					
Lumbar epidural administration Continuous infusion[c]	2 (0.2%)	6 to 14 mL/hr	12 to 28 mg/hr	na	na
Thoracic epidural administration Continuous infusion[c]	2 (0.2%)	6 to 14 mL/hr	12 to 28 mg/hr	na	na
Infiltration (eg, minor nerve block)	2 (0.2%)	1 to 100	2 to 200	1 to 5	2 to 6
	5 (0.5%)	1 to 40	5 to 200	1 to 5	2 to 6

[a] The dose for a major nerve block must be adjusted according to site of administration and patient status. Supraclavicular brachial plexus blocks may be associated with a higher frequency of serious adverse reactions, regardless of the local anesthetic used.
[b] Median dose of 21 mg/hour was administered by continuous infusion or incremental injections (top-ups) over a median delivery time of 5.5 hours.
[c] Cumulative doses up to 770 mg of ropivacaine over 24 hours (intraoperative block plus postoperative infusion): Continuous epidural infusion at rates up to 28 mg/hr for 72 hours have been well tolerated in adults, ie, 2016 mg plus surgical dose of ≈ 100 to 150 mg as top-up.
[d] Not available.

When prolonged blocks are used, either through continuous infusion or through repeated bolus administration, the risks of reaching a toxic plasma concentration or inducing local neural injury must be considered. Experience to date indicates that a cumulative dose of up to 770 mg ropivacaine administered over 24 hours is well tolerated in adults when used for postoperative pain management (ie, 2016 mg). Exercise caution when administering ropivacaine for prolonged periods of time (eg, greater than 70 hours in debilitated patients).

➤*Acute pain management:* For treatment of postoperative pain, the following technique can be recommended: If regional anesthesia was not used intraoperatively, then an initial epidural block with 5 to 7 mL ropivacaine is induced via an epidural catheter. Analgesia is maintained with an infusion of ropivacaine, 2 mg/mL (0.2%). Clinical studies have demonstrated that infusion rates of 6 to 14 mL (12 to 28 mg) per hour provide adequate analgesia with nonprogressive motor block. With this technique a significant reduction in the need for opioids was demonstrated. Clinical experience supports the use of ropivacaine epidural infusions for up to 72 hours.

➤*Incompatibilities:* The solubility of ropivacaine is limited at pH above 6. Thus, care must be taken as precipitation may occur if ropivacaine is mixed with alkaline solutions.

➤*Storage/Stability:* Store at controlled room temperature, 20° to 25°C (68° to 77°F).

Disinfecting agents containing heavy metals, which cause release of respective ions (eg, mercury, zinc, copper) should not be used for skin or mucous membrane disinfection since they have been related to incidents of swelling and edema.

When chemical disinfection of the container surface is desired, either isopropyl alcohol (91%) or ethyl alcohol (70%) is recommended. It is recommended that chemical disinfection be accomplished by wiping the ampule or vial stopper thoroughly with cotton or gauze that has been moistened with the recommended alcohol just prior to use. When a container is required to have a sterile outside, a *Sterile Pak* should be chosen. Glass containers may, as an alternative, be autoclaved once. Stability has been demonstrated using a targeted F_0 of 7 minutes at 121°C (249.8°F).

These products are intended for single use and are free from preservatives. Any solution remaining from an opened container should be discarded promptly. In addition, continuous infusion bottles should not be left in place for more than 24 hours.

Ester Local Anesthetics

CHLOROPROCAINE HYDROCHLORIDE

Rx	**Nesacaine** (AstraZeneca)	**Injection:** 1%	In 30 mL multidose vials.[1]
Rx	**Chloroprocaine Hydrochloride** (Bedford)	**Injection:** 2%	In 20 mL single-dose vials.[2]
Rx	**Nesacaine** (AstraZeneca)		In 30 mL multidose vials.[1]
Rx	**Nesacaine-MPF** (AstraZeneca)		In 20 mL single-dose vials.[2]
Rx	**Chloroprocaine Hydrochloride** (Bedford)	**Injection:** 3%	In 20 mL single-dose vials.[2]
Rx	**Nesacaine-MPF** (AstraZeneca)		In 20 mL single-dose vials.[2]

[1] With methylparaben and EDTA.

[2] Preservative-free.

CHLOROPROCAINE HYDROCHLORIDE — INJECTION

For complete prescribing information, refer to the Injectable Local Anesthetics group monograph.

Indications

➤*Infiltration and peripheral nerve block:* Chloroprocaine 1% and 2% injections, in multidose vials with methylparaben preservative. Do not use for lumbar and caudal epidural anesthesia.

➤*Infiltration, peripheral, and central nerve block, including lumbar and caudal epidural block:* Chloroprocaine 2% and 3% injections, in single-dose vials without preservative and without EDTA.

Administration and Dosage

➤*Approved by the FDA:* March 1955.

Use the smallest dose and concentration required to produce the desired result.

➤*Maximum dosage:* The maximum single recommended doses of chloroprocaine in adults are: without epinephrine, 11 mg/kg, not to exceed a maximum total dose of 800 mg; with epinephrine (1:200,000), 14 mg/kg, not to exceed a maximum total dose of 1,000 mg.

➤*Administration:* Administer as a single injection or continuously through an indwelling catheter. Avoid rapid injection of a large volume of local anesthetic injection through the catheter. Consider fractional doses when feasible. Do not use for subarachnoid administration.

➤*Test dose for caudal and lumbar epidural block:* In order to guard against adverse experiences sometimes noted following unintended penetration of the subarachnoid space, the following procedure modifications are recommended: Use an adequate test dose (3 mL of 3% chloroprocaine injection without preservatives or 5 mL of 2% chloroprocaine injection without preservatives) prior to induction of complete block. Repeat this test dose if the patient is moved in such a fashion as to have displaced the epidural catheter. Allow adequate time for onset of anesthesia following administration of each test dose. Avoid the rapid injection of a large volume of local anesthetic injection through the catheter. Consider fractional doses.

In the event of the known injection of a large volume of local anesthetic injection into the subarachnoid space, after suitable resuscitation and if the catheter is in place, consider attempting the recovery of drug by draining a moderate amount of cerebrospinal fluid (such as 10 mL) through the epidural catheter.

➤*Caudal and lumbar epidural block (chloroprocaine without preservatives):* For caudal anesthesia, the initial dose is 15 to 25 mL of a 2% or 3% solution. Repeated doses may be given at 40- to 60-minute intervals.

For lumbar epidural anesthesia, 2 to 2.5 mL per segment of a 2% or 3% solution can be used. The usual total volume of chloroprocaine injection without preservatives is from 15 to 25 mL. Repeated doses 2 to 6 mL less than the original dose may be given at 40- to 50-minute intervals.

The above dosages are recommended as a guide for use in the average adult. Maximum dosages of all local anesthetics must be individualized after evaluating the size and physical condition of the patient and the rate of systemic absorption from a particular injection site.

➤*Infiltration and peripheral nerve block (chloroprocaine with or without preservatives):*

Suggested Chloroprocaine Doses for Infiltration and Peripheral Nerve Block

Anesthetic procedure	Concentration	Volume (mL)	Total dose (mg)
Mandibular	2%	2 to 3 mL	40 to 60 mg
Infraorbital	2%	0.5 to 1 mL	10 to 20 mg
Brachial plexus	2%	30 to 40 mL	600 to 800 mg
Digital (without epinephrine)	1%	3 to 4 mL	30 to 40 mg
Pudendal	2%	10 mL each side	400 mg
Paracervical	1%	3 mL per each of 4 sites	up to 120 mg

➤*Pediatric dosage:* The maximum dose is determined by the child's age and weight and should not exceed 11 mg/kg (5 mg/lb). Concentrations of 0.5% to 1% are suggested for infiltration and 1% to 1.5% for nerve block. In order to guard against systemic toxicity, use the lowest effective concentration and lowest effective dose at all times. Some of the lower concentrations for use in infants and smaller children are not available in prepackaged containers; it will be necessary to dilute available concentrations with the amount of 0.9% sodium chloride injection necessary to obtain the required final concentration of chloroprocaine injection.

➤*Dosage adjustment:* Reduce dosage for children, elderly, and debilitated patients with cardiac and/or liver disease.

➤*Preparation of epinephrine injections:* To prepare a 1:200,000 epinephrine-chloroprocaine injection, add 0.1 mL of a 1:1,000 epinephrine injection to 20 mL of chloroprocaine injection without preservatives.

➤*Incompatibility:* Chloroprocaine is incompatible with caustic alkalis and their carbonates, soaps, silver salts, iodine, and iodides.

➤*Storage/Stability:* Keep from freezing. Protect from light. Store at controlled room temperature, 15° to 30°C (59° to 86°F). Discard unused chloroprocaine injection without preservatives remaining in vial after use because contains no preservatives (eg, methylparaben). Chloroprocaine injection is slightly photosensitive and may become discolored after prolonged exposure to light. Store these vials in the original outer containers, protected from direct sunlight. Do not administer discolored injection. If exposed to low temperatures, chloroprocaine injection may deposit crystals of chloroprocaine, which will redissolve with shaking when returned to room temperature. Do not use the product if it contains undissolved (eg, particulate) material.

PROCAINE HYDROCHLORIDE

Rx	**Novocain** (Abbott)	**Injection:** 1%	In 2 mL *Uni-Amps*, 6 mL single-dose amps,[1] and 30 mL multidose vials.[2]
Rx	**Procaine HCl** (Various, eg, IDE)	**Injection:** 2%	In 30 mL multidose vials.[3]
Rx	**Novocain** (Abbott)		In 30 mL multidose vials.[2]
Rx	**Novocain** (Abbott)	**Injection:** 10%	In 2 mL *Uni-Amps.*[1]

[1] With acetone sodium bisulfite.

[2] With acetone sodium bisulfite and chlorobutanol.

[3] May contain sodium metabisulfite.

PROCAINE HYDROCHLORIDE — INJECTION

For complete and comparative prescribing information, refer to the Injectable Local Anesthetics group monograph.

Indications

➤*Procaine hydrochloride injection 10%:* For spinal anesthesia.

➤*Procaine hydrochloride injection 1% and 2%:* For the production of local or regional analgesia and anesthesia by local infiltration and peripheral nerve block techniques.

The routes of administration and concentrations are: for local infiltration use 0.25% to 0.5% (via dilution) and for peripheral nerve blocks use 0.5% (via dilution), 1%, and 2% (see Administration and Dosage for additional information).

Administration and Dosage

As with all local anesthetics, the dose of procaine hydrochloride varies and depends upon the area to be anesthetized, the vascularity of the tissues, the number of neuronal segments to be blocked, individual tolerance, and the technique of anesthesia. The lowest dose needed to provide effective anesthesia should be administered. For specific techniques and procedures, refer to standard textbooks.

Dosages of procaine hydrochloride should be reduced for elderly and debilitated patients and patients with cardiac and/or liver disease. The rapid injection of a large volume of local anesthetic solution should be avoided and fractional doses should be used when feasible.

Ester Local Anesthetics

PROCAINE HYDROCHLORIDE — INJECTION

➤*Procaine hydrochloride injection 10%:*

Recommended dosage for spinal anesthesia				
	Procaine HCl injection 10% solution			
Extent of anesthesia	Volume of 10% solution (mL)	Volume of diluent (mL)	Total dose (mg)	Site of injection (lumbar interspace)
Perineum	0.5	0.5	50	4th
Perineum and lower extremities	1	1	100	3rd or 4th
Up to costal margin	2	1	200	2nd, 3rd, or 4th

The diluent may be sterile normal saline, sterile distilled water, spinal fluid; and for hyperbaric technique, sterile dextrose solution.

The usual rate of injection is 1 mL per 5 seconds. Full anesthesia and fixation usually occur in 5 minutes.

Sterilization – The drug in intact ampuls is sterile. The preferred method of destroying bacteria on the exterior of ampuls before opening is heat sterilization (autoclaving). Immersion in antiseptic solution is not recommended.

Single-dose containers and multiple-dose containers of procaine hydrochloride may be sterilized by autoclaving at 15-pound pressure, 121°C (250°F) for 15 minutes. The diluent dextrose may show some brown discoloration due to caramelization. Do not use solutions if crystals, cloudiness, or discoloration is observed. Examine solution carefully before use. Reautoclaving increases likelihood of crystal formation. Do not administer solutions that are discolored or that contain particulate matter. Protect solutions from light.

➤*Procaine hydrochloride injection 1% and 2%:* For infiltration anesthesia, 0.25% or 0.5% solution; 350 mg to 600 mg is generally considered to be a single safe total dose. To prepare 60 mL of a 0.5% solution (5 mg/mL), dilute 30 mL of the 1% solution with 30 mL sodium chloride injection 0.9%. To prepare 60 mL of a 0.25% solution (2.5 mg/mL), dilute 15 mL of the 1% solution with 45 mL sodium chloride injection 0.9%. An anesthetic solution of 0.5 mL to 1 mL of epinephrine 1:1000 per 100 mL may be added for vasoconstrictive effect (1:200,000 to 1:100,000).

For peripheral nerve block, 0.5% solution (up to 200 mL), 1% solution (up to 100 mL), or 2% solution (up to 50 mL). The use of the 2% solution should usually be limited to cases requiring a small volume of anesthetic solution (10 mL to 25 mL). An anesthetic solution of 0.5 mL to 1 mL of epinephrine 1:1000 per 100 mL may be added for vasoconstrictive effect (1:200,000 to 1:100,000).

The usual total dose during one treatment should not exceed 1000 mg.

Pediatric use – In pediatric patients 15 mg/kg of a 0.5% solution for local infiltration is the maximum recommended dose.

➤*Storage / Stability:* Store at controlled room temperature 15° to 30°C (59° to 86°F).

TETRACAINE HYDROCHLORIDE

Rx	**Pontocaine Hydrochloride** (Hospira)	**Injection**: 1%	In 2 mL amps.[1]
		0.2% in 6% dextrose	In 2 mL amps.
		0.3% in 6% dextrose	In 5 mL amps.
		Powder for reconstitution: 20 mg	In *Niphanoid* (instantly soluble) amps.

[1] With acetone sodium bisulfite.

TETRACAINE HYDROCHLORIDE — INJECTION

For complete and comparative prescribing information, refer to the Injectable Local Anesthetics group monograph.

Indications

Tetracaine HCl is indicated for the production of spinal anesthesia for procedures requiring 2 to 3 hours.

Administration and Dosage

As with all anesthetics, the dosage varies and depends upon the area to be anesthetized, the number of neuronal segments to be blocked, individual tolerance, and the technique of anesthesia. The lowest dosage needed to provide effective anesthesia should be administered. For specific techniques and procedures, refer to standard textbooks.

Suggested dosage for spinal anesthesia					
Using Niphanoid			Using 1% solution		
Extent of anesthesia	Dose of Niphanoid (mg)	Volume of spinal fluid (mL)	Dose of solution (mL)	Volume of spinal fluid (mL)	Site of injection (lumbar interspace)
Perineum	5*	1	0.5 (approximately 5 mg)*	0.5	4th
Perineum and lower extremities	10	2	1 (approximately 10 mg)	1	3rd or 4th
Up to coastal margin	15 to 20[1]	3	1.5 to 2 (approximately 15 to 20 mg)[1]	1.5 to 2	2nd, 3rd, or 4th

* For vaginal delivery (saddle block), from 2 mg to 5 mg in dextrose.
[1] Doses exceeding 15 mg are rarely required and should be used only in exceptional cases. Inject solution at rate of about 1 mL per 5 seconds.

The extent and degree of spinal anesthesia depend upon dosage, specific gravity of the anesthetic solution, volume of solution used, force of the injection, level of puncture, position of the patient during and immediately after injection.

When spinal fluid is added to either the Niphanoid or solution, some turbidity results, the degree depending on the pH of the spinal fluid, the temperature of the solution during mixing, as well as the amount of drug and diluent employed. This cloudiness is due to the release of the base from the hydrochloride. Liberation of base (which is completed within the spinal canal) is held to be essential for satisfactory results with any spinal anesthetic.

The specific gravity of spinal fluid at 25°C/25°C (77°F/77°F) varies under normal conditions from 1.0063 to 1.0075. A solution of the instantly soluble form (Niphanoid) in spinal fluid has only a slightly greater specific gravity. The 1% concentration in saline solution has a specific gravity of 1.0060 to 1.0074 at 25°C/25°C (77°F/77°F).

A hyperbaric solution may be prepared by mixing equal volumes of the 1% Solution and Dextrose Solution 10% (which is available in ampuls of 3 mL).

If the Niphanoid form is preferred, it is first dissolved in Dextrose Solution 10% in a ratio of 1 mL dextrose to 10 mg of the anesthetic. Further dilution is made with an equal volume of spinal fluid. The resulting solution now contains 5% dextrose with 5 mg of anesthetic agent per milliliter.

A hypobaric solution may be prepared by dissolving the Niphanoid in Sterile Water for Injection, USP (1 mg per milliliter). The specific gravity of this solution is essentially the same as that of water, 1.000 at 25°C/25°C (77°F/77°F).

Examine ampuls carefully before use. Do not use solution if crystals, cloudiness, or discoloration is observed.

These formulations of tetracaine hydrochloride do not contain preservatives; therefore, unused portions should be discarded and the reconstituted Niphanoid should be used immediately.

➤*Sterilization of ampuls:* The drug in intact ampuls is sterile. The preferred method of destroying bacteria on the exterior of ampuls before opening is heat sterilization (autoclaving). Immersion in antiseptic solution is not recommended.

Autoclave at 15-pound pressure, at 121°C (250°F), for 15 minutes. The Niphanoid form may also be autoclaved in the same way but may lose its snowlike appearance and tend to adhere to the sides of the ampul. This may slightly decrease the rate at which the drug dissolves but does not interfere with its anesthetic potency.

Autoclaving increases likelihood of crystal formation. Unused autoclaved ampuls should be discarded. Under no circumstance should unused ampuls which have been autoclaved be returned to stock.

➤*Storage / Stability:* Protect ampuls from light. Store solution under refrigeration.

COMBINATION LOCAL ANESTHETICS

Rx	**Duocaine** (Amphastar)	**Injection:** 10 mg/mL lidocaine HCl/ 3.75 mg/mL bupivacaine HCl	Preservative-free. In 10 mL single-dose vials. In cartons of 25.

For complete prescribing information, refer to the Injectable Local Anesthetics group monograph.

COMBINATION LOCAL ANESTHETICS — INJECTION

Indications

➤*Surgical anesthesia:* For the production of local or regional anesthesia for ophthalmologic surgery by peripheral nerve block techniques such as parabulbar, retrobulbar, and facial blocks. May be used with or without epinephrine and/or hyaluronidase.

Administration and Dosage

➤*Approved by the FDA:* May 23, 2003.

➤*Peribulbar nerve block:* 6 to 12 mL lidocaine/bupivacaine solution (60 to 120 mg lidocaine and 22 to 45 mg bupivacaine). This technique produces akinesia of the superior oblique muscles, the eyelids, and the orbicularis oculi muscle.

➤*Retrobulbar and facial nerve block:* 2 to 5 mL lidocaine/bupivacaine solution (20 to 50 mg lidocaine and 7 to 18 mg bupivacaine). A portion of the dose is injected retrobulbarly, and the remainder may be used to block the facial nerve.

➤*Maximum dosage:* Individualize maximum dosage limit in each case after evaluating the size and physical status of the patient, as well as the usual rate of systemic absorption from a particular injection site.

For healthy adults, the individual maximum recommended dose of lidocaine/bupivacaine without epinephrine should not exceed 0.18 mL/kg (0.08 mL/lb) of body weight, and, in general, it is recommended that the maximum total dose not exceed 12 mL (120 mg lidocaine and 45 mg bupivacaine). When used with epinephrine, the maximum individual dose should not exceed 0.28 mL/kg (0.14 mL/lb) of body weight, and, in general, it is recommended that the maximum total dose not exceed 20 mL (200 mg lidocaine and 75 mg bupivacaine).

➤*Storage/Stability:* Store at 15° to 25°C (59° to 77°F). Discard unused portion after initial use.

ANTICONVULSANTS

Anticonvulsant drugs include a variety of agents, all possessing the ability to depress abnormal neuronal discharges in the CNS, thus inhibiting seizure activity. Because of differences in pharmacology, therapeutic use, and adverse reaction potential, these agents are discussed in groups as follows:

- Barbiturates
- Hydantoins
- Succinimides
- Oxazolidinediones
- Benzodiazepines
- Adjuvants to anticonvulsants

➤*Warnings:*

Pregnancy – Reports suggest an association between use of anticonvulsant drugs by women with epilepsy and an elevated incidence of birth defects in children born to these women. Data are more extensive with respect to phenytoin and phenobarbital; other reports indicate a possible similar association with other anticonvulsants. Other factors (eg, genetics or the seizure disorder per se) may also contribute to the higher incidence of birth defects. The great majority of mothers receiving anticonvulsant medication deliver healthy infants.

Do not discontinue anticonvulsant drugs in patients in whom the drug is administered to prevent major seizures because of the strong possibility of precipitating status epilepticus with attendant hypoxia and risk to both the mother and the unborn child. Consider discontinuation of anticonvulsants prior to and during pregnancy when the nature, frequency, and severity of the seizures do not pose a serious threat to the patient. It is not known whether even minor seizures constitute some risk to the developing embryo or fetus.

An increase in seizure frequency during pregnancy occurs in a high proportion of patients because of altered phenytoin absorption or metabolism. Periodic measurement of serum phenytoin levels is particularly valuable in the management of pregnant epileptic patients as a guide to an appropriate adjustment of dosage. However, postpartum restoration of the original dosage will probably be indicated.

Reports suggest that maternal ingestion of anticonvulsant drugs, particularly barbiturates and hydantoins, is associated with a neonatal coagulation defect that may cause bleeding during the early (usually within 24 hours of birth) neonatal period. The defect is characterized by decreased levels of vitamin K-dependent clotting factors, and prolongation of either the prothrombin time or the partial thromboplastin time, or both. It has been suggested that prophylactic vitamin K be given to the mother 1 month prior to and during delivery, and to the infant immediately after birth.

In addition to the reports of increased incidence of congenital malformations, such as cleft lip/palate and heart malformations in children of women receiving phenytoin and other antiepileptic drugs, there have been more recent reports of a fetal hydantoin syndrome. This consists of prenatal growth deficiency, microcephaly, and mental deficiency in children born to mothers who have received phenytoin, barbiturates, alcohol, or trimethadione. However, these features are all interrelated and are frequently associated with intrauterine growth retardation from other causes.

There have been isolated reports of malignancies, including neuroblastoma, in children whose mothers received phenytoin during pregnancy.

Seizures – Seizures may be classified based on their clinical form. The following is based on the International Classification of Epileptic Seizures:†

1.) Partial seizures (generally involve 1 hemisphere of the brain at onset)
    a.) Simple (consciousness not impaired)
    b.) With motor symptoms (Jacksonian, adversive)
    c.) With somatosensory or other special sensory symptoms
    d.) With autonomic symptoms
    e.) With psychic symptoms
    f.) Complex (consciousness impaired)
    g.) Simple partial onset followed by impaired consciousness
    h.) Impaired consciousness at onset
    i.) Secondarily generalized
    j.) Simple partial seizures evolving to generalized tonic-clonic seizures
    k.) Complex partial seizures evolving to generalized tonic-clonic seizures
    l.) Simple partial seizures evolving to complex partial seizures, then to generalized tonic-clonic seizures.
2.) Generalized seizures (involve both hemispheres of the brain at onset, consciousness usually impaired)
    a.) Absence
    b.) Typical
    c.) Atypical
    d.) Myoclonic
    e.) Clonic
    f.) Tonic
    g.) Tonic-clonic
    h.) Atonic
3.) Localization-related (focal)
    a.) Idiopathic
    b.) Benign focal epilepsy of childhood
    c.) Symptomatic
    d.) Chronic progressive epilepsia partialis continua
    e.) Temporal-lobe
    f.) Extratemporal
4.) Generalized epilepsy
    a.) Idiopathic
    b.) Benign neonatal convulsions
    c.) Childhood absence
    d.) Juvenile myoclonic
    e.) Other
    f.) Cryptogenic or symptomatic
    g.) West syndrome (infantile spasms)
    h.) Early myoclonic encephalopathy
    i.) Lennox-Gastaut syndrome
    j.) Progressive myoclonic epilepsy
5.) Special syndromes
    a.) Febrile seizures
6.) Unclassified

Withdrawal of anticonvulsants – A long-term prospective study suggests that epileptic adults may remain seizure-free if their anticonvulsant is withdrawn following at least 2 years of a single therapy regimen. Approximately one-third of patients relapsed following withdrawal of the anticonvulsants.

Predictors of relapse include the following: Seizure type (highest relapse rates occurred with complex partial seizures with secondary generalization and generalized seizures).

Number of seizures (higher risk with > 100 seizures before control).

Number of drugs (highest rate with patients taking 2 or 3 drugs).

Treatment duration (longer duration of drug treatment resulted in higher relapse rate).

EEG classification (lower relapse rate with less severe EEG abnormalities).

Type of drug (higher relapse rate following withdrawal of valproic acid).

† Commission on Classification and Terminology of the International League Against Epilepsy. *Epilepsia*. 1981;22:489-501 and 1989;30:389-99.

Anticonvulsants: Indications and Pharmacokinetics

	Drug	Labeled indications	Protein binding (%)	Metabolism/ Excretion	t½ (hrs)	Therapeutic serum levels (mcg/mL)
Barbiturates	Phenobarbital[1] (PB)	Status epilepticus Cortical focal Tonic-clonic	40-60	Liver; 25% eliminated unchanged in urine	53-140	20-40
Hydantoins	Ethotoin	Tonic-clonic Psychomotor	nd	Liver; renal excretion of metabolites	3-9[3]	15-50
	Mephenytoin	Tonic-clonic Psychomotor Focal Jacksonian	nd	Liver	95 (active metabolite)	nd
	Phenytoin	Tonic-clonic Psychomotor Status epilepticus	≈ 90	Liver; renal excretion. < 5% excreted unchanged	Dose-dependent[2]	10-20
Succinimides	Ethosuximide	Absence	0	Liver; 25% excreted unchanged in urine	30 (children 7-9 yrs) 40-60 (adults)	40-100
	Methsuximide	Absence	nd	Liver; < 1% excreted unchanged in urine	< 2 (40, active metabolite)	nd
	Phensuximide	Absence	nd	Urine, bile	8 (active metabolite)	nd
Oxazolidinediones	Trimethadione	Absence	0	Demethylated to dimethadione; 3% excreted unchanged	6-13 days (dimethadione)	≥ 700 (dimethadione)
Benzodiazepines	Clonazepam	Absence Myoclonic Akinetic	50-85	5 metabolites identified; urine is major excretion route	18-60	20-80 ng/ml
	Clorazepate	Partial[4]	97	Hydrolyzed in stomach to desmethyldiazepam (active); metabolized in liver, renally excreted	30-100	nd
	Diazepam	Status epilepticus[4] Convulsive disorders, all forms[4]	97-99	Liver, active metabolites	20-50	nd
	Lamotrigine	Partial (adults)	≈ 55	Glucuronic acid conjugation to inactive metabolites; 94% excreted in urine, 2% in feces.	≈ 33[5]	nd
Adjuncts to anticonvulsants	Carbamazepine	Tonic-clonic Mixed Psychomotor	≈ 75	Liver to active 10, 11–epoxide. 72% excreted in urine, 28% in feces	18-54 (initial) 10-20[5] ≈ 6 (10, 11- epoxide)	4-12
	Felbamate[6]	Partial (adults) Partial/generalized assoc. with Lennox-Gastaut syndrome (children)	22-25	40% to 50% unchanged in urine, 40% as unidentified metabolites and conjugates	20-23	nd[7]
	Gabapentin	Partial (adults) with and without secondary generalization	< 3	Not appreciably metabolized; excreted in urine unchanged	5-7	nd
	Primidone	Tonic-clonic Psychomotor Focal	20-25	Metabolized to PB and PEMA, both active	5-15 (primidone) 10-18 (PEMA) 53-140 (PB)	5-12 (primidone) 15-40 (PB)
	Valproic acid	Absence	80-94	Liver, excreted in urine	6-20	50-150

[1] Other barbiturates are also used as anticonvulsants. See Sedatives/Hypnotics section.
[2] Exhibits dose-dependent, nonlinear pharmacokinetics.
[3] Below 8 mcg/ml; > 8 mcg/ml, t½ not defined due to dose-dependent, nonlinear pharmacokinetics.
[4] Recommended for adjunctive use.
[5] Following multiple administrations (150 mg twice daily) to normal volunteers taking no other medications, lamotrigine induced its own metabolism, resulting in a 25% decrease in half-life compared to values obtained in the same volunteers following a single dose. Evidence gathered from other sources suggests that self-induction may not occur when lamotrigine is given as adjunctive therapy in patients receiving enzyme-inducing antiepileptic drugs (EIAEDs).
[6] Because of cases of aplastic anemia, it has been recommended that the use of this drug be discontinued unless, in the judgment of the physician, continued therapy is warranted. Refer to the specific monograph.
[7] Value of monitoring blood levels not established.

Hydantoins

Refer to the general discussion beginning in the Anticonvulsants introduction.

Indications

Control of grand mal and psychomotor seizures.

➤*Phenytoin:* To prevent and treat seizures occurring during or following neurosurgery.

Parenteral – For the control of status epilepticus of the grand mal type.

➤*Unlabeled uses:* Phenytoin is useful as an antiarrhythmic agent, particularly in cardiac glycoside-induced arrhythmias. (Oral loading dose = 14 mg/kg; oral maintenance = 200 to 400 mg/day. IV loading dose = 50 mg every 5 minutes to total dose of 1 g; IV maintenance dose = 200 to 400 mg/day.) Pharmacokinetic, electrophysiologic and ECG effects of phenytoin are summarized in the Antiarrhythmic Agents monograph.

Phenytoin has been used as an alternative to magnesium sulfate for severe preeclampsia (15 mg/kg IV, given as 10 mg/kg initially and 5 mg/kg 2 hours later).

Phenytoin has been used in the treatment of trigeminal neuralgia (tic douloureux), recessive dystrophic epidermolysis bullosa and junctional epidermolysis bullosa.

Actions

➤*Pharmacology:* The primary site of action of the hydantoins appears to be the motor cortex, where the spread of seizure activity is inhibited. Possibly by promoting sodium efflux from neurons, hydantoins tend to stabilize the threshold against hyperexcitability caused by excessive stimulation or environmental changes capable of reducing membrane sodium gradient. This includes the reduction of post-tetanic potentiation at synapses. Loss of posttetanic potentiation prevents cortical seizure foci from detonating adjacent cortical areas. Hydantoins reduce the maximal activity of brain stem centers responsible for the tonic phase of grand mal seizures.

Phenytoin is available as phenytoin acid (chewable tablets, suspension) or phenytoin sodium (capsules, injection); phenytoin sodium contains 92% phenytoin.

➤*Pharmacokinetics:*

Absorption / Distribution – Phenytoin is slowly absorbed from the small intestine. Rate and extent of absorption varies and is dependent on the product formulation. Bioavailability may differ among products of different manufacturers. Oral phenytoin sodium extended reaches peak plasma levels in 12 hours; phenytoin sodium prompt peaks within 1.5 to 3 hours. Administration IM results in precipitation of phenytoin at the injection site, resulting in slow and erratic absorption, which may continue for up to 5 days or more; 50% to 75% of an IM dose is absorbed within 24 hours. Plasma levels vary and are significantly lower than those achieved with an equal oral dose. Plasma protein binding is 87% to 93% and is lower in uremic patients and neonates. Volume of distribution averages 0.6 L/kg.

Phenytoin's therapeutic plasma concentration is 10 to 20 mcg/ml, although many patients achieve complete seizure control at lower serum concentrations. At plasma concentrations > 20 mcg/ml, far-lateral nystagmus may occur and at concentrations > 30 and 40 mcg/ml, ataxia and gross mental changes are usually seen.

Metabolism / Excretion – Phenytoin is metabolized in the liver to inactive hydroxylated metabolites and excreted in the urine by tubular secretion. The metabolism of phenytoin is capacity-limited and shows saturability. The major metabolite is 5–(p–hydroxyphenyl)-5–phenylhydantoin (p–HPPH); 1% to 5% is excreted unchanged. Because the elimination of p–HPPH glucuronide is rate-limited by its formation from phenytoin, measurement of the metabolite in urine can be used to assess the rate of phenytoin metabolism, patient compliance or bioavailability. Elimination is exponential (first-order) at plasma concentrations < 10 mcg/ml, and plasma half-life ranges from 6 to 24 hours. Dose-dependent elimination is apparent at higher concentrations, and half-life increases; values of 20 to 60 hours may be found at therapeutic levels. A genetically determined limitation in ability to metabolize phenytoin has occurred. Good correlation is generally seen between total phenytoin plasma concentration and therapeutic effects. Serum level monitoring is essential.

Contraindications

Hypersensitivity to hydantoins.

➤*Phenytoin:* Because of its effect on ventricular automaticity, do not use phenytoin in sinus bradycardia, sino-atrial block, second and third degree AV block or in patients with Adams-Stokes syndrome.

Warnings

➤*Abrupt withdrawal:* Abrupt withdrawal in epileptic patients may precipitate status epilepticus. Reduce dosage, discontinue or substitute other anticonvulsant medication gradually.

➤*Other seizures:* Hydantoins are not indicated in seizures due to hypoglycemia or other metabolic causes. Perform appropriate diagnostic procedures.

➤*Phenytoin:* Use with caution in hypotension and severe myocardial insufficiency.

➤*Hypersensitivity reactions:* In the event of an allergic or hypersensitivity reaction, rapid substitution of alternative therapy may be necessary. Alternative therapy should be an anticonvulsant not belonging to the hydantoin chemical class. Phenytoin hypersensitivity reactions are not typical; they may present as one of many different syndromes (eg, lymphoma, hepatitis, Stevens-Johnson syndrome) and may include such symptoms as fever, rash, arthralgias or lymphadenopathy.

➤*Hepatic function impairment:* Biotransformation of hydantoins occurs in the liver; elderly patients or those with impaired liver function or severe illness may show early signs of toxicity. Discontinue drug if hepatic dysfunction occurs.

Induced abnormalities – Phenytoin-induced hepatitis is one of the more commonly reported hypersensitivity syndromes.

➤*Pregnancy:* Refer to information for use during pregnancy in the Anticonvulsants introduction. If megaloblastic anemia occurs during gestation, consider folic acid therapy.

➤*Lactation:* These drugs are excreted in breast milk. Because of the potential for serious adverse reactions in nursing infants, decide whether to discontinue nursing or to discontinue the drug.

Precautions

➤*Hematologic effects:* Perform blood counts and urinalyses when therapy is begun and at monthly intervals for several months thereafter. Blood dyscrasias have occurred. Avoid use in combination with other drugs known to adversely affect the hematopoietic system. Be alert for general malaise, sore throat, fever, mucous membrane bleeding, glandular swelling, petechiae, epistaxis, easy bruising, cutaneous reactions and other symptoms indicative of blood dyscrasias. Signs of marked depression of the blood count indicate the need for drug withdrawal.

Some evidence suggests that hydantoins may interfere with folic acid metabolism, precipitating megaloblastic anemia.

➤*Dermatologic effects:* Discontinue these drugs if a skin rash appears. If the rash is exfoliative, purpuric or bullous, do not resume use. If the rash is milder (measles-like or scarlatiniform), resume therapy after the rash has completely disappeared. If rash recurs upon reinstitution of therapy, further medication is contraindicated.

➤*Lymph node hyperplasia:* Lymph node hyperplasia has been associated with hydantoins, and may represent a hypersensitivity reaction. Rarely, this may progress to frank malignant lymphoma. If lymph node enlargement occurs, attempt to substitute another anticonvulsant drug or drug combination.

Differentiate lymphadenopathy from other lymph gland pathology. Lymphadenopathy which simulates Hodgkin's disease has been observed. If a lymphoma-like syndrome develops, withdraw the drug and observe the patient closely for regression of signs and symptoms before resuming treatment.

Monoclonal gammopathy and multiple myeloma have occurred during prolonged phenytoin therapy.

➤*Hyperglycemia:* Hyperglycemia, resulting from the drug's inhibitory effect on insulin release, has occurred. Hydantoins may also raise blood sugar levels in hyperglycemic persons.

➤*Cardiovascular:* Death from cardiac arrest has occurred after too-rapid IV administration, sometimes preceded by marked QRS widening. Observe the patient closely when the drug is administered IV when possible SA node depression exists. Administer cautiously in the presence of advanced AV block. Do not exceed an IV infusion rate of 50 mg/minute.

➤*Grand mal and petit mal seizures:* Drugs that control grand mal seizures are not effective for petit mal seizures. Therefore, if both conditions are present, combined drug therapy is needed.

➤*Slow metabolism:* A small percentage of individuals treated with hydantoins metabolize the drug slowly. Slow metabolism may be due to limited enzyme availability and lack of induction. It appears to be genetically determined. Metabolism of phenytoin is dose-dependent.

➤*Osteomalacia:* Osteomalacia has been associated with phenytoin therapy.

➤*Acute intermittent porphyria:* Administer hydantoins cautiously to patients with acute intermittent porphyria.

Drug Interactions

The following drug interactions have occurred with the use of phenytoin; however, they may occur when using any of the hydantoins.

➤*Increased pharmacologic effects:* Increased pharmacologic effects of hydantoins may occur when the following drugs are administered concurrently. Mechanisms of these interactions may include:

Hydantoin Drug Interactions: Increased Hydantoin Effects

Inhibit metabolism		Displace anticonvulsant	Unknown
Allopurinol Amiodarone Benzodiazepines Chloramphenicol Cimetidine Disulfiram Ethanol (acute ingestion) Fluconazole Isoniazid	Metronidazole Miconazole Omeprazole Phenacemide Phenylbutazone Succinimides Sulfonamides Trimethoprim Valproic acid[2]	Salicylates[1] Tricyclic antidepressants Valproic acid[2]	Chlorpheniramine Ibuprofen Phenothiazines

[1] **Salicylates** displace phenytoin from its plasma protein binding sites in a dose-dependent manner; no significant change occurs in the free phenytoin level.
[2] **Valproic acid** affects phenytoin disposition in different ways. Displacement of phenytoin from plasma proteins increases the free fraction and decreases total phenytoin levels; the concentration of unbound phenytoin is not significantly altered. Increased levels may result from inhibition of phenytoin metabolism. Conversely, phenytoin increases metabolism of valproic acid.

➤*Decreased pharmacologic effects:* Decreased pharmacologic effects of hydantoins may occur when the following drugs are administered concurrently. Mechanisms of these interactions may include:

Hydantoin Drug Interactions: Decreased Hydantoin Effects		
Increase metabolism	Decrease absorption	Unknown
Barbiturates[1]	Antacids	Antineoplastics
Carbamazepine[2]	Charcoal	Folic acid[3]
Diazoxide	Sucralfate	Influenza virus vaccine[4]
Ethanol (chronic ingestion)		Loxapine
Rifampin		Nitrofurantoin
Theophylline		Pyridoxine

[1] **Barbiturates'** effect on phenytoin is variable and unpredictable. Addition of phenytoin generally increases phenobarbital serum concentrations. Individual monitoring is needed, especially when starting or stopping either drug.
[2] **Carbamazepine's** effect on phenytoin is variable. Carbamazepine serum levels may also be decreased.
[3] See also Drug/Food interactions.
[4] **Influenza virus vaccine** may increase, decrease, or have no effect on total serum phenytoin concentrations.

➤*Phenytoin:* Phenytoin may decrease the pharmacologic effects of the following drugs:

Hydantoin Drug Interactions: Decreased Effects of Other Drugs		
Increased metabolism by phenytoin		Other
Acetaminophen[1]	Haloperidol	Cyclosporine
Amiodarone	Methadone	Dopamine
Carbamazepine	Metyrapone[2]	Furosemide
Cardiac glycosides	Mexiletine	Levodopa
Corticosteroids	Oral contraceptives	Levonorgestrel
Dicumarol	Quinidine	Mebendazole
Disopyramide	Theophylline	Nondepolarizing muscle relaxants
Doxycycline	Valproic acid	Phenothiazines
Estrogens		Sulfonylureas

[1] Although the therapeutic effects of acetaminophen may be reduced by concomitant phenytoin use, the potential hepatotoxicity of acetaminophen may be increased, especially with chronic phenytoin use.
[2] See also Drug/Lab test interactions.

Hydantoin Drug Interactions			
Precipitant drug	Object drug*		Descriptions
Clonazepam	Phenytoin	↓↑	Plasma levels of clonazepam or phenytoin may be decreased with concomitant use, or phenytoin toxicity may occur.
Phenytoin	Clonazepam	↓	
Corticosteroid	Phenytoin	↓	Corticosteroid use may mask systemic manifestations of phenytoin hypersensitivity reactions.
Phenytoin	Dopamine	↓	Five critically ill patients requiring dopamine to maintain blood pressure developed severe hypotension when IV phenytoin was administered.
Phenytoin	Lithium	↑	Lithium toxicity may be increased by coadministration of phenytoin. Marked neurologic symptoms were reported despite normal serum levels of lithium.
Phenytoin	Meperidine	↑	Meperidine's analgesic effectiveness may be decreased, while the toxic effects could be increased by phenytoin. The hepatic metabolism of meperidine is increased, but the formation of normeperidine, a potentially toxic metabolite, is increased.
Phenytoin	Primidone	↑	Primidone's pharmacologic effects may be increased by phenytoin administration; toxicity has occurred. The metabolic conversion of primidone to phenobarbital and phenylethylmalonamide (PEMA) may also be increased. Monitor serum concentrations of primidone and primidone metabolites following alterations in hydantoin therapy.
Phenytoin	Warfarin	↑	Warfarin may be displaced by phenytoin; in one report, a patient died of bleeding complications.

Hydantoin Drug Interactions			
Precipitant drug	Object drug*		Descriptions
Phenytoin Carbamazepine	Cisatracurium Besylate	↓	Resistance to the neuromuscular blocking action of nondepolarizing agents has been demonstrated in patients chronically administered phenytoin or carbamazepine. Slightly shorter durations of neuromuscular block may be anticipated and infusion rate requirements may be higher.

* ↑ = Object drug increased. ↓ = Object drug decreased.

➤*Drug/Lab test interactions:* Phenytoin may interfere with the **metyrapone** and the 1 mg **dexamethasone** tests. Discontinuing hydantoins prior to metyrapone testing would be ideal, but not practical; consider doubling the oral metyrapone dose.

➤*Drug/Food interactions:* Several case reports and single-dose studies suggest that enteral nutritional therapy may decrease phenytoin concentrations; however, this has not been substantiated. Monitor phenytoin concentrations. Consider giving phenytoin 2 hours before and after the enteral feeding, or stopping the enteral therapy for 2 hours before and after phenytoin administration.

Long-term phenytoin therapy may result in folate deficiency, possibly progressing to megaloblastic anemia (rare).

Adverse Reactions

➤*Cardiovascular:*

Phenytoin IV – Cardiovascular collapse; CNS depression; hypotension (when the drug is administered rapidly IV). Rate of administration is very important; do not exceed 50 mg/minute. Severe cardiotoxic reactions and fatalities have occurred with atrial and ventricular conduction depression and ventricular fibrillation, most commonly in elderly or gravely ill patients.

➤*CNS:*

Most common – Nystagmus; ataxia; dysarthria; slurred speech; mental confusion; dizziness; insomnia; transient nervousness; motor twitchings; diplopia; fatigue; irritability; drowsiness; depression; numbness; tremor; headache. These side effects may disappear by reducing dosage. Psychotic disturbances and increased seizures have occurred, but a definite causal relationship is uncertain. Choreoathetosis following IV phenytoin infusion has occurred.

➤*Dermatologic:* Manifestations sometimes accompanied by fever have included scarlatiniform, morbilliform, maculopapular, urticarial and nonspecific rashes; a morbilliform rash is the most common. Rashes are more frequent in children and young adults. Serious forms which may be fatal include bullous, exfoliative or purpuric dermatitis, lupus erythematosus syndrome, Stevens-Johnson syndrome and toxic epidermal necrolysis. Hirsutism and alopecia have occurred.

➤*Endocrine:* Diabetes insipidus; hyperglycemia.

➤*GI:* Nausea; vomiting; diarrhea; constipation. Administration of the drug with or immediately after meals may help prevent GI discomfort.

Gingival hyperplasia – Gingival hyperplasia occurs frequently with phenytoin; incidence may be reduced by good oral hygiene, including gum massage, frequent brushing and appropriate dental care.

➤*Hepatic:* Toxic hepatitis and liver damage may occur and rarely can be fatal. Hypersensitivity reactions with hepatic involvement include hepatocellular degeneration and fatal hepatocellular necrosis. Hepatitis, jaundice and nephrosis have been reported, but a definite cause and effect relationship has not been established. See Warnings.

➤*Hematologic:* Hematopoietic complications, some fatal, include thrombocytopenia, leukopenia, granulocytopenia, agranulocytosis and pancytopenia. Macrocytosis and megaloblastic anemia usually respond to folic acid therapy. Eosinophilia; monocytosis; leukocytosis; simple anemia; hemolytic anemia; aplastic anemia; ecchymosis.

➤*Lab test abnormalities:* Phenytoin may decrease serum thyroxine and free thyroxine concentrations. Although these decreases are generally not associated with clinical hypothyroidism, some patients may develop goiter or hypothyroidism.

➤*Respiratory:* Pneumonia; pharyngitis; sinusitis; hyperventilation; rhinitis; apnea; aspiration pneumonia; asthma; dyspnea; atelectasis; increased cough/sputum; epistaxis; hypoxia; pneumothorax; hemoptysis; bronchitis; chest pain; pulmonary fibrosis.

➤*Special senses:* Tinnitus; diplopia; taste perversion; amblyopia; deafness; visual field defect; eye pain; conjunctivitis; photophobia; hyperacusis; mydriasis; parosmia; ear pain; taste loss.

➤*Miscellaneous:* Polyarthropathy; hyperglycemia; weight gain; chest pain; edema; IgA depression; fever; photophobia; conjunctivitis; gynecomastia; periarteritis nodosa; pulmonary fibrosis; soft tissue injury at the injection site with and without extravasation of IV phenytoin; lymph node hyperplasia (see Precautions).

Connective tissue system – Coarsening of the facial features; enlargement of the lips; Peyronie's disease.

Overdosage

➤*Symptoms:* The lethal dose in adults is estimated to be 2 to 5 g. Initial symptoms are nystagmus, ataxia and dysarthria; the patient may then become comatose and hypotensive, with pupils unresponsive. At plasma concentrations > 20 mcg/ml, far-lateral nystagmus may occur and at concentrations > 30 mcg/ml, ataxia is usually seen. Significantly diminished mental capacity occurs at levels > 40 mcg/ml. Death is due to respiratory and circulatory depression.

➤*Treatment:* Treatment is nonspecific; there is no known antidote. Refer to General Management of Acute Overdosage. Consider hemodialysis, since phenytoin is not completely bound to plasma proteins. Total exchange transfusion has been utilized in the treatment of severe intoxication in children.

Patient Information

Take medication with food to reduce GI upset.

Phenytoin suspension must be thoroughly shaken immediately prior to use.

Do not discontinue medication abruptly or change dosage, except on advice of physician.

Maintain good oral hygiene (regular brushing and flossing) while taking phenytoin. Inform dentist of medication usage.

Patients should carry identification (*Medic Alert*) indicating medication usage and epilepsy.

May cause drowsiness, dizziness or blurred vision; alcohol may intensify these effects. Observe caution while driving or performing other tasks requiring alertness, coordination or physical dexterity. Notify physician if drowsiness, slurred speech or impaired coordination (ataxia) occurs.

Do not use capsules which are discolored.

➤*Diabetic patients:* Monitor urine sugar regularly and report any abnormalities to physician.

Notify physician if any of the following occurs: Skin rash; severe nausea or vomiting; swollen glands; bleeding, swollen or tender gums; yellowish discoloration of the skin or eyes; joint pain; unexplained fever; sore throat; unusual bleeding or bruising; persistent headache; malaise; any indication of an infection or bleeding tendency; pregnancy.

ETHOTOIN

Rx	**Peganone** (Ovation)	**Tablets:** 250 mg	Lactose. White, scored. In 100s.

ETHOTOIN — ORAL

For complete and comparative prescribing information, refer to the Hydantoins group monograph.

Indications

➤*Seizures:* For the control of tonic-clonic (grand mal) and complex partial (psychomotor) seizures.

Administration and Dosage

Ethotoin tablets are administered orally in 4 to 6 divided doses daily. The drug should be taken after food, and doses should be spaced as evenly as practicable. Initial dosage should be conservative. For adults, the initial daily dose should be 1 g or less, with subsequent gradual dosage increases over a period of several days. The optimum dosage must be determined on the basis of individual response. The usual adult maintenance dosage is 2 to 3 g daily. Less than 2 g daily has been found ineffective in most adults.

Pediatric dosage depends upon the age and weight of the patient. The initial dosage should not exceed 750 mg daily. The usual maintenance dose in children ranges from 500 mg to 1 g daily, although occasionally 2 or (rarely) 3 g daily may be necessary.

➤*Concomitant therapy:* If a patient is receiving another antiepileptic drug, it should not be discontinued when ethotoin therapy is begun. Reduce the dosage of the other drug gradually as the dosage of ethotoin is increased. Ethotoin may eventually replace the other drug or the optimal dosage of both antiepileptics may be established.

Ethotoin is compatible with all commonly employed antiepileptic medications, with the possible exception of phenacemide. In tonic-clonic (grand mal) seizures, use of the drug with phenobarbital may be beneficial. Ethotoin may be used in combination with drugs such as trimethadione or paramethadione, as an adjunct in those patients with absence (petit mal) associated with tonic-clonic (grand mal).

➤*Storage/Stability:* Store below 25°C (77°F).

FOSPHENYTOIN SODIUM

Rx	**Cerebyx** (Parke-Davis)	**Injection:** 150 mg (100 mg phenytoin sodium)	In 2 ml vials.
		750 mg (500 mg phenytoin sodium)	In 10 ml vials.

FOSPHENYTOIN SODIUM — INJECTION

For complete and comparative prescribing information, refer to the Hydantoins group monograph.

Indications

➤*Seizures:* For short-term parenteral administration when other means of phenytoin administration are unavailable, inappropriate or deemed less advantageous. The safety and effectiveness of fosphenytoin sodium in this use has not been systematically evaluated for more than 5 days.

Fosphenytoin sodium can be used for the control of generalized convulsive status epilepticus and prevention and treatment of seizures occurring during neurosurgery. It can also be substituted, short-term, for oral phenytoin.

Administration and Dosage

The dose, concentration in dosing solutions, and infusion rate of IV fosphenytoin sodium is expressed as phenytoin sodium equivalents (PE) to avoid the need to perform molecular weight-based adjustments when converting between fosphenytoin and phenytoin sodium doses. Fosphenytoin sodium should always be prescribed and dispensed in phenytoin sodium equivalent units (PE). Fosphenytoin sodium has important differences in administration from those for parenteral phenytoin sodium (see below).

Products with particulate matter or discoloration should not be used. Prior to IV infusion, dilute fosphenytoin sodium in 5% dextrose or 0.9% saline solution for injection to a concentration ranging from 1.5 to 25 mg PE/mL.

➤*Status epilepticus:* The loading dose of fosphenytoin sodium is 15 to 20 mg PE/kg administered at 100 to 150 mg PE/min.

Because of the risk of hypotension, fosphenytoin should be administered no faster than 150 mg PE/min. Continuous monitoring of the electrocardiogram, blood pressure, and respiratory function is essential and the patient should be observed throughout the period where maximal serum phenytoin concentrations occur, ≈ 10 to 20 minutes after the end of fosphenytoin sodium infusions.

Because the full antiepileptic effect of phenytoin, whether given as fosphenytoin sodium or parenteral phenytoin, is not immediate, other measures, including concomitant administration of an IV benzodiazepine, will usually be necessary for the control of status epilepticus.

The loading dose should be followed by maintenance doses of fosphenytoin sodium, or phenytoin either orally or parenterally.

If administration of fosphenytoin sodium does not terminate seizures, the use of other anticonvulsants and other appropriate measures should be considered.

IM fosphenytoin sodium should not be used in the treatment of status epilepticus because therapeutic phenytoin concentrations may not be reached as quickly as with IV administration. If IV access is impossible, loading doses of fosphenytoin sodium have been given by the IM route for other indications.

➤*Nonemergent loading and maintenance dosing:* The loading dose of fosphenytoin sodium is 10 to 20 mg PE/kg given IV or IM. The rate of administration for IV fosphenytoin sodium should be no greater than 150 mg PE/min. Continuous monitoring of the electrocardiogram, blood pressure, and respiratory function is essential and the patient should be observed throughout the period where maximal serum phenytoin concentrations occur, ≈ 10 to 20 minutes after the end of fosphenytoin sodium infusions.

The initial daily maintenance dose of fosphenytoin sodium is 4 to 6 mg PE/kg/day.

➤*IM or IV substitution for oral phenytoin therapy:* Fosphenytoin sodium can be substituted for oral phenytoin sodium therapy at the same total daily dose.

Dilantin capsules are ≈ 90% bioavailable by the oral route. Phenytoin, supplied as fosphenytoin sodium, is 100% bioavailable by both the IM and IV routes. For this reason, plasma phenytoin concentrations may increase modestly when IM or IV fosphenytoin sodium is substituted for oral phenytoin sodium therapy.

The rate of administration for IV fosphenytoin sodium should be no greater than 150 mg PE/min.

In controlled trials, IM fosphenytoin sodium was administered as a single daily dose utilizing either 1 or 2 injection sites. Some patients may require more frequent dosing.

➤*Special populations:*

Renal or hepatic disease function impairment – Due to an increased fraction of unbound phenytoin in patients with renal or hepatic disease, or in those with hypoalbuminemia, the interpretation of total phenytoin plasma concentrations should be made with caution. Unbound phenytoin concentrations may be more useful in these patient populations. After IV fosphenytoin sodium administration to patients with renal or hepatic disease, or in those with hypoalbuminemia, fosphenytoin clearance to phenytoin may be increased without a similar increase in phenytoin clearance. This has the potential to increase the frequency and severity of adverse events.

Elderly – Age does not have a significant impact on the pharmacokinetics of fosphenytoin following fosphenytoin sodium administration. Phenytoin clearance is decreased slightly in elderly patients and lower or less frequent dosing may be required.

➤*Storage/Stability:* Store under refrigeration at 2° to 8°C (36° to 46°F). The product should not be stored at room temperature for more than 48 hours. Vials that develop particulate matter should not be used.

PHENYTOIN SODIUM

Rx	**Phenytoin Sodium** (Elkins-Sinn)	**Injection:** 50 mg/ml (46 mg phenytoin)[1]	In 2 and 5 ml *Dosette* amps, 2 ml *Dosette* vials and 5 ml vials.

[1] With propylene glycol and alcohol.

PHENYTOIN SODIUM — PARENTERAL

For complete prescribing information, refer to the Hydantoins group monograph.

Administration and Dosage

Phenytoin sodium contains 92% phenytoin.

➤*IV administration:* The addition of phenytoin solution to an IV infusion is not recommended due to lack of solubility and resultant precipitation.

Inject parenteral phenytoin slowly and directly into a large vein through a large-gauge needle or IV catheter.

Do not exceed an IV infusion rate of 50 mg/minute in adults or 1 to 3 mg/kg/minute in neonates. There is a relatively small margin between full therapeutic effect and minimally toxic doses. Monitor ECG and blood pressure continuously. In status epilepticus, the IV route is preferred because of the delay in absorption with IM administration.

Follow each IV injection with an injection of sterile saline through the same needle or IV catheter to avoid local venous irritation due to alkalinity of the solution. Avoid continuous infusion.

PHENYTOIN SODIUM — PARENTERAL

Soft tissue irritation and injury, with and without extravasation of IV phenytoin, have occurred at the injection site.

Although not recommended, some studies indicate that an IV infusion of phenytoin may be feasible if proper precautions are observed, such as a suitable vehicle (eg, Sodium Chloride 0.9% or Lactated Ringer's injection), appropriate concentration, preparing the infusion shortly before administration and using an inline filter.

➤*IM administration:* Avoid the IM route due to erratic absorption of phenytoin and pain and muscle damage at the injection site. When IM administration is required for a patient previously stabilized orally, compensating dosage adjustments are necessary to maintain therapeutic plasma levels; an IM dose 50% greater than the oral dose is necessary. When returned to oral administration, reduce the dose by 50% of the original oral dose for 1 week to prevent excessive plasma levels due to sustained release from IM tissue sites. Determine serum drug levels when possible drug interactions are suspected.

If the patient requires > 1 week of IM therapy, consider alternative routes (eg, gastric intubation), using oral preparations. For periods < 1 week, the patient shifted back from IM administration should receive ½ the original oral dose for the same period of time the patient received IM therapy. Monitor plasma levels.

➤*Status epilepticus:* In adults, administer loading dose of 10 to 15 mg/kg slowly. Follow by maintenance doses of 100 mg orally or IV every 6 to 8 hours. For neonates and children, oral absorption of phenytoin is unreliable; IV loading dose is 15 to 20 mg/kg in divided doses of 5 to 10 mg/kg. If administration does not terminate the seizure, consider the use of other anticonvulsants, IV barbiturates, general anesthesia or other measures.

➤*Neurosurgery (prophylactic dosage):* 100 to 200 mg IM at ≈ 4 hour intervals during surgery and the postoperative period.

➤*Storage / Stability:* The solution is suitable for use as long as it remains free of haziness and precipitate. Upon refrigeration or freezing, a precipitate might form; this will dissolve again after the solution is allowed to stand at room temperature. The solution is still suitable for use. Use only a clear solution. A faint yellow color may develop, but has no effect on the potency of the solution.

PHENYTOIN

Rx	**Dilantin Infatab** (Parke-Davis)	**Tablets, chewable**: 50 mg	(P-D 007). Saccharin, sucrose. Yellow, scored. Triangular. In 100s and UD 100s.
Rx	**Phenytoin Sodium** (Various, eg, Major, Parmed, Zenith)	**Capsules**: 100 mg phenytoin sodium (92 mg phenytoin)	In 100s, 1000s and UD 100s.
Rx	**Dilantin Kapseals** (Parke-Davis)	**Capsules, extended release**: 30 mg phenytoin sodium (27.6 mg phenytoin)	Lactose, sucrose. (P-D 365). Transparent w/pink band. In 100s.
Rx	**Phenytoin Sodium** (Various, eg, Goldline, Major)	**Capsules, extended release**: 100 mg phenytoin sodium (92 mg phenytoin)	Clear. In 100s and 1000s.
Rx	**Dilantin Kapseals** (Parke-Davis)		Lactose, sucrose. (DILANTIN 100 mg). Transparent w/orange band. In 100s, 1000s and UD 100s.
Rx	**Phenytek** (Bertek)	**Capsules, extended release**: 200 mg phenytoin sodium	(BERTEK 670). Blue. In 30s and 100s.
Rx	**Phenytek** (Bertek)	**Capsules, extended release**: 300 mg phenytoin sodium	(BERTEK 750). Blue. In 30s and 100s.
Rx	**Phenytoin** (Alpharma)	**Suspension, oral**: 125 mg/5 ml	≤ 0.6% alcohol, sucrose. In 240 ml.
Rx	**Dilantin-125** (Parke-Davis)		≤ 0.6% alcohol, sucrose. Orange-vanilla flavor. In 240 ml.

PHENYTOIN — ORAL

For complete and comparative prescribing information, refer to the Hydantoins group monograph.

Indications

➤*Seizures:* For the control of generalized tonic-clonic (grand mal) and complex partial (psychomotor, temporal lobe) seizures and prevention and treatment of seizures occurring during or following neurosurgery.

Administration and Dosage

➤*Approved by the FDA:* September 25, 1992.

Serum concentrations should be monitored in changing from *Dilantin Kapseals* to prompt phenytoin sodium capsules, USP and from the sodium salt to the free acid form of phenytoin.

*Dilantin Kapseals*and phenytoin parenteral are formulated with the sodium salt of phenytoin. The free acid form of phenytoin is used in *Dilantin-125* oral suspension and *Dilantin Infatabs*. Because there is approximately an 8% increase in drug content with the free acid form over that of the sodium salt, dosage adjustments and serum level monitoring may be necessary when switching from a product formulated with the free acid to a product formulated with the sodium salt and vice versa.

➤*General:* Dosage should be individualized to provide maximum benefit. In some cases, serum blood level determinations may be necessary for optimal dosage adjustments. The clinically effective serum level is usually 10 to 20 mcg/mL. With recommended dosage, a period of 7 to 10 days may be required to achieve steady-state blood levels with phenytoin and changes in dosage (increase or decrease) should not be carried out at intervals shorter than 7 to 10 days.

➤*Adult Dosage:*

Dilantin Kapseals –

Divided daily dosage: Patients who have received no previous treatment may be started on one 100 mg *Dilantin Kapseal* 3 times daily and the dosage then adjusted to suit individual requirements. For most adults, the satisfactory maintenance dosage will be 1 capsule 3 to 4 times a day. An increase up to 2 capsules 3 times a day may be made, if necessary.

Once-a-day dosage: In adults, if seizure control is established with divided doses of three 100 mg *Dilantin Kapseals* daily, once-a-day dosage with 300 mg of *Dilantin Kapseals* may be considered. Studies comparing divided doses of 300 mg with a single daily dose of this quantity indicated absorption, peak plasma levels, biologic half-life, difference between peak and minimum values, and urinary recovery were equivalent. Once-a-day dosage offers a convenience to the individual patient or to nursing personnel for institutionalized patients and is intended to be used only for patients requiring this amount of drug daily. A major problem in motivating noncompliant patients may also be lessened when the patient can take this drug once a day. However, patients should be cautioned not to miss a dose, inadvertently.

Only *Dilantin Kapseals* are recommended for once-a-day dosing. Inherent differences in dissolution characteristics and resultant absorption rates of phenytoin due to different manufacturing procedures and/or dosage forms preclude such recommendation for other phenytoin products. When a change in the dosage form or brand is prescribed, careful monitoring of phenytoin serum levels should be carried out.

Loading dose: Some authorities have advocated use of an oral loading dose of phenytoin in adults who require rapid steady-state serum levels and where IV administration is not desirable. This dosing regimen should be reserved for patients in a clinic or hospital setting where phenytoin serum levels can be closely monitored. Patients with a history of renal or liver disease should not receive the oral loading regimen.

Initially, 1 g of phenytoin capsules is divided into 3 doses (400 mg, 300 mg, 300 mg) and administered at 2-hour intervals. Normal maintenance dosage is then instituted 24 hours after the loading dose, with frequent serum level determinations.

Dilantin Infatabs – Patients who have received no previous treatment may be started on 2 *Dilantin Infatabs* 3 times daily, and the dose is then adjusted to suit individual requirements. For most adults, the satisfactory maintenance dosage will be 6 to 8 tablets daily; an increase to 12 tablets daily may be made, if necessary.

Dilantin Infatabs are not for once-a-day dosing. *Dilantin Infatabs* can be either chewed thoroughly before being swallowed or swallowed whole.

Dilantin-125 – Patients who have received no previous treatment may be started on 1 teaspoonful (5 mL) of *Dilantin-125* oral suspension 3 times daily, and the dose is then adjusted to suit individual requirements. An increase to 5 teaspoonfuls daily may be made, if necessary.

➤*Children:*

Dilantin Kapseals – Initially, 5 mg/kg/day in 2 or 3 equally divided doses, with subsequent dosage individualized to a maximum of 300 mg daily. A recommended daily maintenance dosage is usually 4 to 8 mg/kg. Children over 6 years old and adolescents may require the minimum adult dose (300 mg/day).

Dilantin Infatabs – Initially, 5 mg/kg/day in 2 or 3 equally divided doses, with subsequent dosage individualized to a maximum of 300 mg daily. A recommended daily maintenance dosage is usually 4 to 8 mg/kg. Children over 6 years old and adolescents may require the minimum adult dose (300 mg/day).

If the daily dosage cannot be divided equally, the larger dose should be given before retiring.

Dilantin-125 – Initially, 5 mg/kg/day in 2 or 3 equally divided doses, with subsequent dosage individualized to a maximum of 300 mg daily. A recommended daily maintenance dosage is usually 4 to 8 mg/kg. Children over 6 years old and adolescents may require the minimum adult dose (300 mg/day).

➤*Storage / Stability:*

Dilantin Infatabs and *Dilantin Kapseals* – Store below 30°C (86°F). Protect from light and moisture.

Dilantin-125 Oral Suspension – Store at controlled room temperature 20° to 25°C (68° to 77°F). Protect from freezing and light.

Refer to the general discussion beginning in the Anticonvulsants introduction.

Indications

Control of absence (petit mal) seizures.

➤*Methsuximide:* For petit mal seizures when refractory to other drugs.

Actions

➤*Pharmacology:* Succinimides suppress the paroxysmal three cycle per second spike and wave activity associated with lapses of consciousness common in absence (petit mal) seizures. The frequency of epileptiform attacks is reduced, apparently by motor cortex depression and elevation of the threshold of the CNS to convulsive stimuli.

➤*Pharmacokinetics:*

Absorption/Distribution – These agents are readily absorbed from the GI tract. Peak serum levels of ethosuximide are achieved in 3 to 7 hours; peak levels of methsuximide and phensuximide are reached in 1 to 4 hours. Therapeutic serum concentrations of ethosuximide range from 40 to 100 mcg/ml.

Metabolism/Excretion – Ethosuximide is extensively metabolized to inactive metabolites; ≈ 20% is excreted unchanged via the kidneys. The plasma half-life is 30 hours in children and 60 hours in adults. Less than 1% of a dose of methsuximide is recovered unchanged in urine; plasma half-lives range from 2.6 to 4 hours. Phensuximide is excreted in urine and in bile; half-life is ≈ 4 hours.

Contraindications

Hypersensitivity to succinimides.

Warnings

➤*Hematologic effects:* Blood dyscrasias, some fatal, have occurred; therefore, perform periodic blood counts. Should signs or symptoms of infection (eg, sore throat, fever) develop, consider blood counts at that point.

➤*Lupus:* Cases of systemic lupus erythematosus have occurred.

➤*Renal/Hepatic function impairment:* Succinimides have produced morphological and functional changes in animal liver. Abnormal liver and renal function have been reported in humans. For this reason, administer with extreme caution to patients with known liver or renal disease. Perform periodic urinalyses and liver function studies for all patients receiving these drugs.

➤*Pregnancy:* Refer to information for use during pregnancy in the Anticonvulsant introduction.

Precautions

➤*Grand mal seizures:* Succinimides, when used alone in mixed types of epilepsy, may increase the frequency of grand mal seizures in some patients.

➤*Dosage changes/other medication:* It is important to proceed slowly when increasing or decreasing dosage, and when adding or eliminating other medication. Abrupt withdrawal of anticonvulsant medication may precipitate absence (petit mal) status.

➤*Acute intermittent porphyria:* Use phensuximide with caution.

Drug Interactions

Succinimide Drug Interactions

Precipitant drug	Object drug*		Description
Succinimides	Hydantoins	↑	Serum hydantoin levels may be increased.
Succinimides	Primidone	↓	Lower primidone and phenobarbital levels may occur.
Valproic acid	Succinimides	↔	Both increases and decreases in succinimide levels have occurred.

* ↑ = Object drug increased. ↓ = Object drug decreased.
↔ = Undetermined clinical effect.

Adverse Reactions

The following have been reported with one or more of the succinimides:

➤*CNS:* Drowsiness; ataxia; dizziness; irritability; nervousness; headache; blurred vision; myopia; photophobia; hiccoughs; euphoria; dream-like state; lethargy; hyperactivity; fatigue; insomnia. Drowsiness, ataxia and dizziness are the most frequent **methsuximide** side effects.

➤*Dermatologic:* Pruritus; urticaria; Stevens-Johnson syndrome; pruritic erythematous rashes; skin eruptions; erythema multiforme; systemic lupus erythematosus; alopecia; hirsutism.

➤*GI:* (frequent): Nausea; vomiting; vague gastric upset; cramps; anorexia; diarrhea; weight loss; epigastric and abdominal pain; constipation.

➤*GU:* Urinary frequency, renal damage, hematuria (**phensuximide**), vaginal bleeding; microscopic hematuria.

➤*Hematologic:* Eosinophilia; granulocytopenia; leukopenia; agranulocytosis; monocytosis; pancytopenia, with or without bone marrow suppression.

➤*Psychiatric:* Confusion; instability; mental slowness; depression; hypochondriacal behavior; sleep disturbances; night terrors; aggressiveness; inability to concentrate. These effects may be noted particularly in patients who have previously exhibited psychological abnormalities. There have been rare reports of paranoid psychosis, suicidal behavior, auditory hallucinations, increased libido and increased state of depression.

➤*Miscellaneous:* Periorbital edema; hyperemia; muscle weakness; swelling of the tongue; gum hypertrophy.

Overdosage

The therapeutic range of ethosuximide serum levels is 40 to 100 mcg/ml, although levels as high as 150 mcg/ml have occurred without signs of toxicity. Methsuximide levels > 40 mcg/ml have caused toxicity; coma has been seen at levels of 150 mcg/ml.

➤*Symptoms:*

Acute overdosage – Confusion; sleepiness; unsteadiness; flaccid muscles; coma with slow, shallow respiration; hypotension; cyanosis; hypo- or hyperthermia; absent reflexes; nausea; vomiting; CNS depression including coma with respiratory depression.

Chronic overdosage – Skin rash; confusion; ataxia; dizziness; drowsiness; hangover; depression; irritability; poor judgment; periorbital edema; proteinuria; hepatic dysfunction; fatal bone marrow aplasia; delayed onset of coma; nausea; vomiting; muscular weakness; hematuria; casts; nephrosis.

➤*Treatment:* Treatment includes usual supportive measures. Refer to General Management of Acute Overdosage. Charcoal hemoperfusion may be indicated. Hemodialysis may be useful for ethosuximide. Forced diuresis and exchange transfusions are ineffective.

Patient Information

If GI upset occurs, take with food or milk.

Do not discontinue medication abruptly or change dosage, except on advice of physician.

Patients should carry identification (Medic Alert) indicating medication usage and epilepsy.

May cause drowsiness, dizziness or blurred vision; alcohol may exacerbate these effects. Use caution while driving or performing other tasks requiring alertness, coordination or physical dexterity.

Notify physician if any of the following occurs: Skin rash, joint pain, unexplained fever, sore throat, unusual bleeding or bruising, drowsiness, dizziness, blurred vision or pregnancy.

➤*Phensuximide:* Phensuximide may discolor the urine pink, red or red-brown. This is not harmful.

ETHOSUXIMIDE

Rx	**Ethosuximide** (Sidmak)	**Capsules**: 250 mg	In 100s.
Rx	**Zarontin** (Parke-Davis)		Sorbitol. (PD 237). In 100s.
Rx	**Ethosuximide** (Copley)	**Syrup**: 250 mg/5 ml	Saccharin, sucrose. Raspberry flavor. In 483 ml.
Rx	**Zarontin** (Parke-Davis)		Raspberry flavor. Saccharin, sucrose. In pt.

ETHOSUXIMIDE — ORAL

For complete and comparative prescribing information, refer to the Succinimides group monograph.

Indications

➤*Epilepsy:* For the control of absence (petit mal) epilepsy.

Administration and Dosage

➤*Approved by the FDA:* July 30, 1993.

➤*Patients 3 to 6 years of age:* 250 mg per day.

➤*Patients 6 years of age and older:* 500 mg per day.

➤*Dosage adjustment:* The dose thereafter must be individualized according to the patient's response. Dosage should be increased by small increments. One useful method is to increase the daily dose by 250 mg every 4 to 7 days until control is achieved with minimal side effects. Dosages exceeding 1.5 g daily, in divided doses, should be administered only under the strictest supervision of the physician. The optimal dose for most pediatric patients is 20 mg/kg/day. This dose has given average plasma levels within the accepted therapeutic range of 40 to 100 mcg/mL. Subsequent dose schedules can be based on effectiveness and plasma level determinations.

➤*Concomitant therapy:* Ethosuximide may be administered in combination with other anticonvulsants when other forms of epilepsy coexist with absence (petit mal).

➤*Storage/Stability:*

Capsule – Store at 25°C (77°F); excursions permitted to 15° to 30°C (59° to 86°F) [see USP controlled room temperature].

Syrup – Store below 30°C (86°F). Protect from freezing and light.

Succinimides

METHSUXIMIDE

Rx	**Celontin** (Parke-Davis)	**Capsules:** 150 mg	In 100s.
		300 mg	In 100s.

METHSUXIMIDE — ORAL

For complete and comparative prescribing information, refer to the Succinimides group monograph.

Indications

➤*Seizures:* For the control of absence (petit mal) seizures that are refractory to other drugs.

Administration and Dosage

Optimum dosage of methsuximide must be determined by trial. A suggested dosage schedule is 300 mg per day for the first week. If required, dosage may be increased thereafter at weekly intervals by 300 mg per day for the 3 weeks following to a daily dosage of 1.2 g. Because therapeutic effect and tolerance vary among patients, therapy with methsuximide must be individualized according to the response of each patient. Optimal dosage is that amount of methsuximide which is barely sufficient to control seizures so that side effects may be kept to a minimum. The smaller capsule (150 mg) facilitates administration to small children.

➤*Concomitant therapy:* Methsuximide may be administered in combination with other anticonvulsants when other forms of epilepsy coexist with absence (petit mal).

➤*Storage/Stability:* Store at 25°C (77°F); excursions permitted to 15° to 30°C (59° to 86°F) [see USP Controlled Room Temperature].

Protect from light and moisture. Protect from excessive heat 40°C (104°F).

Sulfonamides

ZONISAMIDE

Rx	**Zonisamide** (Various, eg, Barr, Mutual)	**Capsules:** 25 mg	In 30s, 60s, 100s, 250s, 500s, and 1,000s.
Rx	**Zonegran** (Eisai)		(ZONEGRAN 25). White. In 100s.
Rx	**Zonisamide** (Various, eg, Barr, Mutual)	**Capsules:** 50 mg	In 30s, 60s, 100s, 250s, 500s, and 1,000s.
Rx	**Zonegran** (Eisai)		(ZONEGRAN 50). White/Gray. In 100s.
Rx	**Zonisamide** (Various, eg, Barr, Dr. Reddy's, Mutual, UDL, Wockhardt)	**Capsules:** 100 mg	May contain lactose. In 30s, 60s, 100s, 250s, 500s, 1,000s, and UD 100s.
Rx	**Zonegran** (Eisai)		(ZONEGRAN 100). White/Red. In 100s.

ZONISAMIDE — ORAL

Indications

➤*Seizures:* As adjunctive therapy in the treatment of partial seizures in adults with epilepsy.

Administration and Dosage

➤*Approved by the FDA:* March 27, 2000.

Safety and efficacy in pediatric patients less than 16 years of age have not been established. Zonisamide should be administered once or twice daily, using 25, 50, or 100 mg capsules. Zonisamide is given orally and can be taken with or without food. Capsules should be swallowed whole.

➤*Adults over 16 years of age:* The prescriber should be aware that, because of the long half-life of zonisamide, up to 2 weeks may be required to achieve steady-state levels upon reaching a stable dose or following dosage adjustment. Although the regimen described below is one that has been shown to be tolerated, the prescriber may wish to prolong the duration of treatment at the lower doses in order to fully assess the effects of zonisamide at steady state, noting that many of the side effects of zonisamide are more frequent at doses of 300 mg/day and above. Although there is some evidence of greater response at doses above 100 to 200 mg/day, the increase appears small and formal dose-response studies have not been conducted.

The initial dose should be 100 mg daily. After 2 weeks, the dose may be increased to 200 mg/day for at least 2 weeks. It can be increased to 300 mg/day and 400 mg/day, with the dose stable for at least 2 weeks to achieve steady state at each level. Evidence from controlled trials suggests that zonisamide doses of 100 to 600 mg/day are effective, but there is no suggestion of increasing response above 400 mg/day. There is little experience with doses greater than 600 mg/day.

➤*Renal or hepatic function impairment:* Because zonisamide is metabolized in the liver and excreted by the kidneys, patients with renal or hepatic disease should be treated with caution, and might require slower titration and more frequent monitoring. Single 300 mg zonisamide doses were administered to 3 groups of volunteers. Group 1 was a healthy group with a creatinine clearance ranging from 70 to 152 mL/min. Group 2 and group 3 had creatinine clearances ranging from 14.5 to 59 mL/min and 10 to 20 mL/min, respectively. Zonisamide renal clearance decreased with decreasing renal function (3.42, 2.5, 2.23 mL/min, respectively). Marked renal impairment (creatinine clearance less than 20 mL/min) was associated with an increase in zonisamide AUC of 35%. The pharmacokinetics of zonisamide in patients with impaired liver function have not been studied.

➤*Storage/Stability:* Store at 25°C (77°F), excursions permitted to 15° to 30°C (59° to 86°F), in a dry place and protected from light.

Actions

➤*Pharmacology:* The precise mechanism(s) by which zonisamide exerts its antiseizure effect is unknown. Zonisamide demonstrated anticonvulsant activity in several experimental models. In animals, zonisamide was effective against tonic extension seizures induced by maximal electroshock but ineffective against clonic seizures induced by subcutaneous pentylenetetrazol. Zonisamide raised the threshold for generalized seizures in the kindled rat model and reduced the duration of cortical focal seizures induced by electrical stimulation of the visual cortex in cats. Furthermore, zonisamide suppressed both interictal spikes and the secondarily generalized seizures produced by cortical application of tungstic acid gel in rats or by cortical freezing in cats. The relevance of these models to human epilepsy is unknown.

Zonisamide may produce these effects through action at sodium and calcium channels. In vitro pharmacological studies suggest that zonisamide blocks sodium channels and reduces voltage-dependent, transient inward currents (T-type Ca^{2+} currents), consequently stabilizing neuronal membranes and suppressing neuronal hypersynchronization. In vitro binding studies have demonstrated that zonisamide binds to the GABA/benzodiazepine receptor ionophore complex in an allosteric fashion which does not produce changes in chloride flux. Other in vitro studies have demonstrated that zonisamide (10 to 30 mcg/mL) suppresses synaptically driven electrical activity without affecting postsynaptic GABA or glutamate responses (cultured mouse spinal cord neurons) or neuronal or glial uptake of [^{3}H]-GABA (rat hippocampal slices). Thus, zonisamide does not appear to potentiate the synaptic activity of GABA. In vivo microdialysis studies demonstrated that zonisamide facilitates both dopaminergic and serotonergic neurotransmission. Zonisamide also has weak carbonic anhydrase inhibiting activity, but this pharmacologic effect is not thought to be a major contributing factor in the antiseizure activity of zonisamide.

➤*Pharmacokinetics:*

Absorption – Following a 200 to 400 mg oral zonisamide dose, peak plasma concentrations (range, 2 to 5 mcg/mL) in healthy volunteers occur within 2 to 6 hours. In the presence of food, the time to maximum concentration is delayed, occurring at 4 to 6 hours, but food has no effect on the bioavailability of zonisamide. Zonisamide extensively binds to erythrocytes, resulting in an 8-fold higher concentration of zonisamide in red blood cells (RBC) than in plasma. The pharmacokinetics of zonisamide are dose proportional in the range of 200 to 400 mg, but the C_{max} and AUC increase disproportionately at 800 mg, perhaps due to saturable binding of zonisamide to RBC. Once a stable dose is reached, steady state is achieved within 14 days. The elimination half-life of zonisamide in plasma is about 63 hours. The elimination half-life of zonisamide in RBC is approximately 105 hours.

Distribution – The apparent volume of distribution (V/F) of zonisamide is about 1.45 L/kg following a 400 mg oral dose. Zonisamide, at concentrations of 1 to 7 mcg/mL, is approximately 40% bound to human plasma proteins. Protein binding of zonisamide is unaffected in the presence of therapeutic concentrations of phenytoin, phenobarbital or carbamazepine.

Metabolism/Excretion – Following oral administration of ^{14}C-zonisamide to healthy volunteers, only zonisamide was detected in plasma. Zonisamide is excreted primarily in urine as parent drug and as the glucuronide of a metabolite. Following multiple dosing, 62% of the ^{14}C dose was recovered in the urine, with 3% in the feces by day 10. Zonisamide undergoes acetylation to form N-acetyl zonisamide and reduction to form the open ring metabolite, 2-sulfamoylacetyl phenol (SMAP). Of the excreted dose, 35% was recovered as zonisamide, 15% as N-acetyl zonisamide, and 50% as the glucuronide of SMAP. Reduction of zonisamide to SMAP is mediated by cytochrome P450 isozyme 3A4 (CYP3A4). Zonisamide does not induce its own metabolism. Plasma clearance of zonisamide is approximately 0.3 to 0.35 mL/min/kg in patients not receiving enzyme-inducing antiepilepsy drugs (AEDs). The clearance of zonisamide is increased to 0.5 mL/min/kg in patients concurrently on enzyme-inducing AEDs.

Renal clearance is about 3.5 mL/min. The clearance of an oral dose of zonisamide from RBC is 2 mL/min.

ZONISAMIDE — ORAL

Special populations –

Renal function impairment: See Warnings for more information.

Hepatic function impairment: See Warnings for more information.

Contraindications

Zonisamide is contraindicated in patients who have demonstrated hypersensitivity to sulfonamides or zonisamide.

Warnings

➤*Potentially fatal reactions to sulfonamides:* Fatalities have occurred, although rarely, as a result of severe reactions to sulfonamides (zonisamide is a sulfonamide) including Stevens-Johnson syndrome, toxic epidermal necrolysis, fulminant hepatic necrosis, agranulocytosis, aplastic anemia, and other blood dyscrasias. Such reactions may occur when a sulfonamide is readministered irrespective of the route of administration. If signs of hypersensitivity or other serious reactions occur, discontinue zonisamide immediately. Specific experience with sulfonamide-type adverse reaction to zonisamide is described below.

➤*Serious skin reactions:* Consideration should be given to discontinuing zonisamide in patients who develop an otherwise unexplained rash. If the drug is not discontinued, patients should be observed frequently. Seven deaths from severe rash (ie, Stevens-Johnson syndrome [SJS] and toxic epidermal necrolysis [TEN]) were reported in the first 11 years of marketing in Japan. All of the patients were receiving other drugs in addition to zonisamide. In postmarketing experience from Japan, a total of 49 cases of SJS or TEN have been reported, a reporting rate of 46 per million patient-years of exposure. Although this rate is greater than background, it is probably an underestimate of the true incidence because of under-reporting. There were no confirmed cases of SJS or TEN in the US, European, or Japanese development programs.

In the US and European randomized controlled trials, 6 of 269 (2.2%) zonisamide patients discontinued treatment because of rash compared to none on placebo. Across all trials during the US and European development, rash that led to discontinuation of zonisamide was reported in 1.4% of patients (12 events per 1000 patient-years of exposure). During Japanese development, serious rash or rash that led to study drug discontinuation was reported in 2% of patients (27.8 events per 1000 patient years). Rash usually occurred early in treatment, with 85% reported within 16 weeks in the US and European studies and 90% reported within 2 weeks in the Japanese studies. There was no apparent relationship of dose to the occurrence of rash.

➤*Serious hematologic events:* Two confirmed cases of aplastic anemia and 1 confirmed case of agranulocytosis were reported in the first 11 years of marketing in Japan, rates greater than generally accepted background rates. There were no cases of aplastic anemia and 2 confirmed cases of agranulocytosis in the US, European, or Japanese development programs. There is inadequate information to assess the relationship, if any, between dose and duration of treatment and these events.

➤*Seizures on withdrawal:* As with other AEDs, abrupt withdrawal of zonisamide in patients with epilepsy may precipitate increased seizure frequency or status epilepticus. Dose reduction or discontinuation of zonisamide should be done gradually.

➤*Cognitive/neuropsychiatric adverse reactions:* Use of zonisamide was frequently associated with central nervous system-related adverse reactions. The most significant of these can be classified into 3 general categories:

1.) Psychiatric symptoms, including depression and psychosis.
2.) Psychomotor slowing, difficulty with concentration, and speech or language problems, in particular, word-finding difficulties.
3.) Somnolence or fatigue.

In placebo-controlled trials, 2.2% of patients discontinued zonisamide or were hospitalized for depression compared to 0.4% of placebo patients, while 1.1% of zonisamide and 0.4% of placebo patients attempted suicide. Among all epilepsy patients treated with zonisamide, 1.4% were discontinued and 1% were hospitalized because of reported depression or suicide attempts. In placebo-controlled trials, 2.2% of patients discontinued zonisamide or were hospitalized due to psychosis or psychosis-related symptoms compared to none of the placebo patients. Among all epilepsy patients treated with zonisamide, 0.9% were discontinued and 1.4% were hospitalized because of reported psychosis or related symptoms.

Psychomotor slowing and difficulty with concentration occurred in the first month of treatment and were associated with doses above 300 mg/day. Speech and language problems tended to occur after 6 to 10 weeks of treatment and at doses above 300 mg/day. Although in most cases these reactions were of mild to moderate severity, they at times led to withdrawal from treatment.

Somnolence and fatigue were frequently reported CNS adverse reactions during clinical trials with zonisamide. Although in most cases these events were of mild to moderate severity, they led to withdrawal from treatment in 0.2% of the patients enrolled in controlled trials. Somnolence and fatigue tended to occur within the first month of treatment. Somnolence and fatigue occurred most frequently at doses of 300 to 500 mg/day. Patients should be cautioned about this possibility and special care should be taken by patients if they drive, operate machinery, or perform any hazardous task.

➤*Renal/Hepatic function impairment:* Single 300 mg zonisamide doses were administered to 3 groups of volunteers. Group 1 was a healthy group with a creatinine clearance ranging from 70 to 152 mL/min. Group 2 and group 3 had creatinine clearances ranging from 14.5 to 59 mL/min and 10 to 20 mL/min, respectively. Zonisamide renal clearance decreased with decreasing renal function (3.42, 2.5, 2.23 mL/min, respectively). Marked renal impairment (creatinine clearance less than 20 mL/min) was associated with an increase in zonisamide AUC of 35%. The pharmacokinetics of zonisamide in patients with impaired liver function have not been studied. Somnolence is commonly reported, especially at higher doses of zonisamide. Zonisamide is metabolized by the liver and eliminated by the kidneys; caution should therefore be exercised when administering zonisamide to patients with hepatic and renal dysfunction.

➤*Mutagenesis:* Zonisamide increased mutation frequency in Chinese hamster lung cells in the absence of metabolic activation. Zonisamide was not mutagenic or clastogenic in Ames test, mouse lymphoma assay, sister chromatid exchange test, and human lymphocyte cytogenetics assay in vitro, and the rat bone marrow cytogenetics assay in vivo.

➤*Fertility impairment:* Rats treated with zonisamide (20, 60, or 200 mg/kg) before mating and during the initial gestation phase showed signs of reproductive toxicity (decreased corpora lutea, implantations, and live fetuses) at all doses. The low dose in this study is approximately 0.5 times the maximum recommended human dose (MRHD) on a mg/m^2 basis. The effect of zonisamide on human fertility is unknown.

➤*Elderly:* Single dose pharmacokinetic parameters are similar in elderly and young healthy volunteers. Clinical studies of zonisamide did not include sufficient numbers of subjects aged 65 years and over to determine whether they respond differently from younger subjects. Other reported clinical experience has not identified differences in responses between the elderly and younger patients. In general, dose selection for an elderly patient should be cautious, usually starting at the low end of the dosing range, reflecting the greater frequency of decreased hepatic, renal, or cardiac function, and of concomitant disease or other drug therapy.

➤*Pregnancy: Category C.* Zonisamide was teratogenic in mice, rats, and dogs and embryolethal in monkeys when administered during the period of organogenesis. Fetal abnormalities or embryo-fetal deaths occurred in these species at zonisamide dosage and maternal plasma levels similar to or lower than therapeutic levels in humans, indicating that use of this drug in pregnancy entails a significant risk to the fetus. A variety of external, visceral, and skeletal malformations was produced in animals by prenatal exposure to zonisamide. Cardiovascular defects were prominent in both rats and dogs.

There are no adequate and well-controlled studies in pregnant women. Zonisamide should be used during pregnancy only if the potential benefit justifies the potential risk to the fetus.

Teratogenic – Women of childbearing potential who are given zonisamide should be advised to use effective contraception. Zonisamide was teratogenic in mice, rats, and dogs and embryolethal in monkeys when administered during the period of organogenesis. A variety of fetal abnormalities, including cardiovascular defects, and embryo-fetal deaths occurred at maternal plasma levels similar to or lower than therapeutic levels in humans. These findings suggest that the use of zonisamide during pregnancy in humans may present a significant risk to the fetus. It cannot be said with any confidence, however, that even mild seizures do not pose some hazards to the developing fetus. Zonisamide should be used during pregnancy only if the potential benefit justifies the potential risk to the fetus.

Labor and delivery – The effect of zonisamide on labor and delivery in humans is not known.

➤*Lactation:* It is not known whether zonisamide is excreted in human milk. Because many drugs are excreted in human milk and because of the potential for serious adverse reactions in nursing infants from zonisamide, a decision should be made whether to discontinue nursing or to discontinue the drug, taking into account the importance of the drug to the mother. Zonisamide should be used in nursing mothers only if the benefits outweigh the risks.

➤*Children:* The safety and effectiveness of zonisamide in children younger than 16 years of age have not been established. Cases of oligohidrosis and hyperpyrexia have been reported.

Oligohidrosis and hyperthermia in pediatric patients – Oligohidrosis, sometimes resulting in heat stroke and hospitalization, is seen in association with zonisamide in pediatric patients.

During the preapproval development program in Japan, 1 case of oligohidrosis was reported in 403 pediatric patients, an incidence of 1 case per 285 patient-years of exposure. While there were no cases reported in the US or European development programs, less than 100 pediatric patients participated in these trials.

In the first 11 years of marketing in Japan, 38 cases were reported, an estimated reporting rate of about 1 case per 10,000 patient-years of exposure. In the first year of marketing in the US, 2 cases were reported, an estimated reporting rate of about 12 cases per 10,000 patient-years of exposure. These rates are underestimates of the true incidence because of underreporting. There has been 1 report of heat stroke in an 18-year-old patient in the US.

Decreased sweating and an elevation in body temperature above normal characterized these cases. Many cases were reported after exposure to elevated environmental temperatures. Heat stroke, requiring hospitalization, was diagnosed in some cases. There have been no reported deaths.

Pediatric patients appear to be at an increased risk for zonisamide-associated oligohidrosis and hyperthermia. Patients, especially pediatric patients, treated with zonisamide should be monitored closely for evidence of decreased sweating and increased body temperature, especially in warm or hot weather. Caution should be used when zonisamide is prescribed with other drugs that predispose patients to heat-related disorders; these drugs include, but are not limited to, carbonic anhydrase inhibitors and drugs with anticholinergic activity.

ZONISAMIDE — ORAL

Precautions

➤*Creatine phosphokinase (CPK) elevation and pancreatitis:* In the postmarketing setting, the following rare adverse events have been observed (less than 1:1000):

If patients taking zonisamide develop severe muscle pain and/or weakness, either in the presence or absence of a fever, markers of muscle damage should be assessed, including serum CPK and aldolase levels. If elevated, in the absence of another obvious cause (eg, trauma, grand mal seizures), tapering and/or discontinuance of zonisamide should be considered and appropriate treatment initiated.

Patients taking zonisamide that manifest clinical signs and symptoms of pancreatitis should have pancreatic lipase and amylase levels monitored. If pancreatitis is evident, in the absence of another obvious cause, tapering and/or discontinuation of zonisamide should be considered and appropriate treatment initiated.

➤*Kidney stones:* Among the 991 patients treated during the development of zonisamide, 40 patients (4%) with epilepsy receiving zonisamide developed clinically possible or confirmed kidney stones (eg, clinical symptomatology, sonography), a rate of 34 per 1000 patient-years of exposure (40 patients with 1168 years of exposure). Of these, 12 were symptomatic, and 28 were described as possible kidney stones based on sonographic detection. In 9 patients, the diagnosis was confirmed by a passage of a stone or by a definitive sonographic finding. The rate of occurrence of kidney stones was 28.7 per 1000 patient-years of exposure in the first 6 months, 62.6% per 1000 patient-years of exposure between 6 and 12 months, and 24.3% per 1000 patient-years of exposure after 12 months of use. There are no normative sonographic data available for either the general population or patients with epilepsy. The clinical significance of the sonographic finding is unknown. The analyzed stones were composed of calcium or urate salts. In general, increasing fluid intake and urine output can help reduce the risk of stone formation, particularly in those with predisposing risk factors. It is unknown, however, whether these measures will reduce the risk of stone formation in patients treated with zonisamide.

➤*Effect on renal function:* In several clinical studies, zonisamide was associated with a statistically significant 8% mean increase from baseline of serum creatinine and blood urea nitrogen (BUN) compared to essentially no change in the placebo patients. The increase appeared to persist over time but was not progressive; this has been interpreted as an effect on glomerular filtration rate (GFR). There were no episodes of unexplained acute renal failure in clinical development in the US, Europe, or Japan. The decrease in GFR appeared within the first 4 weeks of treatment. In a 30-day study, the GFR returned to baseline within 2 to 3 weeks of drug discontinuation. There is no information about reversibility, after drug discontinuation, of the effects on GFR after long-term use. Zonisamide should be discontinued in patients who develop acute renal failure or a clinically significant sustained increase in the creatinine/BUN concentration. Zonisamide should not be used in patients with renal failure (estimated GFR less than 50 mL/min) as there has been insufficient experience concerning drug dosing and toxicity.

➤*Sudden unexplained death in epilepsy:* During the development of zonisamide, 9 sudden unexplained deaths occurred among 991 patients with epilepsy receiving zonisamide for whom accurate exposure data are available. This represents an incidence of 7.7 deaths per 1000 patient years. Although this rate exceeds that expected in a healthy population, it is within the range of estimates for the incidence of sudden unexplained deaths in patients with refractory epilepsy not receiving zonisamide (ranging from 0.5 per 1000 patient-years for the general population of patients with epilepsy, to 2 to 5 per 1000 patient-years for patients with refractory epilepsy. Higher incidences range from 9 to 15 per 1000 patient-years among surgical candidates and surgical failures). Some of the deaths could represent seizure-related deaths in which the seizure was not observed.

➤*Status epilepticus:* Estimates of the incidence of treatment emergent status epilepticus in zonisamide treated patients are difficult because a standard definition was not employed. Nonetheless, in controlled trials, 1.1% of patients treated with zonisamide had an event labeled as status epilepticus compared to none of the patients treated with placebo. Among patients treated with zonisamide across all epilepsy studies (controlled and uncontrolled), 1% of patients had an event reported as status epilepticus.

➤*Lab test abnormalities:* In several clinical studies, zonisamide was associated with a mean increase in the concentration of serum creatinine and blood urea nitrogen (BUN) of approximately 8% over the baseline measurement. Consideration should be given to monitoring renal function periodically. Zonisamide was associated with an increase in serum alkaline phosphatase. In the randomized, controlled trials, a mean increase of approximately 7% over baseline was associated with zonisamide compared to a 3% mean increase in placebo-treated patients. These changes were not statistically significant. The clinical relevance of these changes is unknown.

➤*Hazardous tasks:* Patients should be cautioned about the possibility of drowsiness and fatigue, and special care should be taken by patients if they drive, operate machinery, or perform any hazardous task.

Drug Interactions

➤*Effects of other drugs on zonisamide pharmacokinetics:* Drugs that induce liver enzymes increase the metabolism and clearance of zonisamide and decrease its half-life. The half-life of zonisamide following a 400 mg dose in patients concurrently on enzyme-inducing AEDs such as phenytoin, carbamazepine, or phenobarbital was between 27 to 38 hours; the half-life of zonisamide in patients concurrently on the non-enzyme-inducing AED, valproate, was 46 hours. Concurrent medication with drugs that either induce or inhibit CYP3A4 would be expected to alter serum concentrations of zonisamide.

Adverse Reactions

The most commonly observed adverse reactions associated with the use of zonisamide in controlled clinical trials that were not seen at an equivalent frequency among placebo-treated patients were somnolence, anorexia, dizziness, headache, nausea, and agitation/irritability.

In controlled clinical trials, 12% of patients receiving zonisamide as adjunctive therapy discontinued due to an adverse reaction compared to 6% receiving placebo. Approximately 21% of the 1336 patients with epilepsy who received zonisamide in clinical studies discontinued treatment because of an adverse reaction. The adverse reactions most commonly associated with discontinuation were somnolence, fatigue or ataxia (6%), anorexia (3%), difficulty concentrating (2%), difficulty with memory, mental slowing, nausea/vomiting (2%), and weight loss (1%). Many of these adverse reactions were dose-related.

➤*Adverse reaction incidence in controlled clinical trials:* The table below lists treatment-emergent adverse reaction that occurred in at least 2% of patients treated with zonisamide in controlled clinical trials that were numerically more common in the zonisamide group. In these studies, either zonisamide or placebo was added to the patient's current AED therapy. Adverse reactions were usually mild or moderate in intensity.

Incidence (%) of Treatment-Emergent Adverse Reactions in Placebo-Controlled, Add-On Trials (Reactions that Occurred in at Least 2% of Zonisamide-Treated Patients and Occurred More Frequently in Zonisamide-Treated than Placebo-Treated Patients)

Body system/preferred term	Zonisamide (n = 269) %	Placebo (n = 230) %
CNS		
Agitation/irritability	9%	4%
Depression	6%	3%
Dizziness	13%	7%
Speech abnormalities	5%	2%
Difficulty in verbal expression	2%	< 1%
Ataxia	6%	1%
Nystagmus	4%	2%
Paresthesia	4%	1%
Confusion	6%	3%
Difficulty concentrating	6%	2%
Difficulty with memory	6%	2%
Mental slowing	4%	2%
Schizophrenic/schizophreniform behavior	2%	0%
Somnolence	17%	7%
Fatigue	8%	6%
Tiredness	7%	5%
Insomnia	6%	3%
Anxiety	3%	2%
Nervousness	2%	1%
Dermatologic		
Rash	3%	2%
GI		
Anorexia	13%	6%
Nausea	9%	6%
Diarrhea	5%	2%
Dyspepsia	3%	1%
Constipation	2%	1%
Dry mouth	2%	1%
Hematologic/lymphatic		
Ecchymosis	2%	1%
Metabolic/nutritional		
Weight loss	3%	2%
Respiratory		
Rhinitis	2%	1%
Special senses		
Diplopia	6%	3%
Taste perversion	2%	0%
Miscellaneous		
Headache	10%	8%
Abdominal pain	6%	3%
Flu syndrome	4%	3%

Sulfonamides

ZONISAMIDE — ORAL

➤*Other adverse reactions observed during clinical trials:* Reactions are further classified within each category and listed in order of decreasing frequency as follows: Frequent occurring in at least 1:100 patient; infrequent occurring in 1:100 to 1:1000 patients; rare occurring in fewer than 1:1000 patients.

Cardiovascular –
Infrequent: Palpitation, tachycardia, vascular insufficiency, hypotension, hypertension, thrombophlebitis, syncope, bradycardia.
Rare: Atrial fibrillation, heart failure, pulmonary embolus, ventricular extrasystoles.

CNS –
Frequent: Tremor, convulsion, abnormal gait, hyperesthesia, incoordination.
Infrequent: Hypertonia, twitching, abnormal dreams, vertigo, libido decreased, neuropathy, hyperkinesia, movement disorder, dysarthria, cerebrovascular accident, hypotonia, peripheral neuritis, paraesthesia, reflexes increased.
Rare: Circumoral paresthesia, dyskinesia, dystonia, encephalopathy, facial paralysis, hypokinesia, hyperesthesia, myoclonus, oculogyric crisis.

Dermatologic –
Frequent: Pruritus.
Infrequent: Maculopapular rash, acne, alopecia, dry skin, sweating, eczema, urticaria, hirsutism, pustular rash, vesiculobullous rash.

GI –
Frequent: Vomiting.
Infrequent: Flatulence, gingivitis, gum hyperplasia, gastritis, gastroenteritis, stomatitis, cholelithiasis, glossitis, melena, rectal hemorrhage, ulcerative stomatitis, gastro-duodenal ulcer, dysphagia, gum hemorrhage.
Rare: Cholangitis, hematemesis, cholecystitis, cholestatic jaundice, colitis, duodenitis, esophagitis, fecal incontinence, mouth ulceration.

GU –
Frequent: Urinary frequency, dysuria, urinary incontinence, hematuria, impotence, urinary retention, urinary urgency, amenorrhea, polyuria, nocturia.
Rare: Albuminuria, enuresis, bladder pain, bladder calculus, gynecomastia, mastitis, menorrhagia.

Hematologic / Lymphatic –
Infrequent: Leukopenia, anemia, immunodeficiency, lymphadenopathy.
Rare: Thrombocytopenia, microcytic anemia, petechia.

Metabolic / Nutritional –
Infrequent: Peripheral edema, weight gain, edema, thirst, dehydration.
Rare: Hypoglycemia, hyponatremia, increased lactic dehydrogenase, increased AST, increased ALT.

Musculoskeletal –
Infrequent: Leg cramps, myalgia, myasthenia, arthralgia, arthritis.

Psychiatric –
Infrequent: Euphoria.

Respiratory –
Frequent: Pharyngitis, cough increased.
Infrequent: Dyspnea.
Rare: Apnea, hemoptysis.

Special senses –
Frequent: Amblyopia, tinnitus.
Infrequent: Conjunctivitis, parosmia, deafness, visual field defect, glaucoma.
Rare: Photophobia, iritis.

Miscellaneous –
Frequent: Accidental injury, asthenia.
Infrequent: Chest pain, flank pain, malaise, allergic reaction, face edema, neck rigidity.
Rare: Lupus erythematosus.

Overdosage

➤*Symptoms:* Experience with zonisamide daily doses over 800 mg/day is limited. During zonisamide clinical development, 3 patients ingested unknown amounts of zonisamide as suicide attempts, and all 3 were hospitalized with CNS symptoms. One patient became comatose and developed bradycardia, hypotension, and respiratory depression; the zonisamide plasma level was 100.1 mcg/mL measured 31 hours post-ingestion. Zonisamide plasma levels fell with a half-life of 57 hours, and the patient became alert 5 days later.

➤*Treatment:* No specific antidotes for zonisamide overdosage are available. Following a suspected recent overdose, emesis should be induced or gastric lavage performed with the usual precautions to protect the airway. General supportive care is indicated, including frequent monitoring of vital signs and close observation. Zonisamide has a long half-life (approximately 105 hours). Due to the low protein binding of zonisamide (40%), renal dialysis may not be effective. A poison control center should be contacted for information on the management of zonisamide overdosage.

Patient Information

Patients should be advised as follows:

1.) Zonisamide may produce drowsiness, especially at higher doses. Patients should be advised not to drive a car or operate other complex machinery until they have gained experience on zonisamide sufficient to determine whether it affects their performance.
2.) Patients should contact their physicians immediately if a skin rash develops or seizures worsen.
3.) Patients should contact their physicians immediately if they develop signs or symptoms, such as sudden back pain, abdominal pain, or blood in the urine, that could indicate a kidney stone. Increasing fluid intake and urine output may reduce the risk of stone formation, particularly in those with predisposing risk factors for stones.
4.) Patients should contact their physicians immediately if a child has been taking zonisamide and is not sweating as usual with or without a fever.
5.) Because zonisamide can cause hematological complications, patients should contact their physicians immediately if they develop a fever, sore throat, oral ulcers, or easy bruising.
6.) As with other AEDs, patients should contact their physicians if they intend to become pregnant or are pregnant during zonisamide therapy. Patients should notify their physicians if they intend to breastfeed or are breastfeeding infants.
7.) Patients should contact their physicians if they develop severe muscle pain and/or weakness.

Benzodiazepines

CLONAZEPAM

Refer to the general discussion beginning in the Anticonvulsants introduction. For prescribing information, refer to the Clonazepam monograph in the Antianxiety Agents section.

CLORAZEPATE DIPOTASSIUM

Refer to the general discussion beginning in the Anticonvulsants introduction. For prescribing information, refer to the Clorazepate Dipotassium monograph in the Antianxiety Agents section.

DIAZEPAM

Refer to the general discussion beginning in the Anticonvulsants introduction. For prescribing information, refer to the Diazepam monographs in the Antianxiety Agents section.

LORAZEPAM

Refer to the general discussion beginning in the Anticonvulsants introduction. For prescribing information, refer to the lorazepam monograph in the Antianxiety section.

CARBAMAZEPINE

Rx	**Carbamazepine** (Caraco)	**Tablets**: 100 mg	(539). Pink, capsule shape. In 100s, 500s, and 1,000s.
Rx	**Carbamazepine** (Various, eg, Caraco, Ivax, Taro, Teva, TorPharm, UDL)	**Tablets**: 200 mg	May contain corn starch, lactose. In 100s, 500s, 1000s, and UD 100s and 300s.
Rx	**Epitol** (Teva)		Lactose. (Epitol 93-93). White, scored. In 100s.
Rx	**Tegretol** (Novartis)		(Tegretol 27 27). Pink, scored. Capsule shape. In 100s, 1000s, and UD 100s.
Rx	**Carbamazepine** (Caraco)	**Tablets**: 300 mg	(535). Pink, capsule shape. In 100s, 500s, and 1,000s.
		400 mg	(536). Pink, capsule shape. In 100s, 500s, and 1,000s.
Rx	**Carbamazepine** (Various, eg, Caraco, Ivax, Shire, Taro, Teva, UDL)	**Tablets, chewable**: 100 mg	May contain corn starch, sorbitol, sucrose. In 100s, 500s, 1,000s and UD 50s and 100s.
Rx	**Tegretol** (Novartis)		Sucrose. (Tegretol 52 52). Pink, red-speckled, scored. In 100s and UD 100s.
Rx	**Tegretol-XR** (Novartis)	**Tablets, extended-release**: 100 mg	Mannitol. (T 100 mg). Yellow. In 100s.
		200 mg	Mannitol. (T 200 mg). Pink. In 100s.
		400 mg	Mannitol. (T 400 mg). Brown. In 100s.
Rx	**Carbatrol** (Shire)	**Capsules, extended-release**: 100 mg	Lactose. (Shire). Bluish green. In 14s and 120s.
Rx	**Equetro** (Shire)		Lactose. (SPD417 100 mg). Yellow opaque/bluish green opaque. In 120s.
Rx	**Carbatrol** (Shire)	**Capsules, extended-release**: 200 mg	Lactose. (Shire). Lt. gray and bluish green. In 30s and 120s.
Rx	**Equetro** (Shire)		Lactose. (SPD417 200 mg). Yellow opaque/blue opaque. In 120s.
Rx	**Carbatrol** (Shire)	**Capsules, extended-release**: 300 mg	Lactose. (Shire). Black and bluish green. In 30s and 120s.
Rx	**Equetro** (Shire)		Lactose. (SPD417 300 mg). Yellow opaque/blue. In 120s.
Rx	**Carbamazepine** (Various, eg, Alpharma, Taro)	**Suspension**: 100 mg per 5 mL	May contain saccharin, sorbitol, sucrose, parabens. In 450 mL and UD 10 mL.
Rx	**Tegretol** (Novartis)		Sorbitol, sucrose. Citrus/vanilla flavor. In 450 mL.
Rx	**Carbamazepine** (Alpharma)	200 mg per 10 mL	Sorbitol, sucrose. Citrus/vanilla flavor. In 10 mL dose cups.

CARBAMAZEPINE — ORAL

Refer to the general discussion beginning in the Anticonvulsants introduction.

WARNING

Aplastic anemia and agranulocytosis have been reported in association with the use of carbamazepine. Data from a population-based case-control study demonstrate that the risk of developing these reactions is 5 to 8 times greater than in the general population. However, the overall risk of these reactions in the untreated general population is low, approximately 6 patients per 1 million per year for agranulocytosis and 2 patients per 1 million per year for aplastic anemia.

Although reports of transient or persistent decreased platelet or white blood cell counts are not uncommon in association with the use of carbamazepine, data are not available to accurately estimate their incidence or outcome. However, the vast majority of the cases of leukopenia have not progressed to the more serious conditions of aplastic anemia or agranulocytosis.

Because of the very low incidence of agranulocytosis and aplastic anemia, the vast majority of minor hematologic changes observed while monitoring patients on carbamazepine are unlikely to signal the occurrence of either abnormality. Nonetheless, obtain complete pretreatment hematological testing as a baseline. If a patient in the course of treatment exhibits low or decreased white blood cell or platelet counts, monitor the patient closely. Consider discontinuation of the drug if any evidence of significant bone marrow depression develops.

Indications

➤*Bipolar I disorder (Equetro only)*: For the treatment of acute manic and mixed episodes associated with bipolar I disorder.

➤*Epilepsy (except Equetro)*: For use as an anticonvulsant drug. Evidence supporting the efficacy of carbamazepine as an anticonvulsant was derived from active, drug-controlled studies that enrolled patients with the following seizure types:

- Partial seizures with complex symptomatology (psychomotor, temporal lobe). Patients with these seizures appear to show greater improvement than those with other types.
- Generalized tonic-clonic seizures (grand mal).
- Mixed seizure patterns that include the above, or other partial or generalized seizures. Absence seizures (petit mal) do not appear to be controlled by carbamazepine.

➤*Trigeminal neuralgia (except Equetro)*: Treatment of pain associated with true trigeminal neuralgia. Beneficial results have also been reported in glossopharyngeal neuralgia. This drug is not a simple analgesic; do not use for the relief of trivial aches or pains.

➤*Unlabeled uses:* Restless leg syndrome; alternative/adjunctive treatment for certain symptoms associated with borderline personality disorder; alternative to benzodiazepines for managing alcohol withdrawal; adjunctive therapy for schizophrenia; treatment of postherpetic neuralgia

Rectal administration of carbamazepine has been used when oral dosing is interrupted for short periods of time (not for status epilepticus).

Administration and Dosage

➤*Approved by the FDA:* August 14, 1986.

Monitoring of blood levels has increased the efficacy and safety of anticonvulsants. Dosage should be adjusted to the needs of the individual patient. A low initial daily dosage with a gradual increase is advised. As soon as adequate control is achieved, the dosage may be reduced very gradually to the minimum effective level. This medication should be taken with meals.

➤*Bipolar I disorder (Equetro only)*: The recommended initial dose is 400 mg/day given in divided doses, twice daily. The dose should be adjusted in 200 mg daily increments to achieve optimal clinical response. Doses higher than 1,600 mg/day have not been studied.

➤*Epilepsy:*

Children younger than 6 years of age –

Initial: 10 to 20 mg/kg/day twice daily or 3 times daily as tablets or 4 times daily as suspension. Increase the dosage weekly to achieve optimal clinical response, administered 3 times daily or 4 times daily.

Maintenance: Ordinarily, optimal clinical response is achieved at daily doses below 35 mg/kg. If satisfactory clinical response has not been achieved, plasma levels should be measured to determine whether or not they are in the therapeutic range. No recommendation regarding the safety of carbamazepine for use at doses above 35 mg/kg per 24 hours can be made.

Combination therapy: May be used alone or with other anticonvulsants. When added to existing anticonvulsant therapy, the drug should be added gradually while the other anticonvulsants are maintained or gradually decreased, except phenytoin, which may have to be increased.

Children 6 to 12 years of age –

Initial: Either 100 mg twice daily for tablets or ER tablets, or 2.5 mL 4 times daily for suspension (200 mg/day). Increase at weekly intervals by adding up to 100 mg/day using a twice-daily regimen of carbamazepine ER tablets or a 3-times-daily or 4-times-daily regimen of the other formulations until the optimal response is obtained. Dosage generally should not exceed 1,000 mg daily.

Maintenance: Adjust dosage to the minimum effective level, usually 400 to 800 mg daily.

Adults and children older than 12 years of age –

Initial: Either 200 mg twice daily for tablets and ER tablets, or 5 mL 4 times daily for suspension (400 mg/day). Increase at weekly intervals by adding up to 200 mg/day using a twice-daily regimen of carbamazepine ER tablets or a 3-times-daily or 4-times-daily regimen of the other formulations until the optimal response is obtained. Dosage generally should not exceed 1,000 mg daily in children 12 to 15 years of age, and 1,200 mg daily in patients older than 15 years of age. Doses up to 1,600 mg daily have been used in adults in rare instances.

Maintenance – Adjust dosage to the minimum effective level, usually 800 to 1,200 mg daily.

➤*Epilepsy (Carbatrol only):*

Adults and children older than 12 years of age –

Initial: 200 mg twice daily. Increase at weekly intervals by adding up to 200 mg/day until the optimal response is obtained. Dosage generally should

CARBAMAZEPINE — ORAL

not exceed 1,000 mg/day in children 12 to 15 years of age and 1,200 mg daily in patients older than 15 years of age. Doses up to 1,600 mg daily have been used in adults.

Maintenance: Adjust dosage to the minimum effective level, usually 800 to 1,200 mg/day.

Children younger than 12 years of age – Children taking total daily doses of immediate-release carbamazepine 400 mg or greater may be converted to the same total daily dose of carbamazepine ER capsules, using a twice-daily regimen. Ordinarily, optimal clinical response is achieved at daily doses below 35 mg/kg. If satisfactory clinical response has not been achieved, plasma levels should be measured to determine whether or not they are in the therapeutic range. No recommendation regarding the safety of carbamazepine for use at doses above 35 mg/kg per 24 hours can be made.

Combination therapy – Carbamazepine may be used alone or with other anticonvulsants. When added to existing anticonvulsant therapy, the drug should be added gradually while the other anticonvulsants are maintained or gradually decreased, except phenytoin, which may have to be increased.

➤*Trigeminal neuralgia:*

Initial – On the first day, either 100 mg twice daily for tablets or ER tablets, or 2.5 mL 4 times daily for suspension, for a total daily dose of 200 mg. This daily dose may be increased by up to 200 mg/day using increments of 100 mg every 12 hours for tablets or ER tablets, or 50 mg (2.5 mL) 4 times for suspension, only as needed to achieve freedom from pain. Do not exceed 1,200 mg daily.

Maintenance – Control of pain can be maintained in most patients with 400 to 800 mg daily. However, some patients may be maintained on as little as 200 mg daily, while others may require as much as 1,200 mg daily. At least once every 3 months throughout the treatment period, attempts should be made to reduce the dose to the minimum effective level or even to discontinue the drug.

➤*Trigeminal neuralgia (Carbatrol only):*

Initial – On the first day, start with one 200 mg capsule. This daily dose may be increased by up to 200 mg/day every 12 hours only as needed to achieve freedom from pain. Do not exceed 1,200 mg daily.

Maintenance – Control of pain can be maintained in most patients with 400 to 800 mg daily. However, some patients may be maintained on as little as 200 mg daily, while others may require as much as 1,200 mg daily. At least once every 3 months throughout the treatment period, attempts should be made to reduce the dose to the minimum effective level or even to discontinue the drug.

Carbamazepine Dosage Information

	Initial dose			Subsequent dose			Maximum daily dose		
Indication	Tablets	ER tablets	Suspension	Tablets	ER tablets	Suspension	Tablets	ER tablets	Suspension
Epilepsy									
Under 6 years	10 to 20 mg/kg/day twice daily or 3 times daily		10 to 20 mg/kg/day 4 times daily	Increase weekly to achieve optimal clinical response, 3 or 4 times daily		Increase weekly to achieve optimal clinical response, 3 or 4 times daily	35 mg/kg per 24 hours		35 mg/kg per 24 hours
6 to 12 years of age	100 mg twice daily (200 mg/day)	100 mg twice daily (200 mg/day)	2.5 mL 4 times daily (200 mg/day)	Add up to 100 mg/day at weekly intervals, 3 or 4 times daily	Add 100 mg/day at weekly intervals, twice daily	Add up to 5 mL (100 mg)/day at weekly intervals, 3 or 4 times daily	1,000 mg per 24 hours		
Over 12 years	200 mg twice daily (400 mg/day)	200 mg twice daily (400 mg/day)	5 mL 4 times daily (400 mg/day)	Add up to 200 mg/day at weekly intervals, 3 or 4 times daily	Add up to 200 mg/day at weekly intervals, twice daily	Add up to 10 mL (200 mg)/day at weekly intervals, 3 or 4 times daily	1,000 mg per 24 hours (12 to 15 years); 1,200 mg per 24 hours (> 15 years); 1,600 mg per 24 hours (adults, in rare instances)		
Trigeminal neuralgia	100 mg twice daily (200 mg/day)	100 mg twice daily (200 mg/day)	2.5 mL 4 times daily (200 mg/day)	Add up to 200 mg/day in increments of 100 mg every 12 hours	Add up to 200 mg/day in increments of 100 mg every 12 hours	Add up to 10 mL (200 mg/day) in increments of 50 mg (2.5 mL) 4 times daily	1,200 mg per 24 hours		

➤*Suspension:* Carbamazepine suspension in combination with liquid chlorpromazine or thioridazine results in precipitate formation, and, in the case of chlorpromazine, there has been a report of a patient passing an orange rubbery precipitate in the stool following coadministration of the 2 drugs. Because the extent to which this occurs with other liquid medications is not known, carbamazepine suspension should not be administered simultaneously with other liquid medications or diluents.

Since a given dose of carbamazepine suspension will produce higher peak levels than the same dose given as the tablet, it is recommended to start with low doses (children 6 to 12 years of age: 2.5 mL 4 times daily) and increase slowly to avoid unwanted side effects.

Conversion from tablets to suspension – Patients should be converted by administering the same number of mg/day in smaller, more frequent doses (ie, twice-daily tablets to 3-times-daily suspension).

➤*Conversion from conventional tablets to ER tablets:* Carbamazepine is available as an ER formulation for twice-a-day administration. When converting patients from carbamazepine conventional tablets to carbamazepine ER tablets, the same total daily mg dose of carbamazepine ER tablets should be administered. Carbamazepine ER tablets must be swallowed whole and never crushed or chewed. Carbamazepine ER tablets should be inspected for chips or cracks. Damaged tablets or tablets without a release portal should not be consumed. Carbamazepine ER tablet coating is not absorbed and is excreted in the feces; these coatings may be noticeable in the stool.

➤*Conversion from conventional tablets to ER capsules:* Carbamazepine is an ER formulation for twice-a-day administration. When converting patients from immediate-release carbamazepine to carbamazepine ER capsules, the same total daily mg dose of carbamazepine should be administered.

Carbamazepine capsules may be opened and the beads sprinkled over food, such as a teaspoon of applesauce or other similar food products, if this method of administration is preferred. Carbamazepine capsules and their contents should not be crushed or chewed. Carbamazepine can be taken with or without meals.

➤*Storage/Stability:*

Chewable tablets and tablets – Do not store chewable tablets or tablets above 30°C (86°F). Protect from light and moisture. Dispense in a tight, light-resistant container.

ER tablets – Store ER tablets at controlled room temperature, 15° to 30°C (59° to 86°F). Protect from moisture. Dispense in tight container.

ER capsules – Store at 25°C (77°F); excursions permitted from 15° to 30°C (59° to 86°F). Protect from light.

Suspension – Shake suspension well before using. Do not administer suspension simultaneously with other liquid medicinal agents or diluents. Do not store suspension above 30°C (86°F). Dispense in a tight, light-resistant container.

CARBAMAZEPINE — ORAL

Actions

➤*Pharmacology:* The mechanism(s) of action of carbamazepine in the treatment of bipolar disorder has not been elucidated. Although numerous pharmacological effects of carbamazepine have been described in the published literature (eg, modulation of ion channels [sodium and calcium], receptor-mediated neurotransmission [GABAergic, glutamatergic, and monoaminergic], and intracellular signaling pathways in experimental preparations), the contribution of these effects to the efficacy of carbamazepine in bipolar disorder is unknown.

Carbamazepine has demonstrated anticonvulsant properties in rats and mice with electrically and chemically induced seizures. It appears to act by reducing polysynaptic responses and blocking the posttetanic potentiation. Carbamazepine greatly reduces or abolishes pain induced by stimulation of the infraorbital nerve in cats and rats. It depresses thalamic potential and bulbar and polysynaptic reflexes, including the linguomandibular reflex in cats. Carbamazepine is chemically unrelated to other anticonvulsants or other drugs used to control the pain of trigeminal neuralgia. The mechanism of action remains unknown.

The principal metabolite, carbamazepine-10,11-epoxide, has anticonvulsant activity as demonstrated in several in vivo animal models of seizures. Though clinical activity for the epoxide has been postulated, the significance of its activity with respect to the safety and efficacy of carbamazepine has not been established.

➤*Pharmacokinetics:*

Absorption – In clinical studies, carbamazepine suspension, conventional tablets, and ER tablets delivered equivalent amounts of drug to the systemic circulation. However, the suspension was absorbed somewhat faster, and the ER tablet slightly slower, than the conventional tablet. The bioavailability of the ER tablet was 89% compared to suspension. Following a twice-daily dosage regimen, the suspension provides higher peak levels and lower trough levels than those obtained from the conventional tablet for the same dosage regimen.

On the other hand, following a 3-times-daily dosage regimen, carbamazepine suspension affords steady-state plasma levels comparable with carbamazepine tablets given twice daily when administered at the same total mg daily dose. Following a twice-daily dosage regimen, ER carbamazepine tablets afford steady-state plasma levels comparable with conventional carbamazepine tablets given 4 times daily, when administered at the same total mg daily dose.

ER capsules: Taken every 12 hours, carbamazepine ER capsules provide steady-state plasma levels comparable with immediate-release carbamazepine tablets given every 6 hours, when administered at the same total mg daily dose. Following a single 200 mg oral ER dose of carbamazepine, peak plasma concentration was 1.9 ± 0.3 mcg/mL and the time to reach the peak was 19 ± 7 hours. Following chronic administration (800 mg every 12 hours), the peak levels were 11 ± 2.5 mcg/mL, and the time to reach the peak was 5.9 ± 1.8 hours. The pharmacokinetics of carbamazepine ER capsules is linear over the single dose range of 200 to 800 mg.

ER capsules:

• *Food effect* – A high-fat meal diet increased the rate of absorption of a single 400 mg dose (mean t_{max} was reduced from 24 hours, in the fasting state, to 14 hours, and C_{max} increased from 3.2 to 4.3 mcg/mL) but not the extent (AUC) of absorption. The elimination half-life remains unchanged between fed and fasting state. The multiple-dose study conducted in the fed state showed that the steady-state C_{max} values were within the therapeutic concentration range. The pharmacokinetic profile of ER carbamazepine was similar when given by sprinkling the beads over applesauce, compared with the intact capsule administered in the fasted state.

Distribution – Carbamazepine in blood is 76% bound to plasma proteins. Plasma levels of carbamazepine are variable, and may range from 0.5 to 25 mcg/mL, with no apparent relationship to the daily intake of the drug. Usual adult therapeutic levels are between 4 and 12 mcg/mL. In polytherapy, the concentration of carbamazepine and concomitant drugs may be increased or decreased during therapy, and drug effects may be altered.

Following chronic oral administration of suspension, plasma levels peak at approximately 1.5 hours, compared with 4 to 5 hours after administration of conventional carbamazepine tablets, and 3 to 12 hours after administration of ER carbamazepine tablets. The cerebrospinal fluid/serum ratio is 0.22, similar to the 24% unbound carbamazepine in serum.

Metabolism/Excretion – Because carbamazepine induces its own metabolism, the half-life is also variable. Autoinduction is completed after 3 to 5 weeks of a fixed dosing regimen. Initial half-life values range from 25 to 65 hours, decreasing to 12 to 17 hours on repeated doses. Carbamazepine is metabolized in the liver. Cytochrome P-450 3A4 was identified as the major isoform responsible for the formation of carbamazepine-10, 11-epoxide from carbamazepine.

After oral administration of ^{14}C-carbamazepine, 72% of the administered radioactivity was found in the urine and 28% in the feces. This urinary radioactivity was composed largely of hydroxylated and conjugated metabolites, with only 3% of unchanged carbamazepine.

ER capsules: Following a single ER dose of carbamazepine, the average half-life ranged from 35 to 40 hours and 12 to 17 hours on repeated dosing. The apparent oral clearance following a single dose was 25 ± 5 mL/min and, following multiple dosing, 80 ± 30 mL/min.

Carbamazepine-10,11-epoxide: Carbamazepine-10,11-epoxide is considered to be an active metabolite of carbamazepine. Following a single 200 mg oral ER dose of carbamazepine, the peak plasma concentration of carbamazepine-10,11-epoxide was 0.11 ± 0.012 mcg/mL, and the time to reach the peak was 36 ± 6 hours. Following chronic administration of an ER dose of carbamazepine (800 mg every 12 hours), the peak levels of carbamazepine-10,11-epoxide were 2.2 ± 0.9 mcg/mL, and the time to reach the peak was 14 ± 8 hours. The plasma half-life of carbamazepine-10,11-epoxide following administration of carbamazepine is 34 ± 9 hours. Following a single oral dose of ER carbamazepine (200 to 800 mg), the AUC and C_{max} of carbamazepine-10,11-epoxide were less than 10% of carbamazepine. Following multiple dosing of ER carbamazepine (800 to 1,600 mg daily for 14 days), the AUC and C_{max} of carbamazepine-10,11-epoxide were dose-related, ranging from 15.7 mcg•hr/mL and 1.5 mcg/mL at 800 mg/day to 32.6 mcg•hr/mL and 3.2 mcg/mL at 1,600 mg/day, respectively, and were less than 30% of carbamazepine. Carbamazepine-10,11-epoxide is 50% bound to plasma proteins.

Special populations –

Children: The pharmacokinetic parameters of carbamazepine disposition are similar in children and in adults. However, there is a poor correlation between plasma concentrations of carbamazepine and carbamazepine dose in children. Carbamazepine is more rapidly metabolized to carbamazepine-10,11-epoxide (a metabolite shown to be equipotent to carbamazepine as an anticonvulsant in animal screens) in the younger age groups than in adults. In children younger than 15 years of age, there is an inverse relationship between carbamazepine-10,11-epoxide/carbamazepine ratio and increasing age (in 1 report, from 0.44 in children younger than 1 year of age to 0.18 in children between 10 and 15 years of age).

Contraindications

Bone marrow depression, acute intermittent porphyria, hypersensitivity to the drug, or known sensitivity to any of the tricyclic compounds (eg, amitriptyline, desipramine, imipramine, protriptyline, nortriptyline). Likewise, on theoretical grounds its use with monoamine oxidase (MAO) inhibitors is not recommended. Before administration of carbamazepine, discontinue MAO inhibitors for a minimum of 14 days, or longer if the clinical situation permits.

Warnings

➤*Minor pain:* This drug is not a simple analgesic. Do not use it for the relief of minor aches or pains.

➤*Hematologic:* Patients with histories of adverse hematologic reaction to any drug may be particularly at risk.

➤*Dermatologic:* Severe dermatologic reactions, including toxic epidermal necrolysis (Lyell syndrome) and Stevens-Johnson syndrome, have been reported with carbamazepine. These reactions have been extremely rare. However, a few fatalities have been reported.

➤*Discontinuation:* In patients with seizure disorder, do not discontinue carbamazepine abruptly because of the strong possibility of precipitating status epilepticus with attendant hypoxia and threat to life.

➤*Anticholinergic effects:* Carbamazepine has shown mild anticholinergic activity; therefore, closely observe patients with increased intraocular pressure during therapy.

➤*CNS effects:* Because of the relationship of the drug to other tricyclic compounds, keep in mind the possibility of activation of a latent psychosis and, in elderly patients, of confusion or agitation.

➤*Hepatic effects:* Hepatic effects, ranging from slight elevations in liver enzymes to rare cases of hepatic failure, have been reported. In some cases, hepatic effects may progress despite discontinuation of the drug. Given that carbamazepine is primarily metabolized in the liver, it is prudent to proceed with caution in patients with hepatic dysfunction.

➤*Hypersensitivity reactions:* Multiorgan hypersensitivity reactions occurring days to weeks or months after initiating treatment have been reported in rare cases. Consider discontinuation of carbamazepine if any evidence of hypersensitivity develops.

Hypersensitivity reactions to carbamazepine have been reported in patients who previously experienced such reactions to anticonvulsants, including phenytoin and phenobarbital. Obtain a history of hypersensitivity reactions for the patient and the immediate family members. If positive, use caution in prescribing carbamazepine.

➤*Carcinogenesis:* Carbamazepine, when administered to Sprague-Dawley rats for 2 years in the diet at doses of 25, 75, and 250 mg/kg/day (low dose approximately 0.2 times the maximum human daily dose of 1,200 mg on a mg/m^2 basis), resulted in a dose-related increase in the incidence of hepatocellular tumors in females and of benign interstitial cell adenomas in the testes of males. Carbamazepine must, therefore, be considered to be carcinogenic in Sprague-Dawley rats.

➤*Fertility impairment:* Testicular atrophy occurred in rats receiving carbamazepine orally from 4 to 52 weeks at dosage levels of 50 to 400 mg/kg/day. Additionally, rats receiving carbamazepine in the diet for 2 years at dosage levels of 25, 75, and 250 mg/kg/day had a dose-related incidence of testicular atrophy and aspermatogenesis. In dogs, it produced a brownish discoloration, presumably a metabolite, in the urinary bladder at dosage levels of 50 mg/kg and higher. Relevance of these findings to humans is unknown.

➤*Elderly:* Because of the relationship of the drug to other tricyclic compounds, keep in mind the possibility of activation of a latent psychosis and, in elderly patients, of confusion or agitation.

➤*Pregnancy: Category D.* Carbamazepine can cause fetal harm when administered to a pregnant woman.

Epidemiological data suggest that there may be an association between the use of carbamazepine during pregnancy and congenital malformations, including spina bifida. There have been reports in association with carbamazepine of other congenital anomalies and developmental disorders (eg, craniofacial defects, cardiovascular malformations and anomalies involving various body systems). Weigh the benefits of therapy against the risks in treating or counseling women of childbearing potential. If this drug

CARBAMAZEPINE — ORAL

is used during pregnancy or if the patient becomes pregnant while taking this drug, apprise the patient of the potential hazard to the fetus.

Retrospective case reviews suggest that, compared with monotherapy, there may be a higher prevalence of teratogenic effects associated with the use of anticonvulsants in combination therapy. Therefore, if therapy is to be continued, monotherapy may be preferable for pregnant women.

In humans, transplacental passage of carbamazepine is rapid (30 to 60 minutes) and the drug is accumulated in the fetal tissues, with higher levels found in the liver and kidneys than in the brain and lungs.

Do not discontinue antiepileptic drugs abruptly in patients in whom the drug is administered to prevent major seizures because of the strong possibility of precipitating status epilepticus with attendant hypoxia and threat to life. In individual cases where the severity and frequency of the seizure disorder are such that removal of medication does not pose a serious threat to the patient, discontinuation of the drug may be considered prior to and during pregnancy, although it cannot be said with any confidence that even minor seizures do not pose some hazard to the developing embryo or fetus.

There have been a few cases of neonatal seizures or respiratory depression associated with maternal carbamazepine and other concomitant anticonvulsant drug use. A few cases of neonatal vomiting, diarrhea, or decreased feeding have also been reported in association with maternal carbamazepine use. These symptoms may represent a neonatal withdrawal syndrome.

➤*Lactation:* Carbamazepine and its epoxide metabolite are transferred to breast milk. The ratio of the concentration in breast milk to that in maternal plasma is about 0.4 for carbamazepine and about 0.5 for the epoxide. The estimated doses given to the newborn during breast-feeding are in the range of 2 to 5 mg daily for carbamazepine and 1 to 2 mg daily for the epoxide. The concentrations of carbamazepine and its epoxide metabolite are approximately 50% of the maternal plasma concentration.

Because of the potential for serious adverse reactions in breast-feeding infants from carbamazepine, decide whether to discontinue breast-feeding or to discontinue the drug, taking into account the importance of the drug to the mother.

Precautions

➤*Monitoring:* Obtain complete pretreatment blood counts, including platelets and possibly reticulocytes and serum iron, as a baseline. Monitoring of blood levels may be useful, in cases of dramatic increase in seizure frequency, for verification of drug compliance, assessing safety, and determining the cause of toxicity, including when more than one medication is being used. If a patient in the course of treatment exhibits low or decreased white blood cell or platelet counts, monitor the patient closely. Consider discontinuation of the drug if any evidence of significant bone marrow depression develops.

Baseline and periodic evaluations of liver function, particularly in patients with histories of liver disease, must be performed during treatment with this drug because liver damage may occur. Discontinue carbamazepine, based on clinical judgment, if indicated by newly occurring or worsening clinical or laboratory evidence of liver dysfunction or hepatic damage, or in the case of active liver disease.

Baseline and periodic eye examinations, including slit-lamp, funduscopy, and tonometry, are recommended because many phenothiazines and related drugs have been shown to cause eye changes.

Baseline and periodic complete urinalysis and blood urea nitrogen (BUN) determinations are recommended for patients treated with this agent because of observed renal dysfunction.

Increases in total cholesterol, LDL, and HDL have been observed is some patients taking anticonvulsants. Therefore, periodic evaluation of these parameters is also recommended.

➤*Hyponatremia:* Hyponatremia has been reported in association with carbamazepine use, either alone or in combination with other drugs.

➤*Suicide (Equetro only):* The possibility of suicide attempt is inherent in bipolar disorder and close supervision of high risk patients should accompany drug therapy. Write prescriptions for carbamazepine for the smallest quantity consistent with good patient management in order to reduce the risk of overdosage.

➤*Absence seizures:* Use carbamazepine with caution in patients with a mixed seizure disorder that includes atypical absence seizures, since in these patients carbamazepine has been associated with increased frequency of generalized convulsions.

➤*Special risk:* Prescribe therapy only after critical benefit-to-risk appraisal in patients with a history of cardiac, hepatic, or renal damage; adverse hematologic or hypersensitivity reaction to other drugs, including reactions to other anticonvulsants or interrupted courses of therapy with carbamazepine.

➤*Hazardous tasks:* Because dizziness and drowsiness may occur, caution patients about the hazards of operating machinery or automobiles or engaging in other potentially dangerous tasks requiring alertness, coordination, or physical dexterity.

Drug Interactions

Carbamazepine Drug Interactions

Precipitant drug	Object drug[a]		Description
Acetazolamide	Carbamazepine	↑	Carbamazepine plasma levels may be increased. Adjust the dose of carbamazepine as needed.
Antimalarials (eg, chloroquine, mefloquine)	Carbamazepine	↓	Chloroquine and mefloquine may antagonize the activity of carbamazepine. Adjust the dose of carbamazepine as needed.
Azole antifungals (eg, itraconazole, ketoconazole)	Carbamazepine	↑	Carbamazepine plasma levels may be increased. Closely monitor carbamazepine levels when an azole antifungal is started or stopped. Serum itraconazole levels may be decreased in the presence of carbamazepine.
Carbamazepine	Azole antifungals (eg, itraconazole)	↓	
Cimetidine	Carbamazepine	↑	Carbamazepine plasma levels may be increased; toxicity may result. Interaction appears to be of greater clinical importance when cimetidine is added to carbamazepine during the first 4 weeks of therapy.
Cisplatin	Carbamazepine	↓	Carbamazepine plasma levels may be decreased. Monitor carbamazepine levels closely.
Dalfopristin	Carbamazepine	↑	Carbamazepine plasma levels may be increased resulting in possible toxicity.
Danazol	Carbamazepine	↑	Carbamazepine plasma levels may be increased, resulting in an increase in pharmacologic and toxic effects. Avoid coadministration is possible.
Delavirdine	Carbamazepine	↑	Carbamazepine plasma levels may be increased. Monitor carbamazepine levels closely. Coadministration may lead to loss of virologic response and possible resistance to delavirdine or to the class of nonnucleoside reverse transcriptase inhibitors.
Carbamazepine	Delavirdine	↓	
Diltiazem	Carbamazepine	↑	Carbamazepine plasma levels may be increased; toxicity may result. Monitor serum carbamazepine levels and observe the patient.
Doxorubicin	Carbamazepine	↓	Carbamazepine plasma levels may be decreased. Monitor carbamazepine levels.
Felbamate	Carbamazepine	↓	Carbamazepine plasma levels may be decreased. An average decrease of 25% in carbamazepine levels has been reported. Felbamate levels may be decreased, possibly resulting in loss of effectiveness.
Carbamazepine	Felbamate		
Haloperidol	Carbamazepine	↑	The therapeutic effects of carbamazepine may be increased. Consider adjusting the dose of carbamazepine as indicated. Haloperidol serum levels and efficacy may be decreased by carbamazepine. A 60% decrease in levels has been reported.
Carbamazepine	Haloperidol	↓	
Isoniazid	Carbamazepine	↑	Isoniazid is suspected to inhibit carbamazepine metabolism. Carbamazepine toxicity may result. Carbamazepine may increase isoniazid degradation to hepatic metabolites, isoniazid toxicity may result.
Carbamazepine	Isoniazid	↑	
Loratadine	Carbamazepine	↑	Carbamazepine plasma levels may be increased. Closely monitor carbamazepine levels.

CARBAMAZEPINE — ORAL

Carbamazepine Drug Interactions

Precipitant drug	Object drug[a]		Description
Macrolides (eg, clarithromycin, erythromycin, troleandomycin)	Carbamazepine	↑	Carbamazepine plasma levels may be increased. Avoid combination if possible.
MAO inhibitors (eg, isocarboxazid, phenelzine)	Carbamazepine	↑	Coadministration is contraindicated. Discontinue MAO inhibitor at least 14 days prior to administration of carbamazepine.
Carbamazepine	MAO inhibitors (eg, isocarboxazid, phenelzine)		
Nefazodone	Carbamazepine	↑	Carbamazepine plasma levels may be increased. Lower nefazodone levels may result. Coadministration is contraindicated.
Carbamazepine	Nefazodone	↓	
Niacin (eg, niacinamide, nicotinamide)	Carbamazepine	↑	Carbamazepine plasma levels may be increased. Monitor carbamazepine levels and adjust the dose accordingly.
Phenobarbital	Carbamazepine	↓	Carbamazepine plasma levels may be decreased. Monitor serum concentrations of both drugs.
Phenytoin	Carbamazepine	↓	Carbamazepine plasma levels may be decreased. Monitor serum concentrations of both drugs regularly, and adjust their dosages appropriately. Phenytoin plasma levels may increase or decrease in the presence of carbamazepine.
Carbamazepine	Phenytoin	↔	
Primidone	Carbamazepine	↓	Carbamazepine plasma levels may be decreased. Primidone plasma levels may be increased or decreased. Monitor serum concentrations of both drugs regularly, and adjust their doses appropriately.
Carbamazepine	Primidone	↔	
Protease inhibitors (eg, amprenavir, indinavir)	Carbamazepine	↑	Carbamazepine plasma levels may be increased, increasing the risk of toxicity. Monitor serum carbamazepine levels. Antiretroviral treatment failure may occur.
Carbamazepine	Protease inhibitors (eg, amprenavir, indinavir)	↓	
Propoxyphene	Carbamazepine	↑	Increases in carbamazepine levels between 45% and 77% have been reported. Avoid coadministration if possible.
Quinine	Carbamazepine	↑	Carbamazepine plasma levels may be increased. Monitor carbamazepine levels and adjust the dose as needed.
Quinupristin	Carbamazepine	↑	Carbamazepine plasma levels may be increased. Monitor carbamazepine levels closely.
Rifampin	Carbamazepine	↓	Carbamazepine plasma levels may be decreased. Monitor serum carbamazepine levels and observe patient.
Selective serotonin reuptake inhibitors (SSRIs) (eg, fluoxetine, fluvoxamine)	Carbamazepine	↑	Carbamazepine plasma levels may be increased, producing possible toxicity. Monitor carbamazepine serum concentrations closely. Plasma levels of the SSRIs may be decreased. Closely monitor the response of the patient and be prepared to adjust the dose of the SSRI.
Carbamazepine	SSRIs (eg, citalopram, sertraline)	↓	
Succinimides (eg, methsuximide)	Carbamazepine	↓	Carbamazepine plasma level may be decreased. Succinimide levels may be decreased.
Carbamazepine	Succinimides (eg, ethosuximide, methsuximide)	↓	
Theophylline	Carbamazepine	↓	Carbamazepine plasma levels may be decreased. Theophylline levels may be decreased or increased. Monitor carbamazepine and theophylline levels. Adjust doses accordingly.
Carbamazepine	Theophylline	↔	
Tricyclic antidepressants (eg, amitriptyline, desipramine, nortriptyline)	Carbamazepine	↑	Carbamazepine toxicity was reported in one patient on concomitant desipramine. Carbamazepine may induce hepatic metabolism of tricyclic antidepressants.
Carbamazepine	Tricyclic antidepressants (eg, amitriptyline, desipramine, nortriptyline)	↓	
Valproate	Carbamazepine	↑	Carbamazepine plasma levels may be increased. Decreased valproate levels with possible loss of seizure control. Observe patient for seizure activity and toxicity for at least one month after starting or stopping either drug.
Carbamazepine	Valproate	↓	
Verapamil	Carbamazepine	↑	Carbamazepine plasma levels may be increased. Carbamazepine dose may need to be decreased 40% to 50% with coadministration.
Zileuton	Carbamazepine	↑	Carbamazepine plasma levels may be increased.
Carbamazepine	Acetaminophen	↓	Carbamazepine may increase the metabolism of acetaminophen, increasing the risk of acetaminophen-induced hepatotoxicity and/or decreasing its effectiveness.
Carbamazepine	Anticoagulants (eg, dicumarol, warfarin)	↓	The anticoagulant effect may be reduced during coadministration. Monitor prothrombin times when starting or stopping carbamazepine therapy.
Carbamazepine	Antipsychotics (eg, aripiprazole, clozapine, olanzapine, quetiapine, risperidone, ziprasidone)	↓	Coadministration may reduce the plasma levels of these antipsychotics. A single case of neuroleptic malignant syndrome has been reported with clozapine.
Carbamazepine	Benzodiazepines (eg, alprazolam, clonazepam, clobazam, diazepam, lorazepam, midazolam, triazolam)	↓	The pharmacological effects of benzodiazepines may be reduced. Monitor patient response.
Carbamazepine	Bupropion	↓	Carbamazepine increased the hepatic P-450 metabolism of bupropion and has been reported to decrease bupropion peaks 87% and AUC 90%.
Carbamazepine	Buspirone	↓	Plasma levels of buspirone may be decreased. Monitor patient response.
Carbamazepine	Clomipramine	↑	Carbamazepine increases the plasma levels of clomipramine.
Carbamazepine	Cyclosporine	↓	Plasma level of cyclosporine may be decreased, resulting in a reduction of pharmacologic effects. Monitor cyclosporine levels and observe patient for signs of rejection or toxicity.
Carbamazepine	Doxycycline	↓	Carbamazepine may decrease the half-life and serum levels of doxycycline, possibly reducing its therapeutic efficacy.
Carbamazepine	Felodipine	↓	Pharmacologic effects of felodipine may be decreased.

CARBAMAZEPINE — ORAL

Carbamazepine Drug Interactions			
Precipitant drug	Object drug[a]		Description
Carbamazepine	Glucocorticoids (eg, hydrocortisone)	⬇	Plasma levels of glucocorticoids may be reduced.
Carbamazepine	HMG-CoA reductase inhibitors (eg, atorvastatin, simvastatin)	⬇	Plasma concentration of certain HMG-CoA reductase inhibitors may be reduced, decreasing the therapeutic effect (resulting in hypercholesterolemia). Closely monitor the clinical response of the patient.
Carbamazepine	Lamotrigine	⬇	Serum lamotrigine levels may be decreased 40%.
Carbamazepine	Levothyroxine	⬇	Plasma levels of levothyroxine may be decreased. Monitor thyroid-stimulating hormone.
Carbamazepine	Lithium	⬆	Increased CNS toxicity may occur during concomitant therapy. Monitor serum lithium levels and adjust dose accordingly.
Carbamazepine	Methadone	⬇	Pharmacologic effects of methadone may be decreased. A higher dose of methadone may be required.
Carbamazepine	Mirtazapine	⬇	Plasma levels of mirtazapine may be decreased. Monitor patient response.
Carbamazepine	Nondepolarizing muscle relaxants (eg, atracurium, tubocurarine)	⬇	Nondepolarizing muscle relaxants may have shorter than expected duration or be less effective. Monitor patient for reduced muscle relaxant effectiveness and increase the dose of the nondepolarizing muscle relaxant accordingly.
Carbamazepine	Oral contraceptives (eg, Ortho-Novum)	⬇	Breakthrough bleeding has been reported with coadministration, and the reliability of the oral contraceptive may be adversely affected.
Carbamazepine	Oxcarbazepine	⬇	Plasma levels of oxcarbazepine may be decreased.
Carbamazepine	Praziquantel	⬇	Serum praziquantel may be decreased, possibly leading to treatment failures. It may be necessary to increase the dose of praziquantel during coadministration.
Carbamazepine	Tiagabine	⬇	Plasma levels of tiagabine may be decreased.
Carbamazepine	Topiramate	⬇	Carbamazepine may decrease the pharmacologic effects of topiramate.
Carbamazepine	Tramadol	⬇	Plasma levels of tramadol may be decreased.
Carbamazepine	Voriconazole	⬇	Voriconazole plasma levels may be reduced. Coadministration is contraindicated.
Carbamazepine	Zonisamide	⬇	Plasma levels of zonisamide may be reduced.

[a] ⬆ = Object drug increased. ⬇ = Object drug decreased.
⟷ = Undetermined clinical effect.

➤*Drug/Lab test interactions:* Thyroid function tests have been reported to show decreased values when carbamazepine is administered alone.

Interference with some pregnancy tests has been reported.

➤*Drug/Food interactions:*

Grapefruit juice – Serum carbamazepine levels may be elevated. Avoid coadministration of carbamazepine and grapefruit products.

Adverse Reactions

If adverse reactions are of such severity that the drug must be discontinued, be aware that abrupt discontinuation of any anticonvulsant drug in a responsive epileptic patient may lead to seizures or even status epilepticus with its life-threatening hazards.

The most severe adverse reactions have been observed in the hemopoietic system, the skin, liver, and the cardiovascular system.

The most frequently observed adverse reactions, particularly during the initial phases of therapy, are dizziness, drowsiness, unsteadiness, nausea, and vomiting. To minimize the possibility of such reactions, initiate therapy at the lowest dosage recommended.

Carbamazepine ER Adverse Reactions Reported in Bipolar I Disorder Trials (Incidence ≥ 5% and at least Twice Placebo)		
Adverse Reaction	Carbamazepine (n = 251)	Placebo (n = 248)
CNS		
Ataxia	15%	0%
Dizziness	44%	12%
Somnolence	32%	13%
Dermatologic		
Pruritus	8%	2%
GI		
Dry mouth	8%	3%
Nausea	29%	10%
Vomiting	18%	3%
Special senses		
Amblyopia[a]	6%	2%
Speech disorder	6%	0%

[a] Reported as blurred vision.

Carbamazepine Adverse Reactions (*Equetro* Only) (Incidence ≥ 5%)	
Adverse reaction	% events reported
CNS	
Amnesia[a]	8%
Anxiety	7%
Ataxia	5%
Depression[b]	7%
Dizziness	16%
Manic depressive reaction	7%
Somnolence	12%
Dermatologic	
Pruritus	5%
Rash	13%
GI	
Constipation	5%
Diarrhea	10%
Dyspepsia	10%
Nausea	10%
Miscellaneous	
Accidental injury	7%
Asthenia	8%
Back pain	5%
Chest pain	5%
Headache	22%
Infection	12%
Pain	12%

[a] Amnesia includes poor memory, forgetfulness, and memory disturbance.
[b] Depression includes suicidal ideation.

Other significant adverse reactions seen in less than 5% of patients from the bipolar I disorder trials include the following: abnormal liver function tests, allergic reaction, alopecia, bronchitis, depersonalization and extrapyramidal symptoms, diplopia, ear pain, edema, infections (fungal, viral, bacterial), insomnia, leukopenia, lymphadenopathy, manic reaction, nervousness, peripheral edema, pharyngitis, photosensitivity reaction, rhinitis, sinusitis, suicide attempt, and urinary tract infection.

The following additional adverse reactions have been reported:

➤*Cardiovascular:* Adenopathy or lymphadenopathy, aggravation of coronary artery disease, aggravation of hypertension, arrhythmias and AV block, congestive heart failure, edema, hypotension, syncope and collapse, thromboembolism, and thrombophlebitis. Some of these cardiovascular complications have resulted in fatalities. Myocardial infarction has been associated with other tricyclic compounds.

➤*CNS:* Abnormal involuntary movements, blurred vision, confusion, depression with agitation, disturbances of coordination, dizziness, drowsiness, fatigue, headache, hyperacusis, nystagmus, oculomotor disturbances, peripheral neuritis and paresthesias, speech disturbances, talkativeness, tinnitus, transient diplopia, and visual hallucinations. There have been reports of associated paralysis and other symptoms of cerebral arterial insufficiency, but the exact relationship of these reactions to the drug has not been established. Isolated cases of neuroleptic malignant syndrome have been reported with concomitant use of psychotropic drugs.

➤*Dermatologic:* Aggravation of disseminated lupus erythematosus, alopecia, alterations in skin pigmentation, diaphoresis, erythema multiforme and nodosum, exfoliative dermatitis, photosensitivity reactions, pruritic and erythematous rashes, purpura, Stevens-Johnson syndrome, toxic epidermal

CARBAMAZEPINE — ORAL

necrolysis (Lyell syndrome), and urticaria. In certain cases, discontinuation of therapy may be necessary. Isolated cases of hirsutism have been reported, but a causal relationship is not clear.

➤*Endocrine:* Given its anticonvulsant properties, carbamazepine may reduce thyroid function, as has been reported with other anticonvulsants.

➤*GI:* Anorexia, constipation, diarrhea, gastric distress and abdominal pain, nausea, pancreatitis, vomiting, and dryness of the mouth and pharynx, including glossitis and stomatitis.

Pancreatitis.

➤*GU:* Acute urinary retention, azotemia, impotence, oliguria with elevated blood pressure, renal failure, and urinary frequency. Albuminuria, elevated BUN, glycosuria, and microscopic deposits in the urine have also been reported.

➤*Hematologic:* Acute intermittent porphyria, agranulocytosis, aplastic anemia, bone marrow depression, eosinophilia, leukocytosis, leukopenia, pancytopenia, and thrombocytopenia.

➤*Hepatic:* Abnormalities in liver function tests, cholestatic and hepatocellular jaundice, hepatitis, very rare cases of hepatic failure.

➤*Hypersensitivity:* Multiorgan hypersensitivity reactions occurring days to weeks or months after initiating treatment have been reported in rare cases. Signs or symptoms may include, but are not limited to, abnormal liver function tests, arthralgia, disorders mimicking lymphoma, eosinophilia, fever, hepatosplenomegaly, leukopenia, lymphadenopathy, skin rashes, and vasculitis. These signs and symptoms may occur in various combinations and not necessarily concurrently. Signs and symptoms may initially be mild. Various organs, including but not limited to, liver, skin, immune system, lungs, kidneys, pancreas, myocardium, and colon, may be affected.

➤*Metabolic:* Chills and fever. Inappropriate antidiuretic hormone (ADH) secretion syndrome has been reported. Cases of frank water intoxication, with decreased serum sodium (hyponatremia) and confusion, have been reported in association with carbamazepine use. Decreased levels of plasma calcium have been reported.

➤*Musculoskeletal:* Aching joints and muscles, and leg cramps.

➤*Ophthalmic:* Scattered punctate cortical lens opacities, as well as conjunctivitis, have been reported. Although a direct causal relationship has not been established, many phenothiazines and related drugs have been shown to cause eye changes.

➤*Respiratory:* Pulmonary hypersensitivity characterized by dyspnea, fever, pneumonitis, or pneumonia.

➤*Miscellaneous:* Isolated cases of a lupus erythematosus-like syndrome have been reported. There have been occasional reports of elevated levels of cholesterol, HDL cholesterol, and triglycerides in patients taking anticonvulsants.

A case of aseptic meningitis, accompanied by myoclonus and peripheral eosinophilia, has been reported in a patient taking carbamazepine in combination with other medications. The patient was successfully dechallenged, and the meningitis reappeared upon rechallenge with carbamazepine.

Overdosage

➤*Lowest known lethal dose:*

Adults – 3.2 g (a 24-year-old woman died of a cardiac arrest and a 24-year-old man died of pneumonia and hypoxic encephalopathy).

Children – 4 g (a 14-year-old girl died of a cardiac arrest), 1.6 g (a 3-year-old girl died of aspiration pneumonia).

➤*Highest known doses survived (ER carbamazepine only):*

Adults – 30 g (31-year-old woman).

Children – 10 g (6-year-old boy); small children, 5 g (3-year-old girl). Oral LD_{50} in animals (mg/kg): Mice, 1,100 to 3,750; rats, 3,850 to 4,025; rabbits, 1,500 to 2,680; guinea pigs, 920.

➤*Symptoms:* The first signs and symptoms appear after 1 to 3 hours. Neuromuscular disturbances are the most prominent. Cardiovascular disorders are generally milder, and severe cardiac complications occur only when very high doses (greater than 60 g) have been ingested.

Respiration – Irregular breathing, and respiratory depression.

Cardiovascular system – Tachycardia, hypotension or hypertension, shock, and conduction disorders.

Nervous system and muscles – Impairment of consciousness ranging in severity to deep coma. Convulsions, especially in small children. Motor restlessness, muscular twitching, tremor, athetoid movements, opisthotonos, ataxia, drowsiness, dizziness, mydriasis, nystagmus, adiadochokinesia, ballism, psychomotor disturbances, and dysmetria. Initial hyperreflexia, followed by hyporeflexia.

GI tract – Nausea and vomiting.

Kidneys and bladder – Anuria or oliguria, and urinary retention.

Laboratory findings – Isolated instances of overdosage have included leukocytosis, reduced leukocyte count, glycosuria, and acetonuria. Electroencephalogram (EEG) may show dysrhythmias.

➤*Treatment:*

Elimination of the drug –

Activated charcoal: The primary method for gastric decontamination of carbamazepine overdose is use of activated charcoal. Administration of activated charcoal prior to hospital assessment has the potential to significantly reduce drug absorption. There is no specific antidote. In overdose, absorption of carbamazepine may be prolonged and delayed. More than 1 dose of activated charcoal may be beneficial in patients that have evidence of continued absorption (eg, rising serum carbamazepine levels).

Gastric lavage: For substantial recent ingestions, gastric lavage may also be considered. Even when more than 4 hours have elapsed following ingestion of the drug, repeatedly irrigate the stomach, especially if the patient has also consumed alcohol.

Measures to accelerate elimination – The data on use of dialysis to enhance elimination in carbamazepine are scarce. Dialysis, particularly high flux or high efficiency hemodialysis, may be considered in patients with severe carbamazepine poisoning associated with renal failure or in cases of status epilepticus, or where there are rising serum drug levels and worsening clinical status despite appropriate supportive care and gastric decontamination. For severe cases of carbamazepine overdose unresponsive to other measures, charcoal hemoperfusion may be used to enhance drug clearance. Replacement transfusion is indicated in severe poisoning in small children.

Respiratory depression – Keep the airways free; resort, if necessary, to endotracheal intubation, artificial respiration, and administration of oxygen.

Hypotension, shock – Keep the patient's legs raised and administer a plasma expander. If blood pressure fails to rise despite measures taken to increase plasma volume, consider use of vasoactive substances.

Convulsions – Diazepam or barbiturates.

Diazepam/Barbiturates: Diazepam or barbiturates may aggravate respiratory depression (especially in children), hypotension, and coma. However, do not use barbiturates if drugs that inhibit MAO have also been taken by the patient either in overdosage or in recent therapy (within 1 week).

Monitoring – Respiration, cardiac function (ECG monitoring), blood pressure, body temperature, pupillary reflexes, and monitor kidney and bladder function for several days.

Hematologic abnormalities – If evidence of significant bone marrow depression develops, the following recommendations are suggested: Stop the drug. Perform daily CBC, platelet, and reticulocyte counts. Do a bone marrow aspiration and trephine biopsy immediately and repeat with sufficient frequency to monitor recovery.

Special periodic studies might be helpful as follows: White cell and platelet antibodies. ^{59}Fe-ferrokinetic studies. Peripheral blood cell typing. Cytogenetic studies on marrow and peripheral blood. Bone marrow culture studies for colony-forming units. Hemoglobin electrophoresis for A_2 and F hemoglobin. Serum folic acid and B_{12} levels.

A fully developed aplastic anemia will require appropriate, intensive monitoring and therapy, for which specialized consultation should be sought.

Patient Information

Apprise patients of the early toxic signs and symptoms of a potential hematologic problem, as well as dermatologic, hypersensitivity, or hepatic reactions. These symptoms may include, but are not limited to, fever, sore throat, rash, ulcers in the mouth, easy bruising, lymphadenopathy, petechial or purpuric hemorrhage, and in the case of liver reactions, anorexia, nausea/vomiting, or jaundice. Advise the patient that, because these signs and symptoms may signal a serious reaction, they must report any occurrence immediately to a health care provider. In addition, advise the patient to report these signs and symptoms even if mild or occurring after extended use.

Advise patients that carbamazepine may produce drowsiness, dizziness, or blurred vision; advise patients to observe caution while driving or performing other tasks requiring alertness, coordination, or physical dexterity.

Advise patients to notify their health care providers if any of the following occurs: unusual bleeding or bruising, fever, sore throat, rash or ulcers in the mouth, lymphadenopathy, and petechial or purpuric hemorrhage, and, in the case of liver reactions, anorexia, nausea/vomiting, or jaundice.

Advise patients to take the medication with food; however, the ER capsules can be taken with or without food.

Inform patients that the ER tablet coating is not absorbed and is excreted in the feces; these coatings may be noticeable in the stool.

Inform patients not to administer carbamazepine suspension simultaneously with other liquid medications.

Advise patients that if they are taking the suspension, to shake it well before administering.

Inform patients that the capsule formulation may be opened and the beads sprinkled over food, such as applesauce or other similar foods. Inform patients not to crush or chew the capsule.

Inform patients not to use carbamazepine in combination with any other medications containing carbamazepine.

Advise patients to use caution if alcohol is taken in combination with carbamazepine therapy, because of possible additive sedative effect.

Carbamazepine may interact with some drugs. Therefore, advise patients to report to their doctors the use of any other prescription or nonprescription medication or herbal product.

ACETAZOLAMIDE

Refer to the general discussion beginning in the Anticonvulsants introduction. For complete prescribing information, refer to the Acetazolamide monograph in the Renal and Genitourinary Agents.

OXCARBAZEPINE

Rx	**Trileptal** (Novartis)	**Tablets**: 150 mg	(T/D C/G). Yellow, oval, scored. Film-coated. In 100s, 1000s, and UD 100s.
		300 mg	(TE/TE CG/CG). Yellow, oval, scored. Film-coated. In 100s, 1000s, and UD 100s.
		600 mg	(TF/TF CG/CG). Yellow, oval, scored. Film-coated. In 100s, 1000s, and UD 100s.
		Suspension: 300 mg/5 mL	Saccharin, sorbitol, ethanol. In 250 mL with dosing syringe and adapter.

OXCARBAZEPINE — ORAL

Indications

➤*Epilepsy:* For use as monotherapy or adjunctive therapy in the treatment of partial seizures in adults and children 4 to 16 years of age with epilepsy.

➤*Unlabeled uses:* Alternative treatment for bipolar disorder.

Administration and Dosage

➤*Approved by the FDA:* January 17, 2000.

Give all dosing in a twice-daily regimen. Oxcarbazepine may be taken with or without food.

➤*Adults:*

Adjunctive therapy – Initiate treatment with a dose of 600 mg/day, given in a twice-daily regimen. If clinically indicated, the dose may be increased by a maximum of 600 mg/day at approximately weekly intervals; the recommended daily dose is 1200 mg/day. Daily doses more than 1200 mg/day show somewhat greater effectiveness in controlled trials, but most patients were not able to tolerate the 2400 mg/day dose, primarily because of CNS effects. Closely observe and monitor the plasma levels of the concomitant antiepileptic drugs (AEDs) during the period of oxcarbazepine titration, as these plasma levels may be altered, especially at oxcarbazepine doses greater than 1200 mg/day.

Conversion to monotherapy – Patients receiving concomitant AEDs may be converted to monotherapy by initiating treatment with oxcarbazepine at 300 mg twice daily while simultaneously initiating the reduction of the concomitant AEDs' dose. Withdraw the concomitant AEDs over 3 to 6 weeks, while reaching the maximum dose of oxcarbazepine in approximately 2 to 4 weeks. Oxcarbazepine may be increased as clinically indicated by a maximum increment of 600 mg/day at approximate weekly intervals to achieve the recommended daily dose of 2400 mg/day. A daily dose of 1200 mg/day has been shown in 1 study to be effective in patients in whom monotherapy has been initiated with oxcarbazepine.

Initiation of monotherapy – Initiate at a dose of 600 mg/day (given in a twice-daily regimen). Increase by 300 mg/day every third day to a dose of 1200 mg/day. Controlled trials in these patients examined the effectiveness of a 1200 mg/day dose; a dose of 2400 mg/day has been shown to be effective in patients converted from other AEDs to oxcarbazepine monotherapy.

➤*Pediatric patients 4 to 16 years of age:*

Adjunctive therapy – Initiate at a daily dose of 8 to 10 mg/kg not to exceed 300 mg twice daily. Achieve the target maintenance dose of oxcarbazepine over 2 weeks, according to patient weight, using the following table.

Weight (kg)	Target maintenance dose (mg/day)
20 to 29	900
29.1 to 39	1200
> 39	1800

In the clinical trial in which the intention was to reach these target doses, the median daily dose was 31 mg/kg with a range of 6 to 51 mg/kg.

Conversion to monotherapy – Patients receiving concomitant AEDs may be converted to monotherapy by initiating treatment at approximately 8 to 10 mg/kg/day given in a twice-daily regimen, while simultaneously initiating the reduction of the dose of the concomitant AEDs. The concomitant AEDs can be completely withdrawn over 3 to 6 weeks, while oxcarbazine may be increased as clinically indicated by a maximum increment of 10 mg/kg/day at approximately weekly intervals to achieve the recommended daily dose.

Initiation of monotherapy – Patients not currently being treated with antiepileptic drugs may have monotherapy initiated with oxcarbazine. Initiate at a dose of 8 to 10 mg/kg/day given in a twice daily regimen. Increase the dose by 5 mg/kg/day every third day to the recommended daily dose shown in the table below.

Maintenance Doses of Oxcarbazine for Children During Monotherapy	
Weight (kg)	Dose (mg/day)
20	600 to 900
25	900 to 1200
30	900 to 1200
35	900 to 1500
40	900 to 1500
45	1200 to 1500
50	1200 to 1800
55	1200 to 1800
60	1200 to 2100
65	1200 to 2100
70	1500 to 2100

➤*Renal function impairment (Ccr less than 30 mL/min):* Initiate therapy at one-half the usual starting dose (300 mg/day), and increase slowly to achieve the desired clinical response.

➤*Storage/Stability:* Store at 25°C (77°F); excursions permitted to 15° to 30°C (59° to 86°F). Dispense in tight container.

Store oral suspension in the original container. Shake well before using. Use within 7 weeks of first opening the bottle.

Actions

➤*Pharmacology:* Oxcarbazepine activity is primarily exerted through the 10-monohydroxy metabolite (MHD) of oxcarbazepine. The precise mechanism by which oxcarbazepine and MHD exert their antiseizure effect is unknown; however, in vitro electrophysiological studies indicate that they produce blockade of voltage-sensitive sodium channels, resulting in stabilization of hyperexcited neural membranes, inhibition of repetitive neuronal firing, and diminution of propagation of synaptic impulses. These actions are thought to be important in the prevention of seizure spread in the intact brain. In addition, increased potassium conductance and modulation of high-voltage activated calcium channels may contribute to the anticonvulsant effects of the drug. No significant interactions of oxcarbazepine or MHD with brain neurotransmitters or modulator receptor sites have been demonstrated.

➤*Pharmacokinetics:*

Absorption – Following oral administration of oxcarbazepine, it is completely absorbed and extensively metabolized to its pharmacologically active MHD metabolite. After single dose administration of the tablets and suspension to healthy male volunteers under fasted conditions, the median T_{max} was 4.5 (range, 3 to 13 hours and 6 hours, respectively). Food does not effect the rate or extent of oxcarbazepine absorption.

Steady-state plasma concentrations of MHD are reached within 2 to 3 days in patients when oxcarbazine is given twice a day. At steady state, the pharmacokinetics of MHD are linear and show dose proportionality over the dose range of 300 to 2400 mg/day.

Distribution – The apparent volume of distribution of MHD is 49 L. Approximately 40% of MHD is bound to serum proteins, predominantly to albumin. Binding is independent of the serum concentration within the therapeutically relevant range. Oxcarbazepine and MHD do not bind to alpha-1-acid glycoprotein.

Metabolism – Oxcarbazepine is rapidly reduced by cytosolic enzymes in the liver to its MHD, which is primarily responsible for the pharmacological effect of oxcarbazepine. MHD is metabolized further by conjugation with glucuronic acid. Minor amounts (ie, 4% of the dose) are oxidized to the pharmacologically inactive 10,11-dihydroxy metabolite (DHD).

Excretion – The half-life of the parent drug is approximately 2 hours, while the half-life of MHD is approximately 9 hours. Oxcarbazepine is excreted from the body mostly in the form of metabolites, predominantly by the kidneys. More than 95% of the dose appears in the urine, with less than 1% as unchanged oxcarbazepine. Fecal excretion accounts for less than 4% of the administered dose. Approximately 80% of the dose is excreted in the urine either as glucuronides of MHD (49%) or as unchanged MHD (27%); the inactive DHD accounts for approximately 3%, and conjugates of MHD and oxcarbazepine account for 13% of the dose.

Special populations –

Renal function impairment: When oxcarbazepine is administered as a single 300 mg dose in renally impaired patients (Ccr less than 30 mL/min), the elimination half-life of MHD is prolonged to 19 hours, with a 2-fold increase in AUC.

Elderly: Following administration of single (300 mg) and multiple (600 mg/day) doses of oxcarbazine to elderly volunteers (60 to 82 years of age), the maximum plasma concentrations and AUC values of MHD were 30% to 60% higher than in younger volunteers (18 to 32 years of age). Comparisons of Ccr in young and elderly volunteers indicate that the difference was caused by age-related reductions in Ccr.

Children: After a single-dose administration of 5 to 15 mg/kg of oxcarbazepine, the dose-adjusted AUC values of MHD were 30% to 40% lower in children younger than 8 years of age than in children older than 8 years of age. The clearance in children older than 8 years of age approaches that of adults.

Contraindications

Known hypersensitivity to oxcarbazepine or any of its components.

Warnings

➤*Hyponatremia:* Clinically significant hyponatremia (sodium less than 125 mmol/L) generally occurred during the first 3 months of treatment with oxcarbazepine, although there were patients who first developed a serum sodium less than 125 mmol/L more than 1 year after initiation of therapy. Most patients who developed hyponatremia were asymptomatic, but patients in the clinical trials were frequently monitored. Some had their oxcarbazepine dose reduced or discontinued or had their fluid intake restricted for hyponatremia. Whether or not these maneuvers prevented the occurrence of more severe events is unknown. Cases of symptomatic hyponatremia have been reported during postmarketing use. In clinical trials,

OXCARBAZEPINE — ORAL

patients whose treatment with oxcarbazepine was discontinued because of hyponatremia generally experienced normalization of serum sodium within a few days without additional treatment.

Measure serum sodium levels for patients during maintenance treatment with oxcarbazepine, particularly if the patient is receiving other medications known to decrease serum sodium levels (eg, drugs associated with inappropriate ADH secretion) or if symptoms possibly indicating hyponatremia develop (eg, nausea, malaise, headache, lethargy, confusion, obtundation, or increase in seizure frequency or severity).

➤*History of hypersensitivity reaction to carbamazepine:* Approximately 25% to 30% of patients who have had hypersensitivity reactions to carbamazepine will experience a hypersensitivity reaction with oxcarbazepine. Treat with oxcarbazepine only if the potential benefit justifies the potential risk.

➤*Renal function impairment:* There is a linear correlation between Ccr and the renal clearance of MHD (see Administration and Dosage).

➤*Carcinogenesis:* In mice, a dose-related increase in the incidence of hepatocellular adenomas was observed at oxcarbazepine doses of at least 70 mg/kg/day or approximately 0.1 times the maximum recommended human dose (MRHD) on a mg/m^2 basis. In rats, the incidence of hepatocellular carcinomas was increased in females treated with oxcarbazepine at doses at least 25 mg/kg/day (0.1 times the MRHD on a mg/m^2 basis), and incidences of hepatocellular adenomas or carcinomas were increased in males and females treated with MHD at doses of 600 mg/kg/day (2.4 times the MRHD on a mg/m^2 basis) and at least 250 mg/kg/day (equivalent to the MRHD on a mg/m^2 basis), respectively. There was an increase in the incidence of benign testicular interstitial cell tumors in rats at 250 mg oxcarbazepine/kg/day and at least 250 mg MHD/kg/day, and an increase in the incidence of granular cell tumors in the cervix and vagina in rats at 600 mg MHD/kg/day.

➤*Mutagenesis:* Oxcarbazepine increased mutation frequencies in the Ames test in vitro in the absence of metabolic activation in 1 of 5 bacterial strains. Oxcarbazepine and MHD produced increases in chromosomal aberrations and polyploidy in the Chinese hamster ovary assay in vitro in the absence of metabolic activation.

➤*Fertility impairment:* In a fertility study in which rats were administered MHD (50, 150, or 450 mg/kg) orally prior to and during mating and early gestation, estrous cyclicity was disrupted and numbers of corpora lutea, implantations, and live embryos were reduced in females receiving the highest dose (approximately 2 times the MRHD on a mg/m^2 basis).

➤*Elderly:* Following administration of single (300 mg) and multiple (600 mg/day) doses of oxcarbazepine to elderly volunteers (60 to 82 years of age), the maximum plasma concentrations and AUC values of MHD were 30% to 60% higher than in younger volunteers (18 to 32 years of age). Comparisons of Ccr in young and elderly volunteers indicate that the difference was caused by age-related reductions in Ccr.

➤*Pregnancy: Category C.* Increased incidences of fetal structural abnormalities and other manifestations of developmental toxicity (embryolethality, growth retardation) were observed in the offspring of animals treated with either oxcarbazepine or MHD during pregnancy at doses similar to the MRHD.

When pregnant rats were given oxcarbazepine (30, 300, or 1000 mg/kg) orally throughout the period of organogenesis, increased incidences of fetal malformations (craniofacial, cardiovascular, and skeletal) and variations were observed at the intermediate and high doses (approximately 1.2 to 4 times, respectively, the MRHD on a mg/m^2 basis). Increased embryofetal death and decreased fetal body weights were seen at the high dose. Doses of at least 300 mg/kg were also maternally toxic (decreased body weight gain, clinical signs), but there is no evidence to suggest that teratogenicity was secondary to the maternal effects.

In a study in which pregnant rabbits were orally administered MHD (20, 100, or 200 mg/kg) during organogenesis, embryofetal mortality was increased at the highest dose (1.5 times the MRHD on a mg/m^2 basis). This dose produced only minimal maternal toxicity.

In a study in which female rats were dosed orally with oxcarbazepine (25, 50, or 150 mg/kg) during the latter part of gestation and throughout the lactation period, a persistent reduction in body weights and altered behavior (decreased activity) were observed in offspring exposed to the highest dose (0.6 times the MRHD on a mg/m^2 basis). Oral administration of MHD (25, 75, or 250 mg/kg) to rats during gestation and lactation resulted in a persistent reduction in offspring weights at the highest dose (equivalent to the MRHD on a mg/m^2 basis).

Oxcarbazepine and its metabolite are transferred through the placenta.

There are no adequate and well-controlled clinical studies of oxcarbazepine in pregnant women; however, it is closely related structurally to carbamazepine, which is considered to be teratogenic in humans. Therefore, it is likely that oxcarbazepine is a human teratogen. Use during pregnancy only if the potential benefit justifies the potential risk to the fetus.

➤*Lactation:* Oxcarbazepine and its active metabolite MHD are excreted in human breast milk. A milk-to-plasma concentration ratio of 0:5 was found for both. Because of the potential for serious adverse reactions, decide whether to discontinue nursing or to discontinue the drug in nursing women, taking into account the importance of the drug to the mother.

➤*Children:* Oxcarbazepine has been shown to be effective as adjunctive therapy or monotherapy for partial seizures in patients 4 to 16 years of age.

Precautions

➤*CNS effects:* Oxcarbazepine has been associated with cognitive symptoms including psychomotor slowing, difficulty with concentration, and speech or language problems; somnolence or fatigue; and coordination abnormalities, including ataxia and gait disturbances.

➤*Withdrawal of AEDs:* Withdraw gradually to minimize the potential of increased seizure frequency.

➤*Lab test abnormalities:* Serum sodium levels less than 125 mmol/L have been observed in patients treated with oxcarbazepine. Experience from clinical trials indicates that serum sodium levels return toward normal when the oxcarbazepine dosage is reduced or discontinued or when the patient is treated conservatively (eg, fluid restriction).

Laboratory data from clinical trials suggest that oxcarbazepine use was associated with decreases in T_4, without changes in T_3 or TSH.

Drug Interactions

➤*Cytochrome P450:* Oxcarbazepine inhibits CYP2C19 and induces CYP3A4/5 with potentially important effects on plasma concentrations of other drugs. In addition, several AEDs that are cytochrome P450 inducers can decrease plasma concentrations of oxcarbazepine and MHD.

Oxcarbazepine and its pharmacologically active MHD have little or no capacity to function as inhibitors for most of the human cytochrome P450 enzymes evaluated (CYP1A2, CYP2A6, CYP2C9, CYP2D6, CYP2E1, CYP4A9, and CYP4A11), with the exception of CYP2C19 and CYP3A4/5. Although inhibition of CYP3A4/5 by oxcarbazepine and MHD did occur at high concentrations, it is not likely to be of clinical significance. However, the inhibition of CYP2C19 by oxcarbazepine and MHD is clinically relevant.

In vitro, the UDP-glucuronyl transferase level was increased, indicating induction of this enzyme. Increases of 22% with MHD and 47% with oxcarbazepine were observed. As MHD, the predominant plasma substrate, is only a weak inducer of UDP-glucuronyl transferase, it is unlikely to have an effect on drugs that are mainly eliminated by conjugation through UDP-glucuronyl transferase (eg, valproic acid).

In addition, oxcarbazepine and MHD induce a subgroup of the cytochrome P450 3A family (CYP3A4 and CYP3A5) responsible for the metabolism of dihydropyridine calcium antagonists and oral contraceptives, resulting in a lower plasma concentration of these drugs.

As binding of MHD to plasma proteins is low (40%), clinically significant interactions with other drugs through competition for protein-binding sites are unlikely.

Strong inducers of CYP450 enzymes (ie, carbamazepine, phenytoin, phenobarbital) have been shown to decrease the plasma levels of MHD.

Oxcarbazepine Drug Interactions

Precipitant drug	Object drug*		Description
Carbamazepine	Oxcarbazepine	⬇	Concurrent use of carbamazepine and oxcarbazepine decreased MHD[1] concentration by ≈ 40%.
Phenobarbital	Oxcarbazepine	⬇	Administration of phenobarbital with oxcarbazepine decreased MHD[1] concentrations ≈ 25% while phenobarbital concentrations increased ≈ 14%.
Oxcarbazepine	Phenobarbital	⬆	
Phenytoin	Oxcarbazepine	⬇	Coadministration of phenytoin with oxcarbazepine (600 to 1800 mg/day) caused a 30% decrease in MHD[1] AUC. Higher doses of oxcarbazepine (> 1200 to 2400 mg/day) increased phenytoin concentrations up to 40%. A decrease in phenytoin dose may be required when given with oxcarbazepine in doses > 1200 mg/day.
Oxcarbazepine	Phenytoin	⬆	
Oxcarbazepine	Felodipine	⬇	The AUC of felodipine decreased by 28% when repeatedly administered in combination with oxcarbazepine.
Oxcarbazepine	Oral contraceptives	⬇	The mean AUC of ethinyl estradiol decreased by 48% to 52% and the mean AUC of levonorgestrel decreased by 32% to 52% when administered in combination with oxcarbazepine.
Valproic acid	Oxcarbazepine	⬇	Concurrent use of valproic acid and oxcarbazepine decreased MHD[1] concentrations ≈ 18%.
Oxcarbazepine	Lamotrigine	⬇	Oxcarbazepine administration reduced serum concentrations of lamotrigine 29%. Adjust the dose of lamotrigine as needed.
Verapamil	Oxcarbazepine	⬇	Verapamil administration resulted in a 20% decrease of oxcarbazepine (MHD)[1] plasma levels.

* ⬆ = Object drug increased. ⬇ = Object drug decreased.
[1] MHD = pharmacologically active 10-monohydroxy metabolite of oxcarbazepine.

OXCARBAZEPINE — ORAL

Adverse Reactions

Oxcarbazepine (OXC) Adverse Reactions in Adults (%)								
	Patients on Adjunctive Therapy Treated with Oxcarbazepine (mg/day)				Patients on Monotherapy Previously Treated with Other AEDs (mg/day)		Patients on Monotherapy Not Previously Treated with Other AEDs (mg/day)	
Adverse reactions	OXC 600 (n = 163)	OXC 1200 (n = 171)	OXC 2400 (n = 126)	Placebo (n = 166)	OXC 2400 (n = 86)	OXC 300 (n = 86)	OXC (n = 55)	Placebo (n = 49)
CNS								
Headache	32	28	26	23	31	15	13	10
Dizziness	26	32	49	13	28	8	22	6
Somnolence	20	28	36	12	19	5		
Anxiety					7	5		
Ataxia	9	17	31	5	7	1	5	0
Vertigo	6	12	15	2	3	0		
Abnormal gait	5	10	17	1				
Insomnia	4	2	3	1	6	3		
Tremor	3	8	16	5	6	3	4	0
Amnesia					5	1	4	2
Convulsions aggravated					5	2		
Emotional lability					3	2		
Hypoesthesia					3	1		
Nervousness	2	4	2	1	7	0	5	2
Agitation	1	1	2	1				
Abnormal coordination	1	3	2	1	2	1	4	2
Abnormal EEG	0	0	2	0				
Speech disorder	1	1	3	0	2	0		
Confusion	1	1	2	1	7	0		
Cranial injury nos[1]	1	0	2	1				
Dysmetria	1	2	3	0				
Abnormal thinking	0	2	4	0				
Dermatologic								
Acne	1	2	2	0				
Hot flushes					2	1		
Purpura					2	0		
Rash							4	2
GI								
Nausea	15	25	29	10	22	7	16	12
Vomiting	13	25	36	5	15	5	7	6
Abdominal pain	10	13	11	5	5	3		
Anorexia					5	3		
Dry mouth					3	0		
Rectum hemorrhage					2	0		
Toothache					2	1		
Diarrhea	5	6	7	6	7	5	7	2
Dyspepsia	5	5	6	2	6	1	5	4
Constipation	2	2	6	4			5	0
Gastritis	2	1	2	1				
GU								
Urinary tract infection					5	1		
Micturition frequency					2	1		
Vaginitis					2	0		
Metabolic/Nutritional								
Hyponatremia	3	1	2	1	5	0		
Thirst					2	0		
Musculoskeletal								
Muscle weakness	1	2	2	0				
Back pain							4	2
Sprains/Strains	0	2	2	1				
Respiratory								
Rhinitis	2	4	5	4				
Upper respiratory tract infection					10	5	7	0
Coughing					5	0		
Bronchitis					3	0		
Pharyngitis					3	0		
Epistaxis							4	0
Chest infection							4	0
Sinusitis							4	2

OXCARBAZEPINE — ORAL

Oxcarbazepine (OXC) Adverse Reactions in Adults (%)								
	Patients on Adjunctive Therapy Treated with Oxcarbazepine (mg/day)				Patients on Monotherapy Previously Treated with Other AEDs (mg/day)		Patients on Monotherapy Not Previously Treated with Other AEDs (mg/day)	
Adverse reactions	OXC 600 (n = 163)	OXC 1200 (n = 171)	OXC 2400 (n = 126)	Placebo (n = 166)	OXC 2400 (n = 86)	OXC 300 (n = 86)	OXC (n = 55)	Placebo (n = 49)
Special senses								
Diplopia	14	30	40	5	12	1		
Nystagmus	7	20	26	5	2	0		
Taste perversion					5	0		
Earache					2	1		
Ear infection nos[1]					2	0		
Abnormal vision	6	14	13	4	14	2	4	0
Abnormal accommodation	0	0	2	0				
Miscellaneous								
Fatigue	15	12	15	7	21	5		
Fever					3	0		
Allergy					2	0		
Generalized edema					2	1		
Chest pain					2	0		
Asthenia	6	3	6	5				
Edema, legs	2	1	2	1				
Weight increase	1	2	2	1				
Abnormal feeling	0	1	2	0				
Falling down nos[1]							4	0
Lymphadenopathy					2	0		
Hypotension	0	1	2	0				
Infection viral					7	5		
Infection					2	0		

[1] nos = not otherwise specified

Adjunctive therapy/monotherapy in adults previously treated with other AEDs – The most commonly observed (at least 5%) adverse experiences seen in association with oxcarbazepine and substantially more frequent than in placebo-treated patients were the following: Dizziness, somnolence, diplopia, fatigue, nausea, vomiting, ataxia, abnormal vision, abdominal pain, tremor, dyspepsia, abnormal gait.

Approximately 23% of 1537 adult patients discontinued treatment because of an adverse experience. The adverse experiences most commonly associated with discontinuation were the following: Dizziness (6.4%), diplopia (5.9%), ataxia (5.2%), vomiting (5.1%), nausea (4.9%), somnolence (3.8%), headache (2.9%), fatigue (2.1%), abnormal vision (2.1%), tremor (1.8%), abnormal gait (1.7%), rash (1.4%), hyponatremia (1%).

Monotherapy in adults not previously treated with other AEDs – Approximately 9% of 295 adult patients discontinued treatment because of an adverse experience. The adverse experiences most commonly associated with discontinuation were the following: Dizziness, nausea, rash (1.7%); headache (1.4%).

Pediatric Patients on Adjunctive/Monotherapy Previously Treated with Other AEDs (≥ 2%)		
Adverse reactions	OXC (n = 171)	Placebo (n = 139)
CNS		
Headache	31	19
Somnolence	31	13
Dizziness	28	8
Ataxia	13	4
Emotional lability	8	4
Abnormal gait	8	3
Tremor	6	4
Speech disorder	3	1
Impaired concentration	2	1
Convulsions	2	1
Involuntary muscle contractions	2	1
Vertigo	2	0
Dermatologic		
Bruising	4	2
Increased sweating	3	0
GI		
Vomiting	33	14
Nausea	19	5
Constipation	4	1
Dyspepsia	2	0

Pediatric Patients on Adjunctive/Monotherapy Previously Treated with Other AEDs (≥ 2%)		
Adverse reactions	OXC (n = 171)	Placebo (n = 139)
Respiratory		
Rhinitis	10	9
Pneumonia	2	1
Special senses		
Diplopia	17	1
Abnormal vision	13	1
Nystagmus	9	1
Miscellaneous		
Fatigue	13	9
Allergy	2	0
Asthenia	2	1

Adjunctive therapy/monotherapy in pediatric patients previously treated with other AEDs – The most commonly observed (at least 5%) adverse experiences seen in association with oxcarbazepine in pediatric patients were similar to those seen in adults.

Approximately 11% of the 456 pediatric patients discontinued treatment because of an adverse experience. The adverse experiences most commonly associated with discontinuation were the following: Somnolence (2.4%); vomiting (2%); ataxia (1.8%); diplopia, dizziness (1.3%); fatigue, nystagmus (1.1%).

Monotherapy in pediatric patients not previously treated with other AEDs – Approximately 9.2% of 152 pediatric patients discontinued treatment because of an adverse experience. The adverse experiences most commonly associated (at least 1%) with discontinuation were rash (5.3%) and maculopapular rash (1.3%).

➤*Cardiovascular:* Bradycardia; cardiac failure; cerebral hemorrhage; hypertension; postural hypotension; palpitation; syncope; tachycardia.

➤*CNS:* Aggressive reaction; amnesia; anguish; anxiety; apathy; aphasia; aura; aggravated convulsions; delirium; delusion; depressed level of consciousness; dysphonia; dystonia; emotional lability; euphoria; extrapyramidal disorder; feeling drunk; hemiplegia; hyperkinesia; hyperreflexia; hypoesthesia; hypokinesia; hyporeflexia; hypotonia; hysteria; decreased/increased libido; manic reaction; migraine; involuntary muscle contractions; nervousness; neuralgia; oculogyric crisis; panic disorder; paralysis; paroniria; personality disorder; psychosis; ptosis; stupor; tetany.

➤*Dermatologic:* Acne; alopecia; angioedema; bruising; contact dermatitis; eczema; facial rash; flushing; folliculitis; heat rash; hot flushes; photosensitivity reaction; genital pruritus; psoriasis; purpura; erythematous rash; maculopapular rash; vitiligo; urticaria.

➤*GI:* Increased appetite; blood in stool; cholelithiasis; colitis; duodenal ulcer; dysphagia; enteritis; eructation; esophagitis; flatulence; gastric ulcer;

OXCARBAZEPINE — ORAL

gingival bleeding; gum hyperplasia; hematemesis; rectum hemorrhage; hemorrhoids; hiccough; dry mouth; biliary pain; hypochondrium pain right; retching; sialoadenitis; stomatitis; ulcerative stomatitis.

➤*GU:* Dysuria; hematuria; intermenstrual bleeding; leukorrhea; menorrhagia; micturition frequency; renal pain; urinary tract pain; polyuria; priapism; renal calculus.

➤*Hematologic:* Leukopenia; thrombocytopenia.

➤*Lab test abnormalities:* Increased gamma-GT; hyperglycemia; hypocalcemia; hypoglycemia; hypokalemia; elevated liver enzymes; increased serum transaminase.

➤*Respiratory:* Asthma; dyspnea; epistaxis; laryngismus; pleurisy.

➤*Special senses:* Abnormal accommodation; cataract; conjunctival hemorrhage; eye edema; hemianopia; mydriasis; otitis externa; photophobia, scotoma; taste perversion; tinnitus; xerophthalmia.

➤*Miscellaneous:* Fever; malaise; precordial chest pain; rigors; weight decrease; hypertonia muscle; procedure dental oral; procedure female reproductive; procedure musculoskeletal; procedure skin; systemic lupus erythematosus.

Postmarketing – The following adverse events not seen in controlled clinical trials have been observed in named patient programs or post-marketing experience.

➤*Dermatologic:* Erythema multiforme; Stevens-Johnson syndrome; toxic epidermal necrolysis.

➤*Miscellaneous:* Multiorgan hypersensitivity disorders characterized by features such as rash, fever, lymphadenopathy, abnormal liver function tests, eosinophilia, and arthralgia.

Isolated cases of overdose with oxcarbazepine have been reported. The maximum dose taken was approximately 24,000 mg. All patients recovered with symptomatic treatment.

➤*Treatment:* There is no specific antidote. Administer symptomatic and supportive treatment as appropriate. Consider removal of the drug by gastric lavage and/or inactivation by administering activated charcoal.

Patient Information

Inform patients that approximately 25% to 30% of patients who have exhibited hypersensitivity reactions to carbamazepine may experience hypersensitivity reactions to oxcarbazepine.

Additional nonhormonal forms of contraception are recommended when using oxcarbazepine because of a reduction in hormonal contraceptive efficacy.

Advise patients to exercise caution if alcohol is taken in combination with oxcarbazepine therapy because of a possible additive sedative effect.

Oxcarbazepine may cause dizziness and somnolence. Accordingly, advise patients not to drive or operate machinery until they have gained sufficient experience on oxcarbazepine to gauge whether it adversely affects their ability to drive or operate machinery.

FELBAMATE

Rx	**Felbatol**[1] (Wallace Labs)	**Tablets**: 400 mg	Lactose. (Wallace 0430). Yellow, scored. Capsule shape. In 100s and UD 100s.
		600 mg	Lactose. (Wallace 0431). Peach, scored. Capsule shape. In 100s and UD 100s.
		Suspension : 600 mg/5 ml	Sorbitol, parabens, saccharin. In 240 and 960 ml.

[1] It has been recommended that use of this drug be discontinued if aplastic anemia or hepatic failure occurs unless, in the judgment of the physician, continued therapy is warranted. See Warning box. For further information contact Wallace Labs at 800–526–3840.

FELBAMATE — ORAL

Refer to the general discussion beginning in the Anticonvulsants introduction.

WARNING

Felbamate should not be used by patients until there has been a complete discussion of the risks and the patient, parent, or guardian has provided written informed consent.

Aplastic anemia – The use of felbamate is associated with a marked increase in the incidence of aplastic anemia. Accordingly, felbamate should only be used in patients whose epilepsy is so severe that the risk of aplastic anemia is deemed acceptable in light of the benefits conferred by its use. Ordinarily, a patient should not be placed on or continued on felbamate without consideration of appropriate expert hematologic consultation.

Among felbamate treated patients, aplastic anemia (pancytopenia in the presence of a bone marrow largely depleted of hematopoietic precursors) occurs at an incidence that may be more than a 100-fold greater than that seen in the untreated population (ie, 2 to 5 per million persons per year). The risk of death in patients with aplastic anemia generally varies as a function of its severity and etiology; current estimates of the overall case fatality rate are in the range of 20% to 30%, but rates as high as 70% have been reported in the past.

There are too few felbamate associated cases, and too little known about them to provide a reliable estimate of the syndrome's incidence or its case fatality rate or to identify the factors, if any, that might conceivably be used to predict who is at greater or lesser risk.

In managing patients on felbamate, it should be borne in mind that the clinical manifestation of aplastic anemia may not be seen until after a patient has been on felbamate for several months (eg, onset of aplastic anemia among felbamate exposed patients for whom data are available has ranged from 5 to 30 weeks). However, the injury to bone marrow stem cells that is held to be ultimately responsible for the anemia may occur weeks to months earlier. Accordingly, patients who are discontinued from felbamate remain at risk for developing anemia for a variable, and unknown, period afterwards.

It is not known whether or not the risk of developing aplastic anemia changes with duration of exposure. Consequently, it is not safe to assume that a patient who has been on felbamate without signs of hematologic abnormality for long periods of time is without risk.

It is not known whether the dose of felbamate affects the incidence of aplastic anemia.

It is not known whether or not concomitant use of antiepileptic drugs or other drugs affects the incidence of aplastic anemia.

Aplastic anemia typically develops without premonitory clinical or laboratory signs, the full blown syndrome presenting with signs of infection, bleeding, or anemia. Accordingly, routine blood testing cannot be reliably used to reduce the incidence of aplastic anemia, but, it will, in some cases, allow the detection of the hematologic changes before the syndrome declares itself clinically. Felbamate should be discontinued if any evidence of bone marrow depression occurs.

WARNING (cont.)

Hepatic failure – Evaluation of postmarketing experience suggests that acute liver failure is associated with the use of felbamate. The reported rate in the US has been about 6 cases of liver failure leading to death or transplant per 75,000 patient years of use. This rate is an underestimate because of under reporting, and the true rate could be considerably greater than this. For example, if the reporting rate is 10%, the true rate would be 1 case per 1250 patient years of use.

Of the cases reported, about 67% resulted in death or liver transplantation, usually within 5 weeks of the onset of signs and symptoms of liver failure. The earliest onset of severe hepatic dysfunction followed subsequently by liver failure was 3 weeks after initiation of felbamate. Although some reports described dark urine and nonspecific prodromal symptoms (eg, anorexia, malaise, and gastrointestinal symptoms), in other reports it was not clear if any prodromal symptoms preceded the onset of jaundice.

It is not known whether or not the risk of developing hepatic failure changes with duration of exposure.

It is not known whether or not the dosage of felbamate affects the incidence of hepatic failure.

It is not known whether concomitant use of other antiepileptic drugs or other drugs affect the incidence of hepatic failure.

Felbamate should not be prescribed for anyone with a history of hepatic dysfunction.

Treatment with felbamate should be initiated only in individuals without active liver disease and with normal baseline serum transaminases. It has not been proved that periodic serum transaminase testing will prevent serious injury but it is generally believed that early detection of drug-induced hepatic injury along with immediate withdrawal of the suspect drug enhances the likelihood for recovery. There is no information available that documents how rapidly patients can progress from normal liver function to liver failure, but other drugs known to be hepatotoxins can cause liver failure rapidly (eg, from normal enzymes to liver failure in 2 to 4 weeks). Accordingly, monitoring of serum transaminase levels (AST and ALT) is recommended at baseline and periodically thereafter. While the more frequent the monitoring the greater the chances of early detection, the precise schedule for monitoring is a matter of clinical judgement.

Felbamate should be discontinued if either serum AST or serum ALT levels become increased greater than or equal to 2 times the upper limit of normal, or if clinical signs and symptoms suggest liver failure. Patients who develop evidence of hepatocellular injury while on felbamate and are withdrawn from the drug for any reason should be presumed to be at increased risk for liver injury if felbamate is reintroduced. Accordingly, such patients should not be considered for retreatment.

Indications

➤*Seizures:* Felbamate is not indicated as a first-line antiepileptic treatment. Felbamate is recommended for use only in those patients who respond

FELBAMATE — ORAL

inadequately to alternative treatments and whose epilepsy is so severe that a substantial risk of aplastic anemia or liver failure is deemed acceptable in light of the benefits conferred by its use.

If these criteria are met and the patient has been fully advised of the risk and has provided written, informed consent, felbamate can be considered for either monotherapy or adjunctive therapy in the treatment of partial seizures, with and without generalization, in adults with epilepsy and as adjunctive therapy in the treatment of partial and generalized seizures associated with Lennox-Gastaut syndrome in children.

Administration and Dosage

➤*Approved by the FDA:* July 29, 1993.

Felbamate has been studied as monotherapy and adjunctive therapy in adults and as adjunctive therapy in children with seizures associated with Lennox-Gastaut syndrome. As felbamate is added to or substituted for existing antiepileptic drugs (AEDs), it is strongly recommended to reduce the dosage of those AEDs in the range of 20% to 33% to minimize side effects.

Felbamate should be used with caution in patients with renal dysfunction. Adjunctive therapy with medications that affect felbamate plasma concentrations, especially AEDs, may warrant further reductions in felbamate daily doses in patients with renal dysfunction.

➤*Adults (greater than or equal to 14 years of age):* The majority of patients received 3600 mg/day in clinical trials evaluating its use as both monotherapy and adjunctive therapy.

Monotherapy (initial therapy) – Felbamate has not been systematically evaluated as initial monotherapy. Initiate felbamate at 1200 mg/day in divided doses 3 or 4 times daily. The prescriber is advised to titrate previously untreated patients under close clinical supervision, increasing the dosage in 600 mg increments every 2 weeks to 2400 mg/day based on clinical response and thereafter to 3600 mg/day if clinically indicated.

Conversion to monotherapy – Initiate felbamate at 1200 mg/day in divided doses 3 or 4 times daily. Reduce the dosage of concomitant AEDs by one-third at initiation of felbamate therapy. At week 2, increase the felbamate dosage to 2400 mg/day while reducing the dosage of other AEDs up to an additional one-third of their original dosage. At week 3, increase the felbamate dosage up to 3600 mg/day and continue to reduce the dosage of other AEDs as clinically indicated.

Adjunctive therapy – Felbamate should be added at 1200 mg/day in divided doses 3 or 4 times daily while reducing present AEDs by 20% in order to control plasma concentrations of concurrent phenytoin, valproic acid, phenobarbital, and carbamazepine and its metabolites. Further reductions of the concomitant AEDs dosage may be necessary to minimize side effects due to drug interactions. Increase the dosage of felbamate by 1200 mg/day increments at weekly intervals to 3600 mg/day. Most side effects seen during felbamate adjunctive therapy resolve as the dosage of concomitant AEDs is decreased.

Felbamate Dosage Table (Adults)			
	Week 1	Week 2	Week 3
Dosage reduction of concomitant AEDs	Reduce original dose by 20% to 33%]*	Reduce original dose by up to an additional 1/3*	Reduce as clinically indicated
Felbamate dosage	1200 mg/day initial dose	2400 mg/day therapeutic dosing range	3600 mg/day therapeutic dosing range

* See Adjunctive and Conversion to monotherapy sections.

While the above felbamate conversion guidelines may result in a felbamate 3600 mg/day dose within 3 weeks, in some patients titration to a 3600 mg/day felbamate dose has been achieved in as little as 3 days with appropriate adjustment of other AEDs.

➤*Children with Lennox-Gastaut syndrome (ages 2 to 14 years):*

Adjunctive therapy – Felbamate should be added at 15 mg/kg/day in divided doses 3 or 4 times daily while reducing present AEDs by 20% in order to control plasma levels of concurrent phenytoin, valproic acid, phenobarbital, and carbamazepine and its metabolites. Further reductions of the concomitant AEDs dosage may be necessary to minimize side effects due to drug interactions. Increase the dosage of felbamate by 15 mg/kg/day increments at weekly intervals to 45 mg/kg/day. Most side effects seen during felbamate adjunctive therapy resolve as the dosage of concomitant AEDs is decreased.

➤*Storage/Stability:* Shake suspension well before using. Store at controlled room temperature 20° to 25°C (68° to 77°F). Dispense in tight container.

Actions

➤*Pharmacology:* The mechanism by which felbamate exerts its anticonvulsant activity is unknown, but in animal test systems designed to detect anticonvulsant activity, felbamate has properties in common with other marketed anticonvulsants. Felbamate is effective in mice and rats in the maximal electroshock test, the subcutaneous pentylenetetrazol seizure test, and the subcutaneous picrotoxin seizure test. Felbamate also exhibits anticonvulsant activity against seizures induced by intracerebroventricular administration of glutamate in rats and N-methyl-D,L-aspartic acid in mice. Protection against maximal electroshock-induced seizures suggests that felbamate may reduce seizure spread, an effect possibly predictive of efficacy in generalized tonic-clonic or partial seizures. Protection against pentylenetetrazol-induced seizures suggests that felbamate may increase seizure threshold, an effect considered to be predictive of potential efficacy in absence seizures.

Receptor-binding studies in vitro indicate that felbamate has weak inhibitory effects on GABA-receptor binding, benzodiazepine receptor binding, and is devoid of activity at the MK-801 receptor binding site of the NMDA receptor-ionophore complex. However, felbamate does interact as an antagonist at the strychnine-insensitive glycine recognition site of the NMDA receptor-ionophore complex. Felbamate is not effective in protecting chick embryo retina tissue against the neurotoxic effects of the excitatory amino acid agonists NMDA, kainate, or quisqualate in vitro.

The monocarbamate, p-hydroxy, and 2-hydroxy metabolites were inactive in the maximal electroshock-induced seizure test in mice. The monocarbamate and p-hydroxy metabolites had only weak (0.2 to 0.6) activity compared with felbamate in the subcutaneous pentylenetetrazol seizure test. These metabolites did not contribute significantly to the anticonvulsant action of felbamate.

➤*Pharmacokinetics:*

Absorption – Felbamate is well-absorbed after oral administration. Over 90% of the radioactivity after a dose of 1000 mg ^{14}C felbamate was found in the urine. Absolute bioavailability (oral vs parenteral) has not been measured. The tablet and suspension were each shown to be bioequivalent to the capsule used in clinical trials, and pharmacokinetic parameters of the tablet and suspension are similar. There was no effect of food on absorption of the tablet; the effect of food on absorption of the suspension has not been evaluated.

Distribution – The apparent volume of distribution was 756 ± 82 mL/kg after a 1200 mg dose. Felbamate C_{max} and AUC are proportionate to dose after single and multiple doses over a range of 100 to 800 mg single doses and 1200 to 3600 mg daily doses. C_{min} (trough) blood levels are also dose proportional. Multiple-daily doses of 1200, 2400, and 3600 mg gave C_{min} values of 30 ± 5, 55 ± 8, and 83 ± 21 mcg/mL (n = 10 patients). Linear and dose proportional pharmacokinetics were also observed at doses above 3600 mg/day up to the maximum dose studied of 6000 mg/day. Felbamate gave dose proportional steady-state peak plasma concentrations in children age 4 to 12 over a range of 15, 30, and 45 mg/kg/day with peak concentrations of 17, 32, and 49 mcg/mL.

Binding of felbamate to human plasma protein was independent of felbamate concentrations between 10 and 310 mcg/mL. Binding ranged from 22% to 25%, mostly to albumin, and was dependent on the albumin concentration.

Metabolism – Following oral administration, felbamate is the predominant plasma species (about 90% of plasma radioactivity). About 40% to 50% of absorbed dose appears unchanged in urine, and an additional 40% is present as unidentified metabolites and conjugates. About 15% is present as parahydroxyfelbamate, 2-hydroxyfelbamate, and felbamate monocarbamate, none of which have significant anticonvulsant activity.

Excretion – Felbamate is excreted with a terminal half-life of 20 to 23 hours, which is unaltered after multiple doses. Clearance after a single 1200 mg dose is 26 ± 3 mL/hr/kg, and after multiple-daily doses of 3600 mg is 30 ± 8 mL/hr/kg.

Special populations –

Renal function impairment: Felbamate's single-dose monotherapy pharmacokinetic parameters were evaluated in 12 otherwise healthy individuals with renal impairment. Reduced felbamate clearance and a longer half-life were associated with diminishing renal function.

Contraindications

Hypersensitivity to felbamate, its ingredients, or other carbamates; history of any blood dyscrasia or hepatic dysfunction.

Warnings

➤*Aplastic anemia:* The use of felbamate is associated with a marked increase in the incidence of aplastic anemia. Accordingly, felbamate should only be used in patients whose epilepsy is so severe that the risk of aplastic anemia is deemed acceptable in light of the benefits conferred by its use. Ordinarily, a patient should not be placed on or continued on felbamate without consideration of appropriate expert hematologic consultation.

See the Warning box for more information.

➤*Discontinuation:* Antiepileptic drugs should not be suddenly discontinued because of the possibility of increasing seizure frequency.

➤*Hepatic failure:* See the Warning box for more information.

➤*Renal function impairment:* A study in otherwise healthy individuals with renal dysfunction indicated that prolonged half-life and reduced clearance of felbamate are associated with diminishing renal function. Felbamate should be used with caution in patients with renal dysfunction. Adjunctive therapy with medications that affect felbamate plasma concentrations, especially AEDs, may warrant further reductions in felbamate daily doses in patients with renal dysfunction.

➤*Hepatic function impairment:* See the Warning box for more information.

➤*Carcinogenesis:* Carcinogenicity studies were conducted in mice and rats. Mice received felbamate as a feed admixture for 92 weeks at doses of 300, 600, and 1200 mg/kg and rats were also dosed by feed admixture for 104 weeks at doses of 30, 100, and 300 (males) or 10, 30, and 100 (females) mg/kg. The maximum doses in these studies produced steady-state plasma concentrations that were equal to or less than the steady-state plasma concentrations in epileptic patients receiving 3600 mg/day. There was a statistically significant increase in hepatic cell adenomas in high-dose male and female mice and in high-dose female rats. Hepatic hypertrophy was significantly increased in a dose-related manner in mince, primarily males, but also in females. Hepatic hypertrophy was not found in female rats. The relationship between the occurrence of benign hepatocellular adenomas and the finding of liver hypertrophy resulting from liver enzyme induction has not been examined. There was a statistically significant increase in benign

FELBAMATE — ORAL

interstitial cell tumors of the testes in high-dose male rats receiving felbamate. The relevance of these findings to humans is unknown.

As a result of the synthesis process, felbamate could contain small amounts of 2 known animal carcinogens, the genotoxic compound ethyl carbamate (urethane) and the nongenotoxic compound methyl carbamate. It is theoretically possible that a 50 kg patients receiving 3600 mg of felbamate could be exposed to up to 0.72 mcg of urethane and 1800 mcg of methyl carbamate. These daily doses are approximately 1/35,000 (urethane) and 1/5,500 (methyl carbamate) on a mg/m^2 basis, of the dose levels shown to be carcinogenic in rodents. Any presence of these 2 compounds in felbamate used in the lifetime carcinogenicity studies was inadequate to cause tumors.

➤*Elderly:* No systemic studies in geriatric patients have been conducted. Clinical studies of felbamate did not include sufficient numbers of patients aged 65 years and older to determine whether they respond differently from younger patients. Other reported clinical experience has not identified differences in responses between the elderly and younger patients. In general, dosage selection for an elderly patient should be cautious, usually starting at the low end of the dosing range, reflecting the greater frequency of hepatic, renal, or cardiac function, and of concomitant disease or other drug therapy.

➤*Pregnancy: Category C.* The incidence of malformations was not increased compared to control in offspring of rats or rabbits given doses up to 13.9 times (rat) and 4.2 times (rabbit) the human daily dose on a mg/kg basis, or 3 times (rat) and less than 2 times (rabbit) the human daily doses on a mg/m^2 basis. However, in rats, there was a decrease in pup weight and an increase in pup deaths during lactation. The cause for these deaths is not known. The no-effect dose for rat pup mortality was 6.9 times the human dose on a mg/kg basis or 1.5 times the human dose.

Placental transfer of felbamate occurs in rat pups. There are, however, no studies in pregnant women. Because animal reproduction studies are not always predictive of human response, this drug should be used during pregnancy only if clearly needed.

➤*Lactation:* Felbamate has been detected in human milk. The effect on the nursing infant is unknown. In rats, there was a decrease in pup weight and an increase in pup deaths during lactation. The cause for these deaths is not known.

➤*Children:* The safety and efficacy of felbamate in children other than those with Lennox-Gastaut syndrome have not been established.

Precautions

➤*Monitoring:* Full hematologic evaluations should be performed before felbamate therapy, frequently during therapy, and for a significant period of time after discontinuation of felbamate therapy. While it might appear prudent to perform frequent CBCs in patients continuing on felbamate, there is no evidence that such monitoring will allow early detection of marrow suppression before aplastic anemia occurs. Complete pretreatment blood counts, including platelets and reticulocytes, should be obtained as a baseline. If any hematologic abnormalities are detected during the course of treatment, immediate consultation with a hematologist is advised. Felbamate should be discontinued if any evidence of bone marrow depression occurs.

Treatment with felbamate should be initiated only in individuals without active liver disease and with normal baseline serum transaminases. It has not been proved that periodic serum transaminase testing will prevent serious injury but it is generally believed that early detection of drug-induced hepatic injury along with immediate withdrawal of the suspect drug enhances the likelihood for recovery. There is no information available that documents how rapidly patients can progress from normal liver function to liver failure, but other drugs known to be hepatotoxins can cause liver failure rapidly (eg, from normal enzymes to liver failure in 2 to 4 weeks). Accordingly, monitoring of serum transaminase levels (AST and ALT) is recommended at baseline and periodically thereafter. While the more frequent the monitoring the greater the chances of early detection, the precise schedule for monitoring is a matter of clinical judgement. If significant, confirmed liver abnormalities are detected during the course of felbamate treatment, felbamate should be discontinued immediately with continued liver function monitoring until values return to normal.

Drug Interactions

➤*Other antiepileptic drugs:* As felbamate is added to or substituted for existing antiepileptic drugs (AEDs), it is strongly recommended to reduce the dosage of those AEDs in the range of 20% to 33% to minimize side effects. Adjunctive therapy with medications that affect felbamate plasma concentrations, especially AEDs, may warrant further reductions in felbamate daily doses in patients with renal dysfunction. The net effect of these interactions is summarized in the following table:

AED coadministered	AED concentration	Felbamate concentration
Phenytoin	↑	↓
Valproate	↑	↔**
Carbamazepine (CBZ)	↓	↓
*CBZ epoxide	↑	
Phenobarbital	↑	↓

* Not administered, but an active metabolite of carbamazepine.
** No significant effect.

➤*Specific effects of felbamate on other antiepileptic drugs:*

Phenytoin – Felbamate causes an increase in steady-state phenytoin plasma concentrations. In 10 otherwise healthy subjects with epilepsy ingesting phenytoin, the steady-state trough (C_{min}) phenytoin plasma concentration was 17 ± 5 mcg/mL. The steady-state C_{min} increased to 21 ± 5 mcg/mL when 1200 mg/day of felbamate was coadministered. Increasing the felbamate dose to 1800 mg/day in 6 of these subjects increased the steady-state phenytoin C_{min} to 25 ± 7 mcg/mL. In order to maintain phenytoin levels, limit adverse experiences, and achieve the felbamate dose of 3600 mg/day, a phenytoin dose reduction of approximately 40% was necessary for 8 of these 10 subjects.

In a controlled clinical trial, a 20% reduction of the phenytoin dose at the initiation of felbamate therapy resulted in phenytoin levels comparable to those prior to felbamate administration.

Carbamazepine – Felbamate causes a decrease in the steady-state carbamazepine plasma concentrations and an increase in the steady-state carbamazepine epoxide plasma concentration. In 9 otherwise healthy subjects with epilepsy ingesting carbamazepine, the steady-state trough (C_{min}) carbamazepine concentration was 8 ± 2 mcg/mL. The carbamazepine steady-state C_{min} decreased 31% to 5 ± 1 mcg/mL when felbamate (3000 mg/day, divided into 3 doses) was coadministered. Carbamazepine epoxide steady-state C_{min} concentrations increased 57% from 1 ± 0.3 to 1.6 ± 0.4 mcg/mL with the addition of felbamate.

Valproate – Felbamate causes an increase in steady-state valproate concentrations. In 4 subjects with epilepsy ingesting valproate, the steady-state trough (C_{min}) valproate plasma concentration was 63 ± 16 mcg/mL. The steady-state C_{min} increased to 78 ± 14 mcg/mL when 1200 mg/day of felbamate was coadministered. Increasing the felbamate dose to 2400 mg/day increased the steady-state valproate C_{min} to 96 ± 25 mcg/mL. Corresponding values for free valproate C_{min} concentrations were 7 ± 3, 9 ± 4, and 11 ± 6 mcg/mL for 0, 1200, and 2400 mg/day felbamate, respectively. The ratios of the AUCs of unbound valproate to the AUCs of the total valproate were 11.1%, 13%, and 11.5%, with coadministration of 0, 1200, and 2400 mg/day of felbamate, respectively. This indicates that the protein binding of valproate did not change appreciably with increasing doses of felbamate.

Phenobarbital – Coadministration of felbamate with phenobarbital causes an increase in phenobarbital plasma concentrations. In 12 otherwise healthy male volunteers ingesting phenobarbital, the steady-state trough (C_{min}) phenobarbital concentration was 14.2 mcg/mL. The steady-state C_{min} concentration increased to 17.8 mcg/mL when 2400 mg/day of felbamate was coadministered for 1 week.

➤*Effects of other antiepileptic drugs on felbamate:*

Phenytoin – Phenytoin causes an approximate doubling of the clearance of felbamate at steady state and, therefore, the addition of phenytoin causes an approximately 45% decrease in the steady-state trough concentrations of felbamate as compared to the same dose of felbamate given as monotherapy.

Carbamazepine – Carbamazepine causes an approximately 50% increase in the clearance of felbamate at steady state and, therefore, the addition of carbamazepine results in an approximately 40% decrease in the steady-state trough concentrations of felbamate as compared to the same dose of felbamate given as monotherapy.

Phenobarbital – It appears that phenobarbital may reduce plasma felbamate concentrations. Steady-state plasma felbamate concentrations were found to be 29% lower than the mean concentrations of a group of newly diagnosed subjects with epilepsy also receiving 2400 mg of felbamate a day.

➤*Oral contraceptives:* A group of 24 nonsmoking, healthy white female volunteers established on an oral contraceptive regimen containing 30 mcg ethinyl estradiol and 75 mcg gestodene for at least 3 months received 2400 mg/day of felbamate from midcycle (day 15) to midcycle (day 14) of 2 consecutive oral contraceptive cycles. Felbamate treatment resulted in a 42% decrease in the gestodene $AUC_{(0-24)}$, but no clinically relevant effect was observed on the pharmacokinetic parameters of ethinyl estradiol. No volunteer showed hormonal evidence of ovulation, but 1 volunteer reported intermenstrual bleeding during felbamate treatment.

Adverse Reactions

➤*Most common adverse reactions in adults:* The most common adverse reactions seen in association with felbamate in adults during monotherapy are anorexia, vomiting, insomnia, nausea, and headache. The most common adverse reactions seen in association with felbamate in adults during adjunctive therapy are anorexia, vomiting, insomnia, nausea, dizziness, somnolence, and headache.

➤*Most common adverse reactions seen in children:* The most common adverse reactions seen in association with felbamate in children during adjunctive therapy are anorexia, vomiting, insomnia, headache, and somnolence.

➤*Dropout rate due to adverse reactions:* The dropout rate because of adverse reactions or intercurrent illnesses among adult felbamate patients was 12% (120/977). The dropout rate because of adverse reactions or intercurrent illnesses among pediatric felbamate patients was 6% (22/357). In adults, the body systems associated with causing these withdrawals in order of frequency were the following: Digestive (4.3%), psychological (2.2%), whole body (1.7%), neurological (1.5%), and dermatological (1.5%). In children, the body systems associated with causing these withdrawals in order of frequency were the following: Digestive (1.7%), neurological (1.4%), dermatological (1.4%), psychological (1.1%), and whole body (1%). In adults, specific reactions with an incidence of greater than or equal to 1% associated with causing these withdrawals, in order of frequency were the following: Anorexia (1.6%), nausea (1.4%), rash (1.2%), and weight decrease (1.1%). In children, specific reactions with an incidence of greater than or equal to 1% associated with causing these withdrawals, in order of frequency was rash (1.1%).

➤*Incidence in clinical trials:*

Adults: Incidence in controlled clinical trials (monotherapy studies in adults) – The table that follows enumerates adverse reactions that occurred at an incidence of greater than or equal to 2% among 58 adult

FELBAMATE — ORAL

patients who received felbamate monotherapy at dosages of 3600 mg/day in double-blind controlled trials. Reported adverse reactions were classified using standard WHO-based dictionary terminology.

Felbamate Adverse Reactions in Adults		
Adverse reaction	Felbamate* (n = 58) %	Low dose valproate** (n = 50) %
Miscellaneous		
Fatigue	6.9%	4%
Weight decrease	3.4%	0%
Face edema	3.4%	0%
CNS		
Insomnia	8.6%	4%
Headache	6.9%	18%
Anxiety	5.2%	2%
Dermatological		
Acne	3.4%	0%
Rash	3.4%	0%
GI		
Dyspepsia	8.6%	2%
Vomiting	8.6 %	2%
Constipation	6.9%	2%
Diarrhea	5.2%	0%
ALT increased	5.2%	2%
Metabolic/nutritional		
Hypophosphatemia	3.4%	0%
Respiratory		
Upper respiratory tract infection	8.6%	4%
Rhinitis	6.9%	0%
Special senses		
Diplopia	3.4%	4%
Otitis media	3.4%	0%
GU		
Intramenstrual bleeding	3.4%	0%
Urinary tract infection	3.4%	2%

* 3600 mg/day.
** 15 mg/kg/day.

Incidence in controlled add-on clinical studies in adults – The table that follows enumerates adverse reactions that occurred at an incidence of greater than or equal to 2% among 114 adult patients who received felbamate adjunctive therapy in add-on controlled trials at dosages up to 3600 mg/day. Reported adverse reactions were classified using standard WHO-based dictionary terminology.

Many adverse reactions that occurred during adjunctive therapy may be a result of drug interactions. Adverse reactions during adjunctive therapy typically resolved with conversion to monotherapy, or with adjustment of the dosage of other antiepileptic drugs.

Felbamate Adverse Reactions in Adults		
Adverse reaction	Felbamate (n = 114) %	Placebo (n = 43) %
Miscellaneous		
Fatigue	16.8%	7%
Fever	2.6%	4.7%
Chest pain	2.6%	0%
CNS		
Headache	36.8%	9.3%
Somnolence	19.3%	7%
Dizziness	18.4%	14%
Insomnia	17.5%	7%
Nervousness	7%	2.3%
Tremor	6.1%	2.3%
Anxiety	5.3%	4.7%
Gait abnormal	5.3%	0%
Depression	5.3%	0%
Paraesthesia	3.5%	2.3%
Ataxia	3.5%	0%
Dry mouth	2.6%	0%
Stupor	2.6%	0%
Dermatological		
Rash	3.5%	4.7%
GI		
Nausea	34.2%	2.3%
Anorexia	19.3%	2.3%
Vomiting	16.7%	4.7%
Dyspepsia	12.3%	7%
Constipation	11.4%	2.3%
Diarrhea	5.3%	2.3%
Abdominal pain	5.3%	0%
ALT increased	3.5%	0%
Musculoskeletal		
Myalgia	2.6%	0%
Respiratory		
Upper respiratory tract infection	5.3%	7%
Sinusitis	3.5%	0%
Pharyngitis	2.6%	0%
Special senses		
Diplopia	6.1%	0%
Taste perversion	6.1%	0%
Vision abnormal	5.3%	2.3%

Children: Incidence in a controlled add-on trial in children with Lennox-Gastaut syndrome – The table that follows enumerates adverse reactions that occurred more than once among 31 pediatric patients who received felbamate up to 45 mg/kg/day or a maximum of 3600 mg/day. Reported adverse reactions were classified using standard WHO-based dictionary terminology.

Felbamate Adverse Reactions in Children		
Adverse reaction	Felbamate (n = 31) %	Placebo (n = 27) %
Miscellaneous		
Fever	22.6%	11.1%
Fatigue	9.7%	3.7%
Weight decrease	6.5%	0%
Pain	6.5%	0%
CNS		
Somnolence	48.4%	11.1%
Insomnia	16.1%	14.8%
Nervousness	16.1%	18.5%
Gait abnormal	9.7%	0%
Headache	6.5%	18.5%
Thinking abnormal	6.5%	3.7%
Ataxia	6.5%	3.7%
Urinary incontinence	6.5%	7.4%
Emotional lability	6.5%	0%
Miosis	6.5%	0%
Dermatological		
Rash	9.7%	7.4%
GI		
Anorexia	54.8%	14.8%
Vomiting	38.7%	14.8%
Constipation	12.9%	0%
Hiccup	9.7%	3.7%
Nausea	6.5%	0%
Dyspepsia	6.5%	3.7%
Hematologic		
Purpura	12.9%	7.4%
Leukopenia	6.5%	0%
Respiratory		
Upper respiratory tract infection	45.2%	25.9%
Pharyngitis	9.7%	3.7%
Coughing	6.5%	0%
Special senses		
Otitis media	9.7%	0%

➤*Other reactions observed in association with the administration of felbamate:* In the paragraphs that follow, the adverse clinical reactions, other than those in the preceding tables, that occurred in a total of 977 adults and 357 children exposed to felbamate and that are reasonably associated with its use are presented. They are listed in order of decreasing

FELBAMATE — ORAL

frequency. Because the reports cite reactions observed in open-label and uncontrolled studies, the role of felbamate in their causation cannot be reliably determined.

Reactions are classified within body system categories and enumerated in order of decreasing frequency using the following definitions: Frequent adverse reactions are defined as those occurring on 1 or more occasions in at least 1/100 patients; infrequent adverse reactions are those occurring in 1/100 to 1/1000 patients; and rare reactions are those occurring in fewer than 1/1000 patients.

Reaction frequencies are calculated as the number of patients reporting an event divided by the total number of patients (n = 1334) exposed to felbamate.

Cardiovascular – Frequent: Palpitation, tachycardia. Rare: Supraventricular tachycardia.

CNS – Frequent: Agitation, psychological disturbance, aggressive reaction. Infrequent: Hallucination, euphoria, suicide attempt, migraine.

Dermatologic – Frequent: Pruritus. Infrequent: Urticaria, bullous eruption. Rare: Buccal mucous membrane swelling, Stevens-Johnson syndrome.

GI – Frequent: AST increased. Infrequent: Esophagitis, appetite increased. Rare: GGT elevated.

Hematologic – Infrequent: Lymphadenopathy, leukopenia, leukocytosis, thrombocytopenia, granulocytopenia. Rare: Antinuclear factor test positive, qualitative platelet disorder, agranulocytosis.

Metabolic/Nutritional – Infrequent: Hypokalemia, hyponatremia, LDH increased, alkaline phosphatase increased, hypophosphatemia. Rare: Creatinine phosphokinase increased.

Musculoskeletal – Infrequent: Dystonia.

Special senses – Rare: Photosensitivity allergic reaction.

Miscellaneous – Frequent: Weight increase, asthenia, malaise, influenza-like symptoms. Rare: Anaphylactoid reaction, chest pain substernal.

➤*Postmarketing:*

Cardiovascular – Atrial fibrillation, atrial arrhythmia, cardiac arrest, torsade de pointes, cardiac failure, hypotension, hypertension, flushing, thrombophlebitis, ischemic necrosis, gangrene, peripheral ischemia, bradycardia, Henoch-Schönlein purpura (vasculitis).

CNS – Delusion, paralysis, mononeuritis, cerebrovascular disorder, cerebral edema, coma, manic reaction, encephalopathy, paranoid reaction, nystagmus, choreoathetosis, extrapyramidal disorder, confusion, psychosis, status epilepticus, dyskinesia, dysarthria, respiratory depression, apathy, concentration impaired.

Dermatologic – Abnormal body odor, sweating, lichen planus, livedo reticularis, alopecia, toxic epidermal necrolysis.

GI – Hepatitis, hepatic failure, GI hemorrhage, hyperammonemia, pancreatitis, hematemesis, gastritis, rectal hemorrhage, flatulence, gingival bleeding, acquired megacolon, ileus, intestinal obstruction, enteritis, ulcerative stomatitis, glossitis, dysphagia, jaundice, gastric ulcer, gastric dilatation, gastroesophageal reflux.

GU – Menstrual disorder, acute renal failure, hepatorenal syndrome, hematuria, urinary retention, nephrosis, vaginal hemorrhage, abnormal renal function, dysuria, placental disorder.

Hematologic – Increased and decreased prothrombin time, anemia, hypochromic anemia, aplastic anemia, pancytopenia, hemolytic uremic syndrome, increased mean corpuscular volume (MCV) with and without anemia, coagulation disorder, embolism-limb, disseminated intravascular coagulation, eosinophilia, hemolytic anemia, leukemia, including myelogenous leukemia, and lymphoma, including T-cell and B-cell lymphoproliferative disorders.

Metabolic/Nutritional – Hypernatremia, hypoglycemia, SIADH, hypomagnesemia, dehydration, hyperglycemia, hypocalcemia.

Musculoskeletal – Arthralgia, muscle weakness, involuntary muscle contraction, rhabdomyolysis.

Respiratory – Dyspnea, pneumonia, pneumonitis, hypoxia, epistaxis, pleural effusion, respiratory insufficiency, pulmonary hemorrhage, asthma.

Special senses – Hemianopsia, decreased hearing, conjunctivitis.

Miscellaneous – Neoplasm, sepsis, LE syndrome, SIDS, sudden death, edema, hypothermia, rigors, hyperpyrexia.

Fetal disorders: Fetal death, microcephaly, genital malformation, anencephaly, encephalocele.

Overdosage

➤*Symptoms:* Four subjects inadvertently received felbamate as adjunctive therapy in dosages ranging from 5400 to 7200 mg/day for durations between 6 and 51 days. One subject who received 5400 mg/day as monotherapy for 1 week reported no adverse reactions. Another subject attempted suicide by ingesting 12,000 mg of felbamate in a 12-hour period. The only adverse reactions reported were mild gastric distress and a resting heart rate of 100 bpm. No serious adverse reactions have been reported.

➤*Treatment:* General supportive measures should be employed if overdosage occurs. It is not known whether felbamate is dialyzable.

Patient Information

Patients should be informed that the use of felbamate is associated with aplastic anemia and hepatic failure, potentially fatal conditions acutely or over a long term.

The physician should obtain written, informed consent prior to initiation of felbamate therapy.

➤*Aplastic anemia:* Aplastic anemia in the general population is relatively rare. The absolute risk for the individual patient is not known with any degree of reliability, but patients on felbamate may be at more than a 100-fold greater risk for developing the syndrome than the general population.

The long term outlook for patients with aplastic anemia is variable. Although many patients are apparently cured, others require repeated transfusions and other treatments for relapses, and some, although surviving for years, ultimately develop serious complications that sometimes prove fatal (eg, leukemia).

At present there is no way to predict who is likely to get aplastic anemia, nor is there a documented effective means to monitor the patient so as to avoid or reduce the risk. Patients with a history of any blood dyscrasia should not receive felbamate.

Patients should be advised to be alert for signs of infection, bleeding, easy bruising, or signs of anemia (eg, fatigue, weakness, lassitude) and should be advised to report to the physician immediately if any such signs or symptoms appear.

➤*Hepatic failure:* Hepatic failure in the general population is relatively rare. The absolute risk for an individual patient is not known with any degree of reliability but patients on felbamate are at a greater risk for developing hepatic failure than the general population.

At present, there is no way to predict who is likely to develop hepatic failure; however, patients with a history of hepatic dysfunction should not be started on felbamate.

Patients should be advised to follow their physician's directives for liver function testing both before starting felbamate and at frequent intervals while taking felbamate.

Patients should be advised to be alert for signs of liver dysfunction (eg, jaundice, anorexia, gastrointestinal complaints, malaise) and to report them to their doctor immediately if they should occur.

GABAPENTIN

Rx	**Gabapentin** (Ivax)	**Tablets**: 100 mg	Lactose. (4440 100). White. In 100s, 200s, 500s, 5,000s, and UD 100s.
Rx	**Gabarone** (Ivax		Lactose. (4440/100). White. In 100s, 500s, 5,000s, and UD 100s.
Rx	**Gabapentin** (Ivax)	**Tablets**: 300 mg	Lactose. (4441 300). White. In 100s, 200s, 500s, 2,000s, and UD 100s.
Rx	**Gabarone** (Ivax)		Lactose. (4441/300). White. In 100s, 500s, 2,000s, and UD 100s.
Rx	**Gabapentin** (Ivax)	**Tablets**: 400 mg	Lactose. (4442 400). White, oval. In 100s, 200s, 500s, 1,000s, and UD 100s.
Rx	**Gabarone** (Ivax)		Lactose. (4442/400). White, oval. In 100s, 500s, 1,000s, and UD 100s.
Rx	**Gabapentin** (Various, eg, Greenstone, Ivax, Purepac)	**Tablets**: 600 mg	May contain lactose. In 100s, 500s, 1,000s, and UD 100s.
Rx	**Neurontin** (Pfizer)		Talc. (Neurontin 600). White, elliptical. Film-coated. In 100s, 500s, and UD 50s.
Rx	**Gabapentin** (Various, eg, Greenstone, Ivax, Purepac)	**Tablets**: 800 mg	May contain lactose. In 100s, 500s, 1,000s, and UD 100s.
Rx	**Neurontin** (Pfizer)		Talc. (Neurontin 800). White, elliptical. Film-coated. In 100s, 500s, and UD 50s.
Rx	**Gabapentin** (Various, eg, American Health, Greenstone, Teva)	**Capsules**: 100 mg	In 100s, 500s, and UD 50s.
Rx	**Neurontin** (Pfizer)		Lactose, talc. (PD Neurontin/100 mg). White. In 100s and UD 50s.
Rx	**Gabapentin** (Various, eg, American Health, Greenstone, Teva)	**Capsules**: 300 mg	In 100s, 500s, and UD 50s.
Rx	**Neurontin** (Pfizer)		Lactose, talc. (PD Neurontin/300 mg). Yellow. In 100s and UD 50s.

GABAPENTIN

Rx	**Gabapentin** (Various, eg, American Health, Greenstone, Teva)	**Capsules:** 400 mg	In 100s, 500s, and UD 50s.
Rx	**Neurontin** (Pfizer)		Lactose, talc. (PD Neurontin/400 mg). Orange. In 100s and UD 50s.
Rx	**Neurontin** (Pfizer)	**Solution, oral:** 250 mg per 5 mL	Xylitol. Cool strawberry anise flavor. In 470 mL.

GABAPENTIN — ORAL

Refer to the general discussion beginning in the Anticonvulsants introduction.

Indications

➤*Postherpetic neuralgia:* For the management of postherpetic neuralgia in adults.

➤*Epilepsy:* As adjunctive therapy in the treatment of partial seizures with and without secondary generalization in patients over 12 years of age with epilepsy. Gabapentin is also indicated as adjunctive therapy in the treatment of partial seizures in pediatric patients age 3 to 12 years.

➤*Unlabeled uses:* Treatment of tremors associated with multiple sclerosis; neuropathic pain; bipolar disorder; migraine prophylaxis; hot flashes; treatment of various painful neuralgias (such as trigeminal neuralgia) and neuropathies (such as diabetic peripheral neuropathy).

Administration and Dosage

➤*Approved by the FDA:* December 30, 1993.

Gabapentin is given orally with or without food.

If gabapentin is discontinued and/or an alternate anticonvulsant medication is added to the therapy, this should be done gradually over a minimum of 1 week.

➤*Postherpetic neuralgia:* In adults with postherpetic neuralgia, gabapentin therapy may be initiated as a single 300 mg dose on day one, 600 mg/day on day 2 (divided twice daily), and 900 mg/day on day 3 (divided 3 times daily). The dose can subsequently be titrated up as needed for pain relief to a daily dose of 1800 mg (divided 3 times daily). In clinical studies, efficacy was demonstrated over a range of doses from 1800 mg/day to 3600 mg/day with comparable effects across the dose range. Additional benefit of using doses greater than 1800 mg/day was not demonstrated.

➤*Epilepsy:* Gabapentin is recommended for add-on therapy in patients 3 years of age and older. Effectiveness in children below the age of 3 years has not been established.

➤*Patients greater than 12 years of age:* The effective dose of gabapentin is 900 to 1800 mg/day and given in divided doses (3 times a day) using 300 or 400 mg capsules or 600 or 800 mg tablets. The starting dose is 300 mg 3 times a day. If necessary, the dose may be increased using 300 or 400 mg capsules or 600 or 800 mg tablets 3 times a day up to 1800 mg/day. Dosages up to 2400 mg/day have been well tolerated in long-term clinical studies. Doses of 3600 mg/day have also been administered to a small number of patients for a relatively short duration, and have been well tolerated. The maximum time between doses in the 3-times-a-day schedule should not exceed 12 hours.

➤*Children age 3 to 12 years:* The starting dose should range from 10 to 15 mg/kg/day in 3 divided doses, and the effective dose reached by upward titration over a period of approximately 3 days. The effective dose of gabapentin in patients 5 years of age and older is 25 to 35 mg/kg/day and given in divided doses (3 times a day). The effective dose in pediatric patients ages 3 and 4 years is 40 mg/kg/day and given in divided doses (3 times a day). Gabapentin may be administered as the oral solution, capsule, or tablet, or using combinations of these formulations. Dosages up to 50 mg/kg/day have been well-tolerated in a long-term clinical study. The maximum time interval between doses should not exceed 12 hours.

➤*Renal function impairment:*

Gabapentin Dosage Based on Renal Function

Renal function creatinine clearance (mL/min)	Total daily dose range (mg/day)	Dose regimen (mg)				
≥ 60	900 to 3600	300 mg 3 times daily	400 mg 3 times daily	600 mg 3 times daily	800 mg 3 times daily	1200 mg 3 times daily
> 30 to 59	400 to 1400	200 mg twice daily	300 mg twice daily	400 mg twice daily	500 mg twice daily	700 mg twice daily
> 15 to 29	200 to 700	200 mg every day	300 mg every day	400 mg every day	500 mg every day	700 mg every day
15[a]	100 to 300	100 mg once daily	125 mg once daily	150 mg once daily	200 mg once daily	300 mg once daily
		Post-hemodialysis supplemental dose (mg)[b]				
Hemodialysis		125 mg[b]	150 mg[b]	200 mg[b]	250 mg[b]	350 mg[b]

[a] For patients with Ccr less than 15 mL/min, reduce daily dose in proportion to creatinine clearance (eg, patients with a creatinine clearance of 7.5 mL/min should receive one-half the daily dose that patients with a Ccr of 15 mL/min receive).

[b] For patients on hemodialysis, the maintenance dose should be based upon the estimates of Ccr as indicated in the upper portion of the table and a supplemental post-hemodialysis dose administered after each 4 hours of hemodialysis as indicated in the lower portion of the table.

The use of gabapentin in patients less than 12 years of age with compromised renal function has not been studied.

➤*Elderly:* Because elderly patients are more likely to have decreased renal function, care should be taken in dose selection, and dose should be adjusted based on creatinine clearance values in these patients.

➤*Storage / Stability:* Store at 25°C (77°F); excursions permitted to 15° to 30°C (59° to 86°F).

Oral solution – Store refrigerated, 2° to 8°C (36° to 46°F).

Actions

➤*Pharmacology:* The mechanism by which gabapentin exerts its analgesic action is unknown, but in animal models of analgesia, gabapentin prevents allodynia (pain-related behavior in response to a normally innocuous stimulus) and hyperalgesia (exaggerated response to painful stimuli). In particular, gabapentin prevents pain-related responses in several models of neuropathic pain in rats or mice (eg, spinal nerve ligation models, streptozocin-induced diabetes model, spinal cord injury model, acute herpes zoster infection model). Gabapentin also decreases pain-related responses after peripheral inflammation (carrageenan footpad test, late phase of formalin test). Gabapentin did not alter immediate pain-related behaviors (rat tail flick test, formalin footpad acute phase, acetic acid abdominal constriction test, footpad heat irradiation test). The relevance of these models to human pain is not known.

The mechanism by which gabapentin exerts its anticonvulsant action is unknown, but in animal test systems designed to detect anticonvulsant activity, gabapentin prevents seizures as do other marketed anticonvulsants. Gabapentin exhibits antiseizure activity in mice and rats in both the maximal electroshock and pentylenetetrazole seizure models and other preclinical models (eg, strains with genetic epilepsy). The relevance of these models to human epilepsy is not known.

Gabapentin is structurally related to the neurotransmitter GABA (gamma-aminobutyric acid) but it does not interact with GABA receptors, it is not converted metabolically into GABA or a GABA agonist, and it is not an inhibitor of GABA uptake or degradation. Gabapentin was tested in radioligand binding assays at concentrations up to 100 mcM and did not exhibit affinity for a number of other common receptor sites, including benzodiazepine, glutamate, N-methyl-D-aspartate (NMDA), quisqualate, kainate, strychnine-insensitive or strychnine-sensitive glycine, alpha 1, alpha 2, or beta adrenergic, adenosine A1 or A2, cholinergic muscarinic or nicotinic, dopamine D1 or D2, histamine H1, serotonin S1 or S2, opiate mu, delta or kappa, voltage-sensitive calcium channel sites labeled with nitrendipine or diltiazem, or at voltage-sensitive sodium channel sites with batrachotoxinin A 20-alpha-benzoate. Furthermore, gabapentin did not alter the cellular uptake of dopamine, noradrenaline, or serotonin.

In vitro studies with radiolabeled gabapentin have revealed a gabapentin binding site in areas of rat brain including neocortex and hippocampus. A high-affinity binding protein in animal brain tissue has been identified as an auxiliary subunit of voltage-activated calcium channels. However, functional correlates of gabapentin binding, if any, remain to be elucidated.

➤*Pharmacokinetics:*

Absorption – Gabapentin bioavailability is not dose-proportional (ie, as dose is increased, bioavailability decreases). Bioavailability of gabapentin is approximately 60%, 47%, 34%, 33%, and 27% following 900, 1200, 2400, 3600, and 4800 mg/day given in 3 divided doses, respectively. Food has only a slight effect on the rate and extent of absorption of gabapentin (14% increase in AUC and C_{max}).

Distribution – Less than 3% of gabapentin circulates unbound to plasma protein. The apparent volume of distribution of gabapentin after 150 mg intravenous administration is 58 ± 6 L (Mean ± SD). In patients with epilepsy, steady-state predose (C_{min}) concentrations of gabapentin in cerebrospinal fluid were approximately 20% of the corresponding plasma concentrations.

Excretion – Gabapentin is eliminated from the systemic circulation by renal excretion as unchanged drug. Gabapentin is not appreciably metabolized in humans.

Gabapentin elimination half-life is 5 to 7 hours and is unaltered by dose or following multiple dosing. Gabapentin elimination rate constant, plasma clearance, and renal clearance are directly proportional to creatinine clearance. In elderly patients, and in patients with impaired renal function, gabapentin plasma clearance is reduced. Gabapentin can be removed from plasma by hemodialysis.

Special populations –

Renal function impairment: Subjects (n = 60) with renal insufficiency (mean creatinine clearance ranging from 13 to 114 mL/min) were administered single 400 mg oral doses of gabapentin. The mean gabapentin half-life ranged from about 6.5 hours (patients with creatinine clearance greater than 60 mL/min) to 52 hours (creatinine clearance less than 30 mL/min) and gabapentin renal clearance from about 90 mL/min (greater than 60 mL/min group) to about 10 mL/min (less than 30 mL/min). Mean plasma clearance (CL/F) decreased from approximately 190 mL/min to 20 mL/min. Pediatric patients with renal insufficiency have not been studied. Dosage adjustment in patients with compromised renal function is necessary.

GABAPENTIN — ORAL

Elderly: The effect of age was studied in subjects 20 to 80 years of age. Apparent oral clearance (CL/F) of gabapentin decreased as age increased, from about 225 mL/min in those under 30 years of age to about 125 mL/min in those over 70 years of age. Renal clearance (CLr) and CLr adjusted for body surface area also declined with age; however, the decline in the renal clearance of gabapentin with age can largely be explained by the decline in renal function. Reduction of gabapentin dose may be required in patients who have age-related compromised renal function. Because elderly patients are more likely to have decreased renal function, care should be taken in dose selection, and dose should be adjusted based on creatinine clearance values in these patients.

Children: Gabapentin pharmacokinetics were determined in 48 pediatric subjects between the ages of 1 month and 12 years following a dose of approximately 10 mg/kg. Peak plasma concentrations were similar across the entire age group and occurred 2 to 3 hours postdose. In general, pediatric subjects between 1 month and less than 5 years of age achieved approximately 30% lower exposure (AUC) than that observed in those 5 years of age and older. Accordingly, oral clearance normalized per body weight was higher in the younger children. Apparent oral clearance of gabapentin was directly proportional to creatinine clearance. Gabapentin elimination half-life averaged 4.7 hours and was similar across the age groups studied.

A population pharmacokinetic analysis was performed in 253 pediatric subjects between 1 month and 13 years of age. Patients received 10 to 65 mg/kg/day given 3 times daily. Apparent oral clearance (CL/F) was directly proportional to creatinine clearance and this relationship was similar following a single dose and at steady state. Higher oral clearance values were observed in children less than 5 years of age compared to those observed in children 5 years of age and older, when normalized per body weight. The clearance was highly variable in infants less than 1 year of age. The normalized CL/F values observed in pediatric patients 5 years of age and older were consistent with values observed in adults after a single dose. The oral volume of distribution normalized per body weight was constant across the age range.

Hemodialysis: In a study in anuric subjects (n = 11), the apparent elimination half-life of gabapentin on nondialysis days was about 132 hours; during dialysis the apparent half-life of gabapentin was reduced to 3.8 hours. Hemodialysis thus has a significant effect on gabapentin elimination in anuric subjects. Dosage adjustment in patients undergoing hemodialysis is necessary.

Contraindications

Hypersensitivity to the drug or its ingredients.

Warnings

➤*Neuropsychiatric adverse reactions in children 3 to 12 years of age:* Gabapentin use in pediatric patients with epilepsy 3 to 12 years of age is associated with the occurrence of central nervous system related adverse events. The most significant of these can be classified into the following categories: Emotional lability (primarily behavioral problems); Hostility, including aggressive behaviors; Thought disorder, including concentration problems and change in school performance; Hyperkinesia (primarily restlessness and hyperactivity). Among the gabapentin-treated patients, most of the events were mild to moderate in intensity.

In controlled trials in pediatric patients 3 to 12 years of age the incidence of these adverse events was: Emotional lability 6% (gabapentin-treated patients) vs 1.3% (placebo-treated patients); hostility 5.2% vs 1.3%; hyperkinesia 4.7% vs 2.9%; and thought disorder 1.7% vs 0%. One of these events, a report of hostility, was considered serious. Discontinuation of gabapentin treatment occurred in 1.3% of patients reporting emotional lability and hyperkinesia and 0.9% of gabapentin-treated patients reporting hostility and thought disorder. One placebo-treated patient (0.4%) withdrew due to emotional lability.

➤*Withdrawal precipitated seizure:* Antiepileptic drugs should not be abruptly discontinued because of the possibility of increasing seizure frequency.

In the placebo-controlled studies in patients greater than 12 years of age, the incidence of status epilepticus in patients receiving gabapentin was 0.6% (3 of 543) vs 0.5% in patients receiving placebo (2 of 378). Among the 2074 patients greater than 12 years of age treated with gabapentin across all studies (controlled and uncontrolled) 31 (1.5%) had status epilepticus. Of these, 14 patients had no history of status epilepticus either before treatment or while on other medications. Because adequate historical data are not available, it is impossible to say whether or not treatment with gabapentin is associated with a higher or lower rate of status epilepticus than would be expected to occur in a similar population not treated with gabapentin.

➤*Sudden and unexplained deaths:* During the course of premarketing development of gabapentin, 8 sudden and unexplained deaths were recorded among a cohort of 2203 patients treated (2103 patient-years of exposure).

Some of these could represent seizure-related deaths in which the seizure was not observed (eg, at night). This represents an incidence of 0.0038 deaths per patient-year. Although this rate exceeds that expected in a healthy population matched for age and sex, it is within the range of estimates for the incidence of sudden unexplained deaths in patients with epilepsy not receiving gabapentin (ranging from 0.0005 for the general population of epileptics to 0.003 for a clinical trial population similar to that in the gabapentin program, to 0.005 for patients with refractory epilepsy). Consequently, whether these figures are reassuring or raise further concern depends on comparability of the populations reported upon to the gabapentin cohort and the accuracy of the estimates provided.

In standard preclinical in vivo lifetime carcinogenicity studies, an unexpectedly high incidence of pancreatic acinar adenocarcinomas was identified in male, but not female, rats. The clinical significance of this finding is unknown. Clinical experience during gabapentin's premarketing development provides no direct means to assess its potential for inducing tumors in humans.

In clinical studies in adjunctive therapy in epilepsy comprising 2085 patient-years of exposure in patients greater than 12 years of age, new tumors were reported in 10 patients (2 breast, 3 brain, 2 lung, 1 adrenal, 1 non-Hodgkin's lymphoma, 1 endometrial carcinoma in situ), and preexisting tumors worsened in 11 patients (9 brain, 1 breast, 1 prostate) during or up to 2 years following discontinuation of gabapentin. Without knowledge of the background incidence and recurrence in a similar population not treated with gabapentin, it is impossible to know whether the incidence seen in this cohort is or is not affected by treatment.

➤*Elderly:* Clinical studies of gabapentin in epilepsy did not include sufficient numbers of subjects aged 65 and over to determine whether they responded differently from younger subjects. Other reported clinical experience has not identified differences in responses between the elderly and younger patients. In general, dose selection for an elderly patient should be cautious, usually starting at the low end of the dosing range, reflecting the greater frequency of decreased hepatic, renal, or cardiac function, and of concomitant disease or other drug therapy.

See Actions for more information.

➤*Pregnancy: Category C.* Gabapentin has been shown to be fetotoxic in rodents, causing delayed ossification of several bones in the skull, vertebrae, forelimbs, and hindlimbs. These effects occurred when pregnant mice received oral doses of 1000 or 3000 mg/kg/day during the period of organogenesis, or approximately equal to 1 to 4 times the maximum dose of 3600 mg/day given to epileptic patients on a mg/m^2 basis. The no-effect level was 500 mg/kg/day or approximately ½ of the human dose on a mg/m^2 basis.

When rats were dosed prior to and during mating, and throughout gestation, pups from all dose groups (500, 1000 and 2000 mg/kg/day) were affected. These doses are equivalent to less than approximately 1 to 5 times the maximum human dose on a mg/m^2 basis. There was an increased incidence of hydroureter and/or hydronephrosis in rats in a study of fertility and general reproductive performance at 2000 mg/kg/day with no effect at 1000 mg/kg/day, in a teratology study at 1500 mg/kg/day with no effect at 300 mg/kg/day, and in a perinatal and postnatal study at all doses studied (500, 1000 and 2000 mg/kg/day). The doses at which the effects occurred are approximately 1 to 5 times the maximum human dose of 3600 mg/day on a mg/m^2 basis; the no-effect doses were approximately 3 times (Fertility and General Reproductive Performance study) and approximately equal to (Teratogenicity study) the maximum human dose on a mg/m^2 basis. Other than hydroureter and hydronephrosis, the etiologies of which are unclear, the incidence of malformations was not increased compared to controls in offspring of mice, rats, or rabbits given doses up to 50 times (mice), 30 times (rats), and 25 times (rabbits) the human daily dose on a mg/kg basis, or 4 times (mice), 5 times (rats), or 8 times (rabbits) the human daily dose on a mg/m^2 basis.

In a teratology study in rabbits, an increased incidence of postimplantation fetal loss occurred in dams exposed to 60, 300 and 1500 mg/kg/day, or less than approximately ¼ to 8 times the maximum human dose on a mg/m^2 basis. There are no adequate and well-controlled studies in pregnant women. This drug should be used during pregnancy only if the potential benefit justifies the potential risk to the fetus.

➤*Lactation:* Gabapentin is secreted into human milk following oral administration. A nursed infant could be exposed to a maximum dose of approximately 1 mg/kg/day of gabapentin. Because the effect on the nursing infant is unknown, gabapentin should be used in women who are nursing only if the benefits clearly outweigh the risks.

➤*Children:* Safety and effectiveness of gabapentin in the management of postherpetic neuralgia in pediatric patients have not been established. Effectiveness as adjunctive therapy in the treatment of partial seizures in pediatric patients below the age of 3 years has not been established.

Precautions

➤*Monitoring:* Clinical trials data do not indicate that routine monitoring of clinical laboratory parameters is necessary for the safe use of gabapentin. The value of monitoring gabapentin blood concentrations has not been established. Gabapentin may be used in combination with other antiepileptic drugs without concern for alteration of the blood concentrations of gabapentin or of other antiepileptic drugs.

➤*Hazardous tasks:* Patients should be advised that gabapentin may cause dizziness, somnolence and other symptoms and signs of CNS depression. Accordingly, they should be advised neither to drive a car nor to operate other complex machinery until they have gained sufficient experience on gabapentin to gauge whether or not it affects their mental and/or motor performance adversely.

Drug Interactions

Gabapentin is not appreciably metabolized nor does it interfere with the metabolism of commonly coadministered antiepileptic drugs.

GABAPENTIN — ORAL

Gabapentin Drug Interactions			
Precipitant drug	Object drug*		Description
Antacids	Gabapentin	↓	Antacids reduced the bioavailability of gabapentin by about 20%. This decrease in bioavailability was about 5% when gabapentin was given 2 hours after the antacid. It is recommended that gabapentin be taken at least 2 hours following antacid administration.
Cimetidine	Gabapentin	↑	The mean apparent oral clearance of gabapentin fell by 14% and Ccr fell by 10% with concurrent cimetidine. Thus, cimetidine seemed to alter the renal excretion of gabapentin and creatinine. This small decrease in gabapentin excretion is not expected to be of clinical importance.
Hydrocodone	Gabapentin	↑	Coadministration increases gabapentin AUC values by 14%. Coadministration decreases hydrocodone C_{max} and AUC values in a dose-dependent manner. C_{max} and AUC values were 3% and 4% lower, respectively, after administration of 125 mg gabapentin and 21% to 22% lower, respectively after administration of 500 mg gabapentin. The mechanism for this interaction and the magnitude of interaction at other doses is unknown.
Gabapentin	Hydrocodone	↓	
Morphine	Gabapentin	↑	Coadministration of 60 mg morphine 2 hours prior to administration of 600 mg gabapentin resulted in an increase in gabapentin AUC by 44%. The magnitude of interaction at other doses is unknown.
Gabapentin	Contraceptives, oral	↑	The C_{max} of norethindrone was 13% higher when coadministered with gabapentin; this interaction is not expected to be of clinical importance.
Naproxen	Gabapentin	↑	Coadministration (n = 18) of naproxen sodium capsules (250 mg) with gabapentin (125 mg) appears to increase the amount of gabapentin absorbed by 12% to 15%. Gabapentin had no effect on naproxen pharmacokinetic parameters. These doses are lower than the therapeutic doses for both drugs. The magnitude of interaction within the recommended dose ranges of either drug is not known.

* ↑ = Object drug increased. ↓ = Object drug decreased.

➤*Drug/Lab test interactions:* Because false positive readings were reported with the *Ames N-Multistix SG* dipstick test for urinary protein when gabapentin was added to other antiepileptic drugs, the more specific sulfosalicylic acid precipitation procedure is recommended to determine the presence of urine protein.

Adverse Reactions

➤*Postherpetic neuralgia:* The most commonly observed adverse events associated with the use of gabapentin in adults, not seen at an equivalent frequency among placebo-treated patients, were dizziness, somnolence, and peripheral edema.

In the 2 controlled studies in postherpetic neuralgia, 16% of the 336 patients who received gabapentin and 9% of the 227 patients who received placebo discontinued treatment because of an adverse event. The adverse events that most frequently led to withdrawal in gabapentin-treated patients were dizziness, somnolence, and nausea.

Incidence in controlled clinical trials – The following table lists treatment-emergent signs and symptoms that occurred in at least 1% of gabapentin-treated patients with postherpetic neuralgia participating in placebo-controlled trials and that were numerically more frequent in the gabapentin group than in the placebo group. Adverse events were usually mild to moderate in intensity.

Treatment-Emergent Adverse Event Incidence in Controlled Trials in Postherpetic Neuralgia (Events in at Least 1% of Gabapentin-Treated Patients and Numerically More Frequent than in the Placebo Group)		
Body system/ preferred term	Gabapentin (n = 336) %	Placebo (n = 227) %
Miscellaneous		
Asthenia	5.7%	4.8%
Infection	5.1%	3.5%
Headache	3.3%	3.1%
Accidental injury	3.3%	1.3%
Abdominal pain	2.7%	2.6%
GI		
Diarrhea	5.7%	3.1%
Dry mouth	4.8%	1.3%
Constipation	3.9%	1.8%
Nausea	3.9%	3.1%
Vomiting	3.3%	1.8%
Flatulence	2.1%	1.8%
Metabolic/nutritional		
Peripheral edema	8.3%	2.2%
Weight gain	1.8%	0%
Hyperglycemia	1.2%	0.4%
CNS		
Dizziness	28%	7.5%
Somnolence	21.4%	5.3%
Ataxia	3.3%	0%
Thinking abnormal	2.7%	0%
Abnormal gait	1.5%	0%
Incoordination	1.5%	0%
Amnesia	1.2%	0.9%
Hypesthesia	1.2%	0.9%
Respiratory		
Pharyngitis	1.2%	0.4%
Dermatologic		
Rash	1.2%	0.9%
Special senses		
Amblyopia[a]	2.7%	0.9%
Conjunctivitis	1.2%	0%
Diplopia	1.2%	0%
Otitis media	1.2%	0%

[a] Reported as blurred vision.

Other events in more than 1% of patients but equally or more frequent in the placebo group included pain, tremor, neuralgia, back pain, dyspepsia, dyspnea, and flu syndrome.

➤*Epilepsy:* The most commonly observed adverse events associated with the use of gabapentin in combination with other antiepileptic drugs in patients greater than 12 years of age, not seen at an equivalent frequency among placebo-treated patients, were somnolence, dizziness, ataxia, fatigue, and nystagmus. The most commonly observed adverse events reported with the use of gabapentin in combination with other antiepileptic drugs in pediatric patients 3 to 12 years of age, not seen at an equal frequency among placebo-treated patients, were as follows:

1.) Emotional lability (primarily behavioral problems)
2.) Hostility, including aggressive behaviors
3.) Thought disorder, including concentration problems and change in school performance
4.) Hyperkinesia (primarily restlessness and hyperactivity).

Approximately 7% of the 2074 patients greater than 12 years of age and approximately 7% of the 449 pediatric patients 3 to 12 years of age who received gabapentin in premarketing clinical trials discontinued treatment because of an adverse event. The adverse events most commonly associated with withdrawal in patients greater than 12 years of age were somnolence (1.2%), ataxia (0.8%), fatigue (0.6%), nausea and/or vomiting (0.6%), and dizziness (0.6%). The adverse events most commonly associated with withdrawal in pediatric patients were emotional lability (1.6%), hostility (1.3%), and hyperkinesia (1.1%).

GABAPENTIN — ORAL

Incidence in controlled clinical trials –

Treatment-Emergent Adverse Reaction Incidence in Controlled Add-On Trials in Patients > 12 Years of Age (Events in at Least 1% of Gabapentin Patients and Numerically More Frequent than in the Placebo Group)

Body system/ adverse reaction	Gabapentin[a] (n = 543) %	Placebo[a] (n = 378) %
Miscellaneous		
Fatigue	11%	5%
Weight increase	2.9%	1.6%
Back pain	1.8%	0.5%
Peripheral edema	1.7%	0.5%
Cardiovascular		
Vasodilatation	1.1%	0.3%
GI		
Dyspepsia	2.2%	0.5%
Mouth or throat dry	1.7%	0.5%
Constipation	1.5%	0.8%
Dental abnormalities	1.5%	0.3%
Increased appetite	1.1%	0.8%
Hematologic/lymphatic		
Leukopenia	1.1%	0.5%
Musculoskeletal		
Myalgia	2%	1.9%
Fracture	1.1%	0.8%
CNS		
Somnolence	19.3%	8.7%
Dizziness	17.1%	6.9%
Ataxia	12.5%	5.6%
Nystagmus	8.3%	4%
Tremor	6.8%	3.2%
Nervousness	2.4%	1.9%
Dysarthria	2.4%	0.5%
Amnesia	2.2%	0%
Depression	1.8%	1.1%
Thinking abnormal	1.7%	1.3%
Twitching	1.3%	0.5%
Coordination abnormal	1.1%	0.3%
Respiratory		
Rhinitis	4.1%	3.7%
Pharyngitis	2.8%	1.6%
Coughing	1.8%	1.3%
Dermatologic		
Abrasion	1.3%	0%
Pruritus	1.3%	0.5%
GU		
Impotence	1.5%	1.1%
Special senses		
Diplopia	5.9%	1.9%
Amblyopia[b]	4.2%	1.1%
Laboratory test abnormalities		
WBC decreased	1.1%	0.5%

[a] Plus background antiepileptic drug therapy.

[b] Amblyopia was often described as blurred vision. Other events in greater than 1% of patients greater than 12 years of age but equally or more frequent in the placebo group included the following: Headache, viral infection, fever, nausea and/or vomiting, abdominal pain, diarrhea, convulsions, confusion, insomnia, emotional lability, rash, acne.

Among the treatment-emergent adverse events occurring at an incidence of at least 10% of gabapentin-treated patients, somnolence and ataxia appeared to exhibit a positive dose-response relationship. The table below lists treatment-emergent signs and symptoms that occurred in at least 2% of gabapentin-treated patients age 3 to 12 years of age with epilepsy participating in placebo-controlled trials and were numerically more common in the gabapentin group. Adverse events were usually mild to moderate in intensity.

Gabapentin Adverse Reactions in Children

Adverse reaction	Gabapentin[a] (n = 119)	Placebo[a] (n = 128)
Miscellaneous		
Viral infection	10.9%	3.1%
Fever	10.1%	3.1%
Weight increase	3.4%	0.8%
Fatigue	3.4%	1.6%
GI		
Nausea/vomiting	8.4%	7%
CNS		
Somnolence	8.4%	4.7%
Hostility	7.6%	2.3%
Emotional lability	4.2%	1.6%
Dizziness	2.5%	1.6%
Hyperkinesia	2.5%	0.8%
Respiratory		
Bronchitis	3.4%	0.8%
Respiratory tract infection	2.5%	0.8%

[a] Plus background antiepileptic drug therapy.

Other events in more than 2% of children 3 to 12 years of age but equally or more frequent in the placebo group included the following: Pharyngitis, upper respiratory tract infection, headache, rhinitis, convulsions, diarrhea, anorexia, coughing, and otitis media.

➤*Other adverse events observed during clinical trials in adults and adolescents with epilepsy:* Events are further classified within body system categories and enumerated in order of decreasing frequency using the following definitions: Frequent adverse events are defined as those occurring in at least 1/100 patients; infrequent adverse events are those occurring in 1/100 to 1/1000 patients; rare events are those occurring in fewer than 1/1000 patients.

Cardiovascular – Hypertension (frequent); hypotension, angina pectoris, peripheral vascular disorder, palpitation, tachycardia, migraine, murmur (infrequent); atrial fibrillation, heart failure, thrombophlebitis, deep thrombophlebitis, myocardial infarction, cerebrovascular accident, pulmonary thrombosis, ventricular extrasystoles, bradycardia, premature atrial contraction, pericardial rub, heart block, pulmonary embolus, hyperlipidemia, hypercholesterolemia, pericardial effusion, pericarditis (rare).

CNS – Vertigo, hyperkinesia, paresthesia, decreased or absent reflexes, increased reflexes, anxiety, hostility (frequent); CNS tumors, syncope, dreaming abnormal, aphasia, hypesthesia, intracranial hemorrhage, hypotonia, dysesthesia, paresis, dystonia, hemiplegia, facial paralysis, stupor, cerebellar dysfunction, positive Babinski sign, decreased position sense, subdural hematoma, apathy, hallucination, decrease or loss of libido, agitation, paranoia, depersonalization, euphoria, feeling high, doped-up sensation, suicidal, psychosis (infrequent); choreoathetosis, orofacial dyskinesia, encephalopathy, nerve palsy, personality disorder, increased libido, subdued temperament, apraxia, fine motor control disorder, meningismus, local myoclonus, hyperesthesia, hypokinesia, mania, neurosis, hysteria, antisocial reaction, suicide gesture (rare).

Dermatologic – Alopecia, eczema, dry skin, increased sweating, urticaria, hirsutism, seborrhea, cyst, herpes simplex (infrequent); herpes zoster, skin discolor, skin papules, photosensitivity reaction, leg ulcer, scalp seborrhea, psoriasis, desquamation, maceration, skin nodules, subcutaneous nodule, melanosis, skin necrosis, local swelling (rare).

Endocrine – Hyperthyroid, hypothyroid, goiter, hypoestrogen, ovarian failure, epididymitis, swollen testicle, cushingoid appearance (rare).

GI – Anorexia, flatulence, gingivitis (frequent); glossitis, gum hemorrhage, thirst, stomatitis, increased salivation, gastroenteritis, hemorrhoids, bloody stools, fecal incontinence, hepatomegaly (infrequent); dysphagia, eructation, pancreatitis, peptic ulcer, colitis, blisters in mouth, tooth discolor, perleche, salivary gland enlarged, lip hemorrhage, esophagitis, hiatal hernia, hematemesis, proctitis, irritable bowel syndrome, rectal hemorrhage, esophageal spasm (rare).

GU – Hematuria, dysuria, urination frequency, cystitis, urinary retention, urinary incontinence, vaginal hemorrhage, amenorrhea, dysmenorrhea, menorrhagia, breast cancer, inability to climax, ejaculation abnormal (infrequent); kidney pain, leukorrhea, pruritus genital, renal stone, acute renal failure, anuria, glycosuria, nephrosis, nocturia, pyuria, urination urgency, vaginal pain, breast pain, testicle pain (rare).

Hematologic / Lymphatic – Purpura most often described as bruises resulting from physical trauma (frequent); anemia, thrombocytopenia, lymphadenopathy (infrequent); WBC count increased, lymphocytosis, non-Hodgkin's lymphoma, bleeding time increased (rare).

Musculoskeletal – Arthralgia (frequent); tendinitis, arthritis, joint stiffness, joint swelling, positive Romberg test (infrequent); costochondritis, osteoporosis, bursitis, contracture (rare).

Respiratory – Pneumonia (frequent); epistaxis, dyspnea, apnea (infrequent); mucositis, aspiration pneumonia, hyperventilation, hiccup, laryngitis, nasal obstruction, snoring, bronchospasm, hypoventilation, lung edema (rare).

GABAPENTIN — ORAL

Special senses – Abnormal vision (frequent); cataract, conjunctivitis, eyes dry, eye pain, visual field defect, photophobia, bilateral or unilateral ptosis, eye hemorrhage, hordeolum, hearing loss, earache, tinnitus, inner ear infection, otitis, taste loss, unusual taste, eye twitching, ear fullness (infrequent); eye itching, abnormal accommodation, perforated ear drum, sensitivity to noise, eye focusing problem, watery eyes, retinopathy, glaucoma, iritis, corneal disorders, lacrimal dysfunction, degenerative eye changes, blindness, retinal degeneration, miosis, chorioretinitis, strabismus, eustachian tube dysfunction, labyrinthitis, otitis externa, odd smell (rare).

➤*Miscellaneous:* Asthenia, malaise, face edema (frequent); allergy, generalized edema, weight decrease, chill (infrequent); strange feelings, lassitude, alcohol intolerance, hangover effect (rare).

➤*Clinical trials in children with epilepsy:*

CNS – Aura disappeared, occipital neuralgia.

GI – Hepatitis.

Hematologic/Lymphatic – Coagulation defect.

Psychiatric – Sleep walking.

Respiratory – Pseudocroup, hoarseness.

Miscellaneous – Dehydration, infectious mononucleosis.

➤*Clinical trials in adults with neuropathic pain of various etiologies:* Events are further classified within body system categories and enumerated in order of decreasing frequency using the following definitions: Frequent adverse events are defined as those occurring in at least 1/100 patients; infrequent adverse events are those occurring in 1/100 to 1/1000 patients; rare events are those occurring in fewer than 1/1000 patients.

Cardiovascular – Hypertension, syncope, palpitation, migraine, hypotension, peripheral vascular disorder, cardiovascular disorder, cerebrovascular accident, congestive heart failure, myocardial infarction, vasodilatation (infrequent); angina pectoris, heart failure, increased capillary fragility, phlebitis, thrombophlebitis, varicose vein (rare).

CNS – Confusion, depression (frequent); vertigo, nervousness, paresthesia, insomnia, neuropathy, libido decreased, anxiety, depersonalization, reflexes decreased, speech disorder, abnormal dreams, dysarthria, emotional lability, nystagmus, stupor, circumoral paresthesia, euphoria, hyperesthesia, hypokinesia (infrequent); agitation, hypertonia, libido increased, movement disorder, myoclonus, vestibular disorder (rare).

Dermatologic – Pruritus, skin ulcer, dry skin, herpes zoster, skin disorder, fungal dermatitis, furunculosis, herpes simplex, psoriasis, sweating, urticaria, vesiculobullous rash (infrequent); acne, hair disorder, maculopapular rash, nail disorder, skin carcinoma, skin discoloration, skin hypertrophy (rare).

Endocrine – Diabetes mellitus (infrequent).

GI – Gastroenteritis, increased appetite, gastrointestinal disorder, oral moniliasis, gastritis, tongue disorder, thirst, tooth disorder, abnormal stools, anorexia, liver function tests abnormal, periodontal abscess (infrequent); cholecystitis, cholelithiasis, duodenal ulcer, fecal incontinence, gamma glutamyl transpeptidase increased, gingivitis, intestinal obstruction, intestinal ulcer, melena, mouth ulceration, rectal disorder, rectal hemorrhage, stomatitis (rare).

GU – Urinary tract infection, dysuria, impotence, urinary incontinence, vaginal moniliasis, breast pain, menstrual disorder, polyuria, urinary retention (infrequent); cystitis, ejaculation abnormal, swollen penis, gynecomastia, nocturia, pyelonephritis, swollen scrotum, urinary frequency, urinary urgency, urine abnormality (rare).

Hematologic/Lymphatic – Ecchymosis, anemia (infrequent); lymphadenopathy, lymphoma-like reaction, prothrombin decreased (rare).

Metabolic/Nutritional – Edema, gout, hypoglycemia, weight loss (infrequent); alkaline phosphatase increased, diabetic ketoacidosis, lactic dehydrogenase increased (rare).

Musculoskeletal – Arthritis, arthralgia, myalgia, arthrosis, leg cramps, myasthenia (infrequent); shin bone pain, joint disorder, tendon disorder (rare).

Respiratory – Cough increased, bronchitis, rhinitis, sinusitis, pneumonia, asthma, lung disorder, epistaxis (infrequent); hemoptysis, voice alteration (rare).

Special senses – Abnormal vision, ear pain, eye disorder, taste perversion, deafness (infrequent); conjunctival hyperemia, diabetic retinopathy, eye pain, fundi with microhemorrhage, retinal vein thrombosis, taste loss (rare).

Miscellaneous – Chest pain, cellulitis, malaise, neck pain, face edema, allergic reaction, abscess, chills, chills and fever, mucous membrane disorder (infrequent); body odor, cyst, fever, hernia, abnormal BUN value, lump in neck, pelvic pain, sepsis, viral infection (rare).

➤*Postmarketing:* In addition to the adverse experiences reported during clinical testing of gabapentin, the following adverse experiences have been reported in patients receiving marketed gabapentin. These adverse experiences have not been listed above and data are insufficient to support an estimate of their incidence or to establish causation. The listing is alphabetized: Angioedema, blood glucose fluctuation, elevated liver function tests, erythema multiforme, fever, hyponatremia, jaundice, Stevens-Johnson syndrome.

Overdosage

➤*Symptoms:* A lethal dose of gabapentin was not identified in mice and rats receiving single oral doses as high as 8000 mg/kg. Signs of acute toxicity in animals included ataxia, labored breathing, ptosis, sedation, hypoactivity, or excitation.

Acute oral overdoses of gabapentin up to 49 g have been reported. In these cases, double vision, slurred speech, drowsiness, lethargy and diarrhea were observed. All patients recovered with supportive care.

➤*Treatment:* Gabapentin can be removed by hemodialysis. Although hemodialysis has not been performed in the few overdose cases reported, it may be indicated by the patient's clinical state or in patients with significant renal impairment.

Patient Information

Patients should be instructed to take gabapentin only as prescribed.

Patients should be advised that gabapentin may cause dizziness, somnolence and other symptoms and signs of CNS depression. Accordingly, they should be advised neither to drive a car nor to operate other complex machinery until they have gained sufficient experience on gabapentin to gauge whether or not it affects their mental and/or motor performance adversely.

Patients who require concomitant treatment with morphine may experience increases in gabapentin concentrations. Patients should be carefully observed for signs of CNS depression, such as somnolence, and the dose of gabapentin or morphine should be reduced appropriately.

PREGABALIN — ORAL

c-v	**Lyrica** (Pfizer)	**Capsules:** 25 mg	Lactose. (PGN 25). White. In 90s.
		50 mg	Lactose. (PGN 50). White. In 90s.
		75 mg	Lactose. (PGN 75). White/Orange. In 90s.
		100 mg	Lactose. (PGN 100). Orange. In 90s.
		150 mg	Lactose. (PGN 150). White. In 90s.
		200 mg	Lactose. (PGN 200). Lt. orange. In 90s.
		225 mg	Lactose. (PGN 225). White/Lt. orange. In 90s.
		300 mg	Lactose. (PGN 300). White/Orange. In 90s.

PREGABALIN — ORAL

Indications

➤*Neuropathic pain associated with diabetic peripheral neuropathy:* For management of neuropathic pain associated with diabetic peripheral neuropathy.

➤*Partial-onset seizures:* Adjunctive therapy for adult patients with partial-onset seizures.

➤*Postherpetic neuralgia:* For the management of postherpetic neuralgia.

Administration and Dosage

➤*Approved by the FDA:* June 10, 2005.

➤*Neuropathic pain associated with diabetic peripheral neuropathy:* The maximum recommended dose of pregabalin is 100 mg 3 times a day (300 mg/day) in patients with creatinine clearance (Ccr) of at least 60 mL/min. Dosing should begin at 50 mg 3 times a day (150 mg/day) and may be increased to 300 mg/day within 1 week based on efficacy and tolerability. Because pregabalin is eliminated primarily by renal excretion, the dose should be adjusted for patients with reduced renal function.

Although pregabalin was also studied at 600 mg/day, there is no evidence that this dose confers additional significant benefit and this dose was less well tolerated. In view of the dose-dependent adverse effects, treatment with doses above 300 mg/day are not recommended.

➤*Partial-onset seizures:* Pregabalin, at doses of 150 to 600 mg/day, has been shown to be effective as adjunctive therapy in the treatment of partial-onset seizures in adults. The total daily dose should be divided and given 2 or 3 times daily. The efficacy and adverse reaction profiles of pregabalin have been shown to be dose related. In general, it is recommended that patients be started on a total daily dose no greater than 150 mg/day (75 mg 2 times a day, or 50 mg 3 times a day). Based on individual patient response and tolerability, the dose may be increased to a maximum dose of 600 mg/day.

The efficacy of add-on pregabalin in patients taking gabapentin has not been evaluated in controlled trials. Consequently, dosing recommendations for the use of pregabalin with gabapentin cannot be offered.

➤*Postherpetic neuralgia:* The recommended dose of pregabalin is 75 to 150 mg 2 times a day, or 50 to 100 mg 3 times a day (150 to 300 mg/day) in patients with Ccr of at least 60 mL/min. Dosing should begin at 75 mg

PREGABALIN — ORAL

2 times a day, or 50 mg 3 times a day (150 mg/day) and may be increased to 300 mg/day within 1 week based on efficacy and tolerability. Because pregabalin is eliminated primarily by renal excretion, the dose should be adjusted for patients with reduced renal function.

Patients who do not experience sufficient pain relief following 2 to 4 weeks of treatment with 300 mg/day and who are able to tolerate pregabalin may be treated with up to 300 mg 2 times a day or 200 mg 3 times a day (600 mg/day). In view of the dose-dependent adverse effects and the higher rate of treatment discontinuation caused by adverse reactions, dosing above 300 mg/day should be reserved only for those patients who have ongoing pain and are tolerating 300 mg daily.

➤*Renal function impairment:* In view of dose-dependent adverse reactions and because pregabalin is eliminated primarily by renal excretion, the dose should be adjusted in patients with reduced renal function. Dosage adjustment in patients with renal impairment should be based on Ccr, as indicated in the following table. To use this dosing table, an estimate of the patient's Ccr in mL/min is needed. Ccr in mL/min may be estimated from serum creatinine (mg/dL) determination using the Cockcroft and Gault equation.

For patients undergoing hemodialysis, pregabalin daily dose should be adjusted based on renal function. In addition to the daily dose adjustment, a supplemental dose should be given immediately following every 4-hour hemodialysis treatment (see the following table).

Pregabalin Dosage Based on Renal Function

Ccr (mL/min)	Total pregabalin daily dose (mg/day)[a]			Dose regimen
≥ 60	150	300	600	2 divided doses or 3 divided doses
30 to 60	75	150	300	2 divided doses or 3 divided doses
15 to 30	25 to 50	75	150	Single daily dose or 2 divided doses
< 15	25	25 to 50	75	Single daily dose
Supplementary dosage following hemodialysis (mg)[b]				
Patients on the 25 mg single daily dose regimen: Take 1 supplemental dose of 25 or 50 mg.				
Patients on the 25 to 50 mg single daily dose regimen: Take 1 supplemental dose of 50 or 75 mg.				
Patients on the 75 mg single daily dose regimen: Take 1 supplemental dose of 100 or 150 mg.				

[a] Total daily dose (mg/day) should be divided as indicated by dose regimen to provide mg/dose.
[b] Supplementary dose is a single additional dose.

➤*Storage/Stability:* Store at 25°C (77°F); excursions permitted to 15° to 30°C (59° to 86°F).

Actions

➤*Pharmacology:* Pregabalin binds with high affinity to the alpha$_2$-delta site (an auxiliary subunit of voltage-gated calcium channels) in CNS tissues. Although the mechanism of action of pregabalin is unknown, results with genetically modified mice and with compounds structurally related to pregabalin (such as gabapentin) suggest that binding to the alpha$_2$-delta subunit may be involved in pregabalin's antinociceptive and antiseizure effects in animal models. In vitro, pregabalin reduces the calcium-dependent release of several neurotransmitters, possibly by modulation of calcium channel function.

While pregabalin is a structural derivative of the inhibitory neurotransmitter gamma-aminobutyric acid (GABA), it does not bind directly to GABA$_A$, GABA$_B$, or benzodiazepine receptors, does not augment GABA$_A$ responses in cultured neurons, does not alter rat brain GABA concentration or have acute effects on GABA uptake or degradation. However, in cultured neurons prolonged application of pregabalin increases the density of GABA transporter protein and increases the rate of functional GABA transport. Pregabalin does not block sodium channels, is not active at opiate receptors, and does not alter cyclooxygenase enzyme activity. It is inactive at serotonin and dopamine receptors and does not inhibit dopamine, serotonin, or noradrenaline reuptake.

➤*Pharmacokinetics:*

Absorption/Distribution – Following oral administration of pregabalin under fasting conditions, peak plasma concentrations occur within 1.5 hours. Pregabalin oral bioavailability is 90% or more and is independent of dose. Following single- (25 to 300 mg) and multiple-dose (75 to 900 mg/day) administration, maximum plasma concentrations (C_{max}) and area under the plasma concentration-time curve (AUC) values increase linearly. Following repeated administration, steady state is achieved within 24 to 48 hours. Multiple-dose pharmacokinetics can be predicted from single-dose data.

The rate of pregabalin absorption is decreased when given with food, resulting in a decrease in C_{max} of approximately 25% to 30% and an increase in time of maximal concentration (T_{max}) to approximately 3 hours. However, administration of pregabalin with food has no clinically relevant effect on the total absorption of pregabalin. Therefore, pregabalin can be taken with or without food.

Pregabalin does not bind to plasma proteins. The apparent volume of distribution of pregabalin following oral administration is approximately 0.5 L/kg. Pregabalin is a substrate for system L transporter, which is responsible for the transport of large amino acids across the blood-brain barrier. Although there are no data in humans, pregabalin has been shown to cross the blood-brain barrier in mice, rats, and monkeys. In addition, pregabalin has been shown to cross the placenta in rats and is present in the milk of lactating rats.

Metabolism/Excretion – Pregabalin undergoes negligible metabolism in humans. Following a dose of radiolabeled pregabalin, approximately 90% of the administered dose was recovered in the urine as unchanged pregabalin. The N-methylated derivative of pregabalin, the major metabolite of pregabalin found in urine, accounted for 0.9% of the dose. In preclinical studies, pregabalin (S-enantiomer) did not undergo racemization to the R-enantiomer in mice, rats, rabbits, or monkeys.

Pregabalin is eliminated from the systemic circulation primarily by renal excretion as unchanged drug, with a mean elimination half-life of 6.3 hours in subjects with normal renal function. Mean renal clearance was estimated to be 67 to 80.9 mL/min in young healthy subjects. Because pregabalin is not bound to plasma proteins, this clearance rate indicates that renal tubular reabsorption is involved. Pregabalin elimination is nearly proportional to Ccr.

Special populations –

Renal function impairment: Pregabalin clearance is nearly proportional to Ccr. Dosage reduction in patients with renal dysfunction is necessary. Pregabalin is effectively removed from plasma by hemodialysis. Following a 4-hour hemodialysis treatment, plasma pregabalin concentrations are reduced approximately 50%. For patients on hemodialysis, dosing must be modified.

Elderly: Pregabalin oral clearance tended to decrease with increasing age. This decrease in pregabalin oral clearance is consistent with age-related decreases in Ccr. Reduction of pregabalin dose may be required in patients who have age-related compromised renal function.

Contraindications

Hypersensitivity to pregabalin or any of its components.

Warnings

➤*Discontinuation:* As with all antiepileptic drugs, withdraw pregabalin gradually to minimize the potential of increased seizure frequency in patients with seizure disorders. If pregabalin is discontinued, this should be done gradually over a minimum of 1 week.

Following abrupt or rapid discontinuation of pregabalin, some patients reported symptoms including insomnia, nausea, headache, and diarrhea. Taper pregabalin gradually over a minimum of 1 week rather than discontinuing abruptly.

➤*Renal function impairment/Hemodialysis:* See Actions for more information.

➤*Carcinogenesis:* In standard preclinical, in vivo, lifetime carcinogenicity studies of pregabalin, an unexpectedly high incidence of hemangiosarcoma was identified in 2 different strains of mice. The clinical significance of this finding is unknown. Clinical experience during pregabalin's premarketing development provides no direct means to assess its potential for inducing tumors in humans.

In clinical studies across various patient populations, comprising 6,396 patient-years of exposure in patients older than 12 years of age, new or worsening preexisting tumors were reported in 57 patients. Without knowledge of the background incidence and recurrence in similar populations not treated with pregabalin, it is impossible to know whether the incidence seen in these cohorts is or is not affected by treatment.

A dose-dependent increase in the incidence of malignant vascular tumors (hemangiosarcomas) was observed in 2 strains of mice (B6C3F1 and CD-1) given pregabalin (200, 1,000, or 5,000 mg/kg) in the diet for 2 years. Plasma pregabalin exposure (AUC) in mice receiving the lowest dose that increased hemangiosarcomas was approximately equal to the human exposure at the maximum recommended human dose (MRHD) of 600 mg/day. A no-effect dose for induction of hemangiosarcomas in mice was not established. No evidence of carcinogenicity was seen in 2 studies in Wistar rats following dietary administration of pregabalin for 2 years at doses (50, 150, or 450 mg/kg in males and 100, 300, or 900 mg/kg in females) that were associated with plasma exposures in males and females up to approximately 14 and 24 times, respectively, human exposure at the MRHD.

➤*Fertility impairment:* In fertility studies in which male rats were orally administered pregabalin (50 to 2,500 mg/kg) prior to and during mating with untreated females, a number of adverse reproductive and developmental effects were observed. These included decreased sperm counts and sperm motility, increased sperm abnormalities, reduced fertility, increased preimplantation embryo loss, decreased litter size, decreased fetal body weights, and an increased incidence of fetal abnormalities. Effects on sperm and fertility parameters were reversible in studies of this duration (3 to 4 months). The no-effect dose for male reproductive toxicity in these studies (100 mg/kg) was associated with a plasma pregabalin exposure (AUC) approximately 3 times human exposure at the MRHD of 600 mg/day.

In addition, adverse effects on reproductive organ (testes, epididymides) histopathology were observed in male rats exposed to pregabalin (500 to 1,250 mg/kg) in general toxicology studies of 4 weeks or greater duration. The no-effect dose for male reproductive organ histopathology in rats (250 mg/kg) was associated with a plasma exposure approximately 8 times human exposure at the MRHD.

In a fertility study in which female rats were given pregabalin (500, 1,250, or 2,500 mg/kg) orally prior to and during mating and early gestation, disrupted estrous cyclicity and an increased number of days to mating were seen at all doses, and embryolethality occurred at the highest dose. The low dose in this study produced a plasma exposure approximately 9 times that in humans receiving the MRHD. A no-effect dose for female reproductive toxicity in rats was not established.

PREGABALIN — ORAL

➤*Elderly:* Because pregabalin is eliminated primarily by renal excretion, adjust the dose for elderly patients with renal impairment.

➤*Pregnancy: Category C.* Increased incidences of fetal structural abnormalities and other manifestations of developmental toxicity, including lethality, growth retardation, and nervous and reproductive system functional impairment, were observed in the offspring of rats and rabbits given pregabalin during pregnancy, at doses that produced plasma pregabalin exposures (AUC) at least 5 times human exposure at the MRHD of 600 mg/day.

There are no adequate and well-controlled studies in pregnant women. Use pregabalin during pregnancy only if the potential benefit justifies the potential risk to the fetus.

Labor and delivery – The effects of pregabalin on labor and delivery in pregnant women are unknown. In the prenatal-postnatal study in rats, pregabalin prolonged gestation and induced dystocia at exposures greater than or equal to 50 times the mean human exposure ($AUC_{(0-24)}$ of 123 mcg•h/mL) at the maximum recommended clinical dose of 600 mg/day.

➤*Lactation:* It is not known if pregabalin is excreted in human milk; it is, however, present in the milk of rats. Because many drugs are excreted in human milk, and because of the potential for tumorigenicity shown for pregabalin in animal studies, decide whether to discontinue breast-feeding or to discontinue the drug, taking into account the importance of the drug to the mother.

➤*Children:* The safety and efficacy of pregabalin in children have not been established.

Precautions

➤*Dizziness/Somnolence:* Pregabalin causes dizziness and somnolence. Inform patients that pregabalin-related dizziness and somnolence may impair their ability to perform tasks such as driving or operating machinery.

In the pregabalin-controlled trials, dizziness was experienced by 29% of pregabalin-treated patients compared with 9% of placebo-treated patients; somnolence was experienced by 22% of pregabalin-treated patients compared with 8% of placebo-treated patients. Dizziness and somnolence generally began shortly after the initiation of pregabalin therapy and occurred more frequently at higher doses. Dizziness and somnolence were the adverse reactions most frequently leading to withdrawal (4% each) from controlled studies. In pregabalin-treated patients reporting these adverse reactions in short-term, controlled studies, dizziness persisted until the last dose in 31% and somnolence persisted until the last dose in 46% of patients.

➤*Ophthalmological effects:* In controlled studies, a higher proportion of patients treated with pregabalin reported blurred vision (6%) than did patients treated with placebo (2%), which resolved in a majority of cases with continued dosing. Less than 1% of patients discontinued pregabalin treatment because of vision-related reactions (primarily blurred vision).

Prospectively planned ophthalmologic testing, including visual acuity testing, formal visual field testing, and dilated funduscopic examination, was performed in more than 3,600 patients. In these patients, visual acuity was reduced in 7% of patients treated with pregabalin, and 5% of placebo-treated patients. Visual field changes were detected in 13% of pregabalin-treated patients and 12% of placebo-treated patients. Funduscopic changes were observed in 2% of pregabalin-treated patients and 2% of placebo-treated patients.

Although the clinical significance of the ophthalmologic findings is unknown, inform patients to notify their health care provider if changes in vision occur. If visual disturbance persists, consider further assessment. Consider more frequent assessment for patients who are already routinely monitored for ocular conditions.

➤*Weight gain:* Pregabalin treatment caused weight gain. In pregabalin-controlled clinical trials of up to 13 weeks, a gain of 7% or more over baseline weight was observed in 8% of pregabalin-treated patients and 2% of placebo-treated patients. Few patients treated with pregabalin (0.2%) withdrew from controlled trials because of weight gain. Pregabalin-associated weight gain was related to dose and duration of exposure but did not appear to be associated with baseline body mass index (BMI), gender, or age. Weight gain was not limited to patients with edema.

Although weight gain was not associated with clinically important changes in blood pressure in short-term controlled studies, the long-term cardiovascular effects of pregabalin-associated weight gain are unknown.

Among diabetic patients, pregabalin-treated patients gained an average of 1.6 kg (range, −16 to 16 kg), compared with an average 0.3 kg (range, −10 to 9 kg) weight gain in placebo patients. In a cohort of 333 diabetic patients who received pregabalin for at least 2 years, the average weight gain was 5.2 kg.

➤*Peripheral edema:* Pregabalin treatment caused edema, primarily described as peripheral edema. In short-term trials of patients without clinically significant heart or peripheral vascular disease, there was no apparent association between peripheral edema and cardiovascular complications such as hypertension or congestive heart failure (CHF). Peripheral edema was not associated with laboratory changes suggestive of deterioration in renal or hepatic function.

In controlled clinical trials, the incidence of peripheral edema was 6% in the pregabalin group compared with 2% in the placebo group. In controlled clinical trials, 0.6% of pregabalin patients and no placebo patients withdrew because of peripheral edema.

Higher frequencies of weight gain and peripheral edema were observed in patients taking both pregabalin and a thiazolidinedione antidiabetic agent compared with patients taking either drug alone. The majority of patients using thiazolidinedione antidiabetic agents in the overall safety database were participants in studies of pain associated with diabetic peripheral neuropathy. In this population, peripheral edema was reported in 3% (2 of 60) of patients who were using thiazolidinedione antidiabetic agents only, 8% (69 of 859) of patients who were treated with pregabalin only, and 19% (23 of 120) of patients who were on both pregabalin and thiazolidinedione antidiabetic agents. Similarly, weight gain was reported in 0% (0 of 60) of patients on thiazolidinediones only; 4% (35 of 859) of patients on pregabalin only; and 7.5% (9 of 120) of patients on both drugs.

➤*CHF:* Because there are limited data on CHF patients with New York Heart Association (NYHA) Class III or IV cardiac status, use pregabalin with caution in these patients.

➤*Creatine kinase elevations:* Pregabalin treatment was associated with creatine kinase elevations. Mean changes in creatine kinase from baseline to the maximum value were 60 units/L for pregabalin-treated patients and 28 units/L for the placebo patients. In all controlled trials across multiple patient populations, 2% of patients on pregabalin and 1% of placebo patients had a value of creatine kinase at least 3 times the upper limit of normal (ULN). Three pregabalin-treated subjects had events reported as rhabdomyolysis in premarketing clinical trials. The relationship between these myopathy events and pregabalin is not completely understood because the cases had documented factors that may have caused or contributed to these events. Instruct patients to promptly report unexplained muscle pain, tenderness, or weakness, particularly if these muscle symptoms are accompanied by malaise or fever. Discontinue pregabalin treatment if myopathy is diagnosed or suspected or if markedly elevated creatine kinase levels occur.

➤*Decreased platelet count:* Pregabalin treatment was associated with a decrease in platelet count. Pregabalin-treated subjects experienced a mean maximal decrease in platelet count of 20×10^3/mcL, compared with 11×10^3/mcL in placebo patients. In the overall database of controlled trials, 2% of placebo patients and 3% of pregabalin patients experienced a potentially clinically significant decrease in platelets, defined as 20% below baseline value and less than 150×10^3/mcL. In randomized controlled trials, pregabalin was not associated with an increase in bleeding-related adverse reactions.

➤*PR interval prolongation:* Pregabalin treatment was associated with mild PR interval prolongation. In analyses of clinical trial electrocardiogram (ECG) data, the mean PR interval increase was 3 to 6 msec at pregabalin doses greater than or equal to 300 mg/day. This mean change difference was not associated with an increased risk of PR increase 25% or more from baseline, an increased percentage of subjects with on-treatment PR greater than 200 msec, or an increased risk of adverse reactions of second- or third-degree AV block.

Drug Interactions

➤*Drug/Food interactions:* See Actions for more information.

Adverse Reactions

➤*Adverse reactions most commonly leading to discontinuation in all controlled clinical studies:* In controlled trials of all populations combined, 14% of patients treated with pregabalin and 7% of patients treated with placebo discontinued prematurely because of adverse reactions. In the pregabalin treatment group, the adverse reactions most frequently leading to discontinuation were dizziness (4%) and somnolence (3%). In the placebo group, 1% of patients withdrew because of dizziness and less than 1% withdrew because of somnolence. Other adverse reactions that led to discontinuation from controlled trials more frequently in the pregabalin group compared with the placebo group were ataxia, confusion, asthenia, thinking abnormal, blurred vision, incoordination, and peripheral edema (1% each).

➤*Most common adverse reactions in all controlled clinical studies:* In controlled trials of all patient populations combined, dizziness, somnolence, dry mouth, edema, blurred vision, weight gain, and "thinking abnormal" (primarily difficulty with concentration/attention) were more commonly reported by subjects treated with pregabalin than by subjects treated with placebo (5% or more and twice the rate of that seen in placebo).

➤*Controlled studies with neuropathic pain associated with diabetic peripheral neuropathy:*

Adverse reactions leading to discontinuation – In clinical trials in patients with neuropathic pain associated with diabetic peripheral neuropathy, 9% of patients treated with pregabalin and 4% of patients treated with placebo discontinued prematurely because of adverse reactions. In the pregabalin treatment group, the most common reasons for discontinuation caused by adverse reactions were dizziness (3%) and somnolence (2%). In comparison, less than 1% of placebo patients withdrew because of dizziness and somnolence. Other reasons for discontinuation from the trials, occurring with greater frequency in the pregabalin group than in the placebo group, were asthenia, confusion, and peripheral edema. Each of these reactions led to withdrawal in approximately 1% of patients.

Most common adverse reactions – The following table lists all adverse reactions, regardless of causality, occurring in 1% or more of patients with neuropathic pain associated with diabetic neuropathy in the combined pregabalin group for which the incidence was greater in this combined pregabalin group than in the placebo group. A majority of pregabalin-treated patients in clinical studies had adverse reactions with a maximum intensity of "mild" or "moderate."

PREGABALIN — ORAL

Adverse Reactions in Neuropathic Pain Associated with Diabetic Peripheral Neuropathy (≥ 1%)						
Adverse reaction	75 mg/day (n = 77)	150 mg/day (n = 212)	300 mg/day (n = 321)	600 mg/day (n = 369)	All pregabalin (n = 979)	Placebo (n = 459)
CNS						
Abnormal gait	1%	0%	1%	3%	1%	0%
Amnesia	3%	1%	0%	2%	1%	0%
Ataxia	6%	1%	2%	4%	3%	1%
Confusion	0%	1%	2%	3%	2%	1%
Dizziness	8%	9%	23%	29%	21%	5%
Euphoria	0%	0%	3%	2%	2%	0%
Incoordination	1%	0%	2%	2%	2%	0%
Nervousness	0%	1%	1%	1%	1%	0%
Neuropathy	9%	2%	2%	5%	4%	3%
Somnolence	4%	6%	13%	16%	12%	3%
Thinking abnormal[a]	1%	0%	1%	3%	2%	0%
Tremor	1%	1%	1%	2%	1%	0%
Vertigo	1%	2%	2%	4%	3%	1%
GI						
Constipation	0%	2%	4%	6%	4%	2%
Dry mouth	3%	2%	5%	7%	5%	1%
Flatulence	3%	0%	2%	3%	2%	1%
Metabolic/Nutritional						
Edema	0%	2%	4%	2%	2%	0%
Hypoglycemia	1%	3%	2%	1%	2%	1%
Peripheral edema	4%	6%	9%	12%	9%	2%
Weight gain	0%	4%	4%	6%	4%	0%
Respiratory						
Dyspnea	3%	0%	2%	2%	2%	1%
Special senses						
Abnormal vision	1%	0%	1%	1%	1%	0%
Blurry vision[b]	3%	1%	3%	6%	4%	2%
Miscellaneous						
Accidental injury	5%	2%	2%	6%	4%	3%
Asthenia	4%	2%	4%	7%	5%	2%
Back pain	0%	2%	1%	2%	2%	0%
Chest pain	4%	1%	1%	2%	2%	1%
Face edema	0%	1%	1%	2%	1%	0%

[a] Thinking abnormal primarily consists of events related to difficulty with concentration/attention but also includes events related to cognition and language problems and slowed thinking.
[b] Investigator term; summary level term is amblyopia.

➤*Controlled studies in postherpetic neuralgia:*

Adverse reactions leading to discontinuation – In clinical trials in patients with postherpetic neuralgia, 14% of patients treated with pregabalin and 7% of patients treated with placebo discontinued prematurely because of adverse reactions. In the pregabalin treatment group, the most common reasons for discontinuation caused by adverse reactions were dizziness (4%) and somnolence (3%). In comparison, less than 1% of placebo patients withdrew because of dizziness and somnolence. Other reasons for discontinuation from the trials, occurring in greater frequency in the pregabalin group than in the placebo group, were confusion (2%), as well as peripheral edema, asthenia, ataxia, and abnormal gait (1% each).

Most common adverse reactions – The following table lists all adverse reactions, regardless of causality, occurring in 1% or more of patients with neuropathic pain associated with postherpetic neuralgia in the combined pregabalin group for which the incidence was greater in this combined pregabalin group than in the placebo group. In addition, a reaction is included, even if the incidence in the all pregabalin group is not greater than in the placebo group, if the incidence of the reaction in the 600 mg/day group is more than twice that in the placebo group. A majority of pregabalin-treated patients in clinical studies had adverse reactions with a maximum intensity of "mild" or "moderate."

Adverse Reactions in Neuropathic Pain Associated with Postherpetic Neuralgia (≥ 1%)						
Adverse reaction	75 mg/day (n = 84)	150 mg/day (n = 302)	300 mg/day (n = 312)	600 mg/day (n = 154)	All pregabalin (n = 852)	Placebo (n = 398)
CNS						
Abnormal gait	0%	2%	4%	8%	4%	1%
Amnesia	0%	1%	1%	4%	2%	0%
Ataxia	1%	2%	5%	9%	5%	1%
Confusion	1%	2%	3%	7%	3%	0%
Dizziness	11%	18%	31%	37%	26%	9%
Headache	5%	9%	5%	8%	7%	5%
Incoordination	2%	2%	1%	3%	2%	0%
Somnolence	8%	12%	18%	25%	16%	5%
Speech disorder	0%	0%	1%	3%	1%	0%
Thinking abnormal[a]	0%	2%	1%	6%	2%	2%
GI						
Constipation	4%	5%	5%	5%	5%	2%
Dry mouth	7%	7%	6%	15%	8%	3%
Flatulence	2%	1%	2%	3%	2%	1%
Vomiting	1%	1%	3%	3%	2%	1%
GU						
Urinary incontinence	0%	1%	1%	2%	1%	0%
Metabolic/Nutritional						
Edema	0%	1%	2%	6%	2%	1%
Peripheral edema	0%	8%	16%	16%	12%	4%
Weight gain	1%	2%	5%	7%	4%	0%
Musculoskeletal						
Myasthenia	1%	1%	1%	1%	1%	0%
Respiratory						
Bronchitis	0%	1%	1%	3%	1%	1%
Special senses						
Abnormal vision	0%	1%	2%	5%	2%	0%
Blurry vision[b]	1%	5%	5%	9%	5%	3%
Diplopia	0%	2%	2%	4%	2%	0%
Eye disorder	0%	1%	1%	2%	1%	0%
Miscellaneous						
Accidental injury	4%	3%	3%	5%	3%	2%
Face edema	0%	2%	1%	3%	2%	1%
Flu syndrome	1%	2%	2%	1%	2%	1%
Infection	14%	8%	6%	3%	7%	4%
Pain	5%	4%	5%	5%	5%	4%

[a] Thinking abnormal primarily consists of events related to difficulty with concentration/attention but also includes events related to cognition and language problems and slowed thinking.
[b] Investigator term; summary level term is amblyopia.

➤*Controlled add-on studies in partial-onset seizures:*

Adverse reactions leading to discontinuation – Approximately 15% of patients receiving pregabalin and 6% of patients receiving placebo in add-on epilepsy trials discontinued prematurely because of adverse reactions. In the pregabalin treatment group, the adverse reactions most frequently leading to discontinuation were dizziness (6%), ataxia (4%), and somnolence (3%). In comparison, less than 1% of patients in the placebo group withdrew because of each of these reactions. Other adverse reactions that led to discontinuation of at least 1% of patients in the pregabalin group and at least twice as frequently compared with the placebo group were asthenia, diplopia, blurred vision, thinking abnormal, nausea, tremor, vertigo, headache, and confusion (which each led to withdrawal in 2% or less of patients).

Most common adverse reactions – The following table lists all dose-related adverse reactions, regardless of causality, occurring in at least 2% of all pregabalin-treated patients. Dose-relatedness was defined as the incidence of the adverse reaction in the 600 mg/day group was at least 2% greater than the rate in both the placebo and 150 mg/day groups. In these studies, 758 patients received pregabalin and 294 patients received placebo for up to 12 weeks. Because patients were also treated with 1 to 3 other antiepileptic drugs, it is not possible to determine whether the following adverse reactions can be ascribed to pregabalin alone, or the combination of pregabalin and other antiepileptic drugs. A majority of pregabalin-treated patients in these studies had adverse reactions with a maximum intensity of "mild" or "moderate."

Pregabalin Adverse Reactions (≥ 2%)					
Adverse reaction	150 mg/day (n = 185)	300 mg/day (n = 90)	600 mg/day (n = 395)	All pregabalin (n = 670[a])	Placebo (n = 294)
CNS					
Abnormal gait	1%	3%	5%	4%	0%
Amnesia	3%	2%	6%	5%	2%
Ataxia	6%	10%	20%	15%	4%
Confusion	1%	2%	5%	4%	2%
Dizziness	18%	31%	38%	32%	11%
Incoordination	1%	3%	6%	4%	1%
Myoclonus	1%	0%	4%	2%	0%
Somnolence	11%	18%	28%	22%	11%
Speech disorder	1%	2%	7%	5%	1%
Thinking abnormal[b]	4%	8%	9%	8%	2%
Tremor	3%	7%	11%	8%	4%
Twitching	0%	4%	5%	4%	1%

PREGABALIN — ORAL

Pregabalin Adverse Reactions (≥ 2%)					
Adverse reaction	150 mg/day (n = 185)	300 mg/day (n = 90)	600 mg/day (n = 395)	All pregabalin (n = 670[a])	Placebo (n = 294)
GI					
Constipation	1%	1%	7%	4%	2%
Dry mouth	1%	2%	6%	4%	1%
Increased appetite	2%	3%	6%	5%	1%
Metabolic/Nutritional					
Peripheral edema	3%	3%	6%	5%	2%
Weight gain	5%	7%	16%	12%	1%
Special senses					
Abnormal vision	3%	1%	5%	4%	1%
Blurred vision[c]	5%	8%	12%	10%	4%
Diplopia	5%	7%	12%	9%	4%
Miscellaneous					
Accidental injury	7%	11%	10%	9%	5%
Pain	3%	2%	5%	4%	3%

[a] Excludes patients who received the 50 mg dose in study E1.
[b] Thinking abnormal primarily consists of events related to difficulty with concentration/attention but also includes events related to cognition and language problems and slowed thinking.
[c] Investigator term; summary level term is amblyopia.

Adverse reactions occurring in at least 2% of patients with partial-onset seizures in the combined pregabalin group for which the incidence was greater in this combined pregabalin group than in the placebo group, but did not show dose-relatedness, include the following: asthenia, chest pain, infection, nervousness, nystagmus, paresthesias, visual field defect, and vomiting.

➤*Other adverse reactions:*

Cardiovascular – Deep thrombophlebitis, heart failure, hypotension, postural hypotension, retinal vascular disorder, syncope (0.1% to 1%); ST depressed, ventricular fibrillation (less than 0.1%).

CNS – Anxiety, depersonalization, hypertonia, hypesthesia, libido decreased, nystagmus, paresthesia, stupor, twitching (1% or more); abnormal dreams, agitation, apathy, aphasia, circumoral paresthesia, dysarthria, hallucinations, hostility, hyperalgesia, hyperesthesia, hyperkinesia, hypokinesia, hypotonia, libido increased, myoclonus, neuralgia (0.1% to 1%); addiction, cerebellar syndrome, cogwheel rigidity, coma, delirium, delusions, dysautonomia, dyskinesia, dystonia, encephalopathy, extrapyramidal syndrome, Guillain-Barre syndrome, hypalgesia, intracranial hypertension, manic reaction, paranoid reaction, peripheral neuritis, psychotic depression, schizophrenic reaction, torticollis, trismus (less than 0.1%).

Dermatologic – Pruritus (1% or more); alopecia, dry skin, eczema, hirsutism, skin ulcer, urticaria, vesiculobullous rash (0.1% to 1%); angioedema, exfoliative dermatitis, Lichenoid dermatitis, melanosis, petechial rash, purpuric rash, pustular rash, skin atrophy, skin necrosis, skin nodule, Stevens-Johnson syndrome, subcutaneous nodule (less than 0.1%).

GI – Abdominal pain, gastroenteritis, increased appetite (1% or more); cholecystitis, cholelithiasis, colitis, dysphagia, esophagitis, gastritis, GI hemorrhage, melena, mouth ulceration, pancreatitis, rectal hemorrhage, tongue edema (0.1% to 1%); aphthous stomatitis, esophageal ulcer (less than 0.1%).

GU – Anorgasmia, impotence, urinary frequency, urinary incontinence (1% or more); abnormal ejaculation, albuminuria, amenorrhea, dysmenorrhea, dysuria, hematuria, kidney calculus, leukorrhea, menorrhagia, metrorrhagia, nephritis, oliguria, urinary retention (0.1% to 1%); acute kidney failure, balanitis, bladder neoplasm, cervicitis, dyspareunia, epididymitis, female lactation, glomerulitis (less than 0.1%).

Hematologic/Lymphatic – Ecchymosis (1% or more); anemia, eosinophilia, hypochromic anemia, leukocytosis, leukopenia, lymphadenopathy, thrombocytopenia (0.1% to 1%); myelofibrosis, polycythemia, prothrombin decreased, purpura, thrombocythemia (less than 0.1%).

Metabolic/Nutritional – Glucose tolerance decreased, urate crystalluria (less than 0.1%).

Musculoskeletal – Arthralgia, leg cramps, myalgia, myasthenia (1% or more); arthrosis (0.1% to 1%); generalized spasm (less than 0.1%).

Respiratory – Apnea, atelectasis, bronchiolitis, hiccup, laryngismus, lung edema, lung fibrosis, yawn (less than 0.1%).

Special senses – Conjunctivitis, diplopia, otitis media, tinnitus (1% or more); abnormality of accommodation, blepharitis, dry eyes, eye hemorrhage, hyperacusis, photophobia, retinal edema, taste loss, taste perversion (0.1% to 1%); anisocoria, blindness, corneal ulcer, exophthalmos, extraocular palsy, iritis, keratitis, keratoconjunctivitis, miosis, mydriasis, night blindness, ophthalmoplegia, optic atrophy, papilledema, parosmia, ptosis, uveitis (less than 0.1%).

Miscellaneous – Allergic reaction, fever (1% or more); abscess, cellulitis, chills, malaise, neck rigidity, overdose, pelvic pain, photosensitivity reaction, suicide attempt (0.1% to 1%); anaphylactoid reaction, ascites, granuloma, hangover effect, intentional injury, retroperitoneal fibrosis, shock, suicide (less than 0.1%).

Overdosage

➤*Symptoms:* There is limited experience with overdose of pregabalin. The highest reported accidental overdose of pregabalin during the clinical development program was 8,000 mg, and there were no notable clinical consequences. In clinical studies, some patients took as much as 2,400 mg/day. The types of adverse reactions experienced by patients exposed to higher doses (900 mg or more) were not clinically different from those of patients administered recommended doses of pregabalin.

➤*Treatment:* There is no specific antidote for overdose with pregabalin. If indicated, elimination of unabsorbed drug may be attempted by emesis or gastric lavage; observe usual precautions to maintain the airway. General supportive care of the patient is indicated, including monitoring of vital signs and observation of the clinical status of the patient. A certified poison control center should be contacted for up-to-date information on the management of overdose with pregabalin.

Although hemodialysis has not been performed in the few known cases of overdose, it may be indicated by the patient's clinical state or in patients with significant renal impairment. Standard hemodialysis procedures result in significant clearance of pregabalin (approximately 50% in 4 hours).

Patient Information

Counsel patients that pregabalin may cause dizziness, somnolence, blurred vision, and other CNS signs and symptoms. Accordingly, advise them not to drive, operate complex machinery, or engage in other hazardous activities until they have gained sufficient experience on pregabalin to gauge whether or not it affects their mental, visual, and/or motor performance adversely.

Counsel patients that pregabalin may cause visual disturbances. Inform patients to notify their health care provider if changes in vision occur.

Advise patients to take pregabalin as prescribed. Abrupt or rapid discontinuation may result in insomnia, nausea, headache, or diarrhea.

Counsel patients that pregabalin may cause edema and weight gain.

Advise patients that concomitant treatment with pregabalin and a thiazolidinedione antidiabetic agent may lead to an additive effect on edema and weight gain. For patients with preexisting cardiac conditions, this may increase the risk of heart failure.

Instruct patients to promptly report unexplained muscle pain, tenderness, or weakness, particularly if accompanied by malaise or fever.

Inform patients who require concomitant treatment with CNS depressants such as opiates or benzodiazepines that they may experience additive CNS side effects, such as somnolence.

Tell patients to avoid consuming alcohol while taking pregabalin because it may potentiate the impairment of motor skills and sedation of alcohol.

Instruct patients to notify their health care provider if they become pregnant or intend to become pregnant during therapy, and to notify their health care provider if they are breast-feeding or intend to breast-feed during therapy.

Inform men being treated with pregabalin who plan to father a child of the potential risk of male-mediated teratogenicity. In preclinical studies in rats, pregabalin was associated with an increased risk of male-mediated teratogenicity. The clinical significance of this finding is uncertain.

Instruct diabetic patients to pay particular attention to skin integrity while being treated with pregabalin. Some animals treated with pregabalin developed skin ulcerations, although no increased incidence of skin lesions associated with pregabalin was observed in clinical trials.

LAMOTRIGINE

Rx	**Lamictal** (GlaxoSmithKline)	**Tablets**: 25 mg	Lactose. (Lamictal 25). White, shield shape, scored. In 100s.
		100 mg	Lactose. (Lamictal 100). Peach, shield shape, scored. In 100s.
		150 mg	Lactose. (Lamictal 150). Cream, shield shape, scored. In 60s.
		200 mg	Lactose. (Lamictal 200). Blue, shield shape, scored. In 60s.
Rx	**Lamictal** (GlaxoSmithKline)	**Tablets, chewable dispersible**: 2 mg	Saccharin. (LTG 2). White to off-white. Black currant flavor. In 30s.
Rx	**Lamotrigine** (Teva)	**Tablets, chewable dispersible**: 5 mg	Saccharin. (TEVA 5715). White to off white, caplet-shaped. Black currant flavor. In 100s.
Rx	**Lamictal** (GlaxoSmithKline)		Saccharin. (GX CL2). White to off-white. Caplet shaped. Black currant flavor. In 100s.
Rx	**Lamotrigine** (Teva)	**Tablets, chewable dispersible**: 25 mg	Saccharin. (TEVA 57 16) White, elliptical-shaped. Black currant flavor. In 100s.
Rx	**Lamictal** (GlaxoSmithKline)		Saccharin. (GX CL5). White, elliptical. Black currant flavor. In 100s.

LAMOTRIGINE — ORAL

Refer to the general discussion beginning in the Anticonvulsants introduction.

WARNING

Serious rashes requiring hospitalization and discontinuation of treatment have been reported in association with the use of lamotrigine. The incidence of these rashes, which have included Stevens-Johnson syndrome, is approximately 0.8% (8 per 1,000) in pediatric patients (younger than 16 years of age) receiving lamotrigine as adjunctive therapy for epilepsy and 0.3% (3 per 1,000) in adults on adjunctive therapy for epilepsy. In clinical trials of bipolar and other mood disorders, the rate of serious rash was 0.08% (0.8 per 1,000) in adult patients receiving lamotrigine as initial monotherapy and 0.13% (1.3 per 1,000) in adult patients receiving lamotrigine as adjunctive therapy. In a prospectively followed cohort of 1,983 pediatric patients with epilepsy taking adjunctive lamotrigine, there was 1 rash-related death. In worldwide postmarketing experience, rare cases of toxic epidermal necrolysis or rash-related death have been reported in adult and pediatric patients, but those numbers are too few to permit a precise estimate of the rate.

Because the rate of serious rash is greater in pediatric patients than in adults, it bears emphasis that lamotrigine is approved only for use in pediatric patients younger than 16 years of age who have seizures associated with the Lennox-Gastaut syndrome or in patients with partial seizures.

Other than age, no factors have been identified that are known to predict the risk of occurrence or the severity of rash associated with lamotrigine. It is suggested, although not yet proven, that the risk of rash may also be increased by coadministration of lamotrigine with valproate (includes valproic acid and divalproex sodium), exceeding the recommended initial dose of lamotrigine, or exceeding the recommended dose escalation for lamotrigine. However, cases have been reported in the absence of these factors.

Nearly all cases of life-threatening rashes associated with lamotrigine have occurred within 2 to 8 weeks of treatment initiation. However, isolated cases have been reported after prolonged treatment (eg, 6 months). Accordingly, duration of therapy cannot be relied upon as a means to predict the potential risk heralded by the first appearance of a rash.

Although benign rashes also occur with lamotrigine, it is not possible to predict reliably which rashes will prove to be serious or life-threatening. Accordingly, lamotrigine should ordinarily be discontinued at the first sign of rash, unless the rash is clearly not drug related. Discontinuation of treatment may not prevent a rash from becoming life-threatening or permanently disabling or disfiguring.

Indications

➤*Epilepsy:*

Adjunctive therapy – As adjunctive therapy for partial seizures in adults and pediatric patients (2 years of age and older), and for generalized seizures of Lennox-Gastaut syndrome in adult and pediatric patients (2 years of age and older).

Monotherapy – For conversion to monotherapy in adults with partial seizures who are receiving treatment with carbamazepine, phenytoin, phenobarbital, primidone, or valproate as the single antiepileptic drug (AED). Safety and efficacy of lamotrigine have not been established as initial monotherapy; for conversion to monotherapy from AEDs other than carbamazepine, phenytoin, phenobarbital, primidone, or valproate; or for simultaneous conversion to monotherapy from 2 or more concomitant AEDs.

Safety and efficacy in patients younger than 16 years of age, other than those with partial seizures and the generalized seizures of Lennox-Gastaut syndrome, have not been established.

➤*Bipolar disorder:* For the maintenance treatment of bipolar I disorder to delay the time to occurrence of mood episodes (depression, mania, hypomania, mixed episodes) in patients treated for acute mood episodes with standard therapy. The efficacy of lamotrigine in the acute treatment of mood episodes has not been established.

➤*Unlabeled uses:* Management of adults with generalized tonic-clonic seizures, adults and children with absence seizures, juvenile myoclonic epilepsy, and temporal lobe seizures.

Administration and Dosage

➤*Approved by the FDA:* December 27, 1994.

➤*General dosing considerations:* The risk of nonserious rash is increased when the recommended initial dose and/or the rate of dose escalation of lamotrigine is exceeded. It is suggested, although not yet proven, that the risk of severe, potentially life-threatening rash may be increased by coadministration of lamotrigine with valproate, exceeding the recommended initial dose of lamotrigine, or exceeding the recommended dose escalation for lamotrigine. However, cases have been reported in the absence of these factors. Therefore, it is important that the dosing recommendations be followed closely.

It is recommended that lamotrigine not be restarted in patients who discontinued due to rash associated with prior treatment with lamotrigine, unless the potential benefits clearly outweigh the risks. If the decision is made to restart a patient who has discontinued lamotrigine, the need to restart with the initial dosing recommendations should be assessed. The greater the interval of time since the previous dose, the greater consideration should be given to restarting with the initial dosing recommendations. If a patient has discontinued lamotrigine for a period of more than 5 half-lives, it is recommended that initial dosing recommendations and guidelines be followed. The half-life of lamotrigine is affected by other concomitant medications. The apparent clearance of lamotrigine is affected by the coadministration of AEDs. Lamotrigine is eliminated more rapidly in patients who have been taking hepatic enzyme inducing antiepileptic drugs (EIAEDs), including carbamazepine, phenytoin, phenobarbital, and primidone.

➤*Epilepsy:*

Adjunctive therapy with lamotrigine for epilepsy – This section provides specific dosing recommendations for patients 2 to 12 years of age and patients older than 12 years of age. Within each of these age-groups, specific dosing recommendations are provided depending upon whether or not the patient is receiving valproate (see the following tables). In addition, the section provides a discussion of dosing for those patients receiving concomitant AEDs that have not been systematically evaluated in combination with lamotrigine.

For the following dosing guidelines for lamotrigine, EIAEDs include phenytoin, carbamazepine, phenobarbital, and primidone.

Children 2 to 12 years of age: Recommended dosing guidelines for lamotrigine added to an AED regimen containing valproate and for lamotrigine added to EIAEDs are summarized in the following table.

The smallest available strength of lamotrigine chewable tablets is 2 mg, and only whole tablets should be administered. If the calculated dose cannot be achieved using whole tablets, the dose should be rounded down to the nearest whole tablet.

- *Lamotrigine added to oxcarbazepine or levetiracetam, or to AEDs for which the interaction with lamotrigine is not known –*

Lamotrigine Added to an AED Regimen Containing Valproate in Patients 2 to 12 Years of Age			
Weeks 1 and 2	0.15 mg/kg/day in 1 or 2 divided doses, rounded down to the nearest whole tablet. Only whole tablets should be used for dosing.		
Weeks 3 and 4	0.3 mg/kg/day in 1 or 2 divided doses, rounded down to the nearest whole tablet		
Weight-based dosing can be achieved by using the following guide:			
If the patient's weight is:		Give this daily dose, using the most appropriate combination of lamotrigine 2 mg and 5 mg tablets:	
Greater than	and less than	Weeks 1 and 2	Weeks 3 and 4
6.7 kg	14 kg	2 mg every other day	2 mg/day
14.1 kg	27 kg	2 mg/day	4 mg/day
27.1 kg	34 kg	4 mg/day	8 mg/day
34.1 kg	40 kg	5 mg/day	10 mg/day
Usual maintenance dosage: 1 to 5 mg/kg/day (maximum 200 mg/day in 1 or 2 divided doses). To achieve the usual maintenance dosages, subsequent dosages should be increased every 1 to 2 weeks as follows: Calculate 0.3 mg/kg/day, round this amount down to the nearest whole tablet, and add this amount to the previously administered daily dose. The usual maintenance dosage in patients adding lamotrigine to valproate alone ranges from 1 to 3 mg/kg/day. Maintenance dosages in patients weighing less than 30 kg may need to be increased by as much as 50%, based on clinical response.			

Lamotrigine Added to Carbamazepine, Phenytoin, Phenobarbital, or Primidone[a] (Without Valproate) in Patients 2 to 12 Years of Age	
Weeks 1 and 2	0.6 mg/kg/day in 2 divided doses, rounded down to the nearest whole tablet
Weeks 3 and 4	1.2 mg/kg/day in 2 divided doses, rounded down to the nearest whole tablet
Usual maintenance dosage: 5 to 15 mg/kg/day (maximum 400 mg/day in 2 divided doses). To achieve the usual maintenance dosage, subsequent doses should be increased every 1 to 2 weeks as follows: Calculate 1.2 mg/kg/day, round this amount down to the nearest whole tablet, and add this amount to the previously administered daily dose. Maintenance dosages in patients weighing less than 30 kg may need to be increased by as much as 50%, based on clinical response.	

[a] Rifampin has also been shown to increase the apparent clearance of lamotrigine.

➤*Patients older than 12 years of age:* Recommended dosing guidelines for lamotrigine added to valproate are summarized in the following first table. Recommended dosing guidelines for lamotrigine added to EIAEDs are summarized in the following second table.

Lamotrigine added to oxcarbazepine or levetiracetam, or to AEDs for which the interaction with lamotrigine is not known – Oxcarbazepine and levetiracetam do not affect the apparent clearance of lamotrigine. Specific dosing guidelines for the addition of lamotrigine to oxcarbazepine or levetiracetam have not been studied in clinical trials. The effect of AEDs other than those already specified on the metabolism of lamotrigine is not currently known. Therefore, no specific dosing guidelines can be provided in that situation. Conservative starting doses and dose escalations (as with concomitant valproate) would be prudent; maintenance dosing would be expected to fall between the maintenance dose with valproate, which decreases the apparent clearance of lamotrigine, and the maintenance dose without valproate, but with carbamazepine, phenytoin, phenobarbital, or primidone, which increases the apparent clearance of lamotrigine.

LAMOTRIGINE — ORAL

Lamotrigine Added to an AED Regimen Containing Valproate in Patients Older Than 12 Years of Age	
Weeks 1 and 2	25 mg every other day
Weeks 3 and 4	25 mg every day
Usual maintenance dosage: 100 to 400 mg/day (1 or 2 divided doses). To achieve maintenance, dosages may be increased by 25 to 50 mg/day every 1 to 2 weeks. The usual maintenance dosage in patients adding lamotrigine to valproate alone ranges from 100 to 200 mg/day.	

Lamotrigine Added to Carbamazepine, Phenytoin, Phenobarbital, or Primidone[a] (Without Valproate) in Patients Older Than 12 Years of Age	
Weeks 1 and 2	50 mg/day
Weeks 3 and 4	100 mg/day in 2 divided doses
Usual maintenance dosage: 300 to 500 mg/day (in 2 divided doses). To achieve maintenance, dosages may be increased by 100 mg/day every 1 to 2 weeks.	

Conversion from adjunctive therapy with carbamazepine, phenytoin, phenobarbital, primidone, or valproate as the single AED to monotherapy with lamotrigine in patients 16 years of age and older with epilepsy – The goal of the transition regimen is to effect the conversion to monotherapy with lamotrigine under conditions that ensure adequate seizure control while mitigating the risk of serious rash associated with the rapid titration of lamotrigine.

The recommended maintenance dosage of lamotrigine as monotherapy is 500 mg/day given in 2 divided doses.

To avoid an increased risk of rash, the recommended initial dose and subsequent dose escalations of lamotrigine should not be exceeded.

Conversion from adjunctive therapy with carbamazepine, phenytoin, phenobarbital, or primidone to monotherapy with lamotrigine – After achieving a dosage of 500 mg/day of lamotrigine according to the guidelines in the previous table, the concomitant AED should be withdrawn by 20% decrements each week over a 4-week period. The regimen for the withdrawal of the concomitant AED is based on experience gained in the controlled monotherapy clinical trial.

Conversion from adjunctive therapy with valproate to monotherapy with lamotrigine – The conversion regimen involves 4 steps. First, achieve a dosage of 200 mg/day of lamotrigine according the guidelines in the "Lamotrigine Added to an AED Regimen Containing Valproate in Patients Older Than 12 Years of Age" table. Second, while keeping the lamotrigine dosage at 200 mg/day, valproate should be gradually decreased to a dosage of 500 mg/day by decrements no greater than 500 mg/day per week. This dosage regimen is then maintained for 1 week. Third, lamotrigine should then be increased to 300 mg/day while valproate is simultaneously decreased to 250 mg/day. This regimen should be maintained for 1 week. Fourth, valproate should then be discontinued completely and lamotrigine increased by 100 mg/day every week until the recommended monotherapy dosage of 500 mg/day is reached (see the following table).

Conversion from Adjunctive Therapy with Valproate to Monotherapy with Lamotrigine in Patients 16 Years of Age and Older

	Lamotrigine	Valproate
Step 1	Achieve a dosage of 200 mg/day according to guidelines in the "Lamotrigine Added to an AED Regimen Containing Valproate in Patients Older Than 12 Years of Age" table (if not already on 200 mg/day).	Maintain previous stable dose.
Step 2	Maintain at 200 mg/day	Decrease to 500 mg/day by decrements no greater than 500 mg/day per week and then maintain the dose of 500 mg/day for 1 week
Step 3	Increase to 300 mg/day and maintain for 1 week	Simultaneously decrease to 250 mg/day and maintain for 1 week
Step 4	Increase by 100 mg/day every week to achieve maintenance dose of 500 mg/day	Discontinue

Conversion from adjunctive therapy with AEDs other than carbamazepine, phenytoin, phenobarbital, primidone, or valproate to monotherapy with lamotrigine – No specific dosing guidelines can be provided for conversion to monotherapy with lamotrigine with AEDs other than carbamazepine, phenobarbital, phenytoin, primidone, or valproate.

Usual maintenance dosage for epilepsy – The usual maintenance dosages identified are derived from dosing regimens employed in the placebo-controlled adjunctive studies in which the efficacy of lamotrigine was established. In patients receiving multidrug regimens employing carbamazepine, phenytoin, phenobarbital, or primidone without valproate, maintenance dosages of adjunctive lamotrigine as high as 700 mg/day have been used. In patients receiving valproate alone, maintenance dosages of adjunctive lamotrigine as high as 200 mg/day have been used. The advantage of using dosages above those recommended has not been established in controlled trials.

➤*Target plasma levels for patients with epilepsy:* A therapeutic plasma concentration range has not been established for lamotrigine. Dosing of lamotrigine should be based on therapeutic response.

➤*Discontinuation strategy for patients with epilepsy:* For patients receiving lamotrigine in combination with other AEDs, a reevaluation of all AEDs in the regimen should be considered if a change in seizure control or an appearance or worsening of adverse reactions is observed.

If a decision is made to discontinue therapy with lamotrigine, a step-wise reduction of dose over at least 2 weeks (approximately 50% per week) is recommended unless safety concerns require a more rapid withdrawal.

Discontinuing carbamazepine, phenytoin, phenobarbital, or primidone should prolong the half-life of lamotrigine; discontinuing valproate should shorten the half-life of lamotrigine.

➤*Bipolar disorder:* The goal of maintenance treatment with lamotrigine is to delay the time to occurrence of mood episodes (depression, mania, hypomania, mixed episodes) in patients treated for acute mood episodes with standard therapy. The target dosage of lamotrigine is 200 mg/day (100 mg/day in patients taking valproate, which decreases the apparent clearance of lamotrigine, and 400 mg/day in patients not taking valproate and taking either carbamazepine, phenytoin, phenobarbital, primidone, or rifampin, which increase the apparent clearance of lamotrigine). In the clinical trials, dosages up to 400 mg/day as monotherapy were evaluated; however, no additional benefit was seen at 400 mg/day compared with 200 mg/day. Accordingly, dosages above 200 mg/day are not recommended. Treatment with lamotrigine is introduced, based on concurrent medications, according to the regimen outlined in the following table. If other psychotropic medications are withdrawn following stabilization, the dose of lamotrigine should be adjusted. For patients discontinuing valproate, the dose of lamotrigine should be doubled over a 2-week period in equal weekly increments (see table: Adjustments to Lamotrigine Dosing for Patients with Bipolar Disorder Following Discontinuation of Psychotropic Medications). For patients discontinuing carbamazepine, phenytoin, phenobarbital, primidone, or rifampin, the dose of lamotrigine should remain constant for the first week and then should be decreased by half over a 2-week period in equal weekly decrements (see table: Adjustments to Lamotrigine Dosing for Patients with Bipolar Disorder Following Discontinuation of Psychotropic Medications). The dose of lamotrigine may then be further adjusted to the target dose (200 mg) as clinically indicated.

If other drugs are subsequently introduced, the dose of lamotrigine may need to be adjusted. In particular, the introduction of valproate requires reduction in the dose of lamotrigine.

To avoid an increased risk of rash, the recommended initial dose and subsequent dose escalations of lamotrigine should not be exceeded.

Escalation Regimen for Lamotrigine for Patients with Bipolar Disorder[a]

	For patients not taking carbamazepine, phenytoin, phenobarbital, primidone, or rifampin[b] and not taking valproate[c]	For patients taking valproate	For patients taking carbamazepine, phenytoin, phenobarbital, primidone, or rifampin[b] and not taking valproate[c]
Weeks 1 and 2	25 mg/day	25 mg every other day	50 mg/day
Weeks 3 and 4	50 mg/day	25 mg/day	100 mg/day in divided doses
Week 5	100 mg/day	50 mg/day	200 mg/day in divided doses
Week 6	200 mg/day	100 mg/day	300 mg/day in divided doses
Week 7	200 mg/day	100 mg/day	Up to 400 mg/day in divided doses

[a] See Drug Interactions for a description of known drug interactions.
[b] Carbamazepine, phenytoin, phenobarbital, primidone, and rifampin have been shown to increase the apparent clearance of lamotrigine.
[c] Valproate has been shown to decrease the apparent clearance of lamotrigine.

Adjustments to Lamotrigine Dosing for Patients with Bipolar Disorder Following Discontinuation of Psychotropic Medications[a]

	Discontinuation of psychotropic drugs (excluding valproate, carbamazepine, phenytoin, phenobarbital, primidone, rifampin[b], or valproate[c])	After discontinuation of valproate[c]	After discontinuation of carbamazepine, phenytoin, phenobarbital, primidone, or rifampin[b]
		Current lamotrigine dosage 100 mg/day	Current lamotrigine dosage 400 mg/day
Week 1	Maintain current lamotrigine dosage	150 mg/day	400 mg/day

LAMOTRIGINE — ORAL

Adjustments to Lamotrigine Dosing for Patients with Bipolar Disorder Following Discontinuation of Psychotropic Medications[a]			
	Discontinuation of psychotropic drugs (excluding valproate, carbamazepine, phenytoin, phenobarbital, primidone, rifampin[b], or valproate[c])	After discontinuation of valproate[c]	After discontinuation of carbamazepine, phenytoin, phenobarbital, primidone, or rifampin[b]
		Current lamotrigine dosage 100 mg/day	Current lamotrigine dosage 400 mg/day
Week 2	Maintain current lamotrigine dosage	200 mg/day	300 mg/day
Week 3 onward	Maintain current lamotrigine dosage	200 mg/day	200 mg/day

[a] See Drug Interactions for a description of known drug interactions.
[b] Carbamazepine, phenytoin, phenobarbital, primidone, and rifampin have been shown to increase the apparent clearance of lamotrigine.
[c] Valproate has been shown to decrease the apparent clearance of lamotrigine.

There is no body of evidence available to answer the question of how long the patient should remain on lamotrigine therapy. Systematic evaluation of the efficacy of lamotrigine in patients with either depression or mania who responded to standard therapy during an acute 8 to 16 week treatment phase and were then randomized to lamotrigine or placebo for up to 76 weeks of observation for affective relapse demonstrated a benefit of such maintenance treatment. Nevertheless, patients should be periodically reassessed to determine the need for maintenance treatment.

Discontinuation strategy in bipolar disorder – As with other AEDs, lamotrigine should not be abruptly discontinued. In the controlled clinical trials, there was no increase in the incidence, type, or severity of adverse reactions following abrupt termination of lamotrigine. In clinical trials in patients with bipolar disorder, 2 patients experienced seizures shortly after abrupt withdrawal of lamotrigine. However, there were confounding factors that may have contributed to the occurrence of seizures in these bipolar patients. Discontinuation of lamotrigine should involve a step-wise reduction of dose over at least 2 weeks (approximately 50% per week) unless safety concerns require a more rapid withdrawal.

➤*Coadministration with oral contraceptives:*

Starting lamotrigine in women taking oral contraceptives – Although oral contraceptives have been shown to increase the clearance of lamotrigine, no adjustments to the recommended dose escalation guidelines for lamotrigine should be necessary solely based on the use of oral contraceptives. Therefore, dose escalation should follow the recommended guidelines based on whether lamotrigine is added to valproate, lamotrigine is added to carbamazepine, phenytoin, phenobarbital, primidone, or rifampin, or lamotrigine is added in the absence of valproate, carbamazepine, phenytoin, phenobarbital, primidone, or rifampin.

➤*Adjustments to the maintenance dose of lamotrigine:*

Taking or starting oral contraceptives – For women not taking carbamazepine, phenytoin, phenobarbital, primidone, or rifampin, the maintenance dose of lamotrigine may need to be increased by as much as 2 fold over the recommended target maintenance dose, according to clinical response. For women taking lamotrigine in addition to carbamazepine, phenytoin, phenobarbital, primidone, or rifampin, no adjustment should be necessary.

Stopping oral contraceptives – For women not taking carbamazepine, phenytoin, phenobarbital, primidone, or rifampin, the maintenance dose of lamotrigine may need to be decreased by as much as 50% of the maintenance dose with concurrent oral contraceptives, according to clinical response. For women taking lamotrigine in addition to carbamazepine, phenytoin, phenobarbital, primidone or rifampin, no adjustment should be necessary.

➤*Coadministration with other hormonal contraceptive preparations or hormone replacement therapy:* Although the effect of other hormonal contraceptive preparations or hormone replacement therapy on the pharmacokinetics of lamotrigine has not been evaluated, the effect may be similar to oral contraceptives. Therefore, similar adjustments to the dosage of lamotrigine may be needed, based on clinical response.

➤*Special populations:*

Renal function impairment – Initial doses of lamotrigine should be based on patients' AED regimen; reduced maintenance doses may be effective for patients with significant renal functional impairment. Few patients with severe renal impairment have been evaluated during chronic treatment with lamotrigine. Because there is inadequate experience in this population, lamotrigine should be used with caution in these patients.

Hepatic function impairment – Experience in patients with hepatic impairment is limited. Based on a clinical pharmacology study in 24 patients with moderate to severe liver dysfunction, the following general recommendations can be made. Initial, escalation, and maintenance doses should generally be reduced by approximately 50% in patients with moderate (Child-Pugh grade B) and 75% in patients with severe (Child-Pugh grade C) hepatic impairment. Escalation and maintenance doses should be adjusted according to clinical response.

➤*Administration of lamotrigine chewable dispersible tablets:* Lamotrigine chewable dispersible tablets may be swallowed whole, chewed, or dispersed in water or diluted fruit juice. If the tablets are chewed, consume a small amount of water or diluted fruit juice to aid in swallowing.

To disperse lamotrigine chewable dispersible tablets, add the tablets to a small amount of liquid (5 mL, or enough to cover the medication). Approximately 1 minute later, when the tablets are completely dispersed, swirl the solution and consume the entire quantity immediately. No attempt should be made to administer partial quantities of the dispersed tablets.

➤*Storage/Stability:* Store at 25°C (77°F) in a dry place; excursions permitted to 15° to 30°C (59° to 86°F).

Actions

➤*Pharmacology:* The precise mechanism(s) by which lamotrigine exerts its anticonvulsant action are unknown. In animal models designed to detect anticonvulsant activity, lamotrigine was effective in preventing seizure spread in the maximum electroshock (MES) and pentylenetetrazol (scMet) tests, and prevented seizures in the visually and electrically evoked after-discharge (EEAD) tests for antiepileptic activity. The relevance of these models to human epilepsy, however, is not known.

One proposed mechanism of action of lamotrigine, the relevance of which remains to be established in humans, involves an effect on sodium channels. In vitro pharmacological studies suggest that lamotrigine inhibits voltage-sensitive sodium channels, thereby stabilizing neuronal membranes and consequently modulating presynaptic transmitter release of excitatory amino acids (eg, glutamate, aspartate).

Lamotrigine also displayed inhibitory properties in the kindling model in rats both during kindling development and in the fully kindled state. The relevance of this animal model to specific types of human epilepsy is unclear.

➤*Pharmacokinetics:*

Absorption – Lamotrigine is rapidly and completely absorbed after oral administration with negligible first-pass metabolism (absolute bioavailability, 98%). The bioavailability is not affected by food. Peak plasma concentrations occur anywhere from 1.4 to 4.8 hours following drug administration. Lamotrigine chewable/dispersible tablets were found to be equivalent, whether they were administered as dispersed in water, chewed and swallowed, or swallowed as whole, to lamotrigine compressed tablets in terms of rate and extent of absorption.

Distribution – Estimates of the mean apparent volume of distribution (Vd/F) of lamotrigine following oral administration ranged from 0.9 to 1.3 L/kg. Vd/F is independent of dose and is similar following single and multiple doses in both patients with epilepsy and in healthy volunteers.

Data from in vitro studies indicate that lamotrigine is approximately 55% bound to human plasma proteins at plasma lamotrigine concentrations from 1 to 10 mcg/mL (10 mcg/mL is 4 to 6 times the trough plasma concentration observed in the controlled efficacy trials). Because lamotrigine is not highly bound to plasma proteins, clinically significant interactions with other drugs through competition for protein binding sites are unlikely. The binding of lamotrigine to plasma proteins did not change in the presence of therapeutic concentrations of phenytoin, phenobarbital, or valproate. Lamotrigine did not displace other AEDs (carbamazepine, phenytoin, phenobarbital) from protein binding sites.

Metabolism/Excretion – Lamotrigine is metabolized predominantly by glucuronic acid conjugation; the major metabolite is an inactive 2-N-glucuronide conjugate. After oral administration of 240 mg of ^{14}C-lamotrigine (15 mcCi) to 6 healthy volunteers, 94% was recovered in the urine and 2% was recovered in the feces. The radioactivity in the urine consisted of unchanged lamotrigine (10%), the 2-N-glucuronide (76%), a 5-N-glucuronide (10%), a 2-N-methyl metabolite (0.14%), and other unidentified minor metabolites (4%).

Enzyme induction: Following multiple administrations (150 mg twice daily) to healthy volunteers taking no other medications, lamotrigine induced its own metabolism, resulting in a 25% decrease in $t_{½}$ and a 37% increase in apparent plasma clearance (Cl/F) at steady state compared with values obtained in the same volunteers following a single dose. Evidence gathered from other sources suggests that self-induction by lamotrigine may not occur when lamotrigine is given as adjunctive therapy in patients receiving carbamazepine, phenytoin, phenobarbital, primidone, or rifampin.

The pharmacokinetics of lamotrigine have been studied in patients with epilepsy, healthy young and elderly volunteers, and volunteers with chronic renal failure. Lamotrigine pharmacokinetic parameters for adult and pediatric patients and healthy volunteers are summarized in the following tables.

Mean[a] Lamotrigine Pharmacokinetic Parameters in Healthy Volunteers and Adult Patients with Epilepsy				
Adult study population	Number of subjects	T_{max} (h)	$t_{½}$ (h)	Cl/F (mL/min/kg)
Healthy volunteers taking no other medications:				
Single-dose lamotrigine	179	2.2 (0.25 to 12)	32.8 (14 to 103)	0.44 (0.12 to 1.1)
Multiple-dose lamotrigine	36	1.7 (0.5 to 4)	25.4 (11.6 to 61.6)	0.58 (0.24 to 1.15)
Healthy volunteers taking valproate:				
Single-dose lamotrigine	6	1.8 (1 to 4)	48.3 (31.5 to 88.6)	0.3 (0.14 to 0.42)
Multiple-dose lamotrigine	18	1.9 (0.5 to 3.5)	70.3 (41.9 to 113.5)	0.18 (0.12 to 0.33)
Patients with epilepsy taking valproate only:				
Single-dose lamotrigine	4	4.8 (1.8 to 8.4)	58.8 (30.5 to 88.8)	0.28 (0.16 to 0.4)
Patients with epilepsy taking EIAEDs[b] plus valproate:				
Single-dose lamotrigine	25	3.8 (1 to 10)	27.2 (11.2 to 51.6)	0.53 (0.27 to 1.04)
Patients with epilepsy taking EIAEDs[b]:				

LAMOTRIGINE — ORAL

Mean[a] Lamotrigine Pharmacokinetic Parameters in Healthy Volunteers and Adult Patients with Epilepsy				
Adult study population	Number of subjects	T_{max} (h)	t½ (h)	Cl/F (mL/min/kg)
Single-dose lamotrigine	24	2.3 (0.5 to 5)	14.4 (6.4 to 30.4)	1.1 (0.51 to 2.22)
Multiple-dose lamotrigine	17	2 (0.75 to 5.93)	12.6 (7.5 to 23.1)	1.21 (0.66 to 1.82)

[a] The majority of the parameter means determined in each study had coefficients of variation between 20% and 40% for half-life and Cl/F and between 30% and 70% for T_{max}. The overall mean values were calculated from individual study means that were weighted based on the number of volunteers/patients in each study. The number in parentheses after each parameter mean represent the range of individual volunteer/patient values across studies.
[b] Carbamazepine, phenobarbital, phenytoin, and primidone have been shown to increase the apparent clearance of lamotrigine. Oral contraceptives and rifampin have also been shown to increase the apparent clearance of lamotrigine.

Special populations –
Renal function impairment: Twelve volunteers with chronic renal failure (mean creatinine clearance, 13 mL/min; range, 6 to 23) and another 6 individuals undergoing hemodialysis were each given a single 100 mg dose of lamotrigine. The mean plasma half-lives determined in the study were 42.9 hours (chronic renal failure), 13 hours (during hemodialysis), and 57.4 hours (between hemodialysis) compared with 26.2 hours in healthy volunteers. On average, approximately 20% (range, 5.6 to 35.1) of the amount of lamotrigine present in the body was eliminated by hemodialysis during a 4-hour session.

Hepatic function impairment: The pharmacokinetics of lamotrigine following a single 100 mg dose of lamotrigine were evaluated in 24 subjects with moderate to severe hepatic dysfunction and compared with 12 subjects without hepatic impairment. The median apparent clearance of lamotrigine was 0.31, 0.24, or 0.1 mL/kg/min in patients with grade A, B, or C (Child-Pugh classification) hepatic impairment, respectively, compared with 0.34 mL/kg/min in the healthy controls. Median half-life of lamotrigine was 36, 60, or 110 hours in patients with grade A, B, or C hepatic impairment, respectively, versus 32 hours in healthy controls.

Elderly: The pharmacokinetics of lamotrigine following a single 150 mg of lamotrigine were evaluated in 12 elderly volunteers between the ages of 65 and 76 years (mean creatinine clearance, 61 mL/min; range, 33 to 108). The mean half-life of lamotrigine in these subjects was 31.2 hours (range, 24.5 to 43.4 hours) and the mean clearance was 0.4 mL/min/kg (range, 0.26 to 0.48 mL/min/kg).

Children: Population pharmacokinetic analyses involving patients 2 to 18 years of age demonstrated that lamotrigine clearance was influenced predominantly by total body weight and concurrent AED therapy. The oral clearance of lamotrigine was higher, on a body weight basis, in pediatric patients than in adults. Weight-normalized lamotrigine clearance was higher in those subjects weighing less than 30 kg, compared with those weighing greater than 30 kg. Accordingly, patients weighing less than 30 kg may need an increase of as much as 50% in maintenance doses, based on clinical response, as compared with subjects weighing more than 30 kg being administered the same AEDs. These analyses also revealed that, after accounting for body weight, lamotrigine clearance was not significantly influenced by age. Thus, the same weight-adjusted doses should be administered to children irrespective of differences in age. Concomitant AEDs which influence lamotrigine clearance in adults were found to have similar effects in children.

Mean Lamotrigine Pharmacokinetic Parameters in Children with Epilepsy				
Pediatric study population	Number of subjects	T_{max} (h)	t½ (h)	Cl/F (mL/min/kg)
10 months to 5.3 years of age:				
Patients taking EIAEDs[a]	10	3 (1 to 5.9)	7.7 (5.7 to 11.4)	3.62 (2.44 to 5.28)
Patients taking AEDs with no known effect on the apparent clearance of lamotrigine	7	5.2 (2.9 to 6.1)	19 (12.9 to 27.1)	1.2 (0.75 to 2.42)
Patients taking valproate only	8	2.9 (1 to 6)	44.9 (29.5 to 52.5)	0.47 (0.23 to 0.77)
5 to 11 years of age:				
Patients taking EIAEDs[a]	7	1.6 (1 to 3)	7 (3.8 to 9.8)	2.54 (1.35 to 5.58)
Patients taking EIAEDs[a] plus valproate	8	3.3 (1 to 6.4)	19.1 (7 to 31.2)	0.89 (0.39 to 1.93)
Patients taking valproate only[b]	3	4.5 (3 to 6)	65.8 (50.7 to 73.7)	0.24 (0.21 to 0.26)
13 to 18 years of age:				
Patients taking EIAEDs[a]	11	[c]	[c]	1.3
Patients taking EIAEDs[a] plus valproate	8	[c]	[c]	0.5
Patients taking valproate only	4	[c]	[c]	0.3

[a] Carbamazepine, phenobarbital, phenytoin, and primidone have been shown to increase the apparent clearance of lamotrigine. Oral contraceptives and rifampin have also been shown to increase the apparent clearance of lamotrigine.
[b] Two subjects were included in the calculation for mean T_{max}.
[c] Parameter not estimated.

Gender: The clearance of lamotrigine is not affected by gender. However, during dose escalation of lamotrigine in one clinical trial in patients with epilepsy on a stable dose of valproate (N = 77), mean trough lamotrigine concentrations, unadjusted for weight, were 24% to 45% higher (0.3 to 1.7 mcg/mL) in women than in men.

Race: The apparent oral clearance of lamotrigine was 25% lower in non-white patients than white patients.

Contraindications

Hypersensitivity to the drug or its ingredients.

Warnings

➤*Serious rash:* See the Warning box.

Children – The incidence of serious rash associated with hospitalization and discontinuation of lamotrigine in a prospectively followed cohort of pediatric patients with epilepsy was approximately 0.8% (16 of 1,983). When these 14 cases were reviewed by 3 expert dermatologists, there was considerable disagreement as to their proper classification. To illustrate, 1 dermatologist considered none of the cases to be Stevens-Johnson syndrome; another assigned 7 of the 14 to this diagnosis. There was 1 rash-related death in this 1,983 patient cohort. Additionally, there have been rare cases of toxic epidermal necrolysis with and without permanent sequelae or death in US and foreign postmarketing experience. It bears emphasis, accordingly, that lamotrigine is only approved for use in those patients younger than 16 years of age who have partial seizures or generalized seizures associated with the Lennox-Gastaut syndrome.

There is evidence that the inclusion of valproate in a multidrug regimen increases the risk of serious, potentially life-threatening rash in pediatric patients. In pediatric patients who used valproate concomitantly, 1.2% (6 of 482) experienced a serious rash, compared with 0.6% (6 of 952) patients not taking valproate.

Adults – Serious rash associated with hospitalization and discontinuation of lamotrigine occurred in 0.3% (11 of 3,348) of adult patients who received lamotrigine in premarketing clinical trials of epilepsy. In the bipolar and other mood disorders clinical trials, the rate of serious rash was 0.08% (1 of 1,233) of adult patients who received lamotrigine as initial monotherapy and 0.13% (2 of 1,538) of adult patients who received lamotrigine as adjunctive therapy. No fatalities occurred among these individuals. However, in worldwide postmarketing experience, rare cases of rash-related death have been reported, but their numbers are too few to permit a precise estimate of the rate.

Among the rashes leading to hospitalization were Stevens-Johnson syndrome, toxic epidermal necrolysis, angioedema, and a rash associated with a variable number of the following systemic manifestations: fever, lymphadenopathy, facial swelling, hematologic, and hepatologic abnormalities.

There is evidence that the inclusion of valproate in a multidrug regimen increases the risk of serious, potentially life-threatening rash in adults. Specifically, of 584 patients administered lamotrigine with valproate in clinical trials, 6 (1%) were hospitalized in association with rash; in contrast, 4 (0.16%) of 2,398 clinical trial patients and volunteers administered lamotrigine in the absence of valproate were hospitalized.

Other examples of serious and potentially life-threatening rash that did not lead to hospitalization also occurred in premarketing development. Among these, 1 case was reported to be Stevens-Johnson-like.

See the Warning box.

➤*Acute multiorgan failure:* Multiorgan failure, which in some cases has been fatal or irreversible, has been observed in patients receiving lamotrigine. Fatalities associated with multiorgan failure and various degrees of hepatic failure have been reported in 2 of 3,796 adult patients and 4 of 2,435 pediatric patients who received lamotrigine in clinical trials. No such fatalities have been reported in bipolar patients in clinical trials. Rare fatalities from multiorgan failure have also been reported in compassionate plea and postmarketing use. The majority of these deaths occurred in association with other serious medical events, including status epilepticus and overwhelming sepsis, and hantavirus, making it difficult to identify the initial cause.

Additionally, 3 patients (a 45-year-old woman, a 3 ½-year-old boy, and an 11-year-old girl) developed multiorgan dysfunction and disseminated intravascular coagulation 9 to 14 days after lamotrigine was added to their AED regimens. Rash and elevated transaminases were also present in all patients and rhabdomyolysis was noted in 2 patients. Both pediatric patients were receiving concomitant therapy with valproate, while the adult patient was being treated with carbamazepine and clonazepam. All patients subsequently recovered with supportive care after treatment with lamotrigine was discontinued.

➤*Blood dycrasias:* There have been reports of blood dyscrasias that may or may not be associated with the hypersensitivity syndrome. These have included neutropenia, leukopenia, anemia, thrombocytopenia, pancytopenia, and, rarely, aplastic anemia and pure red cell aplasia.

LAMOTRIGINE — ORAL

➤*Withdrawal seizures:* As with other AEDs, lamotrigine should not be abruptly discontinued. In patients with epilepsy, there is a possibility of increasing seizure frequency. In clinical trials in patients with bipolar disorder, 2 patients experienced seizures shortly after abrupt withdrawal of lamotrigine. However, there were confounding factors that may have contributed to the occurrence of seizures in these bipolar patients. Unless safety concerns require a more rapid withdrawal, taper the dose of lamotrigine over a period of at least 2 weeks.

➤*Hypersensitivity reactions:* Hypersensitivity reactions, some fatal or life threatening, have also occurred. Some of these reactions have included clinical features of multiorgan failure/dysfunction, including hepatic abnormalities and evidence of disseminated intravascular coagulation. It is important to note that early manifestations of hypersensitivity (eg, fever, lymphadenopathy) may be present even though a rash is not evident. If such signs or symptoms are present, evaluate the patient immediately. Discontinue lamotrigine if an alternative etiology for the signs or symptoms cannot be established.

Prior to initiation of treatment with lamotrigine, instruct the patient that a rash or other signs or symptoms of hypersensitivity (eg, fever, lymphadenopathy) may herald a serious medical event and that the patient should report any such occurrence to a health care provider immediately.

➤*Renal function impairment:* A study in individuals with severe chronic renal failure (mean creatinine clearance, 13 mL/min) not receiving other AEDs indicated that the t½ of unchanged lamotrigine is prolonged relative to individuals with normal renal function. Until adequate numbers of patients with severe renal impairment have been evaluated during chronic treatment with lamotrigine, use lamotrigine with caution in these patients, generally administering a reduced maintenance dose for patients with significant impairment.

➤*Hepatic function impairment:* See Administration and Dosage for more information.

➤*Elderly:* Clinical studies of lamotrigine did not include sufficient numbers of subjects 65 years of age and older to determine whether they respond differently from younger subjects. In general, dose selection for an elderly patient should be cautious, usually starting at the low end of the dosing range, reflecting the greater frequency of decreased hepatic, renal, or cardiac function, and of concomitant disease or other drug therapy.

➤*Pregnancy: Category C.* No evidence of teratogenicity was found in mice, rats, or rabbits when lamotrigine was orally administered to pregnant animals during the period of organogenesis at doses up to 1.2, 0.5, and 1.1 times, respectively, on a mg/m^2 basis, the highest usual human maintenance dosage (ie, 500 mg/day). However, maternal toxicity and secondary fetal toxicity producing reduced fetal weight and/or delayed ossification were seen in mice and rats, but not in rabbits at these doses. Teratology studies were also conducted using bolus intravenous administration of the isethionate salt of lamotrigine in rats and rabbits. In rat dams administered an intravenous dose at 0.6 times the highest usual human maintenance dosage, the incidence of intrauterine death without signs of teratogenicity was increased.

A behavioral teratology study was conducted in rats dosed during the period of organogenesis. At day 21 postpartum, offspring of dams receiving 5 mg/kg/day or higher displayed a significantly longer latent period for open field exploration and a lower frequency of rearing. In a swimming maze test performed on days 39 to 44 postpartum, time to completion was increased in offspring of dams receiving 25 mg/kg/day. These dosages represent 0.1 and 0.5 times the clinical dose on a mg/m^2 basis, respectively.

When pregnant rats were orally dosed at 0.1, 0.14, or 0.3 times the highest human maintenance dosage (on a mg/m^2 basis) during the latter part of gestation (days 15 to 20), maternal toxicity and fetal death were seen. In dams, food consumption and weight gain were reduced, and the gestation period was slightly prolonged (22.6 vs 22 days in the control group). Stillborn pups were found in all 3 drug-treated groups with the highest number in the high-dose group. Postnatal death was also seen, but only in the 2 highest doses, and occurred between day 1 and 20. Some of these deaths appear to be drug-related and not secondary to the maternal toxicity. A no-observed-effect level (NOEL) could not be determined for this study.

Although lamotrigine was not found to be teratogenic in the above studies, lamotrigine decreases fetal folate concentrations in rats, an effect known to be associated with teratogenesis in animals and humans. There are no adequate and well-controlled studies in pregnant women. Because animal reproduction studies are not always predictive of human response, use this drug during pregnancy only if the potential benefit justifies the potential risk to the fetus.

As with other antiepileptic drugs, physiological changes during pregnancy may affect lamotrigine concentrations or therapeutic effect. There have been reports of decreased lamotrigine concentrations during pregnancy and restoration of prepartum concentrations after delivery. Dosage adjustments may be necessary to maintain clinical response.

Pregnancy exposure registry – To facilitate monitoring fetal outcomes of pregnant women exposed to lamotrigine, health care providers are encouraged to register patients, before fetal outcome (eg, ultrasound, results of amniocentesis, birth) is known, and can obtain information by calling the pregnancy registry at 1-800-336-2176 (toll-free). Patients can enroll themselves in the North American Antiepileptic Drug Pregnancy Registry by calling 1-888-233-2334.

➤*Lactation:* Preliminary data indicate that lamotrigine passes into human milk. Because the effects on the infant exposed to lamotrigine by this route are unknown, breast-feeding while taking lamotrigine is not recommended.

➤*Children:* Lamotrigine is indicated as adjunctive therapy for partial seizures in patients older than 2 years of age and for the generalized seizures of Lennox-Gastaut syndrome. Safety and efficacy for other uses in patients with epilepsy younger than 16 years of age have not been established. Safety and efficacy in patients younger than 18 years of age with bipolar disorder have not been established.

Precautions

➤*Monitoring:* The value of monitoring plasma concentrations of lamotrigine has not been established. Because of the possible pharmacokinetic interactions between lamotrigine and other drugs including AEDs, monitoring of the plasma levels of lamotrigine and concomitant drugs may be indicated, particularly during dosage adjustments. In general, exercise clinical judgment regarding monitoring of plasma levels of lamotrigine and other antiseizure drugs and whether or not dosage adjustments are necessary.

➤*Dermatological events:* Serious rashes associated with hospitalization and discontinuation of lamotrigine have been reported. Rare deaths have been reported, but their numbers are too few to permit a precise estimate of the rate. There are suggestions, yet to be proven, that the risk of rash may also be increased by: Coadministration of lamotrigine with valproate; exceeding the recommended initial dose of lamotrigine; exceeding the recommended dose escalation for lamotrigine. However, cases have been reported in the absence of these factors.

In epilepsy clinical trials, approximately 10% of all patients exposed to lamotrigine developed a rash. In the bipolar disorder clinical trials, 14% of patients exposed to lamotrigine developed a rash. Rashes associated with lamotrigine do not appear to have unique identifying features. Typically, rash occurs in the first 2 to 8 weeks following treatment initiation. However, isolated cases have been reported after prolonged treatment (eg, 6 months). Accordingly, duration of therapy cannot be relied upon as a means to predict the potential risk heralded by the first appearance of a rash.

Although most rashes resolved even with continuation of treatment with lamotrigine, it is not possible to predict reliably which rashes will prove to be serious or life threatening. Accordingly, lamotrigine should ordinarily be discontinued at the first sign of rash, unless the rash is clearly not drug related. Discontinuation of treatment may not prevent a rash from becoming life threatening or permanently disabling or disfiguring.

It is recommended that lamotrigine not be restarted in patients who discontinued due to rash associated with prior treatment with lamotrigine unless the potential benefits clearly outweigh the risks. If the decision is made to restart a patient who has discontinued lamotrigine, assess the need to restart with the initial dosing recommendations. The greater the interval of time since the previous dose, the greater consideration should be given to restarting with the initial dosing recommendations. If a patient has discontinued lamotrigine for a period of more than 5 half-lives, it is recommended that initial dosing recommendations and guidelines be followed. The half-life of lamotrigine is affected by other concomitant medications.

➤*Use in patients with epilepsy:*

Sudden unexplained death in epilepsy (SUDEP) – During the premarketing development of lamotrigine, 20 sudden and unexplained deaths were recorded among a cohort of 4,700 patients with epilepsy (5,747 patient-years of exposure).

Some of these could represent seizure-related deaths in which the seizure was not observed (eg, at night). This represents an incidence of 0.0035 deaths per patient-year. Although this rate exceeds that expected in a healthy population matched for age and gender, it is within the range of estimates for the incidence of sudden unexplained deaths in patients with epilepsy not receiving lamotrigine (ranging from 0.0005 for the general population of patients with epilepsy, to 0.004 for a recently studied clinical trial population similar to that in the clinical development program for lamotrigine, to 0.005 for patients with refractory epilepsy). Consequently, whether these figures are reassuring or suggest concern depends on the comparability of the populations reported upon to the cohort receiving lamotrigine and the accuracy of the estimates provided. Probably most reassuring is the similarity of estimated SUDEP rates in patients receiving lamotrigine and those receiving another AED that underwent clinical testing in a similar population at about the same time. Importantly, that drug is chemically unrelated to lamotrigine. This evidence suggests, although it certainly does not prove, that the high SUDEP rates reflect population rates, not a drug effect.

Status epilepticus – Valid estimates of the incidence of treatment emergent status epilepticus among patients treated with lamotrigine are difficult to obtain because reporters participating in clinical trials did not all employ identical rules for identifying cases. At a minimum, 7 of 2,343 adult patients had episodes that could unequivocally be described as status. In addition, a number of reports of variably defined episodes of seizure exacerbation (eg, seizure clusters, seizure flurries) were made.

➤*Use in patients with bipolar disorder:*

Acute treatment of mood episodes – Safety and efficacy of lamotrigine in the acute treatment of mood episodes have not been established.

Suicide – The possibility of a suicide attempt is inherent in bipolar disorder. Accompany drug therapy with close supervision of high-risk patients. Write prescriptions for lamotrigine for the smallest quantity of tablets consistent with good patient management, in order to reduce the risk of overdose. Overdoses have been reported for lamotrigine, some of which have been fatal. Overdose has resulted in ataxia, nystagmus, increased seizures, decreased level of consciousness, coma, and intraventricular conduction delay.

➤*Addition of lamotrigine to a multidrug regimen that includes valproate (dosage reduction):* Because valproate reduces the clearance of lamotrigine, the dosage of lamotrigine in the presence of valproate is less than half of that required in its absence.

LAMOTRIGINE — ORAL

➤*Melanin-containing tissues:* Because lamotrigine binds to melanin, it could accumulate in melanin-rich tissues over time. This raises the possibility that lamotrigine may cause toxicity in these tissues after extended use. Although ophthalmological testing was performed in 1 controlled clinical trial, the testing was inadequate to exclude subtle effects or injury occurring after long-term exposure. Moreover, the capacity of available tests to detect potentially adverse consequences, if any, of lamotrigine's binding to melanin is unknown.

Accordingly, although there are no specific recommendations for periodic ophthalmological monitoring, be aware of the possibility of long-term ophthalmologic effects.

➤*Special risk:* Clinical experience with lamotrigine in patients with concomitant illness is limited. Caution is advised when using lamotrigine in patients with diseases or conditions that could affect metabolism or elimination of the drug, such as renal, hepatic, or cardiac functional impairment. Hepatic metabolism to the glucuronide followed by renal excretion is the principal route of elimination of lamotrigine.

Drug Interactions

➤*Effects of other drugs on the pharmacokinetics of lamotrigine:*
Folate inhibitors – Lamotrigine is an inhibitor of dihydrofolate reductase. Be aware of this action when prescribing other medications that inhibit folate metabolism.

Lamotrigine Drug Interactions

Precipitant drug	Object drug[a]		Description
Acetaminophen	Lamotrigine	⬇	Serum lamotrigine concentrations may be reduced, producing a decrease in therapeutic effects. With chronic administration of acetaminophen, if an interaction is suspected, it may be necessary to adjust the dose of lamotrigine.
Carbamazepine	Lamotrigine	⬇	Lamotrigine concentration is decreased by approximately 40%. Carbamazepine-exposed levels may be increased.
Lamotrigine	Carbamazepine	⬆	
Contraceptives, oral	Lamotrigine	⬇	Coadministration of ethinyl estradiol/levonorgestrel with lamotrigine increased the clearance of lamotrigine by approximately 20-fold. Similar effects may be seen with hormone replacement therapy.
Primidone Phenobarbital	Lamotrigine	⬇	Lamotrigine concentration is decreased approximately 40%.
Phenytoin	Lamotrigine	⬇	Lamotrigine concentration is decreased approximately 40%.
Rifamycins	Lamotrigine	⬇	Lamotrigine plasma levels may be reduced. Adjust the dose of lamotrigine as needed.
Succinimides (eg, ethosuximide)	Lamotrigine	⬇	Lamotrigine serum concentrations may be reduced, decreasing the therapeutic effects. Adjust the dose of lamotrigine as needed.
Valproic acid	Lamotrigine	⬆	The addition of valproic acid increased lamotrigine steady-state concentration more then 2-fold. Trough steady-state valproic acid concentration decreased by approximately 25% when lamotrigine was added in 1 study. Another study showed no change in valproic acid concentrations.
Lamotrigine	Valproic acid	⬇	

[a] ⬆ = Object drug increased. ⬇ = Object drug decreased.

Adverse Reactions

Serious rash – See Warning box.

➤*Adjunctive therapy in adults with epilepsy:* The most commonly observed (greater than or equal to 5%) adverse reactions seen in association with lamotrigine during adjunctive therapy in adults and not seen at an equivalent frequency among placebo-treated patients were dizziness, ataxia, somnolence, headache, diplopia, blurred vision, nausea, vomiting, and rash. Dizziness, diplopia, ataxia, blurred vision, nausea, and vomiting were dose related. Dizziness, diplopia, ataxia, and blurred vision occurred more commonly in patients receiving carbamazepine with lamotrigine than in patients receiving other AEDs with lamotrigine. Clinical data suggest a higher incidence of rash, including serious rash, in patients receiving concomitant valproate than in patients not receiving valproate.

Approximately 11% of the 3,378 adult patients who received lamotrigine as adjunctive therapy in premarketing clinical trials discontinued treatment because of an adverse reaction. The adverse reactions most commonly associated with discontinuation were rash (3%), dizziness (2.8%), and headache (2.5%). In a dose response study in adults, the rate of discontinuation of lamotrigine for dizziness, ataxia, diplopia, blurred vision, nausea, and vomiting was dose related.

Incidence in controlled adjunctive clinical studies in adults with epilepsy –

Lamotrigine Adverse Reactions in Adults[a]

Adverse reaction[b]	Lamotrigine (n = 711)	Placebo (n = 419)
CNS		
Anxiety	4%	3%
Ataxia	22%	6%
Concentration disturbance	2%	1%
Convulsion	3%	1%
Depression	4%	3%
Dizziness	38%	13%
Headache	29%	19%
Incoordination	6%	2%
Insomnia	6%	2%
Irritability	3%	2%
Somnolence	14%	7%
Speech disorder	3%	0%
Tremor	4%	1%
Dermatologic		
Pruritus	3%	2%
Rash	10%	5%
GI		
Abdominal pain	5%	4%
Anorexia	2%	1%
Constipation	4%	3%
Diarrhea	6%	4%
Dyspepsia	5%	2%
Nausea	19%	10%
Tooth disorder	3%	2%
Vomiting	9%	4%
GU		
Female patients only	(n = 365)	(n = 207)
Amenorrhea	2%	1%
Dysmenorrhea	7%	6%
Vaginitis	4%	1%
Musculoskeletal		
Arthralgia	2%	0%
Respiratory		
Increased cough	8%	6%
Pharyngitis	10%	9%
Rhinitis	14%	9%
Special senses		
Blurred vision	16%	5%
Diplopia	28%	7%
Vision abnormality	3%	1%
Miscellaneous		
Fever	6%	4%
Flu syndrome	7%	6%
Neck pain	2%	1%
Reaction aggravated (seizure exacerbation)	2%	1%

[a] Patients in these adjunctive studies were receiving 1 to 3 of the following concomitant AEDs (carbamazepine, phenytoin, phenobarbital, or primidone) in addition to lamotrigine or placebo. Patients may have reported multiple adverse reactions during the study or at discontinuation; thus, patients may be included in more than 1 category.
[b] Adverse reactions reported by at least 2% of patients treated with lamotrigine are included.

In a randomized, parallel study comparing placebo and 300 and 500 mg/day of lamotrigine, some of the more common drug-related adverse reactions were dose related (see the following table).

Lamotrigine Dose-Related Adverse Reactions

Adverse reaction	Placebo (n = 73)	Lamotrigine 300 mg (n = 71)	Lamotrigine 500 mg (n = 72)
Ataxia	10%	10%	28%[ab]
Blurred vision	10%	11%	25%[ab]
Diplopia	8%	24%[a]	49%[ab]
Dizziness	27%	31%	54%[ab]
Nausea	11%	18%	25%[a]
Vomiting	4%	11%	18%[a]

[a] Significantly greater than placebo group ($P < 0.05$).
[b] Significantly greater than group receiving lamotrigine 300 mg ($P < 0.05$).

Other reactions that occurred in more than 1% of patients but equally or more frequently in the placebo group included: asthenia, back pain, chest pain, flatulence, menstrual disorder, myalgia, paresthesia, respiratory disorder, and urinary tract infection.

➤*Monotherapy in adults with epilepsy:* The most commonly observed (greater than or equal to 5%) adverse reactions seen in association with the use of lamotrigine during the monotherapy phase of the controlled trial in adults not seen at an equivalent rate in the control group were vomiting, coordination abnormality, dyspepsia, nausea, dizziness, rhinitis, anxiety, insomnia, infection, pain, weight decrease, chest pain, and dysmenorrhea.

LAMOTRIGINE — ORAL

The most commonly observed (greater than or equal to 5%) adverse reactions associated with the use of lamotrigine during the conversion to monotherapy (add-on) period, not seen at an equivalent frequency among low-dose valproate-treated patients, were dizziness, headache, nausea, asthenia, coordination abnormality, vomiting, rash, somnolence, diplopia, ataxia, accidental injury, tremor, blurred vision, insomnia, nystagmus, diarrhea, lymphadenopathy, pruritus, and sinusitis.

Approximately 10% of the 420 adult patients who received lamotrigine as monotherapy in premarketing clinical trials discontinued treatment because of an adverse reaction. The adverse reactions most commonly associated with discontinuation were rash (4.5%), headache (3.1%), and asthenia (2.4%).

Incidence in a controlled monotherapy trial in adults with partial seizures –

Lamotrigine Adverse Reactions in Adults[a]		
Adverse reaction[b]	Lamotrigine monotherapy[c] (n = 43)	Low-dose valproate[d] monotherapy (n = 44)
CNS		
Anxiety	5%	0%
Coordination abnormality	7%	0%
Dizziness	7%	0%
Insomnia	5%	2%
GI		
Dyspepsia	7%	2%
Nausea	7%	2%
Vomiting	9%	0%
GU		
Women only	(n = 21)	(n = 28)
Dysmenorrhea	5%	0%
Metabolic/Nutritional		
Weight decrease	5%	2%
Respiratory		
Rhinitis	7%	2%
Miscellaneous		
Chest pain	5%	2%
Infection	5%	2%
Pain	5%	0%

[a] Patients in these studies were converted to lamotrigine or valproate monotherapy from adjunctive therapy with carbamazepine or phenytoin. Patients may have reported multiple adverse reactions during the study; thus, patients may be included in more than 1 category.
[b] Adverse reactions reported by at least 5% of patients are included.
[c] Up to 500 mg/day.
[d] 1,000 mg/day.

➤*Adverse reactions that occurred with a frequency of less than 5% and greater than 2% of patients receiving lamotrigine:*

CNS – Amnesia, ataxia, decreased reflexes, depression, hypesthesia, increased reflexes, irritability, libido increase, nystagmus, suicidal ideation.

Dermatologic – Contact dermatitis, dry skin, sweating.

GI – Anorexia, dry mouth, peptic ulcer, rectal hemorrhage.

Metabolic/Nutritional – Peripheral edema.

Respiratory – Bronchitis, dyspnea, epistaxis.

Special senses – Vision abnormality.

Miscellaneous – Asthenia, fever.

Adjunctive therapy in children with epilepsy – The most commonly observed (greater than or equal to 5%) adverse reactions seen in association with the use of lamotrigine as adjunctive treatment in pediatric patients and not seen at an equivalent rate in the control group were infection, rash, vomiting, fever, somnolence, bronchitis, accidental injury, dizziness, diarrhea, abdominal pain, nausea, ataxia, tremor, asthenia, diplopia, and flu syndrome.

In 339 patients 2 to 16 years of age, 4.2% of patients on lamotrigine and 2.9% of patients on placebo discontinued due to adverse reactions. The most commonly reported adverse reactions that led to discontinuation were rash for patients treated with lamotrigine and deterioration of seizure control for patients treated with placebo.

Approximately 11.5% of the 1,081 pediatric patients who received lamotrigine as adjunctive therapy in premarketing clinical trials discontinued treatment because of an adverse reaction. The adverse reactions most commonly associated with discontinuation were rash (4.4%), reaction aggravated (1.7%), and ataxia (0.6%).

➤*Incidence in a controlled adjunctive trial in children with epilepsy:*

Lamotrigine Adverse Reactions in Children		
Adverse reaction	Lamotrigine (n = 168)	Placebo (n = 171)
Cardiovascular		
Hemorrhage	2%	1%
CNS		
Ataxia	11%	3%
Convulsions	2%	1%
Dizziness	14%	4%
Emotional lability	4%	2%
Gait abnormality	4%	2%
Nervousness	2%	1%
Somnolence	17%	15%
Thinking abnormality	3%	2%
Tremor	10%	1%
Vertigo	2%	1%
Dermatologic		
Eczema	2%	1%
Pruritus	2%	1%
Rash	14%	12%
GI		
Abdominal pain	10%	5%
Constipation	4%	2%
Diarrhea	11%	9%
Dyspepsia	2%	1%
Nausea	10%	2%
Tooth disorder	2%	1%
Vomiting	20%	16%
GU		
Penis disorder (men only)	2% (n = 93)	0% (n = 92)
Urinary tract infection	3%	0%
Hematologic/Lymphatic		
Lymphadenopathy	2%	1%
Metabolic		
Edema	2%	0%
Respiratory		
Bronchitis	7%	5%
Bronchospasm	2%	1%
Increased cough	7%	6%
Pharyngitis	14%	11%
Sinusitis	2%	1%
Special senses		
Blurred vision	4%	1%
Diplopia	5%	1%
Ear disorder	2%	1%
Visual abnormality	2%	0%
Miscellaneous		
Accidental injury	14%	12%
Asthenia	8%	4%
Facial edema	2%	1%
Fever	15%	14%
Flu syndrome	7%	6%
Infection	20%	17%
Pain	5%	4%
Photosensitivity	2%	0%

➤*Bipolar disorder:* The most commonly observed (greater than or equal to 5%) adverse reactions seen in association with the use of lamotrigine as monotherapy (100 to 400 mg/day) in bipolar disorder in the 2 double-blind, placebo-controlled trials of 18 months' duration, and numerically more frequent than in placebo-treated patients are included in the following table. Adverse reactions that occurred in at least 5% of patients and were numerically more common during the dose escalation phase of lamotrigine in these trials (when patients may have been receiving concomitant medications) compared with the monotherapy phase were headache (25%), rash (11%), dizziness (10%), diarrhea (8%), dream abnormality (6%), and pruritus (6%).

During the monotherapy phase of the double-blind, placebo-controlled trials of 18 months' duration, 13% of 227 patients who received lamotrigine (100 to 400 mg/day), 16% of 190 patients who received placebo, and 23% of 166 patients who received lithium discontinued therapy because of an adverse reaction. The adverse reactions which most commonly led to discontinuation of lamotrigine were rash (3%) and mania/hypomania/mixed mood adverse reactions (2%). Approximately 16% of 2,401 patients who received lamotrigine (50 to 500 mg/day) for bipolar disorder in premarketing trials discontinued therapy because of an adverse reaction; most commonly due to rash (5%) and mania/hypomania/mixed mood adverse reactions (2%).

➤*Incidence in controlled clinical studies of lamotrigine for the maintenance treatment of bipolar I disorder:*

LAMOTRIGINE — ORAL

Lamotrigine Adverse Reactions in Adults[a]		
Adverse reaction[b]	Lamotrigine (n = 227)	Placebo (n = 190)
CNS		
Insomnia	10%	6%
Somnolence	9%	7%
Xerostomia (dry mouth)	6%	4%
Dermatologic		
Rash (nonserious)[c]	7%	5%
GI		
Abdominal pain	6%	3%
Constipation	5%	2%
Nausea	14%	11%
Vomiting	5%	2%
Respiratory		
Exacerbation of cough	5%	3%
Pharyngitis	5%	4%
Rhinitis	7%	4%
Miscellaneous		
Back pain	8%	6%
Fatigue	8%	5%

[a] Patients in these studies were converted to lamotrigine (100 to 400 mg/day) or placebo monotherapy from add-on therapy with other psychotropic medications. Patients may have reported multiple adverse reactions during the study; thus, patients may be included in more than 1 category.
[b] Adverse reactions reported by at least 5% of patients are included.
[c] In the overall bipolar and other mood disorders clinical trials, the rate of serious rash was 0.08% (1 of 1,233) of adult patients who received lamotrigine as initial monotherapy and 0.13% (2 of 1,538) of adult patients who received lamotrigine as adjunctive therapy.

These adverse reactions were usually mild to moderate in intensity.

Other reactions that occurred in 5% or more patients but equally or more frequently in the placebo group included dizziness, mania, headache, infection, influenza, pain, accidental injury, diarrhea, and dyspepsia.

➤*Adverse reactions that occurred with a frequency of less than 5% and greater than 1% of patients receiving lamotrigine:*
Cardiovascular – Migraine.

CNS – Abnormal thoughts, agitation, amnesia, depression, dream abnormality, dyspraxia, emotional lability, hypoesthesia.

GI – Flatulence.

GU – Urinary frequency.

Metabolic/Nutritional – Edema, weight gain.

Musculoskeletal – Arthralgia, myalgia.

Respiratory – Sinusitis.

Miscellaneous – Fever, neck pain.

➤*Adverse reactions following abrupt discontinuation:* In the 2 maintenance trials, there was no increase in the incidence, severity, or type of adverse reactions in bipolar disorder patients after abruptly terminating lamotrigine therapy. In clinical trials in patients with bipolar disorder, 2 patients experienced seizures shortly after abrupt withdrawal of lamotrigine. However, there were confounding factors that may have contributed to the occurrence of seizures in these bipolar patients. Discontinuation of lamotrigine should involve a step-wise reduction of dose over at least 2 weeks (approximately 50% per week) unless safety concerns require a more rapid withdrawal.

➤*Mania/Hypomania/Mixed episodes:* During the double-blind, placebo-controlled clinical trials in bipolar I disorder in which patients were converted to lamotrigine monotherapy (100 to 400 mg/day) from other psychotropic medications and followed for durations up to 18 months, the rate of manic or hypomanic or mixed mood episodes reported as adverse reactions was 5% for patients treated with lamotrigine (n = 227), 4% for patients treated with lithium (n = 166), and 7% for patients treated with placebo (n = 190). In all bipolar controlled trials combined, adverse reactions of mania (including hypomania and mixed mood episodes) were reported in 5% of patients treated with lamotrigine (n = 956), 3% of patients treated with lithium (n = 280), and 4% of patients treated with placebo (n = 803).

➤*Other adverse reactions observed during all clinical trials for adult and children with epilepsy or bipolar disorder and other mood disorders:*
Cardiovascular – Flushing, hot flashes, hypertension, palpitations, postural hypotension, syncope, tachycardia, and vasodilation (0.1% to 1%). Angina pectoris, atrial fibrillation, deep thrombophlebitis, ECG abnormality, and myocardial infarction (less than 0.1%).

CNS – Confusion and paresthesia (1% or more). Akathisia, apathy, aphasia, CNS depression, depersonalization, dysarthria, dyskinesia, euphoria, hallucinations, hostility, hyperkinesia, hypertonia, libido decreased, memory decrease, mind racing, movement disorder, myoclonus, panic attack, paranoid reaction, personality disorder, psychosis, sleep disorder, stupor, and suicide ideation (0.1% to 1%). Cerebrovascular accident, cerebellar syndrome, cerebral sinus thrombosis, choreoathetosis, CNS stimulation, delirium, delusions, dystonia, dysphoria, extrapyramidal syndrome, faintness, grand mal convulsions, hemiplegia, hyperalgesia, hyperesthesia, hypokinesia, hypotonia, manic depression reaction, muscle spasm, neurosis, paralysis, and peripheral neuritis (less than 0.1%).

Dermatologic – Acne, alopecia, hirsutism, maculopapular rash, skin discoloration, and urticaria (0.1% to 1%). Angioedema, erythema, erythema multiforme, exfoliative dermatitis, fungal dermatitis, herpes zoster, leukoderma, petechial rash, pustular rash, seborrhea, Stevens-Johnson syndrome, and vesiculobullous rash (less than 0.1%).

Endocrine – Goiter and hypothyroidism (less than 0.1%).

GI – Abnormal liver function tests, dysphagia, eructation, gastritis, gingivitis, increased appetite, increased salivation, and mouth ulceration (0.1% to 1%); GI hemorrhage, glossitis, gum hemorrhage, gum hyperplasia, hematemesis, hemorrhagic colitis, hepatitis, melena, stomach ulcer, stomatitis, thirst, and tongue edema (less than 0.1%).

GU – Abnormal ejaculation, breast pain, hematuria, impotence, menorrhagia, polyuria, urinary abnormality, and urinary incontinence (0.1% to 1%). Acute kidney failure, anorgasmia, breast abscess, breast neoplasm, creatinine increase, cystitis, dysuria, epididymitis, female lactation, kidney failure, kidney pain, nocturia, urinary retention, urinary urgency, and vaginal moniliasis (less than 0.1%).

Hematologic/Lymphatic – Ecchymosis and leukopenia (0.1% to 1%). Anemia, eosinophilia, fibrin decrease, fibrinogen decrease, iron deficiency anemia, leukocytosis, lymphocytosis, macrocytic anemia, petechia, and thrombocytopenia (less than 0.1%).

Metabolic/Nutritional – Aspartate transaminase increased (0.1% to 1%). Alcohol intolerance, alkaline phosphatase increase, alanine transaminase increased, bilirubinemia, gamma-glutamyl transpeptidase increase, general edema, and hyperglycemia (less than 0.1%).

Musculoskeletal – Arthritis, leg cramps, myasthenia, and twitching (0.1% to 1%). Bursitis, joint disorder, muscle atrophy, pathological fracture, and tendinous contracture (less than 0.1%).

Respiratory – Yawn (0.1% to 1%). Hiccup and hyperventilation (less than 0.1%).

Special senses – Amblyopia (1% or more). Abnormality of accommodation, conjunctivitis, dry eyes, ear pain, photophobia, taste perversion, and tinnitus (0.1% to 1%). Deafness, lacrimation disorder, oscillopsia, parosmia, ptosis, strabismus, taste loss, uveitis, and visual field defect (less than 0.1%).

Miscellaneous – Allergic reaction, chills, halitosis, and malaise (0.1% to 1%). Abdomen enlarged, abscess, and suicide/suicide attempt (less than 0.1%).

➤*Postmarketing:*
CNS – Exacerbation of parkinsonian symptoms in patients with preexisting Parkinson's disease, tics.

GI – Esophagitis.

Hematologic/Lymphatic – Agranulocytosis, aplastic anemia, disseminated intravascular coagulation, hemolytic anemia, neutropenia, pancytopenia, red cell aplasia.

Hepatic – Pancreatitis.

Hypersensitivity – Hypersensitivity reaction.

Musculoskeletal – Rhabdomyolysis has been observed in patients experiencing hypersensitivity reactions.

Respiratory – Apnea.

Miscellaneous – Lupus-like reaction, multiorgan failure, progressive immunosuppression, vasculitis.

Overdosage

➤*Symptoms:* Overdoses involving quantities up to 15 g have been reported for lamotrigine, some of which have been fatal. Overdose has resulted in ataxia, nystagmus, increased seizures, decreased level of consciousness, coma, and intraventricular conduction delay.

➤*Treatment:* There are no specific antidotes for lamotrigine. Following a suspected overdose, hospitalization of the patient is advised. General supportive care is indicated, including frequent monitoring of vital signs and close observation of the patient. If indicated, perform gastric lavage; take the usual precautions to protect the airway. Lamotrigine is rapidly absorbed. It is uncertain whether hemodialysis is an effective means of removing lamotrigine from the blood. In 6 renal failure patients, about 20% of the amount of lamotrigine in the body was removed by hemodialysis during a 4-hour session. Contact a poison control center for information on the management of overdosage of lamotrigine.

Patient Information

Prior to initiation of treatment with lamotrigine, instruct the patient that a rash or other signs or symptoms of hypersensitivity (eg, fever, lymphadenopathy) may herald a serious medical event and that the patient should report any such occurrence to a health care provider immediately. In addition, patients should notify their health care provider if worsening of seizure control occurs.

Advise patients that lamotrigine may cause dizziness, somnolence, and other symptoms and signs of CNS depression. Accordingly, advise patients neither to drive a car nor to operate other complex machinery until they have gained sufficient experience on lamotrigine to gauge whether or not it adversely affects their mental or motor performance.

Advise patients to notify their health care provider if they become pregnant or intend to become pregnant during therapy. Advise patients to notify their physicians if they intend to breast-feed or are breast-feeding an infant.

LAMOTRIGINE — ORAL

Advise women to notify their health care provider if they plan to start or stop use of oral contraceptives or other female hormonal preparations. Also advise women to promptly notify their health care provider if they experience changes in menstrual pattern (eg, breakthrough bleeding) while receiving lamotrigine in combination with these medications.

Inform patients of the availability of patient information, and instruct them to read it prior to taking lamotrigine.

LEVETIRACETAM

Rx	**Keppra** (UCB Pharma)	**Tablets:** 250 mg	(ucb 250). Blue, oblong, scored. Film-coated. In 120s.
		500 mg	(ucb 500). Yellow, oblong, scored. Film-coated. In 120s.
		750 mg	(ucb 750). Orange, oblong, scored. Film-coated. In 120s.
		Oral solution: 100 mg/mL	Dye free. Parabens. Grape flavor. In 480 mL.

LEVETIRACETAM — ORAL

Refer to the general discussion beginning in the Anticonvulsants introduction.

Indications

➤*Seizures:* Adjunctive therapy in the treatment of partial onset seizures in adults with epilepsy.

Administration and Dosage

➤*Approved by the FDA:* November 30, 1999.

Treatment should be initiated with a daily dose of 1000 mg/day, given as twice-daily dosing (500 mg twice daily). Additional dosing increments may be given (1000 mg/day additional every 2 weeks) to a maximum recommended daily dose of 3000 mg. Doses greater than 3000 mg/day have been used in open-label studies for periods of 6 months and longer. There is no evidence that doses greater than 3000 mg/day confer additional benefit.

➤*Renal function impairment:* Levetiracetam dosing must be individualized according to the patient's renal function status. Recommended doses and adjustment for dose are shown in the information below.

Levetiracetam Dosing Adjustment Regimen for Patients with Impaired Renal Function

Group	Creatinine clearance (mL/min)	Dosage (mg)	Frequency
Normal	> 80	500 to 1500	Every 12 hours
Mild	50 to 80	500 to 1000	Every 12 hours
Moderate	30 to 50	250 to 750	Every 12 hours
Severe	< 30	250 to 500	Every 12 hours
ESRD patients using dialysis	-	500 to 1000	Every 24 hours[a]

[a] Following dialysis, a 250 to 500 mg supplemental dose is recommended.

➤*Storage/Stability:* Store at 25°C (77°F); excursions permitted to 15° to 30°C (59° to 86°F).

Actions

➤*Pharmacology:* The precise mechanism(s) by which levetiracetam exerts its antiepileptic effect is unknown. The antiepileptic activity of levetiracetam was assessed in a number of animal models of epileptic seizures. Levetiracetam did not inhibit single seizures induced by maximal stimulation with electrical current or different chemoconvulsants and showed only minimal activity in submaximal stimulation and in threshold tests. Protection was observed, however, against secondarily generalized activity from focal seizures induced by pilocarpine and kainic acid, 2 chemoconvulsants that induce seizures that mimic some features of human complex partial seizures with secondary generalization. Levetiracetam also displayed inhibitory properties in the kindling model in rats, another model of human complex partial seizures, both during kindling development and in the fully kindled state. The predictive value of these animal models for specific types of human epilepsy is uncertain.

In vitro and in vivo recordings of epileptiform activity from the hippocampus have shown that levetiracetam inhibits burst firing without affecting normal neuronal excitability, suggesting that levetiracetam may selectively prevent hypersynchronization of epileptiform burst firing and propagation of seizure activity.

➤*Pharmacokinetics:*

Absorption/Distribution – Absorption of levetiracetam is rapid, with peak plasma concentrations occurring in about an hour following oral administration in fasted subjects. The oral bioavailability of levetiracetam tablets is 100% and the tablets and oral solution are bioequivalent in rate and extent of absorption. Food does not affect the extent of absorption of levetiracetam, but it decreases C_{max} by 20% and delays t_{max} by 1.5 hours. The pharmacokinetics of levetiracetam are linear over the dose range of 500 to 5000 mg. Steady state is achieved after 2 days of multiple, twice-daily dosing. Levetiracetam and its major metabolite are less than 10% bound to plasma proteins; clinically significant interactions with other drugs through competition for protein-binding sites are therefore unlikely.

Metabolism – Levetiracetam is not extensively metabolized in humans. The major metabolic pathway is the enzymatic hydrolysis of the acetamide group, which produces the carboxylic acid metabolite, ucb L057 (24%) and is not dependent on any liver cytochrome P450 isoenzymes. The major metabolite is inactive in animal seizure models. Two minor metabolites were identified as the product of hydroxylation of the 2-oxo-pyrrolidine ring (2% of dose) and opening of the 2-oxo-pyrrolidine ring in position 5 (1% of dose). There is no entantiomeric interconversion of levetiracetam or its major metabolite.

Excretion – Levetiracetam plasma half-life in adults is 7 ± 1 hour and is unaffected by either dose or repeated administration. Levetiracetam is eliminated from the systemic circulation by renal excretion as unchanged drug which represents 66% of administered dose. The total body clearance is 0.96 mL/min/kg, and the renal clearance is 0.6 mL/min/kg. The mechanism of excretion is glomerular filtration with subsequent partial tubular reabsorption. The metabolite ucb L057 is excreted by glomerular filtration and active tubular secretion with a renal clearance of 4 mL/min/kg. Levetiracetam elimination is correlated to creatinine clearance. Levetiracetam clearance is reduced in patients with impaired renal function.

Special populations –

Renal function impairment: The disposition of levetiracetam was studied in subjects with varying degrees of renal function. Total body clearance of levetiracetam is reduced in patients with impaired renal function by 40% in the mild group (Ccr = 50 to 80 mL/min), 50% in the moderate group (Ccr = 30 to 50 mL/min), and 60% in the severe renal impairment group (Ccr less than 30 mL/min). Clearance of levetiracetam is correlated with creatinine clearance.

In anuric (end-stage renal disease) patients, the total body clearance decreased 70% compared to healthy subjects (Ccr greater than 80 mL/min). Approximately 50% of the pool of levetiracetam in the body is removed during a standard 4-hour hemodialysis procedure.

Dosage should be reduced in patients with impaired renal function receiving levetiracetam, and supplemental doses should be given to patients after dialysis.

Hepatic function impairment: In subjects with mild (Child-Pugh class A) to moderate (Child-Pugh class B) hepatic impairment, the pharmacokinetics of levetiracetam were unchanged. In patients with severe hepatic impairment (Child-Pugh class C), total body clearance was 50% that of healthy subjects, but decreased renal clearance accounted for most of the decrease. No dose adjustment is needed for patients with hepatic impairment.

Elderly: Pharmacokinetics of levetiracetam were evaluated in 16 elderly subjects (age 61 to 88 years) with creatinine clearance ranging from 30 to 74 mL/min. Following oral administration of twice-daily dosing for 10 days, total body clearance decreased by 38%, and the half-life was 2.5 hours longer in the elderly compared to healthy adults. This is most likely due to the decrease in renal function in these subjects.

Children: Pharmacokinetics of levetiracetam were evaluated in 24 pediatric patients (age 6 to 12 years) after single dose (20 mg/kg). The body weight adjusted apparent clearance of levetiracetam was approximately 40% higher than in adults.

Gender: Levetiracetam C_{max} and AUC were 20% higher in women (n = 11) compared to men (n = 12). However, clearances adjusted for body weight were comparable.

Contraindications

Hypersensitivity to levetiracetam or any of the inactive ingredients.

Warnings

➤*Neuropsychiatric adverse reactions:*

Somnolence/fatigue – In controlled trials of patients with epilepsy, 14.8% of levetiracetam-treated patients reported somnolence, compared to 8.4% of placebo patients. There was no clear dose response up to 3000 mg/day. In a study where there was no titration, about 45% of patients receiving 4000 mg/day reported somnolence. The somnolence was considered serious in 0.3% of the treated patients, compared to 0% in the placebo group. About 3% of levetiracetam-treated patients discontinued treatment due to somnolence, compared to 0.7% of placebo patients. In 1.4% of treated patients, and in 0.9% of placebo patients, the dose was reduced, while 0.3% of the treated patients were hospitalized due to somnolence.

Asthenia – In controlled trials of patients with epilepsy, 14.7% of treated patients reported asthenia, compared to 9.1% of placebo patients. Treatment was discontinued in 0.8% of treated patients as compared to 0.5% of placebo patients. In 0.5% of treated patients, and in 0.2% of placebo patients, the dose was reduced.

Coordination difficulties – A total of 3.4% of levetiracetam treated patients experienced coordination difficulties, (reported as either ataxia, abnormal gait, or incoordination) compared to 1.6% of placebo patients. A total of 0.4% of patients in controlled trials discontinued levetiracetam treatment due to ataxia, compared to 0% of placebo patients. In 0.7% of treated patients, and in 0.2% of placebo patients, the dose was reduced due to coor-

LEVETIRACETAM — ORAL

dination difficulties, while 1 of the treated patients was hospitalized due to worsening of preexisting ataxia.

Somnolence, asthenia and coordination difficulties occurred most frequently within the first 4 weeks of treatment.

Psychotic symptoms – In controlled trials of patients with epilepsy, 5 (0.7%) of levetiracetam-treated patients experienced psychotic symptoms compared to 1 (0.2%) placebo patient. Two (0.3%) levetiracetam-treated patients were hospitalized, and their treatment was discontinued. Both events, reported as psychosis, developed within the first week of treatment and resolved within 1 to 2 weeks following treatment discontinuation. Two other events, reported as hallucinations, occurred after 1 to 5 months and resolved within 2 to 7 days while the patients remained on treatment. In 1 patient experiencing psychotic depression occurring with in a month, symptoms resolved within 45 days while the patient continued treatment. A total of 13.3% of levetiracetam patients experienced other behavioral symptoms (reported as aggression, agitation, anger, hostility, anxiety, apathy, emotional lability, depersonalization, depression, irritability) compared to 6.2% of placebo patients. Approximately half of these patients reported these events within the first 4 weeks. A total of 1.7% of treated patients discontinued treatment due to these events, compared to 0.2% of placebo patients. The treatment dose was reduced in 0.8% of treated patients and in 0.5% of placebo patients. A total of 0.8% of treated patients had a serious behavioral event (compared to 0.2% of placebo patients) and were hospitalized.

In addition, 4 (0.5%) of treated patients attempted suicide compared to 0% of placebo patients. One of these patients successfully committed suicide. In the other 3 patients, the events did not lead to discontinuation or dose reduction. The events occurred after patients had been treated for between 4 weeks and 6 months.

➤*Withdrawal precipitated seizures:* Antiepileptic drugs, including levetiracetam, should be withdrawn gradually to minimize the potential of increased seizure frequency.

➤*Hypersensitivity reactions:* This product should not be administered to patients who have previously exhibited hypersensitivity to levetiracetam or any of the inactive ingredients in levetiracetam tablets.

➤*Renal function impairment:* See Actions for more information.

➤*Elderly:* Levetiracetam is known to be substantially excreted by the kidney, and the risk of adverse reactions to this drug may be greater in patients with impaired renal function. Because elderly patients are more likely to have decreased renal function, care should be taken in dose selection, and it may be useful to monitor renal function.

➤*Pregnancy: Category C.* In animal studies, levetiracetam produced evidence of developmental toxicity at doses similar to or greater than human therapeutic doses.

Administration to female rats throughout pregnancy and lactation was associated with increased incidences of minor fetal skeletal abnormalities and retarded offspring growth pre- or postnatally at doses greater than or equal to 350 mg/kg/day (approximately equivalent to the maximum recommended human dose of 3000 mg [MRHD] on a mg/m^2 basis) and with increased pup mortality and offspring behavioral alterations at a dose of 1800 mg/kg/day (6 times the MRHD on a mg/m^2 basis). The developmental, no-effect dose was 70 mg/kg/day (0.2 times the MRHD on a mg/m^2 basis). There was no overt maternal toxicity at the doses used in this study.

Treatment of pregnant rabbits during the period of organogenesis resulted in increased embryofetal mortality and increased incidences of minor fetal skeletal abnormalities at doses greater than or equal to 600 mg/kg/day (approximately 4 times MRHD on a mg/m^2 basis) and in decreased fetal weights and increased incidences of fetal malformations at a dose of 1800 mg/kg/day (12 times the MRHD on a mg/m^2 basis). The developmental, no-effect dose was 200 mg/kg/day (1.3 times the MRHD on a mg/m^2 basis). Maternal toxicity was also observed at 1800 mg/kg/day.

When pregnant rats were treated during the period of organogenesis, fetal weights were decreased and the incidence of fetal skeletal variations was increased at a dose of 3600 mg/kg/day (12 times the MRHD). One-thousand two hundred (1200) mg/kg/day (4 times the MRHD) was a developmental, no-effect dose. There was no evidence of maternal toxicity in this study.

There are no adequate and well-controlled studies in pregnant women. Levetiracetam should be used during pregnancy only if the potential benefit justifies the potential risk to the fetus.

➤*Lactation:* Levetiracetam is excreted in breast milk. Because of the potential for serious adverse reactions in nursing infants from levetiracetam, a decision should be made whether to discontinue nursing or discontinue the drug, taking into account the importance of the drug to the mother.

➤*Children:* Safety and efficacy in patients below the age of 16 years have not been established.

Precautions

➤*Lab test abnormalities:* Although most laboratory tests are not systematically altered with levetiracetam treatment, there have been relatively infrequent abnormalities seen in hematologic parameters and liver function tests.

Hematologic abnormalities – Minor, but statistically significant, decreases compared to placebo in total mean RBC count (0.03 × 10^6/mm^2), mean hemoglobin (0.09 g/dL), and mean hematocrit (0.38%), were seen in levetiracetam-treated patients in controlled trials.

A total of 3.2% of treated and 1.8% of placebo patients had at least 1 possibly significant (less than or equal to 2.8 × 10^9/L) decreased WBC, and 2.4% of treated and 1.4% of placebo patients had at least 1 possibly significant (less than or equal to 1 × 10^9/L) decreased neutrophil count. Of the treated patients with a low neutrophil count, all but 1 rose towards or to baseline with continued treatment. No patient was discontinued secondary to low neutrophil counts.

Hepatic abnormalities – There were no meaningful changes in mean liver function tests (LFT) in controlled trials; lesser LFT abnormalities were similar in drug and placebo-treated patients in controlled trials (1.4%). No patients were discontinued from controlled trials for LFT abnormalities except for 1 (0.07%) epilepsy patient receiving open treatment.

➤*Hazardous tasks:* Patients should be advised that levetiracetam may cause dizziness and somnolence. Accordingly, patients should be advised not to drive or operate machinery or engage in other hazardous activities until they have gained sufficient experience on levetiracetam to gauge whether it adversely affects their performance of these activities.

Drug Interactions

None known.

Adverse Reactions

In well-controlled clinical studies, the most frequently reported adverse reactions associated with the use of levetiracetam in combination with other AEDs, not seen at an equivalent frequency among placebo-treated patients, were somnolence, asthenia, infection and dizziness.

Levetriacetam Adverse Reactions (≥ 1%)

Adverse reaction	Levetiracetam (n = 769)	Placebo (n = 439)
Miscellaneous		
Asthenia	15%	9%
Headache	14%	13%
Infection	13%	8%
Pain	7%	6%
GI		
Anorexia	3%	2%
CNS		
Amnesia	2%	1%
Anxiety	2%	1%
Ataxia	3%	1%
Depression	4%	2%
Dizziness	9%	4%
Emotional lability	2%	0%
Hostility	2%	1%
Nervousness	4%	2%
Paresthesia	2%	1%
Somnolence	15%	8%
Vertigo	3%	1%
Respiratory		
Increased cough	2%	1%
Pharyngitis	6%	4%
Rhinitis	4%	3%
Sinusitis	2%	1%
Special senses		
Diplopia	2%	1%

Other events reported by greater than or equal to 1% of patients treated with levetiracetam but as or more frequent in the placebo group were as follows: Abdominal pain, accidental injury, amblyopia, arthralgia, back pain, bronchitis, chest pain, confusion, constipation, convulsion, diarrhea, drug level increased, dyspepsia, ecchymosis, fever, flu syndrome, gastroenteritis, gingivitis, grand mal convulsion, fungal infection, insomnia, nausea, otitis media, rash, thinking abnormal, tremor, urinary tract infection, vomiting, and weight gain.

Time course of onset of adverse reactions – Of the most frequently reported adverse reactions, asthenia, somnolence and dizziness appeared to occur predominantly during the first 4 weeks of treatment with levetiracetam.

Discontinuation or dose reduction in well-controlled clinical studies – In well-controlled clinical studies, 15% of patients receiving levetiracetam and 11.6% receiving placebo either discontinued or had a dose reduction as a result of an adverse reaction. The adverse reactions most commonly associated (greater than 1%) with discontinuation or dose reduction in either treatment group are presented in the table below:

Levetiracetam Adverse Reactions Most Commonly Associated with Discontinuation or Dose Reduction

Adverse reaction	Number (%) Levetiracetam (n = 769)	Placebo (n = 439)
Asthenia	10 (1.3%)	3 (0.7%)
Convulsion	23 (3%)	15 (3.4%)

LEVETIRACETAM — ORAL

Levetiracetam Adverse Reactions Most Commonly Associated with Discontinuation or Dose Reduction		
	Number (%)	
Adverse reaction	Levetiracetam (n = 769)	Placebo (n = 439)
Dizziness	11 (1.4%)	0
Somnolence	34 (4.4%)	7 (1.6%)
Rash	0	5 (1.1%)

➤*Postmarketing:* In addition to the adverse experiences listed above, the following have been reported in patients receiving marketed levetiracetam worldwide. The listing is alphabetized: Leukopenia, neutropenia, pancytopenia, and thrombocytopenia. These adverse experiences have not been listed above, and data are insufficient to support an estimate of their incidence or to establish causation.

Overdosage

➤*Symptoms:* The highest known dose of levetiracetam received in the clinical development program was 6000 mg/day. Other than drowsiness, there were no adverse reactions in the few known cases of overdose in clinical trials. Cases of somnolence, agitation, aggression, depressed level of consciousness, respiratory depression, and coma were observed with levetiracetam overdoses in postmarketing use.

➤*Treatment:* There is no specific antidote for overdose with levetiracetam. If indicated, elimination of unabsorbed drug should be attempted by emesis or gastric lavage; usual precautions should be observed to maintain airway. General supportive care of the patient is indicated including monitoring of vital signs and observation of the clinical status of patient. A certified poison control center should be contacted for up-to-date information on the management of overdose with levetiracetam.

Hemodialysis – Standard hemodialysis procedures result in significant clearance of levetiracetam (approximately 50% in 4 hours) and should be considered in cases of overdose. Although hemodialysis has not been performed in the few known cases of overdose, it may be indicated by the patient's clinical state or in patients with significant renal impairment.

Patient Information

Patients should be advised to notify their physician if they become pregnant or intend to become pregnant during therapy.

Patients should be advised that levetiracetam may cause dizziness and somnolence. Accordingly, patients should be advised not to drive or operate machinery or engage in other hazardous activities until they have gained sufficient experience on levetiracetam to gauge whether it adversely affects their performance of these activities.

PRIMIDONE

Rx	**Primidone** (Lannett)	**Tablets:** 50 mg	In 100s, 500s, and 1000s.
Rx	**Mysoline** (Xcel Pharm.)		Lactose. (Mysoline 50 M). White, scored. Square. In 100s and 500s.
Rx	**Primidone** (Various, eg, Danbury, Lannett, Major)	**Tablets:** 250 mg	In 100s, 500s, and 1000s.
Rx	**Mysoline** (Xcel Pharm)		Lactose. (Mysoline 250 M). Yellow, scored. Square. In 100s, 1000s, and UD 100s.

PRIMIDONE — ORAL

Refer to the general discussion beginning in the Anticonvulsants introduction.

Indications

➤*Seizures:* Primidone, used alone or concomitantly with other anticonvulsants, is indicated in the control of grand mal, psychomotor, and focal epileptic seizures. It may control grand mal seizures refractory to other anticonvulsant therapy.

➤*Unlabeled uses:* Benign familial tremor (essential tremor, 750 mg/day).

Administration and Dosage

➤*Adults and children 8 years of age and older:* Patients 8 years of age and older who have received no previous treatment may be started on primidone according to the following regimen using either 50 mg or scored 250 mg primidone tablets: Days 1 to 3: 100 to 125 mg at bedtime; Days 4 to 6: 100 to 125 mg twice daily (morning and evening); Days 7 to 9: 100 to 125 mg 3 times daily (morning, noon, evening); Day 10 to maintenance: 250 mg 3 times daily (morning, noon, evening).

For most adults and children 8 years of age and over, the usual maintenance dosage is three to four 250 mg primidone tablets daily in divided doses (250 mg 3 times daily or 4 times daily). If required, an increase to five or six 250 mg tablets daily may be made, but daily doses should not exceed 500 mg 4 times daily

Dosage should be individualized to provide maximum benefit. In some cases, serum blood level determinations of primidone may be necessary for optimal dosage adjustment. The clinically effective serum level for primidone is between 5 to 12 mcg/mL.

➤*In patients already receiving other anticonvulsants:* Primidone should be started at 100 to 125 mg at bedtime and gradually increased to maintenance level as the other drug is gradually decreased. This regimen should be continued until satisfactory dosage level is achieved for the combination, or the other medication is completely withdrawn. When therapy with primidone alone is the objective, the transition from concomitant therapy should not be completed in less than 2 weeks.

➤*Children younger than 8 years of age.* For children under 8 years of age, the following regimen may be used: Days 1 to 3: 50 mg at bedtime; Days 4 to 6: 50 mg twice daily; Days 7 to 9: 100 mg twice daily; Day 10 to maintenance: 125 mg 3 times daily to 250 mg 3 times daily.

For children under 8 years of age, the usual maintenance dosage is 125 to 250 mg 3 times daily or, 10 to 25 mg/kg/day in divided doses.

➤*Storage/Stability:* Store at controlled room temperature 15° to 30°C (59° to 86°F). Dispense in a well-closed container.

Actions

➤*Pharmacology:* Primidone raises electro- or chemoshock seizure thresholds or alters seizure patterns in experimental animals. The mechanism(s) of primidone's antiepileptic action is not known.

Primidone per se has anticonvulsant activity, as do its 2 metabolites, phenobarbital and phenylethylmalonamide (PEMA). In addition to its anticonvulsant activity, PEMA potentiates the anticonvulsant activity of phenobarbital in experimental animals.

Contraindications

Porphyria; hypersensitivity to phenobarbital, a metabolite of primidone.

Warnings

➤*Withdrawal precipitated seizures:* The abrupt withdrawal of antiepileptic medication may precipitate status epilepticus.

➤*Therapeutic efficacy:* The therapeutic efficacy of a dosage regimen takes several weeks before it can be assessed.

➤*Pregnancy: Category D.* The effects of primidone in human pregnancy and nursing infants are unknown. Recent reports suggest an association between the use of anticonvulsant drugs by women with epilepsy and an elevated incidence of birth defects in children born to these women. Data are more extensive with respect to diphenylhydantoin and phenobarbital, but these are also the most commonly prescribed anticonvulsants; less systematic or anecdotal reports suggest a possible similar association with the use of all known anticonvulsant drugs.

The reports suggesting an elevated incidence of birth defects in children of drug-treated epileptic women cannot be regarded as adequate to prove a definite cause-and-effect relationship. There are intrinsic methodologic problems in obtaining adequate data on drug teratogenicity in humans; the possibility also exists that other factors leading to birth defects (eg, genetic factors, the epileptic condition itself), may be more important than drug therapy. The majority of mothers on anticonvulsant medication deliver healthy infants. It is important to note that anticonvulsant drugs should not be discontinued in patients in whom the drug is administered to prevent major seizures because of the strong possibility of precipitating status epilepticus with attendant hypoxia and threat to life. In individual cases where the severity and frequency of the seizure disorders are such that the removal of medication does not pose a serious threat to the patient, discontinuation of the drug may be considered prior to and during pregnancy, although it cannot be said with any confidence that even minor seizures do not pose some hazard to the developing embryo or fetus.

The prescribing physician will wish to weigh these considerations in treating or counseling epileptic women of childbearing potential.

Neonatal hemorrhage, with a coagulation defect resembling vitamin K deficiency, has been described in newborns whose mothers were taking primidone and other anticonvulsants. Pregnant women under anticonvulsant therapy should receive prophylactic vitamin K_1 therapy for 1 month prior to, and during, delivery.

➤*Lactation:* There is evidence that in mothers treated with primidone, the drug appears in the milk in substantial quantities. Since tests for the presence of primidone in biological fluids are too complex to be carried out in the average clinical laboratory. It is suggested that the presence of undue somnolence and drowsiness in nursing newborns of primidone-treated mothers be taken as an indication that nursing should be discontinued.

Precautions

➤*Monitoring:* Since primidone therapy generally extends over prolonged periods, a complete blood count and a sequential multiple analysis-12 (SMA-12) test should be made every 6 months.

PRIMIDONE — ORAL

Drug Interactions

Primidone Drug Interactions			
Precipitant drug	Object drug*		Description
Carbamazepine	Primidone	↓	Concomitant primidone and carbamazepine may result in decreased primidone, its metabolite phenobarbital, and carbamazepine serum concentrations.
Primidone	Carbamazepine		
Hydantoins (eg, phenytoin)	Primidone	↑	Hydantoins may increase serum primidone and its metabolites. Patients on concomitant treatment with hydantoins and primidone should be monitored closely following any alteration in hydantoin therapy.
Succinimides (eg, ethosuximide, methsuximide)	Primidone	↓	Coadministration of primidone and a succinimide may result in lower primidone and phenobarbital serum concentrations.
Valproic Acid	Primidone	↑	Plasma primidone concentrations may be elevated, increasing the pharmacologic and adverse effects. Primidone dosage may need to be decreased in some patients.
Primidone	Anticoagulants (eg, warfarin sodium)	↓	Primidone reduces the effect of anticoagulants. Monitor anticoagulation dose and tailor doses as needed.
Primidone	Beta-blockers (eg, propranolol)	↓	Pharmacokinetic effects of certain beta-blockers may be reduced. Consider a higher beta-blocker dose during coadministration of primidone.
Primidone	Corticosteroids (eg, prednisone)	↓	Decreased effect of corticosteroid may be observed. If possible, avoid this combination.
Primidone	Doxycycline	↓	Coadministration may decrease doxycycline half-life and serum levels, possibly resulting in a decreased therapeutic effect. These effects may persist for weeks following primidone discontinuation. Consider an alternate tetracycline.
Primidone	Estrogens Oral contraceptives	↓	AUC of estrogen may be decreased. Contraceptive failure has been reported. Alternate contraception methods are recommended.
Primidone	Ethanol	↑	Impaired hand-eye coordination, additive CNS effects, and death have been noted upon acute ingestion. Chronic ethanol ingestion may manifest as drug tolerance. Avoid concomitant use.
Primidone	Felodipine	↓	Pharmacologic effects of felodipine may be decreased. Patients receiving long-term treatment with both drugs may require higher doses of felodipine.
Primidone	Methadone	↓	The actions of methadone may be reduced. Patients receiving chronic methadone treatment may experience opiate withdrawal symptoms. A higher dose of methadone may be required during coadministration with primidone.
Primidone	Metronidazole	↓	Therapeutic failure of metronidazole has been observed. May need to use higher initial metronidazole doses in patients also receiving primidone.
Primidone	Nifedipine	↓	Decreased serum nifedipine concentrations, possibly reducing efficacy have been observed. Titrate dose according to response. A larger nifedipine dose may be needed.
Primidone	Quinidine	↓	Primidone appears to produce decreased quinidine serum concentrations and a decreased quinidine elimination half-life.
Primidone	Theophyllines	↓	Decreased theophylline levels, possibly resulting in reduced therapeutic effects have been observed. Increased theophylline dosages may be required with use of primidone.

*↑ = Object drug increased. ↓ = Object drug decreased.

Adverse Reactions

The most frequently occurring early side effects are ataxia and vertigo. These tend to disappear with continued therapy, or with reduction of initial dosage. Occasionally, the following have been reported: Nausea, anorexia, vomiting, fatigue, hyperirritability, emotional disturbances, sexual impotency, diplopia, nystagmus, drowsiness, and morbilliform skin eruptions. Granulocytopenia, agranulocytosis, and red-cell hypoplasia and aplasia, have been reported rarely. These and, occasionally, other persistent or severe side effects may necessitate withdrawal of the drug. Megaloblastic anemia may occur as a rare idiosyncrasy to primidone and to other anticonvulsants. The anemia responds to folic acid without necessity of discontinuing medication.

TIAGABINE HCl

Rx	**Gabitril Filmtabs** (Cephalon)	**Tablets:** 2 mg	Lactose. (C 402). Orange-peach. In 100s.
		4 mg	Lactose. (C 404). Yellow. In 100s.
		12 mg	Lactose. (C 412). Green. Ovaloid. In 100s.
		16 mg	Lactose. (C 416). Blue. Ovaloid. In 100s.

TIAGABINE HYDROCHLORIDE — ORAL

Indications

➤*Partial seizures:* Tiagabine is indicated as adjunctive therapy in adults and children at least 12 years of age in the treatment of partial seizures.

Administration and Dosage

➤*Approved by the FDA:* September 30, 1997.

➤*Concomitant antiepilepsy therapy:* The blood level of tiagabine obtained after a given dose depends on whether the patient also is receiving a drug that induces the metabolism of tiagabine. The presence of an inducer means that the attained blood level will be substantially reduced. Dosing should take the presence of concomitant medications into account.

Tiagabine is given orally and should be taken with food. Do not use a loading dose of tiagabine. Dose titration: Rapid escalation and/or large dose increments of tiagabine should not be used. Dosage adjustment of tiagabine should be considered whenever a change in patient's enzyme-inducing status occurs as a result of the addition, discontinuation, or dose change of the enzyme-inducing agent.

All patients – The following dosing recommendations apply to all patients taking tiagabine:

➤*Patients taking enzyme-inducing antiepilepsy drugs (AEDs):* The following dosing recommendations apply to patients who are already taking enzyme-inducing AEDs (eg, carbamazepine, phenytoin, primidone, phenobarbital). Such patients are considered induced patients when administering tiagabine.

Children 12 to 18 years of age – In adolescents 12 to 18 years of age, tiagabine should be initiated at 4 mg once daily. Modification of concomitant AEDs is not necessary unless clinically indicated. The total daily dose of tiagabine may be increased by 4 mg at the beginning of week 2. Thereafter, the total daily dose may be increased by 4 to 8 mg at weekly intervals until clinical response is achieved, or up to 32 mg/day. The total daily dose should be given in divided doses 2 to 4 times daily. Dosages above 32 mg/day have been tolerated in a small number of adolescent patients for a relatively short duration.

Adults older than 18 years of age – In adults, tiagabine should be initiated at 4 mg once daily. Modification of concomitant AEDs is not necessary, unless clinically indicated. The total daily dose of tiagabine may be increased by 4 to 8 mg at weekly intervals until clinical response is achieved, or up to 56 mg/day. The total daily dose should be given in divided doses 2 to 4 times daily. Dosages above 56 mg/day have not been systematically evaluated in adequate and well-controlled clinical trials.

TIAGABINE HYDROCHLORIDE — ORAL

Experience is limited in patients taking total daily doses above 32 mg using twice daily dosing. A typical dosing titration regimen for patients taking enzyme-inducing AEDs (induced patients) is provided in the following table.

Typical Dosing Titration Regimen of Tiagabine for Induced Patients		
Week	Initiation and titration schedule	Total daily dose
Week 1	Initiate at 4 mg once daily	4 mg/day
Week 2	Increase total daily dose by 4 mg	8 mg/day (in 2 divided doses)
Week 3	Increase total daily dose by 4 mg	12 mg/day (in 3 divided doses)
Week 4	Increase total daily dose by 4 mg	16 mg/day (in 2 to 4 divided doses)
Week 5	Increase total daily dose by 4 to 8 mg	20 to 24 mg/day (in 2 to 4 divided doses)
Week 6	Increase total daily dose by 4 to 8 mg	24 to 32 mg/day (in 2 to 4 divided doses)
Usual adult maintenance dose	32 to 56 mg/day in 2 to 4 divided doses	

➤*Patients not taking an enzyme-inducing AED (12 years of age and older):* The following dosing recommendations apply to patients who are taking only non–enzyme-inducing AEDs. Such patients are considered noninduced patients.

Following a given dose of tiagabine, the estimated plasma concentration in the noninduced patients is more than twice that in patients receiving enzyme-inducing agents. Use in noninduced patients requires lower doses of tiagabine. These patients may also require a slower titration of tiagabine compared with that of induced patients.

➤*Hepatic function impairment:* Patients with impaired liver function may require reduced initial and maintenance doses of tiagabine and/or longer dosing intervals compared with patients with normal hepatic function.

➤*Storage/Stability:* Store tablets at controlled room temperature, between 20° to 25°C (68° to 77°F). Protect from light and moisture.

Actions

➤*Pharmacology:* The precise mechanism by which tiagabine exerts its antiseizure effect is unknown, although it is believed to be related to its ability, documented in in vitro experiments, to enhance the activity of gamma-aminobutyric acid (GABA), the major inhibitory neurotransmitter in the central nervous system. These experiments have shown that tiagabine binds to recognition sites associated with the GABA uptake carrier. It is thought that, by this action, tiagabine blocks GABA uptake into presynaptic neurons, permitting more GABA to be available for receptor binding on the surfaces of postsynaptic cells. Inhibition of GABA uptake has been shown for synaptosomes, neuronal cell cultures, and glial cell cultures. In rat-derived hippocampal slices, tiagabine has been shown to prolong GABA-mediated inhibitory postsynaptic potentials. Tiagabine increases the amount of GABA available in the extracellular space of the globus pallidus, ventral palladum, and substantia nigra in rats at the ED_{50} and ED_{85} doses for inhibition of pentylenetetrazol-induced tonic seizures. This suggests that tiagabine prevents the propagation of neural impulses that contribute to seizures by a GABA-ergic action.

➤*Pharmacokinetics:*

Absorption/Distribution – In epilepsy clinical trials, most patients were receiving hepatic enzyme-inducing agents (eg, carbamazepine, phenytoin, primidone, phenobarbital). The pharmacokinetic profile in induced patients is significantly different from the noninduced population.

Tiagabine is well absorbed, with food slowing absorption rate but not altering the extent of absorption. Absorption of tiagabine is rapid, with peak plasma concentrations occurring at approximately 45 minutes after an oral dose in the fasting state. Tiagabine is nearly completely absorbed (more than 95%), with an absolute oral bioavailability of about 90%. Tiagabine is well absorbed, with food slowing absorption rate but not altering the extent of absorption. A high-fat meal decreases the absorption rate (mean T_{max} prolonged to 2.5 hours, mean C_{max} reduced by about 40%) but not the extent (area under the curve [AUC]) of tiagabine absorption. In all clinical trials, tiagabine was given with meals.

The pharmacokinetics of tiagabine are linear over the single dose range of 2 to 24 mg. Following multiple dosing, steady state is achieved within 2 days.

Tiagabine is 96% bound to human plasma proteins, mainly to serum albumin and α_1-acid glycoprotein over the concentration range of 10 to 10,000 ng/mL. While the relationship between tiagabine plasma concentrations and clinical response is not currently understood, trough plasma concentrations observed in controlled clinical trials at dosages from 30 to 56 mg/day ranged from less than 1 to 234 ng/mL.

Metabolism/Excretion – Although the metabolism of tiagabine has not been fully elucidated, in vivo and in vitro studies suggest that at least 2 metabolic pathways for tiagabine have been identified in humans: 1) thiophene ring oxidation leading to the formation of 5-oxo-tiagabine, and 2) glucuronidation. The 5-oxo-tiagabine metabolite does not contribute to the pharmacologic activity of tiagabine.

Based on in vitro data, tiagabine is likely to be metabolized primarily by the 3A isoform subfamily of hepatic cytochrome P-450 (CYP3A), although contributions to the metabolism of tiagabine from CYP1A2, CYP2D6, or CYP2C19 have not been excluded.

Approximately 2% of an oral dose of tiagabine is excreted unchanged, with 25% and 63% of the remaining dose excreted into the urine and feces, respectively, primarily as metabolites, at least 2 of which have not been identified. The mean systemic plasma clearance is 109 mL/min (coefficient of variation [CV] = 23%) and the average elimination half-life for tiagabine in healthy subjects ranged from 7 to 9 hours. The elimination half-life decreased 50% to 65% in hepatic enzyme-induced patients with epilepsy compared with noninduced patients with epilepsy.

The systemic clearance of tiagabine in induced patients is approximately 60% greater, resulting in considerably lower plasma concentrations and an elimination half-life of 2 to 5 hours. Given this difference in clearance, the systemic exposure after a dosage of 32 mg/day in an induced population is expected to be comparable with the systemic exposure after a dosage of 12 mg/day in a noninduced population. Similarly, the systemic exposure after a dosage of 56 mg/day in an induced population is expected to be comparable with the systemic exposure after a dosage of 22 mg/day in a noninduced population.

A diurnal effect on the pharmacokinetics of tiagabine was observed. Mean steady-state C_{min} values were 40% lower in the evening than in the morning. Tiagabine steady-state AUC values were also found to be 15% lower after the evening tiagabine dose compared with the AUC after the morning dose.

Special populations –

Hepatic function impairment: In patients with moderate hepatic impairment (Child-Pugh class B), clearance of unbound tiagabine was reduced by about 60%.

See Administration and Dosage for more information.

Children: Tiagabine has not been investigated in adequate and well-controlled clinical trials in patients younger than 12 years of age. The apparent clearance and volume of distribution of tiagabine per unit body surface area or per kg were fairly similar in 25 children (age, 3 to 10 years) and in adults taking enzyme-inducing AEDs (eg, carbamazepine, phenytoin). In children who were taking a non-inducing AED (eg, valproate), the clearance of tiagabine based upon body weight and body surface area was 2- and 1.5-fold higher, respectively, than in noninduced adults with epilepsy.

Contraindications

Hypersensitivity to the drug or its ingredients.

Warnings

➤*Seizures in patients without epilepsy:* Postmarketing reports have shown that tiagabine use has been associated with new onset seizures and status epilepticus in patients without epilepsy. Dose may be an important predisposing factor in the development of seizures, although seizures have been reported in patients taking daily doses of tiagabine as low as 4 mg. In most cases, patients were using concomitant medications (eg, antidepressants, antipsychotics, stimulants, narcotics) that are thought to lower the seizure threshold. Some seizures occurred near the time of a dose increase, even after periods of prior stable dosing.

The tiagabine dosing recommendations in current labeling for treatment of epilepsy were based on use in patients 12 years of age and older with partial seizures, most of whom were taking enzyme-inducing antiepileptic drugs (eg, carbamazepine, phenytoin, primidone, phenobarbital), which lower plasma levels of tiagabine by inducing its metabolism. Use of tiagabine without enzyme-inducing antiepileptic drugs results in blood levels about twice those attained in the studies on which current dosing recommendations are based.

In nonepileptic patients who develop seizures while on tiagabine treatment, discontinue tiagabine and evaluate patients for an underlying seizure disorder.

➤*Withdrawal seizures:* As a rule, do not abruptly discontinue AEDs because of the possibility of increasing seizure frequency. In a placebo-controlled, double-blind, dose-response study designed, in part, to investigate the capacity of tiagabine to induce withdrawal seizures, study drug was tapered over a 4-week period after 16 weeks of treatment. Patients' seizure frequency during this 4-week withdrawal period was compared with their baseline seizure frequency (before study drug). For each partial seizure type, for all partial seizure types combined, and for secondarily generalized tonic-clonic seizures, more patients experienced increases in their seizure frequencies during the withdrawal period in the 3 tiagabine groups than in the placebo group. The increase in seizure frequency was not affected by dose. Withdraw tiagabine gradually to minimize the potential of increased seizure frequency, unless safety concerns require a more rapid withdrawal.

➤*Cognitive/Neuropsychiatric adverse reactions:* Adverse reactions most often associated with the use of tiagabine were related to the CNS. The most significant of these can be classified into 2 general categories:

1.) Impaired concentration, speech or language problems, and confusion (effects on thought processes).
2.) Somnolence and fatigue (effects on level of consciousness).The majority of these reactions were mild to moderate. In controlled clinical trials, these reactions led to discontinuation of treatment with tiagabine in 6% (31 of 494) of patients compared with 2% (5 of 275) of the placebo-treated patients. A total of 1.6% (8 of 494) of the tiagabine-treated patients in the controlled trials were hospitalized secondary to the occurrence of these reactions, compared with 0% of the placebo-treated patients. Some of these reactions were dose related and usually began during initial titration.

Additionally, there have been postmarketing reports of patients who have experienced cognitive/neuropsychiatric symptoms, some accompanied by

TIAGABINE HYDROCHLORIDE — ORAL

EEG abnormalities such as generalized spike and wave activity, that have been reported as nonconvulsant status epilepticus. Some reports describe recovery following reduction of dose or discontinuation of tiagabine.

See Precautions for more information.

➤*Status epilepticus:* In the 3 double-blind, placebo-controlled, parallel-group studies (studies 1, 2, and 3), the incidence of any type of status epilepticus (simple, complex, or generalized tonic-clonic) in patients receiving tiagabine was 0.8% (4 of 494 patients) vs 0.7% (2 of 275 patients) receiving placebo. Among the patients treated with tiagabine across all epilepsy studies (controlled and uncontrolled), 5% had some form of status epilepticus. Of the 5%, 57% of patients experienced complex partial status epilepticus. A critical risk factor for status epilepticus was the presence of a history of this condition; 33% of patients with a history of status epilepticus had recurrence during tiagabine treatment. Because adequate information about the incidence of status epilepticus in a similar population of patients with epilepsy who have not received treatment with tiagabine is not available, it is impossible to state whether or not treatment with tiagabine is associated with a higher or lower rate of status epilepticus than would be expected to occur in a similar population not treated with tiagabine.

➤*Sudden unexpected death in epilepsy (SUDEP):* There have been as many as 10 cases of sudden unexpected deaths during the clinical development of tiagabine among 2,531 patients with epilepsy (3,831 patient-years of exposure).

This represents an estimated incidence of 0.0026 deaths/patient-year. This rate is within the range of estimates for the incidence of sudden and unexpected deaths in patients with epilepsy not receiving tiagabine (ranging from 0.0005 for the general population with epilepsy, 0.003 to 0.004 for clinical trial populations similar to that in the clinical development program for tiagabine, to 0.005 for patients with refractory epilepsy). The estimated SUDEP rates in patients receiving tiagabine are also similar to those observed in patients receiving other AEDs, chemically unrelated to tiagabine, who underwent clinical testing in similar populations at about the same time. This evidence suggests that the SUDEP rates reflect population rates, not a drug effect.

➤*Hepatic function impairment:* Because the clearance of tiagabine is reduced in patients with liver disease, dosage reduction may be necessary in these patients.

➤*Carcinogenesis:* In rats, a study of the potential carcinogenicity associated with tiagabine administration showed that 200 mg/kg/day (AUC, 36 to 100 times that at the maximum recommended human dosage [MRHD] of 56 mg/day) for 2 years resulted in small, but statistically significant increases in the incidences of hepatocellular adenomas in females and Leydig cell tumors of the testis in males. The significance of these findings relative to the use of tiagabine in humans is unknown. The no effect dosage for induction of tumors in this study was 100 mg/kg/day (17 to 50 times the exposure at the MRHD). No statistically significant increases in tumor formation were noted in mice at dosages up to 250 mg/kg/day (20 times the MRHD on a mg/m^2 basis).

➤*Mutagenesis:* Tiagabine produced an increase in structural chromosome aberration frequency in human lymphocytes in vitro in the absence of metabolic activation. No increase in chromosomal aberration frequencies was demonstrated in this assay in the presence of metabolic activation.

➤*Pregnancy: Category C.* Tiagabine has been shown to have adverse effects on embryo-fetal development, including teratogenic effects, when administered to pregnant rats and rabbits at doses greater than the human therapeutic dose.

An increased incidence of malformed fetuses (various craniofacial, appendicular, and visceral defects) and decreased fetal weights were observed following oral administration of 100 mg/kg/day to pregnant rats during the period of organogenesis. This dosage is approximately 16 times the MRHD of 56 mg/day, based on body surface area (mg/m^2). Maternal toxicity (transient weight loss/reduced maternal weight gain during gestation) was associated with this dosage, but there is no evidence to suggest that the teratogenic effects were secondary to the maternal effects. No adverse maternal or embryo-fetal effects were seen at a dosage of 20 mg/kg/day (3 times the MRHD on a mg/m^2 basis).

Decreased maternal weight gain, increased resorption of embryos, and increased incidences of fetal variations, but not malformations, were observed when pregnant rabbits were given 25 mg/kg/day (8 times the MRHD on a mg/m^2 basis) during organogenesis. The no effect level for maternal and embryo-fetal toxicity in rabbits was 5 mg/kg/day (equivalent to the MRHD on a mg/m^2 basis).

When female rats were given tiagabine 100 mg/kg/day during late gestation and throughout parturition and lactation, decreased maternal weight gain during gestation, an increase in stillbirths, and decreased postnatal offspring viability and growth were found. There are no adequate and well-controlled studies in pregnant women. Use tiagabine during pregnancy only if clearly needed.

➤*Lactation:* Studies in rats have shown that tiagabine and/or its metabolites are excreted in the milk of that species. Levels of excretion of tiagabine or its metabolites in human milk have not been determined and effects on the breast-feeding infant are unknown. Use tiagabine in women who are breast-feeding only if the benefits clearly outweigh the risks.

➤*Children:* Safety and efficacy in children younger than 12 years of age have not been established. The pharmacokinetics of tiagabine were evaluated in children 3 to 10 years of age.

See Actions for more information.

Precautions

➤*Monitoring:* A therapeutic range for tiagabine plasma concentrations has not been established. In controlled trials, trough plasma concentrations observed among patients randomized to doses of tiagabine that were statistically significantly more effective than placebo ranged from less than 1 to 234 ng/mL (median, 10th and 90th percentiles are 23.7, 5.4, and 69.8 ng/mL, respectively). Because of the potential for pharmacokinetic interactions between tiagabine and drugs that induce or inhibit hepatic metabolizing enzymes, it may be useful to obtain plasma levels of tiagabine before and after changes are made in the therapeutic regimen.

➤*Concomitant use with non-enzyme-inducing AEDs:* Virtually all experience with tiagabine has been obtained in patients receiving at least 1 concomitant enzyme-inducing AED, which lowers the plasma levels of tiagabine. Use in noninduced patients requires lower doses of tiagabine. These patients may also require a slower titration of tiagabine compared with that of induced patients. Patients taking a combination of inducing and noninducing drugs (eg, carbamazepine, valproate) should be considered to be induced. Patients not receiving hepatic enzyme-inducing agents are referred to as noninduced patients.

➤*Generalized weakness:* Moderately severe to incapacitating generalized weakness has been reported after administration of tiagabine in 28 of 2,531 (approximately 1%) patients with epilepsy. The weakness resolved in all cases after a reduction in dose or discontinuation of tiagabine.

➤*Ophthalmic effects:* When dogs received a single dose of radiolabeled tiagabine, there was evidence of residual binding in the retina and uvea after 3 weeks (the latest time point measured). Although not directly measured, melanin binding is suggested. The ability of available tests to detect potentially adverse consequences, if any, of the binding of tiagabine to melanin-containing tissue is unknown and there was no systematic monitoring for relevant ophthalmological changes during the clinical development of tiagabine. However, long-term (up to 1 year) toxicological studies of tiagabine in dogs showed no treatment-related ophthalmoscopic changes and macro- and microscopic examinations of the eye were unremarkable. Accordingly, although there are no specific recommendations for periodic ophthalmologic monitoring, be aware of the possibility of long-term ophthalmologic effects.

➤*Serious rash:* Four patients treated with tiagabine during the product's premarketing clinical testing developed what were considered to be serious rashes. In 2 patients, the rash was described as maculopapular; in 1 it was described as vesiculobullous; and in the fourth case, a diagnosis of Stevens-Johnson syndrome was made. In none of the 4 cases is it certain that tiagabine was the primary, or even a contributory, cause of the rash. Nevertheless, drug associated rash can, if extensive and serious, cause irreversible morbidity, even death.

➤*Lab test abnormalities:*

EEG abnormalities – Patients with a history of spike and wave discharges on EEG have been reported to have exacerbations of their EEG abnormalities associated with cognitive/neuropsychiatric events. This raises the possibility that these clinical reactions may, in some cases, be a manifestation of underlying seizure activity. In the documented cases of spike and wave discharges on EEG with cognitive/neuropsychiatric reactions, patients usually continued tiagabine, but required dosage adjustment.

➤*Hazardous tasks:* Advise patients that tiagabine may cause dizziness, somnolence, and other symptoms and signs of CNS depression. Accordingly, advise patients not to drive or operate other complex machinery until they have gained sufficient experience on tiagabine to gauge whether or not it affects their mental or motor performance adversely. Because of the possible additive depressive effects, use caution when patients are taking other CNS depressants in combination with tiagabine.

Drug Interactions

In evaluating the potential for interactions among coadministered AEDs, whether or not an AED induces or does not induce metabolic enzymes is an important consideration. Carbamazepine, phenytoin, primidone, and phenobarbital are generally classified as enzyme-inducers; valproate and gabapentin are not. Tiagabine is considered to be a non-enzyme-inducing AED.

Tiagabine Drug Interactions

Precipitant drug	Object drug[a]		Description
Carbamazepine Phenobarbital Phenytoin Primidone	Tiagabine	↓	Tiagabine clearance is 60% greater in patients taking carbamazepine, phenytoin, phenobarbital, or primidone with or without other enzyme-inducing AEDs. Adjust dose accordingly.
Highly protein-bound drugs	Tiagabine	↔	Tiagabine is 96% bound to plasma protein and, therefore, has the potential to interact with other highly protein-bound drugs. Such an interaction can potentially lead to higher free fractions of either drug.
Tiagabine	Highly protein-bound drugs		

TIAGABINE HYDROCHLORIDE — ORAL

Tiagabine Drug Interactions			
Precipitant drug	Object drug[a]		Description
Valproate	Tiagabine	↔	Tiagabine causes a slight decrease (approximately 10%) in steady-sate valproate concentrations. Valproate significantly decreased tiagabine binding in vitro from 96.3% to 94.8%, which resulted in an increase of approximately 40% in the free tiagabine. The clinical relevance is unknown.
Tiagabine	Valproate		

[a] ↓ = Object drug decreased. ↔ = Undetermined clinical effect.

➤*Drug/Food interactions:* See Actions for more information.

Adverse Reactions

The most commonly observed adverse reactions in placebo-controlled, parallel-group, add-on epilepsy trials associated with the use of tiagabine in combination with other AEDs not seen at an equivalent frequency among placebo-treated patients were dizziness/light-headedness, asthenia/lack of energy, somnolence, nausea, nervousness/irritability, tremor, abdominal pain, and thinking abnormal/difficulty with concentration or attention.

Tiagabine Adverse Reactions (≥ 1%)[a]		
Adverse reaction	Tiagabine (n = 494)	Placebo (n = 275)
Cardiovascular		
Vasodilation	2%	1%
CNS		
Abnormal gait	3%	2%
Agitation	1%	0%
Asthenia	20%	14%
Ataxia	5%	3%
Confusion	5%	3%
Depression	3%	1%
Difficulty with concentration/attention	6%	2%
Difficulty with memory	4%	3%
Dizziness	27%	15%
Emotional lability	3%	2%
Hostility	2%	1%
Insomnia	6%	4%
Language problems	2%	0%
Nervousness	10%	3%
Nystagmus	2%	1%
Paresthesia	4%	2%
Somnolence	18%	15%
Speech disorder	4%	2%
Tremor	9%	3%
Dermatologic		
Pruritus	2%	0%
Rash	5%	4%
GI		
Diarrhea	7%	3%
Increased appetite	2%	0%
Mouth ulceration	1%	0%
Nausea	11%	9%
Vomiting	7%	4%
Musculoskeletal		
Myasthenia	1%	0%
Respiratory		
Cough increased	4%	3%
Pharyngitis	7%	4%
Miscellaneous		
Abdominal pain	7%	3%
Pain (unspecified)	5%	3%

[a] Patients in these add-on studies were receiving 1 to 3 concomitant enzyme-inducing AEDs in addition to tiagabine or placebo. Patients may have reported multiple adverse reactions; thus, patients may be included in more than one category.

Other reactions reported by 1% or more of patients treated with tiagabine but equally or more frequent in the placebo group were as follows: accidental injury, chest pain, constipation, flu syndrome, rhinitis, anorexia, back pain, dry mouth, flatulence, ecchymosis, twitching, fever, amblyopia, conjunctivitis, urinary tract infection, urinary frequency, infection, dyspepsia, gastroenteritis, nausea and vomiting, myalgia, diplopia, headache, anxiety, acne, sinusitis, and incoordination.

Study 1 was a dose-response study including doses of 32 and 56 mg. The following table shows adverse reactions reported at a rate of at least 5% in at least 1 tiagabine group and more frequent than in the placebo group. Among these reactions, depression, nervousness, tremor, difficulty with concentration/attention, and, perhaps, asthenia exhibited a positive relationship to dose.

Tiagabine Adverse Reactions (≥ 5%) in Study 1[a]			
Adverse reaction	Tiagabine 56 mg (n = 57)	Tiagabine 32 mg (n = 88)	Placebo (n = 91)
CNS			
Abnormal gait	5%	5%	3%
Asthenia	23%	18%	15%
Ataxia	9%	6%	6%
Depression	7%	1%	0%
Difficulty with concentration/attention	14%	7%	3%
Dizziness	28%	31%	12%
Hostility	5%	5%	2%
Insomnia	5%	6%	3%
Nervousness	14%	11%	6%
Somnolence	19%	21%	17%
Tremor	21%	14%	1%
GI			
Diarrhea	2%	10%	6%
GU			
Urinary tract infection	5%	0%	2%
Hematologic and lymphatic			
Ecchymosis	0%	6%	1%
Musculoskeletal			
Myalgia	5%	2%	3%
Respiratory			
Pharyngitis	7%	8%	6%
Special senses			
Amblyopia	4%	9%	8%
Miscellaneous			
Abdominal pain	5%	7%	4%
Accidental injury	21%	15%	20%
Flu syndrome	9%	6%	3%
Infection	19%	10%	12%
Pain	7%	2%	3%

[a] Patients in this study were receiving 1 to 3 concomitant enzyme-inducing AEDs in addition to tiagabine or placebo. Patients may have reported multiple adverse reactions; thus, patients may be included in more than one category.

➤*Other adverse reactions observed during all clinical trials:*

Cardiovascular – Hypertension, palpitation, syncope, and tachycardia (at least 1%). Angina pectoris, cerebral ischemia, electrocardiogram abnormal, hemorrhage, hypotension, myocardial infarct, pallor, peripheral vascular disorder, phlebitis, postural hypotension, and thrombophlebitis (0.1% to 1%).

CNS – Depersonalization, dysarthria, euphoria, hallucination, hyperkinesia, hypertonia, hypesthesia, hypokinesia, hypotonia, migraine, myoclonus, paranoid reaction, personality disorder, reflexes decreased, stupor, twitching, and vertigo (at least 1%). Abnormal dreams, apathy, choreoathetosis, circumoral paresthesia, CNS neoplasm, coma, delusions, dystonia, encephalopathy, hemiplegia, leg cramps, libido decreased, libido increased, movement disorder, neuritis, neurosis, paralysis, peripheral neuritis, psychosis, reflexes increased, and suicide attempt (0.1% to 1%).

Dermatologic – Alopecia, dry skin, and sweating (at least 1%). Contact dermatitis, eczema, exfoliative dermatitis, furunculosis, herpes simplex, herpes zoster, hirsutism, maculopapular rash, psoriasis, skin benign neoplasm, skin carcinoma, skin discolorations, skin nodules, skin ulcer, subcutaneous nodule, urticaria, and vesiculobullous rash (0.1% to 1%).

Endocrine – Goiter and hypothyroidism (0.1% to 1%).

GI – Gingivitis and stomatitis (at least 1%). Abnormal stools, cholecystitis, cholelithiasis, dry mouth, dysphagia, eructation, esophagitis, fecal incontinence, gastritis, GI hemorrhage, glossitis, gum hyperplasia, hepatomegaly, increased salivation, liver function tests abnormal, melena, periodontal abscess, rectal hemorrhage, thirst, tooth caries, and ulcerative stomatitis (0.1% to 1%).

GU – Dysmenorrhea, dysuria, metrorrhagia, urinary incontinence, and vaginitis (at least 1%). Abortion, amenorrhea, breast enlargement, breast pain, cystitis, fibrocystic breast, hematuria, impotence, kidney failure, menorrhagia, nocturia, polyuria, pyelonephritis, salpingitis, suspicious Pap smear, urethritis, urinary retention, urinary urgency, and vaginal hemorrhage (0.1% to 1%).

TIAGABINE HYDROCHLORIDE — ORAL

Hematologic/Lymphatic – Lymphadenopathy (at least 1%). Anemia, erythrocytes abnormal, leukopenia, petechia, and thrombocytopenia (0.1% to 1%).

Metabolic/Nutritional – Edema, peripheral edema, weight gain, and weight loss (at least 1%). Dehydration, hypercholesteremia, hyperglycemia, hyperlipemia, hypoglycemia, hypokalemia, and hyponatremia (0.1% to 1%).

Musculoskeletal – Arthralgia (at least 1%). Arthritis, arthrosis, bursitis, generalized spasm, leg cramps, and tendinous contracture (0.1% to 1%).

Respiratory – Bronchitis, dyspnea, epistaxis, and pneumonia (at least 1%). Apnea, asthma, hemoptysis, hiccups, hyperventilation, laryngitis, respiratory disorder, and voice alteration (0.1% to 1%).

Special senses – Abnormal vision, ear pain, otitis media, and tinnitus (at least 1%). Blepharitis, blindness, deafness, eye pain, hyperacusis, keratoconjunctivitis, otitis externa, parosmia, photophobia, taste loss, taste perversion, and visual field defect (0.1% to 1%).

Miscellaneous – Allergic reaction, chest pain, chills, cyst, malaise, and neck pain (at least 1%). Abscess, cellulitis, facial edema, halitosis, hernia, neck rigidity, neoplasm, pelvic pain, photosensitivity reaction, sepsis, and sudden death (0.1% to 1%).

Overdosage

➤*Symptoms:* Human experience of acute overdose with tiagabine is limited. Eleven patients in clinical trials took single doses of tiagabine up to 800 mg. All patients fully recovered, usually within 1 day. The most common symptoms reported after overdose included somnolence, impaired consciousness, agitation, confusion, speech difficulty, hostility, depression, weakness, and myoclonus. One patient who ingested a single dose of 400 mg experienced generalized tonic-clonic status epilepticus, which responded to intravenous phenobarbital.

From postmarketing experience, there have been no reports of fatal overdoses involving tiagabine alone (doses up to 720 mg), although a number of patients required intubation and ventilatory support as part of the management of their status epilepticus. Overdoses involving multiple drugs, including tiagabine, have resulted in fatal outcomes. Symptoms most often accompanying tiagabine overdose, alone or with other drugs, have included seizures, including status epilepticus in patients with and without underlying seizure disorders, nonconvulsive status epilepticus, coma, ataxia, confusion, somnolence, drowsiness, impaired speech, agitation, lethargy, myoclonus, spike wave stupor, tremors, disorientation, vomiting, hostility, and temporary paralysis. Respiratory depression was seen in a number of patients, including children, in the context of seizures.

➤*Treatment:* There is no specific antidote for overdose with tiagabine. If indicated, elimination of unabsorbed drug should be achieved by gastric lavage; observe usual precautions to maintain the airway. General supportive care of the patient is indicated, including monitoring of vital signs and observation of clinical status of the patient. Because tiagabine is mostly metabolized by the liver and is highly protein bound, dialysis is unlikely to be beneficial. Consult a certified poison control center for up-to-date information on the management of overdose with tiagabine.

Patient Information

Advise patients that tiagabine may cause dizziness, somnolence, and other symptoms and signs of CNS depression. Accordingly, advise patients not to drive or operate other complex machinery until they have gained sufficient experience on tiagabine to gauge whether or not it affects their mental or motor performance adversely. Because of the possible additive depressive effects, advise patients to use caution when taking other CNS depressants in combination with tiagabine.

Because teratogenic effects were seen in the offspring of rats exposed to maternally toxic doses of tiagabine and because experience in humans is limited, advise patients to notify their health care providers if they become pregnant or intend to become pregnant during therapy.

Because of the possibility that tiagabine may be excreted in breast milk, advise patients to notify those providing care to themselves and their children if they intend to breast-feed or are breast-feeding an infant.

If the patient forgets to take the prescribed dose of tiagabine at the scheduled time, advise the patient not to attempt to make up for the missed dose by increasing the next dose. If a patient has missed multiple doses, advise the patient to refer back to his or her health care provider for possible retitration as clinically indicated.

TOPIRAMATE

Rx	**Topamax** (Ortho-McNeil)	**Tablets**: 25 mg	Lactose. (TOP 25). White. In 60s.
		50 mg	Lactose. (TOPAMAX 50). Light-yellow. In 60s.
		100 mg	Lactose. (TOPAMAX 100). Yellow. In 60s.
		200 mg	Lactose. (TOPAMAX 200). Salmon. In 60s.
		Capsules, sprinkle: 15 mg	Sucrose. (TOP 15 mg). White/clear. In 60s.
		25 mg	Sucrose. (TOP 25 mg). White/clear. In 60s.

TOPIRAMATE — ORAL

Refer to the general discussion beginning in the Anticonvulsants introduction.

Indications

➤*Epilepsy, monotherapy:* As initial monotherapy in patients 10 years of age and older with partial onset or primary generalized tonic-clonic seizures.

➤*Epilepsy, adjunctive therapy:* As adjunctive therapy for adults and children 2 to 16 years of age with partial onset seizures or primary generalized tonic-clonic seizures and in patients 2 years of age and older with seizures associated with Lennox-Gastaut syndrome.

➤*Migraine:* For adults for the prophylaxis of migraine headache. The usefulness of topiramate in the acute treatment of migraine headache has not been studied.

➤*Unlabeled uses:* Adjunctive therapy for bipolar disorder, alcohol and cocaine dependence, binge eating disorder, bulimia nervosa, cluster headaches, infantile spasms, weight loss in obesity, and smoking.

Administration and Dosage

➤*Approved by the FDA:* December 24, 1996.

Topiramate can be taken without regard to meals.

It is not necessary to monitor topiramate plasma concentrations to optimize topiramate therapy. Because of the bitter taste, tablets should not be broken.

➤*Epilepsy, monotherapy:* The recommended dosage for topiramate monotherapy in adults and children 10 years of age and older is 400 mg/day in 2 divided doses. Approximately 58% of patients randomized to 400 mg/day achieved this maximal dosage in the monotherapy controlled trial; the mean dosage achieved in the trial was 275 mg/day. The dosage should be achieved by titrating according to the following schedule:

Topiramate Monotherapy Titration

	Morning dose	Evening dose
Week 1	25 mg	25 mg
Week 2	50 mg	50 mg
Week 3	75 mg	75 mg
Week 4	100 mg	100 mg
Week 5	150 mg	150 mg
Week 6	200 mg	200 mg

➤*Epilepsy, adjunctive therapy:*

Adults (17 years of age and older): partial seizures, primary generalized tonic-clonic seizures, or Lennox-Gastaut syndrome – The recommended total daily dosage of topiramate as adjunctive therapy in adults with partial seizures is 200 to 400 mg/day in 2 divided doses, and 400 mg/day in 2 divided doses as adjunctive treatment in adults with primary generalized tonic-clonic seizures. It is recommended that therapy be initiated at 25 to 50 mg/day followed by titration to an effective dosage in increments of 25 to 50 mg/week. Titrating in increments of 25 mg/week may delay the time to reach an effective dosage. Daily doses above 1,600 mg have not been studied.

In a study of primary generalized tonic-clonic seizures, the initial titration rate was slower than in previous studies; the assigned dose was reached at the end of 8 weeks.

Children (2 to 16 years of age): partial seizures, primary generalized tonic-clonic seizures, or Lennox-Gastaut syndrome – The recommended total daily dose of topiramate as adjunctive therapy for patients with partial seizures, primary generalized tonic-clonic seizures, or seizures associated with Lennox-Gastaut syndrome is approximately 5 to 9 mg/kg/day in 2 divided doses. Begin titration at 25 mg (or less, based on a range of 1 to 3 mg/kg/day) nightly for the first week. Then increase the dosage at 1- or 2-week intervals by increments of 1 to 3 mg/kg/day (administered in 2 divided doses), to achieve optimal clinical response. Guide dose titration by clinical outcome.

In the study of primary generalized tonic-clonic seizures, the initial titration rate was slower than in previous studies; the assigned dosage of 6 mg/kg/day was reached at the end of 8 weeks.

➤*Migraine:* The recommended total daily dose of topiramate as treatment for prophylaxis of migraine headache is 100 mg/day administered in 2 divided doses. The recommended titration rate for topiramate for migraine prophylaxis to 100 mg/day is:

Topiramate Migraine Titration

	Morning Dose (mg)	Evening Dose (mg)
Week 1	None	25
Week 2	25	25
Week 3	25	50
Week 4	50	50

Guide dose titration rate by clinical outcome. If required, longer intervals between dose adjustments can be used.

TOPIRAMATE — ORAL

➤*Concomitant therapy:* On occasion, the addition of topiramate to phenytoin may require an adjustment of the phenytoin dose to achieve optimal clinical outcome.

Addition or withdrawal of phenytoin and/or carbamazepine during adjunctive therapy with topiramate may require adjustment of the topiramate dose.

➤*Sprinkle capsules:* Topiramate capsules may be swallowed whole or administered by carefully opening the capsule and sprinkling the entire contents on a small amount (teaspoon) of soft food. This drug/food mixture should be swallowed immediately and not chewed. Do not store for future use.

➤*Renal function impairment:* In renally impaired subjects (creatinine clearance [Ccr] less than 70 mL/min per 1.73 m^2), one half of the usual adult dose is recommended. Such patients will require a longer time to reach steady state at each dose.

➤*Hemodialysis:* Topiramate is cleared by hemodialysis at a rate that is 4 to 6 times greater than a healthy individual. Accordingly, a prolonged period of dialysis may cause topiramate concentration to fall below that required to maintain an antiseizure effect. To avoid rapid drops in topiramate plasma concentration during hemodialysis, a supplemental dose of topiramate may be required. The actual adjustment should take into account the following: the duration of dialysis period, clearance rate of the dialysis system being used, and effective renal clearance of topiramate in the patient being dialyzed.

➤*Hepatic function impairment:* In hepatically impaired patients, topiramate plasma concentrations may be increased. The mechanism is not well understood.

➤*Storage / Stability:* Protect from moisture. Store topiramate tablets in tightly closed containers at controlled room temperature (15° to 30°C; 59° to 86°F). Store topiramate capsules in tightly closed containers at or below 25°C (77°F).

Actions

➤*Pharmacology:* The precise mechanism by which topiramate exerts its anticonvulsant and migraine prophylaxis effects are unknown; however, preclinical studies have revealed 4 properties that may contribute to topiramate's efficacy for epilepsy and migraine prophylaxis. Electrophysiological and biochemical evidence suggests that topiramate, at pharmacologically relevant concentrations, blocks voltage-dependent sodium channels, augments the activity of the neurotransmitter gamma-aminobutyrate at some subtypes of the gamma-aminobutyric acid (GABA)-A receptor, antagonizes the AMPA/kainate subtype of the glutamate receptor, and inhibits the carbonic anhydrase enzyme, particularly isozymes II and IV.

➤*Pharmacokinetics:*

Absorption / Distribution – Absorption of topiramate is rapid, with peak plasma concentrations occurring at approximately 2 hours following a 400 mg oral dose. The relative bioavailability of topiramate from the tablet formulation is about 80% compared with a solution. The bioavailability of topiramate is not affected by food.

The pharmacokinetics of topiramate are linear, with dose-proportional increases in plasma concentration over the dosage range studied (200 to 800 mg/day). Steady state is reached in about 4 days in patients with normal renal function. Topiramate is 15% to 41% bound to human plasma proteins over the blood concentration range of 0.5 to 250 mcg/mL. The fraction bound decreased as blood concentration increased.

Carbamazepine and phenytoin do not alter the binding of topiramate. Sodium valproate, at 500 mcg/mL (a concentration 5 to 10 times higher than considered therapeutic for valproate) decreased the protein binding of topiramate from 23% to 13%. Topiramate does not influence the binding of sodium valproate.

Metabolism / Excretion – Topiramate is not extensively metabolized and is primarily eliminated unchanged in the urine (approximately 70% of an administered dose). Six metabolites have been identified in humans, none of which constitute greater than 5% of an administered dose. The metabolites are formed via hydroxylation, hydrolysis, and glucuronidation. There is evidence of renal tubular reabsorption of topiramate. In rats given probenecid to inhibit tubular reabsorption along with topiramate, a significant increase in renal clearance of topiramate was observed. This interaction has not been evaluated in humans. Overall, oral plasma clearance (CL/F) is approximately 20 to 30 mL/min in humans following oral administration.

The mean plasma elimination half-life is 21 hours after single or multiple doses.

Special populations –

Renal function impairment: The clearance of topiramate was reduced by 42% in moderately renally impaired (Ccr 30 to 69 mL/min per 1.73 m^2) and by 54% in severely renally impaired subjects (Ccr less than 30 mL/min per 1.73 m^2) compared with normal renal function subjects (Ccr greater than 70 mL/min per 1.73 m^2). Because topiramate is presumed to undergo significant tubular reabsorption, it is uncertain whether this experience can be generalized to all situations of renal impairment. It is conceivable that some forms of renal disease could differentially affect glomerular filtration rate and tubular reabsorption, resulting in a clearance of topiramate not predicted by Ccr. In general, however, one half the usual starting and maintenance dose is recommended in patients with moderate or severe renal impairment.

Hepatic function impairment: In hepatically impaired subjects, the clearance of topiramate may be decreased; the mechanism underlying the decrease is not well understood.

Elderly: The pharmacokinetics of topiramate in elderly subjects (65 to 85 years of age, n = 16) were evaluated in a controlled clinical study. The elderly subject population had reduced renal function (Ccr 20% lower) compared with young adults. Following a single oral 100 mg dose, maximum plasma concentration for elderly and young adults was achieved at approximately 1 to 2 hours. Reflecting the primary renal elimination of topiramate, topiramate plasma and renal clearance were reduced 21% and 19%, respectively, in elderly subjects, compared with young adults. Similarly, topiramate half-life was longer (13%) in the elderly. Reduced topiramate clearance resulted in slightly higher maximum plasma concentration (23%) and area under the curve (AUC; 25%) in elderly subjects than observed in young adults. Topiramate clearance is decreased in the elderly only to the extent that renal function is reduced. As recommended for all patients, dosage adjustment may be indicated in the elderly when impaired renal function (Ccr less than or equal to 70 mL/min per 1.73 m^2) is evident. It may be useful to monitor renal function in the elderly patient.

Children: Pharmacokinetics of topiramate were evaluated in patients 4 to 17 years of age receiving 1 or 2 other antiepileptic drugs (AEDs). Pharmacokinetic profiles were obtained after 1 week at dosages of 1, 3, and 9 mg/kg/day. Clearance was independent of dose.

Children have a 50% higher clearance and consequently shorter elimination half-life than adults. Consequently, the plasma concentration for the same mg/kg dose may be lower in children compared with adults. As in adults, hepatic enzyme-inducing AEDs decrease the steady-state plasma concentrations of topiramate.

Hemodialysis: Topiramate is cleared by hemodialysis. Using a high-efficiency, counterflow, single pass-dialysate hemodialysis procedure, topiramate dialysis clearance was 120 mL/min with blood flow through the dialyzer at 400 mL/min. This high clearance (compared with 20 to 30 mL/min total oral clearance in healthy adults) will remove a clinically significant amount of topiramate from the patient over the hemodialysis treatment period. Therefore, a supplemental dose may be required.

Bioequivalency – The sprinkle formulation is bioequivalent to the immediate-release tablet formulation and, therefore, may be substituted as a therapeutic equivalent.

Contraindications

Hypersensitivity to any component of this product.

Warnings

➤*Metabolic acidosis:* Hyperchloremic, non-anion gap, metabolic acidosis (ie, decreased serum bicarbonate below the normal reference range in the absence of chronic respiratory alkalosis) is associated with topiramate treatment. This metabolic acidosis is caused by renal bicarbonate loss due to the inhibitory effect of topiramate on carbonic anhydrase. Such electrolyte imbalance has been observed with the use of topiramate in placebo-controlled clinical trials and in the postmarketing period. Generally, topiramate-induced metabolic acidosis occurs early in treatment, although cases can occur at any time during treatment. Bicarbonate decrements are usually mild to moderate (average decrease of 4 mEq/L at daily doses of 400 mg in adults and at approximately 6 mg/kg/day in children); rarely, patients can experience severe decrements to values less than 10 mEq/L. Conditions or therapies that predispose to acidosis (eg, renal disease, severe respiratory disorders, status epilepticus, diarrhea, surgery, ketogenic diet, drugs) may be additive to the bicarbonate-lowering effects of topiramate.

Some manifestations of acute or chronic metabolic acidosis may include hyperventilation, nonspecific symptoms such as fatigue and anorexia, or more severe sequelae including cardiac arrhythmias or stupor. Chronic, untreated metabolic acidosis may increase the risk for nephrolithiasis or nephrocalcinosis, and also may result in osteomalacia (referred to as rickets in children) and/or osteoporosis with an increased risk for fractures. Chronic metabolic acidosis in children also may reduce growth rates. A reduction in growth rate may eventually decrease the maximal height achieved. The effect of topiramate on growth and bone-related sequelae has not been systematically investigated.

Measurement of baseline and periodic serum bicarbonate during topiramate treatment is recommended. If metabolic acidosis develops and persists, consider reducing the dose or discontinuing topiramate (using dose tapering). If the decision is made to continue patients on topiramate in the face of persistent acidosis, consider alkali treatment.

Adults – In adults, the incidence of persistent treatment-emergent decreases in serum bicarbonate (levels of less than 20 mEq/L at 2 consecutive visits or at the final visit) in controlled clinical trials for adjunctive treatment of epilepsy was 32% for 400 mg/day, and 1% for placebo. Metabolic acidosis has been observed at dosages as low as 50 mg/day. The incidence of persistent treatment-emergent decreases in serum bicarbonate in adults in the epilepsy controlled clinical trial for monotherapy was 15% for 50 mg/day and 25% for 400 mg/day. The incidence of a markedly abnormally low serum bicarbonate (ie, absolute value less than 17 mEq/L and more than 5 mEq/L decrease from pretreatment) in the adjunctive therapy trials was 3% for 400 mg/day and 0% for placebo and in the monotherapy trial was 1% for 50 mg/day and 7% for 400 mg/day. Serum bicarbonate levels have not been systematically evaluated at daily dosages more than 400 mg/day.

The incidence of persistent treatment-emergent decreases in serum bicarbonate in placebo-controlled trials for adults for prophylaxis of migraine was 44% for 200 mg/day, 39% for 100 mg/day, 23% for 50 mg/day, and 7% for placebo. The incidence of a markedly abnormally low serum bicarbonate (ie, absolute value less than 17 mEq/L and more than 5 mEq/L decrease from pretreatment) in these trials was 11% for 200 mg/day, 9% for 100 mg/day, 2% for 50 mg/day, and less than 1% for placebo.

Children – In pediatric patients (younger than 16 years of age), the incidence of persistent treatment-emergent decreases in serum bicarbonate in placebo-controlled trials for adjunctive treatment of Lennox-Gastaut syndrome or refractory partial onset seizures was 67% for topiramate (at approximately 6 mg/kg/day), and 10% for placebo. The incidence of a markedly abnormally low serum bicarbonate (ie, absolute value less than

TOPIRAMATE — ORAL

17 mEq/L and more than 5 mEq/L decrease from pretreatment) in these trials was 11% for topiramate and 0% for placebo. Cases of moderately severe metabolic acidosis have been reported in patients as young as 5 months old, especially at daily dosages more than 5 mg/kg/day.

In children (10 up to 16 years of age), the incidence of persistent treatment-emergent decreases in serum bicarbonate in the epilepsy-controlled clinical trial for monotherapy was 7% for 50 mg/day and 20% for 400 mg/day. The incidence of a markedly abnormally low serum bicarbonate (ie, absolute value less than 17 mEq/L and greater than 5 mEq/L decreased from pretreatment) in this trial was 4% for 50 mg/day and 4% for 400 mg/day.

➤*Acute myopia and secondary angle closure glaucoma:* A syndrome consisting of acute myopia associated with secondary angle closure glaucoma has been reported in patients receiving topiramate. Symptoms include acute onset of decreased visual acuity and/or ocular pain. Ophthalmologic findings can include myopia, anterior chamber shallowing, ocular hyperemia (redness), and increased intraocular pressure. Mydriasis may or may not be present. This syndrome may be associated with supracillary effusion resulting in anterior displacement of the lens and iris, with secondary angle closure glaucoma. Symptoms typically occur within 1 month of initiating topiramate therapy. In contrast to primary narrow-angle glaucoma, which is rare in patients younger than 40 years of age, secondary angle closure glaucoma associated with topiramate has been reported in children as well as adults. The primary treatment to reverse symptoms is discontinuation of topiramate as rapidly as possible, according to the judgement of the treating health care provider. Other measures in conjunction with discontinuation of topiramate may be helpful.

Elevated intraocular pressure of any etiology, if left untreated, can lead to serious sequelae including permanent vision loss.

➤*Oligohidrosis and hyperthermia:* Oligohidrosis (decreased sweating), infrequently resulting in hospitalization, has been reported in association with topiramate use. Decreased sweating and an elevation in body temperature above normal characterized these cases. Some of the cases were reported after exposure to elevated environmental temperatures.

The majority of the reports have been in children. Closely monitor patients, especially pediatric patients, treated with topiramate for evidence of decreased sweating and increased body temperature, especially in hot weather. Use caution when topiramate is prescribed with other drugs that predispose patients to heat-related disorders; these drugs include, but are not limited to, other carbonic anhydrase inhibitors and drugs with anticholinergic activity.

➤*Withdrawal of AEDs:* Gradually withdraw AEDs, including topiramate, to minimize the potential of increased seizure frequency.

➤*CNS effects:*

Adults – Adverse reactions most often associated with the use of topiramate were related to the CNS and were observed in the epilepsy and migraine populations. In adults, the most frequent of these can be classified into 3 general categories:

1.) Cognitive-related dysfunction (eg, confusion, psychomotor slowing, difficulty with concentration/attention, difficulty with memory, speech or language problems, particularly, word-finding difficulties).
2.) Psychiatric/behavioral disturbances (eg, depression, mood problems).
3.) Somnolence or fatigue.

Cognitive-related dysfunction – The majority of cognitive-related adverse reactions were mild to moderate in severity, and they frequently occurred in isolation. Rapid titration rate and higher initial dose were associated with higher incidences of these reactions. Many of these reactions contributed to withdrawal from treatment.

In the original add-on epilepsy controlled trials (using rapid titration, such as 100 to 200 mg/day weekly increments), the proportion of patients who experienced 1 or more cognitive-related adverse reactions was 42% for 200 mg/day, 41% for 400 mg/day, 52% for 600 mg/day, 56% for 800 and 1,000 mg/day, and 14% for placebo. These dose-related adverse reactions began with a similar frequency in the titration or in the maintenance phase, although in some patients the reactions began during titration and persisted into the maintenance phase. Some patients who experienced 1 or more cognitive-related adverse reactions in the titration phase had a dose-related recurrence of these reactions in the maintenance phase.

In the monotherapy epilepsy controlled trial, the proportion of patients who experienced 1 or more cognitive-related adverse reactions was 19% for topiramate 50 mg/day and 26% for 400 mg/day.

In the 6-month migraine prophylaxis controlled trials using a slower titration regimen (25 mg/day weekly increments), the proportion of patients who experienced 1 or more cognitive-related adverse reactions was 19% for topiramate 50 mg/day, 22% for 100 mg/day, 28% for 200 mg/day, and 10% for placebo. These dose-related adverse reactions typically began in the titration phase and often persisted into the maintenance phase but infrequently began in the maintenance phase. Some patients experienced a recurrence of 1 or more of these cognitive adverse reactions and this recurrence was typically in the titration phase. A relatively small proportion of topiramate-treated patients experienced more than 1 concurrent cognitive adverse reaction. The most common cognitive adverse reactions occurring together included difficulty with memory along with difficulty with concentration/attention, difficulty with memory along with language problems, and difficulty with concentration/attention along with language problems. Rarely, topiramate-treated patients experienced 3 concurrent cognitive reactions.

Psychiatric/Behavioral disturbances – Depression or mood problems were dose-related for the add-on epilepsy and migraine populations.

In the double-blind phases of clinical trials with topiramate in approved and investigational indications, suicide attempts occurred at a rate of 3 per 1,000 patient years (13 reactions per 3,999 patient years) on topiramate vs 0 (0 reactions per 1,430 patient years) on placebo. One completed suicide was reported in a bipolar disorder trial in a patient on topiramate.

Somnolence/Fatigue – These adverse reactions were most frequently reported during clinical trials of topiramate for adjunctive epilepsy. For the adjunctive epilepsy population, the incidence of somnolence did not differ substantially between 200 and 1,000 mg/day, but the incidence of fatigue was dose-related and increased at dosages above 400 mg/day. For the monotherapy epilepsy population in the 50 mg/day and 400 mg/day groups, the incidence of somnolence was dose-related (9% for the 50 mg/day group and 15% for the 400 mg/day group) and the incidence of fatigue was comparable in both treatment groups (14% each). For the migraine population, fatigue and somnolence were dose-related and more common in the titration phase.

Additional nonspecific CNS reactions commonly observed with topiramate in the add-on epilepsy population include dizziness or ataxia.

Children – In double-blind adjunctive therapy and monotherapy epilepsy clinical studies, the incidences of cognitive/neuropsychiatric adverse reactions in children were generally lower than previously observed in adults. These reactions included psychomotor slowing, difficulty with concentration/attention, speech disorders/related speech problems, and language problems. The most frequently reported neuropsychiatric reactions in children during adjunctive therapy double-blind studies were somnolence and fatigue. The most frequently reported neuropsychiatric events in children in the 50 mg/day and 400 mg/day groups during the monotherapy double-blind study were headache, dizziness, anorexia, and somnolence.

No patients discontinued treatment due to any adverse reactions in the adjunctive epilepsy double-blind trials. In the monotherapy epilepsy double-blind trials, 1 child (2%) in the 50 mg/day group and 7 children (12%) in the 400 mg/day group discontinued treatment due to adverse reactions. The most common adverse reaction associated with discontinuation of therapy was difficulty with concentration/attention; all occurred in the 400 mg/day group.

➤*Sudden unexplained death in epilepsy (SUDEP):* During the course of premarketing development of topiramate tablets, 10 sudden and unexplained deaths were recorded among a cohort of treated patients (2,796 subject years of exposure). This represents an incidence of 0.0035 deaths/patient year. Although this rate exceeds that expected in a healthy population matched for age and sex, it is within the range of estimates for the incidence of sudden unexplained deaths in patients with epilepsy not receiving topiramate (ranging from 0.0005 for the general population of patients with epilepsy, to 0.003 for a clinical trial population similar to that in the topiramate program, to 0.005 for patients with refractory epilepsy).

➤*Renal function impairment:* The major route of elimination of unchanged topiramate and its metabolites is via the kidney. Dosage adjustment may be required in patients with reduced renal function.

➤*Hepatic function impairment:* In hepatically impaired patients, administer topiramate with caution as the clearance of topiramate may be decreased.

➤*Carcinogenesis:* An increase in urinary bladder tumors was observed in mice given topiramate (20, 75, and 300 mg/kg) in the diet for 21 months. The elevated bladder tumor incidence, which was statistically significant in males and females receiving 300 mg/kg, was primarily due to the increased occurrence of a smooth muscle tumor considered histomorphologically unique to mice. Plasma exposures in mice receiving 300 mg/kg were approximately 0.5 to 1 times steady state exposures measured in patients receiving topiramate monotherapy at the recommended human dose (RHD) of 400 mg, and 1.5 to 2 times steady state topiramate exposures in patients receiving 400 mg of topiramate plus phenytoin. The relevance of this finding to human carcinogenic risk is uncertain. No evidence of carcinogenicity was seen in rats following oral administration of topiramate for 2 years at doses up to 120 mg/kg (approximately 3 times the RHD on a mg/m^2 basis).

➤*Elderly:* In clinical trials, 3% of patients were older than 60 years of age. No age-related difference in efficacy or adverse effects were evident. However, clinical studies of topiramate did not include sufficient numbers of subjects 65 years of age and older to determine whether they respond differently than younger subjects. Dosage adjustment may be necessary for elderly with impaired renal function (Ccr less than or equal to 70 mL/min per 1.73 m^2) due to reduced clearance of topiramate.

➤*Pregnancy: Category C.* Topiramate has demonstrated selective developmental toxicity, including teratogenicity, in experimental animal studies. When oral doses of 20, 100, or 500 mg/kg were administered to pregnant mice during the period of organogenesis, the incidence of fetal malformations (primarily craniofacial defects) was increased at all doses. The low dose is approximately 0.2 times the RHD (400 mg/day) on a mg/m^2 basis. Fetal body weights and skeletal ossification were reduced at 500 mg/kg in conjunction with decreased maternal body weight gain.

In rat studies (oral doses of 20, 100, and 500 mg/kg or 0.2, 2.5, 30, and 400 mg/kg), the frequency of limb malformations (ectrodactyly, micromelia, and amelia) was increased among the offspring of dams treated with 400 mg/kg (10 times the RHD on a mg/m^2 basis) or greater during the organogenesis period of pregnancy. Embryotoxicity (reduced fetal body weights, increased incidence of structural variations) was observed at doses as low as 20 mg/kg (0.5 times the RHD on a mg/m^2 basis). Clinical signs of maternal toxicity were seen at 400 mg/kg and above, and maternal body weight gain was reduced during treatment with 100 mg/kg or more.

In rabbit studies (20, 60, and 180 mg/kg or 10, 35, and 120 mg/kg orally during organogenesis), embryo/fetal mortality was increased at 35 mg/kg (2 times the RHD on a mg/m^2 basis) or greater, and teratogenic effects (primarily rib and vertebral malformations) were observed at 120 mg/kg (6 times the RHD on a mg/m^2 basis). Evidence of maternal toxicity (decreased body weight gain, clinical signs, and/or mortality) was seen at greater than or equal to 35 mg/kg or more.

TOPIRAMATE — ORAL

When female rats were treated during the latter part of gestation and throughout lactation (0.2, 4, 20, and 100 mg/kg or 2, 20, and 200 mg/kg), offspring exhibited decreased viability and delayed physical development at 200 mg/kg (5 times the RHD on a mg/m^2 basis) and reductions in preweaning and/or postweaning body weight gain 2 mg/kg (0.05 times the RHD on a mg/m^2 basis) and above. Maternal toxicity (decreased body weight gain, clinical signs) was evident at 100 mg/kg or more.

In a rat embryo/fetal development study with a postnatal component (0.2, 2.5, 30, or 400 mg/kg during organogenesis; noted above), pups exhibited delayed physical development at 400 mg/kg (10 times the RHD on a mg/m^2 basis) and persistent reductions in body weight gain at 30 mg/kg (1 times the RHD on a mg/m^2 basis) and higher.

There are no studies using topiramate in pregnant women. Use topiramate during pregnancy only if the potential benefit outweighs the potential risk to the fetus.

In postmarketing experience, cases of hypospadias have been reported in male infants exposed in utero to topiramate, with or without other anticonvulsants; however, a causal relationship with topiramate has not been established.

➤*Lactation:* Topiramate is excreted in the milk of lactating rats. The excretion of topiramate in human milk has not been evaluated in controlled studies. Limited observations in patients suggest an extensive secretion of topiramate into breast milk. Because many drugs are excreted in human milk and because the potential for serious adverse reactions in nursing infants to topiramate is unknown, weigh the potential benefit to the mother against the potential risk to the infant when considering recommendations regarding breast-feeding.

➤*Children:* Safety and efficacy in children younger than 2 years of age have not been established for the adjunctive therapy treatment of partial onset seizures, primary generalized tonic-clonic seizures, or seizures associated with Lennox-Gastaut syndrome. Safety and efficacy in children younger than 10 years of age have not been established for the monotherapy treatment of epilepsy. Topiramate is associated with metabolic acidosis. Chronic untreated metabolic acidosis in children may cause osteomalacia (rickets) and may reduce growth rates. A reduction in growth rate may eventually decrease the maximal height achieved. The effect of topiramate on growth and bone-related sequelae has not been systematically investigated.

Safety and efficacy in children have not been established for the prophylaxis treatment of migraine headache.

Precautions

➤*Monitoring:* Measurement of baseline and periodic serum bicarbonate during topiramate treatment is recommended. Closely monitor patients, especially pediatric patients, treated with topiramate for evidence of decreased sweating and increased body temperature, especially in hot weather.

➤*Hyperammonemia and encephalopathy associated with concomitant valproic acid use:* Concomitant administration of topiramate and valproic acid has been associated with hyperammonemia with or without encephalopathy in patients who have tolerated either drug alone. Clinical symptoms of hyperammonemic encephalopathy often include acute alterations in level of consciousness and/or cognitive function with lethargy or vomiting. In most cases, symptoms and signs abated with discontinuation of either drug. This adverse reaction is not due to a pharmacokinetic interaction.

It is not known if topiramate monotherapy is associated with hyperammonemia.

Patients with inborn errors of metabolism or reduced hepatic mitochondrial activity may be at an increased risk for hyperammonemia with or without encephalopathy. Although not studied, an interaction of topiramate and valproic acid may exacerbate existing defects or unmask deficiencies in susceptible people.

In patients who develop unexplained lethargy, vomiting, or changes in mental status, consider hyperammonemic encephalopathy and measure an ammonia level.

➤*Kidney stones:* A total of 32 out of 2,086 (1.5%) of adults exposed to topiramate during its adjunctive epilepsy therapy development reported the occurrence of kidney stones, an incidence about 2 to 4 times that expected in a similar, untreated population. In the double-blind monotherapy epilepsy study, a total of 4/319 (1.3%) of adults exposed to topiramate reported the occurrence of kidney stones. As in the general population, the incidence of stone formation among topiramate-treated patients was higher in men. Kidney stones also have been reported in children.

An explanation for the association of topiramate and kidney stones may lie in the fact that topiramate is a weak carbonic anhydrase inhibitor. Carbonic anhydrase inhibitors (eg, acetazolamide, dichlorphenamide), promote stone formation by reducing urinary citrate excretion and by increasing urinary pH. The concomitant use of topiramate with other carbonic anhydrase inhibitors or potentially in patients on a ketogenic diet may create a physiological environment that increases the risk of kidney stone formation, and should therefore be avoided.

Increased fluid intake increases the urinary output, lowering the concentration of substances involved in stone formation. Hydration is recommended to reduce new stone formation.

➤*Paresthesia:* Paresthesia (usually tingling of the extremities), an effect associated with the use of other carbonic anhydrase inhibitors, appears to be a common effect of topiramate. Paresthesia was more frequently reported in the monotherapy epilepsy trials and migraine prophylaxis trials versus the adjunctive therapy trials in epilepsy. In the majority of instances, paresthesia did not lead to treatment discontinuation.

Drug Interactions

Topiramate Drug Interactions

Precipitant Drug	Object Drug[a]		Description
Carbamazepine	Topiramate	⬇	Carbamazepine may increase the metabolism of topiramate, causing a 40% decrease in serum concentrations. Adjust dose if needed.
Carbonic anhydrase inhibitors (eg, acetazolamide)	Topiramate	⬆	Because topiramate is also a carbonic anhydrase inhibitor, concomitant use may increase the risk for renal stone formation. Avoid concurrent use.
Topiramate	Carbonic anhydrase inhibitors (eg, acetazolamide)		
Hydantoins (eg, phenytoin)	Topiramate	⬇	Hydantoins may increase the metabolism of topiramate, causing a 48% decrease in serum concentration. Topiramate may decrease the metabolism of phenytoin causing a 25% increase in serum concentrations in some patients. Adjust dose if needed.
Topiramate	Hydantoins (eg, phenytoin)	⬆	
Hydrochlorothiazide	Topiramate	⬆	Concomitant administration increased topiramate C_{max} by 27% and AUC by 29%. Adjust topiramate dose accordingly.
Lamotrigine	Topiramate	⬆	Coadministration produced a 15% increase in topiramate concentration.
Metformin	Topiramate	⬆	Coadministration caused decreased topiramate plasma clearance and metformin C_{max} and AUC to increase by 18% and 25%, respectively, and clearance to decrease 20%. The clinical significance of these effects is not known.
Topiramate	Metformin		
Pioglitazone	Topiramate	⬇	Topiramate's active hydroxy-metabolite had a decrease in C_{max} and AUC by 13% and 16% respectively; as well as a 60% decrease in C_{max} and AUC of active keto-metabolite. Monitor carefully. Pioglitazone AUC decreased by 15%.
Topiramate	Pioglitazone		
Valproic acid	Topiramate	⬇	Coadministration caused a 14% decrease in topiramate serum concentrations and an 11% decrease in valproic acid serum concentrations. Administration has been associated with hyperammonemia with and without encephalopathy.
Topiramate	Valproic acid		
Topiramate	Alcohol, CNS depressants	⬆	Use topiramate with extreme caution because of the potential to cause CNS depression, as well as other cognitive and/or neuropsychiatric adverse reactions.
Topiramate	Amitriptyline	⬆	Amitriptyline plasma concentrations may increase. Adjust amitriptyline dose as needed.
Topiramate	Oral contraceptives, estrogen	⬇	When given as adjunctive therapy with valproic acid, topiramate reduced the ethinyl estradiol AUC by 18% to 30% and plasma concentrations by 15% to 25%. Oral contraceptive efficacy may be reduced. Consider alternate method of contraception or increasing the estrogen dose.
Topiramate	Digoxin	⬇	Serum digoxin AUC was decreased by 12% when given with topiramate. The clinical relevance of this observation has not been established.
Topiramate	Lithium	⬇	Lithium AUC and C_{max} decreased by 20%.

TOPIRAMATE — ORAL

Topiramate Drug Interactions			
Precipitant Drug	Object Drug[a]		Description
Topiramate	Risperidone	⬇	Concurrent administration produced a 25% decrease in exposure to risperidone. Monitor closely.

[a] ⬆ = Object drug increased. ⬇ = Object drug decreased.

Adverse Reactions

The data described in the following sections were obtained using topiramate tablets.

➤*Epilepsy, monotherapy:* The adverse reactions in the controlled trial that occurred most commonly in adults in the 400 mg/day group and at a rate higher than the 50 mg/day group were: paresthesia, weight decrease, somnolence, anorexia, dizziness, and difficulty with memory not otherwise specified (NOS) (see the following table).

The adverse reactions in the controlled trial that occurred most commonly in children (10 to up to 16 years of age) in the 400 mg/day group and at a rate higher than the 50 mg/day group were: weight decrease, upper respiratory tract infection, paresthesia, anorexia, diarrhea, and mood problems (see the second following table).

Approximately 21% of the 159 adult patients in the 400 mg/day group who received topiramate as monotherapy in the controlled clinical trial discontinued therapy due to adverse reactions. Adverse reactions associated with discontinuing therapy (2% or more) included depression, insomnia, difficulty with memory (NOS), somnolence, paresthesia, psychomotor slowing, dizziness, and nausea.

Approximately 12% of the 57 children in the 400 mg/day group who received topiramate as monotherapy in the controlled clinical trial discontinued therapy due to adverse reactions. Adverse reactions associated with discontinuing therapy (5% or more) included difficulty with concentration/attention.

Topiramate Adverse Reactions in the Monotherapy Epilepsy Trial in Adults (≥ 2%)[a]

Adverse reaction	Topiramate 50 mg/day (N = 160)	Topiramate 400 mg/day (N = 159)
CNS		
Anxiety	4	6
Ataxia	3	4
Cognitive problem NOS	1	4
Confusion	3	4
Depression	7	9
Difficulty with concentration/attention	7	8
Difficulty with memory NOS	5	10
Dizziness	13	14
Hypertonia	0	3
Hypoaesthesia	4	5
Insomnia	8	9
Mood problems	2	5
Paresthesia	21	40
Psychomotor slowing	3	5
Somnolence	9	15
Dermatologic		
Acne	2	3
Pruritus	1	4
Rash	1	4
GI		
Anorexia	4	14
Constipation	1	4
Diarrhea	5	6
Dry mouth	1	3
Gastritis	0	3
Gastroesophageal reflux	1	2
Taste perversion	3	5
GU		
Cystitis	1	3
Dysuria	0	2
Libido decreased	0	3
Micturition frequency	0	2
Renal calculus	0	3
Urinary tract infection	1	2
Vaginal hemorrhage	0	3
Metabolic/Nutritional		
Weight decrease	6	16
Respiratory		
Bronchitis	3	4
Dyspnea	1	2
Rhinitis	2	4
Miscellaneous		
Anemia	1	2
Asthenia	4	6
Chest pain	1	2
Gamma-GT increased	1	3
Infection	2	3
Infection viral	6	8
Leg pain	2	3

[a] Values represent the percentage of patients reporting a given adverse reaction. Patients may have reported more than 1 adverse reaction during the study and can be included in more than 1 adverse reaction category.

Topiramate Adverse Reactions in the Monotherapy Epilepsy Trial in Children (≥ 5%)[a]

Adverse reaction	Topiramate 50 mg/day (N = 57)	Topiramate 400 mg/day (N = 57)
CNS		
Cognitive problems NOS	0	7
Difficulty with concentration/attention	4	9
Mood problems	2	11
Nervousness	4	5
Paresthesia	2	16
Dermatologic		
Alopecia	2	5
GI		
Anorexia	11	14
Diarrhea	5	11
Respiratory		
Bronchitis	2	7
Rhinitis	2	7
Sinusitis	2	5
Upper respiratory tract infection	16	18
Metabolic/Nutritional		
Weight decrease	7	21
Miscellaneous		
Fever	0	9
Infection	2	7
Infection viral	4	9

[a] Values represent the percentage of patients reporting a given adverse reaction. Patients may have reported more than 1 adverse reaction during the study and can be included in > 1 adverse reaction category.

➤*Epilepsy, adjunctive therapy:* The most commonly observed adverse reactions associated with the use of topiramate at dosages of 200 to 400 mg/day in controlled trials in adults with partial onset seizures, primary generalized tonic-clonic seizures, or Lennox-Gastaut syndrome, that were seen at greater frequency in topiramate-treated patients and did not appear to be dose related were as follows: somnolence, dizziness, ataxia, speech disorders and related speech problems, psychomotor slowing, abnormal vision, difficulty with memory, paresthesia, and diplopia. The most common dose-related adverse reactions at dosages of 200 to 1,000 mg/day were as follows: fatigue, nervousness, difficulty with concentration or attention, confusion, depression, anorexia, language problems, anxiety, mood problems, and weight decrease.

Adverse reactions associated with the use of topiramate at dosages of 5 to 9 mg/kg/day in controlled trials in children with partial onset seizures, primary generalized tonic-clonic seizures, or Lennox-Gastaut syndrome, that were seen at greater frequency in topiramate-treated patients were fatigue, somnolence, anorexia, nervousness, difficulty with concentration/attention, difficulty with memory, aggressive reaction, and weight decrease.

In controlled clinical trials in adults, 11% of patients receiving topiramate 200 to 400 mg/day as adjunctive therapy discontinued due to adverse reactions. This rate appeared to increase at dosages more than 400 mg/day. Adverse reactions associated with discontinuing therapy included somnolence, dizziness, anxiety, difficulty with concentration or attention, fatigue, and paresthesia and increased at dosages above 400 mg/day. None of the pediatric patients who received topiramate adjunctive therapy at 5 to 9 mg/kg/day in controlled clinical trials discontinued due to adverse reactions.

Approximately 28% of the 1,757 adults with epilepsy who received topiramate at dosages of 200 to 1,600 mg/day in clinical studies discontinued treatment because of adverse reactions; an individual patient could have reported more than 1 adverse reaction. These adverse reactions were the following: Psychomotor slowing (4%), difficulty with memory (3.2%), fatigue (3.2%), confusion (3.1%), somnolence (3.2%), difficulty with concentration/attention (2.9%), anorexia (2.7%), depression (2.6%), dizziness (2.5%), weight decrease (2.5%), nervousness (2.3%), ataxia (2.1%), and paresthesia (2%). Approximately 11% of the 310 children who received topiramate at dosages up to 30 mg/kg/day discontinued due to adverse reactions. Adverse reactions associated with discontinuing therapy included aggravated convulsions (2.3%), difficulty with concentration/attention (1.6%), language problems (1.3%), personality disorder (1.3%), and somnolence (1.3%).

Incidence in epilepsy controlled clinical trials (adjunctive therapy): Partial onset seizures, primary generalized tonic-clonic seizures, and Lennox-Gastaut syndrome – The following table lists treatment-emergent adverse reactions that occurred in at least 1% of adults treated with topiramate 200 to 400 mg/day in controlled trials that were numerically more common at this dose than in the patients treated with placebo. In general, most patients who experienced adverse reactions during the first 8 weeks of these trials no longer experienced them by their last visit. The fourth table lists treatment emergent adverse reactions that occurred in at least 1% of children treated with topiramate 5 to 9 mg/kg in controlled trials that were numerically more common than in patients treated with placebo.

Other adverse reactions (adjunctive therapy epilepsy) – Other events that occurred in more than 1% of adults treated with 200 to 400 mg of topiramate in placebo-controlled epilepsy trials but with equal or greater frequency in the placebo group were: anxiety, convulsions aggravated, coughing, diarrhea, dysmenorrhea, eye pain, fever, headache, injury, insomnia, muscle weakness, pain, personality disorder, rash, upper respiratory tract infection, and vomiting.

Topiramate Adverse Reactions in Add-on Epilepsy Trials in Adults (≥ 1%)[a,b]

		Topiramate dosage (mg/day)	
Adverse reaction[c]	Placebo (n = 291)	200 to 400 mg/day (n = 183)	600 to 1,000 mg/day (n = 414)
CNS			
Agitation	2%	3%	3%
Aggressive reaction	2%	3%	3%
Apathy	1%	1%	3%
Asthenia	1%	6%	3%
Ataxia	7%	16%	14%
Cognitive problems	1%	3%	3%
Confusion	5%	11%	14%
Coordination abnormal	2%	4%	4%
Depersonalization	1%	1%	2%
Depression	5%	5%	13%
Difficulty with concentration/attention	2%	6%	14%
Difficulty with memory	3%	12%	14%
Dizziness	15%	25%	32%
Emotional lability	1%	3%	3%
Fatigue	13%	15%	30%
Gait abnormal	1%	3%	2%
Hypoesthesia	1%	2%	1%
Language problems	1%	6%	10%
Mood problems	2%	4%	9%
Muscle contractions involuntary	1%	2%	2%
Nervousness	6%	16%	19%
Nystagmus	7%	10%	11%
Paresthesia	4%	11%	19%
Psychomotor slowing	2%	13%	21%
Rigors	0%	1%	< 1%
Somnolence	12%	29%	28%
Speech disorders/related speech problems	2%	13%	11%
Stupor	0%	2%	1%
Tremor	6%	9%	9%
Vertigo	1%	1%	2%
Dermatologic			
Rash erythematous	< 1%	1%	< 1%
Skin disorder	< 1%	2%	1%
Sweating increased	< 1%	1%	< 1%
GI			
Abdominal pain	4%	6%	7%
Anorexia	4%	10%	12%
Constipation	2%	4%	3%
Dry mouth	1%	2%	4%
Dyspepsia	6%	7%	6%
Gastroenteritis	1%	2%	1%
GI disorder	< 1%	1%	0%
Gingivitis	< 1%	1%	1%
Nausea	8%	10%	12%
GU			
Amenorrhea	1%	2%	2%
Breast pain	2%	4%	0%
Hematuria	1%	2%	< 1%
Libido decreased	1%	2%	< 1%
Menorrhagia	0%	2%	1%
Menstrual disorder	1%	2%	1%
Micturition frequency	1%	1%	2%
Prostatic disorder	< 1%	2%	0%
Urinary incontinence	< 1%	2%	1%
Urinary tract infection	1%	2%	3%
Urine abnormal	0%	1%	< 1%
Hematologic			
Epistaxis	1%	2%	1%
Leukopenia	1%	2%	1%
Metabolic/Nutritional			
Edema	1%	2%	1%
Weight decrease	3%	9%	13%
Musculoskeletal			
Myalgia	1%	2%	2%
Skeletal pain	0%	1%	0%
Respiratory			
Dyspnea	1%	1%	2%
Pharyngitis	2%	6%	3%
Rhinitis	6%	7%	6%
Sinusitis	4%	5%	6%
Special senses			
Abnormal vision	2%	13%	10%
Diplopia	5%	10%	10%
Hearing decreased	1%	2%	1%
Taste perversion	0%	2%	4%
Miscellaneous			
Allergy	1%	2%	3%
Back pain	4%	5%	3%
Body odor	0%	1%	0%
Chest pain	3%	4%	2%
Hot flushes	1%	2%	1%
Infection	1%	2%	1%
Influenza-like symptoms	2%	3%	4%
Leg pain	2%	2%	4%

TOPIRAMATE — ORAL

Topiramate Adverse Reactions in Add-on Epilepsy Trials in Adults (≥ 1%)[a,b]			
		Topiramate dosage (mg/day)	
Adverse reaction [c]	Placebo (n = 291)	200 to 400 mg/day (n = 183)	600 to 1,000 mg/day (n = 414)
Moniliasis	< 1%	1%	0%
Viral infection	1%	2%	< 1%

[a] Patients in these add-on trials were receiving 1 to 2 concomitant AEDs in addition to topiramate or placebo.
[b] Values represent the percentage of patients reporting a given adverse reaction. Patients may have reported more than 1 adverse reaction during the study and can be included in more than 1 adverse reaction category.
[c] Adverse reactions reported by at least 1% of patients in the topiramate 200 to 400 mg/day group and more common than in the placebo group are listed in this table.

Partial onset seizures in adults (add-on therapy) – Study 119 was a randomized, double-blind, placebo-controlled, parallel group study with 3 treatment arms: 1) placebo; 2) topiramate 200 mg/day with a 25 mg/day starting dosage, increased by 25 mg/day each week for 8 weeks until the 200 mg/day maintenance dosage was reached; and 3) topiramate 200 mg/day with a 50 mg/day starting dosage, increased by 50 mg/day each week for 4 weeks until the 200 mg/day maintenance dosage was reached. All patients were maintained on concomitant carbamazepine with or without another concomitant AED.

The incidence of adverse reactions (see the following table) did not differ significantly between the 2 topiramate regimens. Because the frequencies of adverse reactions reported in this study were markedly lower than those reported in the previous epilepsy studies, they cannot be directly compared with data obtained in other studies.

Topiramate Treatment-emergent Adverse Reactions in Add-on Therapy in Adults with Partial Onset Seizures (≥ 1%)[a,b]		
Adverse reaction[c]	Placebo (n = 92)	Topiramate dosage 200 mg/day (n = 171)
Cardiovascular		
Hypertension	0%	2%
CNS		
Aggressive reaction	0%	2%
Difficulty with concentration/attention	0%	5%
Difficulty with memory	1%	2%
Dizziness	4%	7%
Fatigue	4%	9%
Hypesthesia	0%	2%
Insomnia	3%	4%
Language problems	0%	2%
Leg cramps	0%	2%
Nervousness	2%	9%
Paresthesia	2%	9%
Somnolence	9%	15%
Tremor	2%	3%
GI		
Abdominal pain	3%	5%
Anorexia	7%	9%
Constipation	0%	4%
Diarrhea	1%	2%
Dry mouth	0%	2%
Dyspepsia	0%	2%
GU		
Cystitis	0%	2%
Metabolic/Nutritional		
Weight decrease	4%	8%
Respiratory		
Rhinitis	0%	4%
Special senses		
Diplopia	0%	2%
Tinnitus	0%	2%
Vision abnormal	0%	2%
Miscellaneous		
Chest pain	1%	2%

[a] Patients in these add-on trials were receiving 1 to 2 concomitant AEDs in addition to topiramate or placebo.
[b] Values represent the percentage of patients reporting a given adverse reaction. Patients may have reported > 1 adverse reaction during the study and can be included in > 1 adverse reaction category.
[c] Adverse reactions reported by ≥ 2% of patients in the topiramate 200 mg/day group and more common than in the placebo group are listed in this table.

Topiramate Dose-related Adverse Reactions in Add-on Trials in Adults with Partial Onset Seizures[a]				
		Topiramate dosage (mg/day)		
Adverse reaction	Placebo (n = 216)	200 mg/day (n = 45)	400 mg/day (n = 68)	600 to 1,000 mg/day (n = 414)
CNS				
Anxiety	6%	2%	3%	10%
Confusion	4%	9%	10%	14%
Depression	6%	9%	7%	13%
Difficulty with concentration/ attention	1%	7%	9%	14%
Fatigue	13%	11%	12%	30%
Language problems	< 1%	2%	9%	10%
Mood problems	2%	0%	6%	9%
Nervousness	7%	13%	18%	19%
GI				
Anorexia	4%	4%	6%	12%
Miscellaneous				
Weight decrease	3%	4%	9%	13%

[a] Dose-response studies were not conducted for other adult indications or for pediatric indications. The following table lists treatment-emergent adverse reactions that occurred in at least 1% of children treated with topiramate 5 to 9 mg/kg in controlled trials that were numerically more common than in patients treated with placebo.

Topiramate Adverse Reactions in Add-on Epilepsy Trials in Children (≥ 1%)[a,b]		
Adverse reaction	Placebo (n = 101)	Topiramate (n = 98)
Cardiovascular		
Bradycardia	0%	1%
Hypertension	0%	1%
CNS		
Aggressive reaction	4%	9%
Ataxia	2%	6%
Confusion	3%	4%
Convulsions grand mal	0%	1%
Difficulty with concentration/attention	2%	10%
Difficulty with memory NOS	0%	5%
Dizziness	2%	4%
Fatigue	5%	16%
Gait abnormal	5%	8%
Hyperkinesia	4%	5%
Hyporeflexia	0%	2%
Insomnia	7%	8%
Nervousness	7%	14%
Neurosis	0%	1%
Paresthesia	0%	1%
Personality disorder (behavior problems)	9%	11%
Psychomotor slowing	2%	3%
Somnolence	16%	26%
Speech disorders/ related speech problems	2%	4%

TOPIRAMATE — ORAL

Topiramate Adverse Reactions in Add-on Epilepsy Trials in Children (≥ 1%)[a,b]		
Adverse reaction	Placebo (n = 101)	Topiramate (n = 98)
Dermatologic		
Alopecia	1%	2%
Dermatitis	0%	2%
Eczema	0%	1%
Hypertrichosis	1%	2%
Rash erythematous	0%	2%
Seborrhea	0%	1%
Skin discoloration	0%	1%
Skin disorder	2%	3%
GI		
Anorexia	15%	24%
Appetite increased	0%	1%
Constipation	4%	5%
Dysphagia	0%	1%
Fecal incontinence	0%	1%
Flatulence	0%	1%
Gastroenteritis	2%	3%
Gastroesophageal reflux	0%	1%
Glossitis	0%	1%
Gum hyperplasia	0%	1%
Nausea	5%	6%
Saliva increased	4%	6%
GU		
Leukorrhea	0%	2%
Nocturia	0%	1%
Urinary incontinence	2%	4%
Hematologic		
Epistaxis	1%	4%
Hematoma	0%	1%
Leukopenia	0%	2%
Purpura	4%	8%
Prothrombin increased	0%	1%
Thrombocytopenia	0%	1%
Metabolic/Nutritional		
Hypoglycemia	0%	1%
Thirst	1%	2%
Weight decrease	1%	9%
Weight increase	0%	1%
Ophthalmic		
Abnormal vision	1%	2%
Diplopia	0%	1%
Eye abnormality	1%	2%
Lacrimation abnormal	0%	1%
Myopia	0%	1%
Respiratory		
Pneumonia	1%	5%
Respiratory disorder	0%	1%
Miscellaneous		
Allergic reaction	1%	2%
Back pain	0%	1%
Injury	13%	14%
Pallor	0%	1%
Viral infection	3%	7%

[a] Patients in these add-on trials were receiving 1 to 2 concomitant AEDs in addition to topiramate or placebo.
[b] Values represent the percentage of patients reporting a given adverse reaction. Patients may have reported > 1 adverse reaction during the study and can be included in > 1 adverse reaction category.

➤*Other adverse reactions observed during epilepsy trials:* Other reactions that occurred in greater than 1% of adults treated with topiramate 200 to 400 mg in placebo-controlled trials but with equal or greater frequency in the placebo group were as follows: headache, injury, anxiety, rash, pain, convulsions aggravated, coughing, fever, diarrhea, vomiting, muscle weakness, insomnia, personality disorder, dysmenorrhea, upper respiratory tract infection, and eye pain.

➤*Other adverse reactions observed during all epilepsy clinical trials:*
Cardiovascular – Angina pectoris, atrioventricular (AV) block, deep vein thrombosis, electroencephalogram (EEG) abnormal, flushing, hypotension, phlebitis, postural hypotension, syncope, vasodilation (0.1% to 1%); pulmonary embolism, vasospasm (less than 0.1%).

CNS – Euphoria, hallucination, hypertonia, psychosis, suicide attempt (1% or more); abnormal dreaming, apraxia, delirium, delusion, dyskinesia, dysphonia, dystonia, encephalopathy, hyperesthesia, neuropathy, neurosis, paranoia, paranoid reaction, ptosis, scotoma (0.1% to 1%); cerebellar syndrome, manic reaction, tongue paralysis, upper motor neuron lesion (less than 1%).

Dermatologic – Acne (1% or more); abnormal hair texture, photosensitivity reaction, urticaria (0.1% to 1%); chloasma (less than 0.1%).

GI – Vomiting (1% or more); abdomen enlarged, esophagitis, gastritis, hemorrhoids, melena, stomatitis (0.1% to 1%); tongue edema (less than 1%).

GU – Dysuria, impotence, renal calculus (1% or more); albuminuria, breast discharge, ejaculation disorder, oliguria, polyuria, renal pain, urinary retention (0.1% to 1%;) increased libido (less than 1%).

Hematologic / Lymphatic – Anemia, eosinophilia, gingival bleeding, granulocytopenia, lymphopenia, lymphadenopathy, thrombocythemia (0.1% to 1%); lymphocytosis, marrow depression, pancytopenia, polycythemia (less than 0.1%).

Hepatic – ALT, AST, and gamma-glutamyl transferase (GT) increased (0.1% to 1%).

Metabolic / Nutritional – Dehydration (1% or more); acidosis, face edema, hyperglycemia, hyperlipidemia, hypocalcemia, hypokalemia, increased alkaline phosphatase, xerophthalmia (0.1% to 1%); diabetes mellitus, hyperchloremia, hypernatremia, hypocholesterolemia, hyponatremia, hypophosphatemia, increased creatinine (less than 0.1%).

Musculoskeletal – Arthralgia (1% or more); arthrosis (0.1% to 1%).

Ophthalmic – Conjunctivitis (1% or more); abnormal accommodation, photophobia, strabismus, visual field defect (0.1% to 1%), iritis, mydriasis (less than 0.1%).

Special senses – Parosmia, taste loss (0.1% to 1%).

Miscellaneous – Alcohol intolerance (less than 0.1%).

➤*Migraine:* The following table includes those adverse reactions reported for patients in the placebo-controlled trials where the incidence rate in any topiramate treatment group was at least 2% and was greater than that for placebo patients.

Topiramate Adverse Reactions in Migraine Trials (≥ 2%)[a]				
		Topiramate dosage (mg/day)		
Adverse reaction	Placebo (n = 445)	50 mg/day (n = 235)	100 mg/day (n = 386)	200 mg/day (n = 514)
CNS				
Aggravated depression	1%	1%	2%	2%
Agitation	1%	2%	2%	1%
Anxiety	3%	4%	5%	6%
Asthenia	1%	< 1%	2%	2%
Ataxia	< 1%	1%	2%	1%
Cognitive problems NOS	1%	< 1%	2%	2%
Confusion	2%	2%	3%	4%
Depression	4%	3%	4%	6%
Difficulty with concentration/ attention	2%	3%	6%	10%
Difficulty with memory NOS	2%	7%	7%	11%
Dizziness	10%	8%	9%	12%
Fatigue	11%	14%	15%	19%
Hypoesthesia	2%	6%	7%	8%
Insomnia	5%	6%	7%	6%
Involuntary muscle contractions	1%	2%	2%	4%
Language problems	2%	7%	6%	7%
Mood problems	2%	3%	6%	5%
Nervousness	2%	4%	4%	4%
Paresthesia	6%	35%	51%	49%
Psychomotor slowing	1%	3%	2%	4%
Somnolence	5%	8%	7%	10%
Speech disorders/ related speech problems	< 1%	1%	< 1%	2%

TOPIRAMATE — ORAL

Topiramate Adverse Reactions in Migraine Trials (≥ 2%)[a]				
		Topiramate dosage (mg/day)		
Adverse reaction	Placebo (n = 445)	50 mg/day (n = 235)	100 mg/day (n = 386)	200 mg/day (n = 514)
Dermatologic				
Pruritus	2%	4%	2%	2%
GI				
Abdominal pain	5%	6%	6%	7%
Anorexia	6%	9%	15%	14%
Diarrhea	4%	9%	11%	11%
Dyspepsia	3%	4%	5%	3%
Dry mouth	2%	2%	3%	5%
Gastroenteritis	1%	3%	3%	2%
Nausea	8%	9%	13%	14%
Vomiting	2%	1%	2%	3%
GU				
Ejaculation premature	0%	3%	0%	0%
Libido decreased	1%	1%	1%	2%
Menstrual disorder	2%	3%	2%	2%
Renal calculus	0%	0%	1%	2%
Urinary tract infection	2%	4%	2%	4%
Metabolic/Nutritional				
Thirst	< 1%	2%	2%	1%
Weight decrease	1%	6%	9%	11%
Musculoskeletal				
Arthralgia	2%	7%	3%	1%
Ophthalmic				
Abnormal vision	< 1%	1%	2%	3%
Blurred vision[b]	2%	4%	2%	4%
Conjunctivitis	1%	1%	2%	1%
Respiratory				
Bronchitis	2%	3%	3%	3%
Coughing	2%	2%	4%	3%
Dyspnea	2%	1%	3%	2%
Pharyngitis	4%	5%	6%	2%
Rhinitis	1%	1%	2%	2%
Sinusitis	6%	10%	6%	8%
Upper respiratory tract infection	12%	13%	14%	12%
Special senses				
Otitis media	< 1%	2%	1%	1%
Taste loss	< 1%	1%	1%	2%
Taste perversion	1%	15%	8%	12%
Tinnitus	1%	< 1%	1%	2%
Miscellaneous				
Allergy	< 1%	2%	< 1%	< 1%
Influenza-like symptoms	< 1%	< 1%	< 1%	2%
Injury	7%	9%	6%	6%
Neoplasm NOS	< 1%	2%	< 1%	< 1%
Viral infection	3%	4%	4%	3%

[a] Values represent the percentage of patients reporting a given adverse reaction. Patients may have reported > 1 adverse reaction during the study and can be included in > 1 adverse reaction category.
[b] Blurred vision was the most common term considered as vision abnormal. Blurred vision was an included term that accounted for ≥ 50% of reactions coded as vision abnormal, a preferred term.

Of the 1,135 patients exposed to topiramate in the placebo-controlled studies, 25% discontinued due to adverse reactions, compared with 10% of the 445 placebo patients. The adverse reactions associated with discontinuing therapy in the topiramate-treated patients included paresthesia (7%), fatigue (4%), nausea (4%), difficulty with concentration/attention (3%), insomnia (3%), anorexia (2%), and dizziness (2%).

Patients treated with topiramate experienced mean percent reductions in body weight that were dose-dependent. This change was not seen in the placebo group. Mean changes of 0%, −2%, −3%, and −4% were seen for the placebo group, topiramate 50, 100, and 200 mg groups, respectively.

The following table shows adverse reactions that were dose-dependent. Several CNS adverse reactions, including some that represented cognitive dysfunction, were dose-related. The most common dose-related adverse reactions were paresthesia, fatigue, nausea, anorexia, dizziness, difficulty with memory, diarrhea, weight decrease, difficulty with concentration/attention, and somnolence.

Topiramate Dose-related Adverse Reactions from Migraine Trials[a]				
		Topiramate dosage (mg/day)		
Adverse reaction	Placebo (n = 445)	50 mg/day (n = 235)	100 mg/day (n = 386)	200 mg/day (n = 514)
CNS				
Anxiety	3%	4%	5%	6%
Confusion	2%	2%	3%	4%
Depression	4%	3%	4%	6%
Difficulty with concentration/ attention	2%	3%	6%	10%
Difficulty with memory NOS	2%	7%	7%	11%
Dizziness	10%	8%	9%	12%
Fatigue	11%	14%	15%	19%
Hypoesthesia	2%	6%	7%	8%
Involuntary muscle contractions	1%	2%	2%	4%
Mood problems	2%	3%	6%	5%
Paresthesia	6%	35%	51%	49%
Somnolence	5%	8%	7%	10%
GI				
Anorexia	6%	9%	15%	14%
Diarrhea	4%	9%	11%	11%
Dry mouth	2%	2%	3%	5%
Nausea	8%	9%	13%	14%
GU				
Renal calculus	0%	0%	1%	2%
Metabolic/Nutritional				
Weight decrease	1%	6%	9%	11%
Ophthalmic				
Abnormal vision	< 1%	1%	2%	3%

[a] The incidence rate of the adverse reaction in the 200 mg/day group was ≥ 2% than the rate in both the placebo group and the 50 mg/day group.

➤*Other adverse reactions observed during migraine clinical trials:* The following additional adverse reactions that were not described earlier were reported by greater than 1% of the 1,367 topiramate-treated patients in the controlled clinical trials:

CNS – Headache, migraine aggravated, sensory disturbance, tremor, vertigo.

Dermatologic – Alopecia, rash.

GI – Constipation, gastroesophageal reflux, tooth disorder.

GU – Genital moniliasis, intermenstrual bleeding.

Hematologic – Epistaxis.

Musculoskeletal – Myalgia.

Ophthalmic – Abnormal accommodation, eye pain.

Respiratory – Asthma, pneumonia.

Miscellaneous – Allergic reaction, chest pain, infection, pain.

➤*Postmarketing:* In addition to the adverse reactions reported during clinical testing of topiramate, the following adverse reactions have been reported worldwide in patients receiving topiramate post-approval. These adverse reactions have not been listed above and data are insufficient to support an estimate of their incidence or to establish causation. The listing is alphabetized as follows: bullous skin reactions (including erythema multiforme, Stevens-Johnson syndrome, toxic epidermal necrolysis), hepatic failure (including fatalities), hepatitis, pancreatitis, pemphigus, and renal tubular acidosis.

Overdosage

➤*Symptoms:* Overdoses of topiramate have been reported. Signs and symptoms included convulsions, drowsiness, speech disturbance, blurred vision, diplopia, mentation impaired, lethargy, abnormal coordination, stupor, hypotension, abdominal pain, agitation, dizziness, and depression. The clinical consequences were not severe in most cases, but deaths have been reported after poly-drug overdoses involving topiramate.

Topiramate overdose has resulted in severe metabolic acidosis.

TOPIRAMATE — ORAL

A patient who ingested a dose between 96 and 110 g was admitted to a hospital with coma lasting 20 to 24 hours followed by full recovery after 3 to 4 days.

➤*Treatment:* In acute topiramate overdose, if the ingestion is recent, immediately empty the stomach by lavage. Activated charcoal has been shown to adsorb topiramate in vitro. Treatment should be supportive. Hemodialysis is an effective means of removing topiramate from the body.

Patient Information

Tell patients taking topiramate to seek immediate medical attention if they experience blurred vision or periorbital pain.

Tell patients, especially children, treated with topiramate to watch for evidence of decreased sweating and increased body temperature, especially in hot weather.

Instruct patients, particularly those with predisposing factors, to maintain an adequate fluid intake in order to minimize the risk of renal stone formation.

Warn patients about the potential for somnolence, dizziness, confusion, and difficulty concentrating and advise them not to drive or operate machinery until they have gained sufficient experience on topiramate to gauge whether it adversely affects their mental or motor performance.

Consider additional food intake if the patient is losing weight while on this medication.

➤*How to take topiramate capsules, a guide for patients and caregivers:* Your doctor has given you a prescription for topiramate capsules. Here are your instructions for taking this medication. Please read these instructions prior to use.

To take with food – You may sprinkle the contents of topiramate on a small amount (teaspoon) of soft food, such as applesauce, custard, ice cream, oatmeal, pudding, or yogurt.

Hold the capsule upright so that you can read the word "TOP".

Carefully twist off the clear portion of the capsule. You may find it best to do this over the small portion of the food onto which you will be pouring the sprinkles.

Sprinkle all of the capsule's contents onto a spoonful of soft food, taking care to see that the entire prescribed dosage is sprinkled onto the food.

Be sure the patient swallows the entire spoonful of the sprinkle/food mixture immediately. Avoid chewing. It may be helpful to have the patient drink fluids immediately in order to make sure all of the mixture is swallowed.

Never store any sprinkle/food mixture for use at a later time.

To take without food – Topiramate may also be swallowed as whole capsules. For more information about topiramate, ask your doctor or pharmacist.

VALPROIC ACID and DERIVATIVES

Rx	**Valproic Acid** (Various, eg, Qualitest, Sidmak, UDL, Upsher Smith, Vangard, Watson)	**Capsules**: 250 mg (as valproic acid)	In 10s, 30s, 31s, and 100s.
Rx	**Depakene** (Abbott)		Parabens, corn oil. (Depakene). Orange. In 100s.
Rx	**Depakote** (Abbott)	**Tablets, delayed-release (enteric-coated)**: 125 mg (as divalproex sodium)	Talc. Salmon pink. In 100s and *Abbo-Pac* UD 100s.
		250 mg (as divalproex sodium)	Talc. Peach. In 100s, 500s, and *Abbo-Pac* UD 100s.
		500 mg (as divalproex sodium)	Talc. Lavender. In 100s, 500s, and *Abbo-Pac* UD 100s.
Rx	**Depakote ER** (Abbott)	**Tablets, extended-release**: 250 mg (as divalproex sodium)	Lactose. (a HF). White, oval. In 60s, 100s, 500s, and *Abbo-Pac* UD 100s.
		500 mg (as divalproex sodium)	Lactose, polydextrose. (a HC). Gray, oval. In 100s, 500s, and *Abbo-Pac* UD 100s.
Rx	**Depakote** (Abbott)	**Capsules, sprinkle**: 125 mg (as divalproex sodium)	White/Blue. In 100s and *Abbo-Pac* UD 100s.
Rx	**Valproic Acid** (Various, eg, Alpharma, Hi-Tech, Major, Morton Grove, Pharmaceutical Associates, Qualitest, Teva, Xactdose)	**Syrup**: 250 mg (as sodium valproate)/5 mL	In 473 mL.
Rx	**Depakene** (Abbott)		Parabens, sorbitol, sucrose. In 473 mL.
Rx	**Valproate Sodium** (Bedford)	**Injection**: 100 mg/mL (as valproate sodium)	Preservative free. In 5 mL single-dose vials.
Rx	**Depacon** (Abbott)		EDTA. Preservative free. In 5 mL single-dose vials.

VALPROIC ACID — ORAL

Refer to the general discussion beginning in the Anticonvulsants introduction.

WARNING

Hepatotoxicity – Hepatic failure resulting in fatalities has occurred in patients receiving valproic acid. Experience has indicated that children under the age of 2 years are at a considerably increased risk of developing fatal hepatotoxicity, especially those on multiple anticonvulsants, those with congenital metabolic disorders, those with severe seizure disorders accompanied by mental retardation, and those with organic brain disease. When valproic acid products are used in this patient group, they should be used with extreme caution and as a sole agent. The benefits of therapy should be weighed against the risks. Above this age group, experience in epilepsy has indicated that the incidence of fatal hepatotoxicity decreases considerably in progressively older patient groups.

These incidents usually have occurred during the first 6 months of treatment. Serious or fatal hepatotoxicity may be preceded by nonspecific symptoms such as malaise, weakness, lethargy, facial edema, anorexia, and vomiting. In patients with epilepsy, a loss of seizure control may also occur. Patients should be monitored closely for appearance of these symptoms. Liver function tests should be performed prior to therapy and at frequent intervals thereafter, especially during the first 6 months.

Teratogenicity – Valproate can produce teratogenic effects such as neural tube defects (eg, spina bifida). Accordingly, the use of valproate products in women of childbearing potential requires that the benefits of its use be weighed against the risk of injury to the fetus.

Pancreatitis – Cases of life-threatening pancreatitis have been reported in both children and adults receiving valproate. Some of the cases have been described as hemorrhagic with a rapid progression from initial symptoms to death. Cases have been reported shortly after initial use as well as after several years of use. Patients and guardians should be warned that abdominal pain, nausea, vomiting, or anorexia can be symptoms of pancreatitis that require prompt medical evaluation. If pancreatitis is diagnosed, valproate should ordinarily be discontinued. Alternative treatment for the underlying medical condition should be initiated as clinically indicated.

Indications

➤*Complex partial seziures:* As monotherapy and adjunctive therapy in the treatment of patients with complex partial seizures and pediatric patients 10 years of age and older that occur either in isolation or in association with other types of seizures.

➤*Simple and complex absence seizures:* For use as sole and adjunctive therapy in the treatment of simple and complex absence seizures, and adjunctively in patients with multiple seizure types which include absence seizures.

➤*Unlabeled uses:* This medication may be effective alone or in combination in the treatment of absence, myoclonic, and grand mal seizures. It may also be effective in patients with intractable status epilepticus who have not responded to other therapies (adults, 200 to 1200 mg every 6 hours rectally with phenytoin and phenobarbital; children, 15 to 20 mg/kg). For minor incontinence after ileoanal anastomosis (subchronic administration).

Administration and Dosage

➤*Approved by the FDA:* July 1, 1986.

The capsules should be swallowed without chewing to avoid local irritation of the mouth and throat.

Valproic acid is administered orally. As the valproic acid dosage is titrated upward, concentrations of phenobarbital, carbamazepine, or phenytoin may be affected.

➤*Complex partial seizures:*

Monotherapy (initial therapy) – Valproic acid has not been systematically studied as initial therapy. Patients should initiate therapy at 10 to 15 mg/kg/day. The dosage should be increased by 5 to 10 mg/kg/week to achieve optimal clinical response. Ordinarily, optimal clinical response is achieved at daily doses below 60 mg/kg/day. If satisfactory clinical response has not been achieved, plasma levels should be measured to determine whether or not they are in the usually accepted therapeutic range (50 to 100 mcg/mL). No recommendation regarding the safety of valproate for use at doses above 60 mg/kg/day can be made.

The probability of thrombocytopenia increases significantly at total trough valproate plasma concentrations above 110 mcg/mL in females and 135 mcg/mL in males. The benefit of improved seizure control with higher doses should be weighed against the possibility of a greater incidence of adverse reactions.

Conversion to monotherapy – Patients should initiate therapy at 10 to 15 mg/kg/day. The dosage should be increased by 5 to 10 mg/kg/week to achieve optimal clinical response. Ordinarily, optimal clinical response is achieved at daily doses below 60 mg/kg/day. If satisfactory clinical response

VALPROIC ACID — ORAL

has not been achieved, plasma levels should be measured to determine whether or not they are in the usually accepted therapeutic range (50 to 100 mcg/mL). No recommendation regarding the safety of valproate for use at doses above 60 mg/kg/day can be made. Concomitant antiepilepsy drug (AED) dosage can ordinarily be reduced by approximately 25% every 2 weeks. This reduction may be started at initiation of valproic acid therapy, or delayed by 1 to 2 weeks if there is a concern that seizures are likely to occur with a reduction. The speed and duration of withdrawal of the concomitant AED can be highly variable, and patients should be monitored closely during this period for increased seizure frequency.

Adjunctive therapy – Valproic acid may be added to the patient's regimen at a dosage of 10 to 15 mg/kg/day. The dosage may be increased by 5 to 10 mg/kg/week to achieve optimal clinical response. Ordinarily, optimal clinical response is achieved at daily doses below 60 mg/kg/day. If satisfactory clinical response has not been achieved, plasma levels should be measured to determine whether or not they are in the usually accepted therapeutic range (50 to 100 mcg/mL). No recommendation regarding the safety of valproate for use at doses above 60 mg/kg/day can be made. If the total daily dose exceeds 250 mg, it should be given in divided doses.

➤*Simple and complex absence seizures:* The recommended initial dose is 15 mg/kg/day, increasing at 1-week intervals by 5 to 10 mg/kg/day until seizures are controlled or side effects preclude further increases. The maximum recommended dosage is 60 mg/kg/day. If the total daily dose exceeds 250 mg, it should be given in divided doses.

A good correlation has not been established between daily dose, serum concentrations, and therapeutic effect. However, therapeutic valproate serum concentrations for most patients with absence seizures is considered to range from 50 to 100 mcg/mL. Some patients may be controlled with lower or higher serum concentrations.

Antiepilepsy drugs should not be abruptly discontinued in patients in whom the drug is administered to prevent major seizures because of the strong possibility of precipitating status epilepticus with attendant hypoxia and threat to life.

The following table is a guide for the initial daily dose of valproic acid (15 mg/kg/day):

Weight		Total daily dose	Number of capsules or teaspoonfuls of syrup		
kg	lb	mg	Dose 1	Dose 2	Dose 3
10 to 24.9	22 to 54.9	250	0	0	1
25 to 39.9	55 to 87.9	500	1	0	1
40 to 59.9	88 to 131.9	750	1	1	1
60 to 74.9	132 to 164.9	1,000	1	1	2
75 to 89.9	165 to 197.9	1,250	2	1	2

➤*General dosing advice:*

Elderly – Due to a decrease in unbound clearance of valproate and possibly a greater sensitivity to somnolence in the elderly, the starting dose should be reduced in these patients. Dosage should be increased more slowly and with regular monitoring for fluid and nutritional intake, dehydration, somnolence, and other adverse events. Dose reductions or discontinuation of valproate should be considered in patients with decreased food or fluid intake and in patients with excessive somnolence. The ultimate therapeutic dose should be achieved on the basis of both tolerability and clinical response.

Food – Patients who experience GI irritation may benefit from administration of the drug with food or by slowly building up the dose from an initial low level.

➤*Storage/Stability:* Store capsules at 15° to 25°C (59° to 77°F). Store syrup below 30°C (86°F).

Actions

➤*Pharmacology:*

Pharmacodynamics – The mechanisms by which valproate exerts its antiepileptic effects have not been established. It has been suggested that its activity in epilepsy is related to increased brain concentrations of gamma-aminobutyric acid (GABA).

➤*Pharmacokinetics:*

Absorption – Equivalent oral doses of divalproex sodium products and valproic acid capsules deliver equivalent quantities of valproate ion systemically. Although the rate of valproate ion absorption may vary with the formulation administered (liquid, solid, or sprinkle), conditions of use (eg, fasting, postprandial) and the method of administration (ie, whether the contents of the capsule are sprinkled on food or the capsule is taken intact), these differences should be of minor clinical importance under the steady-state conditions achieved in chronic use in the treatment of epilepsy.

However, it is possible that differences among the various valproate products in t_{max} and C_{max} could be important upon initiation of treatment. For example, in single-dose studies, the effect of feeding had a greater influence on the rate of absorption of the divalproex sodium tablet (increase in t_{max} from 4 to 8 hours) than on the absorption of the divalproex sodium sprinkle capsules (increase in t_{max} from 3.3 to 4.8 hours).

While the absorption rate from the GI tract and fluctuation in valproate plasma concentrations vary with dosing regimen and formulation, the efficacy of valproate as an anticonvulsant in chronic use is unlikely to be affected. Experience employing dosing regimens from once a day to 4 times a day, as well as studies in primate epilepsy models involving constant rate infusion, indicate that total daily systemic bioavailability (extent of absorption) is the primary determinant of seizure control and that differences in the ratios of plasma peak to trough concentrations between valproate formulations are inconsequential from a practical clinical standpoint.

Distribution –

Protein binding: The plasma protein binding of valproate is concentration dependent, and the free fraction increases from approximately 10% at 40 mcg/mL to 18.5% at 130 mcg/mL. Protein binding of valproate is reduced in the elderly, in patients with chronic hepatic diseases, in patients with renal impairment, and in the presence of other drugs (eg, aspirin). Conversely, valproate may displace certain protein-bound drugs (eg, phenytoin, carbamazepine, warfarin, tolbutamide).

CNS distribution: Valproate concentrations in cerebrospinal fluid (CSF) approximate unbound concentrations in plasma (about 10% of total concentration).

Metabolism – Valproate is metabolized almost entirely by the liver. In adult patients on monotherapy, 30% to 50% of an administered dose appears in urine as a glucuronide conjugate. Mitochondrial β-oxidation is the other major metabolic pathway, typically accounting for over 40% of the dose. Usually, less than 15% to 20% of the dose is eliminated by other oxidative mechanisms. Less than 3% of an administered dose is excreted unchanged in urine.

The relationship between dose and total valproate concentration is nonlinear; concentration does not increase proportionally with the dose, but rather, increases to a lesser extent due to saturable plasma protein binding. The kinetics of unbound drug are linear.

Excretion – Mean plasma clearance and volume of distribution for total valproate are 0.56 L/hr/1.73 m^2 and 11 L/1.73 m^2, respectively. Mean plasma clearance and volume of distribution for free valproate are 4.6 L/hr/1.73 m^2 and 92 L/1.73 m^2. Mean terminal half-life for valproate monotherapy ranged from 9 to 16 hours following oral dosing regimens of 250 to 1000 mg.

The estimates cited apply primarily to patients who are not taking drugs that affect hepatic metabolizing enzyme systems. For example, patients taking enzyme-inducing antiepileptic drugs (eg, carbamazepine, phenytoin, phenobarbital) will clear valproate more rapidly. Because of these changes in valproate clearance, monitoring of antiepileptic concentrations should be intensified whenever concomitant antiepileptics are introduced or withdrawn.

Special populations –

Renal function impairment: A slight reduction (27%) in the unbound clearance of valproate has been reported in patients with renal failure (creatinine clearance less than 10 mL/minute); however, hemodialysis typically reduces valproate concentrations by about 20%. Therefore, no dosage adjustment appears to be necessary in patients with renal failure. Protein binding in these patients is substantially reduced; thus, monitoring total concentrations may be misleading.

Hepatic function impairment: Liver disease impairs the capacity to eliminate valproate. In 1 study, the clearance of free valproate was decreased by 50% in 7 patients with cirrhosis and by 16% in 4 patients with acute hepatitis, compared with 6 healthy subjects. In that study, the half-life of valproate was increased from 12 to 18 hours. Liver disease is also associated with decreased albumin concentrations and larger unbound fractions (2- to 2.6-fold increase) of valproate. Accordingly, monitoring of total concentrations may be misleading since free concentrations may be substantially elevated in patients with hepatic disease whereas total concentrations may appear to be normal.

Elderly: The capacity of elderly patients (age range, 68 to 89 years) to eliminate valproate has been shown to be reduced compared to younger adults (age range, 22 to 26). Intrinsic clearance is reduced by 39%; the free fraction is increased by 44%. Accordingly, the initial dosage should be reduced in the elderly.

Children:

- *Neonates* – Children within the first 2 months of life have a markedly decreased ability to eliminate valproate compared to older children and adults. This is a result of reduced clearance (perhaps due to delay in development of glucuronosyltransferase and other enzyme systems involved in valproate elimination) as well as increased volume of distribution (in part due to decreased plasma protein binding). For example, in 1 study, the half-life in children less than 10 days ranged from 10 to 67 hours compared to a range of 7 to 13 hours in children greater than 2 months.
- *Children* – Pediatric patients (ie, between 3 months and 10 years) have 50% higher clearances expressed on weight (ie, mL/min/kg) than do adults. Over the age of 10 years, children have pharmacokinetic parameters that approximate those of adults.

Contraindications

Hepatic disease or significant hepatic dysfunction; hypersensitivity to the drug; known urea cycle disorders (UCD). Hyperammonemic encephalopathy, sometimes fatal, has been reported following initiation of valproate therapy in patients with urea cycle disorders, a group of uncommon genetic abnormalities, particularly ornithine transcarbamylase deficiency.

Warnings

➤*Pancreatitis:* See the Warning box for more information.

➤*Urea cycle disorders (UCD):* Hyperammonemic encephalopathy, sometimes fatal, has been reported following initiation of valproate therapy in patients with urea cycle disorders, a group of uncommon genetic abnormalities, particularly ornithine transcarbamylase deficiency. Prior to the initiation of valproate therapy, evaluation for UCD should be considered in the following patients: Those with a history of unexplained encephalopathy or coma, encephalopathy associated with a protein load, pregnancy-related or postpartum encephalopathy, unexplained mental retardation, or history of elevated plasma ammonia or glutamine; those with cyclical vomiting and lethargy, episodic extreme irritability, ataxia, low blood urea nitrogen (BUN), or protein avoidance; those with a family history of UCD or a family history of unexplained infant deaths (particularly males); those with other

VALPROIC ACID — ORAL

signs or symptoms of UCD. Patients who develop symptoms of unexplained hyperammonemic encephalopathy while receiving valproate therapy should receive prompt treatment (including discontinuation of valproate therapy) and be evaluated for underlying urea cycle disorders. In patients who develop unexplained lethargy and vomiting or changes in mental status, hyperammonemic encephalopathy should be considered and an ammonia level should be measured. If ammonia is increased, valproate therapy should be discontinued.

➤*Somnolence in the elderly:* In a double-blind, multicenter trial of valproate in elderly patients wth dementia (mean age = 83 years), doses were increased by 125 mg/day to a target dose of 20 mg/kg/day. A significantly higher proportion of valproate patients had somnolence compared to placebo, and although not statistically significant, there was a higher proportion of patients with dehydration. Discontinuations for somnolence were also significantly higher than with placebo. In some patients with somnolence (approximately one-half), there was associated reduced nutritional intake and weight loss. There was a trend for the patients who experienced these events to have a lower baseline albumin concentration, lower valproate clearance, and a higher BUN. In elderly patients, dosage should be increased more slowly and with regular monitoring for fluid and nutritional intake, dehydration, somnolence and other adverse reactions. Dose reductions or discontinuation of valproate should be considered in patients with decreased food or fluid intake and in patients with excessive somnolence.

➤*Thrombocytopenia:* The frequency of adverse reactions (particularly elevated liver enzymes and thrombocytopenia) may be dose related. In a clinical trial of divalproex sodium as monotherapy in patients with epilepsy, 34/126 patients (27%) receiving approximately 50 mg/kg/day on average, had at least 1 value of platelets less than or equal to 75 times 10^9/L. Approximately half of these patients had treatment discontinued, with return of platelet counts to normal. In the remaining patients, platelet counts normalized with continued treatment. In this study, the probability of thrombocytopenia appeared to increase significantly at total valproate concentrations of greater than or equal to 110 mcg/mL (females) or greater than or equal to 135 mcg/mL (males). The therapeutic benefit which may accompany the higher doses should therefore be weighed against the possibility of a greater incidence of adverse effects.

➤*Renal function impairment:* A slight reduction (27%) in the unbound clearance of valproate has been reported in patients with renal failure (creatinine clearance less than 10 mL/min); however, hemodialysis typically reduces valproate concentrations by about 20%. Therefore, no dosage adjustment appears to be necessary in patients with renal failure. Protein binding in these patients is substantially reduced; thus, monitoring total concentrations may be misleading.

➤*Hepatic function impairment:* See the Warning box for more information.

The drug should be discontinued immediately in the presence of significant hepatic dysfunction, suspected or apparent. In some cases, hepatic dysfunction has progressed in spite of discontinuation of drug.

➤*Carcinogenesis:* Valproic acid was administered orally to Sprague-Dawley rats and ICR (HA/ICR) mice at doses of 80 and 170 mg/kg/day (approximately 10% to 50% of the maximum human daily dose on a mg/m^2 basis) for 2 years. A variety of neoplasms were observed in both species. The chief findings were a statistically significant increase in the incidence of SC fibrosarcomas in high dose male rats receiving valproic acid and a statistically significant dose-related trend for benign pulmonary adenomas in male mice receiving valproic acid. The significance of these findings for humans is unknown.

➤*Mutagenesis:* Valproate was not mutagenic in an in vitro bacterial assay (Ames test), did not produce dominant lethal effects in mice, and did not increase chromosome aberration frequency in an in vivo cytogenetic study in rats.

Increased frequencies of sister chromatid exchange (SCE) have been reported in a study of epileptic children taking valproate, but this association was not observed in another study conducted in adults. There is some evidence that increased SCE frequencies may be associated with epilepsy. The biological significance of an increase in SCE frequency is not known.

➤*Fertility impairment:* Chronic toxicity studies in juvenile and adult rats and dogs demonstrated reduced spermatogenesis and testicular atrophy at oral doses of 400 mg/kg/day or greater in rats (approximately equivalent to or greater than the maximum human daily dose on a mg/m^2 basis) and 150 mg/kg/day or greater in dogs (approximately 1.4 the maximum human daily dose or greater on a mg/m^2 basis). Segment I fertility studies in rats have shown oral doses up to 350 mg/kg/day (approximately equal to the maximum human daily dose on a mg/m^2 basis) for 60 days to have no effect on fertility. The effect of valproate on testicular development and on sperm production and fertility in humans is unknown.

➤*Elderly:* No patients above 65 years of age were enrolled in double-blind prospective clinical trials of mania associated with bipolar illness. In a case-review study of 583 patients, 72 patients (12%) were greater than 65 years of age. A higher percentage of patients above 65 years of age reported accidental injury, infection, pain, somnolence, and tremor. Discontinuation of valproate was occasionally associated with the latter 2 events. It is not clear whether these events indicate additional risk or whether they result from preexisting medical illness and concomitant medication use among these patients.

➤*Pregnancy:* *Category D.* According to published and unpublished reports, valproic acid may produce teratogenic effects in the offspring of human females receiving the drug during pregnancy.

There are multiple reports in the clinical literature which indicate that the use of antiepileptic drugs during pregnancy results in an increased incidence of birth defects in the offspring. Although data are more extensive with respect to trimethadione, paramethadione, phenytoin, and phenobarbital, reports indicate a possible similar association with the use of other antiepileptic drugs. Therefore, antiepilepsy drug should be administered to women of childbearing potential only if they are clearly shown to be essential in the management of their seizures.

The incidence of neural tube defects in the fetus may be increased in mothers receiving valproate during the first trimester of pregnancy. The Centers for Disease Control (CDC) has estimated the risk of spina bifida to be approximately 1% to 2%.

Other congential anomalies (eg, craniofacial defects, cardiovascular malformations, anomalies involving various body systems), compatible and incompatible with life, have been reported. Sufficient data to determine the incidence of these congential anomalies is not available.

The higher incidence of congenital anomalies in antiepileptic drug-treated women with seizure disorders cannot be regarded as a cause and effect relationship. There are intrinsic methodologic problems in obtaining adequate data on drug teratogenicity in humans; genetic factors or the epileptic condition itself, may be more important than drug therapy in contributing to congenital anomalies.

Patients taking valproate may develop clotting abnormalities. A patient who had low fibrinogen when taking multiple anticonvulsants including valproate gave birth to an infant with afibrinogenemia who subsequently died of hemorrhage. If valproate is used in pregnancy, the clotting parameters should be monitored carefully.

Hepatic failure, resulting in the death of a newborn and of an infant, have been reported following the use of valproate during pregnancy.

Animal studies have demonstrated valproate-induced teratogenicity. Increased frequencies of malformations, as well as intrauterine growth retardation and death, have been observed in mice, rats, rabbits, and monkeys following prenatal exposure to valproate. Malformations of the skeletal system are the most common structural abnormalities produced in experimental animals, but neural tube closure defects have been seen in mice exposed to maternal plasma valproate concentrations exceeding 230 mcg/mL (2.3 times the upper limit of human therapeutic range) during susceptible periods of embryonic development. Administration of an oral dose of 200 mg/kg/day or greater (50% of the maximum human daily dose or greater on a mg/m^2 basis) to pregnant rats during organogenesis produced malformations (skeletal, cardiac, and urogenital) and growth retardation in the offspring. These doses resulted in peak maternal plasma valproate levels of approximately 340 mcg/mL or greater (3.4 times the upper limit of the human therapeutic range or greater). Behavioral deficits have been reported in the offspring of rats given a dose of 200 mg/kg/day thoughout most of the pregnancy. An oral dose of 350 mg/kg/day (approximately 2 times the maximum human daily dose on a mg/m^2 basis) produced skeletal and visceral malformations in rabbits exposed during organogenesis. Skeletal malformations, growth retardation, and death were observed in rhesus monkeys following administraton of an oral dose of 200 mg/kg/day (equal to the maximum human daily dose on a mg/m^2 basis) during organogenesis. This dose resulted in peak maternal plasma valproate levels of approximately 280 mcg/mL (2.8 times the upper limit of the human therapeutic range).

The prescribing physician will wish to weigh the benefits of therapy against the risks in treating or counseling women of childbearing potential. If this drug is used during pregnancy, or if the patient becomes pregnant while taking this drug, the patient should be apprised of the potential hazard to the fetus.

Antiepileptic drugs should not be discontinued abruptly in patients in whom the drug is administered to prevent major seizures because of the strong possibility of precipitating status epilepticus with attendant hypoxia and threat to life. In individual cases where the severity and frequency of the seizure disorder are such that the removal of medication does not pose a serious threat to the patient, discontinuation of the drug may be considered prior to and during pregnancy, although it cannot be said with any confidence that even minor seizures do not pose some hazard to the developing embryo or fetus.

Tests to detect neural tube and other defects using current accepted procedures should be considered a part of routine prenatal care in childbearing women receiving valproate.

➤*Lactation:* Valproate is excreted in breast milk. Concentrations in breast milk have been reported to be 1% to 10% of serum concentrations. It is not known what effect this would have on a nursing infant. Consideration should be given to discontinuing nursing when valproic acid is administered to a nursing woman.

➤*Children:* See the Warning box for more information.

Younger children, especially those receiving enzyme-inducing drugs, will require larger maintenance doses to attain targeted total and unbound valproic acid concentrations.

The variability in free fraction limits the clinical usefulness of monitoring total serum valproic acid concentrations. Interpretation of valproic acid concentrations in children should include consideration of factors that affect hepatic metabolism and protein binding.

The basic toxicology and pathologic manifestations of valproate sodium in neonatal (4-day-old) and juvenile (14-day-old) rats are similar to those seen in young adult rats. However, additional findings, including renal alterations in juvenile rats and renal alterations and retinal dysplasia in neonatal rats, have been reported. These findings occurred at 240 mg/kg/day, a dosage approximately equivalent to the human maximum recommended daily dose on a mg/m^2 basis. They were not seen at 90 mg/kg, or 40% of the maximum human daily dose on a mg/m^2 basis.

VALPROIC ACID — ORAL

Precautions

➤*Monitoring:* Since valproate may interact with concurrently administered drugs which are capable of enzyme induction, periodic plasma concentration determinations of valproate and concomitant drugs are recommended during the early course of therapy.

There are in vitro studies that suggest valproate stimulates the replication of the HIV and CMV viruses under certain experimental conditions. The clinical consequence, if any, is not known. Additionally, the relevance of these in vitro findings is uncertain for patients receiving maximally suppressive antiretroviral therapy. Nevertheless, these data should be borne in mind when interpreting the results from regular monitoring of the viral load in HIV-infected patients receiving valproate or when following CMV-infected patients clinically.

➤*Hepatic dysfunction:* See the Warning box for more information.

➤*Pancreatitis:* See Warnings for more information.

➤*Hyperammonemia:* See Warnings for more information.

Asymptomatic elevations of ammonia are more common and when present, require close monitoring of plasma ammonia levels. If the elevation persists, discontinuation of valproate therapy should be considered.

➤*Thrombocytopenia:* See Warnings for more information.

➤*Lab test abnormalities:* Valproate is partially eliminated in the urine as a keto-metabolite which may lead to a false interpretation of the urine ketone test.

There have been reports of altered thyroid function tests associated with valproate. The clinical significance of these is unknown.

➤*Hazardous tasks:* Since valproic acid products may produce CNS depression, especially when combined with another CNS depressant (eg, alcohol), patient should be advised not to engage in hazardous activities, such as driving an automobile or operating dangerous machinery, until it is known that they do not become drowsy from the drug.

Drug Interactions

Valproic Acid Drug Interactions

Precipitant drug	Object drug*		Description
Charcoal	Valproic acid	↓	Valproic acid absorption is decreased.
Chlorpromazine	Valproic acid	↑	Valproate t½ and trough levels may increase, clearance may decrease.
Cholestyramine	Valproic acid	↓	Serum concentrations and bioavailability of valproic acid may be reduced, resulting in a decrease in therapeutic effects. Administer valproic acid at least 3 hours before, but not within 3 hours following cholestyramine.
Cimetidine	Valproic acid	↑	Small but potentially significant decrease in valproate clearance and increase in t½.
Erythromycin	Valproic acid	↑	Erythromycin may increase serum valproic acid concentrations, producing valproic acid toxicity.
Felbamate	Valproic acid	↑	Coadministration revealed a 35% increase in mean peak valproate levels.
Rifampin	Valproic acid	↓	In 1 study, rifampin increased the oral clearance of valproate by 40%.
Salicylates (eg, aspirin)	Valproic acid	↑	Salicylates may displace valproic acid from protein binding sites and may also alter the metabolic pathways. Monitor serum concentrations.
Valproic acid	Tricyclic antidepressants	↑	Plasma concentrations and side effects of the tricyclic antidepressant may be increased. Coadministration resulted in a 21% decrease in the plasma clearance of amitriptyline and a 34% decrease in the net clearance of nortriptyline.
Valproic acid	Carbamazepine	↑	Variable changes in carbamazepine concentrations with increased levels of the active metabolite; decreased valproic acid levels with possible loss of seizure control may occur.
Carbamazepine	Valproic acid	↓	
Valproic acid	Clonazepam	↔	Concomitant use may induce absence status in patients with a history of absence type seizures.
Valproic acid	Diazepam	↑	Valproate displaces diazepam from its plasma albumin binding sites and inhibits its metabolism.
Valproic acid	Ethosuximide	↑↓	Increases and decreases in ethosuximide blood levels and decreases in valproic acid levels have been reported. Valproic acid appears to inhibit the metabolism of ethosuximide.
Ethosuximide	Valproic acid	↓	
Valproic acid	Lamotrigine	↑	Serum valproic acid concentrations may be decreased while lamotrigine levels increase. In one study, coadministration increased the half-life of lamotrigine from 26 to 70 hours. Lamotrigine dose should be reduced.
Lamotrigine	Valproic acid	↓	
Valproic acid	Barbiturates	↑	Valproic acid may decrease hepatic metabolism of barbiturates. Barbiturate dosage may need to be decreased in some patients.
Valproic acid	Hydantoins (eg, phenytoin)	↑	Increased action of phenytoin, even at therapeutic levels; increased metabolism of valproic acid with decreased pharmacologic effects may occur.
Hydantoins (eg, phenytoin)	Valproic acid	↓	
Valproic acid	Tolbutamide	↔	The unbound fraction of tolbutamide may be increased from 20% to 50%. The clinical relevance of this displacement is unknown.
Valproic acid	Warfarin	↑	The potential exists for valproate to displace warfarin from protein binding sites. Monitor coagulation tests.
Valproic acid	Zidovudine	↑	Zidovudine clearance was decreased by 38% in 6 HIV-seropositive patients.

* ↑ = Object drug increased. ↓ = Object drug decreased.
↔ = Undetermined clinical effect.

➤*Effects of coadministered drugs on valproate clearance:* Drugs that affect the level of expression of hepatic enzymes, particularly those that elevate levels of glucuronosyltransferases, may increase the clearance of valproate. For example, phenytoin, carbamazepine, and phenobarbital (or primidone) can double the clearance of valproate. Thus, patients on monotherapy will generally have longer half-lives and higher concentrations than patients receiving polytherapy with antiepilepsy drugs.

See Precautions for more information.

Adverse Reactions

Epilepsy – The data described in the following section were obtained using divalproex sodium (divalproex sodium) tablets:

Based on a placebo-controlled trial of adjunctive therapy for treatment of complex partial seizures, divalproex sodium was generally well tolerated with most adverse events rated as mild to moderate in severity. Intolerance was the primary reason for discontinuation in the divalproex sodium-treated patients (6%), compared to 1% of placebo-treated patients.

The following information lists treatment-emergent adverse events which were reported by greater than or equal to 5% of divalproex sodium-treated patients and for which the incidence was greater than in the placebo group, in a placebo-controlled trial of adjunctive therapy for the treatment of complex partial seizures. Since patients were also treated with other antiepilepsy drugs, it is not possible, in most cases, to determine whether the following adverse events can be ascribed to divalproex sodium alone, or the combination of divalproex sodium and other antiepilepsy drugs.

Adverse Reactions Reported by ≥ 5% of Patients Treated with Valproic Acid During Placebo-controlled Trial of Adjunctive Therapy for Complex Partial Seizures

Adverse reaction	Valproic acid (%) (n = 77)	Placebo (%) (n = 70)
Miscellaneous		
Headache	31%	21%
Asthenia	27%	7%
Fever	6%	4%
Alopecia	6%	1%
Weight loss	6%	0%

VALPROIC ACID — ORAL

Adverse Reactions Reported by ≥ 5% of Patients Treated with Valproic Acid During Placebo-controlled Trial of Adjunctive Therapy for Complex Partial Seizures

Adverse reaction	Valproic acid (%) (n = 77)	Placebo (%) (n = 70)
GI		
Nausea	48%	14%
Vomiting	27%	7%
Abdominal pain	23%	6%
Diarrhea	13%	6%
Anorexia	12%	0%
Dyspepsia	8%	4%
Constipation	5%	1%
CNS		
Somnolence	27%	11%
Tremor	25%	6%
Dizziness	25%	13%
Diplopia	16%	9%
Amblyopia/ blurred vision	12%	9%
Ataxia	8%	1%
Nystagmus	8%	1%
Emotional lability	6%	4%
Thinking abnormal	6%	0%
Amnesia	5%	1%
Respiratory		
Flu syndrome	12%	9%
Infection	12%	6%
Bronchitis	5%	1%
Rhinitis	5%	4%

Treatment-emergent adverse reactions which were reported by greater than or equal to 5% of patients in the high-dose divalproex sodium group – The following table lists treatment-emergent adverse reactions which were reported by greater than or equal to 5% of patients in the high-dose divalproex sodium group, and for which the incidence was greater than in the low-dose group, in a controlled trial of divalproex sodium monotherapy treatment of complex partial seizures. Since patients were being titrated off another antiepilepsy drug during the first portion of the trial, it is not possible, in many cases, to determine whether the following adverse reactions can be ascribed to divalproex sodium alone, or the combination of divalproex sodium and other antiepilepsy drugs.

Adverse Reactions Reported by ≥ 5% of Patients in the High-dose Group in the Controlled Trial of Valproic Acid Monotherapy for Complex Partial Seizures[1]

Adverse reaction	High dose (%) (n = 131)	Low dose (%) (n = 134)
Miscellaneous		
Asthenia	21%	10%
GI		
Nausea	34%	26%
Diarrhea	23%	19%
Vomiting	23%	15%
Abdominal pain	12%	9%
Anorexia	11%	4%
Dypepsia	11%	10%
Hematologic/lymphatic		
Thrombocytopenia	24%	1%
Ecchymosis	5%	4%
Metabolic/nutritional		
Weight gain	9%	4%
Peripheral edema	8%	3%
CNS		
Tremor	57%	19%
Somnolence	30%	18%
Dizziness	18%	13%
Insomnia	15%	9%
Nervousness	11%	7%
Amnesia	7%	4%
Nystagmus	7%	1%
Depression	5%	4%
Respiratory		
Infection	20%	13%
Pharyngitis	8%	2%
Dyspnea	5%	1%
Dermatologic		
Alopecia	24%	13%
Special senses		
Amblyopia/ blurred vision	8%	4%
Tinnitus	7%	1%

[1] Headache was the only adverse reaction that occurred in greater than or equal to 5% of patients in the high-dose group and at an equal or greater incidence in the low-dose group.

➤*Adverse reactions reported by greater than 1% but less than 5%:* The following additional adverse reactions were reported by greater than 1% but less than 5% of the 358 patients treated with divalproex sodium in the controlled trials of complex partial seizures:

Cardiovascular – Tachycardia, hypertension, palpitation.

CNS – Anxiety, confusion, abnormal gait, paresthesia, hypertonia, incoordination, abnormal dreams, personality disorder.

Dermatologic – Rash, pruritus, dry skin.

GI – Increased appetite, flatulence, hematemesis, eructation, pancreatitis, periodontal abscess.

GU – Urinary incontinence, vaginitis, dysmenorrhea, amenorrhea, urinary frequency.

Hematologic / Lymphatic – Petechia.

Metabolic / Nutritional – AST increased, ALT increased.

Musculoskeletal – Myalgia, twitching, arthralgia, leg cramps, myasthenia.

Respiratory – Sinusitis, cough increased, pneumonia, epistaxis.

Special senses – Taste perversion, abnormal vision, deafness, otitis media.

Miscellaneous – Back pain, chest pain, malaise.

➤*Other patient populations:* Adverse reactions that have been reported with all dosage forms of valproate from epilepsy trials, spontaneous reports, and other sources are listed below by body system.

CNS – Sedative effects have occurred in patients receiving valproate alone but occur most often in patients receiving combination therapy. Sedation usually abates upon reduction of other antiepileptic medication. Tremor (may be dose related), hallucinations, ataxia, headache, nystagmus, diplopia, asterixis, "spots before eyes", dysarthria, dizziness, confusion, hypesthesia, vertigo, incoordination, and parkinsonism have been reported with the use of valproate. Rare cases of coma have occurred in patients receiving valproic acid alone or in conjunction with phenobarbital. In rare instances, encephalopathy with or without fever has developed shortly after the introduction of valproate monotherapy without evidence of hepatic dysfunction or inappropriately high plasma valproate levels. Although recovery has been described following drug withdrawal, there have been fatalities in patients with hyperammonemic encephalopathy, particularly in patients with underlying urea cycle disorders.

See Warnings for more information.

Several reports have noted reversible cerebral atrophy and dementia in association with valproate therapy.

Dermatologic – Transient hair loss, skin rash, photosensitivity, generalized pruritus, erythema multiforme, and Stevens-Johnson syndrome. Rare cases of toxic epidermal necrolysis have been reported including a fatal case in a 6-month-old infant taking valproate and several other concomitant medications. An additional case of toxic epidermal necrosis resulting in death was reported in a 35-year-old patient with AIDS taking several concomitant medications and with a history of multiple cutaneous drug reactions.

Endocrine – Irregular menses, secondary amenorrhea, breast enlargement, galactorrhea, and parotid gland swelling, abnormal thyroid function tests.

There have been rare spontaneous reports of polycystic ovary disease. A cause-and-effect relationship has not been established.

GI – The most commonly reported side effects at the initiation of therapy are nausea, vomiting, and indigestion. These effects are usually transient and rarely require discontinuation of therapy. Diarrhea, abdominal cramps, and constipation have been reported. Both anorexia with some weight loss and increased appetite with weight gain have also been reported. The administration of delayed-release divalproex sodium may result in reduction of gastrointestinal side effects in some patients.

Pancreatic: Patients and guardians should be warned that abdominal pain, nausea, vomiting, or anorexia can be symptoms of pancreatitis that require prompt medical evaluation. If pancreatitis is diagnosed, valproate should ordinarily be discontinued. Alternative treatment for the underlying medical condition should be initiated as clinically indicated.

VALPROIC ACID — ORAL

GU – Enuresis and urinary tract infection.

Hematologic – Thrombocytopenia and inhibition of the secondary phase of platelet aggregation may be reflected in altered bleeding time, petechiae, bruising, hematoma formation, epistaxis, and frank hemorrhage. Relative lymphocytosis, macrocytosis, hypofibrinogenemia, leukopenia, eosinophilia, anemia including macrocytic with or without folate deficiency, bone marrow suppression, pancytopenia, aplastic anemia, and acute intermittent porphyria.

Hepatic – Minor elevations of transaminases (eg, AST, ALT) and LDH are frequent and appear to be dose related. Occasionally, laboratory test results include increases in serum bilirubin and abnormal changes in other liver function tests. These results may reflect potentially serious hepatotoxicity. Serious or fatal hepatotoxicity may be preceded by nonspecific symptoms such as malaise, weakness, lethargy, facial edema, anorexia, and vomiting. In patients with epilepsy, a loss of seizure control may also occur. Patients should be monitored closely for appearance of these symptoms.

Metabolic – Hyperammonemia, hyponatremia, and inappropriate ADH secretion. In patients who develop unexplained lethargy and vomiting or changes in mental status, hyperammonemic encephalopathy should be considered, and an ammonia level should be measured. If ammonia is increased, valproate therapy should be discontinued.

There have been rare reports of Fanconi's syndrome occurring chiefly in children.

Decreased carnitine concentrations have been reported although the clinical relevance is undetermined.

Hyperglycinemia has occurred and was associated with a fatal outcome in a patient with preexistent nonketotic hyperglycinemia.

Musculoskeletal – Weakness.

Psychiatric – Emotional upset, depression, psychosis, aggression, hyperactivity, hostility, and behavioral deterioration.

Special senses – Hearing loss, either reversible or irreversible, has been reported; however, a cause and effect relationship has not been established. Ear pain has also been reported.

Miscellaneous – Anaphylaxis, edema of the extremities, lupus erythematosus, bone pain, cough increased, pneumonia, otitis media, bradycardia, cutaneous vasculitis, and fever.

➤*Mania:* Although valproic acid has not been evaluated for safety and efficacy in the treatment of manic episodes associated with bipolar disorder, the following adverse reactions not listed above were reported by 1% or more of patients from 2 placebo-controlled clinical trials of divalproex sodium tablets.

Cardiovascular – Hypotension, postural hypotension, vasodilation.

CNS – Agitation, catatonic reaction, hypokinesia, reflexes increased, tardive dyskinesia, vertigo.

Dermatologic – Furunculosis, maculopapular rash, seborrhea.

GI – Fecal incontinence, gastroenteritis, glossitis.

GU – Dysuria.

Musculoskeletal – Arthrosis.

Special senses – Conjunctivitis, dry eyes, eye pain.

Miscellaneous – Chills, neck pain, neck rigidity.

➤*Migraine:* Although valproic acid has not been evaluated for safety and efficacy in the treatment of prophylaxis of migraine headaches, the following adverse reactions not listed above were reported by 1% or more of patients from 2 placebo-controlled clinical trials of divalproex sodium tablets:

GI – Dry mouth, stomatitis.

GU – Cystitis, metrorrhagia, and vaginal hemorrhage.

Miscellaneous – Face edema.

Overdosage

➤*Symptoms:* Overdosage with valproate may result in somnolence, heart block, and deep coma. Fatalities have been reported; however, patients have recovered from valproate levels as high as 2120 mcg/mL.

➤*Treatment:* In overdose situations, the fraction of drug not bound to protein is high, and hemodialysis or tandem hemodialysis plus hemoperfusion may result in significant removal of drug. The benefit of gastric lavage or emesis will vary with the time since ingestion. General supportive measures should be applied with particular attention to the maintenance of adequate urinary output.

Naloxone has been reported to reverse the CNS-depressant effects of valproate overdosage. Because naloxone could theoretically also reverse the antiepileptic effects of valproate, it should be used with caution in patients with epilepsy.

Patient Information

Patients and guardians should be warned that abdominal pain, nausea, vomiting, or anorexia can be symptoms of pancreatitis and, therefore, require further medical evaluation promptly.

Patients should be informed of the signs and symptoms associated with hyperammonemic encephalopathy and be told to inform the prescriber if any of these symptoms occur. In patients who develop unexplained lethargy and vomiting or changes in mental status, hyperammonemic encephalopathy should be considered, and an ammonia level should be measured. If ammonia is increased, valproate therapy should be discontinued.

Since valproic acid products may produce CNS depression, especially when combined with another CNS depressant (eg, alcohol), patient should be advised not to engage in hazardous activities, such as driving an automobile or operating dangerous machinery, until it is known that they do not become drowsy from the drug.

Patients and guardians should be warned that malaise, weakness, lethargy, facial edema, anorexia, and vomiting can be symptoms of hepatotoxicity and, therefore, require further medical evaluation promptly.

The incidence of neural tube defects in the fetus may be increased in mothers receiving valproate during the first trimester of pregnancy. The Centers for Disease Control (CDC) has estimated the risk of spina bifida to be approximately 1% to 2%.

The prescribing physician will wish to weigh the benefits of therapy against the risks in treating or counseling women of childbearing potential. If this drug is used during pregnancy, or if the patient becomes pregnant while taking this drug, the patient should be apprised of the potential hazard to the fetus.

DIVALPROEX SODIUM — ORAL

WARNING

Felbamate should not be used by patients until there has been a complete discussion of the risks and the patient, parent, or guardian has provided written informed consent.

Aplastic anemia – The use of felbamate is associated with a marked increase in the incidence of aplastic anemia. Accordingly, felbamate should only be used in patients whose epilepsy is so severe that the risk of aplastic anemia is deemed acceptable in light of the benefits conferred by its use. Ordinarily, a patient should not be placed on or continued on felbamate without consideration of appropriate expert hematologic consultation.

Among felbamate treated patients, aplastic anemia (pancytopenia in the presence of a bone marrow largely depleted of hematopoietic precursors) occurs at an incidence that may be more than a 100-fold greater than that seen in the untreated population (ie, 2 to 5 per million persons per year). The risk of death in patients with aplastic anemia generally varies as a function of its severity and etiology; current estimates of the overall case fatality rate are in the range of 20% to 30%, but rates as high as 70% have been reported in the past.

There are too few felbamate associated cases, and too little known about them to provide a reliable estimate of the syndrome's incidence or its case fatality rate or to identify the factors, if any, that might conceivably be used to predict who is at greater or lesser risk.

In managing patients on felbamate, it should be borne in mind that the clinical manifestation of aplastic anemia may not be seen until after a patient has been on felbamate for several months (eg, onset of aplastic anemia among felbamate exposed patients for whom data are available has ranged from 5 to 30 weeks). However, the injury to bone marrow stem cells that is held to be ultimately responsible for the anemia may occur weeks to months earlier. Accordingly, patients who are discontinued from felbamate remain at risk for developing anemia for a variable, and unknown, period afterwards.

WARNING (cont.)

It is not known whether or not the risk of developing aplastic anemia changes with duration of exposure. Consequently, it is not safe to assume that a patient who has been on felbamate without signs of hematologic abnormality for long periods of time is without risk.

It is not known whether the dose of felbamate affects the incidence of aplastic anemia.

It is not known whether or not concomitant use of antiepileptic drugs or other drugs affects the incidence of aplastic anemia.

An information sheet describing the teratogenic potential of valproate is available for patients.

Pancreatitis – Cases of life-threatening pancreatitis have been reported in both children and adults receiving valproate. Some of the cases have been described as hemorrhagic with a rapid progression from initial symptoms to death. Cases have been reported shortly after initial use and after several years of use. Patients and guardians should be warned that abdominal pain, nausea, vomiting, and anorexia can be symptoms of pancreatitis that require prompt medical evaluation. If pancreatitis is diagnosed, valproate should ordinarily be discontinued. Alternative treatment for the underlying medical condition should be initiated as clinically indicated.

Indications

➤*Epilepsy (sprinkle capsules, delayed-release tablets and extended-release tablets):* As monotherapy or adjunctive therapy in the treatment of adult patients with complex partial seizures that occur either in isolation or in association with other types of seizures.

For use as sole and adjunctive therapy in the treatment of simple and complex absence seizures in adult patients, and adjunctively in adult patients with multiple seizure types that include absence seizures.

Divalproex sodium sprinkle capsules and delayed-release tablets are administered orally. Divalproex sodium capsules and delayed-release tablets are indicated as monotherapy and adjunctive therapy in complex partial seizures in adults and pediatric patients down to the age of 10 years, and in

DIVALPROEX SODIUM — ORAL

simple and complex absence seizures. Divalproex sodium extended-release tablets are indicated as monotherapy and adjunctive therapy in complex partial seizures in adult patients only. As the divalproex sodium dosage is titrated upward, concentrations of phenobarbital, carbamazepine, and phenytoin may be affected.

➤*Complex partial seizures:* Divalproex sodium capsules and delayed-release tablets are indicated for complex partial seizures in adults and children greater than or equal to 10 years of age. Divalproex sodium tablets are indicated for complex partial seizures in adult patients only.

➤*Migraine (delayed-release and extended-release tablets):* For prophylaxis of migraine headaches. There is no evidence that divalproex sodium is useful in the acute treatment of migraine headaches. Because valproic acid may be a hazard to the fetus, divalproex sodium should be considered for women of childbearing potential only after this risk has been thoroughly discussed with the patient and weighed against the potential benefits of treatment.

Before using divalproex sodium (DR and ER), women who can become pregnant should consider the fact that divalproex sodium (DR and ER) has been associated with birth defects, in particular, with spina bifida and other defects related to failure of the spinal canal to close normally. Although the incidence is unknown in migraine patients treated with divalproex sodium (DR and ER), approximately 1% to 2% of children born to women with epilepsy taking divalproex sodium (DR and ER) in the first 12 weeks of pregnancy had these defects (based on data from the Centers for Disease Control, a US agency based in Atlanta). The incidence in the general population is 0.1% to 0.2%.

➤*Mania (delayed-release and extended-release tablets):* For the treatment of the manic episodes (delayed-release) and acute manic or mixed episodes, with or without psychotic features (extended-release), associated with bipolar disorder. A manic episode is a distinct period of abnormally and persistently elevated, expansive, or irritable mood. Typical symptoms of mania include pressure of speech, motor hyperactivity, reduced need for sleep, flight of ideas, grandiosity, poor judgement, aggressiveness, and possible hostility. A mixed episode is characterized by the criteria for a manic episode in conjunction with those for a major depressive episode (depressed mood, loss of interest or pleasure in nearly all activities).

➤*Unlabeled uses:* Divalproex sodium may be effective alone or in combination in the treatment of absence, myoclonic, and grand mal seizures. It may also be effective in patients with intractable status epilepticus who have not responded to other therapies. Divalproex sodium may be effective for minor incontinence after ileoanal anastomosis (subchronic administration).

Administration and Dosage

➤*Approved by the FDA:* March 10, 1983.

Antiepilepsy drugs should not be abruptly discontinued in patients in whom the drug is administered to prevent major seizures because of the strong possibility of precipitating status epilepticus with attendant hypoxia and threat to life.

In epileptic patients previously receiving valproic acid therapy, divalproex sodium delayed-release tablets and divalproex sodium sprinkle capsules should be initiated at the same daily dose and dosing schedule. After the patient is stabilized on divalproex sodium delayed-release tablets and divalproex sprinkle capsules, a dosing schedule of 2 or 3 times a day may be elected in selected patients.

➤*Extended-release tablets:* Divalproex sodium extended-release tablets are for once-a-day oral administration. Divalproex sodium extended-release tablets should be swallowed whole and should not be crushed or chewed.

Mania – 25/mg/kg/day given once daily. The dose should be increased as rapidly as possible to achieve the lowest therapeutic dose, which produces the desired clinical effect or the desired range of plasma concentrations. In placebo-controlled clinical trials of acute mania, patients were dosed to a clinical response with a trough plasma concentration between 85 and 125 mcg/mL. The maximum recommended dosage is 60 mg/kg/day.

Migraine – 500 mg once daily for 1 week, thereafter increasing to 1000 mg once daily. Although doses other than 1000 mg once daily of divalproex sodium extended-release have not been evaluated in patients with migraine, the effective dose range of divalproex sodium delayed-release tablets in these patients is 500 to 1000 mg/day. As with other valproate products, doses of divalproex sodium extended-release should be individualized and dose adjustment may be necessary. If a patient requires smaller dose adjustments than that available with divalproex sodium extended-release tablets, divalproex sodium delayed-release tablets should be used instead.

Epilepsy –

Conversion from divalproex sodium to divalproex sodium extended-release: In adult patients with epilepsy previously receiving divalproex sodium delayed-release, divalproex sodium extended-release should be administered once daily, using a dose 8% to 20% higher than the total daily dose of divaloproex sodium delayed-release (see information below). For patients whose divalproex sodium delayed-release total daily dose can not be directly converted to divalproex sodium extended-release, consideration may be given at the clinician's discretion to increase the patient's divalproex sodium delayed-release total daily dose to the next higher dosage before converting to the appropriate total daily dose of divalproex sodium extended-release.

• *Dose conversion* – The following guidelines may be used when converting a patient from divalproex sodium delayed-release to divalproex sodium extended-release:

- A total daily dose of 500 to 625 mg divalproex sodium converts to 750 mg divalproex sodium extended-release.
- A total daily dose of 750 to 875 mg divalproex sodium converts to 1000 mg divalproex sodium extended-release.
- A total daily dose of 1000 to 1125 mg divalproex sodium converts to 1250 mg divalproex sodium extended-release.
- A total daily dose of 1250 to 1375 mg divalproex sodium converts to 1500 mg divalproex sodium extended-release.
- A total daily dose of 1500 to 1625 mg divalproex sodium converts to 1750 mg divalproex sodium extended-release.
- A total daily dose of 1750 mg divalproex sodium converts to 2000 mg divalproex sodium extended-release.
- A total daily dose of 1875 to 2000 mg divalproex sodium converts to 2250 mg divalproex sodium extended-release.
- A total daily dose of 2125 to 2250 mg divalproex sodium converts to 2500 mg divalproex sodium extended-release.
- A total daily dose of 2375 mg divalproex sodium converts to 2750 mg divalproex sodium extended-release.
- A total daily dose of 2500 to 2750 mg divalproex sodium converts to 3000 mg divalproex sodium extended-release.
- A total daily dose of 2875 mg divalproex sodium converts to 3250 mg divalproex sodium extended-release.
- A total daily dose of 3000 mg to 3125 mg divalproex sodium converts to 3500 mg divalproex sodium extended-release.

Total daily doses of 500 mg, 750 mg, and 1000 mg divalproex sodium cannot be directly converted to an 8% to 20% higher total daily dose of divalproex sodium extended-release because the required dosing strengths of divalproex sodium extended-release are not available. Consideration may be given at the clinician's discretion to increase the patient's divalproex sodium total daily dose to the next higher dosage before converting to the appropriate total daily dose of divalproex sodium extended-release.

There are insufficient data to allow a conversion factor recommendation for patients with divalproex sodium doses above 3125 mg/day.

Compliance – Patients should be informed to take divalproex sodium extended-release every day as prescribed. If a dose is missed it should be taken as soon as possible, unless it is almost time for the next dose. If a dose is skipped, the patient should not double the next dose.

➤*Delayed-release:*

Mania – 750 mg daily, orally in divided doses. The dose should be increased as rapidly as possible to achieve the lowest therapeutic dose, which produces the desired clinical effect or the desired range of plasma concentrations. In placebo-controlled clinical trials of acute mania, patients were dosed to a clinical response with a trough plasma concentration between 50 and 125 mcg/mL. Maximum concentrations were generally achieved within 14 days (delayed-release). The maximum recommended dosage is 60 mg/kg/day.

There is no body of evidence available from controlled trials to guide a clinician in the longer-term management of a patient who improves during divalproex sodium treatment of an acute manic episode. While it is generally agreed that pharmacological treatment beyond an acute response in mania is desirable, both for maintenance of the initial response and for prevention of new manic episodes, there are no systemically obtained data to support the benefits of divalproex sodium in such long-term treatment. Although there are no efficacy data that specifically address longer-term antimanic treatment with divalproex sodium, the safety of divalproex sodium in long-term use is supported by data from record reviews involving approximately 360 patients treated with divalproex sodium for greater than or equal to 3 months.

Migraine – 250 mg orally, twice daily. Some patients may benefit from doses up to 1000 mg/day. In the clinical trials, there was no evidence that higher doses led to greater efficacy.

➤*Sprinkle capsules, delayed-release tablets and extended-release tablets:*

Monotherapy (initial therapy) – Divalproex sodium has not been systematically studied as initial therapy. Initiate therapy orally at 10 to 15 mg/kg/day. The dosage should be increased by 5 to 10 mg/kg/week to achieve optimal clinical response. Ordinarily, optimal clinical response is achieved at daily doses less than 60 mg/kg/day. If satisfactory clinical response has not been achieved, plasma levels should be measured to determine whether or not they are in the usually accepted therapeutic range (50 to 100 mcg/mL). No recommendation regarding the safety of valproate for use at doses greater than 60 mg/kg/day can be made.

Conversion to monotherapy – Initiate therapy orally at 10 to 15 mg/kg/day. The dosage should be increased by 5 to 10 mg/kg/week to achieve optimal clinical response. Ordinarily, optimal clinical response is achieved at daily doses below 60 mg/kg/day. If satisfactory clinical response has not been achieved, plasma levels should be measured to determine whether or not they are in the usually accepted therapeutic range (50 to 100 mcg/mL). No recommendation regarding the safety of valproate for use at doses greater than 60 mg/kg/day can be made. Concomitant antiepilepsy drug (AED) dosage can ordinarily be reduced by approximately 25% every 2 weeks. This reduction may be started at initiation of divalproex sodium therapy, or delayed by 1 to 2 weeks if there is a concern that seizures are likely to occur with a reduction. The speed and duration of withdrawal of the concomitant AED can be highly variable, and patients should be monitored closely during this period for increased seizure frequency.

Adjunctive therapy – Divalproex sodium may be added to the patient's regimen at a dosage of 10 to 15 mg/kg/day. The dosage may be increased by 5 to 10 mg/kg/week to achieve optimal clinical response. Ordinarily, optimal clinical response is achieved at daily doses below 60 mg/kg/day. If satisfactory clinical response has not been achieved, plasma levels should be measured to determine whether or not they are in the usually accepted

DIVALPROEX SODIUM — ORAL

therapeutic range (50 to 100 mcg/mL). No recommendation regarding the safety of valproate for use at doses greater than 60 mg/kg/day can be made. If the total daily dose exceeds 250 mg, it should be given in divided doses.

Simple and complex absence seizures – 15 mg/kg/day, increasing at 1-week intervals by 5 to 10 mg/kg/day until seizures are controlled or side effects preclude further increases. The maximum recommended dosage is 60 mg/kg/day. If the total daily dose exceeds 250 mg, it should be given in divided doses.

A good correlation has not been established between daily dose, serum concentrations, and therapeutic effect. However, therapeutic valproate serum concentrations for most patients with absence seizures is considered to range from 50 to 100 mcg/mL. Some patients may be controlled with lower or higher serum concentrations.

➤*General dosing advice:*

Elderly patients – Due to a decrease in unbound clearance of valproate and possibly a sensitivity to somnolence in the elderly, the starting dose of divalproex sodium should be reduced in these patients. Starting doses in the elderly lower than 250 mg can only be achieved by the use of divalproex sodium delayed-release tablets. Dosage should be increased more slowly and with regular monitoring for fluid and nutritional intake, dehydration, somnolence, and other adverse events. Dose reductions or discontinuation of valproate should be considered in patients with decreased food or fluid intake and in patients with excessive somnolence. The ultimate therapeutic dose should be achieved on the basis of both tolerability and clinical response.

GI irritation – Patients who experience GI irritation may benefit from administration of the drug with food or by slowly building up the dose from an initial low level.

Sprinkle capsules –

Administration: Divalproex sodium sprinkle capsules may be swallowed whole or may be administered by carefully opening the capsule and sprinkling the entire contents on a small amount (teaspoonful) of soft food such as applesauce or pudding. The drug/food mixture should be swallowed immediately (avoid chewing) and not stored for future use. Each capsule is oversized to allow ease of opening.

➤*Storage/Stability:*

Sprinkle capsules – Store capsules below 25°C (77°F).

Delayed-release tablets – Store tablets below 30°C (86°F).

Extended-release tablets – Store tablets at 25°C (77°F); excursions permitted to 15° to 30°C (59° to 86°F).

Actions

➤*Pharmacology:* Divalproex sodium dissociates to the valproate ion in the GI tract. The mechanisms by which valproate exerts its therapeutic effects have not been established. It has been suggested that its activity in epilepsy is related to increased brain concentrations of gamma-aminobutyric acid (GABA).

➤*Pharmacokinetics:*

Absorption –

Sprinkle capsules and delayed-release tablets: Equivalent oral doses of divalproex sodium products and valproic acid capsules deliver equivalent quantities of valproate ion systemically. Although the rate of valproate ion absorption may vary with the formulation administered (ie, liquid, solid, or sprinkle), conditions of use (eg, fasting, postprandial) and the method of administration (eg, whether the contents of the capsule are sprinkled on food or the capsule is taken intact), these differences should be of minor clinical importance under the steady state conditions achieved in chronic use in the treatment of epilepsy.

However, it is possible that differences among the various valproate products in t_{max} and C_{max} could be important upon initiation of treatment. For example, in single-dose studies, the effect of feeding had a greater influence on the rate of absorption of the tablet (increase in t_{max} from 4 to 8 hours) than on the absorption of the sprinkle capsules (increase in t_{max} from 3.3 to 4.8 hours).

While the absorption rate from the GI tract and fluctuation in valproate plasma concentrations vary with dosing regimen and formulation, the efficacy of valproate as an anticonvulsant in chronic use is unlikely to be affected. Experience employing dosing regimens from once a day to 4 times daily, as well as studies in primate epilepsy models involving constant rate infusion, indicate that total daily systemic bioavailability (extent of absorption) is the primary determinant of seizure control and that differences in the ratios of plasma peak to trough concentrations between valproate formulations are inconsequential from a practical clinical standpoint.

Coadministration of oral valproate products with food and substitution among the various divalproex sodium and valproic acid formulations should cause no clinical problems in the management of patients with epilepsy. Nonetheless, any changes in dosage administration, or the addition or discontinuance of concomitant drugs should ordinarily be accompanied by close monitoring of clinical status and valproate plasma concentrations.

Extended-release tablets: The absolute bioavailability of divalproex sodium extended-release tablets administered as a single dose after a meal was approximately 90% relative to IV infusion.

When given in equal total daily doses, the bioavailability of divalproex sodium extended-release is less than that of divalproex sodium delayed-release tablets. In 5 multiple-dose studies in healthy subjects (n = 82) and in subjects with epilepsy (n = 86), when administered under fasting and nonfasting conditions, divalproex sodium extended-release given once daily produced an average bioavailability of 89% relative to an equal total daily dose of divalproex sodium delayed-release given twice daily, 3 times daily, or 4 times daily. The median time to maximum plasma valproate concentrations (C_{max}) after divalproex sodium extended-release administration ranged from 4 to 17 hours. After multiple once-daily dosing of divalproex sodium extended-release, the peak-to-trough fluctuation in plasma valproate concentrations was 10% to 20% lower than that of regular divalproex sodium given twice daily, 3 times daily, or 4 times daily.

Distribution –

Protein binding: The plasma protein binding of valproate is concentration dependent, and the free fraction increases from approximately 10% at 40 mcg/mL to 18.5% at 130 mcg/mL. Protein binding of valproate is reduced in the elderly, in patients with chronic hepatic diseases, in patients with renal impairment, and in the presence of other drugs (eg, aspirin). Conversely, valproate may displace certain protein-bound drugs (eg, phenytoin, carbamazepine, warfarin, tolbutamide).

CNS distribution: Valproate concentrations in cerebrospinal fluid (CSF) approximate unbound concentrations in plasma (approximately 10% of total concentration).

Metabolism – Valproate is metabolized almost entirely by the liver. In adult patients on monotherapy, 30% to 50% of an administered dose appears in urine as a glucuronide conjugate. Mitochondrial β-oxidation is the other major metabolic pathway, typically accounting for greater than 40% of the dose. Usually, less than 15% to 20% of the dose is eliminated by other oxidative mechanisms. Less than 3% of an administered dose is excreted unchanged in urine.

The relationship between dose and total valproate concentration is nonlinear; concentration does not increase proportionally with the dose, but rather, increases to a lesser extent due to saturable plasma protein binding. The kinetics of unbound drug are linear.

Excretion – Mean plasma clearance and volume of distribution for total valproate are 0.56 L/hr/1.73 m^2 and 11 L/1.73 m^2, respectively. Mean plasma clearance and volume of distribution for free valproate are 4.6 L/hr/1.73 m^2 and 92 L/1.73 m^2. Mean terminal half-life for valproate monotherapy ranged from 9 to 16 hours following oral dosing regimens of 250 to 1000 mg.

The estimates cited apply primarily to patients who are not taking drugs that affect hepatic-metabolizing enzyme systems. For example, patients taking enzyme-inducing antiepileptic drugs (carbamazepine, phenytoin, and phenobarbital) will clear valproate more rapidly. Because of these changes in valproate clearance, monitoring of antiepileptic concentrations should be intensified whenever concomitant antiepileptics are introduced or withdrawn.

Special populations –

Renal function impairment: A slight reduction (27%) in the unbound clearance of valproate has been reported in patients with renal failure (creatinine clearance less than 10 mL/min); however, hemodialysis typically reduces valproate concentrations by approximately 20%. Therefore, no dosage adjustment appears to be necessary in patients with renal failure. Protein binding in these patients is substantially reduced; thus, monitoring total concentrations may be misleading.

Hepatic function impairment: Liver disease impairs the capacity to eliminate valproate. In 1 study, the clearance of free valproate was decreased by 50% in 7 patients with cirrhosis and by 16% in 4 patients with acute hepatitis, compared with 6 healthy subjects. In that study, the half-life of valproate was increased from 12 to 18 hours. Liver disease is also associated with decreased albumin concentrations and larger unbound fractions (2- to 2.6-fold increase) of valproate. Accordingly, monitoring of total concentrations may be misleading since free concentrations may be substantially elevated in patients with hepatic disease whereas total concentrations may appear to be normal.

Elderly: The capacity of elderly patients (age range, 68 to 89 years) to eliminate valproate has been shown to be reduced compared to younger adults (age range, 22 to 26). Intrinsic clearance is reduced by 39%; the free fraction is increased by 44%. Accordingly, the initial dosage should be reduced in the elderly. Starting doses in the elderly lower than 250 mg can only be achieved by the use of divalproex sodium delayed-release tablets. Dosage should be increased more slowly and with regular monitoring for fluid and nutritional intake, dehydration, somnolence, and other adverse events.

Children:

• *Neonates* – Children within the first 2 months of life have a markedly decreased ability to eliminate valproate compared to older children and adults. This is a result of reduced clearance (perhaps due to delay in development of glucuronosyltransferase and other enzyme systems involved in valproate elimination) as well as increased volume of distribution (in part due to decreased plasma protein binding). For example, in 1 study, the half-life in children less than 10 days of age ranged from 10 to 67 hours compared to a range of 7 to 13 hours in children greater than 2 months.

• *Children* – Children (ie, between 3 months and 10 years) have 50% higher clearances expressed on weight (ie, mL/min/kg) than do adults. Over the age of 10 years, children have pharmacokinetic parameters that approximate those of adults.

Contraindications

Hepatic disease or significant hepatic dysfunction; hypersensitivity to the drug; known urea cycle disorders.

Warnings

➤*Pancreatitis:* Cases of life-threatening pancreatitis have been reported in both children and adults receiving valproate. Some of the cases have been described as hemorrhagic, with rapid progression from initial symptoms to death. Some cases have occurred shortly after initial use and after several years of use. The rate based upon the reported cases exceeds that expected in the general population and there have been cases in which pancreatitis recurred after rechallenge with valproate. In clinical trials, there were 2 cases of pancreatitis without alternative etiology in 2416 patients, representing 1044 patient-years experience. Patients and guardians should be

DIVALPROEX SODIUM — ORAL

warned that abdominal pain, nausea, vomiting, and anorexia can be symptoms of pancreatitis that require prompt medical evaluation. If pancreatitis is diagnosed, valproate should ordinarily be discontinued. Alternative treatment for the underlying medical condition should be initiated as clinically indicated.

➤*Urea cycle disorders:* Divalproex sodium is contraindicated in patients with known urea cycle disorders.

Hyperammonemic encephalopathy, sometimes fatal, has been reported following initiation of valproate therapy in patients with urea cycle disorders, a group of uncommon genetic abnormalities, particularly ornithine transcarbamylase deficiency. Prior to the initiation of valproate therapy, evaluation for UCD should be considered in the following patients:

Those with a history of unexplained encephalopathy or coma, encephalopathy associated with a protein load, pregnancy-related or postpartum encephalopathy, unexplained mental retardation, or history of elevated plasma ammonia or glutamine.

Those with cyclical vomiting and lethargy, episodic extreme irritability, ataxia, low blood urea nitrogen (BUN), or protein avoidance.

Those with a family history of UCD or a family history of unexplained infant deaths (particularly males).

Those with other signs and symptoms of UCD. Patients who develop symptoms of unexplained hyperammonemic encephalopathy while receiving valproate therapy should receive prompt treatment (including discontinuation of valproate therapy) and be evaluated for underlying urea cycle disorders.

➤*Thrombocytopenia:* The frequency of adverse reactions (particularly elevated liver enzymes and thrombocytopenia) may be dose related. In a clinical trial of divalproex sodium as monotherapy in patients with epilepsy, 34/126 patients (27%) receiving approximately 50 mg/kg/day on average, had at least 1 value of platelets less than or equal to 75 × 10^9/L. Approximately half of these patients had treatment discontinued, with return of platelet counts to normal. In the remaining patients, platelet counts normalized with continued treatment. In this study, the probability of thrombocytopenia appeared to increase significantly at total valproate concentrations of greater than or equal to 110 mcg/mL (females) or greater than or equal to 135 mcg/mL (males). The therapeutic benefit that may accompany the higher doses should therefore be weighed against the possibility of a greater incidence of adverse reactions.

➤*Hepatic function impairment:* Hepatic failure resulting in fatalities has occurred in patients receiving valproic acid. These incidents usually have occurred during the first 6 months of treatment. Serious or fatal hepatotoxicity may be preceded by nonspecific symptoms such as malaise, weakness, lethargy, facial edema, anorexia, and vomiting. In patients with epilepsy, a loss of seizure control may also occur. Patients should be monitored closely for appearance of these symptoms.

Caution should be observed when administering divalproex sodium products to patients with a history of hepatic disease. Patients on multiple anticonvulsants, children, those with congenital metabolic disorders, those with severe seizure disorders accompanied by mental retardation, and those with organic brain disease may be at particular risk. Experience has indicated that children younger than 2 years of age are at a considerably increased risk of developing fatal hepatotoxicity, especially those with the aforementioned conditions. When divalproex sodium is used in this patient group, it should be used with extreme caution and as a sole agent. The benefits of therapy should be weighed against the risks. Above this age group, experience in epilepsy has indicated that the incidence of fatal hepatotoxicity decreases considerably in progressively older patient groups. The use of divalproex sodium extended-release tablets in children is not recommended.

The drug should be discontinued immediately in the presence of significant hepatic dysfunction, suspected or apparent. In some cases, hepatic dysfunction has progressed in spite of discontinuation of drug.

➤*Carcinogenesis:* Valproic acid was administered orally to Sprague-Dawley rats and ICR (HA/ICR) mice at doses of 80 and 170 mg/kg/day (approximately 10% to 50% of the maximum human daily dose on a mg/m^2 basis) for 2 years. A variety of neoplasms were observed in both species. The chief findings were a statistically significant increase in the incidence of subcutaneous fibrosarcomas in high-dose male rats receiving valproic acid and a statistically significant dose-related trend for benign pulmonary adenomas in male mice receiving valproic acid. The significance of these findings for humans is unknown.

➤*Mutagenesis:* Increased frequencies of sister chromatid exchange (SCE) have been reported in a study of epileptic children taking valproate, but this association was not observed in another study conducted in adults. There is some evidence that increased SCE frequencies may be associated with epilepsy. The biological significance of an increase in SCE frequency is not known.

➤*Fertility impairment:* Chronic toxicity studies in juvenile and adult rats and dogs demonstrated reduced spermatogenesis and testicular atrophy at oral doses of 400 mg/kg/day or greater in rats (approximately equivalent to or greater than the maximum human daily dose on a mg/m^2 basis) and 150 mg/kg/day or greater in dogs (approximately 1.4 times the maximum human daily dose or greater on a mg/m^2 basis). Segment I fertility studies in rats have shown oral doses up to 350 mg/kg/day (approximately 3.5 times the maximum human daily dose on a mg/m^2 basis for ER tablets and approximately equal to the maximum human daily dose on a mg/m^2 basis) for 60 days to have no effect on fertility. The effect of valproate on testicular development and on sperm production and fertility in humans is unknown.

➤*Elderly:*

Somnolence – In a double-blind, multicenter trial of valproate in elderly patients with dementia (mean age = 83 years), doses were increased by 125 mg/day to a target dose of 20 mg/kg/day. A significantly higher proportion of valproate patients had somnolence compared to placebo, and although not statistically significant, there was a higher proportion of patients with dehydration. Discontinuations for somnolence were also significantly higher than with placebo. In some patients with somnolence (approximately one-half), there was associated reduced nutritional intake and weight loss. There was a trend for the patients who experienced these events to have a lower baseline albumin concentration, lower valproate clearance, and a higher blood urea nitrogen (BUN). In elderly patients, dosage should be increased more slowly and with regular monitoring for fluid and nutritional intake, dehydration, somnolence, and other adverse events. Dose reductions or discontinuation of valproate should be considered in patients with decreased food or fluid intake and in patients with excessive somnolence. The ultimate therapeutic dose should be achieved on the basis of both tolerability and clinical response. No patients greater than 65 years of age were enrolled in double-blind prospective clinical trials of mania associated with bipolar illness using divalproex sodium DR tablets. In a case review study of 583 patients, 72 patients (12%) were greater than 65 years of age. A higher percentage of patients greater than 65 years of age reported accidental injury, infection, pain, somnolence, and tremor. Discontinuation of valproate was occasionally associated with the latter 2 events. It is not clear whether these events indicate additional risk or whether they result from preexisting medical illness and concomitant medication use among these patients.

A study of elderly patients with dementia revealed drug-related somnolence and discontinuation. The starting dose should be reduced in these patients, and dosage reductions or discontinuation should be considered in patients with excessive somnolence. Starting doses in the elderly lower than 250 mg can only be achieved by the use of divalproex sodium delayed-release tablets. Dosage should be increased more slowly and with regular monitoring for fluid and nutritional intake, dehydration, somnolence, and other adverse events.

➤*Pregnancy: Category D.* According to published and unpublished reports, valproic acid may produce teratogenic effects in the offspring of human females receiving the drug during pregnancy.

The data described below were gained almost exclusively from women who received valproate to treat epilepsy. There are multiple reports in the clinical literature which indicate that the use of antiepileptic drugs during pregnancy results in an increased incidence of birth defects in the offspring. Although data are more extensive with respect to trimethadione, paramethadione, phenytoin, and phenobarbital, reports indicate a possible similar association with the use of other antiepileptic drugs. Therefore, antiepilepsy drugs should be administered to women of childbearing potential only if they are clearly shown to be essential in the management of their seizures.

The incidence of neural tube defects in the fetus may be increased in mothers receiving valproate during the first trimester of pregnancy. The Centers for Disease Control and Prevention (CDC) has estimated the risk of valproic acid exposed women having children with spina bifida to be approximately 1% to 2%.

Other congenital anomalies (eg, craniofacial defects, cardiovascular malformations, anomalies involving various body systems), compatible and incompatible with life, have been reported. Sufficient data to determine the incidence of these congenital anomalies is not available.

The higher incidence of congenital anomalies in antiepileptic drug-treated women with seizure disorders cannot be regarded as a cause-and-effect relationship. There are intrinsic methodologic problems in obtaining adequate data on drug teratogenicity in humans; genetic factors or the epileptic condition itself, may be more important than drug therapy in contributing to congenital anomalies.

Patients taking valproate may develop clotting abnormalities. A patient who had low fibrinogen when taking multiple anticonvulsants including valproate gave birth to an infant with afibrinogenemia who subsequently died of hemorrhage. If valproate is used in pregnancy, the clotting parameters should be monitored carefully.

Hepatic failure, resulting in the death of a newborn and of an infant, have been reported following the use of valproate during pregnancy.

Animal studies have demonstrated valproate-induced teratogenicity. Increased frequencies of malformations, as well as intrauterine growth retardation and death, have been observed in mice, rats, rabbits, and monkeys following prenatal exposure to valproate. Malformations of the skeletal system are the most common structural abnormalities produced in experimental animals, but neural tube closure defects have been seen in mice exposed to maternal plasma valproate concentrations exceeding approximately 230 mcg/mL (2.3 times the upper limit of the human therapeutic range for epilepsy) during susceptible periods of embryonic development. Administration of an oral dose of 200 mg/kg/day or greater (50% of the maximum human daily dose or greater on a mg/m^2 basis) to pregnant rats during organogenesis produced malformations (skeletal, cardiac, and urogenital) and growth retardation in the offspring. These doses resulted in peak maternal plasma valproate levels of approximately 340 mcg/mL or greater (3.4 times the upper limit of the human therapeutic range for epilepsy or greater). Behavioral deficits have been reported in the offspring of rats given a dose of 200 mg/kg/day throughout most of pregnancy. An oral dose of 350 mg/kg/day (approximately 2 times the maximum human daily dose on a mg/m^2 basis) produced skeletal and visceral malformations in rabbits exposed during organogenesis. Skeletal malformations, growth retardation, and death were observed in rhesus monkeys following administration of an oral dose of 200 mg/kg/day (approximately 4 times the maximum human daily dose on a mg/m^2 basis for ER tablets; equal to the maximum human daily dose on a mg/m^2 basis for DR tablets and sprinkle capsules) during organogenesis. This dose resulted in peak maternal plasma valproate levels of approximately 280 mcg/mL (2.8 times the upper limit of the human therapeutic range for epilepsy).

DIVALPROEX SODIUM — ORAL

Antiepileptic drugs should not be discontinued abruptly in patients in whom the drug is administered to prevent major seizures because of the strong possibility of precipitating status epilepticus with attendant hypoxia and threat to life. In individual cases where the severity and frequency of the seizure disorder are such that the removal of medication does not pose a serious threat to the patient, discontinuation of the drug may be considered prior to and during pregnancy, although it cannot be said with any confidence that even minor seizures do not pose some hazard to the developing embryo or fetus.

Tests to detect neural tube and other defects using currently accepted procedures should be considered a part of routine prenatal care in childbearing women receiving valproate.

➤*Lactation:* Valproate is excreted in breast milk. Concentrations in breast milk have been reported to be 1% to 10% of serum concentrations. It is not known what effect this would have on a nursing infant. Consideration should be given to discontinuing nursing when divalproex sodium is administered to a nursing woman.

➤*Children:* Experience has indicated that children younger than 2 years of age are at a considerably increased risk of developing fatal hepatotoxicity, especially those on multiple anticonvulsants, those with congenital metabolic disorders, those with severe seizure disorders accompanied by mental retardation, and those with organic brain disease. When divalproex sodium is used in this patient group, it should be used with extreme caution and as a sole agent. The benefits of therapy should be weighed against the risks. Above the age of 2 years, experience in epilepsy has indicated that the incidence of fatal hepatotoxicity decreases considerably in progressively older patient groups.

Younger children, especially those receiving enzyme-inducing drugs, will require larger maintenance doses to attain targeted total and unbound valproic acid concentrations.

The variability in free fraction limits the clinical usefulness of monitoring total serum valproic acid concentrations. Interpretation of valproic acid concentrations in children should include consideration of factors that affect hepatic metabolism and protein binding.

The safety and efficacy of divalproex sodium for the treatment of acute mania has not been studied in individuals younger than 18 years of age.

The safety and efficacy of divalproex sodium for the prophylaxis of migraines has not been studied in individuals younger than 16 years of age.

Extended-release tablets – Safety and efficacy of divalproex sodium extended-release in the prophylaxis of migraine headaches and for the treatment of epilepsy in pediatric patients have not been established. Because of the known risks of valproate therapy in pediatric patients when used for other conditions, the use of divalproex sodium extended-release in this population is not recommended.

Precautions

➤*Monitoring:* Liver function tests should be performed prior to therapy and at frequent intervals thereafter, especially during the first 6 months. However, physicians should not rely totally on serum biochemistry since these tests may not be abnormal in all instances, but should also consider the results of careful interim medical history and physical examination.

It is recommended that patients receiving divalproex sodium be monitored for platelet count and coagulation parameters prior to planned surgery.

Since divalproex sodium may interact with concurrently administered drugs which are capable of enzyme induction, periodic plasma concentration determinations of valproate and concomitant drugs are recommended during the early course of therapy.

Because of changes in valproate clearance, monitoring of valproate and concomitant drug concentrations should be increased whenever enzyme-inducing drugs are introduced or withdrawn.

Asymptomatic elevations of ammonia are more common and when present, require close monitoring of plasma ammonia levels. If the elevation persists, discontinuation of valproate therapy should be considered.

➤*Hyperammonemia:* Hyperammonemia has been reported in association with valproate therapy and may be present despite normal liver function tests. In patients who develop unexplained lethargy and vomiting or changes in mental status, hyperammonemic encephalopathy should be considered, and an ammonia level should be measured. If ammonia is increased, valproate therapy should be discontinued. Appropriate interventions for treatment of hyperammonemia should be initiated, and such patients should undergo investigation for underlying urea cycle disorders. Divalproex sodium is contraindicated in patients with known urea cycle disorders.

➤*Thrombocytopenia:* Because of reports of thrombocytopenia, inhibition of the secondary phase of platelet aggregation, and abnormal coagulation parameters, (eg, low fibrinogen), platelet counts and coagulation tests are recommended before initiating therapy and at periodic intervals. In a clinical trial of divalproex sodium as monotherapy in patients with epilepsy, 34/126 patients (27%) receiving approximately 50 mg/kg/day on average, had at least 1 value of platelets less than or equal to 75 × 10^9/L. Approximately half of these patients had treatment discontinued, with return of platelet counts to normal. In the remaining patients, platelet counts normalized with continued treatment. In this study, the probability of thrombocytopenia appeared to increase significantly at total valproate concentrations of greater than or equal to 110 mcg/mL (females) or greater than or equal to 135 mcg/mL (males). Evidence of hemorrhage, bruising, or a disorder of hemostasis/coagulation is an indication for reduction of the dosage or withdrawal of therapy.

➤*Psychiatric disorders:* Suicidal ideation may be a manifestation of certain psychiatric disorders, and may persist until significant remission of symptoms occurs. Close supervision of high-risk patients should accompany initial drug therapy.

➤*Lab test abnormalities:* There have been reports of altered thyroid function tests associated with valproate. The clinical significance of these is unknown.

➤*Hazardous tasks:* Since divalproex sodium products may produce CNS depression, especially when combined with another CNS depressant (eg, alcohol), patients should be advised not to engage in hazardous activities, such as driving an automobile or operating dangerous machinery, until it is known that they do not become drowsy from the drug.

Drug Interactions

Valproic Acid Drug Interactions

Precipitant drug	Object drug*		Description
Charcoal	Valproic acid	↓	Valproic acid absorption is decreased.
Chlorpromazine	Valproic acid	↑	Valproate t½ and trough levels may increase, clearance may decrease.
Cholestyramine	Valproic acid	↓	Serum concentrations and bioavailability of valproic acid may be reduced, resulting in a decrease in therapeutic effects. Administer valproic acid at least 3 hours before, but not within 3 hours following cholestyramine.
Cimetidine	Valproic acid	↑	Small but potentially significant decrease in valproate clearance and increase in $t\frac{1}{2}$.
Erythromycin	Valproic acid	↑	Erythromycin may increase serum valproic acid concentrations, producing valproic acid toxicity.
Felbamate	Valproic acid	↑	Coadministration revealed a 35% increase in mean peak valproate levels.
Rifampin	Valproic acid	↓	In 1 study, rifampin increased the oral clearance of valproate by 40%.
Salicylates (eg, aspirin)	Valproic acid	↑	Salicylates may displace valproic acid from protein binding sites and may also alter the metabolic pathways. Monitor serum concentrations.
Valproic acid	Tricyclic antidepressants	↑	Plasma concentrations and side effects of the tricyclic antidepressant may be increased. Coadministration resulted in a 21% decrease in the plasma clearance of amitriptyline and a 34% decrease in the net clearance of nortriptyline.
Valproic acid	Carbamazepine	↑	Variable changes in carbamazepine concentrations with increased levels of the active metabolite; decreased valproic acid levels with possible loss of seizure control may occur.
Carbamazepine	Valproic acid	↓	
Valproic acid	Clonazepam	↔	Concomitant use may induce absence status in patients with a history of absence type seizures.
Valproic acid	Diazepam	↑	Valproate displaces diazepam from its plasma albumin binding sites and inhibits its metabolism.
Valproic acid	Ethosuximide	↑↓	Increases and decreases in ethosuximide blood levels and decreases in valproic acid levels have been reported. Valproic acid appears to inhibit the metabolism of ethosuximide.
Ethosuximide	Valproic acid	↓	
Valproic acid	Lamotrigine	↑	Serum valproic acid concentrations may be decreased while lamotrigine levels increase. In one study, coadministration increased the half-life of lamotrigine from 26 to 70 hours. Lamotrigine dose should be reduced.
Lamotrigine	Valproic acid	↓	

DIVALPROEX SODIUM — ORAL

Valproic Acid Drug Interactions			
Precipitant drug	Object drug*		Description
Valproic acid	Barbiturates	↑	Valproic acid may decrease hepatic metabolism of barbiturates. Barbiturate dosage may need to be decreased in some patients.
Valproic acid	Hydantoins (eg, phenytoin)	↑	Increased action of phenytoin, even at therapeutic levels; increased metabolism of valproic acid with decreased pharmacologic effects may occur.
Hydantoins (eg, phenytoin)	Valproic acid	↓	
Valproic acid	Tolbutamide	↔	The unbound fraction of tolbutamide may be increased from 20% to 50%. The clinical relevance of this displacement is unknown.
Valproic acid	Warfarin	↑	The potential exists for valproate to displace warfarin from protein binding sites. Monitor coagulation tests.
Valproic acid	Zidovudine	↑	Zidovudine clearance was decreased by 38% in 6 HIV-seropositive patients.

* ↑ = Object drug increased. ↓ = Object drug decreased.
↔ = Undetermined clinical effect.

➤*Effects of coadministered drugs on valproate clearance:* Drugs that affect the level of expression of hepatic enzymes, particularly those that elevate levels of glucuronosyltransferases, may increase the clearance of valproate. For example, phenytoin, carbamazepine, and phenobarbital (or primidone) can double the clearance of valproate. Thus, patients on monotherapy will generally have longer half-lives and higher concentrations than patients receiving polytherapy with antiepilepsy drugs.

➤*Drug/Lab test interactions:* Valproate is partially eliminated in the urine as a keto-metabolite which may lead to a false interpretation of the urine ketone test.

Adverse Reactions

➤*Epilepsy (sprinkle capsules, delayed-release tablets and extended-release tablets):* Based on a placebo-controlled trial of adjunctive therapy for treatment of complex partial seizures, divalproex sodium was generally well tolerated with most adverse events rated as mild to moderate in severity. Intolerance was the primary reason for discontinuation in the divalproex sodium-treated patients (6%), compared to 1% of placebo-treated patients.

The following table lists treatment-emergent adverse reactions that were reported by greater than or equal to 5% of divalproex sodium-treated patients and for which the incidence was greater than in the placebo group, in the placebo-controlled trial of adjunctive therapy for treatment of complex partial seizures. Since patients were also treated with other antiepilepsy drugs, it is not possible, in most cases, to determine whether the following adverse events can be ascribed to divalproex sodium alone, or the combination of divalproex sodium and other antiepilepsy drugs.

Adverse Reactions Reported by ≥ 5% of Patients Treated with Divalproex Sodium (Sprinkle Capsules and Delayed-Release Tablets) during Placebo-controlled Trial of Adjunctive Therapy for Complex Partial Seizures		
Adverse event	Divalproex sodium (%) (n = 77)	Placebo (%) (n = 70)
Miscellaneous		
Headache	31%	21%
Asthenia	27%	7%
Fever	6%	4%
GI		
Nausea	48%	14%
Vomiting	27%	7%
Abdominal pain	23%	6%
Diarrhea	13%	6%
Anorexia	12%	0%
Dyspepsia	8%	4%
Constipation	5%	1%
CNS		
Somnolence	27%	11%
Tremor	25%	6%
Dizziness	25%	13%
Diplopia	16%	9%
Amblyopia/ blurred vision	12%	9%
Ataxia	8%	1%
Nystagmus	8%	1%
Emotional lability	6%	4%
Thinking abnormal	6%	0%
Amnesia	5%	1%
Respiratory		
Flu syndrome	12%	9%
Infection	12%	6%
Bronchitis	5%	1%
Rhinitis	5%	4%
Miscellaneous		
Alopecia	6%	1%
Weight loss	6%	0%

Complex partial seizures (greater than or equal to 5%): The following table lists treatment-emergent adverse reactions that were reported by greater than or equal to 5% of patients in the high-dose divalproex sodium group, and for which the incidence was greater than in the low-dose group, in a controlled trial of divalproex sodium monotherapy treatment of complex partial seizures. Since patients were being titrated off another antiepilepsy drug during the first portion of the trial, it is not possible, in many cases, to determine whether the following adverse events can be ascribed to divalproex sodium alone, or the combination of divalproex sodium and other antiepilepsy drugs.

Adverse Reactions Reported by ≥5% of Patients in the High-dose Group in the Controlled Trial of Divalproex Sodium (Sprinkle Capsules and Delayed-release Tablets) Monotherapy for Complex Partial Seizures[1]		
Adverse reaction	High dose (%) (n = 131)	Low dose (%) (n = 134)
Miscellaneous		
Asthenia	21%	10%
GI		
Nausea	34%	26%
Diarrhea	23%	19%
Vomiting	23%	15%
Abdominal pain	12%	9%
Anorexia	11%	4%
Dyspepsia	11%	10%
Hemic/lymphatic		
Thrombocytopenia	24%	1%
Ecchymosis	5%	4%
Metabolic/nutritional		
Weight gain	9%	4%
Peripheral edema	8%	3%
CNS		
Tremor	57%	19%
Somnolence	30%	18%
Dizziness	18%	13%
Insomnia	15%	9%
Nervousness	11%	7%
Amnesia	7%	4%
Nystagmus	7%	1%
Depression	5%	4%
Respiratory		
Infection	20%	13%
Pharyngitis	8%	2%
Dyspnea	5%	1%
Dermatologic		
Alopecia	24%	13%
Special senses		
Ambylopia/ blurred vision	8%	4%
Tinnitus	7%	1%

[1] Headache was the only adverse reaction that occurred in greater than or equal to 5% of patients in the high-dose group and at an equal or greater incidence in the low-dose group.

DIVALPROEX SODIUM — ORAL

➤*Additional adverse reactions in treatment of complex partial seizures (delayed-release tablets and sprinkle capsules):* The following additional adverse events were reported by greater than 1% but less than 5% of the 358 patients treated with divalproex sodium in the controlled trials of complex partial seizures:

Cardiovascular – Tachycardia; hypertension; palpitation.

CNS – Anxiety; confusion; abnormal gait; paresthesia; hypertonia; incoordination; abnormal dreams; personality disorder.

Dermatologic – Rash; pruritus; dry skin.

GI – Increased appetite; flatulence; hematemesis; eructation; pancreatitis; periodontal abscess.

GU – Urinary incontinence; vaginitis; dysmenorrhea; amenorrhea; urinary frequency.

Hematologic/Lymphatic – Petechia.

Metabolic/Nutritional – AST increased; ALT increased.

Musculoskeletal – Myalgia; twitching; arthralgia; leg cramps; myasthenia.

Respiratory – Sinusitis; cough increased; pneumonia; epistaxis.

Special senses – Taste perversion; abnormal vision; deafness; otitis media.

Miscellaneous – Back pain; chest pain; malaise.

➤*Mania (delayed-release tablets):* The incidence of treatment-emergent events has been ascertained based on combined data from 2 placebo-controlled clinical trials of divalproex sodium in the treatment of manic episodes associated with bipolar disorder. The adverse events were usually mild or moderate in intensity, but sometimes were serious enough to interrupt treatment. In clinical trials, the rates of premature termination due to intolerance were not statistically different between placebo, divalproex sodium, and lithium carbonate. A total of 4%, 8%, and 11% of patients discontinued therapy due to intolerance in the placebo, divalproex sodium, and lithium carbonate groups, respectively.

The following table summarizes those adverse events reported for patients in these trials where the incidence rate in the divalproex sodium-treated group was greater than 5% and greater than the placebo incidence, or where the incidence in the divalproex sodium-treated group was statistically significantly greater than the placebo group. Vomiting was the only event that was reported by significantly ($P \leq 0.05$) more patients receiving divalproex sodium compared to placebo.

Adverse Events Reported by > 5% of Divalproex Sodium-treated Patients During Placebo-controlled Trials of Acute Mania[1]

Adverse event	Divalproex sodium (n = 89)	Placebo (n = 97)
Nausea	22%	15%
Somnolence	19%	12%
Dizziness	12%	4%
Vomiting	12%	3%
Asthenia	10%	7%
Abdominal pain	9%	8%
Dyspepsia	9%	8%
Rash	6%	3%

[1] The following adverse events occurred at an equal or greater incidence for placebo than for divalproex sodium: Back pain, headache, constipation, diarrhea, tremor, and pharyngitis.

➤*Additional adverse reactions in the treatment of mania (delayed-release tablets):* The following additional adverse events were reported by greater than 1% but less than 5% of the 89 divalproex sodium-treated patients in controlled clinical trials:

Cardiovascular – Hypertension; hypotension; palpitations; postural hypotension; tachycardia; vasodilation.

CNS – Abnormal dreams; abnormal gait; agitation; ataxia; catatonic reaction; confusion; depression; diplopia; dysarthria; hallucinations; hypertonia; hypokinesia; insomnia; paresthesia; reflexes increased; tardive dyskinesia; thinking abnormalities; vertigo.

Dermatologic – Alopecia; discoid lupus erythematosis; dry skin; furunculosis; maculopapular rash; seborrhea.

GI – Anorexia; fecal incontinence; flatulence; gastroenteritis; glossitis; periodontal abscess.

GU – Dysmenorrhea; dysuria; urinary incontinence.

Hematologic/Lymphatic – Ecchymosis.

Metabolic/Nutritional – Edema; peripheral edema.

Musculoskeletal – Arthralgia; arthrosis; leg cramps; twitching.

Respiratory – Dyspnea; rhinitis.

Special senses – Amblyopia; conjunctivitis; deafness; dry eyes; ear pain; eye pain; tinnitus.

Miscellaneous – Chest pain; chills; chills and fever; fever; neck pain; neck rigidity.

➤*Mania (extended-release tablets):*

Cardiovascular – Arrhythmia, hypotension, postural hypotension.

CNS – Agitation, catatonic reaction, dysarthria, hallucinations, hypokinesia, psychosis, increased reflexes, sleep disorder, tardive dyskinesia.

Dermatologic – Discoid lupus erythematosis, erythema nodosum, furunculosis, maculopapular rash, seborrhea, sweating, vesiculobullous rash.

GI – Dysphagia, fecal incontinence, gastroenteritis, glossitis, gum hemorrhage, mouth ulceration.

GU – Cystitis, menstrual disorder.

Hematologic/Lymphatic – Anemia, increased bleeding time, leukopenia.

Metabolic/Nutritional – Hypoproteinemia.

Musculoskeletal – Arthrosis.

Respiratory – Hiccup.

Special senses – Conjunctivitis, dry eyes, eye disorder, eye pain, photophobia, taste perversion.

Miscellaneous – Chills, chills and fever, increased drug level, neck rigidity.

➤*Mania (sprinkle capsules):* Although divalproex sodium sprinkle capsules have not been evaluated for safety and efficacy in the treatment of manic episodes associated with a bipolar disorder, the following adverse reactions not listed above were reported by 1% or more of patients from 2 placebo-controlled clinical trials of divalproex sodium tablets:

Cardiovascular – Hypotension, postural hypotension, vasodilation.

CNS – Agitation, catatonic reaction, hypokinesia, reflexes increased, tardive dyskinesia, vertigo.

GI – Fecal incontinence, gastroenteritis, glossitis.

GU – Dysuria.

Dermatologic – Furunculosis, maculopapular rash, seborrhea.

Musculoskeletal – Arthrosis.

Special senses – Conjunctivitis, dry eyes, eye pain.

Miscellaneous – Chills, neck pain, neck rigidity.

➤*Migraine (delayed-release tablets):* Based on 2 placebo-controlled clinical trials and their long-term extension, divalproex sodium was generally well tolerated with most adverse reactions rated as mild to moderate in severity. Of the 202 patients exposed to divalproex sodium in the placebo-controlled trials, 17% discontinued for intolerance. This is compared to a rate of 5% for the 81 placebo patients. Including the long-term extension study, the adverse events reported as the primary reason for discontinuation by greater than or equal to 1% of 248 divalproex sodium-treated patients were alopecia (6%), nausea or vomiting (5%), weight gain (2%), tremor (2%), somnolence (1%), elevated AST and ALT (1%), and depression (1%). The following table includes adverse reactions reported for patients in the placebo-controlled trials where the incidence rate in the divalproex sodium delayed-release group was greater than 5% and was greater than that for placebo patients.

Adverse Events Reported by > 5% of Divalproex Sodium Delayed-release-treated Patients during Migraine Placebo-controlled Trials with a Greater Incidence than Patients Taking Placebo[1]

Adverse reaction	Divalproex sodium delayed-release (n = 202)	Placebo (n = 81)
	GI	
Nausea	31%	10%
Dyspepsia	13%	9%
Diarrhea	12%	7%
Vomiting	11%	1%
Abdominal pain	9%	4%
Increased appetite	6%	4%
	CNS	
Asthenia	20%	9%
Somnolence	17%	5%
Dizziness	12%	6%
Tremor	9%	0%
	Miscellaneous	
Weight gain	8%	2%
Back pain	8%	6%
Alopecia	7%	1%

[1] The following adverse events occurred in greater than 5% of divalproex sodium delayed-release-treated patients and at a greater incidence for placebo than for divalproex sodium delayed-release: Flu syndrome and pharyngitis.

➤*Additional adverse reactions in the treatment of migraine (delayed-release tablets):* The following additional adverse events were reported by greater than 1% but not more than 5% of the 202 divalproex sodium-treated patients in the controlled clinical trials.

Cardiovascular – Vasodilatation.

CNS – Abnormal dreams; amnesia; confusion; depression; emotional lability; insomnia; nervousness; paresthesia; speech disorder; thinking abnormalities; vertigo.

DIVALPROEX SODIUM — ORAL

Dermatologic – Pruritus; rash.

GI – Anorexia; constipation; dry mouth; flatulence; gastrointestinal disorder (unspecified); stomatitis.

GU – Cystitis; metrorrhagia; vaginal hemorrhage.

Hematologic/Lymphatic – Ecchymosis.

Metabolic/Nutritional – Peripheral edema; AST increased; ALT increased.

Musculoskeletal – Leg cramps; myalgia.

Respiratory – Cough increased; dyspnea; rhinitis; sinusitis.

Special senses – Conjunctivitis; ear disorder; taste perversion; tinnitus.

Miscellaneous – Chest pain; chills; face edema; malaise.

➤*Migraine (sprinkle capsules):* Although divalproex sodium sprinkle capsules have not been evaluated for safety and efficacy in the treatment of prophylaxis of migraine headaches, the following adverse reactions not listed above were reported by 1% or more of patients from 2 placebo-controlled trials of divalproex sodium tables:

GI – Dry mouth, stomatitis.

GU – Cystitis, metrorrhagia, and vaginal hemorrhage.

Miscellaneous – Face edema.

➤*Migraine (extended-release tablets):* Based on the results of 1 multicenter, randomized, double-blind, placebo-controlled clinical trial, divalproex sodium extended-release was well tolerated in the prophylactic treatment of migraine headache. Of the 122 patients exposed to divalproex sodium extended-release in the placebo-controlled study; 8% discontinued for adverse reactions, compared to 9% for the 115 placebo patients. The following table includes adverse events reported for patients in the placebo-controlled trials where the incidence rate in the divalproex sodium extended-release group was greater than 5% and was greater than that for placebo patients.

Adverse Events Reported by > 5% of Divalproex Sodium Extended-release-treated Patients Treated during Migraine Placebo-controlled Trials with a Greater Incidence than Patients Taking Placebo[1]

Adverse reaction	Divalproex sodium extended-release (n = 122)	Placebo (n = 115)
GI		
Nausea	15%	9%
Dyspepsia	7%	4%
Diarrhea	7%	3%
Vomiting	7%	2%
Abdominal pain	7%	5%
CNS		
Somnolence	7%	2%
Miscellaneous		
Infection	15%	14%

[1] The following adverse events occurred in greater than 5% of divalproex sodium extended-release-treated patients and a greater incidence for placebo than for divalproex sodium extended-release: Asthenia and flu syndrome.

➤*Additional adverse events in the treatment of migraine (extended-release tablets):* The following additional adverse events were reported by greater than 1% but not more than 5% of divalproex sodium extended-release-treated patients with a greater incidence than placebo in the placebo-controlled clinical trial for migraine prophylaxis:

CNS – Abnormal gait; dizziness; hypertonia; insomnia; nervousness; tremor; vertigo.

Dermatologic – Rash.

GU – Increased appetite; tooth disorder.

Metabolic/Nutritional – Edema; weight gain.

Respiratory – Pharyngitis; rhinitis.

Special senses – Tinnitus.

Miscellaneous – Accidental injury; viral infection.

➤*Other patient populations (all doseforms):* Adverse events that have been reported with all dosage forms of valproate from epilepsy trials, spontaneous reports, and other sources are listed below by body system.

CNS – Sedative effects have occurred in patients receiving valproate alone but occur most often in patients receiving combination therapy. Sedation usually abates upon reduction of other antiepileptic medication. Tremor (may be dose-related), hallucinations, ataxia, headache, nystagmus, diplopia, asterixis, "spots before eyes", dysarthria, dizziness, confusion, hypesthesia, vertigo, incoordination, and parkinsonism. Rare cases of coma have occurred in patients receiving valproate alone or in conjunction with phenobarbital. In rare instances encephalopathy with fever has developed shortly after the introduction of valproate monotherapy without evidence of hepatic dysfunction or inappropriately high plasma levels. Although recovery has been described following drug withdrawal, there have been fatalities in patients with hyperammonemic encephalopathy, particularly in patients with underlying urea cycle disorders. Divalproex sodium is contraindicated in patients with known urea cycle disorders.

Several reports have noted reversible cerebral atrophy and dementia in association with valproate therapy.

Dermatologic – Transient hair loss, skin rash, photosensitivity, generalized pruritus, erythema multiforme, and Stevens-Johnson syndrome. Rare cases of toxic epidermal necrolysis have been reported including a fatal case in a 6 month old infant taking valproate and several other concomitant medications. An additional case of toxic epidermal necrosis resulting in death was reported in a 35-year-old patient with AIDS taking several concomitant medications and had with a history of multiple cutaneous drug reactions.

Endocrine – Irregular menses, secondary amenorrhea, breast enlargement, galactorrhea, and parotid gland swelling. Abnormal thyroid function tests.

There have been rare spontaneous reports of polycystic ovary disease. A cause and effect relationship has not been established.

GI – The most commonly reported side effects at the initiation of therapy are nausea, vomiting, and indigestion. These effects are usually transient and rarely require discontinuation of therapy. Diarrhea, abdominal cramps, and constipation have been reported. Both anorexia with some weight loss and increased appetite with weight gain have also been reported. The administration of delayed-release divalproex sodium may result in reduction of GI side effects in some patients.

GU – Enuresis and urinary tract infection.

Hematologic – Thrombocytopenia and inhibition of the secondary phase of platelet aggregation may be reflected in altered bleeding time, petechiae, bruising, hematoma formation, epistaxis, and frank hemorrhage. Relative lymphocytosis, macrocytosis, hypofibrinogenemia, leukopenia, eosinophilia, anemia including macrocytic with or without folate deficiency, bone marrow suppression, pancytopenia, aplastic anemia, and acute intermittent porphyria.

Hepatic – Minor elevations of transaminases (eg, AST and ALT) and LDH are frequent and appear to be dose-related. Occasionally, laboratory test results include increases in serum bilirubin and abnormal changes in other liver function tests. These results may reflect potentially serious hepatotoxicity.

Metabolic – Hyperammonemia, hyponatremia, and inappropriate ADH secretion.

There have been rare reports of Fanconi's syndrome occurring chiefly in children.

Decreased carnitine concentrations have been reported although the clinical relevance is undetermined.

Hyperglycinemia has occurred and was associated with a fatal outcome in a patient with preexistent nonketotic hyperglycinemia.

Musculoskeletal – Weakness.

Psychiatric – Emotional upset; depression; psychosis; aggression; hyperactivity; hostility; behavioral deterioration.

Special senses – Hearing loss, either reversible or irreversible, has been reported; however, a cause and effect relationship has not been established. Ear pain has also been reported.

Miscellaneous – Anaphylaxis; edema of the extremities; lupus erythematosus; bone pain; cough increased; pneumonia; otitis media; bradycardia; cutaneous vasculitis; fever; acute pancreatitis including fatalities.

Overdosage

➤*Symptoms:* Overdosage with valproate may result in somnolence, heart block, and deep coma. Fatalities have been reported; however patients have recovered from valproate levels as high as 2120 mcg/mL.

➤*Treatment:* In overdose situations, the fraction of drug not bound to protein is high and hemodialysis or tandem hemodialysis plus hemoperfusion may result in significant removal of drug. The benefit of gastric lavage or emesis will vary with the time since ingestion. General supportive measures should be applied with particular attention to the maintenance of adequate urinary output.

Naloxone has been reported to reverse the CNS-depressant effects of valproate overdosage. Because naloxone could theoretically also reverse the antiepileptic effects of valproate, it should be used with caution in patients with epilepsy.

Patient Information

Patients and guardians should be warned that abdominal pain, nausea, vomiting, and anorexia can be symptoms of pancreatitis and, therefore, require further medical evaluation promptly.

Patients should be informed of the signs and symptoms associated with hyperammonemic encephalopathy and be told to inform the prescriber if any of these symptoms occurs. In patients who develop unexplained lethargy and vomiting or changes in mental status, hyperammonemic encephalopathy should be considered and an ammonia level should be measured. If ammonia is increased, valproate therapy should be discontinued.

The specially coated particles in divalproex sodium sprinkle capsules have been observed in the stool, but this occurrence has not been associated with clinically significant effects.

➤*Migraine patients:* Since divalproex sodium has been associated with certain types of birth defects, female patients of childbearing age considering the use of divalproex sodium for the prevention of migraine should be advised to read the enclosed patient information labeling that comes with their medications.

DIVALPROEX SODIUM — ORAL

➤*Delayed- and extended-release tablets:*

Pregnancy – Before using divalproex sodium (DR and ER), women who can become pregnant should consider the fact that divalproex sodium (DR and ER) has been associated with birth defects, in particular, with spina bifida and other defects related to failure of the spinal canal to close normally. Although the incidence is unknown in migraine patients treated with divalproex sodium (DR and ER), approximately 1% to 2% of children born to women with epilepsy taking divalproex sodium (DR and ER) in the first 12 weeks of pregnancy had these defects (based on data from the Centers for Disease Control, a US agency based in Atlanta). The incidence in the general population is 0.1% to 0.2%.

The prescribing physician will wish to weigh the benefits of therapy against the risks in treating or counseling women of childbearing potential. If this drug is used during pregnancy, or if the patient becomes pregnant while taking this drug, the patient should be apprised of the potential hazard to the fetus.

Women taking divalproex sodium (DR and ER) for the prevention of migraine who are planning to get pregnant should discuss with their doctor temporarily stopping divalproex sodium (DR and ER), before and during their pregnancies.

If you become pregnant while taking divalproex sodium (DR and ER) for the prevention of migraine, you should contact your doctor immediately.

Divalproex sodium (DR and ER) tablets should be taken exactly as they are prescribed by your doctor to get the most benefits from divalproex sodium (DR and ER) and reduce the risk of side effects.

If you have taken more than the prescribed dose of divalproex sodium (DR and ER), contact your hospital emergency room or local poison center immediately.

This medication was prescribed for your particular condition. Do not use it for another condition or give the drug to others.

VALPROATE SODIUM — INJECTION

Refer to the general discussion beginning in the Anticonvulsants introduction.

WARNING

Hepatotoxicity – Hepatic failure resulting in fatalities has occurred in patients receiving valproic acid and its derivatives. Experience has indicated that children less than 2 years of age are at a considerably increased risk of developing fatal hepatotoxicity, especially those on multiple anticonvulsants, those with congenital metabolic disorders, those with severe seizure disorders accompanied by mental retardation, and those with organic brain disease. When valproate sodium injection is used in this patient group, it should be used with extreme caution and as a sole agent. The benefits of therapy should be weighed against the risks. Above this age group, experience in epilepsy has indicated that the incidence of fatal hepatotoxicity decreases considerably in progressively older patient groups.

These incidents usually have occurred during the first 6 months of treatment. Serious or fatal hepatotoxicity may be preceded by nonspecific symptoms such as malaise, weakness, lethargy, facial edema, anorexia, and vomiting. In patients with epilepsy, a loss of seizure control may also occur. Patients should be monitored closely for appearance of these symptoms. Liver function tests should be performed prior to therapy and at frequent intervals thereafter, especially during the first 6 months.

Teratogenicity – Valproate can produce teratogenic effects such as neural tube defects (eg, spina bifida). Accordingly, the use of valproate products in women of childbearing potential requires that the benefits of its use be weighed against the risk of injury to the fetus.

Pancreatitis – Cases of life-threatening pancreatitis have been reported in both children and adults receiving valproate. Some of the cases have been described as hemorrhagic with a rapid progression from initial symptoms to death. Cases have been reported shortly after initial use as well as after several years of use. Patients and guardians should be warned that abdominal pain, nausea, vomiting, or anorexia can be symptoms of pancreatitis that require prompt medical evaluation. If pancreatitis is diagnosed, valproate should ordinarily be discontinued. Alternative treatment for the underlying medical condition should be initiated as clinically indicated.

Indications

As an intravenous alternative in patients for whom oral administration of valproate products is temporarily not feasible in the following conditions:

➤*Complex partial seizures:* As monotherapy and adjunctive therapy in the treatment of patients with complex partial seizures that occur either in isolation or in association with other types of seizures.

➤*Simple and complex absence seizures:* For use as sole and adjunctive therapy in the treatment of patients with simple and complex absence seizures, and adjunctively in patients with multiple seizure types that include absence seizures.

➤*Unlabeled uses:* May be effective alone or in combination in the treatment of absence, myoclonic, and grand mal seizures. It may also be effective in patients with intractable status epilepticus who have not responded to other therapies (adults: 200 to 1200 mg every 6 hours rectally with phenytoin and phenobarbital; children: 15 to 20 mg/kg). For minor incontinence after ileoanal anastomosis (subchronic administration).

Administration and Dosage

➤*Approved by the FDA:* December 30, 1996.

Valproate sodium injection is for intravenous use only.

Use of valproate sodium injection for periods of greater than 14 days has not been studied. Patients should be switched to oral valproate products as soon as it is clinically feasible.

Valproate sodium injection should be administered as a 60-minute infusion (but not greater than 20 mg/min) with the same frequency as the oral products, although plasma concentration monitoring and dosage adjustments may be necessary.

➤*Initial exposure to valproate:* The following dosage recommendations were obtained from studies utilizing oral divalproex sodium products.

Complex partial seizures – For adults and children 10 years of age or older.

Monotherapy (initial therapy): Valproate sodium injection has not been systematically studied as initial therapy. Patients should initiate therapy at 10 to 15 mg/kg/day. The dosage should be increased by 5 to 10 mg/kg/week to achieve optimal clinical response. Ordinarily, optimal clinical response is achieved at daily doses below 60 mg/kg/day. If satisfactory clinical response has not been achieved, plasma levels should be measured to determine whether or not they are in the usually accepted therapeutic range (50 to 100 mcg/mL). No recommendation regarding the safety of valproate for use at doses above 60 mg/kg/day can be made.

Conversion to monotherapy: Patients should initiate therapy at 10 to 15 mg/kg/day. The dosage should be increased by 5 to 10 mg/kg/week to achieve optimal clinical response. Ordinarily, optimal clinical response is achieved at daily doses below 60 mg/kg/day. If satisfactory clinical response has not been achieved, plasma levels should be measured to determine whether or not they are in the usually accepted therapeutic range (50 to 100 mcg/mL). No recommendation regarding the safety of valproate for use at doses above 60 mg/kg/day can be made. Concomitant antiepilepsy drug (AED) dosage can ordinarily be reduced by approximately 25% every 2 weeks. This reduction may be started at initiation of valproate sodium injection therapy, or delayed by 1 to 2 weeks if there is a concern that seizures are likely to occur with a reduction. The speed and duration of withdrawal of the concomitant AED can be highly variable, and patients should be monitored closely during this period for increased seizure frequency.

Adjunctive therapy: Valproate sodium injection may be added to the patient's regimen at a dosage of 10 to 15 mg/kg/day. The dosage may be increased by 5 to 10 mg/kg/week to achieve optimal clinical response. Ordinarily, optimal clinical response is achieved at daily doses below 60 mg/kg/day. If satisfactory clinical response has not been achieved, plasma levels should be measured to determine whether or not they are in the usually accepted therapeutic range (50 to 100 mcg/mL). No recommendation regarding the safety of valproate for use at doses above 60 mg/kg/day can be made. If the total daily dose exceeds 250 mg, it should be given in divided doses.

Simple and complex absence seizures – The recommended initial dose is 15 mg/kg/day, increasing at 1-week intervals by 5 to 10 mg/kg/day until seizures are controlled or side effects preclude further increases. The maximum recommended dosage is 60 mg/kg/day. If the total daily dose exceeds 250 mg, it should be given in divided doses.

A good correlation has not been established between daily dose, serum concentrations, and therapeutic effect. However, therapeutic valproate serum concentrations for most patients with absence seizures is considered to range from 50 to 100 mcg/mL. Some patients may be controlled with lower or higher serum concentrations.

Antiepilepsy drugs should not be abruptly discontinued in patients in whom the drug is administered to prevent major seizures because of the strong possibility of precipitating status epilepticus with attendant hypoxia and threat to life.

➤*Replacement therapy:* When switching from oral valproate products, the total daily dose of valproate sodium injection should be equivalent to the total daily dose of the oral valproate product, and should be administered as a 60 minute infusion (but not greater than 20 mg/min) with the same frequency as the oral products, although plasma concentration monitoring and dosage adjustments may be necessary. Patients receiving doses near the maximum recommended daily dose of 60 mg/kg/day, particularly those not receiving enzyme-inducing drugs, should be monitored more closely. If the total daily dose exceeds 250 mg, it should be given in a divided regimen. However, the equivalence shown between valproate sodium injection and oral valproate products (divalproex sodium) at steady state was only evaluated in an every 6 hour regimen. Whether, when valproate sodium injection is given less frequently (ie, 2 or 3 times a day), trough levels fall below those that result from an oral dosage form given via the same regimen, is unknown. For this reason, when valproate sodium injection is given 2 or 3 times a day, close monitoring of trough plasma levels may be needed.

➤*General dosing advice:*

Elderly – The capacity of elderly patients (age range, 68 to 89 years) to eliminate valproate has been shown to be reduced compared to younger adults (age range, 22 to 26 years). Intrinsic clearance is reduced by 39%; the free fraction is increased by 44%). Due to a decrease in unbound clearance of valproate and possibly a greater sensitivity to somnolence in the elderly, the starting dose should be reduced in these patients. Dosage should be increased more slowly and with regular monitoring for fluid and nutritional intake, dehydration, somnolence, and other adverse events. Dose reductions or discontinuation of valproate should be considered in patients with decreased food or fluid intake and in patients with excessive somnolence. The ultimate therapeutic dose should be achieved on the basis of both tolerability and clinical response.

VALPROATE SODIUM — INJECTION

➤*Administration:* Rapid infusion of valproate sodium injection has been associated with an increase in adverse events. Infusion times of less than 60 minutes or rates of infusion greater than 20 mg/min have not been studied in patients with epilepsy.

Valproate sodium injection should be administered intravenously as a 60-minute infusion, as noted above. It should be diluted with at least 50 mL of a compatible diluent. Any unused portion of the vial contents should be discarded.

Parenteral drug products should be inspected visually for particulate matter and discoloration prior to administration whenever solution and container permit.

➤*Compatibility and stability:* Valproate sodium injection was found to be physically compatible and chemically stable in the following parenteral solutions for at least 24 hours when stored in glass or polyvinyl chloride (PVC) bags at controlled room temperature 15° to 30°C (59° to 86°F):

- Dextrose (5%) injection.
- Sodium chloride (0.9%) injection.
- Lactated ringer's injection.

➤*Storage/Stability:* Store vials at controlled room temperature 15° to 30°C (59° to 86°F). No preservatives have been added. Unused portion of container should be discarded.

Actions

➤*Pharmacology:* The mechanisms by which valproate exerts its therapeutic effects have not been established. It has been suggested that its activity in epilepsy is related to increased brain concentrations of gamma-aminobutyric acid (GABA).

➤*Pharmacokinetics:*

Absorption –

Bioavailability: Equivalent doses of intravenous (IV) valproate and oral valproate products are expected to result in equivalent C_{max}, C_{min}, and total systemic exposure to the valproate ion. However, the rate of valproate ion absorption may vary with the formulation used. These differences should be of minor clinical importance under the steady state conditions achieved in chronic use in the treatment of epilepsy.

Administration of divalproex sodium tablets and IV valproate (given as a 1-hour infusion), 250 mg every 6 hours for 4 days to 18 healthy male volunteers resulted in equivalent AUC, C_{max}, C_{min} at steady state, as well as after the first dose. The t_{max} after IV valproate sodium injection occurs at the end of the 1-hour infusion, while the t_{max} after oral dosing with divalproex sodium occurs at approximately 4 hours. Because the kinetics of unbound valproate are linear, bioequivalence between valproate sodium injection and divalproex sodium up to the maximum recommended dose of 60 mg/kg/day can be assumed. The AUC and C_{max} resulting from administration of IV valproate 500 mg as a single 1-hour infusion and a single 500 mg dose of valproic acid syrup to 17 healthy male volunteers were also equivalent.

Patients maintained on valproic acid doses of 750 mg to 4250 mg daily (given in divided doses every 6 hours) as oral divalproex sodium alone (n = 24) or with another stabilized antiepileptic drug (carbamazepine [n = 15], phenytoin [n = 11], or phenobarbital [n = 1]), showed comparable plasma levels for valproic acid when switching from oral divalproex sodium to IV valproate (1-hour infusion).

Eleven healthy volunteers were given single infusions of 1000 mg IV valproate over 5, 10, 30 and 60 minutes in a 4-period crossover study. Total valproate concentrations were measured; unbound concentrations were not measured. After the 5-minute infusions (mean rate of 2.8 mg/kg/min), mean C_{max} was 145 ± 32 mcg/mL, while after the 60-minute infusions, mean C_{max} was 115 ± 8 mcg/mL. Ninety to 120 minutes after infusion initiation, total valproate concentrations were similar for all 4 rates of infusion. Because protein binding is nonlinear at higher total valproate concentrations, the corresponding increase in unbound C_{max} at faster infusion rates will be greater.

Distribution –

Protein binding: The plasma protein binding of valproate is concentration dependent and the free fraction increases from approximately 10% at 40 mcg/mL to 18.5% at 130 mcg/mL. Protein binding of valproate is reduced in the elderly, in patients with chronic hepatic diseases, in patients with renal impairment, and in the presence of other drugs (eg, aspirin). Conversely, valproate may displace certain protein-bound drugs (eg, phenytoin, carbamazepine, warfarin, tolbutamide).

CNS distribution: Valproate concentrations in cerebrospinal fluid (CSF) approximate unbound concentrations in plasma (about 10% of total concentration).

Metabolism – Valproate is metabolized almost entirely by the liver. In adult patients on monotherapy, 30% to 50% of an administered dose appears in urine as a glucuronide conjugate. Mitochondrial β-oxidation is the other major metabolic pathway, typically accounting for over 40% of the dose. Usually, less than 15% to 20% of the dose is eliminated by other oxidative mechanisms. Less than 3% of an administered dose is excreted unchanged in urine.

The relationship between dose and total valproate concentration is nonlinear; concentration does not increase proportionally with the dose, but rather, increases to a lesser extent due to saturable plasma protein binding. The kinetics of unbound drug are linear.

Excretion – Mean plasma clearance and volume of distribution for total valproate are 0.56 L/hr/1.73 m^2 and 11 L/1.73 m^2, respectively. Mean terminal half-life for valproate monotherapy after a 60-minute intravenous infusion of 1000 mg was 16 ± 3 hours.

The estimates cited apply primarily to patients who are not taking drugs that affect hepatic metabolizing enzyme systems. For example, patients taking enzyme-inducing antiepileptic drugs (carbamazepine, phenytoin, and phenobarbital) will clear valproate more rapidly. Because of these changes in valproate clearance, monitoring of antiepileptic concentrations should be intensified whenever concomitant antiepileptics are introduced or withdrawn.

Special populations –

Renal function impairment: A slight reduction (27%) in the unbound clearance of valproate has been reported in patients with renal failure (creatinine clearance less than 10 mL/min); however, hemodialysis typically reduces valproate concentrations by about 20%. Therefore, no dosage adjustment appears to be necessary in patients with renal failure. Protein binding in these patients is substantially reduced; thus, monitoring total concentrations may be misleading.

Hepatic function impairment: Liver disease impairs the capacity to eliminate valproate. In one study, the clearance of free valproate was decreased by 50% in 7 patients with cirrhosis and by 16% in 4 patients with acute hepatitis, compared with 6 healthy subjects. In that study, the half-life of valproate was increased from 12 to 18 hours. Liver disease is also associated with decreased albumin concentrations and larger unbound fractions (2- to 2.6-fold increase) of valproate. Accordingly, monitoring of total concentrations may be misleading since free concentrations may be substantially elevated in patients with hepatic disease whereas total concentrations may appear to be normal.

Elderly: See Administration and Dosage for more information.

Children:

- *Neonates –* Children within the first 2 months of life have a markedly decreased ability to eliminate valproate compared to older children and adults. This is a result of reduced clearance (perhaps due to delay in development of glucuronosyltransferase and other enzyme systems involved in valproate elimination) as well as increased volume of distribution (in part due to decreased plasma protein binding). For example, in one study, the half-life in children under 10 days ranged from 10 to 67 hours compared to a range of 7 to 13 hours in children greater than 2 months of age.
- *Children –* Pediatric patients (ie, between 3 months and 10 years of age) have 50% higher clearances expressed on weight (ie, mL/min/kg) than do adults. Over the age of 10 years, children have pharmacokinetic parameters that approximate those of adults.

Contraindications

Hepatic disease or significant hepatic dysfunction; hypersensitivity to the drug; known urea cycle disorders. Hyperammonemic encephalopathy, sometimes fatal, has been reported following initiation of valproate therapy in patients with urea cycle disorders, a group of uncommon genetic abnormalities, particularly ornithine transcarbamylase deficiency.

Warnings

➤*Hepatotoxicity:* See the Warning box for more information.

The drug should be discontinued immediately in the presence of significant hepatic dysfunction, suspected or apparent. In some cases, hepatic dysfunction has progressed in spite of discontinuation of drug.

➤*Pancreatitis:* Cases of life-threatening pancreatitis have been reported in both children and adults receiving valproate. Some of the cases have been described as hemorrhagic with rapid progression from initial symptoms to death. Some cases have occurred shortly after initial use as well as after several years of use. The rate based upon the reported cases exceeds that expected in the general population and there have been cases in which pancreatitis recurred after rechallenge with valproate. In clinical trials, there were 2 cases of pancreatitis without alternative etiology in 2416 patients, representing 1044 patient-years experience. Patients and guardians should be warned that abdominal pain, nausea, vomiting, and/or anorexia can be symptoms of pancreatitis that require prompt medical evaluation. If pancreatitis is diagnosed, valproate should ordinarily be discontinued. Alternative treatment for the underlying medical condition should be initiated as clinically indicated.

➤*Urea cycle disorders:* Hyperammonemic encephalopathy, sometimes fatal, has been reported following initiation of valproate therapy in patients with urea cycle disorders, a group of uncommon genetic abnormalities, particularly ornithine transcarbamylase deficiency. Prior to the initiation of valproate therapy, evaluation for UCD should be considered in the following patients: Those with a history of unexplained encephalopathy or coma, encephalopathy associated with a protein load, pregnancy-related or postpartum encephalopathy, unexplained mental retardation, or history of elevated plasma ammonia or glutamine; those with cyclical vomiting and lethargy, episodic extreme irritability, ataxia, low BUN, or protein avoidance; those with a family history of UCD or a family history of unexplained infant deaths (particularly males); those with other signs or symptoms of UCD. Patients who develop symptoms of unexplained hyperammonemic encephalopathy while receiving valproate therapy should receive prompt treatment (including discontinuation of valproate therapy) and be evaluated for underlying urea cycle disorders.

➤*Somnolence in the elderly:* In a double-blind, multicenter trial of valproate in elderly patients with dementia (mean age = 83 years), doses were increased by 125 mg/day to a target dose of 20 mg/kg/day. A significantly higher proportion of valproate patients had somnolence compared to placebo, and although not statistically significant, there was a higher proportion of patients with dehydration. Discontinuations for somnolence were also significantly higher than with placebo. In some patients with somnolence (approximately 50%), there was associated reduced nutritional intake and weight loss. There was a trend for the patients who experienced these events to have a lower baseline albumin concentration, lower valproate clearance, and a higher BUN. In elderly patients, dosage should be increased more slowly and with regular monitoring for fluid and nutritional

VALPROATE SODIUM — INJECTION

intake, dehydration, somnolence, and other adverse events. Dose reductions or discontinuation of valproate should be considered in patients with decreased food or fluid intake and in patients with excessive somnolence. The ultimate therapeutic dose should be achieved on the basis of both tolerability and clinical response.

➤*Thrombocytopenia:* The frequency of adverse effects (particularly elevated liver enzymes and thrombocytopenia) may be dose related. In a clinical trial of divalproex sodium as monotherapy in patients with epilepsy, 34/126 patients (27%) receiving approximately 50 mg/kg/day on average, had at least 1 value of platelets less than or equal to 75×10^9/L. Approximately half of these patients had treatment discontinued, with return of platelet counts to normal. In the remaining patients, platelet counts normalized with continued treatment. In this study, the probability of thrombocytopenia appeared to increase significantly at total valproate concentrations of greater than or equal to 110 mcg/mL (females) or greater than or equal to 135 mcg/mL (males). The therapeutic benefit which may accompany the higher doses should therefore be weighed against the possibility of a greater incidence of adverse effects.

➤*Posttraumatic seizures:* A study was conducted to evaluate the effect of IV valproate in the prevention of posttraumatic seizures in patients with acute head injuries. Patients were randomly assigned to receive either IV valproate given for 1 week (followed by oral valproate products for either 1 or 6 months per random treatment assignment) or IV phenytoin given for 1 week (followed by placebo). In this study, the incidence of death was found to be higher in the 2 groups assigned to valproate treatment compared to the rate in those assigned to the IV phenytoin treatment group (13% vs 8.5%, respectively). Many of these patients were critically ill with multiple or severe injuries, and evaluation of the causes of death did not suggest any specific drug-related causation. Further, in the absence of a concurrent placebo control during the initial week of intravenous therapy, it is impossible to determine if the mortality rate in the patients treated with valproate was greater or less than that expected in a similar group not treated with valproate, or whether the rate seen in the IV phenytoin treated patients was lower than would be expected. Nonetheless, until further information is available, it seems prudent not to use valproate sodium injection in patients with acute head trauma for the prophylaxis of posttraumatic seizures.

➤*Carcinogenesis:* Valproic acid was administered orally to Sprague-Dawley rats and ICR (HA/ICR) mice at doses of 80 and 170 mg/kg/day (approximately 10 to 50% of the maximum human daily dose on a mg/m^2 basis) for 2 years. A variety of neoplasms were observed in both species. The chief findings were a statistically significant increase in the incidence of subcutaneous fibrosarcomas in high dose male rats receiving valproic acid and a statistically significant dose-related trend for benign pulmonary adenomas in male mice receiving valproic acid. The significance of these findings for humans is unknown.

➤*Fertility impairment:* Chronic toxicity studies in juvenile and adult rats and dogs demonstrated reduced spermatogenesis and testicular atrophy at oral doses of 400 mg/kg/day or greater in rats (approximately equivalent to or greater than the maximum human daily dose on a mg/m^2 basis) and 150 mg/kg/day or greater in dogs (approximately 1.4 times the maximum human daily dose or greater on a mg/m^2 basis). Segment I fertility studies in rats have shown oral doses up to 350 mg/kg/day (approximately equal to the maximum human daily dose on a mg/m^2 basis) for 60 days to have no effect on fertility. The effect of valproate on testicular development and on sperm production and fertility in humans is unknown.

➤*Pregnancy: Category D.* According to published and unpublished reports, valproic acid may produce teratogenic effects in the offspring of human females receiving the drug during pregnancy.

There are multiple reports in the clinical literature which indicate that the use of antiepilepsy drugs during pregnancy results in an increased incidence of birth defects in the offspring. Although data are more extensive with respect to trimethadione, paramethadione, phenytoin, and phenobarbital, reports indicate a possible similar association with the use of other antiepilepsy drugs. Therefore, antiepilepsy drugs should be administered to women of childbearing potential only if they are clearly shown to be essential in the management of their seizures.

The incidence of neural tube defects in the fetus may be increased in mothers receiving valproate during the first trimester of pregnancy. The Centers for Disease Control (CDC) has estimated the risk of valproic acid exposed women having children with spina bifida to be approximately 1% to 2%.

Other congenital anomalies (eg, craniofacial defects, cardiovascular malformations and anomalies involving various body systems), compatible and incompatible with life, have been reported. Sufficient data to determine the incidence of these congenital anomalies is not available.

The higher incidence of congenital anomalies in antiepilepsy drug-treated women with seizure disorders cannot be regarded as a cause and effect relationship. There are intrinsic methodologic problems in obtaining adequate data on drug teratogenicity in humans; genetic factors or the epileptic condition itself, may be more important than drug therapy in contributing to congenital anomalies.

Patients taking valproate may develop clotting abnormalities. A patient who had low fibrinogen when taking multiple anticonvulsants including valproate gave birth to an infant with afibrinogenemia who subsequently died of hemorrhage. If valproate is used in pregnancy, the clotting parameters should be monitored carefully.

Hepatic failure, resulting in the death of a newborn and of an infant, have been reported following the use of valproate during pregnancy.

Animal studies have demonstrated valproate-induced teratogenicity. Increased frequencies of malformations, as well as intrauterine growth retardation and death, have been observed in mice, rats, rabbits, and monkeys following prenatal exposure to valproate. Malformations of the skeletal system are the most common structural abnormalities produced in experimental animals, but neural tube closure defects have been seen in mice exposed to maternal plasma valproate concentrations exceeding 230 mcg/mL (2.3 times the upper limit of the human therapeutic range) during susceptible periods of embryonic development. Administration of an oral dose of 200 mg/kg/day or greater (50% of the maximum human daily dose or greater on a mg/m^2 basis) to pregnant rats during organogenesis produced malformations (skeletal, cardiac, and urogenital) and growth retardation in the offspring. These doses resulted in peak maternal plasma valproate levels of approximately 340 mcg/mL or greater (3.4 times the upper limit of the human therapeutic range or greater). Behavioral deficits have been reported in the offspring of rats given a dose of 200 mg/kg/day throughout most of pregnancy. An oral dose of 350 mg/kg/day (2 times the maximum human daily dose on a mg/m^2 basis) produced skeletal and visceral malformations in rabbits exposed during organogenesis. Skeletal malformations, growth retardation, and death were observed in rhesus monkeys following administration of an oral dose of 200 mg/kg/day (equal to the maximum human daily dose on a mg/m^2 basis) during organogenesis. This dose resulted in peak maternal plasma valproate levels of approximately 280 mcg/mL (2.8 times the upper limit of the human therapeutic range).

The prescribing physician will wish to weigh the benefits of therapy against the risks in treating or counseling women of childbearing potential. If this drug is used during pregnancy, or if the patient becomes pregnant while taking this drug, the patient should be apprised of the potential hazard to the fetus.

Tests to detect neural tube and other defects using current accepted procedures should be considered a part of routine prenatal care in childbearing women receiving valproate.

➤*Lactation:* Valproate is excreted in breast milk. Concentrations in breast milk have been reported to be 1% to 10% of serum concentrations. It is not known what effect this would have on a nursing infant. Consideration should be given to discontinuing nursing when valproate is administered to a nursing woman.

➤*Children:* Experience with oral valproate has indicated that pediatric patients less than 2 years of age are at a considerably increased risk of developing fatal hepatotoxicity, especially those on multiple anticonvulsants, those with congenital metabolic disorders, those with severe seizure disorders accompanied by mental retardation, and those with organic brain disease. The safety of valproate sodium injection has not been studied in individuals below the age of 2 years. If a decision is made to use valproate sodium injection in this age group, it should be used with extreme caution and as a sole agent. The benefits of therapy should be weighed against the risks. Above the age of 2 years, experience in epilepsy has indicated that the incidence of fatal hepatotoxicity decreases considerably in progressively older patient groups.

Younger children, especially those receiving enzyme-inducing drugs, will require larger maintenance doses to attain targeted total and unbound valproic acid concentrations.

The variability in free fraction limits the clinical usefulness of monitoring total serum valproic acid concentrations. Interpretation of valproic acid concentrations in children should include consideration of factors that affect hepatic metabolism and protein binding.

The basic toxicology and pathologic manifestations of valproate sodium in neonatal (4-day-old) and juvenile (14-day-old) rats are similar to those seen in young adult rats. However, additional findings, including renal alterations in juvenile rats and renal alterations and retinal dysplasia in neonatal rats, have been reported. These findings occurred at 240 mg/kg/day, a dosage approximately equivalent to the human maximum recommended daily dose on a mg/m^2 basis. They were not seen at 90 mg/kg, or 40% of the maximum human daily dose on a mg/m^2 basis.

Precautions

➤*Monitoring:* Because of reports of thrombocytopenia, inhibition of the secondary phase of platelet aggregation, and abnormal coagulation parameters (eg, low fibrinogen), platelet counts and coagulation tests are recommended before initiating therapy and at periodic intervals. It is recommended that patients receiving valproate sodium injection be monitored for platelet count and coagulation parameters prior to planned surgery. In a clinical trial of divalproex sodium as monotherapy in patients with epilepsy, 34/126 patients (27%) receiving approximately 50 mg/kg/day on average, had at least 1 value of platelets less than or equal to 75×10^9/L. Approximately half of these patients had treatment discontinued, with return of platelet counts to normal. In the remaining patients, platelet counts normalized with continued treatment. In this study, the probability of thrombocytopenia appeared to increase significantly at total valproate concentrations of greater than or equal to 110 mcg/mL (females) or greater than or equal to 135 mcg/mL (males). Evidence of hemorrhage, bruising, or a disorder of hemostatis/coagulation is an indication for reduction of the dosage or withdrawal of therapy.

Since valproate sodium injection may interact with concurrently administered drugs which are capable of enzyme induction (eg, rifampin, phenobarbital, phenytoin, carbamazepine), periodic plasma concentration determinations of valproate and concomitant drugs are recommended during the early course of therapy.

Patients should be monitored closely for appearance of these symptoms. Liver function tests should be performed prior to therapy and at frequent intervals thereafter, especially during the first 6 months of valproate therapy. However, physicians should not rely totally on serum biochemistry since these tests may not be abnormal in all instances, but should also consider the results of careful interim medical history and physical examination.

➤*Hepatic function impairment:* See the Warning box for more information.

➤*Pancreatitis:* See the Warning box for more information.

VALPROATE SODIUM — INJECTION

➤*Hyperammonemia:* See Warnings for more information.

➤*Lab test abnormalities:* Valproate is partially eliminated in the urine as a keto-metabolite which may lead to a false interpretation of the urine ketone test.

There have been reports of altered thyroid function tests associated with valproate. The clinical significance of these is unknown.

There are in vitro studies that suggest valproate stimulates the replication of the HIV and CMV viruses under certain experimental conditions. The clinical consequence, if any, is not known. Additionally, the relevance of these in vitro findings is uncertain for patients receiving maximally suppressive antiretroviral therapy. Nevertheless, these data should be borne in mind when interpreting the results from regular monitoring of the viral load in HIV-infected patients receiving valproate or when following CMV infected patients clinically.

➤*Hazardous tasks:* Since valproate sodium injection may produce CNS depression, especially when combined with another CNS depressant (eg, alcohol), patients should be advised not to engage in hazardous activities, such as driving an automobile or operating dangerous machinery, until it is known that they do not become drowsy from the drug.

Drug Interactions

Valproic Acid Drug Interactions

Precipitant drug	Object drug*		Description
Charcoal	Valproic acid	↓	Valproic acid absorption is decreased.
Chlorpromazine	Valproic acid	↑	Valproate t½ and trough levels may increase, clearance may decrease.
Cholestyramine	Valproic acid	↓	Serum concentrations and bioavailability of valproic acid may be reduced, resulting in a decrease in therapeutic effects. Administer valproic acid at least 3 hours before, but not within 3 hours following cholestyramine.
Cimetidine	Valproic acid	↑	Small but potentially significant decrease in valproate clearance and increase in $t\frac{1}{2}$.
Erythromycin	Valproic acid	↑	Erythromycin may increase serum valproic acid concentrations, producing valproic acid toxicity.
Felbamate	Valproic acid	↑	Coadministration revealed a 35% increase in mean peak valproate levels.
Rifampin	Valproic acid	↓	In 1 study, rifampin increased the oral clearance of valproate by 40%.
Salicylates (eg, aspirin)	Valproic acid	↑	Salicylates may displace valproic acid from protein binding sites and may also alter the metabolic pathways. Monitor serum concentrations.
Valproic acid	Tricyclic antidepressants	↑	Plasma concentrations and side effects of the tricyclic antidepressant may be increased. Coadministration resulted in a 21% decrease in the plasma clearance of amitriptyline and a 34% decrease in the net clearance of nortriptyline.
Valproic acid	Carbamazepine	↑	Variable changes in carbamazepine concentrations with increased levels of the active metabolite; decreased valproic acid levels with possible loss of seizure control may occur.
Carbamazepine	Valproic acid	↓	
Valproic acid	Clonazepam	↔	Concomitant use may induce absence status in patients with a history of absence type seizures.
Valproic acid	Diazepam	↑	Valproate displaces diazepam from its plasma albumin binding sites and inhibits its metabolism.
Valproic acid	Ethosuximide	↑↓	Increases and decreases in ethosuximide blood levels and decreases in valproic acid levels have been reported. Valproic acid appears to inhibit the metabolism of ethosuximide.
Ethosuximide	Valproic acid	↓	
Valproic acid	Lamotrigine	↑	Serum valproic acid concentrations may be decreased while lamotrigine levels increase. In one study, coadministration increased the half-life of lamotrigine from 26 to 70 hours. Lamotrigine dose should be reduced.
Lamotrigine	Valproic acid	↓	
Valproic acid	Barbiturates	↑	Valproic acid may decrease hepatic metabolism of barbiturates. Barbiturate dosage may need to be decreased in some patients.
Valproic acid	Hydantoins (eg, phenytoin)	↑	Increased action of phenytoin, even at therapeutic levels; increased metabolism of valproic acid with decreased pharmacologic effects may occur.
Hydantoins (eg, phenytoin)	Valproic acid	↓	
Valproic acid	Tolbutamide	↔	The unbound fraction of tolbutamide may be increased from 20% to 50%. The clinical relevance of this displacement is unknown.
Valproic acid	Warfarin	↑	The potential exists for valproate to displace warfarin from protein binding sites. Monitor coagulation tests.
Valproic acid	Zidovudine	↑	Zidovudine clearance was decreased by 38% in 6 HIV seropositive patients.

* ↑ = Object drug increased. ↓ = Object drug decreased. ↔ = Undetermined clinical effect.

➤*Effects of coadministered drugs on valproate clearance:* Drugs that affect the level of expression of hepatic enzymes, particularly those that elevate levels of glucuronosyltransferases, may increase the clearance of valproate. For example, phenytoin, carbamazepine, and phenobarbital (or primidone) can double the clearance of valproate. Thus, patients on monotherapy will generally have longer half-lives and higher concentrations than patients receiving polytherapy with antiepilepsy drugs.

See Precautions for more information.

Adverse Reactions

The adverse events that can result from valproate sodium injection use include all of those associated with oral forms of valproate. The following describes experience specifically with valproate sodium injection. Valproate sodium injection has been generally well tolerated in clinical trials involving 111 healthy adult male volunteers and 352 patients with epilepsy, given at doses of 125 to 6000 mg (total daily dose). A total of 2% of patients discontinued treatment with valproate sodium injection due to adverse events. The most common adverse events leading to discontinuation were 2 cases each of nausea/vomiting and elevated amylase. Other adverse events leading to discontinuation were hallucinations, pneumonia, headache, injection site reaction, and abnormal gait. Dizziness and injection site pain were observed more frequently at a 100 mg/min infusion rate than at rates up to 33 mg/min. At a 200 mg/min rate, dizziness and taste perversion occurred more frequently than at a 100 mg/min rate. The maximum rate of infusion studied was 200 mg/min.

Adverse reactions reported by at least 0.5% of all subjects/patients in clinical trials of valproate sodium are summarized in the table below.

Adverse Reactions Reported During Studies of Valproate Sodium

Adverse reaction	n = 463
Miscellaneous	
Chest pain	1.7%
Headache	4.3%
Injection site inflammation	0.6%
Injection site pain	2.6%
Injection site reaction	2.4%
Pain (unspecified)	1.3%
Cardiovascular	
Vasodilation	0.9%
Dermatologic	
Sweating	0.9%
GI	
Abdominal pain	1.1%
Diarrhea	0.9%
Nausea	3.2%
Vomiting	1.3%

VALPROATE SODIUM — INJECTION

Adverse Reactions Reported During Studies of Valproate Sodium	
Adverse reaction	n = 463
CNS	
Dizziness	5.2%
Euphoria	0.9%
Hypesthesia	0.6%
Nervousness	0.9%
Paresthesia	0.9%
Somnolence	1.7%
Tremor	0.6%
Respiratory	
Pharyngitis	0.6%
Special senses	
Taste perversion	1.9%

In a separate clinical safety trial, 112 patients with epilepsy were given infusions of valproate sodium (up to 15 mg/kg) over 5 to 10 minutes (1.5 to 3 mg/kg/min). The common adverse events (greater than 2%) were somnolence (10.7%), dizziness (7.1%), paresthesia (7.1%), asthenia (7.1%), nausea (6.3%) and headache (2.7%). While the incidence of these adverse events was generally higher than in the table (experience encompassing the standard, much slower infusion rates), eg, somnolence (1.7%), dizziness (5.2%), paresthesia (0.9%), asthenia (0%), nausea (3.2%), and headache (4.3%), a direct comparison between the incidence of adverse events in the 2 cohorts cannot be made because of differences in patient populations and study designs.

Ammonia levels have not been systematically studied after IV valproate, so that an estimate of the incidence of hyperammonemia after IV valproate sodium cannot be provided. Hyperammonemia with encephalopathy has been reported in 2 patients after infusions of valproate sodium.

➤*Epilepsy:* Based on a placebo-controlled trial of adjunctive therapy for treatment of complex partial seizures, divalproex sodium was generally well tolerated with most adverse events rated as mild to moderate in severity. Intolerance was the primary reason for discontinuation in the divalproex sodium-treated patients (6%), compared to 1% of placebo-treated patients.

The table below lists treatment-emergent adverse events which were reported by greater than or equal to 5% of divalproex sodium-treated patients and for which the incidence was greater than in the placebo group, in the placebo-controlled trial of adjunctive therapy for treatment of complex partial seizures. Since patients were also treated with other antiepilepsy drugs, it is not possible, in most cases, to determine whether the following adverse events can be ascribed to divalproex sodium alone, or the combination of divalproex sodium and other antiepilepsy drugs.

Adverse Reactions Reported by ≥ 5% of Patients Treated with Divalproex Sodium During Placebo-controlled Trial of Adjunctive Therapy for Complex Partial Seizures

Adverse reaction	Divalproex sodium (%) (n = 77)	Placebo (%) (n = 70)
Body as a whole		
Headache	31%	21%
Asthenia	27%	7%
Fever	6%	4%
GI		
Nausea	48%	14%
Vomiting	27%	7%
Abdominal pain	23%	6%
Diarrhea	13%	6%
Anorexia	12%	0%
Dyspepsia	8%	4%
Constipation	5%	1%
CNS		
Somnolence	27%	11%
Tremor	25%	6%
Dizziness	25%	13%
Diplopia	16%	9%
Amblyopia/ blurred vision	12%	9%
Ataxia	8%	1%
Nystagmus	8%	1%
Emotional lability	6%	4%
Thinking abnormal	6%	0%
Amnesia	5%	1%
Respiratory		
Flu syndrome	12%	9%
Infection	12%	6%
Bronchitis	5%	1%
Rhinitis	5%	4%
Miscellaneous		
Alopecia	6%	1%
Weight loss	6%	0%

The table below lists treatment-emergent adverse events which were reported by greater than or equal to 5% of patients in the high-dose divalproex sodium group, and for which the incidence was greater than in the low-dose group, in a controlled trial of divalproex sodium monotherapy treatment of complex partial seizures. Since patients were being titrated off another antiepilepsy drug during the first portion of the trial, it is not possible, in many cases, to determine whether the following adverse events can be ascribed to divalproex sodium alone, or the combination of divalproex sodium and other antiepilepsy drugs.

Adverse Reactions Reported by ≥ 5% of Patients in the High Dose Group in the Controlled Clinical Trial of Divalproex Sodium Monotherapy for Complex Partial Seizures[1]

Adverse reaction	High dose (%) (n = 131)	Low dose (%) (n = 134)
Miscellaneous		
Asthenia	21%	10%
GI		
Nausea	34%	26%
Diarrhea	23%	19%
Vomiting	23%	15%
Abdominal pain	12%	9%
Anorexia	11%	4%
Dyspepsia	11%	10%
Hemic/lymphatic system		
Thrombocytopenia	24%	1%
Ecchymosis	5%	4%
Metabolic/nutritional		
Weight gain	9%	4%
Peripheral edema	8%	3%
CNS		
Tremor	57%	19%
Somnolence	30%	18%
Dizziness	18%	13%
Insomnia	15%	9%
Nervousness	11%	7%
Amnesia	7%	4%
Nystagmus	7%	1%
Depression	5%	4%
Respiratory		
Infection	20%	13%
Pharyngitis	8%	2%
Dyspnea	5%	1%
Dermatologic		
Alopecia	24%	13%
Special senses		
Amblyopia/ blurred vision	8%	4%
Tinnitus	7%	1%

[1] Headache was the only adverse event that occurred in greater than or equal to 5% of patients in the high-dose group and at an equal or greater incidence in the low-dose group.

➤*Adverse reactions (greater than 1% but less than 5%):* The following additional adverse events were reported by greater than 1% but less than 5% of the 358 patients treated with divalproex sodium in the controlled trials of complex partial seizures:

Cardiovascular – Tachycardia, hypertension, palpitation.

CNS – Anxiety, confusion, abnormal gait, paresthesia, hypertonia, incoordination, abnormal dreams, personality disorder.

Dermatologic – Rash, pruritus, dry skin.

VALPROATE SODIUM — INJECTION

GI – Increased appetite, flatulence, hematemesis, eructation, pancreatitis, periodontal abscess.

GU – Urinary incontinence, vaginitis, dysmenorrhea, amenorrhea, urinary frequency.

Hematologic/Lymphatic – Petechia.

Metabolic/Nutritional – AST increased, ALT increased.

Musculoskeletal – Myalgia, twitching, arthralgia, leg cramps, myasthenia.

Respiratory – Sinusitis, cough increased, pneumonia, epistaxis.

Special senses – Taste perversion, abnormal vision, deafness, otitis media.

Miscellaneous – Back pain, chest pain, malaise.

➤*Other patient populations:* Adverse events that have been reported with all dosage forms of valproate from epilepsy trials, spontaneous reports, and other sources are listed below by body system.

CNS – Sedative effects have occurred in patients receiving valproate alone but occur most often in patients receiving combination therapy. Sedation usually abates upon reduction of other antiepileptic medication. Tremor (may be dose-related), hallucinations, ataxia, headache, nystagmus, diplopia, asterixis, "spots before eyes", dysarthria, dizziness, confusion, hypesthesia, vertigo, incoordination, and parkinsonism have been reported with the use of valproate. Rare cases of coma have occurred in patients receiving valproate alone or in conjunction with phenobarbital. In rare instances, encephalopathy with or without fever, has developed shortly after the introduction of valproate monotherapy without evidence of hepatic dysfunction or inappropriately high plasma valproate levels. Although recovery has been described following drug withdrawal, there have been fatalities in patients with hyperammonemic encephalopathy, particularly in patients with underlying urea cycle disorders. Hyperammonemic encephalopathy, sometimes fatal, has been reported following initiation of valproate therapy in patients with urea cycle disorders, a group of uncommon genetic abnormalities, particularly ornithine transcarbamylase deficiency.

Several reports have noted reversible cerebral atrophy and dementia in association with valproate therapy.

GI – The most commonly reported side effects at the initiation of therapy are nausea, vomiting, and indigestion. These effects are usually transient and rarely require discontinuation of therapy. Diarrhea, abdominal cramps, and constipation have been reported. Both anorexia with some weight loss and increased appetite with weight gain have also been reported. The administration of delayed-release divalproex sodium may result in reduction of gastrointestinal side effects in some patients using oral therapy.

Pancreatic: Cases of life-threatening pancreatitis have been reported in both children and adults receiving valproate. Some of the cases have been described as hemorrhagic with a rapid progression from initial symptoms to death. Cases have been reported shortly after initial use as well as after several years of use. Patients and guardians should be warned that abdominal pain, nausea, vomiting, or anorexia can be symptoms of pancreatitis that require prompt medical evaluation. If pancreatitis is diagnosed, valproate should ordinarily be discontinued. Alternative treatment for the underlying medical condition should be initiated as clinically indicated.

Dermatologic – Transient hair loss, skin rash, photosensitivity, generalized pruritus, erythema multiforme, and Stevens-Johnson syndrome. Rare cases of toxic epidermal necrolysis have been reported including a fatal case in a 6-month-old infant taking valproate and several other concomitant medications. An additional case of toxic epidermal necrosis resulting in death was reported in a 35-year-old patient with AIDS taking several concomitant medications and with a history of multiple cutaneous drug reactions.

Endocrine – Irregular menses, secondary amenorrhea, breast enlargement, galactorrhea, and parotid gland swelling; abnormal thyroid function tests.

There have been rare spontaneous reports of polycystic ovary disease. A cause and effect relationship has not been established.

GU – Enuresis and urinary tract infection.

Hematologic – Thrombocytopenia and inhibition of the secondary phase of platelet aggregation may be reflected in altered bleeding time, petechiae, bruising, hematoma formation, epistaxis, and frank hemorrhage. Evidence of hemorrhage, bruising, or a disorder of hemostatis/coagulation is an indication for reduction of the dosage or withdrawal of therapy. Relative lymphocytosis, macrocytosis, hypofibrinogenemia, leukopenia, eosinophilia, anemia including macrocytic with or without folate deficiency, bone marrow suppression, pancytopenia, aplastic anemia, and acute intermittent porphyria.

Hepatic – Minor elevations of transaminases (eg, AST, ALT) and LDH are frequent and appear to be dose-related. Occasionally, laboratory test results include increases in serum bilirubin and abnormal changes in other liver function tests. These results may reflect potentially serious hepatotoxicity.

Metabolic – Hyperammonemia, hyponatremia, and inappropriate ADH secretion.

There have been rare reports of Fanconi's syndrome occurring chiefly in children.

Decreased carnitine concentrations have been reported although the clinical relevance is undetermined.

Hyperglycinemia has occurred and was associated with a fatal outcome in a patient with preexistent nonketotic hyperglycinemia.

Musculoskeletal – Weakness.

Psychiatric – Emotional upset, depression, psychosis, aggression, hyperactivity, hostility, and behavioral deterioration.

Special senses – Hearing loss, either reversible or irreversible, has been reported; however, a cause and effect relationship has not been established. Ear pain has also been reported.

Miscellaneous – Anaphylaxis, edema of the extremities, lupus erythematosus, bone pain, cough increased, pneumonia, otitis media, bradycardia, cutaneous vasculitis, and fever.

➤*Mania:* Although valproate sodium injection has not been evaluated for safety and efficacy in the treatment of manic episodes associated with bipolar disorder, the following adverse events not listed above were reported by 1% or more of patients from 2 placebo-controlled clinical trials of divalproex sodium tablets.

Cardiovascular – Hypotension, postural hypotension, vasodilation.

CNS – Agitation, catatonic reaction, hypokinesia, reflexes increased, tardive dyskinesia, vertigo.

Dermatologic – Furunculosis, maculopapular rash, seborrhea.

GI – Fecal incontinence, gastroenteritis, glossitis.

GU – Dysuria.

Musculoskeletal – Arthrosis.

Special senses – Conjunctivitis, dry eyes, eye pain.

Miscellaneous – Chills, neck pain, neck rigidity.

➤*Migraine:* Although valproate sodium injection has not been evaluated for safety and efficacy in the prophylactic treatment of migraine headaches, the following adverse events not listed above were reported by 1% or more of patients from 2 placebo-controlled clinical trials of divalproex sodium tablets.

GI – Dry mouth, stomatitis.

GU – Cystitis, metrorrhagia, and vaginal hemorrhage.

Miscellaneous – Face edema.

Overdosage

➤*Symptoms:* Overdosage with valproate may result in somnolence, heart block, and deep coma. Fatalities have been reported; however, patients have recovered from valproate serum concentrations as high as 2120 mcg/mL.

➤*Treatment:* In overdose situations, the fraction of drug not bound to protein is high and hemodialysis or tandem hemodialysis plus hemoperfusion may result in significant removal of drug. General supportive measures should be applied with particular attention to the maintenance of adequate urinary output.

Naloxone has been reported to reverse the CNS-depressant effects of valproate overdosage. Because naloxone could theoretically also reverse the antiepilepsy effects of valproate, it should be used with caution in patients with epilepsy.

Patient Information

Patients and guardians should be warned that abdominal pain, nausea, vomiting, or anorexia can be symptoms of pancreatitis and, therefore, require further medical evaluation promptly.

Patients should be informed of the signs and symptoms associated with hyperammonemic encephalopathy and be told to inform the prescriber if any of these symptoms occur. In patients who develop unexplained lethargy and vomiting or changes in mental status, hyperammonemic encephalopathy should be considered, and an ammonia level should be measured. If ammonia is increased, valproate therapy should be discontinued.

Since valproate sodium injection may produce CNS depression, especially when combined with another CNS depressant (eg, alcohol), patients should be advised not to engage in hazardous activities, such as driving an automobile or operating dangerous machinery, until it is known that they do not become drowsy from the drug.

The prescribing physician will wish to weigh the benefits of therapy against the risks in treating or counseling women of childbearing potential. If this drug is used during pregnancy, or if the patient becomes pregnant while taking this drug, the patient should be apprised of the potential hazard to the fetus.

There are multiple reports in the clinical literature which indicate that the use of antiepilepsy drugs during pregnancy results in an increased incidence of birth defects in the offspring. Although data are more extensive with respect to trimethadione, paramethadione, phenytoin, and phenobarbital, reports indicate a possible similar association with the use of other antiepilepsy drugs. Therefore, antiepilepsy drugs should be administered to women of childbearing potential only if they are clearly shown to be essential in the management of their seizures.

ATRACURIUM BESYLATE

Rx	**Atracurium Besylate** (Bedford Labs)	**Injection:** 10 mg/mL[a]	In 5 mL single-dose and 10 mL multi-dose vials.[b]
Rx	**Tracrium** (GlaxoWellcome)		In 5 mL single-use and 10 mL multi-dose vials.[c]

[a] With benzenesulfonic acid.
[b] With 0.9% benzyl alcohol in multi-dose vials.
[c] With 0.9% benzyl alcohol.

ATRACURIUM BESYLATE — INJECTION

Indications

As an adjunct to general anesthesia, to facilitate endotracheal intubation and to provide skeletal muscle relaxation during surgery or mechanical ventilation.

Administration and Dosage

➤*Approved by the FDA:* November 23, 1983.

Atracurium besylate should not be administered before unconsciousness has been induced. Atracurium besylate should not be mixed in the same syringe, or administered simultaneously through the same needle, with alkaline solutions (eg, barbiturate solutions).

Administer intravenously. Do not give by intramuscular administration. Intramuscular administration may result in tissue irritation and there are no clinical data to support this route of administration.

Use a peripheral nerve stimulator to monitor twitch suppression and recovery.

➤*Bolus doses for intubation and maintenance of neuromuscular block:*

Adults – A dose of atracurium besylate of 0.4 to 0.5 mg/kg (1.7 to 2.2 times the ED_{95}), given as an intravenous bolus injection, is the recommended initial dose for most patients. With this dose, good or excellent conditions for nonemergency intubation can be expected in 2 to 2.5 minutes in most patients, with maximum neuromuscular block achieved approximately 3 to 5 minutes after injection. Clinically required neuromuscular block generally lasts 20 to 35 minutes under balanced anesthesia. Under balanced anesthesia, recovery to 25% of control is achieved approximately 35 to 45 minutes after injection, and recovery is usually 95% complete approximately 60 minutes after injection.

Atracurium besylate is potentiated by isoflurane or enflurane anesthesia. The same initial dose of atracurium besylate of 0.4 to 0.5 mg/kg may be used for intubation prior to administration of these inhalation agents; however, if atracurium besylate is first administered under steady state of isoflurane or enflurane, the initial dose of atracurium besylate should be reduced by approximately one third (ie, to 0.25 to 0.35 mg/kg) to adjust for the potentiating effects of these anesthetic agents. With halothane, which has only a marginal (approximately 20%) potentiating effect on atracurium besylate, smaller dosage reductions may be considered.

Doses of atracurium besylate of 0.08 to 0.10 mg/kg are recommended for maintenance of neuromuscular block during prolonged surgical procedures. The first maintenance dose will generally be required 20 to 45 minutes after the initial injection of atracurium besylate, but the need for maintenance doses should be determined by clinical criteria. Because atracurium besylate lacks cumulative effects, maintenance doses may be administered at relatively regular intervals for each patient, ranging approximately from 15 to 25 minutes under balanced anesthesia, slightly longer under isoflurane or enflurane. Higher doses of atracurium besylate (up to 0.2 mg/kg) permit maintenance dosing at longer intervals.

Children – No dosage adjustments of atracurium besylate are required for children 2 years of age or older. A dose of atracurium besylate 0.3 to 0.4 mg/kg is recommended as the initial dose for infants (1 month to 2 years of age) under halothane anesthesia. Maintenance doses may be required with slightly greater frequency in infants and children than in adults.

Special considerations – An initial dose of atracurium besylate of 0.3 to 0.4 mg/kg, given slowly or in divided doses over 1 minute, is recommended for adults, adolescents, children, or infants with significant cardiovascular disease and for adults, adolescents, children, or infants with any history (eg, severe anaphylactoid reactions or asthma) suggesting a greater risk of histamine release.

Dosage reductions must be considered also in patients with neuromuscular disease, severe electrolyte disorders, or carcinomatosis in which potentiation of neuromuscular block or difficulties with reversal have been demonstrated. There has been no clinical experience with atracurium besylate in these patients, and no specific dosage adjustments can be recommended. No dosage adjustments of atracurium besylate are required for patients with renal disease.

An initial dose of atracurium besylate of 0.3 to 0.4 mg/kg is recommended for adults following the use of succinylcholine for intubation under balanced anesthesia. Further reductions may be desirable with the use of potent inhalation anesthetics. The patient should be permitted to recover from the effects of succinylcholine prior to administration of atracurium besylate. Insufficient data are available for recommendation of a specific initial dose of atracurium besylate for administration following the use of succinylcholine in children and infants.

➤*Use by continuous infusion:*

Infusion in the operating room (OR) – After administration of a recommended initial bolus dose of atracurium besylate (0.3 to 0.5 mg/kg), a diluted solution of atracurium besylate can be administered by continuous infusion to adults and pediatric patients aged 2 or more years for maintenance of neuromuscular block during extended surgical procedures.

Infusion of atracurium besylate should be individualized for each patient. The rate of administration should be adjusted according to the patient' response as determined by peripheral nerve stimulation. Accurate dosing is best achieved using a precision infusion device.

Infusion of atracurium besylate should be initiated only after early evidence of spontaneous recovery from the bolus dose. An initial infusion rate of 9 to 10 mcg/kg/min may be required to rapidly counteract the spontaneous recovery of neuromuscular function. Thereafter, a rate of 5 to 9 mcg/kg/min should be adequate to maintain continuous neuromuscular block in the range of 89% to 99% in most pediatric and adult patients under balanced anesthesia. Occasional patients may require infusion rates as low as 2 mcg/kg per minute or as high as 15 mcg/kg per minute.

The neuromuscular blocking effect of atracurium besylate administered by infusion is potentiated by enflurane or isoflurane and, to a lesser extent, by halothane. Reduction in the infusion rate of atracurium besylate should, therefore, be considered for patients receiving inhalation anesthesia. The infusion rate of atracurium besylate should be reduced by approximately one-third in the presence of steady-state enflurane or isoflurane anesthesia; smaller reductions should be considered in the presence of halothane.

In patients undergoing cardiopulmonary bypass with induced hypothermia, the rate of infusion of atracurium besylate required to maintain adequate surgical relaxation during hypothermia (25° to 28°C; 77° to 82.4°F) has been shown to be approximately half the rate required during normothermia.

Spontaneous recovery from neuromuscular block following discontinuation of infusion of atracurium besylate may be expected to proceed at a rate comparable to that following administration of a single bolus dose.

Infusion in the intensive care unit (ICU) – The principles for infusion of atracurium besylate in the OR are also applicable to use in the ICU.

An infusion rate of 11 to 13 mcg/kg/min (range, 4.5 to 29.5) should provide adequate neuromuscular block in adult patients in an ICU. Limited information suggests that infusion rates required for pediatric patients in the ICU may be higher than in adult patients. There may be wide interpatient variability in dosage requirements and these requirements may increase or decrease with time (see Precautions). Following recovery from neuromuscular block, readministration of a bolus dose may be necessary to quickly reestablish neuromuscular block prior to reinstitution of the infusion.

➤*Infusion rate tables:* The amount of infusion solution required per minute will depend upon the concentration of atracurium besylate in the infusion solution, the desired dose of atracurium besylate, and the patient' weight. The following tables provide guidelines for delivery, in mL/hr (equivalent to microdrops/min when 60 microdrops = 1 mL), of solutions of atracurium besylate in concentrations of 0.2 mg/mL (20 mg in 100 mL) or 0.5 mg/mL (50 mg in 100 mL) with an infusion pump or a gravity flow device.

Infusion Rates of Atracurium Besylate for a Concentration of 0.2 mg/mL

	Drug delivery rate (mcg/kg per minute)								
	5	6	7	8	9	10	11	12	13
Patient weight (kg)	Infusion delivery rate (mL/h)								
30	45	54	63	72	81	90	99	108	117
35	53	63	74	84	95	105	116	126	137
40	60	72	84	96	108	120	132	144	156
45	68	81	95	108	122	135	149	162	176
50	75	90	105	120	135	150	165	180	195
55	83	99	116	132	149	165	182	198	215
60	90	108	126	144	162	180	198	216	234
65	98	117	137	156	176	195	215	234	254
70	105	126	147	168	189	210	231	252	273
75	113	135	158	180	203	225	248	270	293
80	120	144	168	192	216	240	264	288	312
90	135	162	189	216	243	270	297	324	351
100	150	180	210	240	270	300	330	360	390

ATRACURIUM BESYLATE — INJECTION

Infusion Rates of Atracurium Besylate for a Concentration of 0.5 mg/mL									
	Drug delivery rate (mcg/kg per minute)								
	5	6	7	8	9	10	11	12	13
Patient weight (kg)	Infusion delivery rate (mL/h)								
30	18	22	25	29	32	36	40	43	47
35	21	25	29	34	38	42	46	50	55
40	24	29	34	38	43	48	53	58	62
45	27	32	38	43	49	54	59	65	70
50	30	36	42	48	54	60	66	72	78
55	33	40	46	53	59	66	73	79	86
60	36	43	50	58	65	72	79	86	94
65	39	47	55	62	70	78	86	94	101
70	42	50	59	67	76	84	92	101	109
75	45	54	63	72	81	90	99	108	117
80	48	58	67	77	86	96	106	115	125
90	54	65	76	86	97	108	119	130	140
100	60	72	84	96	108	120	132	144	156

➤*Compatibility and admixtures:* Infusion solutions of atracurium besylate may be prepared by admixing atracurium besylate injection with an appropriate diluent such as 5% dextrose injection; 0.9% sodium chloride injection; or 5% dextrose and 0.9% sodium chloride injection. Infusion solutions should be used within 24 hours of preparation. Unused solutions should be discarded. Solutions containing 0.2 or 0.5 mg/mL atracurium besylate in the above diluents may be stored either under refrigeration or at room temperature for 24 hours without significant loss of potency. Care should be taken during admixture to prevent inadvertent contamination. Visually inspect prior to administration.

Spontaneous degradation of atracurium besylate has been demonstrated to occur more rapidly in Lactated Ringer's solution than in 0.9% sodium chloride solution. Therefore, it is recommended that Lactated Ringer' injection not be used as a diluent in preparing solutions of atracurium besylate for infusion.

Atracurium besylate injection, which has an acid pH, should not be mixed with alkaline solutions (eg, barbiturate solutions) in the same syringe or administered simultaneously during intravenous infusion through the same needle. Depending on the resultant pH of such mixtures, atracurium besylate may be inactivated and a free acid may be precipitated.

➤*Storage/Stability:* Atracurium besylate injection should be refrigerated at 2° to 8°C (36° to 46°F) to preserve potency. Do not freeze. Upon removal from refrigeration to room temperature storage conditions (25°C; 77°F), use atracurium besylate injection within 14 days even if re-refrigerated.

Actions

➤*Pharmacology:* Atracurium besylate is a nondepolarizing skeletal muscle relaxant. Nondepolarizing agents antagonize the neurotransmitter action of acetylcholine by binding competitively with cholinergic receptor sites on the motor end-plate. This antagonism is inhibited, and neuromuscular block reversed, by acetylcholinesterase inhibitors such as neostigmine, edrophonium, and pyridostigmine.

The duration of neuromuscular block produced by atracurium besylate is approximately one-third to one-half the duration of block by d-tubocurarine, metocurine, and pancuronium at initially equipotent doses. As with other nondepolarizing neuromuscular blockers, the time to onset of paralysis decreases and the duration of maximum effect increases with increasing doses of atracurium besylate.

Hemodynamic – Atracurium besylate is a less potent histamine releaser than d-tubocurarine or metocurine. Histamine release is minimal with initial doses of atracurium besylate up to 0.5 mg/kg, and hemodynamic changes are minimal within the recommended dose range. A moderate histamine release and significant falls in blood pressure have been seen following 0.6 mg/kg of atracurium besylate. The histamine and hemodynamic responses were poorly correlated. The effects were generally short-lived and manageable, but the possibility of substantial histamine release in sensitive individuals or in patients in whom substantial histamine release would be especially hazardous (eg, patients with significant cardiovascular disease) must be considered.

➤*Pharmacokinetics:*

Absorption – The pharmacokinetics of atracurium besylate in humans are essentially linear within the 0.3 to 0.6 mg/kg dose range.

Metabolism/Excretion – The duration of neuromuscular block produced by atracurium besylate does not correlate with plasma pseudocholinesterase levels and is not altered by the absence of renal function. This is consistent with the results of in vitro studies that have shown that atracurium besylate is inactivated in plasma via 2 nonoxidative pathways; ester hydrolysis, catalyzed by nonspecific esterases; and Hofmann elimination, a nonenzymatic chemical process that occurs at physiological pH. Some placental transfer occurs in humans.

The elimination half-life is approximately 20 minutes.

Radiolabel studies demonstrated that atracurium besylate undergoes extensive degradation in cats, and that neither kidney nor liver plays a major role in its elimination. Biliary and urinary excretion were the major routes of excretion of radioactivity (totaling greater than 90% of the labeled dose within 7 hours of dosing), of which atracurium besylate represented only a minor fraction. The metabolites in bile and urine were similar, including products of Hofmann elimination and ester hydrolysis.

Contraindications

Known hypersensitivity to atracurium besylate. Use of atracurium besylate from multiple-dose vials containing benzyl alcohol as a preservative is contraindicated in patients with a known hypersensitivity to benzyl alcohol.

Warnings

➤*Administration:* Atracurium besylate should be used only by those skilled in airway management and respiratory support. Equipment and personnel must be immediately available for endotracheal intubation and support of ventilation, including administration of positive pressure oxygen. Adequacy of respiration must be assured through assisted or controlled ventilation. Anticholinesterase reversal agents should be immediately available.

Do not give atracurium besylate by intramuscular administration.

➤*Mutagenesis:* Atracurium was evaluated in a battery of 3 short-term mutagenicity tests. It was nonmutagenic in both the Ames *Salmonella* assay at concentrations up to 1000 mcg/plate, and in a rat bone marrow cytogenicity assay at up to paralyzing doses. A positive response was observed in the mouse lymphoma assay under conditions (80 and 100 mcg/mL, in the absence of metabolic activation) that killed over 80% of the treated cells; there was no mutagenicity at 60 mcg/mL and lower, concentrations that killed up to half of the treated cells. A far weaker response was observed in the presence of metabolic activation at concentrations (1200 mcg/mL and higher) that also killed over 80% of the treated cells.

➤*Elderly:* Since marketing in 1983, uncontrolled clinical experience and limited data from controlled trials have not identified differences in effectiveness, safety, or dosage requirements between healthy elderly and younger patients; however, as with other neuromuscular blocking agents, the use of a peripheral nerve stimulator to monitor neuromuscular function is suggested.

➤*Pregnancy: Category C.*

Teratogenic – Atracurium besylate has been shown to be potentially teratogenic in rabbits when given in doses up to approximately one-half the human dose. There are no adequate and well-controlled studies in pregnant women. Atracurium besylate should be used during pregnancy only if the potential benefit justifies the potential risk to the fetus.

Atracurium besylate was administered subcutaneously on days 6 through 18 of gestation to nonventilated Dutch rabbits. Treatment groups were given either 0.15 mg/kg once daily or 0.10 mg/kg twice daily. Lethal respiratory distress occurred in 2 animals given 0.15 mg/kg and in 1 animal given 0.10 mg/kg, with transient respiratory distress or other evidence of neuromuscular block occurring in 10 of 19 and in 4 of 20 of the animals given 0.15 mg/kg and 0.10 mg/kg, respectively. There was an increased incidence of certain spontaneously occurring visceral and skeletal anomalies or variations in 1 or both treated groups when compared to nontreated controls. The percentage of male fetuses was lower (41% vs 51%) and the postimplantation losses were increased (15% vs 8%) in the group given 0.15 mg/kg once daily when compared to the controls; the mean numbers of implants (6.5 vs 4.4) and healthy live fetuses (5.4 vs 3.8) were greater in this group when compared to the control group.

Labor and delivery – Atracurium besylate (0.3 mg/kg) has been administered to 26 pregnant women during delivery by cesarean section. No harmful effects were attributable to atracurium besylate in any of the neonates, although small amounts of atracurium besylate were shown to cross the placental barrier. The possibility of respiratory depression in the neonate should always be considered following cesarean section during which a neuromuscular blocking agent has been administered. In patients receiving magnesium sulfate, the reversal of neuromuscular block may be unsatisfactory and the dose of atracurium besylate should be lowered as indicated.

➤*Lactation:* It is not known whether this drug is excreted in human milk. Because many drugs are excreted in human milk, caution should be exercised when atracurium besylate is administered to a nursing woman.

➤*Children:* Safety and effectiveness in pediatric patients below the age of 1 month have not been established.

Precautions

➤*Benzyl alcohol:* Atracurium besylate injection 10 mL multiple-dose vials contain benzyl alcohol. In neonates, benzyl alcohol has been associated with an increased incidence of neurological and other complications that are sometimes fatal. Atracurium besylate injection 5 mL single-use vials do not contain benzyl alcohol (see Children).

➤*Long-term use in intensive care unit (ICU):* When there is a need for long-term mechanical ventilation, the benefits-to-risk ratio of neuromuscular block must be considered. The long-term (1 to 10 days) infusion of atracurium besylate during mechanical ventilation in the ICU has been evaluated in several studies. Average infusion rates of 11 to 13 mcg/kg/min (range, 4.5 to 29.5) were required to achieve adequate neuromuscular block. These data suggest that there is wide interpatient variability in dosage requirements. In addition, these studies have shown that dosage requirements may decrease or increase with time. Following discontinuation of infusion of atracurium besylate in these ICU studies, spontaneous recovery of 4 twitches in a train-of-4 occurred in an average of approximately 30 minutes (range, 15 to 75 minutes) and spontaneous recovery to a train-of-4 ratio

ATRACURIUM BESYLATE — INJECTION

more than 75% (the ratio of the height of the fourth to the first twitch in a train-of-4) occurred in an average of approximately 60 minutes (range, 32 to 108 minutes).

Little information is available on the plasma levels and clinical consequences of atracurium metabolites that may accumulate during days to weeks of atracurium administration in ICU patients. Laudanosine, a major biologically active metabolite of atracurium without neuromuscular blocking activity, produces transient hypotension and, in higher doses, cerebral excitatory effects (generalized muscle twitching and seizures) when administered to several species of animals. There have been rare spontaneous reports of seizures in ICU patients who have received atracurium or other agents. These patients usually had predisposing causes (such as head trauma, cerebral edema, hypoxic encephalopathy, viral encephalitis, uremia). There are insufficient data to determine whether or not laudanosine contributes to seizures in ICU patients.

Whenever the use of atracurium besylate or any neuromuscular blocking agent is contemplated in the ICU, it is recommended that neuromuscular transmission be monitored continuously during administration with the help of a nerve stimulator. Additional doses of atracurium besylate or any other neuromuscular blocking agent should not be given before there is a definite response to T_1 or to the first twitch. If no response is elicited, infusion administration should be discontinued until a response returns.

Hemofiltration has a minimal effect on plasma levels of atracurium and its metabolites, including laudanosine. The effects of hemodialysis and hemoperfusion on plasma levels of atracurium and its metabolites are unknown.

➤*Risk of bradycardia:* Since atracurium besylate has no clinically significant effects on heart rate in the recommended dosage range, it will not counteract the bradycardia produced by many anesthetic agents or vagal stimulation. As a result, bradycardia during anesthesia may be more common with atracurium besylate than with other muscle relaxants.

➤*Special risk:*

Burn patients – Resistance to nondepolarizing neuromuscular blocking agents may develop in burn patients. Increased doses of nondepolarizing muscle relaxants may be required in burn patients and are dependent on the time elapsed since the burn injury and the size of the burn.

Malignant hyperthermia (MH) – Multiple factors in anesthesia practice are suspected of triggering malignant hyperthermia (MH), a potentially fatal hypermetabolic state of skeletal muscle. Halogenated anesthetic agents and succinylcholine are recognized as the principal pharmacologic triggering agents in MH-susceptible patients; however, since MH can develop in the absence of established triggering agents, the clinician should be prepared to recognize and treat MH in any patient scheduled for general anesthesia. Reports of MH have been rare in cases in which atracurium besylate has been used. In studies of MH-susceptible animals (swine) and in a clinical study of MH-susceptible patients, atracurium besylate did not trigger this syndrome.

Myasthenia gravis, Eaton-Lambert syndrome, or other neuromuscular diseases – Atracurium besylate may have profound effects in patients with myasthenia gravis, Eaton-Lambert syndrome, or other neuromuscular diseases in which potentiation of nondepolarizing agents has been noted. The use of a peripheral nerve stimulator is especially important for assessing neuromuscular block in these patients. Similar precautions should be taken in patients with severe electrolyte disorders or carcinomatosis.

Histamine release – Although atracurium besylate is a less potent histamine releaser than d-tubocurarine or metocurine, the possibility of substantial histamine release in sensitive individuals must be considered. Special caution should be exercised in administering atracurium besylate to patients in whom substantial histamine release would be especially hazardous (eg, patients with clinically significant cardiovascular disease) and in patients with any history (eg, severe anaphylactoid reactions or asthma) suggesting a greater risk of histamine release. In these patients, the recommended initial dose of atracurium besylate is lower (0.3 to 0.4 mg/kg) than for other patients and should be administered slowly or in divided doses over 1 minute.

Drug Interactions

Atracurium Drug Interactions

Precipitant drug	Object drug*		Description
Diuretics	Atracurium	↑	The neuromuscular blocking effects of atracurium may be increased by thiazide diuretics. Hypokalemia enhances the neuromuscular blockade, possibly by hyperpolarizing the end-plate membrane, increasing resistance to depolarization.
General anesthetics (enflurane, isoflurane, halothane) Antibiotics (eg, aminoglycosides, polypeptide antibiotics) Lithium Verapamil Procainamide Quinidine	Atracurium	↑	These medications may enhance the neuromuscular blocking action of atracurium. Neuromuscular blockade was prolonged 20% by halothane and 35% by enflurane and isoflurane.
Magnesium sulfate	Atracurium	↑	When administered for the management of toxemia of pregnancy, may enhance neuromuscular blockade of pancuronium. However, in one patient, reversal of neuromuscular blockade was not affected by magnesium sulfate.
Other muscle relaxants	Atracurium	↔	If administered during the same procedure, consider the possibility of a synergistic or antagonist effect.
Phenytoin Theophylline	Atracurium	↓	Phenytoin and theophylline may cause resistance to, or reversal of, the neuromuscular blocking action of atracurium.
Succinylcholine	Atracurium	↑	Succinylcholine does not enhance duration, but quickens onset and may increase depth of atracurium-induced neuromuscular blockade.
Acetylcholinesterase inhibitors (eg, neostigmine, edrophonium and pyridostigmine	Atracurium	↓	Antagonism is inhibited and neuromuscular block is reversed by acetylcholinesterase inhibitors.
Corticosteroids	Atracurium	↑	Prolonged weakness may occur.

* ↑ = Object drug increased. ↓ = Object drug decreased. ↔ = Undetermined effect.

Adverse Reactions

➤*Observed in controlled clinical studies:* Atracurium besylate was well tolerated and produced few adverse reactions during extensive clinical trials. Most adverse reactions were suggestive of histamine release. In studies including 875 patients, atracurium besylate was discontinued in only 1 patient (who required treatment for bronchial secretions), and 6 other patients required treatment for adverse reactions attributable to atracurium besylate (wheezing in 1, hypotension in 5). Of the 5 patients who required treatment for hypotension, 3 had a history of significant cardiovascular disease. The overall incidence rate for clinically important adverse reactions, therefore, was 7/875 or 0.8%. The table below includes all adverse reactions reported attributable to atracurium besylate during clinical trials with 875 patients.

Atracurium Adverse Reactions

	Initial dose of atracurium besylate (mg/kg)			
	0 to 0.3 (mg/kg)	0.31 to 0.5* (mg/kg)	≥ 0.6 (mg/kg)	Total (mg/kg)
Adverse reaction	(n = 485)	(n = 366)	(n = 24)	(n = 875)
Skin flush	1%	8.7%	29.2%	5%
Erythema	0.6%	0.5%	0%	0.6%
Itching	0.4%	0%	0%	0.2%
Wheezing/bronchial secretions	0.2%	0.3%	0%	0.2%
Hives	0.2%	0%	0%	0.1%

* Includes the recommended initial dosage range for most patients.

Most adverse reactions were of little clinical significance unless they were associated with significant hemodynamic changes. The table below summarizes the incidences of substantial vital sign changes noted during clinical trials of atracurium besylate with 530 patients, without cardiovascular disease, in whom these parameters were assessed.

ATRACURIUM BESYLATE — INJECTION

Percent of Patients Showing > 30% Vital Sign Changes Following Administration of Atracurium Besylate

	Initial atracurium besylate dose (mg/kg)			
	0 to 0.3 (mg/kg)	0.31 to 0.5* (mg/kg)	≥ 0.6 (mg/kg)	Total (mg/kg)
Vital sign change	(n = 365)	(n = 144)	(n = 21)	(n = 530)
Mean arterial pressure				
Increase	1.9%	2.8%	0%	2.1%
Decrease	1.1%	2.1%	14.3%	1.9%
Heart rate				
Increase	1.6%	2.8%	4.8%	2.1%
Decrease	0.8%	0%	0%	0.6%

* Includes the recommended initial dosage range for most patients.

➤*Observed in clinical practice:* Based on initial clinical practice experience in approximately 3 million patients who received atracurium besylate in the US and in the United Kingdom, spontaneously reported adverse reactions were uncommon (approximately 0.01% to 0.02%). The following adverse reactions are among the most frequently reported, but there are insufficient data to support an estimate of their incidence:

Allergic – Allergic reactions (anaphylactic or anaphylactoid responses) which, in rare instances, were severe (eg, cardiac arrest).

Cardiovascular – Hypotension, vasodilatation (flushing), tachycardia, bradycardia.

CNS – There have been rare spontaneous reports of seizures in ICU patients following long-term infusion of atracurium to support mechanical ventilation. There are insufficient data to define the contribution, if any, of atracurium or its metabolite laudanosine (see Precautions).

Local – Rash, urticaria, reaction at injection site.

Musculoskeletal – Inadequate block, prolonged block.

Respiratory – Dyspnea, bronchospasm, laryngospasm.

Overdosage

➤*Symptoms:* There has been limited experience with overdosage of atracurium besylate. The possibility of iatrogenic overdosage can be minimized by carefully monitoring muscle twitch response to peripheral nerve stimulation. Excessive doses of atracurium besylate can be expected to produce enhanced pharmacological effects. Overdosage may increase the risk of histamine release and cardiovascular effects, especially hypotension.

Three pediatric patients (3 weeks, 4 and 5 months of age) unintentionally received doses of 0.8 mg/kg to 1 mg/kg of atracurium besylate. The time to 25% recovery (50 to 55 minutes) following these doses, which were 5 to 6 times the ED_{95} dose, was moderately longer than the corresponding time observed following doses 20 to 2.5 times the atracurium besylate ED_{95} dose in infants (22 to 36 minutes). Cardiovascular changes were minimal. Nonetheless the possibility of cardiovascular changes must be considered in the case of overdose.

An adult patient (17 years of age) unintentionally received an initial dose of 1.3 mg/kg of atracurium besylate. The time from injection to 25% recovery (83 minutes) was approximately twice that observed following maximum recommended doses in adults (35 to 45 minutes). The patient experienced moderate hemodynamic changes (13% increase in mean arterial pressure and 27% increase in heart rate) which persisted for 40 minutes and did not require treatment.

➤*Treatment:* If cardiovascular support is necessary, this should include proper positioning, fluid administration, and the use of vasopressor agents if necessary. The patient's airway should be assured, with manual or mechanical ventilation maintained as necessary. A longer duration of neuromuscular block may result from overdosage and a peripheral nerve stimulator should be used to monitor recovery. Recovery may be facilitated by administration of an anticholinesterase reversing agent such as neostigmine, edrophonium, or pyridostigmine, in conjunction with an anticholinergic agent such as atropine or glycopyrrolate. The appropriate monographs should be consulted for prescribing information.

CISATRACURIUM BESYLATE

Rx	**Nimbex** (GlaxoWellcome)	**Injection:** 2 mg/ml	In 5 and 10[1] ml vials.
		10 mg/ml	In 20 ml vials.

[1] Contains 0.9% benzyl alcohol as a preservative.

CISATRACURIUM BESYLATE — INJECTION

Indications

For inpatients and outpatients as an adjunct to general anesthesia, to facilitate tracheal intubation, and to provide skeletal muscle relaxation during surgery or mechanical ventilation in the ICU.

Administration and Dosage

➤*Approved by the FDA:* December 15, 1995.

Cisatracurium besylate should only be administered IV.

The dosage information provided below is intended as a guide only. Individualize doses of cisatracurium. The use of a peripheral nerve stimulator will permit the most advantageous use of cisatracurium, minimize the possibility of overdosage or underdosage, and assist in the evaluation of recovery.

➤*Adults:*

Initial doses – One of 2 intubating doses of cisatracurium besylate may be chosen, based on the desired time to tracheal intubation and the anticipated length of surgery. In addition to the dose of neuromuscular-blocking agent, the presence of coinduction agents (eg, fentanyl, midazolam) and the depth of anesthesia are factors that can influence intubation conditions. Doses of 0.15 ($3 \times ED_{95}$ and 0.2 ($4 \times ED_{95}$) mg/kg cisatracurium, as components of a propofol/nitrous oxide/oxygen induction-intubation technique, may produce generally good or excellent conditions for intubation in 2 and 1.5 minutes, respectively. Similar intubation conditions may be expected when these doses of cisatracurium are administered as components of a thiopental/nitrous oxide/oxygen induction-intubation technique. In 2 intubation studies using thiopental or propofol and midazolam and fentanyl as coinduction agents, excellent intubation conditions were most frequently achieved with the 0.2 mg/kg compared to 0.15 mg/kg dose of cisatracurium. The clinically effective durations of action for 0.15 and 0.2 mg/kg cisatracurium during propofol anesthesia are 55 minutes (range, 44 to 74 minutes) and 61 minutes (range, 41 to 81 minutes), respectively. Lower doses may result in a longer time for the development of satisfactory intubation conditions. Doses up to $8 \times ED_{95}$ cisatracurium have been safely administered to healthy adult patients and patients with serious cardiovascular disease. These larger doses are associated with longer clinically effective durations of action.

Because slower times to onset of complete neuromuscular block were observed in elderly patients and patients with renal dysfunction, extending the interval between administration of cisatracurium, and the intubation attempt for these patients may be required to achieve adequate intubation conditions.

A dose of 0.03 mg/kg cisatracurium besylate is recommended for maintenance of neuromuscular block during prolonged surgical procedures. Maintenance doses of 0.03 mg/kg each sustain neuromuscular block for approximately 20 minutes. Maintenance dosing is generally required 40 to 50 minutes following an initial dose of 0.15 mg/kg cisatracurium and 50 to 60 minutes following an initial dose of 0.2 mg/kg cisatracurium, but the need for maintenance doses should be determined by clinical criteria. For shorter or longer durations of action, smaller or larger maintenance doses may be administered.

Isoflurane or enflurane administered with nitrous oxide/oxygen to achieve 1.25 MAC (minimum alveolar concentration) may prolong the clinically effective duration of action of initial and maintenance doses. The magnitude of these effects may depend on the duration of administration of the volatile agents. Fifteen to 30 minutes of exposure to 1.25 MAC isoflurane or enflurane had minimal effects on the duration of action of initial doses of cisatracurium and, therefore, no adjustment to the initial dose should be necessary when cisatracurium is administered shortly after initiation of volatile agents. In long surgical procedures during enflurane or isoflurane anesthesia, less frequent maintenance dosing or lower maintenance doses of cisatracurium may be necessary. No adjustments to the initial dose of cisatracurium are required when used in patients receiving propofol anesthesia.

➤*Children:*

Initial doses – The recommended dose of cisatracurium for children 2 to 12 years of age is 0.1 to 0.15 mg/kg administered over 5 to 10 seconds during either halothane or opioid anesthesia. When administered during stable opioid/nitrous oxide/oxygen anesthesia, 0.1 mg/kg cisatracurium produces maximum neuromuscular block in an average of 2.8 minutes (range, 1.8 to 6.7 minutes) and clinically effective block for 28 minutes (range, 21 to 38 minutes). When administered during stable opioid/nitrous oxide/oxygen anesthesia, 0.15 mg/kg cisatracurium produces maximum neuromuscular block in about 3 minutes (range, 1.5 to 8 minutes) and clinically effective block (time to 25% recovery) for 36 minutes (range, 29 to 46 minutes).

Infants –

Initial doses: The recommended dose of cisatracurium for intubation of infants 1 month to 23 months is 0.15 mg/kg administered over 5 to 10 seconds during either halothane or opioid anesthesia. When administered during stable opioid/nitrous oxide/oxygen anesthesia, 0.15 mg/kg cisatracurium produces maximum neuromuscular block in about 2 minutes (range, 1.3 to 3.4 minutes) and clinically effective block (time to 25% recovery) for about 43 minutes (range, 34 to 58 minutes).

➤*Use by continuous infusion:*

Infusion in the operating room (OR) – After administration of an initial bolus dose of cisatracurium, a diluted solution of cisatracurium can be administered by continuous infusion to adults and children aged 2 or more years for maintenance of neuromuscular block during extended surgical procedures. Individualize infusion of cisatracurium besylate for each patient. Adjust the rate of administration according to the patient's response as

CISATRACURIUM BESYLATE — INJECTION

determined by peripheral nerve stimulation. Accurate dosing is best achieved using a precision infusion device.

Initiate infusion of cisatracurium besylate only after early evidence of spontaneous recovery from the initial bolus dose. An initial infusion rate of 3 mcg/kg/min may be required to rapidly counteract the spontaneous recovery of neuromuscular function. Thereafter, a rate of 1 to 2 mcg/kg/min should be adequate to maintain continuous neuromuscular block in the range of 89% to 99% in most pediatric and adult patients under opioid/nitrous oxide/oxygen anesthesia.

Consider reduction of the infusion rate by up to 30% to 40% when cisatracurium is administered during stable isoflurane or enflurane anesthesia (administered with nitrous oxide/oxygen at the 1.25 MAC level). Greater reductions in the infusion rate of cisatracurium may be required with longer durations of administration of isoflurane or enflurane.

The rate of infusion of atracurium required to maintain adequate surgical relaxation in patients undergoing coronary artery bypass surgery with induced hypothermia (25° to 28°C; 77° to 82.4°F) is approximately half the rate required during normothermia. Based on the structural similarity between cisatracurium and atracurium, a similar effect on the infusion rate of cisatracurium may be expected.

Spontaneous recovery from neuromuscular block following discontinuation of infusion of cisatracurium may be expected to proceed at a rate comparable to that following administration of a single bolus dose.

Infusion in the intensive care unit (ICU) – The principles for infusion of cisatracurium besylate in the operating room are also applicable to use in the ICU. An infusion rate of approximately 3 mcg/kg/min (range, 0.5 to 10.2 mcg/kg/min) should provide adequate neuromuscular block in adult patients in the ICU. There may be wide interpatient variability in dosage requirements and these may increase or decrease with time. Following recovery from neuromuscular block, readministration of a bolus dose may be necessary to quickly reestablish neuromuscular block prior to reinstitution of the infusion.

Infusion rate tables – The amount of infusion solution required per minute will depend upon the concentration of cisatracurium in the infusion solution, the desired dose of cisatracurium, and the patient's weight. The contribution of the infusion solution to the fluid requirements of the patient also must be considered. The tables below provide guidelines for delivery, in mL/hr (equivalent to microdrops/minute when 60 microdrops = 1 mL), of cisatracurium solutions in concentrations of 0.1 mg/mL (10 mg/100 mL) or 0.4 mg/mL (40 mg/100 mL).

Infusion Rates of Cistracurium for Maintenance of Neuromuscular Block during Opioid/Nitrous Oxide/Oxygen Anesthesia for a Concentration of 0.1 mg/mL

Patient weight (kg)	Drug delivery rate (mcg/kg/min)				
	1	1.5	2	3	5
	Infusion delivery rate (mL/hr)				
10	6	9	12	18	30
45	27	41	54	81	135
70	42	63	84	126	210
100	60	90	120	180	300

Infusion Rates of Cistracurium for Maintenance of Neuromuscular Block during Opioid/Nitrous Oxide/Oxygen Anesthesia for a Concentration of 0.4 mg/mL

Patient weight (kg)	Drug delivery rate (mcg/kg/min)				
	1	1.5	2	3	5
	Infusion delivery rate (mL/hr)				
10	1.5	2.3	3	4.5	7.5
45	6.8	10.1	13.5	20.3	33.8
70	10.5	15.8	21	31.5	52.5
100	15	22.5	30	45	75

➤*Compatibility and admixtures:*

Y-site administration – Cisatracurium injection is acidic (pH = 3.25 to 3.65) and may not be compatible with alkaline solution having a pH greater than 8.5 (eg, barbiturate solutions).

Studies have shown that cisatracurium besylate injection is compatible with the following: 5% Dextrose Injection; 0.9% Sodium Chloride Injection; 5% Dextrose and 0.9% Sodium Chloride Injection; Sufentanil citrate injection, diluted as directed; Alfentanil hydrochloride injection, diluted as directed; Fentanyl citrate injection, diluted as directed; Midazolam hydrochloride injection, diluted as directed; Droperidol injection, diluted as directed.

Cisatracurium injection is not compatible with propofol injection or ketorolac injection for Y-site administration. Studies of other parenteral products have not been conducted.

➤*Storage / Stability:* Cisatracurium injection should be refrigerated at 2° to 8°C (36° to 46°F) in the carton to preserve potency. Protect from light. Do not freeze. Upon removal from refrigeration to room temperature storage conditions (25°C/77°F), use cisatracurium injection within 21 days, even if rerefrigerated.

Dilution stability – Cisatracurium injection diluted in 5% Dextrose Injection; 0.9% Sodium Chloride Injection, or 5% Dextrose and 0.9% Sodium Chloride Injection to 0.1 mg/mL may be stored either under refrigeration or at room temperature for 24 hours without significant loss of potency. Dilutions to 0.1 mg/mL or 0.2 mg/mL in 5% Dextrose and Lactated Ringer's Injection may be stored under refrigeration for 24 hours.

Do not dilute cisatracurium injection in Lactated Ringer's Injection due to chemical instability.

Actions

➤*Pharmacology:*

Pharmacodynamics – Cisatracurium binds competitively to cholinergic receptors on the motor end-plate to antagonize the action of acetylcholine, resulting in block of neuromuscular transmission. This action is antagonized by acetylcholinesterase inhibitors such as neostigmine.

➤*Pharmacokinetics:*

Distribution – The volume of distribution of cisatracurium is limited by its large molecular weight and high polarity. The V_{ss} (volume of distribution at steady state) was equal to 145 mL/kg in healthy 19- to 64-year-old surgical patients receiving opioid anesthesia. The V_{ss} was 21% larger in similar patients receiving inhalation anesthesia.

Metabolism – The degradation of cisatracurium is largely independent of liver metabolism. Results from in vitro experiments suggest that cisatracurium undergoes Hofmann elimination (a pH- and temperature-dependent chemical process) to form laudanosine and the monoquaternary acrylate metabolite. The monoquaternary acrylate undergoes hydrolysis by nonspecific plasma esterases to form the monoquaternary alcohol (MQA) metabolite. The MQA metabolite can also undergo Hofmann elimination but at a much slower rate than cisatracurium. Laudanosine is further metabolized to desmethyl metabolites that are conjugated with glucuronic acid and excreted in the urine.

Organ-independent Hofmann elimination is the predominant pathway for the elimination of cisatracurium. The liver and kidney play a minor role in the elimination of cisatracurium but are primary pathways for the elimination of metabolites. Therefore, the t½β values of metabolites (including laudanosine) are longer in patients with kidney or liver dysfunction, and metabolite concentrations may be higher after long-term administration. Most importantly, C_{max} values of laudanosine are significantly lower in healthy surgical patients receiving infusions of cisatracurium than in patients receiving infusions of atracurium (mean ± SD C_{max}: 60 ± 52 and 342 ± 93 ng/mL, respectively).

Excretion – Mean clearance (CL) values for cisatracurium ranged from 4.5 to 5.7 mL/min/kg in studies of healthy surgical patients. Compartmental pharmacokinetic modeling suggests that approximately 80% of the CL is accounted for by Hofmann elimination and the remaining 20% by renal and hepatic elimination. These findings are consistent with the low magnitude of interpatient variability in CL (16%) estimated as part of the population PK/PD analyses and with the recovery of parent and metabolites in urine. Following ^{14}C-cisatracurium administration to 6 healthy male patients, 95% of the dose was recovered in the urine (mostly as conjugated metabolites) and 4% in the feces; less than 10% of the dose was excreted as unchanged parent drug in the urine. In 12 healthy surgical patients receiving nonradiolabeled cisatracurium who had Foley catheters placed for surgical management, approximately 15% of the dose was excreted unchanged in the urine.

In studies of healthy surgical patients, mean t½β values of cisatracurium ranged from 22 to 29 minutes and were consistent with the t½β of cisatracurium in vitro (29 minutes). The mean ± SD t½β values of laudanosine were 3.1 ± 0.4 and 3.3 ± 2.1 hours in healthy surgical patients receiving cisatracurium besylate (n = 10) or atracurium (n = 10), respectively. During IV infusions of cisatracurium besylate, peak plasma concentrations (C_{max}) of laudanosine and the MQA metabolite are approximately 6% and 11% of the parent compound, respectively.

Special populations –

Renal function impairment: Results from a conventional pharmacokinetic study of cisatracurium in 13 healthy adult patients and 15 patients with end-stage renal disease (ESRD) undergoing elective surgery are summarized below. The pharmacokinetic/pharmacodynamic parameters of cisatracurium were similar in healthy adult patients and ESRD patients. The times to 90% block were approximately 1 minute slower in ESRD patients following 0.1 mg/kg cisatracurium. There were no differences in the durations or rates of recovery of cisatracurium between ESRD and healthy adult patients.

The t½β values of metabolites are longer in patients with renal failure and concentrations may be higher after long-term administration.

Population pharmacokinetic analyses revealed that patients with creatinine clearances less than or equal to 70 mL/min had slower rates of equilibration between plasma concentrations and neuromuscular block than patients with normal renal function; this change was associated with slightly slower (approximately 40 seconds) predicted times to 90% T_1 suppression in patients with renal dysfunction following 0.1 mg/kg cisatracurium. There was no clinically significant alteration in the recovery profile of cisatracurium besylate in patients with renal dysfunction. The recovery profile of cisatracurium is unchanged in the presence of renal or hepatic failure, which is consistent with predominantly organ-independent elimination.

Hepatic function impairment: The information summarizes the conventional pharmacokinetic analysis from a study of cisatracurium in 13 patients with end-stage liver disease undergoing liver transplantation and

CISATRACURIUM BESYLATE — INJECTION

11 healthy adult patients undergoing elective surgery. The slightly larger volumes of distribution in liver transplant patients were associated with slightly higher plasma clearances of cisatracurium. The parallel changes in these parameters resulted in no difference in t½β values. There were no differences in k_{eo} or EC_{50} between patient groups. The times to maximum block were approximately 1 minute faster in liver transplant patients than in healthy adult patients receiving 0.1 mg/kg cisatracurium. These minor differences in pharmacokinetics were not associated with clinically significant differences in the recovery profile of cisatracurium.

The t½β values of metabolites are longer in patients with hepatic disease, and concentrations may be higher after long-term administration.

Elderly: The results of conventional pharmacokinetic analysis from a study of 12 healthy elderly patients and 12 healthy young adult patients receiving a single IV dose of 0.1 mg/kg cisatracurium are summarized below. Plasma clearances of cisatracurium were not affected by age; however, the volumes of distribution were slightly larger in elderly patients than in young patients, resulting in slightly longer t½β values for cisatracurium. The rate of equilibration between plasma cisatracurium concentrations and neuromuscular block was slower in elderly patients than in young patients (mean ± SD k_{eo}: 0.071 ± 0.036 and 0.105 ± 0.021 $minutes^{-1}$, respectively); there was no difference in the patient sensitivity to cisatracurium-induced block, as indicated by EC_{50} values (mean ± SD EC_{50}: 91 ± 22 and 89 ± 23 ng/mL, respectively). These changes were consistent with the 1-minute slower times to maximum block in elderly patients receiving 0.1 mg/kg cisatracurium, when compared to young patients receiving the same dose. The minor differences in pharmacokinetic/pharmacodynamic parameters of cisatracurium between elderly patients and young patients were not associated with clinically significant differences in the recovery profile of cisatracurium.

Children: The population pharmacokinetics/pharmacodynamics of cisatracurium were described in 20 healthy pediatric patients during halothane anesthesia, using the same model developed for healthy adult patients. The CL was higher in healthy pediatric patients (5.89 mL/min/kg) than in healthy adult patients (4.57 mL/min/kg) during opioid anesthesia. The rate of equilibration between plasma concentrations and neuromuscular block, as indicated by k_{eo}, was faster in healthy pediatric patients receiving halothane anesthesia (0.133 $minutes^{-1}$) than in healthy adult patients receiving opioid anesthesia (0.0575 $minutes^{-1}$). The EC_{50} in healthy pediatric patients (125 ng/mL) was similar to the value in healthy adult patients (141 ng/mL) during opioid anesthesia. The minor differences in the pharmacokinetic/pharmacodynamic parameters of cisatracurium were associated with a faster time to onset and a shorter duration of cisatracurium-induced neuromuscular block in pediatric patients.

Other patient factors: Population pharmacokinetic/pharmacodynamic analyses revealed that gender and obesity were associated with statistically significant effects on the pharmacokinetics or pharmacodynamics of cisatracurium; these factors were not associated with clinically significant alterations in the predicted onset or recovery profile of cisatracurium. The use of inhalation agents was associated with a 21% larger V_{ss}, a 78% larger k_{eo}, and a 15% lower EC_{50} for cisatracurium. These changes resulted in a slightly faster (approximately 45 seconds) predicted time to 90% T_1 suppression in patients receiving 0.1 mg/kg cisatracurium during inhalation anesthesia than in patients receiving the same dose of cisatracurium during opioid anesthesia; however, there were no clinically significant differences in the predicted recovery profile of cisatracurium between patient groups.

Additional pharmacokinetic data – The neuromuscular-blocking activity of cisatracurium besylate is due to parent drug. Cisatracurium plasma concentration-time data following IV bolus administration are best described by a 2-compartment open model (with elimination from both compartments) with an elimination half-life (t½β) of 22 minutes, a plasma clearance (CL) of 4.57 mL/min/kg, and a V_{ss} of 145 mL/kg. Cisatracurium undergoes organ-independent Hofmann elimination (a chemical process dependent on pH and temperature) to form the monoquaternary acrylate metabolite and laudanosine, neither of which has any neuromuscular-blocking activity. Following administration of radiolabeled cisatracurium, 95% of the dose was recovered in the urine; less than 10% of the dose was excreted as unchanged parent drug. Laudanosine, a metabolite of cisatracurium (and atracurium) has been noted to cause transient hypotension and, in higher doses, cerebral excitatory effects when administered to several animal species. The relationship between CNS excitation and laudanosine concentrations in humans has not been established. Because cisatracurium is 3 times more potent than atracurium, and lower doses are required, the corresponding laudanosine concentrations following cisatracurium are one-third of those that would be expected following an equipotent dose of atracurium.

Contraindications

Hypersensitivities to cisatracurium or other bis-benzylisoquinolinium agents. Use of cisatracurium from vials containing benzyl alcohol as a preservative is contraindicated in patients with a known hypersensitivity to benzyl alcohol.

Warnings

➤*Administration:* Administer cisatracurium in carefully adjusted dosage by or under the supervision of experienced clinicians who are familiar with the drug's actions and the possible complications of its use. Do not administer the drug unless personnel and facilities for resuscitation and life support (tracheal intubation, artificial ventilation, oxygen therapy), and an antagonist of cisatracurium besylate are immediately available. It is recommended that a peripheral nerve stimulator be used to measure neuromuscular function during the administration of cisatracurium besylate in order to monitor drug effect, determine the need for additional doses, and confirm recovery from neuromuscular block.

Cisatracurium besylate has no known effect on consciousness, pain threshold, or cerebration. To avoid distress to the patient, do not induce neuromuscular block before unconsciousness.

➤*Renal/Hepatic function impairment:* See Actions for more information.

➤*Mutagenesis:* Cisatracurium was evaluated in a battery of 4 short-term mutagenicity tests. It was nonmutagenic in the Ames *Salmonella* assay, a rat bone marrow cytogenetic assay, and an in vitro human lymphocyte cytogenetics assay. As was the case with atracurium, the mouse lymphoma assay was positive both in the presence and absence of exogenous metabolic activation (rat liver S-9). In the absence of S-9, cisatracurium was positive at in vitro cisatracurium concentrations of 40 mcg/mL and higher. The highest nonmutagenic concentration (30 mcg/mL) and incubation time (4 hours) resulted in an AUC approximately 120 times that noted in clinical studies and approximately 8.5 times the mean peak clinical concentration noted. In the presence of S-9, cisatracurium was positive at a cisatracurium concentration of 300 mcg/mL but not at lower or higher concentrations.

➤*Elderly:* Of the total number of subjects in clinical studies of cisatracurium, 57 were 65 years and over, 63 were 70 years and over, and 15 were 80 years and over. The geriatric population included a subset of patients with significant cardiovascular disease. No overall differences in safety or effectiveness were observed between these subjects and younger subjects, and other reported clinical experience has not identified differences in responses between elderly and younger subjects, but greater sensitivity of some older individuals to cisatracurium cannot be ruled out.

See Actions for more information.

➤*Pregnancy: Category B.*

Teratogenic – There are no adequate and well-controlled studies of cisatracurium in pregnant women. Because animal studies are not always predictive of human response, use cisatracurium during pregnancy only if clearly needed.

➤*Lactation:* It is not known whether cisatracurium besylate is excreted in human milk. Because many drugs are excreted in human milk, exercise caution following administration of cisatracurium besylate to a nursing woman.

➤*Children:* Cisatracurium besylate has not been studied in children below the age of 1 month. Intubation of the trachea in patients 1 to 4 years old was facilitated more reliably when cisatracurium besylate was used in combination with halothane than when opioids and nitrous oxide were used for induction of anesthesia.

Precautions

➤*Monitoring:* Whenever the use of cisatracurium or any other neuromuscular-blocking agent in the ICU is contemplated, monitor neuromuscular function during administration with a nerve stimulator. Do not give additional doses of cisatracurium or any other neuromuscular-blocking agent before there is a definite response to nerve stimulation. If no response is elicited, discontinue infusion administration until a response returns.

➤*Benzyl alcohol:* The 10 mL multiple-dose vials of cisatracurium besylate contain benzyl alcohol. In newborn infants, benzyl alcohol has been associated with an increased incidence of neurological and other complications which are sometimes fatal. Single-use vials (5 mL and 20 mL) of cisatracurium besylate do not contain benzyl alcohol.

Because of its intermediate onset of action, cisatracurium is not recommended for rapid sequence endotracheal intubation.

➤*Special risk:* Acid-base or serum electrolyte abnormalities may potentiate or antagonize the action of neuromuscular-blocking agents.

Long-term use in the ICU – Long-term infusion (up to 6 days) of cisatracurium during mechanical ventilation in the ICU has been safely used in 2 studies. Dosage requirements may increase or decrease with time.

Whenever the use of cisatracurium or any other neuromuscular-blocking agent in the ICU is contemplated, monitor neuromuscular function during administration with a nerve stimulator. Do not give additional doses of cisatracurium or any other neuromuscular-blocking agent before there is a definite response to nerve stimulation. If no response is elicited, discontinue infusion administration until a response returns.

Malignant hyperthermia (MH) – In a study of MH-susceptible pigs, cisatracurium besylate (highest dose 2,000 mcg/kg equivalent to 3 × ED_{95} in pigs and 40 × ED_{95} in humans) did not trigger MH. Cisatracurium has not been studied in MH-susceptible patients. Because MH can develop in the absence of established triggering agents, be prepared to recognize and treat MH in any patient undergoing general anesthesia.

Neuromuscular-blocking agents may have a profound effect in patients with neuromuscular diseases (eg, myasthenia gravis, the myasthenic syndrome). In these and other conditions in which prolonged neuromuscular block is a possibility (eg, carcinomatosis), the use of a peripheral nerve stimulator and a dose of not more than 0.02 mg/kg cisatracurium is recommended to assess the level of neuromuscular block and to monitor dosage requirements.

Burn patients – Patients with burns have been shown to develop resistance to nondepolarizing neuromuscular-blocking agents, including atracurium. The extent of altered response depends upon the size of the burn and the time elapsed since the burn injury. Cisatracurium has not been studied in patients with burns; however, based on its structural similarity to atracurium, the possibility of increased dosing requirements and shortened duration of action must be considered if cisatracurium besylate is administered to burn patients.

CISATRACURIUM BESYLATE — INJECTION

Hemiparesis/Paraparesis – Patients with hemiparesis or paraparesis also may demonstrate resistance to nondepolarizing muscle relaxants in the affected limbs. To avoid inaccurate dosing, perform neuromuscular monitoring on a nonparetic limb.

Drug Interactions

➤*Succinylcholine:* Cisatracurium has been used safely following varying degrees of recovery from succinylcholine-induced neuromuscular block. Administration of 0.1 mg/kg (2 × ED_{95}) cisatracurium at 10% or 95% recovery following an intubating dose of succinylcholine (1 mg/kg) produced greater than or equal to 95% neuromuscular block. The time to onset of maximum block following cisatracurium is approximately 2 minutes faster with prior administration of succinylcholine. Prior administration of succinylcholine had no effect on the duration of neuromuscular block following initial or maintenance bolus doses of cisatracurium. Infusion requirements of cisatracurium in patients administered succinylcholine prior to infusions of cisatracurium were comparable to or slightly greater than when succinylcholine was not administered.

➤*General anesthetics:* Isoflurane or enflurane administered with nitrous oxide/oxygen to achieve 1.25 MAC (minimum alveolar concentration) may prolong the clinically effective duration of action of initial and maintenance doses of cisatracurium and decrease the required infusion rate of cisatracurium. The magnitude of these effects may depend on the duration of administration of the volatile agents. Fifteen to 30 minutes of exposure to 1.25 MAC isoflurane or enflurane had minimal effects on the duration of action of initial doses of cisatracurium and, therefore, no adjustment to the initial dose should be necessary when cisatracurium is administered shortly after initiation of volatile agents. In long surgical procedures during enflurane or isoflurane anesthesia, less frequent maintenance dosing, lower maintenance doses, or reduced infusion rates of cisatracurium besylate may be necessary. The average infusion rate requirement may be decreased by as much as 30% to 40%.

➤*Other drugs:* Other drugs which may enhance the neuromuscular-blocking action of nondepolarizing agents such as cisatracurium include certain antibiotics (eg, aminoglycosides, tetracyclines, bacitracin, polymyxins, lincomycin, clindamycin, colistin, sodium colistemethate), magnesium salts, lithium, local anesthetics, procainamide, and quinidine.

➤*Phenytoin and carbamazepine:* Resistance to the neuromuscular-blocking action of nondepolarizing neuromuscular blocking agents has been demonstrated in patients chronically administered phenytoin or carbamazepine. While the effects of chronic phenytoin or carbamazepine therapy on the action of cisatracurium are unknown, slightly shorter durations of neuromuscular block may be anticipated and infusion rate requirements may be higher.

Adverse Reactions

➤*Observed in clinical trials of surgical patients:* Adverse reactions were uncommon among the 945 surgical patients who received cisatracurium in conjunction with other drugs in US and European clinical studies in the course of a wide variety of procedures in patients receiving opioid, propofol, or inhalation anesthesia. The following adverse reactions were judged by investigators during the clinical trials to have a possible causal relationship to administration of cisatracurium:

Incidence less than 1% –
Cardiovascular: Bradycardia (0.4%), hypotension (0.2%), flushing (0.2%).
Dermatologic: Rash (0.1%).
Respiratory: Bronchospasm (0.2%).

➤*Observed in clinical trials of ICU patients:* Adverse reactions were uncommon among the 68 ICU patients who received cisatracurium in conjunction with other drugs in US and European clinical studies. One patient experienced bronchospasm. In 1 of the 2 ICU studies, a randomized and double-blind study of ICU patients using TOF neuromuscular monitoring, there were 2 reports of prolonged recovery (167 and 270 minutes) among 28 patients administered cisatracurium and 13 reports of prolonged recovery (range, 90 minutes to 33 hours) among 30 patients administered vecuronium.

➤*Postmarketing:* In addition to adverse reactions reported from clinical trials, the following reactions have been identified during postapproval use of cisatracurium in conjunction with 1 or more anesthetic agents in clinical practice. Because they are reported voluntarily from a population of unknown size, estimates of frequency cannot be made. These reactions have been chosen for inclusion due to a combination of their seriousness, frequency of reporting, or potential causal connection to cisatracurium.

Hypersensitivity – Histamine release, hypersensitivity reactions including anaphylactic or anaphylactoid responses which, in rare instances, were severe. There are rare reports of wheezing, laryngospasm, bronchospasm, rash, and itching following administration of cisatracurium in children. These reported adverse events were not serious, and their etiology could not be established with certainty.

Musculoskeletal – Prolonged neuromuscular block, inadequate neuromuscular block, muscle weakness, and myopathy.

Overdosage

➤*Treatment:* Overdosage with neuromuscular-blocking agents may result in neuromuscular block beyond the time needed for surgery and anesthesia. The primary treatment is maintenance of a patient airway and controlled ventilation until recovery of normal neuromuscular function is ensured. Once recovery from neuromuscular block begins, further recovery may be facilitated by administration of an anticholinesterase agent (eg, neostigmine, edrophonium) in conjunction with an appropriate anticholinergic agent.

Do not administer antagonists (such as neostigmine and edrophonium) when complete neuromuscular block is evident or suspected. The use of a peripheral nerve stimulator to evaluate recovery and antagonism of neuromuscular block is recommended.

Administration of 0.04 to 0.07 mg/kg neostigmine at approximately 10% recovery from neuromuscular block (range, 0% to 15%) produced 95% recovery of the muscle twitch response and a T_4:T_1 ratio greater than or equal to 70% in an average of 9 to 10 minutes. The times from 25% recovery of the muscle twitch response to a T_4:T_1 ratio greater than or equal to 70% following these doses of neostigmine averaged 7 minutes. The mean 25% to 75% recovery index following reversal was 3 to 4 minutes.

Administration of 1 mg/kg edrophonium at approximately 25% recovery from neuromuscular block (range, 16% to 30%) produced 95% recovery and a T_4:T_1 ratio greater than or equal to 70% in an average of 3 to 5 minutes.

Evaluate patients administered antagonists for evidence of adequate clinical recovery (eg, 5-second head lift and grip strength). Ventilation must be supported until no longer required.

The onset of antagonism may be delayed in the presence of debilitation, cachexia, carcinomatosis, and the concomitant use of certain broad spectrum antibiotics, or anesthetic agents and other drugs that enhance neuromuscular block or separately cause respiratory depression. Under such circumstances the management is the same as that of prolonged neuromuscular block.

MIVACURIUM CHLORIDE

Rx	**Mivacron** (Abbott Hospital)	**Injection:** 2 mg/ml	In 5 and 10 ml single use vials in Water for Injection.

MIVACURIUM CHLORIDE — INJECTION

Indications

For inpatients and outpatients, as an adjunct to general anesthesia, to facilitate tracheal intubation and to provide skeletal muscle relaxation during surgery or mechanical ventilation.

Administration and Dosage

➤*Approved by the FDA:* January 22, 1992.

Mivacurium chloride should only be administered intravenously.

When using mivacurium chloride or other neuromuscular blocking agents to facilitate tracheal intubation, it is important to recognize that the most important factors affecting intubation are the depth of general anesthesia and the level of neuromuscular block. Satisfactory intubating conditions can usually be achieved before complete neuromuscular block is attained if there is adequate anesthesia.

The use of a peripheral nerve stimulator will permit the most advantageous use of mivacurium chloride, minimize the possibility of overdosage or underdosage, and assist in the evaluation of recovery. When using a stimulator to monitor onset of neuromuscular block, clinical studies have shown that all 4 twitches of the train-of-four response may be present, with little or no fade, at the times recommended for intubation. Therefore, as with other neuromuscular blocking agents, it is important to use other criteria, such as clinical evaluation of the status of relaxation of jaw muscles and vocal cords, in conjunction with peripheral muscle twitch monitoring, to guide the appropriate time of intubation.

The onset of conditions suitable for tracheal intubation occurs earlier after a conventional intubating dose of succinylcholine than after recommended doses of mivacurium chloride.

➤*Adults:*

Initial doses – Doses of 0.15 mg/kg administered over 5 to 15 seconds, 0.20 mg/kg administered over 30 seconds, or 0.25 mg/kg administered in divided doses (0.15 mg/kg followed in 30 seconds by 0.1 mg/kg) are recommended for facilitation of tracheal intubation for most patients.

Mivacurium Recommended Initial Dosing Regimens for Adults

Dosing paradigm*	Anesthetic induction technique studied	Time to generally good to excellent intubating condition
0.15 mg/kg IV (over 5 to 15 seconds)	Thiopental/opioid/N_2O/O_2 or propofol/opioid	2.5 to 3 minutes after completion of dose
0.2 mg/kg IV (over 30 seconds)	Thiopental/opioid/N_2O/O_2 or propofol/opioid	2 to 2.5 minutes after completion of dose
0.25 mg/kg IV (0.15 mg/kg followed in 30 seconds by 0.1 mg/kg)	Propofol/opioid	1.5 to 2 minutes after completion of 0.15 mg/kg dose

* Dosing instituted after induction of adequate general anesthesia.

MIVACURIUM CHLORIDE — INJECTION

The purpose of slowed or divided dosing of mivacurium chloride at doses above 0.15 mg/kg is to minimize the transient decreases in blood pressure observed in some patients given these doses over 5 to 15 seconds. The quality of intubation conditions does not significantly differ for the times and doses of mivacurium chloride recommended above, but the onset of suitable intubation conditions may be reached earlier with higher doses. The choice of a particular dose and regimen should be based on individual circumstances and patient requirements (see Pharmacokinetics: Individualization of Dosages).

In patients with clinically significant cardiovascular disease and in patients with any history suggesting a greater sensitivity to the release of histamine or other mediators (eg, asthma), the dose of mivacurium chloride should be 0.15 mg/kg or less, administered over 60 seconds (see Precautions). No data are available on the use of doses of mivacurium chloride above 0.15 mg/kg in patients with clinically significant kidney or liver disease.

Clinically effective neuromuscular block may be expected to last for 15 to 20 minutes (range, 9 to 38) and spontaneous recovery may be expected to be 95% complete in 25 to 30 minutes (range, 16 to 41) following 0.15 mg/kg mivacurium chloride administered to patients receiving opioid/nitrous oxide/oxygen anesthesia. The expected duration of clinically effective block and time to 95% spontaneous recovery following 0.2 mg/kg mivacurium chloride are ≈ 20 and 30 minutes, respectively, and following 0.25 mg/kg mivacurium chloride are ≈ 25 and 35 minutes. Initiation of maintenance dosing during opioid/nitrous oxide/oxygen anesthesia is generally required approximately 15, 20, and 25 minutes following initial doses of 0.15, 0.2, and 0.25 mg/kg mivacurium chloride, respectively. Maintenance doses of 0.1 mg/kg each provide approximately 15 minutes of additional clinically effective block. For shorter or longer durations of action, smaller or larger maintenance doses may be administered.

The neuromuscular blocking action of mivacurium chloride is potentiated by isoflurane or enflurane anesthesia. Recommended initial doses of mivacurium chloride may be used to facilitate tracheal intubation prior to the administration of these agents; however, if mivacurium chloride is first administered after establishment of stable-state isoflurane or enflurane anesthesia (administered with nitrous oxide/oxygen to achieve 1.25 MAC), the initial dose of mivacurium chloride may be reduced by as much as 25%. Greater reductions in the dose of mivacurium chloride may be required with higher concentrations of enflurane or isoflurane. With halothane, which has only a minimal potentiating effect on mivacurium chloride, a smaller dosage reduction may be considered.

Continuous infusion – Continuous infusion of mivacurium chloride may be used to maintain neuromuscular block. Upon early evidence of spontaneous recovery from an initial dose, an initial infusion rate of 9 to 10 mcg/kg/min is recommended. If continuous infusion is initiated simultaneously with the administration of an initial dose, a lower initial infusion rate should be used (eg, 4 mcg/kg/min). In either case, the initial infusion rate should be adjusted according to the response to peripheral nerve stimulation and to clinical criteria. On average, an infusion rate of 5 to 7 mcg/kg/min (range, 1 to 15) may be expected to maintain neuromuscular block within the range of 89% to 99% for extended periods in adults receiving opioid/nitrous oxide/oxygen anesthesia. In some patients, particularly those with higher infusion requirements (more than 8 mcg/kg/min) during the first 30 minutes, the infusion rate required to maintain 89% to 99% T_1 suppression may decrease gradually (by ≥ 30%) with time over a 4- to 6-hour period of infusion (see Pharmacology). Reduction of the infusion rate by up to 35% to 40% should be considered when mivacurium chloride is administered during stable-state conditions of isoflurane or enflurane anesthesia (administered with nitrous oxide/oxygen to achieve 1.25 MAC). Greater reductions in the infusion rate of mivacurium chloride may be required with greater concentrations of enflurane or isoflurane. With halothane, smaller reductions in infusion rate may be required.

➤*Children:*

Initial doses – Dosage requirements for mivacurium chloride on a mg/kg basis are higher in children than in adults. Onset and recovery of neuromuscular block occur more rapidly in children than in adults.

The recommended dose of mivacurium chloride for facilitating tracheal intubation in children 2 to 12 years of age is 0.2 mg/kg administered over 5 to 15 seconds. When administered during stable opioid/nitrous oxide/oxygen anesthesia, 0.2 mg/kg of mivacurium chloride produces maximum neuromuscular block in an average of 1.9 minutes (range, 1.3 to 3.3) and clinically effective block for 10 minutes (range, 6 to 15). Maintenance doses are generally required more frequently in children than in adults. Administration of doses of mivacurium chloride above the recommended range (more than 0.2 mg/kg) is associated with transient decreases in MAP in some children. Mivacurium chloride has not been studied in pediatric patients below the age of 2 years.

Continuous infusion – Children require higher infusion rates of mivacurium chloride than adults. During opioid/nitrous oxide/oxygen anesthesia the infusion rate required to maintain 89% to 99% neuromuscular block averages 14 mcg/kg/min (range, 5 to 31). The principles for infusion of mivacurium chloride in adults are also applicable to children.

➤*Special populations:*

Renal or hepatic impairment – A dose of 0.15 mg/kg mivacurium chloride is recommended for facilitation of tracheal intubation in patients with renal or hepatic impairment. However, the clinically effective duration of block produced by this dose may be about 1.5 times longer in patients with end-stage kidney disease and about 3 times longer in patients with end-stage liver disease than in patients with normal renal and hepatic function. Infusion rates should be decreased by as much as 50% in patients with hepatic disease depending on the degree of hepatic impairment (see Warnings). No infusion rate adjustments are necessary in patients with renal impairment.

Conditions causing potentiation of or resistance to neuromuscular block – As with other neuromuscular blocking agents, mivacurium chloride may have profound neuromuscular blocking effects in cachectic or debilitated patients, patients with neuromuscular diseases, and patients with carcinomatosis. In these or other patients in whom potentiation of neuromuscular block or difficulty with reversal may be anticipated, the initial dose should be decreased. A test dose of not more than 0.015 to 0.020 mg/kg, which represents the lower end of the dose-response curve for mivacurium chloride, is recommended in such patients.

Burns: While patients with burns are known to develop resistance to nondepolarizing neuromuscular blocking agents, they may also have reduced plasma cholinesterase activity. Consequently, in these patients, a test dose of not more than 0.015 to 0.020 mg/kg mivacurium chloride is recommended, followed by additional appropriate dosing guided by the use of a neuromuscular block monitor.

Cardiovascular disease: In patients with clinically significant cardiovascular disease, the initial dose of mivacurium chloride should be 0.15 mg/kg or less, administered over 60 seconds.

Obesity: Obese patients (patients weighing ≥ 30% more than their ideal body weight) dosed on the basis of actual body weight, thereby receiving a larger dose than if dosed on the basis of ideal body weight, had a greater probability of experiencing a decrease of ≥ 30% in MAP. Therefore, in obese patients, the initial dose should be determined using the patient's ideal body weight (IBW), according to the following formulas:

- *Men* – IBW in kg (106 [6 × inches in height above 5 feet])/2.2.
- *Women* – IBW in kg (100 [5 × inches in height above 5 feet])/2.2.

Allergy and sensitivity: In patients with any history suggestive of a greater sensitivity to the release of histamine or related mediators (eg, asthma), the initial dose of mivacurium chloride should be 0.15 mg/kg or less, administered over 60 seconds.

➤*Infusion rate tables:* For adults and children, the amount of infusion solution required per hour depends upon the clinical requirements of the patient, the concentration of mivacurium chloride in the infusion solution, and the patient's weight. The contribution of the infusion solution to the fluid requirements of the patient must be considered. The table below provides guidelines for delivery in mL/hr (equivalent to microdrops/min when 60 microdrops = 1 mL) of mivacurium chloride injection (2 mg/mL).

Infusion Rates for Maintenance of Neuromuscular Block During Opioid/Nitrous Oxide/Oxygen Anesthesia Using Mivacurium Chloride Injection (2 mg/mL)

	Drug delivery rate (mcg/kg/min)									
Patient weight (kg)	4	5	6	7	8	10	14	16	18	20
	Infusion delivery rate (mL/hr)									
10	1.2	1.5	1.8	2.1	2.4	3	4.2	4.8	5.4	6
15	1.8	2.3	2.7	3.2	3.6	4.5	6.3	7.2	8.1	9
20	2.4	3	3.6	4.2	4.8	6	8.4	9.6	10.8	12
25	3	3.8	4.5	5.3	6	7.5	10.5	12	13.5	15
35	4.2	5.3	6.3	7.4	8.4	10.5	14.7	16.8	18.9	21
50	6	7.5	9	10.5	12	15	21	24	27	30
60	7.2	9	10.8	12.6	14.4	18	25.2	28.8	32.4	36
70	8.4	10.5	12.6	14.7	16.8	21	29.4	33.6	37.8	42
80	9.6	12	14.4	16.8	19.2	24	33.6	38.4	43.2	48
90	10.8	13.5	16.2	18.9	21.6	27	37.8	43.2	48.6	54
100	12	15	18	21	24	30	42	48	54	60

➤*Mivacurium chloride injection compatibility and admixtures: Y-site administration:* Mivacurium chloride injection may not be compatible with alkaline solutions having a pH greater than 8.5 (eg, barbiturate solutions). Studies have shown that mivacurium chloride injection is compatible with: 5% Dextrose Injection, USP; 0.9% Sodium Chloride Injection, USP; 5% Dextrose and 0.9% Sodium Chloride Injection, USP; Lactated Ringer's Injection, USP; 5% Dextrose in Lactated Ringer's Injection; Sufentanil citrate injection, diluted as directed; Alfentanil hydrochloride injection, diluted as directed; Fentanyl citrate injection, diluted as directed; Midazolam hydrochloride injection, diluted as directed; Droperidol injection, diluted as directed.

➤*Dilution stability:* Mivacurium chloride injection diluted to 0.5 mg mivacurium per mL in 5% Dextrose Injection USP, 5% Dextrose and 0.9% Sodium Chloride Injection USP, 0.9% Sodium Chloride Injection USP, Lactated Ringer's Injection USP, or 5% Dextrose in Lactated Ringer's injection is physically and chemically stable when stored in PVC (polyvinyl chloride) bags at 5° to 25°C (41° to 77°F) for up to 24 hours. Aseptic techniques should be used to prepare the diluted product. Admixtures of mivacurium chloride should be prepared for single patient use only and used within 24 hours of preparation. The unused portion of diluted mivacurium chloride should be discarded after each case.

➤*Storage/Stability:* Store mivacurium chloride injection at room temperature of 15° to 25°C (59° to 77°F). Avoid exposure to direct ultraviolet light. Do not freeze.

MIVACURIUM CHLORIDE — INJECTION

Actions

➤*Pharmacology:*

Pharmacodynamics – The time to maximum neuromuscular block is similar for recommended doses of mivacurium chloride and intermediate-acting agents (eg, atracurium), but longer than for the ultra-short-acting agent, succinylcholine. The clinically effective duration of action of mivacurium chloride (a mixture of three stereoisomers) is one-third to one-half that of intermediate-acting agents and 2 to 2.5 times that of succinylcholine.

In children (2 to 12 years), mivacurium chloride has a higher ED_{95} (0.1 mg/kg), faster onset, and shorter duration of action than in adults. The mean time for spontaneous recovery of the twitch response from 25% to 75% of control amplitude is about 5 minutes (n = 4) following an initial dose of 0.2 mg/kg mivacurium chloride. Recovery following reversal is faster in children than in adults.

➤*Pharmacokinetics:*

Absorption – Mivacurium chloride is a mixture of isomers that do not interconvert in vivo. The cis-trans and trans-trans isomers (92% to 96% of the mixture) are equipotent. The steady-state concentrations of the cis-trans and trans-trans isomers doubled after the infusion rate was increased from 5 to 10 mcg/kg/min, indicating that their pharmacokinetics is dose-proportional.

Stereoisomer Pharmacokinetic Parameters* of Mivacurium in ASA Physical Status I to II Adult Patients/* (n = 18) During Opioid/Nitrous Oxide/Oxygen Anesthesia**

Parameter	trans-trans isomer	cis-trans isomer
Elimination half-life (t½ min)	2 (1 to 3.6)	1.8 (0.8 to 4.8)
Volume of distribution***/** (mL/kg)	147 (67 to 254)	276 (79 to 772)
Plasma clearance (mL/min/kg)	53 (26 to 98)	99 (44 to 199)

* Values shown are mean (range).
**/* Ages 31 to 48 years.
***/** Volume of distribution during the terminal elimination phase.

The cis-cis isomer (6% of the mixture) has approximately one-tenth the neuromuscular blocking potency of the trans-trans and cis-trans isomers in cats. Neuromuscular blocking effects due to the cis-cis isomer cannot be ruled out in humans; however, modeling of clinical pharmacokinetic-pharmacodynamic data suggests that the cis-cis isomer produces minimal (less than 5%) neuromuscular block during a 2-hour infusion. In studies of ASA Physical Status I-II patients receiving infusions of mivacurium chloride lasting as long as 4 to 6 hours, the 5% to 25% and the 25% to 75% recovery indices were independent of the duration of infusion, suggesting that the cis-cis isomer does not affect the rate of post-infusion recovery.

Distribution – The volume of distribution of cis-trans and trans-trans isomers in healthy surgical patients is relatively small, reflecting limited tissue distribution. The volume of distribution of cis-cis isomers is also small and averaged 335 mL/kg (range, 192 to 523) in the 18 healthy surgical patients whose data are displayed above. The protein binding of mivacurium has not been determined due to its rapid hydrolysis by plasma cholinesterase.

Metabolism – Enzymatic hydrolysis by plasma cholinesterase is the primary mechanism for inactivation of mivacurium and yields a quaternary alcohol and a quaternary monoester metabolite. Tests in which these two metabolites were administered to cats and dogs suggest that each metabolite is unlikely to produce clinically significant neuromuscular, autonomic, or cardiovascular effects following administration of mivacurium chloride.

The mean ± S.D. in vitro t½ values of the trans-trans and the cis-trans isomers were 1.3 ± 0.3 and 0.8 ± 0.2 minutes, respectively, in human plasma from healthy male (n = 5) and female (n = 5) volunteers. The mean in vivo t½ values for the more potent trans-trans and cis-trans isomers in healthy surgical patients were similar to those found in vitro, suggesting that hydrolysis by plasma cholinesterase is the predominant elimination pathway for these isomers. The mean ± S.D. in vitro t½ of the less potent cis-cis isomer was 276 ± 130 minutes, while the mean ± S.D. in vivo t½ for the cis-cis isomer in healthy surgical patients was 53 ± 20 minutes. These data suggest that in vivo, pathways other than hydrolysis by plasma cholinesterase contribute to the elimination of the cis-cis isomer

Excretion – The clearance (CL) values of the two more potent isomers, cis-trans and trans-trans, are very high and are dependent on plasma cholinesterase activity. The combination of high CL and low distribution volume results in t½ values of ≈ 2 minutes for the two more potent isomers. The short t½ and high CL of the more potent isomers are consistent with the short duration of action of mivacurium chloride.

The CL of the less-potent cis-cis isomer is not dependent on plasma cholinesterase. The mean ± S.D. CL was 4.6 ± 1.1 mL/min/kg and t½ was 53 ± 20 minutes in the 18 healthy surgical patients whose data are displayed above.

Renal and biliary excretion of unchanged mivacurium are minor elimination pathways; urine and bile are important elimination pathways for the two metabolites.

Special populations –

Renal function impairment: An early clinical trial showed that the clinically effective duration of action of 0.15 mg/kg mivacurium chloride was about 1.5 times longer in kidney transplant patients than in healthy patients, presumably due to reduced clearance of one or more isomers. A second study was conducted in 7 patients with mild to moderate renal impairment, 8 patients with severe renal dysfunction (not undergoing transplantation), and 11 patients with normal renal function. This study showed that the pharmacokinetics of the more potent (cis-trans and trans-trans) isomers were not statistically significantly affected by renal impairment or failure. However, the CL of the cis-cis isomer was lower and the t½ values of the cis-cis isomer and metabolites were longer in patients with renal impairment or failure than in patients with normal renal function. The second study also showed that there were no differences in the average infusion rate required to produce 89% to 99% T_1 suppression, nor were there any differences in the post-infusion recovery profile among these populations. A third study in a similar population showed that patients with renal dysfunction had a longer duration and a slower rate of recovery than patients with normal renal function. This study did, however, confirm that there were no differences in the average infusion rate required to produce 89% to 99% T_1 suppression in these patient populations. Therefore, although there were minor differences in the pharmacokinetics of the cis-cis isomer and metabolites, there were no clinically significant differences in the infusion rate requirements of mivacurium chloride in patients with mild, moderate, or severe renal dysfunction receiving infusions of mivacurium chloride for an average of 1 to 2 hours; however, the duration may be longer and the rate of recovery may be slower following administration of mivacurium chloride in some patients with renal dysfunction.

Hepatic function impairment: The clinically effective duration of action of 0.15 mg/kg mivacurium chloride was 3 times longer in 8 patients with end-stage liver disease (undergoing liver transplantation) than in 8 healthy patients and is likely related to the markedly decreased plasma cholinesterase activity (30% of healthy patient values) that could decrease the clearance of the trans-trans and cis-trans isomers.

A separate study compared the pharmacokinetics and pharmacodynamics of mivacurium in patients with mild or moderate cirrhosis to healthy adults with normal hepatic function. Although the number of patients in each group is small, the CL values of the more potent isomers, trans-trans and cis-trans, are lower in patients with mild or moderate cirrhosis as expected based on the marked decreases in plasma cholinesterase activity in this population.

Elderly: Two pharmacokinetic/pharmacodynamic studies of mivacurium chloride have been conducted in elderly patients. The first study compared the pharmacokinetics and pharmacodynamics of mivacurium in 19 elderly patients with those in 20 adult patients receiving infusions for as long as 4 to 6 hours. The average infusion rate required to produce 89% to 99% T_1 suppression was slightly (≈ 14%) lower in elderly patients. This difference is not regarded as clinically important, but is most likely secondary to differences in pharmacokinetics (ie, a lower CL of the cis-trans and trans-trans isomers in elderly patients). The rate of post-infusion spontaneous recovery was not dependent on duration of infusion and appeared to be comparable in these elderly patients and adult patients.

The second study showed no clinically important differences in the pharmacokinetics of the individual isomers nor the ED_{95} determined for 36 young adult patients (18 to 40 years) and 35 elderly patients (≥ 65years) during opioid/nitrous oxide/oxygen anesthesia. Following infusions for up to 3.5 hours in these patients, the rate of spontaneous recovery was slightly (≈ 2 to 4 minutes, on average) slower in the elderly patients than in young adult patients.

In an earlier study of the pharmacodynamics of 0.1 mg/kg mivacurium chloride administered to 8 elderly patients (68 to 77 years) and 9 adult patients (18 to 49 years) during N_2O/O_2 isoflurane anesthesia, the time to onset was approximately 1.5 minutes slower in elderly patients than in adult patients. In addition, the clinical duration was slightly (≈ 3 minutes, on average) longer in elderly patients than in adult patients; these differences are not considered clinically important.

Although these studies showed conflicting findings, in general, the clearances of the more potent isomers are most likely lower in elderly patients. This difference does not lead to clinically important differences in the ED_{95} of mivacurium chloride or the infusion rate of mivacurium chloride required to produce 95% T_1 suppression in elderly patients. However, the time to onset may be slower, the duration may be slightly longer, and the rate of recovery may be slightly slower.

Contraindications

Hypersensitivity to mivacurium chloride or other benzylisoquinolinium agents, as manifested by reactions such as urticaria or severe respiratory distress or hypotension. Use of mivacurium chloride from multiple-dose vials containing benzyl alcohol as a preservative is contraindicated in patients with a known hypersensitivity to benzyl alcohol.

Warnings

➤*Administration:* Mivacurium chloride should be administered in carefully adjusted dosage by or under the supervision of experienced clinicians who are familiar with the drug actions and the possible complications of its use. The drug should not be administered unless personnel and facilities for resuscitation and life support (tracheal intubation, artificial ventilation, oxygen therapy), and an antagonist of mivacurium chloride are immediately available. It is recommended that a peripheral nerve stimulator be used to measure neuromuscular function during the administration of mivacurium chloride in order to monitor drug effect, determine the need for additional drug, and confirm recovery from neuromuscular block.

➤*Renal/Hepatic function impairment:* The possibility of prolonged neuromuscular block must be considered when mivacurium chloride is used in patients with renal or hepatic disease. Most patients with chronic hepatic disease such as hepatitis, liver abscess, and cirrhosis of the liver exhibit a

MIVACURIUM CHLORIDE — INJECTION

marked reduction in plasma cholinesterase activity. Patients with acute or chronic renal disease may also show a reduction in plasma cholinesterase activity.

➤*Elderly:* Mivacurium chloride was safely administered during clinical trials to 64 elderly (≥ 65 years) patients, including 31 patients with significant cardiovascular disease (see Precautions). The time to onset may be slower, the duration may be slightly longer, and the rate of recovery may be slightly slower in elderly patients (see Pharmacokinetics).

➤*Pregnancy: Category C.*

Teratogenic – There are no adequate and well-controlled studies of mivacurium chloride in pregnant women. Because animal studies are not always predictive of human response, and the doses used were subparalyzing, mivacurium chloride should be used during pregnancy only if the potential benefit justifies the potential risk to the fetus.

➤*Lactation:* It is not known whether any of the stereoisomers of mivacurium are excreted in human milk. Because many drugs are excreted in human milk, caution should be exercised following administration of mivacurium chloride to a nursing woman.

➤*Children:* Mivacurium chloride has not been studied in pediatric patients below the age of 2 years (see Pharmacokinetics and Administration and Dosage for clinical experience and recommendations for use in children 2 to 12 years of age).

Precautions

➤*Benzyl alcohol:* Multiple-dose vials of mivacurium chloride contain benzyl alcohol. In newborn infants, benzyl alcohol has been associated with an increased incidence of neurological and other complications which are sometimes fatal. Single-use vials do not contain benzyl alcohol.

➤*Reduced plasma cholinesterase activity:* The possibility of prolonged neuromuscular block following administration of mivacurium chloride must be considered in patients with reduced plasma cholinesterase (pseudocholinesterase) activity.

Plasma cholinesterase activity may be diminished in the presence of genetic abnormalities of plasma cholinesterase (eg, patients heterozygous or homozygous for the atypical plasma cholinesterase gene), pregnancy, liver or kidney disease, malignant tumors, infections, burns, anemia, decompensated heart disease, peptic ulcer, or myxedema. Plasma cholinesterase activity may also be diminished by chronic administration of oral contraceptives, glucocorticoids, or certain monoamine oxidase inhibitors and by irreversible inhibitors of plasma cholinesterase (eg, organophosphate insecticides, echothiophate, and certain antineoplastic drugs).

Mivacurium chloride has been used safely in patients heterozygous for the atypical plasma cholinesterase gene. At doses of 0.10 to 0.2 mg/kg mivacurium chloride, the clinically effective duration of action was 8 to 11 minutes longer in patients heterozygous for the atypical gene than in genotypically normal patients.

As with succinylcholine, patients homozygous for the atypical plasma cholinesterase gene (1 in 2500 patients) are extremely sensitive to the neuromuscular blocking effect of mivacurium chloride. In 3 such adult patients, a small dose of 0.03 mg/kg (approximately the $ED_{10\text{-}20}$ in genotypically normal patients) produced complete neuromuscular block for 26 to 128 minutes. Once spontaneous recovery had begun, neuromuscular block in these patients was antagonized with conventional doses of neostigmine. One adult patient, who was homozygous for the atypical plasma cholinesterase gene, received a dose of 0.18 mg/kg mivacurium chloride and exhibited complete neuromuscular block for about 4 hours. Response to post-tetanic stimulation was present after 4 hours, all 4 responses to train-of-four stimulation were present after 6 hours, and the patient was extubated after 8 hours. Reversal was not attempted in this patient.

➤*Malignant hyperthermia (MH):* In a study of MH-susceptible pigs, mivacurium chloride did not trigger MH. Mivacurium chloride has not been studied in MH-susceptible patients. Because MH can develop in the absence of established triggering agents, the clinician should be prepared to recognize and treat MH in any patient undergoing general anesthesia.

➤*Special risk:* Although mivacurium chloride (a mixture of 3 stereoisomers) is not a potent histamine releaser, the possibility of substantial histamine release must be considered. Release of histamine is related to the dose and speed of injection.

Caution should be exercised in administering mivacurium chloride to patients with clinically significant cardiovascular disease and patients with any history suggesting a greater sensitivity to the release of histamine or related mediators (eg, asthma). In such patients, the initial dose of mivacurium chloride should be 0.15 mg/kg or less, administered over 60 seconds; assurance of adequate hydration and careful monitoring of hemodynamic status are important.

Obese patients may be more likely to experience clinically significant transient decreases in MAP than non-obese patients when the dose of mivacurium chloride is based on actual rather than ideal body weight. Therefore, in obese patients, the initial dose should be determined using the patient's ideal body weight.

Neuromuscular blocking agents may have a profound effect in patients with neuromuscular diseases (eg, myasthenia gravis and the myasthenic syndrome). In these and other conditions in which prolonged neuromuscular block is a possibility (eg, carcinomatosis), the use of a peripheral nerve stimulator and a dose of not more than 0.015 to 0.02 mg/kg mivacurium chloride is recommended to assess the level of neuromuscular block and to monitor dosage requirements.

Mivacurium chloride has not been studied in patients with burns. Resistance to nondepolarizing neuromuscular blocking agents may develop in patients with burns, depending upon the time elapsed since the injury and the size of the burn. Patients with burns may have reduced plasma cholinesterase activity which may offset this resistance.

Acid-base or serum electrolyte abnormalities may potentiate or antagonize the action of neuromuscular blocking agents. The action of neuromuscular blocking agents may be enhanced by magnesium salts administered for the management of toxemia of pregnancy.

Drug Interactions

➤*Succinylcholine:* Although mivacurium chloride (a mixture of 3 stereoisomers) has been administered safely following succinylcholine-facilitated tracheal intubation, the interaction between mivacurium chloride and succinylcholine has not been systematically studied. Prior administration of succinylcholine can potentiate the neuromuscular blocking effects of nondepolarizing agents. Evidence of spontaneous recovery from succinylcholine should be observed before the administration of mivacurium chloride.

➤*General anesthetics:* Isoflurane and enflurane (administered with nitrous oxide/oxygen to achieve 1.25 MAC) decrease the ED_{50} of mivacurium chloride by as much as 25% (see Clinical Pharmacology: Pharmacodynamics and Pharmacokinetics: Individualization of Dosages). These agents may also prolong the clinically effective duration of action and decrease the average infusion requirement of mivacurium chloride by as much as 35% to 40%. A greater potentiation of the neuromuscular blocking effects of mivacurium chloride may be expected with higher concentrations of enflurane or isoflurane. Halothane has little or no effect on the ED_{50}, but may prolong the duration of action and decrease the average infusion requirement by as much as 20%.

➤*Other drugs:* Other drugs which may enhance the neuromuscular blocking action of nondepolarizing agents such as mivacurium chloride include certain antibiotics (eg, aminoglycosides, tetracyclines, bacitracin, polymyxins, lincomycin, clindamycin, colistin, and sodium colistimethate), magnesium salts, lithium, local anesthetics, procainamide, and quinidine. The neuromuscular blocking effect of mivacurium chloride may be enhanced by drugs that reduce plasma cholinesterase activity (eg, chronically administered oral contraceptives, glucocorticoids, or certain monoamine oxidase inhibitors) or by drugs that irreversibly inhibit plasma cholinesterase (see Precautions).

➤*Phenytoin or carbamazepine:* Resistance to the neuromuscular blocking action of nondepolarizing neuromuscular blocking agents has been demonstrated in patients chronically administered phenytoin or carbamazepine. While the effects of chronic phenytoin or carbamazepine therapy on the action of mivacurium chloride are unknown, slightly shorter durations of neuromuscular block may be anticipated and infusion rate requirements may be higher.

Adverse Reactions

➤*Observed in clinical trials:* Mivacurium chloride (a mixture of 3 stereoisomers) was well tolerated during extensive clinical trials in inpatients and outpatients. Prolonged neuromuscular block, which is an important adverse experience associated with neuromuscular blocking agents as a class, was reported as an adverse experience in 3 of 2074 patients administered mivacurium chloride. The most commonly reported adverse experience following the administration of mivacurium chloride was transient, dose-dependent cutaneous flushing about the face, neck, or chest. Flushing was most frequently noted after the initial dose of mivacurium chloride and was reported in about 25% of adult patients who received 0.15 mg/kg mivacurium chloride over 5 to 15 seconds. When present, flushing typically began within 1 to 2 minutes after the dose of mivacurium chloride and lasted for 3 to 5 minutes. Of 105 patients who experienced flushing after 0.15 mg/kg mivacurium chloride, 2 patients also experienced mild hypotension that was not treated, and 1 patient experienced moderate wheezing that was successfully treated.

Overall, hypotension was infrequently reported as an adverse experience in the clinical trials of mivacurium chloride. One of 332 (0.3%) healthy adults who received 0.15 mg/kg mivacurium chloride over 5 to 15 seconds and none of 37 cardiac surgery patients who received 0.15 mg/kg mivacurium chloride over 60 seconds were treated for a decrease in blood pressure in association with the administration of mivacurium chloride. One to two percent of healthy adults given ≥ 0.2 mg/kg mivacurium chloride over 5 to 15 seconds, 2% to 3% of healthy adults given 0.2 mg/kg over 30 seconds, none of 100 healthy adults given 0.25 mg/kg as a divided dose (0.15 mg/kg followed in 30 seconds by 0.1 mg/kg), and 2% to 4% of cardiac surgery patients given ≥ 0.2 mg/kg over 60 seconds were treated for a decrease in blood pressure. None of the 63 children who received the recommended dose of 0.2 mg/kg mivacurium chloride was treated for a decrease in blood pressure in association with the administration of mivacurium chloride.

➤*Incidence more than 1%:*

Cardiovascular – Flushing (16%).

➤*Incidence less than 1%:*

Cardiovascular – Hypotension, tachycardia, bradycardia, cardiac arrhythmia, phlebitis.

CNS – Dizziness.

Dermatologic – Rash, urticaria, erythema, injection site reaction.

Musculoskeletal – Muscle spasms.

Respiratory – Bronchospasm, wheezing, hypoxemia.

Miscellaneous – Prolonged drug effect.

MIVACURIUM CHLORIDE — INJECTION

➤*Postmarketing:*

Allergic – Allergic reactions which, in rare instances, were severe.

Cardiovascular – Hypotension (rarely severe), flushing.

Dermatologic – Rash.

Musculoskeletal – Diminished drug effect, prolonged drug effect.

Respiratory – Bronchospasm.

Overdosage

➤*Symptoms:* Overdosage with neuromuscular blocking agents may result in neuromuscular block beyond the time needed for surgery and anesthesia.

➤*Treatment:* The primary treatment is maintenance of a patent airway and controlled ventilation until recovery of normal neuromuscular function is assured. Once evidence of recovery from neuromuscular block is observed, further recovery may be facilitated by administration of an anticholinesterase agent (eg, neostigmine, edrophonium) in conjunction with an appropriate anticholinergic agent. Overdosage may increase the risk of hemodynamic side effects, especially decreases in blood pressure. If needed, cardiovascular support may be provided by proper positioning of the patient, fluid administration, or vasopressor agent administration.

Antagonists (such as neostigmine) should not be administered when complete neuromuscular block is evident or suspected. The use of a peripheral nerve stimulator to evaluate recovery and antagonism of neuromuscular block is recommended.

Administration of 0.03 to 0.064 mg/kg neostigmine or 0.5 mg/kg edrophonium at ≈ 10% recovery from neuromuscular block (range, 1 to 15) produced 95% recovery of the muscle twitch response and a T_4/T_1 ratio ≥ 75% in about 10 minutes. The times from 25% recovery of the muscle twitch response to T_4/T_1 ratio ≥ 75% following these doses of antagonists averaged about 7 to 9 minutes. In comparison, average times for spontaneous recovery from 25% to T_4/T_1 ≥ 75% were 12 to 13 minutes.

Patients administered antagonists should be evaluated for adequate clinical evidence of antagonism, eg, 5-second head lift and grip strength. Ventilation must be supported until no longer required.

Antagonism may be delayed in the presence of debilitation, carcinomatosis, and the concomitant use of certain broad spectrum antibiotics, or anesthetic agents and other drugs which enhance neuromuscular block or separately cause respiratory depression (see Drug Interactions). Under such circumstances the management is the same as that of prolonged neuromuscular block.

ROCURONIUM BROMIDE

Rx	**Zemuron** (Organon)	**Injection:** 10 mg/mL	In 5 mL and 10 mL multi-dose vials.

ROCURONIUM BROMIDE — INJECTION

Indications

For inpatients and outpatients as an adjunct to general anesthesia to facilitate both rapid sequence and routine tracheal intubation, and to provide skeletal muscle relaxation during surgery or mechanical ventilation.

Administration and Dosage

➤*Approved by the FDA:* March 17, 1994.

It is recommended that clinicians administering neuromuscular blocking agents such as rocuronium bromide employ a peripheral nerve stimulator to monitor drug response, determine the need for additional relaxant and adequacy of spontaneous recovery or antagonism.

➤*Rapid sequence intubation:* In appropriately premedicated and adequately anesthetized patients, rocuronium bromide injection 0.6 to 1.2 mg/kg will provide excellent or good intubating conditions in most patients in less than 2 minutes. Intubating conditions were assessed in 230 patients in 6 clinical trials where anesthesia was induced with either thiopental (3 to 6 mg/kg) or propofol (1.5 to 2.5 mg/kg) in combination with either fentanyl (2 to 5 mcg/kg) or alfentanil (1 mg). Most of the patients also received a premedication such as midazolam or temazepam. Most patients had intubation attempted within 60 to 90 seconds of administration of rocuronium bromide injection 0.6 mg/kg or succinylcholine 1 to 1.5 mg/kg. Excellent or good intubating conditions were achieved in 119/120 (99% [95% confidence interval 95% to 99.9%]) patients receiving rocuronium bromide and in 108/110 (98% [94% to 99.8%]) patients receiving succinylcholine. The duration of action of rocuronium bromide 0.6 mg/kg is longer than succinylcholine and at this dose is approximately equivalent to the duration of other intermediate acting neuromuscular blocking drugs.

➤*Dose for tracheal intubation:* The recommended initial dose regardless of anesthetic technique is 0.6 mg/kg. Neuromuscular block sufficient for intubation (greater than or equal to 80% block) is attained in a median (range) time of 1 (0.4 to 6) minute(s) and most patients have intubation completed within 2 minutes. Maximum blockade is achieved in most patients in less than 3 minutes. This dose may be expected to provide 31 (15 to 85) minutes of clinical relaxation under opioid/nitrous oxide/oxygen anesthesia. Under halothane, isoflurane, and enflurane anesthesia, some extension of the period of clinical relaxation should be expected.

A lower dose of rocuronium bromide injection (0.45 mg/kg) may be used. Neuromuscular block sufficient for intubation (greater than or equal to 80% block) is attained in a median (range) time of 1.3 (0.8 to 6.2) minute(s) and most patients have intubation completed within 2 minutes. Maximum blockade is achieved in most patients in less than 4 minutes. This dose may be expected to provide 22 (12 to 31) minutes of clinical relaxation under opioid/nitrous oxide/oxygen anesthesia. Patients receiving this low dose of 0.45 mg/kg who achieve less than 90% block (about 16% of these patients) may have a more rapid time to 25% recovery, 12 to 15 minutes.

Should there be reason for the selection of a larger bolus dose in individual patients, initial doses of 0.9 or 1.2 mg/kg can be administered during surgery under opioid/nitrous oxide/oxygen anesthesia without adverse effects to the cardiovascular system. These doses will provide greater than or equal to 80% block in most patients in less than 2 minutes, with maximum blockade occurring in most patients in less than 3 minutes. Doses of 0.9 and 1.2 mg/kg may be expected to provide 58 (27 to 111) and 67 (38 to 160) minutes, respectively, of clinical relaxation under opioid/nitrous oxide/oxygen anesthesia.

➤*Maintenance dosing:* Maintenance doses of 0.1, 0.15, and 0.2 mg/kg rocuronium bromide injection, administered at 25% recovery of control T_1 (defined as 3 twitches of train-of-four), provide a median (range) of 12 (2 to 31), 17 (6 to 50) and 24 (7 to 69) minutes of clinical duration under opioid/nitrous oxide/oxygen anesthesia. In all cases, dosing should be guided based on the clinical duration following initial dose or prior maintenance dose and not administered until recovery of neuromuscular function is evident. A clinically insignificant cumulation of effect with repetitive maintenance dosing has been observed.

➤*Use by continuous infusion:* Infusion at an initial rate of 0.01 to 0.012 mg/kg/min of rocuronium bromide injection should be initiated only after early evidence of spontaneous recovery from an intubating dose. Due to rapid redistribution and the associated rapid spontaneous recovery, initiation of the infusion after substantial return of neuromuscular function (less than 10% of control T_1), may necessitate additional bolus doses to maintain adequate block for surgery.

Upon reaching the desired level of neuromuscular block, the infusion of rocuronium bromide must be individualized for each patient. The rate of administration should be adjusted according to the patient's twitch response as monitored with the use of a peripheral nerve stimulator. In clinical trials, infusion rates have ranged from 0.004 to 0.016 mg/kg/min.

Inhalation anesthetics, particularly enflurane and isoflurane may enhance the neuromuscular blocking action of nondepolarizing muscle relaxants. In the presence of steady-state concentrations of enflurane or isoflurane, it may be necessary to reduce the rate of infusion by 30% to 50%, at 45 to 60 minutes after the intubating dose.

Spontaneous recovery and reversal of neuromuscular blockade following discontinuation of rocuronium bromide infusion may be expected to proceed at rates comparable to that following comparable total doses administered by repetitive bolus injections.

Infusion rates of rocuronium bromide can be individualized for each patient using the following information as guidelines:

Infusion Rates Using Rocuronium Bromide Injection (0.5 mg/mL)*

Patient weight		Drug delivery rate (mcg/kg/min)									
		4	5	6	7	8	9	10	12	14	16
(kg)	(lbs)	Infusion delivery rate (mL/h)									
10	22	4.8	6	7.2	8.4	9.6	10.8	12	14.4	16.8	19.2
15	33	7.2	9	10.8	12.6	14.4	16.2	18	21.6	25.2	28.8
20	44	9.6	12	14.4	16.8	19.2	21.6	24	28.8	33.6	38.4
25	55	12	15	18	21	24	27	30	36	42	48
35	77	16.8	21	25.2	29.4	33.6	37.8	42	50.4	58.8	67.2
50	110	24	30	36	42	48	54	60	72	84	96
60	132	28.8	36	43.2	50.4	57.6	64.8	72	86.4	100.8	115.2
70	154	33.6	42	50.4	58.8	67.2	75.6	84	100.8	117.6	134.4
80	176	38.4	48	57.6	67.2	76.8	86.4	96	115.2	134.4	153.6
90	198	43.2	54	64.8	75.6	86.4	97.2	108	129.6	151.2	172.8
100	220	48	60	72	84	96	108	120	144	168	192

* 50 mg rocuronium bromide in 100 mL solution.

ROCURONIUM BROMIDE — INJECTION

Infusion Rates Using Rocuronium Bromide Injection (1 mg/mL)**

Patient weight		Drug delivery rate (mcg/kg/min)									
		4	5	6	7	8	9	10	12	14	16
(kg)	(lbs)	Infusion delivery rate (mL/h)									
10	22	2.4	3	3.6	4.2	4.8	5.4	6	7.2	8.4	9.6
15	33	3.6	4.5	5.4	6.3	7.2	8.1	9	10.8	12.6	14.4
20	44	4.8	6	7.2	8.4	9.6	10.8	12	14.4	16.8	19.2
25	55	6	7.5	9	10.5	12	13.5	15	18	21	24
35	77	8.4	10.5	12.6	14.7	16.8	18.9	21	25.2	29.4	33.6
50	110	12	15	18	21	24	27	30	36	42	48
60	132	14.4	18	21.6	25.2	28.8	32.4	36	43.2	50.4	57.6
70	154	16.8	21	25.2	29.4	33.6	37.8	42	50.4	58.8	67.2
80	176	19.2	24	28.8	33.6	38.4	43.2	48	57.6	67.2	76.8
90	198	21.6	27	32.4	37.8	43.2	48.6	54	64.8	75.6	86.4
100	220	24	30	36	42	48	54	60	72	84	96

** 100 mg rocuronium bromide in 100 mL solution.

➤*Children:* Initial doses of 0.6 mg/kg in pediatric patients under halothane anesthesia produce excellent to good intubating conditions within 1 minute. The median (range) time to maximum block was 1 (0.5 to 3.3) minute(s). This dose will provide a median (range) time of clinical relaxation of 41 (24 to 68) minutes in 3 months to 1 year-old infants and 27 (17 to 41) minutes in 1 to 12 year-old pediatric patients. Maintenance doses of 0.075 to 0.125 mg/kg, administered upon return of T_1 to 25% of control, provide clinical relaxation for 7 to 10 minutes.

Spontaneous recovery proceeds at approximately the same rate in infants (3 months to 1 year) as in adults, but is more rapid in pediatric patients (1 to 12 years) than adults. A continuous infusion of rocuronium bromide injection initiated at a rate of 0.012 mg/kg/min upon return of T_1 to 10% of control (one twitch present in the train-of-four), may also be used to maintain neuromuscular blockade in pediatric patients. The infusion of rocuronium bromide must be individualized for each patient. The rate of administration should be adjusted according to the patient's twitch response as monitored with the use of a peripheral nerve stimulator. Spontaneous recovery and reversal of neuromuscular blockade following discontinuation of rocuronium bromide infusion may be expected to proceed at rates comparable to that following similar total exposure to single bolus doses.

➤*Obesity:* In obese patients, the initial dose of rocuronium bromide injection 0.6 mg/kg should be based upon the patient's actual body weight (ABW) rather than ideal body weight (IBW). In one clinical trial in obese patients, rocuronium bromide 0.6 mg/kg was dosed according to ABW (n = 12) or IBW (n = 11). Obese patients dosed according to IBW had a longer time to maximum block, a shorter clinical duration of 25 (14 to 29) minutes, and did not achieve intubating conditions comparable to those dosed based on ABW.

➤*Elderly:* See Warnings for more information.

➤*Renal or hepatic function impairment:* No differences from patients with normal hepatic and kidney function were observed for onset time at a dose of 0.6 mg/kg rocuronium bromide injection. When compared to patients with normal renal and hepatic function, the mean clinical duration is similar in patients with end-stage renal disease undergoing renal transplant, and is about 1.5 times longer in patients with hepatic disease. Patients with renal failure may have a greater variation in duration of effect.

➤*Compatibility:* Rocuronium bromide injection is compatible in solution with: 0.9% NaCl solution, Sterile Water for Injection, 5% glucose in water, Lactated Ringers, 5% glucose in saline. Use within 24 hours of mixing with these solutions.

Infusion solutions of rocuronium bromide can be prepared by mixing rocuronium bromide with an appropriate infusion solution such as 5% glucose in water or Lactated Ringers. Unused portions of infusion solutions should be discarded.

Rocuronium bromide, which has an acid pH, should not be mixed with alkaline solutions (eg, barbiturate solutions) in the same syringe or administered simultaneously during intravenous infusion through the same needle.

➤*Storage/Stability:* Rocuronium bromide injection should be stored under refrigeration, 2° to 8°C (36° to 46°F). Do not freeze. Upon removal from refrigeration to room temperature storage conditions (25°C; 77°F), use rocuronium bromide within 60 days. Use opened vials of rocuronium bromide within 30 days.

Actions

➤*Pharmacology:* Rocuronium bromide injection is a nondepolarizing neuromuscular blocking agent with a rapid to intermediate onset depending on dose and intermediate duration. It acts by competing for cholinergic receptors at the motor end-plate. This action is antagonized by acetylcholinesterase inhibitors, such as neostigmine and edrophonium.

Histamine release – In studies of histamine release, clinically significant concentrations of plasma histamine occurred in 1 of 88 patients. Clinical signs of histamine release (flushing, rash, or bronchospasm) associated with the administration of rocuronium bromide injection were assessed in clinical trials and reported in 9 of 1137 (0.8%) patients.

➤*Pharmacokinetics:*

Distribution – Following IV administration of rocuronium bromide injection, plasma levels of rocuronium follow a 3 compartment open model. The rapid distribution half-life is 1 to 2 minutes and the slower distribution half-life is 14 to 18 minutes. Rocuronium is approximately 30% bound to human plasma proteins. In geriatric and other adult surgical patients undergoing either opioid/nitrous oxide/oxygen or inhalational anesthesia the observed pharmacokinetic profile was essentially unchanged.

Mean (SD) Pharmacokinetic Parameters in Adults (n = 22; ages 27 to 58 years) and Geriatric (n = 20; ≥ 65 years of age) during Opioid/Nitrous Oxide/Oxygen Anesthesia

PK parameters	Adults (ages 27 to 58 years)	Geriatrics (≥ 65 years of age)
Clearance (L/kg/h)	0.25 (0.08)	0.21 (0.06)
Volume of distribution at steady state (L/kg)	0.25 (0.04)	0.22 (0.03)
t½ β elimination (hours)	1.4 (0.4)	1.5 (0.4)

Metabolism/Excretion – Studies of distribution, metabolism, and excretion in cats and dogs indicate that rocuronium is eliminated primarily by the liver. The rocuronium analog 17-desacetyl-rocuronium, a metabolite, has been rarely observed in the plasma or urine of humans administered single doses of 0.5 to 1 mg/kg with or without a subsequent infusion (for up to 12 hour) of rocuronium. In the cat, 17-desacetyl-rocuronium has approximately one-twentieth the neuromuscular blocking potency of rocuronium. The effects of renal failure and hepatic disease on the pharmacokinetics and pharmacodynamics of rocuronium in humans are consistent with these findings.

Special populations –

Children: The clinical duration of effects of rocuronium bromide injection did not vary with age in patients 3 months to 8 years of age. The terminal half-life and other pharmacokinetic parameters of rocuronium in these pediatric patients are presented in the following table:

Mean (Sd) Pharmacokinetic Parameters of Rocuronium in Pediatric Patients (ages 3 to < 12 months, n = 6; 1 to < 3 years, n = 5; 3 to < 8 years, n = 7) During Halothane Anesthesia

PK parameters	Patient age range		
	3 to < 12 months	1 to < 3 years	3 to < 8 years
Clearance (L/kg/h)	0.35 (0.08)	0.32 (0.07)	0.44 (0.16)
Volume of distribution at steady state (L/kg)	0.3 (0.04)	0.26 (0.06)	0.21 (0.03)
t½ β elimination (h)	1.3 (0.5)	1.1 (0.7)	0.8 (0.3)

Renal/Hepatic function impairment: In general, patients undergoing cadaver kidney transplant have a small reduction in clearance which is offset pharmacokinetically by a corresponding increase in volume, such that the net effect is an unchanged plasma half-life. Patients with demonstrated liver cirrhosis have a marked increase in their volume of distribution resulting in a plasma half-life approximately twice that of patients with normal hepatic function. The information below shows the pharmacokinetic parameters in subjects with either impaired renal or hepatic function.

Mean (SD) pharmacokinetic parameters in adults with normal renal and hepatic function (n = 10, ages 23 to 65), renal transplant patients (n = 10, ages 21 to 45) and hepatic dysfunction patients (n = 9, ages 31 to 67) during isoflurane anesthesia

PK parameters	Normal renal and hepatic function	Renal transplant patients	Hepatic dysfunction patients
Clearance (L/kg/h)	0.16 (0.05)*	0.13 (0.04)	0.13 (0.06)
Volume of distribution at steady state (L/kg)	0.26 (0.03)	0.34 (0.11)	0.53 (0.14)
t½ β elimination (h)	2.4 (0.8)*	2.4 (1.1)	4.3 (2.6)

* Differences in the calculated t½ β and Cl between this study and the study in young adults vs geriatrics (≥ 65 years) is related to the different sample populations and aesthetic techniques.

The net result of these findings is that subjects with renal failure have clinical durations that are similar to but somewhat more variable than the duration that one would expect in subjects with normal renal function. Hepatically impaired patients, due to the large increase in volume, may demonstrate clinical durations approaching 1.5 times that of subjects with normal hepatic function. In both populations the clinician should individualize the dose to the needs of the patient (see Individualization of dosage).

Tissue redistribution accounts for most (about 80%) of the initial amount of rocuronium administered. As tissue compartments fill with continued dosing

ROCURONIUM BROMIDE — INJECTION

(4 to 8 hours), less drug is redistributed away from the site of action and, for an infusion-only dose, the rate to maintain neuromuscular blockade falls to about 20% of the initial infusion rate. The use of a loading dose and a smaller infusion rate reduces the need for adjustment of dose.

Contraindications

Hypersensitivity to rocuronium bromide.

Warnings

➤*Administration:* See Administration and Dosage for more information.

Rocuronium bromide has no known effect on consciousness, pain threshold, or cerebration. Therefore, its administration must be accompanied by adequate anesthesia or sedation.

➤*Hypersensitivity reactions:* There have been rare reports of severe anaphylactic reactions to rocuronium bromide injection, including some that have been life-threatening. Clinicians should be prepared for the possibility of these reactions and take the necessary precautions, including the immediate availability of emergency treatment.

➤*Hepatic function impairment:* Since rocuronium bromide injection is primarily excreted by the liver it should be used with caution in patients with clinically significant hepatic disease. Rocuronium bromide 0.6 mg/kg has been studied in a limited number of patients (n = 9) with clinically significant hepatic disease under steady-state isoflurane anesthesia. After rocuronium bromide 0.6 mg/kg, the median (range) clinical duration of 60 (35 to 166) minutes was moderately prolonged compared to 42 minutes in patients with normal hepatic function. The median recovery time of 53 minutes was also prolonged in patients with cirrhosis compared to 20 minutes in patients with normal hepatic function. Four (4) of 8 patients with cirrhosis who received rocuronium bromide 0.6 mg/kg under opioid/nitrous oxide/oxygen anesthesia did not achieve complete block. These findings are consistent with the increase in volume of distribution at steady state observed in patients with significant hepatic disease. If used for rapid sequence induction in patients with ascites, an increased initial dosage may be necessary to assure complete block. Duration will be prolonged in these cases. The use of doses higher than 0.6 mg/kg has not been studied.

➤*Elderly:* Rocuronium bromide injection was administered to 140 geriatric patients (65 years of age or older) in US clinical trials and 128 geriatric patients in European clinical trials. The observed pharmacokinetic profile for geriatric patients (n = 20) was similar to that for other adult surgical patients. Onset time and duration of action were slightly longer for geriatric patients (n = 43) in clinical trials. Geriatric patients (65 years of age and older) exhibited a slightly prolonged median (range) clinical duration of 46 (22 to 73), 62 (49 to 75), and 94 (64 to 138) minutes under opioid/nitrous oxide/oxygen anesthesia following doses of 0.6, 0.9 and 1.2 mg/kg, respectively. Maintenance doses of 0.1 and 0.15 mg/kg rocuronium bromide injection, administered at 25% recovery of T_1, provide approximately 13 and 33 minutes of clinical duration under opioid/nitrous oxide/oxygen anesthesia. The median (range) rate of spontaneous recovery of T_1 from 25% to 75% in geriatric patients is 17 (7 to 56) minutes which is not different from that in other adults (13 minutes for other adults).

➤*Pregnancy: Category C.* Developmental toxicology studies have been performed in pregnant, conscious, nonventilated rabbits and rats. Inhibition of neuromuscular function was the endpoint for high-dose selection. The maximum tolerated dose served as the high-dose and was administered intravenously 3 times a day to rats (0.3 mg/kg, 15% to 30% of human intubation dose of 0.6 to 1.2 mg/kg based on the body surface unit of mg/m^2) from day 6 to 17 and to rabbits (0.02 mg/kg, 25% human dose) from day 6 to 18 of pregnancy. High-dose treatment caused acute symptoms of respiratory dysfunction due to the pharmacological activity of the drug. Teratogenicity was not observed in these animal species. The incidence of late embryonic death was increased at the high dose in rats most likely due to oxygen deficiency. Therefore, this finding probably has no relevance for humans because immediate mechanical ventilation of the intubated patient will effectively prevent embryo-fetal hypoxia. However, there are no adequate and well-controlled studies in pregnant women. Rocuronium bromide injection should be used during pregnancy only if the potential benefit justifies the potential risk to the fetus.

➤*Children:* The use of rocuronium bromide injection in children less than 3 months of age and greater than 14 years of age has not been studied.

Precautions

➤*Long-term use in ICU:* Rocuronium bromide injection has not been studied for long-term use in the ICU. As with other nondepolarizing neuromuscular blocking drugs, apparent tolerance to rocuronium bromide may develop rarely during chronic administration in the ICU. While the mechanism for development of this resistance is not known, receptor up-regulation may be a contributing factor. It is strongly recommended that neuromuscular transmission be monitored continuously during administration and recovery with the help of a nerve stimulator. Additional doses of rocuronium bromide or any other neuromuscular blocking agent should not be given until there is a definite response (1 twitch of the train-of-four) to nerve stimulation. Prolonged paralysis or skeletal muscle weakness may be noted during initial attempts to wean from the ventilator patients who have chronically received neuromuscular blocking drugs in the ICU. Therefore, rocuronium bromide should only be used in this setting if, in the opinion of the prescribing physician, the specific advantages of the drug outweigh the risk.

➤*Malignant hyperthermia (MH):* In an animal study in MH-susceptible swine, the administration of rocuronium bromide injection did not appear to trigger malignant hyperthermia. Rocuronium bromide has not been studied in MH-susceptible patients. Because rocuronium bromide is always used with other agents, and the occurrence of malignant hyperthermia during anesthesia is possible even in the absence of known triggering agents, clinicians should be familiar with early signs, confirmatory diagnosis and treatment of malignant hyperthermia prior to the start of any anesthetic.

➤*Altered circulation time:* Conditions associated with slower circulation time (eg, cardiovascular disease or advanced age) may be associated with a delay in onset time. Because higher doses of rocuronium bromide injection produce a longer duration of action, the initial dosage should usually not be increased in these patients to reduce onset time; instead, when feasible, more time should be allowed for the drug to achieve onset of effect.

➤*Pulmonary hypertension:* Rocuronium bromide injection may be associated with increased pulmonary vascular resistance so caution is appropriate in patients with pulmonary hypertension or valvular heart disease. In 1 clinical trial, 10 patients with clinically significant cardiovascular disease undergoing coronary artery bypass graft received an initial dose of 0.6 mg/kg rocuronium bromide injection. Neuromuscular block was maintained during surgery with bolus maintenance doses of 0.3 mg/kg. Following induction, continuous 0.008 mg/kg/min infusion of rocuronium bromide produced relaxation sufficient to support mechanical ventilation for 6 to 12 hours in the surgical intensive care unit (SICU) while the patients were recovering from surgery. Hypertension and tachycardia were reported in some patients but these occurrences were less frequent in patients receiving beta or calcium channel blocking drugs. In 7 of these 10 patients rocuronium bromide was associated with transient increases (greater than or equal to 30%) in pulmonary vascular resistance. In another clinical trial of 17 patients undergoing abdominal aortic surgery, transient increases (greater than or equal to 30%) in pulmonary vascular resistance were observed in 4 of 17 patients receiving rocuronium bromide 0.6 or 0.9 mg/kg.

➤*Special risk:* Resistance to nondepolarizing agents, consistent with up-regulation of skeletal muscle acetylcholine receptors, is associated with burns, disuse atrophy, denervation, and direct muscle trauma. Receptor up-regulation may also contribute to the resistance to nondepolarizing muscle relaxants which sometimes develops in patients with cerebral palsy, patients chronically receiving anticonvulsant agents such as carbamazepine or phenytoin or with chronic exposure to nondepolarizing agents.

Other nondepolarizing neuromuscular blocking agents have been found to exhibit profound neuromuscular blocking effects in cachectic or debilitated patients, patients with neuromuscular diseases, and patients with carcinomatosis. In these or other patients in whom potentiation of neuromuscular block or difficulty with reversal may be anticipated, a decrease from the recommended initial dose should be considered.

Severe acid-base or electrolyte abnormalities may potentiate or cause resistance to the neuromuscular blocking action of rocuronium bromide injection. No data are available in such patients and no dosing recommendations can be made. Rocuronium bromide-induced neuromuscular blockade was modified by alkalosis and acidosis in experimental pigs. Both respiratory and metabolic acidosis prolonged the recovery time. The potency of rocuronium bromide was significantly enhanced in metabolic acidosis and alkalosis, but was reduced in respiratory alkalosis. In addition, experience with other drugs has suggested that acute (eg, diarrhea) or chronic (eg, adrenocortical insufficiency) electrolyte imbalance may alter neuromuscular blockade. Since electrolyte imbalance and acid-base imbalance are usually mixed, either enhancement or inhibition may occur. Magnesium salts, administered for the management of toxemia of pregnancy, may enhance neuromuscular blockade.

In patients with myasthenia gravis or myasthenic (Eaton-Lambert) syndrome, small doses of nondepolarizing neuromuscular blocking agents may have profound effects. In such patients, a peripheral nerve stimulator and use of a small test dose may be of value in monitoring the response to administration of muscle relaxants.

Burns – Patients with burns are known to develop resistance to nondepolarizing neuromuscular blocking agents, probably due to up-regulation of postsynaptic skeletal muscle cholinergic receptors.

Drug Interactions

Rocuronium Drug Interactions

Precipitant drug	Object drug*		Description
Antibiotics (eg, aminoglycosides, vancomycin, tetracyclines, bacitracin, polymyxin, colistin, sodium colistimethate)	Rocuronium	↑	Coadministration may enhance the neuromuscular blocking action of rocuronium.
Azathioprine	Rocuronium	↓	Azathioprine has caused reversal of neuromuscular blocking effects when coadministered with other nondepolarizing muscle relaxants. Consider this possibility for rocuronium.
Carbamazepine	Rocuronium	↓	Rocuronium may have shorter than expected duration or be less effective when given with carbamazepine.

ROCURONIUM BROMIDE — INJECTION

Rocuronium Drug Interactions			
Precipitant drug	Object drug*		Description
Diuretics	Rocuronium	↔	Diuretics may lead to electrolyte imbalances, which in turn, may modify neuromuscular blockade (see Precautions).
Inhalational anesthetics (eg, halothane, enflurane, isoflurane)	Rocuronium	↑	The use of these drugs with rocuronium will enhance neuromuscular blockade. Potentiation is most prominent with enflurane followed by isoflurane.
Ketamine	Rocuronium	↑	Ketamine has enhanced the actions of other nondepolarizing muscle relaxants, contributing to profound and severe respiratory depression. Consider this possibility for rocuronium.
Magnesium sulfate	Rocuronium	↑	Magnesium sulfate, administered for toxemia of pregnancy, may potentiate the actions of rocuronium.
Phenytoin	Rocuronium	↓	Rocuronium may have shorter than expected duration or be less effective when given with phenytoin.
Quinidine	Rocuronium	↑	The use of quinidine during recovery from use of other muscle relaxants suggests that recurrent paralysis may occur. Consider this possibility for rocuronium.
Succinylcholine	Rocuronium	↑	Prior administration enhances the neuromuscular blocking effect of rocuronium and its duration of action. If succinylcholine is used before rocuronium, delay administration of rocuronium until recovery from succinylcholine has been observed.
Theophyllines	Rocuronium	↓	Theophyllines have produced a dose-dependent reversal of neuromuscular blocking effects with other nondepolarizing muscle relaxants. Consider this possibility for rocuronium.
Verapamil	Rocuronium	↑	Verapamil has caused enhanced effects of other nondepolarizing muscle relaxants. Respiratory depression may be prolonged. Consider this possibility for rocuronium.

* ↑ = Object drug increased. ↓ = Object drug decreased.
↔ = Undetermined clinical effect.

➤*Drug/Lab test interactions:* None known.

Adverse Reactions

In the European studies, the most commonly reported adverse reactions were transient hypotension (2%) and hypertension (2%); it is in greater frequency than the US studies (0.1% and 0.1%). Changes in heart rate and blood pressure were defined differently from the US studies in which changes in cardiovascular parameters were not considered as adverse events unless judged by the investigator as unexpected, clinically significant, or thought to be histamine related.

In clinical practice, there have been rare reports, primarily from European sources, of severe allergic reactions (anaphylactic and anaphylactoid reactions and shock) with rocuronium bromide injection including some that have been life-threatening and rarely fatal.

Rocuronium Adverse Reactions (< 1%)	
Cardiovascular	Arrhythmia, abnormal electrocardiogram, tachycardia
GI	Nausea, vomiting
Respiratory	Asthma (bronchospasm, wheezing, or rhonchi), hiccup
Dermatologic	Rash, injection site edema, pruritus

Overdosage

➤*Symptoms:* No cases of significant accidental or intentional overdose with rocuronium bromide injection have been reported. Overdosage with neuromuscular blocking agents may result in neuromuscular block beyond the time needed for surgery and anesthesia.

➤*Treatment:* Antagonists (such as neostigmine) should not be administered prior to the demonstration of some spontaneous recovery from neuromuscular blockade. The use of a nerve stimulator to document recovery and antagonism of neuromuscular blockade is recommended.

Patients should be evaluated for adequate clinical evidence of antagonism (eg, 5 sec head lift, adequate phonation, ventilation, and upper airway maintenance). Ventilation must be supported until no longer required.

Antagonism may be delayed in the presence of debilitation, carcinomatosis, and concomitant use of certain broad spectrum antibiotics, or anesthetic agents and other drugs which enhance neuromuscular blockade or separately cause respiratory depression. Under such circumstances the management is the same as that of prolonged neuromuscular blockade.

The primary treatment is maintenance of a patent airway and controlled ventilation until recovery of normal neuromuscular function is assured. Once evidence of recovery from neuromuscular block is observed, further recovery may be facilitated by administration of an anticholinesterase agent (eg, neostigmine, edrophonium) in conjunction with an appropriate anticholinergic agent (see Antagonism of neuromuscular blockade).

PANCURONIUM BROMIDE

Rx	**Pancuronium Bromide** (Various, eg, Elkins-Sinn, Gensia Sicor)	**Injection:** 1 mg/mL	In 10 mL vials.[1]
		2 mg/mL	In 2 and 5 mL vials, amps.[1]

[1] With benzyl alcohol.

PANCURONIUM BROMIDE — INJECTION

WARNING

This drug should be administered by adequately trained individuals familiar with its actions, characteristics, and hazards.

Indications

As an adjunct to general anesthesia to facilitate tracheal intubation and to provide skeletal muscle relaxation during surgery or mechanical ventilation.

Administration and Dosage

Pancuronium bromide injection is for IV use only. This drug should be administered by or under the supervision of experienced clinicians familiar with the use of neuromuscular blocking agents. Dosage must be individualized in each case. The dosage information that follows is derived from studies based upon units of drug per unit of body weight and is intended to serve as a guide only. Since potent inhalational anesthetics or prior use of succinylcholine may enhance the intensity and duration of pancuronium bromide, the lower end of the recommended initial dosage range may suffice when pancuronium bromide is first used after intubation with succinylcholine and/or after maintenance doses of volatile liquid inhalational anesthetics are started. To obtain maximum clinical benefits of pancuronium bromide injection and to minimize the possibility of overdosage, the monitoring of muscle twitch response to a peripheral nerve stimulator is advised.

➤*Adults:* In adults under balanced anesthesia the initial IV dosage range is 0.04 to 0.1 mg/kg. Later incremental doses starting at 0.01 mg/kg may be used. These increments slightly increase the magnitude of the blockade and significantly increase the duration of blockade, because a significant number of myoneural junctions are still blocked when there is a clinical need for more drug.

If pancuronium bromide injection is used to provide skeletal muscle relaxation for endotracheal intubation, a bolus dose of 0.06 to 0.1 mg/kg is recommended. Conditions satisfactory for intubation are usually present within 2 to 3 minutes.

➤*Children:* Dose response studies in children indicate that, with the exception of neonates, dosage requirements are the same as for adults. Neonates are especially sensitive to nondepolarizing neuromuscular blocking agents, such as pancuronium bromide injection, during the first month of life. It is recommended that a test dose of 0.02 mg/kg be given first in this group to measure responsiveness.

PANCURONIUM BROMIDE — INJECTION

➤*Cesarean section:* The dosage to provide relaxation for intubation and operation is the same as for general surgical procedures. The dosage to provide relaxation, following usage of succinylcholine for intubation, is the same as for general surgical procedures.

➤*Compatibility:* Pancuronium bromide injection is compatible in solution with 0.9% Sodium Chloride Injection, 5% Dextrose Injection, 5% Dextrose and Sodium Chloride Injection, and Lactated Ringer's Injection.

When mixed with the above solutions in glass or plastic containers, pancuronium bromide injection will remain stable in solution for 48 hours with no alteration in potency or pH, no decomposition is observed, and there is no adsorption to either the glass or plastic container.

➤*Storage/Stability:* Both concentrations of pancuronium bromide injection will maintain full clinical potency for 6 months if kept at a room temperature of 18° to 22°C (65° to 72°F); or for 36 months when refrigerated at 2° to 8°C (36° to 46°F).

Actions

➤*Pharmacology:* Pancuronium bromide is a nondepolarizing neuromuscular blocking agent possessing all of the characteristic pharmacological actions of this class of drugs (curariform). It acts by competing for cholinergic receptors at the motor end-plate. The antagonism to acetylcholine is inhibited and neuromuscular block is reversed by anticholinesterase agents such as pyridostigmine, neostigmine, and edrophonium. Pancuronium bromide is ≈ ⅓ less potent than vecuronium and ≈ 5 times as potent as d-tubocurarine: the duration of neuromuscular blockage produced by pancuronium bromide is longer than that of vecuronium at initially equipotent doses.

The most characteristic circulatory effects of pancuronium, studied under halothane anesthesia, are a moderate rise in heart rate, mean arterial pressure, and cardiac output; systemic vascular resistance is not changed significantly and central venous pressure may fall slightly. The heart rate rise is inversely related to the rate immediately before administration of pancuronium, is blocked by prior administration of atropine, and appears unrelated to the concentration of halothane or dose of pancuronium.

➤*Pharmacokinetics:* The elimination half-life of pancuronium has been reported to range between 89 to 161 minutes. The volume of distribution ranges from 241 to 280 mL/kg and plasma clearance is ≈ 1.1 to 1.9 mL/minute/kg. Approximately 40% of the total dose of pancuronium has been recovered in urine as unchanged pancuronium and its metabolites while ≈ 11% has been recovered in bile. As much as 25% of an injected dose may be recovered as 3-hydroxy metabolite, which is half as potent a blocking agent as pancuronium. Less than 5% of the injected dose is recovered as 17-hydroxy metabolite and 3, 17-dihydroxy metabolite, which have been judged to be ≈ 50 times less potent than pancuronium. Pancuronium exhibits strong binding to gamma globulin and moderate binding to albumin. Approximately 13% is unbound to plasma protein. In patients with cirrhosis the volume of distribution is increased by ≈ 50%, the plasma clearance is decreased by ≈ 22% and the elimination half-life is doubled. Similar results were noted in patients with biliary obstruction, except that plasma clearance was less than half the normal rate. The initial total dose to achieve adequate relaxation may thus be high in patients with hepatic and/or biliary tract dysfunction, while the duration of action is greater than usual.

The elimination half-life is doubled and the plasma clearance is reduced by ≈ 60% in patients with renal failure. The volume of distribution is variable, and in some cases elevated. The rate of recovery of neuromuscular blockade, as determined by peripheral nerve stimulation, is variable and sometimes very much slower than normal.

Renal function impairment – A major portion of pancuronium, as well as an active metabolite, are recovered in urine. The elimination half-life is doubled and the plasma clearance is reduced in patients with renal failure; at the same time, the rate of recovery of neuromuscular blockade is variable and sometimes very much slower than normal. This information should be taken into consideration if pancuronium is selected, for other reasons, to be used in a patient with renal failure.

Contraindications

Pancuronium bromide injection is contraindicated in patients known to be hypersensitive to the drug.

Warnings

➤*Administration:* See Administration and Dosage for more information.

➤*Hepatic function impairment:* The doubled elimination half-life and reduced plasma clearance determined in patients with hepatic and/or biliary tract disease, as well as limited data showing that recovery time is prolonged an average of 65% in patients with biliary tract obstruction, suggests that prolongation of neuromuscular blockage may occur. At the same time, these conditions are characterized by an ≈ 50% increase in volume of distribution of pancuronium, suggesting that the total initial dose to achieve adequate relaxation may in some cases be high. The possibility of slower onset, higher total dosage, and prolongation of neuromuscular blockage must be taken into consideration when pancuronium is used in these patients (see Pharmacokinetics).

➤*Pregnancy: Category C.* Animal reproduction studies have not been performed. It is not known whether pancuronium bromide can cause fetal harm when administered to a pregnant woman or can affect reproduction capacity. Pancuronium bromide should be given to a pregnant woman only if the administering clinician decides that the benefits outweigh the risks.

Pancuronium bromide may be used in operative obstetrics (Cesarean section), but reversal of pancuronium may be unsatisfactory in patients receiving magnesium sulfate for toxemia of pregnancy, because magnesium salts enhance neuromuscular blockade. Dosage should usually be reduced, as indicated, in such cases. It is also recommended that the interval between use of pancuronium and delivery be reasonably short to avoid clinically significant placental transfer.

➤*Children:* See Administration and Dosage for more information.

The prolonged use of pancuronium bromide for the management of neonates undergoing mechanical ventilation has been associated in rare cases with severe skeletal muscle weakness that may first be noted during attempts to wean such patients from the ventilator; such patients usually receive other drugs such as antibiotics that may enhance neuromuscular blockade. Microscopic changes consistent with disuse atrophy have been noted at autopsy. Although a cause-and-effect relationship has not been established, the benefits-to-risk ratio must be considered when there is a need for neuromuscular blockade to facilitate long-term mechanical ventilation of neonates.

Rare cases of unexplained, clinically significant methemoglobinemia have been reported in premature neonates undergoing emergency anesthesia and surgery that included combined use of pancuronium, fentanyl, and atropine. A direct cause-and-effect relationship between the combined use of these drugs and the reported cases of methemoglobinemia has not been established.

Precautions

➤*Monitoring:* Use of a peripheral nerve stimulator will usually be of value for monitoring of neuromuscular blocking effect, avoiding overdosage and assisting in evaluation of recovery.

➤*Long-term use in ICU:* In the intensive care unit, in rare cases, long-term use of neuromuscular blocking drugs to facilitate mechanical ventilation may be associated with prolonged paralysis or skeletal muscle weakness, that may be first noted during attempts to wean such patients from the ventilator. Typically, such patients receive other drugs such as broad spectrum antibiotics, narcotics and steroids and may have electrolyte imbalance and diseases that lead to electrolyte imbalance, hypoxic episodes of varying duration, acid-base imbalance, and extreme debilitation, any of which may enhance the actions of a neuromuscular blocking agent. Additionally, patients immobilized for extended periods frequently develop symptoms consistent with disuse muscle atrophy. Therefore, when there is a need for long-term mechanical ventilation, the benefits-to-risk ratio of neuromuscular blockade must be considered.

Under the above conditions, appropriate monitoring, such as use of a peripheral nerve stimulator, to assess the degree of neuromuscular blockade, may preclude inadvertent excess dosing.

➤*Severe obesity or neuromuscular disease:* Patients with severe obesity or neuromuscular disease may pose airway and ventilatory problems requiring special care before, during, and after the use of neuromuscular blocking agents such as pancuronium bromide.

➤*CNS:* Pancuronium bromide has no known effect on consciousness, the pain threshold, or cerebration. Administration should be accompanied by adequate anesthesia or sedation.

➤*Special risk:* Although pancuronium bromide injection has been used successfully in many patients with preexisting pulmonary, hepatic, or renal disease, caution should be exercised in these situations.

In patients who are known to have myasthenia gravis or the myasthenic (Eaton-Lambert) syndrome, small doses of pancuronium bromide may have profound effects. In such patients, a peripheral nerve stimulator and use of a small test dose may be of value in monitoring the response to administration of muscle relaxants.

Conditions associated with slower circulation time (cardiovascular disease, old age, edematous states resulting in increased volume of distribution) may contribute to a delay in onset time; therefore dosage should not be increased.

Electrolyte imbalance and diseases that lead to electrolyte imbalance, such as adrenal cortical insufficiency, have been shown to alter neuromuscular blockade. Depending on the nature of the imbalance, either enhancement or inhibition may be expected.

Drug Interactions

➤*Succinylcholine:* Prior administration of succinylcholine may enhance the neuromuscular blocking effect of pancuronium bromide and increase its duration of action. If succinylcholine is used before pancuronium bromide, the administration of pancuronium bromide should be delayed until the patient starts recovering from succinylcholine-induced neuromuscular blockade.

If a small dose of pancuronium bromide is given ≥ 3 minutes prior to the administration of succinylcholine, in order to reduce the incidence and intensity of succinylcholine-induced fasciculations, this dose may induce a degree of neuromuscular block sufficient to cause respiratory depression in some patients.

➤*Other nondepolarizing neuromuscular blocking agents:* Other nondepolarizing neuromuscular blocking agents (vecuronium, atracurium, d-tubocurarine, metocurine, and gallamine) behave in a clinically similar fashion to pancuronium bromide. The combination of pancuronium bromide-metocurine and pancuronium bromide-d-tubocurarine are significantly more potent than the additive effects of each of the individual drugs given alone; however, the duration of blockade of these combinations is not prolonged. There are insufficient data to support concomitant use of pancuronium and the other 3 muscle relaxants mentioned above in the same patient.

➤*Inhalational anesthetics:* Use of volatile inhalational anesthetics such as enflurane, isoflurane, and halothane with pancuronium bromide will

PANCURONIUM BROMIDE — INJECTION

enhance neuromuscular blockade. Potentiation is most prominent with use of enflurane and isoflurane.

With the above agents, the intubating dose of pancuronium bromide may be the same as with balanced anesthesia unless the inhalational anesthetic has been administered for a sufficient time at a sufficient dose to have reached clinical equilibrium. The relatively long duration of action of pancuronium should be taken into consideration when the drug is selected for intubation in these circumstances.

Clinical experience and animal experiments suggest that pancuronium should be given with caution to patients receiving chronic tricyclic antidepressant therapy who are anesthetized with halothane because severe ventricular arrhythmias may result from this combination. The severity of the arrhythmias appear in part related to the dose of pancuronium.

➤*Antibiotics:* Parenteral or intraperitoneal administration of high doses of certain antibiotics may intensify, or produce neuromuscular block on their own. The following antibiotics have been associated with various degrees of paralysis: Aminoglycosides (such as neomycin, streptomycin, kanamycin, gentamicin, and dihydrostreptomycin); tetracyclines; bacitracin, polymyxin B, colistin, and sodium colistimethate. If these or other newly introduced antibiotics are used preoperatively or in conjunction with pancuronium bromide, unexpected prolongation of neuromuscular block should be considered a possibility.

➤*Magnesium salts:* Magnesium salts, administered for the management of toxemia of pregnancy, may enhance the neuromuscular blockade.

➤*Other:* Experience concerning injection of quinidine during recovery from use of other muscle relaxants suggests that recurrent paralysis may occur. This possibility must also be considered for pancuronium bromide.

Adverse Reactions

➤*Cardiovascular:* See discussion of circulatory effects in Pharmacology.

➤*Dermatologic:* An occasional transient rash is noted accompanying the use of pancuronium bromide.

➤*GI:* Salivation is sometimes noted during very light anesthesia, especially if no anticholinergic premedication is used.

➤*Musculoskeletal:* The most frequent adverse reaction to nondepolarizing blocking agents as a class consists of an extension of the drug's pharmacological action beyond the time period needed. This may vary from skeletal muscle weakness to profound and prolonged skeletal muscle paralysis resulting in respiratory insufficiency or apnea (see Warnings, Children).

Inadequate reversal of the neuromuscular blockade is possible with pancuronium bromide as with all curariform drugs. These adverse experiences are managed by manual or mechanical ventilation until recovery is judged adequate.

Prolonged paralysis and skeletal muscle weakness have been reported after long-term use to support mechanical ventilation in the intensive care unit.

➤*Miscellaneous:* Although histamine release is not a characteristic action of pancuronium bromide, rare hypersensitivity reactions such as bronchospasm, flushing, redness, hypotension, tachycardia, and other reactions possibly mediated by histamine release have been reported.

Overdosage

➤*Symptoms:* Residual neuromuscular blockade beyond the time period needed may occur with pancuronium bromide as with other neuromuscular blockers. This may be manifested by skeletal muscle weakness, decreased respiratory reserve, low tidal volume, or apnea.

➤*Treatment:* A peripheral nerve stimulator may be used to assess the degree of residual neuromuscular blockade and help to differentiate residual neuromuscular blockade from other causes of decreased respiratory reserve.

Pyridostigmine bromide, neostigmine, or edrophonium, in conjunction with atropine or glycopyrrolate, will usually antagonize the skeletal muscle relaxant action of pancuronium bromide. Satisfactory reversal can be judged by adequacy of skeletal muscle tone and by adequacy of respiration. A peripheral nerve stimulator may also be used to monitor restoration of twitch response.

Failure of prompt reversal (within 30 minutes) may occur in the presence of extreme debilitation, carcinomatosis, and with concomitant use of certain broad spectrum antibiotics, or anesthetic agents and other drugs that enhance neuromuscular blockade or cause respiratory depression of their own. Under such circumstances, the management is the same as that of prolonged neuromuscular blockade. Ventilation must be supported by artificial means until the patient has resumed control of his respiration. Prior to the use of reversal agents, reference should be made to the specific monograph of the reversal agent.

VECURONIUM BROMIDE

Rx	**Vecuronium Bromide** (Various, eg, Abbott, Baxter, Bedford)	**Powder for Injection:** 10 mg[1]	In 10 mL vials.
Rx	**Norcuron** (Organon)		In 10 mL vials with and without diluent.[2]
Rx	**Vecuronium Bromide** (Various, eg, Abbott, Baxter, Bedford)	**Powder for Injection:** 20 mg[1]	In 20 mL vials.
Rx	**Norcuron** (Organon)		In 20 mL vials without diluent.

[1] May contain mannitol.

[2] Contains 0.9% benzyl alcohol.

VECURONIUM BROMIDE — INJECTION

WARNING

This drug should be administered by adequately trained individuals familiar with its actions, characteristics, and hazards.

Indications

As an adjunct to general anesthesia, to facilitate endotracheal intubation, and to provide skeletal muscle relaxation during surgery or mechanical ventilation.

Administration and Dosage

Vecuronium bromide for injection is for intravenous use only.

To obtain maximum clinical benefits of vecuronium and to minimize the possibility of overdosage, the monitoring of muscle twitch response to peripheral nerve stimulation is advised.

The recommended initial dose of vecuronium bromide is 0.08 to 0.1 mg/kg (1.4 to 1.75 times the ED_{90}) given as an intravenous bolus injection. This dose can be expected to produce good or excellent nonemergency intubation conditions in 2.5 to 3 minutes after injection. Under balanced anesthesia, clinically required neuromuscular blockade lasts approximately 25 to 30 minutes, with recovery to 25% of control achieved approximately 25 to 40 minutes after injection and recovery to 95% of control achieved approximately 45 to 65 minutes after injection. In the presence of potent inhalation anesthetics, the neuromuscular blocking effect of vecuronium is enhanced. If vecuronium is first administered more than 5 minutes after the start of inhalation agent or when steady state has been achieved, the initial vecuronium bromide dose may be reduced by approximately 15% (ie, 0.06 to 0.085 mg/kg).

Prior administration of succinylcholine may enhance the neuromuscular blocking effect and duration of action of vecuronium. If intubation is performed using succinylcholine, a reduction of initial dose of vecuronium bromide to 0.04 to 0.06 mg/kg with inhalation anesthesia and 0.05 to 0.06 mg/kg with balanced anesthesia may be required.

During prolonged surgical procedures, maintenance doses of 0.01 to 0.015 mg/kg of vecuronium bromide are recommended; after the initial injection of vecuronium, the first maintenance dose will generally be required within 25 to 40 minutes. However, clinical criteria should be used to determine the need for maintenance doses.

Since vecuronium lacks clinically important cumulative effects, subsequent maintenance doses, if required, may be administered at relatively regular intervals for each patient, ranging approximately from 12 to 15 minutes under balanced anesthesia, slightly longer under inhalation agents (if less frequent administration is desired, higher maintenance doses may be administered).

Should there be reason for the selection of larger doses in individual patients, initial doses ranging from 0.15 mg/kg up to 0.28 mg/kg have been administered during surgery under halothane anesthesia without ill effects to the cardiovascular system being noted as long as ventilation is properly maintained (see Pharmacology).

➤*Use by continuous infusion:* After an intubating dose of 80 to 100 mcg/kg, a continuous infusion of 1 mcg/kg/min can be initiated approximately 20 to 40 minutes later. Infusion of vecuronium bromide should be initiated only after early evidence of spontaneous recovery from the bolus dose. Long-term intravenous infusion to support mechanical ventilation in the intensive care unit has not been studied sufficiently to support dosing recommendations (see Precautions).

The infusion of vecuronium bromide should be individualized for each patient. The rate of administration should be adjusted according to the patient's twitch response as determined by peripheral nerve stimulation. An initial rate of 1 mcg/kg/min is recommended, with the rate of the infusion adjusted thereafter to maintain a 90% suppression of twitch response. Average infusion rates may range from 0.8 to 1.2 mcg/kg/min.

Inhalation anesthetics, particularly enflurane and isoflurane, may enhance the neuromuscular blocking action of nondepolarizing muscle relaxants. In the presence of steady state concentrations of enflurane or isoflurane, it may be necessary to reduce the rate of infusion 25% to 60%, 45 to 60 minutes after the intubating dose. Under halothane anesthesia it may not be necessary to reduce the rate of infusion.

Spontaneous recovery and reversal of neuromuscular blockade following discontinuation of vecuronium infusion may be expected to proceed at rates comparable to that following a single bolus dose (see Pharmacology).

Infusion rates of vecuronium bromide can be individualized for each patient using the following table:

VECURONIUM BROMIDE — INJECTION

Drug delivery rate (mcg/kg/min)	Infusion delivery rate (mL/kg/min)	
	0.1 mg/mL*	0.2 mg/mL**
0.7	0.007	0.0035
0.8	0.008	0.004
0.9	0.009	0.0045
1	0.01	0.005
1.1	0.011	0.0055
1.2	0.012	0.006
1.3	0.013	0.0065

* 10 mg of vecuronium bromide in 100 mL solution.
** 20 mg of vecuronium bromide in 100 mL solution.

The following table is a guideline for mL/min delivery for a solution of 0.1 mg/mL (10 mg in 100 mL) with an infusion pump:

Vecuronium Bromide Infusion Rate (mL/min)							
Amount of drug (mcg/kg/min)	Patient weight (kg)						
	40	50	60	70	80	90	100
0.7	0.28	0.35	0.42	0.49	0.56	0.63	0.7
0.8	0.32	0.4	0.48	0.56	0.64	0.72	0.8
0.9	0.36	0.45	0.54	0.63	0.72	0.81	0.9
1	0.4	0.5	0.6	0.7	0.8	0.9	1
1.1	0.44	0.55	0.66	0.77	0.88	0.99	1.1
1.2	0.48	0.6	0.72	0.84	0.96	1.08	1.2
1.3	0.52	0.65	0.75	0.91	1.04	1.17	1.3

➤*Note:* If a concentration of 0.2 mg/mL is used (20 mg in 100 mL), the rate should be decreased by one-half.

➤*Children:* Older children (10 to 17 years of age) have approximately the same dosage requirements (mg/kg) as adults and may be managed the same way. Younger children (1 to 10 years of age) may require a slightly higher initial dose and may also require supplementation slightly more often than adults.

Infants under one year of age but older than 7 weeks are moderately more sensitive to vecuronium on a mg/kg basis than adults and take about 1-½ times as long to recover. Information presently available does not permit recommendation on usage in neonates. There are insufficient data concerning continuous infusion of vecuronium in children; therefore, no dosing recommendations can be made.

➤*Preparation:* Vecuronium bromide for injection 10 mg is dissolved by adding 10 mL of Sterile Water for Injection to a vial, resulting in a solution of 1 mg/mL.

Vecuronium bromide for injection 20 mg is dissolved by adding 20 mL of Sterile Water for Injection to a vial, resulting in a solution of 1 mg/mL.

The drug should be completely dissolved before the solution is withdrawn. The solution is then added to a compatible infusion solution (see Use by continuous infusion).

➤*Compatibility:* Vecuronium bromide is compatible in solution with: Sodium Chloride Injection 0.9%, Dextrose Injection 5%, Sterile Water for Injection, Dextrose 5% and Sodium Chloride Injection, and Lactated Ringer's Injection. Use within 24 hours of mixing with the above solutions.

➤*After reconstitution:* Unused portions of infusion solutions should be discarded.

When reconstituted with Bacteriostatic Water for Injection, USP – Contains benzyl alcohol which is not for use in newborns. Use within 5 days. May be stored at room temperature or refrigerated.

If reconstituted with Sterile Water for Injection, USP or other compatible I.V. solutions – Refrigerate vial. Single use only. Use within 24 hours. Discard unused portion.

➤*Storage/Stability:* Store at controlled room temperature 15° to 30°C (59° to 86°F). Protect from light.

Actions

➤*Pharmacology:* Vecuronium bromide is a nondepolarizing neuromuscular blocking agent possessing all of the characteristic pharmacological actions of this class of drugs (curariform). It acts by competing for cholinergic receptors at the motor-end plate. The antagonism to acetylcholine is inhibited, and neuromuscular block is reversed by acetylcholinesterase inhibitors such as neostigmine, edrophonium, and pyridostigmine. Vecuronium is about ⅓ more potent than pancuronium; the duration of neuromuscular blockade produced by vecuronium is shorter than that of pancuronium at initially equipotent doses. The time to onset of paralysis decreases and the duration of maximum effect increases with increasing vecuronium doses. The use of a peripheral nerve stimulator is recommended in assessing the degree of muscular relaxation with all neuromuscular blocking drugs. The ED_{90} (dose required to produce 90% suppression of the muscle twitch response with balanced anesthesia) has averaged 0.057 mg/kg (0.049 to 0.062 mg/kg in various studies). An initial vecuronium bromide dose of 0.08 to 0.1 mg/kg generally produces first depression of twitch in approximately 1 minute, good or excellent intubation conditions within 2.5 to 3 minutes, and maximum neuromuscular blockade within 3 to 5 minutes of injection in most patients.

➤*Pharmacokinetics:* At clinical doses of 0.04 to 0.1 mg/kg, 60% to 80% of vecuronium is usually bound to plasma protein. The distribution half-life following a single intravenous dose (range 0.025 to 0.28 mg/kg) is approximately 4 minutes. Elimination half-life over this sample dosage range is approximately 65 to 75 minutes in healthy surgical patients and in renal failure patients undergoing transplant surgery.

In late pregnancy, elimination half-life may be shortened to approximately 35 to 40 minutes. The volume of distribution at steady state is approximately 300 to 400 mL/kg; systemic rate of clearance is approximately 3 to 4.5 mL/minute/kg. In man, urine recovery of vecuronium varies from 3% to 35% within 24 hours. Data derived from patients requiring insertion of a T-tube in the common bile duct suggests that 25% to 50% of a total intravenous dose of vecuronium may be excreted in bile within 42 hours. Only unchanged vecuronium has been detected in human plasma following use during surgery. In addition, its 3-desacetylmetabolite has been rarely detected in human plasma following prolonged clinical use in the ICU (see Precautions). One metabolite, 3-desacetyl vecuronium, has been recovered in the urine of some patients in quantities that account for up to 10% of injected dose; 3-desacetyl vecuronium has also been recovered by T-tube in some patients accounting for up to 25% of the injected dose.

This metabolite has been judged by animal screening (dogs and cats) to have 50% or more of the potency of vecuronium; equipotent doses are of approximately the same duration as vecuronium in dogs and cats. Biliary excretion accounts for about half the dose of vecuronium within 7 hours in the anesthetized rat. Circulatory bypass of the liver (cat preparation) prolongs recovery from vecuronium. Limited data derived from patients with cirrhosis or cholestasis suggests that some measurements of recovery may be doubled in such patients. In patients with renal failure, measurements of recovery do not differ significantly from similar measurements in healthy patients.

Contraindications

Known hypersensitivity to vecuronium.

Warnings

➤*Administration:* Vecuronium should be administered in carefully adjusted dosage by or under the supervision of experienced clinicians who are familiar with its actions and the possible complications that might occur following its use. The drug should not be administered unless facilities for intubation, artificial respiration, oxygen therapy, and reversal agents are immediately available. The clinician must be prepared to assist or control respiration. To reduce the possibility of prolonged neuromuscular blockade and other possible complications that might occur following long-term use in the ICU, vecuronium or any other neuromuscular blocking agent should be administered in carefully adjusted doses by or under the supervision of experienced clinicians who are familiar with its actions and who are familiar with appropriate peripheral nerve stimulator muscle monitoring techniques (see Precautions). In patients who are known to have myasthenia gravis or the myasthenic (Eaton-Lambert) syndrome, small doses of vecuronium may have profound effects. In such patients, a peripheral nerve stimulator and use of a small test dose may be of value in monitoring the response to administration of muscle relaxants.

➤*Renal function impairment:* Vecuronium is well tolerated without clinically significant prolongation of neuromuscular blocking effect in patients with renal failure who have been optimally prepared for surgery by dialysis. Under emergency conditions in anephric patients some prolongation of neuromuscular blockade may occur; therefore, if anephric patients cannot be prepared for non-elective surgery, a lower initial dose of vecuronium should be considered.

➤*Hepatic function impairment:* Experience in patients with cirrhosis or cholestasis has revealed prolonged recovery time in keeping with the role the liver plays in vecuronium metabolism and excretion. Data currently available do not permit dosage recommendations in patients with impaired liver function.

➤*Pregnancy: Category C.* Animal reproduction studies have not been conducted with vecuronium. It is also not known whether vecuronium can cause fetal harm when administered to a pregnant woman or can affect reproduction capacity. Vecuronium bromide should be given to a pregnant woman only if clearly needed.

➤*Children:* Infants under 1 year of age but older than 7 weeks, also tested under halothane anesthesia, are moderately more sensitive to vecuronium on a mg/kg basis than adults and take about 1-½ times as long to recover. Information presently available does not permit recommendations for usage in neonates.

Precautions

➤*Altered circulation time:* Conditions associated with slower circulation time in cardiovascular disease, old age, edematous states resulting in increased volume of distribution may contribute to a delay in onset time; therefore, dosage should not be increased.

➤*Long-term use in ICU:* In the intensive care unit, long-term use of neuromuscular blocking drugs to facilitate mechanical ventilation may be associated with prolonged paralysis and/or skeletal muscle weakness that may be first noted during attempts to wean such patients from the ventilator. Typically, such patients receive other drugs such as broad spectrum antibiotics, narcotics, and/or steroids and may have electrolyte imbalance and diseases which lead to electrolyte imbalance, hypoxic episodes of varying duration, acid-base imbalance, and extreme debilitation, any of which may

VECURONIUM BROMIDE — INJECTION

enhance the actions of a neuromuscular blocking agent. Additionally, patients immobilized for extended periods frequently develop symptoms consistent with disuse muscle atrophy. The recovery picture may vary from regaining movement and strength in all muscles, to initial recovery of movement of the facial and small muscles of the extremities, and then to the remaining muscles. In rare cases recovery may be over an extended period of time and may even, on occasion, involve rehabilitation. Therefore, when there is a need for long-term mechanical ventilation, the benefits-to-risk ratio of neuromuscular blockade must be considered.

Continuous infusion or intermittent bolus dosing to support mechanical ventilation, has not been studied sufficiently to support dosage recommendations. In the intensive care unit, appropriate monitoring, with the use of a peripheral nerve stimulator to assess the degree of neuromuscular blockade is recommended to help preclude possible prolongation of the blockade. Whenever the use of vecuronium or any other neuromuscular blocking agent is contemplated in the ICU, it is recommended that neuromuscular transmission be monitored continuously during administration and recovery with the help of a nerve stimulator. Additional doses of vecuronium or any other neuromuscular blocking agent should not be given before there is a definite response to t_1 or to the first twitch. If no response is elicited, infusion administration should be discontinued until a response returns.

➤*Severe obesity or neuromuscular disease:* Patients with severe obesity or neuromuscular disease may pose airway and/or ventilatory problems requiring special care before, during, and after the use of neuromuscular blocking agents such as vecuronium.

➤*Malignant hyperthermia:* Many drugs used in anesthetic practice are suspected of being capable of triggering a potentially fatal hypermetabolism of skeletal muscle known as malignant hyperthermia. There are insufficient data derived from screening in susceptible animals (swine) to establish whether or not vecuronium is capable of triggering malignant hyperthermia.

Drug Interactions

➤*Succinylcholine:* Prior administration of succinylcholine may enhance the neuromuscular blocking effect of vecuronium and its duration of action. If succinylcholine is used before vecuronium, the administration of vecuronium should be delayed until the succinylcholine effect shows signs of wearing off. With succinylcholine as the intubating agent, initial doses of 0.04 to 0.06 mg/kg of vecuronium bromide may be administered to produce complete neuromuscular block with clinical duration of action of 25 to 30 minutes.

➤*Other nondepolarizing neuromuscular blocking agents:* Other nondepolarizing neuromuscular blocking agents (pancuronium, d-tubocurarine, metocurine, and gallamine) act in the same fashion as does vecuronium; therefore, these drugs and vecuronium may manifest an additive effect when used together. There are insufficient data to support concomitant use of vecuronium and other competitive muscle relaxants in the same patient.

➤*Inhalational anesthetics:* Use of volatile inhalational anesthetics such as enflurane, isoflurane, and halothane with vecuronium will enhance neuromuscular blockade. Potentiation is most prominent with use of enflurane and isoflurane. With the above agents, the initial dose of vecuronium may be the same as with balanced anesthesia unless the inhalational anesthetic has been administered for a sufficient time at a sufficient dose to have reached clinical equilibrium (see Pharmacology).

➤*Antibiotics:* Parenteral/intraperitoneal administration of high doses of certain antibiotics may intensify or produce neuromuscular block on their own. The following antibiotics have been associated with various degrees of paralysis: Aminoglycosides (such as neomycin, streptomycin, kanamycin, gentamicin, and dihydrostreptomycin); tetracyclines; bacitracin; polymyxin B; colistin; and sodium colistimethate. If these or other newly introduced antibiotics are used in conjunction with vecuronium, unexpected prolongation of neuromuscular block should be considered a possibility.

➤*Other:* Experience concerning injection of quinidine during recovery from use of other muscle relaxants suggests that recurrent paralysis may occur. This possibility must also be considered for vecuronium. Vecuronium induced neuromuscular blockade has been counteracted by alkalosis and enhanced by acidosis in experimental animals (cats). Electrolyte imbalance and diseases which lead to electrolyte imbalance, such as adrenal cortical insufficiency, have been shown to alter neuromuscular blockade. Depending on the nature of the imbalance, either enhancement or inhibition may be expected. Magnesium salts, administered for the management of toxemia of pregnancy, may enhance the neuromuscular blockade.

Adverse Reactions

Prolonged to profound extensions of paralysis and/or muscle weakness as well as muscle atrophy have been reported after long-term use to support mechanical ventilation in the intensive care unit (see Precautions). The administration of vecuronium has been associated with rare instances of hypersensitivity reactions (bronchospasm, hypotension and/or tachycardia, sometimes associated with acute urticaria or erythema).

Overdosage

➤*Symptoms:* The possibility of iatrogenic overdosage can be minimized by carefully monitoring muscle twitch response to peripheral nerve stimulation.

Excessive doses of vecuronium produce enhanced pharmacological effects. Residual neuromuscular blockade beyond the time period needed may occur with vecuronium as with other neuromuscular blockers. This may be manifested by skeletal muscle weakness, decreased respiratory reserve, low tidal volume, or apnea. A peripheral nerve stimulator may be used to assess the degree of residual neuromuscular blockade from other causes of decreased respiratory reserve.

Respiratory depression may be due either wholly or in part to other drugs used during the conduct of general anesthesia such as narcotics, thiobarbiturates, and other central nervous system depressants.

➤*Treatment:* Under such circumstances the primary treatment is maintenance of a patent airway and manual or mechanical ventilation until complete recovery of normal respiration is assured. Pyridostigmine, neostigmine, or edrophonium in conjunction with atropine or glycopyrrolate will usually antagonize the skeletal muscle relaxant action of vecuronium. Satisfactory reversal can be judged by adequacy of skeletal muscle tone and by adequacy of respiration. A peripheral nerve stimulator may also be used to monitor restoration of twitch height. Failure of prompt reversal (within 30 minutes) may occur in the presence of extreme debilitation, carcinomatosis, and with concomitant use of certain broad spectrum antibiotics, or anesthetic agents and other drugs which enhance neuromuscular blockade or cause respiratory depression of their own. Under such circumstances, the management is the same as that of prolonged neuromuscular blockade. Ventilation must be supported by artificial means until the patient has resumed control of his respiration. Prior to the use of reversal agents, reference should be made to the specific package insert of the reversal agent.

SUCCINYLCHOLINE CHLORIDE

Rx	**Anectine** (GlaxoWellcome)	**Injection:** 20 mg/ml	In 10 ml vials.[1]
Rx	**Quelicin** (Abbott)		In 5 ml *Abboject* (single-dose) syringe and 10 ml vials.[2]
Rx	**Quelicin** (Abbott)	**Injection:** 50 mg/ml	In 10 ml amps.
Rx	**Anectine Flo-Pack** (GlaxoWellcome)	**Powder for infusion:** 500 mg	In vials.
		Powder for infusion: 1 g	In vials.

[1] With methylparaben.
[2] With methyl- and propylparabens.
[3] With benzyl alcohol.

SUCCINYLCHOLINE CHLORIDE — INJECTION

WARNING

There have been rare reports of acute rhabdomyolysis with hyperkalemia followed by ventricular dysrhythmias, cardiac arrest, and death after the administration of succinylcholine to apparently healthy children who were subsequently found to have undiagnosed skeletal muscle myopathy, most frequently Duchenne's muscular dystrophy.

This syndrome often presents as peaked T-waves and sudden cardiac arrest within minutes after the administration of the drug in healthy appearing children (usually, but not exclusively, males, and most frequently 8 years of age or younger). There have also been reports in adolescents.

Therefore, when a healthy appearing infant or child develops cardiac arrest soon after administration of succinylcholine not felt to be due to inadequate ventilation, oxygenation, or anesthetic overdose, immediate treatment for hyperkalemia should be instituted. This should include administration of intravenous calcium, bicarbonate, and glucose with insulin, with hyperventilation. Due to the abrupt onset of this syndrome, routine resuscitative measures are likely to be unsuccessful. However, extraordinary and prolonged resuscitative efforts have resulted in successful resuscitation in some reported cases. In addition, in the presence of signs of malignant hyperthermia, appropriate treatment should be instituted concurrently.

Since there may be no signs or symptoms to alert the practitioner to which patients are at risk, it is recommended that the use of succinylcholine in children should be reserved for emergency intubation or instances where immediate securing of the airway is necessary, eg, laryngospasm, difficult airway, full stomach, or for intramuscular use when a suitable vein is inaccessible.

Indications

As an adjunct to general anesthesia, to facilitate tracheal intubation, and to provide skeletal muscle relaxation during surgery or mechanical ventilation.

SUCCINYLCHOLINE CHLORIDE — INJECTION

Administration and Dosage

➤*Adults:*

Short surgical procedures – The average dose required to produce neuromuscular blockade and to facilitate tracheal intubation is 0.6 mg/kg succinylcholine injection given intravenously. The optimum dose will vary among individuals and may be from 0.3 to 1.1 mg/kg for adults. Following administration of doses in this range, neuromuscular blockade develops in about 1 minute; maximum blockade may persist for about 2 minutes, after which recovery takes place within 4 to 6 minutes. However, very large doses may result in more prolonged blockade. A 5- to 10-mg test dose may be used to determine the sensitivity of the patient and the individual recovery time.

Long surgical procedures – The dose of succinylcholine administered by infusion depends upon the duration of the surgical procedure and the need for muscle relaxation. The average rate for an adult ranges between 2.5 and 4.3 mg per minute.

Solutions containing from 1 to 2 mg per mL succinylcholine have commonly been used for continuous infusion. The more dilute solution (1 mg per mL) is probably preferable from the standpoint of ease of control of the rate of administration of the drug and, hence, of relaxation. This IV solution containing 1 mg per mL may be administered at a rate of 0.5 mg (0.5 mL) to 10 mg (10 mL) per minute to obtain the required amount of relaxation. The amount required per minute will depend upon the individual response as well as the degree of relaxation required. Avoid overburdening the circulation with a large volume of fluid. It is recommended that neuromuscular function be carefully monitored with a peripheral nerve stimulator when using succinylcholine by infusion in order to avoid overdose, detect development of Phase II block, follow its rate of recovery, and assess the effects of reversing agents.

Intermittent IV injections of succinylcholine may also be used to provide muscle relaxation for long procedures. An IV injection of 0.3 to 1.1 mg/kg may be given initially, followed, at appropriate intervals, by further injections of 0.04 to 0.07 mg/kg to maintain the degree of relaxation required.

➤*Pediatrics:* For emergency tracheal intubation or in instances where immediate securing of the airway is necessary, the IV dose of succinylcholine is 2 mg/kg for infants and small children; for older children and adolescents the dose is 1 mg/kg.

See the Warning box for more information.

Intravenous bolus administration of succinylcholine in infants or children may result in profound bradycardia or, rarely, asystole. As in adults, the incidence of bradycardia in children is higher following a second dose of succinylcholine. The occurrence of bradyarrhythmias may be reduced by pretreatment with atropine.

➤*Intramuscular use:* If necessary, succinylcholine may be given intramuscularly to infants, older children, or adults when a suitable vein is inaccessible. A dose of up to 3 to 4 mg/kg may be given, but not more than 150 mg total dose should be administered by this route. The onset of effect of succinylcholine given intramuscularly is usually observed in about 2 to 3 minutes.

➤*Compatibility and admixtures:* Succinylcholine is acidic (pH 3.5) and should not be mixed with alkaline solutions having a pH more than 8.5 (eg, barbiturate solutions). Admixtures containing 1 to 2 mg/mL may be prepared by adding 1 g succinylcholine (the contents of one succinylcholine sterile powder *Flo-Pack* unit containing 1 g succinylcholine chloride) to 1000 or 500 mL sterile solution, such as 5% Dextrose Injection, USP or 0.9% Sodium Chloride Injection, USP. Admixtures of succinylcholine must be used within 24 hours after preparation. Aseptic techniques should be used to prepare the diluted product. Admixtures of succinylcholine should be prepared for single patient use only. The unused portion of diluted succinylcholine should be discarded.

➤*Storage / Stability:*

Multiple-dose 10 ml vials – For immediate injection of single doses: 20 mg in each mL. Store in refrigerator at 2° to 8°C (36° to 46°F). The multidose vials are stable for up to 14 days at room temperature without significant loss of potency.

500 and 1000 mg succinylcholine chloride powder vials – For IV solutions only. Does not require refrigeration. Store at 15° to 25°C (59° to 77°F). Solutions of succinylcholine must be used within 24 hours after preparation. Discard unused solutions.

Actions

➤*Pharmacology:* Succinylcholine is a depolarizing skeletal muscle relaxant. As does acetylcholine, it combines with the cholinergic receptors of the motor end plate to produce depolarization. This depolarization may be observed as fasciculations. Subsequent neuromuscular transmission is inhibited so long as adequate concentration of succinylcholine remains at the receptor site. Onset of flaccid paralysis is rapid (less than 1 minute after IV administration), and with single administration lasts approximately 4 to 6 minutes.

Succinylcholine is rapidly hydrolyzed by plasma cholinesterase to succinylmonocholine (which possesses clinically insignificant depolarizing muscle relaxant properties) and then more slowly to succinic acid and choline (see Precautions). About 10% of the drug is excreted unchanged in the urine. The paralysis following administration of succinylcholine is progressive, with differing sensitivities of different muscles. This initially involves consecutively the levator muscles of the face, muscles of the glottis, and finally, the intercostals and the diaphragm and all other skeletal muscles.

Depending on the dose and duration of succinylcholine administration, the characteristic depolarizing neuromuscular block (Phase I block) may change to a block with characteristics superficially resembling a nondepolarizing block (Phase II block). This may be associated with prolonged respiratory muscle paralysis or weakness in patients who manifest the transition to Phase II block. When this diagnosis is confirmed by peripheral nerve stimulation, it may sometimes be reversed with anticholinesterase drugs such as neostigmine (see Precautions). Anticholinesterase drugs may not always be effective. If given before succinylcholine is metabolized by cholinesterase, anticholinesterase drugs may prolong rather than shorten paralysis.

Succinylcholine has no direct effect on the myocardium. Succinylcholine stimulates both autonomic ganglia and muscarinic receptors which may cause changes in cardiac rhythm, including cardiac arrest. Changes in rhythm, including cardiac arrest, may also result from vagal stimulation, which may occur during surgical procedures, or from hyperkalemia, particularly in children (see Warnings, Children). These effects are enhanced by halogenated anesthetics.

Succinylcholine causes an increase in intraocular pressure immediately after its injection and during the fasciculation phase, and slight increases which may persist after onset of complete paralysis (see Warnings).

Succinylcholine may cause slight increases in intracranial pressure immediately after its injection and during the fasciculation phase (see Precautions).

As with other neuromuscular blocking agents, the potential for releasing histamine is present following succinylcholine administration. Signs and symptoms of histamine-mediated release such as flushing, hypotension, and bronchoconstriction are, however, uncommon in normal clinical usage.

Contraindications

Personal or familial history of malignant hyperthermia; skeletal muscle myopathies; hypersensitivity to the drug; in patients after the acute phase of injury following major burns, multiple trauma, extensive denervation of skeletal muscle, or upper motor neuron injury, because succinylcholine administered to such individuals may result in severe hyperkalemia which may result in cardiac arrest. The risk of hyperkalemia in these patients increases over time and usually peaks at 7 to 10 days after the injury. The risk is dependent on the extent and location of the injury. The precise time of onset and the duration of the risk period are not known.

Warnings

➤*Administration:* Succinylcholine should be used only by those skilled in the management of artificial respiration and only when facilities are instantly available for tracheal intubation and for providing adequate ventilation of the patient, including the administration of oxygen under positive pressure and the elimination of carbon dioxide. The clinician must be prepared to assist or control respiration.

To avoid distress to the patient, succinylcholine should not be administered before unconsciousness has been induced. In emergency situations, however, it may be necessary to administer succinylcholine before unconsciousness is induced.

➤*Hyperkalemia:* Succinylcholine should be administered with *great caution* to patients suffering from electrolyte abnormalities and those who may have massive digitalis toxicity, because in these circumstances succinylcholine may induce serious cardiac arrhythmias or cardiac arrest due to hyperkalemia.

Great caution should be observed if succinylcholine is administered to patients during the acute phase of injury following major burns, multiple trauma, extensive denervation of skeletal muscle, or upper motor neuron injury. The risk of hyperkalemia in these patients increases over time and usually peaks at 7 to 10 days after the injury. The risk is dependent on the extent and location of the injury. The precise time of onset and the duration of the risk period are undetermined. Patients with chronic abdominal infection, subarachnoid hemorrhage, or conditions causing degeneration of central and peripheral nervous systems should receive succinylcholine with *great caution* because of the potential for developing severe hyperkalemia.

➤*Malignant hyperthermia:* Succinylcholine administration has been associated with acute onset of malignant hyperthermia, a potentially fatal hypermetabolic state of skeletal muscle. The risk of developing malignant hyperthermia following succinylcholine administration increases with the concomitant administration of volatile anesthetics. Malignant hyperthermia frequently presents as intractable spasm of the jaw muscles (masseter spasm) which may progress to generalized rigidity, increased oxygen demand, tachycardia, tachypnea and profound hyperpyrexia. Successful outcome depends on recognition of early signs, such as jaw muscle spasm, acidosis, or generalized rigidity to initial administration of succinylcholine for tracheal intubation, or failure of tachycardia to respond to deepening anesthesia. Skin mottling, rising temperature, and coagulopathies may occur later in the course of the hypermetabolic process. Recognition of the syndrome is a signal for discontinuance of anesthesia, attention to increased oxygen consumption, correction of acidosis, support of circulation, assurance of adequate urinary output, and institution of measures to control rising temperature. Intravenous dantrolene sodium is recommended as an adjunct to supportive measures in the management of this problem. Consult literature references and the dantrolene prescribing information for additional information about the management of malignant hyperthermic crisis. Continuous monitoring of temperature and expired CO_2 is recommended as an aid to early recognition of malignant hyperthermia.

➤*Cardiac effects:* In both adults and children, the incidence of bradycardia, which may progress to asystole, is higher following a second dose of succinylcholine. The incidence and severity of bradycardia is higher in children

SUCCINYLCHOLINE CHLORIDE — INJECTION

than in adults. Pretreatment with anticholinergic agents (eg, atropine) may reduce the occurrence of bradyarrhythmias.

➤*Ocular effects:* Succinylcholine causes an increase in intraocular pressure. It should not be used in instances in which an increase in intraocular pressure is undesirable (eg, narrow angle glaucoma, penetrating eye injury) unless the potential benefit of its use outweighs the potential risk.

➤*Pregnancy: Category C.* Animal reproduction studies have not been conducted with succinylcholine chloride. It is also not known whether succinylcholine can cause fetal harm when administered to a pregnant woman or can affect reproduction capacity. Succinylcholine should be given to a pregnant woman only if clearly needed.

Plasma cholinesterase levels are decreased by approximately 24% during pregnancy and for several days postpartum. Therefore, a higher proportion of patients may be expected to show increased sensitivity (prolonged apnea) to succinylcholine when pregnant than when nonpregnant.

Labor and delivery – Succinylcholine is commonly used to provide muscle relaxation during delivery by cesarean section. While small amounts of succinylcholine are known to cross the placental barrier, under normal conditions the quantity of drug that enters fetal circulation after a single dose of 1 mg/kg to the mother should not endanger the fetus. However, since the amount of drug that crosses the placental barrier is dependent on the concentration gradient between the maternal and fetal circulations, residual neuromuscular blockade (apnea and flaccidity) may occur in the neonate after repeated high doses to, or in the presence of atypical plasma cholinesterase in, the mother.

➤*Lactation:* It is not known whether succinylcholine is excreted in human milk. Because many drugs are excreted in human milk, caution should be exercised following succinylcholine administration to a nursing woman.

➤*Children:* See the Warning box for more information.

There may be no signs or symptoms to alert the practitioner to which patients are at risk. A careful history and physical may identify developmental delays suggestive of a myopathy. A preoperative creatine kinase could identify some but not all patients at risk. Due to the abrupt onset of this syndrome, routine resuscitative measures are likely to be unsuccessful. Careful monitoring of the electrocardiogram may alert the practitioner to peaked T-waves (an early sign). Administration of IV calcium, bicarbonate, and glucose with insulin, with hyperventilation have resulted in successful resuscitation in some of the reported cases. Extraordinary and prolonged resuscitative efforts have been effective in some cases. In addition, in the presence of signs of malignant hyperthermia, appropriate treatment should be initiated concurrently. Since it is difficult to identify which patients are at risk, it is recommended that the use of succinylcholine in children should be reserved for emergency intubation or instances where immediate securing of the airway is necessary, eg, laryngospasm, difficult airway, full stomach, or for intramuscular use when a suitable vein is inaccessible.

Precautions

➤*Phase II block:* When succinylcholine is given over a prolonged period of time, the characteristic depolarization block of the myoneural junction (Phase I block) may change to a block with characteristics superficially resembling a nondepolarizing block (Phase II block). Prolonged respiratory muscle paralysis or weakness may be observed in patients manifesting this transition to Phase II block. The transition from Phase I to Phase II block has been reported in 7 of 7 patients studied under halothane anesthesia after an accumulated dose of 2 to 4 mg/kg succinylcholine (administered in repeated, divided doses). The onset of Phase II block coincided with the onset of tachyphylaxis and prolongation of spontaneous recovery. In another study, using balanced anesthesia (N_2O/O_2 /narcotic-thiopental) and succinylcholine infusion, the transition was less abrupt, with great individual variability in the dose of succinylcholine required to produce Phase II block. Of 32 patients studied, 24 developed Phase II block. Tachyphylaxis was not associated with the transition to Phase II block, and 50% of the patients who developed Phase II block experienced prolonged recovery.

When Phase II block is suspected in cases of prolonged neuromuscular blockade, positive diagnosis should be made by peripheral nerve stimulation prior to administration of any anticholinesterase drug. Reversal of Phase II block is a medical decision which must be made upon the basis of the individual, clinical pharmacology, and the experience and judgment of the physician. The presence of Phase II block is indicated by fade of responses to successive stimuli (preferably "train-of-four"). The use of an anticholinesterase drug to reverse Phase II block should be accompanied by appropriate doses of an anticholinergic drug to prevent disturbances of cardiac rhythm. After adequate reversal of Phase II block with an anticholinesterase agent, the patient should be continually observed for at least 1 hour for signs of return of muscle relaxation. Reversal should not be attempted unless: (1) a peripheral nerve stimulator is used to determine the presence of Phase II block (since anticholinesterase agents will potentiate succinylcholine-induced Phase I block), and (2) spontaneous recovery of muscle twitch has been observed for at least 20 minutes and has reached a plateau with further recovery proceeding slowly; this delay is to ensure complete hydrolysis of succinylcholine by plasma cholinesterase prior to administration of the anticholinesterase agent. Should the type of block be misdiagnosed, depolarization of the type initially induced by succinylcholine (ie, Phase I block) will be prolonged by an anticholinesterase agent.

➤*Reduced plasma cholinesterase activity:* Succinylcholine should be used carefully in patients with reduced plasma cholinesterase (pseudocholinesterase) activity. The likelihood of prolonged neuromuscular block following administration of succinylcholine must be considered in such patients (see Administration and Dosage).

Plasma cholinesterase activity may be diminished in the presence of genetic abnormalities of plasma cholinesterase (eg, patients heterozygous or homozygous for atypical plasma cholinesterase gene), pregnancy, severe liver or kidney disease, malignant tumors, infections, burns, anemia, decompensated heart disease, peptic ulcer, or myxedema. Plasma cholinesterase activity may also be diminished by chronic administration of oral contraceptives, glucocorticoids, or certain monoamine oxidase inhibitors, and by irreversible inhibitors of plasma cholinesterase (eg, organophosphate insecticides, echothiophate, and certain antineoplastic drugs).

Patients homozygous for atypical plasma cholinesterase gene (1 in 2500 patients) are extremely sensitive to the neuromuscular blocking effect of succinylcholine. In these patients, a 5- to 10-mg test dose of succinylcholine may be administered to evaluate sensitivity to succinylcholine, or neuromuscular blockade may be produced by the cautious administration of a 1 mg/mL solution of succinylcholine by slow IV infusion. Apnea or prolonged muscle paralysis should be treated with controlled respiration.

➤*Special risk:* Succinylcholine should be employed with caution in patients with fractures or muscle spasm because the initial muscle fasciculations may cause additional trauma.

Succinylcholine may cause a transient increase in intracranial pressure; however, adequate anesthetic induction prior to administration of succinylcholine will minimize this effect.

Succinylcholine may increase intragastric pressure, which could result in regurgitation and possible aspiration of stomach contents.

Neuromuscular blockade may be prolonged in patients with hypokalemia or hypocalcemia.

Drug Interactions

Drugs which may enhance the neuromuscular blocking action of succinylcholine include: Promazine, oxytocin, aprotinin, certain non-penicillin antibiotics, quinidine, β-adrenergic blockers, procainamide, lidocaine, trimethaphan, lithium carbonate, magnesium salts, quinine, chloroquine, diethylether, isoflurane, desflurane, metoclopramide, and terbutaline. The neuromuscular blocking effect of succinylcholine may be enhanced by drugs that reduce plasma cholinesterase activity (eg, chronically administered oral contraceptives, glucocorticoids, or certain monoamine oxidase inhibitors) or by drugs that irreversibly inhibit plasma cholinesterase.

If other neuromuscular blocking agents are to be used during the same procedure, the possibility of a synergistic or antagonistic effect should be considered.

Adverse Reactions

Adverse reactions to succinylcholine consist primarily of an extension of its pharmacological actions. Succinylcholine causes profound muscle relaxation resulting in respiratory depression to the point of apnea; this effect may be prolonged. Hypersensitivity reactions, including anaphylaxis, may occur in rare instances. The following additional adverse reactions have been reported.

➤*Cardiovascular:* Cardiac arrest, arrhythmias, bradycardia, tachycardia, hypertension, hypotension.

➤*Musculoskeletal:* Muscle fasciculation, jaw rigidity, postoperative muscle pain, rhabdomyolysis with possible myoglobinuric acute renal failure.

➤*Respiratory:* Prolonged respiratory depression or apnea.

➤*Miscellaneous:* Increased intraocular pressure, hyperkalemia, malignant hyperthermia, excessive salivation, and rash.

Overdosage

➤*Symptoms:* Overdosage with succinylcholine may result in neuromuscular block beyond the time needed for surgery and anesthesia. This may be manifested by skeletal muscle weakness, decreased respiratory reserve, low tidal volume, or apnea.

➤*Treatment:* The primary treatment is maintenance of a patent airway and respiratory support until recovery of normal respiration is assured. Depending on the dose and duration of succinylcholine administration, the characteristic depolarizing neuromuscular block (Phase I) may change to a block with characteristics superficially resembling a nondepolarizing block (Phase II) (see Precautions).

BACLOFEN

Rx	**Baclofen** (Various, eg, Ivax, Watson)	**Tablets:** 10 mg	In 30s, 100s, 250s, 500s, and 1000s.
Rx	**Lioresal** (Novartis)		(Lioresal 1010). White, scored, oval. In 100s and UD 100s.
Rx	**Baclofen** (Various, eg, Ivax, Watson)	**Tablets:** 20 mg	In 30s, 100s, 250s, 500s, and 1000s.
Rx	**Lioresal** (Novartis)		(Lioresal 2020). White, scored, capsule shape. In 100s and UD 100s.
Rx	**Kemstro** (Schwarz)	**Tablets, orally disintegrating:** 10 mg	Mannitol, aspartame, 3.9 mg phenylalanine. (10 SP 351). Scored. Orange flavor. In 100s.
Rx	**Kemstro** (Schwarz)	20 mg	Mannitol, aspartame, 7.9 mg phenylalanine. (20 SP 352). Scored. Orange flavor. In 100s.
Rx	**Lioresal Intrathecal** (Medtronic)	**Intrathecal:** 0.05 mg/mL (50 mcg/mL)	Preservative-free. In single-use amps.
		10 mg/20 mL (500 mcg/mL)	Preservative-free. In single-use amps (1 amp refill kit).
		10 mg/5 mL (2000 mcg/mL)	Preservative-free. In single-use amps (2 or 4 amp refill kits).

BACLOFEN — ORAL

Indications

➤*Spasticity:* For the alleviation of signs and symptoms of spasticity resulting from multiple sclerosis, particularly for the relief of flexor spasms and concomitant pain, clonus, and muscular rigidity. Patients should have reversible spasticity so that baclofen treatment will aid in restoring residual function .Baclofen may also be of some value in patients with spinal cord injuries and other spinal cord diseases.

Baclofen is not indicated in the treatment of skeletal muscle spasm resulting from rheumatic disorders. The efficacy of baclofen in stroke, cerebral palsy, and Parkinson's disease has not been established and, therefore, it is not recommended for these conditions.

➤*Unlabeled uses:* Treatment of trigeminal neuralgia (tic douloureux); intractable hiccups; to reduce choreiform movements in patients with Huntington's chorea; to reduce rigidity in patients with parkinsonism syndrome; to reduce spasticity in patients with cerebral lesions or rheumatic disorders; to reduce spasticity in patients with cerebrovascular stroke; acquired periodic alternating nystagmus; acquired pendular nystagmus; to reduce the number of gastroesophageal reflux episodes (single 40 mg dose); Tourette syndrome in children (20 mg 3 times daily); prophylactic treatment of migraine; neuropathic pain.

Administration and Dosage

➤*Approved by the FDA:* January 20, 1982.

The determination of optimal dosage requires individual titration. Start therapy at a low dosage and increase gradually until optimum effect is achieved (usually between 40 to 80 mg daily).

The following dosage titration schedule is suggested:
- 5 mg 3 times daily for 3 days;
- 10 mg 3 times daily for 3 days;
- 15 mg 3 times daily for 3 days;
- 20 mg 3 times daily for 3 days.

Thereafter additional increases may be necessary but the total daily dose should not exceed a maximum of 80 mg daily (20 mg 4 times daily). The lowest dose compatible with an optimal response is recommended. If benefits are not evident after a reasonable trial period, patients should be slowly withdrawn from the drug (see Warnings).

➤*Storage/Stability:* Do not store above 30°C (86°F). Dispense in tight container (USP).

Actions

➤*Pharmacology:* The precise mechanism of action of baclofen is not fully known. Baclofen is capable of inhibiting both monosynaptic and polysynaptic reflexes at the spinal level, possibly by hyperpolarization of afferent terminals, although actions at supraspinal sites may also occur and contribute to its clinical effect. Although baclofen is an analog of the putative inhibitory neurotransmitter gamma-aminobutyric acid (GABA), there is no conclusive evidence that actions on GABA systems are involved in the production of its clinical effects. In studies with animals, baclofen has been shown to have general CNS-depressant properties as indicated by the production of sedation with tolerance, somnolence, ataxia, and respiratory and cardiovascular depression.

➤*Pharmacokinetics:* Baclofen is rapidly and extensively absorbed and eliminated. Absorption may be dose-dependent, being reduced with increasing doses. Baclofen is excreted primarily by the kidney in unchanged form and there is relatively large intersubject variation in absorption and/or elimination.

Contraindications

Hypersensitivity to baclofen.

Warnings

➤*Abrupt drug withdrawal:* Hallucinations and seizures have occurred on abrupt withdrawal of baclofen. Therefore, except for serious adverse reactions, the dose should be reduced slowly when the drug is discontinued.

➤*Stroke:* Baclofen has not significantly benefited patients with stroke. These patients have also shown poor tolerability to the drug.

➤*Renal function impairment:* Because baclofen is primarily excreted unchanged through the kidneys, it should be given with caution, and it may be necessary to reduce the dosage.

➤*Pregnancy: Category C.* Baclofen has been shown to increase the incidence of omphaloceles (ventral hernias) in fetuses of rats given ≈ 13 times the maximum dose recommended for human use, at a dose that caused significant reductions in food intake and weight gain in dams. This abnormality was not seen in mice or rabbits. There was also an increased incidence of incomplete sternebral ossification in fetuses of rats given ≈ 13 times the maximum recommended human dose, and an increased incidence of unossified phalangeal nuclei of forelimbs and hindlimbs in fetuses of rabbits given ≈ 7 times the maximum recommended human dose. In mice, no teratogenic effects were observed, although reductions in mean fetal weight with consequent delays in skeletal ossification were present when dams were given 17 or 34 times the human daily dose. There are no studies in pregnant women. Baclofen should be used during pregnancy only if the benefit clearly justifies the potential risk to the fetus.

➤*Lactation:* It is not known whether this drug is excreted in human milk. As a general rule, nursing should not be undertaken while a patient is on a drug since many drugs are excreted in human milk.

➤*Children:* Safety and efficacy in children younger than 12 years of age have not been established.

Precautions

➤*Epilepsy:* In patients with epilepsy, the clinical state and electroencephalogram should be monitored at regular intervals, since deterioration in seizure control and EEG have been reported occasionally in patients taking baclofen.

➤*Spasticity:* Baclofen should be used with caution where spasticity is utilized to sustain upright posture and balance in locomotion or whenever spasticity is utilized to obtain increased function.

➤*Ovarian cysts:* Ovarian cysts have been found by palpation in ≈ 4% of the multiple sclerosis patients that were treated with baclofen for up to 1 year. In most cases these cysts disappeared spontaneously while patients continued to receive the drug. Ovarian cysts are estimated to occur spontaneously in ≈ 1% to 5% of the healthy female population.

➤*Hazardous tasks:* Because of the possibility of sedation, patients should be cautioned regarding the operation of automobiles or other dangerous machinery, and activities made hazardous by decreased alertness. Patients should also be cautioned that the CNS effects of baclofen may be additive to those of alcohol and other CNS depressants.

Adverse Reactions

The most common is transient drowsiness (10% to 63%). In one controlled study of 175 patients, transient drowsiness was observed in 63% of those receiving baclofen compared to 36% of those in the placebo group. Other common adverse reactions are dizziness (5% to 15%), weakness (5% to 15%), and fatigue (2% to 4%). Others reported include the following:

➤*Cardiovascular:* Hypotension (0% to 9%). Rare instances of dyspnea, palpitation, chest pain, and syncope.

➤*GI:* Nausea (4% to 12%), constipation (2% to 6%); and, rarely, dry mouth, anorexia, taste disorder, abdominal pain, vomiting, diarrhea, and positive test for occult blood in stool.

➤*GU:* Urinary frequency (2% to 6%); and, rarely, enuresis, urinary retention, dysuria, impotence, inability to ejaculate, nocturia, and hematuria.

➤*Lab test abnormalities:* Increased AST, elevated alkaline phosphatase, and elevation of blood sugar.

➤*Psychiatric:* Confusion (1% to 11%), headache (4% to 8%), insomnia (2% to 7%); and, rarely, euphoria, excitement, depression, hallucinations, paresthesia, muscle pain, tinnitus, slurred speech, coordination disorder, tremor, rigidity, dystonia, ataxia, blurred vision, nystagmus, strabismus, miosis, mydriasis, diplopia, dysarthria, and epileptic seizure.

➤*Miscellaneous:* Instances of rash, pruritus, ankle edema, excessive perspiration, weight gain, and nasal congestion. Some of the CNS and genitourinary symptoms may be related to the underlying disease rather than to drug therapy.

BACLOFEN — ORAL

Overdosage

➤*Symptoms:* Symptoms of overdosage include vomiting, muscular hypotonia, drowsiness, accommodation disorders, coma, respiratory depression, and seizures.

➤*Treatment:* In the alert patient, empty the stomach promptly by induced emesis followed by lavage. In the obtunded patient, secure the airway with a cuffed endotracheal tube before beginning lavage (do not induce emesis). Maintain adequate respiratory exchange, do not use respiratory stimulants.

BACLOFEN — INTRATHECAL INJECTION

WARNING

Abrupt discontinuation of intrathecal baclofen, regardless of the cause, has resulted in sequelae that include high fever, altered mental status, exaggerated rebound spasticity, and muscle rigidity, which in rare cases has advanced to rhabdomyolysis, multiple organ-system failure, and death.

Prevention of abrupt discontinuation of intrathecal baclofen requires careful attention to programming and monitoring of the infusion system, refill scheduling and procedures, and pump alarms. Advise patients and caregivers of the importance of keeping scheduled refill visits and educate them on the early symptoms of baclofen withdrawal. Give special attention to patients at apparent risk (eg, spinal cord injuries at T-6 or above, communication difficulties, history of withdrawal symptoms from oral or intrathecal baclofen). Consult the technical manual of the implantable infusion system for additional postimplant clinician and patient information (see Warnings).

Indications

➤*Severe spasticity:* For use in the management of severe spasticity. Patients should first respond to a screening dose of intrathecal baclofen prior to consideration for long-term infusion via an implantable pump. For spasticity of spinal cord origin, chronic infusion of baclofen intrathecal injection via an implantable pump should be reserved for patients unresponsive to oral baclofen therapy, or those who experience intolerable CNS side effects at effective doses. Patients with spasticity due to traumatic brain injury should wait at least 1 year after the injury before consideration of long-term intrathecal baclofen therapy. Baclofen intrathecal injection is intended for use by the intrathecal route in single bolus test doses (via spinal catheter or lumbar puncture) and, for chronic use, only in implantable pumps approved by the FDA specifically for the administration of baclofen intrathecal injection into the intrathecal space.

Baclofen intrathecal injection therapy may be considered an alternative to destructive neurosurgical procedures. Prior to implantation of a device for chronic intrathecal infusion of baclofen intrathecal, patients must show a response to it in a screening trial.

➤*Unlabeled uses:* To reduce spasticity in patients with cerebral palsy; generalized dystonia associated with cerebral palsy.

Administration and Dosage

➤*Approved by the FDA:* June 17, 1992.

➤*Screening phase:* Prior to pump implantation and initiation of chronic infusion of baclofen intrathecal injection, patients must demonstrate a positive clinical response to a baclofen intrathecal injection bolus dose administered intrathecally in a screening trial. The screening trial employs baclofen intrathecal injection at a concentration of 50 mcg/mL. A 1 mL ampule (50 mcg/mL) is available for use in the screening trial. The screening procedure is as follows. An initial bolus containing 50 mcg in a volume of 1 mL is administered into the intrathecal space by barbotage over a period of not less than 1 minute. The patient is observed over the ensuing 4 to 8 hours. A positive response consists of a significant decrease in muscle tone and/or frequency and/or severity of spasms. If the initial response is less than desired, a second bolus injection may be administered 24 hours after the first. The second screening bolus dose consists of 75 mcg in 1.5 mL. Again, the patient should be observed for an interval of 4 to 8 hours. If the response is still inadequate, a final bolus screening dose of 100 mcg in 2 mL may be administered 24 hours later.

Patients who do not respond to a 100 mcg intrathecal bolus should not be considered candidates for an implanted pump for chronic infusion.

Children – The starting screening dose for children is the same as in adult patients (ie, 50 mcg). However, for very small patients, a screening dose of 25 mcg may be tried first.

Postimplant dose titration period – To determine the initial daily dose of baclofen intrathecal following implant, the screening dose that gave a positive effect should be doubled and administered over a 24-hour period, unless the efficacy of the bolus dose was maintained for more than 8 hours, in which case the starting daily dose should be the screening dose delivered over a 24-hour period. No dose increases should be given in the first 24 hours (ie, until the steady state is achieved).

Adult patients with spasticity of spinal cord origin: After the first 24 hours, for adult patients, the daily dosage should be increased slowly by 10% to 30% increments and only once every 24 hours, until the desired clinical effect is achieved.

Adult patients with spasticity of cerebral origin: After the first 24 hours, the daily dose should be increased slowly by 5% to 15% only once every 24 hours, until the desired clinical effect is achieved.

Children: After the first 24 hours, the daily dose should be increased slowly by 5% to 15% only once every 24 hours, until the desired clinical effect is achieved.

➤*Maintenance therapy:*

Spasticity of spinal cord origin patients – During periodic refills of the pump, the daily dose may be increased by 10% to 40%, but not more than 40%, to maintain adequate symptom control. The daily dose may be reduced by 10% to 20% if patients experience side effects. Most patients require gradual increases in dose over time to maintain optimal response during chronic therapy. A sudden large requirement for dose escalation suggests a catheter complication (ie, catheter kink or dislodgment).

Maintenance dosage for long-term continuous infusion of baclofen intrathecal has ranged from 12 mcg/day to 2003 mcg/day, with most patients adequately maintained on 300 mcg to 800 mcg/day. There is limited experience with daily doses more than 1,000 mcg/day. Determination of the optimal baclofen intrathecal dose requires individual titration. The lowest dose with an optimal response should be used.

Spasticity of cerebral origin patients – During periodic refills of the pump, the daily dose may be increased by 5% to 20%, but not more than 20%, to maintain adequate symptom control. The daily dose may be reduced by 10% to 20% if patients experience side effects. Many patients require gradual increases in dose over time to maintain optimal response during chronic therapy. A sudden large requirement for dose escalation suggests a catheter complication (ie, catheter kink or dislodgment).

Maintenance dosage for long-term continuous infusion of baclofen intrathecal has ranged from 22 mcg/day to 1400 mcg/day, with most patients adequately maintained on 90 mcg to 703 mcg/day. In clinical trials, only 3 of 150 patients required daily doses more than 1,000 mcg/day.

Children – Use same dosing recommendations for patients with spasticity of cerebral origin. Children younger than 12 years of age seemed to require a lower daily dose in clinical trials. Average daily dose for patients younger than 12 years of age was 274 mcg/day, with a range of 24 to 1199 mcg/day. Dosage requirement for children older than 12 years of age does not seem to be different from that of adult patients. Determination of the optimal baclofen intrathecal dose requires individual titration. The lowest dose with an optimal response should be used.

Potential need for dose adjustments in chronic use – During long-term treatment, ≈ 5% (28/627) of patients become refractory to increasing doses. There is not sufficient experience to make firm recommendations for tolerance treatment; however, this "tolerance" has been treated on occasion, in hospital, by a "drug holiday" consisting of the gradual reduction of baclofen intrathecal over a 2- to 4-week period and switching to alternative methods of spasticity management. After the "drug holiday," baclofen intrathecal may be restarted at the initial continuous infusion dose.

➤*Storage/Stability:*

Preparation instructions –

Screening: Use the 1 mL screening ampule only (50 mcg/mL) for bolus injection into the subarachnoid space. For a 50 mcg bolus dose, use 1 mL of the screening ampule. Use 1.5 mL of 50 mcg/mL baclofen intrathecal for a 75 mcg bolus dose. For the maximum screening dose of 100 mcg, use 2 mL of 50 mcg/mL baclofen intrathecal (2 screening ampules).

Maintenance: For patients who require concentrations other than 500 mcg/mL or 2000 mcg/mL, baclofen intrathecal must be diluted.

Baclofen intrathecal must be diluted with sterile preservative free Sodium Chloride for Injection, USP.

Delivery regimen – Baclofen intrathecal is most often administered in a continuous infusion mode immediately following implant. For those patients implanted with programmable pumps who have achieved relatively satisfactory control on continuous infusion, further benefit may be attained using more complex schedules of baclofen intrathecal delivery. For example, patients who have increased spasms at night may require a 20% increase in their hourly infusion rate. Changes in flow rate should be programmed to start 2 hours before the time of desired clinical effect.

Does not require refrigeration. Do not store above 30°C (86°F). Do not freeze. Do not heat sterilize.

Actions

➤*Pharmacology:* The precise mechanism of action of baclofen as a muscle relaxant and antispasticity agent is not fully understood. Baclofen inhibits both monosynaptic and polysynaptic reflexes at the spinal level, possibly by decreasing excitatory neurotransmitter release from primary afferent terminals, although actions at supraspinal sites may also occur and contribute to its clinical effect. Baclofen is a structural analog of the inhibitory neurotransmitter gamma-aminobutyric acid (GABA), and may exert its effects by stimulation of the $GABA^B$ receptor subtype.

Baclofen intrathecal injection when introduced directly into the intrathecal space permits effective CSF concentrations to be achieved with resultant plasma concentrations 100 times less than those occurring with oral administration.

BACLOFEN — INTRATHECAL INJECTION

Pharmacodynamics –

Intrathecal bolus:

• *Adults* – The onset of action is generally 30 minutes to 1 hour after an intrathecal bolus. Peak spasmolytic effect is seen at ≈ 4 hours after dosing and effects may last 4 to 8 hours. Onset, peak response, and duration of action may vary with individual patients depending on the dose and severity of symptoms.

• *Children* – The onset, peak response and duration of action is similar to those seen in adult patients.

Continuous infusion: Baclofen intrathecal injection's antispastic action is first seen at 6 to 8 hours after initiation of continuous infusion. Maximum activity is observed in 24 to 48 hours.

➤*Pharmacokinetics:* The pharmacokinetics of CSF clearance of baclofen intrathecal injection calculated from intrathecal bolus or continuous infusion studies approximates CSF turnover, suggesting elimination is by bulk-flow removal of CSF.

Intrathecal bolus – After a bolus lumbar injection of 50 or 100 mcg baclofen intrathecal injection in 7 patients, the average CSF elimination half-life was 1.51 hours over the first 4 hours and the average CSF clearance was ≈ 30 mL/hr.

Continuous infusion – The mean CSF clearance for baclofen intrathecal injection was ≈ 30 mL/hr in a study involving 10 patients on continuous intrathecal infusion.

Contraindications

Hypersensitivity to baclofen; not recommended for IV, IM, SC, or epidural administration.

Warnings

➤*Administration:* Baclofen intrathecal injection is for use in single bolus intrathecal injections (via a catheter placed in the lumbar intrathecal space or injection by lumbar puncture) and in implantable pumps approved by the FDA specifically for the intrathecal administration of baclofen. Because of the possibility of potentially life-threatening CNS depression, cardiovascular collapse, and/or respiratory failure, physicians must be adequately trained and educated in chronic intrathecal infusion therapy.

The pump system should not be implanted until the patient's response to bolus baclofen intrathecal injection is adequately evaluated. Evaluation (consisting of a screening procedure) requires that baclofen intrathecal injection be administered into the intrathecal space via a catheter or lumbar puncture. Because of the risks associated with the screening procedure and the adjustment of dosage following pump implantation, these phases must be conducted in a medically supervised and adequately equipped environment following the instructions outlined in Administration and Dosage.

Resuscitative equipment should be available. Following surgical implantation of the pump, particularly during the initial phases of pump use, the patient should be monitored closely until it is certain that the patient's response to the infusion is acceptable and reasonably stable.

Extreme caution must be used when filling an FDA-approved implantable pump. Such pumps should only be refilled through the reservoir refill septum. However, some pumps are also equipped with a catheter access port that allows direct access to the intrathecal catheter. Direct injection into this catheter access port may cause a life-threatening overdose.

➤*Withdrawal:* Baclofen withdrawal has been identified during postapproval use of baclofen intrathecal injection. Because this reaction is reported simultaneously from a population of uncertain size, it is not possible to reliably estimate the frequency.

Early symptoms of baclofen withdrawal may include pruritus, hypotension, and paresthesias.

Abrupt withdrawal of intrathecal baclofen, regardless of the cause, has, in rare cases, resulted in a life-threatening syndrome that included high fever, altered mental status, exaggerated rebound spasticity, and muscle rigidity that progressed to rhabdomyolysis, multiple organ-system failure, and death.

All patients receiving intrathecal baclofen therapy are potentially at risk. Some clinical characteristics of the advanced intrathecal baclofen withdrawal syndrome may resemble autonomic dysreflexia, or infection (sepsis), malignant hyperthermia, neuroleptic-malignant syndrome, and other conditions associated with a hypermetabolic state or widespread rhabdomyolysis. A rapid and accurate diagnosis is important in an emergency room or intensive care setting before initiating treatment in order to prevent the potentially life-threatening central nervous and systemic effects of intrathecal baclofen withdrawal. The suggested treatment for intrathecal baclofen withdrawal is the restoration of intrathecal baclofen at or near the same dosage as before therapy was interrupted. However, if restoration of intrathecal delivery is delayed, treatment with GABA-ergic agonist drugs, such as oral or enteral baclofen, or oral, enteral, or IV benzodiazepines may prevent potentially fatal sequelae. Because of the phenomenon of $GABA_B$ receptor down-regulation, oral or enteral baclofen alone should not be relied upon to halt the progression of the intrathecal baclofen withdrawal syndrome.

Careful monitoring of infusion pump function and inspection of the catheter for occlusion or dislodgment can help reduce the risk of abrupt withdrawal of intrathecal baclofen.

➤*Hallucinations:* Hallucinations have occurred after abrupt withdrawal of baclofen intrathecal injection.

➤*Seizures:* Seizures have been reported during overdose and with withdrawal from baclofen intrathecal injection and in patients maintained on therapeutic doses of baclofen intrathecal injection.

➤*Fatalities:*

Spasticity of spinal cord origin – There were 16 deaths reported among the 576 US patients treated with baclofen intrathecal injection in pre- and postmarketing studies evaluated as of December 1992. Because these patients were treated under uncontrolled clinical settings, it is impossible to determine definitively what role, if any, baclofen intrathecal injection played in their deaths.

Spasticity of cerebral origin – There were 3 deaths occurring among the 211 patients treated with baclofen intrathecal in premarketing studies as of March 1996. These deaths were not attributed to the therapy.

➤*Renal function impairment:* Because baclofen is primarily excreted unchanged by the kidneys, it should be given with caution in patients with impaired renal function and it may be necessary to reduce the dosage.

➤*Pregnancy: Category C.* Baclofen given orally has been shown to increase the incidence of omphaloceles (ventral hernias) in fetuses of rats given ≈ 13 times on a mg/kg basis, or 3 times on a mg/m^2 basis, the maximum oral dose recommended for human use; this dose also caused reductions in food intake and weight gain in the dams.

This abnormality was not seen in mice or rabbits. There are no adequate and well-controlled studies in pregnant women. Baclofen should be used during pregnancy only if the potential benefit justifies the potential risk to the fetus.

➤*Lactation:* In mothers treated with oral baclofen in therapeutic doses, the active substance passes into the breast milk. It is not known whether detectable levels of drug are present in breast milk of nursing mothers receiving baclofen intrathecal injection. As a general rule, nursing should be undertaken while a patient is receiving baclofen intrathecal injection only if the potential benefit justifies the potential risks to the infant.

Precautions

➤*Monitoring:* On each occasion that the dosing rate of the pump or the concentration of baclofen intrathecal injection in the reservoir is adjusted, close medical monitoring is required until it is certain that the patient's response to the infusion is acceptable and reasonably stable.

➤*Screening:* Patients should be infection-free prior to the screening trial with baclofen intrathecal injection because the presence of a systemic infection may interfere with an assessment of the patient's response to bolus baclofen intrathecal injection.

➤*Pump implantation:* Patients should be infection-free prior to pump implantation because the presence of infection may increase the risk of surgical complications. Moreover, a systemic infection may complicate dosing.

➤*Pump dose adjustment and titration:* In most patients, it will be necessary to increase the dose gradually over time to maintain effectiveness; a sudden requirement for substantial dose escalation typically indicates a catheter complication (ie, catheter kink, dislodgment).

➤*Additional considerations pertaining to dosage adjustment:* It may be important to titrate the dose to maintain some degree of muscle tone and allow occasional spasms to:

1.) Help support circulatory function;
2.) possibly prevent the formation of deep vein thrombosis;
3.) optimize activities of daily living and ease of care.

Except in overdose related emergencies, the dose of baclofen intrathecal injection should ordinarily be reduced slowly if the drug is discontinued for any reason.

An attempt should be made to discontinue concomitant oral antispasticity medication to avoid possible overdose or adverse drug interactions, either prior to screening or following implant and initiation of chronic baclofen intrathecal injection infusion. Reduction and discontinuation of oral antispasmotics should be done slowly and with careful monitoring by the physician. Abrupt reduction or discontinuation of concomitant antispastics should be avoided.

➤*Need for spasticity:* Careful dose titration of baclofen intrathecal injection is needed when spasticity is necessary to sustain upright posture and balance in locomotion or whenever spasticity is used to obtain optimal function and care.

➤*Psychotic disorders:* Patients suffering from psychotic disorders, schizophrenia, or confusional states should be treated cautiously with baclofen intrathecal injection and kept under careful surveillance, because exacerbations of these conditions have been observed with oral administration.

➤*Ovarian cysts:* A dose-related increase in incidence of ovarian cysts was observed in female rats treated chronically with oral baclofen. Ovarian cysts have been found by palpation in ≈ 4% of the multiple sclerosis patients who were treated with oral baclofen for up to 1 year. In most cases these cysts disappeared spontaneously while patients continued to receive the drug. Ovarian cysts are estimated to occur spontaneously in ≈ 1% to 5% of the healthy female population.

➤*Autonomic dysreflexia:* Baclofen intrathecal injection should be used with caution in patients with a history of autonomic dysreflexia. The presence of nociceptive stimuli or abrupt withdrawal of baclofen intrathecal may cause an autonomic dysreflexic episode.

➤*Hazardous tasks:* Drowsiness has been reported in patients on baclofen intrathecal injection. Patients should be cautioned regarding the operation of automobiles or other dangerous machinery, and activities made hazardous by decreased alertness.

BACLOFEN — INTRATHECAL INJECTION

Drug Interactions

➤*Alcohol and other CNS depressants:* Patients should also be cautioned that the CNS depressant effects of baclofen intrathecal injection may be additive to those of alcohol and other CNS depressants.

Adverse Reactions

➤*Spasticity of spinal cord origin:*

Commonly observed – In pre- and postmarketing clinical trials, the most commonly observed adverse events associated with use of baclofen intrathecal injection that were not seen at an equivalent incidence among placebo-treated patients were somnolence, dizziness, nausea, hypotension, headache, convulsions, and hypotonia.

Discontinuation of treatment – Eight of 474 patients with spasticity of spinal cord origin receiving long-term infusion of baclofen intrathecal injection in pre- and postmarketing clinical studies in the US discontinued treatment due to adverse events. These include pump pocket infections (3), meningitis (2), wound dehiscence (1), gynecological fibroids (1), and pump overpressurization (1) with unknown, if any, sequela. Eleven patients who developed coma secondary to overdose had their treatment temporarily suspended, but all were subsequently restarted and were not, therefore, considered to be true discontinuations.

Fatalities – See Warnings.

➤*Spasticity of spinal cord origin:*

Incidence in controlled trials – Experience with baclofen intrathecal injection obtained in parallel, placebo-controlled, randomized studies provides only a limited basis for estimating the incidence of adverse events because the studies were of very brief duration (up to 3 days of infusion) and involved only a total of 63 patients. The following events occurred among the 31 patients receiving baclofen intrathecal injection in two randomized, placebo-controlled trials: Hypotension (2), dizziness (2), headache (2), dyspnea (1). No adverse events were reported among the 32 patients receiving placebo in these studies.

Adverse events associated with the use of baclofen intrathecal injection reflect experience gained with 576 patients followed prospectively in the US. They received baclofen intrathecal injection for periods of 1 day (screening) (n = 576) to over 8 years (maintenance) (n = 10). The usual screening bolus dose administered prior to pump implantation in these studies was typically 50 mcg. The maintenance dose ranged from 12 to 2003 mcg/day. Because of the open, uncontrolled nature of the experience, a causal linkage between events observed and the administration of baclofen intrathecal injection cannot be reliably assessed in many cases and many of the adverse events reported are known to occur in association with the underlying conditions being treated. Nonetheless, many of the more commonly reported reactions (eg, hypotonia, somnolence, dizziness, paresthesia, nausea/vomiting, headache) appear clearly drug-related.

Adverse experiences reported during all US studies (both controlled and uncontrolled) are shown in the following table. Eight of 474 patients who received chronic infusion via implanted pumps had adverse experiences, which led to a discontinuation of long-term treatment in the pre- and postmarketing studies.

Baclofen Intrathecal Adverse Reactions (≥ 1%)

Adverse reaction	Screening[a] (n = 576)*	Titration[b] (n = 474)*	Maintenance[c] (n = 430)*
Hypotonia	5.4%	13.5%	25.3%
Somnolence	5.7%	5.9%	20.9%
Dizziness	1.7%	1.9%	7.9%
Paresthesia	2.4%	2.1%	6.7%
Nausea and vomiting	1.6%	2.3%	5.6%
Headache	1.6%	2.5%	5.1%
Constipation	0.2%	1.5%	5.1%
Convulsion	0.5%	1.3%	4.7%
Urinary retention	0.7%	1.7%	1.9%
Dry mouth	0.2%	0.4%	3.3%
Accidental injury	0%	0.2%	3.5%
Asthenia	0.7%	1.3%	1.4%
Confusion	0.5%	0.6%	2.3%
Death	0.2%	0.4%	3%
Pain	0%	0.6%	3%
Speech disorder	0%	0.2%	3.5%
Hypotension	1%	0.2%	1.9%
Amblyopia	0.5%	0.2%	2.3%
Diarrhea	0%	0.8%	2.3%
Hypoventilation	0.2%	0.8%	2.1%
Coma	0%	1.5%	0.9%
Impotence	0.2%	0.4%	1.6%
Peripheral edema	0%	0%	2.3%
Urinary incontinence	0%	0.8%	1.4%
Insomnia	0%	0.4%	1.6%
Anxiety	0.2%	0.4%	0.9%
Depression	0%	0%	1.6%
Dyspnea	0.3%	0%	1.2%
Fever	0.5%	0.2%	0.7%
Pneumonia	0.2%	0.2%	1.2%
Urinary frequency	0%	0.6%	0.9%
Urticaria	0.2%	0.2%	1.2%
Anorexia	0%	0.4%	0.9%
Diplopia	0%	0.4%	0.9%
Dysautonomia	0.2%	0.2%	0.9%
Hallucinations	0.3%	0.4%	0.5%
Hypertension	0.2%	0.6%	0.5%

[a] Following administration of test bolus.
[b] 2-month period following implant.
[c] Beyond 2 months following implant.
* n = total number of patients entering each period.
** % = % of patients evaluated.

In addition to the more common (≥ 1%) adverse events reported in the prospectively followed 576 domestic patients in pre- and postmarketing studies, experience from an additional 194 patients exposed to baclofen intrathecal injection from foreign studies has been reported. The following adverse events, not described in the table, and arranged in decreasing order of frequency, and classified by body system, were reported:

Cardiovascular – Postural hypotension; bradycardia; palpitations; syncope; arrhythmia ventricular; deep thrombophlebitis; pallor; tachycardia.

CNS – Abnormal gait; thinking abnormal; tremor; amnesia; twitching; vasodilatation; cerebrovascular accident; nystagmus; personality disorder; psychotic depression; cerebral ischemia; emotional lability; euphoria; hypertonia; ileus; drug dependence; incoordination; paranoid reaction; ptosis.

Dermatologic – Alopecia; sweating.

GI – Flatulence; dysphagia; dyspepsia; gastroenteritis.

GU – Hematuria; kidney failure.

Hematologic/Lymphatic – Anemia.

Metabolic/Nutritional – Weight loss; albuminuria; dehydration; hyperglycemia.

Respiratory – Respiratory disorder; aspiration pneumonia; hyperventilation; pulmonary embolus; rhinitis.

Special senses – Abnormal vision; abnormality of accommodation; photophobia; taste loss; tinnitus.

Miscellaneous – Suicide; lack of drug effect; abdominal pain; hypothermia; neck rigidity; chest pain; chills; face edema; flu syndrome; overdose.

➤*Spasticity of cerebral origin:*

Commonly observed – In premarketing clinical trials, the most commonly observed adverse events associated with use of baclofen intrathecal injection that were not seen at an equivalent incidence among placebo-treated patients included agitation, constipation, somnolence, leukocytosis, chills, urinary retention, and hypotonia.

Discontinuation of treatment – Nine of 211 patients receiving baclofen intrathecal injection in premarketing clinical studies in the US discontinued long-term infusion due to adverse events associated with intrathecal therapy.

The nine adverse events leading to discontinuation were infection (3), CSF leaks (2), meningitis (2), drainage (1), and unmanageable trunk control (1).

Fatalities – See Warnings for more information.

Incidence in controlled trials – Experience with baclofen intrathecal injection obtained in parallel, placebo-controlled, randomized studies provides only a limited basis for estimating the incidence of adverse events because the studies involved a total of 62 patients exposed to a single 50 mcg intrathecal bolus. The following events occurred among the 62 patients receiving baclofen intrathecal injection in 2 randomized, placebo-controlled trials involving cerebral palsy and head injury patients, respectively: Agitation, constipation, somnolence, leukocytosis, nausea, vomiting, nystagmus, chills, urinary retention, and hypotonia.

Events observed during the premarketing evaluation – Adverse events associated with the use of baclofen intrathecal injection reflect experience gained with a total of 211 US patients with spasticity of cerebral origin, of whom 112 were children (younger than 16 years of age at enrollment). They received baclofen intrathecal injection for periods of one day (screening) (n = 211) to 84 months (maintenance) (n = 1). The usual screening bolus dose administered prior to pump implantation in these studies was 50 to 75 mcg. The maintenance dose ranged from 22 to 1400 mcg/day. Doses used in this patient population for long-term infusion are generally lower than those required for patients with spasticity of spinal cord origin.

BACLOFEN — INTRATHECAL INJECTION

Because of the open, uncontrolled nature of the experience, a causal linkage between events observed and the administration of baclofen intrathecal injection cannot be reliably assessed in many cases. Nonetheless, many of the more commonly reported reactions (eg, somnolence, dizziness, headache, nausea, hypotension, hypotonia, coma) appear clearly drug-related.

The most frequent (≥ 1%) adverse events reported during all clinical trials are shown in the following table. Nine patients discontinued long-term treatment due to adverse events.

Baclofen Intrathecal Adverse Reactions (≥ 1%)

Adverse event	Screening[a] (n = 211)*	Titration[b] (n = 153)*	Maintenance[c] (n = 150)*
Hypotonia	2.4%	14.4%	34.7%
Somnolence	7.6%	10.5%	18.7%
Headache	6.6%	7.8%	10.7%
Nausea and vomiting	6.6%	10.5%	4%
Vomiting	6.2%	8.5%	4%
Urinary retention	0.9%	6.5%	8%
Convulsion	0.9%	3.3%	10%
Dizziness	2.4%	2.6%	8%
Nausea	1.4%	3.3%	7.3%
Hypoventilation	1.4%	1.3%	4%
Hypertonia	0%	0.7%	6%
Paresthesia	1.9%	0.7%	3.3%
Hypotension	1.9%	0.7%	2%
Increased salivation	0%	2.6%	2.7%
Back pain	0.9%	0.7%	2%
Constipation	0.5%	1.3%	2%
Pain	0%	0%	4%
Pruritus	0%	0%	4%
Diarrhea	0.5%	0.7%	2%
Peripheral edema	0%	0%	3.3%
Thinking abnormal	0.5%	1.3%	0.7%
Agitation	0.5%	0%	1.3%
Asthenia	0%	0%	2%
Chills	0.5%	0%	1.3%
Coma	0.5%	0%	1.3%
Dry mouth	0.5%	0%	1.3%
Pneumonia	0%	0%	2%
Speech disorder	0.5%	0.7%	0.7%
Tremor	0.5%	0%	1.3%
Urinary incontinence	0%	0%	2%
Urination impaired	0%	0%	2%

[a] Following administration of test bolus.
[b] 2-month period following implant.
[c] Beyond 2 months following implant.
* n = total number of patients entering each period. 211 patients received drug; (1 of 212) received placebo only.

The more common (≥ 1%) adverse events reported in the prospectively followed 211 patients exposed to baclofen intrathecal injection have been reported. In the total cohort, the following adverse events, not described in the table, and arranged in decreasing order of frequency, and classified by body system, were reported:

Cardiovascular – Bradycardia.

CNS – Akathisia; ataxia; confusion; depression; opisthotonos; amnesia; anxiety; hallucinations; hysteria; insomnia; nystagmus; personality disorder; reflexes decreased; vasodilatation.

Dermatologic – Rash; sweating; alopecia; contact dermatitis; skin ulcer.

GI – Dysphagia; fecal incontinence; GI hemorrhage; tongue disorder.

GU – Abnormal ejaculation; kidney calculus; oliguria; vaginitis.

Hematologic/Lymphatic – Leukocytosis; petechial rash.

Respiratory – Apnea; dyspnea; hyperventilation.

Special senses – Abnormality of accommodation.

Miscellaneous – Death; fever; abdominal pain; carcinoma; malaise; hypothermia.

Overdosage

Signs of overdose may appear suddenly or insidiously. Acute massive overdose may present as coma. Less sudden and/or less severe forms of overdose may present with signs of drowsiness, lightheadedness, dizziness, somnolence, respiratory depression, seizures, rostral progression of hypotonia, and loss of consciousness progressing to coma. Should overdose appear likely, the patient should be taken immediately to a hospital for assessment and emptying of the pump reservoir. In cases reported to date, overdose has generally been related to pump malfunction or dosing error.

It is mandatory that the patient, all patient care givers, and the physicians responsible for the patient receive adequate information regarding the risks of this mode of treatment. All medical personnel and care givers should be instructed in 1) the signs and symptoms of overdose, 2) procedures to be followed in the event of overdose and 3) proper home care of the pump and insertion site.

➤*Symptoms:* Drowsiness, lightheadedness, dizziness, somnolence, respiratory depression, seizures, rostral progression of hypotonia, and loss of consciousness progressing to coma of up to 72 hours of duration. In most cases reported, coma was reversible without sequelae after drug was discontinued.

Symptoms of baclofen intrathecal injection overdose were reported in a sensitive adult patient after receiving a 25 mcg intrathecal bolus.

➤*Treatment:* There is no specific antidote for treating overdoses of baclofen intrathecal injection; however, the following steps should ordinarily be undertaken: Residual baclofen intrathecal injection solution should be removed from the pump as soon as possible; patients with respiratory depression should be intubated if necessary, until the drug is eliminated.

Anecdotal reports suggest that IV physostigmine may reverse central side effects, notably drowsiness and respiratory depression. Caution in administering physostigmine is advised, however, because its use has been associated with the induction of seizures, bradycardia, cardiac conduction disturbances.

Adults – Administer 2 mg of physostigmine intramuscularly or intravenously at a slow controlled rate of no more than 1 mg/min. Dosage may be repeated if life-threatening signs, such as arrhythmia, convulsions, or coma.

Children – Administer 0.02 mg/kg physostigmine intramuscularly or intravenously, do not give more than 0.5 mg/min. The dosage may be repeated at 5 to 10 minute intervals until a therapeutic effect is obtained or a maximum dose of 2 mg is attained.

Physostigmine may not be effective in reversing large overdoses and patients may need to be maintained with respiratory support.

If lumbar puncture is not contraindicated, consideration should be given to withdrawing 30 to 40 mL of CSF to reduce CSF baclofen concentration.

CARISOPRODOL

Rx	**Carisoprodol** (Various, eg, Major, Mutual, Parmed, Schein)	**Tablets:** 350 mg	In 30s, 60s, 100s, 500s, 1000s, and UD 100s.
Rx	**Soma** (Wallace)		(Soma 37 Wallace 2001). White. In 100s, 500s, and UD 500s.

CARISOPRODOL — ORAL

Indications

➤*Musculoskeletal conditions:* As an adjunct to rest, physical therapy, and other measures for the relief of discomfort associated with acute, painful musculoskeletal conditions.

Administration and Dosage

The usual adult dosage is one 350 mg tablet, 3 times daily and at bedtime. Use in patients less than 12 years of age is not recommended.

➤*Storage/Stability:* Store at controlled room temperature 15° to 30°C (59° to 86°F). Dispense in a tight, light-resistant, well-closed container.

Actions

➤*Pharmacology:* The mode of action of this drug has not been clearly identified, but may be related to its sedative properties. Carisoprodol does not directly relax tense skeletal muscles in man. Carisoprodol produces muscle relaxation in animals by blocking interneuronal activity in the descending reticular formation and spinal cord.

➤*Pharmacokinetics:* The onset of action is rapid (30 minutes) and effects last 4 to 6 hours.

Contraindications

Acute intermittent porphyria as well as allergic or idiosyncratic reactions to carisoprodol or related compounds such as meprobamate, mebutamate or tybamate.

Warnings

➤*Hypersensitivity reactions:* On very rare occasions, the first dose of carisoprodol has been followed by idiosyncratic symptoms appearing within minutes or hours. Symptoms reported include extreme weakness, transient quadriplegia, dizziness, ataxia, temporary loss of vision, diplopia, mydriasis, dysarthria, agitation, euphoria, confusion, and disorientation. Symptoms usually subside over the course of the next several hours. Supportive and symptomatic therapy, including hospitalization, may be necessary.

CARISOPRODOL — ORAL

➤*Renal/Hepatic function impairment:* Carisoprodol is metabolized in the liver and excreted by the kidney. To avoid excess accumulation, caution should be exercised in administration to patients with compromised liver or kidney function.

➤*Pregnancy: Category C.* Safe usage of this drug in pregnancy has not been established. Therefore, use of this drug in pregnancy or in women of childbearing potential requires that the potential benefits of the drug be weighed against the potential hazards to mother and child.

➤*Lactation:* Safe usage of this drug in lactation has not been established. Therefore, use of this drug in nursing mothers requires that the potential benefits of the drug be weighed against the potential hazards to mother and child.

Carisoprodol is present in breast milk of lactating mothers at concentrations 2 to 4 times that of maternal plasma. This factor should be taken into account when use of the drug is contemplated in breastfeeding patients.

➤*Children:* Because of limited clinical experience, carisoprodol is not recommended for use in patients less than 12 years of age.

Precautions

➤*Drug abuse and dependence:* In dogs, no withdrawal symptoms occurred after abrupt cessation of carisoprodol from dosages as high as 1 g/kg/day. In a study in man, abrupt cessation of 100 mg/kg/day (about 5 times the recommended daily adult dosage) was followed in some subjects by mild withdrawal symptoms such as abdominal cramps, insomnia, chilliness, headache, and nausea. Delirium and convulsions did not occur. In clinical use, psychological dependence and abuse have been rare, and there have been no reports of significant abstinence signs. Nevertheless, the drug should be used with caution in addiction-prone individuals.

➤*Hazardous tasks:* Patients should be warned that this drug may impair the mental or physical abilities required for the performance of potentially hazardous tasks such as driving a motor vehicle or operating machinery.

Drug Interactions

➤*CNS agents:* Since the effects of carisoprodol and alcohol or carisoprodol and other CNS depressants or psychotropic drugs may be additive, appropriate caution should be exercised with patients who take more than one of these agents simultaneously.

Adverse Reactions

➤*Allergic:* Allergic or idiosyncratic reactions occasionally develop. They are usually seen within the period of the first to fourth dose in patients having had no previous contact with the drug. Skin rash, erythema multiforme, pruritus, eosinophilia, and fixed drug eruption with cross reaction to meprobamate have been reported with carisoprodol. Severe reactions have been manifested by asthmatic episodes, fever, weakness, dizziness, angioneurotic edema, smarting eyes, hypotension, and anaphylactoid shock.

➤*Cardiovascular:* Tachycardia, postural hypotension, and facial flushing.

➤*CNS:* Drowsiness and other CNS effects may require dosage reduction. Also observed were dizziness, vertigo, ataxia, tremor, agitation, irritability, headache, depressive reactions, syncope, and insomnia.

➤*GI:* Nausea, vomiting, hiccup, and epigastric distress.

➤*Hematologic:* Leukopenia, in which other drugs or viral infection may have been responsible, and pancytopenia, attributed to phenylbutazone, have been reported. No serious blood dyscrasias have been attributed to carisoprodol.

Overdosage

➤*Symptoms:* Overdosage of carisoprodol has produced stupor, coma, shock, respiratory depression, and, very rarely, death. The effects of an overdosage of carisoprodol and alcohol or other CNS depressants or psychotropic agents can be additive even when one of the drugs has been taken in the usual recommended dosage.

➤*Treatment:* Any drug remaining in the stomach should be removed and symptomatic therapy given. Should respiration or blood pressure become compromised, respiratory assistance, CNS stimulants, and pressor agents should be administered cautiously as indicated.

Carisoprodol is metabolized in the liver and excreted by the kidney. Although carisoprodol overdosage experience is limited, the following types of treatment have been used successfully with the related drug meprobamate: Diuresis, osmotic (mannitol) diuresis, peritoneal dialysis, and hemodialysis (carisoprodol is dialyzable).

Careful monitoring of urinary output is necessary and caution should be taken to avoid overhydration. Observe for possible relapse due to incomplete gastric emptying and delayed absorption. Carisoprodol can be measured in biological fluids by gas chromatography.

CHLORZOXAZONE

Rx	**Chlorzoxazone** (Various, eg, Goldline)	**Tablets:** 250 mg	In 100s and 1000s.
Rx	**Paraflex Caplets** (McNeil Pharm.)		(Paraflex). Peach, capsule shape. In 100s.
Rx	**Remular-S** (Inter. Ethical)		In 100s.
Rx	**Chlorzoxazone** (Various, eg, Goldline, IDE, Royce, Rugby, Schein)	**Tablets:** 500 mg	In 100s, 500s and 1000s.
Rx	**Parafon Forte DSC Caplets** (McNeil Pharm.)		(McNeil Parafon Forte DSC). Lt. green, scored. In 100s, 500s and UD 100s.

CHLORZOXAZONE — ORAL

Indications

➤*Musculoskeletal conditions:* As an adjunct to rest, physical therapy, and other measures for the relief of discomfort associated with acute, painful musculoskeletal conditions. The mode of action of this drug has not been clearly identified, but may be related to its sedative properties. Chlorzoxazone does not directly relax tense skeletal muscles.

Administration and Dosage

➤*Usual adult dose:*

Tablets (500 mg) – 1 tablet 3 or 4 times daily. If adequate response is not obtained with this dose, it may be increased to 1½ tablets (750 mg) 3 or 4 times daily. As improvement occurs, dosage can usually be reduced.

Tablets (250 mg) – 1 tablet (250 mg) 3 or 4 times daily. Initial dosage for painful musculoskeletal conditions should be 2 tablets (500 mg) 3 or 4 times daily. If adequate response is not obtained with this dose, it may be increased to 3 tablets (750 mg) 3 or 4 times daily. As improvement occurs dosage can usually be reduced.

➤*Storage/Stability:* Store at controlled room temperature (15° to 30°C; 59° to 86°F). Dispense in tight, light-resistant container as defined in the official compendium.

Actions

➤*Pharmacology:* Chlorzoxazone is a centrally acting agent for painful musculoskeletal conditions. Data available from animal experiments as well as human study indicate that chlorzoxazone acts primarily at the level of the spinal cord and subcortical areas of the brain where it inhibits multisynaptic reflex arcs involved in producing and maintaining skeletal muscle spasm of varied etiology. The clinical result is a reduction of the skeletal muscle spasm with relief of pain and increased mobility of the involved muscles.

➤*Pharmacokinetics:*

Absorption – Blood levels of chlorzoxazone can be detected in people during the first 30 minutes and peak levels may be reached, in the majority of the subjects, in about 1 to 2 hours after oral administration of chlorzoxazone.

Metabolism/Excretion – Chlorzoxazone is rapidly metabolized and is excreted in the urine, primarily in a conjugated form as the glucuronide. Less than 1% of a dose of chlorzoxazone is excreted unchanged in the urine in 24 hours.

Contraindications

Intolerance to the drug.

Warnings

➤*Hepatotoxicity:* Serious (including fatal) hepatocellular toxicity has been reported rarely. The mechanism is unknown but appears to be idiosyncratic and unpredictable. Factors predisposing patients to this rare event are not known. Patients should be instructed to report early signs or symptoms of hepatotoxicity (eg, fever, rash, anorexia, nausea, vomiting, fatigue, right upper quadrant pain, dark urine, jaundice). Chlorzoxazone should be discontinued immediately and a physician consulted if any of these signs or symptoms develop. Chlorzoxazone use should also be discontinued if a patient develops abnormal liver enzymes (eg, AST, ALT, alkaline phosphatase, bilirubin.)

➤*Hypersensitivity reactions:* Used with caution in patients with known allergies or with a history of allergic reactions to drugs. If a sensitivity reaction occurs such as urticaria, redness, or itching of the skin, the drug should be stopped.

➤*Pregnancy: Category C.* The safe use of chlorzoxazone has not been established with respect to the possible adverse effects upon fetal development. Therefore, it should be used in women of childbearing potential only when, in the judgment of the physician, the potential benefits outweigh the possible risks.

Drug Interactions

➤*CNS agents:* The concomitant use of alcohol or other CNS depressants may have an additive effect.

Adverse Reactions

After extensive clinical use of chlorzoxazone containing products in an estimated 32 million patients, it is apparent that the drug is well tolerated and seldom produces undesirable side effects. Occasional patients may develop

CHLORZOXAZONE — ORAL

gastrointestinal disturbances. It is possible in rare instances that chlorzoxazone may have been associated with GI bleeding. Drowsiness, dizziness, lightheadedness, malaise, or overstimulation may be noted by an occasional patient. Rarely, allergic-type skin rashes, petechiae, or ecchymoses may develop during treatment. Angioneurotic edema or anaphylactic reactions are extremely rare. There is no evidence that the drug will cause renal damage. Rarely, a patient may note discoloration of the urine resulting from a phenolic metabolite of chlorzoxazone. This finding is of no known clinical significance.

Overdosage

➤*Symptoms:* Initially, GI disturbances such as nausea, vomiting, or diarrhea together with drowsiness, dizziness, lightheadedness or headache may occur. Early in the course there may be malaise or sluggishness followed by marked loss of muscle tone, making voluntary movement impossible. The deep tendon reflexes may be decreased or absent. The sensorium remains intact, and there is no peripheral loss of sensation. Respiratory depression may occur with rapid, irregular respiration and intercostal and substernal retraction. The blood pressure is lowered, but shock has not been observed.

➤*Treatment:* Gastric lavage or induction of emesis should be carried out, followed by administration of activated charcoal. Thereafter, treatment is entirely supportive. If respirations are depressed, oxygen and artificial respiration should be employed and a patent airway assured by use of an oropharyngeal airway or endotracheal tube. Hypotension may be counteracted by use of dextran, plasma, concentrated albumin or a vasopressor agent such as norepinephrine. Cholinergic drugs or analeptic drugs are of no value and should not be used.

CYCLOBENZAPRINE HYDROCHLORIDE

Rx	**Cyclobenzaprine Hydrochloride** (Various, eg, Mylan, Patriot, Pliva, Sandoz, Watson)	**Tablets:** 5 mg	May contain lactose. In 30s, 100s, 500s, 1,000s, and UD 30s.
Rx	**Flexeril** (McNeil)		Lactose. (FLEXERIL). Yellow-orange, 5 sided D-shape. Film-coated. In 100s.
Rx	**Cyclobenzaprine Hydrochloride** (Watson)	**Tablets:** 7.5 mg	(WATSON 3330). White. Film-coated. In 30s, 100s, and 1,000s.
Rx	**Cyclobenzaprine Hydrochloride** (Various, eg, Goldline, Major, Moore, Mylan, Parmed, Patriot, Rugby, Sandoz, Schein, Watson)	**Tablets:** 10 mg	May contain lactose. In 30s, 100s, 500s, and 1,000s.
Rx	**Flexeril** (McNeil)		Lactose. Yellow. Film-coated. In 100s.

CYCLOBENZAPRINE HYDROCHLORIDE — ORAL

Indications

➤*Musculoskeletal conditions:* As an adjunct to rest and physical therapy for relief of muscle spasm associated with acute, painful musculoskeletal conditions.

➤*Unlabeled uses:* Adjunct in the management of the fibrositis syndrome.

Administration and Dosage

For most patients, the recommended dose is 5 mg 3 times a day. Based on individual patient response, the dose may be increased to either 7.5 or 10 mg 3 times a day. Use for periods longer than 2 or 3 weeks is not recommended.

➤*Hepatically impaired and elderly patients:* Less frequent dosing should be considered for hepatically impaired or elderly patients.

See Actions for more information.

The plasma concentration of cyclobenzaprine is increased in the elderly. The elderly may also be more at risk for CNS adverse events such as hallucinations and confusion, cardiac events resulting in falls or other sequelae, drug-drug and drug-disease interactions. For these reasons, in the elderly, use only if clearly needed. In such patients cyclobenzaprine should be initiated with a 5 mg dose and titrated slowly upward.

Actions

➤*Pharmacology:* Cyclobenzaprine relieves skeletal muscle spasm of local origin without interfering with muscle function. It is ineffective in muscle spasm due to CNS disease.

Cyclobenzaprine reduced or abolished skeletal muscle hyperactivity in several animal models. Animal studies indicate that cyclobenzaprine does not act at the neuromuscular junction or directly on skeletal muscle. Such studies show that cyclobenzaprine acts primarily within the central nervous system at brain stem as opposed to spinal cord levels, although its action on the latter may contribute to its overall skeletal muscle relaxant activity. Evidence suggests that the net effect of cyclobenzaprine is a reduction of tonic somatic motor activity, influencing both gamma (γ) and alpha (α) motor systems.

Pharmacological studies in animals showed a similarity between the effects of cyclobenzaprine and the structurally related tricyclic antidepressants, including reserpine antagonism, norepinephrine potentiation, potent peripheral and central anticholinergic effects, and sedation. Cyclobenzaprine caused slight to moderate increase in heart rate in animals.

➤*Pharmacokinetics:*

Absorption/Distribution – Estimates of mean oral bioavailability of cyclobenzaprine range from 33% to 55%. Cyclobenzaprine exhibits linear pharmacokinetics over the dose range 2.5 mg to 10 mg, and is subject to enterohepatic circulation. It is highly bound to plasma proteins. Drug accumulates when dosed 3 times a day, reaching steady-state within 3 to 4 days at plasma concentrations about 4-fold higher than after a single dose. At steady state in healthy subjects receiving 10 mg 3 times daily (n = 18), peak plasma concentration was 25.9 ng/mL (range, 12.8 to 46.1 ng/mL), and area under the concentration-time (AUC) curve over an 8-hour dosing interval was 177 ng•hr/mL (range, 80 to 319 ng•hr/mL).

Metabolism/Excretion – Cyclobenzaprine is extensively metabolized, and is excreted primarily as glucuronides via the kidney. Cytochromes P450 3A4, 1A2, and, to a lesser extent, 2D6, mediate N-demethylation, one of the oxidative pathways for cyclobenzaprine. Cyclobenzaprine is eliminated quite slowly, with an effective half-life of 18 hours (range 8 to 37 hours; n = 18); plasma clearance is 0.7 L/min.

Special populations –

Hepatic function impairment: In a pharmacokinetic study of 16 subjects with hepatic impairment (15 mild, 1 moderate per Child-Pugh score), both AUC and C_{max} were approximately double the values seen in the healthy control group. Cyclobenzaprine should be used with caution in subjects with mild hepatic impairment starting with the 5 mg dose and titrating slowly upward. Due to the lack of data in subjects with more severe hepatic insufficiency, the use of cyclobenzaprine in subjects with moderate to severe impairment is not recommended.

Elderly: In a pharmacokinetic study in elderly individuals (greater than or equal to 65 years old), mean (n = 10) steady-state cyclobenzaprine AUC values were approximately 1.7 fold (171 ng•hr/mL, range 96.1 to 255.3) higher than those seen in a group of eighteen younger adults (101.4 ng•hr/mL, range 36.1 to 182.9) from another study. Elderly male subjects had the highest observed mean increase, approximately 2.4 fold (198.3 ng•hr/mL, range 155.6 to 255.3 vs 83.2 ng•hr/mL, range 41.1 to 142.5 for younger males) while levels in elderly females were increased to a much lesser extent, approximately 1.2-fold (143.8 ng•hr/mL, range 96.1 to 196.3 vs 115.9 ng•hr/mL, range 36.1 to 182.9 for younger females) .In light of these findings, therapy with cyclobenzaprine in the elderly should be initiated with a 5 mg dose and titrated slowly upward.

Contraindications

Hypersensitivity to any component of this product; acute recovery phase of MI, and patients with arrhythmias, heart block or conduction disturbances, or congestive heart failure; hyperthyroidism. Concomitant use of monoamine oxidase inhibitors or within 14 days after their discontinuation. Hyperpyretic crisis seizures, and deaths have occurred in patients receiving cyclobenzaprine (or structurally similar tricyclic antidepressants) concomitantly with MAO inhibitor drugs.

Warnings

➤*Similarity to TCAs:* Cyclobenzaprine is closely related to the tricyclic antidepressants (eg, amitriptyline, imipramine). In short-term studies for indications other than muscle spasm associated with acute musculoskeletal conditions, and usually at doses somewhat greater than those recommended for skeletal muscle spasm, some of the more serious CNS reactions noted with the tricyclic antidepressants have occurred. Tricyclic antidepressants have been reported to produce arrhythmias, sinus tachycardia, prolongation of the conduction time leading to myocardial infarction and stroke.

➤*Hepatic function impairment:* See Actions for more information.

➤*Carcinogenesis:* In rats treated with cyclobenzaprine for up to 67 weeks at doses of approximately 5 to 40 times the maximum recommended human dose, pale, sometimes enlarged, livers were noted and there was a dose-related hepatocyte vacuolation with lipidosis. In the higher dose groups this microscopic change was seen after 26 weeks and even earlier in rats which died prior to 26 weeks; at lower doses, the change was not seen until after 26 weeks.

➤*Elderly:* See Actions for more information.

➤*Pregnancy: Category B.* There are no adequate and well-controlled studies in pregnant women. Because animal reproduction studies are not always predictive of human response, this drug should be used during pregnancy only if clearly needed.

➤*Lactation:* It is not known whether this drug is excreted in human milk. Because cyclobenzaprine is closely related to the tricyclic antidepressants, some of which are known to be excreted in human milk, caution should be exercised when cyclobenzaprine is administered to a nursing woman.

➤*Children:* Safety and efficacy in children below 15 years of age have not been established.

Precautions

➤*Special risk:* Because of its atropine-like action, cyclobenzaprine should be used with caution in patients with a history of urinary retention, angle-

CYCLOBENZAPRINE HYDROCHLORIDE — ORAL

closure glaucoma, increased intraocular pressure, and in patients taking anticholinergic medication.

➤*Drug abuse and dependence:* Pharmacologic similarities among the tricyclic drugs require that certain withdrawal symptoms be considered when cyclobenzaprine hydrochloride is administered, even though they have not been reported to occur with this drug. Abrupt cessation of treatment after prolonged administration may produce nausea, headache, and malaise. These are not indicative of addiction.

➤*Hazardous tasks:* Cyclobenzaprine hydrochloride may impair mental or physical abilities required for performance of hazardous tasks, such as operating machinery or driving a motor vehicle.

Drug Interactions

➤*MAO inhibitors:* Cyclobenzaprine may have life-threatening interactions with MAO inhibitors. See Contraindications for more information.

➤*CNS agents:* Cyclobenzaprine may enhance the effects of alcohol, barbiturates, and other CNS depressants.

➤*Guanethidine:* Tricyclic antidepressants may block the antihypertensive action of guanethidine and similarly acting compounds.

➤*Tramadol:* Tricyclic antidepressants may enhance the seizure risk in patients taking tramadol.

➤*NSAIDs:* Concomitant administration of cyclobenzaprine and naproxen or diflunisal was well tolerated with no reported unexpected adverse effects. However, combination therapy of cyclobenzaprine with naproxen was associated with more side effects than therapy with naproxen alone, primarily in the form of drowsiness.

Adverse Reactions

Cyclobenzaprine Adverse Reactions

Adverse reaction	Cyclobenzaprine 5 mg (n = 464)	Cyclobenzaprine 10 mg (n = 249)	Placebo (n = 469)
Drowsiness	29%	38%	10%
Dry mouth	21%	32%	7%
Fatigue	6%	6%	3%
Headache	5%	5%	8%

Adverse reactions which were reported in 1% to 3% of the patients were abdominal pain, acid regurgitation, constipation, diarrhea, dizziness, nausea, irritability, mental acuity decreased, nervousness, upper respiratory tract infection, and pharyngitis.

The adverse reactions reported most frequently with cyclobenzaprine were drowsiness, dry mouth and dizziness. The incidence of these common adverse reactions was lower in the surveillance program than in the controlled clinical studies.

Adverse reaction	Clinical studies with cyclobenzaprine 10 mg	Surveillance program with cyclobenzaprine 10 mg
Drowsiness	39%	16%
Dry mouth	27%	7%
Dizziness	11%	3%

➤*Less frequent adverse reactions:* Adverse reactions which were reported in 1% to 3% of the patients were fatigue/tiredness, asthenia, nausea, constipation, dyspepsia, unpleasant taste, blurred vision, headache, nervousness, and confusion.

The following adverse reactions have been reported in postmarketing experience or with an incidence of less than 1% in patients in clinical trials with the 10 mg tablet:

Cardiovascular – Tachycardia; arrhythmia; vasodilatation; palpitation; hypotension.

CNS – Seizures; ataxia; vertigo; dysarthria; tremors; hypertonia, convulsions; muscle twitching; disorientation; insomnia; depressed mood; abnormal sensations; anxiety; agitation; psychosis; abnormal thinking and dreaming; hallucinations; excitement; paresthesia; diplopia.

Dermatologic – Sweating.

GI – Vomiting; anorexia; diarrhea; GI pain; gastritis; thirst; flatulence; edema of the tongue.

GU – Urinary frequency or retention.

Hepatic – Abnormal liver function and rare reports of hepatitis, jaundice, and cholestasis.

Hypersensitivity – Anaphylaxis; angioedema; pruritus; facial edema; urticaria; rash.

Musculoskeletal – Local weakness.

Special senses – Ageusia; tinnitus.

Miscellaneous – Syncope; malaise.

➤*Causal relationship unknown:*

Cardiovascular – Hypertension; MI; heart block; stroke.

CNS – Decreased or increased libido; abnormal gait; delusions; aggressive behavior; paranoia; peripheral neuropathy; Bell's palsy; alteration in EEG patterns; extrapyramidal symptoms.

Dermatologic – Photosensitization; alopecia.

Endocrine – Inappropriate ADH syndrome.

GI – Paralytic ileus, tongue discoloration; stomatitis; parotid swelling.

GU – Impaired urination; dilatation of urinary tract; impotence; testicular swelling; gynecomastia; breast enlargement; galactorrhea.

Hematologic/Lymphatic – Purpura; bone marrow depression; leukopenia; eosinophilia; thrombocytopenia.

Metabolic/Nutritional – Elevation and lowering of blood sugar levels; weight gain or loss.

Musculoskeletal – Myalgia.

Respiratory – Dyspnea.

Miscellaneous – Chest pain; edema.

Overdosage

➤*Symptoms:* Although rare, deaths may occur from overdosage with cyclobenzaprine. Multiple drug ingestion (including alcohol) is common in deliberate cyclobenzaprine overdose. As management of overdose is complex and changing, it is recommended that the physician contact a poison control center for current information on treatment. Signs and symptoms of toxicity may develop rapidly after cyclobenzaprine overdose; therefore, hospital monitoring is required as soon as possible. The acute oral LD_{50} of cyclobenzaprine is approximately 338 and 425 mg/kg in mice and rats, respectively.

The most common effects associated with cyclobenzaprine overdose are drowsiness and tachycardia. Less frequent manifestations include tremor, agitation, coma, ataxia, hypertension, slurred speech, confusion, dizziness, nausea, vomiting, and hallucinations. Rare but potentially critical manifestations of overdose are cardiac arrest, chest pain, cardiac dysrhythmias, severe hypotension, seizures, and neuroleptic malignant syndrome. Changes in the electrocardiogram, particularly in QRS axis or width, are clinically significant indicators of cyclobenzaprine toxicity.

➤*Treatment:* In order to protect against the rare but potentially critical manifestations described above, obtain an ECG and immediately initiate cardiac monitoring. Protect the patient's airway, establish an intravenous line and initiate gastric decontamination. Observation with cardiac monitoring and observation for signs of CNS or respiratory depression, hypotension, cardiac dysrhythmias and/or conduction blocks, and seizures is necessary. If signs of toxicity occur at any time during this period, extended monitoring is required. Monitoring of plasma drug levels should not guide management of the patient. Dialysis is probably of no value because of low plasma concentrations of the drug.

Gastrointestinal decontamination – All patients suspected of an overdose with cyclobenzaprine should receive gastrointestinal decontamination. This should include large volume gastric lavage followed by activated charcoal. If consciousness is impaired, the airway should be secured prior to lavage and emesis is contraindicated.

Cardiovascular – A maximal limb-lead QRS duration of greater than or equal to 0.1 seconds may be the best indication of the severity of the overdose. Serum alkalinization, to a pH of 7.45 to 7.55, using intravenous sodium bicarbonate and hyperventilation (as needed), should be instituted for patients with dysrhythmias and/or QRS widening. A pH greater than 7.6 or a pCO_2 less than 20 mm Hg is undesirable. Dysrhythmias unresponsive to sodium bicarbonate therapy/hyperventilation may respond to lidocaine, bretylium or phenytoin. Type 1A and 1C antiarrhythmics are generally contraindicated (eg, quinidine, disopyramide, procainamide).

CNS – In patients with CNS depression, early intubation is advised because of the potential for abrupt deterioration. Seizures should be controlled with benzodiazepines or, if these are ineffective, other anticonvulsants (eg, phenobarbital, phenytoin). Physostigmine is not recommended except to treat life-threatening symptoms that have been unresponsive to other therapies, and then only in close consultation with a poison control center.

Patient Information

Avoid alcohol and other CNS depressants.

Cyclobenzaprine, especially when used with alcohol or other CNS depressants, may impair mental or physical abilities required for performance of hazardous tasks, such as operating machinery or driving a motor vehicle.

In the elderly, the frequency and severity of adverse events associated with the use of cyclobenzaprine, with or without concomitant medications, is increased. In elderly patients, cyclobenzaprine hydrochloride should be initiated with a 5 mg dose and titrated slowly upward.

DIAZEPAM

For prescribing information, refer to the Diazepam monograph and the Benzodiazepine group monograph in the Antianxiety Agents section.

METAXALONE

Rx	**Skelaxin** (King)	**Tablets:** 800 mg	(8667 S). Pink, oval, scored. In 100s and 500s.

METAXALONE — ORAL

Indications

➤*Musculoskeletal conditions:* As an adjunct to rest, physical therapy, and other measures for the relief of discomforts associated with acute, painful musculoskeletal conditions.

The mode of action of this drug has not been clearly identified, but may be related to its sedative properties. Metaxalone does not directly relax tense skeletal muscles in humans.

Administration and Dosage

The recommended dose for adults and children older than 12 years of age is two 400 mg tablets (800 mg) or one 800 mg tablet 3 to 4 times a day.

➤*Storage/Stability:* Store at controlled room temperature, between 15° and 30°C (59° and 86°F).

Actions

➤*Pharmacology:* The mechanism of action of metaxalone in humans has not been established, but may be due to general CNS depression. It has no direct action on the contractile mechanism of striated muscle, the motor end plate or the nerve fiber.

➤*Pharmacokinetics:*

Absorption/Distribution – The absolute bioavailability of metaxalone from metaxalone tablets is not known.

Under fasted conditions, mean peak plasma concentrations (C_{max}) of 865.3 ng/mL were achieved within 3.3 ± 1.2 hours (S.D.) after dosing (t_{max}). Metaxalone concentrations declined with a mean terminal half-life ($t_{1/2}$) of 9.2 ± 4.8 hours. The mean apparent oral clearance (CL/F) of metaxalone was 68 ± 34 L/hr.

In the same study, following a standardized high-fat meal, food statistically significantly increased the rate (C_{max}) and extent of absorption ($AUC_{(0-t)}$, AUC_{inf}) of metaxalone. Relative to the fasted treatment the observed increases were 177.5%, 123.5%, and 115.4%, respectively. The mean t_{max} was also increased to 4.3 ± 2.3 hours, whereas the mean $t_{1/2}$ was decreased to 2.4 ± 1.2 hours. This decrease in half-life over that seen in the fasted subjects is felt to be due to the more complete absorption of metaxalone in the presence of a meal resulting in a better estimate of half-life. The mean apparent oral clearance (CL/F) of metaxalone was relatively unchanged relative to fasted administration (59 ± 29 L/hr). Although a higher C_{max} and AUC were observed after the administration of metaxalone with a standardized high-fat meal, the clinical relevance of these effects is unknown.

Metabolism/Excretion – Metaxalone is metabolized by the liver and excreted in the urine as unidentified metabolites. The impact of age, gender, hepatic, and renal disease on the pharmacokinetics of metaxalone has not been determined. In the absence of such information, metaxalone should be used with caution in patients with hepatic or renal impairment and in the elderly.

Contraindications

Hypersensitivity to the drug; tendency to drug-induced, hemolytic, or other anemias; significantly impaired renal or hepatic function.

Warnings

➤*Hepatic function impairment:* Metaxalone should be administered with great care to patients with preexisting liver damage. Serial liver function studies should be performed in these patients.

➤*Pregnancy:* Postmarketing experience has not revealed evidence of fetal injury, but such experience cannot exclude the possibility of infrequent or subtle damage to the human fetus. Safe use of metaxalone has not been established with regard to possible adverse reactions upon fetal development. Therefore, metaxalone tablets should not be used in women who are or may become pregnant and particularly during early pregnancy unless in the judgment of the physician the potential benefits outweigh the possible hazards.

Reproduction studies have been performed in rats and have revealed no evidence of impaired fertility or harm to the fetus due to metaxalone.

➤*Lactation:* It is not known whether this drug is secreted in human milk. As a general rule, nursing should not be undertaken while a patient is on a drug since many drugs are excreted in human milk.

➤*Children:* Safety and efficacy in children less than or equal to 12 years of age have not been established.

Precautions

➤*Hazardous tasks:* Metaxalone may impair mental or physical abilities required for performance of hazardous tasks, such as operating machinery or driving a motor vehicle, especially when used with alcohol or other CNS depressants.

Drug Interactions

➤*CNS agents:* Metaxalone may enhance the effects of alcohol, barbiturates, and other CNS depressants.

➤*Drug/Lab test interactions:* False-positive Benedict's tests, due to an unknown reducing substance, have been noted. A glucose-specific test will differentiate findings.

Adverse Reactions

➤*CNS:* Drowsiness, dizziness, headache, and nervousness or "irritability."

➤*Dermatologic:* Rash, with or without pruritus.

➤*GI:* Nausea, vomiting, GI upset.

➤*Hematologic:* Leukopenia and hemolytic anemia.

➤*Hepatic:* Jaundice.

➤*Hypersensitivity:* Hypersensitivity reaction. Though rare, anaphylactoid reactions have been reported with metaxalone.

Overdosage

➤*Symptoms:* Deaths by deliberate or accidental overdose have occurred with this class of drugs, particularly in combination with antidepressants or alcohol.

When determining the LD_{50} in rats and mice, progressive sedation, hypnosis and finally respiratory failure were noted as the dosage increased. In dogs, no LD_{50} could be determined as the higher doses produced an emetic action in 15 to 30 minutes.

➤*Treatment:* Gastric lavage and supportive therapy. Consultation with a regional poison control center is recommended.

Patient Information

Metaxalone may impair mental or physical abilities required for performance of hazardous tasks, such as operating machinery or driving a motor vehicle, especially when used with alcohol or other CNS depressants.

Avoid alcohol and other CNS depressants.

METHOCARBAMOL

Rx	**Methocarbamol** (Various, eg, Geneva, Lederle, Major, Schein, UDL, Zenith-Goldline)	**Tablets:** 500 mg	In 100s, 500s and UD 100s.
Rx	**Robaxin** (Schwarz Pharma)		Saccharin. (Robaxin AHR). Light orange. In 100s, 500s, *Disco-Pak* 100s.
Rx	**Methocarbamol** (Various, eg, Geneva, Lederle, Major, Schein, UDL, Zenith-Goldline)	**Tablets:** 750 mg	In 60s, 100s, 500s and UD 100s.
Rx	**Robaxin-750** (Schwarz Pharma)		Saccharin. (AHR Robaxin-750). Orange. Capsule-shaped. In 100s, 500s and *Disco–Pak* 100s.
Rx	**Robaxin** (Wyeth-Ayerst)	**Injection:** 100 mg/ml	In 10 ml vials.[a]

[a] In solution of polyethylene glycol 300. After mixing with IV infusion fluids, do not refrigerate.

METHOCARBAMOL — ORAL

Indications

➤*Musculoskeletal conditions:* As an adjunct to rest, physical therapy, and other measures for the relief of discomfort associated with acute, painful musculoskeletal conditions.

Administration and Dosage

➤*500 mg tablets:* The initial dosage in adults is 3 tablets 4 times a day, and maintenance dosage in adults is 2 tablets 4 times a day.

➤*750 mg tablets:* The initial dosage in adults is 2 tablets 4 times a day and maintenance dosage in adults is 1 tablet every 4 hours, or 2 tablets 3 times a day.

A dosage of 6 g/day is recommended for the first 48 to 72 hours of treatment. (For severe conditions 8 g/day may be administered). Thereafter, the dosage can usually be reduced to approximately 4 g/day.

➤*Storage/Stability:* Store at controlled room temperature, 20° to 25°C (68° to 77°F). Protect from light and moisture. Dispense in a tight container.

METHOCARBAMOL — ORAL

Actions

➤*Pharmacology:* The mechanism of action of methocarbamol in humans has not been established, but may be due to CNS depression. It has no direct action on the contractile mechanism of striated muscle, motor end plate, or nerve fiber.

➤*Pharmacokinetics:*

Absorption – Methocarbamol has an onset of action of 30 minutes. Peak plasma levels occur approximately 2 hours after administration of 2 g.

Metabolism/Excretion – The half-life is from 1 to 2 hours; inactive metabolites are excreted in the urine and small amounts in the feces.

Special populations

Renal function impairment: The clearance of methocarbamol in 8 renally impaired patients on maintenance hemodialysis was reduced about 40% compared with 17 healthy subjects, although the mean (± SD) elimination half-life in these 2 groups was similar: 1.2 (± 0.6) vs 1.1 (± 0.3) hours, respectively.

Hepatic function impairment: In 8 patients with cirrhosis secondary to alcohol abuse, the mean total clearance of methocarbamol was reduced approximately 70% compared with that obtained in 8 age-and weight-matched healthy subjects. The mean (± SD) elimination half-life in the cirrhotic patients and the healthy subjects was 3.38 (± 1.62) and 1.11 (± 0.27) hours, respectively. The percent of methocarbamol bound to plasma proteins was decreased to approximately 40% to 45% compared with 46% to 50% in the healthy subjects.

Elderly: The mean (± SD) elimination half-life of methocarbamol in elderly healthy volunteers (mean (± SD) age, 69 (± 4) years) was slightly prolonged compared with a younger [mean (± SD) age, 53.3 (± 8.8) years), healthy population (1.5 (± 0.4) vs 1.1 (± 0.27) hours, respectively]. The fraction of bound methocarbamol was slightly decreased in the elderly vs younger volunteers (41% to 43% vs 46% to 50%, respectively).

Contraindications

Hypersensitivity to any of the ingredients.

Warnings

➤*Pregnancy:* *Category C.* Safe use of methocarbamol has not been established with regard to possible adverse effects upon fetal development. There have been reports of fetal and congenital abnormalities following in utero exposure of methocarbamol. Therefore, do not use methocarbamol tablets in women who are, or may become, pregnant, particularly during early pregnancy, unless, the potential benefits outweigh the possible hazards.

➤*Lactation:* Methocarbamol or its metabolites are excreted in the milk of dogs. It is not known whether methocarbamol or its metabolites are excreted in human milk. Because many drugs are excreted in human milk, exercise caution when methocarbamol is administered to a nursing woman. As a general rule, breast-feeding should not be undertaken while a patient is on a drug because many drugs are excreted in human milk.

➤*Children:* Safety and efficacy of methocarbamol in children younger than 16 years of age have not been established.

Precautions

➤*Hazardous tasks:* Methocarbamol may impair mental or physical abilities required for performance of hazardous tasks, such as operating machinery or driving a motor vehicle. Caution patients about operating machinery, including automobiles, until they are reasonably certain that methocarbamol therapy does not adversely affect their ability to engage in such activities.

Drug Interactions

➤*Pyridostigmine:* Methocarbamol may inhibit the effect of pyridostigmine bromide. Therefore, use with caution in patients with myasthenia gravis receiving anticholinesterase agents.

➤*CNS agents:* Since methocarbamol may possess a general CNS depressant effect, caution patients receiving methocarbamol about combined effects with alcohol and other CNS depressants.

➤*Drug/Lab test interactions:* Methocarbamol may cause a color interference in certain screening tests for 5-hydroxyindoleacetic acid (5-HIAA) using nitrosonaphthol reagent and in screening tests for urinary vanillylmandelic acid (VMA) using the Gitlow method.

Adverse Reactions

➤*Cardiovascular:* Bradycardia, flushing, hypotension, syncope, thrombophlebitis.

➤*CNS:* Amnesia, confusion, diplopia, dizziness or light-headedness, drowsiness, insomnia, mild muscular incoordination, nystagmus, sedation, seizures (including grand mal), vertigo.

➤*Dermatologic:* Pruritus, rash, urticaria.

➤*GI:* Dyspepsia, jaundice (including cholestatic jaundice), nausea, vomiting.

➤*Hematologic/Lymphatic:* Leukopenia.

➤*Immunologic:* Hypersensitivity reactions.

➤*Special senses:* Blurred vision, conjunctivitis, nasal congestion, metallic taste.

➤*Miscellaneous:* Anaphylactic reaction, angioneurotic edema, fever, headache.

Overdosage

➤*Symptoms:* Limited information is available in the acute toxicity of methocarbamol. Overdose of methocarbamol is frequently in conjunction with alcohol or other CNS depressants and includes the following symptoms: nausea, drowsiness, blurred vision, hypotension, seizures, and coma. One adult survived the deliberate ingestion of 22 to 30 g of methocarbamol without serious toxicity. Another adult survived a dose of 30 to 50 g. The principle symptom in both cases was extreme drowsiness. Treatment was symptomatic and recovery was uneventful.

➤*Treatment:* Management of overdose includes symptomatic and supportive treatment. Supportive measures include maintenance of an adequate airway, monitoring urinary output and vital signs, and administration of IV fluids if necessary. The usefulness of hemodialysis in managing overdose is unknown.

In postmarketing experience, deaths have been reported with an overdose of methocarbamol alone or in the presence of other CNS depressants, alcohol, or psychotropic drugs.

Patient Information

This drug may cause drowsiness, dizziness, or light-headedness. Observe caution while driving or performing other tasks requiring alertness, coordination, or physical dexterity. Avoid alcohol and other CNS depressants.

METHOCARBAMOL — INJECTION

Indications

➤*Musculoskeletal conditions:* As an adjunct to rest, physical therapy, and other measures for the relief of discomfort associated with acute, painful, musculoskeletal conditions.

The mode of action of this drug has not been clearly identified, but may be related to its sedative properties. Methocarbamol does not directly relax tense skeletal muscles.

Administration and Dosage

For IV and IM use only. Total adult dosage should not exceed 30 mL (3 vials) a day for more than 3 consecutive days except in the treatment of tetanus. A like course may be repeated after a lapse of 48 hours if the condition persists. Dosage and frequency of injection should be based on the severity of the condition being treated and therapeutic response noted.

For the relief of symptoms of moderate degree, 10 mL (1 vial) may be adequate. Ordinarily this injection need not be repeated, as the administration of the oral form will usually sustain the relief initiated by the injection. For the severest cases or in postoperative conditions in which oral administration is not feasible, 20 to 30 mL (2 to 3 vials) may be required.

➤*Directions for IV use:* May be administered undiluted directly into the vein at a maximum rate of 3 mL/min. It may also be added to an IV drip of sodium chloride injection (sterile isotonic sodium chloride solution for parenteral use) or 5% dextrose injection (sterile 5% dextrose solution); 1 vial given as a single dose should not be diluted to more than 250 mL for IV infusion. After mixing with IV infusion fluids, do not refrigerate. Care should be exercised to avoid vascular extravasation of this hypertonic solution, which may result in thrombophlebitis. It is preferable that the patient be in a recumbent position during and for at least 10 to 15 minutes following the injection.

➤*Directions for IM use:* When the IM route is indicated, not more than 5 mL (one-half vial) should be injected into each gluteal region. The injections may be repeated at 8 hour intervals, if necessary. When satisfactory relief of symptoms is achieved, it can usually be maintained with tablets.

Not recommended for subcutaneous administration.

➤*Special directions for use in tetanus:* There is clinical evidence which suggests that methocarbamol may have a beneficial effect in the control of the neuromuscular manifestations of tetanus. It does not, however, replace the usual procedure of debridement, tetanus antitoxin, penicillin, tracheotomy, attention to fluid balance, and supportive care. Methocarbamol should be added to the regimen as soon as possible.

For adults – Inject 1 or 2 vials directly into the tubing of the previously inserted indwelling needle. An additional 10 mL or 20 mL may be added to the infusion bottle so that a total of up to 30 mL (3 vials) is given as the initial dose. Rate of injection should not exceed 3 mL/min, (one 10 mL vial in approximately 3 minutes). Since methocarbamol injectable is hypertonic, vascular extravasation must be avoided. A recumbent position will reduce the likelihood of side reactions.This procedure should be repeated every 6 hours until conditions allow for the insertion of a nasogastric tube. Crushed methocarbamol tablets suspended in water or saline may then be given through this tube. Total daily oral doses up to 24 g may be required as judged by patient response.

For children – A minimum initial dose of 15 mg/kg is recommended. This dosage may be repeated every 6 hours as indicated. The maintenance dosage may be given by injection into tubing or by IV infusion with an appropriate quantity of fluid. See directions for IV use.

➤*Storage/Stability:* Store at controlled room temperature, between 20° and 25°C (68° and 77°F). After mixing with IV infusion fluids, do not refrigerate.

METHOCARBAMOL — INJECTION

Actions

➤*Pharmacology:* The mechanism of action in humans has not been established, but may be due to general CNS depression. It has no direct action on the contractile mechanism of striated muscle, the motor end plate, or the nerve fiber.

➤*Pharmacokinetics:*

Special populations –

Renal function impairment: The clearance of methocarbamol in renally impaired patients on maintenance hemodialysis was reduced about 40% compared to a healthy population, although the mean elimination half-life in these 2 groups was similar (1.2 vs 1.1 hours, respectively).

Hepatic function impairment: In patients with cirrhosis secondary to alcohol abuse, the mean total clearance of methocarbamol was reduced approximately 70% compared to a healthy population (11.9 L/hr), and the mean elimination half-life was extended to approximately 3.4 hours. The fraction of methocarbamol bound to plasma proteins was decreased to approximately 40% to 45% compared to 46% to 50% in an age- and weight-matched healthy population.

Contraindications

Hypersensitive to methocarbamol or to any of the injection components; known or suspected renal pathology. This caution is necessary because of the presence of polyethylene glycol 300 in the vehicle.

A much larger amount of polyethylene glycol 300 than is present in recommended doses of methocarbamol injectable is known to have increased preexisting acidosis and urea retention in patients with renal impairment. Although the amount present in this preparation is well within the limits of safety, caution dictates this contraindication.

Warnings

➤*Pregnancy: Category C.*

Teratogenic – Animal reproduction studies have not been conducted with methocarbamol. It is also not known whether methocarbamol can cause fetal harm when administered to a pregnant woman or can affect reproduction capacity. Methocarbamol should be given to a pregnant woman only if clearly needed.

Safe use of methocarbamol has not been established with regard to possible adverse effects upon fetal development. There have been very rare reports of fetal and congenital abnormalities following in utero exposure to methocarbamol. Therefore, methocarbamol should not be used in women who are or may become pregnant and particularly during early pregnancy unless in the judgment of the physician the potential benefits outweigh the possible hazards.

➤*Lactation:* Methocarbamol or its metabolites are excreted in the milk of dogs; however, it is not known whether methocarbamol or its metabolites are excreted in human milk. Because many drugs are excreted in human milk, caution should be exercised when methocarbamol injectable is administered to a nursing woman.

➤*Children:* Safety and effectiveness of methocarbamol in children have not been established except in tetanus. A minimum initial dose of 15 mg/kg is recommended. This dosage may be repeated every 6 hours as indicated. The maintenance dosage may be given by injection into tubing or by IV infusion with an appropriate quantity of fluid.

Precautions

➤*Administration:* As with other agents administered either intravenously or intramuscularly, careful supervision of dose and rate of injection should be observed. Rate of injection should not exceed 3 mL/min, (one 10 mL vial in approximately 3 minutes). Since methocarbamol injectable is hypertonic, vascular extravasation must be avoided. A recumbent position will reduce the likelihood of side reactions.

Blood aspirated into the syringe does not mix with the hypertonic solution. This phenomenon occurs with many other IV preparations. The blood may be safely injected with the methocarbamol, or the injection may be stopped when the plunger reaches the blood, whichever the physician prefers.

The total dosage should not exceed 30 mL (3 vials) a day for more than 3 consecutive days except in the treatment of tetanus.

➤*Special risk:* Caution should be observed in using the injectable form in patients with suspected or known seizure disorders.

➤*Hazardous tasks:* Methocarbamol may impair mental or physical abilities required for performance of hazardous tasks, such as operating machinery or driving a motor vehicle. Patients should be cautioned about operating machinery, including automobiles, until they are reasonably certain that methocarbamol therapy does not adversely affect their ability to engage in such activities.

Drug Interactions

➤*CNS agents:* Since methocarbamol may possess a general CNS depressant effect, patients receiving methocarbamol injectable should be cautioned about combined effects with alcohol and other CNS depressants.

➤*Pyridostigmine:* Methocarbamol may inhibit the effect of pyridostigmine bromide. Therefore, use with caution in patients with myasthenia gravis receiving anticholinesterase agents.

➤*Drug/Lab test interactions:* Methocarbamol may cause a color interference in certain screening tests for 5-hydroxy-indoleacetic acid (5-HIAA) using nitrosonaphthol reagent and in screening tests for urinary vanillylmandelic acid (VMA) using the Gitlow method.

Adverse Reactions

The following adverse reactions have been reported coincident with the administration of methocarbamol. Some events may have been due to an overly rapid rate of IV injection.

➤*Cardiovascular:* Bradycardia, flushing, hypotension, syncope, thrombophlebitis .In most cases of syncope there was spontaneous recovery. In others, epinephrine, injectable steroids, or injectable antihistamines were employed to hasten recovery.

➤*CNS:* Amnesia, confusion, diplopia, dizziness or lightheadedness, drowsiness, insomnia, mild muscular incoordination, nystagmus, seizures (including grand mal), vertigo. The onset of convulsive seizures during IV administration of methocarbamol has been reported in patients with seizure disorders. The psychic trauma of the procedure may have been a contributing factor. Although several observers have reported success in terminating epileptiform seizures with methocarbamol injectable, its administration to patients with epilepsy is not recommended.

➤*Dermatologic:* Pruritus, rash, urticaria.

➤*GI:* Dyspepsia, jaundice (including cholestatic jaundice), nausea and vomiting.

➤*Hematologic/Lymphatic:* Leukopenia.

➤*Local:* Pain and sloughing at the site of injection.

➤*Ophthalmic:* Blurred vision, conjunctivitis with nasal congestion.

➤*Special senses:* Metallic taste.

➤*Miscellaneous:* Anaphylactic reaction, fever, headache.

Overdosage

➤*Symptoms:* Limited information is available on the acute toxicity of methocarbamol. Overdose is frequently in conjunction with alcohol or other CNS depressants and includes the following symptoms: Nausea, drowsiness, blurred vision, hypotension, seizures, and coma. One adult survived the deliberate ingestion of 22 to 30 g of methocarbamol without serious toxicity. Another adult survived a dose of 30 to 50 g. The principal symptom in both cases was extreme drowsiness. Treatment was symptomatic and recovery was uneventful.

➤*Treatment:* Management of overdose includes symptomatic and supportive treatment. Supportive measures include maintenance of an adequate airway, monitoring urinary output and vital signs, and administration of IV fluids if necessary. The usefulness of hemodialysis in managing overdose is unknown.

Patient Information

Patients should be cautioned that methocarbamol may cause drowsiness or dizziness, which may impair their ability to operate motor vehicles or machinery.

Because methocarbamol may possess a general CNS-depressant effect, patients should be cautioned about combined effects with alcohol and other CNS depressants.

ORPHENADRINE CITRATE

Rx	**Orphenadrine Citrate** (Various)	**Tablets:** 100 mg	In 30s, 100s, 500s and 1000s.
Rx	**Orphenadrine Citrate** (Apothecon)	**Tablets, sustained release:** 100 mg	Lactose. (INV 336). White. In 100s and 500s.
Rx	**Norflex** (3M Pharm)		(3M 221). White. In 100s and 500s.
Rx	**Orphenadrine Citrate** (Various, eg, Rugby)	**Injection:** 30 mg per ml	In 2 ml amps and 10 ml vials.
Rx	**Banflex** (Forest Pharm.)		In 10 ml vials.
Rx	**Flexon** (Various, eg, Keene)		In 10 ml vials.
Rx	**Norflex** (3M Pharm)		In 2 ml amps.[1]

[1] With sodium bisulfite.

ORPHENADRINE CITRATE — ORAL

Indications

➤*Musculoskeletal conditions:* As an adjunct to rest, physical therapy, and other measures for the relief of discomfort associated with acute painful musculoskeletal conditions.

➤*Unlabeled uses:* At bedtime in the treatment of quinine-resistant leg cramps.

Administration and Dosage

➤*Approved by the FDA:* June 19, 1998.

➤*Adults:* Two tablets per day; 1 in the morning and 1 in the evening.

➤*Storage/Stability:* Store at controlled room temperature 15° to 30°C (59° to 86°F).

Actions

➤*Pharmacology:* The mode of therapeutic action has not been clearly identified, but may be related to its analgesic properties. Orphenadrine also possesses anticholinergic actions.

➤*Pharmacokinetics:*

Absorption – Peak plasma levels occur 2 hours after administration of 100 mg orphenadrine; duration of action is 4 to 6 hours.

Metabolism/Excretion – The half-life is ≈ 14 hours for the parent drug, and 2 to 25 hours for metabolites. Excretion is via urine and feces. Most of orphenadrine is degraded to eight known metabolites.

Contraindications

Glaucoma, pyloric or duodenal obstruction, stenosing peptic ulcers, prostatic hypertrophy or obstruction of the bladder neck, cardio-spasm (megaesophagus) and myasthenia gravis; hypersensitivity to the drug.

Warnings

➤*Pregnancy: Category C.* Animal reproduction studies have not been conducted with orphenadrine. It is also not known whether orphenadrine can cause fetal harm when administered to a pregnant woman or can affect reproduction capacity. Orphenadrine should be given to a pregnant woman only if clearly needed.

➤*Children:* Safety and efficacy in children have not been established.

Precautions

➤*Long-term therapy:* Safety of continuous long-term therapy has not been established. Therefore, if orphenadrine is prescribed for prolonged use, periodic monitoring of blood, urine, and liver function values is recommended.

➤*Cardiac disease:* Use with caution in patients with tachycardia, cardiac decompensation, coronary insufficiency, cardiac arrhythmias.

➤*Hazardous tasks:* Some patients may experience transient episodes of lightheadedness, dizziness, or syncope. Orphenadrine may impair the ability of the patient to engage in potentially hazardous activities such as operating machinery or driving a motor vehicle; ambulatory patients should therefore be cautioned accordingly.

Drug Interactions

Orphenadrine Drug Interactions

Precipitant drug	Object drug*		Description
Amantadine	Orphenadrine	⬆	Anticholinergic effects may be increased.
Orphenadrine	Haloperidol	⬌	Worsening of schizophrenic symptoms, decreased haloperidol levels and development of tardive dyskinesia may occur.
Orphenadrine	Phenothiazines	⬇	Therapeutic effects of phenothiazines may be decreased.
Orphenadrine	Propoxyphene	⬌	Confusion, anxiety, and tremors have been reported in few patients receiving propoxyphene and orphenadrine concomitantly. As these symptoms may be simply due to an additive effect, reduction of dosage or discontinuation of 1 or both agents is recommended in such cases.

* ⬆ = Object drug increased. ⬇ = Object drug decreased. ⬌ = Undetermined effect.

Adverse Reactions

Adverse reactions of orphenadrine are mainly due to the mild anticholinergic action of orphenadrine, and are usually associated with higher dosage. Dryness of the mouth is usually the first adverse effect to appear. When the daily dose is increased, possible adverse effects include: Tachycardia, palpitation, urinary hesitancy or retention, blurred vision, dilatation of pupils, increased ocular tension, weakness, nausea, vomiting, headache, dizziness, constipation, drowsiness, hypersensitivity reactions, pruritus, hallucinations, agitation, tremor, gastric irritation, and rarely urticaria and other dermatoses. Infrequently, an elderly patient may experience some degree of mental confusion. These adverse reactions can usually be eliminated by reduction in dosage. Very rare cases of aplastic anemia associated with the use of orphenadrine tablets have been reported. No causal relationship has been established.

ORPHENADRINE CITRATE — INJECTION

Indications

➤*Musculoskeletal conditions:* As an adjunct to rest, physical therapy, and other measures for the relief of discomfort associated with acute painful musculoskeletal conditions.

The mode of action of the drug has not been clearly identified, but may be related to its analgesic properties. Orphenadrine citrate does not directly relax tense skeletal muscles.

Administration and Dosage

➤*Approved by the FDA:* March 15, 1982.

➤*Adults:* One 2 mL ampul (60 mg) IV or IM; may be repeated every 12 hours. Relief may be maintained by 1 orphenadrine extended-release tablet twice daily.

➤*Storage/Stability:* Store at controlled room temperature 15° to 30°C (59° to 86°F).

Actions

➤*Pharmacology:* The mode of therapeutic action has not been clearly identified, but may be related to its analgesic properties. Orphenadrine also possesses anticholinergic actions.

Contraindications

Glaucoma, pyloric or duodenal obstruction, stenosing peptic ulcers, prostatic hypertrophy or obstruction of the bladder neck, cardio-spasm (megaesophagus) and myasthenia gravis; hypersensitivity to the drug.

Warnings

➤*Pregnancy: Category C.* Animal reproduction studies have not been conducted with orphenadrine. It is also not known whether orphenadrine can cause fetal harm when administered to a pregnant woman or can affect reproduction capacity. Orphenadrine should be given to a pregnant woman only if clearly needed.

➤*Children:* Safety and efficacy in children have not been established.

Precautions

➤*Long-term therapy:* Safety of continuous long-term therapy has not been established. Therefore, if orphenadrine is prescribed for prolonged use, periodic monitoring of blood, urine and liver function values is recommended.

➤*Cardiac disease:* Use with caution in patients with tachycardia, cardiac decompensation, coronary insufficiency, or cardiac arrhythmias.

➤*Hazardous tasks:* Some patients may experience transient episodes of lightheadedness, dizziness or syncope. Orphenadrine may impair the ability of the patient to engage in potentially hazardous activities such as operating machinery or driving a motor vehicle; ambulatory patients should therefore be cautioned accordingly.

➤*Sulfite sensitivity:* Orphenadrine injection contains sodium bisulfite, a sulfite that may cause allergic-type reactions including anaphylactic symptoms and life-threatening or less severe asthmatic episodes in certain susceptible people. The overall prevalence of sulfite sensitivity in the general population is unknown and probably low. Sulfite sensitivity is seen more frequently in asthmatic than nonasthmatic people.

Drug Interactions

Orphenadrine Drug Interactions

Precipitant drug	Object drug*		Description
Amantadine	Orphenadrine	⬆	Anticholinergic effects may be increased.
Orphenadrine	Haloperidol	⬌	Worsening of schizophrenic symptoms, decreased haloperidol levels and development of tardive dyskinesia may occur.
Orphenadrine	Phenothiazines	⬇	Therapeutic effects of phenothiazines may be decreased.

ORPHENADRINE CITRATE — INJECTION

Orphenadrine Drug Interactions			
Precipitant drug	Object drug*		Description
Orphenadrine	Propoxyphene	↔	Confusion, anxiety and tremors have been reported in few patients receiving propoxyphene and orphenadrine concomitantly. As these symptoms may be simply due to an additive effect, reduction of dosage or discontinuation of one or both agents is recommended in such cases.

* ↑ = Object drug increased. ↓ = Object drug decreased. ↔ = Undetermined effect.

Adverse Reactions

Adverse reactions of orphenadrine are mainly due to the mild anticholinergic action of orphenadrine, and are usually associated with higher dosage. Dryness of the mouth is usually the first adverse effect to appear. When the daily dose is increased, possible adverse effects include: Tachycardia, palpitation, urinary hesitancy or retention, blurred vision, dilatation of pupils, increased ocular tension, weakness, nausea, vomiting, headache, dizziness, constipation, drowsiness, hypersensitivity reactions, pruritus, hallucinations, agitation, tremor, gastric irritation, and rarely urticaria and other dermatoses. Infrequently, an elderly patient may experience some degree of mental confusion. These adverse reactions can usually be eliminated by reduction in dosage. Very rare cases of aplastic anemia associated with the use of orphenadrine tablets have been reported. No causal relationship has been established.

➤*Hypersensitivity:* Rare instances of anaphylactic reaction have been reported associated with the intramuscular injection of orphenadrine citrate injection.

TIZANIDINE HYDROCHLORIDE

Rx	**Tizanidine Hydrochloride** (Various, eg, Par, Teva)	**Tablets:** 2 mg (as base)	In 150s and 300s.
Rx	**Zanaflex** (Acorda Therapeutics[a])		Lactose. (A592). White, scored. In 150s.
Rx	**Tizanidine Hydrochloride** (Various, eg, Eon, Par, Teva)	**Tablets:** 4 mg (as base)	In 150s, 300s, and 1000s.
Rx	**Zanaflex** (Acorda Therapeutics[a])		Lactose. (A594). White, scored. In 150s.
Rx	**Zanaflex** (Acorda Therapeutics[a])	**Capsules:** 2 mg (as base)	Sugar spheres. (2 mg). Blue opaque. In 150s.
		4 mg (as base)	Sugar spheres. (4 mg). Opaque white/lt. blue. In 150s.
		6 mg (as base)	Sugar spheres. (6 mg). Opaque lt. blue. In 150s.

[a] Acorda Therapeutics, 15 Skyline Drive, Hawthorne, NY 10532; (914) 347-4300, fax (914) 347-4560

TIZANIDINE HYDROCHLORIDE — ORAL

Indications

➤*Muscle spasticity:* For the acute and intermittent management of increased muscle tone associated with spasticity.

Administration and Dosage

➤*Approved by the FDA:* November 27, 1996.

➤*Dosage:* A single oral dose of 8 mg tizanidine reduces muscle tone in patients with spasticity for a period of several hours. The effect peaks at ≈ 1 to 2 hours and dissipates between 3 to 6 hours. Effects are dose-related.

Although single doses of < 8 mg have not been demonstrated to be effective in controlled clinical studies, the dose-related nature of tizanidine's common adverse events make it prudent to begin therapy with single oral doses of 4 mg. Increase the dose gradually (2 to 4 mg steps) to optimum effect (satisfactory reduction of muscle tone at a tolerated dose).

The dose can be repeated at 6– to 8–hour intervals, as needed, to a maximum of three doses in 24 hours. Do not exceed 36 mg/day.

Experience with single doses exceeding 8 mg and daily doses exceeding 24 mg is limited. There is essentially no experience with repeated, single, daytime doses > 12 mg or total daily doses > 36 mg.

➤*Administration:* Food has complex effects on tizanidine pharmacokinetics, which differ with the different formulations. These pharmacokinetic differences may result in clinically significant differences when 1) switching administration of the tablet between the fed or fasted state, 2) switching administration of the capsule between the fed or fasted state, 3) switching between the tablet and capsule in the fed state, or 4) switching between the intact capsule and sprinkling the contents of the capsule on applesauce. These changes may result in increased adverse events or delayed/more rapid onset of activity, depending upon the nature of the switch. For this reason, the prescriber should be thoroughly familiar with the changes in kinetics associated with these different conditions (see Pharmacokinetics).

➤*Storage/Stability:* Store at controlled room temperature, between 15° and 30°C (59° and 86°F).

Dispense in a tight, light-resistant container with a child-resistant closure (as required).

Actions

➤*Pharmacology:* Tizanidine is an agonist at α_2 adrenergic receptor sites and presumably reduces spasticity by increasing presynaptic inhibition of motor neurons. In animal models, tizanidine has no direct effect on skeletal muscle fibers or the neuromuscular junction, and no major effect on monosynaptic spinal reflexes. The effects of tizanidine are greatest on polysynaptic pathways. The overall effect of these actions is thought to reduce facilitation of spinal motor neurons.

The imidazoline chemical structure of tizanidine is related to that of the antihypertensive drug clonidine and other α_2 adrenergic agonists. Pharmacological studies in animals show similarities between the 2 compounds, but tizanidine was found to have 1/10 to one-fiftieth (1/50) of the potency of clonidine in lowering blood pressure.

➤*Pharmacokinetics:*

Absorption – Following oral administration, tizanidine is essentially completely absorbed and has a half-life of approximately 2.5 hours (coefficient of variation [CV] = 33%). Following administration of tizanidine, peak plasma concentrations occurred at 1.5 hours (CV = 40%) after dosing. Food increases C_{max} by approximately one-third and shortens time to peak concentration by approximately 40 minutes, but the extent of tizanidine absorption is not affected. Tizanidine has linear pharmacokinetics over a dose of 1 to 20 mg.

Following oral administration of the tablet (in the fasted state), tizanidine has peak plasma concentrations occurring 1 hour after dosing with a half-life of approximately 2 hours.

When two 4 mg tablets are administered with food the mean maximal plasma concentration is increased by approximately 30%, and the median time to peak plasma concentration is increased by 25 minutes, to 1 hour and 25 minutes.

Food also increases the extent of absorption of the tablets.

Distribution – Tizanidine is widely distributed throughout the body; mean steady-state volume of distribution is 2.4 L/kg (CV = 21%) following IV administration in healthy adult volunteers.

Tizanidine is approximately 30% bound to plasma proteins, independent of concentration over the therapeutic range.

Metabolism/Excretion – The absolute oral bioavailability of tizanidine is approximately 40% (CV = 24%), due to extensive first-pass metabolism in the liver; approximately 95% of an administered dose is metabolized. Tizanidine metabolites are not known to be active; their half-lives range from 20 to 40 hours.

Following single and multiple oral dosing of ^{14}C-tizanidine, an average of 60% and 20% of total radioactivity was recovered in the urine and feces, respectively.

Special populations –

Age: No specific pharmacokinetic study was conducted to investigate age effects. Cross-study comparison of pharmacokinetic data following single dose administration of 6 mg tizanidine showed that younger subjects cleared the drug 4 times faster than the elderly subjects. Tizanidine has not been evaluated in children.

Renal impairment: Tizanidine clearance is reduced by greater than 50% in elderly patients with renal insufficiency (creatinine clearance less than 25 mL/min) compared to healthy elderly subjects; this would be expected to lead to a longer duration of clinical effect. Tizanidine should be used with caution in renally impaired patients. In these patients, during titration, the individual doses should be reduced. If higher doses are required, individual doses rather than dosing frequency should be increased. These patients should be monitored closely for the onset or increase in severity of the common adverse reactions (dry mouth, somnolence, asthenia and dizziness) as indicators of potential overdose.

Race: Pharmacokinetic differences due to race have not been studied.

Contraindications

Tizanidine HCl is contraindicated in patients with known hypersensitivity to tizanidine HCl or its ingredients.

Warnings

➤*Chronic and multiple dosing:* Clinical experience with long-term use of tizanidine at doses of 8 to 16 mg single doses or total daily doses of 24 to 36 mg is limited. Approximately 75 patients have been exposed to individual doses of greater than or equal to 12 mg for at least 1 year or more and approximately 80 patients have been exposed to total daily doses of 30 to 36 mg/day for at least 1 year or more. There is essentially no long-term experience with single, daytime doses of 16 mg. Because long-term clinical study experience at high doses is limited, only those adverse reactions with a relatively high incidence are likely to have been identified.

TIZANIDINE HYDROCHLORIDE — ORAL

➤*Hypotension:* Tizanidine is an α_2-adrenergic agonist (eg, clonidine) and can produce hypotension. In a single-dose study where blood pressure was monitored closely after dosing, two-thirds of patients treated with 8 mg of tizanidine had a 20% reduction in either the diastolic or systolic blood pressure (BP). The reduction was seen within 1 hour after dosing, peaked 2 to 3 hours after dosing and was associated, at times, with bradycardia, orthostatic hypotension, lightheadedness/dizziness and rarely syncope. The hypotensive effect is dose related and has been measured following single doses of greater than or equal to 2 mg.

The chance of significant hypotension may possibly be minimized by titration of the dose and by focusing attention on signs and symptoms of hypotension prior to dose advancement. In addition, patients moving from a supine to a fixed upright position may be at increased risk for hypotension and orthostatic effects.

Caution is advised when tizanidine is to be used in patients receiving concurrent antihypertensive therapy and should not be used with other α_2 adrenergic agonists.

➤*Sedation:* In the multiple-dose, controlled clinical studies, 48% of patients receiving any dose of tizanidine reported sedation as an adverse event. In 10% of these cases, the sedation was rated as severe compared to less than 1% in the placebo-treated patients. Sedation may interfere with everyday activity.

The effect appears to be dose related. In a single-dose study, 92% of the patients receiving 16 mg, when asked, reported that they were drowsy during the 6-hour study. This compares to 76% of the patients on 8 mg and 35% of the patients on placebo. Patients began noting this effect 30 minutes following dosing. The effect peaked 1.5 hours following dosing. Of the patients who received a single dose of 16 mg, 51% continued to report drowsiness 6 hours following dosing compared to 13% in the patients receiving placebo or 8 mg of tizanidine.

In the multiple dose studies, the prevalence of patients with sedation peaked following the first week of titration and then remained stable for the duration of the maintenance phase of the study.

➤*Hallucinosis/psychotic-like symptoms:* Tizanidine use has been associated with hallucinations. Formed, visual hallucinations or delusions have been reported in 5 of 170 patients (3%) in 2 North American controlled clinical studies. These 5 cases occurred within the first 6 weeks. Most of the patients were aware that the events were unreal. One patient developed psychoses in association with the hallucinations. One patient among these 5 continued to have problems for at least 2 weeks following discontinuation of tizanidine.

➤*Renal function impairment:* Tizanidine should be used with caution in patients with renal insufficiency (creatinine clearance less than 25 mL/min), as clearance is reduced by greater than 50%. In these patients, during titration, the individual doses should be reduced. If higher doses are required, individual doses rather than dosing frequency should be increased. These patients should be monitored closely for the onset or increase in severity of the common adverse reactions (dry mouth, somnolence, asthenia and dizziness) as indicators of potential overdose.

➤*Hepatic function impairment:* Monitoring of aminotransferase levels is recommended during the first 6 months of treatment (eg, baseline, 1, 3 and 6 months) and periodically thereafter, based on clinical status. Because of the potential toxic hepatic effect of tizanidine, the drug should be used only with extreme caution in patients with impaired hepatic function.

➤*Fertility impairment:* Tizanidine did not affect fertility in male rats at doses of 10 mg/kg, approximately 2.7 times the MRHD on a mg/m^2 basis, and in females at doses of 3 mg/kg, approximately equal to the maximum recommended human dose on a mg/m^2 basis; fertility was reduced in males receiving 30 mg/kg (8 times the maximum recommended human dose on a mg/m^2 basis) and in females receiving 10 mg/kg (2.7 times the MRHD on a mg/m^2 basis). At these doses, maternal behavioral effects and clinical signs were observed including marked sedation, weight loss, and ataxia.

➤*Elderly:* Tizanidine should be used with caution in elderly patients because clearance is decreased 4-fold.

➤*Pregnancy: Category C.* Reproduction studies performed in rats at a dose of 3 mg/kg, equal to the maximum recommended human dose on a mg/m^2 basis, and in rabbits at 30 mg/kg, 16 times the maximum recommended human dose on a mg/m^2 basis, did not show evidence of teratogenicity. Tizanidine at doses that are equal to and up to 8 times the maximum recommended human dose on a mg/m^2 basis increased gestation duration in rats. Prenatal and postnatal pup loss was increased and developmental retardation occurred. Postimplantation loss was increased in rabbits at doses of 1 mg/kg or greater, greater than or equal to 0.5 times the MRHD on a mg/m^2 basis. Tizanidine has not been studied in pregnant women. Tizanidine should be given to pregnant women only if clearly needed.

➤*Lactation:* It is not known whether tizanidine is excreted in human milk; although, as a lipid-soluble drug, it might be expected to pass into breast milk.

➤*Children:* There are no adequate and well-controlled studies to document the safety and efficacy of tizanidine in children.

Precautions

➤*Monitoring:* Monitoring of aminotransferase levels is recommended during the first 6 months of treatment (eg, baseline, 1, 3 and 6 months) and periodically thereafter, based on clinical status. Because of the potential toxic hepatic effect of tizanidine, the drug should be used only with extreme caution in patients with impaired hepatic function.

➤*Cardiovascular:* Prolongation of the QT interval and bradycardia were noted in chronic toxicity studies in dogs at doses equal to the maximum human dose on a mg/m^2 basis. ECG evaluation was not performed in the controlled clinical studies. Reduction in pulse rate has been noted in association with decreases in blood pressure in the single-dose controlled study. In a single-dose study where blood pressure was monitored closely after dosing, two-thirds of patients treated with 8 mg of tizanidine had a 20% reduction in either the diastolic or systolic blood pressure (BP). The reduction was seen within 1 hour after dosing, peaked 2 to 3 hours after dosing and was associated, at times, with bradycardia, orthostatic hypotension, lightheadedness/dizziness and rarely syncope. The hypotensive effect is dose related and has been measured following single doses of greater than or equal to 2 mg.

➤*Ophthalmic:* Dose-related retinal degeneration and corneal opacities have been found in animal studies at doses equivalent to approximately the maximum recommended dose on a mg/m^2 basis. There have been no reports of corneal opacities or retinal degeneration in the clinical studies.

➤*Use in women taking oral contraceptives:* Tizanidine should be used with caution in women taking oral contraceptives, as clearance of tizanidine is reduced by approximately 50% in such patients. In these patients, during titration, the individual doses should be reduced.

➤*Discontinuing therapy:* If therapy needs to be discontinued, especially in patients who have been receiving high doses for long periods, the dose should be decreased slowly to minimize the risk of withdrawal and rebound hypertension, tachycardia, and hypertonia.

➤*Drug abuse and dependence:* Tizanidine is closely related to clonidine, which is often abused in combination with narcotics and is known to cause symptoms of rebound upon abrupt withdrawal. Three cases of rebound symptoms on sudden withdrawal of tizanidine have been reported. The case reports suggest that these patients were also misusing narcotics. Withdrawal symptoms included hypertension, tachycardia, hypertonia, tremor, and anxiety. As with clonidine, withdrawal is expected to be more likely in cases where high doses are used, especially for prolonged periods.

Drug Interactions

➤*Acetaminophen:* Tizanidine delayed the t_{max} of acetaminophen by 16 minutes. Acetaminophen did not affect the pharmacokinetics of tizanidine.

➤*Alcohol:* Alcohol increased the AUC of tizanidine by approximately 20% while also increasing its C_{max} by approximately 15%. This was associated with an increase in side effects of tizanidine. The CNS-depressant effects of tizanidine and alcohol are additive.

➤*Oral contraceptives:* No specific pharmacokinetic study was conducted to investigate interaction between oral contraceptives and tizanidine, but retrospective analysis of population pharmacokinetic data following single and multiple dose administration of 4 mg tizanidine showed that women concurrently taking oral contraceptives had 50% lower clearance of tizanidine than women not on oral contraceptives.

Adverse Reactions

➤*Discontinuation of treatment:* Forty-five of 264 (17%) patients receiving tizanidine and 13 of 261 (5%) patients receiving placebo in 3 multiple-dose, placebo-controlled clinical studies discontinued treatment for adverse reactions. When patients withdrew from the study, they frequently had more than 1 reason for discontinuing. The adverse reactions most frequently leading to withdrawal of tizanidine-treated patients in the controlled clinical studies were asthenia (weakness, fatigue or tiredness) (3%), somnolence (3%), dry mouth (3%), increased spasm or tone (2%) and dizziness (2%).

➤*Most frequent adverse reactions:* In multiple-dose, placebo-controlled, clinical studies involving 264 patients with spasticity, the most frequent adverse reactions were dry mouth, somnolence/sedation, asthenia (weakness, fatigue or tiredness) and dizziness. Three-quarters of the patients rated the events as mild to moderate, and one-quarter of the patients rated the events as being severe. These events appeared to be dose related.

➤*Adverse reactions reported in controlled studies:*

Tizanidine Adverse Reactions (≥ 2%)

Reaction	Placebo (n = 261)	Tizanidine HCl (n = 264)
Dry mouth	10%	49%
Somnolence	10%	48%
Asthenia (weakness, fatigue or tiredness)	16%	41%
Dizziness	4%	16%
Urinary tract infection	7%	10%
Infection	5%	6%
Constipation	1%	4%
Liver function tests abnormal	< 1%	3%
Vomiting	0%	3%
Speech disorder	0%	3%
Amblyopia (blurred vision)	< 1%	3%
Urinary frequency	2%	3%
Flu syndrome	2%	3%

TIZANIDINE HYDROCHLORIDE

Tizanidine Adverse Reactions (≥ 2%)		
Reaction	Placebo (n = 261)	Tizanidine HCl (n = 264)
ALT increased	< 1%	3%
Dyskinesia	0%	3%
Nervousness	< 1%	3%
Pharyngitis	1%	3%
Rhinitis	2%	3%

In the single-dose, placebo-controlled study involving 142 patients with spasticity, the patients were specifically asked if they had experienced any of the 4 most common adverse reactions: Dry mouth, somnolence (drowsiness), asthenia (weakness, fatigue or tiredness) and dizziness. In addition, hypotension and bradycardia were observed. The occurrence of these adverse reactions were summarized in the table below. Other reactions were, in general, reported at a rate of less than or equal to 2%.

Single-Dose, Placebo-Controlled Study (Common Adverse Reactions Reported)			
Reaction	Placebo (n = 48)	Tizanidine 8 mg (n = 45	Tizanidine 16 mg (n = 49)
Somnolence	31%	78%	92%
Dry mouth	35%	76%	88%
Asthenia (weakness, fatigue or tiredness)	40%	67%	78%
Dizziness	4%	22%	45%
Hypotension	0%	16%	33%
Bradycardia	0%	2%	10%

➤*Other adverse reactions observed during the evaluation of tizanidine:*

Cardiovascular – Vasodilatation, postural hypotension, syncope, migraine, arrhythmia (infrequent); angina pectoris, coronary artery disorder, heart failure, myocardial infarct, phlebitis, pulmonary embolus, ventricular extrasystoles, ventricular tachycardia (rare).

CNS – Depression, anxiety, paresthesia (frequent); tremor, emotional lability, convulsion, paralysis, thinking abnormal, vertigo, abnormal dreams, agitation, depersonalization, euphoria, migraine, stupor, dysautonomia, neuralgia (infrequent); dementia, hemiplegia, neuropathy (rare).

Dermatologic – Rash, sweating, skin ulcer (frequent); pruritus, dry skin, acne, alopecia, urticaria (infrequent); exfoliative dermatitis, herpes simplex, herpes zoster, skin carcinoma (rare).

GI – Abdomen pain, diarrhea, dyspepsia (frequent); dysphagia, cholelithiasis, fecal impaction, flatulence, gastrointestinal hemorrhage, hepatitis, melena (infrequent); gastroenteritis, hematemesis, hepatoma, intestinal obstruction, liver damage (rare).

GU – Urinary urgency, cystitis, menorrhagia, pyelonephritis, urinary retention, kidney calculus, enlarged uterine fibroids, vaginal monillasis, vaginitis (infrequent); albuminuria, glycosuria, hematuria, metrorrhagia (rare).

Hematologic/Lymphatic – Ecchymosis, hypercholesteremia, anemia, hyperlipemia, leukopenia, leukocytosis, sepsis (infrequent); petechia, purpura, thrombocythemia, thrombocytopenia (rare).

Metabolic/Nutritional – Edema, hypothyroidism, weight loss (infrequent); adrenal cortex insufficiency, hyperglycemia, hypokalemia, hyponatremia, hypoproteinemia, respiratory acidosis (rare).

Musculoskeletal – Myasthenia, back pain (frequent); pathological fracture, arthralgia, arthritis, bursitis (infrequent).

Respiratory – Sinusitis, pneumonia, bronchitis (infrequent); asthma (rare).

Special senses – Ear pain, tinnitus, deafness, glaucoma, conjunctivitis, eye pain, optic neuritis, otitis media, retinal hemorrhage, visual field defect (infrequent); iritis, keratitis, optic atrophy (rare).

Miscellaneous – Fever (frequent); allergic reaction, moniliasis, malaise, abscess, neck pain, sepsis, cellulitis, death, overdose (infrequent); carcinoma, congenital anomaly, suicide attempt (rare).

Overdosage

➤*Symptoms:* One significant overdosage of tizanidine has been reported. Attempted suicide by a 46-year-old male with multiple sclerosis resulted in coma very shortly after the ingestion of one hundred 4 mg tizanidine tablets. Pupils were not dilated and nystagmus was not present. The patient had marked respiratory depression with Cheyne-Stokes respiration.

➤*Treatment:* Gastric lavage and forced diuresis with furosemide and mannitol were instituted. The patient recovered several hours later without sequelae. Laboratory findings were normal.

Should overdosage occur, basic steps to ensure the adequacy of an airway and the monitoring of cardiovascular and respiratory systems should be undertaken. In general, symptoms resolve within 1 to 3 days following discontinuation of tizanidine and administration of appropriate therapy. Due to the similar mechanism of action, symptoms and management of tizanidine overdose are similar to those following clonidine overdose. For the most recent information concerning the management of overdose, contact a poison control center.

Patient Information

Patients should be advised of the limited clinical experience with tizanidine both in regard to duration of use and the higher doses required to reduce muscle tone.

Because of the possibility of tizanidine lowering blood pressure, patients should be warned about the risk of clinically significant orthostatic hypotension. In a single-dose study where blood pressure was monitored closely after dosing, two-thirds of patients treated with 8 mg of tizanidine had a 20% reduction in either the diastolic or systolic blood pressure (BP). The reduction was seen within 1 hour after dosing, peaked 2 to 3 hours after dosing and was associated, at times, with bradycardia, orthostatic hypotension, lightheadedness/dizziness and rarely syncope. The hypotensive effect is dose related and has been measured following single doses of greater than or equal to 2 mg. Patients should also be instructed that the sedation may be additive when tizanidine hydrochloride is taken in conjunction with drugs (baclofen, benzodiazepines) or substances (eg, alcohol) that act as CNS depressants.

Because of the possibility of sedation, patients should be warned about performing activities requiring alertness, such as driving a vehicle or operating machinery.

Patients should be advised of the change in the absorption profile of tizanidine if taken with food and the potential changes in efficacy and adverse effect profiles that may result.

Patients should be advised not to stop tizanidine suddenly as rebound hypertension and tachycardia may occur.

Tizanidine HCl should be used with caution where spasticity is utilized to sustain posture and balance in locomotion or whenever spasticity is utilized to obtain increased function.

DANTROLENE SODIUM

Rx	**Dantrium** (Procter & Gamble Pharm.)	**Capsules:** 25 mg	(Dantrium 25 mg 0149 0030). Lactose. Orange and light brown. In 100s, 500s and UD 100s.
		50 mg	(Dantrium 50 mg 0149 0031). Lactose. Orange and dark brown. In 100s.
		100 mg	(Dantrium 100 mg 0149 0033). Lactose. Orange and light brown. In 100s and UD 100s.
Rx	**Dantrium Intravenous** (Procter & Gamble Pharm.)	**Powder for Injection:** 20 mg/vial. (≈ 0.32 mg/ml after reconstitution)	With 3 g mannitol per vial. In 70 ml vials.

DANTROLENE SODIUM — ORAL

WARNING

Dantrolene has a potential for hepatotoxicity; do not use in conditions other than those recommended. Symptomatic hepatitis (fatal and nonfatal) has been reported at various dose levels of the drug. The incidence reported in patients taking up to 400 mg/day is much lower than in those taking doses of 800 mg or more per day. Even sporadic short courses of these higher dose levels within a treatment regimen markedly increased the risk of serious hepatic injury. Liver dysfunction as evidenced by blood chemical abnormalities alone (liver enzyme elevations) has been observed in patients exposed to dantrolene for varying periods of time. Overt hepatitis has occurred at varying intervals after initiation of therapy, but has been most frequently observed between the third and 12th month of therapy. The risk of hepatic injury appears to be greater in females, in patients over 35 years of age, and in patients taking other medication(s) in addition to dantrolene. Use dantrolene only in conjunction with appropriate monitoring of hepatic function including frequent determination of AST or ALT. If no observable benefit is derived from the administration of dantrolene after a total of 45 days, discontinue therapy. Prescribe the lowest possible effective dose for the individual patient.

Indications

➤*Chronic spasticity:* Controlling the manifestations of clinical spasticity resulting from upper motor neuron disorders (eg, spinal cord injury, stroke, cerebral palsy, or multiple sclerosis). It is of particular benefit to the patient whose functional rehabilitation has been retarded by the sequelae of spasticity. Such patients must have presumably reversible spasticity where relief of spasticity will aid in restoring residual function. Dantrolene is not indicated in the treatment of skeletal muscle spasm resulting from rheumatic disorders.

➤*Malignant hyperthermia:* Preoperatively, to prevent or attenuate the development of signs of malignant hyperthermia in known, or strongly suspected, malignant hyperthermia-susceptible patients who require anesthesia and/or surgery. Currently accepted clinical practices in the management of such patients must still be adhered to (careful monitoring for early signs of malignant hyperthermia, minimizing exposure to triggering mechanisms, and prompt use of IV dantrolene and indicated supportive measures should signs of malignant hyperthermia appear); see also the package insert for dantrolene IV.

Administer oral dantrolene following a malignant hyperthermic crisis to prevent recurrence of the signs of malignant hyperthermia.

➤*Unlabeled uses:* Exercise-induced muscle pain; neuroleptic malignant syndrome; heat stroke.

Administration and Dosage

➤*Approved by the FDA:* January 15, 1974.

➤*Chronic spasticity:* It is important that the dosage be titrated and individualized for maximum effect. The lowest dose compatible with optimal response is recommended.

In view of the potential for liver damage in long-term dantrolene use, stop therapy if benefits are not evident within 45 days.

Adults – The following gradual titration schedule is suggested. Some patients will not respond until higher daily dosage is achieved. Maintain each dosage level for 7 days to determine the patient's response. If no further benefit is observed at the next higher dose, decrease the dosage to the previous lower dose. Begin with 25 mg once daily for 7 days; then increase to 25 mg 3 times daily for 7 days; then increase to 50 mg 3 times daily for 7 days with a final dosage of 100 mg 3 times daily.

Therapy with a dose 4 times daily may be necessary for some individuals. Do not use doses higher than 100 mg 4 times daily.

Children – The following gradual titration schedule is suggested. Some patients will not respond until higher daily dosage is achieved. Maintain each dosage level for 7 days to determine the patient's response. If no further benefit is observed at the next higher dose, decrease the dosage to the previous lower dose. Start with 0.5 mg/kg once daily for 7 days; then increase to 0.5 mg/kg 3 times daily for 7 days; then increase to 1 mg/kg 3 times daily for 7 days with a final dosage of 2 mg/kg 3 times daily. Therapy with a dose 4 times daily may be necessary for some individuals.

Do not use doses higher than 100 mg 4 times daily.

➤*Malignant hyperthermia:*

Preoperatively – Administer 4 to 8 mg/kg/day of oral dantrolene in 3 or 4 divided doses for 1 or 2 days prior to surgery, with the last dose being given approximately 3 to 4 hours before scheduled surgery with a minimum of water.

This dosage will usually be associated with skeletal muscle weakness and sedation (sleepiness or drowsiness); adjustment can usually be made within the recommended dosage range to avoid incapacitation or excessive GI irritation (including nausea and/or vomiting).

Post-crisis follow-up – Oral dantrolene should also be administered following a malignant hyperthermia crisis, in doses of 4 to 8 mg/kg/day in 4 divided doses, for a 1- to 3-day period to prevent recurrence of the manifestations of malignant hyperthermia.

➤*Storage/Stability:* Avoid excessive heat (over 40°C [104°F]).

Actions

➤*Pharmacology:* In isolated nerve-muscle preparation, dantrolene has been shown to produce relaxation by affecting the contractile response of the skeletal muscle at a site beyond the myoneural junction, directly on the muscle itself. In skeletal muscle, dantrolene dissociates the excitation-contraction coupling, probably by interfering with the release of Ca^{++} from the sarcoplasmic reticulum. This effect appears to be more pronounced in fast muscle fibers as compared to slow ones, but generally affects both. A CNS effect occurs, with drowsiness, dizziness, and generalized weakness occasionally present. Although dantrolene does not appear to directly affect the CNS, the extent of its indirect effect is unknown.

Clinical experience in the management of fulminant human malignant hyperthermia, as well as experiments conducted in malignant hyperthermia-susceptible swine, have revealed that the administration of IV dantrolene, combined with indicated supportive measures, is effective in reversing the hypermetabolic process of malignant hyperthermia. Known differences between human and swine malignant hyperthermia are minor. The prophylactic administration of oral or IV dantrolene to malignant hyperthermia-susceptible swine will attenuate or prevent the development of signs of malignant hyperthermia in a manner dependent upon the dosage of dantrolene administered and the intensity of the malignant hyperthermia triggering stimulus. Limited clinical experience with the administration of oral dantrolene to patients judged malignant hyperthermia susceptible, when combined with clinical experience in the use of IV dantrolene for the treatment of malignant hyperthermia and data derived from the above cited animal model experiments, suggests that oral dantrolene will also attenuate or prevent the development of signs of human malignant hyperthermia, provided that currently accepted practices in the management of such patients are adhered to; IV dantrolene should also be available for use should the signs of malignant hyperthermia appear.

➤*Pharmacokinetics:* The absorption of dantrolene after oral administration in humans is incomplete and slow but consistent, and dose-related blood levels are obtained. The duration and intensity of skeletal muscle relaxation is related to the dosage and blood levels. The mean biologic half-life of dantrolene in adults is 8.7 hours after a 100 mg dose. Specific metabolic pathways in the degradation and elimination of dantrolene in human subjects have been established. Metabolic patterns are similar in adults and children. In addition to the parent compound, dantrolene, which is found in measurable amounts in blood and urine, the major metabolites noted in body fluids are the 5-hydroxy analog and the acetamido analog. Since dantrolene is probably metabolized by hepatic microsomal enzymes, enhancement of its metabolism by other drugs is possible. However, neither phenobarbital nor diazepam appears to affect dantrolene metabolism.

Contraindications

Active hepatic disease, such as hepatitis and cirrhosis; where spasticity is utilized to sustain upright posture and balance in locomotion or whenever spasticity is utilized to obtain or maintain increased function.

Warnings

➤*Long-term use:* Long-term safety has not been established. Chronic studies in rats, dogs, and monkeys at dosages higher than 30 mg/kg/day showed growth or weight depression and signs of hepatopathy and possible occlusion nephropathy, all of which were reversible upon cessation of treatment.

➤*Hepatotoxicity:* It is important to recognize that fatal and nonfatal liver disorders of an idiosyncratic or hypersensitivity type may occur with dantrolene therapy.

At the start of dantrolene therapy, it is desirable to do liver function studies (AST, ALT, alkaline phosphatase, total bilirubin) for a baseline or to establish whether there is preexisting liver disease. If baseline liver abnormalities exist and are confirmed, there is a clear possibility that the potential for dantrolene hepatoxicity could be enhanced, although such a possibility has not yet been established.

Perform liver function studies (eg, AST or ALT) at appropriate intervals during dantrolene therapy. If such studies reveal abnormal values, therapy should generally be discontinued. Consider reinitiation or continuation of therapy only where benefits of the drug have been of major importance to the patient. Some patients have revealed a return to normal laboratory values in the face of continued therapy while others have not.

If symptoms compatible with hepatitis, accompanied by abnormalities in liver function tests or jaundice appear, discontinue dantrolene. If caused by dantrolene and detected early, the abnormalities in liver function characteristically have reverted to normal when the drug was discontinued.

Dantrolene therapy has been reinstituted in a few patients who have developed clinical and/or laboratory evidence of hepatocellular injury. If such reinstitution of therapy is done, attempt it only in patients who clearly need dantrolene and only after previous symptoms and laboratory abnormalities have cleared. Hospitalize the patient and restart the drug in very small and gradually increasing doses. Perform laboratory monitoring frequently, and withdraw the drug immediately if there is any indication of recurrent liver involvement. Some patients have reacted with unmistakable signs of liver abnormality upon administration of a challenge dose, while others have not.

Use dantrolene with particular caution in females and in patients over 35 years of age in view of apparent greater likelihood of drug-induced, potentially fatal, hepatocellular disease in these groups.

➤*Carcinogenesis:* Sprague-Dawley female rats fed dantrolene for 18 months at dosage levels of 15, 30, and 60 mg/kg/day showed an increased incidence of benign and malignant mammary tumors compared with concur-

DANTROLENE SODIUM — ORAL

rent controls. At the highest dose level, there was an increase in the incidence of benign hepatic lymphatic neoplasms. In a 30-month study at the same dose levels also in Sprague-Dawley rats, dantrolene produced a decrease in the time of onset of mammary neoplasms. Female rats at the highest dose level showed an increased incidence of hepatic lymphangiomas and hepatic angiosarcomas.

The only drug-related effect seen in a 30-month study in Fischer-344 rats was a dose-related reduction in the time of onset of mammary and testicular tumors. A 24-month study in HaM/ICR mice revealed no evidence of carcinogenic activity. Carcinogenicity in humans cannot be fully excluded, so this possible risk of chronic administration must be weighed against the benefits of the drug (ie, after a brief trial) for the individual patient.

➤*Mutagenesis:* Dantrolene has produced positive results in the Ames *S. typhimurium* bacterial mutagenesis assay in the presence and absence of a liver-activating system.

➤*Pregnancy: Category C.* Dantrolene has been shown to be embryocidal in the rabbit and has been shown to decrease pup survival in the rat when given at doses 7 times the human oral dose. There are no adequate and well-controlled studies in pregnant women. Use dantrolene capsules during pregnancy only if the potential benefit justifies the potential risk to the fetus.

Labor and delivery – In 1 non-randomized open-label study, 21 term pregnant patients received prophylactic oral dantrolene 100 mg per day for 2 to 10 days prior to delivery. Dantrolene readily crossed the placenta with maternal and fetal whole blood levels approximately equal at delivery; neonatal levels then fell approximately 50% per day for 2 days before declining sharply. No neonatal respiratory and neuromuscular side effects were detected at low dose. More data, at higher doses, are needed before more definitive conclusions can be made.

➤*Lactation:* Do not use dantrolene in nursing mothers.

➤*Children:* The long-term safety of dantrolene in children under the age of 5 years of age has not been established. Because of the possibility that adverse effects of the drug could become apparent only after many years, a benefit-risk consideration of the long-term use of dantrolene is particularly important in children.

Precautions

➤*Special risk:* Use dantrolene with caution in patients with impaired pulmonary function, particularly those with obstructive pulmonary disease, and in patients with severely impaired cardiac function due to myocardial disease. Use with caution in patients with a history of liver disease or dysfunction.

➤*Hazardous tasks:* Caution patients against driving a motor vehicle or participating in hazardous occupations while taking dantrolene. Exercise caution in the concomitant administration of tranquilizing agents.

➤*Photosensitivity:* Dantrolene might possibly evoke a photosensitivity reaction; caution patients about exposure to sunlight while taking it.

Drug Interactions

Dantrolene Drug Interactions

Precipitant drug	Object drug*		Description
Dantrolene	CNS agents	↑	Drowsiness may occur with dantrolene therapy, and the concomitant administration of CNS depressants such as sedatives and tranquilizing agents may result in further drowsiness.
Dantrolene	Vecuronium	↑	Administration of dantrolene may potentiate vecuronium-induced neuromuscular block.
Dantrolene	Verapamil	↑	Hyperkalemia and myocardial depression occurred in one patient during concurrent use.
Clofibrate	Dantrolene	↓	Plasma protein binding of dantrolene may be reduced.
Estrogens	Dantrolene	↑	Although a definite drug interaction is not established, hepatotoxicity occurred more often in women older than 35 years of age receiving these agents concurrently.
Warfarin	Dantrolene	↓	Plasma protein binding of dantrolene may be reduced.

* ↑ = Object drug increased. ↓ = Object drug decreased.

Adverse Reactions

The most frequently occurring side effects of dantrolene have been diarrhea, dizziness, drowsiness, fatigue, general malaise, and weakness. These are generally transient, occurring early in treatment, and can often be obviated by beginning with a low dose and increasing dosage gradually until an optimal regimen is established. Diarrhea may be severe and may necessitate temporary withdrawal of dantrolene therapy. If diarrhea recurs upon readministration of dantrolene, therapy should probably be withdrawn permanently.

Other less frequent side effects, listed according to system are:

➤*Cardiovascular:* Erratic blood pressure; heart failure; phlebitis; tachycardia.

➤*CNS:* Alteration of taste; diplopia; drooling; headache; insomnia; lightheadedness; seizure; speech disturbance; visual disturbance.

➤*Dermatologic:* Abnormal hair growth; acne-like rash; eczematoid eruption; pruritus; sweating; urticaria.

➤*GI:* Abdominal cramps; anorexia; constipation, rarely progressing to signs of intestinal obstruction; gastric irritation; GI bleeding; nausea and/or vomiting; swallowing difficulty.

➤*GU:* Crystalluria; difficult erection; difficult urination and/or urinary retention; hematuria; increased urinary frequency; urinary incontinence and/or nocturia.

➤*Hematologic:* Aplastic anemia; leukopenia; lymphocytic lymphoma; thrombocytopenia.

➤*Hepatic:* Hepatitis.

➤*Hypersensitivity:* Anaphylaxis; pleural effusion with pericarditis.

➤*Musculoskeletal:* Backache; myalgia.

➤*Psychiatric:* Increased nervousness; mental confusion; mental depression.

➤*Respiratory:* Feeling of suffocation; respiratory depression.

➤*Special senses:* Excessive tearing.

➤*Miscellaneous:* Chills and fever. The published literature has included some reports of dantrolene use in patients with neuroleptic malignant syndrome (NMS). Dantrolene capsules are not indicated for the treatment of NMS and patients may expire despite treatment with dantrolene capsules.

Overdosage

➤*Symptoms:* Symptoms that may occur in case of overdose include, but are not limited to, muscular weakness and alterations in the state of consciousness (eg, lethargy, coma), vomiting, diarrhea, and crystalluria.

➤*Treatment:* For acute overdosage, employ general supportive measures along with immediate gastric lavage.

Administer IV fluids in fairly large quantities to avert the possibility of crystalluria. Maintain an adequate airway and keep artificial resuscitation equipment at hand. Institute electrocardiographic monitoring, and observe the patient carefully. To date, no experience has been reported with dialysis and its value in dantrolene overdosage is not known.

Patient Information

Caution patients against driving a motor vehicle or participating in hazardous occupations while taking dantrolene. Exercise caution in the concomitant administration of tranquilizing agents.

DANTROLENE SODIUM — INJECTION

WARNING

Dantrolene has a potential for hepatotoxicity. Do not use in conditions other than those recommended. The incidence of symptomatic hepatitis (fatal and nonfatal) reported in patients taking up to 400 mg/day is much lower than in those taking ≥ 800 mg/day. Even sporadic short courses of these higher dose levels within a treatment regimen markedly increased the risk of serious hepatic injury. Liver dysfunction, as evidenced by liver enzyme elevations, has been observed in patients exposed to the drug for varying periods of time. Overt hepatitis has been most frequently observed between the third and twelfth months of therapy. Risk of hepatic injury appears to be greater in females, in patients older than 35 years of age and in patients taking other medications in addition to dantrolene.

Monitor hepatic function, including frequent determinations of AST or ALT. If no observable benefit is derived from therapy after 45 days, discontinue use.

Use the lowest possible effective dose for each patient.

Indications

➤*Malignant hyperthermia:* Along with appropriate supportive measures, for the management of the fulminant hypermetabolism of skeletal muscle characteristic of malignant hyperthermia crises in patients of all ages. Dantrolene IV should be administered by continuous rapid IV push as soon as the malignant hyperthermia reaction is recognized (ie, tachycardia, tachypnea, central venous desaturation, hypercarbia, metabolic acidosis, skeletal muscle rigidity, increased utilization of anesthesia circuit carbon dioxide absorber, cyanosis and mottling of the skin, and, in many cases, fever).

Dantrolene IV is also indicated preoperatively, and sometimes postoperatively, to prevent or attenuate the development of clinical and laboratory signs of malignant hyperthermia in individuals judged to be malignant hyperthermia-susceptible.

➤*Unlabeled uses:* Exercise-induced muscle pain; neuroleptic malignant syndrome; heat stroke.

Administration and Dosage

As soon as the malignant hyperthermia reaction is recognized, all anesthetic agents should be discontinued; the administration of 100% oxygen is recommended. Dantrolene IV should be administered by continuous rapid IV push beginning at a minimum dose of 1 mg/kg, and continuing until symptoms subside or the maximum cumulative dose of 10 mg/kg has been reached.

If the physiologic and metabolic abnormalities reappear, the regimen may be repeated. It is important to note that administration of dantrolene IV should be continuous until symptoms subside. The effective dose to reverse the crisis is directly dependent upon the individual's degree of susceptibility to malignant hyperthermia, the amount and time of exposure to the triggering agent, and the time elapsed between onset of the crisis and initiation of treatment.

➤*Children:* Experience to date indicates that the dose of dantrolene IV for children is the same as for adults.

➤*Preoperatively:* May be administered preoperatively to patients judged malignant hyperthermia-susceptible as part of the overall patient management to prevent or attenuate the development of clinical and laboratory signs of malignant hyperthermia.

➤*Dantrolene IV:* The recommended prophylactic dose of dantrolene IV is 2.5 mg/kg, starting approximately 1¼ hours before anticipated anesthesia and infused over approximately 1 hour. This dose should prevent or attenuate the development of clinical and laboratory signs of malignant hyperthermia provided that the usual precautions, such as avoidance of established malignant hyperthermia-triggering agents, are followed.

Additional dantrolene IV may be indicated during anesthesia and surgery because of the appearance of early clinical and/or blood gas signs of malignant hyperthermia or because of prolonged surgery (see Pharmacology and Warnings). Additional doses must be individualized.

➤*Post-crisis follow-up:* Dantrolene capsules, 4 to 8 mg/kg/day, in 4 divided doses should be administered for 1 to 3 days following a malignant hyperthermia crisis to prevent recurrence of the manifestations of malignant hyperthermia.

IV dantrolene may be used postoperatively to prevent or attenuate the recurrence of signs of malignant hyperthermia when oral dantrolene administration is not practical. The IV dose of dantrolene in the postoperative period must be individualized, starting with greater than or equal to 1 mg/kg as the clinical situation dictates.

➤*Preparation:* Each vial of dantrolene IV should be reconstituted by adding 60 mL of sterile water for injection USP (without a bacteriostatic agent), and the vial shaken until the solution is clear. The 5% Dextrose Injection USP, 0.9% Sodium Chloride Injection USP, and other acidic solutions are not compatible with dantrolene IV and should not be used. The contents of the vial must be protected from direct light and used within 6 hours after reconstitution. Store reconstituted solutions at controlled room temperature (15° to 30°C; 59° to 86°F). Reconstituted dantrolene IV should not be transferred to large glass bottles for prophylactic infusion due to precipitate formation observed with the use of some glass bottles as reservoirs. For prophylactic infusion, the required number of individual vials of dantrolene IV should be reconstituted as outlined above. The contents of individual vials are then transferred to a larger volume sterile IV plastic bag. However, it is recommended that the prepared infusion be inspected carefully for cloudiness and/or precipitation prior to dispensing and administration. Such solutions should not be used. While stable for 6 hours, it is recommended that the infusion be prepared immediately prior to the anticipated dosage administration time. Parenteral drug products should be inspected visually for particulate matter and discoloration prior to administration.

➤*Storage/Stability:* Store unreconstituted product at controlled room temperature (15°C to 30°C; 59°F to 86°F) and avoid prolonged exposure to light.

Actions

➤*Pharmacology:* In isolated nerve-muscle preparation, dantrolene has been shown to produce relaxation by affecting the contractile response of the muscle at a site beyond the myoneural junction. In skeletal muscle, dantrolene dissociates the excitation-contraction coupling, probably by interfering with the release of Ca^{++} from the sarcoplasmic reticulum. The administration of IV dantrolene to human volunteers is associated with loss of grip strength and weakness in the legs, as well as subjective CNS complaints (see Patient Information). Information concerning the passage of dantrolene across the blood-brain barrier is not available.

In the anesthetic-induced malignant hyperthermia syndrome, evidence points to an intrinsic abnormality of skeletal muscle tissue. In affected humans, it has been postulated that "triggering agents" (eg, general anesthetics and depolarizing neuromuscular blocking agents) produce a change within the cell which results in an elevated myoplasmic calcium. This elevated myoplasmic calcium activates acute cellular catabolic processes that cascade to the malignant hyperthermia crisis.

It is hypothesized that addition of dantrolene to the "triggered" malignant hyperthermic muscle cell re-establishes a normal level of ionized calcium in the myoplasm. Inhibition of calcium release from the sarcoplasmic reticulum by dantrolene re-establishes the myoplasmic calcium equilibrium, increasing the percentage of bound calcium. In this way, physiologic, metabolic, and biochemical changes associated with the malignant hyperthermia crisis may be reversed or attenuated. Experimental results in malignant hyperthermia-susceptible swine show that prophylactic administration of IV or oral dantrolene prevents or attenuates the development of vital sign and blood gas changes characteristic of malignant hyperthermia in a dose-related manner. The efficacy of IV dantrolene in the treatment of human and porcine malignant hyperthermia crisis, when considered along with prophylactic experiments in malignant hyperthermia-susceptible swine, lends support to prophylactic use of oral or IV dantrolene in malignant hyperthermia-susceptible humans. When prophylactic IV dantrolene is administered as directed, whole blood concentrations remain at a near steady state level for greater than or equal to 3 hours after the infusion is completed. Clinical experience has shown that early vital sign and/or blood gas changes characteristic of malignant hyperthermia may appear during or after anesthesia and surgery despite the prophylactic use of dantrolene and adherence to currently accepted patient management practices. These signs are compatible with attenuated malignant hyperthermia and respond to the administration of additional IV dantrolene (see Administration and Dosage). The administration of the recommended prophylactic dose of IV dantrolene to healthy volunteers was not associated with clinically significant cardiorespiratory changes.

➤*Pharmacokinetics:* Specific metabolic pathways for the degradation and elimination of dantrolene in humans have been established. Dantrolene is found in measurable amounts in blood and urine. Its major metabolites in body fluids are 5-hydroxy dantrolene and an acetylamino metabolite of dantrolene. Another metabolite with an unknown structure appears related to the latter. Dantrolene may also undergo hydrolysis and subsequent oxidation forming nitrophenylfuroic acid.

The mean biologic half-life of dantrolene after IV administration is variable, between 4 to 8 hours under most experimental conditions. Based on assays of whole blood and plasma, slightly greater amounts of dantrolene are associated with red blood cells than with the plasma fraction of blood. Significant amounts of dantrolene are bound to plasma proteins, mostly albumin, and this binding is readily reversible.

Contraindications

None.

Warnings

➤*Malignant hyperthermia:* The use of dantrolene IV in the management of malignant hyperthermia crisis is not a substitute for previously known supportive measures. These measures must be individualized, but it will usually be necessary to discontinue the suspect triggering agents, attend to increased oxygen requirements, manage the metabolic acidosis, institute cooling when necessary, monitor urinary output, and monitor for electrolyte imbalance.

Since the effect of disease state and other drugs on dantrolene-related skeletal muscle weakness, including possible respiratory depression, cannot be predicted, patients who receive IV dantrolene preoperatively should have vital signs monitored.

If patients judged malignant hyperthermia-susceptible are administered IV or oral dantrolene preoperatively, anesthetic preparation must still follow a standard malignant hyperthermia-susceptible regimen, including the avoidance of known triggering agents. Monitoring for early clinical and metabolic signs of malignant hyperthermia is indicated because attenuation of malignant hyperthermia, rather than prevention, is possible. These signs usually call for the administration of additional IV dantrolene.

➤*Hepatotoxicity:* See the Warning box for more information.

DANTROLENE SODIUM — INJECTION

➤*Carcinogenesis:* Sprague-Dawley female rats fed dantrolene for 18 months at dosage levels of 15, 30, and 60 mg/kg/day showed an increased incidence of benign and malignant mammary tumors compared with concurrent controls. At the highest dose levels, there was an increase in the incidence of benign hepatic lymphatic neoplasms. In a 30-month study at the same dose levels also in Sprague-Dawley rats, dantrolene produced a decrease in the time of onset of mammary neoplasms. Female rats at the highest dose level showed an increased incidence of hepatic lymphangiomas and hepatic angiosarcomas.

The only drug-related effect seen in a 30-month study in Fischer-344 rats was a dose-related reduction in the time of onset of mammary and testicular tumors. A 24-month study in HaM/ICR mice revealed no evidence of carcinogenic activity.

➤*Mutagenesis:* Dantrolene has produced positive results in the Ames *S. typhimurium* bacterial mutagenesis assay in the presence and absence of a liver activating system.

➤*Elderly:* Clinical studies of dantrolene sodium intravenous did not include sufficient numbers of subjects aged 65 and over to determine whether they respond differently from younger subjects. Other reported clinical experience has not identified differences in response between the elderly and younger patients. In general, dose selection for an elderly patient should be cautious reflecting the greater frequency of decreased hepatic, renal, or cardiac function, and of concomitant disease or other drug therapy.

➤*Pregnancy: Category C.* Dantrolene has been shown to be embryocidal in the rabbit and has been shown to decrease pup survival in the rat when given at doses 7 times the human oral dose. There are no adequate and well-controlled studies in pregnant women. Dantrolene IV should be used during pregnancy only if the potential benefit justifies the potential risk to the fetus.

Labor and delivery – In one uncontrolled study, 100 mg/day of prophylactic oral dantrolene was administered to term pregnant patients awaiting labor and delivery. Dantrolene readily crossed the placenta, with maternal and fetal whole blood levels approximately equal at delivery; neonatal levels then fell approximately 50% per day for 2 days before declining sharply. No neonatal respiratory and neuromuscular side effects were detected at low dose. More data, at higher doses, are needed before more definitive conclusions can be made.

Precautions

➤*Extravasation:* Care must be taken to prevent extravasation of dantrolene solution into the surrounding tissues due to the high pH of the IV formulation.

➤*Mannitol:* When mannitol is used for prevention or treatment of late renal complications of malignant hyperthermia, the 3 g of mannitol needed to dissolve each 20 mg vial of IV dantrolene should be taken into consideration.

Drug Interactions

Dantrolene Drug Interactions

Precipitant drug	Object drug*		Description
Dantrolene	Verapamil	⬆	Hyperkalemia and myocardial depression occurred in one patient during concurrent use.
Dantrolene	Vecuronium	⬆	Administration of dantrolene may potentiate vecuronium-induced neuromuscular block.
Clofibrate	Dantrolene	⬇	Plasma protein binding of dantrolene may be reduced.
Estrogens	Dantrolene	⬆	Although a definite drug interaction is not established, hepatotoxicity occurred more often in women older than 35 years of age receiving these agents concurrently.
Warfarin	Dantrolene	⬇	Plasma protein binding of dantrolene may be reduced.

* ⬆ = Object drug increased. ⬇ = Object drug decreased.

Adverse Reactions

There have been occasional reports of death following malignant hyperthermia crisis even when treated with IV dantrolene; incidence figures are not available (the predantrolene mortality of malignant hyperthermia crisis was approximately 50%). Most of these deaths can be accounted for by late recognition, delayed treatment, inadequate dosage, lack of supportive therapy, intercurrent disease, and/or the development of delayed complications such as renal failure or disseminated intravascular coagulopathy. In some cases there are insufficient data to completely rule out therapeutic failure of dantrolene.

There are rare reports of fatality in malignant hyperthermia crisis, despite initial satisfactory response to IV dantrolene, which involves patients who could not be weaned from dantrolene after initial treatment.

The administration of IV dantrolene to human volunteers is associated with loss of grip strength and weakness in the legs, as well as drowsiness and dizziness.

The following adverse reactions are in approximate order of severity:

- There are rare reports of pulmonary edema developing during the treatment of malignant hyperthermia crisis in which the diluent volume and mannitol needed to deliver IV dantrolene possibly contributed.
- There have been reports of thrombophlebitis following administration of IV dantrolene; actual incidence figures are not available. There have been rare reports of urticaria and erythema possibly associated with the administration of IV dantrolene.
- There has been one case of anaphylaxis.

None of the serious reactions occasionally reported with long-term oral dantrolene use, such as hepatitis, seizures, and pleural effusion with pericarditis, have been reasonably associated with short-term dantrolene IV therapy.

The following events have been reported in patients receiving oral dantrolene: Aplastic anemia, leukopenia, lymphocytic lymphoma, and heart failure.

The published literature has included some reports of dantrolene use in patients with neuroleptic malignant syndrome (NMS). Dantrolene IV is not indicated for the treatment of NMS and patients may expire despite treatment with dantrolene IV.

Overdosage

➤*Symptoms:* Symptoms that may occur in case of overdose include, but are not limited to, muscular weakness and alterations in the state of consciousness (eg, lethargy, coma), vomiting, diarrhea, and crystalluria.

➤*Treatment:* For acute overdosage, general supportive measures should be employed.

IV fluids should be administered in fairly large quantities to avert the possibility of crystalluria. An adequate airway should be maintained and artificial resuscitation equipment should be at hand. Electrocardiographic monitoring should be instituted, and the patient carefully observed. The value of dialysis in dantrolene overdose is not known.

Patient Information

Based upon data in human volunteers, it will sometimes be appropriate to tell patients who receive dantrolene IV that decrease in grip strength and weakness of leg muscles, especially walking down stairs, can be expected postoperatively. In addition, symptoms such as "lightheadedness" may be noted. Since some of these symptoms may persist for up to 48 hours, patients must not operate an automobile or engage in other hazardous activity during this time. Caution is also indicated at meals on the day of administration because difficulty swallowing and choking has been reported. Caution should be exercised in the concomitant administration of tranquilizing agents.

SKELETAL MUSCLE RELAXANT COMBINATIONS

Rx	**Methocarbamol w/ASA** (Various, eg, Moore, Par)	**Tablets**: 400 mg methocarbamol and 325 mg aspirin. *Dose: 2 tablets 4 times daily*	In 15s, 30s, 40s, 100s, 500s and 1000s.
Rx	**Carisoprodol Compound** (Various, eg, Moore, Rugby)	**Tablets**: 200 mg carisoprodol and 325 mg aspirin. *Dose: 1 or 2 tablets 4 times daily*	In 15s, 30s, 40s, 100s, 500s and 1000s.
Rx	**Sodol Compound** (Major)		In 100s and 500s.
Rx	**Soma Compound** (Wallace)		(Soma C Wallace-2103). White and orange. In 100s, 500s and UD 500s.
c-iii	**Carisoprodol, Aspirin, and Codeine Phosphate** (Various, eg, Amide)	**Tablets**: 200 mg carisoprodol, 325 mg aspirin, and 16 mg codeine phosphate. *Dose: 1 or 2 tablets 4 times daily*	In 100s and 500s.
c-iii	**Soma Compound w/Codeine** (Medpointe)		(Soma CC Wallace-2403). White and yellow. In 100s.[1]
Rx	**Flexaphen** (Trimen)	**Capsules**: 250 mg chlorzoxazone and 300 mg acetaminophen. *Dose: 2 capsules 4 times daily*	Tan. In 100s.
Rx	**Lobac** (Seatrace)	**Capsules**: 200 mg salicylamide, 20 mg phenyltoloxamine and 300 mg acetaminophen. *Dose: 2 capsules 4 times daily*	(Seatrace). Eggshell. In 24s and 100s.
Rx	**Norgesic** (3M Pharm)	**Tablets**: 25 mg orphenadrine citrate, 385 mg aspirin and 30 mg caffeine. *Dose: 1 or 2 tablets 3 or 4 times daily*	(NORGESIC 3M). Green, white and yellow. In 100s, 500s and UD 100s.
Rx	**Orphengesic** (Par)		Lactose. (Par 472). Bilayered white/green. In 100s and 500s.
Rx	**Orphengesic Forte** (Par)	**Tablets**: 50 mg orphenadrine citrate, 770 mg aspirin and 60 mg caffeine. *Dose: ½ or 1 tablet 3 or 4 times daily*	Lactose. (Par 473). Bilayered white/green, capsule shape, scored. In 100s and 500s.

[1] With sodium metabisulfite.

SKELETAL MUSCLE RELAXANT COMBINATIONS — ORAL

Indications

➤*Uses:* The methocarbamol and aspirin combinations and the carisoprodol and aspirin (with or without codeine) combinations are indicated as adjuncts to rest, physical therapy and other measures for relief of discomfort associated with acute, painful musculoskeletal conditions. The other combinations are classified as *"probably effective"* for this indication. Components of these combinations include:

MUSCLE RELAXANTS – Methocarbamol; Chlorzoxazone; Carisoprodol; Orphenadrine Citrate; (see individual monographs).

ANALGESICS – Acetaminophen; Aspirin; Codeine; (see individual monographs).

CAFFEINE – Caffeine (see individual monograph), used as a CNS stimulant, also has minor analgesic activity.

Precautions

➤*Sulfite sensitivity:* Some of these products contain sulfites, which may cause allergic-type reactions (eg, hives, itching, wheezing, anaphylaxis) in certain susceptible people. Although the overall prevalence of sulfite sensitivity in the general population is probably low, it is seen more frequently in asthmatics or in atopic nonasthmatic people. Specific products containing sulfites are identified in the product listings.

ANTIPARKINSON AGENTS

➤*Parkinson's Disease:* Parkinsonism is a neurological disease with a variety of origins characterized by tremor, rigidity, akinesia, and disorders of posture and equilibrium. The onset is slow and progressive with symptoms advancing over months to years.

Although the biochemical basis of parkinsonism is complex, the primary defect appears to be an imbalance of neurotransmitters (ie, a relative excess of acetylcholine and a deficiency/absence of dopamine in the basal ganglia). Other central neurotransmitters may have some modifying influence on these primary substances. This defect may be part of a more generalized, structural, and enzymatic defect.

Currently, therapy for Parkinson's disease is palliative, as there is no cure for this disease. The goal of therapy is to provide maximum relief from the symptoms and to attempt to maintain the independence and mobility of the patient.

Drug therapy of Parkinson's disease is aimed at correcting or modifying these neurotransmitter defects by inhibiting the effects of acetylcholine or enhancing the effects of dopamine.

➤*Anticholinergic agents:* Centrally-acting anticholinergics tend to diminish the characteristic tremor. Patients with minimal involvement who are functioning relatively well may not require medication. However, as the disease progresses, the anticholinergics may be considered.

➤*Dopaminergic agents:* Dopamine deficiency appears to be the central feature of the pathogenesis of parkinsonism. **Levodopa**, the immediate precursor of dopamine, directly increases dopamine content in the brain; it is currently the most effective treatment for parkinsonism. Other drugs are available that also affect the dopamine content of the brain: **Bromocriptine** and **pergolide** directly stimulate dopamine receptors. Pergolide is 10 to 1000 times more potent than bromocriptine on a milligram per milligram basis; **amantadine** may increase dopamine at the receptor either by releasing intact striatal dopamine stores or by blocking neuronal dopamine reuptake; **selegiline** increases dopaminergic activity through inhibition of monoamine oxidase type B; however, other mechanisms may exist such as interference of dopamine reuptake at the synapse.

Levodopa is used for symptomatic patients with moderate disabilities; therapy is usually initiated with a combination of levodopa and carbidopa (a dopa decarboxylase inhibitor that prevents peripheral metabolism of levodopa). Unfortunately, the response to levodopa gradually diminishes after 2 to 5 years in most patients, at which time the dopaminergic agonists, bromocriptine or pergolide, selegiline, or amantadine may be added to the drug regimen. Amantadine may also be used in patients with minimal involvement when the patients cannot tolerate an anticholinergic drug.

The table below summarizes the drug therapy available for parkinsonism:

Drug Therapy for Parkinsonism

	Indications					
Drugs	Postencephalitic	Arteriosclerotic	Idiopathic	Drug/chemical induced	Adjunct to Levodopa/Carbidopa	Usual daily dose range (mg)
Anticholinergics						
Benztropine	✓	✓	✓	✓		0.5-6.5
Biperiden	✓	✓	✓	✓		2-8
Diphenhydramine	✓	✓	✓	✓		10-400
Ethopropazine	✓	✓	✓	✓		50-600
Procyclidine	✓	✓	✓	✓		7.5-20
Trihexyphenidyl	✓	✓	✓	✓	✓	1-15
Dopaminergic Agents						
Amantadine	✓	✓	✓	✓		200-400
Bromocriptine	✓		✓			12.5-100
Carbidopa/Levodopa	✓		✓	✓[1]		10/100- 200/2000
Levodopa	✓	✓	✓	✓[1]		500-8000
Pergolide					✓	1-5
Selegiline					✓	10

[1] Not effective in drug-induced extrapyramidal symptoms.

Indications

Adjunctive therapy in all forms of parkinsonism (postencephalitic, arteriosclerotic and idiopathic) and in the control of drug-induced extrapyramidal disorders. Refer to individual drug monographs for specific indications of individual agents.

Administration and Dosage

Dosage depends upon the age of the patient, etiology of the disease, and individual responsiveness. The dosage required for treatment of drug-induced extrapyramidal symptoms will depend on the severity of the side effects. Maintain flexible dosage to permit individualized dosing. In general, younger and postencephalitic patients require and tolerate somewhat higher doses than older patients and those with arteriosclerotic or idiopathic-type parkinsonism.

Give before or after meals, as determined by patient's reaction. Postencephalitic patients (more prone to excessive salivation) may prefer to take it after meals and may, in addition, require small amounts of atropine. If the mouth dries excessively, take before meals, unless it causes nausea. If taken after meals, thirst can be allayed by mint candies, chewing gum, or water.

Actions

➤*Pharmacology:* The anticholinergic agents, although generally less effective than levodopa, are useful in the treatment of all forms of parkinsonism: Postencephalitic, arteriosclerotic, idiopathic, and drug-induced extrapyramidal symptoms. They reduce the incidence and severity of akinesia, rigidity, and tremor by ≈ 20%; secondary symptoms such as drooling are also reduced. In addition to suppressing central cholinergic activity, these agents may also inhibit the reuptake and storage of dopamine at central dopamine receptors, thereby prolonging the action of dopamine.

The naturally occurring belladonna alkaloids (atropine, scopolamine, hyoscyamine) are active anticholinergic agents; however, they have largely been replaced by synthetic agents (eg, benztropine, trihexyphenidyl) with a more selective CNS activity. Peripheral anticholinergic side effects (eg, urinary retention, tachycardia, constipation) frequently limit the size of dosages utilized.

Antihistamines (eg, diphenhydramine) with central anticholinergic effects are also used; they may have a lower incidence of peripheral side effects than the belladonna alkaloids or synthetic derivatives. These agents are generally better tolerated by elderly patients. Some antihistamines provide mild antiparkinson effects, and are useful for initiating therapy in patients with minimal symptoms. Because of their sedative effects, the antihistamines may be useful in certain patients with insomnia.

In spite of limited efficacy, anticholinergics are useful in mild cases of Parkinson's disease where risks and demands of levodopa therapy are not warranted.

➤*Pharmacokinetics:* Little pharmacokinetic data are available for these agents. The following table lists some of the available parameters.

Various Antiparkinson Anticholinergic Pharmacokinetic Parameters

Anticholinergic	Time to peak concentration (hrs)	Peak concentration (mcg/L)	Half-life (hrs)	Oral bioavailability (%)
Benztropine[1]				
Biperiden	1-1.5	4-5	18.4-24.3	29
Diphenhydramine	2-4	65-90	4-15	50-72
Procyclidine	1.1-2	80	11.5-12.6	52-97
Trihexyphenidyl	1-1.3	87.2	5.6-10.2	≈ 100

[1] No data available.

Contraindications

Hypersensitivity to any component; glaucoma, particularly angle-closure glaucoma (simple type glaucomas do not appear to be adversely affected); pyloric or duodenal obstruction; stenosing peptic ulcers; prostatic hypertrophy or bladder neck obstructions; achalasia (megaesophagus); myasthenia gravis; megacolon.

➤*Benztropine:* Children < 3 years of age; use with caution in older children.

Warnings

➤*Ophthalmic:* Incipient narrow-angle glaucoma may be precipitated by these drugs. Perform gonioscopy and closely monitor intraocular pressures at regular intervals.

➤*Elderly:* Geriatric patients, particularly > 60 years of age, frequently develop increased sensitivity to anticholinergic drugs and require strict dosage regulation. Occasionally, mental confusion and disorientation may occur; agitation, hallucinations, and psychotic-like symptoms may develop.

➤*Pregnancy: Category C.* Safety for use during pregnancy has not been established. Use only when clearly needed and when the potential benefits outweigh the potential hazards to the fetus.

➤*Lactation:* Safety for use in the nursing mother has not been established. An inhibitory effect on lactation may occur. Although infants are particularly sensitive to anticholinergic agents, no adverse effects have been reported in nursing infants whose mothers were taking atropine.

➤*Children:* Safety and efficacy for use in children have not been established.

Precautions

➤*Concomitant conditions:* Use caution in patients with tachycardia, cardiac arrhythmias, hypertension, hypotension, prostatic hypertrophy (particularly in the elderly), or any tendency toward urinary retention, liver or kidney disorders, and obstructive disease of the GI or GU tract.

➤*CNS:* When used to treat extrapyramidal reactions resulting from phenothiazines in psychiatric patients, antiparkinson agents may exacerbate mental symptoms and precipitate a toxic psychosis. The possibility of antiparkinson agents masking the development of persistent extrapyramidal symptoms with prolonged phenothiazine therapy has not been investigated. Whether to administer prophylactic anticholinergics to prevent drug-induced extrapyramidal effects is controversial.

In addition, 19% to 30% of patients given anticholinergics develop depression, confusion, delusions, or hallucinations. Also, **benztropine** given in large doses or to susceptible patients may cause weakness and inability to move particular muscle groups. Dosage may have to be adjusted.

Tardive dyskinesia – Tardive dyskinesia may appear in some patients on long-term therapy with phenothiazines and related agents, or may occur after therapy has been discontinued. Antiparkinson agents do not alleviate the symptoms of tardive dyskinesia and, in some instances, may aggravate such symptoms.

➤*Heat illness:* Give with caution during hot weather, especially when given concomitantly with other atropine-like drugs to the elderly, the chronically ill, alcoholics, those who have CNS disease, and those who work in a hot environment. Anhidrosis may occur more readily when some disturbance of sweating already exists. Decrease dosage so that the ability to maintain body heat equilibrium by perspiration is not impaired. Severe anhidrosis and fatal hyperthermia have occurred.

➤*Dry mouth:* If dry mouth is so severe that there is difficulty in swallowing or speaking, or if loss of appetite and weight occurs, reduce dosage or discontinue the drug temporarily.

➤*Abuse potential:* Some patients may use these agents for mood elevations or psychedelic experiences. Cannabinoids, barbiturates, opiates, and alcohol may have additive effects with anticholinergics. It is important to be aware of this potential abuse situation.

➤*Hazardous tasks:* May impair mental or physical abilities; patients should observe caution while driving or performing other tasks requiring alertness.

Drug Interactions

Anticholinergic Drug Interactions

Precipitant drug	Object drug*		Description
Amantadine	Anticholinergics	⬆	Amantadine and anticholinergic coadministration may result in an increased incidence of anticholinergic side effects. These effects disappear when the anticholinergic dose is reduced.
Anticholinergics	Digoxin	⬆	Digoxin serum levels may be increased by anticholinergics when digoxin is administered as a slow dissolution oral tablet.
Anticholinergics	Haloperidol	⬇	Haloperidol and anticholinergic coadministration may result in worsening of schizophrenic symptoms, decreased haloperidol serum concentrations, and development of tardive dyskinesia.
Anticholinergics	Levodopa	⬇	Anticholinergics may decrease gastric motility resulting in increased gastric deactivation of levodopa and decreased intestinal absorption, possibly leading to a reduction in levodopa's efficacy. Other reports refute these findings.
Anticholinergics	Phenothiazines	⬇	The pharmacologic/therapeutic actions of phenothiazines may be reduced by concurrent anticholinergics. An increase in the incidence of anticholinergic side effects has occurred.
Phenothiazines	Anticholinergics	⬆	

* ⬆ = Object drug increased. ⬇ = Object drug decreased.

Adverse Reactions

➤*Cardiovascular:* Tachycardia; palpitations; hypotension; postural hypotension; mild bradycardia.

➤*CNS:* Disorientation; confusion; memory loss; hallucinations; psychoses; agitation; nervousness; delusions; delirium; paranoia; euphoria; excitement; lightheadedness; dizziness; headache; listlessness; depression; drowsiness; weakness; giddiness; paresthesia; heaviness of the limbs.

➤*GI:* Dry mouth; acute suppurative parotitis; nausea; vomiting; epigastric distress; constipation; dilation of the colon; paralytic ileus; development of duodenal ulcer.

➤*Hypersensitivity:* Skin rash; urticaria; other dermatoses.

➤*Musculoskeletal:* Muscular weakness; muscular cramping.

➤*Ophthalmic:* Blurred vision; mydriasis; diplopia; increased intraocular tension; angle-closure glaucoma; dilation of pupils.

➤*Renal:* Urinary retention; urinary hesitancy; dysuria.

➤*Miscellaneous:* Elevated temperature; flushing; numbness of fingers; decreased sweating, hyperthermia, heat stroke (see Precautions); difficulty in achieving or maintaining an erection.

Overdosage

➤*Symptoms:* Characterized by the adverse reactions and may also include the following: Circulatory collapse; cardiac arrest; respiratory depression or arrest; CNS depression preceded or followed by stimulation; intensification of mental symptoms or toxic psychosis in mentally ill patients treated with neuroleptic drugs (eg, phenothiazines); shock; coma; stupor; seizures; convulsions; ataxia; anxiety; incoherence; hyperactivity; combativeness; anhidrosis; hyperpyrexia; fever; hot, dry, flushed skin; dry mucous membranes; dysphagia; foul-smelling breath; decreased bowel sounds; dilated and sluggish pupils.

➤*Treatment:* Immediately following acute ingestion, remove remaining drug from stomach by inducing emesis or by gastric lavage (contraindicated in precomatose, convulsive or psychotic states). Activated charcoal is an effective adsorbent.

Treatment of overdosage is symptomatic. To relieve the peripheral effects, 5 mg of pilocarpine may be given orally at repeated intervals.

Artificial respiration and oxygen therapy may be needed for respiratory depression. A short-acting barbiturate or diazepam may be used for CNS excitement or convulsions; use with caution to avoid subsequent depression; institute supportive care for depression. Urinary retention may require catheterization. Hyperpyrexia is best treated with alcohol sponges, ice bags, or other cold applications. To counteract mydriasis and cycloplegia, a local miotic may be used. Darken room for photophobia. Treat circulatory collapse with fluids and vasopressors. The relapse intervals lengthen as the anticholinergic agent is metabolized; observe patient for 8 to 12 hours after last relapse.

Physostigmine salicylate reverses most cardiovascular and CNS effects of overdosage. In *adults,* 1 to 2 mg IM or IV given slowly (no more than 1 mg/min) is effective. In *children,* start with 0.02 mg/kg IM or by slow IV injection (no more than 0.5 mg/min). If necessary, repeat at 5- to 10-minute intervals until a therapeutic effect or a maximum dose of 2 mg is attained. Avoid rapid injection to reduce the possibility of physostigmine-induced convulsions. Give physostigmine cautiously. It can precipitate seizures, cholinergic crisis, bradyarrhythmias, and asystole. Use in a setting where advanced life support is available.

Patient Information

If GI upset occurs, may be taken with food.

May cause drowsiness, dizziness, or blurred vision; observe caution while driving or performing other tasks requiring alertness until response to drug is known.

Avoid alcohol and other CNS depressants.

May cause dry mouth; sucking hard candy, adequate fluid intake, or good oral hygiene may relieve this symptom. Difficult urination or constipation may occur; constipation may be relieved by use of stool softeners. Notify physician if effects persist.

Notify physician if rapid or pounding heartbeat, confusion, eye pain or rash occurs.

Use caution in hot weather. This medication may increase susceptibility to heat stroke.

BELLADONNA ALKALOIDS

Refer to the general discussion in the Antiparkinson Agents introduction. Prescribing information begins in the Antiparkinson Agent Anticholinergics group monograph. For complete prescribing information on the belladonna alkaloids (atropine, scopolamine HBr, hyoscyamine sulfate and levorotatory alkaloids of belladonna) see Gastrointestinal Anticholinergics/Antispasmodics monograph.

BENZTROPINE MESYLATE

Rx	**Benztropine Mesylate** (Various, eg, Harber, Moore, Par, Parmed, Rugby)	**Tablets:** 0.5 mg	In 100s and UD 100s.
Rx	**Cogentin** (MSD)		(MSD 21). White, scored. In 100s.
Rx	**Benztropine Mesylate** (Various, eg, Goldline, Moore, Purepac, Rugby, Vangard)	**Tablets:** 1 mg	In 100s, 1000s and UD 100s.
Rx	**Benztropine Mesylate** (Various, eg, Goldline, Moore, Purepac, Rugby, Vangard)	**Tablets:** 2 mg	In 100s, 1000s and UD 100s.
Rx	**Cogentin** (MSD)	**Injection:** 1 mg/ml	In 2 ml amps.

BENZTROPINE MESYLATE — ORAL

Refer to the general discussion in the Antiparkinson Agents introduction. Complete and comparative prescribing information begins in the Antiparkinson Agent Anticholinergics group monograph.

Indications

➤*Extrapyramidal disorders:* Useful also in the control of extrapyramidal disorders (except tardive dyskinesia; antiparkinsonism agents do not alleviate the symptoms of tardive dyskinesia and, in some instances, may aggravate them. Benztropine is not recommended for use in patients with tardive dyskinesia.) due to neuroleptic drugs (eg, phenothiazines).

➤*Parkinsonism:* For use as an adjunct in the therapy of all forms of parkinsonism.

Administration and Dosage

Because of cumulative action, initiate therapy with a low dose; increase gradually at 5- or 6-day intervals to the smallest amount necessary for optimal relief. Make increases in increments of 0.5 mg, to a maximum of 6 mg, or until optimal results are obtained without excessive adverse reactions.

➤*Postencephalitic and idiopathic parkinsonism:* The usual daily dose is 1 to 2 mg, with a range of 0.5 to 6 mg, orally or parenterally.

As with any agent used in parkinsonism, dosage must be individualized according to age, weight, and the type of parkinsonism being treated. Generally, older patients and thin patients cannot tolerate large doses. Most patients with postencephalitic parkinsonism need fairly large doses and tolerate them well. Patients with a poor mental outlook are usually poor candidates for therapy.

In idiopathic parkinsonism, therapy may be initiated with a single daily dose of 0.5 to 1 mg at bedtime. In some patients, this will be adequate; in others 4 to 6 mg per day may be required.

In postencephalitic parkinsonism, therapy may be initiated in most patients with 2 mg a day in 1 or more doses. In highly sensitive patients, therapy may be initiated with 0.5 mg at bedtime and increased as necessary.

Some patients experience greatest relief by taking the entire dose at bedtime; others react more favorably to divided doses 2 to 4 times a day. Frequently, 1 dose per day is sufficient and divided doses may be unnecessary or undesirable.

The long duration of action of this drug makes it particularly suitable for bedtime medication. Its effects may last throughout the night, enabling patients to turn in bed during the night, and to rise in the morning more easily.

When benztropine is started, do not abruptly terminate therapy with other antiparkinsonian agents. If the other agents are to be reduced or discontinued, it must be done gradually. Many patients obtain greatest relief with combination therapy.

Benztropine may be used concomitantly with carbidopa-levodopa, or with levodopa, in which case periodic dosage adjustment may be required in order to maintain optimum response.

Give before or after meals, as determined by patient's reaction. Postencephalitic patients (more prone to excessive salivation) may prefer to take it after meals and may, in addition, require small amounts of atropine. If the mouth dries excessively, take before meals unless it causes nausea. If taken after meals, thirst can be allayed by mint candies, chewing gum, or water.

➤*Drug-induced extrapyramidal disorders:* In treating extrapyramidal disorders due to neuroleptic drugs (eg, phenothiazines), the recommended dosage is 1 to 4 mg once or twice per day orally or parenterally. Dosage must be individualized according to the need of the patient. Some patients require more than recommended; others do not need as much.

In acute dystonic reactions, 1 to 2 mL of the injection usually relieves the condition quickly. After that, the tablets, 1 to 2 mg twice per day, usually prevent recurrence.

When extrapyramidal disorders develop soon after initiation of treatment with neuroleptic drugs (eg, phenothiazines), they are likely to be transient. One to 2 mg of benztropine tablets 2 or 3 times a day usually provides relief within 1 or 2 days. After 1 or 2 weeks, withdraw the drug to determine the continued need for it. If such disorders recur, benztropine can be reinstituted.

Certain drug-induced extrapyramidal disorders that develop slowly may not respond to benztropine.

➤*Storage/Stability:* Store at controlled room temperature, 15° to 30° C (59° to 86° F). Dispense in a well-closed container.

BENZTROPINE MESYLATE — INJECTION

Refer to the general discussion in the Antiparkinson Agents introduction. Complete and comparative prescribing information begins in the Antiparkinson Agent Anticholinergics group monograph.

Indications

➤*Parkinsonism:* This medication is indicated for use as an adjunct in the therapy of all forms of parkinsonism.

➤*Extrapyramidal disorders:* Benztropine mesylate injection is also useful in the control of extrapyramidal disorders (except tardive dyskinesia) due to neuroleptic drugs (eg, phenothiazines). Tardive dyskinesia may appear in some patients on long-term therapy with phenothiazines and related agents, or may occur after therapy with these drugs has been discontinued. Antiparkinsonism agents do not alleviate the symptoms of tardive dyskinesia, and in some instances may aggravate them. Benztropine mesylate is not recommended for use in patients with tardive dyskinesia.

Administration and Dosage

Since there is no significant difference in onset of effect after IV or IM injection, usually there is no need to use the IV route. The drug is quickly effective after either route, with improvement sometimes noticeable a few minutes after injection. In emergency situations, when the condition of the patient is alarming, 1 to 2 mL of the injection normally will provide quick relief. If the parkinsonian effect begins to return, the dose can be repeated.

Because of cumulative action, therapy should be initiated with a low dose which is increased gradually at 5- or 6-day intervals to the smallest amount necessary for optimal relief. Increases should be made in increments of 0.5 mg, to a maximum of 6 mg, or until optimal results are obtained without excessive adverse reactions.

➤*Postencephalitic and idiopathic parkinsonism:* The usual daily dose is 1 to 2 mg, with a range of 0.5 to 6 mg parenterally.

As with any agent used in parkinsonism, dosage must be individualized according to age and weight and the type of parkinsonism being treated. Generally, older patients, and thin patients cannot tolerate large doses. Most patients with postencephalitic parkinsonism need fairly large doses and tolerate them well. Patients with a poor mental outlook are usually poor candidates for therapy.

In idiopathic parkinsonism, therapy may be initiated with a single daily dose of 0.5 to 1 mg at bedtime. In some patients, this will be adequate; in others, 4 to 6 mg a day may be required.

In postencephalitic parkinsonism, therapy may be initiated in most patients with 2 mg a day in 1 or more doses. In highly sensitive patients, therapy may be initiated with 0.5 mg at bedtime, and increased as necessary.

Some patients experience greatest relief when given the entire dose at bedtime; others react more favorably to divided doses, 2 to 4 times a day. Frequently, 1 dose a day is sufficient, and divided doses may be unnecessary or undesirable.

The long duration of action of this drug makes it particularly suitable for bedtime medication when its effects may last throughout the night, enabling patients to turn in bed during the night more easily, and to rise in the morning.

When benztropine mesylate is started, do not terminate therapy with other antiparkinsonian agents abruptly. If the other agents are to be reduced or discontinued, it must be done gradually. Many patients obtain greatest relief with combination therapy.

Benztropine mesylate may be used concomitantly with carbidopa-levodopa, or with levodopa, in which case periodic dosage adjustment may be required in order to maintain optimum response.

➤*Drug-induced extrapyramidal disorders :* In treating extrapyramidal disorders due to neuroleptic drugs (eg, phenothiazines), the recommended dosage is 1 to 4 mg once or twice a day parenterally. Dosage must be individualized according to the need of the patient. Some patients require more than recommended; others do not need as much.

In acute dystonic reactions, 1 to 2 mL of the injection usually relieves the condition quickly.

When extrapyramidal disorders develop soon after initiation of treatment with neuroleptic drugs (eg, phenothiazines), they are likely to be transient. One to 2 mg of benztropine mesylate 2 or 3 times a day usually provides relief within 1 or 2 days. After 1 or 2 weeks, the drug should be withdrawn to determine the continued need for it. If such disorders recur, benztropine mesylate can be reinstituted.

Certain drug-induced extrapyramidal disorders that develop slowly may not respond to benztropine mesylate.

BIPERIDEN

Rx	**Akineton** (Par)	**Tablets:** 2 mg (as HCl)	(11). White, scored. In 100s and 1000s.

BIPERIDEN HYDROCHLORIDE — ORAL

Refer to the general discussion in the Antiparkinson Agents introduction. Complete and comparative prescribing information begins in the Antiparkinson Agent Anticholinergics group monograph.

Indications

➤*Extrapyramidal disorders:* Control of extrapyramidal disorders secondary to neuroleptic drug therapy (eg, phenothiazines).

➤*Parkinsonism:* As an adjunct in the therapy of all forms of parkinsonism (idiopathic, postencephalitic, arteriosclerotic).

Administration and Dosage

➤*Drug-induced extrapyramidal symptoms:* One tablet 1 to 3 times daily.

➤*Parkinson's disease:* The usual beginning dose is 1 tablet 3 or 4 times daily. The dosage should be individualized with the dose titrated upward to a maximum of 8 tablets (16 mg) per 24 hours.

➤*Storage/Stability:* Store at 25°C (77°F); excursions permitted to 15° to 30°C (59° to 86°F). Dispense in tight, light-resistant container.

DIPHENHYDRAMINE

For complete prescribing information and product availability, see the Diphenhydramine monograph in the Antihistamines section and the Antihistamines group monograph. Also refer to the general discussion in the Antiparkinson Agents introduction and the Antiparkinson Agent Anticholinergics group monograph.

PROCYCLIDINE

Rx	**Kemadrin** (Glaxo Wellcome)	**Tablets:** 5 mg	(Kemadrin S3A). White, scored. In 100s.

PROCYCLIDINE HYDROCHLORIDE — ORAL

Refer to the general discussion in the Antiparkinson Agents introduction. Complete and comparative prescribing information begins in the Antiparkinson Agent Anticholinergics group monograph.

Indications

➤*Parkinsonism:* Procyclidine hydrochloride is indicated in the treatment of parkinsonism including the postencephalitic, arteriosclerotic, and idiopathic types. Partial control of the parkinsonism symptoms is the usual therapeutic accomplishment. Procyclidine hydrochloride is usually more effective in the relief of rigidity than tremor; but tremor, fatigue, weakness, and sluggishness are frequently beneficially influenced. It can be substituted for all the previous medications in mild and moderate cases. For the control of more severe cases, other drugs may be added to procyclidine therapy as indications warrant.

➤*Extrapyramidal disorders:* Clinical reports indicate that procyclidine often successfully relieves the symptoms of extrapyramidal dysfunction (dystonia, dyskinesia, akathisia, and parkinsonism) which accompany the therapy of mental disorders with phenothiazine and rauwolfia compounds. In addition to minimizing the symptoms induced by tranquilizing drugs, the drug effectively controls sialorrhea resulting from neuroleptic medication. At the same time, freedom from the side effects induced by tranquilizer drugs, as provided by the administration of procyclidine, permits a more sustained treatment of the patient's mental disorder.

Administration and Dosage

➤*For parkinsonism:* The dosage of the drug for the treatment of parkinsonism depends upon the age of the patient, the etiology of the disease, and individual responsiveness. Therefore, the dosage must remain flexible to permit adjustment to the individual tolerance and requirements of each patient. In general, younger and postencephalitic patients require and tolerate a somewhat higher dosage than older patients and those with arteriosclerosis.

For patients who have received no other therapy – The usual dose of procyclidine hydrochloride for initial treatment is 2.5 mg administered 3 times daily after meals. If well tolerated, this dose may be gradually increased to 5 mg 3 times a day and occasionally 5 mg given before retiring. In some cases smaller doses may be employed with good therapeutic results.

Occasionally a patient is encountered who cannot tolerate a bedtime dose of the drug. In such cases it may be desirable to adjust dosage so that the bedtime dose is omitted and the total daily requirement is administered in three equal daytime doses. It is best administered during or after meals to minimize the development of side reactions.

To transfer patients to procyclidine hydrochloride from other therapy – Patients who have been receiving other drugs may be transferred to procyclidine hydrochloride. This is accomplished gradually by substituting 2.5 mg 3 times a day for all or part of the original drug. The dose of procyclidine is then increased as required while that of the other drug is correspondingly omitted or decreased until complete replacement is achieved. The total daily dosage may then be adjusted to the level that produces maximum benefit.

➤*For drug-induced extrapyramidal symptoms:* For treatment of symptoms of extrapyramidal dysfunction induced by tranquilizer drugs during the therapy of mental disorders, the dosage of procyclidine hydrochloride will depend on the severity of side effects associated with tranquilizer

PROCYCLIDINE HYDROCHLORIDE — ORAL

administration. In general, the larger the dosage of the tranquilizer, the more severe will be the associated symptoms, including rigidity and tremors. Accordingly, the drug dosage should be adjusted to suit the needs of the individual patient and to provide maximum relief of the induced symptoms. A convenient method to establish the daily dosage of procyclidine is to begin with the administration of 2.5 mg 3 times daily. This may be increased by 2.5 mg daily increments until the patient obtains relief of symptoms. In most cases excellent results will be obtained with 10 to 20 mg daily.

➤*Storage/Stability:* Store at 15° to 25°C (59° to 77°F) in a dry place.

TRIHEXYPHENIDYL HYDROCHLORIDE

Rx	**Trihexyphenidyl Hydrochloride** (Various, eg, Balan, Bolar, Danbury, Moore, Raway, Schein)	**Tablets:** 2 mg	In 30s, 100s, 250s, 1000s and UD 100s.
Rx	**Trihexy-2** (Geneva)		White. In 100s and 1000s.
Rx	**Trihexyphenidyl Hydrochloride** (Various, eg, Balan, Bolar, Danbury, Lannett, Moore, Schein)	**Tablets:** 5 mg	In 100s, 250s, 1000s and UD 100s.
Rx	**Trihexy-5** (Geneva)		White. In 100s and 1000s.
Rx	**Trihexyphenidyl Hydrochloride** (Versapharm)	**Elixir:** 2 mg per 5 mL	5% alcohol, parabens, sorbitol. Lime-peppermint flavor. In 473 mL.

TRIHEXYPHENIDYL HYDROCHLORIDE — ORAL

Refer to the general discussion in the Antiparkinson Agents introduction. Complete prescribing information begins in the Antiparkinson Agent Anticholinergics group monograph.

Indications

➤*Extrapyramidal disorders:* Trihexyphenidyl HCl is indicated as an adjunct in the treatment of all forms of parkinsonism (postencephalitic, arteriosclerotic, and idiopathic). It is often useful as adjuvant therapy when treating these forms of parkinsonism with levodopa.

➤*Parkinsonism:* It is indicated for the control of extrapyramidal disorders caused by central nervous system drugs such as the dibenzoxazepines, phenothiazines, thioxanthenes, and butyrophenones.

Administration and Dosage

Dosage should be individualized. The initial dose should be low and then increased gradually, especially in patients older than 60 years of age. Whether trihexyphenidyl HCl may best be given before or after meals should be determined by the way the patient reacts. Postencephalitic patients, who are usually more prone to excessive salivation, may prefer to take it after meals and may, in addition, require small amounts of atropine which, under such circumstances, is sometimes an effective adjuvant. If trihexyphenidyl HCl tends to dry the mouth excessively, it may be better to take it before meals, unless it causes nausea. If taken after meals, the thirst sometimes induced can be allayed by mint candies, chewing gum or water.

The total daily intake of trihexyphenidyl HCl tablets and elixir are tolerated best if divided into 3 doses and taken at mealtimes. High doses (greater than 10 mg daily) may be divided into 4 parts, with 3 doses administered at mealtimes and the fourth at bedtime.

➤*Idiopathic parkinsonism:* As initial therapy for parkinsonism, 1 mg of trihexyphenidyl HCl in tablet form may be administered the first day. The dose may then be increased by 2 mg increments at intervals of 3 to 5 days, until a total of 6 to 10 mg is given daily. The total daily dose will depend upon what is found to be the optimal level. Many patients derive maximum benefit from this daily total of 6 to 10 mg, but some patients, chiefly those in the postencephalitic group, may require a total daily dose of 12 to 15 mg.

➤*Drug-induced parkinsonism:* The size and frequency of dose of trihexyphenidyl HCl needed to control extrapyramidal reactions to commonly employed tranquilizers, notably the phenothiazines, thioxanthenes, and butyrophenones, must be determined empirically. The total daily dosage usually ranges between 5 and 15 mg although, in some cases, these reactions have been satisfactorily controlled on as little as 1 mg daily. It may be advisable to commence therapy with a single 1 mg dose. If the extrapyramidal manifestations are not controlled in a few hours, the subsequent doses may be progressively increased until satisfactory control is achieved. Satisfactory control may sometimes be more rapidly achieved by temporarily reducing the dosage of the tranquilizer on instituting trihexyphenidyl HCl therapy and then adjusting dosage of both drugs until the desired ataractic effect is retained without onset of extrapyramidal reactions.

It is sometimes possible to maintain the patient on a reduced trihexyphenidyl HCl dosage after the reactions have remained under control for several days. Instances have been reported in which these reactions have remained in remission for long periods after trihexyphenidyl HCl therapy was discontinued.

➤*Concomitant use of trihexyphenidyl HCl with levodopa:* When trihexyphenidyl HCl is used concomitantly with levodopa, the usual dose of each may need to be reduced. Careful adjustment is necessary, depending on side effects and degree of symptom control. Trihexyphenidyl HCl dosage of 3 to 6 mg daily, in divided doses, is usually adequate.

➤*Concomitant use of trihexyphenidyl HCl with other parasympathetic inhibitors:* Trihexyphenidyl HCl may be substituted, in whole or in part, for other parasympathetic inhibitors. The usual technique is partial substitution initially, with progressive reduction in the other medication as the dose of trihexyphenidyl HCl is increased.

➤*Storage/Stability:* Store at controlled room temperature 15° to 30°C (59° to 86°F). Do not freeze.

AMANTADINE HYDROCHLORIDE

For prescribing information, refer to the Antiviral Agents monograph. Also refer to the general discussion in the Antiparkinson Agents introduction.

BROMOCRIPTINE MESYLATE

Rx	**Bromocriptine Mesylate** (Mylan)	**Tablets**: 2.5 mg (as base)	Lactose, EDTA. (M 42). White to off-white, scored. In 30s and 100s.
Rx	**Parlodel SnapTabs** (Sandoz)		(Parlodel 2½). White, scored. In 30s and 100s.
Rx	**Bromocriptine Mesylate** (Mylan)	**Capsules**: 5 mg (as base)	Lactose, alcohols. (MYLAN 7096). Opaque lt. brown, ivory opaque. In 30s and 100s.
Rx	**Parlodel** (Sandoz)		(Parlodel 5 mg). Caramel/White. In 30s & 100s.

BROMOCRIPTINE MESYLATE — ORAL

Also refer to the general discussion in the Antiparkinson Agents introduction.

Indications

➤*Hyperprolactinemia (associated dysfunctions):* Bromocriptine mesylate is indicated for the treatment of dysfunctions associated with hyperprolactinemia including amenorrhea with or without galactorrhea, infertility, or hypogonadism. Bromocriptine mesylate treatment is indicated in patients with prolactin-secreting adenomas, which may be the basic underlying endocrinopathy contributing to the above clinical presentations. Reduction in tumor size has been demonstrated in both male and female patients with macroadenomas. In cases where adenectomy is elected, a course of bromocriptine mesylate therapy may be used to reduce the tumor mass prior to surgery.

➤*Acromegaly:* Bromocriptine mesylate therapy is indicated in the treatment of acromegaly. Bromocriptine mesylate therapy, alone or as adjunctive therapy with pituitary irradiation or surgery, reduces serum growth hormone by 50% or more in approximately half of patients treated, although not usually to normal levels.

Since the effects of external pituitary radiation may not become maximal for several years, adjunctive therapy with bromocriptine mesylate offers potential benefit before the effects of irradiation are manifested.

➤*Parkinson's disease:* Bromocriptine mesylate tablets or capsules are indicated in the treatment of the signs and symptoms of idiopathic or postencephalitic Parkinson's disease. As adjunctive treatment to levodopa (alone or with a peripheral decarboxylase inhibitor), bromocriptine mesylate therapy may provide additional therapeutic benefits in those patients who are currently maintained on optimal dosages of levodopa, those who are beginning to deteriorate (develop tolerance) to levodopa therapy, and those who are experiencing "end of dose failure" on levodopa therapy. Bromocriptine mesylate therapy may permit a reduction of the maintenance dose of levodopa and, thus may ameliorate the occurrence or severity of adverse reactions associated with long-term levodopa therapy such as abnormal involuntary movements (eg, dyskinesias) and the marked swings in motor function ("on-off" phenomenon). Continued efficacy of bromocriptine mesylate therapy during treatment of more than 2 years has not been established.

Data are insufficient to evaluate potential benefit from treating newly diagnosed Parkinson's disease with bromocriptine mesylate. Studies have shown, however, significantly more adverse reactions (notably nausea, hallucinations, confusion and hypotension) in bromocriptine mesylate treated patients than in levodopa/carbidopa treated patients. Patients unresponsive to levodopa are poor candidates for bromocriptine mesylate therapy.

Administration and Dosage

➤*Recommendation:* It is recommended that bromocriptine mesylate be taken with food. Patients should be evaluated frequently during dose escalation to determine the lowest dosage that produces a therapeutic response.

➤*Hyperprolactinemic indications:* The initial dosage of bromocriptine mesylate is ½ to one 2.5 mg tablet daily. An additional 2.5 mg tablet may be added to the treatment regimen as tolerated every 2 to 7 days until an optimal therapeutic response is achieved. The therapeutic dosage ranged from 2.5 to 15 mg daily in adults studied clinically.

Based on limited data in children of age 11 to 15 years, the initial dose is ½ to one 2.5 mg tablet daily. Dosing may need to be increased as tolerated until a therapeutic response is achieved. The therapeutic dosage ranged from 2.5 to 10 mg daily in children with prolactin-secreting pituitary adenomas.

In order to reduce the likelihood of prolonged exposure to bromocriptine mesylate should an unsuspected pregnancy occur, a mechanical contraceptive should be used in conjunction with bromocriptine mesylate therapy until normal ovulatory menstrual cycles have been restored. Contraception may then be discontinued in patients desiring pregnancy.

Thereafter, if menstruation does not occur within 3 days of the expected date, bromocriptine mesylate therapy should be discontinued and a pregnancy test performed.

➤*Acromegaly:* Virtually all acromegalic patients receiving therapeutic benefit from bromocriptine mesylate also have reductions in circulating levels of growth hormone. Therefore, periodic assessment of circulating levels of growth hormone will, in most cases, serve as a guide in determining the therapeutic potential of bromocriptine mesylate. If, after a brief trial with bromocriptine mesylate therapy, no significant reduction in growth hormone levels has taken place, careful assessment of the clinical features of the disease should be made, and if no change has occurred, dosage adjustment or discontinuation of therapy should be considered.

The initial recommended dosage is ½ to one 2.5 mg bromocriptine mesylate tablet on retiring (with food) for 3 days. An additional ½ to 1 tablet should be added to the treatment regimen as tolerated every 3 to 7 days until the patient obtains optimal therapeutic benefit. Patients should be reevaluated monthly and the dosage adjusted based on reductions of growth hormone or clinical response. The usual optimal therapeutic dosage range of bromocriptine mesylate varies from 20 to 30 mg/day in most patients. The maximal dosage should not exceed 100 mg/day.

Patients treated with pituitary irradiation should be withdrawn from bromocriptine mesylate therapy on a yearly basis to assess both the clinical effects of radiation on the disease process as well as the effects of bromocriptine mesylate therapy. Usually a 4- to 8-week withdrawal period is adequate for this purpose. Recurrence of the signs/symptoms or increases in growth hormone indicate the disease process is still active and further courses of bromocriptine mesylate should be considered.

➤*Parkinson's disease:* The basic principle of bromocriptine mesylate therapy is to initiate treatment at a low dosage and, on an individual basis, increase the daily dosage slowly until a maximum therapeutic response is achieved. The dosage of levodopa during this introductory period should be maintained, if possible. The initial dose of bromocriptine mesylate is ½ of a 2.5 mg tablet twice daily with meals. Assessments are advised at 2-week intervals during dosage titration to ensure that the lowest dosage producing an optimal therapeutic response is not exceeded. If necessary, the dosage may be increased every 14 to 28 days by 2.5 mg/day with meals. Should it be advisable to reduce the dosage of levodopa because of adverse reactions, the daily dosage of bromocriptine mesylate, if increased, should be accomplished gradually in small (2.5 mg) increments.

The safety of bromocriptine mesylate has not been demonstrated in dosages exceeding 100 mg/day.

➤*Storage/Stability:* Store below 25°C (77°F) in a tight, light-resistant container.

Actions

➤*Pharmacology:* Bromocriptine mesylate is a dopamine receptor agonist, which activates post-synaptic dopamine receptors. The dopaminergic neurons in the tuberoinfundibular process modulate the secretion of prolactin from the anterior pituitary by secreting a prolactin inhibitory factor (thought to be dopamine); in the corpus striatum the dopaminergic neurons are involved in the control of motor function. Clinically, bromocriptine mesylate significantly reduces plasma levels of prolactin in patients with physiologically elevated prolactin as well as in patients with hyperprolactinemia. The inhibition of physiological lactation as well as galactorrhea in pathological hyperprolactinemic states is obtained at dose levels that do not affect secretion of other tropic hormones from the anterior pituitary. Experiments have demonstrated that bromocriptine induces long lasting stereotyped behavior in rodents and turning behavior in rats having unilateral lesions in the substantia nigra. These actions, characteristic of those produced by dopamine, are inhibited by dopamine antagonists and suggest a direct action of bromocriptine on striatal dopamine receptors.

Bromocriptine mesylate is a nonhormonal, nonestrogenic agent that inhibits the secretion of prolactin in humans, with little or no effect on other pituitary hormones, except in patients with acromegaly, where it lowers elevated blood levels of growth hormone in the majority of patients.

In about 75% of cases of amenorrhea and galactorrhea, bromocriptine mesylate therapy suppresses the galactorrhea completely, or almost completely, and reinitiates normal ovulatory menstrual cycles.

Menses are usually reinitiated prior to complete suppression of galactorrhea; the time for this on average is 6 to 8 weeks. However, some patients respond within a few days, and others may take up to 8 months.

Galactorrhea may take longer to control depending on the degree of stimulation of the mammary tissue prior to therapy. At least a 75% reduction in secretion is usually observed after 8 to 12 weeks. Some patients may fail to respond even after 12 months of therapy.

In many acromegalic patients, bromocriptine mesylate produces a prompt and sustained reduction in circulating levels of serum growth hormone.

Bromocriptine mesylate produces its therapeutic effect in the treatment of Parkinson's disease, a clinical condition characterized by a progressive deficiency in dopamine synthesis in the substantia nigra, by directly stimulating the dopamine receptors in the corpus striatum. In contrast, levodopa exerts its therapeutic effect only after conversion to dopamine by the neurons of the substantia nigra, which are known to be numerically diminished in this patient population.

➤*Pharmacokinetics:*

Absorption/Distribution – The pharmacokinetics and metabolism of bromocriptine in human subjects were studied with the help of radioactively labeled drug. Twenty-eight percent (28%) of an oral dose was absorbed from the gastrointestinal tract. The blood levels following a 2.5 mg dose were in the range of 2 to 3 ng equivalents/mL. Plasma levels were in the range of 4 to 6 ng equivalents/mL indicating that the red blood cells did not contain

BROMOCRIPTINE MESYLATE — ORAL

appreciable amounts of drug or metabolites. In vitro experiments showed that the drug was 90% to 96% bound to serum albumin.

Metabolism/Excretion – Bromocriptine was completely metabolized prior to excretion. The major route of excretion of absorbed drug was via the bile. Only 2.5% to 5.5% of the dose was excreted in the urine. Almost all (84.6%) of the administered dose was excreted in the feces in 120 hours.

Contraindications

Uncontrolled hypertension and sensitivity to any ergot alkaloids. In patients being treated for hyperprolactinemia bromocriptine mesylate should be withdrawn when pregnancy is diagnosed. In the event that bromocriptine mesylate is reinstituted to control a rapidly expanding macroadenoma and a patient experiences a hypertensive disorder of pregnancy, the benefit of continuing bromocriptine mesylate must be weighed against the possible risk of its use during a hypertensive disorder of pregnancy. When bromocriptine mesylate is being used to treat acromegaly, prolactinoma, or Parkinson's disease in patients who subsequently become pregnant, a decision should be made as to whether the therapy continues to be medically necessary or can be withdrawn. If it is continued, the drug should be withdrawn in those who may experience hypertensive disorders of pregnancy (including eclampsia, preeclampsia, or pregnancy-induced hypertension) unless withdrawal of bromocriptine mesylate is considered to be medically contraindicated.

The drug should not be used during the postpartum period in women with a history of coronary artery disease and other severe cardiovascular conditions unless withdrawal is considered medically contraindicated. If the drug is used in the postpartum period the patient should be observed with caution.

Warnings

➤*Pituitary tumors:* Since hyperprolactinemia with amenorrhea/galactorrhea and infertility has been found in patients with pituitary tumors, a complete evaluation of the pituitary is indicated before treatment with bromocriptine mesylate.

Symptomatic hypotension can occur in patients treated with bromocriptine mesylate for any indication. In postpartum studies with bromocriptine mesylate, decreases in supine systolic and diastolic pressures of greater than 20 mm Hg and 10 mm Hg, respectively, have been observed in almost 30% of patients receiving bromocriptine mesylate. On occasion, the drop in supine systolic pressure was as much as 50 to 59 mm Hg. While hypotension during the start of therapy with bromocriptine mesylate occurs in some patients, in postmarketing experience in the US in postpartum patients 89 cases of hypertension have been reported, sometimes at the initiation of therapy, but often developing in the second week of therapy; seizures have been reported in 72 cases (including 4 cases of status epilepticus), both with and without the prior development of hypertension; 30 cases of stroke have been reported mostly in postpartum patients whose prenatal and obstetric courses had been uncomplicated. Many of these patients experiencing seizures or strokes reported developing a constant and often progressively severe headache hours to days prior to the acute event. Some cases of strokes and seizures were also preceded by visual disturbances (blurred vision, and transient cortical blindness). Nine cases of acute myocardial infarction have been reported.

Although a causal relationship between bromocriptine mesylate administration and hypertension, seizures, strokes, and myocardial infarction in postpartum women has not been established, use of the drug for prevention of physiological lactation, or in patients with uncontrolled hypertension is not recommended. In patients being treated for hyperprolactinemia bromocriptine mesylate should be withdrawn when pregnancy is diagnosed. In the event that bromocriptine mesylate is reinstituted to control a rapidly expanding macroadenoma and a patient experiences a hypertensive disorder of pregnancy, the benefit of continuing bromocriptine mesylate must be weighed against the possible risk of its use during a hypertensive disorder of pregnancy. When bromocriptine mesylate is being used to treat acromegaly or Parkinson's disease in patients who subsequently become pregnant, a decision should be made as to whether the therapy continues to be medically necessary or can be withdrawn. If it is continued, the drug should be withdrawn in those who may experience hypertensive disorders of pregnancy (including eclampsia, preeclampsia, or pregnancy-induced hypertension) unless withdrawal of bromocriptine mesylate is considered to be medically contraindicated. Because of the possibility of an interaction between bromocriptine mesylate and other ergot alkaloids, the concomitant use of these medications is not recommended. Particular attention should be paid to patients who have recently received other drugs that can alter the blood pressure. Periodic monitoring of the blood pressure, particularly during the first weeks of therapy is prudent. If hypertension, severe, progressive, or unremitting headache (with or without visual disturbance), or evidence of CNS toxicity develops, drug therapy should be discontinued and the patient should be evaluated promptly.

➤*Pulmonary effects:* Long-term treatment (6 to 36 months) with bromocriptine mesylate in doses ranging from 20 to 100 mg/day has been associated with pulmonary infiltrates, pleural effusion and thickening of the pleura in a few patients. In those instances in which bromocriptine mesylate treatment was terminated, the changes slowly reverted towards normal.

➤*Carcinogenesis:* A 74-week study was conducted in mice using dietary levels of bromocriptine mesylate equivalent to oral doses of 10 and 50 mg/kg/day. A 100-week study in rats was conducted using dietary levels equivalent to oral doses of 1.7, 9.8, and 44 mg/kg/day. The highest doses tested in mice and rats were approximately 2.5 and 4.4 times, respectively, the maximum human dose administered in controlled clinical trials (100 mg/day) based on body surface area. Malignant uterine tumors, endometrial and myometrial, were found in rats as follows: 0/50 control females, 2/50 females given 1.7 mg/kg daily, 7/49 females given 9.8 mg/kg daily, and 9/50 females given 44 mg/kg daily. The occurrence of these neoplasms is probably attributable to the high estrogen/progesterone ratio which occurs in rats as a result of the prolactin-inhibiting action of bromocriptine mesylate. The endocrine mechanisms believed to be involved in the rats are not present in humans. There is no known correlation between uterine malignancies occurring in bromocriptine-treated rats and human risk. In contrast to the findings in rats, the uteri from mice killed after 74 weeks treatment did not exhibit evidence of drug-related changes.

➤*Fertility impairment:* Increased perinatal loss was produced in the subgroups of female rats, sacrificed on day 21 postpartum after mating with males treated with the highest dose (50 mg/kg).

➤*Pregnancy: Category B.* If pregnancy occurs during bromocriptine mesylate administration, careful observation of these patients is mandatory. Prolactin-secreting adenomas may expand and compression of the optic or other cranial nerves may occur, emergency pituitary surgery becoming necessary. In most cases, the compression resolves following delivery. Reinitiation of bromocriptine mesylate treatment has been reported to produce improvement in the visual fields of patients in whom nerve compression has occurred during pregnancy. The safety of bromocriptine mesylate treatment during pregnancy to the mother and fetus has not been established.

Since pregnancy may occur prior to reinitiation of menses, a pregnancy test is recommended at least every 4 weeks during the amenorrheic period, and, once menses are reinitiated, every time a patient misses a menstrual period. Treatment with bromocriptine mesylate should be discontinued as soon as pregnancy has been established. Patients must be monitored closely throughout pregnancy for signs and symptoms that may signal the enlargement of a previously undetected or existing prolactin-secreting tumor. Discontinuation of bromocriptine mesylate treatment in patients with known macroadenomas has been associated with rapid regrowth of tumor and increase in serum prolactin in most cases.

Administration of 10 to 30 mg/kg of bromocriptine to 2 strains of rats on days 6 to 15 post coitum as well as a single dose of 10 mg/kg on day 5 post coitum interfered with nidation. Three mg/kg given on days 6 to 15 were without effect on nidation, and did not produce any anomalies. In animals treated from day 8 to 15 post coitum (ie, after implantation), 30 mg/kg produced increased prenatal mortality in the form of increased incidence of embryonic resorption. One anomaly, aplasia of spinal vertebrae and ribs, was found in the group of 262 fetuses derived from the dams treated with 30 mg/kg bromocriptine. No fetotoxic effects were found in offspring of dams treated during the peri- or post-natal period.

Two studies were conducted in rabbits (2 strains) to determine the potential to interfere with nidation. Dose levels of 100 or 300 mg/kg/day from day 1 to day 6 post coitum did not adversely affect nidation. The high dose was approximately 63 times the maximum human dose administered in controlled clinical trials (100 mg/day), based on body surface area. In New Zealand white rabbits some embryo mortality occurred at 300 mg/kg which was a reflection of overt maternal toxicity. Three studies were conducted in 2 strains of rabbits to determine the teratological potential of bromocriptine at dose levels of 3, 10, 30, 100, and 300 mg/kg given from day 6 to day 18 post coitum. In 2 studies with the Yellow-silver strain, cleft palate was found in 3 and 2 fetuses at maternally toxic doses of 100 and 300 mg/kg, respectively. One control fetus also exhibited this anomaly. In the third study conducted with New Zealand white rabbits using an identical protocol, no cleft palates were produced.

Information concerning 1276 pregnancies in women taking bromocriptine has been collected. In the majority of cases, bromocriptine was discontinued within 8 weeks into pregnancy (mean, 28.7 days); however, 8 patients received the drug continuously throughout pregnancy. The mean daily dose for all patients was 5.8 mg (range, 1 to 40 mg).

Of these 1276 pregnancies, there were 1088 full-term deliveries (4 stillborn), 145 spontaneous abortions (11.4%), and 28 induced abortions (2.2%). Moreover, 12 extrauterine gravidities and 3 hydatidiform moles (twice in the same patient) caused early termination of pregnancy. These data compare favorably with the abortion rate (11% to 25%) cited for pregnancies induced by clomiphene citrate, menopausal gonadotropin, and chorionic gonadotropin.

Although spontaneous abortions often go unreported, especially prior to 20 weeks of gestation, their frequency has been estimated to be 15%.

➤*Lactation:* Bromocriptine mesylate should not be used during lactation in postpartum women.

➤*Children:* The safety and effectiveness of bromocriptine for the treatment of prolactin-secreting pituitary adenomas have been established in patients age 16 years to adult. No data are available for bromocriptine use in pediatric patients under the age of 8 years. A single 8-year-old patient treated with bromocriptine for prolactin-secreting pituitary macroadenoma has been reported without therapeutic response.

The use of bromocriptine for the treatment of prolactin-secreting adenomas in pediatric patients in the age group 11 to under 16 years is supported by evidence from well-controlled trials in adults, with additional data in a limited number (n = 14) of children and adolescents 11 to 15 years of age with prolactin-secreting pituitary macro- and microadenomas who have been treated with bromocriptine. Of the 14 reported patients, 9 had successful outcomes, 3 partial responses, and 2 failed to respond to bromocriptine treatment. Chronic hypopituitarism complicated macroadenoma treatment in 5 of the responders, both in patients receiving bromocriptine alone and in those who received bromocriptine in combination with surgical treatment or pituitary irradiation.

Safety and effectiveness of bromocriptine in pediatric patients have not been established for any other indication listed.

Precautions

➤*Hyperprolactinemic states:* Visual field impairment is a known complication of macroprolactinoma. Effective treatment with bromocriptine mesylate leads to a reduction in hyperprolactinaemia and often to a resolution of the

BROMOCRIPTINE MESYLATE — ORAL

visual impairment. In some patients, however, a secondary deterioration of visual fields may subsequently develop despite normalized prolactin levels and tumor shrinkage, which may result from traction on the optic chiasm which is pulled down into the now partially empty sella. In these cases, the visual field defect may improve on reduction of bromocriptine dosage while there is some elevation of prolactin and some tumor re-expansion. Monitoring of visual fields in patients with macroprolactinoma is therefore recommended for an early recognition of secondary field loss due to chiasmal herniation and adaptation of drug dosage.

The relative efficacy of bromocriptine mesylate versus surgery in preserving visual fields is not known. Patients with rapidly progressive visual field loss should be evaluated by a neurosurgeon to help decide on the most appropriate therapy. Since pregnancy is often the therapeutic objective in many hyperprolactinemic patients presenting with amenorrhea/galactorrhea and hypogonadism (infertility), a careful assessment of the pituitary is essential to detect the presence of a prolactin-secreting adenoma. Patients not seeking pregnancy, or those harboring large adenomas, should be advised to use contraceptive measures, other than oral contraceptives, during treatment with bromocriptine mesylate.

➤*Acromegaly:* Cold-sensitive digital vasospasm has been observed in some acromegalic patients treated with bromocriptine mesylate. The response, should it occur, can be reversed by reducing the dose of bromocriptine mesylate and may be prevented by keeping the fingers warm. Cases of severe gastrointestinal bleeding from peptic ulcers have been reported, some fatal. Although there is no evidence that bromocriptine mesylate increases the incidence of peptic ulcers in acromegalic patients, symptoms suggestive of peptic ulcer should be investigated thoroughly and treated appropriately. Patients with a history of peptic ulcer or gastrointestinal bleeding should be observed carefully during treatment with bromocriptine mesylate.

Possible tumor expansion while receiving bromocriptine mesylate therapy has been reported in a few patients. Since the natural history of growth hormone secreting tumors is unknown, all patients should be carefully monitored and, if evidence of tumor expansion develops, discontinuation of treatment and alternative procedures considered.

➤*Parkinson's disease:* Safety during long-term use for more than 2 years at the doses required for parkinsonism has not been established.

As with any chronic therapy, periodic evaluation of hepatic, hematopoietic, cardiovascular, and renal function is recommended. Symptomatic hypotension can occur and, therefore, caution should be exercised when treating patients receiving antihypertensive drugs.

High doses of bromocriptine mesylate may be associated with confusion and mental disturbances. Since parkinsonian patients may manifest mild degrees of dementia, caution should be used when treating such patients.

Bromocriptine mesylate administered alone or concomitantly with levodopa may cause hallucinations (visual or auditory). Hallucinations usually resolve with dosage reduction; occasionally, discontinuation of bromocriptine mesylate is required. Rarely, after high doses, hallucinations have persisted for several weeks following discontinuation of bromocriptine mesylate.

As with levodopa, caution should be exercised when administering bromocriptine mesylate to patients with a history of myocardial infarction who have a residual atrial, nodal, or ventricular arrhythmia.

Retroperitoneal fibrosis has been reported in a few patients receiving long-term therapy (2 to 10 years) with bromocriptine mesylate in doses ranging from 30 to 140 mg daily.

➤*Special risk:* Safety and efficacy of bromocriptine mesylate have not been established in patients with renal or hepatic disease. Care should be exercised when administering bromocriptine mesylate therapy concomitantly with other medications known to lower blood pressure.

The drug should be used with caution in patients with a history of psychosis or cardiovascular disease. If acromegalic patients or patients with prolactinoma or Parkinson's disease are being treated with bromocriptine mesylate during pregnancy, they should be cautiously observed, particularly during the postpartum period if they have a history of cardiovascular disease.

➤*Hazardous tasks:* When initiating therapy, all patients receiving bromocriptine mesylate should be cautioned with regard to engaging in activities requiring rapid and precise responses, such as driving an automobile or operating machinery since dizziness (8% to 16%), drowsiness (8%), faintness, fainting (8%), and syncope (less than 1%) have been reported early in the course of therapy.

Drug Interactions

Bromocriptine Drug Interactions

Precipitant drug	Object drug*		Description
Erythromycin	Bromocriptine	↑	Bromocriptine levels may be increased, possibly increasing pharmacologic and toxic effects.
Phenothiazines	Bromocriptine	↓	Efficacy of bromocriptine, when used for prolactin-secreting tumors, may be inhibited.
Sympathomimetics Isometheptene Phenylpropanolamine	Bromocriptine	↑	In several case reports, bromocriptine side effects were exacerbated during concurrent use of these agents, including ventricular tachycardia and cardiac dysfunction.

* ↑ = Object drug increased. ↓ = Object drug decreased.

The risk of using bromocriptine mesylate in combination with other drugs has not been systematically evaluated, but alcohol may potentiate the side effects of bromocriptine mesylate. Bromocriptine mesylate may interact with dopamine antagonists, butyrophenones, and certain other agents. Compounds in these categories result in a decreased efficacy of bromocriptine mesylate: Phenothiazines, haloperidol, metoclopramide, pimozide. Concomitant use of bromocriptine mesylate with other ergot alkaloids is not recommended.

Adverse Reactions

➤*Acromegaly:* The most frequent adverse reactions encountered in acromegalic patients treated with bromocriptine mesylate were nausea (18%), constipation (14%), postural/orthostatic hypotension (6%), anorexia (4%), dry mouth/nasal stuffiness (4%), indigestion/dyspepsia (4%), digital vasospasm (3%), drowsiness/tiredness (3%), and vomiting (2%).

Less frequent adverse reactions (less than 2%) were gastrointestinal bleeding, dizziness, exacerbation of Raynaud's syndrome, headache and syncope. Rarely (less than 1%) hair loss, alcohol potentiation, faintness, lightheadedness, arrhythmia, ventricular tachycardia, decreased sleep requirement, visual hallucinations, lassitude, shortness of breath, bradycardia, vertigo, paresthesia, sluggishness, vasovagal attack, delusional psychosis, paranoia, insomnia, heavy headedness, reduced tolerance to cold, tingling of ears, facial pallor, and muscle cramps have been reported.

➤*Hyperprolactinemic indications:* The incidence of adverse effects is quite high (69%) but these are generally mild to moderate in degree. Therapy was discontinued in approximately 5% of patients because of adverse effects. These in decreasing order of frequency are nausea (49%), headache (19%), dizziness (17%), fatigue (7%), lightheadedness (5%), vomiting (5%), abdominal cramps (4%), nasal congestion (3%), constipation (3%), diarrhea (3%), and drowsiness (3%).

A slight hypotensive effect may accompany bromocriptine mesylate treatment. The occurrence of adverse reactions may be lessened by temporarily reducing dosage to ½ tablet 2 or 3 times daily. A few cases of cerebrospinal fluid rhinorrhea have been reported in patients receiving bromocriptine mesylate for treatment of large prolactinomas. This has occurred rarely, usually only in patients who have received previous transsphenoidal surgery, pituitary radiation, or both, and who were receiving bromocriptine mesylate for tumor recurrence. It may also occur in previously untreated patients whose tumor extends into the sphenoid sinus.

➤*Parkinson's disease:* In clinical trials in which bromocriptine was administered with concomitant reduction in the dose of levodopa/carbidopa, the most common newly appearing adverse reactions were nausea, abnormal involuntary movements, hallucinations, confusion, "on-off" phenomenon, dizziness, drowsiness, faintness/fainting, vomiting, asthenia, abdominal discomfort, visual disturbance, ataxia, insomnia, depression, hypotension, shortness of breath, constipation, and vertigo.

Less common adverse reactions which may be encountered include anorexia, anxiety, blepharospasm, dry mouth, dysphagia, edema of the feet and ankles, erythromelalgia, epileptiform seizure, fatigue, headache, lethargy, mottling of skin, nasal stuffiness, nervousness, nightmares, paresthesia, skin rash, urinary frequency, urinary incontinence, urinary retention, and rarely, signs and symptoms of ergotism such as tingling of fingers, cold feet, numbness, muscle cramps of feet and legs or exacerbation of Raynaud's syndrome.

Pleural and pericardial effusions, pleural, and pulmonary fibrosis and retroperitoneal fibrosis and constrictive pericarditis have been reported rarely in patients treated with bromocriptine mesylate.

Abnormalities in laboratory tests may include elevations in blood urea nitrogen, AST, ALT, GGPT, CPK, alkaline phosphatase and uric acid, which are usually transient and not of clinical significance.

➤*Postpartum patients:* In postpartum studies with bromocriptine mesylate 23% of postpartum patients treated had at least 1 side effect, but they were generally mild to moderate in degree. Therapy was discontinued in approximately 3% of patients. The most frequently occurring adverse reactions were headache (10%), dizziness (8%), nausea (7%), vomiting (3%), fatigue (1%), syncope (0.7%), diarrhea (0.4%), and cramps (0.4%). Decreases in blood pressure (greater than or equal to 20 mm Hg systolic and greater than or equal to 10 mm Hg diastolic) occurred in 28% of patients at least once during the first 3 postpartum days; these were usually of a transient nature. Reports of fainting in the puerperium may possibly be related to this effect. In postmarketing experience in the US serious adverse reactions reported include 72 cases of seizures (including 4 cases of status epilepticus), 30 cases of stroke, and 9 cases of myocardial infarction among postpartum patients. Seizure cases were not necessarily accompanied by the development of hypertension. An unremitting and often progressively severe headache, sometimes accompanied by visual disturbance, often preceded by hours to days many cases of seizure or stroke. Most patients had shown no evidence of any of the hypertensive disorders of pregnancy including eclampsia, preeclampsia or pregnancy induced hypertension. One stroke case was associated with sagittal sinus thrombosis, and another was associated with cerebral and cerebellar vasculitis. One case of myocardial infarction was associated with unexplained disseminated intravascular coagulation and a second occurred in conjunction with use of another ergot alkaloid. The relationship of these adverse reactions to bromocriptine mesylate administration has not been established.

Overdosage

➤*Symptoms:* The most commonly reported signs and symptoms associated with acute bromocriptine mesylate overdose are nausea, vomiting, constipation, diaphoresis, dizziness, pallor, severe hypotension, malaise, confusion, lethargy, drowsiness, delusions, hallucinations, and repetitive yawning. The lethal dose has not been established and the drug has a very wide margin of

BROMOCRIPTINE MESYLATE — ORAL

safety. However, 1 death occurred in a patient who committed suicide with an unknown quantity of bromocriptine mesylate and chloroquine.

➤*Treatment:* Treatment of overdose consists of removal of the drug by emesis (if conscious), gastric lavage, activated charcoal, or saline catharsis. Careful supervision and recording of fluid intake and output is essential. Hypotension should be treated by placing the patient in the Trendelenburg position and administering IV fluids. If satisfactory relief of hypotension cannot be achieved by using the above measures to their fullest extent, vasopressors should be considered.

Patient Information

During clinical trials, dizziness (8% to 16%), drowsiness (8%), faintness, fainting (8%), and syncope (less than 1%) have been reported early in the course of bromocriptine mesylate therapy.

In postmarketing reports, bromocriptine mesylate has been associated with somnolence, and episodes of sudden sleep onset, particularly in patients with Parkinson's disease. Sudden onset of sleep during daily activities, in some cases without awareness or warning signs, has been reported very rarely. All patients receiving bromocriptine mesylate should be cautioned with regard to activities requiring rapid and precise responses, such as driving a car or operating machinery.

Patients receiving bromocriptine mesylate for hyperprolactinemic states associated with macroadenoma or those who have had previous transsphenoidal surgery, should be told to report any persistent watery nasal discharge to their physician. Patients receiving bromocriptine mesylate for treatment of a macroadenoma should be told that discontinuation of drug may be associated with rapid regrowth of the tumor and recurrence of their original symptoms.

CARBIDOPA

Rx	**Lodosyn**[1] (Bristol-Myers Squibb Primary Care)	**Tablets:** 25 mg carbidopa	(MSD 129). Orange, scored. In 100s.

[1] Most patients may be maintained on carbidopa/levodopa combination products. *Lodosyn* is available to physicians for use in patients requiring individual titration of carbidopa and levodopa.

CARBIDOPA — ORAL

Carbidopa is used only with levodopa. See levodopa monograph. Also refer to the general discussion in the Antiparkinson Agents introduction.

Indications

For use with carbidopa-levodopa or with levodopa in the treatment of the symptoms of idiopathic Parkinson's disease (paralysis agitans), postencephalitic parkinsonism, and symptomatic parkinsonism which may follow injury to the nervous system by carbon monoxide intoxication and/or manganese intoxication.

For use with carbidopa-levodopa in patients for whom the dosage of carbidopa-levodopa provides less than adequate daily dosage (usually 70 mg daily) of carbidopa.

For use with levodopa in the occasional patient whose dosage requirement of carbidopa and levodopa necessitates separate titration of each entity.

Carbidopa is used with carbidopa-levodopa or with levodopa to permit the administration of lower doses of levodopa with reduced nausea and vomiting, more rapid dosage titration, and with a somewhat smoother response. However, patients with markedly irregular ("on-off") responses to levodopa have not been shown to benefit from the addition of carbidopa.

Since carbidopa prevents the reversal of levodopa effects caused by pyridoxine, supplemental pyridoxine (vitamin B_6), can be given to patients when they are receiving carbidopa and levodopa concomitantly or as carbidopa-levodopa.

Although the administration of carbidopa permits control of parkinsonism and Parkinson's disease with much lower doses of levodopa, there is no conclusive evidence at present that this is beneficial other than in reducing nausea and vomiting, permitting more rapid titration, and providing a somewhat smoother response to levodopa.

Certain patients who responded poorly to levodopa alone have improved when carbidopa and levodopa were given concurrently. This was most likely due to decreased peripheral decarboxylation of levodopa rather than to a primary effect of carbidopa on the peripheral nervous system. Carbidopa has not been shown to enhance the intrinsic efficacy of levodopa.

In considering whether to give carbidopa with carbidopa-levodopa or with levodopa to patients who have nausea or vomiting, the physician should be aware that, while many patients may be expected to improve, some may not. Since one cannot predict which patients are likely to improve, this can only be determined by a trial of therapy. It should be further noted that in controlled trials comparing carbidopa and levodopa with levodopa alone, about half the patients with nausea or vomiting on levodopa alone improved spontaneously despite being retained on the same dose of levodopa during the controlled portion of the trial.

➤*Unlabeled uses:* Carbidopa is used to reduce the peripheral metabolism of the L-5-hydroxtryptophan (L-5HTP) when used to treat post-anoxic intention myoclonus.

Administration and Dosage

Whether given with carbidopa-levodopa or with levodopa, the optimal daily dosage of carbidopa must be determined by careful titration. Most patients respond to a 1:10 proportion of carbidopa and levodopa, provided the daily dosage of carbidopa is 70 mg or more a day. The maximum daily dosage of carbidopa should not exceed 200 mg, since clinical experience with larger dosages is limited. If the patient is taking carbidopa-levodopa, the amount of carbidopa in carbidopa-levodopa should be considered when calculating the total amount of carbidopa to be administered each day.

➤*Patients receiving carbidopa-levodopa who require additional carbidopa:* Some patients taking carbidopa-levodopa may not have adequate reduction in nausea and vomiting when the dosage of carbidopa is less than 70 mg a day, and the dosage of levodopa is less than 700 mg a day. When these patients are taking carbidopa-levodopa 10-100 (which contains 10 mg of carbidopa and 100 mg of levodopa), 25 mg of carbidopa may be given with the first dose of carbidopa-levodopa each day. Additional doses of 12.5 mg or 25 mg may be given during the day with each dose of carbidopa-levodopa. When patients are taking carbidopa-levodopa 25-250 (which contains 25 mg of carbidopa and 250 mg of levodopa) or carbidopa-levodopa 25-100 (which contains 25 mg of carbidopa and 100 mg of levodopa), 25 mg of carbidopa may be given with any dose of carbidopa-levodopa as required for optimum therapeutic response. The maximum daily dosage of carbidopa, given as carbidopa and as carbidopa-levodopa, should not exceed 200 mg.

➤*Patients requiring individual titration of carbidopa and levodopa dosage:* Although carbidopa-levodopa is the preferred method of carbidopa and levodopa administration, there may be an occasional patient who requires individually titrated doses of these 2 drugs. In these patients, carbidopa should be initiated at a dosage of 25 mg 3 or 4 times a day. The 2 drugs should be given at the same time, starting with no more than one-fifth (20%) to one-fourth (25%) of the previous or recommended daily dosage of levodopa when given without carbidopa. In patients already receiving levodopa therapy, at least 12 hours should elapse between the last dose of levodopa and initiation of therapy with carbidopa and levodopa. A convenient way to initiate therapy in these patients is in the morning following a night when the patient has not taken levodopa for at least 12 hours. Physicians who prescribe separate doses of carbidopa and levodopa should be thoroughly familiar with the directions for use of each drug.

➤*Dosage adjustment:* Dosage of carbidopa may be adjusted by adding or omitting one-half or one tablet a day. Because both therapeutic and adverse responses occur more rapidly with combined therapy than when only levodopa is given, patients should be monitored closely during the dose adjustment period. Specifically, involuntary movements will occur more rapidly when carbidopa and levodopa are given concomitantly than when levodopa is given without carbidopa. The occurrence of involuntary movements may require dosage reduction. Blepharospasm may be a useful early sign of excess dosage in some patients.

Current evidence indicates other standard antiparkinsonian drugs may be continued while carbidopa and levodopa are being administered. However, the dosage of such other standard antiparkinsonian drugs may require adjustment.

➤*Interruption of therapy:* Sporadic cases of a symptom complex resembling neuroleptic malignant syndrome (NMS) have been associated with dose reductions and withdrawal of carbidopa-levodopa or carbidopa-levodopa sustained release. Patients should be observed carefully if abrupt reduction or discontinuation of carbidopa-levodopa or carbidopa-levodopa sustained-release is required, especially if the patient is receiving neuroleptics (see Warnings).

If general anesthesia is required, therapy may be continued as long as the patient is permitted to take fluids and medication by mouth. When therapy is interrupted temporarily, the patient should be observed for symptoms resembling NMS, and the usual daily dosage may be resumed as soon as the patient is able to take medication orally.

Actions

➤*Pharmacology:* Current evidence indicates that symptoms of Parkinson's disease are related to depletion of dopamine in the corpus striatum. Administration of dopamine is ineffective in the treatment of Parkinson's disease apparently because it does not cross the blood-brain barrier. However, levodopa, the metabolic precursor of dopamine, does cross the blood-brain barrier, and presumably is converted to dopamine in the brain. This is thought to be the mechanism whereby levodopa relieves symptoms of Parkinson's disease.

Pharmacodynamics – When levodopa is administered orally it is rapidly decarboxylated to dopamine in extracerebral tissues so that only a small portion of a given dose is transported unchanged to the central nervous system. For this reason, large doses of levodopa are required for adequate therapeutic effect and these may often be accompanied by nausea and other adverse reactions, some of which are attributable to dopamine formed in extracerebral tissues.

The incidence of levodopa-induced nausea and vomiting is less when carbidopa is used with levodopa than when levodopa is used without carbidopa. In many patients this reduction in nausea and vomiting will permit more rapid dosage titration.

Carbidopa inhibits decarboxylation of peripheral levodopa. Carbidopa has not been demonstrated to have any overt pharmacodynamic actions in the recommended doses. It does not appear to cross the blood-brain barrier readily and does not affect the metabolism of levodopa within the central nervous system at doses of carbidopa that are recommended for maximum effective inhibition of peripheral decarboxylation of levodopa.

Since its decarboxylase-inhibiting activity is limited primarily to extracerebral tissues, administration of carbidopa with levodopa makes more levodopa available for transport to the brain. However, since levodopa and

CARBIDOPA — ORAL

carbidopa compete with certain amino acids for transport across the gut wall, the absorption of levodopa and carbidopa may be impaired in some patients on a high protein diet.

➤*Pharmacokinetics:* Carbidopa reduces the amount of levodopa required to produce a given response by about 75% and, when administered with levodopa, increases both plasma levels and the plasma half-life of levodopa, and decreases plasma and urinary dopamine and homovanillic acid.

In clinical pharmacologic studies, simultaneous administration of separate tablets of carbidopa and levodopa produced greater urinary excretion of levodopa in proportion to the excretion of dopamine when compared to the two drugs administered at separate times.

Supplemental pyridoxine (vitamin B_6) can be given to patients when they are receiving carbidopa and levodopa concomitantly or as carbidopa-levodopa sustained-release or carbidopa-levodopa. Previous reports in the medical literature cautioned that high doses of vitamin B_6 should not be taken by patients on levodopa therapy alone because exogenously administered pyridoxine would enhance the metabolism of levodopa to dopamine. The introduction of carbidopa to levodopa therapy, which inhibits the peripheral decarboxylation of levodopa to dopamine, counteracts the metabolic-enhancing effect of pyridoxine.

Contraindications

Hypersensitivity to any component of this drug.

Nonselective monoamine oxidase (MAO) inhibitors are contraindicated for use with levodopa or carbidopa-levodopa combination products with or without carbidopa. These inhibitors must be discontinued at least 2 weeks prior to initiating therapy with levodopa. Carbidopa-levodopa or levodopa may be administered concomitantly with the manufacturer's recommended dose of an MAO inhibitor with selectivity for MAO type B (eg, selegiline HCl).

Levodopa or carbidopa-levodopa products, with or without carbidopa, are contraindicated in patients with narrow-angle glaucoma.

Because levodopa or carbidopa-levodopa products, with or without carbidopa, may activate a malignant melanoma, they should not be used in patients with suspicious, undiagnosed skin lesions or a history of melanoma.

Warnings

➤*Use with levodopa:* When carbidopa is to be given to patients being treated with levodopa, give the two drugs at the same time, starting with no more than 20% to 25% of the previous daily dosage of levodopa. At least 8 hours should elapse between the last dose of levodopa and initiation of therapy with carbidopa and levodopa.

Carbidopa has no antiparkinsonian effect when given alone. It is indicated for use with carbidopa-levodopa or levodopa. Carbidopa does not decrease adverse reactions due to central effects of levodopa.

➤*CNS effects:* As with levodopa, concomitant administration of carbidopa and levodopa may cause involuntary movements and mental disturbances. These reactions are thought to be due to increased brain dopamine following administration of levodopa. All patients should be observed carefully for the development of depression with concomitant suicidal tendencies. Patients with past or current psychoses should be treated with caution. Because carbidopa permits more levodopa to reach the brain and, thus, more dopamine to be formed, dyskinesias may occur at lower levodopa dosages and sooner with concomitant use of carbidopa and levodopa or carbidopa-levodopa combination products than with levodopa alone. The occurrence of dyskinesias may require levodopa dosage reduction.

➤*Neuroleptic malignant syndrome (NMS):* Sporadic cases of a symptom complex resembling NMS have been reported in association with dose reductions or withdrawal of certain antiparkinsonian agents such as levodopa, carbidopa-levodopa or carbidopa-levodopa sustained-release. Therefore, patients should be observed carefully when the dosage of levodopa is reduced abruptly or discontinued, especially if the patient is receiving neuroleptics.

NMS is an uncommon but life-threatening syndrome characterized by fever or hyperthermia. Neurological findings, including muscle rigidity, involuntary movements, altered consciousness, mental status changes; other disturbances, such as autonomic dysfunction, tachycardia, tachypnea, sweating, hyper- or hypotension; laboratory findings, such as creatine phosphokinase elevation, leukocytosis, myoglobinuria, and increased serum myoglobin, have been reported.

The early diagnosis of this condition is important for the appropriate management of these patients. Considering NMS as a possible diagnosis and ruling out other acute illnesses (eg, pneumonia, systemic infection) is essential. This may be especially complex if the clinical presentation includes both serious medical illness and untreated or inadequately treated extrapyramidal signs and symptoms (EPS). Other important considerations in the differential diagnosis include central anticholinergic toxicity, heat stroke, drug fever, and primary central nervous system (CNS) pathology.

The management of NMS should include:

1.) Intensive symptomatic treatment and medical monitoring.
2.) Treatment of any concomitant serious medical problems for which specific treatments are available. Dopamine agonists, such as bromocriptine, and muscle relaxants, such as dantrolene, are often used in the treatment of NMS; however, their effectiveness has not been demonstrated in controlled studies.

➤*Pregnancy: Category C.* There are no adequate and well-controlled studies with carbidopa in pregnant women. It has been reported from individual cases that levodopa crosses the human placental barrier, enters the fetus, and is metabolized. Carbidopa concentrations in fetal tissue appeared to be minimal. Carbidopa should be used during pregnancy only if the potential benefit justifies the potential risk to the fetus.

Carbidopa, at doses as high as 120 mg/kg/day, was without teratogenic effects in the mouse or rabbit. In the rabbit, but not in the mouse, carbidopa-levodopa produced visceral anomalies, similar to those seen with levodopa alone, at approximately 7 times the maximum recommended human dose. The teratogenic effect of levodopa in rabbits was unchanged by the concomitant administration of carbidopa.

➤*Lactation:* It is not known whether carbidopa or levodopa is excreted in human milk. Because many drugs are excreted in human milk, and because of their potential for serious adverse reactions in nursing infants, a decision should be made whether to discontinue nursing or to discontinue the drug, taking into account the importance of the drug to the nursing woman.

➤*Children:* Safety and effectiveness in pediatric patients have not been established, and use of the drug in patients below the age of 18 is not recommended.

Precautions

➤*Monitoring:* As with levodopa alone, periodic evaluations of hepatic, hematopoietic, cardiovascular, and renal function are recommended during extended concomitant therapy with carbidopa and levodopa, or with carbidopa and carbidopa-levodopa, or any combination of these drugs.

➤*Special risk:* Patients with chronic wide-angle glaucoma may be treated cautiously with carbidopa and levodopa or carbidopa-levodopa, or any combination of these drugs, just as with levodopa alone, provided the intraocular pressure is well controlled and the patient is monitored carefully for changes in intraocular pressure during therapy.

Levodopa, with or without carbidopa, should be administered cautiously to patients with severe cardiovascular or pulmonary disease, bronchial asthma, renal, hepatic, or endocrine disease.

Care should be exercised in administering levodopa, with or without carbidopa, to patients with a history of myocardial infarction who have residual atrial, nodal, or ventricular arrhythmias. In such patients, cardiac function should be monitored with particular care during the period of initial dosage adjustment, in a facility with provisions for intensive cardiac care.

As with levodopa alone there is a possibility of upper gastrointestinal hemorrhage in patients with a history of peptic ulcer.

➤*Lab test abnormalities:* Abnormalities in laboratory tests may include elevations of liver function tests such as alkaline phosphatase, AST, ALT, lactic dehydrogenase, and bilirubin. Abnormalities in blood urea nitrogen and positive Coombs test have also been reported. Commonly, levels of blood urea nitrogen, creatinine, and uric acid are lower during concomitant administration of carbidopa and levodopa than with levodopa alone.

Drug Interactions

➤*Antihypertensive agents:* Symptomatic postural hypotension has occurred when carbidopa, given with levodopa or carbidopa-levodopa combination products, was added to the treatment of a patient receiving antihypertensive drugs. Therefore, when therapy with carbidopa, given with or without levodopa or carbidopa-levodopa combination products, is started, dosage adjustment of the antihypertensive drug may be required.

➤*Monoamine oxidase inhibitors:* For patients receiving monoamine oxidase inhibitors. Concomitant therapy with selegiline and carbidopa-levodopa may be associated with severe orthostatic hypotension not attributable to carbidopa-levodopa alone.

➤*Tricyclic antidepressants:* There have been rare reports of adverse reactions, including hypertension and dyskinesia, resulting from the concomitant use of tricyclic antidepressants and carbidopa-levodopa preparations.

➤*Dopamine D_2 receptor antagonists and isoniazid:* Dopamine D_2 receptor antagonists (eg, phenothiazines, butyrophenones, risperidone) and isoniazid may reduce the therapeutic effects of levodopa. In addition, the beneficial effects of levodopa in Parkinson's disease have been reported to be reversed by phenytoin and papaverine. Patients taking these drugs with carbidopa and levodopa or carbidopa-levodopa combination products should be carefully observed for loss of therapeutic response.

➤*Iron salts:* Iron salts may reduce the bioavailability of carbidopa and levodopa. The clinical relevance is unclear.

➤*Metoclopramide:* Although metoclopramide may increase the bioavailability of levodopa by increasing gastric emptying, metoclopramide may also adversely affect disease control by its dopamine receptor antagonistic properties.

➤*Drug/Lab test interactions:* Levodopa and carbidopa-levodopa combination products may cause a false-positive reaction for urinary ketone bodies when a test tape is used for determination of ketonuria. This reaction will not be altered by boiling the urine specimen. False-negative tests may result with the use of glucose-oxidase methods of testing for glucosuria.

Adverse Reactions

Carbidopa has not been demonstrated to have any overt pharmacodynamic actions in the recommended doses. The only adverse reactions that have been observed have been with concomitant use of carbidopa with other drugs such as levodopa, and with carbidopa-levodopa combination products.

When carbidopa is administered concomitantly with levodopa or carbidopa-levodopa combination products, the most common adverse reactions have included dyskinesias such as choreiform, dystonic, and other involuntary movements, and nausea. Other adverse reactions reported with carbidopa when administered concomitantly with levodopa alone or carbidopa-levodopa combination products were psychotic episodes including delusions, hallucinations, and paranoid ideation, depression with or without development of suicidal tendencies, and dementia. Convulsions also have occurred; however, a causal relationship with concomitant use of carbidopa and levodopa has not been established.

CARBIDOPA — ORAL

The following other adverse reactions have been reported with levodopa and carbidopa-levodopa combination products. These same adverse reactions may also occur when carbidopa is administered with these products.

➤*Cardiovascular:* Cardiac irregularities, hypertension, myocardial infarction, hypotension including orthostatic hypotension, palpitation, phlebitis, syncope.

➤*CNS:* Agitation, anxiety, ataxia, blepharospasm (which may be taken as an early sign of excess dosage; consideration of dosage reduction may be made at this time), bradykinetic episodes ("on-off" phenomenon), confusion, decreased mental acuity, disorientation, euphoria, dizziness, dream abnormalities including nightmares, extrapyramidal disorder, falling, gait abnormalities, headache, increased tremor, insomnia, memory impairment, muscle twitching, nervousness, numbness, paresthesia, peripheral neuropathy, somnolence, trismus, activation of latent Horner's syndrome.

➤*Dermatologic:* Flushing, increased sweating, malignant melanoma (see Contraindications), rash, alopecia, dark sweat.

➤*GI:* Anorexia, bruxism, burning sensation of the tongue, constipation, dark saliva, development of duodenal ulcer, diarrhea, dry mouth, dyspepsia, dysphagia, flatulence, gastrointestinal bleeding, gastrointestinal pain, heartburn, hiccups, sialorrhea, taste alterations, vomiting.

➤*GU:* Dark urine, priapism, urinary frequency, urinary incontinence, urinary retention, urinary tract infection.

➤*Hematologic:* Hemolytic and non-hemolytic anemia, leukopenia, thrombocytopenia, agranulocytosis.

➤*Hypersensitivity:* Angioedema, urticaria, pruritus and Henoch-Schonlein purpura, bullous lesions (including pemphigus-like reactions).

➤*Lab test abnormalities:* Abnormalities in alkaline phosphatase, AST, ALT, lactic dehydrogenase, bilirubin, blood urea nitrogen (BUN), Coombs test; elevated serum glucose; decreased hemoglobin and hematocrit; decreased white blood cell count and serum potassium; increased serum creatinine and uric acid; white blood cells, bacteria and blood in the urine; protein and glucose in the urine.

➤*Metabolic:* Edema, weight gain, weight loss.

➤*Musculoskeletal:* Back pain, leg pain, muscle cramps, shoulder pain.

➤*Respiratory:* Upper respiratory tract infection, dyspnea, pharyngeal pain, cough.

➤*Special senses:* Oculogyric crises, diplopia, blurred vision, dilated pupils.

➤*Miscellaneous:* Bizarre breathing patterns, faintness, hoarseness, hot flashes, malaise, neuroleptic malignant syndrome, sense of stimulation, abdominal pain and distress, asthenia, chest pain, fatigue.

Overdosage

No reports of overdose with carbidopa have been received. Management of overdosage with carbidopa is the same as that with levodopa or carbidopa-levodopa preparations.

In the event of overdosage, general supportive measures should be employed, along with immediate gastric lavage. Intravenous fluids should be administered judiciously, and an adequate airway maintained. Electrocardiographic monitoring should be instituted and the patient carefully observed for the development of arrhythmias; if required, appropriate antiarrhythmic therapy should be given. The possibility that the patient may have taken other drugs as well as carbidopa should be taken into consideration. To date, no experience has been reported with dialysis; hence, its value in overdosage is not known. Pyridoxine is not effective in reversing the actions of carbidopa.

Based on studies in which high doses of levodopa or carbidopa were administered, a significant proportion of rats and mice given single oral doses of levodopa of approximately 1500 to 2000 mg/kg are expected to die. A significant proportion of infant rats of both sexes are expected to die at a dose of 800 mg/kg. A significant proportion of rats are expected to die after treatment with similar doses of carbidopa. The addition of carbidopa in a 1:10 ratio with levodopa increases the dose at which a significant proportion of mice are expected to die to 3360 mg/kg.

LEVODOPA

Rx	**Larodopa** (Roche)	**Tablets:** 100 mg	(LARODOPA 100). Pink, scored. In 100s.

LEVODOPA — ORAL

Refer to the general discussion in the Antiparkinson Agents introduction.

Indications

➤*Parkinsonism:* Levodopa is indicated in the treatment of idiopathic Parkinson's disease (Paralysis Agitans), postencephalitic parkinsonism, symptomatic parkinsonism which may follow injury to the nervous system by carbon monoxide intoxication, and manganese intoxication. It is indicated in those elderly patients believed to develop parkinsonism in association with cerebral arteriosclerosis.

➤*Unlabeled uses:* Levodopa has been used with some benefit to relieve herpes zoster (shingles) pain and restless legs syndrome.

Administration and Dosage

The optimal daily dose of levodopa, ie, the dose producing maximal improvement with tolerated side effects, must be determined and carefully titrated for each individual patient. The usual initial dosage is 0.5 g to 1 g daily, divided into 2 or more doses with food.

The total daily dosage is then increased gradually in increments not more than 0.75 g every 3 to 7 days as tolerated. The usual optimal therapeutic dosage should not exceed 8 g. The exceptional patient may carefully be given more than 8 g as required.

In some patients, a significant therapeutic response may not be obtained until 6 months of treatment.

In the event general anesthesia is required, levodopa therapy may be continued as long as the patient is able to take fluids and medication by mouth. If therapy is temporarily interrupted, the usual daily dosage may be administered as soon as the patient is able to take oral medication. Whenever therapy has been interrupted for longer periods, dosage should again be adjusted gradually; however, in many cases the patient can be rapidly titrated to his/her previous therapeutic dosage.

Actions

➤*Pharmacology:* Evidence indicates that the symptoms of Parkinson's disease are related to depletion of striatal dopamine. Since dopamine apparently does not cross the blood-brain barrier, its administration is ineffective in the treatment of Parkinson's disease. However, levodopa, the levorotatory isomer of dihydroxyphenylalanine (dopa) which is the metabolic precursor of dopamine, does cross the blood-brain barrier. Presumably it is converted into dopamine in the basal ganglia. This is generally thought to be the mechanism whereby oral levodopa acts in relieving the symptoms of Parkinson's disease.

➤*Pharmacokinetics:* The major urinary metabolites of levodopa in man appear to be dopamine and homovanillic acid (HVA). In 24-hour urine samples, HVA accounts for 13% to 42% of the ingested dose of levodopa.

Contraindications

Monoamine oxidase (MAO) inhibitors and levodopa should not be given concomitantly and these inhibitors must be discontinued 2 weeks prior to initiating therapy with levodopa. Levodopa is contraindicated in patients with known hypersensitivity to the drug and in narrow angle glaucoma.

Warnings

➤*CNS effects:* All patients should be carefully observed for the development of depression with concomitant suicidal tendencies. Psychotic patients should be treated with caution.

➤*Pyridoxine:* Pyridoxine hydrochloride (vitamin B_6) in oral doses of 10 mg to 25 mg rapidly reverses the toxic and therapeutic effects of levodopa. This should be considered before recommending vitamin preparations containing pyridoxine hydrochloride (vitamin B_6).

➤*Pregnancy: Category C.* The safety of levodopa in women who are or who may become pregnant has not been established; hence it should be given only when the potential benefits have been weighed against possible hazards to mother and child. Studies in rodents have shown that levodopa at dosages in excess of 200 mg/kg/day has an adverse effect on fetal and postnatal growth and viability.

➤*Lactation:* Levodopa should not be used in nursing mothers.

➤*Children:* Safety and effectiveness in pediatric patients have not been established.

Precautions

➤*Monitoring:* Periodic evaluations of hepatic, hematopoietic, cardiovascular and renal function are recommended during extended therapy in all patients.

➤*Glaucoma:* Patients with chronic wide-angle glaucoma may be treated cautiously with levodopa, provided the intraocular pressure is well controlled and the patient monitored carefully for changes in intraocular pressure during therapy.

➤*Special risk:* Levodopa should be administered cautiously to patients with severe cardiovascular or pulmonary disease, bronchial asthma, renal, hepatic or endocrine disease.

Care should be exercised in administering levodopa to patients with a history of myocardial infarction who have residual atrial, nodal or ventricular arrhythmias. If levodopa is necessary in this type of patient, it should be used in a facility with a coronary care unit or an intensive care unit.

One must be on the alert for the possibility of upper gastrointestinal hemorrhage in those patients with a history of active peptic ulcer disease.

Drug Interactions

➤*Antihypertensive agents:* Postural hypotensive episodes have been reported as adverse reactions. Therefore, levodopa should be administered cautiously to patients on antihypertensive drug, and it may be necessary to adjust the dosage of the antihypertensive drugs.

LEVODOPA — ORAL

Levodopa Drug Interactions

Precipitant drug	Object drug*		Description
Antacids	Levodopa	↑	Levodopa bioavailability may be increased, possibly increasing its efficacy.
Anticholinergics	Levodopa	↓	Increased gastric deactivation and decreased intestinal absorption of levodopa may occur.
Benzodiazepines	Levodopa	↓	Levodopa's therapeutic value may be attenuated.
Hydantoins	Levodopa	↓	Levodopa's effectiveness may be reduced.
Methionine	Levodopa	↓	Levodopa's effectiveness may be reduced.
Metoclopramide	Levodopa	↔	Levodopa's bioavailability may be increased; levodopa may decrease the effects of metoclopramide on gastric emptying and lower esophageal pressure.
MAO inhibitors	Levodopa	↑	Hypertensive reactions occur with levodopa and MAOI coadministration. Avoid concurrent use. The MAO-type B inhibitor selegiline is used with levodopa and is not associated with such a reaction.
Papaverine	Levodopa	↓	Levodopa's effectiveness may be reduced.
Pyridoxine	Levodopa	↓	Levodopa's effectiveness is reduced.
Tricyclic antidepressants	Levodopa	↓	Delayed absorption and decreased bioavailability of levodopa may occur. Hypertensive episodes have occurred.

* ↑ = Object drug increased ↓ = Object drug decreased ↔ = Undetermined effect

➤*Drug/Lab test interactions:* The Coombs test has occasionally become positive during extended therapy. Elevations of uric acid have occurred with the colorimetric method, but not with the uricase method.

➤*Drug/Food interactions:* In six of nine patients, meals reduced the peak plasma concentrations of levodopa by 29%; the peak was delayed by 34 minutes. A protein-restricted diet may also help minimize the "fluctuations" (decreased response to levodopa at the end of each day or at various times of day) that occur in some patients.

Adverse Reactions

The most serious adverse reactions associated with the administration of levodopa having frequent occurrences are: Adventitious movements such as choreiform and/or dystonic movements. Other serious adverse reactions with a lower incidence are:

➤*Cardiovascular:* Cardiac irregularities and/or palpitations, orthostatic hypotensive episodes, bradykinetic episodes (the "on-off" phenomena).

➤*GU:* Urinary retention.

➤*Psychiatric:* Mental changes including paranoid ideation and psychotic episodes, depression with or without the development of suicidal tendencies, dementia.

➤*Miscellaneous:* Rarely, gastrointestinal bleeding, development of duodenal ulcer, hypertension, phlebitis, hemolytic anemia, agranulocytosis and convulsions have been observed. (The causal relationship between convulsions and levodopa has not been established.)

Adverse reactions of a less serious nature having a relatively frequent occurrence are the following: Anorexia, nausea and vomiting with or without abdominal pain and distress, dry mouth, dysphagia, sialorrhea, ataxia, increased hand tremor, headache, dizziness, numbness, weakness and faintness, bruxism, confusion, insomnia, nightmares, hallucinations and delusions, agitation and anxiety, malaise, fatigue and euphoria. Occurring with a lesser order of frequency are the following: Muscle twitching and blepharospasm (which may be taken as an early sign of overdosage; consideration of dosage reduction may be made at this time), trismus, burning sensation of the tongue, bitter taste, diarrhea, constipation, flatulence, flushing, skin rash, increased sweating, bizarre breathing patterns, urinary incontinence, diplopia, blurred vision, dilated pupils, hot flashes, weight gain or loss, dark sweat and/or urine.

Rarely, oculogyric crises, sense of stimulation, hiccups, development of edema, loss of hair, hoarseness, priapism and activation of latent Horner's syndrome have been observed.

Leukopenia has occurred and requires cessation, at least temporarily, of levodopa administration. The Coombs' test has occasionally become positive during extended therapy. Elevations of uric acid have been noted when colorimetric method was used but not when uricase method was used.

➤*Lab test abnormalities:* Elevations of blood urea nitrogen, SGOT, SGPT, LDH, bilirubin, alkaline phosphatase or protein-bound iodine have been reported; and the significance of this is not known. Occasional reductions in WBC, hemoglobin and hematocrit have been noted.

Overdosage

For acute overdosage general supportive measures should be employed, along with immediate gastric lavage. Intravenous fluids should be administered judiciously and an adequate airway maintained.

Electrocardiographic monitoring should be instituted and the patient carefully observed for the possible development of arrhythmias; if required, appropriate antiarrhythmic therapy should be given. Consideration should be given to the possibility of multiple drug ingestion by the patient. To date, no experience has been reported with dialysis; hence its value in levodopa overdosage is not known. Although pyridoxine hydrochloride (vitamin B_6) has been reported to reverse the anti-Parkinson effects of levodopa, its usefulness in the management of acute overdosage has not been established.

LEVODOPA AND CARBIDOPA

Rx	**Carbidopa and Levodopa** (Various, eg, Endo, Lemmon, Purepac, Teva, UDL)	**Tablets**: 10 mg carbidopa, 100 mg levodopa	In 100s, 500s, and 1,000s.
Rx	**Sinemet-10/100** (Bristol-Myers Squibb)		(647 SINEMET). Dark blue, scored, oval. In 100s and UD 100s.
Rx	**Carbidopa and Levodopa** (Various, eg, Endo, Ivax, Lemmon, Purepac, Teva, UDL)	**Tablets**: 25 mg carbidopa, 100 mg levodopa	In 100s, 500s, and 1,000s.
Rx	**Sinemet-25/100** (Bristol-Myers Squibb)		(650 SINEMET). Yellow, scored, oval. In 100s and UD 100s.
Rx	**Carbidopa and Levodopa** (Various, eg, Endo, Lemmon, Purepac, Teva, UDL)	**Tablets**: 25 mg carbidopa, 250 mg levodopa	In 100s, 500s, and 1,000s.
Rx	**Sinemet-25/250** (Bristol-Myers Squibb)		(654 SINEMET). Light blue, scored, oval. In 100s and UD 100s.
Rx	**Parcopa** (Schwarz Pharma)	**Tablets, orally disintegrating**: 10 mg carbidopa, 100 mg levodopa	3.4 mg phenylalanine, aspartame, mannitol. (10/100 SP 341). Blue, scored. Mint flavor. In 100s.
		25 mg carbidopa, 100 mg levodopa	3.4 mg phenylalanine, aspartame, mannitol. (25/100 SP 342). Yellow, scored. Mint flavor. In 100s.
		25 mg carbidopa, 250 mg levodopa	8.4 mg phenylalanine, aspartame, mannitol. (25/250 SP 343). Blue, scored. Mint flavor. In 100s.
Rx	**Carbidopa and Levodopa** (Various, eg, Apotex, Mylan, UDL)	**Tablets, extended-release**: 25 mg carbidopa, 100 mg levodopa	In 100s and 500s.
Rx	**Sinemet CR** (Bristol-Myers Squibb)		(601 SINEMET CR). Pink, oval. In 100s, 500s, and UD 100s.
Rx	**Carbidopa and Levodopa** (Various, eg, Apotex, Mylan, UDL)	**Tablets, extended-release**: 50 mg carbidopa, 200 mg levodopa	In 100s and 500s.
Rx	**Sinemet CR** (Bristol-Myers Squibb)		(521 SINEMET CR). Peach, scored, oval. In 100s, 500s, and UD 100s.

LEVODOPA AND CARBIDOPA — ORAL

These agents are used in combination because carbidopa inhibits decarboxylation of levodopa and makes more levodopa available for transport to the brain. For complete information on each of the components, refer to the individual monographs. Also refer to the general discussion in the Antiparkinson Agents introduction.

Indications

➤*Parkinsonism:* Treatment of symptoms of idiopathic Parkinson disease (paralysis agitans), postencephalitic parkinsonism, and symptomatic parkinsonism that may follow injury to the nervous system by carbon monoxide and/or manganese intoxication.

Levodopa and carbidopa are indicated in these conditions to permit the administration of lower doses of levodopa with reduced nausea and vomiting, more rapid dosage titration, a somewhat smoother response, and with supplemental pyridoxine (vitamin B_6).

Administration and Dosage

Determine the optimum daily dose by careful titration in each patient. Extended-release tablets may be administered as whole or half tablets that should not be crushed or chewed.

➤*Patients not receiving levodopa:*

Immediate-release tablets – One tablet of carbidopa 25 mg/levodopa 100 mg 3 times daily or carbidopa 10 mg/levodopa 100 mg 3 or 4 times daily. Dosage may be increased by 1 tablet every day or every other day, as necessary, until a dosage of 8 tablets a day is reached.

Tablets of the 2 ratios (eg, 1:4, 25/100 or 1:10, 10/100 and 25/250) may be given separately or combined as needed to provide the optimum dosage.

Provide at least carbidopa 70 to 100 mg per day. When more carbidopa is required, substitute one 25/100 tablet for each 10/100 tablet. When more levodopa is required, substitute the 25/250 tablet for the 25/100 or 10/100 tablet. If necessary, the dosage of 25/250 may be increased by one-half or 1 tablet every day or every other day to a maximum of 8 tablets a day. Experience with total daily dosages of carbidopa greater than 200 mg is limited.

Extended-release tablets – In patients with mild to moderate disease, the initial recommended dose is one 50/200 tablet twice daily at intervals of 6 hours or more. Doses and dosing intervals may be increased or decreased based on response. Most patients have been adequately treated with a dose that provides 400 to 1,600 mg of levodopa per day (divided doses) at intervals of 4 to 8 hours while awake. Higher doses (2,400 mg or more of levodopa per day) and shorter intervals (less than 4 hours) have been used but are not usually recommended. If an interval of less than 4 hours is used and/or if the divided doses are not equal, give the smaller doses at the end of the day. Allow at least a 3-day interval between dosage adjustments.

➤*Patients currently treated with levodopa:* Discontinue levodopa at least 12 hours before therapy with levodopa/carbidopa. Substitute the combination drug at a dosage that will provide approximately 25% of the previous levodopa dosage.

Immediate-release tablets – Suggested starting dosage is 1 tablet of carbidopa 25 mg/levodopa 250 mg 3 or 4 times daily for patients taking more than levodopa 1,500 mg or carbidopa 25 mg/levodopa 100 mg for patients taking less than levodopa 1,500 mg.

Extended-release tablets – In patients with mild to moderate disease, the initial dose is usually one 50/200 extended-release tablet twice daily.

➤*Patients currently treated with conventional carbidopa/levodopa preparations:* Substitute dosage with extended-release tablets at an amount that provides approximately 10% more levodopa per day, although this may need to be increased to a dosage that provides up to 30% more levodopa per day. Use intervals of 4 to 8 hours while awake.

Guidelines for Initial Conversion From Immediate-Release to Extended-Release (50/100 mg Tablets)	
Immediate-release total daily levodopa dose (mg)	Extended-release (50/100 mg tablets) suggested dosage regimen
300 to 400	200 mg twice daily
500 to 600	300 mg twice daily or 200 mg 3 times daily
700 to 800	Total of 800 mg in 3 or more divided doses (eg, 300 mg am, 300 mg early pm, and 200 mg later pm)
900 to 1,000	Total of 1,000 mg in 3 or more divided doses (eg, 400 mg am, 400 mg early pm, and 200 mg later pm)

➤*Combination therapy:* Other antiparkinson drugs can be given concurrently; dosage adjustment may be necessary.

Immediate-release tablets – Immediate-release tablets (25/100 or 10/100) can be added to the dosage regimen of extended-release tablets in selected patients with advanced disease who need additional levodopa.

➤*Administration of orally disintegrating tablets:* Just prior to administration, gently remove the tablet from the bottle with dry hands. Immediately place the tablet on top of the tongue where it will dissolve in seconds, then swallow with saliva. Administration with liquid is not necessary.

➤*Storage/Stability:* Protect from moisture and light. Avoid storing extended-release tablets above 30°C (86°F). Store disintegrating tablets between 20° to 25°C (68° to 86°F); excursions permitted between 15° to 30°C (59° to 86°F).

Actions

➤*Pharmacokinetics:* The extended-release formulation is designed to release the ingredients over a 4- to 6-hour period. There is less variation in plasma levodopa levels than with the conventional formulation. However, the extended-release form is less systemically bioavailable (70% to 75%) and may require increased daily doses to achieve the same level of symptomatic relief. The half-life of levodopa may be prolonged following the extended-release form because of continuous absorption. In elderly subjects, the mean time to peak levodopa concentration was 2 hours for extended-release versus 0.5 hours for conventional. The maximum levodopa concentration of levodopa following the extended-release form was approximately 35% of the conventional form.

Warnings

➤*CNS effects:* Certain adverse CNS effects (eg, dyskinesias) will occur at lower dosages and sooner during therapy with levodopa and carbidopa than with levodopa alone.

Drug Interactions

➤*Drug/Food interactions:* Administration of a single dose of the extended-release form with food increased the extent of levodopa availability by 50% and increased peak levodopa concentrations by 25%.

Adverse Reactions

In clinical trials, the adverse reaction profile of the extended-release form did not differ substantially from that of the conventional form.

ENTACAPONE

Rx	**Comtan** (Novartis)	**Tablets:** 200 mg	Mannitol, sucrose. (COMTAN). Film-coated. Oval, brownish-orange. In 10s, 100s, and 500s.

ENTACAPONE — ORAL

Indications

➤*Parkinsonism:* Entacapone is indicated as an adjunct to levodopa/carbidopa to treat patients with idiopathic Parkinson's Disease who experience the signs and symptoms of end-of-dose "wearing-off".

Entacapone's effectiveness has not been systematically evaluated in patients with idiopathic Parkinson's Disease who do not experience end-of-dose "wearing-off".

Administration and Dosage

➤*Approved by the FDA:* October 22, 1999.

The recommended dose of entacapone is one 200 mg tablet administered concomitantly with each levodopa/carbidopa dose to a maximum of 8 times daily (200 mg × 8 = 1600 mg per day). Clinical experience with daily doses above 1600 mg is limited.

Entacapone should always be administered in association with levodopa/carbidopa. Entacapone has no antiparkinsonian effect of its own.

In clinical trials, the majority of patients required a decrease in daily levodopa dose if their daily dose of levodopa had been ≥ 800 mg, or if patients had moderate or severe dyskinesias before beginning treatment.

To optimize an individual patient's response, reductions in daily levodopa dose or extending the interval between doses may be necessary. In clinical trials, the average reduction in daily levodopa dose was about 25% in those patients requiring a levodopa dose reduction. (More than 58% of patients with levodopa doses above 800 mg daily required such a reduction.)

Entacapone can be combined with both the immediate and sustained release formulations of levodopa/carbidopa.

Entacapone may be taken with or without food.

➤*Hepatic function impairment:* See Actions for more information.

➤*Withdrawing patients from entacapone:* Rapid withdrawal or abrupt reduction in the entacapone dose could lead to emergence of signs and symptoms of Parkinson's disease, and may lead to Hyperpyrexia and Confusion, a symptom complex resembling the neuroleptic malignant syndrome. This syndrome should be considered in the differential diagnosis for any patient who develops a high fever or severe rigidity. If a decision is made to discontinue treatment with entacapone, patients should be monitored closely and other dopaminergic treatments should be adjusted as needed. Although tapering entacapone has not been systematically evaluated, it seems prudent to withdraw patients slowly if the decision to discontinue treatment is made.

➤*Storage/Stability:* Store at 25°C (77°F) excursions permitted to 15 to 30°C (59 to 86°F).

Actions

➤*Pharmacology:* Entacapone is a selective and reversible inhibitor of catechol-O-methyltransferase (COMT).

ENTACAPONE — ORAL

The mechanism of action of entacapone is believed to be through its ability to inhibit COMT and alter the plasma pharmacokinetics of levodopa. When entacapone is given in conjunction with levodopa and an aromatic amino acid decarboxylase inhibitor, such as carbidopa, plasma levels of levodopa are greater and more sustained than after administration of levodopa and an aromatic amino acid decarboxylase inhibitor alone. It is believed that at a given frequency of levodopa administration, these more sustained plasma levels of levodopa result in more constant dopaminergic stimulation in the brain, leading to greater effects on the signs and symptoms of Parkinson's disease. The higher levodopa levels also lead to increased levodopa adverse effects, sometimes requiring a decrease in the dose of levodopa.

In animals, while entacapone enters the CNS to a minimal extent, it has been shown to inhibit central COMT activity. In humans, entacapone inhibits the COMT enzyme in peripheral tissues. The effects of entacapone on central COMT activity in humans have not been studied.

➤*Pharmacokinetics:*

Absorption – Entacapone is rapidly absorbed, with a T_{max} of approximately 1 hour. The absolute bioavailability following oral administration is 35%. Food does not affect the pharmacokinetics of entacapone.

Distribution – The volume of distribution of entacapone at steady state after IV injection is small (20 L). Entacapone does not distribute widely into tissues due to its high plasma protein binding. Based on in vitro studies, the plasma protein binding of entacapone is 98% over the concentration range of 0.4 to 50 mcg/ml. Entacapone binds mainly to serum albumin.

Metabolism/Excretion – Entacapone is almost completely metabolized prior to excretion, with only a very small amount (0.2% of dose) found unchanged in urine. The main metabolic pathway is isomerization to the cis-isomer, followed by direct glucuronidation of the parent and cis-isomer; the glucuronide conjugate is inactive. After oral administration of a ^{14}C-labeled dose of entacapone, 10% of labeled parent and metabolite is excreted in urine and 90% in feces.

Entacapone pharmacokinetics are linear over the dose range of 5 to 800 mg, and are independent of levodopa/carbidopa coadministration. The elimination of entacapone is biphasic, with an elimination half-life of 0.4 to 0.7 h based on the β-phase and 2.4 h based on the γ-phase. The γ-phase accounts for approximately 10% of the total AUC. The total body clearance after IV administration is 850 ml/min. After a single 200 mg dose of entacapone, the C_{max} is approximately 1.2 mcg/ml.

Special populations –

Hepatic function impairment: A single 200 mg dose of entacapone, without levodopa/dopa decarboxylase inhibitor coadministration, showed approximately twofold higher AUC and C_{max} values in patients with a history of alcoholism and hepatic impairment (n = 10) compared to normal subjects (n = 10). All patients had biopsy-proven liver cirrhosis caused by alcohol. According to Child-Pugh grading, 7 patients with liver disease had mild hepatic impairment and 3 patients had moderate hepatic impairment. As only about 10% of the entacapone dose is excreted in urine as parent compound and conjugated glucuronide, biliary excretion appears to be the major route of excretion of this drug. Consequently, entacapone should be administered with care to patients with biliary obstruction.

Contraindications

Hypersensitivity to the drug or its ingredients.

Warnings

➤*Renal function impairment:* In a 1 year toxicity study, entacapone (plasma exposure 20 times that in humans receiving the maximum recommended daily dose of 1600 mg) caused an increased incidence in male rats of nephrotoxicity that was characterized by regenerative tubules, thickening of basement membranes, infiltration of mononuclear cells and tubular protein casts. These effects were not associated with changes in clinical chemistry parameters, and there is no established method for monitoring for the possible occurrence of these lesions in humans. Although this toxicity could represent a species-specific effect, there is not yet evidence that this is so.

➤*Hepatic function impairment:* Patients with hepatic impairment should be treated with caution. The AUC and C_{max} of entacapone approximately doubled in patients with documented liver disease compared to controls.

➤*Carcinogenesis:* Two-year carcinogenicity studies of entacapone were conducted in mice and rats. Rats were treated once daily by oral gavage with entacapone doses of 20, 90, or 400 mg/kg. An increased incidence of renal tubular adenomas and carcinomas was found in male rats treated with the highest dose of entacapone. Plasma exposures (AUC) associated with this dose were approximately 20 times higher than estimated plasma exposures of humans receiving the maximum recommended daily dose of entacapone (MRDD = 1600 mg). Mice were treated once daily by oral gavage with doses of 20, 100 or 600 mg/kg of entacapone (0.05, 0.3, and 2 times the MRDD for humans on a mg/m^2 basis). Because of a high incidence of premature mortality in mice receiving the highest dose of entacapone, the mouse study is not an adequate assessment of carcinogenicity. Although no treatment related tumors were observed in animals receiving the lower doses, the carcinogenic potential of entacapone has not been fully evaluated. The carcinogenic potential of entacapone administered in combination with levodopa/carbidopa has not been evaluated.

➤*Mutagenesis:* Entacapone was mutagenic and clastogenic in the in vitro mouse lymphoma/thymidine kinase assay in the presence and absence of metabolic activation, and was clastogenic in cultured human lymphocytes in the presence of metabolic activation. Entacapone, either alone or in combination with levodopa/carbidopa, was not clastogenic in the in vivo mouse micronucleus test or mutagenic in the bacterial reverse mutation assay (Ames test).

➤*Pregnancy: Category C.* In embryofetal development studies, entacapone was administered to pregnant animals throughout organogenesis at doses of up to 1000 mg/kg/day in rats and 300 mg/kg/day in rabbits. Increased incidences of fetal variations were evident in litters from rats treated with the highest dose, in the absence of overt signs of maternal toxicity. The maternal plasma drug exposure (AUC) associated with this dose was approximately 34 times the estimated plasma exposure in humans receiving the maximum recommended daily dose (MRDD) of 1600 mg. Increased frequencies of abortions and late/total resorptions and decreased fetal weights were observed in the litters of rabbits treated with maternotoxic doses of 100 mg/kg/day (plasma AUCs 0.4 times those in humans receiving the MRDD) or greater. There was no evidence of teratogenicity in these studies.

However, when entacapone was administered to female rats prior to mating and during early gestation, an increased incidence of fetal eye anomalies (macrophthalmia, microphthalmia, anophthalmia) was observed in the litters of dams treated with doses of 160 mg/kg/day (plasma AUCs 7 times those in humans receiving the MRDD) or greater, in the absence of maternotoxicity. Administration of up to 700 mg/kg/day (plasma AUCs 28 times those in humans receiving the MRDD) to female rats during the latter part of gestation and throughout lactation, produced no evidence of developmental impairment in the offspring.

There is no experience from clinical studies regarding the use of entacapone in pregnant women. Therefore, entacapone should be used during pregnancy only if the potential benefit justifies the potential risk to the fetus.

➤*Lactation:* In animal studies, entacapone was excreted into maternal rat milk.

It is not known whether entacapone is excreted in human milk. Because many drugs are excreted in human milk, caution should be exercised when entacapone is administered to a nursing woman.

➤*Children:* There is no identified potential use of entacapone in pediatric patients.

Precautions

➤*Hypotension/syncope:* Dopaminergic therapy in Parkinson's disease patients has been associated with orthostatic hypotension. Entacapone enhances levodopa bioavailability and, therefore, might be expected to increase the occurrence of orthostatic hypotension. In entacapone clinical trials, however, no differences from placebo were seen for measured orthostasis or symptoms of orthostasis. Orthostatic hypotension was documented at least once in 2.7% and 3% of the patients treated 200 mg entacapone and placebo, respectively. A total of 4.3% and 4% of the patients treated with 200 mg entacapone and placebo, respectively, reported orthostatic symptoms at some time during their treatment and also had at least one episode of orthostatic hypotension documented (however, the episode of orthostatic symptoms itself was not accompanied by vital sign measurements). Neither baseline treatment with dopamine agonists or selegiline, nor the presence of orthostasis at baseline, increased the risk of orthostatic hypotension in patients treated with entacapone compared to patients on placebo.

In the large controlled trials, approximately 1.2% and 0.8% of 200 mg entacapone and placebo patients, respectively, reported at least 1 episode of syncope. Reports of syncope were generally more frequent in patients in both treatment groups who had an episode of documented hypotension (although the episodes of syncope, obtained by history, were themselves not documented with vital sign measurement).

➤*Diarrhea:* In clinical trials, diarrhea developed in 60 of 603 (10.0%) and 16 of 400 (4.0%) of patients treated with 200 mg entacapone and placebo, respectively. In patients treated with entacapone diarrhea was generally mild to moderate in severity (8.6%) but was regarded as severe in 1.3%. Diarrhea resulted in withdrawal in 10 of 603 (1.7%) patients, (1.2%) with mild and moderate diarrhea and 3 (0.5%) with severe diarrhea. Diarrhea generally resolved after discontinuation of entacapone. Two patients with diarrhea were hospitalized. Typically, diarrhea presents within 4 to 12 weeks after entacapone is started, but it may appear as early as the first week and as late as many months after the initiation of treatment.

➤*Hallucinations:* Dopaminergic therapy in Parkinson's disease patients has been associated with hallucinations. In clinical trials, hallucinations developed in approximately 4% of patients treated with 200 mg entacapone or placebo. Hallucinations led to drug discontinuation and premature withdrawal from clinical trials in 0.8% and 0% of patients treated with 200 mg entacapone and placebo, respectively. Hallucinations led to hospitalization in 1% and 0.3% of patients in the 200 mg entacapone and placebo groups, respectively.

➤*Dyskinesia:* Entacapone may potentiate the dopaminergic side effects of levodopa and may cause or exacerbate preexisting dyskinesia. Although decreasing the dose of levodopa may ameliorate this side effect, many patients in controlled trials continued to experience frequent dyskinesias despite a reduction in their dose of levodopa. The rates of withdrawal for dyskinesia were 1.5% and 0.8% for 200 mg entacapone and placebo, respectively.

➤*Other events reported with dopaminergic therapy:* The events listed below are rare events known to be associated with the use of drugs that increase dopaminergic activity, although they are most often associated with the use of direct dopamine agonists:

Rhabdomyolysis – Cases of severe rhabdomyolysis have been reported with entacapone use. The complicated nature of these cases makes it impossible to determine what role, if any, entacapone played in their pathogenesis. Severe prolonged motor activity including dyskinesia may account for rhabdomyolysis. One case, however, included fever and alteration of consciousness. It is therefore possible that the rhabdomyolysis may be a result of the syndrome described in Hyperpyrexia and Confusion (see below).

ENTACAPONE — ORAL

Hyperpyrexia and confusion – Cases of a symptom complex resembling the neuroleptic malignant syndrome characterized by elevated temperature, muscular rigidity, altered consciousness, and elevated creatine phosphokinase have been reported in association with the rapid dose reduction or withdrawal of other dopaminergic drugs. Several cases with similar signs and symptoms have been reported in association with entacapone therapy, although no information about dose manipulation is available. The complicated nature of these cases makes it difficult to determine what role, if any, entacapone may have played in their pathogenesis. No cases have been reported following the abrupt withdrawal or dose reduction of entacapone treatment during clinical studies.

Withdrawing patients from entacapone – See Administration and Dosage for more information.

Fibrotic complications – Cases of retroperitoneal fibrosis, pulmonary infiltrates, pleural effusion, and pleural thickening have been reported in some patients treated with ergot derived dopaminergic agents. These complications may resolve when the drug is discontinued, but complete resolution does not always occur. Although these adverse events are believed to be related to the ergoline structure of these compounds, whether other, nonergot derived drugs (eg, entacapone) that increase dopaminergic activity can cause them is unknown. It should be noted that the expected incidence of fibrotic complications is so low that even if entacapone caused these complications at rates similar to those attributable to other dopaminergic therapies, it is unlikely that it would have been detected in a cohort of the size exposed to entacapone. Four cases of pulmonary fibrosis were reported during clinical development of entacapone; 3 of these patients were also treated with pergolide and 1 with bromocriptine. The duration of treatment with entacapone ranged from 7 to 17 months.

Drug Interactions

Entacapone Drug Interactions

Precipitant drug	Object drug*		Description
MAO Inhibitors	Entacapone	↑	MAO and COMT are the 2 major enzyme systems involved in catecholamine metabolism. Therefore, it is theoretically possible that the combination of entacapone and a non-selective MAO inhibitor (eg, phenelzine, tranylcypromine) would result in inhibition of the majority of the pathways responsible for normal catecholamine metabolism. For this reason, patients should ordinarily not be treated concomitantly with entacapone and a non-selective MAO inhibitor (see Warnings). Entacapone may be taken concomitantly with a selective MAO-B inhibitor (eg, selegiline).
Probenecid Cholestyramine Erythromycin Rifampicin Ampicillin Chloramphenicol	Entacapone	↑	As most entacapone excretion is via the bile, exercise caution when drugs known to interfere with biliary excretion, glucuronidation, and intestinal beta-glucuronidase are given concurrently with entacapone.
Entacapone	Isoproterenol Epinephrine Norepinephrine Dopamine Dobutamine Methyldopa Apomorphine Isoetherine Bitolterol	↑	Administer drugs known to be metabolized by COMT (ie, isoproterenol, epinephrine, norepinephrine, dopamine, dobutamine, methyldopa, apomorphine, isoetherine, bitolterol) with caution in patients receiving entacapone regardless of the route of administration (including inhalation), as their interaction may result in increased heart rates, possibly arrhythmias, and excessive changes in blood pressure.

* ↑ = Object drug increased.

➤*Drugs metabolized by catechol-O-methyltransferase (COMT):* When a single 400 mg dose of entacapone was given together with intravenous isoprenaline (isoproterenol) and epinephrine without coadministered levodopa/dopa decarboxylase inhibitor, the overall mean maximal changes in heart rate during infusion were about 50% and 80% higher than with placebo, for isoprenaline and epinephrine, respectively.

Therefore, drugs known to be metabolized by COMT, such as isoproterenol, epinephrine, norepinephrine, dopamine, dobutamine, alpha-methyldopa, apomorphine, isoetharine, and bitolterol should be administered with caution in patients receiving entacapone regardless of the route of administration (including inhalation), as their interaction may result in increased heart rates, possibly arrhythmias, and excessive changes in blood pressure.

Ventricular tachycardia was noted in one 32 year old healthy male volunteer in an interaction study after epinephrine infusion and oral entacapone administration. Treatment with propranolol was required. A causal relationship to entacapone administration appears probable but cannot be attributed with certainty.

➤*Levodopa and its metabolites:* When 200 mg entacapone is administered together with levodopa/carbidopa, it increases the area under the curve (AUC) of levodopa by approximately 35% and the elimination half life of levodopa is prolonged from 1.3 h to 2.4 h. In general, the average peak levodopa plasma concentration and the time of its occurrence (T_{max} of 1 hour) are unaffected. The onset of effect occurs after the first administration and is maintained during long-term treatment. Studies in Parkinson's disease patients suggest that the maximal effect occurs with 200 mg entacapone. Plasma levels of 3-OMD are markedly and dose-dependently decreased by entacapone when given with levodopa/carbidopa.

Adverse Reactions

The most commonly observed adverse events (> 5%) in the double-blind, placebo-controlled trials (n = 1003) associated with the use of entacapone and not seen at an equivalent frequency among the placebo-treated patients were: Dyskinesia/hyperkinesia, nausea, urine discoloration, diarrhea, and abdominal pain.

Approximately 14% of the 603 patients given entacapone in the double-blind, placebo-controlled trials discontinued treatment due to adverse events compared to 9% of the 400 patients who received placebo. The most frequent causes of discontinuation in decreasing order are: psychiatric reasons (2% vs 1%), diarrhea (2% vs 0%), dyskinesia/hyperkinesia (2% vs 1%), nausea (2% vs 1%), abdominal pain (1% vs 0%), and aggravation of Parkinson's Disease symptoms (1% vs 1%).

➤*Adverse event incidence in controlled clinical studies:* Listed below are treatment emergent adverse events that occurred in at least 1% of patients treated with entacapone participating in the double-blind, placebo-controlled studies and that were numerically more common in the entacapone group, compared to placebo. In these studies, either entacapone (n = 603) or placebo (n = 400) was added to levodopa/carbidopa (or levodopa/benserazide).

Summary of Patients with Adverse Events after Start of Trial Drug Administration at least 1% in Entacapone Group and > Placebo

System organ class, preferred term	Entacapone (n = 603) % of patients	Placebo (n = 400) % of patients
Dermatologic		
Sweating increased	2%	1%
Musculoskeletal		
Back pain	2%	1%
CNS		
Dyskinesia	25%	15%
Hyperkinesia	10%	5%
Hypokinesia	9%	8%
Dizziness	8%	6%
Special senses		
Taste perversion	1%	0%
Psychiatric disorders		
Anxiety	2%	1%
Somnolence	2%	0%
Agitation	1%	0%
GI		
Nausea	14%	8%
Diarrhea	10%	4%
Abdominal pain	8%	4%
Constipation	6%	4%
Vomiting	4%	1%
Mouth dry	3%	0%
Dyspepsia	2%	1%
Flatulence	2%	0%
Gastritis	1%	0%
Gastrointestinal disorders nos	1%	0%
Respiratory		
Dyspnea	3%	1%
Hematologic		
Purpura	2%	1%
GU		
Urine discoloration	10%	0%
Miscellaneous		
Back pain	4%	2%
Fatigue	6%	4%
Asthenia	2%	1%

ENTACAPONE — ORAL

Summary of Patients with Adverse Events after Start of Trial Drug Administration at least 1% in Entacapone Group and > Placebo		
System organ class, preferred term	Entacapone (n = 603) % of patients	Placebo (n = 400) % of patients
Resistance mechanism disorders		
Infection bacterial	1%	0%

Overdosage

➤*Symptoms:* There have been no reported cases of either accidental or intentional overdose with entacapone tablets. However, COMT inhibition by entacapone treatment is dose-dependent. A massive overdose of entacapone may theoretically produce a 100% inhibition of the COMT enzyme in people, thereby preventing the metabolism of endogenous and exogenous catechols.

The highest single dose of entacapone administered to humans was 800 mg, resulting in a plasma concentration of 14.1 mcg/ml. The highest daily dose given to humans was 2400 mg, administered in one study as 400 mg 6 times daily with levodopa/carbidopa for 14 days in 15 Parkinson's disease patients, and in another study as 800 mg tid for 7 days in 8 healthy volunteers. At this daily dose, the peak plasma concentrations of entacapone averaged 2 mcg/ml (at 45 min, compared to 1 and 1.2 mcg/ml with 200 mg entacapone at 45 min). Abdominal pain and loose stools were the most commonly observed adverse events during this study. Daily doses as high as 2000 mg entacapone have been administered as 200 mg 10 times daily with levodopa/carbidopa or levodopa/benserazide for at least 1 year in 10 patients, for at least 2 years by 8 patients and for at least 3 years in 7 patients. Overall, however, clinical experience with daily doses above 1600 mg is limited.

The range of lethal plasma concentrations of entacapone based on animal data was 80 to 130 mcg/ml in mice. Respiratory difficulties, ataxia, hypoactivity, and convulsions were observed in mice after high oral (gavage) doses.

➤*Treatment:* Management of entacapone overdose is symptomatic; there is no known antidote to entacapone. Hospitalization is advised, and general supportive care is indicated. There is no experience with hemodialysis or hemoperfusion, but these procedures are unlikely to be of benefit, because entacapone is highly bound to plasma proteins. An immediate gastric lavage and repeated doses of charcoal over time may hasten the elimination of entacapone by decreasing its absorption/reabsorption from the GI tract. The adequacy of the respiratory and circulatory systems should be carefully monitored and appropriate supportive measures employed. The possibility of drug interactions, especially with catechol-structured drugs, should be borne in mind.

Patient Information

Patients should be instructed to take entacapone only as prescribed.

Patients should be informed that hallucinations can occur.

Patients should be advised that they may develop postural (orthostatic) hypotension with or without symptoms such as dizziness, nausea, syncope, and sweating. Hypotension may occur more frequently during initial therapy. Accordingly, patients should be cautioned against rising rapidly after sitting or lying down, especially if they have been doing so for prolonged periods, and especially at the initiation of treatment with entacapone.

Patients should be advised that they should neither drive a car nor operate other complex machinery until they have gained sufficient experience on entacapone to gauge whether or not it affects their mental or motor performance adversely. Because of the possible additive sedative effects, caution should be used when patients are taking other CNS depressants in combination with entacapone.

Patients should be informed that nausea may occur, especially at the initiation of treatment with entacapone.

Patients should be advised of the possibility of an increase in dyskinesia.

Patients should be advised that treatment with entacapone may cause a change in the color of their urine (a brownish orange discoloration) that is not clinically relevant. In controlled trials, 10% of patients treated with entacapone reported urine discoloration compared to 0% of placebo patients.

Although entacapone has not been shown to be teratogenic in animals, it is always given in conjunction with levodopa/carbidopa, which is known to cause visceral and skeletal malformations in the rabbit. Accordingly, patients should be advised to notify their physicians if they become pregnant or intend to become pregnant during therapy (see Warnings).

Entacapone is excreted into maternal milk in rats. Because of the possibility that entacapone may be excreted into human maternal milk, patients should be advised to notify their physicians if they intend to breastfeed or are breastfeeding an infant.

➤*Laboratory tests:* Entacapone is a chelator of iron. The impact of entacapone on the body's iron stores is unknown; however, a tendency towards decreasing serum iron concentrations was noted in clinical trials. In a controlled clinical study serum ferritin levels (as marker of iron deficiency and subclinical anemia) were not changed with entacapone compared to placebo after one year of treatment and there was no difference in rates of anemia or decreased hemoglobin levels.

CARBIDOPA, LEVODOPA, AND ENTACAPONE

Rx	**Stalevo 50** (Novartis)	**Tablets**: 12.5 mg carbidopa, 50 mg levodopa, and 200 mg entacapone	Mannitol, sucrose. (LCE 50). Film-coated. Round, bi-convex, brownish- or greyish-red. In 100s and 250s.
Rx	**Stalevo 100** (Novartis)	25 mg carbidopa, 100 mg levodopa, and 200 mg entacapone	Mannitol, sucrose. (LCE 100). Film-coated. Oval, brownish- or greyish-red. In 100s and 250s.
Rx	**Stalevo 150** (Novartis)	37.5 mg carbidopa, 150 mg levodopa, and 200 mg entacapone	Mannitol, sucrose. (LCE 150). Film-coated. Ellipse shape, brownish- or greyish-red. In 100s and 250s.

CARBIDOPA, LEVODOPA, AND ENTACAPONE — ORAL

For complete prescribing information on each of the components refer to the individual monographs. Also refer to the general discussion in the Antiparkinson Agents introduction.

Indications

➤*Parkinson disease:* To treat patients with idiopathic Parkinson disease; to substitute (with equivalent strength of each of the 3 components) for immediate release carbidopa/levodopa and entacapone previously administered as individual products; to replace immediate release carbidopa/levodopa therapy (without entacapone) when patients experience the signs and symptoms of end-of-dose "wearing-off" (only for patients taking a total daily dose of levodopa of 600 mg or less and not experiencing dyskinesias).

Administration and Dosage

➤*Approved by the FDA:* June 13, 2003.

Do not fractionate individual tablets and administer only 1 tablet at each dosing interval. Individualize therapy and adjust according to the desired therapeutic response.

Use carbidopa, levodopa, and entacapone combination as a substitute for patients already stabilized on equivalent doses of carbidopa/levodopa and entacapone. Some patients who have been stabilized on a given dose of carbidopa/levodopa may be treated with carbidopa, levodopa, and entacapone combination if a decision has been made to add entacapone.

The optimum daily dosage of carbidopa, levodopa, and entacapone combination must be determined by careful titration in each patient. Carbidopa, levodopa, and entacapone combination tablets are available in 3 strengths, each in a 1:4 ratio of carbidopa to levodopa and combined with 200 mg of entacapone in a standard release formulation.

Studies show that peripheral dopa decarboxylase is saturated by carbidopa at approximately 70 to 100 mg/day. Patients receiving less than this amount of carbidopa are more likely to experience nausea and vomiting. Experience with total daily dosages of carbidopa greater than 200 mg is limited.

Clinical experience with daily doses above 1600 mg of entacapone is limited. It is recommended that no more than 1 carbidopa, levodopa, and entacapone combination tablet be taken at each dosing administration. Thus, the maximum recommended daily dose of carbidopa, levodopa, and entacapone combination is 8 tablets/day.

➤*Transferring patients currently treated with carbidopa/levodopa and entacapone to carbidopa, levodopa, and entacapone combination tablet:*

Carbidopa/levodopa – There is no experience in transferring patients currently treated with formulation of carbidopa/levodopa other than immediate release carbidopa/levodopa with a 1:4 ratio (controlled release formulations, or standard release presentations with a 1:10 ratio of carbidopa/levodopa) and entacapone to carbidopa, levodopa, and entacapone combination.

Entacapone – Patients who are currently treated with entacapone 200 mg tablet with each dose of standard release carbidopa/levodopa, can be directly switched to the corresponding strength of carbidopa, levodopa, and entacapone combination containing the same amounts of levodopa and carbidopa. For example, patients receiving 1 tablet of standard release carbidopa/levodopa 25/100 mg and 1 tablet of entacapone 200 mg at each administration can be switched to a single *Stalevo 100* tablet (containing 25 mg of carbidopa, 100 mg of levodopa, and 200 mg of entacapone).

➤*Transferring patients not currently treated with entacapone tablets from carbidopa/levodopa to carbidopa, levodopa, and entacapone combination tablets:* In patients with Parkinson disease who experience the signs and symptoms of end-of-dose "wearing-off" on their current standard release carbidopa/levodopa treatment, clinical experience shows that patients with a history of moderate or severe dyskinesias or taking more than 600 mg/day of levodopa are likely to require a reduction in daily levodopa dose when entacapone is added to their treatment. Since dose adjustment of the individual components is impossible with fixed dose products, it is recommended that patients first be titrated individually with a carbidopa/levodopa product (ratio 1:4) and an entacapone product, and then transferred to a corresponding dose of carbidopa, levodopa, and entacapone combination once the patient's status has stabilized.

In patients who take a total daily levodopa dose up to 600 mg and who do not have dyskinesias, an attempt can be made to transfer to the correspond-

CARBIDOPA, LEVODOPA, AND ENTACAPONE — ORAL

ing daily dose of carbidopa, levodopa, and entacapone combination. However, even in these patients, a reduction of carbidopa/levodopa or entacapone may be necessary, and the provider is reminded that this may not be possible with carbidopa, levodopa, and entacapone combination. Because entacapone prolongs and enhances the effects of levodopa, individualize therapy and adjust if necessary according to the desired therapeutic response.

➤*Maintenance therapy:* Individualize therapy and adjust for each patient according to the desired therapeutic response.

When less levodopa is required, reduce the total daily dosage of carbidopa/levodopa by decreasing the strength of carbidopa, levodopa, and entacapone combination at each administration or by decreasing the frequency of administration by extending the time between doses.

When more levodopa is required, take the next higher strength of carbidopa, levodopa, and entacapone combination and/or increase the frequency of doses, up to a maximum of 8 times daily and not to exceed the maximum daily dose recommendations as outlined above.

➤*Addition of other antiparkinsonian medications:* Standard drugs for Parkinson disease may be used concomitantly while carbidopa, levodopa, and entacapone combination is being administered, although dosage adjustments may be required.

➤*Interruption of therapy:* Sporadic cases of a symptom complex resembling Neuroleptic Malignant Syndrome (NMS) have been associated with dose reductions and withdrawal of levodopa preparations. Observe patients carefully if abrupt reduction or discontinuation of carbidopa, levodopa, and entacapone combination is required, especially if the patient is receiving neuroleptics.

If general anesthesia is required, carbidopa, levodopa, and entacapone combination may be continued as long as the patient is permitted to take fluids and medication by mouth. If therapy is interrupted temporarily, observe the patient for symptoms resembling NMS, and the usual daily dosage may be administered as soon as the patient is able to take oral medication.

➤*Hepatic function impairment:* Treat patients with hepatic impairment with caution. The AUC and C_{max} of entacapone approximately doubled in patients with documented liver disease, compared with controls. However, these studies were conducted with single-dose entacapone without levodopa/dopa decarboxylase inhibitor coadministration, and therefore the effects of liver disease on the kinetics of chronically administered entacapone have not been evaluated.

➤*Storage/Stability:* Store at 25°C (77°F); excursions permitted to 15° to 30°C (59° to 86°F).

PERGOLIDE MESYLATE

Rx	**Pergolide Mesylate** (Ivax, Par)	**Tablets:** 0.05 mg	May contain lactose. In 100s.
Rx	**Permax** (Amarin)		May contain lactose. (A024). Ivory, rectangular, scored. In 30s.
Rx	**Pergolide Mesylate** (Ivax, Par, UDL)	**Tablets:** 0.25 mg	May contain lactose. (7159). Mottled green, capsule shape, scored. In 100s.
Rx	**Permax** (Amarin)		Lactose. (A025). Green, rectangular, scored. In 100s.
Rx	**Pergolide Mesylate** (Ivax, UDL, Par)	**Tablets:** 1 mg	May contain lactose. In 100s.
Rx	**Permax** (Amarin)		Lactose. (A026). Pink, rectangular, scored. In 100s.

PERGOLIDE MESYLATE — ORAL

Indications

➤*Parkinson disease:* Adjunctive treatment to levodopa/carbidopa in the management of the signs and symptoms of Parkinson disease.

Evidence to support the efficacy of pergolide as an antiparkinson adjunct was obtained in a multicenter study enrolling 376 patients with mild to moderate Parkinson disease who were intolerant to levodopa/carbidopa as manifested by moderate to severe dyskinesia and/or on-off phenomena. On average, the patients evaluated had been on levodopa/carbidopa for 3.9 years (range, 2 days to 16.8 years). The administration of pergolide permitted a 5% to 30% reduction in the daily dose of levodopa. On average, these patients treated with pergolide maintained an equivalent or better clinical status than they exhibited at baseline.

➤*Unlabeled uses:* Management of restless legs syndrome.

Administration and Dosage

➤*Approved by the FDA:* December 30, 1988.

Administration of pergolide should be initiated with a daily dose of 0.05 mg for the first 2 days. The dosage should then be gradually increased by 0.1 or 0.15 mg/day every third day over the next 12 days of therapy. The dosage may then be increased by 0.25 mg/day every third day until an optimal therapeutic dosage is achieved.

Pergolide is usually administered in divided doses 3 times daily. During dosage titration, the dosage of concurrent levodopa/carbidopa may be cautiously decreased.

In clinical studies, the mean therapeutic daily dose of pergolide was 3 mg. The average concurrent daily dose of levodopa/carbidopa (expressed as levodopa) was approximately 650 mg. The efficacy of pergolide at dosages above 5 mg/day has not been systematically evaluated.

➤*Storage/Stability:* Store at controlled room temperature, 25°C (77°F); excursions permitted to 15° to 30°C (59° to 86°F).

Actions

➤*Pharmacology:* Pergolide is a potent dopamine receptor agonist. Pergolide is 10 to 1,000 times more potent than bromocriptine on a milligram per milligram basis in various in vitro and in vivo test systems. Pergolide inhibits the secretion of prolactin in humans; it causes a transient rise in serum concentrations of growth hormone and a decrease in serum concentrations of luteinizing hormone. In Parkinson disease, pergolide is believed to exert its therapeutic effect by directly stimulating postsynaptic dopamine receptors in the nigrostriatal system.

➤*Pharmacokinetics:*

Absorption – Information on oral systemic bioavailability of pergolide is unavailable because of the lack of a sufficiently sensitive assay to detect the drug after the administration of a single dose. However, following oral administration of ^{14}C radiolabeled pergolide, approximately 55% of the administered radioactivity can be recovered from the urine and 5% from expired CO_2, suggesting that a significant fraction is absorbed. Nothing can be concluded about the extent of presystemic clearance, if any.

Distribution – Data on postabsorption distribution of pergolide are unavailable.

Pergolide is approximately 90% bound to plasma proteins. This extent of protein binding may be important to consider when pergolide is coadministered with other drugs known to affect protein binding.

Metabolism – At least 10 metabolites have been detected, including N-despropylpergolide, pergolide sulfoxide, and pergolide sulfone. Pergolide sulfoxide and pergolide sulfone are dopamine agonists in animals. The other detected metabolites have not been identified and it is not known whether any other metabolites are active pharmacologically.

Excretion – The major route of excretion is the kidney.

Contraindications

Hypersensitivity to this drug or other ergot derivatives.

Warnings

➤*Falling asleep during activities of daily living:* Patients treated with pergolide have reported falling asleep while engaged in activities of daily living, including the operation of motor vehicles, which sometimes resulted in accidents. Although many of these patients reported somnolence while on pergolide, some perceived that they had no warning signs such as excessive drowsiness, and believed that they were alert immediately prior to the event. Some of these events were reported as late as 1 year after the initiation of treatment.

Somnolence is a common occurrence in patients receiving pergolide. Many clinical experts believe that falling asleep while engaged in activities of daily living always occurs in a setting of preexisting somnolence, although patients may not give such a history. For this reason, continually reassess patients for drowsiness or sleepiness, especially because some of the events occur well after the start of treatment. Also be aware that patients may not acknowledge drowsiness or sleepiness until directly questioned about drowsiness or sleepiness during specific activities.

Before initiating treatment with pergolide, advise patients of the potential to develop drowsiness and ask patients about factors that may increase the risk with pergolide such as concomitant sedating medications or the presence of sleep disorders. If a patient develops significant daytime sleepiness or episodes of falling asleep during activities that require participation (eg, conversations, eating), pergolide should ordinarily be discontinued. If a decision is made to continue pergolide, advise patients to not drive and to avoid other potentially dangerous activities.

While dose reduction may reduce the degree of somnolence, there is insufficient information to establish that dose reduction will eliminate episodes of patients falling asleep while engaged in activities of daily living.

➤*Symptomatic hypotension:* In clinical trials, approximately 10% of patients taking pergolide with levodopa versus 7% taking placebo with levodopa experienced symptomatic orthostatic and/or sustained hypotension, especially during initial treatment. With gradual dosage titration, tolerance to the hypotension usually develops. Therefore, it is important to warn patients of the risk, begin therapy with low doses, and increase the dosage in carefully adjusted increments over a period of 3 to 4 weeks.

➤*CNS effects:* In controlled trials, pergolide with levodopa caused hallucinosis in about 14% of patients as opposed to 3% taking placebo with levodopa. This was of sufficient severity to cause discontinuation of treatment in about 3% of those enrolled; tolerance to this untoward effect was not observed.

PERGOLIDE MESYLATE — ORAL

➤*Fatalities:* In a placebo-controlled trial, 2 of 187 patients treated with placebo died, compared with 1 of 189 patients treated with pergolide. Of the 2,299 patients treated with pergolide in premarketing studies evaluated as of October 1988, 143 died while on the drug or shortly after discontinuing it. Because the patient population under evaluation was elderly, ill, and at high risk for death, it seems unlikely that pergolide played any role in these deaths, but the possibility that pergolide shortens survival of patients cannot be excluded with absolute certainty.

In particular, a case-by-case review of the clinical course of the patients who died failed to disclose any unique set of signs, symptoms, or laboratory results that would suggest that treatment with pergolide caused their deaths. Sixty-eight percent of the patients who died were 65 years of age or older. No death (other than a suicide) occurred within the first month of treatment; most of the patients who died had been on pergolide for years. A relative frequency of the causes of death by organ system are as follows: pulmonary failure/pneumonia, 35%; cardiovascular, 30%; cancer, 11%; unknown, 8.4%; infection, 3.5%; extrapyramidal syndrome, 3.5%; stroke, 2.1%; dysphagia, 2.1%; injury, 1.4%; suicide, 1.4%; dehydration, 0.7%; glomerulonephritis, 0.7%.

➤*Serious inflammation and fibrosis:* There have been rare reports of pulmonary fibrosis, pleuritis, pleural effusion, pleural fibrosis, pericarditis, pericardial effusion, cardiac valvulopathy involving 1 or more valves, or retroperitoneal fibrosis in patients taking pergolide. In some cases, symptoms or manifestations of cardiac valvulopathy improved after discontinuation of pergolide.

Specific risk factors predisposing patients to developing fibrosis with ergot alkaloids have not been identified. Before initiating treatment with pergolide, carefully weigh therapeutic benefits against potential risks, taking into account the risk-benefit assessment of other ergot and nonergot antiparkinson medication. Use with caution in patients with a history of these conditions, particularly those patients who experienced the events while taking ergot derivatives. Carefully monitor patients with a history of such events clinically and with appropriate radiographic and laboratory studies while they are taking pergolide. If a patient develops a fibrotic condition while on pergolide, discontinue the drug.

➤*Carcinogenesis:* A 2-year carcinogenicity study was conducted in mice using dietary levels of pergolide equivalent to oral dosages of 0.6, 3.7, and 36.4 mg/kg/day in males and 0.6, 4.4, and 40.8 mg/kg/day in females. A 2-year study in rats was conducted using dietary levels equivalent to oral dosages of 0.04, 0.18, and 0.88 mg/kg/day in males and 0.05, 0.28, and 1.42 mg/kg/day in females. The highest dosages tested in the mice and rats were approximately 340 and 12 times the maximum human oral dosage administered in controlled clinical trials (6 mg/day equivalent to 0.12 mg/kg/day).

A low incidence of uterine neoplasms occurred in both rats and mice. Endometrial adenomas and carcinomas were observed in rats. Endometrial sarcomas were observed in mice. The occurrence of these neoplasms is probably attributable to the high estrogen/progesterone ratio that would occur in rodents as a result of the prolactin-inhibiting action of pergolide. The endocrine mechanisms believed to be involved in the rodents are not present in humans. However, even though there is no known correlation between uterine malignancies occurring in pergolide-treated rodents and human risk, there are no human data to substantiate this conclusion.

➤*Mutagenesis:* Pergolide was evaluated for mutagenic potential in a battery of tests that included an Ames bacterial mutation assay, a DNA repair assay in cultured rat hepatocytes, an in vitro mammalian cell-point-mutation assay in cultured L5178Y cells, and a determination of chromosome alteration in bone marrow cells of Chinese hamsters. A weak mutagenic response was noted in the mammalian cell-point-mutation assay only after metabolic activation with rat liver microsomes. No mutagenic effects were obtained in the 2 other in vitro assays and in the in vivo assay. The relevance of these findings in humans is unknown.

➤*Fertility impairment:* A fertility study in male and female mice showed that fertility was maintained at 0.6 and 1.7 mg/kg/day but decreased at 5.6 mg/kg/day. Prolactin has been reported to be involved in stimulating and maintaining progesterone levels required for implantation in mice and, therefore, the impaired fertility at the high dose may have occurred because of depressed prolactin levels.

➤*Elderly:* Of the total number of subjects in clinical studies of pergolide, 78 were 65 years of age and older. There were no apparent differences in efficacy between these subjects and younger subjects. There was an increased incidence of confusion, somnolence, and peripheral edema in patients 65 years of age and older. Other reported clinical experience has not identified differences in responses between the elderly and younger patients, but greater sensitivity of some older individuals cannot be ruled out. This drug is known to be substantially excreted by the kidney, and the risk of toxic reactions to this drug may be greater in patients with impaired renal function. Because elderly patients are more likely to have decreased renal function, take care in dose selection; it may be useful to monitor renal function.

➤*Pregnancy: Category B.* There are no adequate and well-controlled studies in pregnant women. Among women who received pergolide for endocrine disorders in premarketing studies, there were 33 pregnancies that resulted in healthy babies and 6 pregnancies that resulted in congenital abnormalities (3 major, 3 minor); a causal relationship has not been established. Because human data are limited and because animal reproduction studies are not always predictive of human response, use this drug during pregnancy only if clearly needed.

Reproduction studies were conducted in mice at dosages of 5, 16, and 45 mg/kg/day and in rabbits at dosages of 2, 6, and 16 mg/kg/day. The highest dosages tested in mice and rabbits were 375 and 133 times the 6 mg/day maximum human dose administered in controlled clinical trials. In these studies, there was no evidence of harm to the fetus due to pergolide.

➤*Lactation:* It is not known whether this drug is excreted in human milk. The pharmacologic action of pergolide suggests that it may interfere with lactation. Because many drugs are excreted in human milk and because of the potential for serious adverse reactions to pergolide in breast-feeding infants, decide whether to discontinue breast-feeding or the drug, taking into account the importance of the drug to the mother.

➤*Children:* Safety and efficacy in pediatric patients have not been established.

Precautions

➤*Monitoring:* No specific laboratory tests are deemed essential for the management of patients on pergolide. Periodic routine evaluation of all patients, however, is appropriate.

➤*Cardiac effects:* In a study comparing pergolide and placebo, patients taking pergolide were found to have significantly more episodes of atrial premature contractions and sinus tachycardia.

➤*Discontinuation of therapy:* The use of pergolide in patients on levodopa may cause and/or exacerbate preexisting states of confusion and hallucinations and preexisting dyskinesia. Also, the abrupt discontinuation of pergolide in patients receiving it chronically as an adjunct to levodopa may precipitate the onset of hallucinations and confusion; these may occur within a span of several days. Undertake discontinuation of pergolide gradually whenever possible, even if the patient is to remain on levodopa.

➤*Neuroleptic malignant syndrome (NMS):* A symptom complex resembling NMS (characterized by elevated temperature, muscular rigidity, altered consciousness, and autonomic instability), with no other obvious etiology, has been reported in association with rapid dose reduction of, withdrawal of, or changes in antiparkinson therapy, including pergolide.

➤*Special risk:*

Cardiac dysrhythmias – Exercise caution when administering pergolide to patients prone to cardiac dysrhythmias.

Drug Interactions

➤*Dopamine antagonists:* Dopamine antagonists, such as the neuroleptics (phenothiazines, butyrophenones, thioxanthines) or metoclopramide, ordinarily should not be administered concurrently with pergolide (a dopamine agonist); these agents may diminish the efficacy of pergolide.

➤*Protein binding:* Because pergolide is approximately 90% bound to plasma proteins, exercise caution if pergolide is coadministered with other drugs known to affect protein binding.

Adverse Reactions

➤*Most common:* In premarketing clinical trials, the most commonly observed adverse reactions associated with use of pergolide that were not seen at an equivalent incidence among placebo-treated patients were nervous system complaints, including dyskinesia, hallucinations, somnolence, and insomnia; digestive complaints, including nausea, constipation, diarrhea, and dyspepsia; and respiratory system complaints, including rhinitis.

➤*Discontinuation:* Twenty-seven percent of approximately 1,200 patients receiving pergolide for treatment of Parkinson disease in premarketing clinical trials in the United States and Canada discontinued treatment because of adverse reactions. The reactions most commonly causing discontinuation were related to the nervous system (15.5%), primarily hallucinations (7.8%) and confusion (1.8%).

➤*Fatalities:* In a placebo-controlled trial, 2 of 187 patients treated with placebo died, compared with 1 of 189 patients treated with pergolide. Of the 2,299 patients treated with pergolide in premarketing studies evaluated as of October 1988, 143 died while on the drug or shortly after discontinuing it. Because the patient population under evaluation was elderly, ill, and at high risk for death, it seems unlikely that pergolide played any role in these deaths, but the possibility that pergolide shortens survival of patients cannot be excluded with absolute certainty.

In particular, a case-by-case review of the clinical course of the patients who died failed to disclose any unique set of signs, symptoms, or laboratory results that would suggest that treatment with pergolide caused their deaths. Sixty-eight percent of the patients who died were 65 years of age or older. No death (other than a suicide) occurred within the first month of treatment; most of the patients who died had been on pergolide for years. A relative frequency of the causes of death by organ system are pulmonary failure/pneumonia, 35%; cardiovascular, 30%; cancer, 11%; unknown, 8.4%; infection, 3.5%; extrapyramidal syndrome, 3.5%; stroke, 2.1%; dysphagia, 2.1%; injury, 1.4%; suicide, 1.4%; dehydration, 0.7%; glomerulonephritis, 0.7%.

➤*Adverse reactions in controlled clinical trials:* The following table enumerates adverse reactions that occurred at a frequency of 1% or more among patients taking pergolide who participated in premarketing controlled clinical trials comparing pergolide with placebo. In a double-blind, controlled study of 6 months' duration, patients with Parkinson disease were continued on levodopa/carbidopa and randomly assigned to receive either pergolide or placebo as additional therapy.

These figures cannot be used to predict the incidence of adverse reactions in the course of usual medical practice where patient characteristics and other factors differ from those that prevailed in the clinical trials. Similarly, the cited frequencies cannot be compared with figures obtained from other clinical investigations involving different treatments, uses, and investigators. The cited figures, however, do provide some basis for estimating the relative contribution of drug and nondrug factors to the adverse reaction incidence rate in the population studied.

PERGOLIDE MESYLATE — ORAL

Adverse Reactions in Controlled Clinical Trials		
Adverse reaction	Pergolide (n = 189)	Placebo (n = 187)
Cardiovascular		
Arrhythmia	1.1%	< 1%
Hypertension	1.6%	1.1%
Hypotension	2.1%	< 1%
Myocardial infarction (MI)	1.1%	< 1%
Palpitation	2.1%	< 1%
Postural hypotension	9%	7%
Syncope	2.1%	1.1%
Vasodilatation	3.2%	< 1%
CNS		
Abnormal dreams	2.7%	4.3%
Abnormal gait	1.6%	1.6%
Akathisia	1.6%	0%
Akinesia	1.1%	1.1%
Anxiety	6.4%	4.3%
Confusion	11.1%	9.6%
Depression	3.2%	5.4%
Dizziness	19.1%	13.9%
Dyskinesia	62.4%	24.6%
Dystonia	11.6%	8%
Extrapyramidal syndrome	1.6%	1.1%
Hallucinations	13.8%	3.2%
Headache	5.3%	6.4%
Hypertonia	1.1%	0%
Incoordination	1.6%	< 1%
Insomnia	7.9%	3.2%
Neuralgia	1.1%	< 1%
Paresthesia	1.6%	3.2%
Personality disorder	2.1%	< 1%
Psychosis	2.1%	0%
Somnolence	10.1%	3.7%
Speech disorder	1.1%	1.6%
Tremor	4.2%	7.5%
Dermatologic		
Rash	3.2%	2.1%
Sweating	2.1%	2.7%
GI		
Abdominal pain	5.8%	2.1%
Anorexia	4.8%	2.7%
Constipation	10.6%	5.9%
Diarrhea	6.4%	2.7%
Dry mouth	3.7%	< 1%
Dyspepsia	6.4%	2.1%
Nausea	24.3%	12.8%
Vomiting	2.7%	1.6%
GU		
Hematuria	1.1%	< 1%
Urinary frequency	2.7%	6.4%
Urinary tract infection	2.7%	3.7%
Hematologic/Lymphatic		
Anemia	1.1%	< 1%
Metabolic/Nutritional		
Edema	1.6%	0%
Peripheral edema	7.4%	4.3%
Weight gain	1.6%	0%

Adverse Reactions in Controlled Clinical Trials		
Adverse reaction	Pergolide (n = 189)	Placebo (n = 187)
Musculoskeletal		
Arthralgia	1.6%	2.1%
Back pain	1.6%	2.1%
Bursitis	1.6%	< 1%
Myalgia	1.1%	< 1%
Neck pain	2.7%	1.6%
Twitching	1.1%	0%
Respiratory		
Dyspnea	4.8%	1.1%
Epistaxis	1.6%	< 1%
Hiccup	1.1%	0%
Rhinitis	12.2%	5.4%
Special senses		
Abnormal vision	5.8%	5.4%
Diplopia	2.1%	0%
Eye disorder	1.1%	0%
Taste perversion	1.6%	0%
Miscellaneous		
Asthenia	4.2%	4.8%
Chest pain	3.7%	2.1%
Chills	1.1%	0%
Face edema	1.1%	0%
Flu syndrome	3.2%	2.1%
Infection	1.1%	0%
Injury, accident	5.8%	7%
Pain	7%	2.1%
Surgical procedure	1.6%	< 1%

➤*Other adverse reactions:* This section reports event frequencies evaluated as of October 1988 for adverse reactions occurring in a group of approximately 1,800 patients who took multiple doses of pergolide. The conditions and duration of exposure to pergolide varied greatly, involving well-controlled studies as well as experience in open and uncontrolled clinical settings. In the absence of appropriate controls in some of the studies, a causal relationship between these reactions and treatment with pergolide cannot be determined.

The following enumeration by organ system describes reactions in terms of their relative frequency of reporting in the database.

Cardiovascular – Congestive heart failure, hypertension, palpitations, postural hypotension, syncope, vasodilatations (at least 1%).

Abnormal electrocardiogram, angina pectoris, atrial fibrillation, atrioventricular block, bradycardia, cerebral ischemia, cerebrovascular accident, heart arrest, MI, pulmonary embolus, shock tachycardia, thrombophlebitis, varicose vein, ventricular extrasystoles, ventricular tachycardia (0.1% to 1%).

Cerebral hemorrhage, heart block, pericarditis, pulmonary hypertension, vasculitis (less than 0.1%).

CNS – Abnormal dreams, abnormal gait, abnormal thinking, akinesia, amnesia, anxiety, choreoathetosis, confusion, depression, dizziness, dyskinesia, dystonia, extrapyramidal syndrome, hallucinations, headache, incoordination, insomnia, nervousness, paranoid reaction, paresthesia, personality disorder, psychosis, somnolence, tremor (at least 1%).

Acute brain syndrome, agitation, akathisia, apathy, ataxia, coma, delusions, emotional lability, euphoria, hostility, hyperkinesia, hypertonia, hypokinesia, hypotonia, libido decreased, libido increased, manic reaction, meningitis, myoclonus, neuralgia, neuropathy, neurosis, paralysis, seizure, torticollis, vertigo (0.1% to 1%).

Brain edema, facial paralysis, hallucinations and confusion after abrupt discontinuation, hemiplegia, intracranial hypertension, migraine, myelitis, neuritis, stupor (less than 0.1%).

Dermatologic – Rash, sweating (at least 1%).

Acne, alopecia, dry skin, eczema, fungal dermatitis, herpes simplex, herpes zoster, hirsutism, pruritus, seborrhea, skin carcinoma, skin discoloration, skin ulcer (0.1% to 1%).

Lichenoid dermatitis, skin benign neoplasm, skin nodule, subcutaneous nodule, vesiculobullous rash (less than 0.1%).

Endocrine – Adenoma, antidiuretic hormone inappropriate, diabetes mellitus, hypothyroidism (0.1% to 1%).

Endocrine disorder, thyroid adenoma (less than 0.1%).

GI – Abdominal pain, constipation, diarrhea, dry mouth, dyspepsia, dysphagia, nausea, vomiting (at least 1%).

Abnormal liver function tests, cholelithiasis, enlarged abdomen, eructation, esophagitis, flatulence, gastritis, gastroenteritis, gingivitis, hematemesis, hepatitis, hepatomegaly, increased appetite, intestinal obstruction, melena,

PERGOLIDE MESYLATE — ORAL

nausea and vomiting, periodontal abscess, salivary gland enlargement, stomach ulcer, thirst, tooth caries (0.1% to 1%).

Acute abdominal syndrome, aphthous stomatitis, cholecystitis, colitis, duodenitis, esophageal ulcer, fecal incontinence, glossitis, jaundice, pancreatitis, peptic ulcer, sialadenitis (less than 0.1%).

GU – Dysmenorrhea, hematuria, urinary frequency, urinary incontinence, urinary tract infection (at least 1%).

Abortion, breast carcinoma, breast pain, carcinoma, cervical carcinoma cystitis, dysuria, fibrocystic breast, impotence, kidney calculus, kidney failure, lactation, menopause, menorrhagia, metrorrhagia, pelvic pain, priapism, pyuria, salpingitis, urinary retention, urolithiasis, uterine hemorrhage, vaginal hemorrhage, vaginitis (0.1% to 1%).

Amenorrhea, bladder breast engorgement, epididymitis, hypogonadism, leukorrhea, nephrosis, pyelonephritis, urethral pain, uricaciduria, withdrawal bleeding (less than 0.1%).

Hematologic/Lymphatic – Anemia (at least 1%).

Cyanosis, leukocytosis, leukopenia, lymphadenopathy, megaloblastic anemia, petechia, thrombocytopenia (0.1% to 1%).

Acute lymphoblastic leukemia, eosinophilia, lymphocytosis, polycythemia, purpura, splenomegaly, thrombocythemia (less than 0.1%).

Metabolic/Nutritional – Peripheral edema, weight gain, weight loss (at least 1%).

Dehydration, gout, hypercholesterolemia, hyperglycemia, hypoglycemia, hypokalemia, iron deficiency anemia (0.1% to 1%).

Acidosis, cachexia, electrolyte imbalance, hyperuricemia (less than 0.1%).

Musculoskeletal – Arthralgia, back pain, myalgia, neck pain, twitching (at least 1%).

Arthritis, bone pain, bone sarcoma, myositis, tenosynovitis (0.1% to 1%).

Muscle atrophy, osteomyelitis, osteoporosis (less than 0.1%).

Ophthalmic – Abnormal vision, diplopia (at least 1%).

Conjunctivitis, eye hemorrhage, eye pain, glaucoma, photophobia, visual field defect (0.1% to 1%).

Blindness, cataract, retinal detachment, retinal vascular disorder (less than 0.1%).

Respiratory – Cough increased, dyspnea, pharyngitis, pneumonia, rhinitis (at least 1%).

Apnea, asthma, bronchitis, emphysema, epistaxis, hemoptysis, hiccup, hyperventilation, laryngitis, lung edema, pleural effusion, sinusitis, voice alteration (0.1% to 1%).

Carcinoma of lung, hemothorax, hypoventilation, hypoxia, larynx edema, lung fibrosis, pneumothorax (less than 0.1%).

Special senses – Deafness, ear pain, otitis media, taste perversion, tinnitus (0.1% to 1%).

Miscellaneous – Accidental injury, asthenia, chest pain, fever, flu syndrome, pain (at least 1%).

Abscess, cellulitis, chills, facial edema, hernia, hypothermia malaise, jaw pain, moniliasis, neoplasm, sepsis (0.1% to 1%).

Lupus erythematosus syndrome (less than 0.1%).

➤*Postmarketing:* Voluntary reports of adverse reactions temporally associated with pergolide that have been received since market introduction and may have no causal relationship with the drug include NMS.

Overdosage

➤*Symptoms:* There is no clinical experience with massive overdosage. The largest overdose involved a young hospitalized adult patient who was not being treated with pergolide but intentionally took 60 mg of the drug. He experienced vomiting, hypotension, and agitation. Another patient receiving a daily dose of 7 mg of pergolide unintentionally took 19 mg/day for 3 days, after which his vital signs were normal but he experienced severe hallucinations. Within 36 hours of resumption of the prescribed dosage level, the hallucinations stopped. One patient unintentionally took 14 mg/day for 23 days instead of her prescribed 1.4 mg/day dosage. She experienced severe involuntary movements and tingling in her arms and legs. Another patient who inadvertently received 7 mg instead of the prescribed 0.7 mg experienced palpitations, hypotension, and ventricular extrasystoles. The highest total daily dose (prescribed for several patients with refractory Parkinson disease) has exceeded 30 mg.

Animal studies indicate that the manifestations of overdosage in humans might include nausea, vomiting, convulsions, decreased blood pressure, and CNS stimulation. The oral median lethal doses in mice and rats were 54 and 15 mg/kg, respectively.

➤*Treatment:* To obtain up-to-date information about the treatment of overdose, your certified regional poison control center is a good resource. In managing overdosage, consider the possibility of multiple drug overdoses, interaction among drugs, and unusual drug kinetics in your patient.

Management of overdosage may require supportive measures to maintain arterial blood pressure. Monitor cardiac function; an antiarrhythmic agent may be necessary. If signs of CNS stimulation are present, a phenothiazine or other butyrophenone neuroleptic agent may be indicated; the efficacy of such drugs in reversing the effects of overdose has not been assessed.

Protect the patient's airway and support ventilation and perfusion. Meticulously monitor and maintain, within acceptable limits, the patient's vital signs, blood gases, serum electrolytes, etc. Absorption of drugs from the GI tract may be decreased by giving activated charcoal, which, in many cases, is more effective than emesis or lavage; consider charcoal instead of or in addition to gastric emptying. Repeated doses of charcoal over time may hasten elimination of some drugs that have been absorbed. Safeguard the patient's airway when employing gastric emptying or charcoal.

There is no experience with dialysis or hemoperfusion, and these procedures are unlikely to be of benefit.

Patient Information

Because pergolide may cause somnolence and the possibility of falling asleep during activities of daily living, caution patients about operating hazardous machinery, including automobiles, until they are reasonably certain that pergolide therapy does not affect them adversely. Advise patients that if they experience increased somnolence or new episodes of falling asleep during activities of daily living (eg, watching television, riding in a car) at any time during treatment, they should not drive or participate in potentially dangerous activities until they have contacted their health care provider. Due to the possible additive sedative effects, use caution when patients are taking other CNS depressants in combination with pergolide.

Inform patients and their families of the common adverse consequences of the use of pergolide and the risk of hypotension.

Advise patients to notify their health care provider if they become pregnant or intend to become pregnant during therapy.

Advise patients to notify their health care provider if they are breast-feeding an infant.

RASAGILINE

Rx	**Azilect** (Teva)	**Tablets:** 0.5 mg	Mannitol. (GIL 0.5). White. In 30s.
		1 mg	Mannitol. (GIL 1). White. In 30s.

RASAGILINE — ORAL

Indications

➤*Parkinson disease:* For the treatment of the signs and symptoms of idiopathic Parkinson disease as initial monotherapy and as adjunct therapy to levodopa.

The effectiveness of rasagiline was demonstrated in patients with early Parkinson disease who were receiving rasagiline as monotherapy and who were not receiving any concomitant dopaminergic therapy. The effectiveness of rasagiline as adjunct therapy was demonstrated in patients with Parkinson disease who were treated with levodopa.

Administration and Dosage

➤*Approved by the FDA:* May 17, 2006.

Tyramine-rich foods, beverages, or dietary supplements and amines (from nonprescription cough/cold medications) should be avoided to prevent a possible hypertensive crisis/"cheese reaction" during rasagiline treatment.

➤*Monotherapy:* The recommended rasagiline dosage for the treatment of Parkinson disease patients is 1 mg administered once daily.

➤*Adjunctive therapy:* The recommended initial dosage is 0.5 mg administered once daily. If a sufficient clinical response is not achieved, the dosage may be increased to 1 mg administered once daily.

Change of levodopa dose in adjunct therapy – When rasagiline is used in combination with levodopa, a reduction of the levodopa dosage may be considered based upon individual response. During the controlled trials of rasagiline as adjunct therapy to levodopa, levodopa dosage was reduced in some patients. In clinical studies, dosage reduction of levodopa was allowed within the first 6 weeks if dopaminergic side effects, including dyskinesia and hallucinations, emerged. In study 1, levodopa dosage reduction occurred in 8% of patients in the placebo group and in 16% and 17% of patients in the 0.5 and 1 mg/day rasagiline groups, respectively. In those patients who had levodopa dosage reduced, the dose was reduced on average by about 7%, 9%, and 13% in the placebo, 0.5 mg/day, and 1 mg/day groups, respectively. In study 2, levodopa dosage reduction occurred in 6% of patients in the placebo group and in 9% in the rasagiline 1 mg/day group. In patients who had their levodopa dosage reduced, the dose was reduced on average by about 13% and 11% in the placebo and the rasagiline groups, respectively.

➤*Hepatic function impairment:* Rasagiline plasma concentrations will increase in patients with hepatic function impairment. Patients with mild hepatic function impairment should use rasagiline 0.5 mg daily. Rasagiline should not be used in patients with moderate or severe hepatic function impairment.

➤*Concomitant ciprofloxacin and other CYP1A2 inhibitors:* Rasagiline plasma concentrations are expected to double in patients taking concomitant ciprofloxacin and other CYP1A2 inhibitors. Therefore, patients taking concomitant ciprofloxacin or other CYP1A2 inhibitors should use rasagiline 0.5 mg daily.

➤*Storage/Stability:* Store at 25°C (77°F); excursions permitted to 15° to 30°C (59° to 86°F).

SELEGILINE HYDROCHLORIDE (L-Deprenyl)

Rx	**Selegiline HCl** (Various, eg, Endo Labs)	**Tablets:** 5 mg	In 60s and 500s.
Rx	**Carbex** (Du Pont Pharma)		Lactose. (E620). White, oval. In 60s.
Rx	**Eldepryl** (Somerset)	**Capsules:** 5 mg	Lactose. (Eldepryl 5mg). Aqua blue. In 60s and 300s.
Rx	**Emsam** (Bristol-Myers Squibb)	**Transdermal system:** 6 mg/24 hr (20 mg/20 cm^2)	In box of 30s.
		9 mg/24 hr (30 mg/30 cm^2)	In box of 30s.
		12 mg/24 hr (40 mg/40 cm^2)	In box of 30s.

SELEGILINE HYDROCHLORIDE — ORAL

Refer to the general discussion in the Antiparkinson Agents introduction.

Indications

➤*Parkinsonism:* Selegiline hydrochloride is indicated as an adjunct in the management of Parkinsonian patients being treated with levodopa/carbidopa who exhibit deterioration in the quality of their response to this therapy. There is no evidence from controlled studies that selegiline has any beneficial effect in the absence of concurrent levodopa therapy.

Administration and Dosage

Selegiline hydrochloride is intended for administration to Parkinsonian patients receiving levodopa/carbidopa therapy who demonstrate a deteriorating response to this treatment. The recommended regimen for the administration of selegiline hydrochloride is 10 mg/day administered as divided doses of 5 mg each taken at breakfast and lunch. There is no evidence that additional benefit will be obtained from the administration of higher doses. Moreover, higher doses should ordinarily be avoided because of the increased risk of side effects.

After 2 to 3 days of selegiline treatment, an attempt may be made to reduce the dose of levodopa/carbidopa. A reduction of 10% to 30% was achieved with the typical participant in the domestic placebo controlled trials who was assigned to selegiline treatment. Further reductions of levodopa/carbidopa may be possible during continued selegiline therapy.

➤*Storage/Stability:* Store at controlled room temperature 15° to 30°C (59° to 86°F). Dispense contents in a tight, light-resistant container.

Actions

➤*Pharmacology:* The mechanisms accounting for selegiline's beneficial adjunctive action in the treatment of Parkinson's disease are not fully understood. Inhibition of monoamine oxidase, type B, activity is generally considered to be of primary importance; in addition, there is evidence that selegiline may act through other mechanisms to increase dopaminergic activity.

Selegiline is best known as an irreversible inhibitor of monoamine oxidase (MAO), an intracellular enzyme associated with the outer membrane of mitochondria. Selegiline inhibits MAO by acting as a "suicide" substrate for the enzyme; that is, it is converted by MAO to an active moiety which combines irreversibly with the active site or the enzyme's essential FAD cofactor. Because selegiline has greater affinity for type B than for type A active sites, it can serve as a selective inhibitor of MAO type B if it is administered at the recommended dose.

It is important to be aware that selegiline may have pharmacological effects unrelated to MAO-B inhibition. As noted above, there is some evidence that it may increase dopaminergic activity by other mechanisms, including interfering with dopamine re-uptake at the synapse. Effects resulting from selegiline administration may also be mediated through its metabolites. Two of its three principal metabolites, amphetamine and methamphetamine, have pharmacological actions of their own; they interfere with neuronal uptake and enhance release of several neurotransmitters (eg, norepinephrine, dopamine, serotonin). However, the extent to which these metabolites contribute to the effects of selegiline are unknown.

➤*Pharmacokinetics:*

Absorption/Distribution – Single oral dose studies do not predict multiple-dose kinetics. At steady state the peak plasma level of selegiline is 4-fold that obtained following a single dose. Metabolite concentrations increase to a lesser extent, averaging 2 fold that seen after a single dose.

The bioavailability of selegiline is increased 3- to 4-fold when it is taken with food.

Metabolism – The absolute bioavailability of selegiline following oral dosing is not known; however, selegiline undergoes extensive metabolism (presumably attributable to presystemic clearance in gut and liver). The major plasma metabolites are N-desmethylselegiline, L-amphetamine and L-methamphetamine. Only N-desmethylselegiline has MAO-B inhibiting activity. The peak plasma levels of these metabolites following a single oral dose of 10 mg are from 4 to almost 20 times greater than that of the maximum plasma concentration of selegiline (1 ng/mL). The maximum concentrations of amphetamine and methamphetamine, however, are far below those ordinarily expected to produce clinically important effects.

Excretion – The extent of systemic exposure to selegiline at a given dose varies considerably among individuals. Estimates of systemic clearance of selegiline are not available. Following a single oral dose, the mean elimination half-life of selegiline is 2 hours. Under steady state conditions the elimination half-life increases to 10 hours.

Special populations –

Age: Although a general conclusion about the effects of age on the pharmacokinetics of selegiline is not warranted because of the size of the sample evaluated (12 subjects > 60 years of age, 12 subjects between the ages of 18 to 30), systemic exposure was about twice as great in older as compared to a younger population given a single oral dose of 10 mg.

Contraindications

Hypersensitivity to this drug; use with meperidine. This contraindication is often extended to other opioids (see Drug Interactions).

Warnings

➤*Maximum dose:* Selegiline should not be used at daily doses exceeding those recommended (10 mg/day) because of the risks associated with non-selective inhibition of MAO (see Pharmacology).

The selectivity of selegiline for MAO-B may not be absolute even at the recommended daily dose of 10 mg a day. Rare cases of hypertensive reactions associated with ingestion of tyramine-containing foods have been reported in patients taking the recommended daily dose of selegiline. The selectivity is further diminished with increasing daily doses. The precise dose at which selegiline becomes a non-selective inhibitor of all MAO is unknown, but may be in the range of 30 to 40 mg a day.

➤*Levodopa:* Some patients given selegiline may experience an exacerbation of levodopa associated side effects, presumably due to the increased amounts of dopamine with super sensitive, post synaptic receptors. These effects may often be mitigated by reducing the dose of levodopa/carbidopa by ≈ 10% to 30%.

The decision to prescribe selegiline should take into consideration that the MAO system of enzymes is complex and incompletely understood and there is only a limited amount of carefully documented clinical experience with selegiline. Consequently, the full spectrum of possible responses to selegiline may not have been observed in premarketing evaluation of the drug. It is advisable, therefore, to observe patients closely for atypical responses.

➤*Pregnancy: Category C.* No teratogenic effects were observed in a study of embryo-fetal development in Sprague-Dawley rats at oral doses of 4, 12, and 36 mg/kg or 4, 12, and 35 times the human therapeutic dose on a mg/m^2 basis. No teratogenic effects were observed in a study of embryo-fetal development in New Zealand White rabbits at oral doses of 5, 25 and 50 mg/kg or 10, 48 and 95 times the human therapeutic dose on a mg/m^2 basis. However, in this study, the number of litters produced at the 2 higher doses was less than recommended for assessing teratogenic potential. In the rat study, there was a decrease in fetal body weight at the highest dose tested. In the rabbit study, increases in total resorptions and % post-implantation loss, and a decrease in the number of live fetuses per dam occurred at the highest dose tested. In a peri- and postnatal development study in Sprague-Dawley rats (oral doses of 4, 16, and 64 mg/kg or 4, 15, and 62 times the human therapeutic dose on a mg/m^2 basis), an increase in the number of stillbirths and decreases in the number of pups per dam, pup survival, and pup body weight (at birth an throughout the lactation period) were observed at the two highest doses. At the highest dose tested, no pups born alive survived to day 4 postpartum. Postnatal development at the highest dose tested in dams could not be evaluated because of the lack of surviving pups. The reproductive performance of the untreated offspring was not assessed.

There are no adequate and well-controlled studies in pregnant women. Selegiline should be used during pregnancy only if the potential benefit justifies the potential risk to the fetus.

➤*Lactation:* It is not known whether selegiline hydrochloride is excreted in human milk. Because many drugs are excreted in human milk, consideration should be given to discontinuing the use of all but absolutely essential drug treatments in nursing women.

➤*Children:* The effects of selegiline hydrochloride in pediatric patients have not been evaluated.

Precautions

➤*Monitoring:* No specific laboratory tests are deemed essential for the management of patients on selegiline hydrochloride. Periodic routine evaluation of all patients, however, is appropriate.

Drug Interactions

➤*Meperidine:* The occurrence of stupor, muscular rigidity, severe agitation, and elevated temperature has been reported in some patients receiving the combination of selegiline and meperidine. Symptoms usually resolve over days when the combination is discontinued. This is typical of the interaction of meperidine and MAOIs. Other serious reactions (including severe agitation, hallucinations, and death) have been reported in patients receiving this combination.

➤*Sympathomimetics:* One case of hypertensive crisis has been reported in a patient taking the recommended doses of selegiline and a sympathomimetic medication (ephedrine).

➤*Tricyclic antidepressants and SSRIs:* Severe CNS toxicity associated with hyperpyrexia and death have been reported with the combination of tricyclic antidepressants and non-selective MAOIs (phenelzine, tranylcypro-

SELEGILINE HYDROCHLORIDE — ORAL

mine). A similar reaction has been reported for a patient on amitriptyline and selegiline. Another patient receiving protriptyline and selegiline developed tremors, agitation and restlessness followed by unresponsiveness and death 2 weeks after selegiline was added. Related adverse events including hypertension, syncope, asystole, diaphoresis, seizures, changes in behavioral and mental status, and muscular rigidity have also been reported in some patients receiving selegiline and various tricyclic antidepressants.

Serious, sometimes fatal, reactions with signs and symptoms that may include hyperthermia, rigidity, myoclonus, autonomic instability with rapid fluctuations of the vital signs, and mental status changes that include extreme agitation progressing to delirium and coma have been reported with patients receiving a combination of fluoxetine hydrochloride and non-selective MAOIs. Similar signs have been reported in some patients on the combination of selegiline (10 mg a day) and selective serotonin reuptake inhibitors including fluoxetine, sertraline and paroxetine.

Since the mechanisms of these reactions are not fully understood, it seems prudent, in general, to avoid this combination of selegiline and tricyclic antidepressants as well as selegiline and selective serotonin reuptake inhibitors. At least 14 days should elapse between discontinuation of selegiline and initiation of treatment with a tricyclic antidepressant or selective serotonin reuptake inhibitors. Because of the long half lives of fluoxetine and its active metabolite, at least 5 weeks (perhaps longer, especially if fluoxetine has been prescribed chronically or at higher doses) should elapse between discontinuation of fluoxetine and initiation of treatment with selegiline.

➤*L-amphetamine and L-methamphetamine:* The maximum concentrations of amphetamine and methamphetamine, are far below those ordinarily expected to produce clinically important effects.

Adverse Reactions

The importance and severity of various reactions reported often cannot be ascertained. One index of relative importance, however, is whether or not a reaction caused treatment discontinuation. In prospective premarketing studies, the following events led, in decreasing order of frequency, to discontinuation of treatment with selegiline: Nausea, hallucinations, confusion, depression, loss of balance, insomnia, orthostatic hypotension, increased akinetic involuntary movements, agitation, arrhythmia, bradykinesia, chorea, delusions, hypertension, new or increased angina pectoris, and syncope. Events reported only once as a cause of discontinuation are ankle edema, anxiety, burning lips/mouth, constipation, drowsiness/lethargy, dystonia, excess perspiration, increased freezing, GI bleeding, hair loss, increased tremor, and weight loss.

➤*Incidence of treatment-emergent adverse experiences in the placebo-controlled clinical trial:*

Selegiline Adverse Reactions

Adverse event	Number of patients
Selegiline hydrochloride (n = 49)	
Nausea	10
Dizziness/lightheadedness/fainting	7
Abdominal pain	4
Confusion	3
Hallucinations	3
Dry mouth	3
Vivid dreams	2
Dyskinesias	2
Headache	2
Reporting events placebo (n = 50)	
Nausea	3
Dizziness/lightheadedness/fainting	1
Abdominal pain	2
Confusion	0
Hallucinations	1
Dry mouth	1
Vivid dreams	0
Dyskinesias	5
Headache	1

The following events were reported once in either or both groups.

Selegiline Adverse Reactions

Adverse event	Number of patients
Selegiline hydrochloride (n = 49)	
Ache, generalized	1
Anxiety, tension	1
Anemia	0
Diarrhea	1
Hair loss	0
Insomnia	1
Lethargy	1
Leg pain	1
Low back pain	1
Malaise	0
Palpitations	1
Urinary retention	1
Weight loss	1
Reporting events placebo (n = 50)	
Ache, generalized	0
Anxiety/tension	1
Anemia	1
Diarrhea	0
Hair loss	1
Insomnia	1
Lethargy	0
Leg pain	0
Low back pain	0
Malaise	1
Palpitations	0
Urinary retention	0
Weight loss	0

➤*All prospectively monitored clinical investigations:* In all prospectively monitored clinical investigations, enrolling ≈ 920 patients, the following adverse events, classified by body system, were reported (effects followed by an * indicate events reported only at doses > 10 mg/day:

Cardiovascular – Orthostatic hypotension, hypertension, arrhythmia, palpitations, new or increased angina pectoris, hypotension, tachycardia, peripheral edema, sinus bradycardia, and syncope.

CNS –

Motor/coordination/extrapyramidal: Increased tremor, loss of balance, restlessness, blepharospasm, increased bradykinesia, facial grimace, falling down, heavy leg, muscle twitch*, myoclonic jerks*, stiff neck, tardive dyskinesia, dystonic symptoms, dyskinesia, involuntary movements, freezing, festination, increased apraxia, and muscle cramps.

Autonomic nervous system: Dry mouth, blurred vision, and sexual dysfunction.

Pain/altered sensation: Headache, back pain, leg pain, tinnitus, migraine, supraorbital pain, throat burning, ache, chills, numbness of toes/fingers, and taste disturbance.

Dermatologic – Increased sweating, diaphoresis, facial hair, hair loss, hematoma, rash, and photosensitivity.

GI – Nausea/vomiting, constipation, weight loss, anorexia, poor appetite, dysphagia, diarrhea, heartburn, rectal bleeding, bruxism*, and GI bleeding (exacerbation of preexisting ulcer disease).

GU – Slow urination, transient anorgasmia*, nocturia, prostate hypertrophy, urinary hesitancy, urinary retention, decreased penile sensation*, and urinary frequency.

Psychiatric – Hallucinations, dizziness, confusion, anxiety, depression, drowsiness, behavior/mood change, dreams/nightmares, tiredness, delusions, disorientation, lightheadedness, impaired memory*, increased energy*, transient high*, hollow feeling, lethargy/malaise, apathy, overstimulation, vertigo, personality change, sleep disturbance, restlessness, weakness, and transient irritability.

Miscellaneous – Asthma, diplopia, shortness of breath, and speech affected.

➤*Postmarketing:* The following experiences were described in spontaneous postmarketing reports. These reports do not provide sufficient information to establish a clear causal relationship with the use of selegiline hydrochloride.

CNS – Seizure in dialyzed chronic renal failure patient on concomitant medications.

Overdosage

➤*Symptoms:* No specific information is available about clinically significant overdoses with selegiline hydrochloride. However, experience gained during selegiline's development reveals that some individuals exposed to doses of 600 mg d,l-selegiline suffered severe hypotension and psychomotor agitation.

Since the selective inhibition of MAO-B by selegiline hydrochloride is achieved only at doses in the range recommended for the treatment of Parkinson's disease (eg, 10 mg/day), overdoses are likely to cause significant inhibition of both MAO-A and MAO-B. Consequently, the signs and symptoms of overdose may resemble those observed with marketed non-selective MAO inhibitors [eg, tranylcypromine, isocarboxazide and phenelzine].

Overdose with non-selective MAO inhibition –

Note: This section is provided for reference it does not describe events that have actually been observed with selegiline in overdose. Characteristically, signs and symptoms of non-selective MAOI overdose may not appear immediately. Delays of up to 12 hours between ingestion of drug and the appearance of signs may occur. Importantly, the peak intensity of the syndrome may not be reached for upwards of a day following the overdose. Death has been reported following overdosage. Therefore, immediate hospitalization, with continuous patient observation and monitoring for a period of at least 2 days following the ingestion of such drugs in overdose, is strongly recommended.

The clinical picture of MAOI overdose varies considerably; its severity may be a function of the amount of drug consumed. The central nervous and cardiovascular systems are prominently involved.

Signs and symptoms of overdosage may include, alone or in combination, any of the following: Drowsiness, dizziness, faintness, irritability, hyperactivity, agitation, severe headache, hallucinations, trismus, opisthotonus,

SELEGILINE HYDROCHLORIDE — ORAL

convulsions, and coma; rapid and irregular pulse, hypertension, hypotension and vascular collapse; precordial pain, respiratory depression and failure, hyperpyrexia, diaphoresis, and cool, clammy skin.

➤*Treatment:* Treatment of overdose with non-selective MAOIs is symptomatic and supportive. Induction of emesis or gastric lavage with instillation of charcoal slurry may be helpful in early poisoning, provided the airway has been protected against aspiration. Signs and symptom of CNS stimulation, including convulsions, should be treated with diazepam, given slowly by IV. Phenothiazine derivatives and CNS stimulants should be avoided. Hypotension and vascular collapse should be treated with IV fluids and, if necessary, blood pressure titration with an intravenous infusion of a dilute pressor agent. It should be noted that adrenergic agents may produce a markedly increased pressor response.

Respiration should be supported by appropriate measures, including management of the airway, use of supplemental oxygen, and mechanical ventilatory, as required.

Body temperature should be monitored closely. Intensive management of hyperpyrexia may be required. Maintenance of fluid and electrolyte balance is essential.

Patient Information

Patients should be advised of the possible need to reduce levodopa dosage after the initiation of selegiline hydrochloride therapy.

Patients (or their families if the patient is incompetent) should be advised not to exceed the daily recommended dose of 10 mg. The risk of using higher daily doses of selegiline should be explained, and a brief description of the "cheese reaction" provided. Rare hypertensive reactions with selegiline at recommended doses associated with dietary influences have been reported.

Consequently, it may be useful to inform patients (or their families) about the signs and symptoms associated with MAOI induced hypertensive reactions. In particular, patients should be urged to report, immediately, any severe headache or other atypical or unusual symptoms not previously experienced.

SELEGILINE — TRANSDERMAL SYSTEM

WARNING

Suicidality in children and adolescents – Antidepressants increased the risk of suicidal thinking and behavior (suicidality) in short-term studies in children and adolescents with major depressive disorder (MDD) and other psychiatric disorders. Anyone considering the use of selegiline transdermal system or any other antidepressant in a child or adolescent must balance this risk with the clinical need. Observe closely patients who are started on therapy for clinical worsening, suicidality, or unusual changes in behavior. Advise families and caregivers for the need for close observation and communication with the prescriber. Selegiline transdermal system is not approved for use in children.

Pooled analyses of short-term (4 to 16 weeks) placebo-controlled trials of 9 antidepressant drugs (SSRIs and others) in children and adolescents with MDD, obsessive compulsive disorder (OCD), or other psychiatric disorders (a total of 24 trials involving over 4,400 patients) have revealed a greater risk of adverse reactions representing suicidal thinking or behavior (suicidality) during the first few months of treatment in those receiving antidepressants. The average risk of such reactions in patients receiving antidepressants was 4%, twice the placebo risk of 2%. No suicides occurred in these trials.

Indications

➤*Major depressive disorder (MDD):* For the treatment of MDD.

Administration and Dosage

➤*Approved by the FDA:* February 27, 2006.

➤*Administration:* Apply to dry, intact skin on the upper torso (below the neck and above the waist), upper thigh, or the outer surface of the upper arm once every 24 hours.

➤*Initial treatment:* The recommended starting dose and target dose is 6 mg/24 hours. It has been systematically evaluated and shown to be effective in a dose range of 6 mg/24 hours to 12 mg/24 hours. However, the trials were not designed to assess if higher doses are more effective than the lowest effective dose of 6 mg/24 hours.

➤*Dosage adjustments:* Based on clinical judgment, if dose increases are indicated for individual patients, they should occur in dose increments of 3 mg/24 hours (up to a maximum dose of 12 mg/24 hours) at intervals of no less than 2 weeks. As with all antidepressant drugs, full antidepressant effect may be delayed.

➤*Food/Drug interactions:* Inform patients to avoid tyramine-rich foods and beverages beginning on the first day of 9 mg/24 hours or 12 mg/24 hours treatment and should continue to be avoided for 2 weeks after a dose reduction to 6 mg/24 hours or following the discontinuation of 9 mg/24 hours or 12 mg/24 hours.

➤*Special populations:*

Renal/Hepatic function impairment – No dosage adjustment is required for patients with mild to moderate renal or hepatic impairment.

Elderly – The recommended dose for elderly patients (greater than or equal to 65 years of age) is 6 mg/24 hours daily. Dose increases, in the elderly, should be made with caution and closely observe patients for postural changes in blood pressure throughout treatment.

➤*Maintenance:* It is generally agreed that episodes of depression require several months or longer of sustained pharmacologic therapy. The benefit of maintaining depressed patients on therapy at a dose of 6 mg/24 hours after achieving a responder status for an average duration of about 25 days was demonstrated in a controlled trial. Periodically reevaluate the long-term usefulness of the drug for the individual patient.

➤*Storage/Stability:* Store at 20° to 25°C (68° to 77°F). Do not store outside of the sealed pouch. Apply immediately upon removal from the protective pouch. Discard in household trash in a manner that prevents accidental application or ingestion by children, pets, or others.

TOLCAPONE

Rx	**Tasmar** (Roche)	**Tablets:** 100 mg	Lactose. (Tasmar 100 Roche). Beige, hexagonal, biconvex. Film coated. In 90s.
		200 mg	Lactose. (Tasmar 200 Roche). Reddish brown, hexagonal, biconvex. Film coated. In 90s.

TOLCAPONE — ORAL

Refer to the general discussion in the Antiparkinson Agents introduction.

WARNING

Because of the risk of potentially fatal, acute fulminant liver failure, tolcapone should ordinarily be used in patients with Parkinson's disease on l-dopa/carbidopa who are experiencing symptom fluctuations and are not responding satisfactorily to or are not appropriate candidates for other adjunctive therapies.

Because of the risk of liver injury and because tolcapone, when it is effective, provides an observable symptomatic benefit, the patient who fails to show substantial clinical benefit within 3 weeks of initiation of treatment, should be withdrawn from tolcapone.

Tolcapone therapy should not be initiated if the patient exhibits clinical evidence of liver disease or 2 ALT or AST values greater than the upper limit of normal. Patients with severe dyskinesia or dystonia should be treated with caution.

Patients who develop evidence of hepatocellular injury while on tolcapone and are withdrawn from the drug for any reason may be at increased risk for liver injury if tolcapone is reintroduced. Accordingly, such patients should not ordinarily be considered for retreatment.

Cases of severe hepatocellular injury, including fulminant liver failure resulting in death, have been reported in postmarketing use. As of October 1998, 3 cases of fatal fulminant hepatic failure have been reported from approximately 60,000 patients providing about 40,000 patient years of worldwide use. This incidence may be 10- to 100– fold higher than the background incidence in the general population. Underreporting of cases may lead to significant underestimation of the increased risk associated with the use of tolcapone.

A prescriber who elects to use tolcapone in the face of the increased risk of liver injury is strongly advised to monitor patients for evidence of emergent liver injury. Patients should be advised of the need for self-monitoring for both the classical signs of liver disease (eg, clay-colored stools, jaundice) and the nonspecific ones (eg, fatigue, loss of appetite, lethargy).

Although a program of frequent laboratory monitoring for evidence of hepatocellular injury is deemed essential, it is not clear that baseline and periodic monitoring of liver enzymes will prevent the occurrence of fulminant liver failure. However, it is generally believed that early detection of drug-induced hepatic injury along with immediate withdrawal of the suspect drug enhances the likelihood for recovery. It is also widely held, without a robust body of evidence, that patients with preexisting hepatic disease are more vulnerable of hepatotoxins. Accordingly, the following live-monitoring program is recommended.

Before starting treatment with tolcapone, the physician should conduct appropriate tests to exclude the presence of liver disease. In patients determined to be appropriate candidates for treatment with tolcapone, serum glutamic-pyruvic transaminase (ALT) and serum glutamic-oxaloacetic transaminase (AST) levels should be determined at baseline and then every 2 weeks for the first year of therapy, every 4 weeks for the next 6 months, and then every 8 weeks thereafter. If the dose is increased to 200 mg 3 times daily, liver enzyme monitoring should take place before increasing the dose and then be reinitiated at the frequency above.

Tolcapone should be discontinued if ALT or AST exceeds the upper limit of normal (ULN) or if clinical signs and symptoms suggest the onset of hepatic failure (eg, persistent nausea, fatigue, lethargy, anorexia, jaundice, dark urine, pruritus, right upper quadrant tenderness).

Indications

➤*Parkinsonism:* Tolcapone is indicated as an adjunct to levodopa and carbidopa for the treatment of the signs and symptoms of idiopathic Parkinson's disease. Because of the risk of potentially fatal, acute, fulminant liver failure, tolcapone should ordinarily be used in patients with Parkinson's disease on l-dopa/carbidopa who are experiencing symptom fluctuations and are not responding satisfactorily to or are not appropriate candidates for other adjunctive therapies. Because of the risk of liver injury and because tolcapone, when it is effective, provides an observable symptomatic benefit, the patient who fails to show substantial clinical benefit within 3 weeks of initiation of treatment, should be withdrawn from tolcapone.

Administration and Dosage

➤*Approved by the FDA:* January 29, 1998.

Treatment with tolcapone should always be initiated at a dose of 100 mg 3 times daily, always as an adjunct to levodopa/carbidopa therapy. The recommended daily dose of tolcapone is also 100 mg 3 times daily. In clinical trials, elevations in ALT occurred more frequently at the dose of 200 mg 3 times daily. While it is unknown whether the risk of acute fulminant liver failure is increased at the 200 mg dose, it would be prudent to use 200 mg only if the anticipated incremental clinical benefit is justified. If a patient fails to show the expected incremental benefit on the 200 mg dose after a total of 3 weeks of treatment (regardless of dose), tolcapone should be discontinued.

In clinical trials, the first dose of the day of tolcapone was always taken together with the first dose of the day of levodopa/carbidopa, and the subsequent doses of tolcapone were given approximately 6 and 12 hours later.

In clinical trials, the majority of patients required a decrease in their daily levodopa dose if their daily dose of levodopa was over 600 mg or if patients had moderate or severe dyskinesias before beginning treatment.

To optimize an individual patient's response, reductions in daily levodopa dose may be necessary. In clinical trials, the average reduction in daily levodopa dose was about 30% in those patients requiring a levodopa dose reduction. (Greater than 70% of patients with levodopa doses over 600 mg daily required such a reduction.)

Tolcapone can be combined with both the immediate and sustained-release formulations of levodopa/carbidopa.

Tolcapone may be taken with or without food.

➤*Hepatic function impairment:* Tolcapone therapy should not be initiated if any patient with liver disease or 2 ALT or AST values greater than the ULN.

➤*Withdrawing patients from tolcapone:* As with any dopaminergic drug, withdrawal or abrupt reduction in the tolcapone dose may lead to emergence of signs and symptoms of Parkinson's disease or hyperpyrexia and confusion, a syndrome complex resembling the neuroleptic malignant syndrome. If a decision is made to discontinue treatment with tolcapone, then it is recommended to closely monitor the patient and adjust other dopaminergic treatments as needed. This syndrome should be considered in the differential diagnosis for any patient who develops a high fever or severe rigidity. Tapering tolcapone has not been systematically evaluated. As the duration of catechol-O-methyltransferase (COMT) inhibition with tolcapone is generally 5 to 6 hours on average, decreasing the frequency of dosage to twice or once a day may not in itself prevent withdrawal effects.

➤*Storage/Stability:* Store at controlled room temperature 20° to 25°C (68° to 77°F) in tight containers.

Actions

➤*Pharmacology:* Tolcapone is a selective and reversible inhibitor of COMT.

The precise mechanism of action of tolcapone is unknown, but it is believed to be related to its ability to inhibit COMT and alter the plasma pharmacokinetics of levodopa. When tolcapone is given in conjunction with levodopa and an aromatic amino acid decarboxylase inhibitor, such as carbidopa, plasma levels of levodopa are more sustained than after administration of levodopa and an aromatic amino acid decarboxylase inhibitor alone. It is believed that these sustained plasma levels of levodopa result in more constant dopaminergic stimulation in the brain, leading to greater effects on the signs and symptoms of Parkinson's disease in patients as well as increased levodopa adverse reactions, sometimes requiring a decrease in the dose of levodopa. Tolcapone enters the CNS to a minimal extent, but has been shown to inhibit central COMT activity in animals.

➤*Pharmacokinetics:*

Absorption – Tolcapone is rapidly absorbed, with a t_{max} of approximately 2 hours. The absolute bioavailability following oral administration is about 65%. Food given within 1 hour before and 2 hours after dosing of tolcapone decreases the relative bioavailability by 10% to 20%.

Distribution – The steady-state volume of distribution of tolcapone is small (9 L). Tolcapone does not distribute widely into tissues due to its high plasma protein binding. The plasma protein binding of tolcapone is approximately 99.9% over the concentration range of 0.32 to 210 mcg/mL. In vitro experiments have shown that tolcapone binds mainly to serum albumin.

Metabolism/Excretion – Tolcapone is almost completely metabolized prior to excretion, with only a very small amount (0.5% of dose) found unchanged in urine. The main metabolic pathway of tolcapone is glucuronidation; the glucuronide conjugate is inactive. In addition, the compound is methylated by COMT to 3-O-methyl-tolcapone. Tolcapone is metabolized to a primary alcohol (hydroxylation of the methyl group), which is subsequently oxidized to the carboxylic acid. In vitro experiments suggest that the oxidation may be catalyzed by cytochrome P450 3A4 and P450 2A6. The reduction to an amine and subsequent N-acetylation occur to a minor extent. After oral administration of a ^{14}C-labeled dose of tolcapone, 60% of labeled material is excreted in urine and 40% in feces.

Tolcapone is a low-extraction-ratio drug (extraction ratio = 0.15) with a moderate systemic clearance of about 7 L/hr.

Special populations –

Hepatic function impairment: A study in patients with hepatic impairment has shown that moderate, noncirrhotic liver disease had no impact on the pharmacokinetics of tolcapone. In patients with moderate cirrhotic liver disease (Child-Pugh class B), however, clearance and volume of distribution of unbound tolcapone was reduced by almost 50%. This reduction may increase the average concentration of unbound drug by 2-fold (see Administration and Dosage). Tolcapone therapy should not be initiated if the patient exhibits clinical evidence of active liver disease or 2 ALT or AST values greater than the ULN. Tolcapone pharmacokinetics are linear over the dose range of 50 to 400 mg, independent of levodopa/carbidopa coadministration. The elimination half-life of tolcapone is 2 to 3 hours and there is no significant accumulation. With 3-times-daily dosing of 100 or 200 mg, C_{max} is approximately 3 mcg/mL and 6 mcg/mL, respectively.

Contraindications

Liver disease; patients who were withdrawn from tolcapone because of evidence of tolcapone-induced hepatocellular injury; or hypersensitivity to the drug or its ingredients; history of nontraumatic rhabdomyolysis or hyperpyrexia and confusion possibly related to medication.

Warnings

➤*Hepatic failure:* In controlled phase 3 trials, increases to greater than 3 times the ULN in ALT or AST occurred in approximately 1% of patients at 100 mg 3 times daily and 3% of patients at 200 mg 3 times daily. Females were more likely than males to have an increase in liver enzymes (approximately 5% vs 2%). Approximately one-third of patients with elevated enzymes had diarrhea. Increases to greater than 8 times the ULN in liver

TOLCAPONE — ORAL

enzymes occurred in 0.3% at 100 mg 3 times daily and 0.7% at 200 mg 3 times daily. Elevated enzymes led to discontinuation in 0.3% and 1.7% of patients treated with 100 mg 3 times daily and 200 mg 3 times daily, respectively. Elevations usually occurred within 6 weeks to 6 months of starting treatment. In about half the cases with elevated liver enzymes, enzyme levels returned to baseline values within 1 to 3 months while patients continued tolcapone treatment. When treatment was discontinued, enzymes generally declined within 2 to 3 weeks but in some cases took as long as 1 to 2 months to return to normal.

➤*Renal toxicity:* When rats were dosed daily for 1 or 2 years (exposures 6 times the human exposure or greater) there was a high incidence of proximal tubule cell damage consisting of degeneration, single cell necrosis, hyperplasia, karyocytomegaly and atypical nuclei. These effects were not associated with changes in clinical chemistry parameters, and there is no established method for monitoring for the possible occurrence of these lesions in humans. Although it has been speculated that these toxicities may occur as the result of a species-specific mechanism, experiments which would confirm that theory have not been conducted.

➤*Hepatic function impairment:* Because of the risk of liver injury, tolcapone therapy should not be initiated in any patient with liver disease. For similar reasons, treatment should not be initiated in patients who have 2 ALT or AST values greater than the upper limit of normal or any other evidence of hepatocellular dysfunction.

➤*Carcinogenesis:* Carcinogenicity studies in which tolcapone was administered in the diet were conducted in mice and rats. Mice were treated for 80 (female) or 95 (male) weeks with doses of 100, 300 and 800 mg/kg/day, equivalent to 0.8, 1.6 and 4 times human exposure (AUC = 80 mcg•hr/mL) at the recommended daily clinical dose of 600 mg. Rats were treated for 104 weeks with doses of 50, 250 and 450 mg/kg/day. Tolcapone exposures were 1, 6.3 and 13 times the human exposure in male rats and 1.7, 11.8 and 26.4 times the human exposure in female rats. There was an increased incidence of uterine adenocarcinomas in female rats at exposure equivalent to 26.4 times the human exposure. There was evidence of renal tubular injury and renal tubular tumor formation in rats. A low incidence of renal tubular cell adenomas occurred in middle- and high-dose female rats; tubular cell carcinomas occurred in middle- and high-dose male and high-dose female rats, with a statistically significant increase in high-dose males. Exposures were equivalent to 6.3 (males) or 11.8 (females) times the human exposure or greater; no renal tumors were observed at exposures of 1 (males) or 1.7 (females) times the human exposure. Minimal-to-marked damage to the renal tubules, consisting of proximal tubule cell degeneration, single cell necrosis, hyperplasia and karyocytomegaly, occurred at the doses associated with renal tumors. Renal tubule damage, characterized by proximal tubule cell degeneration and the presence of atypical nuclei, as well as 1 adenocarcinoma in a high-dose male, were observed in a 1-year study in rats receiving doses of tolcapone of 150 and 450 mg/kg/day. These histopathological changes suggest the possibility that renal tumor formation might be secondary to chronic cell damage and sustained repair, but this relationship has not been established, and the relevance of these findings to humans is not known. There was no evidence of carcinogenic effects in the long-term mouse study. The carcinogenic potential of tolcapone in combination with levodopa/carbidopa has not been examined.

➤*Mutagenesis:* Tolcapone was clastogenic in the in vitro mouse lymphoma/thymidine kinase assay in the presence of metabolic activation. Tolcapone was not mutagenic in the Ames test, the in vitro V79/HPRT gene mutation assay, or the unscheduled DNA synthesis assay. It was not clastogenic in an in vitro chromosomal aberration assay in cultured human lymphocytes, or in an in vivo micronucleus assay in mice.

➤*Pregnancy: Category C.* Tolcapone, when administered alone during organogenesis, was not teratogenic at doses of up to 300 mg/kg/day in rats or up to 400 mg/kg/day in rabbits (5.7 times and 15 times the recommended daily clinical dose of 600 mg, on a mg/m^2 basis, respectively). In rabbits, however, an increased rate of abortion occurred at a dose of 100 mg/kg/day (3.7 times the daily clinical dose on a mg/m^2 basis) or greater. Evidence of maternal toxicity (decreased weight gain, death) was observed at 300 mg/kg in rats and 400 mg/kg in rabbits. When tolcapone was administered to female rats during the last part of gestation and throughout lactation, decreased litter size and impaired growth and learning performance in female pups were observed at a dose of 250/150 mg/kg/day (dose reduced from 250 to 150 mg/kg/day during late gestation due to high rate of maternal mortality; equivalent to 4.8/2.9 times the clinical dose on a mg/m^2 basis).

Tolcapone is always given concomitantly with levodopa/carbidopa, which is known to cause visceral and skeletal malformations in rabbits. The combination of tolcapone (100 mg/kg/day) with levodopa/carbidopa (80/20 mg/kg/day) produced an increased incidence of fetal malformations (primarily external and skeletal digit defects) compared to levodopa/carbidopa alone when pregnant rabbits were treated throughout organogenesis. Plasma exposures to tolcapone (based on AUC) were 0.5 times the expected human exposure, and plasma exposures to levodopa were 6 times higher than those in humans under therapeutic conditions. In a combination embryofetal development study in rats, fetal body weights were reduced by the combination of tolcapone (10, 30, and 50 mg/kg/day) and levodopa/carbidopa (120/30 mg/kg/day) and by levodopa/carbidopa alone. Tolcapone exposures were 0.5 times expected human exposure or greater: levodopa exposures were 21 times the expected human exposure or greater. The high dose of 50 mg/kg/day of tolcapone given alone was not associated with reduced fetal body weight (plasma exposures of 1.4 times the expected human exposure).

There is no experience from clinical studies regarding the use of tolcapone in pregnant women. Therefore, tolcapone should be used during pregnancy only if the potential benefit justifies the potential risk to the fetus.

➤*Lactation:* In animal studies, tolcapone was excreted into maternal rat milk. It is not known whether tolcapone is excreted in human milk. Because many drugs are excreted in human milk, caution should be exercised when tolcapone is administered to a nursing woman.

➤*Children:* There is no identified potential use of tolcapone in pediatric patients.

Precautions

➤*Monitoring:* Although a program of frequent laboratory monitoring for evidence of hepatocellular injury is deemed essential, it is not clear that baseline and periodic monitoring of liver enzymes will prevent the occurrence of fulminant liver failure. However, it is generally believed that early detection of drug-induced hepatic injury along with immediate withdrawal of the suspect drug enhances the likelihood for recovery. It is also widely held, without a robust body of evidence, that patients with preexisting hepatic disease are more vulnerable to hepatotoxins. Accordingly, the following liver-monitoring program is recommended.

Before starting treatment with tolcapone, the physician should conduct appropriate tests to exclude the presence of liver disease. In patients determined to be appropriate candidates for treatment with tolcapone, serum glutamic-pyruvic transaminase (ALT) and serum glutamic-oxaloacetic transaminase (AST) levels should be determined at baseline and then every 2 weeks for the first year of therapy, every 4 weeks for the next 6 months and then every 8 weeks thereafter.

If the dose is increased to 200 mg 3 times daily, liver enzyme monitoring should take place before increasing the dose and then be reinitiated at the frequency above.

Tolcapone should be discontinued if ALT or AST exceeds the upper limit of normal or if clinical signs and symptoms suggest the onset of hepatic failure (eg, persistent nausea, fatigue, lethargy, anorexia, jaundice, dark urine, pruritus, right upper quadrant tenderness).

➤*Hypotension/syncope:* Dopaminergic therapy in Parkinson's disease patients has been associated with orthostatic hypotension. Tolcapone enhances levodopa bioavailability and, therefore, may increase the occurrence of orthostatic hypotension. In tolcapone clinical trials, orthostatic hypotension was documented at least once in 8%, 14% and 13% of the patients treated with placebo, 100, and 200 mg tolcapone 3 times daily, respectively. A total of 2%, 5% and 4% of the patients treated with placebo, 100 and 200 mg tolcapone 3 times daily, respectively, reported orthostatic symptoms at some time during their treatment and also had at least 1 episode of orthostatic hypotension documented (however, the episode of orthostatic symptoms itself was invariably not accompanied by vital sign measurements). Patients with orthostasis at baseline were more likely than patients without symptoms to have orthostatic hypotension during the study, irrespective of treatment group. In addition, the effect was greater in tolcapone-treated patients than in placebo-treated patients. Baseline treatment with dopamine agonists or selegiline did not appear to increase the likelihood of experiencing orthostatic hypotension when treated with tolcapone. Approximately 0.7% of the patients treated with tolcapone (5% of patients who were documented to have had at least one episode of orthostatic hypotension) eventually withdrew from treatment due to adverse events presumably related to hypotension.

In controlled phase 3 trials, approximately 5%, 4%, and 3% of tolcapone 200 mg 3 times daily, 100 mg 3 times daily and placebo patients, respectively, reported at least 1 episode of syncope. Reports of syncope were generally more frequent in patients in all 3 treatment groups who had an episode of documented hypotension (although the episodes of syncope, obtained by history, were themselves not documented with vital sign measurement) compared to patients who did not have any episodes of documented hypotension.

➤*Diarrhea:* In clinical trials, diarrhea developed in approximately 8%, 16%, and 18% of patients treated with placebo, 100 and 200 mg tolcapone 3 times daily, respectively. While diarrhea was generally regarded as mild to moderate in severity, approximately 3% to 4% of patients on tolcapone had diarrhea which was regarded as severe. Diarrhea was the adverse event which most commonly led to discontinuation, with approximately 1%, 5%, and 6% of patients treated with placebo, 100, and 200 mg tolcapone 3 times daily, respectively, withdrawing from the trials prematurely. Discontinuing tolcapone for diarrhea was related to the severity of the symptom. Diarrhea resulted in withdrawal in approximately 8%, 40%, and 70% of patients with mild, moderate and severe diarrhea, respectively. Although diarrhea generally resolved after discontinuation of tolcapone, it led to hospitalization in 0.3%, 0.7%, and 1.7% of patients in the placebo, 100, and 200 mg tolcapone 3-times-daily groups.

Typically, diarrhea presents 6 to 12 weeks after tolcapone is started, but it may appear as early as 2 weeks and as late as many months after the initiation of treatment. Clinical trial data suggested that diarrhea associated with tolcapone use may sometimes be associated with anorexia (decreased appetite).

It is recommended that all cases of persistent diarrhea should be followed up with an appropriate workup (including occult blood samples).

➤*Hallucinations:* In clinical trials, hallucinations developed in approximately 5%, 8%, and 10% of patients treated with placebo, 100 and 200 mg tolcapone 3 times daily, respectively. Hallucinations led to drug discontinuation and premature withdrawal from clinical trials in 0.3%, 1.4%, and 1% of patients treated with placebo, 100 and 200 mg tolcapone 3 times daily, respectively. Hallucinations led to hospitalization in 0%, 1.7%, and 0% of patients in the placebo, 100 mg and 200 mg tolcapone 3 times daily groups, respectively.

In general, hallucinations present shortly after the initiation of therapy with tolcapone (typically within the first 2 weeks). Clinical trial data suggest that hallucinations associated with tolcapone use may be responsive to levodopa dose reduction. Patients whose hallucinations resolved had a mean levodopa dose reduction of 175 to 200 mg (20% to 25%) after the onset of the halluci-

TOLCAPONE — ORAL

nations. Hallucinations were commonly accompanied by confusion and to a lesser extent sleep disorder (insomnia) and excessive dreaming.

➤*Dyskinesia:* Tolcapone may potentiate the dopaminergic side effects of levodopa and may cause or exacerbate preexisting dyskinesia. Although decreasing the dose of levodopa may ameliorate this side effect, many patients in controlled trials continued to experience frequent dyskinesias despite a reduction in their dose of levodopa. The rates of withdrawal for dyskinesia were 0%, 0.3%, and 1% for placebo, 100, and 200 mg tolcapone 3 times daily, respectively.

➤*Rhabdomyolysis:* Cases of severe rhabdomyolysis, with 1 case of multi-organ system failure rapidly progressing to death, have been reported. The complicated nature of these cases makes it impossible to determine what role, if any, tolcapone played in their pathogenesis. Severe prolonged motor activity including dyskinesia may account for rhabdomyolysis. Some cases, however, included fever, alteration of consciousness and muscular rigidity. It is possible, therefore, that the rhabdomyolysis may be a result of the syndrome described in Hyperpyrexia and confusion (see Events reported with dopaminergic therapy).

➤*Hematuria:* The rates of hematuria in placebo-controlled trials were approximately 2%, 4%, and 5% in placebo, 100, and 200 mg tolcapone 3 times daily, respectively. The etiology of the increase with tolcapone has not always been explained (for example, by urinary tract infection or warfarin therapy). In placebo-controlled trials in the United States (n = 593) rates of microscopically confirmed hematuria were ≈ 3%, 2%, and 2% in placebo, 100 mg and 200 mg tolcapone 3 times daily, respectively.

➤*Events reported with dopaminergic therapy:* The events listed below are known to be associated with the use of drugs that increase dopaminergic activity, although they are most often associated with the use of direct dopamine agonists. While cases of hyperpyrexia and confusion have been reported in association with tolcapone withdrawal (see information below), the expected incidence of fibrotic complications is so low that even if tolcapone caused these complications at rates similar to those attributable to other dopaminergic therapies, it is unlikely that even a single example would have been detected in a cohort of the size exposed to tolcapone.

Hyperpyrexia and confusion – In clinical trials, 4 cases of a symptom complex resembling the neuroleptic malignant syndrome (characterized by elevated temperature, muscular rigidity, and altered consciousness), similar to that reported in association with the rapid dose reduction or withdrawal of other dopaminergic drugs, have been reported in association with the abrupt withdrawal or lowering of the dose of tolcapone. In 3 of these cases, creatine phosphokinase (CPK) was elevated as well. One patient died, and the other 3 patients recovered over periods of approximately 2, 4, and 6 weeks. Rare cases of this symptom complex have been reported during marketed use. These cases are of a complicated nature including the concomitant administration of several medications affecting brain monoaminergic (ie, MAO-I, tricyclic and selective serotonin reuptake inhibitors) and anticholinergic systems. It is difficult, therefore, to determine what role, if any, tolcapone played in the pathogenesis. It may, therefore, be prudent to be particularly cautious if several concomitant medications of these types are used.

Fibrotic complications – Cases of retroperitoneal fibrosis, pulmonary infiltrates, pleural effusion, and pleural thickening have been reported in some patients treated with ergot derived dopaminergic agents. While these complications may resolve when the drug is discontinued, complete resolution does not always occur. Although these adverse events are believed to be related to the ergoline structure of these compounds, whether other, nonergot-derived drugs (eg, tolcapone) that increase dopaminergic activity can cause them is unknown.

Three cases of pleural effusion, one with pulmonary fibrosis, occurred during clinical trials. These patients were also on concomitant dopamine agonists (pergolide or bromocriptine) and had a history of cardiac disease or pulmonary pathology (nonmalignant lung lesion).

➤*Special risk:* Tolcapone therapy should not be initiated if the patient exhibits clinical evidence of active liver disease or 2 ALT or AST values greater than the ULN. Patients with severe dyskinesia or dystonia should be treated with caution. Patients with severe renal impairment should be treated with caution.

➤*Hazardous tasks:* Patients should be advised that they should neither drive a car nor operate other complex machinery until they have gained sufficient experience on tolcapone to gauge whether or not it affects their mental or motor performance adversely. Because of the possible additive sedative effects, caution should be used when patients are taking other CNS depressants in combination with tolcapone.

Drug Interactions

➤*Monamine oxidase (MAO) inhibitors:* MAO and COMT are the 2 major enzyme systems involved in the metabolism of catecholamines. It is theoretically possible, therefore, that the combination of tolcapone and a nonselective MAO inhibitor (eg, phenelzine, tranylcypromine) would result in inhibition of the majority of the pathways responsible for normal catecholamine metabolism. For this reason, patients should ordinarily not be treated concomitantly with tolcapone and a nonselective MAO inhibitor.

Tolcapone can be taken concomitantly with a selective MAO-B inhibitor (eg, selegiline).

➤*Drugs metabolized by COMT:* Tolcapone may influence the pharmacokinetics of drugs metabolized by COMT. However, no effects were seen on the pharmacokinetics of the COMT substrate carbidopa. The effect of tolcapone on the pharmacokinetics of other drugs of this class such as a-methyldopa, dobutamine, apomorphine, and isoproterenol has not been evaluated. A dose reduction of such compounds should be considered when they are coadministered with tolcapone.

➤*Effect of tolcapone on the metabolism of other drugs:* Due to its affinity to cytochrome P450 2C9 in vitro, tolcapone may interfere with drugs, whose clearance is dependent on this metabolic pathway, such as tolbutamide and warfarin. However, in an in vivo interaction study, tolcapone did not change the pharmacokinetics of tolbutamide. Therefore, clinically relevant interactions involving cytochrome P450 2C9 appear unlikely. Similarly, tolcapone did not affect the pharmacokinetics of desipramine, a drug metabolized by cytochrome P450 2D6, indicating that interactions with drugs metabolized by that enzyme are unlikely. Since clinical information is limited regarding the combination of warfarin and tolcapone, coagulation parameters should be monitored when these 2 drugs are coadministered.

➤*Drugs that increase catecholamines:* When tolcapone is administered together with levodopa/carbidopa, it increases the relative bioavailability (AUC) of levodopa by approximately 2-fold. This is due to a decrease in levodopa clearance resulting in a prolongation of the terminal elimination half-life of levodopa (from approximately 2 to 3.5 hours). In general, the average peak levodopa plasma concentration (C_{max}) and the time of its occurrence (t_{max}) are unaffected. The onset of effect occurs after the first administration and is maintained during long-term treatment. Studies in healthy volunteers and Parkinson's disease patients have confirmed that the maximal effect occurs with 100 to 200 mg tolcapone. Plasma levels of 3-OMD are markedly and dose-dependently decreased by tolcapone when given with levodopa/carbidopa.

Population pharmacokinetic analyses in patients with Parkinson's disease have shown the same effects of tolcapone on levodopa plasma concentrations that occur in healthy volunteers.

When tolcapone was given together with levodopa/carbidopa and desipramine, there was no significant change in blood pressure, pulse rate and plasma concentrations of desipramine. Overall, the frequency of adverse events increased slightly. These adverse reactions were predictable based on the known adverse reactions to each of the 3 drugs individually. Therefore, caution should be exercised when desipramine is administered to Parkinson's disease patients being treated with tolcapone and levodopa/carbidopa.

Adverse Reactions

Cases of severe hepatocellular injury, including fulminant liver failure resulting in death, have been reported in postmarketing use. As of October, 1998, 3 cases of fatal fulminant hepatic failure have been reported from approximately 60,000 patients providing about 40,000 patient years of worldwide use. This incidence may be 10- to 100-fold higher than the background incidence in the general population.

The most commonly observed adverse reactions (> 5%) in the double-blind, placebo-controlled trials (n = 892) associated with the use of tolcapone not seen at an equivalent frequency among the placebo-treated patients were dyskinesia, nausea, sleep disorder, dystonia, excessive dreaming, anorexia, muscle cramps, orthostatic complaints, somnolence, diarrhea, confusion, dizziness, headache, hallucination, vomiting, constipation, fatigue, upper respiratory tract infection, falling, increased sweating, urinary tract infection, xerostomia, abdominal pain, urine discoloration.

Approximately 16% of the 592 patients who participated in the double-blind, placebo-controlled trials discontinued treatment due to adverse events compared to 10% of the 298 patients who received placebo. Diarrhea was by far the most frequent cause of discontinuation (approximately 6% in tolcapone patients vs 1% on placebo).

➤*Adverse reaction incidence in controlled clinical studies:*

Summary of Patients with Adverse Reactions after Start of Trial Drug Administration (at least 1% in Tolcapone Group and at least 1 Tolcapone Dose Group Greater than Placebo)

	Placebo	Tolcapone 3 times daily	
	(n = 298)	100 mg (n = 296)	200 mg (n = 298)
Adverse reactions	(%)	(%)	(%)
Dyskinesia	20%	42%	51%
Nausea	18%	30%	35%
Sleep disorder	18%	24%	25%
Dystonia	17%	19%	22%
Dreaming excessive	17%	21%	16%
Anorexia	13%	19%	23%
Muscle cramps	17%	17%	18%
Orthostatic complaints	14%	17%	17%
Somnolence	13%	18%	14%
Diarrhea	8%	16%	18%
Confusion	9%	11%	10%
Dizziness	10%	13%	6%
Headache	7%	10%	11%
Hallucination	5%	8%	10%
Vomiting	4%	8%	10%
Constipation	5%	6%	8%
Fatigue	6%	7%	3%

TOLCAPONE — ORAL

Summary of Patients with Adverse Reactions after Start of Trial Drug Administration (at least 1% in Tolcapone Group and at least 1 Tolcapone Dose Group Greater than Placebo)			
	Placebo	Tolcapone 3 times daily	
		100 mg	200 mg
	(n = 298)	(n = 296)	(n = 298)
Adverse reactions	(%)	(%)	(%)
Upper respiratory tract infection	3%	5%	7%
Falling	4%	4%	6%
Sweating increased	2%	4%	7%
Urinary tract infection	4%	5%	5%
Xerostomia	2%	5%	6%
Abdominal pain	3%	5%	6%
Syncope	3%	4%	5%
Urine discoloration	1%	2%	7%
Dyspepsia	2%	4%	3%
Influenza	2%	3%	4%
Dyspnea	2%	3%	3%
Balance loss	2%	3%	2%
Flatulence	2%	2%	4%
Hyperkinesia	1%	3%	2%
Chest pain	1%	3%	1%
Hypotension	1%	2%	2%
Paresthesia	2%	3%	1%
Stiffness	1%	2%	2%
Arthritis	1%	2%	1%
Chest discomfort	1%	1%	2%
Hypokinesia	1%	1%	3%
Micturition disorder	1%	2%	1%
Neck pain	1%	2%	2%
Burning	0%	2%	1%
Sinus congestion	0%	2%	1%
Agitation	0%	1%	1%
Dermal bleeding	0%	1%	1%
Irritability	0%	1%	1%
Mental deficiency	0%	1%	1%
Hyperactivity	0%	1%	1%
Malaise	0%	1%	0%
Panic reaction	0%	1%	0%
Tumor, skin	0%	1%	0%
Cataract	0%	1%	0%
Euphoria	0%	1%	0%
Fever	0%	0%	1%
Alopecia	0%	1%	0%
Eye inflamed	0%	1%	0%
Hypertonia	0%	0%	1%
Tumor, uterus	0%	1%	0%

Other events reported by greater than or equal to 1% of patients treated with tolcapone but that were equally or more frequent in the placebo group were arthralgia, limb pain, anxiety, micturition frequency, fractures, vision blurred, pneumonia, paresis, lethargy, asthenia, peripheral edema, abnormal gait, taste alteration, weight decrease and sinusitis.

Effects of gender and age on adverse reactions – Experience in clinical trials have suggested that patients older than 75 years of age may be more likely to develop hallucinations than patients younger than 75 years of age, while patients older than 75 may be less likely to develop dystonia. Females may be more likely to develop somnolence than males.

➤*Other adverse reactions observed during all trials in patients with Parkinson's disease:* All reported events that occurred at least twice (or once for serious or potentially serious events), except those already listed above, trivial events and terms too vague to be meaningful are included, without regard to determination of a causal relationship to tolcapone.

Events are further classified within body system categories and enumerated in order of decreasing frequency using the following definitions: Frequent adverse reactions are defined as those occurring in at least 1/100 patients; infrequent adverse reactions are defined as those occurring in between 1/100 and 1/1000 patients; and rare adverse reactions are defined as those occurring in fewer than 1/1000 patients.

Cardiovascular – Palpitation (frequent); hypertension, vasodilation, angina pectoris, heart failure, atrial fibrillation, tachycardia, migraine, aortic stenosis, arrythmia, arteriospasm, bradycardia, cerebral hemorrhage, coronary artery disorder, heart arrest, myocardial infarct, myocardial ischemia, pulmonary embolus (infrequent); arteriosclerosis, cardiovascular disorder, pericardial effusion, thrombosis (rare).

CNS – Depression, hypesthesia, tremor, speech disorder, vertigo, emotional lability (frequent); neuralgia, amnesia, extrapyramidal syndrome, hostility, increased libido, manic reaction, nervousness, paranoid reaction, cerebral ischemia, cerebrovascular accident, delusions, decreased libido, neuropathy, apathy, choreoathetosis, myoclonus, psychosis, abnormal thinking, twitching (infrequent); antisocial reaction, delirium, encephalopathy, hemiplegia, meningitis (rare).

Dermatologic – Rash (frequent); herpes zoster, pruritus, seborrhea, skin discoloration, eczema, erythema multiforme, skin disorder, furunculosis, herpes simplex, urticaria (infrequent).

Endocrine – Diabetes mellitus (infrequent).

GI – Tooth disorder (frequent); dysphagia, gastrointestinal hemorrhage, gastroenteritis, mouth ulceration, increased salivation, abnormal stools, esophagitis, cholelithiasis, colitis, tongue disorder, rectal disorder (infrequent); cholecystitis, duodenal ulcer, gastrointestinal carcinoma, stomach atony (rare).

GU – Urinary incontinence, impotence (frequent); prostatic disorder, dysuria, nocturia, polyuria, urinary retention, urinary tract disorder, hematuria, kidney calculus, prostatic carcinoma, breast neoplasm, oliguria, uterine atony, uterine disorder, vaginitis (infrequent); bladder calculus, ovarian carcinoma, uterine hemorrhage (rare).

Hematologic/Lymphatic – Anemia (infrequent); leukemia, thrombocytopenia (rare).

Metabolic/Nutritional – Edema, hypercholesteremia, thirst, dehydration (infrequent).

Musculoskeletal – Myalgia (frequent); tenosynovitis, arthrosis, joint disorder (infrequent).

Respiratory – Bronchitis, pharyngitis (frequent); increased cough, rhinitis, asthma, epistaxis, hyperventilation, laryngitis, hiccup (infrequent); apnea, hypoxia, lung edema (rare).

Special senses – Tinnitus (frequent); diplopia, ear pain, eye hemorrhage, eye pain, lacrimation disorder, otitis media, parosmia (infrequent); glaucoma (rare).

Miscellaneous – Flank pain, accidental injury, abdominal pain, infection (frequent); hernia, pain, allergic reaction, cellulitis, infection fungal, viral infection, carcinoma, chills, infection bacterial, neoplasm, abscess, face edema, surgical procedure (infrequent); death (rare).

Overdosage

➤*Symptoms:* The highest dose of tolcapone administered to humans was 800 mg 3 times daily, with and without levodopa/carbidopa coadministration. This was in a 1-week study in elderly, healthy volunteers. The peak plasma concentrations of tolcapone at this dose were on average 30 mcg/mL (compared to 3 mcg/mL and 6 mcg/mL with 100 and 200 mg tolcapone, respectively). Nausea, vomiting and dizziness were observed, particularly in combination with levodopa/carbidopa.

➤*Treatment:* Hospitalization is advised. General supportive care is indicated. Based on the physicochemical properties of the compound, hemodialysis is unlikely to be of benefit.

Patient Information

Tolcapone should not be used by patients until there has been a complete discussion of the risks and the patient has provided written informed consent.

Patients should be informed of the clinical signs and symptoms that suggest the onset of hepatic injury (eg, persistent nausea, fatigue, lethargy, anorexia, jaundice, dark urine, pruritus, right upper quadrant tenderness). If symptoms of hepatic failure occur, patients should be advised to contact their physicians immediately.

Patients should be informed that hallucinations can occur.

Patients should be informed of the need to have regular blood tests to monitor liver enzymes.

Patients should be advised that they may develop postural (orthostatic) hypotension with or without symptoms such as dizziness, nausea, syncope, and sometimes sweating. Hypotension may occur more frequently during initial therapy. Accordingly, patients should be cautioned against rising rapidly after sitting or lying down, especially if they have been doing so for prolonged periods, and especially at the initiation of treatment with tolcapone.

Patients should be advised that they should neither drive a car nor operate other complex machinery until they have gained sufficient experience on tolcapone to gauge whether or not it affects their mental or motor performance adversely. Because of the possible additive sedative effects, caution should be used when patients are taking other CNS depressants in combination with tolcapone.

Patients should be informed that nausea may occur, especially at the initiation of treatment with tolcapone.

Patients should be advised of the possibility of an increase in dyskinesia or dystonia.

Although tolcapone has not been shown to be teratogenic in animals, it is always given in conjunction with levodopa/carbidopa, which is known to cause visceral and skeletal malformations in the rabbit. Accordingly,

TOLCAPONE — ORAL

patients should be advised to notify their physicians if they become pregnant or intend to become pregnant during therapy.

Tolcapone is excreted into maternal milk in rats. Because of the possibility that tolcapone may be excreted into human maternal milk, patients should be advised to notify their physicians if they intend to breastfeed or are breastfeeding an infant.

DOPAMINE RECEPTOR AGONISTS, NON-ERGOT

For additional information, refer to the Antiparkinson Agents introduction.

Indications

➤*Parkinson's disease:* For the treatment of the signs and symptoms of idiopathic Parkinson's disease.

Actions

➤*Pharmacology:* **Pramipexole** and **ropinirole**, non-ergot dopamine agonists for Parkinson's disease, have high relative in vitro specificity and full intrinsic activity at the D_2 subfamily of dopamine receptors, binding with higher affinity to D_3 than to D_2 or D_4 receptor subtypes. The relevance of D_3 receptor binding in Parkinson's disease is unknown. Ropinirole also has moderate in vitro affinity for opioid receptors, and its metabolites have negligible in vitro affinity for dopamine D_1, $5HT_1$, $5HT_2$, benzodiazepine, GABA, muscarinic, $alpha_1$-, $alpha_2$- and beta-adrenoreceptors.

The precise mechanism of action as a treatment for Parkinson's disease is unknown, although it is believed to be related to stimulation of dopamine receptors in the striatum.

➤*Pharmacokinetics:* Non-ergot dopamine agonists are rapidly absorbed, reaching peak concentrations in ≈ 1 to 2 hours. They are extensively distributed throughout the body with a volume of distribution of ≈ 500 L. **Pramipexole** also distributes into red blood cells with an erythrocyte-to-plasma ratio of ≈ 2. Steady-state concentrations of non-ergot dopamine agonists are achieved within 2 days after dosing. Urinary excretion is the major route of elimination with > 88% of the dose recovered in the urine.

Select Pharmacokinetic Parameters of Non-Ergot Dopamine Receptor Agonists

	Absolute bioavailability (%)	Protein binding (%)	Half-life (hrs)[1]	Clearance (ml/min)	P450 metabolism
Pramipexole	> 90	15	8 (12)	400	None; ≈ 90% excreted unchanged
Ropinirole	55	30 to 40	6	783	Extensive (CYP1A2); 1 to 2% excreted unchanged

[1] In elderly patients > 65 years of age.

Food – Food does not affect the extent of absorption but increases the time to achieve maximum plasma levels by 1 hour for pramipexole and 2.5 hours for ropinirole.

Special populations – Adjustment of initial doses based on gender, weight or age is not necessary because therapy is initiated at subtherapeutic doses and gradually titrated for optimal therapeutic effect.

Smoking – Cigarette smoking is expected to increase the clearance of ropinirole since CYP1A2 is known to be induced by smoking.

Renal impairment – The clearance of **pramipexole** was decreased ≈ 75% in patients with severe renal impairment (CCl ≈ 20 ml/min) and was 60% lower in patients with moderate renal impairment (CCl ≈ 40 ml/min). Use a lower initial and maintenance dose of pramipexole in these patients.

No dosage adjustment for **ropinirole** is necessary for patients with moderate renal impairment (CCl 30 to 50 ml/min). The effects of severe renal impairment have not been studied.

Hepatic impairment – Plasma levels of **ropinirole** may increase and clearance may decrease; titrate ropinirole with caution in patients with impaired hepatic function.

Contraindications

Hypersensitivity to the product or any of its components.

Warnings

➤*Symptomatic hypotension:* Dopamine agonists appear to impair the systemic regulation of blood pressure, with resulting orthostatic hypotension especially during dose escalation. Parkinson's disease patients appear to have impaired capacity to respond to an orthostatic challenge. Therefore, these patients require careful monitoring for signs and symptoms of orthostatic hypotension while being treated with dopaminergic agonists, especially during dose escalation.

➤*Syncope:* Syncope, sometimes associated with bradycardia, was observed in association with **ropinirole** therapy. In patients with early Parkinson's disease treated with ropinirole (without levodopa), 11.5% had syncope compared with 1.4% on placebo. Most of these cases occurred > 4 weeks after initiation of therapy of ropinirole and were usually associated with a recent increase in dose.

Of 208 patients being treated with both **levodopa** and **ropinirole** in advanced Parkinson's disease trials, syncope was reported in 2.9% vs 1.7% with placebo.

➤*Hallucinations:* Hallucinations were observed in a greater number of patients receiving dopaminergics than placebo. In early Parkinson's disease, hallucinations were observed in ≈ 5% to 9% of treated patients vs ≈ 1.5% to 2.5% for the placebo group. In patients with advanced Parkinson's disease receiving concomitant levodopa, hallucinations were observed in ≈ 10% to 16.5% of patients receiving dopaminergics vs ≈ 4% receiving placebo.

Elderly – Age appears to increase the risk of hallucinations attributable to dopaminergics. Elderly patients (> 65 years of age) with early and advanced Parkinson's disease have experienced hallucinations ≈ 7 and ≈ 5 times more often, respectively, than their younger counterparts when treated with dopaminergics.

➤*Renal function impairment:* Reduce initial and maintenance doses of **pramipexole** for patients with moderate to severe renal impairment (see Administration and Dosage).

➤*Fertility impairment:* A significant increase in testicular Leydig cell adenomas was observed in male rats treated with **ropinirole** at all doses tested (eg, ≥ 1.5 mg/kg [0.6 times the maximum recommended human dose on a mg/m² basis]). The relevance of this occurrence to humans is of questionable significance. An increase in benign uterine endometrial polyps at a dose of 50 mg/kg/day (10 times the maximum recommended human dose on a mg/m² basis) was observed in female mice treated with ropinirole.

➤*Elderly:* The incidence of hallucinations appears to increase with age (see Hallucinations in Warnings).

➤*Pregnancy: Category C.* There are no adequate and well-controlled studies in pregnant women. In animals, **ropinirole** has been shown to have adverse effects on embryo-fetal development, including teratogenic effects, decreased fetal body weight, increased fetal death and digital malformation. Use during pregnancy only if the potential benefit outweighs the potential risk to the fetus.

➤*Lactation:* Treatment with these agents has resulted in an inhibition of prolactin secretion in humans. It is not known whether these drugs are excreted in breast milk. Decide whether to discontinue nursing or the drug, taking into account the importance of the drug to the mother.

➤*Children:* Safety and efficacy have not been established.

Precautions

➤*Monitoring:* Monitor for signs and symptoms of orthostatic hypotension (see Warnings).

➤*Dyskinesia:* Dopamine receptor agonists may potentiate the dopaminergic side effects of levodopa and may cause or exacerbate preexisting dyskinesia. Decreasing the dose of levodopa may ameliorate this side effect.

➤*Retinal pathology:* Pathologic changes (degeneration and loss of photoreceptor cells) were observed in the retinas of albino rats receiving dopamine receptor agonists in a 2-year study. The potential significance of this effect in humans has not been established, but cannot be disregarded because disruption of a mechanism that is universally present in vertebrates (eg, disk shedding) may be involved.

➤*Withdrawal-emergent hyperpyrexia and confusion:* Although not reported with these specific agents, a symptom complex resembling the neuroleptic malignant syndrome (characterized by elevated temperature, muscular rigidity, altered consciousness and autonomic instability) with no other obvious etiology, has occurred in association with rapid dose reduction, withdrawal of or changes in antiparkinsonian dopaminergic therapy.

➤*Fibrotic complication:* Cases of retroperitoneal fibrosis, pulmonary infiltrates, pleural effusion and pleural thickening have occurred in some patients treated with ergot-derived dopaminergic agents. While these complications may resolve when the drug is discontinued, complete resolution does not always occur.

Although these adverse events are believed to be related to the ergoline structure of these compounds, whether non-ergot-derived dopamine agonists can cause these reactions is unknown.

➤*CNS effects:* Use concomitant CNS depressants with caution because of the possible additive sedative effects.

➤*Rhabdomyolysis:* A single case of rhabdomyolysis occurred in a 49-year-old male with advanced Parkinson's disease treated with **pramipexole**. The patient was hospitalized with an elevated CPK (10,631 IU/L). The symptoms resolved with discontinuation of the medication.

➤*Binding to melanin:* **Ropinirole** binds to melanin-containing tissues (eg, eyes, skin) in pigmentated rats. After a single dose, long-term retention of the drug was demonstrated with a half-life in the eye of 20 days. It is not known if ropinirole accumulates in these tissues over time.

DOPAMINE RECEPTOR AGONISTS, NON-ERGOT

Drug Interactions

Non-Ergot Dopamine Receptor Agonist Drug Interactions			
Precipitant drug	Object drug*		Description
Non-ergot dopamine agonists	Levodopa	⬆	Concomitant administration increased levodopa C_{max} (20% to 40%); pramipexole C_{max} decreased from 2.5 to 0.5 hours.
Cimetidine	Pramipexole	⬆	Cimetidine caused a 50% increase in pramipexole AUC and a 40% increase in its half-life.
Estrogen	Ropinirole	⬆	Estrogens (mainly ethinyl estradiol, 0.6 to 3 mg over a 4-month to 23-year period) reduced the oral clearance of ropinirole by 36% in 16 patients. Dosage adjustment may not be needed because ropinirole is titrated to effect. However, dose adjustment may be required if estrogen therapy is stopped or started during treatment with ropinirole.
Ciprofloxacin	Ropinirole	⬆	Coadministration with ciprofloxacin, an inhibitor of CYP1A2, increased ropinirole AUC by 84% on average and C_{max} by 60%.
Drugs eliminated via renal secretion (eg, cimetidine, ranitidine, diltiazem, triamterene, verapamil, quinidine, quinine)	Pramipexole	⬆	Coadministration of drugs that are secreted by the cationic transport system may decrease the oral clearance of pramipexole by ≈ 20%.
Inhibitors of CYP1A2 (eg, cimetidine, ciprofloxacin, diltiazem, enoxacin, erythromycin, fluvoxamine, mexiletine, norfloxacin, tacrine)	Ropinirole	⬆	Potential exists for substrates or inhibitors of CYP1A2 to alter ropinirole's clearance. If therapy with a potent CYP1A2 inhibitor is stopped or started during ropinirole treatment, dose adjustment may be required.
Dopamine antagonists (eg, phenothiazines, butyrophenones, thioxanthenes, metoclopramide)	Nonergot dopamine agonists	⬇	Because these agents are dopamine agonists, it is possible that dopamine antagonists, such as the neuroleptics, may diminish their effectiveness.

* ⬆ = Object drug increased. ⬇ = Object drug decreased.

➤*Drug/Food interactions:* **Pramipexole** and **ropinirole** T_{max} are increased by ≈ 1 and 2.5 hours, respectively, when taken with food, although the extent of absorption is not affected.

Adverse Reactions

➤*Early Parkinson's disease (without levodopa):* The most commonly observed adverse events (> 5%) shared by the non-ergot dopamine receptor agonists were nausea, dizziness, somnolence, dyspepsia, constipation, asthenia and hallucinations.

Approximately 24% of **ropinirole**-treated patients discontinued treatment because of adverse events vs 13% for placebo. The most common adverse events for discontinuing therapy were nausea (6.4%); dizziness (3.8%); aggravated Parkinson's disease, hallucinations, somnolence, vomiting, headache (1.3%). In **pramipexole** studies, ≈ 12% of treated patients vs 11% in the placebo group discontinued therapy because of adverse events. Hallucinations (3.1%); dizziness, nausea (2.1%); somnolence, extrapyramidal syndrome (1.6%); headache and confusion (1.3%) were the most common reason for discontinuation.

Non-Ergot Dopamine Receptor Agonist Adverse Reactions in Early Parkinson's Disease (without Levodopa)[1] (%)		
Adverse reaction	Pramipexole (n = 388)	Ropinirole (n = 157)
Autonomic nervous system		
Increased sweating	-	6
Dry mouth	-	5
Flushing	-	3
Cardiovascular		
Syncope	-	12
Orthostatic symptoms	-	6
Hypertension	-	5
Palpitations	-	3
Atrial fibrillation	-	2
Extrasystoles	-	2
Hypotension	-	2
Tachycardia	-	2
CNS		
Dizziness	25	40
Somnolence	22	40
Insomnia	17	-
Hallucinations[2]	9	5
Confusion	4	5
Amnesia	4	3
Hypesthesia	3	4
Yawning	-	3
Dystonia	2	-
Akathisia	2	-
Thinking abnormalities	2	-
Hyperkinesia	-	2
Impaired concentration	-	2
Vertigo	-	2
Decreased libido	1	-
Myoclonus	1	-
GI		
Nausea	28	60
Constipation	14	-
Vomiting	-	12
Dyspepsia	-	10
Abdominal pain	-	6
Anorexia	4	4
Flatulence	-	3
Dysphagia	2	-
Metabolic/Nutritional		
Peripheral edema	5	4
Decreased weight	2	0
Respiratory		
Pharyngitis	-	6
Rhinitis	-	4
Sinusitis	-	4
Bronchitis	-	3
Dyspnea	-	3
Special senses		
Abnormal vision	3	6
Eye abnormality	-	3
Xerophthalmia	-	2
Miscellaneous		
Asthenia	14	6
Fatigue	-	11
Viral infection	-	11
Pain	-	8
Edema	5	7
Urinary tract infection	-	5
Chest pain	-	4
Malaise	2	3
Fever	1	-
Impotence	2	3
Peripheral ischemia	-	3
Increased alkaline phosphatase	-	3

[1] Data pooled from separate studies; not necessarily comparable.
[2] See Warnings.

➤*Advanced Parkinson's disease (with levodopa):* The most commonly observed adverse events (> 5%) shared by the non-ergot dopamine receptor agonists were dyskinesia, dizziness, extrapyramidal syndrome/aggravated

DOPAMINE RECEPTOR AGONISTS, NON-ERGOT

Parkinsonism, somnolence, insomnia, injury, hallucinations, confusion, urinary frequency/infection, constipation and dry mouth.

Approximately 24% of patients treated with **ropinirole** and levodopa discontinued therapy because of adverse events vs 18% of patients given placebo and levodopa. The most common adverse events causing discontinuation of treatment were dizziness (2.9%); dyskinesia, vomiting, confusion (2.4%); nausea, hallucinations, anxiety (1.9%) and increased sweating (1.4%). In patients treated with **pramipexole** and levodopa, ≈ 12% discontinued therapy as a result of adverse reactions vs 16% in the placebo group. Therapy was discontinued most often because of hallucinations (2.7%); orthostatic hypotension (2.3%); dyskinesia (1.9%); extrapyramidal syndrome (1.5%); dizziness and confusion (1.2%).

Non-Ergot Dopamine Receptor Agonist Adverse Reactions in Advanced Parkinson's Disease (with Levodopa)[1] (%)

Adverse reaction	Pramipexole (n=260)	Ropinirole (n=208)
Cardiovascular		
Postural hypotension	53	2
Syncope	-	3
CNS		
Dyskinesia	47	34
Extrapyramidal syndrome	28	-
Insomnia	27	-
Dizziness	26	26
Somnolence	9	20
Hallucinations	17	10
Headache	-	17
Dream abnormalities	11	3
Confusion	10	9
Falls	-	10
Dystonia	8	-
Gait abnormalities/hypokinesia	7	5
Hypertonia	7	-
Amnesia	6	5
Tremor/twitching	2	6
Nervousness	-	5
Paresthesia	-	5
Akathisia	3	-
Thinking abnormalities	3	-
Paresis	-	3
Paranoid reaction	2	-
Delusions	1	-
Sleep disorders	1	-
GI		
Nausea	-	30
Constipation	10	6
Abdominal pain	-	9
Vomiting	-	7
Diarrhea	-	5
Dysphagia	-	2
Flatulence	-	2
Increased saliva	-	2
GU		
Urinary frequency	6	-
Urinary tract infection	4	6
Urinary incontinence	2	2
Pyuria	-	2
Metabolic/Nutritional		
Peripheral edema	2	-
Increased creatine PK	1	-
Musculoskeletal		
Arthritis	3	3
Twitching	2	6
Bursitis	2	-
Myasthenia	1	-

Non-Ergot Dopamine Receptor Agonist Adverse Reactions in Advanced Parkinson's Disease (with Levodopa)[1] (%)

Adverse reaction	Pramipexole (n=260)	Ropinirole (n=208)
Respiratory		
Pneumonia	2	9
Dyspnea	4	3
Rhinitis	3	-
Special senses		
Accommodation abnormalities	4	-
Vision abnormalities	3	-
Diplopia	1	-
Miscellaneous		
Accidental injury	17	-
Asthenia	10	-
Dry mouth	7	5
Increased sweating	-	7
Increased drug level	-	-
Pain	-	-
General edema	4	-
Chest pain	3	-
Malaise	3	-
Skin disorders	2	-
Anemia	-	2
Weight decrease	-	2

[1] Data pooled from separate studies; not necessarily comparable.

Overdosage

There is no clinical experience with massive overdosage. One patient with a 10-year history of schizophrenia took **pramipexole** 11 mg/day for 2 days (two to three times the recommended daily dose). No adverse events were reported related to the increased dose. Blood pressure remained stable, although pulse rate increased to between 100 and 120 beats/minute. Of ten patients ingesting > 24 mg/day, one experienced mild oro-facial dyskinesia, another experienced intermittent nausea. Other symptoms reported with accidental overdoses were: Agitation, increased dyskinesia, grogginess, sedation, orthostatic hypotension, chest pain, confusion, vomiting and nausea. The largest overdose reported was 435 mg taken over a 7-day period (62.1 mg/day).

➤*Treatment:* There is no known antidote for overdosage of a dopamine agonist. If signs of CNS stimulation are present, a phenothiazine or other butyrophenone neuroleptic agent may be indicated; the efficacy of such drugs in reversing the effects of overdosage has not been assessed. Management of overdose may require general supportive measures along with gastric lavage, IV fluids and ECG monitoring. A negligible amount of **pramipexole** is removed by dialysis. Refer to General Management of Acute Overdosage.

Patient Information

Inform patients that hallucinations can occur and that the elderly are at a higher risk than younger patients with Parkinson's disease.

Patients may develop postural hypotension with or without symptoms such as dizziness, nausea, fainting or blackouts and sometimes sweating. Hypotension may occur more frequently during initial therapy. Accordingly, caution patients against rising rapidly after sitting or lying down, especially if they have been doing so for prolonged periods and at the initiation of treatment with pramipexole.

Advise patients that they may experience somnolence and that they should neither drive a car nor operate other complex machinery until they have gained sufficient experience with the drug to gauge whether or not it affects their mental or motor performance adversely. Inform patients of the possible additive sedative effects when taken in combination with other CNS depressants.

Because **ropinirole** has been shown to have adverse effects on embryo-fetal development, advise patients to notify their physician if they become pregnant or intend to become pregnant during therapy.

Advise patients to notify their physicians if they intend to breastfeed or are breastfeeding an infant.

If patients develop nausea, advise them that taking this medication with food may reduce the occurrence of nausea.

PRAMIPEXOLE

Rx	**Mirapex** (Boehringer Ingelheim)	**Tablets:** 0.125 mg	(U 2). White. In 63s.
		0.25 mg	(UU 44). White, scored. Oval. In 90s.
		0.5 mg	Mannitol. (UU 88). White, scored. Oval. In 90s and UD 100s.
		1 mg	(UU 66). White, scored. In 90s.
		1.5 mg	(UU 3737). White, scored. In 90s.

PRAMIPEXOLE DIHYDROCHLORIDE — ORAL

For complete and comparative prescribing information, refer to the Dopamine Receptor Agonists, Non-Ergot group monograph.

Indications

Pramipexole dihydrochloride tablets are indicated for the treatment of the signs and symptoms of idiopathic Parkinson's disease.

The effectiveness of pramipexole dihydrochloride was demonstrated in randomized, controlled trials in patients with early Parkinson's disease who were not receiving concomitant levodopa therapy as well as in patients with advanced disease on concomitant levodopa.

Administration and Dosage

➤*Approved by the FDA:* July 2, 1997.

In all clinical studies, dosage was initiated at a subtherapeutic level to avoid intolerable adverse effects and orthostatic hypotension. Gradually titrate pramipexole in all patients. Increase the dosage to achieve a maximum therapeutic effect, balanced against the principal side effects of dyskinesia, hallucinations, somnolence, and dry mouth.

➤*Dosing in patients with healthy renal function:*

Initial treatment – Gradually increase dosages from a starting dose of 0.375 mg/day given in 3 divided doses, and do not increase more frequently than every 5 to 7 days. A suggested ascending dosage schedule that was used in clinical studies is shown in the following table:

Ascending Dosage Schedule of Pramipexole		
Week	Dosage (mg)	Total daily dose (mg)
1	0.125 mg 3 times daily	0.375 mg
2	0.25 mg 3 times daily	0.75 mg
3	0.5 mg 3 times daily	1.5 mg
4	0.75 mg 3 times daily	2.25 mg
5	1 mg 3 times daily	3 mg
6	1.25 mg 3 times daily	3.75 mg
7	1.5 mg 3 times daily	4.5 mg

Maintenance treatment – Pramipexole tablets were effective and well tolerated over a dosage range of 1.5 to 4.5 mg/day administered in equally divided doses 3 times/day with or without concomitant levodopa (approximately 800 mg/day).

In a fixed-dose study in early Parkinson's disease patients, doses of 3 mg, 4.5 mg, and 6 mg/day of pramipexole were not shown to provide any significant benefit beyond that achieved at a daily dose of 1.5 mg/day. However, in the same fixed-dose study, the following adverse events were dose related: postural hypotension, nausea, constipation, somnolence, and amnesia. The frequency of these events was generally 2-fold greater than placebo for pramipexole doses greater than 3 mg/day. The incidence of somnolence reported with pramipexole at a dose of 1.5 mg/day was comparable to placebo.

When pramipexole is used in combination with levodopa, consider a reduction of the levodopa dosage. In a controlled study in advanced Parkinson's disease, the dosage of levodopa was reduced by an average of 27% from baseline.

➤*Patients with renal impairment:*

Pramipexole Dosage in Renal Function Impairment		
Renal status	Starting dose (mg)	Maximum dose (mg)
Normal to mild impairment (Ccr > 60 mL/min)	0.125 mg 3 times a day	1.5 mg 3 times a day
Moderate impairment (Ccr = 35 to 59 mL/min)	0.125 mg twice a day	1.5 mg twice a day
Severe impairment (Ccr = 15 to 34 mL/min)	0.125 mg once daily	1.5 mg once daily
Very severe impairment (Ccr < 15 mL/min and hemodialysis patients)	The use of pramipexole has not been adequately studied in this group of patients.	

➤*Discontinuation of treatment:* It is recommended that pramipexole be discontinued over a period of 1 week; in some studies, however, abrupt discontinuation was uneventful.

➤*Storage / Stability:* Store at 25°C (77°F); excursions permitted to 15° to 30°C (59° to 86°F). Protect from light.

ROPINIROLE HYDROCHLORIDE

Rx	**Requip** (GlaxoSmithKline)	**Tablets:** 0.25 mg	Lactose. (SB 4890). White, pentagonal, film-coated *Tiltab* with beveled edges. In 100s.
		0.5 mg	Lactose. (SB 4891). Yellow, pentagonal, film-coated *Tiltab* with beveled edges. In 100s.
		1 mg	Lactose. (SB 4892). Green, pentagonal, film-coated *Tiltab* with beveled edges. In 100s.
		2 mg	Lactose. (SB 4893). Pale yellowish pink, pentagonal, film-coated *Tiltab* with beveled edges. In 100s.
		3 mg	Lactose. (SB 4895). Pale to moderate reddish-purple, pentagonal, film-coated *Tiltab* with beveled edges. In 100s.
		4 mg	Lactose. (SB 4896). Pale brown, pentagonal, film-coated *Tiltab* with beveled edges. In 100s.
		5 mg	Lactose. (SB 4894). Blue, pentagonal, film-coated *Tiltab* with beveled edges. In 100s.

ROPINIROLE HYDROCHLORIDE — ORAL

Indications

➤*Parkinson disease:* Ropinirole is indicated for the treatment of the signs and symptoms of idiopathic Parkinson disease.

The efficacy of ropinirole was demonstrated in randomized, controlled trials in patients with early Parkinson disease who were not receiving concomitant levodopa therapy as well as in patients with advanced disease on concomitant levodopa.

➤*Restless legs syndrome (RLS):* Ropinirole is indicated for the treatment of moderate to severe primary RLS.

Key diagnostic criteria for RLS are as follows: an urge to move the legs, usually accompanied or caused by uncomfortable and unpleasant leg sensations; symptoms begin or worsen during periods of rest or inactivity such as lying or sitting; symptoms are partially or totally relieved by movement such as walking or stretching at least as long as the activity continues; and symptoms are worse or occur only in the evening or night. Difficulty falling asleep may frequently be associated with moderate to severe RLS.

Administration and Dosage

➤*Approved by the FDA:* September 23, 1997.

➤*General dosing considerations for Parkinson disease and RLS:* Ropinirole can be taken with or without food. Patients may be advised that taking ropinirole with food may reduce the occurrence of nausea. However, this has not been established in controlled clinical trials. If a significant interruption in therapy with ropinirole has occurred, retitration of therapy may be warranted.

➤*Parkinson disease dosage:* In all clinical studies, dosage was initiated at a subtherapeutic level and gradually titrated to therapeutic response. The dosage should be increased to achieve a maximum therapeutic effect, balanced against the principal side effects of nausea, dizziness, somnolence, and dyskinesia.

The recommended starting dose for Parkinson disease is 0.25 mg 3 times daily. Based on individual patient response, dosage should then be titrated with weekly increments as described in the following table. After week 4, if necessary, daily dosage may be increased by 1.5 mg/day on a weekly basis up to a dose of 9 mg/day, and then by up to 3 mg/day weekly to a total dose of 24 mg/day. Doses greater than 24 mg/day have not been tested in clinical trials.

Ascending Dose Schedule of Ropinirole for Parkinson Disease		
Week	Dosage	Total daily dose
1	0.25 mg 3 times daily	0.75 mg
2	0.5 mg 3 times daily	1.5 mg
3	0.75 mg 3 times daily	2.25 mg
4	1 mg 3 times daily	3 mg

When ropinirole is administered as adjunct therapy to levodopa, the concurrent dose of levodopa may be decreased gradually as tolerated. Levodopa dosage reduction was allowed during the advanced Parkinson disease (with levodopa) study if dyskinesias or other dopaminergic effects occurred. Overall, reduction of levodopa dose was sustained in 87% of ropinirole-treated patients and in 57% of patients on placebo. On average, the levodopa dose was reduced by 31% in ropinirole-treated patients.

Ropinirole for patients with Parkinson disease should be discontinued gradually over a 7-day period. The frequency of administration should be

ROPINIROLE HYDROCHLORIDE — ORAL

reduced from 3 times daily to twice daily for 4 days. For the remaining 3 days, the frequency should be reduced to once daily prior to complete withdrawal of ropinirole.

➤*RLS dosage:* In all clinical trials, the dose for ropinirole was initiated at 0.25 mg once daily, 1 to 3 hours before bedtime. Patients were titrated based on clinical response and tolerability.

The recommended adult starting dosage for RLS is 0.25 mg once daily, 1 to 3 hours before bedtime. After 2 days, the dosage can be increased to 0.5 mg once daily and to 1 mg once daily at the end of the first week of dosing, then as shown in the following table as needed to achieve efficacy. For RLS, the safety and efficacy of doses greater than 4 mg once daily have not been established.

Dose Titration Schedule of Ropinirole for RLS

Day/Week	Dosage to be taken once daily, 1 to 3 hours before bedtime
Days 1 and 2	0.25 mg
Days 3 to 7	0.5 mg
Week 2	1 mg
Week 3	1.5 mg
Week 4	2 mg
Week 5	2.5 mg
Week 6	3 mg
Week 7	4 mg

In clinical trials of patients being treated for RLS with doses up to 4 mg once daily, ropinirole was discontinued without a taper.

➤*Elderly:* Pharmacokinetic studies demonstrated a reduced clearance of ropinirole in the elderly. Dose adjustment is not necessary because the dose is individually titrated to clinical response.

➤*Hepatic function impairment:* The pharmacokinetics of ropinirole have not been studied in patients with hepatic impairment. Because patients with hepatic impairment may have higher plasma levels and lower clearance, ropinirole should be titrated with caution in these patients.

➤*Storage/Stability:* Protect from light and moisture. Close container tightly after each use. Store at controlled room temperature 20° to 25°C (68° to 77°F).

APOMORPHINE HYDROCHLORIDE

Rx	**Apokyn** (Mylan Bertek)	**Injection:** 10 mg/mL	Sodium metabisulfite. 2 mL glass ampules and 3 mL cartridges.

APOMORPHINE HYDROCHLORIDE — INJECTION

For complete and comparative prescribing information, refer to the Dopamine Receptor Agonists, Non-Ergot group monograph.

Indications

➤*Parkinson disease:* Apomorphine injection is indicated for the acute, intermittent treatment of hypomobility, "off" episodes ("end-of-dose wearing off" and unpredictable "on/off" episodes) associated with advanced Parkinson's disease. Apomorphine injection has been studied as an adjunct to other medications.

Administration and Dosage

➤*Approved by the FDA:* April 20, 2004.

The prescribed dose of apomorphine injection should always be expressed in mL to avoid confusion and doses greater than 0.6 mL (6 mg) are not recommended. Patients and caregivers must receive detailed instructions in the preparation and injection of doses, with particular attention paid to the correct use of the dosing pen.

Apomorphine injection is indicated for subcutaneous administration only. Apomorphine injection should not be initiated without use of a concomitant antiemetic. At the recommended doses of apomorphine, severe nausea and vomiting can be expected. Most antiemetic experience is with trimethobenzamide and this should generally be used. Trimethobenzamide (300 mg 3 times daily orally) should be started 3 days prior to the initial dose of apomorphine and continued at least during the first 2 months of therapy.

Based on reports of profound hypotension and loss of consciousness when apomorphine was administered with ondansetron, the concomitant use of apomorphine with drugs of the $5HT_3$ antagonist class (including, for example, ondansetron, granisetron, dolasetron, palonosetron, and alosetron) is contraindicated.

The dose of apomorphine injection must be titrated on the basis of effectiveness and tolerance, starting at 0.2 mL (2 mg) and up to a maximum recommended dose of 0.6 mL (6 mg) as follows:

Patients in an "off" state should be given a 0.2 mL (2 mg) test dose in a setting where blood pressure can be closely monitored by medical personnel. Both supine and standing blood pressure should be checked predose and at 20, 40, and 60 minutes post dose. Patients who develop clinically significant orthostatic hypotension in response to this test dose of apomorphine should not be considered candidates for treatment with apomorphine injection. If the patient tolerates the 0.2 mL (2 mg) dose, and responds, the starting dose should be 0.2 mL (2 mg) used on an as needed basis to treat existing "off" episodes. If needed, the dose can be increased in 0.1 mL (1 mg) increments every few days on an outpatient basis.

Beyond this, the general principle guiding dosing (described in detail below) is to determine a dose (0.3 mL or 0.4 mL) that the patient will tolerate as a test dose under monitored conditions, and then begin an outpatient dosing trial (periodically assessing both efficacy and tolerability) using a dose 0.1 mL (1 mg) lower than the tolerated test dose.

For patients who tolerate the test dose of 0.2 mL (2 mg) but achieve no response, a dose of 0.4 mL (4 mg) may be administered at the next observed "off" period, but no sooner than 2 hours after the initial test dose of 0.2 mL (2 mg). Both supine and standing blood pressure should be checked predose and at 20, 40, and 60 minutes post dose. If the patient tolerates a test dose of 0.4 mL (4 mg) the starting dose should be 0.3 mL (3 mg) used on an as-needed basis to treat existing "off" episodes. If needed, the dose can be increased in 0.1 mL (1 mg) increments every few days on an outpatient basis. If a patient does not tolerate a test dose of 0.4 mL (4 mg), a test dose of 0.3 mL (3 mg) may be administered during a separate "off" period, no sooner than 2 hours after the test dose of 0.4 mL (4 mg). Both supine and standing blood pressure should be checked predose and at 20, 40, and 60 minutes post dose. If the patient tolerates the 0.3 mL (3 mg) test dose, the starting dose should be 0.2 mL (2 mg) used on an as needed basis to treat existing "off" episodes. If needed, and the 0.2 mL (2 mg) dose is tolerated, the dose can be increased to 0.3 mL (3 mg) after a few days. In such a patient, the dose should ordinarily not be increased to 0.4 mL (4 mg) on an out-patient basis.

Most patients studied in the apomorphine development program responded to 0.3 mL to 0.6 mL (3 mg to 6 mg). There is no evidence from controlled trials that doses greater than 0.6 mL (6 mg) give an increased effect and these doses are not recommended. The average frequency of dosing was 3 times per day in the development program, and there is limited experience with single doses greater than 0.6 mL (6 mg), dosing more than 5 times per day and with total daily doses greater than 2 mL (20 mg).

If a single dose of apomorphine is ineffective for a particular "off" period, a second dose should not be given for that "off" episode. The efficacy of a second dose for a single "off" episode has not been systematically studied and the safety of redosing has not been characterized.

➤*Interruption of therapy:* Patients who have a significant interruption in therapy (more than a week) should be restarted on a 0.2 mL (2 mg) dose and gradually titrated to effect.

➤*Hepatic function impairment:* When dosing patients with mild and moderate hepatic impairment, caution should be exercised due to the increased C_{max} and AUC in these patients.

➤*Renal function impairment:* For patients with mild and moderate renal impairment, the testing dose and subsequently the starting dose should be reduced to 0.1 mL (1 mg).

➤*Storage/Stability:* Store at 25°C (77°F). Excursions permitted to 15° to 30°C (59° to 86°F).

Indications

➤*Myasthenia gravis:* Treatment of myasthenia gravis.

➤*Urinary retention:* The prevention and treatment of postoperative distention and urinary retention after mechanical obstruction has been excluded.

➤*Reversal of nondepolarizing muscle relaxants:* Reversal of nondepolarizing muscle relaxants (**pyridostigmine** and **neostigmine**).

➤*Unlabeled uses:* Diagnosis of myasthenia gravis (0.022 mg/kg/dose IM × 1).

Actions

➤*Pharmacology:* These drugs facilitate transmission of impulses across the myoneural junction by inhibiting the destruction of acetylcholine by cholinesterase. They differ in duration of action and in adverse effects. Equivalent doses, onset and duration of action are summarized below.

Drug	Route	Equivalent Dosage (mg)	Onset (min)	Duration (hours)	Indications
Ambenonium	PO	5-10	20-30	3-8	Myasthenia gravis
Edrophonium	IM	10	2-10	0.17-0.67	Diagnosis myasthenia gravis
	IV	10	< 1	0.08-0.33	Diagnosis myasthenia gravis;[1] Nondepolarizing muscle relaxant antagonist
Neostigmine	PO	15	45-75	2-4	Myasthenia gravis
	IM	1.5	20-30	2-4	Myasthenia gravis
	IV	0.5	4-8	2-4	Diagnosis myasthenia gravis; Nondepolarizing muscle relaxant antagonist
Pyridostigmine	PO	60	20-30	3-6	Myasthenia gravis
	IM	2	< 15	2-4	Myasthenia gravis
	IV	2	2-5	2-4	Myasthenia gravis; Nondepolarizing muscle relaxant antagonist

[1] Also used to evaluate treatment requirements in myasthenia gravis.

Contraindications

Hypersensitivity to anticholinesterases; mechanical intestinal and urinary obstructions; peritonitis (**neostigmine**); history of reaction to bromides (**neostigmine** and **pyridostigmine**).

Warnings

➤*Use with caution:* Use with caution in patients with bronchial asthma, epilepsy, bradycardia, recent coronary occlusion, vagotonia, hyperthyroidism, cardiac arrhythmias or peptic ulcer. Treat transient bradycardia with atropine sulfate. Isolated instances of cardiac and respiratory arrest, believed to be vagotonic effects, have occurred. When large doses are given, prior or simultaneous injection of atropine sulfate may be advisable. Use separate syringes.

➤*Cholinergic/Myasthenic crisis:* Overdosage may result in cholinergic crisis, characterized by increasing muscle weakness that, through involvement of the respiratory muscles, may lead to death. Myasthenic crisis because of an increase in disease severity is also accompanied by extreme muscle weakness and may be difficult to distinguish from cholinergic crisis. Differentiation is extremely important; use **edrophonium** and clinical judgment.

Treatment of the two conditions differs radically: Myasthenic crisis requires more intensive anticholinesterase therapy; cholinergic crisis calls for withdrawal of all drugs of this type and immediate use of atropine. Have a syringe containing 1 mg of atropine sulfate immediately available to be given IV to counteract severe cholinergic reactions. Use atropine to abolish or blunt GI side effects or other muscarinic reactions; however, such use may lead to inadvertent induction of cholinergic crisis by masking signs of overdosage.

➤*Used as antagonists to nondepolarizing muscle relaxants:* Obtain adequate recovery of voluntary respiration and neuromuscular transmission prior to discontinuing respiratory assistance. Observe continuously. If there is doubt concerning adequacy of recovery from the nondepolarizing muscle relaxant, continue artificial ventilation.

➤*Supervision:* Great care and supervision are required with **ambenonium.** Because ambenonium has a more prolonged action than other antimyasthenic drugs, simultaneous use with other cholinergics is contraindicated except under strict supervision. Therefore, when a patient is to be given the drug, suspend use of all other cholinergics until the patient has been stabilized.

➤*Hypersensitivity reactions:* Because of possible hypersensitivity in an occasional patient, have atropine and epinephrine readily available when using parenteral therapy.

➤*Pregnancy:* (*Category C* – neostigmine.) Safety for use during pregnancy has not been established. Transient muscular weakness occurred in ≈ 20% of infants born to mothers treated with these drugs during pregnancy. Use only when clearly needed and when the potential benefits outweigh the potential hazards to the fetus.

Anticholinesterase drugs may cause uterine irritability and induce premature labor when given IV to pregnant women near term.

➤*Lactation:* **Pyridostigmine** is excreted in breast milk. Because they are ionized at physiologic pH, **ambenonium** and **neostigmine** would not be expected to be excreted in breast milk.

➤*Children:* Safety and efficacy for use of **neostigmine** in children are not established.

Precautions

➤*Anticholinesterase insensitivity:* Anticholinesterase insensitivity may develop for brief or prolonged periods. Carefully monitor the patient; respiratory assistance may be needed. Reduce or withhold dosages until the patient again becomes sensitive.

Drug Interactions

Anticholinesterase Muscle Stimulants Drug Interactions

Precipitant drug	Object drug*		Description
Anticholinesterase muscle stimulants	Anticholinesterase drugs	↑	Exercise caution in patients with myasthenic symptoms who are receiving other anticholinesterase muscle stimulants. Because symptoms of anticholinesterase overdose (cholinergic crisis) may mimic underdosage (myasthenic weakness), the condition may be worsened.
Anticholinesterase muscle stimulants	Succinylcholine	↑	Neuromuscular blocking effects may be increased. Prolonged respiratory depression with extended periods of apnea may occur. Provide respiratory support as needed.
Aminoglycoside antibiotics (eg, neomycin, streptomycin, kanamycin)	Anticholinesterase muscle stimulants	↑	Aminoglycoside antibiotics have a mild but definite nondepolarizing blocking action which may accentuate neuromuscular block.
Local and general anesthetics Antiarrhythmics	Anticholinesterase muscle stimulants	↓	Use cautiously, if at all, in patients with myasthenia gravis. The neostigmine dose may have to be increased accordingly.
Atropine Belladonna derivatives	Anticholinesterase muscle stimulants	↑	Routine administration of these agents may suppress the parasympathomimetic (muscarinic) symptoms of excessive GI stimulation leaving only the more serious symptoms of fasciculation and paralysis of voluntary muscles as signs of overdosage.
Corticosteroids	Anticholinesterase muscle stimulants	↓	May decrease the anticholinesterase effects of these agents. Conversely, anticholinesterase effects may increase after stopping corticosteroids. Provide respiratory support as needed.
Depolarizing muscle relaxants (eg, succinylcholine, decamethonium)	Anticholinesterase muscle stimulants	↑	Neostigmine may prolong the Phase I block of these drugs. Use these drugs in myasthenic patients only when definitely indicated. Carefully adjust the anticholinesterase dosage.
Magnesium	Anticholinesterase muscle stimulants	↓	Magnesium has a direct depressant effect on skeletal muscle, and it may antagonize the beneficial effects of anticholinesterase therapy.
Mecamylamine	Anticholinesterase muscle stimulants	↑	Do not administer to patients receiving this ganglionic blocking agent.
Methocarbamol	Anticholinesterase muscle stimulants	↓	A single case report indicates this drug may have impaired the effect of **pyridostigmine** in a patient with myasthenia gravis.

* ↑ = Object drug increased. ↓ = Object drug decreased.

Adverse Reactions

➤*Cardiovascular:* Arrhythmias (especially bradycardia); fall in cardiac output leading to hypotension; tachycardia; AV block; nodal rhythm; nonspecific EKG changes; cardiac arrest; syncope.

➤*CNS:* Convulsions; dysarthria; dysphonia; dizziness; loss of consciousness; drowsiness; headache.

➤*Dermatologic:* Skin rash (**pyridostigmine** and **neostigmine**; subsides upon discontinuance); thrombophlebitis (IV).

➤*GI:* Increased salivary, gastric and intestinal secretions; nausea; vomiting; dysphagia; increased peristalsis; diarrhea; abdominal cramps; flatulence.

➤*Hypersensitivity:* Allergic reactions and anaphylaxis.

➤*Musculoskeletal:* Weakness; fasciculations; muscle cramps and spasms; arthralgia.

➤*Respiratory:* Increased tracheobronchial secretions; laryngospasm; bronchiolar constriction; respiratory muscle paralysis; central respiratory paralysis; dyspnea; respiratory depression; respiratory arrest; bronchospasm.

➤*Miscellaneous:* Urinary frequency and incontinence; urinary urgency; diaphoresis; rash; urticaria; flushing; alopecia (**pyridostigmine**).

Overdosage

➤*Symptoms:* When the drug produces overstimulation, the clinical picture is one of increasing parasympathomimetic action that is more or less characteristic when not masked by the use of atropine. Signs and symptoms of overdosage, including cholinergic crises, vary considerably. They are usually manifested by increasing GI stimulation with epigastric distress, abdominal cramps, diarrhea and vomiting, excessive salivation, pallor, cold sweating, urinary urgency, blurring of vision and eventually fasciculation and paralysis of voluntary muscles, including those of the tongue (thick tongue and difficulty in swallowing), shoulder, neck and arms. Miosis, increase in blood pressure with or without bradycardia and subjective sensations of internal trembling, and often severe anxiety and panic may complete the picture. A cholinergic crisis is usually differentiated from the weakness and paralysis of myasthenia gravis insufficiently treated by cholinergic drugs by the fact that myasthenic weakness is not accompanied by any of the above signs and symptoms, except the last two subjective ones (anxiety and panic).

➤*Treatment:* Because the warning of overdosage is minimal, the existence of a narrow margin between the first appearance of side effects and serious toxic effects must be borne in mind constantly. If signs of overdosage occur (excessive GI stimulation, excessive salivation, miosis and more serious fasciculations of voluntary muscles), discontinue temporarily all cholinergic medication and administer from 0.5 to 1 mg (1/120 to 1/60 grain) of atropine IV. A total atropine dose of 5 to 10 mg or more may be required. Give other supportive treatment as indicated (artificial respiration, tracheotomy, oxygen, etc).

Patient Information

Notify physician if nausea, vomiting, diarrhea, sweating, increased salivary secretions, irregular heartbeat, muscle weakness, severe abdominal pain or difficulty in breathing occurs.

AMBENONIUM CHLORIDE

Rx	**Mytelase** (Sanofi Winthrop)	**Tablets:** 10 mg	Scored. In 100s.

AMBENONIUM CHLORIDE — ORAL

For complete and comparative prescribing information, refer to the Anticholinesterase Muscle Stimulants group monograph.

Indications

➤*Myasthenia gravis:* The treatment of myasthenia gravis.

Administration and Dosage

The oral dose must be individualized according to the patient's response because the disease varies widely in its severity in different patients and because patients vary in their sensitivity to cholinergic drugs. Since the point of maximum therapeutic effectiveness with optimal muscle strength and no gastrointestinal disturbances is a highly critical one, the close supervision of a physician familiar with the disease is necessary.

Because its action is longer, administration of ambenonium chloride is necessary only every three or four hours, depending on the clinical response. Usually medication is not required throughout the night, so that the patient can sleep uninterruptedly.

For the patient with moderately severe myasthenia, from 5 mg to 25 mg of ambenonium chloride three or four times daily is an effective dose. In some patients a 5 mg dose is effective, whereas other patients require as much as from 50 mg to 75 mg per dose. The physician should start with a 5 mg dose, carefully observing the effect of the drug on the patient. The dosage may then be increased gradually to determine the effective and safe dose. The longer duration of action of ambenonium chloride makes it desirable to adjust dosage at intervals of one to two days to avoid drug accumulation and overdosage.

In addition to individual variations in dosage requirements, the amount of cholinergic medication necessary to control symptoms may fluctuate in each patient, depending on his activity and the current status of the disease, including spontaneous remission. A few patients have required greater doses for adequate control of myasthenic symptoms, but increasing the dosage above 200 mg daily requires exacting supervision of a physician well aware of the signs and treatment of overdosage with cholinergic medication.

Edrophonium may be used to evaluate the adequacy of the maintenance dose of anticholinesterase medication. Edrophonium 2 mg is administered intravenously one hour after the last anticholinesterase dose. A transient increase in strength occurring about 30 seconds later and lasting 3 to 5 minutes indicates insufficient maintenance dose. If the dose is adequate or excessive, no change or a transient decrease in strength will occur, sometimes accompanied by muscarinic symptoms.

See the edrophonium monograph.

➤*Storage/Stability:* Store at room temperature up to 25° C (77° F).

EDROPHONIUM CHLORIDE

Rx	**Enlon** (Ohmeda)	**Injection:** 10 mg/ml	In 15 ml vials.[1]
Rx	**Reversol** (Organon)		In 10 ml vials (25s).[1]
Rx	**Tensilon** (ICN)		In 1 ml amps,[2] 10 ml vials.[1]

[1] With 0.45% phenol and 0.2% sodium sulfite.

[2] With 0.2% sodium sulfite.

EDROPHONIUM CHLORIDE — INJECTION

Complete and comparative prescribing information for these products begins in the Anticholinesterase Muscle Stimulants group monograph.

Indications

➤*Myasthenia gravis:* Edrophonium chloride is recommended for the differential diagnosis of myasthenia gravis and as an adjunct in the evaluation of treatment requirements in this disease. It may also be used for evaluating emergency treatment in myasthenic crises. Because of its brief duration of action, it is not recommended for maintenance therapy in myasthenia gravis.

➤*Curare antagonist:* Edrophonium chloride is also useful whenever a curare antagonist is needed to reverse the neuromuscular block produced by curare, tubocurarine, gallamine triethiodide or dimethyl-tubocurarine. It is not effective against decamethonium bromide and succinylcholine chloride. It may be used adjunctively in the treatment of respiratory depression caused by curare overdosage.

Administration and Dosage

➤*Approved by the FDA:* August 6, 1985.

➤*Edrophonium chloride test in the differential diagnosis of myasthenia gravis:*

Adult dosage –

Intravenous: A tuberculin syringe containing 1 mL (10 mg) of edrophonium chloride is prepared with an intravenous needle, and 0.2 mL (2 mg) is injected intravenously within 15 to 30 seconds. The needle is left in situ. Only if no reaction occurs after 45 seconds is the remaining 0.8 mL (8 mg) injected. If a cholinergic reaction (muscarinic side effects, skeletal muscle fasciculations and increased muscle weakness) occurs after injection of 0.2 mL (2 mg), the test is discontinued and atropine sulfate, 0.4 mg to 0.5 mg, is administered intravenously. After one-half hour the test may be repeated.

Intramuscular dosage: In adults with inaccessible veins, dosage for intramuscular injection is 1 mL (10 mg) of edrophonium chloride. Subjects who demonstrate hyperreactivity to this injection (cholinergic reaction), should be retested after one-half hour with 0.2 mL (2 mg) of edrophonium chloride intramuscularly to rule out false-negative reactions.

Pediatric dose –

Intravenous: The intravenous testing dose of edrophonium chloride in children weighing up to 75 lbs is 0.1 mL (1 mg); above this weight, the dose is 0.2 mL (2 mg). If there is no response after 45 seconds, it may be titrated up to 0.5 mL (5 mg) in children under 75 lbs, given in increments of 0.1 mL (1 mg) every 30 to 45 seconds and up to 1 mL (10 mg) in heavier children. In infants, the recommended dose is 0.05 mL (0.5 mg).

Intramuscular: Because of technical difficulty with intravenous injection in children, the intramuscular route may be used. In children weighing up to 75 lbs, 0.2 mL (2 mg) is injected intramuscularly. In children weighing more than 75 lbs, 0.5 mL (5 mg) is injected intramuscularly. All signs which would appear with the intravenous test appear with the intramuscular test except that there is a delay of 2 to 10 minutes before a reaction is noted. Alternatively, the following schedule is recommended: Total dose is 0.2 mg/kg. Give 0.04 mg/kg initially as a test dose, then 1 mg increments if no reaction occurs within 1 minute. Maximum dose is 10 mg total.

➤*Edrophonium chloride test for evaluation of treatment requirements in myasthenia gravis:* The recommended dose is 0.1 mL to 0.2 mL (1 mg to 2 mg) of edrophonium chloride, administered intravenously 1 hour after oral intake of the drug being used in treatment. Response will be myasthenic in the undertreated patient, adequate in the controlled patient, and

EDROPHONIUM CHLORIDE — INJECTION

cholinergic in the overtreated patient. Responses to edrophonium chloride in myasthenic and nonmyasthenic individuals are summarized in the following chart.

	Myasthenic[a]	Adequate[b]	Cholinergic[c]
Muscle strength (ptosis, diplopia, dysphonia, dysphagia, dysarthria, respiration, limb strength)	Increased	No change	Decreased
Fasciculations (orbicularis oculi, facial muscles, limb muscles)	Absent	Present or absent	Present or absent
Side reactions (lacrimation diaphoresis, salivation, abdominal cramps, nausea, vomiting, diarrhea)	Absent	Minimal	Severe

[a] Myasthenic response occurs in untreated myasthenics and may serve to establish diagnosis; in patients under treatment, indicates that therapy is inadequate.
[b] Adequate response is observed in treated patients when therapy is stabilized; a typical response in healthy individuals. In addition to this response in non-myasthenics, the phenomenon of forced lid closure is often observed in psychoneurotics.
[c] Cholinergic response seen in myasthenics who have been overtreated with anticholinesterase drugs.

➤*Edrophonium chloride test in crisis:* The term crisis is applied to the myasthenic whenever severe respiratory distress with objective ventilatory inadequacy occurs and the response to medication is not predictable. This state may be secondary to a sudden increase in severity of myasthenia gravis (myasthenic crisis), or to overtreatment with anticholinesterase drugs (cholinergic crisis).

When a patient is apneic, controlled ventilation must be secured immediately in order to avoid cardiac arrest and irreversible central nervous system damage. No attempt is made to test with edrophonium chloride until respiratory exchange is adequate.

➤*Dosage used at this time is most important:* If the patient is cholinergic, edrophonium chloride will cause increased oropharyngeal secretions and further weakness in the muscles of respiration. If the crisis is myasthenic, the test clearly improves respiration and the patient can be treated with longer-acting intravenous anticholinesterase medication. When the test is performed, there should not be more than 0.2 mL (2 mg) edrophonium chloride in the syringe. An intravenous dose of 0.1 mL (1 mg) is given initially. The patient's heart action is carefully observed. If, after an interval of 1 minute, this dose does not further impair the patient, the remaining 0.1 mL (1 mg) can be injected. If no clear improvement of respiration occurs after 0.2 mL (2 mg) dose, it is usually wisest to discontinue all anticholinesterase drug therapy and secure controlled ventilation by tracheostomy with assisted respiration.

➤*For use as a curare antagonist:* Edrophonium chloride should be administered by intravenous injection in 1 mL (10 mg) doses given slowly over a period of 30 to 45 seconds so that the onset of cholinergic reaction can be detected. This dosage may be repeated whenever necessary. The maximal dose for any one patient should be 4 mL (40 mg). Because of its brief effect, edrophonium chloride should not be given prior to the administration of curare, tubocurarine, gallamine triethiodide or dimethyl-tubocurarine; it should be used at the time when its effect is needed. When given to counteract curare overdosage, the effect of each dose on the respiration should be carefully observed before it is repeated, and assisted ventilation should always be employed.

➤*Storage / Stability:* Edrophonium chloride injection should be stored at controlled room temperature 15° to 30°C (59° to 86°F).

EDROPHONIUM CHLORIDE/ATROPINE SULFATE

Rx	**Enlon-Plus** (Ohmeda)	**Injection:** 10 mg edrophonium chloride and 0.14 mg atropine sulfate	In 5 ml amps[1] and 15 ml multidose vials.[2]

[1] With 2 mg sodium sulfite.
[2] With 2 mg sodium sulfite and 4.5 mg phenol.

EDROPHONIUM CHLORIDE/ATROPINE SULFATE — INJECTION

Complete prescribing information for these products begins in the Anticholinesterase Muscle Stimulants monograph.

Indications

➤*Antagonist of nondepolarizing neuromuscular blocking agents:* As a reversal agent or antagonist of nondepolarizing neuromuscular blocking agents.

➤*Curare overdosage:* Adjunctively in the treatment of respiratory depression caused by curare overdosage.

Not effective against depolarizing neuromuscular blocking agents. Not recommended for use in the differential diagnosis of myasthenia gravis.

Administration and Dosage

➤*Approved by the FDA:* November 6, 1991.

Dosages of edrophonium and atropine injection range from 0.05 to 0.1 ml/kg given slowly over 45 seconds to 1 minute at a point of at least 5% recovery of twitch response to neuromuscular stimulation (95% block). The dosage delivered is 0.5 to 1 mg/kg edrophonium and 0.007 to 0.014 mg/kg atropine. A total dosage of 1 mg/kg edrophonium should rarely be exceeded. Monitor response carefully and secure assisted or controlled ventilation. Satisfactory reversal permits adequate voluntary respiration and neuromuscular transmission (as tested with a peripheral nerve stimulator). Recurarization has not been reported after satisfactory reversal has been attained.

➤*Storage / Stability:* Store between 15° to 26°C (59° to 78°F).

NEOSTIGMINE

Rx	**Neostigmine Methylsulfate** (Various)	**Injection:** 1:1000	In 10 ml vials.
Rx	**Prostigmin** (ICN)		In 10 ml vials.[1]
Rx	**Neostigmine Methylsulfate** (Various)	**Injection:** 1:2000	In 1 ml amps and 10 ml vials.
Rx	**Prostigmin** (ICN)		In 1 ml amps[2] and 10 ml vials.[1]
Rx	**Neostigmine Methylsulfate** (Various)	**Injection:** 1:4000	In 1 ml amps.
Rx	**Prostigmin** (ICN)		In 1 ml amps.[2]

[1] With 0.45% phenol.
[2] With 0.2% methyl and propylparabens.

NEOSTIGMINE METHYLSULFATE — INJECTION

For complete and comparative prescribing information, refer to the Anticholinesterase Muscle Stimulants group monograph.

Indications

Neostigmine methylsulfate is indicated for:

- The symptomatic control of myasthenia gravis when oral therapy is impractical.
- The prevention and treatment of postoperative distention and urinary retention after mechanical obstruction has been excluded.
- Reversal of effects of nondepolarizing neuromuscular blocking agents (eg, tubocurarine, metocurine, gallamine, or pancuronium) after surgery.

Administration and Dosage

➤*Symptomatic control of myasthenia gravis:* One mL of the 1:2000 solution (0.5 mg) subcutaneously or intramuscularly. Subsequent doses should be based on the individual patient's response. In most patients, however, oral treatment with neostigmine methylsulfate tablets, 15 mg each, is adequate for control of symptoms.

➤*Prevention of postoperative distention and urinary retention:* One mL of the 1:4000 solution (0.25 mg) subcutaneously or intramuscularly as soon as possible after operation; repeat every 4 to 6 hours for 2 or 3 days.

➤*Treatment of postoperative distention:* One mL of the 1:2000 solution (0.5 mg) subcutaneously or intramuscularly, as required.

➤*Treatment of urinary retention:* One mL of the 1:2000 solution (0.5 mg) subcutaneously or intramuscularly. If urination does not occur within 1 hour, the patient should be catheterized. After the patient has voided, or the bladder has been emptied, continue the 0.5 mg injections every 3 hours for at least 5 injections.

➤*Reversal of effects of nondepolarizing neuromuscular-blocking agents:* When neostigmine methylsulfate is administered intravenously, it is recommended that atropine sulfate (0.6 to 1.2 mg) also be given intravenously using separate syringes. Some authorities have recommended that the atropine be injected several minutes before the neostigmine methylsulfate rather than concomitantly. The usual dose is 0.5 to 2 mg neostigmine methylsulfate given by slow intravenous injection, repeated as required. Only in exceptional cases should the total dose of neostigmine methylsulfate exceed 5 mg. It is recommended that the patient be well ventilated and a

NEOSTIGMINE METHYLSULFATE — INJECTION

patent airway maintained until complete recovery of normal respiration is assured. The optimum time for administration of the drug is during hyperventilation when the carbon dioxide level of the blood is low. It should never be administered in the presence of high concentrations of halothane or cyclopropane. In cardiac cases and severely ill patients, it is advisable to filtrate the exact dose of neostigmine methylsulfate required, using a peripheral nerve stimulator device. In the presence of bradycardia, the pulse rate should be increased to about 80/minute with atropine before administering neostigmine methylsulfate.

Parenteral drug products should be inspected visually for particulate matter and discoloration prior to administration, whenever solution and container permit.

PYRIDOSTIGMINE BROMIDE

Rx	**Pyridostigmine Bromide** (Various, eg, Geneva, Watson)	**Tablets:** 60 mg	Scored. In 100s and 500s.
Rx	**Mestinon** (ICN)		Lactose. (MESTINON 60 ICN). Scored. In 100s and 500s.
Rx	**Mestinon** (ICN)	**Tablets, extended-release:** 180 mg	(ICN-M180). Scored. In 30s.
Rx	**Mestinon** (ICN)	**Syrup:** 60 mg/5mL	Sucrose, sorbitol, 5% alcohol. Raspberry flavor. In 480 mL.
Rx	**Mestinon** (ICN)	**Injection:** 5 mg/mL[1]	In 2 mL amps.

[1] With 0.2% parabens and 0.02% sodium citrate.

PYRIDOSTIGMINE BROMIDE — ORAL

For complete and comparative prescribing information, refer to the Anticholinesterase Muscle Stimulants group monograph.

Indications

➤*Myasthenia gravis:* Pyridostigmine bromide is useful in the treatment of myasthenia gravis.

➤*Unlabeled uses:*

Treatment of myasthenia gravis in children – 7 mg/kg/24 hours orally divided into 5 or 6 doses.

Administration and Dosage

➤*Dosage:* The size and frequency of the dosage must be adjusted to the needs of the individual patient.

Adults – The average dose is 600 mg/day of syrup or conventional tablets, spaced to provide maximum relief.

Extended-release tablets – 180 to 540 mg once or twice daily will usually be sufficient to control symptoms. Individual needs vary markedly. Use dosage intervals of greater than or equal to 6 hours. Do not crush or chew. For optimum control, rapidly acting conventional tablets or syrup may also be needed in conjunction with extended-release therapy.

➤*Note:* For information on a diagnostic test for myasthenia gravis, and for the evaluation and stabilization of therapy, please see the monograph for edrophonium chloride.

➤*Storage/Stability:* Store at controlled room temperature 15° to 30°C (59° to 86°F). Dispense in tight containers.

PYRIDOSTIGMINE BROMIDE — INJECTION

For complete and comparative prescribing information, refer to the Anticholinesterase Muscle Stimulants group monograph.

Indications

Pyridostigmine bromide injectable is useful in the treatment of myasthenia gravis and as a reversal agent or antagonist to nondepolarizing muscle relaxants such as curariform drugs and gallamine triethiodide.

Administration and Dosage

➤*For myasthenia gravis:* To supplement oral dosage, pre- and postoperatively, during labor and postpartum, during myasthenic crisis, or whenever oral therapy is impractical, ≈ 1/30 of the oral dose of pyridostigmine bromide may be given parenterally, either by IM or very slow IV injection. The patient must be closely observed for cholinergic reactions, particularly if the IV route is used.

Neonates of myasthenic mothers may have transient difficulty in swallowing, sucking and breathing. Injectable pyridostigmine bromide may be indicated, by symptomatology and use of the edrophonium chloride test, until pyridostigmine bromide syrup can be taken. To date the world literature consists of < 100 neonate patients. Of these only 5 were treated with injectable pyridostigmine, with the vast majority of the remaining neonates receiving neostigmine. Dosage requirements of pyridostigmine bromide injectable are minute, ranging from 0.05 mg to 0.15 mg/kg of body weight given IM. It is important to differentiate between cholinergic and myasthenic crises in neonates.

Pyridostigmine bromide given parenterally 1 hour before completion of second stage labor enables patients to have adequate strength during labor and provides protection to infants in the immediate postnatal state.

Note – For information on a diagnostic test for myasthenia gravis, and on the evaluation and stabilization of therapy, please see monograph on edrophonium chloride.

➤*For reversal of nondepolarizing muscle relaxants:* When pyridostigmine bromide injectable is given IV to reverse the action of muscle relaxant drugs, it is recommended that atropine sulfate (0.6 to 1.2 mg) also be given IV immediately prior to the pyridostigmine bromide. Side effects, notably excessive secretions and bradycardia, are thereby minimized. Usually 10 or 20 mg of pyridostigmine bromide will be sufficient for antagonism of the effects of the nondepolarizing muscle relaxants. Although full recovery may occur within 15 minutes in most patients, others may require a half hour or more. Satisfactory reversal can be evident by adequate voluntary respiration, respiratory measurements, and use of a peripheral nerve stimulator device. It is recommended that the patient be well ventilated and a patent airway maintained until complete recovery of normal respiration is assured. Once satisfactory reversal has been attained, recurarization has not been reported.

Failure of pyridostigmine bromide injectable to provide prompt (within 30 minutes) reversal may occur, eg, in the presence of extreme debilitation, carcinomatosis, or with concomitant use of certain broad spectrum antibiotics or anesthetic agents, notably ether. Under these circumstances ventilation must be supported by artificial means until the patient has resumed control of his respiration.

GUANIDINE HYDROCHLORIDE

Rx	**Guanidine HCl** (Key)	**Tablets:** 125 mg	Mannitol. (KEY 74). In 100s.

GUANIDINE HYDROCHLORIDE — ORAL

Indications

➤*Myasthenic syndrome of Eaton-Lambert:* Guanidine is indicated for the reduction of the symptoms of muscle weakness and easy fatigability associated with the myasthenic syndrome of Eaton-Lambert. It is not indicated for treating myasthenia gravis. The Eaton-Lambert syndrome is ordinarily differentiated from myasthenia gravis by the usual association of the syndrome with small cell carcinoma of the lung, but myography may be necessary to make the diagnosis.

Administration and Dosage

Initial dosage is usually between 10 and 15 mg/kg of body weight per day in 3 or 4 divided doses. This dosage may be gradually increased to a total daily dosage of 35 mg/kg of body weight per day or up to the development of side effects. As individual tolerance is highly variable, the dosage must be carefully titrated. Once a tolerable dose has been established it should be continued. Occasionally removal of the primary neoplastic lesion may result in improvement of symptoms, permitting the discontinuance of guanidine.

➤*Storage/Stability:* Store between 15° and 30°C (59° and 86°F).

Actions

➤*Pharmacology:* Guanidine apparently acts by enhancing the release of acetylcholine following a nerve impulse. It also appears to slow the rates of depolarization and repolarization of muscle cell membranes.

Contraindications

Guanidine is contraindicated in individuals with a history of intolerance or allergy to this drug.

Warnings

➤*Bone-marrow suppression:* Fatal bone-marrow suppression, apparently dose related, can occur with guanidine.

➤*Lactation:* Because guanidine is excreted in milk, patients on this drug should discontinue breast feeding.

➤*Children:* Since there is inadequate experience in children who have received this drug, safety and efficacy in children have not been established.

GUANIDINE HYDROCHLORIDE — ORAL

Precautions

➤*Monitoring:* Baseline blood studies should be followed by frequent red and white blood cell and differential counts. The drug should be discontinued upon appearance of bone-marrow suppression. Concurrent therapy with other drugs that may cause bone-marrow suppression should be avoided.

Renal function may be affected in some patients receiving guanidine. Patients should therefore have regular urine examinations and serum creatinine determinations while taking this drug.

Physicians should be given adequate precautions pertaining to the gastrointestinal side effects and the possibility of induced behavior disorders.

Treatment should not be continued longer than necessary.

Adverse Reactions

Anemia, leukopenia, and thrombocytopenia resulting from bone-marrow depression attributable to guanidine have been reported. Other adverse reactions that have been observed are:

➤*Cardiovascular:* Palpitation, tachycardia, atrial fibrillation, hypotension.

➤*CNS:* Paresthesia of lips, face, hands, feet; cold sensations in hands and feet; nervousness, lightheadedness, jitteriness, increased irritability; tremor, trembling sensation; ataxia.

➤*Dermatologic:* Rash, flushing or pink complexion; folliculitis; petechiae, purpura, ecchymoses; sweating; skin eruptions; dryness and scaling of the skin.

➤*GI:* Dry mouth; gastric irritation; anorexia; nausea; diarrhea; abdominal cramping. Gastrointestinal side effects may preclude the use of guanidine as a desired form of therapy.

➤*Hepatic:* Abnormal liver function tests.

➤*Psychiatric:* Emotional lability; psychotic state; confusion; mood changes and hallucinations.

➤*Renal:* Elevation of blood creatinine; uremia; chronic, interstitial nephritis, acute interstitial nephritis, and renal tubular necrosis.

➤*Miscellaneous:* Sore throat, fever.

Overdosage

Mild gastrointestinal disorders, such as anorexia, increased peristalsis, or diarrhea are early warnings that tolerance is being exceeded. These symptoms may be relieved by atropine, but nevertheless note should be taken of these symptoms and dosage reductions considered. Slight numbness or tingling of the lips and fingertips shortly after taking a dose of guanidine has been reported. This per se is not an indication to discontinue treatment and/or reduce dosage.

Severe guanidine intoxication is characterized by nervous hyperirritability, fibrillary tremors and convulsive contractions of muscle, salivation, vomiting, diarrhea, hypoglycemia, and circulatory disturbances. Administration of intravenous calcium gluconate may control the neuromuscular and convulsive symptoms and provide some relief of other toxic manifestations.

Atropine is more effective than calcium in relieving the G.I. symptoms, circulatory disturbances, and changes in blood sugar.

DISULFIRAM

Rx	**Antabuse** (Odyssey)	**Tablets:** 250 mg	Lactose. (OP 706). In 100s.

DISULFIRAM — ORAL

WARNING

Disulfiram should never be administered to a patient when he is in a state of alcohol intoxication, or without his full knowledge. The physician should instruct relatives accordingly.

Indications

➤*Alcoholism:* Disulfiram is an aid in the management of selected chronic alcohol patients who want to remain in a state of enforced sobriety so that supportive and psychotherapeutic treatment may be applied to best advantage.

Administration and Dosage

➤*Approved by the FDA:* December 8, 1983.

Disulfiram should never be administered until the patient has abstained from alcohol for at least 12 hours.

➤*Initial dosage schedule:* In the first phase of treatment, a maximum of 500 mg daily is given in a single dose for 1 to 2 weeks. Although usually taken in the morning, disulfiram may be taken on retiring by patients who experience a sedative effect. Alternatively, to minimize, or eliminate, the sedative effect, dosage may be adjusted downward.

➤*Maintenance regimen:* The average maintenance dose is 250 mg daily (range, 125 to 500 mg). It should not exceed 500 mg daily.

Occasionally patients, while seemingly on adequate maintenance doses of disulfiram, report that they are able to drink alcoholic beverages with impunity and without any symptomatology. All appearances to the contrary, such patients must be presumed to be disposing of their tablets in some manner without actually taking them. Until such patients have been observed reliably taking their daily disulfiram tablets (preferably crushed and well mixed with liquid), it cannot be concluded that disulfiram is ineffective.

➤*Duration of therapy:* The daily, uninterrupted administration of disulfiram must be continued until the patient is fully recovered socially and a basis for permanent self-control is established. Depending on the individual patient, maintenance therapy may be required for months or even years.

➤*Trial with alcohol:* During early experience with disulfiram, it was thought advisable for each patient to have at least 1 supervised alcohol-drug reaction. More recently, the test reaction has been largely abandoned. Furthermore, such a test reaction should never be administered to a patient over 50 years of age. A clear, detailed and convincing description of the reaction is felt to be sufficient in most cases.

However, where a test reaction is deemed necessary, the suggested procedure is as follows:

After the first 1 to 2 weeks' therapy with 500 mg daily, a drink of 15 mL (½ oz) of 100 proof whiskey, or equivalent, is taken slowly. This test dose of alcoholic beverage may be repeated once only, so that the total dose does not exceed 30 mL (1 oz) of whiskey. Once a reaction develops, no more alcohol should be consumed. Such tests should be carried out only when the patient is hospitalized, or comparable supervision and facilities, including oxygen, are available.

➤*Management of disulfiram-alcohol reaction:* In severe reactions, whether caused by an excessive test dose or by the patient's unsupervised ingestion of alcohol, supportive measures to restore blood pressure and treat shock should be instituted. Other recommendations include oxygen, carbogen (95% oxygen and 5% carbon dioxide), vitamin C intravenously in massive doses (1 g) and ephedrine sulfate. Antihistamines have also been used intravenously. Potassium levels should be monitored, particularly in patients on digitalis, since hypokalemia has been reported.

➤*Storage/Stability:* Store at controlled room temperature 15° to 30°C (59° to 86°F).

Actions

➤*Pharmacology:* Disulfiram produces a sensitivity to alcohol which results in a highly unpleasant reaction when the patient under treatment ingests even small amounts of alcohol.

Disulfiram blocks the oxidation of alcohol at the acetaldehyde stage. During alcohol metabolism following disulfiram intake, the concentration of acetaldehyde occurring in the blood may be 5 to 10 times higher than that found during metabolism of the same amount of alcohol alone.

Accumulation of acetaldehyde in the blood produces a complex of highly unpleasant symptoms referred to hereinafter as the disulfiram-alcohol reaction. This reaction, which is proportional to the dosage of both disulfiram and alcohol, will persist as long as alcohol is being metabolized. Disulfiram does not appear to influence the rate of alcohol elimination from the body.

➤*Pharmacokinetics:* Disulfiram is absorbed slowly from the gastrointestinal tract and is eliminated slowly from the body. One (or even 2) weeks after a patient has taken his last dose of disulfiram, ingestion of alcohol may produce unpleasant symptoms.

Prolonged administration of disulfiram does not produce tolerance; the longer a patient remains on therapy, the more exquisitely sensitive he becomes to alcohol.

Contraindications

Patients who are receiving or have recently received metronidazole, paraldehyde, alcohol, or alcohol-containing preparations (eg, cough syrups, tonics and the like); the presence of severe myocardial disease or coronary occlusion, psychoses, and hypersensitivity to disulfiram or to other thiuram derivatives used in pesticides and rubber vulcanization.

Warnings

➤*Use with caution:* See the Warning box for more information.

The patient must be fully informed of the disulfiram-alcohol reaction. He must be strongly cautioned against surreptitious drinking while taking the drug, and he must be fully aware of the possible consequences. He should be warned to avoid alcohol in disguised forms (ie, in sauces, vinegars, cough mixtures, and even in aftershave lotions and back rubs). He should also be warned that reactions may occur with alcohol up to 14 days after ingesting disulfiram.

It is suggested that every patient under treatment carry an identification card stating that he is receiving disulfiram and describing the symptoms most likely to occur as a result of the disulfiram-alcohol reaction. In addition, this card should indicate the physician or institution to be contacted in an emergency.

➤*Disulfiram-alcohol reaction:* Disulfiram plus alcohol, even small amounts, produce flushing, throbbing in head and neck, throbbing headache, respiratory difficulty, nausea, copious vomiting, sweating, thirst, chest pain, palpitation, dyspnea, hyperventilation, tachycardia, hypotension, syncope, marked uneasiness, weakness, vertigo, blurred vision, and confusion. In severe reactions there may be respiratory depression, cardiovascular collapse, arrhythmias, myocardial infarction, acute congestive heart failure, unconsciousness, convulsions, and death.

The intensity of the reaction varies with each individual, but is generally proportional to the amounts of disulfiram and alcohol ingested. Mild reactions may occur in the sensitive individual when the blood alcohol concentration is increased to as little as 5 to 10 mg per 100 mL. Symptoms are fully developed at 50 mg per 100 mL, and unconsciousness usually results when the blood alcohol level reaches 125 to 150 mg.

The duration of the reaction varies from 30 to 60 minutes, to several hours in the more severe cases, or as long as there is alcohol in the blood.

➤*Special risk:* Because of the possibility of an accidental disulfiram-alcohol reaction, disulfiram should be used with extreme caution in patients with any of the following conditions: Diabetes mellitus, hypothyroidism, epilepsy, cerebral damage, chronic and acute nephritis, hepatic cirrhosis or insufficiency.

➤*Hepatic toxicity:* Hepatic toxicity including hepatic failure resulting in transplantation or death have been reported. Severe and sometimes fatal hepatitis associated with disulfiram therapy may develop even after many months of therapy. Hepatic toxicity has occurred in patients with or without prior history of abnormal liver function. Patients should be advised to immediately notify their physician of any early symptoms of hepatitis, such as fatigue, weakness, malaise, anorexia, nausea, vomiting, jaundice, or dark urine.

➤*Hypersensitivity reactions:* Patients with a history of rubber contact dermatitis should be evaluated for hypersensitivity to thiuram derivatives before receiving disulfiram. Hypersensitivity to thiuram derivatives is a containdication for use of disulfiram.

➤*Elderly:* A determination has not been made whether controlled clinical studies of disulfiram included sufficient numbers of subjects aged 65 and over to define a difference in response from younger subjects. Other reported clinical experience has not identified differences in responses between the elderly and younger patients. In general, dose selection for an elderly patient should be cautious, usually starting at the low end of the dosing range, reflecting the greater frequency of decreased hepatic, renal or cardiac function, and of concomitant disease or other drug therapy.

➤*Pregnancy: Category C.* The safe use of this drug in pregnancy has not been established. Therefore, disulfiram should be used during pregnancy only when, in the judgement of the physician, the probable benefits outweigh the possible risks.

➤*Lactation:* It is not known whether this drug is excreted in human milk. Since many drugs are so excreted, disulfiram should not be given to nursing mothers.

➤*Children:* Safety and effectiveness in children have not been established.

Precautions

➤*Monitoring:* Baseline and follow-up liver function tests (10 to 14 days) are suggested to detect any hepatic dysfunction that may result with disulfiram therapy. In addition, a complete blood count and serum chemistries, including liver function tests, should be monitored.

➤*Ethylene dibromide:* Patients taking disulfiram tablets should not be exposed to ethylene dibromide or its vapors. This precaution is based on preliminary results of animal research currently in progress that suggest a toxic interaction between inhaled ethylene dibromide and ingested disulfiram resulting in a higher incidence of tumors and mortality in rats. A correlation between this finding and humans, however, has not been demonstrated.

Drug Interactions

➤*Nitrite:* In rats, simultaneous ingestion of disulfiram and nitrite in the diet for 78 weeks has been reported to cause tumors, and it has been suggested that disulfiram may react with nitrites in the rat stomach to form a nitrosamine, which is tumorigenic. Disulfiram alone in the rat's diet did not lead to such tumors. The relevance of this finding to humans is not known at this time.

DISULFIRAM — ORAL

Precipitant drug	Object drug*		Description
Isoniazid	Disulfiram	↑	Observe patients receiving isoniazid and disulfiram for the appearance of unsteady gait or marked changes in behavior; discontinue disulfiram or reduce the dose if such signs appear.
Metronidazole	Disulfiram	↑	Patients may exhibit acute toxic psychosis or confusional state when taking metronidazole in combination with disulfiram, requiring discontinuation of 1 or both of the agents.
Disulfiram	Alcohol	↑	Disulfiram causes a severe alcohol-intolerance reaction (eg, flushing and increased respiration, pulse rate, and cardiac output). Death has been reported. Avoid alcohol in all forms. See Warnings.
Disulfiram	Benzodiazepines	↑	Disulfiram decreases the plasma clearance of benzodiazepines metabolized by oxidation, possibly resulting in increased CNS depressant actions. When benzodiazepine therapy is indicated, use oxazepam, temazepam, or lorazepam since they are metabolized by glucuronidation.
Disulfiram	Caffeine	↑	Cardiovascular and CNS stimulation effects of caffeine may be increased by disulfiram.
Disulfiram	Chlorzoxazone	↑	Disulfiram inhibits the hepatic metabolism of chlorzoxazone. Decrease the dose of chlorzoxazone if increased CNS depression occur.
Disulfiram	Cocaine	↑	Cardiovascular side effects of cocaine may be increased when used concurrently with disulfiram.
Disulfiram	Hydantoins (eg, phenytoin)	↑	Serum hydantoin levels may be increased by disulfiram, resulting in an increase in the pharmacologic and toxic effects. Monitor hydantoin levels and adjust the dosage as needed.
Disulfiram	Theophyllines	↑	Disulfiram may inhibit the metabolism of the theophylline, thus increasing its effects. Monitor the theophylline level and adjust dose accordingly.
Disulfiram	Tricyclic antidepressants	↑	Tricyclic antidepressants and disulfiram coadministration may result in acute organic brain syndrome. The bioavailability of the antidepressant may also be increased.
Disulfiram	Warfarin	↑	Disulfiram may increase the anticoagulant effect of warfarin. Monitor prothrombin time and adjust the warfarin dosage as necessary.

* ↑ = Object drug increased.

Adverse Reactions

Optic neuritis, peripheral neuritis, polyneuritis, and peripheral neuropathy may occur following administration of disulfiram.

Multiple cases of hepatitis, including both cholestatic and fulminant hepatitis, as well as hepatic failure resulting in transplantation or death, have been reported with administration of disulfiram.

Occasional skin eruptions are, as a rule, readily controlled by concomitant administration of an antihistaminic drug.

In a small number of patients, a transient mild drowsiness, fatigability, impotence, headache, acneform eruptions, allergic dermatitis, or a metallic or garlic-like aftertaste may be experienced during the first 2 weeks of therapy. These complaints usually disappear spontaneously with the continuation of therapy, or with reduced dosage.

Psychotic reactions have been noted, attributable in most cases to high dosage, combined toxicity (with metronidazole or isoniazid), or to the unmasking of underlying psychoses in patients stressed by the withdrawal of alcohol.

➤*Disulfiram-Alcohol interaction:* See Warnings for more information.

Overdosage

No specific information is available on the treatment of overdosage with disulfiram. It is recommended that the physician contact the local poison control center.

ACAMPROSATE CALCIUM

Rx	**Campral** (Forest)	**Tablets, delayed release:** 333 mg	(333). White. Enteric-coated. In 180s, 1,080s, and Dose Pak 180s.

ACAMPROSATE CALCIUM — ORAL

Indications

➤*Alcoholism:* For the maintenance of abstinence from alcohol in patients with alcohol dependence who are abstinent at treatment initiation. Treatment with acamprosate should be part of a comprehensive management program that includes psychosocial support.

The efficacy of acamprosate in promoting abstinence has not been demonstrated in subjects who have not undergone detoxification and not achieved alcohol abstinence prior to beginning acamprosate treatment. The efficacy of acamprosate in promoting abstinence from alcohol in polysubstance abusers has not been adequately assessed.

Administration and Dosage

➤*Approved by the FDA:* July 29, 2004.

The recommended dose of acamprosate is two 333 mg tablets (each dose should total 666 mg) taken 3 times daily. Although dosing may be done without regard to meals, dosing with meals was employed during clinical trials and is suggested as an aid to compliance in those patients who regularly eat 3 meals daily. A lower dose may be effective in some patients.

Initiate treatment with acamprosate as soon as possible after the period of alcohol withdrawal, when the patient has achieved abstinence, and maintain treatment if the patient relapses. Acamprosate should be used as part of a comprehensive psychosocial treatment program.

➤*Renal function impairment:* For patients with moderate renal impairment (creatinine clearance [Ccr] 30 to 50 mL/min), a starting dose of one 333 mg tablet taken 3 times daily is recommended. Do not give acamprosate to patients with severe renal impairment (Ccr 30 mL/min or less).

➤*Storage/Stability:* Store at 25°C (77°F); excursions permitted to 15° to 30°C (59° to 86°F).

Actions

➤*Pharmacology:* The mechanism of action of acamprosate in the maintenance of alcohol abstinence is not completely understood. Chronic alcohol exposure is hypothesized to alter the normal balance between neuronal excitation and inhibition. In vitro and in vivo studies in animals have provided evidence to suggest acamprosate may interact with glutamate and gamma-aminobutyric acid (GABA) neurotransmitter systems centrally, and have led to the hypothesis that acamprosate restores this balance.

Pharmacodynamic studies have shown that acamprosate reduces alcohol intake in alcohol-dependent animals in a dose-dependent manner and that this effect appears to be specific to alcohol and the mechanisms of alcohol dependence.

Acamprosate has negligible observable central nervous system (CNS) activity in animals outside of its effects on alcohol dependence, exhibiting no anticonvulsant, antidepressant, or anxiolytic activity.

Acamprosate is not known to cause alcohol aversion and does not cause a disulfiram-like reaction as a result of ethanol ingestion.

➤*Pharmacokinetics:*

Absorption – The absolute bioavailability of acamprosate after oral administration is approximately 11%. Steady-state plasma concentrations of acamprosate are reached within 5 days of dosing. Steady-state peak plasma concentrations after acamprosate doses of two 333 mg tablets 3 times daily average 350 ng/mL and occur at 3 to 8 hours postdose. Coadministration of acamprosate with food decreases bioavailability as measured by C_{max} and AUC by approximately 42% and 23%, respectively. The food effect on absorption is not clinically significant and no adjustment of dose is necessary.

Distribution – The volume of distribution for acamprosate following intravenous administration is estimated to be 72 to 109 L (approximately 1 L/kg). Plasma protein binding of acamprosate is negligible.

Metabolism – Acamprosate does not undergo metabolism.

ACAMPROSATE CALCIUM — ORAL

Excretion – After oral dosing of two 333 mg acamprosate tablets, the terminal half-life ranges from approximately 20 to 33 hours. Following oral administration of acamprosate, the major route of excretion is via the kidneys as acamprosate.

Special populations –

Renal function impairment: Peak plasma concentrations after administration of a single dose of two 333 mg acamprosate tablets to patients with moderate or severe renal impairment were approximately 2- and 4-fold higher, respectively, compared with healthy subjects. Similarly, elimination half-life was approximately 1.8- and 2.6-fold longer, respectively, compared with healthy subjects. There is a linear relationship between Ccr values and total apparent plasma clearance, renal clearance, and plasma half-life of acamprosate.

See Administration and Dosage for more information.

Elderly: The pharmacokinetics of acamprosate have not been evaluated in an elderly population. However, because renal function diminishes in elderly patients and acamprosate is excreted unchanged in urine, acamprosate plasma concentrations are likely to be higher in the elderly population compared with younger adults.

Contraindications

Hypersensitivity to acamprosate or any of its components; severe renal impairment (Ccr 30 mL/min or less).

Warnings

➤*Renal function impairment:* See Administration and Dosage for more information.

➤*Elderly:* This drug is known to be substantially excreted by the kidney, and the risk of toxic reactions to this drug may be greater in patients with impaired renal function. Because elderly patients are more likely to have decreased renal function, use care in dose selection; it may be useful to monitor renal function.

➤*Pregnancy: Category C.* Acamprosate has been shown to be teratogenic in rats when given in doses approximately equal to the human dose (on a mg/m^2 basis) and in rabbits when given in doses approximately 3 times the human dose (on a mg/m^2 basis). Acamprosate produced a dose-related increase in the number of fetuses with malformations in rats at oral doses of 300 mg/kg/day or greater (approximately equal to the daily oral MRHD on a mg/m^2 basis). The malformations included hydronephrosis, malformed iris, retinal dysplasia, and retroesophageal subclavian artery. No findings were observed at an oral dose of 50 mg/kg/day (approximately one fifth the daily oral MRHD on a mg/m^2 basis). An increased incidence of hydronephrosis also was noted in Burgundy Tawny rabbits at oral doses of 400 mg/kg/day or greater (approximately 3 times the daily oral MRHD on a mg/m^2 basis). No developmental effects were observed in New Zealand white rabbits at oral doses up to 1,000 mg/kg/day (approximately 8 times the daily oral MRHD on a mg/m^2 basis). The findings in animals should be considered in relation to known adverse developmental effects of ethyl alcohol, which include the characteristics of fetal alcohol syndrome (eg, craniofacial dysmorphism, intrauterine and postnatal growth retardation, retarded psychomotor and intellectual development) and milder forms of neurological and behavioral disorders in humans. There are no adequate and well-controlled studies in pregnant women. Use acamprosate during pregnancy only if the potential benefit justifies the potential risk to the fetus.

A study conducted in pregnant mice that were administered acamprosate by the oral route starting on day 15 of gestation through the end of lactation on postnatal day 28 demonstrated an increased incidence of stillborn fetuses at doses of 960 mg/kg/day or greater (approximately 2 times the daily oral MRHD on a mg/m^2 basis). No effects were observed at a dose of 320 mg/kg/day (approximately one half the daily MRHD on a mg/m^2 basis).

➤*Lactation:* In animal studies, acamprosate was excreted in the milk of lactating rats dosed orally with acamprosate. The concentration of acamprosate in milk compared with blood was 1.3:1. It is not known whether acamprosate is excreted in human milk. Because many drugs are excreted in human milk, exercise caution when acamprosate is administered to a woman who is breastfeeding.

➤*Children:* The safety and efficacy of acamprosate have not been established in children.

Precautions

➤*Withdrawal symptoms:* Use of acamprosate does not eliminate or diminish withdrawal symptoms.

➤*Suicide:* In controlled clinical trials of acamprosate, adverse events of a suicidal nature (eg, suicidal ideation, suicide attempts, completed suicides) were infrequent overall, but were more common in acamprosate-treated patients than in patients treated with placebo (1.4% vs 0.5% in studies of 6 months or less; 2.4% vs 0.8% in year-long studies). Completed suicides occurred in 3 of 2,272 (0.13%) patients in the pooled acamprosate group from all controlled studies and 2 of 1,962 patients (0.1%) in the placebo group. Adverse events coded as "depression" were reported at similar rates in acamprosate-treated and placebo-treated patients. Although many of these events occurred in the context of alcohol relapse, no consistent pattern of relationship between the clinical course of recovery from alcoholism and the emergence of suicidality was identified. The interrelationship of alcohol dependence, depression, and suicidality is well-recognized and complex. Monitor alcohol-dependent patients, including those patients being treated with acamprosate, for the development of symptoms of depression or suicidal thinking. Alert families and caregivers of patients being treated with acamprosate of the need to monitor patients for the emergence of symptoms of depression or suicidality, and to report such symptoms to the patient's health care provider.

Drug Interactions

➤*Naltrexone:* Coadministration of naltrexone with acamprosate produced a 25% increase in AUC and a 33% increase in the C_{max} of acamprosate. No adjustment of dosage is recommended in such patients.

Adverse Reactions

➤*Adverse events leading to discontinuation:* In placebo-controlled trials of 6 months or less, 8% of acamprosate-treated patients discontinued treatment because of an adverse event, compared with 6% of patients treated with placebo. In studies longer than 6 months, the discontinuation rate caused by adverse events was 7% in both the placebo-treated and the acamprosate-treated patients. Only diarrhea was associated with the discontinuation of more than 1% of patients (2% of acamprosate-treated vs 0.7% of placebo-treated patients). Other events, including nausea, depression, and anxiety, while accounting for discontinuation in less than 1% of patients, were nevertheless more commonly cited in association with discontinuation in acamprosate-treated patients than in placebo-treated patients.

➤*Common adverse events reported in controlled trials:*

Acamprosate Adverse Events (≥ 3%)				
	Number of patients (%) with events			
Adverse reaction	Acamprosate 1,332 mg/day n = 397	Acamprosate 1,998 mg/day[1] n = 1,539	Acamprosate pooled[2] n = 2,019	Placebo n = 1,706
Number (%) of patients with an AE	248 (62%)	910 (59%)	1,231 (61%)	955 (56%)
CNS	150 (38%)	417 (27%)	598 (30%)	500 (29%)
Anxiety[b]	32 (8%)	80 (5%)	118 (6%)	98 (6%)
Depression	33 (8%)	63 (4%)	102 (5%)	87 (5%)
Dizziness	15 (4%)	49 (3%)	67 (3%)	44 (3%)
Dry mouth	13 (3%)	23 (1%)	36 (2%)	28 (2%)
Insomnia	34 (9%)	94 (6%)	137 (7%)	121 (7%)
Paresthesia	11 (3%)	29 (2%)	40 (2%)	34 (2%)
Dermatologic	26 (7%)	150 (10%)	187 (9%)	169 (10%)
Pruritus	12 (3%)	68 (4%)	82 (4%)	58 (3%)
Sweating	11 (3%)	27 (2%)	40 (2%)	39 (2%)
GI	85 (21%)	440 (29%)	574 (28%)	344 (20%)
Anorexia	20 (5%)	35 (2%)	57 (3%)	44 (3%)
Diarrhea	39 (10%)	257 (17%)	329 (16%)	166 (10%)
Flatulence	4 (1%)	55 (4%)	63 (3%)	28 (2%)
Nausea	11 (3%)	69 (4%)	87 (4%)	58 (3%)
Miscellaneous	121 (30%)	513 (33%)	685 (34%)	517 (30%)
Accidental injury[a]	17 (4%)	44 (3%)	70 (3%)	52 (3%)
Asthenia	29 (7%)	79 (5%)	114 (6%)	93 (5%)
Pain	6 (2%)	56 (4%)	65 (3%)	55 (3%)

[a] Includes events coded as "fracture" by sponsor.
[b] Includes events coded as "nervousness" by sponsor.
[1] Includes 258 patients treated with acamprosate 2,000 mg/day, using a different dosage strength and regimen.
[2] Includes all patients in the first 2 columns as well as 83 patients treated with acamprosate 3,000 mg/day, using a different dosage strength and regimen.

➤*Other adverse events:* Events are further categorized by body system and listed in order of decreasing frequency according to the following definitions: frequent adverse events are those occurring in at least 1/100 patients (only those not already listed in the summary of adverse events in controlled trials appear in this listing); infrequent adverse events are those occurring in 1/100 to 1/1000 patients; rare events are those occurring in fewer than 1/1000 patients.

Cardiovascular – Frequent: hypertension, palpitation, syncope, vasodilatation; Infrequent: angina pectoris, hemorrhage, hypotension, myocardial infarct, phlebitis, postural hypotension, tachycardia, varicose vein; Rare: cardiomyopathy, deep thrombophlebitis, heart failure, mesenteric arterial occlusion, shock.

CNS – Frequent: abnormal thinking, amnesia, headache, libido decrease, somnolence, tremor; Infrequent: abnormal dreams, agitation, apathy, confusion, convulsion, hallucinations, hostility, hypesthesia, libido increase, migraine, neuralgia, neurosis, suicidal ideation, vertigo, withdrawal syndrome; Rare: alcohol craving, depersonalization, encephalopathy, hyperkinesia, increased salivation, manic reaction, paranoid reaction, psychosis, torticollis, twitching.

Dermatologic – Frequent: rash; Infrequent: acne, alopecia, dry skin, eczema, exfoliative dermatitis, maculopapular rash, urticaria, vesiculobullous rash; Rare: psoriasis.

Endocrine – Rare: goiter, hypothyroidism.

GI – Frequent: abdominal pain, constipation, dyspepsia, increased appetite, vomiting; Infrequent: abnormal liver function tests, dysphagia, eructation, esophagitis, gastritis, gastroenteritis, gastrointestinal hemorrhage, hematemesis, hepatitis, liver cirrhosis, nausea and vomiting, pancreatitis, rectal hemorrhage; Rare: carcinoma of liver, cholecystitis, colitis, duodenal ulcer, enlarged abdomen, melena, mouth ulceration, stomach ulcer.

ACAMPROSATE CALCIUM — ORAL

GU – Frequent: impotence; Infrequent: abnormal sexual function, metrorrhagia, urinary frequency, urinary incontinence, urinary tract infection, vaginitis; Rare: abnormal ejaculation, hematuria, kidney calculus, menorrhagia, nocturia, polyuria, urinary urgency.

Hematologic / Lymphatic – Infrequent: anemia, ecchymosis, eosinophilia, lymphocytosis, thrombocytopenia; Rare: leukopenia, lymphadenopathy, monocytosis.

Lab test abnormalities – Infrequent: ALT increase, AST increase; Rare: alkaline phosphatase increase, creatinine increase, lactic dehydrogenase increase.

Metabolic / Nutritional – Frequent: peripheral edema, weight gain; Infrequent: avitaminosis, bilirubinemia, diabetes mellitus, gout, hyperglycemia, hyperuricemia, thirst, weight loss; Rare: hyponatremia.

Musculoskeletal – Frequent: arthralgia, myalgia; Infrequent: leg cramps; Rare: myopathy, rheumatoid arthritis.

Respiratory – Frequent: bronchitis, cough increase, dyspnea, pharyngitis, rhinitis; Infrequent: asthma, epistaxis, pneumonia; Rare: laryngismus, pulmonary embolus.

Special senses – Frequent: abnormal vision, taste perversion; Infrequent: amblyopia, deafness, tinnitus; Rare: diplopia, ophthalmitis, photophobia.

Miscellaneous – Frequent: back pain, chest pain, chills, flu syndrome, infection, suicide attempt; Infrequent: abscess, allergic reaction, fever, hernia, intentional injury, intentional overdose, malaise, neck pain; Rare: ascites, facial edema, photosensitivity reaction, sudden death.

➤*Postmarketing:* Although no causal relationship to acamprosate has been found, the serious adverse event of acute kidney failure has been reported to be temporally associated with acamprosate treatment in at least 3 patients and is not described elsewhere in the labeling.

Overdosage

➤*Symptoms:* In all reported cases of acute overdosage with acamprosate (total reported doses of up to 56 g acamprosate), the only symptom that could be reasonably associated with acamprosate was diarrhea. Hypercalcemia has not been reported in cases of acute overdose. Consider a risk of hypercalcemia in chronic overdosage only.

➤*Treatment:* Treatment of overdose should be symptomatic and supportive.

Patient Information

Any psychoactive drug may impair judgment, thinking, or motor skills. Caution patients about operating hazardous machinery, including automobiles, until they are reasonably certain that acamprosate therapy does not affect their ability to engage in such activities.

Advise patients to notify their physician if they become pregnant or intend to become pregnant during therapy.

Advise patients to notify their physician if they are breastfeeding.

Advise patients to continue acamprosate therapy as directed, even in the event of relapse. Remind them to discuss any renewed drinking with their physician.

Advise patients that acamprosate has been shown to help maintain abstinence only when used as a part of a treatment program that includes counseling and support.

SMOKING DETERRENTS

Nicotine

Indications

As an aid to smoking cessation for the relief of nicotine withdrawal symptoms. Use as part of a comprehensive behavioral smoking-cessation program.

➤*Unlabeled uses:* In 2 children, use of nicotine polacrilex gum and haloperidol improved symptoms (eg, tics) of Tourette's syndrome. Further study is needed.

Administration and Dosage

Withdrawal from nicotine in addicted individuals is characterized by craving, nervousness, restlessness, irritability, mood lability, anxiety, drowsiness, sleep disturbances, impaired concentration, increased appetite, minor somatic complaints (headache, myalgia, constipation, fatigue), and weight gain. Nicotine toxicity is characterized by nausea, abdominal pain, vomiting, diarrhea, diaphoresis, flushing, dizziness, disturbed hearing/vision, confusion, weakness, palpitations, altered respiration, and hypotension.

The following table includes dosing, duration of therapy, and availability information for nicotine replacement therapy products.

Nicotine Replacement Pharmacotherapy			
Type of therapy	Dosage	Duration	Availability
Gum	< 24 cigarettes/day: 2 mg gum up to 24 pieces/day	up to 12 weeks	*otc*
	> 25 cigarettes/day: 4 mg gum up to 24 pieces/day		
Inhaler	6 to 16 cartridges/day	up to 6 months	*Rx* only
Transdermal patch	21 mg/24 hr 14 mg/24 hr 7 mg/24 hr	4 to 6 weeks then 2 weeks then 2 weeks	*otc*
	15 mg/16 hr	6 weeks	
Nasal spray	8 to 40 doses/day	3 to 6 months	*Rx* only

Actions

➤*Pharmacology:* Nicotine, the chief alkaloid in tobacco products, binds stereoselectively to acetylcholine receptors at the autonomic ganglia, in the adrenal medulla, at neuromuscular junctions, and in the brain. Two types of CNS effects are believed to be the basis of nicotine's positively reinforcing properties. A stimulating effect, exerted mainly in the cortex via the locus ceruleus, produces increased alertness and cognitive performance. A "reward" effect via the "pleasure system" in the brain is exerted in the limbic system. At low doses the stimulant effects predominate, while at high doses the reward effects predominate. Intermittent IV administration of nicotine activates neurohormonal pathways, releasing acetylcholine, norepinephrine, dopamine, serotonin, vasopressin, beta-endorphin, growth hormone, and adrenocorticotropic hormone (ACTH).

The cardiovascular effects of nicotine include peripheral vasoconstriction, tachycardia, and elevated blood pressure. Acute and chronic tolerance to nicotine develops from smoking tobacco or ingesting nicotine preparations. Acute tolerance (a reduction in response for a given dose) develops rapidly (< 1 hour), but at distinct rates for different physiologic effects (eg, skin temperature, heart rate, subjective effects). Withdrawal symptoms, such as cigarette craving, can be reduced in some individuals by plasma nicotine levels lower than those for smoking.

Nicotine polacrilex contains nicotine bound to an ion exchange resin in a chewing gum base. The **nicotine transdermal system** is a multilayered unit containing nicotine as the active agent that provides systemic delivery of nicotine for up to 24 hours (*Nicotrol*, up to 16 hours) following its application to intact skin.

➤*Pharmacokinetics:*

Absorption / Distribution –

Nicotine: Nicotine as tobacco smoke is absorbed rapidly through the lungs. Nicotine is a weak base; absorption through mucous membranes depends on pH. Nicotine gum is buffered at an alkaline pH to increase absorption through the buccal mucosa. The volume of distribution of IV nicotine is ≈ 2 to 3 L/kg. Plasma protein binding is < 5%.

Gum: The nicotine is bound to an ion exchange resin and is released only during chewing; nicotine will not be released in significant amounts if the gum is swallowed. The blood level of nicotine will depend upon the vigor and duration of chewing. The trough level of nicotine obtained by smoking 1 cigarette/hour is ≈ 2 times that of chewing one 2 mg piece of gum.

Transdermal: Following application, ≈ 68% of the nicotine released from the system enters the systemic circulation. The remainder of the nicotine released from the system is lost via evaporation from the edge. All systems are labeled by the actual amount of nicotine absorbed by the patient.

After application, plasma concentrations rise rapidly, plateau within 2 to 12 hours, and then slowly decline until the system is removed, after which they decline more rapidly. Following the second daily application, steady-state plasma nicotine concentrations are achieved and are on average 25% to 30% higher compared with single-dose applications. Plasma nicotine concentrations are proportional to dose and are similar for all sites of application on the upper body and upper outer arm.

Half-hourly smoking of cigarettes produces average plasma nicotine concentrations of ≈ 44 ng/mL. Average plasma nicotine concentrations from transdermal nicotine are ≈ 5 to 17 ng/mL.

Inhaler: Most of the nicotine released from the inhaler is deposited in the mouth with only a fraction of the dose released (< 5%) reaching the lower respiratory tract. Eight deep inhalations over 20 minutes releases on average 4 mg of nicotine content from each cartridge, of which 2 mg is systemically absorbed. Peak plasma concentrations are typically reached within 15 minutes after inhalation ends. Absorption of nicotine through the buccal mucosa is relatively slow. Nicotine arterial plasma concentration peaks and declines seen with cigarette smoking are not achieved with the inhaler. After use of a single inhaler, the arterial nicotine concentration rises slowly to an average of 6 ng/mL in contrast to those of a cigarette, which increase rapidly and reach a mean C_{max} of ≈ 49 ng/mL within 5 minutes.

Intermittent use of the nicotine inhaler typically produces nicotine plasma levels of 6 to 8 ng/mL, corresponding to ≈ 33% of those achieved with cigarette smoking.

Nasal spray: Following administration of 2 sprays of nicotine nasal spray (1 mg), ≈ 53% enters the systemic circulation. Plasma concentrations of nicotine rise rapidly, reaching maximum venous concentrations of 12 ng/mL in 15 minutes. The apparent absorption half-life of nicotine is ≈ 3 minutes. There is a wide variation among subjects in the plasma nicotine concentrations for the spray. Peak nicotine concentrations similar to whose seen after smoking 1 cigarette (17 ng/mL) were seen in 20% of subjects after a 1 mg dose of spray.

Metabolism / Excretion –

Nicotine: Nicotine is rapidly and extensively metabolized by the liver. More than 20 metabolites have been identified, all of which are believed to be less active than the parent compound. The primary plasma metabolite, cotinine, has a half-life of 15 to 20 hours, and concentrations that exceed nicotine by 10-fold. About 10% of the nicotine absorbed is excreted unchanged in the urine. This may be increased up to 30% with high urinary flow rates and urine pH < 5. The half-life of nicotine averages 1 to 2 hours. Nicotine accumulates in the body over 6 to 9 hours of regular smoking. Thus, smoking results in a nicotine exposure that lasts 24 hours a day. Persistence of nicotine in the brain results in changes in nicotinic receptors in the brain. Changes in receptor numbers or function are presumably the substrate for nicotine withdrawal syndrome.

Transdermal: Following removal of transdermal nicotine, plasma nicotine concentrations decline exponentially with an apparent mean half-life of 3 to 4 hours due to continued absorption from the skin depot. Most nonsmoking patients will have nondetectable nicotine concentrations in 10 to 12 hours.

Nicotine Pharmacokinetics					
Parameter	Smoking	Gum	Transdermal	Nasal spray	Inhaler
Time to peak levels (hours)	ND[1]	0.25 to 0.5	2 to 12	0.25	0.25
Peak plasma level (ng/mL)	44	5 to 10	5 to 17	12	6
Half-life (hours)	15 to 20[2]	3 to 4	3 to 4	1 to 2	ND

[1] No data.
[2] Refers to cotinine, the primary plasma metabolite of nicotine.

Contraindications

Hypersensitivity to nicotine or any components of the products, including menthol.

Warnings

➤*Nicotine risks:* Nicotine from any source can be toxic and addictive. Smoking causes lung disease, cancer, and heart disease, and may adversely affect pregnant women or the fetus. For any smoker, with or without concomitant disease or pregnancy, the risk of nicotine replacement in a smoking cessation program should be weighed against the hazard of continued smoking, and the likelihood of achieving cessation of smoking without nicotine replacement.

➤*Renal/Hepatic function impairment:* Because nicotine is extensively metabolized and its total system clearance is dependent on liver blood flow, anticipate some influence of hepatic impairment on drug kinetics (reduced clearance). Only severe renal impairment should affect clearance of nicotine or its metabolites from circulation.

➤*Carcinogenesis:* Nicotine does not appear to be a carcinogen in laboratory animals. Nicotine and its metabolites increased the incidences of tumors in the cheek pouches of hamsters and forestomach of rats, respectively, when given in combination with tumor-initiators. One study, which could not be replicated, suggested that cotinine, the primary metabolite of nicotine, may cause lymphoreticular sarcoma in the large intestine of rats.

➤*Fertility impairment:* In rats and rabbits, implantation can be delayed or inhibited by a reduction in DNA synthesis that appears to be caused by nicotine. Studies have shown a decrease in litter size in rats treated with nicotine during gestation.

➤*Elderly:* Nicotine **inhaler** and **nasal spray** therapy appeared to be as effective in elderly patients ≥ 60 years of age as in younger smokers.

➤*Pregnancy: Category D* (**inhaler, spray, transdermal patch**); *Category C* (**gum**). Tobacco smoke contains nicotine, hydrogen cyanide, and carbon monoxide. The harmful effects of cigarette smoking on maternal and fetal health are clearly established. These include low birth weight (21% to 39% of all infants), an increased risk of spontaneous abortion, increased perinatal mortality, and decreased placental perfusion. Smoking causes a decrease in the oxygen-carrying capacity of hemoglobin when carbon monoxide passes through the placenta. Nicotine causes vasoconstriction and decreased placenta blood flow. Smoking interferes with the body's ability to process essential vitamins and minerals, resulting in decreased intestinal synthesis of vitamin B_{12}, calcium loss from bones, and decreased usage of vitamin C. In general, smokers have a nutrient-poor diet. Smoking during pregnancy increases the risk of ectopic pregnancy, spontaneous abortion, preterm birth, premature rupture of membranes, placenta previa, abruptio placenta, and chorioamnionitis.

No association has been found between maternal smoking and congenital anomalies; however, nicotine and cotinine are found in higher concentrations in infants whose mothers smoke.

Second-hand smoking is an increasing concern for its potential effects on infants and siblings. There is an association between maternal smoking and sudden infant death syndrome, but it is unclear whether it is from in utero exposure or postnatal passive exposure, or both.

Nicotine was shown to produce skeletal abnormalities in the offspring of mice when toxic doses were given to the dams.

A nicotine bolus (up to 2 mg/kg) to pregnant rhesus monkeys caused acidosis, hypercarbia, and hypotension (fetal and maternal concentrations were ≈ 20 times those achieved after smoking 1 cigarette in 5 minutes). Fetal breathing movements were reduced in the fetal lamb after IV injection of 0.25 mg/kg nicotine to the ewe (equivalent to smoking 1 cigarette every 20 seconds for 5 minutes). Uterine blood flow was reduced ≈ 30% after infusion of 0.1 mcg/kg/min nicotine to pregnant rhesus monkeys (equivalent to smoking ≈ 6 cigarettes every minute for 20 minutes).

The inhaler and nasal spray do not deliver hydrogen cyanide and carbon monoxide. However, because they do deliver nicotine, it is presumed that the inhaler and the nasal spray can cause fetal harm when administered to a pregnant woman. The effect of nicotine delivered by the inhaler and nasal spray has not been examined in pregnancy and the specific effects of nicotine inhaler and nasal spray therapy on fetal development are unknown. Spontaneous abortion during nicotine replacement therapy has been reported; as with smoking, nicotine as a contributing factor cannot be excluded. Pregnant smokers should be encouraged to attempt cessation using education and behavioral interventions before using pharmacological approaches. If the inhaler or nasal spray are used during pregnancy, or if the patient becomes pregnant while using it, the patient should be apprised of the potential hazard to the fetus. Inhaler and spray therapy should be used during pregnancy only if the likelihood of smoking cessation justifies the potential risk of using it by the pregnant patient who might continue to smoke.

➤*Lactation:* Nicotine and cotinine pass freely into breast milk up to 2 hours after maternal smoking; the milk to plasma ratio averages 2.9. Nicotine is absorbed orally. An infant has the ability to clear nicotine by hepatic first-pass clearance; however, the efficiency of removal is probably lowest at birth. Nicotine concentrations in milk can be expected to be lower with **inhaler** and **nasal spray** nicotine therapy when used as directed than with cigarette smoking, as maternal plasma nicotine concentrations are generally reduced with nicotine replacement. Decide whether to discontinue nursing or to discontinue the drug, weighing the risk of exposure of the infant to nicotine from replacement therapy against the risks associated with the infant's exposure to nicotine from continued smoking by the mother and from nicotine therapy alone or in combination with continued smoking.

➤*Children:* Safety and efficacy in children/adolescents < 18 years of age who smoke have not been evaluated.

Cigarette smoke contains many compounds including carbon monoxide, dioxin, cyanide, and cadmium. Studies have shown residual effects beyond the neonatal period, including growth deficits, and deficiencies in intellectual, emotional, and behavioral development. These manifest as poor auditory responsiveness, fine motor tremors, hypertonicity, and decreases in verbal comprehension.

The amounts of nicotine that are tolerated by adult smokers can produce symptoms of poisoning and could prove fatal if inhaled, ingested, or bucally absorbed by children or pets. An inhaler or nasal spray cartridge container contains ≈ 60% (6 mg) of its initial drug content when discarded. Therefore, caution patients to keep the used and unused systems out of the reach of children and pets.

Precautions

➤*General:* Urge the patient to stop smoking completely when initiating nicotine replacement therapy. Inform patients that if they continue to smoke while using the product, they may experience adverse effects due to peak nicotine levels higher than those experienced from smoking alone. If there is a clinically significant increase in cardiovascular or other effects attributable to nicotine, the treatment should be discontinued. Physicians should anticipate that concomitant medications may need dosage adjustment (see Drug Interactions). Sustained use (> 6 months) of inhaler or nasal spray by patients who stop smoking has not been studied and is not recommended (see Drug Abuse and Dependence).

➤*Bronchospastic disease:* The **inhaler** has not been specifically studied in asthma or chronic pulmonary disease. Nicotine is an airway irritant and might cause bronchospasm. The inhaler should be used with caution in patients with bronchospastic disease. Other forms of nicotine replacement might be preferable in patients with severe bronchospastic airway disease.

Asthma, bronchospasm, and reactive airway disease exacerbation of bronchospasm in patients with pre-existing asthma has been reported. Use of the **nasal spray** in patients with severe reactive airway disease is not recommended.

➤*Nasal disorders:* Use of the **nasal spray** is not recommended in patients with known chronic nasal disorders (eg, allergy, rhinitis, nasal polyps, sinusitis) because such use has not been adequately studied. The effect of the nasal spray on the nasal mucosa topical application of either nicotine or tobacco products is irritating to the nasal mucosa and physicians should consider both the risks and benefits to the patient before initiating or continuing nasal spray therapy. The effect of the nasal spray on the nasal mucosa was studied in 39 cigarette smokers who used the nasal spray for 1 month. When compared with baseline, random biopsies taken after 4 weeks of treatment revealed 1 patient with persistence of pre-existing dysplasia and 1 patient with a newly found dysplasia. In both, dysplasia was not seen after a recovery period of 8 weeks. Forty-two patients who used the nasal spray for > 6 months underwent follow-up ear, nose, and throat examinations 1 to 3 months after discontinuing the use of the spray. Many reported local irritant effects of the spray during spray use, but none showed persistent mucosal injury that the examining physician could attribute to use of the product. The clinical significance of these findings is not known, but extended use of the product > 6 months is not recommended.

➤*Cardiovascular:* Weigh the benefits against the risks of nicotine in patients with certain cardiovascular and peripheral vascular diseases. Specifically, screen and evaluate patients with coronary heart disease (history of MI or angina pectoris), serious cardiac arrhythmias, or vasospastic diseases (Buerger's disease, Prinzmetal variant angina, Raynaud's phenomena) before nicotine is prescribed. There have been occasional reports of tachycardia and palpitations associated with nicotine replacement therapy; therefore, if cardiovascular symptoms occur, discontinue the drug. Generally, do not use during the immediate post-MI period, nor in patients with serious arrhythmias or with severe or worsening angina pectoris.

Accelerated hypertension – Nicotine therapy constitutes a risk factor for development of malignant hypertension in patients with accelerated hypertension. **Inhaler** therapy should be used with caution in these patients and only when the benefits of including nicotine replacement in a smoking cessation program outweigh the risks.

➤*Endocrine:* Because of the action of nicotine on the adrenal medulla (release of catecholamines), use with caution in patients with hyperthyroidism, pheochromocytoma, or insulin-dependent diabetes.

➤*Oral/GI:* Because nicotine delays healing in peptic ulcer disease, use in patients with active or inactive peptic ulcer only when benefits of including nicotine in a smoking cessation program outweigh risks.

➤*Dental:* When used over an extended time, nicotine **gum** may cause severe occlusal stress due to its heavier viscosity than ordinary chewing gum. Nicotine gum may cause loosening of inlays or fillings, can stick to dentures, and cause damage to oral mucosa and natural teeth. Hard, sugarless candy between doses of gum is recommended to help provide oral stimulation required by some patients. Temporol mandibular joint dysfunction and pain have also been reported with excessive chewing.

➤*Drug abuse and dependence:*

Inhaler – The nicotine inhaler is likely to have a low abuse potential based on slower absorption, smaller fluctuations, and lower blood levels of nicotine when compared with cigarettes. However, nicotine withdrawal symptoms were noted in clinical trials during tapering and discontinuation of the nicotine inhaler. Dependence can occur from transference of tobacco-related nicotine dependence to the inhaler. The use of the inhaler for > 6 months is not recommended. Encourage patients to withdraw gradually from therapy after 3 months of usage to minimize the risk of dependence. If necessary, dose reduction can be gradually achieved over a 6- to 12-week period.

Nasal spray – Nicotine nasal spray has a dependence potential intermediate between other nicotine-based therapies and cigarettes. The nasal spray is distinct from other nicotine-based smoking cessation therapies in its greater speed of onset, greater capacity of self-titration of dose, and frequent, rapid fluctuations of plasma nicotine concentration. Dependence on nicotine nasal spray occurred during clinical trials. Feelings of dependency were reported by 32% of active spray users and 13% of placebo spray users. Such dependence may represent transference of tobacco-related nicotine dependence to the nasal spray. Some patients (15% to 20%) used the active spray for longer than recommended (6 to 12 months) and 5% used a higher dose than recommended. Some patients experienced anxiety after discontinuing the spray and some reported craving the spray rather than cigarettes.

Drug Interactions

Smoking cessation, with or without nicotine substitutes, may alter response to concomitant medication in ex-smokers.

Cigarette smoking is an inducer of CYP1A2 enzymes, the primary mechanism for drug interactions. For drugs whose metabolism is stimulated by enzyme inducers, the dose may need to be increased upon initiation of inducer (smoking) therapy and decreased when the inducer (smoking) is discontinued.

Smoking Drug Interactions

Precipitant drug	Object drug*		Description
Smoking	Alcohol	↓	May decrease the rate of absorption and peak serum concentration.
Smoking	Benzodiazepines (diazepam, chlordiazepoxide)	↓	Smoking may decrease sedation and drowsiness probably by CNS stimulation.
Smoking	Beta adrenergic blockers	↓	Sympathetic activation by nicotine may decrease end-organ responsiveness. Beta blockers may be less effective for blood pressure and heart rate control in smokers.
Smoking	Caffeine Clozapine Fluvoxamine Olanzapine Tacrine Theophylline	↓	Smoking is an inducer of CYP1A2 enzymes. It can increase clearance and decrease AUC, mean plasma concentration, half-life, and volume of distribution.
Smoking	Clorazepate Lidocaine (oral)	↓	Smoking can decrease AUC.
Smoking	Estradiol	↓	Smoking can increase 2-hydroxylation with possible antiestrogenic effects.
Smoking	Flecanide Imipramine	↓	Can increase clearance and decrease serum concentrations.
Smoking	Heparin	↓	Smoking can increase clearance and decrease half-life. The smoker may require higher doses of heparin.
Smoking	Insulin	↓	Smoking can cause decreased SC absorption resulting in higher insulin requirements for smokers.
Smoking	Mexiletine	↓	Smoking may increase oral clearance and decrease half-life.
Smoking	Opioids (dextropropoxyphene, pentazocine)	↓	Smoking can decrease the analgesic effect; therefore, smokers may require higher doses for analgesia.
Smoking	Propranolol	↓	Smoking can increase oral clearance.

Smoking Drug Interactions

Precipitant drug	Object drug*		Description
Smoking Nicotine	Catecholamines Cortisol	↑	Smoking and nicotine can increase circulating cortisol and catecholamines. Therapy with adrenergic agonists or adrenergic blockers may need to be adjusted upon changes in nicotine therapy or smoking status.

* ↑ = Object drug increased. ↓ = Object drug decreased.

➤*Nasal spray:* The extent of absorption and peak plasma concentration is slightly reduced in patients with the common cold/rhinitis. In addition, the time to peak concentration is prolonged. The use of a nasal vasoconstrictor such as xylometazoline in patients with rhinitis will further prolong the time to peak.

Adverse Reactions

Assessment of adverse events in patients who participated in controlled clinical trials is complicated by the occurrence of signs and symptoms of nicotine withdrawal in some patients and nicotine excess in others. The incidence of adverse events is compounded by the many minor complaints that smokers commonly have, continued smoking by many patients, and the local irritation from the active drug and placebo.

➤*Inhaler:*

Nicotine Inhaler Adverse Reactions (%)

Adverse reaction	Drug	Placebo
Local irritation (mouth, throat)	40	18
Coughing	32	12
Rhinitis	23	16
Dyspepsia	18	9
Headache	26	15

Local – Taste complaints, pain in jaw and neck, tooth disorders, sinusitis (≥ 3%).

Miscellaneous – Influenza-like symptoms, pain, back pain, allergy, paresthesias, flatulence, fever (≥ 3%).

Withdrawal: Dizziness, anxiety, sleep disorder, depression, withdrawal syndrome, drug dependence, fatigue, myalgia (≥ 3%).

Nicotine-related: Nausea, diarrhea, hiccough (≥ 3%).

Smoking-related: Chest discomfort, bronchitis, hypertension (≥ 3%).

➤*Nasal spray:*

Common smoker complaints: Chest tightness, dyspepsia, paresthesias in limbs, constipation, and stomatitis.

Withdrawal symptoms: Anxiety, irritability, restlessness, cravings, dizziness, impaired concentration, weight increase, emotional lability, somnolence, fatigue, increased sweating, insomnia (≥ 5%); confusion, depression, apathy, tremor, increased appetite, incoordination, increased dreaming (< 5%).

Local irritation: Moderate-to-severe in 94% of patients during the first 2 days of treatment, declining to 81% after 3 weeks of treatment (rated moderate-to-mild); runny nose; throat irritation; watering eyes; sneezing; cough; nasal congestion; subjective comments related to the taste or usage of the dosage form; sinus irritation; transient epistaxis; eye irritation; transient changes in sense of smell; pharyngitis; paresthesias of the nose, mouth, or head; numbness of the nose or mouth; burning of the nose or eyes; earache; facial flushing; transient changes in sense of taste; hoarseness; nasal ulcer or blister.

Dependence: Feelings of dependence and calming were reported by more patients on active spray than placebo.

Others (not attributable to intercurrent illness):

Nicotine Nasal Spray Adverse Reactions (> 1%)

Adverse reaction	Drug	Placebo
Headache	18	15
Back pain	6	4
Dyspnea	5	8
Nausea	5	5
Arthralgia	5	1
Menstrual disorder	4	4
Palpitation	4	4
Flatulence	4	3
Tooth disorder	4	1
Gum disorder	4	1
Myalgia	3	4
Abdominal pain	3	3
Confusion	3	3
Acne	3	1
Dysmenorrhea	3	0
Pruritus	2	3

CNS – Aphasia, amnesia, migraine, numbness (< 1%).

GI – Dry mouth, hiccough, diarrhea (< 1%).

Respiratory – Bronchitis, bronchospasm, increased sputum (< 1%).

Miscellaneous – Peripheral edema, pain, allergy, purpura, rash, abnormal vision (< 1%).

➤*Gum:*

Miscellaneous – Injury to mouth, teeth, or dental work; belching; increased salivation; mild jaw muscle ache; sore mouth or throat.

➤*Transdermal:*

Miscellaneous – Erythema, pruritus, and/or burning at the application site.

Overdosage

➤*Symptoms:* Signs and symptoms of acute nicotine poisoning include the following: Pallor, cold sweat, nausea, salivation, vomiting, abdominal pain, diarrhea, headache, dizziness, disturbed hearing and vision, tremor, mental confusion, weakness. Prostration, hypotension, and respiratory failure may ensue with large overdoses. Lethal doses produce convulsions quickly; death follows as a result of peripheral or central respiratory paralysis or, less frequently, cardiac failure. The oral minimum acute lethal dose for nicotine in adult humans is reported to be 40 to 60 mg.

➤*Treatment:* Large oral nicotine ingestions cause vomiting, and the consequences of an overdose will vary. Institute gastric lavage and/or activated charcoal (with protected airway) when appropriate. Avoid syrup of ipecac.

Other supportive measures include diazepam or barbiturates for seizures, atropine for excessive bronchial secretions or diarrhea, respiratory support for respiratory failure, and vigorous fluid support for hypotension and cardiovascular collapse.

Nasal spray – A full bottle of nicotine nasal spray contains 100 mg of nicotine and would be expected to be irritating if sprayed in the eyes, mouth, or ears. Treat eye exposure with copious water irrigation for 20 minutes.

Inhaler – One cartridge of nicotine inhaler contains 10 mg of nicotine, of which, ≈ 4 mg is delivered nicotine. It is unlikely that an excessive nicotine overdose will occur via inhalation, but should such an overdose occur, the patient should contact a physician immediately. Refer patients ingesting nicotine inhaler cartridges to a health care facility for management. Administer repeated doses of activated charcoal as long as the cartridge remains in the GI tract because the cartridge will continue to release nicotine for many hours. The cartridge can be identified with a radiogram.

Transdermal – Remove the patch, flush the skin with water, and dry. Do not use soap, which may increase nicotine absorption. If the patch has been ingested, administer activated charcoal. In an unconscious patient, secure an airway before administering activated charcoal via a nasogastric tube. As long as the patch remains in the GI tract, administer repeated doses of charcoal because the patch will continue to release nicotine. A saline cathartic or sorbitol may be added to the first dose of activated charcoal to enhance passage of the patch.

NICOTINE TRANSDERMAL SYSTEM

	Product/Distributor	Dose absorbed in 24 hours (mg/day)	How supplied
otc	**Nicotine Transdermal System Step 1** (Various, eg, Novartis, Watson)	21	In 7 and 30 systems per box.
otc	**Nicotine Transdermal System Step 2** (Various, eg, Novartis, Watson)	14	In 7 and 30 systems per box.
otc	**Nicotine Transdermal System Step 3** (Various, eg, Novartis, Watson)	7	In 7 and 30 systems per box.
otc	**Nicoderm CQ Step 1** (GlaxoSmithKline Consumer)	21	In 7 and 14 systems per box; original and clear patches.
otc	**Nicoderm CQ Step 2** (GlaxoSmithKline Consumer)	14	In 14 systems per box; original and clear patches.
otc	**Nicoderm CQ Step 3** (GlaxoSmithKline Consumer)	7	In 14 systems per box; original and clear patches.
otc	**Nicotrol Step 1** (Pharmacia)	15[1]	In 7s and 14s.
otc	**Nicotrol Step 2** (Pharmacia)	10[1]	In 7s and 14s.
otc	**Nicotrol Step 3** (Pharmacia)	5[1]	In 7s and 14s.

[1] Dose absorbed in 16 hours.

NICOTINE — TRANSDERMAL

For complete and comparative prescribing information, refer to the Nicotine group monograph.

Indications

➤*Smoking cessation:* Nicotine transdermal system is indicated for the reduction of withdrawal symptoms, including nicotine craving, associated with quitting smoking.

Administration and Dosage

➤*Approved by the FDA:* November 1991.

➤*Directions:* Patients under 18 years of age should ask a doctor before use. Before using this product, patients should read the user's guide for complete directions and other information. Patients should stop smoking completely prior to beginning use of the patch.

Persons who smoke greater than 10 cigarettes/day should use the transdermal system according to the 10-week schedule below:

21, 14, 7 mg patches –

Step 1	Step 2	Step 3
Use one 21 mg patch/day	Use one 14 mg patch/day	Use one 7 mg patch/day
Weeks 1 to 6	Weeks 7 to 8	Weeks 9 to 10

15, 10, 5 mg patches:

Step 1	Step 2	Step 3
Use one 15 mg patch/day for 6 weeks	Use one 10 mg patch/day for 2 weeks	Use one 5 mg patch/day for 2 weeks
Weeks 1 to 6	Weeks 7 to 8	Weeks 9 to 10

Persons who smoke 10 or fewer cigarettes per day should not use step 1. These patients should start with step 2 for 6 weeks, then step 3 for 2 weeks and should then stop. Steps 2 and 3 allow one to gradually reduce his level of nicotine. Completing the full program will increase the chances of quitting successfully.

Patients should apply 1 new patch every 24 hours on skin that is dry, clean and hairless and should follow these instructions:

1.) Remove backing from patch and immediately press onto skin (upper arm or hip). Hold for 10 seconds.
2.) Wash hands after applying or removing patch. Throw away the patch in the enclosed disposal tray. See user's guide for safety and handling.
3.) Wear the patch for 16 or 24 hours. Patients who crave cigarettes upon awakening should wear the patch for 24 hours.
4.) If vivid dreams or other sleep disturbances occur, remove the patch at bedtime and apply a new one in the morning. The used patch should be removed and a new one applied to a different skin site at the same time each day.
5.) Do not wear more than 1 patch at a time.
6.) Do not cut patch in half or into smaller pieces.
7.) Do not leave patch on for more than 24 hours because it may irritate the skin and lose strength after 24 hours.
8.) Stop using the patch at the end of 10 weeks. When starting the program with step 2, stop using the patch at the end of 8 weeks. If the need to use the patch is still present, consult a physician.

➤*Storage/Stability:* Nicotine transdermal system should be stored at 20° to 25°C (68° to 77°F).

This medication should be kept out of the reach of children and pets. Used patches have enough nicotine to poison children and pets.

NICOTINE POLACRILEX (Nicotine resin complex)

otc	**Commit** (GlaxoSmithKline Consumer)	**Lozenge**: 2 mg nicotine (as polacrilex) per lozenge	Aspartame[1] and mannitol. In 72s.
		4 mg nicotine (as polacrilex) per lozenge	Aspartame[1] and mannitol. In 72s.
otc	**Nicotine Gum** (Various, eg, Rugby)	**Chewing gum**: 2 mg nicotine (as polacrilex) per square	In 48s and 108s.
otc	**Nicorette** (GlaxoSmithKline Consumer)		In orange, mint, and original flavors. In 48s, 108s, and 168s.
otc	**Nicotine Gum** (Various, eg, Rugby)	**Chewing gum**: 4 mg nicotine (as polacrilex) per square.	In 48s and 108s.
otc	**Nicorette** (GlaxoSmithKline Consumer)		In orange, mint, and original flavors. In 48s, 108s, and 168s.

[1] Contains 3.4 mg phenylalanine.

NICOTINE POLACRILEX — ORAL

For complete and comparative prescribing information, refer to the Nicotine group monograph.

Indications

➤*Smoking cessation:* Nicotine polacrilex is indicated for the reduction of withdrawal symptoms, including nicotine craving, associated with quitting smoking.

Administration and Dosage

➤*Approved by the FDA:* January 1984.

Advise the patient to stop smoking completely when beginning to use the gum or lozenges.

Patients less than 18 years of age should ask a doctor before use.

➤*Gum:* For persons who smoke less than 25 cigarettes a day, use 2 mg nicotine gum. For persons who smoke 25 cigarettes a day or more, start with the 4 mg nicotine gum. Refer to the dosing schedule below.

Instruct the patient to chew gum slowly until it tingles, then park it between the cheek and gum. When the tingle is gone, instruct the patient to begin chewing again until the tingle returns. Repeat the process until most of the tingle is gone (about 30 minutes).

Advise the patient not to eat or drink for 15 minutes before chewing the nicotine gum or while chewing a piece. To improve the chances of quitting, chew at least 9 pieces per day for the first 6 weeks. If there are strong and frequent cravings, use a second piece within the hour. However, do not continuously use 1 piece after another because this may cause hiccoughs, heartburn, nausea, or other side effects.

Stop using the nicotine gum at the end of 12 weeks. If the need to use nicotine gum is still present, consult a physician.

➤*Lozenges:* If the patient smokes his/her first cigarette more than 30 minutes after waking up, use 2 mg nicotine lozenges. If the patient smokes his/her first cigarette within 30 minutes of waking up, use 4 mg nicotine lozenges. Refer to the dosing schedule below.

Nicotine lozenge is a medicine and must be used a certain way to get the best results.

Instruct the patient to place the lozenge in the mouth and allow it to slowly dissolve (about 20 to 30 minutes). Minimize swallowing. Advise the patient not to chew or swallow the lozenge. The patient may feel a warm or tingling sensation. Advise the patient to occasionally move the lozenge from one side of the mouth to the other until completely dissolved.

Advise the patient not to eat or drink 15 minutes before using or while the lozenge is in the mouth. To improve the chances of quitting, use at least 9 lozenges/day for the first 6 weeks. Do not use more than 1 lozenge at a time or continuously use 1 lozenge after another because this may cause hiccoughs, heartburn, nausea, or other side effects.

Do not use more than 5 lozenges in 6 hours. Do not use more than 20 lozenges/day.

Stop using the nicotine lozenges at the end of 12 weeks. If you still feel the need to use nicotine lozenges, consult a physician.

➤*Dosing schedule:*

Weeks 1 to 6 – 1 piece of gum or lozenge every 1 to 2 hours.

Weeks 7 to 9 – 1 piece of gum or lozenge every 2 to 4 hours.

Weeks 10 to 12 – 1 piece of gum or lozenge every 4 to 8 hours.

➤*Disposal:*

Gum – Place used chewing pieces in a wrapper and dispose of in such a way to prevent its access by children or pets. Pieces of nicotine gum may have enough nicotine to make children or pets sick. In case of overdose, contact a medical professional or a poison control center.

Lozenges – Nicotine lozenges may have enough nicotine to make children or pets sick. If you need to remove the lozenge, wrap it in paper and throw away in the trash. In case of overdose, contact a medical professional or a poison control center.

➤*Storage/Stability:* Store at 20° to 25°C (68° to 77°F). Protect from light.

NICOTINE INHALATION SYSTEM

Rx	**Nicotrol Inhaler** (Pharmacia)	**Inhaler**: 4 mg delivered (10 mg/cartridge)	Kit contains mouthpiece, storage trays each containing 6 cartridges, plastic storage case, and patient information leaflet. In 42s and 168s.

NICOTINE — INHALATION SYSTEM

For complete prescribing information, refer to the Nicotine group monograph.

Indications

➤*Smoking cessation:* As an aid in smoking cessation for the relief of nicotine withdrawal symptoms. Inhaler therapy is recommended for use as part of a comprehensive behavioral smoking cessation program.

Administration and Dosage

➤*Approved by the FDA:* May 2, 1997.

Patients must desire to stop smoking and should be instructed to stop smoking completely as they begin using the inhaler.

➤*Initial dosage:* The initial dosage of the nicotine inhaler is individualized. Patients may self-titrate to the level of nicotine they require. Most successful patients in the clinical trials used between 6 and 16 cartridges per day. Best effect was achieved by frequent continuous puffing (20 minutes). The recommended duration of treatment is 3 months, after which patients may be weaned from the inhaler by gradual reduction of the daily dose over the following 6 to 12 weeks.

Encourage patients to use at least 6 cartridges/day at least for the first 3 to 6 weeks of treatment. In clinical trials, the average daily dose was more than 6 (range, 3 to 18) cartridges for patients who successfully quit smoking. Additional doses may be needed to control the urge to smoke with a maximum of 16 cartridges daily for up to 12 weeks. Regular use of the inhaler during the first week of treatment may help patients adapt to the irritant effects of the product. Some patients may exhibit signs or symptoms of nicotine withdrawal or excess that will require an adjustment of the dosage.

➤*Gradual reduction of dose (up to 12 weeks):* Most patients will need to gradually discontinue the use of the inhaler after the initial treatment period. Gradual reduction of dose may begin after 12 weeks of initial treatment and may last for up to 12 weeks. Recommended strategies for discontinuing use include suggesting to patients that they use the product less frequently, keep a tally of daily usage, try to meet a steadily reducing target, or set a planned "quit date" for stopping use of the product.

➤*Individualization of dosage:* The goal of the inhaler therapy is complete abstinence. If a patient is unable to stop smoking by the fourth week of therapy, discontinue treatment.

Treat patients who are successfully abstinent on the inhaler at the selected dosage for up to 12 weeks, then gradually reduce use of the inhaler over the next 6 to 12 weeks. Some patients may not require gradual reduction of dosage and may abruptly stop treatment successfully. The safe use of this product for more than 6 months has not been established.

Controlled clinical trials of nicotine products suggest that palpitations, nausea, and sweating are more often symptoms of nicotine excess, whereas anxiety, nervousness, and irritability are more often symptoms of nicotine withdrawal.

➤*Safety and handling:* See patient information sheet for instructions on handling and disposal. After using the inhaler, carefully separate the mouthpiece, remove the used cartridge, and throw it away, out of the reach of children and pets. Store the mouthpiece in the plastic storage case for further use. The mouthpiece is reusable and should be cleaned regularly with soap and water.

➤*Storage/Stability:* Store at room temperature not to exceed 25°C (77°F). Protect cartridges from light.

NICOTINE NASAL SPRAY

Rx	**Nicotrol NS** (Pharmacia)	**Spray pump:** 0.5 mg nicotine/actuation (10 mg/mL)	Parabens, EDTA. Each unit has a glass container mounted with metered spray pump (delivers ≈ 200 applications). In 10 mL bottles.

NICOTINE — NASAL SPRAY

For complete prescribing information, refer to the Nicotine group monograph.

Indications

➤*Smoking cessation:* As an aid to smoking cessation for the relief of nicotine withdrawal symptoms. The nasal spray should be used as a part of a comprehensive behavioral smoking cessation program.

Safety and efficacy of continued use of nicotine nasal spray for periods longer than 6 months have not been adequately studied and such use is not recommended.

Administration and Dosage

➤*Approved by the FDA:* March 22, 1996.

Instruct patients to stop smoking completely when they begin using the product. Instruct them not to sniff, swallow, or inhale through the nose as the spray is being administered. They should also be advised to administer the spray with the head tilted back slightly.

➤*Dosage:* Each actuation of the nasal spray delivers a metered 50 mcL spray containing 0.5 mg nicotine. One dose is 1 mg of nicotine (2 sprays, 1 in each nostril). Start patients with 1 or 2 doses per hour, which may be increased up to a maximum recommended dose of 40 mg (80 sprays, somewhat less than ½ of the bottle) per day. For best results, encourage patients to use at least the recommended minimum of 8 doses/day, as less is unlikely to be effective. In clinical trials, the patients who successfully quit smoking used the product heavily when nicotine withdrawal was at its peak, sometimes up to the recommended maximum of 40 doses/day (in heavier smokers).

Nicotine Nasal Spray Dosing Recommendations

Maximum recommended duration of treatment	Recommended doses/hr	Maximum doses/hr	Maximum doses/day
3 months	1 to 2[1]	5	40

[1] One dose = 2 sprays (1 in each nostril). One dose delivers 1 mg of nicotine to the nasal mucosa.

➤*Discontinuation:* No tapering strategy has been shown to be optimal in clinical studies. Many patients simply stopped using the spray at their last clinic visit. Recommended strategies for discontinuation of use include suggesting the following to patients: Use only ½ a dose (1 spray) at a time, use the spray less frequently, keep a tally of daily usage, try to meet a steadily reducing usage target, skip a dose by not medicating every hour, or set a planned "quit date" for stopping use of the spray.

➤*Individualization of dosage:* The goal of the nasal spray therapy is complete abstinence. If a patient is unable to stop smoking by the fourth week of therapy, discontinue treatment. Regular use of the spray during the first week of treatment may help patients adapt to the irritant effects of the spray. Patients who are successfully abstinent on the nasal spray should be treated at the selected dosage for up to 8 weeks, following which use of the spray should be discontinued over the next 4 to 6 weeks. Some patients may not require gradual reduction of dosage and may abruptly stop treatment successfully. Treatment with the nasal spray for longer periods has not been shown to improve outcome, and the safety of use for periods longer than 6 months has not been established.

Controlled clinical trials of nicotine products suggest that palpitations, nausea, and sweating are more often symptoms of nicotine excess; whereas anxiety, nervousness, and irritability are more often symptoms of nicotine withdrawal.

➤*Safety and handling:* Take care in handling the nasal spray during periods of opening and closing the container. It may break if dropped. If this occurs, the spill should be cleaned up immediately with an absorbent cloth/paper towel. Take care to avoid contact of the solution with the skin and wash the area several times. Should even a small amount of the nasal spray come in contact with the skin, lips, mouth, eyes, or ears, immediately rinse the affected areas with water. Dispose of used bottles with the child-resistant cap in place. Used bottles should be disposed of in such a way as to prevent access by children or pets.

➤*Storage/Stability:* Store at room temperature not to exceed 30°C (86°F).

BUPROPION HYDROCHLORIDE

Refer to the Antidepressants section for complete prescribing information.

RILUZOLE

Rx	**Rilutek** (Rhone-Poulenc Rorer)	**Tablets:** 50 mg	(RPR 202). White. Capsule shape. Film coated. In 60s.

RILUZOLE— ORAL

Indications

➤*Amyotrophic lateral sclerosis:* Riluzole is indicated for the treatment of patients with amyotrophic lateral sclerosis (ALS). Riluzole extends survival or time to tracheostomy.

Administration and Dosage

➤*Approved by the FDA:* December 12, 1995.

The recommended dose for riluzole is 50 mg every 12 hours. No increased benefit can be expected from higher daily doses, but adverse reactions are increased.

Riluzole tablets should be taken at least an hour before, or 2 hours after, a meal to avoid a food-related decrease in bioavailability.

➤*Storage/Stability:* Store at controlled room temperature 20° to 25°C (68° to 77°F) and protect from bright light.

Keep out of the reach of children.

Actions

➤*Pharmacology:* The mode of action of riluzole is unknown. Its pharmacological properties include the following, some of which may be related to its effect: An inhibitory effect on glutamate release, inactivation of voltage-dependent sodium channels, and ability to interfere with intracellular events that follow transmitter binding at excitatory amino acid receptors. Riluzole has also been shown, in a single study, to delay median time to death in a transgenic mouse model of ALS. These mice express human superoxide dismutase bearing one of the mutations found in one of the familial forms of human ALS.

It is also neuroprotective in various in vivo experimental models of neuronal injury involving excitotoxic mechanisms. In in vitro tests, riluzole protected cultured rat motor neurons from the excitotoxic effects of glutamic acid and prevented the death of cortical neurons induced by anoxia.

Due to its blockade of glutamatergic neurotransmission, riluzole also exhibits myorelaxant and sedative properties in animal models at doses of 30 mg/kg (about 20 times the recommended human daily dose) and anticonvulsant properties at a dose of 2.5 mg/kg (about 2 times the recommended human daily dose).

➤*Pharmacokinetics:*

Absorption/Distribution – Riluzole is well-absorbed (approximately 90%), with average absolute oral bioavailability of about 60% (CV = 30%). Pharmacokinetics are linear over a dose range of 25 to 100 mg given every 12 hours. A high-fat meal decreases absorption, reducing AUC by about 20% and peak blood levels by about 45%. The mean elimination half-life of riluzole is 12 hours (CV = 35%) after repeated doses. With multiple-dose administration, riluzole accumulates in plasma by about 2-fold, and steady-state is reached in less than 5 days. Riluzole is 96% bound to plasma proteins, mainly to albumin and lipoproteins over the clinical concentration range. The 50 mg market tablet was equivalent, with respect to AUC, to the tablet used in the dose ranging clinical trials, while the C_{max} was approximately 30% higher. Both tablets have been used in clinical trials. However, if doses greater than those recommended are given, it is likely that higher plasma levels will be achieved, the safety of which has not been established. No increased benefit can be expected from higher daily doses, but adverse reactions are increased.

Metabolism/Excretion – Riluzole is extensively metabolized to 6 major and a number of minor metabolites, not all of which have been identified. Some metabolites appear pharmacologically active in in vitro assays. The metabolism of riluzole is mostly hepatic and consists of cytochrome P450-dependent hydroxylation and glucuronidation.

There is marked interindividual variability in the clearance of riluzole, probably attributable to variability of CYP 1A2 activity, the principal isozyme involved in N-hydroxylation.

In vitro studies using liver microsomes show that hydroxylation of the primary amine group producing N-hydroxyriluzole is the main metabolic pathway in human, monkey, dog and rabbit. In humans, cytochrome P450 1A2 is the principal isozyme involved in N-hydroxylation. In vitro studies predict that CYP2D6, CYP2C19, CYP3A4 and CYP2E1 are unlikely to contribute significantly to riluzole metabolism in humans. Whereas direct glucuroconjugation of riluzole (involving the glucurotransferase isoform UGT-HP4) is very slow in human liver microsomes, N-hydroxyriluzole is readily conjugated at the hydroxylamine group resulting in the formation of O– (greater than 90%) and N-glucuronides.

Following a single 150 mg dose of ^{14}C-riluzole to 6 healthy males, 90% and 5% of the radioactivity was recovered in the urine and feces, respectively, over a period of 7 days. Glucuronides accounted for more than 85% of the metabolites in urine. Only 2% of a riluzole dose was recovered in the urine as unchanged drug.

Special populations –

Gender: CYP1A2 activity has been reported to be lower in women than in men. Therefore, a gender effect on riluzole kinetics may be expected in women, resulting in higher blood concentrations of riluzole and its metabolites. No gender effect on favorable or adverse effects of riluzole was seen in controlled trials, however.

Race: Clearance of riluzole in Japanese subjects native to Japan was found to be 50% lower as compared to white patients after normalizing for body weight. Although it is not clear if this difference is due to genetic or environmental factors (eg, smoking, alcohol, coffee, dietary preferences), it is possible that Japanese subjects may possess a lower capacity (oxidative or conjugative) for metabolizing riluzole. There are no studies, however, of lower doses in Japanese subjects.

Hepatic and renal disease: Since riluzole is extensively metabolized and subsequently excreted in the urine, it is likely that functional hepatic and renal impairment will reduce the clearance of riluzole and its metabolites and give higher plasma levels.

Contraindications

Riluzole is contraindicated in patients who have a history of severe hypersensitivity reactions to riluzole or any of the tablet components.

Warnings

➤*Neutropenia:* Among approximately 4000 patients given riluzole for ALS, there were 3 cases of marked neutropenia (absolute neutrophil count less than 500/mm^3), all seen within the first 2 months of riluzole treatment. In 1 case, neutrophil counts rose on continued treatment. In a second case, counts rose after therapy was stopped. A third case was more complex, with marked anemia as well as neutropenia and the etiology of both is uncertain. Patients should be warned to report any febrile illness to their physicians. The report of a febrile illness should prompt treating physicians to check white blood cell counts.

➤*Hepatic effects:* Riluzole, even in patients without a history of liver disease, causes serum aminotransferase elevations. Experience in almost 800 ALS patients indicates that about 50% of riluzole-treated patients will experience at least one ALT/SGPT level above the upper limit of normal, about 8% will have elevations greater than 3 × ULN, and about 2% of patients will have elevations greater than 5 X ULN. A single non-ALS patient with epilepsy treated with concomitant carbamazepine and phenobarbital experienced marked, rapid elevations of liver enzymes with jaundice (ALT 26 × ULN, AST 17 × ULN, and bilirubin 11 × ULN) 4 months after starting riluzole; these returned to normal 7 weeks after treatment discontinuation.

Maximum increases in serum ALT usually occurred within 3 months after the start of riluzole therapy and were usually transient when less than 5 times ULN. In trials, if ALT levels were less than 5 times ULN, treatment continued, and ALT levels usually returned to below 2 times ULN within 2 to 6 months. Treatment in studies was discontinued, however, if ALT levels exceeded 5 × ULN, so that there is no experience with continued treatment of ALS patients once ALT values exceed 5 times ULN. There were rare instances of jaundice.

Liver chemistries should be monitored.

➤*Renal/Hepatic function impairment:* Riluzole should be prescribed with care in patients with current evidence or history of abnormal liver function indicated by significant abnormalities in serum transaminase (ALT; AST), bilirubin, or gamma-glutamate transferase (GGT) levels. Since riluzole is extensively metabolized and subsequently excreted in the urine, it is likely that functional hepatic and renal impairment will reduce the clearance of riluzole and its metabolites and give higher plasma levels. Baseline elevations of several LFTs (especially elevated bilirubin) should preclude the use of riluzole.

➤*Mutagenesis:* The genotoxic potential of riluzole was evaluated in the bacterial mutagenicity (Ames) test, the mouse lymphoma mutation assay in L5178Y cells, the in vitro chromosomal aberration assay in human lymphocytes and the in vivo rat cytogenetic assay and in vivo mouse micronucleus assay in bone marrow. There was no evidence of mutagenic or clastogenic potential in the Ames test, the mouse lymphoma assay, or the in vivo assays in the mouse and rat. There was an equivocal clastogenic response in the in vitro lymphocyte chromosomal aberration assay.

➤*Fertility impairment:* Riluzole impaired fertility when administered to male and female rats prior to and during mating at an oral dose of 15 mg/kg or 1.5 times the maximum daily dose on a mg/m^2 basis.

➤*Elderly:* Age-related compromised renal and hepatic function may cause a decrease in clearance of riluzole. In controlled clinical trials, about 30% of patients were over 65 years. There were no differences in adverse reactions between younger and older patients.

➤*Pregnancy:* *Category C.* Oral administration of riluzole to pregnant animals during the period of organogenesis caused embryotoxicity in rats and rabbits at doses of 27 mg/kg and 60 mg/kg, respectively, or 2.6 and 11.5 times, respectively, the recommended maximum human daily dose on a mg/m^2 basis. Evidence of maternal toxicity was also observed at these doses.

When administered to rats prior to and during mating (males and females) and throughout gestation and lactation (females), riluzole produced adverse effects on pregnancy (decreased implantations, increased intrauterine death) and offspring viability and growth at an oral dose of 15 mg/kg or 1.5 times the maximum daily dose on a mg/m^2 basis. There are no adequate and well-controlled studies in pregnant women. Riluzole should be used during pregnancy only if the potential benefit justifies the potential risk to the fetus.

➤*Lactation:* In rat studies, ^{14}C-riluzole was detected in maternal milk. It is not known whether riluzole is excreted in human breast milk. Because many drugs are excreted in human milk, and because the potential for serious adverse reactions in nursing infants from riluzole is unknown, women should be advised not to breastfeed during treatment with riluzole.

➤*Children:* The safety and the efficacy of riluzole in pediatric patients have not been established.

RILUZOLE— ORAL

Precautions

➤*Monitoring:* It is recommended that serum aminotransferases, including ALT levels, be measured before and during riluzole therapy. Serum ALT levels should be evaluated every month during the first 3 months of treatment, every 3 months during the remainder of the first year, and periodically thereafter. Serum ALT levels should be evaluated more frequently in patients who develop elevations. Baseline elevations of several LFTs (especially elevated bilirubin) should preclude the use of riluzole. Riluzole, even in patients without a history of liver disease, causes serum aminotransferase elevations. Experience in almost 800 ALS patients indicates that about 50% of riluzole-treated patients will experience at least one ALT level above the upper limit of normal, about 8% will have elevations greater than 3 × ULN, and about 2% of patients will have elevations greater than 5 X ULN. A single non-ALS patient with epilepsy treated with concomitant carbamazepine and phenobarbital experienced marked, rapid elevations of liver enzymes with jaundice (ALT 26 × ULN, AST 17 × ULN, and bilirubin 11 × ULN) 4 months after starting riluzole; these returned to normal 7 weeks after treatment discontinuation.

As noted in Warnings, there is no experience with continued treatment of patients once ALT exceeds 5 × ULN. If a decision is made to continue to treat these patients, frequent monitoring (at least weekly) of complete liver function is recommended. Treatment should be discontinued if ALT exceeds 10 × ULN or if clinical jaundice develops. Because there is no experience with rechallenge of patients who have had riluzole discontinued for ALT greater than 5 × ULN, no recommendations about restarting riluzole can be made.

➤*Hematologic effects:* In the 2 controlled trials in patients with ALS, the frequency with which values for hemoglobin, hematocrit, and erythrocyte counts fell below the lower limit of normal was greater in riluzole-treated patients than in placebo-treated patients; however, these changes were mild and transient. The proportions of patients observed with abnormally low values for these parameters showed a dose-response relationship. Only 1 patient was discontinued from treatment because of severe anemia. The significance of this finding is unknown.

➤*Special risk:* Riluzole should be used with caution in patients with concomitant liver or renal insufficiency. In particular, in cases of riluzole-induced hepatic injury manifested by elevated liver enzymes, the effect of the hepatic injury on riluzole metabolism is unknown.

Riluzole should be used with caution in elderly patients whose hepatic or renal functions may be compromised due to age. Also, females and Japanese patients may possess a lower metabolic capacity to eliminate riluzole compared to males and white subjects, respectively.

➤*Hazardous tasks:* Patients should be warned about the potential for dizziness, vertigo, or somnolence and advised not to drive or operate machinery until they have gained sufficient experience on riluzole to gauge whether or not it affects their mental or motor performance adversely.

Drug Interactions

➤*CYP450 system:* In vitro studies using human liver microsomal preparations suggest that CYP1A2 is the principal isozyme involved in the initial oxidative metabolism of riluzole and, therefore, potential interactions may occur when riluzole is given concurrently with agents that affect CYP1A2 activity. Potential inhibitors of CYP1A2 (eg, caffeine, phenacetin, theophylline, amitriptyline, quinolones) could decrease the rate of riluzole elimination, while inducers of CYP1A2 (eg, cigarette smoke, charcoal-broiled food, rifampicin, omeprazole) could increase the rate of riluzole elimination.

Potential interactions may occur when riluzole is given concurrently with other agents which are also metabolized primarily by CYP1A2 (eg, theophylline, caffeine, tacrine). Currently, it is not known whether riluzole has any potential for enzyme induction in humans.

Adverse Reactions

The most commonly observed adverse associated with the use of riluzole more frequently than placebo-treated patients were asthenia, nausea, dizziness, decreased lung function, diarrhea, abdominal pain, pneumonia, vomiting, vertigo, circumoral paresthesia, anorexia, and somnolence. Asthenia, nausea, dizziness, diarrhea, anorexia, vertigo, somnolence, and circumoral paresthesia were dose related.

Approximately 14% (n = 141) of the 982 individuals with ALS who received riluzole in premarketing clinical trials discontinued treatment because of an adverse experience. Of those patients who discontinued due to adverse events, the most commonly reported were nausea, abdominal pain, constipation, and ALT elevations. In a dose-response study in ALS patients, the rates of discontinuation of riluzole for asthenia, nausea, abdominal pain, and ALT elevation were dose related.

➤*Incidence in controlled ALS clinical studies:* The table below lists treatment-emergent signs and symptoms that occurred in at least 2% of patients with ALS treated with riluzole (n = 794) participating in placebo-controlled trials and were numerically greater in the patients treated with riluzole 100 mg/day than with placebo or for which a dose response relationship is suggested.

Adverse Reactions Occurring in Placebo-Controlled Clinical Trials

	Percent of patients reporting events			
Body system/adverse reaction	Riluzole 50 mg/day (n = 237)	Riluzole 100 mg/day (n = 313)	Riluzole 200 mg/day (n = 244)	Placebo (n = 320)
Cardiovascular				
Hypertension	6.8%	5.1%	3.3%	4.1%
Palpitation	0.4%	0.6%	1.2%	0.9%
Phlebitis	0.4%	1.0%	0.8%	0.3%
Postural hypotension	0.8%	0%	1.6%	0.6%
Tachycardia	1.3%	2.6%	2%	1.3%
CNS				
Circumoral paresthesia	1.3%	1.6%	3.3%	0%
Depression	4.2%	4.5%	6.1%	5.0%
Dizziness	5.1%	3.8%	12.7%	2.5%
Dry mouth	3%	3.5%	2.0%	3.4%
Hypertonia	5.9%	6.1%	5.3%	5.9%
Insomnia	2.1%	3.5%	2.9%	3.4%
Somnolence	0.8%	1.9%	4.1%	1.3%
Vertigo	2.5%	1.9%	4.5%	0.9%
Dermatologic				
Alopecia	0%	1.0%	1.2%	0.6%
Eczema	0.8%	1.6%	1.6%	0.6%
Exfoliative dermatitis	0%	0.6%	1.2%	0%
Pruritus	3.8%	3.8%	2.5%	3.1%
GI				
Anorexia	3.8%	3.2%	8.6%	3.8%
Diarrhea	5.5%	2.9%	9%	3.1%
Dyspepsia	2.5%	3.8%	6.1%	5%
Flatulence	2.5%	2.6%	2%	1.9%
Nausea	12.2%	16.3%	20.5%	10.6%
Oral moniliasis	0.4%	0.6%	1.2%	0.3%
Stomatitis	0.8%	1%	1.2%	0%
Tooth disorder	0%	1%	1.2%	0.3%
Vomiting	4.2%	4.2%	4.5%	1.6%
GU				
Dysuria	0%	1%	1.2%	0.3%
Urinary tract infection	2.5%	2.6%	4.5%	2.2%
Metabolic/nutritional				
Peripheral edema	4.2%	2.9%	3.3%	2.2%
Weight loss	4.6%	4.8%	3.7%	4.7%
Musculoskeletal				
Arthralgia	5.1%	3.5%	1.6%	3.4%
Respiratory				
Decreased lung function	13.1%	10.2%	16%	9.4%
Rhinitis	8.9%	6.4%	7.8%	6.3%
Increased cough	2.1%	2.6%	3.7%	1.6%
Sinusitis	0.4%	1%	1.6%	0.9%
Miscllaneous				
Asthenia	14.8%	19.2%	20.1%	12.2%
Headache	8%	7.3%	7%	6.6%
Abdominal pain	6.8%	5.1%	7.8%	3.8%
Back pain	1.7%	3.2%	4.1%	2.5%
Aggravation reaction	0.4%	1.3%	2%	0.9%
Malaise	0.4%	0.6%	1.2%	0%

➤*Other adverse events observed:* Other events which occurred in more than 2% of patients treated with riluzole 100 mg/day but equally or more frequently in the placebo group included accidental injury, apnea, bronchitis, constipation, death, dysphagia, dyspnea, flu syndrome, heart arrest, increased sputum, pneumonia, and respiratory disorder.

The overall adverse event profile for riluzole was similar between females and males, and was independent of age. Because the largest nonwhite racial subgroup was only 2% of patients exposed to riluzole (18/794) in placebo-controlled trials, there are insufficient data to support a statement regarding the distribution of adverse experience reports by race. In ALS studies, dizziness did occur more commonly in females (11%) than in males (4%). There was not a difference between females and males in the rates of discontinuation of riluzole for individual adverse experiences.

➤*Other adverse events observed during all clinical trials:* Events are further classified within body system categories and enumerated in order of decreasing frequency using the following definitions: Frequent adverse events are defined as those occurring in at least 1/100 patients; infrequent adverse events are those occurring in 1/100 to 1/1000 patients; rare adverse events are those occurring in fewer than 1/1000 patients.

In the following information, an event in which the frequency is less than or equal to placebo is marked with an asterisk.

Cardiovascular –

Infrequent: Syncope*, hypotension, heart failure, migraine, peripheral vascular disease, angina pectoris*, myocardial infarction*, ventricular extrasystoles, cerebral hemorrhage, atrial fibrillation*, bundle branch block, congestive heart failure, pericarditis, lower extremity embolus, myocardial ischemia*, shock*.

RILUZOLE— ORAL

Rare: Bradycardia, cerebral ischemia, hemorrhage, mesenteric artery occlusion, subarachnoid hemorrhage, supraventricular tachycardia*, thrombosis, ventricular fibrillation, ventricular tachycardia.

CNS –

Frequent: Agitation*, tremor.

Infrequent: Hallucinations, personality disorder*, abnormal thinking*, coma, paranoid reaction*, manic reaction, ataxia, extrapyramidal syndrome, hypokinesia, urinary retention, emotional lability, delusions, apathy, hypesthesia, incoordination, confusion*, convulsion, leg cramps, amnesia, dysarthria, increased libido, stupor, subdural hematoma, abnormal gait, delirium, depersonalization, facial paralysis, hemiplegia, decreased libido, myoclonus.

Rare: Abnormal dreams, acute brain syndrome, CNS depression, dementia, cerebral embolism, euphoria*, hypotonia, ileus*, peripheral neuritis, psychosis*, psychotic depression, schizophrenic reaction, trismus, wristdrop.

Dermatologic –

Infrequent: Skin ulceration, urticaria, psoriasis, seborrhea*, skin disorder, fungal dermatitis*.

Rare: Angioedema, contact dermatitis, erythema multiforme, furunculosis*, skin moniliasis, skin granuloma, skin nodule.

Endocrine –

Infrequent: Diabetes mellitus, thyroid neoplasia.

Rare: Diabetes insipidus, parathyroid disorder.

GI –

Infrequent: Increased appetite, intestinal obstruction*, fecal impaction, GI hemorrhage, GI ulceration, gastritis*, fecal incontinence, jaundice, hepatitis, glossitis, gum hemorrhage*, pancreatitis, tenesmus, esophageal stenosis.

Rare: Cheilitis*, cholecystitis, hematemesis, melena*, biliary pain, proctitis, pseudomembranous enterocolitis, enlarged salivary gland, tongue discoloration, tooth caries.

GU –

Infrequent: Urinary urgency, urine abnormality, urinary incontinence, kidney calculus, hematuria, impotence, prostate carcinoma, kidney pain, metrorrhagia, priapism.

Rare: Amenorrhea, breast abscess, breast pain, nephritis*, nocturia, pyelonephritis, enlarged uterine fibroids, uterine hemorrhage, vaginal moniliasis.

Hematologic / Lymphatic –

Infrequent: Anemia*, leukocytosis, leukopenia, ecchymosis.

Rare: Neutropenia, aplastic anemia, cyanosis, hypochromic anemia, iron deficiency anemia, lymphadenopathy, petechiae*, purpura.

Lab test abnormalities –

Infrequent: Increased gamma glutamyl transferase, abnormal liver function/tests, increased alkaline phosphatase, positive direct Coombs test, increased gamma globulins.

Rare: Increased lactic dehydrogenase.

Metabolic / Nutritional –

Infrequent: Gout*, respiratory acidosis, edema, thirst*, hypokalemia, hyponatremia, weight gain*.

Rare: Generalized edema, hypercalcemia, hypercholesteremia.

Musculoskeletal –

Infrequent: Arthrosis, myasthenia*, bone neoplasm.

Rare: Bone necrosis, osteoporosis, tetany.

Respiratory –

Infrequent: Hiccup, pleural disorder*, asthma, epistaxis, hemoptysis, yawn, hyperventilation*, lung edema*, hypoventilation*, lung carcinoma, hypoxia, laryngitis, pleural effusion, pneumothorax*, respiratory moniliasis, stridor.

Special senses –

Infrequent: Amblyopia, ophthalmitis.

Rare: Blepharitis, cataract, deafness, diplopia*, ear pain, glaucoma, hyperacusis, photophobia, taste loss, vestibular disorder.

Miscellaneous –

Frequent: Hostility*.

Infrequent: Abscess*, sepsis*, photosensitivity reaction*, cellulitis, face edema*, hernia, peritonitis, attempted suicide, injection site reaction, chills*, flu syndrome, intentional injury, enlarged abdomen, neoplasm.

Rare: Acrodynia, hypothermia, moniliasis*, rheumatoid arthritis.

Overdosage

➤*Symptoms:* Experience with riluzole overdose in humans is limited. Methemoglobinemia of undetermined origin has been reported in association with a riluzole overdose many times the recommended daily dose. This was rapidly reversible after treatment with methylene blue. The estimated oral median lethal dose is 94 mg/kg and 39 mg/kg for male mice and rats, respectively.

➤*Treatment:* No specific antidote or information on treatment of overdosage with riluzole is available. In the event of overdose, riluzole therapy should be discontinued immediately. Treatment should be supportive and directed toward alleviating symptoms.

Patient Information

Patients should be advised to report any febrile illness to their physicians The report of a febrile illness should prompt treating physicians to check white blood cell counts.

Patients and caregivers should be advised that riluzole should be taken on a regular basis and at the same time of the day (eg, in the morning and evening) each day. If a dose is missed, take the next tablet as originally planned.

Patients should be warned about the potential for dizziness, vertigo, or somnolence and advised not to drive or operate machinery until they have gained sufficient experience on riluzole to gauge whether or not it affects their mental or motor performance adversely.

Whether alcohol increases the risk of serious hepatotoxicity with riluzole is unknown; therefore, patients being treated with riluzole should be discouraged from drinking excessive amounts of alcohol.

Patients should also be made aware that riluzole should be stored at temperatures between 20° to 25°C (68° to 77°F) and protected from bright light. Riluzole must be kept out of the reach of children.

PHYSICAL ADJUNCTS

HYALURONIC ACID DERIVATIVES

Rx	**Euflexxa** (Ferring)	**Solution:** 10 mg sodium hyaluronate per mL[a]	In 2 mL prefilled syringes.
Rx	**Hyalgan** (Sanofi-Synthelabo)	**Solution:** 20 mg sodium hyaluronate per 2 mL[b]	In 2 mL vials and prefilled syringes.
Rx	**Supartz** (Smith & Nephew)	**Solution:** 25 mg sodium hyaluronate per 2.5 mL[c]	In 2.5 mL prefilled syringe.
Rx	**Synvisc** (Wyeth)	**Solution:** 16 mg hylan polymers (hylan G-F 20) per 2 mL[d]	In 2 mL glass syringe with 3 disposable syringes.
Rx	**Orthovisc** (Ortho Biotech)	**Injection:** 30 mg hyaluronan,[e] 18 mg sodium chloride	In 2 mL single use vials.

[a] Molecular weight is 2,400,000 to 3,600,000 daltons.
[b] Molecular weight is 500,000 to 730,000 daltons.
[c] Molecular weight is 620,000 to 1,170,000 daltons.
[d] Molecular weight is 6,000,000 daltons on average.
[e] Molecular weight is 1,000,000 to 2,900,000 daltons.

HYALURONIC ACID DERIVATIVES

Sodium hyaluronate is also used as an ophthalmic agent. For complete prescribing information, refer to the individual monograph in the Ophthalmics section.

Indications

➤*Osteoarthritis symptoms:* For the treatment of pain in osteoarthritis of the knee in patients who have failed to respond adequately to conservative nonpharmacologic therapy and simple analgesics (eg, acetaminophen).

Administration and Dosage

➤*Approved by the FDA:* May 28, 1997.

Administer 2 mL (2.5 mL for *Supartz*) by intra-articular injection in affected knee once weekly for the recommended number of injections per treatment cycle. If treatment is bilateral, use a separate 2 mL (2.5 mL for *Supartz*) vial/syringe for each knee. Do not prepare injection site with skin disinfectants containing quarternary ammonium salts; precipitation of drug can occur. Do not give other intra-articular injectables concomitantly (see Warnings).

➤*Treatment cycle:*

Euflexxa – Give a dose of 2 mL injected intra-articularly into the affected knee at weekly intervals for 3 weeks for a total of 3 injections. Remove joint effusion if present.

Hyalgan – Give a total of 5 injections/treatment cycle using a 20 gauge needle. Inject local anesthetic (eg, lidocaine) SC prior to administration. Studies with a follow-up period of 60 days have shown that patients may experience benefit with 3 injections given at weekly intervals.

Supartz – Give a total of 5 injections/treatment cycle using a 22 to 23 gauge needle. Injection of a local anesthetic (eg, lidocaine) SC prior to administration may be recommended.

Synvisc – Give a total of 3 injections/treatment cycle using an 18 to 22 gauge needle. Remove synovial fluid or effusion before each injection.

Orthovisc – Inject into the knee joint in a series of intra-articular injections 1 week apart for 3 or 4 injections.

➤*Joint effusion:* If present, remove effusion before administering therapy. Do not use the same syringe for removing fluid and injecting hyaluronic acid derivatives. However, use the same needle for injecting **hylan G-F 20**.

➤*Storage / Stability:*

Euflexxa – For single use only. Do not resterilize. Twenty to 30 minutes before use, remove the product box from the refrigerator, remove the blister pack from the box, and allow the syringe to come to room temperature. Be sure to return any syringes not intended for use to the refrigerator. Store refrigerated at 2° to 8°C (36° to 46°F). Protect from light. Do not freeze.

HYALURONIC ACID DERIVATIVES

Hyalgan and *Supartz* – Products are intended for single use; use immediately once opened and discard any unused portion. Store in original package below 25°C (less than 77°F); do not freeze.

Synvisc – Products are intended for single use; use immediately once opened and discard any unused portion. Store in original package below 30°C (less than 86°F); protect from light; do not freeze.

Actions

➤*Pharmacology:* Hyaluronic acid is a naturally occurring polysaccharide of the glycosaminoglycan family containing repeating disaccharide units of sodium-glucuronate-N-acetylglucosamine. Certain disease states can affect the integrity and rheology of synovial fluid and in the case of osteoarthritis (OA), decrease its viscosity and elasticity. This results from both a decrease in the molecular size and concentration of hyaluronan within the synovial fluid. Intra-articular viscosupplementation with hyaluronic acid, high molecular weight fractions of purified natural sodium hyaluronate, and cross-linked polymers of hyaluronan known as hylans are aimed at improving the elasticity and viscosity of synovial fluid for the treatment of OA. Exact mechanism(s) of action of hyaluronic acid derivatives is/are unknown.

➤*Pharmacokinetics:* The molecular weight of the agent may have an effect on its half-life. The higher the molecular weight, the longer the half-life may be. Higher molecular weights also appear to lead to increased elasticity of the synovial fluid.

Contraindications

Hypersensitivity to hyaluronan or any components of the product; infections or skin diseases in the area of the injection site; concomitant skin disinfectants containing quarternary ammonium salts (see Warnings).

Warnings

➤*Quarternary ammonium salts:* Avoid concomitant use of disinfectants for skin preparation containing quarternary ammonium salts; precipitation of drug may occur.

➤*Intra-articular administration:* Administer by intra-articular injection only. Avoid intravascular, extra-articular, synovial tissue and capsule administration; rare systemic adverse events have been reported with **hylan G-F 20**. Safety and efficacy of intra-articular administration in locations other than the knee and for conditions other than osteoarthritis have not been established. Use **hylan G-F 20** with caution when evidence of lymphatic or venous stasis exists in treatment leg. The safety and efficacy of **hylan G-F 20** in severely inflamed knee joints have not been established.

Do not coadminister with other intra-articular injectables. Safety and efficacy have not been established and may be altered by dilutional effects.

➤*Inflammatory arthritis:* Transient increases in inflammation in the injected knee following injections with **sodium hyaluronate** have been reported in some patients with inflammatory arthritis (eg, rheumatoid or gouty arthritis).

➤*Hypersensitivity reactions:* Anaphylactoid reactions have occurred with **sodium hyaluronate**. The incidents resolved with favorable outcomes upon discontinuation of therapy. Five allergic reactions were reported in the **sodium hyaluronate** group. All 5 events were classified as mild to moderate. These were: Hayfever, reaction on face and neck, cutaneous reaction on forearms and knees, and an undefined mild allergy reaction. No anaphylactic reactions were observed.

➤*Pregnancy:* Safety and efficacy have not been established in pregnant women. Give to a pregnant woman only if potential benefits outweigh the potential risks.

➤*Lactation:* It is not known if hyaluronic acid derivatives are excreted in breast milk. Safety and efficacy have not been established in lactating women. Exercise caution when administering to a breastfeeding woman.

➤*Children:* Safety and efficacy have not been established.

Precautions

➤*Avian allergies:* These products are extracted from chicken/rooster combs. Use caution in patients allergic to avian proteins, feathers, and egg products.

➤*Joint effusion:* Remove joint effusion before using hyaluronic acid derivatives.

➤*Latex sensitivity:* Administer **hylan G-F 20** with caution to patients with a possible history of latex sensitivity, because the packaging contains dry natural rubber.

➤*Treatment cycle:* The efficacy of a single treatment cycle of less than the recommended number of injections has not been established; 5 injections of *Hylagan*, 5 injections of *Supartz*, 3 injections of *Synvisc*. Safety and efficacy of repeat cycles have not been established.

Adverse Reactions

➤*Hyalgan*:

CNS – Headache (18%).

GI – GI complaints (29%, severe in 2.4%).

Local – Injection site pain (23%); skin reaction, including ecchymosis and rash (14%); joint pain and swelling (13%, severe in 1.2%); pruritus (7%); positive bacterial cultures of aspirated effusion from the treated knee (1.2%).

➤*Supartz*:

CNS – Headache (4.4%); dizziness (1% to 4%).

GI – Abdominal pain, diarrhea, dyspepsia, nausea (1% to 4%).

Local – Injection site reaction, including application/injection site reaction, injection site inflammation, and purpura (5.7%); injection site pain (4.2%).

Musculoskeletal – Arthralgia (17.8%); arthropathy/arthrosis/arthritis (11%).

Respiratory – Upper respiratory infection, sinusitis, bronchitis, rhinitis (1% to 4%).

Miscellaneous – Back pain (6.5%); pain, non-specific (6%); flu-like symptoms, UTI, inflicted injury, leg pain, discomfort in legs, fall (1% to 4%).

➤*Synvisc*:

Dermatologic – Rash, thorax and back (2%); pruritus (2%).

Musculoskeletal – Calf cramps, muscle pain.

Local – Knee pain or swelling (2.2% of injections, 7.2% of patients).

Miscellaneous – Ankle edema, tonsillitis with nausea, low back sprain, hemorrhoid problems, tachyarrhythmia, phlebitis with varicosities.

➤*Postmarketing:*

Hyalgan –

Fever: Seven cases of fever were reported, in which 3 were associated with local reactions; pyogenic arthritis was ruled out for all 3 cases. All fever patients discontinued treatment and all resolved.

Shock: One patient reported incident of shock (hypotensive crisis). The incident resolved and treatment was continued.

Synvisc –

CNS: Headache, dizziness, chills, paresthesia, malaise (rare).

Dermatological: Rash; itching; hives (rare).

Local: The most common adverse events reported have been pain, swelling, and/or effusion in the injected knee. In some cases the effusion was considerable and caused pronounced pain. In some instances, patients have presented with knees that were tender, warm, and red. It is important to rule out infection or cystalline arthopathies in such cases. Synovial fluid aspirates of varying volumes have revealed a range of cell counts, from very few to over 50,000 cells/mm^3. Reported treatments included symptomatic therapy (eg, rest, ice, heat, elevation, simple analgesics, NSAIDs) and/or arthrocentesis. Intra-articular corticosteroids have been used when infection was excluded. Rarely, arthroscopy has been performed. The occurrence of post-injection effusion may be associated with patient history of effusion, advanced stage of disease, and/or the number of injections a patient receives. Reactions generally abate within a few days. Clinical benefit from the treatment may still occur after such reactions.

Miscellaneous: Nausea, fever, muscle cramps, peripheral edema, flushing facial edema, intra-articular infections, respiratory difficulties, thrombocytopenia (rare).

Patient Information

Provide patients with a copy of Patient Information sheet prior to use.

Inform patients that transient pain/swelling of the treated joint may occur.

Advise patients to avoid strenuous or prolonged (more than 1 hour) weight-bearing activities (eg, jogging, tennis) within 48 hours following treatment.

Advise patients receiving **hylan G-F 20** that transient effusion may occur. In some cases the effusion may be considerable and cause pronounced pain; advise patients to consult with physician if swelling is extensive.

HYALURONIC ACID DERIVATIVES, DERMAL

Rx	**Hylaform** (Inamed Aesthetics)	**Gel for injection**: 5.5 mg/mL (as hylan B)	In single-use, prefilled syringes.
Rx	**Restylane** (Medicis Aesthetics)	**Gel for injection**: 20 mg/mL	In single-use, prefilled syringes.

HYALURONIC ACID — INJECTION

Indications

➤*Facial wrinkles and folds:* Hyaluronic acid injection is indicated for mid-to-deep dermal implantation for the correction of moderate to severe facial wrinkles and folds, such as nasolabial folds.

Administration and Dosage

➤*Approved by the FDA:* December 12, 2003.

➤*Directions for use:*

Treatment procedure –

1.) It is necessary to counsel the patient and discuss the appropriate indication, risks, benefits and expected responses to the hyaluronic acid injection treatment. Advise the patient of the necessary precautions before commencing with the procedure.
2.) Assess the patient's need for pain management.
3.) Clean the area to be treated with alcohol or another suitable antiseptic solution.

HYALURONIC ACID — INJECTION

4.) Before injecting, press the rod carefully until a small droplet is visible at the tip of the needle.
5.) Hyaluronic acid injection is administered using a thin gauge needle (30 G × ½″). The needle is inserted at an approximate angle of 30° parallel to the length of the wrinkle or fold. The bevel of the needle should face upwards and the substance should be injected into the middle of the dermis. Tip: For mid-dermis placement, the contour of the needle should be visible but not the color of it. If hyaluronic acid injection is injected too deep or intramuscularly, the duration of the effect will be shorter. If hyaluronic acid injection is injected too superficially this may result in visible lumps and/or grayish discoloration.
6.) Inject hyaluronic acid injection applying even pressure on the plunger rod while slowly pulling the needle backwards. The wrinkle should be lifted and eliminated by the end of the injection. It is important that the injection is stopped just before the needle is pulled out of the skin to prevent material from leaking out or ending up too superficially in the skin.
7.) Only correct to 100% of the desired volume effect. Do not overcorrect. With cutaneous contour deformities the best results are obtained if the defect can be manually stretched to the point where it is eliminated. The degree and duration of the correction depend on the character of the defect treated, the tissue stress at the implant site, the depth of the implant in the tissue and the injection technique. Markedly indurated defects may be difficult to correct.
8.) The injection technique with regard to the depth of injection and the administered quantity may vary. The linear threading technique, serial puncture injections, or a combination of the 2 have been used with success.
9.) When the injection is completed, the treated site should be gently massaged so that it conforms to the contour of the surrounding tissues. If an overcorrection has occurred, massage the area firmly between your fingers or against an underlying superficial bone to obtain optimal results.
10.) If so called "blanching" is observed (ie, the overlying skin turns a whitish color), the injection should be stopped immediately and the area massaged until it returns to a normal color.
11.) If the wrinkle needs further treatment, the same procedure should be repeated with several punctures of the skin until a satisfactory result is obtained. Additional treatment with hyaluronic acid injection may be necessary to achieve the desired correction. With patients who have localized swelling, the degree of correction is sometimes difficult to judge at the time of treatment. In these cases, it is better to invite the patient to a touch-up session after 1 to 2 weeks.
12.) Typical usage for each treatment session is less than 2 mL per treatment site.
13.) If the treated area is swollen directly after the injection, an ice pack can be applied on the site for a short period.
14.) Patients may have mild to moderate injection site reactions, which typically resolve in few days.

➤*Storage / Stability:* Store at a temperature of up to 25°C (77°F). Do not freeze and protect from sunlight. Refrigeration is not needed.

Do not resterilize hyaluronic acid injection as this may damage or alter the product.Do not use if the package is damaged. Immediately return the damaged product to the manufacturer.

Contraindications

Hyaluronic acid injection is contraindicated for patients with severe allergies manifested by a history of anaphylaxis, or history or presence of multiple severe allergies. Hyaluronic acid injection contains trace amounts of gram-positive bacterial proteins, and is contraindicated for patients with a history of allergies to such material. Hyaluronic acid injection is contraindicated for use in breast augmentation, and for implantation into bone, tendon, ligament, or muscle. Hyaluronic acid injection must not be implanted into blood vessels. Implantation of hyaluronic acid injection into dermal vessels may cause vascular occlusion, infarction, or embolic phenomena.

Warnings

➤*Skin eruptions:* Use of hyaluronic acid injection at specific sites in which an active inflammatory process (skin eruptions such as cysts, pimples, rashes, or hives) or infection is present should be deferred until the inflammatory process has been controlled.

➤*Injection site reactions:* Injection site reaction to hyaluronic acid injection has been observed as consisting mainly of short-term inflammatory symptoms starting early after treatment and with less than 7 days duration.

➤*Superficial necrosis:* Localized superficial necrosis may occur after injection in the glabellar area. It is thought to result from the injury, obstruction, or compromise of blood vessels.

➤*Hypersensitivity reactions:* Hypersensitivity as an inflammatory reaction to hyaluronic acid injection has been observed with swelling, redness, tenderness, induration, and, rarely, acneform papules at the injection site.

➤*Pregnancy:* The safety of hyaluronic acid injection for use during pregnancy has not been established.

➤*Lactation:* The safety of hyaluronic acid injection for use in breastfeeding females has not been established.

➤*Children:* The safety of hyaluronic acid injection for use in patients under 18 years has not been established.

Precautions

Based on US clinical studies, patients should be limited to 1.5 mL per treatment site. The safety of injecting greater amounts has not been established.

The safety or effectiveness of hyaluronic acid injection for the treatment of anatomic regions other than naso-labial folds has not been established in controlled clinical studies.

➤*Long-term use:* Long-term safety and effectiveness of hyaluronic acid injection beyond 1 year have not been investigated in clinical trials.

➤*Infection:* As with all transcutaneous procedures, hyaluronic acid injection implantation carries a risk of infection. Standard precautions associated with injectable materials should be followed.

➤*Keloid formation and hypertrophic scarring:* The safety of hyaluronic acid injection in patients with increased susceptibility to keloid formation and hypertrophic scarring has not been studied. Hyaluronic acid injection should not be used in patients with known susceptibility to keloid formation or hypertrophic scarring.

➤*Photosensitivity / Cold weather:* The patient should be informed that he or she should minimize exposure of the treated area to excessive sun and UV lamp exposure and extreme cold weather until any initial swelling and redness has resolved.

➤*Other skin treatment:* If laser treatment, chemical peeling or any other procedure based on active dermal response is considered after treatment with hyaluronic acid injection there is a possible risk of eliciting an inflammatory reaction at the implant site. This also applies if hyaluronic acid injection is administered before the skin has healed completely after such a procedure.

➤*Special risk:* Hyaluronic acid injection should be used with caution in patients on immunosuppressive therapy.

Patients who are using substances that reduce coagulation, such as aspirin and nonsteroidal anti-inflammatory drugs (NSAIDs) may, as with any injection, experience increased bruising or bleeding at injection sites.

Adverse Reactions

In a study of 138 patients at 6 centers, adverse events reported in hyaluronic acid injection patient diaries during 14 days after treatment are reported in the following table. Patients in the study received hyaluronic acid injections in 1 side of the face, and a bovine collagen dermal filler (*Zyplast*) in the other side of the face:

Maximum Intensity of Symptoms after Initial Treatment, Patient Diary

	Hyaluronic acid injection side	*Zyplast* side	Hyaluronic acid injection side				*Zyplast* side			
	Total reporting symptoms	Total reporting symptoms	None	Mild	Moderate	Severe	None	Mild	Moderate	Severe
	n (%)	n (%)	n (%)	n (%)	n (%)	n (%)	n (%)	n (%)	n (%)	n (%)
Bruising	72 (52.2%)	67 (48.6%)	63 (45.6%)	32 (23.2%)	35 (25.4%)	5 (3.6%)	68 (49.3%)	43 (31.2%)	23 (16.7%)	1 (0.7%)
Redness	117 (84.8%)	117 (84.8%)	17 (12.3%)	56 (40.6%)	54 (39.1%)	7 (5.1%)	17 (12.3%)	72 (52.2%)	37 (26.8%)	8 (5.8%)
Swelling	130 (87%)	102 (73.9%)	14 (10.1%)	54 (39.1%)	61 (44.2%)	5 (3.6%)	32 (23.2%)	65 (47.1%)	35 (25.4%)	2 (1.4%)
Pain	79 (57.2%)	58 (42%)	55 (39.9%)	40 (29%)	34 (24.6%)	5 (3.6%)	76 (55.1%)	46 (33.3%)	10 (7.2%)	2 (1.4%)
Tenderness	107 (77.5%)	89 (64.5%)	27 (19.6%)	60 (43.5%)	43 (31.2%)	4 (2.9%)	45 (32.6%)	70 (50.7%)	17 (12.3%)	2 (1.4%)
Itching	42 (30.4%)	33 (23.9%)	91 (65.9%)	31 (22.5%)	11 (8%)	0 (0)	101 (73.2%)	27 (19.6%)	6 (4.4%)	0 (0)
Other	34 (24.6%)	33 (23.9%)	93 (67.4%)	14 (10.1%)	15 (10.9%)	5 (3.6%)	94 (68.1%)	20 (14.5%)	10 (7.2%)	3 (2.2%)

Events are reported as local events; because of the design (split-face) of the study, causality of the systemic adverse events cannot be assigned.

HYALURONIC ACID — INJECTION

Duration of Adverse Events after Initial Treatment, Patient Diary										
	Hyaluronic acid injection side	*Zyplast* side	Hyaluronic acid injection side				*Zyplast* side			
	Total reporting symptoms	Total reporting symptoms	Number of days				Number of days			
			1	2 to 7	8 to 13	14+	1	2 to 7	8 to 13	14+
	n (%)	n (%)	n (%)	n (%)	n (%)	n (%)	n (%)	n (%)	n (%)	n (%)
Bruising	72 (52.2%)	67 (48.6%)	7 (5.1%)	56 (40.6%)	6 (4.4%)	3 (2.2%)	7 (5.1%)	53 (38.4%)	5 (3.6%)	2 (1.4%)
Redness	117 (84.8%)	117 (84.8%)	19 (13.8%)	68 (49.3%)	18 (13%)	12 (8.7%)	19 (13.8%)	71 (51.4%)	15 (10.9%)	12 (8.7%)
Swelling	120 (87%)	102 (73.9%)	16 (11.6%)	84 (60.9%)	16 (11.6%)	4 (2.9%)	14 (10.1%)	70 (50.7%)	16 (11.6%)	2 (1.4%)
Pain	79 (57.2%)	58 (42%)	29 (21%)	48 (34.8%)	2 (1.4%)	0 (0)	31 (22.5%)	25 (18.1%)	1 (0.7%)	1 (0.7%)
Tenderness	107 (77.5%)	89 (64.5%)	21 (15.2%)	78 (56.5%)	6 (4.4%)	2 (1.4%)	27 (19.6%)	54 (39.1%)	6 (4.4%)	2 (1.4%)
Itching	42 (30.4%)	33 (23.9%)	11 (8%)	25 (18.1%)	6 (4.4%)	0 (0)	8 (5.8%)	22 (15.9%)	3 (2.2%)	0 (0)
Other	34 (24.6%)	33 (23.9%)	7 (5.1%)	23 (16.7%)	3 (2.2%)	1 (0.7%)	10 (7.2%)	15 (10.9%)	6 (4.4%)	2 (1.4%)

Other Adverse Events Reported in the Randomized Study from Physician Case Report Forms	
Description of adverse event type (WHO preferred term)	N (n = 138)
Inflicted injury	8
Sinusitis	7
Upper respiratory tract infection	6
Acne	5
Back pain	3
Depression	3
Depression aggravated	3
Tooth disorder	4
Bronchitis	2
Pneumonia	2
Dermatitis contact	2
Allergic reaction*	2
Arthralgia	2
Osteoporosis	2
Headache	2
Migraine	2

Other Adverse Events Reported in the Randomized Study from Physician Case Report Forms	
Description of adverse event type (WHO preferred term)	N (n = 138)
Herpes simplex	2
Hypercholesterolemia	2
Urinary incontinence	2

* One case of seasonal allergy, and 1 reaction to make-up in the peri-orbital area.

➤*Postmarketing adverse reactions:* In postmarketing surveillance in other countries, presumptive bacterial infections, inflammatory adverse events, allergic adverse events, and necrosis have been reported. Reported treatments have included systemic steroids, systemic antibiotics, and IV administrations of medications. Additionally, inflammatory reaction to hyaluronic acid injection has been observed with swelling, redness, tenderness, induration, and, rarely, acneform papules at the injection site with onset at 1 to several weeks after the initial treatment in previously unexposed individuals, and in less than 7 days following treatment in patients known to have been previously exposed. Average duration of this effect is 2 weeks. The manufacturer is conducting a post-approval study to determine the likelihood of hypersensitivity reactions for patients receiving hyaluronic acid injections.

Adverse reactions should be reported to the manufacturer at 1-866-222-1480.

HYALURONIDASE

Rx	**Vitrase** (ISTA Pharmaceuticals)	**Powder for injection, lyophilized:** 6,200 units (ovine source)	Lactose 5 mg. Preservative free. In single-use 5 mL vials with 1 mL syringe and 5 mcg filter needle.
Rx	**Amphadase** (Amphastar)	**Solution for injection**: 150 units/mL (bovine source)	Contains no more than 0.1 mg thimerosal. In 2 mL vials.
Rx	**Hydase** (PrimaPharm)		In 1 mL single-use vials.[a]
Rx	**Hylenex** (Baxter Anesthesia)	**Solution for injection**: 150 units/mL (recombinant human)	In 1 mL single-dose vials.[b]
Rx	**Vitrase** (ISTA Pharmaceuticals)	**Solution for injection**: 200 units/mL (ovine source)	Lactose 0.93 mg. Preservative free. In single-use 2 mL vials.

[a] With 8.5 mg sodium chloride, 1 mg EDTA, 0.4 mg calcium chloride, monobasic sodium phosphate buffer, sodium hydroxide.

[b] With 8.5 mg sodium chloride, 1.8 mg sodium phosphate dibasic dihydrate, 4.2 mg sodium hydroxide, 1 mg human serum albumin, 1 mg EDTA, 0.4 mg calcium chloride dihydrate.

HYALURONIDASE — INJECTION

Indications

➤*Absorption and dispersion of injected drugs:* As an adjuvant to increase the absorption and dispersion of other injected drugs.

➤*Hypodermoclysis:* For hypodermoclysis.

➤*Subcutaneous urography:* As an adjunct in subcutaneous urography for improving resorption of radiopaque agents.

➤*Unlabeled uses:* Treatment of vitreous hemorrhage and diabetic retinopathy.

Administration and Dosage

➤*Approved by the FDA:* March 22, 1950.

Administer hyaluronidase only as discussed below because its effects relative to absorption and dispersion of other drugs are not produced when it is administered intravenously (IV).

➤*Absorption and dispersion of injected drugs:* Absorption and dispersion of other injected drugs may be enhanced by adding 50 to 300 units, most typically hyaluronidase 150 units, to the injection solution.

When considering the administration of any other drug with hyaluronidase, it is recommended that appropriate references first be consulted to determine the usual precautions for the use of the other drug (eg, when epinephrine is injected along with hyaluronidase, observe precautions for the use of epinephrine in cardiovascular disease, thyroid disease, diabetes, digital nerve block, ischemia of the fingers and toes, etc).

➤*Incompatibilities:* Before adding hyaluronidase to a solution containing another drug, it is recommended that appropriate references be consulted regarding physical or chemical incompatibilities.

Furosemide, benzodiazepines, and phenytoin have been found to be incompatible with hyaluronidase.

➤*Hypodermoclysis:* One-hundred fifty units (*Vitrase* lyophilized powder for injection, *Hydase*, and *Amphadase* solution for injection) or 200 units (*Vitrase* solution for injection) will facilitate absorption of 1,000 mL or more of solution. As with all parenteral fluid therapy, observe effect closely, with same precautions for restoring fluid and electrolyte balance as in IV injections. Carefully adjust the dose, the rate of injection, and the type of solution (eg, saline, glucose, Ringer's) to the individual patient. When solutions devoid of inorganic electrolytes are given by hypodermoclysis, hypovolemia may occur. This may be prevented by using solutions containing adequate amounts of inorganic electrolytes or controlling the volume and speed of administration.

Children (3 years of age and younger) – Hyaluronidase may be added to small volumes of solution (up to 200 mL), such as small clysis for infants or solutions of drugs for subcutaneous injection. For infants and children younger than 3 years of age, limit the volume of a single clysis to 200 mL; in premature infants or during the neonatal period, do not exceed a daily dosage of 25 mL/kg of body weight; the rate of administration should not be greater than 2 mL/min. For older patients, the rate and volume of administration should not exceed those employed for IV infusion.

HYALURONIDASE — INJECTION

Administration – Insert needle with aseptic precautions. With tip lying free and movable between skin and muscle, begin clysis; fluid should start in readily without pain or lump. Then inject hyaluronidase into rubber tubing close to needle. An alternate method is to inject hyaluronidase under the skin prior to clysis.

➤*Subcutaneous urography:* The subcutaneous route of administration of urographic contrast media is indicated when IV administration cannot be successfully accomplished, particularly in infants and small children. With the patient prone, hyaluronidase 75 units is injected subcutaneously over each scapula, followed by injection of the contrast medium at the same sites.

➤*Reconstitution / Dilution:*

Hyaluronidase lyophilized powder – Reconstitute hyaluronidase in the vial to a concentration of 1,000 units/mL of sodium chloride injection by adding 6.2 mL of solution to the vial. Prior to administration, further dilute the reconstituted solution to the desired concentration, commonly 150 units/mL (see the following table). Use the resulting solution immediately after preparation.

A 1 mL syringe and a 5 micron filter needle are supplied in the hyaluronidase kit. Following reconstitution as described above, apply the 5 micron filter needle to the 1 mL syringe. Draw the desired amount of hyaluronidase into the syringe, and dilute according to the following table. Remove the filter needle and apply a needle appropriate for the intended injection.

Desired Concentration	Amount of Hyaluronidase Reconstituted Solution (1,000 units/mL)	Additional Sodium Chloride Injection
50 units/mL	0.05 mL	0.95 mL
75 units/mL	0.075 mL	0.925 mL
150 units/mL	0.15 mL	0.85 mL
300 units/mL	0.3 mL	0.7 mL

Hyaluronidase 200 units / mL solution – Draw the desired amount of hyaluronidase into the syringe to obtain the target hyaluronidase activity according to the following table.

Amount of Hyaluronidase Solution (200 units/mL) Withdrawn Per Target Hyaluronidase Activity	
Target hyaluronidase activity (units)	Volume withdrawn from vial (mL)
50 units	0.25 mL
75 units	0.38 mL
150 units	0.75 mL
200 units	1 mL

➤*Storage / Stability:*

Hyaluronidase lyophilized powder – Store unopened vial in refrigerator at 2° to 8°C (35° to 46°F). After reconstitution, store at controlled room temperature 20° to 25°C (68° to 77°F), and use within 6 hours. Protect from light.

Hyaluronidase solution – Store unopened vial in refrigerator at 2° to 8°C (35° to 46°F). Protect from light. Do not freeze.

Actions

➤*Pharmacology:* Hyaluronidase is a spreading or diffusing substance that modifies the permeability of connective tissue through the hydrolysis of hyaluronic acid, a polysaccharide found in the intercellular ground substance of connective tissue, and of certain specialized tissues, such as the umbilical cord and vitreous humor. Hyaluronic acid also is present in the capsules of type A and C hemolytic streptococci. Hyaluronidase hydrolyzes hyaluronic acid by splitting the glucosaminidic bond between C_1 of the glucosamine moiety and C_4 of glucuronic acid. This temporarily decreases the viscosity of the cellular cement and promotes diffusion of injected fluids or of localized transudates or exudates, thus facilitating their absorption.

Hyaluronidase cleaves glycosidic bonds of hyaluronic acid and, to a variable degree, some other acid mucopolysaccharides of the connective tissue. The activity is measured in vitro by monitoring the decrease in the amount of an insoluble serum albumen-hyaluronic acid complex as the enzyme cleaves the hyaluronic acid component.

When no spreading factor is present, material injected subcutaneously spreads very slowly, but hyaluronidase causes rapid spreading, provided local interstitial pressure is adequate to furnish the necessary mechanical impulse. Such an impulse normally is initiated by injected solutions. The rate of diffusion is proportionate to the amount of enzyme, and the extent is proportionate to the volume of solution.

Knowledge of the mechanisms involved in the disappearance of injected hyaluronidase is limited. It is known, however, that the blood of a number of mammalian species brings about the inactivation of hyaluronidase. Studies have demonstrated that hyaluronidase is antigenic; repeated injections of relatively large amounts of this enzyme may result in the formation of neutralizing antibodies.

The reconstitution of the dermal barrier removed by intradermal injection of hyaluronidase (20, 2, 0.2, 0.02, and 0.002 units/mL) to adult humans indicated that, at 24 hours, the restoration of the barrier is incomplete and inversely related to the dosage of enzyme; at 48 hours, the barrier is completely restored in all treated areas.

Results from an experimental study in humans on the influence of hyaluronidase in bone repair support the conclusion that this enzyme alone, in the usual clinical dosage, does not deter bone healing.

Contraindications

Hypersensitivity to hyaluronidase or any other ingredient in the formulation is a contraindication to the use of this product.

Warnings

➤*Uses:* Do not use hyaluronidase to enhance the absorption and dispersion of dopamine and/or alpha-agonist drugs.

Do not use hyaluronidase to reduce the swelling of bites or stings.

➤*Infection / skin inflammation:* Do not inject hyaluronidase into or around an infected or acutely inflamed area because of the danger of spreading a localized infection.

➤*Administration:* Do not use hyaluronidase for IV injections because the enzyme is rapidly inactivated.

Do not apply hyaluronidase directly to the cornea.

➤*Hypersensitivity reactions:* Discontinue hyaluronidase if sensitization occurs.

➤*Fertility impairment:* Long-term animal studies have not been performed to assess whether hyaluronidase impaired fertility; however, it has been reported that testicular degeneration may occur with the production of organ-specific antibodies against this enzyme following repeated injections. Human studies on the effect of intravaginal hyaluronidase in sterility caused by oligospermia indicated that hyaluronidase may have aided conception. Thus, it appears that hyaluronidase may not adversely affect fertility in females.

➤*Elderly:* No overall differences in safety or effectiveness have been observed between elderly and younger adult patients.

➤*Pregnancy: Category C.* No adequate and well-controlled animal studies have been conducted with hyaluronidase to determine reproductive effects. No adequate and well-controlled studies have been conducted with hyaluronidase in pregnant women. Use hyaluronidase during pregnancy only if clearly needed.

Labor and delivery – Administration of hyaluronidase during labor was reported to cause no complications: no increase in blood loss or differences in cervical trauma were observed. It is not known whether hyaluronidase has an effect on the fetus if used during labor; the effect of hyaluronidase on the later growth, development, and functional maturation of the infant is unknown.

➤*Lactation:* It is not known whether hyaluronidase is excreted in human milk. Because many drugs are excreted in human milk, exercise caution when hyaluronidase is administered to a breast-feeding woman.

➤*Children:* Hyaluronidase may be added to small volumes of solution (up to 200 mL), such as a small clysis for infants or solutions of drugs for subcutaneous injection. Keep in mind the potential for chemical or physical incompatibilities.

For infants and children younger than 3 years of age, limit the volume of a single clysis to 200 mL; in premature infants or during the neonatal period, do not exceed a daily dosage of 25 mL/kg of body weight; the rate of administration should not be greater than 2 mL/min. For older patients, the rate and volume of administration should not exceed those employed for IV infusion.

During hypodermoclysis, take special care in children to avoid overhydration by controlling the rate and total volume of the clysis.

Precautions

➤*Skin testing:* A preliminary skin test for hypersensitivity to hyaluronidase can be performed. This skin test is made by an intradermal injection of approximately 0.02 mL solution (3 or 4 units of a 150 or 200 unit/mL solution, respectively). A positive reaction consists of a wheal with pseudopods appearing within 5 minutes and persisting for 20 to 30 minutes and accompanied by localized itching. Transient vasodilation at the site of the test (ie, erythema) is not a positive reaction.

Drug Interactions

Patients receiving large doses of salicylates, cortisone, adrenocorticotropic hormone (ACTH), estrogens, or antihistamines may require larger amounts of hyaluronidase for equivalent dispersing effect because these drugs apparently render tissues partly resistant to the action of hyaluronidase.

➤*Local anesthetic:* When hyaluronidase is added to a local anesthetic agent, it hastens the onset of analgesia and tends to reduce the swelling caused by local infiltration. However, the wider spread of the local anesthetic solution increases its absorption; this shortens its duration of action and tends to increase the incidence of systemic reaction.

Adverse Reactions

The most frequently reported adverse reactions have been local injection-site reactions. Hyaluronidase has been reported to enhance the adverse reactions associated with coadministered drug products. Edema has been reported most frequently in association with hypodermoclysis. Allergic reactions (eg, urticaria, angioedema) have been reported in less than 0.1% of patients receiving hyaluronidase. Anaphylactic-like reactions following retrobulbar block or IV injections have occurred rarely.

Overdosage

➤*Symptoms:* Symptoms of toxicity consist of local edema or urticaria, erythema, chills, nausea, vomiting, dizziness, tachycardia, and hypotension.

➤*Treatment:* Discontinue the enzyme and initiate supportive measures immediately.

POLY-L-LACTIC ACID

Rx	**Sculptra** (Dermik Laboratories)	**Powder for injection** (freeze dried)	Single-use vials.

POLY-L-LACTIC ACID — INJECTION

Indications

➤*Facial fat loss (lipoatrophy):* For restoration and/or correction of the signs of facial fat loss (lipoatrophy) in people with human immunodeficiency virus.

Administration and Dosage

➤*Approved by the FDA:* August 3, 2004.

➤*Individualization of treatment:* The quantity of poly-L-lactic acid and the number of injection sessions will vary by patient. Treatment for severe facial fat loss typically requires the injection of 1 vial of poly-L-lactic acid per cheek area per injection session. A typical treatment course for severe facial fat loss involves 3 to 6 injection sessions, with the sessions separated by 2 or more weeks. Full effects of the treatment course are evident within weeks to months. Reevaluate the patient no sooner than 2 weeks after each injection session to determine if additional correction is needed. Advise patients that supplemental injection sessions may be required to maintain an optimal treatment effect.

➤*Reconstitution:* Poly-L-lactic acid is reconstituted in the following way:

1.) Remove the flip-off cap from the vial and clean the penetrable stopper of the vial with an antiseptic. If the vial, seal, or flip-off cap are damaged, do not use, and call the manufacturer.
2.) Attach an 18-gauge sterile needle to a sterile, single-use 5 mL syringe.
3.) Draw 3 to 5 mL SWFI into the 5 mL syringe.
4.) Introduce the 18-gauge sterile needle into the stopper of the vial and slowly add all SWFI into the vial.
5.) Let the vial stand for at least 2 hours to ensure complete hydration; do not shake during this period. Poly-L-lactic acid can be stored at room temperature up to 30°C (86°F) during and after hydration. Refrigeration is not required.
6.) After waiting at least 2 hours, agitate the vial until a uniform translucent suspension is obtained. A single vial swirling agitator may be used. Agitate product immediately prior to use. The reconstituted product is usable within 72 hours of reconstitution. Discard any material remaining after use or after 72 hours following reconstitution.
7.) Clean the penetrable stopper of the vial with an antiseptic, and use a new, 18-gauge sterile needle to withdraw an appropriate amount of the suspension (typically 1 mL) into a single-use 1 to 3 mL sterile syringe. Do not store the reconstituted product in the syringe.
8.) Replace the 18-gauge needle with a 26-gauge sterile needle before injecting the product into the deep dermis or subcutaneous layer. Do not inject poly-L-lactic acid using needles of an internal diameter smaller than 26-gauge.
9.) To withdraw remaining contents of the vial, repeat steps 6 through 8.

➤*Patient treatment:*

Dermal plane – Inject poly-L-lactic acid into the deep dermis or subcutaneous layer to avoid superficial injections. In order to control the injection depth of poly-L-lactic acid, stretch and pull the skin opposite to the direction of the injection to create a firm injection surface. Introduce the 26-gauge sterile needle, bevel up, into the skin at an angle of approximately 30 to 40 degrees, until the desired skin depth is reached. A change in tissue resistance is evident when the needle traverses the dermal-subcutaneous junction. If the needle is inserted at too shallow an angle (ie, into the mid or superficial [papillary] dermis), the bevel of the needle may be visible through the skin. If the product is injected too superficially, it will be evident as immediate or slightly delayed blanching in the injected area. If this occurs, remove the needle and gently massage the treatment area.

Injecting: Threading or tunneling –

Technique: When the appropriate dermal plane is reached, lower the needle angle to advance the needle in that dermal plane. Prior to depositing poly-L-lactic acid in the skin, perform a reflux maneuver to ensure that a blood vessel has not been entered. Using the threading or tunneling technique, deposit a thin trail of poly-L-lactic acid in the tissue plane as the needle is withdrawn. To avoid deposition in the superficial skin, stop deposition before the needle bevel is visible in the skin.

Volume per injection: Limit the volume of poly-L-lactic acid to approximately 0.1 to 0.2 mL per each individual injection. Note that in areas such as the cheek, approximately 20 injections may be required to cover the targeted area.

Volume per treatment area: The volume of product injected per treatment area will vary depending on the surface area to be treated. Treatment of an entire cheek typically requires injection of 1 vial of poly-L-lactic acid per cheek per injection session. Multiple injections (typically administered in a grid or cross-hatched pattern) may be required to cover the targeted area. The total number of injections and, thus, total volume of poly-L-lactic acid injected will vary based on the surface area to be corrected, not on the depth or severity of the deficiency to be corrected.

Depot injection –

Technique: The depot technique is most appropriate for injections into areas of thin skin at the level of the upper zygoma or temples. When using this technique, poly-L-lactic acid is injected as a small bolus. For the upper zygoma, it is injected under the orbicularis oculi muscle. For the temples, it is injected in the temporal fascia.

Volume per injection: Reduce the volume of poly-L-lactic acid to approximately 0.05 mL/injection. Following each injection, massage the area.

Massage during the injection session – Periodically massage the treatment areas during the injection session to evenly distribute the product.

Degree of correction – The depressed area should never be overcorrected (overfilled) in an injection session. Limited correction of the treatment area allows for the gradual improvement of the depressed area over several weeks as the treatment effect occurs. Typically, patients will experience some degree of edema associated with the injection procedure itself, which will give the appearance of a full correction by the end of the injection session (within approximately 30 minutes). Inform the patient that the injection-related edema typically resolves in several hours to a few days, resulting in the "reappearance" of the original contour deficiency.

Posttreatment care – Immediately following an injection session with poly-L-lactic acid, redness, swelling, or bruising may be noted in the treatment area. After the injection session, apply an ice pack (avoiding any direct contact of the ice with the skin) to the treatment area in order to reduce swelling. It is important to thoroughly massage the treatment area to evenly distribute the product. Instruct the patient to periodically massage the treatment area for several days after the injection session to promote a natural-looking correction.

Posttreatment assessment – During the first injection session with poly-L-lactic acid, only a limited correction should be made. Do not overcorrect (overfill). Evaluate the patient no sooner than 2 weeks after the injection session to determine if additional correction is needed. The original skin depression may initially reappear, but the depression should gradually improve within several weeks as the treatment effect of poly-L-lactic acid occurs. Advise the patient of the potential need for additional injection sessions at the first consultation.

➤*Storage/Stability:* Store poly-L-lactic acid at room temperature, up to 30°C (86°F). Do not freeze. Refrigeration is not required.

Each vial of poly-L-lactic acid is packaged for single-use only. Do not resterilize.

If the vial, seal, or the flip-off cap are damaged, do not use and contact the manufacturer.

Contraindications

Hypersensitivity to any of the components of the product.

Warnings

➤*Skin inflammation/infection:* Defer use of poly-L-lactic acid in any person with active skin inflammation or infection in or near the treatment area until the inflammatory or infectious process has been controlled.

➤*Administration:* Poly-L-lactic acid should only be used by health care providers with expertise in the correction of volume deficiencies in patients with human immunodeficiency virus after fully familiarizing themselves with the product, the product educational materials, and the entire package insert.

Use poly-L-lactic acid in the deep dermis or subcutaneous layer. Avoid superficial injections. Take special care when using poly-L-lactic acid in areas of thin skin.

Safety and effectiveness of treatment in the periorbital area have not been established.

Do not overcorrect (overfill) a contour deficiency because the depression should gradually improve within several weeks as the treatment effect of poly-L-lactic acid occurs.

Take special care to avoid injection into the blood vessels. An introduction into the vasculature may occlude the vessels and could cause infarction or embolism.

As with all injections, patients treated with anticoagulants may run the risk of a hematoma or localized bleeding at the injection site.

➤*Local effects:* Injection procedure reactions to poly-L-lactic acid have been observed, consisting mainly of hematoma, bruising, edema, discomfort, inflammation, and erythema. The most common device-related adverse effect was the delayed occurrence of subcutaneous papules, which were confined to the injection site and were typically palpable, asymptomatic, and nonvisible.

➤*Keloid formation or hypertrophic scarring:* The safety of using poly-L-lactic acid in patients with increased susceptibility to keloid formation and hypertrophic scarring has not been studied. Dermik will conduct a postapproval study to determine the likelihood of keloid formation and hypertrophic scars in patients with human immunodeficiency virus receiving poly-L-lactic acid injections.

➤*Pregnancy:* The safety of poly-L-lactic acid for use during pregnancy has not been established.

➤*Lactation:* The safety of poly-L-lactic acid for use in breastfeeding females has not been established.

➤*Children:* The safety of poly-L-lactic acid for use in patients younger than 18 years of age has not been established.

Precautions

➤*Long-term use:* Long-term safety and effectiveness of poly-L-lactic acid beyond 2 years have not been investigated. Dermik is conducting a postapproval study to evaluate the safety and effectiveness of poly-L-lactic acid beyond 2 years.

POLY-L-LACTIC ACID — INJECTION

➤*Risk of infection:* As with all transcutaneous procedures, poly-L-lactic acid injection carries a risk of infection. Follow standard precautions associated with injectable materials.

➤*Photosensitivity:* Inform the patient that he or she should minimize exposure of the treatment area to excessive sun and UV lamp exposure until any initial swelling and redness has resolved.

Drug Interactions

No studies of interactions of poly-L-lactic acid with drugs or other substances or implants have been made.

Adverse Reactions

Adverse event data from 4 clinical studies that included 277 patients are summarized in the following tables.

Number of Patients with Treatment-Related Adverse Events Observed in Clinical Studies with 2-Year Follow-Up			
	VEGA study (N = 50)	C&W study[c] (N = 29)	Average duration (days)
Injection procedure-related adverse events			
Bruising	3 (6%)	11(38%)	6
Discomfort	0	3 (10%)	3
Edema	2 (4%)	2 (7%)	3
Erythema	0	3 (10%)	3
Hematoma	14 (28%)	0	17
Inflammation	0	3 (10%)	3
Device-related adverse events			Average onset[b] (months)
Injection-site subcutaneous papule[a]	26 (52%)	9 (31%)	7

[a] Subcutaneous papules refer to lesions of 5 mm or less, typically palpable, asymptomatic, and nonvisible.
[b] Onset data available from VEGA study only. Duration not noted for subcutaneous papules because most were ongoing at study completion.
[c] Safety data were collected post hoc for 27 of the patients at approximately 2 years from study start.

Number of Patients with Treatment-Related Adverse Events Observed in Clinical Studies with 1-Year Follow-Up		
	APEX 002 study (N = 99)	Blue Pacific study (N = 99)
Injection procedure-related adverse events		
Bruising	1 (1%)	30 (30%)
Discomfort	19 (19%)	15 (15%)
Edema	3 (3%)	17 (17%)
Erythema	0	3 (3%)
Device-related adverse events		
Injection-site subcutaneous papule	6 (6%)	13 (13%)

The duration of the adverse events in the table above was not collected. The most common device-related adverse effect was the delayed occurrence of subcutaneous papules, which were confined to the injection site and were typically palpable, asymptomatic, and nonvisible. The study protocols did not include evaluation of treatment for subcutaneous papules; therefore, no information is available on how the papules were treated. In the VEGA study, the average onset of subcutaneous papules was 7 months after initial injection (range, 0.3 to 25 months). Subcutaneous papules resolved spontaneously in 6 of 26 patients (24%) during the study. No information of onset and duration of papules is available from the Chelsea & Westminster study.

Treatment-related adverse events, not included in the previous 2 tables, observed in clinical studies with a frequency of less than 5% were fever, injection-site bleeding, injection-site induration, injection-site infection, injection-site lesion, and injection-site tenderness.

➤*Postmarketing:*

CNS – Fatigue, lack of effectiveness, malaise.

Dermatologic – Application-site discharge, ectropion, hypertrophy of skin, injection-site abscess, injection-site atrophy, injection-site fat atrophy, injection-site granuloma, injection-site reaction, skin rash, skin roughness, telangiectasias, visible nodules with or without inflammation or dyspigmentation.

Miscellaneous – Aching joints, allergic reaction, angioedema, brittle nails, colitis not otherwise specified, hair breakage, hypersensitivity reaction, photosensitivity reaction, Quincke edema.

Patient Information

To report any adverse reactions, call the manufacturer.

Within the first 24 hours, patients should apply an ice pack (avoiding any direct contact of the ice with the skin) to the treatment area to reduce swelling. Poly-L-lactic acid may cause redness, swelling, or bruising when first injected into the skin, typically resolving in hours to 1 week. Hematoma also may occur, typically resolving in hours to approximately 2 weeks. Instruct patients to report worsening or prolonged symptoms or signs to the health care provider. The original skin depression may initially reappear, but the depression should gradually improve within several weeks as the treatment effect of poly-L-lactic acid occurs. The health care provider will assess the need for additional poly-L-lactic acid injection sessions after 2 or more weeks.

Instruct patients to massage the treatment area daily, for several days following any injection session.

Treatment with poly-L-lactic acid can result in small papules in the treatment area. These subcutaneous papules are typically not visible and asymptomatic and may be noticed only upon pressing on the treatment area. However, visible nodules, sometimes with redness or color change to the skin, have been reported. Advise patients to report any side effects to their health care provider.

Make-up may be applied a few hours posttreatment if no complications are present (eg, open wounds, bleeding, redness, swelling).

Instruct patients to minimize exposure of the treatment area to excessive sun and UV lamp exposure until any initial swelling and redness has resolved.

BOTULINUM TOXINS

BOTULINUM TOXIN TYPE A

Rx	**Botox** (Allergan)	**Powder for Injection (vacuum dried)**: 100 units of *Clostridium botulinum* toxin type A neurotoxin complex[a]	Preservative-free. 0.5 mg albumin (human), 0.9 mg sodium chloride. In single-use vials.
Rx	**Botox Cosmetic** (Allergan)		Preservative-free. 0.5 mg albumin (human), 0.9 mg sodium chloride. In single-use vials.

[a] One unit corresponds to the calculated median lethal intraperitoneal dose (LD_{50}) in mice.

BOTULINUM TOXIN TYPE A — INJECTION

Indications

➤*Axillary hyperhidrosis (Botox only)*: For the treatment of severe primary axillary hyperhidrosis that is inadequately managed with topical agents.

➤*Cervical dystonia (CD) (Botox only)*: For the treatment of CD in adults to decrease the severity of abnormal head position and neck pain associated with CD.

➤*Glabellar lines (Botox Cosmetic only)*: For the temporary improvement in the appearance of moderate to severe glabellar lines associated with corrugator and/or procerus muscle activity in adult patients 65 years of age and younger.

➤*Strabismus and blepharospasm associated with dystonia (Botox only)*: For the treatment of strabismus and blepharospasm associated with dystonia, including benign essential blepharospasm or VII nerve disorders in patients 12 years of age and older.

➤*Unlabeled uses:* Treatment of hemifacial spasms, spasmodic torticollis (ie, clonic twisting of the head), oromandibular dystonia, spasmodic dysphonia (laryngeal dystonia), and for other dystonias (eg, writer's cramp, focal task-specific dystonias). Botulinum toxin is being assessed in the treatment of head and neck tremor unresponsive to pharmacologic therapy. Designated an orphan drug for the treatment of dynamic muscle contracture in pediatric cerebral palsy patients.

Other reported uses of botulinum toxin type A include the following: acquired nystagmus, oscillopsia, tremor, tics, detrusor sphincter dyssynergia, achalasia, anismus/vaginismus, cosmesis, hyperhidrosis, myofacial pain, temporomandibular joint dysfunction, cervicogenic headache, spasticity, sialorrhea, and gustatory sweating.

Administration and Dosage

➤*Approved by the FDA:* December 1989.

➤*CD (Botox only):*

Patients with a known history of tolerance – The phase 3 study enrolled patients who had extended histories of receiving and tolerating

BOTULINUM TOXIN TYPE A — INJECTION

botulinum toxin type A injections, with prior individualized adjustment of dose. The mean botulinum toxin type A dose administered to patients in the phase 3 study was 236 units (25th to 75th percentile range, 198 to 300 units). The botulinum toxin type A dose was divided among the affected muscles. Tailor dosing in initial and sequential treatment sessions to the individual patient based on the patient's head and neck position, localization of pain, muscle hypertrophy, patient response, and adverse event history.

Patients without prior use – The initial dose for a patient without prior use of botulinum toxin type A should be at a lower dose, with subsequent dosing adjusted based on individual response. Limiting the total dose injected into the sternocleidomastoid muscles to 100 units or less may decrease the occurrence of dysphagia. A 25, 27 or 30 gauge needle may be used for superficial muscles, and a longer 22 gauge needle may be used for deeper musculature. Localization of the involved muscles with electromyographic guidance may be useful.

Clinical improvement generally begins within the first 2 weeks after injection, with maximum clinical benefit at approximately 6 weeks postinjection. In the phase 3 study, most subjects were observed to have returned to pretreatment status by 3 months posttreatment.

➤*Primary axillary hyperhidrosis (Botox* only): The recommended dose is 50 units per axilla. Define the hyperhidrotic area to be injected using standard staining techniques (eg, Minors Iodine-Starch Test). Botulinum toxin type A is reconstituted with 0.9% non-preserved sterile saline (100 units/4 mL). Using a 30 gauge needle, 50 units of botulinum toxin type A (2 mL) is injected intradermally in 0.1 to 0.2 mL aliquots to each axilla evenly distributed in multiple sites (10 to 15) approximately 1 to 2 cm apart.

Administer repeat injections for hyperhidrosis when the clinical effect of a previous injection diminishes.

Minor's Iodine Starch Test procedure – Patients should shave underarms and abstain from use of over-the-counter deodorants or antiperspirants for 24 hours prior to the test. Patient should be resting comfortably without exercise, hot drinks, etc for approximately 30 minutes prior to the test. Dry the underarm area and then immediately paint it with iodine solution. Allow the area to dry, then lightly sprinkle the area with starch powder. Gently blow off any excess starch powder. The hyperhidrotic area will develop a deep blue-black color over approximately 10 minutes.

Each injection site has a ring of effect of up to approximately 2 cm in diameter. To minimize the area of no effect, the injection sites should be evenly spaced.

Each dose is injected to a depth of approximately 2 mm and at a 45° angle to the skin surface with the bevel side up to minimize leakage and to ensure the injections remain intradermal.

If injection sites are marked in ink, do not inject botulinum toxin type A directly through the ink mark to avoid a permanent tattoo effect.

➤*Blepharospasm (Botox* only): For blepharospasm, reconstituted botulinum toxin type A is injected using a sterile, 27 to 30 gauge needle without electromyographic guidance. The initial recommended dose is 1.25 to 2.5 units (0.05 to 0.1 mL volume at each site) injected into the medial and lateral pretarsal orbicularis oculi of the upper lid and into the lateral pretarsal orbicularis oculi of the lower lid. Avoiding injection near the levator palpebrae superioris may reduce the complication of ptosis. Avoiding medial lower lid injections, and thereby reducing diffusion into the inferior oblique, may reduce the complication of diplopia. Ecchymosis occurs easily in the soft eyelid tissues. This can be prevented by applying pressure at the injection site immediately after the injection.

In general, the initial effect of the injections is seen within 3 days and reaches a peak at 1 to 2 weeks posttreatment. Each treatment lasts approximately 3 months, following which the procedure can be repeated. At repeat treatment sessions, the dose may be increased up to 2-fold if the response from the initial treatment is considered insufficient (usually defined as an effect that does not last longer than 2 months). However, there appears to be little benefit obtainable from injecting more than 5 units per site. Some tolerance may be found when botulinum toxin type A is used in treating blepharospasm if treatments are given any more frequently than every 3 months, and is rare to have the effect be permanent.

The cumulative dose of botulinum toxin type A treatment in a 30-day period should not exceed 200 units.

➤*Strabismus (Botox* only): The volume of botulinum toxin type A injected for treatment of strabismus should be between 0.05 to 0.15 mL per muscle.

Botulinum toxin type A is intended for injection into extraocular muscles utilizing the electrical activity recorded from the tip of the injection needle as a guide to placement within the target muscle. Do not attempt injection without surgical exposure or electromyographic guidance. Physicians should be familiar with electromyographic technique.

To prepare the eye for botulinum toxin type A injection, it is recommended that several drops of a local anesthetic and an ocular decongestant be given several minutes prior to injection.

➤*Doses:* The initial listed doses of the reconstituted botulinum toxin type A typically create paralysis of injected muscles beginning 1 to 2 days after injection and increasing in intensity during the first week. The paralysis lasts for 2 to 6 weeks and gradually resolves over a similar time period. Overcorrections lasting over 6 months have been rare. About one half of patients will require subsequent doses because of inadequate paralytic response of the muscle to the initial dose, or because of mechanical factors such as large deviations or restrictions, or because of the lack of binocular motor fusion to stabilize the alignment.

1.) Initial doses in units. Use the lower listed doses for treatment of small deviations. Use the larger doses only for large deviations.
   a.) For vertical muscles, and for horizontal strabismus of less than 20 prism diopters: 1.25 to 2.5 units in any 1 muscle.
   b.) For horizontal strabismus of 20 to 50 prism diopters: 2.5 to 5 units in any 1 muscle.
   c.) For persistent VI nerve palsy of 1 month or longer duration: 1.25 to 2.5 units in the medial rectus muscle.

2.) Subsequent doses for residual or recurrent strabismus.
   a.) It is recommended that patients be re-examined 7 to 14 days after each injection to assess the effect of that dose.
   b.) Patients experiencing adequate paralysis of the target muscle that require subsequent injections should receive a dose comparable to the initial dose.
   c.) Subsequent doses for patients experiencing incomplete paralysis of the target muscle may be increased up to 2-fold compared with the previously administered dose.
   d.) Do not administer subsequent injections until the effects of the previous dose have dissipated as evidenced by substantial function in the injected and adjacent muscles.
   e.) The maximum recommended dose as a single injection for any 1 muscle is 25 units.

➤*Dilution technique (Botox* only): Prior to injection, reconstitute vacuum-dried botulinum toxin type A with sterile normal saline without a preservative; 0.9% sodium chloride injection is the recommended diluent. Draw up the proper amount of diluent in the appropriate size syringe, and slowly inject the diluent into the vial. Discard the vial if a vacuum does not pull the diluent into the vial. Gently mix botulinum toxin type A with the saline by rotating the vial. Record the date and time of reconstitution on the space on the label. Administer botulinum toxin type A within 4 hours after reconstitution.

These dilutions are calculated for an injection volume of 0.1 mL. A decrease or increase in the botulinum toxin type A dose is also possible by administering a smaller or larger injection volume from 0.05 mL (50% decrease in dose) to 0.15 mL (50% increase in dose).

Dilution Table	
Diluent added (0.9% sodium chloride injection)	Resulting dose
	Units per 0.1 mL
1 mL	10 units
2 mL	5 units
4 mL	2.5 units
8 mL	1.25 units

➤*Glabellar lines (Botox Cosmetic* only): For IM injection only. Botulinum toxin type A (cosmetic) is to be reconstituted with 0.9% sterile, non-preserved saline (100 units in 2.5 mL saline) prior to IM injection. Once opened and reconstituted, it should be stored in a refrigerator (2° to 8°C; 35.6° to 46.4°F) and used within 4 hours. The resulting formulation will be 4 units per 0.1 mL and a total treatment dose of 20 units in 0.5 mL. The duration of activity of botulinum toxin type A (cosmetic) for glabellar lines is approximately 3 to 4 months. The safety and effectiveness of more frequent dosing with botulinum toxin type A (cosmetic) has not been clinically evaluated and is not recommended.

Dilution technique – Using a 21 gauge needle and an appropriately sized syringe, draw up a total of 2.5 mL of 0.9% sterile saline without a preservative. Insert the needle at a 45° angle and slowly inject into the botulinum toxin type A (cosmetic) vial. Discard the vial if a vacuum does not pull the diluent into the vial. Gently rotate the vial and record the date and time of reconstitution on the space on the label.

Draw at least 0.5 mL of the properly reconstituted toxin into the sterile syringe, preferably a tuberculin syringe and expel any air bubbles in the syringe barrel. Remove the needle used to reconstitute the product and attach a 30 gauge needle. Confirm the patency of the needle.

Injection technique – Glabellar facial lines arise from the activity of the corrugator and orbicularis oculi muscles. These muscles move the brow medially, and the procerus and depressor supercilii pull the brow inferiorly. This creates a frown or "furrowed brow". The location, size, and use of the muscles vary markedly among individuals. Lines induced by facial expression occur perpendicular to the direction of action of contracting facial muscles. An effective dose for facial lines is determined by gross observation of the patient's ability to activate the superficial muscles injected.

In order to reduce the complication of ptosis, take the following steps:
- Avoid injection near the levator palpebrae superioris, particularly in patients with larger brow depressor complexes.
- Place lateral corrugator injections at least 1 cm above the bony supraorbital ridge.
- Ensure the injected volume/dose is accurate and, where feasible, kept to a minimum.
- Do not inject toxin closer than 1 cm above the central eyebrow.

Using a 30 gauge needle, inject a dose of 0.1 mL into each of 5 sites, 2 in each corrugator muscle and 1 in the procerus muscle for a total dose of 20 units. Typically the initial doses of reconstituted botulinum toxin type A (cosmetic) induce chemical denervation of the injected muscles 1 to 2 days after injection, increasing in intensity during the first week.

➤*Storage/Stability:* Botulinum toxin type A is supplied in a single-use vial. Store unopened vials in a refrigerator (2° to 8°C [36.5° to 46.4°F]) for up to 24 months. Administer within 4 hours of reconstitution; during this time period, store reconstituted botulinum toxin type A in a refrigerator (2° to 8°C [36.5° to 46.4°F]). Reconstituted botulinum toxin type A should be clear, colorless, and free of particulate matter. Discard any remaining solution. Do not freeze reconstituted botulinum toxin type A.

BOTULINUM TOXIN TYPE A — INJECTION

During these 4 hours, store reconstituted botulinum toxin type A in a refrigerator (2° to 8°C [36° to 46°F]). Reconstituted botulinum toxin type A should be clear, colorless and free of particulate matter. Inspect parenteral drug products visually for particulate matter and discoloration prior to administration and whenever the solution and the container permit.

Carefully dispose of all vials, including expired vials, or equipment used with the drug as is done with all medical waste.

Actions

➤*Pharmacology:* Botulinum toxin type A blocks neuromuscular transmission by binding to acceptor sites on motor nerve or sympathetic terminals, entering the nerve terminals, and inhibiting the release of acetylcholine. This inhibition occurs as the neurotoxin cleaves SNAP-25, a protein integral to the successful docking and release of acetylcholine from vesicles situated within nerve endings. When injected IM at therapeutic doses, botulinum toxin type A produces partial chemical denervation of the muscle resulting in a localized reduction in muscle activity. In addition, the muscle may atrophy, axonal sprouting may occur, and extrajunctional acetylcholine receptors may develop. There is evidence that reinnervation of the muscle may occur, thus slowly reversing muscle denervation produced by botulinum toxin type A. When injected intradermally, botulinum toxin type A produces temporary chemical denervation of the sweat gland, resulting in local reduction in sweating.

➤*Pharmacokinetics:* Botulinum toxin type A is not expected to be present in the peripheral blood at measurable levels following IM or intradermal injection at the recommended doses. The recommended quantities of neurotoxin administered at each treatment session are not expected to result in systemic, overt distant clinical effects (ie, muscle weakness) in patients without other neuromuscular dysfunction. However, sub-clinical systemic effects have been shown by single-fiber electromyography after IM doses of botulinum toxins appropriate to produce clinically observable local muscle weakness.

These side effects may be caused by local spread of toxin from the injection site or misplaced injections.

Clinical studies have reported changes in clinical electromyographic parameters (ie, jitter) in muscles distant to the site of botulinum toxin type A (cosmetic) injection. This may indicate spread of the toxin via circulation, retro- or ortho-grade axonal transport, or some action of the toxin at a third, central, or unidentified site.

Contraindications

Infection at the proposed injection site(s); hypersensitivity to any ingredient in the formulation.

Warnings

➤*Administration:* Do not exceed the recommended dosage and frequency of administration for botulinum toxin type A. Risks resulting from administration at higher dosages are not known.

➤*Cardiovascular events:* There have also been rare reports following administration of botulinum toxin type A for other indications of adverse events involving the cardiovascular system, including arrhythmia and myocardial infarction, some with fatal outcomes. Some of these patients had risk factors including preexisting cardiovascular disease.

➤*Dysphagia:* Dysphagia is a commonly reported adverse event following treatment of CD patients with all botulinum toxins. In these patients, there are reports of rare cases of dysphagia severe enough to warrant the insertion of a gastric feeding tube. There are also rare case reports where subsequent to the finding of dysphagia a patient developed aspiration pneumonia and died.

➤*Neuropathic disorders:* Exercise caution when administering botulinum toxin type A to individuals with peripheral motor neuropathic diseases (eg, amyotrophic lateral sclerosis, or motor neuropathy) or neuromuscular junctional disorders (eg, myasthenia gravis or Lambert-Eaton syndrome). Patients with neuromuscular disorders may be at increased risk of clinically significant systemic effects including severe dysphagia and respiratory compromise from typical doses of botulinum toxin type A. Published medical literature has reported rare cases of administration of a botulinum toxin to patients with known or unrecognized neuromuscular disorders where the patients have shown extreme sensitivity to the systemic effects of typical clinical doses. In some of these cases, dysphagia has lasted several months and required placement of a gastric feeding tube.

➤*Albumin:* This product contains albumin, a derivative of human blood. Based on effective donor screening and product manufacturing processes, it carries an extremely remote risk for transmission of viral diseases. A theoretical risk for transmission of Creutzfeldt-Jakob disease (CJD) also is considered extremely remote. No cases of transmission of viral diseases or CJD have ever been identified for albumin.

➤*Hypersensitivity reactions:* Serious and/or immediate hypersensitivity reactions have been rarely reported. These reactions include anaphylaxis, urticaria, soft tissue edema, and dyspnea. One fatal case of anaphylaxis for another indication has been reported in which lidocaine was used as the diluent, and consequently the causal agent cannot be reliably determined. If such a reaction occurs, discontinue further injection and institute appropriate medical therapy immediately.

If an anaphylactic reaction occurs, epinephrine should be available or other precautionary methods taken as necessary.

➤*Fertility impairment:* The reproductive no observed effect level (NOEL) following IM injection of 0, 4, 8, and 16 units/kg was 4 units/kg in male rats and 8 units/kg in female rats. Higher doses were associated with dose-dependent reductions in fertility in male rats (where limb weakness resulted in the inability to mate), and testicular atrophy or an altered estrous cycle in female rats. There were no adverse effects on the viability of the embryos.

➤*Elderly:* There were too few patients older than 75 years of age to enable any comparisons. In general, dose selection for an elderly patient should be cautious, usually starting at the low end of the dosing range, reflecting the greater frequency of decreased hepatic, renal, or cardiac function, and of concomitant disease or other drug therapy.

➤*Pregnancy: Category C.* In a range finding study in rabbits, daily injection of 0.125 units/kg/day (days 6 to 18 of gestation) and 2 units/kg (days 6 and 13 of gestation) produced severe maternal toxicity, abortions, and/or fetal malformations. Higher doses resulted in death of the dams. The rabbit appears to be a very sensitive species to botulinum toxin type A.

When pregnant mice and rats were injected IM during the period of organogenesis, the development NOEL of botulinum toxin type A was 4 units/kg. Higher doses (8 or 16 units/kg) were associated with reductions in fetal body weights and/or delayed ossification which may be reversible.

There are no adequate and well-controlled studies of botulinum toxin type A in pregnant women. Because animal reproductive studies are not always predictive of human response, administer botulinum toxin type A during pregnancy only if the potential benefit justifies the potential risk to the fetus. If this drug is used during pregnancy, or if the patient becomes pregnant while taking this drug, apprise the patient of the potential risks, including abortion or fetal malformations, which have been observed in rabbits.

Administration of *Botox* cosmetic is not recommended during pregnancy.

➤*Lactation:* It is not known whether this drug is excreted in human milk. Because many drugs are excreted in human milk, exercise caution when botulinum toxin type A is administered to a breast—feeding woman.

➤*Children:*

Botox – Safety and effectiveness in children younger than 12 years of age have not been established for blepharospasm or strabismus, or younger than 16 years of age for CD or 18 years of age for hyperhidrosis.

Botox Cosmetic – Use of botulinum toxin type A (cosmetic) is not recommended in children.

Precautions

➤*Safe and effective use:* The safe and effective use of botulinum toxin type A depends upon proper storage of the product, selection of the correct dose, and proper reconstitution and administration techniques. Physicians administering botulinum toxin type A must understand the relevant neuromuscular or orbital anatomy of the area involved and any alterations to the anatomy caused by prior surgical procedures. An understanding of standard electromyographic techniques is also required for treatment of strabismus and may be useful for the treatment of CD.

➤*Injection site:* Use caution when botulinum toxin type A treatment is used in the presence of inflammation at the proposed injection site(s) or when excessive weakness or atrophy is present in the target muscle(s).

➤*Blepharospasm:* Reduced blinking from botulinum toxin type A injection of the orbicularis muscle can lead to corneal exposure, persistent epithelial defect, and corneal ulceration, especially in patients with VII nerve disorders. One case of corneal perforation in an aphakic eye requiring corneal grafting has occurred because of this effect. Careful testing of corneal sensation in eyes previously operated upon, avoidance of injection into the lower lid area to avoid ectropion, and vigorous treatment of any epithelial defect should be employed. This may require protective drops, ointment, therapeutic soft contact lenses, or closure of the eye by patching or other means.

Inducing paralysis in 1 or more extraocular muscles may produce spatial disorientation, double vision, or past pointing. Covering the affected eye may alleviate these symptoms.

➤*Botox:*

CD – Patients with smaller neck muscle mass and patients who require bilateral injections into the sternocleidomastoid muscle have been reported to be at greater risk for dysphagia. Limiting the dose injected into the sternocleidomastoid muscle may reduce the occurrence of dysphagia. Injections into the levator scapulae may be associated with an increased risk of upper respiratory tract infection and dysphagia.

Primary axillary hyperhidrosis – Evaluate patients for potential causes of secondary hyperhidrosis (eg, hyperthyroidism) to avoid symptomatic treatment of hyperhidrosis without the diagnosis and/or treatment of the underlying disease. The safety and effectiveness of botulinum toxin type A for hyperhidrosis in other body areas have not been established. Weakness of hand muscles and blepharoptosis may occur in patients who receive botulinum toxin type A for palmar hyperhidrosis and facial hyperhidrosis, respectively.

Strabismus – During the administration of botulinum toxin type A for the treatment of strabismus, retrobulbar hemorrhages sufficient to compromise retinal circulation have occurred from needle penetrations into the orbit. It is recommended that appropriate instruments to decompress the orbit be accessible. Ocular (globe) penetrations by needles have also occurred. An ophthalmoscope to diagnose this condition should be available. Inducing paralysis in 1 or more extraocular muscles may produce spatial disorientation, double vision, or past pointing. Covering the affected eye may alleviate these symptoms.

➤*Botox* cosmetic: Use caution when botulinum toxin type A (cosmetic) treatment is used in patients who have an inflammatory skin problem at the injection site, marked facial asymmetry, ptosis, excessive dermatochalasis, deep dermal scarring, thick sebaceous skin, or the inability to substantially lessen glabellar lines by physically spreading them apart as these patients were excluded from the phase 3 safety and efficacy trials. As with any injec-

BOTULINUM TOXIN TYPE A — INJECTION

tion, procedure-related injury could occur. An injection could result in localized infection, pain, inflammation, tenderness, swelling, erythema, and/or bleeding/bruising. Use caution in patients who have bleeding disorders or are taking anticoagulants. Needle-related pain and/or anxiety may result in vasovagal responses (eg, syncope, hypotension). Take care when injecting near vulnerable anatomic structures.

Administration – Injection intervals of botulinum toxin type A (cosmetic) should be no more frequent than every 3 months and should be performed using the lowest effective dose.

Drug Interactions

Coadministration of botulinum toxin type A and aminoglycosides or other agents interfering with neuromuscular transmission (eg, curare-like nondepolarizing blockers, lincosamides, polymyxins, quinidine, magnesium sulfate, anticholinesterases, succinylcholine chloride) should only be performed with caution because the effect of the toxin may be potentiated.

The effect of administering different botulinum neurotoxin serotypes at the same time or within several months of each other is unknown. Excessive neuromuscular weakness may be exacerbated by administration of another botulinum toxin prior to the resolution of the effects of a previously administered botulinum toxin.

Adverse Reactions

➤*Botox*: There have been rare spontaneous reports of death, sometimes associated with dysphagia, pneumonia, and/or other significant debility or anaphylaxis, after treatment with botulinum toxin.

There have also been rare reports of adverse reactions involving the cardiovascular system, including arrhythmia and myocardial infarction, some with fatal outcomes. Some of these patients had risk factors including cardiovascular disease. The exact relationship of these reactions to the botulinum toxin injection has not been established.

The following reactions have been reported since the drug has been marketed and a causal relationship to the botulinum toxin injected is unknown: skin rash (including erythema multiforme, urticaria, and psoriasiform eruption), pruritus, and allergic reaction.

In general, adverse reactions occur within the first week following injection of botulinum toxin type A, and while generally transient, may have a duration of several months. Localized pain, tenderness, or bruising may be associated with the injection. Local weakness of the injected muscle(s) represents the expected pharmacological action of botulinum toxin. However, weakness of adjacent muscles may also occur because of spread of toxin.

CD – In CD patients evaluated for safety in double-blind and open-label studies following injection of botulinum toxin type A, the most frequently reported adverse reactions were dysphagia (19%), upper respiratory infection (12%), neck pain (11%), and headache (11%).

Other reactions reported in 2% to 10% of patients in any 1 study in decreasing order of incidence include increased cough, flu syndrome, back pain, rhinitis, dizziness, hypertonia, soreness at injection site, asthenia, oral dryness, speech disorder, fever, nausea, and drowsiness. Stiffness, numbness, diplopia, ptosis, and dyspnea have been reported rarely.

Dysphagia and symptomatic general weakness may be attributable to an extension of the pharmacology of botulinum toxin type A resulting from the spread of the toxin outside the injected muscles.

The most common severe adverse reaction associated with the use of botulinum toxin type A injection in patients with CD is dysphagia, with about 20% of these cases also reporting dyspnea. Most dysphagia is reported as mild or moderate in severity. However, it may rarely be associated with more severe signs and symptoms.

Additionally, reports in the literature include a case of a female patient who developed brachial plexopathy 2 days after injection of botulinum toxin type A 120 units for the treatment of CD, and reports of dysphonia in patients who have been treated for CD.

Primary axillary hyperhidrosis – The most frequently reported adverse events (3% to 10% of patients) following injection of botulinum toxin type A in double-blind studies included injection site pain and hemorrhage, nonaxillary sweating, infection, pharyngitis, flu syndrome, headache, fever, neck or back pain, pruritus, and anxiety.

Blepharospasm – In a study of blepharospasm patients who received an average dose per eye of 33 units (injected at 3 to 5 sites) of the currently manufactured botulinum toxin type A, the most frequently reported treatment-related adverse reactions were ptosis (20.8%), superficial punctate keratitis (6.3%), and eye dryness (6.3%).

In this study, the rate for ptosis in the current botulinum toxin type A-treated group (20.8% of patients) was significantly higher than the original botulinum toxin type A treated group (4% of patients) ($P = 0.014\%$). All of these reactions were mild or moderate except for 1 case of ptosis which was rated severe.

Other reactions reported in prior clinical studies in decreasing order of incidence include irritation, tearing, lagophthalmos, photophobia, ectropion, keratitis, diplopia and entropion, diffuse skin rash, and local swelling of the eyelid skin lasting for several days following eyelid injection.

In 2 cases of VII nerve disorder (1 case of an aphakic eye), reduced blinking from botulinum toxin type A injection of the orbicularis muscle led to serious corneal exposure, persistent epithelial defect, and corneal ulceration. Perforation occurred in the aphakic eye and required corneal grafting.

A report of acute angle-closure glaucoma 1 day after receiving an injection of botulinum toxin for blepharospasm was received, with recovery 4 months later after laser iridotomy and trabeculectomy. Focal facial paralysis, syncope, and exacerbation of myasthenia gravis have also been reported after treatment of blepharospasm.

Strabismus – Extraocular muscles adjacent to the injection site can be affected, causing ptosis or vertical deviation, especially with higher doses of botulinum toxin type A. The incidence rates of these adverse effects in 2,058 adults who received a total of 3,650 injections for horizontal strabismus are 15.7% and 16.9%, respectively.

Inducing paralysis in 1 or more extraocular muscles may produce spatial disorientation, double vision, or past-pointing. Covering the affected eye may alleviate these symptoms.

The incidence of ptosis was 0.9% after inferior rectus injection and 37.7% after superior rectus injection.

Ptosis (0.3%) and vertical deviation greater than 2 prism diopters (2.1%) were reported to persist for over 6 months in a larger series of 5587 injections of horizontal muscles in 3104 patients.

In these patients, the injection procedure itself caused 9 scleral perforations. A vitreous hemorrhage occurred in 1 case and later cleared. No retinal detachment or visual loss occurred in any case. Sixteen retrobulbar hemorrhages occurred without visual loss. Decompression of the orbit after 5 minutes was done to restore retinal circulation in 1 case. Five eyes had pupillary change consistent with ciliary ganglion damage (Adie's pupil).

One patient developed anterior segment ischemia after receiving botulinum toxin type A injection into the medial rectus muscle under direct visualization for esotropia.

Immunogenicity – Formation of neutralizing antibodies to botulinum toxin type A may reduce the effectiveness of botulinum toxin type A treatment by inactivating the biological activity of the toxin. The rate of formation of neutralizing antibodies in patients receiving botulinum toxin type A has not been well studied.

In the phase 3 CD study that enrolled only patients with a history of receiving botulinum toxin type A for multiple treatment sessions, at study entry there were 192 patients with antibody assay results, of whom 33 (17%) had a positive assay for neutralizing activity. There were 96 patients in the randomized period of the phase 3 study with valid assays at both study entry and end and who were neutralizing activity negative at entry. Of these 96, two patients (2%) converted to positive for neutralizing activity. Both of these converting patients were among the 52 who had received 2 botulinum toxin type A treatments between the 2 assays; none were in the group randomized to placebo in the controlled comparison period of the study.

In the randomized period of the CD study, patients in the botulinum toxin type A group whose baseline assays were neutralizing antibody negative showed improvements on CDSS (n = 64, mean CDSS change −2.1) while patients whose baseline assays were neutralizing antibody positive did not (n = 14, mean CDSS change +1.1). However, in uncontrolled studies there are also individual patients who are perceived as continuing to respond to treatments despite the presence of neutralizing activity. Not all patients who become nonresponsive to botulinum toxin type A after an initial period of clinical response have demonstrable levels of neutralizing activity.

However, in uncontrolled studies there are also individual patients who are perceived as continuing to respond to treatments despite the presence of neutralizing activity. Not all patients who become nonresponsive to botulinum toxin type A after an initial period of clinical response have demonstrable levels of neutralizing activity.

One patient among the 445 hyperhidrosis patients with analyzed specimens showed the presence of neutralizing antibodies.

The data reflect the patients whose test results were considered positive or negative for neutralizing activity to botulinum toxin type A in a mouse protection assay. The results of these tests are highly dependent on the sensitivity and specificity of the assay. Additionally, the observed incidence of neutralizing activity in an assay may be influenced by several factors including sample handling, concomitant medications, and underlying disease. For these reasons, comparison of the incidence of neutralizing activity to botulinum toxin type A with the incidence reported to other products may be misleading.

The critical factors for neutralizing antibody formation have not been well characterized. The results from some studies suggest that botulinum toxin type A injections at more frequent intervals or at higher doses may lead to greater incidence of antibody formation. The potential for antibody formation may be minimized by injecting with the lowest effective dose given at the longest feasible intervals between injections.

➤*Botox Cosmetic*: The most serious adverse reactions reported for other indications studied include rare, spontaneous reports of death, sometimes associated with dysphagia, pneumonia, and/or other significant debility, after treatment with botulinum toxin. There have also been rare reports of adverse reactions involving the cardiovascular system, including arrhythmia and myocardial infarction, some with fatal outcomes. Some of these patients had risk factors including preexisting cardiovascular disease. In addition, there have been rare reports of seizures or convulsions, mostly in patients who are predisposed to experiencing these events. The exact relationship of these reactions to the botulinum toxin injection has not been established. Additionally, a report of acute angle closure glaucoma 1 day after receiving an injection of botulinum toxin for blepharospasm was received, with recovery 4 months later after laser iridotomy and trabeculectomy. Focal facial paralysis, syncope, and exacerbation of myasthenia gravis have also been reported after treatment of blepharospasm.

In general, adverse events occur within the first week following injection and, while generally transient, may have a duration of several months or, in rare cases, longer.

Glabellar lines – In clinical trials of botulinum toxin type A (cosmetic) the most frequently reported adverse reactions following injection of botulinum

BOTULINUM TOXIN TYPE A — INJECTION

toxin type A (cosmetic) were headache, respiratory infection, flu syndrome, blepharoptosis, and nausea.

Less frequently occurring (less than 3%) adverse reactions included pain in the face, erythema at the injection site, and muscle weakness. While local weakness of the injected muscle(s) is representative of the expected pharmacological action of botulinum toxin, weakness of adjacent muscles may occur as a result of the spread of toxin. These reactions are thought to be associated with the injection and occurred within the first week. The reactions were generally transient but may last several months or, in some cases, longer.

In the open-label, repeat injection study, blepharoptosis was reported for 2.1% (8 of 373) of subjects in the first treatment cycle and 1.2% (4 of 343) of subjects in the second treatment cycle. Adverse reactions of any type were reported for 49.1% (183 of 373) of subjects overall. The most frequently reported of these adverse reactions in the open-label study included respiratory infection, headache, flu syndrome, blepharoptosis, pain, and nausea.

Randomized, Double-Blind Studies: Rates of Adverse Reactions Reported by > 2 or More Subjects in the Botulinum Toxin Type A (Cosmetic) Group, by Treatment Group

Adverse reaction [in order of decreasing frequency for botulinum toxin type A (cosmetic)]	Botulinum toxin type A (cosmetic) (n = 405)	Placebo (n = 130)
Overall	177 (43.7%)	54 (41.5%)
Cardiovascular		
Hypertension	4 (1%)	0 (0%)
CNS		
Anxiety	3 (0.7%)	0 (0%)
Dizziness	5 (1.2%)	2 (1.5%)
Paresthesia	4 (1%)	1 (0.8%)
Twitch	3 (0.7%)	0 (0%)
Dermatologic		
Erythema	7 (1.7%)	2 (1.5%)
Irritation skin	3 (0.7%)	0 (0%)
Skin tightness	4 (1%)	0 (0%)
GI		
Dyspepsia	4 (1%)	0 (0%)
Liver function abnormal	3 (0.7%)	2 (1.5%)
Nausea	12 (3%)	3 (2.3%)
Tooth disorder	4 (1%)	0 (0%)
GU		
Infection urinary tract	4 (1%)	1 (0.8%)
Hemic and lymphatic		
Ecchymosis	7 (1.7%)	3 (2.3%)
Musculoskeletal		
Muscle weakness	8 (2%)	0 (0%)
Respiratory		
Bronchitis	6 (1.5%)	1 (0.8%)
Dyspnea	3 (0.7%)	0 (0%)
Infection	14 (3.5%)	5 (3.8%)
Infection sinus	3 (0.7%)	2 (1.5%)
Laryngitis	3 (0.7%)	0 (0%)
Pharyngitis	5 (1.2%)	2 (1.5%)
Rhinitis	3 (0.7%)	2 (1.5%)
Sinusitis	6 (1.5%)	1 (0.8%)
Special senses		
Blepharoptosis	13 (3.2%)	0 (0%)
Miscellaneous		
Edema at injection site	6 (1.5%)	3 (2.3%)
Flu syndrome	8 (2%)	2 (1.5%)
Headache	54 (13.3%)	23 (17.7%)
Injury accidental	3 (0.7%)	1 (0.8%)
Pain in back	4 (1%)	3 (2.3%)
Pain in face	9 (2.2%)	1 (0.8%)
Pain at injection site	7 (1.7%)	1 (0.8%)

In published literature of the use of botulinum toxin type A for facial lines, there has been a single reported incident of diplopia, which resolved completely in 3 weeks. Transient ptosis, the most frequently reported complication, has been reported in the literature in approximately 5% of patients.

Immunogenicity – Treatment with botulinum toxin type A (cosmetic) for cosmetic purposes may result in the formation of antibodies that may reduce the effectiveness of subsequent treatments with botulinum toxin type A (cosmetic) for glabellar lines or botulinum toxin type A for other indications. Formation of neutralizing antibodies to botulinum toxin type A may reduce the effectiveness of botulinum toxin type A (cosmetic) treatment of the appearance of glabellar lines and the effectiveness of botulinum toxin type A in the treatment of other clinical indications such as CD, blepharospasm and strabismus by inactivating the biological activity of the toxin. The rate of formation of neutralizing antibodies in patients receiving botulinum toxin type A (cosmetic) has not been well studied.

The critical factors for neutralizing antibody formation have not been well characterized. The results from some studies suggest that botulinum toxin type A injections at more frequent intervals or at higher doses may lead to greater incidence of antibody formation. The potential for antibody formation may be minimized by injecting with the lowest effective dose given at the longest feasible intervals between injections.

Passive adverse reaction surveillance – The following adverse reactions have been identified since the drug has been marketed: allergic reaction; brachial plexopathy; flu-like symptoms, such as chest discomfort, fever, malaise, myalgia, and sweating; focal facial paralysis; gastrointestinal disturbances, including abdominal pain, diarrhea, loss of appetite, nausea, and vomiting; headache; pruritus; and skin rash (including erythema multiforme, urticaria, and psoriasiform eruption). Because these reactions are reported voluntarily from a population of uncertain size, it is not always possible to reliably estimate their frequency or establish a causal relationship to botulinum toxin.

Between January 1, 1990 and December 2003, there have been spontaneous reports of serious adverse reactions documented as being related to the reported cosmetic use of botulinum toxin type A, including syncope, anaphylactic reaction, myasthenia gravis, decreased hearing, ear noise and localized numbness, blurred vision and retinal vein occlusion, glaucoma, and vertigo with nystagmus.

Reporting adverse reactions – Report adverse reactions following use of botulinum toxin type A (cosmetic) to the Pharmacovigilance Department, Allergan Inc. (1-800-433-8871). Adverse reactions may also be reported to the US Department of Health and Human Services (DHHS) adverse event reporting system. Report forms and reporting requirement information can be obtained from adverse event reporting system (AERS) through a toll-free number 1-800-822-7967.

Overdosage

➤*Symptoms:* Signs and symptoms of overdose are not apparent immediately following injection. If accidental injection or oral ingestion occurs, the person should be medically supervised for up to several weeks for signs or symptoms of systemic weakness or muscle paralysis.

➤*Treatment:* An antitoxin is available in the event of immediate knowledge of an overdose or misinjection. The antitoxin will not reverse any botulinum toxin induced muscle weakness effects already apparent by the time of antitoxin administration.

Patient Information

Advise patients or caregivers to seek immediate medical attention if swallowing, speech, or respiratory disorders arise.

Inform patients with CD of the possibility of experiencing dysphagia, which is typically mild to moderate, but could be severe. Rare consequences of severe dysphagia include aspiration, dyspnea, pneumonia, and the need to reestablish an airway.

As with any treatment with the potential to allow previously sedentary patients to resume activities, caution the sedentary patient to resume activity gradually following the administration of botulinum toxin type A.

BOTULINUM TOXIN TYPE B

Rx	**Myobloc** (Elan Pharm)	**Solution, injectable:**[1] 5000 U/mL	Preservative free. In 3.5 mL single-use vials.[2]

[1] One unit corresponds to the calculated median lethal intraperitoneal dose (LD_{50}) in mice.

[2] With 0.05% human serum albumin, 0.01 M sodium succinate, 0.1 M sodium chloride.

BOTULINUM TOXIN TYPE B — INJECTION

Indications

➤*Cervical dystonia (CD):* For the treatment of patients with CD to reduce the severity of abnormal head position and neck pain associated with CD.

Administration and Dosage

➤*Approved by the FDA:* December 11, 2000.

➤*Cervical dystonia:* The recommended initial dose of botulinum toxin type B for patients with a history of tolerating botulinum toxin injections is 2500 to 5000 U divided among affected muscles. Give patients without a history of tolerating botulinum toxin injections a lower initial dose. Optimize subsequent dosing according to the patient's individual response. The duration of effect in patients responding to botulinum toxin type B treatment has been observed in studies to be between 12 and 16 weeks at doses of 5000 U or 10,000 U. Botulinum toxin type B should be administered by physicians familiar and experienced in the assessment and management of patients with CD. Units of biological activity of botulinum toxin type B cannot be compared with or converted into units of any other botulinum toxin.

➤*Storage/Stability:* Store under refrigeration at 2° to 8°C (36° to 46°F) for up to 21 months. Do not freeze. Do not shake. After dilution with normal saline, the product must be used within 4 hours as the formulation does not contain a preservative.

Actions

➤*Pharmacology:* Botulinum toxin type B injectable solution is a sterile liquid formulation of a purified neurotoxin that acts at the neuromuscular junction to produce flaccid paralysis. The neurotoxin is produced by fermentation of the bacterium *Clostridium botulinum* type B (Bean strain).

Contraindications

Known hypersensitivity to any ingredient in the formulation.

Warnings

➤*Neuropathic disorders:* Exercise caution when administering botulinum toxin type B to individuals with peripheral motor neuropathic diseases (eg, amyotrophic lateral sclerosis, motor neuropathy) or neuromuscular junctional disorders (eg, myasthenia gravis, Lambert-Eaton syndrome). Patients with neuromuscular disorders may be at increased risk of clinically significant systemic effects including severe dysphagia and respiratory compromise from typical doses of botulinum toxin type B. Published medical literature has reported rare cases of administration of a botulinum toxin to patients with known or unrecognized neuromuscular disorders where the patients have shown extreme sensitivity to the systemic effects of typical clinical doses. In some cases, dysphagia has lasted months and required placement of a gastric feeding tube.

➤*Botulism:* There were no documented cases of botulism resulting from the IM injection of botulinum toxin type B in patients with CD treated in clinical trials. However, if botulism is clinically suspected, hospitalization for the monitoring of systemic weakness or paralysis and respiratory function (incipient respiratory failure) may be required.

➤*Dysphagia:* Dysphagia is a commonly reported adverse event following treatment with all botulinum toxins in cervical dystonia patients. In the medical literature, there are reports of rare cases of dysphagia severe enough to warrant the insertion of a gastric feeding tube. There are also rare case reports where subsequent to the finding of dysphagia, a patient developed aspiration pneumonia and died.

➤*Viral diseases:* This product contains albumin, a derivative of human blood. Based on effective donor screening and product manufacturing processes, it carries an extremely remote risk for transmission of viral diseases. A theoretical risk for transmission of Creutzfeldt-Jakob disease (CJD) also is considered extremely remote. No cases of transmission of viral diseases or CJD have ever been identified with albumin.

➤*Pregnancy: Category C.* Animal reproduction studies have not been conducted with botulinum toxin type B. It is also not known whether it can cause fetal harm when administered to a pregnant woman or can affect reproduction capacity. Give botulinum toxin type B to a pregnant woman only if clearly needed.

➤*Lactation:* It is not known if this drug is excreted in human milk. Exercise caution when botulinum toxin type B is administered to a nursing woman.

➤*Children:* Safety and efficacy in pediatric patients have not been established.

Precautions

Only 9 subjects without a history of tolerating injections of type A botulinum toxin have been studied. Initiate treatment of botulinum toxin naive patients at lower doses. During repeated treatment studies, 446 subjects were followed with periodic ELISAbased evaluations for development of antibody responses against botulinum toxin type B. Of these patients, 12% had positive ELISAassays at baseline. Patients began to develop new ELISAresponses after a single treatment session with botulinum toxin type B. By 6 months after initiating treatment, estimates for ELISApositive rate were 20%, which continued to rise to 36% at 1 year and 50% positive ELISA status at 18 months. Serum neutralizing activity was primarily not seen in patients until after 6 months. Estimated rates of development were 10% at 1 year and 18% at 18 months in the overall group of patients, based on analysis of samples from ELISApositive individuals. The clinical significance of development of antibodies has not been determined.

Drug Interactions

Coadminister botulinum toxin type B and aminoglycosides or other agents interfering with neuromuscular transmission (eg, curare-like compounds) with caution as the effect of the toxin may be potentiated.

The effect of administering different botulinum neurotoxin serotypes at the same time or within < 4 months of each other is unknown. However, neuromuscular paralysis may be potentiated by coadministration or overlapping administration of different botulinum toxin serotypes.

Adverse Reactions

The most commonly reported adverse events associated with botulinum toxin type B treatment in all studies were dry mouth, dysphagia, dyspepsia, and injection site pain. Dry mouth and dysphagia were the adverse reactions most frequently resulting in discontinuation of treatment. There was an increased incidence of dysphagia with increased dose in the sternocleidomastoid muscle. The incidence of dry mouth showed some dose-related increase with doses injected into the splenius capitis, trapezius, and sternocleidomastoid muscles.

Only 9 subjects without a history of tolerating injections of type A botulinum toxin have been studied. Adverse event rates have not been adequately evaluated in these patients.

Botulinum Toxin Type B Adverse Reactions Following Single Treatment Session (%)

Adverse reaction	Dosing groups 2500 U (n = 31)	5000 U (n = 67)	10,000 U (n = 106)	Placebo (n = 104)
CNS				
Dizziness	3	3	6	2
Neck pain related to CD	0	16	17	16
Headache	10	16	11	8
Torticollis	0	4	8	7
Pain related to CD/Torticollis	10	4	7	4
GI				
Dry mouth	3	12	34	3
Dysphagia	16	10	25	3
Dyspepsia	3	0	10	5
Nausea	10	3	8	5
Miscellaneous				
Injection site pain	16	12	15	9
Infection	13	19	15	15
Pain	6	6	13	10
Flu syndrome	6	9	8	4
Arthralgia	0	1	7	5
Back pain	3	4	7	3
Cough increased	3	6	7	3
Myasthenia	3	4	6	3
Asthenia	3	0	6	4
Accidental injury	0	4	5	4
Rhinitis	3	1	5	6

The following additional adverse events were reported in ≥ 2% of patients:

➤*CNS:* Headache related to injection; migraine; anxiety; tremor; hyperesthesia; somnolence; confusion; pain related to CD/torticollis; vertigo.

➤*Dermatologic:* Pruritus; ecchymosis

➤*GI:* GI disorder; vomiting; glossitis; stomatitis; tooth disorder.

➤*GU:* Urinary tract infection; cystitis; vaginal moniliasis.

➤*Metabolic/Nutritional:* Peripheral edema; edema; hypercholesterolemia.

➤*Musculoskeletal:* Arthritis; joint disorder.

➤*Respiratory:* Dyspnea; lung disorder; pneumonia.

➤*Special senses:* Amblyopia; otitis media; abnormal vision; taste perversion; tinnitus.

➤*Miscellaneous:* Allergic reaction; fever; chest pain; chills; hernia; malaise; abscess; cyst; neoplasm; viral infection; vasodilation.

Overdosage

➤*Symptoms:* Symptoms of overdose are not likely to present immediately following injection(s). Should a patient ingest the product or be accidently overdosed, monitor the patient for up to several weeks for signs and symptoms of systemic weakness or paralysis.

➤*Treatment:* In the event of an overdose, an antitoxin may be adminstered. Contact Elan Pharmaceuticals (888) 638-7605 for additional information and your State Health Department to process a request for antitoxin through the Centers for Disease Control and Prevention in Atlanta, GA. The antitoxin will not reverse any botulinum toxin induced muscle weakness effects already apparent by the time of antitoxin administration.

BISMUTH SUBSALICYLATE, METRONIDAZOLE AND TETRACYCLINE HCl COMBINATION

Rx	**Helidac** (Procter & Gamble)	**Tablets:** 262.4 mg bismuth subsalicylate	(PG 11). Pink, chewable. In 8s.
		250 mg metronidazole	(PG 10). White. In 4s.
		Capsules: 500 mg tetracycline	(PG 12). Pale orange and white. In 4s.

BISMUTH SUBSALICYLATE, METRONIDAZOLE AND TETRACYCLINE HCl COMBINATION — ORAL

For more information, refer to the *H. pylori* Treatment Guidelines and individual monographs.

Administration and Dosage

➤*Adults:* Take 525 mg bismuth subsalicylate, 250 mg metronidazole, and 500 mg tetracycline plus an H_2 antagonist 4 times daily at meals and at bedtime for 14 days. Chew and swallow the bismuth subsalicylate tablets. Swallow the metronidazole tablet and tetracycline capsule whole with a full glass of water (8 ounces). Take concomitantly prescribed H_2 antagonist therapy as directed.

Ingestion of adequate amounts of fluid, particularly with the bedtime dose of tetracycline HCl, is recommended to reduce the risk of esophageal irritation and ulceration.

Missed doses can be made up by continuing the normal dosing schedule until the medication is gone. Do not take double doses. If more than 4 doses are missed, contact the physician.

LANSOPRAZOLE, AMOXICILLIN, AND CLARITHROMYCIN COMBINATION

Rx	**Prevpac** (TAP Pharmaceuticals)	**Daily administration pack:** Two 30 mg *Prevacid* (lansoprazole) capsules, four 500 mg *Trimox* (amoxicillin) capsules, and two 500 mg *Biaxin* (clarithromycin) tablets.

LANSOPRAZOLE, AMOXICILLIN, AND CLARITHROMYCIN COMBINATION — ORAL

For more information, refer to the *H. pylori* Treatment Guidelines and individual monographs.

Indications

➤*Eradication of H. pylori:* Eradication of *H. pylori* to reduce risk of duodenal ulcer recurrence.

Administration and Dosage

➤*Adults:* 30 mg lansoprazole, 1 g amoxicillin, and 500 mg clarithromycin administered together twice daily (morning and evening) for 14 days.

Do not use in patients with creatinine clearance less than 30 mL/min.

HISTAMINE H_2 ANTAGONISTS

Indications

➤*Benign gastric ulcer:* For the short-term treatment of active, benign gastric ulcer. **Ranitidine** is also indicated for the maintenance therapy after the healing of acute ulcer.

➤*Duodenal ulcer:* For the short-term treatment of active duodenal ulcer and maintenance therapy after the healing of active ulcer.

➤*Gastroesophageal reflux disease (GERD):*

Cimetidine (oral only) – For the treatment of erosive esophagitis diagnosed by endoscopy.

Famotidine – For the short-term treatment of GERD and esophagitis due to GERD, including erosive or ulcerative disease diagnosed by endoscopy.

Nizatidine – For the treatment of endoscopically diagnosed esophagitis, including erosive and ulcerative esophagitis, and associated heartburn due to GERD.

Ranitidine – For the treatment of GERD and endoscopically diagnosed erosive esophagitis; for the maintenance of healing of erosive esophagitis.

➤*GI bleeding (intravenous [IV] cimetidine only):* For the prevention of upper GI bleeding in critically ill patients.

➤*Pathological hypersecretory conditions* (**cimetidine, famotidine, ranitidine**): For the treatment of pathological hypersecretory conditions (eg, Zollinger-Ellison syndrome, systemic mastocytosis, multiple endocrine adenomas).

➤*Heartburn (OTC products only):* For the relief of heartburn associated with acid indigestion and sour stomach; for the prevention of heartburn associated with acid indigestion and sour stomach brought on by certain foods and beverages.

➤*Unlabeled uses:* As part of a multidrug regimen to eradicate *Helicobacter pylori* in the treatment of peptic ulcer; in the perioperative setting to suppress gastric acid secretion, prevent stress ulcers, and prevent aspiration pneumonitis; in combination with histamine H_1 antagonists in the treatment of certain types of urticaria.

Cimetidine – Treatment of cutaneous warts (data are conflicting); prevention of paclitaxel hypersensitivity (IV cimetidine); to reduce the incidence of GI hemorrhage associated with stress-related ulcers (IV cimetidine).

Famotidine – Prevention of paclitaxel hypersensitivity (IV famotidine); prevention of recurrent bleeding after successful endoscopic treatment of bleeding peptic ulcer (IV famotidine); to reduce the incidence of GI hemorrhage associated with stress-related ulcers (IV famotidine).

Ranitidine – Prevention of paclitaxel hypersensitivity (IV ranitidine); as prophylaxis to reduce the incidence of nonsteroidal anti-inflammatory drug (NSAID)-induced duodenal ulcer; to reduce the incidence of GI hemorrhage associated with stress-related ulcers (IV ranitidine).

Histamine H_2 Antagonists: Summary of Indications[a]

✓ – Labeled x – Unlabeled	Cimetidine	Famotidine	Nizatidine	Ranitidine
Benign gastric ulcer				
Treatment	✓	✓	✓	✓
Maintenance				✓
Duodenal ulcer				
Treatment	✓	✓	✓	✓
Maintenance	✓	✓	✓	✓
GERD (including erosive esophagitis)	✓	✓	✓	✓
Erosive esophagitis, maintenance				✓
Pathological hypersecretory conditions	✓	✓		✓
Peptic ulcer[c]	x	x	x	x
Prevent aspiration pneumonitis	x	x	x	x
Prevent NSAID-induced duodenal ulcer				x
Prevent paclitaxel hypersensitivity	x (IV)	x (IV)		x (IV)
Prevent of stress ulcers	x	x	x	x
Prevent upper GI bleeding	✓ (IV)			
Reduce incidence of GI hemorrhage associated with stress-related ulcers	x (IV)	x (IV)		x (IV)
Reduce recurrent peptic ulcer bleeding (after endoscopy)		x (IV)		
Relieve and prevent heartburn/acid indigestion/sour stomach	✓[b]	✓[b]	✓[b]	✓[b]
Suppress gastric acid secretion perioperatively	x	x	x	x
Treat certain types of urticaria[d]	x	x	x	x
Treat cutaneous warts	x			

[a] For more detailed information, see the preceding paragraphs and individual drug monographs.
[b] OTC use only.
[c] As part of a multidrug regimen to eradicate *H. pylori.*
[d] In combination with histamine H_1 antagonists.

Actions

➤*Pharmacology:* Histamine H_2 antagonists (also known as H_2 blockers) competitively and reversibly inhibit the action of histamine at the histamine H_2 receptors, including receptors on the gastric parietal cells. These agents are not anticholinergic.

Cimetidine –

Antisecretory activity:

• *Nocturnal* – Cimetidine 800 mg at bedtime reduces mean hourly hydrogen ion (H^+) activity by more than 85% over 8 hours in duodenal ulcer patients, with no effect on daytime acid secretion. The 1600 mg bedtime dose produces 100% inhibition of mean hourly H^+ activity over an 8-hour period in duodenal ulcer patients, but also reduces H^+ activity by 35% for an additional 5 hours the next morning. Both the 400 mg twice daily and 300 mg

4 times daily dosages decrease nocturnal acid secretion in a dose-related manner, 47% to 83% over 6 to 8 hours and 54% over 9 hours, respectively.

• *Food stimulated* – By the first hour after a standard meal, 300 mg inhibited gastric acid secretion in duodenal ulcer patients by at least 50% and during the next 2 hours by at least 75%. A 300 mg breakfast dose continued for at least 4 hours, with partial suppression of the rise in gastric acid secretion following lunch in duodenal ulcer patients.

Total pepsin output is also reduced as a result of the decrease in volume of gastric juice. Cimetidine 300 mg inhibited the rise in intrinsic factor concentration produced by betazole, but some intrinsic factor was secreted at all times.

• *24-hour mean activity* – Dosages of 800 mg at bedtime, 400 mg twice daily, and 300 mg 4 times daily all provide a similar, moderate (less than 60%) level of 24-hour acid suppression. However, the 800 mg at bedtime regimen exerts its entire effect on nocturnal acid, and does not affect daytime gastric physiology.

Famotidine – The acid concentration and volume of gastric secretion are suppressed, while changes in pepsin secretion are proportional to volume output. Exocrine pancreatic function is not affected. After oral use, the onset of antisecretory effect occurred within 1 hour; the maximum effect was dose-dependent, occurring within 1 to 3 hours. Duration of secretion inhibition by doses of 20 and 40 mg was 10 and 12 hours, respectively.

After IV administration, the maximum effect was achieved within 30 minutes. Single IV doses of 10 and 20 mg inhibited nocturnal secretion for 10 and 12 hours, respectively.

There is no cumulative effect with repeated doses. The nocturnal intragastric pH was raised by evening doses of 20 and 40 mg to mean values of 5 and 6.4, respectively. When famotidine was given after breakfast, the basal daytime interdigestive pH at 3 and 8 hours after 20 or 40 mg was raised to about 5.

Nizatidine – Nizatidine significantly inhibited nocturnal gastric acid secretion for up to 12 hours. Total pepsin output was reduced in proportion to the reduced volume of gastric secretions. Oral administration of 75 to 300 mg of nizatidine increased betazole-stimulated secretion of intrinsic factor.

Ranitidine – Basal, nocturnal, and betazole-stimulated secretion are most sensitive to inhibition by ranitidine, responding almost completely to doses of 100 mg or less. Ranitidine does not affect pepsin secretion or pentagastrin-stimulated intrinsic factor secretion. Other pharmacological actions include an increase in gastric nitrate-reducing organisms; small, transient, dose-related increases in serum prolactin after IV bolus injections of 100 mg or more, and possible impairment of vasopressin release. No effect on prolactin levels has been noted with recommended oral or IV doses.

➤*Pharmacokinetics:*

Pharmacokinetic Properties of Histamine H_2 Antagonists

H_2 receptor antagonist	Bioavailability (%)	T_{max} (h)[a]	Peak plasma concentration[b] (mcg/mL)	Half-life (h)	Protein binding (%)	Volume of distribution (L/kg)	Elimination (%) Urine, unchanged	
							Oral	IV
Cimetidine	≈ 60 (oral)	0.75 to 1.5 (oral)	2 to 3 (400 mg oral dose)	≈ 2[c]	13 to 25	≈ 1	48	75
Famotidine	40 to 45 (oral)	1 to 3	–	2.5 to 3.5[d]	15 to 20	≈ 1.3	25 to 30	65 to 70
Nizatidine	> 70	0.5 to 3	0.7 to 1.8/ 1.4 to 3.6 (150/300 mg dose)	1 to 2[d]	≈ 35	0.8-1.5	60	NA[e]
Ranitidine	50 (oral) (90 to 100 IM)[f]	2 to 3 (oral) (0.25 IM)	0.44 to 0.55 (oral) (0.58 IM)	2.5 to 3 (oral)[d] 2 to 2.5 (IV)[d]	15	1.3	30	≈70

[a] T_{max} = time to maximum concentration.
[b] Dose-dependent.
[c] Increased in renal and hepatic impairment and in the elderly.
[d] Increased in renal impairment.
[e] NA = not applicable.
[f] IM = intramuscular. Additional pharmacokinetic data for these agents are discussed individually.

Cimetidine – Absorption may be decreased by antacids. Both oral and parenteral administration provide comparable periods of effective serum levels. Blood concentrations remain above those required to provide 80% inhibition of basal gastric acid secretion for 4 to 5 hours following a 300 mg dose. Cimetidine is widely distributed. Following oral administration, the drug is extensively metabolized, the sulfoxide being the major metabolite. Hemodialysis reduces the level of circulating cimetidine.

Famotidine – Plasma levels after multiple doses of famotidine are similar to those after single doses. Famotidine is eliminated by renal (65% to 70%) and metabolic (30% to 35%) routes. The only metabolite identified is the S-oxide.

Nizatidine – Plasma concentrations 12 hours after administration are less than 10 mcg/L. Plasma clearance is 40 to 60 L/h. Because of the short half-life and rapid clearance, drug accumulation would not be expected in individuals with normal renal function who take either 300 mg at bedtime or 150 mg twice daily. Nizatidine exhibits dose proportionality over the recommended dose range.

Antacids consisting of aluminum and magnesium hydroxides with simethicone decrease nizatidine absorption by about 10%. With food, area under the curve (AUC) and maximum concentration increase by about 10%.

In humans, less than 7% of an oral dose is metabolized as N2-monodesmethylnizatidine, an H_2-receptor antagonist. Other likely metabolites are the N2-oxide (less than 5% of the dose) and the S-oxide (less than 6% of the dose). More than 90% of an oral dose of nizatidine is excreted in the urine within 12 hours. Renal clearance is approximately 500 mL/min, which indicates excretion by active tubular secretion. Less than 6% is eliminated in the feces.

Ranitidine – Absorption of oral ranitidine is not significantly impaired by the administration of food or antacids. Hepatic metabolism results in 3 metabolites. Maintenance of serum concentrations necessary to inhibit 50% of stimulated gastric acid secretion (36 to 94 ng/mL) is 12 hours orally (6 to 8 hours IV). However, blood levels bear no consistent relationship to dose or degree of acid inhibition.

Contraindications

Hypersensitivity to individual agents or to other histamine H_2 antagonists (cross-sensitivity has been observed).

Warnings

➤*Carcinogenesis:* A statistically significant increase in benign Leydig cell tumor incidence was seen in rats that received 378 and 950 mg/kg/day **cimetidine**. The tumors were common in control groups as well as treated groups, and the difference became apparent only in aged rats.

➤*Benzyl alcohol:* Benzyl alcohol contained in some of these products as a preservative, has been associated with a fatal "gasping syndrome" in premature infants.

➤*Phenylketonurics:* Inform with phenylketonuria patients that some of these products contain phenylalanine.

➤*Hypersensitivity reactions:* Rare cases of anaphylaxis have occurred, as well as rare episodes of hypersensitivity (eg, bronchospasm, laryngeal edema, rash, eosinophilia). Refer to Management of Acute Hypersensitivity Reactions.

➤*Renal function impairment:* Because these agents are excreted primarily via the kidneys, decreased clearance may occur; reduced dosage may be necessary (see Administration and Dosage). Since CNS adverse effects have been reported in patients with moderate and severe renal insufficiency, longer intervals between doses or lower doses may need to be used in patients with moderate (creatinine clearance [Ccr] less than 50 mL/min) or severe ([Ccr] less than 10 mL/min) renal insufficiency to adjust for the longer elimination half-life of famotidine.

➤*Hepatic function impairment:* Observe caution. Decreased clearance may occur; these agents are partly metabolized in the liver. In normal renal function with uncomplicated hepatic dysfunction, **nizatidine** disposition is similar to that in healthy individuals.

➤*Elderly:* Safety and efficacy appear similar to those of younger patients; however, the elderly may have reduced renal function. Exercise caution in dose selection.

➤*Pregnancy: Category B.* Cimetidine crosses the placenta. There are no adequate and well controlled studies with these agents in pregnant women. Use only when clearly needed and when the potential benefits outweigh the potential hazards to the fetus.

➤*Lactation:*

Cimetidine – Cimetidine is excreted in breast milk. However, the American Academy of Pediatrics considers cimetidine to be compatible with breast-feeding.

Famotidine – Famotidine is excreted in the breast milk of rats. Transient growth depression was seen in young rats suckling from mothers treated with maternotoxic doses of at least 600 times the usual human dose. Famotidine is detectable in human milk. Because of the potential for serious adverse reactions in breast-feeding infants, decide whether to discontinue breast-feeding or the drug, taking into account the importance of the drug to the mother.

Ranitidine – Ranitidine is excreted in breast milk. Exercise caution when administering to a breast-feeding mother.

Nizatidine – Studies have shown that 0.1% of an oral dose of nizatidine is excreted in breast milk in proportion to plasma concentrations. Because of the growth depression in pups reared by lactating rats treated with nizatidine, decide whether to discontinue breast-feeding or the drug, taking into account the importance of the drug to the mother.

➤*Children:*

Cimetidine – Safety and efficacy are limited. **Cimetidine** is not recommended for children younger than 16 years of age, unless anticipated benefits outweigh potential risks. In very limited experience, cimetidine 20 to 40 mg/kg/day has been used. OTC use is not recommended in children younger than 12 years of age.

Famotidine – Efficacy has been established. See individual monograph for suggested dosages.

Nizatidine – Efficacy in patients younger than 12 years of age has not been established.

Ranitidine – Safety and efficacy of ranitidine have been established in infants and children from 1 month to 16 years of age for treatment of duodenal and gastric ulcers, GERD, and erosive esophagitis; and for the maintenance of healed duodenal and gastric ulcer. Safety and efficacy in pediatric patients for the treatment of pathological hypersecretory conditions or the maintenance of healing of erosive esophagitis have not been established. Safety and efficacy in neonates (younger than 1 month of age) have not been established.

Precautions

➤*Gastric malignancy:* Symptomatic response to these agents does not preclude gastric malignancy. Rare reports of transient healing of gastric ulcers has occurred with **cimetidine** despite subsequently documented malignancy. Follow gastric ulcer patients closely.

➤*CNS effects:* Reversible CNS effects (eg, mental confusion, agitation, psychosis, depression, anxiety, hallucinations, disorientation) have occurred. For **cimetidine**, these confusional states usually developed within 2 to 3 days after initiation of therapy and cleared within 3 to 4 days following discontinuation. Advancing age (50 years of age and older) and preexisting liver and/or renal disease appear to be contributing factors.

➤*Hepatic effects:* Occasionally, reports of hepatocellular, cholestatic, or mixed hepatitis, with or without jaundice, have occurred with **ranitidine**. In such circumstances, immediately discontinue ranitidine. These events are usually reversible, but in rare circumstances death has occurred. Rare cases of hepatic failure have also been reported. In normal volunteers, ALT values were increased to at least twice the pretreatment levels in 6 of 12 subjects receiving 100 mg 4 times daily IV for 7 days, and in 4 of 24 subjects receiving 50 mg 4 times a day IV for 5 days. In patients receiving IV ranitidine at dosages of 100 mg 4 times daily or higher for periods of 5 days or longer, monitor ALT daily (from day 5) for the remainder of IV therapy. For more information regarding other histamine H_2 antagonists causing hepatic effects, see Adverse Reactions.

Laboratory test monitoring – Laboratory test monitoring for liver abnormalities is appropriate.

➤*Porphyria:* Rare reports suggest that **ranitidine** may precipitate acute porphyric attacks in patients with acute porphyria. Avoid using ranitidine in patients with a history of acute porphyria.

➤*Rapid IV administration:* Rapid IV administration of **cimetidine** has been followed by rare instances of cardiac arrhythmias and hypotension. Bradycardia in association with rapid administration of IV **ranitidine** may occur rarely, usually in patients predisposed to cardiac rhythm disturbances.

➤*Antiandrogenic effect:* **Cimetidine** has a weak antiandrogenic effect. Gynecomastia in patients treated for 1 month or more may occur. In patients with pathological hypersecretory states, this occurred in approximately 4% of cases; in all others, the incidence was approximately 0.3% to 1%. No evidence of endocrine dysfunction was found; the condition remained unchanged or returned to normal with continuing treatment. (Also see Adverse Reactions.)

➤*Immunocompromised patients:* Decreased gastric acidity, including that produced by acid-suppressing agents such as histamine H_2 antagonists, may increase the possibility of strongyloidiasis.

Drug Interactions

➤*Cytochrome P-450:* **Cimetidine** reduces the hepatic metabolism of drugs metabolized via the cytochrome P-450 pathway, delaying elimination and increasing serum levels. Drugs metabolized by hepatic microsomal enzymes, particularly those of low therapeutic ratio or in patients with renal or hepatic impairment, may require dosage adjustment. **Ranitidine** (which weakly binds to cytochrome P-450 in vitro), **famotidine**, and **nizatidine** do not inhibit the cytochrome P-450–linked oxygenase enzyme system in the liver. Drug interactions with these agents mediated by inhibition of hepatic metabolism are not expected. However, some interactions may occur with these agents (see table).

Histamine H_2 Antagonist Drug Interactions

Precipitant drug	Object drug[a]		Description
H_2 antagonists Cimetidine	Amiodarone	⬆	Coadministration may increase amiodarone and its active metabolite. Monitor closely.
H_2 antagonists Cimetidine Ranitidine	Benzodiazepines	⬆	Coadministration of cimetidine or ranitidine with benzodiazepines that undergo oxidative metabolism may increase the serum levels of these benzodiazepines (eg, alprazolam, chlordiazepoxide, clorazepate, diazepam, flurazepam, midazolam, triazolam). Ranitidine has been shown to increase triazolam plasma concentrations.
H_2 antagonists Cimetidine	Beta-blockers (ie, metoprolol, propranolol, timolol)	⬆	Cimetidine may reduce the hepatic metabolism of beta-blockers metabolized by CYP-450 (ie, metoprolol, propranolol, timolol). Monitor closely and adjust the beta-blocker dose accordingly.
H_2 antagonists Cimetidine Ranitidine	Calcium channel blockers (ie, diltiazem, nifedipine)	⬆	Cimetidine may reduce the hepatic metabolism of nifedipine. Monitor closely and adjust the nifedipine dose accordingly. Cimetidine and ranitidine increased diltiazem concentrations.
H_2 antagonists Cimetidine	Carbamazepine	⬆	Cimetidine may inhibit carbamazepine hepatic metabolism. Monitor carbamazepine levels and adjust dose as needed.
H_2 antagonists Cimetidine	Carmustine	⬆	Cimetidine may enhance the myelosuppressive effects of carmustine. Avoid coadministration if possible.
H_2 antagonists	Cephalosporins (ie, cefpodoxime, cefuroxime, cephalexin)	⬇	H_2 antagonists may possibly decrease the bioavailability of certain cephalosporins.
H_2 antagonists Cimetidine	Chloroquine	⬆	Cimetidine may inhibit the hepatic metabolism of chloroquine.
H_2 antagonists Cimetidine	Dofetilide	⬆	Cimetidine may increase dofetilide concentrations, increasing the risk of ventricular arrhythmias including torsades de pointes. Coadministration is contraindicated.
H_2 antagonists	Ethanol	⬆	Coadministration may increase ethanol concentrations. Data are conflicting.
H_2 antagonists Cimetidine	Hydantoins (eg, phenytoin)	⬆	Cimetidine may reduce the hepatic metabolism of hydantoins, thereby increasing blood levels. Monitor closely and adjust the hydantoin dose accordingly.
H_2 antagonists	Iron Salts	⬇	Oral absorption of iron may be impaired. Consider administering iron preparations at least 1 hour before H_2 antagonists.
H_2 antagonists	Ketoconazole	⬇	Alteration of gastric pH may affect the absorption of ketoconazole.
H_2 antagonists Cimetidine	Lidocaine	⬆	Cimetidine may reduce the hepatic metabolism of lidocaine, causing increased adverse effects.
H_2 antagonists Cimetidine	Metformin	⬆	Coadministration may increase metformin concentrations. Monitor closely.
H_2 antagonists Cimetidine	Metronidazole	⬆	Cimetidine may reduce the hepatic metabolism of metronidazole, thereby increasing blood levels. Data are conflicting.
H_2 antagonists Cimetidine	Moricizine	⬆	Cimetidine may inhibit the hepatic metabolism of moricizine. Monitor closely, especially electrocardiogram.
H_2 antagonists Cimetidine	Pentoxifylline	⬆	Cimetidine may inhibit the hepatic metabolism of pentoxifylline.
H_2 antagonists Cimetidine	Praziquantel	⬆	Plasma concentrations of praziquantel may be elevated. Observe closely.
H_2 antagonists Cimetidine Ranitidine	Procainamide	⬆	Increased procainamide concentrations may occur. Avoid coadministration with cimetidine if possible. Monitor closely.
H_2 antagonists Cimetidine	Quinidine	⬆	Increased quinidine concentrations may occur. Avoid coadministration if possible. Monitor closely.
H_2 antagonists Nizatidine	Salicylates	⬆	Increased serum salicylate levels occurred when nizatidine was coadministered to patients receiving very high daily doses of aspirin (3,900 mg).

Histamine H_2 Antagonist Drug Interactions			
Precipitant drug	Object drug[a]		Description
H_2 antagonists Cimetidine	Sildenafil	↑	Sildenafil plasma concentrations may be elevated.
H_2 antagonists Cimetidine	Selective serotonin reuptake inhibitors	↑	Serum levels of certain SSRIs may be increased.
H_2 antagonists Cimetidine	St. John's wort	↑	Cimetidine may increase the levels of hypericin.
H_2 antagonists Cimetidine Ranitidine	Sulfonylureas	↑	Reduced clearance of sulfonylureas may occur. Monitor blood glucose and adjust dose as needed.
H_2 antagonists Cimetidine	Theophyllines	↑	Cimetidine may reduce the hepatic metabolism of theophyllines. Monitor theophylline levels closely and adjust dose as needed.
H_2 antagonists Cimetidine	Tricyclic antidepressants	↑	Cimetidine may reduce the hepatic metabolism of certain tricyclic antidepressants. Monitor closely and adjust the dose as needed.
H_2 antagonists Cimetidine Ranitidine	Warfarin	↑	The effects of warfarin may be increased. Monitor anticoagulation parameters closely and adjust warfarin dose as needed.

[a] ↑ = Object drug increased. ↓ = Object drug decreased.

➤*Drug/Lab test interactions:* False-positive tests for urobilinogen with *Multistix* may occur during **nizatidine** therapy. False-positive tests for urine protein with *Multistix* may occur during **ranitidine** therapy; testing with sulfosalicylic acid is recommended.

➤*Drug/Food interactions:* Food may increase bioavailability of **famotidine** and **nizatidine**; this is of no clinical consequence.

Adverse Reactions

Histamine H_2 Antagonist Adverse Reactions[a]				
Adverse reaction	Cimetidine	Famotidine	Nizatidine	Ranitidine
CNS				
Agitation/Anxiety	[b]	[b]	1.8%	rare
Confusional states[c]	[b]	[b]	rare	rare
Depression	[b]	[b]		rare
Dizziness	1%	1.3%	4.6%	rare
Hallucinations	[b]	[b]		rare
Headache	2.1% to 3.5%[d]	4.7%	16.6%	[b,d]
Insomnia		[b]	2.7%	rare
Somnolence/ Fatigue	1%	[b]	1.9%	rare
Dermatologic				
Alopecia	rare[c]	[b]		rare
Erythema multiforme	rare			rare
Exfoliative dermatitis/ erythroderma	rare		[b]	
Pruritus/Urticaria		[b]	1.7%/0.5%	
Rash	[b]	[b]	1.9%	[b]
GI				
Abdominal discomfort		[b]		[b]
Cholestatic/Hepatocellular effects	rare[c]	[b]	rare	[b]
Constipation		1.2%		[b]
Diarrhea	1%	1.7%	7.2%	[b]
Nausea		[b]	[b]	[b]
Pancreatitis	rare[c]			rare
Vomiting		[b]		[b]
Hematologic				
Agranulocytosis	rare	rare		rare
Granulocytopenia				rare[c]
Immune hemolytic/ aplastic anemia	rare			rare
Leukopenia		rare		rare[c]
Pancytopenia	rare	rare		rare
Thrombocytopenia	rare	rare	[b]	[b,c]
Miscellaneous				
Arthralgia	rare[c]	[b]		rare
Decreased libido		[b]	[b]	[b]
Gynecomastia	0.3% to 4%	rare	rare	[b]
Hypersensitivity reactions	rare[c]	[b]	rare	rare
Impotence	[b,c]	rare	[b]	[b]
Transient pain at injection site		[b]	NA	[b]

[a] Data are pooled from separate studies and are not necessarily comparable.
[b] Occurs, no incidence reported or not well established.
[c] Reversible.
[d] May be severe.

In addition to the adverse reactions listed in the table, the following have been reported:

Cimetidine –

Cardiovascular: Rare cases of bradycardia, tachycardia and atrioventricular (AV) heart block have been reported with histamine H_2 antagonists. Rare instances of cardiac arrhythmias and hypotension have been reported following the rapid administration of cimetidine injection by IV bolus.

CNS: Reversible confusional states (see Precautions).

Dermatologic: Very rarely, cases of severe generalized skin reactions including Stevens-Johnson syndrome, epidermal necrolysis, erythema multiforme, exfoliative dermatitis and generalized exfoliative erythroderma have been reported with histamine H_2 antagonists.

GU: Gynecomastia (see Precautions). Reversible impotence has been reported in patients with pathological hypersecretory disorders (eg, Zollinger-Ellison syndrome) receiving cimetidine, particularly in high doses, for at least 12 months (range, 12 to 79 months; mean, 38 months). However, in large-scale surveillance studies at regular dosage, the incidence has not exceeded that commonly reported in the general population.

Small, possibly dose-related increases in plasma creatinine, presumably due to competition for renal tubular secretion, are not uncommon and do not signify deteriorating renal function. Rare cases of interstitial nephritis and urinary retention, which cleared on withdrawal of the drug, have been reported.

Hematologic: Decreased white blood cell counts (approximately 1 per 100,000 patients), including agranulocytosis (approximately 3 per million patients), have been reported, including a few reports of recurrence on rechallenge. Most of these reports were in patients who had serious concomitant illnesses and received drugs and/or treatment known to produce neutropenia.

Hepatic: Dose-related increases in serum transaminase have been reported. In most cases they did not progress with continued therapy and returned to normal at the end of therapy. There have been rare reports of cholestatic or mixed cholestatic-hepatocellular effects. These were usually reversible. Because of the predominance of cholestatic features, severe parenchymal injury is considered highly unlikely. However, as in the occasional liver injury with other histamine H_2 antagonists, in exceedingly rare circumstances fatal outcomes have been reported. There has been reported a single case of biopsy-proven periportal hepatic fibrosis in a patient receiving cimetidine.

Musculoskeletal: There have been rare reports of reversible myalgia; exacerbation of joint symptoms in patients with preexisting arthritis has also been reported. Such symptoms have usually been alleviated by a reduction in the dosage of cimetidine. Rare cases of polymyositis have been reported, but no causal relationship has been established.

Miscellaneous: Rare cases of fever and allergic reactions including anaphylaxis and hypersensitivity vasculitis, which cleared on withdrawal of the drug, have been reported. There have been extremely rare reports of strongyloidiasis hyperinfection in immunocompromised patients.

Famotidine –

Cardiovascular: Arrhythmia, AV block, palpitation.

CNS: Generalized tonic-clonic seizure; paresthesia; psychic disturbances, which were reversible in cases for which follow-up was obtained (see Precautions).

Dermatologic: Acne, dry skin, flushing; toxic epidermal necrolysis (very rare).

GI: Anorexia, cholestatic jaundice, dry mouth, liver enzyme abnormalities.

Hypersensitivity: Anaphylaxis, angioedema, conjunctival injection, orbital or facial edema, rash, urticaria.

Musculoskeletal: Musculoskeletal pain including muscle cramps.

Respiratory: Bronchospasm.

Special Senses: Taste disorder, tinnitus.

Miscellaneous: Asthenia, fatigue, fever.

• *Children* – In a clinical study in 35 pediatric patients younger than 1 year of age with GERD symptoms (eg, vomiting [spitting up], irritability [fussing]), agitation was observed in 5 patients on famotidine that resolved when the medication was discontinued.

Nizatidine –

Cardiovascular: In clinical pharmacology studies, short episodes of asymptomatic ventricular tachycardia occurred in 2 individuals administered nizatidine and in 3 untreated subjects.

CNS: Rare cases of reversible mental confusion have been reported (see Precautions).

Dermatologic: Sweating; vasculitis has been reported rarely.

GU: Clinical pharmacology studies and controlled clinical trials showed no evidence of antiandrogenic activity due to nizatidine.

Hematologic: Anemia; fatal thrombocytopenia was reported in a patient who was treated with nizatidine and another histamine H_2 antagonist. On previous occasions, this patient had experienced thrombocytopenia while taking other drugs. Rare cases of thrombocytopenic purpura have been reported.

Hepatic: Hepatocellular injury, evidenced by elevated liver enzyme tests (AST, ALT, or alkaline phosphatase), occurred in some patients and was possibly or probably related to nizatidine. In some cases, there was marked elevation of AST, ALT enzymes (greater than 500 units/L) and, in a single instance, ALT was greater than 2,000 units/L. The overall rate of occurrences of elevated liver enzymes and elevations to 3 times the upper limit of normal, however, did not significantly differ from the rate of liver enzyme abnormalities in placebo-treated patients. All abnormalities were reversible after discontinuation of nizatidine. Since market introduction, hepatitis and jaundice have been reported. Rare cases of cholestatic or mixed hepatocellular and cholestatic injury with jaundice have been reported with reversal of the abnormalities after discontinuation of nizatidine.

Miscellaneous: As with other histamine H_2 antagonists, rare cases of anaphylaxis following administration of nizatidine have been reported. Rare episodes of hypersensitivity reactions (eg, bronchospasm, laryngeal edema, rash, eosinophilia) have been reported. Serum sickness-like reactions have occurred rarely in conjunction with nizatidine use. Hyperuricemia unassociated with gout or nephrolithiasis was reported. Eosinophilia and fever have been reported.

• *Children* – In controlled clinical trials in pediatric patients (2 to 18 years of age), nizatidine was found to be generally safe and well tolerated. The principal adverse reactions (greater than 5%) were pyrexia, nasopharyngitis, diarrhea, vomiting, irritability, nasal congestion, and cough. Most adverse reactions were mild or moderate in severity. Mild elevations in serum transaminase (1 to 2 times the upper limit of normal) were noted in some patients. One subject experienced a seizure by electroencephalogram diagnosis after taking nizatidine oral solution 2.5 mg/kg twice daily for 23 days.

Ranitidine –

Cardiovascular: As with other histamine H_2 antagonists, rare reports of arrhythmias such as tachycardia, bradycardia, AV block, and premature ventricular beats. Bradycardia in association with rapid administration of ranitidine injection has been reported rarely, usually in patients with factors predisposing to cardiac rhythm disturbances.

CNS: Rarely, malaise and vertigo. Rare cases of reversible mental confusion (see Precautions), agitation, depression, and hallucinations have been reported, predominantly in severely ill elderly patients. Rare cases of reversible blurred vision suggestive of a change in accommodation have been reported. Rare reports of reversible involuntary motor disturbances have been received.

Dermatologic: Rare cases of vasculitis.

Endocrine: Controlled studies in animals and humans have shown no stimulation of any pituitary hormone by ranitidine and no antiandrogenic activity, and cimetidine-induced gynecomastia and impotence in hypersecretory patients have resolved when ranitidine has been substituted.

Hepatic: There have been occasional reports of hepatocellular, cholestatic, or mixed hepatitis, with or without jaundice. In such circumstances, immediately discontinue ranitidine. These events are usually reversible, but in rare circumstances death has occurred. Rare cases of hepatic failure have also been reported. In normal volunteers, ALT values were increased to at least twice the pretreatment levels in 6 of 12 subjects receiving 100 mg 4 times daily IV for 7 days, and in 4 of 24 subjects receiving 50 mg 4 times daily IV for 5 days (see Precautions).

Musculoskeletal: Rare reports of myalgias.

Miscellaneous: Rare cases of hypersensitivity reactions (eg, bronchospasm, fever, rash, eosinophilia), anaphylaxis, angioneurotic edema, and small increases in serum creatinine. Transient pain at the site of IM injection has been reported. Transient local burning or itching has been reported with IV administration of ranitidine.

Overdosage

➤*Symptoms:* Toxic doses in animals are associated with rapid respiration or respiratory failure, tachycardia, muscular tremors, vomiting, restlessness, pallor of mucous membranes or redness of mouth and ears, hypotension, and collapse.

Reported ingestions of up to 20 g of **cimetidine** have been associated with transient adverse reactions similar to those encountered in normal clinical experience. Two deaths have occurred in adults who reportedly ingested more than 40 g on a single occasion.

Famotidine dosages of up to 640 mg/day have been given to patients with pathological hypersecretory conditions with no serious adverse effects.

Reported acute ingestions of up to 18 g of **ranitidine** have been associated with transient adverse reactions similar to those encountered in normal clinical experience. In addition, abnormalities of gait and hypotension have been reported.

➤*Treatment:* Symptomatic and supportive. Remove unabsorbed material from the GI tract, monitor the patient, and employ supportive therapy. Refer to General Management of Acute Overdosage.

The ability of hemodialysis to remove **nizatidine** from the body has not been conclusively demonstrated; however, due to its large volume of distribution, nizatidine is not expected to be efficiently removed from the body by this method.

Patient Information

Advise patients to inform their health care provider or pharmacist of any concomitant drug therapy, especially when taking **cimetidine**.

These agents may be taken without regard to meals.

➤*OTC:* Patients should not take maximum daily dose for longer than 2 weeks continuously except under the advice and supervision of a health care provider.

CIMETIDINE

otc	**Cimetidine** (Various, eg, Ivax, Mylan, Teva)	**Tablets**: 200 mg	In 30s and 50s.
otc	**Acid Reducer 200** (Major)		In 30s.
otc	**Tagamet HB 200** (GlaxoSmith-Kline Consumer)		In 6s, 30s, and 50s.
Rx	**Cimetidine** (Various, eg, Endo, Major, Mylan, Novopharm, Schein)	**Tablets**: 200 mg	In 100s, 500s, and 1,000s.
Rx	**Cimetidine** (Various, eg, Ivax, Major, Mylan)	**Tablets**: 300 mg	In 100s, 500s, and 1,000s.
Rx	**Tagamet** (GlaxoSmithKline)		(Tagamet 300 SB). Light green. In 100s.
Rx	**Cimetidine** (Various, eg, Endo, Ivax, Major, Mylan)	**Tablets**: 400 mg	In 60s, 100s, 500s, and 1,000s.
Rx	**Tagamet** (GlaxoSmithKline)		(Tagamet 400 SB). Light green. Capsule shape. In 60s.
Rx	**Cimetidine** (Various, eg, Ivax, Mylan)	**Tablets**: 800 mg	In 30s, 100s, and 250s.
Rx	**Tagamet** (GlaxoSmithKline)		(Tagamet 800 SB). Light green. Oval. In 30s.
Rx	**Cimetidine** (Various, eg, Roxane, Teva)	**Oral solution**: 300 mg (as hydrochloride) per 5 mL	May contain alcohol, parabens, saccharin, sorbitol. In 240 and 480 mL and UD 5 mL.
Rx	**Cimetidine** (Various, eg, Hospira, Stada)	**Injection**: 150 mg (as hydrochloride) per mL	In 2 mL single-dose vials and 8 mL multidose vials.[a]
Rx	**Cimetidine in 0.9% Sodium Chloride** (Hospira)	**Injection (premixed)**: 6 mg (as hydrochloride) per mL	In 50 mL single-dose flexible container.

[a] May contain 9 mg/mL benzyl alcohol as a preservative.

CIMETIDINE — ORAL

For complete and comparative prescribing information, refer to the Histamine H_2 Antagonists group monograph.

Indications

➤*Benign gastric ulcer:* Short-term treatment.

➤*Duodenal ulcer:* Short-term treatment and maintenance therapy.

➤*Gastroesophageal reflux disease (GERD), erosive (oral only):* For the treatment of erosive esophagitis diagnosed by endoscopy.

➤*Pathological hypersecretory conditions:* For the treatment of pathological hypersecretory conditions (eg, Zollinger-Ellison syndrome, systemic mastocytosis, multiple endocrine adenomas).

➤*Heartburn (OTC only):* For the relief of heartburn associated with acid indigestion and sour stomach; for the prevention of heartburn associated with acid indigestion and sour stomach brought on by certain food and beverages.

➤*Unlabeled uses:* As part of a multidrug regimen to eradicate *Helicobacter pylori* in the treatment of peptic ulcer; in the perioperative setting to sup-

CIMETIDINE — ORAL

press gastric acid secretion, prevent stress ulcers, and prevent aspiration pneumonitis; in combination with histamine H_1 antagonists in the treatment of certain types of urticaria; treatment of cutaneous warts (data are conflicting).

Administration and Dosage

➤*Approved by the FDA:* 1977.

➤*Benign gastric ulcer:* For short-term treatment, 800 mg at bedtime or 300 mg 4 times a day with meals and at bedtime. The preferred regimen is 800 mg at bedtime based on convenience and lowered potential for drug interaction. There is no information concerning usefulness of treatment periods longer than 8 weeks.

➤*Duodenal ulcer:*

Short-term treatment – 800 mg at bedtime. Alternate regimens are 300 mg 4 times a day with meals and at bedtime, or 400 mg twice a day. Give antacids as needed for pain relief. However, simultaneous administration with antacids is not recommended, since antacids have been reported to interfere with the absorption of cimetidine. While healing often occurs during the first few weeks, continue treatment for 4 to 6 weeks unless healing is demonstrated by endoscopy. It has been shown that patients who have an endoscopically demonstrated ulcer larger than 1 cm and who are also heavy smokers (one pack of cigarettes or more a day) are more difficult to heal. There is some evidence that suggests more rapid healing can be achieved in this subpopulation with a dose of 1,600 mg at bedtime.

Maintenance therapy – 400 mg at bedtime.

➤*GERD, erosive:*

Adults – 1,600 mg daily in divided doses (800 mg twice daily or 400 mg 4 times a day) for 12 weeks. Use beyond 12 weeks has not been established.

➤*Pathological hypersecretory conditions:* 300 mg 4 times a day with meals and at bedtime. If necessary, give higher doses more often. Individualize dosage. Do not exceed 2400 mg/day; continue as long as clinically indicated.

➤*Heartburn (OTC only):* To relieve symptoms, 200 mg with water as symptoms occur or as directed, up to twice daily (up to 400 mg in 24 hours). To prevent symptoms, 200 mg with a glass of water right before or any time up to 30 minutes before eating food or drinking beverages that cause heartburn. Patients should not take the maximum dose for longer than 2 weeks continuously unless otherwise directed by a health care provider.

Children – Do not give to children younger than 12 years of age unless otherwise directed.

➤*Renal function impairment:* In severe renal impairment, accumulation may occur. Use the lowest dose; 300 mg every 12 hours orally or IV has been recommended. According to the patient's condition, dosage frequency may be increased to every 8 hours or even further with caution. Hemodialysis reduces the level of circulating cimetidine. Give the dose at the end of hemodialysis. When liver impairment is also present, further dosage reductions may be necessary.

➤*Storage/Stability:* Store between 15° and 30°C (59° and 86°F); dispense in a tight, light-resistant container.

CIMETIDINE — INJECTION

For complete and comparative prescribing information, refer to the Histamine H_2 Antagonists group monograph.

Indications

➤*Benign gastric ulcer:* Short-term treatment.

➤*Duodenal ulcer:* Short-term treatment and maintenance therapy.

➤*GI bleeding (intravenous [IV] only):* For the prevention of upper GI bleeding in critically ill patients.

➤*Pathological hypersecretory conditions:* For the treatment of pathological hypersecretory conditions (ie, Zollinger-Ellison syndrome, systemic mastocytosis, multiple endocrine adenomas).

➤*Unlabeled uses:* As part of a multidrug regimen to eradicate *Helicobacter pylori* in the treatment of peptic ulcer; in the perioperative setting to suppress gastric acid secretion, prevent stress ulcers, and prevent aspiration pneumonitis; in combination with histamine H_1 antagonists in the treatment of certain types of urticaria; treatment of cutaneous warts (data are conflicting); prevention of paclitaxel hypersensitivity (IV only); to reduce the incidence of GI hemorrhage associated with stress-related ulcers (IV only).

Administration and Dosage

➤*Approved by the FDA:* 1977.

➤*Parenteral:* For hospitalized patients with pathological hypersecretory conditions or intractable ulcers, or patients unable to take oral medication. The usual dosage is 300 mg every 6 to 8 hours. If it is necessary to increase dosage, do so by more frequent administration of a 300 mg dose, not to exceed 2,400 mg/day. Concomitant antacids should be given as needed for relief of pain.

GI bleeding – Continuous IV infusion of 50 mg/hour. Patients with creatinine clearance less than 30 mL/min should receive half the recommended dose. Treatment beyond 7 days has not been studied.

Gastroesophageal reflux disease (GERD) – The doses and regimen for parenteral administration in patients with GERD have not been established.

Cimetidine injection (150 mg/mL) –
Intramuscular: Administer undiluted.
IV injection: Dilute cimetidine 300 mg injection in 0.9% sodium chloride injection or other compatible IV solution to a total volume of 20 mL and inject over a period of at least 5 minutes.

Intermittent IV infusion: Dilute cimetidine 300 mg in at least 50 mL of 5% dextrose injection or another compatible IV solution and infuse over a period of 15 to 20 minutes.

Continuous IV infusion: 37.5 mg/h (900 mg/day). For patients requiring more rapid elevation of gastric pH, continuous infusion may be preceded by a 150 mg loading dose administered by IV infusion (see the previous paragraph). Dilute cimetidine 900 mg injection in a compatible IV solution for constant rate infusion over a 24 hour period. Cimetidine injection may be diluted in 100 to 1,000 mL; however, a volumetric pump is recommended if the volume for 24-hour infusion is less than 250 mL.

Cimetidine in 0.9% sodium chloride (premixed) –
Intermittent IV infusion: Administer over 15 to 20 minutes.
• *Continuous IV infusion* – 37.5 mg/h (900 mg/day). For patients requiring more rapid elevation of gastric pH, continuous infusion may be preceded by a 150 mg loading dose administered by IV infusion (see the previous paragraph). A volumetric pump is recommended if the volume for 24-hour infusion is less than 250 mL.

➤*Renal function impairment:* In severe renal impairment, accumulation may occur. Use the lowest dose; 300 mg every 12 hours orally or IV has been recommended. According to the patient's condition, dosage frequency may be increased to every 8 hours or even further with caution. Hemodialysis reduces the level of circulating cimetidine. Give the dose at the end of hemodialysis. When liver impairment is also present, further dosage reductions may be necessary.

➤*Admixture incompatibilities:* Do not add other drugs to premixed cimetidine in 0.9% sodium chloride injection.

➤*Storage/Stability:*

Cimetidine injection – Store vials at controlled room temperature 15° to 30°C (59° to 86°F). Do not refrigerate. When added to or diluted with most commonly used IV solutions (eg, 0.9% sodium chloride injection, 5% or 10% dextrose injection, Ringer's lactate solution, 5% sodium bicarbonate injection), cimetidine injection should not be used after more than 48 hours of storage at room temperature.

Cimetidine in 0.9% sodium chloride – Avoid excessive heat. Store at room temperature (25°C; 77°F).

RANITIDINE

otc	**Ranitidine** (Various, eg, Ivax, Major)	**Tablets**: 75 mg (as base)	In 10s, 20s, 30s, and 60s.
otc sf	**Zantac 75** (Pfizer Consumer Healthcare)		(Z 75). In 4s, 10s, 20s, 30s, 60s, 80s, and 100s.
otc sf	**Zantac 150 Maximum Strength** (Pfizer Consumer Healthcare)	**Tablets**: 150 mg (as base)	(Z). In 8s, 24s, 50s, and 65s.
Rx	**Ranitidine** (Various, eg, Apotex, Ivax, Ranbaxy, Teva, UDL, Watson)	**Tablets**: 150 mg (as base)	In 60s, 100s, 500s, 1,000s, 5,000s, and UD 100s.
Rx	**Zantac** (GlaxoSmithKline)		(Zantac 150 Glaxo). Peach, 5-sided. Film-coated. In 60s, 180s, 500s, 1,000s, and UD 100s.
Rx	**Ranitidine** (Various, eg, Apotex, Ivax, Ranbaxy, Teva, Watson)	**Tablets**: 300 mg (as base)	In 30s, 100s, 250s.
Rx	**Zantac** (GlaxoSmithKline)		(Zantac 300 Glaxo). Yellow, capsule shape. Film-coated. In 30s, 250s, and UD 100s.
Rx	**Zantac EFFERdose** (GlaxoSmithKline)	**Tablets, effervescent**: 25 mg (as base)	(GS 25C). White/pale yellow. In 60s.[a]
		150 mg (as base)	(Zantac 150 427). White/pale yellow. In 60s.[b]

RANITIDINE

Rx	**Ranitidine** (Various, eg, Par)	**Capsules**: 150 mg (as base)	In 60s and 500s.
		300 mg (as base)	In 30s and 100s.
Rx	**Zantac** (GlaxoSmithKline)	**Syrup**: 15 mg (as base) per mL	7.5% alcohol, saccharin, sorbitol, parabens. Peppermint flavor. In 480 mL.
Rx	**Zantac** (GlaxoSmithKline)	**Injection (premixed)**: 1 mg (as base) per mL	Preservative free. In premixed 50 mL single-dose plastic containers.[c]
Rx	**Ranitidine** (Bedford)	**Injection**: 25 mg (as base) per mL	In 2 mL single-dose vials and 6 mL multidose vials.[d]
Rx	**Zantac** (GlaxoSmithKline)		In 2 mL single-dose vials and 6 mL multidose vials.[d]

[a] With aspartame, 2.81 mg phenylalanine, and 30.52 mg sodium/tablet.
[b] With aspartame, 16.84 mg phenylalanine, and 183.12 mg sodium/tablet
[c] Premixed in 0.45% sodium chloride.
[d] With 5 mg/mL phenol.

RANITIDINE — ORAL

For complete and comparative prescribing information, refer to the Histamine H_2 Antagonists group monograph.

Indications

➤*Benign gastric ulcer:* For the short-term treatment of active, benign gastric ulcer and maintenance therapy after the healing of acute ulcer.

➤*Duodenal ulcer:* For the short-term treatment of active duodenal ulcer and maintenance therapy after the healing of acute ulcers.

➤*Erosive esophagitis:* For the treatment of endoscopically diagnosed erosive esophagitis; for the maintenance of healing of erosive esophagitis.

➤*Gastroesophageal reflux disease (GERD):* For the treatment of GERD.

➤*Pathological hypersecretory conditions:* For the treatment of pathological hypersecretory conditions (eg, Zollinger-Ellison syndrome, systemic mastocytosis).

➤*Heartburn (OTC only):* For the relief of heartburn associated with acid indigestion and sour stomach; for the prevention of heartburn associated with acid indigestion and sour stomach brought on by certain foods and beverages.

➤*Unlabeled uses:* As part of a multidrug regimen to eradicate *Helicobacter pylori* in the treatment of peptic ulcer; in the perioperative setting to suppress gastric acid secretion, prevent stress ulcers, and prevent aspiration pneumonitis; in combination with histamine H_1 antagonists in the treatment of certain types of urticaria; as prophylaxis to reduce the incidence of nonsteroidal anti-inflammatory drug (NSAID)-induced duodenal ulcer.

Administration and Dosage

➤*Approved by the FDA:* June 1983.

➤*Adults:*

Benign gastric ulcer –
Treatment: 150 mg twice daily.
Maintenance: 150 mg at bedtime.

Duodenal ulcer –
Treatment: 150 mg orally twice daily. An alternate dosage of 300 mg once daily after the evening meal or at bedtime can be used for patients in whom dosing convenience is important; 100 mg twice daily is as effective as the 150 mg dose in inhibiting gastric acid secretion.
Maintenance: 150 mg at bedtime.

Erosive esophagitis –
Treatment: 150 mg 4 times daily.
Maintenance: 150 mg twice daily.

GERD – 150 mg twice daily.

Pathological hypersecretory conditions – 150 mg orally twice a day. More frequent doses may be necessary. Individualize dosage and continue as long as indicated. Dosages up to 6 g/day have been used for severe disease.

Heartburn (OTC only)
Treatment: For relief of symptoms, swallow 1 tablet with a glass of water.
Prevention: To prevent symptoms, swallow 1 tablet with a glass of water 30 to 60 minutes before eating food or drinking beverages that cause heartburn.
Maintenance: Can be used up to twice daily (up to 2 tablets in 24 hours).

➤*Children:* The safety and efficacy of ranitidine have been established in children from 1 month to 16 years of age. There is insufficient information about the pharmacokinetics of ranitidine in neonatal patients less than 1 month of age to make dosing recommendations. Do not give OTC ranitidine to children younger than 12 years of age unless directed by a health care provider.

Active duodenal and gastric ulcers –
Treatment: 2 to 4 mg/kg twice daily to a maximum of 300 mg/day.
Maintenance: 2 to 4 mg/kg once daily to a maximum of 150 mg/day.

GERD and erosive esophagitis – Although limited data exist for these conditions in pediatric patients, published literature supports a dosage of 5 to 10 mg/kg/day, usually given as 2 divided doses.

➤*Preparation:*

Zantac EFFERdose 25 mg tablets – Dissolve 1 tablet in no less than 5 mL (1 teaspoonful) of water in an appropriate measuring cup. Wait until the tablet is completely dissolved before administering the solution to the infant/child. The solution may be administered by medicine dropper for infants. Tablet should not be chewed, swallowed whole, or dissolved on the tongue.

Zantac EFFERdose 150 mg tablets – Dissolve each dose in approximately 6 to 8 oz of water before drinking. Tablet should not be chewed, swallowed whole, or dissolved on the tongue.

➤*Renal function impairment (creatinine clearance less than 50 mL/min):* 150 mg orally every 24 hours. The frequency of dosing may be increased to every 12 hours or further with caution. Hemodialysis reduces the level of circulating ranitidine. Adjust dosage timing so that a scheduled dose coincides with the end of hemodialysis.

➤*Elderly:* Elderly patients are more likely to have decreased renal function; therefore, exercise caution in dose selection. It also may be useful to monitor renal function.

➤*Concomitant antacids:* Concomitant antacids should be given as needed for pain relief to patients with active duodenal ulcer; active, benign gastric ulcer; hypersecretory states; GERD; and erosive esophagitis.

➤*Storage/Stability:*

Tablets – Store between 15° and 30°C (59° and 86°F) in a dry place. Protect from light. Replace cap securely after each opening.

Effervescent tablets and granules – Store between 2° and 30°C (36° and 86°F).

Syrup – Store between 4° and 25°C (39° and 77°F). Dispense in a tight, light-resistant containers.

RANITIDINE — INJECTION

For complete and comparative prescribing information, refer to the Histamine H_2 Antagonists group monograph.

Indications

➤*Intravenous (IV):* Indicated in some hospitalized patients with pathological hypersecretory conditions or intractable duodenal ulcers, or as an alternative to the oral dosage form for short-term use in patients who are unable to take oral medication.

➤*Unlabeled uses:* As part of a multidrug regimen to eradicate *Helicobacter pylori* in the treatment of peptic ulcer; in the perioperative setting to suppress gastric acid secretion, prevent stress ulcers, and prevent aspiration pneumonitis; in combination with histamine H_1 antagonists in the treatment of certain types of urticaria; prevention of paclitaxel hypersensitivity (IV ranitidine); as prophylaxis to reduce the incidence of nonsteroidal anti-inflammatory drug (NSAID)-induced duodenal ulcer; reduce the incidence of GI hemorrhage associated with stress-related ulcers (IV ranitidine).

Administration and Dosage

➤*Approved by the FDA:* June 1983.

➤*Parenteral:*

Intramuscular – 50 mg (2 mL) every 6 to 8 hours. (No dilution necessary.)

Intermittent bolus – 50 mg (2 mL) every 6 to 8 hours. Dilute 50 mg in 0.9% sodium chloride or other compatible IV solution to a concentration no greater than 2.5 mg/mL (20 mL). Inject at a rate no greater than 4 mL/min (5 minutes).

Intermittent IV infusion – 50 mg (2 mL) every 6 to 8 hours. Dilute 50 mg in 5% dextrose injection or other compatible IV solution to a concentration no greater than 0.5 mg/mL (100 mL) and infuse at a rate no greater than 5 to 7 mL/min (15 to 20 minutes), or use 50 mL of 1 mg/mL premixed solution and infuse over 15 to 20 minutes; do not exceed 400 mg/day.

Premixed injection – Requires no dilution and should be infused over 15 to 20 minutes. Administer by slow IV drip infusion only. Do not introduce additives into the solution. If used with a primary IV fluid system, discontinue primary solution during premixed infusion.

Continuous IV infusion – Add ranitidine injection to 5% dextrose injection or other compatible IV solution (see Storage/Stability). Deliver at a rate of 6.25 mg/h (eg, 150 mg [6 mL] ranitidine injection in 250 mL of 5% dextrose injection at 10.7 mL/h).

For Zollinger-Ellison patients, dilute ranitidine injection in 5% dextrose injection or other compatible IV solution (see Storage/Stability) to a concentration of 2.5 mg/mL or less. Start the infusion at a rate of 1 mg/kg/h. If after 4 hours either the measured gastric acid output is greater than 10 mEq/h or the patient becomes symptomatic, adjust the dose upwards in 0.5 mg/kg/h increments and remeasure the acid output. Doses up to 2.5 mg/kg/h and infusion rates as high as 220 mg/h have been used.

➤*Children:* The recommended IV dose in pediatric patients is for a total daily dose of 2 to 4 mg/kg, to be divided and administered every 6 to 8 hours up to a maximum of 50 mg given every 6 to 8 hours. Limited data in neonatal patients (less than 1 month of age) receiving extracorporeal membrane oxygenation have shown that a dose of 2 mg/kg is usually sufficient to

RANITIDINE — INJECTION

increase gastric pH to greater than 4 for at least 15 hours. Therefore, consider doses of 2 mg/kg given every 12 to 24 hours or as a continuous infusion.

➤*Renal function impairment (creatinine clearance less than 50 mL/min):* 50 mg parenterally every 18 to 24 hours. The frequency of dosing may be increased to every 12 hours or further with caution. Hemodialysis reduces the level of circulating ranitidine. Adjust dosage timing so that a scheduled dose coincides with the end of hemodialysis.

➤*Elderly:* Elderly patients are more likely to have decreased renal function; therefore, exercise caution in dose selection. It also may be useful to monitor renal function.

➤*Concomitant antacids:* Concomitant antacids should be given as needed for pain relief to patients with active duodenal ulcer; active, benign gastric ulcer; hypersecretory states; gastroesophageal reflux disease; and erosive esophagitis.

➤*Ranitidine injection premixed in flexible plastic containers instructions for use:* To open, tear outer wrap at notch and remove solution container. Check for minute leaks by squeezing container firmly. If leaks are found, discard unit as sterility may be impaired.

Preparation for administration – Use aseptic technique.

1.) Close flow control clamp of administration set.
2.) Remove cover from outlet port at bottom of container.
3.) Insert piercing pin of administration set into port with a twisting motion until the pin is firmly seated.
4.) Suspend container from hanger.
5.) Squeeze and release drip chamber to establish proper fluid level in chamber during infusion of ranitidine injection premixed.
6.) Open flow control clamp to expel air from set. Close clamp.
7.) Attach set to venipuncture device. If device is not indwelling, prime and make venipuncture.
8.) Perform venipuncture.
9.) Regulate rate of administration with flow control clamp.

Ranitidine injection premixed in flexible plastic containers is to be administered by slow IV drip infusion only. Additives should not be introduced into this solution. If used with a primary IV fluid system, the primary solution should be discontinued during ranitidine HCl injection premixed infusion.

Do not administer unless solution is clear and container is undamaged.

Do not use flexible plastic container in series connections.

➤*Renal function impairment:* The administration of ranitidine as a continuous infusion has not been evaluated in patients with impaired renal function. On the basis of experience with a group of subjects with severely impaired renal function treated with ranitidine, the recommended dosage in patients with a creatinine clearance less than 50 mL/min is 50 mg every 18 to 24 hours. Should the patient's condition require, the frequency of dosing may be increased to every 12 hours or even further with caution. Hemodialysis reduces the level of circulating ranitidine. Ideally, the dosing schedule should be adjusted so that the timing of a scheduled dose coincides with the end of hemodialysis.

Elderly patients are more likely to have decreased renal function, therefore, caution should be exercised in dose selection, and it may be useful to monitor renal function (see Warnings, Elderly in the Histamine H_2 Antagonists group monograph).

➤*Storage/Stability:*

Stability –

Parenteral: Undiluted ranitidine injection tends to exhibit a yellow color that may intensify over time without adversely affecting potency. Ranitidine injection is stable for 48 hours at room temperature when added to or diluted with most commonly used IV solutions (eg, 0.9% sodium chloride injection, 5% or 10% dextrose injection, Ringer's lactate injection, 5% sodium bicarbonate injection).

Store the premixed injection between 2° and 25°C (36° and 77°F) and the injection between 4° and 25°C (39° and 77°F). Protect from light. Ranitidine injection premixed in flexible plastic containers is sterile through the expiration date on the label when stored under recommended conditions.

Note – Parenteral drug products should be inspected visually for particulate matter and discoloration before administration whenever solution and container permit.

Injection – Ranitidine injection premixed, 50 mg/50 mL, in 0.45% sodium chloride, is available as a sterile, premixed solution for IV administration in single-dose, flexible plastic containers. It contains no preservatives.

Exposure of pharmaceutical products to heat should be minimized. Avoid excessive heat; however, brief exposure up to 40°C (104°F) does not adversely affect the product. Protect from freezing.

NIZATIDINE

otc	**Axid AR** (Wyeth Consumer)	**Tablets:** 75 mg	(AXID AR). In 12s and 30s.
Rx	**Nizatidine** (Various, eg, Eon, Ivax, Mylan, Par)	**Capsules:** 150 mg	In 60s, 100s, 500s, 1000s, and UD 100s.
Rx	**Axid Pulvules** (Reliant)		(Lilly 3144/Axid 150 mg). Yellow. In 60s, 500s, and *Identi-Dose* 100s and 620s.
Rx	**Nizatidine** (Various, eg, Eon, Ivax, Mylan, Par)	**Capsules:** 300 mg	In 30s, 100s, and 500s.
Rx	**Axid Pulvules** (Reliant)		(Lilly 3145/Axid 300 mg). Yellow/brown. In 30s.
Rx	**Axid** (Braintree)	**Oral solution:** 15 mg/mL	Parabens, saccharin, sucrose. Clear yellow. Bubble gum flavor. In 480 mL.

NIZATIDINE — ORAL

For complete and comparative prescribing information, refer to the Histamine H_2 Antagonists group monograph.

Indications

➤*Benign gastric ulcer:* For the treatment of active benign ulcer for up to 8 weeks.

➤*Duodenal ulcer:* For the treatment of active ulcer for up to 8 weeks and maintenance therapy after healing of active ulcer.

➤*Gastroesophageal reflux disease (GERD):* For the treatment of endoscopically diagnosed esophagitis, including erosive and ulcerative esophagitis, and associated heartburn due to GERD.

➤*Heartburn (OTC only):* For the relief of heartburn, acid indigestion, and sour stomach and prevention of these symptoms brought on by consuming food and beverages.

Administration and Dosage

➤*Approved by the FDA:* April 1988.

For adult use only (12 years of age or older for oral solution and OTC).

➤*Benign gastric ulcer:* 300 mg given either as 150 mg twice daily or 300 mg once daily at bedtime.

➤*Duodenal ulcer:*

Acute therapy – 300 mg once daily at bedtime. An alternative dosage regimen is 150 mg twice daily. Most heal in 4 weeks.

Maintenance therapy – 150 mg once daily at bedtime.

➤*GERD:* 150 mg twice daily.

➤*Heartburn (OTC only):* Can be used up to twice daily (up to 2 tablets in 24 hours).

Relief – For relief of symptoms, 1 tablet with a full glass of water.

Prevention – For prevention of symptoms, 1 tablet with a full glass of water right before eating or up to 60 minutes before consuming food and beverages that cause heartburn.

➤*Moderate to severe renal insufficiency:*

Nizatidine Dosage in Renal Insufficiency

Creatinine clearance	Dosage: Active duodenal ulcer, GERD, benign gastric ulcer	Dosage: Maintenance therapy
20 to 50 mL/min	150 mg/day	150 mg every other day
< 20 mL/min	150 mg every other day	150 mg every 3 days

➤*Storage/Stability:*

Capsules – Store at controlled room temperature 20° to 25°C (68° to 77°F) in a tightly closed container.

Solution – Store at 25°C (77°F); excursions are permitted to 15° to 30°C (59° to 86°F). Dispense in a tight, light-resistant container.

FAMOTIDINE

otc	**Famotidine** (Ivax)	**Tablets**: 10 mg	In 18s, 30s, 50s, and 70s.
otc	**Pepcid AC** (J & J Merck)		(Pepcid AC). In 2s, 6s, 18s, 30s, 60s, and 90s.
Rx	**Famotidine** (Various, eg, Ivax, Teva, UDL)	**Tablets**: 20 mg	May contain lactose. In 30s, 100s, 500s, 1,000s, UD 100s, and *Robot-Ready* 25s.
Rx	**Pepcid** (Merck)		(MSD 963 PEPCID). Beige, U-shape. Film-coated. In 1,000s, 10,000s, unit-of-use 30s, 90s, and 100s, UD 100s, and *Uniblister* 31s.
otc	**Pepcid AC Maximum Strength** (J & J Merck)		In 25s.
Rx	**Famotidine** (Various, eg, Ivax, Par, Teva)	**Tablets**: 40 mg	May contain lactose. In 30s, 100s, 500s, 1,000s, and UD 100s.
Rx	**Pepcid** (Merck)		(MSD 964 PEPCID). Lt. brownish orange, U-shape. Film-coated. In 1,000s, 10,000s, unit of use 30s, 90s, and 100s, UD 100s, and *Uniblister* 31s.
otc	**Pepcid AC** (J & J Merck)	**Gelcaps**: 10 mg	(PEPCID AC). In 30s, 50s, 60s, and 90s.
otc	**Pepcid AC** (J & J Merck)	**Tablets, chewable**: 10 mg	Aspartame, lactose, mannitol, 1.4 mg phenylalanine. (PEPCID AC). In 6s, 18s, 30s, 50s, 60s, and 68s.
Rx	**Pepcid RPD** (Merck)	**Tablets, orally disintegrating**: 20 mg	Aspartame, mannitol, 1.05 mg phenylalanine. Mint flavor. Pale rose, hexagonal. In UD 30s and 100s.
		40 mg	Aspartame, mannitol, 2.1 mg phenylalanine. Mint flavor. Pale rose, hexagonal. In UD 30s and 100s.
Rx	**Pepcid** (Merck)	**Powder for oral suspension**: 40 mg per 5 mL when reconstituted	Parabens, sucrose. Cherry-banana-mint flavor. In bottles of 400 mg.
Rx	**Famotidine** (Various, eg, American Pharma, Baxter, Bedford, Hospira)	**Injection**: 10 mg/mL	May contain mannitol or benzyl alcohol. In 1 and 2 mL single-dose vials and 4, 20, and 50 mL multidose vials.
Rx	**Pepcid** (Merck)		Mannitol. In 2 mL single-dose vials[a] and 4 and 20 mL multidose vials.[b]
Rx	**Famotidine** (Baxter)	**Injection (premixed)**: 20 mg per 50 mL	In 50 mL single-dose *Galaxy* containers.
Rx	**Pepcid** (Merck)		Preservative free. In 50 mL single-dose *Galaxy* containers.

[a] Preservative free.

[b] With 0.9% benzyl alcohol.

FAMOTIDINE — ORAL

For complete and comparative prescribing information, refer to the Histamine H_2 Antagonists group monograph.

Indications

➤*Benign gastric ulcer:* For the short-term treatment (up to 8 weeks) of active benign gastric ulcer.

➤*Duodenal ulcer:* For the short-term treatment (up to 8 weeks) of active duodenal ulcer and maintenance therapy after healing of active ulcer.

➤*Gastroesophageal reflux disease (GERD):* For the short-term treatment (up to 6 weeks) of GERD and esophagitis due to GERD, including erosive or ulcerative disease diagnosed by endoscopy.

➤*Pathological hypersecretory conditions:* For the treatment of pathological hypersecretory conditions (eg, Zollinger-Ellison syndrome).

➤*Heartburn (OTC only):* For the relief of heartburn associated with acid indigestion and sour stomach; for the prevention of heartburn associated with acid indigestion and sour stomach brought on by certain foods and beverages.

➤*Unlabeled uses:* As part of a multidrug regimen to eradicate *Helicobacter pylori* in the treatment of peptic ulcer; in the perioperative setting to suppress gastric acid secretion, prevent stress ulcers, and prevent aspiration pneumonitis; in combination with histamine H_1 antagonists in the treatment of certain types of urticaria.

Administration and Dosage

➤*Approved by the FDA:* October 1986.

➤*Duodenal ulcer:*

Acute therapy – 40 mg/day at bedtime. Most heal in 4 weeks; there is rarely reason to use full dosage for more than 6 to 8 weeks. 20 mg twice daily is also effective.

Maintenance therapy – 20 mg once a day at bedtime.

➤*Benign gastric ulcer:*

Acute therapy – 40 mg once a day at bedtime.

➤*Pathological hypersecretory conditions:* Individualize dosage. The adult starting dosage is 20 mg every 6 hours; some patients may require a higher starting dose. Continue as long as clinically indicated. Dosages up to 160 mg every 6 hours have been administered to some adult patients with severe Zollinger-Ellison syndrome.

➤*GERD:* 20 mg twice daily for up to 6 weeks. For esophagitis including erosions and ulcerations and accompanying symptoms due to GERD, 20 or 40 mg twice daily for up to 12 weeks.

➤*Children:* Studies suggest the following starting dosages in pediatric patients 1 to 16 years of age.

Peptic ulcer – 0.5 mg/kg/day orally at bedtime or divided twice daily up to 40 mg/day.

GERD with or without esophagitis including erosions and ulcerations – 1 mg/kg/day orally divided twice daily up to 40 mg twice daily.

While published uncontrolled studies suggest efficacy of famotidine in the treatment of GERD and peptic ulcer, data in pediatric patients are insufficient to establish percent response with dose and duration of therapy. Therefore, individualize treatment duration (initially based on adult duration recommendations) and dose based on clinical response and/or pH determination (gastric or esophageal) and endoscopy. Published uncontrolled clinical studies in pediatric patients 1 to 16 years of age have employed dosages up to 1 mg/kg/day for peptic ulcer and 2 mg/kg/day for GERD with or without esophagitis including erosions and ulcerations.

➤*Infants:*

GERD – Studies suggest the following starting dosages in pediatric patients younger than 1 year of age: 0.5 mg/kg/dose of oral suspension for the treatment of GERD for up to 8 weeks once daily in patients younger than 3 months of age, and 0.5 mg/kg/dose twice daily in patients 3 months to younger than 1 year of age. Patients should also be receiving conservative measures (eg, thickened feedings). The use of IV famotidine in pediatric patients younger than 1 year of age with GERD has not been adequately studied.

➤*Heartburn, acid indigestion, and sour stomach (OTC only):*

Acute therapy – 10 or 20 mg with water.

Prevention – 10 or 20 mg 15 to 60 minutes before eating food or drinking a beverage that is expected to cause symptoms.

Use – Can be used up to twice daily (up to 2 tablets in 24 hours). Patients should not take the maximum dose for more than 2 weeks continuously unless otherwise directed by their health care provider.

Children – Do not give to children younger than 12 years of age unless otherwise directed.

➤*Oral suspension:* Famotidine oral suspension may be substituted for famotidine tablets in any of these indications. Each 5 mL contains 40 mg of famotidine after constitution of the powder with 46 mL of purified water as directed.

➤*Directions for preparing famotidine oral suspension:* Prepare suspension at time of dispensing. Slowly add 46 mL of purified water. Shake vigorously for 5 to 10 seconds immediately after adding the water and immediately before use.

➤*Stability of famotidine oral suspension:* Unused constituted oral suspension should be discarded after 30 days.

➤*Concomitant use of antacids:* Antacids may be given concomitantly if needed.

➤*Renal function impairment:* In adult patients with moderate (creatinine clearance less than 50 mL/min) or severe (creatinine clearance less than 10 mL/min) renal insufficiency, the elimination half-life of famotidine is increased. For patients with severe renal insufficiency, it may exceed 20 hours, reaching approximately 24 hours in anuric patients. Since CNS adverse reactions have been reported in patients with moderate and severe renal insufficiency, to avoid excess accumulation of the drug in patients with moderate or severe renal insufficiency, the dose of famotidine may be reduced by half or the dosing interval may be prolonged to 36 to 48 hours as indicated by the patient's clinical response.

Based on the comparison of pharmacokinetic parameters for famotidine in adults and pediatric patients, dosage adjustment in pediatric patients with moderate or severe renal insufficiency should be considered.

FAMOTIDINE — ORAL

➤*OTC:* For adults and children 12 years of age and older, famotidine is available in these forms: gelcaps, tablets, and chewable tablets. The decision to choose gelcaps, tablets, or chewable tablets is a matter of personal choice. Famotidine oral provides various forms to meet the specific preferences of each individual person. Some find the tablets easier to swallow while others prefer gelcaps, and some prefer to chew the chewable tablets.

Adults and children 12 years of age and older –
Gelcaps and tablets: To relieve symptoms, instruct patients to swallow 1 gelcap or tablet with a glass of water.

To prevent symptoms, instruct patients to swallow 1 gelcap or tablet with a glass of water at any time from 15 to 60 minutes before eating food or drinking beverages that cause heartburn.

Patients should not use more than 2 gelcaps or tablets in 24 hours.

Chewable tablets: Patients should not swallow tablets whole; they should be chewed completely.

To relieve symptoms, instruct patients to chew 1 chewable tablet.

To prevent symptoms, instruct patients to chew 1 chewable tablet at any time from 15 to 60 minutes before eating food or drinking beverages that cause heartburn.

Patients should not use more than 2 chewable tablets in 24 hours.

Children younger than 12 years of age – Consult a health care provider.

➤*Storage/Stability:*

Tablets/Oral suspension dry powder and suspension – Store at 25°C (77°F); excursions are permitted to 15° to 30°C (59° to 86°F). Protect suspension from freezing. Discard unused suspension after 30 days.

OTC products – Store at 20° to 30°C (68° to 86°F). Protect from moisture.

FAMOTIDINE — INJECTION

For complete and comparative prescribing information, refer to the Histamine H_2 Antagonists group monograph.

Indications

➤*Benign gastric ulcer:* For the short-term treatment (up to 8 weeks) of active benign gastric ulcer.

➤*Duodenal ulcer:* For the short-term treatment (up to 8 weeks) of active duodenal ulcer and maintenance therapy after healing of active ulcer.

➤*Pathological hypersecretory conditions:* For the treatment of pathological hypersecretory conditions (eg, Zollinger-Ellison syndrome).

➤*Gastroesophageal reflux disease (GERD):* For the short-term treatment (up to 6 weeks) of GERD and esophagitis due to GERD, including erosive or ulcerative disease diagnosed by endoscopy.

➤*Intravenous (IV):* For use in some hospitalized patients with pathological hypersecretory conditions or intractable ulcers, or as an alternative to the oral dosage forms for short-term use in patients who are unable to take oral medication.

➤*Unlabeled uses:* As part of a multidrug regimen to eradicate *Helicobacter pylori* in the treatment of peptic ulcer; in the perioperative setting to suppress gastric acid secretion, prevent stress ulcers, and prevent aspiration pneumonitis; in combination with histamine H_1 antagonists in the treatment of certain types of urticaria; prevention of paclitaxel hypersensitivity (IV famotidine); prevention of recurrent bleeding after successful endoscopic treatment of bleeding peptic ulcer (IV famotidine); to reduce the incidence of GI hemorrhage associated with stress-related ulcers (IV famotidine).

As part of a premedication regimen with diphenhydramine and IV dexamethasone to reduce or prevent paclitaxel-related hypersensitivity reactions.

Administration and Dosage

➤*Approved by the FDA:* November 4, 1986.

➤*Parenteral:*

IV – In some hospitalized patients with pathological hypersecretory conditions or intractable ulcers, or in patients unable to take oral medication, give famotidine IV 20 mg every 12 hours. Doses and regimen for GERD are not established.

Children – Individualize dosage. Starting dose in pediatric patients 1 to 16 years of age is 0.25 mg/kg IV (injected over a period of at least 2 minutes or as a 15-minute infusion) every 12 hours, up to 40 mg/day.

The starting dose in pediatric patients younger than 1 year of age is 0.5 mg/kg/dose of famotidine oral suspension for the treatment of GERD for up to 8 weeks once daily in patients younger than 3 months of age and 0.5 mg/kg/dose twice daily in patients 3 months to less than 1 year of age. Patients should also be receiving conservative measures (eg, thickened feedings). The use of IV famotidine in pediatric patients younger than 1 year of age with GERD has not been adequately studied.

Preparation of IV solutions – Dilute 2 mL famotidine IV (solution containing 10 mg/mL) with 0.9% sodium chloride injection or other compatible IV solution to a total volume of either 5 or 10 mL and inject over not less than 2 minutes.

Preparation of IV infusion solutions – Famotidine IV may also be administered as an infusion, 2 mL diluted with 100 mL of 5% dextrose or other compatible solution, and infused over 15 to 30 minutes. A premixed solution is also available containing famotidine premixed with 0.9% sodium chloride, and it should be infused over 15 to 30 minutes.

➤*Renal function impairment:* To avoid excess accumulation of the drug in patients with moderate (creatinine clearance less than 50 mL/min) or severe renal insufficiency (creatinine clearance less than 10 mL/min) the dose may be reduced to half the dose or the dosing interval may be prolonged to 36 to 48 hours, as indicated by patient response.

➤*Concomitant use of antacids:* Antacids may be given concomitantly if needed.

➤*Storage/Stability:* Solution is stable for 7 days at room temperature when added to or diluted with most commonly used IV solutions (eg, water for injection, 0.9% sodium chloride injection, 5% or 10% dextrose injection, Ringer's lactate injection, 5% sodium bicarbonate injection). When added to or diluted with 5% sodium bicarbonate injection, a precipitate may form at higher concentrations of famotidine injection (more than 0.2 mg/mL). Although diluted famotidine injection has been shown to be stable for 7 days at room temperature, there are no data on the maintenance of sterility after dilution. Therefore, it is recommended that if not used immediately after preparation, diluted solutions of famotidine injection should be refrigerated and used within 48 hours.

Store injection vials (non-premixed) at 2° to 8°C (36° to 46°F). Store premixed injection at room temperature (25°C; 77°F). Avoid exposure of the premixed product to excessive heat; brief exposure to temperatures up to 35°C (95°F) does not adversely affect the product. If solution freezes, bring to room temperature; allow sufficient time to solubilize all the components.

HISTAMINE H_2 ANTAGONIST COMBINATIONS

otc	**Pepcid Complete** (J & J Merck)	**Tablets, chewable:** 10 mg famotidine, 800 mg calcium carbonate, 165 mg magnesium hydroxide	Lactose, sugar. (P). Mint flavor. In 5s, 15s, 25s, and 50s.

HISTAMINE H_2 ANTAGONIST COMBINATIONS — ORAL

For complete prescribing information, refer to the Histamine H_2 Antagonists group monograph.

Indications

➤*Heartburn:* For the relief of heartburn associated with acid indigestion and sour stomach.

Administration and Dosage

➤*12 years of age and older:* To relieve symptoms, chew 1 tablet before swallowing. Instruct patients not to use more than 2 tablets in 24 hours and not to swallow tablets whole; they should be chewed completely.

➤*Storage/Stability:* Store at 25° to 30°C (77° to 86°F).

PROTON PUMP INHIBITORS

Indications

Proton Pump Inhibitors - Summary of Indications[a]

Indication ✓ = Labeled X = Unlabeled	Esomeprazole	Lansoprazole	Omeprazole	Pantoprazole	Rabeprazole
Duodenal ulcer		✓[b]	✓	X	✓
Duodenal ulcer associated with *Helicobacter pylori* (in combination with antibiotics)	✓	✓[b]	✓[c]	X	✓
Gastric ulcer		✓[b]	✓[c]	X	X
Erosive esophagitis	✓	✓	✓	✓	✓
GERD[d] in adults	✓	✓[b]	✓	✓	✓
GERD in children		X	X		

Proton Pump Inhibitors - Summary of Indications[a]					
Indication ✓ = Labeled X = Unlabeled	Esomeprazole	Lansoprazole	Omeprazole	Pantoprazole	Rabeprazole
H. pylori gastritis in children[e]		X	X		
Hypersecretory conditions (eg, Zollinger-Ellison syndrome)		✓[b]	✓[c]	✓	✓
GERD-related laryngitis			X		
To improve pancreatic enzyme absorption in cystic fibrosis patients with intestinal malabsorption		X	X		

[a] For more detailed information, see the information below and the individual drug monographs.
[b] Oral only.
[c] Except omeprazole oral suspension.
[d] Gastroesophageal reflux disease.
[e] In combination with amoxicillin and clarithromycin.

➤*Duodenal ulcer (lansoprazole, omeprazole, rabeprazole):* For short-term treatment of active duodenal ulcer. Lansoprazole also is indicated to maintain the healing of duodenal ulcers.

➤*Duodenal ulcer associated with H. pylori infection:* For treatment of patients with *H. pylori* infection and duodenal ulcer to eradicate *H. pylori*.

Dual therapy – In combination with clarithromycin (**omeprazole**) or amoxicillin (**lansoprazole**).

Triple therapy (esomeprazole, lansoprazole, omeprazole, rabeprazole) – In combination with clarithromycin and amoxicillin.

➤*Erosive esophagitis (esomeprazole, lansoprazole, omeprazole, pantoprazole, rabeprazole):* For short-term treatment and maintenance of healing of erosive esophagitis.

➤*Gastric ulcer (lansoprazole, omeprazole):* For short-term treatment of active benign gastric ulcer. Lansoprazole also is indicated for the healing and reducing the risk of nonsteroidal anti-inflammatory agent (NSAID)-associated gastric ulcers in patients who continue NSAID use.

➤*GERD (esomeprazole, lansoprazole, omeprazole, pantoprazole, rabeprazole):* For the treatment of heartburn and other symptoms associated with GERD.

➤*Hypersecretory conditions (lansoprazole, omeprazole, pantoprazole, rabeprazole):* For the long-term treatment of pathological hypersecretory conditions (eg, Zollinger-Ellison syndrome, multiple endocrine adenomas, systemic mastocytosis).

Actions

➤*Pharmacology:* **Omeprazole**, **esomeprazole**, **lansoprazole**, **rabeprazole**, and **pantoprazole** belong to a class of antisecretory compounds, the substituted benzimidazoles, that do not exhibit anticholinergic or histamine H_2 antagonistic properties, but that suppress gastric acid secretion by specific inhibition of the H^+/K^+ ATPase enzyme system at the secretory surface of the gastric parietal cell. Because this enzyme system is the "acid (proton) pump" within the gastric mucosa, these agents have been characterized as gastric acid pump inhibitors; they block the final step of acid production. This effect is dose-related and inhibits basal and stimulated acid secretion regardless of the stimulus.

Serum gastrin levels increase parallel with inhibition of acid secretion. No further increase in serum gastrin occurs with continued treatment. Gastrin values usually returned to pretreatment levels within 24 hours (IV pantoprazole), 1 to 2 weeks (omeprazole), 4 weeks (esomeprazole, lansoprazole), or 3 months (oral pantoprazole) after discontinuation of therapy.

➤*Pharmacokinetics:*

Absorption / Distribution – Most of these oral agents contain enteric-coated granules. Absorption of these agents is rapid and begins only after the granules leave the stomach.

Peak plasma concentrations of AUC and **omeprazole** are approximately proportional with doses up to 40 mg, but because of saturable first-pass effect, a greater than linear response occurs with doses greater than 40 mg.

The **esomeprazole** C_{max} increases proportionally when the dose is increased, and there is a 3-fold increase in the AUC from 20 to 40 mg. The AUC after administration of a single 40 mg dose of esomeprazole is decreased by 43% to 53% after food intake compared with fasting conditions.

C_{max} and AUC of **lansoprazole** are diminished by approximately 50% to 70% if the drug is given 30 minutes after food as opposed to the fasting condition. The AUC after administration of a single 40 mg dose of esomeprazole is decreased by 43% to 53% after food intake compared with fasting conditions. Esomeprazole should be taken at least 1 hour before meals. When **pantoprazole** is given with food, its T_{max} is highly variable and may increase significantly. Absorption may be delayed up to 2 hours or longer; however, the C_{max} and AUC of pantoprazole are not altered. When **rabeprazole** is administered with a high-fat meal, its T_{max} is variable and may delay its absorption up to 4 hours or longer; however, the C_{max} and AUC are not significantly altered.

Metabolism / Excretion – These agents are extensively metabolized by the liver. Several metabolites have been identified. These metabolites have very little or no antisecretory activity. The plasma elimination half-life of proton pump inhibitors does not reflect duration of suppression of gastric acid secretion. Thus, the plasma elimination half-life is less than 2 hours while the acid inhibitory effect lasts more than 24 hours, apparently because of prolonged binding to the parietal H^+/K^+ ATPase enzyme. When the drug is discontinued, secretory activity returns over 1 to 5 days.

Little unchanged drug is excreted in urine. Approximately 33% of **lansoprazole** and the majority of **omeprazole** (approximately 77%), **esomeprazole** (approximately 80%), **rabeprazole** (approximately 90%), and **pantoprazole** (approximately 71%) is eliminated in urine. The remainder of the dose is excreted in feces. This implies a significant biliary excretion of the metabolites of omeprazole and lansoprazole.

Proton Pump Inhibitors Pharmacokinetics					
Parameter	Esomeprazole	Lansoprazole	Omeprazole[a]	Pantoprazole	Rabeprazole
Bioavailability (%)	≈ 64 (single dose) ≈ 90 (multiple dose)	> 80	30 to 40	≈ 77 (oral)	≈ 52
T_{max} (h)	≈ 1.5	1.7	0.5 to 3.5	≈ 2.5 (oral)	2 to 5
Protein binding (%)	97	97	≈ 95	≈ 98	96.3
Half-life (h)	≈ 1 to 1.5	≈ 1.5 (oral) ≈ 1.3 (IV)	0.5 to 1	≈ 1	1 to 2
Total body clearance (mL/min)		≈ 185 (IV)	500 to 600	≈ 127 to 233 (IV)	
Onset (h)		1 to 3	≤ 1		≤ 1
Duration (h)		> 24	72	> 24	

[a] Capsules.

Special populations –

Renal function impairment: In patients with chronic renal impairment (Ccr, 10 to 62 mL/min/1.73 m^2), the disposition of **omeprazole** was similar to that in healthy volunteers but with a slight increase in bioavailability. Because urinary excretion is a primary route of elimination of omeprazole metabolites, their elimination slowed in proportion to the decreased Ccr. However, no dosage adjustment is necessary.

In patients with severe renal insufficiency, plasma protein binding decreased by 1% to 1.5% after administration of 60 mg **lansoprazole**. Patients with renal insufficiency had a shortened elimination half-life and decreased total AUC (free and bound). However, AUC for free lansoprazole in plasma was not related to the degree of renal impairment, and C_{max} and T_{max} were not different from subjects with healthy kidneys.

Hepatic function impairment: In patients with severe hepatic insufficiency, the **esomeprazole** AUC was 2 to 3 times higher.

In patients with chronic hepatic disease, the bioavailability of **omeprazole** increased to approximately 100%, reflecting decreased first-pass effect; plasma half-life increased to nearly 3 hours. Plasma clearance averaged 70 mL/min, compared with 500 to 600 mL/min in healthy subjects.

In patients with various degrees of chronic hepatic disease, the mean plasma half-life of **lansoprazole** was prolonged from 1.5 hours to 3.2 to 7.2 hours. An increase in mean AUC of up to 500% was observed at steady state in hepatically impaired patients compared with healthy subjects. Consider dose reduction in patients with severe hepatic disease.

In patients with chronic, mild to moderate hepatic disease, the AUC of **rabeprazole** doubled, the elimination half-life increased 2- to 3-fold, and the total body clearance decreased to less than half compared with healthy patients after a 20 mg oral dose.

In patients with mild to severe hepatic impairment, maximum **pantoprazole** concentrations increased 1.5-fold, serum half-life increased 7 to 9 hours, and AUC increased 5- to 7-fold compared with healthy subjects; however, these values were no greater than those observed in slow CYP2C19 metabolizers.

Elderly: In the elderly, the elimination rate of **omeprazole** was somewhat decreased and bioavailability was increased. Omeprazole was 76% bioavailable with a 40 mg oral dose in elderly volunteers versus 58% in young volunteers. Nearly 70% of the dose was recovered in urine as metabolites; no unchanged drug was detected. The plasma clearance of omeprazole was 250 mL/min and its plasma half-life averaged 1 hour. However, no dosage adjustment is necessary.

The **esomeprazole** AUC and C_{max} values were slightly higher (25% and 18%, respectively) in the elderly compared with younger subjects.

The clearance of **lansoprazole** is decreased in the elderly, with elimination half-life increased by approximately 50% to 100%. Because the mean half-life in the elderly remains between 1.9 to 2.9 hours, repeated once-daily dosing does not result in accumulation of lansoprazole.

In healthy elderly subjects receiving 20 mg **rabeprazole** once daily for 7 days, AUC values doubled and C_{max} increased by 60% compared with a younger control group.

In elderly subjects receiving **pantoprazole**, the AUC increased by 43% and the C_{max} increased by 26% compared with younger subjects.

Race: An increase in AUC of **omeprazole** of approximately 4-fold was noted in Asian subjects compared with white subjects. Consider dose adjustment for Asian subjects, particularly where maintenance of healing of erosive esophagitis is indicated.

The mean AUCs of **lansoprazole** in Asian subjects were approximately twice those seen in pooled US data; however, the interindividual variability was high. The C_{max} values were comparable.

In healthy Japanese men, the **rabeprazole** AUC was approximately 50% to 60% greater than values derived from pooled data from healthy men in the United States.

Contraindications

Hypersensitivity to any component of the formulation; substituted benzimidazoles (**rabeprazole**, **esomeprazole**).

Warnings

➤*Gastritis:* Atrophic gastritis has been noted occasionally in gastric corpus biopsies from patients treated long-term with **esomeprazole** and **omeprazole**.

Patients with healed GERD were treated for up to 40 months with **rabeprazole** and monitored with serial gastric biopsies. Patients with *H. pylori* infection at baseline had mild or moderate inflammation of the gastric body or mild inflammation in the gastric antrum. At baseline, 8% of patients had atrophy of glands in the gastric body and 15% had atrophy in the gastric antrum. At endpoint, 15% of patients had atrophy of glands in the gastric body and 11% had atrophy in the gastric antrum. Approximately 4% of patients had intestinal metaplasia at some point during follow-up, but no consistent changes were seen.

➤*Hepatic effects:* Mild, transient transaminase elevations have been observed in IV **pantoprazole** clinical studies. The clinical significance is unknown.

➤*Hypersensitivity reactions:* Anaphylaxis has been reported with the use of IV **pantoprazole**. This may require emergency medical treatment.

➤*Hepatic function impairment:* In patients with various degrees of chronic hepatic disease, the mean plasma half-life of **lansoprazole** was prolonged from 1.5 to 3.2 to 7.2 hours, and an increase in the mean AUC of up to 500% was observed at steady state.

In patients with chronic hepatic disease, the bioavailability and plasma half-life of **omeprazole** increased and the plasma clearance decreased.

In patients with chronic mild to moderate compensated cirrhosis of the liver, **rabeprazole** AUC was approximately doubled, elimination half-life was 2- to 3-fold higher, and the total body clearance was decreased to less than half.

In patients with severe hepatic insufficiency, the **esomeprazole** AUC was 2 to 3 times higher.

➤*Carcinogenesis:* In two 24-month carcinogenicity studies in rats, **esomeprazole** and **omeprazole** at daily doses approximately 0.7 to 57 times the human dose produced gastric enterochromaffin-like (ECL) cell carcinoids in a dose-related manner in male and female rats; the incidence was markedly higher in female rats that had higher blood levels of omeprazole. In addition, ECL cell hyperplasia was present in all treated groups of both sexes.

Gastric biopsy specimens from the body of the stomach from approximately 150 patients treated continuously with **lansoprazole** for 1 year or longer have not shown evidence of gastric ECL cell effects similar to those seen in rat studies. Longer-term data are needed to rule out the possibility of an increased risk of development of gastric tumors in patients receiving long-term lansoprazole therapy. In male rats, lansoprazole produced a dose-related increase of testicular interstitial cell adenomas. Lansoprazole also produced an increased incidence of liver tumors (hepatocellular adenoma plus carcinoma) in mice.

In a study with rats, **rabeprazole** produced gastric ECL cell hyperplasia in male and female rats and ECL cell carcinoid tumors in female rats at all test doses (lowest dose was 0.1 times the human exposure at the recommended dose for GERD). In greater than 400 patients treated with 10 or 20 mg/day rabeprazole for up to 1 year, the incidence of ECL hyperplasia increased with time and dose. No patient developed the adenomatoid, dysplastic, or neoplastic changes of ECL cells in the gastric mucosa, and no patient developed the carcinoid tumors observed in rats.

In a 24-month study with rats treated with oral **pantoprazole** 0.1 to 40 times the human exposure of a 50 kg person dosed at 40 mg/day on a body surface basis, dose-related ECL cell hyperplasia and benign and malignant neuroendocrine cell tumors were observed. Other GI tumors, as well as tumors of the liver and thyroid gland, also were observed. Other studies in rats and mice have produced similar findings. In 39 patients treated with 40 to 240 mg/day pantoprazole for up to 5 years, a moderate increase in ECL cell density was observed starting after the first year of use. The effect appeared to plateau after 4 years.

➤*Mutagenesis:* **Rabeprazole** was positive in the Ames test, the Chinese hamster ovary cell forward gene mutation test, and the mouse lymphoma cell forward gene mutation test. Its demethylated metabolite also was positive in the Ames test.

Omeprazole was positive for clastogenic effects in an in vitro human lymphocyte chromosomal aberration assay, in 1 of 2 in vivo mouse micronucleus tests, and in an in vivo bone marrow cell chromosomal aberration assay.

Esomeprazole and **lansoprazole** were positive in the in vitro human lymphocyte chromosome aberration test.

Pantoprazole was positive in the in vitro human lymphocyte chromosomal aberration assays, in 1 of 2 mouse micronucleus tests for clastogenic effects, and in the in vitro Chinese hamster ovarian cell forward mutation assay for mutagenic effects.

➤*Elderly:* The elimination rate of **omeprazole** was somewhat decreased in the elderly and the bioavailability increased (see Pharmacokinetics).

The clearance of **lansoprazole** is decreased in the elderly, with an approximately 50% to 100% increase of elimination half-life (see Pharmacokinetics).

AUC values and C_{max} of **esomeprazole**, **rabeprazole**, and oral **pantoprazole** were increased in elderly subjects compared with healthy controls (see Pharmacokinetics), but no dosage adjustment is recommended.

➤*Pregnancy: Category C* (**omeprazole**); *Category B* (**esomeprazole**, **lansoprazole**, **rabeprazole**, **pantoprazole**). In rabbits, doses 5.5 to 56 times the human dose of omeprazole produced dose-related increases in embryolethality, fetal resorptions, and pregnancy disruptions. In rats, dose-related embryo/fetal toxicity and postnatal developmental toxicity were observed in offspring of parents treated with approximately 5.6 to 56 times the human dose.

Sporadic reports have been received of congenital abnormalities occurring in infants born to women who have received omeprazole during pregnancy.

An expert review of published data on experiences with omeprazole use during pregnancy by the Teratogen Information System (TERIS) concluded that therapeutic doses during pregnancy are unlikely to pose a substantial teratogenic risk (the quantity and quality of data were assessed as fair).

However, there are no adequate and well-controlled studies in pregnant women. Use during pregnancy only if the potential benefit justifies the risk to the fetus.

➤*Lactation:* The excretion of **esomeprazole** in milk has not been studied, however **omeprazole** concentrations have been measured in the breast milk of women. Omeprazole has been measured in the breast milk of women. The peak concentration of omeprazole in breast milk was less than 7% of the peak serum concentration. **Lansoprazole** and **pantoprazole** and their metabolites are excreted in the milk of rats. Decreased body weight gain of rat pups was observed when **rabeprazole** was administered to rats in late gestation and during lactation at doses of approximately 195 times the human dose for body surface area. Because of the potential for serious adverse reactions in nursing infants, and because of the potential for tumorigenicity shown in rat carcinogenicity studies, decide whether to discontinue nursing or to discontinue the drug, taking into account the importance of the drug to the mother.

➤*Children:* The safety and efficacy of **esomeprazole**, **pantoprazole**, and **rabeprazole** in children have not been established. The safety and efficacy of **lansoprazole** have been established in pediatric patients 1 to 17 years of age for short-term treatment of symptomatic GERD and erosive esophagitis. The safety and efficacy of lansoprazole in patients younger than 1 year of age have not been established. The safety and efficacy of **omeprazole** have been established in the 2 to 16 years of age group for the treatment of acid-related GI diseases, including the treatment of symptomatic GERD and the treatment and maintenance of healing of erosive esophagitis. The safety and efficacy of omeprazole have not been established for pediatric patients younger than 2 years of age.

Precautions

➤*Gastric malignancy:* Symptomatic response to therapy with proton pump inhibitors does not preclude the presence of gastric malignancy.

➤*Vitamin B_{12} deficiency:* Generally, daily treatment with any acid-suppressing medications over a long period of time (ie, longer than 3 years) may lead to malabsorption of cyanocobalamin (vitamin B_{12}) caused by hypo- or achlorhydria. Rare reports of cyanocobalamin deficiency occurring with acid-suppressing therapy have been reported in the literature. Consider this possibility if clinical symptoms consistent with cyanocobalamin deficiency are observed.

Drug Interactions

Proton pump inhibitors cause a profound and long-lasting inhibition of gastric acid secretion; therefore, **esomeprazole**, **lansoprazole**, **omeprazole**, **pantoprazole**, and **rabeprazole** may interfere with the absorption of drugs where gastric pH is an important determinant of bioavailability (eg, ketoconazole, ampicillin, iron salts, digoxin, cyanocobalamin).

➤*CYP450 system:* There have been reports of interactions between **omeprazole** and certain drugs metabolized via the CYP450 system (eg, cyclosporine, disulfiram, benzodiazepines). **Esomeprazole**, **lansoprazole**, **pantoprazole**, and **rabeprazole** are extensively metabolized by CYP2C19 and CYP3A4. In clinical trials, antacids were used concomitantly with these agents.

Proton Pump Inhibitor Drug Interactions

Precipitant drug	Object drug*		Description
Clarithromycin	Proton pump inhibitors Esomeprazole Omeprazole Rabeprazole	↑	Serum concentrations of clarithromycin and the proton pump inhibitor may be increased. Based upon available data, no special action is needed.
Proton pump inhibitors Esomeprazole Omeprazole	Clarithromycin		

Proton Pump Inhibitor Drug Interactions			
Precipitant drug	Object drug*		Description
Sucralfate	Proton pump inhibitors Lansoprazole	⬇	Coadministration delayed the absorption and the bioavailability of the proton pump inhibitor. Take the proton pump inhibitor at least 30 minutes prior to sucralfate.
Proton pump inhibitors	Azole antifungals (eg, itraconazole, ketoconazole)	⬇	The bioavailability of certain azole antifungals may be decreased because of a possible reduction in tablet dissolution in the presence of a high gastric pH. Avoid concomitant administration if possible.
Proton pump inhibitors Esomeprazole Omeprazole	Benzodiazepines	⬆	The oxidative metabolism of certain benzodiazepines (eg, diazepam, triazolam) may be decreased, thus reducing the clearance, prolonging the half-life, and increasing the serum levels of the benzodiazepines. Reduce the benzodiazepine dosage or increase the dosing interval.
Proton pump inhibitors Omeprazole	Cilostazol	⬆	Concurrent use may increase cilostazol plasma concentrations, increasing the therapeutic and adverse effects. Consider dosage adjustment of cilostazol.
Proton pump inhibitors	Digoxin	⬆	Coadministration may increase serum digoxin levels. The magnitude of this change would not be expected to be clinically important in most patients.
Proton pump inhibitors Omeprazole	Hydantoins (eg, phenytoin)	⬆	Serum hydantoin levels may be increased because of omeprazole inhibiting the oxidative hepatic metabolism of hydantoins. Consider monitoring serum hydantoin levels and adjust dosage as needed.
Proton pump inhibitors	Salicylates	⬆	Enteric-coated salicylates may dissolve more rapidly, increasing gastric side effects.
Proton pump inhibitors Omeprazole	Sulfonylureas	⬆	Concurrent use may increase the serum sulfonylurea concentration, increasing the hypoglycemic effects. Based upon available data, no special action is needed.
Proton pump inhibitors	Warfarin	⬆	Postmarketing reports of changes in prothrombin measures have been received among patients on concomitant warfarin and a proton pump inhibitor. Monitor international normalized ratio (INR) and prothrombin time.

* ⬆ = Object drug increased. ⬇ = Object drug decreased.

➤*Drug/Food interactions:* When 20 mg **omeprazole** capsules were administered with applesauce, the C_{max} was reduced 25% without a significant change in AUC; however, the clinical significance is unknown. When omeprazole oral suspension is administered 1 hour after a meal, C_{max} and AUC are reduced by 63% and 24%, respectively. It is recommended that omeprazole capsules are administered before meals and the oral suspension administered on an empty stomach 1 hour before a meal. The AUC after administration of a single 40 mg dose of **esomeprazole** is decreased by 43% to 53% after food intake compared with fasting conditions. Esomeprazole should be taken at least 1 hour before eating. Both C_{max} and AUC of **lansoprazole** are diminished by approximately 50% to 70% if the drug is given 30 minutes after food as opposed to the fasting condition; therefore, lansoprazole should be taken before eating. When **pantoprazole** is given with food, its T_{max} is highly variable and may increase significantly. Absorption may be delayed up to 2 hours or longer; however, the C_{max} and AUC of pantoprazole are not altered and pantoprazole may be taken without regard to timing of meals. When **rabeprazole** is administered with a high fat meal, its T_{max} is variable and may delay its absorption up to 4 hours or longer; however, the C_{max} and AUC are not significantly altered and rabeprazole may be taken without regard to timing of meals.

Adverse Reactions

Omeprazole is generally well tolerated. In clinical trials of 3096 patients (including duodenal ulcer, Zollinger-Ellison syndrome and resistant ulcer patients), the following adverse experiences occurred in 1% or more of patients:

Selected Adverse Reactions: Omeprazole vs Ranitidine			
Adverse reaction	Omeprazole (n = 465)	Ranitidine (n = 195)	Placebo (n = 64)
CNS			
Asthenia	1.1%	1.5%	1.6%
Dizziness	1.5%	2.6%	0%
Headache	6.9%	7.7%	6.3%
GI			
Abdominal pain	2.4%	2.1%	3.1%
Constipation	1.1%	0%	0%
Diarrhea	3%	2.1%	3.1%
Nausea	2.2%	4.1%	3.1%
Vomiting	1.5%	1.5%	4.7%
Miscellaneous			
Back pain	1.1%	0.5%	0%
Cough	1.1%	1.5%	0%
Rash	1.5%	0%	0%
Upper respiratory tract infection	1.9%	2.6%	1.6%

In general, **lansoprazole** treatment has been well tolerated in short- and long-term trials. The following adverse events were reported in 1% or more of patients: Diarrhea (3.8%); abdominal pain (2.1%); nausea (1.3%); constipation (1%). Headache occurred at a greater than 1% incidence but was more common with placebo. The incidence of diarrhea is similar between placebo and 15 mg and 30 mg lansoprazole patients (2.9%, 1.4%, and 4.2%, respectively), but higher with lansoprazole 60 mg (7.4%). The most commonly reported adverse event during maintenance therapy was diarrhea.

In clinical trials with **rabeprazole**, the only adverse event occurring in greater than 1% of patients and appearing with greater frequency than placebo was headache (2.4% vs placebo 1.6%).

The following adverse events occurred in 1% or more of patients treated with **pantoprazole**: Abdominal pain, ALT increased, anxiety, arthralgia, asthenia, back pain, bronchitis, chest pain, constipation, cough increased, diarrhea, dizziness, dyspepsia, dyspnea, eructation, flatulence, flu syndrome, gastroenteritis, GI disorder, headache, hyperglycemia, hyperlipemia, hypertonia, infection, insomnia, liver function tests abnormal, migraine, nausea, neck pain, pain, pharyngitis, rash, rectal disorder, rhinitis, sinusitis, upper respiratory tract infection, urinary frequency, urinary tract infection, and vomiting. The following adverse events occurred in greater than 1% of patients treated with IV pantoprazole: Abdominal pain, constipation, diarrhea, dyspepsia, headache, injection site reaction (including thrombophlebitis and abscess), insomnia, nausea, rhinitis.

The following adverse reactions occurred in less than 1% of patients:

➤*Cardiovascular:*

Esomeprazole – Hypertension, tachycardia.

Lansoprazole – Angina, arrythmia, bradycardia, cerebrovascular accident/cerebral infarction, hypertension/hypotension, myocardial infarction, palpitations, shock (circulatory failure), syncope, tachycardia, vasodilation.

Omeprazole – Bradycardia, chest pain or angina, elevated blood pressure, palpitation, tachycardia.

Pantoprazole – Abnormal electrocardiogram, angina pectoris, arrhythmia, atrial fibrillation/flutter, cardiovascular disorder, congestive heart failure, hemorrhage, hypertension, hypotension, myocardial infarction, myocardial ischemia, palpitation, syncope, tachycardia, thrombophlebitis, thrombosis, vasodilatation.

Rabeprazole – Angina pectoris, bundle branch block, electrocardiogram abnormal, hypertension, myocardial infarction, palpitation, sinus bradycardia, syncope, tachycardia; bradycardia, pulmonary embolus, QTc prolongation, supraventricular tachycardia, thrombophlebitis, vasodilation, and ventricular tachycardia (less than or equal to 0.1%).

➤*CNS:*

Esomeprazole – Apathy, appetite increased, asthenia, confusion, depression aggravated, dizziness, fatigue, hypertonia, hypesthesia, insomnia, migraine, migraine aggravated, nervousness, paresthesia, sleep disorder, somnolence, tremor, vertigo.

Lansoprazole – Abnormal dreams, agitation, amnesia, anxiety, apathy, asthenia, confusion, convulsion, depersonalization, depression, diplopia, dizziness, emotional lability, hallucinations, hemiplegia, hostility aggravated, hyperkinesia, hypertonia, hypesthesia, insomnia, libido decreased/increased, migraine, nervousness, neurosis, paresthesia, sleep disorder, somnolence, thinking abnormality, tremor, vertigo.

Omeprazole – Aggression, anxiety, apathy, confusion, depression, dream abnormalities, fatigue, hallucinations, hemifacial dysesthesia, insomnia, nervousness, paresthesia, somnolence, tremors, vertigo.

Pantoprazole – Abnormal dreams, confusion, convulsion, depression, dysarthia, emotional lability, hallucinations, hyperkinesia, hypesthesia, libido decreased, nervousness, neuralgia, neuritis, neuropathy, paresthesia, reflexes decreased, sleep disorder, somnolence, thinking abnormal, tremor, vertigo.

Rabeprazole – Abnormal dreams, anxiety, asthenia, convulsion, depression, dizziness, hypertonia, insomnia, libido decreased, migraine, nervousness, neuralgia, neuropathy, paresthesia, somnolence, tremor, vertigo; agitation, amnesia, confusion, extrapyramidal syndrome, hyperkinesia (less than or equal to 0.1%).

➤*Dermatologic:*

Esomeprazole – Acne, angioedema, dermatitis, pruritus, pruritus ani, rash, rash erythematous, rash maculopapular, skin inflammation, sweating increased, urticaria.

Lansoprazole – Acne, alopecia, contact dermatitis, dry skin, fixed eruption, hair disorder, maculopapular rash, nail disorder, pruritus, rash, skin carcinoma, skin disorder, sweating, urticaria.

Omeprazole – Rash and, rarely, cases of severe generalized skin reactions including toxic epidermal necrolysis (some fatal), Stevens-Johnson syndrome, and erythema multiforme (some severe); alopecia, angioedema, dry skin, hyperhidrosis, pruritus purpura and/or petechiae (some with rechallenge), skin inflammation, urticaria.

Pantoprazole – Acne, alopecia, contact dermatitis, dry skin, eczema, fungal dermatitis, hemorrhage, herpes simplex, herpes zoster, lichenoid dermatitis, maculopapular rash, pruritus, skin disorder, skin ulcer, sweating, urticaria.

Rabeprazole – Alopecia, pruritus, rash, sweating, urticaria; dry skin, herpes zoster, psoriasis, skin discoloration (less than or equal to 0.1%).

➤*GI:*

Esomeprazole – Abdomen enlarged, anorexia, bowel irregularity, constipation aggravated, dyspepsia, dysphagia, epigastric pain, eructation, esophageal disorder, frequent stools, gastroenteritis, GI dysplasia, GI hemorrhage, GI symptoms not otherwise specified, melena, mouth disorder, pharynx disorder, rectal disorder, tongue disorder, tongue edema, ulcerative stomatitis, vomiting.

Lansoprazole – Abdomen enlarged, abnormal stools, anorexia, bezoar, cardiospasm, cholelithiasis, colitis, diarrhea, dry mouth, dyspepsia, dysphagia, enteritis, eructation, esophageal stenosis, esophageal ulcer, esophagitis, fecal discoloration, flatulence, gastric nodules/fundic gland polyps, gastritis, gastroenteritis, GI anomaly, GI disorder, GI hemorrhage, glossitis, gum hemorrhage, hematemesis, increased appetite, increased salivation, melena, mouth ulceration, nausea, oral moniliasis, rectal disorder, rectal hemorrhage, stomatitis, tenesmus, tongue disorder, ulcerative colitis, ulcerative stomatitis, vomiting.

Omeprazole – Abdominal swelling, anorexia, dry mouth, esophageal candidiasis, fecal discoloration, flatulence, gastric fundic gland polyps (rare, reversible), irritable colon, mucosal atrophy of the tongue, pancreatitis (some fatal).

Pantoprazole – Anorexia, aphthous stomatitis, cardiospasm, colitis, dry mouth, duodenitis, dysphagia, enteritis, esophageal hemorrhage, esophagitis, GI carcinoma, GI hemorrhage, GI moniliasis, gingivitis, glossitis, halitosis, hematemesis, increased appetite, melena, mouth ulceration, oral moniliasis, periodontal abscess, periodontitis, rectal hemorrhage, stomach ulcer, stomatitis, stools abnormal, tongue discoloration, ulcerative colitis.

Rabeprazole – Abdomen enlarged, abdominal pain, abnormal stools, anorexia, cholecystitis, cholelithiasis, colitis, constipation, diarrhea, dry mouth, dyspepsia, dysphagia, eructation, esophagitis, flatulence, gastroenteritis, gingivitis, glossitis, increased appetite, melena, mouth ulceration, nausea, pancreatitis, proctitis, rectal hemorrhage, stomatitis, vomiting; bloody diarrhea, cholangitis, duodenitis, GI hemorrhage, salivary gland enlargement (less than or equal to 0.1%).

➤*GU:*

Esomeprazole – Abnormal urine, albuminuria, cystitis, dysmenorrhea, dysuria, fungal infection, genital moniliasis, glycosuria, hematuria, impotence, menstrual disorder, micturition frequency, moniliasis, polyuria, vaginitis.

Lansoprazole – Abnormal menses, albuminuria, breast enlargement, breast pain, breast tenderness, dysmenorrhea, dysuria, glycosuria, gynecomastia, hematuria, impotence, kidney calculus, kidney pain, leukorrhea, menorrhagia, menstrual disorder, penis disorder, polyuria, testis disorder, urethral pain, urinary frequency, urinary tract infection, urinary urgency, urination impaired, vaginitis.

Omeprazole – Glycosuria, gynecomastia, hematuria, interstitial nephritis (some with positive rechallenge), microscopic pyuria, proteinuria, testicular pain, urinary tract infection, urinary frequency.

Pantoprazole – Albuminuria, balanitis, breast pain, cystitis, dysmenorrhea, dysuria, epididymitis, glycosuria, hematuria, impotence, kidney calculus, kidney pain, nocturia, prostatic disorder, pyelonephritis, scrotal edema, urethral pain, urethritis, urinary tract disorder, urination impaired, vaginitis.

Rabeprazole – Cystitis, dysmenorrhea, dysuria, kidney calculus, metrorrhagia, polyuria, urinary frequency; breast enlargement, hematuria, impotence, leukorrhea, menorrhagia, orchitis, urinary incontinence, urine abnormality (less than or equal to 0.1%).

➤*Esomeprazole:* Anemia, anemia hypochromic, cervical lymphadenopathy, epistaxis, leukocytosis, leukopenia, thrombocytopenia.

Anemia, anemia hypochromic, cervical lymphadenopathy, epistaxis, leukocytosis, leukopenia, thrombocytopenia.

Lansoprazole – Anemia, hemolysis, lymphadenopathy.

Omeprazole – Agranulocytosis (some fatal), anemia, hemolytic anemia, leukocytosis, neutropenia, pancytopenia (rare), thrombocytopenia.

Pantoprazole – Anemia, ecchymosis, eosinophilia, hypochromic anemia, iron deficiency anemia, leukocytosis, leukopenia, thrombocytopenia.

Rabeprazole – Anemia, ecchymosis, hypochromic anemia, lymphadenopathy.

➤*Hepatic:*

Esomeprazole – Bilirubinemia, hepatic function abnormal.

Omeprazole – Overt liver disease has occurred rarely, including hepatocellular, cholestatic, or mixed hepatitis, liver necrosis (some fatal), hepatic failure (some fatal), and hepatic encephalopathy.

Pantoprazole – Biliary pain, cholecystitis, cholelithiasis, cholestatic jaundice, hepatitis, hyperbilirubinemia.

Rabeprazole – Hepatic encephalopathy, hepatitis, hepatoma, liver fatty deposit.

➤*Lab test abnormalities:*

Esomeprazole – Increased alkaline phosphatase, ALT, AST, creatinine, hemoglobin, platelets, potassium, serum gastrin, sodium, thyroid stimulating hormone, thyroxine, total bilirubin, uric acid, and white blood cell count.

Decreased hemoglobin, platelets, potassium, sodium, thyroxine, and white blood cell count.

Lansoprazole – Abnormal bilirubinemia, eosinophilia, hyperlipemia, liver function tests, RBC; increased AST, ALT, alkaline phosphatase, creatinine, gastrin levels, GGTP, globulins, glucocorticoids, LDH; increased/decreased/abnormal WBC, platelets; increased/decreased cholesterol electrolytes.

Urine abnormalities such as albuminuria, glycosuria, and hematuria also were reported.

Omeprazole – Increased alkaline phosphatase, ALT, AST, bilirubin, elevated serum creatinine, γ-glutamyl transpeptidase.

Pantoprazole – Abnormal laboratory test; increased alkaline phosphatase, ALT, AST, creatinine, glycosuria, hypercholesterolemia, hyperuricemia, γ-glutamyl transpeptidase.

Rabeprazole – Abnormal erythrocytes, liver function tests, platelets, urine, WBC; increased ALT, creatine phosphokinase, prostatic specific antigen; albuminuria, hypercholesteremia, hyperglycemia, hyperlipemia, hypokalemia, hyponatremia, leukocytosis, leukorrhea.

➤*Metabolic/Nutritional:*

Esomeprazole – Facial edema, generalized edema, goiter, hyperuricemia, hyponatremia, leg edema, peripheral edema, thirst, vitamin B12 deficiency, weight gain/loss.

Lansoprazole – Dehydration, diabetes mellitus, edema, goiter, gout, hyperglycemia/hypoglycemia, hypothyroidism, peripheral edema, thirst, weight gain/loss.

Omeprazole – Hyponatremia, hypoglycemia, peripheral edema, weight gain.

Pantoprazole – Dehydration, diabetes mellitus, facial edema, generalized edema, goiter, gout, peripheral edema, thirst, weight gain/loss.

Rabeprazole – Dehydration, edema, facial edema, gout, hyperthyroidism, hypothyroidism, peripheral edema, thirst, weight gain/loss.

➤*Musculoskeletal:*

Esomeprazole – Arthralgia, arthritis aggravated, arthropathy, cramps, fibromyalgia syndrome, hernia, polymyalgia rheumatica.

Lansoprazole – Arthralgia, arthritis, bone disorder, joint disorder, leg cramps, musculoskeletal pain, myalgia, myasthenia, synovitis.

Omeprazole – Joint pain, leg pain, muscle cramps, muscle weakness, myalgia.

Pantoprazole – Arthritis, arthrosis, bone disorder/pain, bursitis, joint disorder, leg cramps, myalgia, tenosynovitis.

Rabeprazole – Arthritis, arthrosis, bone pain, bursitis, leg cramps, myalgia; twitching (less than 0.1% or equal to).

➤*Respiratory:*

Esomeprazole – Asthma aggravated, coughing, dyspnea, hiccup, larynx edema, pharyngitis, rhinitis, sinusitis.

Lansoprazole – Asthma, bronchitis, cough increased, dyspnea, epistaxis, hemoptysis, hiccup, laryngeal neoplasia, pharyngitis, pleural disorder, pneumonia, respiratory disorder, rhinitis, sinusitis, stridor, upper respiratory inflammation/infection.

Omeprazole – Epistaxis, pharyngeal pain.

Pantoprazole – Asthma, epistaxis, hiccup, laryngitis, lung disorder, pneumonia, voice alteration.

Rabeprazole – Asthma, dyspnea, epistaxis, hiccup, hyperventilation, laryngitis; apnea, hypoventilation (less than or equal to 0.1%).

➤*Special senses:*

Esomeprazole – Conjunctivitis, earache, otitis media, parosmia, taste loss, taste perversion, tinnitus, visual field defect, vision abnormal.

Lansoprazole – Abnormal vision, blurred vision, conjunctivitis, deafness, dry eyes, ear disorder, eye pain, otitis media, parosmia, photophobia, retinal degeneration, taste loss, taste perversion, tinnitus, visual field defect.

Omeprazole – Anterior ischemic optic neuropathy, blurred vision, double vision, dry eye syndrome, taste perversion, tinnitus, ocular irritation, optic atrophy, optic neuritis.

Pantoprazole – Abnormal vision, amblyopia, cataract specified, deafness, diplopia, ear pain, extraocular palsy, glaucoma, otitis externa, retinal vascular disorder, taste perversion, tinnitus.

Rabeprazole – Abnormal vision, amblyopia, cataract, dry eyes, glaucoma, otitis media, tinnitus; blurred vision, corneal opacity, diplopia, deafness, eye pain, retinal degeneration, strabismus (less than or equal to 0.1%).

➤*Miscellaneous:*

Esomeprazole – Allergic reaction, back pain, chest pain, chest pain substernal, fever, flu-like disorder, flushing, hot flushes, malaise, pain, rigors.

Lansoprazole – Allergic reaction, back pain, candidiasis, carcinoma, chest pain (not otherwise specified), chills, fever, flu syndrome, halitosis, infection (not otherwise specified), malaise, neck pain, neck rigidity, pain, pelvic pain.

Omeprazole – Allergic reactions, including, rarely anaphylaxis, fever, pain, malaise.

Pantoprazole – Abscess, allergic reaction, chest pain substernal, chills, cyst, fever, heat stroke, hernia, malaise, moniliasis, neck rigidity, neoplasm, nonspecified drug reaction, photosensitivity reaction.

Rabeprazole – Allergic reaction, asthenia, chest pain substernal, chills, fever, malaise, neck rigidity, photosensitivity reaction; face edema, hangover effect (less than or equal to 0.1%).

➤*Postmarketing:*

Esomeprazole – Anaphylactic reaction.

Lansoprazole – Agranulocytosis, anaphylactoid-like reaction, aplastic anemia, hemolytic anemia, hepatotoxicity, leukopenia, neutropenia, pancreatitis, pancytopenia, severe dermatologic reactions including erythema multiforme, Stevens-Johnson syndrome, thrombocytopenia, thrombotic thrombocytopenic purpura, toxic epidermal necrolysis (some fatal); speech disorder, urinary retention, vomiting.

Pantoprazole – Anaphylaxis (including anaphylactic shock); angioedema (Quincke edema); anterior ischemic optic neuropathy; elevated CPK (creatine phosphokinase); severe dermatologic reactions, including erythema multiforme, Stevens-Johnson syndrome, and toxic epidermal necrolysis (some fatal); hepatocellular damage leading to jaundice and hepatic failure; interstitial nephritis; pancreatitis; pancytopenia; and rhabdomyolysis. Confusion, hypokinesia, speech disorder, increased salivation, vertigo, nausea, tinnitus, and blurred vision.

Rabeprazole – Agranulocytosis, anaphylaxis, angioedema, bullous and other drug eruptions of the skin, coma, delirium, disorientation, erythema multiforme, hemolytic anemia, hyperammonemia, interstitial nephritis, interstitial pneumonia, jaundice, leukopenia, pancytopenia, rhabdomyolysis, severe dermatologic reactions including toxic epidermal necrolysis (some fatal), Stevens-Johnson syndrome, sudden death, thrombocytopenia, TSH elevations; Increases in prothrombin time/INR in patients treated with concomitant warfarin have been reported.

Overdosage

➤*Symptoms:* Overdosage with **omeprazole** has been reported. Doses ranged up to 2,400 mg (120 times the usual recommended dose). Symptoms were transient and included blurred vision, confusion, diaphoresis, drowsiness, dry mouth, flushing, headache, nausea, tachycardia, and vomiting. No serious clinical outcome has been reported. No specific antidote for omeprazole overdosage is known.

In 1 overdose case, a patient consumed 600 mg of **lansoprazole** with no adverse reaction.

There has been no experience with large overdoses of **rabeprazole**. The maximum reported overdose was 80 mg. There were no signs or symptoms associated with any overdose. Patients with Zollinger-Ellison syndrome have been treated with up to 120 mg/day.

Two reports of overdose with 400 and 600 mg of **pantoprazole** have been reported with no adverse effects observed. There has been 1 report of suicide involving an overdose of 560 mg pantoprazole; however, the death was more reasonably attributed to other drugs ingested.

➤*Treatment:* **Omeprazole**, **esomeprazole**, **lansoprazole**, **pantoprazole**, and **rabeprazole** are extensively protein bound and are not readily dialyzable. Treatment should be symptomatic and supportive. Refer to General Management of Acute Overdosage.

Patient Information

Take **omeprazole**, **esomeprazole**, and **lansoprazole** before meals. Take **rabeprazole** and **pantoprazole** without regard to meals.

Do not open, crush or chew omeprazole or esomeprazole capsules; do not chew or crush omeprazole tablets or lansoprazole products; do not chew, crush or split rabeprazole or pantoprazole tablets.

Antacids may be used while taking proton pump inhibitors.

ESOMEPRAZOLE MAGNESIUM

Rx	**Nexium** (AstraZeneca)	**Capsules, delayed release**[a]: 20 mg (as base)	Sugar spheres, talc. (NEXIUM 20 mg). Amethyst. In 90s, 1,000s, unit-of-use 30s, and UD 100s.
		40 mg (as base)	Sugar spheres, talc. (NEXIUM 40 mg). Amethyst. In 90s, 1,000s, unit-of-use 30s, and UD 100s.
Rx	**Nexium I.V.** (AstraZeneca)	**Powder for injection, freeze dried**: 20 mg	Single-use vials. EDTA. In 10s.
		40 mg	Single-use vials. EDTA. In 10s.

[a] Contains enteric-coated pellets.

ESOMEPRAZOLE MAGNESIUM — ORAL

For complete and comparative prescribing information, refer to the Proton Pump Inhibitors group monograph.

Indications

➤*Healing of erosive esophagitis:* For the short-term treatment (4 to 8 weeks) in the healing and symptomatic resolution of diagnostically confirmed erosive esophagitis. For those patients who have not healed after 4 to 8 weeks of treatment, consider an additional 4- to 8-week course of esomeprazole.

➤*Maintenance of healing of erosive esophagitis:* To maintain symptom resolution and healing of erosive esophagitis. Controlled studies do not extend beyond 6 months.

➤*Symptomatic gastroesophageal reflux disease (GERD):* For treatment of heartburn and other symptoms associated with GERD.

➤*Risk reduction of nonsteroidal anti-inflammatory drug (NSAID)-associated gastric ulcer:* For the reduction in the occurrence of gastric ulcers associated with continuous NSAID therapy in patients at risk for developing gastric ulcers. Patients are considered to be at risk because of their age (60 years of age and older) and/or documented history of gastric ulcers. Controlled studies do not extend beyond 6 months.

➤*Helicobacter pylori eradication to reduce the risk of duodenal ulcer recurrence:*

Triple therapy (esomeprazole plus amoxicillin and clarithromycin) – In combination with amoxicillin and clarithromycin for the treatment of patients with *H. pylori* infection and duodenal ulcer disease (active or history of within the past 5 years) to eradicate *H. pylori*. Eradication of *H. pylori* has been shown to reduce the risk of duodenal ulcer recurrence. In patients who fail therapy, perform susceptibility testing. If resistance to clarithromycin is demonstrated or susceptibility testing is not possible, institute alternative antimicrobial therapy.

Administration and Dosage

➤*Approved by the FDA:* February 20, 2001.

Following are the recommended adult dosages. Esomeprazole delayed-release capsules should be swallowed whole and taken at least 1 hour before eating.

➤*Difficulty swallowing:* For patients who have difficulty swallowing capsules, 1 tablespoon of applesauce can be added to an empty bowl and the esomeprazole delayed-release capsule can be opened, and the pellets inside the capsule carefully emptied onto the applesauce. Pellets should be mixed with the applesauce and then swallowed immediately. The applesauce used should not be hot and should be soft enough to be swallowed without chewing. Pellets should not be chewed or crushed. Do not store the pellet/applesauce mixture for future use.

➤*Administration per nasogastric (NG) tube:* For patients who have an NG tube in place, esomeprazole delayed-release capsules can be opened and the intact granules emptied into a 60 mL syringe and mixed with 50 mL of water. Replace the plunger and shake the syringe vigorously for 15 seconds. Hold the syringe with the tip up and check for granules remaining in the tip. Attach the syringe to a NG tube and deliver the contents of the syringe through the NG tube into the stomach. After administering the granules, the NG tube should be flushed with additional water. Do not administer the pellets if they have dissolved or disintegrated.

The suspension must be used immediately after preparation.

Recommended Adult Dosage Schedule of Esomeprazole

Indication	Dose	Frequency
GERD		
Healing of erosive esophagitis	20 or 40 mg	Once daily for 4 to 8 weeks[a]
Maintenance of healing of erosive esophagitis	20 mg	Once daily[b]
Symptomatic GERD	20 mg	Once daily for 4 weeks[c]
Risk reduction of NSAID-associated gastric ulcer	20 or 40 mg	Once daily for up to 6 months[b]
H. pylori eradication to reduce the risk of duodenal ulcer recurrence		
Triple therapy		
Esomeprazole	40 mg	Once daily for 10 days
Amoxicillin	1,000 mg	Twice daily for 10 days
Clarithromycin	500 mg	Twice daily for 10 days
Pediatric use (12 to 17 years of age)		
Short-term treatment of GERD	20 or 40 mg	Once daily for up to 8 weeks

[a] The majority of patients are healed within 4 to 8 weeks. For patients who do not heal after 4 to 8 weeks, consider an additional 4 to 8 weeks of treatment.
[b] Controlled studies did not extend beyond 6 months.
[c] If symptoms do not resolve completely after 4 weeks, consider an additional 4 weeks of treatment.

➤*Special populations:*

Elderly – The area under the curve (AUC) and C_{max} values were slightly higher (25% and 18%, respectively) in the elderly compared with younger subjects at steady state. Dosage adjustment based on age is not necessary.

ESOMEPRAZOLE MAGNESIUM — ORAL

Hepatic function impairment – No dosage adjustment is necessary in patients with mild to moderate liver function impairment (Child-Pugh class A/B). For patients with severe liver function impairment (Child-Pugh class C), do not exceed a dose of esomeprazole 20 mg.

Gender – The AUC and C_{max} values were slightly higher (13%) in women than men at steady state. Dosage adjustment based on gender is not necessary.

➤*Storage / Stability:* Store at 25°C (77°F); excursions permitted to 15° to 30°C (59° to 86°F). Keep the container tightly closed. Dispense in a tight container if the product package is subdivided.

ESOMEPRAZOLE SODIUM — INJECTION

Indications

➤*Gastroesophageal reflux disease (GERD) with a history of erosive esophagitis:* For the short-term treatment (up to 10 days) of GERD patients with a history of erosive esophagitis as an alternative to oral therapy when therapy with esomeprazole capsules is not possible or appropriate.

Administration and Dosage

➤*Approved by the FDA:* March 31, 2005.

➤*Dosage:* Either 20 or 40 mg of esomeprazole given once daily by IV injection (no less than 3 minutes) or IV infusion (10 to 30 minutes).

➤*Duration of treatment:* Safety and efficacy of esomeprazole injection as a treatment of GERD patients with a history of erosive esophagitis for more than 10 days have not been demonstrated.

➤*Hepatic function impairment:* No dosage adjustment is necessary in patients with mild to moderate liver function impairment (Child-Pugh classes A and B). For patients with severe liver function impairment (Child-Pugh class C), a dose of 20 mg of esomeprazole should not be exceeded.

➤*Preparation for IV use / administration:*

IV injection (20 or 40 mg) over no less than 3 minutes – The freeze-dried powder should be reconstituted with 5 mL of sodium chloride 0.9% injection. Withdraw 5 mL of the reconstituted solution and administer as an IV injection over no less than 3 minutes.

IV infusion (20 or 40 mg) over 10 to 30 minutes – A solution for IV infusion is prepared by first reconstituting the contents of 1 vial with 5 mL of sodium chloride 0.9% injection, Ringer's lactate injection, or dextrose 5% injection and further diluting the resulting solution to a final volume of 50 mL. The solution (admixture) should be administered as an IV infusion over a period of 10 to 30 minutes.

Diluent	Administer within:
Sodium chloride 0.9% injection	12 hours
Ringer's lactate injection	12 hours
Dextrose 5% injection	6 hours

Parenteral drug products should be inspected visually for particulate matter and discoloration prior to administration whenever solution and container permit.

Admixture incompatibilities – Esomeprazole injection should not be coadministered with any other medications through the same IV site and/or tubing. The IV line should always be flushed with either sodium chloride 0.9% injection, Ringer's lactate injection, or dextrose 5% injection prior to and after administration of esomeprazole injection.

➤*Storage / Stability:* Store at 25°C (77°F); excursions permitted to 15° to 30°C (59° to 86°F). Protect from light. Store in carton until time of use.

IV injection – Store the reconstituted solution at room temperature, up to 30°C (86°F), and administer within 12 hours after reconstitution. No refrigeration is required.

IV infusion – Store the admixture at room temperature, up to 30°C (86°F), and administer within the designated time period as listed in the preceding table. No refrigeration is required.

➤*Pharmacology:* Esomeprazole is a proton pump inhibitor that suppresses gastric acid secretion by specific inhibition of the H^+/K^+-ATPase in the gastric parietal cell. The S- and R-isomers of omeprazole are protonated and converted in the acidic compartment of the parietal cell forming the active inhibitor, the achiral sulphenamide. By acting specifically on the proton pump, esomeprazole blocks the final step in acid production, thus reducing gastric acidity. This effect is dose-related up to a daily dose of 20 to 40 mg and leads to inhibition of gastric acid secretion.

➤*Pharmacokinetics:*

Absorption – The pharmacokinetic profile of esomeprazole 20 and 40 mg injection was determined in 24 healthy volunteers for the 20 mg dose and 38 healthy volunteers for the 40 mg dose following once-daily administration of 20 and 40 mg of esomeprazole injection by constant rate over 30 minutes for 5 days. The results are shown in the following table.

Pharmacokinetic Parameters of Esomeprazole Following IV Dosing for 5 Days[a]

Parameter	Esomeprazole IV 20 mg	Esomeprazole IV 40 mg
AUC[b] (mcmol•h/L)	5.11 (3.96:6.61)	16.21 (14.46:18.16)
C_{max}[c] (mcmol/L)	3.86 (3.16:4.72)	7.51 (6.93:8.13)
t½ (h)	1.05 (0.9:1.22)	1.41 (1.3:1.52)

[a] Values represent the geometric mean (95% CI).
[b] AUC = area under the curve.
[c] C_{max} = maximum concentration of drug.

Distribution – Esomeprazole is 97% bound to plasma proteins. Plasma protein binding is constant over the concentration range of 2 to 20 mcmol/L. The apparent volume of distribution at steady state in healthy volunteers is approximately 16 L.

Metabolism – Esomeprazole is extensively metabolized in the liver by the cytochrome P-450 (CYP) enzyme system. The metabolites of esomeprazole lack antisecretory activity. The major part of esomeprazole's metabolism is dependent upon the CYP2C19 isoenzyme, which forms the hydroxy and desmethyl metabolites. The remaining amount is dependent on CYP3A4, which forms the sulphone metabolite. CYP2C19 isoenzyme exhibits polymorphism in the metabolism of esomeprazole because some 3% of white patients and 15% to 20% of Asian patients lack CYP2C19 and are termed poor metabolizers. At steady state, the ratio of AUC in poor metabolizers to AUC in the rest of the population (extensive metabolizers) is approximately 2.

Following administration of equimolar doses, the S- and R-isomers are metabolized differently by the liver, resulting in higher plasma levels of the S-isomer than the R-isomer.

Excretion – Esomeprazole is excreted as metabolites primarily in urine but also in feces. Less than 1% of parent drug is excreted in the urine. Esomeprazole is completely eliminated from plasma and there is no accumulation during once-daily administration. The plasma elimination half-life of esomeprazole IV is approximately 1.1 to 1.4 hours and is prolonged with an increasing dose of esomeprazole IV.

Special populations –

Hepatic function impairment: In oral studies, the steady-state pharmacokinetics of esomeprazole obtained after administration of 40 mg once daily to 4 patients each with mild (Child-Pugh A), moderate (Child-Pugh class B), and severe (Child-Pugh class C) liver function impairment were compared with those obtained in 36 male and female GERD patients with healthy liver function. In patients with mild and moderate hepatic function impairment, the AUCs were within the range that could be expected in patients with healthy liver function. In patients with severe hepatic function impairment, the AUCs were 2 to 3 times higher than in the patients with healthy liver function. No dosage adjustment is recommended for patients with mild to moderate hepatic function impairment (Child-Pugh classes A and B). However, in patients with severe hepatic function impairment (Child-Pugh class C), do not exceed a dosage of 20 mg once daily.

Known hypersensitivity to any component of the formulation or to substituted benzimidazoles.

➤*Carcinogenesis:* The carcinogenic potential of esomeprazole was assessed using omeprazole studies. In two 24-month oral carcinogenicity studies in rats, omeprazole at daily doses of 1.7, 3.4, 13.8, 44, and 140.8 mg/kg/day (about 0.7 to 57 times the human dose of 20 mg/day expressed on a body surface area [BSA] basis) produced gastric ECL cell carcinoids in a dose-related manner in both male and female rats; the incidence of this effect was markedly higher in female rats, which had higher blood levels of omeprazole. Gastric carcinoids seldom occur in the untreated rat. In addition, ECL cell hyperplasia was present in all treated groups of both sexes. In one of these studies, female rats were treated with omeprazole 13.8 mg/kg/day (about 5.6 times the human dose on a body surface area basis) for 1 year, and then followed for an additional year without the drug. No carcinoids were seen in these rats. An increased incidence of treatment-related ECL cell hyperplasia was observed at the end of 1 year (94% treated vs 10% controls). By the second year, the difference between treated and control rats was much smaller (46% vs 26%), but still showed more hyperplasia in the treated group. Gastric adenocarcinoma was seen in 1 rat (2%). No similar tumor was seen in male or female rats treated for 2 years. For this strain of rat, no similar tumor has been noted historically, but a finding involving only 1 tumor is difficult to interpret. A 78-week oral mouse carcinogenicity study of omeprazole did not show increased tumor occurrence, but the study was not conclusive.

➤*Mutagenesis:* Esomeprazole was positive in the in vitro human lymphocyte chromosome aberration test. Omeprazole was positive in the in vitro human lymphocyte chromosome aberration test, the in vivo mouse bone marrow cell chromosome aberration test, and the in vivo mouse micronucleus test.

➤*Pregnancy: Category B.*

Teratogenic – Teratology studies have been performed in rats at oral doses up to 280 mg/kg/day (about 57 times the human dose on a BSA basis) and in rabbits at oral doses up to 86 mg/kg/day (about 35 times the human dose on a BSA basis) and have revealed no evidence of impaired fertility or harm to the fetus caused by esomeprazole. There are, however, no adequate and well-controlled studies in pregnant women. Because animal reproduction studies are not always predictive of human response, use this drug during pregnancy only if clearly needed.

In rabbits, omeprazole in a dosage range of 6.9 to 69.1 mg/kg/day (about 5.5 to 56 times the human dose on a BSA basis) produced dose-related increases in embryo lethality, fetal resorptions, and pregnancy disruptions. In rats, dose-related embryo/fetal toxicity and postnatal developmental toxicity were observed in offspring resulting from parents treated with omeprazole at 13.8 to 138 mg/kg/day (about 5.6 to 56 times the human doses on a BSA basis). There are no adequate and well-controlled studies in pregnant women. Sporadic reports have been received of congenital abnormalities occurring in infants born to women who have received omeprazole during pregnancy.

ESOMEPRAZOLE SODIUM — INJECTION

➤*Lactation:* The excretion of esomeprazole in milk has not been studied. However, esomeprazole concentrations have been measured in the breast milk of a woman following oral administration of 20 mg. Because esomeprazole is likely to be excreted in human milk, because of the potential for serious adverse reactions in breast-feeding infants from esomeprazole, and because of the potential for tumorigenicity shown for omeprazole in rat carcinogenicity studies, decide whether to discontinue breast-feeding or the drug, taking into account the importance of the drug to the mother.

➤*Children:* Safety and efficacy in children have not been established.

➤*Gastric malignancy:* Symptomatic response to therapy with esomeprazole does not preclude the presence of gastric malignancy.

➤*Gastritis:* Atrophic gastritis has been noted occasionally in gastric corpus biopsies from patients treated long term with omeprazole, of which esomeprazole is an enantiomer.

➤*Discontinue therapy:* Discontinue treatment with esomeprazole injection as soon as the patient is able to resume treatment with esomeprazole capsules.

Esomeprazole (Injection) Drug Interactions			
Precipitant Drug	Object Drug[a]		Description
Esomeprazole	Digoxin Iron salts Ketoconazole	⬇	Esomeprazole inhibits gastric acid secretion. Therefore, esomeprazole may interfere with the absorption of drugs in which gastric pH is an important determinant of bioavailability.
Esomeprazole	Warfarin	⬆	Postmarketing reports of changes in prothrombin measures, such as an increase in INR and prothrombin time, have been received among patients on concomitant warfarin and esomeprazole therapy. Monitor INR and prothrombin time.

[a] ⬆ = Object drug increased. ⬇ = Object drug decreased.

The safety of esomeprazole IV is based on results from clinical trials conducted in 3 different populations, including patients with symptomatic GERD with or without a history of erosive esophagitis (n = 206), patients with erosive esophagitis (n = 246), and healthy subjects (n = 204). Adverse reactions occurring in greater than 1% of patients treated with esomeprazole IV (n = 359) in trials, irrespective of the relationship to esomeprazole, are listed below by body system.

IV treatment with esomeprazole 20 and 40 mg administered as an injection or as an infusion was found to have a safety profile similar to that of oral administration of esomeprazole 20 and 40 mg.

➤*CNS:* Dizziness (2.5%); headache (10.9%).

➤*Dermatologic:* Pruritus (1.1%).

➤*GI:* Abdominal pain (5.8%); constipation (2.5%); diarrhea, dry mouth (3.9%); dyspepsia (6.4%); flatulence (10.3%); nausea (6.4%).

➤*Local:* Application site reaction (1.7%), including mild focal erythema and pruritus at IV insertion site.

➤*Respiratory:* Respiratory infection (1.1%); sinusitis (1.7%).

➤*Miscellaneous:* Reactions associated with test procedures (23.1%).

➤*Lab test abnormalities:* The following potentially clinically significant laboratory changes in clinical trials, irrespective of relationship to esomeprazole, were reported in less than or equal to 1% of patients: increased creatinine, uric acid, total bilirubin, alkaline phosphatase, ALT, AST, hemoglobin, white blood cell count, platelets, serum gastrin, potassium, sodium, thyroxine, and thyroid stimulating hormone. Decreases were seen in hemoglobin, white blood cell count, platelets, potassium, sodium, and thyroxine.

➤*Symptoms:* The minimum lethal dose of esomeprazole in rats after bolus administration was 310 mg/kg (about 62 times the human dose on a BSA basis). The major signs of acute toxicity were reduced motor activity, changes in respiratory frequency, tremor, ataxia, and intermittent clonic convulsions.

There have been some reports of overdosage with oral esomeprazole. Reports have been received of overdosage with oral omeprazole in humans. Doses ranged up to 2,400 mg (120 times the usual recommended clinical dose). Manifestations were variable, but included confusion, drowsiness, blurred vision, tachycardia, nausea, diaphoresis, flushing, headache, dry mouth, and other adverse reactions similar to those seen in normal clinical experience.

➤*Treatment:* No specific antidote for esomeprazole is known. Because esomeprazole is extensively protein bound, it is not expected to be removed by dialysis. In the event of overdosage, treatment should be symptomatic and supportive.

As with the management of any overdose, consider the possibility of multiple drug ingestion. For current information on treatment of any drug overdose, contact the National Poison Control Center at 1-800-222-1222.

LANSOPRAZOLE

Rx	**Prevacid** (TAP Pharm)	**Tablets, orally disintegrating, delayed-release**[a]: 15 mg	Mannitol, lactose, aspartame, 2.5 mg phenylalanine. White to yellowish-white with orange to dark brown speckles. Strawberry flavor. In UD 30s.
		30 mg	Mannitol, lactose, aspartame, 5.1 mg phenylalanine. White to yellowish-white with orange to dark brown speckles. Strawberry flavor. In UD 30s.
		Capsules, delayed-release[a]: 15 mg	Sugar spheres, sucrose. (PREVACID 15). Pink/Green. In 1000s, unit-of-use 30s, and UD 100s.
		30 mg	Sugar spheres, sucrose. (PREVACID 30). Pink/Black. In 100s, 1,000s, and UD 100s.
		Granules for oral suspension, delayed-release[a]: 15 mg	Sugar, mannitol, docusate sodium. Strawberry flavor. In UD 30s.
		30 mg	Sugar, mannitol, docusate sodium. Strawberry flavor. In UD 30s.
Rx	**Prevacid IV** (TAP Pharm)	**Powder for injection, lyophilized**: 30 mg/vial	60 mg mannitol, 10 mg meglumine. In single-dose vials with in-line (1.2 micron) filters.

[a] Contains enteric-coated granules.

LANSOPRAZOLE — ORAL

For complete and comparative prescribing information, refer to the Proton Pump Inhibitors group monograph. Refer to the Penicillins and Macrolides group monographs for complete prescribing information for amoxicillin and clarithromycin.

Indications

➤*Short-term treatment of active duodenal ulcer:* Short-term treatment (up to 4 weeks) for healing and symptom relief of active duodenal ulcer.

➤*H. pylori eradication to reduce the risk of duodenal ulcer recurrence:*

Triple therapy –

Lansoprazole/amoxicillin/clarithromycin: For the treatment of patients with *Helicobacter pylori* infection and duodenal ulcer disease (active or 1-year history of a duodenal ulcer) to eradicate *H. pylori*. Eradication of *H. pylori* has been shown to reduce the risk of duodenal ulcer recurrence.

Dual therapy –

Lansoprazole/amoxicillin: For the treatment of patients with *H. pylori* infection and duodenal ulcer disease (active or 1-year history of a duodenal ulcer) who are either allergic or intolerant to clarithromycin or in whom resistance to clarithromycin is known or suspected. Eradication of *H. pylori* has been shown to reduce the risk of duodenal ulcer recurrence.

➤*Maintenance of healed duodenal ulcers:* To maintain healing of duodenal ulcers. Controlled studies do not extend beyond 12 months.

➤*Short-term treatment of active benign gastric ulcer:* For short-term treatment (up to 8 weeks) for healing and symptom relief of active benign gastric ulcer.

➤*Healing of NSAID associated gastric ulcer:* For the treatment of NSAID-associated gastric ulcer in patients who continue NSAID use. Controlled studies did not extend beyond 8 weeks.

➤*Risk reduction of NSAID (associated gastric ulcer):* For reducing the risk of NSAID-associated gastric ulcers in patients with a history of a documented gastric ulcer who require the use of an NSAID. Controlled studies did not extend beyond 12 weeks.

➤*Gastroesophageal reflux disease (GERD):*

Short-term treatment of symptomatic GERD – For the treatment of heartburn and other symptoms associated with GERD.

Erosive esophagitis – For short-term treatment (up to 8 weeks) for healing and symptomatic relief of all grades of erosive esophagitis; to maintain healing of erosive esophagitis.

➤*Maintenance of healing of erosive esophagitis:* To maintain healing of erosive esophagitis. Controlled studies did not extend beyond 12 months.

➤*Pathological hypersecretory conditions including Zollinger-Ellison syndrome:* For the long-term treatment of pathological hypersecretory conditions, including Zollinger-Ellison syndrome.

Administration and Dosage

➤*Approved by the FDA:* May 10, 1995.

Take oral formulations before meals.

Do not crush or chew lansoprazole oral products.

➤*Duodenal ulcer:*

Short-term treatment – 15 mg once daily for 4 weeks.

LANSOPRAZOLE — ORAL

Maintenance – 15 mg once daily to maintain healing of duodenal ulcers.

Associated with H. pylori –

Dual therapy: 30 mg lansoprazole plus 1 g amoxicillin both taken 3 times/day (every 8 hours) for 14 days for patients intolerant or resistant to clarithromycin.

Triple therapy: 30 mg lansoprazole plus 500 mg clarithromycin and 1 g amoxicillin all taken twice daily (every 12 hours) for 10 or 14 days.

➤*Erosive esophagitis:*

Adults and children 12 to 17 years of age –

Short-term treatment: 30 mg once daily for up to 8 weeks. For adults who do not heal within 8 weeks (5% to 10%), it may be helpful to give an additional 8 weeks of treatment. If there is a recurrence of erosive esophagitis, consider an additional 8-week course.

Maintenance (adults): 15 mg once daily to maintain healing of erosive esophagitis.

Children 1 to 11 years of age (short-term treatment) –

30 kg or less: 15 mg/day for up to 12 weeks. The lansoprazole dose was increased (up to 30 mg twice daily) in some pediatric patients after 2 or more weeks of treatment if they remained symptomatic. For pediatric patients unable to swallow an intact capsule, see Difficulty swallowing.

Over 30 kg: 30 mg/day for up to 12 weeks. The lansoprazole dose was increased (up to 30 mg twice daily) in some pediatric patients after 2 or more weeks of treatment if they remained symptomatic. For pediatric patients unable to swallow an intact capsule, see Difficulty swallowing.

➤*Gastric ulcer:*

Short-term treatment – 30 mg once daily for up to 8 weeks.

Associated with NSAIDs –

Healing: 30 mg once daily for up to 8 weeks. Controlled studies did not extend beyond indicated duration.

Risk reduction: 15 mg once daily for up to 12 weeks. Controlled studies did not extend beyond indicated duration.

➤*GERD:*

Adults and children 12 to 17 years of age – 15 mg once daily for up to 8 weeks.

Children 1 to 11 years of age (short-term treatment) –

30 kg or less: 15 mg/day for up to 12 weeks. The lansoprazole dose was increased (up to 30 mg twice daily) in some pediatric patients after 2 or more weeks of treatment if they remained symptomatic. For pediatric patients unable to swallow an intact capsule, see Difficulty swallowing.

Over 30 kg: 30 mg/day for up to 12 weeks. The lansoprazole dose was increased (up to 30 mg twice daily) in some pediatric patients after 2 or more weeks of treatment if they remained symptomatic. For pediatric patients unable to swallow an intact capsule, see Difficulty swallowing.

➤*Hypersecretory conditions, including Zollinger-Ellison syndrome:* Individualize dosage. Recommended adult starting dose is 60 mg once daily. Dosages up to 90 mg twice daily have been administered. Administer daily dosages greater than 120 mg in divided doses. Some patients with Zollinger-Ellison syndrome have been treated with lansoprazole for longer than 4 years.

➤*Hepatic function impairment:* Consider dosage adjustment in patients with severe liver disease.

➤*Nasogastric (NG) tube:*

Capsules – For patients who have an NG tube in place, lansoprazole capsules can be opened and the intact granules mixed in 40 mL apple juice. Do not use other liquids. Inject through the NG tube into the stomach. After administering the granules, flush the NG tube with additional apple juice to clear the tube.

Orally disintegrating tablets – For administration via a NG tube, place a 15 mg tablet in a syringe and draw up 4 mL water, or place a 30 mg tablet in a syringe and draw up 10 mL water. Shake gently to allow for a quick dispersal. After the tablet has dispersed, inject through the NG tube into the stomach within 15 minutes. Refill the syringe with approximately 5 mL of water, shake gently, and flush the NG tube.

➤*Difficulty swallowing:*

Capsules – For patients who have difficulty swallowing capsules, lansoprazole can be opened and the intact granules contained within can be sprinkled on 1 tablespoon of applesauce, *Ensure* pudding, cottage cheese, yogurt, or strained pears and swallowed immediately. Alternatively, the delayed-release capsules may be emptied into a small volume of apple, orange, or tomato juice (60 mL; approximately 2 oz), mixed briefly, and swallowed immediately. To ensure complete delivery of the dose, rinse the glass with 2 or more volumes of juice and swallow the contents immediately. Use in other foods and liquids has not been studied clinically and, therefore, is not recommended.

Oral suspension – Empty packet contents into 2 tablespoons of water. Do not use other liquids or foods. Stir well and drink immediately. If any material remains after drinking, add more water, stir, and drink immediately. Do not give through enteral administration tubes.

Orally disintegrating tablets – Place the tablet on the tongue. Allow it to disintegrate with or without water until the particles can be swallowed. The tablet typically disintegrates in less than 1 minute. *SoluTabs* are not designed to be swallowed intact or chewed.

For administration via oral syringe, place a 15 mg tablet in an oral syringe and draw up approximately 4 mL of water, or place a 30 mg tablet in oral syringe and draw up approximately 10 mL of water. Shake gently to allow for a quick dispersal. After the tablet has dispersed, administer the contents within 15 minutes. Refill the syringe with approximately 2 mL (5 mL for the 30 mg tablet) of water, shake gently, and administer any remaining contents.

➤*Storage/Stability:* Store at 25°C (77°F); excursions permitted to 15 to 30°C (59 to 86°F). Store in a tight container protected from moisture.

LANSOPRAZOLE — INJECTION

For complete and comparative prescribing information, refer to the Proton Pump Inhibitors group monograph.

Indications

➤*Erosive esophagitis:* When patients are unable to take the oral formulations, lansoprazole IV for injection is indicated as an alternative for the short-term treatment (up to 7 days) of all grades of erosive esophagitis. Once the patient is able to take medications orally, therapy can be switched to an oral formulation of lansoprazole for a total of 6 to 8 weeks. The safety and efficacy of lansoprazole as an initial treatment of erosive esophagitis have not been demonstrated. Refer to full prescribing information for the oral formulations of lansoprazole.

Administration and Dosage

➤*Approved by the FDA:* May 27, 2004.

Lansoprazole must be reconstituted with 5 mL of Sterile Water for Injection. Failure to reconstitute with Sterile Water may result in formation of precipitation/particulates. Administer lansoprazole admixtures IV using the in-line filter provided. The filter must be used to remove precipitate that may form when the reconstituted drug product is mixed with IV solutions. Studies have shown that filtration does not alter the amount of drug that is available for administration (see instructions below).

➤*Reconstitution in vial:*

1.) Inject 5 mL of only Sterile Water for Injection into a 30 mg vial of lansoprazole IV for injection. The resulting solution will contain lansoprazole 6 mg/mL (30 mg per 5 mL).
2.) Mix gently until the powder is dissolved.

The pH of this reconstituted solution is approximately 11. The reconstituted solution can be held for 1 hour when stored at 25°C (77°F) prior to further dilution.

➤*Preparation of admixture:* Dilute the reconstituted solution in either 50 mL of 0.9% Sodium Chloride Injection, Lactated Ringer's Injection, or 5% Dextrose Injection.

Store the admixture at 25°C (77°F), and administer within the designated time period as listed in the following table. No refrigeration is required.

Diluent	pH	Administer within:
0.9% Sodium Chloride Injection	Approximately 10.2	24 hours
Lactated Ringer's Injection	Approximately 10	24 hours
5% Dextrose Injection	Approximately 9.5	12 hours

➤*Instructions for priming and use of filter:*

To prime filter –

1.) Prime administration set in usual manner and close administration set clamp.
2.) Connect luer adapter of administration set to filter inlet using a twisting motion. Avoid overtightening.
3.) Hold filter below the level of solution container.
4.) Open administration set clamp and slowly prime filter.
5.) Close administration set clamp. Verify no air bubbles are present on patient side of filter.
6.) If air bubbles are observed, open set clamp slightly to reestablish flow then gently tap filter housing. Observe that no air bubbles are present and close clamp.
7.) Connect to patient and regulate flow. Filter may be primed using a syringe and saline.
8.) The administration set can then be connected to inlet of filter.

Precautions with use of filter – Follow instructions carefully:

Use aseptic technique. This medication is for single use only. Do not resterilize or reuse. Do not use if package is damaged.

If repositioning of filter is required, loosen luer locking collar, reposition, then retighten locking collar firmly.

Maximum working pressure is 1,500 mm Hg (30 psi, 2 bar). When the working limits of the filter are exceeded, investigate and correct causes of the added resistance.

The internal volume of the filter is approximately 0.7 mL.

Close the administration set clamp during solution container change.

It is recommended that this filter is changed at 24 hours.

Pumps should not be used downstream of filter.

➤*Administration:*

In-line filter must be used.

Administer IV over 30 minutes.

A dedicated line is not required; however, flush the IV line before and after administration of lansoprazole IV for injection with either 0.9% Sodium Chloride Injection, Lactated Ringer's Injection, or 5% Dextrose Injection.

Do not administer with other drugs or diluents as this may cause incompatibilities.

➤*Treatment of erosive esophagitis:* The recommended adult dose (when patients are unable to take the oral therapy) is 30 mg of lansoprazole (1 vial of lansoprazole IV for injection) per day administered by IV infusion over 30 minutes for up to 7 days. Once the patient is able to take medications orally, therapy can be switched to an oral lansoprazole formulation for a

LANSOPRAZOLE — INJECTION

total of 6 to 8 weeks (refer to full prescribing information for the oral formulations of lansoprazole).

Hepatic function impairment – For patients with severe liver disease, consider dosage adjustment.

➤*Storage/Stability:* Store lansoprazole IV at 25°C (77°F); excursions permitted to 15° to 30°C (59° to 86°F). Protect from light. Use carton to protect contents from light.

OMEPRAZOLE

otc	**Prilosec OTC**[a] (Procter and Gamble)	**Tablets, delayed-release**: 20 mg	Sucrose, talc. In 14s, 28s, and 42s.
Rx	**Omeprazole** (Various, eg, Kremers-Urban, Mylan)	**Capsules, delayed-release**[b]: 10 mg	In 30s and 100s.
Rx	**Prilosec** (AstraZeneca)		Lactose, mannitol. (606 PRILOSEC 10). Apricot and amethyst. In 1,000s and unit-of-use 30s.
Rx	**Omeprazole** (Various, eg, Allscripts, H.J. Harkins, Kremers-Urban, Lek, Mylan)	**Capsules, delayed-release**[b]: 20 mg	In 30s and 100s.
Rx	**Prilosec** (AstraZeneca)		Lactose, mannitol. (742 PRILOSEC 20). Amethyst. In 1,000s and unit-of-use 30s.
Rx	**Prilosec** (AstraZeneca)	**Capsules, delayed-release**[b]: 40 mg	Lactose, mannitol. (743 PRILOSEC 40). Apricot and amethyst. In 100s, 1,000s, and unit-of-use 30s.

[a] As omeprazole magnesium.

[b] Contains enteric-coated granules.

OMEPRAZOLE — ORAL

For complete and comparative prescribing information, refer to the Proton Pump Inhibitors group monograph. Refer to the Penicillins and Macrolides group monographs for complete prescribing information for amoxicillin and clarithromycin.

Indications

➤*Duodenal ulcer (Rx only):* For short-term treatment of active duodenal ulcer.

➤*Duodenal ulcer associated with H. pylori (Rx only):* In combination with clarithromycin to eradicate *H. pylori* . In patients with a 1-year history of duodenal ulcers or active duodenal ulcers, use in combination with clarithromycin and amoxicillin to eradicate *H. pylori*. Eradication of *H. pylori* has been shown to reduce the risk of duodenal ulcer recurrence.

➤*Erosive esophagitis (Rx only):* For short-term treatment (4 to 8 weeks) of erosive esophagitis diagnosed by endoscopy; to maintain healing of erosive esophagitis.

➤*Gastric ulcer (Rx only):* For short-term treatment (4 to 8 weeks) of active benign gastric ulcer.

➤*Gastroesophageal reflux disease (GERD) (Rx only):* For the treatment of heartburn and other symptoms associated with GERD.

➤*Heartburn (OTC):* To treat frequent heartburn (occurs 2 or more days a week); not intended for immediate relief.

➤*Hypersecretory conditions:* For long-term treatment of hypersecretory conditions (eg, Zollinger-Ellison syndrome, multiple endocrine adenomas, systemic mastocytosis).

➤*Unlabeled uses:* GERD-related laryngitis.

Treatment of GERD in infants and children (1 mg/kg/day once or twice daily); in combination with antibiotics (eg, amoxicillin, clarithromycin) for the eradication of *H. pylori* in children with *H. pylori*-induced gastritis; to improve pancreatic enzyme absorption in cystic fibrosis patients with intestinal malabsorption.

Alternate-day dosing has been shown to be effective in maintaining ulcer or GERD remission after patients have been healed via a shorter course of daily therapy.

Administration and Dosage

➤*Approved by the FDA:* September 14, 1989

➤*Adults:*

Duodenal ulcer –

Treatment: 20 mg/day. Most patients heal within 4 weeks, although some may require an additional 4 weeks of therapy.

Associated with H. pylori:

• *Triple therapy (omeprazole/clarithromycin/amoxicillin)* – Omeprazole 20 mg plus clarithromycin 500 mg plus amoxicillin 1,000 mg each given twice daily for 10 days. If an ulcer is present at the initiation of therapy, continue omeprazole 20 mg once daily for an additional 18 days.

• *Dual therapy (omeprazole/clarithromycin)* – Omeprazole 40 mg once daily plus clarithromycin 500 mg 3 times/day for 14 days. If an ulcer is present at the initiation of therapy, continue omeprazole 20 mg for an additional 14 days.

Among patients who fail therapy, omeprazole with clarithromycin is more likely to be associated with the development of clarithromycin resistance as compared with triple therapy. In patients who fail therapy, susceptibility testing should be done. If resistance to clarithromycin is demonstrated or susceptibility testing is not possible, alternative antimicrobial therapy should be instituted.

➤*Erosive esophagitis:*

Treatment – 20 mg/day for 4 to 8 weeks.

Maintenance – 20 mg/day. Controlled studies do not extend beyond 12 months.

➤*Gastric ulcer:* 40 mg once a day for 4 to 8 weeks.

➤*GERD:*

GERD without esophageal lesions – 20 mg/day for up to 4 weeks.

GERD with erosive esophagitis – 20 mg/day for 4 to 8 weeks. The efficacy of omeprazole used for more than 8 weeks in patients with GERD has not been established. In the rare patient not responding to 8 weeks of treatment, an additional 4 weeks of treatment may help. If there is recurrence of erosive esophagitis or GERD, an additional 4- to 8-week course of omeprazole may be considered.

➤*Heartburn (OTC):* Swallow 1 tablet with a glass of water once daily before eating in the morning. Take every day for 14 days. It may take 1 to 4 days for full effect, although some patients get complete relief within 24 hours. The 14-day course may be repeated every 4 months. Maximum dose is 1 tablet in 24 hours.

➤*Pathological hypersecretory conditions:* Individualize dosage. Initial adult dose is 60 mg/day. Continue for as long as clinically indicated. Dosages up to 120 mg 3 times/day have been administered. Administer daily doses greater than 80 mg in divided doses. Some patients with Zollinger-Ellison syndrome have been treated continuously for more than 5 years.

➤*Children:* For the treatment of GERD or other acid-related disorders, the recommended dose for children 2 years of age and older is as follows: omeprazole 10 mg for patients weighing less than 20 kg, and omeprazole 20 mg for patients weighing 20 kg or more. On a per kg basis, the doses of omeprazole required to heal erosive esophagitis are greater than those for adults.

➤*Difficulty swallowing:* For patients who have difficulty swallowing capsules, add 1 tablespoon of applesauce to an empty bowl, open the omeprazole capsule, and empty the pellets onto the applesauce. Mix the pellets with the applesauce and swallow immediately with cool water to ensure complete swallowing of the pellets. Do not heat or chew the applesauce. Do not chew or crush the pellets. Do not store the pellet/applesauce mixture for future use.

➤*Administration:* Take on an empty stomach at least 1 hour before a meal. Do not crush or chew the capsule; swallow whole. Do not chew or crush the tablets.

➤*Hepatic function impairment:* Consider dose adjustment, particularly when maintenance of healing of erosive esophagitis is indicated, for patients with hepatic function impairment.

➤*Race:* Consider dose adjustment in Asian patients, particularly when maintenance of healing of erosive esophagitis is indicated.

➤*Storage/Stability:*

Tablets – Store tablets at 20° to 25°C (68° to 77°F). Keep product out of high heat and humidity, and protect from moisture.

Capsules – Store capsules at 15° to 30°C (59° to 86°F) in a tight container. Protect from light and moisture.

PANTOPRAZOLE SODIUM

Rx	**Protonix** (Wyeth-Ayerst)	**Tablets, delayed-release**: 20 mg (as base)	Mannitol. (P20). Yellow, oval. In 90s.
		40 mg (as base)	Mannitol. (PROTONIX). Yellow, oval. In 90s, 100s, 1,000s, and *Redipak* blister strips of 10.
Rx	**Protonix I.V.** (Wyeth-Ayerst)	**Powder for injection, freeze-dried**: 40 mg (as base)/vial	EDTA. In vials.

PANTOPRAZOLE SODIUM — ORAL

For comparative prescribing information, refer to the Proton Pump Inhibitors group monograph.

Indications

➤*Maintenance of healing of erosive esophagitis:* For maintenance of healing of erosive esophagitis and reduction in relapse rates of daytime and nighttime heartburn symptoms in patients with gastroesophageal reflux disease (GERD). Controlled studies did not extend beyond 12 months.

➤*Pathological hypersecretory conditions including Zollinger-Ellison syndrome:* For the long-term treatment of pathological hypersecretory conditions, including Zollinger-Ellison syndrome.

➤*Short-term treatment of erosive esophagitis associated with gastroesophageal reflux disease (GERD):* For the short-term treatment (up to 8 weeks) in the healing and symptomatic relief of erosive esophagitis. For those patients who have not healed after 8 weeks of treatment, an additional 8 week course of pantoprazole may be considered.

Administration and Dosage

➤*Approved by the FDA:* February 2, 2000.

➤*Treatment of erosive esophagitis:* 40 mg once daily for up to 8 weeks. For those patients who have not healed after 8 weeks of treatment, an additional 8-week course of pantoprazole may be considered.

➤*Maintenance of healing of erosive esophagitis:* One 40 mg delayed-release tablet, taken daily.

➤*Pathological hypersecretory conditions including Zollinger-Ellison syndrome:* The dosage of pantoprazole in patients with pathological hypersecretory conditions varies with the individual patient. The recommended adult starting dosage is 40 mg twice daily. Adjust dosage regimens to individual patient needs and continue for as long as clinically indicated. Dosages up to 240 mg daily have been administered. Some patients have been treated continuously with pantoprazole for more than 2 years.

➤*Administration:* Swallow whole, with or without food in the stomach. If patients are unable to swallow a 40 mg tablet, two 20 mg tablets may be taken. Concomitant administration of antacids does not affect the absorption of pantoprazole.

Caution patients that pantoprazole delayed-release tablets should not be split, chewed, or crushed.

➤*Storage / Stability:* Store pantoprazole delayed-release tablets at 20° to 25°C (68° to 77°F); excursion permitted to 15° to 30°C (59° to 86°F).

PANTOPRAZOLE SODIUM — INJECTION

For complete and comparative prescribing information, refer to the Proton Pump Inhibitors group monograph.

Indications

➤*Treatment of GERD associated with a history of erosive esophagitis:* For short-term treatment (7 to 10 days) of patients having gastroesophageal reflux disease (GERD) with a history of erosive esophagitis, as an alternative to oral therapy in patients who are unable to continue taking pantoprazole sodium delayed-release tablets. Safety and efficacy of pantoprazole sodium for injection as an initial treatment for GERD with a history of erosive esophagitis have not been demonstrated.

➤*Pathological hypersecretion associated with Zollinger-Ellison syndrome:* For the treatment of pathological hypersecretory conditions associated with Zollinger-Ellison syndrome or other neoplastic conditions.

Administration and Dosage

➤*Administration:* Administer pantoprazole sodium for injection IV through a dedicated line, using the filter provided. The filter must be used to remove precipitate that may form when the drug product is reconstituted or mixed with IV solutions. Studies have shown that filtration does not alter the amount of drug that is available for administration. If administration through a Y-site is desirable, the in-line filter must be positioned below the Y-site that is closest to the patient. Flush the IV line before and after administration of pantoprazole sodium for injection with either 5% Dextrose Injection, 0.9% Sodium Chloride Injection, or Lactated Ringer's Injection. Do not administer pantoprazole sodium for injection simultaneously through the same line with other IV solutions.

Discontinue treatment with pantoprazole sodium for injection as soon as the patient is able to resume treatment with pantoprazole sodium delayed-release tablets. Also, data on the safe and effective dosing for conditions other than those described, such as life-threatening upper GI bleeds, are not available. Pantoprazole sodium injection 40 mg once daily does not raise gastric pH to levels sufficient to contribute to the treatment of such life-threatening conditions.

Parenteral routes of administration other than IV are not recommended.

➤*Treatment of GERD associated with a history of erosive esophagitis:* The recommended adult dose, as an alternative to continued oral therapy, is pantoprazole 40 mg given once daily by IV infusion for 7 to 10 days. Safety and efficacy of pantoprazole sodium IV for injection as a treatment of patients having GERD with a history of erosive esophagitis for more than 10 days have not been demonstrated.

15-minute infusion – Reconstitute pantoprazole sodium for injection with 10 mL of 0.9% Sodium Chloride Injection, and further dilute (admix) with 100 mL of 5% Dextrose Injection, 0.9% Sodium Chloride Injection, or Lactated Ringer's Injection, to a final concentration of approximately 0.4 mg/mL. The reconstituted solution may be stored for up to 2 hours at room temperature prior to further dilution; the admixed solution may be stored for up to 12 hours at room temperature prior to IV infusion. Neither the reconstituted solution nor the admixed solution needs to be protected from light.

Administer admixtures IV over a period of approximately 15 minutes at a rate of approximately 7 mL/min using the filter provided.

2-minute infusion – Reconstitute pantoprazole sodium IV for injection with 10 mL of 0.9% Sodium Chloride Injection, to a final concentration of approximately 4 mg/mL. The reconstituted solution may be stored for up to 2 hours at room temperature prior to IV infusion and does not need to be protected from light. Administer IV over a period of at least 2 minutes using the filter provided.

➤*Pathological hypersecretion associated with Zollinger-Ellison syndrome:* The dosage of pantoprazole sodium for injection in patients with pathological hypersecretory conditions associated with Zollinger-Ellison Syndrome or other neoplastic conditions varies with individual patients. The recommended adult dosage is 80 mg every 12 hours. The frequency of dosing can be adjusted to individual patient needs based on acid output measurements. In those patients who need a higher dosage, 80 mg every 8 hours is expected to maintain acid output below 10 mEq/h. Daily doses higher than 240 mg or administered for more than 6 days have not been studied. Perform transition from oral to IV and from IV to oral formulations of gastric acid inhibitors in such a manner to ensure continuity of effect of suppression of acid secretion. Patients with Zollinger-Ellison Syndrome may be vulnerable to serious clinical complications of increased acid production even after a short period of loss of effective inhibition.

15-minute infusion – Reconstitute each vial of pantoprazole sodium IV for injection with 10 mL of 0.9% Sodium Chloride Injection. Combine the contents of the 2 vials and further dilute (admix) with 80 mL of 5% Dextrose Injection, 0.9% Sodium Chloride Injection, or Lactated Ringer's Injection, to a total volume of 100 mL, with a final concentration of approximately 0.8 mg/mL. The reconstituted solution may be stored for up to 2 hours at room temperature prior to further dilution; the admixed solution may be stored for up to 12 hours at room temperature prior to IV infusion. Neither the reconstituted solution nor the admixed solution need to be protected from light.

Administer pantoprazole sodium IV for injection over a period of approximately 15 minutes at a rate of approximately 7 mL/min using the filter provided.

2-minute infusion – Reconstitute pantoprazole sodium IV for injection with 10 mL of 0.9% Sodium Chloride Injection per vial to a final concentration of approximately 4 mg/mL. The reconstituted solution may be stored for up to 2 hours at room temperature prior to IV infusion and does not need to be protected from light. Administer the total volume from both vials IV over a period of at least 2 minutes using the filter provided.

➤*Storage / Stability:* Store pantoprazole sodium for injection vials at 2° to 8°C (36° to 46°F), and protect from light. Do not freeze the reconstituted product.

Store the provided in-line filters at room temperature.

RABEPRAZOLE SODIUM

Rx	**Aciphex** (Eisai)	**Tablets, delayed-release:** 20 mg	Mannitol. (ACIPHEX 20). Lt. yellow. Enteric-coated. In 30s, 90s, and UD 100s.

RABEPRAZOLE SODIUM — ORAL

For complete and comparative prescribing information, refer to the Proton Pump Inhibitors group monograph. Refer to the Penicillins and Macrolides group monographs for complete prescribing information for amoxicillin and clarithromycin.

Indications

➤*Healing of erosive or ulcerative gastroesophageal reflux disease (GERD):* Short-term (4 to 8 weeks) treatment in the healing and symptomatic relief of erosive or ulcerative GERD. For those patients who have not healed after 8 weeks of treatment, an additional 8-week course of rabeprazole sodium may be considered.

➤*Maintenance of healing of erosive or ulcerative GERD:* For maintaining healing and reduction in relapse rates of heartburn symptoms in patients with erosive or ulcerative GERD. Controlled studies do not extend beyond 12 months.

➤*Treatment of symptomatic GERD:* For the treatment of daytime and nighttime heartburn and other symptoms associated with GERD.

➤*Healing of duodenal ulcers:* For short-term (less than or equal to 4 weeks) treatment in the healing and symptomatic relief of duodenal ulcers. Most patients heal within 4 weeks.

➤*Treatment of pathological hypersecretory conditions, including Zollinger-Ellison syndrome:* For the long-term treatment of pathological hypersecretory conditions, including Zollinger-Ellison syndrome.

RABEPRAZOLE SODIUM — ORAL

Administration and Dosage

➤*Approved by the FDA:* August 19, 1999.

➤*Healing of erosive or ulcerative GERD:* 20 mg once daily for 4 to 8 weeks (see Indications). For those patients who have not healed after 8 weeks of treatment, an additional 8-week course of rabeprazole sodium may be considered.

➤*Maintenance of healing of erosive or ulcerative GERD:* 20 mg once daily (see Indications).

➤*Treatment of symptomatic GERD:* 20 mg once daily for 4 weeks (see Indications). If symptoms do not resolve completely after 4 weeks, an additional course of treatment may be considered.

➤*Healing of duodenal ulcers:* 20 mg once daily after the morning meal for a period up to 4 weeks (see Indications). Most patients with duodenal ulcer heal within 4 weeks. A few patients may require additional therapy to achieve healing.

➤*Treatment of pathological hypersecretory conditions including Zollinger-Ellison syndrome:* The dosage of rabeprazole sodium in patients with pathologic hypersecretory conditions varies with the individual patient. The recommended adult oral starting dose is 60 mg once daily. Doses should be adjusted to individual patient needs and should continue for as long as clinically indicated. Some patients may require divided doses. Doses up to 100 mg daily and 60 mg twice daily have been administered. Some patients with Zollinger-Ellison syndrome have been treated continuously with rabeprazole sodium for up to 1 year. No dosage adjustment is necessary in elderly patients, in patients with renal disease, or in patients with mild to moderate hepatic impairment. Administration of rabeprazole to patients with mild to moderate liver impairment resulted in increased exposure and decreased elimination. Due to the lack of clinical data on rabeprazole in patients with severe hepatic impairment, caution should be exercised in those patients.

Administration – Rabeprazole sodium tablets should be swallowed whole. The tablets should not be chewed, crushed, or split.

➤*Storage/Stability:* Store at 25°C (77°F); excursions permitted to 15° to 30°C (59° to 86°F). Protect from moisture.

PROTON PUMP INHIBITOR COMBINATION

Rx	**Zegerid** (Santarus)[a]	**Capsules, immediate-release**: 20 mg omeprazole/1,100 mg sodium bicarbonate	(Santarus 20). Light blue and white. In 30s.
		40 mg omeprazole/1,100 mg sodium bicarbonate	(Santarus 40). Dark blue and white. In 30s.
		Powder for oral suspension: 20 mg omeprazole/1,680 sodium bicarbonate	Sucrose, sucralose, xylitol, xanthan gum. In 30 unit-dose packets.
		40 mg omeprazole/1,680 sodium bicarbonate	Sucrose, sucralose, xylitol, xanthan gum. In 30 unit-dose packets.

[a] Santarus, Inc., 10590 West Ocean Air Drive, Suite 200, San Diego, CA 92130; 858–314–5701; http://www.santarus.com.

OMEPRAZOLE/SODIUM BICARBONATE — ORAL

For complete and comparative prescribing information, refer to the Proton Pump Inhibitors group monograph. Also see the Sodium Bicarbonate monograph

Indications

➤*Benign gastric ulcer:* For short-term treatment (4 to 8 weeks) of active benign gastric ulcer

➤*Duodenal ulcer:* For short-term treatment of active duodenal ulcer. Most patients heal within 4 weeks. Some patients may require an additional 4 weeks of therapy.

➤*Gastroesophageal reflux disease (GERD):*

Symptomatic GERD – For the treatment of heartburn and other symptoms associated with GERD.

Erosive esophagitis – For the short-term treatment (4 to 8 weeks) of erosive esophagitis that has been diagnosed by endoscopy.

The efficacy of omeprazole/sodium bicarbonate used for longer than 8 weeks in these patients has not been established. In the rare instance of a patient not responding to 8 weeks of treatment, it may be helpful to give up to an additional 4 weeks of treatment. If there is recurrence of erosive esophagitis or GERD symptoms (eg, heartburn), additional 4 to 8 week courses of omeprazole may be considered.

➤*Maintenance of healing of erosive esophagitis:* To maintain healing of erosive esophagitis. Controlled studies do not extend beyond 12 months.

➤*Reduction of risk of upper GI bleeding in critically ill patients:* Omeprazole/sodium bicarbonate 40 mg/1,680 mg powder for oral suspension is indicated for the reduction of risk of upper GI bleeding in critically ill patients.

Administration and Dosage

Omeprazole/sodium bicarbonate is available as a capsule and as a powder for oral suspension in 20 and 40 mg strengths for adult use. Directions for use for each indication are summarized in the following table.

Since the 20 and 40 mg oral suspension packets contain the same amount of sodium bicarbonate (1,680 mg), 2 packets of 20 mg are not equivalent to one 40 mg packet of omeprazole/sodium bicarbonate; therefore, two 20 mg packets of omeprazole/sodium bicarbonate should not be substituted for one 40 mg packet of omeprazole/sodium bicarbonate.

Since the 20 and 40 mg capsules contain the same amount of sodium bicarbonate (1,100 mg), 2 capsules of 20 mg are not equivalent to one 40 mg capsule of omeprazole/sodium bicarbonate; therefore, two 20 mg capsules of omeprazole/sodium bicarbonate should not be substituted for one 40 mg capsule of omeprazole/sodium bicarbonate .

Omeprazole/sodium bicarbonate should be taken on an empty stomach at least 1 hour before a meal.

For patients receiving continuous nasogastric/orogastric (NG/OG) tube feeding, enteral feeding should be suspended approximately 3 hours before and 1 hour after administration of omeprazole/sodium bicarbonate powder for oral suspension.

Recommended Doses of Omeprazole/Sodium Bicarbonate for Adults 18 Years of Age and Older

Indication	Recommended dose	Frequency
Active duodenal ulcer	20 mg	Once daily for 4 weeks[a]
Benign gastric ulcer	40 mg	Once daily for 4 to 8 weeks
GERD		
Symptomatic GERD (with no esophageal erosions)	20 mg	Once daily for up to 4 weeks
Erosive esophagitis	20 mg	Once daily for 4 to 8 weeks
Maintenance of healing of erosive esophagitis	20 mg	Once daily
Reduction of risk of upper GI bleeding in critically ill patients (40 mg oral suspension only)	40 mg	40 mg initially followed by 40 mg 6 to 8 hours later and 40 mg daily thereafter for 14 days

[a] Most patients heal within 4 weeks. Some patients may require an additional 4 weeks of therapy.

➤*Administration of capsules:* Omeprazole/sodium bicarbonate capsules should be swallowed intact with water. Do not use other liquids. Do not open capsule and sprinkle contents onto food.

➤*Preparation and administration of suspension:* Empty packet contents into a small cup containing 1 to 2 tablespoons of water. Do not use other liquids or foods. Stir well and drink immediately. Refill cup with water and drink. If omeprazole/sodium bicarbonate is to be administered through a NG/OG tube, the suspension should be constituted with approximately 20 mL of water. Do not use other liquids or foods. Stir well and administer immediately. An appropriately-sized syringe should be used to instill the suspension in the tube. The suspension should be washed through the tube with 20 mL of water.

➤*Storage/Stability:* Store at 25°C (77°F); excursions permitted to 15° to 30°C (59° to 86°F).

SUCRALFATE

SUCRALFATE

Rx	**Sucralfate** (Various, eg, Eon Labs, Major, Martec, Teva)	**Tablets:** 1 g	In 100s and 500s.
Rx	**Carafate** (Axcan Scandipharm)		(Carafate 1712). Light pink, oblong, scored. In 100s, 120s, and 500s.
Rx	**Sucralfate** (Precision Dose)	**Suspension:** 1 g/10 mL	Methylparaben, sorbitol. In 10 mL unit dose cups.
Rx	**Carafate** (Axcan Scandipharm)		Sorbitol, methylparaben. In 415 mL.

SUCRALFATE — ORAL

Indications

➤*Active duodenal ulcer:* Short-term treatment (up to 8 weeks) of active duodenal ulcer.

➤*Maintenance therapy for duodenal ulcer:* For duodenal ulcer patients at reduced dosage after healing of acute ulcers.

➤*Unlabeled uses:* Sucralfate has been used in the following conditions: Accelerating healing of gastric ulcers; long-term treatment of gastric ulcers; treatment of reflux and peptic esophagitis; treatment of NSAID- and aspirin-induced GI symptoms and mucosal damage; prevention of stress ulcers and GI bleeding in critically ill patients. Because increased gastric pH may be implicated in causing nosocomial infections in critically ill patients, sucralfate may offer an advantage over antacids and histamine H_2 antagonists in stress ulcer prophylaxis.

Sucralfate in suspension has also been used in treatment of oral and esophageal ulcers due to radiation, chemotherapy and sclerotherapy.

Administration and Dosage

➤*Approved by the FDA:* December 16, 1993.

➤*Active duodenal ulcer:* 1 g (10 mL or 2 teaspoons of the oral suspension) 4 times a day on an empty stomach.

Antacids may be prescribed as needed for relief of pain but should not be taken within one-half hour before or after sucralfate.

While healing with sucralfate may occur during the first week or two, treatment should be continued for 4 to 8 weeks unless healing has been demonstrated by x-ray or endoscopic examination.

➤*Maintenance therapy:* 1 g twice a day.

➤*Storage / Stability:*

Oral suspension – Store at controlled room temperature 20° to 25°C (68° to 77°F). Shake well before using.

Actions

➤*Pharmacokinetics:* Sucralfate is only minimally absorbed from the gastrointestinal tract. The small amounts of the sulfated disaccharide that are absorbed are excreted primarily in the urine.

Although the mechanism of sucralfate's ability to accelerate healing of duodenal ulcers remains to be fully defined, it is known that it exerts its effect through a local, rather than systemic, action. The following observations also appear pertinent:

1.) Studies in human subjects and with animal models of ulcer disease have shown that sucralfate forms an ulcer-adherent complex with proteinaceous exudate at the ulcer site.
2.) In vitro, a sucralfate-albumin film provides a barrier to diffusion of hydrogen ions.
3.) In human subjects, sucralfate given in doses recommended for ulcer therapy inhibits pepsin activity in gastric juice by 32%.
4.) In vitro, sucralfate absorbs bile salts.

These observations suggest that sucralfate's antiulcer activity is the result of formation of an ulcer-adherent complex that covers the ulcer site and protects it against further attack by acid, pepsin, and bile salts. There are approximately 14 to 16 mEq of acid-neutralizing capacity per 1 g dose of sucralfate.

Contraindications

There are no known contraindications to the use of sucralfate.

Warnings

➤*Pregnancy: Category B.*

There are no adequate and well-controlled studies in pregnant women. Because animal reproduction studies are not always predictive of human response, this drug should be used during pregnancy only if clearly needed.

➤*Lactation:* It is not known whether this drug is excreted in human milk. Because many drugs are excreted in human milk, caution should be exercised when sucralfate is administered to a nursing woman.

➤*Children:* Safety and effectiveness in pediatric patients have not been established.

Precautions

➤*Ulcer recurrence:* Duodenal ulcer is a chronic, recurrent disease. While short-term treatment with sucralfate can result in complete healing of the ulcer, a successful course of treatment with sucralfate should not be expected to alter the posthealing frequency or severity of duodenal ulceration.

➤*Renal function impairment:* When sucralfate is administered orally, small amounts of aluminum are absorbed from the gastrointestinal tract. Concomitant use of sucralfate with other products that contain aluminum, such as aluminum-containing antacids, may increase the total body burden of aluminum. Patients with normal renal function receiving the recommended doses of sucralfate and aluminum-containing products adequately excrete aluminum in the urine. Patients with chronic renal failure or those receiving dialysis have impaired excretion of absorbed aluminum. In addition, aluminum does not cross dialysis membranes because it is bound to albumin and transferrin plasma proteins. Aluminum accumulation and toxicity (aluminum osteodystrophy, osteomalacia, encephalopathy) have been described in patients with renal impairment. Sucralfate should be used with caution in patients with chronic renal failure.

Drug Interactions

Sucralfate Drug Interactions

Precipitant drug	Object drug*		Description
Sucralfate	Antacids, aluminum-containing	⬆	The total body burden of aluminum may be increased with sucralfate coadministration. See Warnings.
Sucralfate	Anticoagulants	⬇	A decrease in the hypoprothrombinemic effect of warfarin may occur.
Sucralfate	Diclofenac	⬇	The pharmacologic effects of diclofenac may be decreased.
Sucralfate	Digoxin	⬇	Serum digoxin levels may be reduced, decreasing the therapeutic effects.
Sucralfate	Histamine H_2 antagonists Cimetidine Ranitidine	⬇	Bioavailability of the histamine H_2 antagonists may be decreased. Administering the histamine H_2 antagonist ≥ 2 hours before sucralfate may eliminate the interaction.
Sucralfate	Hydantoins	⬇	Phenytoin absorption may be decreased.
Sucralfate	Ketoconazole	⬇	Ketoconazole bioavailability may be decreased.
Sucralfate	Levothyroxine	⬇	The effects of levothyroxine may be decreased.
Sucralfate	Penicillamine	⬇	Penicillamine's effectiveness may be lessened or negated.
Sucralfate	Quinidine	⬇	Serum quinidine levels may be reduced, decreasing the therapeutic effects.
Sucralfate	Quinolones	⬇	Bioavailability of the quinolones may be decreased. Administering the quinolone ≥ 2 hours before sucralfate may eliminate the interaction.
Sucralfate	Tetracycline	⬇	Tetracycline bioavailability may be decreased.
Sucralfate	Theophylline	⬇	Theophylline bioavailability may be decreased.

* ⬆ = Object drug increased. ⬇ = Object drug decreased.

Adverse Reactions

Constipation was the most frequent complaint (2%). Other adverse effects reported in less than 0.5% of the patients are listed below by body system:

➤*CNS:* Dizziness, insomnia, sleepiness, vertigo.

➤*Dermatologic:* Pruritus, rash.

➤*GI:* Diarrhea, nausea, vomiting, gastric discomfort, indigestion, flatulence, dry mouth.

➤*Miscellaneous:* Back pain, headache.

➤*Postmarketing experience with sucralfate:* Postmarketing reports of hypersensitivity reactions, including urticaria (hives), angioedema, respiratory difficulty, rhinitis, laryngospasm, and facial swelling have been reported in patients receiving sucralfate tablets. Similar events were reported with sucralfate suspension. However, a causal relationship has not been established.

Bezoars have been reported in patients treated with sucralfate. The majority of patients had underlying medical conditions that may predispose to bezoar formation (such as delayed gastric emptying) or were receiving concomitant enteral tube feedings.

Inadvertent injection of insoluble sucralfate and its insoluble excipients has led to fatal complications, including pulmonary and cerebral emboli. Sucralfate is not intended for intravenous administration.

Overdosage

➤*Symptoms:* Acute oral toxicity studies in animals, however, using doses up to 12 g/kg body weight, could not find a lethal dose. Sucralfate is only minimally absorbed from the gastrointestinal tract. Risks associated with acute overdosage should, therefore, be minimal. In rare reports describing sucralfate overdose, most patients remained asymptomatic. Those few reports where adverse events were described included symptoms of dyspepsia, abdominal pain, nausea, and vomiting.

➤*Treatment:* Due to limited experience in humans with overdosage of sucralfate, no specific treatment recommendations can be given.

MISOPROSTOL

Rx	**Misoprostol** (Various, eg, Greenstone)	**Tablets:** 100 mcg	(G 5007). White. In unit-of-use 60s and 120s.
Rx	**Cytotec** (Pfizer)		(SEARLE 1451). White. In UD 100s and unit-of-use 60s and 120s.
Rx	**Misoprostol** (Various, eg, Greenstone)	**Tablets:** 200 mcg	(G 5008). White, hexagonal. In unit-of-use 60s and 100s.
Rx	**Cytotec** (Pfizer)		(SEARLE 1461). White, hexagonal. In UD 100s and unit-of-use 60s and 100s.

MISOPROSTOL — ORAL

WARNING

Misoprostol administration to women who are pregnant can cause abortion, premature birth, or birth defects. Uterine rupture has been reported when misoprostol was administered in pregnant women to induce labor or to induce abortion beyond the eighth week of pregnancy (see Warnings, Pregnancy, Labor and delivery). Misoprostol should not be taken by pregnant women to reduce the risk of ulcers induced by nonsteroidal anti-inflammatory drugs (NSAIDs) (see Contraindications, Warnings, and Precautions).

Patients must be advised of the abortifacient property and warned not to give the drug to others.

Misoprostol should not be used for reducing the risk of NSAID-induced ulcer in women of childbearing potential unless the patient is at high risk of complications from gastric ulcers associated with use of the NSAID, or is a high risk of developing gastric ulceration. In such patients, misoprostol may be prescribed if the patient:

- Has had a negative serum pregnancy test within 2 weeks prior to beginning therapy.
- Is capable of complying with effective contraceptive measures.
- Has received both oral and written warnings of the hazards of misoprostol, the risk of possible contraception failure, and the danger to other women of childbearing potential should the drug be taken by mistake.
- Will begin misoprostol only on the second or third day of the next normal menstrual period.

Indications

Misoprostol is indicated for the prevention of NSAID-induced gastric ulcers in patients at high risk of complications from gastric ulcer (eg, the elderly and patients with concomitant debilitating disease) as well as patients at high risk of developing gastric ulceration, such as patients with a history of ulcer. Misoprostol has not been shown to prevent duodenal ulcers in patients taking NSAIDs. Misoprostol should be taken for the duration of NSAID therapy. Misoprostol has been shown to prevent gastric ulcers in controlled studies of 3 months' duration. It had no effect, compared to placebo, on GI pain or discomfort associated with NSAID use.

➤*Unlabeled uses:*

Cervical ripening and labor induction – Vaginal misoprostol has been proven safe and effective for cervical ripening and labor induction. However, vaginal misoprostol is associated with a higher frequency of excessive uterine contractility and intervention (see Warnings).

Pregnancy termination – Misoprostol has been used in combination with mifepristone for pregnancy termination. Patients taking mifepristone must take 400 mcg misoprostol orally 2 days after taking mifepristone unless a complete abortion has already been confirmed before that time.

Postpartum hemorrhage – Vaginal administration of misoprostol for the treatment of serious postpartum hemorrhage in the presence of uterine atony (see Warnings).

Chronic, idiopathic constipation – Short-term trials have shown an acceleration of intestinal transit in healthy individuals and in those with chronic constipation. Improvement in stool frequency in patients with chronic constipation has been seen with treatment doses of 200 mcg 2 to 4 times/day.

Administration and Dosage

➤*Approved by the FDA:* 1988.

➤*Recommended adult oral dose:* The recommended adult oral dose of misoprostol for the prevention of NSAID-induced gastric ulcers is 200 mcg 4 times daily with food. If this dose cannot be tolerated, a dose of 100 mcg can be used. Misoprostol should be taken for the duration of NSAID therapy as prescribed by the physician. Misoprostol should be taken with a meal, and the last dose of the day should be at bedtime.

➤*Renal impairment:* Adjustment of the dosing schedule in renally impaired patients is not routinely needed, but dosage can be reduced if the 200 mcg dose is not tolerated (see Pharmacokinetics).

➤*Storage/Stability:* Store at or below 25°C (77°F), in a dry area.

Actions

➤*Pharmacology:* Misoprostol has both antisecretory (inhibiting gastric acid secretion) and (in animals) mucosal protective properties. NSAIDs inhibit prostaglandin synthesis, and a deficiency of prostaglandins within the gastric mucosa may lead to diminishing bicarbonate and mucus secretion and may contribute to the mucosal damage caused by these agents. Misoprostol can increase bicarbonate and mucus production, but in man this has been shown at doses 200 mcg and above that are also antisecretory. It is therefore not possible to tell whether the ability of misoprostol to prevent gastric ulcer is the result of its antisecretory effect, its mucosal protective effect, or both.

In vitro studies on canine parietal cells using tritiated misoprostol acid as the ligand have led to the identification and characterization of specific prostaglandin receptors. Receptor binding is saturable, reversible, and stereospecific. The sites have a high affinity for misoprostol, for its acid metabolite, and for other E type prostaglandins, but not for F or I prostaglandins and other unrelated compounds, such as histamine or cimetidine. Receptor-site affinity for misoprostol correlates well with an indirect index of antisecretory activity. It is likely that these specific receptors allow misoprostol taken with food to be effective topically, despite the lower serum concentrations attained.

Misoprostol produces a moderate decrease in pepsin concentration during basal conditions, but not during histamine stimulation. It has no significant effect on fasting or postprandial gastrin nor on intrinsic factor output.

Effects on gastric acid secretion – Misoprostol, over the range of 50 to 200 mcg, inhibits basal and nocturnal gastric acid secretion, and acid secretion in response to a variety of stimuli, including meals, histamine, pentagastrin, and coffee. Activity is apparent 30 minutes after oral administration and persists for at least 3 hours. In general, the effects of 50 mcg were modest and shorter-lived, and only the 200 mcg dose had substantial effects on nocturnal secretion or on histamine and meal-stimulated secretion.

Uterine effects – Misoprostol has been shown to produce uterine contractions that may endanger pregnancy (see Warning Box). In studies in women undergoing elective termination of pregnancy during the first trimester, misoprostol caused partial or complete expulsion of the uterine contents in 11% of the subjects and increased uterine bleeding in 41%.

Other pharmacologic effects – Misoprostol does not produce clinically significant effects on serum levels of prolactin, gonadotropins, thyroid-stimulating hormone, growth hormone, thyroxine, cortisol, gastrointestinal hormones (somatostatin, gastrin, vasoactive intestinal polypeptide, and motilin), creatinine, or uric acid. Gastric emptying, immunologic competence, platelet aggregation, pulmonary function, or the cardiovascular system are not modified by recommended doses of misoprostol.

➤*Pharmacokinetics:*

Absorption – Misoprostol is extensively absorbed, and undergoes rapid de-esterification to its free acid, which is responsible for its clinical activity and, unlike the parent compound, is detectable in plasma. The alpha side chain undergoes beta oxidation and the beta side chain undergoes omega oxidation followed by reduction of the ketone to give prostaglandin F analogs.

In healthy volunteers, misoprostol is rapidly absorbed after oral administration with a t_{max} of misoprostol acid of 12 ± 3 minutes and a terminal half-life of 20 to 40 minutes.

Distribution – There is high variability of plasma levels of misoprostol acid between and within studies but mean values after single doses show a linear relationship with dose over the range of 200 to 400 mcg. No accumulation of misoprostol acid was noted in multiple dose studies; plasma steady state was achieved within 2 days.

Metabolism – Maximum plasma concentrations of misoprostol acid are diminished when the dose is taken with food, and total availability of misoprostol acid is reduced by use of concomitant antacid. Clinical trials were conducted with concomitant antacid, however, so this effect does not appear to be clinically important.

Mean ± SD	C_{max} (pg/mL)	$AUC_{(0-4)}$ (pg•hr/mL)	t_{max} (min)
Fasting	811 ± 317	417 ± 135	14 ± 8
With antacid	689 ± 315	349 ± 108*	20 ± 14
With high-fat breakfast	303 ± 176*	373 ± 111	64 ± 79*

* Comparisons with fasting results statistically significant, $P < 0.05$.

Excretion – After oral administration of radiolabeled misoprostol, about 80% of detected radioactivity appears in urine. Pharmacokinetic studies in patients with varying degrees of renal impairment showed an approximate doubling of $t_{½}$, C_{max}, and AUC compared to healthy patients, but no clear correlation between the degree of impairment and AUC. In subjects over 64 years of age, the AUC for misoprostol acid is increased. No routine dosage adjustment is recommended in older patients or patients with renal impairment, but dosage may need to be reduced if the usual dose is not tolerated.

Misoprostol does not affect the hepatic mixed function oxidase (cytochrome P450) enzyme systems in animals.

Drug interaction and pharmacokinetic studies – Drug interaction studies between misoprostol and several nonsteroidal anti-inflammatory drugs showed no effect on the kinetics of ibuprofen or diclofenac, and a 20% decrease in aspirin AUC, not thought to be clinically significant.

Pharmacokinetic studies also showed a lack of drug interaction with antipyrine and propranolol when these drugs were given with misoprostol. Misoprostol given for 1 week had no effect on the steady state pharmacokinetics of diazepam when the 2 drugs were administered 2 hours apart.

The serum protein binding of misoprostol acid is less than 90% and is concentration-independent in the therapeutic range.

MISOPROSTOL — ORAL

Contraindications

See Warning Box. Misoprostol should not be taken by pregnant women to reduce the risk of ulcers induced by NSAIDs.

Misoprostol should not be taken by anyone with a history of allergy to prostaglandins.

Warnings

See Warning Box.

➤*Carcinogenesis:* There was no evidence of an effect of misoprostol on tumor occurrence or incidence in rats receiving daily doses up to 150 times the human dose for 24 months. Similarly, there was no effect of misoprostol on tumor occurrence or incidence in mice receiving daily doses up to 1000 times the human dose for 21 months.

➤*Mutagenesis:* The mutagenic potential of misoprostol was tested in several in vitro assays, all of which were negative.

➤*Fertility impairment:* Misoprostol, when administered to breeding male and female rats at doses 6.25 times to 625 times the maximum recommended human therapeutic dose, produced dose-related pre- and postimplantation losses and a significant decrease in the number of live pups born at the highest dose. These findings suggest the possibility of a general adverse effect on fertility in males and females.

➤*Elderly:* There were no significant differences in the safety profile of misoprostol in approximately 500 ulcer patients who were 65 years of age or older compared with younger patients.

➤*Pregnancy: Category X.*

Teratogenic – See Warning Box. Congenital anomalies sometimes associated with fetal death have been reported subsequent to the unsuccessful use of misoprostol as an abortifacient but the drug's teratogenic mechanism has not been demonstrated. Several reports in the literature associate the use of misoprostol during the first trimester of pregnancy with skull defects, cranial nerve palsies, facial malformations, and limb defects.

Misoprostol in not fetotoxic or teratogenic in rats and rabbits at doses 625 and 63 times the human dose, respectively.

Nonteratogenic – See Warning Box. Misoprostol may endanger pregnancy (may cause abortion) and thereby cause harm to the fetus when administered to a pregnant woman. Misoprostol may produce uterine contractions, uterine bleeding, and expulsion of the products of conception. Abortions caused by misoprostol may be incomplete. If a woman is or becomes pregnant while taking this drug to reduce the risk of NSAID-induced ulcers, the drug should be discontinued and the patient apprised of the potential hazard to the fetus.

Labor and delivery – Misoprostol can induce or augment uterine contractions. Vaginal administration of misoprostol, outside of its approved indication, has been used as a cervical ripening agent, for the induction of labor and for treatment of serious postpartum hemorrhage in the presence of uterine atony. A major adverse effect of the obstetrical use of misoprostol is hyperstimulation of the uterus that may progress to uterine tetany with marked impairment of uteroplacental blood flow, uterine rupture (requiring surgical repair, hysterectomy, or salpingo-oophorectomy), or amniotic fluid embolism. Pelvic pain, retained placenta, severe genital bleeding, shock, fetal bradycardia, and fetal and maternal death have been reported.

There may be an increased risk of uterine tachysystole, uterine rupture, meconium passage, meconium staining of amniotic fluid, and Cesarean delivery due to uterine hyperstimulation with the use of higher doses of misoprostol; including the manufactured 100 mcg tablet. The risk of uterine rupture increases with advancing gestational ages and with prior uterine surgery, including Cesarean delivery. Grand multiparity also appears to be a risk factor for uterine rupture.

The effect of misoprostol on the later growth, development, and functional maturation of the child when misoprostol is used for cervical ripening or induction of labor have not been established. Information on misoprostol's effect on the need for forceps delivery or other intervention is unknown.

➤*Lactation:* It is unlikely that misoprostol is excreted in human milk since it is rapidly metabolized throughout the body. However, it is not known if the active metabolite (misoprostol acid) is excreted in human milk. Therefore, misoprostol should not be administered to nursing mothers because the potential excretion of misoprostol acid could cause significant diarrhea in nursing infants.

➤*Children:* Safety and effectiveness of misoprostol in pediatric patients have not been established.

Drug Interactions

See Pharmacokinetics. Misoprostol has not been shown to interfere with the beneficial effects of aspirin on signs and symptoms of rheumatoid arthritis. Misoprostol does not exert clinically significant effects on the absorption, blood levels, and antiplatelet effects of therapeutic doses of aspirin. Misoprostol has no clinically significant effect on the kinetics of diclofenac or ibuprofen.

➤*Animal toxicology:* A reversible increase in the number of normal surface gastric epithelial cells occurred in the dog, rat, and mouse. No such increase has been observed in humans administered misoprostol for up to 1 year.

An apparent response of the female mouse to misoprostol in long-term studies at 100 to 1000 times the human dose was hyperostosis, mainly of the medulla of sternebrae. Hyperostosis did not occur in long-term studies in the dog and rat and has not been seen in humans treated with misoprostol.

Adverse Reactions

The following have been reported as adverse reactions in subjects receiving misoprostol:

➤*GI:* In subjects receiving misoprostol 400 or 800 mcg daily in clinical trials, the most frequent gastrointestinal adverse reactions were diarrhea and abdominal pain. The incidence of diarrhea at 800 mcg in controlled trials in patients on NSAIDs ranged from 14% to 40% and in all studies (over 5000 patients) averaged 13%. Abdominal pain occurred in 13% to 20% of patients in NSAID trials and about 7% in all studies, but there was no consistent difference from placebo.

Diarrhea was dose-related and usually developed early in the course of therapy (after 13 days), usually was self-limiting (often resolving after 8 days), but sometimes required discontinuation of misoprostol (2% of the patients). Rare instances of profound diarrhea leading to severe dehydration have been reported. Patients with an underlying condition such as inflammatory bowel disease, or those in whom dehydration, were it to occur, would be dangerous, should be monitored carefully if misoprostol is prescribed. The incidence of diarrhea can be minimized by administering after meals and at bedtime, and by avoiding coadministration of misoprostol with magnesium-containing antacids.

➤*GU:* Women who received misoprostol during clinical trials reported the following gynecological disorders: Spotting (0.7%), cramps (0.6%), hypermenorrhea (0.5%), menstrual disorder (0.3%) and dysmenorrhea (0.1%). Postmenopausal vaginal bleeding may be related to misoprostol administration. If it occurs, diagnostic workup should be undertaken to rule out gynecological pathology. There have been reports in which intravaginal administration of misoprostol in pregnant women resulted in rupture of the uterus and death of the infant (see Warning Box).

➤*Additional adverse reactions (incidence greater than 1%):*

Miscellaneous – In clinical trials, the following adverse reactions were reported by more than 1% of the subjects receiving misoprostol and may be causally related to the drug: Nausea (3.2%), flatulence (2.9%), headache (2.4%), dyspepsia (2%), vomiting (1.3%), and constipation (1.1%). However, there were no significant differences between the incidences of these events for misoprostol and placebo.

➤*Adverse reactions (infrequent):* The following adverse reactions were infrequently reported. Causal relationships between misoprostol and these reactions have not been established but cannot be excluded:

Cardiovascular – Chest pain, edema, diaphoresis, hypotension, hypertension, arrhythmia, phlebitis, increased cardiac enzymes, and syncope.

CNS – Anxiety, change in appetite, depression, drowsiness, dizziness, thirst, impotence, loss of libido, sweating increase, neuropathy, neurosis, and confusion.

Dermatologic – Dermatitis, alopecia, and pallor.

GI – GI bleeding, GI inflammation/infection, rectal disorder, abnormal hepatobiliary function, gingivitis, reflux, dysphagia, and amylase increase.

GU – Polyuria, dysuria, hematuria, and urinary tract infection.

Hypersensitivity – Anaphylaxis.

Metabolic – Glycosuria, gout, increased nitrogen, and increased alkaline phosphatase.

Respiratory – Upper respiratory tract infection, bronchitis, bronchospasm, dyspnea, pneumonia, and epistaxis.

Special senses – Abnormal taste, abnormal vision, conjunctivitis, deafness, tinnitus, and earache.

Miscellaneous – Aches/pains, asthenia, fatigue, fever, rigors, weight changes, and breast pain.

Musculoskeletal – Arthralgia, myalgia, muscle cramps, stiffness, and back pain.

Hematologic – Anemia, abnormal differential, thrombocytopenia, purpura, and ESR increased.

Overdosage

➤*Symptoms:* The toxic dose of misoprostol in humans has not been determined. Cumulative total daily doses of 1600 mcg have been tolerated, with only symptoms of GI discomfort being reported. In animals, the acute toxic effects are diarrhea, gastrointestinal lesions, focal cardiac necrosis, hepatic necrosis, renal tubular necrosis, testicular atrophy, respiratory difficulties, and depression of the CNS. Clinical signs that may indicate an overdose are sedation, tremor, convulsions, dyspnea, abdominal pain, diarrhea, fever, palpitations, hypotension, or bradycardia. Symptoms should be treated with supportive therapy.

➤*Treatment:* It is not known if misoprostol acid is dialyzable. However, because misoprostol is metabolized like a fatty acid, it is unlikely that dialysis would be appropriate treatment for overdosage.

Patient Information

See Warning Box.

Women of childbearing potential using misoprostol to decrease the risk of NSAID-induced ulcers should be told that they must not be pregnant when misoprostol therapy is initiated, and they must use an effective contraception method while taking misoprostol.

Misoprostol is intended for administration along with NSAIDs, including aspirin, to decrease the chance of developing an NSAID-induced gastric ulcer.

Misoprostol should be taken only according to the directions given by a physician.

MISOPROSTOL — ORAL

If the patient has questions about or problems with misoprostol, the physician should be contacted promptly.

The patient should not give misoprostol to anyone else. Misoprostol has been prescribed for the patient's specific condition, may not be the correct treatment for another person, and may be dangerous to the other person if she is or were to become pregnant.

The misoprostol package the patient receives from the pharmacist will include information containing patient information. The patient should read this information before taking misoprostol and each time the prescription is renewed because the information may have been revised.

Keep out of reach of children.

➤*Special note for women:* Misoprostol may cause abortion (sometimes incomplete), premature labor, or birth defects if given to pregnant women.

Misoprostol is available only as a unit-of-use package that includes patient information.

Misoprostol is being prescribed by your doctor to decrease the chance of getting stomach ulcers related to the arthritis/pain medication that you take.

Do not take misoprostol to reduce the risk of NSAID-induced ulcers if you are pregnant (see Warning Box). Misoprostol can cause abortion (sometimes incomplete that could lead to dangerous bleeding and require hospitalization and surgery), premature birth, or birth defects. It is also important to avoid pregnancy while taking this medication and for at least 1 month or through 1 menstrual cycle after you stop taking it. Misoprostol has been reported to cause the uterus to rupture (tear) when given after the eighth week of pregnancy. Rupturing (tearing) of the uterus can result in severe bleeding, hysterectomy, or maternal or fetal death.

If you become pregnant during misoprostol therapy, stop taking misoprostol and contact your physician immediately. Remember than even if you are on a means of birth control it is still possible to become pregnant. Should this occur, stop taking misoprostol and contact your physician immediately.

Misoprostol may cause diarrhea, abdominal cramping, or nausea in some people. In most cases these problems develop during the first few weeks of therapy and stop after about a week. You can minimize possible diarrhea by making sure you take misoprostol with food.

Because these side effects are usually mild to moderate and usually go away in a matter of days, most patients can continue to take misoprostol. If you have prolonged difficulty (more than 8 days), or if you have severe diarrhea, cramping or nausea, call your doctor.

Take misoprostol only according to the directions given by your physician.

Do not give misoprostol to anyone else. It has been prescribed for your specific condition, may not be the correct treatment for another person, and would be dangerous if the other person were pregnant.

The information does not cover all possible side effects of misoprostol. The patient information does not address the side effects of your arthritis/pain medication. See your doctor if you have questions.

ANTACIDS

Indications

➤*Hyperacidity:* Symptomatic relief of upset stomach associated with hyperacidity (heartburn, gastroesophageal reflux, acid indigestion, and sour stomach); hyperacidity associated with peptic ulcer and gastric hyperacidity.

➤*Aluminum carbonate:* Treatment, control, or management of hyperphosphatemia or for use with a low phosphate diet to prevent formation of phosphate urinary stones.

➤*Calcium carbonate:* Treating calcium deficiency states (ie, postmenopausal/senile osteoporosis). See Calcium monograph in Minerals and Electrolytes, Oral section.

➤*Magnesium oxide:* Treatment of magnesium deficiencies or magnesium depletion from malnutrition, restricted diet, alcoholism, or magnesium-depleting drugs.

➤*Unlabeled uses:* Antacids with aluminum and magnesium hydroxides or aluminum hydroxide alone effectively prevent significant stress ulcer bleeding. Antacids are also effective in treatment and maintenance of duodenal ulcer and may be effective in treating gastric ulcer. Antacids are also recommended, initially, for gastroesophageal reflux disease.

Aluminum hydroxide has been used to reduce phosphate absorption in hyperphosphatemia in patients with chronic renal failure.

Calcium carbonate may also be used to bind phosphate.

Administration and Dosage

Administration and dosage depends on the condition being treated and the agent being used. See individual products for specific information.

Liquid doseforms are usually preferred because of their rapid action and greater activity; however, tablets may be more acceptable and convenient, particularly when patients are away from home or where the liquid would be inconvenient to carry. Other doseforms are available but do not appear to offer any significant advantage.

Actions

➤*Pharmacology:* Antacids neutralize gastric acidity, resulting in an increase in the pH of the stomach and duodenal bulb. Additionally, by increasing the gastric pH above 4, they inhibit the proteolytic activity of pepsin. Antacids do not "coat" the mucosal lining, but may have a local astringent effect. Antacids also increase the lower esophageal sphincter tone. Aluminum ions inhibit smooth muscle contraction, thus inhibiting gastric emptying. Use aluminum-containing products with caution in patients with gastric outlet obstruction.

A systemic antacid (eg, sodium bicarbonate) is readily absorbed and capable of producing systemic electrolyte disturbances and alkalosis. A nonsystemic antacid forms compounds that are not absorbed to a significant extent and thus does not exert an appreciable systemic effect unless use is chronic, high-dose, or the patient has confounding pathology. However, nonsystemic antacids may alter urinary pH in some patients.

Acid neutralizing capacity (ANC) – ANC is a consideration in selecting an antacid. It varies for commercial antacid preparations and is expressed as mEq/mL. Milliequivalents of ANC is defined by the mEq of HCl required to keep an antacid suspension at pH 3.5 for 10 minutes in vitro. An antacid must neutralize ≥ 5 mEq/dose. Also, any ingredient must contribute ≥ 25% of the total ANC of a given product to be considered an antacid. Antacids with high ANC are usually more effective in vivo. Sodium bicarbonate and calcium carbonate have the greatest neutralizing capacity but are not suitable for chronic therapy because of systemic effects. Suspensions have greater neutralizing capacity than powders or tablets. For maximum effectiveness, chew tablets thoroughly. If ingested in the fasting state, antacids reduce acidity for approximately 20 to 40 minutes because of rapid gastric emptying. If ingested 1 hour after meals, they reduce gastric acidity for at least 3 hours.

Alginic acid – Alginic acid, an ingredient found with sodium bicarbonate in some antacid products, is not an antacid; however, in the presence of saliva, it reacts with sodium bicarbonate to form sodium alginate. Its protective effect is due to its foaming, viscous, and floating properties.

Phosphate binding – Aluminum-containing antacids bind with phosphate ions in the intestine to form insoluble aluminum phosphate, which is excreted in the feces. This is of value in treating hyperphosphatemia of chronic renal failure. Calcium carbonate can also suppress phosphate concentrations. The aluminum salt with useful phosphate binding capacity is aluminum hydroxide.

Warnings

➤*Sodium content:* Sodium content of antacids may be significant. Patients with hypertension, CHF, marked renal failure, or those on restricted or low-sodium diets should use a low-sodium preparation. The sodium content of most commercial antacid preparations is found in the product listings.

➤*"Acid rebound":* Antacids may cause dose-related rebound hyperacidity because they may increase gastric secretion or serum gastrin levels. Early data implicated calcium carbonate as the only agent that caused "acid rebound;" however, it is now clear that most antacids may result in this effect. In addition, the effect may not be clinically significant because the "acid rebound" may be compensated for by buffers in the antacid.

➤*Milk-alkali syndrome:* Milk-alkali syndrome, an acute illness with symptoms of headache, nausea, irritability, and weakness, or a chronic illness with alkalosis, hypercalcemia, and possibly, renal impairment, has occurred following the concurrent use of high-dose calcium carbonate and sodium bicarbonate.

➤*Hypophosphatemia:* Prolonged use of aluminum-containing antacids may result in hypophosphatemia in normophosphatemic patients if phosphate intake is not adequate. In its more severe forms, hypophosphatemia can lead to anorexia, malaise, muscle weakness, and osteomalacia.

➤*Renal function impairment:* Use magnesium-containing products with caution, particularly when more than 50 mEq magnesium is given daily. Hypermagnesemia and toxicity may occur because of decreased clearance of the magnesium ion. Approximately 5% to 20% of orally administered magnesium salts can be systemically absorbed.

Prolonged use of aluminum-containing antacids in patients with renal failure may result in or worsen dialysis osteomalacia. Elevated tissue aluminum levels contribute to the development of the dialysis encephalopathy and osteomalacia syndromes. Small amounts of aluminum are absorbed from the GI tract and renal excretion of aluminum is impaired in renal failure. Aluminum is not well removed by dialysis because it is bound to albumin and transferrin, which do not cross dialysis membranes. As a result, aluminum is deposited in bone, and dialysis osteomalacia may develop when large amounts of aluminum are ingested orally by patients with impaired renal function.

➤*Pregnancy:* A pregnant woman should consult a physician before using an antacid.

Precautions

➤*GI hemorrhage:* Use aluminum hydroxide with care in patients who have recently suffered massive upper GI hemorrhage.

➤*Lipid effects:* In 1 study, administration of an aluminum hydroxide-containing antacid reduced LDL cholesterol by 18.5% after 4 months in hypercholesterolemic patients. Although HDL was also reduced (to a lesser extent), the HDL/LDL ratio increased by 13%. Similar results were noted in a smaller pilot study. In another study, calcium carbonate reduced LDL by 4.4% and increased HDL by 4.1%. Further studies are needed to determine the role of antacids in hypercholesterolemia.

➤*Buffered aspirin solutions:* Caution against use of these antacid/analgesic combinations in chronic pain syndromes. Alkalinization of urine accelerates aspirin excretion, and systemic alkalosis and increased sodium load may occur.

Drug Interactions

Antacid Drug Interactions

Drug	Antacid[a]				
	Aluminum salts	Calcium salts	Magnesium salts	Sodium bicarbonate	Magnesium-aluminum combinations
Allopurinol	↓				
Amphetamines				↑	
Benzodiazepines	↑		↓	↓	↓
Captopril					↓
Chloroquine	↓		↓		
Corticosteroids	↓		↓		↓
Dicumarol			↑		
Diflunisal	↓				
Digoxin	↓		↓		
Ethambutol	↓				
Flecainide				↑	
Fluoroquinolones		↓			↓
Histamine H_2 antagonists	↓		↓		↓
Hydantoins		↓	↓		↓
Iron salts	↓	↓	↓	↓	↓
Isoniazid	↓				
Ketoconazole				↓	↓
Levodopa					↑
Lithium				↓	
Methenamine				↓	
Methotrexate				↓	
Nitrofurantoin			↓		
Penicillamine	↓		↓		↓
Phenothiazines	↓		↓		↓
Quinidine		↑	↑	↑	↑
Salicylates		↓		↓	↓
Sodium polystyrene sulfonate					‡[b]
Sulfonylureas			↑	↓	↑
Sympathomimetics				↑	
Tetracyclines	↓	↓	↓	↓	↓
Thyroid hormones	↓				
Ticlopidine	↓		↓		↓
Valproic acid					↑

[a] Pharmacologic effect increased (↑) or decreased (↓) by antacids.
[b] Concomitant use may cause metabolic alkalosis in patients with renal impairment.

Antacids may interfere with drugs by:

1.) Increasing the gastric pH altering disintegration, dissolution, solubility, ionization and gastric emptying time. Absorption of weakly acidic drugs is decreased, possibly resulting in decreased drug effect (eg, digoxin, phenytoin, chlorpromazine, isoniazid). Weakly basic drug absorption is increased possibly resulting in toxicity or adverse reactions (eg, pseudoephedrine, levodopa).
2.) Adsorbing or binding drugs to their surface resulting in decreased bioavailability (eg, tetracycline). Magnesium trisilicate and magnesium hydroxide have the greatest ability to adsorb drugs; calcium carbonate and aluminum hydroxide have an intermediate ability to adsorb drugs.
3.) Increasing urinary pH affecting the rate of drug elimination. The effect is inhibition of the excretion of basic drugs (eg, quinidine, amphetamines) and enhanced excretion of acidic drugs (eg, salicylates). Sodium bicarbonate has the most pronounced effect on urinary pH.

Staggering the administration times of the interacting drug and the antacid by ≥ 2 hours will often help avoid undesirable drug interactions. Refer to individual product monographs for information.

Adverse Reactions

Magnesium-containing antacids – Laxative effect as saline cathartic may cause diarrhea; hypermagnesemia in renal failure patients (see Warnings).

Aluminum-containing antacids – Constipation (may lead to intestinal obstruction); aluminum-intoxication, osteomalacia and hypophosphatemia (see Precautions); accumulation of aluminum in serum, bone and the CNS (aluminum accumulation may be neurotoxic); encephalopathy.

Antacids – Dose-dependent rebound hyperacidity and milk-alkali syndrome (see Warnings).

Patient Information

➤*Chewable tablets:* Thoroughly chew before swallowing. Follow with a glass of water.

➤*Effervescent tablets:* Allow to completely dissolve in water. Allow most of the bubbling to stop before drinking.

➤*Drug interaction precaution:* Antacids may interact with certain prescription drugs. If you are presently taking a prescription drug, do not take an antacid without checking with your physician or pharmacist.

Magnesium-containing products may act as a saline cathartic in larger doses and produce a laxative effect and may cause diarrhea; aluminum and calcium-containing products may cause constipation. Magnesium/aluminum antacid mixtures are used to avoid bowel function changes.

Notify physician if relief is not obtained or if there are any symptoms that suggest bleeding, such as black tarry stools or "coffee ground" vomitus.

Taking too much of these products can cause the stomach to secrete excess stomach acid. Consult your physician or pharmacist about the appropriate dose. Do not use the maximum dosage of antacids for more than 2 weeks, except under the supervision of a physician.

MAGNESIA (Magnesium Hydroxide)

otc	**Phillips' Chewable** (Bayer Consumer)	**Tablets, chewable:** 311 mg	Sucrose. Mint flavor. In 100s and 200s.
otc	**Milk of Magnesia** (Various, eg, Geneva, Goldline, Rugby, UDL)	**Liquid:** 400 mg per 5 mL	In 360 mL, pt and gal, UD 15 and 30 mL.
otc	**Phillips' Milk of Magnesia** (Sterling Health)		Original, mint and cherry flavors. In 120, 360 and 780 mL.
otc sf	**Dulcolax** (Boehringer Ingelheim)		Original and mint flavors. In 355 mL.
otc	**Concentrated Phillips' Milk of Magnesia** (Sterling Health)	**Liquid:** 800 mg per 5 mL	Sorbitol, sugar. Strawberry flavor. In 240 mL.

MAGNESIUM HYDROXIDE — ORAL

For complete prescribing information, refer to the Laxatives group monograph.

Indications

➤*Laxative:* For relief of occasional constipation. This product generally produces bowel movement in ½ to 6 hours.

➤*Antacid:* For the temporary relief of heartburn, upset stomach, sour stomach, or acid indigestion.

➤*Rectal/bowel examinations:* Certain saline laxative are used to evacuate the colon for rectal and bowel examinations.

Administration and Dosage

➤*As a laxative:* Drink a full glass (240 mL; 8 ounces) of liquid following each dose. The dose may be taken as a single daily dose or in divided doses. Shake well before using.

Adults and children 12 years of age and over –
Milk of magnesia concentrate: 10 to 20 mL (2 to 4 tsp).
Milk of magnesia liquid: 30 to 60 mL (2 to 4 tbsp).
Chewable tablets: Chew 6 to 8 tablets. Take before bedtime, followed by a full glass (8 ounces) of water.

Children 6 to under 12 years of age –
Milk of magnesia concentrate: Oral dosage is 5 to 10 mL (1 to 2 tsp).

MAGNESIUM HYDROXIDE — ORAL

Milk of magnesia liquid: Oral dosage is 15 to 30 mL (1 to 2 tbsp).

Chewable tablets: Chew 3 to 4 tablets. Take preferably before bedtime followed by a full glass (240 mL; 8 ounces) of water.

Children 2 (3 for chewable tablets) to under 6 years of age –

Milk of magnesia concentrate: Oral dosage is 5 mL (1 tsp) or as directed by a physician. The dose may be taken as a single daily dose or in divided doses.

Milk of magnesia liquid: Oral dosage is 5 to 15 mL (1 to 3 tsp) or as directed by a physician.

Chewable tablets: Chew 1 to 2 tablets. Take preferably before bedtime followed by a full glass (240 mL; 8 ounces) of water.

Children under 2 (3 for chewable tablets) years of age –

Milk of magnesia concentrate and liquid: Consult a physician.

Chewable tablets: Consult a physician.

➤*As an antacid:* Do not take more than 60 mL (12 tsp) in 24 hours.

Do not use the maximum dosage for more than 2 weeks.

Shake well before using.

Chewable tablets –

Adults: Chew 2 to 4 tablets. Take up to 4 times a day or as directed.

Children 7 to 14 years: Chew 1 tablet. Take up to 4 times a day or consult a physician.

Adults and children 12 years of age and over –

Milk of magnesia concentrate: Oral dosage is 5 mL (1 tsp) with a little water up to 4 times daily or as directed by a physician.

Milk of magnesia liquid: Oral dosage is 5 to 15 mL (1 to 3 tsp) with a little water up to 4 times daily or as directed by a physician.

Children under 12 years of age –

Milk of magnesia concentrate and liquid: Consult a physician.

➤*Storage/Stability:* Keep tightly closed. Store at controlled room temperature, 20° to 25°C (68° to 77°F). Protect from freezing.

Keep out of the reach of children.

Chewable tablets – Store at room temperature 15° to 30°C (59° to 86°F) in a dry place.

Avoid excessive heat and freezing.

ALUMINUM HYDROXIDE

	Product	Form/Strength	Description	Sodium[a] (mg)	ANC[a] (mEq)
otc	**Alu-Tab** (3M Pharm)	**Tablets**: 500 mg	Green. Film coated. In 250s.		10.6
otc	**Amphojel** (Wyeth-Ayerst)	**Tablets**: 600 mg	(Wyeth). Saccharin. In 100s.		
otc	**Alu-Cap** (3M Pharm)	**Capsules**: 400 mg	Red/green. In 100s.		8.5
otc	**Dialume** (RPR)	**Capsules**: 500 mg	In 500s.	≤ 1.2	
otc	**Aluminum Hydroxide Gel** (Various, eg, Goldline, Pharm Assoc, Rugby, UDL)	**Suspension**: 320 mg per 5 mL	In 360 and 480 mL, UD 15 and 30 mL.		
otc	**Concentrated Aluminum Hydroxide Gel** (Roxane)	**Suspension**: 450 mg per 5 mL	Peppermint flavor. In 500 mL and UD 30 mL.	1-2	
		675 mg per 5 mL	Creamsicle flavor. In 180 and 500 mL, UD 20 and 30 mL.		
otc	**Concentrated Aluminum Hydroxide Gel** (Various, eg, Pharm Assoc, Roxane)	**Liquid**: 600 mg per 5 mL	In 30, 180 and 480 mL.		
otc	**AlternaGEL** (J & J-Merck)		Parabens, sorbitol. In 150 and 360 mL.		

[a] Acid neutralizing capacity and sodium content per capsule, tablet, or 5 mL.

ALUMINUM HYDROXIDE — ORAL

For complete and comparative prescribing information, refer to the Antacids group monograph.

Indications

Uncomplicated peptic ulcer and gastric hyperacidity.

Administration and Dosage

➤*Tablets/Capsules:* 500 to 1,500 mg 3 to 6 times daily, between meals and at bedtime.

➤*Liquid:* 5 to 10 mL between meals, at bedtime or as directed by a physician.

➤*Maximum dose:*

Suspension – 5 to 30 mL as needed between meals and at bedtime or as directed.

Do not take more than 9 tablets or capsules in a 24-hour period, or use maximum dosage of this product for more than 2 weeks, except under the advice and supervision of a physician.

CALCIUM CARBONATE

For prescribing information, see the Calcium monograph in the Nutrients and Nutritional Agents. Also refer to the Antacids group monograph.

MAGNESIUM OXIDE

	Product	Form/Strength	Description	ANC[a] (mEq)
otc	**Mag-Ox 400** (Blaine)	**Tablets**: 400 mg	In 100s, 1000s and UD 100s.	
otc	**Magnesium Oxide** (Various, eg, Breckenridge, Cypress, Plus Pharma)		In 120s and 400s.	
otc	**Maox 420** (Manne Co)	**Tablets**: 420 mg	Tartrazine. In 250s and 1000s.	21
otc	**Magnesium Oxide** (Various, eg, Major)	**Tablets**: 500 mg	In 100s.	
otc	**Mag-Caps** (Genesis)	**Capsules**: ≈ 140 mg (85 mg elemental magnesium	In 100s.	
otc	**Uro-Mag** (Blaine)	**Capsules**: 140 mg	In 100s and 1000s.	

[a] Acid neutralizing capacity per capsule or tablet.

MAGNESIUM OXIDE — ORAL

For complete and comparative prescribing information, refer to the Antacids group monograph.

Indications

➤*Tablets:* Dietary supplement to increase daily intake of magnesium and for the relief of acid indigestion and upset stomach.

➤*Capsules:* Adult dietary supplement to increase daily intake of magnesium.

➤*Unlabeled uses:* A pyridoxine/magnesium oxide combination has been used to prevent recurrence of calcium oxalate kidney stones.

Administration and Dosage

➤*Tablets:*

As a dietary supplement for adults – Take 1 to 2 tablets daily or as directed by a physician.

As an antacid for adults – Take 1 tablet 2 times a day or as directed by a physician.

➤*Capsules:*

As a dietary supplement for adults – Take 4 or 5 capsules daily or as directed by a physician.

➤*Storage/Stability:* Store tablets and capsules at controlled room temperature 15° to 30°C (59° to 86°F). Keep out of the reach of children.

MAGALDRATE (Aluminum Magnesium Hydroxide Sulfate)

otc	**Riopan** (Whitehall)	**Suspension:** 540 mg per 5 mL	Saccharin, sorbitol. Mint flavor. In 360 mL.
otc	**Magaldrate** (Various, eg, Moore)	**Liquid:** 540 mg per 5 mL	In 355 mL.
otc	**Iosopan** (Goldline)		In 355 mL.

MAGALDRATE — ORAL

For complete and comparative prescribing information, refer to the Antacids group monograph.

Indications

Magaldrate relieves heartburn, sour stomach, acid indigestion, and upset stomach associated with these symptoms.

It is also indicated for treating hyperphosphatemia, hypocalcemia, and hypomagnesemia.

Administration and Dosage

Shake well before use.

➤*Dosage:* Adults and children 12 years and over, take 5 to 10 mL (1 to 2 teaspoonfuls) between meals and at bedtime, but not more than 80 mL (16 teaspoonfuls) in a 24-hour period.

Do not use the maximum dosage for more than 2 weeks.

➤*Storage / Stability:* Store at room temperature or refrigerate.

Protect from freezing. Keep tightly closed.

Keep out of reach of children.

SODIUM BICARBONATE

For prescribing information, see the Sodium Bicarbonate monograph in the Systemic Alkalinizers section of the Nutrients and Nutritional Agents chapter. Also refer to the Antacids group monograph.

SODIUM CITRATE

				Sodium[a] (mg)
otc	**Citra pH** (ValMed)	**Solution:** 450 mg	Sucrose. Clear. In 30 mL.	105.67

[a] Sodium content per 5 mL.

SODIUM CITRATE DIHYDRATE — ORAL

For complete and comparative prescribing information, refer to the Antacids group monograph.

Indications

Sodium citrate dihydrate is indicated for the quick relief of acid indigestion, sour stomach or heartburn.

Administration and Dosage

➤*Administration:* Use the contents of 1 unit dose cup (30 mL) daily or as directed by a physician. Taste is enhanced if chilled before use.

➤*Dosage:* Do not take more than 120 mL (8 tablespoonfuls) in a 24-hour period or use the maximum dosage of this product for more than 2 weeks, except under the advice and supervision of a physician. This product may have a laxative effect. Do not use this product except under the advice and supervision of a physician if you are on a sodium restricted diet. Each 30 mL contains 634 mg sodium.

➤*Storage / Stability:* Keep this and all drugs out of the reach of children.

Antacid Combinations

CAPSULES AND TABLETS

Content given in mg per tablet or gelcap. 23 mg sodium = 1 mEq.

	Product & distributor	Aluminum Hydroxide	Magnesium Hydroxide	Calcium Carbonate	Other Content	Sodium (mg)	How supplied
otc	**Rolaids Tablets** (Pfizer Consumer)		110	550	Dextrose, sucrose		Chewable. Peppermint, spearmint, and cherry flavors. In 12s, 36s, 150s, 250s, and 300s.
otc	**Mylanta Antacid Gelcaps** (J&J/Merck)		125	550	Benzyl alcohol, parabens		In 24s, 50s, and 100s.
otc	**Rolaids Extra Strength Tablets** (Pfizer Consumer)		135	675	Dextrose, sucrose		Chewable. Cool strawberry, freshmint, fruit, and tropical punch flavors. In 10s, 30s, and 100s.
otc	**Rolaids Multi-Symptom Tablets** (Pfizer Consumer)		135	675	60 mg simethicone, dextrose, sucrose		Chewable. Cool mint and berry flavors. In 10s, 30s, and 60s.
otc	**Mylanta Ultra Tabs** (J&J/Merck)		300	700	Sugar, sorbitol		Chewable. Cool mint and cherry creme flavors. In 35s and 70s and 3 roll packs.
otc	**Mintox Tablets** (Major)	200	200		Saccharin		Chewable. Mint flavor. In ´00s.
otc *sf*	**Titralac Extra Strength Tablets** (3M Pharm.)			750	Saccharin	0.6	Chewable. Spearmint flavor. In 100s.
otc	**Maalox Max Maximum Strength Tablets** (Novartis)			1,000	60 mg simethicone, 400 mg calcium, dextrose		Chewable. In wild berry, lemon, and assorted fruit flavors. In 35s, 65s, and 90s.
otc	**Mylagen Gelcaps** (Goldline)			311	232 mg magnesium carbonate		In 24s.
otc	**Gas-Ban** (Roberts Med)			300	40 mg simethicone		In UD 8s and 1000s.
otc	**Gas-X with Maalox Extra Strength Tablets** (Novartis))			500	125 mg simethicone, dextrose		Chewable. Wild berry and orange flavors. In 8s and 24s.
otc *sf*	**Calglycine Antacid** (Rugby)			420	150 mg glycine.		In 250s and 1000s.
otc *sf*	**Titralac Tablets** (3M Pharm.)				Saccharin	0.3	Chewable. Spearmint flavor. In 40s, 100s and 1000s.
otc	**Titralac Plus Tablets** (3M Pharm.)				21 mg simethicone, saccharin	1.1	Chewable. (TITRALAC PLUS). Spearmint flavor. In 100s.
otc	**Foamicon Tablets** (Invamed)	80			Alginic acid, sodium bicarbonate, 20 mg magnesium trisilicate, calcium stearate, sugar, sucrose	18.4	Chewable. White. In 100s.
otc	**Gaviscon Tablets** (SK-Beecham)				Alginic acid, sodium bicarbonate, 20 mg magnesium trisilicate, sucrose, calcium stearate	18.4	Chewable. (GAVISCON 1175). In 30s and 100s.
otc	**Double Strength Gaviscon-2 Tablets** (SK-Beecham)	160			Alginic acid, sodium bicarbonate, 40 mg magnesium trisilicate, sucrose	36.8	Chewable. In 48s.
otc	**Gaviscon Extra Strength Antacid** (GlaxoSmithKline Consumer Healthcare)				105 mg magnesium carbonate, acesulfame K, alginic acid, corn syrup, mannitol, sodium bicarbonate, sucrose, calcium stearate	29.9	Chewable. Cherry flavor. In 30s and 100s.
otc	**Extra Strength Alenic Alka Tablets** (Rugby)				105 mg magnesium carbonate	29.9	Chewable. Butterscotch flavor. In 100s.
otc	**Extra Strength Genaton Tablets** (Goldline)				105 mg magnesium carbonate, alginic acid, sodium bicarbonate, sucrose, calcium stearate	29.9	Chewable. In 100s.
otc	**Almacone Tablets** (Rugby)	200	200		20 mg simethicone		Chewable. Yellow/white Peppermint flavor. In 100s and 1000s.
otc	**Trial AG Tablets** (Zee Medical)				25 mg simethicone, sucrose, mannitol		Lemon flavor. In 20s.
otc	**Gelusil Tablets** (Parke-Davis)				25 mg simethicone, sorbitol, sugar	< 5	Chewable. (P-D GELUSIL 034). Peppermint flavor. In 100s.
otc	**Mintox Plus Tablets** (Major)				25 mg simethicone, saccharin, sucrose		Chewable. In 100s.
otc	**Calcium Rich Rolaids Tablets** (Warner-Lambert)		80	412		0.4	Chewable. Original, cherry, spearmint and assorted fruit flavors. In 12s, 36s, 75s and 150s.

Antacid Combinations

CAPSULES AND TABLETS

	Product & distributor	Aluminum Hydroxide	Magnesium Hydroxide	Calcium Carbonate	Other Content	Sodium (mg)	How supplied
otc	**Advanced Formula Di-Gel Tablets** (Schering-Plough)		128	280	20 mg simethicone, sucrose		Chewable. Mint and lemon-orange flavors. In 30s, 60s. and 90s.
otc	**Riopan Plus Tablets** (Whitehall)				480 mg magaldrate, 20 mg simethicone, sorbitol, sucrose		Chewable. Cool mint flavor. In 50s and 100s.
otc	**Riopan Plus Double Strength Tablets** (Whitehall)				1080 mg magaldrate, 20 mg simethicone, saccharin, sorbitol, sucrose		Chewable. Cool mint flavor. In 60s

Refer to the general discussion of these products in the Antacids group monograph.

LIQUIDS

Content given in mg per 5 mL. 23 mg sodium = 1 mEq.

	Product & Distributor	Aluminum Hydroxide	Magnesium Hydroxide	Calcium Carbonate	Other Content	Sodium (mg)	How Supplied
otc	**Maalox Regular Strength Liquid** (Novartis)	200	200		20 mg simethicone, parabens, saccharin, sorbitol		In mint and cherry flavors. In 148, 355, and 769 mL.
otc	**Mylanta Regular Strength Liquid** (J&J Merck)				20 mg simethicone, parabens, saccharin, sorbitol		In original, cherry, and mint flavors. In 150 mL (original), 360 mL (all flavors), and 720 mL (original and cherry).
otc	**Alamag Suspension** (Goldline)	225	200		Sorbitol, sucrose, parabens	< 1.25	Mint flavor. In 355 mL.
otc	**Alamag Plus Suspension** (Goldline)				25 mg simethicone, parabens, saccharin, sorbitol		Lemon flavor. In 355 mL.
otc	**Mintox Suspension** (Major)				Parabens, saccharin, sorbitol	1.4	Mint flavor. In 355 and 780 mL.
otc	**RuLox Suspension** (Rugby)						Mint flavor. In 360 and 769 mL and gal.
otc	**Aludrox Suspension** (Wyeth-Ayerst)	307	103		Simethicone, saccharin, sorbitol, parabens		In 355 mL.
otc	**Mylanta Extra Strength Liquid** (J&J/Merck)	400	400		40 mg simethicone, parabens, saccharin, sorbitol	2 mg sodium	Cherry and mint flavors. In 360 and 480 mL.
otc	**Extra Strength Mintox Plus Liquid** (Major)	500	450		40 mg simethicone, parabens, saccharin, sorbitol		Lemon Swiss creme flavor. In 355 mL.
otc	**Simaal Gel 2 Liquid** (Schein)	500	400		40 mg simethicone		In 360 mL.
otc	**Gaviscon Extra Strength Relief Formula Liquid** (SK-Beecham)	254			237.5 mg magnesium carbonate, parabens, EDTA, saccharin, sorbitol, simethicone, sodium alginate		Cool mint flavor. In 355 mL.
otc	**Alenic Alka Liquid** (Rugby)	31.7			137.3 mg magnesium carbonate, sodium alginate, EDTA, saccharin, sorbitol, parabens	13	Spearmint flavor. In 355 mL.
otc	**Gaviscon Liquid** (SK-Beecham)				119.3 mg magnesium carbonate, sodium alginate, EDTA, saccharin, sorbitol, parabens	13	Cool mint flavor. In 177 and 355 mL.
otc	**Marblen Liquid** (Fleming)			520	400 mg magnesium carbonate		Peach/Apricot flavor. In 473 mL.
otc *sf*	**Titralac Plus Liquid** (3M Personal Health Care)			500	20 mg simethicone, parabens, saccharin, sorbitol	0.15	Mint flavor. In 360 mL.
otc	**Almacone Liquid** (Rugby)	200	200		20 mg simethicone		In 360 mL and gal.
otc	**Di-Gel Liquid** (Schering-Plough)				20 mg simethicone, saccharin, sorbitol, parabens		Mint and lemon-orange flavors. In 180 and 360 mL.
otc	**Mi-Acid Liquid** (Major)				20 mg simethicone, parabens, sorbitol		In 355 and 780 mL.
otc	**Mylagen Liquid** (Goldline)				20 mg simethicone, parabens, sorbitol, sucrose	< 1.25	In 355 mL.
otc	**Mygel Suspension** (Geneva)				20 mg simethicone		In 360 mL.
otc	**Mylanta** (J&J-Merck)				20 mg simethicone, sorbitol, parabens, saccharin (lemon, mint, cherry only)		Original, lemon, mint, and cherry flavors. In 150 (original), 355 (original, cherry, lemon, mint), and 720 (original, cherry) mL.
otc	**Alumina, Magnesia, and Simethicone Suspension** (Roxane)	213	200		20 mg simethicone, parabens, sorbitol		In UD 15 and 30 mL.

Antacid Combinations

LIQUIDS

	Product & Distributor	Aluminum Hydroxide	Magnesium Hydroxide	Calcium Carbonate	Other Content	Sodium (mg)	How Supplied
otc	**Gas Ban DS Liquid** (Roberts)	400	400		40 mg simethicone		In 150 mL.
otc	**Mygel II Suspension** (Geneva)				40 mg simethicone		In 360 mL.
otc	**Almacone II Double Strength Liquid** (Rugby)				40 mg simethicone, saccharin, sorbitol		In 360 mL and gal.
otc	**Mylagen II Liquid** (Goldline)				40 mg simethicone, parabens, sorbitol, sucrose	< 1.25	In 355 mL.
otc	**Mi-Acid II Liquid** (Major)				40 mg simethicone, parabens, sorbitol		In 355 mL.
otc	**RuLox Plus Suspension** (Rugby)	500	450		40 mg simethicone, saccharin, sorbitol, parabens		Lemon creme flavor. In 355 mL.
otc	**Iosopan Plus Liquid** (Goldline)				540 mg magaldrate, 40 mg simethicone		In 355 mL.
otc	**Magaldrate Plus Suspension** (Various, eg, Moore)				540 mg magaldrate, 40 mg simethicone		In 360 mL.
otc	**Mylanta Supreme** (Johnson & Johnson/Merck)		135	400	Saccharin, sorbitol.		Mint, lemon, and cherry flavors. In 355 mL.

Refer to the general discussion of these products in the Antacids group monograph.

POWDERS AND EFFERVESCENT TABLETS

Content given per dose or tablet.

	Product and Distributor	Sodium Bicarbonate (mg)	Other Content	Sodium (mg)	How Supplied
otc	**Bromo Seltzer Effervescent Granules** (Warner-Lambert)	2781	325 mg acetaminophen, 2224 mg citric acid (when dissolved, forms 2848 mg sodium citrate), sugar	761	In 127.5 g.
otc	**Sparkles Effervescent Granules** (Lafayette)	2000	1500 mg citric acid, simethicone		In UD 50s.
otc	**Gold Alka-Seltzer Effervescent Tablets** (Bayer)	958[a]	832 mg citric acid, 312 mg potassium bicarbonate	311	In 20s and 36s.
otc	**Original Alka-Seltzer Effervescent Tablets** (Bayer)	1700	325 mg aspirin, 1000 mg citric acid, 9 mg phenylalanine	506	Aspartame. Lemon-lime flavor. In 24s.
otc	**Zee-Seltzer Effervescent Tablets** (Zee Medical)	1916	325 mg aspirin, 1000 mg citric acid	524	In 12s.
otc	**Original Alka-Seltzer Effervescent Tablets** (Bayer)	1916[a]	325 mg aspirin, 1000 mg citric acid	567	In 36s.
otc	**Extra Strength Alka-Seltzer Effervescent Tablets** (Bayer)	1985[a]	500 mg aspirin, 1000 mg citric acid	588	In 12s and 24s.

[a] Heat-treated.

Refer to the general discussion of these products in the Antacids group monograph.

Indications

The general uses for these agents are listed below. Refer to the individual product listings for specific indications.

➤*Peptic ulcer:* Adjunctive therapy for peptic ulcer. These agents suppress gastric acid secretion. There is no conclusive evidence they aid in the healing of a peptic ulcer, decrease the rate of recurrence or prevent complications. Anticholinergics are used much less frequently in modern ulcer management.

➤*Other GI conditions:* Functional GI disorders (diarrhea, pylorospasm, hypermotility, neurogenic colon), irritable bowel syndrome (spastic colon, mucous colitis), acute enterocolitis, ulcerative colitis, diverticulitis, mild dysenteries, pancreatitis, splenic flexure syndrome and infant colic.

➤*Biliary tract:* For spastic disorders of the biliary tract. Given in conjunction with a narcotic analgesic.

➤*Urogenital tract:* Uninhibited hypertonic neurogenic bladder.

➤*Bradycardia:* Atropine is used in the suppression of vagally mediated bradycardias.

➤*Preoperative medication:* Atropine, scopolamine, hyoscyamine and glycopyrrolate are used as preanesthetic medication to control bronchial, nasal, pharyngeal, and salivary secretions; and to block cardiac vagal inhibitory reflexes during induction of anesthesia and intubation. Scopolamine is used for preanesthetic sedation and for obstetric amnesia.

➤*Antidotes for poisoning by cholinergic drugs:* Atropine is used for poisoning by organophosphorus insecticides, chemical warfare nerve gases and as an antidote for mushroom poisoning due to muscarine in certain species such as *Amanita muscaria* (see Pralidoxime Chloride monograph).

➤*Miscellaneous uses:* Calming delirium; motion sickness (scopolamine), see Antiemetic/Antivertigo Agents group monograph; parkinsonism, see Antiparkinson Agents group monograph.

➤*Unlabeled uses:*

Bronchial asthma – Atropine and related agents are effective in some patients with cholinergic-mediated bronchospasm. Use in chronic lung disease is not generally recommended; these agents reduce bronchial secretions resulting in decreased fluidity and thickening of residual secretion.

Glycopyrrolate may be effective in the treatment of bronchial asthma; doses of 1 mg (nebulization) and 1.3 mg (solution) have been used.

Actions

➤*Pharmacology:* Anticholinergics are also known as antimuscarinic drugs. In addition to the Anticholinergics/Antispasmodics discussed below, related drugs include: Anticholinergic Antiparkinson Agents, Cycloplegic Mydriatics and Urinary Anticholinergics. See specific monographs.

GI anticholinergics are used primarily to decrease motility (smooth muscle tone) in GI, biliary and urinary tracts and for antisecretory effects. Antispasmodics, related compounds, decrease GI motility by acting on smooth muscle.

Gastrointestinal Anticholinergic/Antispasmodic Dosage

Drug	Adult Dosage	
	Oral	Parenteral
Anticholinergics Atropine	0.4-0.6 mg	0.4-0.6 mg
Scopolamine		0.32-0.65 mg
L-hyoscyamine	0.125-0.25 mg tid-qid (0.375 to 0.7 mg q 12 h – sustained release)	0.25-0.5 mg q 4 h
L-alkaloids of belladonna	0.25-0.5 mg tid	
Belladonna alkaloids	0.18-0.3 mg tid-qid	
Quaternary Anticholinergics Methscopolamine bromide	2.5 mg ac; 2.5-5 mg hs	
Clidinium bromide	2.5-5 mg tid-qid	
Glycopyrrolate	1-2 mg bid-tid	0.1-0.2 mg tid-qid
Mepenzolate bromide	25-50 mg qid	
Methantheline bromide	50-100 mg q 4-6 h	
Propantheline bromide	7.5-15 mg tid; 30 mg hs	
Tridihexethyl chloride	25-50 mg tid-qid	
Antispasmodics Dicyclomine HCl	20-40 mg qid	20 mg qid

These agents inhibit the muscarinic actions of acetylcholine at postganglionic parasympathetic neuroeffector sites including smooth muscle, secretory glands and CNS sites. Large doses may block nicotinic receptors at the autonomic ganglia and at the neuromuscular junction.

Specific anticholinergic responses are dose-related. Small doses inhibit salivary and bronchial secretions and sweating; moderate doses dilate the pupil, inhibit accommodation and increase heart rate (vagolytic effect); larger doses decrease motility of GI and urinary tracts; very large doses inhibit gastric acid secretion.

➤*Pharmacokinetics:*

Absorption/Distribution –

Belladonna alkaloids: Belladonna alkaloids are rapidly absorbed after oral use. They readily cross blood-brain barrier, and affect the CNS. The major difference between these agents is that atropine at usual therapeutic doses is a stimulant, whereas scopolamine is a CNS depressant. Undesirable peripheral and central effects occur at doses sufficient to control GI motility and gastric acid secretion.

Atropine has a half-life of about 2.5 hours; 94% of a dose is eliminated through the urine in 24 hours.

Quaternary anticholinergics: Synthetic or semisynthetic derivatives structurally related to the belladonna alkaloids, they are poorly and unreliably absorbed orally. Because they do not cross the blood-brain barrier, CNS effects are negligible. They are also less likely to affect the pupil or ciliary muscle of the eye. Duration of action is more prolonged than alkaloids. In addition, they may cause some degree of ganglionic blockade; neuromuscular blockade may occur at toxic doses.

Antispasmodics: The tertiary ammonium compounds have little or no antimuscarinic activity, and therefore, no significant effect on gastric acid secretion. They exhibit a nonspecific direct relaxant effect on smooth muscle.

Contraindications

➤*Hypersensitivity:* Hypersensitivity to anticholinergic drugs; patients hypersensitive to belladonna or to barbiturates may be hypersensitive to **scopolamine**.

➤*Ocular:* Narrow-angle glaucoma; adhesions (synechiae) between the iris and lens.

➤*Cardiovascular:* Tachycardia; unstable cardiovascular status in acute hemorrhage; myocardial ischemia.

➤*GI:* Obstructive disease (eg, achalasia, pyloroduodenal stenosis or pyloric obstruction, cardiospasm); paralytic ileus; intestinal atony of the elderly or debilitated; severe ulcerative colitis; toxic megacolon complicating ulcerative colitis; hepatic disease.

➤*GU:* Obstructive uropathy (eg, bladder neck obstruction due to prostatic hypertrophy); renal disease.

➤*Musculoskeletal:* Myasthenia gravis.

➤*Asthma:* **Atropine** is contraindicated in asthma patients.

➤*Dicyclomine:* Infants younger than 6 months of age (see Warnings).

Warnings

➤*Heat prostration:* Heat prostration can occur with anticholinergic drug use (fever and heat stroke due to decreased sweating) in the presence of a high environmental temperature.

➤*Diarrhea:* Diarrhea may be an early symptom of incomplete intestinal obstruction, especially in patients with ileostomy or colostomy. Treatment of diarrhea with these drugs is inappropriate and possibly harmful.

➤*Parkinsonism:* Vomiting, malaise, sweating and salivation may occur in patients with parkinsonism upon sudden withdrawal of large doses of **scopolamine**.

➤*Anticholinergic psychosis:* Anticholinergic psychosis has been reported in sensitive individuals given anticholinergic drugs. CNS signs and symptoms include confusion, disorientation, short-term memory loss, hallucinations, dysarthria, ataxia, coma, euphoria, decreased anxiety, fatigue, insomnia, agitation and mannerisms, and inappropriate affect. These CNS signs and symptoms usually resolve 12 to 24 hours after drug discontinuation.

➤*Gastric ulcer:* Gastric ulcer may produce a delay in gastric emptying time and may complicate therapy (antral stasis).

➤*Elderly:* Elderly patients may react with excitement, agitation, drowsiness and other untoward manifestations to even small doses of anticholinergic drugs.

➤*Pregnancy: Category B* (**glycopyrrolate**, parenteral); *Category C* (**hyoscyamine**, **atropine**, **scopolamine**, **isopropamide**, **propantheline**, **methantheline**). Hyoscyamine crosses the placenta; atropine and scopolamine cross the placenta rapidly after IV use. Effects on the fetus depend on maturity of its parasympathetic nervous system. In neonates, scopolamine may depress respiration and contribute to neonatal hemorrhage due to reduction in vitamin K-dependent clotting factors.

Safety for use during pregnancy has not been established. Use only when clearly needed and when the potential benefits outweigh the potential hazards to the fetus.

Labor and delivery – **Scopolamine** does not affect uterine contractions during labor or increase duration of labor. It crosses the placenta but has not been reported to affect the fetus adversely.

➤*Lactation:* **Hyoscyamine** is excreted in breast milk; other anticholinergics (especially **atropine**) may be excreted in milk, causing infant toxicity, and may reduce milk production. Documentation is lacking or conflicting. Generally, do not use in nursing women.

➤*Children:* Safety and efficacy are not established. **Hyoscyamine** has been used in infant colic. Safety and efficacy of **glycopyrrolate** in children younger than 12 years of age are not established for peptic ulcer.

There are reports of infants in the first 3 months of life, administered **dicyclomine** syrup, who experienced respiratory distress, seizures, syncope, asphyxia, pulse rate fluctuations, muscular hypotonia, and coma. These symptoms occurred within minutes of ingestion and lasted 20 to 30 minutes; this suggests that they were a consequence of local irritation or aspiration rather than a pharmacologic effect. A few deaths have been reported in infants ≤ 3 months of age. Two of these were associated with excessively high dicyclomine blood levels. Dicyclomine is contraindicated in infants younger than 6 months of age.

Precautions

➤*Use with caution in the following:*

Cardiovascular – Coronary heart disease; CHF; cardiac arrhythmias; tachycardia; hypertension.

GI – Hepatic disease; early evidence of ileus, as in peritonitis; ulcerative colitis (large doses may suppress intestinal motility and precipitate or aggravate toxic megacolon); hiatal hernia associated with reflux esophagitis (anticholinergics may aggravate it).

GU – Renal disease; prostatic hypertrophy. Patients with prostatism can have dysuria and may require catheterization.

Ocular – Glaucoma; light irides. If there is mydriasis and photophobia, wear dark glasses. Use caution in the elderly because of increased incidence of glaucoma.

Pulmonary – Debilitated patients with chronic lung disease; reduction in bronchial secretions can lead to inspissation and formation of bronchial plugs. Use cautiously in patients with asthma or allergies.

Miscellaneous – Autonomic neuropathy; hyperthyroidism.

In pain or severe anxiety, scopolamine is usually given with analgesics or sedatives to avoid behavioral disturbances. Risk of hyperpyrexia is increased in patients with fever. In elderly patients, confusional states are more common.

➤*Special risk:* Use cautiously in infants, small children, and people with Down's syndrome, brain damage, or spastic paralysis.

➤*Hazardous tasks:* Patients should use caution while driving or performing other tasks requiring alertness, coordination, or physical dexterity.

➤*Tartrazine sensitivity:* Some of these products contain tartrazine (FD&C yellow #5), which may cause allergic-type reactions (including bronchial asthma) in susceptible individuals. Although the incidence of sensitivity is low, it is frequently seen in patients who also have aspirin hypersensitivity. Specific products containing tartrazine are identified in the product listings.

➤*Sulfite sensitivity:* Some of these products contain sulfites that may cause allergic-type reactions (including anaphylactic symptoms and life-threatening or less severe asthmatic episodes) in certain susceptible persons. The overall prevalence of sulfite sensitivity in the general population is unknown and probably low. It is seen more frequently in asthmatic or atopic nonasthmatic persons.

Drug Interactions

➤*Amantadine:* Coadministration of anticholinergics may result in an increase in anticholinergic side effects. Consider decreasing the anticholinergic dose.

➤*Atenolol:* The pharmacologic effects may be increased by concurrent anticholinergic administration. **Metoprolol** and **propranolol** were not affected in 2 studies.

➤*Digoxin:* Pharmacologic effects may be increased by anticholinergic coadministration. This may be product specific, (ie, slow-dissolving digoxin tablets interact whereas digoxin capsules and elixir are not affected). However, because USP standards require a minimum dissolution rate, tablets available in the US are not likely to be affected.

➤*Phenothiazines:* The antipsychotic effectiveness may be decreased by anticholinergic coadministration. Anticholinergic side effects may also be increased by concurrent therapy. Adjust the phenothiazine dose as necessary.

➤*Tricyclic antidepressants:* Anticholinergic coadministration may increase anticholinergic side effects (eg, dry mouth, constipation, urinary retention) because of an additive effect. A tricyclic antidepressant with less anticholinergic activity may be beneficial.

Adverse Reactions

➤*Cardiovascular:* Palpitations; bradycardia (following low doses of **atropine**); tachycardia (after higher doses).

➤*CNS:* Headache; flushing; nervousness; drowsiness; weakness; dizziness; confusion; insomnia; fever (especially in children); mental confusion or excitement especially in elderly patients with even small doses. Large doses may produce CNS stimulation (restlessness, tremor). In the presence of pain, **scopolamine** may produce excitement, restlessness, hallucinations, or delirium. Parenteral **dicyclomine** may cause temporary lightheadedness.

➤*Dermatologic:* Severe allergic reactions including anaphylaxis, urticaria, and other dermal manifestations. Local irritation may occur with parenteral **dicyclomine.**

➤*GI:* Xerostomia; altered taste perception; nausea; vomiting; dysphagia; heartburn; constipation; bloated feeling; paralytic ileus.

➤*GU:* Urinary hesitancy and retention; impotence.

➤*Ophthalmic:* Blurred vision; mydriasis; photophobia; cycloplegia; increased intraocular pressure; dilated pupils

➤*Miscellaneous:* Suppression of lactation; nasal congestion; decreased sweating.

Overdosage

➤*Symptoms:*

GI – Dry mouth; thirst; vomiting; nausea; abdominal distention; difficulty swallowing.

CNS – Theoretically, a curare-like action may occur (ie, neuromuscular blockade leading to muscular weakness and paralysis); CNS stimulation; delirium; drowsiness; restlessness; anxiety; stupor; fever; disorientation; dizziness; headache; seizures; hallucinations; ataxia; convulsions; coma; psychotic behavior; other signs of an acute organic psychosis.

Cardiovascular – Circulatory failure; rapid pulse and respiration; vasodilation; tachycardia with weak pulse; hypertension; hypotension; respiratory depression; palpitations.

GU – Urinary urgency with difficulty in micturition.

Ocular – Blurred vision; photophobia; dilated pupils.

Miscellaneous – Leukocytosis; flushed hot dry skin; rash; respiratory failure.

Children – Children, especially those with Down's syndrome, spastic paralysis, or brain damage, are more sensitive than adults to toxic effects.

➤*Treatment:* Induce emesis or perform gastric lavage, then administer activated charcoal slurry, and supportive and symptomatic therapy, as indicated. See also General Management of Acute Overdosage.

Physostigmine by slow IV injection of 0.2 to 4 mg has been used to reverse anticholinergic effects. Because physostigmine is rapidly metabolized, the patient may relapse into coma after 1 to 2 hours; repeat doses as necessary to a total of 6 mg (2 mg in children). However, profound bradycardia, asystole, and seizures may occur (see Antidotes monograph). The role of physostigmine is not clear; avoid it if other therapeutic agents successfully reverse cardiac dysrhythmias.

Neostigmine methylsulfate 0.25 to 2.5 mg IV, repeated as needed, may be given.

Diazepam, short-acting barbiturates, IV sodium thiopental (2% solution), or chloral hydrate (100 to 200 mL of a 2% solution) by rectal infusion may control excitement. **Hyoscyamine** is dialyzable, but hemodialysis is ineffective for atropine poisoning. Treat hyperpyrexia with physical cooling measures.

If the curare-like effect progresses to paralysis of respiratory muscles, institute artificial respiration and maintain until effective respiratory action returns.

Patient Information

Usually taken 30 to 60 minutes before a meal.

May cause drowsiness, dizziness, or blurred vision; patients should observe caution while driving or performing other tasks requiring alertness.

Notify physician if rash, flushing, or eye pain occurs.

May cause dry mouth, difficulty in urination, constipation or increased sensitivity to light; notify physician if these effects persist or become severe.

Belladonna Alkaloids

L-HYOSCYAMINE SULFATE

Rx	**Anaspaz** (Ascher)	**Tablets**: 0.125 mg	(225/295). In 100s and 500s.
Rx	**ED-SPAZ** (Edwards)		White, scored. In 100s.
Rx	**Levsin** (Schwarz Pharma)		(SCHWARZ 531). White, scored. In 100s and 500s.
Rx	**Cystospaz** (PolyMedica)	**Tablets**: 0.15 mg	(W 2225). Blue. In 100s.
Rx	**Hyoscyamine Sulfate** (Kremers Urban)	**Tablets, sublingual**: 0.125 mg	(KU 102). White, scored, beveled. Peppermint flavor. In 100s.
Rx	**A-Spas S/L** (Hyrex)		White. In 100s.
Rx	**Levsin/SL** (Schwarz Pharma)		(Schwarz 532). Blue-green, scored. Octagonal. Peppermint flavor. In 100s and 500s.
Rx	**Symax-SL** (Capellon)		(SL 125). Green. In 100s.
Rx	**Hyoscyamine Sulfate** (Various, eg, Econolab, Ethex, Global, Goldline)	**Tablets, extended-release**: 0.375 mg	In 100s and 1000s.
Rx	**Levbid** (Schwarz Pharma)		(SP538). Orange, scored. Capsule shape. In 100s.
Rx	**Symax-SR** (Capellon)	**Tablets, sustained- release**: 0.375 mg	(SR 375). Green, scored, capsule shape. In 100s.

L-HYOSCYAMINE SULFATE

Rx	**Symax Duotab** (Capellon)	**Tablets, extended-release**: 0.375 mg (0.125 mg immediate-release, 0.25 mg extended-release)	(SYMAX DUOTAB). Purple/White, capsule-shape, bilayered. In 90s.
Rx	**Neosol** (Breckenridge)	**Tablets, orally disintegrating**: 0.125 mg	Mint flavor. White. In 100s.
Rx	**NuLev** (Schwarz Pharma)		Aspartame, mannitol. 1.7 mg phenylalanine. (SP 111). White. Mint flavor. In 100s.
Rx	**Symax FasTab** (Capellon)		Lactose. mannitol. (FT). Green. Peppermint flavor. In 100s.
Rx	**Mar-Spas** (Marnel)	**Tablets, orally disintegrating**: 0.25 mg	Aspartame, 3.5 mg phenylalanine. (4 4). Spearmint flavor. White, scored, capsule-shape. In 100s.
Rx	**Hyoscyamine Sulfate** (Ethex)	**Capsules, extended release**: 0.375 mg	In 100s.
Rx	**Hyoscyamine Sulfate** (Various, eg, Breckenridge)	**Capsules, timed release**: 0.375 mg	In 100s.
Rx	**Levsinex Timecaps** (Schwarz Pharma)		(SCHWARZ 537). Brown/clear. In 100s and 500s.
Rx	**Hyoscyamine Sulfate** (Goldline)	**Solution**: 0.125 mg/mL	5% alcohol. In 15 mL w/dropper.
Rx	**Levsin Drops** (Schwarz Pharma)		5% alcohol. Sorbitol. Orange flavor. In 15 mL.
Rx	**Levsin** (Schwarz Pharma)	**Elixir**: 0.125 mg/5 mL	20% alcohol. Sorbitol. Orange flavor. In pt.
Rx	**Levsin** (Schwarz Pharma)	**Injection**: 0.5 mg/mL	In 1 mL amps and 10 mL[1] vials.
Rx	**IB-Stat** (InKine)	**Oral spray**: 0.125 mg/mL (0.125 mg/spray)	5.3% alcohol, liquid sugar, methylparaben, sorbitol. In 30 mL.

[1] With 1.5% benzyl alcohol and 0.1% sodium metabisulfite.

HYOSCYAMINE SULFATE – ORAL

For complete and comparative prescribing information, refer to the Gastrointestinal Anticholinergics/Antispasmodics group monograph.

Indications

➤*GI:* To aid in the control of gastric secretion, visceral spasm, hypermotility in spastic colitis, spastic bladder, pylorospasm, and associated abdominal cramps. To relieve symptoms in functional intestinal disorders (eg, mild dysenteries and diverticulitis), infant colic, and biliary colic. As adjunctive therapy in peptic ulcer; irritable bowel syndrome (irritable colon, spastic colon, mucous colitis, acute enterocolitis, functional GI disorders); neurogenic bowel disturbances including splenic flexure syndrome and neurogenic colon; to reduce pain and hypersecretion in pancreatitis.

➤*Respiratory tract:* As a "drying agent" in the relief of symptoms of acute rhinitis.

➤*CNS:* In parkinsonism to reduce rigidity and tremors and to control associated sialorrhea and hyperhidrosis. May be used for poisoning by anticholinesterase agents.

➤*GU:* Cystitis; renal colic.

➤*Cardiovascular:* Certain cases of partial heart block associated with vagal activity.

Administration and Dosage

Adjust dosage according to the conditions and severity of symptoms.

➤*Regular tablets and sublingual tablets:* Hyoscyamine sublingual tablets are formulated for sublingual administration; however, the tablets may be chewed or taken orally.

Adults and pediatric patients 12 years of age and older – 1 to 2 tablets every 4 hours or as needed. Do not exceed 12 tablets in 24 hours.

Pediatric patients 2 to younger than 12 years of age – One-half to 1 tablet every 4 hours or as needed. Do not exceed 6 tablets in 24 hours.

➤*Orally disintegrating tablets:* Place hyoscyamine orally disintegrating tablets on tongue, allowing the tablet to rapidly disintegrate and be swallowed. Hyoscyamine orally disintegrating tablets may be taken with or without water.

Mar-Spas (only) –

Adults and adolescent patients 12 years of age and older: ½ to 1 tablet 3 to 4 times a day, 30 minutes to 1 hour before meals and at bedtime. Not recommended for children under 12 years of age.

All other disintegrating tablets –

Adults and pediatric patients 12 years of age and older: 1 to 2 tablets every 4 hours or as needed. Do not exceed 12 tablets in 24 hours.

Pediatric patients 2 to younger than 12 years of age: One-half to 1 tablet every 4 hours or as needed. Do not exceed 6 tablets in 24 hours.

➤*Extended-release tablets:*

Adults and pediatric patients 12 years of age and older – 1 to 2 tablets every 12 hours. Tablets are scored and may be broken to allow for dose titration if needed. Do not crush or chew tablets. Do not exceed 4 tablets in 24 hours.

➤*Sustained release tablets:* Tablets should be swallowed whole.

Adults and adolescents – 1 tablet 2 times per day in the morning and at bedtime. Increase the dosage, if necessary, to obtain desired response.

Elderly: The elderly may be more sensitive to the effects of the usual adult dose.

Children 2 years of age and older – 1 tablet 2 times per day in the morning and at bedtime. Do not exceed 2 tablets in 24 hours.

Children younger than 2 years of age – Use is not recommended.

➤*Extended-release and timed release capsules:*

Adults and children 12 years of age and older – 1 to 2 capsules every 12 hours. Dosage may be adjusted to 1 capsule every 8 hours if needed. Do not crush or chew capsules. Do not exceed 4 capsules in 24 hours.

➤*Oral solution:*

Adults and pediatric patients 12 years of age and older – 1 to 2 mL every 4 hours or as needed. Do not exceed 12 mL in 24 hours.

Pediatric patients 2 to younger than 12 years of age – 0.25 to 1 mL every 4 hours or as needed. Do not exceed 6 mL in 24 hours.

Pediatric patients younger than 2 years of age – The following dosage guide is based upon body weight. The doses may be repeated every 4 hours or as needed.

Body weight	Usual dose	Do not exceed in 24 hours
3.4 kg (7.5 lb)	4 drops	24 drops
5 kg (11 lb)	5 drops	30 drops
7 kg (15 lb)	6 drops	36 drops
10 kg (22 lb)	8 drops	48 drops

➤*Elixir:*

Adults and pediatric patients 12 years of age and older – 1 to 2 teaspoonfuls every 4 hours or as needed. Do not exceed 12 teaspoonfuls in 24 hours.

Pediatric patients 2 to younger than 12 years of age – Please see the following dosage guide based on body weight. The doses may be repeated every 4 hours or as needed. Do not exceed 6 teaspoonfuls in 24 hours.

Body weight	Usual dose
10 kg (22 lb)	1/4 tsp (1.25 mL)
20 kg (44 lb)	1/2 tsp (2.5 mL)
40 kg (88 lb)	3/4 tsp (3.75 mL)
50 kg (110 lb)	1 tsp (5 mL)

➤*Oral spray:*

Adults and pediatric patients 12 years of age and older – 1 to 2 mL (1 to 2 sprays) every 4 hours or as needed. Do not exceed 12 mL (12 sprays) in 24 hours.

➤*Storage/Stability:* Store at controlled room temperature 15° to 30°C (59° to 86°F).

Orally disintegrating tablets – Store at 25°C (77°F); excursions permitted to 15° to 30°C (59° to 86°F). Protect from moisture. Dispense in tight, light-resistant container.

Oral spray – Dispense in original container with metered sprayer.

HYOSCYAMINE SULFATE — INJECTION

For complete and comparative prescribing information, refer to the Gastrointestinal Anticholinergics/Antispasmodics group monograph.

Indications

➤*GI:* To aid in the control of gastric secretion, visceral spasm, hypermotility in spastic colitis, spastic bladder, pylorospasm, and associated abdominal cramps. To relieve symptoms in functional intestinal disorders (eg, mild dysenteries and diverticulitis), infant colic, and biliary colic. As adjunctive therapy in peptic ulcer; irritable bowel syndrome (irritable colon, spastic colon, mucous colitis, acute enterocolitis, functional GI disorders); neurogenic bowel disturbances including splenic flexure syndrome and neurogenic colon; to reduce pain and hypersecretion in pancreatitis.

➤*Respiratory tract:* As a "drying agent" in the relief of symptoms of acute rhinitis.

➤*CNS:* In parkinsonism to reduce rigidity and tremors and to control associated sialorrhea and hyperhidrosis. May be used for poisoning by anticholinesterase agents.

➤*GU:* Cystitis; renal colic.

➤*Cardiovascular:* Certain cases of partial heart block associated with vagal activity.

➤*Parenteral:* Reduces duodenal motility to facilitate the diagnostic radiologic procedure, hypotonic duodenography. May also improve radiologic visibility of the kidneys.

➤*Preoperative medication:* Parenteral hyoscyamine is indicated as a preoperative antimuscarinic to reduce salivary, tracheobronchial, and pharyngeal secretions; to reduce volume and acidity of gastric secretions; to block cardiac vagal inhibitory reflexes during induction of anesthesia and intubation. Hyoscyamine protects against peripheral muscarinic effects such as bradycardia and excessive secretions produced by halogenated hydrocarbons and cholinergic agents such as physostigmine, neostigmine, and pyridostigmine given to reverse actions of curariform agents.

Administration and Dosage

➤*Gastrointestinal disorders:* The usual adult recommended dose is 0.5 to 1 mL (0.25 to 0.5 mg). Some patients may need only a single dose; others may require administration 2, 3, or 4 times a day at 4-hour intervals.

➤*Diagnostic procedures:* The usual adult recommended dose is 0.5 to 1 mL (0.25 to 0.5 mg) administered IV 5 to 10 minutes prior to the diagnostic procedure.

➤*Anesthesia:*

Adults and pediatric patients over 2 years of age – As a preanesthetic medication, the recommended dose is 5 mcg (0.005 mg) per kg of body weight. This dose is usually given 30 to 60 minutes prior to the anticipated time of induction of anesthesia or at the time the preanesthetic narcotic or sedatives are administered.

Hyoscyamine injection may be used during surgery to reduce drug-induced bradycardia. It should be administered IV in increments of 0.25 mL and repeated as needed.

To achieve reversal of neuromuscular blockade, the recommended dose is 0.2 mg (0.4 mL) hyoscyamine injection for every 1 mg neostigmine or the equivalent dose of physostigmine or pyridostigmine.

➤*Administration:* The dose may be administered subcutaneously, IM, or IV without dilution. As with all parenteral drug products, visually inspect hyoscyamine injection for particulate matter and discoloration prior to administration whenever solution and container permit.

➤*Storage/Stability:* Store at controlled room temperature 15° to 30°C (59° to 86°F).

ATROPINE SULFATE

Rx	**Sal-Tropine** (Hope)	**Tablets:** 0.4 mg	In 100s.
Rx	**Atropine Sulfate** (Hospira)	**Injection:** 0.05 mg/mL	In 5 mL Abboject syringes.
Rx	**Atropine Sulfate** (Hospira)	**Injection:** 0.1 mg/mL	In 5 and 10 mL Abboject syringes.
Rx	**Atropine Sulfate** (Various, eg, Elkins-Sinn, GlaxoWellcome-,Loch, Moore, Schein, Vortech)	**Injection:** 0.3 mg/mL	In 1 and 30 mL vials.
		0.4 mg/mL	In 1 mL amps and 1, 20, and 30 mL vials.
		0.5 mg/mL	In 1 and 30 mL vials and 5 mL syringes.
		0.8 mg/mL	In 0.5 and 1 mL amps and 0.5 mL syringes.
		1 mg/mL	In 1 mL amps and vials and 10 mL syringes.
Rx	**AtroPen** (Meridian Medical Technologies)	**Injection:** 0.5 mg	Glycerin, phenol. In pre-filled auto-injectors.
		1 mg	Glycerin, phenol. In pre-filled auto-injectors.
		2 mg	Glycerin, phenol. In pre-filled auto-injectors.

ATROPINE SULFATE — ORAL

For complete and comparative prescribing information, refer to the Gastrointestinal Anticholinergics/Antispasmodics group monograph. For information on the Atropine Sulfate Ophthalmic preparations, refer to the individual monograph.

Indications

Atropine sulfate is used to reduce salivation and bronchial secretions.

The antispasmodic action of atropine sulfate is useful in pylorospasm and other spastic conditions of the gastrointestinal tract. For ureteral and biliary colic, concomitant use of atropine and morphine may be indicated.

Administration and Dosage

The usual oral adult dose of atropine is 0.4 mg.

Suggested doses for children are as follows: 7-16 pounds - 0.1 mg; 17-24 pounds - 0.15 mg; 24-40 pounds - 0.2 mg; 40-65 pounds - 0.3 mg; 65-90 pounds - 0.4 mg; over 90 pounds - 0.4 mg.

These doses may be exceeded in certain cases.

ATROPINE SULFATE — INJECTION

For complete and comparative prescribing information, refer to the Gastrointestinal Anticholinergics/Antispasmodics group monograph. For information on the Atropine Sulfate Ophthalmic preparations, refer to the individual monograph.

Indications

Antisialogogue for preanesthetic medication to prevent or reduce secretions of the respiratory tract.

Treatment of parkinsonism. Rigidity and tremor are relieved by the apparently selective depressant action.

Restore cardiac rate and arterial pressure during anesthesia when vagal stimulation produced by intra-abdominal surgical traction causes a sudden decrease in pulse rate and cardiac action.

Lessen the degree of atrioventricular heart block when increased vagal tone is a major factor in the conduction defect as in some cases due to digitalis.

Overcome severe bradycardia and syncope due to a hyperactive carotid sinus reflex.

Antidote (with external cardiac massage) for cardiovascular collapse from the injudicious use of a choline ester (cholinergic) drug, pilocarpine, physostigmine, or isoflurophate.

Relieve pylorospasm, hypertonicity of small intestine, and hypermotility of colon.

Relax the spasm of biliary and ureteral colic and bronchial spasm.

Relaxation of the upper GI tract and colon during hypertonic radiography.

Diminish the tone of the detrusor muscle of the urinary bladder in the treatment of urinary tract disorders.

Control the crying and laughing episodes in patients with brain lesions.

In cases of closed head injuries that cause acetylcholine to be released or to be present in cerebrospinal fluid, which in turn causes abnormal EEG patterns, stupor, and neurological signs.

Relieve hypertonicity of the uterine muscle.

Management of peptic ulcer.

Control rhinorrhea of acute rhinitis or hay fever.

➤*Poisoning:* Treatment of anticholinesterase poisoning from organophosphorus insecticides; as an antidote for mushroom poisoning due to muscarine, in certain species such as *Amanita muscaria*.

For the treatment of poisoning by susceptible organophosphorus nerve agents having cholinesterase activity as well as organophosphorus or carbamate insecticides. Also intended as initial treatment of the muscarinic symptoms of insecticide or nerve agent poisonings (generally breathing difficulties due to increased secretions). Pralidoxime chloride may serve as an important adjunct to atropine therapy.

ATROPINE SULFATE — INJECTION

Administration and Dosage

➤*Adults:* 0.4 to 0.6 mg.

➤*Children:*

Atropine Dosage Recommendations in Children		
Weight		Dose
lb	kg	mg
7 to 16	3.2 to 7.3	0.1
16 to 24	7.3 to 10.9	0.15
24 to 40	10.9 to 18.1	0.2
40 to 65	18.1 to 29.5	0.3
65 to 90	29.5 to 40.8	0.4
> 90	40.8	0.4 to 0.6

➤*Hypotonic radiography:* 1 mg IM.

➤*Surgery:* Give SC, IM or IV. The average adult dose is 0.5 mg (range 0.4 to 0.6 mg). As an antisialogogue, it is usually injected IM prior to induction of anesthesia. In children, it has been suggested to use a dose of 0.01 mg/kg to a maximum of 0.4 mg, repeated every 4 to 6 hours as needed. A recommended infant dose is 0.04 mg/kg (infants less than 5 kg) or 0.03 mg/kg (infants more than 5 kg), repeated every 4 to 6 hours as needed. During surgery, the drug is given IV when reduction in pulse rate and cessation of cardiac action are due to increased vagal activity. However, if the anesthetic is cyclopropane, use doses less than 0.4 mg and give slowly to avoid production of ventricular arrhythmia. Usual doses reduce severe bradycardia and syncope associated with hyperactive carotid sinus reflex.

➤*Bradyarrhythmias:* The usual IV adult dosage ranges from 0.4 to 1 mg every 1 to 2 hours as needed; larger doses, up to a maximum of 2 mg, may be required. In children, IV dosage ranges from 0.01 to 0.03 mg/kg. Atropine is also a specific antidote for cardiovascular collapse resulting from injudicious administration of choline ester. When cardiac arrest has occurred, external cardiac massage or other method of resuscitation is required to distribute the drug after IV injection.

➤*Poisoning:* In anticholinesterase poisoning from exposure to insecticides, give large doses of ≥ 2 to 3 mg parenterally; repeat until signs of atropine intoxication appear. In "rapid" type of mushroom poisoning, give in doses sufficient to control parasympathomimetic signs before coma and cardiovascular collapse supervene.

AtroPen – Primary protection against exposure to chemical nerve agent and insecticide poisoning is the wearing of protective garments including masks, designed specifically for this use. Individuals should not rely solely upon the availability of antidotes such as atropine and pralidoxime to provide complete protection from chemical nerve agent and insecticide poisoning. Immediate evacuation from the contaminated environment is essential. Decontamination of the poisoned individual should occur as soon as possible. If dermal exposure has occurred, clothing should be removed and the hair and skin washed thoroughly with sodium bicarbonate or alcohol as soon as possible.

The *AtroPen* Auto-injector should be administered as soon as symptoms of organophosphorus. or carbamate poisoning appear (eg, usually tearing, excessive oral secretions, wheezing, muscle fasciculations). In moderate to severe poisoning, the administration of more than 1 *AtroPen* may be required until atropinization is achieved (flushing, mydriasis, tachycardia, dryness of the mouth and nose).

No more than 3 *AtroPen* injections should be used unless the patient is under the supervision of a trained medical provider. Different dose strengths of the *AtroPen* are available depending on the recipient's age and weight.

AtroPen Dosing	
Patient group	Dose strength
Adults and children weighing more than 90 lbs (generally over 10 years of age)	2 mg
Children weighing 40 to 90 lbs (generally 4 to 10 years of age)	1 mg
Children weighing 15 to 40 lbs (generally 6 months to 4 years of age)*	0.5 mg

* Children weighing less than 15 lbs (generally younger than 6 months of age) should ordinarily not be treated with the *AtroPen* auto-injector. Atropine doses for these children should be individualized at doses of 0.05 mg/kg.

Concomitant therapy: In severe poisonings, it may also be desirable to concurrently administer an anticonvulsant if seizure is suspected in the unconscious individual since the classic tonic-clonic jerking may not be apparent due to the effects of the poison. In poisonings due to organophosphorus nerve agents and insecticides, it also may be helpful to concurrently administer a cholinesterase reactivator such as pralidoxime chloride.

Pralidoxime (if used) is most effective if administered immediately or soon after the poisoning. Generally, little is accomplished if pralidoxime is given more than 36 hours after termination of exposure unless the poison is known to age slowly or re-exposure is possible, such as in delayed continuing GI absorption of ingested poisons. Fatal relapses, thought to be due to delayed absorption, have been reported after initial improvement. Continued administration for several days may be useful in such patients.

An anticonvulsant such as diazepam may be administered to treat convulsions if suspected in the unconscious individual. The effects of nerve agents and some insecticides can mask the motor signs of a seizure.

Mild symptoms: One *AtroPen* is recommended if 2 or more of the following mild symptoms of nerve agent (nerve gas) or insecticide exposure appear in situations where exposure is known or suspected:

- Blurred vision, miosis
- Excessive unexplained teary eyes
- Excessive unexplained runny nose
- Increased salivation such as sudden unexplained excessive drooling
- Chest tightness or difficulty breathing
- Tremors throughout the body or muscular twitching
- Nausea and/or vomiting
- Unexplained wheezing or coughing
- Acute onset of stomach cramps
- Tachycardia or bradycardia

Severe symptoms: Two additional *AtroPen* injections given in rapid succession are recommended 10 minutes after receiving the first *AtroPen* injection if the victim develops any of the following severe symptoms. If possible, a person other than the victim should administer the second and third *AtroPen* injections. If a victim is encountered who is either unconscious or has any of the severe symptoms, immediately administer 3 *AtroPen* injections into the victim's mid-lateral thigh in rapid succession using the appropriate weight-based *AtroPen* dose.

- Strange or confused behavior
- Severe difficulty breathing or severe secretions from the lungs/airway
- Severe muscular twitching and general weakness
- Involuntary urination and defecation (feces)
- Convulsions
- Unconsciousness

Emergency care of the severely poisoned individual should include removal of oral and bronchial secretions, maintenance of a patent airway, supplemental oxygen and, if necessary, artificial ventilation. In general, atropine should not be used until cyanosis has been overcome since atropine may produce ventricular fibrillation and possible seizures in the presence of hypoxia.

Close supervision of all moderately to severely poisoned patients is indicated for at least 48 to 72 hours.

Administration:

1.) Snap the grooved end of the plastic sleeve down and over the yellow safety cap. Remove the *AtroPen* from the plastic sleeve. Do not place fingers on the green tip.
2.) Firmly grasp the *AtroPen* with the green tip pointed down.
3.) Pull off the yellow safety cap with your other hand.
4.) Aim and firmly jab the green tip straight down (a 90° angle) against the outer thigh. The *AtroPen* device will then activate and deliver the medicine. It is okay to inject through clothing, but make sure pockets at the injection site are empty. Very thin people and small children also should be injected in the thigh, but before giving the *AtroPen*, bunch up the thigh to provide a thicker area for injection.
5.) Hold the auto-injector firmly in place for at least 10 seconds to allow the injection to finish.
6.) Remove the *AtroPen* and massage the injection site for several seconds. If the needle is not visible, check to be sure the yellow safety cap has been removed, and repeat steps 3 and 5, but press harder.

➤*Storage/Stability:* Store at controlled room temperature 15° to 30°C (59° to 86°F).

AtroPen – Store at 25°C (77°F); excursions permitted to 15° to 30°C (59° to 86°F). Keep from freezing; protect from light.

SCOPOLAMINE HBr (Hyoscine HBr)

Rx	**Scopace** (Hope Pharm)	**Tablets, soluble:** 0.4 mg	(Hope 301). White. In 100s.
Rx	**Scopolamine HBr** (Various, eg, Loch)	**Injection:** 0.3 mg/mL	In 1 mL vials.
Rx	**Scopolamine HBr** (Various, eg, GlaxoWellcome)	**Injection:** 0.4 mg/mL	In 0.5 mL amps and 1 mL vials.
Rx	**Scopolamine HBr** (GlaxoWellcome)	**Injection:** 0.86 mg/mL	In 0.5 mL amps.[1]
Rx	**Scopolamine HBr** (Various, eg, Loch)	**Injection:** 1 mg/mL	In 1 mL vials.

[1] With alcohol and mannitol.

Belladonna Alkaloids

SCOPOLAMINE HYDROBROMIDE — ORAL

For complete and comparative prescribing information, refer to the Gastrointestinal Anticholinergics/Antispasmodics group monograph. See also the Antiemetic/Antivertigo Agents monograph.

Indications

Scopolamine HBr tablets are used as an anticholinergic, CNS depressant; in the symptomatic treatment of postencephalitic parkinsonism and paralysis agitans; in spastic states; and, locally as a substitute for atropine in ophthalmology.

Scopolamine hydrobromide inhibits excessive motility and hypertonus of the GI tract in such conditions as the irritable colon syndrome, mild dysentery, diverticulitis, pylorospasm, and cardiospasm. It may also prevent motion sickness.

➤*Unlabeled uses:* Treatment of postoperative and chemotherapy-induced nausea and vomiting.

Administration and Dosage

➤*Dosage:* The dosage range for scopolamine is 0.4 to 0.8 mg. The dosage may be cautiously increased in parkinsonism and spastic states.

➤*Storage/Stability:* Store at controlled room temperature 15° to 30°C (59° to 86°F).

SCOPOLAMINE HBr — INJECTION

For complete and comparative prescribing information, refer to the Gastrointestinal Anticholinergics/Antispasmodics group monograph. See also the Antiemetic/Antivertigo Agents monograph.

Indications

Scopolamine HBr injection is indicated as a sedative and tranquilizing depressant to the central nervous system. In its peripheral actions, scopolamine differs from atropine in that it is a stronger blocking agent for the iris, ciliary body and salivary, bronchial, and sweat glands, but is weaker in its action on the heart (in which it is incapable of exerting actions in tolerated doses), the intestinal tract and bronchial musculature.

In addition to the usual uses for antimuscarinic drugs, scopolamine is employed for its central depressant actions as a sedative. Frequently, it is given as a preanesthetic medicament for both its sedative-tranquilizing and antisecretory actions. It is an effective antiemetic. It is used in maniacal states, in delirium tremens and in obstetrics. As a mydriatic and cycloplegic, it has a somewhat shorter duration (3 to 7 days) and intraocular pressure is affected less markedly than with atropine.

Administration and Dosage

➤*Adult:* For obstetric amnesia or preoperative sedation, 0.32 to 0.65 mg (320 to 650 mcg).

For sedation or tranquilization, 0.6 mg (600 mcg) 3 or 4 times a day.

Subcutaneous, as an antiemetic, 0.6 to 1 mg.

➤*Pediatric:* Age 6 months to 3 years, 0.1 to 0.15 mg (100 to 150 mcg).

Age 3 to 6 years, 0.2 to 0.3 mg (200 to 300 mcg).

Subcutaneous, as antiemetic, 0.006 mg (6 mcg) per kg.

➤*Dosage equivalents:*

The dosage equivalents for the 1 mg (1,000 mcg)/mL strength vial are as follows –

1 mg (1,000 mcg) = 1 mL.
0.8 mg (800 mcg) = 0.8 mL.
0.6 mg (600 mcg) = 0.6 mL.
0.5 mg (500 mcg) = 0.5 mL.
0.4 mg (400 mcg) = 0.4 mL.
0.3 mg (300 mcg) = 0.3 mL.
0.2 mg (200 mcg) = 0.2 mL.
0.1 mg (100 mcg) = 0.1 mL.

The dosage equivalents for the 0.4 mg (400 mcg)/mL strength vial are as follows –

0.4 mg (400 mcg) = 1 mL
0.0.25 mg (250 mcg) = 0.63 mL.
3 mg (300 mcg) = 0.75 mL
0.2 mg (200 mcg) = 0.5 mL.
0.15 mg (150 mcg) = 0.38 mL.

Belladonna alkaloids provide a therapeutic effect in about 1 or 2 hours with a duration of about 4 hours.

Geriatric and debilitated patients may respond to the usual doses with excitement, agitation, drowsiness, or confusion; lower doses may be required in such patients.

Close supervision is recommended for infants, blondes, people with Down syndrome, and children with spastic paralysis or brain damage, since an increased responsiveness to belladonna alkaloids has been reported in these patients and dosage adjustments are often required.

➤*Administration:* Administration of belladonna alkaloids and barbiturates 30 to 60 minutes before meals is recommended to maximize absorption and, when issued for reducing stomach acid formation, to allow its effect to coincide better with antacid administration following the meal.

➤*Storage/Stability:* Store at controlled room temperature 15° to 30°C (59° to 86°F).

Protect from light. Use only if solution is clear and seal intact.

Parenteral drug products should be inspected visually for particulate matter prior to administration, whenever solution and container permit.

BELLADONNA

Rx	**Belladonna Tincture** (Various, eg, Lilly)	**Liquid:** 27 to 33 mg belladonna alkaloids/100 mL	65% to 70% alcohol. In 120 mL, pt and gal.

BELLADONNA — ORAL

For complete prescribing information, refer to the Gastrointestinal Anticholinergics/Antispasmodics group monograph.

Indications

➤*GI:* As adjunctive therapy in the treatment of peptic ulcer, functional digestive disorders (including spastic, mucous and ulcerative colitis), diarrhea, diverticulitis, pancreatitis.

➤*GU:* Dysmenorrhea, nocturnal enuresis.

➤*CNS:* Parkinsonism (idiopathic and postencephalitic). Large doses may provide some symptomatic relief; tremor, rigidity, sialorrhea and oculogyric crises are reduced; posture, gait and speech are improved.

➤*Other:* Motion sickness; nausea and vomiting of pregnancy.

Administration and Dosage

➤*Belladonna tincture:*

Adults – 0.6 to 1 mL, 3 to 4 times daily.
Children – 0.03 mL/kg (0.8 mL/m^2) 3 times daily.

Quaternary Anticholinergics

METHSCOPOLAMINE BROMIDE

Rx	**Pamine** (Kenwood/Bradley)	**Tablets:** 2.5 mg	White. In 100s and 500s.
Rx	**Pamine Forte** (Kenwood Therapeutics)	**Tablets:** 5 mg	(PAMINE 5). White, oval. In 60s.

METHSCOPOLAMINE BROMIDE — ORAL

For complete and comparative prescribing information, refer to the Gastrointestinal Anticholinergics/Antispasmodics group monograph.

Indications

➤*Peptic ulcer:* Adjunctive therapy for the treatment of peptic ulcer.

Methscopolamine bromide has not been shown to be effective in contributing to the healing of peptic ulcer, decreasing the rate of recurrence or preventing complications.

➤*Unlabeled uses:* Atropine and related agents are effective in some patients with cholinergic-mediated bronchospasm. Use in chronic lung disease is not generally recommended; these agents reduce bronchial secretions resulting in decreased fluidity and thickening of residual secretions.

Administration and Dosage

2.5 mg one-half hour before meals and 2.5 to 5 mg at bedtime. A starting dose of 12.5 mg/day will be clinically effective in most patients without the production of appreciable side effects.

Patients whose dosage has been reduced to eliminate or modify side effects often continue to show adequate response both subjectively in relief of symptoms and objectively as measured by antisecretory effects.

If the patient is having severe symptoms which demand prompt relief, the drug may be started on a dosage of 20 mg/day, administered in doses of 5 mg one-half hour before meals and at bedtime. If very unpleasant side effects develop promptly, the daily dosage should be reduced. If neither symptom-

METHSCOPOLAMINE BROMIDE — ORAL

atic relief nor side effects appear, the daily dosage may be increased. Some patients have tolerated 30 mg/day with no unpleasant reactions.

➤*Storage/Stability:* Store at controlled room temperature 15° to 30°C (59° to 86°F).

GLYCOPYRROLATE

Rx	**Glycopyrrolate** (Rising)	**Tablets:** 1 mg	Lactose. (cor 155). White. In 100s and 1,000s.
Rx	**Robinul** (Horizon)		Lactose. (HPC 200). White, scored. In 100s and 500s.
Rx	**Glycopyrrolate** (Rising)	**Tablets:** 2 mg	Lactose. (cor 156). White. In 100s and 1,000s.
Rx	**Robinul Forte** (Horizon)		Lactose. (Horizon 205). White, scored. In 100s.
Rx	**Glycopyrrolate** (Various, eg, American Regent, Quad, Schein, Texas Drug, VHA)	**Injection:** 0.2 mg per mL	In 1, 2, 5, and 20 mL vials.
Rx	**Robinul** (Robins)		In 1, 2, 5 and 20 mL vials.[a]

[a] With 0.9% benzyl alcohol.

GLYCOPYRROLATE — ORAL

For complete and comparative prescribing information, refer to the Gastrointestinal Anticholinergics/Antispasmodics group monograph.

Indications

➤*Peptic ulcer:* For use as adjunctive therapy in the treatment of peptic ulcer.

➤*Unlabeled uses:* Treatment of sialorrhea (excessive salivation).

Administration and Dosage

The dosage of glycopyrrolate or glycopyrrolate forte should be adjusted to the needs of the individual patient to ensure symptomatic control with a minimum of adverse reactions. The presently recommended maximum daily dosage of glycopyrrolate is 8 mg.

➤*1 mg tablets:* The recommended initial dosage of glycopyrrolate for adults is 1 mg tablet 3 times daily (in the morning, early afternoon, and at bedtime). Some patients may require 2 tablets at bedtime to ensure overnight control of symptoms. For maintenance, a dosage of 1 tablet twice a day is frequently adequate.

➤*2 mg tablets:* The recommended dosage of glycopyrrolate extra-strength for adults is a 2 mg tablet 2 or 3 times daily at equally spaced intervals. Glycopyrrolate tablets are not recommended for use in children younger than 12 years of age.

➤*Storage/Stability:* Store at controlled room temperature, 15° to 30°C (59° to 86°F). Dispense in tight container.

GLYCOPYRROLATE — INJECTION

For complete and comparative prescribing information, refer to the Gastrointestinal Anticholinergics/Antispasmodics group monograph.

Indications

➤*Anesthesia:* Use as a preoperative antimuscarinic to reduce salivary, tracheobronchial, and pharyngeal secretions; to reduce the volume and free acidity of gastric secretions; and to block cardiac vagal inhibitory reflexes during induction of anesthesia and intubation. When indicated, glycopyrrolate injection may be used intraoperatively to counteract drug-induced or vagal traction reflexes with the associated arrhythmias. Glycopyrrolate protects against the peripheral muscarinic effects (eg, bradycardia, excessive secretions) of cholinergic agents such as neostigmine and pyridostigmine given to reverse the neuromuscular blockade due to nondepolarizing muscle relaxants.

➤*Peptic ulcer:* For use in adults as adjunctive therapy for the treatment of peptic ulcer when rapid anticholinergic effect is desired or when oral medication is not tolerated.

Administration and Dosage

Glycopyrrolate injection may be administered IM or IV without dilution in the following indications:

➤*Anesthesia (adults):*

Preanesthetic medication – The recommended dose of glycopyrrolate injection is 0.002 mg (0.01 mL) per pound of body weight by IM injection, given 30 to 60 minutes prior to the anticipated time of induction of anesthesia or at the time the preanesthetic narcotic or sedative is administered.

Intraoperative medication – Glycopyrrolate injection may be used during surgery to counteract drug induced or vagal traction reflexes with the associated arrhythmias (eg, bradycardia). It should be administered IV as single doses of 0.1 mg (0.5 mL) and repeated, as needed, at intervals of 2 to 3 minutes. The usual attempts should be made to determine the etiology of the arrhythmia, and the surgical or anesthetic manipulations necessary to correct parasympathetic imbalance should be performed.

Reversal of neuromuscular blockade – The recommended dose of glycopyrrolate injection is 0.2 mg (1 mL) for each 1 mg of neostigmine or 5 mg of pyridostigmine. In order to minimize the appearance of cardiac side effects, the drugs may be administered simultaneously by IV injection and may be mixed in the same syringe.

➤*Anesthesia (children):*

Preanasthetic medication – The recommended dose of glycopyrrolate injection in children to 12 years of age is 0.002 mg (0.01 mL) per pound of body weight IM, given 30 to 60 minutes prior to the anticipated time of induction of anesthesia or at the time the preanesthetic narcotic or sedative is administered.

Children younger than 2 years of age may require up to 0.004 mg (0.02 mL) per pound of body weight.

Intraoperative medication – Because of the long duration of action of glycopyrrolate injection, if used as preanesthetic medication, additional glycopyrrolate injection for anticholinergic effect intraoperatively is rarely needed; in the event it is required the recommended pediatric dose is 0.002 mg (0.01 mL) per pound of body weight intravenously, not to exceed 0.1 mg (0.5 mL) in a single dose which may be repeated, as needed, at intervals of 2 to 3 minutes. The usual attempts should be made to determine the etiology of the arrhythmia, and the surgical or anesthetic manipulations necessary to correct parasympathetic imbalance should be performed.

Reversal of neuromuscular blockade – The recommended pediatric dose of glycopyrrolate injection is 0.2 mg (1 mL) for each 1 mg of neostigmine or 5 mg of yridostigmine. In order to minimize the appearance of cardiac side effects, the drugs may be administered simultaneously by IV injection and may be mixed in the same syringe.

➤*Peptic ulcer (Adults):*

Peptic ulcer – The usual recommended dose of glycopyrrolate injection is 0.1 mg (0.5 mL) administered at 4-hr intervals, 3 or 4 times daily IV or IM. Where more profound effect is required, 0.2 mg (1 mL) may be given. Some patients may need only a single dose and frequency of administration should be dictated by patient response up to a maximum of 4 times daily. Glycopyrrolate injection is not recommended for peptic ulcers in children younger than 12 years of age (see Warnings).

➤*Incompatibilities:* Glycopyrrolate injection stability is generally dependent upon pH. The pH of the USP product ranges between 2 and 3. Stability decreases rapidly above pH 6.

Glycopyrrolate injection is stable for 48 hours in IV infusion solutions of 5% Dextrose, 10% Dextrose, 0.45% Sodium Chloride, 0.9% Sodium Chloride or Ringer's Injection.

Glycopyrrolate injection is generally physically compatible with drugs having an acid pH (less than 6); however, this would also be dependent on concentration of the drugs and temperature as well as pH.

Glycopyrrolate injection would be expected to be incompatible with drugs having a more alkaline pH (more than 6) such as the barbiturates, diazepam or buffered Lactated Ringer's injection. The latter may be used for administration via the tubing of a running IV infusion.

➤*Storage/Stability:* Store at controlled room temperature 15° to 30°C (59° to 86°F).

Parenteral drug products should be inspected visually for particulate matter and discoloration prior to administration whenever solution and container permit.

MEPENZOLATE BROMIDE

Rx	**Cantil** (Hoechst Marion Roussel)	**Tablets:** 25 mg	Tartrazine. (Merrell 37). Yellow. In 100s.

Quaternary Anticholinergics

MEPENZOLATE BROMIDE — ORAL

For complete and comparative prescribing information, refer to the Gastrointestinal Anticholinergics/Antispasmodics group monograph.

Indications

➤*Peptic ulcer:* Adjunctive therapy in the treatment of peptic ulcer. It has not been shown to be effective in contributing to the healing of peptic ulcer, decreasing the rate of recurrence, or preventing complications.

Administration and Dosage

➤*Dosage:* The usual adult dose is 1 or 2 tablets (25 or 50 mg) 4 times a day preferably with meals and at bedtime. Begin with the lower dosage when possible and adjust subsequently according to the patient's response. Safety and efficacy in pediatric patients have not been established.

➤*Storage / Stability:* Keep tightly closed. Store at room temperature, preferably below 30°C (86°F). Protect from excessive heat. Dispense in tight containers with child-resistant closure.

PROPANTHELINE BROMIDE

Rx	**Pro-Banthine** (Schiapparelli Searle)	**Tablets:** 7.5 mg	(RPC 073). White, sugar coated. In 100s.
Rx	**Propantheline Bromide** (Various, eg, Goldline, Harber, Moore, Par, Richlyn, Roxane)	**Tablets:** 15 mg	In 100s, 500s, 1000s, and UD 100s.
Rx	**Pro-Banthine** (Schiapparelli Searle)		(Searle 601) Peach, sugar coated. In 100s, 500s, and UD 100s.

PROPANTHELINE BROMIDE — ORAL

For complete and comparative prescribing information, refer to the Gastrointestinal anticholinergics/Antispasmodics group monograph.

Indications

➤*Peptic ulcer:* Adjunctive therapy in the treatment of peptic ulcer.

Administration and Dosage

➤*Dosage:* 15 mg taken 30 minutes before each meal and 30 mg at bedtime (a total of 75 mg daily). Subsequent dosage adjustment should be made according to the patient's individual response and tolerance. The administration of one 7.5 mg tablet 3 times a day is convenient for patients with mild manifestations and for geriatric patients and for those of small stature.

➤*Storage / Stability:* Dispense in tight, light-resistant container as defined in the USP/NF.

Antispasmodics

DICYCLOMINE HYDROCHLORIDE

Rx	**Dicyclomine HCl** (Various, eg, Bolar, Goldline, Lederle, Major, Rugby)	**Capsules:** 10 mg	In 30s, 100s, 120s, 1000s, and UD 100s.
Rx	**Bentyl** (Axcan Scandipharm)		(Bentyl 10). In 100s, 500s, and UD 100s.
Rx	**Byclomine** (Major)		In 100s, 250s, 1000s, and UD 100s.
Rx	**Di-Spaz** (Vortech)		In 1000s.
Rx	**Dicyclomine HCl** (Various, eg, Bolar, Goldline, Lederle, Major, Rugby)	**Tablets:** 20 mg	In 15s, 20s, 30s, 100s, 120s, 250s, 1000s, and UD 100s.
Rx	**Bentyl** (Axcan Scandipharm)		(Bentyl 20) In 100s, 500s, 1000s, and UD 100s.
Rx	**Byclomine** (Major)		In 100s, 250s, 1000s, and UD 100s.
Rx	**Dicyclomine HCl** (Various, eg, Moore, Ritchie)	**Capsules** : 20 mg	In 100s, and 1000s.
Rx	**Dicyclomine HCl** (Various, eg, Gen-King, Goldline, Harber, Moore, Qualitest, Rugby)	**Syrup:** 10 mg/5 mL	In 118 mL, pt, and gal.
Rx	**Bentyl** (Axcan Scandipharm)		Saccharin in pt.
Rx	**Dicyclomine HCl** (Various, eg, Baxter, Goldline, Major, Moore, Ritchie, Rugby, Steris)	**Injection:** 10 mg/mL	In 2 and 10 mL vials.
Rx	**Bentyl** (Axcan Scandipharm)		In 2 mL amps and 10 mL vials.
Rx	**Dibent** (Hauck)		In 10 mL vials.
Rx	**Dilomine** (Kay Drug)		In 10 mL vials.
Rx	**Di-Spaz** (Vortech)		In 10 mL vials.
Rx	**Or-Tyl** (Ortega)		In 10 mL vials.

DICYCLOMINE HYDROCHLORIDE — ORAL

For complete and comparative prescribing information, refer to the Gastrointestinal Anticholinergics/Antispasmodics group monograph.

Indications

For the treatment of functional bowel/irritable bowel syndrome (irritable colon, spastic colon, mucous colitis).

Administration and Dosage

➤*Approved by the FDA:* October 15, 1984.

Dosage must be adjusted to individual patient needs.

➤*Adult dose:* The only oral dose clearly shown to be effective is 160 mg/day (in 4 equally divided doses). Since this dose is associated with a significant incidence of side effects, it is prudent to begin with 80 mg/day (in 4 equally divided doses). Depending upon the patient's response during the first week of therapy, the dose should be increased to 160 mg/day unless side effects limit dosage escalation.

If efficacy is not achieved within 2 weeks or side effects require doses below 80 mg/day, the drug should be discontinued. Documented safety data are not available for doses greater than 80 mg daily for periods greater than 2 weeks.

➤*Storage / Stability:* Store at controlled room temperature 15° to 30°C (59° to 86°F). Protect from light, freezing, and moisture.

Dispense in a tight, light-resistant container using a child-resistant closure.

DICYCLOMINE HYDROCHLORIDE — INJECTION

For complete and comparative prescribing information, refer to the Gastrointestinal Anticholinergics/Antispasmodics group monograph.

Indications

For the treatment of functional bowel/irritable bowel syndrome.

Administration and Dosage

➤*Approved by the FDA:* October 15, 1984.

Dosage must be adjusted to individual patient needs.

➤*Adults:* The IM dosage form is to be used temporarily when the patient cannot take oral medication. IM injection is about twice as bioavailable as oral dosage forms; consequently, the recommended IM dose is 80 mg daily (in 4 equally divided doses).

Oral dicyclomine hydrochloride should be started as soon as possible and the IM form should not be used for periods of longer than 1 or 2 days.

Administration – IM injection. Not for IV use.

Aspirate the syringe before injecting to avoid intravascular injection, since thrombosis may occur if the drug is inadvertently injected intravascularly. Parenteral drug products should be inspected visually for particulate matter and discoloration prior to administration, whenever solution and container permit.

➤*Storage / Stability:* Store at room temperature, preferably below 30°C (86°F). Protect from freezing.

Gastrointestinal Anticholinergic Combinations

Refer to the general discussion of these products in the GI Anticholinergics/Antispasmodics group monograph.

Actions

➤*Pharmacology:* Combination anticholinergic preparations may include the following components:

Sedatives and antianxiety agents – See: Barbiturates, Prochlorperazine, Hydroxyzine, Meprobamate, Chlordiazepoxide.

Ergotamine tartrate – Ergotamine tartrate provides inhibition of the sympathetic nervous system.

GI ANTICHOLINERGIC COMBINATIONS, CAPSULES AND TABLETS

Content given per tablet or capsule.

	Product and Distributor	Anticholinergic	Sedative, Antianxiety Agent or Other	Daily Dose (Tablets)	How Supplied
Rx	**Donnatal Extentabs Extended-Release Tablets** (PBM Pharm[a])	0.0582 mg atropine sulfate, 0.0195 mg scopolamine HBr, 0.3111 mg hyoscyamine sulfate	48.6 mg phenobarbital	2 to 3	Lactose, polydextrose. (P421). Green. Film coated. In 100s and 500s.
Rx	**Belladonna Alkaloids w/Phenobarbital Tablets** (Various, eg, Goldline, Major, Westward)	0.0194 mg atropine sulfate, 0.0065 mg scopolamine HBr, 0.1037 mg hyoscyamine HBr or sulfate	16.2 mg phenobarbital	3 to 8	In 50s, 100s, 1,000s and UD 100s.
Rx	**Donnatal Tablets** (PBM Pharm[a])				Lactose. (D Donnatal). White, D shape. In 100s and 1,000s.
Rx	**Hyosophen Tablets** (Rugby)				(Rugby 3920). White, scored. In 100s and 1,000s.
Rx	**Spasmolin Tablets** (Various, eg, Global)				In 100s and 1,000s.
Rx	**Butibel Tablets** (Wallace)	15 mg belladonna extract	15 mg butabarbital sodium	4 to 8	(Butibel 37/046). Red. In 100s.
Rx	**Chlordiazepoxide w/Clidinium Bromide Capsules** (Various, eg, Chelsea Labs, Eon, Goldline, Major, Moore, Schein)	2.5 mg clidinium	5 mg chlordiazepoxide hydrochloride	3 to 8	In 100s, 500s, 1,000s, and UD 100s.
Rx	**Bellamine Tablets** (Major)	0.2 mg levorotatory alkaloids of belladonna	40 mg phenobarbital, 0.6 mg ergotamine tartrate	1 in morning and night	In 100s.
c-iv	**Librax Capsules** (Victory Pharma)	2.5 mg methscopolamine nitrate	5 mg chlordiazepoxide hydrochloride	1 to 2 capsules 3 or 4 times/day before meals and at bedtime[b]	Lactose. (Librax). Opaque green. In 100s.

[a] PBM Pharmaceuticals, Linney House, 204 North Main Street, Gordonsville, VA 22942; (800)485-9828.

[b] Initial dose in geriatric patients should not exceed 2 capsules per day, to be increased gradually.

Refer to the general discussion of these products in the GI Anticholinergics/Antispasmodics group monograph.

GI ANTICHOLINERGIC COMBINATIONS, TABLETS, SUSTAINED RELEASE

Content given per tablet.

	Product and Distributor	Anticholinergic	Sedative or Antianxiety Agent	Other Content	Daily Dose (Tablets)	How Supplied
Rx	**Bel-Phen-Ergot SR Tablets** (Goldline)	0.2 mg l-alkaloids of belladonna	40 mg phenobarbital, 0.6 mg ergotamine tartrate	Lactose	2	In 100s.

Refer to the general discussion of these products in the GI Anticholinergics/Antispasmodics group monograph.

GI ANTICHOLINERGIC COMBINATIONS, LIQUIDS

Content given per 5 mL liquid and 1 mL drops.

	Product and Distributor	Anticholinergic	Sedative	Other Content	Daily Dose	How Supplied
Rx	**Hyosophen Elixir** (Rugby)	0.0194 mg atropine sulfate, 0.0065 mg scopolamine HBr, 0.1037 mg hyoscyamine HBr or sulfate	16.2 mg phenobarbital	23% alcohol, sugar, sorbitol	15 to 40 mL *Children*: 4.5 kg to 45.4 kg - 0.5 to 5 mL q 4 h or 0.75 to 7.5 mL q 6 h, respectively	In 120 mL, pt and gal.
Rx	**Antispasmodic Elixir**[a] (Various, eg, Goldline, Qualitest, RID, UDL)					In 120 mL, pt, and gal.
Rx	**Donnatal Elixir** (PBM Pharm[b])			95% ethyl alcohol, saccharin, sucrose, sorbitol	5 to 10 mL tid or qid. *Children: 4.5 kg* - 0.5 mL every 4 h or 0.75 mL every 6 h; *9.1 kg* - 1 mL every 4 h or 1.5 mL every 6 h; *13.6 kg* - 1.5 mL every 4 h or 2 mL every 6 h; *22.7 kg* - 2.5 mL every 4 h or 3.75 mL every 6 h; *34 kg* - 3.75 mL every 4 h or 5 mL every 6 h; *45 kg* - 5 mL every 4 h or 7.5 mL every 6 h.	Grape flavor. In 118 and 473 mL.
Rx	**Butibel Elixir** (Wallace)	15 mg belladonna extract	15 mg butabarbital sodium	7% alcohol, sucrose, saccharin	20 to 40 mL. *Children* ≥ *6* - 10 mL; *Children* < *6* - 5 to 10 mL	Orange flavor. In pt.
Rx sf	**Antrocol Elixir** (ECR)	0.195 mg atropine sulfate	16 mg phenobarbital	20% alcohol	15 to 40 mL. *Children* - 0.5 mL per 15 lbs every 4 to 6 hours	In pt.

[a] May contain alcohol.

[b] PBM Pharmaceuticals, Linney House, 204 North Main Street, Gordonsville, VA 22942; (800)485-9828.

Refer to the general discussion of these products at the beginning of the GI Anticholinergics/Antispasmodics group monograph.

MESALAMINE (5-aminosalicylic acid, 5-ASA)

Rx	**Asacol** (Procter & Gamble)	**Tablets, delayed release**: 400 mg	Lactose. (Asacol NE). Red-brown. Capsule shape. In 100s.
Rx	**Pentasa** (Shire US)	**Capsules, controlled release**: 250 mg	Sugar. (2010 PENTASA 250 mg). Green/blue. In 240s and UD 80s.
		500 mg	Sugar, talc. (PENTASA 500 mg). Blue. In 120s and UD 80s.
Rx	**Canasa** (Axcan Scandipharm)	**Suppositories**: 500 mg	Hard fat base. Light tan. In 30s.
Rx	**FIV-ASA** (Paddock)		In 30s.
Rx	**Canasa** (Axcan Scandipharm)	**Suppositories**: 1,000 mg	Hard fat base. Light tan. In 30s.
Rx	**Mesalamine** (Various, eg,Clay Park, Teva)	**Enema**: 4 g per 60 mL	May contain EDTA, potassium acetate, potassium metabisulfite, sodium benzoate, white petrolatum. In 7s with lubricated applicator tip.
Rx	**Rowasa** (Solvay)		EDTA, potassium acetate, potassium metabisulfite, sodium benzoate, white petrolatum. In 7s and 28s with lubricated applicator tip.

MESALAMINE — ORAL

Indications

➤*Ulcerative colitis:* The treatment of mildly to moderately active ulcerative colitis and for the maintenance of remission of ulcerative colitis.

Administration and Dosage

➤*Approved by the FDA:* January 31, 1992.

➤*Tablets:* 800 mg 3 times daily for a total dose of 2.4 g/day for 6 weeks.

➤*Capsules:* 1 g 4 times daily for a total dose of 4 g for up to 8 weeks.

➤*Storage / Stability:*

Delayed-release tablets – Store at controlled room temperature 20° to 25°C (68° to 77°F) [See USP].

Controlled-release capsules – Store at controlled room temperature 15° to 30°C (59° to 86°F).

Actions

➤*Pharmacology:* Mesalamine is thought to be the major therapeutically active part of the sulfasalazine molecule in the treatment of ulcerative colitis. Sulfasalazine is converted to equimolar amounts of sulfapyridine (SP) and mesalamine (5-ASA) by bacterial action in the colon. The usual oral dose of sulfasalazine for active ulcerative colitis in adults is 3 to 4 g daily in divided doses, which provides 1.2 to 1.6 g of mesalamine to the colon. The mechanism of action of mesalamine (and sulfasalazine) is unknown, but appears to be topical rather than systemic. Mucosal production of arachidonic acid (AA) metabolites, both through the cyclooxygenase pathways (ie, prostanoids), and through the lipoxygenase pathways (ie, leukotrienes [LTs]) and hydroxyeicosatetraenoic acids (HETEs), is increased in patients with chronic inflammatory bowel disease, and it is possible that mesalamine diminishes inflammation by blocking cyclooxygenase and inhibiting prostaglandin (PG) production in the colon.

➤*Pharmacokinetics:*

Absorption / Distribution –

Delayed-release tablets: Mesalamine delayed-release tablets are coated with an acrylic-based resin that delays release of mesalamine until it reaches the terminal ileum and beyond. This has been demonstrated in human studies conducted with radiological and serum markers. Approximately 28% of the mesalamine in mesalamine delayed-release tablets is absorbed after oral ingestion, leaving the remainder available for topical action and excretion in the feces. Absorption of mesalamine is similar in fasted and fed subjects. The absorbed mesalamine is rapidly acetylated in the gut mucosal wall and by the liver. It is excreted mainly by the kidney as N-acetyl-5-aminosalicylic acid. Mesalamine from orally administered mesalamine delayed-release tablets appears to be more extensively absorbed than the mesalamine released from sulfasalazine. Maximum plasma levels of mesalamine and N-acetyl-5-aminosalicylic acid following multiple mesalamine delayed-release tablet doses are about 1.5 to 2 times higher than those following an equivalent dose of mesalamine in the form of sulfasalazine. Combined mesalamine and N-acetyl-5-aminosalicylic acid AUCs and urine drug dose recoveries following multiple doses of mesalamine delayed-release tablets are about 1.3 to 1.5 times higher than those following an equivalent dose of mesalamine in the form of sulfasalazine. The t_{max} for mesalamine and its metabolite, N-acetyl-5-aminosalicylic acid, is usually delayed, reflecting the delayed release, and ranges from 4 to 12 hours.

Controlled-release capsules: Mesalamine controlled-release capsules are an ethylcellulose-coated, controlled-release formulation of mesalamine designed to release therapeutic quantities of mesalamine throughout the GI tract. Based on urinary excretion data, 20% to 30% of the mesalamine in mesalamine controlled-release capsules is absorbed. In contrast, when mesalamine is administered orally as an unformulated 1 g aqueous suspension, mesalamine is ≈ 80% absorbed. Plasma mesalamine concentration peaked at ≈ 1 mcg/mL 3 hours following a 1 g mesalamine controlled-release capsules dose and declined in a biphasic manner.

Metabolism / Excretion –

Delayed-release tablets: The half-lives of elimination for mesalamine and N-acetyl-5-aminosalicylic acid are usually about 12 hours, but are variable, ranging from 2 to 15 hours. There is a large intersubject variability in the plasma concentrations of mesalamine and N-acetyl-5-aminosalicylic acid and in their elimination half-lives following administration of mesalamine delayed-release tablets.

Controlled-release capsules: The literature describes a mean terminal half-life of 42 minutes for mesalamine following IV administration. Because of the continuous release and absorption of mesalamine from mesalamine controlled-release capsules throughout the GI tract, the true elimination half-life cannot be determined after oral administration. N-acetylmesalamine, the major metabolite of mesalamine, peaked at ≈ 3 hours at 1.8 mcg/mL, and its concentration followed a biphasic decline. Pharmacological activities of N-acetylmesalamine are unknown, and other metabolites have not been identified.

Oral mesalamine pharmacokinetics were nonlinear when mesalamine controlled-release capsules were dosed from 250 mg to 1 g 4 times daily, with steady-state mesalamine plasma concentrations increasing about 9 times, from 0.14 mcg/mL to 1.21 mcg/mL, suggesting saturable first-pass metabolism. N-acetylmesalamine pharmacokinetics were linear.

About 130 mg free mesalamine was recovered in the feces following a single 1 g mesalamine controlled-release capsules dose, which was comparable to the 140 mg of mesalamine recovered from the molar equivalent sulfasalazine tablet dose of 2.5 g. Elimination of free mesalamine and salicylates in feces increased proportionately with mesalamine controlled-release capsules dose. N-acetylmesalamine was the primary compound excreted in the urine (19% to 30%) following mesalamine controlled-release capsules dosing.

Contraindications

Hypersensitivity to salicylates or to any of the components of mesalamine.

Warnings

➤*Renal function impairment:*

Delayed-release tablets – Renal impairment, including minimal change nephropath and acute and chronic interstitial nephritis, has been reported in patients taking mesalamine delayed-release tablets as well as other compounds which contain or are converted to mesalamine. In animal studies (rats, dogs), the kidney is the principal target organ for toxicity. At doses of ≈ 750 mg/kg to 1,000 mg/kg [15 to 20 times the administered recommended human dose (based on a 50 kg person) on a mg/kg basis and 3 to 4 times on a mg/m^2 basis], mesalamine causes renal papillary necrosis. Therefore, caution should be exercised when using mesalamine delayed-release tablets (or other compounds which contain or are converted to mesalamine or its metabolites) in patients with known renal dysfunction or history of renal disease. It is recommended that all patients have an evaluation of renal function prior to initiation of mesalamine delayed-release tablets and periodically while on mesalamine delayed-release tablets therapy.

Controlled-release capsules – Caution should be exercised if mesalamine controlled-release capsules are administered to patients with impaired renal function. Single reports of nephrotic syndrome and interstitial nephritis associated with mesalamine therapy have been described in the foreign literature. There have been rare reports of interstitial nephritis in patients receiving mesalamine controlled-release capsules. In animal studies, a 13-week oral toxicity study in mice, and 13-week and 52-week oral toxicity studies in rats and cynomolgus monkeys have shown the kidney to be the major target organ of mesalamine toxicity. Oral daily doses of 2400 mg/kg in mice and 1150 mg/kg in rats produced renal lesions, including granular and hyaline casts, tubular degeneration, tubular dilation, renal infarct, papillary necrosis, tubular necrosis, and interstitial nephritis. In cynomolgus monkeys, oral daily doses of 250 mg/kg or higher produced nephrosis, papillary edema, and interstitial fibrosis. Patients with preexisting renal disease, increased blood urea nitrogen (BUN) or serum creatinine, or proteinuria should be carefully monitored.

➤*Pregnancy: Category B.*

Mesalamine is known to cross the placental barrier.

Teratogenic – Reproduction studies have been performed in rats at doses up to 1000 mg/kg/day (5900 mg/m^2) and rabbits at doses of 800 mg/kg/day (6856 mg/m^2) and have revealed no evidence of teratogenic effects or harm to the fetus due to mesalamine. There are, however, no adequate and well-controlled studies in pregnant women. Because animal reproduction studies are not always predictive of human response, mesalamine should be used during pregnancy only if clearly needed.

➤*Lactation:* Minute quantities of mesalamine were distributed to breast milk and amniotic fluid of pregnant women following sulfasalazine therapy. When treated with sulfasalazine at a dose equivalent to 1.25 g/day of mesalamine, 0.02 mcg/mL to 0.08 mcg/mL and trace amounts of mesalamine were measured in amniotic fluid and breast milk, respectively. N-acetylmesalamine, in quantities of 0.07 mcg/mL to 0.77 mcg/mL and 1.13 mcg/mL to 3.44 mcg/mL, was identified in the same fluids, respectively.

Caution should be exercised when mesalamine is administered to a nursing woman.

➤*Children:* Safety and efficacy of mesalamine delayed-release tablets or controlled-release capsules in pediatric patients have not been established.

MESALAMINE — ORAL

Precautions

➤*Pyloric stenosis:* Patients with pyloric stenosis may have prolonged gastric retention of mesalamine delayed-release tablets which could delay release of mesalamine in the colon.

➤*Exacerbation of colitis symptoms:* Exacerbation of the symptoms of colitis has been reported in 3% of mesalamine delayed-release tablets-treated patients in controlled clinical trials. This acute reaction, characterized by cramping, abdominal pain, bloody diarrhea, and occasionally by fever, headache, malaise, pruritus, rash, and conjunctivitis, has been reported after the initiation of mesalamine delayed-release tablets as well as other mesalamine products. Symptoms usually abate when mesalamine delayed-release tablets are discontinued.

➤*Hypersensitivity reactions:* Some patients who have experienced a hypersensitivity reaction to sulfasalazine may have a similar reaction to mesalamine delayed-release tablets or to other compounds which contain or are converted to mesalamine.

➤*Hepatic function impairment:* Caution should be exercised if mesalamine controlled-release capsules is administered to patients with impaired hepatic function.

➤*Acute intolerance syndrome (controlled-release):* Mesalamine has been associated with an acute intolerance syndrome that may be difficult to distinguish from a flare of inflammatory bowel disease. Although the exact frequency of occurrence cannot be ascertained, it has occurred in 3% of patients in controlled clinical trials of mesalamine or sulfasalazine. Symptoms include cramping, acute abdominal pain and bloody diarrhea, sometimes fever, headache, and rash. If acute intolerance syndrome is suspected, prompt withdrawal is required. If a rechallenge is performed later in order to validate the hypersensitivity, it should be carried out under close medical supervision at reduced dose and only if clearly needed.

Drug Interactions

There are no known drug interactions.

Adverse Reactions

➤*Delayed-release tablets:* Mesalamine delayed-release tablets have been evaluated in 3685 inflammatory bowel disease patients (most patients with ulcerative colitis) in controlled and open-label studies. Adverse events seen in clinical trials with mesalamine delayed-release tablets have generally been mild and reversible. Adverse events presented in the following sections may occur regardless of length of therapy and similar events have been reported in short- and long-term studies and in the postmarketing setting. In 2 short-term (6 week) placebo-controlled clinical studies involving 245 patients, 155 of whom were randomized to mesalamine delayed-release tablets, five (3.2%) of the mesalamine delayed-release tablets patients discontinued mesalamine delayed-release tablets therapy because of adverse reactions as compared to two (2.2%) of the placebo patients. Adverse reactions leading to withdrawal from mesalamine delayed-release tablets included the following (each in 1 patient): Diarrhea and colitis flare; dizziness, nausea, joint pain, and headache; rash, lethargy and constipation; dry mouth, malaise, lower back discomfort, mild disorientation, mild indigestion and cramping; headache, nausea, malaise, aching, vomiting, muscle cramps, a stuffy head, plugged ears, and fever. Adverse reactions occurring in mesalamine delayed-release tablets-treated patients at a frequency of ≥ 2% in the 2 short-term, double-blind, placebo-controlled trials mentioned above are listed below. Overall, the incidence of adverse events seen with mesalamine delayed-release tablets was similar to placebo.

Frequency (%) of Common Adverse Reactions Reported in Ulcerative Colitis Patients Treated with Mesalamine Tablets or Placebo in Short-Term (6-Week) Double-Blind Controlled Studies

	% of patients with adverse reactions	
Reaction	Placebo (n = 87)	Mesalamine tablets (n = 152)
Headache	36%	35%
Abdominal pain	14%	18%
Eructation	15%	16%
Pain	8%	14%
Nausea	15%	13%
Pharyngitis	9%	11%
Dizziness	8%	8%
Asthenia	15%	7%
Diarrhea	9%	7%
Back pain	5%	7%
Fever	8%	6%
Rash	3%	6%
Dyspepsia	1%	6%
Rhinitis	5%	5%
Arthralgia	3%	5%
Hypertonia	3%	5%
Vomiting	2%	5%
Constipation	1%	5%
Flatulence	7%	3%
Dysmenorrhea	3%	3%
Chest pain	2%	3%
Chills	2%	3%
Flu syndrome	2%	3%
Peripheral edema	2%	3%
Myalgia	1%	3%
Sweating	1%	3%
Colitis exacerbation	0%	3%
Pruritus	0%	3%
Acne	1%	2%
Increased cough	1%	2%
Malaise	1%	2%
Arthritis	0%	2%
Conjunctivitis	0%	2%
Insomnia	0%	2%

Of these adverse reactions, only rash showed a consistently higher frequency with increasing mesalamine delayed-release tablets dose in these studies.

In a 6-month placebo-controlled, maintenance trial involving 264 patients, 177 of whom were randomized to mesalamine delayed-release tablets, six (3.4%) of the mesalamine delayed-release tablets patients discontinued mesalamine delayed-release tablets therapy because of adverse events, as compared to four (4.6%) of the placebo patients. Adverse reactions leading to withdrawal from mesalamine delayed-release tablets included the following (each in 1 patient): Anxiety; headache; pruritus; decreased libido; rheumatoid arthritis; and stomatitis and asthenia.

In the 6-month placebo-controlled, maintenance trial, the incidence of adverse reactions seen with mesalamine delayed-release tablets was similar to that seen with placebo. In addition to reactions listed above, the following adverse reactions occurred in mesalamine delayed-release tablets treated patients at a frequency of ≥ 2% in this study: Abdominal enlargement, anxiety, bronchitis, ear disorder, ear pain, gastroenteritis, GI hemorrhage, infection, joint disorder, migraine, nervousness, paresthesia, rectal disorder, rectal hemorrhage, sinusitis, stool abnormalities, tenesmus, urinary frequency, vasodilation, and vision abnormalities.

In 3342 patients in uncontrolled clinical trials, the following adverse reactions occurred at a frequency of ≥ 5% and appeared to increase in frequency with increasing dose: Asthenia, fever, flu syndrome, pain, abdominal pain, back pain, flatulence, GI bleeding, arthralgia, and rhinitis.

In addition to the adverse reactions listed above, the following events have been reported with mesalamine delayed-release tablets use:

Cardiovascular – Pericarditis (rare), myocarditis (rare).

CNS – Depression, somnolence, emotional lability, hyperesthesia, vertigo, confusion, tremor, peripheral neuropathy (rare), transverse myelitis (rare), Guillain-Barré syndrome (rare).

Dermatologic – Alopecia, psoriasis (rare), pyoderma gangrenosum (rare), dry skin, erythema nodosum, urticaria.

GI – Anorexia, hepatitis (rare), pancreatitis, gastritis, increased appetite, cholecystitis, dry mouth, oral ulcers, perforated peptic ulcer (rare), bloody diarrhea.

GU – Interstitial nephritis (see also Warnings, Renal function impairment), minimal change nephropathy, dysuria, urinary urgency, hematuria, epididymitis, menorrhagia.

Hematologic – Agranulocytosis (rare), aplastic anemia (rare), thrombocytopenia, eosinophilia, leukopenia, anemia, lymphadenopathy.

Lab test abnormalities – Elevated AST or ALT, elevated alkaline phosphatase, elevated serum creatinine and blood urea nitrogen (BUN). Hepatitis has been reported to occur rarely with mesalamine delayed-release tablets. More commonly, asymptomatic elevations of liver enzymes have occurred which usually resolve during continued use or with discontinuation of the drug.

Musculoskeletal – Gout.

Respiratory – Eosinophilic pneumonia, interstitial pneumonitis, asthma exacerbation.

Special senses – Eye pain, taste perversion, blurred vision, tinnitus.

Miscellaneous – Neck pain, facial edema, edema.

➤*Controlled-release capsules:* In combined domestic and foreign clinical trials, more than 2100 patients with ulcerative colitis or Crohn's disease received mesalamine controlled-release capsules therapy. Generally, mesalamine controlled-release capsules therapy was well tolerated. The most common events (ie, ≥ 1%) were diarrhea (3.4%), headache (2%), nausea (1.8%) abdominal pain (1.7%), dyspepsia (1.6%), vomiting (1.5%), and rash (1%).

In 2 domestic placebo-controlled trials involving over 600 ulcerative colitis patients, adverse events were fewer in mesalamine controlled-release capsules-treated patients than in the placebo group (mesalamine controlled-release capsules 14% vs placebo 18%) and were not dose related. Events occurring at ≥ 1% are shown below. Of these, only nausea and vomiting were more frequent in the mesalamine controlled-release capsules group. Withdrawal from therapy due to adverse events was more common on placebo than mesalamine controlled-release capsules (7% vs 4%).

MESALAMINE — ORAL

Adverse Reactions Occurring in More Than 1% of Either Placebo or Mesalamine Controlled-Release Capsule Patients in DomesticPlacebo-Controlled Ulcerative Colitis Trials (Mesalamine Controlled-Release Capsules Comparison with Placebo)		
Reaction	Mesalamine controlled-release capsules (n = 451)	Placebo (n = 173)
Diarrhea	16 (3.5%)	13 (7.5%)
Headache	10 (2.2%)	6 (3.5%)
Nausea	14 (3.1%)	—
Abdominal pain	5 (1.1%)	7 (4%)
Melena (bloody diarrhea)	4 (0.9%)	6 (3.5%)
Rash	6 (1.3%)	2 (1.2%)
Anorexia	5 (1.1%)	2 (1.2%)
Fever	4 (0.9%)	2 (1.2%)
Rectal urgency	1 (0.2%)	4 (2.3%)
Nausea/vomiting	5 (1.1%)	—
Worsening of ulcerative colitis	2 (0.4%)	2 (1.2%)
Acne	1 (0.2%)	2 (1.2%)

Clinical laboratory measurements showed no significant abnormal trends for any test, including measurement of hematologic, liver, and kidney function. The following adverse events, presented by body system, were reported infrequently (ie, less than 1%) during domestic ulcerative colitis and Crohn's disease trials. In many cases, the relationship to mesalamine controlled-release capsules has not been established.

Cardiovascular – Palpitations, pericarditis, vasodilation.

CNS – Depression, dizziness, insomnia, somnolence, paresthesia.

Dermatologic – Acne, alopecia, dry skin, eczema, erythema nodosum, nail disorder, photosensitivity, pruritus, sweating, urticaria.

GI – Abdominal distention, anorexia, constipation, duodenal ulcer, dysphagia, eructation, esophageal ulcer, fecal incontinence, GGTP increase, GI bleeding, increased alkaline phosphatase, LDH increase, mouth ulcer, oral moniliases, pancreatitis, rectal bleeding, APT increase, AST increase, stool abnormalities (color or texture change), thirst.

Miscellaneous – Albuminuria, amenorrhea, amylase increase, arthralgia, asthenia, breast pain, conjunctivitis, ecchymosis, edema, fever, hematuria, hypomenorrhea, Kawasaki-like syndrome, leg cramps, lichen planus, lipase increase, malaise, menorrhagia, metrorrhagia, myalgia, pulmonary infiltrates, thrombocythemia, thrombocytopenia, urinary frequency.

One week after completion of an 8-week ulcerative colitis study, a 72-year-old male, with no history of pulmonary problems, developed dyspnea. The patient was subsequently diagnosed with interstitial pulmonary fibrosis without eosinophilia by 1 physician and bronchiolitis obliterans with organizing pneumonitis by a second physician. A causal relationship between this event and mesalamine therapy has not been established.

Published case reports or spontaneous postmarketing surveillance have described infrequent instances of pericarditis, fatal myocarditis, chest pain and T-wave abnormalities, hypersensitivity pneumonitis, pancreatitis, nephrotic syndrome, interstitial nephritis, hepatitis, aplastic anemia, pancytopenia, leukopenia, or anemia while receiving mesalamine therapy. Anemia can be a part of the clinical presentation of inflammatory bowel disease.

Overdosage

➤*Symptoms:*

Delayed-release tablets – Two cases of pediatric overdosage have been reported. A 3-year-old male who ingested 2 g of mesalamine delayed-release tablets was treated with ipecac and activated charcoal; no adverse reactions occurred. Another 3-year-old male, ≈ 16 kg, ingested an unknown amount of a maximum of 24 g of mesalamine delayed-release tablets crushed in solution (ie, uncoated mesalamine); he was treated with orange juice and activated charcoal, and experienced no adverse reactions. In dogs, single doses of 6 g of mesalamine delayed-release tablets resulted in renal papillary necrosis but were not fatal. This was ≈ 12.5 times the recommended human dose (based on a dose of 2.4 g/day in a 50 kg person). Single oral doses of uncoated mesalamine in mice and rats of 5000 mg/kg and 4595 mg/kg, respectively, or of 3000 mg/kg in cynomolgus monkeys, caused significant lethality.

Controlled-release capsules – There is no clinical experience with mesalamine controlled-release capsules overdosage. Mesalamine controlled-release capsules are an aminosalicylate, and symptoms of salicylate toxicity may be possible, such as the following: Tinnitus, vertigo, headache, confusion, drowsiness, sweating, hyperventilation, vomiting, and diarrhea. Severe intoxication with salicylates can lead to disruption of electrolyte balance and blood pH, hyperthermia, and dehydration.

➤*Treatment:* Since mesalamine is an aminosalicylate, conventional therapy for salicylate toxicity may be beneficial in the event of acute overdosage. This includes prevention of further GI tract absorption by emesis and, if necessary, by gastric lavage. Fluid and electrolyte imbalance should be corrected by the administration of appropriate IV therapy. Adequate renal function should be maintained.

Patient Information

Patients should be instructed to swallow the mesalamine delayed-release tablets whole, taking care not to break the outer coating. The outer coating is designed to remain intact to protect the active ingredient and thus ensure mesalamine availability for action in the colon. In 2% to 3% of patients in clinical studies, intact or partially intact tablets have been reported in the stool. If this occurs repeatedly, patients should contact their physician. Patients with ulcerative colitis should be made aware that ulcerative colitis rarely remits completely, and that the risk of relapse can be substantially reduced by continued administration of mesalamine delayed-release tablets at a maintenance dosage.

MESALAMINE — RECTAL

Indications

Treatment of active mild to moderate distal ulcerative colitis, proctosigmoiditis or proctitis.

Administration and Dosage

➤*Approved by the FDA:* December 24, 1987 (enema); January 5, 2001 (suppositories).

➤*Suppository:* One 500 mg suppository 2 times daily (with possible increase to 3 times daily if inadequate response at 2 weeks) or one 1,000 mg suppository daily at bedtime. Retain the suppository in the rectum for 1 to 3 hours or more if possible to achieve maximum benefit. While the effect may be seen within 3 to 21 days, the usual course of therapy is 3 to 6 weeks depending on symptoms and sigmoidoscopic findings. Studies have suggested the suppositories will delay relapse after the 6-week, short-term treatment.

➤*Enema:* One rectal instillation (4 g) once a day, preferably at bedtime, and retained for approximately 8 hours.

➤*Storage/Stability:*

Rectal suspension enema – Store at controlled room temperature 15° to 30°C (59° to 86°F). Once the foil-wrapped unit of 7 bottles is opened, all enemas should be used promptly as directed by your physician. Contents of enemas removed from the foil pouch may darken with time. Slight darkening will not affect potency; however, enemas with dark brown contents should be discarded.

Suppositories – Store at 19° to 26°C (66° to 79°F).

Note – Mesalamine rectal suspension enema or suppositories will cause staining of direct contact surfaces, including but not limited to fabrics, flooring, painted surfaces, marble, granite, vinyl, and enamel. Take care in choosing a suitable location for administration of this product.

Actions

➤*Pharmacology:* Sulfasalazine is split by bacterial action in the colon into sulfapyridine (SP) and mesalamine (5-ASA). It is thought that the mesalamine component is therapeutically active in ulcerative colitis. The usual oral dose of sulfasalazine for active ulcerative colitis in adults is 2 to 4 g/day in divided doses. Four (4) grams of sulfasalazine provide 1.6 g of free mesalamine to the colon. Each mesalamine suspension enema delivers up to 4 g of mesalamine to the left side of the colon. Each mesalamine suppository delivers 500 mg of mesalamine to the rectum.

The mechanism of action of mesalamine (and sulfasalazine) is unknown, but appears to be topical rather than systemic. Mucosal production of arachidonic acid (AA) metabolites, both through the cyclooxygenase pathways (ie, prostanoids), and through the lipoxygenase pathways (ie, leukotrienes (LTs), (hydroxyeicosatetraenoic acids [HETEs]) is increased in patients with chronic inflammatory bowel disease, and it is possible that mesalamine diminishes inflammation by blocking cyclooxygenase and inhibiting prostaglandin (PG) production in the colon.

Preclinical toxicology – Preclinical studies have shown the kidney to be the major target organ for mesalamine toxicity. Adverse renal function changes were observed in rats after a single 600 mg/kg oral dose, but not after a 200 mg/kg dose. Gross kidney lesions, including papillary necrosis, were observed after a single oral dose greater than 900 mg/kg, and after IV doses of greater than 214 mg/kg. Mice responded similarly. In a 13-week oral (gavage) dose study in rats, the high dose of 640 mg/kg/day mesalamine caused deaths, probably due to renal failure, and dose-related renal lesions (papillary necrosis or multifocal tubular injury) were seen in most rats given the high dose (males and females) as well as in males receiving lower doses of 160 mg/kg/day. Renal lesions were not observed in the 160 mg/kg/day female rats. Minimal tubular epithelial damage was seen in the 40 mg/kg/day males and was reversible. In a 6-month oral study in dogs, the no-observable dose level of mesalamine was 40 mg/kg/day and doses of 80 mg/kg/day and higher caused renal pathology similar to that described for the rat. In a combined 52-week toxicity and 127-week carcinogenicity study in rats, degeneration in kidneys was observed at doses of 100 mg/kg/day and above admixed with diet for 52 weeks, and at 127 weeks increased incidence of kidney degeneration and hyalinization of basement membranes and Bowman's capsule were seen at 100 mg/kg/day and above. In the 12-month eye toxicity study in dogs, keratoconjunctivitis sicca (KCS) occurred at oral doses of 40 mg/kg/day and above. The oral preclinical studies were done with a highly bioavailable suspension where absorption throughout the gastrointestinal tract occurred. The human dose of 4 g represents approximately 80 mg/kg but when mesalamine is given rectally as a suspension, absorption is poor and limited to the distal colon. The extent of absorption is dependent upon the retention time of the drug product, and there is considerable individual variation. Overt renal toxicity has not been observed, but the potential must be considered. Patients on mesalamine rectal suspension enema, especially those on concurrent oral products which

MESALAMINE — RECTAL

liberate mesalamine and those with preexisting renal disease, should be carefully monitored with urinalysis, blood urea nitrogen (BUN) and creatinine studies.

➤*Pharmacokinetics:*

Absorption/Distribution – Mesalamine administered rectally as mesalamine rectal suspension enema is poorly absorbed from the colon and is excreted principally in the feces during subsequent bowel movements. The extent of absorption is dependent upon the retention time of the drug product, and there is considerable individual variation. At steady state, approximately 10% to 30% of the daily 4 g dose can be recovered in cumulative 24-hour urine collections. Other than the kidney, the organ distribution and other bioavailability characteristics of absorbed mesalamine in man are not known. It is known that the compound undergoes acetylation, but whether this process takes place at colonic or systemic sites has not been elucidated.

Metabolism/Excretion – Whatever the metabolic site, most of the absorbed mesalamine is excreted in the urine as the N-acetyl-5-ASA metabolite. The poor colonic absorption of rectally administered mesalamine is substantiated by the low serum concentration of 5-ASA and N-acetyl-5-ASA seen in ulcerative colitis patients after dosage with mesalamine. Under clinical conditions patients demonstrated plasma levels 10 to 12 hours post mesalamine administration of 2 mcg/mL, about two-thirds of which was the N-acetyl metabolite. While the elimination half-life of mesalamine is short (0.5 to 1.5 hours), the acetylated metabolite exhibits a half-life of 5 to 10 hours. In addition, steady-state plasma levels demonstrated a lack of accumulation of either free or metabolized drug during repeated daily administrations.

Contraindications

Mesalamine rectal suspension enema or suppositories are contraindicated for patients known to have hypersensitivity to the drug or any component of this medication.

Warnings

➤*Hypersensitivity reactions:* Mesalamine has been implicated in the production of an acute intolerance syndrome characterized by cramping, acute abdominal pain and bloody diarrhea, sometimes fever, headache and a rash; in such cases prompt withdrawal is required. The patient's history of sulfasalazine intolerance, if any, should be reevaluated. If a rechallenge is performed later in order to validate the hypersensitivity it should be carried out under close supervision and only if clearly needed, giving consideration to reduced dosage. In the literature, 1 patient previously sensitive to sulfasalazine was rechallenged with 400 mg oral mesalamine; within 8 hours she experienced headache, fever, intensive abdominal colic, profuse diarrhea and was readmitted as an emergency. She responded poorly to steroid therapy and 2 weeks later a pancolectomy was required.

In a clinical trial most patients who were hypersensitive to sulfasalazine were able to take mesalamine enemas without evidence of any allergic reaction. Nevertheless, caution should be exercised when mesalamine is initially used in patients known to be allergic to sulfasalazine. These patients should be instructed to discontinue therapy if signs of rash or fever become apparent.

➤*Renal function impairment:* Although renal abnormalities were not noted in the clinical trials with mesalamine rectal suspension enema, the possibility of increased absorption of mesalamine and concomitant renal tubular damage as noted in the preclinical studies must be kept in mind. Patients on mesalamine rectal suspension enema, especially those on concurrent oral products which liberate mesalamine and those with preexisting renal disease, should be carefully monitored with urinalysis, blood urea nitrogen (BUN) and creatinine studies.

➤*Pregnancy: Category B.* Teratologic studies have been performed in rats and rabbits at oral doses up to 5 and 8 times, respectively, the maximum recommended human dose, and have revealed no evidence of harm to the embryo or the fetus. There are, however, no adequate and well controlled studies in pregnant women for either sulfasalazine or 5-ASA. Because animal reproduction studies are not always predictive of human response, 5-ASA should be used during pregnancy only if clearly needed.

➤*Lactation:* It is not known whether mesalamine or its metabolite(s) are excreted in human milk. As a general rule, nursing should not be undertaken while a patient is on a drug since many drugs are excreted in human milk.

➤*Children:* Safety and efficacy in pediatric patients have not been established.

Precautions

➤*Pancolitis:* While using mesalamine rectal suspension enema some patients have developed pancolitis. However, extension of upper disease boundary or flare-ups occurred less often in the mesalamine suspension enema-treated group than in the placebo-treated group.

➤*Pericarditis:* Rare instances of pericarditis have been reported with mesalamine-containing products including sulfasalazine. Cases of pericarditis have also been reported as manifestations of inflammatory bowel disease. In the cases reported with mesalamine rectal suspension enema, there have been positive rechallenges with mesalamine or mesalamine-containing products. In 1 of these cases, however, a second rechallenge with sulfasalazine was negative throughout a 2-month follow-up. Chest pain or dyspnea in patients treated with mesalamine rectal suspension enema should be investigated with this information in mind. Discontinuation of mesalamine rectal suspension enema may be warranted in some cases, but rechallenge with mesalamine can be performed under careful clinical observation should the continued therapeutic need for mesalamine be present.

➤*Sulfite sensitivity:* Mesalamine rectal suspension enema contains potassium metabisulfite, a sulfite that may cause allergic-type reactions including anaphylactic symptoms and life-threatening or less severe asthmatic episodes in certain susceptible people. The overall prevalence of sulfite sensitivity in the general population is unknown but probably low. Sulfite sensitivity is seen more frequently in asthmatic or in atopic nonasthmatic persons. Epinephrine is the preferred treatment for serious allergic or emergency situations even though epinephrine injection contains sodium or potassium metabisulfite with the above-mentioned potential liabilities. The alternatives to using epinephrine in a life-threatening situation may not be satisfactory. The presence of a sulfite(s) in epinephrine injection should not deter the administration of the drug for treatment of serious allergic or other emergency situations.

Adverse Reactions

Mesalamine is usually well tolerated. Most adverse reactions have been mild and transient.

Adverse Reactions Occurring in More Than 0.1% of Mesalamine Rectal Suspension Enema-Treated Patients (Comparison with Placebo)

	Mesalamine (n = 815)		Placebo (n = 128)	
Reaction	n	%	n	%
Abdominal pain/cramps/discomfort	66	8.1%	10	7.81%
Headache	53	6.5%	16	12.5%
Gas/flatulence	50	6.13%	5	3.91%
Nausea	47	5.77%	12	9.38%
Flu	43	5.28%	1	0.78%
Tired/weak/malaise/fatigue	28	3.44%	8	6.25%
Fever	26	3.19%	0	0%
Rash/spots	23	2.82%	4	3.12%
Cold/sore throat	19	2.33%	9	7.03%
Diarrhea	17	2.09%	5	3.91%
Log/joint pain	17	2.09%	1	0.78%
Dizziness	15	1.84%	3	2.34%
Bloating	12	1.47%	2	1.56%
Back pain	11	1.35%	1	0.78%
Pain on insertion of enema tip	11	1.35%	1	0.78%
Hemorrhoids	11	1.35%	0	0%
Itching	10	1.23%	1	0.78%
Rectal pain	10	1.23%	0	0%
Constipation	8	0.98%	4	3.12%
Hair loss	7	0.86%	0	0%
Peripheral edema	5	0.61%	11	8.59%
UTI/urinary burning	5	0.61%	4	3.12%
Rectal pain/soreness/burning	5	0.61%	3	2.34%
Asthenia	1	0.12%	4	3.12%
Insomnia	1	0.12%	3	2.34%

In addition, the following adverse reactions have been identified during postapproval use of products which contain (or are metabolized to) mesalamine in clinical practice: Nephrotoxicity, pancreatitis, fibrosing alveolitis and elevated liver enzymes. Cases of pancreatitis and fibrosing alveolitis have been reported as manifestations of inflammatory bowel disease as well. Published case reports or spontaneous postmarketing surveillance have described rare instances of aplastic anemia, agranulocytosis, thrombocytopenia, or eosinophilia. Anemia, leukocytosis, and thrombocytosis can be part of the clinical presentation of inflammatory bowel disease.

➤*Miscellaneous:*

Hair loss – Mild hair loss characterized by "more hair in the comb" but no withdrawal from clinical trials has been observed in 7 of 815 mesalamine patients but none of the placebo-treated patients. In the literature, there are at least 6 additional patients with mild hair loss who received either mesalamine or sulfasalazine. Retreatment is not always associated with repeated hair loss.

Overdosage

There have been no documented reports of serious toxicity in man resulting from massive overdosing with mesalamine. Under ordinary circumstances, mesalamine absorption from the colon is limited.

Patient Information

➤*Rectal suspension enema:* Best results are achieved if the bowel is emptied immediately before the medication is given.

Note – Mesalamine rectal suspension enema will cause staining of direct contact surfaces, including but not limited to fabrics, flooring, painted surfaces, marble, granite, vinyl, and enamel. Take care in choosing a suitable location for administration of this product.

Bottles – Remove the bottles from the protective foil pouch by tearing or by using scissors as shown, being careful not to squeeze or puncture bottles. Mesalamine rectal suspension is an off-white to tan colored suspension. Once the foil-wrapped unit of seven bottles is opened, all enemas should be used promptly as directed by your physician. Contents of enemas removed from the foil pouch may darken with time. Slight darkening will not affect potency; however, enemas with dark brown contents should be discarded.

Prepare the medication for administration – Shake the bottle well to make sure that the medication is thoroughly mixed.

Remove the protective sheath from the applicator tip. Hold the bottle at the neck so as not to cause any of the medication to be discharged.

MESALAMINE — RECTAL

Assume the correct body position – Best results are obtained by lying on the left side with the left leg extended and the right leg flexed forward for balance.

An alternative to lying on the left side is the "knee-chest" position.

Administer the medication – Gently insert the lubricated applicator tip into the rectum to prevent damage to the rectal wall, pointed slightly toward the navel.

Grasp the bottle firmly, then tilt slightly so that the nozzle is aimed toward the back, squeeze slowly to instill the medication. Steady hand pressure will discharge most of the medication. After administering, withdraw and discard the bottle.

Remain in position for at least 30 minutes to allow thorough distribution of the medication internally. Retain the medication all night, if possible.

➤*Suppositories:*

Note – Mesalamine suppositories will cause staining of direct contact surfaces, including but not limited to fabrics, flooring, painted surfaces, marble, granite, vinyl, and enamel. Take care in choosing a suitable location for administration of this product.

1.) Detach 1 suppository from strip of suppositories.
2.) Hold suppository upright and carefully remove the foil wrapper.
3.) Avoid excessive handling of suppository, which is designed to melt at body temperature.
4.) Insert suppository completely into rectum with gentle pressure, pointed end first.

OLSALAZINE SODIUM

Rx	**Dipentum** (Celltech)	**Capsules:** 250 mg	(Dipentum 250 mg). Beige. In 100s and 500s.

OLSALAZINE SODIUM — ORAL

Indications

➤*Ulcerative colitis:* Maintenance of remission of ulcerative colitis in patients who are intolerant of sulfasalazine.

Administration and Dosage

➤*Approved by the FDA:* July 31, 1990.

➤*Dosage:* 1 g/day in 2 divided doses.

➤*Storage/Stability:* Store at 25°C (77°F). Excursions permitted to 15° to 30°C (59° to 86°F).

Actions

➤*Pharmacology:* The conversion of olsalazine to mesalamine (5-ASA) in the colon is similar to that of sulfasalazine, which is converted into sulfapyridine and mesalamine. It is thought that the mesalamine component is therapeutically active in ulcerative colitis. The usual dose of sulfasalazine for maintenance of remission in patients with ulcerative colitis is 2 g daily, which would provide approximately 0.8 g of mesalamine to the colon. More than 0.9 g of mesalamine would usually be made available in the colon from 1 g of olsalazine.

The mechanism of action of mesalamine (and sulfasalazine) is unknown, but appears to be topical rather than systemic. Mucosal production of arachidonic acid (AA) metabolites, both through the cyclooxygenase pathways (ie, prostanoids) and through the lipoxygenase pathways (ie, leukotrienes [LTs] and hydroxyelcosatetraenoic acids [HETEs]) is increased in patients with chronic inflammatory bowel disease, and it is possible that mesalamine diminishes inflammation by blocking cyclooxygenase and inhibiting prostaglandin (PG) production in the colon.

➤*Pharmacokinetics:*

Absorption – After oral administration, olsalazine has limited systemic bioavailability. Based on oral dosing studies, approximately 2.4% of a single 1 g oral dose is absorbed.

Distribution – The pharmacokinetics of olsalazine are similar in both healthy volunteers and in patients with ulcerative colitis. Maximum serum concentrations of olsalazine appear after approximately 1 hour, and are low (eg, 1.6 to 6.2 mcmol/L) even after a 1 g single dose. Olsalazine has a very short serum half-life, approximately 0.9 hours. Olsalazine is greater than 99% bound to plasma proteins. It does not interfere with protein binding of warfarin.

Total recovery of oral ^{14}C-labeled olsalazine in animals and humans ranges from 90% to 97%.

Metabolism – Approximately 0.1% of an oral dose of olsalazine is metabolized in the liver to olsalazine-O-sulfate (olsalazine-S). Olsalazine-S, in contrast to olsalazine, has a half-life of 7 days. Olsalazine-S accumulates to steady state within 2 to 3 weeks.

Patients on daily doses of 1 g olsalazine for 2 to 4 years show a stable plasma concentration of olsalazine-S (3.3 to 12.4 mcmol/L). Olsalazine-S is greater than 99% bound to plasma proteins. Its long half-life is mainly due to slow dissociation from the protein binding site. Less than 1% of both olsalazine and olsalazine-S appears undissociated in plasma.

5-aminosalicylic acid (5-ASA): Serum concentrations of 5-ASA are detected after 4 to 8 hours. The peak levels of 5-ASA after an oral dose of 1 g olsalazine are low (ie, 0 to 4.3 mcmol/L). Of the total 5-ASA found in the urine, more than 90% is in the form of N-acetyl-5-ASA (Ac-5-ASA). Only small amounts of 5-ASA are detected.

N-acetyl-5-ASA (Ac-5-ASA), the major metabolite of 5-ASA found in plasma and urine, is acetylated (deactivated) in at least 2 sites, the colonic epithelium and the liver. Ac-5-ASA is found in the serum, with peak values of 1.7 to 8.7 mcmol/L after a single 1 g dose.

Excretion – Less than 1% of olsalazine is recovered in the urine. The remaining 98% to 99% of an oral dose will reach the colon where each molecule is rapidly converted into 2 molecules of 5-aminosalicylic acid (5-ASA) by colonic bacteria and the low prevailing redox potential found in this environment. The liberated 5-ASA is absorbed slowly resulting in very high local concentrations in the colon.

Approximately 20% of the total 5-ASA is recovered in the urine, where it is found almost exclusively as Ac-5-ASA. The remaining 5-ASA is partially acetylated and is excreted in the feces. From fecal dialysis, the concentration of 5-ASA in the colon following olsalazine has been calculated to be 18 to 49 mmol/L. No accumulation of 5-ASA or Ac-5-ASA in plasma has been detected. 5-ASA and Ac-5-ASA are 74% and 81%, respectively, bound to plasma proteins.

Contraindications

Hypersensitivity to salicylates.

Warnings

➤*Renal function impairment:* Although renal abnormalities were not reported in clinical trials with olsalazine, there have been rare reports from postmarketing experience. Therefore, the possibility of renal tubular damage due to absorbed mesalamine or its n-acetylated metabolite must be kept in mind, particularly for patients with preexisting renal disease. In these patients, monitoring with urinalysis, BUN, and creatinine determinations is advised.

➤*Carcinogenesis:* In a 2-year oral rat carcinogenicity study, olsalazine was tested in male and female Wistar rats at daily doses of 200, 400, and 800 mg/kg/day (approximately 10 to 40 times the human maintenance dose, based on a patient weight of 50 kg and a human dose of 1 g). Urinary bladder transitional cell carcinomas were found in 3 male rats (6%, P = 0.022, exact trend test) receiving 40 times the human dose and were not found in untreated male controls. In the same study, urinary bladder transitional cell carcinoma and papilloma occurred in 2 untreated control female rats (2%). No such tumors were found in any of the female rats treated at doses up to 40 times the human dose.

In an 18 month oral mouse carcinogenicity study, olsalazine was tested in male and female CD-1 mice at daily doses of 500, 1,000, and 2,000 mg/kg/day (approximately 25 to 100 times the human maintenance dose). Liver hemangiosarcomata were found in 2 male mice (4%) receiving olsalazine at 100 times the human dose, while no such tumor occurred in the other treated male mice groups or any of the treated female mice. The observed incidence of this tumor is within the 4% incidence in historical controls.

➤*Elderly:* In general, elderly patients should be treated with caution due to the greater frequency of decreased hepatic, renal, or cardiac function, coexistence of other diseases, as well as concomitant drug therapy.

➤*Pregnancy: Category C.*

Olsalazine has been shown to produce fetal developmental toxicity as indicated by reduced fetal weights, retarded ossifications, and immaturity of the fetal visceral organs when given during organogenesis to pregnant rats in doses 5 to 20 times the human dose (100 to 400 mg/kg). There are no adequate and well-controlled studies in pregnant women. Olsalazine should be used during pregnancy only if the potential benefit justifies the potential risk to the fetus.

➤*Lactation:* Oral administration of olsalazine to lactating rats in doses 5 to 20 times the human dose produced growth retardation in their pups. It is not known whether this drug is excreted in human milk. Because many drugs are excreted in human milk, caution should be exercised when olsalazine is administered to a breast-feeding woman.

➤*Children:* Safety and efficacy in children have not been established.

Precautions

➤*Monitoring:* Monitoring with urinalysis, BUN, and creatinine determinations is advised in patients with preexisting renal disease.

➤*Diarrhea:* Overall, approximately 17% of subjects receiving olsalazine in clinical studies reported diarrhea sometime during therapy. This diarrhea resulted in withdrawal of treatment in 6% of patients. This diarrhea appears to be dose related, although it may be difficult to distinguish from the underlying symptoms of the disease.

➤*Exacerbation of colitis symptoms:* Exacerbation of the symptoms of colitis thought to have been caused by mesalamine or sulfasalazine has been noted.

Drug Interactions

➤*Warfarin:* Increased prothrombin time in patients taking concomitant warfarin has been reported.

OLSALAZINE SODIUM — ORAL

Adverse Reactions

Adverse reactions resulting in withdrawal from controlled studies		
Adverse reaction	Olsalazine (n = 441)	Placebo (n = 208)
Diarrhea/loose stools	26 (5.9%)	10 (4.8%)
Nausea	3	2
Abdominal pain	5 (1.1%)	0
Rash/itching	5 (1.1%)	0
Headache	3	0
Heartburn	2	0
Rectal bleeding	1	0
Insomnia	1	0
Dizziness	1	0
Anorexia	1	0
Light-headedness	1	0
Depression	1	0
Miscellaneous	4 (0.9%)	3 (1.4%)
Total number of patients withdrawn	46 (10.4%)	14 (6.7%)

Comparative incidence (%) of adverse reactions reported by 1% or more of ulcerative colitis patients treated with olsalazine or placebo in double-blind controlled studies		
Adverse reaction	Olsalazine (n = 441) %	Placebo (n = 208) %
GI		
Abdominal pain/cramps	10.1%	7.2%
Anorexia	1.3%	1.9%
Bloating	1.5%	1.4%
Diarrhea	11.1%	6.7%
Dyspepsia	4%	4.3%
Increased blood in stools	-	3.4%
Nausea	5%	3.9%
Stomatitis	1%	-
Vomiting	1%	-
CNS		
Fatigue/drowsiness/lethargy	1.8%	2.9%
Headache	5%	4.8%
Insomnia	-	2.4%
Vertigo/dizziness	1%	-
Psychiatric		
Depression	1.5%	-
Dermatologic		
Itching	1.3%	-
Rash	2.3%	1.4%
Musculoskeletal		
Arthralgia/joint pain	4%	2.9%
Miscellaneous		
Upper respiratory tract infection	1.5%	-

➤*Other clinical trials:* Over 2500 patients have been treated with olsalazine in various controlled and uncontrolled clinical studies. In these as well as in the postmarketing experience, olsalazine was administered mainly to patients intolerant to sulfasalazine. There have been rare reports of the following adverse reactions in patients receiving olsalazine. These were often difficult to distinguish from possible symptoms of the underlying disease or from the effects of prior or concomitant therapy. A causal relationship to the drug has not been demonstrated for some of these reactions.

Cardiovascular – Pericarditis; second-degree heart block; interstitial pulmonary disease; hypertension; orthostatic hypotension; peripheral edema; chest pains; tachycardia; palpitations; bronchospasm; shortness of breath.

A patient who developed thyroid disease 9 days after starting olsalazine was given propranolol and radioactive iodine and subsequently developed shortness of breath and nausea. The patient died 5 days later with signs and symptoms of acute diffuse myocarditis.

CNS – Chills; depression; fatigue; headache; insomnia; irritability; mood swings; paresthesia; tremors; fever; rigors; vertigo; dizziness; drowsiness; lethargy.

Dermatologic – Erythema nodosum; photosensitivity; erythema; hot flashes; rash/itching; alopecia.

GI – Pancreatitis; diarrhea with dehydration; increased blood in stool; rectal bleeding; flare in symptoms; rectal discomfort; epigastric discomfort; flatulence.

In a double-blind, placebo-controlled study, increased frequency and severity of diarrhea were reported in patients randomized to olsalazine 500 mg twice daily with concomitant pelvic radiation.

GU – Frequency; dysuria; hematuria; proteinuria; nephrotic syndrome; interstitial nephritis; impotence; menorrhagia.

Hematologic – Leukopenia; neutropenia; lymphopenia; eosinophilia; thrombocytopenia; anemia; hemolytic anemia; reticulocytosis.

Hepatic – Rare cases of granulomatous hepatitis and nonspecific, reactive hepatitis have been reported in patients receiving olsalazine. Additionally, a patient developed mild cholestatic hepatitis during treatment with sulfasalazine and experienced the same symptoms 2 weeks later after the treatment was changed to olsalazine. Withdrawal of olsalazine led to complete recovery in these cases.

Lab test abnormalities – ALT or AST elevated beyond the normal range.

Musculoskeletal – Muscle cramps.

Respiratory – Upper respiratory tract infection.

Special senses – Tinnitus; dry mouth; dry eyes; watery eyes; blurred vision.

➤*Postmarketing reports:* The following events have been identified during postapproval use of products that contain (or are metabolized to) mesalamine in clinical practice. Because they are reported voluntarily from a population of unknown size, estimates of frequency cannot be made. These events have been chosen for inclusion due to a combination of seriousness, frequency of reporting, or potential causal connection to mesalamine.

Reports of hepatotoxicity, including elevated liver function tests (AST, ALT, GGT, LDH, alkaline phosphatase, bilirubin), jaundice, cholestatic jaundice, cirrhosis, and possible hepatocellular damage including liver necrosis and liver failure. Some of these cases were fatal. One case of Kawasaki-like syndrome that included hepatic function changes was also reported.

Overdosage

Symptoms of acute toxicity were decreased motor activity and diarrhea in all species tested and in addition, vomiting in dogs.

➤*Animal toxicology:* Preclinical subacute and chronic toxicity studies in rats have shown the kidney to be the major target organ of olsalazine toxicity. At an oral daily dose of greater than or equal to 400 mg/kg, olsalazine treatment produced nephritis and tubular necrosis in a 4-week study; interstitial nephritis and tubular calcinosis in a 6-month study, and renal fibrosis, mineralization, and transitional cell hyperplasia in a 1-year study.

Patient Information

Patients should be instructed to take olsalazine with food. The drug should be taken in evenly divided doses. Patients should be informed that approximately 17% of subjects receiving olsalazine during clinical studies reported diarrhea sometime during therapy. If diarrhea occurs, patients should contact their physician.

BALSALAZIDE DISODIUM

Rx	**Colazal** (Salix)	**Capsules:** 750 mg	≈ 86 mg sodium. (CZ). Beige. In 280s.

BALSALAZIDE DISODIUM — ORAL

Indications

➤*Ulcerative colitis:* Balsalazide disodium is indicated for the treatment of mildly to moderately active ulcerative colitis. Safety and efficacy of balsalazide disodium beyond 12 weeks have not been established.

Administration and Dosage

➤*Approved by the FDA:* July 18, 2000.

➤*Dosage:* For treatment of active ulcerative colitis the usual dose in adults is 3 balsalazide disodium 750 mg capsules to be taken 3 times a day for a total daily dose of 6.75 g for a duration of 8 weeks. Some patients in the clinical trials required treatment for up to 12 weeks.

➤*Storage/Stability:* Store at 25°C (77°F); excursions permitted to 15° to 30°C (59° to 86°F).

Actions

➤*Pharmacology:* Balsalazide disodium is delivered intact to the colon where it is cleaved by bacterial azoreduction to release equimolar quantities of mesalamine, which is the therapeutically active portion of the molecule, and 4-aminobenzoyl-β-alanine. The recommended dose of 6.75 g/day, for the treatment of active disease, provides 2.4 g of free 5-aminosalicylic acid to the colon.

The 4-aminobenzoyl-β-alanine carrier moiety released when balsalazide disodium is cleaved is only minimally absorbed and largely inert. The mechanism of action of 5-aminosalicylic acid is unknown, but appears to be topical rather than systemic. Mucosal production of arachidonic acid metabolites, both through the cyclooxygenase pathways (ie, prostanoids), and through the lipoxygenase pathways (ie, leukotrienes and hydroxyeicosatetraenoic acids) is increased in patients with chronic inflammatory bowel disease, and it is possible that 5-aminosalicylic acid diminishes inflammation by blocking production of arachidonic acid metabolites in the colon.

BALSALAZIDE DISODIUM — ORAL

➤*Pharmacokinetics:*

Absorption – In healthy individuals, the systemic absorption of intact balsalazide was very low and variable. The mean C_{max} occurs approximately 1 to 2 hours after single oral doses of 1.5 g or 2.25 g. The absolute bioavailability of this compound was not determined. In a study of ulcerative colitis patients receiving balsalazide, 1.5 g twice daily, for over 1 year, systemic drug exposure, based on mean AUC values, was up to 60 times greater (8 ng•hr/mL to 480 ng•hr/mL) after equivalent multiple doses of 1.5 g twice daily when compared to healthy subjects who received the same dose. There was a large intersubject variability in the plasma concentration of balsalazide vs time profiles in all studies, thus its half-life could not be determined. The effect of food intake on the absorption of this compound was not studied.

Distribution – The binding of balsalazide to human plasma proteins was ≥ 99%.

Metabolism – Balsalazide disodium capsules contain granules of balsalazide disodium which are insoluble in acid and designed to be delivered to the colon intact. Upon reaching the colon, bacterial azoreductases cleave the compound to release 5-aminosalicylic acid, the therapeutically active portion of the molecule, and 4-aminobenzoyl-β-alanine.

The products of the azoreduction of this compound, 5-aminosalicylic acid and 4-aminobenzoyl-β-alanine, and their N-acetylated metabolites have been identified in plasma, urine, and feces.

Excretion – Less than 1% of an oral dose was recovered as parent compound, 5-aminosalicylic acid or 4-aminobenzoyl-β-alanine in the urine of healthy subjects after single and multiple doses of balsalazide disodium, while up to 25% of the dose was recovered as the N-acetylated metabolites. In a study with 10 healthy volunteers, 65% of a single 2.25 g dose of balsalazide disodium was recovered as 5-aminosalicylic acid, 4-aminobenzoyl-β-alanine, and the N-acetylated metabolites in feces, while less than 1% of the dose was recovered as parent compound.

In a study that examined the disposition of balsalazide in patients who were taking 3 to 6 g of balsalazide disodium daily for more than 1 year and who were in remission from ulcerative colitis, less than 1% of an oral dose was recovered as intact balsalazide in the urine. Less than 4% of the dose was recovered as 5-aminosalicylic acid, while virtually no 4-aminobenzoyl-β-alanine was detected in urine. The urinary recovery of the N-acetylated metabolites comprised 20% to 25% of the balsalazide dose. No fecal recovery studies were performed in this population.

Contraindications

Hypersensitivity to salicylates or to any of the components of balsalazide disodium capsules or balsalazide metabolites.

Warnings

➤*Renal function impairment:* There have been no reported incidents of renal impairment in patients taking balsalazide disodium. At doses up to 2,000 mg/kg (approximately 21 times the recommended 6.75 g/day dose on a mg/kg basis for a 70 kg person), balsalazide disodium had no nephrotoxic effects in rats or dogs. Renal toxicity has been observed in animals and patients given other mesalamine products. Therefore, caution should be exercised when administering balsalazide disodium to patients with known renal dysfunction or a history of renal disease.

➤*Mutagenesis:* Balsalazide disodium was not genotoxic in the following in vitro or in vivo tests: Ames test human lymphocyte chromosomal aberration test, mouse lymphoma cell (L5178Y/TK+/−) forward mutation test, or mouse micronucleus test. However, it was genotoxic in the in vitro Chinese hamster lung cell (CH V79/HGPRT) forward mutation test. 4-aminobenzoyl-β-alanine, a metabolite of balsalazide disodium, was not genotoxic in the Ames test and the mouse lymphoma cell (L5178Y/TK+/−) forward mutation test, but was positive in the human lymphocyte chromosomal aberration test. N-acetyl-4-aminobenzoyl-β-alanine, a conjugated metabolite of balsalazide disodium, was not genotoxic in the Ames test, the mouse lymphoma cell (L5178Y/TK+/−) forward mutation tests, or the human lymphocyte chromosomal aberration test.

➤*Pregnancy:* Category B.

Teratogenic – Reproduction studies were performed in rats and rabbits at oral doses up to 2 g/kg/day, 2.4 and 4.7 times the recommended human dose based on body surface area for the rat and rabbit, respectively, and revealed no evidence of impaired fertility or harm to the fetus due to balsalazide disodium. There are, however, no adequate and well-controlled studies in pregnant women. Because animal reproduction studies are not always predictive of human response, this drug should be used during pregnancy only if clearly needed.

➤*Lactation:* It is not known whether balsalazide disodium is excreted in human milk. Because many drugs are excreted in human milk, caution should be exercised when balsalazide disodium is administered to a breastfeeding woman.

➤*Children:* Safety and efficacy of balsalazide disodium in pediatric patients have not been established.

Precautions

➤*Exacerbation of colitis symptoms:* Of the 259 patients treated with balsalazide disodium 6.75 g/day in controlled clinical trials of active disease, exacerbation of the symptoms of colitis, possibly related to drug use, has been reported by 3 patients.

➤*Pyloric stenosis:* Patients with pyloric stenosis may have prolonged gastric retention of balsalazide disodium capsules.

Drug Interactions

➤*Oral antibiotics:* No drug interaction studies have been conducted for balsalazide disodium; however the use of orally administered antibiotics could, theoretically, interfere with the release of mesalamine in the colon.

Adverse Reactions

Over 1,000 patients received treatment with balsalazide disodium in domestic and foreign clinical trials. In 4 controlled clinical trials patients receiving a balsalazide disodium dose of 6.75 g/day most frequently reported the following reactions (reporting frequency ≥ 3%), headache (8%), abdominal pain (6%), diarrhea (5%), nausea (5%), vomiting (4%), respiratory tract infection (4%), and arthralgia (4%). Withdrawal from therapy due to adverse reactions was comparable among patients on balsalazide disodium and placebo.

Adverse reactions reported by 1% or more of patients who participated in the 4 well-controlled, Phase 3 trials are presented by treatment group.

Adverse reactions occurring in at least 1% of balsalazide disodium and ulcerative colitis patients in controlled trials		
Adverse reaction	Balsalazide disodium 6.75 g/day (n = 259)	Placebo (n = 35)
Abdominal pain	16 (6%)	1 (3%)
Anorexia	4 (2%)	
Arthralgia	9 (4%)	-
Back pain	4 (2%)	1 (3%)
Constipation	3 (1%)	
Coughing	4 (2%)	-
Cramps	3 (1%)	-
Diarrhea	14 (5%)	1 (3%)
Dizziness	3 (1%)	2 (6%)
Dry mouth	3 (1%)	-
Dyspepsia	5 (2%)	-
Fatigue	6 (2%)	-
Flatulence	5 (2%)	-
Fever	5 (2%)	-
Flu-like disorder	3 (1%)	-
Frequent stools	3 (1%)	1 (3%)
Headache	22 (8%)	3 (9%)
Insomnia	6 (2%)	-
Myalgia	3 (1%)	-
Nausea	14 (5%)	2 (6%)
Pain	4 (2%)	1 (3%)
Pharyngitis	4 (2%)	-
Rectal bleeding	5 (2%)	1 (3%)
Respiratory	9 (4%)	5 (14%)
Rhinitis	6 (2%)	-
Sinusitis	3 (1%)	1 (3%)
Urinary tract	3 (1%)	-
Vomiting	11 (4%)	2 (6%)

The number of placebo patients is too small for valid comparisons. Some adverse reactions, such as abdominal pain, fatigue, and nausea were reported more frequently in women subjects than in men. Abdominal pain, rectal bleeding, and anemia can be part of the clinical presentation of ulcerative colitis.

➤*Infrequently reported adverse reactions:* The following adverse reactions, presented by body system, have also been infrequently reported by patients taking balsalazide disodium during clinical trials (n = 513) for the treatment of active acute ulcerative colitis or from foreign postmarketing reports. In most cases no relationship to balsalazide disodium has been established.

Cardiovascular – Bradycardia, deep venous thrombosis, hypertension, leg ulcer, palpitations, pericarditis.

CNS – Aphasia, dysphonia, gait abnormal, hypertonia, hypoesthesia, paresis, spasm generalized, tremor.

Dermatologic – Alopecia, angioedema, dermatitis, dry skin, erythema nodosum, erythematous rash, pruritus, pruritus ani, psoriasis, skin ulceration.

GI – Amylase increased, bowel irregularity, colitis ulcerative aggravated, diarrhea with blood, diverticulosis, epigastric pain, eructation, fecal incontinence, feces abnormal, gastroenteritis, giardiasis, glossitis, hemorrhoids, melena, neoplasm benign, pancreatitis, ulcerative stomatitis, stools frequent, tenesmus, tongue discoloration.

GU – Menstrual disorder, hematuria, interstitial nephritis, micturition frequency, polyuria, pyuria.

Hematologic – Anemia, epistaxis, fibrinogen plasma increase, hemorrhage, prothrombin decrease, prothrombin increase, thrombocythemia.

Hepatic – Bilirubin increase, hepatic function abnormal, SGOT increase, SGPT increase.

Immunologic – Abscess, immunoglobulins decrease, infection, moniliasis, viral infection.

Lymphatic – Eosinophilia, granulocytopenia, leukocytosis, leukopenia, lymphadenopathy, lymphoma-like disorder, lymphopenia.

BALSALAZIDE DISODIUM — ORAL

Metabolic/Nutritional – Creatinine phosphokinase increased, hypocalcemia, hypokalemia, hypoproteinemia, LDH increase, weight decrease, weight increase.

Musculoskeletal – Arthritis, arthropathy, stiffness in legs.

Psychiatric – Anxiety, depression, nervousness, somnolence.

Respiratory – Bronchospasm, dyspnea, hemoptysis.

Special senses – Conjunctivitis, earache, ear infection, iritis, parosmia, taste perversion, tinnitus, vision abnormal.

Miscellaneous – Abdomen enlarged, asthenia, chest pain, chills, edema, hot flushes, malaise.

➤*Postmarketing reports:* The following reactions have been identified during postapproval use in clinical practice, of products which contain (or are metabolized to) mesalamine. Because they are reported voluntarily from a population of unknown size, estimates of frequency cannot be made. These reactions have been chosen for inclusion due to a combination of seriousness, frequency of reporting, or potential causal connection to mesalamine.

Hepatic – Reports of hepatotoxicity, including elevated liver function tests (AST, ALT, GGT, LDH, alkaline phosphatase, bilirubin), jaundice, cholestatic jaundice, cirrhosis, hepatocellular damage including liver necrosis and liver failure. Some of these cases were fatal, however, no fatalities associated with these reactions were reported in balsalazide disodium clinical trials. One case of Kawasaki-like syndrome, which included hepatic function changes, was also reported, however; this event was not reported in balsalazide disodium clinical trials.

Overdosage

No case of overdose has occurred with balsalazide disodium. A 3-year-old boy is reported to have ingested 2 g of another mesalamine product. He was treated with ipecac and activated charcoal with no adverse reactions.

If an overdose occurs with balsalazide disodium use, treatment should be supportive, with particular attention to correction of electrolyte abnormalities.

SULFASALAZINE

Rx	**Sulfasalazine** (Various, eg, Mutual Pharm, Watson)	**Tablets:** 500 mg	In 50s, 100s, 500s, and 1,000s.
Rx	**Azulfidine** (Pfizer)		(101 KPh). Gold, scored. In 100s, 300s, and UD 100s.
Rx	**Sulfasalazine** (Greenstone)	**Tablets, delayed-release:** 500 mg	(104). Gold, elliptical. Enteric coated. In 100s and 300s.
Rx	**Azulfidine EN-tabs** (Pfizer)		(102 KPh). Gold, elliptical. Enteric coated. In 100s and 300s.

SULFASALAZINE — ORAL

Indications

➤*Tablets and delayed-release tablets:* Treatment of mild-to-moderate ulcerative colitis, and as adjunctive therapy in severe ulcerative colitis, and for the prolongation of the remission period between acute attacks of ulcerative colitis.

➤*Delayed-release tablets:* Treatment of patients with rheumatoid arthritis who have responded inadequately to salicylates or other nonsteroidal anti-inflammatory drugs (NSAIDs) (eg, an insufficient therapeutic response to, or intolerance of, an adequate trial of full doses of 1 or more nonsteroidal anti-inflammatory drugs).

Sulfasalazine delayed-release tablets are also indicated in the treatment of pediatric patients with polyarticular-course juvenile rheumatoid arthritis who have responded inadequately to salicylates or other NSAIDs.

Sulfasalazine enteric-coated, delayed-release tablets are particularly indicated in patients with ulcerative colitis who cannot take uncoated sulfasalazine tablets because of GI intolerance, and in whom there is evidence that this intolerance is not primarily the result of high blood levels of sulfapyridine and its metabolites (eg, patients experiencing nausea and vomiting with the first few doses of the drug, or patients in whom a reduction in dosage does not alleviate the adverse GI effects).

In patients with rheumatoid arthritis or juvenile rheumatoid arthritis, continue rest and physiotherapy as indicated. Unlike anti-inflammatory drugs, sulfasalazine delayed-release tablets do not produce an immediate response. Concurrent treatment with analgesics or NSAIDs is recommended at least until the effect of sulfasalazine delayed-release tablets is apparent.

➤*Unlabeled uses:* Ankylosing spondylitis; Crohn disease; granulomatous colitis; regional enteritis.

Administration and Dosage

➤*Approved by the FDA:* April 6, 1983.

Adjust dosage to each individual's response and tolerance.

Instruct patients to take sulfasalazine tablets in evenly divided doses, preferably after meals, and to swallow the tablets whole.

Some patients may be sensitive to treatment with sulfasalazine. Various desensitization-like regimens have been reported to be effective in 34 of 53 patients, 7 of 8 patients, and 19 of 20 patients. These regimens suggest starting with a total daily dose of 50 to 250 mg sulfasalazine initially, and doubling it every 4 to 7 days thereafter until the desired therapeutic level is achieved. If the symptoms of sensitivity recur, discontinue sulfasalazine. Do not attempt desensitization in patients who have a history of agranulocytosis or who have experienced an anaphylactoid reaction while on a previous course of sulfasalazine therapy.

➤*Ulcerative colitis:* The response of acute ulcerative colitis to sulfasalazine can be evaluated by clinical criteria, including the presence of fever, weight changes, and degree and frequency of diarrhea and bleeding, as well as by sigmoidoscopy and the evaluation of biopsy samples. It is often necessary to continue medication even when clinical symptoms, including diarrhea, have been controlled. When endoscopic examination confirms satisfactory improvement, reduce dosage of sulfasalazine to a maintenance level. If diarrhea recurs, increase dosage to previously effective levels.

If symptoms of gastric intolerance (eg, anorexia, nausea, vomiting) occur after the first few doses of sulfasalazine, they are probably due to increased serum levels of total sulfapyridine, and may be alleviated by halving the daily dose of sulfasalazine and subsequently increasing it gradually over several days. If gastric intolerance continues, stop the drug for 5 to 7 days, then reintroduce at a lower daily dose.

Initial therapy –

Adults: 3 to 4 g daily in evenly divided doses with dosage intervals not exceeding 8 hours. It may be advisable to initiate therapy with a lower dosage (eg, 1 to 2 g daily) to reduce possible GI intolerance. If daily doses exceeding 4 g are required to achieve the desired therapeutic effect, keep in mind the increased risk of toxicity.

Children 6 years of age and older: 40 to 60 mg/kg of body weight in each 24-hour period, divided into 3 to 6 doses.

Maintenance therapy –

Adults: 2 g daily.

Children 6 years of age and older: 30 mg/kg of body weight in each 24-hour period, divided into 4 doses.

➤*Adult rheumatoid arthritis:*

Delayed-release tablets – 2 g daily in 2 evenly divided doses. It is advisable to initiate therapy with a lower dosage of sulfasalazine delayed-release tablets (eg, 0.5 to 1 g daily) to reduce possible GI intolerance. A suggested dosing schedule is given below.

Suggested Dosing Schedule for Adult Rheumatoid Arthritis

Week of treatment	Number of sulfasalazine delayed-release tablets	
	Morning	Evening
1	-	1
2	1	1
3	1	2
4	2	2

In rheumatoid arthritis, the effect of sulfasalazine can be assessed by the degree of improvement in the number and extent of actively inflamed joints. A therapeutic response has been observed as early as 4 weeks after starting treatment with sulfasalazine delayed-release tablets, but treatment for 12 weeks may be required in some patients before clinical benefit is noted. Consideration can be given to increasing the daily dose of sulfasalazine delayed-release tablets to 3 g if the clinical response after 12 weeks is inadequate. Careful monitoring is recommended for doses over 2 g/day.

➤*Juvenile rheumatoid arthritis (polyarticular course):*

Delayed-release tablets – Children 6 years of age and older should take 30 to 50 mg/kg of body weight daily in 2 evenly divided doses. Typically, the maximum dose is 2 g/day. To reduce possible GI intolerance, begin with a quarter to a third of the planned maintenance dose and increase weekly until reaching the maintenance dose at 1 month.

➤*Storage/Stability:* Store at 25°C (77°F); excursions permitted to 15° to 30°C (59° to 86°F).

Actions

➤*Pharmacokinetics:*

Absorption – In vivo studies have indicated that the absolute bioavailability of orally administered SSZ is less than 15% for parent drug. In the intestine, SSZ is metabolized by intestinal bacteria to SP and 5-ASA. Of the 2 species, SP is relatively well absorbed from the intestine and highly metabolized, while 5-ASA is much less well absorbed.

Following oral administration of 1 g of SSZ to 9 healthy males, less than 15% of a dose of SSZ is absorbed as parent drug. Detectable serum concentrations of SSZ have been found in healthy subjects within 90 minutes after the ingestion. Maximum concentrations of SSZ occur between 3 and 12 hours postingestion, with the mean peak concentration (6 mcg/mL) occurring at 6 hours.

In comparison, peak plasma levels of both SP and 5-ASA occur approximately 10 hours after dosing. This longer time to peak is indicative of GI transit to the lower intestine, where bacteria-mediated metabolism occurs. SP apparently is well absorbed from the colon, with an estimated bioavailability of 60%. In this same study, 5-ASA is much less well absorbed from the GI tract, with an estimated bioavailability of 10% to 30%.

SULFASALAZINE — ORAL

Distribution – Following IV injection, the calculated volume of distribution (Vd_{ss}) for SSZ was 7.5 ± 1.6 L. SSZ is highly bound to albumin (greater than 99.3%), while SP is only about 70% bound to albumin. Acetylsulfapyridine (AcSP), the principal metabolite of SP, is approximately 90% bound to plasma proteins.

Metabolism – As mentioned above, SSZ is metabolized by intestinal bacteria to SP and 5-ASA. Approximately 15% of a dose of SSZ is absorbed as parent and is metabolized to some extent in the liver to the same 2 species. The observed plasma half-life for IV sulfasalazine is 7.6 ± 3.4 hours. The primary route of metabolism of SP is via acetylation to form AcSP. The rate of metabolism of SP to AcSP is dependent upon acetylator phenotype. In fast acetylators, the mean plasma half-life of SP is 10.4 hours, while in slow acetylators, it is 14.8 hours. SP can also be metabolized to 5-hydroxysulfapyridine (SPOH) and N-acetyl-5-hydroxy-sulfapyridine. 5-ASA is primarily metabolized in both the liver and intestine to N-acetyl-5-aminosalicylic acid via a nonacetylation, phenotype-dependent route. Due to low plasma levels produced by 5-ASA after oral administration, reliable estimates of plasma half-life are not possible.

Excretion – Absorbed SP and 5-ASA and their metabolites are primarily eliminated in the urine either as free metabolites or as glucuronide conjugates. The majority of 5-ASA stays within the colonic lumen and is excreted as 5-ASA and acetyl-5-ASA with the feces. The calculated clearance of SSZ following IV administration was 1 L/h. Renal clearance was estimated to account for 37% of total clearance.

Special populations –

Elderly: Elderly patients with rheumatoid arthritis showed a prolonged plasma half-life for SSZ, SP, and their metabolites. The clinical impact of this is unknown.

Children: Small studies have been reported in the literature in children down to the age of 4 years with ulcerative colitis and inflammatory bowel disease. In these populations, relative to adults, the pharmacokinetics of SSZ and SP correlated poorly with either age or dose.

Acetylator status: The metabolism of SP to AcSP is mediated by polymorphic enzymes such that 2 distinct populations of slow and fast metabolizers exist. Approximately 60% of the white population can be classified as belonging to the slow acetylator phenotype. These subjects will display a prolonged plasma half-life for SP (14.8 vs 10.4 hours) and an accumulation of higher plasma levels of SP than fast acetylators. The clinical implication of this is unclear; however, in a small pharmacokinetic trial where acetylator status was determined, subjects who were slow acetylators of SP showed a higher incidence of adverse reactions.

Contraindications

Hypersensitivity to sulfasalazine, its metabolites, sulfonamides, or salicylates; intestinal or urinary obstruction; porphyria.

Warnings

➤*Deaths:* Deaths associated with the administration of sulfasalazine have been reported from hypersensitivity reactions, agranulocytosis, aplastic anemia, other blood dyscrasias, renal and liver damage, irreversible, neuromuscular and CNS changes, and fibrosing alveolitis.

➤*Blood dyscrasis:* Only administer sulfasalazine to patients with blood dyscrasis after critical appraisal.

The presence of clinical signs such as sore throat, fever, pallor, purpura, or jaundice may be indications for serious blood disorders.

➤*Hypersensitivity reactions:* Give sulfasalazine with caution to patients with severe allergy or bronchial asthma. Adequate fluid intake must be maintained in order to prevent crystalluria and stone formation. Observe patients with glucose-6-phosphate dehydrogenase deficiency closely for signs of hemolytic anemia. This reaction is frequently dose related. If toxic or hypersensitivity reactions occur, discontinue the drug immediately.

➤*Renal/Hepatic function impairment:* Use sulfasalazine only after a critical appraisal in patients with hepatic or renal damage.

➤*Carcinogenesis:* Two-year oral carcinogenicity studies were conducted in male and female F344/N rats and B6C3F1 mice. Sulfasalazine was tested at 84 (496 mg/m^2), 168 (991 mg/m^2), and 337.5 (1,991 mg/m^2) mg/kg/day doses in rats. A statistically significant increase in the incidence of urinary bladder transitional cell papillomas was observed in male rats. In female rats, 2 (4%) of the 337.5 mg/kg rats had transitional cell papilloma of the kidney. The increased incidence of neoplasms in the urinary bladder and kidney of rats was also associated with an increase in the renal calculi formation and hyperplasia of transitional cell epithelium. For the mouse study, sulfasalazine was tested at 675 (2,025 mg/m^2), 1,350 (4,050 mg/m^2) and 2,700 (8,100 mg/m^2) mg/kg/day. The incidence of hepatocellular adenoma or carcinoma in male and female mice was significantly greater than the control at all doses tested.

➤*Mutagenesis:* Sulfasalazine did not show mutagenicity in the bacterial reverse mutation assay (Ames test) or in the L51784 mouse lymphoma cell assay at the HGPRT gene. However, sulfasalazine showed equivocal mutagenic response in the micronucleus assay of mouse and rat bone marrow and mouse peripheral RBC and in the sister chromatid exchange, chromosomal aberration, and micronucleus assays in lymphocytes obtained from humans.

➤*Fertility impairment:* Impairment of male fertility was observed in reproductive studies performed in rats at a dose of 800 mg/kg/day (4,800 mg/m^2). Oligospermia and infertility have been described in men treated with sulfasalazine. Withdrawal of the drug appears to reverse these effects.

➤*Pregnancy:* Category B.

Teratogenic – Reproduction studies have been performed in rats and rabbits at doses up to 6 times the human dose and have revealed no evidence of impaired female fertility or harm to the fetus due to sulfasalazine. There are, however, no adequate and well-controlled studies in pregnant women. Because animal reproduction studies are not always predictive of human response, use this drug during pregnancy only if clearly needed.

Nonteratogenic – Sulfasalazine and sulfapyridine pass the placental barrier. Although sulfapyridine has been shown to have poor bilirubin-displacing capacity, keep in mind the potential for kernicterus in newborns.

A case of agranulocytosis has been reported in an infant whose mother was taking both sulfasalazine and prednisone throughout pregnancy.

➤*Lactation:* Exercise caution when sulfasalazine is administered to a breast-feeding mother. Sulfonamides are excreted in the milk. In the newborn, they compete with bilirubin for binding sites on the plasma proteins and may cause kernicterus. Insignificant amounts of uncleaved sulfasalazine have been found in milk, whereas the sulfapyridine levels in milk are about 30% to 60% of those in the maternal serum. Sulfapyridine has been shown to have a poor bilirubin-displacing capacity.

➤*Children:* The safety and efficacy of sulfasalazine in pediatric patients below the age of 2 years with ulcerative colitis have not been established.

Delayed-release tablets – The safety and efficacy of sulfasalazine for the treatment of the signs and symptoms of polyarticular-course juvenile rheumatoid arthritis in pediatric patients aged 6 to 16 years is supported by evidence from adequate and well-controlled studies in adult rheumatoid arthritis patients. The extrapolation from adults with rheumatoid arthritis to children with polyarticular-course juvenile rheumatoid arthritis is based on similarities in disease and response to therapy between these 2 patient populations. Published studies support the extrapolation of safety and efficacy for sulfasalazine to polyarticular-course juvenile rheumatoid arthritis.

It has been reported that the frequency of adverse reactions in patients with systemic-course of juvenile arthritis is high. Use in children with systemic-course juvenile rheumatoid arthritis has frequently resulted in a serum sickness-like reaction. This reaction is often severe and presents as fever, nausea, vomiting, headache, rash, and abnormal liver function tests. Treatment of systemic-course juvenile rheumatoid arthritis with sulfasalazine is not recommended.

Precautions

➤*Monitoring:* Perform complete blood counts, including differential white cell count and liver function tests, before starting sulfasalazine and every second week during the first 3 months of therapy. During the second 3 months, do the same tests once monthly and thereafter once every 3 months, and as clinically indicated. Do urinalysis and an assessment of renal function periodically during treatment with sulfasalazine.

The determination of serum sulfapyridine levels may be useful since concentrations greater than 50 mcg/mL appear to be associated with an increased incidence of adverse reactions.

➤*Undisintegrated tablets:* Isolated instances have been reported when sulfasalazine delayed-release tablets have passed undisintegrated. If this is observed, discontinue the administration of sulfasalazine delayed-release tablets immediately.

Drug Interactions

Sulfasalazine Drug Interactions

Precipitant drug	Object drug[a]		Description
Sulfasalazine	Cyclosporine	⬇⬆	Cyclosporine serum levels may be decreased. The risk of nephrotoxicity may be increased.
Sulfasalazine	Digoxin	⬇	Reduced absorption of digoxin has been reported when coadministered with sulfasalazine.
Sulfasalazine	Folic acid	⬇	Reduced GI absorption of folic acid has been reported when coadministered with sulfasalazine. Periodically monitor patients taking sulfasalazine. If folate deficiency is noted, potential treatment measures include increasing dietary folate, giving sulfasalazine between meals, and administering additional folic acid or folinic acid.
Sulfasalazine	Methotrexate	⬆	Sulfonamides (eg, sulfasalazine) may displace methotrexate from protein binding and decrease renal clearance, therefore increasing the risk of methotrexate-induced bone marrow suppression. Monitor for hematologic toxicity. In addition, the overall toxicity profile of this combination revealed an increased incidence of GI adverse reactions, especially nausea.

SULFASALAZINE — ORAL

Sulfasalazine Drug Interactions			
Precipitant drug	Object drug[a]		Description
Sulfasalazine	Sulfonylureas (eg, glipizide)	↑	Sulfonamides (eg, sulfasalazine) may impair hepatic metabolism of sulfonylureas or alter plasma protein binding. Monitor blood glucose and decrease the sulfonylurea dose as necessary.
Sulfasalazine	Thiopurines (eg, azathioprine, mercaptopurine)	↑	The risk of leukopenia may be increased due to inhibition of the thiopurine-metabolizing enzyme by sulfasalazine. Closely monitor leukocyte counts.
Sulfasalazine	Warfarin	↑	Anticoagulant effect of warfarin may be increased. Monitor closely.

[a] ↑ = Object drug increased. ↓ = Object drug decreased.

Adverse Reactions

➤*Most common adverse reactions:*

Miscellaneous – The most common adverse reactions associated with sulfasalazine in ulcerative colitis are anorexia, headache, nausea, vomiting, gastric distress, and apparently reversible oligospermia. These occur in about one-third of the patients. Less frequent adverse reactions are skin rash, pruritus, urticaria, fever, Heinz body anemia, hemolytic anemia, and cyanosis which may occur at a frequency of 1 in every 30 patients or less. Experience suggests that with a daily dosage of 4 g of more, or total serum sulfapyridine levels above 50 mcg/mL, the incidence of adverse reactions tends to increase.

Delayed-release tablets: Similar adverse reactions are associated with sulfasalazine use in adult rheumatoid arthritis, although there was a greater incidence of some reactions. In rheumatoid arthritis studies, the following common adverse reactions were noted: nausea (19%), dyspepsia (13%), rash (13%), headache (9%), abdominal pain (8%), vomiting (8%), fever (5%), dizziness (4%), stomatitis (4%), pruritus (4%), abnormal liver function tests (4%), leukopenia (3%), and thrombocytopenia (1%). One report showed a 10% rate of immunoglobulin suppression, which was slowly reversible and rarely accompanied by clinical findings.

In general, the adverse reactions in juvenile rheumatoid arthritis patients are similar to those seen in patients with adult rheumatoid arthritis except for a high frequency of serum sickness-like syndrome in systemic-course juvenile rheumatoid arthritis (see Warnings, Children). One clinical trial showed an approximate 10% rate of immunoglobulin suppression.

➤*Less common or rare adverse reactions:* Although the following listing includes a few adverse reactions that have not been reported with this specific drug, the pharmacological similarities among the sulfonamides require that each of these reactions be considered when sulfasalazine is administered.

CNS – Transverse myelitis, convulsions, meningitis, transient lesions of the posterior spinal column, cauda equina syndrome, Guillain-Barre syndrome, peripheral neuropathy, mental depression, vertigo, hearing loss, insomnia, ataxia, hallucinations, tinnitus and drowsiness.

GI – Hepatitis, pancreatitis, bloody diarrhea, impaired folic acid absorption, impaired digoxin absorption, stomatitis, diarrhea, abdominal pains, and neutropenic enterocolitis.

Hematologic –

Blood dyscrasias: Aplastic anemia, agranulocytosis, leukopenia, megaloblastic (macrocytic) anemia, purpura, thrombocytopenia, hypoprothrombinemia, methemoglobinemia, congenital neutropenia, and myleodysplastic syndrome.

Hypersensitivity – Erythema multiforme (Stevens-Johnson syndrome); exfoliative dermatitis; epidermal necrolysis (Lyell's syndrome) with corneal damage; anaphylaxis; serum sickness syndrome; pneumonitis with or without eosinophilia; vasculitis; fibrosing alveolitis; pleuritis; pericarditis with or without tamponade; allergic myocarditis; polyarteritis nodosa; lupus erythematosus-like syndrome; hepatitis and hepatic necrosis with or without immune complexes; fulminant hepatitis, sometimes leading to liver transplantation; parapsoriasis varioliformis acuta (Mucha-Haberman syndrome); rhabdomyolysis; photosensitization; arthralgia; periorbital edema; conjunctival and scleral injection; and alopecia.

Renal – Toxic nephrosis with oliguria and anuria, nephritis, nephrotic syndrome, hematuria, crystalluria, proteinuria, and hemolytic-uremic syndrome.

Miscellaneous – Urine discoloration and skin discoloration.

The sulfonamides bear certain chemical similarities to some goitrogens, diuretics (acetazolamide and the thiazides), and oral hypoglycemic agents. Goiter production, diuresis, and hypoglycemia have occurred rarely in patients receiving sulfonamides. Cross sensitivity may exist with these agents. Rats appear to be especially susceptible to the goitrogenic effects of sulfonamides, and long-term administration has produced thyroid malignancies in this species.

➤*Postmarketing reports:*

GI – Reports of hepatotoxicity, including elevated liver function tests (AST, ALT, gamma-glutamyl transferase [GGT], lactic dehydrogenase [LDH], alkaline phosphatase, bilirubin), jaundice, cholestatic jaundice, cirrhosis, and possible hepatocellular damage including liver necrosis and liver failure. Some of these cases were fatal. One case of Kawasaki-like syndrome, which included hepatic function changes, was also reported.

Overdosage

➤*Symptoms:* There is evidence that the incidence and severity of toxicity following overdosage are directly related to the total serum sulfapyridine concentration. Symptoms of overdosage may include nausea, vomiting, gastric distress, and abdominal pains. In more advanced cases, CNS symptoms (eg, drowsiness, convulsions) may be observed. Serum sulfapyridine concentrations may be used to monitor the progress of recovery from overdosage.

There are no documented reports of deaths due to ingestion of large single doses of sulfasalazine. It has not been possible to determine the LD_{50} in laboratory animals such as mice, since the highest oral daily dose of sulfasalazine which can be given (12 g/kg) is not lethal; a single oral dose of 12 g/kg was not lethal to mice. Doses of regular sulfasalazine tablets of 16 g/day have been given to patients without mortality.

➤*Treatment:* Gastric lavage or emesis plus catharsis as indicated. Alkalinize urine. If kidney function is normal, force fluids. If anuria is present, restrict fluids and salt, and treat appropriately. Catherization of the ureters may be indicated for complete renal blockage by crystals. The low molecular weight of sulfasalazine and its metabolites may facilitate their removal by dialysis.

Patient Information

Inform patients of the possibility of adverse reactions and of the need for careful medical supervision. The occurrence of sore throat, fever, pallor, purpura, or jaundice may indicate a serious blood disorder. Should any of these occur, the patient should seek medical advice.

Instruct patients to take sulfasalazine in evenly divided doses preferably after meals. Swallow the enteric-coated tablets whole. Additionally, advise patients that sulfasalazine may produce an orange-yellow discoloration of the urine or skin.

➤*Ulcerative colitis:* Patients with ulcerative colitis should be made aware that ulcerative colitis rarely remits completely, and that the risk of relapse can be substantially reduced by continued administration of sulfasalazine tablets at a maintenance dosage.

➤*Delayed-release tablets:*

Rheumatoid arthritis – Rheumatoid arthritis rarely remits. Therefore, continued administration of sulfasalazine is indicated. Patients requiring sulfasalazine should follow up with their physicians to determine the need for continued administration.

LUBIPROSTONE

Rx	Amitiza (Sucampo Pharm/Takeda Pharm)[a]	Capsules: 24 mcg	Sorbitol. (SPI). Orange, oval. In 100s.

[a] Sucampo Pharmaceuticals Inc., 4733 Bethesda Ave., Ste. 450, Bethesda, MD 20814; 301-961-3400; http://www.sucampo.com.

LUBIPROSTONE — ORAL

Indications

➤*Chronic idiopathic constipation:* For the treatment of chronic idiopathic constipation in adults.

Administration and Dosage

➤*Approved by the FDA:* January 31, 2006.

➤*Dosage:* 24 mcg taken twice daily orally with food. Health care providers and patients should periodically assess the need for continued therapy.

➤*Storage/Stability:* Store at 25°C (77°F); excursions permitted to 15° to 30°C (59° to 86°F).

Actions

➤*Pharmacology:* Chronic idiopathic constipation is generally defined by infrequent or difficult passage of stool. The signs and symptoms associated with chronic idiopathic constipation (eg, abdominal pain or discomfort, bloating, straining, hard or lumpy stools) may be the result of abnormal colonic motility that can delay the transit of intestinal contents and impede the evacuation of rectal contents. One approach to the treatment of chronic idiopathic constipation is the secretion of fluid into the abdominal lumen through the activation of chloride channels in the apical membrane of the GI epithelium.

Lubiprostone is a locally acting chloride channel activator that enhances a chloride-rich intestinal fluid secretion without altering sodium and potassium concentrations in the serum. Lubiprostone acts by specifically activat-

LUBIPROSTONE — ORAL

ing ClC-2, which is a normal constituent of the apical membrane of the human intestine, in a protein kinase A-independent fashion. By increasing intestinal fluid secretion, lubiprostone increases motility in the intestine, thereby increasing the passage of stool and alleviating symptoms associated with chronic idiopathic constipation. Patch clamp cell studies in human cell lines have indicated that the majority of the beneficial biological activity of lubiprostone and its metabolites is observed only on the apical (luminal) portion of the GI epithelium.

➤*Pharmacokinetics:*

Absorption – Lubiprostone has low systemic availability following oral administration and concentrations of lubiprostone in plasma are below the level of quantitation (10 pg/mL). Therefore, standard pharmacokinetic parameters such as area under the curve (AUC), maximum effective plasma concentration (C_{max}), and half-life cannot be reliably calculated. However, the pharmacokinetic parameters of M3 (only measurable active metabolite) have been characterized.

Peak plasma levels of M3, after a single, oral dose of lubiprostone 24 mcg occur at approximately 1.14 hours. The C_{max} was 41.9 pg/mL, and the mean AUC was 59.1 pg•h/mL. AUC of M3 increases dose proportionally after single doses of lubiprostone 24 and 144 mcg.

Food effect: A study was conducted with a single dose of ^{3}H-labeled lubiprostone 72 mcg to evaluate the potential of a food effect on lubiprostone absorption, metabolism, and excretion. Pharmacokinetic parameters of total radioactivity demonstrated that C_{max} decreased by 55% while $AUC_{0-\infty}$ was unchanged when lubiprostone was administered with a high-fat meal. The clinical relevance of the effect of food on the pharmacokinetics of lubiprostone is not clear. However, lubiprostone was administered with food in a majority of clinical trials.

Distribution – In vitro protein binding studies indicate lubiprostone is approximately 94% bound to human plasma proteins. Studies in rats with radiolabeled lubiprostone indicate minimal distribution beyond the GI tissues. Concentrations of radiolabeled compound at 48 hours postadministration were minimal in all tissues.

Metabolism – The results of human and animal studies indicate that lubiprostone is rapidly and extensively metabolized by 15-position reduction, α-chain β-oxidation, and ω-chain ω-oxidation. These biotransformations are not mediated by the hepatic cytochrome P-450 system but rather appear to be mediated by the ubiquitously expressed carbonyl reductase. M3, a metabolite of lubiprostone in humans and animals, is formed by the reduction of the carbonyl group at the 15-hydroxy moiety that consists of α-hydroxy and β-hydroxy epimers. M3 makes up less than 10% of the dose of radiolabeled lubiprostone. Animal studies have shown that metabolism of lubiprostone rapidly occurs within the stomach and jejunum, most likely in the absence of any systemic absorption. This is presumed to be the case in humans as well.

Excretion – Lubiprostone could not be detected in plasma; however, M3 has a half-life ranging from 0.9 to 1.4 hours. After a single, oral dose of ^{3}H-labeled lubiprostone 72 mcg, 60% of total administered radioactivity was recovered in the urine within 24 hours and 30% of total administered radioactivity was recovered in the feces by 168 hours. Lubiprostone and M3 are only detected in trace amounts in feces in humans.

Contraindications

Known hypersensitivity to the drug or any of its excipients, and in patients with a history of mechanical GI obstruction.

Warnings

➤*GI obstruction:* Evaluate patients with symptoms suggestive of mechanical GI obstruction prior to initiating lubiprostone treatment.

➤*Carcinogenesis:* Two 2-year oral (gavage) carcinogenicity studies (1 in Crl:B6C3F1 mice and 1 in Sprague-Dawley rats) were conducted with lubiprostone In the 2-year carcinogenicity study in mice, lubiprostone dosages of 25, 75, 200, and 500 mcg/kg/day (approximately 2, 6, 17, and 42 times the recommended human dose, respectively, based on body surface area) were used. In the 2-year rat carcinogenicity study, lubiprostone dosages of 20, 100, and 400 mcg/kg/day (approximately 3, 17, and 68 times the recommended human dosage, respectively, based on body surface area) were used. In the mouse carcinogenicity study, there was no significant increase in any tumor incidences. There was a significant increase in the incidence of interstitial cell adenoma of the testes in male rats at the 400 mcg/kg/day dosage. In female rats, treatment with lubiprostone produced hepatocellular adenoma at the 400 mcg/kg/day dosage.

➤*Pregnancy: Category C.*

Teratogenic – Teratology studies with lubiprostone have been conducted in rats at oral dosages up to 2,000 mcg/kg/day (approximately 332 times the recommended human dosage, based on body surface area), and in rabbits at oral dosages of up to 100 mcg/kg/day (approximately 33 times the recommended human dosage, based on body surface area). Lubiprostone was not teratogenic in rats and rabbits.

In guinea pigs, lubiprostone caused fetal loss at repeated dosages of 10 and 25 mcg/kg/day (approximately 2 and 6 times the human dosage, respectively, based on body surface area) administered on days 40 to 53 of gestation.

There are no adequate and well controlled studies in pregnant women. However, during clinical testing of lubiprostone at 24 mcg twice daily, 4 women became pregnant. Per protocol, lubiprostone was discontinued upon pregnancy detection. Three of the 4 women delivered healthy babies. The fourth woman was monitored for 1 month following discontinuation of study drug, at which time the pregnancy was progressing as expected; the patient was subsequently lost to follow-up.

Only use lubiprostone during pregnancy if the potential benefit justifies the potential risk to the fetus. If a woman is or becomes pregnant while taking the drug, apprise the patient of the potential hazard to the fetus. Women who could become pregnant should have a negative pregnancy test prior to beginning therapy with lubiprostone and should be capable of complying with effective contraceptive measures.

➤*Lactation:* It is not known whether lubiprostone is excreted in human milk. Because many drugs are excreted in human milk and because of the potential for serious adverse reactions in breast-feeding infants from lubiprostone, decide whether to discontinue breast-feeding or the drug, taking into account the importance of the drug to the mother.

➤*Children:* Lubiprostone has not been studied in children.

Precautions

➤*GI effects:* Lubiprostone may cause nausea. If this occurs, coadministration of food with lubiprostone may reduce symptoms of nausea. Do not administer lubiprostone to patients that have severe diarrhea. Patients should be aware of the possible occurrence of diarrhea during treatment.

Drug Interactions

None known.

Adverse Reactions

In clinical trials, 1,429 patients received lubiprostone 24 mcg twice daily or placebo. The following table presents data for the adverse reactions that were reported in at least 1% of patients who received lubiprostone and that occurred more frequently on study drug than placebo. It should be noted that the placebo data presented are from short-term exposure (4 weeks or less) whereas the lubiprostone data are cumulative data that were collected over 3- or 4-week, 6-month, and 12-month observational periods, and that some conditions are common among otherwise healthy patients over a 6-and 12-month observational period.

Lubiprostone Adverse Reactions

Adverse reaction	Placebo (n = 316)	Lubiprostone 24 mcg daily (n = 29)	Lubiprostone 24 mcg twice daily (n = 1,113)	Lubiprostone at any active dose[a] (n = 1,175)
Cardiovascular				
Hypertension	0%	0%	1%	0.9%
CNS				
Anxiety	0.3%	0%	1.4%	1.4%
Depression	0%	0%	1.4%	1.4%
Dizziness	1.3%	3.4%	4.1%	4%
Fatigue	1.9%	6.9%	2.3%	2.5%
Headache	6.6%	3.4%	13.2%	13%
Hypesthesia	0%	3.4%	0.5%	0.6%
Insomnia	0.6%	0%	1.4%	1.4%
GI				
Abdominal discomfort	0%	3.4%	1.5%	1.5%
Abdominal distension	2.2%	0%	7.1%	6.8%
Abdominal pain	2.8%	3.4%	6.7%	6.8%
Abdominal pain, lower	0.6%	0%	1.9%	1.8%
Abdominal pain, upper	1.9%	0%	2.2%	2.1%
Constipation	0.9%	0%	1.1%	1%
Diarrhea	0.9%	10.3%	13.2%	13.2%
Dry mouth	0.3%	0%	1.5%	1.4%
Dyspepsia	1.3%	0%	2.9%	2.7%
Flatulence	1.9%	3.4%	6.1%	5.9%
Gastroenteritis viral	0%	3.4%	1%	1%
Gastroesophageal reflux disease	0.6%	0%	1.8%	1.7%
Loose stools	0%	0%	3.4%	3.2%
Nausea	5.1%	17.2%	31.1%	30.9%
Stomach discomfort	0.3%	0%	1.1%	1%
Vomiting	0.9%	0%	4.6%	4.4%
GU				
Urinary tract infection	1.9%	3.4%	4.4%	4.3%
Metabolic				
Weight increased	0%	0%	1%	0.9%
Musculoskeletal				
Arthralgia	0.3%	0%	3.1%	3%
Back pain	0.9%	3.4%	2.3%	2.3%
Muscle cramp	0%	0%	1%	0.9%
Pain in extremity	0%	3.4%	1.9%	1.9%
Respiratory				
Bronchitis	0.3%	3.4%	1.6%	1.7%
Cough	0.6%	0%	1.6%	1.5%

LUBIPROSTONE — ORAL

Lubiprostone Adverse Reactions				
Adverse reaction	Placebo (n = 316)	Lubiprostone 24 mcg daily (n = 29)	Lubiprostone 24 mcg twice daily (n = 1,113)	Lubiprostone at any active dose[a] (n = 1,175)
Dyspnea	0%	3.4%	2.4%	2.5%
Nasopharyngitis	2.2%	0%	2.9%	2.7%
Pharyngolaryngeal pain	2.2%	0%	1.7%	1.6%
Sinusitis	1.6%	0%	4.9%	4.8%
Upper respiratory tract infection	0.9%	0%	3.7%	3.6%
Miscellaneous				
Chest discomfort	0%	3.4%	1.6%	1.6%
Chest pain	0%	0%	1.1%	1%
Edema peripheral	0.3%	0%	3.8%	3.6%
Influenza	0.6%	0%	2%	1.9%
Pyrexia	0.3%	0%	1.1%	1%
Viral infection	0.3%	3.4%	0.5%	0.6%

[a] Includes patients dosed at 24 mcg daily, 24 mcg twice daily, and 24 mcg three times daily.

➤*Nausea:* Among constipated patients, 31.1% of those receiving lubiprostone 24 mcg twice daily reported nausea. Of those patients, 3.4% reported severe nausea and 8.7% discontinued treatment due to nausea. It should be noted that the incidence of nausea increased in a dose-dependent manner with the lowest overall incidence for nausea seen at the 24 mcg daily dose (17.2%). Further analysis of nausea has shown that long-term exposure to lubiprostone does not appear to place patients at elevated risk for experiencing nausea. In the open-label, long-term studies, patients were allowed to titrate the dosage of lubiprostone down to 24 mcg daily from 24 mcg twice daily if experiencing nausea. It should also be noted that nausea decreased when lubiprostone was administered with food and that, across all dosage groups, the rate of nausea was substantially lower among constipated men (13.2%) and constipated elderly patients (18.6%) when compared with the overall rate (30.9%). No patients in the trials were hospitalized due to nausea.

➤*Diarrhea:* Among constipated patients, 13.2% of those receiving lubiprostone 24 mcg twice daily reported diarrhea. Of those patients, 3.4% reported severe diarrhea and 2.2% discontinued treatment due to diarrhea. The incidence of diarrhea did not appear to be dose-dependent. No serious adverse reactions were reported for electrolyte imbalance in the 6 clinical trials and no clinically significant changes were seen in serum electrolyte levels while patients were receiving lubiprostone.

➤*Other adverse reactions:* The following list of adverse reactions include those that were considered by the investigator to be possibly related to lubiprostone and reported more frequently (more than 0.2%) on lubiprostone than placebo and those that lead to discontinuation more frequently (at least 0.2%) on lubiprostone than placebo. Although the reactions reported occurred during treatment with lubiprostone, they were not necessarily attributed to dosing of lubiprostone.

Cardiovascular – Flushing, palpitations.

CNS – Asthenia, nervousness, paraesthesia, syncope, tremor, vertigo.

Dermatologic – Hyperhidrosis, rash, urticaria.

GI – Abnormal bowel sounds, dysgeusia, fecal incontinence, frequent bowel movements, retching, watery stools.

Metabolic/Nutritional – Decreased appetite, edema.

Respiratory – Asthma, painful respiration, throat tightness.

Miscellaneous – Malaise, pain, rigors.

Overdosage

➤*Symptoms:* There have been 2 confirmed reports of overdosage with lubiprostone. The first report involved a 3-year-old child who accidentally ingested 7 to 8 capsules of lubiprostone 24 mcg and fully recovered. The second report was a study subject who self-administered a total of lubiprostone 96 mcg daily for 8 days. The subject experienced no adverse reactions during this time. Additionally, in a definitive phase 1 cardiac repolarization study, 51 patients administered a single, oral dose of lubiprostone 144 mcg, which is 6 times the normal single administration dose. Thirty-nine of the 51 patients experienced an adverse reaction.

The adverse reactions reported in more than 1% of this group included the following: nausea (45.1%); vomiting (27.5%); diarrhea (25.5%); dizziness (17.6%); loose or watery stools (13.7%); headache (11.8%); retching (7.8%); abdominal pain (5.9%); flushing or hot flush (5.9%); dyspnea, pallor, stomach discomfort, syncope (3.9%); anorexia, asthenia, chest discomfort, dry mouth, hyperhidrosis, skin irritation, upper abdominal pain, and vasovagal episode (2%).

Patient Information

Lubiprostone may cause nausea. If this occurs, coadministration of food with lubiprostone may reduce symptoms of nausea. Do not administer lubiprostone to patients who have severe diarrhea. Patients should be aware of the possible occurrence of diarrhea during treatment. If the diarrhea becomes severe, patients should consult their health care provider.

TEGASEROD MALEATE

Rx	**Zelnorm** (Novartis)	**Tablets:** 2 mg	Lactose. (NVR DL). In UD 60s.
		6 mg	Lactose. (NVR EH). In 60s, 500s, and UD 60s.

TEGASEROD MALEATE — ORAL

Indications

➤*IBS with constipation:* Tegaserod is indicated for the short-term treatment of women with irritable bowel syndrome (IBS) whose primary bowel symptom is constipation.

The safety and efficacy of tegaserod in men with IBS with constipation have not been established.

➤*Chronic idiopathic constipation:* Tegaserod is indicated for the treatment of patients younger than 65 years of age with chronic idiopathic constipation. The efficacy of tegaserod in patients 65 years of age and older with chronic idiopathic constipation has not been established.

The efficacy of tegaserod for the treatment of IBS with constipation or chronic idiopathic constipation has not been studied beyond 12 weeks.

Administration and Dosage

➤*Approved by the FDA:* July 24, 2002.

➤*IBS with constipation:* The recommended dosage of tegaserod is 6 mg taken twice daily orally before meals for 4 to 6 weeks. For those women who respond to therapy at 4 to 6 weeks, an additional 4- to 6-week course can be considered.

➤*Chronic idiopathic constipation:* The recommended dosage of tegaserod is 6 mg taken twice daily orally before meals. Physicians and patients should periodically assess the need for continued therapy.

➤*Storage/Stability:* Store at 25°C (77°F); excursions permitted to 15° to 30°C (59° to 86°F). Protect from moisture.

Actions

➤*Pharmacology:* IBS with constipation and chronic idiopathic constipation are both lower GI dysmotility disorders. Clinical investigations have shown that both motor and sensory functions of the gut appear to be altered in patients suffering from IBS, while in patients with chronic idiopathic constipation, reduced intestinal motility is the predominant cause of the condition. Both the enteric nervous system, which acts to integrate and process information in the gut, and 5-hydroxytryptamine (5-HT, serotonin) are thought to represent key elements in the etiology of IBS and idiopathic constipation. Approximately 95% of serotonin is found throughout the GI tract, primarily stored in enterochromaffin cells but also in enteric nerves acting as a neurotransmitter. Serotonin has been shown to be involved in regulating motility, visceral sensitivity, and intestinal secretion. Investigations suggest an important role of serotonin type 4 (5-HT_4) receptors in the maintenance of GI functions in humans. 5-HT_4 receptor mRNA has been found throughout the human GI tract.

Tegaserod is a 5-HT_4 receptor partial agonist that binds with high affinity at human 5-HT_4 receptors, whereas it has no appreciable affinity for 5-HT_3 or dopamine receptors. It has moderate affinity for 5-HT_1 receptors. Tegaserod, by acting as an agonist at neuronal 5-HT_4 receptors, triggers the release of further neurotransmitters such as calcitonin gene-related peptide from sensory neurons. The activation of 5-HT_4 receptors in the GI tract stimulates the peristaltic reflex and intestinal secretion, as well as inhibits visceral sensitivity. In vivo studies showed that tegaserod enhanced basal motor activity and normalized impaired motility throughout the GI tract. In addition, studies demonstrated that tegaserod moderated visceral sensitivity during colorectal distension in animals.

➤*Pharmacokinetics:*

Absorption – Peak plasma concentrations are reached approximately 1 hour after oral dosing. The absolute bioavailability of tegaserod when administered to fasting subjects is approximately 10%. The pharmacokinetics are dose proportional over the 2 to 12 mg range given twice daily for 5 days. There was no clinically relevant accumulation of tegaserod in plasma when a 6 mg twice daily dose was given for 5 days. The recommended dosage of tegaserod is 6 mg taken twice daily orally before meals for 4 to 6 weeks. For those patients who respond to therapy at 4 to 6 weeks, an additional 4- to 6-week course can be considered.

Food effects: When the drug is administered with food, the bioavailability of tegaserod is reduced 40% to 65% and C_{max} approximately 20% to 40%. Similar reductions in plasma concentration occur when tegaserod is administered to subjects within 30 minutes prior to a meal, or 2.5 hours after a meal. T_{max} of tegaserod is prolonged from approximately 1 to 2 hours when taken following a meal, but decreased to 0.7 hours when taken 30 minutes prior to a meal.

TEGASEROD MALEATE — ORAL

Distribution – Tegaserod is approximately 98% bound to plasma proteins, predominantly alpha-1-acid glycoprotein. Tegaserod exhibits pronounced distribution into tissues following intravenous dosing with a volume of distribution at steady state of 368 ± 223 L.

Metabolism – Tegaserod is metabolized mainly via 2 pathways. The first is a presystemic acid catalyzed hydrolysis in the stomach followed by oxidation and conjugation, which produces the main metabolite of tegaserod, 5-methoxyindole-3-carboxylic acid glucuronide. The main metabolite has negligible affinity for 5-HT_4 receptors in vitro. In humans, systemic exposure to tegaserod was not altered at neutral gastric pH values. The second metabolic pathway of tegaserod is direct glucuronidation, which leads to generation of 3 isomeric N-glucuronides.

Excretion – The plasma clearance of tegaserod is 77 ± 15 L/h with an estimated terminal half-life (½) of 11 ± 5 hours following intravenous dosing. Approximately two thirds of the oral dose of tegaserod is excreted unchanged in the feces, with the remaining one third excreted in the urine, primarily as the main metabolite.

Special populations –

Renal function impairment: No change in the pharmacokinetics of tegaserod was observed in subjects with severe renal impairment requiring hemodialysis (creatinine clearance less than or equal to 15 mL/min/1.73 m^2). C_{max} and area under the curve (AUC) of the main pharmacologically inactive metabolite of tegaserod, 5-methoxy-indole-3-carboxylic acid glucuronide, increased 2- and 10-fold, respectively, in subjects with severe renal impairment compared with healthy controls. No dosage adjustment is required in patients with mild-to-moderate renal impairment. Tegaserod is not recommended in patients with severe renal impairment.

Hepatic function impairment: In subjects with mild hepatic impairment, mean AUC was 31% higher and C_{max} was 16% higher compared with subjects with normal hepatic function. No dosage adjustment is required in patients with mild impairment; however, caution is recommended when using tegaserod in this patient population. Tegaserod has not adequately been studied in patients with moderate and severe hepatic impairment, and is therefore not recommended in these patients.

Elderly: In a clinical pharmacology study conducted to assess the pharmacokinetics of tegaserod administered to healthy young (18 to 40 years of age) and healthy elderly (65 to 85 years of age) subjects, peak plasma concentration and exposure were 22% and 40% greater, respectively, in elderly women than young women but still within the variability seen in tegaserod pharmacokinetics in healthy subjects. Based on an analysis across several pharmacokinetic studies in healthy subjects, there is no age effect on the pharmacokinetics of tegaserod when allowing for body weight as a covariate. Therefore, dose adjustment in elderly patients who have IBS with constipation is not necessary.

Contraindications

Severe renal impairment; moderate or severe hepatic impairment; a history of bowel obstruction, symptomatic gallbladder disease, suspected sphincter of Oddi dysfunction, or abdominal adhesions; and a known hypersensitivity to the drug or any of its excipients.

Warnings

➤*Diarrhea:* Serious consequences of diarrhea including hypovolemia, hypotension, and syncope have been reported in the clinical studies and during marketed use of tegaserod. In some cases, these complications have required hospitalization for rehydration. Discontinue tegaserod immediately in patients who develop severe diarrhea, hypotension, or syncope. Do not initiate tegaserod in patients who are currently experiencing or frequently experience diarrhea.

➤*Carcinogenesis:* In mice, dietary administration of tegaserod for 104 weeks produced mucosal hyperplasia and adenocarcinoma of small intestine at 600 mg/kg/day (approximately 83 to 110 times the human exposure at 6 mg twice daily based on plasma $AUC_{0\text{-}24\ h}$). There was no evidence of carcinogenicity at a lower dose of 200 mg/kg/day (approximately 24 to 35 times the human exposure at 6 mg twice daily based on plasma $AUC_{0\text{-}24\ h}$) or 60 mg/kg/day (approximately 3 to 4 times the human exposure at 6 mg twice daily based on plasma $AUC_{0\text{-}24\ h}$).

➤*Elderly:*

Chronic idiopathic constipation – Patients 65 years of age and older who received tegaserod experienced a higher incidence of diarrhea and discontinuations because of diarrhea than patients younger than 65 years of age.

➤*Pregnancy: Category B.* Reproduction studies have been performed in rats at oral doses up to 100 mg/kg/day (approximately 15 times the human exposure at 6 mg twice daily based on plasma $AUC_{0\text{-}24\ h}$) and rabbits at oral doses up to 120 mg/kg/day (approximately 51 times the human exposure at 6 mg twice daily based on plasma $AUC_{0\text{-}24\ h}$) and have revealed no evidence of impaired fertility or harm to the fetus caused by tegaserod. Because animal reproduction studies are not always predictive of human response, use this drug during pregnancy only if clearly needed.

➤*Lactation:* Tegaserod and its metabolites are excreted in the milk of lactating rats with a high milk to plasma ratio. It is not known whether tegaserod is excreted in human milk. Many drugs, which are excreted in human milk, have potential for serious adverse reactions in nursing infants. Based on the potential for tumorigenicity shown for tegaserod in the mouse carcinogenicity study, decide whether to discontinue breast-feeding or to discontinue the drug, taking into account the importance of the drug to the mother.

➤*Children:* Tegaserod has not been studied in pediatric patients.

Precautions

➤*Discontinue therapy:* Immediately discontinue tegaserod in patients with new or sudden worsening of abdominal pain or symptoms of ischemic colitis, such as rectal bleeding and bloody diarrhea.

➤*Ischemic colitis:* Ischemic colitis and other forms of intestinal ischemia have been reported in patients receiving tegaserod during marketed use of the drug. In some cases, hospitalization was required. Discontinue tegaserod immediately in patients who develop symptoms of ischemic colitis, such as rectal bleeding, bloody diarrhea, or new or worsening abdominal pain. Promptly evaluate patients experiencing these symptoms and have appropriate diagnostic testing performed. Do not resume treatment with tegaserod in patients who develop findings consistent with ischemic colitis or other forms of intestinal ischemia.

Drug Interactions

Tegaserod Drug Interactions

Precipitant drug	Object drug[a]		Description
Tegaserod	Digoxin	⬇	Coadministration reduced peak plasma concentrations and exposure of digoxin approximately 15%. This reduction of bioavailability is not considered clinically relevant and, therefore, a dose adjustment is unlikely to be required.
Tegaserod	Oral contraceptives	⬇	Coadministration reduced peak concentrations and exposure of levonorgestrel 8%. This is not expected to alter the risk of ovulation and, therefore, no alteration in contraceptive therapy is necessary.

[a] ⬇ = Object drug decreased.

➤*Drug/Food interactions:* When the drug is administered with food, the bioavailability of tegaserod is reduced by 40% to 65% and C_{max} approximately 20% to 40%. Similar reductions in plasma concentration occur when tegaserod is administered to subjects within 30 minutes prior to a meal or 2.5 hours after a meal. T_{max} of tegaserod is prolonged from approximately 1 to 2 hours when taken following a meal, but decreases to 0.7 hours when taken 30 minutes prior to a meal.

Adverse Reactions

➤*IBS with constipation:* The following adverse experiences were reported in 1% or more of patients who received tegaserod and occurred more frequently on tegaserod than placebo:

Tegaserod Adverse Reactions Occurring in ≥ 1% of IBS with Constipation Patients

Adverse reaction	Tegaserod 6 mg twice daily (n = 1,327)	Placebo (n = 1,305)
CNS		
Dizziness	4%	3%
Headache	15%	12%
Migraine	2%	1%
GI		
Abdominal pain	12%	11%
Diarrhea	9%	4%
Flatulence	6%	5%
Nausea	8%	7%
Musculoskeletal		
Arthropathy	2%	1%
Back pain	5%	4%
Miscellaneous		
Accidental trauma	3%	2%
Leg pain	1%	< 1%

➤*Chronic idiopathic constipation:*

Tegaserod Adverse Reactions Occurring in ≥ 1% of Chronic Idiopathic Constipation Patients

Adverse reaction	Tegaserod 6 mg twice daily (n = 881)	Tegaserod 2 mg twice daily (n = 861)	Placebo (n = 861)
CNS			
Dizziness	2%	1%	2%
Fatigue	1%	1%	1%
Headache, aggravated	1%	1%	0%
Insomnia	2%	1%	1%
Dermatologic			
Pruritus	0%	1%	0%
Rash	1%	1%	0%

TEGASEROD MALEATE — ORAL

Tegaserod Adverse Reactions Occurring in ≥ 1% of Chronic Idiopathic Constipation Patients			
Adverse reaction	Tegaserod 6 mg twice daily (n = 881)	Tegaserod 2 mg twice daily (n = 861)	Placebo (n = 861)
GI			
Abdominal distension	4%	3%	4%
Abdominal pain	5%	6%	5%
Abdominal pain, upper	2%	2%	2%
Diarrhea	7%	4%	3%
Nausea	5%	5%	4%
Vomiting	2%	1%	1%
GU			
Dysmenorrhea	1%	2%	1%
Urinary tract infection	1%	2%	1%
Musculoskeletal			
Back pain	3%	2%	3%
Myalgia	1%	1%	1%
Respiratory			
Pharyngitis	1%	1%	1%
Sinus congestion	1%	0%	1%
Sinusitis	3%	3%	2%
Upper respiratory tract infection	4%	3%	2%
Miscellaneous			
Fungal infection	0%	1%	1%

➤*Diarrhea:*

IBS with constipation – In the phase 3 clinical studies, 8.8% of patients receiving tegaserod reported diarrhea as an adverse experience compared to 3.8% of patients receiving placebo. Diarrhea can be a pharmacologic response to tegaserod. The majority of the tegaserod patients reporting diarrhea had a single episode. In most cases, diarrhea occurred within the first week of treatment. Typically, diarrhea resolved with continued therapy. Overall, the discontinuation rate from the studies because of diarrhea was 1.6% among the tegaserod-treated patients. In clinical studies, a small number of patients (0.04%) experienced clinically significant diarrhea including hospitalization, hypovolemia, hypotension, and need for IV fluids.

Chronic idiopathic constipation – In the 2 phase 3 studies, 6.6% of patients treated with tegaserod 6 mg twice daily and 4.2 % of patients treated with tegaserod 2 mg twice daily reported diarrhea as an adverse reaction versus 3% of patients receiving placebo.

The diarrhea episodes experienced by patients treated with tegaserod occurred early after initiation of treatment (median, 5.5 days), were of short duration (median, 2.5 days) and occurred only once in the majority of patients.

Typically, diarrhea resolved with continued therapy; only 0.9% of patients treated with tegaserod 6 mg twice daily discontinued the study because of diarrhea (compared with 0.3% in the tegaserod 2 mg twice daily group and 0.2% in the placebo group).

➤*Abdominal surgeries, including cholecystectomy:* An increase in abdominal surgeries was observed on tegaserod (9 of 2,965; 0.3%) vs placebo (3 of 1,740; 0.2%) in the phase 3 IBS clinical studies. The increase was primarily caused by a numerical imbalance in cholecystectomies reported in patients treated with tegaserod (5 of 2,965; 0.17%) vs placebo (1 of 1,740; 0.06%). In chronic idiopathic constipation clinical trials, there was no increase in the frequency of abdominal and pelvic surgeries in active vs placebo groups: 9 of 1,752; 0.5% on tegaserod vs 8 of 861; 0.9% on placebo. A causal relationship between abdominal surgeries and tegaserod has not been established.

➤*Other adverse reactions:* The following list of adverse reactions includes those from phase 3 clinical studies (6 mg twice daily or 2 mg twice daily) that were reported more frequently (greater than 0.2%) in patients on tegaserod than placebo; or that were considered by the investigator to be possibly related to tegaserod and reported more frequently (greater than 0.1%) on tegaserod than placebo; or that lead to discontinuation more frequently (greater than or equal to 0.1% and in more than 1 patient) on tegaserod than placebo. The list also contains those serious adverse reactions from all clinical trials in patients treated with tegaserod 6 mg twice daily or 2 mg twice daily that were either considered by the investigator as possibly drug related, or occurred in at least 2 more patients on tegaserod than on placebo. Although the reactions reported occurred during treatment with tegaserod, they were not necessarily caused by it.

Cardiovascular – Angina pectoris, supraventricular tachycardia, syncope, flushing, hypotension.

CNS – Depression, restlessness, sleep disorder, vertigo.

GI – Hemorrhoids, proctalgia, stomach discomfort, fecal incontinence, IBS, dyspepsia, gastroesophageal reflux, gastritis.

GU – Breast carcinoma, menorrhagia, miscarriage.

Hepatic – Cholecystectomy, cholelithiasis.

Metabolic/Nutritional – Increased appetite, peripheral edema.

Ophthalmic – Visual disturbance.

Respiratory – Dyspnea, pharyngolaryngeal pain.

Miscellaneous – Chest pain, hypersensitivity reactions, creatinine phosphokinase increased, increased eosinophil count, low neutrophil count.

➤*Postmarketing:* Voluntary reports of adverse reactions occurring with the use of tegaserod include those listed below. Because these cases are reported voluntarily from a population of unknown size, estimates of frequency cannot be made. No causal relationship between these events and tegaserod use has been established.

Postmarketing reports of diarrhea, which can be a pharmacologic response to tegaserod, have also been received.

Cardiovascular – Hypotension, syncope.

GI – Bile duct stone, gangrenous bowel, ischemic colitis, mesenteric ischemia, rectal bleeding, suspected sphincter of Oddi spasm.

Hypersensitivity – Allergic reaction including rash, urticaria, pruritus, and serious allergic type I reactions.

Hepatic – Cholecystitis with elevated transaminases.

Metabolic – Electrolyte disorders, hypovolemia.

Overdosage

➤*Symptoms:* There have been no reports of human overdosage with tegaserod. Single oral doses of 120 mg of tegaserod were administered to 3 healthy volunteers in 1 study. All 3 subjects developed diarrhea and headache. Two of these subjects also reported intermittent abdominal pain, and 1 developed orthostatic hypotension. In 28 healthy subjects exposed to doses of tegaserod of 90 to 180 mg/day for several days, adverse reactions were diarrhea (100%), headache (57%), abdominal pain (18%), flatulence (18%), nausea (7%), and vomiting (7%).

➤*Treatment:* Based on the large distribution volume and high protein binding of tegaserod, it is unlikely that tegaserod could be removed by dialysis. In cases of overdosage, treat symptomatically and institute supportive measures as appropriate.

Patient Information

Advise patients to take tegaserod before a meal.

Advise patients to stop tegaserod treatment and consult their health care provider if they experience new or worsening abdominal pain with or without rectal bleeding.

Inform patients of the possible occurrence of diarrhea during therapy. Diarrhea can be a pharmacologic response to tegaserod. The majority of the tegaserod patients reporting diarrhea had a single episode. In most cases, diarrhea occurred within the first week of treatment. Typically, diarrhea resolved with continued therapy. Advise patients to consult their health care provider if they experience severe diarrhea, or if the diarrhea is accompanied by severe cramping, abdominal pain, or dizziness. Do not initiate therapy with tegaserod if the patient is currently experiencing or frequently experiences diarrhea.

LAXATIVES

Indications

➤*Constipation:* Treatment of constipation.

➤*Rectal/Bowel examinations:* Certain stimulant, lubricant, and saline laxatives are used to evacuate the colon for rectal and bowel examinations.

➤*Prophylaxis:* Laxatives, generally **fecal softeners** or **mineral oil**, are useful prophylactically in patients who should not strain during defecation (ie, following anorectal surgery, MI).

➤*Psyllium:* Useful in patients with irritable bowel syndrome and diverticular disease.

➤*Polycarbophil:* For constipation or diarrhea associated with conditions such as irritable bowel syndrome and diverticulosis; acute nonspecific diarrhea.

➤*Mineral oil (enema):* Relief of fecal impaction.

➤*Docusate sodium:* Prevention of dry, hard stools.

➤*Unlabeled uses:* **Psyllium** appears to be useful in the reduction of cholesterol levels as an adjunct to a dietary program.

Actions

➤*Pharmacology:* Laxatives function by promoting active electrolyte secretion, decreasing water and electrolyte absorption, increasing intraluminal osmolarity, or increasing hydrostatic pressure in the gut.

Pharmacologic Actions of Laxatives					
	Laxatives	Onset of action (h)	Site of action	Mechanism of action	Comments
Saline	Dibasic sodium phosphate[a,b] Magnesium citrate Magnesium hydroxide Magnesium sulfate Monobasic sodium phosphate[a,b] Sodium biphosphate[a]	0.5 to 3	Small and large intestine	Attract/Retain water in intestinal lumen, increasing intraluminal pressure; cholecystokinin release.	May alter fluid and electrolyte balance. Sulfate salts are considered the most potent.
Stimulant/Irritant	Cascara	6 to 8	Colon	Direct action on intestinal mucosa or nerve plexus; alters water and electrolyte secretion.	May prefer castor oil when more complete evacuation is required.
	Bisacodyl tablets Casanthranol Senna	6 to 10			
	Bisacodyl suppository	0.25 to 1			
Bulk-producing	Methylcellulose Polycarbophil Psyllium	12 to 72	Small and large intestine	Holds water in stool to increase bulk-stimulating peristalsis; forms emollient gel.	Safe; minimal side effects. Take with plenty of water (240 mL/dose).
Emollient	Mineral oil	6 to 8	Colon	Retards colonic absorption of fecal water; softens stool.	May decrease absorption of fat-soluble vitamins.
Fecal softeners/ Surfactants	Docusate[c]	12 to 72	Small and large intestine	Facilitates admixture of fat and water to soften stool.	Beneficial in anorectal conditions in which passage of a firm stool is painful.
Hyperosmotic	Glycerin suppository	0.25 to 1	Colon	Local irritation; hyperosmotic action.	Sodium stearate in preparation causes local irritation.
	Lactulose	24 to 48	Colon	Osmotic effect retains fluid in the colon, lowering the pH and increasing colonic peristalsis.	Also indicated in portal-systemic encephalopathy.
Miscellaneous	Castor oil	2 to 6	Small intestine	Direct action on intestinal mucosa or nerve plexus; alters water and electrolyte secretion.	Castor oil is converted to ricinoleic acid (active component) in the gut.

[a] Onset of action for rectal preparations is 2 to 15 minutes.
[b] Colon is site of action for rectal preparations.
[c] Site of action for potassium salt is in the colon.

Calcium polycarbophil is a hydrophilic agent. As a bulk laxative, it retains free water within the intestinal lumen and indirectly opposes dehydrating forces of the bowel, promoting well-formed stools. In diarrhea, when the intestinal mucosa is incapable of absorbing water at normal rates, it absorbs free fecal water, forming a gel and producing formed stools. Thus, in diarrhea and constipation, it works by restoring a more normal moisture level and providing bulk.

Lactulose, a synthetic disaccharide analog of lactose containing galactose and fructose, decreases blood ammonia concentrations and reduces the degree of portal-systemic encephalopathy.

The human GI tissue does not have an enzyme capable of hydrolysis of this disaccharide; as a result, oral doses pass to the colon virtually unchanged. After reaching the colon, lactulose is metabolized by bacteria resulting in the formation of lactic acid, formic acid, acetic acid, and carbon dioxide. These products produce an increased osmotic pressure and slightly acidify the colonic contents, resulting in an increase in stool water content and stool softening. Because the colonic contents are more acidic than the blood, ammonia can migrate from the blood into the colon. The acid colonic contents convert NH_3 to the ammonium ion $[NH_4]^+$, trapping it and preventing its absorption. The laxative action of the lactulose metabolites then expels the trapped ammonium ion from the colon.

➤*Pharmacokinetics:* **Lactulose** is poorly absorbed. When given orally, only small amounts reach the blood. Urinary excretion is ≤ 3% and is essentially complete within 24 hours. Lactulose does not exert its effect until it reaches the colon. Transit time through the colon may be slow; therefore, 24 to 48 hours may be required to produce a normal bowel movement.

Contraindications

Hypersensitivity to any ingredient; nausea, vomiting, or other symptoms of appendicitis; fecal impaction; intestinal obstruction; undiagnosed abdominal pain; patients who require a low galactose diet (**lactulose**).

Do not give **docusate sodium** if **mineral oil** is being given.

Warnings

➤*Constipation:* Prior to using laxatives, consider living habits affecting bowel function, including disease state and drug history. Treatment and prevention of constipation include the following: Adequate fluid intake (4 to 6 glasses [8 oz] of water daily), proper dietary habits including increasing fiber intake, responding to the urge to defecate, and daily exercise. Restrict self-medication to short-term therapy of constipation; chronic use of laxatives (particularly stimulants) may lead to dependence.

Agents That May Cause Constipation	
Prostaglandin synthesis inhibitors	Non-potassium sparing diuretics
Anticholinergics	Ganglionic blockers
Antihistamines	Iron preparations
Phenothiazines	Barium sulfate
Tricyclic antidepressants	Clonidine
Benztropine	Polystyrene sodium sulfonate
Trihexyphenidyl	Antacids containing either calcium
Opiates	carbonate or aluminum hydroxide

➤*Fluid and electrolyte balance:* Excessive laxative use may lead to significant fluid and electrolyte imbalance. Monitor patients periodically.

Preparations containing sodium should be used cautiously by individuals on a sodium-restricted diet, and in the presence of edema, CHF, renal failure, or borderline hypertension.

Megacolon, bowel obstruction, imperforate anus, or CHF – Do not use **sodium phosphate** and **sodium biphosphate** in these patients; hypernatremic dehydration may occur.

Abuse/Dependency – Chronic use of laxatives may result in fluid and electrolyte imbalances, steatorrhea, osteomalacia, diarrhea, cathartic colon, and liver disease. Also known as laxative abuse syndrome (LAS), it is difficult to diagnose. It is often seen in women with depression, personality disorders, or anorexia nervosa. Many agents can be detected in urine or stool samples; however, it is important to follow up negative test results if LAS is suspected, because patients may be intermittent abusers or change laxative products frequently.

Cathartic colon – Cathartic colon, a poorly functioning colon, results from the chronic abuse of stimulant cathartics.

➤*Melanosis coli:* Melanosis coli is a darkened pigmentation of the colonic mucosa resulting from chronic use of anthraquinone derivatives (**casanthrol, cascara sagrada, senna**).

➤*Lipid pneumonitis:* Lipid pneumonitis may result from oral ingestion and aspiration of **mineral oil**, especially when patient reclines. The young, elderly, and debilitated are at greatest risk.

➤*Electrocautery procedures:* A theoretical hazard may exist for patients being treated with **lactulose** who may undergo electrocautery procedures during proctoscopy or colonoscopy. Accumulation of H_2 gas in significant concentration in the presence of an electrical spark may result in an explosion. Although this complication has not been reported with lactulose, patients should have a thorough bowel cleansing with a nonfermentable solution. Insufflation of CO_2 as an additional safeguard may be pursued, but is considered a redundant measure.

➤*Renal function impairment:* Up to 20% of the magnesium in magnesium salts may be absorbed. Use caution with products containing phosphate, sodium, magnesium, or potassium salts in the presence of renal dysfunction. Use **sodium phosphate** and **sodium biphosphate** with caution in these patients; hyperphosphatemia, hypernatremia, acidosis, and hypocalcemia may occur.

➤*Pregnancy: Category B.* (**Lactulose, magnesium sulfate**). *Category C.* (**Casanthranol, cascara sagrada, danthron, docusate sodium, docusate calcium, docusate potassium, mineral oil, senna**). Do not use **castor oil** during pregnancy; its irritant effect may induce premature labor. Mineral oil may decrease absorption of fat-soluble vitamins. Improper use of saline cathartics can lead to dangerous electrolyte imbalance. If needed, limit use to bulk-forming or surfactant laxatives.

➤*Lactation:* Anthraquinone derivatives (eg, **casanthranol, cascara sagrada, danthron**) are excreted in breast milk resulting in a potential increased incidence of diarrhea in the nursing infant. Magnesium emulsions administered orally did not affect the stools of nursing infants, although magnesium content in breast milk was slightly elevated compared with untreated patients. Sennosides A and B (eg, **senna**) are not excreted in breast milk. It is not known whether **docusate calcium, docusate potassium, docusate sodium, lactulose**, and **mineral oil** are excreted in breast milk.

➤*Children:* Administer with caution. Dosage is product specific. Do not administer enemas to children younger than 2 years of age. Infants receiving **lactulose** may develop hyponatremia and dehydration.

Precautions

➤*Monitoring:* In the overall management of portal-systemic encephalopathy, there is serious underlying liver disease with complications such as electrolyte disturbance (eg, hypokalemia, hypernatremia), which may require other specific therapy. Elderly, debilitated patients who receive **lactulose** for more than 6 months should have serum electrolytes (potassium, chloride) and carbon dioxide measured periodically.

➤*Diabetic patients:* **Lactulose** syrup contains galactose (less than 1.6 g/15 mL) and lactose (less than 1.2 g/15 mL). Use with caution in these individuals.

➤*Concomitant laxative use:* Do not use other laxatives, especially during the initial phase of therapy for portal-systemic encephalopathy; the resulting loose stools may falsely suggest adequate lactulose dosage.

➤*Rectal bleeding or failure to respond:* Rectal bleeding or failure to respond to therapy may indicate a serious condition, which may require further medical attention.

➤*Urine discoloration:* Discoloration of acidic urine to yellow-brown or black may occur with **cascara sagrada** or **senna**. Pink-red, red-violet, or red-brown discoloration of alkaline urine may occur with cascara sagrada or senna.

➤*Impaction or obstruction:* Impaction or obstruction may be caused by bulk-forming agents if temporarily arrested in their passage through the alimentary canal (eg, patients with esophageal strictures). Administer bulk-forming agents with plenty of fluid (240 mL/dose).

➤*Melanosis coli:* Anthraquinone derivatives (**casanthrol, cascara sagrada**, and **senna**) may cause melanosis coli, a harmless discoloring of colonic mucosa, persisting ≤ 6 months following discontinuation.

➤*Tartrazine sensitivity:* Some of these products contain tartrazine, which may cause allergic-type reactions (including bronchial asthma) in susceptible individuals. Although the incidence of tartrazine sensitivity in the general population is low, it is frequently seen in patients who also have aspirin hypersensitivity. Specific products containing tartrazine are identified in the product listings.

Drug Interactions

Laxative Drug Interactions

Precipitant drug	Object drug[a]		Description
Surfactants (eg, docusate)	Mineral oil	↑	When concomitantly administered, surfactants (eg, docusate) may increase mineral oil absorption.
Milk Antacids H_2 antagonists Protein pump inhibitors	Bisacodyl	↑	Avoid administration 1 to 2 hours before bisacodyl tablets; concomitant administration may cause the enteric coating to dissolve, resulting in gastric lining irritation or dyspepsia.
Mineral oil	Lipid-soluble vitamins	↓	Absorption of lipid-soluble vitamins may decrease during prolonged mineral oil administration.
Neomycin and other anti-infectives	Lactulose	↔	Reports conflict about concomitant use of lactulose syrup. The elimination of certain colonic bacteria may interfere with desired degradation of lactulose and prevent acidification of colonic contents. Monitor patient if concomitant oral anti-infectives are given.
Antacids	Lactulose	↓	Nonabsorbable antacids given concurrently with lactulose may inhibit the desired lactulose-induced drop in colonic pH.

[a] ↑ = Object drug increased. ↓ = Object drug decreased.
↔ = Undetermined clinical effect.

Adverse Reactions

Diarrhea; nausea; vomiting; perianal irritation; fainting; bloating; flatulence; cramps.

Obstruction of the esophagus, stomach, small intestine, and colon has occurred when bulk-forming laxatives are administered without adequate fluids or in patients with intestinal stenosis.

Large doses of **mineral oil** may cause anal seepage, resulting in itching (pruritus ani), rectal inflammation, and perianal discomfort.

Lactulose – Gaseous distention with flatulence, belching, abdominal discomfort such as cramping (≈ 20%); nausea; vomiting. Excessive dosage can lead to diarrhea.

Overdosage

There have been no reports of accidental **lactulose** overdose. It is expected that diarrhea and abdominal cramps would be the major symptoms; discontinue the drug.

Patient Information

Direct attention to proper dietary fiber intake, adequate fluids, and regular exercise.

Do not use in the presence of abdominal pain, nausea, or vomiting.

Laxative use is only a temporary measure; do not use more than 1 week. When regularity returns, discontinue use. Prolonged, frequent, or excessive use may result in dependence or electrolyte imbalance.

Notify physician if unrelieved constipation, rectal bleeding, or symptoms of electrolyte imbalance (eg, muscle cramps or pain, weakness, dizziness) occur.

Pink-red, red-violet, red-brown, yellow-brown, or black discoloration of urine may occur with **cascara sagrada** or **senna**.

Refrigerate **magnesium citrate** solutions to improve taste.

➤*Mineral oil:* Preferably administered on an empty stomach.

➤*Bisacodyl tablets:* Swallow whole; do not take within 1 to 2 hours of antacids, prescription or *otc* H_2 antagonists, proton pump inhibitors, or milk.

➤*Lactulose:* May be mixed with fruit juice, water, or milk to increase palatability.

May cause belching, flatulence, or abdominal cramps; notify physician if these effects become bothersome or if diarrhea occurs.

Do not take other laxatives while on lactulose therapy.

In the event that unusual diarrheal condition occurs, contact your physician.

SALINE LAXATIVES

otc	**Phillips'** (Bayer HealthCare)	**Tablets:** 500 mg magnesium (as oxide)	Polyvinyl alcohol. In 24s.
otc	**Epsom Salt** (Various, eg, Humco)	**Granules:** Magnesium sulfate. *Dose:* Adults ≥ 12 years - 5 to 10 mL in ½ glass of water. Children 6 to 12 years - 2.5 to 5 mL in ½ glass of water.	In 120 g and 1 and 4 lbs.
otc	**Milk of Magnesia – Concentrated** (Roxane)	**Suspension:** Equiv. to 30 mL milk of magnesia *Dose:* 10 to 20 mL.	In 100 and 400 mL and UD 10 mL.

SALINE LAXATIVES

otc	**Phillips' Milk of Magnesia, Concentrated** (Bayer)	**Suspension:** Magnesium hydroxide 800 mg/5 mL *Dose:* Adults and children ≥ 12 years – 15 to 30 mL. Children 6 to 11 years - 7.5 to 15 mL Children 2 to 5 years - 2.5 to 7.5 mL	Sorbitol, sugar. Strawberry creme flavor. In 240 mL.
otc	**Milk of Magnesia** (Various, eg, Geneva, Goldline, Humco, Roxane, Rugby, URL)	**Suspension:** Magnesium hydroxide 400 mg/5 mL *Dose:* Adults and children ≥ 12 years - 30 to 60 mL/day, taken with liquid. Children 6 to 11 years - 15 to 30 mL/day Children 2 to 5 years - 5 to 15 mL/day	In 180, 360, 480 mL and UD 30 mL, gallon
otc	**Phillips' Milk of Magnesia** (Bayer)		Saccharin (mint); sorbitol, sugar (cherry). Mint, cherry, and regular flavors. In 120, 360, and 780 mL.
otc sf	**Magnesium Citrate Solution** (Humco)	**Solution:** 1.75 g magnesium citrate/30 mL *Dose:* Adults and children ≥ 12 years - ½ to 1 bottle Children 6 to 12 years - ⅓ to ½ bottle	Saccharin. Cherry and lemon flavors. In 296 mL.
otc sf	**Fleet Phospho-soda** (Fleet)	**Solution:** 2.4 g monobasic sodium phosphate and 0.9 g dibasic sodium phosphate/5 mL *Dose:* Adults and children ≥ 12 years - 20 to 45 mL/day Children 10 to 11 years - 10 to 20 mL/day Children 5 to 9 years - 5 to 10 mL/day	556 mg sodium/5 mL. Saccharin. Regular and ginger-lemon flavors. In 45, 90, and 240 mL.

For complete and comparative prescribing information, refer to the Laxatives group monograph.

Irritant or Stimulant Laxatives

CASCARA SAGRADA

otc	**Cascara Sagrada** (Various, eg, Rugby)	**Tablets:** 325 mg *Dose:* Adults and children ≥ 12 years - 1 tablet/day	In 100s and 1000s.
otc	**Aromatic Cascara Fluidextract** (Various, eg, Goldline, Hi-Tech Pharmacal Co., Inc., Rugby)	**Liquid:** *Dose:* Adults and children ≥ 12 years - 2 to 6 mL single daily dose	19% alcohol. In 473 mL.
otc	**Cascara Aromatic** (Humco)	**Liquid:** *Dose:* Adults and children ≥ 12 years of age- 2.5 to 5 mL in a single daily dose Children 2 to younger than 12 years of age - ⅕ to ½ teaspoonful	18% alcohol. In 120 and 473 mL.

For complete and comparative prescribing information, refer to the Laxatives group monograph.

SENNOSIDES

otc	**Dr. Edwards' Olive** (Oakhurst)	**Tablets:** 8.6 mg sennosides (from senna concentrate) *Dose:* Adults - 2 tablets a day, not to exceed 4 tablets twice daily Children 6 to 12 y -1 tablet a day, not to exceed 2 tablets twice daily	In 75s.
otc	**Senexon** (Rugby)	**Tablets:** 8.6 mg sennosides *Dose:* Adults and children ≥ 12 y - 2 tablets once or twice daily Children 6 to younger than 12 y - 1 tablet once or twice/day	Lactose. In 100s and 1,000s.
otc	**Senna-Gen** (Zenith-Goldline)	**Tablets:** 8.6 mg sennosides *Dose:* Adults and children ≥ 12 y - 2 to 4 tablets once or twice daily Children 6 to younger than 12 y - 1 to 2 tablets once or twice daily Children 2 to younger than 6 y - ½ to 1 tablet once or twice daily	Lactose. In 100s and 1,000s.
otc	**Senna Concentrate** (Akyma)	**Tablets:** 8.6 mg sennosides *Dose:* Adults and children ≥ 12 y - 2 tablets once a day, not to exceed 4 tablets twice a day Children 6 to younger than 12 y - 1 tablet once a day, not to exceed 2 tablets twice a day Children 2 to younger than 6 y - ½ tablet once a day, not to exceed 1 tablet twice a day	Lactose. In 1,000s.
otc	**ex•lax** (Novartis Consumer)	**Tablets:** 15 mg sennosides *Dose:* Adults and children ≥ 12 y - 2 tablets once or twice daily with water Children 6 to younger than 12 y - 1 tablet once or twice daily with water	Sucrose. (ex-lax 1). In 8s, 30s, and 60s.
otc	**ex•lax chocolated** (Novartis Consumer)	**Tablets:** 15 mg sennosides *Dose:* Adults and children ≥ 12 y - 2 tablets once or twice daily with water Children 6 to younger than 12 y - 1 tablet once or twice daily with water	Sugar, oil, dry milk. Chocolated. In 6s, 18s, and 48s.
otc	**Lax-Pills** (G & W Labs)	**Tablets:** 15 mg sennosides *Dose:* Adults and children ≥ 12 y - 2 tablets once or twice daily with water Children 6 to younger than 12 y - 1 tablet once or twice daily with water	In blister pack 30s and 60s.
otc	**SenokotXTRA** (Purdue Fredrick)	**Tablets:** 17 mg sennosides *Dose:* Adults and children ≥ 12 y - Start with 1 tablet/day, not to exceed 2 tablets twice/day Children 6 to younger than 12 y - Start with ½ tablet/day, not to exceed 1 tablet twice/day	Lactose. In 12s and 36s.
otc	**Lax-Pills** (G & W Labs)	**Tablets:** 25 mg sennosides *Dose:* Adults and children ≥ 12 years - 2 tablets once or twice daily with water Children 6 to younger than 12 years - 1 tablet once or twice daily with water	In blister pack 24s and 48s.
otc	**Maximum Relief ex•lax** (Novartis Consumer)	**Tablets:** 25 mg sennosides *Dose:* Adults and children ≥ 12 y - 2 tablets once or twice daily with water Children 6 to younger than 12 y - 1 tablet once or twice daily with water	Sucrose. (ex-lax 1). In 24s and 48s.
otc	**Black Draught** (Lee Pharmaceuticals)	**Tablets:** 6 mg sennosides *Dose:* Adults and children ≥ 12 y - 2 tablets once or twice/day Children 6 to younger than 12 y - 1 tablet once or twice/day	Sucrose. In 30s.
		Tablets, chewable: 10 mg sennosides *Dose:* Adults and children ≥ 12 y - 2 tablets once or twice daily Children 6 to younger than 12 y - 1 tablet once or twice/day	Sugar. In 30s.
		Granules: 20 mg sennosides/5 mL *Dose:* Adults and children ≥ 12 y - As a tea: ¼ to ½ cup	Tartrazine, sucrose. In 22.5 g.

SENNOSIDES

otc	**Senokot** (Purdue Frederick)	**Tablets**: 8.6 mg sennosides *Dose:* Adults and children ≥ 12 y - Start with 2 tablets/day, not to exceed 4 tablets twice/day Children 6 to younger than 12 y - Start with 1 tablet/day, not to exceed 2 tablets twice/day Children 2 to younger than 6 y - ½ tablet/day, not to exceed 1 tablet twice/day	Lactose. In 10s, 20s, 50s, 100s, 1,000s, and UD 100s.
		Granules: 15 mg/5 mL sennosides *Dose:* Adults and children ≥ 12 y - Start with 1 tsp/day, not to exceed 2 tsp twice/day Children 6 to younger than 12 y - ½ tsp/day, not to exceed 1 tsp twice/day Children 2 to younger than 6 y - ¼ tsp/day, not to exceed ½ tsp twice/day	Sucrose. In 56, 170, and 340 g.
		Syrup: 8.8 mg/5 mL sennosides *Dose:* Adults and children ≥ 12 y - 2 to 3 tsp/day, not to exceed 3 tsp twice/day Children 6 to younger than 12 y - 1 to 1½ tsp/day, not to exceed 1½ tsp twice/day Children 2 to younger than 6 y - ½ to ¾ tsp/day, not to exceed ¾ tsp twice/day	Alcohol free. Parabens, sucrose. In 59 and 237 mL.
otc	**Senna** (Pharmaceutical Associates)	**Syrup**: 176 mg/5 mL senna leaf extract *Dose*: Adults and children ≥ 12 y - 10 to 15 mL once/day not to exceed 15 mL twice/day Children 6 to younger than 12 y - 5 to 7.5 mL once/day not to exceed 7.5 mL twice/day Children 2 to younger than 6 y - 2.5 to 3.75 mL once/day not to exceed 3.75 mL twice/day	Glycerin, parabens, sucrose. In 237 mL.
otc	**Evac-u-gen** (Lee Pharmaceuticals)	**Tablets, chewable**: 10 mg sennosides *Dose:* Adults - 2 tablets once or twice daily Children ≥ 6 y - 1 tablet once or twice/day	Sugar. In 35s.
otc	**Senexon** (Rugby)	**Liquid**: 8.8 mg sennosides/5 mL *Dose:* Adults and children ≥ 12 y - 10 to 15 mL once a day, not to exceed 15 mL twice a day Children 6 to younger than 12 y - 5 to 7.5 mL once a day, not to exceed 7.5 mL twice a day Children 2 to younger than 6 y - 2.5 to 3.75 mL once a day, not to exceed 3.75 mL twice a day	Parabens, sucrose. In 237 mL.
otc	**Fletcher's Castoria** (Mentholatum)	**Liquid**: 33.3 mg/mL senna concentrate *Dose:* Children 6 to 15 y -10 to 15 mL ≤ 2 times/day Children 2 to 5 y - 5 to 10 mL ≤ 2 times/day	Alcohol free. Sucrose, parabens. In 74 and 150 mL.
otc	**Little Tummys Laxative Drops** (Vetco Inc.)	**Drops, oral**: 8.8 mg/mL sennosides *Dose:* Children 6 to younger than 12 y - 1 to 1.5 mL once a day, not to exceed 1.5 mL twice a day Children 2 to younger than 6 y - 0.5 to 0.75 mL once a day, not to exceed 0.75 mL twice a day	Alcohol free. Parabens, sorbitol. In 30 mL with dropper.

SENNOSIDES — ORAL

For complete and comparative prescribing information, refer to the Laxatives group monograph.

BISACODYL

otc	**Bisacodyl** (Various, eg, Global Source, Major, UDL, URL)	**Tablets, enteric-coated**: 5 mg	In 25s, 50s, 100s, 1,000s, and UD 100s.
otc	**Alophen** (Numark)		Sugar. In 100s.
otc	**Bisa-Lax** (Bergen Brunswig)		In 25s and 50s.
otc	**Dulcolax** (Boehringer Ingelheim)		Lactose, sucrose, parabens. (BI 12). In 10s, 25s, 50s, and 100s.
otc	**Fleet Laxative** (Fleet)		Sucrose. In 25s and 100s.
otc	**Modane** (Savage Labs)		Lactose. In 100s.
otc	**Bisac-Evac** (G & W Labs)		In 25s.
otc	**Caroid** (Mentholatum Co.)		Sugar. In 100s.
otc	**Correctol** (Schering-Plough)		Talc, lactose, sugar. (Correctol). In 30s, 60s, and 90s.
otc	**Feen-a-mint** (Schering-Plough)		Talc, lactose, sugar. (Feen-a-mint). In 30s.
otc	**Doxidan** (Pharmacia)	**Tablets, delayed-release**: 10 mg	In 10s, 30s, and 90s.
otc	**Bisacodyl** (Various, eg, Global Source, URL)	**Suppositories**: 10 mg	In 12s, 16s, and 100s.
otc	**Bisacodyl Uniserts** (Upsher-Smith)		In 12s.
otc	**Bisa-Lax** (Bergen Brunswig)		Hydrogenated vegetable oil. In 50s.
otc	**Bisac-Evac** (G & W Labs)		In 8s, 12s, 50s, 100s, 500s, and 1,000s.
otc	**Dulcolax** (Boehringer Ingelheim)		In 4s, 8s, 16s, and 50s.
otc	**Fleet Laxative** (Fleet)		In 4s, 12s, 50s, and 100s.
otc	**Dulcolax Bowel Prep Kit** (Boehringer Ingelheim)	**Tablets**: 5 mg	Docusate sodium, lactose, parabens, sucrose. In 4s.
		Suppository: 10 mg	Hydrogenated vegetable oil. In 1s.

BISACODYL — ORAL

For complete and comparative prescribing information, refer to the Laxatives group monograph.

Indications

This medication is used to relieve occasional constipation (irregularity).

➤*Enteric-coated tablets:* Expect results in 8 to 12 hours if taken at bedtime or within 6 hours if taken before breakfast.

➤*Regular tablets and delayed-release tablets:* Bisacodyl generally causes a bowel movement in 6 to 12 hours.

Administration and Dosage

Do not administer tablets within 1 hour after taking an antacid or milk.

Do not chew or crush tablets.

Follow dosage below or as directed by a doctor.

➤*Enteric-coated 5 mg tablets:*

Adults and children 12 years of age and over – Take 2 or 3 tablets (usually 2) in a single dose once daily.

Children 6 to under 12 years of age – Take 1 tablet once daily.

Children under 6 years of age – Oral administration is not recommended due to the requirement to swallow tablets whole. Consult a physician.

➤*Regular 5 mg tablets and delayed-release 5 mg tablets:*

Adults and children 12 years of age and over – Take 1 to 3 tablets (usually 2) in a single daily dose.

Children 6 to under 12 years of age – Take 1 tablet in a single daily dose.

Children under 6 years – Ask a doctor.

➤*Storage/Stability:* Keep out of the reach of children.

Enteric-coated tablets – Store bisacodyl enteric-coated tablets at controlled room temperature 15° to 30°C (59° to 86°F). Avoid excessive humidity. Do not use if carton is opened or if blister unit is torn, broken, or shows any signs of tampering.

Regular tablets – Do not expose to temperatures above 30°C (86°F). Avoid excessive humidity.

Delayed-release tablets – Store at room temperature 15° to 30°C (59° to 86°F). Do not expose to temperatures above 30°C (86°F).

Irritant or Stimulant Laxatives

BISACODYL — RECTAL

For complete and comparative prescribing information, refer to the Laxatives group monograph.

Indications

➤*Suppositories:* This medication is indicated for relief of occasional constipation and irregularity. This medication stimulates bowel movement in 15 minutes to 1 hour.

➤*Enema:* This preparation is indicated for relief of occasional constipation or bowel cleansing before rectal examinations in adults and children 12 years of age and older.

Administration and Dosage

➤*Suppositories:* Remove foil wrap. Lie on side and gently insert suppository pointed end first towards the navel and well up into rectum. Make sure suppository touches the bowel wall. Retain suppository for at least 15 to 20 minutes.

Adults and children 12 years of age and older – Use 1 suppository.

Children under 12 years of age – One-half suppository.

➤*Enema:*

Directions –

Left side position: Lie on left side with knee bent and arms resting comfortably.

Knee-chest position: Kneel, then lower head and chest forward until left side of face is resting on surface with left arm folded comfortably. How to use this enema:

1.) Remove protective shield from enema tip before inserting.
2.) With steady pressure, gently insert enema tip into rectum with a slight side-to-side movement, with tip pointing toward navel. Insertion may be easier if the person receiving enema bears down, as if having a bowel movement. This helps relax the muscles around the anus.
3.) Do not force the enema tip into the rectum, as this may cause injury.
4.) Squeeze bottle until nearly all the liquid is gone. It is not necessary to empty the bottle completely, as it contains more liquid than needed.
5.) Remove enema tip from rectum and maintain position until urge to evacuate is strong, 5 to 20 minutes, if possible.

Single daily dose:

- *Adults and children 12 years of age and over* – 1 bottle.
- *Children under 12 years of age* – Do not use.

➤*Storage/Stability:*

Suppositories – Bisacodyl suppositories should be stored below 25°C (77°F). Therefore, they may be stored in the refrigerator if the room temperature exceeds 25°C (77°F) in order to help keep suppositories from softening. Allow the product to return to room temperature before using.

Keep out of the reach of children.

Bulk-Producing Laxatives

PSYLLIUM

otc	**Metamucil** (Procter & Gamble)	**Capsules:** 0.52 g psyllium husk *Dose:* Adults 12 years of age and older - 2 to 6 capsules for increasing daily fiber intake; 6 capsules for cholesterol-lowering use. Take with 8 oz liquid (swallow 1 capsule at a time) up to tid.	In 100s and 160s.
otc sf	**Fiberall Tropical Fruit Flavor** (Heritage Consumer)	**Powder:** 3.5 g psyllium hydrophilic mucilloid per dose *Dose:* 1 rounded teaspoon (5 to 5.9 g) in 6 oz cool water or juice once daily followed immediately by ½ glass of water. After 1 week, may take ≤ 3 servings/day.	Aspartame. In 454 g and UD 10 g packets.
otc	**Fiberall Orange Flavor** (Heritage Consumer)		Aspartame. In 480 g.
otc	**Genfiber** (Goldline Consumer)	**Powder:** 3.4 g psyllium hydrophilic mucilloid fiber and 14 calories per dose. *Dose:* Adults - 1 rounded teaspoon in 8 oz liquid 1 to 3 times/day. Children 6 to 12 years of age - ½ rounded teaspoon in 8 oz liquid 1 to 3 times/day.	Dextrose. In 595 g.
otc	**Genfiber, Orange Flavor** (Goldline Consumer)	**Powder:** 3.4 g psyllium hydrophilic mucilloid per dose. *Dose:* Adults - 1 rounded tablespoon in 8 oz liquid 1 to 3 times/day. Children 6 to 12 years of age - ½ rounded tablespoon in 8 oz liquid 1 to 3 times/day.	Sucrose. Orange flavor. In 397 g.
otc	**Natural Psyllium Fiber** (Plus Pharma)	**Powder:** 3.4 g psyllium hydrophilic mucilloid fiber, 3 mg sodium, and 25 calories per dose. *Dose:* Adults - 1 rounded teaspoon in 8 oz liquid 2 to 3 times/day.	Dextrose. In 368 g.
otc	**Natural Psyllium Fiber, Orange** (Plus Pharma)	**Powder:** 3.4 g psyllium hydrophilic mucilloid fiber, 3 mg sodium, and 25 calories per dose. *Dose:* Adults - 1 rounded teaspoon in 8 oz liquid 2 to 3 times/day.	Sucrose. Orange flavor. In 368 g.
otc sf	**Hydrocil Instant** (Numark)	**Powder:** 3.5 g psyllium hydrophilic mucilloid/dose *Dose:* 1 level scoopful (3.7 g) in liquid	In 250 g.
otc sf	**Konsyl** (Konsyl Pharm.)	**Powder:** 6 g psyllium. *Dose:* 1 packet or rounded teaspoon (6 g) in liquid	In 300 and 450 g and UD 6 g packets.
otc sf	**Konsyl Easy Mix Formula** (Konsyl Pharm.)	**Powder:** 6 g psyllium, 4.4 mg Na, 48 mg Ca, 4 mg P, 0.06 mg Zn, 42 mg K, 0.35 g carbohydrates, 4 calories/5 mL *Dose:* 1 teaspoon (5 mL) or 6.3 g packet	In 200 g and packets.
otc	**Metamucil Orange Flavor, Smooth Texture** (Procter & Gamble)	**Powder:** ≈ 3.4 g psyllium husk, 5 mg sodium, 12 g carbohydrates, and 45 calories per dose *Dose:* Adults and children 12 years of age or older - 1 rounded tablespoon in liquid, 1 to 3 times a day. Children 6 to 12 years of age - ½ adult dose	Sucrose. In 420, 630, and 1368 g, and 100 UD single-dose packs (100s).
otc sf	**Metamucil, Sugar Free, Smooth Texture** (Procter & Gamble)	**Powder:** ≈ 3.4 g psyllium husk, 5 g carbohydrates, 4 mg sodium, and 20 calories per dose *Dose:* Adults and children 12 years of age and older - 1 rounded teaspoon in liquid, 1 to 3 times a day. Children 6 to 12 years of age - ½ adult dose	In 425 g and packets of 30s or 100s.
otc sf	**Metamucil, Sugar Free, Orange Flavor, Smooth Texture** (Procter & Gamble)	**Powder:** ≈ 3.4 mg psyllium husk, 5 g carbohydrates, 5 mg sodium, 20 calories per dose. *Dose:* Adults and children 12 years of age and older - 1 rounded teaspoon in liquid 1 to 3 times a day. Children 6 to 12 years of age - ½ adult dose	Aspartame, 25 mg phenylalanine per dose. In 210, 420, 630, and 660 g.
otc	**Metamucil Orange Flavor, Original Texture** (Procter & Gamble)	**Powder:** ≈ 3.4 g psyllium husk, 10 g carbohydrates, 5 mg sodium, 40 calories/dose *Dose:* Adults and children 12 years of age and older - 1 rounded tablespoon in 8 oz liquid ≤ 3 times/day Children 6 to 12 years of age - ½ adult dose	Sucrose. In 210, 420, 538, and 630 g.
otc	**Metamucil Original Texture** (Procter & Gamble)	**Powder:** ≈ 3.4 g psyllium husk, 6 g carbohydrates, 3 mg sodium, 25 calories/dose *Dose:* Adults and children 12 years of age and older - 1 rounded teaspoon in 8 oz liquid ≤ 3 times/day Children 6 to 12 years of age - ½ adult dose	Sucrose. In 822 g and packets of 30.
otc	**Reguloid, Orange** (Rugby)	**Powder:** ≈ 3.4 g psyllium mucilloid/tablespoon *Dose:* Adults and children 12 years of age and older - 1 rounded tablespoon, 1 to 3 times daily in 8 oz liquid. Children 6 to 12 years of age - ½ adult dose	Sucrose. Orange flavor. In 369 and 540 g.
otc sf	**Reguloid, Sugar Free Orange** (Rugby)	**Powder:** ≈ 3.4 g psyllium hydrophilic mucilloid per rounded teaspoon *Dose:* Adults and children 12 years of age and older - 1 rounded teaspoon in 8 oz liquid, 1 to 3 times/day. Children 6 to 12 years of age - ½ adult dose in 8 oz liquid 1 to 3 times/day	Aspartame, 30 mg phenylalanine per dose. In 284 and 426 g

Bulk-Producing Laxatives

PSYLLIUM

otc sf	**Regulold, Sugar Free Regular** (Rugby)	**Powder:** ≈ 3.4 g psyllium hydrophilic mucilloid per dose *Dose:* Adults and children 12 years of age and older - 1 rounded teaspoon in 8 oz liquid, 1 to 3 times/day. Children 6 to 12 years of age - ½ adult dose in 8 oz liquid 1 to 3 times a day.	Aspartame, 6 mg phenylalanine per dose. In 284 and 426 g.
otc	**Natural Fiber Laxative** (Apothecary)	**Powder:** ≈ 3.4 g psyllium hydrophilic mucilloid/7 g dose. 14 calories/dose. *Dose:* Adults and children 12 years of age and older - 7 g 1 to 3 times/day Children 6 to 12 years of age - ½ adult dose	Sodium free. In 390 g.
otc	**Syllact** (Wallace)	**Powder:** 3.3 g psyllium seed husks and ≈ 14 calories per rounded teaspoon *Dose:* Adults and children 12 years of age and older - 1 rounded teaspoon in 8 oz liquid, 1 to 3 times daily. Children 6 to younger than 12 years of age – ½ to 1 rounded teaspoon in 8 oz liquid 1 to 3 times/day	Dextrose, saccharin, parabens. Fruit flavor. In 284 g.
otc	**Konsyl-D** (Konsyl Pharm.)	**Powder:** 3.4 g psyllium, 14 calories per rounded teaspoon *Dose:* Adults and children 12 years of age and older - 1 teaspoon 1 to 3 times/day Children 6 to younger than 12 years of age - ½ teaspoon 1 to 3 times/day	Dextrose. In 325 and 500 g and UD 6.5 g.
otc	**Reguloid** (Rugby)		Dextrose. 14 calories per rounded teaspoon. In 369 and 540 g.
otc	**Perdiem Fiber Therapy** (Novartis Consumer Health)	**Granules:** 4.03 g psyllium, 1.8 mg sodium, 36.1 mg potassium and 4 calories/rounded teaspoon (6 g) *Dose:* Adults - 1 to 2 rounded teaspoons with 8 oz liquid, once or twice daily. Do not chew. Children 7 to 11 years of age - 1 rounded teaspoon with 8 oz liquid once or twice daily	Sucrose. Dye free. Mint flavor. In 100 and 250 g.
otc	**Serutan** (Menley & James)	**Granules:** 2.5 g psyllium and less than 0.03 g sodium per heaping teaspoon *Dose:* Adults - 1 to 3 heaping teaspoon on cereal or other food, 1 to 3 times daily. Children 6 to 12 years of age - ½ to 1½ heaping teaspoon with 8 oz liquid.	Saccharin, sugar. In 170 and 540 g.
otc	**Metamucil** (Procter & Gamble)	**Wafers:** ≈ 3.4 g psyllium husk/dose, 17 g carbohydrates, 20 mg sodium, 5 g fat, 120 calories/dose *Dose:* Adults and children 12 years of age and older - 2 wafers w/8 oz liquid ≤ 3 times/day Children 6 to 12 years of age - 1 wafer w/8 oz liquid ≤ 3 times/day	Sugar, fructose, molasses, sucrose. Cinnamon spice and apple crisp flavors. In 24s

PSYLLIUM — ORAL

For complete and comparative prescribing information, refer to the Laxatives group monograph.

POLYCARBOPHIL

otc	**Equalactin** (Numark)	**Tablets, chewable:** 625 mg calcium polycarbophil (equivalent to 500 mg polycarbophil)	Citrus flavor. In 24s and 48s.
otc	**Konsyl Fiber** (Konsyl)	**Tablets:** 500 mg polycarbophil	In 90s.
otc	**Fiber-Lax** (Rugby)	**Tablets:** 625 mg calcium polycarbophil (equivalent to 500 mg polycarbophil)	In 60s, 90s, and 500s.
otc	**Bulk Forming Fiber Laxative** (Goldline Consumer)		Film-coated. In 60s.
otc	**FiberCon** (Lederle)		Calcium carbonate. (LL F66). In 36s, 60s, 90s, and 150s.

POLYCARBOPHIL — ORAL

For complete and comparative prescribing information, refer to the Laxatives group monograph.

Indications

Polycarbophil promotes normal function of the bowel by increasing bulk volume and water content of the stool. This product generally produces a bowel movement in 12 to 72 hours.

Administration and Dosage

Continued use for 1 to 3 days is normally required to provide full benefit. Dosage may vary according to diet, exercise, previous laxative use, or severity of constipation.

➤*Adults and children 12 years of age and older:* Swallow 2 tablets 1 to 4 times a day.

➤*Children 6 to 12 years of age:* Swallow 1 tablet 1 to 3 times a day.

➤*Children under 6 years of age:* Consult a physician.

➤*Administration:* A full glass (8 fl oz; 240 mL) of liquid should be taken with each dose. Taking this product without adequate fluid may cause it to swell and block your throat or esophagus and may cause choking. Do not take this product if you have difficulty swallowing. Do not take more than the maximum daily dose.

➤*Storage/Stability:* Store at controlled room temperature 15° to 30°C (59° to 86°F). Protect contents from moisture. Keep this and all medicines out of the reach of children.

MISCELLANEOUS BULK-PRODUCING LAXATIVES

otc	**Citrucel** (GlaxoSmithKline)	**Powder:** 2 g methylcellulose per heaping tbsp	Sucrose. Orange flavor. In 480 and 840 g.
otc sf	**Citrucel Sugar Free** (GlaxoSmithKline)	**Powder:** 2 g methylcellulose, 52 mg phenylalanine per leveled scoop	Aspartame. Orange flavor. In 245 and 480 g.
otc	**Citrucel** (GlaxoSmithKline)	**Tablets:** 500 mg methylcellulose	Maltodextrin. (CIT). Capsule shape. In 164s.
otc	**Unifiber** (Niche)	**Powder:** Powdered cellulose	In 150, 270, and 480 g.
otc	**Maltsupex** (Wallace)	**Powder:** 8 g malt soup extract per level scoop	In 227 and 454 g.

MISCELLANEOUS BULK-PRODUCING LAXATIVES

For complete and comparative prescribing information, refer to the Laxatives group monograph.

Administration and Dosage

Take with a full glass of water; encourage additional fluid intake.

➤*Citrucel:*

Adults and children ≥ 12 years of age – 1 heaping tbsp (19 g) or 1 packet (10.7 g) in 8 oz cold water, 1 to 3 times daily.

Children 6 years of age to younger than 12 years of age – ½ the adult dose in 8 oz cold water, once daily.

➤*Unifiber:* Dose is 1 tbsp into a glass with 3 or 4 oz. of fruit juice, milk, or water, or mix with soft foods such as applesauce, mashed potatoes, or pudding. Can be taken up to 3 times daily if needed or as recommended by a doctor.

➤*Maltsupex:*

Tablets – Adults, 12 to 36 g/day. Initially, 4 tablets 4 times daily (at meals and bedtime).

Bulk-Producing Laxatives

MISCELLANEOUS BULK-PRODUCING LAXATIVES

Powder – Adults, up to 32 g twice daily for 3 or 4 days, then 16 to 32 g at bedtime. Children 6 to 12 years, up to 16 g twice daily for 3 or 4 days; 2 to 6 years, 8 g twice daily for 3 or 4 days. For infants younger than 2 years of age, consult a doctor.

Liquid – Adults, 2 tbsp twice daily for 3 or 4 days, then 1 to 2 tbsp at bedtime. Children 6 to 12 years, 1 tbsp twice daily for 3 or 4 days; 2 to 6 years, ½ tbsp twice daily for 3 or 4 days. For infants younger than 2 years of age, consult a doctor.

Emollients

MINERAL OIL

otc	**Mineral Oil** (Various, eg, Fleet, Paddock)	**Liquid**: Mineral oil	In 180 and 473 mL.
otc	**Kondremul Plain** (Heritage Consumer Prod.)	**Emulsion**: Mineral oil	Irish moss, acacia, glycerin. In 480 mL.

MINERAL OIL — ORAL

For complete and comparative prescribing information, refer to the Laxatives group monograph.

Fecal Softeners/Surfactants

DOCUSATE SODIUM (Dioctyl Sodium Sulfosuccinate; DSS)

otc	**ex-lax Stool Softener** (Novartis Consumer Health)	**Tablets**: 100 mg *Dose:* Adults and children ≥ 12 years - 100 to 300 mg/day Children 2 to younger than 12 years - 100 mg/day	Methylparabens. Caplet shape. In 40s.
otc	**Dioctyn** (Dixon-Shane)	**Tablets**: 100 mg *Dose:* Adults and children ≥ 12 years - 100 to 200 mg at bedtime Children 6 to 12 years - 100 mg at bedtime	Sorbitol. In 1,000s.
otc	**Colace** (Purdue)	**Capsules**: 50 mg *Dose:* Adults and children ≥ 12 years - 50 to 300 mg/day Children 6 to 12 years - 50 to 150 mg/day	(RPC 052). In 30s, 60s, and UD 100s.
otc	**Colace** (Purdue)	**Capsules**: 100 mg *Dose:* Adults and children ≥ 12 years - 100 to 300 mg/day Children 6 to 12 years - 100 mg/day Children 2 to 6 years - Products vary. Consult product labeling for specific guidelines.	In 30s, 60s, 250s, 1,000s, and UD 100s.
otc	**D-S-S** (Magno-Humphries)		In 100s.
otc	**Non-Habit Forming Stool Softener** (Rugby)		Sorbitol, parabens. In 100s and 1000s.
otc	**Stool Softener** (Rugby)		Lactose, tartrazine. In 1000s.
otc	**Regulax SS** (Republic)		In 60s, 100s, and 1000s.
otc	**Docusate Sodium** (Various, eg, Geneva, UDL, URL)	**Capsules**: 250 mg *Dose:* Adults and children ≥ 12 years - 250 mg/day	In 100s and 1000s, and UD 100s.
otc	**Stool Softener** (Rugby)		Lactose. In 1000s.
otc	**Docusate Sodium** (UDL)	**Capsules, soft gel**: 50 mg *Dose:* Adults and children ≥ 12 years - 50 to 300 mg/day Children 2 to younger than 12 years - 50 mg/day	In 100s and UD 100s.
otc	**Docusate Sodium** (Various, eg, Goldline Consumer, UDL, URL)	**Capsules, soft gel**: 100 mg *Dose:* Adults and children ≥ 12 years - 100 to 300 mg/day Children 6 to younger than 12 years - 100 mg/day Children 2 to 6 years - Products vary. Consult product labeling for specific guidelines.	In 100s, 1000s, and UD 100s and 300s.
otc	**D.O.S.** (Goldline Consumer)		Parabens. In 100s and 1000s.
otc	**Dulcolax Stool Softener** (Boehringer Ingelheim Consumer)		Sorbitol, glycerin. In 25s.
otc	**Genasoft** (Goldline Consumer)		Methylparaben. In 60s.
otc	**Phillips' Liqui-Gels** (Bayer Consumer)		Parabens, sorbitol. (Phillips). In 10s, 30s, and 50s.
otc	**Sof-lax** (Fleet)		5 mg sodium/gelcap. In 60s.
otc	**Docusate Sodium** (Various, eg, Schein)	**Capsules, soft gel**: 250 mg *Dose:* Adults and children ≥ 12 years - 250 mg/day	In 100s.
otc	**Stool Softener** (Rugby)		Sorbitol, parabens. In 100s and 1000s.
otc	**D.O.S.** (Goldline Consumer)		Oblong. Red-orange. In 100s and 500s.
otc	**Docusate Sodium** (Roxane)	**Syrup**: 50 mg per 15 mL *Dose:* Adults and children ≥ 12 years - 50 to 100 mg Children 6 to 12 years - 50 mg Children 3 to 5 years - 33 mg	Saccharin, sucrose, parabens. In UD 15 and 30 mL (100s).
otc	**Docu** (Hi-Tech Pharmacal Co.)	**Syrup**: 20 mg per 5 mL *Dose:* Adults and children ≥ 12 years - 60 to 180 mg/day Children 6 to 12 years - 40 mg 1 to 3 times/day Children 3 to 6 years - 20 to 60 mg/day	5% alcohol. In 480 mL.

DOCUSATE SODIUM (Dioctyl Sodium Sulfosuccinate; DSS)

otc	**Diocto** (Various, eg, Alpharma)	**Syrup**: 60 mg per 15 mL	In 480 mL. *Dose:* Adults and children ≥ 12 years - 60 to 360 mg/day Children 2 to 12 years - Dosage varies. Consult product labeling for specific guidelines. Generally, 40 to 150 mg/day.
otc	**Colace** (Purdue)		≤ 1% alcohol. Menthol, parabens, sucrose. In 237 and 473 mL. *Dose:* Adults and children ≥ 12 years - 60 to 300 mg/day Children 6 to 12 years - 40 to 120 mg/day Children 3 to 6 years - 20 to 60 mg/day Children younger than 3 years of age- 10 to 40 mg/day
otc	**Silace** (Silarx)		≤ 1% alcohol. In 473 mL. *Dose:* Adults and children ≥ 12 years - 60 to 180 mg/day Children 6 to 12 years - 40 mg 1 to 3 times/day
otc	**Docusate Sodium** (Roxane)	**Syrup**: 100 mg/30 mL *Dose:* Adults and children ≥ 12 years - 50 to 100 mg Children 6 to 12 years - 50 mg Children 3 to 5 years - 33 mg	Saccharin, sucrose, parabens. In UD 15 and 30 mL (100s).
otc	**Silace** (Silarx)	**Liquid**: 10 mg/mL *Dose:* Adults and children ≥ 12 years - 50 to 200 mg/day (5 to 20 mL) Children 6 to younger than 12 years - 40 to 120 mg/day (4 to 12 mL) Children 3 to younger than 6 years - 20 to 60 mg/day (2 to 6 mL)	Parabens. In 473 mL.
otc	**Diocto** (Various, eg, Goldline Consumer, Rugby)	**Liquid**: 150 mg per 15 mL	In 480 mL. *Dose:* Adults and children ≥ 12 years - 50 to 350 mg/day Children 2 to younger than 12 years - Dosage varies. Consult product labeling for specific guidelines. Generally, 20 to 150 mg/day.
otc	**Colace** (Purdue)		Parabens. In 30 and 480 mL. *Dose:* Children 3 to 6 years - 20 mg 1 to 3 times/day
otc	**Docu** (Hi-Tech Pharmacal Co.)		In 480 mL. *Dose:* Adults and children older than 12 years - 50 to 200 mg/day Children 6 to 12 years - 40 to 120 mg/day Children 3 to 6 years - 20 to 60 mg/day

DOCUSATE SODIUM — ORAL

For complete and comparative prescribing information, refer to the Laxatives group monograph.

Indications

➤*Docusate sodium tablets and capsules:* Relief of occasional constipation (irregularity), especially for sensitive systems. This stimulant-free formula generally works within 12 to 72 hours after the first dose.

➤*Docusate sodium syrup and liquid:* Useful in constipation due to hard stools in painful anorectal conditions, in cardiac and other conditions in which maximum ease of passage is desirable to avoid difficult or painful defecation, and when peristaitic stimulants are contraindicated.

Administration and Dosage

➤*Tablets:* Take docusate sodium stool softener tablets with a glass of water at any time.

Adults and children 12 years of age and older – Take 1 to 3 tablets (100 to 300 mg) daily as needed.

Children 2 to less than 12 years of age – Take 1 tablet (100 mg) daily. This dose may be taken as a single daily dose or in divided doses.

Children younger than 2 years of age – Consult a doctor.

➤*Docusate sodium 50 mg capsules:*

Adults and children 12 years of age and older – Take 1 to 6 capsules (50 to 300 mg) which may be taken as a single daily dose or in divided doses.

Children 2 to less than 12 years of age – Take 1 capsule (50 mg) daily.

Children younger than 2 years of age – Consult a doctor. Each capsule contains approximately 2.7 mg of sodium. The maximum daily dose (6 capsules, 300 mg) is considered very low sodium.

➤*Docusate sodium 100 mg capsules:*

Adults and children 12 years of age and older – Take 100 to 300 mg/day.

Children 6 to 12 years of age – Take 100 mg/day.

Children 2 to 6 years of age – Products vary. Consult product labeling for specific guidelines.

➤*Docusate sodium 250 mg capsules:*

Adults and children 12 years of age and older – Take 250 mg/day.

➤*Docusate sodium syrup 20 mg/5 mL:*

Adults and children 12 years of age and older – Take 15 to 45 mL (60 to 180 mg) daily.

Children 6 to 12 years of age – Take 30 mL (40 mg) 1 to 3 times daily.

Children 3 to 6 years of age – Take 15 to 45 mL (20 to 60 mg) daily.

Children 2 years of age or younger – Take as directed by physician. Shake well before using. Take each dose with a full glass of water or liquid (may be taken with fruit juice). Drink increased fluids. The higher doses are recommended for initial therapy. Dosage should be adjusted to individual response. The effect on stools is usually apparent 1 to 3 days after the first dose. To mask taste, the syrup may be given in a half a glass of milk or fruit juice or in infant formula.

➤*Docusate sodium syrup 50 mg/15 mL:*

Adults and children 12 years of age or older – Take 50 to 100 mg.

Children 6 to 12 years of age – Take 50 mg.

Children 3 to 5 years of age – Take 33 mg.

➤*Docusate sodium syrup 100 mg/30 mL:*

Adults and children 12 years of age or older – Take 50 to 100 mg.

Children 6 to 12 years of age – Take 50 mg.

Children 3 to 5 years of age – Take 33 mg.

➤*Docusate sodium liquid 50 mg/5 mL:*

Adults and older children – Take 50 to 200 mg (5 to 20 mL).

Children 6 to 12 years of age – Take 40 to 120 mg (4 to 12 mL).

Children 3 to 6 years of age – Take 20 to 60 mg (2 to 6 mL).

Infants and children younger than 3 years of age – Take as prescribed by a physician. The higher doses are recommended for initial therapy. Dosage should be adjusted to individual response. The effect on stools is usually apparent 1 to 3 days after the first dose. Shake well before using. Give in ½ glass of milk or fruit juice or in infant formula. For retention or flushing enemas, add 50 to 100 mg (5 to 10 mL) to the enema fluid.

➤*Storage/Stability:*

Tablets and capsules – Store in a dry place at controlled room temperature 15° to 30°C (59° to 86°F). Protect from moisture.

Syrup and liquid – Store at controlled room temperature 15° to 30°C (59° to 86°F). Protect from excessive temperatures. Dispense in tight, light-resistant container as described in official compendia. See label of container for number and expiration date.

Fecal Softeners/Surfactants

DOCUSATE CALCIUM (Dioctyl Calcium Sulfosuccinate)

otc	**Docusate Calcium** (Various)	**Capsules**: 240 mg	In 100s, 500s, and UD 100s and 300s.
otc	**Stool Softener** (Apothecary)		In 50s.
otc	**Stool Softener DC** (Rugby)		Sorbitol, parabens. In 100s, 500s, and 1000s.
otc	**Sulfolax** (Major)	**Capsules, soft gel**: 240 mg	Sorbitol, parabens. In 100s.
otc	**Surfak Liquigels** (Pharmacia & Upjohn)		Sorbitol, parabens. Red. In 10s, 30s, 100s, 500s, and UD 100s.
otc	**DC Softgels** (Goldline)		In 100s and 500s.

DOCUSATE CALCIUM — ORAL

For complete and comparative prescribing information, refer to the Laxatives group monograph.

Indications

➤*Constipation:* Docusate calcium, a stool softener, is indicated for the relief of occasional constipation. It is used for the prevention of dry, hard stools.

➤*Prophylaxis:* Fecal softeners are useful prophylactically in patients who should not strain during defecation (ie, following anorectal surgery, MI).

Administration and Dosage

➤*Adults and children 12 years of age and older:* One capsule by mouth daily for several days or until bowel movements are normal. For use in children younger than 12 years of age, consult a physician.

➤*Storage/Stability:* Store at room temperature in a dry place.

Hyperosmotic Agents

GLYCERIN

otc	**Glycerin** (Various, eg, Apothecary)	**Suppositories** : Glycerin	**Adults**: In 10s, 12s, 25s, 50s, and 100s.
			Pediatric: In 10s, 12s, and 25s.
otc	**Sani-Supp** (G & W Labs)		**Adults**: In 10s, 25s, and 50s.
			Pediatric: In 10s and 25s.
otc	**Colace** (Purdue)		**Adults**: In 12s, 24s, 48s, and 100s.
otc	**Colace Infant/Child** (Purdue)		**Pediatric**: In 12s and 24s.
otc	**Fleet Babylax** (Fleet)	**Liquid**: 4 mL per applicator	In 6 applicators.

GLYCERIN — RECTAL

For complete and comparative prescribing information, refer to the Laxatives group monograph.

Indications

➤*Constipation:* For relief of occasional constipation. This product generally produces a bowel movement within 15 minutes to 1 hour.

Administration and Dosage

➤*Suppositories:*
- Remove foil wrapper.
- Insert 1 suppository into rectum and retain for about 15 minutes.
- It need not melt to produce laxative action.

Note – Do not exceed 1 suppository daily or as directed by a doctor.

Do not use in children less than 2 years of age before consulting a physician.

➤*Pediatric rectal liquid:*

Single daily dosage –
Children 2 to under 6 years of age: 1 unit or as directed by a doctor.
Children under 2 years of age: Consult a doctor.

Directions –
Left side position: Place child on left side with knees bent and arms resting comfortably.
Knee-chest position: Have child kneel, then lower head and chest forward until left side of face is resting on the surface with left arm folded comfortably.

Removal of shield – Hold unit upright, grasping bulb of unit with fingers. Grasp orange protective shield with the other hand, pull gently to remove. With steady pressure, gently insert tip into rectum with a slight side-to-side movement, with tip pointing toward the navel. Discontinue use if resistance is encountered. Forcing the tip can result in injury. Squeeze the bulb until nearly all the liquid is expelled. While continuing to squeeze the bulb, remove the tip from the rectum and discard unit. It is not necessary to empty the unit completely. The unit contains more than the amount of liquid needed for effective use. A small amount of liquid will remain in the unit after squeezing.

➤*Storage/Stability:* Avoid excessive heat.

Keep out of reach of children.

LACTULOSE

Rx	**Lactulose** (Various, eg, Zenith Goldline)	**Solution**: 10 glactulose per 15 mL. (< 1.6 g galactose, < 1.2 g lactose and ≤ 1.2 g of other sugars).	In 237, 473, 960, and 1893 mL.
Rx	**Cephulac** (Hoechst-Marion Roussel)		In 473 mL, 1.9 L, and UD 30 mL.
Rx	**Cholac** (Alra)		In 30, 240, 480, 960, 1920, and 3785 mL.
Rx	**Constulose** (Alpharma)		In 237 and 946 mL.
Rx	**Enulose** (Alpharma)		In 473 mL and 1.89 L.
Rx	**Kristalose** (Bertek)	**Crystals for reconstitution**: Lactulose (< 0.3 g galactose and lactose/10 g).	In 10 g (30s) and 20 g (30s).

LACTULOSE — ORAL

For complete and comparative prescribing information, refer to the Laxatives group monograph.

Indications

➤*Constipation:* For the treatment of constipation. In patients with a history of chronic constipation, lactulose therapy increases the number of bowel movements per day and the number of days on which bowel movements occur.

➤*Portal-systemic encephalopathy (solution only):* For the prevention and portal-systemic encephalopathy, including the stages of hepatic precoma and coma.

Administration and Dosage

➤*Approved by the FDA:* March 25, 1976.

➤*Treatment of constipation:* Twenty-four to 48 hours may be required to produce a normal bowel movement.

Solution – The usual dose is 15 to 30 mL, containing 10 to 20 g of lactulose daily. The dose may be increased to 60 mL daily if necessary.

Crystals – The usual dose is 10 to 20 g of lactulose daily. The dose may be increased to 40 g daily if necessary.

➤*Prevention and treatment of portal-systemic encephalopathy:*

Adults – The usual adult oral dosage is 30 to 45 mL containing 20 to 30 g of lactulose 3 or 4 times daily. The dosage may be adjusted every day or two (as needed) to produce 2 or 3 soft stools daily. Hourly doses of 30 to 45 mL may be used to induce the rapid laxation indicated in the initial phase of the therapy of portal-systemic encephalopathy. When the laxative effect has been achieved, the dose of lactulose may then be reduced to the recommended daily dose. Improvement in the patient's condition may occur within 24 hours, but may not begin before 48 hours or even later.

Continuous long-term therapy is indicated to lessen the severity and prevent the recurrence of portal-systemic encephalopathy. The dose of lactulose for this purpose is the same as the recommended daily dose.

Pediatric – Very little information on the use of lactulose in young children and adolescents has been recorded. As with adults, the subjective goal in proper treatment is to produce 2 or 3 soft stools daily. On the basis of information available, the recommended initial daily oral dose in infants is 2.5 to 10 mL in divided doses. For older children and adolescents, the total daily

Hyperosmotic Agents

LACTULOSE — ORAL

dose is 40 to 90 mL. If the initial dose causes diarrhea, reduce the dose immediately. If diarrhea persists, discontinue lactulose.

➤*Solution:* Some patients have found that lactulose solution may be more acceptable when mixed with fruit juice, water, or milk.

➤*Crystals for reconstitution:*

Directions for preparation – Dissolve contents of packet in half a glass (120 mL) of water.

When lactulose crystals are dissolved in water, the resulting solution may be colorless to a slightly pale yellow.

➤*Storage/Stability:* Store at controlled room temperature 15° to 30°C (59° to 86°F), preferably below 30°C (86°F). Do not freeze.

Solution – Dispense in a tight, light-resistant container with a child-resistant closure.

Under recommended storage conditions, a normal darkening of color may occur. Such darkening is characteristic of sugar solutions and does not affect therapeutic action. Prolonged exposure to temperatures greater than 30°C (86°F) or to direct light may cause extreme darkening and turbidity, which may be pharmaceutically objectionable. If this condition develops, do not use.

Prolonged exposure to freezing temperatures may cause change to a semi-solid, too viscous to pour. Viscosity will return to normal upon warming to room temperature.

LACTULOSE — RECTAL

For complete and comparative prescribing information, refer to the Laxatives group monograph.

Indications

➤*Portal-systemic encephalopathy:* For the prevention and treatment of portal-systemic encephalopathy, including the stages of hepatic precoma and coma.

Administration and Dosage

➤*Approved by the FDA:* July 26, 1988.

When the adult patient is in the impending coma or coma stage of portal-systemic encephalopathy and the danger of aspiration exists, or when the necessary endoscopic or intubation procedures physically interfere with the administration of the recommended oral doses, lactulose solution may be given as a retention enema via a rectal balloon catheter. Do not use cleansing enemas containing soap suds or other alkaline agents.

Mix lactulose solution 300 mL with water or physiologic saline 700 mL and retain for 30 to 60 minutes. This lactulose enema may be repeated every 4 to 6 hours. If this lactulose enema is inadvertently evacuated too promptly, it may be repeated immediately.

The goal of treatment is reversal of the coma stage in order that the patient may be able to take oral medication. Reversal of coma may take place within 2 hours of the first enema in some patients. Start lactulose given orally in the recommended doses before lactulose by enema is stopped entirely.

➤*Storage/Stability:* Store at controlled room temperature 2° to 30°C (36° to 86°F). Do not freeze.

Under recommended storage conditions, a normal darkening of color may occur. Such darkening is characteristic of sugar solutions and does not affect therapeutic action. Prolonged exposure to temperatures above 30°C (86°F) or to direct light may cause extreme darkening and turbidity that may be pharmaceutically objectionable. If this condition develops, do not use.

Prolonged exposure to freezing temperatures may cause change to a semi-solid, too viscous to pour. Viscosity will return to normal upon warming to room temperature.

Enemas

MISCELLANEOUS ENEMAS

otc	**Fleet** (Fleet)	**Disposable enema:** 7 g dibasic sodium phosphate and 19 g monobasic sodium phosphate per 118 mL delivered dose (4.4 g sodium per dose) *Dose:* Adults – 118 mL. Children 2 to younger than 12 years – 59 mL.	In squeeze bottles. **Pediatric:** In 66 mL. **Adult:** In 133 mL.
otc	**Fleet Bisacodyl** (Fleet)	**Disposable enema:** 10 mg bisacodyl per 30 mL delivered dose *Dose:* Adults and children ≥ 12 years – 30 mL.	In 37 mL squeeze bottles.
otc	**Fleet Mineral Oil** (Fleet)	**Disposable enema:** Mineral oil *Dose:* Adults and children ≥ 12 years – 118 mL. Children 2 to younger than 12 years – 59 mL.	In 133 mL plastic squeeze bottles.
otc	**Therevac-SB** (Jones Medical)	**Disposable enema:** 283 mg docusate sodium in a base of soft soap, polyethylene glycol, and 275 mg glycerin per 4 mL ampule *Dose:* 4 mL.	In UD 30s.
otc	**Therevac-Plus** (Jones Medical)	**Disposable enema:** 283 mg docusate sodium, 275 mg glycerin, and 20 mg benzocaine in a base of soft soap, polyethylene glycol per 4 mL ampule *Dose:* 4 mL.	In 50s and UD 30s.

For complete prescribing information, refer to the Laxatives group monograph. For Bisacodyl prescribing information, see the Bisacodyl Rectal monograph in the Irritant or Stimulant Laxatives section.

MINERAL OIL — RECTAL

For complete and comparative prescribing information, refer to the Laxatives group monograph.

CO_2-RELEASING SUPPOSITORIES

otc	**Ceo-Two** (Beutlich)	**Suppositories:** Sodium bicarbonate and potassium bitartrate in a water-soluble polyethylene glycol base. Before inserting, moisten suppository with warm water.	In 10s.

For complete and comparative prescribing information, refer to the Laxatives group monograph.

Bowel Evacuants

POLYETHYLENE GLYCOL-ELECTROLYTE SOLUTION (PEG-ES)

Rx	**CoLyte** (Schwarz Pharma)	**Powder for Oral Solution:** 1 gal: 227.1 g PEG 3350, 21.5 g sodium sulfate, 6.36 g sodium bicarb, 5.53 g NaCl, 2.82 g KCl.	Regular and pineapple flavors. In bottles.
		4 L: 240 g PEG 3350, 22.72 g sodium sulfate, 6.72 g sodium bicarb, 5.84 g NaCl, 2.98 g KCl.	Citrus berry, lemon lime, cherry, and pineapple flavors. In bottles.
Rx	**GoLYTELY** (Braintree Labs.)	**Powder for Oral Solution:** 236 g PEG 3350, 22.74 g sodium sulfate, 6.74 g sodium bicarb, 5.86 g NaCl, 2.97 g KCl.	In disposable jugs.
		227.1 g PEG 3350, 21.5 g sodium sulfate, 6.36 g sodium bicarb, 5.53 g NaCl, 2.82 g KCl.	In packets.
Rx	**NuLytely** (Braintree Labs.)	**Powder for Reconstitution:** 420 g PEG 3350, 5.72 g sodium bicarb, 11.2 g NaCl, 1.48 g KCl.	Cherry, lemon-lime, and orange flavors. In 4 L disposable jugs.
Rx	**OCL** (Abbott)	**Oral Solution:** 146 mg NaCl, 168 mg sodium bicarb, 1.29 g sodium sulfate decahydrate, 75 mg KCl, 6 g PEG 3350, 30 mg polysorbate 80/100 mL.	In 1500 mL (3 pack).

POLYETHYLENE GLYCOL-ELECTROLYTE SOLUTION (PEG-ES) — ORAL

For complete prescribing information, refer to the Laxatives group monograph.

Indications

For bowel cleansing prior to GI examination.

➤*Unlabeled uses:* PEG electrolyte solutions are useful in the management of acute iron overdose in children. In a 33-month-old, 2953 mL/kg was administered over 5 days.

Administration and Dosage

The patient should fast 3 to 4 hours prior to ingestion of the solution; do not give solid foods less than 2 hours before solution is administered.

One method is to schedule patients for midmorning exam, allowing 3 hours for drinking and 1 hour to complete bowel evacuation. Another method is to give the solution the evening before the exam, particularly if the patient is to have a barium enema. No foods, except clear liquids, are permitted after solution administration.

➤*Adults:* Dosage is 4 L of oral solution prior to GI exam. May be given via a nasogastric tube to patients unwilling or unable to drink the preparation. Drink 240 mL every 10 minutes until 4 L are consumed or until the rectal effluent is clear. Rapid drinking of each portion is preferred to drinking small amounts continuously. Nasogastric tube administration is at the rate of 20 to 30 mL/min (1.2 to 1.8 L/hour). The first bowel movement should occur in ≈ 1 hour.

➤*Preparation of solution:* Tap water may be used to reconstitute the solution. Shake container vigorously several times to ensure that the powder is completely dissolved. Do not add flavorings or additional ingredients to solution before use.

After reconstitution to 4 L volume with water, the solution contains PEG 3350 17.6 mmol/L, sodium 125 mmol/L, sulfate 40 mmol/L (*Colyte*80 mmol/L), chloride 35 mmol/L, bicarbonate 20 mmol/L, and potassium 10 mmol/L.

➤*Storage/Stability:* Refrigerate reconstituted solution (chilling before administration improves palatability); use within 48 hours.

Actions

➤*Pharmacology:* Oral solution induces diarrhea, which rapidly cleanses the bowel, usually within 4 hours. Polyethylene glycol 3350 (PEG 3350) and the electrolyte concentration result in virtually no net absorption or excretion of ions or water. Large volumes may be given without significant changes in water or electrolyte balance.

Contraindications

GI obstruction; gastric retention; bowel perforation; toxic colitis, megacolon, or ileus.

Warnings

➤*Pregnancy:* Category C. Safety has not been established. Use only when clearly needed and when the benefits outweigh the potential hazards to the fetus.

➤*Children:* Safety and efficacy for use in children have not been established.

Several studies in infants and children from 3 to 14 years of age showed PEG-electrolyte solutions are safe and effective in bowel evacuation.

Precautions

➤*Regurgitation/Aspiration:* Observe unconscious or semiconscious patients with impaired gag reflex and those who are otherwise prone to regurgitation or aspiration during use, especially if given via a nasogastric tube. If GI obstruction or perforation is suspected, rule out these contraindications before administration.

➤*GI problems:* If a patient experiences severe bloating, distention, or abdominal pain, slow or temporarily discontinue administration until symptoms abate.

➤*Severe ulcerative colitis:* Use with caution.

Drug Interactions

Oral medication given within 1 hour of start of therapy may be flushed from the GI tract and not absorbed.

Adverse Reactions

Nausea, abdominal fullness, and bloating are the most common adverse reactions (occurring in up to 50% of patients). Abdominal cramps, vomiting, and anal irritation occur less frequently. These adverse reactions are transient. Isolated cases of urticaria, rhinorrhea, and dermatitis have been reported, which may represent allergic reactions.

POLYETHYLENE GLYCOL (PEG) SOLUTION

Rx	**GlycoLax** (Kremers Urban)	**Powder for Oral Solution:** 17 g PEG 3350	In 14 single-dose packets.
Rx	**Polyethylene Glycol** (Braintree)	**Powder for Oral Solution:** 255 g PEG 3350	In 16 oz.
Rx	**GlycoLax** (Kremers Urban)		In 16 oz w/dosing cup.
Rx	**MiraLax** (Braintree)		In 14 oz.
Rx	**Polyethylene Glycol** (Braintree)	**Powder for Oral Solution:** 527 g PEG 3350	In 32 oz.
Rx	**GlycoLax** (Kremers Urban)		In 24 oz w/dosing cup.
Rx	**MiraLax** (Braintree)		In 26 oz.

POLYETHYLENE GLYCOL 3350 — ORAL

For complete and comparative prescribing information, refer to the Laxatives group monograph.

Indications

➤*Constipation:* For the treatment of occasional constipation. This product should be used for 2 weeks or less or as directed by a physician.

Administration and Dosage

The usual dose is 17 g (about 1 heaping tbsp) of powder per day (or as directed by physician) in 8 ounces of water. Each bottle of polyethylene glycol is supplied with a measuring cap marked to contain 17 g of laxative powder when filled to the indicated line.

Two to 4 days (48 to 96 hours) may be required to produce a bowel movement.

Polyethylene glycol should be administered dissolved in ≈ 8 ounces of water.

➤*Storage/Stability:* Store at 25°C (77°F); excursions permitted to 15° to 30°C (59° to 86°F) (see USP Controlled Room Temperature).

MISCELLANEOUS BOWEL EVACUANTS

otc	**X-Prep Liquid** (Gray)	Senna extract, parabens, 50 g sugar. Alcohol free. In 74 mL.
otc	**Tridrate Bowel Cleansing System** (Lafayette)	19 g magnesium citrate. 3 bisacodyl tablets (5 mg each). 1 bisacodyl suppository (10 mg).
otc	**X-Prep Bowel Evacuant Kit-1** (Gray)	74 mL **X-Prep** liquid: Extract of senna concentrate, 50 g sugar, sucrose, parabens. Alcohol-free. 2 **Senokot-S** tablets: Standardized senna concentrate and 50 mg docusate sodium per tablet, lactose. 1 **Rectolax** suppository: 10 mg bisacodyl.
otc	**Fleet Prep Kit 1** (Fleet)	45 mL **Phospho-soda** (21.6 g monobasic sodium phosphate and 8.1 g dibasic sodium phosphate). 4 bisacodyl tablets (5 mg each). Enteric-coated. 1 bisacodyl suppository (10 mg).
otc	**Fleet Prep Kit 2** (Fleet)	45 mL **Phospho-soda** (21.6 g monobasic sodium phosphate and 8.1 g dibasic sodium phosphate). 4 bisacodyl tablets (5 mg each). Enteric-coated. 1 bag enema.
otc	**Fleet Prep Kit 3** (Fleet)	45 mL **Phospho-soda** (21.6 g monobasic sodium phosphate and 8.1 g dibasic sodium phosphate). 4 bisacodyl tablets (5 mg each). Enteric-coated. One 30 mL bisacodyl enema (10 mg).
Rx	**Visicol** (InKine Pharmaceutical)	**Tablets:** 1.102 g sodium phosphate monobasic monohydrate, 0.398 g sodium phosphate dibasic anhydrous (total of 1.5 g sodium phosphate). In 40s.

Bowel Evacuants

MISCELLANEOUS BOWEL EVACUANTS

Rx	**HalfLytely** (Braintree)	2 L bottle **HalfLytely Powder for oral solution**(210 g PEG 3350, 5.6 g sodium chloride, 2.86 g sodium bicarbonate, 0.74 g potassium chloride, lemon-lime flavor). 4 bisacodyl delayed-release tablets (5 mg each). Lactose, sugar, sucrose. Enteric-coated.

For complete and comparative prescribing information, refer to the Laxatives group monograph.

Miscellaneous Laxatives

CASTOR OIL

otc	**Castor Oil** (Various, eg, Humco, Paddock)	**Liquid**: *Dose:* Adults and children > 12 years - 15 to 60 mL/day. Children 2 to younger than 12 years - 5 to 15 mL/day.	In 60, 120, and 480 mL.
otc	**Emulsoil** (Paddock)	**Emulsion**: 95% castor oil with emulsifying agents. *Dose:* Adults and children ≥ 12 years - 15 to 60 mL/day mixed with ½ to 1 glass liquid. Children 2 to younger than 12 years - 5 to 15 mL mixed with ½ to 1 glass liquid.	Butylparaben. In 63 mL.
otc *sf*	**Neoloid** (Kenwood)	**Emulsion**: 36.4% castor oil with 0.1% sodium benzoate, 0.2% potassium sorbate. *Dose:* Adults and children ≥ 12 years - 45 to 60 mL/day. Children 2 to younger than 12 years - 15 to 30 mL/day	Mint flavor. In 118 mL.

CASTOR OIL — ORAL

For complete and comparative prescribing information, refer to the Laxatives group monograph.

Laxative Combinations

LAXATIVE COMBINATIONS, CAPSULES AND TABLETS

		Docusate (mg)	Senna Concentrate (mg)	Casanthranol (mg)	Cascara sagrada (mg)	Psyllium (mg)	Other Content and How Supplied
otc	**Senna Plus Tablets** (Contract Pharmacal)	50[a]	8.6[b]				Tartrazine. In 100s.
otc	**Senna-S** (Akyma)	50[a]	8.6[b]				In 1,000s.
otc	**Senokot-S Tablets** (Purdue Frederick)	50[a]	8.6[b]				Lactose. In 10s, 30s, 60s, 1,000s, and UD 100s.
otc	**PeriColace Tablets** (Purdue)	50[a]	8.6[b]				In 10s, 30s, and 60s.
otc	**ex-lax Gentle Strength Caplets** (Novartis)	65[a]	10[b]				Lactose, methylparaben, polydextrose. (ex-lax). In 24s.
otc	**Docusate w/Casanthranol Caps** (Various, eg, Paddock, Schein, URL)	100[a]		30			In 100s, 1,000s, and UD 100s, 300s, and 600s.
otc	**DSS 100 Plus Capsules** (Magno-Humphries)						In 60s.
otc	**Laxative & Stool Softener** (Rugby)						Parabens, sorbitol. In 100s.
otc	**Peri-Colace Capsules** (Roberts)						Sorbitol, parabens. In 30s, 60s, 250s, 1,000s, and UD 100s.
otc	**Peri-Dos Softgels (Capsules)** (Goldline)						Sorbitol, parabens. Maroon. In 100s and 1,000s.
otc	**Senna Prompt Capsules** (Konsyl)		9			500	In 90s.
otc	**Nature's Remedy Tablets** (Block Drug)				150		100 mg aloe, lactose. In 15s, 30s, and 60s.

[a] As sodium. [b] As sennosides.

LAXATIVE COMBINATIONS — CAPSULES AND TABLETS

For complete prescribing information, refer to the Laxatives group monograph.

Administration and Dosage

➤*Adults:* 1 to 4 capsules/tablets per day. Products vary. Consult product labeling for specific guidelines.

➤*Children younger than 12 years of age:* Products vary. Consult product labeling for specific guidelines.

LAXATIVE COMBINATIONS, LIQUIDS

otc	**Diocto C** (Various, eg, Alpharma, Rugby)	**Syrup**: 60 mg docusate sodium and 30 mg casanthranol per 15 mL	In 480 mL.
otc	**Peri-Colace** (Roberts)		10% alcohol. Sorbitol, sucrose, parabens. In 240 and 480 mL.
otc *sf*	**Liqui-Doss** (Ferndale)	**Emulsion**: Mineral oil in an emulsifying base	Alcohol free. In 60 and 480 mL.
otc	**Haley's M-O** (Bayer)	**Liquid:** ≈ 900 mg magnesium hydroxide and 3.75 mL mineral oil per 15 mL	Saccharin (vanilla creme only). Regular or vanilla creme. In 360 (both) and 780 mL (vanilla creme only).
otc	**Black-Draught** (Monticello)	**Syrup**: 90 mg per 15 mL casanthranol with senna extract, rhubarb, methyl salicylate, and menthol	5% alcohol. Tartrazine, parabens, sucrose, saccharin. In 60 and 150 mL.
otc	**Silace-C** (Silarx)	**Syrup**: 30 mg casanthranol, 60 mg docusate sodium per 15 mL	10% alcohol. In 473 mL.
otc	**Sorbitol Solution** (Various, eg, Geritrex , Spectrum, Upsher-Smith)	**Solution**: 70% w/w D-sorbitol	In 454 mL.

LAXATIVE COMBINATIONS — LIQUIDS

For complete prescribing information, refer to the Laxatives group monograph.

Administration and Dosage

➤*Dose:*

Adults – 5 to 60 mL. Products vary. Consult product labeling for specific guidelines.

Children younger than 12 years of age – Products vary. Consult product labeling for specific guidelines.

LAXATIVE COMBINATIONS, GRANULES

otc	**Perdiem Overnight Relief** (Novartis Consumer Health)	**Granules**: 3.25 g psyllium, 0.74 g senna, 1.8 mg sodium, 35.5 mg potassium, and 4 calories per rounded teaspoonful	Dye free. Sucrose. Mint flavor. In 100, 250, and 400 g.

LAXATIVE COMBINATIONS — GRANULES

For complete prescribing information, refer to the Laxatives group monograph.

Administration and Dosage

➤*Dose:*

Adults and children ≥ 12 years of age – 1 or 2 rounded tsp, 1 to 2 times daily, with ≥ 8 oz cool liquid. Do not chew.

Children 7 to 11 years of age – 1 rounded tsp 1 to 2 times daily with ≥ 8 oz cool liquid. Do not chew.

For severe constipation – May take ≤ 2 rounded tsp every 6 hours, not to exceed 5 tsp/24 hours.

DIFENOXIN HYDROCHLORIDE WITH ATROPINE SULFATE

c-iv	**Motofen** (Carnrick)	**Tablets:** 1 mg difenoxin (as hydrochloride) and 0.025 mg atropine sulfate	Dye free. (C 8674). White, scored. Five-sided. In 50s and 100s.

DIFENOXIN HYDROCHLORIDE WITH ATROPINE SULFATE — ORAL

Indications

Adjunctive therapy in management of acute nonspecific diarrhea and acute exacerbations of chronic functional diarrhea.

Administration and Dosage

➤*Adults:* Recommended starting dose: 2 tablets, then 1 tablet after each loose stool; 1 tablet every 3 to 4 hours as needed. The total dosage during any 24 hour treatment period should not exceed 8 tablets. For diarrhea in which clinical improvement is not observed in 48 hours, continued administration is not recommended. For acute diarrhea and acute exacerbations of functional diarrhea, treatment beyond 48 hours is usually not necessary.

Difenoxin hydrochloride with atropine sulfate is not innocuous; strictly adhere to dosage recommendations.

➤*Children:* Studies in children younger than 12 years of age are inadequate to evaluate safety and efficacy. Contraindicated in children younger than 2 years of age.

Actions

➤*Pharmacology:* Difenoxin is an antidiarrheal agent chemically related to meperidine. Atropine sulfate is present to discourage deliberate overdosage.

Animal studies have shown that difenoxin manifests its antidiarrheal effect by slowing intestinal motility. The mechanism of action is by a local effect on the gastrointestinal wall.

Difenoxin is the principal active metabolite of diphenoxylate and is effective at one-fifth the dosage of diphenoxylate.

➤*Pharmacokinetics:* Difenoxin is rapidly and extensively absorbed orally. Mean peak plasma levels of 160 ng/mL occur within 40 to 60 minutes in most patients following a 2 mg dose. Plasma levels decline to less than 10% of their peak values within 24 hours and to less than 1% of their peak values within 72 hours. This decline parallels the appearance of difenoxin and its metabolites in the urine. Difenoxin is metabolized to an inactive hydroxylated metabolite. Both the drug and its metabolites are excreted, mainly as conjugates, in urine and feces.

Contraindications

Diarrhea associated with organisms that penetrate the intestinal mucosa (eg, toxigenic *E. coli*, *Salmonella* sp, *Shigella*;) and pseudomembranous colitis associated with broad-spectrum antibiotics. Antiperistaltic agents may prolong or worsen diarrhea.

Children younger than 2 years of age because of the decreased margin of safety of drugs in this class in younger age groups.

Hypersensitivity to difenoxin, atropine or any of the inactive ingredients; jaundice.

Warnings

➤*Fluid and electrolyte balance:* The use of this drug does not preclude the administration of appropriate fluid and electrolyte therapy. Dehydration, particularly in children, may further influence the variability of response and may predispose to delayed difenoxin intoxication. Drug-induced inhibition of peristalsis may result in fluid retention in the colon, and this may further aggravate dehydration and electrolyte imbalance. If severe dehydration or electrolyte imbalance is manifested, withhold the drug until appropriate corrective therapy has been initiated.

➤*Ulcerative colitis:* Agents which inhibit intestinal motility or delay intestinal transit time have induced toxic megacolon. Consequently, carefully observe patients with acute ulcerative colitis. Discontinue promptly if abdominal distention occurs or if other untoward symptoms develop.

➤*Liver and kidney disease:* Use with extreme caution in patients with advanced hepato-renal disease and in all patients with abnormal liver function tests since hepatic coma may be precipitated.

➤*Atropine:* A subtherapeutic dose of atropine has been added to difenoxin to discourage deliberate overdosage. A recommended dose is not likely to cause prominent anticholinergic side effects, but avoid in patients in whom anticholinergic drugs are contraindicated. Observe the warnings and precautions for use of anticholinergic agents. In children, signs of atropinism may occur even with recommended doses, particularly in patients with Down's syndrome.

➤*Pregnancy: Category C.* Reproduction studies in rats and rabbits with doses up to 75 times the human therapeutic dose demonstrated no evidence of teratogenesis. Pregnant rats receiving oral doses 20 times the maximum human dose had an increase in delivery time as well as a significant increase in the percent of stillbirths. Neonatal survival in rats was also reduced with most deaths occurring within 4 days of delivery. There are no well controlled studies in pregnant women. Use during pregnancy only if the potential benefit justifies the potential risk to the fetus.

➤*Lactation:* Because of the potential for serious adverse reactions in nursing infants, decide whether to discontinue nursing or to discontinue the drug, taking into account the importance of the drug to the mother.

➤*Children:* Contraindicated in children under 2 years of age. Safety and efficacy in children below the age of 12 have not been established. See Overdosage section for information on hazards from accidental poisoning in children.

Precautions

➤*Drug abuse and dependence:* Addiction to (dependence on) difenoxin is theoretically possible at high dosage. Therefore, do not exceed recommended dosage. Because of the structural and pharmacological similarities of difenoxin to drugs with definite addiction potential, administer with caution to patients receiving addicting drugs, to addiction-prone individuals, or to those whose histories suggest they may increase the dosage on their own initiative.

Drug Interactions

Difenoxin Drug Interactions

Precipitant drug	Object drug*		Description
Difenoxin	Barbiturates, tranquilizers, narcotics, and alcohol	↑	Barbiturates, tranquilizers, narcotics, and alcohol may be potentiated by coadministration of difenoxin. Closely monitor patients.
Difenoxin	MAOIs	↑	Because the chemical structure of difenoxin is similar to meperidine, concurrent use with MAOIs may, in theory, precipitate a hypertensive crisis.

* ↑ = Object drug increased.

Adverse Reactions

Anticholinergic – In view of the small amount of atropine present (0.025 mg/tablet), effects such as dryness of the skin and mucous membranes, flushing, hyperthermia, tachycardia and urinary retention are very unlikely to occur, except perhaps in children.

Many adverse effects reported during clinical investigation are difficult to distinguish from symptoms of diarrheal syndrome. However, the following events have occurred:

➤*CNS:* Dizziness, lightheadedness (5%); drowsiness (4%); headache (2.5%); tiredness, nervousness, insomnia, confusion (less than 1%).

➤*GI:* Nausea (7%), vomiting, dry mouth (3%); epigastric distress, constipation (≤ 1%).

➤*Ophthalmic:* Burning eyes, blurred vision (infrequent).

Overdosage

➤*Symptoms:* Initial signs may include dryness of the skin and mucous membranes, flushing, hyperthermia and tachycardia followed by lethargy or coma, hypotonic reflexes, nystagmus, pinpoint pupils and respiratory depression. Overdosage may result in severe respiratory depression and coma, possibly leading to permanent brain damage or death.

➤*Treatment:* Gastric lavage, establishment of a patent airway and, possibly, mechanically assisted respiration are advised. Refer to General Management of Acute Overdosage.

Naloxone may be used in the treatment of respiratory depression. When administered IV, the onset is generally apparent within 2 minutes. Naloxone may also be administered SC or IM providing a slightly less rapid onset but a more prolonged effect.

Because the duration of action of difenoxin is longer than that of naloxone, improvement of respiration following administration may be followed by recurrent respiratory depression. Continuous observation is necessary until the effect of difenoxin on respiration (which may persist for many hours) has passed. Supplemental IM naloxone doses may be used to produce a longer lasting effect. Treat all possible overdosages as serious; observe for at least 48 hours, preferably under continuous hospital care.

Although signs of overdosage and respiratory depression may not be evident soon after ingestion of difenoxin, respiratory depression may occur 12 to 30 hours later.

Patient Information

Adhere strictly to recommended dosage schedules. Keep out of reach of children since accidental overdosage may result in severe, even fatal, respiratory depression.

May cause dizziness or drowsiness; use caution while driving or performing other tasks requiring alertness, coordination or physical dexterity.

DIPHENOXYLATE HYDROCHLORIDE WITH ATROPINE SULFATE

c-v	**Diphenoxylate hydrochloride w/Atropine Sulfate** (Various, eg, Mylan, Purepac, Rugby, Schein)	**Tablets:** 2.5 mg diphenoxylate hydrochloride and 0.025 mg atropine sulfate	In 100s, 500s, 1000s, 2500s and UD 100s.
c-v	**Logen** (Goldline)		White. In 100s, 500s & 1000s.
c-v	**Lomotil** (Searle)		Sorbitol, sucrose. (Searle 61). White. In 100s, 500s, 1000s, 2500s, UD 100s.
c-v	**Lonox** (Sandoz)		(GG 4). White. In 30s, 100s, 500s, 1,000s & UD 100s.
c-v	**Diphenoxylate hydrochloride w/ Atropine Sulfate** (Various, eg, Goldline, Roxane, Rugby)	**Liquid:** 2.5 mg diphenoxylate hydrochloride and 0.025 mg atropine sulfate per 5 mL	In 60 mL, UD 4 and 10 mL.
c-v	**Lomanate** (Qualitest)		In 60 mL.
c-v	**Lomotil** (Searle)		15% alcohol. Sorbitol. Cherry flavor. In 60 mL w/dropper.

DIPHENOXYLATE HYDROCHLORIDE WITH ATROPINE SULFATE — ORAL

Indications

Adjunctive therapy in the management of diarrhea.

Administration and Dosage

➤*Adults:* Individualize dosage. Initial dose is 5 mg 4 times a day.

➤*Children:* See Warnings. In children 2 to 12 years of age, use liquid form only. The recommended initial dosage is 0.3 to 0.4 mg/kg daily, in 4 divided doses.

Diphenoxylate w/Atropine Pediatric Dosage

Age (years)	Approximate weight kg	Approximate weight lb	Dosage (mL) (4 times daily)
2	11 to 14	24 to 31	1.5 to 3
3	12 to 16	26 to 35	2 to 3
4	14 to 20	31 to 44	2 to 4
5	16 to 23	35 to 51	2.5 to 4.5
6 to 8	17 to 32	38 to 71	2.5 to 5
9 to 12	23 to 55	51 to 121	3.5 to 5

This pediatric schedule is the best approximation of an average dose recommendation which may be adjusted downwards according to the overall nutritional status and degree of dehydration encountered in the sick child.

➤*Reduce dosage:* Reduce dosage as soon as initial control of symptoms is achieved. Maintenance dosage may be as low as ¼ of the initial daily dosage. Do not exceed recommended dosage. Clinical improvement of acute diarrhea is usually observed within 48 hours. If clinical improvement of chronic diarrhea is not seen within 10 days after a maximum daily dose of 20 mg, symptoms are unlikely to be controlled by further use.

Actions

➤*Pharmacology:* Diphenoxylate, a constipating meperidine congener, lacks analgesic activity. High doses (40 to 60 mg) cause opioid activity, (eg, euphoria, suppression of morphine abstinence syndrome, physical dependence after chronic use).

➤*Pharmacokinetics:* Bioavailability of tablet vs liquid is ≈ 90%. Diphenoxylate is rapidly, extensively metabolized to diphenoxylic acid (difenoxine), the active major metabolite. Elimination half-life is ≈ 12 to 14 hrs. An average of 14% of drug and metabolites are excreted over 4 days in urine, 49% in feces. Urinary excretion of unmetabolized drug is less than 1%; difenoxine plus its glucuronide conjugate constitutes ≈ 6%.

Contraindications

Children younger than 2 years of age, due to greater variability of response; hypersensitivity to diphenoxylate or atropine; obstructive jaundice; diarrhea associated with pseudomembranous enterocolitis or enterotoxin-producing bacteria (see Warnings).

Warnings

➤*Diarrhea:* Diphenoxylate may prolong or aggravate diarrhea associated with organisms that penetrate intestinal mucosa (ie, toxigenic *Escherichia coli, Salmonella, Shigella*) or in pseudomembranous enterocolitis associated with broad-spectrum antibiotics. Do not use diphenoxylate in these conditions. In some patients with acute ulcerative colitis, diphenoxylate may induce toxic megacolon. Discontinue therapy if abdominal distention or other untoward symptoms develop.

➤*Fluid/electrolyte balance:* Dehydration, particularly in younger children, may influence variability of response and may predispose to delayed diphenoxylate intoxication. Inhibition of peristalsis may result in fluid retention in the intestine, which may further aggravate dehydration and electrolyte imbalance. If severe dehydration or electrolyte imbalance occurs, withhold the drug until initiating corrective therapy.

➤*Hepatic function impairment:* Use with extreme caution in patients with advanced hepato-renal disease or abnormal liver function; hepatic coma may be precipitated.

➤*Pregnancy: Category C.* There are no adequate and well controlled studies in pregnant women. Use in women of childbearing potential only when clearly needed and when the potential benefits outweigh the potential hazards to the fetus.

➤*Lactation:* Exercise caution when administering to a nursing mother. Diphenoxylic acid may be excreted in breast milk and atropine is excreted in breast milk.

➤*Children:* Use with caution; signs of atropinism may occur with recommended doses, particularly in Down's syndrome patients. Use with caution in young children due to variable response. Not recommended in children younger than 2 years of age.

Precautions

➤*Drug abuse and dependence:* In recommended doses, diphenoxylate has not produced addiction and is devoid of morphine-like subjective effects. At high doses, it exhibits codeine-like subjective effects; therefore, addiction to diphenoxylate is possible. A subtherapeutic dose of atropine may discourage deliberate abuse.

➤*Hazardous tasks:* Patients should use caution while driving or performing other tasks requiring alertness, coordination or physical dexterity.

Drug Interactions

Diphenoxylate Drug Interactions

Precipitant drug	Object drug*		Description
Diphenoxylate	MAOIs	↑	Since the chemical structure of diphenoxylate is similar to meperidine, concurrent use may precipitate hypertensive crises.
Diphenoxylate	Barbiturates, tranquilizers, and alcohol	↑	Diphenoxylate may potentiate the depressant action. Closely observe the patient when these medications are used concomitantly.

* ↑ = Object drug increased.

Adverse Reactions

Atropine effects – Dry skin and mucous membranes, flushing, hyperthermia, tachycardia, urinary retention, especially in children.

➤*CNS:* Dizziness; drowsiness; sedation; headache; malaise; lethargy; restlessness; euphoria; depression; numbness of extremities; confusion.

➤*GI:* Anorexia; nausea; vomiting; abdominal discomfort; paralytic ileus; toxic megacolon; pancreatitis.

➤*Hypersensitivity:* Pruritus; gum swelling; angioneurotic edema; urticaria; anaphylaxis.

Overdosage

➤*Symptoms:* Initial signs include dry skin and mucous membranes, mydriasis, restlessness, flushing, hyperthermia and tachycardia followed by lethargy or coma, hypotonic reflexes, nystagmus and pinpoint pupils. Severe, even fatal, respiratory depression may result. Signs of overdosage and respiratory depression may not be evident soon after ingestion; respiratory depression may occur 12 to 30 hours later.

➤*Treatment:* includes usual supportive measures. Refer to General Management of Acute Overdosage. Gastric lavage, induction of emesis, establishment of a patent airway, and, possibly, mechanically assisted respiration are advised. Use naloxone for respiratory depression (see individual monograph). Diphenoxylate's duration of action is longer than that of naloxone; improved respiration after administration may be followed by recurrent respiratory depression. Consequently, continuous observation for at least 48 hours is necessary until diphenoxylate's effect on respiration has passed. Activated charcoal may significantly decrease bioavailability of diphenoxylate. In non-comatose patients, 100 g activated charcoal slurry can be given immediately after induction of vomiting or gastric lavage.

Patient Information

Do not exceed prescribed dosage. Avoid alcohol and other CNS depressants.

May cause drowsiness or dizziness; use caution while driving or performing other tasks requiring alertness, coordination or physical dexterity.

May cause dry mouth.

Notify physician if diarrhea persists or if fever, palpitations or abnormal distention occur.

LOPERAMIDE HYDROCHLORIDE

otc	**Diar-aid Caplets** (Thompson)	**Tablets**: 2 mg	In 12s.
otc	**Imodium A-D Caplets** (McNeil-CPC)		Lactose. (Imodium Janssen). In 6s and 12s.
otc	**K-Pek II** (Rugby)		Lactose. (122). Capsule shape. In 12s.
Rx	**Loperamide** (Various, eg, Mylan, Novopharm)	**Capsules**: 2 mg	In 100s, 500s and 1000s.
otc	**Neo-Diaral** (Roberts)		In UD 8s and 250s.
otc	**Loperamide** (Various, eg, Barre-National, Roxane)	**Liquid**: 1 mg/5 mL	In 60 and 118 mL.
otc	**Imodium A-D** (McNeil-CPC)		5.25% alcohol. Cherry/licorice flavor. In 60, 90 and 120 mL.
otc	**Imodium A-D** (McNeil Consumer)	**Liquid**: 1 mg/7.5 mL	Mint flavor. In 120 mL.
otc	**Pepto Diarrhea Control** (Procter & Gamble)	**Liquid**: 1 mg/mL	5.25% alcohol, parabens. Cherry flavor. In 60 and 120 mL.

LOPERAMIDE HYDROCHLORIDE — ORAL

Indications

➤*Rx:* Loperamide is indicated for the control and symptomatic relief of acute nonspecific diarrhea and of chronic diarrhea associated with inflammatory bowel disease. Loperamide is also indicated for reducing the volume of discharge from ileostomies.

➤*OTC:* Control of symptoms of diarrhea, including traveler's diarrhea.

➤*Unlabeled uses:* In one study, the combination of loperamide (4 mg loading dose, 2 mg after each loose stool) plus trimethoprim sulfamethoxazole for 3 days resulted in more rapid relief from traveler's diarrhea than either agent alone.

Administration and Dosage

➤*Approved by the FDA:* December 28, 1976.

➤*Rx:* Patients should receive appropriate fluid and electrolyte replacement as needed.

Acute diarrhea –

Adults:

• *Capsules* – The recommended initial dose is 4 mg (2 capsules) followed by 2 mg (1 capsule) after each unformed stool. Daily dosage should not exceed 16 mg (8 capsules). Clinical improvement is usually observed within 48 hours.

Children: Loperamide hydrochloride use is not recommended for children under 2 years of age. In children 2 to 5 years of age (20 kg or less), a nonprescription liquid formulation should be used; for children ages 6 to 12, either loperamide hydrochloride capsules or liquid may be used. For children 2 to 12 years of age, the following schedule for capsules or liquid will usually fulfill initial dosage requirements.

Recommended first day dosage schedule:

• *Children 2 to 5 years (13 to 20 kg)* – 1 mg 3 times a day (3 mg daily dose).

• *Children 5 to 8 years (20 to 30 kg)* – 2 mg twice a day (4 mg daily dose).

• *Children 8 to 12 years (greater than 30 kg)* – 2 mg 3 times a day (6 mg daily dose).

Recommended subsequent daily dosage: Following the first treatment day, it is recommended that subsequent loperamide doses (1 mg/10 kg body weight) be administered only after a loose stool. Total daily dosage should not exceed recommended dosages for the first day.

Chronic diarrhea –

Adults: The recommended initial dose is 4 mg (2 capsules) followed by 2 mg (1 capsule) after each unformed stool until diarrhea is controlled, after which the dosage of loperamide should be reduced to meet individual requirements. When the optimal daily dosage has been established, this amount may then be administered as a single dose or in divided doses.

The average daily maintenance dosage in clinical trials was 4 to 8 mg (2 to 4 capsules). A dosage of 16 mg (8 capsules) was rarely exceeded. If clinical improvement is not observed after treatment with 16 mg per day for at least 10 days, symptoms are unlikely to be controlled by further administration. Loperamide administration may be continued if diarrhea cannot be adequately controlled with diet or specific treatment.

Children: Although loperamide hydrochloride has been studied in a limited number of children with chronic diarrhea, the therapeutic dose for the treatment of chronic diarrhea in a pediatric population has not been established.

➤*OTC:*

Liquid –

Adults and children 12 years of age and older: For adults and children 12 years of age and older, 20 mL (4 teaspoonfuls) after the first loose bowel movement and 10 mL (2 teaspoonfuls) after each subsequent loose bowel movement but no more than 40 mL (8 teaspoonfuls) a day for no more than 2 days.

• *Liquid (1 mg per 7.5 mL formulation)* – 30 mL (6 teaspoonfuls) after the first loose stool; 15 mL (3 teaspoonfuls) after each subsequent loose stool; no more than 60 mL (12 teaspoonfuls) in 24 hours.

Children 9 to 11 years of age (60 to 95 lbs): For children 9 to 11 years of age, 10 mL (2 teaspoonfuls) after the first loose bowel movement and 5 mL (1 teaspoonful) after each subsequent loose bowel movement but no more than 30 mL (6 teaspoonfuls) a day for no more than 2 days.

• *Liquid (1 mg per 7.5 mL formulation)* – 15 mL (3 teaspoonfuls) after first loose stool; 7.5 mL (1.5 teaspoonfuls) after each subsequent loose stool; no more than 45 mL (9 teaspoonfuls) in 24 hours.

Children 6 to 8 years of age (48 to 59 lbs): For children 6 to 8 years of age, 10 mL (2 teaspoonfuls) after the first loose bowel movement and 5 mL (1 teaspoonful) after each subsequent loose bowel movement but no more than 20 mL (4 teaspoonfuls) a day for no more than 2 days.

• *Liquid (1 mg per 7.5 mL formulation)* – 15 mL (3 teaspoonfuls) after first loose stool; 7.5 mL (1.5 teaspoonfuls) after each subsequent loose stool; no more than 30 mL (6 teaspoonfuls) in 24 hours.

Children under 6 years old (up to 47 lbs): Consult a physician. Not intended for use in children under 6 years old.

Tablets – Drink plenty of clear fluids to help prevent dehydration, which may accompany diarrhea. Find right dose on chart. If possible, use weight to dose, otherwise use age.

Adults and children 12 years and older: 2 tablets after the first loose bowel movement; 1 tablet after each subsequent loose bowel movement. No more than 4 tablets a day.

Children 9 to 11 years (60 to 95 lbs): 1 tablet after the first loose bowel movement; ½ tablet after each subsequent loose bowel movement. No more than 3 tablets a day.

Children 6 to 8 years (45 to 59 lbs): 1 tablet after the first loose bowel movement; ½ tablet after each subsequent loose bowel movement. No more than 2 tablets a day.

Children under 6 years (up to 47 lbs): Ask a doctor (not intended for use in children under 6 years old).

➤*Storage / Stability:* Dispense in a tight, light-resistant container using a child-resistant closure.

Capsules and liquid – Store at controlled room temperature 15° to 30°C (59° to 86°F).

Tablets – Store at 15° to 25°C (59° to 77°F).

Actions

➤*Pharmacology:* In vitro and animal studies show that loperamide acts by slowing intestinal motility and by affecting water and electrolyte movement through the bowel. Loperamide inhibits peristaltic activity by a direct effect on the circular and longitudinal muscles of the intestinal wall.

In man, loperamide prolongs the transit time of the intestinal contents. It reduces the daily fecal volume, increases the viscosity and bulk density, and diminishes the loss of fluid and electrolytes. Tolerance to the antidiarrheal effect has not been observed.

➤*Pharmacokinetics:* Clinical studies have indicated that the apparent elimination half-life of loperamide in man is 10.8 hours with a range of 9.1 to 14.4 hours. Plasma levels of unchanged drug remain below 2 ng/mL after the intake of a 2 mg capsule of loperamide. Plasma levels are highest approximately 5 hours after administration of the capsule and 2.5 hours after the liquid. The peak plasma levels of loperamide were similar for both formulations. Of the total excreted in urine and feces, most of the administered drug was excreted in feces.

In those patients in whom biochemical and hematological parameters were monitored during clinical trials, no trends toward abnormality during loperamide therapy were noted. Similarly, urinalyses, EKG and clinical ophthalmological examinations did not show trends toward abnormality.

Contraindications

Loperamide is contraindicated in patients with known hypersensitivity to the drug and in those in whom constipation must be avoided.

Warnings

➤*Acute dysentery:* Loperamide should not be used in the case of acute dysentery, which is characterized by blood in stools and high fever.

➤*Fluid and electrolyte depletion:* Fluid and electrolyte depletion may occur in patients who have diarrhea. In such cases, administration of appropriate fluid and electrolytes is very important. The use of loperamide does not preclude the administration of appropriate fluid and electrolyte therapy.

➤*Toxic megacolon:* In some patients with acute ulcerative colitis, and in pseudomembranous colitis associated with broad-spectrum antibiotics,

LOPERAMIDE HYDROCHLORIDE — ORAL

agents which inhibit intestinal motility or delay intestinal transit time have been reported to induce toxic megacolon.

➤*Discontinue use:* Loperamide therapy should be discontinued promptly if abdominal distention, constipation, or ileus occurs.

➤*Hepatic function impairment:* Patients with hepatic dysfunction should be monitored closely for signs of CNS toxicity because of the apparent large first-pass biotransformation.

➤*Fertility impairment:* Reproduction studies in rats indicated that high doses (150 to 200 times the human dose) could cause marked female infertility and reduced male fertility.

➤*Pregnancy: Category B.* Reproduction studies in rats and rabbits have revealed no evidence of impaired fertility or harm to the fetus at doses up to 30 times the human dose. Higher doses impaired the survival of mothers and nursing young. The studies offered no evidence of teratogenic activity. There are, however, no adequate and well controlled studies in pregnant women. Because animal reproduction studies are not always predictive of human response, this drug should be used during pregnancy only if clearly needed.

➤*Lactation:* It is not known whether this drug is excreted in human milk. Because many drugs are excreted in human milk, caution should be exercised when loperamide is administered to a nursing woman.

➤*Children:* Loperamide should be used with special caution in young children because of the greater variability of response in this age group. Dehydration, particularly in younger children, may further influence the variability of response to loperamide.

Precautions

➤*Monitoring:* Patients with hepatic dysfunction should be monitored closely for signs of CNS toxicity because of the apparent large first-pass biotransformation.

In acute diarrhea, if clinical improvement is not observed in 48 hours, the administration of loperamide should be discontinued.

➤*Drug abuse and dependence:*

Abuse – A specific clinical study designed to assess the abuse potential of loperamide at high doses resulted in a finding of extremely low abuse potential.

Dependence – Studies in morphine-dependent monkeys demonstrated that loperamide hydrochloride at doses above those recommended for humans prevented signs of morphine withdrawal. However, in humans, the naloxone challenge pupil test, which when positive indicates opiate-like effects, performed after a single high dose, or after more than 2 years of therapeutic use of loperamide, was negative. Orally administered loperamide (loperamide formulated with magnesium stearate) is both highly insoluble and penetrates the CNS poorly.

Drug Interactions

There was no evidence in clinical trials of drug interactions with concurrent medications.

Adverse Reactions

The adverse effects reported during clinical investigations of loperamide are difficult to distinguish from symptoms associated with the diarrheal syndrome. Adverse experiences recorded during clinical studies with loperamide were generally of a minor and self-limiting nature. They were more commonly observed during the treatment of chronic diarrhea.

The following patient complaints have been reported and are listed in decreasing order of frequency with the exception of hypersensitivity reactions, which is listed first since it may be the most serious:

- Hypersensitivity reactions (including skin rash) have been reported with loperamide use.
- Abdominal pain, distention or discomfort.
- Nausea and vomiting.
- Constipation.
- Tiredness.
- Drowsiness or dizziness.
- Dry mouth.

In postmarketing experiences, there have been rare reports of paralytic ileus associated with abdominal distention. Most of these reports occurred in the setting of acute dysentery, overdose, and with very young children of less than 2 years of age.

Overdosage

➤*Symptoms:* In cases of overdosage, paralytic ileus and CNS depression may occur. Children may be more sensitive to CNS effects than adults.

➤*Treatment:* Clinical trials have demonstrated that a slurry of activated charcoal administered promptly after ingestion of loperamide hydrochloride can reduce the amount of drug which is absorbed into the systemic circulation by as much as 9-fold. If vomiting occurs spontaneously upon ingestion, a slurry of 100 g of activated charcoal should be administered orally as soon as fluids can be retained.

If vomiting has not occurred, gastric lavage should be performed followed by administration of 100 g of activated charcoal slurry through the gastric tube. In the event of overdosage, patients should be monitored for signs of CNS depression for at least 24 hours. Children may be more sensitive to central nervous system effects than adults. If CNS depression is observed, naloxone may be administered. If responsive to naloxone, vital signs must be monitored carefully for recurrence of symptoms of drug overdose for at least 24 hours after the last dose of naloxone.

In view of the prolonged action of loperamide and the short duration (1 to 3 hours) of naloxone, the patient must be monitored closely and treated repeatedly with naloxone as indicated. Since relatively little drug is excreted in the urine, forced diuresis is not expected to be effective for loperamide overdosage.

In clinical trials an adult who took three 20 mg doses within a 24 hour period was nauseated after the second dose and vomited after the third dose. In studies designed to examine the potential for side effects, intentional ingestion of up to 60 mg of loperamide hydrochloride in a single dose to healthy subjects resulted in no significant adverse effects.

Patient Information

Patients should be advised to check with their physician if their diarrhea does not improve after a couple of days or if they note blood in their stools or develop a fever.

Do not use if you have ever had a rash or other allergic reaction to loperamide hydrochloride. Do not use if you have bloody or black stool. Ask a doctor before use if you have high fever (greater than 38.3°C; 101°F), mucus present in your stool, a history of liver disease, or are taking antibiotics. Stop use and ask a doctor if diarrhea lasts for more than 2 days. If pregnant or breastfeeding, ask a health professional before use. In case of overdose, get medical help or contact a poison control center right away. Do not use for more than 2 days unless directed by a physician.

➤*OTC tablets:* Do not use if you have ever had a rash or other allergic reaction to loperamide hydrochloride. Do not use if you have bloody or black stool.

Ask a doctor of pharmacist before use if you are taking antibiotics. Stop use and ask a doctor if diarrhea lasts for more than 2 days. If pregnant or breastfeeding, ask a health professional before use.

Keep out of reach of children. In case of overdose, get medical help or contact a poison control center right away.

BISMUTH SUBSALICYLATE (BSS)

otc	**Kaopectate** (Pfizer Consumer Health)	**Tablets:** 262 mg	Capsule shape. In 12s and 20s.
otc	**Bismatrol** (Major)	**Tablets, chewable:** 262 mg	Saccharin. In 240 mL.
otc	**Peptic Relief** (Rugby)		Dextrose, sorbitol. In 30s.
otc sf	**Pepto-Bismol** (Procter & Gamble)		< 2 mg sodium/tablet. Saccharin, mannitol. (Pepto-Bismol). Pink. Original and cherry flavors. In 30s and 42s (cherry). In 24s and 42s (original).
otc	**Kaopectate Children's** (Pharmacia)	**Liquid:** 87 mg per 5 mL	Sucrose. Cherry flavor. In 236 mL.
otc	**Pink Bismuth** (Various, eg, Goldline)	**Liquid:** 130 mg per 15 mL	In 240 mL.
otc	**Pink Bismuth** (Various, eg, Goldline)	**Liquid:** 262 mg per 15 mL	In 240 mL.
otc	**Kao-Tin** (Major)		Saccharin, sorbitol. In 236 and 473 mL.
otc	**Kaopectate** (Pharmacia)		Sucrose. In 236 and 355 mL (regular flavor) and 236 and 355 mL (peppermint flavor).
otc	**Peptic Relief** (Rugby)		Saccharin, sorbitol. In 237 mL.
otc sf	**Pepto-Bismol** (Procter & Gamble)		5 mg sodium/15 mL. Saccharin. In 120, 240, 360, and 480 mL.
otc sf	**Pepto-Bismol Maximum Strength** (Procter & Gamble)	**Liquid:** 524 mg per 15 mL	< 5 mg sodium/15 mL. Saccharin. In 120, 240, and 360 mL.

BISMUTH SUBSALICYLATE (BSS)

otc	**Kaopectate Extra Strength** (Pharmacia)	**Liquid**: 525 mg per 15 mL	Sucrose. Peppermint flavor. In 236 mL.
otc	**K-Pek** (Rugby)	**Suspension**: 262 mg per 15 mL	Sugar. In 237 mL.
otc	**Kapectolin** (United Research Laboratories)		Glycerin, saccharin, sorbitol. Mint flavor. In 480 mL.
otc	**Maalox Total Stomach Relief Liquid** (Novartis)	**Suspension**: 525 mg per 15 mL	Parabens, sorbitol, sucralose, and alcohol (peppermint only). In strawberry and peppermint flavors. In 355 mL.

BISMUTH SUBSALICYLATE — ORAL

Indications

To control diarrhea, gas, upset stomach, indigestion, heartburn, nausea; reduce number of bowel movements; help firm stool.

➤*Unlabeled uses:* Bismuth subsalicylate (BSS) has been used to prevent traveler's diarrhea (enterotoxigenic *Escherichia coli*), in doses of 2.1 g/day (2 tablets 4 times daily before meals and at bedtime) for up to 3 weeks during brief periods of high risk. The suspension has also been used (4.2 g/day). BSS has been effective in up to 65% of patients.

Administration and Dosage

Shake well immediately before each use.

For accurate dosing of liquid, use convenient pre-measured dose cup.

Chew or dissolve tablets in mouth.

Repeat dose every 30 minutes to 1 hour, as needed, to a maximum of 8 doses in a 24-hour period.

Drink plenty of clear fluids to help prevent dehydration which may accompany diarrhea.

This medication may cause a temporary and harmless darkening of the tongue or stool.

➤*Dosing:*

Adults and children 12 years of age and older – 2 tablets or 30 mL. Repeat dosage every 30 minutes to 1 hour, as needed, up to 8 doses in 24 hours. Use until diarrhea stops but not more than 2 days.

Children 9 to 11 years of age – For children 9 to 11 years of age, the dose is 1 tablet or 15 mL (1 tablespoonful).

Children 6 to 8 years of age – For children 6 to 8 years of age, the dose is ⅔ tablet or 10 mL (2 teaspoonfuls).

Children 3 to 5 years of age – For children 3 to 5 years of age, the dose is ⅓ tablet or 5 mL (1 teaspoonful).

Children younger than 3 years of age – For children under 3 years of age, ask a doctor.

➤*Storage/Stability:* Store at room temperature 20° to 25°C (68° to 77°F). Avoid excessive heat, 40°C (104°F).

Keep out of reach of children. In case of overdose, get medical help or contact a poison control center right away.

Do not use if inner seal is broken or missing.

Actions

➤*Pharmacology:* BSS appears to have antisecretory and antimicrobial effects in vitro and may have some anti-inflammatory effects. The salicylate moiety provides the antisecretory effect, while the bismuth moiety may exert direct antimicrobial effects against bacterial and viral enteropathogens.

➤*Pharmacokinetics:*

Absorption/Distribution – BSS undergoes chemical dissociation in the GI tract. Two BSS tablets yield 204 mg salicylate. Following ingestion, salicylate is absorbed, with greater than 90% recovered in the urine; plasma levels are similar to levels achieved after a comparable dose of aspirin. Absorption of bismuth is negligible.

Warnings

➤*Reye's syndrome:* Children and teenagers who have or are recovering from chicken pox, flu symptoms, or flu should not use this product. If nausea, vomiting, or fever occur, consult a doctor because these symptoms could be an early sign of Reye's syndrome, a rare but serious illness.

➤*Ringing in the ears:* This product contains salicylates. If taken with other salicylate-containing preparations (such as aspirin) and ringing in the ears occurs, discontinue use.

Precautions

➤*Impaction:* Impaction may occur in infants and debilitated patients.

➤*Radiologic examinations:* May interfere with radiologic examinations of GI tract. Bismuth is radiopaque.

Drug Interactions

Bismuth Subsalicylate (BSS) Drug Interactions

Precipitant drug	Object drug*		Description
BSS	Aspirin	⬆	BSS contains salicylate. If taken with aspirin and ringing of the ears occurs, discontinue use.
BSS	Tetracyclines	⬇	BSS may decrease GI absorption and bioavailability of tetracyclines, reducing their efficacy.

* ⬆ = Object drug increased. ⬇ = Object drug decreased.

Ask a doctor or pharmacist before use if you are taking a prescription drug for anticoagulation (thinning the blood), diabetes, gout, or arthritis

Patient Information

Shake liquid well before using. Chew tablets or allow to dissolve in mouth.

Stool may temporarily appear gray-black.

If diarrhea is accompanied by high fever or continues for more than 2 days, consult physician.

Do not use if you are allergic to salicylates (including aspirin) unless directed by a doctor.

Ask a doctor or pharmacist before use if you are taking a prescription drug for anticoagulation (thinning the blood), diabetes, gout, or arthritis

Do not use for more than 2 days or in the presence of fever, or in children under 3 years of age unless directed by a doctor

If pregnant or breastfeeding, ask a health professional before use.

ANTIDIARRHEAL COMBINATION PRODUCTS

otc	**Kaolin w/Pectin** (Various, eg, Roxane, Wyeth-Ayerst)	**Suspension**: 90 g kaolin, 2 g pectin/30 mL. *Dose:* After each bowel movement *Adults* - 60 to 120 mL/dose. *Children - 6 to 12 years:* 30 to 60 mL/dose. *3 to 6 years:* 15 to 30 mL/dose.	In 180 mL, pt and UD 30 mL.
otc	**Kapectolin** (Various, eg, Goldline, Major)		In 360 mL.
otc	**Parepectolin** (Rhone-Poulenc Rorer)	**Concentrated liquid**: 600 mg attapulgite/15 mL. *Dose:* After each bowel movement up to 7 doses/day. *Adults* – 30 mL/dose. *Children - 6 to 12 years:* 15 mL/dose. *3 to younger than 6 years of age:* 7.5 mL/dose.	Sucrose. In 240 mL.
otc	**K-Pek** (Rugby)	**Suspension**: 750 mg attapulgite/15 mL. *Dose:* After each bowel movement up to 6 doses/day. *≥ 12* – 30 mL. *Children - 6 to younger than 12 years of age:* 15 mL/dose. *3 to younger than 6 years of age:* 7.5 mL/dose.	EDTA, methylparaben. sucrose. In 237 and 473 mL.

ANTIDIARRHEAL COMBINATION PRODUCTS

otc	**Kaodene Non-Narcotic** (Pfeiffer)	**Liquid**: 3.9 g kaolin, 194.4 mg pectin/ 30 mL, bismuth subsalicylate. *Dose:* 1 to 3 doses/day or after each loose stool. *Adults* – 45 mL/dose. *Children - 6 to 12 years:* 22.5 mL/dose. *3 to 6 years:* 15 mL/dose.	Alcohol free. Sucrose. In 120 mL.
otc	**Diasorb** (Columbia)	**Tablets**: 750 mg activated attapulgite. *Dose:* After each bowel movement up to 3 doses/day. *Adults* - 4/dose. *Children – 6 to 12 years:* 2/dose. *3 to 6 years:* 1/dose.	Sorbitol. In 24s.
		Liquid: 750 mg activated attapulgite/ 5 mL. *Dose:* After each bowel movement up to 3 doses/day. *Adults* – 20 mL/dose. *Children – 6 to 12 years:* 10 mL/dose. *3 to 6 years:* 5 mL/dose.	Sugar free. Sorbitol, saccharin. Cola flavor. In 120 mL.
otc	**Kaopectate Maximum Strength** (Upjohn)	**Caplets**: 750 mg attapulgite. *Dose:* After each bowel movement up to 6 doses/day. *Adults* - 2/dose. *Children - 6 to 12 years:* 1/dose.	Sucrose. In 12s and 20s.

ANTIDIARRHEAL COMBINATION PRODUCTS — ORAL

Indications

For the symptomatic treatment of diarrhea by reducing intestinal motility or adsorbing fluid.

Warnings

➤*Diarrhea from other causes:* Do not use antiperistaltic agents for diarrhea associated with pseudomembranous enterocolitis or in diarrhea caused by toxigenic bacteria.

➤*Salicylate absorption:* Salicylate absorption may occur from bismuth subsalicylate; therefore, observe caution in patients with bleeding disorders or salicylate sensitivity and in children.

➤*Ingredients:* The use of the ingredients in combination in the following products as nonspecific antidiarrheal agents has, to a large extent, been empiric. Adequate controlled clinical studies demonstrating the efficacy of these antidiarrheal combinations are lacking. The FDA has determined that the following ingredients are *not* generally recognized as safe and effective and are misbranded when present in *otc* antidiarrheal preparations: Aluminum hydroxide, atropine sulfate, calcium carbonate, carboxymethylcellulose, glycine, homatropine methylbromide, hyoscyamine sulfate, *Lactobacillus acidophilus* and *bulgaricus*, opium (powdered and tincture), paregoric, phenyl salicylate, scopolamine hydrobromide and zinc phenolsulfonate.

In 1986, in the tentative final monograph for these agents, the FDA considered attapulgite a Category I agent (safe and effective) and placed kaolin and pectin in Category III (insufficient data to permit classification). Recently, however, an FDA advisory committee recommended that the FDA reverse the classifications, making attapulgite Category III and kaolin and pectin Category I. Further studies are pending.

Activated attapulgite, kaolin and **pectin** are used for their adsorbent and protectant actions.

Bismuth salts have antacid and adsorbent properties.

ANTIFLATULENTS

SIMETHICONE

otc	**Phazyme** (Reed & Carnrick)	**Tablets**: 60 mg	Enteric coated inner core. In 50s, 100s and 1000s.
otc	**Phazyme 95** (GlaxoSmithKline Consumer)	**Tablets**: 95 mg	Enteric coated inner core. In 50s, 100s, 500s and Consumer Pak 10s.
otc	**Degas** (Invamed)	**Tablets, chewable**: 80 mg	Sucrose. In 100s.
otc	**Gas Relief** (Rugby)		In 100s.
otc	**Gax-X** (Sandoz)		(Gas-X). White, scored. In 12s, 30s.
otc	**Genasyme** (Goldline)		In 100s.
otc	**Mylanta Gas** (J&J/Merck)		Mint flavor. In 100s.
otc	**Extra Strength Gas-X** (Sandoz)	**Tablets, chewable**: 125 mg	(Gas-X). Yellow, scored. In 18s.
otc	**Gas Relief** (Rugby)		Dextrose, sugar, sorbitol. In 60s and 100s.
otc	**Mylanta Gas Maximum Strength** (J&J/Merck)		Mint and cherry flavors. In 12s, 24s, and 60s.
otc	**Phazyme 125** (GlaxoSmithKline Consumer)	**Capsules**: 125 mg	(Phazyme 125). Red. In 50s.
otc	**Phazyme** (GlaxoSmithKline Consumer)	**Capsules**: 180 mg	In 12s.
otc	**Gas-X Extra Strength** (Sandoz)	**Capsules, softgel**: 125 mg	Sorbitol. In 10s and 30s.
otc	**Mylanta Gas Maximum Strength** (J&J/Merck)		Peppermint oil. In 24s.
otc	**Simethicone** (Various)	**Drops**: 40 mg per 0.6 mL	In 30 mL w/calibrated oral syringe.
otc	**Flatulex** (Dayton)		In 30 mL w/calibrated dropper.
otc	**Genasyme Drops** (Goldline)		Hydroxypropyl methylcellulose, saccharin calcium, sodium benzoate, sodium citrate. In 30 mL.
otc	**Mylicon** (J&J/Merck)		In 30 mL dropper bottle.

SIMETHICONE — ORAL

Indications

➤*Gas retention:* For relief of painful symptoms (ie, pressure, bloating, discomfort) of excess gas in the stomach and intestines. Used as an adjunct in the treatment of many conditions in which gas retention may be a problem, such as postoperative gaseous distention, air swallowing, functional dyspepsia, peptic ulcer, spastic or irritable colon, or diverticulosis.

➤*Unlabeled uses:* Simethicone has been used for treating the symptoms of infant colic. It is generally administered with meals.

Administration and Dosage

➤*Softgel capsules and tablets:* Swallow with water 1 or 2 capsules or tablets as needed after meals and at bedtime. Do not exceed 500 mg in 24 hours except under the advice and supervision of a physician.

➤*Chewable tablets:* Chew thoroughly and swallow 1 or 2 chewable tablets as needed after meals and at bedtime. Do not exceed 500 mg in 24 hours except under the advice and supervision of a physician.

➤*Drops:* Shake well before using.

Adults – 40 to 80 mg as needed after meals and at bedtime.

Children 2 to 12 years of age or greater than 24 pounds – 40 mg (0.6 mL) as needed after meals and at bedtime.

Children younger than 2 years of age or less than 24 pounds – 20 mg (0.3 mL).

All dosages may be repeated as needed, after meals and at bedtime, or as directed by a physician. Do not exceed 12 doses per day.

Fill enclosed dropper to recommended dosage level and dispense liquid slowly into the infant's mouth, toward the inner cheek. The dosage can also be mixed with 1 oz of cool water, infant formula, or other suitable liquids.

➤*Storage/Stability:* Store at room temperature. Protect from excessive moisture and heat.

Actions

➤*Pharmacology:* The defoaming action relieves flatulence by dispersing and preventing the formation of mucus-surrounded gas pockets in the GI tract. It acts in the stomach and intestines to change the surface tension of gas bubbles, enabling them to coalesce; thus, gas is freed and eliminated more easily by belching or passing flatus.

Warnings

➤*Drops:* Do not use if printed plastic overwrap or printed neck wrap is missing or broken. Do not exceed 12 doses per day unless directed by a physician.

➤*Children:* Keep this and all drugs out of the reach of children.

Drug Interactions

No known drug interactions.

Overdosage

In case of overdosage, contact a physician or poison control center immediately.

CHARCOAL

otc	**Charcoal Plus DS** (Kramer)	**Tablets:** 250 mg	Sorbitol. In 120s.
otc	**Charcoal** (Various, eg, Nature's Bounty, Rugby)	**Capsules:** 260 mg	In 50s and 100s.
otc	**CharcoCaps** (Requa)		In 8s, 36s and 100s.

CHARCOAL — ORAL

Indications

For relief of intestinal gas, diarrhea and GI distress associated with indigestion and accompanying cramps or odor.

For the prevention of nonspecific pruritus associated with kidney dialysis treatment.

For use as an antidote in poisonings, see individual monograph in the Endocrine/Metabolic chapter.

Administration and Dosage

Usual adult dosage is 500 to 520 mg after meals or at first sign of discomfort. Repeat as needed, up to 5 g daily.

Actions

➤*Pharmacology:* Charcoal is an adsorbent, detoxicant and soothing agent. It reduces the volume of intestinal gas and relieves related discomfort.

Warnings

➤*Diarrhea:* If diarrhea persists for more than 2 days or is accompanied by fever, consult physician.

➤*High dosage or prolonged use:* High dosage or prolonged use does not cause side effects or harm the patient's nutritional state.

➤*Children:* Do not use in children younger than 3 years of age.

Drug Interactions

Activated charcoal can adsorb drugs while they are in the GI tract. Therefore, take charcoal 2 hours before, or 1 hour after other medication.

Charcoal Drug Interactions

Precipitant drug	Object drug*			Description
Charcoal	Acetaminophen Barbiturates Carbamazepine Digitoxin Digoxin Furosemide Glutethimide Hydantoins Methotrexate Nizatidine Phenothiazines	Phenylbutazones Propoxyphene Salicylates Sulfones Sulfonylureas Tetracyclines Theophyllines Tricyclic antidepressants Valproic acid	⬇	Charcoal can reduce absorption of these drugs and actually remove them from the systemic circulation which may reduce the effectiveness of a given agent. Charcoal is also used as an antidote for drug overdoses (refer to the individual monograph in the Endocrine/Metabolic chapter).

* ⬇ = Object drug decreased.

CHARCOAL AND SIMETHICONE

otc	**Flatulex** (Dayton)	**Tablets:** 250 mg activated charcoal and 80 mg simethicone	Green. In 100s.

CHARCOAL AND SIMETHICONE — ORAL

Indications

For the relief of gas pain and associated symptoms.

Administration and Dosage

1 tablet 3 times daily and at bedtime.

Actions

➤*Pharmacology:* Charcoal reduces the volume of gas. Simethicone disperses and prevents the formation of mucus-surrounded gas pockets, and allows for their elimination. For further information on simethicone, refer to the individual monograph.

LIPASE INHIBITORS

ORLISTAT

Rx	**Xenical** (Roche)	**Capsules:** 120 mg	(Roche XENICAL 120). Dark blue. In 90s.

ORLISTAT — ORAL

Indications

➤*Obesity management:* Orlistat is indicated for obesity management including weight loss and weight maintenance when used in conjunction with a reduced-calorie diet. Orlistat is also indicated to reduce the risk for weight regain after prior weight loss. Orlistat is indicated for obese patients with an initial body mass index (BMI) greater than or equal to 30 kg/m^2 or greater than or equal to 27 kg/m^2 in the presence of other risk factors (eg, hypertension, diabetes, dyslipidemia).

Body mass index (BMI) is calculated by dividing weight in kilograms by height in meters squared. For example, a person who weighs 180 lbs and is 5'5" would have a BMI of 30.

Administration and Dosage

➤*Approved by the FDA:* April 23, 1999.

The recommended dose of orlistat is one 120 mg capsule 3 times daily with each main meal containing fat (during or up to 1 hour after the meal).

The patient should be on a nutritionally balanced, reduced-calorie diet that contains approximately 30% of calories from fat. The daily intake of fat, carbohydrate, and protein should be distributed over 3 main meals. If a meal is occasionally missed or contains no fat, the dose of orlistat can be omitted.

Because orlistat has been shown to reduce the absorption of some fat-soluble vitamins and beta-carotene, counsel patients to take a multivitamin containing fat-soluble vitamins to ensure adequate nutrition. The supplement should be taken at least 2 hours before or after the administration of orlistat, such as at bedtime.

Doses higher than 120 mg 3 times daily have not been shown to provide additional benefit.

Based on fecal fat measurements, the effect of orlistat is seen as soon as 24 to 48 hours after dosing. Upon discontinuation of therapy, fecal fat content usually returns to pretreatment levels within 48 to 72 hours.

The safety and efficacy of orlistat beyond 2 years have not been determined at this time.

➤*Storage/Stability:* Store at 25°C (77°F); excursions permitted to 15° to 30°C (59° to 86°F). Keep bottle tightly closed.

Actions

➤*Pharmacology:* Orlistat is a reversible inhibitor of lipases. It exerts its therapeutic activity in the lumen of the stomach and small intestine by forming a covalent bond with the active serine residue site of gastric and pancreatic lipases. The inactivated enzymes are thus unavailable to hydrolyze dietary fat in the form of triglycerides into absorbable free fatty acids and monoglycerides. As undigested triglycerides are not absorbed, the resulting caloric deficit may have a positive effect on weight control. Systemic absorption of the drug is therefore not needed for activity. At the recommended therapeutic dose of 120 mg 3 times daily, orlistat inhibits dietary fat absorption by approximately 30%.

➤*Pharmacokinetics:*

Absorption – Systemic exposure to orlistat is minimal. Following oral dosing with 360 mg ^{14}C-orlistat, plasma radioactivity peaked at approximately 8 hours; plasma concentrations of intact orlistat were near the limits of detection (less than 5 ng/mL). In therapeutic studies involving monitoring of plasma samples, detection of intact orlistat in plasma was sporadic and concentrations were low (less than 10 ng/mL or 0.02 mcM), without evidence of accumulation, and consistent with minimal absorption.

The average absolute bioavailability of intact orlistat was assessed in studies with male rats at oral doses of 150 and 1,000 mg/kg/day and in male dogs at oral doses of 100 and 1,000 mg/kg/day and found to be 0.12%, 0.59% in rats and 0.7%, 1.9% in dogs, respectively.

Distribution – In vitro orlistat was greater than 99% bound to plasma proteins (lipoproteins and albumin were major binding proteins). Orlistat minimally partitioned into erythrocytes.

Metabolism – Based on animal data, it is likely that the metabolism of orlistat occurs mainly within the gastrointestinal wall. Based on an oral ^{14}C-orlistat mass balance study in obese patients, 2 metabolites, M1 (4-member lactone ring hydrolyzed) and M3 (M1 with N-formyl leucine moiety cleaved), accounted for approximately 42% of total radioactivity in plasma. M1 and M3 have an open beta-lactone ring and extremely weak lipase inhibitory activity (1,000- and 2,500-fold less than orlistat, respectively). In view of this low inhibitory activity and the low plasma levels at the therapeutic dose (average of 26 ng/mL and 108 ng/mL for M1 and M3, respectively, 2 to 4 hours after a dose), these metabolites are considered pharmacologically inconsequential. The primary metabolite M1 had a short half-life (approximately 3 hours) whereas the secondary metabolite M3 disappeared at a slower rate (half-life approximately 13.5 hours). In obese patients, steady-state plasma levels of M1, but not M3, increased in proportion to orlistat doses.

Excretion – Following a single oral dose of 360 mg ^{14}C-orlistat in both healthy weight and obese subjects, fecal excretion of the unabsorbed drug was found to be the major route of elimination. Orlistat and its M1 and M3 metabolites were also subject to biliary excretion. Approximately 97% of the administered radioactivity was excreted in feces; 83% of that was found to be unchanged orlistat. The cumulative renal excretion of total radioactivity was less than 2% of the given dose of 360 mg ^{14}C-orlistat. The time to reach complete excretion (fecal plus urinary) was 3 to 5 days. The disposition of orlistat appeared to be similar between healthy weight and obese subjects. Based on limited data, the half-life of the absorbed orlistat is in the range of 1 to 2 hours.

Contraindications

Chronic malabsorption syndrome or cholestasis; hypersensitivity to orlistat or to any component of this product.

Warnings

➤*Causes of obesity:* Exclude organic causes of obesity (eg, hypothyroidism) before prescribing orlistat.

➤*Pregnancy:* Category B.

Teratogenic –

The incidence of dilated cerebral ventricles was increased in the mid- and high-dose groups of the rat teratology study. These doses were 6 and 23 times the daily human dose calculated on a body surface area (mg/m^2) basis for the mid- and high-dose levels, respectively. This finding was not reproduced in 2 additional rat teratology studies at similar doses.

There are no adequate and well-controlled studies of orlistat in pregnant women. Because animal reproductive studies are not always predictive of human response, orlistat is not recommended for use during pregnancy.

➤*Lactation:* It is not known if orlistat is secreted in human milk. Therefore, orlistat should not be taken by nursing women.

➤*Children:* The safety and efficacy of orlistat have been evaluated in obese adolescent patients aged 12 to 16 years. Orlistat has not been studied in pediatric patients younger than 12 years of age.

Precautions

➤*Dietary guidelines:* Advise patients to adhere to dietary guidelines. Gastrointestinal events may increase when orlistat is taken with a diet high in fat (greater than 30% total daily calories from fat). The daily intake of fat should be distributed over 3 main meals. If orlistat is taken with any one meal very high in fat, the possibility of gastrointestinal effects increases.

➤*Multivitamin supplement:* Strongly encourage patients to take a multivitamin supplement that contains fat-soluble vitamins to ensure adequate nutrition because orlistat has been shown to reduce the absorption of some fat-soluble vitamins and beta-carotene. In addition, the levels of vitamin D and beta-carotene may be low in obese patients compared with nonobese subjects. Give the supplement once a day at least 2 hours before or after the administration of orlistat, such as at bedtime.

Incidence of Low Vitamin Values on 2 or More Consecutive Visits (Nonsupplemented Adult Patients with Normal Baseline Values [First and Second Year])

	Placebo[a]	Orlistat[a]
Vitamin A	1%	2.2%
Vitamin D	6.6%	12%
Vitamin E	1%	5.8%
Beta-carotene	1.7%	6.1%

[a] Treatment designates placebo plus diet or orlistat plus diet.

Incidence of Low Vitamin Values on 2 or More Consecutive Visits (Pediatric Patients with Normal Baseline Values[a])

	Placebo[b]	Orlistat[b]
Vitamin A	0%	0%
Vitamin D	0.7%	1.4%
Vitamin E	0%	0%
Beta-carotene	0.8%	1.5%

[a] All patients were treated with vitamin supplementation throughout the course of the study.
[b] Treatment designates placebo plus diet or orlistat plus diet.

➤*Special risk:* Some patients may develop increased levels of urinary oxalate following treatment with orlistat. Exercise caution when prescribing orlistat to patients with a history of hyperoxaluria or calcium oxalate nephrolithiasis.

Diabetic patients – Weight-loss induction by orlistat may be accompanied by improved metabolic control in diabetics, which might require a reduction in dose of oral hypoglycemic medication (eg, sulfonylureas, metformin) or insulin.

➤*Drug abuse and dependence:* As with any weight-loss agent, the potential exists for misuse of orlistat in inappropriate patient populations (eg, patients with anorexia nervosa or bulimia).

Drug Interactions

Orlistat Drug Interactions

Precipitant drug	Object drug*		Description
Orlistat	Cyclosporine	↔	Because changes in cyclosporine absorption have been reported with variations in dietary intake, caution is advised in the concomitant use of orlistat plus diet in patients receiving cyclosporine therapy.

ORLISTAT — ORAL

Orlistat Drug Interactions			
Precipitant drug	Object drug*		Description
Orlistat	Fat-soluble vitamins	⬇	A pharmacokinetic interaction study showed a 30% reduction in beta-carotene supplement absorption when concomitantly administered with orlistat. Orlistat inhibited absorption of a vitamin E acetate supplement by ≈ 60%. The effect on the absorption of supplemental vitamin D, vitamin A, and nutritionally derived vitamin K is not known at this time.
Orlistat	Warfarin	⬌	In 12 healthy-weight subjects, administration of orlistat 120 mg 3 times a day for 16 days did not result in any change in either warfarin pharmacokinetics or pharmacodynamics. Although undercarboxylated osteocalcin, a marker of vitamin K nutritional status, was unaltered with orlistat administration, vitamin K levels tended to decline in subjects taking orlistat. Therefore, as vitamin K absorption may be decreased with orlistat, monitor patients on chronic stable doses of warfarin who are prescribed orlistat closely for changes in coagulation parameters.

* ⬇ = Object drug decreased. ⬆ = Object drug increased.
⬌ = Undetermined clinical effect.

Adverse Reactions

➤*Commonly observed adverse reactions (based on first-year and second-year data orlistat 120 mg 3 times daily vs placebo):* Gastrointestinal symptoms were the most commonly observed treatment-emergent adverse events associated with the use of orlistat in double-blind, placebo-controlled clinical trials and are primarily a manifestation of the mechanism of action. (Commonly observed is defined as an incidence of greater than or equal to 5% and an incidence in the orlistat 120 mg group that is at least twice that of placebo.)

Commonly Observed Adverse Reactions				
	Year 1		Year 2	
	Orlistat[a]	Placebo[a]	Orlistat[a]	Placebo[a]
	% of patients	% of patients	% of patients	% of patients
Adverse reaction	(n = 1,913)	(n = 1,466)	(n = 613)	(n = 524)
Fatty/oily stool	20%	2.9%	5.5%	0.6%
Fecal incontinence	7.7%	0.9%	1.8%	0.2%
Fecal urgency	22.1%	6.7%	2.8%	1.7%
Flatus with discharge	23.9%	1.4%	2.1%	0.2%
Increased defecation	10.8%	4.1%	2.6%	0.8%
Oily evacuation	11.9%	0.8%	2.3%	0.2%
Oily spotting	26.6%	1.3%	4.4%	0.2%

[a] Treatment designates orlistat 3 times daily plus diet or placebo plus diet.

These and other commonly observed adverse reactions were generally mild and transient, and they decreased during the second year of treatment. In general, the first occurrence of these events was within 3 months of starting therapy. Overall, approximately 50% of all episodes of GI adverse events associated with orlistat treatment lasted for less than 1 week, and a majority lasted for no more than 4 weeks. However, GI adverse events may occur in some individuals over a period of 6 months or longer.

➤*Discontinuation of treatment:* In controlled clinical trials, 8.8% of patients treated with orlistat discontinued treatment due to adverse events, compared with 5% of placebo-treated patients. For orlistat, the most common adverse events resulting in discontinuation of treatment were gastrointestinal.

➤*Incidence in controlled clinical trials:*

Other Treatment-Emergent Adverse Reactions from 7 Placebo-Controlled Clinical Trials (≥ 2%)				
	Year 1		Year 2	
	Orlistat[a]	Placebo[a]	Orlistat[a]	Placebo[a]
Body system/ adverse reaction	% of patients (n = 1,913)	% of patients (n = 1,466)	% of patients (n = 613)	% of patients (n = 524)
Cardiovascular				
Pedal edema	-	-	2.8%	1.9%
CNS				
Dizziness	5.2%	5%	-	-
Headache	30.6%	27.6%	-	-
Dermatological				
Dry skin	2.1%	1.4%	-	-
Rash	4.3%	4%	-	-
GI				
Abdominal pain/ discomfort	25.5%	21.4%	-	-
Gingival disorder	4.1%	2.9%	2%	1.5%
Infectious diarrhea	5.3%	4.4%	-	-
Nausea	8.1%	7.3%	3.6%	2.7%
Rectal pain/ discomfort	5.2%	4%	3.3%	1.9%
Tooth disorder	4.3%	3.1%	2.9%	2.3%
Vomiting	3.8%	3.5%	-	-
GU				
Menstrual irregularity, female	9.8%	7.5%	-	-
Urinary tract infection	7.5%	7.3%	5.9%	4.8%
Vaginitis, female	3.8%	3.6%	2.6%	1.9%
Hearing and vestibular disorders				
Otitis	4.3%	3.4%	2.9%	2.5%
Musculoskeletal				
Arthritis	5.4%	4.8%	-	-
Back pain	13.9%	12.1%	-	-
Joint disorder	2.3%	2.2%	-	-
Myalgia	4.2%	3.3%	-	-
Pain, lower extremities	-	-	10.8%	10.3%
Tendonitis	-	-	2%	1.9%
Psychiatric				
Depression	-	-	3.4%	2.5%
Psychiatric anxiety	4.7%	2.9%	2.8%	2.1%
Respiratory				
Ear, nose, and throat symptoms	2%	1.6%	-	-
Influenza	39.7%	36.2%	-	-
Lower respiratory tract infection	7.8%	6.6%	-	-
Upper respiratory tract infection	38.1%	32.8%	26.1%	25.8%
Miscellaneous				
Fatigue	7.2%	6.4%	3.1%	1.7%
Sleep disorder	3.9%	3.3%	-	-

[a] Treatment designates orlistat 120 mg 3 times daily plus diet or placebo plus diet. None reported at a frequency greater than or equal to 2% and greater than placebo.

➤*Other clinical studies or postmarketing surveillance:* Rare cases of hypersensitivity have been reported with the use of orlistat. Signs and symptoms have included pruritus, rash, urticaria, angioedema, and anaphylaxis.

Preliminary data from a orlistat and cyclosporine drug interaction study indicate a reduction in cyclosporine plasma levels when orlistat was coadministered with cyclosporine.

➤*Pediatric patients:* In clinical trials with orlistat in adolescent patients ages 12 to 16 years, the profile of adverse reactions was generally similar to that observed in adults.

Overdosage

Single doses of 800 mg orlistat and multiple doses of up to 400 mg 3 times daily for 15 days have been studied in healthy-weight and obese subjects without significant adverse findings.

Should a significant overdose of orlistat occur, it is recommended that the patient be observed for 24 hours. Based on human and animal studies, systemic effects attributable to the lipase-inhibiting properties of orlistat should be rapidly reversible.

Patient Information

Read the patient information before starting treatment with orlistat and each time your prescription is renewed.

METOCLOPRAMIDE

Rx	**Metoclopramide HCl** (Various, eg, Goldline, Invamed, Major)	**Tablets:** 5 mg as (monohydrochloride monohydrate)	In 100s, 500s and 1000s.
Rx	**Reglan** (Schwarz Pharma)		Lactose. (Reglan 5 AHR). Green. Elliptical. In 100s and *Dis-Co* UD 100s.
Rx	**Metoclopramide HCl** (Various, eg, Geneva, Goldline, Invamed, Major, Martec, Parmed, Rugby, Schein, Warner-C)	**Tablets:** 10 mg (as monohydrochloride monohydrate)	In 100s, 500s, 1000s, 2500s and UD 100s.
Rx	**Maxolon** (SK-Beecham)		Lactose. (BMP 192). Blue, scored. In 100s.
Rx	**Reglan** (Schwarz Pharma)		(Reglan AHR 10). Pink, scored. Capsule shape. In 100s, 500s and *Dis-Co* UD 100s.
Rx	**Metoclopramide HCl** (Various, eg, Goldline, Major, Roxane, Rugby, Warner-C)	**Syrup:** 5 mg/5 mL (as monohydrochloride monohydrate)	In 480 mL and UD 10 mL.
Rx	**Metoclopramide HCl** (Various, eg, DuPont, Smith & Nephew SoloPak)	**Injection:** 5 mg/mL (as monohydrochloride monohydrate)	In 2, 10, 20 and 30 mL vials and 2 mL amps.
Rx	**Octamide PFS** (Adria)		Preservative free. In 2, 10 and 30 mL single-dose vials.
Rx	**Reglan** (Wyeth-Ayerst)		Preservative free. In 2 and 10 mL amps and 2, 10 and 30 mL vials.

METOCLOPRAMIDE HYDROCHLORIDE — ORAL

See also the Antiemetic/Antivertigo monograph.

Indications

➤*Symptomatic gastroesophageal reflux (GER):* Short-term (4 to 12 weeks) therapy for adults with symptomatic, documented GER who fail to respond to conventional therapy.

The principal effect of metoclopramide is on symptoms of postprandial and daytime heartburn with less observed effect on nocturnal symptoms. If symptoms are confined to particular situations, such as following the evening meal, consider use of metoclopramide as single doses prior to the provocative situation, rather than using the drug throughout the day. Healing of esophageal ulcers and erosions has been endoscopically demonstrated at the end of a 12-week trial using dosage of 15 mg 4 times daily. Because there is no documented correlation between symptoms and healing of esophageal lesions, patients with documented lesions should be monitored endoscopically.

➤*Diabetic gastroparesis (diabetic gastric stasis):* For the relief of symptoms associated with acute and recurrent diabetic gastric stasis. The usual manifestations of delayed gastric emptying (eg, nausea, vomiting, heartburn, persistent fullness after meals, anorexia) appear to respond to metoclopramide within different time intervals. Significant relief of nausea occurs early and continues to improve over a 3-week period. Relief of vomiting and anorexia may precede the relief of abdominal fullness by 1 week or more.

➤*Unlabeled uses:* Used to improve lactation. Dosage of 30 to 45 mg/day have increased milk secretion, possibly by elevating serum prolactin levels.

Studies have indicated some potential value of metoclopramide in the following conditions: nausea and vomiting of a variety of etiologies (uncontrolled studies report 80% to 90% efficacy), including emesis during pregnancy and labor; gastric ulcer; anorexia nervosa (due to GI stimulation); improvement in patient response to ergotamine, analgesics, and sedatives in migraine, perhaps by enhancing absorption of the other medications; treatment of postoperative gastric bezoars (10 mg 3 or 4 times daily); diabetic cystoparesis (atonic bladder); esophageal variceal bleeding; radiation-induced emesis.

Administration and Dosage

➤*Approved by the FDA:* July 29, 1985.

➤*For the relief of symptomatic gastroesophageal reflux disease (GERD):* 10 to 15 mg of metoclopramide orally up to 4 times daily 30 minutes before each meal and at bedtime, depending upon symptoms being treated and clinical response. If symptoms occur only intermittently or at specific times of the day, use of metoclopramide in single doses up to 20 mg prior to the provoking situation may be preferred rather than continuous treatment. Occasionally, patients (such as elderly patients) who are more sensitive to the therapeutic or adverse effects of metoclopramide will require only 5 mg per dose.

Experience with esophageal erosions and ulcerations is limited, but healing has thus far been documented in 1 controlled trial using 4 times daily therapy at 15 mg/dose; use this regimen when lesions are present, so long as it is tolerated. Because of the poor correlation between symptoms and endoscopic appearance of the esophagus, therapy directed at esophageal lesions is best guided by endoscopic evaluation.

Therapy longer than 12 weeks has not been evaluated and cannot be recommended.

➤*For the relief of symptoms associated with diabetic gastroparesis (diabetic gastric stasis):* 10 mg of metoclopramide 30 minutes before each meal and at bedtime for 2 to 8 weeks, depending upon response and the likelihood of continued well-being upon drug discontinuation.

Determine the initial route of administration by the severity of the presenting symptoms. If only the earliest manifestations of diabetic gastric stasis are present, initiate oral administration of metoclopramide. However, if severe symptoms are present, begin therapy with metoclopramide injection (IM or IV) (consult labeling of the injection prior to initiating parenteral administration).

Administration of metoclopramide for injection up to 10 days may be required before symptoms subside, at which time oral administration may be instituted. Since diabetic gastric stasis is frequently recurrent, reinstitute metoclopramide therapy at the earliest manifestation.

➤*Use in patients with renal or hepatic impairment:* Since metoclopramide is excreted principally through the kidneys, initiate therapy in patients whose creatinine clearance is less than 40 mL/min at approximately one-half the recommended dosage. Depending upon clinical efficacy and safety considerations, the dosage may be increased or decreased as appropriate.

It is unlikely that dosage would need to be adjusted to compensate for losses through dialysis.

Metoclopramide undergoes minimal hepatic metabolism, except for simple conjugation. Its safe use has been described in patients with advanced liver disease whose renal function was healthy.

➤*Storage / Stability:* Tablets should be stored at controlled room temperature 15° to 30°C (59° to 86°F).

Dispense in a tight, light-resistant container.

This product is light-sensitive. Inspect before use and discard if either color or particulate is observed.

Actions

➤*Pharmacology:* Metoclopramide stimulates motility of the upper GI tract without stimulating gastric, biliary, or pancreatic secretions. Its mode of action is unclear. It seems to sensitize tissues to the action of acetylcholine. The effect of metoclopramide on motility is not dependent on intact vagal innervation, but it can be abolished by anticholinergic drugs.

Metoclopramide increases the tone and amplitude of gastric (especially antral) contractions, relaxes the pyloric sphincter and the duodenal bulb, and increases peristalsis of the duodenum and jejunum, resulting in accelerated gastric emptying and intestinal transit. It increases the resting tone of the lower esophageal sphincter. It has little, if any, effect on the motility of the colon or gallbladder.

In patients with GER and lower esophageal sphincter pressure (LESP), single oral doses of metoclopramide produce dose-related increases in LESP. Effects begin at about 5 mg and increase through 20 mg (the largest dose tested). The increase in LESP from a 5 mg dose lasts about 45 minutes and that of 20 mg lasts between 2 and 3 hours. Increased rate of stomach emptying has been observed with single oral doses of 10 mg.

The antiemetic properties of metoclopramide appear to be a result of its antagonism of central and peripheral dopamine receptors. Dopamine produces nausea and vomiting by stimulation of the medullary chemoreceptor trigger zone (CTZ), and metoclopramide blocks stimulation of the CTZ by agents like levodopa or apomorphine which are known to increase dopamine levels or to possess dopamine-like effects. Metoclopramide also abolishes the slowing of gastric emptying caused by apomorphine.

Like the phenothiazines and related drugs, which are also dopamine antagonists, metoclopramide produces sedation and may produce extrapyramidal reactions, although these are comparatively rare. Metoclopramide inhibits the central and peripheral effects of apomorphine, induces release of prolactin, and causes a transient increase in circulating aldosterone levels, which may be associated with transient fluid retention.

The onset of pharmacological action of metoclopramide is 30 to 60 minutes following an oral dose; pharmacological effects persist for 1 to 2 hours.

In pediatric patients, the pharmacodynamics of metoclopramide following oral administration are highly variable and a concentration-effect relationship has not been established.

➤*Pharmacokinetics:*

Absorption / Distribution – Metoclopramide is rapidly and well absorbed. Relative to an IV dose of 20 mg, the absolute oral bioavailability of metoclopramide is 80% ± 15.5% as demonstrated in a crossover study of 18 subjects. Peak plasma concentrations occur at about 1 to 2 hours after a single oral dose. Similar time to peak is observed after individual doses at steady state.

METOCLOPRAMIDE HYDROCHLORIDE — ORAL

In a single dose study of 12 subjects, the area under the drug concentration-time curve (AUC) increases linearly with doses from 20 to 100 mg. Peak concentrations increase linearly with dose, time to peak concentrations remain the same, whole body clearance is unchanged, and the elimination rate remains the same. The average elimination half-life in individuals with normal renal function is 5 to 6 hours. Linear kinetic processes adequately describe the absorption and elimination of metoclopramide.

The drug is not extensively bound to plasma proteins (about 30%). The whole body volume of distribution is high (about 3.5 L/kg), which suggests extensive distribution of drug to the tissues.

Excretion – Approximately 85% of the radioactivity of an orally administered dose appears in the urine within 72 hours. Of the 85% eliminated in the urine, about half is present as free or conjugated metoclopramide.

Special populations –

Renal function impairment: Renal impairment affects the clearance of metoclopramide. In a study with patients with varying degrees of renal impairment, a reduction in creatinine clearance was correlated with a reduction in plasma clearance, renal clearance, nonrenal clearance, and increase in elimination half-life. The kinetics of metoclopramide in the presence of renal impairment remained linear, however. The reduction in clearance as a result of renal impairment suggests that a downward adjustment maintenance dosage should be done to avoid drug accumulation.

Adult Pharmacokinetic Data	
Parameter	Value
Vd (L/kg)	≈ 3.5
Plasma protein binding	≈ 30%
t ½ (h)	5 to 6
Oral bioavailability	80% ± 15.5%

Children: In pediatric patients, the pharmacodynamics of metoclopramide following oral and IV administration are highly variable and a concentration-effect relationship has not been established.

In an open-label study, 6 pediatric patients (age range, 3.5 weeks to 5.4 months) with GER received metoclopramide 0.15 mg/kg oral solution every 6 hours for 10 doses. The mean peak plasma concentration of metoclopramide after the tenth dose was 2-fold (56.8 mcg/L) higher compared with that observed after the first dose (29 mcg/L), indicating drug accumulation with repeated dosing. After the tenth dose, the mean time to reach peak concentrations (2.2 hours), half-life (4.1 hours), clearance (0.67 L/h/kg), and volume of distribution (4.4 L/kg) of metoclopramide were similar to those observed after the first dose. In the youngest patient (age, 3.5 weeks), metoclopramide half-life after the first and the tenth dose (23.1 and 10.3 hours, respectively) was significantly longer compared with other infants due to reduced clearance. This may be attributed to immature hepatic and renal systems at birth.

Pediatric Pharmacokinetic Studies					
Reference	Dose, route	t ½ (hr)	Cl (L/hr/kg)	Vd (L/kg)	C_{max} (mcg/L)
[a]	0.15 mg/kg oral soln, multiple dose	4.1[b,c]	0.67 ± 0.14	4.4 ± 0.65 (Vd area)	1st dose = 29 ± 2.3 10th dose = 56.8 ± 10.5

[a] Kearns, GL, et al. *J Pediatric Gastroenterol Nutr.* 1988; 7:823-829.
[b] Data presented as means ± SEM.
[c] SEM not available.

Contraindications

Do not use metoclopramide whenever stimulation of GI motility might be dangerous, (eg, in the presence of GI hemorrhage, mechanical obstruction, or perforation).

Metoclopramide is contraindicated in patients with pheochromocytoma because the drug may cause a hypertensive crisis, probably due to release of catecholamines from the tumor. Such hypertensive crises may be controlled by phentolamine.

Metoclopramide is contraindicated in patients with known sensitivity or intolerance to the drug.

Do not use metoclopramide in epileptics or patients receiving other drugs that are likely to cause extrapyramidal reactions, because the frequency and severity of seizures or extrapyramidal reactions may be increased.

Warnings

➤*Depression:* Mental depression has occurred in patients with and without a history of depression. Symptoms have ranged from mild to severe and have included suicidal ideation and suicide. Give metoclopramide to patients with a history of depression only if the expected benefits outweigh the potential risks.

➤*Extrapyramidal symptoms (EPS):* Extrapyramidal symptoms, manifested primarily as acute dystonic reactions, occur in approximately 1 in 500 patients treated with the usual adult dosages of 30 to 40 mg/day of metoclopramide. These usually are seen during the first 24 to 48 hours of treatment with metoclopramide, occur more frequently in pediatric patients and adult patients younger than 30 years of age, and are even more frequent at the higher doses. These symptoms may include involuntary movements of limbs and facial grimacing, torticollis, oculogyric crisis, rhythmic protrusion of tongue, bulbar type of speech, trismus, or dystonic reactions resembling tetanus. Rarely, dystonic reactions may present as stridor and dyspnea, possibly due to laryngospasm. If these symptoms should occur, inject 50 mg diphenhydramine hydrochloride IM and they usually will subside. Benztropine mesylate 1 to 2 mg IM may also be used to reverse these reactions.

➤*Parkinsonian-like symptoms:* Parkinsonian-like symptoms have occurred, more commonly within the first 6 months after beginning treatment with metoclopramide, but occasionally after longer periods. These symptoms generally subside within 2 to 3 months following discontinuance of metoclopramide. Give patients with preexisting Parkinson disease metoclopramide cautiously, if at all, because such patients may experience exacerbation of Parkinsonian symptoms when taking metoclopramide.

➤*Tardive dyskinesia:* Tardive dyskinesia, a syndrome consisting of potentially irreversible, involuntary, dyskinetic movements, may develop in patients treated with metoclopramide. Although the prevalence of the syndrome appears to be highest among the elderly, especially elderly women, it is impossible to predict which patients are likely to develop the syndrome. Both the risk of developing the syndrome and the likelihood that it will become irreversible are believed to increase with the duration of treatment and the total cumulative dose.

Less commonly, the syndrome can develop after relatively brief treatment periods at low doses; in these cases, symptoms appear more likely to be reversible.

There is no known treatment for established cases of tardive dyskinesia, although the syndrome may remit, partially or completely, within several weeks to months after metoclopramide is withdrawn. Metoclopramide itself, however, may suppress (or partially suppress) the signs of tardive dyskinesia, thereby masking the underlying disease process. The effect of this symptomatic suppression upon the long-term course of the syndrome is unknown. Therefore, the use of metoclopramide for the symptomatic control of tardive dyskinesia is not recommended.

➤*Carcinogenesis:* A 77-week study was conducted in rats with oral doses up to approximately 40 times the maximum recommended human daily dose. Metoclopramide elevates prolactin levels and the elevation persists during chronic administration. Tissue culture experiments indicate that approximately one-third of human breast cancers are prolactin dependent in vitro, a factor of potential importance if the prescription of metoclopramide is contemplated in a patient with previously detected breast cancer. Although disturbances such as galactorrhea, amenorrhea, gynecomastia, and impotence have been reported with prolactin-elevating drugs, the clinical significance of elevated serum prolactin levels is unknown for most patients. An increase in mammary neoplasms has been found in rodents after chronic administration of prolactin-stimulating neuroleptic drugs and metoclopramide. Neither clinical studies nor epidemiologic studies conducted to date, however, have shown an association between chronic administration of these drugs and mammary tumorigenesis; the available evidence is too limited to be conclusive at this time.

➤*Pregnancy: Category B.*

There are no adequate and well-controlled studies in pregnant women. Because animal reproduction studies are not always predictive of human response, this drug should be used during pregnancy only if clearly needed.

➤*Lactation:* Metoclopramide is excreted in human milk. Exercise caution when metoclopramide is administered to a nursing mother.

➤*Children:* Safety and effectiveness in pediatric patients have not been established except to facilitate small bowel intubation.

Care should be exercised in administering metoclopramide to neonates because prolonged clearance may produce excessive serum concentrations. In addition, neonates have reduced levels of nicotinamide adenine dinucleotide-methemoglobin reductase that, in combination with the aforementioned pharmacokinetic factors, make neonates more susceptible to methemoglobinemia.

The safety profile of metoclopramide in adults cannot be extrapolated to pediatric patients. Dystonias and other extrapyramidal reactions associated with metoclopramide are more common in the pediatric population than in adults.

Precautions

➤*Special risk:* In 1 study in hypertensive patients, IV-administered metoclopramide was shown to release catecholamines; hence, exercise caution when metoclopramide is used in patients with hypertension.

Because metoclopramide produces a transient increase in plasma aldosterone, certain patients, especially those with cirrhosis or congestive heart failure, may be at risk of developing fluid retention and volume overload. If these side effects occur at any time during metoclopramide therapy, discontinue the drug.

Anastomosis or closure of the gut – Giving a promotility drug such as metoclopramide theoretically could put increased pressure on suture lines following a gut anastomosis or closure. Although adverse events related to this possibility have not been reported to date, consider and weigh the possibility when deciding whether to use metoclopramide or nasogastric suction in the prevention of postoperative nausea and vomiting.

➤*Hazardous tasks:* Metoclopramide may impair the mental or physical abilities required for the performance of hazardous tasks such as operating machinery or driving a motor vehicle.

METOCLOPRAMIDE HYDROCHLORIDE — ORAL

Drug Interactions

Metoclopramide Drug Interactions

Precipitant drug	Object drug*		Description
Metoclopramide	Alcohol	↑	Metoclopramide increases the rate of absorption of alcohol by decreasing the time it takes alcohol to reach the small intestine where it is rapidly absorbed.
Metoclopramide	Cimetidine	↓	Bioavailability of cimetidine may be reduced due to decreased absorption as a result of faster gastric transit time.
Metoclopramide	Cyclosporine	↑	A faster gastric emptying time may allow for an increase in cyclosporine absorption, possibly increasing its immunosuppressive and toxic effects.
Metoclopramide	Digoxin	↓	Digoxin absorption, plasma levels and therapeutic effects may be decreased. The capsule, elixir and tablets with a high dissolution rate are least affected.
Metoclopramide	Levodopa	↑	These agents have opposite effects on dopamine receptors. The bioavailability of levodopa may be increased, and levodopa may decrease the effects of metoclopramide on gastric emptying and lower esophageal pressure. Metoclopramide is relatively contraindicated in Parkinson's disease patients.
Levodopa	Metoclopramide	↓	
Metoclopramide	MAO inhibitors	↑	Since metoclopramide releases catecholamines in patients with essential hypertension, use cautiously, if at all, in patients receiving MAO inhibitors.
Metoclopramide	Succinylcholine	↑	By inhibiting plasma cholinesterase, metoclopramide may increase the neuromuscular blocking effects of succinylcholine.
Anticholinergics Narcotic analgesics	Metoclopramide	↓	The effects of metoclopramide on GI motility are antagonized by these agents.

* ↑ = Object drug increased. ↓ = Object drug decreased.

The effects of metoclopramide on GI motility are antagonized by anticholinergic drugs and narcotic analgesics. Additive sedative effects can occur when metoclopramide is given with alcohol, sedatives, hypnotics, narcotics, or tranquilizers.

Absorption of drugs from the stomach may be diminished (eg, digoxin) by metoclopramide, whereas the rate or extent of absorption of drugs from the small bowel may be increased (eg, acetaminophen, tetracycline, levodopa, ethanol, cyclosporine).

Gastroparesis (gastric stasis) may be responsible for poor diabetic control in some patients. Exogenously administered insulin may begin to act before food has left the stomach and lead to hypoglycemia. Because the action of metoclopramide will influence the delivery of food to the intestines and thus the rate of absorption, insulin dosage or timing of dosage may require adjustment.

Adverse Reactions

➤*Allergic:* A few cases of rash, urticaria, or bronchospasm, especially in patients with a history of asthma. Rarely, angioneurotic edema, including glossal or laryngeal edema.

➤*Cardiovascular:* Hypotension, hypertension, supraventricular tachycardia, bradycardia, fluid retention, acute congestive heart failure, and possible AV block.

➤*CNS:* Restlessness, drowsiness, fatigue, and lassitude occur in approximately 10% of patients receiving the most commonly prescribed dosage of 10 mg 4 times daily. Insomnia, headache, confusion, dizziness, or mental depression with suicidal ideation occur less frequently. There are isolated reports of convulsive seizures without clear-cut relationship to metoclopramide. Rarely, hallucinations have been reported.

EPS – Acute dystonic reactions, the most common type of EPS associated with metoclopramide, occur in approximately 0.2% of patients (1 in 500) treated with 30 to 40 mg/day. Symptoms include involuntary movements of limbs, facial grimacing, torticollis, oculogyric crisis, rhythmic protrusion of tongue, bulbar type of speech, trismus, opisthotonus (tetanus-like reactions), and, rarely, stridor and dyspnea, possibly due to laryngospasm; ordinarily, these symptoms are readily reversed by diphenhydramine.

Parkinsonian-like symptoms – Parkinsonian-like symptoms may include bradykinesia, tremor, cogwheel rigidity, mask-like faces.

Tardive dyskinesia – Tardive dyskinesia most frequently is characterized by involuntary movements of the tongue, face, mouth, or jaw, and sometimes by involuntary movements of the trunk or extremities; movements may be choreoathetotic in appearance.

Motor restlessness (akathisia) may consist of feelings of anxiety, agitation, jitteriness, and insomnia, as well as the inability to sit still, pacing, and foot-tapping. These symptoms may disappear spontaneously or respond to a reduction in dosage.

➤*Endocrine:* Galactorrhea, amenorrhea, gynecomastia, impotence secondary to hyperprolactinemia. Fluid retention secondary to transient elevation of aldosterone.

➤*GI:* Nausea and bowel disturbances, primarily diarrhea.

➤*Hematologic:* A few cases of neutropenia, leukopenia, or agranulocytosis, generally without clear-cut relationship to metoclopramide. Methemoglobinemia, especially with overdosage in neonates.

Sulfhemoglobinemia in adults.

➤*Hepatic:* Rarely, cases of hepatotoxicity, characterized by such findings as jaundice and altered liver function tests, when metoclopramide was administered with other drugs with known hepatotoxic potential.

➤*Renal:* Urinary frequency and incontinence.

➤*Miscellaneous:* Visual disturbances. Porphyria. Rare occurrences of neuroleptic malignant syndrome (NMS) have been reported. This potentially fatal syndrome is comprised of the symptom complex of hyperthermia, altered consciousness, muscular rigidity, and autonomic dysfunction.

Overdosage

➤*Symptoms:* Symptoms of overdosage may include drowsiness, disorientation, and extrapyramidal reactions.

Unintentional overdose due to misadministration has been reported in infants and children with the use of metoclopramide oral solution. While there was no consistent pattern to the reports associated with these overdoses, events included seizures, extrapyramidal reactions, and lethargy.

Methemoglobinemia has occurred in premature and full-term neonates who were given overdoses of metoclopramide (1 to 4 mg/kg/day orally, IM or IV for 1 to 3 or more days). Methemoglobinemia has not been reported in neonates treated with 0.5 mg/kg/day in divided doses. Methemoglobinemia can be reversed by the IV administration of methylene blue.

➤*Treatment:* Anticholinergic or antiparkinson drugs or antihistamines with anticholinergic properties may be helpful in controlling the extrapyramidal reactions. Symptoms are self-limiting and usually disappear within 24 hours.

Hemodialysis removes relatively little metoclopramide, probably because of the small amount of the drug in blood relative to tissues. Similarly, continuous ambulatory peritoneal dialysis does not remove significant amounts of drug. It is unlikely that dosage would need to be adjusted to compensate for losses through dialysis. Dialysis is not likely to be an effective method of drug removal in overdose situations.

Patient Information

Metoclopramide may impair the mental or physical abilities required for the performance of hazardous tasks such as operating machinery or driving a motor vehicle. Caution the ambulatory patient.

METOCLOPRAMIDE HYDROCHLORIDE — INJECTION

See also the Antiemetic/Antivertigo monograph.

Indications

➤*Diabetic gastroparesis (diabetic gastric stasis):* For the relief of symptoms associated with acute and recurrent diabetic gastric stasis. The usual manifestations of delayed gastric emptying (eg, nausea, vomiting, heartburn, persistent fullness after meals, anorexia) appear to respond to metoclopramide within different time intervals. Significant relief of nausea occurs early and continues to improve over a 3-week period. Relief of vomiting and anorexia may precede the relief of abdominal fullness by 1 week or more.

➤*Prevention of nausea and vomiting associated with emetogenic cancer chemotherapy:* For the prophylaxis of vomiting associated with emetogenic cancer chemotherapy.

➤*Prevention of postoperative nausea and vomiting:* For the prophylaxis of postoperative nausea and vomiting in those circumstances where nasogastric suction is undesirable.

➤*Small bowel intubation:* To facilitate small bowel intubation in adults and pediatric patients in whom the tube does not pass the pylorus with conventional maneuvers.

➤*Radiological examination:* To stimulate gastric emptying and intestinal transit of barium in cases where delayed emptying interferes with radiological examination of the stomach and/or small intestine.

➤*Unlabeled uses:* Used to improve lactation. Doses of 30 to 45 mg/day have increased milk secretion, possibly by elevating serum prolactin levels.

Studies have indicated some potential value of metoclopramide in the following conditions: nausea and vomiting of a variety of etiologies (uncontrolled studies report 80% to 90% efficacy), including emesis during pregnancy and labor; gastric ulcer; anorexia nervosa (due to GI stimulation);

METOCLOPRAMIDE HYDROCHLORIDE — INJECTION

to improve patient response to ergotamine, analgesics, and sedatives in migraine, perhaps by enhancing absorption of the other medications; treatment of postoperative gastric bezoars (10 mg 3 or 4 times daily); diabetic cystoparesis (atonic bladder); esophageal variceal bleeding; radiation-induced emesis.

Administration and Dosage

➤*For the relief of symptoms associated with diabetic gastroparesis (diabetic gastric stasis):* If only the earliest manifestations of diabetic gastric stasis are present, oral administration of metoclopramide may be initiated. However, if severe symptoms are present, therapy should begin with metoclopramide (intramuscular [IM] or intravenous [IV]). Doses of 10 mg may be administered slowly by the IV route over a 1- to 2-minute period.

Administration of metoclopramide injection up to 10 days may be required before symptoms subside, at which time oral administration of metoclopramide may be instituted.

➤*For the prevention of nausea and vomiting associated with emetogenic cancer chemotherapy:* For doses in excess of 10 mg, metoclopramide injection should be diluted in 50 mL of a parenteral solution.

The preferred parenteral solution is sodium chloride injection (normal saline), which, when combined with metoclopramide injection, can be stored frozen for up to 4 weeks. Metoclopramide injection is degraded when admixed and frozen with dextrose 5% in water. Metoclopramide injection diluted in sodium chloride injection, dextrose 5% in water, dextrose 5% in 0.45% sodium chloride, Ringer injection, or Ringer lactate injection may be stored up to 48 hours (without freezing) after preparation if protected from light. All dilutions may be stored unprotected from light under normal light conditions up to 24 hours after preparation.

Make IV infusions slowly over a period of not less than 15 minutes, 30 minutes before beginning cancer chemotherapy and repeat every 2 hours for 2 doses, then every 3 hours for 3 doses.

The initial 2 doses should be 2 mg/kg if highly emetogenic drugs such as cisplatin or dacarbazine are used alone or in combination. For less emetogenic regimens, 1 mg/kg dose may be adequate.

If extrapyramidal symptoms (EPS) occur, inject diphenhydramine hydrochloride 50 mg IM, and EPS usually will subside.

➤*For the prevention of postoperative nausea and vomiting:* Give metoclopramide injection IM near the end of surgery. The usual adult dose is 10 mg; however, doses of 20 mg may be used.

➤*To facilitate small bowel intubation:* If the tube has not passed the pylorus with conventional maneuvers in 10 minutes, a single dose (undiluted) may be administered slowly by the IV route over a 1- to 2-minute period.

The recommended single dose is:

Pediatric patients older than 14 years of age and adults – Metoclopramide base 10 mg.

Pediatric patients (6 to 14 years of age) – Metoclopramide base 2.5 to 5 mg.

Pediatric patients (younger than 6 years of age) – Metoclopramide base 0.1 mg/kg.

➤*To aid in radiological examinations:* In patients where delayed gastric emptying interferes with radiological examination of the stomach and/or small intestine, a single dose may be administered slowly by the IV route over a 1- to 2-minute period.

The recommended single dose is:

Pediatric patients older than 14 years of age and adults – Metoclopramide base 10 mg.

Pediatric patients (6 to 14 years of age) – Metoclopramide base 2.5 to 5 mg.

Pediatric patients (younger than 6 years of age) – Metoclopramide base 0.1 mg/kg.

➤*Renal function impairment:* Because metoclopramide is excreted principally through the kidneys, in those patients whose creatinine clearance is below 40 mL/min, initiate therapy at approximately one half the recommended dosage. Depending upon clinical efficacy and safety considerations, the dosage may be increased or decreased as appropriate.

➤*Admixture compatibilities:* Metoclopramide injection is compatible for mixing and injection with the following doseforms to the extent indicated below:

Physically and chemically compatible up to 48 hours – Cimetidine hydrochloride, mannitol, potassium acetate, potassium phosphate.

Physically compatible up to 48 hours – Ascorbic acid, benztropine mesylate, cytarabine, dexamethasone sodium phosphate, diphenhydramine hydrochloride, doxorubicin hydrochloride, heparin sodium, hydrocortisone sodium phosphate, lidocaine hydrochloride, multivitamin infusion (must be refrigerated). Vitamin B complex with ascorbic acid.

Physically compatible up to 24 hours (do not use if precipitation occurs) – Clindamycin phosphate, cyclophosphamide, insulin.

Conditionally compatible (use within 1 hour after mixing or may be infused directly into the same running IV line) – Ampicillin sodium, cisplatin, erythromycin lactobionate, methotrexate sodium, penicillin G potassium, tetracycline hydrochloride.

Incompatible (do not mix) – Cephalothin sodium, chloramphenicol sodium, sodium bicarbonate.

➤*Storage/Stability:* Store vials in carton until used. Do not store open single-dose vials for later use, as they contain no preservative.

This product is light sensitive. Inspect before use and discard if either color or particulate is observed.

Dilutions may be stored unprotected from light under normal light conditions up to 24 hours after preparation.

Store at controlled room temperature 20° to 25°C (68° to 77°F).

Actions

➤*Pharmacology:* Metoclopramide stimulates motility of the upper GI tract without stimulating gastric, biliary, or pancreatic secretions. Its mode of action is unclear. It seems to sensitize tissues to the action of acetylcholine. The effect of metoclopramide on motility is not dependent on intact vagal innervation, but it can be abolished by anticholinergic drugs.

Metoclopramide increases the tone and amplitude of gastric (especially antral) contractions, relaxes the pyloric sphincter and the duodenal bulb, and increases peristalsis of the duodenal and jejunum resulting in accelerated gastric emptying and intestinal transit. It increases the resting tone of the lower esophageal sphincter. It has little, if any, effect on the motility of the colon or gallbladder.

In patients with gastroesophageal reflux (GER) and low LESP (lower esophageal sphincter pressure), single oral doses of metoclopramide produce dose-related increases in LESP. Effects begin at about 5 mg and increase through 20 mg (the largest dose tested). The increase in LESP from a 5 mg dose lasts about 45 minutes and that of 20 mg lasts between 2 and 3 hours. Increased rate of stomach emptying has been observed with single oral doses of 10 mg.

The antiemetic properties of metoclopramide appear to be a result of its antagonism of central and peripheral dopamine receptors. Dopamine produces nausea and vomiting by stimulation of the medullary chemoreceptor trigger zone (CTZ), and metoclopramide blocks stimulation of the CTZ by agents like levodopa or apomorphine, which are known to increase dopamine levels or to possess dopamine-like effects. Metoclopramide also abolishes the slowing of gastric emptying caused by apomorphine.

Like the phenothiazines and related drugs, which are also dopamine antagonists, metoclopramide produces sedation and may produce extrapyramidal reactions, although these are comparatively rare. Metoclopramide inhibits the central and peripheral effects of apomorphine, induces release of prolactin and causes a transient increase in circulating aldosterone levels, which may be associated with transient fluid retention.

➤*Pharmacokinetics:*

Absorption/Distribution – The onset of pharmacological action of metoclopramide is 1 to 3 minutes following an IV dose, 10 to 15 minutes following IM administration. Similar time to peak is observed after individual doses at steady state. Pharmacological effects persist for 1 to 2 hours.

In a single dose study of 12 subjects, the area under the drug concentration-time curve increases linearly with doses from 20 to 100 mg. Peak concentrations increase linearly with dose, time to peak concentrations remains the same, whole body clearance is unchanged, and the elimination rate remains the same.

The drug is not extensively bound to plasma proteins (about 30%). The whole body volume of distribution is high (about 3.5 L/kg) which suggests extensive distribution of drug to the tissues.

Metabolism/Excretion – The average elimination half-life in individuals with normal renal function is 5 to 6 hours. Linear kinetic processes adequately describe the absorption and elimination of metoclopramide.

Approximately 85% of the radioactivity of an orally administered dose appears in the urine within 72 hours. Of the 85% eliminated in the urine, about half is present as free or conjugated metoclopramide.

Special populations –

Renal function impairment: Renal impairment affects the clearance of metoclopramide. In a study with patients with varying degrees of renal impairment, a reduction in creatinine clearance was correlated with a reduction in plasma clearance, renal clearance, non-renal clearance, and increase in elimination half-life. The kinetics of metoclopramide in the presence of renal impairment remained linear, however. The reduction in clearance as a result of renal impairment suggests that adjustment downward of maintenance dosage should be done to avoid drug accumulation.

Adult Pharmacokinetic Data

Parameter	Value
Vd (L/kg)	≈ 3.5
Plasma protein binding	≈ 30%
$t_{1/2}$ (h)	5 to 6
Oral bioavailability	80% ± 15.5%

Children: In pediatric patients, the pharmacodynamics of metoclopramide following oral and IV administration are highly variable and a concentration-effect relationship has not been established.

Single IV doses of metoclopramide 0.22 to 0.46 mg/kg (mean, 0.35 mg/kg) were administered over 5 minutes to 9 pediatric cancer patients receiving chemotherapy (mean age, 11.7 years; range, 7 to 14 years) for prophylaxis of cytotoxic-induced vomiting. The metoclopramide plasma concentrations extrapolated to time zero ranged from 65 to 395 mcg/L (mean, 152 mcg/L). The mean elimination half-life, clearance, and volume of distribution of metoclopramide were 4.4 hours (range, 1.7 to 8.3 hours), 0.56 L/h/kg (range, 0.12 to 1.2 L/h/kg), and 3 L/kg (range, 1 to 4.8 L/kg), respectively.

In another study, 9 pediatric cancer patients (age range, 1 to 9 years) received 4 to 5 IV infusions (over 30 minutes) of metoclopramide at a dose of

METOCLOPRAMIDE HYDROCHLORIDE — INJECTION

2 mg/kg to control emesis. After the last dose, the peak serum concentrations of metoclopramide ranged from 1,060 to 5,680 mcg/L. The mean elimination half-life, clearance, and volume of distribution of metoclopramide were 4.5 hours (range, 2 to 12.5 hours), 0.37 L/h/kg (range, 0.1 to 1.24 L/h/kg), and 1.93 L/kg (range, 0.95 to 5.5 L/kg), respectively.

Pediatric Pharmacokinetic Studies

Reference	Dose, route	t½(h)	Cl (L/h/kg)	Vd (L/kg)	C_{max} (mcg/L)
a	0.35 mg/kg IV over 5 minutes	4.4 ± 0.56	0.56 ± 0.1	3 ± 0.38 (Dose/Cp0)	152 ± 31
b	2 mg/kg 30 minutes IV infusion 4 to 5 times within 9.5 hours	4.5[c]	0.37[c]	1.93[c]	1,060 to 5,680[c]

[a] Bateman, DN, et al. *Br J Clin Pharmac.* 1983;15:557-559.
[b] Ford, C. *Clin Pharmac Ther.* 1988;43:196.
[c] SEM not available.

Contraindications

Do not use metoclopramide whenever stimulation of GI motility might be dangerous (eg, in the presence of GI hemorrhage, mechanical obstruction, perforation).

Metoclopramide is contraindicated in patients with pheochromocytoma because the drug may cause a hypertensive crisis, probably due to release of catecholamines from the tumor. Such hypertensive crises may be controlled by phentolamine.

Metoclopramide is contraindicated in patients with known sensitivity or intolerance to the drug.

Do not use metoclopramide in epileptics or patients receiving other drugs that are likely to cause extrapyramidal reactions, because the frequency and severity of seizures or extrapyramidal reactions may be increased.

Warnings

➤*Depression:* Mental depression has occurred in patients with and without history of depression. Symptoms have ranged from mild to severe and have included suicidal ideation and suicide. Only give metoclopramide to patients with a history of depression if the expected benefits outweigh the potential risks.

➤*Extrapyramidal symptoms (EPS):* EPS, manifested primarily as acute dystonic reactions, occur in approximately 1 in 500 patients treated with the usual adult dosages of metoclopramide 30 to 40 mg/day. These usually are seen during the first 24 to 48 hours of treatment with metoclopramide, occur more frequently in pediatric patients and adult patients less than 30 years of age and are even more frequent at the higher doses used in prophylaxis of vomiting due to cancer chemotherapy. These symptoms may include involuntary movements of limbs and facial grimacing, torticollis, oculogyric crisis, rhythmic protrusion of tongue, bulbar type of speech, trismus, or dystonic reactions resembling tetanus. Rarely, dystonic reactions may present as stridor and dyspnea, possibly due to laryngospasm. If these symptoms should occur, inject diphenhydramine hydrochloride 50 mg IM, and they usually will subside. Benztropine mesylate 1 to 2 mg IM may also be used to reverse these reactions.

➤*Parkinsonian-like symptoms:* Parkinsonian-like symptoms have occurred, more commonly within the first 6 months after beginning treatment with metoclopramide, but occasionally after longer periods. These symptoms generally subside within 2 to 3 months following discontinuance of metoclopramide. Give patients with preexisting Parkinson disease metoclopramide cautiously, if at all, because such patients may experience exacerbation of parkinsonian symptoms when taking metoclopramide.

➤*Tardive dyskinesia:* Tardive dyskinesia, a syndrome consisting of potentially irreversible, involuntary, dyskinetic movements may develop in patients treated with metoclopramide. Although the prevalence of the syndrome appears to be highest among the elderly, especially elderly women, it is impossible to predict which patients are likely to develop the syndrome. Both the risk of developing the syndrome and the likelihood that it will become irreversible are believed to increase with the duration of treatment and the total cumulative dose.

Less commonly, the syndrome can develop after relatively brief treatment periods at low doses; in these cases, symptoms appear more likely to be reversible.

There is no known treatment for established cases of tardive dyskinesia although the syndrome may remit, partially or completely, within several weeks-to-months after metoclopramide is withdrawn. Metoclopramide itself, however, may suppress (or partially suppress) the signs of tardive dyskinesia, thereby masking the underlying disease process. The effect of this symptomatic suppression upon the long-term course of the syndrome is unknown. Therefore, the use of metoclopramide for the symptomatic control of tardive dyskinesia is not recommended.

➤*Neuroleptic malignant syndrome (NMS):* There have been rare reports of an uncommon but potentially fatal symptom complex sometimes referred to as NMS associated with metoclopramide. Clinical manifestations of NMS include hyperthermia, muscle rigidity, altered consciousness, and evidence of autonomic instability (irregular pulse or blood pressure, tachycardia, diaphoresis and cardiac arrhythmias).

The diagnostic evaluation of patients with this syndrome is complicated. In arriving at a diagnosis, it is important to identify cases where the clinical presentation includes both serious medical illness (eg, pneumonia, systemic infection) and untreated or inadequately treated extrapyramidal signs and symptoms (EPS). Other important considerations in the differential diagnosis include central anticholinergic toxicity, heat stroke, malignant hyperthermia, drug fever, and primary CNS pathology.

The management of NMS includes the following:

1.) Immediate discontinuation of metoclopramide and other drugs not essential to concurrent therapy.
2.) Intensive symptomatic treatment and medical monitoring.
3.) Treatment of any concomitant serious medical problems for which specific treatments are available. Bromocriptine and dantroline sodium have been used in treatment of NMS, but their effectiveness has not been established.

➤*Carcinogenesis:* A 77-week study was conducted in rats in oral doses up to about 40 times the maximum recommended human daily dose. Metoclopramide elevates prolactin levels and the elevation persists during chronic administration. Tissue culture experiments indicate that approximately one-third of human breast cancers are prolactin-dependent in vitro, a factor of potential importance if the prescription of metoclopramide is contemplated in a patient with previously detected breast cancer. Although disturbances such as galactorrhea, amenorrhea, gynecomastia, and impotence have been reported with prolactin-elevating drugs, the clinical significance of elevated serum prolactin levels is unknown for most patients. An increase in mammary neoplasms has been found in rodents after chronic administration of prolactin-stimulating neuroleptic drugs and metoclopramide. Neither clinical studies nor epidemiologic studies conducted to date, however, have shown an association between chronic administration of these drugs and mammary tumorigenesis; the available evidence is too limited to be conclusive at this time.

➤*Elderly:* The risk of developing parkinsonian-like side effects increases with ascending dose. Geriatric patients should receive the lowest dose of metoclopramide that is effective. If parkinsonian-like symptoms develop in a geriatric patient receiving metoclopramide, metoclopramide should generally be discontinued before initiating any specific anti-parkinsonian agent.

The elderly may be at greater risk for tardive dyskinesia.

Sedation has been reported in metoclopramide users. Sedation may cause confusion and manifest as oversedation in elderly.

Renal function impairment – Metoclopramide is known to be substantially excreted by the kidney, and the risk of toxic reactions to this drug may be greater in patients with impaired renal function.

For these reasons, dose selection for an elderly patient should be cautious, usually starting at the low end of the dosing range, reflecting the greater frequency of decreased renal function, concomitant disease, or other drug therapy in the elderly.

➤*Pregnancy: Category B.*

There are no adequate and well-controlled studies in pregnant women. Because animal reproduction studies are not always predictive of human response, use this drug during pregnancy only if clearly needed.

➤*Lactation:* Metoclopramide is excreted in human milk. Exercise caution when metoclopramide is administered to a breastfeeding mother.

➤*Children:* Safety and efficacy in pediatric patients have not been established except as stated to facilitate small bowel intubation.

Exercise care in administering metoclopramide to neonates because prolonged clearance may produce excessive serum concentrations (see Pharmacokinetics).

In addition, neonates have reduced levels of NADH-cytochrome b_5 reductase which, in combination with the aforementioned pharmacokinetic factors, make neonates more susceptible to methemoglobinemia.

The safety profile of metoclopramide in adults cannot be extrapolated to pediatric patients. Dystonias and other extrapyramidal reactions associated with metoclopramide are more common in the pediatric population than in adults.

Precautions

➤*Administration:* IV injections of undiluted metoclopramide should be made slowly allowing 1 to 2 minutes for 10 mg because a transient but intense feeling of anxiety and restlessness, followed by drowsiness, may occur with rapid administration.

IV administration of metoclopramide injection, diluted in a parenteral solution, should be made slowly over a period of not less than 15 minutes.

➤*Anastomosis or closure of the gut:* Giving a promotility drug such as metoclopramide theoretically could put increased pressure on suture lines following a gut anastomosis or closure. Although adverse reactions related to this possibility have not been reported to date, consider and weigh the possibility when deciding whether to use metoclopramide or nasogastric suction in the prevention of postoperative nausea and vomiting.

➤*Special risk:* In 1 study in hypersensitive patients, IV administered metoclopramide was shown to release catecholamines; hence, exercise caution when metoclopramide is used in patients with hypertension.

Because metoclopramide produces a transient increase in plasma aldosterone, certain patients, especially those with cirrhosis or congestive heart failure, may be at risk of developing fluid retention and volume overload. If these side effects occur at any time during metoclopramide therapy, discontinue the drug.

Patients with NADH-cytochrome b_5 reductase deficiency are at an increased risk of developing methemoglobinemia or sulfhemoglobinemia when metoclopramide is administered. In patients with glucose-6-phosphate dehydrogenase (G6PD) deficiency who experience metoclopramide-induced methemoglobinemia, methylene blue treatment is not recommended.

METOCLOPRAMIDE HYDROCHLORIDE — INJECTION

➤*Hazardous tasks:* Metoclopramide may impair the mental and/or physical abilities required for the performance of hazardous tasks such as operating machinery or driving a motor vehicle. Caution the ambulatory patient accordingly.

Drug Interactions

Metoclopramide Drug Interactions

Precipitant drug	Object drug*		Description
Metoclopramide	Alcohol	↑	Metoclopramide increases the rate of absorption of alcohol by decreasing the time it takes alcohol to reach the small intestine where it is rapidly absorbed.
Metoclopramide	Cimetidine	↓	Bioavailability of cimetidine may be reduced due to decreased absorption as a result of faster gastric transit time.
Metoclopramide	Cyclosporine	↑	A faster gastric emptying time may allow for an increase in cyclosporine absorption, possibly increasing its immunosuppressive and toxic effects.
Metoclopramide	Digoxin	↓	Digoxin absorption, plasma levels and therapeutic effects may be decreased. The capsule, elixir and tablets with a high dissolution rate are least affected.
Metoclopramide	Levodopa	↑	These agents have opposite effects on dopamine receptors. The bioavailability of levodopa may be increased, and levodopa may decrease the effects of metoclopramide on gastric emptying and lower esophageal pressure. Metoclopramide is relatively contraindicated in Parkinson's disease patients.
Levodopa	Metoclopramide	↓	
Metoclopramide	MAO inhibitors	↑	Since metoclopramide releases catecholamines in patients with essential hypertension, use cautiously, if at all, in patients receiving MAO inhibitors.
Metoclopramide	Succinylcholine	↑	By inhibiting plasma cholinesterase, metoclopramide may increase the neuromuscular blocking effects of succinylcholine.
Anticholinergics Narcotic analgesics	Metoclopramide	↓	The effects of metoclopramide on GI motility are antagonized by these agents.

* ↑ = Object drug increased. ↓ = Object drug decreased.

The effects of metoclopramide on GI motility are antagonized by anticholinergic drugs and narcotic analgesics. Additive sedative effects can occur when metoclopramide is given with alcohol, sedatives, hypnotics, narcotics, or tranquilizers.

Absorption of drugs from the stomach may be diminished (eg, digoxin) by metoclopramide, whereas the rate and/or extent of absorption of drugs from the small bowel may be increased (eg, acetaminophen, tetracycline, levodopa, ethanol, cyclosporine).

Gastroparesis (gastric stasis) may be responsible for poor diabetic control in some patients. Exogenously administered insulin may begin to act before food has left the stomach and lead to hypoglycemia. Because the action of metoclopramide will influence the delivery of food to the intestines and thus the rate of absorption, insulin dosage or timing of dosage may require adjustment.

Adverse Reactions

➤*Allergic:* A few cases of rash, urticaria, or bronchospasm, especially in patients with a history of asthma. Rarely, angioneurotic edema, including glossal or laryngeal edema.

➤*Cardiovascular:* Hypotension, hypertension, supraventricular tachycardia, bradycardia, fluid retention, acute congestive heart failure, and possible atrioventricular (AV) block.

➤*CNS:* Restlessness, drowsiness, fatigue, and lassitude may occur in patients receiving the recommended prescribed dose of metoclopramide injection. Insomnia, headache, confusion, dizziness, or mental depression with suicidal ideation occur. In cancer chemotherapy patients being treated with 1 to 2 mg/kg per dose, incidence of drowsiness is about 70%. There are isolated reports of convulsive seizures without clear-cut relationship to metoclopramide. Rarely, hallucinations have been reported.

EPS – Acute dystonic reactions, the most common type of EPS associated with metoclopramide, occur in approximately 0.2% of patients (1 in 500) treated with 30 to 40 mg of metoclopramide per day. In cancer chemotherapy patients receiving 1 to 2 mg/kg per dose, the incidence is 2% in patients older than 30 to 35 years of age, and 25% or higher in pediatric patients and adult patients younger than 30 years of age who have not had prophylactic administration of diphenhydramine. Symptoms include involuntary movements of limbs, facial grimacing, torticollis, oculogyric crisis, rhythmic protrusion of tongue, bulbar type of speech, trismus, opisthotonus (tetanus-like reactions) and, rarely, stridor and dyspnea, possibly due to laryngospasm; ordinarily these symptoms are readily reversed by diphenhydramine.

Parkinsonian-like symptoms – Parkinsonian-like symptoms may include bradykinesia, tremor, cogwheel rigidity, mask-like facies.

Tardive dyskinesia – Tardive dyskinesia most frequently is characterized by involuntary movements of the tongue, face, mouth or jaw, and sometimes by involuntary movements of the trunk and/or extremities; movements may be choreoathetotic in appearance.

Motor restlessness (akathisia) may consist of feelings of anxiety, agitation, jitteriness, and insomnia, as well as inability to sit still, pacing, and foot tapping. These symptoms may disappear spontaneously or respond to a reduction in dosage.

NMS – Rare occurrences of NMS have been reported. This potentially fatal syndrome is comprised of the symptom complex of hyperthermia, muscular rigidity, altered consciousness, and autonomic instability.

➤*Endocrine:* Galactorrhea, amenorrhea, gynecomastia, impotence secondary to hyperprolactinemia. Fluid retention secondary to transient elevation of aldosterone.

➤*GI:* Nausea and bowel disturbances, primarily diarrhea.

➤*Hematologic:* A few cases of neutropenia, leukopenia, or agranulocytosis, generally without clear-cut relationship to metoclopramide. Methemoglobinemia in adults and especially with overdosage in neonates. Sulfhemoglobinemia in adults.

➤*Hepatic:* Rarely, cases of hepatotoxicity, characterized by such findings as jaundice and altered liver function tests, when metoclopramide was administered with other drugs with known hepatotoxic potential.

➤*Renal:* Urinary frequency and incontinence.

➤*Miscellaneous:* Visual disturbances, porphyria.

Transient flushing of the face and upper body, without alterations in vital signs, following high IV doses.

Overdosage

➤*Symptoms:* Symptoms of overdosage may include drowsiness, disorientation, and extrapyramidal reactions. Anticholinergic or antiparkinson drugs or antihistamines with anticholinergic properties may be helpful in controlling the extrapyramidal reactions. Symptoms are self-limiting and usually disappear within 24 hours.

Unintentional overdose due to misadministration has been reported in infants and children with the use of metoclopramide syrup. While there was no consistent pattern to the reports associated with these overdoses, events included seizures, extrapyramidal reactions, and lethargy.

➤*Treatment:* Hemodialysis removes relatively little metoclopramide, probably because of the small amount of the drug in blood relative to tissues. Similarly, continuous ambulatory peritoneal dialysis does not remove significant amounts of drug. It is unlikely that dosage would need to be adjusted to compensate for losses through dialysis. Dialysis is not likely to be an effective method of drug removal in overdose situations.

Methemoglobinemia has occurred in premature and full-term neonates who were given overdoses of metoclopramide (1 to 4 mg/kg/day orally, IM or IV for 1 to 3 or more days). Methemoglobinemia can be reversed by the IV administration of methylene blue. However, methylene blue may cause hemolytic anemia in patients with G6PD deficiency, which may be fatal.

Patient Information

Metoclopramide may impair the mental and/or physical abilities required for the performance of hazardous tasks such as operating machinery, driving a motor vehicle, or performing other tasks requiring alertness, coordination, or physical dexterity. Caution the ambulatory patient accordingly.

Notify your doctor if involuntary movement of eyes, face, or limbs occurs.

DEXPANTHENOL (Dextro-Pantothenyl Alcohol)

Rx	**Dexpanthenol** (Various)	**Injection:** 250 mg per mL	In 10 mL and 2 mL vials.
Rx	**Ilopan** (Adria)		In UD *Stat-Pak* 2 mL disp. syringes.[1]

[1] Syringes contain no more than 0.5% chlorobutanol.

DEXPANTHENOL — INJECTION

Indications

Prophylactic use immediately after major abdominal surgery to minimize the possibility of paralytic ileus. Intestinal atony causing abdominal distention; postoperative or postpartum retention of flatus, or postoperative delay in resumption of intestinal motility; paralytic ileus.

Administration and Dosage

For the prevention of postoperative adynamic ileus the dose is 250 mg (1 mL) or 500 mg (2 mL) IM. May repeat in 2 hrs and then every 6 hrs until all danger of adynamic ileus has passed.

For the treatment of adynamic ileus, the dose is 500 mg (2 mL) IM. May repeat in 2 hrs and then every 6 hrs as needed.

For IV administration, dexpanthenol injection 2 mL (500 mg) may be mixed with bulk IV solutions such as glucose or Lactated Ringer's and slowly infused by IV.

➤*Storage/Stability:* Store at controlled room temperature 15° to 30°C (59°to 86°F). Protect from freezing or excessive heat.

Actions

➤*Pharmacology:* Pantothenic acid is a precursor of coenzyme A, which serves as a cofactor for a variety of enzyme-catalyzed reactions involving transfer of acetyl groups. The final step in the synthesis of acetylcholine consists of the choline acetylase transfer of acetyl group from acetylcoenzyme A to choline. Acetylcholine is the neurohumoral transmitter in the parasympathetic system and as such maintains the normal functions of the intestine. Decrease in acetylcholine content would result in decreased peristalsis and in extreme cases adynamic ileus. The pharmacological mode of action of the drug is unknown.

➤*Pharmacokinetics:* Pharmacokinetics data in humans is unavailable.

Contraindications

There are no known contraindications to the use of dexpanthenol injection.

Warnings

➤*Administration:* Administration of dexpanthenol injection directly into the vein is not advised (See Dosage and Administration).

➤*Hypersensitivity reactions:* If any signs of a hypersensitivity reaction appear, dexpanthenol injection should be discontinued.

There have been rare instances of allergic reactions of unknown cause during the concomitant use of dexpanthenol injection with drugs such as antibiotics, narcotics and barbiturates.

➤*Pregnancy: Category C.*

Dexpanthenol injection should be given to a pregnant woman only if clearly needed.

➤*Lactation:* It is not known whether this drug is excreted in human milk. Because many drugs are excreted in human milk, caution should be exercised when dexpanthenol injection is administered to a nursing woman.

➤*Children:* Safety and effectiveness in children have not been established.

Precautions

➤*Mechanical obstruction:* If ileus is a secondary consequence of mechanical obstruction, primary attention should be directed to the obstruction. The management of adynamic ileus includes the correction of any fluid and electrolyte imbalance (especially hypokalemia), anemia and hypoproteinemia, treatment of infection, avoidance where possible of drugs which are known to decrease gastrointestinal motility and decompression of the GI tract when considerably distended by nasogastric suction or use of a long intestinal tube.

Drug Interactions

The effects of succinylcholine appeared to have been prolonged in a woman administered dexpanthenol. (See Warnings).

Dexpanthenol Drug Interactions

Precipitant drug	Object drug*		Description
Dexpanthenol	Antibiotics, barbiturates, or narcotics	↑	Allergic reactions have occurred rarely during concomitant use of dexpanthenol.
Dexpanthenol	Succinylcholine	↑	Temporary respiratory difficulty occurred following dexpanthenol administration 5 minutes after succinylcholine was discontinued. Succinylcholine's effects appeared to have been prolonged. Do not administer within 1 hour of succinylcholine.

* ↑ = Object drug increased.

Adverse Reactions

➤*Allergic:* There have been a few reports of allergic reactions and single reports of several other adverse events in association with the administration of dexpanthenol. A causal relationship is uncertain. One patient experienced itching, tingling, difficulty in breathing. Another patient had red patches of skin. Two patients had generalized dermatitis and one patient urticaria.

➤*Cardiovascular:* One patient experienced a noticeable but slight drop in blood pressure after administration of dexpanthenol while in the recovery room.

➤*GI:* One patient experienced intestinal colic ½ hr after the drug was administered.

➤*Respiratory:* One patient experienced temporary respiratory difficulty following administration of dexpanthenol injection 5 minutes after succinylcholine was discontinued.

➤*Miscellaneous:* Two patients vomited following administration and two patients had diarrhea 10 days post-surgery and after dexpanthenol injection.

One elderly patient became agitated after administration of the drug.

DIGESTIVE ENZYMES

Content given per capsule, tablet, or 0.7 g powder.

	Product and Distributor[a]	Lipase (USP units)	Protease (USP units)	Amylase (USP units)	How Supplied
			PANCREATIN		
Rx	**Ku-Zyme Capsules**[b] (Schwarz Pharma)	1,200	15,000	15,000	(SCHWARZ 4122). Yellow/White. In 100s.
Rx	**Kutrase Capsules**[b] (Schwarz Pharma)	2,400	30,000	30,000	(SCHWARZ 4175). Green/White. In 100s.
			PANCRELIPASE		
Rx	**Pancrease MT 4 Capsules**[b] (McNeil)	4,000	12,000	12,000	(McNEIL PANCREASE MT 4). Yellow/Clear. Enteric-coated microtablets. In 100s.
Rx	**Pancrecarb MS-4 Delayed-Release Capsules**[b] (Digestive Care)	4,000	25,000	25,000	(DCI PANCRECARB MS-4). Clear. Enteric-coated microspheres. In 100s.
Rx	**Pancrelipase Capsules**[b] (Various, eg, Global)	4,500	25,000	20,000	Enteric-coated microspheres. In 100s and 250s.
Rx	**Panocaps Delayed-Release Capsules**[b] (Breckenridge)				Sucrose. (B 406). Clear/White. Enteric-coated microspheres. In 100s and 250s.
Rx	**Lipram 4500 Delayed-Release Capsules**[b] (Global)				(0115 7035). White. Enteric-coated microspheres. In 100s and 250s.
Rx	**Pancrease Capsules**[b] (McNeil)				Sucrose. Dye free. (McNEIL Pancrease). White/Clear. Enteric-coated microspheres. In 100s and 250s.
Rx	**Ultrase Capsules**[b] (Axcan Scandipharm)				Sugar. (ULTRASE). White. Enteric-coated microspheres. In 100s.
Rx	**Creon 5 Delayed-Release Capsules**[b] (Solvay)	5,000	18,750	16,600	(SOLVAY 1205). Orange/Blue. Enteric-coated *Minimicrospheres.* In 100s and 250s.
Rx	**Lipram-CR5 Delayed-Release Capsules**[b] (Global)				(0115 7057). Natural/White. Enteric-coated microspheres. In 100s and 250s.

DIGESTIVE ENZYMES

	Product and Distributor[a]	Lipase (USP units)	Protease (USP units)	Amylase (USP units)	How Supplied
Rx	**Pancrelipase Tablets**[b] (Various, eg, Contract Pharmacal)	8,000	30,000	30,000	May contain lactose. In 100s and 500s.
Rx	**Ku-Zyme HP Capsules**[b] (Schwarz Pharma)				Lactose. (SCHWARZ 525). White. In 100s.
Rx	**Panokase Tablets**[b] (Breckenridge)				Lactose. In 100s and 500s.
Rx	**Plaretase 8000 Tablets**[b] (Ethex)				(ETH 416). Tan. In 100s and 500s.
Rx	**Viokase 8 Tablets**[b] (Axcan Scandipharm)				Lactose. (VIOKASE 9111). Tan. In 100s and 500s.
Rx	**Pancrecarb MS-8 Delayed-Release Capsules**[b] (Digestive Care)	8,000	45,000	40,000	(DCI PANCRECARB MS-8). Clear. Enteric-coated microspheres. In 100s and 250s.
otc sf	**PAN-2400 Capsules** (Bio-Tech)	9,816	60,214	75,900	Preservative free. In 100s.
Rx	**Lipram-PN10 Delayed-Release Capsules**[b] (Global)	10,000	30,000	30,000	(0115 7040). Natural/Brown. Enteric-coated microspheres. In 100s.
Rx	**Pancrease MT 10 Capsules**[b] (McNeil)				(McNEIL PANCREASE MT 10). Pink/Clear. Enteric-coated microtablets. In 100s.
Rx	**Creon 10 Delayed-Release Capsules**[b] (Solvay)	10,000	37,500	33,200	(SOLVAY 1210). Brown/Natural. Enteric-coated *Minimicrospheres.* In 100s and 250s.
Rx	**Lipram-CR10 Delayed-Release Capsules**[b] (Global)				(0115 7036). Brown/Flesh. Enteric-coated microspheres. In 100s and 250s.
Rx	**Palcaps 10 Delayed-Release Capsules**[b] (Breckenridge)				Sucrose. (B 410). Clear/Brown opaque. Enteric-coated microspheres. In 100s and 250s.
Rx	**Lipram-UL12 Delayed-Release Capsules**[b] (Global)	12,000	39,000	39,000	(0115 7042). Natural/White. Enteric-coated microspheres. In 100s.
Rx	**Ultrase MT 12 Capsules**[b] (Axcan Scandipharm)				(ULTRASE MT12). White/Yellow. Enteric-coated minitablets. In 100s.
Rx	**Pancrelipase Capsules**[b] (Various, eg, Mutual)	16,000	48,000	48,000	Enteric-coated microspheres. In 100s and 250s.
Rx	**Panocaps MT 16 Delayed-Release Capsules**[b] (Breckenridge)				Sucrose. (B 407). Clear/Orange opaque. Enteric-coated microspheres. In 100s.
Rx	**Lipram-PN16 Delayed-Release Capsules**[b] (Global)				(0115 7023). Flesh. Enteric-coated microspheres. In 100s.
Rx	**Pancrease MT 16 Capsules**[b] (McNeil)				(McNEIL PANCREASE MT 16). Salmon/Clear. Enteric-coated microtablets. In 100s.
Rx	**Pancrecarb MS-16 Delayed-Release Capsules**[b] (Digestive Care)	16,000	52,000	52,000	(DCI PANCRECARB MS-16). Clear. Enteric-coated microspheres. In 100s and 250s.
Rx	**Pancrelipase Tablets**[b] (Various, eg, Contract Pharmacal)	16,000	60,000	60,000	May contain lactose. In 100s and 500s.
Rx	**Viokase 16 Tablets**[b] (Axcan Scandipharm)				Lactose. (V^{16} 9116). Tan, oval. In 100s and 500s.
Rx	**Viokase Powder**[b,c] (Axcan Scandipharm)	16,800	70,000	70,000	Lactose. In 227 g.
Rx	**Lipram-UL18 Delayed-Release Capsules**[b] (Global)	18,000	58,500	58,500	(0115 7041). Flesh/White. Enteric-coated microspheres. In 100s.
Rx	**Ultrase MT 18 Capsules**[b] (Axcan Scandipharm)				(ULTRASE MT18). Gray/White. Enteric-coated minitablets. In 100s.
Rx	**Lipram-PN20 Delayed-Release Capsules**[b] (Global)	20,000	44,000	56,000	(0115 7055). Flesh/Natural. Enteric-coated microspheres. In 100s.
Rx	**Pancrease MT 20 Capsules**[b] (McNeil)				(McNEIL/PANCREASE MT 20). White. Enteric-coated microtablets. In 100s.
Rx	**Panocaps MT 20 Delayed-Release Capsules**[b] (Breckenridge)				Sucrose. (B 408). Yellow opaque/white opaque. Enteric-coated microspheres. In 100s.
Rx	**Lipram-UL20 Delayed-Release Capsules**[b] (Global)	20,000	65,000	65,000	(0115 7043). Brown. Enteric-coated microspheres. In 100s and 500s.
Rx	**Ultrase MT 20 Capsules**[b] (Axcan Scandipharm)				(ULTRASE MT20). Light gray/yellow. Enteric-coated minitablets. In 100s and 500s.
Rx	**Creon 20 Delayed-release Capsules**[b] (Solvay)	20,000	75,000	66,400	(SOLVAY 1220). Orange/Natural. Enteric-coated *Minimicrospheres.* In 100s and 250s.
Rx	**Lipram-CR20 Delayed-Release Capsules**[b] (Global)				(0115 7024). Brown/White. Enteric-coated microspheres. In 100s and 250s.
Rx	**Palcaps 20 Delayed-Release Capsules**[b] (Breckenridge)				Sucrose. (B 411). Clear/Orange opaque. Enteric-coated microspheres. In 100s and 250s.

[a] Product tables do not imply bioequivalence (see page xi). Also refer to Bioequivalency (in Administration and Dosage).

[b] Porcine-derived enzymes.

[c] Amount in ¼ teaspoon.

DIGESTIVE ENZYMES – ORAL

Indications

Enzyme replacement therapy in patients with deficient exocrine pancreatic secretions, such as in cystic fibrosis, chronic pancreatitis, postpancreatectomy, ductal obstructions caused by cancer of the pancreas or common bile duct, pancreatic insufficiency, and for steatorrhea of malabsorption syndrome and postgastrectomy (Billroth II and Total) or post-GI surgery (eg, Billroth II gastroenterostomy).

Presumptive test for pancreatic function, especially in pancreatic insufficiency caused by chronic pancreatitis.

Administration and Dosage

➤*Bioequivalency:* These products are not bioequivalent and cannot be interchanged without physician supervision. Variability not only occurs at the product level, but may also be clinically significant from one batch of product to the next.

Pancrelipase capsules and tablets are required to contain between 90% and 150% of the labeled lipase activity. Pancrelipase delayed-release capsules are required to contain between 90% and 165% of the labeled lipase activity, and not less than 90% of amylase and protease labeled activities. No USP standards have currently been identified for pancreatin capsules.

➤*Enzyme supplementation.* Take capsules or tablets with meals or snacks. Adjust dosage based on severity of the exocrine pancreatic enzyme deficiency. The number of tablets, capsules, or dosage given with meals or snacks should be estimated by assessing which dose minimizes steatorrhea and maintains good nutritional status. Dose increases, if required, should be made slowly, with careful monitoring of response and symptomatology.

To protect enteric coating, do not crush or chew the microspheres or microtablets. Where swallowing of capsules is difficult, they may be opened and shaken onto a small quantity of soft non-hot food (eg, applesauce, gelatin) that does not require chewing. Swallow immediately without chewing as the proteolytic action may cause irritation of the mucosa. Follow with a glass of juice or water to ensure complete swallowing of the microspheres/microtablets. Microsphere contact with foods having a pH greater than 5.5 can dissolve the enteric coating.

➤*Ku-Zyme, Pancrecarb, Ultrase, Ultrase MT:* Initiate with 1 or 2 capsules with each meal or snack.

➤*Kutrase:* Take 1 capsule with each meal or snack.

➤*Ku-Zyme HP:* Take 1 to 3 capsules with each meal or snack. In severe deficiencies, increase the dose to 8 capsules with meals or increase the frequency to hourly intervals if nausea, cramps, or diarrhea do not occur.

DIGESTIVE ENZYMES - ORAL

➤*Pancrease, Pancrease MT 4, Panocaps, Panocaps MT:*

Infants (up to 12 months) – 2,000 to 4,000 lipase units/120 mL of formula or breast milk.

Under 4 years of age – Initiate with 1,000 lipase units/kg/meal up to a maximum of 2,500 lipase units/kg/meal

Over 4 years of age – Initiate with 400 lipase units/kg/meal up to a maximum of 2,500 lipase units/kg/meal. The total daily dose reflects approximately 3 meals and 2 to 3 snacks/day. If doses greater than 2,500 lipase units/kg/meal are required, then further investigation is warranted to rule out other causes of malabsorption. Doses greater than 2,500 lipase units/kg/meal should be used with caution and only if they are documented to be effective by 3-day fecal fat measures. It is unknown if doses this high are safe.

➤*Pancrelipase, Lipram:*

Children 6 months to less than 1 year of age – 2,000 lipase units/meal.

Children 1 to 6 years of age – 4,000 to 8,000 lipase units with each meal and 4,000 units with snacks.

Children 7 to 12 years of age – 4,000 to 12,000 lipase units with each meal and with snacks.

Adults – 4,000 to 20,000 lipase units with each meal and with snacks.

➤*Creon 5:*

Adults and children over 6 years of age – Usual starting dose is 2 to 4 capsules/meal or snack.

Children under 6 years of age – The exact dosage should be selected based on clinical experience with this age group. Initiate with 1 to 2 capsules/meal or snack.

Cystic fibrosis patients – Usual doses are 1,500 to 3,000 lipase units/kg/meal. Doses in excess of 6,000 lipase units/kg/meal are not recommended.

➤*Creon 10, Palcaps 10:*

Adults and children over 6 years of age – Usual starting dose is 1 to 2 capsules per meal or snack.

Children under 6 years of age – Usual starting dose is up to 1 capsule per meal or snack.

Cystic fibrosis patients – Usual doses are 1,500 to 3,000 lipase units/kg/meal. Doses in excess of 6,000 lipase units/kg/meal are not recommended.

➤*Creon 20, Palcaps 20:*

Adults and children over 6 years of age – Typical starting dose is 1 capsule/meal or snack.

Children under 6 years of age – Select the exact dosage based on clinical experience for this age group.

Cystic fibrosis patients – Usual doses are 1,500 to 3,000 lipase units/kg/meal. Doses in excess of 6,000 lipase units/kg/meal are not recommended.

➤*Panokase, Plaretase, Viokase (tablets):*

Cystic fibrosis and chronic pancreatitis patients – Dose ranges from 8,000 to 32,000 lipase units (1 to 4 tablets [*Plaretase, Panokase, Viokase 8*] or 1 to 2 tablets [*Viokase 16*]). Take with meals.

Pancreatectomy or obstruction of pancreatic ducts – Take 1 to 2 tablets (*Plaretase, Panokase, Viokase 8*) or 1 tablet (*Viokase 16*) every 2 hours.

➤*Viokase (powder):*

Cystic fibrosis – Take 0.7 g (¼ tsp) with meals.

➤*PAN-2400:* One capsule or more daily.

➤*Storage/Stability:*

Creon, Ku-Zyme, Kutrase, Palcaps, Ultrase, Ultrase MT – Store at controlled room temperature 15° to 25°C (59° to 86°F) in a dry place. Protect from high humidity. Do not refrigerate.

Ku-Zyme HP, Lipram, Pancrease, Pancrease MT, Pancrecarb, Pancrelipase, Panocaps, Panocaps MT, Panokase, Plaretase, Viokase – Store at room temperature not exceeding 25°C (77°F) in a dry place. Protect from high humidity. Store in tight containers. Do not refrigerate.

PAN-2400 – Store tightly closed in a cool dry place.

Actions

➤*Pharmacology:* Digestive enzymes (pancreatic enzymes) hydrolyze fats to glycerol and fatty acids, change proteins into peptides and amino acids, and starch into dextrins and maltose. These agents exert their primary actions in the duodenum and upper jejunum. Once the digestive enzymes accomplish their catalytic function to hydrolyze food, the digestive enzymes may be inactivated by anti-enzymes, excreted by intestinal mucosa, or by protease digestion. The digested enzyme fragments may be absorbed from the intestine and subsequently excreted in the urine. The inactivated enzymes are excreted in the feces. Fat malabsorption (steatorrhea) and protein maldigestion occur when the pancreas loses more than 90% of its ability to produce digestive enzymes. The resultant diarrhea and malabsorption can be reasonably managed if 30,000 lipase units are delivered to the duodenum during a 4-hour period with and after a meal, representing approximately 10% of the normal pancreatic output.

The USP defines standards for 2 pancreatic enzyme preparations, pancreatin and pancrelipase. Pancreatin (a substance containing principally amylase, lipase, and protease) contains not less than 2 USP units of lipase activity, and not less than 25 USP units of amylase as well as protease activity. Pancrelipase (a substance containing principally lipase, and also containing amylase and protease) contains not less than 24 USP units of lipase activity, and not less than 100 USP units of amylase as well as protease activity.

Contraindications

Hypersensitivity to pork protein or enzymes; acute pancreatitis; acute exacerbations of chronic pancreatic diseases.

Warnings

➤*Colonic strictures:* Cases of fibrotic strictures in the colon have been reported primarily in cystic fibrosis patients with the use of enzyme supplements, generally at dosages above the recommended range. Some cases required surgery, including resection of the bowel. If symptoms suggestive of GI obstruction occur, consider the possibility of bowel strictures.

➤*Treatment failure:* Treatment failures have been reported in cystic fibrosis patients when brand name products were replaced by a generic substitution. Use care and monitor closely when switching patients from one product to another.

➤*Replacement therapy:* Pancreatic exocrine replacement therapy should not delay or supplant treatment of the primary disorder.

➤*Pregnancy:* *Category B* (*Pancrease, Pancrease MT*). Reproduction studies have been conducted in rats and rabbits at doses 0.44 and 0.35 times the maximum daily human dose, respectively, and have revealed no evidence of impaired fertility or harm to the fetus caused by *Pancrease MT*. However, there are no adequate and well-controlled studies in pregnant women. Use during pregnancy only if clearly needed.

Category C (*Creon, Ku-Zyme, Ku-Zyme HP, Kutrase, Lipram, Pancrelipase, Panokase, Plaretase, Ultrase, Ultrase MT, Viokase*). It is not known whether the drug can cause fetal harm when administered to a pregnant woman or can affect reproduction capacity. Give to a pregnant woman only if clearly needed. The enteric coating component, diethyl phthalate, has been teratogenic in rats with high intraperitoneal dosing.

➤*Lactation:* It is not known whether pancreatin is excreted in breast milk. Exercise caution when administering to a nursing mother.

➤*Children:* Colonic strictures, particularly in children with cystic fibrosis, have been associated with doses generally above the recommended dosing range (see Warnings). Patients currently receiving doses above 2,500 lipase units/kg/meal or 4,000 lipase units/g fat/day should be re-evaluated and the dosage either immediately decreased or titrated downward to the lowest effective clinical dose as assessed by 3-day fecal fat excretion.

Precautions

➤*Excessive doses:* Excessive doses may cause nausea, abdominal cramps, or diarrhea. Extremely high doses have been associated with hyperuricosuria and hyperuricemia.

➤*Pork sensitivity:* Use pork products with caution in patients sensitive to pork. Discontinue use if symptoms of sensitivity appear and initiate symptomatic and supportive treatment if necessary. Individuals previously sensitized to trypsin, pancreatin, or pancrelipase may have allergic reactions.

➤*Irritation of skin/mucous membranes:* Do not spill powder on hands because it may irritate skin. The dust of finely powdered concentrates irritates the nasal mucosa and the respiratory tract. Inhalation of airborne powder can precipitate an asthma attack. Asthma also can occur in patients sensitized to pancreatic enzyme concentrates.

Drug Interactions

Digestive Enzymes Drug Interactions

Precipitant drug	Object drug*		Description
Antacids	Digestive enzymes	⬇	Calcium carbonate or magnesium hydroxide may negate the beneficial effect of the enzymes.
Digestive enzymes	Folic acid	⬇	Impaired folic acid absorption by oral pancreatic enzymes may lead to folic acid deficiency.
Digestive enzymes	Iron	⬇	The serum iron response to oral iron may be decreased by concomitant pancreatic extracts.

* ⬇ = Object drug decreased.

Adverse Reactions

The most frequently reported adverse reactions are GI in nature. Less frequently, allergic-type reactions also have been observed. Other adverse reactions reported include the following: Colonic structures; diarrhea; abdominal pain; intestinal obstruction; vomiting; intestinal stenosis; constipation; dermatitis; flatulence; nausea; melena; weight decrease; pain; bloating; cramping. Perianal irritation and, rarely, inflammation with large doses may occur with pancreatin. Extremely high doses have been associated with hyperuricemia and hyperuricosuria.

Overdosage

Overdosage may cause diarrhea or transient intestinal upset. No acute toxic reactions have been reported.

Patient Information

Take before or with meals. Take with plenty of fluids.

Do not inhale powder dosage form or powder from capsules because it may irritate skin or mucous membranes.

To protect enteric coating, do not crush or chew the microspheres/tablets in the enteric-coated capsule formulations.

Do not switch products without consulting your physician.

URSODIOL (Ursodeoxycholic acid)

Rx	**Ursodiol** (Watson)	**Capsules:** 300 mg	(Watson 3159). White. In 100s.
Rx	**Actigall** (Watson)		(ACTIGALL 300 mg). White and pink. In 100s.
Rx	**URSO 250** (Axcan Pharma)	**Tablets:** 250 mg	(URS785). Elliptical, white. Film-coated. In 100s and 500s.
Rx	**URSO Forte** (Axcan Pharma)	**Tablets:** 500 mg	(URS790). Elliptical, white. Film-coated. In 100s and 500s.

URSODIOL — ORAL

Indications

➤*Capsules:* For patients with radiolucent, noncalcified gallbladder stones less than 20 mm in greatest diameter in whom elective cholecystectomy would be undertaken except for the presence of increased surgical risk caused by systemic disease, advanced age, idiosyncratic reaction to general anesthesia, or for those patients who refuse surgery. Safety for use of ursodiol beyond 24 months is not established.

For the prevention of gallstone formation in obese patients experiencing rapid weight loss.

➤*Tablets:* For the treatment of patients with primary biliary cirrhosis (PBC).

Administration and Dosage

➤*Approved by the FDA:* December 31, 1987.

➤*Capsules:*

Gallstone dissolution – The recommended dose for ursodiol capsule treatment of radiolucent gallbladder stones is 8 to 10 mg/kg/day given in 2 or 3 divided doses.

Obtain ultrasound images of the gallbladder at 6-month intervals for the first year of ursodiol therapy to monitor gallstone response. If gallstones appear to have dissolved, continue ursodiol therapy and confirm dissolution on a repeat ultrasound examination within 1 to 3 months. Most patients who eventually achieve complete stone dissolution will show partial or complete dissolution at the first on-treatment reevaluation. If partial stone dissolution is not seen by 12 months of ursodiol therapy, the likelihood of success is greatly reduced.

Gallstone prevention – The recommended dosage of ursodiol capsules for gallstone prevention in patients undergoing rapid weight loss is 600 mg/day (300 mg twice daily).

➤*Tablets:* The recommended adult dosage for ursodiol tablets in the treatment of PBC is 13 to 15 mg/kg/day administered in 2 to 4 divided doses with food. Adjust dosing regimen according to each patient's need at the discretion of the health care provider.

➤*Storage/Stability:*

Capsules – Store at 25°C (77°F); excursions permitted to 15° to 30°C (59° to 86°F). Dispense in a tight container.

Tablets – Store at 20°C to 25°C (68° to 77°F). Dispense in a tight container.

Actions

➤*Pharmacology:* Ursodiol is normally present as a minor fraction of the total bile acids in humans (5%).

Ursodiol suppresses hepatic synthesis and secretion of cholesterol and also inhibits intestinal absorption of cholesterol. It appears to have little inhibitory effect on synthesis and secretion into bile of endogenous bile acids and does not appear to affect secretion of phospholipids into bile.

Although insoluble in aqueous media, cholesterol can be solubilized in at least 2 different ways in the presence of dihydroxy bile acids. In addition to solubilizing cholesterol in micelles, ursodiol acts by an apparently unique mechanism to cause dispersion of cholesterol as liquid crystals in aqueous media. Thus, even though administration of high doses (eg, 15 to 18 mg/kg/day) does not result in a concentration of ursodiol higher than 60% of the total bile acid pool, ursodiol-rich bile effectively solubilizes cholesterol. The overall effect of ursodiol is to increase the concentration level at which saturation of cholesterol occurs.

The various actions of ursodiol combine to change the bile of patients with gallstones from cholesterol-precipitating to cholesterol-solubilizing, thus resulting in bile conducive to cholesterol stone dissolution.

➤*Pharmacokinetics:*

Absorption/Distribution –

Capsules: About 90% of a therapeutic dose of ursodiol is absorbed in the small bowel after oral administration. After absorption, ursodiol enters the portal vein and undergoes efficient extraction from portal blood by the liver (there is a large "first-pass" effect) where it is conjugated with either glycine or taurine and is then secreted into the hepatic bile ducts. Ursodiol in bile is concentrated in the gallbladder and expelled into the duodenum in gallbladder bile via the cystic and common ducts by gallbladder contractions provoked by physiologic responses to eating. Only small quantities of ursodiol appear in the systemic circulation and very small amounts are excreted into urine. The sites of the drug's therapeutic actions are in the liver, bile, and gut lumen. With repeated dosing, bile ursodeoxycholic acid concentrations reach steady state in about 3 weeks.

After ursodiol dosing is stopped, the concentration of the bile acid in bile falls exponentially, declining to about 5% to 10% of its steady-state level in about 1 week.

Tablets: Following oral administration, the majority of ursodiol is absorbed by passive diffusion and its absorption is incomplete. Once absorbed, ursodiol undergoes hepatic extraction to the extent of about 50% in the absence of liver disease. As the severity of liver disease increases, the extent of extraction decreases. In the liver, ursodiol is conjugated with glycine or taurine, then secreted into bile. These conjugates of ursodiol are absorbed in the small intestine by passive and active mechanisms. The conjugates also can be deconjugated in the ileum by intestinal enzymes, leading to the formation of free ursodiol that can be reabsorbed and reconjugated in the liver.

In healthy subjects, at least 70% of ursodiol (unconjugated) is bound to plasma protein. No information is available on the binding of conjugated ursodiol to plasma protein in healthy subjects or PBC patients. Its volume of distribution has not been determined, but is expected to be small because the drug is mostly distributed in the bile and small intestine.

Metabolism/Excretion –

Capsules: Beyond conjugation, ursodiol is not altered or catabolized appreciably by the liver or intestinal mucosa. A small proportion of orally administered drug undergoes bacterial degradation with each cycle of enterohepatic circulation. Ursodiol can be both oxidized and reduced at the 7-carbon, yielding either 7-keto-lithocholic acid or lithocholic acid, respectively. Further, there is some bacterially catalyzed deconjugation of glyco- and tauro-ursodeoxycholic acid in the small bowel. Free ursodiol, 7-keto-lithocholic acid, and lithocholic acid are relatively insoluble in aqueous media and larger proportions of these compounds are lost from the distal gut into the feces. Reabsorbed free ursodiol is reconjugated by the liver. Eighty percent (80%) of lithocholic acid formed in the small bowel is excreted in the feces, but the 20% that is absorbed is sulfated at the 3-hydroxyl group in the liver to relatively insoluble lithocholyl conjugates that are excreted into bile and lost in feces. Absorbed 7-keto-lithocholic acid is stereospecifically reduced in the liver to chenodiol.

Lithocholic acid, when administered chronically to animals, causes cholestatic liver injury and can cause death from liver failure in certain species unable to form sulfate conjugates. Lithocholic acid is formed by 7-dehydroxylation of the dihydroxy bile acids (ursodiol and chenodiol) in the gut lumen. The 7-dehydroxylation reaction appears to be alpha-specific (chenodiol is more efficiently 7-dehydroxylated than ursodiol) and, for equimolar doses of ursodiol and chenodiol, levels of lithocholic acid appearing in bile are lower with the former. Humans and chimpanzees can sulfate lithocholic acid. Although liver injury has not been associated with ursodiol therapy, a reduced capacity to sulfate may exist in some individuals. Nonetheless, such a deficiency has not yet been clearly demonstrated and must be extremely rare, given the several thousand patient-years of clinical experience with ursodiol.

Tablets: Nonabsorbed ursodiol passes into the colon where it is mostly 7-dehydroxylated to lithocholic acid. Some ursodiol is epimerized to chenodiol (CDCA) via a 7-oxa intermediate. Chenodiol also undergoes 7-dehydroxylation to lithocholic acid. These metabolites are poorly soluble and excreted in the feces. A small portion of lithocholic acid is reabsorbed, conjugated in the liver with glycine or taurine, and sulfated at the 3 position. The resulting sulfated lithocholic acid conjugates are excreted in bile and then lost in feces.

Ursodiol is excreted primarily in the feces. With treatment, urinary excretion increases, but remains lower than 1% except in severe cholestatic liver disease.

During chronic administration of ursodiol, it becomes a major biliary and plasma bile acid. At a chronic dose of 13 to 15 mg/kg/day, ursodiol constitutes 30% to 50% of biliary and plasma bile acids.

Contraindications

Hypersensitivity or intolerance to ursodiol or any of the components of the formulations.

Ursodiol will not dissolve calcified cholesterol stones, radiopaque stones, or radiolucent bile pigment stones. Hence, patients with such stones are not candidates for ursodiol therapy.

Patients with compelling reasons for cholecystectomy including unremitting acute cholecystitis, cholangitis, biliary obstruction, gallstone pancreatitis, or biliary-GI fistula are not candidates for ursodiol therapy.

Allergy to bile acids.

Warnings

➤*Carcinogenesis:*

Capsules: Ursodeoxycholic acid was tested in 2-year oral carcinogenicity studies in CD-1 mice and Sprague-Dawley rats at daily doses of 50, 250, and 1,000 mg/kg/day. It was not tumorigenic in mice. In the rat study, it produced statistically significant dose-related increased incidences of pheochromocytomas of adrenal medulla in males (P = 0.014, Peto trend test) and females (P = 0.004, Peto trend test). A 78-week rat study employing intrarectal instillation of lithocholic acid and tauro-deoxycholic acid, metabolites of ursodiol and chenodiol, has been conducted. These bile acids alone did not produce any tumors. A tumor-promoting effect of both metabolites was observed when they were coadministered with a carcinogenic agent. Results of epidemiologic studies suggest that bile acids might be involved in the pathogenesis of human colon cancer in patients who had undergone a cholecystectomy, but direct evidence is lacking.

Tablets: In a life-span (126 to 138 weeks) oral carcinogenicity study, Sprague-Dawley rats were treated with doses of 33 to 300 mg/kg/day (0.4 to 3.2 times the recommended maximum human dose based on body surface area). Ursodiol produced a significantly (P less than 0.5, Fisher's exact test) increased incidence of pheochromocytomas of the adrenal medulla in females of the highest dose group.

In a 103-week oral carcinogenicity study of lithocholic acid, a metabolite of ursodiol, doses up to 250 mg/kg/day in mice and 500 mg/kg/day in rats did not produce any tumors. In a 78-week rat study, intrarectal instillation of lithocholic acid (1 mg/kg/day) for 13 months did not produce colorectal tumors. A tumor-promoting effect was observed when it was administered after a single intrarectal dose of a known carcinogen N-methyl-N'-nitro-N-nitrosoguanidine. On the other hand, in a 32-week rat study, ursodiol at a daily dose of 240 mg/kg (1,440 mg/m^2, 2.6 times the maximum recommended human dose based on body surface area) suppressed the colonic carcinogenic effect of another known carcinogen azoxymethane.

➤*Mutagenesis:*
Capsules: Ursodiol is not mutagenic in the Ames test. Dietary administration of lithocholic acid to chickens is reported to cause hepatic adenomatous hyperplasia.

➤*Fertility impairment:*
Capsules: Studies employing 100- to 200-fold the human dose in rats have shown some reduction in fertility rate and litter size.

➤*Elderly:*
Capsules – Small differences in efficacy and greater sensitivity of some elderly individuals taking ursodiol cannot be ruled out. Therefore, it is recommended that dosing proceed with caution in this population.

➤*Pregnancy: Category B.*

There have been no adequate and well-controlled studies of the use of ursodiol in pregnant women, but inadvertent exposure of 4 women to therapeutic doses of the drug in the first trimester of pregnancy during the ursodiol trials led to no evidence of effects on the fetus or newborn baby. Although it seems unlikely, the possibility that ursodiol can cause fetal harm cannot be ruled out; hence, the drug is not recommended for use during pregnancy.

➤*Lactation:* It is not known whether ursodiol is excreted in human milk. Because many drugs are excreted in human milk, exercise caution when ursodiol is administered to a breastfeeding mother.

➤*Children:* The safety and effectiveness of ursodiol in pediatric patients have not been established.

Precautions

➤*Monitoring:* Abnormalities in liver enzymes have not been associated with ursodiol therapy and, in fact, ursodiol has been shown to decrease liver enzyme levels in liver disease. However, patients given ursodiol should have AST and ALT measured at the initiation of therapy and thereafter as indicated by the particular clinical circumstances.

Patients with variceal bleeding, hepatic encephalopathy, ascites, or in need of an urgent liver transplant should receive appropriate specific treatment.

Hepatic effects – Ursodiol therapy has not been associated with liver damage. Lithocholic acid, a naturally occurring bile acid, is known to be a liver-toxic metabolite. This bile acid is formed in the gut from ursodiol less efficiently and in smaller amounts than that seen from chenodiol. Lithocholic acid is detoxified in the liver by sulfation and, although man appears to be an efficient sulfater, it is possible that some patients may have a congenital or acquired deficiency in sulfation, thereby predisposing them to lithocholate-induced liver damage.

Drug Interactions

Ursodiol Drug Interactions

Precipitant drug	Object drug[a]		Description
Antacids	Ursodiol	⬇	Aluminum-based antacids adsorb bile acids in vitro and interfere with the action of ursodiol by reducing its absorption.
Bile acid sequestrants	Ursodiol	⬇	Cholestyramine and colestipol may interfere with the action of ursodiol by reducing its absorption.
Clofibrate Estrogens Oral Contraceptives	Ursodiol	⬇	These agents (and perhaps other lipid-lowering drugs) increase hepatic cholesterol secretion, and encourage cholesterol gallstone formation and hence may counteract the effectiveness of ursodiol.

[a] ⬇ = Object drug decreased.

Adverse Reactions

➤*Capsules:*

Gallstone dissolution (≥ 5%)				
	Ursodiol 8 to 10 mg/kg/day (n = 155)		Placebo (n = 159)	
Adverse reaction	n	%	n	%
CNS				
Fatigue	7	4.5%	8	5%
Headache	28	18.1%	34	21.4%
Insomnia	3	1.9%	8	5%
GI				
Abdominal pain	67	43.2%	70	44%
Cholecystitis	8	5.2%	7	4.4%
Constipation	15	9.7%	14	8.8%
Diarrhea	42	27.1%	34	21.4%
Dyspepsia	26	16.8%	18	11.3%
Flatulence	12	7.7%	12	7.5%
GI disorder	6	3.9%	8	5%
Nausea	22	14.2%	27	17%
Vomiting	15	9.7%	11	6.9%
GU				
Urinary tract infection	10	6.5%	7	4.4%
Musculoskeletal				
Arthralgia	12	7.7%	24	15.1%
Arthritis	9	5.8%	4	2.5%
Back pain	11	7.1%	18	11.3%
Myalgia	9	5.8%	9	5.7%
Respiratory				
Bronchitis	10	6.5%	6	3.8%
Coughing	11	7.1%	7	4.4%
Pharyngitis	13	8.4%	5	3.1%
Rhinitis	8	5.2%	11	6.9%
Sinusitis	17	11%	18	11.3%
Upper respiratory tract infection	24	15.5%	21	13.2%
Miscellaneous				
Allergy	8	5.2%	7	4.4%
Chest pain	5	3.2%	10	6.3%
Infection, viral	30	19.4%	41	25.8%

Gallstone prevention				
	Ursodiol 600 mg (n = 322)		Placebo (n = 325)	
Adverse reaction	n	%	n	%
CNS				
Dizziness	53	16.5%	42	12.9%
Fatigue	25	7.8%	33	10.2%
Headache	80	24.8%	78	24%
Dermatologic				
Alopecia	17	5.3%	8	2.5%
GI				
Abdominal pain	20	6.2%	39	12%
Constipation	85	26.4%	72	22.2%
Diarrhea	81	25.2%	68	20.9%
Flatulence	15	4.7%	24	7.4%
Nausea	56	17.4%	43	13.2%
Vomiting	44	13.7%	44	13.5%
GU				
Dysmenorrhea	18	5.6%	19	5.8%
Musculoskeletal				
Back pain	38	11.8%	21	6.5%
Musculoskeletal pain	19	5.9%	15	4.6%
Respiratory				
Pharyngitis	10	3.1%	19	5.8%
Sinusitis	17	5.3%	18	5.5%
Upper respiratory tract infection	40	12.4%	35	10.8%
Miscellaneous				
Infection viral	29	9%	29	8.9%
Influenza-like symptoms	21	6.5%	19	5.8%

➤*Tablets:* The following table summarizes the adverse reactions observed in the 2 placebo-controlled clinical trials.

	Visit at 12 months		Visit at 24 months	
	UDCA[b]	Placebo	UDCA[b]	Placebo
Adverse reactions[a]	n (%)	n (%)	n (%)	n (%)
Diarrhea	-	-	1 (1.32%)	-
Elevated creatinine	-	-	1 (1.32%)	-
Elevated blood glucose	1 (1.18%)	-	1 (1.32%)	-
Leukopenia	-	-	2 (2.63%)	-
Peptic ulcer	-	-	1 (1.32%)	-
Skin rash	-	-	2 (2.63%)	-

[a] Those adverse reactions occurring at the same or higher incidence in the placebo group as in the UDCA group have been deleted from this table (this includes diarrhea and thrombocytopenia at 12 months, nausea/vomiting, fever, and other toxicity).
[b] UDCA = Ursodeoxycholic acid = ursodiol.

URSODIOL — ORAL

In a randomized, crossover study in 60 PBC patients, 4 patients (6.7%) experienced 1 serious adverse reaction each (diabetes mellitus, cyst, and breast neoplasm [experienced by 2 patients]). No deaths occurred in the study. Forty-three patients (71.7%) experienced at least 1 treatment-emergent adverse reaction (TEAE) during the study. The most common (greater than 5%) TEAEs were asthenia (11.7%), dyspepsia (10%), peripheral edema (8.3%), hypertension (8.3%), nausea (8.3%), GI disorders, chest pain, and pruritus (5%). Seven patients (11.6%) reported 9 events that were judged as possibly or probably related to study medication. These 9 TEAEs included abdominal pain and asthenia (1 patient), nausea (3 patients), dyspepsia (2 patients) and anorexia and esophagitis (1 patient each). One patient on the twice-daily regimen (total dose 1,000 mg) withdrew due to nausea. All of these 9 TEAEs except esophagitis were observed with the twice-daily regimen at a total daily dose of 1,000 mg or greater.

Overdosage

➤*Symptoms:* Neither accidental nor intentional overdosage with ursodiol has been reported. Doses of ursodiol in the range of 16 to 20 mg/kg/day have been tolerated by 7 patients for 6 to 37 months without symptoms. The LD_{50} for ursodiol in rats is over 5,000 mg/kg given over 7 to 10 days and over 7,500 mg/kg for mice.

Single oral doses of ursodiol at 10, 5, and 10 g/kg in mice, rats, and dogs, respectively, were not lethal. A single oral dose of ursodiol at 1.5 g/kg was lethal in hamsters. Symptoms of acute toxicity were salivation and vomiting in dogs, and ataxia, dyspnea, ptosis, agonal convulsions, and coma in hamsters.

➤*Treatment:* The most likely manifestation of severe overdose with ursodiol would likely be diarrhea, which should be treated symptomatically.

MOUTH AND THROAT PRODUCTS

NYSTATIN

For prescribing information, see the Nystatin monograph in the Antifungal Agents section of the Anti-Infective Agents chapter.

CLOTRIMAZOLE

Rx	**Clotrimazole** (Various, eg, Roxane)	**Troches:** 10 mg	In 70s, 140s, 500s, and UD 70s.
Rx	**Mycelex** (Bayer)		(MYCELEX 10). White. In 70s and 140s.

CLOTRIMAZOLE — ORAL

For information on topical and vaginal clotrimazole, refer to individual monographs.

Indications

➤*Treatment of oropharyngeal candidiasis:* For the local treatment of oropharyngeal candidiasis. The diagnosis should be confirmed by a KOH smear or culture prior to treatment.

➤*Prophylaxis of oropharyngeal candidiasis:* Prophylactically to reduce the incidence of oropharyngeal candidiasis in patients immunocompromised by conditions that include chemotherapy, radiotherapy, or steroid therapy utilized in the treatment of leukemia, solid tumors, or renal transplantation. There are no data from adequate and well-controlled trials to establish the safety and efficacy of this product for prophylactic use in patients immunocompromised by etiologies other than those listed in the previous sentence.

Administration and Dosage

➤*Approved by the FDA:* June 17, 1983.

Clotrimazole troches are administered only as a lozenge that must be slowly dissolved in the mouth. The recommended dose is 1 troche 5 times a day for 14 consecutive days. Only limited data are available on the safety and effectiveness of the clotrimazole troche after prolonged administration; therefore, therapy should be limited to short term use, if possible.

For prophylaxis to reduce the incidence of oropharyngeal candidiasis in patients immunocompromised by conditions that include chemotherapy, radiotherapy, or steroid therapy utilized in the treatment of leukemia, solid tumors, or renal transplantation, the recommended dose is one troche three times daily for the duration of chemotherapy or until steroids are reduced to maintenance levels.

➤*Storage/Stability:* Store below 30°C (86°F). Avoid freezing.

Actions

➤*Pharmacology:* Clotrimazole is a broad-spectrum antifungal agent that inhibits the growth of pathogenic yeasts by altering the permeability of cell membranes. The action of clotrimazole is fungistatic at concentrations of drug up to 20 mcg/mL and may be fungicidal in vitro against *Candida albicans* and other species of the genus *Candida* at higher concentrations. No single-step or multiple-step resistance to clotrimazole has developed during successive passages of *Candida albicans* in the laboratory; however, individual organism tolerance has been observed during successive passages in the laboratory. Such in vitro tolerance has resolved once the organism has been removed from the antifungal environment.

After oral administration of a 10 mg clotrimazole troche to healthy volunteers, concentrations sufficient to inhibit most species of *Candida* persist in saliva for up to three hours following the ≈ 30 minutes needed for a troche to dissolve. The long term persistence of drug in saliva appears to be related to the slow release of clotrimazole from the oral mucosa to which the drug is apparently bound. Repetitive dosing at three hour intervals maintains salivary levels above the minimum inhibitory concentrations of most strains of *Candida*; however, the relationship between in vitro susceptibility of pathogenic fungi to clotrimazole and prophylaxis or cure of infections in humans has not been established.

In another study, the mean serum concentrations were 4.98 ± 3.7 and 3.23 ± 1.4 nanograms/mL of clotrimazole at 30 and 60 minutes, respectively, after administration as a troche.

Contraindications

Hypersensitivity to clotrimazole or any of its components.

Warnings

➤*Systemic mycoses:* Clotrimazole troches are not indicated for the treatment of systemic mycoses including systemic candidiasis.

➤*Pregnancy: Category C.* Clotrimazole has been shown to be embryotoxic in rats and mice when given in doses 100 times the adult human dose (in mg/kg), possibly secondary to maternal toxicity. The drug was not teratogenic in mice, rabbits, and rats when given in doses up to 200, 180, and 100 times the human dose.

Clotrimazole given orally to mice from nine weeks before mating through weaning at a dose 120 times the human dose was associated with impairment of mating, decreased number of viable young, and decreased survival to weaning. No effects were observed at 60 times the human dose. When the drug was given to rats during a similar time period at 50 times the human dose, there was a slight decrease in the number of pups per litter and decreased pup viability.

There are no adequate and well controlled studies in pregnant women. Clotrimazole troches should be used during pregnancy only if the potential benefit justifies the potential risk to the fetus.

➤*Children:* Safety and effectiveness of clotrimazole in children below the age of 3 years have not been established; therefore, its use in such patients is not recommended.

The safety and efficacy of the prophylactic use of clotrimazole troches in children have not been established.

Precautions

➤*Monitoring:* Abnormal liver function tests have been reported in patients treated with clotrimazole troches; elevated SGOT levels were reported in about 15% of patients in the clinical trials. In most cases the elevations were minimal and it was often impossible to distinguish effects of clotrimazole from those of other therapy and the underlying disease (malignancy in most cases). Periodic assessment of hepatic function is advisable particularly in patients with preexisting hepatic impairment.

Since patients must be instructed to allow each troche to dissolve slowly in the mouth in order to achieve maximum effect of the medication, they must be of such an age and physical or mental condition to comprehend such instructions.

Adverse Reactions

Abnormal liver function tests have been reported in patients treated with clotrimazole troches; elevated SGOT levels were reported in about 15% of patients in the clinical trials.

Nausea, vomiting, unpleasant mouth sensations and pruritus have also been reported with the use of the troche.

CHLORHEXIDINE GLUCONATE

Rx	**PerioChip** (Astra)	**Chip:** 2.5 mg	Glycerin, hydrolyzed gelatin. Orange-brown, rectangular (rounded at 1 end). In 10s.
Rx	**Chlorhexidine Gluconate** (Xttrium)	**Oral Rinse:** 0.12%	In 473 mL.[a]
Rx	**Peridex** (Procter & Gamble)		In 480 mL.[a]
Rx	**PerioGard** (Colgate Oral)		In 473 mL with 15 mL dose cup.[a]

[a] With 11.6% alcohol, saccharin.

CHLORHEXIDINE GLUCONATE — ORAL

Indications

➤*Chip:* As an adjunct to scaling and root planing procedures for reduction of pocket depth in patients with adult periodontitis. Chlorhexidine gluconate chip may be used as a part of a periodontal maintenance program, which includes good oral hygiene and scaling and root planing.

➤*Rinse:* For use between dental visits as part of a professional program for the treatment of gingivitis as characterized by redness and swelling of the gingivae, including gingival bleeding upon probing. Chlorhexidine gluconate oral rinse has not been tested among patients with acute necrotizing ulcerative gingivitis (ANUG). For patients having coexisting gingivitis and periodontitis, see Precautions.

Administration and Dosage

➤*Approved by the FDA:* January 14, 1994.

➤*Chip:* One chip is inserted into a periodontal pocket with probing pocket depth (PD) ≥ 5 mm. Up to 8 chlorhexidine gluconate chips may be inserted in a single visit. Treatment is recommended to be administered once every 3 months in pockets with PD remaining ≥ 5 mm.

The periodontal pocket should be isolated and the surrounding area dried prior to chip insertion. The chlorhexidine gluconate chip should be grasped using forceps (such that the rounded end points away from the forceps) and inserted into the periodontal pocket to its maximum depth. If necessary, the chlorhexidine gluconate chip can be further maneuvered into position using the tips of the forceps or a flat instrument. The chlorhexidine gluconate chip does not need to be removed since it biodegrades completely.

In the unlikely event of chlorhexidine gluconate chip dislodgment (in the 2 pivotal clinical trials, only 8 chips were reported lost), several actions are recommended, depending on the day of chlorhexidine gluconate chip loss. If dislodgment occurs ≥ 7 days after placement, the dentist should consider the subject to have received a full course of treatment. If dislodgment occurs within 48 hours after placement, a new chlorhexidine gluconate chip should be inserted. If dislodgment occurs more than 48 hours after placement, the dentist should not replace the chlorhexidine gluconate chip, but reevaluate the patient at 3 months and insert a new chlorhexidine gluconate chip if the pocket depth has not been reduced to less than 5 mm.

➤*Rinse:* Therapy should be initiated directly following a dental prophylaxis. Patients using chlorhexidine gluconate oral rinse should be reevaluated and given a thorough prophylaxis at intervals no longer than 6 months.

Recommended use is twice daily oral rinsing for 30 seconds, morning and evening after toothbrushing. Usual dosage is ½ fl. oz. (marked on dosage cup) of undiluted chlorhexidine gluconate oral rinse. Patients should be instructed not to rinse with water or other mouthwashes, brush teeth, or eat immediately after using the rinse. The rinse is not intended for ingestion and should be expectorated after rinsing.

➤*Storage / Stability:*

Chip – Store in a refrigerator between 2° to 8°C (36° to 46°F).

Rinse – Store above freezing (0°C; 32°F).

Actions

➤*Pharmacology:*

Rinse – Chlorhexidine gluconate oral rinse provides antimicrobial activity during oral rinsing. The clinical significance of 0.12% chlorhexidine gluconate oral rinse's antimicrobial activities is not clear. Microbiological sampling of plaque has shown a general reduction of counts of certain assayed bacteria, both aerobic and anaerobic, ranging from 54% to 97% through 6 months of use.

Use of a chlorhexidine gluconate oral rinse in a 6-month clinical study did not result in any significant changes in bacterial resistance, overgrowth of potentially opportunistic organisms or other adverse changes in the oral microbial ecosystem. Three months after chlorhexidine gluconate use was discontinued, the number of bacteria in plaque had returned to baseline levels and the resistance of plaque bacteria to chlorhexidine gluconate was equal to that at baseline.

➤*Pharmacokinetics:*

Chip – Chlorhexidine gluconate chip releases chlorhexidine in vitro in a biphasic manner, initially releasing ≈ 40% of the chlorhexidine within the first 24 hours and then releasing the remaining chlorhexidine in an almost linear fashion for 7 to 10 days. This enzymatic release rate assay is an experimental collagenase assay that differs from the Regulatory Specification's Agar Release Rate Assay. This release profile may be explained as an initial burst effect, dependent on diffusion of chlorhexidine from the chip, followed by a further release of chlorhexidine as a result of enzymatic degradation.

In an in vivo study of 18 evaluable adult patients, there were no detectable plasma or urine levels of chlorhexidine following the insertion of 4 chlorhexidine gluconate chips under clinical conditions. The concentration of chlorhexidine released from the chlorhexidine gluconate chip was determined in the gingival crevicular fluid (GCF) of these same subjects. In these subjects, a highly variable biphasic release profile for chlorhexidine was demonstrated, with GCF levels 4 hours after chip insertion (mean: 1444 ± 783 mcg/mL), followed by a second peak at 72 hours (mean: 1902 ± 1073 mcg/mL). In a second study involving the insertion of 1 chlorhexidine gluconate chip under clinical conditions, the mean GCF level of chlorhexidine peaked at 1088 ± 678 mcg/mL at 4 hours. The mean GCF levels then declined in a highly erratic fashion to levels of 482 ± 447 mcg/mL at 72 hours without producing a true second peak. The results of these studies confirm a high degree of intersubject variability in chlorhexidine release from the chlorhexidine gluconate chip matrix in vivo that was not seen in vitro. Due to the nature and clinical use of the chlorhexidine gluconate chip dosage form, dose proportionality was not and would not be expected to be demonstrated between the 2 studies.

Rinse – Pharmacokinetic studies with a 0.12% chlorhexidine gluconate oral rinse indicate ≈ 30% of the active ingredient is retained in the oral cavity following rinsing. This retained drug is slowly released into the oral fluids. Studies conducted on human subjects and animals demonstrate chlorhexidine gluconate is poorly absorbed from the GI tract. The mean plasma level of chlorhexidine gluconate reached a peak of 0.206 mcg/g in humans 30 minutes after they ingested a 300 mg dose of the drug. Detectable levels of chlorhexidine gluconate were not present in the plasma of these subjects 12 hours after the compound was administered. Excretion of chlorhexidine gluconate occurred primarily through the feces (≈ 90%). Less than 1% of the chlorhexidine gluconate ingested by these subjects was excreted in the urine.

➤*Microbiology:* Chlorhexidine gluconate is active against a broad spectrum of microbes. The chlorhexidine molecule, due to its positive charge, reacts with the microbial cell surface, destroys the integrity of the cell membrane, penetrates into the cell, precipitates the cytoplasm, and the cell dies. Studies with chlorhexidine gluconate chip showed reductions in the numbers of the putative periodontopathic organisms *Porphyromonas (Bacteriodes) gingivalis*, *Prevotella (Bacteriodes) intermedia*, *Bacteriodes forsythus*, and *Campylobacter rectus* (*Wolinella recta*) after placement of the chip. No overgrowth of opportunistic organisms or other adverse changes in the oral microbial ecosystem were noted. The relationship of the microbial findings to clinical outcome has not been established.

Contraindications

Hypersensitivity to chlorhexidine gluconate or other formula ingredients.

Warnings

➤*Calculus deposits:* The effect of chlorhexidine gluconate oral rinse on periodontitis has not been determined. An increase in supragingival calculus was noted in clinical testing with users of chlorhexidine gluconate oral rinse compared with control users. It is not known if chlorhexidine gluconate use results in an increase in subgingival calculus. Calculus deposits should be removed by a dental prophylaxis at intervals not greater than 6 months. Hypersensitivity and generalized allergic reactions have occurred (see Contraindications).

➤*Pregnancy:*

Chip – *Category C.*

While chlorhexidine is known to be very poorly absorbed from the GI tract, it may be absorbed following placement within a periodontal pocket. Therefore, it is unclear whether these data are relevant to clinical use of chlorhexidine gluconate chip. In clinical studies, placement of 4 chlorhexidine gluconate chips within periodontal pockets resulted in plasma concentrations of chlorhexidine that were at or below the limit of detection. However, it is not known whether chlorhexidine gluconate chip can cause fetal harm when administered to a pregnant woman or can affect reproductive capacity. Chlorhexidine gluconate chip should be used in a pregnant woman only if clearly needed.

Rinse – *Category B.*

Adequate and well-controlled studies in pregnant women have not been done. Because animal reproduction studies are not always predictive of human response, this drug should be used during pregnancy only if clearly needed.

➤*Lactation:* It is not known whether this drug is excreted in human milk. Because many drugs are excreted in human milk, caution should be exercised when chlorhexidine gluconate is administered to a nursing woman.

➤*Children:* Clinical safety and efficacy of chlorhexidine gluconate oral rinse have not been established in children younger than 18 years of age.

Precautions

➤*Abscessed periodontal pocket:* The use of chlorhexidine gluconate chip in an acutely abscessed periodontal pocket has not been studied and therefore is not recommended. Management of patients with periodontal disease should include consideration of potentially contributing medical disorders, such as cancer, diabetes, and immunocompromised status.

➤*Gingivitis and periodontitis:* For patients having coexisting gingivitis and periodontitis, the presence or absence of gingival inflammation following treatment with chlorhexidine gluconate oral rinse should not be used as a major indicator of underlying periodontitis.

➤*Staining:* Chlorhexidine gluconate oral rinse can cause staining of oral surfaces, such as tooth surfaces, restorations, and the dorsum of the tongue. Not all patients will experience a visually significant increase in tooth staining. In clinical testing, 56% of the chlorhexidine gluconate oral rinse users exhibited a measurable increase in facial anterior stain, compared to 35% of control users after 6 months; 15% of the chlorhexidine gluconate users developed what was judged to be heavy stain, compared to 1% of control users after 6 months. Stain will be more pronounced in patients who have heavier accumulations of unremoved plaque.

Stain resulting from the use of chlorhexidine gluconate oral rinse does not adversely affect health of the gingivae or other oral tissues. Stain can be removed from most tooth surfaces by conventional professional prophylactic techniques. Additional time may be required to complete the prophylaxis.

Discretion should be used when prescribing to patients with anterior facial restorations with rough surfaces or margins. If natural stain cannot be removed from these surfaces by a dental prophylaxis, patients should be excluded from chlorhexidine gluconate oral rinse treatment if permanent

CHLORHEXIDINE GLUCONATE — ORAL

discoloration is unacceptable. Stain in these areas may be difficult to remove by dental prophylaxis and on rare occasions may necessitate replacement of these restorations.

➤*Taste perception alteration:* Some patients may experience an alteration in taste perception while undergoing treatment with a chlorhexidine gluconate oral rinse. Rare instances of permanent taste alteration following chlorhexidine gluconate oral rinse use have been reported via postmarketing surveillance.

Adverse Reactions

➤*Chip:* The most frequently observed adverse events in the 2 pivotal clinical trials were toothache, upper respiratory tract infection, and headache. Toothache was the only adverse reaction that was significantly higher (P = 0.042) in the chlorhexidine gluconate chip group when compared to placebo. Most oral pain or sensitivity occurred within the first week of the initial chip placement following SRP procedures, was mild to moderate in nature, and spontaneously resolved within days. These reactions were observed less frequently with subsequent chip placement at 3 and 6 months.

Adverse events (frequency ≥ 1% for the chlorhexidine gluconate group) reported from 2 five-center US clinical trials

	Chlorhexidine gluconate chip (n = 225)		Placebo chip (n = 222)	
Adverse reaction	n	%	n	%
All patients with adverse events	193	85.8%	189	85.1%
Toothache*	114	50.7%	92	41.4%
Upper respiratory tract infection	64	28.4%	58	26.1%
Headache	61	27.1%	61	27.5%
Sinusitis	31	13.8%	29	13.1%
Influenza-like symptoms	17	7.6%	21	9.5%
Back pain	15	6.7%	25	11.3%
Tooth disorder**	14	6.2%	15	6.8%
Bronchitis	14	6.2%	7	3.2%
Abscess	13	5.8%	13	5.9%
Pain	11	4.9%	11	5%
Allergy	9	4%	13	5.9%
Myalgia	9	4%	9	4.1%
Gum hyperplasia	8	3.6%	5	2.3%
Pharyngitis	8	3.6%	5	2.3%
Arthralgia	7	3.1%	13	5.9%
Dysmenorrhea	7	3.1%	13	5.9%
Dyspepsia	7	3.1%	6	2.7%
Rhinitis	6	2.7%	11	5%
Coughing	6	2.7%	7	3.2%
Arthrosis	6	2.7%	4	1.8%
Hypertension	5	2.2%	6	2.7%
Stomatitis ulcerative	5	2.2%	1	0.5%
Tendinitis	5	2.2%	1	0.5%

* Includes dental, gingival or mouth pain, tenderness, aching, throbbing, soreness, and discomfort or sensitivity.
** Includes broken, cracked or fractured teeth, mobile teeth, and lost bridges, crowns, or fillings.

➤*Rinse:* The most common side effects associated with chlorhexidine gluconate oral rinses are an increase in staining of teeth and other oral surfaces, an increase in calculus formation, and an alteration in taste perception (see Precautions). Oral irritation and local allergy-type symptoms have been spontaneously reported as side effects associated with use of chlorhexidine gluconate rinse. The following oral mucosal side effects were reported during placebo-controlled adult clinical trials: Aphthous ulcer, grossly obvious gingivitis, trauma, ulceration, erythema, desquamation, coated tongue, keratinization, geographic tongue, mucocele, and short frenum. Each occurred at a frequency of less than 1%.

Among postmarketing reports, the most frequently reported oral mucosal symptoms associated with chlorhexidine gluconate oral rinse are stomatitis, gingivitis, glossitis, ulcer, dry mouth, hypesthesia, glossal edema, and paresthesia.

Minor irritation and superficial desquamation of the oral mucosa have been noted in patients using chlorhexidine gluconate oral rinses.

There have been cases of parotid gland swelling and inflammation of the salivary glands (sialadentitis) reported in patients using chlorhexidine gluconate oral rinse.

Overdosage

Ingestion of 1 or 2 ounces of chlorhexidine gluconate oral rinse by a small child (≈ 10 kg body weight) might result in gastric distress, including nausea, or signs of alcohol intoxication. Medical attention should be sought if more than 4 ounces of chlorhexidine gluconate oral rinse is ingested by a small child or if signs of alcohol intoxication develop.

Patient Information

Patients should avoid dental floss at the site of chlorhexidine gluconate chip insertion for 10 days after placement, because flossing might dislodge the chip. All other oral hygiene may be continued as usual. No restrictions regarding dietary habits are needed. Dislodging of the chlorhexidine gluconate chip is uncommon; however, patients should be instructed to notify the dentist promptly if the chlorhexidine gluconate chip dislodges. Patients should also be advised that, although some mild to moderate sensitivity is normal during the first week after placement of chlorhexidine gluconate chip, they should notify the dentist promptly if pain, swelling, or other problems occur.

CARBAMIDE PEROXIDE (Urea Peroxide)

otc	**Cankaid Liquid** (Dickinson)	**Solution:** 10% in anhydrous glycerol	EDTA. In 22.5 mL.
otc	**Gly-Oxide Liquid** (GlaxoSmithKline)	**Solution:** 10%	In 15 and 60 mL.
otc	**Orajel Perioseptic** (Del)	**Liquid:** 15%	Saccharin, sorbitol, EDTA, methylparaben, ethyl alcohol. In 240 mL.

CARBAMIDE PEROXIDE — ORAL

Indications

➤*Liquid:*

Oral hygiene – For everyday use, to improve oral hygiene as an aid to regular brushing or when regular brushing is inadequate or impossible (eg, total care geriatrics). Carbamide peroxide kills germs to reduce mouth odors and odors on dental appliances. Carbamide peroxide penetrates between teeth and other areas of the mouth to flush out food particles ordinary brushing can miss. Carbamide peroxide also helps remove stains on dental appliances to improve appearance.

Specific dental problems – For temporary (problem) use, carbamide peroxide cleanses canker sores and minor wounds or gum inflammation resulting from minor dental procedures, dentures, orthodontic appliances, accidental injury or other irritations of the mouth and gums. Carbamide peroxide can also be used to guard against the risk of infections in the mouth and gums.

Administration and Dosage

Do not dilute. Replace tip on bottle or tube when not in use.

➤*Liquid:*

Adults and children 2 years of age and older – Apply several drops directly from bottle onto affected area; spit out after 2 to 3 minutes. Use up to 4 times daily after meals and at bedtime or as directed by your dentist or doctor, or place 10 drops on tongue, mix with saliva, swish for several minutes, and then spit out. Supervise use by children younger than 12 years of age.

Children younger than 2 years of age – Consult a dentist or doctor.

➤*For everyday use:* Apply carbamide peroxide to the toothbrush (it will sink into the brush), cover with toothpaste, brush normally, and spit out. Or you may follow the directions above for temporary use.

➤*Storage/Stability:* Protect from excessive heat and direct sunlight.

Actions

➤*Pharmacology:* Carbamide peroxide releases oxygen to help gently remove unhealthy tissue, then cleanse and soothe canker sores and minor wounds and inflammations. It also inhibits odor-forming bacteria.

Warnings

➤*Monitoring:* Severe or persistent oral inflammation, denture irritation, or gingivitis may be serious. If these conditions or unexpected side effects occur, consult a dentist or health care provider immediately. Avoid contact with eyes.

CARBAMIDE PEROXIDE — ORAL

➤*Children:* Do not use for children younger than 2 years of age unless directed by a dentist or health care provider. Supervise children younger than 12 years of age in the use of this product.

Keep out of reach of children. In case of accidental overdose, seek professional assistance or contact poison control immediately.

Patient Information

Severe or persistent oral inflammation, denture irritation, or gingivitis may be serious. If these or unexpected side effects occur, consult health care provider or dentist promptly.

Discontinue use if condition persists or worsens.

PILOCARPINE HYDROCHLORIDE

Rx	**Pilocarpine Hydrochloride** (Various, eg, Purepac, Sandoz)	**Tablets:** 5 mg	In 100s.
Rx	**Salagen** (MGI Pharma)		(MGI 705). White. Film-coated. In 100s.
Rx	**Salagen** (MGI Pharma)	**Tablets:** 7.5 mg	(SAL 7.5). Blue. Film-coated. In 100s.

PILOCARPINE HYDROCHLORIDE — ORAL

For information on the ophthalmic use of pilocarpine, refer to the individual monograph in the Ophthalmics chapter.

Indications

➤*Dry mouth:* Treatment of symptoms of dry mouth from salivary gland hypofunction caused by radiotherapy for cancer of the head and neck; treatment of symptoms of dry mouth in patients with Sjogren's syndrome.

➤*Unlabeled uses:* Relief of dry mouth in patients with graft-versus-host disease (GVHD).

Administration and Dosage

➤*Approved by the FDA:* March 22, 1994.

➤*Head and neck cancer patients:* The recommended dose for the initiation of treatment is 5 mg 3 times/day. Adjust dosage according to therapeutic response and tolerability. The usual dosage range is 3 to 6 tablets or 15 to 30 mg/day (not to exceed 2 tablets/dose). Although early improvement may be realized, at least 12 weeks of uninterrupted therapy may be necessary to assess whether a beneficial response will be achieved. The incidence of the most common adverse events increases with dose. Use the lowest dose that is tolerated and effective for maintenance.

➤*Sjogren's syndrome:* 5 mg 4 times/day. Efficacy was established by 6 weeks of use.

➤*Hepatic function impairment:* The starting dose in patients with moderate hepatic impairment should be 5 mg twice daily, followed by adjustment based on therapeutic response and tolerability. Patients with mild hepatic insufficiency do not require dosage reductions. The use of pilocarpine in patients with severe hepatic insufficiency is not recommended.

➤*Storage/Stability:* Store at controlled room temperature (15° to 30°C; 59° to 86°F).

Actions

➤*Pharmacology:* Pilocarpine is a cholinergic parasympathomimetic agent exerting a broad spectrum of pharmacologic effects with predominant muscarinic action. Pilocarpine in appropriate dosage can increase secretion by the exocrine glands. The sweat, salivary, lacrimal, gastric, pancreatic, intestinal glands, and the mucous cells of the respiratory tract may be stimulated. Dose-related smooth muscle stimulation of the intestinal tract may cause increased tone, increased motility, spasm, and tenesmus. Bronchial smooth muscle tone may increase. The tone and motility of urinary tract, gallbladder, and biliary duct smooth muscle may be enhanced. Pilocarpine may have paradoxical effects on the cardiovascular system. The expected effect of a muscarinic agonist is vasodepression, but administration of pilocarpine may produce hypertension after a brief episode of hypotension. Bradycardia and tachycardia have been reported with use of pilocarpine.

➤*Pharmacokinetics:*

Special populations –

Hepatic function impairment: In patients with mild to moderate hepatic impairment (n = 12), administration of a single 5 mg dose resulted in a 30% decrease in total plasma clearance and a doubling of exposure (as measured by AUC). Peak plasma levels also were increased by about 30% and half-life was increased to 2.1 hours.

Elderly: In 5 healthy elderly female volunteers, the mean C_{max} and AUC were approximately twice that of elderly males and young healthy male volunteers. In a study in 12 healthy male volunteers, there was a dose-related increase in unstimulated salivary flow following single 5 and 10 mg oral doses. The stimulatory effect was time-related with an onset at 20 minutes and peak at 1 hour with a duration of 3 to 5 hours.

In a multiple-dose pharmacokinetic study in male volunteers following 2 days of 5 or 10 mg oral pilocarpine given at 8 am, noon, and 6 pm, the mean elimination half-life was 0.76 and 1.35 hours for the 5 and 10 mg doses, respectively. T_{max} was 1.25 and 0.85 hours and C_{max} was 15 and 41 ng/mL, respectively. The AUC was 33 and 108 ng•h/mL, respectively, following the last 6-hour dose.

Inactivation of pilocarpine is thought to occur at neuronal synapses and probably in plasma. Pilocarpine and its minimally active or inactive degradation products, including pilocarpic acid, are excreted in the urine.

When taken with a high-fat meal, there was a decrease in the rate of absorption of pilocarpine. Mean T_{max} was 1.47 and 0.87 hours and mean C_{max} was 51.8 and 59.2 ng/mL for fed and fasted states, respectively.

Contraindications

Uncontrolled asthma; hypersensitivity to pilocarpine; when miosis is undesirable (eg, in acute iritis and in narrow-angle [angle closure] glaucoma).

Warnings

➤*Cardiovascular disease:* Patients with significant cardiovascular disease may be unable to compensate for transient changes in hemodynamics or rhythm induced by pilocarpine. Pulmonary edema has been reported as a complication of pilocarpine toxicity from high ocular doses given for acute angle-closure glaucoma. Administer pilocarpine with caution and under close medical supervision in patients with significant cardiovascular disease.

The dose-related cardiovascular effects of pilocarpine include hypotension, hypertension, bradycardia, and tachycardia.

➤*Ocular effects:* Ocular formulations of pilocarpine have caused visual blurring, which may result in decreased visual acuity, especially at night and in patients with central lens changes, and impairment of depth perception. Advise caution while driving at night or performing hazardous activities in reduced lighting.

➤*Pulmonary disease:* Pilocarpine increases airway resistance, bronchial smooth muscle tone, and bronchial secretions. Administer with caution and under close medical supervision in patients with controlled asthma, chronic bronchitis, or chronic obstructive pulmonary disease requiring pharmacologic therapy.

➤*Hepatic function impairment:* Based on decreased plasma clearance observed in patients with moderate hepatic impairment, the starting dose in these patients should be 5 mg twice daily, followed by adjustment based on therapeutic response and tolerability. Patients with mild hepatic insufficiency (Child-Pugh score of 5 to 6) do not require dosage reductions. To date, pharmacokinetic studies in subjects with severe hepatic impairment (Child-Pugh score of 10 to 15) have not been carried out. The use of pilocarpine in these patients is not recommended.

➤*Carcinogenesis:* In rats, a dosage of 18 mg/kg/day, which yielded a systemic exposure approximately 100 times larger than the maximum systemic exposure observed clinically, resulted in a statistically significant increase in the incidence of benign pheochromocytomas in both males and females and a statistically significant increase in the incidence of hepatocellular adenomas in female rats.

➤*Fertility impairment:* Oral administration of pilocarpine to male and female rats at a dosage of 18 mg/kg/day, which yielded a systemic exposure approximately 100 times larger than the maximum systemic exposure observed clinically, resulted in impaired reproductive function, including reduced fertility, decreases sperm motility, and morphologic evidence of abnormal sperm. It is unclear whether the reduction in fertility was due to effects on male animals, female animals, or males and females. In dogs, exposure to pilocarpine at a dosage of 3 mg/kg/day (approximately 3 times the maximum recommended human dose when compared on the basis of body surface area (mg/m^2) estimates) for 6 months resulted in evidence of impaired spermatogenesis. The data obtained in these studies suggest that pilocarpine may impair the fertility of male and female humans. Administer pilocarpine tablets to individuals who are attempting to conceive a child only if the potential benefit justifies potential fertility impairment.

➤*Elderly:* In placebo-controlled trials in Sjogren's syndrome patients, the mean age of patients was approximately 55 years of age (range, 21 to 85 years of age). The adverse events reported by those over 65 years of age and those 65 years of age and younger were comparable except for notable trends for urinary frequency, diarrhea, and dizziness.

➤*Pregnancy: Category C.* Pilocarpine was associated with a reduction in mean fetal body weight and an increase in the incidence of skeletal variations when given to pregnant rats at a dosage of 90 mg/kg/day (approximately 26 times the maximum recommended dose for a 50 kg human). These effects may have been secondary to maternal toxicity. In another study, oral administration of pilocarpine to female rats during gestation and lactation at a dosage of 36 mg/kg/day (approximately 10 times the maximum recommended dose for a 50 kg human when compared on the basis of body surface area (mg/m^2) estimates) resulted in an increased incidence of stillbirths; decreased neonatal survival and reduced mean body weight of pups were observed at dosages of 18 mg/kg/day (approximately 5 times the maximum recommended dose for a 50 kg human when compared on the basis of body surface area (mg/m^2) estimates) and above. There are no adequate and well-controlled studies in pregnant women. Use during pregnancy only if the potential benefit justifies the potential risk to the fetus.

➤*Lactation:* It is not known whether this drug is excreted in breast milk. Because of the potential for serious adverse reactions in nursing infants, decide whether to discontinue nursing or to discontinue the drug, taking into account the importance of the drug to the mother.

➤*Children:* Safety and efficacy in children have not been established.

PILOCARPINE HYDROCHLORIDE — ORAL

Precautions

➤*Toxicity:* Pilocarpine toxicity is characterized by an exaggeration of its parasympathomimetic effects. These may include the following: Headache; visual disturbance; lacrimation; sweating; respiratory distress; GI spasm; nausea; vomiting; diarrhea; AV block; tachycardia; bradycardia; hypotension; hypertension; shock; mental confusion; cardiac arrhythmia; tremors.

➤*Biliary tract:* Administer with caution to patients with known or suspected cholelithiasis or biliary tract disease. Contractions of the gallbladder or biliary smooth muscle could precipitate complications including cholecystitis, cholangitis, and biliary obstruction.

➤*Renal colic:* Pilocarpine may increase ureteral smooth muscle tone and could theoretically precipitate renal colic (or ureteral reflux), particularly in patients with nephrolithiasis.

➤*Psychiatric disorder:* Cholinergic agonists may have dose-related CNS effects. Consider this when treating patients with underlying cognitive or psychiatric disturbances.

Drug Interactions

Pilocarpine (Oral) Drug Interactions

Precipitant drug	Object drug*		Description
Pilocarpine	Anticholinergics	⬇	Pilocarpine may antagonize the anticholinergic effects of drugs used concomitantly. Consider these effects when anticholinergic properties may be contributing to the therapeutic effect of concomitant medication (eg, atropine, inhaled ipratropium).
Pilocarpine	Beta blockers	⬆	Use coadministration with caution because of possible conduction disturbances.

* ⬆ = Object drug increased. ⬇ = Object drug decreased.

➤*Drug/Food interactions:* The rate of absorption of pilocarpine is decreased when taken with a high-fat meal. Maximum concentration is decreased and time to reach maximum concentration is increased.

Adverse Reactions

➤*Head and neck cancer patients:*

Pilocarpine Adverse Reactions (%)

Adverse reaction	Placebo (n = 152)	Pilocarpine 5 mg tid (n = 141)	Pilocarpine 10 mg tid (n = 121)	Pilocarpine 5 or 10 mg tid (n = 212)
Sweating	9	29	68	-
Nausea	4	6	15	-
Rhinitis	7	5	14	-
Diarrhea	5	4	7	-
Chills	< 1	3	15	-
Flushing	3	8	13	-
Urinary frequency	7	9	12	-
Dizziness	4	5	12	-
Asthenia	3	6	12	-
Headache	8	-	-	11
Dyspepsia	5	-	-	7
Lacrimation	8	-	-	6
Edema	4	-	-	5
Abdominal pain	4	-	-	4
Amblyopia	2	-	-	4
Vomiting	1	-	-	4
Pharyngitis	8	-	-	3
Hypertension	1	-	-	3

The following events were reported at dosages of 7.5 to 30 mg/day (1% to 2%) – Abnormal vision, conjunctivitis, dysphagia, epistaxis, myalgias, pruritus, rash, sinusitis, tachycardia, taste perversion, tremor, voice alteration.

The following events also were reported (less than 1%). Causal relation is unknown. –

Cardiovascular: Bradycardia; ECG abnormality; palpitations; syncope.

CNS: Anxiety; confusion; depression; abnormal dreams; hyperkinesia; hypesthesia; nervousness; paresthesias; speech disorder; twitching.

GI: Anorexia; increased appetite; esophagitis; GI disorder; tongue disorder.

GU: Dysuria; metrorrhagia; urinary impairment.

Hematologic: Leukopenia; lymphadenopathy.

Respiratory: Increased sputum; stridor; yawning.

Special senses: Deafness; eye pain; glaucoma.

Miscellaneous: Body odor; hypothermia; mucous membrane abnormality; seborrhea. In long-term treatment of 2 patients with underlying cardiovascular disease, 1 experienced an MI and the other an episode of syncope.

➤*Sjogren's syndrome patients:* The adverse events reported by those over 65 years of age and those 65 years of age and younger were comparable except for notable trends for urinary frequency, diarrhea, and dizziness. The incidences of urinary frequency and diarrhea in the elderly were about double those in the nonelderly. The incidence of dizziness was about 3 times as high in the elderly as in the nonelderly. These adverse experiences were not considered to be serious. In the 2 placebo-controlled studies, the most common adverse events related to drug use were sweating, urinary frequency, chills, and vasodilation (flushing). The most commonly reported reason for patient discontinuation of treatment was sweating. Expected pharmacologic effects of pilocarpine include the following adverse experiences.

Pilocarpine Adverse Experiences (%)

Adverse event	5 mg qid (20 mg/day) (n = 255)	Placebo qid (n = 253)
Sweating	40	7
Urinary frequency	10	4
Nausea	9	9
Flushing	9	2
Rhinitis	7	8
Diarrhea	6	7
Chills	4	2
Increased salivation	3	0
Asthenia	2	2
Headache	13	19
Flu syndrome	9	9
Dyspepsia	7	7
Dizziness	6	7
Pain	4	2
Sinusitis	4	5
Abdominal pain	3	4
Vomiting	3	1
Pharyngitis	2	5
Rash	2	3
Infection	2	6

The following events were reported in Sjogren's syndrome patients at incidences of 1% to 2% at dosing of 20 mg/day: Accidental injury; allergic reaction; back pain; blurred vision; constipation; increased cough; edema; epistaxis; face edema; fever; flatulence; glossitis; lab test abnormalities, including chemistry, hematology, and urinalysis; myalgia; palpitation; pruritus; somnolence; stomatitis; tachycardia; tinnitus; urinary incontinence, urinary tract infection; vaginitis.

The following events were reported rarely in Sjogren's syndrome patients (fewer than 1%) at dosing of 10 to 30 mg/day. Causal relation is unknown.

Cardiovascular: Angina pectoris, arrhythmia, ECG abnormality, hypotension, hypertension, intracranial hemorrhage, migraine, MI.

CNS: Abnormal dreams, abnormal thinking, aphasia, confusion, depression, emotional lability, hyperkinesia, hypesthesia, insomnia, leg cramps, nervousness, paresthesias, tremor.

Dermatologic: Alopecia, contact dermatitis, dry skin, eczema, erythema nodosum, exfoliative dermatitis, herpes simplex, skin ulcer, vesiculobullous rash.

GI: Abnormal liver function tests, anorexia, bilirubinemia, cholelithiasis, colitis, dry mouth, eructation, gastritis, gastroenteritis, GI disorder, gingivitis, hepatitis, increased sputum, melena, nausea and vomiting, pancreatitis, parotid gland enlargement, salivary gland enlargement, taste loss, tongue disorder, tooth disorder.

GU: Breast pain, dysuria, mastitis, menorrhagia, metrorrhagia, ovarian disorder, pyuria, salpingitis, urethral pain, urinary urgency, vaginal hemorrhage, vaginal moniliasis.

Hematologic: Abnormal WBC, abnormal platelets, hematuria, lymphadenopathy, thrombocythemia, thrombocytopenia, thrombosis.

Metabolic/Nutritional: Hypoglycemia, peripheral edema.

Musculoskeletal: Arthralgia, arthritis, bone disorder, myasthenia, pathological fracture, spontaneous bone fracture, tendon disorder, tenosynovitis.

Respiratory: Bronchitis, dyspnea, hiccough, laryngismus, laryngitis, pneumonia, viral infection, voice alteration.

Special senses: Abnormal vision, cataract, conjunctivitis, dry eyes, ear disorder, ear pain, eye disorder, eye hemorrhage, glaucoma, lacrimation disorder, retinal disorder, taste perversion.

Miscellaneous: Chest pain, cyst, death, moniliasis, neck pain, neck rigidity, photosensitivity reaction.

The following adverse experiences have been reported rarely with ocular pilocarpine: AV block, agitation, ciliary congestion, confusion, delusion, depression, dermatitis, eyelid twitching, iris cysts, macular hole, malignant glaucoma, middle ear disturbance, shock, and visual hallucination.

Overdosage

Pilocarpine fatal overdosage resulting from poisoning has been reported at doses presumed to be greater than 100 mg in 2 hospitalized patients; 100 mg is considered potentially fatal. Treat overdosage with atropine titration (0.5 to 1 mg SC or IV) and use supportive measures to maintain respiration and circulation. Epinephrine (0.3 to 1 mg SC or IM) also may be of value in the presence of severe cardiovascular depression or bronchoconstriction. Refer to General Management of Acute Overdosage. It is not known if pilocarpine is dialyzable.

Patient Information

Inform patients that pilocarpine may cause visual disturbances, especially at night, that could impair their ability to drive safely.

If a patient sweats excessively while taking pilocarpine and cannot drink enough liquid, have the patient consult a physician. Dehydration may develop.

CEVIMELINE HYDROCHLORIDE

Rx	Evoxac (Daiichi Pharm.)	Capsules: 30 mg	Lactose. White. In 100s and 500s.

CEVIMELINE HYDROCHLORIDE — ORAL

Indications

➤*Dry mouth:* For the treatment of symptoms of dry mouth in patients with Sjögren's syndrome.

Administration and Dosage

➤*Approved by the FDA:* January 11, 2000.

➤*Dosage:* 30 mg 3 times a day. There is insufficient safety and efficacy information to support doses greater than 30 mg 3 times daily.

➤*Storage/Stability:* Store at 25°C (77°F); excursion permitted to 15° to 30°C (59°to 86° F).

Actions

➤*Pharmacology:*

Pharmacodynamics – Cevimeline hydrochloride is a cholinergic agonist which binds to muscarinic receptors. Muscarinic agonists in sufficient dosage can increase secretion of exocrine glands, such as salivary and sweat glands and increase tone of the smooth muscle in the GI and urinary tracts.

➤*Pharmacokinetics:*

Absorption – After administration of a single 30 mg capsule, cevimeline hydrochloride was rapidly absorbed with a mean time to peak concentration of 1.5 to 2 hours. No accumulation of active drug or its metabolites was observed following multiple-dose administration. When administered with food, there is a decrease in the rate of absorption, with a fasting T_{max} of 1.53 hours and a T_{max} of 2.86 hours after a meal; the peak concentration is reduced by 17.3%. Single oral doses across the clinical dose range are dose proportional.

Distribution – Cevimeline hydrochloride has a volume of distribution of ≈ 6 L/kg and is less than 20% bound to human plasma proteins. This suggests that cevimeline hydrochloride is extensively bound to tissues; however, the specific binding sites are unknown.

Metabolism – Isozymes CYP2D6 and CYP3A3/4 are responsible for the metabolism of cevimeline hydrochloride. After 24 hours, 86.7% of the dose was recovered (16% unchanged, 44.5% as cis and trans-sulfoxide, 22.3% of the dose as glucuronic acid conjugate and 4% of the dose as N-oxide of cevimeline hydrochloride). Approximately 8% of the trans-sulfoxide metabolite is then converted into the corresponding glucuronic acid conjugate and eliminated. Cevimeline hydrochloride did not inhibit cytochrome P450 isozymes 1A2, 2A6, 2C9, 2C19, 2D6, 2E1, and 3A4.

Excretion – The mean half-life of cevimeline is 5 ± 1 hours. After 24 hours, 84% of a 30 mg dose of cevimeline hydrochloride was excreted in urine. After 7 days, 97% of the dose was recovered in the urine and 0.5% was recovered in the feces.

Contraindications

Uncontrolled asthma, hypersensitivity to cevimeline hydrochloride, and when miosis is undesirable (eg, in acute iritis and in narrow-angle [angle-closure] glaucoma).

Warnings

➤*Cardiovascular disease:* Cevimeline hydrochloride can potentially alter cardiac conduction or heart rate. Patients with significant cardiovascular disease may potentially be unable to compensate for transient changes in hemodynamics or rhythm induced by cevimeline hydrochloride. Cevimeline hydrochloride should be used with caution and under close medical supervision in patients with a history of cardiovascular disease evidenced by angina pectoris or myocardial infarction (MI).

➤*Pulmonary disease:* Cevimeline hydrochloride can potentially increase airway resistance, bronchial smooth muscle tone, and bronchial secretions. Cevimeline hydrochloride should be administered with caution and with close medical supervision to patients with controlled asthma, chronic bronchitis, or chronic obstructive pulmonary disease.

➤*Ocular:* Ophthalmic formulations of muscarinic agonists have been reported to cause visual blurring which may result in decreased visual acuity, especially at night and in patients with central lens changes, and to cause impairment of depth perception. Caution should be advised while driving at night or performing hazardous activities in reduced lighting.

➤*Carcinogenesis:* Lifetime carcinogenicity studies were conducted in CD-1 mice and F-344 rats. A statistically significant increase in the incidence of adenocarcinomas of the uterus was observed in female rats that received cevimeline hydrochloride at a dosage of 100 mg/kg/day (≈ 8 times the maximum human exposure based on comparison of AUC data). No other significant differences in tumor incidence were observed in either mice or rats.

➤*Fertility impairment:* Cevimeline hydrochloride did not adversely affect the reproductive performance or fertility of male Sprague-Dawley rats when administered for 63 days prior to mating and throughout the period of mating at dosages up to 45 mg/kg/day (≈ 5 times the maximum recommended dose for a 60 kg human following normalization of the data on the basis of body surface area estimates). Females that were treated with cevimeline hydrochloride at dosages up to 45 mg/kg/day from 14 days prior to mating through day 7 of gestation exhibited a statistically significantly smaller number of implantations than did control animals.

➤*Elderly:* Although clinical studies of cevimeline hydrochloride included subjects over the age of 65, the numbers were not sufficient to determine whether they respond differently from younger subjects. Special care should be exercised when cevimeline hydrochloride treatment is initiated in an elderly patient, considering the greater frequency of decreased hepatic, renal, or cardiac function, and of concomitant disease or other drug therapy in the elderly.

➤*Pregnancy:* Category C.

Cevimeline hydrochloride was associated with a reduction in the mean number of implantations when given to pregnant Sprague-Dawley rats from 14 days prior to mating through day 7 of gestation at a dosage of 45 mg/kg/day (≈ 5 times the maximum recommended dose for a 60 kg human when compared on the basis of body surface area estimates). This effect may have been secondary to maternal toxicity. There are no adequate and well-controlled studies in pregnant women. Cevimeline hydrochloride should be used during pregnancy only if the potential benefit justifies the potential risk to the fetus.

➤*Lactation:* It is not known whether this drug is secreted in human milk. Because many drugs are excreted in human milk, and because of the potential for serious adverse reactions in nursing infants from cevimeline hydrochloride, a decision should be made whether to discontinue nursing or discontinue the drug, taking into account the importance of the drug to the mother.

➤*Children:* Safety and effectiveness in pediatric patients have not been established.

Precautions

➤*Toxicity:* Cevimeline hydrochloride toxicity is characterized by an exaggeration of its parasympathomimetic effects. These may include headache, visual disturbance, lacrimation, sweating, respiratory distress, GI spasm, nausea, vomiting, diarrhea, atrioventricular block, tachycardia, bradycardia, hypotension, hypertension, shock, mental confusion, cardiac arrhythmia, and tremors.

➤*Special risk:* Cevimeline hydrochloride should be administered with caution to patients with a history of nephrolithiasis or cholelithiasis. Contractions of the gallbladder or biliary smooth muscle could precipitate complications such as cholecystitis, cholangitis and biliary obstruction. An increase in the ureteral smooth muscle tone could theoretically precipitate renal colic or ureteral reflux in patients with nephrolithiasis.

➤*Hazardous tasks:* Ophthalmic formulations of muscarinic agonists have been reported to cause visual blurring which may result in decreased visual acuity, especially at night and in patients with central lens changes, and to cause impairment of depth perception. Caution should be advised while driving at night or performing hazardous activities in reduced lighting.

Drug Interactions

Drugs which inhibit CYP2D6 and CYP3A3/4 also inhibit the metabolism of cevimeline hydrochloride. Cevimeline hydrochloride should be used with caution in individuals known or suspected to be deficient in CYP2D6 activity, based on previous experience, as they may be at a higher risk of adverse events. In an in vitro study cytochrome P450 isozymes 1A2, 2A6, 2C9, 2C19, 2D6, 2E1, and 3A4 were not inhibited by exposure to cevimeline hydrochloride.

Cevimeline Drug Interactions

Precipitant drug	Object drug*		Description
Cevimeline	Beta blockers	⬆	Administer cevimeline with caution to patients taking beta adrenergic antagonists because of the possibility of conduction disturbances.
Cevimeline	Parasympathomimetics	⬆	Drugs with parasympathomimetic effects administered concurrently with cevimeline may be expected to have additive effects.
Cevimeline	Antimuscarinics	⬇	Cevimeline might interfere with desirable antimuscarinic effects of drugs used concomitantly.

* ⬆ = Object drug increased. ⬇ = Object drug decreased.

➤*Drug/Food interactions:* See Actions for more information.

Adverse Reactions

The following adverse events associated with muscarinic agonism were observed in the clinical trials of cevimeline hydrochloride in Sjögren's syndrome patients:

Adverse event	Cevimeline 30 mg (3 times daily) n = 533*	Placebo (3 times daily) n = 164
Excessive sweating	18.7%	2.4%
Nausea	13.8%	7.9%
Rhinitis	11.2%	5.4%
Diarrhea	10.3%	10.3%
Excessive salivation	2.2%	0.6%

CEVIMELINE HYDROCHLORIDE — ORAL

Adverse event	Cevimeline 30 mg (3 times daily) n = 533*	Placebo (3 times daily) n = 164
Urinary frequency	0.9%	1.8%
Asthenia	0.5%	0%
Flushing	0.3%	0.6%
Polyuria	0.1%	0.6%

* N is the total number of patients exposed to the dose at any time during the study.

In addition, the following adverse events (≥ 3% incidence) were reported in the Sjögren's clinical trials:

Adverse event	Cevimeline 30 mg (3 times daily) n = 533 *	Placebo (3 times daily) n = 164
Headache	14.4%	20.1%
Sinusitis	12.3%	10.9%
Upper respiratory tract infection	11.4%	9.1%
Dyspepsia	7.8%	8.5%
Abdominal pain	7.6%	6.7%
Urinary tract infection	6.1%	3%
Coughing	6.1%	3%
Pharyngitis	5.2%	5.4%
Vomiting	4.6%	2.4%
Injury	4.5%	2.4%
Back pain	4.5%	4.2%
Rash	4.3%	6%
Conjunctivitis	4.3%	3.6%
Dizziness	4.1%	7.3%
Bronchitis	4.1%	1.2%
Arthralgia	3.7%	1.8%
Surgical intervention	3.3%	3%
Fatigue	3.3%	1.2%
Pain	3.3%	3%
Skeletal pain	2.8%	1.8%
Insomnia	2.4%	1.2%
Hot flushes	2.4%	0%
Rigors	1.3%	1.2%
Anxiety	1.3%	1.2%

* N is the total number of patients exposed to the dose at any time during the study.

The following events were reported in Sjögren's patients at incidences of less than 3% and ≥ 1%: Constipation, tremor, abnormal vision, hypertonia, peripheral edema, chest pain, myalgia, fever, anorexia, eye pain, ear ache, dry mouth, vertigo, salivary gland pain, pruritus, influenza-like symptoms, eye infection, post-operative pain, vaginitis, skin disorder, depression, hiccup, hyporeflexia, infection, fungal infection, sialoadenitis, otitis media, erythematous rash, pneumonia, edema, salivary gland enlargement, allergy, gastroesophageal reflux, eye abnormality, migraine, tooth disorder, epistaxis, flatulence, tooth ache, ulcerative stomatitis, anemia, hypoesthesia, cystitis, leg cramps, abscess, eructation, moniliasis, palpitation, increased amylase, xerophthalmia, allergic reaction.

The following events were reported rarely in treated Sjögren's patients (less than 1%) (causal relation is unknown):

➤*Cardiovascular:* Abnormal ECG, heart disorder, heart murmur, aggravated hypertension, hypotension, arrhythmia, extrasystoles, t wave inversion, tachycardia, supraventricular tachycardia, angina pectoris, myocardial infarction, pericarditis, pulmonary embolism, peripheral ischemia, superficial phlebitis, purpura, deep thrombophlebitis, vascular disorder, vasculitis, hypertension.

➤*CNS:* Carpal tunnel syndrome, coma, abnormal coordination, dysesthesia, dyskinesia, dysphonia, aggravated multiple sclerosis, involuntary muscle contractions, neuralgia, neuropathy, paresthesia, speech disorder, agitation, confusion, depersonalization, aggravated depression, abnormal dreaming, emotional lability, manic reaction, paroniria, somnolence, abnormal thinking, hyperkinesia, hallucination.

➤*Dermatologic:* Acne, alopecia, burn, dermatitis, contact dermatitis, lichenoid dermatitis, eczema, furunculosis, hyperkeratosis, lichen planus, nail discoloration, nail disorder, onychia, onychomycosis, paronychia, photosensitivity reaction, rosacea, scleroderma, seborrhea, skin discoloration, dry skin, skin exfoliation, skin hypertrophy, skin ulceration, urticaria, verruca, bullous eruption, cold clammy skin, basal cell carcinoma, squamous carcinoma.

➤*Endocrine:* Increased glucocorticoids, goiter, hypothyroidism.

➤*GI:* Appendicitis, increased appetite, ulcerative colitis, diverticulitis, duodenitis, dysphagia, enterocolitis, gastric ulcer, gastritis, gastroenteritis, gastrointestinal hemorrhage, gingivitis, glossitis, rectum hemorrhage, hemorrhoids, ileus, irritable bowel syndrome, melena, mucositis, esophageal stricture, esophagitis, oral hemorrhage, peptic ulcer, periodontal destruction, rectal disorder, stomatitis, tenesmus, tongue discoloration, tongue disorder, geographic tongue, tongue ulceration, dental caries.

➤*GU:* Epididymitis, prostatic disorder, abnormal sexual function, amenorrhea, female breast neoplasm, malignant female breast neoplasm, female breast pain, positive cervical smear test, dysmenorrhea, endometrial disorder, intermenstrual bleeding, leukorrhea, menorrhagia, menstrual disorder, ovarian cyst, ovarian disorder, genital pruritus, uterine hemorrhage, vaginal hemorrhage, atrophic vaginitis, albuminuria, bladder discomfort, increased blood urea nitrogen, dysuria, hematuria, micturition disorder, nephrosis, nocturia, increased nonprotein nitrogen, pyelonephritis, renal calculus, abnormal renal function, renal pain, strangury, urethral disorder, abnormal urine, urinary incontinence, decreased urine flow, pyuria.

➤*Hematologic:* Thrombocytopenic purpura, thrombocythemia, thrombocytopenia, hypochromic anemia, eosinophilia, granulocytopenia, leucopenia, leukocytosis, cervical lymphadenopathy, lymphadenopathy.

➤*Hepatic:* Cholelithiasis, increased gamma-glutamyl transferase, increased hepatic enzymes, abnormal hepatic function, viral hepatitis, increased serum AST, increased serum ALT.

➤*Immunologic:* Cellulitis, herpes simplex, herpes zoster, bacterial infection, viral infection, genital moniliasis, sepsis.

➤*Metabolic/Nutritional:* Dehydration, diabetes mellitus, hypercalcemia, hypercholesterolemia, hyperglycemia, hyperlipemia, hypertriglyceridemia, hyperuricemia, hypoglycemia, hypokalemia, hyponatremia, thirst.

➤*Musculoskeletal:* Arthritis, aggravated arthritis, arthropathy, femoral head avascular necrosis, bone disorder, bursitis, costochondritis, plantar fasciitis, muscle weakness, osteomyelitis, osteoporosis, synovitis, tendinitis, tenosynovitis, aggravated rheumatoid arthritis, lupus erythematosus rash, lupus erythematosus syndrome.

➤*Respiratory:* Asthma, bronchospasm, chronic obstructive airway disease, dyspnea, hemoptysis, laryngitis, nasal ulcer, pleural effusion, pleurisy, pulmonary congestion, pulmonary fibrosis, respiratory disorder.

➤*Special senses:* Deafness, decreased hearing, motion sickness, parosmia, taste perversion, blepharitis, cataract, corneal opacity, corneal ulceration, diplopia, glaucoma, anterior chamber eye hemorrhage, keratitis, keratoconjunctivitis, mydriasis, myopia, photopsia, retinal deposits, retinal disorder, scleritis, vitreous detachment, tinnitus.

➤*Miscellaneous:* Aggravated allergy, precordial chest pain, abnormal crying, hematoma, leg pain, edema, periorbital edema, activated pain trauma, pallor, changed sensation temperature, weight decrease, weight increase, choking, mouth edema, syncope, malaise, face edema, substernal chest pain, fall, food poisoning, heat stroke, joint dislocation, post-operative hemorrhage.

In 1 subject with lupus erythematosus receiving concomitant multiple drug therapy, a highly elevated ALT level was noted after the fourth week of cevimeline hydrochloride therapy. In 2 other subjects receiving cevimeline hydrochloride in the clinical trials, very high AST levels were noted. The significance of these findings is unknown.

Additional adverse events – Additional adverse events (relationship unknown) which occurred in other clinical studies (patient population different from Sjögren's patients) are as follows:

Cholinergic syndrome, blood pressure fluctuation, cardiomegaly, postural hypotension, aphasia, convulsions, abnormal gait, hyperesthesia, paralysis, abnormal sexual function, enlarged abdomen, change in bowel habits, gum hyperplasia, intestinal obstruction, bundle branch block, increased creatine phosphokinase, electrolyte abnormality, glycosuria, gout, hyperkalemia, hyperproteinemia, increased lactic dehydrogenase (LDH), increased alkaline phosphatase, failure to thrive, abnormal platelets, aggressive reaction, amnesia, apathy, delirium, delusion, dementia, illusion, impotence, neurosis, paranoid reaction, personality disorder, hyperhemoglobinemia, apnea, atelectasis, yawning, oliguria, urinary retention, distended vein, lymphocytosis.

Overdosage

➤*Treatment:* Management of the signs and symptoms of acute overdosage should be handled in a manner consistent with that indicated for other muscarinic agonists; general supportive measures should be instituted. If medically indicated, atropine, an anticholinergic agent, may be of value as an antidote for emergency use in patients who have had an overdose of cevimeline hydrochloride. If medically indicated, epinephrine may also be of value in the presence of severe cardiovascular depression or bronchoconstriction. It is not known if cevimeline hydrochloride is dialyzable.

Patient Information

Patients should be informed that cevimeline hydrochloride may cause visual disturbances, especially at night, that could impair their ability to drive safely.

If a patient sweats excessively while taking cevimeline hydrochloride, dehydration may develop. The patient should drink extra water and consult a health care provider.

SALIVA SUBSTITUTES

otc	**Saliva Substitute** (Roxane)	**Solution:** Sorbitol, sodium carboxymethylcellulose, methylparaben	In 120 mL bottle.
otc	**Moi-Stir** (Kingswood)	**Solution:** Dibasic sodium phosphate, magnesium, calcium chloride, sodium chloride, and potassium chlorides, sorbitol, sodium carboxymethylcellulose, parabens	In 120 mL spray.
otc	**Moi-Stir Swabsticks** (Kingswood)	**Swabsticks:** Dibasic sodium phosphate, magnesium, calcium chloride, sodium chloride, and potassium chlorides, sorbitol, sodium carboxymethylcellulose, parabens	In packets (3s).
otc	**Entertainer's Secret** (KLI Corp)	**Solution:** Sodium carboxymethylcellulose, potassium chloride, dibasic sodium phosphate, parabens, aloe vera gel, glycerin	In 60 mL spray.
otc	**Salivart** (Gebauer)	**Solution:** Sodium carboxymethylcellulose, sorbitol, sodium chloride, potassium chloride, calcium chloride, magnesium chloride, dibasic potassium phosphate, nitrogen (as propellant)	Preservative-free. In 75 mL aerosol spray cans.
otc	**MouthKote** (Parnell)	**Solution:** Xylitol, sorbitol, yerba santa, citric acid, ascorbic acid, sodium benzoate, saccharin	Lemon-lime flavor. In 60 and 240 mL spray.
otc	**Numoisyn** (Align[a])	**Lozenges:** 0.3 g sorbitol, polyethylene glycol, malic acid, sodium citrate, calcium phosphate dibasic, hydrogenated cottonseed oil, citric acid, magnesium stearate, silicon dioxide	In 100s.

[a] Align Pharmaceuticals, 5625 Dillard Drive, Suite 201, Cary, NC, 27511; 1-(919) 398-6225; fax 1-(919) 398-6250

SALIVA SUBSTITUTES — ORAL

Indications

➤*Dry mouth and throat:* These products are used as saliva substitutes to relieve dry mouth and throat in xerostomia, which may be caused by the following: Surgery or radiation near the salivary glands; chemotherapy; Sjogren syndrome; Bell palsy; HIV/AIDS; lupus; diabetes; aging; emotional factors; dry throat; scratchy, hoarse voice; medications (eg, antidepressants, antihistamines, antihypertensives); infection or dysfunction of the salivary glands.

Administration and Dosage

Refer to specific product labeling for additional dosage guidelines.

➤*Spray:* Hold close to mouth and spray for one-half second or less to relieve dryness. May be used as often as needed to moisten and lubricate; may swallow or expectorate.

➤*Swabsticks:* Swab and cleanse all intraoral surfaces for 2 to 3 minutes using all 3 disposable swabsticks. Repeat procedure every 3 to 4 hours while awake or more frequently if needed.

➤*Lozenges:* Dissolve slowly in the mouth when needed. To obtain optimal effect, move the lozenge around in the mouth. Repeat as necessary. Do not exceed 16 lozenges in 24 hours.

➤*Storage/Stability:* Store at controlled room temperature, 15° to 30°C (59° to 86°F). Protect from direct sunlight and heat above 38°C (100°F) .

DOXYCYCLINE

For prescribing information, refer to the Doxycycline monograph in the Anti-Infectives, Systemic chapter. Refer to the Tetracyclines group monograph for more information.

MINOCYCLINE HYDROCHLORIDE

For prescribing information, refer to the Minocycline monograph in the Tetracyclines in the Anti-infective chapter.

AMLEXANOX

Rx	**Aphthasol** (Access)	**Paste:** 5%	Benzyl alcohol, mineral oil, petrolatum. In 5 g.

AMLEXANOX — ORAL PASTE

Indications

➤*Aphthous ulcers:* For the treatment of aphthous ulcers in people with normal immune systems.

Administration and Dosage

➤*Approved by the FDA:* December 17, 1996.

The paste should be applied as soon as possible after noticing the symptoms of an aphthous ulcer and should be used 4 times daily, preferably following oral hygiene after breakfast, lunch, dinner, and at bedtime. Squeeze a dab of paste approximately ½ inch (0.5 cm) onto a finger tip. With gentle pressure, dab the paste onto each ulcer in the mouth. Use of the medication should be continued until the ulcer heals. If significant healing or pain reduction has not occurred in 10 days, consult your dentist or physician.

➤*Storage/Stability:* Store at controlled room temperature, 15° to 30°C (59° to 86°F).

Actions

➤*Pharmacology:* The mechanism of action by which amlexanox accelerates healing of aphthous ulcers is unknown. In vitro studies have demonstrated amlexanox to be a potent inhibitor of the formation or release of inflammatory mediators (histamine and leukotrienes) from mast cells, neutrophils and mononuclear cells. Given orally to animals, amlexanox has demonstrated antiallergenic and anti-inflammatory activities and has been shown to suppress both immediate and delayed type hypersensitivity reactions. The relevance of these activities of amlexanox to its effects on aphthous ulcers has not been established.

➤*Pharmacokinetics:* After a single oral application of 100 mg of paste (5 mg amlexanox), maximal serum levels of approximately 120 ng/mL are observed at 2.4 hours. Most of the systemic absorption of amlexanox is via the gastrointestinal tract, and the amount absorbed directly through the active ulcer is not a significant portion of the applied dose. The half-life for elimination was 3.5 ± 1.1 hours in healthy individuals. Approximately 17% of the dose is eliminated into the urine as unchanged amlexanox, a hydroxylated metabolite, and their conjugates. With multiple applications 4 times daily, steady-state levels were reached within 1 week, and no accumulation was observed with up to 4 weeks of use.

Contraindications

Hypersensitivity to amlexanox or other ingredients in the formulation.

Warnings

➤*Elderly:* Clinical studies of amlexanox oral paste did not include sufficient numbers of subjects aged 65 and over to determine whether they respond differently from younger subjects. Other reported clinical experience has not identified differences in responses between the elderly and younger patients. In general, dose selection for an elderly patient should be cautious, usually starting at the low end of the dosing range, reflecting the greater frequency of decreased hepatic, renal, or cardiac function, and of concomitant disease or other drug therapy.

➤*Pregnancy: Category B.*

There are no adequate and well-controlled studies in pregnant women. Because animal reproduction studies are not always predictive of human response, this drug should be used during pregnancy only if clearly needed.

➤*Lactation:* Amlexanox was found in the milk of lactating rats; therefore, caution should be exercised when administering amlexanox oral paste to a nursing woman.

➤*Children:* Safety and effectiveness of amlexanox oral paste in pediatric patients have not been established.

Precautions

➤*Local irritation:* Wash hands immediately after applying amlexanox oral paste directly to ulcers with the finger tips. In the event that a rash or contact mucositis occurs, discontinue use.

Adverse Reactions

Adverse reactions considered related or possibly related to amlexanox oral paste were not reported by more than 5% of patients. Adverse reactions reported by 1% to 2% of patients were transient pain, stinging or burning at the site of application. Infrequent (less than 1%) adverse reactions in the clinical studies were contact mucositis, nausea, and diarrhea.

Overdosage

There are no reports of human ingestion overdosage. Ingestion of a full tube of 5 g of paste would result in systemic exposure well below the maximum nontoxic dose of amlexanox in animals. Gastrointestinal upset such as diarrhea and vomiting could result from an overdose.

SULFURIC ACID/SULFONATED PHENOLICS

Rx	**Debacterol** (Epien Medical[a])	**Liquid:** 30% sulfuric acid and 50% sulfonated phenolics	In 1.5 mL.

[a] Epien Medical, Inc., 4225 White Bear Parkway, Suite 600, St. Paul, MN 55110-3389; (888) 884-4675, (651) 653-3380, fax (651) 653-8569

SULFURIC ACID/SULFONATED PHENOLICS — ORAL

Indications

➤*Ulcerating lesions:* Topical treatment of ulcerating lesions of the oral cavity, such as recurrent aphthous stomatitis (canker sores). Provides relief from pain and discomfort of oral mucosal ulcers.

Not intended for the treatment of vesicular lesions, such as cold sores or fever blisters.

Administration and Dosage

Immediately before applying, thoroughly dry the ulcerated area of oral mucosa that is to be treated using a sterile cotton-tipped applicator or some similar method. After drying the lesion, hold swab with the colored ring end up. Bend the colored ring tip gently to the side until it snaps to release the liquid inside. Liquid flows down into the white tip applicator. Then apply the coated applicator directly to the dried ulcer bed. A very brief stinging sensation is experienced immediately upon application of the liquid to the ulcer. Hold the cotton-tipped applicator in contact with the ulcer for at least 5 seconds while using a rolling motion to thoroughly coat the entire ulcer bed, the ulcer rim, and the surrounding halo of normal mucosa. Do not hold the applicator on the ulcer for more than 10 seconds. The sulfuric acid/sulfonated phenolics liquid will not harm the normal oral mucosa when used as directed. Then thoroughly rinse out the mouth with water and spit out the rinse water. The stinging sensation and ulcer pain will subside almost immediately after the water rinse.

One application per ulcer treatment is usually sufficient. However, if the ulcer pain returns shortly after rinsing with water, it is an indication that some part of the ulcer was not covered with the sulfuric acid/sulfonated phenolics liquid. A second application should then be applied to the ulcer immediately during the same treatment session until it remains pain-free after rinsing. It is not recommended that more than 1 treatment session be performed on any individual mucosal ulcer. Do not reapply the product to the same lesion after it is free of pain.

➤*Storage / Stability:* Store at room temperature, 15° to 30°C (59° to 86°F).

Actions

➤*Pharmacology:* The liquid contains sulfonated phenolics, which are antiseptic agents with topical analgesic properties, and sulfuric acid, which is a tissue denaturant and sterilizing agent, in an aqueous solution.

Contraindications

Known allergy to sulfonated phenolics.

Warnings

➤*Allergy:* Do not use if allergic to sulfonated phenolics.

➤*Prolonged use:* Because of its nature, prolonged use on normal tissue should be avoided. The sulfuric acid/sulfonated phenolics liquid will eventually necrotize and slough all tissue to which it is applied in sufficient volume; apply carefully.

➤*Pregnancy:* Category C.

➤*Children:* Safety and efficacy in children younger than 12 years of age have not been established. Keep out of the reach of children.

Precautions

➤*External use only:* Avoid eye contact.

Adverse Reactions

May cause local irritation upon administration. If excess irritation occurs during use, a rinse with sodium bicarbonate (baking soda) solution will neutralize the reaction (use 2.5 mL in 120 mL of water).

Mouth and Throat Products

Indications

Minor sore throat and minor irritation of the throat or mouth.

Administration and Dosage

Do not use for more than 2 days or in children younger than 2 years of age, unless directed by physician. For dosage guidelines, refer to the specific package labeling.

Actions

➤*Pharmacology:*

Benzocaine and dyclonine – Benzocaine and dyclonine are local anesthetics.

Cetylpyridinium chloride, eucalyptus oil, thymol and hexylresorcinol – Cetylpyridinium chloride, eucalyptus oil, thymol, and hexylresorcinol have antiseptic activity.

Menthol, camphor, capsicum, dyclonine and phenol – Menthol, camphor, capsicum, dyclonine, and phenol are used for their antipruritic, local anesthetic and counterirritant activities.

Hydrocortisone and triamcinolone (corticosteroids) – Hydrocortisone and triamcinolone (corticosteroids) are used for their anti-inflammatory activities.

Warnings

➤*Severe / Persistent sore throat:* Severe and persistent sore throat or sore throat accompanied by high fever, headache, nausea and vomiting may be serious. Consult physician promptly.

Precautions

➤*Tartrazine sensitivity:* Some of these products contain tartrazine (FD&C yellow #5), which may cause allergic-type reactions (including bronchial asthma) in susceptible individuals. Although the incidence of sensitivity is low, it is frequently seen in patients who also have aspirin hypersensitivity. Specific products containing tartrazine are identified in the product listings.

LOZENGES AND TROCHES

otc	**Vicks Children's Chloraseptic** (Richardson-Vicks)	**Lozenges**: 5 mg benzocaine	Corn syrup, sucrose. Grape flavor. In 18s.
otc sf	**Cepacol Maximum Strength** (J.B. Williams)	**Lozenges**: 10 mg benzocaine	Menthol. Cherry and cool mint flavors. In 16s.
otc	**Spec-T** (Apothecon)		Sucrose. In 10s.
otc	**Cēpacol Sore Throat** (Combe)	**Lozenges**: 10 mg benzocaine, 2 mg menthol.	Glucose, sucrose. Menthol flavor. In 18s.
otc	**Cēpacol Sore Throat** (Combe)	**Lozenges**: 10 mg benzocaine, 2.1 mg menthol	Glucose, sucrose. Citrus flavor. In 18s.
otc	**Cēpacol Sore Throat** (Combe)	**Lozenges**: 10 mg benzocaine, 2.6 mg menthol	Glucose, sucrose. Honey-lemon flavor. In 18s.
otc	**Cēpacol Sore Throat** (Combe)	**Lozenges**: 10 mg benzocaine, 3.6 mg menthol	Glucose, sucrose. Cherry flavor. In 18s.
otc sf	**Cēpacol Sore Throat** (Combe)	**Lozenges**: 10 mg benzocaine, 4.5 mg menthol	Sorbitol. Cherry flavor. In 16s.
otc sf	**Mycinettes** (Pfeiffer)	**Lozenges**: 15 mg benzocaine	Sorbitol, saccharin, menthol. Cherry flavor. In 12s.
otc	**Chloraseptic Sore Throat** (Prestige)	**Lozenges**: 6 mg benzocaine, 10 mg menthol	Sucrose. Honey lemon, cherry, menthol flavors. In 18s.
otc sf	**Cylex** (Pharmakon)	**Lozenges**: 15 mg benzocaine, 5 mg cetylpyridinium chloride	Sorbitol. Cherry flavor. In 12s.
otc	**Cēpacol Throat** (J.B. Williams)	**Lozenges**: 0.07% cetylpyridinium chloride, 0.3% benzyl alcohol	Tartrazine. In 27s and 40s.
otc	**Sucrets Children's Sore Throat** (SK-Beecham)	**Lozenges**: 1.2 mg dyclonine hydrochloride	Corn syrup, sucrose. Cherry flavor. In 24s.
otc	**Vapor Lemon Sucrets** (SK-Beecham)	**Lozenges**: 2 mg dyclonine hydrochloride	Sucrose, corn syrup. In 18s.
otc	**Sucrets Maximum Strength** (SK-Beecham)	**Lozenges**: 3 mg dyclonine hydrochloride, menthol	Corn syrup, sucrose. Wintergreen and vapor black cherry flavors. In 24s, 48s, and 55s.
otc	**Cēpacol Sore Throat Post Nasal Drip** (Combe)	**Lozenges**: 3 mg menthol	Glucose, sucrose. Menthol flavor. In 18s.
otc	**Sucrets Sore Throat** (SK-Beecham)	**Lozenges**: 2.4 mg hexylresorcinol	In regular and mentholated flavors. In 24s.

Mouth and Throat Products

LOZENGES AND TROCHES

otc *sf*	**N'ice 'n Clear** (SK-Beecham)	**Lozenges:** 5 mg menthol	Sorbitol. Cool peppermint, cherry eucalyptus, and menthol eucalyptus flavors. In 16s.
otc	**Robitussin Honey Cough** (Whitehall-Robins)		Herbal with natural honey center. Corn syrup, sorbitol, sucrose. In 20s. Honey lemon tea flavor: Corn syrup, sucrose. In 25s.
otc	**Cēpacol Sore Throat Post Nasal Drip** (Combe)	**Lozenges:** 5.4 mg menthol	Glucose, sucrose. Cherry flavor. In 18s.
otc	**Kof-Eze** (Roberts Med)	**Lozenges:** 6 mg menthol	In 4s and 500s.
otc	**Menthol Cough Drops** (Major)	**Lozenges:** 6.5 mg menthol	Eucalyptus oil, glucose syrup, sucrose. In 30s.
otc	**Extra Strength Vicks Cough Drops** (Richardson-Vicks)	**Lozenges:** 8.4 mg menthol	Corn syrup, sucrose. Menthol flavor. In 9s and 30s.
otc	**Extra Strength Vicks Cough Drops** (Richardson-Vicks)	**Lozenges:** 10 mg menthol	Corn syrup, sucrose. Cherry and honey lemon flavors. In 9s and 30s.
otc	**Maximum Strength Halls-Plus** (Warner-Lambert)	**Lozenges:** 10 mg menthol	Corn syrup, sucrose. In regular, cherry, mentholyptus, and honey-lemon flavors. In 10s and 25s.
otc	**Robitussin Cough Drops** (Robins)	**Lozenges:** 7.4 mg menthol, eucalyptus oil	Sucrose, corn syrup. (R). In cherry and menthol eucalyptus flavors. In 9s and 25s.
		10 mg menthol, eucalyptus oil	Sucrose, corn syrup. (R). Honey-lemon flavor. In 9s and 25s.
otc	**Vicks Menthol Cough Drops** (Richardson-Vicks)	**Lozenges:** Menthol, thymol, eucalyptus oil, camphor, tolu balsam	Benzyl alcohol. Menthol flavor. In 14s and 40s.
otc *sf*	**Cēpastat Cherry** (Heritage Consumer Prod.)	**Lozenges:** 14.5 mg phenol, menthol	Saccharin, sorbitol. Cherry flavor. In 18s.
otc *sf*	**Cēpastat Extra Strength** (Heritage Consumer Prod.)	**Lozenges:** 29 mg phenol, menthol, eucalyptus oil	Sorbitol. In 18s.
otc	**Get Better Bear Sore Throat Pops** (Whitehall)	**Lozenge on a stick:** 19 mg pectin	Corn syrup, sucrose, parabens. Cherry and grape flavors. In 10s.
otc	**Cēpacol Anesthetic** (J.B. Williams)	**Troches:** 10 mg benzocaine, 0.07% cetylpyridinium chloride	Tartrazine. In 18s and 24s.
otc *sf*	**Hall's Sugar Free Mentho-Lyptus** (Warner-Lambert)	**Tablets:** 5 mg menthol, 2.8 mg eucalyptus oil	Citrus blend and black cherry flavors. In 25s.
		Tablets: 6 mg menthol, 2.8 mg eucalyptus oil	Mountain menthol flavor. In 25s.

MOUTHWASHES AND SPRAYS

otc	**TiSol** (Parnell)	**Solution:** 1% benzyl alcohol, 0.04% menthol, 0.9% isotonic NaCl	EDTA, sorbitol. In 237 mL.
Rx	**OraMagicRx** (MPM Medical)	**Powder for oral rinse:** *AloemannonPlus* (high molecular weight complex carbohydrates, mannons, and low molecular weight constituents extracted from aloe vera L), citric acid, lemon/lime flavor, maltodextrin, potassium benzoate, potassium sorbate, xanthan, xylitol	Alcohol free. In 25 and 37.5 g.
otc	**FreshBurst Listerine** (GlaxoWellcome)	**Rinse:** 0.064% thymol, 0.092% eucalyptol, 0.06% methyl salicylate, 0.042% menthol, 21.6% alcohol	Sorbitol, saccharin. In 250 mL.
otc	**Scope** (Procter & Gamble)	**Rinse:** Cetylpyridinium chloride, 67.9% SD alcohol 38-F	Tartrazine, saccharin. Original mint and wintergreen flavors. In 90, 180, 360, 720, 1,080, and 1,440 mL.
otc *sf*	**Sucrets** (SK-Beecham)	**Throat spray:** 0.1% dyclonine hydrochloride, 10% alcohol	Sorbitol. Mint and cherry flavors. In 90 and 180 mL.
otc	**Cēpacol Sore Throat** (Combe)	**Spray:** 0.1% dyclonine hydrochloride, 33% glycerin	Menthol. Cherry, honey-lemon, citrus, menthol, and sugar-free cherry flavors. In 118 mL.
otc	**N'ice** (SK-Beecham)	**Throat spray:** 0.12% menthol, 25% glycerin, 23% alcohol	Glucose, saccharin, sorbitol. Peppermint flavor. In 180 mL.
otc *sf*	**Chloraseptic Kids Sore Throat** (Prestige)	**Throat spray:** 0.5% phenol	Saccharin. Alcohol free. Grape flavor. In 177 mL.
otc *sf*	**Triaminic Sore Throat** (Novartis Consumer Health)		Alcohol free. Saccharin, sorbitol. Grape flavor. In 118 mL.
otc *sf*	**Chloraseptic Sore Throat** (Prestige)	**Throat spray:** 1.4% phenol	Saccharin. Alcohol free. Cherry, soothing citrus, menthol, and cool mint flavors. In 177 mL.
otc *sf*	**Sore Throat Spray** (Major)		Alcohol free. Saccharin. Cherry and menthol flavors. In 177 mL.
otc *sf*	**Phenaseptic** (Rugby)		Saccharin. Cherry flavor. In 177 mL.
otc *sf*	**Green Throat Spray** (Clay-Park Labs)		Alcohol free. Glycerin, saccharin. In 473 mL.
otc *sf*	**Red Throat Spray** (Clay-Park Labs)		Alcohol free. Glycerin, saccharin. In 177 mL.
otc	**Cheracol Sore Throat** (Roberts)	**Throat spray:** 1.4% phenol, 12.5% alcohol	Sorbitol, saccharin. Cherry flavor. In 180 mL.
otc *sf*	**Mycinette** (Pfeiffer)	**Throat spray:** 1.4% phenol, 0.3% alum (aluminum ammonium sulfate)	Alcohol free. Regular, cherry, mint, and cool blue menthol flavors. In 180 mL.
otc	**Throto-Ceptic** (S.S.S. Company)	**Spray/Gargle:** 1.4% phenol, 0.5% alum (aluminum ammonium sulfate)	Mint, cherry, cool blue menthol, or regular flavors. In 171 mL.
otc *sf*	**Vicks Chloraseptic** (Procter & Gamble)	**Mouthrinse/Gargle:** 1.4% phenol	Alcohol free. Saccharin. Menthol flavor. In 355 mL.

MOUTHWASHES AND SPRAYS

otc	**Bioténe with Calcium** (Laclede)	**Mouthwash**: Propylene glycol, xylitol, hydrogenated starch hydrosylate, poloxamer 407, hydroxyethylcellulose, sodium benzoate, peppermint, benzoic acid, zinc gluconate, aloe vera, calcium lactate, lactoferrin, lysozyme, lactoperoxidase, potassium thiocyanate, glucose oxidase	Alcohol free. In 474 mL.
otc *sf*	**Choice DM Gentle Care** (Bristol-Myers Squibb)	**Mouthwash**: Sorbitol, poloxamer 407, sodium, saccharin, flavor, cetylpyridinium chloride, citric acid, blue 1, yellow 5	Alcohol free. Fresh mint flavor. In 500 mL.
otc	**Listerine, Natural Citrus** (Pfizer Consumer)	**Mouthwash**: 0.064% thymol, 0.092% eucalyptol, 0.06% methyl salicylate, 0.042% menthol, 21.6% alcohol	Sorbitol, sucralose. In 250 and 500 mL and 1 and 1.5 L.
otc	**Listerine, Tartar Control** (Pfizer Consumer)	**Mouthwash**: 0.064% thymol, 0.092% eucalyptol, 0.06% methyl salicylate, 0.042% menthol, 21.6% alcohol	Sorbitol, sucrose. Wintermint flavor. In 250 and 500 mL and 1 and 1.5 L.
otc	**Listermint Arctic Mint** (GlaxoWellcome)	**Mouthwash**: Glycerin, poloxamer 335, PEG 600, sodium lauryl sulfate, sodium benzoate, benzoic acid, zinc chloride	Saccharin. In 946 mL.
otc	**Cēpacol** (J.B. Williams)	**Mouthwash**: 0.05% cetylpyridinium chloride, 14% alcohol	Tartrazine, saccharin. In 360, 540, 720, and 960 mL.
otc	**Plax** (Pfizer Consumer Health)	**Mouthwash**: Sorbitol solution, 8.7% alcohol, tetrasodium pyrophosphate, benzoic acid, flavor, poloxamer 407, sodium benzoate, sodium lauryl sulfate, sodium saccharin, xanthan gum	Original, mint sensation, and softmint flavors. In 118, 237, 473, and 710 mL.
otc	**Listerine** (GlaxoWellcome)	**Mouthwash**: 0.06% thymol, 0.09% eucalyptol, 0.06% methyl salicylate, 0.04% menthol, 26.9% alcohol (regular flavor), 21.6% alcohol (cool mint flavor)	Sorbitol, saccharin (Cool Mint). Regular, cool mint flavors. In 90, 180, 360, 540, 720, 960, and 1,440 mL.
otc	**Phylorinol** (Schaffer)	**Mouthwash**: 0.6% phenol, methyl salicylate	Alcohol free. Sorbitol. In 240 mL.
otc	**Oral Wound Rinse** (Carrington Laboratories)	**Mouthwash**: Acemannan hydrogel	Fructose. In 7.4 g
otc	**Tonsiline** (Oakhurst)	**Mouthwash**: 4% alcohol, glycerin, sucrose, iron chloride, flavor, magnesium carbonate, tolu balsam, sodium saccharide	In 118 mL.

MISCELLANEOUS MOUTH AND THROAT PREPARATIONS

otc	**Dent's Extra Strength Toothache Gum** (C.S. Dent)	**Gum**: 20% benzocaine	In 1 g.
otc	**Baby Orajel** (Del Pharm)	**Liquid**: 7.5% benzocaine	Parabens, saccharin, sorbitol. Very berry flavor. In 13.3 mL.
otc sf	**Tanac Roll-On** (Del Pharm)	**Liquid**: 5% benzocaine, 0.12% benzalkonium chloride	Saccharin. In 8.8 mL.
otc	**Anbesol** (Whitehall)	**Liquid**: 6.3% benzocaine, 0.5% phenol, 70% alcohol, menthol, camphor, povidone-iodine	In 9 and 22 mL.
otc	**Orasol** (Goldline)	**Liquid**: 6.3% benzocaine, 0.5% phenol, 70% alcohol, povidone-iodine	In 14.79 mL.
otc	**Tanac** (Del Pharm)	**Liquid**: 10% benzocaine, 0.12% benzalkonium chloride	Saccharin. In 13 mL.
otc	**Dent-O-Kain/20** (Geritrex)	**Liquid**: 20% benzocaine	Benzyl alcohol, saccharin. In 9 mL.
otc	**Maximum Strength Orajel** (Del Pharm)	**Liquid**: 20% benzocaine, 44.2% ethyl alcohol, phenol	Tartrazine, saccharin. In 13.3 mL.
otc sf	**Orajel Mouth-Aid** (Del Pharm)	**Liquid**: 20% benzocaine, 0.1% cetylpyridinium chloride, 70% ethyl alcohol, povidone	Tartrazine, saccharin. In 13.3 mL.
otc	**Maximum Strength Anbesol** (Whitehall)	**Liquid**: 20% benzocaine, 60% alcohol, polyethylene glycol	Saccharin. In 9 mL.
otc	**Dent's Maximum Strength Toothache Drops** (C.S. Dent)	**Liquid**: 20% benzocaine, 74% alcohol, eugenol, 0.09% chlorobutanol anhydrous	In 3.7 mL.
otc	**Double-Action Toothache Kit** (C.S. Dent)	**Liquid**: Benzocaine, 74% alcohol, 0.09% chlorobutanol anhydrous	Also contains *Maranox Pain Relief Tablets* containing 325 mg acetaminophen. In 8 tablets with 3.7 mL drops.
otc	**Red Cross Toothache** (Mentholatum)	**Liquid**: 85% eugenol, sesame oil	In 3.7 mL with cotton pellets and tweezers.
otc sf	**Ulcerease** (Med-Derm)	**Liquid**: 0.6% liquefied phenol, glycerin, sodium bicarbonate, sodium borate	Alcohol free. In 180 mL.
otc	**Phylorinol** (Schaffer)	**Liquid**: 0.6% phenol, boric acid, strong iodine solution, sodium copper chlorophyll	Sorbitol. In 240 mL.
otc	**Curasore** (S.S.S. Company)	**Liquid**: 1% pramoxine hydrochloride	Ethyl alcohol, ethyl ether. In 15 mL.
otc	**Orasept** (Pharmakon Labs)	**Liquid**: 12.16% tannic acid, 1.53% methylbenzethonium Cl, 53.31% denatured ethyl alcohol, camphor, menthol, benzyl alcohol, spearmint oil and oil of Cassia	In 15 mL.
otc	**Kank-a** (Blistex)	**Liquid/Film**: 20% benzocaine, benzoin compound tincture, SD alcohol 38b, benzyl alcohol, castor oil	Saccharin. In 9.9 mL.
otc	**Benzodent** (Procter & Gamble)	**Ointment**: 20% benzocaine	In 30 g.
otc	**Blistex** (Blistex)	**Ointment**: 0.5% camphor, 0.5% phenol, 1% allantoin, lanolin	Mineral oil base. In 4.2 and 10.5 g.
otc	**Lip Medex** (Blistex)	**Ointment**: Petrolatum, 1% camphor, 0.54% phenol, cocoa butter, lanolin	In 210 g.
otc	**Orajel P.M. Nighttime Formula Toothache Pain Relief** (Del Pharm)	**Cream**: 20% benzocaine, menthol, methyl salicylate, saccharin	In 5.4 g.
otc	**Abreva** (SmithKline Beecham Consumer)	**Cream**: 10% docosanol, benzyl alcohol, light mineral oil	In 2 g.
otc	**Numzit Teething** (Goody's)	**Lotion**: 0.2% benzocaine, 12.1% alcohol, 0.02% saccharin, 2% glycerin, 0.5% kelgin MU	Methylparaben, saccharin. In 15 mL.
otc sf	**Babee Teething** (Pfeiffer)	**Lotion**: 2.5% benzocaine, 0.02% cetalkonium chloride, camphor, eucalyptol, menthol	Dye free. Alcohol. In 15 mL.
otc	**Pfeiffer's Cold Sore** (Pfeiffer)	**Lotion**: 7% gum benzoin, camphor, menthol, eucalyptol, 85% alcohol	In 15 mL.
otc	**Dent's Lotion-Jel** (C.S. Dent)	**Lotion/Gel**: Benzocaine	In 6 g.
otc	**Banadyne-3** (Norstar)	**Solution**: 4% lidocaine, menthol 1%, 45% alcohol	In 7.5 mL.
otc	**Peroxyl Dental Rinse** (Colgate)	**Solution**: 1.5% hydrogen peroxide, 6% alcohol	Mint flavor. In 240 mL and pint.
otc	**Amosan** (Oral-B)	**Powder**: Sodium peroxyborate monohydrate (derived from sodium perborate)	Saccharin. Peppermint, menthol, and vanilla flavors. In 1.7 g UD packets (20s and 40s).
otc	**hda Toothache Gel** (S.S.S. Company)	**Gel**: 6.5% benzocaine	Benzyl alcohol, glycerin. In 15 mL bottle with applicator.
otc	**Baby Anbesol** (Whitehall)	**Gel**: 7.5% benzocaine	EDTA, saccharin. In 7.2 g.
otc	**Baby Orajel** (Del Pharm)	**Gel**: 7.5% benzocaine	Saccharin, sorbitol. Alcohol free. In 9.45 g.
otc	**Baby Orajel Nighttime** (Del Pharm)	**Gel**: 10% benzocaine	Alcohol free. Saccharin, sorbitol. Cherry flavor. In 6 g.
otc sf	**Orajel/d** (Del Pharm)	**Gel**: 10% benzocaine	Saccharin. In 9.45 g.
otc	**Numzident** (Goody's)	**Gel**: 10% benzocaine, 47.86% PEG 400 NF, 10% PEG 3350 NF	Saccharin. Cherry-vanilla flavor. In 15 g.
otc	**Zilactin-B Medicated** (Zila)	**Gel**: 10% benzocaine, 76% alcohol	In 7.5 g.
otc sf	**Orajel Brace-aid** (Del Pharm)	**Gel**: 20% benzocaine	Saccharin. In 14.1 g.
otc	**SensoGARD** (Block)	**Gel**: 20% benzocaine	Parabens. In 0.5 g.

MISCELLANEOUS MOUTH AND THROAT PREPARATIONS

otc	**Maximum Strength Orajel** (Del Pharm)	**Gel**: 20% benzocaine	Saccharin. In 9.45 g.
otc	**Maximum Strength Anbesol** (Whitehall)	**Gel**: 20% benzocaine, 60% alcohol, carbomer 934P, polyethylene glycol	Saccharin. In 7.2 g.
otc sf	**Orajel Mouth-Aid** (Del Pharm)	**Gel**: 20% benzocaine, 0.02% benzalkonium chloride, 0.1% zinc chloride	Saccharin. In 9.45 g.
otc	**Baby Orajel Tooth & Gum Cleanser** (Del Pharm)	**Gel**: 2% poloxamer 407, 0.12% simethicone	Parabens, saccharin, sorbitol. In 14.2 g.
otc	**Numzit Teething** (Goody's)	**Gel**: 7.5% benzocaine, 0.018% peppermint oil, 0.09% clove leaf oil, 66.2% PEG-400, 26.1% PEG-3350	0.036% saccharin. In 14.1 g.
otc sf	**Anbesol** (Whitehall)	**Gel**: 6.3% benzocaine, 0.5% phenol, 70% alcohol, camphor	In 7.5 g.
otc	**Toothache Gel** (Roberts Med)	**Gel**: Benzocaine, oil of cloves, benzyl alcohol, propylene glycol	In 15 g.
otc	**Probax** (Fischer)	**Gel**: 2% propolis, petrolatum, mineral oil, lanolin	In 3.5 g.
otc	**Tanac** (Del Pharm)	**Gel**: 1% dyclonine hydrochloride, 0.5% allantoin, petrolatum, lanolin	In 9.45 g.
otc	**Zilactin** (Blairex Labs)	**Gel**: 10% benzyl alcohol	Salicylic acid, hydroxypropylcellulose. In 7 g.
otc	**Rembrandt Canker Pain Relief Kit** (Den-Mat Corp.)	**Gel**: 5% benzocaine **Rinse**: Methylparaben, saccharin **Paste**: 0.15% fluoride ion from sodium monofluorophosphate w/v ½.	In 28 g. In 37 mL. In 34 g.
otc	**Orabase-B** (Colgate)	**Paste**: 20% benzocaine, mineral oil	In 5 and 15 g.
Rx	**Orabase HCA** (Colgate)	**Paste**: 0.5% hydrocortisone acetate, 5% polyethylene, mineral oil	In 5 g.
Rx	**Kenalog in Orabase** (Apothecon)	**Paste**: 0.1% triamcinolone acetonide	In 5 g.
Rx	**Oralone Dental** (Thames)	**Paste**: 0.1% triamcinolone acetonide	In 5 g.
otc	**Orabase-Plain** (Colgate)	**Paste**: Plasticized hydrocarbon gel	In 5 and 15 g.
otc	**Tanac Dual Core** (Del Pharm)	**Stick**: 7.5% benzocaine, 6% tannic acid, 0.75% octyl dimethyl PABA, 0.2% allantoin, 0.12% benzalkonium chloride	Cetyl alcohol, butylparaben. In 2.84 g stick.
otc	**Blistex** (Blistex)	**Lip balm**: 0.5% camphor, 0.5% phenol, 1% allantoin, 2% dimethicone, 6.6% padimate O, 2.5% oxybenzone, petrolatum	SPF 10. Parabens. In 4.5 g.
otc	**Herpecin-L** (Campbell Labs)	**Lip balm**: Allantoin, padimate O	In 2.8 g.
otc	**Blistex** (Blistex)	**Lip balm**: 1% camphor, 1% menthol, 0.5% phenol, petrolatum, cocoa butter, lanolin, mixed waxes, oil of cloves	In 0.25 and 0.38 oz.
otc	**Chap Stick Medicated Lip Balm** (Robins)	**Lip balm**: 1% camphor, 0.6% menthol, 0.5% phenol, petrolatum, mineral oil, cocoa butter, lanolin	Parabens. In jars (7 g), squeezable tubes (10 g), and sticks (4.2 g).
otc	**3 in 1 Toothache Relief** (C.S. Dent)	**Gum, Liquid, Lotion/Gel**: Benzocaine	In family first-aid packs.
otc	**Chloraseptic Kids Sore Throat** (Medtech)	**Strips**: 2 mg benzocaine, 2 mg menthol	Glycerin, sucralose. In 20s.

PREPARATIONS FOR SENSITIVE TEETH

otc	**Denquel Sensitive Teeth** (Procter & Gamble)	**Toothpaste**: 5% potassium nitrate	Mint flavor. In 48, 90 and 135 g.
otc	**Sensodyne Cool Gel** (Block)	**Toothpaste**: Potassium nitrate, sodium fluoride	Saccharin, sorbitol, parabens. In 28.3 g.
otc	**Sensodyne-F** (Block)	**Toothpaste**: Potassium nitrate, sodium monofluorophosphate	Saccharin, sorbitol. In 72 and 138 g.
otc	**Sensodyne-SC** (Block)	**Toothpaste**: 10% strontium Cl hexahydrate	Saccharin, sorbitol, parabens. In 26 g.
otc	**Sensitivity Protection Crest** (Procter & Gamble)	**Toothpaste**: Sodium fluoride, potassium nitrate	Mint flavor. In 175 g.
otc	**Sensodyne Fresh Mint** (Block)	**Toothpaste**: Potassium nitrate, sodium monofluorophosphate	Sorbitol, saccharin. In 26 g.
Rx	**Triamcinolone Acetonide Dental 0.1%** (Various, eg, Qualitest, Taro)	**Paste**: 0.1% triamcinolone acetonide	In 5 g.

DENTAL PREPARATIONS FOR SENSITIVE TEETH — ORAL

Administration and Dosage

These toothpastes are specially formulated to replace regular toothpaste for people with sensitive teeth. Use daily as in regular dental care.

CHLOROPHYLL DERIVATIVES (Chlorophyllin)

otc sf	**Chlorophyll** (Freeda)	**Tablets:** 20 mg chlorophyll	In 100s, 250s and 500s.
otc	**PALS** (Palisades)	**Tablets:** 100 mg chlorophyllin copper complex	In 100s.
otc	**Chloresium** (Rystan)	**Tablets:** 14 mg chlorophyllin copper complex	In 100s and 1000s.
otc	**Derifil** (Integra LifeSciences)	**Tablets:** 100 mg chlorophyllin copper complex sodium	6 mg sodium, dextrose. (D). Dark green, scored. Film coated. In 30s, 100s, and 1,000s.
otc	**Chloresium** (Rystan)	**Solution:** 0.2% chlorophyllin copper complex in an isotonic saline solution	In 240 mL and qt.
otc	**Chloresium** (Rystan)	**Ointment:** 0.5% water-soluble chlorophyllin copper complex in a hydrophilic base	In 30 and 120 g and lb.

CHLOROPHYLL DERIVATIVES (Chlorophyllin) – ORAL AND TOPICAL

Refer to the Dermatologicals chapter for additional information.

Indications

➤*Oral:* To control fecal odors in colostomy, ileostomy or incontinence; also for certain breath and body odors.

➤*Topical:* To promote normal healing, relieve pain and inflammation, and reduce malodors in wounds, burns, surface ulcers, cuts, abrasions and skin irritations.

Administration and Dosage

➤*Topical:*

Ointment – Apply generously and cover with gauze, linen or other appropriate dressing. Change no more often than every 48 to 72 hours.

Solution – Apply full strength as continuous wet dressing.

➤*Oral:*

Adults and children (older than 12 years of age) – 1 to 2 tablets/day; may be increased to 3 tablets/day.

Children (younger than 12 years of age) – Consult physician.

➤*Ostomies:* In ostomies, take tablets orally or place in the appliance.

Warnings

➤*Diarrhea:* If cramping or diarrhea occur, reduce the dosage.

Adverse Reactions

Oral – No toxic effects have been reported. A temporary mild laxative effect may occur; the stool is commonly stained dark green.

Topical – Sensitivity reactions are extremely rare; only a few instances of slight itching or irritation have been reported.

BISMUTH SUBGALLATE

otc	**Devrom** (Parthenon)	**Tablets:** 200 mg	Lactose, sugar. Chewable. In 100s.

BISMUTH SUBGALLATE – ORAL

Indications

To control fecal odors in colostomy, ileostomy or incontinence.

Administration and Dosage

Take 1 or 2 tablets 3 times daily with meals. Chew or swallow whole.

Adverse Reactions

A temporary darkening of the tongue or stool may occur.

ANORECTAL PREPARATIONS

The anorectal preparations are used primarily for the symptomatic relief of the discomfort associated with hemorrhoids and perianal itching or irritation. In addition to the products specifically listed in this section, many of the Topical Local Anesthetics and Topical Corticosteroids may also be used locally in anorectal therapy (see specific monographs in the Dermatologics chapter).

Active Ingredients

The various components of these products are briefly discussed below. For complete information on specific indications, contraindications, precautions and adverse effects of ingredients, refer to the appropriate monographs as indicated.

➤*Hydrocortisone:* Hydrocortisone (see additional monographs in the Endocrine/Metabolic and Dermatologics chapters) reduces inflammation, itching and swelling.

➤*Local anesthetics:* Local anesthetics (benzocaine, pramoxine) temporarily relieve pain, itching and irritation. The most frequent adverse effects of topical local anesthetic use are allergic reactions (eg, burning, itching). Their safety and efficacy when used intrarectally require further evaluation (see additional monographs in the Dermatologics chapter).

➤*Vasoconstrictors:* Vasoconstrictors (ephedrine, phenylephrine) reduce swelling and congestion of anorectal tissues. They relieve local itching by a slight anesthetic effect. These agents are not effective in stopping bleeding from venous tissues.

➤*Astringents:* Astringents (witch hazel, zinc oxide) coagulate the protein in skin cells, protecting the underlying tissue and decreasing the cell volume. They lessen mucus and other secretions, and relieve anorectal irritation and inflammation.

➤*Antiseptics:* Antiseptics (benzalkonium chloride, phenylmercuric nitrate) are not of therapeutic value when applied to the anorectal area. There is no convincing evidence that they prevent infection in the anorectal area. Many are present as preservatives.

➤*Emollients/protectants:* Emollients (glycerin, lanolin, mineral oil, petrolatum, zinc oxide, cocoa butter, shark liver oil, bismuth salts) form a physical barrier on the skin and lubricate tissues, preventing irritation of the anorectal area and water loss from the stratum corneum. Many of these substances are used as bases and carriers of pharmacologically active compounds.

➤*Counterirritants:* Counterirritants (camphor) evoke a feeling of comfort, cooling, tingling or warmth and distract the perception of pain and itching.

➤*Keratolytics:* Keratolytics (resorcinol) cause desquamation and sloughing of epidermal surface cells and may help to expose underlying tissue to therapeutic agents.

➤*Wound-healing agents:* Wound-healing agents (balsam peru, skin respiratory factor or srf, yeast cell derivative) are claimed to promote wound healing or tissue repair. Effectiveness of these compounds has not been conclusively demonstrated.

➤*Anticholinergic agents:* Anticholinergic agents inhibit the action of acetylcholine. Because these agents produce their action systemically, they are not effective in ameliorating local symptoms of anorectal disease.

Patient Information

Maintain normal bowel function by proper diet, adequate fluid intake and regular exercise.

Products for external use only are not to be used intrarectally. Apply external products sparingly after, rather than before, a bowel movement. If possible, wash, rinse and dry the area before use.

Avoid excessive laxative use.

Stool softeners or bulk laxatives may be useful adjunctive therapy.

In general, patients with conditions such as diabetes, hypertension, hyperthyroidism or cardiovascular disease should not use products containing vasoconstrictors.

Products containing resorcinol should not be used on open wounds.

If anorectal symptoms do not improve in 7 days, or if bleeding, protrusion, seepage or pain occurs, consult a physician.

STEROID-CONTAINING PRODUCTS

Rx	**Lidocaine/Hydrocortisone Rectal** (River's Edge)	**Cream**: 0.5% hydrocortisone acetate, 3% lidocaine HCl	Alcohols, aluminum sulfate, glycerin, lt. mineral oil, parabens, petrolatum. In 7 g single-use units with applicator.
Rx	**Proctocort** (Salix)	**Cream**: 1% hydrocortisone	Stearyl and cetyl alcohols. In 28.35 g.
Rx	**Dermol HC** (Dermol)		Mineral oil, lanolin and cetyl alcohols, parabens. In 30 g.
Rx	**Analpram-HC** (Ferndale)	**Cream**: 1% hydrocortisone acetate, 1% pramoxine HCl	Cetyl alcohol, 0.1% potassium sorbate, 0.1% sorbic acid. In 30 g.
Rx	**ProctoCream-HC** (Schwarz Pharma)		In 30 g.
Rx	**Analpram-HC** (Ferndale)	**Cream**: 2.5% hydrocortisone acetate, 1% pramoxine HCl	0.1% potassium sorbate, 0.1 % sorbic acid, cetyl alcohol. In 30 g.
Rx	**Anusol-HC** (Salix)	**Cream**: 2.5% hydrocortisone	Petrolatum, EDTA, benzyl and stearyl alcohols. In 30 g.
Rx	**ProctoCream-HC** (Schwarz Pharma)	**Cream**: 2.5% hydrocortisone	Glycerin, stearyl alcohol, benzyl alcohol. In 30 g.
Rx	**HC Pramoxine** (Veracity[a])	**Cream**: 2.5% hydrocortisone acetate and 1% pramoxine hydrochloride	Cetyl alcohol. In 28 g.
Rx	**Dermol HC** (Dermol)	**Cream**: 2.5% hydrocortisone	Mineral oil, lanolin and cetyl alcohols, parabens. In 30 g.
Rx	**Analpram-HC** (Ferndale)	**Lotion**: 2.5% hydrocortisone acetate, 1% pramoxine hydrochloride	Hydrophilic. Alcohol, glycerin. In 60 mL.
Rx	**Dermol HC** (Dermol)	**Ointment**: 1% hydrocortisone	Mineral oil, white petrolatum. In 30 g.
Rx	**Cortifoam** (Schwarz Pharma)	**Aerosol Foam**: 10% hydrocortisone acetate	Parabens. 90 mg/applicatorful. In 14 applications.
Rx	**Proctofoam-HC** (Schwarz Pharma)	**Aerosol Foam**: 1% hydrocortisone acetate, 1% pramoxine HCl	Parabens, cetyl alcohol, stearyl alcohol. In 10 g (≥ 14 applications) w/applicator.
Rx	**Pramoxine HC** (Rugby)		Parabens, cetyl alcohol. In 10 g with applicator.
Rx	**Proctocort** (Salix)	**Suppositories**: 30 mg hydrocortisone acetate	In hydrogenated vegetable oil base. In 12s and 24s.
Rx	**Hydrocortisone Acetate** (Various, eg, Able, Clay-Park, Cypress, Major, Paddock)	**Suppositories**: 25 mg hydrocortisone acetate	In 12s and 24s.
Rx	**Anucort-HC** (G & W)		Vegetable oil. In 12, 24s and 100s.
Rx	**Anusol-HC** (Salix)		In a hydrogenated vegetable oil base. In 12s and 24s.
Rx	**Cort-Dome High Potency** (Bayer)		In 12s.
Rx	**Hemril-HC Uniserts** (Upsher-Smith)		Vegetable oil. In 12s.
Rx	**Hemorrhoidal HC** (Various, eg, Schein, Geneva, Goldline)		In 12s, 24s, 50s, 100s & UD 12s.

[a] Veracity Pharmaceuticals, 6601 Lyons Road, Suite E-7, Coconut Creek, FL 33073; (954) 426-4199, fax (954) 426-1905

Refer to the general discussion of these products in the Anorectal Preparations Introduction.

LOCAL ANESTHETIC-CONTAINING PRODUCTS

otc	**Tronolane** (Lee)	**Cream**: 1% pramoxine hydrochloride	5% zinc oxide, cetyl alcohol, parabens. In 30 and 60 g.
otc	**Americaine** (Novartis Consumer)	**Ointment**: 20% benzocaine	In 22.5 g.
otc	**Medicone** (Lee)	**Ointment**: 20% benzocaine	Mineral oil, white petrolatum. In 30 g.
otc	**Tucks** (Pfizer Consumer Health)	**Ointment**: 1% pramoxine hydrochloride	12.5% zinc oxide, 46.6% mineral oil and cocoa butter. In 30 g with applicator.
otc	**ProctoFoam NS** (Schwarz Pharma)	**Aerosol Foam**: 1% pramoxine hydrochloride	In 15 g with applicator.
otc	**Fleet Pain Relief** (Fleet)	**Pads**: 1% pramoxine hydrochloride, 12% glycerin	In 100s.

Refer to the general discussion of these products in the Anorectal Preparations Introduction. Also see Benzocaine and Pramoxine Hydrochloride monographs in the Local Anesthetics, Topical, section of the Dermatological Agents chapter.

PERIANAL HYGIENE PRODUCTS

otc	**Balneol Perianal Cleansing** (Solvay)	**Lotion**: Mineral oil, lanolin oil	Methylparaben. In 120 mL.
otc	**Sensi-Care Perineal Skin Cleanser Solution** (ConvaTec)	**Solution**: Sodium C_{12-14} olefin sulfonate, disodium cocoamphodiacetate.	Aloe vera. In 120 and 240 mL.
otc	**Bodi Kleen** (Geritrex)	**Spray**: Triethanolamine lauryl sulfate, 2-phenoxy-ethanol, hexylene glycol, aloe vera gel	In 8 oz.
otc	**Tucks Take-Alongs** (Parke-Davis)	**Pads**: 50% witch hazel and 10% glycerin with 0.003% benzalkonium Cl	In 12s.
otc	**Fleet Medicated Wipes** (Fleet)	**Pads**: 50% hamamelis water, 7% alcohol, 10% glycerin, benzalkonium chloride and methylparaben	In 100s.
otc	**Preparation H Cleansing** (Whitehall)	**Tissues**: Propylene glycol, phenoxyethanol	Alcohol free. Parabens, citric acid. In 15s and 40s.

Refer to the general discussion of these products in the Anorectal Preparations Introduction.

MISCELLANEOUS ANORECTAL COMBINATION PRODUCTS

otc	**Preparation H Cooling Gel** (Whitehall-Robins)	**Gel:** 50% witch hazel, 0.25% phenylephrine hydrochloride. 7.5% alcohol, EDTA, parabens.	In 51 g.
otc	**Preparation H** (Whitehall-Robins)	**Cream:** 18% petrolatum, 12% glycerin, 3% shark liver oil, 0.25% phenylephrine hydrochloride, cetyl alcohol, stearyl alcohol, EDTA, lanolin, parabens	In 27 and 54 g.
		Ointment: 71.9% petrolatum, 14% mineral oil, 3% shark liver oil, 0.25% phenylephrine hydrochloride, corn oil, glycerin, lanolin, lanolin alcohol, parabens, tocopherol	In 30 and 60 g.
otc	**Formulation R** (G & W)	**Cream:** 18% petrolatum, 12% glycerin, 0.25% phenylephrine hydrochloride	In 52 g.
		Ointment: 71.9% petrolatum, 14% mineral oil, 0.25% phenylephrine hydrochloride	Parabens. In 28.4 and 56.8 g.
otc	**Hem-Prep** (G & W)	**Ointment:** 0.025% phenylephrine hydrochloride, 11% zinc oxide, white petrolatum	In 42.5 g
otc	**Hemorrhoidal Ointment** (Cardinal Health)	**Ointment:** 0.25% phenylephrine hydrochloride, 3% shark liver oil, 71.9% petrolatum, 14% mineral oil	Benzoic acid, glycerin, lanolin, lanolin alcohol, parabens, thyme oil. In 57 g.
otc	**Preparation H** (Whitehall)	**Suppositories:** 3% shark liver oil, 79% cocoa butter, corn oil, EDTA, parabens and tocopherol	In 12s, 24s, 36s, and 48s.
otc	**Wyanoids Relief Factor** (Wyeth)	**Suppositories:** 79% cocoa butter, 3% shark liver oil, corn oil, EDTA, parabens and tocopherol	In 12s.
otc	**Nupercainal** (Ciba Consumer)	**Suppositories:** 2.1 g cocoa butter, 0.25 g zinc oxide and sodium bisulfite	In 12s and 24s.
otc	**Tucks** (Pfizer Consumer Health)	**Suppositories:** 51% topical starch	Benzyl alcohol, hydrogenated vegetable oil, vitamin E. In 12s and 24s.
otc	**Hemril Uniserts** (Upsher-Smith)	**Suppositories:** 2.25% bismuth subgallate, 1.75% bismuth resorcin compound, 1.2% benzyl benzoate, 11% zinc oxide, 1.8% balsam peru in hydrolyzed vegetable oil base	In 12s and 50s.
otc	**Rectagene** (Pfeiffer)	**Suppositories:** Live yeast cell derivative supplying 2,000 units Skin Respiratory Factor per ounce and shark liver oil in a cocoa butter base	In 12s.
otc	**Rectagene** II (Pfeiffer)	**Suppositories:** 2.25% bismuth subgallate, 1.75% bismuth resorcin compound, 1.2% benzyl benzoate, 1.8% peruvian balsam, 11% zinc oxide, bismuth subiodide, calcium phosphate in a hydrogenated vegetable oil base	In 12s.
otc	**Pazo Hemorrhoid** (Bristol-Myers)	**Suppositories:** 3.8 mg ephedrine sulfate, 96.5 mg zinc oxide, vegetable oil	In 12s and 24s.
otc	**Hem-Prep** (G & W)	**Suppositories:** 0.25% phenylephrine hydrochloride, 11% zinc oxide	In 12s.
otc	**Anu-Med** (Major)	**Suppositories:** 0.25% phenylephrine hydrochloride, 88.7% hard fat	Corn starch, parabens. In 12s.
otc	**Tronolane** (Ross)	**Suppositories:** 11% zinc oxide, 95% hard fat	In 10s and 20s.
otc	**Hemorid For Women** (Thompson Medical)	**Cream:** 30% white petrolatum, 20% mineral oil, 1% pramoxine hydrochloride, 0.25% phenylephrine hydrochloride, aloe vera gel, parabens, cetyl and stearyl alcohols	In 28.3 g.

Refer to the general discussion of these products in the Anorectal Preparations Introduction.

Indications

➤*Oral:* In the treatment of mildly to moderately severe infections caused by penicillin-sensitive microorganisms.

➤*Penicillinase-resistant penicillins:* The percentage of staphylococcal isolates resistant to **penicillin G** outside the hospital is increasing, approximating the high percentage found in the hospital. Therefore, use a penicillinase-resistant penicillin as initial therapy for any suspected staphylococcal infection until culture and sensitivity results are known.

When treatment is initiated before definitive culture and sensitivity results are known, consider that these agents are only effective in the treatment of infections caused by pneumococci, group A beta-hemolytic streptococci, and penicillin G-resistant and penicillin G-sensitive staphylococci.

➤*Parenteral:* In patients with severe infection or when there is nausea, vomiting, gastric dilatation, cardiospasm, or intestinal hypermotility. Parenteral aqueous **penicillin G** (eg, potassium, sodium) is the dosage form of choice in severe infections caused by penicillin-sensitive microorganisms when rapid and high penicillin serum levels are required.

For specific labeled indications, refer to individual drug monographs.

Administration and Dosage

Therapy may be initiated prior to obtaining results of bacteriologic studies when there is reason to believe the causative organisms may be susceptible. Once results are known, adjust therapy.

Dosage for any individual patient must take into consideration the severity of infection, the susceptibility of the organisms causing the infection and the status of the patient's host defense mechanism. Duration of therapy depends on the severity of the infection.

Continue treatment of all infections for a minimum of 48 to 72 hours beyond the time that the patient becomes asymptomatic or evidence of bacterial eradication has been obtained, unless single-dose therapy is employed. A minimum of 10 days treatment is recommended for any infection caused by group A beta-hemolytic streptococci to prevent the occurrence of acute rheumatic fever or acute glomerulonephritis.

Patients with a history of rheumatic fever or chorea and receiving continuous prophylaxis may harbor increased numbers of penicillin-resistant organisms.

Actions

➤*Pharmacology:* Penicillins are bactericidal antibiotics that include natural and semisynthetic derivatives. These agents contain the 6-β-aminopenicillanic acid nucleus and have a similar mechanism of action. All penicillins share cross-allergenicity. Significant differences among agents include: resistance to gastric acid inactivation; resistance to inactivation by penicillinase; spectrum of antimicrobial activity. In addition to the prototype **penicillin G**, this class includes an acid-stable penicillin G derivative (**penicillin V**), penicillinase-resistant penicillins, the aminopenicillins, and the extended spectrum derivatives. Several of these penicillins also are available in combination with agents that inactivate β-lactamase enzymes (eg, clavulanic acid, sulbactam), thereby extending the antibiotic spectrum to include many bacteria normally resistant to it and to other β-lactam antibiotics (see Pharmacokinetics). The available combinations include **ampicillin/sulbactam**, **amoxicillin/potassium clavulanate**, **ticarcillin/potassium clavulanate**, and **piperacillin/tazobactam sodium**.

Penicillins

	Routes of administration	Penicillinase-resistant	Acid stable	% Protein bound	May be taken with meals
Natural					
Penicillin G	IM-IV	no	no	60%	†[a]
Penicillin V	Oral	no	no	80%	yes
Penicillinase-resistant					
Dicloxacillin	Oral	yes	yes	98%	no
Nafcillin	IM-IV-Oral	yes	yes	87% to 90%	no
Oxacillin	IM-IV-Oral	yes	yes	94%	no
Aminopenicillins					
Amoxicillin	Oral	no	yes	20%	yes
Amoxicillin/potassium clavulanate	Oral	yes	yes	18%/25%	yes
Ampicillin	IM-IV-Oral	no	yes	20%	no
Ampicillin/sulbactam	IM-IV	yes	†[a]	28%/38%	†[a]
Extended-spectrum					
Carbenicillin	Oral	no	yes	50%	no
Piperacillin	IM-IV	no	†[a]	16%	†[a]
Piperacillin/tazobactam sodium	IV	yes	†[a]	30%/30%	†[a]
Ticarcillin	IM-IV	no	†[a]	45%	†[a]
Ticarcillin/potassium clavulanate	IV	yes	†[a]	45%/9%	†[a]

[a] Available only for intramuscular (IM) or intravenous (IV) use.

Mechanism – Penicillins inhibit the biosynthesis of cell wall mucopeptide. They are bactericidal against sensitive organisms when adequate concentrations are reached, and they are most effective during the stage of active multiplication. Inadequate concentrations may produce only bacteriostatic effects.

➤*Pharmacokinetics:*

Absorption – Because gastric acidity, stomach emptying time and other factors affecting absorption may vary considerably, serum levels may be reduced to nontherapeutic levels in certain individuals. **Penicillin V** shows less individual variation than **penicillin G** and has become the only natural penicillin available for oral administration. **Nafcillin**'s oral absorption is inferior to **oxacillin** and **dicloxacillin**. **Ampicillin** and **carbenicillin** indanyl have good GI absorption, but amoxicillin is more completely absorbed.

Absorption of most penicillins is affected by food; these medications are best taken on an empty stomach, 1 hour before or 2 hours after meals. Penicillin V may be given with meals; however blood levels may be slightly higher when given on an empty stomach. Amoxicillin tablets and **amoxicillin/potassium clavulanate** may be given without regard to meals.

Peak serum levels occur approximately 1 hour after oral use. After a 500 mg oral dose, peak serum concentrations for oxacillin and dicloxacillin range from 5 to 7, 7.5 to 14.4, and 10 to 17 mcg/mL, respectively. One hour after a 1 g oral nafcillin dose, average serum concentration was 1.19 mcg/mL (range, 0 to 3.12). IM injections of 1 g nafcillin, 560 mg oxacillin, and 1 g **methicillin** produced peak serum levels in 0.5 to 1 hour of 7.61, 15, and 17 mcg/mL, respectively.

Parenteral penicillin G (sodium and potassium) gives rapid and high but transient blood levels; derivatives provide prolonged penicillin blood levels with IM use. **Procaine penicillin G**, an equimolecular suspension of procaine and penicillin G, must be given IM; it dissolves slowly at the injection site and plateaus in about 4 hours; levels decline gradually over 15 to 20 hours. **Benzathine penicillin G** also must be given IM only; is absorbed very slowly from the injection site and is hydrolyzed to penicillin G; hence, serum levels are much lower but more prolonged, sustaining serum levels for up to 4 weeks.

Distribution – Penicillins are bound to plasma proteins, primarily albumin, in varying degrees (see table in Pharmacology section). They diffuse readily into most body tissues and fluids, including kidneys, liver, lungs, heart, skin, synovial fluid, intestines, bile, peritoneal fluid, bronchial and wound secretions, bone, prostate, pericardial and ascitic fluids, spleen and other tissues. Penetration into cerebrospinal fluid (CSF), the brain, and the eye occurs only with inflammation. CSF levels usually do not exceed 5% of penicillin G's peak serum concentration. Penicillins cross the placenta and appear in amniotic fluid and cord serum.

Excretion – Penicillins are excreted largely unchanged in the urine by glomerular filtration and active tubular secretion. Nonrenal elimination includes hepatic inactivation and excretion in bile; this is only a minor route for all penicillins except **nafcillin** and oxacillin. Excretion by renal tubular secretion can be delayed by coadministration of probenecid. Excretion is delayed in neonates and infants. Elimination half-life of most penicillins is short (1.4 h or less). Impaired renal function prolongs the serum half-life of penicillins eliminated primarily by renal excretion. The half-life is not greatly affected for nafcillin, oxacillin, and **dicloxacillin** because of increased biotransformation and biliary excretion. Because **piperacillin** is excreted by biliary and renal routes, it can be used safely in appropriate dosage in patients with severe renal impairment and in the treatment of hepatobiliary infections.

β-lactamase inhibitors: (Clavulanic acid, sulbactam, and tazobactam). These have weak antimicrobial activity but irreversibly inactivate bacterial β-lactamase enzymes. Used with β-lactam antibiotics, they protect antibiotics from inactivation by β-lactamase-producing organisms.

Clavulanic acid – Used in combination with **amoxicillin** and **ticarcillin**, it inhibits plasmid-mediated β-lactamases (eg, *Haemophilus influenzae*, *Neisseria gonorrheae*, *Escherichia coli*, *Salmonella*, *Shigella*, staphylococci) and chromosomal-mediated β-lactamases (eg, *Klebsiella*, *Bacteroides fragilis*, *Legionella*). It does not inhibit β-lactamases produced by *Enterobacter*, *Serratia*, *Morganella*, *Citrobacter*, *Pseudomonas*, or *Acinetobacter* species.

Clavulanic acid is well absorbed orally and widely distributed to many body tissues. Half-life is approximately 1 hour; 35% to 45% is excreted unchanged in the urine during the first 6 hours after administration. Probenecid does not alter renal excretion of clavulanic acid.

Sulbactam – Another β-lactamase inhibitor, this extends the bacterial spectrum of ampicillin to include such β-lactamase-producing organisms as *S. aureus*, *H. influenzae*, *B. fragilis*, and most strains of *E. coli*.

Tazobactam – This is a penicillanic acid sulfone β-lactamase inhibitor and has poor activity against chromosomal β-lactamases of Enterobacteriaceae but has good activity against many of the plasmid β-lactamases. Tazobactam extends the spectrum but does not increase the activity of **piperacillin** against *Pseudomonas aeruginosa*. The currently recommended piperacillin dose in **piperacillin/tazobactam** is less than the recommended dose of piperacillin when used alone for serious infections and may prove ineffective in the treatment of some *P. aeruginosa* infections. The manufacturer recommends concomitant aminoglycoside therapy when treating *P. aeruginosa* nosocomial pneumonia.

➤*Microbiology:* The following table indicates the organisms that are generally susceptible to the penicillins in vitro:

Organisms Generally Susceptible to Penicillins

	Organisms	Natural penicillins		Penicillinase-resistant			Aminopenicillins				Extended spectrum				
	✓ = Generally susceptible	Penicillin G	Penicillin V	Dicloxacillin	Nafcillin	Oxacillin	Amoxicillin	Ampicillin	Amoxicillin/potassium clavulanate	Ampicillin/sulbactam	Carbenicillin	Piperacillin	Ticarcillin	Ticarcillin/potassium clavulanate	Piperacillin/tazobactam sodium
Gram-positive	Staphylococci	✓[a]	✓[a]	✓	✓	✓	✓[a]	✓[a]	✓	✓	✓[a]	✓[a]	✓[a]	✓	
	Staphylococcus aureus	✓[a]	✓[a]	✓	✓	✓			✓	✓	✓[a]	✓[a]	✓[a]	✓	✓
	Staphylococcus epidermidis														✓[b]
	Streptococci	✓	✓					✓		✓					
	Streptococcus pneumoniae	✓	✓	✓	✓	✓	✓	✓	✓	✓	✓	✓	✓	✓	✓[c]
	Beta-hemolytic streptococci	✓	✓		✓		✓	✓	✓	✓	✓	✓	✓	✓	
	Enterococcus (Streptococcus) faecalis	✓[d]	✓				✓	✓	✓	✓	✓	✓	✓	✓	✓
	Streptococcus viridans	✓	✓		✓		✓	✓	✓	✓		✓		✓	
	Corynebacterium diphtheriae	✓	✓												
	Bacillus anthracis	✓	✓					✓		✓					
	Streptococcus agalactiae													✓	
	Streptococcus pyogenes													✓	
	Erysipelothrix rhusiopathiae	✓													
	Listeria monocytogenes	✓	✓				✓	✓		✓					
Gram-negative	*Escherichia coli*	✓					✓	✓	✓	✓	✓	✓	✓	✓	✓
	Haemophilus influenzae						✓	✓	✓	✓	✓	✓[c]	✓	✓	✓
	Haemophilus parainfluenzae														
	Eikenella corrodens								✓						
	Bacteroides melaninogenicus														✓
	Pseudomonas sp.													✓	
	Klebsiella sp.								✓	✓		✓		✓	✓
	Neisseria gonorrhoeae	✓[a]	✓				✓	✓	✓	✓	✓	✓	✓	✓	✓
	Neisseria meningitidis	✓						✓	✓	✓		✓	✓	✓	✓[c]
	Proteus mirabilis	✓					✓	✓	✓	✓	✓	✓	✓	✓	✓
	Salmonella sp.	✓						✓		✓	✓	✓	✓	✓	
	Shigella sp.	✓						✓		✓		✓			
	Morganella morganii									✓	✓	✓	✓	✓	✓
	Proteus vulgaris									✓	✓	✓	✓	✓	✓
	Providencia rettgeri									✓	✓	✓	✓	✓	
	Providencia stuartii									✓				✓	
	Enterobacter sp.	✓							✓	✓	✓	✓	✓	✓	
	Citrobacter sp.										✓	✓	✓	✓	
	Pseudomonas aeruginosa										✓	✓	✓	✓	✓
	Serratia sp.										✓	✓	✓	✓	✓
	Acinetobacter sp.									✓		✓		✓	
	Streptobacillus moniliformis	✓	✓												
	Moraxella (Branhamella) catarrhalis								✓	✓		✓		✓	✓
Anaerobic	*Clostridium* sp.	✓	✓				✓	✓	✓	✓	✓	✓	✓	✓	✓
	Peptococcus sp.	✓	✓				✓	✓	✓	✓	✓	✓	✓	✓	
	Peptostreptococcus sp.	✓	✓				✓		✓	✓	✓	✓	✓	✓	
	Bacteroides sp.	✓[e]							✓	✓	✓	✓	✓	✓	✓
	Fusobacterium sp.	✓							✓	✓	✓	✓	✓	✓	✓
	Eubacterium sp.	✓										✓		✓	
	Treponema pallidum	✓	✓												
	Actinomyces bovis	✓	✓									✓			
	Veillonella sp.											✓	✓	✓	

[a] Nonpenicillinase-producing.
[b] Nonmethicillin/oxacillin-resistant strains.
[c] Nonbeta-lactamase-producing.
[d] Bacteriostatic effect.
[e] Many strains of *B. fragilis* are resistant.

Contraindications

History of hypersensitivity to penicillins, cephalosporins, imipenem, or β-lactamase inhibitors (**piperacillin/tazobactam**).

Do not treat severe pneumonia, empyema, bacteremia, pericarditis, meningitis and purulent or septic arthritis with an oral penicillin during the acute stage.

History of **amoxicillin/clavulanate** potassium-associated cholestatic jaundice/hepatic dysfunction (amoxicillin/clavulanate potassium only).

Warnings

➤*Bleeding abnormalities:* **Ticarcillin** or **piperacillin** may induce hemorrhagic manifestations associated with abnormalities of coagulation tests (eg, bleeding time, prothrombin time, platelet aggregation). Upon withdrawal of the drug, bleeding should cease and coagulation abnormalities revert to normal. Observe patients with renal impairment, in whom excretion of these drugs is delayed, for prolonged bleeding manifestations.

➤*Cystic fibrosis:* These patients have a higher incidence of side effects (eg, fever, rash) when treated with extended spectrum penicillins (eg, **piperacillin, carbenicillin**). This may be caused by the higher IgE, IgG and eosinophil levels in this population.

➤*Hypersensitivity reactions:* Serious and occasionally fatal immediate hypersensitivity reactions have occurred. The incidence of anaphylactic shock is between 0.015% and 0.04%. Anaphylactic shock resulting in death has occurred in approximately 0.002% of the patients treated. Although anaphylaxis is more frequent following parenteral therapy, it may occur with oral use. Accelerated reactions (including urticaria and laryngeal edema) and delayed reactions (serum sickness-like reactions) may also occur. These reactions are likely to be immediate and severe in penicillin-sensitive individuals with a history of atopic conditions (see Adverse Reactions).

Hypersensitivity myocarditis – This is not dose-dependent and may occur at any time during treatment. The initial reaction involves rash, fever, and eosinophilia. The second stage reflects cardiac involvement. Sinus tachycardia, ST-T changes, slight increase in cardiac enzymes (creatine phosphokinase), and cardiomegaly.

An urticarial rash, not representing a true penicillin allergy, occasionally occurs with **ampicillin** (9%). This reaction is more frequent in patients on allopurinol (14% to 22.4%), patients with lymphatic leukemia (90%), and in those with infectious mononucleosis (43% to 100%). Typically, the rash appears 7 to 10 days after the start of oral ampicillin therapy and remains for a few days to a week after drug discontinuance. In most cases, the rash is maculopapular, pruritic, and generalized.

Before therapy, inquire about previous hypersensitivity reactions to penicillins, cephalosporins, and other allergens.

Desensitization: Patients with a positive skin test to one of the penicillin determinants can be desensitized, which is a relatively safe procedure. This is recommended in instances when penicillin must be given (eg, neurosyphilis, congenital syphilis, syphilis in pregnancy) where no proven alternatives exist. This can be done orally, IV, or subcutaneously; however, oral is thought to be safest and easiest. Various protocols are described, but each protocol utilizes the same principles, which involve gradually increasing doses of penicillin, increasing each dose every 15 to 20 minutes. For example, one oral protocol using **penicillin V** uses 14 total doses, each dose given 15 minutes apart. The units per dose are doubled at each interval (eg, 100, 200, 400, 800) for a total cumulative dose of 1.3 million units over 4 hours. After desensitization, maintain patients on penicillin for the duration of therapy.

Cross-allergenicity with cephalosporins: Individuals with a history of penicillin hypersensitivity have experienced severe reactions when treated with a cephalosporin. The incidence of cross-allergenicity between penicillins and cephalosporins is estimated to range from 5% to 16%; however, it is possible the incidence is much lower, possibly 3% to 7%.

Urticaria, other skin rashes and serum sickness-like reactions may be controlled by antihistamines and, if necessary, corticosteroids. Discontinue use unless the condition being treated is life-threatening and amenable only to penicillin therapy. Serious anaphylactoid reactions require emergency measures. (See Management of Acute Hypersensitivity Reactions).

➤*Renal function impairment:* Because **carbenicillin** is primarily excreted by the kidney, patients with severe renal impairment (creatinine clearance [Ccr] less than 10 mL/min) will not achieve the therapeutic urine levels of carbenicillin.

In patients with Ccr 10 to 20 mL/min, it may be necessary to adjust dosage to prevent accumulation of the drug.

Reduce the dosage of **penicillin G** in patients with severe renal impairment, with additional modifications when hepatic disease accompanies the renal impairment.

➤*Pregnancy: Category B.* There are no adequate or well-controlled studies in pregnant women. Penicillins cross the placenta. Use during pregnancy only if clearly needed.

Labor and delivery – Oral aminopenicillins are poorly absorbed during labor. It is not known whether use has immediate or delayed adverse effects on the fetus or alters normal labor.

➤*Lactation:* Penicillins are excreted in breast milk in low concentrations; use may cause diarrhea, candidiasis, or allergic response in the nursing infant. **Ampicillin** use by breast-feeding mothers may lead to sensitization of infants; therefore, decide whether to discontinue breast-feeding or ampicillin, taking into account the importance of the drug to the mother.

➤*Children:* Safety and efficacy of **carbenicillin**, **piperacillin**, and the β-lactamase inhibitor/penicillin combinations have not been established in infants and children younger than 12 years of age. Penicillins are excreted largely unchanged by the kidney. Because of incompletely developed renal function in infants, the rate of elimination will be slow. Penicillinase-resistant penicillins (especially **methicillin**) may not be completely excreted, with abnormally high blood levels resulting. Oral aminopenicillins are not absorbed as well in neonates as in adults. Use caution in administering to newborns and evaluate organ system function frequently. Frequent blood levels are advisable, with dosage adjustments when necessary. Monitor all newborns closely for clinical and laboratory evidence of toxic or adverse effects.

Precautions

➤*Monitoring:* Perform bacteriologic studies to determine causative organisms and their susceptibility so that appropriate therapy is administered.

Obtain blood cultures, white blood cell (WBC) and differential cell counts prior to initiation of therapy and at least weekly during therapy with penicillinase-resistant penicillins. Measure AST and ALT during therapy to monitor for liver function abnormalities.

Perform periodic urinalysis, blood-urea nitrogen (BUN), and creatinine determinations during therapy with penicillinase-resistant penicillins, and consider dosage alterations if these values become elevated. If renal impairment is known or suspected, reduce the total dosage and monitor blood levels to avoid possible neurotoxic reactions.

Monitoring is particularly important in newborns, infants and when high dosages are used.

➤*Streptococcal infections:* Therapy must be sufficient to eliminate the organism (a minimum of 10 days); otherwise, sequelae (eg, endocarditis, rheumatic fever) may occur. Take cultures after treatment to confirm that streptococci have been eradicated.

➤*Sexually transmitted diseases:* When treating gonococcal infections in which primary and secondary syphilis are suspected, perform proper diagnostic procedures, including darkfield examinations and monthly serological tests for at least 4 months. All cases of penicillin-treated syphilis should receive clinical and serological examinations every 6 months for 2 to 3 years. Test all syphilis patients for HIV infection.

➤*Resistance:* The number of strains of staphylococci resistant to penicillinase-resistant penicillins has been increasing; widespread use of penicillinase-resistant penicillins may result in an increasing number of resistant staphylococcal strains. Interpret resistance to any penicillinase-resistant penicillin as evidence of clinical resistance to all. Cross-resistance with cephalosporin derivatives also occurs frequently.

➤*Pseudomembranous colitis:* This has occurred with the use of broad spectrum antibiotics because of overgrowth of *Clostridia* sp; therefore, it is important to consider its diagnosis in patients who develop diarrhea in association with antibiotic use. Mild cases may respond to drug discontinuation alone. Manage moderate to severe cases with fluid, electrolyte, and protein supplementation. If it is not relieved by drug withdrawal, or when it is severe, oral vancomycin is the treatment of choice.

➤*Procaine sensitivity:* If sensitivity to the procaine in **penicillin G procaine** is suspected, inject 0.1 mL of a 1% to 2% procaine solution intradermally. Development of erythema, wheal, flare, or eruption indicates procaine sensitivity; treat by the usual methods. Do not use procaine penicillin preparations.

➤*Parenteral administration:* Inadvertent intravascular administration, including direct intra-arterial injection or injection immediately adjacent to arteries, has resulted in severe neurovascular damage, including transverse myelitis with permanent paralysis, gangrene requiring amputation of digits and more proximal portions of extremities, and necrosis and sloughing at and surrounding the injection site. Such severe effects have occurred following injections into the buttock, thigh, and deltoid areas. Other serious complications include immediate pallor, mottling, or cyanosis of the extremity, both distal and proximal to the injection site, followed by bleb formation; severe edema requiring anterior or posterior compartment fasciotomy in the lower extremity. These severe effects have most often occurred in infants and small children. Promptly consult a specialist if any evidence of a compromise of the blood supply occurs at, proximal to, or distal to the site of injection.

Quadriceps femoris fibrosis and atrophy have occurred following repeated IM injections of penicillin preparations into the anterolateral thigh.

Take particular care with IV administration because of the possibility of thrombophlebitis. Higher than recommended IV doses of most of the penicillins may cause neuromuscular excitability or convulsions.

Avoid subcutaneous and fat layer injections; pain and induration may occur. If these occur, apply an ice pack.

➤*Electrolyte imbalance:* Administer **aqueous penicillin G** IV in high doses (more than 10 million units) slowly because of electrolyte imbalance from either the potassium or sodium content. When sodium restriction is necessary (eg, cardiac patients), make periodic electrolyte determinations and monitor cardiac status.

Patients given continuous IV therapy with **potassium penicillin G** in high dosage (more than 10 million units daily) may suffer severe or even fatal potassium poisoning, particularly if renal insufficiency is present. Hyperreflexia, convulsions, coma, cardiac arrhythmias, and cardiac arrest may be indicative of this syndrome. High dosage of **sodium salts of penicillins** may result in or aggravate congestive heart failure because of high sodium intake. Individuals with liver disease or those receiving cytotoxic therapy or diuretics rarely demonstrated a decrease in serum potassium concentrations with high doses of **piperacillin**.

Sodium penicillin G contains 2 mEq sodium per million units, **potassium penicillin G** contains 1.7 mEq potassium and 0.3 mEq sodium per million units. The sodium content of other IV penicillin derivatives is listed below:

Sodium Content of IV Penicillins

Penicillin	Maximum recommended daily dose (g)	Sodium content (mEq/g)[a]	Sodium (mEq/day)[a,b]
Ampicillin sodium	14	2.9 to 3.1	40.6 to 43.4
Nafcillin sodium	6	2.9	17.4
Oxacillin sodium	6	2.5 to 3.1	15 to 18.6
Piperacillin sodium	24	1.85	44.4
Piperacillin/tazobactam sodium	12	2.35	28.2
Ticarcillin disodium	18	5.2 to 6.5	93.6 to 117

[a] 1 mEq sodium equals 23 mg.
[b] Based on maximum daily dose.

Hypokalemia – This has occurred in a few patients receiving **ticarcillin** and **piperacillin**. It may also occur in patients with low potassium reserves and in patients receiving cytotoxic therapy or diuretics. Monitor serum potassium and supplement when necessary.

➤*Superinfection:* Use of antibiotics (especially prolonged or repeated therapy) may result in bacterial or fungal overgrowth of nonsusceptible organisms. Such overgrowth may lead to a secondary infection. Take appropriate measures if this occurs.

Indwelling IV catheters encourage superinfections.

➤*Tartrazine sensitivity:* Some of these products contain tartrazine, which may cause allergic-type reactions (including bronchial asthma) in susceptible individuals. Although the incidence of tartrazine sensitivity in the general population is low, it is frequently seen in patients who also have aspirin hypersensitivity. Specific products containing tartrazine are identified in the product listings.

➤*Sulfite sensitivity:* Some of these products contain sodium formaldehyde sulfoxylate, a sulfite that may cause allergic-type reactions including anaphylactic symptoms and life-threatening or less severe asthmatic episodes in certain susceptible people. The overall prevalence of sulfite sensitivity in the general population is unknown and probably low. Sulfite sensitivity is seen more frequently in asthmatic than in nonasthmatic people.

Drug Interactions

Penicillin Drug Interactions

Precipitant drug	Object drug[a]		Description
Penicillins, parenteral	Aminoglycosides, parenteral	↔	Although these agents are often used together to achieve a synergistic action, certain penicillins may inactivate certain aminoglycosides in vitro. Do not mix in the same IV solution. Also, oral neomycin may reduce the serum concentrations of oral penicillin.
Penicillins, parenteral	Anticoagulants	↑	Large IV doses of penicillins can increase bleeding risks of anticoagulants by prolonging bleeding time. Conversely, nafcillin and dicloxacillin have been associated with warfarin resistance.
Penicillins, oral	Beta blockers	↔	Ampicillin may reduce the bioavailability of atenolol. Case reports indicated that beta blockers may potentiate anaphylactic reactions of penicillin.
Penicillins	Contraceptives, oral	↓	The efficacy of oral contraceptives may be reduced and increased breakthrough bleeding may occur. Although infrequently reported, contraceptive failure is possible; the use of an additional form of contraception during penicillin therapy is advisable.
Penicillins, parenteral	Heparin	↑	An increased risk of bleeding may occur, possibly because of additive effects.
Allopurinol	Ampicillin	↑	The rate of ampicillin-induced skin rash appears much higher when coadministered with allopurinol than with either drug by itself (see Warnings).
Chloramphenicol	Penicillins	↔	Synergistic effects may develop, but antagonism has been reported in animal studies.
Erythromycin	Penicillins	↔	In vitro tests and clinical studies have demonstrated both antagonism and synergism with coadministration.
Tetracyclines	Penicillins	↓	The bacteriostatic action of tetracycline derivatives may impair the bactericidal effects of penicillins.
Nafcillin	Cyclosporine	↓	Administered concomitantly subtherapeutic cyclosporine levels have been reported. When used concomitantly in organ transplant patients, the cyclosporine levels should be monitored.
Piperacillin	Vecuronium	↑	Piperacillin when used concomitantly with vecuronium has been implicated in the prolongation of the neuromuscular blockade of vecuronium. It is expected that the neuromuscular blockade produced by any of the non-depolarizing muscle relaxants could be prolonged in the presence of piperacillin.

Penicillin Drug Interactions

Precipitant drug	Object drug[a]		Description
Aspirin, phenylbutazone, sulfonamides, indomethacin, thiazide diuretics, furosemide, ethacrynic acid	Penicillin G	↑	These drugs may compete with penicillin G for renal tubular secretion and thus prolong the serum half-life of penicillin.
Probenecid	Penicillins (renally excreted)	↑	Probenecid administered concomitantly with piperacillin/tazobactam prolongs the half-life of piperacillin by 21% and tazobactam by 71%. Carbenicillin indanyl sodium blood levels may be increased and prolonged by concurrent administration of probenecid.

[a] ↑ = Object drug increased. ↓ = Object drug decreased. ↔ = Undetermined clinical effect.

➤*Drug/Lab test interactions:* False-positive **urine glucose** reactions may occur with penicillin therapy if Clinitest, Benedict's Solution or Fehling's Solution are used. It is recommended that enzymatic glucose oxidase tests (such as *Clinistix* or *Tes-Tape*) be used. Positive *Coombs' tests* have occurred. Positive direct antiglobulin tests (DAT) have been reported after large IV doses of **piperacillin**; **clavulanic acid** has also been reported to cause a positive DAT. High urine concentrations of some penicillins may produce false-positive protein reactions (pseudoproteinuria) with the following methods: Sulfosalicylic acid and boiling test, acetic acid test, biuret reaction, and nitric acid test. The bromphenol blue (*Multi-Stix*) reagent strip test has been reported to be reliable.

➤*Drug/Food interactions:* Absorption of most penicillins is affected by food; these medications are best taken on an empty stomach, 1 hour before or 2 hours after meals. **Penicillin V** may be given with meals; however, blood levels may be slightly higher when taken on an empty stomach. **Amoxicillin** and **amoxicillin/potassium clavulanate** tablets may be given without regard to meals.

Adverse Reactions

➤*Cardiovascular:* Cardiac arrest, cerebrovascular accident, hypotension, palpitations, pulmonary embolism, pulmonary hypertension, syncope, tachycardia, vasovagal reaction, vasodilation.

➤*CNS:* Penicillins have caused neurotoxicity (manifested as convulsions and seizures, hallucinations, lethargy, neuromuscular hyperirritability) when given in large IV doses, especially in patients with renal failure. Mental disturbances including agitation, anxiety, combativeness, confusion, depression, hallucinations, seizures, weakness, and expressed "fear of impending death" have been reported in individuals following single-dose therapy for gonorrhea with **penicillin G procaine**, which may have been a reaction to procaine. Reactions have been transient, lasting from 15 to 30 minutes. Dizziness, fatigue, insomnia, reversible hyperactivity, and prolonged muscle relaxation have occurred.

➤*GI:* Abdominal pain or cramp, abnormal taste sensation, black "hairy" tongue, diarrhea or bloody diarrhea, dry mouth, enterocolitis, epigastric distress, flatulence, furry tongue, gastritis, glossitis, nausea, sore mouth or tongue, rectal bleeding, stomatitis, vomiting; pseudomembranous colitis, intestinal necrosis (see Precautions). Incidence of symptoms, particularly diarrhea, is less with **amoxicillin** than with **ampicillin**.

➤*GU:* hematuria, impotence, neurogenic bladder, priapism, proteinuria, renal failure, vaginitis.

➤*Hematologic/Lymphatic:*

Bleeding abnormalities – Hemorrhagic manifestations associated with abnormalities of coagulation tests such as clotting and prothrombin time have occurred and are more likely to occur in patients with renal failure (see Warnings). Agranulocytosis; anemia; bone marrow depression; decrease in WBC and lymphocyte counts; eosinophilia; granulocytopenia; hemolytic anemia; increase in lymphocytes, monocytes, basophils, and platelets; leukopenia; lymphadenopathy; neutropenia; prolongation of bleeding and prothrombin time; reduction in hemoglobin or hematocrit; thrombocytopenia; thrombocytopenic purpura. These reactions are usually reversible on discontinuation of therapy and are believed to be hypersensitivity phenomena. A slight thrombocytosis occurred in less than 1% of patients treated with **amoxicillin and clavulanate potassium**. Atypical lymphocytosis has been observed in one pediatric patient receiving **ampicillin/sulbactam sodium**.

➤*Hypersensitivity:* Adverse reactions (estimated incidence, 0.7% to 10%) are more likely to occur in individuals with previously demonstrated hypersensitivity. In penicillin-sensitive individuals with a history of allergy, asthma, or hay fever, the reactions may be immediate and severe (see Warnings).

Allergic symptoms include allergic vasculitis, angioneurotic edema, asthenia, bronchospasm, death, erythema multiforme (rarely, Stevens-Johnson syndrome), headache, hypotension, laryngeal edema, laryngospasm, maculopapular to exfoliative dermatitis, pain, prostration, pruritus, reactions resembling serum sickness (arthralgia, arthritis, chills, edema, fever, malaise), skin rashes, urticaria, vascular collapse, vesicular eruptions.

➤*Local:* atrophy; deep vein thrombosis; ecchymosis; hematomas; pain (accompanied by induration) at the site of injection; skin ulcer; neurovascular reactions including warmth, vasospasm, pallor, mottling, gangrene, numbness of the extremities, cyanosis of the extremities and neurovascular damage. Vein irritation and phlebitis can occur, particularly when undiluted solution is injected directly into the vein. Tissue necrosis due to extravasated **nafcillin** has been successfully modified with hyaluronidase.

➤*Renal:* Interstitial nephritis (eg, hematuria, hyaline casts, oliguria, proteinuria, pyuria) and nephropathy are infrequent and usually associated with high doses of parenteral penicillins; however, this has occurred with all of the penicillins. Such reactions are hypersensitivity responses and are usually associated with fever, skin rash, and eosinophilia. Elevations of creatinine or BUN may occur.

➤*Miscellaneous:* Anorexia; apnea; blindness; blurred vision; diaphoresis; dyspnea; exacerbation of arthritis; hypoxia; joint disorder; myoglobinuria; periostitis; rhabdomyolysis; hyperthermia, itchy eyes, transient hepatitis, and cholestatic jaundice (rare); sciatic neuritis caused by IM injection of penicillin. The Jarisch-Herxheimer reaction has been reported in the treatment of syphilis.

➤*Lab test abnormalities:* Elevations of AST, ALT, bilirubin, and LDH have been noted in patients receiving semisynthetic penicillins (particularly **oxacillin**); such reactions are more common in infants. Elevations of serum alkaline phosphatase and hypernatremia, and reduction in serum potassium, albumin, total proteins, and uric acid may occur. Decreased hemoglobin, hematocrit, red blood cell counts, WBC, neutrophils, lymphocytes, platelets, and increased lymphocytes, monocytes, basophils, eosinophils and platelets; increased BUN and creatinine; presence of RBCs and hyaline casts in urine (**ampicillin sodium/sulbactam sodium**). Evidence indicates glutamic oxaloacetic transaminase (GOT) is released at the site of IM injection of **ampicillin**. Increased amounts of this enzyme in the blood do not necessarily indicate liver involvement.

Hemorrhagic manifestations associated with abnormalities of coagulation tests such as clotting and prothrombin time have occurred and are more likely to occur in patients with renal failure (see Warnings).

Overdosage

➤*Symptoms:* Penicillin overdosage can result in neuromuscular hyperexcitability or convulsive seizures. Dose-related toxicity may arise with the use of massive doses of IV penicillins (40 to 100 million units/day), particularly in patients with severe renal impairment. Manifestations may include agitation, confusion, asterixis, hallucinations, stupor, coma, multifocal myoclonus, seizures and encephalopathy. Hyperkalemia is also possible.

➤*Treatment:* In case of overdosage, discontinue penicillin, treat symptomatically and institute supportive measures as required. Refer to General Management of Acute Overdosage. If necessary, hemodialysis may be used to reduce blood levels of **penicillin**, although the degree of effectiveness of this procedure is questionable. Hemodialysis does not accelerate the rate of clearance of **nafcillin** from the blood. The metabolic by-products of **carbenicillin indanyl sodium**, **indanyl sulfate** and **glucuronide**, as well as free **carbenicillin**, are dialyzable. In renal function impairment, aminopenicillins can be removed by hemodialysis, but not peritoneal dialysis. The molecular weight, degree of protein binding and pharmacokinetic profile of **sulbactam** and **clavulanic acid** suggest these compounds may also be removed by hemodialysis.

Patient Information

Complete full course of therapy.

Take on an empty stomach 1 hour before or 2 hours after meals. Absorption of **penicillin V** and **amoxicillin** tablets and **amoxicillin/potassium clavulanate** is not significantly affected by food.

Take at even intervals, preferably around the clock.

Notify physician if skin rash, itching, hives, severe diarrhea, shortness of breath, wheezing, black "hairy"tongue, sore throat, nausea, vomiting, fever, swollen joints, or any unusual bleeding or bruising occurs.

Discard any liquid forms of **penicillin** after 7 days if stored at room temperature or after 14 days if refrigerated.

Natural Penicillins

PENICILLIN G (AQUEOUS)

Rx	**Penicillin G Potassium** (Baxter)	**Injection, premixed, frozen:** 1,000,000 units	In 50 mL *Galaxy* containers.
		2,000,000 units	In 50 mL *Galaxy* containers.
		3,000,000 units	In 50 mL *Galaxy* containers.
Rx	**Pfizerpen** (Pfizer)	**Powder for Injection:** 5,000,000 units	≈ 6.8 mg sodium (0.3 mEq), 65.6 mg potassium (1.68 mEq)/million units. In vials.
		Powder for Injection: 20,000,000 units per vial	≈ 6.8 mg sodium (0.3 mEq), 65.6 mg potassium (1.68 mEq)/million units. In vials.

PENICILLIN G (AQUEOUS) — INJECTION

For complete and comparative prescribing information, refer to the Penicillins group monograph.

Administration and Dosage

➤*Infants:* Preferably administered IV as 15- to 30-minute infusions.

Older than 7 days old – 75,000 units/kg/day in divided doses every 8 hours (meningitis – 200,000 to 300,000 units/kg/day every 6 hours).

Younger than 7 days old – 50,000 units/kg/day in divided doses every 12 hours; group B streptococcus – 100,000 units/kg/day; meningitis – 100,000 to 150,000 units/kg/day).

Streptococci in groups A, C, G, H, L and M are very sensitive to penicillin G. Some group D organisms are sensitive to the high serum levels obtained with aqueous penicillin G.

Penicillin G injection should be administered by IV infusion.

Parenteral Penicillin G Use and Dosages in Adults	
Indications	Adult dosage
Labeled uses:	
Meningococcal meningitis/septicemia:	24 million units/day; 1 to 2 million units IM every 2 hours; or 20 to 30 million units/day continuous IV drip for 14 days or until afebrile for 7 days; or 200,000 to 300,000 units/kg/day every 2 to 4 hours in divided doses for a total of 24 doses
Actinomycosis:	
For cervicofacial cases	1 to 6 million units/day
For thoracic and abdominal disease	10 to 20 million units/day IV every 4 to 6 hours for 6 weeks. May be followed by oral penicillin V, 500 mg 4 times daily for 2 to 3 months
Clostridial infections:	
Botulism (adjunctive therapy to antitoxin), gas gangrene and tetanus (adjunctive therapy to human tetanus immune globulin)	20 million units/day every 4 to 6 hours as adjunct to antitoxin
Fusospirochetal infections: Severe infections of oropharynx, lower respiratory tract and genital area	5 to 10 million units/day every 4 to 6 hours
Rat-bite fever (Spirillum minus, Streptobacillus moniliformis), Haverhill fever:	12 to 20 million units/day every 4 to 6 hours for 3 to 4 weeks
Listeria infections (Listeria monocytogenes):	
Meningitis (adults)	15 to 20 million units/day every 4 to 6 hours for 2 weeks
Endocarditis (adults)	15 to 20 million units/day every 4 to 6 hours for 4 weeks
Pasteurella infections (Pasteurella multocida): Bacteremia and meningitis	4 to 6 million units/day every 4 to 6 hours for 2 weeks
Erysipeloid (Erysipelothrix rhusiopathiae): Endocarditis	12 to 20 million units/day every 4 to 6 hours for 4 to 6 weeks
Diphtheria: Adjunct to antitoxin to prevent carrier state	2 to 3 million units/day in divided doses every 4 to 6 hours for 10 to 12 days
Anthrax: (B. anthracis is often resistant)	Minimum 5 million units/day; 12 to 20 million units/day have been used

PENICILLIN G (AQUEOUS) — INJECTION

Parenteral Penicillin G Use and Dosages in Adults

Indications	Adult dosage
Serious streptococcal infections (S. pneumoniae):	
Empyema, pneumonia, pericarditis, endocarditis, meningitis	5 to 24 million units/day in divided doses every 4 to 6 hours
Syphilis:[1]	
Neurosyphilis[1]	18 to 24 million units/day IV (3 to 4 million units every 4 hours) for 10 to 14 days. Many recommend benzathine penicillin G 2.4 million units IM weekly for 3 weeks following the completion of this regimen
Disseminated gonococcal infections: (eg, meningitis, endocarditis, arthritis)	10 million units/day every 4 to 6 hours, with the exception of meningococcal meningitis/septicemia, ie, every 2 hours
Unlabeled uses:	
Lyme disease (Borrelia burgdorferi):	
Erythema chronicum migrans	Use oral penicillin V
Neurologic complications (eg, meningitis, encephalitis)	200,000 to 300,000 units/kg/day (up to 20 million units) IV for 10 to 14 days
Carditis	200,000 to 300,000 units/kg/day (up to 20 million units) IV for 10 days with cardiac monitoring and a temporary pacemaker for complete heart block
Arthritis	200,000 to 300,000 units/kg/day (up to 20 million units) IV for 10 to 20 days

[1] CDC 1998 Sexually Transmitted Diseases Treatment Guidelines. *Morbidity and Mortality Weekly Report* 1997 Jan 23;47 (No. RR-1):1-118.

Parenteral Penicillin G Use and Dosages in Children

Indications	Pediatric dosage
Serious streptococcal infections, such as pneumonia and endocarditis (*S. pneumoniae*) and meningococcus:	150,000 units/kg/day divided in equal doses every 4 to 6 hours; duration depends on infecting organism and type of infection
Meningitis caused by susceptible strains of pneumococcus and meningococcus:	250,000 units/kg/day divided in equal doses every 4 hours for 7 to 14 days depending on the infecting organism (maximum dose of 12 to 20 million units/day)
Disseminated gonococcal infections (penicillin-susceptible strains):	*Weight < 45 kg:*
Arthritis	100,000 units/kg/day in 4 equally divided doses for 7 to 10 days
Meningitis	250,000 units/kg/day in equal doses every 4 hours for 10 to 14 days
Endocarditis	250,000 units/kg/day in equal doses every 4 hours for 4 weeks
	Weight ≥ 45 kg:
Arthritis, meningitis, endocarditis	10 million units/day in 4 equally divided doses with the duration of therapy depending on the type of infection
Syphilis (congenital and neurosyphilis) after the newborn period:	200,000 to 300,000 units/kg/day (administered as 50,000 units/kg every 4 to 6 hours) for 10 to 14 days
Congenital syphilis:[a] Symptomatic or asymptomatic infants	*Infants:* 50,000 units/kg/dose IV every 12 hours the first 7 days, thereafter every 8 hours for total of 10 days. *Children:* 50,000 units/kg every 4 to 6 hours for 10 days.
Diphtheria (adjunctive therapy to antitoxin and for prevention of carrier state):	150,000 to 250,000 units/kg/day in equal doses every 6 hours for 7 to 10 days
Rat-bite fever; Haverhill fever (with endocarditis caused by S. moniliformis):	150,000 to 250,000 units/kg/day in equal doses every 4 hours for 4 weeks

[a] CDC 1998 Sexually Transmitted Diseases Treatment Guidelines. *Morbidity and Mortality Weekly Report* 1997 Jan 23;47 (No. RR-1):1-118.

➤*Renal function impairment:* Penicillin G is relatively nontoxic and dosage adjustments are generally required only in cases of severe renal impairment. The recommended dosage regimen is as follows:

Creatinine clearance less than 10 mL/min; administer a full loading dose followed by one-half of the loading dose every 8 to 10 hours.

Uremic patients with a creatinine clearance more than 10 mL/min; administer a full loading dose followed by one-half of the loading dose every 4 to 5 hours.

➤*Rheumatic fever:* Because alpha-hemolytic streptococci resistant to penicillin may be found when patients are receiving continuous oral penicillin for secondary prevention of rheumatic fever, prophylactic agents other than penicillin may be prescribed in addition to their continuous rheumatic fever prophylactic regimen.

➤*Potassium and sodium content:* Penicillin G potassium contains 1.7 mEq potassium and 0.3 mEq sodium per million units; penicillin G sodium contains 2 mEq sodium per million units.

Give recommended daily dosage IM or by continuous IV infusion.

➤*IM:* Keep total volume of injection small. The IM route is the preferred route of administration. Solutions containing ≤ 100,000 units/mL may be used with a minimum of discomfort. Use greater concentrations as required.

➤*Continuous IV infusion:* When larger doses are required, administer aqueous solutions by means of continuous IV infusion. Determine volume and rate of fluid administration required by the patient in a 24-hour period. Add appropriate daily dosage to this fluid.

➤*Intrapleural or other local infusion:* If fluid is aspirated, give infusion in a volume equal to one fourth or one half the amount of fluid aspirated; otherwise, prepare as for the IM injection.

➤*Intrathecal use:* Must be highly individualized. Use only with full consideration of the possible irritating effects of penicillin when used by this route. The preferred route of therapy in bacterial meningitis is IV, supplemented by IM injection. It has been suggested that intrathecal use has no place in therapy.

➤*Admixture compatibility/incompatibility:* Depending on the route of administration, use sterile water for injection, isotonic sodium chloride injection, or dextrose injection. Penicillins are rapidly inactivated in the presence of carbohydrate solutions at alkaline pH.

➤*Storage/Stability:* The dry powder is stable and does not require refrigeration. Sterile solutions may be kept in the refrigerator for 1 week without loss of potency. Solutions prepared for IV infusion are stable at room temperature for at least 24 hours.

Premixed, frozen solution – Thaw frozen container at room temperature (25°C; 77°F) or in a refrigerator (5°C; 41°F). Do not force thaw by immersion in water baths or by microwave irradiation.

The thawed solution is stable for 24 hours at room temperature or for 14 days under refrigeration. Do not refreeze thawed antibiotics.

PENICILLIN G PROCAINE, INJECTABLE

Rx	**Penicillin G Procaine** (Monarch)	**Injection:** 600,000 units/vial	In 1 mL *Tubex.*[a]
		Injection: 1,200,000 units/vial	In 2 mL *Tubex.*[a]

[a] With parabens and povidone.

PENICILLIN G PROCAINE — INJECTION

For complete and comparative prescribing information, refer to the Penicillins group monograph.

Indications

In the treatment of moderately severe infections in both adults and pediatric patients due to penicillin-G-susceptible microorganisms that are susceptible to the low and persistent serum levels common to this particular dosage form in the indications listed below. Therapy should be guided by bacteriological studies (including susceptibility tests) and by clinical response.

When high, sustained serum levels are required, aqueous penicillin G, either IM or IV, should be used. The following infections will usually respond to adequate dosages of IM penicillin G procaine: Moderately severe to severe infections of the upper respiratory tract, skin and soft-tissue infections, scarlet fever, and erysipelas due to susceptible streptococci (group A, without bacteremia).

➤*Streptococcal infections:* Streptococci in groups A, C, G, H, L, and M are very sensitive to penicillin G. Other groups, including group D (enterococcus), are resistant. Aqueous penicillin is recommended for streptococcal infections with bacteremia.

➤*Respiratory tract infection:* Moderately severe infections of the respiratory tract due to susceptible pneumococci.

Severe pneumonia, empyema, bacteremia, pericarditis, meningitis, peritonitis, and arthritis of pneumococcal etiology are better treated with aqueous penicillin G during the acute stage.

➤*Skin and soft tissue infection:* Moderately severe infections of the skin and soft tissues due to susceptible staphylococci (penicillin G-susceptible).

Reports indicate an increasing number of strains of staphylococci resistant to penicillin G, emphasizing the need for culture and sensitivity studies in treating suspected staphylococcal infections. Indicated surgical procedures should be performed.

➤*Fusospirochetosis:* Fusospirochetosis (Vincent's gingivitis and pharyngitis). Moderately severe infections of the oropharynx due to susceptible fusiform bacilli and spirochetes.

Necessary dental care should be accomplished in infections involving the gum tissue.

➤*Syphilis:* Syphilis (all stages) due to susceptible *Treponema pallidum.*

➤*Beta-lactamase producing bacteria:* This drug should not be used in the treatment of beta-lactamase producing organisms that include most strains of *Neisseria gonorrhea.*

➤*Yaws, bejel, and pinta:* Yaws, bejel, and pinta due to susceptible organisms.

➤*Diphtheria:* Penicillin G procaine is an adjunct to antitoxin for prevention of the carrier stage of diphtheria due to susceptible *C. diphtheriae.*

➤*Anthrax:* To reduce the incidence or progression of the disease following exposure to aerosolized *Bacillus anthracis.*

➤*Rat-bite fever:* Rat-bite fever due to susceptible *Streptobacillus moniliformis* and *Spirillum minus* organisms.

➤*Erysipeloid:* Erysipeloid due to susceptible *Erysipelothrix rhusiopathiae.*

➤*Endocarditis:* Subacute bacterial endocarditis, only in extremely sensitive infections, due to susceptible group A streptococci.

Administration and Dosage

➤*Method of administration:* Do not inject into or near an artery or nerve. Injection into or near a nerve may result in permanent neurologic damage.

Inadvertent intravascular administration, including inadvertent direct intra-arterial injection or injection immediately adjacent to arteries, of penicillin G procaine and other penicillin preparations has resulted in severe neurovascular damage, including transverse myelitis with permanent paralysis, gangrene requiring amputation of digits and more proximal portions of extremities, and necrosis and sloughing at and surrounding the injection site. Such severe effects have been reported following injections into the buttock, thigh, and deltoid areas. Other serious complications of suspected intravascular administration which have been reported include immediate pallor, mottling, or cyanosis of the extremity, both distal and proximal to the injection site, followed by bleb formation; severe edema requiring anterior or posterior compartment fasciotomy in the lower extremity. The above-described severe effects and complications have most often occurred in infants and small children. Prompt consultation with an appropriate specialist is indicated if any evidence of compromise of the blood supply occurs at, proximal to, or distal to the site of injection.

Quadriceps femoris fibrosis and atrophy have been reported following repeated IM injections of penicillin preparations into the anterolateral thigh.

Penicillin G procaine (aqueous) is for IM injection only.

Administer by deep IM injection in the upper, outer quadrant of the buttock. In neonates, infants and small children, the midlateral aspect of the thigh may be preferable. When doses are repeated, vary the injection site.

Because of the high concentration of suspended material in this product, the needle may be blocked if the injection is not made at a slow, steady rate.

➤*Pneumonia (pneumococcal), moderately severe (uncomplicated):* 600,000 to 1,000,000 units/day.

➤*Streptococcal infections (group A), moderately severe to severe tonsillitis, erysipelas, scarlet fever, upper respiratory tract, skin and soft tissue:* 600,000 to 1,000,000 units/day for 10-day minimum.

➤*Staphylococcal infections, moderately severe to severe:* 600,000 to 1,000,000 units/day.

In pneumonia, streptococcal (group A) and staphylococcal infections in pediatric patients under 60 pounds – 300,000 units/day.

➤*Bacterial endocarditis (group A streptococci) only in extremely sensitive infections:* 600,000 to 1,000,000 units/day.

Penicillin G procaine is not recommended for prophylaxis against bacterial endocarditis. For prophylaxis against bacterial endocarditis in patients with congenital heart disease or rheumatic or other acquired valvular heart disease when undergoing dental procedures or surgical procedures of the upper respiratory tract, use penicillin V. For patients unable to take oral medications, aqueous penicillin G procaine is recommended.

➤*Syphilis:*

Primary, secondary, and latent with a negative spinal fluid in adults and pediatric patients over 12 years of age – 600,000 units/day for 8 days; total 4,800,000 units.

Late (tertiary, neurosyphilis, and latent syphilis with positive spinal-fluid examination or no spinal-fluid examination) – 600,000 units/day for 10 to 15 days; total 6 to 9 million units.

Congenital syphilis under 70 lb body weight – 50,000 units/kg/day for 10 days.

Yaws, bejel, and pinta – Treatment as for syphilis in corresponding stage of disease.

➤*Diphtheria:*

Adjunctive therapy with antitoxin – 300,000 to 600,000 units/day.

Diphtheria carrier state – 300,000 units/day for 10 days.

➤*Anthrax:*

Anthrax, cutaneous – 600,000 to 1,000,000 units/day.

Anthrax, inhalational (postexposure) – 1,200,000 units every 12 hours in adults, 25,000 units/kg of body weight (maximum 1,200,000 units) every 12 hours in children. The available safety data for penicillin G procaine at this dose would best support a duration of therapy of 2 weeks or less. Treatment for inhalational anthrax (postexposure) must be continued for a total of 60 days. Physicians must consider the risks and benefits of continuing administration of penicillin G procaine for more than 2 weeks or switching to an effective alternative treatment.

➤*Fusospirochetosis:*

Vincent's infection – 600,000 to 1,000,000 units/day.

➤*Erysipeloid:* 600,000 to 1,000,000 units/day.

➤*Rat-bite fever:*

Streptobacillus moniliformis and Spirillum minus (rat-bite fever) – 600,000 to 1,000,000 units/day.

➤*Storage/Stability:* Store in a refrigerator, 2° to 8°C (36° to 46°F). Keep from freezing.

PENICILLIN G BENZATHINE, INTRAMUSCULAR

Rx	**Bicillin L-A** (Monarch)	**Injection:** 600,000 units/dose	In 1 mL *Tubex*[a]
		1,200,000 units/dose	In 2 mL *Tubex*[a]
		2,400,000 units/dose	In 4 mL prefilled syringe.[a]
Rx	**Permapen** (Roerig)	**Injection:** 1,200,000 units/dose	In 2 mL *Isoject*[b]

[a] With povidone and parabens.

[b] With polyvinylpyrrolidone and parabens.

PENICILLIN G BENZATHINE — INTRAMUSCULAR

For complete and comparative prescribing information, refer to the Penicillins group monograph.

Indications

Treatment of infections due to penicillin G-sensitive microorganisms that are susceptible to the low and very prolonged serum levels common to this particular dosage form. Therapy should be guided by bacteriological studies (including sensitivity tests) and by clinical response.

The following infections will usually respond to adequate dosage of IM penicillin G benzathine:

➤*Respiratory infections:* Mild-to-moderate infections of the upper respiratory tract due to susceptible streptococci.

PENICILLIN G BENZATHINE — INTRAMUSCULAR

➤*Venereal infections:* Syphilis, yaws, bejel, and pinta.

➤*Prophylaxis of rheumatic fever and chorea:* Prophylaxis with penicillin G benzathine has proven effective in preventing recurrence of these conditions. It has also been used as follow-up prophylactic therapy for rheumatic heart disease and acute glomerulonephritis.

Administration and Dosage

➤*Streptococcal (group A):*

Upper respiratory tract infections (ie, pharyngitis). –
Adults: A single injection of 1,200,000 units.
Older pediatric patients: A single injection of 900,000 units.
Infants and pediatric patients less than 60 lbs: 300,000 to 600,000 units.

➤*Venereal infection:*

Syphilis –
Primary, secondary, and latent: 2,400,000 units (1 dose).
Late (tertiary and neuro-syphilis): 2,400,000 units at 7-day intervals for 3 doses.

Congenital –
Younger than 2 years of age: 50,000 untis/kg/body weight.
2 to 12 years of age: Adjust dosage based on adult dosage schedule.

Yaws, bejel, and pinta – 1,200,000 units (1 injection).

➤*Prophylaxis for rheumatic fever and glomerulonephritis:* Following an acute attack, penicillin G benzathine (parenteral) may be given in doses of 1,200,000 units once a month or 600,000 units every 2 weeks.

➤*Method of administration:* Penicillin G benzathine is intended for IM injection only. Do not inject into or near an artery or nerve, or intravenously or admix with other IV solutions (see Warnings).

Administer by deep intramuscular injection in the upper, outer quadrant of the buttock. In neonates, infants and small children, the midlateral aspect of the thigh may be preferable. When doses are repeated, vary the injection site.

Because of the high concentration of suspended material in this product, the needle may be blocked if the injection is not made at a slow, steady rate.

Penicillin G Benzathine Uses and Dosages

Organisms/Infections	Dosage
Streptococcal (group A): Upper respiratory tract infections	*Adults:* 1.2 million units IM as a single injection *Older children:* 900,000 units IM as a single injection *Infants and children (< 60 lbs; 27 kg):* 300,000 to 600,000 units
Syphilis:[1] *Early syphilis* - Primary, secondary, or latent syphilis	*Adults:* 2.4 million units IM in single dose *Children:* 50,000 units/kg IM, up to adult dosage
Gummas and cardiovascular syphilis[1] - Latent	*Adults:* 2.4 million units IM once weekly for 3 weeks *Children:* 50,000 units/kg IM, up to adult dosage
Neurosyphilis[1]	Aqueous penicillin G, 18 to 24 million units/day IV (3 to 4 million units every 4 hours) for 10 to 14 days. Many recommend benzathine penicillin G, 2.4 million IM units once/week for up to 3 weeks following completion of this regimen. or Procaine penicillin G, 2.4 million units/day IM *plus* probenecid 500 mg orally 4 times daily, both for 10 to 14 days. Many recommend benzathine penicillin G, 2.4 million units IM once/week for up to 3 weeks following completion of this regimen.
Syphilis in pregnancy[1]	Dosage schedule appropriate for stage of syphilis recommended for nonpregnant patients.
Congenital syphilis	*Children < 2 years of age:* 50,000 units/kg/body weight *Children 2 to 12 years of age:* Adjust dosage based on adult dosage schedule.
Yaws, bejel, and pinta	1.2 million units IM in a single dose
Prophylaxis for rheumatic fever and glomerulonephritis	Following an acute attack, may be given IM in doses of 1.2 million units once a month or 600,000 units every 2 weeks

[1] CDC 2002 Sexually Transmitted Diseases Treatment Guidelines. *MMWR Morbid Mortal Wkly Rept.* 2002;51(RR-6):1-82.

➤*Storage/Stability:* Store in a refrigerator 2° to 8°C (36° to 46°F). Keep from freezing.

PENICILLIN G BENZATHINE/PENICILLIN G PROCAINE

Rx	**Bicillin C-R** (Monarch)	**Injection:** 600,000 units/dose (300,000 units each penicillin G benzathine and penicillin G procaine)	In 1 mL *Tubex*[a]
		1,200,000 units/dose (600,000 units each penicillin G benzathine and penicillin G procaine)	In 2 mL *Tubex*[a]
		2,400,000 units/dose (1,200,000 units each penicillin G benzathine and penicillin G procaine)	In 4 mL syringe.[a]
Rx	**Bicillin C-R 900/300** (Monarch)	**Injection:** 1,200,000 units/dose (900,000 units penicillin G benzathine and 300,000 units penicillin G procaine)	In 2 mL *Tubex*[a]

[a] With parabens, lecithin, and povidone.

PENICILLIN G BENZATHINE/PENICILLIN G PROCAINE — INJECTION

For complete and comparative prescribing information, refer to the Penicillins group monograph.

WARNING

Not for intravenous (IV) use. Do not inject IV or admix with other IV solutions. There have been reports of inadvertent IV administration of penicillin G benzathine, which has been associated with cardiorespiratory arrest and death. Prior to administration of this drug, carefully read the labeling.

Indications

Treatment of moderately severe infections due to penicillin G–susceptible microorganisms that are susceptible to serum levels common to this particular dosage form. Therapy should be guided by bacteriological studies (including susceptibility testing) and by clinical response.

Treatment of the following in adults and children (*Bicillin C-R 900/300* is only indicated in children):

➤*Streptococcal infections:* Moderately severe to severe infections of the upper respiratory tract, scarlet fever, erysipelas, and skin and soft tissue infections due to susceptible streptococci.

Streptococci in groups A, C, G, H, L, and M are very sensitive to penicillin G. Other groups, including group D (enterococci), are resistant. Penicillin G sodium or potassium is recommended for streptococcal infections with bacteremia.

➤*Pneumococcal infections:* Moderately severe pneumonia and otitis media due to susceptible pneumococci.

Severe pneumonia, empyema, bacteremia, pericarditis, meningitis, peritonitis, and arthritis of pneumococcal etiology are better treated with penicillin G sodium or potassium during the acute stage.

➤*High serum levels:* When high, sustained serum levels are required, use penicillin G sodium or potassium, either intramuscular (IM) or IV.

➤*Venereal diseases:* Do not use this drug in the treatment of venereal diseases, including syphilis, gonorrhea, yaws, bejel, and pinta.

Administration and Dosage

➤*Approved by the FDA:* Prior to January 1, 1982.

➤*Streptococcal infections group A:* Infections of the upper respiratory tract, skin and soft-tissue infections, scarlet fever, and erysipelas.

Bicillin C-R 900/300 – A single injection of *Bicillin C-R 900/300* is usually sufficient for the treatment of group A streptococcal infections in children.

Bicillin C-R – Treatment is usually given at a single session using multiple IM sites when indicated.
1.) Adults and children (over 60 lbs [27 kg]): 2,400,000 units.
2.) Children (30 to 60 lbs [14 to 27 kg]): 900,000 to 1,200,000 units.
3.) Children (under 30 lbs [14 kg]): 600,000 units.

Alternative dosing – An alternative dosage schedule may be used, giving one half the total dose on day 1 and one half on day 3. This will also ensure

PENICILLIN G BENZATHINE/PENICILLIN G PROCAINE — INJECTION

the penicillinemia required over a 10-day period; however, this alternate schedule should be used only when the health care provider can be assured of the patient's cooperation.

➤*Pneumococcal infections (except pneumococcal meningitis):*

Bicillin C-R – The dose should be repeated every 2 or 3 days until the temperature is normal for 48 hours. Other forms of penicillin may be necessary for severe cases.

1.) Adults: 1,200,000 units IM
2.) Children: 600,000 units IM

Bicillin C-R 900/300 – One *Tubex* cartridge of *Bicillin C-R 900/300* repeated at 2- or 3-day intervals until the temperature is normal for 48 hours. Other forms of penicillin may be necessary for severe cases.

➤*Administration:* See the Warning box for more information.

Administer by deep IM injection in the upper, outer quadrant of the buttock. In neonates, infants and small children, the midlateral aspect of the thigh may be preferable. When doses are repeated, vary the injection site.

➤*Storage/Stability:* Store in a refrigerator at 2° to 8°C (36° to 46°F). Keep from freezing.

PENICILLIN V (Phenoxymethyl Penicillin)

Rx	**Penicillin VK** (Various, eg, Teva)	**Tablets**: 250 mg	In 100s, and 1000s.
Rx	**Veetids** (Geneva)		Lactose. (BL V1). White. Film-coated. In 100s and 1000s.
Rx	**Penicillin VK** (Various, eg, Teva)	**Tablets**: 500 mg	In 100s and 500s.
Rx	**Veetids** (Geneva)		Lactose. (BL V2). White. Film-coated. In 100s and 1000s.
Rx	**Penicillin VK** (Various, eg, Teva)	**Powder for Oral Solution**: 125 mg/5 mL when reconstituted	In 100 and 200 mL.
Rx	**Veetids** (Geneva)		DL-menthol, saccharin, sucrose. In 100 and 200 mL.
Rx	**Penicillin VK** (Various, eg, Teva)	**Powder for Oral Solution**: 250 mg/5 mL when reconstituted	In 100 and 200 mL.
Rx	**Veetids** (Geneva)		DL-menthol, saccharin, sucrose. In 100 and 200 mL.

PENICILLIN V POTASSIUM — ORAL

For complete and comparative prescribing information, refer to the Penicillins group monograph.

Indications

Treatment of mild to moderately severe infections due to penicillin G-sensitive microorganisms. Therapy should be guided by bacteriologic studies (including sensitivity tests) and by clinical response.

Severe pneumonia, empyema, bacteremia, pericarditis, meningitis, and arthritis should not be treated with penicillin V during the acute stage.

Indicated surgical procedures should be performed.

➤*Streptococcal infections (without bacteremia):* The following infections will usually respond to adequate dosage of penicillin V. Mild-to-moderate infections of the upper respiratory tract, scarlet fever, and mild erysipelas due to susceptible streptococci.

Streptococci in groups A, C, G, H, L, and M are very sensitive to penicillin. Other groups, including group D (*enterococcus*), are resistant.

➤*Pneumococcal infections:* Mild to moderately severe infections of the respiratory tract, including otitis media, due to susceptible pneumococci.

➤*Staphylococcal infections-penicillin G-sensitive:* Mild infections of the skin and soft tissues due to susceptible staphylococci.

➤*Fusospirochetosis (Vincent's gingivitis and pharyngitis):* Reports indicate an increasing number of strains of staphylococci resistant to penicillin G, emphasizing the need for culture and sensitivity studies in treating suspected staphylococcal infections.

➤*For the prevention of recurrence following rheumatic fever and/or chorea:* Prophylaxis with oral penicillin on a continuing basis has proven effective in preventing recurrence of these conditions.

➤*Unlabeled uses:*

Penicillin V Uses and Dosages for Adults and Children > 12 Years of Age

Organisms/Infections	Dosage
Labeled uses:	
Streptococcal infections: Mild to moderately severe infections of the upper respiratory tract, including scarlet fever and mild erysipelas	125 to 250 mg orally every 6 to 8 hours for 10 days
Pharyngitis in children	25 to 50 mg/kg/day divided every 6 hours for 10 days
Pneumococcal infections: Mild to moderately severe respiratory tract infections including otitis media	250 to 500 mg orally every 6 hours until afebrile at least 2 days
Staphylococcal infections: Mild infections of skin and soft tissue	250 to 500 mg orally every 6 to 8 hours
Fusospirochetosis (Vincent's infection) of the oropharynx: Mild to moderately severe infections	250 to 500 mg orally every 6 to 8 hours
For prevention of recurrence following rheumatic fever or chorea	125 to 250 mg orally 2 times/day on a continuing basis
Unlabeled uses:	
Prophylactic treatment of children with sickle cell anemia or splenectomy: To reduce the incidence of *S. pneumoniae* septicemia	*3 months to 5 years of age:* 125 mg orally 2 times/day *> 5 years of age:* 250 mg BID
Actinomycosis	Penicillin G 10 to 20 mg/day IV for 4 to 6 week, then Penicillin V 2 to 4 g/day for 6 to 12 months
Early Lyme disease (Borrelia burgdorferi): Erythema migrans	500 mg orally 4 times a day for 10 to 20 days
Anthrax: Postexposure prophylaxis - Confirmed or suspected exposure to *Bacillus anthracis*	*Adults:* 7.5 mg/kg orally 4 times/day *Children < 9 years of age:* 50 mg/kg/day orally divided 4 times/day Continue prophylaxis until exposure to *B. anthracis* has been excluded. If exposure is confirmed and vaccine is available, continue prophylaxis for 4 weeks and until 3 doses of vaccine have been administered or for 30 to 60 days if vaccine if not available.

Administration and Dosage

The dosage of penicillin V should be determined according to the sensitivity of the causative microorganisms and the severity of infection, and adjusted to the clinical response of the patient.

The usual dosage recommendations for adults and children 12 years of age and older are as follows:

➤*Streptococcal infections:* 125 to 250 mg (200,000 to 400,000 units) every 6 to 8 hours for 10 days.

➤*Pneumococcal infections:* 250 to 500 mg (400,000 to 800,000 units) every 6 hours until the patient has been afebrile for at least 2 days.

➤*Staphylococcal infections:* 250 to 500 mg (400,000 to 800,000 units) every 6 to 8 hours.

➤*Fusospirochetosis (Vincent's infection) of the oropharynx:* 250 to 500 mg (400,000 to 800,000 units) every 6 to 8 hours.

➤*Prevention of rheumatic fever/chorea:* For the prevention of recurrence following rheumatic fever and/or chorea: 125 to 250 mg (200,000 to 400,000 units) twice daily on a continuing basis.

➤*Storage/Stability:*

Solution – After reconstitution, solution must be stored in a refrigerator. Discard any unused portion after 14 days.

Tablets – Dispense in a tight container. Keep tightly closed.

NAFCILLIN SODIUM INJECTION

Rx	**Nafcillin Sodium** (Sandoz)	**Powder for injection**: 1 g (as base)	In *Add-Vantage* vials.
		2 g (as base)	In *Add-Vantage* vials.
Rx	**Nafcillin Injection** (Baxter)	**Injection**: 1 g (as base)	In premixed, frozen 50 mL single-dose *Galaxy* containers.
		2 g (as base)	In premixed, frozen 100 mL in single-dose *Galaxy* containers.

NAFCILLIN SODIUM — INJECTION

For complete and comparative prescribing information, refer to the Penicillins group monograph.

Indications

➤*Staphylococcal infections:* Treatment of infections caused by penicillinase-producing staphylococci which have demonstrated susceptibility to the drug. Culture and susceptibility tests should be performed initially to determine the causative organism and its susceptibility to the drug.

To initiate therapy in suspected cases of resistant staphylococcal infections prior to the availability of susceptibility test results. Nafcillin should not be used in infections caused by organisms susceptible to penicillin G. If the susceptibility tests indicate that the infection is due to an organism other than a resistant *Staphylococcus*, therapy should not be continued with nafcillin sodium.

Administration and Dosage

➤*Approved by the FDA:* August 2, 1984.

➤*Dose:* The usual IV dosage for adults is 500 mg every 4 hours. For severe infections, 1 g every 4 hours is recommended.

➤*Duration:* Duration of therapy varies with the type and severity of infection as well as the overall condition of the patient; therefore, determine duration by the clinical and bacteriological response of the patient. In severe staphylococcal infections, continue nafcillin therapy for at least 14 days. Continue therapy for at least 48 hours after the patient has become afebrile, and asymptomatic and cultures are negative. The treatment of endocarditis and osteomyelitis may require a longer duration of therapy.

➤*Nafcillin in Galaxy containers:*

Administration – Administer slowly over at least 30 to 60 minutes to minimize the risk of vein irritation and extravasation.

Do not use plastic containers in series connections. Such use could result in air embolism because of residual air being drawn from the primary container before administration of the fluid from the secondary container is complete.

Preparation – Thaw frozen container at room temperature (25°C or 77°F) or under refrigeration (5°C or 41°F). Do not force thaw by immersion in water baths or by microwave irradiation.

Components of the solution may precipitate in the frozen state and will dissolve upon reaching room temperature with little or no agitation. Agitate after solution has reached room temperature. If after visual inspection the solution remains cloudy or if an insoluble precipitate is noted or if any seals or outlet ports are not intact, discard the container.

➤*Nafcillin powder for injection:*

Administration – For IV use only. The drug concentration and the rate and volume of the infusion should be adjusted so that the total dose of nafcillin is administered before the drug loses its stability in the solution in use. This route of administration should be used for relatively short-term therapy (24 to 48 hours) because of the occasional occurrence of thrombophlebitis particularly in elderly patients.

Preparation – Vials in the *ADD-Vantage Drug Delivery System* are to be used with *ADD-Vantage* diluent containers of 0.9% sodium chloride injection 50 and 100 mL. See manufacturer's instructions for reconstitution and administration instructions.

➤*Hepatic / Renal function impairment:* For patients with hepatic insufficiency and renal failure, measure nafcillin serum levels and adjust dosage accordingly.

➤*Elderly:* With IV administration, particularly in elderly patients, take care because of the possibility of thrombophlebitis.

➤*Admixture incompatibility:* Do not add supplementary medication to nafcillin injection.

➤*Storage / Stability:*

Galaxy containers – Store at or below −20°C (−4°F). The thawed 1 and 2 g solutions are stable for 21 days under refrigeration (5°C or 41°F) or 72 hours at room temperature (25°C or 77°F). Do not refreeze.

Vials – Store at 20° to 25°C (68° to 77°F). At concentrations ranging from 10 to 40 mg/mL in 0.9% sodium chloride injection or 5% dextrose injection, nafcillin will have utility times of 24 hours at room temperature (25°C; 77F).

OXACILLIN SODIUM

Rx	**Oxacillin Sodium** (Various, eg, Geneva)	**Powder for Oral Solution**: 250 mg/5 mL when reconstituted	In 100 mL.
		Powder for Injection: 500 mg	In vials.
		Powder for Injection: 1 g	In vials, *ADD-Vantage* vials, and piggyback vials.
		Powder for Injection: 2 g	In vials, *ADD-Vantage* vials, and piggyback vials.
		Powder for Injection: 10 g	In bulk vials.

OXACILLIN SODIUM — ORAL

For complete and comparative prescribing information, refer to the Penicillins group monograph.

Indications

➤*Staphylococcal infections:* In the treatment of infections caused by penicillinase-producing staphylococci which have demonstrated susceptibility to the drugs. Culture and susceptibility tests should be performed initially to determine the causative organism and its sensitivity to the drug.

To initiate therapy in suspected cases of resistant staphylococcal infections prior to the availability of laboratory test results. Oxacillin sodium should not be used in infections caused by organisms susceptible to penicillin G. If the susceptibility tests indicate that the infection is due to an organism other than a resistant staphylococcus, therapy should not be continued with oxacillin sodium.

Administration and Dosage

➤*Duration:* Duration of therapy varies with the type and severity of infection as well as the overall condition of the patient, therefore, it should be determined by the clinical and bacteriological response of the patient. In severe staphylococcal infections, therapy with oxacillin sodium should be continued for at least 14 days. Therapy should be continued for at least 48 hours after the patient has become afebrile, asymptomatic, and cultures are negative. The treatment of endocarditis and osteomyelitis may require a longer term of therapy.

➤*Concomitant medications:* Coadministration of oxacillin sodium and probenecid increases and prolongs serum penicillin levels. Probenecid decreases the apparent volume of distribution and slows the rate of excretion by competitively inhibiting renal tubular secretion of penicillin. Penicillin-probenecid therapy is generally limited to those infections where very high serum levels of penicillin are necessary.

Oral preparations of oxacillin sodium should not be used as initial therapy in serious, life-threatening infections. Occasionally patients will not absorb therapeutic amount of orally administered penicillin. Oral therapy with oxacillin sodium may be used to follow-up the previous use of a parenteral agent as soon as the clinical condition warrants.

➤*Dosages for mild to moderate and severe infections:*

Adults – For adults with mild to moderate infections, the dose is 500 mg of oxacillin every 4 to 6 hours.

For adults with severe infections, the dose is 1 g every 4 to 6 hours (follow-up of parenteral therapy).

Children – For children with mild to moderate infections, the dose is 50 mg/kg/day (for patients weighing less than 40 kg [88 lbs]) in equally divided doses every 6 hours.

For children with severe infections, the dose is 100 mg/kg/day (for patients weighing less than 40 kg [88 lbs]) in equally divided doses every 4 to 6 hours (follow-up of parenteral therapy).

➤*Directions for dispensing oral solution:* Prepare these formulations at the time of dispensing. For ease in preparation, add water to the bottle in 2 portions, and shake well after each addition. Add the total amount of water as directed on the labeling of the package being dispensed. The reconstituted formulation is stable for 3 days at room temperature or 14 days under refrigeration.

➤*Storage / Stability:* The reconstituted formulation is stable for 3 days at room temperature or 14 days under refrigeration.

Penicillinase-Resistant Penicillins

OXACILLIN SODIUM — INJECTION

For complete and comparative prescribing information, refer to the Penicillins group monograph.

Indications

➤*Staphylococcal infections:* In the treatment of infections caused by penicillinase-producing staphylococci which have demonstrated susceptibility to the drug. Cultures and susceptibility tests should be performed initially to determine the causative organism and their susceptibility to the drug.

To initiate therapy in suspected cases of resistant staphylococcal infections prior to the availability of laboratory test results. Oxacillin should not be used in infections caused by organisms susceptible to penicillin G. If the susceptibility tests indicate that the infection is due to an organism other than a resistant staphylococcus, therapy should not be continued with oxacillin.

Administration and Dosage

➤*Approved by the FDA:* December 23, 1986.

Oxacillin injection supplied as a premixed frozen solution is to be administered as a continuous or intermittent intravenous infusion.

➤*Dosage:*

Usual Dose Recommendation	
Adults	Pediatric patients less than 40 kg (88 lbs)
250 to 500 mg IV every 4 to 6 hours (mild to moderate infections)	50 mg/kg/day IV in equally divided doses every 6 hours (mild to moderate infections)
1 g IV every 4 to 6 hours (severe infections)	100 mg/kg/day IV in equally divided doses every 4 to 6 hours (severe infections)

➤*Duration:* Duration of therapy varies with the type of severity of infection as well as the overall condition of the patient, therefore, it should be determined by the clinical and bacteriological response of the patient. In severe staphylococcal infections, therapy with oxacillin should be continued for at least 14 days. Therapy should be continued for at least 48 hours after the patient has become afebrile, asymptomatic, and cultures are negative. Treatment of endocarditis and osteomyelitis may require a longer term of therapy.

➤*Concomitant medications:* Coadministration of oxacillin and probenecid increases and prolongs serum penicillin levels. Probenecid decreases the apparent volume of distribution and slows the rate of excretion by competitively inhibiting renal tubular secretion of penicillin. Penicillin-probenecid therapy is generally limited to those infections where very high serum levels of penicillin are necessary.

➤*Elderly:* With intravenous administration, particularly in elderly patients, care should be taken because of the possibility of thrombophlebitis.

➤*Admixture incompatibility:* Do not add supplementary medication to oxacillin injection.

➤*Plastic containers:* Do not use plastic containers in series connections. Such use could result in air embolism due to residual air being drawn from the primary container before administration of the fluid from the secondary container is complete.

➤*Storage / Stability:* Store in a freezer capable of maintaining a temperature at or below −20°C (−4°F).

Directions for use of Galaxy plastic container – Thaw at room temperature (25°C; 77°F) or under refrigeration (5°C; 41°F). [Do not force thaw by immersion in water baths or by microwave irradiation]. Components of the solution may precipitate in the frozen state and will dissolve upon reaching room temperature with little or no agitation. Potency is not affected. Mix after solution has reached room temperature. Check for minute leaks by squeezing bag firmly. If leaks are found, discard solution as sterility may be impaired. Do not use if the solution is cloudy or precipitated or if seals are not intact. The thawed solution is stable for 21 days under refrigeration or 48 hours at room temperature. Do not refreeze.

Use sterile equipment.

DICLOXACILLIN SODIUM

Rx	**Dicloxacillin Sodium** (Various, eg, Teva)	**Capsules:** 250 mg	In 40s, 100s, 500s, and UD 100s.
		500 mg	In 30s, 40s, 50s, 100s, 500s, and UD 100s.

DICLOXACILLIN SODIUM — ORAL

For complete and comparative prescribing information, refer to the Penicillins group monograph.

Indications

➤*Staphylococcal infections:* Treatment of infections caused by penicillinase-producing staphylococci. May be used to initiate therapy when a staphylococcal infection is suspected (see Indications in the group monograph concerning use of penicillinase-resistant penicillins).

Administration and Dosage

Dicloxacillin sodium is best absorbed when taken on an empty stomach, preferably 1 to 2 hours before meals.

Recommended Dosages for Dicloxacillin in Mild to Moderate and Severe Infections			
Adults		Children	
Mild to moderate	Severe	Mild to moderate	Severe
125 mg every 6 hours	250 mg every 6 hours	12.5 mg/kg/day[a] in equally divided doses every 6 hours	25 mg/kg/day[a] in equally divided doses every 6 hours.

[a] Patients weighing less than 40 kg (88 lbs).

➤*Duration:* In severe staphylococcal infections, continue therapy with penicillinase-resistant penicillins for at least 14 days. Continue therapy for at least 48 hours after the patient has become afebrile and asymptomatic and cultures are negative. The treatment of endocarditis and osteomyelitis may require a longer term of therapy.

Treat infections caused by Group A beta-hemolytic streptococci for at least 10 days to help prevent the occurrence of acute rheumatic fever or acute glomerulonephritis.

Penicillin-probenecid therapy generally is limited to those infections where very high serum levels of penicillin are necessary. Do not use oral preparations of the penicillinase-resistant penicillins as initial therapy in serious, life-threatening infections.

Aminopenicillins

AMPICILLIN

Rx	**Ampicillin** (Various, eg, Teva)	**Capsules:** 250 mg (as trihydrate)	In 100s and 500s.
Rx	**Principen** (Geneva)		Lactose. (BRISTOL 7992). Lt. gray/scarlet. In 100s, 500s, and UD 100s.
Rx	**Ampicillin** (Various, eg, Teva)	**Capsules:** 500 mg (as trihydrate)	In 100s and 500s.
Rx	**Principen** (Geneva)		Lactose. (BRISTOL 7993). Lt. gray/scarlet. In 100s, 500s, and UD 100s.
Rx	**Principen** (Geneva)	**Powder for Oral Suspension:** 125 mg/5 mL (as trihydrate) when reconstituted	Sucrose. Fruit flavor. In 100, 150, and 200 mL.
Rx	**Principen** (Geneva)	**Powder for Oral Suspension:** 250 mg/5 mL (as trihydrate) when reconstituted	Sucrose. Fruit flavor. In 100 and 200 mL.
Rx	**Ampicillin Sodium** (Various, eg, APP, Geneva)	**Powder for Injection**[a]: 250 mg	In vials.
Rx	**Ampicillin Sodium** (Various, eg, APP, Geneva)	**Powder for Injection**[a]: 500 mg	In vials.
Rx	**Ampicillin Sodium** (Various, eg, APP)	**Powder for Injection**[a]: 1 g	In vials.
Rx	**Ampicillin Sodium** (Various, eg, APP)	**Powder for Injection**[a]: 2 g	In vials.

[a] Contains approximately 2.9 mEq of sodium/g.

AMPICILLIN — ORAL

For complete and comparative prescribing information, refer to the Penicillins group monograph.

Indications

➤*Genitourinary tract infections, including gonorrhea:* *E. coli*, *P. mirabilis*, enterococci, *Shigella*, *S. typhosa* and other *Salmonella*, and nonpenicillinase-producing *N. gonorrhoeae*.

➤*Respiratory tract infections:* Nonpenicillinase-producing *H. influenzae* and staphylococci, and streptococci including *streptococcus pneumoniae*.

➤*GI tract infections:* *Shigella*, *S. typhosa* and other *Salmonella*, *E. coli*, *P. mirabilis*, and enterococci.

➤*Meningitis:* Due to *N. meningitides*.

Administration and Dosage

➤*Adults, and children weight over 20 kg:*

GI and GU infections – For GU or GI tract infections other than gonorrhea in men and women, the usual dose is 500 mg 4 times a day in equally spaced doses; severe or chronic infections may required larger doses.

Gonorrhea – For the treatment of gonorrhea in both men and women, a single oral dose of 3.5 grams of ampicillin administered simultaneously with 1 gram of probenecid is recommended. Physicians are cautioned to use no less than the above recommended dosage for the treatment of gonorrhea. Follow-up cultures should be obtained from the original site(s) of infection 7 to 14 days after therapy. In women, it is also desirable to obtain culture test-of-cure from both the endocervical and anal canals. Prolonged intensive therapy is needed for complications such as prostatitis and epididymitis.

Respiratory tract infections – For respiratory tract infections, the usual dose is 250 mg 4 times a day in equally spaced doses.

➤*Children weighing 20 kg or less:*

GI or GU infections – For GU or GI tract infections, the usual dose is 100 mg/kg/day total, 4 times a day in equally divided and spaced doses.

Respiratory tract infections – For respiratory tract infections, the usual dose is 50 mg/kg/day total, in equally divided and spaced doses 3 to 4 times daily. Doses for children should not exceed doses recommended for adults.

➤*All patients, irrespective of age and weight:* Larger doses may be required for severe or chronic infections. Although ampicillin is resistant to degradation by gastric acid, it should be administered at least 30 minutes before or 2 hours after meals for maximal absorption. Except for the single dose regimen for gonorrhea referred to above, therapy should be continued for a minimum of 48 to 72 hours after the patient becomes asymptomatic or evidence of bacterial eradication has been obtained. In infections caused by hemolytic strains of streptococci, a minimum of 10 days' treatment is recommended to guard against the risk of rheumatic fever of glomerulonephritis. In the treatment of chronic urinary or gastrointestinal infections, frequent bacteriologic and clinical appraisal is necessary during therapy and may be necessary for several months afterwards. Stubborn infections may require treatment for several weeks. Smaller doses than those indicated above should not be used.

➤*Storage / Stability:*

Capsules – Store at room temperature; avoid excessive heat; keep tightly closed.

Ampicillin for oral suspension – Store at room temperature; after constitution, discard unused portion after 7 days if kept at room temperature or after 14 days if refrigerated; keep bottles tightly closed.

AMPICILLIN — INJECTION

For complete and comparative prescribing information, refer to the Penicillins group monograph.

Indications

➤*Respiratory tract infections:* Caused by *S. pneumoniae*, *Staphylococcus aureus* (penicillinase and non-penicillinase producing), *H. influenzae*, and group A beta-hemolytic streptococci.

➤*Bacterial meningitis:* Caused by *E. coli*, group B streptococci, and other Gram-negative bacteria (*Listeria monocytogenes*, *N. meningitidis*). The addition of an aminoglycoside with ampicillin may increase its effectiveness against gram-negative bacteria.

➤*Septicemia and endocarditis:* Caused by susceptible Gram-positive organisms including *Streptococcus* sp., penicillin G-susceptible staphylococci, and enterococci. Gram-negative sepsis caused by *E. coli. Proteus mirabilis*, and *Salmonella* sp. respond to ampicillin. Endocarditis due to enterococcal strains usually respond to IV therapy. The addition of an aminoglycoside may enhance the effectiveness of ampicillin when treating streptococcal endocarditis.

➤*Urinary tract infections:* Caused by sensitive strains of *E. coli* and *Proteus mirabilis*.

➤*GI infections:* Caused by *Salmonella typhosa* (typhoid fever), other *Salmonella* sp. and *Shigella* sp. (dysentery) usually respond to oral or IV therapy.

It is advisable to reserve the parenteral form of this drug for moderately severe and severe infections and for patients who are unable to take the oral forms. A change to oral ampicillin may be made as soon as appropriate.

Indicated surgical procedures should be performed.

Administration and Dosage

➤*Infections of the respiratory tract and soft tissues:*

Patients weighing 40 kg (88 pounds) or more – 250 to 500 mg every 6 hours.

Patients weighing less than 40 kg (88 pounds) – 25 to 50 mg/kg/day in equally divided doses at 6 to 8 hour intervals.

➤*Infections of the GI and genitourinary tracts (including those caused by Neisseria gonorrhoeae in females):*

Patients weighing 40 kg (88 pounds) or more – 500 mg every 6 hours.

Patients weighing less than 40 kg (88 pounds) – 50 mg/kg/day in equally divided doses at 6 to 8 hour intervals. In the treatment of chronic urinary tract and intestinal infections, frequent bacteriological and clinical appraisal is necessary. Smaller doses than those recommended above should not be used. Higher doses should be used for stubborn or severe infections. In stubborn infections, therapy may be required for several weeks. It may be necessary to continue clinical or bacteriological follow-up for several months after cessation of therapy.

➤*Urethritis in males due to N. gonorrhoeae:*

Adults – Two doses of 500 mg each at an interval of 8 to 12 hours. Treatment may be repeated if necessary or extended if required. In the treatment of complications of gonorrheal urethritis, such as prostatitis and epididymitis, prolonged and intensive therapy is recommended. Cases of gonorrhea with a suspected primary lesion of syphilis should have darkfield examinations before receiving treatment. In all other cases where concomitant syphilis is suspected, monthly serological tests should be made for a minimum of 4 months.

The doses for the preceding infections may be given by either the IM or IV route. A change to oral ampicillin may be made when appropriate.

➤*Bacterial meningitis:*

Adults and children – 150 to 200 mg/kg/day in equally divided doses every 3 to 4 hours. (Treatment may be initiated with IV infusion therapy and continued with IM injections.) The doses for other infections may be given by either the intravenous or intramuscular route.

➤*Septicemia:*

Adults and children – 150 to 200 mg/kg/day. Start with IV administration for at least 3 days and continue with the IM route every 3 to 4 hours. Treatment of all infections should be continued for a minimum of 48 to 72 hours beyond the time that the patient becomes asymptomatic or evidence of bacterial eradication has been obtained. A minimum of 10 days treatment is recommended for any infection caused by group A beta-hemolytic streptococci to help prevent the occurrence of acute rheumatic fever or acute glomerulonephritis.

➤*Preparation for administration:* Use only freshly prepared solutions. IM and IV injections should be administered within 1 hour after preparation, since the potency may decrease significantly after this period.

For IM use – Dissolve contents of a vial with the amount of Sterile Water for Injection or Bacteriostatic Water for Injection listed in the following table.

Preparation of Ampicillin IM Solution

Vial Strength	Amount of diluent to be added (mL)	Approximate available volume (mL)	Approximate concentration (in mg/mL)
250 mg	0.9 mL	1 mL	250 mg/mL
500 mg	1.7 mL	2 mL	250 mg/mL
1 g	3.4 mL	4 mL	250 mg/mL
2 g	6.8 mL	8 mL	250 mg/mL

While ampicillin for injection 1 g and 2 g vials are primarily for IV use, the contents may be administered IM when the 250 mg or 500 mg vials are unavailable. In such instances, dissolve in 3.4 or 6.8 mL Sterile Water for Injection or Bacteriostatic Water for Injection, respectively. The resulting solution will provide a concentration of 250 mg per mL.

For direct IV use – Add 5 mL Sterile Water for Injection or Bacteriostatic Water for Injection to the 250 and 500 mg vials and administer slowly over a 3-to 5-minute period. Ampicillin for injection, 1 g or 2 g, may also be given by direct IV administration. Dissolve in 7.4 or 14.8 mL Sterile Water for Injection or Bacteriostatic Water for Injection, respectively, and administer slowly over at least 10 to 15 minutes. Caution: More rapid administration may result in convulsive seizures.

For administration by IV drip – Reconstitute as directed above (For direct IV use) prior to diluting with IV solution. Stability studies on ampicillin at several concentrations in various IV solutions indicate the drug will lose less than 10% activity at the temperatures noted for the time periods stated.

AMPICILLIN — INJECTION

Room temperature (25°C)		
Diluent	Concentrations	Stability periods
Sterile Water for Injection	up to 30 mg/mL	8 h
Sodium Chloride Injection 0.9%	up to 30 mg/mL	8 h
M/6 Sodium Lactate Injection	up to 30 mg/mL	8 h
5% Dextrose in Water	10 to 20 mg/mL	2 h
5% Dextrose in Water	up to 2 mg/mL	4 h
5% Dextrose and 0.45 NaCl injection	up to 2 mg/mL	4 h
10% Invert Sugar in Water	up to 2 mg/mL	4 h
Lactated Ringer's Injection	up to 30 mg/mL	8 h

Refrigerated 4°C		
Diluent	Concentrations	Stability periods
Sterile Water for Injection	30 mg/mL	48 h
Sterile Water for Injection	up to 20 mg/mL	72 h
Sodium Chloride injection 0.9%	30 mg/mL	48 h
Sodium Chloride injection 0.9%	up to 20 mg/mL	72 h
Lactated Ringer's Injection	up to 30 mg/mL	24 h
M/6 Sodium Lactate Injection	up to 30 mg/mL	8 h
5% Dextrose in Water	up to 20 mg/mL	4 h
5% Dextrose and 0.45 NaCl injection	up to 10 mg/mL	4 h
10% Invert Sugar	up to 20 mg/mL	3 h

Only those solutions listed above should be used for the IV infusion of ampicillin for injection. The concentrations should fall within the range specified. The drug concentration and the rate and volume of the infusion should be adjusted so that the total dose of ampicillin is administered before the drug loses its stability in the solution in use.

➤*Storage/Stability:* Store at controlled room temperature 15° to 30°C (59° to 86°F).

AMPICILLIN SODIUM AND SULBACTAM SODIUM

Rx	**Ampicillin and Sulbactam** (ESI Lederle)	**Powder for injection:** 1.5 g (1 g ampicillin sodium/ 0.5 g sulbactam sodium)	In vials.
Rx	**Unasyn** (Roerig)		In vials, bottles, and *ADD-Vantage* vials.
Rx	**Ampicillin and Sulbactam** (ESI Lederle)	3 g (2 g ampicillin sodium/1 g sulbactam sodium)	In vials.
Rx	**Unasyn** (Roerig)		In vials, bottles, and *ADD-Vantage* vials.
Rx	**Unasyn** (Roerig)	15 g (10 g ampicillin sodium/5 g sulbactam sodium)	In bulk package.

AMPICILLIN SODIUM AND SULBACTAM SODIUM — INJECTION

For complete prescribing information, refer to the Penicillins group monograph.

Indications

➤*Skin and skin structure infections:* Those caused by β-lactamase-producing strains of *Staphylococcus aureus*, *Escherichia coli*†, *Klebsiella*† sp. (including *K. pneumoniae*†), *Proteus mirabilis*†, *Bacteroides fragilis*†, *Enterobacter*† sp. and *Acinetobacter calcoaceticus*†.

➤*Intra-abdominal infections:* Those caused by β-lactamase-producing strains of *E. coli, Klebsiella* sp. (including *K. pneumoniae*†), *Bacteroides* sp. (including *B. fragilis*), *Enterobacter*† sp.

➤*Gynecological infections:* Those caused by β-lactamase-producing strains of *E. coli*† and *Bacteroides* sp.† (including *B. fragilis*†).

While this combination is indicated only for the conditions listed above, infections caused by ampicillin-susceptible organisms also are amenable to treatment because of the ampicillin content. Therefore, mixed infections caused by ampicillin-susceptible organisms and β-lactamase-producing organisms susceptible to this combination should not require the addition of another antibiotic.

Administration and Dosage

Give IV or IM.

➤*Adult:* 1.5 g (1 g ampicillin + 0.5 g sulbactam) to 3 g (2 g ampicillin + 1 g sulbactam) every 6 hours. Do not exceed 4 g/day sulbactam.

➤*Children:* Do not routinely exceed 14 days of IV therapy. Safety and efficacy of IM administration have not been established.

Children 1 year of age or older – 300 mg/kg/day IV (200 mg ampicillin/ 100 mg sulbactam) in divided doses every 6 hours.

Children 40 kg or more – Dose according to adult recommendations; total sulbactam dose should not exceed 4 g/day.

The safety and efficacy of ampicillin/sulbactam sodium have been established for pediatric patients 1 year of age or older for skin and skin structure infections as approved in adults but have not been established for pediatric patients for intra-abdominal infections.

➤*Renal function impairment:* The elimination kinetics of ampicillin and sulbactam are similarly affected; hence, the ratio of one to the other will remain constant despite the renal function. In patients with renal impairment, administer as follows:

Ampicillin/Sulbactam Dosage Guide For Patients With Renal Impairment		
Ccr (mL/min/1.73 m^2)	Half-life (hours)	Recommended dosage
≥ 30	1	1.5 to 3 g q 6 to 8 h
15-29	5	1.5 to 3 g q 12 h
5-14	9	1.5 to 3 g q 24 h

➤*Preparation for IV use:* Reconstitute powder for IV and IM use with any of the compatible diluents described below. Allow solutions to stand after dissolution so that any foaming will dissipate. This permits visual inspection for complete solubilization.

1.5 and 3 g bottles – Reconstitute to desired concentrations (3 to 45 mg/ mL) with any of the following diluents. Discard unused solutions after indicated times.

Preparation of Ampicillin/Sulbactam for IV Use		
Diluent	Maximum concentration (mg/mL)	Stability
Sterile water for injection	45 (30/15)	8h @ 25°C
	45 (30/15)	48 h @ 4°C
	30 (20/10)	72 h @ 4°C
0.9% sodium chloride injection	45 (30/15)	8h @ 25°C
	45 (30/15)	48 h @ 4°C
	30 (20/10)	72 h @ 4°C
5% dextrose injection	30 (20/10)	2h @ 25°C
	30 (20/10)	4 h @ 4°C
	3 (2/1)	4h @ 25°C
Lactated Ringer's injection	45 (30/15)	8 h @ 25°C
	45 (30/15)	24 h @ 4°C
M/6 sodium lactate injection	45 (30/15)	8 h @ 25°C
	45 (30/15)	8 h @ 4°C
5% dextrose in 0.45% saline	3 (2/1)	4 h @ 25°C
	15 (10/5)	4 h @ 4°C
10% invert sugar	3 (2/1)	4 h @ 25°C
	30 (20/10)	3 h @ 4°C

If piggyback bottles are unavailable, use standard vials of sterile powder. Initially, reconstitute with sterile water for injection to yield 375 mg/mL (250 mg ampicillin/125 mg sulbactam/mL). Then immediately dilute to yield 3 to 45 mg/mL (2 to 30 mg ampicillin/1 to 15 mg sulbactam/mL). Inject slowly over at least 10 to 15 minutes or infuse in greater dilutions with 50 to 100 mL diluent over 15 to 30 minutes.

The *ADD-Vantage* system is intended as single-dose for IV administration after dilution with the *ADD-Vantage Flexible Diluent Container* containing 50 mL (1.5 g vial only), 100 mL or 250 mL of 0.9% sodium chloride injection only. Once diluted, the solution is stable at a maximum concentration of 30 (20/10) mg/mL for 8 hours at 25°C, 77°F. Therefore, the final diluted solution should be completely administered within 8 hours to assure proper potency.

➤*Preparation for IM injection:* Reconstitute with sterile water for injection or 0.5% or 2% lidocaine HCl injection. Consult the following table for recommended volumes needed to obtain 375 mg/mL solutions (250 mg ampicillin/125 mg sulbactam/mL). Use only freshly prepared solutions; give within 1 hour after preparation.

Preparation of Ampicillin/Sulbactam for IM Use		
Vial size	Diluent to be added	Withdrawal volume
1.5 g	3.2 mL	4 mL
3 g	6.4 mL	8 mL

† Efficacy for these organisms in this organ system was studied in fewer than 10 infections.
† Efficacy for this organism in this organ system was studied in fewer than 10 infections.

AMPICILLIN SODIUM AND SULBACTAM SODIUM — INJECTION

➤*Admixture incompatibility:* When concomitant aminoglycosides are indicated, reconstitute and administer this product and aminoglycosides separately; aminopenicillins inactivate aminoglycosides in vitro.

➤*Storage / Stability:* Store at or below 30°C (86°F) prior to reconstitution.

AMOXICILLIN

Rx	**Amoxicillin** (Various, eg, Ranbaxy, Teva)	**Tablets, chewable:** 125 mg (as trihydrate)	In 100s.
Rx	**Amoxicillin** (Ranbaxy)	**Tablets, chewable:** 200 mg (as trihydrate)	In 20s.
Rx	**Amoxil** (GlaxoSmithKline)		Aspartame, 1.82 mg phenylalanine. (AMOXIL 200). Pale pink. Cherry-banana-peppermint flavor. In 20s and 100s.
Rx	**Amoxicillin** (Various, eg, Ranbaxy, Teva)	**Tablets, chewable:** 250 mg (as trihydrate)	In 100s, 250s, and 500s.
Rx	**Amoxicillin** (Ranbaxy)	**Tablets, chewable:** 400 mg (as trihydrate)	In 20s and 100s.
Rx	**Amoxil** (GlaxoSmithKline)		Aspartame, 3.64 mg phenylalanine. (AMOXIL 400). Pale pink. Cherry-banana-peppermint flavor. In 20s.
Rx	**Amoxicillin** (Various, eg, Ranbaxy, Teva)	**Tablets:** 500 mg (as trihydrate)	In 20s and 100s.
Rx	**Amoxil** (GlaxoSmithKline)		(Amoxil 500). Pink, capsule shape. Film-coated. In 20s, 100s, and 500s.
Rx	**Amoxicillin** (Various, eg, Ranbaxy, Teva)	**Tablets:** 875 mg (as trihydrate)	In 20s, 100s, and 500s.
Rx	**Amoxil** (GlaxoSmithKline)		(Amoxil 875). Pink, capsule shape, scored. Film-coated. In 20s, 100s, 500s.
Rx	**Amoxicillin** (Various, eg, Ranbaxy, Teva)	**Capsules:** 250 mg (as trihydrate)	In 100s, 500s, and 1000s.
Rx	**Amoxicillin** (Various, eg, Ranbaxy, Teva)	**Capsules:** 500 mg (as trihydrate)	In 50s, 100s, and 500s.
Rx	**Amoxil** (GlaxoSmithKline)		(Amoxil 500). Blue/Pink. In 500s.
Rx	**Amoxil Pediatric Drops** (GlaxoSmithKline)	**Powder for oral suspension:** 50 mg/mL (as trihydrate) when reconstituted	Sucrose. Bubble-gum flavor. In 15 and 30 mL.
Rx	**Amoxicillin** (Various, eg, Teva)	**Powder for oral suspension:** 125 mg/5 mL (as trihydrate) when reconstituted	In 80, 100, and 150 mL.
Rx	**Amoxil** (GlaxoSmithKline)		Sucrose. Strawberry flavor. In 80 and 150 mL.
Rx	**Trimox** (Sandoz)		Sucrose. Raspberry-strawberry flavor. In 80, 100, and 150 mL.
Rx	**Amoxicillin** (Ranbaxy)	**Powder for oral suspension:** 200 mg/5 mL (as trihydrate) when reconstituted	Fruit flavor. In 50, 75, and 100 mL.
Rx	**Amoxil** (GlaxoSmithKline)		Sucrose. Bubble-gum flavor. In 50, 75, and 100 mL.
Rx	**Amoxicillin** (Various, eg, Teva)	**Powder for oral suspension:** 250 mg/5 mL (as trihydrate) when reconstituted	In 80, 100, and 150 mL.
Rx	**Amoxil** (GlaxoSmithKline)		Sucrose. Bubble-gum flavor. In 100 and 150 mL.
Rx	**Amoxicillin** (Ranbaxy)	**Powder for oral suspension:** 400 mg/5 mL (as trihydrate) when reconstituted	Fruit flavor. In 50, 75, and 100 mL.
Rx	**Amoxil** (GlaxoSmithKline)		Sucrose. Bubble-gum flavor. In 50, 75, and 100 mL.
Rx	**DisperMox** (Ranbaxy)	**Tablets for oral suspension:** 200 mg	Aspartame, 5.6 mg phenylalanine. (RX565). Lt. pink, mottled. Strawberry flavor. In 20s, 60s, 1000s, and UD 100s.
		400 mg	Aspartame, 5.6 mg phenylalanine. (RX567). Lt. pink, mottled. Strawberry flavor. In 20s, 60s, 500s, and UD 100s.

AMOXICILLIN — ORAL

For complete and comparative prescribing information, refer to the Penicillins group monograph. For information on amoxicillin therapy in *Helicobacter pylori* infection, refer to the *H. pylori* Agents monographs in the GI chapter.

Indications

In the treatment of infections due to susceptible (only beta-lactamase-negative) strains of the designated microorganisms in the following conditions.

➤*ENT infections:* Infections of the ear, nose, and throat due to *Streptococcus* sp. (alpha- and beta-hemolytic strains only), *Streptococcus pneumoniae*, *Staphylococcus* sp., or *H. influenzae*.

➤*GU tract infections:* Infections of the GU tract due to *E. coli*, *P. mirabilis*, or *E. faecalis*.

➤*Skin and skin structure infections:* Infections of the skin and skin structure due to *Streptococcus* sp. (alpha- and beta-hemolytic strains only), *Staphylococcus* sp., or *E. coli*.

➤*Lower respiratory tract infections:* Infections of the lower respiratory tract due to *Streptococcus* sp. (alpha- and beta-hemolytic strains only), *Streptococcus pneumoniae*, *Staphylococcus* sp. or *H. influenzae*.

➤*Gonorrhea:* Gonorrhea, acute uncomplicated (anogenital and urethral infections) due to *N. gonorrhoeae* (males and females).

➤*H. pylori infections: H. pylori* eradication to reduce the risk of duodenal ulcer recurrence.

➤*Triple therapy (amoxicillin / clarithromycin / lansoprazole):* Amoxicillin, in combination with clarithromycin plus lansoprazole as triple therapy, is indicated for the treatment of patients with *H. pylori* infection and duodenal ulcer disease (active or 1-year history of a duodenal ulcer) to eradicate *H. pylori*. Eradication of *H. pylori* has been shown to reduce the risk of duodenal ulcer recurrence.

➤*Dual therapy (amoxicillin / lansoprazole):* Amoxicillin, in combination with lansoprazole delayed-release capsules as dual therapy, is indicated for the treatment of patients with *H. pylori* infection and duodenal ulcer disease (active or 1-year history of a duodenal ulcer) who are either allergic or intolerant to clarithromycin or in whom resistance to clarithromycin is known or suspected. Eradication of *H. pylori* has been shown to reduce the risk of duodenal ulcer recurrence.

Indicated surgical procedures should be performed.

Administration and Dosage

➤*Approved by the FDA:* August 6, 1984.

➤*Capsules, chewable tablets, and oral suspension:* Amoxicillin capsules, chewable tablets, and oral suspensions of amoxicillin may be given without regard to meals. The 400 mg suspension, the 400 mg chewable tablet and the 875 mg tablet have been studied only when administered at the start of a light meal. However, food-effect studies have not been performed with the 200 mg and 500 mg formulations.

➤*Neonates and infants aged less than or equal to 12 weeks (less than or equal to 3 months):* Due to incompletely developed renal function affecting elimination of amoxicillin in this age group, the recommended upper dose of amoxicillin is 30 mg/kg/day divided every 12 hours.

Adults and Pediatric Patients Older Than 3 Months of Age			
Infection	Severity[a]	Usual adult dose	Usual dose for children > 3 months[b,c]
Ear/nose/throat	Mild/moderate	500 mg every 12 h or 250 mg every 8 h	25 mg/kg/day in divided doses every 12 h or 20 mg/kg/day in divided doses every 8 h
	Severe	875 mg every 12 h or 500 mg every 8 h	45 mg/kg/day in divided doses every 12 h or 40 mg/kg/day in divided doses every 8 h

AMOXICILLIN — ORAL

Adults and Pediatric Patients Older Than 3 Months of Age			
Infection	Severity[a]	Usual adult dose	Usual dose for children > 3 months[b,c]
Lower respiratory tract	Mild/moderate or severe	875 mg every 12 h or 500 mg every 8 h	45 mg/kg/day in divided doses every 12 h or 40 mg/kg/day in divided doses every 8 h
Skin/skin structure	Mild/moderate	500 mg every 12 h or 250 mg every 8 h	25 mg/kg/day in divided doses every 12 h or 20 mg/kg/day in divided doses every 8 h
	Severe	875 mg every 12 h or 500 mg every 8 h	45 mg/kg/day in divided doses every 12 h or 40 mg/kg/day in divided doses every 8 h
GU tract	Mild/moderate	500 mg every 12 h or 250 mg every 8 h	25 mg/kg/day in divided doses every 12 h or 20 mg/kg/day in divided doses every 8 h
	Severe	875 mg every 12 h or 500 mg every 8 h	45 mg/kg/day in divided doses every 12 h or 40 mg/kg/day in divided doses every 8 h
Gonorrhea acute, uncomplicated ano-genital, and urethral infections in males and females		3 g as single oral dose	Prepubertal children: 50 mg/kg amoxicillin, combined with 25 mg/kg probenecid as a single dose. Note: Since probenecid is contraindicated in children under 2 years, do not use this regimen in these cases.

[a] Dosing for infections caused by less susceptible organisms should follow the recommendations for severe infections.
[b] The children's dosage is intended for individuals whose weight is less than 40 kg. Children weighing 40 kg or more should be dosed according to the adult recommendations.
[c] Each strength of the suspension of amoxicillin is available as a chewable tablet for use by older children.

➤*H. pylori eradication to reduce the risk of duodenal ulcer recurrence:*

Triple therapy (amoxicillin/clarithromycin/lansoprazole) – The recommended adult oral dose is 1 g amoxicillin, 500 mg clarithromycin, and 30 mg lansoprazole, all given twice daily (every 12 hours) for 14 days.

Dual therapy (amoxicillin/lansoprazole) – The recommended adult oral dose is 1 g amoxicillin and 30 mg lansoprazole, each given 3 times daily (every 8 hours) for 14 days. Please refer to clarithromycin and lansoprazole monographs for Contraindications and Warnings, and for information regarding dosing in elderly and renally impaired patients.

➤*Renal function impairment:* Patients with impaired renal function do not generally require a reduction in dose unless the impairment is severe. Severely impaired patients with a glomerular filtration rate of less than 30 mL/min should not receive the 875 mg tablet. Patients with a glomerular filtration rate of 10 to 30 mL/min should receive 500 mg or 250 mg every 12 hours, depending on the severity of the infection. Patients with a less than 10 mL/min glomerular filtration rate should receive 500 mg or 250 mg every 24 hours, depending on severity of the infection.

Hemodialysis patients should receive 500 mg or 250 mg every 24 hours, depending on severity of the infection. They should receive an additional dose both during and at the end of dialysis.

There are currently no dosing recommendations for pediatric patients with impaired renal function.

➤*Mixing oral suspension:* Prepare suspension at time of dispensing as follows: Tap bottle until all powder flows freely. Add approximately ⅓ of the total amount of water for reconstitution and shake vigorously to wet powder. Add remainder of the water and again shake vigorously.

➤*Mixing pediatric drops:* Prepare pediatric drops at time of dispensing as follows: Add the required amount of water (see below) to the bottle and shake vigorously. Each mL of suspension will then contain amoxicillin trihydrate equivalent to 50 mg amoxicillin.

The amount of water required for reconstituting amoxicillin pediatric drops is 12 and 23 mL to bottle sizes of 15 and 30 mL, respectively.

➤*Oral suspension:* Shake both oral suspension and pediatric drops well before using. Keep bottle tightly closed. Any unused portion of the reconstituted suspension must be discarded after 14 days. Refrigeration is preferable for all formulations, but may or may not be required. Patients should refer to the package labeling for refrigeration requirements.

➤*Mixing tablets for oral suspension:* Mix 1 tablet in approximately 10 mL of water. Drink entire mixture, rinse with small amount of water, and drink the contents to ensure entire dose is taken. Do not chew or swallow tablets. The tablets will not rapidly dissolve in mouth.

The tablet is not recommended to be mixed with any liquid other than water, as studies have only been conducted using water.

➤*Storage/Stability:* Store 250 mg and 500 capsules and 125 mg and 250 mg unreconstituted powder at or below 20°C (68°F).

Store 200 mg and 400 mg unreconstituted powder, 200 mg and 400 mg chewable tablets, and 500 mg and 875 mg tablets at or below 25°C (77°F). Dispense in a tight container.

Note – Any unused portion of the reconstituted suspension must be discarded after 14 days. Refrigeration is preferable but not required.

AMOXICILLIN AND POTASSIUM CLAVULANATE (Co-amoxiclav)

Rx	**Augmentin** (GlaxoSmithKline)	**Tablets**: 250 mg amoxicillin (as trihydrate) and 125 mg clavulanic acid[a]	0.63 mEq potassium. (Augmentin 250/125). White, oval. Film-coated. In 30s and UD 100s.
Rx	**Amoxicillin, Clavulanate Potassium** (Various, eg, Geneva, Ranbaxy, Teva)	**Tablets**: 500 mg amoxicillin (as trihydrate) and 125 mg clavulanic acid[a]	In 20s.
Rx	**Augmentin** (GlaxoSmithKline)		0.63 mEq potassium. (Augmentin 500/125). White, oval. Film-coated. In 20s and UD 100s.
Rx	**Amoxicillin, Clavulanate Potassium** (Various, eg, Geneva, Lek, Ranbaxy, Teva)	**Tablets**: 875 mg amoxicillin (as trihydrate) and 125 mg clavulanic acid[a]	In 20s.
Rx	**Augmentin** (GlaxoSmithKline)		0.63 mEq potassium. (Augmentin 875). White, capsule shape, scored. In 20s and UD 100s.
Rx	**Augmentin XR** (GlaxoSmithKline)	**Tablets, extended-release**: 1,000 mg amoxicillin and 62.5 mg clavulanic acid	**Unscored tablets:** 0.32 mEq potassium, 1.27 mEq sodium. (AC 1,000/62.5). White, oval. Film-coated. In 28s (7 day XR pack) and 40s (10 day XR pack). **Scored tablets:** 0.32 mEq potassium, 1.27 mEq sodium. (AUGMENTIN XR). White, oval. Film-coated. In 28s (7 day XR pack) and 40s (10 day XR pack).
Rx	**Augmentin** (GlaxoSmithKline)	**Tablets, chewable**: 125 mg amoxicillin (as trihydrate) and 31.25 mg clavulanic acid[a]	0.16 mEq potassium, saccharin, mannitol. (BMP 189). Yellow, mottled. Lemon-lime flavor. In 30s.
Rx	**Amoxicillin, Clavulanate Potassium** (Geneva)	**Tablets, chewable**: 200 mg amoxicillin (as trihydrate) and 28.5 mg clavulanic acid[a]	In UD 20s.
Rx	**Augmentin** (GlaxoSmithKline)		0.14 mEq potassium, saccharin, mannitol, aspartame.[b] (AUGMENTIN 200). Pink, mottled. Cherry-banana flavor. In 20s.
Rx	**Augmentin** (GlaxoSmithKline)	**Tablets, chewable**: 250 mg amoxicillin (as trihydrate) and 62.5 mg clavulanic acid[a]	0.32 mEq potassium, saccharin, mannitol. (BMP 190). Yellow, mottled. Lemon-lime flavor. In 30s.

AMOXICILLIN AND POTASSIUM CLAVULANATE (Co-amoxiclav)

Rx	**Amoxicillin, Clavulanate Potassium** (Geneva)	**Tablets, chewable**: 400 mg amoxicillin (as trihydrate) and 57 mg clavulanic acid[a]	In UD 20s.
Rx	**Augmentin** (GlaxoSmithKline)		0.29 mEq potassium, saccharin, mannitol, aspartame.[c] (AUGMENTIN 400). Pink, mottled. Cherry-banana flavor. In 20s.
Rx	**Augmentin** (GlaxoSmithKline)	**Powder for oral suspension**: 125 mg amoxicillin and 31.25 mg clavulanic acid[a] per 5 mL (after reconstitution)	0.16 mEq potassium per 5 mL, saccharin, mannitol. Banana flavor. In 75, 100, and 150 mL.
Rx	**Amoxicillin, Clavulanate Potassium** (Geneva)	**Powder for oral suspension**: 200 mg amoxicillin and 28.5 mg clavulanic acid[a] per 5 mL (after reconstitution)	In 100 mL.
Rx	**Amoclan** (West-ward)		0.143 mEq potassium per 5 mL, aspartame.[d] Golden syrup and orange flavor. In 50, 75, and 100 mL.
Rx	**Augmentin** (GlaxoSmithKline)		0.14 mEq potassium per 5 mL, saccharin, mannitol, aspartame.[d] Orange-raspberry flavor. In 50, 75, and 100 mL.
Rx	**Augmentin** (GlaxoSmithKline)	**Powder for oral suspension**: 250 mg amoxicillin and 62.5 mg clavulanic acid[a] per 5 mL (after reconstitution)	0.32 mEq potassium per 5 mL, saccharin, mannitol. Orange flavor. In 75, 100, and 150 mL.
Rx	**Amoxicillin, Clavulanate Potassium** (Geneva)	**Powder for oral suspension**: 400 mg amoxicillin and 57 mg clavulanic acid[a] per 5 mL (after reconstitution)	In 100 mL.
Rx	**Amoclan** (West-ward)		0.286 mEq potassium per 5 mL, aspartame.[d] Golden syrup and orange flavor. In 50, 75, and 100 mL.
Rx	**Augmentin** (GlaxoSmithKline)		0.29 mEq potassium per 5 mL, saccharin, mannitol, aspartame.[d] Orange-raspberry flavor. In 50, 75, and 100 mL.
Rx	**Amoxicillin, Clavulanate Potassium** (Various, eg, Ivax, Teva)	**Powder for oral suspension**: 600 mg amoxicillin (as trihydrate) and 42.9 mg clavulanic acid[a] per 5 mL (after reconstitution)	0.23 mEq potassium per 5 mL. May contain aspartame or saccharin. In 75, 125, and 200 mL.
Rx	**Augmentin ES-600** (GlaxoSmithKline)		0.23 mEq potassium per 5 mL, aspartame.[d] Orange-raspberry flavor. In 75 mL.

[a] As the potassium salt.
[b] Contains 2.1 mg phenylalanine.
[c] Contains 4.2 mg phenylalanine.
[d] Contains 7 mg phenylalanine per 5 mL.

AMOXICILLIN AND POTASSIUM CLAVULANATE (Co-amoxiclav) — ORAL

For complete and comparative prescribing information, refer to the Penicillins group monograph.

Indications

➤*Lower respiratory infections:* Those caused by β-lactamase-producing strains of *Haemophilus influenzae* and *Moraxella catarrhalis*.

➤*Otitis media and sinusitis:* Those caused by β-lactamase-producing strains of *H. influenzae* and *M. (Branhamella) catarrhalis*.

➤*Skin and skin structure infections:* Those caused by β-lactamase-producing strains of *Staphylococcus aureus*, *Escherichia coli*, and *Klebsiella* sp.

➤*Urinary tract infections:* Those caused by β-lactamase-producing strains of *Escherichia coli*, *Klebsiella* sp., and *Enterobacter* sp.

➤*Augmentin ES-600*:

Acute otitis media (Augmentin ES-600) – For the treatment of pediatric patients with recurrent or persistent acute otitis media due to *Streptococcus pneumoniae* (penicillin MICs less than or equal to 2 mcg/mL), *H. influenzae* (including β-lactamase-producing strains), *M. catarrhalis* (including β-lactamase-producing strains) characterized by the following risk factors: Antibiotic exposure for acute otitis media within the preceding 3 months, and either of the following:

- Age of 2 years or younger, or
- daycare attendance.

Acute otitis media due to *S. pneumoniae* alone can be treated with amoxicillin. *Augmentin ES-600* is not indicated for the treatment of acute otitis media due to *S. pneumoniae* with penicillin MIC at least 4 mcg/mL.

➤*Augmentin XR:*

Community-acquired pneumonia and acute bacterial sinusitis – For the treatment of patients with community-acquired pneumonia or acute bacterial sinusitis due to confirmed or suspected β-lactamase-producing pathogens (ie, *H. influenzae*, *M. catarrhalis*, *H. parainfluenzae*, *K. pneumoniae*, or methicillin-susceptible *S. aureus*) and *S. pneumoniae* with reduced susceptibility to penicillin (ie, penicillin MICs equal to 2 mcg/mL). *Augmentin XR* is not indicated for the treatment of infections due to *S. pneumoniae* with penicillin MICs 4 mcg/mL or more. Data are limited with regard to infections due to *S. pneumoniae* with penicillin MICs 4 mcg/mL or more. Acute bacterial sinusitis or community-acquired pneumonia due to a penicillin-susceptible strain of *S. pneumoniae* plus a β-lactamase-producing pathogen can be treated with another *Augmentin* product containing lower daily doses of amoxicillin. Acute bacterial sinusitis or community-acquired pneumonia due to *S. pneumoniae* alone can be treated with amoxicillin.

While amoxicillin/potassium clavulanate is indicated only for the conditions listed above, infections caused by ampicillin-susceptible organisms are also amenable to this drug because of its amoxicillin content. Therefore, mixed infections caused by ampicillin-susceptible organisms and β-lactamase-producing organisms susceptible to amoxicillin/potassium clavulanate should not require an additional antibiotic. Therapy may be instituted prior to obtaining the results from bacteriologic and susceptibility studies when there is reason to believe the infection may involve any of the β-lactamase-producing organisms listed above. Once the results are known, adjust therapy.

Administration and Dosage

➤*Augmentin:* May be administered without regard to meals; however, absorption of clavulanate potassium is enhanced when taken at the start of a meal. To minimize the potential for GI intolerance, give the drug at the start of a meal.

Contraindicated in patients with a history of amoxicillin/clavulanate potassium-associated cholestatic jaundice/hepatic dysfunction. Use with caution in patients with evidence of hepatic dysfunction.

Tablet interchangeability – Because the 250 and 500 mg tablets contain the same amount of clavulanic acid (125 mg as potassium salt), two 250 mg tablets are not equivalent to one 500 mg tablet. The 875 mg tablet also contains 125 mg potassium clavulanate. In addition, the 250 mg tablet and 250 mg chewable tablet do not contain the same amount of potassium clavulanate and should not be substituted for each other, as they are not interchangeable.

Dosage –

Adults: One 500 mg tablet every 12 hours or one 250 mg tablet every 8 hours.

- *Suspension* – Adults who have difficulty swallowing may be given the 125 mg/5 mL or 250 mg/5 mL suspension in place of the 500 mg tablet or give 200 mg/5 mL or 400 mg/5 mL suspension in place of the 875 mg tablet.
- *Severe infections and respiratory tract infections* – One 875 mg tablet every 12 hours or one 500 mg tablet every 8 hours.
- *Renal function impairment* – This does not generally require a dose reduction unless impairment is severe. Severely impaired patients with a glomerular filtration rate (GFR) of less than 30 mL/min should not receive the 875 mg tablet. Give patients with a GFR of 10 to 30 mL/min 500 or 250 mg every 12 hours, depending on the severity of infection. Give patients with a GFR less than 10 mL/min 500 or 250 mg every 24 hours, depending on severity of infection. Give hemodialysis patients 500 or 250 mg every 24 hours, and an additional dose both during and at the end of dialysis.
- *Hepatic function impairment* – Dose with caution and monitor hepatic function.

Children –

Younger than 3 months of age: 30 mg/kg/day divided every 12 hours, based on the amoxicillin component. Use of the 125 mg/5 mL oral suspension is recommended.

3 months of age or older: Children's dose is based on amoxicillin content. Refer to the following table. Because of the different amoxicillin to clavulanic acid ratios in the 250 mg tablets (250/125) vs the 250 mg chewable tablets (250/62.5), do not use the 250 mg tablet until the child weighs 40 kg or more.

40 kg or more: Dose according to adult recommendations.

AMOXICILLIN AND POTASSIUM CLAVULANATE (Co-amoxiclav) — ORAL

Amoxicillin/Potassium Clavulanate Dosing in Children ≥ 3 Months of Age		
	Dosing regimen	
Infections	200 mg/5 mL or 400 mg/5 mL (q 12 hr)[a,b]	125 mg/5 mL or 250 mg/5 mL (q 8 hr)[b]
Otitis media,[c] sinusitis, lower respiratory tract infections, severe infections	45 mg/kg/day	40 mg/kg/day
Less severe infections	25 mg/kg/day	20 mg/kg/day

[a] The every-12-hour regimen is associated with significantly less diarrhea; however, the 200 and 400 mg formulations (suspension and chewable tablets) contain aspartame and should not be used by phenylketonurics.
[b] Each strength of the suspension is available as a chewable tablet for use by older children.
[c] Recommended duration is 10 days.

➤*Augmentin ES-600*: *Augmentin ES-600*, 600 mg/5 mL, does not contain the same amount of clavulanic acid (as the potassium salt) as any of the other *Augmentin* suspensions. *Augmentin ES-600* contains 42.9 mg clavulanic acid per 5 mL whereas *Augmentin* 200 mg/5 mL suspension contains 28.5 mg clavulanic acid per 5 mL and the 400 mg/5 mL suspension contains 57 mg clavulanic acid per 5 mL. Therefore, *Augmentin* 200 mg/5 mL and 400 mg/5 mL suspensions should not be substituted for *Augmentin ES-600*, as they are not interchangeable.

Dosage –

Pediatric patients 3 months and older: Based on the amoxicillin component (600 mg/5 mL), the recommended dose of *Augmentin ES-600* is 90 mg/kg/day divided every 12 hours, administered for 10 days (see table below).

Recommended Dose of *Augmentin ES-600*	
Body weight (kg)	Volume of *Augmentin ES-600* providing 90 mg/kg/day
8	3 mL twice daily
12	4.5 mL twice daily
16	6 mL twice daily
20	7.5 mL twice daily
24	9 mL twice daily
28	10.5 mL twice daily
32	12 mL twice daily
36	13.5 mL twice daily

Pediatric patients weighing 40 kg or more: Experience with *Augmentin ES-600* in this group is not available.

Adults: Experience with *Augmentin ES-600* in adults is not available and adults who have difficulty swallowing should not be given *Augmentin ES-600* in place of the *Augmentin* 500 mg or 875 mg tablet.

Hepatic function impairment: Dose hepatically impaired patients with caution and monitor hepatic function at regular intervals.

Preparing oral suspension – Prepare a suspension at time of dispensing as follows: Tap bottle until all the powder flows freely. Add approximately two thirds of the total amount of water for reconstitution and shake vigorously to suspend powder. Add remainder of the water and again shake vigorously.

Administration – To minimize the potential for GI intolerance, take at the start of a meal. Absorption of clavulanate potassium may be enhanced when the drug is administered at the start of a meal.

➤*Augmentin XR*: Take at the start of a meal to enhance the absorption of amoxicillin and minimize the potential for GI intolerance. Absorption of the amoxicillin component is decreased when *Augmentin XR* is taken on an empty stomach.

Dosage – The recommended dose is 4,000 mg/250 mg daily according to the following table.

Augmentin XR Dosing		
Indication	Dose	Duration
Acute bacterial sinusitis	2 tablets q 12 h	10 days
Community-acquired pneumonia	2 tablets q 12 h	7 to 10 days

Tablet interchangeability – *Augmentin* tablets (250 or 500 mg) cannot be used to provide the same dosages as *Augmentin XR* extended-release tablets. This is because *Augmentin XR* contains 62.5 mg clavulanic acid, while the *Augmentin* 250 and 500 mg tablets each contain 125 mg clavulanic acid. In addition, the extended-release tablet provides an extended time course of plasma amoxicillin concentrations compared with immediate-release tablets. Thus, 2 *Augmentin* 500 mg tablets are not equivalent to 1 *Augmentin XR* tablet.

The scored *Augmentin XR* tablets are available for greater convenience for adult patients who have difficulty swallowing. The scored *Augmentin XR* tablet may be broken in half at score line. The scored tablet is not intended to reduce the dosage of medication taken; as stated in the table above, the recommended dose of *Augmentin XR* is 2 tablets twice daily every 12 hours.

Renal function impairment – The pharmacokinetics of *Augmentin XR* have not been studied in patients with renal impairment. *Augmentin XR* is contraindicated in severely impaired patients with a creatinine clearance of less than 30 mL/min and in hemodialysis patients.

Hepatic function impairment – Dose hepatically impaired patients with caution and monitor hepatic function at regular intervals.

Children – Safety and efficacy in pediatric patients younger than 16 years of age have not been established.

➤*Storage/Stability:* Refrigerate reconstituted suspension and discard after 10 days. Shake well before using. Store tablets and dry powder at or below 25°C (77°F); dispense in the original container.

TICARCILLIN DISODIUM

Rx	**Ticar** (GlaxoSmithKline)	**Powder for Injection:** 3 g (of ticarcillin)	In 3 g vials.

TICARCILLIN DISODIUM — INJECTION

For complete and comparative prescribing information, refer to the Penicillins group monograph.

Indications

For the treatment of the following infections: Bacterial septicemia caused by susceptible strains of *Pseudomonas aeruginosa*, *Proteus* species (both indole-positive and indole-negative) and *Escherichia coli*; skin and soft-tissue infections; acute and chronic respiratory tract infections. Though clinical improvement has been shown, bacteriological cures cannot be expected in patients with chronic respiratory disease or cystic fibrosis.

➤*GU tract infections:* Complicated and uncomplicated due to susceptible strains of *Pseudomonas aeruginosa*, *Proteus* species (both indole-positive and indole-negative), *Escherichia coli*, *Enterobacter* and *Streptococcus faecalis* (enterococcus).

➤*Infections due to susceptible anaerobic bacteria:*
- Bacterial septicemia.
- Lower respiratory tract infections such as empyema, anaerobic pneumonitis and lung abscess.
- Intra-abdominal infections such as peritonitis and intra-abdominal abscess (typically resulting from anaerobic organisms resident in the normal GI tract).
- Infections of the female pelvis and genital tract, such as endometritis, pelvic inflammatory disease, pelvic abscess and salpingitis.
- Skin and soft-tissue infections.

Although ticarcillin disodium is primarily indicated in gram-negative infections, its in vitro activity against gram-positive organisms should be considered in treating infections caused by both gram-negative and gram-positive organisms.

➤*Therapy with aminoglycosides:* Based on the in vitro synergism between ticarcillin disodium and gentamicin sulfate, tobramycin sulfate or amikacin sulfate against certain strains of *Pseudomonas aeruginosa*, combined therapy has been successful, using full therapeutic dosages.

Administration and Dosage

➤*Approved by the FDA:* April 4, 1984.

Clinical experience indicates that in serious urinary tract and systemic infections, IV therapy in the higher doses should be used. IM injections should not exceed 2 g/injection.

➤*Adults:*

Ticarcillin Uses and Dosages in Adults	
Bacterial septicemia	200 to 300 mg/kg/day by IV infusion in divided doses every 4 or 6 hours
Respiratory tract infections	(The usual dose is 3 g given every 4 hours [18 g/day] or 4 g given every 6 hours [16 g/day] depending on weight and the severity of the infection.)
Skin and soft tissue infections	
Intra-abdominal infections	
Infections of the female pelvis and genital tract	
Urinary tract infections	
Complicated	150 to 200 mg/kg/day by IV infusion in divided doses every 4 or 6 hours. (Usual recommended dosage for average [70 kg] adults: 3 g 4 times a day)

TICARCILLIN DISODIUM — INJECTION

Ticarcillin Uses and Dosages in Adults	
Uncomplicated	1 g IM or direct IV every 6 hours
Infections complicated by renal insufficiency*	Initial loading dose of 3 g IV followed by IV doses, based on creatinine clearance and type of dialysis, as indicated below:
Creatinine clearance (mL/min)	
Over 60	3 g every 4 hours
30 to 60	2 g every 4 hours
10 to 30	2 g every 8 hours
less than 10	2 g every 12 hours (or 1 g IM every 6 hours)
less than 10 with hepatic dysfunction	2 g every 24 hours (or 1 g IM every 12 hours)
patients on peritoneal dialysis	3 g every 12 hours
patients on hemodialysis	2 g every 12 hours supplemented with 3 g after each dialysis

To calculate creatinine clearance[a] from a serum creatinine value, use the following formula:

$$Ccr = \frac{(140-\text{age})\ (\text{weight in kg})}{72 \times S_{cr}(\text{mg/100 mL})}.$$

This is the calculated creatinine clearance for adult males; for females, it is 15% less.

* The half-life of ticarcillin in patients with renal failure is approximately 13 hours.
[a] Cockcroft, D.W., et al: Prediction of Creatinine Clearance from Serum Creatinine. *Nephron* 16:31-44, 1976.

Ticarcillin Uses and Dosages in Children under 40 kg (88 lbs)	
The daily dose for children should not exceed the adult dosage.	
Bacterial septicemia	200 to 300 mg/kg/day by IV infusion in divided doses every 4 or 6 hours.
Respiratory tract infections	(same as above)
Skin and soft tissue infections	(same as above)
Intra-abdominal infections	(same as above)
Infections of the female pelvis and genital tract	(same as above)
Urinary tract infections	
Complicated	150 to 200 mg/day by IV infusion in divided doses every 4 or 6 hours
Uncomplicated	50 to 100 mg/kg/day IM or direct IV in divided doses every 6 or 8 hours
Infections complicated by renal insufficiency	Clinical data are insufficient to recommend an optimum dose.

➤*Children:* Children weighing more than 40 kg (88 lbs) should receive adult dosages.

➤*Neonates:* In the neonate, for severe infections (sepsis) due to susceptible strains of *Pseudomonas*, *Proteus* and *E. coli*, the following ticarcillin disodium dosages may be given IM or by 10- to 20-minute IV infusion:

Infants under 2,000 g body weight		Infants over 2,000 g body weight	
Aged 0 to 7 days	75 mg/kg/12 hours (150 mg/kg/day)	Aged 0 to 7 days	75 mg/kg/8 hours (225 mg/kg/day)
Aged over 7 days	75 mg/kg/8 hours (225 mg/kg/day)	Aged over 7 days	100 mg/kg/8 hours (300 mg/kg/day)

This dosage schedule is intended to produce peak serum concentrations of 125 to 150 mcg/mL 1 hour after a dose of ticarcillin disodium and trough concentrations of 25 to 50 mcg/mL immediately before the next dose.

➤*Concomitant medications:* Gentamicin, tobramycin or amikacin may be used concurrently with ticarcillin disodium for initial therapy until results of culture and susceptibility studies are known.

Seriously ill patients should receive the higher doses. Ticarcillin disodium has proved to be useful in infections in which protective mechanisms are impaired, such as in acute leukemia and during therapy with immunosuppressive or oncolytic drugs.

➤*Preparation/Administration:*

IM – For initial reconstitution, use Sterile Water for Injection Sodium Chloride Injection or 1% Lidocaine Hydrochloride solution (without epinephrine).

Each gram of ticarcillin disodium should be reconstituted with 2 mL of Sterile Water for Injection, USP, Sodium Chloride Injection or 1% Lidocaine Hydrochloride solution (without epinephrine) and used promptly. Each 2.6 mL of the resulting solution will then contain 1 g of ticarcillin disodium concentration of approximately 385 mg/mL.

Do not use more than 1 g of reconstituted ticarcillin disodium in a single IM injection. As with all IM preparations, ticarcillin disodium should be injected well within the body of a relatively large muscle using usual techniques and precautions.

IV – For initial reconstitution, use Sodium Chloride Injection Dextrose Injection 5% or Lactated Ringer's Injection.

Reconstitute each gram of ticarcillin disodium with 4 mL of the appropriate diluent. After the addition of 4 mL of diluent per gram of ticarcillin disodium, each 1 mL of the resulting solution will have an approximate concentration of 200 mg. Once dissolved, further dilute if desired.

Direct IV injection: In order to avoid vein irritation, administer solution as slowly as possible.

IV infusion: Administer by continuous or intermittent IV drip. Intermittent infusion should be administered over a 30-minute to 2-hour period in equally divided doses.

In order to avoid vein irritation, the solution should be administered as slowly as possible. A dilution of approximately 50 mg/mL or more will further reduce the incidence of vein irritation.

Stability studies in the IV solutions listed below indicate that ticarcillin disodium disodium will provide sufficient activity between 21° and 24°C (70° and 75°F) within the stated time periods at concentrations between 10 mg/mL and 50 mg/mL.

After reconstitution, and prior to administration, ticarcillin disodium, as with other parenteral drugs, should be inspected visually for particulate matter and discoloration.

➤*Admixture incompatibility:* It is recommended that ticarcillin disodium and gentamicin sulfate, tobramycin sulfate or amikacin sulfate not be mixed together in the same IV solution due to the gradual inactivation of gentamicin sulfate, tobramycin sulfate or amikacin sulfate under these circumstances. The therapeutic effect of ticarcillin disodium and these aminoglycoside drugs remains unimpaired when administered separately.

➤*Storage/Stability:*

	Stability period	
IV solution (concentration of 10 mg/mL to 100 mg/mL)	Room temperature, 21° to 24°C (70° to 75°F)	Refrigeration, 4°C (40°F)
Sodium chloride injection	72 h	14 days
Dextrose injection 5%	72 h	14 days
Lactated ringer's injection	48 h	14 days

Refrigerated solutions stored longer than 72 hours should not be used for multidose purposes.

After reconstitution and dilution to a concentration of 10 mg/mL to 100 mg/mL, this solution can be frozen −18°C (0°F) and stored for up to 30 days. The thawed solution must be used within 24 hours.

Unused solutions should be discarded after the time periods mentioned above.

Store dry powder at room temperature or below.

TICARCILLIN AND CLAVULANATE POTASSIUM

Rx	**Timentin** (GlaxoSmithKline)	**Powder for Injection:** 3 g ticarcillin (as disodium) and 0.1 g clavulanic acid (as potassium)[a]	In 3.1 g vials, piggyback bottles, *ADD-Vantage* vials and 31 g pharmacy bulk packages.[b]
		Injection, solution: 3 g ticarcillin (as disodium) and 0.1 g clavulanic acid (as potassium)/100 mL[c]	In 100 mL premixed, frozen *Galaxy* plastic containers.

[a] Contains 4.75 mEq sodium and 0.15 mEq potassium/g.
[b] Pharmacy bulk package contains 30 g ticarcillin (as disodium) and 1 g clavulanic acid.
[c] Contains 18.7 mEq sodium and 0.5 mEq potassium/100 mL.

TICARCILLIN AND CLAVULANATE POTASSIUM — INJECTION

For complete and comparative prescribing information, refer to the Penicillins group monograph.

Indications

➤*Septicemia:* This includes bacteremia caused by β-lactamase-producing strains of *Klebsiella* sp., *Escherichia coli*, *Staphylococcus aureus*, and *Pseudomonas aeruginosa* (and other *Pseudomonas* species).

➤*Lower respiratory tract infections:* Those caused by β-lactamase-producing strains of *S. aureus*, *Haemophilus influenzae*, and *Klebsiella* sp.

➤*Bone and joint infections:* Those caused by β-lactamase-producing strains of *S. aureus*.

➤*Skin and skin structure infections:* Those caused by β-lactamase-producing strains of *S. aureus*, *Klebsiella* sp., and *E. coli*.

TICARCILLIN AND CLAVULANATE POTASSIUM — INJECTION

➤*Urinary tract infections:* Complicated and uncomplicated infections caused by β-lactamase-producing strains of *E. coli*, *Klebsiella* sp., *P. aeruginosa* (and other *Pseudomonas* species), *Citrobacter* sp., *Enterobacter cloacae*, *Serratia marcescens*, *S. aureus*.

➤*Gynecologic infections:* Endometritis caused by β-lactamase-producing strains of *Bacteroides melaninogenicus*, *Enterobacter* sp. (including *E. cloacae*), *E. coli*, *K. pneumoniae*, *S. aureus*, and *Staphylococcus epidermidis*.

➤*Intra-abdominal infections:* Peritonitis caused by β-lactamase-producing strains of *E. coli*, *K. pneumoniae*, and *Bacteroides fragilis* group.

While this combination is indicated only for the conditions listed above, infections caused by ticarcillin-susceptible organisms also are amenable to this combination treatment caused by its ticarcillin content.

Treatment of mixed infections and for presumptive therapy prior to the identification of the causative organisms.

Administration and Dosage

➤*Approved by the FDA:* December 17, 1997.

➤*Duration:* Administer by IV infusion over 30 minutes.

Generally, continue treatment for at least 2 days after signs and symptoms of infection have disappeared. The usual duration is 10 to 14 days; however, difficult and complicated infections may require more prolonged therapy.

Frequent bacteriologic and clinical appraisal is necessary during therapy of chronic urinary tract infections and may be required for several months after therapy has been completed; persistent infections may require treatment for several weeks; do not use doses smaller than those indicated.

In certain infections involving abscess formation, perform appropriate surgical drainage in conjunction with antimicrobial therapy.

➤*Adults:*

Ticarcillin/Clavulanate Potassium Administration in Adults

	Systemic and urinary tract infections	Gynecological infections	
		Moderate	Severe
Adults ≥ 60 kg	3.1 g every 4 to 6 h	200 mg/kg/day every 6 h	300 mg/kg/day every 4 h
Adults < 60 kg	200 to 300 mg/kg/day every 4 to 6 h		

There are no sufficient data to support the use of this product in pediatric patients younger than 3 months of age or for the treatment of septicemia or infections in the pediatric population where the suspected or proven pathogen is *H. influenzae* type b.

➤*Children:*

Dosage Guidelines for Ticarcillin/Clavulanate Potassium in Children ≥ 3 Months of Age

	Mild to moderate infections	Severe infections
Children ≥ 60 kg	3.1 g every 6 h	3.1 g every 4 h
Children < 60 kg (dosed at 50 mg/kg/dose)	200 mg/kg/day every 6 h	300 mg/kg/day every 4 h

➤*Renal function impairment:*

Dosage of Ticarcillin/Clavulanate Potassium in Renal Insufficiency[a]

Ccr (mL/min)	Dosage
> 60	3.1 g every 4 h
30 to 60	2 g every 4 h
10 to 30	2 g every 8 h
< 10	2 g every 12 h
< 10 with hepatic dysfunction	2 g every 24 h
Patients on peritoneal dialysis	3.1 g every 12 h
Patients on hemodialysis	2 g every 12 h supplemented with 3.1 g after each dialysis

[a] Initial loading dose is 3.1 g. Follow with doses based on Ccr and type of dialysis.

➤*Preparation of infusion solution:* Reconstitute by adding approximately 13 mL of Sterile Water for Injection or NaCl Injection. Shake well. The resulting ticarcillin concentration is approximately 200 mg/mL and 6.7 mg/mL clavulanic acid for the 3.1 g dose. Conversely, each 5 mL of the 3.1 g dose reconstituted with approximately 13 mL of diluent will contain approximately 1 g ticarcillin and 33 mg clavulanic acid.

Further dilute the solution with sodium chloride injection, 5% dextrose injection or Lactated Ringer's injection to a concentration between 10 to 100 mg/mL. Administer over 30 minutes by direct infusion or through a Y-type IV infusion set already in place. If this method or the piggyback method is used, temporarily discontinue administering any other solutions during the infusion of ticarcillin and clavulanate potassium.

➤*Admixture incompatibility:* Incompatible with sodium bicarbonate.

When administering in combination with another antimicrobial (eg, an aminoglycoside), administer each drug separately.

➤*Storage/Stability:* The concentrated stock solution (200 mg/mL) is stable for up to 6 hours at room temperature (21° to 23°C; 70° to 75°F) or up to 72 hours under refrigeration (4°C; 40°F); if further diluted to a concentration between 10 and 100 mg/mL with any of the recommended diluents, the following stability periods apply:

Stability and Storage for IV Solution of Ticarcillin/Clavulanate Potassium

		Stability		
Concentration	Compatible diluents	Controlled room temp	Refrigerated	Frozen
10 mg/mL to 100 mg/mL	Sodium chloride injection	24 h	7 days	30 days
	5% dextrose injection	24 h	3 days	7 days
	Lactated Ringer's injection	24 h	7 days	30 days

Unused solutions must be discarded after the time period stated above. Use all thawed solutions within 8 hours. Do not refreeze thawed solutions.

Premixed, frozen solutions – Store at ≤ –20°C (– 4°F). Thaw at room temperature 22°C (72°F) or in a refrigerator 4°C (39°F). Do not force thaw by immersion in water baths or by microwave irradiation. Thawed solution is stable for 7 days if stored under refrigeration or for 24 hours at room temperature. Do not refreeze.

PIPERACILLIN SODIUM

Rx	**Piperacillin Sodium** (American Pharmaceutical Partners)	**Powder for injection:** 2 g (as base)	In vials.[a]
		3 g (as base)	In vials.[a]
		4 g (as base)	In vials.[a]
		40 g	In pharmacy bulk vials.[a]

[a] Contains 1.85 mEq (42.5 mg) sodium/g

PIPERACILLIN SODIUM — INJECTION

For complete and comparative prescribing information, refer to the Penicillins group monograph.

Indications

➤*Combination therapy:* May be administered as single-drug therapy in some situations where normally 2 antibiotics might be employed.

Successfully used with aminoglycosides, especially in patients with impaired host defenses. Both drugs should be used in full therapeutic doses.

For the treatment of serious infections caused by susceptible strains of the designated organisms in the conditions listed below.

➤*Intra-abdominal infections (including hepatobiliary and surgical infections):* Those caused by *Escherichia coli*, *Pseudomonas aeruginosa*, enterococci, *Clostridium* sp, anaerobic cocci, and *Bacteroides* sp, including *B. fragilis*.

➤*Urinary tract infections (UTIs):* Those caused by *E. coli*, *Klebsiella* sp, *P. aeruginosa*, *Proteus* sp, including *P. mirabilis*, and enterococci.

➤*Gynecologic infections (including endometritis, pelvic inflammatory disease, pelvic cellulitis):* Those caused by *Bacteroides* sp including *B. fragilis*, anaerobic cocci, *Neisseria gonorrhoeae*, and enterococci (*S. faecalis*).

➤*Septicemia (including bacteremia):* Caused by *E. coli*, *Klebsiella* sp, *Enterobacter* sp, *Serratia* sp, *P. mirabilis*, *S. pneumoniae*, enterococci, *P. aeruginosa*, *Bacteroides* sp, and anaerobic cocci.

➤*Lower respiratory tract infections:* Those caused by *E. coli*, *Klebsiella* sp, *Enterobacter* sp, *P. aeruginosa*, *Serratia* sp, *Haemophilus influenzae*, *Bacteroides* sp, and anaerobic cocci.

Although improvement has been noted in patients with cystic fibrosis, lasting bacterial eradication may not necessarily be achieved.

➤*Skin and skin structure infections:* Those caused by *E. coli*, *Klebsiella* sp, *Serratia* sp, *Acinetobacter* sp, *Enterobacter* sp, *P. aeruginosa*, indole-positive *Proteus* sp, *P. mirabilis*, *Bacteroides* sp, including *B. fragilis*, anaerobic cocci, and enterococci.

➤*Bone and joint infections:* Those caused by *P. aeruginosa*, enterococci, *Bacteroides* sp, and anaerobic cocci.

➤*Gonococcal infections:* Treatment of uncomplicated gonococcal urethritis.

➤*Streptococcal infections:* Clinically effective for the treatment of infections at various sites caused by *Streptococcus* species including group A β-hemolytic *Streptococcus* and *S. pneumoniae*; however, infections caused by these organisms are ordinarily treated with more narrow spectrum penicillins. Because of its broad spectrum of bactericidal activity against gram-positive and gram-negative aerobic and anaerobic bacteria, piperacillin is

PIPERACILLIN SODIUM — INJECTION

particularly useful for the treatment of mixed infections and presumptive therapy prior to the identification of the causative organisms.

➤*Prophylaxis:* For prophylactic use in surgery, including intra-abdominal (GI and biliary) procedures, vaginal hysterectomy, abdominal hysterectomy, and cesarean section. Effective prophylactic use depends on the time of administration, and piperacillin should be given 30 minutes to 1 hour before the operation so that effective levels can be achieved in the site prior to the procedure.

Stop the prophylactic use of piperacillin within 24 hours, since continuing administration of any antibiotic increases the possibility of adverse reactions, but in the majority of surgical procedures, does not reduce the incidence of subsequent infections. If there are signs of infection, obtain specimens for culture for identification of the causative organism so that appropriate therapy can be instituted.

Administration and Dosage

May be administered IM (except pharmacy bulk package) or IV as a 20- to 30-minute infusion. The usual dosage of piperacillin for injection for serious infections is 3 to 4 g given every 4 to 6 hours as a 20- to 30-minute infusion. For serious infections, use the IV route.

The maximum daily dose for adults is usually 24 g/day, although higher doses have been used.

Limit IM injections to 2 g/injection site. This route of administration has been used primarily in the treatment of patients with uncomplicated gonorrhea and UTIs.

Dosage Recommendations	
Type of infection	Usual total daily dose
Serious infections such as septicemia, nosocomial pneumonia, intra-abdominal infections, aerobic and anaerobic gynecologic infections, and skin and soft tissue infections	12 to 18 g/day IV (200 to 300 mg/kg/day) in divided doses every 4 to 6 hours
Complicated UTIs	8 to 16 g/day IV (125 to 200 mg/kg/day) in divided doses every 6 to 8 hours
Uncomplicated UTIs and most community-acquired pneumonia	6 to 8 g/day IM or IV (100 to 125 mg/kg/day) in divided doses every 6 to 12 hours
Uncomplicated gonorrhea infections	2 g IM[a] as a 1-time dose

[a] One g of probenecid given orally one-half hour prior to injection.

➤*Duration:* The average duration of piperacillin treatment is from 7 to 10 days, except in the treatment of gynecologic infections, in which it is from 3 to 10 days; the duration should be guided by the patient's clinical and bacteriological progress. For most acute infections, continue treatment for at least 48 to 72 hours after the patient becomes asymptomatic. Maintain antibiotic therapy for *S. pyogenes* infections for at least 10 days to reduce the risk of rheumatic fever.

➤*Concomitant therapy:* When piperacillin is given concurrently with aminoglycosides, use both drugs in full therapeutic doses.

➤*Renal function impairment:*

Dosage in Renal Impairment			
Creatinine clearance mL/min	UTI (uncomplicated)	UTI (complicated)	Serious systemic infection
> 40	No dosage adjustment necessary		
20 to 40	No dosage adjustment necessary	9 g/day (3 g every 8 h)	12 g/day (4 g every 8 h)
< 20	6 g/day (3 g every 12 h)	6 g/day (3 g every 12 h)	8 g/day (4 g every 12 h)

For patients on hemodialysis, the maximum daily dose is 6 g/day (2 g every 8 hours). In addition, because hemodialysis removes 30% to 50% of piperacillin in 4 hours, administer 1 g additional dose following each dialysis period.

For patients with renal failure and hepatic insufficiency, measurement of serum levels of piperacillin will provide additional guidance for adjusting dosage.

➤*Prophylaxis:* When possible, administer piperacillin as a 20- to 30-minute infusion just prior to anesthesia. Administration while the patient is awake will facilitate identification of possible adverse reactions during drug infusion.

Indication	First Dose	Second Dose	Third Dose
Intra-abdominal surgery	2 g IV just prior to surgery	2 g during surgery	2 g every 6 h post-op for no more than 24 h
Vaginal hysterectomy	2 g IV just prior to surgery	2 g 6 h after the first dose	2 g 12 h after the first dose
Cesarean section	2 g IV after the cord is clamped	2 g 4 h after the first dose	2 g 8 h after the first dose
Abdomina hysterectomy	2 g IV just prior to surgery	2 g on return to the recovery room	2 g after 6 h

➤*Admixture incompatibilities:* Do not mix piperacillin with an aminoglycoside in a syringe or infusion bottle since this can result in inactivation of the aminoglycoside.

➤*Compatible diluents/IV solutions:* Diluents for reconstitution

- Sterile water for injection
- Bacteriostatic water for injection
- Sodium chloride injection
- Bacteriostatic sodium chloride injection
- Dextrose 5% in water
- Dextrose 5% and 0.9% sodium chloride
- Lidocaine hydrochloride 0.5% to 1% (without epinephrine)

IV solutions

- Dextrose 5% in water
- 0.9% sodium chloride
- Dextrose 5% and 0.9% sodium chloride
- Lactated Ringer's injection
- Dextran 6% in 0.9% sodium chloride

IV admixtures

- Normal saline [+ KCl 40 mEq]
- 5% Dextrose in water [+ KCl 40 mEq]
- 5% Dextrose/normal saline [+ KCl 40 mEq]
- Ringer's injection [+ KCl 40 mEq]
- Lactated Ringer's injection [+ KCl 40 mEq]

➤*Reconstitution directions for bulk vial:* Reconstitute the 40 g vial with 172 mL of suitable diluent (except lidocaine hydrochloride 0.5% to 1% without epinephrine) listed above to achieve a concentration of 1 g per 5 mL.

Withdraw container contents without delay. If this is not possible, a maximum of 4 hours from initial closure entry is permitted to complete fluid transfer operations. Begin this time limit with the introduction of solvent or diluent into the PBP.

Reconstituting directions conventional vials – Reconstitute each gram of piperacillin for injection with at least 5 mL of suitable diluent (except lidocaine hydrochloride 0.5% to 1% without epinephrine) listed above. Shake well until dissolved. Reconstituted solution may be further diluted to the desired volume (eg, 50 or 100 mL) in the above listed IV solutions and admixture.

➤*Directions for administration:*

Intermittent IV infusion – Infuse diluted solution over a period of approximately 30 minutes. During infusion, it is desirable to discontinue the primary IV solution.

IV injection (bolus): Inject reconstituted solution from conventional vials slowly over a 3- to 5-minute period to help avoid vein irritation.

➤*Storage/Stability:* Store at 20° to 25°C (68° to 77°F).

Pharmacy bulk package – After entry, use entire contents of vial promptly. Dispense the entire contents of the vial within 4 hours of initial entry. Never freeze the pharmacy bulk vial after reconstitution.

Conventional vials – Piperacillin is stable in both glass and plastic containers when reconstituted with recommended diluents and when diluted with the IV solutions and IV admixtures listed above.

Use pharmacy vials immediately after reconstitution. Discard any unused portion after 24 hours if stored at room temperature (20° to 25°C [68° to 77°F]), or after 48 hours if stored at refrigerated temperature (2° to 8°C [36° to 46°F]). Do not freeze vials after reconstitution.

Extended-Spectrum Penicillins

PIPERACILLIN SODIUM AND TAZOBACTAM SODIUM

Rx	**Zosyn** (Wyeth)	**Powder for Injection, lyophilized:** 2.25 g (2 g piperacillin/0.25 g tazobactam)	4.69 mEq sodium. Preservative-free. In vials and *ADD-Vantage* vials.
		3.375 g (3 g piperacillin/0.375 g tazobactam)	7.04 mEq sodium. Preservative-free. In vials and *ADD-Vantage* vials.
		4.5 g (4 g piperacillin/0.5 g tazobactam)	9.39 mEq sodium. Preservative-free. In vials and *ADD-Vantage* vials.
		40.5 g (36 g piperacillin/4.5 g tazobactam)	84.5 mEq sodium. Preservative-free. In bulk vials.
		Injection[a]: 2.25 g/50 mL (2 g piperacillin/0.25 g tazobactam)	5.7 mEq sodium. In *Galaxy* containers.
		3.375 g/50 mL (3 g piperacillin/0.375 g tazobactam)	8.6 mEq sodium. In *Galaxy* containers.
		4.5 g/100 mL (4 g piperacillin/0.5 g tazobactam)	11.4 mEq sodium. In *Galaxy* containers.

[a] Supplied as frozen, iso-osmotic solution in single dose plastic containers.

PIPERACILLIN SODIUM AND TAZOBACTAM SODIUM — INJECTION

For complete and comparative prescribing information, refer to the Penicillins group monograph.

Indications

For the treatment of patients with moderate to severe infections caused by piperacillin-resistant, piperacillin/tazobactam susceptible, β-lactamase-producing strains of the microorganisms in the conditions listed below.

➤*Appendicitis (complicated by rupture or abscess) and peritonitis:* Caused by piperacillin-resistant, β-lactamase-producing strains of *Escherichia coli* or these members of the *Bacteroides* group: *B. fragilis*, *B. ovatus*, *B. thetaiotaomicron* or *B. vulgatus*.

➤*Uncomplicated and complicated skin and skin structure infections:* Those including cellulitis, cutaneous abscesses and ischemic/diabetic foot infections caused by piperacillin-resistant, β-lactamase-producing strains of *Staphylococcus aureus*.

➤*Postpartum endometritis or pelvic inflammatory disease:* Caused by piperacillin-resistant, β-lactamase-producing strains of *E. coli*.

➤*Community-acquired pneumonia (moderate severity only):* Caused by piperacillin-resistant, β-lactamase-producing strains of *Haemophilus influenzae*.

➤*Nosocomial pneumonia (moderate to severe):* Caused by piperacillin-resistant, β-lactamase-producing strains of *S. aureus* and by piperacillin/tazobactam-susceptible *Acinetobacter baumanii*, *H. influenzae*, *Klebsiella pneumoniae*, and *Pseudomonas aeruginosa* in combination with an aminoglycoside.

Indicated only for the specified conditions listed above. However, infections caused by piperacillin-susceptible organisms for which piperacillin is effective are also amenable to piperacillin/tazobactam treatment because of its piperacillin content. The treatment of mixed infections caused by piperacillin-susceptible organisms and piperacillin-resistant, β-lactamase-producing organisms susceptible to piperacillin/tazobactam should not require adding another antibiotic. An exception is in the treatment of *P. aeruginosa* in nosocomial pneumonia, which should be treated in combination with an aminoglycoside.

Administration and Dosage

➤*Approved by the FDA:* October 22, 1993.

Administer by IV infusion over 30 minutes. The usual total daily dose for adults is 3.375 g every 6 hours totaling 13.5 g (12 g piperacillin/1.5 g tazobactam) for 7 to 10 days.

➤*Nosocomial pneumonia:* Start with 4.5 g every 6 hours plus an aminoglycoside. The recommended total daily dose is 18 g (16 g piperacillin/2 g tazobactam) for 7 to 14 days. Continue the aminoglycoside in patients from whom *P. aeruginosa* is isolated. If it is not isolated, the aminoglycoside may be discontinued at the discretion of the treating physician as guided by the severity of the infection and the patient's clinical and bacteriological progress.

➤*Renal function impairment:* In patients with renal insufficiency (Ccr 40 mL/min or less), adjust the IV dose to the degree of actual renal function impairment. In patients with nosocomial pneumonia receiving concomitant aminoglycoside therapy, adjust the aminoglycoside dosage according to the manufacturer's recommendations.

Piperacillin Sodium and Tazobactam Sodium Dosage Recommendations[a]

Creatinine clearance (mL/min)	All indications (except nosocomial pneumonia)	Nosocomial pneumonia
> 40	3.375 g every 6 h	4.5 g every 6 h
20-40[b]	2.25 g every 6 h	3.375 g every 6 h
< 20[b]	2.25 g every 8 h	2.25 g every 6 h
Hemodialysis[c]	2.25 g every 12 h	2.25 g every 8 h
CAPD	2.25 g every 12 h	2.25 g every 8 h

[a] Dosage provided is "total" combined piperacillin/tazobactam.
[b] Creatinine clearance for patients not receiving hemodialysis.
[c] Administer 0.75 g following each hemodialysis session on hemodialysis days.

➤*Hemodialysis:* The maximum dose is 2.25 g every 12 hours for all indications other than nosocomial pneumonia and 2.25 g every 8 hours for nosocomial pneumonia. In addition, because hemodialysis removes 30% to 40% of a dose, give one additional 0.75 g dose following each dialysis period. Peritoneal dialysis removes approximately 6% and 21% of the piperacillin and tazobactam doses, respectively. No additional dosage of piperacillin/tazobactam is necessary for continuous ambulatory peritoneal dialysis (CAPD) patients.

➤*Reconstitution:* Reconstitute conventional vials with 5 mL of compatible diluent per gram of piperacillin. Shake well until dissolved. Dilute to at least 50 mL to 150 mL. Administer over a period of at least 30 minutes.

➤*Admixture compatibility/incompatibility:* These include 0.9% sodium chloride for injection, sterile water for injection (maximum recommended volume per dose is 50 mL), 5% dextrose, bacteriostatic saline/parabens, bacteriostatic water/parabens, bacteriostatic saline/benzyl alcohol, and bacteriostatic water/benzyl alcohol. Lactated Ringer's solution is not compatible.

➤*IV compatible solutions:* These include 0.9% sodium chloride for injection, sterile water for injection (maximum recommended volume per dose is 50 mL), 5% dextrose, and 6% dextran in saline.

➤*ADD-Vantage system admixtures:* These include 5% dextrose in water (50 or 100 mL) and 0.9% sodium chloride (50 or 100 mL).

➤*Coadministration infusion:* During the infusion it is desirable to discontinue the primary infusion solution. When cotherapy with aminoglycosides is indicated, reconstitute piperacillin/tazobactam and the aminoglycoside, and administer separately (because of the in vitro inactivation of the aminoglycoside by the penicillin).

➤*Storage/Stability:* Store piperacillin/tazobactam vials and *ADD-Vantage* vials at controlled room temperature (20° to 25°C [68° to 77°F]) prior to reconstitution. Use single-dose vials immediately after reconstitution. Discard any unused portion after 24 hours if stored at room temperature or after 48 hours if stored at refrigerated temperature (2° to 8°C [36° to 46°F]). Do not freeze vials after reconstitution. Stability in the IV bags has been demonstrated for up to 24 hours at room temperature and up to 1 week at refrigerated temperature. Stability in an ambulatory IV infusion pump has been demonstrated for a period of 12 hours at room temperature. Stability with the admixed *ADD-Vantage* system has been demonstrated through 24 hours at room temperature. Do not refrigerate or freeze the admixed *ADD-Vantage* after reconstitution.

CARBENICILLIN INDANYL SODIUM

Rx	**Geocillin** (Roerig)	**Tablets:** 382 mg carbenicillin (118 mg indanyl sodium ester)	Yellow. Film coated. Capsule shape. In 100s and UD 100s.

CARBENICILLIN INDANYL SODIUM — ORAL

For complete and comparative prescribing information, refer to the Penicillins group monograph.

Indications

➤*Urinary tract infections:* In the treatment of acute and chronic infections of the upper and lower urinary tract and in asymptomatic bacteriuria due to susceptible strains of the following organisms: *Escherichia coli*, *Proteus mirabilis*, *Morganella morganii*(formerly *Proteus morganii*), *Providencia rettgeri* (formerly *Proteus rettgeri*), *Proteus vulgaris*, *Pseudomonas*, *Enterobacter* species, and *enterococci*.

➤*Prostatitis:* In the treatment of prostatitis due to susceptible strains of the following organisms: *Escherichia coli*, enterococcus (*S. faecalis*), *Proteus mirabilis*, and *Enterobacter* sp.

Administration and Dosage

Carbenicillin indanyl sodium is available as a coated tablet to be administered orally.

➤*Usual adult dose:*

Urinary tract infections –

Escherichia coli, Proteus species, and Enterobacter species: 1 to 2 tablets 4 times daily.

Pseudomonas and enterococci: 2 tablets 4 times daily.

Prostatitis – 2 tablets 4 times daily.

Indications

For specific approved indications, refer to individual drug monographs.

Administration and Dosage

➤*Duration of therapy:* Continue administration for a minimum of 48 to 72 hours after fever abates or after evidence of bacterial eradication has been obtained. A minimum of 10 days treatment is recommended for group A β-hemolytic streptococci infections to guard against the risk of rheumatic fever or glomerulonephritis.

➤*Perioperative prophylaxis:* Discontinue prophylactic use within 24 hours after the surgical procedure. In surgery where infection may be particularly devastating (eg, open heart surgery, prosthetic arthroplasty), may continue prophylactic use for 3 to 5 days following surgery completion. If there are signs of infection, obtain cultures and perform sensitivity tests so appropriate therapy may be instituted.

Actions

➤*Pharmacology:* Cephalosporins are structurally and pharmacologically related to penicillins. **Cefoxitin** and **cefotetan** (cephamycins) and **loracarbef** (a carbacephem) are included because of their similarity.

Most cephalosporins and related compounds are divided into first, second and third generation agents (see table). Within each group, differentiation is primarily by pharmacokinetics; groups are divided by antibacterial spectrum. In general, progression from first to third generation reveals broadening gram-negative spectrum, loss of efficacy against gram-positive organisms, greater efficacy against resistant organisms and increased cost. However, this classification scheme is becoming less clearly defined as newer agents enter the market. The decision to use a specific agent in the clinical setting should be primarily based on bacterial spectrum, route of administration, side effect profile and indications.

Mechanism – Cephalosporins inhibit mucopeptide synthesis in the bacterial cell wall, making it defective and osmotically unstable. The drugs are usually bactericidal, depending on organism susceptibility, dose, tissue concentrations and the rate at which organisms are multiplying. They are more effective against rapidly growing organisms forming cell walls.

➤*Pharmacokinetics:*

Pharmacokinetic Parameters of Cephalosporins

	Drug	Routes	Half-Life: Normal renal function (minutes)	Half-Life: ESRD[1] (hours)	Half-Life: Hemodialysis (hours)	Protein bound (%)	Recovered unchanged in urine (%)	Peak serum level 1 g IV dose (mcg/ml)	Sodium (mEq/g)
First	Cefadroxil	Oral	78-96	20-25	3-4	20	> 90	—	—
	Cefazolin	IM-IV	90–120	3-7	9-14	80-86	60-80	185	2-2.1
	Cephalexin	Oral	50-80	19-22	4-6	10	> 90	—	—
	Cephapirin	IM-IV	36	1.8-4	1.8	44-50	70	73	2.4
	Cephradine	Oral/IM-IV	48-80	8-15	—	8-17	> 90	86	6[2]
Second	Cefaclor	Oral	35-54	2-3	1.6-2.1	25	60-85	—	—
	Cefmetazole	IM-IV	72-90	—	—	65	85	—	2
	Cefonicid	IM-IV	270	11	—	90	99	221.3	3.7
	Cefotetan	IM-IV	180-276	13-35	5	88-90	51-81	158	3.5
	Cefoxitin	IV	40-60	20	4	73	85	110	2.3
	Cefprozil	Oral	78	5.2-5.9	decreased	36	60	—	—
	Cefuroxime	Oral/IM-IV	80	16-22[3]	3.5	50	66-100	100[4]	2.4[3]
	Loracarbef	Oral	60	32	4	25	> 90	—	—
Third	Cefdinir	Oral	100	16	3.2	60-70	12-18	—	—
	Cefepime	IM-IV	102-138	17-21	11-16	20	85	79	—
	Cefixime	Oral	180-240	11.5	—	65	50	—	—
	Cefoperazone	IM-IV	120	1.3-2.9	2	82-93	20-30	73-153	1.5
	Cefotaxime	IM-IV	60	3-11	2.5	30-40	60	42-102	2.2
	Cefpodoxime[5]	Oral	120-180	9.8	—	21-29	29-33	—	—
	Ceftazidime	IM-IV	114-120	14-30	—	< 10	80-90	69-90	2.3
	Ceftibuten	Oral	144	13.4-22.3	2-4	65	56	—	—
	Ceftizoxime	IM-IV	102	25-30	6	30	80	60-87	2.6
	Ceftriaxone	IM-IV	348-522	15.7	14.7	85-95	33-67	151	3.6

[1] ESRD = End stage renal disease (Ccr < 10 ml/min/1.73 m^2).
[2] Also available in sodium-free form.
[3] Injection only.
[4] Following 1.5 g IV dose.
[5] Extended-spectrum agent.

CEPHALOSPORINS AND RELATED ANTIBIOTICS

Organisms Generally Susceptible to Cephalosporins																								
Organisms		First Generation					Second Generation								Third Generation									
✓ = generally susceptible ‡ = demonstrated in vitro activity		Cefadroxil	Cefazolin	Cephalexin	Cephapirin	Cephradine	Cefaclor	Cefonicid	Cefoxitin	Cefuroxime	Cefmetazole	Cefotetan	Cefprozil	Loracarbef	Cefdinir	Cefepime[1]	Cefixime	Cefoperazone	Cefotaxime	Cefpodoxime[2]	Ceftazidime	Ceftibuten	Ceftizoxime	Ceftriaxone
Gram-positive	Staphylococci[3]	✓	✓	✓[4]	✓	✓	✓[4]	✓[4]	✓	✓	✓	✓	✓	✓	✓[5]	✓[6]		✓	✓[5]	✓[4]	✓		✓	✓
	Staphylococcus aureus														✓[5]									
	Staphylococcus epidermidis									‡				‡	‡[6]									
	Staphylococcus saprophyticus									‡				✓										
	Streptococci, beta-hemolytic	✓	✓	✓	✓	✓	✓	✓	✓	✓	✓	✓	✓	✓		‡	✓	✓	✓	✓	✓		✓	✓
	Streptococcus agalactiae									‡				‡	‡									
	Streptococcus bovis													‡										
	Streptococcus pneumoniae	✓	✓	✓	✓	✓	✓	✓	✓	✓	✓	✓	✓	✓	✓[7]	✓	✓	✓	✓	✓	✓	✓[7]	✓	✓
	Streptococcus pyogenes						✓	✓		✓	✓	✓	✓	✓	✓	✓[8]	✓	✓	✓	✓	✓	✓	✓	✓
	Streptococcus viridans													‡	‡									

CEPHALOSPORINS AND RELATED ANTIBIOTICS

✓ = generally susceptible
‡ = demonstrated in vitro activity

Organisms Generally Susceptible to Cephalosporins																								
Organisms		First Generation					Second Generation								Third Generation									
		Cefadroxil	Cefazolin	Cephalexin	Cephapirin	Cephradine	Cefaclor	Cefonicid	Cefoxitin	Cefuroxime	Cefmetazole	Cefotetan	Cefprozil	Loracarbef	Cefdinir	Cefepime[1]	Cefixime	Cefoperazone	Cefotaxime	Cefpodoxime[2]	Ceftazidime	Ceftibuten	Ceftizoxime	Ceftriaxone
Gram-negative	*Acinetobacter* sp.															‡		✓[4]	✓		‡		✓	‡
	Citrobacter sp.							‡		✓[4]	‡	‡	‡	‡	‡	‡	‡	✓	✓	‡	✓		‡	‡
	Enterobacter sp.		✓[4]					‡		✓[4]	‡	✓				✓		✓	✓		✓		✓	✓
	Escherichia coli	✓	✓	✓	✓	✓	✓	✓	✓	✓	✓	✓	‡	✓	‡	✓	✓	✓	✓	✓	✓		✓	✓
	Haemophilus influenzae		✓	✓	✓	✓	✓[5]	✓[5]	✓[5]	✓[5]	✓[5]	✓[5]	✓[5]	✓[5]	✓[5]	‡[5]	✓[5]	✓[5]	✓[5]	✓[5]	✓[5]	✓[5]	✓[5]	✓[5]
	Haemophilus parainflu-enzae						‡			‡				‡	✓[5]		‡[5]		✓	‡	‡			✓
	Hafnia alvei															‡								
	Klebsiella sp.	✓	✓	✓	✓	✓	✓	✓	✓	✓	✓	✓	‡	‡	‡	✓	‡	✓	✓	✓	✓		✓	✓
	Klebsiella pneumoniae						‡																	
	Moraxella (Branhamella) catarrhalis	‡		‡			✓[5]			‡	‡	‡	✓[5]	✓[5]	✓[5]	‡[5]	✓[5]			✓	✓	✓[5]	‡	
	Morganella (Proteus) morganii							✓	✓	✓[4]	✓	✓				‡		✓	✓		‡		✓	✓
	Neisseria catarrhalis			✓																				
	Neisseria gonorrhoeae						‡	‡	✓	✓	‡	‡	‡	‡[3]			‡	✓[5]	✓	✓[4]	‡		✓	✓
	Neisseria meningitidis									✓								‡	✓		✓		‡	✓
	Pasteurella multocida													‡										
	Proteus inconstans									‡														
	Proteus mirabilis	✓	✓	✓	✓	✓	✓	✓	✓	✓	✓	✓	‡	‡	‡	✓	✓	✓	✓	✓	✓		✓	✓
	Proteus vulgaris							✓	✓		✓	✓				‡	‡	✓	✓	‡	✓		✓	✓
	Providencia sp.								✓	✓	✓	✓				‡	‡		‡		‡		‡	‡
	Providencia rettgeri							✓	✓	✓	‡	✓				‡	‡	✓	✓	‡	‡		✓	‡
	Pseudomonas aerugi-nosa															✓		✓	✓[4]		✓		✓[4]	✓[4]
	Salmonella sp.									✓	‡	‡	‡	‡			‡	‡	‡		‡		‡	‡
	Salmonella typhi																		‡				‡	‡
	Serratia sp.											‡				‡	‡	✓	✓		✓		✓	✓
	Shigella sp.									✓	‡	‡	‡	‡			‡	‡	‡		‡		‡	‡
	Yersinia enterocolitica											✓		‡										

CEPHALOSPORINS AND RELATED ANTIBIOTICS

	Organisms	Organisms Generally Susceptible to Cephalosporins																						
		First Generation					Second Generation								Third Generation									
✓ = generally susceptible ‡ = demonstrated in vitro activity		Cefadroxil	Cefazolin	Cephalexin	Cephapirin	Cephradine	Cefaclor	Cefonicid	Cefoxitin	Cefuroxime	Cefmetazole	Cefotetan	Cefprozil	Loracarbef	Cefdinir	Cefepime[1]	Cefixime	Cefoperazone	Cefotaxime	Cefpodoxime[2]	Ceftazidime	Ceftibuten	Ceftizoxime	Ceftriaxone
Anaerobes	*Bacteroides* sp.						✓		✓	✓	✓	✓[4]	‡					✓	✓		✓[4]		‡	✓
	Bacteroides fragilis								✓		✓	✓						✓	✓				✓	‡
	Clostridium sp.							‡	✓	✓	✓	✓	‡	‡				✓	✓		‡		‡	‡
	Clostridium difficile											‡	‡					‡						
	Eubacterium sp.																	‡						‡
	Fusobacterium sp.							‡		✓	✓	✓	‡	‡				‡	✓				‡	‡
	Peptococcus sp.						‡	‡	✓	✓	‡	✓		‡				✓	✓		‡		✓	‡
	Peptococcus niger						‡							‡										
	Peptostreptococcus sp.						‡	‡	✓	✓	‡	✓	‡	‡				✓	✓	‡	‡		✓	‡
	Porphyromonas asaccharolytica											‡												
	Prevotella bivia											✓												
	Prevotella digiens											✓												
	Prevotella melaninogenica											‡												
	Prevotella oralis											‡												
	Propionibacterium acnes						‡							‡										
	Propionibacterium sp.											‡												
	Veillonella sp.											‡												
Other	*Borrelia burgdorferi*									✓														

[1] Including some β-lactamase-producing strains.
[2] Extended-spectrum agent.
[3] Methicillin-susceptible strains only.
[4] Some strains are resistant.
[5] Penicillin-susceptible strains only.
[6] Lancefield's group *A streptococci.*
[7] Some other references consider this fourth generation.
[8] Coagulase-positive, coagulase-negative, and penicillinase-producing.

—

Absorption **Cephalexin**, **cephradine**, **cefaclor**, **cefixime**, **cefprozil**, **cefadroxil**, **ceftibuten** and **loracarbef** are well absorbed from the GI tract; absorption of these agents (except cefadroxil and cefprozil) may be delayed by food, but the amount absorbed is not affected. Peak plasma levels of loracarbef (capsules) are decreased by food and occur later. After oral administration, **cefuroxime axetil** is absorbed from the GI tract and rapidly hydrolyzed in the intestinal mucosa and blood to cefuroxime. **Cefpodoxime proxetil** is a pro-drug that is absorbed from the GI tract and de-esterified to its active metabolite, cefpodoxime. The absorption of oral cefuroxime and cefpodoxime is increased when given with food. **Cefdinir** may be taken without regard to meals.

Distribution – Cephalosporins are widely distributed to most tissues and fluids. First and second generation agents do not readily enter cerebrospinal fluid (CSF), except **cefuroxime**, even when meninges are inflamed. Third generation compounds (little data for **cefixime**) and cefuroxime readily diffuse into the CSF of patients with inflamed meninges. However, CSF levels of **cefoperazone** are relatively low. No data are available for **cefdinir** human CSF penetration. Therapeutic levels are reached in bone after usual doses of most agents. **Cefazolin** penetrates acutely inflamed bone at higher concentrations than in normal bone.

High concentrations of **ceftriaxone** and **cefoperazone** are attained in bile. Therapeutic levels of **ceftizoxime**, **cefuroxime**, **cefotetan**, **ceftazidime**, **cefoxitin** and **cefonicid** are attained in bile. Bile levels of **cefazolin** can reach or exceed serum levels by up to five times in patients without obstructive biliary disease.

Metabolism/Excretion – **Cefuroxime axetil** is metabolized to free cefuroxime plus acetaldehyde and acetic acid. **Cephapirin** is metabolized to less active compounds; however, desacetylcephapirin contributes to the drug's antibacterial activity. Desacetylcefotaxime, a major metabolite of **cefotaxime**, contributes to the bactericidal activity and increases the spectrum to include anaerobes, specifically *Bacteroides* sp; the synergy with the parent drug appears to extend the dosing interval to 8 to 12 hours because of the prolonged metabolite half-life. **Cefpodoxime proxetil** is a pro-drug that is de-esterified to its active metabolite, cefpodoxime. **Cefdinir** is not appreciably metabolized and is primarily excreted renally. Most cephalosporins and metabolites are primarily excreted renally. **Cefoperazone** is excreted mainly in the bile; peak serum levels and serum half-lives are unchanged, even in patients with severe renal insufficiency. In hepatic dysfunction, serum half-life and urinary excretion are increased.

➤*Microbiology:* Refer to the previous tables for organisms generally susceptible to cephalosporins.

β-lactamase resistance – First generation cephalosporins are generally inactivated by β-lactamase-producing organisms. Newer agents are distinguished by an increasing resistance to β-lactamase inactivation. **Cefonicid**, **cefdinir**, **loracarbef** and **cefixime** have a high degree of stability to some β–lactamases. **Cefoxitin**, **cefuroxime**, **ceftriaxone**, **cefotaxime**,**ceftizoxime**, **cefmetazole** and **cefotetan** have a high degree of stability in the presence of both penicillinases and cephalosporinases produced by gram-negative and gram-positive bacteria. **Cefoperazone**, **cefpodoxime** and **ceftazidime** are highly stable in the presence of β-lactamases produced by most gram-negative pathogens and are active against some organisms that are resistant to other β-lactam antibiotics because of β-lactamase production. **Cefepime** has a broad spectrum of activity against gram-positive and gram-negative bacteria but has a low affinity for chromosomally encoded beta-lactamases. **Cefaclor** is stable in the presence of some β-lactamases. **Cefprozil** has in vitro activity against a broad range of gram-positive and gram-negative bacteria.

Contraindications

Hypersensitivity to cephalosporins or related antibiotics (see Warnings).

Warnings

➤*Cross-allergenicity with penicillin:* Administer cautiously to penicillin-sensitive patients. There is evidence of partial cross-allergenicity; cephalosporins cannot be assumed to be an absolutely safe alternative to penicillin in the penicillin-allergic patient. The estimated incidence of cross-sensitivity is 5% to 16%; however, it is possibly as low as 3% to 7%.

➤*Serum sickness-like reactions:* Erythema multiforme or skin rashesaccompanied by polyarthritis, arthralgia and, frequently, fever have been reported; these reactions usually occurred following a second course of therapy. Signs and symptoms occur after a few days of therapy and resolve a few days after drug discontinuation with no serious sequelae. Antihistamines and corticosteroids may be of benefit in managing symptoms.

➤*Seizures:* Several cephalosporins have been implicated in triggering seizures, particularly in patients with renal impairment when the dosage was not reduced. If seizures associated with drug therapy occur, discontinue the drug. Anticonvulsant therapy can be given if clinically indicated.

➤*Coagulation abnormalities:* **Cefmetazole**, **cefoperazone**, **cefotetan** and **ceftriaxone** may be associated with a fall in prothrombin activity. Those at risk include patients with renal impairment, cancer, impaired vitamin K synthesis or low vitamin K stores (eg, chronic hepatic disease or malnutrition), as well as patients receiving a protracted course of antimicrobial therapy. Monitor prothrombin time for patients at risk and administer exogenous vitamin K as indicated. Vitamin K administration may be necessary if the prothrombin time is prolonged before therapy.

➤*Pseudomembranous colitis:* This occurs with cephalosporins (and other broad spectrum antibiotics); consider this diagnosis in patients who develop diarrhea with antibiotic use. Colitis may range in severity from mild to life-threatening. Treatment alters normal flora of the colon and may permit overgrowth of *Clostridia* species. A toxin produced by *C. difficile* is a primary cause of antibiotic-associated colitis. Cholestyramine and colestipol resins bind the toxin in vitro.

Mild cases of colitis may respond to drug discontinuation alone. Manage moderate-to-severe cases by sigmoidoscopy, bacteriologic studies and with fluid, electrolyte and protein supplementation, as indicated. When the colitis is not relieved by drug discontinuation, or when it is severe, oral vancomycin (see individual monograph) is treatment of choice. Rule out other causes of colitis.

Prescribe broad-spectrum antibiotics with caution in individuals with a history of GI disease, especially colitis.

➤*Immune hemolytic anemia:* This has been observed in patients receiving cephalosporin class antibiotics. Rare cases of severe hemolytic anemia, including fatalities, have been reported in association with cephalosporins. If a patient develops anemia any time within 2 to 3 weeks subsequent to the start of therapy, the diagnosis of cephalosporin-associated anemia should be considered and the drug stopped until the etiology is determined with certainty. Blood transfusions may be administered as needed. Patients who receive prolonged courses of cephalosporins for treatment of infections should have periodic monitoring for signs and symptoms of hemolytic anemia, including a measurement of hematological parameters where appropriate.

➤*Renal function impairment:* Cephalosporins may be nephrotoxic; use with caution in the presence of markedly impaired renal function (creatinine clearance [Ccr] rate of < 50 ml/min/1.73 m^2). In the elderly and in patients with known or suspected renal impairment, monitor carefully prior to and during therapy.

Reduce total daily antibiotic dosage in patients with transient or persistent reduction of urinary output caused by renal insufficiency; high and prolonged serum concentrations can occur in such patients from usual doses. See individual product monographs for information on dosage adjustments in impaired renal function.

➤*Hepatic function impairment:* **Cefoperazone** is extensively excreted in bile. Serum half-life increases 2-fold to 4-fold in patients with hepatic disease or biliary obstruction. If higher dosages are used (> 4 g), monitor serum concentrations.

➤*Elderly:* In elderly patients, dosage adjustments based on decreased renal function may be necessary.

➤*Pregnancy:* *Category B*. Safety for use during pregnancy is not established. Use only when potential benefits outweigh potential hazards to the fetus. Cephalosporins appear safe for pregnant patients, but relatively few controlled studies exist.

These agents cross the placenta; peak umbilical cord concentrations for the various agents range from 3 to 29 mcg/ml following doses of 0.5 to 2 g. These data yielded a maternal:fetal serum ratio range of 0.16 to 1. Drug levels in cord blood after administration of **cefazolin** are ≈ ¼ to ⅓ maternal drug levels. **Cefotetan** reaches therapeutic levels in cord blood.

In addition, the pharmacokinetic parameters of these drugs appear to change in the pregnant woman; tendencies are toward shorter half-lives, lower serum levels, larger volumes of distribution and increased clearance.

➤*Lactation:* Most of these agents are excreted in breast milk in small quantities. Levels range from 0.16 to 4 mcg/ml, or a breast milk:maternal serum ratio of 0.01 to 0.5 following 0.5 to 2 g doses. **Cefdinir** was not detected in breast milk following single 600 mg doses. However, consider these problems for the nursing infant: Modification/alteration of bowel flora; pharmacological effects; interference with interpretation of culture results if a fever/infection workup is needed. **Ceftibuten** has not been studied.

➤*Children:* When using cephalosporins in infants, consider the relative benefit to risk. In neonates, accumulation of cephalosporin antibiotics, with resulting prolongation of drug half-life, has occurred.

In children ≥ 3 months of age, higher doses of **cefoxitin** have been associated with an increased incidence of eosinophilia and elevated AST.

In children ≥ 6 months of age, **ceftizoxime** has been associated with transient elevated levels of eosinophils, AST, ALT and CPK.

Safety and efficacy in children < 1 month (**cefazolin** and **cefaclor** capsule and suspension),< 3 months (**cefuroxime**, **cephapirin** and **cefoxitin**), < 5 months (**cefpodoxime**), < 6 months (**cefdinir**, **loracarbef**, **cefixime**, **ceftozoxime** and **cefprozil**), < 9 months (**oral cephradine**) and < 1 year (**cefepime** and **parenteral cephradine**) have not been established.

Safety and efficacy of **cefaclor** extended release tablets in children < 16 years of age have not been established.

Safety and efficacy of **cefonicid**, **cefmetazole**, **cefoperazone**, **cephalexin** and **cefotetan** in children have not been established.

Precautions

➤*Parenteral use:* Inject IM preparations deep into musculature; properly dilute IV preparations and administer over an appropriate time interval. See individual product monographs. Prolonged or high dosage IV use may be associated with thrombophlebitis; use small IV needles, larger veins and alternate infusion sites.

➤*Gonorrhea:* In the treatment of gonorrhea, all patients should have a serologic test for syphilis. Patients with incubating syphilis (seronegative without clinical signs of syphilis) are likely to be cured by the regimens used for gonorrhea.

➤*Benzyl alcohol:* Some cephalosporin products contain benzyl alcohol. In neonates, benzyl alcohol has been associated with neurological and other complications which are sometimes fatal. Benzyl alcohol-containing cephalosporin products should not be used in neonates.

➤*Superinfection:* Use of antibiotics (especially prolonged or repeated therapy) may result in bacterial or fungal overgrowth of nonsusceptible organisms. Such overgrowth may lead to a secondary infection. Take appropriate measures if this occurs.

Drug Interactions

Cephalosporin Drug Interactions			
Precipitant drug	Object drug*		Description
Cephalosporins Cefazolin Ceftmetazole Cefoperazone Cefotetan	Ethanol	↑	Alcoholic beverages consumed concurrently with or ≤ 72 hours after cefoperazone, cefazolin, cefmetazole or cefotetan may produce acute alcohol intolerance (disulfiram-like reaction). These antibiotics possess a methyltetrazolethiol side chain that may inhibit aldehyde dehydrogenase. The reaction begins within 30 minutes after alcohol ingestion and may subside 30 minutes to several hours afterwards; the reaction may occur ≤ 3 days after the last dose of the antibiotic.
Cephalosporins	Aminoglycosides	↑	Aminoglycoside nephrotoxicity may be potentiated by concurrent use of some cephalosporins, specifically cephalothin. Monitor renal function closely.
Cephalosporins Cefazolin Cefmetazole Cefoperazone Cefotetan	Anticoagulants	↑	Hypoprothrombinemic effects of anticoagulants may be increased by cephalosporins with the methyltetrazolethiol side chain (cefazolin, cefmetazole, cefoperazone, cefotetan). Bleeding complications may occur (see Warnings). Bleeding disorders have occurred with some of the other cephalosporins; therefore, the risk might be increased in anticoagulated patients. The concurrent use of heparin may also theoretically increase the risk of bleeding.
Cephalosporins Cephalothin	Polypeptide antibiotics	↑	The nephrotoxic effects of colistimethate may be increased by cephalothin. Monitor renal function.
Probenecid	Cephalosporins	↑	Probenecid may increase and prolong cephalosporin plasma levels by competitively inhibiting renal tubular secretion. This is most significant for cephalosporins eliminated primarily by tubular secretion.
Antacids	Cephalosporins Cefaclor Cefdinir Cefpodoxime	↓	Plasma concentrations of cefaclor extended release tablets, cefdinir and cefpodoxime may be reduced by coadministration of antacids. If antacids are required during administration of these antibiotics, the cephalosporin should be taken 2 hours before or after the antacid. Cefprozil and ceftibuten do not appear to be affected by coadministration of antacids.
H_2 antagonists	Cephalosporins Cefpodoxime Cefuroxime	↓	Plasma concentrations of cefpodoxime and cefuroxime may be reduced by coadministration of H_2 antagonists, decreasing the antibiotic effect. Cefaclor extended release tablets do not appear to be affected by coadministration of H_2 antagonists.
Iron supplements	Cephalosporins Cefdinir	↓	Iron supplements and foods fortified with iron reduce the absorption of cefdinir by 80% and 30%, respectively. If iron supplements are needed during cefdinir therapy, cefdinir should be taken 2 hours before or after the supplement. Iron-fortified infant formula (2.2 mg elemental iron/6 oz) has no effect on cefdinir absorption.
Loop diuretics	Cephalosporins	↑	Use cephalosporins with caution in patients receiving potent diuretics (eg, loop diuretics). The risk of nephrotoxicity may be increased. Monitor renal function.

* ↑ = Object drug increased. ↓ = Object drug decreased.

➤*Drug/Lab test interactions:* A false-positive reaction for **urine glucose** may occur with Benedict's solution, Fehling's solution or with *Clinitest* tablets, but not with enzyme-based tests such as *Clinistix* and *Tes-Tape*.

Cephradine may cause false-positive reactions in urinary protein tests that use sulfosalicylic acid.

Cefuroxime may cause a false-negative reaction in the ferricyanide test for **blood glucose**.

Cefdinir may cause a false-positive reaction for ketones in urine when measured using nitroprusside but not nitroferricynide.

A false-positive direct *Coombs' test* has occurred in some patients receiving cephalosporins, particularly those with azotemia, in hematologic studies, in transfusion cross-matching procedures when **antiglobulin tests** are performed on the minor side or in Coombs' testing of newborns of mothers receiving cephalosporins before parturition. This reaction is nonimmunological.

Cephalosporins may falsely elevate **urinary 17-ketosteroid** values.

High concentrations of **cephalothin** or **cefoxitin** (> 100 mcg/ml) may interfere with measurement of creatinine levels by the Jaffe reaction and produce false results. Serum samples from patients on cefoxitin should not be analyzed for creatinine if obtained within 2 hours of drug use. **Cefotetan** may affect these measurements.

➤*Drug/Food interactions:* Food increases absorption of **cefpodoxime** and oral **cefuroxime**.

Adverse Reactions

➤*Cardiovascular:* Hypotension; palpitations; chest pain; vasodilation; syncope.

➤*CNS:* Headache; dizziness; vertigo; lethargy; fatigue; paresthesia; confusion; anxiety; hyperactivity; nervousness; insomnia; hypertonia; somnolence. Generalized tonic-clonic seizures, mild hemiparesis and extreme confusion after large doses in renal failure (**cefazolin**).

➤*Dermatologic:* Urticaria; diaphoresis; flushing; cutaneous moniliasis.

➤*GI:* Nausea; vomiting; diarrhea; constipation; anorexia; thirst; glossitis; oral candidiasis and moniliasis; abdominal pain; flatulence; heartburn; gastritis; stomach cramps; eructation; melena; bleeding peptic ulcer; ileus; gall bladder sludge; dyspepsia; colitis, including pseudomembranous colitis, can appear during or after treatment (see Warnings); adverse GI effects after parenteral use of some cephalosporins.

➤*GU:* Transitory elevations in BUN with and without elevated serum creatinine; pyuria; dysuria; vaginitis; vaginal discharge; genito-anal pruritus; genital candidiasis and moniliasis; reversible interstitial nephritis; hematuria; toxic nephropathy; acute renal failure (rare); casts in urine (**ceftriaxone**).

➤*Hematologic:* Eosinophilia; transient neutropenia; lymphocytosis; leukocytosis; leukopenia; thrombocythemia; thrombocytopenia; agranulocytosis; granulocytopenia; hemolytic anemia; bone marrow depression; pancytopenia; decreased platelet function; bleeding in association with hypoprothrombinemia; anemia; aplastic anemia; hemorrhage; transient thrombocytosis; neutropenia caused by an immunologic reaction and characterized by rapid destruction of peripheral neutrophils may require drug discontinuation; transient fluctuations in leukocyte counts, predominantly lymphocytosis; slight decreases in neutrophil count; decreased hemoglobin or hematocrit; disturbances in vitamin K-dependent clotting function (increased PT); increased platelet and increased bleeding. Lymphopenia, monocytosis, basophilia (ceftriaxone, rare and may be accompanied by jaundice, glycosuria, bronchospasm, palpitations and epistaxis).

➤*Hepatic:* Elevated AST, ALT, total bilirubin, alkaline phosphatase, LDH; hepatomegaly; hepatitis; jaundice; cholestasis; cholestatic jaundice; hepatic failure.

➤*Hypersensitivity:* Anaphylaxis; angioedema; Stevens-Johnson syndrome; erythema multiforme; toxic epidermal necrolysis; renal dysfunction; toxic nephropathy; hepatic dysfunction (including cholestasis); aplastic anemia; hemolytic anemia; hemorrhage; erythema; maculopapular rash; urticaria; pruritus.

➤*Local:* Pain; induration; temperature elevation and tenderness from IM injection; sterile abscesses from accidental SC injection; local swelling; inflammation; burning, cellulitis, paresthesia, phlebitis and thrombophlebitis following IV or IM administration.

➤*Musculoskeletal:* Myalgia; arthralgia; rhabdomyolysis; exacerbation of myasthenia gravis (**cefoxitin**).

➤*Respiratory:* Asthma; laryngeal edema; dyspnea; interstitial pneumonitis; bronchitis; bronchospasm; pneumonia; respiratory failure; epistaxis (**ceftriaxone**, rare); rhinitis (**loracarbef**).

➤*Miscellaneous:* Facial edema; swollen tongue; fever; chills; malaise; asthenia; dysgeusia; glucosuria; encephalopathy in renally impaired patients receiving unadjusted dosage regiment (**cefepime**); Jarisch Herxheimer reaction (**cefuroxime**); muscle cramps, stiffness, spasms of neck, pain/tightness in chest, pain/bleeding in urethra, kidney pain, tachycardia, lockjaw-type reaction (**cefuroxime**, single dose for gonorrhea); elevated CPK (IM **ceftizoxime** or **cefaclor** extended release tablets); mild-to-moderate hearing loss reported in some pediatric patients (**cefuroxime**).

Overdosage

➤*Parenteral cephalosporins:* Inappropriately large doses may cause seizures, particularly in renal impairment. Reduce dosage when renal function is impaired. If seizures occur, promptly discontinue drug; administer anticonvulsants if clinically indicated; consider hemodialysis in cases of overwhelming overdosage.

Patient Information

➤*For oral preparations:* Complete full course of therapy.

May cause GI upset; may take with food or milk. Take **cefpodoxime** and **cefuroxime** with food to increase absorption.

A false-positive reaction for urine glucose may occur with the nonspecific urine tests. Use an enzyme-based test.

➤*Cephradine:*

Diabetics – Notify physician before changing diet or dosage of medication.

➤*Phenylketonurics:* **Cefprozil** oral suspension contains phenylalanine 28 mg/5 ml.

➤*Antacids:* Those containing magnesium or aluminum interfere with the absorption of cefdinir. If this type of antacid is required during **cefdinir** therapy, take cefdinir 2 hours before or after the antacid.

CEFPODOXIME PROXETIL

Rx	**Vantin** (Pharmacia & Upjohn)	**Tablets:** 100 mg	Lactose. (U3617). Orange. Film coated. In 20s, 100s and UD 100s.
		200 mg	Lactose. (U3618). Coral red. Film coated. In 20s, 100s and UD 100s.
		Granules for suspension: 50 mg/5 ml	Lactose, sucrose. Lemon creme flavor. In 50, 75 and 100 ml bottles.
		100 mg/5 ml	Lactose, sucrose. Lemon creme flavor. In 50 and 100 ml bottles.

CEFPODOXIME PROXETIL — ORAL

For complete and comparative prescribing information, refer to the Cephalosporins group monograph.

Indications

➤*Acute otitis:* Caused by *Streptococcus pneumoniae*, (excluding penicillin-resistant strains). *Streptococcus pyogenes, Haemophilus influenzae* (including beta-lactamase-producing strains), or *Moraxella* (*Branhamella*) *catarrhalis* (including beta-lactamase producing strains).

➤*Pharyngitis or tonsillitis:* Caused by *Streptococcus pyogenes*. Only penicillin by the IM route of administration has been shown to be effective in the prophylaxis of rheumatic fever. Cefpodoxime proxetil is generally effective in the eradication of streptococci from the oropharynx. However, data establishing the efficacy of cefpodoxime proxetil for the prophylaxis of subsequent rheumatic fever are not available.

➤*Community-acquired pneumonia:* Caused by *S. pneumoniae* or *H. influenzae* (including beta-lactamase-producing strains).

➤*Acute bacterial exacerbation of chronic bronchitis:* Caused by *S. pneumoniae, H. influenzae* (non-beta-lactamase-producing strains only), or *M. catarrhalis*. Data are insufficient at this time to establish efficacy in patients with acute bacterial exacerbations of chronic bronchitis caused by beta-lactamase-producing strains of *H. influenzae*.

➤*Acute, uncomplicated urethral and cervical gonorrhea:* Caused by *Neisseria gonorrhoeae* (including penicillinase-producing strains).

➤*Acute, uncomplicated anorectal infections in women:* Due to *Neisseria gonorrhoeae* (including penicillinase-producing strains).

The efficacy of cefpodoxime in treating male patients with rectal infections caused by *N. gonorrhoeae* has not been established. Data do not support the use of cefpodoxime proxetil in the treatment of pharyngeal infections due to *N. gonorrhoeae* in men or women.

➤*Uncomplicated skin and skin structure infections:* Caused by *Staphylococcus aureus* (including penicillinase-producing strains) or *Streptococcus pyogenes*. Abscesses should be surgically drained as clinically indicated.

In clinical trials, successful treatment of uncomplicated skin and skin structure infections was dose related. The effective therapeutic dose for skin infections was higher than those used in other recommended indications (see Administration and Dosage).

➤*Acute maxillary sinusitis:* Caused by *Haemophilus influenzae* (including beta-lactamase producing strains), *Streptococcus pneumoniae*, and *Moraxella catarrhalis*.

➤*Uncomplicated urinary tract infections (cystitis):* Caused by *Escherichia coli, Klebsiella pneumoniae, Proteus mirabilis*, or *Staphylococcus saprophyticus*.

In considering the use of cefpodoxime proxetil in the treatment of cystitis, cefpodoxime proxetil's lower bacterial eradication rates should be weighed against the increased eradication rates and different safety profiles of some other classes of approved agents.

Administration and Dosage

➤*Approved by the FDA:* August 7, 1992.

➤*Film-coated tablets:* Cefpodoxime proxetil tablets should be administered orally with food to enhance absorption (see Pharmacology).

Adults and adolescents (age 12 years and older)			
Type of infection	Total daily dose	Dose frequency	Duration
Pharyngitis and/ or tonsillitis	200 mg	100 mg every 12 hours	5 to 10 days
Acute community-acquired pneumonia	400 mg	200 mg every 12 hours	14 days
Acute bacterial exacerbations of chronic bronchitis	400 mg	200 mg every 12 hours	10 days
Uncomplicated gonorrhea (men and women) and rectal gonococcal infections (women)	200 mg	single dose	
Skin and skin structure	800 mg	400 mg every 12 hours	7 to 14 days
Acute maxillary sinusitis	400 mg	200 mg every 12 hours	10 days
Uncomplicated urinary tract infection	200 mg	100 mg every 12 hours	7 days

➤*Granules for oral suspension:* Cefpodoxime proxetil oral suspension may be given without regard to food.

Adults and adolescents (age 12 years and older)			
Type of infection	Total daily dose	Dose frequency	Duration
Pharyngitis and/ or tonsillitis	200 mg	100 mg every 12 hours	5 to 10 days
Acute community-acquired pneumonia	400 mg	200 mg every 12 hours	14 days
Uncomplicated gonorrhea (men and women) and rectal gonococcal infections (women)	200 mg	single dose	
Skin and skin structure	800 mg	400 mg every 12 hours	7 to 14 days
Acute maxillary sinusitis	400 mg	200 mg every 12 hours	10 days
Uncomplicated urinary tract infection	200 mg	100 mg every 12 hours	7 days
Infants and pediatric patients (age 2 months through 12 years):			
Acute otitis media	10 mg/kg/day (max 400 mg/day)	5 mg/kg every 12 hours (max 200 mg/dose)	5 days
Pharyngitis and/ or tonsillitis	10 mg/kg/day (max 200 mg/day)	5 mg/kg/dose every 12 hours (max 100 mg/dose)	5 to 10 days
Acute maxillary sinusitis	10 mg/kg/day (max 400 mg/day)	5 mg/kg every 12 hours (max 200 mg/dose)	10 days

➤*Renal function impairment:* For patients with severe renal impairment (< 30 mL/min creatinine clearance), the dosing intervals should be increased to Q 24 hours. In patients maintained on hemodialysis, the dose frequency should be 3 times/week after hemodialysis.

➤*Preparation of suspension:* Direction for mixing are included on the label. After mixing, the suspension should be stored in a refrigerator, 2° to 8°C (36° to 46°F). Shake well before using. Keep container tightly closed. The mixture may be used for 14 days. Discard unused portion after 14 days.

➤*Storage / Stability:* Store tablets at controlled room temperature 20° to 25°C (68° to 77°F) [see USP]. Replace cap securely after each opening. Protect unit dose packs from excessive moisture.

Store unsuspended granules at controlled room temperature 20° to 25°C (68° to 77°F) [see USP]. After mixing, suspension should be stored in a refrigerator, 2° to 8°C (36° to 46°F). The mixture may be used for 14 days. Discard unused portion after 14 days.

CEFACLOR

Rx	**Raniclor** (Ranbaxy)	**Tablets, chewable:** 125 mg	2.8 mg phenylalanine, aspartame, mannitol, tartrazine. (RX 555). Yellow, scored. Fruity flavor. In 20s, 30s, 250s, and UD 100s.
		187 mg	4.2 mg phenylalanine, aspartame, mannitol, tartrazine. (RX 556). Yellow, scored. Fruity flavor. In 20s, 250s, and UD 100s.
		250 mg	5.6 mg phenylalanine, aspartame, mannitol, tartrazine. (RX 557). Yellow, scored. Fruity flavor. In 20s, 30s, 250s, and UD 100s.
		375 mg	8.4 mg phenylalanine, aspartame,Sure. mannitol, tartrazine. (RX 558). Yellow, scored. Fruity flavor. In 20s, 250s, and UD 100s.
Rx	**Cefaclor** (Zenith Goldline)	**Tablets, extended release:** 375 mg	(X 4194 500). Blue, oval. In 100s.
		500 mg	
Rx	**Cefaclor** (Various, eg, Apothecon, Mylan, Rugby, URL)	**Capsules:** 250 mg	In 30s, 100s, 500s, and 1000s.
Rx	**Ceclor Pulvules** (Eli Lilly)		(3061). White and purple. In 15s, 100s and UD 100s.
Rx	**Cefaclor** (Various, eg, Apothecon, Mylan, Rugby, URL)	**Capsules:** 500 mg	In 15s, 100s and 500s.
Rx	**Cefaclor** (Various, eg, Apothecon, Mylan, Rugby, URL, Zenith Goldline)	**Powder for oral suspension:** 125 mg/5 ml	In 75 and 150 ml.
	Ceclor (Eli Lilly)		Sucrose. Strawberry flavor. In 75 and 150 ml.
Rx	**Cefaclor** (Various, eg, Apothecon, Mylan, Rugby, URL, Zenith Goldline)	**Powder for oral suspension:** 187 mg/5 ml	In 50 and 100 ml.
	Ceclor (Eli Lilly)		Sucrose. Strawberry flavor. In 50 and 100 ml.
Rx	**Cefaclor** (Various, eg, Apothecon, Mylan, Rugby, URL, Zenith Goldline)	**Powder for oral suspension:** 250 mg/5 ml	In 75 and 150 ml.
	Ceclor (Eli Lilly)		Sucrose. Strawberry flavor. In 75 and 150 ml.
Rx	**Cefaclor** (Various, eg, Apothecon, Mylan, Rugby, URL, Zenith Goldline)	**Powder for oral suspension:** 375 mg/5 ml	In 50 and 100 ml.
	Ceclor (Eli Lilly)		Sucrose. Strawberry flavor. In 50 and 100 ml.

CEFACLOR — ORAL

For complete and comparative prescribing information, refer to the Cephalosporins group monograph.

Indications

➤*Extended-release tablets:*

Pharyngitis and tonsillitis – Pharyngitis and tonsillitis due to *Streptococcus pyogenes.*

Uncomplicated skin and skin structure infections – Uncomplicated skin and skin structure infections due to *Staphylococcus aureus* (methicillin-susceptible).

Acute bacterial exacerbations of chronic bronchitis – Acute bacterial exacerbations of chronic bronchitis due to *Haemophilus influenzae* (non-β-lactamase-producing strains only), *Moraxella catarrhalis* (including β-lactamase-producing strains) or *Streptococcus pneumoniae.*

Secondary bacterial infections of acute bronchitis – Secondary bacterial infections of acute bronchitis due to *Haemophilus influenzae* (non-β-lactamase-producing strains only), *Moraxella catarrhalis* (including β-lactamase-producing strains), or *Streptococcus pneumoniae.*

➤*Capsules, chewable tablets, and oral suspension:*

Otitis media – Caused by *Streptococcus pneumoniae, Haemophilus influenzae,* staphylococci, and *Streptococcus pyogenes.*

Pharyngitis and tonsillitis – Due to *Streptococcus pyogenes.*

Lower respiratory tract infections – Including pneumonia, caused by *Streptococcus pneumoniae, Haemophilus influenzae,* and *Streptococcus pyogenes.*

Urinary tract infections – Including pyelonephritis and cystitis, caused by *Escherichia coli, Proteus mirabilis, Klebsiella* spp, and coagulase-negative staphylococci.

Administration and Dosage

➤*Extended-release tablets:* Cefaclor extended-release tablets should be administered with meals (ie, at least within 1 hour of eating). The extended-release tablets should not be cut, crushed, or chewed.

Equivalence – 500 mg twice daily of cefaclor extended-release tablets is clinically equivalent to 250 mg 3 times daily of cefaclor immediate-release as a capsule. 500 mg twice daily of cefaclor extended-release tablets is not equivalent to 500 mg 3 times daily of other cefaclor formulations.

Adults (age 16 years and older)			
Type of infection (as qualified in the Indications section)	Total daily dose	Dose and frequency	Duration
Acute bacterialexacerbations of chronic bronchitis due to *H. influenzae* (non-β-lactamase-producing strains only), *Moraxella catarrhalis* (including β-lactamase producing strains) or *Streptococcus pneumoniae*	1000 mg	500 mg every 12 hours	7 days
Secondary bacterial infection of acute bronchitis due to to *H. influenzae* (non-β-lactamase-producing strains only), *Moraxella catarrhalis* (including β-lactamase producing strains) or *S. pneumoniae* (see Indications)	1000 mg	500 mg every 12 hours	7 days
Pharyngitis or tonsillitis due to *S. pyogenes*	750 mg	375 mg every 12 hours	10 days
Uncomplicated skin and skin structure infections due to *S. aureus* (methicillin-susceptible strains) (see Indications)	750 mg	375 mg every 12 hours	7 to 10 days

➤*Capsules, chewable tablets, and oral suspension:*

Adults – The usual adult dosage is 250 mg every 8 hours. For more severe infections (such as pneumonia) or those caused by less susceptible organisms, doses may be doubled.

Capsules: Food does not affect the extent of absorption.

Children – The usual recommended daily dosage for pediatric patients is 20 mg/kg/day in divided doses every 8 hours. In more serious infections, otitis media, and infections caused by less susceptible organisms, 40 mg/kg/day are recommended, with a maximum dosage of 1 g/day.

	Cefaclor suspension	
	20 mg/kg/day	
Weight	125 mg/5 mL	250 mg/5mL
9 kg	2.5 mL 3 times daily	
18 kg	5 mL 3 times daily	2.5 mL 3 times daily

CEFACLOR — ORAL

Weight	Cefaclor suspension 40 mg/kg/day	
	125 mg/5 mL	250 mg/5mL
9 kg	5 mL 3 times daily	2.5 mL 3 times daily
18 kg		5 mL 3 times daily

Twice daily treatment option: For the treatment of otitis media and pharyngitis, the total daily dosage may be divided and administered every 12 hours.

Weight	Cefaclor suspension 20 mg/kg/day (pharyngitis)	
	187 mg/5 mL	375 mg/5 mL
9 kg	2.5 mL twice daily	
18 kg	5 mL twice daily	2.5 mL twice daily

Weight	Cefaclor suspension 40 mg/kg/day (pharyngitis)	
	187 mg/5 mL	375 mg/5 mL
9 kg	5 mL twice daily	2.5 mL twice daily
18 kg		5 mL twice daily

Renal function impairment: Cefaclor may be administered in the presence of impaired renal function. Under such a condition, the dosage usually is unchanged.

In the elderly and in patients with known or suspected renal impairment, monitor carefully prior to and during therapy.

See Actions for more information.

Duration: Continue administration for a minimum of 48 to 72 hours after fever abates or after evidence of bacterial eradication has been obtained. In the treatment of β-hemolytic streptococcal infections, a therapeutic dosage of cefaclor should be administered for at least 10 days to guard against the risk of rheumatic fever or glomerulonephritis.

➤*Storage / Stability:*

Extended-release tablets, chewable tablets, and capsules – Store at controlled room temperature, 15° to 30°C (59° to 86°F).

Oral suspension – Refrigerate suspension after reconstitution; discard after 14 days.

CEPHALEXIN

Rx	**Cephalexin** (Various, eg, Geneva, Lederle, Rugby)	**Capsules:** 250 mg	In 100s, 500s, 1,000s, UD 20s and 100s.
Rx	**Keflex** (Advancis)		(Keflex 250 mg). White/dark green. In 20s and 100s.
Rx	**Keflex** (Advancis)	333 mg	(Kelfex 333 mg). Light green. In 50s.
Rx	**Cephalexin** (Various, eg, Geneva, Lederle, Major, Rugby)	500 mg	In 100s, 250s, 500s, 1,000s, UD 20s and 100s.
Rx	**Keflex** (Advancis)		(Keflex 500 mg). Light green and dark green. In 20s and 100s.
Rx	**Keflex** (Advancis)	750 mg	(Kelfex 750 mg). Dark green. In 50s.
Rx	**Cephalexin** (Various, eg, Barr, Lederle, Zenith-Goldline)	**Tablets:** 250 mg	In 20s, 100s, and 500s.
Rx	**Cephalexin** (Various, eg, Barr, Lederle, Schein, Zenith-Goldline)	500 mg	In 20s, 100s, and 500s.
Rx	**Cephalexin** (Various, eg, Geneva, Lederle, Zenith-Goldline)	**Powder for oral suspension:** 125 mg per 5 mL (after reconstitution)	In 100 and 200 mL.
Rx	**Keflex** (Advancis)		Sucrose. In 100 and 200 mL.
Rx	**Cephalexin** (Various, eg, Barr, Geneva, Lederle, Zenith-Goldline)	250 mg per 5 mL (after reconstitution)	In 100 and 200 mL.
Rx	**Keflex** (Advancis)		Sucrose. In 100 and 200 mL.

CEPHALEXIN — ORAL

For complete and comparative prescribing information, refer to the Cephalosporins group monograph.

Indications

➤*Respiratory tract infections:* Caused by *Streptococcus pneumoniae* and *Streptococcus pyogenes*.

➤*Otitis media:* Caused by *S. pneumoniae*, *Haemophilus influenzae*, *Staphylococcus aureus*, *S. pyogenes*, and *Moraxella catarrhalis*.

➤*Skin and skin structure infections:* Caused by *S. aureus* and/or *S. pyogenes*.

➤*Bone infections:* Caused by *S. aureus* and/or *Proteus mirabilis*.

➤*Genitourinary tract infections:* These include acute prostatitis caused by *Escherichia coli*, *P. mirabilis*, and *Klebsiella pneumoniae*.

Administration and Dosage

➤*Approved by the FDA:* 1969.

➤*Note:* Culture and susceptibility tests should be initiated prior to and during therapy. Renal function studies should be performed when indicated.

To reduce the development of drug-resistant bacteria and maintain the effectiveness of cephalexin and other antibacterial drugs, cephalexin should be used only to treat or prevent infections that are proven or strongly suspected to be caused by susceptible bacteria. When culture and susceptibility information are available, they should be considered in selecting or modifying antibacterial therapy. In the absence of such data, local epidemiology and susceptibility patterns may contribute to the empiric selection of therapy.

➤*Adults:* 1 to 4 g daily in divided doses. The 333 and 750 mg strengths should be administered so that the daily dose is within 1 to 4 g per day. The usual adult dosage is 250 mg every 6 hours. For the following infections, a dosage of 500 mg may be administered every 12 hours: streptococcal pharyngitis, skin and skin structure infections, and uncomplicated cystitis in patients older than 15 years of age. Cystitis therapy should be continued for 7 to 14 days. For more severe infections or those caused by less susceptible organisms, larger doses may be needed. If daily doses of cephalexin greater than 4 g are required, parental cephalosporins, in appropriate doses, should be considered.

➤*Children:* Do not exceed adult recommended doses. The usual recommended daily dose for children is 25 to 50 mg/kg in divided doses. For streptococcal pharyngitis in patients older than 1 year of age and for skin and skin structure infections, the total daily dose may be divided and administered every 12 hours. In severe infections, the dose may be doubled.

Otitis media – 75 to 100 mg/kg/day in 4 divided doses.

β-hemolytic streptococcal infections – Continue treatment for at least 10 days.

➤*Storage / Stability:* Shake the reconstituted suspension well and refrigerate; discard after 14 days. Store the tablets, capsules, and powder for oral suspension at controlled room temperature, 20° to 25°C (68° to 77°F).

CEFADROXIL

Rx	**Cefadroxil** (Various, eg, Major)	**Capsules:** 500 mg[1]	In 100s.
Rx	**Duricef** (Bristol-Myers Squibb)		(PPP 784). In 20s, 50s, 100s and UD 100s.
Rx	**Cefadroxil** (Various, eg, Major)	**Tablets:** 1 g[1]	In 24s, 50s, 100s and 500s.
Rx	**Duricef** (Bristol-Myers Squibb)		(PPP 785). In 50s, 100s, UD 40s and 100s.

CEFADROXIL

Rx	**Duricef** (Bristol-Myers Squibb)	**Powder for oral suspension:** 125 mg/5 ml	Orange-pineapple flavor. In 50 and 100 ml.
		250 mg/5 ml	Sucrose. Orange-pineapple flavor. In 50 and 100 ml.
		500 mg/5 ml	Sucrose. Orange-pineapple flavor. In 75 and 100 ml.

[1] As monohydrate.

CEFADROXIL — ORAL

For complete and comparative prescribing information, refer to the Cephalosporins group monograph.

Indications

➤*Urinary tract infections:* Caused by *E. coli*, *P. mirabilis*, and *Klebsiella* species.

➤*Skin and skin structure infections:* Caused by staphylococci or streptococci.

➤*Pharyngitis or tonsillitis:* Caused by *Streptococcus pyogenes* (group A beta-hemolytic streptococci).

Administration and Dosage

➤*Approved by the FDA:* 1977.

Cefadroxil is acid-stable and may be administered orally without regard to meals. Administration with food may be helpful in diminishing potential GI complaints occasionally associated with oral cephalosporin therapy.

➤*Adults:*

Urinary tract infections – For uncomplicated lower urinary tract infections (ie, cystitis) the usual dosage is 1 or 2 g per day in single (every day) or divided doses (twice daily).

For all other urinary tract infections the usual dosage is 2 g/day in divided doses (twice daily).

Skin and skin structure infections – For skin and skin structure infections, the usual dosage is 1 g/day in single (every day) or divided doses (twice daily).

Pharyngitis and tonsillitis – Treatment of group A beta-hemolytic streptococcal pharyngitis and tonsillitis 1 g per day in single (every day) or divided doses (twice daily) for 10 days.

➤*Children:* For urinary tract infections, the recommended daily dosage for children is 30 mg/kg/day in divided doses every 12 hours. For pharyngitis, tonsillitis, and impetigo, the recommended daily dosage for children is 30 mg/kg/day in a single dose or in equally divided doses every 12 hours. For other skin and skin structure infections, the recommended daily dosage is 30 mg/kg/day in equally divided doses every 12 hours. In the treatment of beta-hemolytic streptococcal infections, a therapeutic dosage of cefadroxil should be administered for at least 10 days.

Daily dosage of cefadroxil oral suspension				
Child's weight				
lbs	kg	125 mg/5 mL	250 mg/5 mL	500 mg/5 mL
10	4.5	5 mL	-	-
20	9.1	10 mL	5 mL	-
30	13.6	15 mL	7.5 mL	-
40	18.2	20 mL	10 mL	5 mL
50	22.7	25 mL	12.5 mL	6.25 mL
60	27.3	30 mL	15 mL	7.5 mL
70 and above	31.8+	-	-	10 mL

➤*Renal function impairment:* In patients with renal impairment, the dosage of cefadroxil should be adjusted according to creatinine clearance rates to prevent drug accumulation. The following schedule is suggested. In adults, the initial dose is 1 g of cefadroxil, and the maintenance dose (based on the creatinine clearance rate [mL/min/1.73 M^2]) is 500 mg at the time intervals listed below.

Creatinine clearances	Dosage interval
0 to 10 mL/min	36 hours
10 to 25 mL/min	24 hours
25 to 50 mL/min	12 hours

➤*Perparation of suspension:* Patients with creatinine clearance rates over 50 mL/min may be treated as if they have healthy renal function.

Directions for mixing are included on the label. After reconstitution, store in the refrigerator. Shake well before using. Keep container tightly closed. Discard unused portion after 14 days.

➤*Storage/Stability:* Store tablets and capsules at controlled room temperature 15° to 30°C (59° to 86°F). Discard unused portion of oral suspension after 14 days.

LORACARBEF

Rx	**Lorabid** (Monarch)	**Pulvules (capsules):** 200 mg	(3170). Blue/gray. In 30s.
		400 mg	(3171). Blue/pink. In 30s.
		Powder for oral suspension: 100 mg/5 ml	Parabens, sucrose. Strawberry bubble gum flavor. In 50, 75 and 100 ml.
		200 mg/5 ml	Parabens, sucrose. Strawberry bubble gum flavor. In 50, 75 and 100 ml.

LORACARBEF — ORAL

For complete and comparative prescribing information, refer to the Cephalosporins group monograph.

Indications

➤*Secondary bacterial infection of acute bronchitis:* Caused by *S. pneumoniae*, *H. influenzae* (including β-lactamase-producing strains), or *M. catarrhalis* (including β-lactamase-producing strains).

➤*Acute bacterial exacerbations of chronic bronchitis:* Caused by *S. pneumoniae*, *H. influenzae* (including β-lactamase-producing strains), or *M. catarrhalis* (including β-lactamase-producing strains).

➤*Pneumonia:* Caused by *S. pneumoniae* or *H. influenzae* (non-β-lactamase-producing strains only).

➤*Otitis media:* Caused by *S. pneumoniae*, *H. influenzae* (including β-lactamase-producing strains), *M. catarrhalis* (including β-lactamase-producing strains), or *S. pyogenes*.

➤*Acute maxillary sinusitis:* Caused by *S. pneumoniae*, *H. influenzae* (non-β-lactamase-producing strains only), or *M. catarrhalis* (including β-lactamase-producing strains).

In a patient population with significant numbers of β-lactamase-producing organisms, loracarbef's clinical cure and bacteriological eradication rates were somewhat less than those observed with a product containing a β-lactamase inhibitor. Loracarbef's decreased potential for toxicity compared to products containing β-lactamase inhibitors along with the susceptibility patterns of the common microbes in a given geographic area should be taken into account when considering the use of an antimicrobial. For information on use in pediatric patients, see Warnings.

➤*Pharyngitis and tonsillitis:* Caused by *S. pyogenes*.

➤*Uncomplicated skin and skin structure infections:* Caused by *S. aureus* (including penicillinase-producing strains) or *S. pyogenes*. Abscesses should be surgically drained as clinically indicated.

➤*Uncomplicated urinary tract infections (cystitis):* Caused by *E. coli* or *S. saprophyticus*. Although treatment of infections due to *S. saprophyticus* in this organ system demonstrated a clinically acceptable overall outcome, efficacy was studied in fewer than 10 infections.

In considering the use of loracarbef in the treatment of cystitis, loracarbef's lower bacterial eradication rates and lower potential for toxicity should be weighed against the increased eradication rates and increased potential for toxicity demonstrated by some other classes of approved agents.

➤*Uncomplicated pyelonephritis:* Caused by *E. coli*.

Administration and Dosage

➤*Approved by the FDA:* December 31, 1991.

Loracarbef is administered orally either at least 1 hour prior to eating or at least 2 hours after eating.

Dosage/Duration of Loracarbef		
Population/infection	Dosage (mg)	Duration (days)
Adults (13 years and older)		
Lower respiratory tract		
Secondary bacterial infection of acute bronchitis	200 to 400 every 12 hours	7
Acute bacterial exacerbation of chronic bronchitis	400 every 12 hours	7
Pneumonia	400 every 12 hours	14
Upper respiratory tract		
Pharyngitis/tonsillitis	200 every 12 hours	10[a]
Sinusitis (see Clinical trials and Indications for further information)	400 every 12 hours	10

LORACARBEF — ORAL

Dosage/Duration of Loracarbef		
Population/infection	Dosage (mg)	Duration (days)
Skin and skin structure		
Uncomplicated skin and skin structure infections	200 every 12 hours	7
Urinary tract		
Uncomplicated cystitis (see Indications for further information)	200 every 24 hours	7
Uncomplicated pyelonephritis	400 every 12 hours	14
Pediatric patients (6 months to 12 years)		
Upper respiratory tract		
Acute otitis media[b] (see Indications for further information)	30 mg/kg/day in divided doses every 12 hours	10
Acute maxillary sinusitis (see Indications)	30 mg/kg/day in divided doses every 12 hours	10
Pharyngitis/tonsillitis	15 mg/kg/day in divided doses every 12 hours	10[a]
Skin and skin structure		
Impetigo	15 mg/kg/day in divided doses every 12 hours	7

[a] In the treatment of infections due to *S. pyogenes*, loracarbef should be administered for at least 10 days.

[b] Otitis media should be treated with the suspension. Clinical studies of otitis media were conducted with the suspension formulation only. The suspension is more rapidly absorbed than the capsules, resulting in higher peak plasma concentrations when administered at the same dose. Therefore, the capsule should not be substituted for the suspension in the treatment of otitis media (see Pharmacology).

Pediatric suspension dosage chart (daily dose 15 mg/kg/day)					
Weight		100 mg/5 mL twice daily		200 mg/5 mL twice daily	
lb	kg	mL	tsp	mL	tsp
15	7	2.6	0.5	-	-
29	13	4.9	1	2.5	0.5
44	20	7.5	1.5	3.8	0.75
57	26	9.8	2	4.9	1

Pediatric suspension dosage chart (daily dose 30 mg/kg/day)					
Weight		100 mg/5 mL twice daily		200 mg/5 mL twice daily	
lb	kg	mL	tsp	mL	tsp
15	7	5.2	1	2.6	0.5
29	13	9.8	2	4.9	1
44	20	-	-	7.5	1.5
57	26	-	-	9.8	2

➤*Renal function impairment:* Loracarbef may be administered to patients with impaired renal function. The usual dose and schedule may be employed in patients with creatinine clearance levels of 50 mL/min or greater. Patients with creatinine clearance between 10 and 49 mL/min may be given half of the recommended dose at the usual dosage interval, or the normal recommended dose at twice the usual dosage interval. Patients with creatinine clearance levels < 10 mL/min may be treated with the recommended dose given every 3 to 5 days; patients on hemodialysis should receive another dose following dialysis.

➤*Storage/Stability:* After mixing, the suspension may be kept at room temperature, 59° to 86°F (15° to 30°C), for 14 days without significant loss of potency. Discard unused portion after 14 days.

CEFPROZIL

Rx	**Cefprozil** (Various, eg, Lupin, Sandoz, Teva)	**Tablets:** 250 mg (as anhydrous)	In 100s.
Rx	**Cefzil** (Bristol-Myers Squibb)		(7720 250). Light orange. Film coated. In 100s and UD 100s.
Rx	**Cefprozil** (Various, eg, Lupin, Sandoz, Teva)	**Tablets:** 500 mg (as anhydrous)	In 50s and 100s.
Rx	**Cefzil** (Bristol-Myers Squibb)		(7721 500). White. Film coated. In 50s, 100s and UD 100s.
Rx	**Cefprozil** (Various, eg, Lupin, Sandoz, Teva)	**Powder for oral suspension:** 125 mg per 5 mL (as anhydrous)	May contain aspartame, sucrose, phenylalanine. In 50, 75, and 100 mL.
Rx	**Cefzil** (Bristol-Myers Squibb)		Aspartame, sucrose, 28 mg per 5 mL phenylalanine. Bubble gum flavor. In 50, 75 and 100 mL.
Rx	**Cefprozil** (Various, eg, Lupin, Sandoz, Teva)	**Powder for oral suspension:** 250 mg per 5 mL (as anhydrous)	May contain aspartame, sucrose, phenylalanine. In 50, 75, and 100 mL.
Rx	**Cefzil** (Bristol-Myers Squibb)		Aspartame, sucrose, 28 mg per 5 mL phenylalanine. Bubble gum flavor. In 50, 75, and 100 mL.

CEFPROZIL — ORAL

For complete and comparative prescribing information, refer to the Cephalosporins group monograph.

Indications

➤*Pharyngitis/tonsillitis:* Caused by *Streptococcus pyogenes*.

➤*Otitis media:* Caused by *Streptococcus pneumoniae, Haemophilus influenzae* (including β-lactamase-producing strains) and *Moraxella (Branhamella) catarrhalis* (including β-lactamase-producing strains.

In the treatment of otitis media due to β-lactamase-producing organisms, cefprozil had bacteriologic eradication rates somewhat lower than those observed with a product containing a specific β-lactamase inhibitor. In considering the use of cefprozil, lower overall eradication rates should be balanced against the susceptibility patterns of the common microbes in a given geographic area and the increased potential for toxicity with products containing β-lactamase inhibitors.

➤*Acute sinusitis:* Caused by *Streptococcus pneumoniae, Haemophilus influenzae* (including β-lactamase-producing strains), and *Moraxella (Branhamella) catarrhalis* (including β-lactamase-producing strains).

➤*Secondary bacterial infection of acute bronchitis and acute bacterial exacerbation of chronic bronchitis:* Caused by *Streptococcus pneumoniae, Haemophilus influenzae* (including β-lactamase-producing strains), and *Moraxella (Branhamella) catarrhalis* (including β-lactamase-producing strains).

➤*Uncomplicated skin and skin structure infections:* Caused by *Staphylococcus aureus* (including penicillinase-producing strains) and *Streptococcus pyogenes*. Abscesses usually require surgical drainage.

Administration and Dosage

➤*Approved by the FDA:* December 23, 1991.

Population/infection	Dosage (mg)	Duration (days)
Adults (13 years and older)		
Upper respiratory tract		
Pharyngitis/tonsillitis	500 mg every 24 hours	10[a]
Acute sinusitis (For moderate to severe infections, the higher dose should be used.)	250 mg every 12 hours or	10
	500 mg every 12 hours	
Lower respiratory tract		
Secondary bacterial infection of acute bronchitis and acute bacterial exacerbation of chronic bronchitis	500 mg every 12 hours	10

CEFPROZIL — ORAL

Population/infection	Dosage (mg)	Duration (days)
Skin and skin structure		
Uncomplicated skin and skin structure infections	250 mg every 12 hours or	10
	500 mg every 24 hours or	
	500 mg every 12 hours	
Children (2 years to 12 years)		
Upper respiratory tract[b]		
Pharyngitis/tonsillitis	7.5 mg/kg every 12 hours	10[a]
Skin and skin structure[b]		
Uncomplicated skin and skin structure infections	20 mg/kg every 24 hours	10
Infants and children (6 months to 12 years)		
Upper respiratory tract[b]		
Otitis media (see Indications)	15 mg/kg every 12 hours	10
Acute sinusitis (For moderate to severe infections, the higher dose should be used.)	7.5 mg/kg every 12 hours or 15 mg/kg	10

[a] In the treatment of infections due to *Streptococcus pyogenes*, cefprozil should be administered for at least 10 days.
[b] Not to exceed recommended adult doses.

➤*Renal impairment:* The following dosage schedule should be used.

Creatinine clearance (mL/min)	Dosage (mg)	Dosing interval
30 to 120	standard	standard
0 to 29*	50% of standard	standard

* Cefprozil is in part removed by hemodialysis; therefore, cefprozil should be administered after the completion of hemodialysis.

➤*Reconstitution for oral suspension:* Prepare the suspension at the time of dispensing; for ease in preparation, add water in 2 portions and shake well after each aliquot. After mixing, store in a refrigerator and discard unused portion after 14 days.

➤*Storage/Stability:*

Tablets – Store at controlled room temperature, 15° to 30°C (59° to 86°F).

Oral suspension – Store at 15° to 25° C (59° to 77°F) prior to constitution. After mixing, store in a refrigerator and discard unused portion after 14 days.

CEFTIBUTEN

Rx	**Cedax** (Shionogi)	**Capsules**: 400 mg	Parabens. (Cedax 400). White. In 20s.
		Powder for oral suspension: 90 mg per 5 mL (after reconstitution)	Sucrose. In 30, 60, 90, and 120 mL.

CEFTIBUTEN — ORAL

For complete and comparative prescribing information, refer to the Cephalosporins group monograph.

Indications

➤*Acute bacterial exacerbations of chronic bronchitis:* Acute bacterial exacerbations of chronic bronchitis due to *Haemophilus influenzae* (including β-lactamase-producing strains), *Moraxella catarrhalis* (including β-lactamase-producing strains), or *Streptococcus pneumoniae* (penicillin-susceptible strains only).

In acute bacterial exacerbations of chronic bronchitis clinical trials where *Moraxella catarrhalis* was isolated from infected sputum at baseline, ceftibuten clinical efficacy was 22% less than control.

➤*Acute bacterial otitis media:* Acute bacterial otitis media due to *Haemophilus influenzae* (including β-lactamase-producing strains), *Moraxella catarrhalis* (including β-lactamase-producing strains), or *Streptococcus pyogenes*.

Although ceftibuten used empirically was equivalent to comparators in the treatment of clinically or microbiologically documented acute otitis media, the efficacy against streptococcus pneumoniae was 23% less than control. Therefore, ceftibuten should be given empirically only when adequate antimicrobial coverage against *Streptococcus pneumoniae* has been previously administered.

➤*Pharyngitis and tonsillitis:* Pharyngitis and tonsillitis due to *Streptococcus pyogenes*.

Administration and Dosage

➤*Approved by the FDA:* December 20, 1995.

Ceftibuten must be administered at least 2 hours before or 1 hour after a meal.

Ceftibuten Dosage and Duration

Type of infection (as qualified in the Indications section)	Daily maximum dose	Dose and frequency	Duration
Adults (12 years of age and older): Acute bacterial exacerbations of chronic bronchitis due to *H. influenzae* (including beta-lactamase-producing strains), *M. catarrhalis* (including beta-lactamase-producing strains), or *Streptococcus pneumoniae* (penicillin-susceptible strains only; see Indications), pharyngitis and tonsillitis due to *S. pyogenes*, acute bacterial otitis media due to *H. influenzae* (including beta-lactamase-producing strains), *M. catarrhalis* (including beta-lactamase-producing strains) or *S. pyogenes* (see Indications).	400 mg	400 mg once daily	10 days
Pediatric patients: Pharyngitis and tonsillitis due to *S. pyogenes*, acute bacterial otitis media due to *H. influenzae* (including beta-lactamase-producing strains), *M. catarrhalis* (including beta-lactamase-producing strains) or *S. pyogenes* (see Indications).	400 mg	9 mg/kg once daily	10 days

Ceftibuten oral suspension pediatric dosage chart

Child's weight	90 mg/5 mL
10 kg/ 22 lbs	1 tsp once daily
20 kg/44 lbs	2 tsp once daily
40 kg/88 lbs	4 tsp once daily

Pediatric patients weighing more than 45 kg should receive the maximum daily dose of 400 mg.

➤*Renal function impairment:* Ceftibuten capsules and ceftibuten oral suspension may be administered at normal doses in the presence of impaired renal function with creatinine clearance of ≥ 50 mL/min. The recommendations for dosing in patients with varying degrees of renal insufficiency are presented in the following table.

CEFTIBUTEN — ORAL

Creatinine clearance (mL/min)	Recommended dosing schedule
> 50	9 mg/kg or 400 mg every 24 hours (normal dosing schedule)
30 to 49	4.5 mg/kg or 200 mg every 24 hours
5 to 29	2.25 mg/kg or 100 mg every 24 hours

➤*Hemodialysis patients:* In patients undergoing hemodialysis 2 or 3 times weekly, a single 400 mg dose of ceftibuten capsules, or a single dose of 9 mg/kg (maximum of 400 mg of ceftibuten) oral suspension may be administered at the end of each hemodialysis session.

➤*Preparation of oral suspension:* Directions for mixing are included on the product label. After mixing, the suspension may be kept for 14 days and must be stored in the refrigerator. Keep tightly closed. Shake well before each use. Discard any unused portion after 14 days.

➤*Storage/Stability:*

Capsules – Store the capsules between 2° and 25°C (36° and 77°F). Replace cap securely after each opening.

Oral suspension – Prior to reconstitution, the powder must be stored between 2° and 25°C (36° and 77°F). Once it is reconstituted, the oral suspension is stable for 14 days when stored in the refrigerator between 2° and 8°C (36° and 46°F).

CEFDINIR

Rx	**Omnicef** (Abbott)	**Capsules:** 300 mg	(OMNICEF). Lavender and turquoise. In 60s.
		Oral suspension: 125 mg and 5 mL	Sucrose. Strawberry-flavored. In 60 and 100 mL.
		250 mg per 5 mL	Sucrose. Strawberry-flavored. In 60 and 100 mL.

CEFDINIR — ORAL

For complete and comparative prescribing information, refer to the Cephalosporins group monograph.

Indications

➤*Adults and adolescents:*

Community-acquired pneumonia – Caused by *Haemophilus influenzae* (including β-lactamase-producing strains), *H. parainfluenzae* (including β-lactamase-producing strains), *Streptococcus pneumoniae* (penicillin-susceptible strains only) and *Moraxella catarrhalis* (including β-lactamase-producing strains).

Acute exacerbations of chronic bronchitis – Caused by *H. influenzae* (including β-lactamase producing strains), *H. parainfluenzae* (including β-lactamase-producing strains), *S. pneumoniae* (penicillin-susceptible strains only) and *M. catarrhalis* (including β-lactamase-producing strains).

Acute maxillary sinusitis – Caused by *H. influenzae* (including β-lactamase-producing strains), *S. pneumoniae* (penicillin-susceptible strains only) and *M. catarrhalis* (including β-lactamase-producing strains).

Pharyngitis/Tonsillitis – Caused by *S. pyogenes.*

Uncomplicated skin and skin structure infections – Caused by *Staphylococcus aureus* (including β-lactamase-producing strains) and *S. pyogenes.*

➤*Children:*

Acute bacterial otitis media – Caused by *H. influenzae* (including β-lactamase-producing strains), *S. pneumoniae* (penicillin-susceptible strains only) and *M. catarrhalis* (including β-lactamase-producing strains).

Pharyngitis/Tonsillitis – Caused by *S. pyogenes.*

Uncomplicated skin and skin structure infections – Caused by *S. aureus* (including β-lactamase-producing strains) and *S. pyogenes.*

Administration and Dosage

➤*Approved by the FDA:* December 4, 1997.

➤*Adults/Adolescents:* The recommended dosage and duration of treatment for infections in adults and adolescents are described in the following chart; the total daily dose for all infections is 600 mg. Once-daily dosing for 10 days is as effective as twice-daily dosing. Once-daily dosing has not been studied in pneumonia or skin infections; therefore, administer capsules twice daily in these infections. Capsules may be taken without regard to meals.

Cefdinir Dosage in Adults and Adolescents (≥ 13 years of age)

Type of infection	Dosage	Duration
Community-acquired pneumonia	300 mg q 12 hrs	10 days
Acute exacerbations of chronic bronchitis	300 mg q 12 hrs or 600 mg q 24 hrs	5 to 10 days 10 days
Acute maxillary sinusitis	300 mg q 12 hrs or 600 mg q 24 hrs	10 days 10 days
Pharyngitis/Tonsillitis	300 mg q 12 hrs or 600 mg q 24 hrs	5 to 10 days 10 days
Uncomplicated skin and skin structure infections	300 mg q 12 hrs	10 days

➤*Children (6 months through 12 years of age):* The recommended dosage and duration of treatment for infections in pediatric patients are described in the following chart; the total daily dose for all infections is 14 mg/kg, up to a maximum dose of 600 mg/day. Once-daily dosing for 10 days is as effective as twice-daily dosing. Once-daily dosing has not been studied in skin infections; therefore, administer oral suspension twice daily in this infection. Oral suspension may be administered without regard to meals.

Cefdinir Dosage in Pediatric Patients (Age 6 Months Through 12 years)

Type of infection	Dosage	Duration
Acute bacterial otitis media	7 mg/kg q 12 h or 14 mg/kg q 24 h	5 to 10 days 10 days
Acute maxillary sinusitis	7 mg/kg q 12 h or 14 mg/kg q 24 h	10 days 10 days
Pharyngitis/Tonsillitis	7 mg/kg q 12 h or 14 mg/kg q 24 h	5 to 10 days 10 days
Uncomplicated skin and skin structure infections	7 mg/kg q 12 h	10 days

Cefdinir for Oral Suspension Pediatric Dosage Chart

Weight			
kg	lb	125 mg per 5 mL	250 mg per 5 mL
9	20	2.5 mL (½ tsp) q 12 h or 5 mL (1 tsp) q 24 h	use 125 mg per 5 mL product
18	40	5 mL (1 tsp) q 12 h or 10 mL (2 tsp) q 24 h	2.5 mL q 12 h or 5 mL q 24 h
27	60	7.5 mL (1½ tsp) q 12 h or 15 mL (3 tsp) q 24 h	3.75 mL q 12 h or 7.5 mL q 24 h
36	80	10 mL (2 tsp) q 12 h or 20 mL (4 tsp) q 24 h	5 mL q 12 h or 10 mL q 24 h
≥ 43[a]	95	12 mL (2½ tsp) q 12 h or 24 mL (5 tsp) q 24 h	6 mL q 12 h or 12 mL q 24 h

[a] Pediatric patients who weigh ≥ 43 kg should receive the maximum daily dose of 600 mg.

➤*Renal function impairment:* For adult patients with creatinine clearance < 30 mL/min, the dose of cefdinir should be 300 mg given once daily.

For pediatric patients with a creatinine clearance of < 30 mL/min/1.73 m^2, the dose of cefdinir should be 7 mg/kg (≤ 300 mg) given once daily.

➤*Hemodialysis:* Hemodialysis removes cefdinir from the body. In patients maintained on chronic hemodialysis, the recommended initial dosage regimen is a 300 mg or 7 mg/kg dose every other day. At the conclusion of each hemodialysis session, 300 mg (or 7 mg/kg) should be given. Subsequent doses (300 mg or 7 mg/kg) are then administered every other day.

➤*Reconstitution of oral suspension:* For the 60 mL bottle, add 38 mL water; for the 100 mL bottle, add 63 mL water. Shake well before each use.

➤*Storage/Stability:*

Capsules and powder for oral suspension – Store at 25°C (77°F); excursions permitted to 15° to 30°C (59° to 86°F).

Reconstituted oral suspension – After mixing, the suspension can be stored at room temperature (25°C; 77°F). The suspension may be used for 10 days, after which any unused portion must be discarded.

CEFAZOLIN SODIUM

Rx	**Cefazolin Sodium** (Apothecon)	**Powder for Injection:**[1] 500 mg	In vials and piggyback vials.
Rx	**Cefazolin Sodium** (Apothecon)	**Powder for Injection:**[1] 1 g	In vials and piggyback vials.
Rx	**Cefazolin Sodium** (Apothecon)	**Powder for Injection:**[1] 5 g	In vials and piggyback vials.
		10 g	In pharmacy bulk packages.
		20 g	In pharmacy bulk packages.

[1] Contains 2.1 mEq sodium/g.

CEFAZOLIN — INJECTION

Indications

Cefazolin is indicated in the treatment of the following serious infections due to susceptible organisms:

➤*Respiratory tract infections:* Due to *Streptococcus pneumoniae*, *Klebsiella* species, *Haemophilus influenzae*, *Staphylococcus aureus* (penicillin-sensitive and penicillin-resistant) and group A beta-hemolytic streptococci.

Injectable benzathine penicillin is considered to be the drug of choice in treatment and prevention of streptococcal infections, including the prophylaxis of rheumatic fever.

Cefazolin is effective in the eradication of streptococci from the nasopharynx; however, data establishing the efficacy of cefazolin in the subsequent prevention of rheumatic fever are not available at present.

➤*Urinary tract infections:* Due to *Escherichia coli*, *Proteus mirabilis*, *Klebsiella* species and some strains of enterobacter and enterococci.

➤*Skin and skin structure infections:* Due to *Staphylococcus aureus* (penicillin-sensitive and penicillin-resistant), group A beta-hemolytic streptococci and other strains of streptococci.

➤*Biliary tract infections:* Due to *Escherichia coli*, various strains of streptococci, *Proteus mirabilis*, *Klebsiella* species and *Staphylococcus aureus*.

➤*Bone and joint infections:* Due to *Staphylococcus aureus*.

➤*Genital infections (ie, prostatitis, epididymitis):* Due to *Escherichia coli*, *Proteus mirabilis*, *Klebsiella* species and some strains of enterococci.

➤*Septicemia:* Due to *Streptococcus pneumoniae*, *Staphylococcus aureus* (penicillin-sensitive and penicillin-resistant), *Proteus mirabilis*, *Escherichia coli* and *Klebsiella* species.

➤*Endocarditis:* Due to *Staphylococcus aureus* (penicillin-sensitive and penicillin-resistant) and group A beta-hemolytic streptococci.

➤*Perioperative prophylaxis:* The prophylactic administration of cefazolin preoperatively, intraoperatively and postoperatively may reduce the incidence of certain postoperative infections in patients undergoing surgical procedures which are classified as contaminated or potentially contaminated (eg, vaginal hysterectomy, and cholecystectomy in high-risk patients such as those greater than 70 years of age, with acute cholecystitis, obstructive jaundice or common duct bile stones).

The perioperative use of cefazolin may also be effective in surgical patients in whom infection at the operative site would present a serious risk (eg, during open-heart surgery and prosthetic arthroplasty).

The prophylactic administration of cefazolin should usually be discontinued within a 24-hour period after the surgical procedure. In surgery where the occurrence of infection may be particularly devastating (eg, open-heart surgery and prosthetic arthroplasty), the prophylactic administration of cefazolin may be continued for 3 to 5 days following the completion of surgery.

Administration and Dosage

➤*Adults:*

Usual adult dosage		
Type of infection	Dose	Frequency
Moderate to severe infections	500 mg to 1 g	every 6 to 8 hours
Mild infections caused by susceptible gram and cocci	250 mg to 500 mg	every 8 hours
Acute, uncomplicated urinary tract infections	1 g	every 12 hours
Pneumococcal pneumonia	500 mg	every 12 hours
Severe, life-threatening infections (eg, endocarditis, septicemia)*	1 g to 1.5 g	every 6 hours

* In rare instances, doses of up to 12 g of cefazolin injection per day have been used.

➤*Perioperative prophylactic use:* To prevent postoperative infection in contaminated or potentially contaminated surgery, recommended doses are:

Preoperative – 1 g IV or IM administered ½ hour to 1 hour prior to the start of surgery.

Intraoperative (greater than or equal to 2 hours) – For lengthy operative procedures (eg, 2 hours or more), 500 mg to 1 g IV or IM during surgery (administration modified depending on the duration of the operative procedure).

Postoperative – 500 mg to 1 g IV or IM every 6 to 8 hours for 24 hours postoperatively.

It is important that the preoperative dose be given just (½ to 1 hour) prior to the start of surgery so that adequate antibiotic levels are present in the serum and tissues at the time of initial surgical incision; and cefazolin injection be administered, if necessary, at appropriate intervals during surgery to provide sufficient levels of the antibiotic at the anticipated moments of greatest exposure to infective organisms.

In surgery where the occurrence of infection may be particularly devastating (eg, open-heart surgery and prosthetic arthroplasty), the prophylactic administration of cefazolin injection may be continued for 3 to 5 days following the completion of surgery.

➤*Renal function impairment:* All reduced dosage recommendations apply after an initial loading dose appropriate to the severity of the infection.

Cefazolin Dosage in Renal Impairment				
		Dose		
Serum creatinine (mg/dl)	Ccr (ml/min)	Mild-to-moderate infection (mg)	Moderate-to-severe infection (mg)	Dosage interval (hrs)
≤ 1.5	≥ 55	250 to 500	500 to 1000	6-8
1.6-3	35-54	250 to 500	500 to 1000	≥ 8
3.1-4.5	11-34	125 to 250	250 to 500	12
≥ 4.6	≤ 10	125 to 250	250 to 500	18-24

➤*Patients undergoing peritoneal dialysis:* In patients undergoing peritoneal dialysis (2 L/hr), cefazolin produced mean serum levels of approximately 10 and 30 mcg/mL after 24 hours' instillation of a dialyzing solution containing 50 mg/L and 150 mg/L, respectively. Mean peak levels were 29 mcg/mL (range 13 to 44 mcg/mL) with 50 mg/L (3 patients), and 72 mcg/mL (range 26 to 142 mcg/mL) with 150 mg/L (6 patients). Intraperitoneal administration of cefazolin is usually well tolerated.

➤*Children:* In pediatric patients, a total daily dosage of 25 to 50 mg per kg (approximately 10 to 20 mg per pound) of body weight, divided into 3 or 4 equal doses, is effective for most mild to moderately severe infections. Total daily dosage may be increased to 100 mg per kg (45 mg per pound) of body weight for severe infections. Since safety for use in premature infants and in neonates has not been established, the use of cefazolin in these patients is not recommended.

Pediatric dosage guidelines					
Weight		25 mg/kg/day divided into 3 doses		25 mg/kg/day divided into 4 doses	
lbs	kg	Approximate single dose (mg) every 8 hours	Volume (mL) needed with dilution of 125 mg/mL	Approximate single dose (mg) every 6 hours	Volume (mL) needed with dilution of 125 mg/mL
10	4.5	40 mg	0.35 mL	30 mg	0.25 mL
20	9	75 mg	0.6 mL	55 mg	0.45 mL
30	13.6	115 mg	0.9 mL	85 mg	0.7 mL
40	18.1	150 mg	1.2 mL	115 mg	0.9 mL
50	22.7	190 mg	1.5 mL	140 mg	1.1 mL
Weight		50 mg/kg/day divided into 3 doses		50 mg/kg/day divided into 4 doses	
lbs	kg	Approximate single dose (mg) every 8 hours	Volume (mL) needed with dilution of 225 mg/mL	Approximate single dose (mg) every 6 hours	Volume (mL) needed with dilution of 225 mg/mL
10	4.5	75 mg	0.35 mL	55 mg	0.25 mL
20	9	150 mg	0.7 mL	110 mg	0.5 mL
30	13.6	225 mg	1 mL	170 mg	0.75 mL
40	18.1	300 mg	1.35 mL	225 mg	1 mL
50	22.7	375 mg	1.7 mL	285 mg	1.25 mL

Renal function impairment – In pediatric patients with mild to moderate renal impairment (creatinine clearance of 70 to 40 mL/min), 60% of the normal daily dose given in equally divided doses every 12 hours should be sufficient. In patients with moderate impairment (creatinine clearance of 40 to 20 mL/min), 25% of the normal daily dose given in equally divided doses every 12 hours should be adequate. Pediatric patients with severe renal impairment (creatinine clearance of 20 to 5 mL/min) may be given 10% of the normal daily dose every 24 hours. All dosage recommendations apply after an initial loading dose.

CEFAZOLIN — INJECTION

➤*Reconstitution:*

Preparation of parenteral solution – Parenteral drug products should be shaken well when reconstituted, and inspected visually for particulate matter prior to administration. If particulate matter is evident in reconstituted fluids, the drug solutions should be discarded. Reconstituted solutions may range in color from pale yellow to yellow without a change in potency.

When reconstituted or diluted according to the instructions below, cefazolin is stable for 24 hours at room temperature or for 10 days if stored under refrigeration (5°C or 41°F).

Single dose vials – For IM injection, IV direct (bolus) injection or IV infusion, reconstitute with Sterile Water for Injection according to the following table. Shake well.

Vial size	Amount of diluent	Approximate concentration	Approximate available volume
500 mg	2 mL	225 mg/mL	2.2 mL
1 g	2.5 mL	330 mg/mL	3 mL

Infusion bottles – Reconstitute with 50 to 100 mL of Sodium Chloride Injection or other IV solution listed under administration. When adding diluent to vial, allow air to escape by using a small vent needle or by pumping the syringe. Shake well. Administer with primary IV fluids, as a single dose.

➤*Administration:*

Intramuscular administration – Reconstitute vials with Sterile Water for Injection according to the dilution information above. Shake well until dissolved. Cefazolin should be injected into a large muscle mass. Pain on injection is infrequent with cefazolin.

Intravenous administration –

Direct (bolus) injection: Following reconstitution according to the above information, further dilute vials with approximately 5 mL Sterile Water for Injection. Inject the solution slowly over 3 to 5 minutes, directly or through tubing for patients receiving parenteral fluids (see list below).

Intermittent or continuous infusion: Dilute reconstituted cefazolin in 50 to 100 mL of one of the following solutions: Sodium Chloride Injection, 5% or 10% Dextrose Injection, 5% Dextrose in Lactated Ringer's Injection, 5% Dextrose and 0.9% Sodium Chloride Injection, 5% Dextrose and 0.45% Sodium Chloride Injection, 5% Dextrose and 0.2% Sodium Chloride Injection, Lactated Ringer's Injection, Invert Sugar 5% or 10% in Sterile Water for Injection, Ringer's Injection, 5% Sodium Bicarbonate Injection.

➤*Storage/Stability:* As with other cephalosporins, cefazolin tends to darken depending on storage conditions; within the stated recommendations, however, product potency is not adversely affected.

Prior to reconstitution, store at 25°C (77°F); excursions permitted to 15° to 30°C (59° to 86°F) and protect from light.

CEFOXITIN SODIUM

Rx	**Cefoxitin** (American Pharmaceutical Partners)	**Powder for Injection:** 1 g	In vials and infusion bottles.
Rx	**Mefoxin** (Merck)		In vials and infusion bottles.[1]
Rx	**Cefoxitin** (American Pharmaceutical Partners)	**Powder for Injection:** 2 g	In vials and infusion bottles.
Rx	**Mefoxin** (Merck)		In vials and infusion bottles.[1]
Rx	**Cefoxitin** (American Pharmaceutical Partners)	**Powder for Injection:** 10 g	In pharmacy bulk packages.
Rx	**Mefoxin** (Merck)		In bulk bottles.[1]
Rx	**Mefoxin** (Merck)	**Injection:** 1 g	Dextrose. Premixed, frozen. In 50 ml plastic containers.
		2 g	Dextrose. Premixed, frozen. In 50 ml plastic containers.

[1] Contains 2.3 mEq sodium/g.

CEFOXITIN SODIUM — INJECTION

For complete and comparative prescribing information, refer to the Cephalosporins group monograph.

Indications

➤*Lower respiratory tract infections:* Including pneumonia and lung abscess, caused by *S. pneumoniae*, other streptococci (excluding enterococci; eg, *E. faecalis* [formerly *Streptococcus faecalis*]), *S. aureus* (including penicillinase-producing strains), *E. coli*, *Klebsiella* species, *Haemophilus influenzae*, and *Bacteroides* species.

➤*Urinary tract infections:* Caused by *E. coli*, *Klebsiella* species, *P. mirabilis*, *Morganella morganii*, *Proteus vulgaris* and *Providencia* species (including *Providencia rettgeri*).

➤*Intra-abdominal infections:* Including peritonitis and intra-abdominal abscess, caused by *E. coli*, *Klebsiella* species, *Bacteroides* species (including *Bacteroides fragilis*), and *Clostridium* species.

➤*Gynecological infections:* Including endometritis, pelvic cellulitis, and pelvic inflammatory disease caused by *E. coli*, *Neisseria gonorrhoeae* (including penicillinase-producing strains), *Bacteroides* species including *B. fragilis*, *Clostridium* species, *P. niger*, *Peptostreptococcus* species, and *Streptococcus agalactiae*.

➤*Chlamydia trachomatis:* See Administration and Dosage for more information.

➤*Septicemia:* Caused by *S. pneumoniae*, *S. aureus* (including penicillinase-producing strains), *E. coli*, *Klebsiella* species, and *Bacteroides* species including *B. fragilis*.

➤*Bone and joint infections:* Caused by *S. aureus* (including penicillinase-producing strains).

➤*Skin and skin structure infections:* Caused by *S. aureus* (including penicillinase-producing strains), *Staphylococcus epidermidis*, *Streptococcus pyogenes* and other streptococci (excluding enterococci [eg, *E. faecalis*] [formerly *S. faecalis*]), *E. coli*, *P. mirabilis*, *Klebsiella* species, *Bacteroides* species including *B. fragilis*, *Clostridium* species, *P. niger*, and *Peptostreptococcus* species.

➤*Perioperative prophylaxis:* For the prophylaxis of infection in patients undergoing uncontaminated GI surgery, vaginal hysterectomy, abdominal hysterectomy, or cesarean section.

Administration and Dosage

➤*Approved by the FDA:* October 18, 1978.

➤*Dosage:*

Adults – 1 to 2 g every 6 to 8 hours. Dosage should be determined by susceptibility of the causative organisms, severity of infection, and the condition of the patient (see the following table).

Cefoxitin Dosage Guidelines for Adults		
Type of infection	Daily dosage	Frequency and route
Uncomplicated forms[a] of infection such as pneumonia, urinary tract infection, cutaneous infection	3 to 4 g	1 g every 6 to 8 hours IV
Moderately severe or severe infections	6 to 8 g	1 g every 4 hours or 2 g every 6 to 8 hours IV
Infections commonly requiring antibiotics in higher dosage (eg, gas gangrene)	12 g	2 g every 4 hours or 3 g every 6 hours IV

[a] Including patients in whom bacteremia is absent or unlikely.

C. trachomatis: If *C. trachomatis* is a suspected pathogen, appropriate antichlamydial coverage should be added, because cefoxitin has no activity against this organism.

Streptococcal infections: Antibiotic therapy for group A beta-hemolytic streptococcal infections should be maintained for at least 10 days to guard against the risk of rheumatic fever or glomerulonephritis.

In staphylococcal and other infections involving a collection of pus, surgical drainage should be carried out where indicated.

Prophylactic use, surgery: Effective prophylactic use depends on the time of administration. Cefoxitin usually should be given 30 minutes to 1 hour before the operation, which is sufficient time to achieve effective levels in the wound during the procedure. Prophylactic administration should usually be stopped within 24 hours since continuing administration of any antibiotic increases the possibility of adverse reactions but, in the majority of surgical procedures, does not reduce the incidence of subsequent infection.

For prophylactic use in uncontaminated GI surgery, vaginal hysterectomy, or abdominal hysterectomy, the following doses are recommended in adults:

2 g administered IV just prior to surgery (approximately 30 minutes to 1 hour before the initial incision) followed by 2 g every 6 hours after the first dose for no more than 24 hours.

Prophylactic use, cesarean section: For patients undergoing cesarean section, either a single 2 g dose administered IV as soon as the umbilical cord is clamped or a 3-dose regimen consisting of 2 g given IV as soon as the umbilical cord is clamped followed by 2 g 4 and 8 hours after the initial dose is recommended.

Renal function impairment: Cefoxitin may be used in patients with reduced renal function with the following dosage adjustments:

In adults with renal insufficiency, an initial loading dose of 1 to 2 g may be given. After a loading dose, the recommendations for maintenance dosage (see information following) may be used as a guide.

CEFOXITIN SODIUM — INJECTION

• *Hemodialysis* – In patients undergoing hemodialysis, the loading dose of 1 to 2 g should be given after each hemodialysis, and the maintenance dose should be given as indicated in the following table.

Maintenance Cefoxitin Dosage in Adults with Renal Impairment			
Renal function	Creatinine clearance (mL/min)	Dose (g)	Frequency
Mild impairment	30 to 50	1 to 2	every 8 to 12 hours
Moderate impairment	10 to 29	1 to 2	every 12 to 24 hours
Severe impairment	5 to 9	0.5 to 1	every 12 to 24 hours
Essentially no function	< 5	0.5 to 1	every 24 to 48 hours

Infants and children 3 months of age or older – The recommended dosage in pediatric patients 3 months of age or older is 80 to 160 mg/kg/day divided into 4 to 6 equal doses. The higher dosages should be used for more severe or serious infections. The total daily dose should not exceed 12 g.

Prophylactic use, surgery (3 months of age or older) – 30 to 40 mg/kg doses may be given at the times designated for adults.

Renal function impairment – In pediatric patients with renal insufficiency, the dosage and frequency of dosage should be modified consistent with the recommendations for adults.

➤*Administration:*

Preparation for administration – The preceding table is provided for convenience in constituting cefoxitin for IV administration.

Vials: 1 g should be constituted with at least 10 mL, and 2 g with 10 or 20 mL, of sterile water for injection, bacteriostatic water for injection, 0.9% sodium chloride injection, or 5% dextrose injection.

Bulk packages: The 10 g bulk packages should be constituted with 43 or 93 mL of sterile water for injection, bacteriostatic water for injection, 0.9% sodium chloride injection, or 5% dextrose injection. Caution: The 10 g bulk stock solution is not for direct infusion.

These primary solutions may be further diluted in 50 to 1,000 mL of the following diluents: 0.9% sodium chloride injection, 5% or 10% dextrose injection, 5% dextrose and 0.9% sodium chloride injection, 5% dextrose injection with 0.2% or 0.45% saline solution, Ringer's lactate injection, 5% dextrose in Ringer's lactate injection, 5% sodium bicarbonate injection, M/6 sodium lactate solution, mannitol 5% and 10%.

Infusion bottles: 1 or 2 g of cefoxitin for infusion may be constituted with 50 or 100 mL of 0.9% sodium chloride injection, or 5% or 10% dextrose injection.

ADD-Vantage vials: Cefoxitin in *ADD-Vantage* vials should be constituted with *ADD-Vantage* diluent containers containing 50 mL or 100 mL of either 0.9% sodium chloride injection or 5% dextrose injection.

Cefoxitin in *ADD-Vantage* vials is for IV use only.

Galaxy containers (PL 2040 plastic) – Thaw frozen container at room temperature, 25°C (77°F), or under refrigeration, 2° to 8°C (36° to 46°F). Do not force thaw by immersion in water baths or by microwave irradiation.

After thawing, check for minute leaks by squeezing container firmly. If leaks are detected, discard solution because sterility may be impaired.

The container should be visually inspected for particulate matter and discoloration prior to administration. Components of the solution may precipitate in the frozen state and will dissolve upon reaching room temperature with little or no agitation. Agitate after solution has reached room temperature.

Do not use if the solution is cloudy or if a precipitate has formed. If any seals or outlet ports are not intact, the container should be discarded. Solutions of cefoxitin tend to darken depending on storage conditions; product potency, however, is not adversely affected.

Additives should not be introduced into this solution.

Caution: Do not use plastic containers in series connections. Such use would result in air embolism due to residual air being drawn from the primary container before administration of the fluid from the secondary container is complete.

➤*Administration of solution:* Cefoxitin may be administered IV after constitution.

IV administration – The IV route is preferable for patients with bacteremia, bacterial septicemia, or other severe or life-threatening infections, or for patients who may be poor risks because of lowered resistance resulting from such debilitating conditions as malnutrition, trauma, surgery, diabetes, heart failure, or malignancy, particularly if shock is present or impending.

Intermittent IV administration: A solution containing 1 or 2 g in 10 mL of sterile water for injection can be injected over a period of 3 to 5 minutes. Using an infusion system, it may also be given over a longer period of time through the tubing system by which the patient may be receiving other IV solutions. However, during infusion of the solution containing cefoxitin, it is advisable to temporarily discontinue administration of any other solutions at the same site.

Continuous IV infusion: For higher doses, solution of cefoxitin may be added to an IV bottle containing 5% dextrose injection, 0.9% sodium chloride injection, or 5% dextrose and 0.9% sodium chloride injection. *Butterfly* or scalp vein-type needles are preferred for this type of infusion.

Premixed IV solution – This premixed solution is for IV use only. Cefoxitin premixed IV solution in *Galaxy* containers (PL 2040 plastic) is to be administered either as a continuous or intermittent infusion using sterile equipment. Scalp vein-type needles are preferred for this type of infusion. It is recommended that the IV administration apparatus be replaced at least once every 48 hours.

Cefoxitin premixed IV solution may be administered through the tubing system by which the patient may be receiving other IV solutions. However, during infusion of the solution containing cefoxitin premixed IV solution, it is advisable to temporarily discontinue administration of any other solutions at the same site.

➤*Admixture incompatibility:* Solutions of cefoxitin, like those of most beta-lactam antibiotics, should not be added to aminoglycoside solutions (eg, gentamicin sulfate, tobramycin sulfate, amikacin sulfate) because of potential interaction. However, cefoxitin and aminoglycosides may be administered separately to the same patient.

➤*Storage/Stability:*

Vials and bulk packages – Cefoxitin powder for injection, as supplied in vials or the bulk package and constituted to 1 g per 10 mL with sterile water for injection, bacteriostatic water for injection, 0.9% sodium chloride injection, or 5% dextrose injection, maintains satisfactory potency for 6 hours at room temperature or for 1 week under refrigeration (less than 5°C; 43°F).

Infusion bottles – Cefoxitin, as supplied in infusion bottles and constituted with 50 to 100 mL of 0.9% sodium chloride injection, or 5% or 10% dextrose injection, maintains satisfactory potency for 24 hours at room temperature or for 1 week under refrigeration (less than 5°C; 43°F).

ADD-Vantage vials – Cefoxitin is supplied in single-dose *ADD-Vantage* vials and should be prepared as directed in the accompanying instructions for use of cefoxitin in *ADD-Vantage* vials using *ADD-Vantage* diluent containers containing 50 mL or 100 mL of either 0.9% sodium chloride injection or 5% dextrose injection. When prepared with either of these diluents, cefoxitin maintains satisfactory potency for 24 hours at room temperature.

After the time periods mentioned previously, any unused solutions should be discarded. Cefoxitin in the dry state should be stored between 2° to 25°C (36° to 77°F). Avoid exposure to temperatures greater than 50°C (122°F). The dry material as well as solutions tend to darken, depending on storage conditions; product potency, however, is not adversely affected.

Cefoxitin premixed IV solution – Store at or below −20°C (−4°F).

Cefoxitin, supplied as frozen, premixed, iso-osmotic solution in *Galaxy* containers (PL 2040 plastic), maintains satisfactory potency after thawing for 24 hours at a room temperature of 25°C (77°F) or 21 days under refrigeration, 2° to 8°C (36° to 46°F). After these periods, any unused solutions should be discarded. Do not refreeze.

CEFUROXIME

Rx	**Cefuroxime Axetil** (Ranbaxy)	**Tablets:** (as axetil) 125 mg	(RX 750). Blue, capsule shape. In 60s and 100s.
Rx	**Ceftin** (GlaxoWellcome)		(Glaxo 395). White. Capsule shape. Film coated. In 20s and UD 100s.
Rx	**Cefuroxime Axetil** (Ranbaxy)	**Tablets:** (as axetil) 250 mg	(RX 751). Blue, capsule shape. In 20s, 60s, and 100s.
Rx	**Ceftin** (GlaxoWellcome)		(Glaxo 387). Light blue. Capsule shape. Film coated. In 10s, 20s, 60s and UD 100s.
Rx	**Cefuroxime Axetil** (Ranbaxy)	**Tablets:** (as axetil) 500 mg	(RX 752). Blue, capsule shape. In 20s, 60s, and 100s.
Rx	**Ceftin** (GlaxoWellcome)		(Glaxo 394). Dark blue. Capsule shape. Film coated. In 20s, 60s and UD 50s.
Rx	**Ceftin** (GlaxoWellcome)	**Suspension:** 125 mg/5 ml (as axetil) when reconstituted	Sucrose. Tutti-frutti flavor. In 50 and 100 ml bottles.
		250 mg/5 ml (as axetil) when reconstituted	Sucrose. Tutti-frutti flavor. In 50 and 100 ml bottles.
Rx	**Cefuroxime Sodium** (Various)	**Powder for Injection:**[1] 750 mg (as sodium).	In 10 ml vials and 100 ml piggyback vials.
Rx	**Zinacef** (GlaxoWellcome)		In vials, infusion pack and *ADD-Vantage* vials.
Rx	**Cefuroxime Sodium** (Various)	**Powder for Injection:**[1] 1.5 g (as sodium)	In 20 ml vials and 100 ml piggyback vials.
Rx	**Zinacef** (GlaxoWellcome)		In vials, infusion packs and *ADD-Vantage* vials.

CEFUROXIME

Rx	**Cefuroxime Sodium** (Various)	**Powder for Injection:**[1] 7.5 g (as sodium)	In pharmacy bulk package.
Rx	**Zinacef** (GlaxoWellcome)		In pharmacy bulk package.
Rx	**Zinacef** (GlaxoWellcome)	**Injection:**[1] 750 mg (as sodium)	Premixed, frozen. In 50 ml.
		1.5 g (as sodium)	Premixed, frozen. In 50 ml.

[1] Contains 2.4 mEq sodium/g.

CEFUROXIME AXETIL — ORAL

For complete and comparative prescribing information, refer to the Cephalosporins group monograph.

Indications

➤*Tablets:*

Pharyngitis/tonsillitis – Caused by *Streptococcus pyogenes*. The usual drug of choice in the treatment and prevention of streptococcal infections, including the prophylaxis of rheumatic fever, is penicillin given by the IM route. Cefuroxime axetil tablets are generally effective in the eradication of streptococci from the nasopharynx; however, substantial data establishing the efficacy of cefuroxime in the subsequent prevention of rheumatic fever are not available. Please also note that in all clinical trials, all isolates had to be sensitive to both penicillin and cefuroxime. There are no data from adequate and well-controlled trials to demonstrate the effectiveness of cefuroxime in the treatment of penicillin-resistant strains of *Streptococcus pyogenes*.

Acute bacterial otitis media – Caused by *Streptococcus pneumoniae*, *Haemophilus influenzae* (including beta-lactamase-producing strains), *Moraxella catarrhalis* (including beta-lactamase-producing strains), or *Streptococcus pyogenes*.

Acute bacterial maxillary sinusitis – Caused by *Streptococcus pneumoniae* or *Haemophilus influenzae* (non-beta-lactamase-producing strains only). In view of the insufficient numbers of isolates of beta-lactamase-producing strains of *Haemophilus influenzae* and *Moraxella catarrhalis* that were obtained from clinical trials with cefuroxime axetil tablets for patients with acute bacterial maxillary sinusitis, it was not possible to adequately evaluate the effectiveness of cefuroxime axetil tablets for sinus infections known, suspected, or considered potentially to be caused by beta-lactamase-producing *Haemophilus influenzae* or *Moraxella catarrhalis*.

Acute bacterial exacerbations of chronic bronchitis and secondary bacterial infections of acute bronchitis – Caused by *Streptococcus pneumoniae*, *Haemophilus influenzae* (beta-lactamase negative strains), or *Haemophilus parainfluenzae* (beta-lactamase negative strains).

Uncomplicated skin and skin-structure infections – Caused by *Staphylococcus aureus* (including beta-lactamase-producing strains) or *Streptococcus pyogenes*.

Uncomplicated urinary tract infections – Caused by *Escherichia coli* or *Klebsiella pneumoniae*.

Uncomplicated gonorrhea, urethral and endocervical – Caused by penicillinase-producing and non-penicillinase-producing strains of *Neisseria gonorrhoeae* and uncomplicated gonorrhea, rectal, in females, caused by non-penicillinase-producing strains of *Neisseria gonorrhoeae*.

Early Lyme disease (erythema migrans) – Caused by *Borrelia burgdorferi*.

➤*Powder for oral suspension:* For the treatment of pediatric patients 3 months to 12 years of age with mild-to-moderate infections caused by susceptible strains of the designated microorganisms in the conditions listed below. The safety and efficacy of cefuroxime axetil for oral suspension in the treatment of infections other than those specifically listed below have not been established either by adequate and well-controlled trials or by pharmacokinetic data with which to determine an effective and safe dosing regimen.

Pharyngitis/tonsillitis – Caused by *Streptococcus pyogenes*. The usual drug of choice in the treatment and prevention of streptococcal infections, including the prophylaxis of rheumatic fever, is penicillin given by the IM route. Cefuroxime axetil for oral suspension is generally effective in the eradication of streptococci from the nasopharynx; however, substantial data establishing the efficacy of cefuroxime in the subsequent prevention of rheumatic fever are not available. Please also note that in all clinical trials, all isolates had to be sensitive to both penicillin and cefuroxime. There are no data from adequate and well-controlled trials to demonstrate the effectiveness of cefuroxime in the treatment of penicillin-resistant strains of *Streptococcus pyogenes*.

Acute bacterial otitis media – Caused by *Streptococcus pneumoniae*, *Haemophilus influenzae* (including beta-lactamase-producing strains), *Moraxella catarrhalis* (including beta-lactamase-producing strains), or *Streptococcus pyogenes*.

Impetigo – Caused by *Staphylococcus aureus* (including beta-lactamase-producing strains) or *Streptococcus pyogenes*.

Administration and Dosage

➤*Approved by the FDA:* December 28, 1987.

➤*Note:* Cefuroxime axetil tablets and powder for oral suspension are not bioequivalent and are not substitutable on a mg/mg basis. Cefuroxime tablets may be administered without regard to meals, and cefuroxime powder for oral suspension must be administered with food.

➤*Tablets:*

Dosage for Cefuroxime Axetil Tablets

Population/infection	Dosage	Duration (days)
Adolescents and adults (13 years and older)		
Pharyngitis/tonsillitis	250 mg twice daily	10
Acute bacterial maxillary sinusitis	250 mg twice daily	10
Acute bacterial exacerbations of chronic bronchitis	250 or 500 mg twice daily	10*
Secondary bacterial infections of acute bronchitis	250 or 500 mg twice daily	5 to 10
Uncomplicated skin and skin-structure infections	250 or 500 mg twice daily	10
Uncomplicated urinary tract infections	250 mg twice daily	7 to 10
Uncomplicated gonorrhea	1000 mg once	single dose
Early lyme disease	500 mg twice daily	20
Pediatric patients (who can swallow tablets whole)		
Acute otitis media	250 mg twice daily	10
Acute bacterial maxillary sinusitis	250 mg twice daily	10

* The safety and effectiveness of cefuroxime administered for less than 10 days in patients with acute exacerbations of chronic bronchitis have not been established.

➤*Oral suspension:* Cefuroxime axetil for oral suspension must be taken with food and may be administered to pediatric patients ranging in age from 3 months to 12 years of age, according to the following dosages.

Shake well each time before using.

Dosage for Cefuroxime Axetil Suspension

Population/infection	Dosage	Daily maximum dose	Duration (days)
Pediatric patients (3 months to 12 years)			
Pharyngitis/tonsillitis	20 mg/kg/day divided twice daily	500 mg	10
Acute otitis media	30 mg/kg/day divided twice daily	1000 mg	10
Acute bacterial maxillary sinusitis	30 mg/kg/day divided twice daily	1000 mg	10
Impetigo	30 mg/kg/day divided twice daily	1000 mg	10

Renal function impairment – The safety and efficacy of cefuroxime axetil in patients with renal failure have not been established. Since cefuroxime is renally eliminated, its half-life will be prolonged in patients with renal failure.

➤*Storage/Stability:*

Tablets – Store the tablets between 15° and 30°C (59° and 86°F). Replace cap securely after each opening. Protect unit-dose packs from excessive moisture.

Oral suspension – Before reconstitution, store dry powder between 2° and 30°C (36° and 86°F). After reconstitution, store suspension between 2° and 25°C (36° and 77°F), in a refrigerator or at room temperature. Discard after 10 days.

CEFUROXIME SODIUM — INJECTION

For complete and comparative prescribing information, refer to the Cephalosporins group monograph.

Indications

➤*Lower respiratory tract infections:* Including pneumonia, caused by *Streptococcus pneumoniae, Haemophilus influenzae* (including ampicillin-resistant strains), *Klebsiella* sp., *Staphylococcus aureus* (penicillinase- and non-penicillinase-producing strains), *Streptococcus pyogenes*, and *Escherichia coli*.

➤*Urinary tract infections:* Caused by *E. coli* and *Klebsiella* sp.

➤*Skin and skin structure infections:* Caused by *S. aureus* (penicillinase- and non-penicillinase-producing strains), *S. pyogenes, E. coli, Klebsiella* sp., and *Enterobacter* sp.

➤*Septicemia:* Caused by *S. aureus* (penicillinase and non penicillinase producing strains), *S. pneumoniae, E. coli, H. influenzae* (including ampicillin-resistant strains), and *Klebsiella* sp.

➤*Meningitis:* Caused by *S. pneumoniae, H. influenzae* (including ampicillin-resistant strains), *Neisseria meningitidis*, and *S. aureus* (penicillinase- and non-penicillinase-producing strains).

➤*Gonorrhea:* Uncomplicated and disseminated gonococcal infections due to *Neisseria gonorrhoeae* (penicillinase- and non-penicillinase-producing strains) in both men and women.

➤*Bone and joint infections:* Caused by *S. aureus* (penicillinase- and non-penicillinase-producing strains).

➤*Mixed infections:* Clinical microbiological studies in skin and skin-structure infections frequently reveal the growth of susceptible strains of both aerobic and anaerobic organisms. Cefuroxime sodium has been used successfully in these mixed infections in which several organisms have been isolated.

In certain cases of confirmed or suspected gram-positive or gram-negative sepsis or in patients with other serious infections in which the causative organism has not been identified, cefuroxime sodium injection may be used concomitantly with an aminoglycoside. The recommended doses of both antibiotics may be given, depending on the severity of the infection and the patient's condition.

➤*Preoperative prohylaxis:* The preoperative prophylactic administration of cefuroxime sodium may prevent the growth of susceptible disease-causing bacteria and thereby may reduce the incidence of certain postoperative infections in patients undergoing surgical procedures (eg, vaginal hysterectomy) that are classified as clean-contaminated or potentially contaminated procedures. Effective prophylactic use of antibiotics in surgery depends on the time of administration. Cefuroxime sodium should usually be given one-half to 1 hour before the operation to allow sufficient time to achieve effective antibiotic concentrations in the wound tissues during the procedure. Repeat the dose intraoperatively if the surgical procedure is lengthy.

Prophylactic administration is usually not required after the surgical procedure ends and should be stopped within 24 hours. In the majority of surgical procedures, continuing prophylactic administration of any antibiotic does not reduce the incidence of subsequent infections but will increase the possibility of adverse reactions and the development of bacterial resistance.

The perioperative use of cefuroxime sodium has also been effective during open heart surgery for surgical patients in whom infections at the operative site would present a serious risk. For these patients it is recommended that therapy with cefuroxime sodium be continued for at least 48 hours after the surgical procedure ends. If an infection is present, obtain specimens for culture for the identification of the causative organism, and institute appropriate antimicrobial therapy.

Administration and Dosage

➤*Approved by the FDA:* October 19, 1983.

➤*Adults:* 750 mg to 1.5 g every 8 hours, usually for 5 to 10 days. In uncomplicated urinary tract infections, skin and skin structure infections, disseminated gonococcal infections, and uncomplicated pneumonia, a 750 mg dose every 8 hours is recommended. In severe or complicated infections, a 1.5 g dose every 8 hours is recommended.

In bone and joint infections, a 1.5 g dose every 8 hours is recommended. In clinical trials, surgical intervention was performed when indicated as an adjunct to therapy with cefuroxime sodium. A course of oral antibiotics was administered when appropriate following the completion of parenteral administration of cefuroxime sodium.

In life-threatening infections or infections due to less susceptible organisms, 1.5 g every 6 hours may be required. In bacterial meningitis, the dosage should not exceed 3 g every 8 hours. The recommended dosage for uncomplicated gonococcal infection is 1.5 g given intramuscularly (IM) as a single dose at 2 different sites together with 1 g of oral probenecid.

➤*Preoperative prophylaxis:* For preventive use for clean-contaminated or potentially contaminated surgical procedures, a 1.5 g dose administered intravenously (IV) just before surgery (approximately one-half to 1 hour before the initial incision) is recommended. Thereafter, give 750 mg IV or IM every 8 hours when the procedure is prolonged.

For preventive use during open heart surgery, a 1.5 g dose administered IV at the induction of anesthesia and every 12 hours thereafter for a total of 6 g is recommended.

➤*Renal function impairment:* A reduced dosage must be employed when renal function is impaired. Dosage should be determined by the degree of renal impairment and the susceptibility of the causative organism (see the following table).

Dosage of Cefuroxime Injection in Adults with Renal Function Impairment		
Creatinine clearance (mL/min)	Dose	Frequency
> 20	750 mg to 1.5 g	every 8 hours
10 to 20	750 mg	every 12 hours
< 10	750 mg	every 24 hours[a]

[a] Because cefuroxime is dialyzable, give patients on hemodialysis a further dose at the end of the dialysis.

➤*Duration of treatment:* As with antibiotic therapy in general, administration of cefuroxime sodium should be continued for a minimum of 48 to 72 hours after the patient becomes asymptomatic or after evidence of bacterial eradication has been obtained; a minimum of 10 days of treatment is recommended in infections caused by *S. pyogenes* in order to guard against the risk of rheumatic fever or glomerulonephritis; frequent bacteriologic and clinical appraisal is necessary during therapy of chronic urinary tract infection and may be required for several months after therapy has been completed; persistent infections may require treatment for several weeks; and doses smaller than those indicated above should not be used. In staphylococcal and other infections involving a collection of pus, carry out surgical drainage where indicated.

➤*Children older than 3 months of age:* Administration of 50 to 100 mg/kg/day in equally divided doses every 6 to 8 hours has been successful for most infections susceptible to cefuroxime sodium. The higher dosage of 100 mg/kg/day (not to exceed the maximum adult dosage) should be used for the more severe or serious infections.

In bone and joint infections, 150 mg/kg/day (not to exceed the maximum adult dosage) is recommended in equally divided doses every 8 hours. In clinical trials, a course of oral antibiotics was administered to pediatric patients following the completion of parenteral administration of cefuroxime sodium.

In cases of bacterial meningitis, a larger dosage of cefuroxime sodium is recommended, 200 to 240 mg/kg/day IV in divided doses every 6 to 8 hours.

Renal function impairment – In pediatric patients with renal impairment, the frequency of dosing should be modified consistent with the recommendations for adults.

➤*Preparation of solution and suspension:*

For IM use – Constitute each 750 mg vial of cefuroxime sodium injection with 3 mL of sterile water for injection. Shake gently to disperse and withdraw completely the resulting suspension for injection.

For IV use – Constitute each 750 mg vial with 8 mL of sterile water for injection. Withdraw completely the resulting solution for injection.

Constitute each 1.5 g vial with 16 mL of sterile water for injection. Withdraw completely the solution for injection.

Constitute the 7.5 g pharmacy bulk vial with 77 mL of sterile water for injection; each 8 mL of the resulting solution contains 750 mg of cefuroxime sodium.

Constitute each 750 mg and 1.5 g infusion pack with 100 mL of sterile water for injection, 5% dextrose injection, 0.9% sodium chloride injection, ⅙ M sodium lactate injection, Ringer injection, Ringer lactate injection, 5% dextrose and 0.9% sodium chloride injection, 5% dextrose injection, 5% dextrose and 0.45% sodium chloride injection, 5% dextrose and 0.225% sodium chloride injection, 10% dextrose injection, and 10% invert sugar in water for injection.

➤*Administration:* After constitution, cefuroxime sodium may be given IV or by deep IM injection into a large muscle mass (eg, gluteus, lateral part of the thigh). Before injecting IM, aspiration is necessary to avoid inadvertent injection into a blood vessel.

➤*IV administration:* The IV route may be preferable for patients with bacterial septicemia or other severe or life-threatening infections or for patients who may be poor risks because of lowered resistance, particularly if shock is present or impending.

Direct intermittent IV administration – For direct intermittent IV administration, slowly inject the solution into a vein over a period of 3 to 5 minutes or give it through the tubing system by which the patient is also receiving other IV solutions.

Intermittent IV infusion – For intermittent IV infusion with a Y-type administration set, dosing can be accomplished through the tubing system by which the patient may be receiving other IV solutions. However, during infusion of the solution containing cefuroxime sodium injection, it is advisable to temporarily discontinue administration of any other solutions at the same site.

Continuous IV infusion – For continuous IV infusion, a solution of cefuroxime sodium injection may be added to an IV infusion pack containing 1 of the following fluids: 0.9% sodium chloride injection, 5% dextrose injection, 10% dextrose injection, 5% dextrose and 0.9% sodium chloride injection, 5% dextrose and 0.45% sodium chloride injection, or ⅙ M sodium lactate injection.

➤*Admixture incompatibility:* Solutions of cefuroxime sodium injection, like those of most beta-lactam antibiotics, should not be added to solutions of aminoglycoside antibiotics because of potential interaction.

However, if concurrent therapy with cefuroxime sodium injection and an aminoglycoside is indicated, each of these antibiotics can be administered separately to the same patient.

➤*Storage/Stability:* Cefuroxime sodium in the dry state should be stored between 15° and 30°C (59° and 86°F) and protected from light.

CEFUROXIME SODIUM — INJECTION

IM – When constituted as directed with sterile water for injection, suspensions of cefuroxime sodium for IM injection maintain satisfactory potency for 24 hours at room temperature and for 48 hours under refrigeration (5°C; 41°F).

After the periods mentioned above any unused suspensions should be discarded.

IV – When the 750 mg, 1.5 g, and 7.5 g pharmacy bulk vials are constituted as directed with sterile water for injection, the solutions of cefuroxime sodium for IV administration maintain satisfactory potency for 24 hours at room temperature and for 48 hours (750 mg and 1.5 g vials) or for 7 days (7.5 mg pharmacy bulk vial) under refrigeration (5°C; 44°F). More dilute solutions, such as 750 mg or 1.5 g plus 100 mL of sterile water for injection, 5% dextrose injection, or 0.9% sodium chloride injection, also maintain satisfactory potency for 24 hours at room temperature and for 7 days under refrigeration.

These solutions may be further diluted to concentrations of between 1 and 30 mg/mL in the following solutions and will lose not more than 10% activity for 24 hours at room temperature or for at least 7 days under refrigeration: 0.9% sodium chloride injection, ⅙ M sodium lactate injection, Ringer's injection, Ringer lactate injection, 5% dextrose and 0.9% sodium chloride injection, 5% dextrose injection, 5% dextrose and 0.45% sodium chloride injection, 5% dextrose and 0.225% sodium chloride injection, 10% dextrose injection, and 10% invert sugar in water for injection.

Discard unused solutions after the time periods previously mentioned.

Cefuroxime sodium injection has also been found compatible for 24 hours at room temperature when admixed in IV infusion with heparin (10 and 50 units/mL) in 0.9% sodium chloride injection and potassium chloride (10 and 40 mEqL) in 0.9% sodium chloride injection. Sodium bicarbonate injection is not recommended for the dilution of cefuroxime sodium.

The 750 mg and 1.5 g cefuroxime sodium *ADD-Vantage* vials, when diluted in 50 or 100 mL of 5% dextrose injection, 0.9% sodium chloride injection, or 0.45% sodium chloride injection, may be stored for up to 24 hours at room temperature or for 7 days under refrigeration.

Frozen stability – Constitute the 750 mg, 1.5 g, or 7.5 g vial as directed for IV administration in the Preparation of Solution and Suspension table. Immediately withdraw the total contents of the 750 mg or 1.5 g vial or 8 or 16 mL from the 7.5 g bulk vial and add to a Baxter *Viaflex Mini-Bag* containing 50 or 100 mL of 0.9% sodium chloride injection or 5% dextrose injection and freeze. Frozen solutions are stable for 6 months when stored at −20°C (4°F). Frozen solutions should be thawed at room temperature and not refrozen. Do not force thaw by immersion in water baths or by microwave irradiation. Thawed solutions may be stored for up to 24 hours at room temperature or for 7 days in a refrigerator.

Cefuroxime sodium powder as well as solutions and suspensions tend to darken, depending on storage conditions, without adversely affecting product potency.

Directions for dispensing (pharmacy bulk package [not for direct infusion]) – The pharmacy bulk package is for use in a pharmacy admixture service only under a laminar flow hood. Entry into the vial must be made with a sterile transfer set or other sterile dispensing device, and the contents dispensed in aliquots using aseptic technique. The use of syringe and needle is not recommended as it may cause leakage. After initial withdrawal use entire contents of vial promptly. Any unused portion must be discarded within 24 hours.

CEFTRIAXONE SODIUM

Rx	**Ceftriaxone Sodium** (Various, eg, Apotex, Baxter, Hospira, Lupin, Sandoz)	**Powder for injection** 250 mg (as base)	In vials.[a]
Rx	**Rocephin** (Roche)		In vials.
Rx	**Ceftriaxone Sodium** (Various, eg, Apotex, Baxter, Hospira, Lupin, Sandoz)	**Powder for injection**: 500 mg (as base)	In vials.[a]
Rx	**Rocephin** (Roche)		In vials.
Rx	**Ceftriaxone Sodium** (Various, eg, Apotex, Baxter, Hospira, Lupin, Sandoz)	**Powder for injection**: 1 g (as base)	In vials.[a]
Rx	**Rocephin** (Roche)		In vials, piggyback vials and *ADD-Vantage* vials.
Rx	**Ceftriaxone Sodium** (Various, eg, Apotex, Baxter, Hospira, Lupin, Sandoz)	**Powder for injection**: 2 g (as base)	In vials.[a]
Rx	**Rocephin** (Roche)		In vials, piggyback vials and *ADD-Vantage* vials.
Rx	**Ceftriaxone** (Various, eg, Apotex, Sandoz)	**Powder for injection**: 10 g (as base)	In bulk containers.[a]
Rx	**Rocephin** (Roche)		In bulk containers.[a]
Rx	**Ceftriaxone Sodium** (Various, eg, Baxter, B. Braun McGaw, Hospira)	**Injection**: 1 g (as base)	May contain dextrose. In 50 mL *ADD-Vantage* vials.[a]
Rx	**Rocephin** (Roche)		Dextrose. Premixed, frozen. In 50 mL plastic containers.
Rx	**Ceftriaxone Sodium** (Various, eg, Baxter, B. Braun McGaw, Hospira)	**Injection**: 2 g (as base)	May contain dextrose. In 50 mL *ADD-Vantage* vials.[a]
Rx	**Rocephin** (Roche)		Dextrose. Premixed, frozen. In 50 mL plastic containers.

[a] Contains 3.6 mEq sodium/g.

CEFTRIAXONE SODIUM — INJECTION

For complete and comparative prescribing information, refer to the Cephalosporins group monograph.

Indications

➤*Lower respiratory tract infections:* Caused by *Streptococcus pneumoniae, Staphylococcus aureus, Haemophilus influenzae, Haemophilus parainfluenzae, Klebsiella pneumoniae, Escherichia coli, Enterobacter aerogenes, Proteus mirabilis* or *Serratia marcescens.*

➤*Acute bacterial otitis media:* Caused by *Streptococcus pneumoniae, Haemophilus influenzae* (including beta-lactamase-producing strains) or *Moraxella catarrhalis* (including beta-lactamase-producing strains). In 1 study, lower clinical cure rates were observed with a single dose of ceftriaxone sodium compared to 10 days of oral therapy. In a second study, comparable cure rates were observed between single dose ceftriaxone sodium and the comparator. The potentially lower clinical cure rate of ceftriaxone sodium should be balanced against the potential advantages of parenteral therapy.

➤*Skin and skin structure infections:* Caused by *Staphylococcus aureus, Staphylococcus epidermidis, Streptococcus pyogenes,* viridans group streptococci, *Escherichia coli, Enterobacter cloacae, Klebsiella oxytoca, Klebsiella pneumoniae, Proteus mirabilis, Morganella morganii* (efficacy for this organism in this organ system was studied in less than 10 infections), *Pseudomonas aeruginosa, Serratia marcescens, Acinetobacter calcoaceticus, Bacteroides fragilis* (efficacy for this organism in this organ system was studied in less than 10 infections) or *Peptostreptococcus* species.

➤*Urinary tract infections (complicated and uncomplicated):* Caused by *Escherichia coli, Proteus mirabilis, Proteus vulgaris, Morganella morganii* or *Klebsiella pneumoniae.*

➤*Uncomplicated gonorrhea (cervical/urethral and rectal):* Caused by *Neisseria gonorrhoeae,* including both penicillinase- and nonpenicillinase-producing strains, and pharyngeal gonorrhea caused by nonpenicillinase-producing strains of *Neisseria gonorrhoeae.*

➤*Pelvic inflammatory disease (PID):* Caused by *Neisseria gonorrhoeae.* Ceftriaxone sodium, like other cephalosporins, has no activity against *Chlamydia trachomatis.* Therefore, when cephalosporins are used in the treatment of patients with pelvic inflammatory disease and *C. trachomatis* is 1 of the suspected pathogens, appropriate antichlamydial coverage should be added.

➤*Bacterial septicemia:* Caused by *Staphylococcus aureus, Streptococcus pneumoniae, Escherichia coli, Haemophilus influenzae* or *Klebsiella pneumoniae.*

➤*Bone and joint infections:* Caused by *Staphylococcus aureus, Streptococcus pneumoniae, Escherichia coli, Proteus mirabilis, Klebsiella pneumoniae* or *Enterobacter* species.

➤*Intra-abdominal infections:* Caused by *Escherichia coli, Klebsiella pneumoniae, Bacteroides fragilis, Clostridium* species (most strains of *C. difficile* are resistant) or *Peptostreptococcus* species.

CEFTRIAXONE SODIUM — INJECTION

➤*Meningitis:* Caused by *Haemophilus influenzae*, *Neisseria meningitidis* or *Streptococcus pneumoniae*. Ceftriaxone sodium has also been used successfully in a limited number of cases of meningitis and shunt infection caused by *Staphylococcus epidermidis* and *Escherichia coli* (efficacy for these 2 organisms in this organ system was studied in less than 10 infections).

➤*Surgical prophylaxis:* The preoperative administration of a single 1 g dose of ceftriaxone sodium may reduce the incidence of postoperative infections in patients undergoing surgical procedures classified as contaminated or potentially contaminated (eg, vaginal or abdominal hysterectomy or cholecystectomy for chronic calculous cholecystitis in high-risk patients, such as those older than 70 years of age, with acute cholecystitis not requiring therapeutic antimicrobials, obstructive jaundice or common duct bile stones) and in surgical patients for whom infection at the operative site would present serious risk (eg, during coronary artery bypass surgery). Although ceftriaxone sodium has been shown to have been as effective as cefazolin in the prevention of infection following coronary artery bypass surgery, no placebo-controlled trials have been conducted to evaluate any cephalosporin antibiotic in the prevention of infection following coronary artery bypass surgery.

When administered prior to surgical procedures for which it is indicated, a single 1 g dose of ceftriaxone sodium provides protection from most infections due to susceptible organisms throughout the course of the procedure.

➤*Unlabeled uses:* Ceftriaxone 2 g/day IV for 14 to 28 days is effective in treating neurologic complications, arthritis and carditis associated with Lyme disease in patients refractory to penicillin G.

Administration and Dosage

➤*Approved by the FDA:* December 21, 1984.

May be administered IV or IM.

➤*Adults:* 1 to 2 g given once a day (or in equally divided doses twice daily) depending on the type and severity of infection. The total daily dose should not exceed 4 g.

If *C. trachomatis* is a suspected pathogen, appropriate antichlamydial coverage should be added, because ceftriaxone sodium has no activity against this organism.

➤*Uncomplicated gonococcal infections:* A single IM dose of 250 mg is recommended.

➤*Surgical prophylaxis:* A single dose of 1 g administered IV ½ to 2 hours before surgery is recommended.

➤*Children:*

Skin and skin structure infections – The recommended total daily dose is 50 to 75 mg/kg given once a day (or in equally divided doses twice daily). The total daily dose should not exceed 2 g.

Acute bacterial otitis media – A single IM dose of 50 mg/kg (not to exceed 1 g) is recommended.

Serious infections other than meningitis – The recommended total daily dose is 50 to 75 mg/kg, given in divided doses every 12 hours. The total daily dose should not exceed 2 g.

➤*Meningitis:* It is recommended that the initial therapeutic dose be 100 mg/kg (not to exceed 4 g). Thereafter, a total daily dose of 100 mg/kg/day (not to exceed 4 g daily) is recommended. The daily dose may be administered once a day (or in equally divided doses every 12 hours). The usual duration of therapy is 7 to 14 days.

➤*Duration:* Generally, ceftriaxone sodium therapy should be continued for at least 2 days after the signs and symptoms of infection have disappeared. The usual duration of therapy is 4 to 14 days; in complicated infections, longer therapy may be required.

➤*Streptococcal infections:* When treating infections caused by *Streptococcus pyogenes*, therapy should be continued for at least 10 days.

➤*Renal/Hepatic function impairment:* No dosage adjustment is necessary for patients with impairment of renal or hepatic function; however, blood levels should be monitored in patients with severe renal impairment (eg, dialysis patients) and in patients with both renal and hepatic dysfunctions, the dose should not exceed 2 g/day without closely monitoring serum concentrations.

➤*Preparation for use:*

IM – Reconstitute ceftriaxone sodium powder with the appropriate diluent.

Inject diluent into vial, shake vial thoroughly to form solution. Withdraw entire contents of vial into syringe to equal total labeled dose.

After reconstitution, each 1 mL of solution contains approximately 250 or 350 mg equivalent of ceftriaxone according to the amount of dilute indicated below. If required, more diluent solutions could be utilized. A 350 mg/mL concentration is not recommended for the 250 mg vial since it may not be possible to withdraw the entire contents. As with all IM preparations, ceftriaxone sodium should be injected well within the body of a relatively large muscle; aspiration helps to avoid unintentional injection into a blood vessel.

Vial Dosage Size	Amount of Diluent to be Added	
	250 mg/mL	350 mg/mL
250 mg	0.9 mL	-
500 mg	1.8 mL	1 mL
1 g	3.6 mL	2.1 mL
2 g	7.2 mL	4.2 mL

IV – Ceftriaxone sodium should be administered IV by infusion over a period of 30 minutes. Concentrations between 10 mg/mL and 40 mg/mL are recommended; however, lower concentrations may be used if desired. Reconstitute vials or "piggyback" bottles with an appropriate IV diluent.

Vial Dosage Size	Amount of Diluent to be Added
250 mg	2.4 mL
500 mg	4.8 mL
1 g	9.6 mL
2 g	19.2 mL

After reconstitution, each 1 mL of solution contains approximately 100 mg equivalent of ceftriaxone. Withdraw entire contents and dilute to the desired concentration with the appropriate IV diluent.

Piggyback Bottle Dosage Size	Amount of Diluent to be Added
1 g	10 mL
2 g	20 mL

After reconstitution, further dilute to 50 mL or 100 mL volumes with the appropriate IV diluent.

➤*Pharmacy bulk package:* The 10 g vial should be reconstituted with 95 mL of an appropriate IV diluent in a suitable work area such as a laminar flow hood. The resulting solution will contain approximately 100 mg/mL of ceftriaxone. This closure may be penetrated only 1 time after reconstitution, using a suitable sterile transfer device or dispensing set which allows measured dispensing of the contents.

After reconstitution of the pharmacy bulk package, unused solutions should be discarded within 24 hours of initial entry. Unused portions of solution held longer than the recommended time periods should be discarded.

Reconstituted bulk solutions should not be used for direct infusion.

➤*Admixture incompatibility:* Ceftriaxone has been shown to be compatible with metronidazole hydrochloride injection. The concentration should not exceed 5 to 7.5 mg/mL metronidazole hydrochloride with ceftriaxone 10 mg/mL as an admixture. The admixture is stable for 24 hours at room temperature only in 0.9% sodium chloride injection or 5% dextrose in water draw. No compatibility studies have been conducted with the *Flagyl IV RUT* (metronidazole) formulation or using other diluents. Metronidazole at concentrations greater than 8 mg/mL will precipitate. Do not refrigerate the admixture as precipitation will occur.

Vancomycin and fluconazole are physically incompatible with ceftriaxone in admixtures. When either of these drugs is to be administered concomitantly with ceftriaxone by intermittent intravenous infusion, it is recommended that they be given sequentially, with thorough flushing of the intravenous lines (with one of the compatible fluids) between the administrations.

After the indicated stability time periods, unused portions of solutions should be discarded.

Ceftriaxone sodium solutions should not be physically mixed with or piggybacked into solutions containing other antimicrobial drugs or into diluent solutions other than those listed above, due to possible incompatibility.

➤*Storage/Stability:* Ceftriaxone sodium sterile powder should be stored at room temperature (25°C [77°F]) or below and protected from light. After reconstitution, protection from normal light is not necessary. The color of solutions ranges from light yellow to amber, depending on the length of storage, concentration and diluent used.

Ceftriaxone sodium IM solutions remain stable (loss of potency less than 10%) for the following time periods:

Diluent	Concentration (mg/mL)	Storage	
		Room Temperature (25°C; 77°F)	Refrigerated (4°C; 39.2°F)
Sterile Water for Injection	100	2 days	10 days
	250, 350	24 hours	3 days
0.9% Sodium Chloride Solution	100	2 days	10 days
	250, 350	24 hours	3 days
5% Dextrose Solution	100	2 days	10 days
	250, 350	24 hours	3 days
Bacteriostatic Water + 0.9% Benzyl Alcohol	100	24 hours	10 days
	250, 350	24 hours	3 days
1% Lidocaine Solution (without epinephrine)	100	24 hours	10 days
	250, 350	24 hours	3 days

Ceftriaxone sodium IV solutions, at concentrations of 10, 20 and 40 mg/ml, remain stable (loss of potency less than 10%) for the following time periods stored in glass or PVC containers:

Diluent	Storage	
	Room Temperature (25°C; 77°F)	Refrigerated (4°C; 39.2°F)
Sterile Water	2 days	10 days
0.9% Sodium Chloride Solution	2 days	10 days
5% Dextrose Solution	2 days	10 days

CEFTRIAXONE SODIUM — INJECTION

	Storage	
Diluent	Room Temperature (25°C; 77°F)	Refrigerated (4°C; 39.2°F)
10% Dextrose Solution	2 days	10 days
5% Dextrose + 0.9% Sodium Chloride Solution*	2 days	Incompatible
5% Dextrose + 0.45% Sodium Chloride Solution	2 days	Incompatible

* Data available for 10 to 40 mg/mL concentrations in this diluent in PVC containers only.

Similarly, ceftriaxone sodium IV solutions, at concentrations of 100 mg/mL, remain stable in the IV piggyback glass containers for the above specified time periods.

The following IV ceftriaxone sodium solutions are stable at room temperature (25°C; 77°F) for 24 hours, at concentrations between 10 mg/mL and 40 mg/mL: Sodium Lactate (PVC container), 10% Invert Sugar (glass container), 5% Sodium Bicarbonate (glass container), *Freamine III* (glass container), *Mormonism* in 5% Dextrose (glass and PVC containers), *Insoluble* in 5% Dextrose (glass container), 5% Mannitol (glass container), 10% Mannitol (glass container).

Ceftriaxone sodium reconstituted with 5% Dextrose or 0.9% Sodium Chloride solution at concentrations between 10 mg/mL and 40 mg/mL, and then stored in frozen state (−20°C; −4°F) in PVC or polyolefin containers, remains stable for 26 weeks. Reconstituted *ADD-Vantage* units, however, should not be stored in a frozen state −20°C (−4°F).

All frozen solutions of ceftriaxone sodium, including those frozen following reconstitution and those supplied premixed as a frozen solution in *Galaxy* containers, should be thawed at room temperature before use. After thawing, unused portions should be discarded. Do not refreeze.

Galaxy containers (PL 2040 plastic) – Ceftriaxone sodium supplied as a frozen, iso-osmotic, sterile, nonpyrogenic solution in *Galaxy* containers (PL 2040 plastic) is for IV administration using sterile equipment.

Store in a freezer capable of maintaining a temperature of −20°C (−4°F).

Thawing of plastic container: Thaw frozen container at room temperature (25°C [77°F]) or under refrigeration (5°C [41°F]). Do not force thaw by immersion in water baths or by microwave irradiation.

Check for minute leaks by squeezing container firmly. If leaks are detected, discard solution as sterility may be impaired.

Do not add supplementary medication.

The container should be visually inspected. Components of the solution may precipitate in the frozen state and will dissolve upon reaching room temperature with little or no agitation. Potency is not affected. Agitate after solution has reached room temperature. If after visual inspection the solution remains cloudy or if an insoluble precipitate is noted or if any seals or outlet ports are not intact, the container should be discarded.

The thawed solution is stable for 21 days under refrigeration (5°C [41°F]) or 72 hours at room temperature (25°C [77°F]). Do not refreeze thawed antibiotics.

		Storage	
Diluent	Concentration	Room Temperature (25°C; 77°F)	Refrigeration (4°C; 39.2°F)
0.9% Sodium Chloride solution	10 mg/mL to 40 mg/mL	2 days	10 days
5% Dextrose Solution	10 mg/mL to 40 mg/mL	2 days	10 days

Reconstituted *ADD-Vantage* units should not be stored in a frozen state (−20°C [−4°F]).

CEFIXIME

Rx	**Suprax** (Lupin Pharma)	**Powder for Oral Suspension:** 100 mg/5 mL	Sucrose. Strawberry flavored. In 50 and 75 mL.

CEFIXIME — ORAL

For complete and comparative prescribing information, refer to the Cephalosporins group monograph.

Indications

➤*Uncomplicated urinary tract infections:* Caused by *Escherichia coli* and *Proteus mirabilis.*

➤*Otitis media:* Caused by *Haemophilus influenzae* (beta-lactamase positive and negative strains), *Moraxella (Branhamella) catarrhalis,* (most of which are beta-lactamase positive) and *S. pyogenes*†.

➤*Pharyngitis and tonsillitis:* Caused by *S. pyogenes.*

➤*Acute bronchitis and acute exacerbations of chronic bronchitis:* Caused by *Streptococcus pneumoniae* and *Haemophilus influenzae* (beta-lactamase positive and negative strains).

Uncomplicated gonorrhea (cervical/urethral) – Caused by *Neisseria gonorrhoeae* (penicillinase- and non-penicillinase-producing strains).

Administration and Dosage

➤*Adults:* Once cefixime oral suspension is reconstituted, the recommended dose of the suspension is 400 mg daily. For the treatment of uncomplicated cervical/urethral gonococcal infections, a single oral dose of 400 mg is recommended.

➤*Children:* 8 mg/kg/day. This may be administered as a single daily dose or may be given in 2 divided doses, as 4 mg/kg every 12 hours.

Pediatric dosage chart

Patient weight (kg)	Dose/day (mg)	Dose/day (mL)	Dose/day (5 mL of suspension)
6.25	50	2.5	0.5
12.5	100	5	1
18.75	150	7.5	1.5
25	200	10	2
31.25	250	12.5	2.5
37.5	300	15	3

Children weighing more than 50 kg or older than 12 years should be treated with the recommended adult dose.

➤*Streptococcal infections:* In the treatment of infections due to *S. pyogenes*, a therapeutic dosage of cefixime should be administered for at least 10 days.

➤*Renal function impairment:* Cefixime oral suspension may be administered in the presence of impaired renal function. Normal dose and schedule may be employed in patients with creatinine clearances of 60 mL/min or greater. Patients whose clearance is between 21 and 60 mL/min, or patients who are on renal hemodialysis may be given 75% of the standard dosage at the standard dosing interval (ie, 300 mg daily). Patients whose clearance is less than 20 mL/min, or patients who are on continuous ambulatory peritoneal dialysis may be given half the standard dosage at the standard dosing interval (ie, 200 mg daily). Neither hemodialysis nor peritoneal dialysis removes significant amounts of drug from the body.

➤*Storage/Stability:*

Prior to reconstitution – Store drug powder at 20° to 25°C (68° to 77°F).

After reconstitution – Store at room temperature or under refrigeration. Discard unused portion after 14 days.

Follow directions for mixing included on the product label. After reconstitution, the suspension may be kept for 14 days either at room temperature, or under refrigeration, without significant loss of potency. Keep tightly closed. Shake well before using.

CEFOPERAZONE SODIUM

Rx	**Cefobid** (Roerig)	**Powder for Injection:**[1] 1 g	In vials and piggyback units.
		2 g	In vials and piggyback units.
		Injection:[1] 1 g	Premixed, frozen. In 50 ml plastic containers.[2]
		2 g	Premixed, frozen. In 50 ml plastic containers.[3]
		10 g	Pharmacy bulk package.

[1] Contains 1.5 mEq sodium/g.
[2] With 2.3 g dextrose hydrous.
[3] With 1.8 g dextrose hydrous.

† Efficacy for this organism in this organ system was studied in fewer than 10 infections.

CEFOPERAZONE SODIUM — INJECTION

For complete and comparative prescribing information, refer to the Cephalosporins group monograph.

Indications

➤*Respiratory tract infections:* Caused by *S. pneumoniae*, *H. influenzae*, *S. aureus* (penicillinase and nonpenicillinase-producing strains), *S. pyogenes*† (group A beta-hemolytic streptococci), *P. aeruginosa*, *Klebsiella pneumoniae*, *E. coli*, *Proteus mirabilis*, and *Enterobacter* species.

➤*Peritonitis and other intra-abdominal infections:* Caused by *E. coli*, *P. aeruginosa*†, and anaerobic gram-negative bacilli (including *Bacteroides fragilis*).

➤*Bacterial septicemia:* Caused by *S. pneumoniae*, *S. agalactiae*†, *S. aureus*, *Pseudomonas aeruginosa*†, *E. coli*, *Klebsiella* spp.†, *Klebsiella pneumoniae*, *Proteus* species (indole-positive and indole-negative), *Clostridium* spp.† and anaerobic gram-positive cocci†.

➤*Skin and skin structure infections:* Caused by *S. aureus* (penicillinase and nonpenicillinase-producing strains), *S. pyogenes*†, and *P. aeruginosa*.

➤*Pelvic inflammatory disease, endometritis:* Including other infections of the female genital tract caused by *N. gonorrhoeae*, *S. epidermidis*†, *S. agalactiae*, *E. coli*, *Clostridium* spp.†, *Bacteroides* species (including *Bacteroides fragilis*), and anaerobic gram-positive cocci.

➤*Urinary tract infections:* Caused by *Escherichia coli* and *Pseudomonas aeruginosa*.

Administration and Dosage

➤*Approved by the FDA:* November 18, 1982.

➤*Dosage:* 2 to 4 g/day administered in equally divided doses every 12 hours.

In severe infections or infections caused by less sensitive organisms, the total daily dose or frequency may be increased. Patients have been successfully treated with a total daily dosage of 6 to 12 g divided into 2, 3 or 4 administrations ranging from 1.5 to 4 g/dose.

In a pharmacokinetic study, a total daily dose of 16 g was administered to severely immunocompromised patients by constant infusion without complications. Steady state serum concentrations were approximately 150 mcg/mL in these patients.

➤*Streptococcal infections:* When treating infections caused by *Streptococcus pyogenes*, therapy should be continued for at least 10 days.

➤*Admixture incompatibility:* Solutions of cefoperazone and aminoglycoside should not be directly mixed, since there is a physical incompatibility between them. If combination therapy with cefoperazone and an aminoglycoside is contemplated (see Indications) this can be accomplished by sequential intermittent IV infusion provided that separate secondary IV tubing is used, and that the primary IV tubing is adequately irrigated with an approved diluent between doses. It is also suggested that cefoperazone be administered prior to the aminoglycoside. In vitro testing of the effectiveness of drug combination(s) is recommended.

➤*Reconstitution:* The following solutions may be used for the initial reconstitution of cefoperazone (sterile cefoperazone):

Solutions for Initial Reconstitution	
5% Dextrose Injection (USP)	0.9% NaCl Injection (USP)
5% Dextrose and 0.9% NaCl Injection (USP)	*Normosol* M and 5% Dextrose Injection
5% Dextrose and 0.2% NaCl Injection (USP)	*Normosol* R
10% Dextrose Injection (USP)	Sterile Water for Injection[1]
Bacteriostatic Water for Injection (Benzyl Alcohol or Parabens) (USP)[1,2]	

[1] Not to be used as a vehicle for IV infusion.
[2] Preparations containing Benzyl Alcohol should not be used in neonates.

General reconstitution procedures – Cefoperazone for IV or IM use may be initially reconstituted with any compatible solution mentioned above. Solutions should be allowed to stand after reconstitution to allow any foaming to dissipate to permit visual inspection for complete solubilization. Vigorous and prolonged agitation may be necessary to solubilize cefoperazone in higher concentrations (above 333 mg cefoperazone/mL). The maximum solubility of cefoperazone (sterile cefoperazone) is approximately 475 mg cefoperazone/mL of compatible diluent.

IV administration – Cefoperazone concentrations between 2 mg/mL and 50 mg/mL are recommended for IV administration.

Vials – Vials of cefoperazone may be initially reconstituted with a minimum of 2.8 mL/ g of cefoperazone of any compatible reconstituting solution appropriate for IV administration described above in the previous information. For ease of reconstitution, the use of 5 mL of compatible solution per gram of cefoperazone is recommended. The entire quantity of the resulting solution should then be withdrawn for further dilution and administration using any of the following vehicles for IV infusion:

Vehicles for IV Infusion	
5% Dextrose Injection (USP)	Lactated Ringer's Injection (USP)
5% Dextrose and Lactated Ringer's Injection	0.9% NaCl Injection (USP)
5% Dextrose and 0.9% NaCl Injection (USP)	*Normosol* M and 5% Dextrose Injection
5% Dextrose and 0.2% NaCl Injection (USP)	*Normosol* R
10% Dextrose Injection (USP)	

The resulting IV solution should be administered in one of the following manners:

Intermittent infusion – Solutions of cefoperazone should be administered over a 15- to 30-minute time period.

Continuous infusion – Cefoperazone can be used for continuous infusion after dilution to a final concentration of between 2 and 25 mg cefoperazone/mL.

IM administration – Any suitable solution listed above may be used to prepare cefoperazone for IM injection. When concentrations of 250 mg/mL or more are to be administered, a lidocaine solution should be used. These solutions should be prepared using a combination of Sterile Water for Injection and 2% lidocaine HCl injection that approximates a 0.5% lidocaine HCl solution. A 2-step dilution process as follows is recommended: First, add the required amount of Sterile Water for Injection and agitate until cefoperazone powder is completely dissolved. Second, add the required amount of 2% lidocaine and mix.

	Final cefoperazone concentration	Step 1 volume of Sterile water	Step 2 volume of 2% lidocaine	Withdrawable volume[1,2]
1 g vial	333 mg/mL	2 mL	0.6 mL	3 mL
	250 mg/mL	2.8 mL	1 mL	4 mL
2 g vial	333 mg/mL	3.8 mL	1.2 mL	6 mL
	250 mg/mL	5.4 mL	1.8 mL	8 mL

[1] There is sufficient excess present to allow for withdrawal of the stated volume.
[2] Final lidocaine concentration will approximate that obtained if a 0.5% Lidocaine HCl solution is used as diluent.

When a diluent other than lidocaine HCl injection is used, reconstitute as follows:

	Cefoperazone concentration	Volume of diluent to be added	Withdrawable volume[1]
1 g vial	333 mg/mL	2.6 mL	3 mL
	250 mg/mL	3.8 mL	4 mL
2 g vial	333 mg/mL	5 mL	6 mL
	250 mg/mL	7.2 mL	8 mL

[1] There is sufficient excess present to allow for withdrawal of the stated volume.

➤*Storage / Stability:* Cefoperazone is to be stored at or below 25°C (77°F) and protected from light prior to reconstitution. After reconstitution, protection from light is not necessary.

The following parenteral diluents and approximate concentrations of cefoperazone provide stable solutions under the following conditions for the indicated time periods. (After the indicated time periods, unused portions of solutions should be discarded.)

Compatibility, Stability, and Storage of Cefoperazone	
Room Temperature (15° to 25°C; 59° to 77°F)	
24 hours	Approximate concentrations
Bacteriostatic Water for Injection (Benzyl Alcohol or Parabens)	300 mg/mL
5% Dextrose Injection	2 mg to 50 mg/mL
5% Dextrose and Lactated Ringer's Injection	2 mg to 50 mg/mL
5% Dextrose and 0.9% Sodium Chloride Injection	2 mg to 50 mg/mL
5% Dextrose and 0.2% Sodium Chloride Injection	2 mg to 50 mg/mL
10% Dextrose Injection	2 mg to 50 mg/mL
Lactated Ringer's Injection	2 mg/mL
0.5% Lidocaine HCl Injection	300 mg/mL
0.9% Sodium Chloride Injection	2 mg to 300 mg/mL
Normosol M and 5% Dextrose Injection	2 mg to 50 mg/mL
Normosol R	2 mg to 50 mg/mL
Sterile Water for Injection	300 mg/mL

† Efficacy of this organism was studied in fewer than 10 infections.

CEFOPERAZONE SODIUM — INJECTION

Compatibility, Stability, and Storage of Cefoperazone	
Room Temperature (15° to 25°C; 59° to 77°F)	
Refrigerator temperature (2° to 8°C; 36° to 46°F)	
5 days	Approximate concentrations
Bacteriostatic Water for Injection (Benzyl Alcohol or Parabens)	300 mg/mL
5% Dextrose Injection	2 mg to 50 mg/mL
5% Dextrose and 0.9% Sodium Chloride Injection	2 mg to 50 mg/mL
5% Dextrose and 0.2% Sodium Chloride Injection	2 mg to 50 mg/mL
Lactated Ringer's Injection	2 mg/mL
0.5% Lidocaine HCl Injection	300 mg/mL
0.9% Sodium Chloride Injection	2 mg to 300 mg/mL
Normosol M and 5% Dextrose Injection	2 mg to 50 mg/mL
Normosol R	2 mg to 50 mg/mL
Sterile Water for Injection	300 mg/mL
Freezer temperature (−20° to −10°C; −4° to 14°F)	
3 weeks	Approximate concentrations
5% Dextrose Injection	50 mg/mL
5% Dextrose and 0.9% Sodium Chloride Injection	2 mg/mL
5% Dextrose and 0.2% Sodium Chloride Injection	2 mg/mL
5 weeks	
0.9% Sodium Chloride Injection	300 mg/mL
Sterile Water for Injection	300 mg/mL

Reconstituted cefoperazone solutions may be stored in glass or plastic syringes, or in glass or flexible plastic parenteral solution containers.

Frozen samples should be thawed at room temperature before use. After thawing, unused portions should be discarded. Do not refreeze.

CEFOTAXIME SODIUM

Rx	**Cefotaxime** (Various, eg, American Pharma, Baxter, Cura)	**Powder for Injection:**[a] 500 mg	In vials, packages of 10.
Rx	**Claforan** (Hoechst Marion Roussel)		In vials, packages of 10.
Rx	**Cefotaxime** (Various, eg, American Pharma, Baxter, Cura)	**Powder for Injection:**[a] 1 g	In vials, packages of 25.
Rx	**Claforan** (Hoechst Marion Roussel)		In vials, packages of 10s, 25s, 50s. Infusion bottles in 10s. *ADD-Vantage* system vials in 25s and 50s.
Rx	**Cefotaxime** (Various, eg, American Pharma, Baxter, Cura)	**Powder for Injection:**[a] 2 g	In vials, packages of 25.
Rx	**Claforan** (Hoechst Marion Roussel)		In vials, packages of 10s, 25s, 50s. Infusion bottles in 10s. *ADD-Vantage* system vials in 25s and 50s.
Rx	**Cefotaxime** (Various, eg, American Pharma, Cura)	**Powder for Injection:**[a] 10 g	In bottles.
Rx	**Claforan** (Hoechst Marion Roussel)		In bottles.
Rx	**Cefotaxime** (Cura)	**Injection:**[a] 1 g	In infusion bottles, packages of 25.
Rx	**Claforan** (Hoechst Marion Roussel)		Premixed, frozen. In 50 mL, package of 12s.
Rx	**Cefotaxime** (Cura)	**Injection:**[a] 2 g	In infusion bottles, packages of 25.
Rx	**Claforan** (Hoechst Marion Roussel)		Premixed, frozen. In 50 mL, package of 12s.

[a] Contains 2.2 mEq sodium/g.

CEFOTAXIME SODIUM — INJECTION

Complete and comparative prescribing information for these products begins in the Cephalosporins group monograph.

Indications

➤*Lower respiratory tract infections:* Including pneumonia, caused by *Streptococcus pneumoniae* (formerly *Diplococcus pneumoniae*), *Streptococcus pyogenes* (efficacy for this organism, in this organ system, has been studied in less than 10 infections [group A streptococci]) and other streptococci (excluding enterococci, [eg, *Enterococcus faecalis*]), *Staphylococcus aureus* (penicillinase and nonpenicillinase producing), *Escherichia coli*, *Klebsiella* species, *Haemophilus influenzae* (including ampicillin-resistant strains), *Haemophilus parainfluenzae*, *Proteus mirabilis*, *Serratia marcescens* (efficacy for this organism, in this organ system, has been studied in less than 10 infections), *Enterobacter* species, and indole-positive *Proteus* and *Pseudomonas* species (including *Pseudomonas aeruginosa*).

➤*Genitourinary infections:* Caused by *Enterococcus* species, *Staphylococcus epidermidis*, *S. aureus* (penicillinase and nonpenicillinase producing; efficacy for this organism, in this organ system, has been studied in less than 10 infections), *Citrobacter* species, *Enterobacter* species, *E. coli*, *Klebsiella* species, *P. mirabilis*, *Proteus vulgaris* (efficacy for this organism, in this organ system, has been studied in less than 10 infections), *Providencia stuartii*, *Morganella morganii* (efficacy for this organism, in this organ system, has been studied in less than 10 infections), *Providencia rettgeri* (efficacy for this organism, in this organ system, has been studied in less than 10 infections), *Serratia marcescens*, and *Pseudomonas* species (including *P. aeruginosa*). Also, uncomplicated gonorrhea (cervical/urethral and rectal) caused by *Neisseria gonorrhoeae*, including penicillinase-producing strains.

➤*Gynecologic infections:* Including pelvic inflammatory disease, endometritis, and pelvic cellulitis, caused by *S. epidermidis*, *Streptococcus* species, *Enterococcus* species, *Enterobacter* species (efficacy for this organism, in this organ system, has been studied in less than 10 infections), *Klebsiella* species (efficacy for this organism, in this organ system, has been studied in less than 10 infections), *E. coli*, *P. mirabilis*, *Bacteroides* species (including *Bacteroides fragilis*; efficacy for this organism, in this organ system, has been studied in less than 10 infections), *Clostridium* species, and anaerobic cocci (including *Peptostreptococcus* and *Peptococcus* species) and *Fusobacterium* species (including *Fusobacterium nucleatum*; efficacy for this organism, in this organ system, has been studied in less than 10 infections).

Cefotaxime, like other cephalosporins, has no activity against *Chlamydia trachomatis*. Therefore, when cephalosporins are used in the treatment of patients with pelvic inflammatory disease and *C. trachomatis* is 1 of the suspected pathogens, add appropriate antichlamydial coverage.

➤*Bacteremia/Septicemia:* Caused by *E. coli*, *Klebsiella* species, and *S. marcescens*, *S. aureus* and *Streptococcus* species (including *S. pneumoniae*).

➤*Skin and skin structure infections:* Caused by *S. aureus* (penicillinase and nonpenicillinase producing), *S. epidermidis*, *S. pyogenes* (group A streptococci) and other streptococci, *Enterococcus* species, *Acinetobacter* species (efficacy for this organism, in this organ system, has been studied in less than 10 infections), *E. coli*, *Citrobacter* species (including *Citrobacter freundii*; efficacy for this organism, in this organ system, has been studied in less than 10 infections), *Enterobacter* species, *Klebsiella* species, *P. mirabilis*, *P. vulgaris* (efficacy for this organism, in this organ system, has been studied in less than 10 infections), *M. morganii*, *P. rettgeri* (efficacy for this organism, in this organ system, has been studied in less than 10 infections), *Pseudomonas* species, *S. marcescens*, *Bacteroides* species, and anaerobic cocci (including *Peptostreptococcus*; efficacy for this organism, in this organ system, has been studied in less than 10 infections) species and *Peptococcus* species.

➤*Intra-abdominal infections:* Including peritonitis caused by *Streptococcus* species (efficacy for this organism, in this organ system, has been studied in less than 10 infections), *E. coli*, *Klebsiella* species, *Bacteroides* species, and anaerobic cocci (including *Peptostreptococcus*; efficacy for this organism, in this organ system, has been studied in less than 10 infections) species and *Peptococcus* (efficacy for this organism, in this organ system, has been studied in less than 10 infections) species, *P. mirabilis* (efficacy for this organism, in this organ system, has been studied in less than 10 infections), and *Clostridium* species (efficacy for this organism, in this organ system, has been studied in less than 10 infections).

➤*Bone or joint infections:* Caused by *S. aureus* (penicillinase and nonpenicillinase producing strains), *Streptococcus* species (including *S. pyogenes*; efficacy for this organism, in this organ system, has been studied in

CEFOTAXIME SODIUM — INJECTION

less than 10 infections), *Pseudomonas* species (including *P. aeruginosa*; efficacy for this organism, in this organ system, has been studied in less than 10 infections), and *P. mirabilis* (efficacy for this organism, in this organ system, has been studied in less than 10 infections).

➤*CNS infections:* Caused by *Neisseria meningitidis*, *H. influenzae*, *S. pneumoniae*, *K. pneumoniae* (efficacy for this organism, in this organ system, has been studied in less than 10 infections), and *E. coli* (efficacy for this organism, in this organ system, has been studied in less than 10 infections).

Although many strains of enterococci (eg, *Streptococcus faecalis*) and *Pseudomonas* species are resistant to cefotaxime in vitro, cefotaxime has been used successfully in treating patients with infections caused by susceptible organisms.

➤*Concomitant aminoglycoside therapy:* In certain cases of confirmed or suspected gram-positive or gram-negative sepsis, or in patients with other serious infections in which the causative organism has not been identified, cefotaxime may be used concomitantly with an aminoglycoside. The dosage recommended in the labeling of both antibiotics may be given and depends on the severity of the infection and the patient's condition. Carefully monitor renal function, especially if higher dosages of the aminoglycosides are to be administered or if therapy is prolonged, because of the potential nephrotoxicity and ototoxicity of aminoglycoside antibiotics. It is possible that nephrotoxicity may be potentiated if cefotaxime is used concomitantly with an aminoglycoside.

➤*Perioperative prophylaxis:* The administration of cefotaxime preoperatively reduces the incidence of certain infections in patients undergoing surgical procedures (eg, abdominal or vaginal hysterectomy, GI and GU tract surgery) that may be classified as contaminated or potentially contaminated.

For patients undergoing GI surgery, preoperative bowel preparation by mechanical cleansing, as well as with a nonabsorbable antibiotic (eg, neomycin), is recommended.

➤*Cesarean section:* In patients undergoing cesarean section, intraoperative (after clamping the umbilical cord) and postoperative use of cefotaxime may also reduce the incidence of certain postoperative infections. The first dose of 1 g is administered intravenously (IV) as soon as the umbilical cord is clamped. The second and third doses should be given as 1 g IV or intramuscularly (IM) at 6 and 12 hours after the first dose.

Administration and Dosage

➤*Approved by the FDA:* December 29, 1983.

➤*Adults:* Dosage and route of administration should be determined by susceptibility of the causative organisms, severity of the infection, and the condition of the patient (see the following table for dosage guidelines). The maximum daily dose should not exceed 12 g.

Premixed injection – Premixed cefotaxime injection is intended for IV administration after thawing.

Powder for injection – Cefotaxime sterile powder for injection may be administered IM or IV after reconstitution.

Guidelines for Dosage of Cefotaxime

Type of infection	Daily dose (grams)	Frequency and route
Gonococcal urethritis/ cervicitis in males and females	0.5	0.5 g IM (single dose)
Rectal gonorrhea in females	0.5	0.5 g IM (single dose)
Rectal gonorrhea in males	1	1 g IM (single dose)
Uncomplicated infections	2	1 g every 12 h IM or IV
Moderate to severe infections	3 to 6	1 to 2 g every 8 h IM or IV
Infections commonly needing antibiotics in higher dosage (eg, septicemia)	6 to 8	2 g every 6 to 8 h IV
Life-threatening infections	≤ 12	2 g every 4 h IV

Perioperative prophylaxis – To prevent postoperative infection in contaminated or potentially contaminated surgery, the recommended dose is a single 1 g IM or IV administered 30 to 90 minutes prior to start of surgery.

Cesarean section – The first dose of 1 g is administered IV as soon as the umbilical cord is clamped. The second and third doses should be given as 1 g IV or IM at 6 and 12 hours after the first dose.

➤*Children:*

Cefotaxime Dosage Guidelines in Pediatric Patients

Age	Weight (kg)	Dosage schedule	Route
0 to 1 week	—	50 mg/kg every 12 hours	IV
1 to 4 weeks	—	50 mg/kg every 8 hours	IV
1 month to 12 years	< 50[a]	50 to 180 mg/kg/day in 4 to 6 divided doses[b]	IV or IM

[a] For children ≥ 50 kg, use adult dosage. Do not exceed adult recommended doses.
[b] Use higher doses for more severe or serious infections, including meningitis.

➤*Renal function impairment:* Because high and prolonged serum antibiotic concentrations can occur from usual doses in patients with transient or persistent reduction of urinary output because of renal insufficiency, the total daily dose should be reduced when cefotaxime is administered to such patients. Continued dosage should be determined by degree of renal impairment, severity of infection, and susceptibility of the causative organism.

Although there is no clinical evidence supporting the necessity of changing the dosage of cefotaxime in patients with even profound renal dysfunction, it is suggested that, until further data are obtained, the dose of cefotaxime be halved in patients with estimated creatinine clearances (Ccr) of less than 20 mL/min/1.73 m^2.

➤*CDC recommended treatment schedules for gonorrhea (Morbidity and Mortality Weekly Report.* 2002;51]:1-80.):

Uncomplicated gonococcal infections of the cervix, urethra, and rectum – 500 mg IM.

Disseminated gonococcal infection – 1 g IV every 8 hours.

Disseminated gonococcal infection and gonococcal scalp abscesses in newborns – 25 mg/kg IV or IM every 12 hours for 7 days, with a duration of 10 to 14 days if meningitis is documented.

➤*Administration:*

IV administration – The IV route is preferable for patients with bacteremia, bacterial septicemia, peritonitis, meningitis, or other severe or life-threatening infections, or for patients who may be poor risks because of lowered resistance resulting from such debilitating conditions as malnutrition, trauma, surgery, diabetes, heart failure, or malignancy, particularly if shock is present or impending.

Intermittent IV – For intermittent IV administration, a solution containing 1 or 2 g in 10 mL of sterile water for injection can be injected over a period of 3 to 5 minutes. Cefotaxime should not be administered over a period of less than 3 minutes. With an infusion system, it may also be given over a longer period of time through the tubing system by which the patient may be receiving other IV solutions. However, during infusion of the solution containing cefotaxime, it is advisable to discontinue temporarily the administration of other solutions at the same site.

Continuous IV – For the administration of higher doses by continuous IV infusion, a solution of cefotaxime may be added to IV bottles containing the solutions discussed in this section.

IM administration – As with all IM preparations, cefotaxime should be injected well within the body of a relatively large muscle, such as the upper outer quadrant of the buttock (ie, gluteus maximus); aspiration is necessary to avoid inadvertent injection into a blood vessel. Individual IM doses of 2 g may be given if the dose is divided and administered in different IM sites.

➤*Duration of treatment:* As with antibiotic therapy in general, administration of cefotaxime should be continued for a minimum of 48 to 72 hours after the patient defervescence or after evidence of bacterial eradication has been obtained. A minimum of 10 days of treatment is recommended for infections caused by group A beta-hemolytic streptococci in order to guard against the risk of rheumatic fever or glomerulonephritis. Frequent bacteriologic and clinical appraisal is necessary during therapy of chronic urinary tract infection and may be required for several months after therapy has been completed. Persistent infections may require treatment of several weeks. Doses smaller than those previously indicated should not be used.

➤*Preparation of solution:* Cefotaxime sterile powder for IM or IV administration should be reconstituted as follows:

Preparation of Cefotaxime Solution

Strength	Diluent (mL)	Withdrawable volume (mL)	Approximate concentration (mg/mL)
500 mg vial[a] (IM)	2	2.2	230
1 g vial[a] (IM)	3	3.4	300
2 g vial[a] (IM)	5	6	330
500 mg vial[a] (IV)	10	10.2	50
1 g vial[a] (IV)	10	10.4	95
2 g vial[a] (IV)	10	11	180
1 g infusion	50 to 100	50 to 100	10 to 20
2 g infusion	50 to 100	50 to 100	20 to 40

[a] In conventional vials.

Shake to dissolve; inspect for particulate matter and discoloration prior to use. Solutions of cefotaxime range from very pale yellow to light amber, depending on concentration, diluent used, and length and condition of storage.

A solution of cefotaxime 1 g in 14 mL of sterile water for injection is isotonic.

➤*IM:* Reconstitute vials with sterile water for injection or bacteriostatic water for injection as previously described.

➤*IV:* Reconstitute vials with at least 10 mL of sterile water for injection. Reconstitute infusion bottles with 50 or 100 mL of 0.9% sodium chloride injection or 5% dextrose injection. For other diluents, see the Compatibility and stability section.

➤*Admixture incompatibility:* Solution of cefotaxime must not be admixed with aminoglycoside solutions. If cefotaxime and aminoglycosides are to be administered to the same patient, they must be administered separately and not as mixed injection.

CEFOTAXIME SODIUM — INJECTION

➤*Directions for use of cefotaxime injection in Galaxy container (PL 2040 plastic):* Cefotaxime injection in *Galaxy* containers (PL 2040 plastic) is for continuous or intermittent infusion using sterile equipment.

Store in a freezer capable of maintaining a temperature of −20°C (−4°F).

Thawing of plastic container – Thaw frozen container at room temperature or under refrigeration (at or below 5°C [41°F]). Do not force thaw by immersion in water baths or by microwave irradiation.

Check for minute leaks by squeezing container firmly. If leaks are detected, discard solution because sterility may be impaired.

Do not add supplementary medication.

Visually inspect the container. Components of the solution may precipitate in the frozen state and will dissolve upon reaching room temperature with little or no agitation. Potency is not affected. Agitate after solution has reached room temperature. If the solution remains cloudy after visual inspection, an insoluble precipitate is noted, or any seals or outlet ports are not intact, discard the container.

The thawed solution is stable for 10 days under refrigeration (at or below 5°C [41°F]) or 24 hours at or below 22°C (72°F). Do not refreeze thawed antibiotics.

Caution: Do not use plastic containers in series connections. Such use could result in air embolism caused by residual air being drawn from the primary container before administration of the fluid from the secondary container is complete.

➤*Preparation of cefotaxime sterile (powder for injection) in ADD-Vantage system:* Cefotaxime sterile powder for injection 1 or 2 g may be reconstituted in 50 or 100 mL of 5% dextrose or 0.9% sodium chloride in the *ADD-Vantage* diluent container. Refer to separate instructions for *ADD-Vantage* system.

➤*Compatibility and stability (powder for injection):* Solutions of cefotaxime sterile powder for injection reconstituted as previously described remain chemically stable (potency remains greater than 90%) as follows when stored in original containers and disposable plastic syringes:

Reconstituted Cefotaxime Stability				
			Stability Under Refrigeration (≤ 5°C; 41°F)	
Strength	Reconstituted Concentration mg/mL	Stability ≤ 22°C; 71.6°F	Original Containers	Plastic Syringes
500 mg vial IM	230	12 hours	7 days	5 days
1 g vial IM	300	12 hours	7 days	5 days
2 g vial IM	330	12 hours	7 days	5 days
500 mg vial IV	50	24 hours	7 days	5 days
1 g vial IV	95	24 hours	7 days	5 days
2 g vial IV	180	12 hours	7 days	5 days
1 g infusion bottle	10-20	24 hours	10 days	
2 g infusion bottle	20-40	24 hours	10 days	

Reconstituted solutions stored in original containers and plastic syringes remain stable for 13 weeks frozen.

Reconstituted solutions may be further diluted up to 1,000 mL with the following solutions and maintain satisfactory potency for 24 hours at or below 22°C (71.6°F), and at least 5 days under refrigeration (at or below 5°C; 41°F): 0.9% sodium chloride injection; 5% or 10% dextrose injection; 5% dextrose and 0.9% sodium chloride injection, 5% dextrose and 0.45% sodium chloride injection; 5% dextrose and 0.2% sodium chloride injection; Ringer's lactate solution; sodium lactate injection (M/6); 10% invert sugar injection, 8.5% *Travasol* amino acid injection without electrolytes.

Solutions of cefotaxime sterile powder for injection reconstituted in 0.9% sodium chloride injection or 5% dextrose injection in *Viaflex* plastic containers maintain satisfactory potency for 24 hours at or below 22°C (71.6°F), 5 days under refrigeration (at or below 5°C; 41°F) and 13 weeks frozen. Solutions of cefotaxime sterile powder for injection sterile reconstituted in 0.9% sodium chloride injection or 5% dextrose injection in the *ADD-Vantage* flexible containers maintain satisfactory potency for 24 hours at or below 22°C (71.6°F). Do not freeze.

➤*Storage/Stability:* Store cefotaxime in the dry state below 30°C (86°F). The dry material as well as solutions tend to darken depending on storage conditions; and protect from elevated temperatures and excessive light.

Store premixed cefotaxime injection at or below −20°C (−4°F).

Cefotaxime solutions exhibit maximum stability in the pH 5 to 7 range. Do not prepare solutions of cefotaxime with diluents having a pH greater than 7.5, such as sodium bicarbonate injection.

CEFTIZOXIME SODIUM

Rx	**Cefizox** (Fujisawa)	**Powder for Injection:**[1,2] 500 mg	In 10 ml single-dose fliptop vials.
		1 g	In 20 ml single-dose fliptop vials and 100 ml piggyback vials.
		2 g	In 20 ml single-dose fliptop vials and 100 ml piggyback vials.
		10 g	In pharmacy bulk package.
		Injection:[2] 1 g	Frozen, premixed. In 50 ml single-dose plastic containers.
		2 g	Frozen, premixed. In 50 ml single-dose plastic containers.

[1] Contains 2.6 mEq sodium/g.
[2] As sodium.

CEFTIZOXIME SODIUM — INJECTION

For complete and comparative prescribing information, refer to the Cephalosporins group monograph.

Indications

➤*Lower respiratory tract infections:* Caused by *Klebsiella* spp.; *Proteus mirabilis; Escherichia coli; Haemophilus influenzae* including ampicillin-resistant strains; *Staphylococcus aureus* (penicillinase- and nonpenicillinase-producing); *Serratia* spp.; *Enterobacter* spp.; *Bacteroides* spp.; and *Streptococcus* spp. including *S. pneumoniae*, but excluding enterococci.

➤*Urinary tract infections:* Caused by *Staphylococcus aureus* (penicillinase- and nonpenicillinase-producing); *Escherichia coli; Pseudomonas* spp. including *P. aeruginosa; Proteus mirabilis; P. vulgaris; Providencia rettgeri* (formerly *Proteus rettgeri*) and *Morganella morganii* (formerly *Proteus morganii*); *Klebsiella* spp.; *Serratia* spp. including *S. marcescens*; and *Enterobacter* spp.

➤*Gonorrhea:* Including uncomplicated cervical and urethral gonorrhea caused by *Neisseria gonorrhoeae*.

➤*Pelvic inflammatory disease:* Caused by *Neisseria gonorrhoeae, Escherichia coli* or *Streptococcus agalactiae*.

Ceftizoxime, like other cephalosporins, has no activity against *Chlamydia trachomatis*. Therefore, when cephalosporins are used in the treatment of patients with pelvic inflammatory disease and *C. trachomatis* is one of the suspected pathogens, appropriate anti-chlamydial coverage should be added.

➤*Intra-abdominal infections:* Caused by *Escherichia coli; Staphylococcus epidermidis; Streptococcus* spp. (excluding enterococci); *Enterobacter* spp.; *Klebsiella* spp.; *Bacteroides* spp. including *B. fragilis*; and anaerobic cocci, including *Peptococcus* spp. and *Peptostreptococcus* spp.

➤*Septicemia:* Caused by *Streptococcus* spp. including *S. pneumoniae* (but excluding enterococci); *Staphylococcus aureus* (penicillinase- and nonpenicillinase-producing); *Escherichia coli; Bacteroides* spp. including *B. fragilis; Klebsiella* spp.; and *Serratia* spp.

➤*Skin and skin structure infections:* Caused by *Staphylococcus aureus* (penicillinase- and nonpenicillinase-producing); *Staphylococcus epidermidis; Escherichia coli; Klebsiella* spp.; *Streptococcus* spp. including *Streptococcus pyogenes* (but excluding enterococci); *Proteus mirabilis; Serratia* spp.; *Enterobacter* spp.; *Bacteroides* spp. including *B. fragilis*; and anaerobic cocci, including *Peptococcus* spp. and *Peptostreptococcus* spp.

➤*Bone and joint infections:* Caused by *Staphylococcus aureus* (penicillinase- and nonpenicillinase-producing); *Streptococcus* spp. (excluding enterococci); *Proteus mirabilis; Bacteroides* spp.; and anaerobic cocci, including *Peptococcus* spp. and *Peptostreptococcus* spp.

➤*Meningitis:* Caused by *Haemophilus influenzae*. Ceftizoxime has also been used successfully in the treatment of a limited number of pediatric and adult cases of meningitis caused by *Streptococcus pneumoniae*.

➤*Mixed infections:* Infections caused by aerobic gram-negative and by mixtures of organisms resistant to other cephalosporins, aminoglycosides, or penicillins have responded to treatment with ceftizoxime.

Administration and Dosage

➤*Approved by the FDA:* September 15, 1983.

The usual adult dosage is 1 or 2 g of ceftizoxime for injection every 8 to 12 hours. Proper dosage and route of administration should be determined by the condition of the patient, severity of the infection, and susceptibility of the causative organisms.

CEFTIZOXIME SODIUM — INJECTION

➤*General guidelines for dosage of ceftizoxime:*

Ceftizoxime Dosage Guidelines in Adults		
Type of infection	Daily dose (g)	Frequency and route
Uncomplicated urinary tract	1	500 mg every 12 hours IM or IV
PID[1]	6	2 g every 8 hours IV
Other sites	2-3	1 g every 8 to 12 hours IM or IV
Severe or refractory	3-6	1 g every 8 hours IM or IV 2 g every 8 to 12 hours IM[1] or IV
Life-threatening [2]	9-12	3 to 4 g every 8 hours IV

[1] Dosages ≤ 2 g every 4 hours have been given.
[2] Divide 2 g IM doses and give in different large muscle masses. For 2 g IM injections, the dose should be divided and administered in different large muscle masses.

Life-threatening infections – Dosages of up to 2 g IV every 4 hours have been given for life-threatening infections.

➤*Urinary tract infections:* Because of the serious nature of urinary tract infections due to *P. aeruginosa* and because many strains of *Pseudomonas* species are only moderately susceptible to ceftizoxime, higher dosage is recommended. Other therapy should be instituted if the response is not prompt.

➤*Gonorrhea:* A single, 1 g IM dose is the usual dose for treatment of uncomplicated gonorrhea.

The IV route may be preferable for patients with bacterial septicemia, localized parenchymal abscesses (such as intra-abdominal abscess), peritonitis, or other severe or life-threatening infections.

In those with normal renal function, the IV dosage for such infections is 2 to 12 g of ceftizoxime for injection daily. In conditions such as bacterial septicemia, 6 to 12 g/day may be given initially by the IV route for several days, and the dosage may then be gradually reduced according to clinical response and laboratory findings.

➤*Children:* Pediatric dosing for patients 6 months or older is 50 mg/kg/dose every 6 to 8 hours.

Dosage may be increased to a total daily dose of 200 mg/kg (not to exceed the maximum adult dose for serious infection).

➤*Renal function impairment:* Modification of ceftizoxime dosage is necessary in patients with impaired renal function. Following an initial loading dose of 500 mg to 1 g IM or IV, the maintenance dosing schedule shown below should be followed. Further dosing should be determined by therapeutic monitoring, severity of the infection, and susceptibility of the causative organisms.

In patients undergoing hemodialysis, no additional supplemental dosing is required following hemodialysis; however, dosing should be timed so that the patient receives the dose (according to the table below) at the end of the dialysis.

Ceftizoxime dosing in patients with impaired renal function is as follows:

Mild impairment (Ccr 50 to 79 mL/min) – 500 mg every 8 hours; 0.75 g to 1.5 g every 8 hours for life-threatening infections.

Moderate to severe impairment (Ccr 5 to 49 mL/min) – 250 to 500 mg every 12 hours; 0.5 g to 1 g every 12 hours for life-threatening infections.

Patients receiving dialysis (Ccr less than 4 mL/min) – 500 mg every 48 hours or 250 mg every 24 hours; 0.5 g to 1 g every 48 hours, or 500 mg every 24 hours for life-threatening infections.

➤*Preparation of parenteral solution:* Reconstituted solutions may range from yellow to amber without changes in potency.

➤*Reconstitution:*

Pharmacy bulk vials – Pharmacy bulk vials are not for direct infusion. Reconstitute before use according to the following table using Sterile Water for Injection. Shake well. Add to parenteral fluids listed below under IV administration.

When 30 mL of diluent is added to a 10 g bulk vial, the approximate available volume is 37 mL, yielding an approximate concentration of 1 g in 3.5 mL. The stability of this solution at room temperature is 16 hours. When 45 mL of diluent is added to a 10 g bulk vial, the approximate available volume is 51 mL, yielding an approximate concentration of 1 g in 5 mL. The stability of this solution at room temperature is 24 hours.

These reconstituted solutions of ceftizoxime are stable for 96 hours if refrigerated (5°C; 41°F).

Pharmacy bulk packages – The container closure of the pharmacy bulk vial may be penetrated only one time after reconstitution, utilizing a suitable sterile transfer device or dispensing set which allows measured distribution of the contents. Since ceftizoxime is a sterile substance which must be reconstituted prior to use, a separate entry into the pharmacy bulk vial may be required. Use of ceftizoxime in pharmacy bulk vials is restricted to a suitable work area, such as a laminar flow hood.

The withdrawal of reconstituted transfer fluid from a pharmacy bulk vial should be accomplished without delay. However, if this is not possible, a maximum time of 4 hours from the initial introduction of the solvent, or diluent, into the pharmacy bulk vial is permitted to complete fluid transfer operations.

Although the ceftizoxime in the transfer fluid is stable for 16 or 24 hours at room temperature, depending on dilution (see Reconstitution) or 96 hours if refrigerated (5°C; 41°F), it is recommended that the transfer fluid/admixture be used promptly.

IM injection: Inject well within the body of a relatively large muscle. Aspiration is necessary to avoid inadvertent injection into a blood vessel. When administering 2 g IM doses, the dose should be divided and given in different large muscle masses.

IV administration: Direct (bolus) injection, slowly over 3 to 5 minutes, directly or through tubing for patients receiving parenteral fluids (see list below). Intermittent or continuous infusion, dilute reconstituted ceftizoxime in 50 to 100 mL of 1 of the following solutions:

- Sodium Chloride Injection.
- 5% or 10% Dextrose Injection.
- 5% Dextrose and 0.9%, 0.45%, or 0.2% Sodium Chloride Injection.
- Ringer's Injection.
- Lactated Ringer's Injection.
- Invert Sugar 10% in Sterile Water for Injection.
- 5% Sodium Bicarbonate in Sterile Water for Injection.
- 5% Dextrose in Lactated Ringer's Injection (only when reconstituted with 4% Sodium Bicarbonate Injection).

In these fluids, ceftizoxime is stable 24 hours at room temperature or 96 hours if refrigerated (5°C; 41°F).

➤*Storage/Stability:* Unreconstituted ceftizoxime should be protected from excessive light, and stored at controlled room temperature 15° to 30°C (59° to 86°F) in the original package until used.

CEFOTETAN DISODIUM

Rx	**Cefotan** (Zeneca)	**Powder for Injection:**[1] 1 g	In *ADD-Vantage* and piggyback vials.[2]
		2 g	In *ADD-Vantage* and piggyback vials.[2]
		10 g	In 100 ml vials
		Injection: 1 g/50 ml	Dextrose. Frozen, iso-osmotic, premixed. In 50 ml single-dose *Galaxy* containers.
		2 g/50 ml	Dextrose. Frozen, iso-osmotic, premixed. In 50 ml single-dose *Galaxy* containers.

[1] Contains 3.5 mEq sodium/g.
[2] Reconstitute only with sodium chloride 0.9% or dextrose injection 5% in the 50, 100 or 250 ml flexible diluent containers.

CEFOTETAN — INJECTION

For complete and comparative prescribing information, refer to the Cephalosporins group monograph.

Indications

➤*Urinary tract infections:* Caused by *E. coli*, *Klebsiella* sp. (including *K. pneumoniae*), *Proteus mirabilis* and *Proteus* sp. (which may include the organisms now called *Proteus vulgaris*, *Providencia rettgeri*, and *Morganella morganii*).

➤*Lower respiratory tract infections:* Caused by *Streptococcus pneumoniae*, *Staphylococcus aureus* (penicillinase- and non-penicillinase-producing strains), *Haemophilus influenzae* (including ampicillin-resistant strains), *Klebsiella* species (including *K. pneumoniae*), *E. coli*, *Proteus mirabilis*, and *Serratia marcescens* (efficacy for this organism in this organism system was studied in < 10 infections).

➤*Skin and skin structure infections:* Due to *Staphylococcus aureus* (penicillinase- and non-penicillinase-producing strains), *Staphylococcus epidermidis*, *Streptococcus pyogenes*, *Streptococcus* species (excluding enterococci), *Escherichia coli*, *Klebsiella pneumoniae*, *Peptococcus niger* (efficacy for this organism in this organism system was studied in < 10 infections), *Peptostreptococcus* species.

➤*Gynecologic infections:* Caused by *Staphylococcus aureus*, (including penicillinase- and non-penicillinase-producing strains), *Staphylococcus epidermidis*, *Streptococcus* species (excluding enterococci), *Streptococcus agalactiae*, *E. coli*, *Proteus mirabilis*, *Neisseria gonorrhoeae*, *Bacteroides* species (excluding *B. distasonis*, *B. ovatus*, *B. thetaiotaomicron*), *Fusobacterium* species (efficacy for this organism in this organism system was studied in < 10 infections), and gram-positive anaerobic cocci (including *Peptococcus* and *Peptostreptococcus* species).

Cefotetan, like other cephalosporins, has no activity against *Chlamydia trachomatis*. Therefore, when cephalosporins are used in the treatment of pelvic inflammatory disease, and *C. trachomatis* is 1 of the suspected pathogens, appropriate antichlamydial coverage should be added.

➤*Intra-abdominal infections:* Caused by *E. coli*, *Klebsiella* species (including *K. pneumoniae*), *Streptococcus* species (excluding enterococci), *Bacteroides* species (excluding *B. distasonis*, *B. ovatus*, *B. thetaiotaomicron*) and *Clostridium* species (efficacy for this organism in this organ system was studied in < 10 infections).

➤*Bone and joint infections:* Caused by *Staphylococcus aureus* (efficacy for this organism in this organ system was studied in < 10 infections).

CEFOTETAN — INJECTION

➤*Preoperative prophylaxis:* The preoperative administration of cefotetan may reduce the incidence of certain postoperative infections in patients undergoing surgical procedures that are classified as clean contaminated or potentially contaminated (eg, cesarean section, abdominal or vaginal hysterectomy, transurethral surgery, biliary tract surgery, and GI surgery).

Administration and Dosage

Cefotetan for injection in *Galaxy* plastic containers should not be used for IM administration.

Cefotetan in the *ADD-Vantage* vial is intended for IV infusion only, after dilution with the appropriate volume of *ADD-Vantage* diluent solution.

➤*Dosage:* The usual adult dosage is 1 or 2 g of cefotetan disodium for injection administered IV or IM or cefotetan injection in the *Galaxy* plastic container (PL 2040) administered IV every 12 hours for 5 to 10 days. Proper dosage and route of administration should be determined by the condition of the patient, severity of the infection, and susceptibility of the causative organism.

General guidelines for dosage of cefotetan		
Type of infection	Daily dose	Frequency and route
Urinary tract	1 to 4 g	500 mg every 12 hours IV or IM
		1 or 2 g every 24 hours IV or IM
Skin and skin structure		
Mild to moderate[a]	2 g	2 g every 24 hours IV
		1 g every 12 hours IV or IM
Severe	4 g	2 g every 12 hours IV
Other sites	2 to 4 g	1 or 2 g every 12 hours IV or IM
Severe	4 g	2 g every 12 hours IV
Life-threatening	6 g[b]	3 g every 12 hour IV

[a] *Klebsiella pneumoniae* skin and skin structure infections should be treated with 1 or 2 g every 12 hours IV or IM.

[b] If *Chlamydia trachomatis* is a suspected pathogen in gynecologic infections, appropriate antichlamydial coverage should be added, since cefotetan has no activity against this organism.

➤*Prophylaxis:* To prevent postoperative infection in clean contaminated or potentially contaminated surgery in adults, the recommended dosage is 1 or 2 g of cefotetan administered once, IV, 30 to 60 minutes prior to surgery. In patients undergoing cesarean section, the dose should be administered as soon as the umbilical cord is clamped.

➤*Renal function impairment:* When renal function is impaired, a reduced dosage schedule must be employed. In the following table, dose is determined by the type and severity of infection, and susceptibility of the causative organism.

Dosage guidelines for patients with impaired renal function		
Creatinine clearance (mL/min)	Dose	Frequency
> 30	Usual recommended dosage*	Every 12 hours
10 to 30	Usual recommended dosage*	Every 24 hours
< 10	Usual recommended dosage*	Every 48 hours

* Dose determined by the type and severity of infection, and susceptibility of the causative organism.

Alternatively, the dosing interval may remain constant at 12-hour intervals, but the dose reduced to one-half the usual recommended dose for patients with a creatinine clearance of 10 to 30 mL/min, and one-quarter the usual recommended dose for patients with a creatinine clearance of < 10 mL/min.

Hemodialysis – Cefotetan is dialyzable and it is recommended that for patients undergoing intermittent hemodialysis, one-fourth of the usual recommended dose be given every 24 hours on days between dialysis and one-half the usual recommended dose on the day of dialysis.

➤*IV administration:* The IV route is preferable for patients with bacteremia, bacterial septicemia, or other severe or life-threatening infections, or for patients who may be poor risks because of lowered resistance resulting from such debilitating conditions as malnutrition, trauma, surgery, diabetes, heart failure, or malignancy, particularly if shock is present or impending.

Intermittent IV administration – For intermittent IV administration, a solution containing 1 or 2 g of cefotetan disodium for injection in Sterile Water for Injection can be injected over a period of 3 to 5 minutes. Using an infusion system, the solution may also be given over a longer period of time through the tubing system by which the patient may be receiving other IV solutions. *Butterfly* or scalp vein-type needles are preferred for this type of infusion. However, during infusion of the solution containing cefotetan disodium for injection, it is advisable to discontinue temporarily the administration of other solutions at the same site.

Galaxy containers – Using an infusion system, cefotetan injection in *Galaxy* plastic container (PL 2040) should be given over 20 to 60 minutes through the tubing system by which the patient may be receiving other IV solutions. *Butterfly* or scalp vein-type needles are preferred for this type of infusion. However, during infusion of the solution containing cefotetan injection in *Galaxy* plastic container (PL 2040), it is advisable to discontinue temporarily the administration of other solutions at the same site.

➤*IM administration:* As with all IM preparations, cefotetan disodium for injection should be injected well within the body of a relatively large muscle such as the upper outer quadrant of the buttock (ie, gluteus maximus); aspiration is necessary to avoid inadvertent injection into a blood vessel.

➤*Admixture incompatibility:* Solutions of cefotetan must not be admixed with solutions containing aminoglycosides. If cefotetan and aminoglycosides are to be administered to the same patient, they must be administered separately and not as a mixed injection. Do not add supplementary medications.

➤*Preparation of solution:*

IV – Reconstitute with Sterile Water for Injection. Shake to dissolve and let stand until clear.

Vial size	Amount of diluent added (mL)	Approximate withdrawable volume (mL)	Approximate average concentration (mg/mL)
1 g	10	10.5	95
2 g	10 to 20	11 to 21	182 to 95

Infusion bottles (100 mL) may be reconstituted with 50 to 100 mL of Dextrose Injection 5% or Sodium Chloride Injection 0.9%. Note: *ADD-Vantage* vials are not to be used in this manner.

ADD-Vantage vials – *ADD-Vantage* vials of cefotetan are to be reconstituted only with Sodium Chloride Injection 0.9% or Dextrose Injection 5% in the 50, 100 or 250 mL flexible diluent containers. Cefotetan supplied in single-use *ADD-Vantage* vials should be prepared as directed.

➤*IM:* Reconstitute with Sterile Water for Injection; Bacteriostatic Water for Injection; Sodium Chloride Injection 0.9%, USP; 0.5% Lidocaine HCl; or 1% Lidocaine HCl. Shake to dissolve and let stand until clear.

Vial size	Amount of diluent added (mL)	Approximate withdrawable volume (mL)	Approximate average concentration (mg/mL)
1 g	2	2.5	400
2 g	3	4	500

➤*Galaxy containers:* Cefotetan injection in *Galaxy* plastic container (PL 2040) is for IV administration only.

Store in a freezer capable of maintaining a temperature of −20°C (−4°F).

Thaw frozen container at room temperature (25°C; 77°F) or in a refrigerator (5°C; 41°F). [Do not force thaw by immersion in water baths or by microwave irradiation.]

➤*Compatibility and stability of cefotetan products:* Frozen samples should be thawed at room temperature before use. After the periods mentioned below, any unused solutions or frozen material should be discarded. Do not refreeze.

➤*Storage/Stability:* Store containers at or below −20°C (−4°F). [See Administration and Dosage, Directions for use of cefotetan injection in *Galaxy* plastic container (PL 2040)].

Cefotetan disodium for injection – Cefotetan disodium for injection reconstituted as described above (see Administration and Dosage, Preparation of solution) maintains satisfactory potency for 24 hours at room temperature (25°C; 77°F), for 96 hours under refrigeration (5°C; 41°F), and for at least 1 week in the frozen state (−20°C; −4°F). After reconstitution and subsequent storage in disposable glass or plastic syringes, cefotetan disodium for injection is stable for 24 hours at room temperature and 96 hours under refrigeration.

ADD-Vantage vials – Ordinarily, *ADD-Vantage* vials should be reconstituted only when it is certain that the patient is ready to receive the drug. However, *ADD-Vantage* vials of cefotetan reconstituted as described in Administration and Dosage, Preparation of solution for *ADD-Vantage* vials, maintain satisfactory potency for 24 hours at room temperature (25°C; 77°F). (Do not refrigerate or freeze cefotetan in *ADD-Vantage* vials.)

Cefotetan injection – The thawed solution in *Galaxy* plastic container (PL 2040) remains chemically stable for 48 hours at room temperature (25°C; 77°F) or for 21 days under refrigeration (5°C; 41°F).

CEFTAZIDIME

Rx	**Fortaz** (GlaxoWellcome)	**Powder for Injection:** 500 mg	In vials.[1]
Rx	**Ceptaz** (GlaxoWellcome)	**Powder for Injection:** 1 g	In vials and infusion packs.[2]
Rx	**Fortaz** (GlaxoWellcome)		In vials, *ADD-Vantage* vials and infusion packs.[1]
Rx	**Tazicef** (SmithKline Beecham/Bristol-Myers Squibb)		In vials, *ADD-Vantage* vials and piggyback vials.[1]
Rx	**Tazidime** (Eli Lilly)		In 20 ml, 100 ml and *ADD-Vantage* vials.[2]
Rx	**Ceptaz** (GlaxoWellcome)	**Powder for Injection:** 2 g	In vials and infusion packs.[2]
Rx	**Fortaz** (GlaxoWellcome)		In vials, *ADD-Vantage* vials and infusion packs.[1]
Rx	**Tazicef** (SmithKline Beecham/Bristol-Myers Squibb)		In vials, *ADD-Vantage* vials and piggyback vials.[1]
Rx	**Tazidime** (Eli Lilly)		In 50 ml, 100 ml and *ADD-Vantage* vials.[2]
Rx	**Fortaz** (GlaxoWellcome)	**Powder for Injection:** 6 g	In bulk package.[1]
Rx	**Tazicef** (SmithKline Beecham/Bristol-Myers Squibb)		In bulk package.[1]
Rx	**Tazidime** (Eli Lilly)		In 100 ml vial.[2]
Rx	**Fortaz** (GlaxoWellcome)	**Injection:** 1 g	Premixed, frozen. In 50 ml.[3]
		2 g	Premixed, frozen. In 50 ml.[4]
Rx	**Tazicef** (SmithKline Beecham/Bristol-Myers Squibb)	**Injection:** 1 g	In *Galaxy* containers.
		2 g	In *Galaxy* containers.

[1] Contains 2.3 mEq sodium/g.
[2] As pentahydrate with L-arginine.
[3] With 2.2 g dextrose hydrous.
[4] With 1.6 g dextrose hydrous.

CEFTAZIDIME — INJECTION

For complete and comparative prescribing information, refer to the Cephalosporins group monograph.

Indications

➤*Lower respiratory tract infections:* Including pneumonia, caused by *Pseudomonas aeruginosa* and other *Pseudomonas* spp.; *Haemophilus influenzae*, including ampicillin-resistant strains; *Klebsiella* spp.; *Enterobacter* spp.; *Proteus mirabilis*; *Escherichia coli*; *Serratia* spp.; *Citrobacter* spp.; *Streptococcus pneumoniae*; and *Staphylococcus aureus* (methicillin-susceptible strains).

➤*Skin and skin-structure infections:* Caused by *Pseudomonas aeruginosa*; *Klebsiella* spp.; *Escherichia coli*; *Proteus* spp.; including *Proteus mirabilis* and indole-positive *Proteus*; *Enterobacter* spp.; *Serratia* spp.; *Staphylococcus aureus* (methicillin-susceptible strains); and *Streptococcus pyogenes* (group A beta-hemolytic streptococci).

➤*Urinary tract infections, complicated and uncomplicated:* Caused by *Pseudomonas aeruginosa*; *Enterobacter* spp.; *Proteus* spp., including *Proteus mirabilis* and indole-positive *Proteus*; *Klebsiella* spp.; and *Escherichia coli*.

➤*Bacterial septicemia:* Caused by *Pseudomonas aeruginosa*, *Klebsiella* spp., *Haemophilus influenzae*, *Escherichia coli*, *Serratia* spp., *Streptococcus pneumoniae*, and *Staphylococcus aureus* (methicillin-susceptible strains).

➤*Bone and joint Infections:* Caused by *Pseudomonas aeruginosa*, *Klebsiella* spp., *Enterobacter* spp., and *Staphylococcus aureus* (methicillin-susceptible strains).

➤*Gynecologic infections:* Including endometritis, pelvic cellulitis, and other infections of the female genital tract caused by *Escherichia coli*.

➤*Intra-abdominal infections:* Including peritonitis caused by *Escherichia coli*, *Klebsiella* spp., and *Staphylococcus aureus* (methicillin-susceptible strains) and polymicrobial infections caused by aerobic and anaerobic organisms and *Bacteroides* spp. (many strains of *Bacteroides fragilis* are resistant).

➤*CNS infections:* Including meningitis, caused by *Haemophilus influenzae* and *Neisseria meningitidis*. Ceftazidime has also been used successfully in a limited number of cases of meningitis due to *Pseudomonas aeruginosa* and *Streptococcus pneumoniae*.

➤*Concomitant therapy:* Ceftazidime may also be used concomitantly with other antibiotics, such as aminoglycosides, vancomycin, and clindamycin; in severe and life-threatening infections; and in the immunocompromised patient. When such concomitant treatment is appropriate, prescribing information in the labeling for the other antibiotics should be followed. The dose depends on the severity of the infection and the patient's condition.

Administration and Dosage

➤*Approved by the FDA:* July 19, 1985.

➤*Dosage:* The usual adult dosage is 1 g administered IV or IM every 8 to 12 hours. The dosage and route should be determined by the susceptibility of the causative organisms, the severity of infection, and the condition and renal function of the patient.

Recommended dosage schedule		
	Dose	Frequency
Adults		
Usual recommended dosage	1 g IV or IM	every 8 to 12 hours
Uncomplicated urinary tract infections	250 mg IV or IM	every 12 hours

Recommended dosage schedule		
	Dose	Frequency
Bone and joint infections	2 g IV	every 12 hours
Complicated urinary tract infections	500 mg IV or IM	every 8 to 12 hours
Uncomplicated pneumonia; mild skin and skin-structure infections	500 mg to 1 g IV or IM	every 8 hours
Serious gynecologic and intra-abdominal infections	2 g IV	every 8 hours
Meningitis	2 g IV	every 8 hours
Very severe life-threatening infections, especially in immunocompromised patients	2 g IV	every 8 hours
Lung infections caused by *Pseudomonas* spp. in patients with cystic fibrosis with healthy renal function*	30 to 50 mg/kg IV to a maximum of 6 g per day	every 8 hours
Neonates (0 to 4 weeks)	30 mg/kg IV	every 12 hours
Infants and children (1 month to 12 years)	30 to 50 mg/kg IV to a maximum of 6 g per day**	every 8 hours

* Although clinical improvement has been shown, bacteriologic cures cannot be expected in patients with chronic respiratory disease and cystic fibrosis.
** The higher dose should be reserved for immunocompromised pediatric patients or pediatric patients with cystic fibrosis or meningitis.

➤*Renal function impairment:* Ceftazidime is excreted by the kidneys, almost exclusively by glomerular filtration. Therefore, in patients with impaired renal function (glomerular filtration rate [GFR] less than 50 mL/min), it is recommended that the dosage of ceftazidime be reduced to compensate for its slower excretion. In patients with suspected renal insufficiency, an initial loading dose of 1 g of ceftazidime may be given. An estimate of GFR should be made to determine the appropriate maintenance dosage. The recommended dosages are presented in the table below.

If the dose recommended in the table above is lower than that recommended for patients with renal insufficiency as outlined in the table below, the lower dose should be used.

Creatinine clearance (mL/min)	Recommended unit dose of ceftazidime	Frequency of dosing
50 to 31	1 g	every 12 hours
30 to 16	1 g	every 24 hours
15 to 6	500 mg	every 24 hours
< 5	500 mg	every 48 hours

In patients with severe infections who would normally receive 6 g ceftazidime daily were it not for renal insufficiency, the unit dose given in the infor-

CEFTAZIDIME — INJECTION

mation above for maintenance dosing in renal insufficiency may be increased by 50% or the dosing frequency may be increased appropriately. Further dosing should be determined by therapeutic monitoring, severity of the infection, and susceptibility of the causative organism.

In pediatric patients as for adults, the creatinine clearance should be adjusted for body surface area or lean body mass, and the dosing frequency should be reduced in cases of renal insufficiency.

Dialysis – In patients undergoing hemodialysis, a loading dose of 1 g is recommended, followed by 1 g after each hemodialysis period.

Ceftazidime can also be used in patients undergoing intraperitoneal dialysis and continuous ambulatory peritoneal dialysis. In such patients, a loading dose of 1 g of ceftazidime may be given, followed by 500 mg every 24 hours. In addition to IV use, ceftazidime can be incorporated in the dialysis fluid at a concentration of 250 mg for 2 L of dialysis fluid.

➤*Preparation for administration:* Ceftazidime may be given IV or by deep IM injection into a large muscle mass such as the upper outer quadrant of the gluteus maximus or lateral part of the thigh. Intra-arterial administration should be avoided (see Precautions).

IM administration – For IM administration, ceftazidime should be constituted with one of the following diluents: Sterile Water for Injection, Bacteriostatic Water for Injection, or 0.5% or 1% Lidocaine Hydrochloride Injection.

IV administration – The IV route is preferable for patients with bacterial septicemia, bacterial meningitis, peritonitis, or other severe or life-threatening infections, or for patients who may be poor risks because of lowered resistance resulting from such debilitating conditions as malnutrition, trauma, surgery, diabetes, heart failure, or malignancy, particularly if shock is present or pending.

Intermittent IV administration: Reconstitute ceftazidime as directed below with Sterile Water for Injection. Slowly inject directly into the vein over a period of 3 to 5 minutes or give through the tubing of an administration set while the patient is also receiving one of the compatible IV fluids (see Storage/Stability).

IV infusion: Reconstitute the 1 gram infusion pack with 100 mL of Sterile Water for Injection or one of the compatible IV fluids listed under the Storage/Stability section. Alternatively, constitute the 500 mg, 1 or 2 gram vial and add an appropriate quantity of the resulting solution to an IV container with one of the compatible IV fluids.

Intermittent IV infusion: Intermittent IV infusion with a Y-type administration set can be accomplished with compatible solutions. However, during infusion of a solution containing ceftazidime, it is desirable to discontinue the other solution.

ADD-Vantage vials are to be constituted only with 50 or 100 mL of 5% Dextrose Injection, 0.9% Sodium Chloride Injection, or 0.45% Sodium Chloride Injection in Abbott *ADD-Vantage* flexible diluent containers (see Instructions for constitution). *ADD-Vantage* vials that have been joined to Abbott *ADD-Vantage* diluent containers and activated to dissolve the drug are stable for 24 hours at room temperature or for 7 days under refrigeration. Joined vials that have not been activated may be used within a 14-day period; this period corresponds to that for use of Abbott *ADD-Vantage* containers following removal of the outer packaging (overwrap).

Freezing solutions of ceftazidime in the *ADD-Vantage* system is not recommended.

➤*Admixture incompatibility:* Solutions of ceftazidime, like those of most beta-lactam antibiotics, should not be added to solutions of aminoglycoside antibiotics because of potential interaction.

However, if concurrent therapy with ceftazidime and an aminoglycoside is indicated, each of these antibiotics can be administered separately to the same patient.

➤*Galaxy containers:* Ceftazidime supplied as a frozen, sterile, iso-osmotic, nonpyrogenic solution in plastic containers is to be administered after thawing either as a continuous or intermittent IV infusion. The thawed solution is stable for 24 hours at room temperature or for 7 days if stored under refrigeration. Do not refreeze.

Thaw container at room temperature (25°C; 77°F) or under refrigeration (5°C; 41°F). Do not force thaw by immersion in water baths or by microwave irradiation. Components of the solution may precipitate in the frozen state and will dissolve upon reaching room temperature with little or no agitation. Potency is not affected. Mix after solution has reached room temperature. Check for minute leaks by squeezing bag firmly. Discard bag if leaks are found as sterility may be impaired. Do not add supplementary medication. Do not use unless solution is clear and seal is intact.

➤*Storage / Stability:*

IM – Ceftazidime, when constituted as directed with Sterile Water for Injection, Bacteriostatic Water for Injection, or 0.5% or 1% Lidocaine Hydrochloride Injection, maintains satisfactory potency for 24 hours at room temperature or for 7 days under refrigeration. Solutions in Sterile Water for Injection that are frozen immediately after constitution in the original container are stable for 3 months when stored at -20°C (-4°F). Once thawed, solutions should not be refrozen. Thawed solutions may be stored for up to 8 hours at room temperature or for 4 days in a refrigerator.

IV – Ceftazidime, when constituted as directed with Sterile Water for Injection, maintains satisfactory potency for 24 hours at room temperature or for 7 days under refrigeration. Solutions in Sterile Water for Injection in the infusion vial or in 0.9% Sodium Chloride Injection in *Viaflex* small-volume containers that are frozen immediately after constitution are stable for 6 months when stored at -20°C (-4°F). Do not force thaw by immersion in water baths or by microwave irradiation. Once thawed, solutions should not be refrozen. Thawed solutions may be stored for up to 24 hours at room temperature or for 7 days in a refrigerator. More concentrated solutions in Sterile Water for Injection in the original container that are frozen immediately after constitution are stable for 3 months when stored at -20°C (-4°F). Once thawed, solutions should not be refrozen. Thawed solutions may be stored for up to 8 hours at room temperature or for 4 days in a refrigerator.

Ceftazidime is compatible with the more commonly used IV infusion fluids. Solutions at concentrations between 1 and 40 mg/mL in 0.9% Sodium Chloride Injection; 1/6 M Sodium Lactate Injection; 5% Dextrose Injection; 5% Dextrose and 0.225% Sodium Chloride Injection; 5% Dextrose and 0.45% Sodium Chloride Injection; 5% Dextrose and 0.9% Sodium Chloride Injection; 10% Dextrose Injection; Ringer's Injection, USP; Lactated Ringer's Injection, USP; 10% Invert Sugar in Water for Injection; and *Normosol-M* in 5% Dextrose Injection may be stored for up to 24 hours at room temperature or for 7 days if refrigerated.

The 1- and 2-g ceftazidime *ADD-Vantage* vials, when diluted in 50 or 100 mL of 5% Dextrose Injection, 0.9% Sodium Chloride Injection, or 0.45% Sodium Chloride Injection, may be stored for up to 24 hours at room temperature or for 7 days under refrigeration.

Ceftazidime is less stable in Sodium Bicarbonate Injection than in other IV fluids. It is not recommended as a diluent. Solutions of ceftazidime in 5% Dextrose Injection and 0.9% Sodium Chloride Injection are stable for at least 6 hours at room temperature in plastic tubing, drip chambers, and volume control devices of common IV infusion sets.

Ceftazidime at a concentration of 4 mg/mL has been found compatible for 24 hours at room temperature or for 7 days under refrigeration in 0.9% Sodium Chloride Injection or 5% Dextrose Injection when admixed with: Cefuroxime sodium 3 mg/mL; heparin 10 or 50 U/mL; or potassium chloride 10 or 40 mEq/L.

As with other cephalosporins, ceftazidime powder as well as solutions tend to darken, depending on storage conditions; within the stated recommendations, however, product potency is not adversely affected.

Ceftazidime in the dry state should be stored between 15° and 30°C (59° and 86°F) and protected from light.

CEFEPIME HYDROCHLORIDE

Rx	**Maxipime** (Dura)	**Powder for Injection:**[1] 500 mg	In 15 ml vial.
		1 g	In 15 ml vials, *ADD-Vantage* vials, and 100 ml piggyback bottles.
		2 g	In 20 ml vials, *ADD-Vantage* vials, and 100 ml piggyback bottles.

[1] Contains arginine.

CEFEPIME HYDROCHLORIDE — INJECTION

For complete and comparative prescribing information, refer to the Cephalosporins group monograph.

Indications

➤*Pneumonia (moderate to severe):* Caused by *Streptococcus pneumoniae*, including cases associated with concurrent bacteremia, *Pseudomonas aeruginosa*, *Klebsiella pneumoniae*, or *Enterobacter* species.

➤*Empiric therapy for febrile neutropenic patients:* As monotherapy for empiric treatment of febrile neutropenic patients. In patients at high risk for severe infection (including patients with a history of recent bone marrow transplantation, with hypotension at presentation, with an underlying hematologic malignancy, or with severe or prolonged neutropenia), antimicrobial monotherapy may not be appropriate. Insufficient data exist to support the efficacy of cefepime monotherapy in such patients.

➤*Uncomplicated and complicated urinary tract infections (including pyelonephritis):* Caused by *Escherichia coli* or *Klebsiella pneumoniae*, when the infection is severe, or caused by *Escherichia coli*, *Klebsiella pneumoniae*, or *Proteus mirabilis*, when the infection is mild to moderate, including cases associated with concurrent bacteremia with these microorganisms.

➤*Uncomplicated skin and skin structure infections:* Caused by *Staphylococcus aureus* (methicillin-susceptible strains only) or *Streptococcus pyogenes*.

➤*Complicated intra-abdominal infections (used in combination with metronidazole):* Caused by *Escherichia coli*, viridans group streptococci, *Pseudomonas aeruginosa*, *Klebsiella pneumoniae*, *Enterobacter* species, or *Bacteroides fragilis*.

Administration and Dosage

➤*Approved by the FDA:* January 18, 1996.

CEFEPIME HYDROCHLORIDE — INJECTION

Cefepime should be administered IV over approximately 30 minutes.

Recommended dosage schedule for cefepime in patients with Ccr greater than 60 mL/min			
Site and type of infection	Dose	Frequency	Duration (days)
Adults			
Moderate to severe pneumonia due to *S. pneumoniae*,[1] *P. aeruginosa*, *K. pneumoniae*, or *Enterobacter* species	1 to 2 g IV	q12h	10
Empiric therapy for febrile neutropenic patients	2 g IV	q8h	7[2]
Mild to moderate uncomplicated or complicated urinary tract infections, including pyelonephritis, due to *E. coli*, *K. pneumoniae*, or *P. mirabilis*[1]	0.5 to 1 g IV/IM[3]	q12h	7 to 10
Severe uncomplicated or complicated UTIs, including pyelonephritis, due to *E. coli* or *K. pneumoniae*[1]	2 g IV	q12h	10
Moderate to severe uncomplicated skin and skin structure infections due to *S. aureus* or *S. pyogenes*	2 g IV	q12h	10
Complicated intra-abdominal infections (used in combination with metronidazole) caused by *E. coli*, viridans group streptococci, *P. aeruginosa*, *K. pneumoniae*, *Enterobacter* species, or *B. fragilis*	2 g IV	q12h	7 to 10
Pediatric patients (2 months up to 16 years): The maximum dose for pediatric patients should not exceed the recommended adult dose. The usual recommended dosage in pediatric patients up to 40 kg in weight for uncomplicated and complicated urinary tract infections (including pyelonephritis), uncomplicated skin and skin structure infections, and pneumonia is 50 mg/kg/dose, administered every 12 hours (50 mg/kg/dose, every 8 hours for febrile neutropenic patients), for durations as given above.			

[1] Including cases associated with concurrent bacteremia.
[2] Or until resolution of neutropenia. In patients whose fever resolves but who remain neutropenic for more than 7 days, the need for continued antimicrobial therapy should be reevaluated frequently.
[3] IM route of administration is indicated only for mild to moderate, uncomplicated, or complicated UTIs due to *E. coli* when the IM route is considered to be a more appropriate route of drug administration.

➤*Renal function impairment:* In patients with impaired renal function (creatinine clearance less than or equal to 60 mL/min), the dose of cefepime should be adjusted to compensate for the slower rate of renal elimination. The recommended initial dose of cefepime should be the same as in patients with healthy renal function except in patients undergoing hemodialysis. The recommended doses of cefepime in patients with renal insufficiency are presented below.

Recommended dosing schedule for cefepime in adult patients (healthy renal function, renal insufficiency, and hemodialysis)				
Ccr (mL/min)	Recommended maintenance schedule			
> 60 normal recommended dosing schedule	500 mg q12h	1 g q12h	2 g q12h	2 g q8h
30 to 60	500 mg q24h	1 g q24h	2 g q24h	2 g q12h
11 to 29	500 mg q24h	500 mg q24h	1 g q24h	2 g q24h
< 11	250 mg q24h	250 mg q24h	500 mg q24h	1 g q24h
CAPD	500 mg q48h	1 g q48h	2 g q48h	2 g q48h
Hemodialysis[1]	1 g on Day 1, then 500 mg q24h thereafter			1 g q24h

[1] On hemodialysis days, cefepime should be administered following hemodialysis. Whenever possible, cefepime should be administered at the same time each day.

In patients undergoing continuous ambulatory peritoneal dialysis (CAPD), cefepime may be administered at normally recommended doses at a dosage interval of every 48 hours. The recommended maintenance schedule based on previously mentioned site and type of infection (see information above) is either 500 mg every 48 hours, 1 g every 48 hours, 2 g every 48 hours, or 2 g every 48 hours.

➤*Dialysis:* In patients undergoing hemodialysis, approximately 68% of the total amount of cefepime present in the body at the start of dialysis will be removed during a 3-hour dialysis period. The dosage of cefepime for hemodialysis patients is 1 g on day 1 followed by 500 mg every 24 hours for the treatment of all infections except febrile neutropenia, which is 1 g every 24 hours. Cefepime should be administered at the same time each day and following the completion of hemodialysis on hemodialysis days.

➤*Children:* Data in pediatric patients with impaired renal function are not available; however, since cefepime pharmacokinetics are similar in adults and pediatric patients, changes in the dosing regimen proportional to those in adults (see previous information) are recommended for pediatric patients.

➤*IV Administration:* For IV infusion, constitute the 1 or 2 g piggyback (100 mL) bottle with 50 or 100 mL of a compatible IV fluid listed in Compatibility and stability. Alternatively, constitute the 500 mg, 1 or 2 g vial, and add an appropriate quantity of the resulting solution to an IV container with one of the compatible IV fluids. The resulting solution should be administered over approximately 30 minutes.

Intermittent IV infusion with a Y-type administration set can be accomplished with compatible solutions. However, during infusion of a solution containing cefepime HCl, it is desirable to discontinue the other solution.

ADD-Vantage vials are to be constituted only with 50 or 100 mL of 5% Dextrose injection or 0.9% Sodium Chloride Injection in Abbott *ADD-Vantage* flexible diluent containers. (See *ADD-Vantage* vial instructions for use.)

➤*IM administration:* For IM administration, cefepime should be constituted with 1 of the following diluents: Sterile Water for Injection, 0.9% Sodium Chloride, 5% Dextrose Injection, 0.5% or 1% Lidocaine HCl, or Sterile Bacteriostatic Water for Injection with parabens or benzyl alcohol.

➤*Storage/Stability:* Cefepime in the dry state should be stored between 2° to 25°C (36° to 77°F) and protected from light.

Compatibility and stability –

IV: Cefepime is compatible at concentrations between 1 and 40 mg/mL with the following IV infusion fluids: 0.9% Sodium Chloride Injection, 5% and 10% Dextrose injection, M/6 Sodium Lactate injection, 5% Dextrose and 0.9% Sodium Chloride injection, Lactated Ringers and 5% Dextrose injection, *Normosol-R*, and *Normosol-M* in 5% Dextrose injection. These solutions may be stored up to 24 hours at controlled room temperature 20° to 25°C (68° to 77°F) or 7 days in a refrigerator 2° to 8°C (36° to 46°F). Cefepime in *ADD-Vantage* vials is stable at concentrations of 10 to 40 mg/mL in 5% Dextrose injection or 0.9% Sodium Chloride injection for 24 hours at controlled room temperature 20° to 25°C (68° to 77°F) or 7 days in a refrigerator 2° to 8°C (36° to 46°F).

Cefepime admixture stability				
			Stability time for	
Cefepime concentration	Admixture and concentration	IV infusion solutions	RT/L[a] (20° to 25°C; 68° to 77°F)	Refrigeration (2° to 8°C; 36° to 46°F)
40 mg/mL	Amikacin 6 mg/mL	NS[b] or D5W[c]	24 hours	7 days
40 mg/mL	Ampicillin 1 mg/mL	D5W[c]	8 hours	8 hours
40 mg/mL	Ampicillin 10 mg/mL	D5W[c]	2 hours	8 hours
40 mg/mL	Ampicillin 1 mg/mL	NS[b]	24 hours	48 hours
40 mg/mL	Ampicillin 10 mg/mL	NS[b]	8 hours	48 hours
4 mg/mL	Ampicillin 40 mg/mL	NS[b]	8 hours	8 hours
4 to 40 mg/mL	Clindamycin phosphate 0.25 to 6 mg/ml	NS[b] or D5W[c]	24 hours	7 days
4 mg/mL	Heparin 10 to 50 units/mL	NS[b] or D5W[c]	24 hours	7 days
4 mg/mL	Potassium chloride 10 to 40 mEq/L	NS[b] or D5W[c]	24 hours	7 days
4 mg/mL	Theophylline 0.8 mg/mL	D5W[c]	24 hours	7 days
1 to 4 mg/mL	na[d]	*Aminosyn* II 4.25% with electrolytes and calcium	8 hours	3 days
0.125 to 0.25 mg/mL	na[d]	*Inpersol* with 4.25% dextrose	24 hours	7 days

[a] RT/L = ambient room temperature and light
[b] NS = 0.9% sodium chloride injection
[c] D5W = 5% dextrose injection
[d] na = not applicable

Admixture incompatibility: Solutions of cefepime HCl, like those of most beta-lactam antibiotics, should not be added to solutions of ampicillin at a concentration greater than 40 mg/mL, and should not be added to metronidazole, vancomycin, gentamicin, tobramycin, netilmicin sulfate or amino-

CEFEPIME HYDROCHLORIDE — INJECTION

phylline because of potential interaction. However, if concurrent therapy with cefepime is indicated, each of these antibiotics can be administered separately.

IM: Cefepime constituted as directed is stable for 24 hours at controlled room temperature 20° to 25°C (68° to 77°F) or for 7 days in a refrigerator 2° to 8°C (36° to 46°F) with the following diluents: Sterile Water for injection, 0.9% Sodium Chloride injection, 5% Dextrose injection, Sterile Bacteriostatic Water for injection with parabens or benzyl alcohol, or 0.5% or 1% lidocaine HCl.

As with other cephalosporins, the color of cefepime powder, as well as its solutions, tend to darken depending on storage conditions; however, when stored as recommended, the product potency is not adversely affected.

CEFDITOREN PIVOXIL

Rx	**Spectracef** (Purdue)	**Tablets:** 200 mg cefditoren (as cefditoren pivoxil)	Mannitol. (TAP 200 mg). White, elliptical. Film-coated. In 20s and 60s.

CEFDITOREN PIVOXIL — ORAL

For complete and comparative prescribing information, refer to the Cephalosporins group monograph.

Indications

For the treatment of mild-to-moderate infections in adults and adolescents (12 years of age or older) that are caused by susceptible strains of the designated microorganisms in the following conditions:

➤*Acute bacterial exacerbation of chronic bronchitis:* Caused by *Haemophilus influenzae* (including β-lactamase-producing strains), *Haemophilus parainfluenzae* (including β-lactamase-producing strains), *Streptococcus pneumoniae* (penicillin-susceptible strains only), or *Moraxella catarrhalis* (including β-lactamase-producing strains).

➤*Community-acquired pneumonia:* Caused by *Haemophilus influenzae* (including β-lactamase-producing strains), *Haemophilus parainfluenzae* (including β-lactamase-producing strains), *Streptococcus pneumoniae* (penicillin-susceptible strains only), or *Moraxella catarrhalis* (including β-lactamase-producing strains).

➤*Pharyngitis/tonsillitis:* Caused by *Streptococcus pyogenes.*

➤*Uncomplicated skin and skin-structure infections:* Caused by *Staphylococcus aureus* (including β-lactamase-producing strains) or *Streptococcus pyogenes.*

Administration and Dosage

➤*Approved by the FDA:* August 29, 2001.

Take cefditoren with meals..

Cefditoren Dosage and Administration in Adults and Adolescents (≥ 12 Years of Age)

Type of infection	Dosage	Duration (days)
Community-acquired pneumonia	400 mg twice daily	14
Acute bacterial exacerbation of chronic bronchitis	400 mg twice daily	10
Pharyngitis/Tonsillitis	200 mg twice daily	
Uncomplicated skin and skin structure infections		

➤*Renal function impairment:* No dose adjustment is necessary for patients with mild renal impairment (Ccr, 50 to 80 mL/min/1.73 m^2). It is recommended that not more than 200 mg twice daily be administered to patients with moderate renal impairment (Ccr, 30 to 49 mL/min/1.73 m^2) and 200 mg once daily be administered to patients with severe renal impairment (Ccr, less than 30 mL/min/1.73 m^2). The appropriate dose in patients with end-stage renal disease has not been determined.

➤*Storage/Stability:* Store at 25°C (77°F); excursions permitted to 15° to 30°C (59° to 86°F). Protect from light and moisture. Dispense in a tight, light-resistant container.

CARBAPENEM

MEROPENEM

Rx	**Merrem I.V.** (AstraZeneca)	**Powder for injection:** 500 mg	In 20 and 30 mL vials.
		1 g	In 20 and 30 mL vials.

MEROPENEM — INJECTION

Indications

➤*Bacterial meningitis (pediatric patients 3 months of age and older only):* Bacterial meningitis caused by *Streptococcus pneumoniae*†, *Haemophilus influenzae* (β-lactamase and non-β-lactamase-producing isolates), and *Neisseria meningitidis.*

Meropenem has been found to be effective in eliminating concurrent bacteremia in association with bacterial meningitis.

➤*Intra-abdominal infections:* Complicated appendicitis and peritonitis caused by viridans group streptococci, *Escherichia coli, Klebsiella pneumoniae, Pseudomonas aeruginosa, Bacteroides fragilis, Bacteroides thetaiotaomicron,* and *Peptostreptococcus* species.

➤*Skin and skin structure infections (SSSIs):* Complicated SSSIs caused by *Staphylococcus aureus* (β-lactamase and non-β-lactamase-producing, methicillin-susceptible isolates only), *Streptococcus pyogenes, Streptococcus agalactiae,* viridans group streptococci, *Enterococcus faecalis* (excluding vancomycin-resistant isolates), *P. aeruginosa, E. coli, Proteus mirabilis, B. fragilis,* and *Peptostreptococcus* species.

➤*Unlabeled uses:* Empiric therapy in febrile neutropenic patients; community-acquired pneumonia.

Administration and Dosage

➤*Approved by the FDA:* June 2, 1996.

➤*Adults:* Meropenem should be administered by intravenous (IV) infusion over approximately 15 to 30 minutes. Doses of 1 g may also be administered as an IV bolus injection (5 to 20 mL) over approximately 3 to 5 minutes.

SSSIs – 500 mg given every 8 hours.

Intra-abdominal infections – 1 g given every 8 hours.

➤*Renal function impairment:* Dosage should be reduced in adult patients with creatinine clearance (Ccr) less than 51 mL/min (see the following table).

Meropenem Dosage Schedule for Adults with Impaired Renal Function

Ccr (mL/min)	Dose (dependent on type of infection)	Dosing interval
≥ 51	Recommended dose (500 mg complicated SSSI and 1 g intra-abdominal)	Every 8 hours
26 to 50	Recommended dose (1,000 mg)	Every 12 hours
10 to 25	½ recommended dose	Every 12 hours
< 10	½ recommended dose	Every 24 hours

There is no experience in pediatric patients with renal impairment.

➤*Children:* For children 3 months of age and older, the meropenem dose is 10, 20, or 40 mg/kg every 8 hours (maximum dose is 2 g every 8 hours), depending on the type of infection (complicated SSSI, intra-abdominal, or meningitis) (see the following table). Pediatric patients weighing more than 50 kg should be administered meropenem at a varying dose depending on the type of infection. Meropenem should be given as IV infusion over approximately 15 to 30 minutes or as an IV bolus injection (5 to 20 mL) over approximately 3 to 5 minutes.

Meropenem Dosage Schedule for Pediatric Patients with Healthy Renal Function

Type of infection	Dose (mg/kg)	Up to a maximum dose	Dosing interval
Complicated SSSI	10	500 mg	Every 8 hours
Intra-abdominal	20	1 g	Every 8 hours
Meningitis	40	2 g	Every 8 hours

Children (more than 50 kg) –

SSSIs: 500 mg every 8 hours for complicated SSSIs.

Intra-abdominal infections: 1 g every 8 hours for intra-abdominal infections.

Meningitis: 2 g every 8 hours for meningitis.

† The efficacy of meropenem as monotherapy in the treatment of meningitis caused by penicillin nonsusceptible isolates of *S. pneumoniae* has not been established.

MEROPENEM — INJECTION

➤*Preparation of solution:*

For IV bolus administration – Constitute injection vials (500 mg and 1 g) with sterile water for injection (see the following table). Shake to dissolve and let stand until clear.

Vial size	Amount of diluent added (mL)	Approximate withdrawable volume (mL)	Approximate average concentration (mg/mL)
500 mg	10	10	50
1 g	20	20	50

For infusion – Infusion vials (500 mg and 1 g) may be directly constituted with a compatible infusion fluid. Alternatively, an injection vial may be constituted, then the resulting solution added to an IV container and further diluted with an appropriate infusion fluid.

Do not use flexible container in series connections.

➤*Compatibility and stability:* Compatibility of meropenem with other drugs has not been established. Meropenem should not be mixed with or physically added to solutions containing other drugs.

Freshly prepared solutions of meropenem should be used whenever possible. However, constituted solutions of meropenem maintain satisfactory potency at controlled room temperature 15° to 25°C (59° to 77°F) or under refrigeration at 4°C (39°F) as described below. Solutions of meropenem should not be frozen.

➤*Storage/Stability:*

Dry powder – The dry powder should be stored at controlled room temperature 20° to 25°C (68° to 77°F).

IV bolus administration – Meropenem injection vials constituted with sterile water for injection for bolus administration (meropenem up to 50 mg/mL) may be stored for up to 2 hours at controlled room temperature 15° to 25°C (59° to 77°F) or for up to 12 hours at 4°C (39°F).

IV infusion administration –

Stability in infusion vials: Meropenem infusion vials constituted with sodium chloride injection 0.9% (meropenem concentrations ranging from 2.5 to 50 mg/mL) are stable for up to 2 hours at controlled room temperature 15° to 25°C (59° to 77°F) or for up to 18 hours at 4°C (39°F). Infusion vials of meropenem constituted with dextrose injection 5% (meropenem concentrations ranging from 2.5 to 50 mg/mL) are stable for up to 1 hour at controlled room temperature 15° to 25°C (59° to 77°F) or for up to 8 hours at 4°C (39°F).

Stability in plastic IV bags: Solutions prepared for infusion (meropenem concentrations ranging from 1 to 20 mg/mL) may be stored in plastic IV bags with diluents as shown in the following table.

Meropenem Stability with Diluents		
Diluent	Number of hours stable at controlled room temperature 15° to 25°C (59° to 77°F)	Number of hours stable at 4°C (39°F)
Sodium chloride injection 0.9%	4	24
Dextrose injection 5%	1	4
Dextrose injection 10%	1	2
Dextrose and sodium chloride injection 5%/0.9%	1	2
Dextrose and sodium chloride injection 5%/0.2%	1	4
Potassium chloride in dextrose injection 0.15%/5%	1	6
Sodium bicarbonate in dextrose injection 0.02%/5%	1	6
Dextrose injection 5% in *Normosol-M*	1	8
Dextrose injection 5% in Ringer's lactate injection	1	4
Dextrose and sodium chloride injection 2.5%/0.45%	3	12
Mannitol injection 2.5%	2	16
Ringer's injection	4	24
Ringer's lactate injection	4	12
Sodium lactate injection 1/6 N	2	24
Sodium bicarbonate injection 5%	1	4

Stability in Baxter Minibag Plus: Solutions of meropenem (concentrations ranging from 2.5 to 20 mg/mL) in *Baxter Minibag Plus* bags with sodium chloride injection 0.9% may be stored for up to 4 hours at controlled room temperatures 15° to 25°C (59° to 77°F) or for up to 24 hours at 4°C (39°F). Solutions of meropenem (concentrations ranging from 2.5 to 20 mg/mL) in *Baxter Minibag Plus* bags with dextrose injection 5% may be stored up to 1 hour at controlled room temperatures 15° to 25°C (59° to 77°F) or for up to 6 hours at 4°C (39°F).

Stability in plastic syringes, tubing, and IV infusion sets: Solutions of meropenem (concentrations ranging from 1 to 20 mg/mL) in water for injection or sodium chloride injection 0.9% (for up to 4 hours) or in dextrose injection 5% (for up to 2 hours) at controlled room temperatures 15° to 25°C (59° to 77°F) are stable in plastic tubing and volume-control devices of common IV infusion sets.

Solutions of meropenem (concentrations ranging from 1 to 20 mg/mL) in water for injection or sodium chloride injection 0.9% (for up to 48 hours) or in dextrose injection 5% (for up to 6 hours) are stable at 4°C (39°F) in plastic syringes.

Actions

➤*Pharmacology:* Meropenem is a broad-spectrum carbapenem antibiotic. It is active against gram-positive and gram-negative bacteria. Meropenem exerts its action by penetrating bacterial cells readily and interfering with the synthesis of vital cell wall components, which leads to cell death. The bactericidal activity of meropenem results from the inhibition of cell wall synthesis. Meropenem readily penetrates the cell wall of most gram-positive and gram-negative bacteria to reach penicillin-binding-protein (PBP) targets.

➤*Pharmacokinetics:*

Absorption – Meropenem has dose-dependent kinetics. At the end of a 30-minute IV infusion of a single dose of meropenem in healthy volunteers, mean peak plasma concentrations are approximately 23 mcg/mL (range, 14 to 26) for the 500 mg dose and 49 mcg/mL (range, 39 to 58) for the 1 g dose. A 5-minute IV bolus injection of meropenem in healthy volunteers results in mean peak plasma concentrations of approximately 45 mcg/mL (range, 18 to 65) for the 500 mg dose and 112 mcg/mL (range, 83 to 140) for the 1 g dose.

Following IV doses of 500 mg, mean plasma concentrations of meropenem usually decline to approximately 1 mcg/mL at 6 hours after administration.

Distribution – Plasma protein binding of meropenem is approximately 2%.

Meropenem penetrates well into most body fluids and tissues, including cerebrospinal fluid (CSF), achieving concentrations matching or exceeding those required to inhibit most susceptible bacteria. After a single IV dose of meropenem, the highest mean concentrations of meropenem were found in tissues and fluids at 1 hour (0.5 to 1.5 hours) after the start of infusion, except where indicated in the tissues and fluids listed in the following table.

Meropenem Concentrations in Selected Tissues (Highest Concentrations Reported)				
Tissue	IV dose (g)	Number of samples	Mean (mcg/mL or mcg/g)[a]	Range (mcg/mL or mcg/g)
Endometrium	0.5	7	4.2	1.7 to 10.2
Myometrium	0.5	15	3.8	0.4 to 8.1
Ovary	0.5	8	2.8	0.8 to 4.8
Cervix	0.5	2	7	5.4 to 8.5
Fallopian tube	0.5	9	1.7	0.3 to 3.4
Skin	0.5	22	3.3	0.5 to 12.6
Interstitial fluid[b]	0.5	9	5.5	3.2 to 8.6
Skin	1	10	5.3	1.3 to 16.7
Interstitial fluid[b]	1	5	26.3	20.9 to 37.4
Colon	1	2	2.6	2.5 to 2.7
Bile	1	7	14.6 (3 h)	4 to 25.7
Gallbladder	1	1		3.9
Peritoneal fluid	1	9	30.2	7.4 to 54.6
Lung	1	2	4.8 (2 h)	1.4 to 8.2
Bronchial mucosa	1	7	4.5	1.3 to 11.1
Muscle	1	2	6.1 (2 h)	5.3 to 6.9
Fascia	1	9	8.8	1.5 to 20
Heart valves	1	7	9.7	6.4 to 12.1
Myocardium	1	10	15.5	5.2 to 25.5
CSF (inflamed)	20 mg/kg[c]	8	1.1 (2 h)	0.2 to 2.8
	40 mg/kg[d]	5	3.3 (3 h)	0.9 to 6.5
CSF (uninflamed)	1	4	0.2 (2 h)	0.1 to 0.3

[a] At 1 hour unless otherwise noted.
[b] Obtained from blister fluid.
[c] In pediatric patients 5 months to 8 years of age.
[d] In pediatric patients 1 month to 15 years of age.

Metabolism – There is 1 metabolite that is microbiologically inactive.

Excretion – In subjects with normal renal function, the elimination half-life of meropenem is approximately 1 hour. Approximately 70% of the IV dose is recovered as unchanged meropenem in the urine over 12 hours, after which little further urinary excretion is detectable. Urinary concentrations of meropenem in excess of 10 mcg/mL are maintained for up to 5 hours after a 500 mg dose. No accumulation of meropenem in plasma or urine was observed with regimens using 500 mg administered every 8 hours or 1 g administered every 6 hours in volunteers with normal renal function.

Special populations –

Renal function impairment: Pharmacokinetic studies with meropenem in patients with renal insufficiency have shown that the plasma clearance of meropenem correlates with Ccr. Dosage adjustments are necessary in subjects with renal impairment. A pharmacokinetic study with meropenem in elderly patients with renal insufficiency has shown a reduction in plasma clearance of meropenem that correlates with age-associated reduction in Ccr.

See Overdosage for more information.

MEROPENEM — INJECTION

Elderly: A pharmacokinetic study with meropenem in elderly patients with renal insufficiency has shown a reduction in plasma clearance of meropenem that correlates with age-associated reduction in creatinine clearance. The mean terminal half-life is prolonged slightly to 1.27 hours.

➤*Microbiology:*

Resistance –

Mechanism of resistance: There are several mechanisms of resistance to carbapenems: 1) decreased permeability of the outer membrane of gram-negative bacteria (due to diminished production of porins) causing reduced bacterial uptake, 2) reduced affinity of the target PBP, 3) increased expression of efflux pump components, and 4) production of antibiotic-destroying enzymes (carbapenemases, metallo-β-lactamases).

Meropenem has been shown to be active against most isolates of the following microorganisms, both in vitro and in clinical infections.

Aerobic and facultative gram-positive microorganisms – E. faecalis (excluding vancomycin-resistant isolates); *S. aureus* (β-lactamase and non-β-lactamase-producing, methicillin-susceptible isolates only); *S. agalactiae*; *S. pyogenes*; Viridans group streptococci; *S. pneumoniae* (penicillin-susceptible isolates only). Note: Penicillin-resistant isolates had meropenem minimum inhibitory concentration (MIC_{90}) values of 1 or 2 mcg/mL, which is above the 0.12 mcg/mL susceptible breakpoint for this species.

Aerobic and facultative gram-negative microorganisms – E. coli; *H. influenzae* (β-lactamase and non-β-lactamase-producing); *K. pneumoniae*; *N. meningitidis*; *P. aeruginosa*; *P. mirabilis*.

Anaerobic microorganisms – B. fragilis; *B. thetaiotaomicron*; *Peptostreptococcus species*.

Contraindications

Known hypersensitivity to any component of this product or to other drugs in the same class or in patients who have demonstrated anaphylactic reactions to beta-lactams.

Warnings

➤*Pseudomembranous colitis:* Pseudomembranous colitis has been reported with nearly all antibacterial agents, including meropenem, and may range in severity from mild to life-threatening. Therefore, it is important to consider this diagnosis in patients who present with diarrhea subsequent to the administration of antibacterial agents.

Treatment with antibacterial agents alters the normal flora of the colon and may permit overgrowth of clostridia. Studies indicate that a toxin produced by *Clostridium difficile* is a primary cause of "antibiotic-associated colitis."

After the diagnosis of pseudomembranous colitis has been established, initiate therapeutic measures. Mild cases of pseudomembranous colitis usually respond to drug discontinuation alone. In moderate to severe cases, consider management with fluids and electrolytes, protein supplementation, and treatment with antibacterial drug clinically effective against *Clostridium difficile* colitis.

➤*Hypersensitivity reactions:* Serious and occasionally fatal hypersensitivity (anaphylactic) reactions have been reported in patients receiving therapy with β-lactams. These reactions are more likely to occur in individuals with a history of sensitivity to multiple allergens.

There have been reports of individuals with a history of penicillin hypersensitivity who have experienced severe hypersensitivity reactions when treated with another β-lactam. Before initiating therapy with meropenem, make careful inquiry concerning previous hypersensitivity reactions to penicillins, cephalosporins, other β-lactams, and other allergens. If an allergic reaction to meropenem occurs, discontinue the drug immediately. Serious anaphylactic reactions require immediate emergency treatment with epinephrine, oxygen, IV steroids, and airway management, including intubation. Other therapy may also be administered as indicated.

➤*Renal function impairment:* In patients with renal dysfunction, thrombocytopenia has been observed but no clinical bleeding has been reported.

See Administration and Dosage for more information.

➤*Elderly:* Of the total number of subjects in clinical studies of meropenem, approximately 1,100 (30%) were 65 years of age and older, while 400 (11%) were 75 years of age and older. Additionally, in a study of 511 patients with complicated SSSIs, 93 (18%) were 65 years of age and older, while 38 (7%) were 75 years of age and older. No overall differences in safety or efficacy were observed between these subjects and younger subjects; spontaneous reports and other reported clinical experience have not identified differences in responses between the elderly and younger patients, but greater sensitivity of some older individuals cannot be ruled out.

A pharmacokinetic study with meropenem in elderly patients with renal insufficiency has shown a reduction in plasma clearance of meropenem that correlates with age-associated reduction in Ccr.

Meropenem is known to be substantially excreted by the kidney, and the risk of toxic reactions to this drug may be greater in patients with impaired renal function. Because elderly patients are more likely to have decreased renal function, take care in dose selection; it may be useful to monitor renal function.

➤*Pregnancy: Category B.*

Reproductive studies have been performed with meropenem in rats at doses of up to 1,000 mg/kg/day, and cynomolgus monkeys at doses of up to 360 mg/kg/day (on the basis of AUC comparisons, approximately 1.8 and 3.7 times, respectively, to the human exposure at the usual dose of 1 g every 8 hours). These studies revealed no evidence of impaired fertility or harm to the fetus caused by meropenem, although there were slight changes in fetal body weight at doses of 250 mg/kg/day (on the basis of AUC comparisons, 0.4 times the human exposure at a dose of 1 g every 8 hours) and above in rats. There are, however, no adequate and well-controlled studies in pregnant women. Because animal reproduction studies are not always predictive of human response, use this drug during pregnancy only if clearly needed.

➤*Lactation:* It is not known whether this drug is excreted in human milk. Because many drugs are excreted in human milk, exercise caution when meropenem is administered to a breast-feeding woman.

➤*Children:* The safety and efficacy of meropenem have been established for children 3 months of age and older.

Precautions

➤*Monitoring:* While meropenem possesses the characteristic low toxicity of the beta-lactam group of antibiotics, periodic assessment of organ system functions, including renal, hepatic, and hematopoietic, is advisable during prolonged therapy.

➤*Reducing drug resistance:* Prescribing meropenem in the absence of a proven or strongly suspected bacterial infection or a prophylactic indication is unlikely to provide benefit to the patient and increases the risk of the development of drug-resistant bacteria.

➤*Seizures:* Seizures and other CNS adverse experiences have been reported during treatment with meropenem. These experiences have occurred most commonly in patients with CNS disorders (eg, brain lesions or history of seizures) or with bacterial meningitis and/or compromised renal function.

During clinical investigations, 2,904 immunocompetent adult patients were treated for infections outside the CNS, with the overall seizure rate being 0.7% (based on 20 patients with this adverse reaction). All meropenem-treated patients with seizures had preexisting contributing factors. Among these are included prior history of seizures or CNS abnormality and concomitant medications with seizure potential. Dosage adjustment is recommended in patients with advanced age and/or reduced renal function.

Close adherence to the recommended dosage regimens is urged, especially in patients with known factors that predispose to convulsive activity. Continue anticonvulsant therapy in patients with known seizure disorders. If focal tremors, myoclonus, or seizures occur, evaluate patients neurologically, place them on anticonvulsant therapy if not already instituted, and reexamine the dosage of meropenem to determine whether it should be decreased or the antibiotic discontinued.

➤*Superinfection:* As with other broad-spectrum antibiotics, prolonged use of meropenem may result in overgrowth of nonsusceptible organisms. Repeated evaluation of the patient is essential. If superinfection does occur during therapy, take appropriate measures.

Drug Interactions

➤*Probenecid:* Probenecid competes with meropenem for active tubular secretion and thus inhibits the renal excretion of meropenem. This led to statistically significant increases in the elimination half-life (38%) and in the extent of systemic exposure (56%). Therefore, the coadministration of probenecid with meropenem is not recommended.

➤*Valproic acid:* There is evidence that meropenem may reduce serum levels of valproic acid to subtherapeutic levels (therapeutic range considered to be total valproate 50 to 100 mcg/mL).

Adverse Reactions

➤*Adult patients:* During clinical investigations, 2,904 immunocompetent adult patients were treated for infections outside the CNS with meropenem (500 or 1,000 mg every 8 hours). Deaths in 5 patients were assessed as possibly related to meropenem; 36 (1.2%) patients had meropenem discontinued because of adverse reactions. Many patients in these trials were severely ill, had multiple background diseases, had physiological impairments, and were receiving multiple other drug therapies. In the seriously ill patient population, it was not possible to determine the relationship between observed adverse reactions and therapy with meropenem.

Local – Local adverse reactions that were reported irrespective of the relationship to therapy with meropenem were as follows: inflammation at the injection site (2.4%), injection-site reaction (0.9%), phlebitis/thrombophlebitis (0.8%), pain at the injection site (0.4%), edema at the injection site (0.2%).

Systemic – Systemic adverse clinical reactions that were reported irrespective of the relationship to meropenem occurring in more than 1% of the patients were diarrhea (4.8%), nausea/vomiting (3.6%), headache (2.3%), rash (1.9%), sepsis (1.6%), constipation (1.4%), apnea (1.3%), shock (1.2%), and pruritus (1.2%).

➤*Additional adverse reactions:*

Cardiovascular – Heart failure, heart arrest, tachycardia, hypertension, myocardial infarction, pulmonary embolus, bradycardia, hypotension, syncope (0.1% to 1%).

CNS – Insomnia, agitation/delirium, confusion, dizziness, seizure, nervousness, paresthesia, hallucinations, somnolence, anxiety, depression, asthenia (0.1% to 1%).

Seizures: See Warnings for more information.

Dermatologic – Urticaria, sweating, skin ulcer (0.1% to 1%).

GI – Oral moniliasis, anorexia, cholestatic jaundice/jaundice, flatulence, ileus, hepatic failure, dyspepsia, intestinal obstruction (0.1% to 1%).

GU – Dysuria, kidney failure, vaginal moniliasis, urinary incontinence (0.1% to 1%).

Hematologic – Bleeding events were seen in 1.2%, as follows: gastrointestinal hemorrhage (0.5%), melena (0.3%), epistaxis (0.2%), hemoperitoneum (0.2%). Anemia, hypochromic anemia, hypervolemia (0.1% to 1%).

MEROPENEM — INJECTION

Metabolic/Nutritional – Peripheral edema, hypoxia (0.1% to 1%).

Respiratory – Respiratory disorder, dyspnea, pleural effusion, asthma, cough increased, lung edema (0.1% to 1%).

Miscellaneous – Pain, abdominal pain, chest pain, fever, back pain, abdominal enlargement, chills, pelvic pain (0.1% to 1%).

➤*Lab test abnormalities:* Adverse laboratory changes that were reported irrespective of relationship to meropenem and occurring in more than 0.2% of the patients were as follows.

Hematologic – Eosinophils increased, hematocrit decreased, hemoglobin decreased, hypokalemia, leukocytosis, platelets increased/decreased, shortened prothrombin time, shortened partial thromboplastin time, white blood cell count decreased.

Hepatic – Increased alkaline phosphatase, ALT, AST, bilirubin, and LDH.

Renal – Increased blood urea nitrogen, increased creatinine.

For patients with varying degrees of renal impairment, the incidence of heart failure, kidney failure, seizure, and shock reported irrespective of relationship to meropenem increased in patients with moderately severe renal impairment (Ccr greater than 10 to 26 mL/min).

Urinalysis: Presence of red blood cells.

➤*Complicated SSSIs:* In a study of complicated SSSI, the type of clinical adverse reactions were similar to those listed above. The patients with the most common adverse reactions with an incidence of more than 5% were: headache (7.8%), nausea (7.8%), constipation (7%), diarrhea (7%), anemia (5.5%), and pain (5.1%). Adverse reactions with an incidence of more than 1% and not listed above include the following: accidental injury, GI disorder, hypoglycemia, peripheral vascular disorder, pharyngitis, pneumonia.

➤*Children:* Meropenem was studied in 515 pediatric patients (3 months of age and older to younger than 13 years of age) with serious bacterial infections (excluding meningitis) at dosages of 10 to 20 mg/kg every 8 hours. The types of clinical adverse reactions seen in these patients are similar to the adults, with the most common adverse reactions reported as possibly, probably, or definitely related to meropenem and their rates of occurrence as follows: diarrhea (3.5%), rash (1.6%), and nausea and vomiting (0.8%).

Meropenem was studied in 321 pediatric patients (3 months of age and older to younger than 17 years of age) with meningitis at a dosage of 40 mg/kg every 8 hours. The types of clinical adverse reactions seen in these patients are similar to the adults, with the most common adverse reactions reported as possibly, probably, or definitely related to meropenem and their rates of occurrence as follows: diarrhea (4.7%), rash (mostly diaper area moniliasis) (3.1%), oral moniliasis (1.9%), glossitis (1%).

Seizures – In the meningitis studies, the rates of seizure activity during therapy were comparable between patients with no CNS abnormalities who received meropenem and those who received comparator agents (either cefotaxime or ceftriaxone). In the meropenem-treated group, 12 of 15 patients with seizures had late-onset seizures (defined as occurring on day 3 or later) versus 7 of 20 in the comparator arm.

Renal –

➤*Postmarketing:*

Dermatologic – Toxic epidermal necrolysis, Stevens-Johnson syndrome, angioedema, erythema multiforme.

Hematologic – Agranulocytosis, leukopenia, neutropenia.

Overdosage

➤*Symptoms:* In mice and rats, large IV doses of meropenem (2,200 to 4,000 mg/kg) have been associated with ataxia, dyspnea, convulsions, and mortalities.

Intentional overdosing of meropenem is unlikely, although accidental overdosing might occur if large doses are given to patients with reduced renal function. The largest dosage of meropenem administered in clinical trials has been 2 g given IV every 8 hours. At this dosage, no adverse pharmacological effects or increased safety risks have been observed.

➤*Treatment:* No specific information is available for the treatment of meropenem overdosage. In the event of an overdose, discontinue meropenem and general give supportive treatment until renal elimination takes place. Meropenem and its metabolite are readily dialyzable and effectively removed by hemodialysis; however, no information is available on the use of hemodialysis to treat overdosage.

Patient Information

Counsel patients only to use antibacterial drugs, including meropenem, to treat bacterial infections. Antibacterial drugs do not treat viral infections (eg, the common cold). When meropenem is prescribed to treat a bacterial infection, tell patients that although it is common to feel better early in the course of therapy, the medication should be taken exactly as directed. Skipping doses or not completing the full course of therapy may (1) decrease the efficacy of the immediate treatment and (2) increase the likelihood that bacteria will develop resistance and will not be treatable by meropenem or other antibacterial drugs in the future.

IMIPENEM-CILASTATIN

Rx	**Primaxin I.V.** (Merck)	**Powder for Injection:** 250 mg imipenem equivalent and 250 mg cilastatin equivalent. Contains 0.8 mEq sodium.	In vials, infusion bottles, and *ADD-Vantage* vials.
		500 mg imipenem equivalent and 500 mg cilastatin equivalent. Contains 1.6 mEq sodium.	In vials, infusion bottles, and *ADD-Vantage* vials.
Rx	**Primaxin I.M.** (Merck)	**Powder for Injection:** 500 mg imipenem equivalent and 500 mg cilastatin equivalent. Contains 1.4 mEq sodium.	In vials.
		750 mg imipenem equivalent and 750 mg cilastatin equivalent. Contains 2.1 mEq sodium.	In vials.

IMIPENEM-CILASTATIN — INJECTION

Indications

➤*IV:* Treatment of serious infections caused by susceptible strains of the designated microorganisms in the conditions listed below:

Lower respiratory tract infections – *Staphylococcus aureus* (penicillinase-producing), *Escherichia coli, Klebsiella* sp., *Enterobacter* sp., *Haemophilus influenzae, Haemophilus parainfluenzae, Acinetobacter* sp., *Serratia marcescens.*

Urinary tract infections (complicated and uncomplicated) – *Enterococcus faecalis, S. aureus* (penicillinase-producing), *E. coli, Klebsiella* sp., *Enterobacter* sp., *Proteus vulgaris, Providencia rettgeri, M. morganii, P. aeruginosa.*

Intra-abdominal infections – *E. faecalis, S. aureus* (penicillinase-producing), *Staphylococcus epidermidis, E. coli, Klebsiella* sp., *Enterobacter* sp., *Proteus* sp., *Morganella morganii, P. aeruginosa, Citrobacter* sp., *Clostridium* sp., *Bacteroides* sp. including *B. fragilis, Fusobacterium* sp., *Peptococcus* sp., *Peptostreptococcus* sp., *Eubacterium* sp., *Propionibacterium* sp., *Bifidobacterium* sp.

Gynecologic infections – *E. faecalis; S. aureus* (penicillinase-producing), *S. epidermidis, Streptococcus agalactiae* (group B streptococcus), *E. coli* , *Klebsiella* sp., *Proteus* sp., *Enterobacter* sp., *Bifidobacterium* sp., *Bacteroides* sp. including *B. fragilis, Gardnerella vaginalis; Peptococcus* sp., *Peptostreptococcus* sp., *Propionibacterium* sp.

Bacterial septicemia – *E. faecalis, S. aureus* (penicillinase-producing), *E. coli, Klebsiella* sp., *P. aeruginosa, Serratia* sp., *Enterobacter* sp., *Bacteroides* sp.

Bone and joint infections – *E. faecalis; S. aureus* (penicillinase-producing), *S. epidermidis, Enterobacter* sp., *P. aeruginosa.*

Skin and skin structure infections – *E. faecalis, S. aureus* (penicillinase-producing), *S. epidermidis, E. coli, Klebsiella* sp., *Enterobacter* sp., *P. vulgaris, P. rettgeri, M. morganii, P. aeruginosa, Serratia* sp., *Citrobacter* sp., *Acinetobacter* sp., *Bacteroides* sp., *Fusobacterium* sp., *Peptococcus* sp., *Peptostreptococcus* sp.

Endocarditis – *S. aureus* (penicillinase-producing).

Polymicrobic infections – Including those in which *S. pneumoniae* (pneumonia, septicemia), *S. pyogenes* (skin and skin structure) or nonpenicillinase-producing *S. aureus* is one of the causative organisms. However, these monobacterial infections are usually treated with narrower spectrum antibiotics (eg, penicillin G). Although clinical improvement has been observed in patients with cystic fibrosis, chronic pulmonary disease, and lower respiratory tract infections caused by *P. aeruginosa*, bacterial eradication may not be achieved.

➤*IM:* Treatment of serious infections of mild-to-moderate severity where IM therapy is appropriate. Not intended for severe or life-threatening infections, including bacterial sepsis or endocarditis, or in major physiological impairments (eg, shock).

Lower respiratory tract infections – Including pneumonia and bronchitis as an exacerbation of COPD that are caused by *S. pneumoniae* and *H. influenzae.*

Intra-abdominal infections – Including acute gangrenous or perforated appendicitis and appendicitis with peritonitis that are caused by group D streptococcus including *E. faecalis*; Streptococcus (viridans group); *E. coli; Klebsiella pneumoniae; P. aeruginosa; Bacteroides* sp. including *B. fragilis, B. distasonis, B. intermedius,* and *B. thetaiotaomicron; Fusobacterium* sp; *Peptostreptococcus* sp.

Skin and skin structure infections – Including abscesses, cellulitis, infected skin ulcers, and wound infections caused by *S. aureus* (including penicillinase-producing strains); *Streptococcus pyogenes*; group D streptococcus including *E. faecalis; Acinetobacter* sp. including *A. calcoaceticus; Citrobacter* sp; *E. coli; Enterobacter cloacae; K. pneumoniae; P. aeruginosa; Bacteroides* sp. including *B. fragilis.*

Gynecologic infections – Including postpartum endomyometritis that are caused by group D streptococcus such as *E. faecalis; E. coli; K. pneumoniae; B. intermedius; Peptostreptococcus* sp.

Infections resistant to other antibiotics (eg, cephalosporins, penicillins, aminoglycosides) have responded to treatment with imipenem.

IMIPENEM-CILASTATIN — INJECTION

Administration and Dosage

Dosage recommendations represent the quantity of imipenem to be administered. An equivalent amount of cilastatin is also present in the solution.

Base the initial dosage on the type or severity of infection and administer in equally divided doses. Base subsequent dosing on severity of illness, degree of susceptibility of the pathogen(s), renal function, weight, and creatinine clearance.

➤*IV:* Give a 125, 250, or 500 mg dose by IV infusion over 20 to 30 min. Infuse a 750 mg or 1 g dose over 40 to 60 min. If nausea develops, slow the infusion rate.

Because of high antimicrobial activity, do not exceed 50 mg/kg/day or 4 g/day, whichever is lower. There is no evidence that higher doses provide greater efficacy.

Imipenem-Cilastatin IV Dosing Schedule for Adults with Normal Renal Function

Type or severity of infection	Fully susceptible organisms[a]	Total daily dose	Moderately susceptible organisms, primarily some strains of *P. aeruginosa*	Total daily dose
Mild	250 mg every 6 h	1 g	500 mg every 6 h	2 g
Moderate	500 mg every 8 h or 500 mg every 6 h	1.5 or 2 g	500 mg every 6 h or 1 g every 8 h	2 or 3 g
Severe, life-threatening	500 mg every 6 h	2 g	1 g every 8 h or 1 g every 6 h	3 or 4 g
Uncomplicated UTI	250 mg every 6 h	1 g	250 mg every 6 h	1 g
Complicated UTI	500 mg every 6 h	2 g	500 mg every 6 h	2 g

[a] Including gram-positive and -negative aerobes and anaerobes

Renal function impairment or body weight less than 70 kg – Patients with creatinine clearance (Ccr) less than 70 mL/min per 1.73 m^2 for IV require dosage adjustment (see table). Safety and efficacy of patients with Ccr less than 20 mL/min per 1.73 m^2 (for IM administration) have not been studied.

From the IV Dosing Schedule for Adults with Normal Renal Function table, determine a total daily dose based on type of infection and organism. Then, using the table below, find the appropriate reduced dosing schedule according to the patient's weight and Ccr.

Reduced IV Dosage in Adult Patients with Impaired Renal Function or Body Weight < 70 kg

Body weight	≥ 70 kg	60 kg	50 kg	40 kg	30 kg
Ccr (mL/min/1.73 m^2)	If total daily dose for normal renal function is 1 g/day, use:				
≥ 71	250 every 6 h	250 every 8 h	125 every 6 h	125 every 6 h	125 every 8 h
41 to 70	250 every 8 h	125 every 6 h	125 every 6 h	125 every 8 h	125 every 8 h
21 to 40	250 every 12 h	250 every 12 h	125 every 8 h	125 every 12 h	125 every 12 h
6 to 20	250 every 12 h	125 every 12 h	125 every 12 h	125 every 12 h	125 every 12 h
	If total daily dose for normal renal function is 1.5 g/day, use:				
≥ 71	500 every 8 h	250 every 6 h	250 every 6 h	250 every 8 h	125 every 6 h
41 to 70	250 every 6 h	250 every 8 h	250 every 8 h	125 every 6 h	125 every 8 h
21 to 40	250 every 8 h	250 every 8 h	250 every 12 h	125 every 8 h	125 every 8 h
6 to 20	250 every 12 h	250 every 12 h	250 every 12 h	125 every 12 h	125 every 12 h
	If total daily dose for normal renal function is 2 g/day, use:				
≥ 71	500 every 6 h	500 every 8 h	250 every 6 h	250 every 6 h	250 every 8 h
41 to 70	500 every 8 h	250 every 6 h	250 every 6 h	250 every 8 h	125 every 6 h
21 to 40	250 every 6 h	250 every 8 h	250 every 8 h	250 every 12 h	125 every 8 h
6 to 20	250 every 12 h	250 every 12 h	250 every 12 h	250 every 12 h	125 every 12 h
	If total daily dose for normal renal function is 3 g/day, use:				
≥ 71	1,000 every 8 h	750 every 8 h	500 every 6 h	500 every 8 h	250 every 6 h
41 to 70	500 every 6 h	500 every 8 h	500 every 8 h	250 every 6 h	250 every 8 h
21 to 40	500 every 8 h	500 every 8 h	250 every 6 h	250 every 8 h	250 every 8 h
6 to 20	500 every 12 h	500 every 12 h	250 every 12 h	250 every 12 h	250 every 12 h
	If total daily dose for normal renal function is 4 g/day, use:				
≥ 71	1,000 every 6 h	1,000 every 8 h	750 every 8 h	500 every 6 h	500 every 8 h
41 to 70	750 every 8 h	750 every 8 h	500 every 6 h	500 every 8 h	250 every 6 h
21 to 40	500 q 6 h	500 q 8 h	500 q 8 h	250 every 6 h	250 every 8 h
6 to 20	500 q 12 h	500 q 12 h	500 q 12 h	250 q 12 h	250 q 12 h

Children –

Pediatric Dosing Guidelines (≥ 3 months old)

≥ 3 months old (non-CNS infections)
15 to 25 mg/kg/dose every 6 hours
Maximum daily dose for fully susceptible organisms is 2 g/day, and for infections with moderately susceptible organisms (primarily some strains of *P. aeruginosa*) is 4 g/day (based on adults studies).
Higher doses (≤ 90 mg/kg/day in older children) have been used in cystic fibrosis patients.

Pediatric Dosing Guidelines (≤ 3 months old)

≤ 3 months old (weighing ≥ 1,500 g; non-CNS infections)
< 1 week old: 25 mg/kg every 12 hours
1 to 4 weeks old: 25 mg/kg every 8 hours
4 weeks to 3 months old: 25 mg/kg every 6 hours

Give doses less than or equal to 500 mg by IV infusion over 15 to 30 minutes. Give doses more than 500 mg by IV infusion over 40 to 60 minutes.

Imipenem-cilastatin IV is not recommended in pediatric patients with CNS infections because of the risk of seizures and in pediatric patients less than 30 kg with impaired renal function, as no data are available.

➤*IM:* Total daily IM dosages more than 1,500 mg/day are not recommended.

Duration of therapy depends on the type and severity of the infection. Generally, continue for greater than or equal to 2 days after signs and symptoms of infection have resolved. Safety and efficacy of treatment more than 14 days have not been established.

Administer by deep IM injection into a large muscle mass (such as the gluteal muscles or lateral part of the thigh) with a 21-gauge 2-inch needle. Aspiration is necessary to avoid inadvertent injection into a blood vessel.

Imipenem-Cilastatin IM Dosage Guidelines in Adults

Type/Location of infection	Severity	Dosage regimen
Lower respiratory tract Skin and skin structure Gynecologic	Mild/Moderate	500 or 750 mg every 12 h depending on the severity of infection
Intra-abdominal	Mild/Moderate	750 mg every 12 h

Children – In mild to moderate infections the recommended dose is 10 to 15 mg/kg every 6 hours.

Hemodialysis – Imipenem-cilastatin is cleared by hemodialysis. Administer after hemodialysis and at 12-hour intervals timed from the end of that dialysis session. For patients on hemodialysis, imipenem-cilastatin is recommended only when the benefits outweigh the potential risk of seizures.

IMIPENEM-CILASTATIN — INJECTION

There is inadequate information to recommend usage for patients undergoing peritoneal dialysis. Carefully monitor dialysis patients, especially those with CNS diseases.

➤*Preparation of solution:*

IV – Reconstitute contents of infusion bottles with 100 ml diluent (see Compatibility).

IM – Prepare with 1% lidocaine solution (without epinephrine). Prepare the 500 mg vial with 2 ml and the 750 mg vial with 3 ml lidocaine.

➤*Compatibility:* Do not mix with or physically add to antibiotics. However, it may be administered concomitantly with other antibiotics (eg, aminoglycosides).

Diluents – Imipenem-cilastatin in infusion bottles and vials, reconstituted as directed with the following diluents, maintains satisfactory potency for 4 hours at room temperature and for 24 hours when refrigerated (5°C; 41°F): 0.9% Sodium Chloride Injection; 5% or 10% Dextrose Injection; 5% Dextrose and 0.9% Sodium Chloride Injection; 5% Dextrose Injection with 0.225% or 0.45% saline solution; 5% Dextrose Injection with 0.15% potassium chloride solution; Mannitol 5% and 10%. Do not freeze solutions.

➤*Storage/Stability:* Store dry powder at less than 25°C (77°F) .

Actions

➤*Pharmacology:* This product is a formulation of imipenem, a thienamycin antibiotic, and cilastatin sodium, the inhibitor of dehydropeptidase 1, which inactivates imipenem when it is administered alone. Cilastatin thereby increases urinary recovery of imipenem and decreases possible renal toxicity associated with excessive intracellular antibiotic accumulation. The bactericidal activity of imipenem results from the inhibition of cell wall synthesis with a high affinity for penicillin binding proteins (PBPs) 1A, 1B, 2, 4, 5, and 6 of *Escherichia coli* and 1A, 1B, 2, 4, and 5 of *Pseudomonas aeruginosa*. The lethal effect is related to binding to PBP 2 and PBP 1B.

➤*Pharmacokinetics:*

Absorption/Distribution –

IV: IV infusion over 20 minutes results in peak plasma levels of imipenem antimicrobial activity of 14 to 24 mcg/ml for the 250 mg dose, 21 to 58 mcg/ml for the 500 mg dose, and 41 to 83 mcg/ml for the 1 g dose. Plasma levels declined to less than 1 mcg/mL in 4 to 6 hours. Peak plasma levels of cilastatin following a 20-minute IV infusion range from 15 to 25 mcg/mL for the 250 mg dose, 31 to 49 mcg/mL for the 500 mg dose, and 56 to 88 mcg/mL for the 1 g dose.

The plasma half-life of each component is approximately 1 hour. Protein binding is 20% for imipenem and 40% for cilastatin. Urine imipenem concentrations more than 10 mcg/mL can be maintained for up to 8 hours at the 500 mg dose.

After a 1 g dose, the following average levels (mcg/ml or mcg/g) of imipenem were measured (usually 1 hour post-dose except where indicated) in the following tissues and fluids: peritoneal 23.9 (2 hours); pleural 22; interstitial 16.4; fallopian tubes 13.6; endometrium 11.1; lung 5.6; bile 5.3 (2.25 hours); myometrium 5; skin, fascia 4.4; vitreous humor 3.4 (3.5 hours); aqueous humor 2.99 (2 hours); CSF (inflamed) 2.6 (2 hours); bone 2.6; sputum 2.1; CSF (uninflamed) 1 (4 hours).

IM: Following IM administration of 500 or 750 mg doses, peak plasma levels of imipenem antimicrobial activity occur within 2 hours and average 10 and 12 mcg/ml, respectively. For cilastatin, peak plasma levels average 24 and 33 mcg/ml, respectively, and occur within 1 hour. When compared with IV administration, imipenem is approximately 75% bioavailable following IM administration while cilastatin is approximately 95% bioavailable. The absorption of imipenem from the IM injection site continues for 6 to 8 hours while that for cilastatin is essentially complete within 4 hours. This prolonged absorption of imipenem following IM use results in an effective plasma half-life of approximately 2 to 3 hours and plasma levels which remain above 2 mcg/ml for at least 6 or 8 hours following a 500 or 750 mg dose, respectively. This plasma profile for imipenem permits IM administration every 12 hours with no accumulation of cilastatin and only slight accumulation of imipenem. Imipenem urine levels remain above 10 mcg/ml for the 12-hour dosing interval following IM administration of 500 or 750 mg doses. Total urinary excretion of imipenem and cilastatin averages 50% and 75%, respectively, following either dose.

Metabolism/Excretion – Imipenem, when administered alone, is metabolized in the kidneys by dehydropeptidase 1 resulting in relatively low levels in urine. Cilastatin, an inhibitor of this enzyme, prevents renal metabolism of imipenem. Within 10 hours of administration, approximately 70% of imipenem and cilastatin is recovered in urine.

➤*Microbiology:* Imipenem has in vitro activity against a wide range of gram-positive and gram-negative organisms. It has a high degree of stability in the presence of beta-lactamases, including penicillinases and cephalosporinases produced by gram-negative and gram-positive bacteria. It is a potent inhibitor of β-lactamases from certain gram-negative bacteria resistant to many beta-lactam antibiotics (eg, *Pseudomonas aeruginosa*, *Serratia* sp., *Enterobacter* sp.).

In vitro, imipenem is active against most strains of clinical isolates in the following microorganisms: Gram-positive aerobes; streptococcus; gram-negative aerobes; gram-positive anaerobes; gram-negative anaerobes.

In vitro tests show imipenem to act synergistically with aminoglycoside antibiotics against some isolates of *Pseudomonas aeruginosa*.

Contraindications

Hypersensitivity to any component of this product.

➤*IM:* Hypersensitivity to local anesthetics of the amide type and in patients with severe shock or heart block due to the use of lidocaine HCl diluent.

➤*IV:* Patients with meningitis (safety and efficacy have not been established).

Warnings

➤*Benzyl alcohol:* As a preservative, it has been associated with toxicity in neonates. While toxicity has not been demonstrated in children more than 3 months old, small pediatric patients in this age range may also be at risk for benzyl alcohol toxicity. Therefore, do not use diluents containing benzyl alcohol when imipenem-cilastatin IV is constituted for administration to pediatric patients in this age range.

➤*Resistance:* As with other beta-lactam antibiotics, some strains of *Pseudomonas aeruginosa* may develop resistance fairly rapidly during treatment with imipenem-cilastatin. During therapy of *P. aeruginosa* infections, perform periodic susceptibility testing when clinically appropriate.

➤*Pseudomembranous colitis:* Consider this diagnosis in patients who present with diarrhea because it has occurred with nearly all antibacterial agents. Treatment with antibacterial agents alters the normal flora of the colon and may permit overgrowth of clostridia. Studies show that a toxin produced by *Clostridium difficile* is a primary cause of "antibiotic-associated colitis." Initiate therapeutic measures after the diagnosis of pseudomembranous colitis has been established. Mild cases respond to the discontinuation of the drug alone. In moderate-to-severe cases, consider management with fluids and electrolytes, protein supplementation, and treatment with an antibacterial drug effective against *C. difficile* colitis.

➤*Hypersensitivity reactions:* Serious and occasionally fatal hypersensitivity (anaphylactic) reactions have occurred with β-lactam therapy and are more apt to occur in people with a sensitivity history to multiple allergens. Patients with a history of penicillin hypersensitivity have experienced severe reactions when treated with another β-lactam. If a reaction occurs, discontinue the drug. Serious reactions require immediate emergency measures (see Management of Acute Hypersensitivity Reactions).

➤*Renal function impairment:* Do not give imipenem-cilastatin IV to patients with creatinine clearance (Ccr) of less than or equal to 5 mL/min per 1.73 m^2 unless hemodialysis is instituted within 48 hours. For patients on hemodialysis, imipenem-cilastatin IV is recommended only when the benefit outweighs the potential risk of seizures.

➤*Pregnancy: Category C.* There are no adequate and well-controlled studies in pregnant women. Use only when potential benefits outweigh potential hazards.

➤*Lactation:* It is not known whether this drug is excreted in breast milk. Exercise caution when administering to a breast-feeding woman.

➤*Children:*

IM – Safety and efficacy in children younger than 12 years old have not been established.

IV – Use in neonates to 16 years of age (with non-CNS infections) is supported by evidence from adequate and well controlled studies. IV use is not recommended in pediatric patients with CNS infections because of the risk of seizures, or in pediatric patients less than 30 kg with impaired renal function because no data are available.

Precautions

➤*Monitoring:* While imipenem-cilastatin has the characteristic low toxicity of the beta-lactam group of antibiotics, periodically assess organ system functions, including renal, hepatic, and hematopoietic, during prolonged therapy.

➤*CNS effects:* Adverse reactions (eg, myoclonic activity, confusional states, seizures) have occurred with the IV formulation, especially when recommended dosages were exceeded. They are most common in patients with CNS disorders (eg, brain lesions, history of seizures) who may also have compromised renal function. However, CNS adverse experiences have been reported in patients who had no recognized or documented underlying CNS disorder or compromised renal function. Closely adhere to recommended dosage and dosage schedules, especially in patients with known factors that predispose to convulsive activity. Continue anticonvulsants in patients with a known seizure disorder. If focal tremors, myoclonus, or seizures occur, neurologically evaluate patient, institute anticonvulsants, re-examine the dose, and determine whether to decrease dosage or discontinue the drug. If these effects occur with the IM formulation, discontinue the drug.

➤*Cross-allergenicity:* Use caution when administering to patients with a history of penicillin allergy due to a possible cross-sensitivity to imipenem-cilastatin.

➤*Superinfection:* Use of antibiotics (especially prolonged or repeated therapy) may result in bacterial or fungal overgrowth of nonsusceptible organisms. Such overgrowth may lead to secondary infection. Take appropriate measures if superinfection occurs.

Drug Interactions

Imipenem-Cilastatin Drug Interactions

Precipitant Drug	Object Drug*		Description
Cyclosporine	Imipenem-Cilastatin	↑	The CNS side effects of both agents may be increased possibly because of additive or synergistic toxicity.
Imipenem-Cilastatin	Cyclosporine	↑	

IMIPENEM-CILASTATIN — INJECTION

Imipenem-Cilastatin Drug Interactions			
Precipitant Drug	Object Drug*		Description
Imipenem-Cilastatin	Ganciclovir	↑	Generalized seizures have occurred with coadministration. Do not use concomitantly.
Probenecid	Imipenem	↑	Coadministration results in only minimal increases in imipenem levels and half-life; do not give probenecid concurrently.

* ↑ = Object drug increased.

Adverse Reactions

➤*IV:*

Lab test abnormalities –

Hepatic: Increased AST, ALT, alkaline phosphatase, bilirubin, and LDH.

Hemic: Increased eosinophils, monocytes, lymphocytes, basophils; decreased neutrophils, agranulocytosis, hemoglobin, hematocrit; increased/decreased WBCs and platelets; positive Coombs' test; abnormal prothrombin time.

Electrolytes: Decreased serum sodium; increased potassium and chloride.

Renal: Increased BUN and creatinine.

Urinalysis: Presence of protein, RBCs, WBCs, casts, bilirubin, or urobilinogen.

Cardiovascular – Hypotension (0.4%); palpitations, tachycardia (less than 0.2%).

CNS – Fever (0.5%); seizures (0.4%); dizziness (0.3%); somnolence (0.2%); encephalopathy, tremor, confusion, myoclonus, paresthesia, vertigo, headache, psychic disturbances including hallucinations (less than 0.2%).

Dermatologic – Rash (0.9%); pruritus (0.3%); urticaria (0.2%); erythema multiforme, Stevens-Johnson syndrome, angioneurotic edema, toxic epidermal necrolysis, flushing, cyanosis, skin texture changes, candidiasis, hyperhidrosis, pruritus vulvae (less than 0.2%).

GI – Nausea (2%); diarrhea (1.8%); vomiting (1.5%); pseudomembranous colitis, hemorrhagic colitis, hepatitis, jaundice, staining of the teeth or tongue, gastroenteritis, abdominal pain, glossitis, tongue papillar hypertrophy, heartburn, pharyngeal pain, increased salivation (less than 0.2%).

Hematologic – Pancytopenia, bone marrow depression, thrombocytopenia, neutropenia, leukopenia, hemolytic anemia (less than 0.2%).

Local – Phlebitis/thrombophlebitis (3.1%); pain (0.7%) and erythema at injection site (0.4%); vein induration (0.2%); infused vein infection (0.1%).

Respiratory – Chest discomfort, dyspnea, hyperventilation, thoracic spine pain (less than 0.2%).

Miscellaneous – Hearing loss, tinnitus, polyarthralgia, taste perversion, asthenia/weakness, drug fever, oliguria/anuria, polyuria, acute renal failure, urine discoloration (less than 0.2%).

Children greater than or equal to 3 months old: Diarrhea (3.9%); rash, phlebitis (2.2%); gastroenteritis, vomiting, IV site irritation, urine discoloration (1.1%).

Newborn to 3 months old: Convulsions (5.9%); diarrhea (3%); oliguria/anuria (2.2%); oral candidiasis, rash, tachycardia (1.5%).

➤*IM:*

Lab test abnormalities –

Hemic: Decreased hemoglobin and hematocrit; eosinophilia; increased/decreased WBCs and platelets; decreased erythrocytes; increased prothrombin time.

Hepatic: Increased AST, ALT, alkaline phosphatase and bilirubin.

Renal: Increased BUN and creatinine.

Urinalysis: Presence of RBCs, WBCs, casts and bacteria in the urine.

Miscellaneous – Pain at the injection site (1.2%); nausea, diarrhea (0.6%); rash (0.4%); vomiting (0.3%).

Overdosage

➤*Treatment:* In the case of overdosage, discontinue the drug. Treat symptomatically and institute supportive measures as required. Refer to General Management of Acute Overdosage. Imipenem-cilastatin is hemodialyzable; however, usefulness of this procedure in the overdosage setting is questionable.

ERTAPENEM

Rx	**Invanz** (Merck)	**Powder for injection, lyophilized:** 1.046 g ertapenem sodium (equivalent to 1 g ertapenem)	6 mEq sodium, 175 mg sodium bicarbonate. In vials.

ERTAPENEM — INJECTION

Indications

Ertapenem is indicated for the treatment of patients with the following moderate to severe infections caused by susceptible isolates of the designated microorganisms.

➤*Acute pelvic infections (API):* Including postpartum endomyometritis, septic abortion, and postsurgical gynecologic infections caused by *Streptococcus agalactiae, Escherichia coli, Bacteroides fragilis, Porphyromonas asaccharolytica, Peptostreptococcus* species, or *Prevotella bivia*.

➤*Community-acquired pneumonia (CAP):* Caused by *Streptococcus pneumoniae* (penicillin-susceptible isolates only), including cases with concurrent bacteremia, *Haemophilus influenzae* (beta-lactamase–negative isolates only), or *Moraxella catarrhalis*.

➤*Complicated intra-abdominal infections (IAI):* Caused by *E. coli, Clostridium clostridioforme, Eubacterium lentum, Peptostreptococcus* species, *B. fragilis, Bacteroides distasonis, Bacteroides ovatus, Bacteroides thetaiotaomicron*, or *Bacteroides uniformis*.

➤*Complicated skin and skin structure infections (SSSI):* Including diabetic foot infections without osteomyelitis caused by *Staphylococcus aureus* (methicillin-susceptible isolates only), *S. agalactiae, Streptococcus pyogenes, E. coli, Klebsiella pneumoniae, Proteus mirabilis, B. fragilis, Peptostreptococcus* species, *P. asaccharolytica*, or *P. bivia*. Ertapenem has not been studied in diabetic foot infections with concomitant osteomyelitis.

➤*Complicated urinary tract infections (UTI):* Including pyelonephritis caused by *E. coli*, including cases with concurrent bacteremia or *K. pneumoniae*.

Administration and Dosage

➤*Approved by the FDA:* November 29, 2001.

➤*Dosage:*

Adults and children 13 years of age and older – 1 g given once a day.

Children 3 months to 12 years of age – 15 mg/kg twice daily (not to exceed 1 g/day). Ertapenem may be administered by intravenous (IV) infusion for up to 14 days or intramuscular (IM) injection for up to 7 days. When administered IV, ertapenem should be infused over a period of 30 minutes.

IM administration of ertapenem may be used as an alternative to IV administration in the treatment of those infections for which IM therapy is appropriate.

The following table presents dosage guidelines for ertapenem.

Ertapenem Dosage Guidelines for Adults and Children with Healthy Renal Function[a] and Body Weight			
Infection[b]	Daily dose (IV or IM) in adults and children 13 years of age and older	Daily dose (IV or IM) in children 3 months to 12 years of age	Recommended duration of total antimicrobial treatment
Complicated IAI	1 g	15 mg/kg twice daily[c]	5 to 14 days
Complicated SSSIs, including diabetic foot infections[d]	1 g	15 mg/kg twice daily[c]	7 to 14 days[e]
CAP	1 g	15 mg/kg twice daily[c]	10 to 14 days[f]
Complicated UTIs, including pyelonephritis	1 g	15 mg/kg twice daily[c]	10 to 14 days[f]
APIs, including postpartum endomyometritis, septic abortion, and postsurgical gynecologic infections	1 g	15 mg/kg twice daily[c]	3 to 10 days

[a] Defined as creatinine clearance (Ccr) greater than 90 mL/min/1.73 m^2.
[b] Caused by the designated pathogens.
[c] Not to exceed 1 g/day.
[d] Ertapenem has not been studied in diabetic foot infections with concomitant osteomyelitis.
[e] Adult patients with diabetic foot infections received up to 28 days of treatment (parenteral or parenteral plus oral switch therapy).
[f] Duration includes a possible switch to an appropriate oral therapy, after at least 3 days of parenteral therapy, once clinical improvement has been demonstrated.

➤*Renal function impairment:* Ertapenem may be used for the treatment of infections in adult patients with renal function impairment. In patients whose Ccr is greater than 30 mL/min/1.73 m^2, no dosage adjustment is necessary.

Adult patients with advanced renal function impairment (Ccr less than or equal to 30 mL/min/1.73 m^2) and end-stage renal function impairment (Ccr less than or equal to 10 mL/min/1.73 m^2) should receive 500 mg daily. There are no data in children with renal function impairment.

ERTAPENEM — INJECTION

➤*Hemodialysis:* When adult patients on hemodialysis are given the recommended daily dose of ertapenem 500 mg within 6 hours prior to hemodialysis, a supplementary dose of 150 mg is recommended following the hemodialysis session. If ertapenem is given at least 6 hours prior to hemodialysis, no supplementary dose is needed. There are no data in patients undergoing peritoneal dialysis or hemofiltration. There are no data in children on hemodialysis.

➤*Preparation of solution:*

Adults and children 13 years of age and older –

IV: Ertapenem must be reconstituted and then diluted prior to administration.

1.) Reconstitute the contents of a 1 g vial of ertapenem with 10 mL of one of the following: water for injection, sodium chloride 0.9% injection, or bacteriostatic water for injection.
2.) Shake well to dissolve and immediately transfer the contents of the reconstituted vial to 50 mL of sodium chloride 0.9% injection.
3.) Complete the infusion within 6 hours of reconstitution.

IM: Ertapenem must be reconstituted prior to administration.

1.) Reconstitute the contents of a 1 g vial of ertapenem with 3.2 mL of lidocaine 1% injection (without epinephrine). Shake the vial thoroughly to form solution.
2.) Immediately withdraw the contents of the vial and administer by deep IM injection into a large muscle mass (eg, the gluteal muscles, lateral part of the thigh).
3.) The reconstituted IM solution should be used within 1 hour after preparation. The reconstituted solution should not be administered IV.

Children 3 months to 12 years of age –

IV: Ertapenem must be reconstituted and then diluted prior to administration.

1.) Reconstitute the contents of a 1 g vial of ertapenem with 10 mL of one of the following: water for injection, sodium chloride 0.9% injection, or bacteriostatic water for injection.
2.) Shake well to dissolve and immediately withdraw a volume equal to 15 mg/kg of body weight (not to exceed 1 g/day) and dilute in sodium chloride 0.9% injection to a final concentration of 20 mg/mL or less.
3.) Complete the infusion within 6 hours of reconstitution.

IM: Ertapenem must be reconstituted prior to administration.

1.) Reconstitute the contents of a 1 g vial of ertapenem with 3.2 mL of lidocaine 1% injection (without epinephrine). Shake vial thoroughly to form solution.
2.) Immediately withdraw a volume equal to 15 mg/kg of body weight (not to exceed 1 g/day) and administer by deep IM injection into a large muscle mass (eg, the gluteal muscles, lateral part of the thigh).
3.) The reconstituted IM solution should be used within 1 hour after preparation. The reconstituted solution should not be administered IV.

Admixture incompatibility – Do not mix or coinfuse ertapenem with other medications. Do not use diluents containing dextrose (α-D-glucose).

Parenteral drug products should be inspected visually for particulate matter and discoloration prior to use, whenever solution and container permit. Solutions of ertapenem range from colorless to pale yellow. Variations of color within this range do not affect the potency of the product.

➤*Storage/Stability:* Do not store the lyophilized powder above 25°C (77°F).

The reconstituted solution, immediately diluted in sodium chloride 0.9% injection, may be stored at room temperature (25°C; 77°F) and used within 6 hours, or stored for 24 hours under refrigeration (5°C; 41°F) and used within 4 hours after removal from refrigeration. Do not freeze.

Actions

➤*Pharmacokinetics:*

Absorption – Average plasma concentrations (mcg/mL) of ertapenem following a single 30-minute infusion of a 1 g IV dose and administration of a single 1 g IM dose in healthy young adults are presented in the following table.

Plasma Concentrations of Ertapenem in Adults After Single-Dose Administration

	Average plasma concentrations (mcg/mL)								
Dose/route	0.5 h	1 h	2 h	4 h	6 h	8 h	12 h	10 h	24 h
1 g IV[a]	155	115	83	48	31	20	9	3	1
1 g IM	33	53	67	57	40	27	13	4	2

[a] Infused at a constant rate over 30 minutes.

The area under the plasma concentration-time curve (AUC) of ertapenem increased less than dose proportional based on total ertapenem concentrations over the 0.5 to 2 g dose range, whereas the AUC increased greater than dose proportional based on unbound ertapenem concentrations. Ertapenem exhibits nonlinear pharmacokinetics because of concentration-dependent plasma protein binding at the proposed therapeutic dose.

There is no accumulation of ertapenem following multiple IV or IM 1 g daily doses in healthy adults.

Average plasma concentrations (mcg/mL) of ertapenem in pediatric patients are presented in the following table.

Plasma Concentrations of Ertapenem in Children After Single IV[a] Dose Administration

Age group	Dose	Average plasma concentrations (mcg/mL)							
		0.5 h	1 h	2 h	4 h	6 h	8 h	12 h	24 h
3 to 23 months									
	15 mg/kg[b]	103.8	57.3	43.6	23.7	13.5	8.2	2.5	—
	20 mg/kg[b]	126.8	87.6	58.7	28.4	—	12	3.4	0.4
	40 mg/kg[c]	199.1	144.1	95.7	58	—	20.2	7.7	0.6
2 to 12 years									
	15 mg/kg[b]	113.2	63.9	42.1	21.9	12.8	7.6	3	—
	20 mg/kg[b]	147.6	97.6	63.2	34.5	—	12.3	4.9	0.5
	40 mg/kg[c]	241.7	152.7	96.3	55.6	—	18.8	7.2	0.6
13 to 17 years									
	20 mg/kg[b]	170.4	98.3	67.8	40.4	—	16	7	1.1
	1 g[d]	155.9	110.9	74.8	—	24	—	6.2	—
	40 mg/kg[c]	255	188.7	127.9	76.2	—	31	15.3	2.1

[a] Infused at a constant rate over 30 minutes.
[b] Up to a maximum dose of 1 g/day.
[c] Up to a maximum dose of 2 g/day.
[d] Based on 3 patients receiving ertapenem 1 g who volunteered for pharmacokinetic assessment in 1 of the 2 safety and efficacy studies.

Ertapenem, reconstituted with lidocaine 1% injection (in saline without epinephrine), is almost completely absorbed following IM administration at the recommended dose of 1 g. The mean bioavailability is approximately 90%. Following 1 g daily IM administration, mean peak plasma concentrations (C_{max}) are achieved in approximately 2.3 hours (T_{max}).

Distribution – Ertapenem is highly bound to human plasma proteins, primarily albumin. In healthy young adults, the protein binding of ertapenem decreases as plasma concentrations increase, from approximately 95% bound at an approximate plasma concentration of less than 100 mcg/mL to approximately 85% bound at an approximate plasma concentration of 300 mcg/mL.

The apparent volume of distribution at steady state (V_{ss}) of ertapenem in adults is approximately 0.12 L/kg, approximately 0.2 L/kg in pediatric patients 3 months to 12 years of age, and approximately 0.16 L/kg in pediatric patients 13 to 17 years of age.

The concentrations of ertapenem achieved in suction-induced skin blister fluid at each sampling point on the third day of 1 g once-daily IV doses are presented in the following table. The ratio of AUC_{0-24} in skin blister fluid/ AUC_{0-24} in plasma is 0.61.

Concentrations (mcg/mL) of Ertapenem in Adult Skin Blister Fluid

0.5 h	1 h	2 h	4 h	8 h	12 h	24 h
7	12	17	24	24	21	8

The concentration of ertapenem in breast milk from 5 lactating women with pelvic infections (5 to 14 days postpartum) was measured at random time points daily for 5 consecutive days following the last 1 g dose of IV therapy (3 to 10 days of therapy). The concentration of ertapenem in breast milk within 24 hours of the last dose of therapy in all 5 women ranged from less than 0.13 (lower limit of quantitation) to 0.38 mcg/mL; peak concentrations were not assessed. By day 5 after discontinuation of therapy, the level of ertapenem was undetectable in the breast milk of 4 women and below the lower limit of quantitation (less than 0.13 mcg/mL) in 1 woman.

Metabolism – In healthy young adults, after infusion of IV radiolabeled ertapenem 1 g, the plasma radioactivity consisted predominantly (94%) of ertapenem. The major metabolite of ertapenem is the inactive ring-opened derivative formed by hydrolysis of the beta-lactam ring.

Excretion – Ertapenem is eliminated primarily by the kidneys. The mean plasma half-life in healthy young adults is approximately 4 hours and the plasma clearance is approximately 1.8 L/h. The mean plasma half-life in pediatric patients 13 to 17 years of age is approximately 4 hours and approximately 2.5 hours in pediatric patients 3 months to 12 years of age.

Following the administration of IV radiolabeled ertapenem 1 g to healthy young adults, approximately 80% is recovered in urine and 10% in feces. Of the 80% recovered in urine, approximately 38% is excreted as unchanged drug and approximately 37% as the ring-opened metabolite.

In healthy young adults given a 1 g IV dose, the mean percentage of the administered dose excreted in urine was 17.4% during 0 to 2 hours postdose, 5.4% during 4 to 6 hours postdose, and 2.4% during 12 to 24 hours postdose.

Special populations –

Renal function impairment: Total and unbound fractions of ertapenem pharmacokinetics were investigated in 26 adult subjects (31 to 80 years of age) with varying degrees of renal function impairment. Following a single IV dose of ertapenem 1 g, the unbound AUC increased 1.5-fold and 2.3-fold in subjects with mild renal function impairment (Ccr 60 to 90 mL/min/1.73 m^2) and moderate renal function impairment (Ccr 31 to 59 mL/min/1.73 m^2), respectively, compared with healthy young subjects (25 to 45 years of age). No dosage adjustment is necessary in patients with Ccr greater than or equal to 31 mL/min/1.73 m^2. The unbound AUC increased 4.4-fold and 7.6-fold in subjects with advanced renal function impairment (Ccr 5 to 30 mL/ min/1.73 m^2) and end-stage renal function impairment (Ccr less than 10 mL/ min/1.73 m^2), respectively, compared with healthy young subjects. The effects of renal function impairment on AUC of total drug were of smaller

ERTAPENEM — INJECTION

magnitude. The recommended dose of ertapenem in patients with Ccr less than or equal to 30 mL/min/1.73 m^2 is 0.5 g every 24 hours.

Following a single 1 g IV dose given immediately prior to a 4-hour hemodialysis session in 5 patients with end-stage renal function impairment, approximately 30% of the dose was recovered in the dialysate. A supplementary dose of 150 mg is recommended if ertapenem is administered within 6 hours prior to hemodialysis. There are no data in pediatric patients with renal function impairment.

Elderly: The impact of age on the pharmacokinetics of ertapenem was evaluated in healthy men (n = 7) and women (n = 7) 65 years of age and older. The total and unbound AUC increased 37% and 67%, respectively, in elderly adults relative to young adults. These changes were attributed to age-related changes in Ccr. No dosage adjustment is necessary for elderly patients with normal (for their age) renal function.

Children: Plasma concentrations of ertapenem are comparable in pediatric patients 13 to 17 years of age and adults following a 1 g once-daily IV dose.

Following the 20 mg/kg dose (up to a maximum dose of 1 g), the pharmacokinetic parameter values in patients 13 to 17 years of age (n = 6) were generally comparable with those in healthy young adults.

Plasma concentrations at the midpoint of the dosing interval following a single 15 mg/kg IV dose of ertapenem in patients 3 months to 12 years of age are comparable with plasma concentrations at the midpoint of the dosing interval following a 1 g once-daily IV dose in adults. The plasma clearance (mL/min/kg) of ertapenem in patients 3 months to 12 years of age is approximately 2-fold higher compared with that in adults. At the 15 mg/kg dose, the AUC value (doubled to model a twice-daily dosing regimen; ie, 30 mg/kg/day exposure) in patients 3 months to 12 years of age was comparable with the AUC value in young healthy adults receiving a 1 g IV dose of ertapenem.

Contraindications

Known hypersensitivity to any component of this product or to other drugs in the same class or in patients who have demonstrated anaphylactic reactions to beta-lactams.

Because of the use of lidocaine as a diluent, ertapenem administered IM is contraindicated in patients with a known hypersensitivity to local anesthetics of the amide type.

Warnings

See Administration and Dosage for more information.

➤*Pseudomembranous colitis:* Pseudomembranous colitis has been reported with nearly all antibacterial agents, including ertapenem, and may range in severity from mild to life-threatening. Therefore, it is important to consider this diagnosis in patients who present with diarrhea subsequent to the administration of antibacterial agents.

After the diagnosis of pseudomembranous colitis has been established, initiate therapeutic measures. Mild cases of pseudomembranous colitis usually respond to drug discontinuation alone. In moderate to severe cases, consider management with fluids and electrolytes, protein supplementation, and treatment with an antibacterial drug clinically effective against *C. difficile* colitis.

➤*Hypersensitivity reactions:* Serious and occasionally fatal hypersensitivity (anaphylactic) reactions have been reported in patients receiving therapy with beta-lactams. These reactions are more likely to occur in individuals with a history of sensitivity to multiple allergens. There have been reports of individuals with a history of penicillin hypersensitivity who have experienced severe hypersensitivity reactions when treated with another beta-lactam. Before initiating therapy with ertapenem, make careful inquiry concerning previous hypersensitivity reactions to penicillins, cephalosporins, other beta-lactams, and other allergens. If an allergic reaction to ertapenem occurs, discontinue the drug immediately. Serious anaphylactic reactions require immediate emergency treatment with epinephrine, oxygen, IV steroids, and airway management, including intubation. Other therapy may also be administered as indicated.

➤*Renal function impairment:* See Actions for more information.

➤*Fertility impairment:* In mice and rats, IV doses of up to 700 mg/kg/day (for mice, approximately 3 times the recommended human dose of 1 g based on body surface area and for rats, approximately 1.2 times the human exposure at the recommended dose of 1 g based on plasma AUCs) resulted in no effects on mating performance, fecundity, fertility, or embryonic survival.

➤*Elderly:* Of the 1,835 patients in phase 2b/3 studies treated with ertapenem, approximately 26% were 65 years of age and older, while approximately 12% were 75 years of age and older. No overall differences in safety or efficacy were observed between these patients and younger patients. Other reported clinical experience has not identified differences in responses between the elderly and younger patients, but greater sensitivity of some older individuals cannot be ruled out.

This drug is known to be substantially excreted by the kidney, and the risk of toxic reactions to this drug may be greater in patients with impaired renal function. Because elderly patients are more likely to have decreased renal function, take care in dose selection, and it may be useful to monitor renal function.

➤*Pregnancy: Category B.*

Teratogenic – In mice and rats given IV doses of up to 700 mg/kg/day (for mice, approximately 3 times the recommended human dose of 1 g based on body surface area and for rats, approximately 1.2 times the human exposure at the recommended dose of 1 g based on plasma AUCs), there was no evidence of developmental toxicity as assessed by external, visceral, and skeletal examination of the fetuses.

In mice given 700 mg/kg/day, slight decreases in average fetal weights and an associated decrease in the average number of ossified sacrocaudal vertebrae were observed. Ertapenem crosses the placental barrier in rats.

There are, however, no adequate and well-controlled studies in pregnant women. Because animal reproduction studies are not always predictive of human response, use this drug during pregnancy only if clearly needed.

➤*Lactation:* Ertapenem is excreted in human breast milk. Exercise caution when administering ertapenem to a breast-feeding women. Administer ertapenem to breast-feeding mothers only when the expected benefit outweighs the risk.

➤*Children:* Safety and efficacy of ertapenem in pediatric patients 3 months to 17 years of age are supported by evidence from adequate and well-controlled studies in adults, pharmacokinetic data in pediatric patients, and additional data from comparator-controlled studies in pediatric patients 3 months to 17 years of age with the following infections: complicated IAI, complicated SSSI, CAP, complicated UTI, and API.

Ertapenem is not recommended in infants younger than 3 months of age; no data are available.

Ertapenem is not recommended in the treatment of meningitis in the pediatric population because of a lack of sufficient cerebrospinal fluid penetration.

Precautions

➤*Monitoring:* While ertapenem possesses toxicity similar to the beta-lactam group of antibiotics, periodic assessment of organ system function, including renal, hepatic, and hematopoietic, is advisable during prolonged therapy.

➤*IM administration:* Use caution when administering ertapenem IM to avoid inadvertent injection into a blood vessel.

Lidocaine is the diluent for IM administration of ertapenem.

➤*Reducing drug resistance:* Prescribing ertapenem in the absence of a proven or strongly suspected bacterial infection or a prophylactic indication is unlikely to provide benefit to the patient and increases the risk of the development of drug-resistant bacteria.

➤*Seizures:* Seizures and other CNS adverse reactions have been reported during treatment with ertapenem.

➤*Superinfection:* As with other antibiotics, prolonged use of ertapenem may result in overgrowth of nonsusceptible organisms. Repeated evaluation of the patient's condition is essential. If superinfection occurs during therapy, take appropriate measures.

Drug Interactions

➤*Probenecid:* When ertapenem is coadministered with probenecid (500 mg every 6 hours), probenecid competes for active tubular secretion and reduces the renal clearance of ertapenem. Based on total ertapenem concentrations, probenecid increased the AUC 25% and reduced the plasma and renal clearances 20% and 35%, respectively. The half-life increased from 4 to 4.8 hours. Because of the small effect on half-life, coadministration of probenecid to extend the half-life of ertapenem is not recommended.

➤*Cytochrome P-450 system/P-glycoprotein–mediated transport:* In vitro studies indicate that ertapenem does not inhibit P-glycoprotein–mediated transport of digoxin or vinblastine and that ertapenem is not a substrate for P-glycoprotein–mediated transport. In vitro studies in human liver microsomes indicate that ertapenem does not inhibit metabolism mediated by any of the following 6 cytochrome P-450 isoforms: 1A2, 2C9, 2C19, 2D6, 2E1, and 3A4. Drug interactions caused by inhibition of P-glycoprotein–mediated drug clearance or cytochrome P-450–mediated drug clearance with the listed isoforms are unlikely.

➤*Valproic acid:* Valproic acid plasma levels may be decreased, leading to loss of seizure control. Monitor valproic acid plasma concentrations and observe the patient for benzine activity.

Adverse Reactions

➤*Adults:* Clinical studies enrolled 1,954 patients treated with ertapenem; in some of the clinical studies, parenteral therapy was followed by a switch to an appropriate oral antimicrobial. Most adverse reactions reported in these clinical studies were described as mild to moderate in severity. Ertapenem was discontinued because of adverse reactions in 4.7% of patients. The following table shows the incidence of adverse reactions reported in greater than or equal to 1% of patients in these studies.

The most common drug-related adverse reactions in patients treated with ertapenem, including those who were switched to therapy with an oral antimicrobial, were diarrhea (5.5%), infused vein complication (3.7%), nausea (3.1%), headache (2.2%), vaginitis in woman (2.1%), phlebitis/thrombophlebitis (1.3%), and vomiting (1.1%).

Ertapenem Adverse Reactions in Adults (≥ 1%)

Adverse reactions	Ertapenem[a] 1 g daily (n = 802)	Piperacillin/Tazobactam[a] 3.375 g every 6 h (n = 774)	Ertapenem[b] 1 g daily (n = 1,152)	Ceftriaxone[b] 1 or 2 g daily (n = 942)
Cardiovascular				
Chest pain	1.5%	1.4%	1%	2.5%
Hypertension	1.6%	1.4%	0.7%	1%
Hypotension	2%	1.4%	1%	1.2%
Tachycardia	1.6%	1.3%	1.3%	0.7%

ERTAPENEM — INJECTION

Ertapenem Adverse Reactions in Adults (≥ 1%)				
Adverse reactions	Ertapenem[a] 1 g daily (n = 802)	Piperacillin/ Tazobactam[a] 3.375 g every 6 h (n = 774)	Ertapenem[b] 1 g daily (n = 1,152)	Ceftriaxone[b] 1 or 2 g daily (n = 942)
CNS				
Altered mental status[c]	5.1%	3.4%	3.3%	2.5%
Anxiety	1.4%	1.3%	0.8%	1.2%
Asthenia/Fatigue	1.2%	0.9%	1.2%	1.1%
Dizziness	2.1%	3%	1.5%	2.1%
Headache	5.6%	5.4%	6.8%	6.9%
Insomnia	3.2%	5.2%	3%	4.1%
Dermatologic				
Erythema	1.6%	1.7%	1.2%	1.2%
Pruritus	2%	2.6%	1%	1.9%
Rash	2.5%	3.1%	2.3%	1.5%
GI				
Abdominal pain	3.6%	4.8%	4.3%	3.9%
Acid regurgitation	1.6%	0.9%	1.1%	0.6%
Constipation	4%	5.4%	3.3%	3.1%
Diarrhea	10.3%	12.1%	9.2%	9.8%
Dyspepsia	1.1%	0.6%	1%	1.6%
Nausea	8.5%	8.7%	6.4%	7.4%
Oral candidiasis	0.1%	1.3%	1.4%	1.9%
Vomiting	3.7%	5.3%	4%	4%
GU				
Vaginitis	1.4%	1%	3.3%	3.7%
Local				
Extravasation	1.9%	1.7%	0.7%	1.1 %
Infused vein complication	7.1%	7.9%	5.4%	6.7%
Phlebitis/ Thrombophlebitis	1.9%	2.7%	1.6%	2%
Respiratory				
Cough	1.6%	1.7%	1.3%	0.5%
Dyspnea	2.6%	1.8%	1%	2.4%
Pharyngitis	0.7%	1.4%	1.1%	0.6%
Rales/Rhonchi	1.1%	1%	0.5%	1%
Respiratory distress	1%	0.4%	0.2%	0.2%
Miscellaneous				
Death	2.5%	1.6%	1.3%	1.6%
Edema/Swelling	3.4%	2.5%	2.9%	3.3%
Fever	5%	6.6%	2.3%	3.4%
Leg pain	1.1%	0.5%	0.4%	0.3%

[a] Includes phase 2b/3 complicated IAI, complicated SSSI, and API studies.
[b] Includes phase 2b/3 CAP and complicated UTI, and phase 2a studies.
[c] Includes agitation, changed mental status, confusion, decreased mental acuity, disorientation, somnolence, or stupor.

In patients treated for complicated IAI, death occurred in 4.7% (15/316) of patients receiving ertapenem and 2.6% (8/307) of patients receiving comparator drug. These deaths occurred in patients with significant comorbidity and/or severe baseline infections. Deaths were considered unrelated to study drugs by investigators.

Seizures – In clinical studies, seizure was reported during study therapy plus a 14-day follow-up period in 0.5% of patients treated with ertapenem, 0.3% of patients treated with piperacillin/tazobactam, and 0% of patients treated with ceftriaxone.

Adverse reactions (greater than 0.1%) – Additional adverse reactions that were reported with ertapenem with an incidence greater than 0.1% within each body system are listed in the following sections:

Cardiovascular – Arrhythmia, asystole, atrial fibrillation, bradycardia, cardiac arrest, heart failure, heart murmur, hematoma, subdural hemorrhage, syncope, ventricular tachycardia.

CNS – Aggressive behavior, depression, hypesthesia, nervousness, paresthesia, seizure, spasm, tremor, vertigo.

Dermatologic – Dermatitis, desquamation, flushing, sweating, urticaria.

GI – Abdominal distention, anorexia, *C. difficile*-associated diarrhea, cholelithiasis, duodenitis, dysphagia, esophagitis, flatulence, gastritis, GI hemorrhage, hemorrhoids, ileus, jaundice, mouth ulcer, pancreatitis, pyloric stenosis, stomatitis.

GU – Bladder dysfunction, hematuria, oliguria/anuria, renal function impairment, urinary retention, vaginal candidiasis, vaginal pruritus, vulvovaginitis.

Respiratory – Asthma, bronchoconstriction, epistaxis, hemoptysis, hiccups, hypoxemia, pharyngeal discomfort, pleural effusion, pleuritic pain, voice disturbance.

Special senses – Taste perversion.

Miscellaneous – Candidiasis, chills, dehydration, facial edema, flank pain, gout, injection-site induration, injection-site pain, malaise, necrosis, pain, septic shock, septicemia, weight loss.

➤*Children:* Clinical studies enrolled 384 patients treated with ertapenem; in some of the clinical studies, parenteral therapy was followed by a switch to an appropriate oral antimicrobial. The overall adverse reaction profile in pediatric patients is comparable with that in adult patients. The following table shows the incidence of adverse reactions reported in 1% or more of pediatric patients in clinical studies. The most common drug-related adverse reactions in pediatric patients treated with ertapenem, including those who were switched to therapy with an oral antimicrobial, were diarrhea (6.5%), infusion-site pain (5.5%), infusion-site erythema (2.6%), and vomiting (2.1%).

Ertapenem Adverse Reactions in Children (≥ 1%)			
Adverse reactions	Ertapenem[a,b] (n = 384)	Ceftriaxone[a] (n = 100)	Ticarcillin/ Clavulanate[b] (n = 24)
CNS			
Dizziness	1.6%	0%	0%
Headache	4.4%	4%	0%
Dermatologic			
Dermatitis	1%	1%	0%
Diaper dermatitis	4.7%	4%	0%
Pruritus	1.6%	0%	0%
Rash	2.9%	2%	8.3%
GI			
Abdominal abscess	1%	0%	4.2%
Abdominal pain	4.7%	3%	4.2%
Constipation	2.3%	0%	0%
Diarrhea	11.7%	17%	4.2%
Loose stools	2.1%	0%	0%
Nausea	1.6%	0%	0%
Upper abdominal pain	1%	2%	0%
Vomiting	10.2%	11%	8.3%
Local			
Infusion-site erythema	3.9%	3%	8.3%
Infusion-site induration	1%	1%	0%
Infusion-site pain	7%	4%	20.8%
Infusion-site phlebitis	1.8%	3%	0%
Infusion-site swelling	1.8%	1%	4.2%
Infusion-site warmth	1.3%	1%	4.2%
Respiratory			
Cough	4.4%	3%	0%
Nasopharyngitis	1.6%	6%	0%
Upper respiratory tract infection	2.3%	3%	0%
Viral pharyngitis	1%	0%	0%
Wheezing	1%	0%	0%
Miscellaneous			
Herpes simplex	1%	1%	4.2%
Hypothermia	1.6%	1%	0%
Pyrexia	4.9%	6%	8.3%

[a] Includes phase 2b complicated SSSI, CAP, and complicated UTI studies in which patients 3 months to 12 years of age received ertapenem 15 mg/kg IV twice daily up to a maximum of 1 g or ceftriaxone 50 mg/kg/day IV in 2 divided doses up to a maximum of 2 g, and patients 13 to 17 years of age received ertapenem 1 g IV daily or ceftriaxone 50 mg/kg/day IV in a single daily dose.
[b] Includes phase 2b API and complicated IAI studies in which patients 3 months to 12 years of age received ertapenem 15 mg/kg IV twice daily up to a maximum of 1 g and patients 13 to 17 years of age received ertapenem 1 g IV daily or ticarcillin/clavulanate 50 mg/kg for patients < 60 kg or ticarcillin/clavulanate 3 g for patients > 60 kg, 4 or 6 times a day.

Adverse reactions (0.5% to 1%) – Additional adverse reactions that were reported with ertapenem with an incidence of less than 1% and greater than 0.5% within each body system are listed in the following sections:

Cardiovascular – Chest pain, phlebitis.

CNS – Insomnia, somnolence.

Dermatologic – Atopic dermatitis, erythematous rash, skin lesion.

ERTAPENEM — INJECTION

GU – Genital rash.

Metabolic/Nutritional – Decreased appetite.

Musculoskeletal – Arthralgia.

Respiratory – Pleural effusion, rhinitis, rhinorrhea.

Miscellaneous – Candidiasis, ear infection, infusion-site pruritus, oral candidiasis.

➤*Lab test abnormalities:*

Adults – Laboratory adverse reactions that were reported during therapy in greater than or equal to 1% of adult patients treated with ertapenem in clinical studies are presented in the following table. Drug-related laboratory adverse reactions that were reported during therapy in greater than or equal to 1% of adult patients treated with ertapenem, including those who were switched to therapy with an oral antimicrobial, in clinical studies were ALT increased (6%), AST increased (5.2%), serum alkaline phosphatase increased (3.4%), platelet count increased (2.8%), and eosinophils increased (1.1%). Ertapenem was discontinued because of laboratory adverse reactions in 0.3% of patients.

Lab Test Abnormalities in Adults (≥ 1%)[a]

Lab test abnormalities	Ertapenem[b] 1 g daily (n[c] = 766)	Piperacillin/ Tazobactam[b] 3.375 g every 6 h (n[c] = 755)	Ertapenem[d] 1 g daily (n[b] = 1,122)	Ceftriaxone[d] 1 or 2 g daily (n[b] = 920)
ALT increased	8.8%	7.3%	8.3%	6.9%
AST increased	8.4%	8.3%	7.1%	6.5%
Eosinophils increased	1.1%	1.1%	2.1%	1.8%
Hematocrit decreased	3%	2.9%	3.4%	2.4%
Hemoglobin decreased	4.9%	4.7%	4.5%	3.5%
Platelet count decreased	1.1%	1.2%	1.1%	1%
Platelet count increased	6.5%	6.3%	4.3%	3.5%
Prothrombin time increased	1.2%	2%	0.3%	0.9%
Segmented neutrophils decreased	1%	0.3%	1.5%	0.8%
Serum albumin decreased	1.7%	1.5%	0.9%	1.6%
Serum alkaline phosphatase increased	6.6%	7.2%	4.3%	2.8%
Serum creatinine increased	1.1%	2.7%	0.9%	1.2%
Serum glucose increased	1.2%	2.3%	1.7%	2%
Serum potassium decreased	1.7%	2.8%	1.8%	2.4%
Serum potassium increased	1.3%	0.5%	0.5%	0.7%
Total serum bilirubin increased	1.7%	1.4%	0.6%	1.1%
Urine red blood cells increased	2.5%	2.9%	1.1%	1%
Urine white blood cells increased	2.5%	3.2%	1.6%	1.1%
White blood cells decreased	0.8%	0.7%	1.5%	1.4%

[a] Number of patients with laboratory adverse reactions/number of patients with the laboratory test.
[b] Includes phase 2b/3 complicated IAI, complicated SSSI, and API studies.
[c] Number of patients with 1 or more laboratory tests.
[d] Includes phase 2b/3 CAP and complicated UTI, and phase 2a studies.

Additional laboratory adverse reactions that were reported during therapy in greater than 0.1% but less than 1% of patients treated with ertapenem in clinical studies include: increases in serum urea nitrogen, direct and indirect serum bilirubin, serum sodium, monocytes, partial thromboplastin time, and urine epithelial cells; decreases in serum bicarbonate.

Children – Laboratory adverse reactions that were reported during therapy in 1% or more of pediatric patients treated with ertapenem in clinical studies are presented in the following table. Drug-related laboratory adverse reactions that were reported during therapy in 2% or more of pediatric patients treated with ertapenem, including those who were switched to therapy with an oral antimicrobial, in clinical studies were neutrophil count decreased (3%), ALT increased (2.2%), and AST increased (2.1%).

Lab Test Abnormalities in Children (≥ 1%)[a]

Lab test abnormalities	Ertapenem (n[b] = 379)	Ceftriaxone (n[b] = 97)	Ticarcillin/ Clavulanate (n[b] = 24)
Alkaline phosphatase increased	1.1%	0%	0%
ALT increased	3.8%	1.1%	4.3%
AST increased	3.8%	1.1%	4.3%
Eosinophil count increased	1.1%	2.1%	0%
Neutrophil count decreased	5.8%	3.1%	0%
Platelet count increased	1.3%	0%	8.7%

[a] Number of patients with laboratory adverse reactions/number of patients with the laboratory test; at least 300 patients had the test.
[b] Number of patients with 1 or more laboratory tests.

Additional laboratory adverse reactions that were reported during therapy in greater than 0.5% but less than 1% of patients treated with ertapenem in clinical studies include: white blood cell count decreased and protein urine present.

Overdosage

➤*Symptoms:* No specific information is available on the treatment of overdosage with ertapenem. Intentional overdosing of ertapenem is unlikely. IV administration of ertapenem at a dose of 2 g over 30 minutes or 3 g over 1 to 2 hours in healthy volunteers resulted in an increased incidence of nausea. In clinical studies in adults, inadvertent administration of three 1 g doses of ertapenem in a 24-hour period resulted in diarrhea and transient dizziness in 1 patient. In pediatric clinical studies, a single IV dose of 40 mg/kg up to a maximum of 2 g did not result in toxicity.

➤*Treatment:* In the event of an overdose, discontinue ertapenem and give general supportive treatment until renal elimination takes place.

Ertapenem can be removed by hemodialysis; the plasma clearance of the total fraction of ertapenem was increased 30% in subjects with end-stage renal function impairment when hemodialysis (4-hour session) was performed immediately following administration. However, no information is available on the use of hemodialysis to treat overdosage.

MONOBACTAMS

AZTREONAM

Rx	**Azactam** (Squibb)	**Powder for Injection (lyophilized cake):** 500 mg[1]	In single-dose 15 ml vials.
		1 g[1]	In single-dose 15 ml vials and single-dose 100 ml infusion bottles.
		2 g[1]	In 30 ml single-dose vials and single-dose 100 ml infusion bottles.

[1] With ≈ 780 mg L–arginine per gram aztreonam.

AZTREONAM — INJECTION

Indications

➤*Urinary tract infections (complicated and uncomplicated):* Including pyelonephritis and cystitis (initial and recurrent) caused by *Escherichia coli*; *Klebsiella pneumoniae*; *Proteus mirabilis*; *Pseudomonas aeruginosa*; *Enterobacter cloacae*; *Klebsiella oxytoca*, *Citrobacter* species and *Serratia marcescens* (efficacy of these organisms in this organ system was studied in less than 10 infections.

➤*Lower respiratory tract infections:* Including pneumonia and bronchitis caused by *Escherichia coli*, *Klebsiella pneumoniae*, *Pseudomonas aeruginosa*, *Haemophilus influenzae*, *Proteus mirabilis*, *Enterobacter* and *Serratia marcescens* (efficacy of this organism in this organ system was studied in less than 10 infections).

AZTREONAM — INJECTION

➤*Septicemia:* *Enterobacter* species; caused by *Escherichia coli*; *Klebsiella pneumoniae*; *Pseudomonas aeruginosa*; *Proteus mirabilis, Serratia marcescens* (efficacy for these organisms in this organ system was studied in less than 10 infections).

➤*Skin and skin-structure infections:* Including those associated with postoperative wounds, ulcers and burns caused by *Escherichia coli, Proteus mirabilis, Serratia marcescens, Enterobacter species, Pseudomonas aeruginosa, Klebsiella pneumoniae* and *Citrobacter* species (efficacy for these organisms in this organ system was studied in fewer than 10 infections).

➤*Intra-abdominal infections:* Including peritonitis caused by *Escherichia coli; Klebsiella* species including *K. pneumoniae; Enterobacter* species including *E. cloacae* (efficacy for E. cloacae in this organ system was studied in less than 10 infections); *Pseudomonas aeruginosa; Citrobacter* species including *C. freundii*, and *Serratia* species including *S. marcescens* (efficacy for the specified organisms and their species in this organ system was studied in less than 10 infections).

➤*Gynecologic infections:* Including endometritis and pelvic cellulitis caused by *Escherichia coli; Klebsiella pneumoniae, Enterobacter*species including *E. cloacae, Proteus mirabilis*.

➤*Surgery:* Aztreonam is indicated for adjunctive therapy to surgery in the management of infections caused by susceptible organisms, including abscesses, infections complicating hollow viscus perforations, cutaneous infections and infections of serous surfaces. Aztreonam is effective against most of the commonly encountered gram-negative aerobic pathogens seen in general surgery.

➤*Concurrent therapy:* Concurrent initial therapy with other antimicrobial agents and aztreonam for injection is recommended before the causative organism(s) is known in seriously ill patients who are also at risk of having an infection due to gram-positive aerobic pathogens. If anaerobic organisms are also suspected as etiologic agents, therapy should be initiated using an anti-anaerobic agent concurrently with aztreonam (see Administration and Dosage). Certain antibiotics (eg, cefoxitin, imipenem) may induce high levels of beta-lactamase in vitro in some gram-negative aerobes such as *Enterobacter* and *Pseudomonas* species, resulting in antagonism to many beta-lactam antibiotics including aztreonam. These in vitro findings suggest that such beta-lactamase inducing antibiotics not be used concurrently with aztreonam. Following identification and susceptibility testing of the causative organism(s), appropriate antibiotic therapy should be continued.

➤*Unlabeled uses:* 1 g IM may be beneficial for acute uncomplicated gonorrhea in patients with penicillin-resistant gonococci, as an alternative to spectinomycin.

Administration and Dosage

➤*Adults:* Aztreonam may be administered intravenously or by IM injection. Dosage and route of administration should be determined by susceptibility of the causative organisms, severity and site of infection, and the condition of the patient.

Aztreonam for Injection Dosage Guidelines

Type of infection	Dose	Frequency (hours)
Adults*		
Urinary tract infections	500 mg or 1 g	8 or 12
Moderately severe systemic infections	1 g or 2 g	8 or 12
Severe systemic or life-threatening infections	2 g	6 or 8
Pediatric patients**		
Mild to moderate infections	30 mg/kg	8
Moderate to severe infections	30 mg/kg	6 or 8

* Maximum recommended dose is 8 g/day.
** Maximum recommended dose is 120 mg/kg/day.

IV route – The IV route is recommended for patients requiring single doses greater than 1 g or those with bacterial septicemia, localized parenchymal abscess (eg, intra-abdominal abscess), peritonitis or other severe systemic or life-threatening infections.

Duration – The duration of therapy depends on the severity of infection. Generally, aztreonam should be continued for at least 48 hours after the patient becomes asymptomatic or evidence of bacterial eradication has been obtained. Persistent infections may require treatment for several weeks. Doses smaller than those indicated should not be used.

➤*Renal function impairment:* Prolonged serum levels of aztreonam may occur in patients with transient or persistent renal insufficiency. Therefore, the dosage of aztreonam should be halved in patients with estimated creatinine clearances between 10 and 30 mL/min/1.73 m^2 after an initial loading dose of 1 or 2 g.

In patients with severe renal failure (creatinine clearance less than 10 mL/min per 1.73 m^2), such as those supported by hemodialysis, the usual dose of 500 mg, 1 g or 2 g should be given initially. The maintenance dose should be one-fourth of the usual initial dose given at the usual fixed interval of 6, 8, or 12 hours. For serious or life-threatening infections, in addition to the maintenance doses, one-eighth of the initial dose should be given after each hemodialysis session.

➤*Elderly:* Renal status is a major determinant of dosage in the elderly; these patients in particular may have diminished renal function. Serum creatinine may not be an accurate determinant of renal status. Therefore, as with all antibiotics eliminated by the kidneys, estimates of creatinine clearance should be obtained, and appropriate dosage modifications made if necessary.

➤*Children:* Aztreonam should be administered intravenously to pediatric patients with normal renal function. There are insufficient data regarding IM administration to children or dosing in children with renal impairment.

➤*Pseudomonal infections:* Because of the serious nature of infections due to *Pseudomonas aeruginosa*, dosage of 2 g every 6 or 8 hours is recommended, at least upon initiation of therapy, in systemic infections caused by this organism in adults.

➤*IV administration:*

Bolus injection – A bolus injection may be used to initiate therapy. The dose should be slowly injected directly into a vein, or the tubing of a suitable administration set, over a period of 3 to 5 minutes (see next paragraph regarding flushing of tubing).

Infusion – With any intermittent infusion of aztreonam and another drug with which it is not pharmaceutically compatible, the common delivery tube should be flushed before and after delivery of aztreonam with any appropriate infusion solution compatible with both drug solutions; the drugs should not be delivered simultaneously. Any aztreonam infusion should be completed within a 20- to 60-minute period. With use of a Y-type administration set, careful attention should be given to the calculated volume of aztreonam solution required so that the entire dose will be infused. A volume control administration set may be used to deliver an initial dilution of Aztreonam (see Preparation of parenteral solutions, for infusion) into a compatible infusion solution during administration; in this case, the final dilution of aztreonam should provide a concentration not exceeding 2% w/v.

➤*IM administration:* The dose should be given by deep injection into a large muscle mass (such as the upper outer quadrant of the gluteus maximus or lateral part of the thigh). Aztreonam is well tolerated and should not be admixed with any local anesthetic agent.

➤*Preparation of parenteral solutions:*

General – Upon the addition of the diluent to the container, contents should be shaken immediately and vigorously. Constituted solutions are not for multiple-dose use; should the entire volume in the container not be used for a single-dose, the unused solution must be discarded.

Depending upon the concentration of aztreonam and diluent used, constituted aztreonam yields a colorless to light straw yellow solution, which may develop a slight pink tint on standing (potency is not affected). Parenteral drug products should be inspected visually for particulate matter and discoloration whenever solution and container permit.

➤*Admixtures compatibilities:* IV infusion solutions of aztreonam not exceeding 2% w/v prepared with Sodium Chloride injection 0.9% or Dextrose injection 5%, to which clindamycin phosphate, gentamicin sulfate, tobramycin sulfate, or cefazolin sodium have been added at concentrations usually used clinically, are stable for up to 48 hours at room temperature or 7 days under refrigeration. Ampicillin sodium admixtures with aztreonam in Sodium Chloride injection 0.9% are stable for 24 hours at room temperature and 48 hours under refrigeration; stability in Dextrose injection 5% is 2 hours at room temperature and 8 hours under refrigeration.

Aztreonam-cloxacillin sodium and aztreonam-vancomycin hydrochloride admixtures are stable in peritoneal dialysis solution (with 4.25% Dextrose) for up to 24 hours at room temperature.

Admixture incompatibility – Aztreonam is incompatible with nafcillin sodium, cephradine, and metronidazole.

Other admixtures are not recommended since compatibility data are not available.

➤*IV solutions:*

For bolus injection – The contents of an aztreonam 15 mL capacity vial should be constituted with 6 to 10 mL Sterile Water for Injection.

For infusion – Contents of the 100 ml capacity bottle should be constituted to a final concentration not exceeding 2% w/v (at least 50 ml of any appropriate infusion solution listed below per gram aztreonam). These solutions may be frozen immediately after constitution in the original container (see Stability below.) If the contents of a 15 mL or 30 mL capacity vial are to be transferred to an appropriate infusion solution, each gram of aztreonam should be initially constituted with at least 3 mL Sterile Water for Injection. Further dilution may be obtained with one of the following IV infusion solutions: 0.9% Sodium Chloride injection; Ringer's injection; Ringer's lactate injection; 5% or 10% Dextrose injection; Dextrose and Sodium Chloride injection, 5%:0.9%, 5%:0.45% or 5%:0.2%; Sodium Lactate injection (M/6 Sodium Lactate); *Ionosol* B and 5% Dextrose; *Isolyte* E; *Isolyte* E with 5% Dextrose; *Isolyte* M with 5% Dextrose; *Normosol*-R; *Normosol*-R and 5% Dextrose; *Normosol*-M and 5% Dextrose; Mannitol injection, 5% or 10%; Lactated Ringer's and 5% Dextrose injection; *Plasma-Lyte* M and 5% Dextrose; 10% *Travert* injection; 10% *Travert* and Electrolyte No. 1 injection; 10% *Travert* and Electrolyte No. 2 injection; 10% *Travert* and Electrolyte No. 3 injection.

➤*IM solutions:* The contents of an aztreonam for injection 15 mL capacity vial should be constituted with at least 3 mL of an appropriate diluent per gram aztreonam. The following diluents may be used: Sterile Water for injection; Sterile Bacteriostatic Water for Injection (with benzyl alcohol or with methyl- and propylparabens); Sodium Chloride injection 0.9%; Bacteriostatic Sodium Chloride injection (with benzyl alcohol).

➤*Storage / Stability:* Store original packages at room temperature; avoid excessive heat.

Stability of IV and IM solutions – Aztreonam solutions for IV infusion at concentrations not exceeding 2% w/v must be used within 48 hours following constitution if kept at controlled room temperature (15° to 30°C; 59° to 86°F) or within 7 days if refrigerated (2° to 8°C; 36° to 46°F).

AZTREONAM — INJECTION

Frozen aztreonam infusion solutions may be stored for up to 3 months at −20°C (−4°F); frozen solutions may be thawed at controlled room temperature or by overnight refrigeration. Solutions that have been thawed and maintained at controlled room temperature or under refrigeration should be used within 24 or 72 hours after removal from the freezer, respectively. Solutions should not be refrozen.

Aztreonam solutions at concentrations exceeding 2% w/v, except those prepared with Sterile Water for Injection or Sodium Chloride injection, should be used promptly after preparation; the 2 excepted solutions must be used within 48 hours if stored at controlled room temperature or within 7 days if refrigerated.

Actions

➤*Pharmacokinetics:*

Absorption/Distribution – Single 30-minute IV infusions of 500 mg, 1 g, and 2 g doses of aztreonam for injection in healthy subjects produced aztreonam peak serum levels of 54, 90, and 204 mcg/mL, respectively, immediately after administration; at 8 hours, serum levels were 1, 3, and 6 mcg/mL, respectively . Single 3-minute IV injections of the same doses resulted in serum levels of 58, 125, and 242 mcg/mL at 5 minutes following completion of injection.

Serum concentrations of aztreonam in healthy subjects following completion of single IM injections of 500 mg and 1 g doses are depicted in the figure below; maximum serum concentrations occur at about 1 hour. After identical single IV or IM doses of aztreonam, the serum concentrations of aztreonam are comparable at 1 hour (1.5 hours from start of IV infusion) with similar slopes of serum concentrations thereafter.

When aztreonam pharmacokinetics were assessed for adult and pediatric patients, they were found to be comparable (down to 9 months old). The serum half-life of aztreonam averaged 1.7 hours (1.5 to 2) in subjects with normal renal function, independent of the dose and route of administration. In healthy subjects, based on a 70 kg person, the serum clearance was 91 mL/min and renal clearance was 56 mL/min; the apparent mean volume of distribution at steady-state averaged 12.6 L, approximately equivalent to extracellular fluid volume.

Average urine concentrations of aztreonam were approximately 1,100, 3,500, and 6,600 mcg/mL within the first 2 hours following single 500 mg, 1 and 2 g IV doses of aztreonam (30 minute infusions), respectively. The range of average concentrations for aztreonam in the 8 to 12 hour urine specimens in these studies was 25 to 120 mcg/mL. After IM injection of single 500 mg and 1 g doses of aztreonam for injection, urinary levels were approximately 500 and 1,200 mcg/mL, respectively, within the first 2 hours, declining to 180 and 470 mcg/mL in the 6 to 8 hour specimens. In healthy subjects, aztreonam is excreted in the urine about equally by active tubular secretion and glomerular filtration. Approximately 60% to 70% of an IV or IM dose was recovered in the urine by 8 hours. Urinary excretion of a single parenteral dose was essentially complete by 12 hours after injection. About 12% of a single IV radiolabeled dose was recovered in the feces. Unchanged aztreonam and the inactive beta-lactam ring hydrolysis product of aztreonam were present in feces and urine.

IV or IM administration of a single 500 mg or 1 g dose of aztreonam every 8 hours for 7 days to healthy subjects produced no apparent accumulation of aztreonam or modification of its disposition characteristics; serum protein binding averaged 56% and was independent of dose. An average of about 6% of a 1 g IM dose was excreted as a microbiologically inactive open beta-lactam ring hydrolysis product (serum half-life approximately 26 hours) of aztreonam in the 0 to 8 hour urine collection on the last day of multiple dosing.

Special populations –

Renal function impairment: In patients with impaired renal function, the serum half-life of aztreonam is prolonged.

Hepatic function impairment: The serum half-life of aztreonam is only slightly prolonged in patients with hepatic function impairment since the liver is a minor pathway of excretion.

Elderly: In a study of healthy elderly male subjects (65 to 75 years of age), the average elimination half-life of aztreonam was slightly longer than in young healthy males.

➤*Microbiology:* Aztreonam exhibits potent and specific activity in vitro against a wide spectrum of gram-negative aerobic pathogens including *Pseudomonas aeruginosa*. The bactericidal action of aztreonam results from the inhibition of bacterial cell wall synthesis due to a high affinity of aztreonam for penicillin binding protein 3 (PBP3). Aztreonam, unlike the majority of beta-lactam antibiotics, does not induce beta-lactamase activity and its molecular structure confers a high degree of resistance to hydrolysis by beta-lactamases (ie, penicillinases, cephalosporinases) produced by most gram-negative and gram-positive pathogens; it is, therefore, usually active against gram-negative aerobic microorganisms that are resistant to antibiotics hydrolyzed by beta-lactamases. It is active against many strains that are multiply-resistant to other antibiotics, such as certain cephalosporins, penicillin, and aminoglycosides. Aztreonam maintains its antimicrobial activity over a pH range of 6 to 8 in vitro, as well as in the presence of human serum and under anaerobic conditions.

Aztreonam has been shown to be active against most strains of the following microorganisms, both in vitro and in clinical infections as described in the Indications section.

Aerobic gram-negative microorganisms – *Citrobacter* species, including *C. freundii*, *Enterobacter* species, including *E. cloacae*, *Escherichia coli*, *Haemophilus influenzae* (including ampicillin-resistant and other penicillinase-producing strains), *Klebsiella oxytoca*, *Klebsiella pneumoniae*, *Proteus mirabilis*, *Pseudomonas aeruginosa*, *Serratia* species, including *S. marcescens*.

Aerobic gram-negative microorganisms –

Aztreonam and aminoglycosides have been shown to be synergistic in vitro against most strains of *P. aeruginosa*, many strains of *Enterobacteriaceae*, and other gram-negative aerobic bacilli.

Alterations of the anaerobic intestinal flora by broad spectrum antibiotics may decrease colonization resistance, thus permitting overgrowth of potential pathogens (eg, Candida and *Clostrium* species). Aztreonam has little effect on the anaerobic intestinal microflora in in vitro studies. *Clostridium difficile* and its cytotoxin were not found in animal models following administration of aztreonam. (See Adverse Reactions.)

Contraindications

Hypersensitivity to aztreonam or any other component in the formulation.

Warnings

➤*Pseudomembranous colitis:* Pseudomembranous colitis has been reported with nearly all antibacterial agents, including aztreonam, and may range in severity from mild to life-threatening. Therefore, it is important to consider this diagnosis in patients who present with diarrhea subsequent to the administration of antibacterial agents.

Treatment with antibacterial agents alters the normal flora of the colon and may permit overgrowth of clostridia. Studies indicate that a toxin produced by *Clostridium difficile* is one primary cause of "antibiotic-associated colitis."

After the diagnosis of pseudomembranous colitis has been established, therapeutic measures should be initiated. Mild cases of pseudomembranous colitis usually respond to drug discontinuation alone. In moderate to severe cases, consideration should be given to management with fluids and electrolytes, protein supplementation, and treatment with an antibacterial drug clinically effective against *C. difficile* colitis.

➤*Toxic epidermal necrolysis:* Rare cases of toxic epidermal necrolysis have been reported in association with aztreonam in patients undergoing bone marrow transplant with multiple risk factors including sepsis, radiation therapy and other concomitantly administered drugs associated with toxic epidermal necrolysis.

➤*Hypersensitivity reactions:* Careful inquiry should be made to determine whether the patient has any history of hypersensitivity reactions to any allergens.

While cross-reactivity of aztreonam with other beta-lactam antibiotics is rare, this drug should be administered with caution to any patient with a history of hypersensitivity to beta-lactams (eg, penicillins, cephalosporins, carbapenems). Treatment with aztreonam can result in hypersensitivity reactions in patients with or without prior exposure to aztreonam. If an allergic reaction to aztreonam occurs, discontinue the drug and institute supportive treatment as appropriate (eg, maintenance of ventilation, pressor amines, antihistamines, corticosteroids). Serious hypersensitivity reactions may require epinephrine and other emergency measures.

➤*Pregnancy: Category B.* Aztreonam crosses the placenta and enters the fetal circulation.

There are no adequate and well-controlled studies in pregnant women. Because animal reproduction studies are not always predictive of human response, aztreonam should be used during pregnancy only if clearly needed.

➤*Lactation:* Aztreonam is excreted in human milk in concentrations that are less than 1% of concentrations determined in simultaneously obtained maternal serum; consideration should be given to temporary discontinuation of nursing and use of formula feedings.

➤*Children:* The safety and efficacy of IV aztreonam for injection have been established in the age groups 9 months to 16 years. Use of aztreonam in these age groups is supported by evidence from adequate and well-controlled studies of aztreonam in adults with additional efficacy, safety, and pharmacokinetic data from noncomparative clinical studies in pediatric patients. Sufficient data are not available for children less than 9 months of age or for the following treatment indications/pathogens: Septicemia and skin and skin-structure infections (where the skin infection is believed or known to be due to *H. influenzae* type B). In children with cystic fibrosis, higher doses of aztreonam may be warranted.

Precautions

➤*Monitoring:* In patients with impaired hepatic or renal function, appropriate monitoring is recommended during therapy. If an aminoglycoside is used concurrently with aztreonam, especially if high dosages of the former are used or if therapy is prolonged, renal function should be monitored because of the potential nephrotoxicity and ototoxicity of aminoglycoside antibiotics.

➤*Superinfection:* The use of antibiotics may promote the overgrowth of nonsusceptible organisms, including gram-positive organisms (*Staphylococcus aureus* and *Streptococcus faecalis*) and fungi. Should superinfection occur during therapy, appropriate measures should be taken.

Drug Interactions

Aztreonam Drug Interactions

Precipitant drug	Object drug*		Description
Probenecid Furosemide	Aztreonam	↑	Concomitant administration causes clinically insignificant increases in aztreonam serum levels.

AZTREONAM — INJECTION

Aztreonam Drug Interactions			
Precipitant drug	Object drug*		Description
Antibiotics (eg, cefoxitin, imipenem)	Aztreonam	⬇	Antibiotics may induce high levels of β-lactamase in vitro in some gram-negative aerobes such as *Enterobacter* and *Pseudomonas* sp, resulting in antagonism to many β-lactam antibiotics including aztreonam. Do not use β-lactamase-inducing antibiotics concurrently with aztreonam.
Aztreonam	Aminoglycosides	⬆	If an aminoglycoside is used concurrently with aztreonam, especially if high dosages of the former are used or if therapy is prolonged, monitor renal function because of potential nephrotoxicity and ototoxicity of aminoglycoside antibiotics.

* ⬆ = Object drug increased. ⬇ = Object drug decreased.

Adverse Reactions

➤*Local:* Local reactions such as phlebitis/thrombophlebitis following IV administration, and discomfort/swelling at the injection site following IM administration occurred at rates of approximately 1.9% and 2.4%, respectively.

➤*Systemic:* Systemic reactions (considered to be related to therapy or of uncertain etiology) occurring at an incidence of 1% to 1.3% include diarrhea, nausea and/or vomiting, and rash. Reactions occurring at an incidence of less than 1% are listed within each body system in order of decreasing severity:

➤*Cardiovascular:* Hypotension; transient ECG changes (ventricular bigeminy and PVC); flushing.

➤*CNS:* Seizure; confusion; vertigo; paresthesia; insomnia; dizziness.

➤*Dermatologic:* Toxic epidermal necrolysis (see Warnings); purpura; erythema multiforme; exfoliative dermatitis; urticaria; petechiae; pruritus; diaphoresis.

➤*GI:* Abdominal cramps; rare cases of *C. difficile*-associated diarrhea, including pseudomembranous colitis, or gastrointestinal bleeding have been reported. Onset of pseudomembranous colitis symptoms may occur during or after antibiotic treatment. (See Warnings.)

➤*GU:* Vaginal candidiasis; vaginitis; breast tenderness.

➤*Hematologic:* Pancytopenia; neutropenia; thrombocytopenia; anemia; eosinophilia; leukocytosis; thrombocytosis.

➤*Hepatic:* Hepatitis; jaundice.

➤*Hypersensitivity:* Anaphylaxis; angioedema; bronchospasm.

➤*Musculoskeletal:* Muscular aches.

➤*Respiratory:* Wheezing; dyspnea; chest pain.

➤*Special senses:* Tinnitus; diplopia; mouth ulcer; altered taste; numb tongue; sneezing; nasal congestion; halitosis.

➤*Miscellaneous:* Weakness; headache; fever; malaise.

➤*Children:* Of the 612 children who were treated with aztreonam for injection in clinical trials, less than 1% required discontinuation of therapy due to adverse events. The following systemic adverse events, regardless of drug relationship, occurred in greater than or equal to 1% of treated patients in domestic clinical trials: Rash (4.3%), diarrhea (1.4%), and fever (1%). These adverse events were comparable to those observed in adult clinical trials.

In 343 children receiving IV therapy, the following local reactions were noted: Pain (12%), erythema (2.9%), induration (0.9%), and phlebitis (2.1%). In the US patient population, pain occurred in 1.5% of patients, while each of the remaining three local reactions had an incidence of 0.5%.

➤*Laboratory adverse reactions:* The following laboratory adverse reactions, regardless of drug relationship, occurred in greater than or equal to 1% of treated patients: increased ALT (6.5%), increased eosinophils (6.3%), increased serum creatinine (5.8%), increased platelets (3.6%), increased AST (3.8%), and neutropenia (3.2%).

Adverse laboratory changes without regard to drug relationship that were reported during clinical trials were:

Hematologic – Increases in prothrombin and partial thromboplastin times, positive Coombs' test.

Hepatic – Elevations of AST, ALT, and alkaline phosphatase; signs or symptoms of hepatobiliary dysfunction occurred in less than 1% of recipients (see above).

Renal – Increases in serum creatinine.

➤*Children:* In US pediatric clinical trials, neutropenia (absolute neutrophil count less than 1,000/mm^3) occurred in 11.3% of patients (8 of 71) less than 2 years of age receiving 30 mg/kg every 6 hours. AST and ALT elevations to greater than 3 times the upper limit of normal were noted in 15% to 20% of patients greater than or equal to 2 years of age receiving 50 mg/kg every 6 hours. The increased frequency of these reported laboratory adverse events may be due to either increased severity of illness treated or higher doses of aztreonam administered.

Overdosage

➤*Treatment:* If necessary, aztreonam may be cleared from the serum by hemodialysis or peritoneal dialysis.

CHLORAMPHENICOL

Rx	**Chloramphenicol Sodium Succinate** (Various)	**Powder for Injection:** 100 mg/ml (as sodium succinate) when reconstituted	1 g in 15 ml vials.
Rx	**Chloromycetin Sodium Succinate** (Parke-Davis)		2.25 mEq sodium per g. In 1 g vials.

CHLORAMPHENICOL SODIUM SUCCINATE — INJECTION

WARNING

Serious and fatal blood dyscrasias (aplastic anemia, hypoplastic anemia, thrombocytopenia, and granulocytopenia) are known to occur after the administration of chloramphenicol. In addition, there have been reports of aplastic anemia attributed to chloramphenicol which later terminated in leukemia. Blood dyscrasias have occurred after both short-term and prolonged therapy with this drug. Chloramphenicol must not be used when less potentially dangerous agents will be effective, as described in Indications. It must not be used in the treatment of trivial infections or where it is not indicated, as in colds, influenza, infections of the throat; or as a prophylactic agent to prevent bacterial infections.

It is essential that adequate blood studies be made during treatment with the drug. While blood studies may detect early peripheral blood changes, such as leukopenia, reticulocytopenia, or granulocytopenia, before they become irreversible, such studies cannot be relied on to detect bone marrow depression prior to development of aplastic anemia. To facilitate appropriate studies and observation during therapy, it is desirable that patients be hospitalized.

Indications

➤*Serious infections:* In accord with the concepts in the Warning Box, chloramphenicol must be used only in those serious infections for which less potentially dangerous drugs are ineffective or contraindicated. However, chloramphenicol may be chosen to initiate antibiotic therapy on the clinical impression that one of the conditions below is believed to be present; in vitro sensitivity tests should be performed concurrently so that the drug may be discontinued as soon as possible if less potentially dangerous agents are indicated by such tests. The decision to continue use of chloramphenicol rather than another antibiotic when both are suggested by in vitro studies to be effective against a specific pathogen should be based upon severity of the infection, susceptibility of the pathogen to the various antimicrobial drugs, efficacy of the various drugs in the infection, and the important additional concepts contained in the Warning Box above.

Serious infections caused by susceptible strains in accordance with the concepts expressed above:

1.) *Salmonella* species.
2.) *H. influenzae*, specially meningeal infections.
3.) Rickettsia.
4.) Lymphogranuloma-psittacosis group.
5.) Various gram-negative bacteria causing bacteremia, meningitis, or other serious gram-negative infections.
6.) Other susceptible organisms which have been demonstrated to be resistant to all other appropriate antimicrobial agents.

➤*Acute infections caused by Salmonella typhi:* It is not recommended for the routine treatment of the typhoid carrier state.

In treatment of typhoid fever some authorities recommend that chloramphenicol be administered at therapeutic levels for 8 to 10 days after the patient has become afebrile to lessen the possibility of relapse.

➤*Cystic fibrosis:* Cystic fibrosis regimens.

Administration and Dosage

➤*Approved by the FDA:* August 25, 1982.

➤*Therapeutic dose:* Chloramphenicol, like other potent drugs, should be prescribed at recommended doses known to have therapeutic activity. Administration of 50 mg/kg/day in divided doses will produce blood levels of the magnitude to which the majority of susceptible microorganisms will respond.

➤*IV administration:* Chloramphenicol sodium succinate is intended for intravenous use only. It has been demonstrated to be ineffective when given intramuscularly.

CHLORAMPHENICOL SODIUM SUCCINATE — INJECTION

1.) Chloramphenicol sodium succinate must be hydrolyzed to its microbiologically active form, and there is a lag in achieving adequate blood levels compared with the base given intravenously.
2.) Patients started on intravenous chloramphenicol sodium succinate should be changed to the oral form of another appropriate antibiotic as soon as practical.

➤*Adults:* Adults should receive 50 mg/kg/day in divided doses at 6-hour intervals. In exceptional cases patients with infections due to moderately resistant organisms may require increased dosage up to 100 mg/kg/day to achieve blood levels inhibiting the pathogen, but these high doses should be decreased as soon as possible.

Renal/hepatic function impairment – Adults with impairment of hepatic or renal function or both may have reduced ability to metabolize and excrete the drug. In instances of impaired metabolic processes, dosages should be adjusted accordingly. (See discussion under Neonates.) Precise control of concentration of the drug in the blood should be carefully followed in patients with impaired metabolic processes by the available microtechniques (information available on request).

➤*Children:* Dosage of 50 mg/kg/day divided into 4 doses at 6-hour intervals yields blood levels in the range effective against most susceptible organisms. Severe infections (eg, bacteremia or meningitis), especially when adequate cerebrospinal fluid concentrations are desired, may require dosage up to 100 mg/kg/day; however, it is recommended that dosage be reduced to 50 mg/kg/day as soon as possible. Children with impaired liver or kidney function may retain excessive amounts of the drug.

Newborn – (See section titled "Gray syndrome" under Adverse Reactions.)

A total of 25 mg/kg/day in 4 equal doses at 6-hour intervals usually produces and maintains concentrations in blood and tissues adequate to control most infections for which the drug is indicated. Increased dosage in these individuals, demanded by severe infections, should be given only to maintain the blood concentration within a therapeutically effective range. After the first 2 weeks of life, full-term neonates ordinarily may receive up to a total of 50 mg/kg/day equally divided into 4 doses at 6-hour intervals. These dosage recommendations are extremely important because blood concentration in all premature and full-term neonates under 2 weeks of age differs from that of other infants neonates. This difference is due to variations in the maturity of the metabolic functions of the liver and the kidneys.

When these functions are immature (or seriously impaired in adults), high concentrations of the drug are found which tend to increase with succeeding doses.

Infants and children with immature metabolic processes – In young infants and other pediatric patients in whom immature metabolic functions are suspected, a dose of 25 mg/kg/day will usually produce therapeutic concentrations of the drug in the blood. In this group particularly, the concentration of the drug in the blood should be carefully followed by microtechniques.

Intravenously as a 10% (100 mg/mL) solution to be injected over at least a 1-minute interval. This is prepared by the addition of 10 mL of an aqueous diluent such as water for injection or 5% dextrose injection.

➤*Storage/Stability:* Store between 15° and 25°C (59° and 77° F).

Actions

➤*Pharmacokinetics:*

Absorption – Chloramphenicol administered orally is absorbed rapidly from the intestinal tract. In controlled studies in adult volunteers using the recommended dosage of 50 mg/kg/day, a dosage of 1 g every 6 hours for 8 doses was given. Using the microbiological assay method, the average peak serum level was 11.2 mcg/mL 1 hour after the first dose. A cumulative effect gave a peak rise to 18.4 mcg/mL after the fifth dose of 1 g. Mean serum levels ranged from 8 to 14 mcg/mL over the 48-hour period.

Distribution – Chloramphenicol diffuses rapidly, but its distribution is not uniform. Highest concentrations are found in liver and kidney, and lowest concentrations are found in brain and cerebrospinal fluid. Chloramphenicol enters cerebrospinal fluid even in the absence of meningeal inflammation, appearing in concentrations about half of those found in the blood. Measurable levels are also detected in pleural and in ascitic fluids, saliva, milk, and in the aqueous and vitreous humors. Transport across the placental barrier occurs with somewhat lower concentration in cord blood of neonates than in maternal blood.

Excretion – Total urinary excretion of chloramphenicol in these studies ranged from a low of 68% to a high of 99% over a 3-day period. From 8% to 12% of the antibiotic excreted is in the form of free chloramphenicol; the remainder consists of microbiologically inactive metabolites, principally the conjugate with glucuronic acid. Since the glucuronide is excreted rapidly, most chloramphenicol detected in the blood is in the microbiologically active free form. Despite the small proportion of unchanged drug excreted in the urine, the concentration of free chloramphenicol is relatively high, amounting to several hundred mcg/mL in patients receiving divided doses of 50 mg/kg/day. Small amounts of active drug are found in bile and feces.

➤*Microbiology:* Chloramphenicol is a broad-spectrum antibiotic originally isolated from *Streptomyces venezuelae*. It inhibits bacterial protein synthesis by interfering with the transfer of activated amino acids from soluble RNA to ribsomes. In vitro, chloramphenicol exerts mainly a bacteriostatic effect on a wide range of gram-negative and gram-positive bacteria. Bacteriological studies should be performed to determine the causative organisms and their susceptibilities to chloramphenicol.

Chloramphenicol has been shown to be active against most strains of the following microorganisms, both in vitro and in clinical infections as described in the Indications.

Aerobic gram-negative microorganisms – *Haemophilus influenzae*; *Salmonella* species, including *Salmonella typhi*

Other microorganisms – Lymphogranuloma-psittacosis group; Rickettsia

Contraindications

History of previous hypersensitivity or toxic reaction to it. It must not be used in the treatment of trivial infections or where it is not indicated, as in colds, influenza, infections of the throat; or as a prophylactic agent to prevent bacterial infections.

Warnings

Repeated courses of chloramphenicol treatment should be avoided if at all possible. Treatment should not be continued longer than required to produce a cure with little or no risk or relapse of the disease.

➤*Renal/Hepatic function impairment:* Excessive blood levels may result from administration of the recommended dose to patients with impaired liver or kidney function. The dosage should be adjusted accordingly, or preferably, the blood concentration should be determined at appropriate intervals.

➤*Pregnancy: Category C.*

Animal reproduction studies have not been conducted with chloramphenicol. There are no adequate and well-controlled studies to establish safety of this drug in pregnancy. It is not known whether chloramphenicol can cause fetal harm when administered to a pregnant woman. Orally administered chloramphenicol has been shown to cross the placental barrier. Because of potential toxic effects on the fetus, chloramphenicol should be given to a pregnant woman only if the potential benefit justifies the potential risk to the fetus.

➤*Lactation:* Chloramphenicol is excreted in human milk following oral administration of the drug. Because of the potential for serious adverse reactions in nursing infants from chloramphenicol, a decision should be made whether to discontinue nursing or to discontinue the drug, taking into account the importance of the drug to the mother.

➤*Children:* Precaution should be used in therapy of premature and full-term neonates and infants to avoid Gray syndrome toxicity. Due to immature metabolic processes in the neonate and infant, excessive blood levels may result from administration of the recommended dose. The dosage should be adjusted accordingly or, preferable, the blood concentration should be determined at appropriate intervals (see Adverse Reactions, Gray syndrome).

See Administration and Dosage for dosing information in the pediatric population.

Precautions

➤*Monitoring:* Baseline blood studies should be followed by periodic blood studies approximately every 2 days during therapy. The drug should be discontinued upon appearance of reticulocytopenia, leukopenia, thrombocytopenia, anemia or any other blood study findings attributable to chloramphenicol. However, it should be noted that such studies do not exclude the possible later appearance of the irreversible type of bone marrow depression.

➤*Superinfection:* The use of this antibiotic, as with other antibiotics, may result in an overgrowth of nonsusceptible organisms, including fungi. If infections caused by nonsusceptible organisms appear during therapy, appropriate measures should be taken.

Drug Interactions

Chloramphenicol Drug Interactions

Precipitant drug	Object drug*		Description
Barbiturates	Chloramphenicol	↓	Decreased chloramphenicol serum levels may occur, and barbiturate clearance may be decreased, resulting in increased levels or toxicity.
Chloramphenicol	Barbiturates	↑	
Rifampin	Chloramphenicol	↓	Concomitant administration may reduce serum chloramphenicol levels, presumably through hepatic enzyme induction.
Chloramphenicol	Anticoagulants	↑	Anticoagulant action may be enhanced.
Chloramphenicol	Cyclophosphamide	↓	Decreased or delayed activation of cyclophosphamide may occur, although it is unclear if a significant decrease in its effect would occur.
Chloramphenicol	Hydantoins	↑	Serum hydantoin levels may be increased, possibly resulting in toxicity. In addition, chloramphenicol levels may be increased or decreased.
Hydantoins	Chloramphenicol	↔	

CHLORAMPHENICOL SODIUM SUCCINATE — INJECTION

Chloramphenicol Drug Interactions

Precipitant drug	Object drug*		Description
Chloramphenicol	Iron salts	↑	Serum iron levels may be increased.
Chloramphenicol	Penicillins	↔	Synergistic effects may develop in the treatment of certain microorganisms, but antagonism may also occur.
Chloramphenicol	Sulfonylureas	↑	Clinical manifestations of hypoglycemia may occur with concurrent use.
Chloramphenicol	Vitamin B_{12}	↓	Hematologic effects of vitamin B_{12} may be decreased in patients with pernicious anemia by concurrent chloramphenicol.

* ↑ = Object drug increased. ↓ = Object drug decreased. ↔ = Undetermined effect.

Concurrent therapy with other drugs that may cause bone marrow depression should be avoided.

Adverse Reactions

➤*CNS:* Headache, mild depression, mental confusion, and delirium have been described in patients receiving chloramphenicol. Optic and peripheral neuritis have been reported, usually following long-term therapy. If this occurs, the drug should be promptly withdrawn.

➤*GI:* Nausea, vomiting, glossitis and stomatitis, diarrhea and enterocolitis may occur in low incidence.

➤*Hematologic:* The most serious adverse effect of chloramphenicol is bone marrow depression. Serious and fatal blood dyscrasias (aplastic anemia, hypoplastic anemia, thrombocytopenia, and granulocytopenia) are known to occur after the administration of chloramphenicol. An irreversible type of marrow depression leading to aplastic anemia with a high rate of mortality is characterized by the appearance weeks or months after therapy of bone marrow aplastic or hypoplasia. Peripherally, pancytopenia is most often observed, but in a small number of cases only 1 or 2 of the 3 major cell types (erythrocytes, leukocytes, platelets) may be depressed.

A reversible type of bone marrow depression, which is dose related, may occur. This type of marrow depression is characterized by vacuolization of the erythroid cells, reduction of reticulocytes and leukopenia, and responds promptly to the withdrawal of chloramphenicol.

An exact determination of the risk of serious and fatal blood dyscrasias is not possible because of lack of accurate information regarding the size of the population at risk, the total number of drug-associated dyscrasias, and the total number of non-drug associated dyscrasias.

Aplastic anemia – In a report to the California State Assembly by the California Medical Association and the State Department of Public Health in January 1967, the risk of fatal aplastic anemia was estimated at 1:24,200 to 1:40,500 based on 2 dosage levels.

There have been reports of aplastic anemia attributed to chloramphenicol which later terminated in leukemia.

Hemoglobinuria Paroxysmal nocturnal hemoglobinuria has been reported.

➤*Hypersensitivity:* Fever, macular and vesicular rashes, angioedema, urticaria, and anaphylaxis may occur. Herxheimer's reactions have occurred during therapy for typhoid fever.

➤*Miscellaneous:* Toxic reactions including fatalities have occurred in the premature and neonate; the signs and symptoms associated with these reactions have been referred to as the Gray syndrome. One case of Gray syndrome has been reported in a neonate born to a mother having received chloramphenicol during labor. One case has been reported in a 3-month-old infant. The following summarizes the clinical and laboratory studies that have been made on these patients:

1.) In most cases, therapy with chloramphenicol had been instituted within the first 48 hours of life.
2.) Symptoms first appeared after 3 to 4 days of continued treatment with high doses of chloramphenicol.
3.) The symptoms appeared in the following order:
   a.) Abdominal distension with or without emesis.
   b.) Progressive pallid cyanosis.
   c.) Vasomotor collapse, frequently accompanied by irregular respiration.
   d.) Death within a few hours of onset of these symptoms.
4.) The progression of symptoms from onset to exitus was accelerated with higher dose schedules.
5.) Preliminary blood serum level studies revealed unusually high concentrations of chloramphenicol (over 90 mcg/mL after repeated doses).
6.) Termination of therapy upon early evidence of the associated symptomatology frequently reversed the process with complete recovery.

QUINOLONES

NALIDIXIC ACID

Rx	**NegGram** (Sanofi Winthrop)	**Tablets:** 500 mg	Scored. In 56s and 500s.

NALIDIXIC ACID — ORAL

Indications

➤*Urinary tract infections:* For the treatment of urinary tract infections (UTIs) caused by susceptible gram-negative microorganisms, including the majority of *Escherichia coli*, *Enterobacter* species, *Klebsiella* species, and *Proteus* species. Perform disc susceptibility testing with the 30 mcg disc prior to administration of the drug and during treatment if clinical response warrants.

Administration and Dosage

➤*Approved by the FDA:* March 6, 1964.

➤*Adults:*

Initial therapy – 1 g administered 4 times/day for 1 or 2 weeks (total daily dose, 4 g).

Prolonged therapy – For prolonged therapy, the total daily dose may be reduced to 2 g after the initial treatment period. Underdosage during initial treatment may predispose to emergence of bacterial resistance.

➤*Children (3 months to 12 years of age):* Until further experience is gained, nalidixic acid should not be administered to infants younger than 3 months of age.

Initial therapy – Dosage in children 12 years of age and younger should be calculated on the basis of body weight. The recommended total daily dose for initial therapy is 55 mg/kg/day (25 mg/lb/day), administered in 4 equally divided doses.

Prolonged therapy – For prolonged therapy, the total daily dose may be reduced to 33 mg/kg/day (15 mg/lb/day). Nalidixic acid 250 mg tablets may be used.

➤*Storage/Stability:* Store tablets at room temperature up to 30°C (86°F).

Actions

➤*Pharmacology:* Nalidixic acid, a bactericidal agent, appears to interfere with deoxyribonucleic acid (DNA) polymerization.

➤*Pharmacokinetics:*

Absorption – After oral administration, nalidixic acid is absorbed rapidly from the GI tract.

Distribution – Peak serum levels of active drug average approximately 20 to 40 mcg/mL (90% protein bound) 1 to 2 hours after administration of a 1 g dose to a fasting healthy individual, with a half-life of about 90 minutes.

Metabolism – After oral administration, nalidixic acid is partially metabolized in the liver. Unchanged nalidixic acid appears in the urine along with an active metabolite, hydroxynalidixic acid, which has antibacterial activity similar to that of nalidixic acid. Other metabolites include glucuronic acid conjugates of nalidixic acid and hydroxynalidixic acid, and the dicarboxylic acid derivative. The hydroxy metabolite represents 30% of the biologically active drug in the blood and 85% in the urine.

Excretion – After oral administration, nalidixic acid is excreted rapidly through the kidney. Approximately 4% of nalidixic acid is excreted in the feces. Traces of nalidixic acid were found in blood and urine of an infant whose mother had received the drug during the last trimester of pregnancy. Peak urine levels of active drug average approximately 150 to 200 mcg/mL 3 to 4 hours after administration, with a half-life of about 6 hours.

➤*Microbiology:* Nalidixic acid has marked antibacterial activity against gram-negative bacteria, including *Enterobacter* species, *E. coli*, *Morganella morganii*, *Proteus mirabilis*, *Proteus vulgaris*, and *Providencia rettgeri*. *Pseudomonas* species generally are resistant to the drug. Nalidixic acid is bactericidal and is effective over the entire urinary pH range. Conventional chromosomal resistance to nalidixic acid taken in full dosage has been reported to emerge in approximately 2% to 14% of patients during treatment; however, bacterial resistance to nalidixic acid has not been shown to be transferable via R factor.

Contraindications

Hypersensitivity to nalidixic acid or to related compounds; infants younger than 3 months of age; porphyria or a history of convulsive disorders; patients undergoing concomitant therapy with melphalan or other related cancer chemotherapeutic alkylating agents because of serious GI toxicity (eg, hemorrhagic ulcerative colitis, intestinal necrosis); lactation.

Warnings

➤*CNS effects:* CNS effects, including convulsions, increased intracranial pressure, and toxic psychosis have been reported with nalidixic acid therapy. Convulsive seizures have been reported with other drugs in this class. Quinolones also may cause CNS stimulation, which may lead to confusion, hallucinations, light-headedness, restlessness, and tremor. Therefore, use nalidixic acid with caution in patients with known or suspected CNS disorders (eg, cerebral arteriosclerosis, epilepsy) or other factors that predispose

NALIDIXIC ACID — ORAL

to seizures. If these reactions occur in patients receiving nalidixic acid, discontinue the drug and institute appropriate measures.

➤*Pseudomembranous colitis:* Pseudomembranous colitis has been reported with nearly all antibacterial agents, including quinolones, and may range in severity from mild to life-threatening. Therefore, it is important to consider this diagnosis in patients who present with diarrhea subsequent to the administration of antibacterial agents.

Treatment with antibacterial agents alters the normal flora of the colon and may permit overgrowth of clostridia. Studies indicate that a toxin produced by *Clostridium difficile* is a primary cause of "antibiotic-associated colitis."

After the diagnosis of pseudomembranous colitis has been established, initiate therapeutic measures. Patients with mild cases of pseudomembranous colitis usually respond to drug discontinuation alone. In moderate to severe cases, consider management with fluids and electrolytes, protein supplementation, and treatment with an antibacterial drug clinically effective against *C. difficile* colitis.

➤*Peripheral neuropathy:* Rare cases of sensory or sensorimotor axonal polyneuropathy affecting small and/or large axons resulting in paresthesias, hypesthesias, dysesthesias, and weakness have been reported in patients receiving quinolones, including nalidixic acid. Discontinue nalidixic acid if the patient experiences symptoms of neuropathy, including burning, numbness, pain, tingling, and/or weakness, or is found to have deficits in light touch, motor strength, pain, position sense, temperature, and/or vibratory sensation in order to prevent the development of an irreversible condition.

➤*Tendon effects:* Ruptures of the Achilles tendon or other tendons, hand, and shoulder that required surgical repair or resulted in prolonged disability have been reported in patients receiving quinolones, including nalidixic acid. Postmarketing surveillance reports indicate that this risk may be increased in patients receiving concomitant corticosteroids, especially in the elderly. Discontinue nalidixic acid if the patient experiences pain, inflammation, or rupture of a tendon. Patients should rest and refrain from exercise until the diagnosis of tendonitis or tendon rupture has been excluded. Tendon rupture may occur during or after therapy with quinolones, including nalidixic acid.

➤*Arthropathy:* Nalidixic acid and other members of the quinolone drug class have been shown to cause arthropathy in juvenile animals.

➤*Hypersensitivity reactions:* Serious and occasionally fatal hypersensitivity (anaphylactoid) reactions, some following the first dose, have been reported in patients receiving quinolone therapy. Some reactions were accompanied by cardiovascular collapse, dyspnea, itching, loss of consciousness, pharyngeal or facial edema, tingling, and urticaria. Only a few patients had a history of hypersensitivity reactions. Serious anaphylactoid reactions required immediate emergency treatment with epinephrine. Administer oxygen, intravenous (IV) steroids, and airway management, including intubation, as indicated.

➤*Carcinogenesis:* In lifetime studies in the rat given nalidixic acid in the diet, there was an increased incidence of preputial gland neoplasms in the treated males and clitoral gland neoplasms in the treated females. Studies in mice in which nalidixic acid was administered in the feed for 2 years, or was given in the feed for 76 weeks, followed by no treatment for 9 weeks, gave equivocal evidence of carcinogenic activity.

➤*Elderly:*

Observe caution when using nalidixic acid in elderly patients. This drug is known to be substantially excreted by the kidney, and the risk of toxic reactions to this drug may be higher in patients with impaired renal function. Because elderly patients are more likely to have decreased renal function, take care in dose selection; it also may be useful to monitor renal function.

➤*Pregnancy:* *Category C.*

Teratogenic – Nalidixic acid has been shown to be teratogenic and embryocidal in rats when given in oral doses 6 times the human dose. Nalidixic acid also prolonged the duration of pregnancy, especially at 4 times the clinical dose. There are no adequate and well-controlled studies in pregnant women. Because nalidixic acid, like other drugs in this class, causes arthropathy in immature animals, use nalidixic acid during pregnancy only if the potential benefit justifies the potential risk to the fetus.

➤*Lactation:* Because nalidixic acid is excreted in breast milk, it is contraindicated during lactation.

➤*Children:* Safety and efficacy in infants younger than 3 months of age have not been established.

Use in patients younger than 18 years of age – Toxicological studies have shown that nalidixic acid and related drugs can produce erosions of the cartilage in weight-bearing joints and other signs of arthropathy in immature animals of most species tested. No such joint lesions have been reported in humans to date. Nevertheless, until the significance of this finding is clarified, only use this drug in patients younger than 18 years of age when the potential benefit justifies the potential risk. If arthralgia occurs, stop treatment with nalidixic acid.

Precautions

➤*Monitoring:* Perform blood cell counts and renal and liver function tests periodically if treatment is continued for more than 2 weeks.

➤*Resistance:* If bacterial resistance to nalidixic acid emerges during treatment, it usually does so within 48 hours, permitting rapid change to another antimicrobial. Therefore, if the clinical response is unsatisfactory or if relapse occurs, repeat cultures and sensitivity tests. Underdosage with nalidixic acid during initial treatment (with less than 4 g/day for adults) may predispose to emergence of bacterial resistance.

Cross-resistance between nalidixic acid and other quinolone derivatives (eg, oxolinic acid, cinoxacin) has been observed. Prescribing nalidixic acid in the absence of a proven or strongly suspected bacterial infection or a prophylactic indication is unlikely to provide benefit to patient and increases the risk of development of drug-resistant bacteria.

➤*Glucose-6-phosphate dehydrogenase deficiency:* Use caution in patients with glucose-6-phosphate dehydrogenase deficiency.

➤*Renal function impairment:* While caution should be used in patients with severe renal failure, therapeutic concentrations of nalidixic acid in the urine, without increased toxicity caused by drug accumulation in the blood, have been observed in patients on full dosage with creatinine clearances (Ccr) as low as 2 to 8 mL/min.

➤*Special risk:* Use nalidixic acid with caution in patients with epilepsy, liver disease, or severe cerebral arteriosclerosis.

➤*Hazardous tasks:* Quinolones may cause dizziness and lightheadedness. Patients should know how they react to nalidixic acid before they operate an automobile or machinery or engage in activities requiring mental alertness or coordination.

➤*Photosensitivity:* Moderate to severe phototoxicity reactions have been observed in patients who are exposed to direct sunlight while receiving nalidixic acid or other members of this drug class. Avoid excessive sunlight. Discontinue therapy if phototoxicity occurs.

Drug Interactions

Nalidixic Acid Drug Interactions

Precipitant drug	Object drug[a]		Description
Nalidixic acid	Theophylline	⬆	Elevated plasma levels of theophylline have been reported. Consider monitoring theophylline plasma levels.
Nalidixic acid	Caffeine	⬆	Quinolones have been shown to interfere with the metabolism of caffeine, which may reduce caffeine clearance and prolong plasma half-life.
Nalidixic acid	Oral anticoagulants (eg, warfarin)	⬆	Nalidixic acid may enhance the effects of warfarin. Monitor prothrombin time closely.
Bacteriostatic agents (eg, chloramphenicol, nitrofurantoin, tetracycline)	Nalidixic acid	⬇	The action of nalidixic acid may be inhibited by the presence of bacteriostatic agents by antagonizing nalidixic acid in vitro.
Probenecid	Nalidixic acid	⬇	Probenecid inhibits tubular secretion of nalidixic acid and may reduce its efficacy while increasing the risk of adverse reactions.
Antacids containing magnesium, aluminum, calcium	Nalidixic acid	⬇	Coadministration may interfere with the absorption of quinolones, resulting in systemic levels lower than desired. Do not take these antacids within 2 hours before or within 2 hours after nalidixic acid.
Sucralfate	Nalidixic acid	⬇	Sucralfate may interfere with the absorption of quinolones, resulting in systemic levels lower than desired. Do not take sucralfate within 2 hours before or within 2 hours after nalidixic acid.
Iron salts	Nalidixic acid	⬇	Iron salts may interfere with the absorption of quinolones, resulting in systemic levels lower than desired. Do not take iron salts within 2 hours before or within 2 hours after nalidixic acid.

NALIDIXIC ACID — ORAL

Nalidixic Acid Drug Interactions			
Precipitant drug	Object drug[a]		Description
Multivitamins containing zinc	Nalidixic acid	⬇	Multivitamins containing zinc may interfere with the absorption of quinolones, resulting in systemic levels lower than desired. Do not take multivitamins containing zinc within 2 hours before or within 2 hours after nalidixic acid.
Didanosine	Nalidixic acid	⬇	Didanosine chewable/buffered tablets or pediatric powder for oral solution may interfere with the absorption of quinolones, resulting in systemic levels lower than desired. Do not take didanosine within 2 hours before or within 2 hours after nalidixic acid.
Quinolones (eg, gatifloxacin, levofloxacin)	Antiarrhythmic agents (eg, amiodarone, quinidine, sotalol)	⬆	The risk of life-threatening cardiac arrhythmias, including torsades de pointes, may be increased.
Nalidixic acid	Melphalan	⬆	Serious GI toxicity has been associated with concomitant use. Nalidixic acid is contraindicated in patients undergoing concomitant therapy with melphalan or other related cancer chemotherapeutic alkylating agents.

[a] ⬆ = Object drug increased. ⬇ = Object drug decreased.

➤*Drug/Lab test interactions:* When Benedict's or Fehling's solution, or *Clinitest Reagent* tablets are used to test the urine of patients taking nalidixic acid, a false-positive reaction for glucose may be obtained, because of the liberation of glucuronic acid from the metabolites excreted. However, a colorimetric test for glucose based on an enzyme reaction (eg, with *Clinistix Reagent Strips* or *Tes-Tape*) does not give a false-positive reaction to the liberated glucuronic acid.

Incorrect values may be obtained for urinary 17-keto and ketogenic steroids in patients receiving nalidixic acid, because of an interaction between the drug and the m-dinitrobenzene used in the usual assay method. In such cases, the Porter-Silber test for 17-hydroxycorticoids may be used.

Adverse Reactions

➤*CNS:* Dizziness, drowsiness, headache, weakness, and vertigo. Toxic psychosis or brief convulsions have been reported rarely, usually following excessive doses. In general, the convulsions have occurred in patients with predisposing factors such as epilepsy or cerebral arteriosclerosis. In infants and children receiving therapeutic doses of nalidixic acid, increased intracranial pressure with bulging anterior fontanel, papilledema, and headache occasionally has been observed. A few cases of sixth cranial nerve palsy have been reported. Although the mechanisms of these reactions are unknown, the signs and symptoms usually disappeared rapidly with no sequelae when treatment was discontinued.

➤*GI:* Abdominal pain; diarrhea; nausea; vomiting.

➤*Hematologic:* Hemolytic anemia, leukopenia, thrombocytopenia, or sometimes associated with glucose 6-phosphate dehydrogenase deficiency (rare).

➤*Hypersensitivity:* Anaphylactoid reaction (including anaphylactic shock), angioedema, arthralgia with joint stiffness and swelling, eosinophilia, pruritus, rash, and urticaria. Erythema multiforme and Stevens-Johnson syndrome have been reported with nalidixic acid and other drugs in this class. Rash was the most frequently reported adverse reaction.

Photosensitivity – Photosensitivity reactions consisting of erythema and bullae on exposed skin surfaces usually resolve completely in 2 weeks to 2 months after nalidixic acid is discontinued; however, bullae may continue to appear with successive exposures to sunlight or with mild skin trauma for up to 3 months after discontinuation of drug.

➤*Ophthalmic:* Reversible subjective visual disturbances without objective findings have occurred infrequently (generally with each dose during the first few days of treatment). These reactions include overbrightness of lights, change in color perception, difficulty in focusing, decrease in visual acuity, and double vision. They usually disappeared promptly when dosage was reduced or therapy was discontinued.

➤*Miscellaneous:* Cholestasis, metabolic acidosis, paresthesia, peripheral neuropathy (rare).

Overdosage

➤*Symptoms:* Convulsions, increased intracranial pressure, metabolic acidosis, or toxic psychosis may occur in patients taking more than the recommended dosage. Lethargy, nausea, and vomiting, also may occur after overdosage.

➤*Treatment:* Reactions are short lived (2 to 3 hours) because the drug is rapidly excreted. If absorption has occurred, increased fluid administration is advisable, and supportive measures such as oxygen and means of artificial respiration should be available. Although anticonvulsant therapy has not been used in the few instances of overdosage reported, it may be indicated in a severe case.

Patient Information

Nalidixic acid may be taken with or without meals. Advise patients to drink fluids liberally and not to take antacids.

Advise patients that quinolones may be associated with hypersensitivity reactions, even following a single dose. Patients should discontinue the drug at the first sign of a skin rash or other allergic reactions.

Quinolones may cause dizziness and light-headedness. Patients should know how they react to nalidixic acid before they operate an automobile or machinery or engage in activities requiring mental alertness or coordination.

Advise patients that quinolones may increase the effects of theophylline and caffeine. There is a possibility of caffeine accumulation when products containing caffeine are consumed while taking quinolones.

Advise patients to avoid excessive sunlight or artificial ultraviolet light while receiving nalidixic acid and to discontinue therapy if phototoxicity occurs.

Advise patients that convulsions have been reported in patients taking quinolones, including nalidixic acid, and to notify their physician before taking this drug if there is a history of this condition.

Advise patients not to take mineral supplements, vitamins with iron or minerals, calcium-, aluminum-, or magnesium-based antacids, sucralfate or didanosine chewable/buffered tablets or the pediatric powder for oral solution within the 2-hour period before or within the 2-hour period after taking nalidixic acid.

Advise patients:
- that nalidixic acid may cause changes in the electrocardiogram (QTc interval prolongation);
- that nalidixic acid should be avoided in patients receiving class IA (eg, quinidine, procainamide) or class 3 (eg, amiodarone, sotalol) antiarrhythmic agents;
- that nalidixic acid should be used with caution in subjects receiving drugs that affect the QTc interval such as cisapride, erythromycin, antipsychotics, and tricyclic antidepressants;
- to inform their physicians of any personal or family history of QTc prolongation or proarrhythmic conditions such as hypokalemia, bradycardia, or recent myocardial ischemia;
- that peripheral neuropathies have been associated with nalidixic acid use. If symptoms of peripheral neuropathy including pain, burning, tingling, numbness, and/or weakness develop, they should discontinue treatment and contact their physicians.

Counsel patients that antibacterial drugs, including nalidixic acid, should only be used to treat bacterial infections; they do not treat viral infections (eg, the common cold). When nalidixic acid is prescribed to treat a bacterial infection, tell patients that, although it is common to feel better early in the course of therapy, they should take the medication exactly as directed. Skipping doses or not completing the full course of therapy may decrease the effectiveness of the immediate treatment and increase the likelihood that bacteria will develop resistance and will not be treatable by nalidixic acid or other antibacterial drugs in the future.

CINOXACIN

Rx	**Cinoxacin** (Biocraft)	**Capsules:** 250 mg	(Biocraft 163). Blue/yellow. In 40s and 100s.
Rx	**Cinoxacin** (Various, eg, Moore, Rugby)	**Capsules:** 500 mg	In 50s and 100s.

CINOXACIN — ORAL

Indications

➤*Urinary tract infections:* For the treatment of initial and recurrent urinary tract infections in adults caused by the following susceptible microorganisms: *Escherichia coli, Proteus mirabilis, Proteus vulgaris, Klebsiella* species (including *K. pneumoniae*), and *Enterobacter* species.

➤*Prophylaxis:* Cinoxacin is effective in preventing urinary tract infections for up to 5 months in women with a history of recurrent urinary tract infections.

Administration and Dosage

➤*Approved by the FDA:* February 28, 1992.

➤*Urinary tract infections:* The usual adult dosage for the treatment of urinary tract infections is 1 g daily, administered orally in 2 or 4 divided doses (500 mg twice daily or 250 mg 4 times daily, respectively) for 7 to 14 days. Administer doses at least 2 hours before or 2 hours after antacids containing magnesium or aluminum, as well as sucralfate, metal cations such as iron, and multivitamin preparations with zinc, or didanosine chewable tablets or the pediatric powder for oral solution. Although susceptible organisms may be eradicated within a few days after therapy has begun, the full treatment course is recommended.

➤*Renal function impairment:* When renal function is impaired, employ a reduced dosage. After an initial dose of 500 mg, use a maintenance dosage schedule.

Maintenance Dosage Guide for Patients with Renal Impairment

Creatinine clearance (mL/min per 1.73 m^2)	Renal function	Dosage
> 80	Normal	500 mg twice daily
80 to 50	Mild impairment	250 mg 3 times daily
50 to 20	Moderate impairment	250 mg twice daily
< 20	Marked impairment	250 mg daily

Administration of cinoxacin to anuric patients is not recommended.

➤*Preventive therapy:* A single dose of 250 mg at bedtime for up to 5 months has been shown to be effective in women with a history of recurrent urinary tract infections.

➤*Storage/Stability:* Store at controlled room temperature 15° to 30°C (59° to 86°F).

Actions

➤*Pharmacokinetics:*

Absorption – Cinoxacin is rapidly absorbed after oral administration. In fluorometric assay, a 500 mg dose produced a peak serum concentration of 15 mcg/mL, which declined to approximately 1 to 2 mcg/mL 6 hours after administration. A 500 mg dose produced an average urine concentration of approximately 300 mcg/mL during the first 4 hours and approximately 100 mcg/mL during the second 4-hour period. These urine concentrations are many times greater than the minimal inhibitory concentration (MIC) of cinoxacin for most gram-negative organisms commonly found in urinary tract infections.

The presence of food did not affect the total absorption of cinoxacin. Peak serum concentrations were reduced by 30%, but the 24-hour urinary recovery of antibacterial activity was unaltered. The mean serum half-life is 1.5 hours.

Metabolism/Excretion – Ninety-seven percent (97%) of a 500 mg oral dose of radiolabeled cinoxacin was recovered in the urine within 24 hours, 60% of which was present as unaltered cinoxacin and the remainder as inactive metabolic products.

Special populations –

Elderly: Twenty geriatric patients (ages 70 to 89, 14 men and 6 women) with creatinine clearance from 58 to 80 mL/min, were given cinoxacin 500 mg every 12 hours for 7 days. Following the first dose of cinoxacin, the mean peak of the serum concentration was 14 mcg/mL. Following the last dose, the mean peak of the serum concentration was 15 mcg/mL. The mean urine concentration after 3 hours was 656 mcg/mL, at 3 to 6 hours was 1,234 mcg/mL, and at 12 hours was 33 mcg/mL. The mean recovery of unaltered cinoxacin from the urine following the first dose and last dose was 55% and 62%, respectively.

➤*Microbiology:* Cinoxacin has in vitro activity against many gram-negative aerobic bacteria, particularly strains of Enterobacteriaceae. Cinoxacin inhibits bacterial deoxyribonucleic acid (DNA) synthesis, is bactericidal, and is active over the entire urinary pH range. Cross-resistance with nalidixic acid has been demonstrated.

Conventional chromosomal resistance to cinoxacin taken at recommended doses has been reported to emerge in approximately 4% of patients during treatment; however, bacterial resistance to cinoxacin has not been shown to be transferable via R-factor.

Cinoxacin has been shown to be active against most strains of the following organisms both in vitro and in clinical initial and recurrent urinary tract infections:

Gram-negative aerobes – *Enterobacter* species; *Escherichia coli*; *Klebsiella* species; *Proteus mirabilis*; *Proteus vulgaris*.

Enterococcus species, *Pseudomonas* species, and *Staphylococcus* species are resistant.

Contraindications

Hypersensitivity to cinoxacin or other quinolones.

Warnings

➤*Arthropathy:* The oral administration of a single 250 mg/kg dose of cinoxacin causes lameness in immature dogs. Histopathological examination of the weightbearing joints of these dogs revealed lesions of the cartilage. Other quinolones also produce erosions of cartilage of weightbearing joints and other signs of arthropathy in immature animals of various species.

➤*CNS effects:* Convulsions and abnormal electroencephalograms have been reported in a few patients receiving quinolone class antimicrobials. No causal relationship has been established. Convulsions, increased intracranial pressure, and toxic psychoses have also been reported in patients receiving other drugs in this class.

Quinolones also may cause central nervous system (CNS) stimulation with tremors, restlessness, lightheadedness, confusion, or hallucinations. If these reactions occur in patients receiving cinoxacin, discontinue the drug and institute appropriate measures. As with all quinolones, use cinoxacin with caution in patients with known or suspected CNS disorders, such as severe cerebral arteriosclerosis, epilepsy, and other factors that predispose to seizures.

➤*Tendon effects:* Achilles and other tendon ruptures that required surgical repair or resulted in prolonged disability have been reported with quinolones. Discontinue cinoxacin if the patient experiences pain, inflammation, or tendon rupture.

➤*Hypersensitivity reactions:* Serious and occasionally fatal hypersensitivity (anaphylactic) reactions, some following the first dose, have been reported in patients receiving quinolone class antimicrobials. Some reactions were accompanied by cardiovascular collapse, loss of consciousness, tingling, pharyngeal or facial edema, dyspnea, urticaria, and itching. Only a few patients had a history of previous hypersensitivity reactions. If an allergic reaction to cinoxacin occurs, discontinue the drug. Serious acute hypersensitivity reactions may require treatment with epinephrine and other resuscitative measures, including oxygen, IV fluids, IV antihistamines, corticosteroids, pressor amines, and airway management as clinically indicated.

➤*Renal function impairment:* Because cinoxacin is eliminated primarily by the kidney, the usual dosage should be lower in patients with reduced renal function.

See Administration and Dosage for more information.

➤*Elderly:* See Actions for more information.

In geriatric patients with reduced renal function, reduce the dosage.

See Administration and Dosage for more information.

In general, dose selection for an elderly patient should be cautious, usually starting at the low end of the dosing range, reflecting the greater frequency of decreased hepatic, renal or cardiac function, and of concomitant disease or other drug therapy.

➤*Pregnancy: Category C.*

Teratogenic –

There are no adequate and well-controlled studies in pregnant women. Use cinoxacin during pregnancy only if the potential benefit justifies the potential risk to the fetus.

➤*Lactation:* It is not known whether cinoxacin is excreted in human milk. Because other drugs in this class are excreted in human milk and because of the potential for serious adverse reactions from cinoxacin in breast-feeding infants, make a decision whether to discontinue breast-feeding or the drug, taking into account the importance of the drug to the mother.

➤*Children:* The safety and effectiveness of cinoxacin in pediatric patients and adolescents less than 18 years of age have not been established. Cinoxacin causes arthropathy in juvenile animals (see above).

Precautions

➤*Monitoring:* As with any potent drug, periodic assessment of organ system function, including renal, hepatic, and hematopoietic function, is advisable during prolonged therapy.

In clinical trials with large doses of quinolones, crystalluria was reported in some volunteers. Although crystalluria is not expected to occur with the usually recommended dosages of cinoxacin, hydrate patients well, and avoid the alkalinization of urine.

CINOXACIN — ORAL

➤*Hazardous tasks:* Cinoxacin can cause dizziness and light-headedness; therefore, patients should know how they react to the drug before operating an automobile or machinery or engaging in an activity requiring mental alertness or coordination.

➤*Photosensitivity:* Moderate to severe phototoxicity reactions have been observed in patients who were exposed to direct sunlight while receiving some members of this drug class. Avoid excessive sunlight. Discontinue therapy if phototoxicity occurs.

Drug Interactions

➤*Theophylline:* Elevated plasma levels of theophylline have been reported with concomitant use of some quinolones. There have been reports of theophylline-related side effects in patients on concomitant theophylline-quinolone therapy. Therefore, consider monitoring of theophylline plasma levels and adjust dosage of theophylline as required.

➤*Caffeine:* Quinolones have also been shown to interfere with the metabolism of caffeine. This may lead to reduced clearance of caffeine and a prolongation of its plasma half-life. Although this interaction has not been reported with cinoxacin, exercise caution when cinoxacin is given concomitantly with caffeine-containing products.

➤*Antacids, sucralfate:* Antacids or sucralfate substantially interfere with the absorption of some quinolones, resulting in low urine levels. Also, concomitant administration of quinolones with products containing iron, multivitamins containing zinc, or didanosine chewable/buffered tablets or the pediatric powder for oral solution may result in low urine levels.

➤*Oral anticoagulants:* Quinolones, including cinoxacin, may enhance the effects of oral anticoagulants, such as warfarin or its derivatives. When these products are administered concomitantly, closely monitor prothrombin time or other suitable coagulation tests.

➤*NSAIDs:* Seizures have been reported in patients taking another quinolone class antimicrobial and the nonsteroidal anti-inflammatory drug fenbufen concurrently. Animal studies also suggest an increased potential for seizures when these 2 drugs are given concomitantly. Fenbufen is not approved in the United States at this time. Physicians are provided this information to increase awareness of the potential for serious interactions when cinoxacin and certain nonsteroidal anti-inflammatory agents are administered concomitantly.

➤*Cyclosporine:* Elevated cyclosporine serum levels have been reported with the concomitant use of quinolones and cyclosporine.

Adverse Reactions

➤*CNS:* The most frequent side effects were dizziness and headache, reported by 1 in 100 patients. Other adverse reactions possibly related to cinoxacin include drowsiness, insomnia, perineal burning, photophobia, tingling sensation, and tinnitus. These were reported by less than 1 in 100 patients.

➤*GI:* Nausea was reported most commonly and occurred in less than 3 in 100 patients. Other side effects, occurring less frequently (1 in 100), were abdominal cramps/pain, anorexia, diarrhea, perverse taste, and vomiting.

➤*Hematologic:* Rare reports of thrombocytopenia.

➤*Hypersensitivity:* Angioedema, edema, eosinophilia, pruritus, rash, urticaria, and were reported by less than 3 in 100 patients. Rare cases of anaphylactic reactions have been reported. Toxic epidermal necrolysis has been reported very rarely. Erythema multiforme and Stevens-Johnson syndrome have been reported with cinoxacin and other drugs in this class.

➤*Lab test abnormalities:* Laboratory values reported to be abnormal were, in descending order of frequency, elevation of BUN (1 in 100), AST, ALT, serum creatinine, and alkaline phosphatase; and reduction in hematocrit/hemoglobin (each less than 1 in 100).

➤*Postmarketing:* The most frequently reported adverse events in postmarketing surveillance of cinoxacin have been anaphylactic reactions and rash. Other frequently reported reactions have been abdominal pain, allergic reactions, headache, nausea, pruritus, and urticaria.

Overdosage

➤*Symptoms:* Symptoms following an overdose of cinoxacin may include anorexia, diarrhea, epigastric distress, nausea, and vomiting. The severity of the epigastric distress and the diarrhea are dose related. Dizziness, headache, insomnia, photophobia, a tingling sensation, and tinnitus have been reported in some patients. If other symptoms are present, they are probably secondary to an underlying disease state, an allergic reaction, or the ingestion of a second medication with toxicity.

➤*Treatment:* In all cases of suspected overdosage, call your regional poison control center to obtain the most up-to-date information about the treatment of overdose. This recommendation is made because, in general, information regarding the treatment of overdosage may change more rapidly than do package inserts.

In managing overdosage, consider the possibility of multiple drug overdoses, interaction among drugs, and unusual drug kinetics in your patient.

Keep patients who have ingested an overdose of cinoxacin well hydrated to prevent crystalluria.

Protect the patient's airway and support ventilation and perfusion. Meticulously monitor and maintain, within acceptable limits, the patient's vital signs, blood gases, serum electrolytes, etc. Absorption of drugs from the gastrointestinal tract may be decreased by giving activated charcoal, which, in many cases, is more effective than emesis or lavage; consider charcoal instead of, or in addition to, gastric emptying. Repeated doses of charcoal over time may hasten elimination of some drugs that have been absorbed. Safeguard the patient's airway when employing gastric emptying or charcoal.

Forced diuresis, peritoneal dialysis, hemodialysis, or charcoal hemoperfusion have not been established as beneficial for an overdose of cinoxacin.

Patient Information

Advise patients that cinoxacin may be taken with or without meals. Patients should drink fluids liberally. Antacids containing magnesium or aluminum, as well as sucralfate, metal cations such as iron, and multivitamin preparations with zinc, or didanosine chewable/buffered tablets or the pediatric powder for oral solution may interfere with the gastrointestinal absorption of cinoxacin. These agents should be taken at least 2 hours before or 2 hours after cinoxacin administration.

Advise patients to avoid excessive sunlight during cinoxacin therapy. If phototoxicity occurs, discontinue cinoxacin therapy.

Cinoxacin may be associated with hypersensitivity reactions following even a single dose. Discontinue the drug at the first sign of skin rash or allergic reaction.

Cinoxacin can cause dizziness and light-headedness; therefore, patients should know how they react to the drug before operating an automobile or machinery or engaging in an activity requiring mental alertness or coordination.

Advise patients that convulsions have been reported in patients taking quinolones, including cinoxacin acid, and that they should notify their physicians before taking this drug if there is a history of this condition.

Advise patients that cinoxacin may increase the effects of theophylline and caffeine. There is a possibility of caffeine accumulation when products containing caffeine are consumed during cinoxacin therapy.

FLUOROQUINOLONES

Indications

For specific approved indications, refer to individual drug monographs.

➤*Unlabeled uses:*

Ciprofloxacin – Ciprofloxacin has been used in children with cystic fibrosis for periods of 10 days to 6 months without documented adverse effects or intolerance.

Gatifloxacin, and moxifloxacin – Gatifloxacin, and moxifloxacin are effective against multidrug-resistant strains of *S. pneumoniae* and, therefore, may be used in pediatric patients who fail initial treatment for acute otitis media and sinusitis.

Ciprofloxacin and norfloxacin – Ciprofloxacin and norfloxacin have been used for the treatment of gastroenteritis in children.

Mycobacterial infections – In children, atypical mycobacterial infections have been satisfactorily treated with ciprofloxacin as part of combination therapy; in vitro, gatifloxacin has been shown to be active against *M. leprae.*

Fluoroquinolones – Fluoroquinolones are used as empiric therapy for low-risk febrile neutropenic pediatric patients. Regimens including fluoroquinolones for tuberculosis have been shown to be equivalent to standard antituberculosis regimens, and these agents are currently suggested for the management of multidrug-resistant infections or in patients with adverse reactions to other agents. The outcome of regimens including quinolones has been poorer in HIV-seropositive patients. Ciprofloxacin and ofloxacin are the quinolones most often evaluated and recommended in mycobacterial diseases.

Actions

➤*Pharmacology:* The fluoroquinolones are synthetic, broad-spectrum antibacterial agents that inhibit DNA gyrase and topoisomerase IV. DNA gyrase is an essential enzyme that is involved in the replication, transcription, and repair of bacterial DNA. Topoisomerase IV is an enzyme known to play a key role in the partitioning of the chromosomal DNA during bacterial cell division. The basic molecule has been modified at the N-1 position, with different groups added to the C-6, C-7, and C-8 positions. The addition of a fluorine atom at position C-6 enhances DNA gyrase inhibitory activity and provides activity against *staphylococci*; addition of a second fluorine group at position C-8 increases absorption and longer half-life; the addition of a piperazine group at position C-7 provides the best gram-negative activity; ring alkylation improves gram-positive activity and half-life; substitution of a methyl group for the piperazine group increases absorption and a longer half-life; and addition of acyclopropyl group at position N-1 and amino group at position C-5 and a fluorine group at C-8 increases activity against mycoplasma and chlamydia.

➤*Pharmacokinetics:*

Pharmacokinetics of Fluoroquinolones

Fluoroquinolone	Bio-avail-ability (%)	Max urine concentra-tion (mcg/mL) (dose)	Mean peak plasma concen-tration (mcg/mL) (dose)	Area under curve (AUC) (mcg • hr/mL) (dose)	Protein binding (%)	t½ (hr)	Urine recovery unchanged (%)
Ciprofloxacin Oral	≈ 70-80	> 200 (250 mg)	1.2 (250 mg) 2.4 (500 mg) 4.3 (750 mg) 5.4 (1000 mg)	4.8 (250 mg) 11.6 (500 mg) 20.2 (750 mg) 30.8 (1000 mg)	20-40	≈ 4	≈ 40-50
IV		> 200 (200 mg) > 400 (400 mg)	4.4 (400 mg)	4.8 (200 mg) 11.6 (400 mg)		≈ 5-6	≈ 50-70
Gatifloxacin[a] Oral	≈ 96		≈ 2 (200 mg single dose) ≈ 3.8 (400 mg single dose) ≈ 4.2 (400 mg multiple dose)	≈ 14.2 (200 mg single dose) ≈ 33 (400 mg single dose) ≈ 34.4 (400 mg multiple dose)	≈ 20	≈ 7.8 (400 mg single dose) ≈7.1 (400 mg multiple dose)	≈ 73.8 (200 mg single dose) ≈72.4 (400 mg single dose) ≈ 80.2 (400 mg multiple dose)
IV			≈ 2.2 (200 mg single dose) ≈ 2.4 (200 mg multiple dose) ≈ 5.5 (400 mg single dose) ≈ 4.6 (400 mg multiple dose)	≈ 15.9 (200 mg single dose) ≈ 16.8 (200 mg multiple dose) ≈ 35.1 (400 mg single dose) ≈ 35.4 (400 mg multiple dose)		≈ 11.1 (200 mg single dose) ≈ 12.3 (200 mg multiple dose) ≈ 7.4 (400 mg single dose) ≈ 13.9 (400 mg multiple dose)	≈ 71.7 (200 mg single dose) ≈ 72.4 (200 mg multiple dose) ≈ 62.3 (400 mg single dose) ≈ 83.5 (400 mg multiple dose)
Levofloxacin	≈ 99		≈ 2.8-11.5 (single dose oral or IV) ≈ 5.7-12.1 (multiple dose oral or IV)	≈ 27.2-110 (single dose oral or IV) ≈ 47.5-108 (multiple dose oral or IV)	≈ 24-38	≈ 6.3-7.5 (single dose oral or IV) ≈ 7-8.8 (multiple dose oral or IV)	≈ 87 (oral)
Lomefloxacin	≈ 95-98	> 300 (400 mg)	0.8 (100 mg) 1.4 (200 mg) 3.2 (400 mg)	5.6 (100 mg) 10.9 (200 mg) 26.1 (400 mg)	≈ 10	≈ 8	≈ 65
Moxifloxacin	≈ 90		4.5 (400 mg)	≈ 48 (400 mg)	≈ 50	≈ 12	≈ 20
Norfloxacin	30-40	≥ 200 (400 mg)	0.8 (200 mg) 1.5 (400 mg) 2.4 (800 mg)		10-15	3-4	26-32
Ofloxacin Oral	≈ 98	≈ 220 (200 mg)	1.5 (200 mg) 2.4 (300 mg) 2.9 (400 mg) 4.6 (400 mg steady-state)	14.1 (200 mg) 21.2 (300 mg) 31.4 (400 mg) 61 (400 mg steady-state)	≈ 32	≈ 9	65-80
IV		nd[b]	2.7 (200 mg) 4 (400 mg)	43.5 (400 mg)	≈ 32	5-10	≈ 65
Sparfloxacin	92	> 12 (400 mg)[c]	≈ 1.3 (400 mg)	≈ 34 (400 mg)	≈ 45	≈ 20	≈ 10

[a] Single dose: AUC (0-∞); Multiple dose: AUC (0-24).
[b] nd = no data.
[c] Following a 400 mg loading dose of sparfloxacin, the mean urine concentration 4 hours postdose was in excess of 12 mcg/mL.

Norfloxacin –

Absorption/Distribution: Absorption is rapid. Food or dairy products may decrease absorption. Steady-state norfloxacin levels will be attained within 2 days of dosing. Urinary concentrations of ≥ 200 mcg/mL are attained 2 to 3 hours after a single 400 mg dose. Mean urinary concentrations of norfloxacin remain above 30 mcg/mL for at least 12 hours following a 400 mg dose. Norfloxacin is least soluble at urinary pH of 7.5; greater solubility occurs at pHs above and below this value.

Metabolism/Excretion: Norfloxacin is eliminated through metabolism, biliary excretion, and renal excretion. Renal excretion occurs by glomerular filtration and tubular secretion, as evidenced by the high rate of renal clearance (≈ 275 mL/min). Within 24 hours of administration, 5% to 8% of the dose is recovered in the urine as 6 less-active metabolites. Fecal recovery accounts for another 30%. In healthy elderly volunteers (65 to 75 years of age), norfloxacin is eliminated more slowly because of decreased renal function. Drug absorption appears unaffected. Disposition of norfloxacin in patients with creatinine clearance (Ccr) rates > 30 mL/min/1.73 m^2 is similar to that in healthy volunteers. In patients with Ccr rates ≤ 30 mL/min/1.73 m^2, the renal elimination decreases so that the effective serum half-life is 6.5 hours; dosage alteration is necessary. See Administration and Dosage.

Ciprofloxacin –

Absorption/Distribution: Ciprofloxacin is rapidly and well absorbed from the GI tract after oral administration with no substantial loss by first-pass metabolism. When given concomitantly with food, there is a delay in the absorption of the drug, resulting in peak concentrations that are closer to 2 hours after dosing rather than 1 hour. However, the overall absorption is not substantially affected. Maximum serum concentrations are attained 1 to 2 hours after oral dosing. Mean concentrations 12 hours after dosing with 250, 500, or 750 mg are 0.1, 0.2, and 0.4 mcg/mL, respectively. Following 60-minute IV infusions of 200 and 400 mg, mean maximum serum concentrations achieved were 2.1 and 4.6 mcg/mL, respectively; concentrations at 12 hours were 0.1 and 0.2 mcg/mL, respectively. Ciprofloxacin is widely distributed throughout the body. Tissue concentrations often exceed serum concentrations in men and women, particularly in genital tissue. The drug diffuses into the cerebrospinal fluid (CSF); however, CSF concentrations are generally < 10% of peak serum concentrations.

Metabolism/Excretion: Four metabolites have been identified in urine which, together, account for ≈ 15% of an oral dose. The metabolites have antimicrobial activity, but are less active than unchanged ciprofloxacin. After IV administration, 3 metabolites have been identified in urine, which account for ≈ 10% of the IV dose. After a 250 mg oral dose, urine concentrations usually exceed 200 mcg/mL during the first 2 hours and are ≈ 30 mcg/mL at 8 to 12 hours after dosing. Following a 200 or 400 mg IV dose, urine concentrations usually exceed 200 and 400 mcg/mL, respectively, during the first 2 hours and are generally > 15 and > 30 mcg/mL, respectively, at 8 to 12 hours after dosing. Urinary ciprofloxacin excretion is virtually complete within 24 hours after dosing. Renal clearance is ≈ 300 mL/min; active tubular secretion plays a significant role. Although bile concentrations are several-fold higher than serum after oral dosing, only a small amount is recovered from the bile. Approximately 20% to 35% of an oral dose is recovered from feces within 5 days after dosing. In patients with reduced renal function, the half-life is slightly prolonged; dosage adjustments may be required. See Administration and Dosage.

Ofloxacin –

Absorption/Distribution: Maximum serum concentrations are achieved 1 to 2 hours after an oral dose. The amount absorbed increases proportionately with the dose. Elimination is biphasic; half-lives are ≈ 4 to 5 hours and 20 to 25 hours, although accumulation at steady state can be estimated using a half-life of 9 hours. Steady-state concentrations are achieved after 4 doses and are ≈ 40% higher than concentrations after single doses. Ofloxacin is widely distributed to body tissues and fluids.

Metabolism/Excretion: Ofloxacin has a pyridobenzoxazine ring that appears to decrease the extent of parent compound metabolism; < 5% of a dose is recovered in the urine as the desmethyl or N-oxide metabolites. Elimination is mainly by renal excretion; 4% to 8% is excreted in the feces. A longer plasma half-life of ≈ 6.4 to 7.4 hours was observed in elderly subjects, compared with 4 to 5 hours for young subjects. Slower elimination is observed in elderly subjects as compared with younger subjects, which may be attributable to the reduced renal function and renal clearance observed in the elderly subjects. Because ofloxacin is known to be substantially excreted by the kidney, and elderly patients are more likely to have decreased renal function, dosage adjustment is necessary for elderly patients with impaired renal function as recommended for all patients. Clearance is reduced in patients with renal function impairment (Ccr ≤ 50 mL/min); dosage adjustment is necessary. See Administration and Dosage.

Lomefloxacin –

Absorption/Distribution: Absorption is rapid. Following coadministration with food, rate of absorption is delayed (time to reach maximum plasma concentration delayed by 41%, maximum concentration decreased by 18%), and the extent of absorption (AUC) is decreased by 12%. At 24 hours postdose, single doses of 200 or 400 mg result in mean plasma levels of 0.1 and 0.24 mcg/mL, respectively. Steady-state concentrations are achieved within 48 hours of initiating once-daily dosing. The mean urine concentration exceeds 35 mcg/mL for ≥ 24 hours after dosing. Urine pH appears to affect the solubility of lomefloxacin, with solubilities ranging from 7.8 mg/mL at pH 5.2, to 2.4 mg/mL at pH 6.5, and 3.03 mg/mL at pH 8.12.

Metabolism/Excretion: Mean renal clearance is 145 mL/min in subjects with normal renal function, which may indicate tubular secretion. Approximately 9% of a dose is recovered in the urine as the glucuronide metabolite; 4 other metabolites have been identified and account for < 0.5% of the dose. Approximately 10% of a dose is recovered unchanged in the feces. In healthy elderly volunteers, plasma clearance was reduced by ≈ 25% and the AUC was increased by ≈ 33%, which may be caused by decreased renal function in this population. In patients with Ccr between 10 and 40 mL/min/1.73 m^2, the mean AUC after a single dose increased 335% over the AUC in patients with Ccr > 80 mL/min/1.73 m^2, and mean half-life increased to 21 hours. In patients with Ccr < 10 mL/min/1.73 m^2, AUC increased 700% and half-life increased to 45 hours. Adjustment of dosage is necessary. See Administration and Dosage.

Levofloxacin –

Absorption: Levofloxacin is rapidly and completely absorbed after oral administration. Peak plasma concentrations are usually attained 1 to 2 hours after oral dosing. Levofloxacin pharmacokinetics are linear and predictable after single and multiple oral/IV dosing regimens. Steady-state is reached within 48 hours following a 500 or 750 mg once-daily dosage regimen. The mean peak and trough concentrations attained following multiple once-daily oral dosage regimens were ≈ 5.7 and 0.5 mcg/mL after the 500 mg doses, and 8.6 and 1.1 mcg/mL after the 750 mg doses, respectively. The mean peak and trough plasma concentrations attained following multiple once-daily IV regimens were ≈ 6.4 and 0.6 mcg/mL after the 500 mg doses and 12.1 and 1.3 mcg/mL after the 750 mg doses, respectively. Oral administration of 500 mg levofloxacin tablet with food slightly prolongs the time to peak concentration by ≈ 1 hour and slightly decreases the peak concentration by ≈ 14%. Therefore, levofloxacin tablets can be administered without regard to food. The plasma concentration profile of levofloxacin after IV administration is similar and comparable in extent of exposure (AUC) to that observed for levofloxacin tablets when equal doses (mg/mg) are administered. Therefore, the oral and IV routes of administration can be considered interchangeable.

Distribution: The mean volume of distribution of levofloxacin generally ranges from 74 to 112 L after single and multiple 500 or 750 mg doses, indicating widespread distribution into body tissues. It reaches peak levels in skin tissues and in blister fluid at ≈ 3 hours after dosing. Levofloxacin also penetrates well into the lung tissues. Lung tissue concentrations were generally 2- to 5-fold higher than plasma concentrations. Levofloxacin is mainly bound to serum albumin and is independent of the drug concentration.

Metabolism: Levofloxacin undergoes limited metabolism and is primarily excreted as unchanged drug in the urine. Less than 4% of the dose was recovered in the feces in 72 hours. Less than 5% of an administered dose was recovered in the urine as the desmethyl and N-oxide metabolites. These metabolites have little relevant pharmacological activity.

Excretion: Levofloxacin is excreted largely as unchanged drug in the urine. The mean apparent total body clearance and renal clearance range from ≈ 144 to 226 mL/min and 96 to 142 mL/min, respectively. Renal clearance in excess of the glomerular filtration rate suggest the tubular secretion of levofloxacin occurs in addition to glomerular filtration.

Sparfloxacin –

Absorption: Sparfloxacin is well absorbed following oral administration. Steady-state concentration was achieved on the first day by giving a loading dose that was double the daily dose. Maximum plasma concentrations for the initial oral 400 mg loading dose were typically achieved between 3 to 6 hours following administration with a mean value of ≈ 4 hours. Maximum plasma concentrations for a 200 mg dose were also achieved between 3 to 6 hours after administration with a mean of ≈ 4 hours. Oral absorption of sparfloxacin is unaffected by administration with milk or food, including high-fat meals.

Distribution: Upon reaching general circulation, it distributes well into the body. The volume of distribution is 3.9 L/kg. It has low plasma protein binding. It penetrates well into body fluids and tissues. The concentrations in the lower respiratory tract tissues and fluids generally exceed the corresponding plasma concentrations.

Metabolism: Sparfloxacin is metabolized by the liver, primarily by phase II glucuronidation, to form a glucuronide conjugate. It does not utilize or interfere with cytochrome P450.

Excretion: The total body clearance and renal clearance of sparfloxacin were 11.4 and 1.5 L/hr respectively. It is excreted in the feces (50%) and urine (50%). The half-life is independent of the administered dose, suggesting the sparfloxacin elimination kinetics is linear.

Moxifloxacin –

Absorption: Moxifloxacin is well absorbed from the GI tract. Coadministration with a high-fat meal (eg, 500 calories from fat) does not affect the absorption of moxifloxacin. Consumption of 1 cup of yogurt with moxifloxacin does not significantly affect the extent or rate of systemic absorption (AUC). The C_{max} is attained 1 to 3 hours after oral dosing. The mean trough concentration is ≈ 0.95 mcg/mL. Plasma concentrations increase proportionally. Steady state is achieved after ≥ 3 days with a 400 mg once-daily regimen.

Distribution: The volume of distribution ranges from 1.7 to 2.7 L/kg. Moxifloxacin is widely distributed throughout the body, with tissue concentrations often exceeding plasma concentrations. The rates of elimination of moxifloxacin from tissue generally parallel the elimination from plasma.

Metabolism/Excretion: Moxifloxacin is metabolized via glucuronide and sulfate conjugation. The cytochrome P450 system is not involved and is not affected by moxifloxacin. The sulfate conjugate (M1) accounts for ≈ 38% of the dose and is eliminated primarily in the feces. Approximately 14% of an oral or IV dose are converted to a glucuronide conjugate (M2), which is excreted exclusively in the urine. A total of 95% of an oral dose is excreted as either unchanged drug or known metabolites. The mean apparent total body clearance and renal clearance are ≈ 12 L/hr and 2.6 L/hr, respectively.

Gatifloxacin –

Absorption: Gatifloxacin is well absorbed from the GI tract after oral administration and can be given without regard to food. Peak plasma concentrations usually occur 1 to 2 hours after oral dosing. The oral and IV routes of administration can be considered interchangeable since the pharmacokinetics of gatifloxacin after 1 hour IV administration are similar to those observed for orally administered gatifloxacin when equal doses are administered. Gatifloxacin pharmacokinetics are linear and time-independent at doses ranging from 200 to 800 mg administered over a period of up to 14 days. Steady-state concentrations are achieved by the third daily oral or IV dose. The mean steady-state peak and trough plasma concentrations attained are ≈ 4.2 mcg/mL and 0.4 mcg/mL, respectively for oral administration 4.6 mcg/mL and 0.4 mcg/mL, respectively for IV administration.

Distribution: Serum protein binding is ≈ 20% and is concentration-independent. Concentrations of gatifloxacin in saliva were approximately equal to those in plasma. The mean volume of distribution of gatifloxacin at steady-state ranged from 1.5 to 2 L/kg. Gatifloxacin was widely distributed throughout the body into many body tissues and fluids. Rapid distribution of gatifloxacin into tissues results in higher gatifloxacin concentrations in most target tissues than in serum.

Metabolism: Gatifloxacin undergoes limited biotransformation in humans with < 1% of the dose excreted in the urine as ethylenediamine and methylethylenediamine metabolites. It does not inhibit cytochrome P450.

Excretion: Gatifloxacin is excreted as unchanged drug primarily by the kidney. Less than 1% of the dose is recovered in the urine as 2 metabolites. The mean elimination half-life ranges from 7 to 14 hours and is independent of dose and route of administration. Renal clearance is independent of dose with mean value ranging from 124 to 161 mL/min. Gatifloxacin undergoes glomerular filtration and tubular secretion. It may also undergo minimal biliary or intestinal elimination, since 5% of the dose was recovered in the feces as unchanged drug.

➤*Microbiology:*

	Organisms Generally Susceptible to Fluoroquinolones In Vitro								
	Organism	Ciprofloxacin	Gatifloxacin	Levofloxacin	Lomefloxacin	Moxifloxacin	Norfloxacin	Ofloxacin	Sparfloxacin
Gram-negative	*Acinetobacter anitritus*								✓[1]
	Acinetobacter iwoffi	✓[1]	✓[1]	✓[1]					✓[1]
	Acinetobacter calcoaceticus							✓[1]	
	Aeromonas hydrophilia	✓[1]			✓[1]				
	Bacteroides distasonis								
	Bacteroides ovatus								
	Bordetella pertussis			✓[1]				✓[1]	
	Campylobacter jejuni	✓[2]							
	Chlamydia trachamotis							✓	
	Citrobacter diversus	✓	✓[1]	✓[1]	✓		✓[1]		✓[1]
	Citrobacter freundii	✓	✓[1]		✓[1]	✓[1]	✓	✓[1]	
	Citrobacter koseri		✓[1]						
	Enterobacter cloacae	✓	✓[1]	✓	✓	✓[1]	✓	✓[1]	✓
	Enterobacter aerogenes	✓[1]	✓[1]	✓[1]	✓[1]		✓	✓	✓[1]
	Enterobacter agglomerans			✓[1]	✓[1]		✓[1]		
	Enterobacter sakazakii			✓[1]					
	Escherichia coli	✓	✓	✓	✓	✓[1]	✓	✓	✓
	Edwardsiella tarda	✓[1]					✓[1]		
	Fusobacterium sp.					✓[1]			
	Gardenella vaginalis							✓	
	Haemophilus ducreyi						✓[1]	✓[1]	
	Haemophilus influenzae	✓	✓	✓	✓	✓		✓	✓
	Haemophilus parainfluenzae	✓	✓	✓	✓[1]	✓			✓
	Hafnia alvei				✓[1]				
	Klebsiella pneumoniae	✓	✓	✓	✓	✓	✓	✓	✓
	Klebsiella oxytoca	✓[1]	✓[1]	✓[1]	✓[1]	✓[1]	✓[1]	✓[1]	✓[1]
	Klebsiella ozaenae				✓[1]				
	Moraxella-catarrhalis	✓[2]	✓	✓	✓	✓		✓[1]	✓
	Morganella morganii	✓	✓[1]	✓[1]	✓[1]	✓	✓[1]	✓[1]	✓[1]
	Mycoplasma hominis							✓[1]	
	Neisseria gonorrhoeae	✓[2]					✓	✓	
	Pasteurella multocida	✓[1]							
	Prevotella sp.					✓[1]			
	Proteus mirabilis	✓		✓	✓	✓[1]	✓	✓	✓[1]
	Proteus vulgaris	✓	✓[1]	✓[1]	✓[1]		✓	✓[1]	✓[1]
	Providencia alcalifaciens				✓[1]		✓[1]		
	Providencia rettgeri	✓		✓[1]	✓[1]		✓[1]	✓[1]	
	Providencia stuartii	✓		✓[1]			✓[1]	✓[1]	
	Pseudomonas aeruginosa	✓		✓[3]	✓[4]		✓	✓[3]	
	Pseudomonas fluorescens			✓[1]			✓[1]		
	Pseudomonas stutzeri						✓[1]		
	Salmonella sp.	✓[5]	✓	✓		✓		✓	✓
	Salmonella typhi	✓							
	Salmonella enteritidis	✓[1]							
	Serratia marcescens	✓		✓[1]	✓[1]		✓	✓[1]	
	Serratia proteomaculans				✓[1]				
	Shigella sp.	✓[5]	✓	✓		✓		✓	✓
	Shigella boydii	✓[2]							
	Shigella dysenteriae	✓[2]							
	Shigella flexneri	✓[2]							
	Shigella sonnei	✓[2]							
	Ureoplasma urealtycium						✓[1]	✓[1]	
	Vibrio parahemolyticus	✓[1]							
	Vibrio vulnificus	✓[1]							
	Vibrio cholerae	✓[1]							
	Yersinia enterocolitica	✓[1]							

Organisms Generally Susceptible to Fluoroquinolones In Vitro									
	Organism	Ciprofloxacin	Gatifloxacin	Levofloxacin	Lomefloxacin	Moxifloxacin	Norfloxacin	Ofloxacin	Sparfloxacin
Gram-positive	*Staphylococcus aureus* methicillin susceptible	✓	✓	✓	✓[1]	✓	✓[6]	✓	✓[6]
	Staphylococcus aureus methicillin resistant				✓[1]				
	Staphylococcus epidermidis methicillin susceptible	✓[6]	✓	✓[1]	✓[1]	✓	✓[6]	✓[1]	✓
	Staphylococcus epidermidis methicillin resistant		✓		✓[1]	✓			
	Staphylococcus hemolyticus	✓							
	Staphylococcus hominis	✓							
	S. saprophyticus	✓	✓[1]	✓	✓		✓	✓[1]	
	Streptococci pyogenes	✓	✓[1]	✓		✓[1]		✓	✓[1]
	Streptococcus viridans			✓[1]					✓[1]
	Streptococcus group c/f, g			✓[1]					
	Streptococcus milleri			✓[1]					
	S. agalactiae			✓[1]		✓	✓		✓[1]
	Enteroccus faecalis	✓[7]		✓[7]			✓		
	Penicillin susceptible		✓	✓		✓		✓	✓
	Penicillin resistant		✓[1]	✓		✓[1]		✓[1]	✓[1]
Atypical bacteria	*Legionella pneumophilia*	✓[1]	✓	✓	✓[1]	✓[1]		✓[1]	✓[1]
	Mycoplasma pneumoniae		✓	✓		✓		✓[1]	✓
	Chlamydia pneumoniae		✓	✓	✓	✓		✓[1]	✓
Anaerobe bacteria	*Bacteroides fragilis*								
	Peptostreptococcus sp.		✓[1]			✓[1]			
	Clostridium perfringes			✓[1]			✓	✓[1]	

[1] Exhibits in vitro MIC of ≤ 1 mcg/mL (ciprofloxacin, sparfloxacin); ≤ 2 mcg/mL (gatifloxacin, levofloxacin, lomefloxacin, moxifloxacin and ofloxacin); ≤ 4 mcg/mL norfloxacin against most (≥ 90%) strains of microorganisms; however, the safety and effectiveness in treating clinical infections due to these microorganisms have not been established in adequate and well-controlled clinical trials.
[2] Oral ciprofloxacin.
[3] As with other drugs in this class, some strains of *P. aeruginosa* may develop resistance fairly rapidly during treatment.
[4] Urinary tract only.
[5] See following text for individual microorganisms.
[6] Does not specify susceptible or resistant.
[7] Many strains are moderately susceptible.

Ciprofloxacin – Most strains of streptococci are only moderately susceptible, as are *Mycobacterium tuberculosis*, *M. fortuitum*, and *Chlamydia trachomatis* (moderate activity). Some strains of *Pseudomonas aeruginosa* may develop resistance fairly rapidly.

Ciprofloxacin does not cross-react with other antimicrobial agents such as beta-lactams or aminoglycosides; however, additive activity may result when it is combined with beta-lactams, aminoglycosides, clindamycin, or metronidazole.

Most strains of *Burkholderia cepacia* and some strains of *Stenotrophomonas maltophilia* are resistant to ciprofloxacin as are most anaerobic bacteria, including *Bacteroides fragilis* and *Clostridium difficile*.

Gatifloxacin – The activity of gatifloxacin against *T. pallidum* has not been evaluated; however, other quinolones are not active against *T. pallidum*.

Levofloxacin – As with other drugs in this class, some strains of *P. aeruginosa* may develop resistance fairly rapidly during treatment with levofloxacin.

Norfloxacin – *Ureoplasma urealyticum* is susceptible in vitro. Resistance to norfloxacin due to spontaneous mutation in vitro is rare (< 1%). Development of resistance is greatest in the following: *P. aeruginosa*; *Klebsiella pneumoniae*; *Acinetobacter* sp.; enterococcus sp. Norfloxacin is not generally active against obligate anaerobes.

Norfloxacin has not been shown to be active against *T. pallidum*.

Ofloxacin – The following organisms are susceptible in vitro:
Anaerobes: Clostridium perfringens; Gardnerella vaginalis.
Other: Chlamydia pneumoniae; C. trachomatis; Mycoplasma pneumoniae; M. hominis; U. urealyticum.

Many strains of other streptococcal sp, enterococcus sp, and anaerobes are resistant. It is not active against *T. pallidum*. Although cross-resistance has been observed between ofloxacin and other fluoroquinolones, some organisms resistant to other quinolones may be susceptible to ofloxacin.

Lomefloxacin – Most group A, B, D, and G streptococci, *S. pneumoniae*, *Pseudomonas cepacia*, *U. urealyticum*, *M. hominis* and anaerobic bacteria are resistant.

Cross-resistance has occurred between lomefloxacin and other quinolone-class antimicrobial agents, but not between lomefloxacin and other antimicrobials, such as aminoglycosides, penicillins, tetracyclines, cephalosporins, or sulfonamides. Lomefloxacin is active in vitro against some strains of cephalosporin- and aminoglycoside-resistant gram-negative bacteria.

Contraindications

Hypersensitivity to fluoroquinolones or the quinolone group; tendinitis or tendon rupture associated with quinolone use; patients receiving disopyramide and amiodarone as well as other QT_c-prolonging antiarrhythmic drugs reported to cause torsade de pointes, such as class IA antiarrhythmic agents (eg, quinidine, procainamide), class III antiarrhythmic agents (eg, sotalol), and bepridil (**sparfloxacin** only); patients with known QT_c prolongation or in patients being treated concomitantly with medications known to produce an increase in the QT_c interval or torsades de pointes (**sparfloxacin**); patients whose lifestyle or employment will not permit compliance with required safety precautions concerning phototoxicity (**sparfloxacin**).

Warnings

➤*Phototoxicity:* Moderate-to-severe phototoxic reactions have occurred in patients exposed to direct or indirect sunlight or to artificial ultraviolet light (eg, sunlamps) during or following treatment with **lomefloxacin**, **sparfloxacin** or **ofloxacin**. These reactions also have occurred in patients exposed to shaded or diffused light, including exposure through glass. Advise patients to discontinue therapy of any fluoroquinolone antibiotic at the first signs or symptoms of a phototoxicity reaction such as a sensation of skin burning, redness, swelling, blisters, rash, itching, or dermatitis.

These reactions have occurred with and without the use of sunscreens or sunblocks and with single doses of lomefloxacin. In a few cases, recovery was prolonged for several weeks. As with some other types of phototoxicity, there is the potential for exacerbation of the reaction on re-exposure to sunlight or artificial ultraviolet light prior to complete recovery from the reaction. In rare cases, reactions have recurred up to several weeks after stopping therapy.

Avoid direct exposure to direct or indirect sunlight (even when using sunscreens or sunblocks) while taking lomefloxacin and other fluoroquinolones for several days following therapy. Discontinue therapy at first signs or symptoms of phototoxicity.

➤*Cardiac toxicity:* **Moxifloxacin** and **gatifloxacin** have been shown to prolong the QT interval of the electrocardiogram in some patients. Avoid in patients with known prolongation of the QT interval, patients with uncorrected hypokalemia, and patients receiving class IA (eg, quinidine, procainamide) or class III (eg, amiodarone, sotalol) antiarrhythmic agents, due to the lack of clinical experience with these drugs in these patient populations.

Increases in the QT_c interval have been observed in healthy volunteers treated with **sparfloxacin**. After a single loading dose of 400 mg, a mean increase in the QT_c interval of 11 msec (2.9%) is seen; at steady-state the mean increase is 7 msec (1.9%). The magnitude of the QT_c effect does not increase with repeated administration, and the QT_c returns to baseline within 48 hours of the last dose.

Avoid the concomitant prescription of medications known to prolong the QT_c interval (eg, erythromycin, terfenadine, astemizole, cisapride, pentamidine, tricyclic antidepressants, some antipsychotics including phenothiazines). **Sparfloxacin** is not recommended for use in patients with proarrhythmic conditions (eg, hypokalemia, significant bradycardia, CHF, myocardial ischemia, atrial fibrillation).

➤*Convulsions:* Increased intracranial pressure, convulsions, and toxic psychosis have occurred. CNS stimulation may also occur, which may lead to tremor, restlessness, lightheadedness, confusion, dizziness, depression, hallucinations, and rarely, suicidal thoughts or acts. Use with caution in patients with known or suspected CNS disorders (eg, severe cerebral arteriosclerosis, epilepsy) or other factors that predispose to seizures or lower the seizure threshold, or in the presence of other risk factors that may predispose to seizures or lower the seizure threshold (eg, certain drug therapy, renal dysfunction). If these reactions occur, stop the drug, and institute appropriate measures.

➤*Tendon rupture / Tendinitis:* Ruptures of the shoulder, hand, and Achilles tendons that required surgical repair or resulted in prolonged disability have been reported with fluoroquinolone antimicrobials. Discontinue therapy if the patient experiences pain, inflammation, or rupture of a tendon. Patients should rest and refrain from exercise until the diagnosis of tendinitis or tendon rupture has been confidently excluded. Tendon rupture can occur at any time during or after therapy.

➤*Syphilis:* **Ofloxacin**, **ciprofloxacin**, **norfloxacin** and **gatifloxacin** are not effective for syphilis. High doses of antimicrobial agents for short periods of time to treat gonorrhea may mask or delay symptoms of incubating syphilis. All patients should have a serologic test for syphilis at the time of gonorrhea diagnosis. Patients treated with ofloxacin, ciprofloxacin, norfloxacin and gatifloxacin should have a follow-up serologic test after 3 months.

➤*Chronic bronchitis due to S. pneumoniae:* **Lomefloxacin** is not indicated for the empiric treatment of acute bacterial exacerbation of chronic bronchitis when it is probable that *S. pneumoniae* is a causative pathogen because it exhibits in vitro resistance to lomefloxacin. Use only if sputum gram stain demonstrates an adequate quality of specimen and there is a predominance of gram-negative and not gram-positive organisms.

➤*Pseudomonas aeruginosa:* In clinical trials of complicated UTIs due to *P. aeruginosa*, 12 of 16 patients had the microorganism eradicated from the urine after therapy with **lomefloxacin**. No patients had concomitant bacteremia. Serum levels of lomefloxacin do not reliably exceed the MIC of *Pseudomonas* isolates. The safety and efficacy of lomefloxacin in treating patients with *Pseudomonas* bacteremia have not been established.

➤*Pseudomembranous colitis:* This has been reported with nearly all antibacterial agents, including fluoroquinolones, and may range from mild to life-threatening in severity. Therefore, it is important to consider this diagnosis in patients who present with diarrhea subsequent to the administration of antibacterial agents. After the diagnosis of pseudomembranous colitis has been established, initiate therapeutic measures. Mild cases of pseudomembranous colitis usually respond to discontinuation of drug alone. In moderate-to-severe cases, consider management with fluid and electrolytes, protein supplementation, and treatment with an antibacterial drug clinically effective against *C. difficile* colitis.

➤*Hypersensitivity reactions:* Serious and occasionally fatal reactions have occurred in patients receiving quinolone therapy, some following the first dose. Some reactions were accompanied by cardiovascular collapse, loss of consciousness, tingling, pharyngeal or facial edema, dyspnea, urticaria, and itching. If an allergic reaction occurs, discontinue the drug. Refer to Management of Acute Hypersensitivity Reactions.

➤*Renal function impairment:* Alteration in dosage regimen is necessary. See Administration and Dosage.

The pharmacokinetic parameters of **moxifloxacin** are not significantly altered by mild, moderate, or severe renal impairment. No dosage adjustment is necessary in patients with renal impairment.

Total **gatifloxacin** clearance was reduced 57% in moderate renal insufficiency and 77% with severe renal insufficiency following administration of a single oral 400 mg dose. Systemic exposure was ≈ 2 times higher in moderate renal insufficiency and 4 times higher in severe renal insufficiency. Reduce the dose of gatifloxacin in patients with a Ccr < 40 mL/min, including patients requiring hemodialysis or continuous ambulatory peritoneal dialysis (CAPD).

In patients with renal impairment, the terminal elimination half-life is lengthened. Single or multiple doses of **sparfloxacin** in patients with varying degrees of renal impairment typically produce plasma concentrations that are twice those observed in patients with normal renal function. Adjust the dosage accordingly.

Clearance of **levofloxacin** is substantially reduced and plasma elimination half-life is prolonged in patients with impaired renal function, requiring dosage adjustments in such patients to avoid accumulation. Neither hemodialysis nor CAPD is effective in removal of levofloxacin from the body, indicating that supplemental doses of levofloxacin are not required following hemodialysis or CAPD.

➤*Carcinogenesis:* Mice exposed to UVA light while receiving **lomefloxacin** developed a phototoxic response. Time to development of skin tumors was 16 weeks; with other quinolones and UVA light, times to skin tumor development ranged from 28 to 52 weeks. Well-differentiated squamous cell carcinomas developed in 92% of mice, which were nonmetastatic and endophytic. Lomefloxacin alone did not result in skin or systemic tumors.

In a study of repeated exposure (5 days/week for 40 weeks) of hairless albino mice to a low dose of solar simulated UV radiation, skin tumors were induced with a median onset time of 43 weeks. As expected for this model, gross appearance of the tumors in this study was consistent with squamous cell carcinoma or its precursors. When **sparfloxacin** (6 or 12.5 mg/kg/day) was administered by the oral route, the median tumor onset time was reduced to 38 and 32 weeks, respectively. This reduction in median onset time was similar to that observed when mice were exposed to a higher dose of solar-simulated UV radiation alone. At a dose level of 12.5 mg/kg/day, mice had skin sparfloxacin concentrations of ≈ 1.8 mcg/g. Following a 400 mg dose of sparfloxacin, skin levels measured in human subjects averaged 5.5 mcg/g. A similar effect on the time to the development of skin tumors has been observed in this mouse strain with some other fluoroquinolone antibiotics. The clinical significance of these findings to humans is unknown.

➤*Elderly:* **Norfloxacin** is eliminated more slowly because of decreased renal function; absorption appears unaffected. The apparent half-life of **ofloxacin** is 6.4 to 7.4 hours, compared with 4 to 5 hours in younger adults; absorption is unaffected. **Lomefloxacin** plasma clearance was reduced by ≈ 25% and the AUC was increased by ≈ 33% in the elderly, which may be due to decreased renal function in this population.

➤*Pregnancy:* *Category C.* There are no adequate and well-controlled studies in pregnant women. Use during pregnancy only if the potential benefit justifies the potential risk to the fetus.

Norfloxacin – Produces embryonic loss in monkeys when given in doses 10 times the maximum human dose.

Ciprofloxacin, moxifloxacin, sparfloxacin, gatifloxacin, levofloxacin, and norfloxacin – Caused lameness in immature dogs due to permanent cartilage lesions, and caused arthropathy in immature animals.

Ofloxacin – Doses equivalent to 10 to 50 times the recommended maximum dose were fetotoxic (ie, decreased fetal body weight, increased fetal mortality) in rats and rabbits, and minor skeletal variations occurred in rats; it also caused arthropathy in immature animals.

Lomefloxacin – Increased incidence of fetal loss in monkeys at ≈ 3 to 6 times the recommended human dose. In rabbits, maternal toxicity and associated fetotoxicity, decreased placental weight and variations of the coccygeal vertebrae occurred at doses 2 times the recommended human dose.

➤*Lactation:* **Norfloxacin** was not detected in breast milk following the administration of 200 mg to nursing mothers; however, this was a low dose. **Ciprofloxacin** is excreted in breast milk. **Ofloxacin**, as a single 200 mg dose, resulted in breast milk concentrations in nursing females that were similar to those found in plasma. **Levofloxacin** has not been measured in breast milk. Based upon data from ofloxacin, it can be presumed that levofloxacin will be excreted in breast milk. **Sparfloxacin** is excreted in breast milk. **Gatifloxacin** and **moxifloxacin** are excreted in the breast milk of rats. It is not known whether **lomefloxacin** or **gatifloxacin** are excreted in breast milk. Because of the potential for serious adverse reactions in nursing infants, decide whether to discontinue nursing or to discontinue the drug, taking into account the importance of the drug to the mother.

➤*Children:* Safety and efficacy of **gatifloxacin**, **levofloxacin**, **moxifloxacin**, **norfloxacin**, **lomefloxacin**, **sparfloxacin**, and **ofloxacin** in children younger than 18 years of age have not been established. **Ciprofloxacin**, **sparfloxacin**, **gatifloxacin**, **levofloxacin**, **moxifloxacin**, **lomefloxacin**, and **ofloxacin** cause arthropathy and osteochondrosis in immature animals. Administration of **norfloxacin**, **moxifloxacin**, and **ciprofloxacin** caused lameness in immature dogs due to permanent cartilage lesions.

Precautions

➤*Monitoring:* Periodic assessment of organ system functions, including renal, hepatic, and hematopoietic, is advisable during prolonged therapy.

➤*Crystalluria:* Needle-shaped crystals were found in the urine of some volunteers who received either placebo or 800 or 1600 mg **norfloxacin**. While crystalluria is not expected to occur under usual conditions with 400 mg twice daily, do not exceed the daily recommended dosage. Crystalluria related to **ciprofloxacin** has occurred only rarely in humans because human urine is usually acidic. Advise the patient to drink sufficient fluids to ensure proper hydration and adequate urinary output. Avoid alkalinity of the urine and do not exceed the recommended daily dose.

➤*Hemolytic reactions:* Rarely, hemolytic reactions have been reported in patients with latent or actual defects in glucose-6-phosphate dehydrogenase activity who take quinolone antibacterial agents, including **norfloxacin**.

➤*Myasthenia gravis:* Quinolones may exacerbate the signs of myasthenia gravis and lead to life-threatening weakness of the respiratory muscles. Exercise caution when using quinolones in patients with myasthenia gravis.

➤*Blood glucose abnormalities:* As with other quinolones, disturbances of blood glucose, including symptomatic hyper- and hypoglycemia, have been reported, usually in diabetic patients receiving concomitant treatment with an oral hypoglycemic agent (eg, glyburide/glibenclamide) or with insulin. In these patients, careful monitoring of blood glucose is recommended. If a hypoglycemic reaction occurs, initiate appropriate therapy immediately.

➤*Phototoxicity:* Reactions, moderate to severe, have occurred in patients who are exposed to direct sunlight while receiving some drugs in this class. See Warnings.

➤*Superinfection:* Use of antibiotics (especially prolonged or repeated therapy) may result in bacterial or fungal overgrowth of nonsusceptible organisms. Such overgrowth may lead to a secondary infection. Take appropriate measures if superinfection occurs.

Drug Interactions

Fluoroquinolone Drug Interactions			
Precipitant drug	Object drug*		Description
Sparfloxacin Gatifloxacin Moxifloxacin	Antiarrhythmic agents (amiodarone, bretylium, disopyramide, procainamide, quinidine, sotalol)	↑	The risk of life-threatening cardiac arrhythmias including torsades de pointes may be increased. The mechanism is unknown. Sparfloxacin is contraindicated in patients receiving class IA and III antiarrhythmic agents.
Sparfloxacin	Astemizole Terfenadine[1]	↑	Sparfloxacin is contraindicated in patients receiving astemizole.
Sparfloxacin	Bepridil Erythromycin Phenothiazine Tricyclic antidepressants	↑	The risk of life-threatening cardiac arrhythmias, including torsades de pointes may be increased. Sparfloxacin is contraindicated in drugs that prolong the QT_c interval.
Cisapride	Sparfloxacin	↑	The rate of sparfloxacin absorption may be accelerated. The risk of cardiovascular side effects may be increased. Sparfloxacin is contraindicated in patients receiving other QT_c-prolonging drugs or drugs reported to cause torsades de pointes.
Fluoroquinolones (eg, ciprofloxacin, norfloxacin, ofloxacin)	Theophyllines	↑	Administration of theophylline with ciprofloxacin has decreased theophylline clearance and increased plasma levels and symptoms of toxicity, including seizures.
Sucralfate	Fluoroquinolones	↓	Decreased GI absorption of quinolones. Avoid simultaneous use; administer sucralfate ≥ 6 hours after the quinolone.
Iron salts	Fluoroquinolones	↓	GI absorption of certain quinolones may be decreased by formation of an iron-quinolone complex. Avoid coadministration of these drugs.
Didanosine	Quinolones	↓	The magnesium and aluminum cations in the buffers present in didanosine tablets decrease the GI absorption of quinolones via chelation. Avoid simultaneous use.
Antacids	Quinolones	↓	Decreased GI absorption of quinolones resulting in decreased serum levels. Avoid simultaneous use.
Ofloxacin	Procainamide	↑	Plasma procainamide concentrations may be increased. Monitor plasma procainamide concentrations and adjust dose accordingly.
Ciprofloxacin Norfloxacin	Caffeine	↑	The hepatic metabolism of caffeine is decreased by certain quinolones; therefore, the pharmacologic effects of caffeine may be increased.
Ciprofloxacin Norfloxacin	Cyclosporine	↑	Increased cyclosporine toxicity. The mechanism is unknown.
Cimetidine	Fluoroquinolones	↑	Cimetidine may interfere with the elimination of the fluoroquinolones.
Nitrofurantoin	Norfloxacin	↓	Antibacterial effect of norfloxacin in the urinary tract may be antagonized.
Probenecid	Norfloxacin Gatifloxacin Lomefloxacin	↑	Diminished urinary excretion of the quinolones have been reported during the concomitant administration with probenecid.
Fluoroquinolones (eg, levofloxacin, norfloxacin)	Anticoagulants	↑	Quinolones decrease the clearance of the R-warfarin, the less active isomer of racemic warfarin. Enoxacin does not affect the clearance of the active S-isomer, and changes in clotting time have not been observed when coadministered. Nevertheless, monitor the prothrombin time when given concomitantly.
NSAIDs	Fluoroquinolones (eg, ofloxacin, levofloxacin)	↑	The concurrent administration of NSAIDs with a quinolone may increase the risk of CNS stimulation and convulsive seizures. Seizures have been reported in patients taking NSAIDs.
Azlocillin	Ciprofloxacin	↑	The clearance of ciprofloxacin is decreased by azlocillin resulting in a higher and prolonged ciprofloxacin serum concentration.

* ↑ = Object drug increased. ↓ = Object drug decreased.
[1] Withdrawn from market.

➤*Drug/Lab test interactions:* **Sparfloxacin** therapy may produce false-negative culture results for *Mycobacterium tuberculosis* by suppression of mycobacterial growth.

➤*Drug/Food interactions:* Food may decrease the absorption of **norfloxacin**. Food delays the absorption of **ciprofloxacin**, resulting in peak concentrations that are closer to 2 hours after dosing rather than 1 hour; however, overall absorption is not substantially affected. Dairy products such as milk and yogurt reduce the absorption of ciprofloxacin; avoid concurrent use. The bioavailability of ciprofloxacin may also be decreased by enteral feedings. Food delays the rate of absorption of **lomefloxacin** (time-to-reach maximum plasma concentration delayed by 41%, maximum concentration decreased by 18%) and decreases the extent of absorption (AUC) by 12%.

Adverse Reactions

Fluoroquinolone Adverse Reactions (%)									
Adverse reaction		Ciprofloxacin[1]	Gatifloxacin	Levofloxacin	Lomefloxacin	Moxifloxacin	Norfloxacin[2]	Ofloxacin[1]	Sparfloxacin
CNS	Headache	1.2	3	0.1-6.4	3.6	2	2-2.8	1-9	4.2-8.1
	Dizziness	< 1	3	0.3-2.7	2.1	3	1.7-2.6	1-5	2-3.8
	Fatigue/Lethargy/Malaise	< 1		< 1-1.2	< 1	> 0.05-< 1	0.3-1	1-3	< 1
	Somnolence/Drowsiness	< 1	< 0.1	< 1	< 1	> 0.05-< 1	0.3-1	1-3	< 1-1.5
	Depression	< 1	< 0.1	< 1	< 1		0.1-0.2	< 1	< 1
	Insomnia	< 1	≥ 0.1-< 3	0.5-4.6	< 1	> 0.05-< 1	0.3-1	3-7	1.9
	Seizures/Convulsions[3]	< 1	< 0.1	< 1	< 1		✓[4]	< 1	
	Confusion	≤ 1	< 0.1	< 1	< 1	> 0.05-< 1	✓[4]	< 1	< 1
	Psychotic reactions	< 1					✓[4]		
	Paresthesia	< 1	≥ 0.1-< 3	< 1	< 1		✓[4]	< 1	< 1
	Hallucinations	< 1	< 0.1	< 1		> 0.05-< 1		< 1	< 1

Fluoroquinolone Adverse Reactions (%)

	Adverse reaction	Ciprofloxacin[1]	Gatifloxacin	Levofloxacin	Lomefloxacin	Moxifloxacin	Norfloxacin[2]	Ofloxacin[1]	Sparfloxacin
Dermatologic	Photosensitivity[3]	< 1			2.3		✓[4]	✓[4]	
	Rash	1.1	≥ 0.1-< 3	0.3-1.2	< 1	> 0.05-< 1	0.3-1	1-3	1.1
	Pruritus	< 1	< 0.1	0.4-1.3	< 1	> 0.05-< 1	0.3-1	1-3	1.8-3.3
	Toxic epidermal necrolysis	< 1					✓[4]		
	Stevens-Johnson syndrome	< 1					✓[4]		
	Exfoliative dermatitis	< 1					✓[4]		
	Hypersensitivity[3]	< 1			< 1		✓[4]	✓[3]	
GI	Nausea	5.2	8	1.3-7.2	3.5	8	2.6-4.2	3-10	4.3-7.6
	Abdominal pain/discomfort/ cramping	≤ 1-1.7	≥ 0.1-< 3	0.4-2.5	1.2	> 0.05-≤ 2	0.3-1.6	1-3	1.8-2.4
	Diarrhea	2.3	4	1-5.6	1.4	6	0.3-1	1-4	3.2-4.6
	Vomiting	≤ 1-2	≥ 0.1-< 3	0.2-2.3	< 1	2	0.3-1	1-4	< 1-1.3
	Dry/painful mouth	< 1		< 1	< 1	> 0.05-< 1	0.3-1	1-3	< 1-1.4
	Dyspepsia/Heartburn	< 1	≥ 0.1-< 3	0.3-2.4	< 1	1	0.3-1	< 1	1.6-2.3
	Constipation	< 1	≥ 0.1-< 3	0.1-3.2	< 1	> 0.05-< 1	0.3-1	1-3	< 1
	Flatulence	< 1	< 0.1	0.4-1.5	< 1		0.3-1	1-3	< 1-1.1
	Pseudomembranous colitis[3]	< 1	< 0.1	< 1	✓[4]		✓[4]	✓[3]	
Miscellaneous	Visual disturbances	< 1			< 1		0.1-0.2	1-3	
	Hearing loss	< 1					✓[4]	< 1	
	Vaginitis	< 1	6	0.7-1.8	< 1	> 0.05-< 1		1-5	< 1
	Hypertension	< 1	< 0.1	< 1	< 1	> 0.05-< 1		< 1	< 1
	Palpitations	< 1	≥ 0.1-< 3	< 1		> 0.05-< 1		< 1	< 1
	Syncope	< 1		< 1	< 1			< 1	
	Chills	< 1	≥ 0.1-< 3		< 1	> 0.05-< 1	0.1-0.2	< 1	< 1
	Edema	< 1	< 0.1	< 1	< 1		0.1-0.2	< 1	
	Fever	< 1	≥ 0.1-< 3	< 1			0.3-1	1-3	< 1
Abnormal laboratory values	↑ ALT/↑ AST	1.9/1.7	< 1		≤ 0.4		1.4/1.4-1.6	≥ 1	2-2.3
	↑ Alkaline phosphatase	0.8	< 1		0.1		1.1	≥ 1	< 1
	↑ LDH	0.4		< 1			✓[4]		
	↑ or ↓ Bilirubin	0.3	< 1		0.1	≥ 2			< 1
	Eosinophilia	0.6			0.1	> 0.05-< 1	0.6-1.5	≥ 1	
	Leukopenia	0.4		< 1	0.1	> 0.05-< 1	1.4	≥ 1	
	↑ or ↓ Platelets	0.1			< 1		1		< 1
	Pancytopenia	0.1							
	↑ ESR/Lymphocytopenia				< 0.1			≥ 1	
	Neutropenia		< 1				1.4	≥ 1	
	↑ Serum creatinine	1.1			0.1		✓[4]	≥ 1	
	↑ BUN	0.9			0.1		✓[4]	≥ 1	
	Crystalluria/Cylinduria/ Candiduria	✓[4]					✓[4]		
	Hematuria	✓[4]						≥ 1	
	Glucosuria/Pyuria						✓[4]	≥ 1	
	Proteinuria/Albuminuria				< 0.1		1	≥ 1	
	↑ γ-glutamyltransferase	< 0.1			< 0.1				
	↑ Serum amylase	< 0.1	< 1						< 1
	↑ Uric acid	< 0.1							
	↑ or ↓ Blood glucose	< 0.1		2.2	< 0.1			≥ 1	< 1
	↓ Hemoglobin/Hematocrit	< 0.1			< 0.1	≥ 2	0.6		
	↑ or ↓ Potassium	✓[4]			0.1				< 1
	Anemia	< 0.1			< 0.1			≥ 1	
	Bleeding/↑ PT	< 0.1			< 0.1				
	↑ Monocytes	< 0.1			0.2				< 1
	Leukocytosis	< 0.1		< 1	0.1			≥ 1	
	↑ Triglycerides/Cholesterol	✓[4]							

[1] Includes data for oral and IV formulations.
[2] From single- and multiple-dose studies.
[3] See Warnings or Precautions.
[4] ✓ = Adverse reaction observed; incidence not reported.

Other adverse reactions listed only for the individual agents:

➤*Ciprofloxacin:*

Cardiovascular – Cardiovascular collapse, arrhythmia, tachycardia, cardiac murmur, hypotension (≤ 1%); angina pectoris, atrial flutter, cardiopulmonary arrest, cerebral thrombosis, MI, ventricular ectopy (< 1%); postural hypotension.

CNS – Restlessness (1.1%); paranoia, toxic psychosis, dysphasia, phobia, depersonalization, unresponsiveness, lightheadedness, anxiety, weakness, manic reaction (≤ 1%); nightmares, irritability, tremor, ataxia, anorexia (< 1%).

Dermatologic – Anaphylactic reactions, erythema multiforme, vasculitis, angioedema, edema of the lips, face, neck, conjunctivae, hands or lower extremities, purpura, cutaneous candidiasis, vesicles, increased perspiration; urticaria, flushing, hyperpigmentation, erythema nodosum (< 1%).

GI – Ileus, jaundice, *C. difficile*-associated diarrhea, pancreatitis, hepatic necrosis, oral ulceration, anorexia (≤ 1%); painful oral mucosa (< 1%).

GU – Renal calculi, hemorrhagic cystitis, frequent urination, gynecomastia, candiduria, crystalluria, cylindruria, hematuria, albuminuria (≤ 1%); acidosis, interstitial nephritis, nephritis, renal failure, polyuria, urinary retention, urethral bleeding (< 1%); vaginal candidiasis.

Hypersensitivity – Hyperpigmentation (< 1%)

Musculoskeletal – Arthralgia, jaw, arm, or back pain, joint stiffness, neck and chest pain, achiness, flare-up of gout (≤ 1%).

Respiratory – Respiratory arrest, respiratory distress, pleural effusion (≤ 1%); bronchospasm, dyspnea, epistaxis, hemoptysis, hiccoughs, laryngeal/pulmonary edema, pulmonary embolism (< 1%).

Special senses – Nystagmus, decreased visual acuity, blurred vision, anosmia (≤ 1%); bad taste in mouth, eye pain, tinnitus, diplopia (< 1%).

Miscellaneous – Thrombophlebitis, injection site burning, pain, pruritus, paresthesia, erythema, swelling (≤ 1%); oral candidiasis, intestinal perforation, GI bleeding, (< 1%); exacerbation of myasthenia gravis; dysphasia; agranulocytosis; cholestatic jaundice.

➤*Gatifloxacin:*

CNS – Abnormal dream, tremor, vasodilatation, vertigo (≥ 0.1% to < 3%); abnormal thinking, agitation, alcohol intolerance, anorexia, anxiety, ataxia, depersonalization, euphoria, hostility, migraine, nervousness, panic attack, paranoia, psychosis, stress (< 0.1%).

Cardiovascular – Bradycardia, breast pain, substernal chest pain, tachycardia (< 0.1%).

Dermatologic – Cheilitis, dry skin, ecchymosis, epistaxis, face edema, hyperesthesia, lymphadenopathy, maculopapular rash, vesiculobullous rash (< 0.1%).

Endocrine – Diabetes mellitus, hyperglycemia, hypoglycemia (< 0.1%).

GI – Glossitis, oral moniliasis, stomatitis, mouth ulcer (≥ 0.1% to < 3%); colitis, dysphagia, gastritis, GI hemorrhage, gingivitis, halitosis, hematemesis, mouth edema, rectal hemorrhage, thirst, tongue edema (< 0.1%).

GU – Dysuria, hematuria (≥ 0.1% to < 3%); metorrhagia (< 0.1%).

Musculoskeletal – Arthralgia, arthritis, asthenia, bone pain, hypertonia, leg cramp, myalgia, myasthenia, neck pain (< 0.1%).

Respiratory – Dyspnea, pharyngitis (≥ 0.1% to < 3%); asthma (bronchospasm), cyanosis, hyperventilation (< 0.1%).

Special senses – Abnormal vision, taste perversion, tinnitus (≥ 0.1% to < 3%); ear pain, eye pain, parosmia, ptosis, taste loss (< 0.1%).

Miscellaneous – Local injection site reaction (redness at injection site) (5%); allergic reaction, back pain, chest pain, peripheral edema, sweating (≥ 0.1% to < 3%); electrolyte abnormalities (< 1%).

➤*Levofloxacin:*

Cardiovascular – Cardiac failure, circulatory failure, hypotension, arrhythmia, atrial fibrillation, bradycardia, cardiac arrest, heart block, supraventricular tachycardia, tachycardia, ventricular fibrillation, angina pectoris, coronary thrombosis, MI, postural hypotension (< 1%).

CNS – Abnormal coordination, coma, hyperkinesia, hypertonia, hypoaesthesia, involuntary muscle contractions, paralysis, speech disorder, stupor, tremor, vertigo (< 1%).

Dermatologic – Erythema nodosum, genital pruritus, increased sweating, skin disorder, skin exfoliation, skin ulceration (< 1%); rash erythematous (0.1%); urticaria (< 1% to 0.1%).

GI – Dysphagia, gastroenteritis, GI hemorrhage, pancreatitis, tongue edema (< 1%).

GU – Abnormal renal function, acute renal failure, face edema, hematuria (< 1%).

Hematologic – Abnormal platelets, embolism (blood clot), epistaxis, purpura, thrombocytopenia, anemia (< 1%).

Hepatic – Abnormal hepatic function, cholelithiasis, hepatic coma, jaundice (< 1%).

Lab test abnormalities – Granulocytopenia, lymphadenopathy, WBC abnormal (not otherwise specified) (< 1%).

Metabolic/Nutritional – Aggravated diabetes mellitus, dehydration, hyperglycemia, hyperkalemia, hypoglycemia, hypokalemia, weight decrease (< 1%).

Musculoskeletal – Arthralgia, arthritis, arthrosis, muscle weakness, myalgia, osteomyelitis, rhabdomyolysis, synovitis, tendinitis (< 1%).

Psychiatric – Abnormal dreaming, aggressive reaction, agitation, anorexia, anxiety, delirium, emotional lability, impaired concentration, impotence, manic reaction, mental deficiency, paranoia, sleep disorder, withdrawal syndrome (< 1%); nervousness (0.1% to < 1%).

Respiratory – ARDS, asthma, coughing, dyspnea, hemoptysis, hypoxia, pleural effusion, respiratory insufficiency (< 1%).

Special senses – Taste perversion (0.2% to 1%); ear disorder (not otherwise specified), tinnitus, abnormal vision, conjunctivitis, diplopia (< 1%).

Miscellaneous – Injection site reaction (3.5%); decreased lymphocytes (2.2%); injection site pain (1.7%); pain (1.4%); sinusitis (1.3%); chest pain (1.2%); back pain, injection site inflammation (1.1%); rhinitis (0.2% to 1%); asthenia, rigors, substernal chest pain, carcinoma, parosmia, ejaculation failure, cerebrovascular disorder, phlebitis (< 1%); fungal infection (0.1% to < 1%); genital moniliasis (0.2% to < 1%); moniliasis (0.1%).

➤*Lomefloxacin:*

Cardiovascular – Hypotension, tachycardia, bradycardia, arrhythmia, extrasystoles, cyanosis, cardiac failure, angina pectoris, MI, pulmonary embolism, cerebrovascular disorder, cardiomyopathy, phlebitis (< 1%).

CNS – Coma, hyperkinesia, tremor, vertigo, nervousness, anorexia, anxiety, agitation, increased appetite, depersonalization, paranoid reaction, paroniria, twitching, hypertonia, confusion, abnormal thinking, concentration impairment (< 1%).

Dermatologic – Urticaria, eczema, skin exfoliation, skin disorder, bullous eruption, acne, skin discoloration, skin ulceration, angioedema (< 1%).

GI – GI inflammation/bleeding, dysphagia, tongue discoloration, stomatitis (< 1%).

GU – Dysuria, hematuria, strangury, micturition disorder, anuria, leukorrhea, intermenstrual bleeding, perineal pain, vaginal moniliasis, orchitis, epididymitis, menstrual disorder (< 1%).

Hematologic – Thrombocythemia, thrombocytopenia, anemia (< 1%).

Respiratory – Dyspnea, respiratory tract infection, epistaxis, respiratory disorder, bronchospasm, cough, increased sputum, stridor, rhinitis, pharyngitis, respiratory depression (< 1%).

Special senses – Earache, tinnitus, conjunctivitis, eye pain, abnormal lacrimation, taste perversion (< 1%).

Miscellaneous – Flushing, increased sweating, back/chest pain, asthenia, facial edema, influenza-like symptoms, decreased heat tolerance, purpura, lymphadenopathy, increased fibrinolysis, thirst, gout, hypoglycemia, leg cramps, arthralgia, myalgia, hot flashes, abnormal liver function, hyperglycemia, viral infection, moniliasis, fungal infection, allergic reaction, anaphylactoid reaction (< 1%); abnormalities of urine specific gravity or serum electrolytes (≤ 0.1%); increased albumin, macrocytosis (< 0.1%).

➤*Moxifloxacin:*

Cardiovascular – Vasodilatation, tachycardia, peripheral edema, hypotension, chest pain (> 0.05% to < 1%).

CNS – Nervousness, anxiety, depersonalization, hypertonia, incoordination, tremor, vertigo, paresthesia (> 0.05% to < 1%).

Dermatologic – Sweating, urticaria, dry skin (> 0.05% to < 1%).

GI – Oral moniliasis, anorexia, stomatitis, gastritis, glossitis, GI disorder, cholestatic jaundice, GGTP increased (> 0.05% to < 1%).

GU – Vaginal moniliasis, cystitis, kidney function abnormal (> 0.05% to < 1%).

Hematologic/Lymphatic – Prothrombin time decrease/increase, thrombocythemia, thrombocytopenia (> 0.05% to < 1%).

Lab test abnormalities – Abnormal liver function test (1%); increased MCH, neutrophils, WBCs, PT ratio, ionized calcium, chloride, albumin, globulin (≥ 2%); decreases in RBCs, neutrophils, eosinophils, basophils, PT ratio, glucose, pO_2, amylase (≥ 2%).

Metabolic/Nutritional – Hyperglycemia, hyperlipidemia, lactic dehydrogenase increased (> 0.05% to < 1%).

Musculoskeletal – Arthralgia, myalgia (> 0.05% to < 1%).

Respiratory – Asthma, dyspnea, cough increased, pneumonia, pharyngitis, rhinitis, sinusitis (> 0.05% to < 1%).

Special senses – Taste perversion (1%); tinnitus, amblyopia (> 0.05% to < 1%).

Miscellaneous – Asthenia, moniliasis, pain, lab test abnormal (not specified), allergic reaction, leg pain, pelvic pain, back pain, infection, hand pain (> 0.05% to < 1%).

➤*Norfloxacin (single- and multiple-dose studies):*

Cardiovascular – Chest pain, MI, palpitation (0.1% to 0.2%).

CNS – Myoclonus; tingling of the fingers (0.3% to 1%); anxiety, sleep disturbances (0.1% to 0.2%).

Dermatologic – Erythema multiforme; erythema, urticaria (0.1% to 0.2%).

GI – Hepatitis; pancreatitis; stomatitis; anorexia, anal/rectal pain, loose stools (0.3% to 1%); abdominal swelling, bitter taste, anorexia, mouth ulcer, renal colic (0.1% to 0.2%).

Musculoskeletal – Arthralgia; back pain (0.3% to 1%); bursitis (0.1% to 0.2%).

Miscellaneous – Hyperhidrosis (0.3% to 1%); asthenia (0.3% to 1.3%); allergies, dysmenorrhea, pruritus ani (0.1% to 0.2%).

➤*Ofloxacin:*

Cardiovascular – Chest pain (1% to 3%); vasodilation, cardiac arrest, hypotension (< 1%).

CNS – Sleep disorders, nervousness (1% to 3%); anxiety, cognitive change, dream abnormality, euphoria, vertigo, tremor (< 1%).

Dermatologic – Angioedema, urticaria, vasculitis (< 1%).

GU – Vaginal discharge (1% to 3%); external genital pruritus in women (1% to 6%); burning/irritation/pain/rash of female genitalia, dysmenorrhea, menorrhagia, metrorrhagia, urinary frequency/pain/retention, dysuria (< 1%).

Respiratory – Cough, rhinorrhea, respiratory arrest (< 1%).

Special senses – Dysgeusia (1% to 3%); photophobia, tinnitus, decreased hearing acuity (< 1%).

Miscellaneous – Decreased appetite, GI distress, pharyngitis, trunk pain (1% to 3%); hyperglycemia, hypoglycemia (≥ 1%); arthralgia, asthenia, diaphoresis, myalgia, thirst, vasculitis, weight loss, extremity pain, epistaxis, pain (< 1%).

➤*Sparfloxacin:*

Cardiovascular – QT_c interval prologation (1.3%); chest pain, electrocardiogram abnormal, tachycardia, sinus bradycardia, PR interval shortened, angina pectoris, arrhythmia, atrial fibrillation, atrial flutter, complete AV block, first degree AV block, second degree AV block, cardiovascular disorder, hemorrhage, migraine, peripheral vascular disorder, supraventricular extrasystoles, ventricular extrasystoles, postural hypotension (< 1%).

CNS – Hypesthesia, nervousness, abnormal dreams, tremor, anxiety, hyperesthesia, hyperkinesia, sleep disorder, hypokinesia, vertigo, abnormal gait, agitation, lightheadedness, emotional lability, euphoria, abnormal thinking, amnesia, twitching (< 1%).

Dermatologic – Photosensitivity reaction (3.6% to 7.9%); rash, cellulitis, face edema, maculopapular rash, dry skin, herpes simplex, sweating, urticaria, vesiculobullous rash, exfoliative dermatitis, acne, alopecia, angioedema, contact dermatitis, fungal dermatitis, furunculosis, pustular rash, skin discoloration, herpes zoster, petechial rash (< 1%).

GI – Anorexia, gingivitis, oral moniliasis, stomatitis, tongue disorder, tooth disorder, gastroenteritis, increased appetite, mouth ulceration (< 1%).

GU – Dysuria, breast pain, dysmenorrhea, hematuria, menorrhagia, nocturia, polyuria, urinary tract infection, kidney pain, leukorrhea, metorrhagia, vulvovaginal disorder (< 1%).

Hematologic – Cyanosis, ecchymosis, lymphadenopathy (< 1%).

Lab test abnormalities – Elevated white blood cells (1.1%); increased/decreased white blood cells, increased aPTT, increased blood urea nitrogen, increased calcium, increased creatinine, increased eosinophils, increased serum lipase, increased neutrophils, increased urine glucose, increased urine protein, increased urine red blood cells, increased urine white blood cells, decreased albumin, decreased creatinine clearance, decreased hematocrit, decreased hemoglobin, decreased lymphocytes, decreased phosphorus, decreased red blood cells, decreased sodium (< 1%).

Metabolic/Nutritional – Gout, peripheral edema, thirst (< 1%).

Musculoskeletal – Arthralgia, arthritis, joint disorder, myalgia, neck pain, rheumatoid arthritis (< 1%).

Respiratory – Asthma, epistaxis, pneumonia, rhinitis, pharyngitis, bronchitis, hemoptysis, sinusitis, cough increased, dyspnea, laryngismus, lung disorder, pleural disorder (< 1%).

Special senses – Taste perversion (1.4%); ear pain, amblyopia, photophobia, tinnitus, conjunctivitis, diplopia, abnormality of accommodation, blepharitis, ear disorder, eye pain, lacrimation disorder, otitis media (< 1%).

Miscellaneous – Vaginal moniliasis (2.8%); asthenia (1.7%); vasodilatation (1%); generalized pain, allergic reaction, back pain, accidental injury, anaphylactoid reaction, infection, mucous membrane disorder (< 1%).

Overdosage

➤*Symptoms:* One patient developed oliguric acute renal failure following ingestion of 21 g of **ciprofloxacin** (serum concentration, 12 mcg/mL). The patient responded to prednisone therapy.

Information on overdosage with **ofloxacin** is limited. One incident of accidental overdosage has been reported. In this case, an adult female received 3 g of ofloxacin IV over 45 minutes. A blood sample obtained 15 minutes after the completion of the infusion revealed an ofloxacin level of 39.3 mcg/mL. In 7 hours, the level had fallen to 16.2 mcg/mL and by 24 hours to 2.7 mcg/mL. During the infusion, the patient developed drowsiness, nausea, dizziness, hot and cold flushes, subjective facial swelling and numbness, slurring of speech, and mild to moderate disorientation. All complaints, except the dizziness, subsided within 1 hour after discontinuation of the infusion. The dizziness, most bothersome while standing, resolved in ≈ 9 hours. Laboratory testing reportedly revealed no clinically significant changes in routine parameters in this patient.

Levofloxacin exhibits a low potential for acute toxicity. Mice, rats, dogs, and monkeys exhibited the following clinical signs after receiving a single high dose of levofloxacin: Ataxia, ptosis, decreased locomotor activity, dyspnea, prostration, tremors, and convulsions. Doses in excess of 1500 mg/kg orally and 250 mg/kg IV produced significant mortality in rodents. In the event of an acute overdosage, the stomach should be emptied. Observe the patient and maintain appropriate hydration. Levofloxacin is not efficiently removed by hemodialysis or peritoneal dialysis.

In case of overdosage, monitor the patient in a suitably equipped medical facility and advise to avoid sun exposure for 5 days. ECG monitoring is recommended because of the possible prolongation of the QT_c interval. There is no known antidote for **sparfloxacin** overdosage. It is not known whether sparfloxacin is dialyzable.

➤*Treatment:* Empty the stomach by inducing vomiting or by gastric lavage. Observe patient carefully and give symptomatic and supportive treatment. Maintain adequate hydration. Refer to General Management of Acute Overdosage.

Only a small amount of **ciprofloxacin** (< 10%) is removed from the body after hemodialysis or peritoneal dialysis. In the event of acute **moxifloxacin** overdosage, the stomach should be emptied and ECG monitoring is recommended because of the possible prolongation of the QT interval. Carefully observe the patient and give supportive treatment. Adequate hydration must be maintained. It is not known whether moxifloxacin is dialyzable. **Ofloxacin**, **norfloxacin**, **gatifloxacin**, **levofloxacin**, and **lomefloxacin** are not efficiently removed by dialysis.

Patient Information

Drink fluids liberally.

Do not take antacids containing magnesium, calcium, or aluminum or products containing citric acid buffered with sodium citrate, iron, magnesium, zinc, or didanosine chewable/buffered tablets or buffered solution, or the pediatric powder for oral solution simultaneously or within 6 hours before or 2 hours (8 hours with **moxifloxacin**) after dosing.

Take **norfloxacin** 1 hour before or 2 hours after meals. **Ciprofloxacin**, **ofloxacin**, **levofloxacin**, **moxifloxacin**, **gatifloxacin**, and **lomefloxacin** can be taken without regard to meals.

Sparfloxacin can be taken with food, milk, or caffeine-containing products.

Ciprofloxacin may increase the effects of theophylline and caffeine. There is a possibility of caffeine accumulation when products containing caffeine are consumed while taking quinolones.

May cause dizziness or lightheadedness; observe caution while driving or performing other tasks requiring alertness, coordination, or physical dexterity. CNS stimulation may occur (eg, tremor, restlessness, confusion); use with caution in patients predisposed to seizures or with other CNS disorders.

Hypersensitivity reactions may occur, even following the first dose; discontinue the drug at the first sign of skin rash or other allergic reaction.

Avoid excessive sunlight/artificial ultraviolet light; discontinue drug if phototoxicity occurs. Avoid re-exposure to sunlight and ultraviolet light. Reactions may recur up to several weeks after stopping therapy. See Warnings.

Discontinue treatment and inform physician if experiencing pain, inflammation, or rupture of a tendon, and to rest and refrain from exercise until the diagnosis of tendinitis or tendon rupture has been confidently excluded.

Discontinue **levofloxacin**, **ofloxacin**, or **gatifloxacin** and consult a physician if patient is diabetic and being treated with insulin or an oral hypoglycemic agent and a hypoglycemic reaction occurs.

Patients should notify their physician if they are taking warfarin; concurrent administration of warfarin and **levofloxacin** has been associated with increases of the International Normalized Ratio (INR) or prothrombin time and clinical episodes of bleeding.

Convulsions have been reported in patients taking quinolones. Notify physician before taking quinolones if there is a history of this condition.

Inform physician if development of symptoms suggestive of pancreatitis including abdominal pain or nausea and vomiting occurs.

Gatifloxacin and **moxifloxacin** may produce changes in the electrocardiogram (QT_c interval prolongation).

Avoid **gatifloxacin** and **moxifloxacin** in patients receiving Class IA (eg, quinidine, procainimide) or Class III (eg, amiodarone, sotalol) antiarrhythmic agents.

Use **gatifloxacin** and **moxifloxacin** with caution in patients receiving drugs that may affect the QT_c interval such as cisapride, erythromycin, antipsychotics, and tricyclic antidepressants.

Inform physician of any personal or family history of QT_c prolongation or proarrhythmic condition such as recent hypokalemia, significant bradycardia, or recent myocardial ischemia.

Inform physician of any other medications when taken concurrently with fluoroquinolones, including OTC medications.

Contact the physician if palpitations or fainting spells occur while taking **gatifloxacin** or **moxifloxacin**.

CIPROFLOXACIN

Rx	**Ciprofloxacin** (Dr. Reddy's)	**Tablets:** 100 mg	(R125). White, oval-shape. Film-coated. In 6s.
Rx	**Cipro** (Bayer)		(CIPRO 100). Yellowish. Film-coated. In *Cipro Cystitis Pack* 6s.
Rx	**Ciprofloxacin** (Various, eg, Barr, Dr. Reddy's, Mylan)	**Tablets:** 250 mg	In 50s, 100s, 500s, and UD 10s.
Rx	**Cipro** (Bayer)		(CIPRO 250). Yellowish. Film-coated. In 50s, 100s, and UD 100s.
Rx	**Ciprofloxacin** (Various, eg, Barr, Dr. Reddy's, Mylan)	**Tablets:** 500 mg	In 50s, 100s, 500s, and UD 10s.
Rx	**Cipro** (Bayer)		(CIPRO 500). Yellowish, capsule shape. Film-coated. In 50s, 100s, and UD 100s.
Rx	**Ciprofloxacin** (Various, eg, Barr, Dr. Reddy's, Mylan)	**Tablets:** 750 mg	In 50s, 100s, 500s, and UD 10s.
Rx	**Cipro** (Bayer)		(CIPRO 750). Yellowish, capsule shape. Film-coated. In 50s, 100s, and UD 100s.
Rx	**Cipro XR** (Bayer)	**Tablets, extended-release:** 500 mg	(BAYER C500 QD). Yellowish, oblong. Film-coated. In 50s and 100s.
		1000 mg	(BAYER C1000 QD). Yellowish, oblong. Film-coated. In 50s, 100s, and UD 30s.
Rx	**Ciprofloxacin** (Barr)	**Powder for oral suspension, oral:** 250 mg/5 mL (5%) (when reconstituted)	Sucrose. Strawberry flavor. Contains a bottle of microcapsules, diluent, and a teaspoon.
Rx	**Cipro** (Bayer)		Sucrose. Strawberry flavor. Contains a bottle of microcapsules, diluent, and a teaspoon.

CIPROFLOXACIN

Rx	**Ciprofloxacin** (Barr)	500 mg/5 mL (10%) (when reconstituted)	Sucrose. Strawberry flavor. Contains a bottle of microcapsules, diluent, and a teaspoon.
Rx	**Cipro** (Bayer)		Sucrose. Strawberry flavor. Contains a bottle of microcapsules, diluent, and a teaspoon.
Rx	**Cipro I.V.** (Bayer)	**Injection**: 200 mg	Lactic acid. In 20 mL vials (1%), 100 mL in 5% dextrose flexible containers (0.2%), and 120 mL bulk packages.
		400 mg	Lactic acid. In 40 mL vials (1%), 200 mL in 5% dextrose flexible containers (0.2%), and 120 mL bulk packages.

CIPROFLOXACIN — ORAL

For complete and comparative prescribing information, refer to the Fluoroquinolones group monograph.

Indications

➤*Immediate-release (IR) tablets and oral suspension:*

Adults –

Acute sinusitis: Acute sinusitis caused by *Haemophilus influenzae, Streptococcus pneumoniae*, or *Moraxella catarrhalis.*

Acute uncomplicated cystitis: Acute uncomplicated cystitis in women caused by *Escherichia coli* or *Staphylococcus saprophyticus.*

Bone and joint infections: Bone and joint infections caused by *Enterobacter cloacae, Serratia marcescens*, or *Pseudomonas aeruginosa.*

Chronic bacterial prostatitis: Chronic bacterial prostatitis caused by *E. coli* or *Proteus mirabilis.*

Complicated intra-abdominal infections: Complicated intra-abdominal infections (used in combination with metronidazole) caused by *E. coli, P. aeruginosa, P. mirabilis, Klebsiella pneumoniae*, or *Bacteroides fragilis.*

Infectious diarrhea: Infectious diarrhea caused by *E. coli* (enterotoxigenic strains), *Campylobacter jejuni, Shigella boydii* (although treatment of infections caused by this organism in this organ system demonstrated a clinically significant outcome, efficacy was studied in fewer than 10 patients), *Shigella dysenteriae, Shigella flexneri*, or *Shigella sonnei* (although treatment of infections caused by this organism in this organ system demonstrated a clinically significant outcome, efficacy was studied in fewer than 10 patients) when antibacterial therapy is indicated.

Lower respiratory tract infections: Lower respiratory tract infections caused by *E. coli, K. pneumoniae, E. cloacae, P. mirabilis, P. aeruginosa, H. influenzae, Haemophilus parainfluenzae*, or *S. pneumoniae*. Also, *M. catarrhalis* for the treatment of acute exacerbations of chronic bronchitis. Although effective in clinical trials, ciprofloxacin is not a drug of first choice in the treatment of presumed or confirmed pneumonia secondary to *S. pneumoniae.*

Skin and skin structure infections: Skin and skin structure infections caused by *E. coli, K. pneumoniae, E. cloacae, P. mirabilis, Proteus vulgaris, Providencia stuartii, Morganella morganii, Citrobacter freundii, P. aeruginosa, Staphylococcus aureus* (methicillin-susceptible), *Staphylococcus epidermidis*, or *Streptococcus pyogenes.*

Typhoid fever: Typhoid fever (enteric fever) caused by *Salmonella typhi*. The efficacy of ciprofloxacin in the eradication of the chronic typhoid carrier state has not been demonstrated.

Uncomplicated cervical and urethral gonorrhea: Uncomplicated cervical and urethral gonorrhea caused by *Neisseria gonorrhoeae.*

Urinary tract infections (UTIs): UTIs caused by *E. coli, K. pneumoniae, E. cloacae, S. marcescens, P. mirabilis, Providencia rettgeri, M. morganii, Citrobacter diversus, C. freundii, P. aeruginosa, S. epidermidis, S. saprophyticus*, or *Enterococcus faecalis.*

Children (1 to 17 years of age) –

Complicated UTIs and pyelonephritis: Complicated UTIs and pyelonephritis caused by *E. coli*. Although effective in clinical trials, ciprofloxacin is not a drug of first choice in the pediatric population because of an increased incidence of adverse reactions compared with controls, including reactions related to joints and/or surrounding tissues. Ciprofloxacin, like other fluoroquinolones, is associated with arthropathy and histopathological changes in weightbearing joints of juvenile animals.

Adults and children –

Inhalational anthrax (postexposure): To reduce the incidence or progression of disease following exposure to aerosolized *Bacillus anthracis*. Ciprofloxacin serum concentrations achieved in humans serve as a surrogate end point reasonably likely to predict clinical benefit and provide the basis for this indication.

➤*Extended-release (ER) tablets:* Ciprofloxacin ER and IR tablets are not interchangeable.

Acute uncomplicated pyelonephritis (AUP) – AUP caused by *E. coli*. The safety and efficacy of ciprofloxacin ER in treating infections other than UTIs have not been demonstrated.

Complicated UTIs – Complicated UTIs caused by *E. coli, K. pneumoniae, E. faecalis, P. mirabilis*, or *P. aeruginosa.*

Uncomplicated UTIs (acute cystitis) – Uncomplicated UTIs (acute cystitis) caused by *E. coli, P. mirabilis, E. faecalis*, or *S. saprophyticus* (treatment of infections caused by this organism in this organ system was studied in fewer than 10 patients).

➤*Unlabeled uses:* Ciprofloxacin has been used in children with cystic fibrosis for periods of 10 days to 6 months without documented adverse reactions or intolerance.

Ciprofloxacin has been used for the treatment of gastroenteritis in children.

Atypical mycobacterial infections have been satisfactorily treated with ciprofloxacin as part of combination therapy.

Ciprofloxacin is recommended for mycobacterial diseases.

Multi-drug-resistant tuberculosis, alternative regimen for tularemia, alternative regimen for cutaneous and GI anthrax, alternative therapy for the plague.

Disseminated gonorrhea (alternative regimen) – 400 mg intravenously (IV) every 12 hours for 24 to 48 hours after improvement begins, then 500 mg orally twice daily for 7 days.

Administration and Dosage

➤*Approved by the FDA:* October 22, 1987.

➤*Concomitant therapy:* Ciprofloxacin should be administered at least 2 hours before or 6 hours after magnesium/aluminum antacids, sucralfate, didanosine chewable/buffered tablets or pediatric powder for oral solution, or other products containing calcium, iron, or zinc.

Ciprofloxacin ER and IR tablets are not interchangeable.

➤*IR tablets and oral suspension:*

Adults – Ciprofloxacin tablets and oral suspension should be administered orally to adults as described in the following table.

Duration: The duration of treatment depends upon the severity of infection. The usual duration is 7 to 14 days; however, for severe and complicated infections, more prolonged therapy may be required.

Ciprofloxacin Dosage Guidelines for Adults

Infection	Severity	Dose	Frequency	Usual durations[a]
Acute sinusitis	Mild/Moderate	500 mg	Every 12 hours	10 days
Bone and joint	Mild/Moderate	500 mg	Every 12 hours	≥ 4 to 6 weeks
	Severe/Complicated	750 mg	Every 12 hours	≥ 4 to 6 weeks
Chronic bacterial prostatitis	Mild/Moderate	500 mg	Every 12 hours	28 days
Lower respiratory tract	Mild/Moderate	500 mg	Every 12 hours	7 to 14 days
	Severe/Complicated	750 mg	Every 12 hours	7 to 14 days
Skin and skin structure	Mild/Moderate	500 mg	Every 12 hours	7 to 14 days
	Severe/Complicated	750 mg	Every 12 hours	7 to 14 days
Urinary tract	Acute uncomplicated	250 mg	Every 12 hours	3 days
	Mild/Moderate	250 mg	Every 12 hours	7 to 14 days
	Severe/Complicated	500 mg	Every 12 hours	7 to 14 days
Infectious diarrhea	Mild/Moderate/Severe	500 mg	Every 12 hours	5 to 7 days
Inhalational anthrax (postexposure)[b]	Adult	500 mg	Every 12 hours	60 days
Intra-abdominal[c]	Complicated	500 mg	Every 12 hours	7 to 14 days
Typhoid fever	Mild/Moderate	500 mg	Every 12 hours	10 days
Urethral and cervical gonococcal infections	Uncomplicated	250 mg	Single dose	Single dose

[a] Generally ciprofloxacin should be continued for at least 2 days after the signs and symptoms of infection have disappeared, except for inhalational anthrax (postexposure).
[b] Drug administration should begin as soon as possible after suspected or confirmed exposure.
[c] Used in conjunction with metronidazole.

CIPROFLOXACIN — ORAL

Conversion of IV to oral dosing in adults – Patients whose therapy is started with IV ciprofloxacin may be switched to ciprofloxacin tablets or oral suspension at the discretion of the health care provider when clinically indicated.

Ciprofloxacin Equivalent AUC[a] Dosing Regimens	
Ciprofloxacin oral dosage	Equivalent ciprofloxacin IV dosage
250 mg tablet every 12 hours	200 mg IV every 12 hours
500 mg tablet every 12 hours	400 mg IV every 12 hours
750 mg tablet every 12 hours	400 mg IV every 8 hours

[a] AUC = area under the curve.

Children – Ciprofloxacin tablets and oral suspension should be administered orally as described in the following table. An increased incidence of adverse reactions compared with controls, including reactions related to joints and/or surrounding tissues, has been observed.

Dosing and initial route of therapy (ie, IV, oral) for complicated UTI or pyelonephritis should be determined by the severity of the infection. In the clinical trial, children with moderate to severe infection were initiated on 6 to 10 mg/kg IV every 8 hours and allowed to switch to oral therapy (10 to 20 mg/kg every 12 hours) at the discretion of the health care provider.

Ciprofloxacin Dosage Guidelines for Children				
Infection	Route of administration	Dose (mg/kg)	Frequency	Total duration
Complicated urinary tract or pyelonephritis (patients from 1 to 17 years of age)	IV	6 to 10 mg/kg (maximum 400 mg/dose; not to be exceeded even in patients weighing > 51 kg)	Every 8 hours	10 to 21 days[a]
	Oral	10 to 20 mg/kg (maximum 750 mg/dose; not to be exceeded even in patients weighing > 51 kg)	Every 12 hours	
Inhalational anthrax (postexposure)[b]	IV	10 mg/kg (maximum 400 mg/dose)	Every 12 hours	60 days
	Oral	15 mg/kg (maximum 500 mg/dose)	Every 12 hours	

[a] The total duration of therapy for complicated UTI and pyelonephritis in the clinical trial was determined by the health care provider. The mean duration of treatment was 11 days (range, 10 to 21 days).

[b] Drug administration should begin as soon as possible after suspected or confirmed exposure to *B. anthracis* spores. This indication is based on a surrogate end point, ciprofloxacin serum concentration achieved in humans, reasonably likely to predict clinical benefit.

➤*ER tablets:* Patients whose therapy is started with ciprofloxacin IV for UTIs may be switched to ciprofloxacin ER tablets at the discretion of the health care provider when clinically indicated.

Ciprofloxacin ER tablets should be administered orally once daily as described in the following table.

Ciprofloxacin ER Dosage Guidelines			
Indication	Unit dose	Frequency	Usual duration
AUP	1,000 mg	Every 24 hours	7 to 14 days
Complicated UTI	1,000 mg	Every 24 hours	7 to 14 days
Uncomplicated UTI (acute cystitis)	500 mg	Every 24 hours	3 days

Administration – Although ciprofloxacin ER tablets may be taken with meals that include milk, coadministration with dairy products alone or with calcium-fortified products, should be avoided because decreased absorption is possible. A 2-hour window between substantial calcium intake (800 mg or more) and dosing with ciprofloxacin ER is recommended. Ciprofloxacin ER should be swallowed whole. Do not split, crush, or chew the tablets.

➤*Renal function impairment:* Ciprofloxacin is eliminated primarily by renal excretion; however, the drug also is metabolized and partially cleared through the biliary system of the liver and through the intestine. These alternate pathways of drug elimination appear to compensate for the reduced renal excretion in patients with renal impairment.

IR tablets and oral suspension – Some modification of dosage is recommended, particularly for patients with severe renal dysfunction. The following table provides dosage guidelines for use in adults with renal impairment.

Ciprofloxacin Dosage in Adults with Renal Function Impairment	
Creatinine clearance (Ccr) (mL/min)	Dose
> 50	See usual dosage in the table above.
30 to 50	250 to 500 mg every 12 hours
5 to 29	250 to 500 mg every 18 hours
Patients on hemodialysis or peritoneal dialysis	250 to 500 mg every 24 hours (after dialysis)

In patients with severe infections and severe renal impairment, a unit dose of 750 mg may be administered at the intervals noted above. Patients should be carefully monitored.

ER tablets – No dosage adjustment is required for patients with uncomplicated UTIs receiving ciprofloxacin 500 mg ER. In patients with complicated UTIs and AUP who have a Ccr of less than 30 mL/min, the dose of ciprofloxacin ER should be reduced from 1,000 to 500 mg daily. For patients on hemodialysis or peritoneal dialysis, administer ciprofloxacin ER after the dialysis procedure is completed.

➤*Preparation of ciprofloxacin oral suspension:* Ciprofloxacin oral suspension is supplied in 5% (ciprofloxacin 5 g in 100 mL) and 10% (ciprofloxacin 10 g in 100 mL) strengths. The drug product is composed of 2 components (microcapsules and diluent), which must be combined prior to dispensing.

One teaspoonful (5 mL) of 5% ciprofloxacin oral suspension equals ciprofloxacin 250 mg.

One teaspoonful (5 mL) of 10% ciprofloxacin oral suspension equals of ciprofloxacin 500 mg.

Appropriate Dosing Volumes of Ciprofloxacin Oral Suspension		
Dose	5%	10%
250 mg	5 mL	2.5 mL
500 mg	10 mL	5 mL
750 mg	15 mL	7.5 mL

1.) The small bottle contains the microcapsules, the large bottle contains the diluent.
2.) Open both bottles. The bottles have a childproof cap; press down according to instructions on the cap while turning to the left.
3.) Pour the microcapsules completely into the large bottle of diluent. Do not add water to the suspension.
4.) Remove the top layer of the diluent bottle label (to reveal the ciprofloxacin oral suspension label).
5.) Close the large bottle completely according to the directions on the cap and shake vigorously for about 15 seconds. The suspension is ready for use.

Ciprofloxacin oral suspension should not be administered through feeding tubes because of its physical characteristics.

Instruct the patient to shake ciprofloxacin oral suspension vigorously each time before use for approximately 15 seconds and not to chew the microcapsules.

➤*Storage/Stability:*

IR tablets – Store below 30°C (86°F).

Oral suspension – Store microcapsules and diluent below 25°C (77°F) and protect from freezing.

Reconstituted product may be stored below 30°C (86°F) for 14 days. Protect from freezing.

ER tablets – Store at 25°C (77°F); excursions permitted to 15° to 30°C (59° to 86°F).

CIPROFLOXACIN — INJECTION

For complete and comparative prescribing information, refer to the Fluoroquinolones group monograph.

Indications

➤*Bacterial infections:* For the treatment of infections caused by susceptible strains of the designated microorganisms in the following conditions and patient populations when the intravenous (IV) administration offers a route of administration advantageous to the patient. If anaerobic organisms are suspected of contributing to the infection, administer appropriate therapy.

➤*Adults:*

Acute sinusitis – Caused by *Haemophilus influenzae*, *Streptococcus pneumoniae*, or *Moraxella catarrhalis*.

CIPROFLOXACIN — INJECTION

Bone and joint infections – Caused by *Enterobacter cloacae*, *Serratia marcescens*, or *Pseudomonas aeruginosa*.

Chronic bacterial prostatitis – Caused by *Escherichia coli* or *Proteus mirabilis*.

Complicated intraabdominal infections (used in conjunction with metronidazole) – Caused by *E. coli*, *P. aeruginosa*, *P. mirabilis*, *Klebsiella pneumoniae*, or *Bacteroides fragilis*.

Empirical therapy for febrile neutropenic patients – In combination with piperacillin sodium.

Lower respiratory tract infections – Caused by *E. coli*, *K. pneumoniae* subspecies *pneumoniae*, *E. cloacae*, *P. mirabilis*, *P. aeruginosa*, *H. influenzae*, *Haemophilus parainfluenzae*, or *S. pneumoniae*. Also, *M. catarrhalis* for the treatment of acute exacerbations of chronic bronchitis.

Although effective in clinical trials, ciprofloxacin is not a drug of first choice in the treatment of presumed or confirmed pneumonia secondary to *S. pneumoniae*.

Nosocomial pneumonia – Caused by *H. influenzae* or *K. pneumoniae*.

Skin and skin structure infections – Caused by *E. coli*, *K. pneumoniae* subspecies *pneumoniae*, *E. cloacae*, *P. mirabilis*, *Proteus vulgaris*, *Providencia stuartii*, *Morganella morganii*, *Citrobacter freundii*, *P. aeruginosa*, *Staphylococcus aureus* (methicillin-susceptible), *Staphylococcus epidermidis*, or *Streptococcus pyogenes*.

Urinary tract infections (UTI) – Caused by *E. coli* (including cases with secondary bacteremia), *K. pneumoniae* subspecies pneumoniae, *E. cloacae*, *S. marcescens*, *P. mirabilis*, *Providencia rettgeri*, *M. morganii*, *Citrobacter diversus*, *C. freundii*, *P. aeruginosa*, *S. epidermidis*, *Staphylococcus saprophyticus*, or *Enterococcus faecalis*.

➤*Children (1 to 17 years of age):*

Complicated UTI and pyelonephritis – Caused by *E. coli*.

See Warnings for more information.

➤*Adults and children:*

Inhalational anthrax (postexposure) – To reduce the incidence or progression of disease following exposure to aerosolized *Bacillus anthracis*.

➤*Unlabeled uses:* Multidrug-resistant tuberculosis; alternative regimen for tularemia; alternative regimen for cutaneous, oropharyngeal, and GI anthrax; alternative therapy for the plague.

Ciprofloxacin has been used in children with cystic fibrosis for periods of 10 days to 6 months without documented adverse reactions or intolerance.

Disseminated gonorrhea (alternative regimen) – 400 mg IV every 12 hours for 24 to 48 hours after improvement begins, then 500 mg orally twice daily for 7 days.

Administration and Dosage

➤*Approved by the FDA:* October 22, 1987 (oral)

➤*Adults:*

Ciprofloxacin Adult Dosage Guidelines				
Infection[a]	Severity	Unit dose	Frequency	Usual duration
Acute sinusitis	Mild/ moderate	400 mg	Every 12 hours	10 days
Bone and joint	Mild/ moderate	400 mg	Every 12 hours	≥ 4 to 6 weeks
	Severe/ complicated	400 mg	Every 8 hours	≥ 4 to 6 weeks
Chronic bacterial prostatitis	Mild/ moderate	400 mg	Every 12 hours	28 days
Empirical therapy in febrile neutropenic patients	Severe	Ciprofloxacin 400 mg	Every 8 hours	7 to 14 days
		Piperacillin 50 mg/kg, not to exceed 24 g/day	Every 4 hours	
Inhalational anthrax (postexposure)[b]		400 mg	Every 12 hours	60 days
Intraabdominal[c]	Complicated	400 mg	Every 12 hours	7 to 14 days
Lower respiratory tract	Mild/ moderate	400 mg	Every 12 hours	7 to 14 days
	Severe/ complicated	400 mg	Every 8 hours	7 to 14 days
Nosocomial pneumonia	Mild/ moderate/ severe	400 mg	Every 8 hours	10 to 14 days
Skin and skin structure	Mild/ moderate	400 mg	Every 12 hours	7 to 14 days
	Severe/ complicated	400 mg	Every 8 hours	7 to 14 days
Urinary tract	Mild/ moderate	200 mg	Every 12 hours	7 to 14 days
	Severe/ complicated	400 mg	Every 12 hours	7 to 14 days

[a] Because of the designated pathogens.
[b] Drug administration should begin as soon as possible after suspected or confirmed exposure. This indication is based on a surrogate end point, ciprofloxacin serum concentrations achieved in humans, reasonably likely to predict clinical benefit. Total duration of ciprofloxacin administration (IV or oral) for inhalational anthrax (postexposure) is 60 days.
[c] Used in conjunction with metronidazole.

Conversion of IV to oral dosing in adults –

Ciprofloxacin Equivalent AUC[a] Dosing Regimens	
Ciprofloxacin oral dosage	Equivalent ciprofloxacin IV dosage
250 mg tablet every 12 hours	200 mg IV every 12 hours
500 mg tablet every 12 hours	400 mg IV every 12 hours
750 mg tablet every 12 hours	400 mg IV every 8 hours

[a] AUC = area under the curve.

➤*Children:* See Indications for more information.

Ciprofloxacin Child Dosage Guidelines				
Infection	Route of administration	Dose (mg/kg)	Frequency	Total duration
Complicated urinary tract or pyelonephritis (patients 1 to 17 years of age)	IV	6 to 10 mg/kg (maximum 400 mg/dose; not to be exceeded even in patients weighing more than 51 kg)	Every 8 hours	10 to 21 days[a]
	Oral	10 to 20 mg/kg (maximum 750 mg/dose; not to be exceeded even in patients weighing more than 51 kg)	Every 12 hours	
Inhalational anthrax (postexposure)[b]	IV	10 mg/kg (maximum 400 mg/dose)	Every 12 hours	60 days
	Oral	15 mg/kg (maximum 500 mg/dose)	Every 12 hours	

[a] The total duration of therapy for complicated UTI and pyelonephritis in the clinical trial was determined by the health care provider. The mean duration of treatment was 11 days (range, 10 to 21 days).
[b] Drug administration should begin as soon as possible after suspected or confirmed exposure to *B. anthracis* spores. This indication is based on a surrogate end point ciprofloxacin achieved in humnas reasonably likely to predict clinical benefit.

➤*Renal function impairment:*

Adults –

Ciprofloxacin Dosage in Renal Function Impairment	
Creatinine clearance (Ccr) (mL/min)	Dosage
> 30	See usual dosage
5 to 29	200 to 400 mg every 18 to 24 hours

➤*Preparation and administration:*

Vials (injection concentrate) – This preparation must be diluted before use. The IV dose should be prepared by aseptically withdrawing the concentrate from the vial of ciprofloxacin IV. This should be diluted with a suitable IV solution to a final concentration of 1 to 2 mg/mL. The resulting solution should be infused over a period of 60 minutes by direct infusion or through a Y-type IV infusion set, which may already be in place.

Compatible IV solutions – Ciprofloxacin injection 1% (10 mg/mL), when diluted with the following IV solutions to concentrations of 0.5 to 2 mg/mL, is stable for up to 14 days at refrigerated or room temperature storage: sodium chloride 0.9% injection, dextrose 5% injection, sterile water for injection, dextrose 10% for injection, dextrose 5% and sodium chloride 0.225% for injection, dextrose 5% and sodium chloride 0.45% for injection, or Ringer's lactate for injection.

Admixture incompatibilities – If the Y-type or the "piggyback" method of administration is used, it is advisable to discontinue temporarily the administration of any other solutions during the infusion of ciprofloxacin. If the concomitant use of ciprofloxacin and another drug is necessary, each drug

CIPROFLOXACIN — INJECTION

should be given separately in accordance with the recommended dosage and route of administration for each drug.

Flexible containers – Ciprofloxacin IV is also available as a 0.2% premixed solution in dextrose 5% in flexible containers of 100 or 200 mL. The solutions in flexible containers do not need to be diluted and may be infused as previously described.

➤*Storage / Stability:* Store vials between 5° and 30°C (41° and 86°F) and flexible containers between 5° and 25°C (41° and 77°F). Protect from light, avoid excessive heat, and protect from freezing.

GATIFLOXACIN

Rx	**Tequin** (Bristol-Myers Squibb)	**Tablets:** 200 mg	(BMS TEQUIN 200). White, almond shape. Film-coated. In 30s and blister pack 100s.
		400 mg	(BMS TEQUIN 400). White, almond shape. Film-coated. In 50s, blister pack 100s, and carton of 3 *Teq-Paqs* (5 tablets each).
		Powder for oral suspension: 200 mg per 5 mL (after reconstitution)	168 mg phenylalanine, parabens, sucrose. Fruit flavor. In 1, 2, 3, and 4 g (25, 50, 75, and 100 mL bottles).
		Injection (concentrate): 400 mg (10 mg/mL)	Preservative-free. In single-use 40 mL vials in 5% dextrose.
		Injection (premix): 200 mg (2 mg/mL)	Preservative-free. In premixed 100 mL flexible containers in 5% dextrose.
		400 mg (2 mg/mL)	Preservative-free. In premixed 200 mL flexible containers in 5% dextrose.

GATIFLOXACIN — ORAL

For complete and comparative prescribing information, refer to the Fluoroquinolones group monograph.

Indications

For the treatment of infections caused by the susceptible strains of the designated microorganisms in the conditions listed below:

➤*Acute bacterial exacerbation of chronic bronchitis:* Caused by *Streptococcus pneumoniae, Haemophilus influenzae, Haemophilus parainfluenzae, Moraxella catarrhalis*, or *Staphylococcus aureus*.

➤*Acute sinusitis:* Caused by *S. pneumoniae* or *H. influenzae*.

➤*Community-acquired pneumonia:* Caused by *S. pneumoniae* (including multidrug-resistant strains [MDRSP])†, *H. influenzae, H. parainfluenzae, M. catarrhalis, S. aureus, Mycoplasma pneumoniae, Chlamydia pneumoniae*, or *Legionella pneumophila*.

➤*Uncomplicated skin and skin structure infections (simple abscesses, furuncles, folliculitis, wound infections, cellulitis):* Caused by *S. aureus* (methicillin-susceptible strains only) or *Streptococcus pyogenes*.

➤*Uncomplicated urinary tract infections (UTIs; cystitis):* Caused by *Escherichia coli, Klebsiella pneumoniae*, or *Proteus mirabilis*.

➤*Complicated UTIs:* Caused by *E. coli, K. pneumoniae*, or *P. mirabilis*.

➤*Pyelonephritis:* Caused by *E. coli*.

➤*Uncomplicated urethral and cervical gonorrhea:* Caused by *Neisseria gonorrhoeae*.

➤*Acute, uncomplicated rectal infections in women:* Caused by *N. gonorrhoeae*.

Administration and Dosage

➤*Approved by the FDA:* December 17, 1999.

Administer gatifloxacin without regard to food, including milk and dietary supplements containing calcium. Administer once every 24 hours.

➤*Concomitant therapy:* Administer oral gatifloxacin at least 4 hours before the administration of ferrous sulfate; dietary supplements containing zinc, magnesium, or iron (such as multivitamins); aluminum/magnesium-containing antacids; or didanosine buffered tablets, buffered solution, or buffered powder for oral suspension.

➤*Switching from IV to oral therapy:* When switching from IV to oral dosage administration, no dosage adjustment is necessary. Patients whose therapy is started with the injection may be switched to tablets when clinically indicated.

➤*Dosage:*

Gatifloxacin Dosage Guidelines

Infection[1]	Daily dose (mg)[2]	Duration
Acute bacterial exacerbation of chronic bronchitis	400	5 days
Acute sinusitis	400	10 days
Community-acquired pneumonia	400	7 to 14 days
Uncomplicated skin and skin structure infections	400	7 to 10 days
Uncomplicated UTIs (cystitis)	400	Single dose
	or 200	3 days
Complicated UTIs	400	7 to 10 days
Acute pyelonephritis	400	7 to 10 days
Uncomplicated urethral gonorrhea in men; endocervical and rectal gonorrhea in women	400	Single dose

[1] Caused by the designated pathogens (see Indications).
[2] For oral or IV routes of administration.

➤*Renal function impairment:* Because gatifloxacin is eliminated primarily by renal excretion, a dosage modification of gatifloxacin is recommended for patients with Ccr less than 40 mL/min, including patients on hemodialysis and on continuous ambulatory peritoneal dialysis (CAPD). The recommended dosage of gatifloxacin follows:

Recommended Dosage of Gatifloxacin in Adult Patients with Renal Impairment

Ccr	Initial dose (mg)	Subsequent dose[1]
≥ 40 mL/min	400	400 mg/day
< 40 mL/min	400	200 mg/day
Hemodialysis	400	200 mg/day
Continuous peritoneal dialysis	400	200 mg/day

[1] Start subsequent dose on day 2 of dosing.

Administer gatifloxacin after a dialysis session for patients on hemodialysis.

Uncomplicated UTIs and gonorrhea – Single 400 mg dose regimen (for the treatment of uncomplicated UTIs and gonorrhea) and 200 mg once daily for 3 days regimen (for the treatment of uncomplicated UTIs) require no dosage adjustment in patients with impaired renal function.

➤*Storage / Stability:* Store at 25°C (77°F); excursions permitted to 15° to 30°C (59° to 86°F).

After reconstitution, the oral suspension is stable for 14 days under refrigeration 2° to 8°C (36° to 46°F). Shake thoroughly prior to each use.

† MDRSP includes isolates previously known as penicillin-resistant *S. pneumoniae* (PRSP), and are strains resistant to 2 or more of the following antibiotics: penicillin (minimum inhibitory concentration [MIC] greater than or equal to 2 mcg/mL), second generation cephalosporins (eg, cefuroxime), macrolides, tetracyclines, and trimethoprim/sulfamethoxazole.

GATIFLOXACIN — INJECTION

For complete and comparative prescribing information, refer to the Fluoroquinolones group monograph.

Indications

For the treatment of infections due to susceptible strains of the designated microorganisms in the following conditions:

➤*Acute bacterial exacerbation of chronic bronchitis:* Due to *Streptococcus pneumoniae, Haemophilus influenzae, Haemophilus parainfluenzae, Moraxella catarrhalis*, or *Staphylococcus aureus*.

➤*Acute sinusitis:* Due to *S. pneumoniae* or *H. influenzae*.

➤*Community-acquired pneumonia:* Due to *S. pneumoniae* (including multidrug-resistant strains [MDRSP])†, *H. influenzae, H. parainfluenzae, M. catarrhalis, S. aureus, Mycoplasma pneumoniae, Chlamydia pneumoniae*, or *Legionella pneumophila*.

➤*Uncomplicated skin and skin structure infections:* Due to *S. aureus* (methicillin-susceptible strains only) or *Streptococcus pyogenes*. Note: An insufficient number of patients with the diagnosis of impetiginous lesions were available for evaluation.

➤*Uncomplicated urinary tract infections (cystitis):* Due to *Escherichia coli, Klebsiella pneumoniae*, or *Proteus mirabilis*.

➤*Complicated urinary tract infections:* Due to *E. coli, K. pneumoniae*, or *P. mirabilis*.

➤*Pyelonephritis:* Due to *E. coli*.

➤*Uncomplicated urethral and cervical gonorrhea:* Due to *Neisseria gonorrhoeae*.

➤*Acute, uncomplicated rectal infections in women:* Due to *N. gonorrhoeae*.

Administration and Dosage

➤*Approved by the FDA:* December 17, 1999.

➤*Dosage:* Doses of gatifloxacin are administered once every 24 hours. These recommendations apply to all patients with a creatinine clearance greater than or equal to 40 mL/min. For patients with a creatinine clearance less than 40 mL/min, see Renal function impairment.

Conversion of IV to oral dosing – When switching from intravenous (IV) to oral dosage administration, no dosage adjustment is necessary. Patients whose therapy is started with gatifloxacin injection may be switched to gatifloxacin tablets when clinically indicated at the discretion of the health care provider.

Gatifloxacin Dosage Guidelines

Infection[1]	Daily dose (mg)[2]	Duration
Acute bacterial exacerbation of chronic bronchitis	400	5 days
Acute sinusitis	400	10 days
Community-acquired pneumonia	400	7 to 14 days
Uncomplicated skin and skin structure infections	400	7 to 10 days
Uncomplicated UTIs (cystitis)	400	Single dose
	or 200	3 days
Complicated UTIs	400	7 to 10 days
Acute pyelonephritis	400	7 to 10 days
Uncomplicated urethral gonorrhea in men; endocervical and rectal gonorrhea in women	400	Single dose

[1] Caused by the designated pathogens (see Indications).
[2] For oral or IV routes of administration.

➤*Renal function impairment:*

Elderly – Give consideration to the possibility that the elderly may have impaired renal function. Because elderly patients are more likely to have decreased renal function, take care in dose selection, and it may be useful to monitor renal function.

Because gatifloxacin is eliminated primarily by renal excretion, a dosage modification of gatifloxacin is recommended for patients with creatinine clearance less than 40 mL/min, including patients on hemodialysis and on continuous ambulatory peritoneal dialysis (CAPD). The recommended dosage of gatifloxacin in adult patients is:

Recommended Dosage of Gatifloxacin in Adult Patients with Renal Impairment

Ccr	Initial dose (mg)	Subsequent dose[1]
≥ 40 mL/min	400	400 mg/day
< 40 mL/min	400	200 mg/day
Hemodialysis	400	200 mg/day
Continuous peritoneal dialysis	400	200 mg/day

[1] Start subsequent dose on day 2 of dosing. Administer gatifloxacin after a dialysis session for patients on hemodialysis.

Uncomplicated urinary tract infections and gonorrhea – Single 400 mg dose gatifloxacin regimen (for the treatment of uncomplicated urinary tract infections and gonorrhea) and 200 mg once daily for 3 days gatifloxacin regimen (for the treatment of uncomplicated urinary tract infections) require no dosage adjustment in patients with impaired renal function.

➤*IV administration:* Administer gatifloxacin injection by IV infusion only. It is not intended for intramuscular (IM), intrathecal, intraperitoneal, or subcutaneous administration.

Single-use vials require dilution prior to administration.

Administer gatifloxacin injection by IV infusion over a period of 60 minutes.

Caution – Avoid rapid or bolus IV infusion.

Preparation for IV administration –

Single-use vials: Gatifloxacin injection is supplied in single-use 40 mL vials (10 mg/mL) containing a concentrated solution of gatifloxacin in 5% dextrose (400 mg of gatifloxacin). Gatifloxacin injection single-use vials must be further diluted with an appropriate solution prior to IV administration. The concentration of the resulting diluted solution should be 2 mg/mL prior to administration.

Compatible IV solutions – Because a hypotonic solution results, do not use water for injection as a diluent when preparing a 2 mg/mL solution from the concentrated solution of gatifloxacin (10 mg/mL). Any of the following IV solutions may be used to prepare a 2 mg/mL gatifloxacin solution: 5% dextrose injection, 0.9% sodium chloride injection, 5% dextrose and 0.9% sodium chloride injection, Ringer's lactate and 5% dextrose injection, 5% sodium bicarbonate injection, *Plasma-Lyte* 56 and 5% dextrose injection (multiple electrolytes and dextrose injection, Type 1), and M/6 sodium lactate injection.

Gatifloxacin solutions at 2 mg/mL also have been shown to be compatible with 20 mEq/L potassium chloride in 5% dextrose and 0.45% sodium chloride injection.

Inspect this IV drug product visually for particulate matter prior to dilution and administration. Discard samples containing visible particles. Because no preservative or bacteriostatic agent is present in this product, aseptic technique must be used in preparation of the final IV solution. The vials are for single use only; discard any unused portion remaining in the vial.

Admixture incompatibilities – Only limited data are available on the compatibility of gatifloxacin IV injection with other IV substances; do not add additives or other medications to gatifloxacin injection in single-use vials or infuse them simultaneously through the same IV line.

If the same IV line is used for sequential infusion of different drugs, flush the line before and after infusion of gatifloxacin injection with an infusion solution compatible with gatifloxacin injection and with any other drug(s) administered via this common line.

If gatifloxacin injection is to be given concomitantly with another drug, give each drug separately in accordance with the recommended dosage and route of administration for each drug.

➤*Premix in single-use flexible containers:* Gatifloxacin injection is also available in ready-to-use 100 and 200 mL flexible bags containing a dilute solution of 200 or 400 mg gatifloxacin in 5% dextrose. No further dilution of this preparation is necessary.

Inspect this IV drug product visually for particulate matter prior to administration. Discard samples containing visible particles.

The premix flexible bags are for single use only; discard any unused portion.

➤*Storage / Stability:*

Single-use vials – Store at 25°C (77°F); excursions permitted to 15° to 30°C (59° to 86°F).

Premix bags – Store at 25°C (77°F); excursions permitted to 15° to 30°C (59° to 86°F). Do not freeze.

Stability following dilution – Gatifloxacin injection, when diluted in a compatible IV fluid to a concentration of 2 mg/mL, is stable for 14 days when stored between 20° and 25°C (68° and 77°F) or when stored under refrigeration between 2° and 8°C (36° and 46°F).

Gatifloxacin injection, when diluted to a concentration of 2 mg/mL in a compatible IV fluid except for 5% sodium bicarbonate injection, may be stored for up to 6 months at −25°C to −10°C (−13°F to 14°F). Frozen solutions may be thawed at controlled room temperature. Solutions that have been thawed are stable for 14 days after removal from the freezer when stored between 20° and 25°C (68° and 77°F) or when stored under refrigeration between 2° and 8°C (36° and 46°F). Do not refreeze solutions.

† MDRSP includes isolates previously known as penicillin-resistant *S. pneumoniae* (PRSP), and are strains resistant to 2 or more of the following antibiotics: penicillin (minimum inhibitory concentration [MIC] greater than or equal to 2 mcg/mL), second generation cephalosporins (eg, cefuroxime), macrolides, tetracyclines, and trimethoprim/sulfamethoxazole.

LEVOFLOXACIN

Rx	**Levaquin** (Ortho-McNeil)	**Tablets:** 250 mg	(LEVAQUIN 250). Terra cotta pink. Film-coated. In 50s and UD 100s.
		500 mg	(LEVAQUIN 500). Peach. Film-coated. In 50s and UD 100s.
		750 mg	(LEVAQUIN 750). White. Film-coated. In 20s, UD 100s, and *Leva-Pak* 5s.
		Oral solution: 25 mg/mL	Benzyl alcohol, glycerin, sucrose. In 480 mL.
		Injection (concentrate): 500 mg (25 mg/mL)	Preservative free. In single-use 20 mL vials in water for injection.
		750 mg (25 mg/mL)	Preservative free. In single-use 30 mL vials in water for injection.
		Injection (premix): 250 mg (5 mg/mL)	Preservative free. In 50 mL premix flexible containers in 5% dextrose solution.
		500 mg (5 mg/mL)	Preservative free. In 100 mL premix flexible containers in 5% dextrose solution.
		750 mg (5 mg/mL)	Preservative free. In 150 mL premix flexible containers in 5% dextrose solution.

LEVOFLOXACIN — ORAL

For complete and comparative prescribing information, refer to the Fluoroquinolones group monograph.

Indications

For the treatment of adults (18 years of age and older) with mild, moderate, and severe infections caused by susceptible strains of the designated microorganisms in the conditions listed below:

➤*Acute bacterial exacerbation of chronic bronchitis:* Caused by *Staphylococcus aureus, Streptococcus pneumoniae, Haemophilus influenzae, Haemophilus parainfluenzae*, or *Moraxella catarrhalis*.

➤*Acute maxillary sinusitis:* Caused by *S. pneumoniae, H. influenzae*, or *M. catarrhalis*.

➤*Acute pyelonephritis (mild to moderate):* Caused by *Escherichia coli*.

➤*Chronic bacterial prostatitis:* Caused by *E. coli, Enterococcus faecalis*, or *Staphylococcus epidermidis*.

➤*Inhalational anthrax (postexposure):* To prevent the development of inhalational anthrax following exposure to *Bacillus anthracis*.

➤*Pneumonia, community-acquired:* Caused by *S. aureus, S. pneumoniae* (including multidrug-resistant strains [MDRSP; strains resistant to 2 or more of the following antibiotics: penicillin (minimal inhibitory concentration [MIC] 2 mcg/mL or more), second-generation cephalosporins (eg, cefuroxime), macrolides, tetracyclines, and trimethoprim/sulfamethoxazole]), *H. influenzae, H. parainfluenzae, Klebsiella pneumoniae, M. catarrhalis, Chlamydia pneumoniae, Legionella pneumophila*, or *Mycoplasma pneumoniae*.

➤*Pneumonia, nosocomial:* Caused by methicillin-susceptible *S. aureus, Pseudomonas aeruginosa, Serratia marcescens, E. coli, K. pneumoniae, H. influenzae*, or *S. pneumoniae*. Use adjunctive therapy as clinically indicated. Where *P. aeruginosa* is a documented or presumptive pathogen, combination therapy with an antipseudomonal β-lactam is recommended.

➤*Skin and skin structure infections (SSSIs), complicated:* Caused by methicillin-susceptible *S. aureus, E. faecalis, Streptococcus pyogenes*, or *Proteus mirabilis*.

➤*SSSIs, uncomplicated (mild to moderate):* Including abscesses, cellulitis, furuncles, impetigo, pyoderma, and wound infections caused by *S. aureus* or *S. pyogenes*.

➤*Urinary tract infections (UTIs), complicated (mild to moderate):* Caused by *E. faecalis, Enterobacter cloacae, E. coli, K. pneumoniae, P. mirabilis*, or *P. aeruginosa*.

➤*UTIs, uncomplicated (mild to moderate):* Caused by *E. coli, K. pneumoniae*, or *Staphylococcus saprophyticus*.

➤*Unlabeled uses:*

Epididymitis (alternative regimen) – 500 mg/day orally for 10 days.

Gonococcal infections, disseminated (alternative regimen) – 250 mg once daily intravenously (IV) for 24 to 48 hours (after improvement begins, then 500 mg/day orally for 7 days).

Gonococcal infections, uncomplicated, of the cervix, urethra, and rectum – 250 mg orally as a single dose plus azithromycin 1 g as a single oral dose or doxycycline 100 mg orally 2 times a day for 7 days if chlamydial infection is not ruled out.

Nongonococcal urethritis (alternative regimen) – 500 mg/day for 7 days.

Pelvic inflammatory disease (alternative regimen) – 500 mg/day orally for 14 days.

Administration and Dosage

➤*Approved by the FDA:* December 20, 1996.

➤*Dosage:* The usual dose of levofloxacin tablets or oral solution (25 mg/mL) is 250, 500, or 750 mg administered orally every 24 hours as indicated by infection and described in the following dosing table. Levofloxacin tablets can be administered without regard to food. It is recommended that levofloxacin oral solution be taken 1 hour before or 2 hours after eating.

Concomitant therapy – Administer oral doses at least 2 hours before or 2 hours after antacids containing magnesium, aluminum, or sucralfate, metal cations such as iron, or multivitamin preparations with zinc or didanosine chewable/buffered tablets or pediatric powder for oral solution.

Levofloxacin Dosing for Patients with Normal Renal Function (Creatinine Clearance [Ccr] > 80 mL/min)

Infection[a]	Unit dose	Frequency	Duration[b]	Daily dose
Acute bacterial exacerbation of chronic bronchitis	500 mg	Every 24 h	7 days	500 mg
Acute maxillary sinusitis	500 mg	Every 24 h	10 to 14 days	500 mg
Acute pyelonephritis	250 mg	Every 24 h	10 days	250 mg
Chronic bacterial prostatitis	500 mg	Every 24 h	28 days	500 mg
Inhalational anthrax (postexposure), adult[c,d]	500 mg	Every 24 h	60 days[d]	500 mg
Pneumonia, community-acquired	500 mg	Every 24 h	7 to 14 days	500 mg
	750 mg[e]	Every 24 h	5 days	750 mg
Pneumonia, nosocomial	750 mg	Every 24 h	7 to 14 days	750 mg
SSSI, complicated	750 mg	Every 24 h	7 to 14 days	750 mg
SSSI, uncomplicated	500 mg	Every 24 h	7 to 10 days	500 mg
UTI, complicated	250 mg	Every 24 h	10 days	250 mg
UTI, uncomplicated	250 mg	Every 24 h	3 days	250 mg

[a] Caused by the designated pathogens.
[b] Sequential therapy (IV to oral) may be instituted at the discretion of the health care provider.
[c] Begin drug administration as soon as possible after suspected or confirmed exposure to aerosolized *B. anthracis*. This indication is based on a surrogate endpoint. Levofloxacin plasma concentrations achieved in humans are reasonably likely to predict clinical benefit.
[d] The safety of levofloxacin in adults for durations of therapy beyond 28 days has not been studied. Only use prolonged levofloxacin therapy in adults when the benefit outweighs the risk.
[e] Efficacy of this alternative regimen has been demonstrated to be effective for infections caused by *S. pneumoniae* (excluding MDRSP), *H. influenzae, H. parainfluenzae, M. pneumoniae*, and *C. pneumoniae*.

Renal function impairment –

Levofloxacin Dosing for Patients with Renal Function Impairment

Renal status	Initial dose	Subsequent dose
Acute bacterial exacerbation of chronic bronchitis/community-acquired pneumonia/acute maxillary sinusitis/uncomplicated SSSI/chronic bacterial prostatitis		
Ccr 50 to 80 mL/min	No dosage adjustment required	
Ccr 20 to 49 mL/min	500 mg	250 mg every 24 h
Ccr 10 to 19 mL/min	500 mg	250 mg every 48 h
Hemodialysis	500 mg	250 mg every 48 h
CAPD[a]	500 mg	250 mg every 48 h
Complicated SSSI/nosocomial pneumonia/community-acquired pneumonia		
Ccr 50 to 80 mL/min	No dosage adjustment required	
Ccr 20 to 49 mL/min	750 mg	750 mg every 48 h
Ccr 10 to 19 mL/min	750 mg	500 mg every 48 h
Hemodialysis	750 mg	500 mg every 48 h
CAPD[a]	750 mg	500 mg every 48 h
Complicated UTI/acute pyelonephritis		
Ccr ≥ 20 mL/min	No dosage adjustment required	
Ccr 10 to 19 mL/min	250 mg	250 mg every 48 h
Uncomplicated UTI	No dosage adjustment required	

[a] CAPD = chronic ambulatory peritoneal dialysis.

➤*Storage/Stability:*

Tablets – Store at 15° to 30°C (59° to 86°F) in a well-closed container.

Oral solution – Store at 25°C (77°F); excursions permitted to 15° to 30°C (59° to 86°F).

LEVOFLOXACIN — INJECTION

For complete and comparative prescribing information, refer to the Fluoroquinolones group monograph.

Indications

For the treatment of adults (18 years of age and older) with mild, moderate, and severe infections caused by susceptible strains of the designated microorganisms in the conditions listed below. Levofloxacin injection is indicated when intravenous (IV) administration offers a route of administration advantageous to the patient (eg, patient cannot tolerate an oral dosage form).

➤*Acute bacterial exacerbation of chronic bronchitis:* Caused by *Staphylococcus aureus, Streptococcus pneumoniae, Haemophilus influenzae, Haemophilus parainfluenzae,* or *Moraxella catarrhalis.*

➤*Acute bacterial sinusitis:* Caused by *S. pneumoniae, H. influenzae,* or *M. catarrhalis.*

➤*Acute pyelonephritis (mild to moderate):* Caused by *Escherichia coli.*

➤*Chronic bacterial prostatitis:* Caused by *E. coli, Enterococcus faecalis,* or *Staphylococcus epidermidis.*

➤*Inhalational anthrax (postexposure):* To prevent the development of inhalational anthrax following exposure to *Bacillus anthracis.*

➤*Pneumonia, community-acquired:* Caused by *S. aureus, S. pneumoniae* (including multidrug-resistant strains [MDRSP; strains resistant to 2 or more of the following antibiotics: penicillin (minimal inhibitory concentration [MIC] 2 mcg/mL or more), second-generation cephalosporins (eg, cefuroxime), macrolides, tetracyclines, and trimethoprim/sulfamethoxazole]), *H. influenzae, H. parainfluenzae, Klebsiella pneumoniae, M. catarrhalis, Chlamydia pneumoniae, Legionella pneumophila,* or *Mycoplasma pneumoniae.*

➤*Pneumonia, nosocomial:* Caused by methicillin-susceptible *S. aureus, Pseudomonas aeruginosa, Serratia marcescens, E. coli, K. pneumoniae, H. influenzae,* or *S. pneumoniae.* Use adjunctive therapy as clinically indicated. Where *P. aeruginosa* is a documented or presumptive pathogen, combination therapy with an antipseudomonal β-lactam is recommended.

➤*Skin and skin structure infections (SSSIs), complicated:* Caused by methicillin-susceptible *S. aureus, E. faecalis, Streptococcus pyogenes,* or *Proteus mirabilis.*

➤*SSSIs, uncomplicated (mild to moderate):* Including abscesses, cellulitis, furuncles, impetigo, pyoderma, and wound infections caused by *S. aureus* or *S. pyogenes.*

➤*Urinary tract infections (UTIs), complicated (mild to moderate):* Caused by *E. faecalis, Enterobacter cloacae, E. coli, K. pneumoniae, P. mirabilis,* or *P. aeruginosa.*

➤*UTIs, uncomplicated (mild to moderate):* Caused by *E. coli, K. pneumoniae,* or *Staphylococcus saprophyticus.*

➤*Unlabeled uses:*

Gonococcal infections, disseminated (alternative regimen) – 250 mg IV once daily for 24 to 48 hours (after improvement begins, then 500 mg/day orally for 7 days).

Pelvic inflammatory disease (alternative regimen) – 500 mg IV once daily for 14 days.

Administration and Dosage

➤*Approved by the FDA:* December 20, 1996.

➤*Dosage:* The usual dose of levofloxacin injection is 250 or 500 mg administered by slow infusion over 60 minutes every 24 hours or 750 mg administered by slow infusion over 90 minutes every 24 hours, as indicated by infection and described by the following dosing recommendations. These recommendations apply to patients with normal renal function (ie, creatinine clearance [Ccr] more than 80 mL/min). For patients with altered renal function, see the second table below.

Levofloxacin Dosing for Patients with Normal Renal Function (Ccr > 80 mL/min)

Infection[a]	Unit dose	Frequency	Duration[b]	Daily dose
Acute bacterial exacerbation of chronic bronchitis	500 mg	Every 24 h	7 days	500 mg
Acute bacterial sinusitis	500 mg	Every 24 h	10 to 14 days	500 mg
	750 mg	Every 24 h	5 days	750 mg
Acute pyelonephritis	250 mg	Every 24 h	10 days	250 mg
Chronic bacterial prostatitis	500 mg	Every 24 h	28 days	500 mg
Inhalational anthrax (postexposure), adult[c,d]	500 mg	Every 24 h	60 days[d]	500 mg
Pneumonia, community-acquired	500 mg	Every 24 h	7 to 14 days	500 mg
	750 mg[e]	Every 24 h	5 days	750 mg
Pneumonia, nosocomial	750 mg	Every 24 h	7 to 14 days	750 mg
SSSI, complicated	750 mg	Every 24 h	7 to 14 days	750 mg
SSSI, uncomplicated	500 mg	Every 24 h	7 to 10 days	500 mg
UTI, complicated	250 mg	Every 24 h	10 days	250 mg
UTI, uncomplicated	250 mg	Every 24 h	3 days	250 mg

[a] Caused by the designated pathogens.
[b] Sequential therapy (IV to oral) may be instituted at the discretion of the health care provider.
[c] Begin drug administration as soon as possible after suspected or confirmed exposure to aerosolized *B. anthracis*. This indication is based on a surrogate endpoint. Levofloxacin plasma concentrations achieved in humans are reasonably likely to predict clinical benefit.
[d] The safety of levofloxacin in adults for durations of therapy beyond 28 days has not been studied. Use prolonged levofloxacin therapy in adults only when the benefit outweighs the risk.
[e] Efficacy of this alternative regimen has been demonstrated to be effective for infections caused by *S. pneumoniae* (excluding MDRSP), *H. influenzae, H. parainfluenzae, M. pneumoniae,* and *C. pneumoniae.*

➤*Renal function impairment:*

Levofloxacin Dosing for Patients with Renal Function Impairment

Renal status	Initial dose	Subsequent dose
Acute bacterial exacerbation of chronic bronchitis/community-acquired pneumonia/acute bacterial sinusitis/uncomplicated SSSI/chronic bacterial prostatitis/inhalational anthrax (post-exposure)		
Ccr 50 to 80 mL/min	No dosage adjustment required	
Ccr 20 to 49 mL/min	500 mg	250 mg every 24 h
Ccr 10 to 19 mL/min	500 mg	250 mg every 48 h
Hemodialysis	500 mg	250 mg every 48 h
CAPD[a]	500 mg	250 mg every 48 h
Complicated SSSI/nosocomial pneumonia/community-acquired pneumonia/acute bacterial sinusitis		
Ccr 50 to 80 mL/min	No dosage adjustment required	
Ccr 20 to 49 mL/min	750 mg	750 mg every 48 h
Ccr 10 to 19 mL/min	750 mg	500 mg every 48 h
Hemodialysis	750 mg	500 mg every 48 h
CAPD[a]	750 mg	500 mg every 48 h
Complicated UTI/acute pyelonephritis		
Ccr ≥ 20 mL/min	No dosage adjustment required	
Ccr 10 to 19 mL/min	250 mg	250 mg every 48 h
Uncomplicated UTI	No dosage adjustment required	

[a] CAPD = chronic ambulatory peritoneal dialysis. When only the serum creatinine is known, the following formula may be used to estimate Ccr: Mean:

Ccr (mL/min) = Weight (kg) × (140 − age)/72 × serum creatinine (mg/dL)
Women: 0.85 × the value calculated for men. The serum creatinine should represent a steady state of renal function.

➤*Preparation/Administration of injection:* Levofloxacin injection should only be administered by IV infusion. It is not for intramuscular, intrathecal, intraperitoneal, or subcutaneous administration.

Avoid rapid or bolus IV infusion. Infuse levofloxacin IV slowly over a period of at least 60 or 90 minutes, depending on the dosage.

Single-use vials require dilution prior to administration.

Levofloxacin injection in single-use vials – Levofloxacin injection is supplied in single-use vials containing a concentrated levofloxacin solution with the equivalent of 500 mg (20 mL vial) and 750 mg (30 mL vial) of levofloxacin in water for injection. The 20 and 30 mL vials contain levofloxacin 25 mg/mL. These single-use vials must be further diluted with an appropriate solution prior to IV administration. The concentration of the resulting diluted solution should be 5 mg/mL prior to administration.

This IV drug product should be inspected visually for particulate matter prior to administration. Samples containing visible particles should be discarded.

Because no preservative or bacteriostatic agent is present in this product, aseptic technique must be used in preparation of the final IV solution. Because the vials are for single-use only, discard any unused portion remaining in the vial. When used to prepare two 250 mg doses from the 20 mL vial containing levofloxacin 500 mg, withdraw the full content of the vial at once using a single-entry procedure, and prepare a second dose and store it for subsequent use.

Admixture incompatibility: Because only limited data are available on the compatibility of levofloxacin IV injection with other IV substances, do not add additives or other medications to levofloxacin injection in single-use vials or infuse simultaneously through the same IV line. If the same IV line is used for sequential infusion of several different drugs, flush the line before and after infusion of levofloxacin injection with an infusion solution compatible with levofloxacin injection and with any other drug administered via this common line.

LEVOFLOXACIN — INJECTION

Levofloxacin IV Dosing Preparation			
Desired dosage strength	Withdraw volume from appropriate vial	Volume of diluent	Infusion time (min)
250 mg	10 mL (20 mL vial)	40 mL	60
500 mg	20 mL (20 mL vial)	80 mL	60
750 mg	30 mL (30 mL vial)	120 mL	90

For example, to prepare a 500 mg dose using the 20 mL vial (25 mg/mL), withdraw 20 mL and dilute with a compatible IV solution to a total volume of 100 mL.

Compatible IV solutions: Any of the following IV solutions may be used to prepare a levofloxacin 5 mg/mL solution with the approximate pH values:

IV Fluids	Final pH of Levofloxacin Solution
0.9% Sodium chloride injection	4.71
5% Dextrose (D5W) injection	4.58
D5W/0.9% sodium chloride injection	4.62
D5W in Ringer's lactate	4.92
Plasma-Lyte 56/D5W injection	5.03
D5W, 0.45% sodium chloride, and 0.15% potassium chloride injection	4.61
Sodium lactate injection (M/6)	5.54

Premix in single-use flexible containers – Levofloxacin injection also is supplied in flexible containers containing a premixed, ready-to-use levofloxacin solution in D5W for single-use. The fill volume is either 50 or 100 mL for the 100 mL flexible container or 150 mL for the 150 mL container. No further dilution of these preparations is necessary. Consequently, each 100 and 150 mL premix flexible container already contains a dilute solution with the equivalent of 250 or 500 mg (100 mL container) and 750 mg of levofloxacin (150 mL container) in D5W. The concentration of each presentation is 5 mg/mL of levofloxacin solution.

Because the premix flexible containers are for single-use only, discard any unused portion.

➤*Storage/Stability:*

IV –

Single-use vial: Store at controlled room temperature (15° to 30°C; 59° to 86°F); protect from light.

Premix: Store at or below 25°C (77°F); however, brief exposure up to 40°C (104°F) does not adversely affect the product. Avoid excessive heat and protect from freezing and light.

Stability of levofloxacin injection following dilution: Levofloxacin injection, when diluted in a compatible IV fluid to a concentration of 5 mg/mL, is stable for 72 hours when stored at or below 25°C (77°F) and for 14 days when stored under refrigeration at 5°C (41°F) in plastic IV containers. Solutions that are diluted in a compatible IV solution and frozen in glass bottles or plastic IV containers are stable for 6 months when stored at −20°C (−4°F). Thaw frozen solutions at room temperature (25°C; 77°F) or in a refrigerator (8°C; 46°F). Do not force thaw by microwave irradiation or water bath immersion. Do not refreeze after initial thawing.

LOMEFLOXACIN HYDROCHLORIDE

Rx	**Maxaquin** (Biovail)	**Tablets:** 400 mg	Lactose. (Maxaquin 400). White, oval, scored. Film-coated. In 20s.

LOMEFLOXACIN — ORAL

For complete and comparative prescribing information, refer to the Fluoroquinolones group monograph.

Indications

For the treatment of adults with mild-to-moderate infections caused by susceptible strains of the designated microorganisms in the conditions listed below.

➤*Acute bacterial exacerbation of chronic bronchitis:* Caused by *Haemophilus influenzae* or *Moraxella catarrhalis.*

➤*Uncomplicated urinary tract infections (cystitis):* Caused by *Escherichia coli, Klebsiella pneumoniae, Proteus mirabilis,* or *Staphylococcus saprophyticus.*

➤*Complicated urinary tract infections:* Caused by *Escherichia coli, Klebsiella pneumoniae, Proteus mirabilis, Pseudomonas aeruginosa, Citrobacter diversus,* or *Enterobacter cloacae.*

➤*Preoperative prevention:* Preoperatively for the prevention of infection in the following situations:

Transrectal prostate biopsy – To reduce the incidence of urinary tract infection, in the early and late postoperative periods (3 to 5 days and 3 to 4 weeks postsurgery).

Transurethral surgical procedures – To reduce the incidence of urinary tract infection in the early postoperative period (3 to 5 days postsurgery).

Administration and Dosage

➤*Administration:* Lomefloxacin may be taken without regard to meals. Sucralfate and antacids containing magnesium or aluminum, or didanosine, chewable/buffered tablets or the pediatric powder for oral solution should not be taken within 4 hours before or 2 hours after taking lomefloxacin. Risk of reaction to solar UVA light may be reduced by taking lomefloxacin at least 12 hours before exposure to the sun (eg, in the evening).

➤*Dosage:*

Recommended Daily Dose of Lomefloxacin				
Infection	Unit dose	Frequency	Duration	Daily dose
Acute bacterial exacerbation of chronic bronchitis	400 mg	Every day	10 days	400 mg

Recommended Daily Dose of Lomefloxacin				
Infection	Unit dose	Frequency	Duration	Daily dose
Uncomplicated cystitis in females caused by *E. coli*	400 mg	Every day	3 days	400 mg
Uncomplicated cystitis caused by *K pneumoniae, P mirabilis,* or *S saprophyticus*	400 mg	Every day	10 days	400 mg
Complicated UTI	400 mg	Every day	14 days	400 mg

➤*Renal function impairment:* Lomefloxacin is primarily eliminated by renal excretion. Approximately 65% of an orally administered dose was excreted in the urine as unchanged drug in patients with healthy renal function. Modification of dosage is recommended in patients with renal dysfunction. In patients with a creatinine clearance greater than 10 mL/min/1.73 m^2 but less than 40 mL/min/1.73 m^2, the recommended dosage is an initial loading dose of 400 mg followed by daily maintenance doses of 200 mg (½ tablet) once daily for the duration of treatment. It is suggested that serial determinations of lomefloxacin levels be performed to determine any necessary alteration in the appropriate next dosing interval.

➤*Dialysis patients:* Hemodialysis removes only a negligible amount of lomefloxacin (3% in 4 hours). Hemodialysis patients should receive an initial loading dose of 400 mg followed by daily maintenance doses of 200 mg (½ tablet) once daily for the duration of treatment.

➤*Preoperative prevention:* The recommended dose of lomefloxacin is described in the following table.

Procedure	Dose	Oral administration
Transrectal prostate biopsy	400 mg single dose	1 to 6 hours prior to procedure
Transurethral surgical procedures*	400 mg single dose	2 to 6 hours prior to procedure

* When preoperative prophylaxis is considered appropriate.

➤*Storage/Stability:* Store at 15° to 25°C (59° to 77°F).

MOXIFLOXACIN HYDROCHLORIDE

Rx	**Avelox** (Bayer)	**Tablets:** 400 mg (as base)	Lactose. (BAYER M400). Red, oblong. Film-coated. In 30s, UD 50s, and *ABC* packs of 5.
Rx	**Avelox I.V.** (Bayer)	**Injection (premix):** 400 mg (as base)	With 0.8% sodium chloride. Preservative-free. In 250 mL latex-free flexible bags.[a]

[a] No further dilution of this preparation is necessary.

MOXIFLOXACIN HYDROCHLORIDE — ORAL

For complete and comparative prescribing information, refer to the Fluoroquinolones group monograph.

Indications

For the treatment of adults (18 years of age or older) with infections caused by susceptible strains of the designated microorganisms in the following conditions:

➤*Acute bacterial exacerbation of chronic bronchitis:* Caused by *Streptococcus pneumoniae, Haemophilus influenzae, Haemophilus parainfluenzae, Klebsiella pneumoniae,* methicillin-susceptible *Staphylococcus aureus,* or *Moraxella catarrhalis.*

➤*Acute bacterial sinusitis:* Caused by *S. pneumoniae, H. influenzae,* or *M. catarrhalis.*

➤*Community-acquired pneumonia:* Caused by *S. pneumoniae* (including multidrug-resistant strains†), *H. influenzae, M. catarrhalis,* methicillin-susceptible *S. aureus, K. pneumoniae, Mycoplasma pneumoniae,* or *Chlamydia pneumoniae.*

➤*Complicated intra-abdominal infections:* Including polymicrobial infections such as abscess caused by *Escherichia coli, Bacteroides fragilis, Streptococcus anginosus, Streptococcus constellatus, Enterococcus faecalis, Proteus mirabilis, Clostridium perfringens, Bacteroides thetaiotaomicron,* or *Peptostreptococcus* species.

➤*Complicated skin and skin structure infections:* Caused by methicillin-susceptible *S. aureus, E. coli, K. pneumoniae,* or *Enterobacter cloacae.*

➤*Uncomplicated skin and skin-structure infections:* Caused by methicillin-susceptible *S. aureus* or *Streptococcus pyogenes.*

Perform appropriate culture and susceptibility tests before treatment in order to isolate and identify organisms causing infection and to determine their susceptibilities to moxifloxacin. Therapy with moxifloxacin may be initiated before results of these tests are known; once results become available, continue appropriate therapy.

To reduce the development of drug-resistant bacteria and maintain the efficacy of moxifloxacin and other antibacterial drugs, use moxifloxacin only to treat or prevent infections that are proven or strongly suspected to be caused by susceptible bacteria. Consider culture and susceptibility information (when available) in selecting or modifying antibacterial therapy. In the absence of such data, local epidemiology and susceptibility patterns may contribute to the empiric selection of therapy.

Administration and Dosage

➤*Approved by the FDA:* December 10, 1999.

The dosage of moxifloxacin is 400 mg orally once every 24 hours. The duration of therapy depends on the type of infection, as described in the following table:

Moxifloxacin Dosing Recommendations

Infection[a]	Daily dose	Duration
Acute bacterial sinusitis	400 mg	10 days
Acute bacterial exacerbation of chronic bronchitis	400 mg	5 days
Community-acquired pneumonia	400 mg	7 to 14 days
Uncomplicated skin and skin-structure infections	400 mg	7 days
Complicated intra-abdominal infections[b]	400 mg	5 to 14 days
Complicated skin and skin structure infections	400 mg	7 to 21 days

[a] Caused by the designated pathogens.
[b] For complicated intra-abdominal infections, therapy should be initiated with the intravenous (IV) formulation.

➤*Storage/Stability:* Store at 25°C (77°F); excursions permitted to 15° to 30°C (59° to 86°F). Avoid high humidity.

MOXIFLOXACIN HYDROCHLORIDE — INJECTION

For complete and comparative prescribing information, refer to the Fluoroquinolones group monograph.

Indications

For the treatment of adults (18 years of age or older) with infections caused by susceptible strains of the designated microorganisms in the following conditions:

➤*Acute bacterial exacerbation of chronic bronchitis:* Caused by *S. pneumoniae, H. influenzae, Haemophilus parainfluenzae, Klebsiella pneumoniae,* methicillin-susceptible*S. aureus,* or *M. catarrhalis.*

➤*Acute bacterial sinusitis:* Caused by *Streptococcus pneumoniae, Haemophilus influenzae,* or *Moraxella catarrhalis.*

➤*Community-acquired pneumonia:* Caused by *S. pneumoniae* (including multidrug-resistant strains†), *H. influenzae, M. catarrhalis,* methicillin-susceptible *S. aureus, K. pneumoniae, Mycoplasma pneumoniae,* or *Chlamydia pneumoniae.*

➤*Complicated intra-abdominal infections:* Including polymicrobial infections such as abscess caused by *Escherichia coli, Bacteroides fragilis, Streptococcus anginosus, Streptococcus constellatus, Enterococcus faecalis, Proteus mirabilis, Clostridium perfringens, Bacteroides thetaiotaomicron,* or *Peptostreptococcus* species.

➤*Complicated skin and skin structure infections:* Caused by methicillin-susceptible *S. aureus, E. coli, K. pneumoniae,* or *E. cloacae.*

➤*Uncomplicated skin and skin-structure infections:* Caused by methicillin-susceptible*S. aureus* or *S. pyogenes.*

Perform appropriate culture and susceptibility tests before treatment in order to isolate and identify organisms causing infection and to determine their susceptibilities to moxifloxacin. Therapy with moxifloxacin may be initiated before results of these tests are known; once results become available, continue appropriate therapy.

To reduce the development of drug-resistant bacteria and maintain the effectiveness of moxifloxacin and other antibacterial drugs, use moxifloxacin only to treat or prevent infections that are proven or strongly suspected to be caused by susceptible bacteria. Consider culture and susceptibility information (when available) in selecting or modifying antibacterial therapy. In the absence of such data, local epidemiology and susceptibility patterns may contribute to the empiric selection of therapy.

Administration and Dosage

➤*Approved by the FDA:* December 10, 1999.

The dose of moxifloxacin is 400 mg as an IV infusion once every 24 hours. The duration of therapy depends on the type of infection, as described in the following table:

Moxifloxacin Dosing Recommendations

Infection[a]	Daily Dose	Duration
Acute bacterial sinusitis	400 mg	10 days
Acute bacterial exacerbation of chronic bronchitis	400 mg	5 days
Community-acquired pneumonia	400 mg	7 to 14 days
Uncomplicated skin and skin-structure infections	400 mg	7 days
Complicated skin and skin-structure infections	400 mg	7 to 21 days
Complicated intra-abdominal infections[b]	400 mg	5 to 14 days

[a] Due to the designated pathogens.
[b] For complicated intra-abdominal infections, therapy should be initiated with the IV formulation.

➤*IV administration:* Administer moxifloxacin by IV infusion only. It is not intended for intra-arterial, intramuscular (IM), intrathecal, intraperitoneal, or subcutaneous administration. Administer moxifloxacin by IV infusion over a period of 60 minutes by direct infusion or through a Y-type IV infusion set that may already be in place. Rapid or bolus IV infusion must be avoided.

Compatibility/incompatibilities – Because only limited data are available on the compatibility of moxifloxacin IV injection with other IV substances, do not add additives or other medications to moxifloxacin IV or infuse them simultaneously through the same IV line. If the same IV line or a Y-type line is used for sequential infusion of other drugs, or if the "piggyback" method of administration is used, flush the line before and after infusion of moxifloxacin IV with an infusion solution compatible with moxifloxacin IV as well as with other drug(s) administered via this common line.

Moxifloxacin IV is compatible with the following IV solutions at ratios from 1:10 to 10:1:0.9% sodium chloride injection, 1M sodium chloride injection, 5% dextrose injection, sterile water for injection, 10% dextrose for injection, Ringer's lactate for injection.

➤*Preparation for administration of moxifloxacin IV injection premix in flexible containers:* No further dilution of this preparation is necessary.

1.) Close flow-control clamp of administration set.
2.) Remove cover from port at bottom of container.
3.) Insert piercing pin from an appropriate transfer set (eg, one that does not require excessive force, such as ISO-compatible administration set) into port with a gentle twisting motion until pin is firmly seated.

Note – Refer to complete directions that have been provided with the administration set.

† MDRSP, multidrug-resistant *S. pneumoniae* includes isolates previously known as PRSP (penicillin-resistant *S. pneumoniae*), and are strains resistant to 2 or more of the following antibiotics: penicillin (minimum inhibitory concentration [MIC] greater than or equal to 2 mcg/mL), second generation cephalosporins (eg, cefuroxime), macrolides, tetracyclines, and trimethoprim/sulfamethoxazole.

MOXIFLOXACIN HYDROCHLORIDE — INJECTION

Visually inspect parenteral drug products for particulate matter prior to administration. Do not use samples containing visible particulates.

➤*Storage/Stability:*

IV solution, premixed bags – The premixed flexible containers are for single use only; discard any unused portion. Store at 25°C (77°F); excursions permitted to 15° to 30°C (59° to 86°F). Do not refrigerate; product precipitates upon refrigeration.

GEMIFLOXACIN

Rx	**Factive** (Oscient[a])	**Tablets:** 320 mg (as base)	(GE 320). White to off-white, oval, scored. Film-coated. In unit of use 5s and 7s and hospital pack 30s.

[a] Oscient Pharmaceuticals, 1000 Winter Street, Ste. 2200, Waltham, MA 02154; (781) 398-2300.

GEMIFLOXACIN MESYLATE — ORAL

For complete prescribing information, refer to the Fluoroquinolones group monograph.

Indications

For the treatment of infections caused by susceptible strains of the designated microorganisms in the conditions listed below.

➤*Acute bacterial exacerbation of chronic bronchitis:* Caused by *Streptococcus pneumoniae, Haemophilus influenzae, Haemophilus parainfluenzae*, or *Moraxella catarrhalis*.

➤*Community-acquired pneumonia (mild to moderate):* Caused by *Streptococcus pneumoniae* (including penicillin-resistant strains, MIC value for penicillin greater than or equal to 2 mcg/mL), *Haemophilus influenzae, Moraxella catarrhalis, Mycoplasma pneumoniae, Chlamydia pneumoniae*, or *Klebsiella pneumoniae*.†

Administration and Dosage

➤*Approved by the FDA:* April 4, 2003.

Can be taken with or without food and should be swallowed whole with a liberal amount of liquid.

➤*Dosage:*

Gemifloxacin Dosage Guidlines

Indication	Dose	Duration
Acute bacterial exacerbation of chronic bronchitis	One 320 mg tablet daily	5 days
Community-acquired pneumonia (of mild to moderate severity)	One 320 mg tablet daily	7 days

➤*Renal function impairment:* Dose adjustment in patients with creatinine clearance greater than 40 mL/min is not required. Modification of the dosage is recommended for patients with creatinine clearance less than or equal to 40 mL/min.

Recommended Doses for Patients with Impaired Renal Function

Creatinine clearance (mL/min)	Dose
> 40	See usual dosage
≤ 40	160 mg every 24 hours

Dialysis – Patients requiring routine hemodialysis or continuous ambulatory peritoneal dialysis (CAPD) should receive 160 mg every 24 hours.

➤*Storage/Stability:* Store at 25°C (77°F); excursions permitted to 15° to 30°C (59° to 86°F). Protect from light.

NORFLOXACIN

Rx	**Noroxin** (Merck)	**Tablets:** 400 mg	(MSD 705 Noroxin). Dark pink, oval. Film coated. In 100s and UD 20s and 100s.

NORFLOXACIN — ORAL

For complete and comparative prescribing information, refer to the Fluoroquinolones group monograph.

Indications

For the treatment of adults with the following infections caused by susceptible strains of the designated microorganisms:

➤*Urinary tract infections:* Uncomplicated urinary tract infections (including cystitis) due to *Enterococcus faecalis, Escherichia coli, Klebsiella pneumoniae, Proteus mirabilis, Pseudomonas aeruginosa, Staphylococcus epidermidis, Staphylococcus saprophyticus, Citrobacter freundii, Enterobacter aerogenes, Enterobacter cloacae, Proteus vulgaris, Staphylococcus aureus*, or *Streptococcus agalactiae*.

Complicated urinary tract infections due to *Enterococcus faecalis, Escherichia coli, Klebsiella pneumoniae, Proteus mirabilis, Pseudomonas aeruginosa*, or *Serratia marcescens*.

➤*Sexually transmitted diseases:* Due to *Neisseria gonorrhoeae*.

➤*Prostatitis:* Prostatitis due to *Escherichia coli*.

Administration and Dosage

➤*Approved by the FDA:* October 31, 1986.

➤*Administration:* Take norfloxacin at least 1 hour before or at least 2 hours after a meal or ingestion of milk or other dairy products. Multivitamins, other products containing iron or zinc, antacids containing magnesium and aluminum, sucralfate, or didanosine chewable/buffered tablets or the pediatric powder for oral solution, should not be taken within 2 hours of administration of norfloxacin. Take norfloxacin with a glass of water. Patients receiving norfloxacin should be well hydrated.

➤*Dosage:*

Recommended Norfloxacin Dosage

Infection	Description	Unit dose	Frequency	Duration	Daily dose
Urinary tract	Uncomplicated urinary tract infections (UTIs) (cystitis) due to *E. coli, K. pneumoniae*, or *P. mirabilis*	400 mg	every 12 hours	3 days	800 mg
	Uncomplicated UTIs due to other indicated organisms	400 mg	every 12 hours	7 to 10 days	800 mg
	Complicated UTIs	400 mg	every 12 hours	10 to 21 days	800 mg
Sexually transmitted diseases	Uncomplicated gonorrhea	800 mg	single dose	1 days	800 mg
Prostatitis	Acute or chronic	400 mg	every 12 hours	28 days	800 mg

➤*Renal function impairment:* Norfloxacin may be used for the treatment of urinary tract infections in patients with renal insufficiency. In patients with a creatinine clearance rate of 30 mL/min/1.73 m^2 or less, the recommended dosage is one 400 mg tablet once daily for the duration given above. At this dosage, the urinary concentration exceeds the minimum inhibitory concentrations (MICs) for most urinary pathogens susceptible to norfloxacin, even when the creatinine clearance is less than 10 mL/min/1.73 m^2.

➤*Elderly:* Elderly patients being treated for urinary tract infections who have a creatinine clearance of greater than 30 mL/min/1.73 m^2 should receive the dosages recommended under Normal renal function.

Elderly patients being treated for urinary tract infections who have a creatinine clearance of 30 mL/min/1.73 m^2 or less should receive 400 mg once daily as recommended under Renal impairment.

➤*Storage/Stability:* Store at 25°C (77°F), excursions permitted to 15° to 30°C (59° to 86°F). Keep container tightly closed.

† MDRSP, multidrug-resistant *S. pneumoniae* includes isolates previously known as PRSP (penicillin-resistant *S. pneumoniae*), and are strains resistant to 2 or more of the following antibiotics: penicillin (minimum inhibitory concentration [MIC] greater than or equal to 2 mcg/mL), second generation cephalosporins (eg, cefuroxime), macrolides, tetracyclines, and trimethoprim/sulfamethoxazole.

OFLOXACIN

Rx	**Ofloxacin** (Various, eg, Par, Ranbaxy)	**Tablets:** 200 mg	In 50s and 100s.
Rx	**Floxin** (Ortho-McNeil)		Lactose. (Floxin 200). Lt. yellow. Film coated. In 50s and UD 6s and 100s.
Rx	**Ofloxacin** (Various, eg, Par, Ranbaxy)	**Tablets:** 300 mg	In 50s and 100s.
Rx	**Floxin** (Ortho-McNeil)		Lactose. (Floxin 300). White. Film coated. In 50s and UD 100s.
Rx	**Ofloxacin** (Various, eg, Par, Ranbaxy)	**Tablets:** 400 mg	In 100s.
Rx	**Floxin** (Ortho-McNeil)		Lactose. (Floxin 400). Pale gold. Film coated. In 100s and UD 100s.

[1] Preservative free.

OFLOXACIN — ORAL

For complete and comparative prescribing information, refer to the Fluoroquinolones group monograph.

Indications

For the treatment of adults with mild to moderate infections (unless otherwise indicated) caused by susceptible strains of the designated microorganisms in the infections listed below.

➤*Acute bacterial exacerbations of chronic bronchitis:* Due to *Haemophilus influenzae* or *Streptococcus pneumoniae.*

➤*Community-acquired pneumonia:* Due to *Haemophilus influenzae* or *Streptococcus pneumoniae.*

➤*Uncomplicated skin and skin structure infections:* Due to *Staphylococcus aureus, Streptococcus pyogenes,* or *Proteus mirabilis.*

➤*Acute, uncomplicated urethral and cervical gonorrhea:* Due to *Neisseria gonorrhoeae.*

➤*Nongonococcal urethritis and cervicitis:* Due to *Chlamydia trachomatis.*

➤*Mixed infections of the urethra and cervix:* Due to *Chlamydia trachomatis* and *Neisseria gonorrhoeae.*

➤*Acute pelvic inflammatory disease (including severe infection):* Due to *Chlamydia trachomatis* or *Neisseria gonorrhoeae.*

➤*Uncomplicated cystitis:* Due to *Citrobacter diversus, Enterobacter aerogenes, Escherichia coli, Klebsiella pneumoniae, Proteus mirabilis,* or *Pseudomonas aeruginosa.*

➤*Complicated urinary tract infections:* Due to *Escherichia coli, Klebsiella pneumoniae, Proteus mirabilis, Citrobacter diversus,* or *Pseudomonas aeruginosa.* Although treatment of infections due to *Citrobacter diversus* and *Pseudomonas aeruginosa* in this organ system demonstrated a clinically significant outcome, efficacy was studied in fewer than 10 patients.

➤*Prostatitis:* Due to *Escherichia coli.*

Administration and Dosage

➤*Approved by the FDA:* December 28, 1990.

➤*Dosage:* The usual dose of ofloxacin tablets is 200 mg to 400 mg orally every 12 hours as described in the following dosing table. These recommendations apply to patients with normal renal function (ie, creatinine clearance greater than 50 mL/min). For patients with altered renal function (ie, creatinine clearance less than or equal to 50 mL/min), see the following.

Ofloxacin Dosage Guidelines

Infection[1]	Unit dose	Frequency	Duration	Daily dose
Acute bacterial exacerbation of chronic bronchitis	400 mg	every 12 hours	10 days	800 mg
Community-acquired pneumonia	400 mg	every 12 hours	10 days	800 mg
Uncomplicated skin and skin structure infections	400 mg	every 12 hours	10 days	800 mg
Acute, uncomplicated urethral and cervical gonorrhea	400 mg	single dose	1 day	400 mg
Nongonococcal cervicitis/urethritis due to *C. trachomatis*	300 mg	every 12 hours	7 days	600 mg
Mixed infection of the urethra and cervix due to *C. trachomatis* and *N. gonorrhoeae*	300 mg	every 12 hours	7 days	600 mg
Acute pelvic inflammatory disease	400 mg	every 12 hours	10 to 14 days	800 mg
Uncomplicated cystitis due to *E. coli* or *K. pneumoniae*	200 mg	every 12 hours	3 days	400 mg
Uncomplicated cystitis due to other approved pathogens	200 mg	every 12 hours	7 days	400 mg
Complicated UTIs	200 mg	every 12 hours	10 days	400 mg
Prostatitis due to *E. coli*	300 mg	every 12 hours	6 weeks	600 mg

[1] Due to the designated pathogens.

➤*Concomitant therapy:* Antacids containing calcium, magnesium, or aluminum; sucralfate; divalent or trivalent cations such as iron; multivitamins containing zinc; or didanosine, chewable/buffered tablets or the pediatric powder for oral solution should not be taken within 2 hours period before or within 2 hours after taking ofloxacin.

➤*Renal function impairment:* Dosage should be adjusted for patients with a creatinine clearance less than or equal to 50 mL/min. After a normal initial dose, dosage should be adjusted as follows:

Ofloxacin Dosage in Impaired Renal Function

Creatinine clearance	Maintenance dose	Frequency
20 to 50 mL/min	The usual recommended unit dose	every 24 hr
< 20 mL/min	Half the usual recommended unit dose	every 24 hr

The serum creatinine should represent a steady-state of renal function.

➤*Hepatic function impairment:* The excretion of ofloxacin may be reduced in patients with severe liver function disorders (eg, cirrhosis with or without ascites). A maximum dose of 400 mg of ofloxacin per day should therefore not be exceeded.

➤*Storage/Stability:* Ofloxacin tablets should be stored in well-closed containers. Store at 20° to 25°C (68° to 77°F).

TETRACYCLINES

Refer to the Gastrointestinal Agents chapter for additional information regarding tetracycline use in periodontitis.

Indications

Refer to individual agents for more specific information.

➤*Gram-negative organisms: Haemophilus ducreyi* (chancroid); *Francisella tularensis* (tularemia); *Yersinia pestis* (plague); *Bartonella bacilliformis* (bartonellosis); *Campylobacter fetus; Vibrio cholerae* (cholera); *Brucella* sp. (brucellosis, may be in conjunction with streptomycin); *Calymmatobacterium granulomatis* (granuloma inguinale).

➤*Infections caused by the following miscellaneous microorganisms: Rickettsiae* (Rocky Mountain spotted fever, typhus fever and the typhus group, Q fever, rickettsialpox, and tick fevers); *Mycoplasma pneumoniae* (PPLO, Eaton agent, respiratory tract infections); *Chlamydia trachomatis* (lymphogranuloma venereum, trachoma [infectious agent not always eliminated], inclusion conjunctivitis, uncomplicated urethral, endocervical, or rectal infections); *Chlamydia psittaci* (psittacosis [ornithosis]); *Borrelia* sp. (relapsing fever); *Ureaplasma urealyticum* (nongonococcal urethritis).

➤*Following susceptibility testing (resistance has been documented): Escherichia coli; Enterobacter aerogenes; Acinetobacter* sp.; *Haemophilus influenzae* (respiratory tract infections); *Klebsiella* sp. (respiratory and urinary infections); *Streptococcus pneumoniae* (upper respiratory tract infections); *S. pyogenes, S. pneumoniae, Mycoplasma pneumoniae* (Eaton agent), and *Klebsiella* sp. (lower respiratory tract infections); *Staphylococcus aureus, S. pyogenes* (skin and skin structure infections); *Bacteroides* and *Shigella* sp.

➤*Alternative therapy for the following infections when penicillin is contraindicated:* Uncomplicated gonorrhea due to *Neisseria gonorrhoeae*-;syphilis due to *Treponema pallidum*; yaws due to *T. pertenue*; *Listeria monocytogenes*; anthrax due to *Bacillus anthracis*; Vincent's infection due to *Fusobacterium fusiforme*; actinomycosis due to *Actinomyces* sp.; *Clostridium* sp.

➤*Acute intestinal amebiasis:* Due to *Entamoeba histolytica* as adjunct to amebicides.

➤*Severe acne (tetracycline, doxycycline, minocycline only):* As adjunctive therapy.

➤*Anthrax, including inhalational anthrax (doxycline only):* To reduce the incidence or progression of disease following exposure to aerosolized *Bacillus anthracis*.

➤*Malaria (doxycycline only):* Prophylaxis of malaria due to *Plasmodium falciparum* in short-term travelers (less than 4 months) to areas with chloroquine and/or pyrimethamine-sulfadoxine resistant strains.

➤*Neisseria meningitidis (minocycline only):* Treatment of asymptomatic meningococcal carriers of *N. meningitidis*.

➤*Note:* Do not use tetracyclines for streptococcal disease unless organism has been shown to be susceptible. Tetracyclines are not the drugs of choice in treatment of any type of staphylococcal infection.

➤*Unlabeled uses:*

Tetracycline – In conjunction with metronidazole for the treatment of extraintestinal amebiasis caused by *E. histolytica*; gonococcal arthritis; early Lyme disease; malaria; ocular rosacea; adjunctive therapy for peptic ulcers due to *Helicobacter pylori* (500 mg 4 times/day).

Doxycycline – Treatment of malaria (100 mg twice daily for 7 days in combination with other antimalarial agents), pleural malignant effusions, alternative agent for nocardiosis in patients who cannot take sulfa medications, ocular rosacea, treatment of traveler's diarrhea, prophylaxis of pneumothorax.

Lyme disease:
- *Tick bite from endemic area* – 200 mg once.
- *Early Lyme disease* – 100 mg twice daily for 14 to 21 days.
- *Carditis (first degree AV block)* – 100 mg twice daily for 14 to 21 days.
- *Facial nerve paralysis* – 100 mg twice daily for 14 to 21 days.
- *Arthritis* – 100 mg twice daily for 30 to 60 days.

CDC recommended treatment schedules for sexually transmitted diseases:
- *Granuloma inguinale (donovanosis)* – 100 mg twice daily for at least 3 weeks.
- *Early syphilis* – 100 mg twice daily for 14 days.
- *Latent syphilis* – 100 mg twice daily for 28 days.
- *Chlamydial infections* –
  Adults and children (8 years of age and older): 100 mg twice daily for 7 days.
- *Pelvic inflammatory disease* – 100 mg orally or IV every 12 hours plus cefotetan 2 g IV every 12 hours or cefoxitin 2 g IV every 6 hours. May discontinue parenteral therapy after 24 hours; continue oral therapy with doxycycline for a total of 14 days.
- *Epididymitis most likely caused by gonococcal or chlamydial infection* – 100 mg twice daily for 10 days plus a single dose of ceftriaxone 250 mg IM.
- *Sexual assault prophylaxis* – 100 mg twice daily for 7 days plus ceftriaxone and metronidazole.

Minocycline – Treatment of early rheumatoid arthritis, gallbladder infections caused by *E. coli*, alternative agent for nocardiosis in patients who cannot take sulfa medications, chronic malignant pleural effusion.

Demeclocycline – Treatment of the syndrome of inappropriate antidiuretic hormone (SIADH).

Administration and Dosage

Avoid rapid IV administration. Thrombophlebitis may result from prolonged IV therapy.

Continue therapy at least 24 to 48 hours after symptoms and fever subside. Treat all infections caused by group A β-hemolytic streptococci for 10 days or more.

Take on an empty stomach, at least 2 hours before or after meals. Absorption and peak plasma levels may be reduced when administered with meals or with dairy products, including milk.

Administer oral tetracyclines with plenty of fluids.

Actions

➤*Pharmacology:* The tetracyclines are bacteriostatic. They exert their antimicrobial effect by reversibly binding to the 30S subunit of the bacterial ribosome, preventing the binding of aminoacyl transfer RNA and inhibiting protein synthesis and thus cell growth. Tetracyclines are active against a wide range of gram-positive and gram-negative organisms and have similar antimicrobial spectra, and cross-resistance is common.

➤*Pharmacokinetics:*

Absorption / Distribution – Tetracyclines are adequately but incompletely absorbed from the GI tract. The percentage absorbed when taken on an empty stomach is lowest for **demeclocycline**, and **tetracycline**, and highest for **doxycycline** and **minocycline**. The extent of absorption is usually decreased by the presence of divalent and trivalent cations and to a variable degree by milk or food (see Drug Interactions). Tetracyclines are bound to plasma proteins in varying degrees.

Penetration of the tetracyclines into most body fluids and tissues is excellent. Tetracyclines are distributed in varying amounts into bile, liver, lung, kidney, prostate, urine, CSF, synovial fluid, mucosa of the maxillary sinus, brain, sputum, and bone. Inflammation of the meninges is not required for passage into the CSF, but concentrations may increase in the presence of inflamed meninges. Tetracyclines cross the placenta and enter the fetal circulation and amniotic fluid.

Metabolism / Excretion – The tetracyclines are concentrated in the bile by the liver. They are excreted in the urine and feces at high concentrations in a biologically active form. Because renal clearance of tetracyclines is by glomerular filtration, excretion is significantly affected by the state of renal function. The renal clearance of **demeclocycline** has been shown to be about half of that of tetracycline. The urinary and fecal recovery of **minocycline** is one half to one third that of other tetracyclines, and minocycline also appears to undergo some metabolism, largely to 9-hydroxyminocycline. **Doxycycline** appears to be excreted extensively by the digestive tract.

Tetracycline Pharmacokinetics

Tetracyclines	Absorption (%)	C_{max} (mcg/mL)	T_{max} (h)	Protein binding (%)	Serum half-life (h)	Excreted in urine (%)
Demeclocycline	60% to 80%	1.5 to 1.7[a]	3 to 4[a]	35% to 90%	16	nd[b]
Doxycycline	90% to 100%	2.6 (hyclate)[c] 3.61 (monohydrate)[c] 3.6 (IV)[d]	2 (hyclate)[c] 2.6 (monohydrate)[c]	80% to 95%	18 to 22	40%
Minocycline	90% to 100%	2.1 to 5.1[e]	1 to 4	75%	11 to 22 (oral) 15 to 23 (IV)	5% to 10%
Tetracycline	60% to 80%	nd	2 to 4	20% to 65%	6 to 12	20% to 55%

[a] 300 mg single oral dose.
[b] nd = no data
[c] 200 mg single oral dose.
[d] 200 mg administered IV over 2 hours.
[e] Single oral dose of two 100 mg pellet-filled capsules.

➤*Microbiology:*

Organisms Generally Susceptible to Tetracyclines[a]

	Organism	Demeclocycline	Doxycycline	Minocycline	Tetracycline
Gram-positive	*Actinomyces* sp.	✓	✓	✓	✓
	Alpha-hemolytic streptococci (Viridans group)		✓	✓	✓
	Bacillus anthracis		✓	✓	✓
	Clostridium sp.	✓	✓	✓	✓
	Enterococcus faecalis[b,c]		✓	✓	✓
	E. faecium		✓	✓	✓
	Listeria monocytogenes	✓	✓	✓	✓
	Propionibacterium acnes		✓	✓	✓
	Staphylococcus aureus[d]	✓	✓	✓	✓
	Streptococcus pneumoniae[b]	✓	✓	✓	✓
	S. pyogenes[b,e]	✓	✓	✓	✓
	Treponema pallidum	✓	✓	✓	✓
	T. pertenue	✓	✓	✓	✓

Organisms Generally Susceptible to Tetracyclines[a]

	Organism	Demeclocycline	Doxycycline	Minocycline	Tetracycline
Gram-negative	*Acinetobacter* sp.[b]	✓	✓	✓	✓
	Bacteroides sp.[b]	✓	✓	✓	✓
	Bartonella bacilliformis	✓	✓	✓	✓
	Borrelia recurrentis	✓	✓	✓	✓
	Brucella sp.	✓	✓	✓	✓
	Calymmatobacterium granulomatis	✓	✓	✓	✓
	Campylobacter fetus	✓	✓	✓	✓
	Enterobacter aerogenes[b]	✓	✓	✓	✓
	Escherichia coli[b]	✓	✓	✓	✓
	Francisella tularensis	✓	✓	✓	✓
	Fusobacterium fusiforme	✓	✓	✓	✓
	Haemophilus ducreyi	✓	✓	✓	✓
	H. influenzae[b]	✓	✓	✓	✓
	Klebsiella sp.[b]	✓	✓	✓	✓
	Neisseria gonorrhoeae	✓	✓	✓	✓
	N. meningitides		✓	✓	
	Shigella sp.[b]	✓	✓	✓	✓
	Vibrio cholerae	✓	✓	✓	✓
	Yersinia pestis	✓	✓	✓	✓
Miscellaneous	*Balantidium coli*		✓	✓	✓
	Chlamydia psittaci	✓	✓	✓	✓
	C. trachomatis	✓	✓	✓	✓
	Entamoeba sp.	✓	✓	✓	✓
	Mycobacterium marinum			✓	
	Mycoplasma pneumoniae	✓	✓	✓	✓
	Plasmodium falciparum[f]		✓		
	Rickettsiae sp.	✓	✓	✓	✓
	Ureaplasma urealyticum		✓	✓	✓

[a] Cross-resistance of these organisms to tetracyclines is common.
[b] Because many strains of gram-negative micro-organisms have been shown to be resistant to tetracyclines, culture and susceptibility testing are recommended.
[c] Up to 74% of *Enterococcus faecalis* have been found to be resistant to tetracyclines.
[d] Tetracyclines are not the drugs of choice in the treatment of any type of staphylococcal infections.
[e] Up to 44% of *Streptococcus pyogenes* have been found to be resistant to tetracycline drugs.
[f] Doxycycline has been found to be active against the asexual erythrocytic form of *Plasmodium falciparum* but not against the gametocytes of *P. falciparum*.

Contraindications

Hypersensitivity to any of the tetracyclines or components of product formulations.

Warnings

➤*Malaria prophylaxis (doxycycline only):* **Doxycycline** offers substantial, but not complete, suppression of the asexual stages of *Plasmodium* strains. It does not suppress *P. falciparum*'s sexual blood stage gametocytes, and patients completing this prophylactic regimen may still transmit the infection to mosquitos outside endemic areas. Advise patients taking doxycycline for malaria prophylaxis as to when prophylaxis should begin and end; that no present-day antimalarial, including doxycycline, guarantees protection against malaria; and to avoid being bitten by mosquitos (eg, wear protective clothing, use effective insect-repellent and mosquito nets).

➤*Pseudomembranous colitis:* Treatment with antibacterial agents alters the normal flora of the colon and may permit overgrowth of clostridia. Pseudomembranous colitis has been reported with nearly all antibacterial agents and may range in severity from mild to life-threatening. It is important to consider this diagnosis in patients who present with diarrhea following subsequent administration of antibacterial agents. Once the diagnosis is established, initiate therapeutic measures. Mild cases usually respond to discontinuation of the drug. Moderate to severe cases may require management with fluids, electrolytes, protein supplementation, and treatment with an antibacterial agent effective against *Clostridium difficile* colitis.

➤*Parenteral therapy:* Reserve for situations in which oral therapy is not indicated. Institute oral therapy as soon as possible. If given IV over prolonged periods, thrombophlebitis may result. IM use produces lower blood levels than recommended oral dosages. If high blood levels are needed rapidly, administer IV.

➤*Nephrogenic diabetes insipidus:* Administration of **demeclocycline** has resulted in appearance of the diabetes insipidus syndrome (eg, polyuria, polydipsia, weakness) in some patients on long-term therapy. The syndrome has been shown to be nephrogenic, dose-dependent, and reversible on discontinuation of therapy.

➤*Hypersensitivity reactions:* Sensitivity reactions are more likely to occur in patients with a history of allergy, asthma, hay fever, or urticaria. Use tetracyclines with caution in these patients. Cross-sensitivity among the tetracyclines is extremely common.

➤*Renal function impairment:* Use tetracyclines with caution in patients with impaired renal function.

If renal impairment exists, even usual doses may lead to excessive systemic accumulation of the tetracyclines (with the exception of **doxycycline**) and possible liver toxicity. Use lower than usual doses; if therapy is prolonged, drug serum level determinations may be advisable. Concurrent use of tetracycline and methoxyflurane has resulted in fatal renal toxicity.

The antianabolic action of tetracyclines may cause an increase in blood urea nitrogen. In significantly impaired renal function, higher serum tetracycline levels may lead to azotemia, hyperphosphatemia, and acidosis. This does not seem to occur with doxycycline.

➤*Hepatic function impairment:* Use tetracyclines with caution in patients with impaired liver function.

In the presence of renal dysfunction, and particularly in pregnancy, IV tetracycline more than 2 g/day has been associated with death secondary to liver failure. When need for intensive treatment outweighs its potential dangers (especially during pregnancy or in known or suspected renal and liver impairment), monitor renal and liver function tests. Serum tetracycline concentrations should not exceed 15 mcg/mL. Do not prescribe other potentially hepatotoxic drugs concomitantly.

Hepatotoxicity has been reported with **minocycline**; therefore, minocycline should be used with caution in patients with hepatic dysfunction and in conjunction with other hepatotoxic drugs.

The hazard of liver toxicity is of particular importance in parenteral administration to pregnant or postpartum patients with pyelonephritis.

➤*Carcinogenesis:* There has been evidence of oncogenic activity in studies with **minocycline** (thyroid tumors) in rats and dogs.

➤*Mutagenesis:* **Tetracycline** has produced positive mutagenic results in mammalian cell assays in vitro.

➤*Fertility impairment:* **Minocycline** has been shown to impair fertility in male rats.

➤*Pregnancy: Category D.* Tetracyclines readily cross the placenta, are found in fetal tissues, and can have toxic effects on the developing fetus (retardation of skeletal development). Evidence of embryotoxicity has also been noted in animals treated early in pregnancy.

A case-control study (18,515 mothers of infants with congenital anomalies and 32,804 mothers of infants with no congenital anomalies) shows a weak but marginally statistically significant association with total malformations and use of **doxycycline** any time during pregnancy. Sixty-three (0.19%) of the controls and 56 (0.3%) of the cases were treated with doxycycline. This association was not seen when the analysis was confined to maternal treatment during the period of organogenesis with the exception of a marginal relationship with neural tube defect based on only 2 exposed cases.

➤*Lactation:* Tetracyclines are excreted in breast milk. Milk:plasma ratios vary between 0.25 and 1.5. Because of the potential for serious adverse reactions, decide whether to discontinue nursing or the drug.

➤*Children:* Generally, do not use tetracyclines in children younger than 8 years of age (except for anthrax, including inhalational) unless other drugs are not likely to be effective or are contraindicated.

Teeth – The use of tetracyclines during the period of tooth development (from the last half of pregnancy through 8 years of age) may cause permanent discoloration (yellow, gray, brown) of teeth. This adverse reaction is more common during long-term use of the drugs, but has been observed following repeated short-term courses. Enamel hypoplasia has also been reported.

Bone – Tetracyclines form a stable calcium complex in any bone-forming tissue. Decreased fibula growth rate occurred in premature infants given oral tetracycline 25 mg/kg every 6 hours. This was reversible when the drug was discontinued.

Precautions

➤*Monitoring:* In sexually transmitted diseases when coexistent syphilis is suspected, perform darkfield examination before starting treatment and repeat the blood serology monthly for at least 4 months.

In long-term therapy, perform periodic laboratory evaluation of organ systems, including hematopoietic, renal, and hepatic studies.

➤*CNS effects:* In adults, pseudotumor cerebri (benign intracranial hypertension) has been associated with tetracycline use. Usual clinical manifestations are headache and blurred vision. Bulging fontanels have been associated with tetracycline use in infants. While both conditions and related symptoms usually resolve soon after tetracycline discontinuation, the possibility for permanent sequelae exists.

➤*Outdated products:* Under no circumstances should outdated tetracyclines be administered; the degradation products of tetracyclines are highly nephrotoxic and have, on occasion, produced a Fanconi-like syndrome.

➤*Hazardous tasks:* Light-headedness, dizziness, or vertigo may occur with tetracyclines. Advise patients to observe caution while driving or performing other tasks requiring alertness. These symptoms may disappear during therapy and always disappear rapidly when the drug is discontinued.

➤*Superinfection:* Use of antibiotics (especially prolonged or repeated therapy) may result in bacterial or fungal overgrowth of nonsusceptible organisms. Such overgrowth may lead to a secondary infection. Take appropriate measures if superinfection occurs. Superinfection of the bowel by staphylococci may be life-threatening.

➤*Photosensitivity:* Photosensitivity manifested by an exaggerated sunburn reaction has been observed in some individuals taking tetracyclines. Advise patients who are apt to be exposed to direct sunlight or ultraviolet light that this reaction can occur with tetracycline drugs, and discontinue treatment at the first evidence of skin erythema.

Exaggerated sunburn reactions are characterized by severe burns of exposed surfaces, resulting from direct exposure to sunlight during therapy with moderate or large doses. Phototoxic reactions are most frequent with demeclocycline and occur less frequently with the other tetracyclines.

➤*Sulfite sensitivity:* Some of these products contain sulfites that may cause allergic-type reactions (eg, anaphylactic symptoms, life-threatening or less severe asthmatic episodes) in certain susceptible people. The overall prevalence of sulfite sensitivity in the general population is unknown and probably low. It is seen more frequently in asthmatic or atopic nonasthmatic people. Specific products containing sulfites are identified in the product listings.

Drug Interactions

Tetracycline Drug Interactions

Precipitant drug	Object drug[a]		Description
Antacids (containing aluminum, calcium or magnesium salts) Iron salts Zinc salts	Tetracyclines	⬇	Tetracyclines administered with aluminum, calcium, magnesium, iron, or zinc salts form an insoluble chelate, thereby decreasing the absorption and serum levels of the tetracycline. Administer tetracyclines at least 2 hours before or after these agents.
Barbiturates	Doxycycline	⬇	Barbiturates increase the hepatic metabolism of doxycycline, therefore decreasing doxycycline's half-life and serum levels. Adjust doxycycline dose as needed. Consider using an alternative tetracycline.
Bismuth salts	Tetracyclines	⬇	Coadministration of bismuth salts in liquid formulations may decrease the serum levels of tetracyclines. Give the bismuth salt 2 hours after the tetracycline.
Carbamazepine	Doxycycline	⬇	Carbamazepine may decrease the half-life and serum levels of doxycycline because of increased hepatic metabolism. Adjust doxycycline dose as needed. Consider using an alternative tetracycline.
Cholestyramine Colestipol	Tetracyclines	⬇	Coadministration may decrease or delay the absorption of tetracyclines, therefore decreasing the serum concentrations. Adjust the tetracycline dose if needed.
Phenytoin Rifamycins	Doxycycline	⬇	Phenytoin and rifamycins appear to induce the metabolism of doxycycline, causing the half-life to be significantly decreased. Increased doxycycline dosage may be needed.
Urinary alkalinizers (eg, sodium lactate, potassium citrate)	Tetracyclines	⬇	Coadministration may result in increased excretion of the tetracyclines and decreased serum levels. Separate administration by 3 to 4 hours; however, this may not be effective, and an increase in tetracycline dose may be necessary if the pH of the urine remains increased.
Tetracyclines	Anticoagulants, oral	⬆	The action of oral anticoagulants may be increased because of the elimination of vitamin K-producing gut bacteria by tetracyclines. Monitor coagulation parameters and adjust anticoagulant dose as needed.
Tetracyclines	Contraceptives, oral	⬇	Tetracyclines may interfere with the enterohepatic recirculation of certain contraceptive steroids, leading to reduced efficacy. Although infrequently reported, contraceptive failure is possible.
Tetracyclines	Digoxin	⬆	Coadministration may result in increased serum levels of digoxin in a small subset of patients (≈ 10%). Monitor digoxin levels and signs of toxicity.
Tetracyclines	Insulin	⬆	The ability of insulin to produce hypoglycemia may be potentiated. In diabetic patients, monitor blood glucose concentrations closely and tailor the insulin regimen as needed.
Tetracyclines	Isotretinoin	⬆	Isotretinoin use has been associated with a number of cases of pseudotumor cerebri, some of which involved coadministration of tetracyclines. Therefore, avoid concomitant use.
Tetracyclines	Methoxyflurane	⬆	Coadministration may enhance the risk for renal toxicity; deaths have been reported. Do not coadminister. If possible seek alternative agents.
Tetracyclines	Penicillins	⬇	The bacteriostatic action of tetracyclines may interfere with the bactericidal activity of penicillins. Consider avoiding this combination if at all possible.
Tetracyclines	Theophyllines	⬆	The incidence of adverse reactions to theophyllines may be increased. Monitor theophylline levels and adjust dose as needed.

[a] ⬆ = Object drug increased. ⬇ = Object drug decreased.

➤*Drug/Lab test interactions:* During **doxycycline** or **minocycline** therapy, false elevations of urinary catecholamine levels may occur because of interference with the fluorescence test.

➤*Drug/Food interactions:* The administration of **demeclocycline** and **tetracycline** with milk and dairy products forms poorly absorbed chelates. A number of studies have reported the serum levels of these tetracyclines, when administered with milk products, to be 50% to 80% lower. Administer the interacting tetracyclines at least 2 hours before or after meals. The inhibitory effect of food and milk on the absorption of **doxycycline** and **minocycline** is considerably less than that observed with the other tetracycline derivatives. These 2 drugs are often administered without regard to meals, but the potential risk of decreased drug efficacy must be weighed against the benefit of treating the infection. The administration of doxycycline with a high-fat meal has been shown to delay the time to peak plasma concentrations by an average 1 hour 20 minutes. Peak plasma concentrations of doxycycline were also decreased by up to 20% with simultaneous ingestion of dairy products or a high-fat, high-protein meal. The peak plasma concentration of minocycline was slightly decreased and delayed by 1 hour when administered with food, compared with dosing under fasting conditions.

Adverse Reactions

The following adverse reactions have been reported with the tetracyclines.

➤*Oral:*

CNS – Bulging fontanel, convulsions, dizziness, headache, hypesthesia, paresthesia, pseudotumor cerebri, sedation, vertigo; myasthenic syndrome (**demeclocycline**; rare).

Dermatologic – Alopecia, balanitis, erythema multiforme, erythema nodosum, fixed drug eruptions, hyperpigmentation of the nails, maculopapular and erythematous rashes, photosensitivity, pruritus, skin and mucus membrane pigmentation, Stevens-Johnson syndrome, toxic epidermal necrolysis, vasculitis; exfoliative dermatitis (rare).

GI – Anorexia, diarrhea, dyspepsia, dysphagia, enamel hypoplasia, enterocolitis, esophageal ulcerations, esophagitis, glossitis, inflammatory lesions (with monilial overgrowth) in the anogenital region, nausea, pancreatitis, pseudomembranous colitis, stomatitis, vomiting; black hairy tongue, bulky loose stools, hoarseness, sore throat (**tetracycline**).

Due to oral **minocycline** and **doxycycline**'s virtually complete absorption, adverse reactions of the lower bowel, particularly diarrhea, have been infrequent.

Hematologic – Anemia, eosinophilia, hemolytic anemia, neutropenia, thrombocytopenia.

Hepatic – Hepatic cholestasis, hepatic toxicity, hyperbilirubinemia, increased liver enzymes; hepatic failure, hepatitis (rare).

Hypersensitivity – Anaphylactoid purpura, anaphylaxis, angioneurotic edema, pericarditis, polyarthralgia, pulmonary infiltrates with eosinophilia, systemic lupus erythematosus exacerbation, urticaria.

Musculoskeletal – Arthralgia, arthritis, bone discoloration, joint stiffness and swelling, myalgia.

Renal – Acute renal failure, dose-related increase in BUN, interstitial nephritis; nephrogenic diabetes insipidus (**demeclocycline**).

Respiratory – Asthma exacerbation, bronchospasm, cough, dyspnea.

Miscellaneous – Brown-black microscopic discoloration of thyroid glands (prolonged therapy), decreased hearing, fever, lupus-like syndrome, secretion discoloration, serum sickness-like syndrome, tooth discoloration, tinnitus, vulvovaginitis.

➤*Parenteral:*

CNS – Bulging fontanels, convulsions, dizziness, headache, hypesthesia, paresthesia, pseudotumor cerebri, sedation, vertigo.

Dermatologic – Alopecia, balanitis, erythema multiforme, erythema nodosum, fixed drug eruptions, hyperpigmentation of the nails, injection site erythema and injection site pain, maculopapular and erythematous rashes, photosensitivity, pruritus, skin and mucus membrane pigmentation, Stevens-Johnson syndrome, toxic epidermal necrolysis, vasculitis; exfoliative dermatitis (rare).

GI – Anorexia, diarrhea, dyspepsia, dysphagia, enamel hypoplasia, enterocolitis, glossitis, inflammatory lesions (with monilial overgrowth) in the anogenital region, pancreatitis, pseudomembranous colitis, nausea, stomatitis, vomiting.

Hematologic – Agranulocytosis, eosinophilia, hemolytic anemia, leukopenia, neutropenia, thrombocytopenia, pancytopenia.

Hepatic – Hepatic cholestasis, hepatitis, hyperbilirubinemia, increased liver enzymes, jaundice, liver failure.

Hypersensitivity – Anaphylactoid purpura, anaphylaxis, angioneurotic edema, exacerbation of systemic lupus erythematosus, myocarditis, pericarditis, pulmonary infiltrates, urticaria.

Musculoskeletal – Arthralgia, arthritis, bone discoloration, joint stiffness and swelling, myalgia, polyarthralgia.

Renal – Dose-related increase in BUN; acute renal failure, interstitial nephritis (**minocycline**).

Respiratory – Asthma exacerbation, bronchospasm, cough, dyspnea.

Miscellaneous – Brown-black microscopic discoloration of thyroid glands (prolonged therapy); hypersensitivity syndrome (cutaneous reaction, eosinophilia, and one or more of the following: fever, hepatitis, lymphadenopathy, myocarditis, nephritis, pericarditis, pneumonitis), lupus-like syndrome, secretion discoloration, serum sickness-like syndrome, tinnitus, tooth discoloration, vulvovaginitis.

Overdosage

➤*Symptoms:* Dizziness, nausea, and vomiting are the most commonly seen adverse reactions in overdosage situations.

➤*Treatment:* Discontinue medication and institute appropriate symptomatic treatment and supportive measures. Tetracyclines are not significantly removed by hemodialysis or peritoneal dialysis.

Patient Information

Advise patients to take medicine on an empty stomach, at least 2 hours before or after meals, with full glass of water (240 mL).

Instruct patients to avoid simultaneous dairy products (milk, cheese), antacids, laxatives, or iron-containing products. If these items must be taken, instruct them to take at least 2 hours before or 2 hours after tetracyclines.

Concurrent use of tetracyclines with oral contraceptives may render oral contraceptives less effective (see Drug Interactions).

Advise patients to avoid prolonged exposure to sunlight or sunlamps; tetracyclines may cause photosensitivity.

Caution patients who experience CNS symptoms about driving vehicles or using hazardous machinery while receiving therapy.

Advised patients to discard unused supplies of tetracycline antibiotics by the expiration date.

TETRACYCLINE HYDROCHLORIDE

Rx	**Tetracycline** (Various, eg, Ivax)	**Capsules:** 250 mg	In 100s, 1000s, and UD 100s.
Rx	**Sumycin '250'** (Par)		Mineral oil, lactose. (SQUIBB 655). Pink. In 100s and 1000s.
Rx	**Tetracycline HCl** (Various, eg, Ivax)	**Capsules:** 500 mg	In 100s, 1000s, and UD 100s.
Rx	**Sumycin '500'** (Par)		Mineral oil, lactose. (SQUIBB 763). Pink/White. In 100s and 500s.
Rx	**Sumycin Syrup** (Par)	**Oral Suspension:** 125 mg/5 mL	Saccharin, sodium metabisulfite, sorbitol, sucrose. Fruit flavor. In 473 mL.

TETRACYCLINE HYDROCHLORIDE — ORAL

Complete and comparative prescribing information for these products begins in the Tetracyclines group monograph.

Indications

➤*Gram-negative organisms: Haemophilus ducreyi* (chancroid); *Francisella tularensis* (tularemia); *Yersinia pestis* (plague); *Bartonella bacilliformis* (bartonellosis); *Campylobacter fetus*; *Vibrio cholerae* (cholera); *Brucella* sp. (in conjunction with streptomycin); *Calymmatobacterium granulomatis* (granuloma inguinale).

➤*Infections caused by the following miscellaneous organisms: Rickettsiae* (Rocky Mountain spotted fever, typhus fever and the typhus group, Q fever, rickettsialpox, tick fevers); *Mycoplasma pneumoniae* (respiratory tract infections); *Chlamydia trachomatis* (lymphogranuloma venereum, trachoma [infectious agent not always eliminated], inclusion conjunctivitis, uncomplicated urethral, endocervical, or rectal infections); *Chlamydia psittaci* (psittacosis [ornithosis]); *Borellia* sp. (relapsing fever); *Ureaplasma urealyticum* (nongonococcal urethritis).

➤*Following susceptibility testing (resistance has been documented) : Escherichia coli*; *Enterobacter aerogenes*; *Acinetobacter* sp.; *Haemophilus influenzae* (upper respiratory tract infections); *Klebsiella* sp. (respiratory and urinary tract infections); *Streptococcus pneumoniae* (upper respiratory infections); *Streptococcus pyogenes*, *S. pneumoniae*, *Mycoplasma pneumoniae* (Eaton agent), and *Klebsiella* sp. (lower respiratory tract infections); *Staphylococcus aureus*, *S. pyogenes* (skin and skin structure infections); *Bacteroides* and *Shigella* sp.

➤*Alternative therapy for the following infections when penicillin is contraindicated:* Uncomplicated gonorrhea due to *Neisseria gonorrhoeae*; syphilis due to *Treponema pallidum*; yaws due to *Treponema pertenue*; *Listeria monocytogenes*; anthrax due to *Bacillus anthracis*; Vincent's infection due to *Fusobacterium fusiforme*; actinomycosis due to *Actinomyces* sp.; *Clostridium* sp.

➤*Acute intestinal amebiasis:* As adjunct to amebicides.

➤*Severe acne:* As adjunctive therapy.

➤*Unlabeled uses:* In conjunction with metronidazole for the treatment of extraintestinal amebiasis caused by *E. histolytica*; gonococcal arthritis; early Lyme disease; malaria; ocular rosacea; adjunctive therapy for peptic ulcers caused by *Helicobacter pylori* (500 mg 4 times/day).

Administration and Dosage

Take with plenty of fluids. Food and some dairy products interfere with the absorption of tetracycline.

TETRACYCLINE HYDROCHLORIDE — ORAL

➤*Adults:* Usual dose: 1 to 2 g/day in 2 or 4 equal doses.

Mild to moderate infections – 500 mg 2 times/day or 250 mg 4 times/day.

Severe infections – 500 mg 4 times/day.

➤*Children (over 8 years of age):* Daily dose is 10 to 20 mg/lb (25 to 50 mg/kg) in 4 equally divided doses.

➤*Brucellosis:* 500 mg 4 times/day for 3 weeks, accompanied by 1 g streptomycin IM twice/day the first week, and once daily the second week.

➤*Syphilis:*

Sumycin only – A total of 30 to 40 g in equally divided doses over 10 to 15 days. Perform close follow-up and laboratory tests.

All except Sumycin –
Early (less than 1 year): 500 mg 4 times/day for 15 days.
More than 1 year duration: 500 mg 4 times/day for 30 days.

CDC recommended treatment schedules for syphilis (penicillin-allergic patients)† –
Early: 500 mg 4 times/day for 14 days.
More than 1 year's duration: 500 mg 4 times/day for 28 days.

➤*Uncomplicated gonorrhea:* 500 mg every 6 hours for 7 days.

➤*Uncomplicated urethral, endocervical, or rectal infections in adults caused by C. trachomatis:* 500 mg 4 times/day for at least 7 days.

➤*Severe acne (long-term therapy):* Initially, 1 g/day in divided doses. For maintenance, give 125 to 500 mg/day. (Alternate-day or intermittent therapy may be adequate in some patients.)

➤*Streptococcal infections:* Treat for at least 10 days.

➤*Concomitant therapy:* Absorption is impaired by antacids containing aluminum, calcium, or magnesium, and preparations containing iron, zinc, or sodium bicarbonate.

➤*Renal function impairment:* Decrease recommended dosages and/or extend dosing intervals in patients with renal impairment.

➤*Storage/Stability:* Keep tightly closed. Protect from light; avoid excessive heat. Store below 30°C (86°F).

Outdated products – Under no circumstances should outdated tetracyclines be administered, as the degradation of tetracyclines are highly nephrotoxic and have, on occasion, produced a Fanconi-like syndrome.

DEMECLOCYCLINE HYDROCHLORIDE

Rx	**Demeclocycline HCl** (Impax)	**Tablets:** 150 mg	Lactose. (G 2111). In 100s and 500s.
Rx	**Declomycin** (ESP Pharma)		(LL D11). Red. Film-coated. In 100s.
Rx	**Demeclocycline HCl** (Impax)	**Tablets:** 300 mg	Lactose. (G 2122). In 48s, 100s, and 500s.
Rx	**Declomycin** (ESP Pharma)		(LL D12). Red. Film-coated. In 48s.

DEMECLOCYCLINE HYDROCHLORIDE — ORAL

Complete and comparative prescribing information for these products begins in the Tetracyclines group monograph.

Indications

➤*Gram-negative organisms:* *Haemophilus ducreyi* (chancroid); *Francisella tularensis*; *Yersinia pestis*; *Bartonella bacilliformis*; *Campylobacter fetus*; *Vibrio cholerae*; *Brucella* sp. (in conjunction with streptomycin); *Calymmatobacterium granulomatis* (granuloma inguinale).

➤*Infections caused by the following miscellaneous organisms:* *Rickettsiae* (Rocky Mountain spotted fever, typhus fever and the typhus group, Q fever, rickettsialpox, tick fevers); *Mycoplasma pneumoniae* (PPLO, Eaton agent); *Chlamydia trachomatis* (lymphogranuloma venereum, trachoma [infectious agent not always eliminated], inclusion conjunctivitis); *Chlamydia psittaci* (psittacosis [ornithosis]); *Calymmatobacterium granulomatis* (granuloma inguinale); *Borellia recurrentis* (relapsing fever); *Bacteroides* sp.

➤*Following susceptibility testing (resistance has been documented)*: *Escherichia coli*; *Enterobacter aerogenes*; *Acinetobacter* sp.; *Haemophilus influenzae* (respiratory tract infections); *Klebsiella* sp. (respiratory and urinary tract infections); *Streptococcus pneumoniae* (upper respiratory infections); *Streptococcus pyogenes*, *S. pneumoniae*, *Mycoplasma pneumoniae* (Eaton agent) and *Klebsiella* sp. (lower respiratory tract infections); *Staphylococcus aureus* (skin and skin structure infections); *Streptococcus pyogenes*; *Shigella* sp.

➤*Alternative therapy for the following infections when penicillin is contraindicated:* *Neisseria gonorrhoeae*; syphilis due to *Treponema pallidum*; yaws due to *Treponema pertenue*; *Listerial monocytogenes*; anthrax due to *Bacillus anthracis*; Vincent's infection due to *Fusobacterium fusiforme*; *Actinomyces* sp.; *Clostridium* sp.

➤*Acute intestinal amebiasis:* As an adjunct to amebicides.

➤*Unlabeled uses:* Treatment of the syndrome of inappropriate antidiuretic hormone (SIADH).

Administration and Dosage

Take with plenty of fluids. Foods and some dairy products interfere with absorption; take demeclocycline at least 1 hour before or 2 hours after meals or dairy products.

➤*Adults:*

Daily dose – 4 divided doses of 150 mg each or 2 divided doses of 300 mg each.

➤*Children (over 8 years of age):*

Usual daily dose – 3 to 6 mg/lb (6.6 to 13.2 mg/kg), depending upon the severity of the disease, divided into 2 or 4 doses.

➤*Gonorrhea patients sensitive to penicillin:* Initially, 600 mg; follow with 300 mg every 12 hours for 4 days to a total of 3 g.

➤*Streptococcal infections:* Treat streptococcal infections for at least 10 days.

➤*Concomitant therapy:* Absorption is impaired by antacids containing aluminum, calcium, or magnesium, and by preparations containing iron. Take demeclocycline at least 1 hour before or 2 hours after these products.

➤*Renal/Hepatic function impairment:* Administer tetracyclines cautiously with renal or hepatic impairment; reduce the recommended dosage and/or extend the dosing interval.

➤*Storage/Stability:* Store at controlled room temperature 20° to 25°C (68° to 77°F).

DOXYCYCLINE

Rx	**Doxycycline** (Lannett Company, Inc.)	**Tablets:** 20 mg (as hyclate)	Lactose. (LCI 1336). White. Film-coated. In 60s, 100s, and 1,000s.
Rx	**Periostat** (CollaGenex)		Lactose. (PS 20). White. In 60s, 100s, and 1000s.
Rx	**Doxycycline** (Lannett Company, Inc.)	**Tablets:** 50 mg (as monohydrate)	Corn starch, lactose. (LCI 1335). Yellow. Film-coated. In 100s.
Rx	**Adoxa** (Bioglan)		(B 728). Yellow. Film-coated. In 100s.
Rx	**Adoxa** (Bioglan)	**Tablets:** 75 mg (as monohydrate)	(B 730). Lt. orange. Film-coated. In 100s and 500s.
Rx	**Doxycycline** (Lannett Company, Inc.)	**Tablets:** 100 mg (as monohydrate)	Corn starch, lactose. (LCI 1338). Yellow. Film-coated. In 50s and 250s.
Rx	**Adoxa** (Bioglan)		(B 729). Yellow. Film-coated. In 50s and 250s.
Rx	**Doxycycline** (Various, eg, Ivax, Watson)	**Tablets:** 100 mg (as hyclate)	In 50s, 100s, 200s, 500s and UD 100s.
Rx	**Vibra-Tabs** (Pfizer)		(VIBRA-TABS PFIZER 099). Salmon. Film-coated. In 50s.
Rx	**Doryx** (Warner Chilcott)	**Tablets, delayed-release:** 75 mg (as hyclate)	Lactose. (D75). White, oval. In 60s.
		100 mg (as hyclate)	Lactose. (D100). White, oval. In 100s.
Rx	**Oracea** (CollaGenex)	**Capsules:** 40 mg (30 mg immediate release and 10 mg delayed release)	Sugar spheres. (CGPI 40). Beige opaque. In 30s.
Rx	**Doxycycline** (Various, eg, Ivax, Watson)	**Capsules:** 50 mg (as hyclate)	In 50s and 500s.

† *MMWR.* 2002 May 10;51 (No. RR-6):1-84.

DOXYCYCLINE

Rx	**Doxycycline Monohydrate** (Watson)	**Capsules**: 50 mg (as monohydrate)	(WATSON 410 50 mg). White/Ivory opaque. In 100s.
Rx	**Monodox** (Oclassen)		(MONODOX 50 M 260). White/ yellow. In 100s.
Rx	**Doxycycline** (Various, eg, Ivax, Watson)	**Capsules**: 100 mg (as hyclate)	In 50s, 500s, and UD 100s.
Rx	**Vibramycin** (Pfizer)		(VIBRA PFIZER 095). Lt. blue. In 50s.
Rx	**Doxycycline Monohydrate** (Watson)	**Capsules**: 100 mg (as monohydrate)	(WATSON 411 100 mg). Ivory/Brown opaque. In 50s and 250s.
Rx	**Monodox** (Oclassen)		(MONODOX 100 M 259). Yellow/brown. In 50s and 250s.
Rx	**Doryx** (Warner Chilcott)	**Capsules, coated pellets**: 75 mg (as hyclate)	(DORYX 75). Orange/Green. In 60s.
		100 mg (as hyclate)	(DORYX WC). Dk. yellow/lt. blue. In 50s.
Rx	**Vibramycin** (Pfizer)	**Powder for Oral Suspension**: 25 mg (as monohydrate) per 5 mL when reconstituted	Parabens, sucrose. Raspberry flavor. In 60 mL.
Rx	**Vibramycin** (Pfizer)	**Syrup**: 50 mg (as calcium) per 5 mL	Parabens, sodium metabisulfite, sorbitol. Apple-raspberry flavor. In 473 mL.
Rx	**Atridox** (CollaGenex)	**Injection**: 42.5 mg (as hyclate, 10%)	In 2 syringe mixing system[1] and blunt cannula.
Rx	**Doxycycline** (Various, eg, Bedford)	**Powder for Injection, lyophilized**: 100 mg (as hyclate)	In vials.
Rx	**Doxy 100** (APP)		300 mg mannitol. In vials.
Rx	**Doxy 200** (APP)	**Powder for Injection, lyophilized**: 200 mg (as hyclate)	600 mg mannitol. In vials.

DOXYCYCLINE CALCIUM — ORAL

Complete and comparative prescribing information for these products begins in the Tetracyclines group monograph.

Indications

➤*Treatment of infections caused by miscellaneous organisms:* Rocky mountain spotted fever, typhus fever and the typhus group; Q fever, rickettsialpox, and tick fevers caused by Rickettsiae; respiratory tract infections caused by *Mycoplasma pneumoniae*; lymphogranuloma venereum caused by *Chlamydia trachomatis*; psittacosis (ornithosis) caused by *Chlamydia psittaci*; trachoma caused by *Chlamydia trachomatis*, although the infectious agent is not always eliminated as judged by immunofluorescence; inclusion conjunctivitis caused by *Chlamydia trachomatis*; uncomplicated urethral, endocervical or rectal infections in adults caused by *Chlamydia trachomatis*; nongonococcal urethritis caused by *Ureaplasma urealyticum*; and relapsing fever due to *Borrelia recurrentis*.

➤*Treatment of infections caused by gram-negative microorganisms:* Chancroid caused by *Haemophilus ducreyi*; plague due to *Yersinia pestis*; tularemia due to *Francisella tulerensis*; cholera caused by *Vibrio cholerae*; campylobacter fetus infections caused by *Campylobacter fetus*; brucellosis due to *Brucella* species (in conjunction with streptomycin); bartonellosis due to *Bartonella bacilliformis*; and granuloma inguinale caused by *Calymmatobacterium granulomatis*.

➤*Following susceptibility testing (resistance has been documented):* *Escherichia coli*; *Enterobacter aerogenes*; *Shigella* species; *Acinetobacter* species; respiratory tract infections caused by *Haemophilus influenzae*; respiratory tract and urinary tract infections caused by *Klebsiella* species; and upper respiratory tract infections caused by *Streptococcus pneumoniae*.

➤*Anthrax including inhalational anthrax:* Due to *Bacillus anthracis*, including inhalational anthrax (postexposure), to reduce the incidence or progression of disease following exposure to aerosolized *Bacillus anthracis*.

➤*Alternative therapy for infections when penicillin is contraindicated:*Uncomplicated gonorrhea caused by *Neisseria gonorrhoeae*; syphilis caused by *Treponema pallidum*; yaws caused by *Treponema pertenue*; listeriosis due to *Listeria monocytogenes*; Vincent's infection caused by *Fusobacterium fusiforme*; actinomycosis caused by *Actinomyces israelii*; and infections caused by *Clostridium* species

➤*Acute intestinal amebiasis:* In acute intestinal amebiasis, doxycycline may be a useful adjunct to amebicides.

➤*Severe acne:* In severe acne, doxycycline may be useful adjunctive therapy.

➤*Malaria prophylaxis:* Doxycycline is indicated for the prophylaxis of malaria due to *Plasmodium falciparum* in short-term travelers (under 4 months) to areas with chloroquine or pyrimethamine-sulfadoxine resistant strains. For adults, the recommended dose is 100 mg daily. For children over 8 years of age, the recommended dose is 2 mg/kg given once daily up to the adult dose. Prophylaxis should begin 1 to 2 days before travel to the malarious area. Prophylaxis should be continued daily during travel in the malarious area and for 4 weeks after the traveler leaves the malarious area.

➤*Unlabeled uses:* Treatment of malaria (100 mg twice daily for 7 days in combination with other antimalarial agents); pleural malignant effusions; alternative agent for nocardiosis in patients who cannot take sulfa medications; ocular rosacea; treatment of traveler's diarrhea; prophylaxis of pneumothorax.

Lyme disease –
Tick bite from endemic area: 200 mg once.
Early Lyme disease: 100 mg twice daily for 14 to 21 days.
Carditis (first degree AV block): 100 mg twice daily for 14 to 21 days.
Facial nerve paralysis: 100 mg twice daily for 14 to 21 days.
Arthritis: 100 mg twice daily for 30 to 60 days.

CDC recommended treatment schedules for sexually transmitted diseases –
Granuloma inguinale (donovanosis): 100 mg twice daily for at least 3 weeks.
Early syphilis: 100 mg twice daily for 14 days.
Latent syphilis: 100 mg twice daily for 28 days.
Chlamydial infections (adults and children 8 years of age and older): 100 mg twice daily for 7 days.
Pelvic inflammatory disease: 100 mg orally or IV every 12 hours plus cefotetan 2 g IV every 12 hours or cefoxitin 2 g IV every 6 hours. May discontinue parenteral therapy after 24 hours; continue oral therapy with doxycycline for a total of 14 days.
Epididymitis most likely caused by gonococcal or chlamydial infection: 100 mg twice daily for 10 days plus a single dose of ceftriaxone 250 mg IM.
Sexual assault prophylaxis: 100 mg twice daily for 7 days plus ceftriaxone and metronidazole.

Administration and Dosage

➤*Administration:* Administration of adequate amounts of non-dairy fluid along with capsule and tablet forms of drugs in the tetracycline class is recommended to wash down the drugs and reduce the risk of esophageal irritation and ulceration.

Absorption and peak plasma levels may be reduced when administered with meals or with dairy products, including milk.

If GI upset occurs, administration with a small amount of a low-fat, low-protein, non-dairy food may reduce upset, but the potential risk of decreased drug efficacy must be weighed against the benefit of treating the infection with this antibiotic.

➤*Adults:* The usual dose of oral doxycycline is 200 mg on the first day of treatment (administered 100 mg every 12 hours) followed by a maintenance dose of 100 mg/day. The maintenance dose may be administered as a single dose or as 50 mg every 12 hours.

Severe infections – In the management of more severe infections (particularly chronic infections of the urinary tract), 100 mg every 12 hours is recommended.

➤*Children older than 8 years of age:* The recommended dosage schedule for children weighing less than or equal to 100 pounds is 2 mg/lb of body weight divided into 2 doses on the first day of treatment, followed by 1 mg/lb of body weight given as a single daily dose or divided into 2 doses, on subsequent days. For more severe infections up to 2 mg/lb of body weight may be used. For children greater than 100 lbs, the usual adult dose should be used.

➤*Streptococcal infections:* When used in streptococcal infections, therapy should be continued for 10 days.

➤*Uncomplicated gonococcal infections in adults (except anorectal infections in men):* 100 mg, by mouth, twice a day for 7 days. As an alternate single visit dose, administer 300 mg immediately followed in 1 hour by a second 300 mg dose.

➤*Uncomplicated urethral, endocervical, or rectal infection in adults caused by Chlamydia trachomatis:* 100 mg by mouth twice a day for 7 days.

➤*Nongonococcal urethritis (NGU) caused by C. trachomatis or U. urealyticum:* 100 mg by mouth twice a day for 7 days.

➤*Syphilis (early):* Patients who are allergic to penicillin should be treated with doxycycline 100 mg by mouth twice a day for 2 weeks.

➤*Syphilis of more than 1 year's duration:* Patients who are allergic to penicillin should be treated with doxycycline 100 mg by mouth twice a day for 4 weeks.

➤*Acute epididymo-orchitis caused by N. gonorrhoeae:* 100 mg, by mouth, twice a day for at least 10 days.

➤*Acute epididymo-orchitis caused by C. trachomatis:* 100 mg, by mouth, twice a day for at least 10 days.

➤*Malaria prophylaxis:* For adults, the recommended dose is 100 mg daily. For children over 8 years of age, the recommended dose is 2 mg/kg given once daily up to the adult dose. Prophylaxis should begin 1 to 2 days

DOXYCYCLINE CALCIUM — ORAL

before travel to the malarious area. Prophylaxis should be continued daily during travel in the malarious area and for 4 weeks after the traveler leaves the malarious area.

➤*Inhalational anthrax (postexposure):*

Adults – 100 mg of doxycycline, by mouth, twice a day for 60 days.

Children – Children weighing less than 100 lbs (45 kg); 1 mg/lb (2.2 mg/kg) of body weight, by mouth, twice a day for 60 days. Children weighing 100 lb or more should receive the adult dose.

➤*CDC recommended treatment schedules for sexually transmitted diseases†:*

Granuloma inguinale (donovanosis) – 100 mg twice daily for at least 3 weeks.

Syphilis in patients allergic to penicillins –
Early syphilis: 100 mg twice daily for 14 days.
Latent syphilis: 100 mg twice daily for 28 days.

Chlamydial infections –
Adults and children (8 years of age or older): 100 mg twice daily for 7 days.

Pelvic inflammatory disease – 100 mg orally or IV every 12 hours plus 2 g cefotetan IV every 12 hours or 2 g cefoxitin IV every 6 hours. May discontinue parenteral therapy after 24 hours; continue oral therapy with doxycycline for a total of 14 days.

Epididymitis most likely caused by gonococcal or chlamydial infection – 100 mg twice daily for 10 days plus a single dose of 250 mg ceftriaxone IM.

Sexual assault prophylaxis – 100 mg twice daily for 7 days plus ceftriaxone and metronidazole.

Lymphogranuloma venereum – 100 mg twice daily for at least 21 days.

Nongonococcal urethritis – 100 mg twice daily for 7 days.

➤*Storage/Stability:* All products are to be stored below 30°C (86°F) and dispensed in tight, light-resistant containers.

DOXYCYCLINE HYCLATE — ORAL

Complete and comparative prescribing information for these products begins in the Tetracyclines group monograph.

Indications

➤*Treatment of infections caused by miscellaneous organisms:* Rocky mountain spotted fever, typhus fever and the typhus group, Q fever, rickettsialpox, and tick fevers caused by Rickettsiae; *Mycoplasma pneumoniae* (PPLO, Eaton's agent); respiratory tract infections caused by *Mycoplasma pneumoniae*; lymphogranuloma venereum caused by *Chlamydia trachomatis* and granuloma inguinale; psittacosis (ornithosis) caused by *Chlamydia psittaci*; trachoma caused by *Chlamydia trachomatis*, although the infectious agent is not always eliminated as judged by immunofluorescence; inclusion conjunctivitis caused by *Chlamydia trachomatis*; uncomplicated urethral, endocervical or rectal infections in adults caused by *Chlamydia trachomatis*; nongonococcal urethritis caused by *Ureaplasma urealyticum*; and relapsing fever due to *Borrelia recurrentis*.

➤*Treatment of the following infections caused by gram-negative microorganisms:* Chancroid caused by *Haemophilus ducreyi*; plague due to *Yersinia pestis* (formerly *Pasteurella pestis*); tularemia due to *Francisella tularensis* (formerly *Pasteurella tularensis*); cholera caused by *Vibrio cholerae* (formerly *Vibrio comma*); campylobacter fetus infections caused by *Campylobacter fetus* (formerly *Vibrio fetus*); brucellosis due to *Brucella* species (in conjunction with streptomycin); Bartonellosis due to *Bartonella bacilliformis*; *Bacteroides* species; and granuloma inguinale caused by *Calymmatobacterium granulomatis*.

➤*Following susceptibility testing (resistance has been documented)* : *Escherichia coli*; *Enterobacter aerogenes* (formerly *Aerobacter aerogenes*); *Shigella* species; *Acinetobacter* species (formerly *Mima* species and *Herellea* species); respiratory tract infections caused by *Haemophilus influenzae*; Respiratory tract and urinary tract infections caused by *Klebsiella* species; upper respiratory tract infections caused by *Streptococcus pneumoniae* (formerly *Diplococcus pneumoniae*); and*Streptococcus* species. Up to 44% of strains of *Streptococcus pyogenes* and 74% of *Streptococcus faecalis* have been found to be resistant to tetracycline drugs. Therefore, tetracyclines should not be used for streptococcal disease unless the organism has been demonstrated to be susceptible. For upper respiratory tract infections due to group A beta-hemolytic streptococci, penicillin is the usual drug of choice, including prophylaxis of rheumatic fever. *Staphylococcus aureus* (respiratory, skin and soft-tissue infections); tetracyclines are not the drug of choice in the treatment of any type of staphylococcal infection.

➤*Anthrax, including inhalational anthrax:* Due to *Bacillus anthracis*, including inhalational anthrax (postexposure), to reduce the incidence or progression of disease following exposure to aerosolized *Bacillus anthracis*.

➤*Alternative therapy when penicillin is contraindicated:* Uncomplicated gonorrhea caused by *Neisseria gonorrhoeae*; syphilis caused by *Treponema pallidum*; yaws caused by *Treponema pertenue*; listeriosis due to *Listeria monocytogenes*; anthrax due to *Bacillus anthracis*; Vincent's infection caused by *Fusobacterium fusiforme*; actinomycosis caused by *Actinomyces israelii*; and infections caused by *Clostridium* species.

➤*Acute intestinal amebiasis:* In acute intestinal amebiasis, doxycycline may be a useful adjunct to amebicides.

➤*Severe acne:* In severe acne, doxycycline may be useful adjunctive therapy.

➤*Trachoma:* Treatment of trachoma, although the infectious agent is not always eliminated, as judged by immunofluorescence.

➤*Inclusion conjunctivitis:* Inclusion conjunctivitis may be treated with oral doxycycline alone, or with a combination of topical agents.

➤*Uncomplicated urethral, endocervical or rectal infections:* Doxycycline is indicated for the treatment of uncomplicated urethral, endocervical or rectal infections in adults caused by *Chlamydia trachomatis*.

➤*Nongonococcal urethritis:* Doxycycline is indicated for the treatment of nongonococcal urethritis caused by *Chlamydia trachomatis* and *Ureaplasma urealyticum* and for the treatment of acute epididymo-orchitis caused by *Chlamydia trachomatis*.

➤*Uncomplicated gonococcal infections:* For the treatment of uncomplicated gonococcal infections in adults (except for anorectal infections in men), the gonococcal arthritis-dermatitis syndrome and acute epididymo-orchitis caused by *N. gonorrhoeae*.

➤*Malaria prophylaxis:* Doxycycline is indicated for the prophylaxis of malaria due to *Plasmodium falciparum* in short-term travelers (under 4 months) to areas with chloroquine or pyrimethamine-sulfadoxine resistant strains.

➤*Periostat* tablets: Doxycycline hyclate is indicated for use as an adjunct to scaling and root planing to promote attachment level gain and to reduce pocket depth in patients with adult periodontitis.

➤*Unlabeled uses:* Treatment of malaria (100 mg twice daily for 7 days in combination with other antimalarial agents); pleural malignant effusions; alternative agent for nocardiosis in patients who cannot take sulfa medications; ocular rosacea; treatment of traveler's diarrhea; prophylaxis of pneumothorax.

Lyme disease –
Tick bite from endemic area: 200 mg once.
Early Lyme disease: 100 mg twice daily for 14 to 21 days.
Carditis (first degree AV block): 100 mg twice daily for 14 to 21 days.
Facial nerve paralysis: 100 mg twice daily for 14 to 21 days.
Arthritis: 100 mg twice daily for 30 to 60 days.

CDC recommended treatment schedules for sexually transmitted diseases –
Granuloma inguinale (donovanosis): 100 mg twice daily for at least 3 weeks.
Early syphilis: 100 mg twice daily for 14 days.
Latent syphilis: 100 mg twice daily for 28 days.
Chlamydial infections (adults and children 8 years of age and older): 100 mg twice daily for 7 days.
Pelvic inflammatory disease: 100 mg orally or IV every 12 hours plus cefotetan 2 g IV every 12 hours or cefoxitin 2 g IV every 6 hours. May discontinue parenteral therapy after 24 hours; continue oral therapy with doxycycline for a total of 14 days.
Epididymitis most likely caused by gonococcal or chlamydial infection: 100 mg twice daily for 10 days plus a single dose of ceftriaxone 250 mg IM.
Sexual assault prophylaxis: 100 mg twice daily for 7 days plus ceftriaxone and metronidazole.

Administration and Dosage

➤*Approved by the FDA:* February 29, 1982.

➤*Concomitant therapy:* Antacids containing aluminum, calcium or magnesium, sodium bicarbonate and iron-containing preparations should not be given to patients using oral tetracyclines.

➤*Adults:* The usual dose of oral doxycycline is 200 mg on the first day of treatment (administered 100 mg every 12 hours) followed by a maintenance dose of 100 mg/day. The maintenance dose may be administered as a single dose or as 50 mg every 12 hours.

In the management of more severe infections (particularly chronic infections of the urinary tract), 100 mg every 12 hours is recommended.

➤*Children older than 8 years of age:* The recommended dosage schedule for children weighing less than or equal to 100 pounds is 2 mg/lb of body weight divided into 2 doses on the first day of treatment, followed by 1 mg/lb of body weight given as a single daily dose or divided into 2 doses, on subsequent days. For more severe infections, up to 2 mg/lb of body weight may be used. For children over 100 lbs, the usual adult dose should be used.

➤*Streptococcal infections:* When used in streptococcal infections, therapy should be continued for 10 days.

➤*Administration:* Administration of adequate amounts of non-dairy fluid with capsule and tablet forms of drugs in the tetracycline class is recommended to wash down the drugs and reduce the risk of esophageal irritation and ulceration.

Absorption and peak plasma levels may be reduced when administered with meals or with dairy products, including milk.

† *MMWR*. 2002 May 10;51 (No. RR-6):1-84.

DOXYCYCLINE HYCLATE — ORAL

If GI upset occurs, administration with a small amount of a low-fat, low-protein, non-dairy food may reduce upset, but the potential risk of decreased drug efficacy must be weighed against the benefit of treating the infection with this antibiotic.

➤*Uncomplicated gonococcal infections in adults (except anorectal infections in men):* 100 mg orally twice a day for 7 days. As an alternate single-visit dose, administer 300 mg immediately followed in 1 hour by a second 300 mg dose. The dose may be administered with food, including carbonated beverage, as required.

➤*Uncomplicated urethral, endocervical, or rectal infection in adults caused by Chlamydia trachomatis:* 100 mg orally twice a day for 7 days.

➤*Nongonococcal urethritis (NGU) caused by C. trachomatis or U. urealyticum:* 100 mg orally twice a day for 7 days.

➤*Syphilis (early):* Patients who are allergic to penicillin should be treated with doxycycline 100 mg by mouth twice a day for 2 weeks.

➤*Syphilis of more than 1 year's duration:* Patients who are allergic to penicillin should be treated with doxycycline 100 mg by mouth twice a day for 4 weeks.

➤*Acute epididymo-orchitis caused by N. gonorrhoeae:* 100 mg orally twice a day for at least 10 days.

➤*Acute epididymo-orchitis caused by C. trachomatis:* 100 mg orally twice a day for at least 10 days.

➤*Prophylaxis of malaria:* For adults, the recommended dose is 100 mg daily. For children over 8 years of age, the recommended dose is 2 mg/kg given once daily up to the adult dose. Prophylaxis should begin 1 to 2 days before travel to the malarious area. Prophylaxis should be continued daily during travel in the malarious area and for 4 weeks after the traveler leaves the malarious area.

➤*Inhalational anthrax (postexposure):*

Adults – 100 mg of doxycycline orally twice a day for 60 days.

Children –
Less than 100 lbs (45 kg): Children weighing less than 100 lbs (45 kg) should take 1 mg/lb (2.2 mg/kg) of body weight, by mouth, twice a day for 60 days.
100 lbs or more: Children weighing 100 lb or more should receive the adult dose.

➤*Coated pellets:*

Primary and secondary syphilis – 300 mg/day in divided doses for at least 10 days.

Sprinkling the capsule contents (coated pellets) on applesauce – Doxycycline hyclate coated pellet capsules may also be administered by carefully opening the capsules and sprinkling the capsule contents onto a spoonful of applesauce. However, any loss of pellets in the transfer would prevent using the dose. The applesauce should be swallowed immediately without chewing and followed with a cool 240 mL glass of water to ensure complete swallowing of the capsule contents. The applesauce should not be hot, and it should be just enough to be swallowed without chewing. In the event that a prepared dose of applesauce and doxycycline hyclate coated pellet capsules cannot be taken immediately, the mixture should be discarded and not stored for later use.

➤*Periostat* tablets: The dosage of *Periostat* differs from that of doxycycline used to treat infections. Exceeding the recommended dosage may result in an increased incidence of side effect, including the development of resistant microorganisms.

Periostat 20 mg twice daily as an adjunct following scaling and root planing may be administered for up to 9 months. *Periostat* should be taken twice daily at 12-hour intervals, usually in the morning and evening. It is recommended that if *Periostat* tablets are taken close to meal times, patients should allow at least 1 hour prior to or 2 hours after meals. Safety beyond 12 months and efficacy beyond 9 months have not been established.

➤*CDC recommended treatment schedules for sexually transmitted diseases†:*

Granuloma inguinale (donovanosis) – 100 mg twice daily for at least 3 weeks.

Syphilis in patients allergic to penicillins –
Early syphilis: 100 mg twice daily for 14 days.
Latent syphilis: 100 mg twice daily for 28 days.

Chlamydial infections –
Adults and children (8 years of age or older): 100 mg twice daily for 7 days.

Pelvic inflammatory disease – 100 mg orally or IV every 12 hours plus 2 g cefotetan IV every 12 hours or 2 g cefoxitin IV every 6 hours. May discontinue parenteral therapy after 24 hours; continue oral therapy with doxycycline for a total of 14 days.

Epididymitis most likely caused by gonococcal or chlamydial infection – 100 mg twice daily for 10 days plus a single dose of 250 mg ceftriaxone IM.

Sexual assault prophylaxis – 100 mg twice daily for 7 days plus ceftriaxone and metronidazole.

Lymphogranuloma venereum – 100 mg twice daily for at least 21 days.

Nongonococcal urethritis – 100 mg twice daily for 7 days.

➤*Storage / Stability:*

Capsules and tablets – Store at controlled room temperature below 30°C (86°F) and dispense in a tight, light-resistant container.

Coated pellets – Store at controlled room temperature below 25°C (77°F).

Periostat tablets – Store at controlled room temperatures of 15° to 30°C (59° to 86°F) and dispense in tight, light-resistant container.

DOXYCYCLINE MONOHYDRATE — ORAL

Complete and comparative prescribing information for these products begins in the Tetracyclines group monograph.

Indications

➤*Treatment of infections caused by miscellaneous organisms:* Rocky mountain spotted fever, typhus fever and the typhus group, Q fever, rickettsialpox, and tick fevers caused by Rickettsiae; respiratory tract infections caused by *Mycoplasma pneumoniae*; lymphogranuloma venereum caused by *Chlamydia trachomatis*; psittacosis (ornithosis) caused by *Chlamydia psittaci*; trachoma caused by *Chlamydia trachomatis*, although the infectious agent is not always eliminated as judged by immunofluorescence; inclusion conjunctivitis caused by *Chlamydia trachomatis*; uncomplicated urethral, endocervical, or rectal infections in adults caused by *Chlamydia trachomatis*; nongonococcal urethritis caused by *Ureaplasma urealyticum*; and relapsing fever due to *Borrelia recurrentis*.

➤*Treatment of the following infections caused by gram-negative microorganisms:* Chancroid caused by *Haemophilus ducreyi*; plague due to *Yersinia pestis* (formerly *Pasteurella pestis*); tularemia due to *Francisella tularensis* (formerly *Pasteurella tularensis*); cholera caused by *Vibrio cholerae* (formerly *Vibrio comma*); campylobacter fetus infections caused by *Campylobacter fetus* (formerly *Vibrio fetus*); brucellosis due to *Brucella* species (in conjunction with streptomycin); bartonellosis due to *Bartonella bacilliformis*; and granuloma inguinale caused by *Calymmatobacterium granulomatis*.

➤*Susceptibility testing (resistance has been documented): Escherichia coli*; *Enterobacter aerogenes* (formerly *Aerobacter aerogenes*); *Shigella* species and *Acinetobacter* species (formerly *Mima* species and *Herellea* species); respiratory tract infections caused by *Haemophilus influenzae*; respiratory tract and urinary tract infections caused by *Klebsiella* species; upper respiratory tract infections caused by *Streptococcus pneumoniae*; and skin and skin structure infections caused by *Staphylococcus aureus*. Doxycycline is not the drug of choice in the treatment of any type of staphylococcal infections.

➤*Anthrax, including inhalational anthrax:* Due to *Bacillus anthracis*, including inhalational anthrax (postexposure): To reduce the incidence or progression of disease following exposure to aerosolized *Bacillus anthracis*.

➤*Alternative therapy when penicillin is contraindicated:* Uncomplicated gonorrhea caused by *Neisseria gonorrhoeae*; syphilis caused by *Treponema pallidum*; yaws caused by *Treponema pertenue*; listeriosis due to *Listeria monocytogenes*; Vincent's infection caused by *Fusobacterium fusiforme*; actinomycosis caused by *Actinomyces israelii*; and infections caused by *Clostridium* species.

➤*Acute intestinal amebiasis:* Doxycycline may be a useful adjunct to amebicides.

➤*Severe acne:* In severe acne, doxycycline may be useful adjunctive therapy.

➤*Malaria prophylaxis:* For the prophylaxis of malaria due to *Plasmodium falciparum* in short-term travelers (under 4 months) to areas with chloroquine or pyrimethamine-sulfadoxine resistant strains.

➤*Unlabeled uses:* Treatment of malaria (100 mg twice daily for 7 days in combination with other antimalarial agents); pleural malignant effusions; alternative agent for nocardiosis in patients who cannot take sulfa medications; ocular rosacea; treatment of traveler's diarrhea; prophylaxis of pneumothorax.

Lyme disease –
Tick bite from endemic area: 200 mg once.
Early Lyme disease: 100 mg twice daily for 14 to 21 days.
Carditis (first degree AV block): 100 mg twice daily for 14 to 21 days.
Facial nerve paralysis: 100 mg twice daily for 14 to 21 days.
Arthritis: 100 mg twice daily for 30 to 60 days.

CDC recommended treatment schedules for sexually transmitted diseases –
Granuloma inguinale (donovanosis): 100 mg twice daily for at least 3 weeks.
Early syphilis: 100 mg twice daily for 14 days.
Latent syphilis: 100 mg twice daily for 28 days.
Chlamydial infections (adults and children 8 years of age and older): 100 mg twice daily for 7 days.
Pelvic inflammatory disease: 100 mg orally or IV every 12 hours plus cefotetan 2 g IV every 12 hours or cefoxitin 2 g IV every 6 hours. May discontinue parenteral therapy after 24 hours; continue oral therapy with doxycycline for a total of 14 days.

† *MMWR*. 2002 May 10;51 (No. RR-6):1-84.

DOXYCYCLINE MONOHYDRATE — ORAL

Epididymitis most likely caused by gonococcal or chlamydial infection: 100 mg twice daily for 10 days plus a single dose of ceftriaxone 250 mg IM.

Sexual assault prophylaxis: 100 mg twice daily for 7 days plus ceftriaxone and metronidazole.

Administration and Dosage

➤*Adults:*

More severe infections – In the management of more severe infections (particularly chronic infections of the urinary tract), 100 mg every 12 hours is recommended.

➤*Children older than 8 years of age:* The recommended dosage schedule for children weighing 100 pounds or less is 2 mg/lb of body weight divided into 2 doses on the first day of treatment, followed by 1 mg/lb of body weight given as a single daily dose or divided into 2 doses, on subsequent days. For more severe infections, up to 2 mg/lb of body weight may be used. For children over 100 lbs, the usual adult dose should be used.

➤*Streptococcal infections:* When used in streptococcal infections, therapy should be continued for 10 days.

➤*Administration:* Absorption and peak plasma levels may be reduced when administered with meals or with dairy products, including milk.

If GI upset occurs, administration with a small amount of a low-fat, low-protein, non-dairy food may reduce upset, but the potential risk of decreased drug efficacy must be weighed against the benefit of treating the infection with this antibiotic.

➤*Uncomplicated gonococcal infections in adults (except anorectal infections in men):* 100 mg, orally, twice a day for 7 days. As an alternate single visit dose, administer 300 mg immediately followed in 1 hour by a second 300 mg dose.

➤*Uncomplicated urethral, endocervical, or rectal infection in adults caused by Chlamydia trachomatis:* 100 mg orally twice a day for 7 days.

➤*Nongonococcal urethritis (NGU) caused by C. trachomatis or U. urealyticum:* 100 mg orally twice a day for 7 days.

➤*Early syphilis:* Patients who are allergic to penicillin should be treated with doxycycline 100 mg orally twice a day for 2 weeks.

➤*Syphilis of more than 1 year's duration:* Patients who are allergic to penicillin should be treated with doxycycline 100 mg orally twice a day for 4 weeks.

➤*Acute epididymo-orchitis caused by N. gonorrhoeae:* 100 mg orally twice a day for at least 10 days.

➤*Acute epididymo-orchitis caused by C. trachomatis:* 100 mg orally twice a day for at least 10 days.

➤*Malaria prophylaxis:* For adults, the recommended dose is 100 mg daily. For children over 8 years of age, the recommended dose is 2 mg/kg given once daily up to the adult dose. Prophylaxis should begin 1 to 2 days before travel to the malarious area. Prophylaxis should be continued daily during travel in the malarious area and for 4 weeks after the traveler leaves the malarious area.

➤*Primary and secondary syphilis:* 300 mg a day in divided doses for at least 10 days.

➤*Inhalational anthrax (postexposure):*

Adults – 100 mg of doxycycline, by mouth, twice a day for 60 days.

Children – Weighing less than 100 lb (45 kg); 1 mg/lb (2.2 mg/kg) of body weight, by mouth, twice a day for 60 days. Children weighing 100 lb or more should receive the adult dose. Administration of adequate amounts of fluid along with capsule and tablet forms of drugs in the tetracycline class is recommended to wash down the drugs and reduce the risk of esophageal irritation and ulceration. Most of these patients took medications immediately before going to bed. Absorption and peak plasma levels may be reduced when administered with meals or with dairy products, including milk. If GI upset occurs, administration with a small amount of a low-fat, low-protein, non-dairy food may reduce upset, but the potential risk of decreased drug efficacy must be weighed against the benefit of treating the infection with this antibiotic. Ingestion of a high-fat meal has been shown to delay the time to peak plasma concentrations by an average of 1 hour and 20 minutes. However, in the same study, food enhanced the average peak concentration by 7.5% and the area under the curve by 5.7%.

➤*CDC recommended treatment schedules for sexually transmitted diseases†:*

Granuloma inguinale (donovanosis) – 100 mg twice daily for at least 3 weeks.

Syphilis in patients allergic to penicillins –
Early syphilis: 100 mg twice daily for 14 days.
Latent syphilis: 100 mg twice daily for 28 days.

Chlamydial infections –
Adults and children (8 years of age or older): 100 mg twice daily for 7 days.

Pelvic inflammatory disease – 100 mg orally or IV every 12 hours plus 2 g cefotetan IV every 12 hours or 2 g cefoxitin IV every 6 hours. May discontinue parenteral therapy after 24 hours; continue oral therapy with doxycycline for a total of 14 days.

Epididymitis most likely caused by gonococcal or chlamydial infection – 100 mg twice daily for 10 days plus a single dose of 250 mg ceftriaxone IM.

Sexual assault prophylaxis – 100 mg twice daily for 7 days plus ceftriaxone and metronidazole.

Lymphogranuloma venereum – 100 mg twice daily for at least 21 days.

Nongonococcal urethritis – 100 mg twice daily for 7 days.

➤*Storage/Stability:* All products are to be stored at controlled room temperature 15° to 30°C (59° to 86°F) and dispensed in tight, light-resistant containers. The unit-dose packs should also be stored in a dry place.

DOXYCYCLINE HYCLATE — INJECTION

Complete and comparative prescribing information for these products begins in the Tetracyclines group monograph.

Indications

➤*Infections caused by miscellaneous organisms: Rickettsiae* (Rocky Mountain spotted fever, typhus fever, and the typhus group, Q fever, rickettsialpox and tick fevers); *Mycoplasma pneumoniae* (PPLO, Eaton Agent); agents of psittacosis and ornithosis; agents of lymphogranuloma venereum and granuloma inguinale; and the spirochetal agent of relapsing fever (*Borrelia recurrentis*).

➤*Infections caused by gram-negative microorganisms: Haemophilus ducreyi* (chancroid); *Pasteurella pestis* and *Pasteurella tularensis*; *Bartonella bacilliformis*; *Bacteroides* species; *Vibrio comma* and *Vibrio fetus*; and *Brucella* species (in conjunction with streptomycin).

➤*Infections following susceptibility testing (resistance has been documented): Escherichia coli*; *Enterobacter aerogenes* (formerly *Aerobacter aerogenes*); *Shigella* species; *Mima* species and *Herellea* species; *Haemophilus influenzae* (respiratory infections); *Klebsiella* species (respiratory and urinary infections); *Diplococcus pneumoniae*.

Staphylococcus aureus, respiratory, skin and soft tissue infections. Tetracyclines are not the drugs of choice in the treatment of any type of staphylococcal infections.

Streptococcus species – Up to 44% of strains of *Streptococcus pyogenes* and 74% of *Streptococcus faecalis* have been found to be resistant to tetracycline drugs. Therefore, tetracyclines should not be used for streptococcal disease unless the organism has been demonstrated to be sensitive.

For upper respiratory tract infections due to group A beta-hemolytic streptococci, penicillin is the usual drug of choice, including prophylaxis of rheumatic fever.

➤*Alternative therapy when penicillin is contraindicated: Neisseria gonorrhoeae* and *N. meningitidis*; *Treponema pallidum* and *Treponema pertenue* (syphilis and yaws); *Listeria monocytogenes*; *Clostridium* species; *Bacillus anthracis*; *Fusobacterium fusiforme* (Vincent's infection); and *Actinomyces* species.

➤*Acute intestinal amebiasis:* In acute intestinal amebiasis, doxycycline may be a useful adjunct to amebicides.

➤*Trachoma:* Doxycycline is indicated in the treatment of trachoma, although the infectious agent is not always eliminated, as judged by immunofluorescence.

➤*Atridox* only: For chronic adult periodontitis for a gain in clinical attachment, reduction in probing depth, and reduction in bleeding on probing.

Administration and Dosage

➤*Approved by the FDA:* December 9, 1983.

Rapid administration is to be avoided. Parenteral therapy is indicated only when oral therapy is not indicated. Oral therapy should be instituted as soon as possible. If IV therapy is given over prolonged periods of time, thrombophlebitis may result.

The usual dosage and frequency of administration of doxycycline IV (100 to 200 mg/day) differs from that of the other tetracyclines (1 to 2 g/day). Exceeding the recommended dosage may result in an increased incidence of side effects.

➤*Streptococcal infections:* Because tetracyclines have been shown to depress plasma prothrombin activity, patients who are on anticoagulant therapy may require downward adjustment of their anticoagulant dosage.

➤*Adults:* The usual dosage of doxycycline IV is 200 mg on the first day of treatment administered in 1 or 2 infusions. Subsequent daily dosage is 100 to 200 mg depending upon the severity of infection, with 200 mg administered in 1 or 2 infusions.

Syphilis – In the treatment of primary and secondary syphilis, the recommended dosage is 300 mg daily for at least 10 days.

Inhalational anthrax – In the treatment of inhalational anthrax if strain is susceptible (postexposure), the recommended dose is 100 mg of doxycycline, twice a day. Parenteral therapy is only indicated when oral therapy is not indicated and should not be continued over a prolonged period of time. Oral therapy should be instituted as soon as possible. Therapy must continue for a total of 60 days.

† *MMWR*. 2002 May 10;51 (No. RR-6):1-84.

DOXYCYCLINE HYCLATE — INJECTION

➤*Children older than 8 years of age:* The recommended dosage schedule for children weighing 100 pounds or less is 2 mg/lb of body weight on the first day of treatment, administered in 1 or 2 infusions. Subsequent daily dosage is 1 to 2 mg/lb of body weight given as 1 or 2 infusions, depending on the severity of the infection. For children over 100 pounds, the usual adult dose should be used.

Inhalational anthrax – In the treatment of inhalational anthrax if strain is susceptible (postexposure), the recommended dose is 1 mg/lb (2.2 mg/kg) of body weight, twice a day in children weighing less than 100 lbs (45 kg). Parenteral therapy is only indicated when oral therapy is not indicated and should not be continued over a prolonged period of time. Oral therapy should be instituted as soon as possible. Therapy must continue for a total of 60 days.

➤*Administration:* The duration of infusion may vary with the dose (100 to 200 mg/day), but is usually 1 to 4 hours. A recommended minimum infusion time for 100 mg of a 0.5 mg/mL solution is 1 hour. Therapy should be continued for at least 24 to 48 hours after symptoms and fever have subsided. The therapeutic antibacterial serum activity will usually persist for 24 hours following recommended dosage. IV solutions should not be injected IM or SC. Caution should be taken to avoid the inadvertent introduction of the IV solution into the adjacent soft tissue.

➤*Preparation of solution:* To prepare a solution containing 10 mg/mL, the contents of the vial should be reconstituted with 10 mL (for the 100 mg/vial container) of Sterile Water for Injection or any of the following 10 IV infusion solutions. Each 100 mg of doxycycline (ie, withdraw entire solution from the 100 mg vial) is further diluted with 100 mL to 1000 mL of the following IV solutions: 0.9% Sodium Chloride Injection; 5% Dextrose Injection; Ringer's Injection; Invert Sugar, 10% in Water; Lactated Ringer's Injection; Dextrose 5% in Lactated Ringer's; *Normosol-M* in D5-W; *Normosol-R* in D5-W; *Plasma-Lyte* 56 in 5% Dextrose; and *Plasma-Lyte* 148 in 5% Dextrose.

This will result in desired concentrations of 0.1 to 1 mg/mL. Concentrations lower than 0.1 mg/mL or higher than 1 mg/mL are not recommended.

➤*Atridox* only: **Doxycycline** injection is a variable-dose product dependent on the size, shape, and number of pockets being treated.

Administration – Doxycycline does not require local anesthesia for placement.

Bend the cannula to resemble a periodontal probe and explore the periodontal pocket in a manner similar to periodontal probing. Keeping the cannula tip near the base of the pocket, express the product into the pocket until the formulation reaches the top of the gingival margin. Withdraw the cannula tip from the pocket. In order to separate the tip from the formulation, turn the tip of the cannula towards the tooth, press the tip against the tooth surface, and pinch the string of formulation from the tip of the cannula. Variations on this technique may be needed to achieve separation between doxycycline and cannula.

If desired, using an appropriate dental instrument, doxycycline may be packed into the pocket. Dipping the edge of the instrument in water before packing will help keep doxycycline from sticking to the instrument and will help speed coagulation of doxycycline. To aid coagulation, put a few drops of water onto the surface of doxycycline once in the pocket. If necessary, add more doxycycline as described above and pack it into the pocket until the pocket is full.

Cover the pockets containing doxycycline with either *Coe-Pak* periodontal dressing or *Octyldent* dental adhesive.

Application of doxycycline may be repeated 4 months after initial treatment.

➤*CDC recommended treatment schedules for sexually transmitted diseases:*

Granuloma inguinale (donovanosis) – 100 mg twice daily for at least 3 weeks.

Syphilis in patients allergic to penicillins –
Early syphilis: 100 mg twice daily for 14 days.
Latent syphilis: 100 mg twice daily for 28 days.

Chlamydial infections –
Adults and children (8 years of age or older): 100 mg twice daily for 7 days.

Pelvic inflammatory disease – 100 mg orally or IV every 12 hours plus 2 g cefotetan IV every 12 hours or 2 g cefoxitin IV every 6 hours. May discontinue parenteral therapy after 24 hours; continue oral therapy with doxycycline for a total of 14 days.

Epididymitis most likely caused by gonococcal or chlamydial infection – 100 mg twice daily for 10 days plus a single dose of 250 mg ceftriaxone IM.

Sexual assault prophylaxis – 100 mg twice daily for 7 days plus ceftriaxone and metronidazole.

Lymphogranuloma venereum – 100 mg twice daily for at least 21 days.

Nongonococcal urethritis – 100 mg twice daily for 7 days.

➤*Storage/Stability:* Store lyophilized product at or below 25°C (77°F) and protect from light.

Atridox – Store at 2° to 8°C (36° to 46°F).

Stability – Doxycycline is stable for 48 hours in solution when diluted with Sodium Chloride Injection or 5% Dextrose Injection to concentrations between 1 and 0.1 mg/mL and stored at 25°C (77°F). Doxycycline in these solutions is stable under fluorescent light for 48 hours, but must be protected from direct sunlight during storage and infusion. Reconstituted solutions (1 to 0.1 mg/mL) may be stored up to 72 hours prior to start of infusion if refrigerated and protected from sunlight and artificial light. Infusion must then be completed within 12 hours. Solutions must be used within these time periods or discarded.

Doxycycline, when diluted with Ringer's injection or Invert Sugar, 10% in Water, or *Normosol-M* in D5-W, or *Normosol-R* in D5-W, or *Plasma-Lyte* 56 in 5% Dextrose, or *Plasma-Lyte* 148 in 5% Dextrose to a concentration between 1 and 0.1 mg/mL, must be completely infused within 12 hours after reconstitution to ensure adequate stability. During infusion, the solution must be protected from direct sunlight. Reconstituted solutions (1 to 0.1 mg/mL) may be stored up to 72 hours prior to start of infusion if refrigerated and protected from sunlight and artificial light. Infusion must then be completed within 12 hours. Solutions must be used within these time periods or discarded.

When diluted with Lactated Ringer's Injection or Dextrose 5% in Lactated Ringer's, infusion of the solution (ca. 1 mg/mL) or lower concentrations (not less than 0.1 mg/mL) must be completed within 6 hours after reconstitution to ensure adequate stability. During infusion, the solution must be protected from direct sunlight. Solutions must be used within this time period or discarded.

Solutions of doxycycline hyclate for injection at a concentration of 10 mg/mL in Sterile Water for Injection, when frozen immediately after reconstitution are stable for 8 weeks when stored at −20°C (−44°F). If the product is warmed, care should be taken to avoid heating it after the thawing is complete. Once thawed, the solution should not be refrozen.

MINOCYCLINE HYDROCHLORIDE

Rx	**Minocycline Hydrochloride** (Par)	**Tablets**: 50 mg (as base)	Lactose. (Par 511). White, capsule shape. Film coated. In 100s and 1,000s.
Rx	**Dynacin** (Medicis)		Lactose. (DYN-50 747). White, capsule shape. Film coated. In 100s and 1,000s.
Rx	**Myrac** (Glades)		Lactose. (STIEFEL 7338). Yellow, oval. Film coated. In 100s.
Rx	**Minocycline Hydrochloride** (Par)	**Tablets**: 75 mg (as base)	Lactose. (Par 512). White, capsule shape. Film coated. In 100s and 1,000s.
Rx	**Dynacin** (Medicis)		Lactose. (DYN-75 748). Gray, capsule shape. Film coated. In 100s and 1,000s.
Rx	**Myrac** (Glades)		Lactose. (STIEFEL 7339). Yellow, oval. Film coated. In 100s.
Rx	**Minocycline Hydrochloride** (Par)	**Tablets**: 100 mg (as base)	Lactose. (Par 513). White, capsule shape. Film coated. In 50s and 1,000s.
Rx	**Dynacin** (Medicis)		Lactose. (DYN-100 749). Dark gray, capsule shape. Film coated. In 50s and 1,000s.
Rx	**Myrac** (Glades)		Lactose. (STIEFEL 7340). Yellow, oval, bisected. Film coated. In 50s.
Rx	**Minocycline Hydrochloride** (Various, eg, Danbury, Global, Ranbaxy, Teva)	**Capsules**: 50 mg (as base)	In 100s.
Rx	**Dynacin** (Medicis)		(0497 DYNACIN 50 mg). White. In 100s, 500s, and 1,000s.
	Minocycline Hydrochloride (Various, eg, Global, Ranbaxy)	**Capsules**: 75 mg (as base)	In 100s.
Rx	**Dynacin** (Medicis)		(0499 DYNACIN 75 mg). Lt. gray. In 100s and 1,000s.
Rx	**Minocycline Hydrochloride** (Various, eg, Danbury, Global, Ranbaxy, Teva)	**Capsules**: 100 mg (as base)	In 50s.
Rx	**Dynacin** (Medicis)		(0498 DYNACIN 100 mg). Dk. gray/white. In 50s, 500s, and 1,000s.
Rx	**Minocin** (Lederle)	**Capsules, pellet filled**: 50 mg (as base)	(M45 Lederle 50 mg). Yellow/Green. In 100s.
		100 mg (as base)	(M46 Lederle 100 mg). Lt. green/Green. In 50s.
		Oral suspension: 50 mg (as base) per 5 mL	5% alcohol, parabens, EDTA, saccharin. Custard flavor. In 60 mL.

MINOCYCLINE HYDROCHLORIDE

Rx	**Arestin** (Cord Logistics)	**Microspheres, sustained-release:** 1 mg (as base)	In UD 12s.

MINOCYCLINE HYDROCHLORIDE — ORAL

Complete and comparative prescribing information for these products begins in the Tetracyclines group monograph.

Indications

➤*Gram-negative organisms: Haemophilus ducreyi* (chancroid); *Francisella tularensis* (tularemia); *Yersinia pestis* (plague); *Bartonella bacilliformis* (bartonellosis); *Campylobacter fetus*; *Vibrio cholerae* (cholera); *Brucella* sp. (in conjunction with streptomycin); *Neisseria gonorrhoeae* (uncomplicated urethritis in men).

➤*Infections caused by the following miscellaneous organisms: Rickettsiae* (Rocky Mountain spotted fever, typhus fever and the typhus group, Q fever, rickettsialpox, tick fevers); *Mycoplasma pneumoniae* (respiratory tract infections); *Chlamydia trachomatis* (lymphogranuloma venereum, trachoma [infectious agent not always eliminated], inclusion conjunctivitis); *Chlamydia psittaci* (psittacosis [ornithosis]); *Borellia recurrentis* (relapsing fever); *Ureaplasma urealyticum* (nongonococcal urethritis).

➤*Following susceptibility testing (resistance has been documented): Escherichia coli*; *Enterobacter aerogenes*; *Acinetobacter* and *Shigella* sp.; *Haemophilus influenzae* (respiratory tract infections); *Klebsiella* sp. (respiratory and urinary tract infections); *Streptococcus pneumoniae* (upper respiratory infections); *Staphylococcus aureus* (skin and skin structure infections).

➤*Alternative therapy for the following infections when penicillin is contraindicated: Neisseria gonorrhoeae* infections; syphilis due to *Treponema pallidum*; yaws due to *Treponema pertenue*; listeriosis due to *Listeria monocytogenes*; anthrax due to *Bacillus anthracis*; Vincent's infection due to *Fusobacterium fusiforme*; actinomycosis due to *Actinomyces israelii*; infections due to *Clostridium* sp.

➤*Acute intestinal amebiasis:* As adjunct to amebicides.

➤*Severe acne:* As adjunctive therapy.

➤*Neisseria meningitidis:* Treatment of asymptomatic meningococcal carriers of *N. meningitidis*.

➤*Unlabeled uses:* Treatment of early rheumatoid arthritis; gallbladder infections caused by *E. coli*; alternative agent for nocardiosis in patients who cannot take sulfa medications; chronic malignant pleural effusion.

Administration and Dosage

May be taken with or without food. Take with plenty of fluids.

➤*Usual dosage:*

Adults – 200 mg initially, followed by 100 mg every 12 hours. If more frequent doses are preferred, give 100 or 200 mg initially; follow with 50 mg, 4 times/day.

Children (over 8 years of age) – Initially, 4 mg/kg; follow with 2 mg/kg every 12 hours.

Syphilis – Administer usual dose over a period of 10 to 15 days. Close follow-up, including laboratory tests, is recommended.

Uncomplicated urethral infections in adults caused by C. trachomatis or Ureaplasma urealyticum – 100 mg every 12 hours for at least 7 days.

Uncomplicated gonococcal urethritis in men – 100 mg every 12 hours for 5 days.

Uncomplicated gonococcal infections except urethritis and anorectal infections in men – 200 mg initially, followed by 100 mg every 12 hours for at least 4 days, with posttherapy cultures within 2 to 3 days.

Meningococcal carrier state – 100 mg every 12 hours for 5 days.

Unlabeled use –

Mycobacterium marinum infections: Although optimal doses are not established, 100 mg every 12 hours for 6 to 8 weeks has been successful in a limited number of cases.

➤*Renal function impairment:* Decrease the recommended dosage and/or increase the dosing intervals in patients with renal impairment. Do not exceed 200 mg *Minocin* in 24 hours in patients with renal impairment.

➤*Storage/Stability:*

Capsules/Suspension – Store at controlled room temperature 15° to 30°C (59° to 86°F). Do not freeze. Protect from light, moisture, and excessive heat.

GLYCYLCYCLINES

TIGECYCLINE

Rx	**Tygacil** (Wyeth)	**Powder for injection, lyophilized:** 50 mg	Preservative-free. In single-dose 5 mL vials.

TIGECYCLINE — INTRAVENOUS

Indications

➤*Bacterial infections:* Tigecycline is indicated for the treatment of infections in patients 18 years of age and older caused by susceptible strains of the designated microorganisms in the following conditions:

Complicated skin and skin structure infections – Complicated skin and skin structure infections caused by *Escherichia coli*, *Enterococcus faecalis* (vancomycin-susceptible isolates only), *Staphylococcus aureus* (methicillin-susceptible and methicillin-resistant isolates), *Streptococcus agalactiae*, *Streptococcus anginosus* group (includes *S. anginosus*, *Streptococcus intermedius*, and *Streptococcus constellatus*), *Streptococcus pyogenes*, and *Bacteroides fragilis*.

Complicated intra-abdominal infections – Complicated intra-abdominal infections caused by *Citrobacter freundii*, *Enterobacter cloacae*, *E. coli*, *Klebsiella oxytoca*, *Klebsiella pneumoniae*, *E. faecalis* (vancomycin-susceptible isolates only), *S. aureus* (methicillin-susceptible isolates only), *S. anginosus* group (includes *S. anginosus*, *S. intermedius*, and *S. constellatus*), *B. fragilis*, *Bacteroides thetaiotaomicron*, *Bacteroides uniformis*, *Bacteroides vulgatus*, *Clostridium perfringens*, and *Peptostreptococcus micros*.

Administration and Dosage

➤*Approved by the FDA:* June 15, 2005.

➤*Dosage:* The recommended dosage regimen for tigecycline is an initial dose of 100 mg, followed by 50 mg every 12 hours. Intravenous (IV) infusions of tigecycline should be administered over approximately 30 to 60 minutes every 12 hours.

➤*Treatment duration:* The recommended duration of treatment with tigecycline for complicated skin and skin structure infections or for complicated intraabdominal infections is 5 to 14 days. The duration of therapy should be guided by the severity and site of the infection, and the patient's clinical and bacteriological progress.

➤*Hepatic function impairment:* No dosage adjustment is warranted in patients with mild to moderate hepatic impairment (Child-Pugh class A and B). In patients with severe hepatic impairment (Child-Pugh class C), the initial dose of tigecycline should be 100 mg, followed by a reduced maintenance dose of 25 mg every 12 hours. Patients with severe hepatic impairment should be treated with caution and monitored for treatment response.

➤*Preparation:* Each vial of tigecycline should be reconstituted with 5.3 mL of 0.9% sodium chloride injection or 5% dextrose injection to achieve a concentration of 10 mg/mL of tigecycline. (Note: Each vial contains a 6% overage. Thus, 5 mL of reconstituted solution is equivalent to 50 mg of the drug.) The vial should be gently swirled until the drug dissolves. Immediately withdraw 5 mL of the reconstituted solution from the vial and add to a 100 mL IV bag for infusion (for a 100 mg dose, reconstitute 2 vials; for a 50 mg dose, reconstitute 1 vial). The maximum concentration in the IV bag should be 1 mg/mL. The reconstituted solution should be yellow to orange in color; if not, the solution should be discarded. Parenteral drug products should be inspected visually for particulate matter and discoloration (eg, green, black) prior to administration. Tigecycline may be stored in the IV bag at room temperature for up to 6 hours, or refrigerated at 2° to 8°C (36° to 46°F) for up to 24 hours.

➤*Administration:* IV infusions of tigecycline should be administered over approximately 30 to 60 minutes every 12 hours. Tigecycline may be administered IV through a dedicated line or through a Y-site. If the same IV line is used for sequential infusion of several drugs, the line should be flushed before and after infusion of tigecycline with either 0.9% sodium chloride injection or 5% dextrose injection. Injection should be made with an infusion solution compatible with tigecycline and with any other drug(s) administered via this common line.

➤*Compatibilities/Incompatibilities:* Compatible IV solutions include 0.9% sodium chloride injection and 5% dextrose injection. When administered through a Y-site, tigecycline is compatible with the following drugs or diluents: dobutamine, dopamine hydrochloride, lidocaine hydrochloride, potassium chloride, ranitidine hydrochloride, Ringer's lactate, and theophylline.

The following drugs should not be administered simultaneously through the same Y-site as tigecycline: amphotericin B, chlorpromazine, methylprednisolone, and voriconazole.

➤*Storage/Stability:* Prior to reconstitution, store tigecycline at 20° to 25°C (68° to 77°F); excursions permitted to 15° to 30°C (59° to 86°F). Reconstituted solution must be immediately transferred and further diluted for IV infusion. Tigecycline may be stored in the IV bag at room temperature for up to 6 hours, or refrigerated at 2° to 8°C (36° to 46°F) for up to 24 hours.

TIGECYCLINE — INTRAVENOUS

Actions

➤*Pharmacology:* Tigecycline, a glycylcycline, inhibits protein translation in bacteria by binding to the 30S ribosomal subunit and blocking entry of amino-acyl tRNA molecules into the A site of the ribosome. This prevents incorporation of amino acid residues into elongating peptide chains.

Glycylcycline class antibiotics are structurally similar to tetracycline class antibiotics and may have similar adverse reactions.

➤*Pharmacokinetics:*

Absorption / Distribution – In a single-dose study, tigecycline 100 mg was administered to subjects prior to undergoing elective surgery or medical procedure for tissue extraction. Concentrations at 4 hours after tigecycline administration were higher in gallbladder (38-fold, n = 6), lung (8.6-fold, n = 1), and colon (2.1-fold, n = 5), and lower in synovial fluid (0.58-fold, n = 5) and bone (0.35 fold, n = 6) relative to serum. The concentration of tigecycline in these tissues after multiple doses has not been studied.

Following the administration of tigecycline 100 mg followed by 50 mg every 12 hours to 33 healthy volunteers, the tigecycline area under the curve (AUC_{0-12h}) (134 mcg•h/mL) in alveolar cells was approximately 78-fold higher than the AUC_{0-12h} in the serum, and the AUC_{0-12h} (2.28 mcg•h/mL) in epithelial lining fluid was approximately 32% higher than the AUC_{0-12h} in serum. The AUC_{0-12h} (1.61 mcg•h/mL) of tigecycline in skin blister fluid was approximately 26% lower than the AUC_{0-12h} in the serum of 10 healthy subjects.

The in vitro plasma protein binding of tigecycline ranges from approximately 71% to 89% at concentrations observed in clinical studies (0.1 to 1 mcg/mL). The steady-state volume of distribution of tigecycline averaged 500 to 700 L (7 to 9 L/kg), indicating tigecycline is extensively distributed beyond the plasma volume and into the tissues.

Metabolism / Excretion – Tigecycline is not extensively metabolized. In vitro studies with tigecycline using human liver microsomes, liver slices, and hepatocytes led to the formation of only trace amounts of metabolites. In healthy male volunteers receiving ^{14}C-tigecycline, tigecycline was the primary ^{14}C labeled material recovered in urine and feces, but a glucuronide, an N-acetyl metabolite, and a tigecycline epimer (each at no more than 10% of the administered dose) were also present.

The recovery of total radioactivity in feces and urine following administration of ^{14}C-tigecycline indicates that 59% of the dose is eliminated by biliary/fecal excretion, and 33% is excreted in urine. Approximately 22% of the total dose is excreted as unchanged tigecycline in urine. Overall, the primary route of elimination for tigecycline is biliary excretion of unchanged tigecycline and its metabolites. Glucuronidation and renal excretion of unchanged tigecycline are secondary routes.

Special populations –

Hepatic function impairment: In a study comparing 10 patients with mild hepatic function impairment (Child-Pugh class A), 10 patients with moderate hepatic impairment (Child-Pugh class B), and 5 patients with severe hepatic impairment (Child-Pugh class C) to 23 age- and weight-matched healthy control subjects, the single-dose pharmacokinetic disposition of tigecycline was not altered in patients with mild hepatic impairment. However, systemic clearance of tigecycline was reduced by 25% and the half-life of tigecycline was prolonged by 23% in patients with moderate hepatic impairment. Systemic clearance of tigecycline was reduced by 55%, and the half-life of tigecycline was prolonged by 43% in patients with severe hepatic impairment. Based on the pharmacokinetic profile of tigecycline, no dosage adjustment is warranted in patients with mild to moderate hepatic impairment. However, in patients with severe hepatic impairment, the initial dose of tigecycline should be 100 mg followed by a reduced maintenance dosage of 25 mg every 12 hours. Treat patients with severe hepatic impairment with caution and monitor them for treatment response.

Elderly: No significant differences in pharmacokinetics were observed between healthy elderly subjects (n = 15, 65 to 75 years of age; n = 13, older than 75 years of age) and younger subjects (n = 18) receiving a single dose of tigecycline 100 mg. Therefore, no dosage adjustment is necessary based on age.

Pharmacokinetic parameters – The mean pharmacokinetic parameters of tigecycline after single and multiple IV doses based on pooled data from clinical pharmacology studies are summarized in the following table. IV infusions of tigecycline were administered over approximately 30 to 60 minutes.

Mean (CV%) Pharmacokinetic Parameters of Tigecycline

Pharmacokinetic Parameter	Single Dose 100 mg (n = 224)	Multiple Dose[a] 50 mg every 12 hours (n = 103)
C_{max} (mcg/mL)[b]	1.45 (22%)	0.87 (27%)
C_{max} (mcg/mL)[c]	0.9 (30%)	0.63 (15%)
AUC (mcg•h/mL)	5.19 (36%)	-
AUC_{0-24h} (mcg•h/mL)	-	4.7 (36%)
C_{min} (mcg/mL)	-	0.13 (59%)
$t_{½}$ (h)	27.1 (53%)	42.4 (83%)
CL (L/h)	21.8 (40%)	23.8 (33%)
CL_r (mL/min)	38 (82%)	51 (58%)
V_{ss} (L)	568 (43%)	639 (48%)

[a] 100 mg initially, followed by 50 mg every 12 hours.
[b] 30-minute infusion.
[c] 60-minute infusion.

➤*Microbiology:* Tigecycline carries a glycylamido moiety attached to the 9-position of minocycline. The substitution pattern is not present in any naturally occurring or semisynthetic tetracycline and imparts certain microbiologic properties to tigecycline. Tigecycline is not affected by the 2 major tetracycline resistance mechanisms, ribosomal protection and efflux. Accordingly, tigecycline has demonstrated in vitro and in vivo activity against a broad spectrum of bacterial pathogens. There has been no cross-resistance observed between tigecycline and other antibiotics. Tigecycline is not affected by resistance mechanisms such as beta-lactamases (including extended spectrum beta-lactamases), target site modifications, macrolide efflux pumps, or enzyme target changes (eg, gyrase/topoisomerase). In vitro studies have not demonstrated antagonism between tigecycline and other commonly used antibacterial drugs. In general, tigecycline is considered bacteriostatic.

Tigecycline has been shown to be active against most strains of the following microorganisms, both in vitro and in clinical infections.

Aerobic facultative gram-positive microorganisms – *E. faecalis* (vancomycin-susceptible isolates only); *S. aureus* (methicillin-susceptible and methicillin-resistant isolates); *S. agalactiae*; *S. anginosus* group (includes *S. anginosus*, *S. intermedius*, and *S. constellatus*); *S. pyogenes*.

Aerobic and facultative gram-negative microorganisms – *C. freundii*; *E. cloacae*; *E. coli*; *K. oxytoca*; *K. pneumoniae*.

Anaerobic microorganisms – *B. fragilis*; *B. thetaiotaomicron*; *B. uniformis*; *B. vulgatus*; *C. perfringens*; *P. micros*.

Contraindications

Known hypersensitivity to tigecycline.

Warnings

➤*Tooth discoloration:* The use of tigecycline during tooth development (last half of pregnancy, infancy, and childhood until the age of 8 years) may cause permanent discoloration of the teeth (yellow-gray-brown). Results of studies in rats with tigecycline have shown bone discoloration. Do not use tigecycline during tooth development unless other drugs are not likely to be effective or are contraindicated.

➤*Pseudomembranous colitis:* Pseudomembranous colitis has been reported with nearly all antibacterial agents and may range in severity from mild to life-threatening. Therefore, it is important to consider this diagnosis in patients who present with diarrhea subsequent to the administration of any antibacterial agent.

Treatment with antibacterial agents alters the flora of the colon and may permit overgrowth of clostridia. Studies indicate that a toxin produced by *Clostridium difficile* is the primary cause of "antibiotic-associated colitis." After the diagnosis of pseudomembranous colitis has been established, initiate therapeutic measures. Mild cases of pseudomembranous colitis usually respond to drug discontinuation alone. In moderate to severe cases, consider management with fluids and electrolytes, protein supplementation, and treatment with an antibacterial drug clinically effective against *C. difficile* colitis.

➤*Hypersensitivity reactions:* Administer tigecycline with caution to patients with known hypersensitivity to tetracycline class antibiotics.

➤*Hepatic function impairment:* See Administration and Dosage for more information.

➤*Elderly:* Of the total number of subjects who received tigecycline in phase 3 clinical studies (n = 1,415), 278 were 65 years of age and older, while 110 were 75 years of age and older. No unexpected overall differences in safety or efficacy were observed between these subjects and younger subjects, but greater sensitivity to adverse reactions of some older individuals cannot be ruled out.

➤*Pregnancy:* *Category D.* Tigecycline may cause fetal harm when administered to a pregnant woman. If the patient becomes pregnant while taking tigecycline, apprise her of the potential hazard to the fetus. Results of animal studies indicate that tigecycline crosses the placenta and is found in fetal tissues. Decreased fetal weights in rats and rabbits (with associated delays in ossification), and fetal loss in rabbits have been observed with tigecycline.

Tigecycline was not teratogenic in the rat or rabbit. In preclinical safety studies, ^{14}C-labeled tigecycline crossed the placenta and was found in fetal tissues, including fetal bony structures. The administration of tigecycline was associated with slight reductions in fetal weights and an increased incidence of minor skeletal anomalies (delays in bone ossification) at exposures of 5 times and 1 times the human daily dose based on AUC in rats and rabbits, respectively. An increased incidence of fetal loss was observed at maternotoxic doses in the rabbits with exposure equivalent to human dose. There are no adequate and well-controlled studies of tigecycline in pregnant women. Use tigecycline during pregnancy only if the potential benefit justifies the potential risk to the fetus.

➤*Lactation:* Results from animal studies using ^{14}C-labeled tigecycline indicate that tigecycline is excreted readily via the milk of lactating rats. Consistent with the limited oral bioavailability of tigecycline, there is little or no systemic exposure to tigecycline in nursing pups as a result of exposure via maternal milk.

It is not known whether this drug is excreted in human milk. Because many drugs are excreted in human milk, exercise caution when tigecycline is administered to a breast-feeding woman.

➤*Children:* Safety and efficacy in children younger than 18 years of age have not been established. Therefore, use in patients younger than 18 years of age is not recommended.

Precautions

➤*Monitoring:* Monitor prothrombin time or other suitable anticoagulation test if tigecycline is administered with warfarin.

➤*Tetracycline class antibiotics:* Glycylcycline class antibiotics are structurally similar to tetracycline class antibiotics and may have similar adverse

TIGECYCLINE — INTRAVENOUS

effects. Such effects may include photosensitivity, pseudotumor cerebri, pancreatitis, and antianabolic action (which has led to increased serum urea nitrogen [BUN], azotemia, acidosis, and hypophosphatemia).

➤*Resistance:* Prescribing tigecycline in the absence of a proven or strongly suspected bacterial infection is unlikely to provide benefit to the patient and increases the risk of the development of drug-resistant bacteria.

➤*Special risk:* Exercise caution when considering tigecycline monotherapy in patients with complicated intraabdominal infections secondary to clinically apparent intestinal perforation. In phase 3 complicated intraabdominal infection studies (n = 1,642), 6 patients treated with tigecycline and 2 patients treated with imipenem/cilastatin presented with intestinal perforations and developed sepsis/septic shock. The 6 patients treated with tigecycline had higher Acute Physiology and Chronic Health Evaluation II (APACHE II) scores (median = 13) vs the 2 patients treated with imipenem/cilastatin (APACHE II scores = 4 and 6). Because of differences in baseline APACHE II scores between treatment groups and small overall numbers, the relationship of this outcome to treatment cannot be established.

➤*Superinfection:* As with other antibacterial drugs, use of tigecycline may result in overgrowth of nonsusceptible organisms, including fungi. Carefully monitor patients during therapy. If superinfection occurs, take appropriate measures.

Drug Interactions

➤*Warfarin:* Monitor prothrombin time or other suitable anticoagulation test if tigecycline is administered with warfarin.

Coadministration of tigecycline (100 mg followed by 50 mg every 12 hours) and warfarin (25 mg single dose) to healthy subjects resulted in a decrease in clearance of R-warfarin and S-warfarin by 40% and 23%, an increase in C_{max} by 38% and 43% and an increase in AUC by 68% and 29%, respectively. Tigecycline did not significantly alter the effects of warfarin on INR. In addition, warfarin did not affect the pharmacokinetic profile of tigecycline.

➤*Oral contraceptives:* Concurrent use of antibacterial drugs with oral contraceptives may render oral contraceptives less effective.

Adverse Reactions

Phase 3 clinical studies enrolled 1,415 patients treated with tigecycline. Tigecycline was discontinued because of treatment-emergent adverse reactions in 5% of patients compared with 4.7% for all comparators (5.3% for vancomycin/aztreonam and 4.4% for imipenem/cilastatin). The following table shows the incidence of treatment-emergent adverse reactions through test of cure reported in at least 2% of patients in these studies regardless of causality.

Tigecycline Adverse Reactions (≥ 2%)

Adverse reactions	Tigecycline[a] (n = 1,415)	Comparators[b] (n = 1,382)
Cardiovascular		
Hypertension	4.9%	5.6 %
Hypotension	2.3%	1.7%
Phlebitis	1.8%	3.8%
CNS		
Dizziness	3.5%	2.7%
Headache	5.9%	6.5%
Insomnia	2.3%	3.3%
Dermatologic		
Pruritus	2.6%	4.1%
Rash	2.4%	4.1%
Sweating	2.3%	1.6%
GI		
Constipation	2.8%	4.1%
Diarrhea	12.7%	10.8%
Dyspepsia	2.9%	1.6%
Nausea	29.5%	15.8%
Vomiting	19.7%	10.8%
Hematologic/Lymphatic		
Anemia	4.2%	4.8%
Leukocytosis	3.7%	2.5%
Thrombocythemia	6.1%	6.2%
Metabolic/Nutritional		
Alkaline phosphatase increased	3.5%	2.6%
Amylase increased	3.1%	1.4%
Bilirubinemia	2.3%	0.9%
BUN increased	2.1%	0.2%
Hyperglycemia	1.8%	2.9%
Hypokalemia	2.1%	2.9%
Hypoproteinemia	4.5%	3%
Lactic dehydrogenase increased	4%	3.5%
ALT increased[c]	5.6%	4.7%
AST increased[c]	4.3%	4.4%
Respiratory		
Cough increased	3.7%	3.8%
Dyspnea	2.9%	2.7%
Pulmonary physical finding	1.9%	2.2%
Miscellaneous		
Abdominal pain	6.8%	5.7%
Abnormal healing	3.5%	2.6%
Abscess	3.2%	2.6%
Asthenia	2.5%	1.7%
Back pain	1.2%	2.3%
Fever	7.1%	9.8%
Infection	8.3%	5.4%
Local reaction to procedure	9%	9.1%
Pain	3.7%	2.9%
Peripheral edema	3.3%	3.3%

[a] 100 mg initially, followed by 50 mg every 12 hours.
[b] Vancomycin/aztreonam, imipenem/cilastatin, linezolid.
[c] LFT abnormalities in tigecycline-treated patients were reported more frequently in the posttherapy period than those in comparator-treated patients, which occurred more often on therapy.

In phase 3 complicated skin and skin structure infections and complicated intraabdominal infections studies, death occurred in 2.3% (32/1,383) of patients receiving tigecycline and 1.6% (22/1,375) of patients receiving comparator drugs; this difference is not statistically significant and relationship to treatment cannot be established. In all treatment groups, mortality was associated with higher baseline comorbidity and/or greater severity of baseline infections.

In phase 3 clinical studies, infection-related serious adverse reactions were more frequently reported for subjects treated with tigecycline (6.7%) vs comparators (4.6%). Significant differences in sepsis/septic shock with tigecycline (1.5%) vs comparators (0.5%) were observed. Because of baseline differences between treatment groups in this subset of patients, the relationship of this outcome to treatment cannot be established. Other reactions included nonsignificant differences in abscess (1.8% vs 1.6%) and infections, including wound infections (1.7% vs 1.1%) for tigecycline vs comparators, respectively.

The most common treatment-emergent adverse reactions were nausea and vomiting, which generally occurred during the first 1 to 2 days of therapy. The majority of cases of nausea and vomiting associated with tigecycline and comparators were either mild or moderate in severity. In patients treated with tigecycline, nausea incidence was 29.5% (19.6% mild, 8.5% moderate, 1.4% severe) and vomiting incidence was 19.7% (12.3% mild, 6.3% moderate, 1.1% severe). In patients treated for complicated skin and skin structure infections, nausea incidence was 35% for tigecycline and 8.9% for vancomycin/aztreonam; vomiting incidence was 20% for tigecycline and 4.2% for vancomycin/aztreonam. In patients treated for complicated intraabdominal infections, nausea incidence was 25.3% for tigecycline and 20.5% for imipenem/cilastatin; vomiting incidence was 19.5% for tigecycline and 15.3% for imipenem/cilastatin.

Discontinuation from tigecycline was most frequently associated with nausea (1.3%) and vomiting (1%). For comparators, discontinuations were most frequently associated with rash (1.1%, vancomycin/aztreonam) and nausea (1%, imipenem/cilastatin).

The following drug-related adverse reactions were reported infrequently (at least 0.2% and less than 2%) in patients receiving tigecycline in phase 3 clinical studies:

➤*Cardiovascular:* Bradycardia, tachycardia, thrombophlebitis, vasodilatation.

➤*CNS:* Somnolence.

➤*GI:* Abnormal stools, anorexia, dry mouth.

➤*GU:* Leukorrhea, vaginal moniliasis, vaginitis.

➤*Hematologic/Lymphatic:* Eosinophilia, increased INR, prolonged activated partial thromboplastin time (aPTT), prolonged prothrombin time, thrombocytopenia.

➤*Hepatic:* Jaundice.

➤*Metabolic/Nutritional:* Hypocalcemia, hypoglycemia, hyponatremia, increased creatinine.

➤*Special senses:* Taste perversion.

➤*Miscellaneous:* Allergic reaction, chills, injection site edema, injection site inflammation, injection site pain, injection site phlebitis, injection site reaction, septic shock.

Overdosage

➤*Symptoms:* IV administration of tigecycline at a single dose of 300 mg over 60 minutes in healthy volunteers resulted in an increased incidence of nausea and vomiting.

In single-dose IV toxicity studies conducted with tigecycline in mice, the estimated median lethal dose (LD_{50}) was 124 mg/kg in men and 98 mg/kg in women. In rats, the estimated LD_{50} was 106 mg/kg for both sexes.

No specific information is available on the treatment of overdosage with tigecycline. In 2-week studies, decreased erythrocytes, reticulocytes, leukocytes, and platelets, in association with bone marrow hypocellularity, have been seen with tigecycline at exposures of 8 and 10 times the human daily dose based on AUC in rats and dogs, respectively. These alterations were shown to be reversible after 2 weeks of dosing. No evidence of photosensitivity was observed in rats following administration of tigecycline.

➤*Treatment:* Tigecycline is not removed in significant quantities by hemodialysis.

Patient Information

Tigecycline may cause fetal harm when administered to a pregnant woman. If the patient becomes pregnant while taking tigecycline, apprise her of the potential hazard to the fetus.

TIGECYCLINE — INTRAVENOUS

Counsel patients that antibacterial drugs, including tigecycline, should only be used to treat bacterial infections. Antibacterial drugs do not treat viral infections (eg, the common cold). When tigecycline is prescribed to treat a bacterial infection, tell patients that although it is common to feel better early in the course of therapy, the medication should be taken exactly as directed. Skipping doses or not completing the full course of therapy may decrease the efficacy of the immediate treatment and increase the likelihood that bacteria will develop resistance and not be treatable by tigecycline or other antibacterial drugs in the future.

MACROLIDES

Indications

General Indications for Macrolides[1]

Indication	Azithromycin	Clarithromycin	Dirithromycin	Erythromycin
Adults				
Pharyngitis/Tonsillitis	✓	✓	✓	
Respiratory tract infections				✓
Acute maxillary sinusitis		✓		
Acute bacterial exacerbation of chronic bronchitis		✓	✓	
Skin and skin structure infections[2]	✓	✓	✓	✓
Pertussis (whooping cough)				✓
Diphtheria				✓
Erythrasma				✓
Intestinal amebiasis				✓
Uncomplicated urethral, endocervical, or rectal infections				✓
Urogenital infections during pregnancy				✓
Nongonococcal urethritis				✓
Primary syphilis				✓
Legionnaire's disease				✓
Rheumatic fever				✓
Bacterial endocarditis				✓
Listeria monocytogenes				✓
Pneumonia		✓		
Community-acquired pneumonia	✓		✓	
Disseminated bacterial infections (TWAR strain)		✓		
Prevention of disseminated *Mycobacterium avium* complex in patients with advanced HIV infection		✓		
Chronic obstructive pulmonary disease	✓			
Genital ulcer disease	✓			
Pelvic inflammatory disease	✓			✓
Urethritis/Cervicitis	✓			
Secondary bacterial infection of acute bronchitis			✓	
Children				
Pharyngitis/Tonsillitis	✓	✓		
Pneumonia		✓		
Community-acquired pneumonia	✓			
Acute maxillary sinusitis		✓		
Acute otitis media	✓	✓		
Skin and skin structure infections[2]		✓		
Disseminated mycobacterial infections		✓		
Prevention of disseminated *Mycobacterium avium* complex disease in patients with advanced HIV infection		✓		
Conjunctivitis of the newborn				✓
Pneumonia of infancy				✓

[1] Causative organisms may vary for each indication for specific macrolides. Refer to individual monographs for this information.

[2] Abscesses usually require surgical drainage.

➤*Note:* The usual drug of choice in the treatment and prevention of streptococcal infections and the prophylaxis of rheumatic fever is penicillin oral/IM. Azithromycin, clarithromycin, and dirithromycin are generally effective in the eradication of *Streptococcus pyogenes* from the nasopharynx; however, data establishing the efficacy of clarithromycin and dirithromycin in the subsequent prevention of rheumatic fever are not available at present. Because some strains are resistant to azithromycin, perform susceptibility tests when patients are treated with azithromycin.

Injectable benzathine penicillin G or oral penicillin V is considered by the American Heart Association to be the drug of choice in the treatment and prevention of streptococcal pharyngitis. For patients allergic to penicillin, erythromycin and azithromycin are effective alternatives. Erythromycin is also an alternative agent for long-term prophylaxis of rheumatic fever in patients allergic to penicillin or sulfadiazine.

➤*Helicobacter pylori double therapy:* Clarithromycin in combination with omeprazole or ranitidine bismuth citrate is indicated for the treatment of patients with an active duodenal ulcer associated with *H. pylori* infection.

➤*Helicobacter pylori triple therapy:* Clarithromycin, lansoprazole, and amoxicillin as combination triple therapy for the treatment of *H. pylori* infection and duodenal ulcer disease (active or 1-year history of duodenal ulcer) to eradicate *H. pylori*.

➤*Unlabeled uses:*

Azithromycin –

Uncomplicated gonococcal infections of the cervix, urethra, and rectum: Caused by *N. gonorrhoeae*.†

Gonococcal pharyngitis: Caused by *N. gonorrhoeae*.

Chlamydial infections: Caused by *C. trachomatis*.

† CDC 1998 Guidelines for Treatment of Sexually Transmitted Diseases. *MMWR* 1998 Jan 23;47(No. 441):1-117.

Erythromycin –
Treponema pallidum: Early syphilis (primary or secondary) for nonpregnant patients for whom compliance with therapy and follow-up can be ensured. In treatment of primary syphilis, examine spinal fluid before treatment and as part of the follow-up after therapy. The use of erythromycin for the treatment of in utero syphilis is not recommended.
Campylobacter jejuni: Erythromycin has been used successfully in prolonged diarrhea associated with campylobacter enteritis.
Lymphogranuloma venereum: Genital, inguinal, or anorectal.
Granuloma inguinale: Caused by *Calymmatobacterium granulomatis*.
Haemophilus ducreyi (chancroid): Treat until ulcers or lymph nodes are healed.

Prior to elective colorectal surgery, to reduce wound complications, erythromycin base with oral neomycin is a popular preoperative combination. Other uses, as alternative to penicillins, include: Anthrax; Vincent's gingivitis; erysipeloid; tetanus; actinomycosis; *Nocardia* infections (with a sulfonamide); *Eikenella corrodens* infections; *Borrelia* infections (including early Lyme disease).

Actions

➤*Pharmacology:* Macrolide antibiotics, which include azithromycin, clarithromycin, dirithromycin, and erythromycin, reversibly bind to the P site of the 50S ribosomal subunit of susceptible organisms and may inhibit RNA-dependent protein synthesis by stimulating the dissociation of peptidyl t-RNA from ribosomes. They may be bacteriostatic or bactericidal, depending on such factors as drug concentration.

Rearrangement of erythromycin's 9-oxime derivative, followed by reduction and N-methylation, yields the ring-expanded derivative azithromycin, an azalide. Alkylation of the hydroxyl group at C-6 yields clarithromycin. The classical erythromycins A, B, C, and D and oleandomycin are 14-membered macrolides; azithromycin is a 15-membered-ring macrolide.

Macrolides are weak bases; their activity increases in alkaline pH. Macrolides enter pleural fluid, ascitic fluid, middle-ear exudates, and sputum. When meninges are inflamed, macrolides may enter the CSF. They are used for respiratory, genital, GI tract, and skin and soft tissue infections, especially when beta-lactam antibiotics or tetracyclines are contraindicated.

Erythromycin base, the active form, is marketed in acid-resistant enteric coated form to retard gastric inactivation. Converting the base to its acid-stable salt (stearate), ester (ethyl succinate and propionate), or salt of an ester (estolate) also improves oral bioavailability. For IV injection, a relatively water-soluble salt, lactobionate, is available.

Dirithromycin is a pro-drug. Available as an enteric coated tablet, it is converted non-enzymatically during intestinal absorption into the microbiologically active moiety erythromycylamine.

➤*Pharmacokinetics:* Despite differing structures, macrolides have similar antibacterial spectrum, mechanisms of action and resistance, but relatively different pharmacokinetics (see table). Macrolides distribute readily into body tissues and fluids. Because of high intracellular concentrations, tissue levels are higher than serum levels.

Various Pharmacokinetic Parameters of Macrolides

Macrolide	Route of administration	Protein binding (%)	Bioavailability (%)	Effect of food	C_{max}* (mcg/mL)	T_{max}* (h)	Half-life (h)	Metabolism	Elimination
Azithromycin	Oral IV	51 (0.02 mcg/L) 7 (2 mcg/L)	≈ 40	Food increases absorption, C_{max} by 23% and suspension by 56%; take on empty stomach.	0.5 1.14[a] 3.63[b]	2.2	68[c]	Some hepatic but mainly excreted unchanged	6% excreted unchanged in urine; primarily excreted unchanged in bile
Clarithromycin	Oral	40 to 70	≈ 50	Food delays onset of absorption and formation of metabolite; does not affect extent of bioavailability. Take without regard to meals.	1 to 3	2 to 3	3 to 7	Metabolized to active metabolite (14-OH clarithromycin)	Primarily renal; rate approximates normal GFR
Dirithromycin	Oral	15 to 30[2]	≈ 10	Take with food or within an hour of having eaten.	0.3 to 0.4[d]	3.9 to 4.1[d]	2 to 36	Nonenzymatic conversion to erythromycylamine	81% to 97% fecal/hepatic[d]
Erythromycin	Oral IV	70-80 (96 estolate)	> 35	Base or stearate: Take on an empty stomach. Estolate, ethylsuccinate, delayed release base: Take without regard to meals.	0.3 to 2	1.6	1.6	Hepatic; demethylation	< 5% (oral) and 12% to 15% (IV) excreted unchanged in urine; significant quantity excreted in bile

* C_{max} = Maximum concentration; T_{max} = Time to reach maximum concentration.
[a] At a concentration of 1 mg/mL.
[b] At a concentration of 2 mg/mL.
[c] Average terminal half-life.
[d] Value listed for erythromycylamine, the active moiety.

Children – In 2 clinical studies, **azithromycin** for oral suspension was dosed at 10 mg/kg on day 1, followed by 5 mg/kg on days 2 through 5 to 2 groups of children (ages 1 to 5 years and 5 to 15 years, respectively). The mean pharmacokinetic parameters at day 5 were C_{max} = 0.216 mcg/mL, T_{max} = 1.9 hours and AUC_{0-24} = 1.822 mcg•h/mL for the 1- to 5-year-old group. Mean pharmacokinetic parameters at day 5 for the 5- to 15-year olds were C_{max} = 0.383 mcg/mL, T_{max} = 2.4 hours and AUC_{0-24} = 3.109 mcg•h/mL.

➤*Microbiology:*

Organisms Generally Susceptible to Macrolides In Vitro

	Organisms (✓ = generally susceptible)	Azithromycin	Clarithromycin	Dirithromycin	Erythromycin
Gram-positive aerobes	*Staphylococcus aureus*	✓	✓	✓	✓
	Streptococcus pyogenes	✓	✓	✓	✓
	Streptococcus pneumoniae	✓	✓	✓	✓
	Streptococcus agalactiae	✓	✓	✓	✓
	Streptococcus sp.	✓	✓	✓	
	Streptococcus viridans	✓	✓	✓	✓
	Listeria monocytogenes			✓	✓
	Corynebacterium diphtheriae				✓
	Corynebacterium minutissimum				✓
Gram-negative aerobes	*Haemophilus influenzae*	✓	✓	✓	†[a]
	Haemophilus ducreyi	✓			
	Moraxella catarrhalis	✓	✓	✓	✓
	Bordetella pertussis	✓	✓	✓	✓
	Legionella pneumophila	✓	✓	✓	✓
	Neisseria gonorrhoeae	✓	✓		
	Pasteurella multocida		✓		

Organisms Generally Susceptible to Macrolides In Vitro					
	Organisms (✓ = generally susceptible)	Azithromycin	Clarithromycin	Dirithromycin	Erythromycin
Anaerobes	*Prevotella* (formerly *Bacteroides*) *bivius*	✓			
	Prevotella (formerly *Bacteroides*) *melaninogenicus*		✓		
	Clostridium perfringens		✓		
	Propionibacterium acnes		✓	✓	
	Peptococcus niger		✓		
	Peptostreptococcus sp.	✓			
Other	*Borrelia burgdorferi*	✓			
	Chlamydia trachomatis	✓	✓		✓
	Mycobacterium kansasii		✓		
	Mycoplasma pneumoniae	✓	✓	✓	✓
	Treponema pallidum	✓			✓
	Ureaplasma urealyticum	✓			✓
	Entamoeba histolytica				✓
	Chlamydia pneumoniae (TWAR strain)	✓	✓		
	Mycoplasma hominis	✓			
	Mycobacterium avium		✓		
	Mycobacterium intracellulare		✓		
	Helicobacter pylori		✓		
	Clostridium tetani				✓

[a] Many strains resistant to erythromycin alone; may be susceptible to erythromycin plus a sulfonamide.

Contraindications

Hypersensitivity to any of the macrolide antibiotics; patients receiving astemizole, cisapride, or pimozide; known, suspected, or potential bacteremias (dirithromycin); preexisting liver disease (erythromycin estolate).

Warnings

➤*Pseudomembranous colitis:* This has occurred with nearly all antibacterial agents and may range in severity from mild to life-threatening. Therefore, it is important to consider this diagnosis in patients who present with diarrhea subsequent to the administration of antibacterial agents.

Treatment with antibacterial agents alters the normal flora of the colon and may permit overgrowth of clostridia. Studies indicate that a toxin produced by *Clostridium difficile* is a primary cause of "antibiotic-associated colitis."

After the diagnosis of pseudomembranous colitis has been established, initiate therapeutic measures. Mild cases of pseudomembranous colitis usually respond to discontinuation of the drug alone. In moderate-to-severe cases, give consideration to management with fluids and electrolytes, protein supplementation and treatment with an antibacterial drug effective against *C. difficile* colitis. When colitis does not improve after discontinuation, or when it is severe, oral vancomycin or metronidazole is the drug of choice; rule out other causes.

➤*Acute porphyria:* Do not use **clarithromycin** in combination with ranitidine bismuth citrate in patients with a history of acute porphyria.

➤*Pneumonia:* Do not use oral **azithromycin** in patients with pneumonia who are judged to be inappropriate for oral therapy because of moderate to severe illness or risk factors such as any of the following: nosocomially acquired infections; known or suspected bacteremia; conditions requiring hospitalization; cystic fibrosis; significant underlying health problems that may compromise patients' ability to respond to their illness (including immunodeficiency or functional asplenia); elderly or debilitated patients.

➤*Cardiac effects:* Ventricular arrhythmias, including ventricular tachycardia and torsades de pointes, in individuals with prolonged QT intervals have been reported with macrolide antibiotics; however, it has not occurred with **azithromycin**.

➤*Bacteremias:* Do not use **dirithromycin** in patients with known, suspected, or potential bacteremias because serum levels are inadequate to provide antibacterial coverage of the blood stream.

➤*Hepatotoxicity:* **Erythromycin** administration has been associated with the infrequent occurrence of cholestatic hepatitis. This effect is most common with erythromycin estolate; however, it has also occurred with other erythromycin salts. Laboratory findings include abnormal hepatic function, peripheral eosinophilia, and leukocytosis. Symptoms may include malaise, nausea, vomiting, abdominal cramps, and fever. Jaundice may or may not be present. In some instances, severe abdominal pain may simulate the pain of biliary colic, pancreatitis, perforated ulcer, or an acute abdominal surgical problem. In other instances, clinical symptoms and results of liver function tests have resembled findings in extrahepatic obstructive jaundice. Although initial symptoms have developed after a few days of treatment, they generally have followed 1 or 2 weeks of continuous therapy. Symptoms reappear promptly, usually within 48 hours after the drug is readministered to sensitive patients. The syndrome seems to result from a form of sensitization, occurs chiefly in adults, and is reversible when medication is discontinued.

➤*Myasthenia gravis:* **Erythromycin** may aggravate the weakness of patients with myasthenia gravis.

➤*Hypersensitivity reactions:* Rare serious allergic reactions, including angioedema, anaphylaxis, and dermatologic reactions including Stevens-Johnson syndrome and toxic epidermal necrolysis have occurred in patients on **azithromycin** therapy. Although rare, fatalities have occurred. Despite initially successful symptomatic treatment of the allergic symptoms, when symptomatic therapy was discontinued, the allergic symptoms recurred soon thereafter in some patients without further azithromycin exposure. These patients required prolonged periods of observation and symptomatic treatment. The relationship of these episodes to the long tissue half-life of azithromycin and subsequent prolonged exposure to antigen is unknown at present.

If an allergic reaction occurs with azithromycin, discontinue and institute appropriate therapy. Physicians should be aware that reappearance of the allergic symptoms may occur when symptomatic therapy is discontinued.

Serious allergic reactions, including anaphylaxis, have occurred with **erythromycin**. Refer to Management of Acute Hypersensitivity Reactions.

➤*Renal / Hepatic function impairment:* **Clarithromycin** is principally excreted via the liver and kidney and may be administered without dosage adjustment to patients with hepatic impairment and normal renal function. However, in the presence of severe renal impairment (creatinine clearance [Ccr] less than 30 mL/min) with or without coexisting hepatic impairment, the dosage should be halved or the dosing intervals doubled. Clarithromycin in combination with ranitidine bismuth citrate therapy is not recommended in patients with Ccr less than 25 mL/min.

Because **azithromycin** is principally eliminated via the liver, exercise caution when administering to patients with impaired hepatic function. There are no data regarding azithromycin usage in patients with renal impairment; thus, exercise caution when prescribing azithromycin in these patients.

The mean peak plasma concentration (C_{max}) and AUC of **dirithromycin** with renal impairment tended to increase as creatinine clearance decreased; however, based on data available to date, no dosage adjustment should be necessary in patients with impaired renal function, including dialysis patients. In patients with mild (Child's Grade A) hepatic impairment, mean peak serum concentration, AUC, and volume of distribution of dirithromycin increased somewhat with multiple-dose administration; however, based on the magnitude of these changes, no dosage adjustment should be necessary in patients with mildly impaired hepatic function. The pharmacokinetics of dirithromycin in patients with moderate or severe hepatic function impairment (Child's Grade B or greater) have not been studied. Because dirithromycin/erythromycylamine is principally eliminated via the liver, administer dirithromycin to such patients only when absolutely necessary.

Erythromycin is principally excreted by the liver. Exercise caution in administering to patients with impaired hepatic function. There have been reports of hepatic dysfunction with or without jaundice.

➤*Elderly:* Maximum concentrations and AUC of **clarithromycin** and 14-OH clarithromycin are increased. These changes in pharmacokinetics parallel known age-related decreases in renal function. In clinical trials, elderly patients did not have an increased incidence of adverse events compared with younger patients. Consider dosage adjustment in elderly patients with severe renal impairment.

Pharmacokinetic parameters in older volunteers (65 to 85 years old) were similar to those in younger volunteers (18 to 40 years old) for the 5-day therapeutic regimen of **azithromycin**. Dosage adjustment does not appear to be necessary for older patients with normal renal and hepatic function receiving treatment with this dosage regimen.

While C_{max} and AUC of **dirithromycin** tended to increase with age, neither was statistically or clinically significantly altered with age. Therefore, based on these pharmacokinetic results, no dosage adjustment should be necessary in elderly patients.

➤*Pregnancy:* (*Category B*: **Azithromycin**, **erythromycin**; *Category C*: **Clarithromycin**, **dirithromycin**). Clarithromycin has adverse reactions on pregnancy outcome or embryo-fetal development in monkeys, rats, mice, and rabbits. Animal studies with dirithromycin demonstrated that fetal weight was significantly depressed at 8 times the maximum recommended human dose with an increased occurrence of incomplete ossification. Erythromycin crosses the placental barrier but fetal levels are low. There are no adequate and well controlled studies in pregnant women. Do not use clarithromycin in pregnant women except in clinical circumstances when no alternative therapy is appropriate. If pregnancy occurs while taking this drug, apprise the patient of the hazard to the fetus. Use clarithromycin and dirithromycin during pregnancy only if the potential benefit justifies the potential risk to the fetus. Use azithromycin and erythromycin only when clearly needed.

➤*Lactation:* **Erythromycin** is excreted in breast milk and may concentrate (observed milk:plasma ratio of 0.5). Although no infant adverse reactions are reported, potential problems for the nursing infant include modification of bowel flora, pharmacological effects, and interference with fever work-ups. Erythromycin is considered compatible with breast-feeding by the American Academy of Pediatrics. It is not known whether **clarithromycin**, **dirithromycin**, or **azithromycin** is excreted in breast milk. Exercise caution when administering to a breast-feeding woman.

➤*Children:* Safety and efficacy of **clarithromycin** in children younger than 6 months of age have not been established. The safety of clarithromycin has not been studied in MAC patients younger than 20 months of age.

Safety and efficacy of **azithromycin** for IV injection in children or adolescents younger than 16 years have not been established. In controlled clinical studies, azithromycin has been administered to children (6 months to 16 years of age) by the oral route.

Safety and efficacy of **azithromycin** in children younger than 6 months of age have not been established for acute otitis media or community-acquired pneumonia.

Safety and efficacy of **azithromycin** in children younger than 2 years of age have not been established for pharyngitis/tonsillitis.

Safety and efficacy of **dirithromycin** in children younger than 12 years of age have not been established.

Precautions

➤*Local IV site reactions:* This has been reported with the IV administration of **azithromycin**. The incidence and severity of these reactions were the same when 500 mg was given over 1 hour (2 mg/mL as 250 mL infusion) or over 3 hours (1 mg/mL as 500 ml infusion). All volunteers who received infusate concentrations more than 2 mg/ml experienced local IV site reactions; therefore, avoid higher concentrations.

➤*Superinfection:* Use of antibiotics (especially prolonged or repeated therapy) may result in bacterial or fungal overgrowth of nonsusceptible organisms. Such overgrowth may lead to a secondary infection. Appropriate measures should be taken if superinfection occurs.

Drug Interactions

Macrolide Antibiotic Drug Interactions

Precipitant Drug	Object Drug[a]		Description
Antacids	Macrolides Azithromycin Dirithromycin Erythromycin	↔	Aluminum- and magnesium-containing antacids reduce peak serum levels but not the extent of azithromycin absorption. When given immediately following antacids, dirithromycin absorption is slightly enhanced. When given immediately prior to antacids, the elimination rate constant of erythromycin may be slightly decreased.
Fluconazole	Macrolides Clarithromycin	↑	Coadministration led to increases in mean steady-state trough levels (33%) and AUC (18%) of clarithromycin.
H_2 antagonist	Macrolides Dirithromycin	↑	When given immediately after H_2 antagonists, dirithromycin absorption is slightly enhanced.
Macrolides Clarithromycin	Ranitidine bismuth citrate	↔	Coadministration resulted in increased plasma ranitidine levels (57%), increased plasma bismuth trough concentrations (48%), and increased 14-OH clarithromycin plasma levels (31%). These effects do not appear to be clinically important.
Ranitidine bismuth citrate	Macrolides Clarithromycin		
Pimozide	Macrolides Azithromycin Clarithromycin Dirithromycin Erythromycin	↑	Coadministration is contraindicated. Two sudden deaths have occurred when clarithromycin was added to ongoing pimozide therapy.
Rifamycins Rifabutin Rifampin	Macrolides Clarithromycin Erythromycin	↓	The antimicrobial effects of the macrolide antibiotic may be decreased while the frequency of GI adverse effects may be increased.
Macrolides Erythromycin	Alfentanil	↑	Alfentanil clearance may be decreased and the elimination half-life increased.
Macrolides Clarithromycin Erythromycin	Anticoagulants, oral	↑	Anticoagulant effects may be potentiated. Until more data are available, it is prudent to monitor anticoagulant function in patients receiving anticoagulants and any macrolide antibiotic.
Macrolides Clarithromycin Erythromycin	Benzodiazepines Alprazolam Diazepam Midazolam Triazolam	↑	The plasma levels of certain benzodiazepines may be elevated, increasing and prolonging the CNS depressant effects. Azithromycin and dirithromycin would not be expected to interact.
Macrolides Erythromycin	Bromocriptine	↑	Bromocriptine serum levels may be elevated, resulting in an increase in the pharmacologic and adverse effects.
Macrolides Clarithromycin Erythromycin	Buspirone	↑	Plasma buspirone concentrations may be elevated, increasing the pharmacologic and adverse effects. Azithromycin and dirithromycin would not be expected to interact.
Macrolides Clarithromycin Erythromycin	Carbamazepine	↑	Increased concentrations of carbamazepine may occur. Azithromycin and dirithromycin would not be expected to interact.
Macrolides Clarithromycin Erythromycin	Cisapride	↑	Coadministration of these drugs is contraindicated. Serious cardiac arrhythmias including ventricular tachycardia, ventricular fibrillation, torsades de pointes, and QT interval prolongation may occur. Azithromycin and dirithromycin would not be expected to interact with cisapride.
Macrolides Azithromycin Clarithromycin Erythromycin	Cyclosporine	↑	Elevated cyclosporine concentrations with increased risk of toxicity (nephrotoxicity, neurotoxicity) may occur. Azithromycin and dirithromycin would not be expected to interact. However, a single case report implied that azithromycin may interact with cyclosporine.
Macrolides Clarithromycin Erythromycin	Digoxin	↑	Serum digoxin concentrations may be elevated because of the effect of the antibiotic on gut flora that metabolize digoxin in ≈ 10% of patients. Carefully monitor patients receiving digoxin and any macrolide antibiotic.
Macrolides Clarithromycin Erythromycin	Disopyramide	↑	Disopyramide plasma levels may be increased. Arrhythmias and increased QT_c intervals have occurred.
Macrolides Clarithromycin Erythromycin	Ergot alkaloids	↑	Acute ergot toxicity characterized by severe peripheral vasospasm and dysesthesia has occurred. Carefully monitor patients receiving ergot alkaloids and any macrolide antibiotic.
Macrolides Erythromycin	Felodipine	↑	Felodipine plasma levels may be elevated, increasing pharmacologic and adverse effects.
Macrolides Erythromycin	Fluoroquinolones Grepafloxacin Sparfloxacin	↑	Sparfloxacin is contraindicated with erythromycin while grepafloxacin is contraindicated unless appropriate cardiac monitoring can be ensured (eg, hospitalized patients). Risk of life-threatening cardiac arrhythmias, including torsades de pointes, may be increased with coadministration.
Macrolides Azithromycin Clarithromycin Erythromycin	HMG-CoA reductase inhibitors	↑	The risk of severe myopathy or rhabdomyolysis may be increased.
Macrolides Erythromycin	Lincosamides	↓	Under some conditions, coadministration may be antagonistic.

Macrolide Antibiotic Drug Interactions			
Precipitant Drug	Object Drug[a]		Description
Macrolides Erythromycin	Methylprednisolone	↑	The clearance of methylprednisolone is greatly reduced. This has been used as a therapeutic advantage to reduce the dose.
Macrolides Clarithromycin	Omeprazole	↑	Coadministration may result in increased plasma levels of omeprazole, clarithromycin, and 14-OH clarithromycin.
Omeprazole	Macrolides Clarithromycin		
Macrolides Erythromycin	Penicillins	↔	Both antagonism and synergism have occurred with coadministration.
Macrolides Clarithromycin Erythromycin	Tacrolimus	↑	Concurrent use may be associated with elevated serum tacrolimus levels, increasing the risk of side effects (eg, nephrotoxicity). Azithromycin and dirithromycin would not be expected to interact.
Macrolides Clarithromycin Erythromycin	Theophylline	↑	Concurrent use may be associated with increased serum theophylline levels. Azithromycin and dirithromycin would not be expected to interact. Monitor serum theophylline levels in patients receiving theophylline and any macrolide antibiotic. In addition, plasma erythromycin levels may be decreased.
Theophylline	Macrolides Erythromycin	↓	
Macrolides Erythromycin	Vinblastine	↑	Risk of vinblastine toxicity (eg, constipation, myalgia, neutropenia) may be increased.
Macrolides Clarithromycin	Zidovudine	↔	Peak serum zidovudine concentrations may be increased or decreased.

[a] ↑ = Object drug increased. ↓ = Object drug decreased.
↔ = Undetermined clinical effect.

➤*Drug/Lab test interactions:* **Erythromycin** interferes with the fluorometric determination of urinary catecholamines.

Erythromycin may interfere with AST determinations if azone-fast violet B or diphenylhydrazine colorimetric determinations are used.

➤*Drug/Food interactions:* Food delays both the onset of **clarithromycin** absorption and the formation of 14-OH clarithromycin (the active metabolite) but does not affect the extent of bioavailability of the tablets. Following administration of the suspension, both the mean peak serum levels and extent of absorption were either decreased or increased when administered to adults or children, respectively. However, clarithromycin tablets and oral suspension may be given without regard to meals.

When **azithromycin** suspension was administered with food, the rate of absorption was increased by 56% while the extent of absorption (AUC) was unchanged. Administration of azithromycin tablets with food increased C_{max} by 23% with no change in AUC.

Administer **dirithromycin** with food or within an hour of eating. The effect of food on bioavailability was evaluated after administration of two 250 mg tablets 1 or 4 hours before food and immediately after a standard breakfast. Results indicated an increase in absorption of erythromycylamine when dirithromycin was administered after food, while a significant decrease in C_{max} (33%) and AUC (31%) occurred when administered 1 hour before food. Dietary fat had little or no effect on the bioavailability of dirithromycin.

Antimicrobial effectiveness of **erythromycin** stearate and certain formulations of erythromycin base may be reduced. Take ≥ 2 hours before or after a meal. Erythromycin estolate and ethylsuccinate and the base in a delayed release form may be administered without regard to meals.

Adverse Reactions

The majority of side effects with **clarithromycin** observed in clinical trials were of a mild and transient nature. Less than 3% of adult patients without mycobacterial infections and < 2% of children without mycobacterial infections discontinued therapy because of drug-related side effects.

Most side effects with **azithromycin** are mild to moderate in severity and are reversible upon discontinuation of the drug. Approximately 0.7% of the patients (adults and children) from the multiple-dose clinical trials discontinued therapy because of treatment-related side effects. Approximately 1.2% of patients discontinued IV therapy and a total of 2.4% discontinued IV or oral therapy because of clinical or laboratory side effects. Most of the side effects leading to discontinuation were related to the GI tract (eg, nausea, vomiting, diarrhea, abdominal pain). Rare, but potentially serious side effects, were angioedema and cholestatic jaundice. In clinical trials conducted in patients with pelvic inflammatory disease, in which 1 to 2 IV doses were given, 2% of women who received monotherapy with azithromycin and 4% who received azithromycin plus metronidazole discontinued therapy because of clinical side effects.

Eighty-seven of 3,299 (2.6%) patients discontinued **dirithromycin** because of adverse reactions. Thirty-five (40%) of the 87 patients who discontinued therapy did so because of nausea or abdominal pain.

Macrolide Adverse Reactions (> 1%)				
Adverse reaction	Azithromycin	Clarithromycin	Dirithromycin	Erythromycin
GI				
Abdominal pain/ discomfort	1.9 to 7	2	9.7	7.5
Abnormal taste	—	3	> 0.1 to < 1	—
Anorexia	1.9	—	> 0.1 to < 1	✓
Diarrhea/loose stools	4.3 to 14	3	7.7	7.3
Dyspepsia	≤ 1	2	2.6	2.1
Flatulence	≤ 1	—	1.5	1.5
GI disorder	—	—	1.6	1.4
Nausea	3 to 18	3	8.3	7.5
Vomiting	≤ 7	—	3	2.8
Injection site reactions				
Local inflammation	3.1	—	—	—
Pain	6.5	—	—	—
Lab test abnormalities				
ALT elevated	1 to 6	< 1	> 0.1 to < 1	—
AST elevated	1 to 6	< 1	> 0.1 to < 1	—
Bicarbonate decreased	—	—	1.4	2
BUN elevated	< 1	4	—	—
Eosinophils increased	—	—	1.2	0.6
GGT elevated	1 to 2	< 1	> 0.1 to < 1	—
LDH elevated	≤ 3	< 1	—	—
Platelet count increased	—	—	3.8	4.8
Potassium elevated	1 to 2	—	2.6	—
Segmented neutrophils increased	—	—	1.2	1.3
Serum CPK elevated	1 to 2	—	1.2	0.9
Serum creatinine elevated	≤ 6	< 1	> 0.1 to < 1	—
Total bilirubin elevated	≤ 3	< 1	> 0.1 to < 1	—
Miscellaneous				
Asthenia	—	—	2	1.9
Dizziness	≤ 1	—	2.3	2.3
Dyspnea	—	—	1.2	1.2
Headache	≤ 1	2	8.6	8.2
Increased cough	—	—	1.5	2.6
Pain (non-specific)	—	—	2.2	1.6
Pruritus	1.9	—	1.2	1

Macrolide Adverse Reactions (> 1%)				
Adverse reaction	Azithromycin	Clarithromycin	Dirithromycin	Erythromycin
Rash	1.9	—	1.4	2.6
Vaginitis	≤ 2.8	—	0.4	0.6
Children				
Abdominal pain	1.9 to 3	3	—	—
Diarrhea/loose stools	2 to 6	6	—	—
Headache	≤ 1	2	—	—
Nausea	1 to 2	—	—	—
Rash	≤ 1.6	3	—	—
Vomiting	1 to 5	6	—	—

[1] ✓ = Event occurred, but incidence is unknown.

The following adverse reactions occurred at an incidence unknown or less than 1%:

Azithromycin – Mucositis; oral moniliasis; melena; cholestatic jaundice; gastritis; chest pain; palpitations; fatigue; somnolence; vertigo; monilia; nephritis; angioedema; photosensitivity; bronchospasm; taste perversion; elevated serum alkaline phosphatase; leukopenia; neutropenia; elevated blood glucose; elevated phosphate; decreased platelet count. Laboratory test abnormalities appeared to be reversible.

Children: Hyperkinesia; dizziness; agitation; nervousness; insomnia; fatigue; fever; malaise; dyspepsia; constipation; anorexia; flatulence; gastritis; conjunctivitis; chest pain; pruritus; urticaria.

Significant abnormalities occurring in children during clinical trials were reported at a frequency of less than 1% but were similar in type to the adult pattern.

Clarithromycin – Elevated alkaline phosphatase; elevated prothrombin time; decreased WBC.

Dirithromycin – Abnormal stools; constipation; gastritis; anorexia; dry mouth; dysphagia; gastroenteritis; mouth ulceration; palpitations; anxiety; depression; nervousness; paresthesias; somnolence; peripheral edema; sweating; syncope; thirst; tinnitus; tremor; vasodilation; dysmenorrhea; urinary frequency; vaginal moniliasis; allergic reaction; amblyopia; dehydration; edema; epistaxis; eye disorder; fever; flu syndrome; hemoptysis; hyperventilation; malaise; myalgia; myasthenia; neck pain; insomnia; increased leukocytes; elevated alkaline phosphatase; decreased platelet count; decreased albumin; decreased chloride; decreased hematocrit; decreased hemoglobin; decreased lymphocytes; decreased segmented neutrophils; decreased phosphorus; decreased serum alkaline phosphatase; decreased serum uric acid; decreased total protein; increased basophils; increased calcium; increased lymphocytes; increased hematocrit; increased hemoglobin; increased monocytes; increased phosphorus; increased uric acid.

Erythromycin – Pseudomembranous colitis; anorexia; ventricular arrhythmias; hepatotoxicity; urticaria; bullous eruptions; eczema; erythema multiforme; Stevens-Johnson syndrome; toxic epidermal necrolysis; allergic reaction; anaphylaxis; insomnia; increased leukocytes.

Local: Venous irritation and phlebitis have occurred with parenteral administration of erythromycin, but the risk of such reactions may be reduced if the infusion is given slowly, in dilute solution, by continuous IV infusion or intermittent infusion over 20 to 60 minutes.

Special senses: There have been isolated reports of reversible hearing loss with erythromycin occurring chiefly in patients with renal or hepatic insufficiency, in the elderly and in those receiving high doses (more than 4 g/day). In rare instances involving IV use, the ototoxic effect has been irreversible.

Overdosage

➤*Symptoms:* The toxic symptoms following an overdose of a macrolide antibiotic may include nausea, vomiting, epigastric distress, and diarrhea.

Hearing loss may occur with **erythromycin**, especially in patients with renal insufficiency.

➤*Treatment:* Forced diuresis, peritoneal dialysis, hemodialysis, or hemoperfusion have not been established as beneficial for an overdose of **dirithromycin**. Hemodialysis has been shown to be ineffective in hastening the elimination of erythromycylamine from plasma in patients with chronic renal failure.

Treatment includes usual supportive measures. Refer to General Management of Acute Overdosage. Induce prompt elimination of unabsorbed drug. Control allergic reactions with conventional therapy as indicated. Hemodialysis and peritoneal dialysis are not particularly effective.

Patient Information

Clarithromycin may be given without regard to meals and may be taken with milk.

Caution patients to take **azithromycin** *suspension* greater than or equal to 1 hour prior to a meal or greater than or equal to 2 hours after a meal. Azithromycin *tablets* can be taken with or without food.

Take **dirithromycin** with food or within 1 hour of eating.

Take **erythromycin** on an empty stomach (greater than or equal to 1 hour before or 2 hours after meals); if GI upset occurs, take with food. Erythromycin estolate, ethylsuccinate and certain brands of erythromycin base enteric coated tablets may be taken without regard to meals; consult the current package literature. Take each erythromycin dose with an adequate amount of water (180 to 240 mL).

Take **erythromycin** at evenly spaced intervals during the day, preferably around the clock. Complete full course of therapy; take until gone.

Caution patients not to take aluminum- and magnesium-containing antacids and oral **azithromycin** simultaneously.

Patients should discontinue the drug immediately and contact a physician if any signs of an allergic reaction occur.

Do not cut, chew, or crush the tablets.

Notify physician if nausea, vomiting, diarrhea or stomach cramps, severe abdominal pain, yellow discoloration of the skin or eyes, darkened urine, pale stools, or unusual tiredness occurs with **erythromycin**.

Shake the suspension well before each use. Do not refrigerate.

CLARITHROMYCIN

Rx	**Clarithromycin** (Teva)	**Tablets**: 250 mg	(93 7157). Yellow, oval. Film-coated. In 60s.
Rx	**Biaxin** (Abbott)		(KT). Yellow, oval. Film-coated. In 60s and *ABBO-PAC* UD 100s.
Rx	**Clarithromycin** (Teva)	**Tablets**: 500 mg	(93 7158). Lt. yellow, oval. Film-coated. In 60s.
Rx	**Biaxin** (Abbott)		(KL). Yellow, oval. Film-coated. In 60s and *ABBO-PAC* UD 100s.
Rx	**Biaxin** (Abbott)	**Granules for oral suspension when reconstituted**: 125 mg/5 mL	Sucrose. Fruit punch flavor. In 50 and 100 mL.
		250 mg/5 mL	Sucrose. Fruit punch flavor. In 50 and 100 mL.
Rx	**Biaxin XL** (Abbott)	**Tablets, extended-release**: 500 mg	Lactose. (KJ). Yellow, oval. Film-coated. In 60s and *BIAXIN XL PAC* blister pack 4 × 14s.
Rx	**Clarithromycin** (Ranbaxy)	**Tablets, extended-release**: 1,000 mg	Lactose. (RB 36). Yellow, oval. Film-coated. In 10s and 500s.

CLARITHROMYCIN — ORAL

For complete and comparative prescribing information, refer to the Macrolides group monograph.

Indications

➤*Tablets and granules:* For the treatment of mild to moderate infections caused by susceptible strains of the designated microorganisms in the following conditions.

Adults –

Pharyngitis/Tonsillitis: Caused by *Streptococcus pyogenes*.

The usual drug of choice in the treatment and prevention of streptococcal infections and the prophylaxis of rheumatic fever is penicillin oral/IM. Clarithromycin is generally effective in the eradication of *S. pyogenes* from the nasopharynx; however, data establishing the efficacy of clarithromycin in the subsequent prevention of rheumatic fever are not available at present.

Acute maxillary sinusitis: Caused by *Haemophilus influenzae*, *Moraxella catarrhalis*, or *S. pneumoniae*.

Acute bacterial exacerbation of chronic bronchitis: Caused by *H. influenzae*, *H. parainfluenzae*, *M. catarrhalis*, or *S. pneumoniae*.

Community-acquired pneumonia: Caused by *H. influenzae*, *Mycoplasma pneumoniae*, *S. pneumoniae*, or *Chlamydia pneumoniae* (TWAR strain).

Uncomplicated skin and skin structure infections: Caused by *Staphylococcus aureus* or *S. pyogenes*. Abscesses usually require surgical drainage.

Disseminated mycobacterial infections: Caused by *Mycobacterium avium* or *M. intracellulare*.

Prevention of disseminated Mycobacterium Avium Complex (MAC) disease: In patients with advanced HIV infection.

Helicobacter pylori dual therapy: Clarithromycin in combination with omeprazole or ranitidine bismuth citrate is indicated for the treatment of patients with an active duodenal ulcer associated with *H. pylori* infection. Regimens that contain clarithromycin as the single antimicrobial agent are more likely to be associated with the development of clarithromycin resis-

CLARITHROMYCIN — ORAL

tance among patients who fail therapy. In patients who fail therapy, susceptibility testing should be done if possible. The eradication of *H. pylori* has been demonstrated to reduce the risk of duodenal ulcer recurrence.

Helicobacter pylori triple therapy: Clarithromycin, lansoprazole or omeprazole, and amoxicillin as combination triple therapy for the treatment of *H. pylori* infection and duodenal ulcer disease (active or 5-year history of duodenal ulcer) to eradicate *H. pylori*.

Children –

Pharyngitis/Tonsillitis: Caused by *S. pyogenes*.

Community-acquired pneumonia: Caused by *M. pneumoniae, S. pneumoniae*, or *C. pneumoniae* (TWAR) strain.

Acute maxillary sinusitis: Caused by *H. influenzae, M. catarrhalis*, or *S. pneumoniae*.

Acute otitis media: Caused by *H. influenzae, M. catarrhalis*, or *S. pneumoniae*.

Uncomplicated skin and skin structure infections: Caused by *S. aureus* or *S. pyogenes*. Abscesses usually require surgical drainage.

Disseminated mycobacterial infections: Caused by *M. avium* or *M. intracellulare*.

Prevention of disseminated MAC disease: In patients with advanced HIV infection.

➤*Extended-release tablets:* Treatment of adults with mild to moderate infection caused by susceptible strains of the designated microorganisms in the conditions listed below.

Acute maxillary sinusitis – Caused by *H. influenzae, M. catarrhalis, S. pneumoniae*.

Acute bacterial exacerbation of chronic bronchitis – Caused by *H. influenzae, H. parainfluenzae, M. catarrhalis*, or *S. pneumoniae*.

Community-acquired pneumonia – Caused by *H. influenzae, H. parainfluenzae, M. catarrhalis, S. pneumoniae, C. pneumoniae* (TWAR), or *M. pneumoniae*.

Administration and Dosage

➤*Approved by the FDA:* October 31, 1991.

Tablets and granules may be given with or without food. Take the extended-release tablets with food. Swallow the extended-release tablets whole and not chewed, broken, or crushed.

➤*Adults:*

Clarithromycin Dosage Guidelines

Infection	Tablets Dosage (every 12 h)	Tablets Duration (days)	Extended-release tablets Dosage (every 24 h)	Extended-release tablets Duration (days)
Pharyngitis/Tonsillitis	250 mg	10	-	-
Acute maxillary sinusitis	500 mg	14	1,000 mg	14
Acute exacerbation of chronic bronchitis caused by:				
H. parainfluenzae	500 mg	7	1,000 mg	7
S. pneumoniae	250 mg	7 to 14	1,000 mg	7
M. catarrhalis	250 mg	7 to 14	1,000 mg	7
H. influenzae	500 mg	7 to 14	1,000 mg	7
Community-acquired pneumonia caused by:				
S. pneumoniae	250 mg	7 to 14	1,000 mg	7
M. pneumoniae	250 mg	7 to 14	1,000 mg	7
H. influenzae	250 mg	7	1,000 mg	7
H. parainfluenzae	-	-	1,000 mg	7
M. catarrhalis	-	-	1,000 mg	7
C. pneumoniae	250 mg	7 to 14	1,000 mg	7
Uncomplicated skin and skin structure infection	250 mg	7 to 14	-	-

➤*H. pylori eradication to reduce the risk of duodenal ulcer recurrence:*

Triple therapy –

Clarithromycin/Lansoprazole/Amoxicillin: 500 mg clarithromycin, 30 mg lansoprazole, and 1 g amoxicillin every 12 hours for 10 or 14 days.

Clarithromycin/Omeprazole/Amoxicillin: 500 mg clarithromycin, 20 mg omeprazole, and 1 g amoxicillin every 12 hours for 10 days. In patients with an ulcer present at the time of initiation of therapy, an additional 18 days of omeprazole 20 mg once daily is recommended for ulcer healing and symptom relief.

Dual therapy –

Clarithromycin/Omeprazole: 500 mg clarithromycin 3 times/day (every 8 hours), and 40 mg omeprazole once daily (every morning) for 14 days. An additional 14 days of 20 mg omeprazole once daily is recommended for ulcer healing and symptom relief.

Clarithromycin/Ranitidine bismuth citrate: 500 mg clarithromycin 2 times/day (every 12 hours) or 3 times/day (every 8 hours), and 400 mg ranitidine bismuth citrate given 2 times/day (every 12 hours) for 14 days. An additional 14 days of ranitidine bismuth citrate 2 times/day is recommended for ulcer healing and symptom relief. This combination is not recommended in patients with a creatinine clearance < 25 mL/min.

➤*Mycobacterial infections:* Recommended as the primary agent for the treatment of disseminated MAC. Use in combination with other antimycobacterial drugs that have shown in vitro activity against MAC or clinical benefit in MAC treatment. Continue clarithromycin therapy for life if clinical and mycobacterial improvements are observed.

Dosage (treatment and prevention) –

Adults: 500 mg twice daily.

Children: 7.5 mg/kg twice daily up to 500 mg twice daily. Doses recommended for pediatric prophylaxis are derived from MAC treatment studies in children. Refer to the Pediatric Dosage table for dosing recommendations.

➤*Children:* Usual recommended daily dosage is 15 mg/kg/day divided every 12 hours for 10 days.

Pediatric Clarithromycin Dosage Guidelines (Based on Body Weight)

Dosing calculated on 7.5 mg/kg every 12 h

Weight kg	Weight lbs	Dose (q 12 hr)	125 mg/5 mL (q 12 hr)	250 mg/5 mL (q 12 hr)
9	20	62.5 mg	2.5 mL	1.25 mL
17	37	125 mg	5 mL	2.5 mL
25	55	187.5 mg	7.5 mL	3.75 mL
33	73	250 mg	10 mL	5 mL

➤*Renal/Hepatic function impairment:* May be administered without dosage adjustment in the presence of hepatic impairment if there is normal renal function. In the presence of severe renal impairment (Ccr < 30 mL/min) with or without coexisting hepatic impairment, halve the dose or double the dosing interval.

➤*Reconstitution of granules:* The following table indicates the volume of water to be added when constituting.

Clarithromycin Granule Reconstitution

Total volume after constitution (mL)	Clarithromycin concentration after constitution	Amount of water to be added (mL)
50	125 mg/5 mL	27
100	125 mg/5 mL	55
50	250 mg/5 mL	27
100	250 mg/5 mL	55

Add half the volume of water to the bottle and shake vigorously. Add the remainder of water to the bottle and shake.

➤*Storage/Stability:*

Tablets and granules – Store at controlled room temperature in a well-closed container. Protect the 250 mg tablets from light.

Extended-release tablets – Store the extended-release tablets at 20° to 25°C (68° to 77°F); excursions permitted to 15° to 30°C (59° to 86°F).

Reconstituted suspension – Shake well before each use. Keep tightly closed. Do not refrigerate. After mixing, store at 15° to 30°C (59° to 86°F), and use within 14 days.

AZITHROMYCIN

Rx	**Zithromax** (Pfizer)	**Tablets**: 250 mg (as dihydrate)	Lactose. (PFIZER 306). Pink, capsule shape. Film coated. In 30s, UD 50s, and *Z-Pak* 6s.
		500 mg (as dihydrate)	Lactose. (PFIZER ZTM500). Pink, capsule shape. Film coated. In 30s, UD 50s, and *TRI-PAK* 3s.
		600 mg (as dihydrate)	Lactose. (PFIZER 308). White, oval. Film coated. In 30s.
		Powder for injection, lyophilized: 500 mg	In 10 mL vials and 10 mL vials with 1 *Vial-Mate* adaptor.
		Powder for oral suspension: 100 mg per 5 mL (as dihydrate) when reconstituted	Sucrose. In 300 mg bottles.
		200 mg per 5 mL (as dihydrate) when reconstituted	Sucrose. In 600, 900, and 1,200 mg bottles.
		1 g/packet (as dihydrate)	Sucrose. In single-dose packets of 3s and 10s.
Rx	**Zmax** (Pfizer)	**Powder for oral suspension**: 167 mg per 5 mL (as dihydrate) when reconstituted	Extended-release microspheres. sucrose, 148 mg sodium. Cherry/Banana flavors. In 2 g bottles.

AZITHROMYCIN — ORAL

For complete prescribing information, refer to the Macrolides group monograph.

Indications

For the treatment of patients with mild to moderate infections caused by susceptible strains of the designated microorganisms in the specific conditions listed below:

➤*Adults:*

Note – Zmax is only indicated for the treatment of acute bacterial sinusitis and community-acquired pneumonia. See below for the designated microorganisms.

Acute bacterial sinusitis – Caused by *Haemophilus influenzae, Moraxella catarrhalis*, or *Streptococcus pneumoniae*.

Chronic obstructive pulmonary disease (COPD) – In patients with acute bacterial exacerbations of COPD caused by *H. influenzae, M. catarrhalis*, or *S. pneumoniae*.

Community-acquired pneumonia – In patients appropriate for oral therapy with community-acquired pneumonia of mild severity caused by *H. influenzae, Chlamydia pneumoniae, Mycoplasma pneumoniae*, or *S. pneumoniae*.

Note: Do not use azithromycin in patients with pneumonia who are judged to be inappropriate for oral therapy because of moderate to severe illness or risk factors such as any of the following: Patients with cystic fibrosis, nosocomially acquired infections, known or suspected bacteremia, patients requiring hospitalization, elderly or debilitated patients, or those with significant underlying health problems that may compromise their ability to respond to their illness (including immunodeficiency or functional asplenia).

Genital ulcer disease – In men with genital ulcer disease caused by *Haemophilus ducreyi* (chancroid).

Note: Do not rely upon azithromycin to treat gonorrhea and syphilis at the recommended dose. Antimicrobial agents used in high doses for short periods of time to treat nongonococcal urethritis may mask or delay the symptoms of incubating gonorrhea and syphilis. Administer a serologic test for syphilis and appropriate cultures for gonorrhea performed at the time of diagnosis to all patients with sexually transmitted urethritis or cervicitis. Initiate appropriate antimicrobial therapy and follow-up tests for these diseases if infection is confirmed.

Pharyngitis/Tonsillitis – As an alternative to first-line therapy in patients with pharyngitis/tonsillitis caused by *Streptococcus pyogenes* in individuals who cannot use first-line therapy.

Skin/Skin structure infections – In patients with uncomplicated skin and skin structure infections caused by *Staphylococcus aureus, S. pyogenes*, or *Streptococcus agalactiae*. Abscesses usually require surgical drainage.

Urethritis/Cervicitis – In patients with urethritis and cervicitis caused by *Chlamydia trachomatis* or *Neisseria gonorrhoeae*.

Prophylaxis of disseminated Mycobacterium avium complex (MAC) disease – Azithromycin taken alone or in combination with rifabutin at its approved dose is indicated for the prevention of disseminated MAC disease in people with advanced HIV infection.

Treatment of disseminated MAC disease – Azithromycin taken in combination with ethambutol is indicated for the treatment of disseminated MAC infections in people with advanced HIV infection.

➤*Children:*

Acute bacterial sinusitis – In children 6 months of age and older with acute bacterial sinusitis caused by *H. influenzae, M. catarrhalis*, or *S. pneumoniae*.

Acute otitis media – In children 6 months of age and older with acute otitis media caused by *H. influenzae, M. catarrhalis*, or *S. pneumoniae*.

Community-acquired pneumonia – In children 6 months of age and older with community-acquired pneumonia caused by *C. pneumoniae, H. influenzae, M. pneumoniae*, or *S. pneumoniae* in patients appropriate for oral therapy.

Note:: Do not use azithromycin in pediatric patients with pneumonia who are judged to be inappropriate for oral therapy because of moderate to severe illness or risk factors such as any of the following: Patients with cystic fibrosis, nosocomially acquired infections, known or suspected bacteremia, patients requiring hospitalization, or those with significant underlying health problems that may compromise their ability to respond to their illness (including immunodeficiency or functional asplenia).

Pharyngitis/Tonsillitis – In children 2 years of age and older and as an alternative to first-line therapy in patients with pharyngitis/tonsillitis caused by *S. pyogenes* in individuals who cannot use first-line therapy.

➤*Unlabeled uses: Helicobacter pylori* infections, *Bartonella* infection, Lyme disease, toxoplasmosis, babesiosis, granuloma inguinale (donovanosis), cryptosporidiosis.

Chlamydial infections – Caused by *C. trachomatis*. CDC treatment recommendations are 1 g azithromycin orally in a single dose. Alternatives include doxycycline, erythromycin base, erythromycin ethylsuccinate, or ofloxacin.

For children with chlamydial infection weighing 45 kg or more but younger than 8 years of age, CDC treatment recommendation is 1 g azithromycin orally in a single dose.

For children 8 years of age and older with chlamydial infection, CDC treatment recommendation is 1 g azithromycin orally in a single dose. Doxycycline is an alternative to azithromycin.

Uncomplicated gonococcal infections of the cervix, urethra, and rectum – Caused by *N. gonorrhoeae*. CDC treatment recommendation is 1 g azithromycin orally in a single dose in combination with 1 of the following: Cefixime, ceftriaxone, ciprofloxacin, or ofloxacin. Doxycycline is an alternative to azithromycin.

Uncomplicated gonococcal infection of the pharynx – CDC treatment recommendation is 1 g azithromycin orally in a single dose in combination with 1 of the following: Ceftriaxone, ciprofloxacin, or ofloxacin. Doxycycline is an alternative to azithromycin.

Prophylaxis after a sexual assault – CDC treatment recommendation is 1 g azithromycin orally in a single dose plus ceftriaxone and metronidazole. Doxycycline is an alternative to azithromycin.

Administration and Dosage

➤*Approved by the FDA:* November 1, 1991.

Tablets and oral suspension (except *Zmax*) can be taken with or without food; however, increased tolerability has been observed when tablets are taken with food. It is recommended that *Zmax* be taken on an empty stomach (at least 1 hour before or 2 hours following a meal. Single-dose 1 g packets are not for pediatric use.

➤*Renal function impairment:* Exercise caution when azithromycin is administered to subjects with severe renal impairment.

➤*Adults:*

Mild to moderate acute bacterial exacerbations of COPD – 500 mg/day for 3 days or 500 mg as a single dose on the first day followed by 250 mg once daily on days 2 through 5.

Community-acquired pneumonia of mild severity, pharyngitis/tonsillitis (as second-line therapy), and uncomplicated skin and skin structure infections – 500 mg as a single dose on the first day followed by 250 mg once daily on days 2 through 5. For community-acquired pneumonia, a single 2 g dose of *Zmax* may be given.

Acute bacterial sinusitis – 500 mg/day for 3 days or 2 g as a single dose of *Zmax*.

Genital ulcer disease caused by H. ducreyi (chancroid) – Single 1 g dose.

Nongonococcal urethritis/cervicitis – Single 1 g dose.

Gonococcal urethritis/cervicitis – Single 2 g dose.

Prevention of disseminated MAC infections – 1,200 mg taken once weekly. This dose of azithromycin may be combined with the approved dosage regimen of rifabutin.

Treatment of disseminated MAC infections – 600 mg/day in combination with ethambutol at the recommended daily dose of 15 mg/kg. Other antimycobacterial drugs that have shown in vitro activity against MAC may be added to the regimen of azithromycin plus ethambutol at the discretion of the physician or health care provider.

➤*Children (6 months of age and older):*

Acute otitis media – 30 mg/kg oral suspension given as a single dose or 10 mg/kg once daily for 3 days or 10 mg/kg as a single dose on the first day, followed by 5 mg/kg on days 2 through 5.

Acute bacterial sinusitis – 10 mg/kg oral suspension once daily for 3 days.

Community-acquired pneumonia – 10 mg/kg oral suspension as a single dose on the first day followed by 5 mg/kg on days 2 through 5.

Azithromycin Pediatric Dosage Guidelines for Otitis Media and Community-Acquired Pneumonia: 5-Day Regimen[a,b]

Weight		Amount of 100 m per 5 mL suspension		Amount of 200 mg per 5 mL suspension		Total mL per treatment course	Total mg per treatment course
kg	lbs	Day 1	Days 2 to 5	Day 1	Days 2 to 5		
5	11	2.5 mL	1.25 mL			7.5 mL	150 mg
10	22	5 mL	2.5 mL			15 mL	300 mg
20	44			5 mL	2.5 mL	15 mL	600 mg
30	66			7.5 mL	3.75 mL	22.5 mL	900 mg
40	88			10 mL	5 mL	30 mL	1,200 mg
≥ 50	≥ 110			12.5 mL	6.25 mL	37.5 mL	1,500 mg

[a] Dosing calculated on 10 mg/kg on day 1, followed by 5 mg/kg on days 2 to 5.
[b] Effectiveness of the 1- or 3-day regimen in children with community-acquired pneumonia has not been established.

Azithromycin Pediatric Dosage Guidelines for Otitis Media and Acute Bacterial Sinusitis: 3-Day Regimen[a,b]

Weight		Amount of 100 mg per 5 mL suspension	Amount of 200 mg per 5 mL suspension	Total mL per treatment course	Total mg per treatment course
kg	lbs	Day 1 to 3	Day 1 to 3		
5	11	2.5 mL		7.5 mL	150 mg
10	22	5 mL		15 mL	300 mg
20	44		5 mL	15 mL	600 mg

AZITHROMYCIN — ORAL

Azithromycin Pediatric Dosage Guidelines for Otitis Media and Acute Bacterial Sinusitis: 3-Day Regimen[a,b]					
Weight		Amount of 100 mg per 5 mL suspension	Amount of 200 mg per 5 mL suspension	Total mL per treatment course	Total mg per treatment course
kg	lbs	Day 1 to 3	Day 1 to 3		
30	66		7.5 mL	22.5 mL	900 mg
40	88		10 mL	30 mL	1,200 mg
≥ 50	≥ 110		12.5 mL	37.5 mL	1,500 mg

[a] Dosing calculated on 10 mg/kg/day.
[b] Effectiveness of the 1- or 5-day regimen in children with acute bacterial sinusitis has not been established.

Azithromycin Pediatric Dosage Guidelines for Otitis Media: 1-Day Regimen[a]				
Weight		Amount of 200 mg per 5 mL suspension	Total mL per treatment course	Total mg per treatment course
kg	lbs	Day 1		
5	11	3.75 mL	3.75 mL	150 mg
10	22	7.5 mL	7.5 mL	300 mg
20	44	15 mL	15 mL	600 mg
30	66	22.5 mL	22.5 mL	900 mg
40	88	30 mL	30 mL	1,200 mg
≥ 50	≥ 110	37.5 mL	37.5 mL	1,500 mg

[a] Dosing calculated on 30 mg/kg as a single dose.

Pharyngitis/Tonsillitis – 12 mg/kg once daily for 5 days. See the following table.

Azithromycin Pediatric Dosage Guidelines for Pharyngitis/Tonsillitis: 5-Day Regimen (≥ 2 years of age)[a]				
Weight		Amount of 200 mg per 5 mL suspension	Total mL per treatment course	Total mg per treatment course
kg	lbs	Day 1 to 5		
8	18	2.5 mL	12.5 mL	500 mg
17	37	5 mL	25 mL	1,000 mg
25	55	7.5 mL	37.5 mL	1,500 mg
33	73	10 mL	50 mL	2,000 mg
40	88	12.5 mL	62.5 mL	2,500 mg

[a] Dosing calculated on 12 mg/kg/day for 5 days.

➤*Preparation for IV administration:* Prepare the initial solution of azithromycin for injection by adding 4.8 mL sterile water for injection to the 500 mg vial and shaking the vial until all of the drug is dissolved. Because azithromycin for injection is supplied under vacuum, it is recommended that a standard 5 mL (nonautomated) syringe be used to ensure that the exact amount of 4.8 mL of sterile water is dispensed. Each mL of reconstituted solution contains 100 mg azithromycin. To provide azithromycin over a concentration range of 1 to 2 mg/mL, transfer 5 mL of the 100 mg/mL azithromycin solution into the appropriate amount of any of the diluents listed below: Normal saline (0.9% sodium chloride); ½ normal saline (0.45% sodium chloride); 5% dextrose in water; lactated Ringer's solution; 5% dextrose in ½ normal saline (0.45% sodium chloride) with 20 mEq KCl; 5% dextrose in lactated Ringer's solution; 5% dextrose in ⅓ normal saline (0.3% sodium chloride); 5% dextrose in ½ normal saline (0.45% sodium chloride); *Normosol-M* in 5% dextrose; *Normosol-R* in 5% dextrose.

➤*Preparation for administration of single 1 g packet:* Thoroughly mix the entire contents of the packet with approximately 60 mL (2 oz) of water. Drink the entire contents immediately; add an additional 60 mL of water, mix, and drink to ensure complete consumption of dosage. Do not use the single-dose packet to administer doses other than 1,000 mg of azithromycin. This packet is not for pediatric use.

➤*Preparation of single 2 g dose bottle:* Reconstitute with 60 mL water. Shake well before dispensing. Suspension should be consumed within 12 hours.

➤*Storage/Stability:*

Tablets – Store tablets between 15° to 30°C (59° to 86°F).

Oral suspension – Store dry powder below 30°C (86°F). Store single-dose packets between 5° and 30°C (41° and 86°F). Store reconstituted oral suspension between 5° and 30°C (41° and 86°F) and use within 10 days. Discard after full dosing is completed. Shake well before each use. Store *Zmax* dry powder at or below 30°C (86°F). Store reconstituted suspension at 25°C (77°F); excursions permitted to 15° to 30°C (59° to 86°F). Do not refrigerate or freeze. Suspension should be consumed within 12 hours.

AZITHROMYCIN — INJECTION

For complete prescribing information, refer to the Macrolides group monograph.

Indications

For the treatment of patients with mild to moderate infections caused by susceptible strains of the designated microorganisms in the specific conditions listed below:

➤*Adults:*

Community-acquired pneumonia – In patients requiring initial IV therapy with community-acquired pneumonia caused by *C. pneumoniae*, *H. influenzae*, *S. pneumoniae*, *M. pneumoniae*, *Legionella pneumophila*, *M. catarrhalis*, and *S. aureus*.

Pelvic inflammatory disease – In patients requiring initial IV therapy with pelvic inflammatory disease caused by *C. trachomatis*, *N. gonorrhoeae*, or *Mycoplasma hominis*. If anaerobic microorganisms are suspected of contributing to the infection, administer an antimicrobial agent with anaerobic activity in combination with azithromycin.

Children – IV azithromycin is not for use in children younger than 16 years of age.

➤*Note:* Penicillin IM is the usual drug of choice in the treatment of *S. pyogenes* infection and the prophylaxis of rheumatic fever. Azithromycin often is effective in the eradication of susceptible strains of *S. pyogenes* from the nasopharynx. Because some strains are resistant to azithromycin, perform susceptibility tests when patients are treated with azithromycin.

➤*Unlabeled uses:* *Helicobacter pylori* infections, *Bartonella* infection, Lyme disease, toxoplasmosis, babesiosis, granuloma inguinale (donovanosis), cryptosporidiosis.

Administration and Dosage

➤*Approved by the FDA:* January 30, 1997.

➤*Renal function impairment:* Exercise caution when azithromycin is administered to subjects with severe renal impairment.

➤*Adults:* Infuse injections over a period of not less than 60 minutes. The infusate concentration and rate of infusion for azithromycin for injection should be 1 mg/mL over 3 hours or 2 mg/mL over 1 hour. Do not administer azithromycin for injection as a bolus or IM injection.

Community-acquired pneumonia – 500 mg as a single daily dose IV for at least 2 days. Follow IV therapy by the oral route at a single daily dose of 500 mg to complete a 7- to 10-day course of therapy.

Pelvic inflammatory disease – 500 mg as a single daily dose IV for 1 or 2 days. Follow IV therapy by the oral route at a single daily dose of 250 mg to complete a 7-day course of therapy. If anaerobic microorganisms are suspected of contributing to the infection, administer an antimicrobial agent with anaerobic activity with azithromycin.

➤*Preparation for IV administration:* Prepare the initial solution of azithromycin for injection by adding 4.8 mL sterile water for injection to the 500 mg vial and shaking the vial until all of the drug is dissolved. Because azithromycin for injection is supplied under vacuum, it is recommended that a standard 5 mL (nonautomated) syringe be used to ensure that the exact amount of 4.8 mL of sterile water is dispensed. Each mL of reconstituted solution contains 100 mg azithromycin. To provide azithromycin over a concentration range of 1 to 2 mg/mL, transfer 5 mL of the 100 mg/mL azithromycin solution into the appropriate amount of any of the diluents listed below: Normal saline (0.9% sodium chloride); ½ normal saline (0.45% sodium chloride); 5% dextrose in water; lactated Ringer's solution; 5% dextrose in ½ normal saline (0.45% sodium chloride) with 20 mEq KCl; 5% dextrose in lactated Ringer's solution; 5% dextrose in ⅓ normal saline (0.3% sodium chloride); 5% dextrose in ½ normal saline (0.45% sodium chloride); *Normosol-M* in 5% dextrose; *Normosol-R* in 5% dextrose.

➤*Storage/Stability:* Reconstituted solution and the diluted solution for injection are stable for 24 hours when stored below 30°C (86°F) for 7 days. The diluted solution for injection is stable when refrigerated at 5°C (41°F).

WARNING

Erythromycin estolate – Hepatic dysfunction with or without jaundice has occurred, chiefly in adults, in association with erythromycin estolate administration. It may be accompanied by malaise, nausea, vomiting, abdominal colic, and fever. In some instances, severe abdominal pain may stimulate an abdominal surgical emergency. If the above findings occur, discontinue erythromycin estolate oral suspension promptly. Erythromycin estolate oral suspension is contraindicated for patients with a known history of sensitivity to this drug and for those with preexisting liver disease.

Indications

To reduce the development of drug-resistant bacteria and maintain the effectiveness, erythromycin should only be used to treat or prevent infections that are proven, or strongly suspected, to be caused by susceptible bacteria. When culture and susceptibility information are available, they should be considered in selecting or modifying antibacterial therapy. In the absence of such data, local epidemiology and susceptibility patterns may contribute to the empiric selection of therapy.

Indicated for treatment of infections caused by susceptible strains of the designated microorganisms in the diseases listed below:

➤*Bacterial endocarditis, prophylaxis:* Oral erythromycin may be used for prevention of bacterial endocarditis in penicillin-allergic patients with prosthetic cardiac valves, most congenital cardiac malformations, surgically constructed systemic pulmonary shunts, rheumatic or other acquired valvular dysfunction, idiopathic hypertrophic subaortic stenosis (IHSS), previous history of bacterial endocarditis, or mitral valve prolapse with insufficiency when undergoing dental procedures or surgical procedures of the upper respiratory tract. However, the American Heart Association no longer recommends its use because of GI upset and complicated pharmacokinetics of various formulations. Practitioners may continue to use erythromycin if they have had success in its use.

➤*Conjunctivitis of the newborn, pneumonia of infancy, urogenital infections during pregnancy:* Caused by *Chlamydia trachomatis* (oral erythromycin only).

➤*Diphtheria:* Adjunct to antitoxin in infections caused by *Corynebacterium diphtheriae*, to prevent establishment of carriers and to eradicate the organism in carriers.

➤*Erythrasma:* Treatment of infections caused by *Corynebacterium minutissimum*.

➤*Intestinal amebiasis:* Caused by *Entamoeba histolytica* (oral erythromycin only). Extra-enteric amebiasis requires treatment with other agents.

➤*Legionnaire disease:* Caused by *Legionella pneumophila*. Although no controlled clinical efficacy studies have been conducted, in vitro and limited preliminary clinical data suggest effectiveness.

➤*Nongonococcal urethritis:* Caused by *Ureaplasma urealyticum* when tetracyclines are contraindicated or not tolerated (oral erythromycin only).

➤*Pelvic inflammatory disease (PID), acute:* Caused by *Neisseria gonorrhoeae*: As an alternative to penicillin in patients with a history of penicillin sensitivity. Patients should have an acrologic test for syphilis before receiving erythromycin as treatment of gonorrhea and a follow-up serologic test for syphilis after 3 months.

➤*Pertussis (whooping cough):* Caused by *Bordetella pertussis*. Effective in eliminating the organism from the nasopharynx of infected patients. May be helpful in the prophylaxis of pertussis in exposed susceptible individuals (oral erythromycin only).

➤*Primary syphilis:* Caused by *Treponema pallidum*: Erythromycin (oral only) as an alternative to penicillin in penicillin-allergic patients.

➤*Respiratory tract infections:* Caused by *Mycoplasma pneumoniae* (Eaton's agent).

➤*Rheumatic fever:* Prevention of initial or recurrent attacks as an alternative in patients who are allergic to penicillins or sulfonamides.

➤*Uncomplicated urethral, endocervical, or rectal infections in adults:* Caused by *C. trachomatis* when tetracyclines are contraindicated or not tolerated.

➤*Upper respiratory tract infections:* Mild to moderate severity caused by: *Streptococcus pyogenes* (group A beta-hemolytic streptococci), *Streptococcus pneumoniae*, or *Haemophilus influenzae* (with concomitant sulfonamides because not all strains of *H. influenzae* are susceptible at the erythromycin concentrations ordinarily achieved).

➤*Listeria: Listeria monocytogenes* infections.

➤*Lower respiratory tract infections:* Mild to moderate severity caused by *S. pyogenes* (group A beta-hemolytic streptococci) or *S. (diplococcus) pneumoniae*.

➤*Skin/Skin structure infections:* Mild to moderate severity caused by *S. pyogenes*; *Staphylococcus aureus* (resistant staphylococci may emerge during treatment).

➤*Unlabeled uses:*

Acne vulgaris – Helpful in decreasing the population of lipophilic bacteria and may also have an anti-inflammatory effect.

Bacillary angiomatosis (immunocompromised patients) – Caused by *Bartonella henselae* or *B. quintana*; as an alternative agent, erythromycin 500 mg 4 times/day.

Campylobacter enteritis – Caused by *Campylobacter jejuni*.

Cellulitis, erysipelas – As an alternative agent for the treatment of cellulitis (erysipelas) of the extremities that is not associated with venous catheter and not diabetes-related.

Chancroid – Caused by *Haemophilus ducreyi*.

Granuloma inguinale (Donovanosis) – Caused by *Calymmatobacterium granulomatis*; as an alternative to doxycycline or trimethoprim-sulfamethoxazole.

Impetigo, ecthyma – As an alternative agent for the treatment of nonbullous lesions.

Inclusion conjunctivitis (adults) – Caused by *C. trachomatis*; as an alternative agent.

Infected wounds, extremity – As an alternative agent for the treatment of mild to moderate, uncomplicated, infected wounds of the extremities.

Leptospirosis – Caused by *Leptospira* species; for the treatment of moderate to severe leptospirosis.

Lyme disease (early) – Caused by *Borrelia burgorferi*; as an alternate agent.

Lymphogranuloma venereum – Caused by *C. trachomatis*; as an alternative to doxycycline.

Relapsing fever – For the treatment of tick-borne relapsing fever and louse-borne relapsing fever.

Tetanus – Caused by *Clostridium tetani*; as an alternative agent.

Administration and Dosage

➤*Oral:* Dosages and product strengths are expressed as erythromycin base equivalents. Because of differences in absorption and biotransformation, varying quantities of each salt form are required to produce the same free erythromycin serum levels. For example, expressed in base equivalents, 400 mg erythromycin ethylsuccinate produces the same free erythromycin serum levels as 250 mg of erythromycin base, stearate, or estolate.

Erythromycin base is inactivated by gastric acids, and therefore is administered as enteric-coated tablets or capsules containing enteric-coated pellets. Erythromycin esters (ie, stearate, ethylsuccinate, estolate) have been formulated to improve acid stability and absorption. Optimal serum levels of erythromycin are reached when erythromycin base or stearate is taken in the fasting state. Erythromycin ethylsuccinate, estolate, and enteric-coated erythromycin may be administered without regard to meals.

Usual dosage –

Adults: 250 mg (or 400 mg ethylsuccinate) every 6 hours, or 500 mg every 12 hours, or 333 mg every 8 hours. May increase up to 4 g/day, according to severity of infection. If twice daily dosage is desired, the recommended dose is 500 mg every 12 hours. Twice daily dosing is not recommended when doses greater than 1 g/day are administered.

Children: 30 to 50 mg/kg/day in divided doses. Proper dosage is determined by age, weight, and severity of infection. When twice daily dosing is desired, half of the total daily dose may be taken every 12 hours. For more severe infections, dosage may be doubled but should not exceed 4 grams.

Erythromycin Uses and Dosages[a]

Indication	Dosage (stated as erythromycin base)	Duration of treatment
Labeled uses:		
Bacterial endocarditis, prophylaxis[b]	*Adults:* 1 g administered 1 h before procedure then 500 mg administered 6 h later	2 doses
	Children: 20 mg/kg administered 1 h before procedure than 10 mg/kg administered 6 h later	
Conjunctivitis of the newborn (*C. trachomatis*)	50 mg/kg/day in 4 divided doses	≥ 14 days
Pneumonia of infancy (*C. trachomatis*)	50 mg/kg/day in 4 divided doses	≥ 21 days (14 days per CDC)[c]
Urogenital infections during pregnancy (*C. trachomatis*)	500 mg 4 times/day or two 333 mg tablets (666 mg) every 8 hours	≥ 7 days
	(For women who are unable to tolerate this regimen, give 250 mg every 6 h or 333 mg every 8 h or 500 mg every 12 hours for ≥ 14 days)	

Erythromycin Uses and Dosages[a]		
Indication	Dosage (stated as erythromycin base)	Duration of treatment
Diphtheria (*C. diphtheriae*)	500 mg 4 times/day[d]	14 days[d] (7 days for cutaneous diphtheria and carriers)[d]
Erythrasma (*C. minutissimum*)	250 mg every 6 h[e]	14 days[e]
Intestinal amebiasis (*E. histolytica*)	*Adults:* 250 mg (or 400 mg as ethylsuccinate) every 6 h or 333 mg every 8 h or 500 mg every 12 h *Children:* 30 to 50 mg/kg/day in equally divided doses.	10 to 14 days
Legionnaire disease (*L. pneumophila*)	1 to 4 grams in divided doses	
Nongonoccal urethritis (*U. urealyticum*)	500 mg 4 times/day or two 333 mg tablets (666 mg) every 8 hours or 800 mg (as ethylsuccinate) every 8 h	≥ 7 days
Pelvic inflammatory disease (acute) (*N. gonorrhoeae*)	500 mg IV every 6 h for 3 days followed by 250 mg orally every 6 h or 333 mg every 8 h for 7 days	10 days
Pertussis (whooping cough) (*B. pertussis*)	40 to 50 mg/kg/day, given in divided doses	5 to 14 days
Primary syphilis (*T. pallidum*)	30 to 40 grams (or 48 to 64 grams as ethylsuccinate) given in divided doses over 10 to 15 days	10 to 15 days
Respiratory tract infections (*M. pneumoniae*)	*Adults:* 250 to 500 mg every 6 h[d] *Children:* 20 to 50 mg/kg/day in 3 or 4 divided doses[d]	14 to 21 days[d]
Rheumatic fever, prevention of initial attack	400 mg every 6 h	10 days
Rheumatic fever, prevention of recurrent attacks	250 mg (or 400 mg as ethylsuccinate) twice daily	Continuous
Uncomplicated urethral, endocervical, or rectal infections (*C. trachomatis*)	Adults: 500 mg 4 times/day or two 333 mg tablets (666 mg) every 8 h or 800 mg (as ethylsuccinate) 4 times/day[c]	≥ 7 days
	Children (≤ 45 kg): 50 mg/kg/day in 4 divided doses[c]	14 days[c]
Upper respiratory tract infections of mild to moderate severity *S. pyogenes* *S. pneumoniae* *H. influenzae*	*Adults:* 250 mg every 6 h or 333 mg every 8 h or 500 mg every 12 h. Max dose is 4 g/day. *Children:* 30 to 50 mg/kg/day in equally divided doses. Max dose is 4 g/day. *H. influenzae* infections should be treated concomitantly with a sulfonamide.	≥ 10 days (for streptococcal infections)
Unlabeled uses:		
Acne vulgaris	250 to 1000 mg/day[d]	
Bacillary angiomatosis (immunocompromised patients):[e] *Bartonella henselae* or *B. quintana*	500 mg 4 times/day	
Campylobacter enteritis[d] (*C. jejuni*)	*Adults:* 250 mg 4 times/day *Children:* 30 to 50 mg/kg/day in divided doses	5 to 7 days
Chancroid[c] (*H. ducreyi*)	500 mg 3 times/day	7 days
Granuloma inguinale (Donavanosis)[c] (*C. granulomatis*)	500 mg 4 times/day	≥ 21 days
Inclusion conjunctivitis (adults) (*C. trachomatis*)	250 mg 4 times/day	1 to 3 weeks
Leptospirosis[d] (*Leptospira* species)	500 mg IV 4 times/day	7 days
Lyme disease[d] (*B. burgdorferi*)	250 mg 4 times/day	
Lymphogranuloma venereum[c] (*C. trachomatis*)	500 mg 4 times/day	21 days
Relapsing fever[d]	*Louse-borne:* 500 mg (single dose)	Single dose
	Tick-borne: 500 mg every 6 h	7 days

[a] Dosages are for adults unless otherwise specified.
[b] Erythromycin is no longer recommended by the American Heart Association for the prevention of bacterial endocarditis. However, practitioners may continue to use erythromycin if they have had success with its use.
[c] CDC 2002 Sexually Transmitted Diseases Treatment Guidelines.
[d] Harrison's Principles of Internal Medicine 14th ed.
[e] The Sanford Guide to Antimicrobial Therapy 2004.

➤*Parenteral:*

Erythromycin IV – This is indicated when oral use is impossible, or when severity of the infection requires immediate high serum levels. Replace IV therapy with oral as soon as possible.

Continuous infusion: This is preferable, but intermittent infusion in 20- to 60-minute periods at intervals of less than or equal to 6 hours also is effective. Because of irritative properties of erythromycin, IV push is unacceptable.

Severe infections – 15 to 20 mg/kg/day. Higher doses, up to 4 g/day, may also be given for severe infections.

Preparation of solution –

Vials: Prepare the initial solution by adding 10 mL sterile water for injection to the 500 mg vial or 20 mL sterile water for injection to the 1 g vial. Use only sterile water for injection as other diluents may cause precipitation during reconstitution. Do not use diluents containing preservatives or inorganic salts. After reconstitution, each mL contains 50 mg erythromycin activity.

Add the initial dilution to one of the following diluents before administration to give a concentration of 1 g/L (1 mg/mL) erythromycin activity for continuous infusion or 1 to 5 mg/mL for intermittent infusion: 0.9% sodium chloride injection; Ringer's lactate injection; *Normosol-R*.

The following solutions may also be used providing they are first buffered with 4% sodium bicarbonate or *Neut* by adding 1 mL of the 4% sodium bicarbonate injection or *Neut* per 100 mL of solution: 5% dextrose injection; 5% dextrose and Lactated Ringer's injection; 5% dextrose and 0.9% sodium chloride injection.

➤*Storage / Stability:*

Erythromycin base and stearate – Store at controlled room temperature 15° to 30°C (59° to 86°F).

Erythromycin estolate – Shake the suspension well before using. Refrigerate to maintain optimum taste. Dispense in a tight, light-resistant container.

Erythromycin ethylsuccinate – Store tablets and granules (prior to mixing) below 30°C (86°F). After reconstitution of the oral suspension, refrigerate (to preserve taste) and use within 10 days. After reconstitution of the oral drops, store at or below 25°C (77°F) and use within 35 days; refrigeration is not required. Store the premixed oral suspension under refrigeration to preserve taste until dispensed. Refrigeration by patient is not required if used within 14 days.

Injection – The *initial* solution is stable for 2 weeks if refrigerated for 24 hours at room temperature. Completely administer the final diluted solution within 8 hours in order to ensure proper potency because it is not suitable for storage.

ERYTHROMYCIN BASE

Rx	**Ery-Tab** (Abbott)	**Tablets, delayed-release:** 250 mg	Enteric-coated. (EC). In 100s, 500s, and UD 100s.
Rx	**Ery-Tab** (Abbott)	**Tablets, delayed-release:** 333 mg	Enteric-coated. (EH). In 100s, 500s, and UD 100s.
Rx	**PCE Dispertab** (Abbott)	**Tablets with polymer-coated particles:** 333 mg	Lactose. (PCE). White with pink speckles. In 60s.
Rx	**Ery-Tab** (Abbott)	**Tablets, delayed-release:** 500 mg	Enteric-coated. (ED). In 100s and UD 100s.
Rx	**PCE Dispertab** (Abbott)	**Tablets with polymer-coated particles:** 500 mg	(EK). White. In 100s.
Rx	**Erythromycin Filmtabs** (Abbott)	**Tablets, film-coated:** 250 mg	(EB). Pink. In 100s, 500s, and UD 100s.
Rx	**Erythromycin Filmtabs** (Abbott)	**Tablets, film-coated:** 500 mg	(EA). Pink. In 100s.
Rx	**Eryc** (FH Faulding & Co. Ltd.)	**Capsules, delayed-release:** 250 mg	Enteric-coated pellets. (Capsule 696). Clear and orange. In 100s.
Rx	**Erythromycin** (Various, eg, Abbott)		Enteric-coated pellets. In 100s and 500s.

ERYTHROMYCIN BASE — ORAL

Complete and comparative prescribing information begins in the Erythromycin group monograph.

ERYTHROMYCIN ESTOLATE

Rx	**Erythromycin Estolate** (Alpharma)	**Suspension:** 125 mg (as base) per 5 mL	May contain EDTA, parabens, saccharin, and sucrose. In 473 mL.
Rx	**Erythromycin Estolate** (Alpharma)	**Suspension:** 250 mg (as base) per 5 mL	May contain EDTA, parabens, saccharin, and sucrose. In 473 mL.

ERYTHROMYCIN ESTOLATE — ORAL

Complete and comparative prescribing information begins in the Erythromycin group monograph.

ERYTHROMYCIN STEARATE

Rx	**Erythrocin Stearate** (Abbott)	**Tablets, film-coated:** 250 mg (as base)	(ES). Pink. In 100s and 500s.
Rx	**Erythrocin Stearate** (Abbott)	**Tablets, film-coated:** 500 mg (as base)	(ET). Pink. In 100s.

ERYTHROMYCIN STEARATE — ORAL

Complete and comparative prescribing information begins in the Erythromycin group monograph.

ERYTHROMYCIN ETHYLSUCCINATE

Rx	**Erythromycin Ethylsuccinate** (Various, eg, Abbott, Mylan)	**Tablets:** 400 mg (as base)	In 100s and 500s.
Rx	**E.E.S. 400** (Abbott)		Sugar. (EE). Pink. Film coated. In 100s, 500s, and UD 100s.
Rx	**Erythromycin Ethylsuccinate** (Various, eg, Abbott)	**Suspension:** 200 mg (as base) per 5 mL	In 473 mL.
Rx	**E.E.S. 200** (Abbott)		Parabens, sucrose. Fruit flavor. In 100 and 473 mL.
Rx	**Erythromycin Ethylsuccinate** (Various, eg, Abbott)	**Suspension:** 400 mg (as base) per 5 mL	In 473 mL.
Rx	**E.E.S. 400** (Abbott)		Parabens, sucrose. Orange flavor. In 100 and 473 mL bottles.
Rx	**EryPed Drops** (Abbott)	**Suspension:** 100 mg (as base) per 2.5 mL	Sucrose. Fruit flavor. In 50 mL.
Rx	**EryPed 200** (Abbott)	**Powder for oral suspension:** 200 mg (as base) per 5 mL when reconstituted	Sucrose. Fruit flavor. In 100, 200 mL, UD 5 mL (100s).
Rx	**E.E.S. Granules** (Abbott)		Sucrose. Cherry flavor. In 100 and 200 mL.
Rx	**EryPed 400** (Abbott)	**Powder for oral suspension:** 400 mg (as base) per 5 mL when reconstituted	Sucrose. Banana flavor. In 60, 100, 200, and UD 5 mL (100s).

ERYTHROMYCIN ETHYLSUCCINATE — ORAL

Complete and comparative prescribing information begins in the Erythromycin group monograph.

ERYTHROMYCIN LACTOBIONATE

Rx	**Erythrocin Lactobionate** (Hospira)	**Powder for injection, lyophilized:** 500 mg (as base)	May contain benzyl alcohol. In vials.
		1 g (as base)	May contain benzyl alcohol. In vials.

ERYTHROMYCIN LACTOBIONATE — INJECTION

Complete and comparative prescribing information begins in the Erythromycin group monograph.

TELITHROMYCIN

Rx	**Ketek** (Aventis)	**Tablets:** 300 mg	(38AV). Lt. orange, oval. Film-coated. In 20s.
		400 mg	(H3647 400). Lt. orange, oval. Film-coated. In 60s, blister pack 10s, and UD 100s.

TELITHROMYCIN — ORAL

Indications

Telithromycin is indicated for the treatment of infections caused by susceptible strains of the designated microorganisms in the following conditions for patients 18 years of age and older.

➤*Acute bacterial exacerbation of chronic bronchitis:* Due to *Streptococcus pneumoniae*, *Haemophilus influenzae*, or *Moraxella catarrhalis*.

➤*Acute bacterial sinusitis:* Due to *S. pneumoniae*, *H. influenzae*, *M. catarrhalis*, or *Staphylococcus aureus*.

➤*Community-acquired pneumonia (CAP) (of mild to moderate severity):* Due to *S. pneumoniae*, (including multidrug-resistant isolates [multidrug-resistant *S. pneumoniae* (MDRSP), includes isolates known as penicillin-resistant *S. pneumoniae* (PRSP), and are isolates resistant to 2 or more of the following antibiotics: penicillin, second-generation cephalosporins (eg, cefuroxime), macrolides, tetracyclines, trimethoprim/sulfamethoxazole]), *H. influenzae*, *M. catarrhalis*, *Chlamydophila pneumoniae*, or *Mycoplasma pneumoniae*.

➤*Unlabeled uses:* Acute tonsillitis/pharyngitis.

Administration and Dosage

➤*Approved by the FDA:* April 1, 2004.

➤*Dosage:* The dosage of telithromycin is 800 mg taken orally once every 24 hours. The duration of therapy depends on the infection type and is described in the following table. Telithromycin can be administered with or without food.

Telithromycin Dosage

Infection	Daily dose and route of administration	Frequency of administration	Duration of treatment
Acute bacterial exacerbation of chronic bronchitis	800 mg oral (two 400 mg tablets)	once daily	5 days
Acute bacterial sinusitis	800 mg oral (two 400 mg tablets)	once daily	5 days
CAP	800 mg oral (two 400 mg tablets)	once daily	7 to 10 days

➤*Renal function impairment:* In the presence of severe renal function impairment (creatinine clearance [Ccr] less than 30 mL/min), including patients who need dialysis, the dosage should be reduced to telithromycin 600 mg once daily. In patients undergoing hemodialysis, telithromycin should be given after the dialysis session on dialysis days.

In the presence of severe renal function impairment (Ccr less than 30 mL/min) with coexisting hepatic function impairment, the dosage should be reduced to telithromycin 400 mg once daily.

➤*Storage/Stability:* Store at 25°C (77°F); excursions are permitted to 15° to 30°C (59° to 86°F).

Actions

➤*Pharmacology:* Telithromycin belongs to the ketolide class of antibacterials and is structurally related to the macrolide family of antibiotics. Telithromycin blocks protein synthesis by binding to domains II and V of 23S ribosomal ribonucleic acid (rRNA) of the 50S ribosomal subunit. By binding at domain II, telithromycin retains activity against gram-positive cocci (eg, *S. pneumoniae*) in the presence of resistance mediated by methylases (erm genes) that alter the domain V binding site of telithromycin. Telithromycin may also inhibit the assembly of nascent ribosomal units.

➤*Pharmacokinetics:*

Absorption – Following oral administration, telithromycin reached maximal concentration (C_{max}) at about 1 hour (range, 0.5 to 4 hours). It has an absolute bioavailability of 57% in both younger and elderly subjects. The rate and extent of absorption are unaffected by food intake; thus, telithromycin tablets can be given without regard to food.

In healthy adult subjects, peak plasma telithromycin concentrations of approximately 2 mcg/mL are attained at a median of 1 hour after an 800 mg oral dose. Steady-state plasma concentrations are reached within 2 to 3 days of once-daily dosing with telithromycin 800 mg. The pharmacokinetics of telithromycin after administration of single and multiple (7 days) once-daily 800 mg doses to healthy adult subjects are shown in the following table.

Mean Telithromycin Pharmacokinetic Parameters

Parameter	Mean (SD[a]) Single dose (n = 18)	Multiple dose (n = 18)
C_{max} (mcg/mL)	1.9 (0.8)	2.27 (0.71)
t_{max}[b] (h) median (min, max)[c]	1 (0.5, 4)	1 (0.5, 3)
$AUC^{d}_{(0-24)}$ (mcg•h/mL)	8.25 (2.6)	12.5 (5.4)
Terminal $t_{½}$[e] (h)	7.16 (1.3)	9.81 (1.9)
$C_{24\,h}$[f] (mcg/mL)	0.03 (0.013)	0.07 (0.051)

[a] SD = Standard deviation.
[b] t_{max} = time to C_{max}.
[c] Median (min, max) values.
[d] AUC = area under concentration vs time curve.
[e] ½ = terminal plasma half-life.
[f] $C_{24\,h}$ = plasma concentration at 24 hours post-dose.

In a patient population, mean peak and trough plasma concentrations were 2.9 mcg/mL (± 1.55; n = 219) and 0.2 mcg/mL (± 0.22; n = 204), respectively, after 3 to 5 days of telithromycin 800 mg once daily.

Distribution – Total in vitro protein binding is approximately 60% to 70% and is primarily due to human serum albumin. Protein binding is not modified in elderly subjects or in patients with hepatic function impairment. The volume of distribution of telithromycin after intravenous (IV) infusion is 2.9 L/kg.

Telithromycin concentrations in bronchial mucosa, epithelial lining fluid, and alveolar macrophages after 800 mg once-daily dosing for 5 days in patients are displayed in the following table.

Telithromycin Tissue Concentrations

Tissue	Hours postdose	Mean concentration (mcg/mL) Tissue or fluid	Plasma	Tissue/Plasma ratio
Bronchial mucosa	2	3.88[a]	1.86	2.11
	12	1.41[a]	0.23	6.33
	24	0.78[a]	0.08	12.11
Epithelial lining fluid	2	14.89	1.86	8.57
	12	3.27	0.23	13.8
	24	0.84	0.08	14.41
Alveolar macrophages	2	65	1.07	55
	8	100	0.605	180
	24	41	0.073	540

[a] Units in mg/kg.

Telithromycin concentration in white blood cells exceeds the concentration in plasma and it is eliminated more slowly from white blood cells than from plasma. Mean white blood cell concentrations of telithromycin peaked at 72.1 mcg/mL at 6 hours, and remained at 14.1 mcg/mL 24 hours after 5 days of repeated dosing of 600 mg once daily. After 10 days of repeated dosing of 600 mg once daily, white blood cell concentrations remained at 8.9 mcg/mL 48 hours after the last dose.

Metabolism/Excretion – In total, metabolism accounts for approximately 70% of the dose. In plasma, the main circulating compound after administration of an 800 mg radiolabeled dose was parent compound, representing 56.7% of the total radioactivity. The main metabolite represented 12.6% of the AUC of telithromycin. Three other plasma metabolites were quantified, each representing 3% or less of the AUC of telithromycin. It is estimated that approximately 50% of its metabolism is mediated by cytochrome P-450 3A4 and the remaining 50% is P-450–independent.

The systemically available telithromycin is eliminated by multiple pathways as follows: 7% of the dose is excreted unchanged in feces by biliary and/or intestinal secretion, 13% of the dose is excreted unchanged in urine by renal excretion, and 37% of the dose is metabolized by the liver. Following oral dosing, the mean terminal elimination half-life of telithromycin is 10 hours.

Special populations –

Renal function impairment: In a multiple-dose study, 36 subjects with varying degrees of renal function impairment received telithromycin 400, 600, or 800 mg once daily for 5 days. There was a 1.4-fold increase in $C_{max,ss}$ and a 1.9-fold increase in $AUC_{(0-24)ss}$ at 800 mg multiple doses in the severely renally impaired group (Ccr less than 30 mL/min), compared with healthy volunteers. Renal excretion may serve as a compensatory elimination pathway for telithromycin in situations in which metabolic clearance is impaired. Patients with severe renal function impairment are prone to conditions that may impair their metabolic clearance. Therefore, in the presence of severe renal function impairment (Ccr less than 30 mL/min), a reduced dosage of telithromycin is recommended.

In a single-dose study in patients with end-stage renal failure on hemodialysis (n = 10), the mean C_{max} and AUC values were similar to healthy subjects when telithromycin was administered 2 hours postdialysis. However, the effect of dialysis on removing telithromycin from the body has not been studied.

Hepatic function impairment: An increase in renal elimination was observed in hepatically impaired patients, indicating that this pathway may compensate for some of the decrease in metabolic clearance. No dosage adjustment is recommended in cases of hepatic function impairment.

Elderly: Pharmacokinetic data show that there is a 1.4-fold increase in exposure (AUC) in 20 patients 65 years of age or older with CAP in a phase 3 study, and a 2-fold increase in exposure (AUC) in 14 subjects 65 years of

TELITHROMYCIN — ORAL

age or older, as compared with subjects younger than 65 years of age in a phase 1 study. No dosage adjustment is required based on age alone.

Multiple insufficiency: The effects of coadministration of ketoconazole in 12 subjects (60 years of age or older) with impaired renal function were studied (Ccr, 24 to 80 mL/min). In this study, when severe renal function impairment (Ccr less than 30 mL/min; n = 2) and concomitant impairment of CYP3A4 metabolism pathway were present, telithromycin exposure ($AUC_{[0-24]}$) was increased by approximately 4- to 5-fold, compared with the exposure in healthy subjects with normal renal function receiving telithromycin alone. In the presence of severe renal function impairment (Ccr less than 30 mL/min) with coexisting hepatic function impairment, a reduced dosage of telithromycin is recommended.

➤*Microbiology:* Telithromycin concentrates in phagocytes, where it exhibits its activity against intracellular respiratory pathogens. In vitro, telithromycin has been shown to demonstrate concentration-dependent bactericidal activity against isolates of *S. pneumoniae* (including multidrug-resistant isolates [MDRSP includes isolates known as PRSP , and are isolates resistant to 2 or more of the following antimicrobials: penicillin, second generation cephalosporins (eg, cefuroxime), macrolides, tetracyclines, trimethoprim/sulfamethoxazole.]).

Resistance – S. aureus and *Streptococcus pyogenes* with the constitutive macrolide-lincosamide–streptogramin B ($cMLS_B$) phenotype are resistant to telithromycin.

Mutants of *S. pneumoniae* derived in the laboratory by serial passage in subinhibitory concentrations of telithromycin have demonstrated resistance based on L22 riboprotein mutations (telithromycin minimum inhibitory concentrations [MICs] are elevated but still within the susceptible range), 1 of 2 reported mutations affecting the L4 riboprotein, and production of K-peptide. The clinical significance of these laboratory mutants is not known.

Cross resistance – Telithromycin does not induce resistance through methylase gene expression in erythromycin-inducibly resistant bacteria, a function of its 3-keto moiety. Telithromycin has not been shown to induce resistance to itself.

Contraindications

History of hypersensitivity to telithromycin and/or any components of telithromycin tablets, or any macrolide antibiotic; coadministration with cisapride or pimozide.

Warnings

➤*Pseudomembranous colitis:* Pseudomembranous colitis has been reported with nearly all antibacterial agents, including telithromycin, and may range in severity from mild to life-threatening. Therefore, it is important to consider this diagnosis in patients who present with diarrhea subsequent to the administration of any antibacterial agents.

Treatment with antibacterial agents alters the flora of the colon and may permit overgrowth of clostridia. Studies indicate that toxin-producing strains of *Clostridium difficile* are the primary cause of "antibiotic-associated colitis."

After the diagnosis of pseudomembranous colitis has been established, initiate therapeutic measures. Mild cases of pseudomembranous colitis usually respond to drug discontinuation alone. In moderate to severe cases, consider management with fluids and electrolytes, protein supplementation, and treatment with an antibacterial drug clinically effective against *C. difficile* colitis.

➤*Cardiac effects:* Telithromycin has the potential to prolong the QTc interval of the electrocardiogram (ECG) in some patients. QTc prolongation may lead to an increased risk for ventricular arrhythmias, including torsades de pointes. Thus, avoid telithromycin use in patients with congenital prolongation of the QTc interval, and in patients with ongoing proarrhythmic conditions such as uncorrected hypokalemia or hypomagnesemia, those with clinically significant bradycardia, and in patients receiving class IA (eg, quinidine, procainamide) or class III (eg, dofetilide) antiarrhythmic agents.

No cardiovascular morbidity or mortality attributable to QTc prolongation occurred with telithromycin treatment in 4,780 patients in clinical efficacy trials, including 204 patients who had a prolonged QTc at baseline.

➤*Myasthenia gravis:* Exacerbations of myasthenia gravis have been reported in patients with myasthenia gravis treated with telithromycin. This has sometimes occurred within a few hours after intake of the first dose of telithromycin. Reports have included life-threatening acute respiratory failure with a rapid onset in patients with myasthenia gravis treated for respiratory tract infections with telithromycin. Telithromycin is not recommended in patients with myasthenia gravis unless no other therapeutic alternatives are available. If other therapeutic alternatives are not available, patients with myasthenia gravis taking telithromycin must be closely monitored. Patients must be advised that if they experience exacerbation of their symptoms, they should discontinue treatment of telithromycin and immediately seek medical attention. Institute supportive measures as medically necessary.

➤*Renal / Hepatic function impairment:* Telithromycin is principally excreted via the liver and kidney. In the presence of severe renal function impairment (Ccr less than 30 mL/min), a reduced dosage of telithromycin is recommended. Telithromycin may be administered without dosage adjustment in the presence of hepatic function impairment.

➤*Fertility impairment:* At doses of 1.8 to 3.6 times the human daily dose, at which signs of parental toxicity were observed, moderate reductions in fertility indices were noted in male and female animals treated with telithromycin.

➤*Elderly:* In all phase 3 clinical trials (n = 4,780), telithromycin was administered to 694 patients who were 65 years of age and older, including 231 patients who were 75 years of age or older.

Efficacy and safety in elderly patients 65 years of age or older were generally similar to those observed in younger patients; however, greater sensitivity of some older individuals cannot be ruled out. No dosage adjustment is required based on age alone.

➤*Pregnancy: Category C.*

At doses higher than the 900 mg/m^2 and 240 mg/m^2 in rats and rabbits, respectively, maternal toxicity may have resulted in delayed fetal maturation.

There are no adequate and well-controlled studies in pregnant women. Use telithromycin during pregnancy only if the potential benefit justifies the potential risk to the fetus.

➤*Lactation:* Telithromycin is excreted in breast milk of rats. Telithromycin may also be excreted in human milk. Because many drugs are excreted in human milk, exercise caution when telithromycin is administered to a breast-feeding mother.

➤*Children:* The safety and efficacy of telithromycin in children have not been established.

Precautions

➤*Hepatic effects:* Hepatic dysfunction, including increased liver enzymes and hepatitis, with or without jaundice, has been reported with the use of telithromycin. These events were generally reversible. Use caution in patients with a history of hepatitis/jaundice associated with the use of telithromycin.

➤*Visual disturbances:* Telithromycin may cause visual disturbances, particularly in slowing the ability to accommodate and the ability to release accommodation. Visual disturbances included blurred vision, difficulty focusing, and diplopia. Most events were mild to moderate; however, severe cases have been reported.

➤*Syncope:* There have been postmarketing adverse reaction reports of syncope usually associated with vagal syndrome.

➤*Hazardous tasks:* Caution patients about the potential effects of visual disturbances and syncope on driving a vehicle, operating machinery, or engaging in other potentially hazardous activities.

➤*Superinfection:* Prescribing telithromycin in the absence of a proven or strongly suspected bacterial infection or a prophylactic indication is unlikely to provide benefit to the patient and increases the risk of the development of drug-resistant bacteria.

Drug Interactions

➤*Cytochrome P-450 system:* Telithromycin is a strong inhibitor of the cytochrome P-450 3A4 system. Coadministration of telithromycin tablets and a drug primarily metabolized by the cytochrome P-450 3A4 enzyme system may result in increased plasma concentration of the drug coadministered with telithromycin that could increase or prolong both the therapeutic and adverse effects. Therefore, appropriate dosage adjustments may be necessary for the drug coadministered with telithromycin. Coadministration of other CYP3A4 inducers, such as phenytoin, carbamazepine, or phenobarbital, is likely to result in subtherapeutic levels of telithromycin and loss of effect.

Telithromycin Drug Interactions

Precipitant drug	Object drug[a]		Description
Azole Antifungals Itraconazole Ketoconazole	Telithromycin	↑	Coadministration with itraconazole resulted in an increase in telithromycin C_{max} and AUC 22% and 54%, respectively. Coadministration with ketoconazole resulted in an increase in telithromycin C_{max} and AUC by 51% and 95%, respectively.
Phenytoin Carbamazepine Phenobarbital	Telithromycin	↓	Coadministration with CYP 3A4 inducers (eg, phenytoin, carbamazepine, phenobarbital) is likely to result in subtherapeutic levels of telithromycin and loss of effect.
Rifampin	Telithromycin	↓	Coadministration of rifampin and telithromycin resulted in a decrease in telithromycin C_{max} and AUC of 79% and 86%, respectively. Avoid coadministration.
Telithromycin	Antiarrhythmic agents (eg, amiodarone, bretylium, disopyramide, dofetilide, procainamide, quinidine, sotalol)	↑	The risk of life-threatening cardiac arrhythmias, including torsades de pointes, may be increased. Avoid coadministration with class IA and class III antiarrhythmic agents.

TELITHROMYCIN — ORAL

Telithromycin Drug Interactions			
Precipitant drug	Object drug[a]		Description
Telithromycin	Benzodiazepines (eg, midazolam)	↑	Coadministration resulted in an increase in midazolam AUC. Monitor closely and adjust midazolam dose as needed. Use with caution with other benzodiazepines that are metabolized by CYP3A4 and undergo a high first-pass effect (eg, triazolam).
Telithromycin	Carbamazepine, cyclosporine, hexobarbital, phenytoin, sirolimus, tacrolimus	↑	Elevation of serum levels of these drugs may be observed when coadministered with telithromycin. Increases or prolongation of the therapeutic and/or adverse reactions of the concomitant drug may be observed.
Telithromycin	Cisapride	↑	Coadministration resulted in a 95% increase in cisapride peak plasma concentrations, resulting in significant increases in QTc interval. Coadministration is contraindicated.
Telithromycin	Digoxin	↑	Coadministration resulted in a 73% and 21% increase in digoxin plasma peak and trough levels, respectively. Monitor digoxin levels and side effects during use with telithromycin therapy.
Telithromycin	Ergot alkaloids	↑	Acute ergot toxicity characterized by severe peripheral vasospasm and dysesthesia has occurred when an ergot alkaloid was given with a macrolide. Without further data, the coadministration of telithromycin and ergot alkaloids is not recommended.
Telithromycin	HMG-CoA reductase inhibitors Simvastatin Atorvastatin Lovastatin	↑	Coadministration resulted in a 5.3- and 8.9-fold increase in simvastatin C_{max} and AUC, respectively. Avoid concurrent use of simvastatin, atorvastatin, or lovastatin with telithromycin.
Telithromycin	Metoprolol	↑	Coadministration resulted in an approximate 38% increase in metoprolol C_{max} and AUC; however, there was no effect on metoprolol elimination half-life. Coadminister with caution in heart failure patients.
Telithromycin	Oral anticoagulants (eg, warfarin)	↑	The anticoagulant effect of oral anticoagulants may be increased. Hemorrhage has occurred. Monitor prothrombin time/INR when coadministering.
Telithromycin	Oral contraceptives	↑	When oral contraceptives containing ethinyl estradiol and levonorgestrel were coadministered with telithromycin, the steady-state AUC of ethinyl estradiol did not change but the steady-state AUC of levonorgestrel was increased 50%.
Telithromycin	Pimozide	↑	Coadministration may lead to increased pimozide plasma levels. Coadministration is contraindicated.
Telithromycin	Sotalol	↓	Coadministration resulted in a decrease in sotalol C_{max} and AUC of 34% and 20%, respectively.
Telithromycin	Tacrolimus	↑	Plasma tacrolimus levels may be elevated, increasing the risk of toxicity.
Telithromycin	Theophylline	↑	Coadministration resulted in an approximate 16% and 17% increase in theophylline C_{max} and AUC, respectively. Coadministration may worsen GI effects such as nausea and vomiting. Take telithromycin and theophylline 1 hour apart to decrease the risk of GI side effects.
Telithromycin	Verapamil	↑	Increased risk of cardiotoxicity. Closely monitor cardiac function.

[a] ↑ = Object drug increased. ↓ = Object drug decreased.

Adverse Reactions

In phase 3 clinical trials, 4,780 patients (n = 2,702 in controlled trials) received daily oral doses of telithromycin 800 mg once daily for 5 days or 7 to 10 days. Most adverse reactions were mild to moderate in severity. In the combined phase 3 studies, discontinuation because of treatment-emergent adverse reactions occurred in 4.4% of telithromycin-treated patients and 4.3% of combined comparator-treated patients. Most discontinuations in the telithromycin group were due to treatment-emergent adverse reactions in the GI body system, primarily diarrhea (0.9% for telithromycin vs 0.7% for comparators) and nausea (0.7% for telithromycin vs 0.5% for comparators).

All and possibly related treatment-emergent adverse reactions occurring in controlled clinical studies in greater than or equal to 2% of all patients are included in the following table:

Telithromycin Adverse Reactions (≥ 2%)				
	All treatment-emergent adverse reactions		Possibly-related treatment-emergent adverse reactions	
Adverse reaction[a]	Telithromycin (n = 2,702)	Comparator[b] (n = 2,139)	Telithromycin (n = 2,702)	Comparator[b] (n = 2,139)
CNS				
Dizziness (excluding vertigo)	3.7%	2.7%	2.8%	1.5%
Headache	5.5%	5.8%	2%	2.5%
GI				
Diarrhea	10.8%	8.6%	10%	8%
Dysgeusia	1.6%	3.6%	1.5%	3.6%
Loose stools	2.3%	1.5%	2.1%	1.4%
Nausea	7.9%	4.6%	7%	4.1%
Vomiting	2.9%	2.2%	2.4%	1.4%

[a] Based on a frequency of all and possibly related treatment-emergent adverse events of 2% or more in telithromycin or comparator groups.
[b] Includes comparators from all controlled phase 3 studies.

➤*Adverse reactions (at least 0.2% and less than 2%):* The following events judged by investigators to be at least possibly drug related were observed infrequently (greater than or equal to 0.2% and less than 2%), in telithromycin-treated patients in the controlled phase 3 studies.

CNS – Dry mouth, fatigue, increased sweating, insomnia, somnolence, vertigo.

Dermatologic – Rash.

GI – Abdominal distension, abdominal pain, anorexia, constipation, dyspepsia, flatulence, gastritis, gastroenteritis, GI upset, glossitis, oral candidiasis, stomatitis, upper abdominal pain, watery stools.

GU – Vaginal candidiasis, vaginitis, vaginosis fungal.

Hematologic – Increased platelet count.

Hepatic – Hepatitis, with or without jaundice, occurred in 0.07% of patients treated with telithromycin, and was reversible.

Lab test abnormalities – Abnormal liver function tests: increased liver enzymes (eg, ALT, AST) and increased transaminases were usually asymptomatic and reversible; ALT elevations above 3 times the upper limit of normal were observed in 1.6%, and 1.7% of patients treated with telithromycin and comparators, respectively.

Special senses – Visual adverse reactions most often included blurred vision, diplopia, or difficulty focusing. Most events were mild to moderate; however, severe cases have been reported. Some patients discontinued therapy because of these adverse reactions. Visual adverse reactions were reported as having occurred after any dose during treatment, but most visual adverse reactions (65%) occurred following the first or second dose. Visual events lasted several hours and recurred upon subsequent dosing in some patients. For patients who continued treatment, some resolved on therapy while others continued to have symptoms until they completed the full course of treatment.

Women and patients younger than 40 years of age experienced a higher incidence of telithromycin-associated visual adverse reactions.

➤*Adverse reactions (less than 0.2%):* Other possibly related clinically relevant events occurring in less than 0.2% of patients treated with telithromycin from the controlled phase 3 studies included anxiety, bradycardia, eczema, elevated blood bilirubin, erythema multiforme, flushing, hypoten-

TELITHROMYCIN — ORAL

sion, increased blood alkaline phosphatase, increased eosinophil count, paresthesia, pruritus, urticaria.

➤*Postmarketing:* In addition to adverse reactions reported from clinical trials, the following events have been reported from worldwide postmarketing experience with telithromycin.

Cardiovascular – Atrial arrhythmias, palpitations.

CNS – Syncope usually associated with vagal syndrome.

GI – Pancreatitis.

Hepatic – Hepatic dysfunction, including increased liver enzymes, and hepatocellular and/or cholestatic hepatitis, with or without jaundice, have been infrequently reported with telithromycin. This hepatic dysfunction may be severe and is usually reversible.

Hypersensitivity – Face edema; rare reports of severe allergic reactions, including angioedema and anaphylaxis.

Musculoskeletal – Muscle cramps, rare reports of exacerbation of myasthenia gravis.

Overdosage

➤*Treatment:* In the event of acute overdosage, empty the stomach by gastric lavage. Carefully monitor the patient (eg, ECG, electrolytes) and give symptomatic and supportive treatment. Maintain adequate hydration. The efficacy of hemodialysis in an overdose situation with telithromycin is unknown.

Patient Information

Telithromycin may cause problems with vision, particularly when looking quickly between objects nearby and objects far away. These events include blurred vision, difficulty focusing, and objects looking doubled. Most events were mild to moderate; however, severe cases have been reported. Problems with vision were reported as having occurred after any dose during treatment, but most occurred following the first or second dose. These problems lasted several hours and in some patients came back with the next dose.

If visual difficulties occur:

- Tell patients to avoid driving a motor vehicle, operating heavy machinery, or engaging in otherwise hazardous activities.
- Inform patients that avoiding quick changes in viewing between objects in the distance and objects nearby may help to decrease the effects of these visual difficulties.
- Tell patients to contact their health care provider if these visual difficulties interfere with their daily activities.

Patients should be aware of the possibility of experiencing syncope (fainting) and its impact on the the ability to drive, especially if they are experiencing vagal symptoms (severe nausea, vomiting, and/or lightheadedness). If patients experience these symptoms, they should avoid driving a motor vehicle, operating heavy machinery, or engaging in otherwise hazardous activities.

Also advise:

- That antibacterial drugs, including telithromycin, should only be used to treat bacterial infections. They do not treat viral infections (eg, the common cold). When telithromycin is prescribed to treat a bacterial infection, tell patients that although it is common to feel better early in the course of therapy, the medication should be taken exactly as directed. Skipping doses or not completing the full course of therapy may (1) decrease the efficacy of the immediate treatment and (2) increase the likelihood that bacteria will develop resistance and will not be treatable by telithromycin or other antibacterial drugs in the future.
- That telithromycin has the potential to produce changes in the ECG (QTc interval prolongation) and that they should report any fainting occurring during drug treatment.
- That telithromycin should be avoided in patients receiving class IA (eg, quinidine, procainamide) or class III (eg, dofetilide) antiarrhythmic agents.
- To inform their health care provider of any personal or family history of QTc prolongation or proarrhythmic conditions, such as uncorrected hypokalemia, or clinically significant bradycardia.
- That telithromycin is not recommended in patients with myasthenia gravis. Patients should inform their health care provider if they have myasthenia gravis.
- That simvastatin, lovastatin, or atorvastatin should be avoided in patients receiving telithromycin. If telithromycin is prescribed, stop therapy with simvastatin, lovastatin, or atorvastatin during the course of treatment.
- That telithromycin tablets can be taken with or without food.
- To inform their health care provider of any other medications taken concurrently with telithromycin, including over-the-counter medications and dietary supplements.

SPECTINOMYCIN

SPECTINOMYCIN

Rx	**Trobicin** (Upjohn)	**Powder for Injection:** 400 mg (as hydrochloride) per mL when reconstituted	In 2 g vial w/ 3.2 mL diluent (w/ 0.9% benzyl alcohol).

SPECTINOMYCIN HYDROCHLORIDE — INJECTION

Indications

➤*Gonorrhea:* Indicated in the treatment of acute gonorrheal urethritis and proctitis in the male and acute gonorrheal cervicitis and proctitis in the female when due to susceptible strains of *Neisseria gonorrhoeae*. Men and women with known recent exposure to gonorrhea should be treated as those known to have gonorrhea.

Administration and Dosage

➤*Administration:* For IM use only. Shake vials vigorously immediately after adding diluent and before withdrawing dose. It is recommended that disposable syringes and needles be used to avoid contamination with penicillin residue, especially when treating patients known to be highly sensitive to penicillin. Use of a 20-gauge needle is recommended.

➤*Dosage:* Intramuscular injections should be made deep into the upper outer quadrant of the gluteal muscle.

Adults (men and women) – Inject 5 mL intramuscularly for a 2 g dose. This is also the recommended dose for patients being treated after failure of previous antibiotic therapy.

In geographic areas where antibiotic resistance is known to be prevalent, initial treatment with 4 g (10 mL) intramuscularly is preferred. The 10 mL injection may be divided between two gluteal injection sites.

➤*Storage/Stability:* Store unreconstituted product at controlled room temperature 20° to 25°C (68° to 77°F) [see USP]. Store prepared suspension at controlled room temperature 20° to 25°C (68° to 77°F) and use within 24 hours.

Actions

➤*Pharmacology:* Spectinomycin hydrochloride is an inhibitor of protein synthesis in the bacterial cell; the site of action is the 30S ribosomal subunit.

In vitro studies have shown spectinomycin hydrochloride to be active against most strains of *Neisseria gonorrhoeae* (minimum inhibitory concentration less than 7.5 to 20 mcg/mL).

➤*Pharmacokinetics:* Spectinomycin is rapidly absorbed after intramuscular injection. A single, 2 g injection produces peak serum concentrations averaging about 100 mcg/mL at one hour; a single, 4 g injection produces peak serum concentrations averaging 160 mcg/mL at two hours. Average serum concentrations of 15 mcg/mL for the 2 g dose and 31 mcg/mL for the 4 g dose were present 8 hours after dosing.

Contraindications

Patients previously found hypersensitive to spectinomycin.

Warnings

➤*Syphilis:* Spectinomycin hydrochloride is not effective in the treatment of syphilis. Antibiotics used in high doses for short periods of time to treat gonorrhea may mask or delay the symptoms of incubating syphilis. Since the treatment of syphilis demands prolonged therapy with any effective antibiotic, patients being treated for gonorrhea should be closely observed clinically. All patients with gonorrhea should have a serologic test for syphilis at the time of diagnosis. Patients treated with spectinomycin hydrochloride should have a follow-up serologic test for syphilis after three months.

➤*Benzyl alcohol:* Contains benzyl alcohol. Benzyl alcohol has been reported to be associated with a fatal "Gasping Syndrome" in premature infants and an increased incidence of neurologic and other complications.

➤*Hypersensitivity reactions:* The usual precautions should be observed with atopic individuals.

➤*Pregnancy: Category B.*

Since there are no controlled studies of spectinomycin in pregnant women, and because animal reproduction studies are not always predictive of human responses, spectinomycin should be used during pregnancy only if clearly needed.

➤*Lactation:* It is not known whether this drug is excreted in human milk. Because many drugs are excreted in human milk, caution should be exercised when spectinomycin is administered to a nursing woman.

➤*Children:* Safety and efficacy in children have not been established.

Precautions

➤*Monitoring:* The clinical effectiveness of spectinomycin sterile powder should be monitored to detect evidence of development of resistance by *Neisseria gonorrhoeae*.

Adverse Reactions

Unless stated otherwise, the following reactions were observed during the single dose clinical trials.

➤*Hypersensitivity:* A few cases of anaphylaxis or anaphylactoid reactions have been reported. If serious allergic reactions occur, the usual agents (epi-

SPECTINOMYCIN HYDROCHLORIDE — INJECTION

nephrine, corticosteroids, and/or antihistamines) should be available for emergency use. In cases of severe anaphylaxis, airway support and oxygen may also be required.

➤*Lab test abnormalities:* During multiple dose subchronic tolerance studies in normal human volunteers, the following were noted: a decrease in hemoglobin, hematocrit and creatinine clearance; elevation of alkaline phosphatase, BUN and ALT.

➤*Local:* Soreness at the injection site.

➤*CNS:* Dizziness, insomnia.

➤*Renal:* In single and multiple dose studies in normal volunteers, a reduction in urine output was noted. Extensive renal function studies demonstrated no consistent changes indicative of renal toxicity.

➤*Miscellaneous:* Urticaria, chills, fever and nausea.

Overdosage

Information on overdosage in humans is not available.

➤*Treatment:* Hemodialysis has been reported to aid in the removal of intravenously administered spectinomycin from the body.

STREPTOGRAMINS

QUINUPRISTIN/DALFOPRISTIN

Rx	**Synercid** (Monarch)	**Injection, lyophilized:** 500 mg (150 mg quinupristin; 350 mg dalfopristin)/10 mL	In 10 mL vials.

QUINUPRISTIN/DALFOPRISTIN — INJECTION

WARNING

One of quinupristin/dalfopristin's approved indications is for the treatment of patients with serious or life-threatening infections associated with vancomycin-resistant *Enterococcus faecium* (VREF) bacteremia. Quinupristin/dalfopristin has been approved for marketing in the US for this indication under the FDA's accelerated approval regulations that allow marketing of products for use in life-threatening conditions when other therapies are not available. Approval of drugs for marketing under these regulations is based upon a demonstrated effect on a surrogate endpoint that is likely to predict clinical benefit.

Approval of this indication is based upon quinupristin/dalfopristin's ability to clear VREF from the bloodstream with clearance of bacteremia considered to be a surrogate end point. No results from well-controlled clinical studies confirm the validity of this surrogate marker. However, a study to verify the clinical benefit of therapy with quinupristin/dalfopristin on traditional clinical endpoints (such as cure of the underlying infection) is presently underway.

Indications

➤*Life-threatening infections:* Treatment of patients with serious or life-threatening infections associated with vancomycin-resistant *Enterococcus faecium* (VREF) bacteremia.

➤*Complicated skin and skin structure infections:* Caused by *Staphylococcus aureus* (methicillin-susceptible) or *Streptococcus pyogenes*.

Administration and Dosage

➤*Approved by the FDA:* September 21, 1999.

Administer by IV infusion in 5% Dextrose in Water solution over a 60-minute period (see Warnings). The recommended dosage for the treatment of infections is described in the table below. An infusion pump or device may be used to control the rate of infusion. If necessary, central venous access (eg, PICC) can be used to administer quinupristin/dalfopristin to decrease the incidence of venous irritation.

Indication	Dose
Vancomycin-resistant *Enterococcus faecium*	7.5 mg/kg every 8 h
Complicated skin and structure infection	7.5 mg/kg every 12 h

The minimum recommended treatment duration for complicated skin and skin structure infections is 7 days. For vancomycin-resistant *E. faecium* infection, base treatment duration on the site and severity of the infection.

➤*Special populations:*

Hepatic function impairment –

Pharmacokinetic data in patients with hepatic cirrhosis (Child Pugh A or B) suggest that dosage reduction may be necessary, but exact recommendations cannot be made at this time.

Children (younger than16 years of age) – Based on a limited number of pediatric patients treated under emergency-use conditions, no dosage adjustment of quinupristin/dalfopristin is required.

➤*Preparation and administration of solution:*

1.) Reconstitute the single dose vial by slowly adding 5 ml of 5% Dextrose in Water or Sterile Water for Injection.
2.) Gently swirl the vial by manual rotation without shaking to ensure dissolution of contents while limiting foam formation.
3.) Allow the solution to sit for a few minutes until all the foam has disappeared. The resulting solution should be clear. Vials reconstituted in this manner will give a solution of 100 mg/ml. Caution: further dilution required before infusion.
4.) According to the patient's weight, add the reconstituted solution to 250 ml of 5% Dextrose solution (approximately 2 mg/ml). An infusion volume of 100 ml may be used for central line infusions.
5.) If moderate-to-severe venous irritation occurs following peripheral administration of quinupristin/dalfopristin diluted in 250 ml of Dextrose 5% in Water, consider increasing the infusion volume to 500 or 750 ml, changing the infusion site, or infusing by a peripherally inserted central catheter (PICC) or a central venous catheter.
6.) Administer the desired dose by IV infusion over 60 minutes.

➤*Admixture compatibility/incompatibility:* Do not dilute with saline solutions because quinupristin/dalfopristin is not compatible with these agents. Do not mix quinupristin/dalfopristin with or physically add to other drugs except for the following drugs, for which compatibility by Y-site injection has been established.

Y-Site Injection Compatibility of Quinupristin/Dalfopristin at 2 mg/mL Concentration

Admixture and concentration	IV infusion solutions for admixture
Aztreonam 20 mg/mL	D5W[a]
Ciprofloxacin 1 mg/mL	D5W
Fluconazole 2 mg/mL	Used as the undiluted solution
Haloperidol 0.2 mg/mL	D5W
Metoclopramide 5 mg/mL	D5W
Potassium Chloride 40 mEq/L	D5W

[a] D5W = 5% Dextrose Injection.

If quinupristin/dalfopristin is to be given concomitantly with another drug, give each drug separately in accordance with the recommended dosage and route of administration for each drug.

With intermittent infusion of quinupristin/dalfopristin and other drugs through a common IV line, flush the line before and after administration with 5% Dextrose in Water solution.

➤*Storage/Stability:*

Before reconstitution – Refrigerate the unopened vials at 2° to 8°C (36° to 46°F).

Reconstituted and infusion solutions – Because quinupristin/dalfopristin contains no antibacterial preservative, reconstitute under strict aseptic conditions (eg, Laminar Air Flow Hood). Dilute the reconstituted solution within 30 minutes. Vials are for single use. The storage time of the diluted solution should be as short as possible to minimize the risk of microbial contamination. Stability of the diluted solution prior to the infusion is established as 5 hours at room temperature or 54 hours if refrigerated 2° to 8°C (36° to 46°F). Do not freeze the solution.

Actions

➤*Pharmacology:* Quinupristin/dalfopristin, a streptogramin antibacterial agent for IV administration, is a sterile, lyophilized formulation of 2 semisynthetic pristinamycin derivatives, quinupristin (derived from pristinamycin I) and dalfopristin (derived from pristinamycin IIA).

The streptogramin components of quinupristin/dalfopristin are present in a ratio of 30 parts quinupristin to 70 parts dalfopristin. These 2 components act synergistically so that quinupristin/dalfopristin's microbiologic in vitro activity is greater than that of the components individually. Quinupristin's and dalfopristin's metabolites also contribute to the antimicrobial activity of quinupristin/dalfopristin. In vitro synergism of the major metabolites with the complementary parent compound has been demonstrated.

Quinupristin/dalfopristin is bacteriostatic against *E. faecium* and bactericidal against strains of methicillin-susceptible and methicillin-resistant staphylococci.

The site of action of quinupristin and dalfopristin is the bacterial ribosome. Dalfopristin inhibits the early phase of protein synthesis while quinupristin inhibits the late phase of protein synthesis.

Resistance – In non-comparative studies, emerging resistance to quinupristin/dalfopristin during treatment of VREF infections occurred. Resistance to quinupristin/dalfopristin is associated with resistance to both components.

➤*Pharmacokinetics:*

Special populations –

Renal function impairment: In patients with creatinine clearance 6 to 28 mL/min, the AUC of quinupristin and dalfopristin in combination with their major metabolites increased approximately 40% and 30%, respectively.

In patients undergoing continuous ambulatory peritoneal dialysis, dialysis clearance for quinupristin, dalfopristin, and their metabolites is negligible. The plasma AUC of unchanged quinupristin and dalfopristin increased

QUINUPRISTIN/DALFOPRISTIN — INJECTION

approximately 20% and 30%, respectively. Because of the high molecular weight of both components, it is unlikely to be removed by hemodialysis.

Hepatic function impairment: In patients with hepatic dysfunction (Child-Pugh scores A and B), the terminal half-life of quinupristin and dalfopristin was not modified. However, the AUC of quinupristin and dalfopristin in combination with their major metabolites increased ≈ 180% and 50%, respectively (see Administration and Dosage).

Obesity (body mass index at least 30): In obese patients, the C_{max} and AUC of quinupristin increased approximately 30% and those of dalfopristin approximately 40%. Quinupristin and dalfopristin are the main active components circulating in the plasma. They are converted to several active major metabolites: 2 conjugated metabolites for quinupristin (1 with glutathione and 1 with cysteine) and 1 non-conjugated metabolite for dalfopristin (formed by drug hydrolysis).

Pharmacokinetic profiles of quinupristin and dalfopristin in combination with their metabolites were determined using a bioassay following multiple 60-minute infusions in 2 groups of healthy young adult male volunteers. Each group received 7.5 mg/kg of quinupristin/dalfopristin IV every 12 hours or every 8 hours for a total of 9 or 10 doses, respectively. The pharmacokinetic parameters were proportional with every-12-hour and every-8-hour dosing: Those of the every-8-hour regimen are shown in the following table.

Mean Steady-State Pharmacokinetic Parameters of Quinupristin and Dalfopristin in Combination with Their Metabolites (Dose = 7.5 mg/kg every 8 h; n = 10)

	C_{max} (mcg/mL)	AUC (mcg•h/mL)	t½ (h)
Quinupristin and metabolites	3.2	7.2	3.07
Dalfopristin and metabolite	7.96	10.57	1.04

The clearances of unchanged quinupristin and dalfopristin are similar (0.72 L/h/kg), and the steady-state volume of distribution is 0.45 and 0.24 L/kg, respectively. The elimination half-life of quinupristin and dalfopristin is approximately 0.85 and 0.7 hours, respectively. The protein binding is moderate.

Penetration of unchanged quinupristin and dalfopristin in noninflammatory blister fluid corresponds to approximately 19% and 11%, respectively, of that estimated in plasma. The penetration into blister fluid of quinupristin and dalfopristin in combination with their major metabolites was in total approximately 40% compared with that in plasma.

In vitro, the transformation of the parent drugs into their major active metabolites occurs by non-enzymatic reactions and is not dependent on cytochrome-P450 or glutathione-transferase enzyme activities. Quinupristin/dalfopristin is a major inhibitor of the activity of cytochrome P450 3A4 isoenzyme (see Warnings). Quinupristin/dalfopristin can interfere with the metabolism of other drug products that are associated with QTc prolongation. However, electrophysiologic studies confirm that quinupristin/dalfopristin does not itself induce QTc prolongation (see Warnings).

Fecal excretion constitutes the main elimination route for both parent drugs and their metabolites (75% to 77% of dose). Urinary excretion accounts for approximately 15% of the quinupristin dose and 19% of the dalfopristin dose. Preclinical data in rats demonstrated that approximately 80% of the dose is excreted in the bile and suggest that in humans, biliary excretion is probably the principal route for fecal elimination.

➤*Microbiology:* Quinupristin/dalfopristin is active against most strains of the following microorganisms both in vitro and in clinical infections.

Aerobic gram-positive microorganisms – Enterococcus faecium (vancomycin-resistant and multi-drug resistant strains only); *Staphylococcus aureus* (methicillin-susceptible strains); *Streptococcus pyogenes*.

Note: Quinupristin/dalfopristin is not active against *Enterococcus faecalis*. Differentiation of enterococcal species is important to avoid misidentification of *E. faecalis* as *E. faecium*.

Contraindications

Hypersensitivity to quinupristin/dalfopristin or prior hypersensitivity to other streptogramins (eg, pristinamycin, virginiamycin).

Warnings

➤*Pseudomembranous colitis:* Pseudomembranous colitis has been reported with nearly all antibacterial agents, including quinupristin/dalfopristin, and may range in severity from mild to life-threatening. Therefore, consider this diagnosis in patients who present with diarrhea subsequent to the administration of antibacterial agents. After the diagnosis of pseudomembranous colitis has been established, initiate therapeutic measures. Mild cases usually respond to drug discontinuation alone. In moderate-to-severe cases, consider managing with fluids and electrolytes, protein supplementation, and treatment with an antibacterial drug clinically effective against *C. difficile* colitis.

➤*Hepatic function impairment:* Following a single 1-hour infusion of quinupristin/dalfopristin (7.5 mg/kg) to patients with hepatic insufficiency, plasma concentrations were significantly increased. However, the effect of dose reduction or increase in dosing interval on the pharmacokinetics of quinupristin/dalfopristin in these patients has not been studied. Therefore, no recommendations can be made at this time regarding the appropriate dose modification.

➤*Mutagenesis:* Dalfopristin was associated with the production of structural chromosome aberrations when tested in the Chinese hamster ovary cell chromosome aberration assay. Quinupristin/dalfopristin were negative in this assay.

➤*Pregnancy: Category B.* There are no adequate and well-controlled studies in pregnant women. Use during pregnancy only if clearly needed.

➤*Lactation:* In lactating rats, quinupristin/dalfopristin was excreted in milk. It is not known whether quinupristin/dalfopristin is excreted in human breast milk. Exercise caution when administering to a breastfeeding woman.

➤*Children:* Quinupristin/dalfopristin has been used in a limited number of pediatric patients under emergency-use conditions at a dose of 7.5 mg/kg every 8 or 12 hours. However, the safety and efficacy in patients younger than 16 years of age have not been established.

Precautions

➤*Venous irritation:* Following completion of a peripheral infusion, flush the vein with 5% Dextrose in Water solution to minimize venous irritation. Do not flush with saline or heparin after quinupristin/dalfopristin administration because of incompatibility concerns. If moderate-to-severe venous irritation occurs following peripheral administration of quinupristin/dalfopristin diluted in 250 mL of Dextrose 5% in Water, consider increasing the infusion volume to 500 or 750 mL, changing the infusion site, or infusing by a peripherally inserted central catheter (PICC) or a central venous catheter. In clinical trials, concomitant administration of hydrocortisone or diphenhydramine did not appear to alleviate venous pain or inflammation.

➤*Rate of infusion:* In animal studies, toxicity was higher when quinupristin/dalfopristin was administered as a bolus compared with slow infusion. However, the safety of an IV bolus has not been studied in humans. Clinical trial experience has been exclusively with an IV duration of 60 minutes and, thus, other infusion rates cannot be recommended.

➤*Arthralgias/Myalgias:* Episodes of arthralgia and myalgia, some severe, have been reported in patients treated with quinupristin/dalfopristin. In some patients, improvement has been noted with a reduction in dose frequency to every 12 hours. In those patients available for follow-up, symptoms resolved following discontinuation of treatment. The etiology of these myalgias and arthralgias is under investigation.

➤*Hyperbilirubinemia:* Elevations of total bilirubin more than 5 times the upper limit of normal were noted in approximately 25% of patients in the noncomparative studies. In some patients, isolated hyperbilirubinemia (primarily conjugated) can occur during treatment, possibly resulting from competition between quinupristin/dalfopristin and bilirubin for excretion. In the comparative trials, elevations in ALT and AST occurred at a similar frequency in both the quinupristin/dalfopristin and comparator groups.

➤*Superinfection:* Use of antibiotics (especially prolonged or repeated therapy) may result in bacterial or fungal overgrowth of nonsusceptible organisms. Such overgrowth may lead to a secondary infection. Appropriate measures should be taken if superinfection occurs.

Drug Interactions

➤*Cytochrome P450 3A4 inhibition:* It is reasonable to expect that the concomitant administration of quinupristin/dalfopristin and other drugs primarily metabolized by the cytochrome P450 3A4 enzyme system may result in increased plasma concentrations of these drugs that could increase or prolong their therapeutic effect or increase adverse reactions (see the following table). Therefore, coadministration with drugs that are cytochrome P450 3A4 substrates and possess a narrow therapeutic window requires caution and monitoring of these drugs whenever possible. Avoid concomitant medications metabolized by the cytochrome P450 3A4 enzyme system that may prolong the QTc interval.

Cyclosporine – Twenty-four subjects given quinupristin/dalfopristin 7.5 mg/kg every 8 hours for 2 days and 300 mg of cyclosporine on day 3 showed an increase of 63% in the AUC of cyclosporine, a 30% increase in C_{max}, a 77% increase in the half-life, and a 34% decrease in clearance. Perform therapeutic level monitoring of cyclosporine when cyclosporine must be used concomitantly with quinupristin/dalfopristin.

Nifedipine/Midazolam – Coadministration of quinupristin/dalfopristin and nifedipine (repeated oral doses) and midazolam (IV bolus dose) in healthy volunteers led to elevated plasma concentrations of these drugs. The C_{max} increased by 18% and 14% (median values) and the AUC increased by 44% and 33% for nifedipine and midazolam, respectively.

Selected Drugs That are Predicted to Have Plasma Concentrations Increased by Quinupristin/Dalfopristin[a]
Anti-HIV (NNRTIs and protease inhibitors): Delavirdine, nevirapine, indinavir, ritonavir
Antineoplastic agents: Vinca alkaloids (eg, vinblastine), docetaxel, paclitaxel
Benzodiazepines: Midazolam, diazepam
Calcium channel blockers: Dihydropyridines (eg, nifedipine), verapamil, diltiazem
Cholesterol-lowering agents: HMG-CoA reductase inhibitors
GI motility agents: Cisapride
Immunosuppressive agents: Cyclosporine, tacrolimus
Steroids: Methylprednisolone
Other: Carbamazepine, quinidine, lidocaine, disopyramide

[a] This list of drugs is not all inclusive.

Adverse Reactions

➤*Comparative trials:* Safety data are available from 5 comparative clinical studies (n = 1,099 quinupristin/dalfopristin; n = 1,095 comparator). One of the deaths in the comparative studies was assessed as possibly related to quinupristin/dalfopristin. The most frequent reasons for discontinuation because of drug-related adverse reactions were as follows:

QUINUPRISTIN/DALFOPRISTIN — INJECTION

Patients Discontinuing Quinupristin/Dalfopristin Therapy (%): All Comparative Studies		
Type	Quinupristin/Dalfopristin (n = 1099)	Comparator (n = 1095)
Venous	9.2	2
Non-venous	9.6	4.3
Rash	1	0.5
Nausea	0.9	0.6
Vomiting	0.5	0.5
Pain	0.5	0
Pruritus	0.5	0.3

Quinupristin/Dalfopristin Adverse Reactions (≥ 1%): All Comparative Studies		
Adverse reaction	Quinupristin/Dalfopristin (n = 1099)	Comparator (n = 1095)
Inflammation at infusion site	42	25
Pain at infusion site	40	23.7
Edema at infusion site	17.3	9.5
Infusion site reaction	13.4	10.1
Nausea	4.6	7.2
Diarrhea	2.7	3.2
Vomiting	2.7	3.8
Rash	2.5	1.4
Thrombophlebitis	2.4	0.3
Headache	1.6	0.9
Pruritus	1.5	1.1
Pain	1.5	0.1

Additional adverse reactions that were possibly or probably related to quinupristin/dalfopristin with an incidence less than 1% are listed below.

Cardiovascular – Palpitation; phlebitis.

CNS – Anxiety; confusion; dizziness; hypertonia; insomnia; leg cramps; paresthesia; vasodilation.

Dermatologic – Maculopapular rash; sweating; urticaria.

GI – Constipation; dyspepsia; oral moniliasis; pancreatitis; pseudomembranous enterocolitis; stomatitis.

GU – Hematuria; vaginitis.

Metabolic – Gout; peripheral edema.

Musculoskeletal – Arthralgia; myalgia; myasthenia.

Respiratory – Dyspnea; pleural effusion.

Miscellaneous – Abdominal pain; worsening of underlying illness; allergic reaction; chest pain; fever; infection.

Patients Discontinuing Quinupristin/Dalfopristin Therapy (%): Skin/Skin Structure Studies		
Type	Quinupristin/Dalfopristin (n = 1,099)	Comparator[a] (n = 1,095)
Venous	12	2
Non-venous	11.8	4
Rash	2	0.9
Nausea	1.1	0
Vomiting	0.9	0
Pain	0.9	0
Pruritus	0.9	0.5

[a] Comparator regimens were oxacillin/vancomycin or cefazolin/vancomycin.

Quinupristin/Dalfopristin Adverse Reactions (%): Skin/Skin Structure Studies		
Adverse reaction	Quinupristin/Dalfopristin (n = 1,099)	Comparator (n = 1,095)
Venous	68	32.7
Pain at infusion site	44.7	17.8
Inflammation at infusion site	38.2	14.7
Edema at infusion site	18	7.2
Infusion site reaction	11.6	3.6
Non-venous	24.7	13.1
Nausea	4	2
Vomiting	3.7	1
Rash	3.1	1.3
Pain	3.1	0.2

There were 8 (1.7%) episodes of thrombus or thrombophlebitis in the quinupristin/dalfopristin arms and none in the comparator arms.

Lab test abnormalities – The following table shows the percentage of patients exhibiting laboratory values above or below the clinically relevant "critical" values during treatment phase.

Lab Test Abnormalities: Quinupristin/Dalfopristin vs Comparator (≥ 0.1%): All Comparative Studies			
Parameter	Critically high or low value	Quinupristin/ Dalfopristin critically high or low	Comparator critically high or low
AST	> 10 × ULN	0.9	0.2
ALT	> 10 × ULN	0.4	0.4
Total bilirubin	> 5 × ULN	0.9	0.2
Conjugated bilirubin	> 5 × ULN	3.1	1.3
LDH	> 5 × ULN	2.6	2.1
Alkaline phosphatase	> 5 × ULN	0.3	0.7
Gamma-GT	> 10 × ULN	1.9	1
CPK	> 10 × ULN	1.6	1.4
Creatinine	≥ 440 mcmol/L	0.1	0.1
BUN	≥ 35.5 mmol/L	0.3	1.2
Blood glucose	> 22.2 mmol/L	1.3	1.3
	< 2.2mmol/L	0.1	0.1
Bicarbonates	> 40 mmol/L	0.3	0.5
	< 10 mmol/L	0.5	0.5
CO_2	> 50 mmol/L	0	0
	< 15 mmol/L	0.2	0
Sodium	> 160 mmol/L	0	0
	< 120 mmol/L	0.5	0.3
Potassium	> 6 mmol/L	0.3	0.6
	< 2 mmol/L	0	0.1
Hemoglobin	< 8 g/dl	2.6	1.6
Hematocrit	> 60%	0.2	0
Platelets	> 1,000,000/mm^3	0.2	0.2
	< 50,000/mm^3	0.6	0.7

➤*Noncomparative trials:* Approximately 33% of patients discontinued therapy in these trials because of adverse events. However, the discontinuation rate because of adverse reactions assessed by the investigator as possibly or probably related to quinupristin/dalfopristin therapy was approximately 5%.

There were 3 prospectively designed non-comparative clinical trials in patients (n = 972) treated with quinupristin/dalfopristin. One of these studies (301) had more complete documentation than the other two (398 and 398B). The most common events probably or possibly related to therapy were the following.

Quinupristin/Dalfopristin Adverse Reactions (%): Noncomparative Studies	
Adverse reaction	
Arthralgia	4.3-7.8
Arthralgia and myalgia	3.3-7.4
Nausea	2.8-4.9
Myalgia	0.95-5.1

The percentage of patients who experienced severe related arthralgia and myalgia was 3.3% and 3.1%, respectively. The percentage of patients who discontinued treatment because of related arthralgia and myalgia was 2.3% and 1.8%, respectively.

Lab test abnormalities – The most frequently observed abnormalities in laboratory studies were in total and conjugated bilirubin, with increases more than 5 times the ULN, regardless of relationship to quinupristin/dalfopristin, reported in 25% and 34.6% of patients, respectively. The percentage of patients who discontinued treatment because of increased total and conjugated bilirubin was 2.7% and 2.3%, respectively. Notably, 46.5% and 59% of patients had high baseline total and conjugated bilirubin levels before study entry.

Miscellaneous – Serious adverse reactions in clinical trials, including noncomparative studies, considered possibly or probably related to quinupristin/dalfopristin administration with an incidence of less than 0.1% include the following: Acidosis; anaphylactoid reaction; apnea; arrhythmia; bone pain; cerebral hemorrhage; cerebrovascular accident; coagulation disorder; convulsion; dysautonomia; encephalopathy; grand mal convulsion; hemolysis; hemolytic anemia; heart arrest; hepatitis; hypoglycemia; hyponatremia; hypoplastic anemia; hypoventilation; hypovolemia; hypoxia; jaundice; mesenteric arterial occlusion; neck rigidity; neuropathy; pancytopenia; paraplegia; pericardial effusion; pericarditis; respiratory distress syndrome; shock; skin ulcer; supraventricular tachycardia; syncope; tremor; ventricular extrasystoles; ventricular fibrillation. Cases of hypotension and GI hemorrhage were reported in less than 0.2% of patients.

QUINUPRISTIN/DALFOPRISTIN — INJECTION

Overdosage

➤*Symptoms:* There are 4 reports of patients receiving quinupristin/dalfopristin at doses up to 3 times that recommended (7.5 mg/kg). No adverse events were considered possibly or probably related to quinupristin/dalfopristin overdose. Signs of acute overdosage may include dyspnea, emesis, tremors, and ataxia as seen in animals given extremely high doses (50 mg/kg) of quinupristin/dalfopristin.

➤*Treatment:* Carefully observe patients who receive an overdose, and give them supportive treatment. Refer to the General Management of Acute Overdosage. Quinupristin/dalfopristin is not removed by peritoneal dialysis or by hemodialysis.

LIPOPEPTIDES

DAPTOMYCIN

Rx	**Cubicin** (Cubist)	**Powder for injection, lyophilized**: 250 mg	Preservative-free. In single-use vials.
		500 mg	Preservative-free. In single-use vials.

DAPTOMYCIN — INJECTION

Indications

➤*Complicated skin and skin structure infection:* For the treatment of complicated skin and skin structure infections caused by susceptible strains of the following gram-positive microorganisms: *Staphylococcus aureus* (including methicillin-resistant strains); *Streptococcus pyogenes*; *Streptococcus agalactiae*; *Streptococcus dysgalactiae* subsp. *equisimilis*; *Enterococcus faecalis* (vancomycin-susceptible strains only).

Combination therapy may be clinically indicated if the documented or presumed pathogens include gram-negative or anaerobic organisms.

➤*S. aureus bloodstream infections:* For the treatment of *S. aureus* bloodstream infections (bacteremia), including those with right-sided infective endocarditis, caused by methicillan-susceptible and methicillin-resistant isolates. Combination therapy may be clinically indicated if the documented or presumed pathogens include gram-negative or anaerobic organisms.

The efficacy of daptomycin for injection in patients with left-sided infective endocarditis due to *S. aureus* has not been demonstrated. The clinical trial of daptomycin in patients with *S. aureus* bloodstream infections included limited data from patients with left-sided infective endocarditis; outcomes in these patients were poor. Daptomycin injection has not been studied in patients with prosthetic valve endocarditis or meningitis.

Patients with persisting or relapsing *S. aureus* infection or poor clinical response should have repeat blood cultures. If a culture is positive for *S. aureus*, perform MIC susceptibility testing of the isolate using a standardized procedure, as well as diagnostic evaluation to rule out sequestered foci of infection.

Administration and Dosage

➤*Approved by the FDA:* September 12, 2003.

➤*Complicated skin and skin structure infections (CSSSI):* Daptomycin 4 mg/kg should be administered over a 30-minute period by intravenous (IV) infusion in 0.9% sodium chloride injection once every 24 hours for 7 to 14 days. In phase 1 and 2 clinical studies, serum creatine phosphokinase (CPK) elevations appeared to be more frequent when daptomycin was dosed more frequently than once daily. Therefore, daptomycin injection should not be dosed more frequently than once a day.

S. aureus bloodstream infections (bacteremia), including those with right-sided endocarditis, caused by methicillin-susceptible and methicillin-resistant strains – Daptomycin 6 mg/kg should be administered over a 30-minute period by IV infusion in 0.9% sodium chloride injection once every 24 hours for a minimum of 2 to 6 weeks. Duration of treatment should be based on the treating health care provider's working diagnosis. There are limited safety data for the use of daptomycin for more than 28 days of therapy. In the phase 3 study, there were a total of 14 patients who were treated with daptomycin for more than 28 days, 8 of whom were treated for 6 weeks or longer.

In phase 1 and 2 clinical studies, CPK elevations appeared to be more frequent when daptomycin was dosed more frequently than once daily. Therefore, daptomycin should not be dosed more frequently than once a day.

Renal function impairment – Because daptomycin is eliminated primarily by the kidney, a dosage modification is recommended for patients with creatinine clearance (CCr) < 30 mL/min, including patients receiving hemodialysis or continuous ambulatory peritoneal dialysis (CAPD), as listed in the following table. When possible, daptomycin should be administered following hemodialysis on hemodialysis days.

Recommended Dosage of Daptomycin Injection in Adult Patients with Renal Function Impairment

Ccr	Dosage regimen (CSSSI)	Dosage regimen (*S. aureus* bloodstream infections)
≥ 30 mL/min	4 mg/kg once every 24 h	6 mg/kg once every 24 h
< 30 mL/min, including hemodialysis or CAPD	4 mg/kg once every 48 h	6 mg/kg once every 48 h

➤*Preparation for administration:* The contents of a daptomycin 500 mg vial should be reconstituted with 10 mL of 0.9% sodium chloride injection. Reconstituted daptomycin should be further diluted with 0.9% sodium chloride injection to be administered by IV infusion over a period of 30 minutes.

➤*Admixture incompatibilities:* Because only limited data are available on the compatibility of daptomycin with other IV substances, additives or other medications should not be added to daptomycin single-use vials or infused simultaneously through the same IV line. If the same IV line is used for sequential infusion of several different drugs, the line should be flushed with a compatible infusion solution before and after infusion with daptomycin.

➤*Compatible IV solutions:* Daptomycin is compatible with 0.9% sodium chloride injection and Ringer's lactate injection. Daptomycin is not compatible with dextrose-containing diluents.

➤*Storage/Stability:* Store original packages at refrigerated temperatures, 2° to 8°C (36° to 46°F); avoid excessive heat. Daptomycin vials are for single use only.

Stability studies have shown that the reconstituted solution is stable in the vial for 12 hours at room temperature or up to 48 hours if stored under refrigeration at 2° to 8°C (36° to 46°F). The diluted solution is stable in the infusion bag for 12 hours at room temperature or 48 hours if stored under refrigeration. The combined time (vial and infusion bag) at room temperature should not exceed 12 hours; the combined time (vial and infusion bag) under refrigeration should not exceed 48 hours.

Actions

➤*Pharmacology:* The mechanism of action of daptomycin is distinct from any other antibiotic. Daptomycin binds to bacterial membranes and causes a rapid depolarization of membrane potential. The loss of membrane potential leads to inhibition of protein, DNA, and RNA synthesis, which results in bacterial cell death.

Animal pharmacology –

Tissue distribution studies in rats have shown that daptomycin is retained in the kidney but does not appear to penetrate across the blood-brain barrier following single and multiple doses.

➤*Pharmacokinetics:*

Absorption –

Mean (SD) Daptomycin Pharmacokinetic Parameters in Healthy Volunteers on Day 7[a]

Dose mg/kg	C_{max} (mcg/mL)	t_{max}[b] (h)	AUC_{0-24} (mcg•h/mL)	t½ (h)	V_d (L/kg)	CL_T (mL/h/kg)	CL_R (mL/h/kg)	Ae_{24} %
4 mg/kg (n = 6)	57.8 (3)	0.8 (0.5, 1)	494 (75)	8.1 (1)	0.096 (0.009)	8.3 (1.3)	4.8 (1.3)	53 (10.8)
6 mg/kg (n = 6)	98.6 (12)	0.5 (0.5, 1)	747 (91)	8.9 (1.3)	0.104 (0.013)	8.1 (1)	4.4 (0.3)	47.4 (11.5)
8 mg/kg (n = 6)	133 (13.5)	0.5 (0.5, 1)	1,130 (117)	9 (1.2)	0.092 (0.012)	7.2 (0.8)	3.7 (0.5)	52.1 (5.19)

[a] C_{max} = Maximum plasma concentration; t_{max} = Time to C_{max}; AUC_{0-24} = Area under concentration-time curve from 0 to 24 hours; t½ = Terminal elimination half-life; V_d = Apparent volume of distribution; CL_T = Systemic clearance; CL_R = Renal clearance; Ae_{24} = Percent of dose recovered in urine over 24 hours as unchanged daptomycin following the first dose.

[b] Median (minimum, maximum).

Daptomycin pharmacokinetics are nearly linear and time-independent at doses up to 6 mg/kg administered once daily for 7 days. Steady-state concentrations are achieved by the third daily dose. The mean (SD) steady-state trough concentrations (days 4 to 8) attained following administration of 4, 6, and 8 mg/kg every 24 hours are 5.9 (1.6), 9.4 (2.5), and 14.9 (2.9) mcg/mL, respectively.

Distribution – Daptomycin is reversibly bound to human plasma proteins, primarily to serum albumin, in a concentration-independent manner. The mean serum protein binding of daptomycin was approximately 92% in healthy adults after the administration of 4 mg/kg or 6 mg/kg. Serum protein binding was not altered as a function of daptomycin concentration, dose, or number of doses received.

In clinical studies, mean serum protein binding in subjects with Ccr greater than or equal to 30 mL/min was comparable to that observed in healthy subjects with normal renal function. However, there was a trend toward decreasing serum protein binding among subjects with Ccr less than 30 mL/min (87.6%), including hemodialysis patients (85.9%) and CAPD patients (83.5%). The protein binding of daptomycin in subjects with hepatic impairment (Child-Pugh B) was similar to healthy adult subjects. The apparent volume of distribution of daptomycin at steady-state in healthy adult subjects was approximately 0.09 L/kg.

DAPTOMYCIN — INJECTION

Metabolism –

It is unlikely that daptomycin will inhibit or induce the metabolism of drugs metabolized by the CYP P450 system. It is unknown whether daptomycin is a substrate of the CYP P450 system.

In 5 healthy young adults, after infusion of radiolabeled ^{14}C-daptomycin, the plasma total radioactivity was similar to the concentration determined by microbiological assay. Inactive metabolites of daptomycin have been detected in the urine, as determined by the difference in total radiolabeled concentrations and microbiologically active concentrations. The site of metabolism has not been identified.

Excretion – Daptomycin is excreted primarily by the kidney. In a mass balance study of 5 healthy subjects using radiolabeled daptomycin, approximately 78% of the administered dose was recovered from urine based on total radioactivity (approximately 52% of the dose based on microbiologically active concentrations) and 5.7% of the dose was recovered from feces (collected for up to 9 days), based on total radioactivity.

Because renal excretion is the primary route of elimination, dosage adjustment is necessary in patients with severe renal insufficiency (Ccr less than 30 mL/min).

Special populations –

Renal function impairment: Population derived pharmacokinetic parameters were determined for patients with skin and skin structure infections and healthy non-infected subjects with varying degrees of renal function (n = 282). Following the administration of a single 4 mg/kg IV dose of daptomycin, the plasma clearance (CL_T) was reduced and the systemic exposure ($AUC_{0-\infty}$) was increased with decreasing renal function (see table below). The mean $AUC_{0-\infty}$ was not markedly different for subjects and patients with Ccr 30 to 80 mL/min as compared to those with normal renal function (Ccr greater than 80 mL/min). The mean $AUC_{0-\infty}$ values for subjects and patients with Ccr less than 30 mL/min and hemodialysis (dosed post dialysis) / CAPD subjects were approximately 2 and 3 times higher, respectively, than the values in individuals with normal renal function. The mean C_{max} ranged from 59.6 mcg/mL to 69.6 mcg/mL in subjects with Ccr greater than or equal to 30 mL/min while those with Ccr less than 30 mL/min ranged from 41.1 mcg/mL to 57.7 mcg/mL. In 11 non-infected adult subjects undergoing dialysis, approximately 15% and 11% of the administered dose was removed by 4 hours of hemodialysis and 48 hours of CAPD, respectively.

Mean (SD) Daptomycin Population Pharmacokinetic Parameters Following a Single 30-Minute Intravenous Infusion of 4 mg/kg to Infected Patients and Non-Infected Subjects with Varying Degrees of Renal Function

Renal function[a]	$AUC_{0-\infty}$ (mcg•h/mL)	t½ (h)	V_{ss} (L/kg)	CL_T (mL/h/kg)
Normal (Ccr > 80 mL/min) (n = 165)	417 (155)	9.39 (4.74)	0.13 (0.05)	10.9 (4)
Mild renal impairment (Ccr 50 to 80 mL/min) (n = 64)	466 (177)	10.75 (8.36)	0.12 (0.05)	9.9 (4)
Moderate renal impairment (Ccr 30 to < 50 mL/min) (n = 24)	560 (258)	14.7 (10.5)	0.15 (0.06)	8.5 (3.4)
Severe renal impairment (Ccr < 30 mL/min) (n = 8)	925 (467)	27.83 (14.85)	0.2 (0.15)	5.9 (3.9)
Hemodialysis and CAPD (n = 21)	1244 (374)	29.81 (6.13)	0.15 (0.04)	3.7 (1.9)

[a] Ccr = Creatinine clearance estimated using the Cockroft-Gault equation with actual body weight.

Elderly: The pharmacokinetics of daptomycin were evaluated in 12 healthy elderly subjects (greater than or equal to 75 years of age) and 11 healthy young matched controls (18 to 30 years of age). Following administration of a single intravenous 4 mg/kg dose, the mean total clearance of daptomycin was reduced approximately 35% and the mean $AUC_{0-\infty}$ increased approximately 58% in elderly subjects compared to young healthy subjects. There were no differences in C_{max}. No dosage adjustment is warranted for elderly patients with normal (for age) renal function.

Obesity: The pharmacokinetics of daptomycin were evaluated in 6 moderately obese (body mass index [BMI] 25 to 39.9 kg/m^2) and 6 extremely obese (BMI greater than or equal to 40 kg/m^2) subjects and controls matched for age, sex, and renal function. Following administration of a single intravenous 4 mg/kg dose based on total body weight, the plasma clearance of daptomycin increased approximately 18% in moderately obese subjects and 46% in extremely obese subjects compared with non-obese controls. The $AUC_{0-\infty}$ of daptomycin increased approximately 30% in moderately obese and 31% in extremely obese subjects compared with non-obese controls. The differences were most likely due to differences in the renal clearance of daptomycin. No dosage adjustment of daptomycin is warranted in obese subjects.

➤*Microbiology:* Daptomycin is an antibacterial agent of a new class of antibiotics, the cyclic lipopeptides. Daptomycin is a natural product which has clinical utility in the treatment of infections caused by aerobic gram-positive bacteria. The in vitro spectrum of activity of daptomycin encompasses most clinically relevant gram-positive pathogenic bacteria. Daptomycin retains potency against antibiotic-resistant gram-positive bacteria, including isolates resistant to methicillin, vancomycin, and linezolid.

Daptomycin exhibits rapid, concentration-dependent bactericidal activity against gram-positive organisms in vitro. This has been demonstrated both by time-kill curves and by MBC/MIC ratios using both dilution methodology.

In vitro studies have demonstrated additive or indifferent interactions of daptomycin with other antibiotics. Antagonism, as determined by kill curve studies, has not been observed. In vitro synergistic interactions occurred with aminoglycosides and β-lactam antibiotics against some isolates of staphylococci and enterococci, including some MRSA isolates.

Contraindications

Hypersensitivity to daptomycin.

Warnings

➤*Pseudomembranous colitis:* Pseudomembranous colitis has been reported with nearly all antibacterial agents, including daptomycin, and may range in severity from mild to life-threatening. Therefore, it is important to consider this diagnosis in patients who present with diarrhea subsequent to the administration of any antibacterial agent.

Treatment with antibacterial agents alters the normal flora of the colon and may permit overgrowth of clostridia. Studies indicated that a toxin produced by *Clostridium difficile* is a primary cause of "antibiotic-associated colitis."

If a diagnosis of pseudomembranous colitis has been established, appropriate therapeutic measures should be initiated. Mild cases of pseudomembranous colitis usually respond to drug discontinuation alone. In moderate to severe cases, consideration should be given to management with fluids and electrolytes, protein supplementation, and treatment with an antibacterial agent clinically effective against *C. difficile*.

➤*Elderly:* Of the 534 patients treated with daptomycin in phase 3 controlled clinical trials of complicated skin and skin structure infection (cSSSI), 27% were 65 years of age or older and 12.4% were 75 years or older. In the 2 phase 3 clinical studies in patients with cSSSI, lower clinical success rates were seen in patients 65 years of age or older compared to those younger than 65 years of age. In addition, treatment-emergent adverse events were more common in patients 65 years old or older than in patients younger than 65 years of age in both cSSSI studies.

➤*Pregnancy:* *Category B.* There are no adequate and well-controlled studies in pregnant women. Because animal reproduction studies are not always predictive of human response, this drug should be used during pregnancy only if clearly needed.

➤*Lactation:* It is not known if daptomycin is excreted in human milk. Caution should be exercised when daptomycin is administered to nursing women.

➤*Children:* Safety and efficacy of daptomycin in patients younger than 18 years of age have not been established.

Precautions

➤*Skeletal muscle:* In phase 3 cSSSI trials, elevations in serum creatine phosphokinase (CPK) were reported as clinical adverse events in 15/534 (2.8%) daptomycin-treated patients, compared to 10/558 (1.8%) comparator-treated patients. Skeletal muscle effects associated with daptomycin were observed in animals.

Patients receiving daptomycin should be monitored for the development of muscle pain or weakness, particularly of the distal extremities. CPK levels should be monitored weekly in patients who receive daptomycin. Patients who develop unexplained elevations in CPK while receiving daptomycin should be monitored more frequently. Among patients with abnormal CPK (greater than 500 units/L) at baseline, 2/19 (10.5%) treated with daptomycin and 4/24 (16.7%) treated with comparator developed further increases in CPK while on therapy. In this same population, no patients developed myopathy. Daptomycin-treated patients with baseline CPK greater than 500 units/L (n = 19) did not experience an increased incidence of CPK elevations or myopathy relative to those treated with comparator (n = 24).

Daptomycin should be discontinued in patients with unexplained signs and symptoms of myopathy in conjunction with CPK elevation greater than 1,000 units/L (approximately 5 × ULN), or in patients without reported symptoms who have marked elevations in CPK (greater than or equal to 10 × ULN). In addition, consideration should be given to temporarily suspending agents associated with rhabdomyolysis, such as HMG-CoA reductase inhibitors, in patients receiving daptomycin.

➤*Neuropathy:* In a small number of patients in phase 1 and phase 2 studies, administration of daptomycin was associated with decreases in nerve conduction velocity and with adverse events (eg, paresthesias, Bell's palsy), possibly reflective of peripheral or cranial neuropathy. Nerve conduction deficits were also detected in a similar number of comparator subjects in these studies.

In phase 3 cSSSI and community-acquired pneumonia (CAP) studies, 7/989 (0.7%) daptomycin-treated patients and 7/1,018 (0.7%) comparator-treated patients experienced paresthesias. New or worsening peripheral neuropathy was not diagnosed in any of these patients. In animals, effects of daptomycin on peripheral nerve were observed (see Animal pharmacology below). Therefore, physicians should be alert to the possibility of signs and symptoms of neuropathy in patients receiving daptomycin.

➤*Superinfection:* The use of antibiotics may promote the overgrowth of nonsusceptible organisms. Should superinfection occur during therapy, appropriate measures should be taken.

DAPTOMYCIN — INJECTION

Drug Interactions

➤*Warfarin:* Concomitant administration of daptomycin (6 mg/kg once every 24 hours for 5 days) and warfarin (25 mg single oral dose) had no significant effect on the pharmacokinetics of either drug, and the INR was not significantly altered. As experience with the concomitant administration of daptomycin and warfarin is limited to volunteer studies, anticoagulant activity in patients receiving daptomycin and warfarin should be monitored for the first several days after initiating therapy with daptomycin.

➤*HMG-CoA reductase inhibitors:* Inhibitors of HMG-CoA reductase may cause myopathy, which is manifested as muscle pain or weakness associated with elevated levels of CPK. There were no reports of skeletal myopathy in a placebo-controlled phase 1 trial in which 10 healthy subjects on stable simvastatin therapy were treated concurrently with daptomycin (4 mg/kg once every 24 hours) for 14 days. Experience with coadministration of HMG-CoA reductase inhibitors and daptomycin in patients is limited, therefore, consideration should be given to temporarily suspending use of HMG-CoA reductase inhibitors in patients receiving daptomycin.

Adverse Reactions

Clinical studies enrolled 1,409 patients treated with daptomycin and 1,185 treated with comparator. Most adverse events reported in these clinical studies were described as mild or moderate in intensity. In phase 3 cSSSI trials, daptomycin was discontinued in 15/534 (2.8%) patients due to an adverse event while comparator was discontinued in 17/558 (3%) patients.

Incidence (%) of Adverse Events that Occurred in ≥ 2% of Patients in Either Daptomycin or Comparator Treatment Groups in Phase 3 cSSSI Studies

Adverse event	Daptomycin (n = 534)	Comparator[a] (n = 558)
GI		
Constipation	6.2%	6.8%
Nausea	5.8%	9.5%
Diarrhea	5.2%	4.3%
Vomiting	3.2%	3.8%
Dyspepsia	0.9%	2.5%
Miscellaneous		
Injection site reactions	5.8%	7.7%
Fever	1.9%	2.5%
CNS		
Headache	5.4%	5.4%
Insomnia	4.5%	5.4%
Dizziness	2.2%	2%
Dermatologic		
Rash	4.3%	3.8%
Pruritus	2.8%	3.8%
Diagnostic investigations		
Abnormal liver function tests	3%	1.6%
Elevated CPK	2.8%	1.8%
Infections		
Fungal infections	2.6%	3.2%
Urinary tract infections	2.4%	0.5%
Cardiovascular		
Hypotension	2.4%	1.4%
Hypertension	1.1%	2%
Renal		
Renal failure	2.2%	2.7%
Hematologic/lymphatic		
Anomia	2.1%	2.3%
Respiratory		
Dyspnea	2.1%	1.6%
Musculoskeletal		
Limb pain	1.5%	2%
Arthralgia	0.9%	2.2%

[a] Comparators included vancomycin (1 g IV every 12 hours) and semi-synthetic penicillins (ie, nafcillin, oxacillin, cloxacillin, flucloxacillin; 4 to 12 g/day in divided doses).

In phase 3 studies of CAP, the death rate and rates of serious cardiorespiratory adverse events were higher in daptomycin-treated patients than in comparator-treated patients. These differences were due to lack of therapeutic effectiveness of daptomycin in the treatment of CAP in patients experiencing these adverse events.

Additional adverse events that occurred in 1% to 2% of patients in either daptomycin- or comparator-treatment groups in the cSSSI studies are as follows: Edema, cellulitis, hypoglycemia, elevated alkaline phosphatase, cough, back pain, abdominal pain, hypokalemia, hyperglycemia, decreased appetite, anxiety, chest pain, sore throat, cardiac failure, confusion, and Candida infections. These events occurred at rates ranging from 0.2% to 1.7% in daptomycin-treated patients and at rates of 0.4% to 1.8% in comparator-treated patients.

➤*Additional adverse events (possibly or probably related) in less than 1% of patients:* Additional drug-related adverse events (possibly or probably related) that occurred in less than 1% of patients receiving daptomycin in cSSSI trials are as follows:

Cardiovascular – Supraventricular arrhythmia.

CNS – Vertigo, mental status change, paraesthesia.

Dermatologic – Eczema.

GI – Abdominal distension, flatulence, stomatitis, jaundice, increased serum lactate dehydrogenase.

Hematologic/Lymphatic – Leukocytosis, thrombocytopenia, thrombocytosis, eosinophilia, increased international normalized ratio (INR).

Metabolic/Nutritional – Hypomagnesemia, increased serum bicarbonate, electrolyte disturbance.

Musculoskeletal – Myalgia, muscle cramps, muscle weakness, osteomyelitis.

Special senses – Taste disturbance, eye irritation.

Miscellaneous – Fatigue, weakness, rigors, discomfort, jitteriness, flushing, hypersensitivity.

➤*Lab test abnormalities:* Elevations in CPK observed in patients treated with daptomycin or comparator were not clinically or statistically significantly different ($P < 0.05$).

Incidence (%) of creatine phosphokinase (CPK) elevations from baseline while on therapy in either daptomycin or comparator treatment groups in phase 3 cSSSI studies

	All patients				Patients with normal CPK at baseline			
	Daptomycin (n = 430)		Comparator (n = 459)		Daptomycin (n = 374)		Comparator (n = 392)	
CPK levels	n	%	n	%	n	%	n	%
No increase	90.7%	390	91.1%	418	91.2%	341	91.1%	357
Maximum value > 1 × ULN[a]	9.3%	40	8.9%	41	8.8%	33	8.9%	35
> 2 × ULN	4.9%	21	4.8%	22	3.7%	14	3.1%	12
> 4 × ULN	1.4%	6	1.5%	7	1.1%	4	1%	4
> 5 × ULN	1.4%	6	0.4%	2	1.1%	4	0%	0
> 10 × ULN	0.5%	2	0.2%	1	0.2%	1	0%	0

[a] ULN (upper limit of normal) is defined as 200 units/L.

In clinical trials, 0.2% of patients treated with daptomycin had symptoms of muscle pain or weakness associated with CPK elevations to greater than 4 times the upper limit of normal. The symptoms resolved within 3 days and CPK returned to normal within 7 to 10 days after discontinuing treatment. In phase 3 comparator-controlled trials, there was no clinically or statistically significant difference ($P < 0.05$) in the frequency of CPK elevations between patients treated with daptomycin and those treated with comparator. CPK elevations in both groups were generally related to medical conditions, for example, skin and skin structure infection, surgical procedures, or intramuscular injections, and were not associated with muscle symptoms.

There were no substantial differences between daptomycin and the comparators in the frequency or distribution of changes in other laboratory parameters, regardless of drug relationship.

Overdosage

➤*Treatment:* In the event of overdosage, supportive care is advised with maintenance of glomerular filtration. Daptomycin is slowly cleared from the body by hemodialysis (approximately 15% recovered over 4 hours) or by peritoneal dialysis (approximately 11% recovered over 48 hours).

VANCOMYCIN

Rx	**Vancocin** (ViroPharma[a])	**Pulvules:** 125 mg	(3125 Vancocin Hydrochloride 125 mg). Blue and brown. In *Identi-Dose* 20s.
		250 mg	(3126 Vancocin Hydrochloride 250 mg). Blue and lavender. In *Identi-Dose* 20s.
Rx	**Vancomycin Hydrochloride** (ESI Lederle)	**Powder for Oral Solution:** 1 g	In bottles.
Rx	**Vancomycin Hydrochloride** (Various, eg, American Pharmaceutical Partners[b], ESI Lederle, Hospira)	**Powder for Injection:** 500 mg	In vials.
Rx	**Vancocin** (ViroPharma[a])		In 10 mL vials and 15 mL *ADD-Vantage* vials.
Rx	**Vancoled** (Lederle)		In vials.
Rx	**Vancomycin Hydrochloride** (Various, eg, American Pharmaceutical Partners[b], ESI Lederle, Hospira)	**Powder for Injection:** 1 g	In vials.
Rx	**Vancoled** (Lederle)		In vials.
Rx	**Vancomycin Hydrochloride** (American Pharm. Partners[b])	**Powder for Injection:** 5 g	In 100 mL vials.
Rx	**Vancoled** (Lederle)		In pharmacy bulk package.
Rx	**Vancomycin Hydrochloride** (American Pharm. Partners[b])	**Powder for Injection:** 10 g	In vials.
Rx	**Vancocin** (ViroPharma[a])		In 100 mL vials.

[a] ViroPharma, Inc., 397 Eagleview Boulevard, Exton, PA 19341; (610) 458-7300, Fax (610) 458-7380.

[b] American Pharmaceutical Partners, Inc., 2045 North Cornell Ave., Melrose Park, IL 60160 (888) 386-1300.

VANCOMYCIN HYDROCHLORIDE — ORAL

Indications

For treatment of enterocolitis caused by *Staphylococcus aureus* (including methicillin-resistant strains) and antibiotic-associated pseudomembranous colitis caused by *C. difficile*. Parenteral administration of vancomycin hydrochloride is not effective for the above indications; therefore, vancomycin hydrochloride must be given orally for these indications. Orally administered vancomycin hydrochloride is not effective for other types of infection.

Administration and Dosage

➤*Adults:* The usual adult total daily dosage is 500 mg to 2 g administered orally in 3 or 4 divided doses for 7 to 10 days.

➤*Children:* The usual daily dosage is 40 mg/kg in 3 or 4 divided doses for 7 to 10 days. The total daily dosage should not exceed 2 g.

➤*Storage/Stability:* Store at controlled room temperature, 59° to 86°F (15° to 30°C).

Actions

➤*Pharmacokinetics:*

Absorption – Vancomycin is poorly absorbed after oral administration. During multiple dosing of 250 mg every 8 hours for 7 doses, fecal concentrations of vancomycin in volunteers exceeded 100 mg/kg in the majority of samples. No blood concentrations were detected and urinary recovery did not exceed 0.76%. Additional data using an oral solution follow. In anephric patients with no inflammatory bowel disease, blood concentrations of vancomycin were barely measurable (0.66 mcg/mL) in 2 of 5 subjects who received 2 g of vancomycin hydrochloride for oral solution daily for 16 days. No measurable blood concentrations were attained in the other 3 patients. With doses of 2 g daily, very high concentrations of drug can be found in the feces (greater than 3,100 mg/kg) and very low concentrations (less than 1 mcg/mL) can be found in the serum of patients with normal renal function who have pseudomembranous colitis. Orally administered vancomycin does not usually enter the systemic circulation even when inflammatory lesions are present. After multiple-dose oral administration of vancomycin, measurable serum concentrations may infrequently occur in patients with active *C. difficile*-induced pseudomembranous colitis, and, in the presence of renal impairment, the possibility of accumulation exists.

➤*Microbiology:* The bactericidal action of vancomycin results primarily from inhibition of cell-wall biosynthesis. In addition, vancomycin alters bacterial-cell-membrane permeability and RNA synthesis. There is no cross-resistance between vancomycin and other antibiotics.

The oral form of vancomycin is effective only for the infections noted in the Indications section. The oral form is not effective for any other type of infection.

Aerobic gram-positive microorganisms – *Staphylococcus aureus* (including methicillin-resistant strains) associated with enterocolitis.

Anaerobic gram-positive microorganisms – *Clostridium difficile* antibiotic-associated pseudomembranous colitis.

Contraindications

Hypersensitivity to this antibiotic.

Warnings

➤*Pregnancy: Category B.*

In a controlled clinical study, the potential ototoxic and nephrotoxic effects of vancomycin hydrochloride on infants were evaluated when the drug was administered intravenously to pregnant women for serious staphylococcal infections complicating intravenous drug abuse. Vancomycin hydrochloride was found in cord blood. No sensorineural hearing loss or nephrotoxicity attributable to vancomycin hydrochloride was noted. One infant whose mother received vancomycin hydrochloride in the third trimester experienced conductive hearing loss that was not attributed to the administration of vancomycin hydrochloride. Because the number of patients treated in this study was limited and vancomycin hydrochloride was administered only in the second and third trimesters, it is not known whether vancomycin hydrochloride causes fetal harm. Because animal reproduction studies are not always predictive of human response, vancomycin hydrochloride should be given to a pregnant woman only if clearly needed.

➤*Lactation:* Vancomycin is excreted in human milk based on information obtained with the intravenous administration of vancomycin hydrochloride. However, systemic absorption of vancomycin is very low following oral administration of vancomycin hydrochloride capsules (see Pharmacokinetics). It is not known whether oral vancomycin is excreted in human milk, as no studies of vancomycin concentration in human milk after oral administration have been done. Caution should be exercised when vancomycin hydrochloride is administered to a nursing woman. Because of the potential for adverse events, a decision should be made whether to discontinue nursing or discontinue the drug, taking into account the importance of the drug to the mother.

➤*Children:* Safety and efficacy in pediatric patients have not been established.

Precautions

➤*Monitoring:* Clinically significant serum concentrations have been reported in some patients who have taken multiple oral doses of vancomycin for active *C. difficile*-induced pseudomembranous colitis; therefore, monitoring of serum concentrations may be appropriate in some instances (eg, in patients with renal insufficiency or colitis).

When patients with underlying renal dysfunction or those receiving concomitant therapy with an aminoglycoside are being treated, serial monitoring of renal function should be performed.

➤*Systemic absorption:* Some patients with inflammatory disorders of the intestinal mucosa may have significant systemic absorption of vancomycin and, therefore, may be at risk for the development of adverse reactions associated with the parenteral administration of vancomycin. (See monograph accompanying the intravenous preparation.) The risk is greater if renal impairment is present. It should be noted that the total systemic and renal clearances of vancomycin are reduced in the elderly.

➤*Ototoxicity:* Ototoxicity has occurred in patients receiving vancomycin hydrochloride. It may be transient or permanent. It has been reported mostly in patients who have been given excessive intravenous doses, who have an underlying hearing loss, or who are receiving concomitant therapy with another ototoxic agent, such as an aminoglycoside. Serial tests of auditory function may be helpful in order to minimize the risk of ototoxicity.

➤*Superinfection:* Use of vancomycin may result in the overgrowth of nonsusceptible organisms. If superinfection occurs during therapy, appropriate measures should be taken.

Adverse Reactions

➤*Hematologic:* Reversible neutropenia, usually starting 1 week or more after onset of intravenous therapy with vancomycin hydrochloride or after a total dose of more than 25 g, has been reported for several dozen patients. Neutropenia appears to be promptly reversible when vancomycin hydrochloride is discontinued. Thrombocytopenia has rarely been reported.

➤*Hypersensitivity:* A condition has been reported that is similar to the IV-induced syndrome with symptoms consistent with anaphylactoid reactions, including hypotension, wheezing, dyspnea, urticaria, pruritus, flushing of the upper body ("red man syndrome"), pain and muscle spasm of the chest and back. These reactions usually resolve within 20 minutes but may persist for several hours.

➤*Renal:* Rarely, renal failure, principally manifested by increased serum creatinine or BUN concentrations, especially in patients given large doses of intravenously administered vancomycin hydrochloride has been reported. Rare cases of interstitial nephritis have been reported. Most of these have occurred in patients who were given aminoglycosides concomitantly or who

VANCOMYCIN HYDROCHLORIDE — ORAL

had preexisting kidney dysfunction. When vancomycin hydrochloride was discontinued, azotemia resolved in most patients.

➤*Special senses:* A few dozen cases of hearing loss associated with intravenously administered vancomycin hydrochloride have been reported. Most of these patients had kidney dysfunction or a preexisting hearing loss or were receiving concomitant treatment with an ototoxic drug. Vertigo, dizziness, and tinnitus have been reported rarely.

➤*Miscellaneous:* Infrequently, patients have been reported to have had anaphylaxis, drug fever, chills, nausea, eosinophilia, rashes (including exfoliative dermatitis), Stevens-Johnson syndrome, toxic epidermal necrolysis, and rare cases of vasculitis in association with the administration of vancomycin hydrochloride.

Overdosage

➤*Treatment:* Supportive care is advised, with maintenance of glomerular filtration. Vancomycin is poorly removed by dialysis. Hemofiltration and hemoperfusion with polysulfone resin have been reported to result in increased vancomycin clearance.

Patient Information

Patients should be counseled that antibacterial drugs including vancomycin hydrochloride should only be used to treat bacterial infections. Antibacterial drugs do not treat viral infections (eg, the common cold). When vancomycin hydrochloride is prescribed to treat a bacterial infection, patients should be told that although it is common to feel better early in the course of therapy, the medication should be taken exactly as directed. Skipping doses or not completing the full course of therapy may (1) decrease the effectiveness of the immediate treatment and (2) increase the likelihood that bacteria will develop resistance and will not be treatable by vancomycin hydrochloride or other antibacterial drugs in the future.

VANCOMYCIN HYDROCHLORIDE — INJECTION

Indications

➤*Staphylococcal infections:* For the treatment of serious or severe infections caused by susceptible strains of methicillin-resistant (beta-lactam-resistant) staphylococci. It is indicated for penicillin-allergic patients, for patients who cannot receive or who have failed to respond to other drugs, including the penicillins or cephalosporins, and for infections caused by vancomycin-susceptible organisms that are resistant to other antimicrobial drugs. Vancomycin hydrochloride is indicated for initial therapy when methicillin-resistant staphylococci are suspected, but after susceptibility data are available, therapy should be adjusted accordingly. Its effectiveness has been documented in other infections due to staphylococci, including septicemia, bone infections, lower respiratory tract infections, and skin and skin structure infections. When staphylococcal infections are localized and purulent, antibiotics are used as adjuncts to appropriate surgical measures.

➤*Endocarditis:*

Staphylococcal – Vancomycin hydrochloride is effective in the treatment of staphylococcal endocarditis.

Streptococcal – Vancomycin hydrochloride has been reported to be effective alone or in combination with an aminoglycoside for endocarditis caused by *Streptococcus viridans* or *S. bovis*. For endocarditis caused by enterococci (eg, *E. faecalis*), vancomycin hydrochloride has been reported to be effective only in combination with an aminoglycoside.

Diphtheroid – Vancomycin hydrochloride has been reported to be effective for the treatment of diphtheroid endocarditis. Vancomycin hydrochloride has been used successfully in combination with either rifampin, an aminoglycoside, or both in early-onset prosthetic valve endocarditis caused by *S. epidermidis* or diphtheroids.

Prophylactic – Although no controlled clinical efficacy studies have been conducted, IV vancomycin has been suggested by the American Heart Association (AHA) and the American Dental Association (ADA) as prophylaxis against bacterial endocarditis in penicillin-allergic patients who have congenital heart disease or rheumatic or other acquired valvular heart disease when these patients undergo dental procedures or surgical procedures of the upper respiratory tract.

➤*Pseudomembranous colitis/Staphylococcal enterocolitis:* The parenteral form of vancomycin hydrochloride may be administered orally for treatment of antibiotic-associated pseudomembranous colitis caused by *C. difficile* and for staphylococcal enterocolitis. Parenteral administration of vancomycin hydrochloride alone is of unproven benefit for these indications. Vancomycin hydrochloride is not effective by the oral route for other types of infection.

Administration and Dosage

➤*Approved by the FDA:* July 13, 1983.

➤*Infusion-related reactions:* Infusion-related events are related to both concentration and rate of administration of vancomycin. Concentrations of no more than 5 mg/mL and rates of no more than 10 mg/min are recommended in adults (see also age-specific recommendations). In selected patients in need of fluid restriction, a concentration up to 10 mg/mL may be used; use of such higher concentrations may increase the risk of infusion-related events. Infusion-related events may occur, however, at any rate or concentration.

➤*Dosage:*

Adults – The usual daily IV dose is 2 g divided either as 500 mg every 6 hours or 1 g every 12 hours. Each dose should be administered at no more than 10 mg/min or over a period of at least 60 minutes, whichever is longer. Other patient factors, such as age or obesity, may call for modification of the usual IV daily dose.

Children – The usual IV dosage of vancomycin hydrochloride is 10 mg/kg/dose given every 6 hours. Each dose should be administered over a period of at least 60 minutes.

Infants and neonates – In neonates and young infants, the total daily IV dosage may be lower. In both neonates and infants, an initial dose of 15 mg/kg is suggested, followed by 10 mg/kg every 12 hours for neonates in the first week of life and every 8 hours thereafter up to the age of 1 month. Each dose should be administered over 60 minutes. Close monitoring of serum concentrations of vancomycin may be warranted in these patients.

➤*Renal function impairment:* Dosage adjustment must be made in patients with impaired renal function. In premature infants and the elderly, greater dosage reductions than expected may be necessary because of decreased renal function. Measurement of vancomycin serum concentrations can be helpful in optimizing therapy, especially in seriously ill patients with changing renal function. Vancomycin serum concentrations can be determined by use of microbiologic assay, radioimmunoassay, fluorescence polarization immunoassay, fluorescence immunoassay, or high-pressure liquid chromatography.

If creatinine clearance can be measured or estimated accurately, the dosage for most patients with renal impairment can be calculated using the following data. The dosage of vancomycin hydrochloride/day in mg is about 15 times the glomerular filtration rate in mL/min.

Dosage for Patients with Impaired Renal Function	
Creatinine clearance	Dose
100 mL/min	1,545 mg per 24 h
90 mL/min	1,390 mg per 24 h
80 mL/min	1,235 mg per 24 h
70 mL/min	1,080 mg per 24 h
60 mL/min	925 mg per 24 h
50 mL/min	770 mg per 24 h
40 mL/min	620 mg per 24 h
30 mL/min	465 mg per 24 h
20 mL/min	310 mg per 24 h
10 mL/min	155 mg per 24 h

The initial dose should be no less than 15 mg/kg, even in patients with mild-to-moderate renal insufficiency.

Anephric patients – The information above is not valid for functionally anephric patients. For such patients, an initial dose of 15 mg/kg of body weight should be given to achieve prompt therapeutic serum concentrations. The dose required to maintain stable concentrations is 1.9 mg/kg every 24 hours. In patients with marked renal impairment, it may be more convenient to give maintenance doses of 250 to 1,000 mg once every several days rather than administering the drug on a daily basis. In anuria, a dose of 1,000 mg every 7 to 10 days has been recommended.

➤*Preparation for administration:* The safety and efficacy of vancomycin administration by the intrathecal (intralumbar or intraventricular) routes have not been assessed.

Intermittent infusion is the recommended method of administration.

➤*Reconstitution:* At the time of use, reconstitute by adding either 10 mL of Sterile Water for Injection to the 500 mg vial or 20 mL of Sterile Water for Injection to the 1 g vial of dry, sterile vancomycin powder. Vials reconstituted in this manner will give a solution of 50 mg/mL. Further dilution is required.

Reconstituted solutions containing 500 mg of vancomycin must be diluted with at least 100 mL of diluent. Reconstituted solutions containing 1 g of vancomycin must be diluted with at least 200 mL of diluent. The desired dose, diluted in this manner, should be administered by intermittent IV infusion over a period of at least 60 minutes.

➤*Compatible diluents:* The following diluents are physically and chemically compatible (with 4 g/L vancomycin hydrochloride): 5% Dextrose Injection, 5% Dextrose Injection and 0.9% Sodium Chloride Injection, Lactated Ringer's Injection, 5% Dextrose and Lactated Ringer's Injection, *Normosol-M* and 5% Dextrose, 0.9% Sodium Chloride Injection, *Isolyte E*, and Acetated Ringer's Injection.

➤*Incompatibilities/Admixture:* Mixtures of solutions of vancomycin and beta-lactam antibiotics have been shown to be physically incompatible. The likelihood of precipitation increases with higher concentrations of vancomycin. It is recommended to adequately flush the IV lines between the administration of these antibiotics. It is also recommended to dilute solutions of vancomycin to 5 mg/mL or less.

Vancomycin solution has a low pH and may cause physical instability of other compounds.

➤*Storage/Stability:* Store at controlled room temperature, 15° to 30°C (59° to 86°F). After reconstitution, the vials may be stored in a refrigerator for 96 hours without significant loss of potency.

Parenteral solutions are stable for 14 days if refrigerated after initial reconstitution. After further dilution, the parenteral solution is stable for 24 hours

VANCOMYCIN HYDROCHLORIDE — INJECTION

at room temperature and for 2 months under refrigeration (less than 6% loss of potency) after dilution with Dextrose 5% or Sodium Chloride 0.9%.

Actions

➤*Pharmacokinetics:*

Absorption – Vancomycin is poorly absorbed after oral administration; it is given IV for therapy of systemic infections. IM injection is painful.

In subjects with healthy kidney function, multiple IV dosing of 1 g of vancomycin (15 mg/kg) infused over 60 minutes produces mean plasma concentrations of approximately 63 mcg/mL immediately after the completion of infusion, mean plasma concentrations of approximately 23 mcg/mL 2 hours after infusion, and mean plasma concentrations of approximately 8 mcg/mL 11 hours after the end of the infusion. Multiple dosing of 500 mg infused over 30 minutes produces mean plasma concentrations of about 49 mcg/mL at the completion of infusion, mean plasma concentrations of about 19 mcg/mL 2 hours after infusion, and mean plasma concentrations of about 10 mcg/mL 6 hours after infusion. The plasma concentrations during multiple dosing are similar to those after a single dose.

Distribution – Vancomycin is approximately 55% serum protein bound as measured by ultrafiltration at vancomycin serum concentrations of 10 to 100 mcg/mL. After IV administration of vancomycin hydrochloride, inhibitory concentrations are present in pleural, pericardial, ascitic, and synovial fluids; in urine; in peritoneal dialysis fluid; and in atrial appendage tissue. Vancomycin hydrochloride does not readily diffuse across normal meninges into the spinal fluid; but, when the meninges are inflamed, penetration into the spinal fluid occurs.

Metabolism/Excretion – The mean elimination half-life of vancomycin from plasma is 4 to 6 hours in subjects with healthy renal function. In the first 24 hours, about 75% of an administered dose of vancomycin is excreted in urine by glomerular filtration. Mean plasma clearance is about 0.058 L/kg/hr, and mean renal clearance is about 0.048 L/kg/h. Renal dysfunction slows excretion of vancomycin. In anephric patients, the average half-life of elimination is 7.5 days. The distribution coefficient is from 0.3 to 0.43 L/kg. There is no apparent metabolism of the drug. About 60% of an intraperitoneal dose of vancomycin administered during peritoneal dialysis is absorbed systemically in 6 hours. Serum concentrations of about 10 mcg/mL are achieved by intraperitoneal injection of 30 mg/kg of vancomycin. Although vancomycin is not effectively removed by either hemodialysis or peritoneal dialysis, there have been reports of increased vancomycin clearance with hemoperfusion and hemofiltration.

Total systemic and renal clearance of vancomycin may be reduced in the elderly.

➤*Microbiology:* The bactericidal action of vancomycin results primarily from inhibition of cell-wall biosynthesis. In addition, vancomycin alters bacterial cell-membrane permeability and ribonucleic acid (RNA) synthesis. There is no cross-resistance between vancomycin and other antibiotics. Vancomycin is active against staphylococci, including *Staphylococcus aureus* and *Staphylococcus epidermidis* (including heterogeneous methicillin-resistant strains); streptococci, including *Streptococcus pyogenes*, *Streptococcus pneumoniae* (including penicillin-resistant strains), *Streptococcus agalactiae*, the viridans group, *Streptococcus bovis*, and enterococci (eg, *Enterococcus faecalis* [formerly *Streptococcus faecalis*]); *Clostridium difficile* (eg, toxigenic strains implicated in pseudomembranous enterocolitis); and diphtheroids. Other organisms that are susceptible to vancomycin in vitro include *Listeria monocytogenes*, *Lactobacillus* species, *Actinomyces* species, *Clostridium* species, and *Bacillus* species.

Synergy – The combination of vancomycin and an aminoglycoside acts synergistically in vitro against many strains of *S. aureus*, nonenterococcal group D streptococci, enterococci, and *Streptococcus* species (viridans group).

Contraindications

Hypersensitivity to this antibiotic.

Warnings

➤*Hypotension:* Rapid bolus administration (eg, over several minutes) may be associated with exaggerated hypotension, and, rarely, cardiac arrest.

Vancomycin hydrochloride should be administered in a dilute solution over a period of not less than 60 minutes to avoid rapid-infusion-related reactions. Stopping the infusion usually results in prompt cessation of these reactions.

➤*Ototoxicity:* Ototoxicity has occurred in patients receiving vancomycin hydrochloride. It may be transient or permanent. It has been reported mostly in patients who have been given excessive doses, who have an underlying hearing loss, or who are receiving concomitant therapy with another ototoxic agent, such as an aminoglycoside.

➤*Pseudomembranous colitis:* Pseudomembranous colitis has been reported with nearly all antibacterial agents, including vancomycin, and may range in severity from mild to life-threatening. Therefore, it is important to consider this diagnosis in patients who present with diarrhea subsequent to the administration of antibacterial agents.

Treatment with antibacterial agents alters the normal flora of the colon and may permit overgrowth of clostridia. Studies indicate that a toxin produced by *Clostridium difficile* is a primary cause of antibiotic-associated colitis. After the diagnosis of pseudomembranous colitis has been established, therapeutic measures should be initiated. Mild cases of pseudomembranous colitis usually respond to drug discontinuation alone. In moderate-to-severe cases, consideration should be given to management with fluids and electrolytes, protein supplementation, and treatment with an antibacterial drug clinically effective against *C. difficile*.

In rare instances, there have been reports of pseudomembranous colitis due to *C. difficile* developing in patients who received IV vancomycin.

➤*Hypersensitivity reactions:* During or soon after the rapid infusion of vancomycin hydrochloride, patients may develop anaphylactoid reactions, including hypotension, wheezing, dyspnea, urticaria, or pruritus. In animal studies, hypotension and bradycardia occurred in dogs receiving an IV infusion of vancomycin hydrochloride, 25 mg/kg, at a concentration of 25 mg/mL and an infusion rate of 13.3 mL/min. The median lethal IV dose is 319 mg/kg in rats and 400 mg/kg in mice. Rapid infusion may also cause flushing of the upper body ("red man syndrome") or pain and muscle spasm of the chest and back. These reactions usually resolve within 20 minutes but may persist for several hours. Such events are infrequent if vancomycin hydrochloride is given by a slow infusion over 60 minutes. In studies of healthy volunteers, infusion-related events did not occur when vancomycin hydrochloride was administered at a rate of less than or equal to 10 mg/min.

➤*Renal function impairment:* Vancomycin should be used with caution in patients with renal insufficiency because the risk of toxicity is appreciably increased by high, prolonged blood concentrations.

See Administration and Dosage for more information.

➤*Elderly:* The natural decrement of glomerular filtration with increasing age may lead to elevated vancomycin serum concentrations if dosage is not adjusted. Vancomycin dosage schedules should be adjusted in elderly patients.

➤*Pregnancy: Category C.* In a controlled clinical study, the potential ototoxic and nephrotoxic effects of vancomycin hydrochloride on infants were evaluated when the drug was administered to pregnant women for serious staphylococcal infections that were complications of their IV drug abuse. Vancomycin hydrochloride was found in cord blood. No sensorineural hearing loss or nephrotoxicity attributable to vancomycin hydrochloride was noted. One infant whose mother received vancomycin hydrochloride in the third trimester experienced conductive hearing loss that was not attributed to the administration of vancomycin hydrochloride. Because the number of patients treated in this study was limited, and vancomycin hydrochloride was administered only in the second and third trimesters, it is not known whether vancomycin hydrochloride causes fetal harm. Vancomycin hydrochloride should be given to a pregnant woman only if clearly needed.

➤*Lactation:* Vancomycin hydrochloride is excreted in human milk. Caution should be exercised when vancomycin hydrochloride is administered to a nursing woman. Because of the potential for adverse reactions, a decision should be made whether to discontinue nursing or to discontinue the drug, taking into account the importance of the drug to the mother.

➤*Children:* In premature neonates and young infants, it may be appropriate to confirm desired vancomycin serum concentrations. Concomitant administration of vancomycin and anesthetic agents has been associated with erythema and histamine-like flushing in pediatric patients. There have been reports that the frequency of infusion-related events (including hypotension, flushing, erythema, urticaria, and pruritus) increases with the concomitant administration of anesthetic agents. Infusion-related events may be minimized by the administration of vancomycin hydrochloride as a 60-minute infusion prior to anesthetic induction.

Precautions

➤*Monitoring:* In order to minimize the risk of nephrotoxicity when treating patients with underlying renal dysfunction or patients receiving concomitant therapy with an aminoglycoside, serial monitoring of renal function should be performed and particular care should be taken in following appropriate dosing schedules.

Serial tests of auditory function may be helpful in order to minimize the risk of ototoxicity.

➤*Neutropenia:* Reversible neutropenia, usually starting 1 week or more after onset of therapy with vancomycin hydrochloride or after a total dosage of greater than 25 g, has been reported in patients receiving vancomycin hydrochloride. Patients who will undergo prolonged therapy with vancomycin hydrochloride or those who are receiving concomitant drugs that may cause neutropenia should have periodic monitoring of the leukocyte count.

➤*Tissue irritation:* Vancomycin hydrochloride is irritating to tissue and must be given by a secure IV route of administration. Pain, tenderness, and necrosis occur with IM injection of vancomycin hydrochloride or with inadvertent extravasation. Thrombophlebitis may occur, the frequency and severity of which can be minimized by administering the drug slowly as a dilute solution (2.5 to 5 g/L) and by rotating the sites of infusion.

➤*Intraperitoneal and intrathecal routes:* The safety and efficacy of vancomycin administration by the intraperitoneal and intrathecal (intralumbar or intraventricular) routes have not been assessed.

Although the safety and efficacy of sterile vancomycin hydrochloride by the intraperitoneal route have not been established, reports reveal that the product has been given by this route during peritoneal dialysis. Administration of sterile vancomycin hydrochloride by the intraperitoneal route during continuous ambulatory peritoneal dialysis has resulted in over 50 reports of chemical peritonitis that developed in some patients within the 12-hour period after administration. To date, all have been self-limited and ranged from cloudy dialysate alone to severe abdominal pain and fever. Most cloudy dialysates were sterile and some contained increased numbers of white blood cells and polymorphonuclear cells. Fluids usually cleared promptly after discontinuation of the sterile vancomycin hydrochloride.

➤*Superinfection:* Prolonged use of vancomycin hydrochloride may result in the overgrowth of nonsusceptible organisms. Careful observation of the patient is essential. If superinfection occurs during therapy, appropriate measures should be taken.

VANCOMYCIN HYDROCHLORIDE — INJECTION

Drug Interactions

Vancomycin Drug Interactions			
Precipitant drug	Object drug[a]		Description
Vancomycin	Aminoglycosides	↑	The risk of nephrotoxicity may be increased above that associated with aminoglycoside use alone.
Vancomycin	Anesthetics	↑	Concomitant use has been associated with erythema and histamine-like flushing in children.
Vancomycin	Neurotoxic/ Nephrotoxic agents	↑	Concurrent or sequential systemic or topical use requires careful monitoring.
Vancomycin	Nondepolarizing muscle relaxants	↑	Neuromuscular blockade may be enhanced.

[a] ↑ = Object drug increased.

➤*Anesthetic agents:* Coadministration of vancomycin and anesthetic agents has been associated with erythema and histamine-like flushing and anaphylactoid reactions. There have been reports that the frequency of infusion-related events (including hypotension, flushing, erythema, urticaria, and pruritus) increases with the concomitant administration of anesthetic agents. Infusion-related events may be minimized by the administration of vancomycin hydrochloride as a 60-minute infusion prior to anesthetic induction.

➤*Other neurotoxic/nephrotoxic drugs:* Concurrent and/or sequential systemic or topical use of other potentially neurotoxic or nephrotoxic drugs, such as amphotericin B, aminoglycosides, bacitracin, polymyxin B, colistin, viomycin, or cisplatin, when indicated, requires careful monitoring.

Adverse Reactions

➤*GI:* See Warnings for more information.

➤*Hematologic:* Reversible neutropenia, usually starting 1 week or more after onset of therapy with vancomycin hydrochloride or after a total dosage of greater than 25 g, has been reported for several dozen patients. Neutropenia appears to be promptly reversible when vancomycin hydrochloride is discontinued. Thrombocytopenia has rarely been reported.

Although a causal relationship has not been established, reversible agranulocytosis (granulocytes less than 500/mm^3) has been reported rarely.

➤*Hypersensitivity:* See Warnings for more information.

➤*Local:* Inflammation at the injection site has been reported.

➤*Renal:*

Nephrotoxicity – Rarely, renal failure, principally manifested by increased serum creatinine or blood urea nitrogen (BUN) concentrations, especially in patients given large doses of vancomycin hydrochloride, has been reported. Rare cases of interstitial nephritis have been reported. Some studies suggest that the incidence of nephrotoxicity is increased in patients given aminoglycosides concomitantly or who had preexisting kidney dysfunction when vancomycin hydrochloride was discontinued; azotemia resolved in most patients.

➤*Special senses:* A few dozen cases of hearing loss associated with vancomycin hydrochloride have been reported. Most of these patients had kidney dysfunction or a preexisting hearing loss or were receiving concomitant treatment with an ototoxic drug. Vertigo, dizziness, and tinnitus have been reported rarely.

➤*Miscellaneous:* Infrequently, patients have been reported to have had anaphylaxis, drug fever, nausea, chills, eosinophilia, rashes (including exfoliative dermatitis), linear IgA bullous dermatosis, Stevens-Johnson syndrome, toxic epidermal necrolysis, and rare cases of vasculitis in association with administration of vancomycin hydrochloride.

➤*Chemical peritonitis:* See Precautions for more information.

Overdosage

➤*Treatment:* Supportive care is advised, with maintenance of glomerular filtration. Vancomycin is poorly removed by dialysis. Hemofiltration and hemoperfusion with polysulfone resin have been reported to result in increased vancomycin clearance. The median lethal IV dose is 319 mg/kg in rats and 400 mg/kg in mice.

OXAZOLIDINONES

LINEZOLID

Rx	**Zyvox** (Pharmacia)	**Tablets:** 400 mg[a]	(ZYVOX 400mg). White, oblong. Film-coated. In 20s, 100s, and UD 30s.
		600 mg[b]	(ZYVOX 600mg). White, capsule-shape. Film-coated. In 20s, 100s, and UD 30s.
		Powder for oral suspension: 100 mg/5 mL[c]	Sucrose, aspartame, mannitol, 20 mg phenylalanine. Orange flavor. 115 mL fill in 240 mL bottle.
		Injection: 2 mg/mL[d]	Sodium citrate. In 100, 200, and 300 mL single-use, ready to use bags.

[a] Sodium content is 1.95 mg per 400 mg tablet (0.1 mEq/tablet).
[b] Sodium content is 2.92 mg per 600 mg tablet (0.1 mEq/tablet).
[c] Sodium content is 8.52 mg per 5 mL (0.4 mEq/5 mL).
[d] Sodium content is 0.38 mg/mL (5 mEq/300 mL bag, 3.3 mEq/200 mL bag, 1.7 mEq/100 mL bag).

LINEZOLID — ORAL

Indications

➤*Vancomycin-resistant enterococcal infections:* Vancomycin-resistant *Enterococcus faecium* infections, including cases with concurrent bacteremia.

➤*Nosocomial pneumonia:* Caused by *Staphylococcus aureus* (methicillin-susceptible and -resistant strains), or *Streptococcus pneumoniae* (penicillin-susceptible strains only). Combination therapy may be clinically indicated if the documented or presumptive pathogens include gram-negative organisms.

➤*Complicated skin and skin structure infections:* Complicated skin and skin structure infections, including diabetic foot infections, without concomitant osteomyelitis, caused by *Staphylococcus aureus* (methicillin-susceptible and -resistant strains), *Streptococcus pyogenes*, or *Streptococcus agalactiae*. Linezolid has not been studied in the treatment of diabetic foot and decubitus ulcers. Combination therapy may be clinically indicated if the documented or presumptive pathogens include gram-negative organisms.

➤*Uncomplicated skin and skin structure infections:* Caused by *Staphylococcus aureus* (methicillin-susceptible strains only) or *Streptococcus pyogenes*.

➤*Community-acquired pneumonia:* Caused by *Streptococcus pneumoniae* (penicillin-susceptible strains only), including cases with concurrent bacteremia, or *Staphylococcus aureus* (methicillin-susceptible strains only).

Due to concerns about inappropriate use of antibiotics leading to an increase in resistant organisms, prescribers should carefully consider alternatives before initiating treatment with linezolid in the outpatient setting.

Administration and Dosage

➤*Approved by the FDA:* April 18, 2000.

Dosage Guidelines for Linezolid			
	Dosage and route of administration		
Infection[a]	Pediatric patients[b] (birth through 11 years of age)	Adults and adolescents (12 years of age and older)	Recommended duration of treatment (consecutive days)
Complicated skin and skin structure infections	10 mg/kg IV or oral[c] every 8 h	600 mg IV or oral[c] every 12 h	10 to 14
Community-acquired pneumonia, including concurrent bacteremia			
Nosocomial pneumonia			
Vancomycin-resistant *Enterococcus faecium* infections, including concurrent bacteremia	10 mg/kg IV or oral[c] every 8 h	600 mg IV or oral[c] every 12 h	14 to 28
Uncomplicated skin and skin structure infections	< 5 years: 10 mg/kg oral[c] every 8 h	Adults: 400 mg oral[c] every 12 h	10 to 14
	5 to 11 years: 10 mg/kg oral[c] every 12 h	Adolescents: 600 mg oral[c] every 12 h	

[a] Due to the designated pathogens.
[b] Neonates less than 7 days: Most pre-term neonates less than 7 days of age (gestational age less than 34 weeks) have lower systemic linezolid clearance values and larger AUC values than many full-term neonates and older infants. These neonates should be initiated with a dosing regimen of 10 mg/kg every 12 hours. Consideration may be given to the use of 10 mg/kg every 8 hours regimen in neonates with a sub-optimal clinical response. All neonatal patients should receive 10 mg/kg every 8 hours by 7 days of life.
[c] Oral dosing using either linezolid tablets or linezolid for oral suspension.

LINEZOLID — ORAL

➤*Methicillin-resistant staphylococcal infections:* Adult patients with infection due to methicillin-resistant *Staphylococcus aureus* (MRSA) should be treated with linezolid 600 mg every 12 hours.

➤*Duration:* In controlled clinical trials, the protocol-defined duration of treatment for all infections ranged from 7 to 28 days. Total treatment duration was determined by the treating physician based on site and severity of the infection, and on the patient's clinical response.

➤*IV to oral conversion:* No dose adjustment is necessary when switching from IV to oral administration. Patients whose therapy is started with linezolid IV injection may be switched to either linezolid tablets or oral suspension at the discretion of the physician, when clinically indicated.

➤*Reconstitution of oral suspension:* Linezolid for oral suspension is supplied as a powder/granule for constitution. Gently tap bottle to loosen powder. Add a total of 123 mL distilled water in 2 portions. After adding the first half, shake vigorously to wet all of the powder. Then add the second half of the water and shake vigorously to obtain a uniform suspension. After constitution, each 5 mL of the suspension contains 100 mg of linezolid. Before using, gently mix by inverting the bottle 3 to 5 times. Do not shake. Store constituted suspension at room temperature. Use within 21 days after constitution.

➤*Storage/Stability:* Store at 25°C (77°F); excursions permitted to 15° to 30°C (59° to 86°F). Protect from light. Keep bottles tightly closed to protect from moisture.

Actions

➤*Pharmacokinetics:*

Absorption – Linezolid is rapidly and extensively absorbed after oral dosing. Maximum plasma concentrations are reached approximately 1 to 2 hours after dosing, and the absolute bioavailability is approximately 100%. Therefore, linezolid may be given orally or IV without dose adjustment.

Linezolid may be administered without regard to the timing of meals. The time to reach the maximum concentration is delayed from 1.5 hours to 2.2 hours and C_{max} is decreased by about 17% when high-fat food is given with linezolid. However, the total exposure measured as $AUC_{0-\infty}$ values is similar under both conditions.

Distribution – Animal and human pharmacokinetic studies have demonstrated that linezolid readily distributes to well-perfused tissues. The plasma protein binding of linezolid is approximately 31% and is concentration-independent. The volume of distribution of linezolid at steady state averaged 40 to 50 L in healthy adult volunteers.

Metabolism – Linezolid is primarily metabolized by oxidation of the morpholine ring, which results in 2 inactive ring-opened carboxylic acid metabolites, the aminoethoxyacetic acid metabolite (A), and the hydroxyethyl glycine metabolite (B). Formation of metabolite B is mediated by a nonenzymatic chemical oxidation mechanism in vitro. Linezolid is not an inducer of cytochrome P450 (CYP) in rats, and it has been demonstrated from in vitro studies that linezolid is not detectably metabolized by human cytochrome P450 and it does not inhibit the activities of clinically significant human CYP isoforms (1A2, 2C9, 2C19, 2D6, 2E1, 3A4).

Excretion – Nonrenal clearance accounts for approximately 65% of the total clearance of linezolid. Under steady-state conditions, approximately 30% of the dose appears in the urine as linezolid, 40% as metabolite B, and 10% as metabolite A. The renal clearance of linezolid is low (average 40 mL/min) and suggests net tubular reabsorption. Virtually no linezolid appears in the feces, while approximately 6% of the dose appears in the feces as metabolite B, and 3% as metabolite A.

A small degree of nonlinearity in clearance was observed with increasing doses of linezolid, which appears to be due to lower renal and nonrenal clearance of linezolid at higher concentrations. However, the difference in clearance was small and was not reflected in the apparent elimination half-life.

Special populations –

Renal function impairment: The pharmacokinetics of the parent drug, linezolid, are not altered in patients with any degree of renal insufficiency; however, the 2 primary metabolites of linezolid may accumulate in patients with renal insufficiency, with the amount of accumulation increasing with the severity of renal dysfunction. The clinical significance of accumulation of these 2 metabolites has not been determined in patients with severe renal insufficiency. Because similar plasma concentrations of linezolid are achieved regardless of renal function, no dose adjustment is recommended for patients with renal insufficiency. However, given the absence of information on the clinical significance of accumulation of the primary metabolites, use of linezolid in patients with renal insufficiency should be weighed against the potential risks of accumulation of these metabolites. Both linezolid and the 2 metabolites are eliminated by dialysis. No information is available on the effect of peritoneal dialysis on the pharmacokinetics of linezolid. Approximately 30% of a dose was eliminated in a 3-hour dialysis session beginning 3 hours after the dose of linezolid was administered; therefore, linezolid should be given after hemodialysis.

Children: The C_{max} and the volume of distribution (V_{ss}) of linezolid are similar regardless of age in pediatric patients. However, clearance of linezolid varies as a function of age. With the exclusion of pre-term neonates less than 1 week of age, clearance is most rapid in the youngest age groups ranging from greater than 1 week old to 11 years, resulting in lower single-dose systemic exposure (AUC) and shorter half-life as compared with adults. As age of pediatric patients increases, the clearance of linezolid gradually decreases, and by adolescence mean clearance values approach those observed for the adult population. There is wider inter-subject variability in linezolid clearance and systemic drug exposure (AUC) across all pediatric age groups as compared with adults.

Similar mean daily AUC values were observed in pediatric patients from birth to 11 years of age dosed every 8 hours relative to adolescents or adults dosed every 12 hours. Therefore, the dosage for pediatric patients up to 11 years of age should be 10 mg/kg every 8 hours. Pediatric patients 12 years and older should receive 600 mg every 12 hours (see Dosage and Administration).

➤*Microbiology:* In clinical trials, resistance to linezolid developed in 6 patients infected with *E. faecium* (4 patients received 200 mg every 12 hours, lower than the recommended dose, and 2 patients received 600 mg every 12 hours). In a compassionate use program, resistance to linezolid developed in 8 patients with *E. faecium* and in 1 patient with *E. faecalis*. All patients had either unremoved prosthetic devices or undrained abscesses. Resistance to linezolid occurs in vitro at a frequency of 1×10^{-9} to 1×10^{-11}. In vitro studies have shown that point mutations in the ′ rRNA are associated with linezolid resistance.

Reports of vancomycin resistant *E. faecium* becoming resistant to linezolid during its clinical use have been published. In one report nosocomial spread of vancomycin- and linezolid-resistant *E. faecium* occurred. There has been a report of *Staphylococcus aureus* (methicillin-resistant) developing resistance to linezolid during its clinical use. The linezolid resistance in these organisms was associated with a point mutation in the 23S rRNA (substitution of thymine for guanine at position 2576) of the organism. When antibiotic-resistant organisms are encountered in the hospital, it is important to emphasize infection control policies. Resistance to linezolid has not been reported in *Streptococcus* spp., including *Streptococcus pneumoniae*.

In vitro studies have demonstrated additivity or indifference between linezolid and vancomycin, gentamicin, rifampin, imipenem-cilastatin, aztreonam, ampicillin, or streptomycin.

Linezolid has been shown to be active against most isolates of the following microorganisms, both in vitro and in clinical infections, as described in Indications.

Aerobic and facultative gram-positive microorganisms –
- *Enterococcus faecium* (vancomycin-resistant strains only).
- *Staphylococcus aureus* (including methicillin-resistant strains).
- *Streptococcus agalactiae*.
- *Streptococcus pneumoniae* (penicillin-susceptible strains only).
- *Streptococcus pyogenes*.

Contraindications

Linezolid formulations are contraindicated for use in patients who have known hypersensitivity to linezolid or any of the other product components.

Warnings

➤*Myelosuppression:* Myelosuppression (including anemia, leukopenia, pancytopenia, and thrombocytopenia) has been reported in patients receiving linezolid. In cases where the outcome is known, when linezolid was discontinued, the affected hematologic parameters have risen toward pretreatment levels. Complete blood counts should be monitored weekly in patients who receive linezolid, particularly in those who receive linezolid for longer than 2 weeks, those with preexisting myelosuppression, those receiving concomitant drugs that produce bone marrow suppression, or those with a chronic infection who have received previous or concomitant antibiotic therapy. Discontinuation of therapy with linezolid should be considered in patients who develop or have worsening myelosuppression.

➤*Pseudomembranous colitis:* Pseudomembranous colitis has been reported with nearly all antibacterial agents, including linezolid, and may range in severity from mild to life-threatening. Therefore, it is important to consider this diagnosis in patients who present with diarrhea subsequent to the administration of any antibacterial agent.

Treatment with antibacterial agents alters the healthy flora of the colon and may permit overgrowth of clostridia. Studies indicated that a toxin produced by *Clostridium difficile* is a primary cause of "antibiotic-associated colitis."

After the diagnosis of pseudomembranous colitis has been established, appropriate therapeutic measures should be initiated. Mild cases of pseudomembranous colitis usually respond to drug discontinuation alone. In moderate-to-severe cases, consideration should be given to management with fluids and electrolytes, protein supplementation, and treatment with an antibacterial agent clinically effective against *Clostridium difficile*.

➤*Fertility impairment:* Linezolid did not affect the fertility or reproductive performance of adult female rats. It reversibly decreased fertility and reproductive performance in adult male rats when given at doses greater than or equal to 50 mg/kg/day, with exposures approximately equal to or greater than the expected human exposure level (exposure comparisons are based on AUCs). The reversible fertility effects were mediated through altered spermatogenesis. Affected spermatids contained abnormally formed and oriented mitochondria and were non-viable. Epithelial cell hypertrophy and hyperplasia in the epididymis was observed in conjunction with decreased fertility. Similar epididymal changes were not seen in dogs.

In sexually mature male rats exposed to drug as juveniles, mildly decreased fertility was observed following treatment with linezolid through most of their period of sexual development (50 mg/kg/day from days 7 to 36 of age, and 100 mg/kg/day from days 37 to 55 of age), with exposures up to 1.7-fold greater than mean AUCs observed in pediatric patients aged 3 months to 11 years. Decreased fertility was not observed with shorter treatment periods, corresponding to exposure in utero through the early neonatal period (gestation day 6 through postnatal day 5), neonatal exposure (postnatal days 5 to 21), or to juvenile exposure (postnatal days 22 to 35). Reversible reductions in sperm motility and altered sperm morphology were observed in rats treated from postnatal day 22 to 35.

➤*Pregnancy: Category C.* Linezolid was not teratogenic in mice or rats at exposure levels 6.5-fold (in mice) or equivalent to (in rats) the expected human exposure level, based on AUCs. However, embryo and fetal toxicities

LINEZOLID — ORAL

were seen. There are no adequate and well-controlled studies in pregnant women. Linezolid should be used during pregnancy only if the potential benefit justifies the potential risk to the fetus.

In mice, embryo and fetal toxicities were seen only at doses that caused maternal toxicity (clinical signs and reduced body weight gain). A dose of 450 mg/kg/day (6.5-fold the estimated human exposure level based on AUCs) correlated with increased postimplantational embryo death, including total litter loss, decreased fetal body weights, and an increased incidence of costal cartilage fusion.

In rats, mild fetal toxicity was observed at 15 and 50 mg/kg/day (exposure levels 0.22-fold to approximately equivalent to the estimated human exposure, respectively, based on AUCs). The effects consisted of decreased fetal body weights and reduced ossification of sternebrae, a finding often seen in association with decreased fetal body weights. Slight maternal toxicity, in the form of reduced body weight gain, was seen at 50 mg/kg/day.

When female rats were treated with 50 mg/kg/day (approximately equivalent to the estimated human exposure based on AUCs) of linezolid during pregnancy and lactation, survival of pups was decreased on postnatal days 1 to 4. Male and female pups permitted to mature to reproductive age, when mated, showed an increase in preimplantation loss.

➤*Lactation:* Linezolid and its metabolites are excreted in the milk of lactating rats. Concentrations in milk were similar to those in maternal plasma. It is not known whether linezolid is excreted in human milk. Because many drugs are excreted in human milk, caution should be exercised when linezolid is administered to a nursing woman.

➤*Children:* The safety and effectiveness of linezolid for the treatment of pediatric patients ranging in age from birth through 11 years has been established.

See Actions for more information.

Recommendations for the dosage regimen for pre-term neonates less than 7 days of age (gestational age less than 34 weeks) are based on pharmacokinetic data from 9 pre-term neonates. Most of these pre-term neonates have lower systemic linezolid clearance values and larger AUC values than many full-term neonates and older infants. Therefore, these pre-term neonates should be initiated with a dosing regimen of 10 mg/kg every 12 hours. Consideration may be given to the use of a 10 mg/kg every 8 hours regimen in neonates with a sub-optimal clinical response. All neonatal patients should receive 10 mg/kg every 8 hours by 7 days of life.

In limited clinical experience, 5 out of 6 (83%) pediatric patients with infections due to gram-positive pathogens with MICs of 4 mcg/mL treated with linezolid had clinical cures. However, pediatric patients exhibit wider variability in linezolid clearance and systemic exposure (AUC) compared with adults. In pediatric patients with a sub-optimal clinical response, particularly those with pathogens with MIC of 4 mcg/mL, lower systemic exposure, site and severity of infection, and the underlying medical condition should be considered when assessing clinical response.

Precautions

➤*Lactic acidosis:* Lactic acidosis has been reported with the use of linezolid. In reported cases, patients experienced repeated episodes of nausea and vomiting. Patients who develop recurrent nausea or vomiting, unexplained acidosis, or a low bicarbonate level while receiving linezolid should receive immediate medical evaluation.

➤*General:* Linezolid has not been studied in patients with uncontrolled hypertension, pheochromocytoma, carcinoid syndrome, or untreated hyperthyroidism.

➤*Duration of therapy:* The safety and efficacy of linezolid formulations given for greater than 28 days have not been evaluated in controlled clinical trials.

➤*Superinfection:* The use of antibiotics may promote the overgrowth of nonsusceptible organisms. Should superinfection occur during therapy, appropriate measures should be taken.

Drug Interactions

Linezolid Drug Interactions

Precipitant drug	Object drug[a]		Description
Linezolid	Adrenergic agents (eg, dopamine and epinephrine)	↑	Linezolid is a reversible, nonselective inhibitor of monoamine oxidase. Therefore, linezolid has the potential for interaction with adrenergic agents. Reduce and titrate initial doses of adrenergic agents, such as dopamine and epinephrine, to achieve the desired response.
Linezolid	Serotonergic agents (eg, fluoxetine, paroxetine, sertraline)	↑	Linezolid has the potential for interaction with serotonergic agents. Because there is limited experience with administration of linezolid and serotonergic agents, physicians should be alert to the possibility of signs and symptoms of serotonin syndrome (eg, hyperpyrexia, cognitive dysfunction) in patients receiving concomitant therapy.

[a] ↑ = Object drug increased.

➤*Monoamine oxidase inhibition:* Linezolid is a reversible, nonselective inhibitor of monoamine oxidase. Therefore, linezolid has the potential for interaction with adrenergic and serotonergic agents.

Adverse Reactions

➤*Adults:* The safety of linezolid formulations was evaluated in 2,046 patients enrolled in 7 phase 3 comparator-controlled clinical trials, who were treated for up to 28 days. In these studies, 85% of the adverse reactions reported with linezolid were described as mild to moderate in intensity. The table below describes the incidence of adverse reactions reported in at least 2% of patients in these trials. The most common adverse reactions in patients treated with linezolid were diarrhea (incidence across studies, 2.8% to 11%), headache (incidence across studies, 0.5% to 11.3%), and nausea (incidence across studies, 3.4% to 9.6%).

Incidence (%) of Adverse Reactions Reported in ≥ 2% of Patients in Comparator-Controlled Clinical Trials with Linezolid Formulations

Adverse reaction	Linezolid (n = 2,046)	All comparators[a] (n = 2,001)
Diarrhea	8.3%	6.3%
Headache	6.5%	5.5%
Nausea	6.2%	4.6%
Vomiting	3.7%	2%
Insomnia	2.5%	1.7%
Constipation	2.2%	2.1%
Rash	2%	2.2%
Dizziness	2%	1.9%
Fever	1.6%	2.1%

[a] Comparators included cefpodoxime proxetil 200 mg orally every 12 hours; ceftriaxone 1 g IV every 12 hours; clarithromycin 250 mg orally every 12 hours; dicloxacillin 500 mg orally every 6 hours; oxacillin 2 g IV every 6 hours; vancomycin 1 g IV every 12 hours.

Other adverse reactions reported in phase 2 and phase 3 studies included oral moniliasis, vaginal moniliasis, hypertension, dyspepsia, localized abdominal pain, pruritus, and tongue discoloration.

Incidence of Drug-Related Adverse Reactions Occurring in > 1% of Patients Treated with Linezolid in Comparator-Controlled Clinical Trials

	Uncomplicated skin and skin structure infections		All other indications	
	Linezolid 400 mg orally every 12 h	Clarithromycin 250 mg orally every 12 h	Linezolid 600 mg every 12 h	All other comparators[a]
Adverse reactions	(n = 548)	(n = 537)	(n = 1498)	(n = 1464)
% of patients with 1 drug-related adverse reaction	25.4%	19.6%	20.4%	14.3%
% of patients discontinuing due to drug-related adverse reactions[b]	3.5%	2.4%	2.1%	1.7%
Diarrhea	5.3%	4.8%	4%	2.7%
Nausea	3.5%	3.5%	3.3%	1.8%
Headache	2.7%	2.2%	1.9%	1%
Taste alteration	1.8%	2%	0.9%	0.2%
Vaginal moniliasis	1.6%	1.3%	1%	0.4%
Fungal infection	1.5%	0.2%	0.1%	< 0.1%
Abnormal liver function tests	0.4%	0%	1.3%	0.5%
Vomiting	0.9%	0.4%	1.2%	0.4%
Tongue discoloration	1.1%	0%	0.2%	0%
Dizziness	1.1%	1.5%	0.4%	0.3%
Oral moniliasis	0.4%	0%	1.1%	0.4%

[a] Comparators included cefpodoxime proxetil 200 mg orally every 12 hours; ceftriaxone 1 g IV every 12 hours; dicloxacillin 500 mg orally every 6 hours; oxacillin 2 g IV every 6 hours; vancomycin 1 g IV every 12 hours.

[b] The most commonly reported drug-related adverse reactions leading to discontinuation in patients treated with linezolid were nausea, headache, diarrhea and vomiting.

➤*Children:* The safety of linezolid formulations was evaluated in 215 pediatric patients ranging in age from birth through 11 years, and in 248 pediatric patients aged 5 through 17 years (146 of these 248 were age 5 through 11 and 102 were age 12 to 17). These patients were enrolled in 2 phase 3 comparator-controlled clinical trials and were treated for up to 28 days. In these studies, 83% and 99%, respectively, of the adverse events reported with linezolid were described as mild to moderate in intensity. In the study of hospitalized pediatric patients (birth through 11 years) with gram-positive infections, who were randomized 2 to 1 (linezolid:vancomycin), mortality was 6% (13/215) in the linezolid arm and 3% (3/101) in the vancomycin arm. However, given the severe underlying illness in the patient population,

LINEZOLID — ORAL

no causality could be established. The following table shows the incidence of adverse events reported in at least 2% of pediatric patients treated with linezolid in these trials.

Incidence (%) of Adverse Events Reported in ≥ 2% of Pediatric Patients Treated with Linezolid in Comparator-Controlled Clinical Trials

Event	Uncomplicated skin and skin structure infections[a]		All other indications[b]	
	Linezolid (n = 248)	Cefadroxil (n = 251)	Linezolid (n = 215)	Vancomycin (n = 101)
Fever	2.9%	3.6%	14.1%	14.1%
Diarrhea	7.8%	8%	10.8%	12.1%
Vomiting	2.9%	6.4%	9.4%	9.1%
Sepsis	0%	0%	8%	7.1%
Rash	1.6%	1.2%	7%	15.2%
Headache	6.5%	4%	0.9%	0%
Anemia	0%	0%	5.6%	7.1%
Thrombocytopenia	0%	0%	4.7%	2%
Upper respiratory tract infection	3.7%	5.2%	4.2%	1%
Nausea	3.7%	3.2%	1.9%	0%
Dyspnea	0%	0%	3.3%	1%
Reaction at site of injection or of vascular catheter	0%	0%	3.3%	5.1%
Trauma	3.3%	4.8%	2.8%	2%
Pharyngitis	2.9%	1.6%	0.5%	1%
Convulsion	0%	0%	2.8%	2%
Hypokalemia	0%	0%	2.8%	3%
Pneumonia	0%	0%	2.8%	2%
Thrombocythemia	0%	0%	2.8%	2%
Cough	2.4%	4%	0.9%	0%
Generalized abdominal pain	2.4%	2.8%	0.9%	2%
Localized abdominal pain	2.4%	2.8%	0.5%	1%
Apnea	0%	0%	2.3%	2%
GI bleeding	0%	0%	2.3%	1%
Generalized edema	0%	0%	2.3%	1%
Loose stools	1.6%	0.8%	2.3%	3%
Localized pain	2%	1.6%	0.9%	0%
Skin disorder	2%	0%	0.9%	1%

[a] Patients 5 through 11 years of age received linezolid 10 mg/kg by mouth every 12 hours or cefadroxil 15 mg/kg by mouth every 12 hours. Patients 12 years or older received linezolid 600 mg by mouth every 12 hours or cefadroxil 500 mg by mouth every 12 hours.
[b] Patients from birth through 11 years of age received linezolid 10 mg/kg IV/by mouth every 8 hours or vancomycin 10 to 15 mg/kg IV every 6 to 24 hours, depending on age and renal clearance.

Incidence (%) of Drug-Related Adverse Reactions Occurring in > 1% of Pediatric Patients (and > 1 Patient) in Either Treatment Group in Comparator-Controlled Clinical Trials

Event	Uncomplicated skin and skin structure infections[a]		All other indications[b]	
	Linezolid (n = 248)	Cefadroxil (n = 251)	Linezolid (n = 215)	Vancomycin (n = 101)
% of patients with ≥ 1 drug-related adverse reaction	19.2%	14.1%	18.8%	34.3%
% of patients discontinuing due to a drug-related adverse reaction	1.6%	2.4%	0.9%	6.1%
Diarrhea	5.7%	5.2%	3.8%	6.1%
Nausea	3.3%	2%	1.4%	0%
Headache	2.4%	0.8%	0%	0%
Loose stools	1.2%	0.8%	1.9%	0%
Thrombocytopenia	0%	0%	1.9%	0%
Vomiting	1.2%	2.4%	1.9%	1%
Generalized abdominal pain	1.6%	1.2%	0%	0%
Localized abdominal pain	1.6%	1.2%	0%	0%
Anemia	0%	0%	1.4%	1%
Eosinophilia	0.4%	0.4%	1.4%	0%
Rash	0.4%	1.2%	1.4%	7.1%
Vertigo	1.2%	0.4%	0%	0%
Oral moniliasis	0%	0%	0.9%	4%
Fever	0%	0%	0.5%	3%
Pruritus at non-application site	0.4%	0%	0%	2%
Anaphylaxis	0%	0%	0%	10.1%[c]

[a] Patients 5 through 11 years of age received linezolid 10 mg/kg by mouth every 12 hours or cefadroxil 15 mg/kg by mouth every 12 hours. Patients 12 years or older received linezolid 600 mg by mouth every 12 hours or cefadroxil 500 mg by mouth every 12 hours.
[b] Patients from birth through 11 years of age received linezolid 10 mg/kg IV/by mouth every 8 hours or vancomycin 10 to 15 mg/kg IV every 6 to 24 hours, depending on age and renal clearance.
[c] These reports were of "red-man syndrome", which were coded as anaphylaxis.

➤*Thrombocytopenia:* Linezolid has been associated with thrombocytopenia when used in doses up to and including 600 mg every 12 hours for up to 28 days. In phase 3 comparator-controlled trials, the percentage of patients who developed a substantially low platelet count (defined as less than 75% of lower limit of normal or baseline) was 2.4% (range among studies was 0.3% to 10%) with linezolid and 1.5% (range among studies was 0.4% to 7%) with a comparator. In a study of hospitalized pediatric patients ranging in age from birth through 11 years, the percentage of patients who developed a substantially low platelet count (defined as less than 75% of lower limit of normal and/or baseline) was 12.9% with linezolid and 13.4% with vancomycin. In an outpatient study of pediatric patients aged from 5 through 17 years, the percentage of patients who developed a substantially low platelet count was 0% with linezolid and 0.4% with cefadroxil. Thrombocytopenia associated with the use of linezolid appears to be dependent on duration of therapy (generally more than 2 weeks of treatment). The platelet counts for most patients returned to the normal range/baseline during the follow-up period. No related clinical adverse reactions were identified in phase 3 clinical trials in patients developing thrombocytopenia. Bleeding events were identified in thrombocytopenic patients in a compassionate use program for linezolid; the role of linezolid in these events cannot be determined.

➤*Lab test abnormalities:*

Percent of Adult Patients who Experienced at Least 1 Substantially Abnormal[a] Hematology Laboratory Value in Comparator-Controlled Clinical Trials with Linezolid

Laboratory assay	Uncomplicated skin and skin structure infections		All other indications	
	Linezolid 400 mg every 12 h	Clarithromycin 250 mg every 12 h	Linezolid 600 mg every 12 h	All other comparators[b]
Hemoglobin (g/dL)	0.9%	0%	7.1%	6.6%
Platelet count (x 10^3/mm^3)	0.7%	0.8%	3%	1.8%
WBC (x 10^3/mm^3)	0.2%	0.6%	2.2%	1.3%
Neutrophils (x 10^3/mm^3)	0%	0.2%	1.1%	1.2%

[a] Less than 75% (less than 50% for neutrophils) of lower limit of normal (LLN) for values normal at baseline; less than 75% (less than 50% for neutrophils) of LLN and of baseline for values abnormal at baseline.
[b] Comparators included cefpodoxime proxetil 200 mg orally every 12 hours; ceftriaxone 1 g IV every 12 hours; dicloxacillin 500 mg orally every 6 hours; oxacillin 2 g IV every 6 hours; vancomycin 1 g IV every 12 hours.

Percent of Adult Patients who Experienced at Least 1 Substantially Abnormal[a] Serum Chemistry Laboratory Value in Comparator-Controlled Clinical Trials with Linezolid

Laboratory assay	Uncomplicated skin and skin structure infections		All other indications	
	Linezolid 400 mg every 12 h	Clarithromycin 250 mg every 12 h	Linezolid 600 mg every 12 h	All other comparators[b]
AST (U/L)	1.7%	1.3%	5%	6.8%
ALT (U/L)	1.7%	1.7%	9.6%	9.3%
LDH (U/L)	0.2%	0.2%	1.8%	1.5%

LINEZOLID — ORAL

Percent of Adult Patients who Experienced at Least 1 Substantially Abnormal[a] Serum Chemistry Laboratory Value in Comparator-Controlled Clinical Trials with Linezolid				
Laboratory assay	Uncomplicated skin and skin structure infections		All other indications	
	Linezolid 400 mg every 12 h	Clarithromycin 250 mg every 12 h	Linezolid 600 mg every 12 h	All other comparators [b]
Alkaline phosphatase (U/L)	0.2%	0.2%	3.5%	3.1%
Lipase (U/L)	2.8%	2.6%	4.3%	4.2%
Amylase (U/L)	0.2%	0.2%	2.4%	2%
Total bilirubin (mg/dL)	0.2%	0%	0.9%	1.1%
BUN (mg/dL)	0.2%	0%	2.1%	1.5%
Creatinine (mg/dL)	0.2%	0%	0.2%	0.6%

[a] Greater than 2 times the upper limit of normal (ULN) for values normal at baseline; greater than 2 times ULN and greater than 2 times baseline for values abnormal at baseline.
[b] Comparators included cefpodoxime proxetil 200 mg orally every 12 hours; ceftriaxone 1 g IV every 12 hours; dicloxacillin 500 mg orally every 6 hours; oxacillin 2 g IV every 6 hours; vancomycin 1 g IV every 12 hours.

Percent of Pediatric Patients who Experienced at Least 1 Substantially Abnormal[a] Hematology Laboratory Value in Comparator-Controlled Clinical Trials with Linezolid				
Laboratory assay	Uncomplicated skin and skin structure infections[b]		All other indications[c]	
	Linezolid	Cefadroxil	Linezolid	Vancomycin
Hemoglobin (g/dL)	0%	0%	15.7%	12.4%
Platelet count ($\times 10^3/mm^3$)	0%	0.4%	12.9%	13.4%
WBC ($\times 10^3/mm^3$)	0.8%	0.8%	12.4%	10.3%
Neutrophils ($\times 10^3/mm^3$)	1.2%	0.8%	5.9%	4.3%

[a] Less than 75% (less than 50% for neutrophils) of lower limit of normal (LLN) for values normal at baseline; less than 75% (less than 50% for neutrophils) of LLN and less than 75% (less than 50% for neutrophils, less than 90% for hemoglobin if baseline less than LLN) of baseline for values abnormal at baseline.
[b] Patients 5 through 11 years of age received linezolid 10 mg/kg orally every 12 hours or cefadroxil 15 mg/kg orally every 12 hours. Patients 12 years or older received linezolid 600 mg orally every 12 hours or cefadroxil 500 mg orally every 12 hours.
[c] Patients from birth through 11 years of age received linezolid 10 mg/kg IV/orally every 8 hours or vancomycin 10 to 15 mg/kg IV every 6 to 24 hours, depending on age and renal clearance.

Percent of Pediatric Patients who Experienced at Least 1 Substantially Abnormal[a] Serum Chemistry Laboratory Value in Comparator-Controlled Clinical Trials with Linezolid				
Laboratory assay	Uncomplicated skin and skin structure infections[b]		All other indications[c]	
	Linezolid	Cefadroxil	Linezolid	Vancomycin
ALT (U/L)	0%	0%	10.1%	12.5%
Lipase (U/L)	0.4%	1.2%	—	—
Amylase (U/L)	—	—	0.6%	1.3%
Total bilirubin (mg/dL)	—	—	6.3%	5.2%
Creatinine (mg/dL)	0.4%	0%	2.4%	1%

[a] Greater than 2 times upper limit of normal (ULN) for values normal at baseline; greater than 2 times ULN and greater than 2 (greater than 1.5 for total bilirubin) times baseline for values abnormal at baseline.
[b] Patients 5 through 11 years of age received linezolid 10 mg/kg orally every 12 hours or cefadroxil 15 mg/kg orally every 12 hours. Patients 12 years or older received linezolid 600 mg orally every 12 hours or cefadroxil 500 mg orally every 12 hours.
[c] Patients from birth through 11 years of age received linezolid 10 mg/kg IV/orally every 8 hours or vancomycin 10 to 15 mg/kg IV every 6 to 24 hours, depending on age and renal clearance.

➤*Postmarketing:* Myelosuppression (including anemia, leukopenia, pancytopenia and thrombocytopenia) has been reported during postmarketing use of linezolid. Neuropathy (peripheral, optic) has been reported in patients treated with linezolid. Lactic acidosis has been reported with the use of linezolid. Although these reports have primarily been in patients treated for longer than the maximum recommended duration of 28 days, these events have also been reported in patients receiving shorter courses of therapy. These events have been chosen for inclusion due to either their seriousness, frequency of reporting, possible causal connection to linezolid, or a combination of these factors. Because they are reported voluntarily from a population of unknown size, estimates of frequency cannot be made and causal relationship cannot be precisely established.

Overdosage

➤*Symptoms:* Clinical signs of acute toxicity in animals were decreased activity and ataxia in rats and vomiting and tremors in dogs treated with 3,000 mg/kg/day and 2,000 mg/kg/day, respectively.

➤*Treatment:* In the event of overdosage, supportive care is advised, with maintenance of glomerular filtration. Hemodialysis may facilitate more rapid elimination of linezolid. In a phase 1 clinical trial, approximately 30% of a dose of linezolid was removed during a 3-hour hemodialysis session beginning 3 hours after the dose of linezolid was administered. Data are not available for removal of linezolid with peritoneal dialysis or hemoperfusion.

Patient Information

Linezolid may be taken with or without food.

Inform doctor of any history of hypertension.

Large quantities of foods or beverages with high tyramine content should be avoided while taking linezolid. Quantities of tyramine consumed should be less than 100 mg/meal. Foods high in tyramine content include those that may have undergone protein changes by aging, fermentation, pickling, or smoking to improve flavor, such as aged cheeses (0 to 15 mg tyramine/ounce); fermented or air-dried meats (0.1 to 8 mg tyramine/ounce); sauerkraut (8 mg tyramine/8 ounces); soy sauce (5 mg tyramine/1 teaspoon); tap beers (4 mg tyramine/12 ounces); red wines (0 to 6 mg tyramine/8 ounces). The tyramine content of any protein-rich food may be increased if stored for long periods or improperly refrigerated.

Inform doctor if taking medications containing pseudoephedrine hydrochloride or phenylpropanolamine hydrochloride, such as cold remedies and decongestants.

Inform doctor if taking serotonin reuptake inhibitors or other antidepressants.

Phenylketonurics: Each 5 mL of the 100 mg/5 mL linezolid for oral suspension contains 20 mg phenylalanine. The other linezolid formulations do not contain phenylalanine. Contact your doctor or pharmacist.

LINEZOLID — INJECTION

Indications

For the treatment of adult patients with the following infections caused by susceptible strains of the designated microorganisms.

➤*Vancomycin-resistant enterococcal infections:* Vancomycin-resistant *Enterococcus faecium* infections, including cases with concurrent bacteremia.

➤*Nosocomial pneumonia:* Caused by *Staphylococcus aureus* (methicillin-susceptible and -resistant strains), or *Streptococcus pneumoniae* (penicillin-susceptible strains only). Combination therapy may be clinically indicated if the documented or presumptive pathogens include gram-negative organisms.

➤*Complicated skin and skin structure infections:* Caused by *Staphylococcus aureus* (methicillin-susceptible and -resistant strains), *Streptococcus pyogenes*, or *Streptococcus agalactiae*. Linezolid has not been studied in the treatment of diabetic foot and decubitus ulcers. Combination therapy may be clinically indicated if the documented or presumptive pathogens include gram-negative organisms.

➤*Uncomplicated skin and skin structure infections:* Caused by *Staphylococcus aureus* (methicillin-susceptible strains only) or *Streptococcus pyogenes*.

➤*Community-acquired pneumonia:* Caused by *Streptococcus pneumoniae* (penicillin-susceptible strains only), including cases with concurrent bacteremia, or *Staphylococcus aureus* (methicillin-susceptible strains only).

Administration and Dosage

➤*Approved by the FDA:* April 18, 2000.

The recommended dosage for linezolid formulations for the treatment of infections is described below. Doses of linezolid are administered every 12 hours.

LINEZOLID — INJECTION

Dosage Guidelines			
	Dosage and route of administration		
Infection[a]	Pediatric patients[b] (birth through 11 years)	Adults and adolescents (12 years and older)	Recommended duration of treatment (consecutive days)
Complicated skin and skin structure infections	10 mg/kg IV or oral[c] every 8 h	600 mg IV or oral [c] every 12 h	10 to 14 days
Community-acquired pneumonia, including concurrent bacteremia			
Nosocomial pneumonia			
Vancomycin-resistant *Enterococcus faecium* infections, including concurrent bacteremia	10 mg/kg IV or oral[c] every 8 h	600 mg IV or oral[c] every 12 h	14 to 28 days
Uncomplicated skin and skin structure infections	< 5 years: 10 mg/kg oral[c] every 8 h 5 to 11 years: 10 mg/kg oral[c] every 12 h	Adults: 400 mg oral[c] every 12 h Adolescents: 600 mg oral[c] every 12 h	10 to 14 days

[a] Due to the designated pathogens.
[b] Neonates younger than 7 days: Most preterm neonates younger than 7 days of age (gestational age younger than 34 weeks) have lower systemic linezolid clearance values and larger AUC values than many full-term neonates and older infants. These neonates should be initiated with a dosing regimen of 10 mg/kg every 12 hours. Consideration may be given to the use of 10 mg/kg every-8-hour regimen in neonates with a suboptimal clinical response. All neonatal patients should receive 10 mg/kg every 8 hours by 7 days of life.
[c] Oral dosing using either linezolid tablets or linezolid for oral suspension.

➤*Methicillin-resistant staphylococcal infections:* Adult patients with infection due to methicillin-resistant *Staphylococcus aureus* (MRSA) should be treated with linezolid 600 mg every 12 hours.

➤*Duration:* In controlled clinical trials, the protocol-defined duration of treatment for all infections ranged from 7 to 28 days. Total treatment duration was determined by the treating physician based on site and severity of the infection, and on the patient's clinical response.

➤*IV to oral conversion:* No dose adjustment is necessary when switching from IV to oral administration. Patients whose therapy is started with linezolid IV injection may be switched to either linezolid tablets or oral suspension at the discretion of the physician, when clinically indicated.

➤*IV administration:* Linezolid IV injection is supplied in single-use, ready-to-use infusion bags. Parenteral drug products should be inspected visually for particulate matter prior to administration. Check for minute leaks by firmly squeezing the bag. If leaks are detected, discard the solution, as sterility may be impaired.

Linezolid IV injection should be administered by IV infusion over a period of 30 to 120 minutes. Do not use this IV infusion bag in series connections. Additives should not be introduced into this solution. If linezolid IV injection is to be given concomitantly with another drug, each drug should be given separately in accordance with the recommended dosage and route of administration for each product. In particular, physical incompatibilities resulted when linezolid IV injection was combined with the following drugs during simulated Y-site administration: Amphotericin B, chlorpromazine hydrochloride, diazepam, pentamidine isethionate, erythromycin lactobionate, phenytoin sodium, and trimethoprim-sulfamethoxazole. Additionally, chemical incompatibility resulted when linezolid IV injection was combined with ceftriaxone sodium.

If the same IV line is used for sequential infusion of several drugs, the line should be flushed before and after infusion of linezolid IV injection with an infusion solution compatible with linezolid IV injection and with any other drug or drugs administered via the common line (see information following).

➤*Compatible IV solutions:* Five percent (5%) dextrose injection, USP; 0.9% Sodium Chloride Injection, USP; Lactated Ringer's Injection, USP.

Keep the infusion bags in the overwrap until ready to use. Store at room temperature. Protect from freezing. Linezolid IV injection may exhibit a yellow color that can intensify over time without adversely affecting potency.

➤*Storage/Stability:* Store at 25°C (77°F); excursions permitted to 15° to 30°C (59° to 86°F). Protect from light. Keep bottles tightly closed to protect from moisture. It is recommended that the infusion bags be kept in the overwrap until ready to use. Protect infusion bags from freezing.

Actions

➤*Pharmacology:* Linezolid is a synthetic, antibacterial agent of a new class of antibiotics, the oxazolidinones, which has clinical utility in the treatment of infections caused by aerobic gram-positive bacteria. The in vitro spectrum of activity of linezolid also includes certain gram-negative bacteria and anaerobic bacteria. Linezolid inhibits bacterial protein synthesis through a mechanism of action different from that of other antibacterial agents; therefore, cross-resistance between linezolid and other classes of antibiotics is unlikely. Linezolid binds to a site on the bacterial 23S ribosomal RNA of the 50S subunit and prevents the formation of a functional 70S initiation complex, which is an essential component of the bacterial translation process. The results of time-kill studies have shown linezolid to be bacteriostatic against enterococci and staphylococci. For streptococci, linezolid was found to be bactericidal for the majority of strains.

➤*Pharmacokinetics:*

Distribution – Animal and human pharmacokinetic studies have demonstrated that linezolid readily distributes to well-perfused tissues. The plasma protein binding of linezolid is approximately 31% and is concentration-independent. The volume of distribution of linezolid at steady-state averaged 40 to 50 L in healthy adult volunteers.

Metabolism – Linezolid is primarily metabolized by oxidation of the morpholine ring, which results in 2 inactive, ring-opened carboxylic acid metabolites: The aminoethoxyacetic acid metabolite (A), and the hydroxyethyl glycine metabolite (B). Formation of metabolite B is mediated by a nonenzymatic chemical oxidation mechanism in vitro. Linezolid is not an inducer of cytochrome P450 (CYP) in rats, and it has been demonstrated from in vitro studies that linezolid is not detectably metabolized by human cytochrome P450 and it does not inhibit the activities of clinically significant human CYP isoforms (1A2, 2C9, 2C19, 2D6, 2E1, 3A4).

Excretion – Nonrenal clearance accounts for approximately 65% of the total clearance of linezolid. Under steady-state conditions, approximately 30% of the dose appears in the urine as linezolid, 40% as metabolite B, and 10% as metabolite A. The renal clearance of linezolid is low (average 40 mL/min) and suggests net tubular reabsorption. Virtually no linezolid appears in the feces, while approximately 6% of the dose appears in the feces as metabolite B, and 3% as metabolite A.

A small degree of nonlinearity in clearance was observed with increasing doses of linezolid, which appears to be due to lower renal and nonrenal clearance of linezolid at higher concentrations. However, the difference in clearance was small and was not reflected in the apparent elimination half-life.

Special populations –

Renal function impairment: The pharmacokinetics of the parent drug, linezolid, are not altered in patients with any degree of renal insufficiency; however, the 2 primary metabolites of linezolid may accumulate in patients with renal insufficiency, with the amount of accumulation increasing with the severity of renal dysfunction (see information following). The clinical significance of accumulation of these 2 metabolites has not been determined in patients with severe renal insufficiency. Because similar plasma concentrations of linezolid are achieved regardless of renal function, no dose adjustment is recommended for patients with renal insufficiency. However, given the absence of information on the clinical significance of accumulation of the primary metabolites, use of linezolid in patients with renal insufficiency should be weighed against the potential risks of accumulation of these metabolites. Both linezolid and the 2 metabolites are eliminated by dialysis. No information is available on the effect of peritoneal dialysis on the pharmacokinetics of linezolid. Approximately 30% of a dose was eliminated in a 3-hour dialysis session beginning 3 hours after the dose of linezolid was administered; therefore, linezolid should be given after hemodialysis.

Hepatic function impairment: The pharmacokinetics of linezolid are not altered in patients (n = 7) with mild-to-moderate hepatic insufficiency (Child-Pugh class A or B). On the basis of the available information, no dose adjustment is recommended for patients with mild-to-moderate hepatic insufficiency. The pharmacokinetics of linezolid in patients with severe hepatic insufficiency have not been evaluated.

Children: The C_{max} and the volume of distribution (V_{ss}) of linezolid are similar regardless of age in pediatric patients. However, clearance of linezolid varies as a function of age. With the exclusion of preterm neonates less than 1 week of age, clearance is most rapid in the youngest age groups ranging from older than 1 week old to 11 years of age, resulting in lower single-dose systemic exposure (AUC) and shorter half-life as compared with adults. As age of pediatric patients increases, the clearance of linezolid gradually decreases, and by adolescence mean clearance values approach those observed for the adult population. There is wider intersubject variability in linezolid clearance and systemic drug exposure (AUC) across all pediatric age groups as compared with adults.

Similar mean daily AUC values were observed in pediatric patients from birth to 11 years of age dosed every 8 hours relative to adolescents or adults dosed every 12 hours. Therefore, the dosage for pediatric patients up to 11 years of age should be 10 mg/kg every 8 hours. Pediatric patients 12 years and older should receive 600 mg every 12 hours.

➤*Microbiology:* In clinical trials, resistance to linezolid developed in 6 patients infected with *E. faecium* (4 patients received 200 mg every 12 hours, lower than the recommended dose, and 2 patients received 600 mg every 12 hours). In a compassionate-use program, resistance to linezolid developed in 8 patients with *E. faecium* and in 1 patient with *E. faecalis*. All patients had either unremoved prosthetic devices or undrained abscesses. Resistance to linezolid occurs in vitro at a frequency of 1×10^{-9} to 1×10^{-11}. In vitro studies have shown that point mutations in the 23S rRNA are associated with linezolid resistance.

Reports of vancomycin-resistant *E. faecium* becoming resistant to linezolid during its clinical use have been published. In 1 report, nosocomial spread of vancomycin- and linezolid-resistant *E. faecium* occurred. There has been a

LINEZOLID — INJECTION

report of *Staphylococcus aureus* (methicillin-resistant) developing resistance to linezolid during its clinical use. The linezolid resistance in these organisms was associated with a point mutation in the 23S rRNA (substitution of thymine for guanine at position 2576) of the organism. When antibiotic-resistant organisms are encountered in the hospital, it is important to emphasize infection control policies. Resistance to linezolid has not been reported in *Streptococcus* spp., including *Streptococcus pneumoniae*.

In vitro studies have demonstrated additivity or indifference between linezolid and vancomycin, gentamicin, rifampin, imipenem-cilastatin, aztreonam, ampicillin, or streptomycin.

Linezolid has been shown to be active against most isolates of the following microorganisms, both in vitro and in clinical infections.

Aerobic and facultative gram-positive microorganisms – *Enterococcus faecium* (vancomycin-resistant strains only); *Staphylococcus aureus* (including methicillin-resistant strains); *Streptococcus agalactiae*; *Streptococcus pneumoniae* (penicillin-susceptible strains only); *Streptococcus pyogenes*.

Contraindications

Hypersensitivity to linezolid or any of the other product components.

Warnings

➤*Myelosuppression:* Myelosuppression (including anemia, leukopenia, pancytopenia, and thrombocytopenia) has been reported in patients receiving linezolid. In cases where the outcome is known, when linezolid was discontinued, the affected hematologic parameters have risen toward pretreatment levels. Complete blood counts should be monitored weekly in patients who receive linezolid, particularly in those who receive linezolid for longer than 2 weeks, those with preexisting myelosuppression, those receiving concomitant drugs that produce bone marrow suppression, or those with a chronic infection who have received previous or concomitant antibiotic therapy. Discontinuation of therapy with linezolid should be considered in patients who develop or have worsening myelosuppression.

➤*Pseudomembranous colitis:* Pseudomembranous colitis has been reported with nearly all antibacterial agents, including linezolid, and may range in severity from mild to life-threatening. Therefore, it is important to consider this diagnosis in patients who present with diarrhea subsequent to the administration of any antibacterial agent.

Treatment with antibacterial agents alters the normal flora of the colon and may permit overgrowth of clostridia. Studies indicated that a toxin produced by *Clostridium difficile* is a primary cause of "antibiotic-associated colitis."

After the diagnosis of pseudomembranous colitis has been established, appropriate therapeutic measures should be initiated. Mild cases of pseudomembranous colitis usually respond to drug discontinuation alone. In moderate-to-severe cases, consideration should be given to management with fluids and electrolytes, protein supplementation, and treatment with an antibacterial agent clinically effective against *Clostridium difficile*.

➤*Fertility impairment:* Linezolid did not affect the fertility or reproductive performance of adult female rats. It reversibly decreased fertility and reproductive performance in adult male rats when given at doses greater than or equal to 50 mg/kg/day, with exposures approximately equal to or greater than the expected human exposure level (exposure comparisons are based on AUCs). The reversible fertility effects were mediated through altered spermatogenesis. Affected spermatids contained abnormally formed and oriented mitochondria and were nonviable. Epithelial cell hypertrophy and hyperplasia in the epididymis was observed in conjunction with decreased fertility. Similar epididymal changes were not seen in dogs.

In sexually mature male rats exposed to drug as juveniles, mildly decreased fertility was observed following treatment with linezolid through most of their period of sexual development (50 mg/kg/day from days 7 to 36 of age, and 100 mg/kg/day from days 37 to 55 of age), with exposures up to 1.7-fold greater than mean AUCs observed in pediatric patients aged 3 months to 11 years. Decreased fertility was not observed with shorter treatment periods, corresponding to exposure in utero through the early neonatal period (gestation day 6 through postnatal day 5), neonatal exposure (postnatal days 5 to 21), or to juvenile exposure (postnatal days 22 to 35). Reversible reductions in sperm motility and altered sperm morphology were observed in rats treated from postnatal day 22 to 35.

➤*Pregnancy: Category C.*

Teratogenic – Linezolid was not teratogenic in mice or rats at exposure levels 6.5-fold (in mice) or equivalent to (in rats) the expected human exposure level, based on AUCs. However, embryo and fetal toxicities were seen (see information following). There are no adequate and well-controlled studies in pregnant women. Linezolid should be used during pregnancy only if the potential benefit justifies the potential risk to the fetus.

Nonteratogenic – In mice, embryo and fetal toxicities were seen only at doses that caused maternal toxicity (clinical signs and reduced body weight gain). A dose of 450 mg/kg/day (6.5-fold the estimated human exposure level based on AUCs) correlated with increased postimplantational embryo death, including total litter loss, decreased fetal body weights, and an increased incidence of costal cartilage fusion.

In rats, mild fetal toxicity was observed at 15 and 50 mg/kg/day (exposure levels 0.22-fold to approximately equivalent to the estimated human exposure, respectively, based on AUCs). The effects consisted of decreased fetal body weights and reduced ossification of sternebrae, a finding often seen in association with decreased fetal body weights. Slight maternal toxicity, in the form of reduced body weight gain, was seen at 50 mg/kg/day.

When female rats were treated with 50 mg/kg/day (approximately equivalent to the estimated human exposure based on AUCs) of linezolid during pregnancy and lactation, survival of pups was decreased on postnatal days 1 to 4. Male and female pups permitted to mature to reproductive age, when mated, showed an increase in preimplantation loss, with a corresponding decrease in fertility.

➤*Lactation:* Linezolid and its metabolites are excreted in the milk of lactating rats. Concentrations in milk were similar to those in maternal plasma. It is not known whether linezolid is excreted in human milk. Because many drugs are excreted in human milk, caution should be exercised when linezolid is administered to a nursing woman.

➤*Children:* The safety and efficacy of linezolid for the treatment of pediatric patients ranging in age from birth through 11 years has been established.

See Actions for more information.

Recommendations for the dosage regimen for preterm neonates less than 7 days of age (gestational age less than 34 weeks) are based on pharmacokinetic data from 9 preterm neonates. Most of these preterm neonates have lower systemic linezolid clearance values and larger AUC values than many full-term neonates and older infants. Therefore, these preterm neonates should be initiated with a dosing regimen of 10 mg/kg every 12 hours. Consideration may be given to the use of a 10 mg/kg every-8-hour regimen in neonates with a suboptimal clinical response. All neonatal patients should receive 10 mg/kg every 8 hours by 7 days of life.

In limited clinical experience, 5 out of 6 (83%) pediatric patients with infections due to gram-positive pathogens with MICs of 4 mcg/mL treated with linezolid had clinical cures. However, pediatric patients exhibit wider variability in linezolid clearance and systemic exposure (AUC) compared with adults. In pediatric patients with a suboptimal clinical response, particularly those with pathogens with MIC of 4 mcg/mL, lower systemic exposure, site and severity of infection, and the underlying medical condition should be considered when assessing clinical response.

Precautions

➤*Monitoring:* Complete blood counts should be monitored weekly in patients who receive linezolid, particularly in those who receive linezolid for longer than 2 weeks, those with preexisting myelosuppression, those receiving concomitant drugs that produce bone marrow suppression, or those with a chronic infection who have received previous or concomitant antibiotic therapy. Discontinuation of therapy with linezolid should be considered in patients who develop or have worsening myelosuppression.

Thrombocytopenia – Thrombocytopenia has been reported in patients receiving linezolid. Platelet counts should be monitored in patients who are at increased risk for bleeding, who have preexisting thrombocytopenia, who receive concomitant medications that may decrease platelet count or function, or who may require longer than 2 weeks of linezolid therapy.

➤*Lactic acidosis:* Lactic acidosis has been reported with the use of linezolid. In reported cases, patients experienced repeated episodes of nausea and vomiting. Patients who develop recurrent nausea or vomiting, unexplained acidosis, or a low bicarbonate level while receiving linezolid should receive immediate medical evaluation.

➤*Duration of therapy:* The safety and efficacy of linezolid formulations given for longer than 28 days have not been evaluated in controlled clinical trials.

➤*Resistance:* Prescribing linezolid in the absence of a proven or strongly suspected bacterial infection or a prophylactic indication is unlikely to provide benefit to the patient and increases the risk of the development of drug-resistant bacteria.

➤*Superinfection:* The use of antibiotics may promote the overgrowth of nonsusceptible organisms. Should superinfection occur during therapy, appropriate measures should be taken.

Drug Interactions

Linezolid Drug Interactions

Precipitant drug	Object drug[a]		Description
Linezolid	Adrenergic agents (eg, dopamine, epinephrine)	↑	Linezolid is a reversible, nonselective inhibitor of monoamine oxidase. Therefore, linezolid has the potential for interaction with adrenergic agents. Reduce and titrate initial doses of adrenergic agents, such as dopamine and epinephrine, to achieve the desired response.
Linezolid	Serotonergic agents (eg, fluoxetine, paroxetine, sertraline)	↑	Linezolid has the potential for interaction with serotonergic agents. Because there is limited experience with administration of linezolid and serotonergic agents, physicians should be alert to the possibility of signs and symptoms of serotonin syndrome (eg, hyperpyrexia, cognitive dysfunction) in patients receiving concomitant therapy.

[a] ↑ = Object drug increased.

➤*Monoamine oxidase inhibition:* Linezolid is a reversible, nonselective inhibitor of monoamine oxidase. Therefore, linezolid has the potential for interaction with adrenergic and serotonergic agents.

LINEZOLID — INJECTION

Adverse Reactions

The safety of linezolid formulations was evaluated in 2,046 patients enrolled in 7 phase 3 comparator-controlled, clinical trials, who were treated for up to 28 days. In these studies, 85% of the adverse reactions reported with linezolid were described as mild to moderate in intensity. The table below shows the incidence of adverse reactions reported in at least 2% of patients in these trials. The most common adverse reactions in patients treated with linezolid were diarrhea (incidence across studies is 2.8% to 11%), headache (incidence across studies is 0.5% to 11.3%), and nausea (incidence across studies is 3.4% to 9.6%).

Incidence (%) of Adverse Reactions Reported in ≥ 2% of Patients in Comparator-Controlled Clinical Trials with Linezolid

Reaction	Linezolid (n = 2,046)	All comparators[a] (n = 2,001)
Diarrhea	8.3%	6.3%
Headache	6.5%	5.5%
Nausea	6.2%	4.6%
Vomiting	3.7%	2%
Insomnia	2.5%	1.7%
Constipation	2.2%	2.1%
Rash	2%	2.2%
Dizziness	2%	1.9%
Fever	1.6%	2.1%

[a] Comparators included cefpodoxime proxetil 200 mg orally every 12 hours; ceftriaxone 1 g IV every 12 hours; clarithromycin 250 mg orally every 12 hours; dicloxacillin 500 mg orally every 6 hours; oxacillin 2 g IV every 6 hours; vancomycin 1 g IV every 12 hours.

Other adverse reactions reported in phase 2 and phase 3 studies included oral moniliasis, vaginal moniliasis, hypertension, dyspepsia, localized abdominal pain, pruritus, and tongue discoloration.

Incidence of Drug-Related Adverse Reactions Occurring in > 1% of Patients Treated with Linezolid in Comparator-Controlled Clinical Trials

Adverse reactions	Uncomplicated skin and skin structure infections		All other indications	
	Linezolid 400 mg orally every 12 h (n = 548)	Clarithromycin 250 mg orally every 12 h (n = 537)	Linezolid 600 mg every 12 h (n = 1,498)	All other comparators[a] (n = 1,464)
% of patients with 1 drug-related adverse reaction	25.4%	19.6%	20.4%	14.3%
% of patients discontinuing due to drug-related adverse reactions[b]	3.5%	2.4%	2.1%	1.7%
Diarrhea	5.3%	4.8%	4%	2.7%
Nausea	3.5%	3.5%	3.3%	1.8%
Headache	2.7%	2.2%	1.9%	1%
Taste alteration	1.8%	2%	0.9%	0.2%
Vaginal moniliasis	1.6%	1.3%	1%	0.4%
Fungal infection	1.5%	0.2%	0.1%	< 0.1%
Abnormal liver function tests	0.4%	0%	1.3%	0.5%
Vomiting	0.9%	0.4%	1.2%	0.4%
Tongue discoloration	1.1%	0%	0.2%	0%
Dizziness	1.1%	1.5%	0.4%	0.3%
Oral moniliasis	0.4%	0%	1.1%	0.4%

[a] Comparators included cefpodoxime proxetil 200 mg orally every 12 hours; ceftriaxone 1 g IV every 12 hours; dicloxacillin 500 mg orally every 6 hours; oxacillin 2 g IV every 6 hours; vancomycin 1 g IV every 12 hours.

[b] The most commonly reported drug-related adverse reactions leading to discontinuation in patients treated with linezolid were nausea, headache, diarrhea, and vomiting.

➤*Children:* The safety of linezolid formulations was evaluated in 215 pediatric patients ranging in age from birth through 11 years, and in 248 pediatric patients aged 5 through 17 years (146 of these 248 were age 5 through 11 and 102 were age 12 to 17). These patients were enrolled in 2 phase 3 comparator-controlled clinical trials and were treated for up to 28 days. In these studies, 83% and 99%, respectively, of the adverse events reported with linezolid were described as mild to moderate in intensity. In the study of hospitalized pediatric patients (birth through 11 years) with gram-positive infections, who were randomized 2 to 1 (linezolid:vancomycin), mortality was 6% (13/215) in the linezolid arm and 3% (3/101) in the vancomycin arm. However, given the severe underlying illness in the patient population, no causality could be established.

Incidence (%) of Adverse Reactions Reported in ≥ 2% of Pediatric Patients Treated with Linezolid in Comparator-Controlled Clinical Trials

Reaction	Uncomplicated skin and skin structure infections[a]		All other indications[b]	
	Linezolid (n = 248)	Cefadroxil (n = 251)	Linezolid (n = 215)	Vancomycin (n = 101)
Fever	2.9%	3.6%	14.1%	14.1%
Diarrhea	7.8%	8%	10.8%	12.1%
Vomiting	2.9%	6.4%	9.4%	9.1%
Sepsis	0%	0%	8%	7.1%
Rash	1.6%	1.2%	7%	15.2%
Headache	6.5%	4%	0.9%	0%
Anemia	0%	0%	5.6%	7.1%
Thrombocytopenia	0%	0%	4.7%	2%
Upper respiratory tract infection	3.7%	5.2%	4.2%	1%
Nausea	3.7%	3.2%	1.9%	0%
Dyspnea	0%	0%	3.3%	1%
Reaction at site of injection or of vascular catheter	0%	0%	3.3%	5.1%
Trauma	3.3%	4.8%	2.8%	2%
Pharyngitis	2.9%	1.6%	0.5%	1%
Convulsion	0%	0%	2.8%	2%
Hypokalemia	0%	0%	2.8%	3%
Pneumonia	0%	0%	2.8%	2%
Thrombocythemia	0%	0%	2.8%	2%
Cough	2.4%	4%	0.9%	0%
Generalized abdominal pain	2.4%	2.8%	0.9%	2%
Localized abdominal pain	2.4%	2.8%	0.9%	2%
Apnea	0%	0%	2.3%	2%
GI bleeding	0%	0%	2.3%	1%
Generalized edema	0%	0%	2.3%	1%
Loose stools	1.6%	0.8%	2.3%	3%
Localized pain	2%	1.6%	0.9%	0%
Skin disorder	2%	0%	0.9%	1%

[a] Patients 5 through 11 years of age received linezolid 10 mg/kg orally every 12 hours or cefadroxil 15 mg/kg orally every 12 hours. Patients 12 years of age or older received linezolid 600 mg orally every 12 hours or cefadroxil 500 mg orally every 12 hours.

[b] Patients from birth through 11 years of age received linezolid 10 mg/kg IV/orally every 8 hours or vancomycin 10 to 15 mg/kg IV every 6 to 24 hours, depending on age and renal clearance.

Incidence (%) of drug-related adverse reactions occurring in more than 1% of pediatric patients (and more than 1 patient) in either treatment group in comparator-controlled clinical trials

Reaction	Uncomplicated skin and skin structure infections[a]		All other indications[b]	
	Linezolid (n = 248)	Cefadroxil (n = 251)	Linezolid (n = 215)	Vancomycin (n = 101)
% of patients with ≥ 1 drug-related adverse reaction	19.2%	14.1%	18.8%	34.3%
% of patients discontinuing due to a drug-related adverse reaction	1.6%	2.4%	0.9%	6.1%
Diarrhea	5.7%	5.2%	3.8%	6.1%
Nausea	3.3%	2%	1.4%	0%
Headache	2.4%	0.8%	0%	0%
Loose stools	1.2%	0.8%	1.9%	0%
Thrombocytopenia	0%	0%	1.9%	0%
Vomiting	1.2%	2.4%	1.9%	1%
Generalized abdominal pain	1.6%	1.2%	0%	0%
Localized abdominal pain	1.6%	1.2%	0%	0%
Anemia	0%	0%	1.4%	1%
Eosinophilia	0.4%	0.4%	1.4%	0%
Rash	0.4%	1.2%	1.4%	7.1%

LINEZOLID — INJECTION

Incidence (%) of drug-related adverse reactions occurring in more than 1% of pediatric patients (and more than 1 patient) in either treatment group in comparator-controlled clinical trials

Reaction	Uncomplicated skin and skin structure infections[a]		All other indications[b]	
	Linezolid (n = 248)	Cefadroxil (n = 251)	Linezolid (n = 215)	Vancomycin (n = 101)
Vertigo	1.2%	0.4%	0%	0%
Oral moniliasis	0%	0%	0.9%	4%
Fever	0%	0%	0.5%	3%
Pruritus at non-application site	0.4%	0%	0%	2%
Anaphylaxis	0%	0%	0%	10.1%[c]

[a] Patients 5 through 11 years of age received linezolid 10 mg/kg orally every 12 hours or cefadroxil 15 mg/kg orally every 12 hours. Patients 12 years or older received linezolid 600 mg orally every 12 hours or cefadroxil 500 mg orally every 12 hours.
[b] Patients from birth through 11 years of age received linezolid 10 mg/kg IV/orally every 8 hours or vancomycin 10 to 15 mg/kg IV every 6 to 24 hours, depending on age and renal clearance.
[c] These reports were of "red-man syndrome," which were coded as anaphylaxis.

➤*Thrombocytopenia:* Linezolid has been associated with thrombocytopenia when used in doses up to and including 600 mg every 12 hours for up to 28 days. In phase 3 comparator-controlled trials, the percentage of patients who developed a substantially low platelet count (defined as less than 75% of lower limit of normal or baseline) was 2.4% (range among studies: 0.3% to 10%) with linezolid and 1.5% (range among studies: 0.4% to 7%) with a comparator. In a study of hospitalized pediatric patients ranging in age from birth through 11 years, the percentage of patients who developed a substantially low platelet count (defined as less than 75% of lower limit of normal or baseline) was 12.9% with linezolid and 13.4% with vancomycin. In an outpatient study of pediatric patients aged from 5 through 17 years of age, the percentage of patients who developed a substantially low platelet count was 0% with linezolid and 0.4% with cefadroxil. Thrombocytopenia associated with the use of linezolid appears to be dependent on duration of therapy, (generally greater than 2 weeks of treatment). The platelet counts for most patients returned to the normal range/baseline during the follow-up period. No related clinical adverse reactions were identified in phase 3 clinical trials in patients developing thrombocytopenia. Bleeding events were identified in thrombocytopenic patients in a compassionate use program for linezolid; the role of linezolid in these events cannot be determined.

➤*Lab test abnormalities:* Changes seen in other laboratory parameters, without regard to drug relationship, revealed no substantial differences between linezolid and the comparators. These changes were generally not clinically significant, did not lead to discontinuation of therapy, and were reversible.

Percent of Adult Patients who Experienced at Least 1 Substantially Abnormal[a] Hematology Laboratory Value in Comparator-Controlled Clinical Trials with Linezolid

Laboratory assay	Uncomplicated skin and skin structure infections		All other indications	
	Linezolid 400 mg every 12 h	Clarithromycin 250 mg every 12 h	Linezolid 600 mg every 12 h	All other comparators [b]
Hemoglobin (g/dL)	0.9%	0%	7.1%	6.6%
Platelet count (x 10^3/mm^3)	0.7%	0.8%	3%	1.8%
WBC (x 10^3/mm^3)	0.2%	0.6%	2.2%	1.3%
Neutrophils (x 10^3/mm^3)	0%	0.2%	1.1%	1.2%

[a] Less than 75% (less than 50% for neutrophils) of lower limit of normal (LLN) for values normal at baseline; less than 75% (less than 50% for neutrophils) of LLN and of baseline for values abnormal at baseline.
[b] Comparators included cefpodoxime proxetil 200 mg orally every 12 hours; ceftriaxone 1 g IV every 12 hours; dicloxacillin 500 mg orally every 6 hours; oxacillin 2 g IV every 6 hours; vancomycin 1 g IV every 12 hours.

Percent of Adult Patients who Experienced at Least 1 Substantially Abnormal[a] Serum Chemistry Laboratory Value in Comparator-Controlled Clinical Trials with Linezolid

Laboratory assay	Uncomplicated skin and skin structure infections		All other indications	
	Linezolid 400 mg every 12 h	Clarithromycin 250 mg every 12 h	Linezolid 600 mg every 12 h	All other comparators[b]
AST (U/L)	1.7%	1.3%	5%	6.8%
ALT (U/L)	1.7%	1.7%	9.6%	9.3%
LDH (U/L)	0.2%	0.2%	1.8%	1.5%
Alkaline phosphatase (U/L)	0.2%	0.2%	3.5%	3.1%
Lipase (U/L)	2.8%	2.6%	4.3%	4.2%
Amylase (U/L)	0.2%	0.2%	2.4%	2%
Total bilirubin (mg/dL)	0.2%	0%	0.9%	1.1%
Blood urea nitrogen (BUN) (mg/dL)	0.2%	0%	2.1%	1.5%
Creatinine (mg/dL)	0.2%	0%	0.2%	0.6%

[a] Greater than 2 x upper limit of normal (ULN) for values normal at baseline; greater than 2 x ULN and greater than 2 x baseline for values abnormal at baseline.
[b] Comparators included cefpodoxime proxetil 200 mg orally every 12 hours; ceftriaxone 1 g IV every 12 hours; dicloxacillin 500 mg orally every 6 hours; oxacillin 2 g IV every 6 hours; vancomycin 1 g IV every 12 hours.

Percent of Pediatric Patients who Experienced at Least 1 Substantially Abnormal[a] Hematology Laboratory Value in Comparator-Controlled Clinical Trials with Linezolid

Laboratory assay	Uncomplicated skin and skin structure infections[b]		All other indications[c]	
	Linezolid	Cefadroxil	Linezolid	Vancomycin
Hemoglobin (g/dL)	0%	0%	15.7%	12.4%
Platelet count (× 10^3/mm^3)	0%	0.4%	12.9%	13.4%
WBC (× 10^3/mm^3)	0.8%	0.8%	12.4%	10.3%
Neutrophils (× 10^3/mm^3)	1.2%	0.8%	5.9%	4.3%

[a] Less than 75% (less than 50% for neutrophils) of lower limit of normal (LLN) for values normal at baseline; less than 75% (less than 50% for neutrophils) of LLN and less than 75% (less than 50% for neutrophils, less than 90% for hemoglobin if baseline less than LLN) of baseline for values abnormal at baseline.
[b] Patients 5 through 11 years of age received linezolid 10 mg/kg orally every 12 hours or cefadroxil 15 mg/kg orally every 12 hours. Patients 12 years or older received linezolid 600 mg orally every 12 hours or cefadroxil 500 mg orally every 12 hours.
[c] Patients from birth through 11 years of age received linezolid 10 mg/kg IV/orally every 8 hours or vancomycin 10 to 15 mg/kg IV every 6 to 24 hours, depending on age and renal clearance.

Percent of Pediatric Patients who Experienced at Least 1 Substantially Abnormal[a] Serum Chemistry Laboratory Value in Comparator-Controlled Clinical Trials with Linezolid

Laboratory assay	Uncomplicated skin and skin structure infections[b]		All other indications[c]	
	Linezolid	Cefadroxil	Linezolid	Vancomycin
ALT (U/L)	0%	0%	10.1%	12.5%
Lipase (U/L)	0.4%	1.2%		
Amylase (U/L)			0.6%	1.3%
Total bilirubin (mg/dL)			6.3%	5.2%
Creatinine (mg/dL)	0.4%	0%	2.4%	1%

[a] Greater than 2 times the upper limit of normal (ULN) for values normal at baseline; greater than 2 times ULN and greater than 2 (greater than 1.5 for total bilirubin) times baseline for values abnormal at baseline.
[b] Patients 5 through 11 years of age received linezolid 10 mg/kg orally every 12 hours or cefadroxil 15 mg/kg orally every 12 hours. Patients 12 years or older received linezolid 600 mg orally every 12 hours or cefadroxil 500 mg orally every 12 hours.
[c] Patients from birth through 11 years of age received linezolid 10 mg/kg IV/orally every 8 hours or vancomycin 10 to 15 mg/kg IV every 6 to 24 hours, depending on age and renal clearance.

➤*Postmarketing:* Myelosuppression (including anemia, leukopenia, pancytopenia, and thrombocytopenia) has been reported during postmarketing use of linezolid. Neuropathy (peripheral, optic) has been reported in patients treated with linezolid. Lactic acidosis has been reported with the use of linezolid. Although these reports have primarily been in patients treated for longer than the maximum recommended duration of 28 days, these events have also been reported in patients receiving shorter courses of therapy. These reactions have been chosen for inclusion due to either their seriousness, frequency of reporting, possible causal connection to linezolid, or a combination of these factors. Because they are reported voluntarily from a population of unknown size, estimates of frequency cannot be made and causal relationship cannot be precisely established.

Overdosage

➤*Symptoms:* Clinical signs of acute toxicity in animals were decreased activity and ataxia in rats and vomiting and tremors in dogs treated with 3,000 mg/kg/day and 2,000 mg/kg/day, respectively.

LINEZOLID — INJECTION

➤*Treatment:* In the event of overdosage, supportive care is advised, with maintenance of glomerular filtration. Hemodialysis may facilitate more rapid elimination of linezolid. In a phase 1 clinical trial, approximately 30% of a dose of linezolid was removed during a 3-hour hemodialysis session beginning 3 hours after the dose of linezolid was administered. Data are not available for removal of linezolid with peritoneal dialysis or hemoperfusion.

Patient Information

Linezolid may be taken with or without food.

Inform your doctor of any history of hypertension.

Large quantities of foods or beverages with high tyramine content should be avoided while taking linezolid. Quantities of tyramine consumed should be less than 100 mg/meal. Foods high in tyramine content include those that may have undergone protein changes by aging, fermentation, pickling, or smoking to improve flavor, such as aged cheeses (0 to 15 mg tyramine/ounce); fermented or air-dried meats (0.1 to 8 mg tyramine/ounce); sauerkraut (8 mg tyramine/8 ounces); soy sauce (5 mg tyramine/teaspoon); tap beers (4 mg tyramine/12 ounces); red wines (0 to 6 mg tyramine/8 ounces). The tyramine content of any protein-rich food may be increased if stored for long periods or improperly refrigerated.

Inform doctor if taking medications containing pseudoephedrine hydrochloride or phenylpropanolamine hydrochloride, such as cold remedies and decongestants.

Inform doctor if taking serotonin reuptake inhibitors or other antidepressants.

Phenylketonurics: Each 5 mL of the 100 mg/5 mL linezolid for oral suspension contains 20 mg phenylalanine. The other linezolid formulations do not contain phenylalanine. Contact your doctor or pharmacist.

Patients should be counseled that antibacterial drugs, including linezolid, should only be used to treat bacterial infections. They do not treat viral infections (eg, the common cold). When linezolid is prescribed to treat a bacterial infection, patients should be told that although it is common to feel better early in the course of therapy, the medication should be taken exactly as directed. Skipping doses or not completing the full course of therapy may decrease the effectiveness of the immediate treatment and increase the likelihood that bacteria will develop resistance and will not be treatable by linezolid or other antibacterial drugs in the future.

LINCOSAMIDES

WARNING

These agents can cause severe and possibly fatal colitis, characterized by severe persistent diarrhea, severe abdominal cramps, and possibly the passage of blood and mucus. Endoscopic examination may reveal pseudomembranous colitis. Toxin(s) produced by *Clostridia* is a primary cause of antibiotic-associated colitis.

When significant diarrhea occurs, discontinue the drug or, if necessary, continue only with close observation of the patient. Large bowel endoscopy is recommended.

Mild colitis may respond to stopping drug. Promptly manage moderate-to-severe cases with fluid, electrolyte, and protein supplements as indicated. Systemic corticosteroids and corticosteroid retention enemas may help relieve the colitis. Also consider other causes such as previous sensitivities to drugs or other allergens.

Antiperistaltic agents such as opiates and diphenoxylate with atropine may prolong or aggravate the condition. Diarrhea, colitis, and pseudomembranous colitis can begin up to several weeks following cessation of therapy.

Vancomycin is effective in antibiotic-associated pseudomembranous colitis produced by *C. difficile*. (See individual monograph for complete information.)

Reserve for serious infections where less toxic antimicrobial agents are inappropriate (see Indications). Do not use in patients with nonbacterial infections (ie, most upper respiratory tract infections).

Indications

➤*Serious infections:* Treatment of serious infections due to susceptible strains of streptococci, pneumococci, and staphylococci. Reserve use for penicillin-allergic patients or when penicillin is inappropriate. Because of the risk of colitis (see Warning Box), consider the nature of the infection and the suitability of less toxic alternatives (eg, erythromycin).

For specific indications, refer to individual monographs.

Actions

➤*Pharmacology:* **Lincomycin** and **clindamycin** (7-deoxy, 7-chloro derivative of lincomycin), known collectively as lincosamides, bind exclusively to the 50S subunit of bacterial ribosomes and suppress protein synthesis. Cross-resistance has been demonstrated between these two agents. Clindamycin is preferred because it is better absorbed and more potent.

➤*Pharmacokinetics:* Administration with food markedly impairs **lincomycin** (but not **clindamycin**) oral absorption. Both agents achieve significant tissue penetration; lincomycin may reach cerebrospinal fluid (CSF) concentration 40% of serum levels with inflamed meninges, but neither crosses well if meninges are normal.

Lincomycin – Levels above the MIC for most gram-positive organisms are maintained with oral doses of 500 mg for 6 to 8 hours and for 14 hours after a 600 mg IV infusion. Following a 600 mg IM dose, detectable levels persist for 24 hours.

Clindamycin – Serum levels exceed MIC for most indicated organisms at least 6 hours after recommended doses. Maintain levels above in vitro MIC for most indicated organisms by giving clindamycin phosphate every 8 to 12 hours to adults, every 6 to 8 hours to children, or by continuous IV infusion. Equilibrium is reached by dose 3.

Select Pharmacokinetic Parameters of Lincosamides

Lincosamides	Bioavailability (%)	Mean peak serum level (mcg/mL)	Time to peak serum level (hours)	Protein binding (%)	Half-life (hours)	Elimination (%) Hepatic	Elimination (%) Unchanged in urine (range)	Elimination (%) Feces
Clindamycin[a]								
Oral	90	2.5	0.75					
IM		6 to 9	1 to 3	≈ 90	2.4 to 3[c]	> 90	10	3.6
IV		7 to 14	0[b]					
Lincomycin								
Oral	20 to 30	1.8 to 5.3	2 to 4				4 (1 to 31)	
IM		9.3 to 18.5	0.5	57-72	4.4 to 6.4	> 90	17.3 (2 to 25)	40
IV		15.9 to 20.9	0				13.8 (5 to 30)	

[a] Clindamycin palmitate and phosphate are rapidly hydrolyzed to the base.
[b] By end of infusion, peak levels are reached.
[c] Increased slightly in patients with markedly reduced renal or hepatic function.

➤*Microbiology:*

Organisms Generally Susceptible to Lincosamides

✔ = generally susceptible

	Microorganism	Lincomycin	Clindamycin
Gram-positive	*Staphylococcus aureus*	✔	✔
	S. epidermidis[a]	✔	✔
	S. albus	✔	
	Streptococcus pneumoniae	✔	✔
	S. pyogenes	✔	✔
	β-hemolytic streptococci	✔	
	S. viridans	✔	✔
	Pneumococci		✔
	Corynebacterium diphtheriae	✔	✔
	Diplococcus pneumoniae	✔	
	Corynebacterium acnes	✔	
	Nocardia asteroides	✔	✔
Anaerobes	*Bacteroides* sp.	✔	✔[b]
	Fusobacterium sp.		✔
	Propionibacterium (same as *C. acnes*)	✔	✔
	Eubacterium sp.	✔	✔
	Actinomyces sp.	✔	✔
	Peptococcus sp.	✔	✔
	Peptostreptococcus sp.	✔	✔
	Microaerophilic streptococci		✔
	Clostridium perfringens	✔	✔
	C. tetani	✔	✔
	Veillonella sp.		✔

[a] Penicillinase and nonpenicillinase.
[b] Including *B. fragilis* and *B. melaninogenicus*.

Contraindications

Hypersensitivity to lincosamides; treatment of minor bacterial or viral infections.

Warnings

➤*Meningitis:* **Clindamycin** does not diffuse adequately into CSF; not for meningitis.

➤*Hypersensitivity reactions:* Use with caution in patients with a history of asthma or significant allergies. If hypersensitivity occurs, discontinue the drug and institute emergency treatment. Refer to Management of Acute Hypersensitivity Reactions.

➤*Renal/Hepatic function impairment:* Cautiously give **clindamycin** to patients with severe renal or hepatic disease accompanied by severe metabolic aberrations; monitor serum clindamycin levels during high-dose therapy. Use of **lincomycin** in preexisting liver disease is not recommended unless special circumstances so indicate.

➤*Elderly:* Older patients with associated severe illness may not tolerate diarrhea well; carefully monitor these patients for changes in bowel frequency.

➤*Pregnancy: Category B* (**clindamycin**). Safety has not been established. **Clindamycin** and **lincomycin** cross the placenta in amounts approximately % and 25% of maternal serum levels, respectively.

➤*Lactation:* **Clindamycin** appears in breast milk in ranges of 0.7 to 3.8 mcg/mL following doses of 150 mg orally to 600 mg IV. **Lincomycin** appears in breast milk in ranges of 0.5 to 2.4 mcg/mL. Breast-feeding is probably best discontinued when taking these agents to avoid potential problems in the infant. However, the American Academy of Pediatrics considers clindamycin to be compatible with breast-feeding.

➤*Children:* **Lincomycin** is not indicated for use in the newborn. When **clindamycin** is administered to newborns and infants, monitor organ system functions. Each mL of clindamycin and lincomycin contains 9.45 mg benzyl alcohol (see Precautions).

Precautions

➤*Monitoring:* For prolonged therapy, perform liver/kidney function tests, blood counts.

➤*IV infusion:* Do NOT inject IV undiluted as a bolus; infuse over at least 10 to 60 minutes as directed in Administration and Dosage.

➤*GI disease:* Use cautiously in patients with GI disease, particularly colitis.

➤*Benzyl alcohol:* Some of these products contain benzyl alcohol which has been associated with fatal "gasping syndrome" in premature infants.

➤*Superinfection:* Use of antibiotics may result in bacterial or fungal overgrowth of nonsusceptible organisms, particularly yeasts. Such overgrowth may lead to a secondary infection. Take appropriate measures if superinfection occurs.

➤*Tartrazine sensitivity:* Some products contain tartrazine, which may cause allergic-type reactions (including bronchial asthma) in susceptible individuals. Although incidence of tartrazine sensitivity in the general population is low, it is frequently seen in patients who also have aspirin hypersensitivity. Refer to product listings.

Drug Interactions

Lincosamide Drug Interactions

Precipitant drug	Object drug[a]		Description
Erythromycin	Lincosamides	↓	Antagonism has occurred in vitro between clindamycin and erythromycin.
Kaolin-Pectin	Lincosamides	↓	GI absorption is decreased for lincomycin and delayed for clindamycin when they are administered with kaolin-pectin antidiarrheals.
Lincosamides	Neuromuscular blockers	↑	The actions of the nondepolarizing neuromuscular blockers may be enhanced, possibly contributing to profound and severe respiratory depression.

[a] ↑ = Object drug increased. ↓ = Object drug decreased.

➤*Drug/Food interactions:* Food impairs the absorption of **lincomycin**; do not take anything by mouth (except water) for 1 to 2 hours before and after lincomycin. **Clindamycin** absorption is not affected by food.

Adverse Reactions

➤*Cardiovascular:* Hypotension, cardiopulmonary arrest after too rapid IV use (rare).

➤*GI:* Diarrhea (clindamycin 2% to 20%); pseudomembranous colitis (clindamycin 0.01% to 10%; more frequent with oral administration); nausea; vomiting; abdominal pain, esophagitis (clindamycin); unpleasant or metallic taste (following higher doses of IV clindamycin); glossitis, stomatitis, pruritus ani (lincomycin).

➤*Hematologic:* Neutropenia; leukopenia; agranulocytosis; thrombocytopenic purpura; aplastic anemia, pancytopenia (rare) (lincomycin).

➤*Hepatic:* Jaundice; liver function test abnormalities (serum transaminase elevations).

➤*Hypersensitivity:* Skin rashes, urticaria, erythema multiforme, some cases resembling Stevens-Johnson syndrome (rare); anaphylaxis; maculopapular rash, generalized morbilliform-like rash (clindamycin); angioneurotic edema, serum sickness (lincomycin).

➤*Local:* Pain following injection. Induration and sterile abscess have occurred after IM injection and thrombophlebitis after IV infusion with clindamycin; give deep IM injections and avoid prolonged use of IV catheters.

➤*Renal:* Dysfunction has been characterized by azotemia, oliguria, and proteinuria (rare).

➤*Special senses:* Tinnitus, vertigo (lincomycin).

➤*Miscellaneous:* Transient eosinophilia, polyarthritis (rare) (clindamycin); vaginitis, exfoliative, vesiculobullous dermatitis (rare) (lincomycin).

Patient Information

May cause diarrhea; notify physician if this occurs. Do not treat diarrhea without notifying the physician.

Take each dose with a full glass of water. Complete full course of therapy.

Do not take anything by mouth (except water) for 1 to 2 hours before and after lincomycin. Clindamycin may be taken without regard to meals.

LINCOMYCIN

Rx	**Lincocin** (Upjohn)	**Capsules:** 500 mg (as hydrochloride)	Lactose. Powder blue and dark blue. In 100s.
Rx	**Lincocin** (Upjohn)	**Injection:** 300 mg (as hydrochloride)/mL	In 2 and 10 mL vials.[a]

[a] With 9.45 mg benzyl alcohol/mL.

LINCOMYCIN — ORAL

For complete and comparartive prescribing information, refer to the Lincosamides group monograph.

WARNING

Pseudomembranous colitis has been reported with nearly all antibacterial agents, including lincomycin, and may range in severity from mild to life-threatening. Therefore, it is important to consider this diagnosis in patients who present with diarrhea subsequent to the administration of antibacterial agents.

Because lincomycin therapy has been associated with severe colitis which may end fatally, it should be reserved for serious infections where less toxic antimicrobial agents are inappropriate, as described in Indications. It should not be used in patients with nonbacterial infections such as most upper respiratory tract infections. Treatment with antibacterial agents alters the normal flora of the colon and may permit overgrowth of clostridia. Studies indicate that a toxin produced by *Clostridium difficile* is one primary cause of "antibiotic-associated colitis."

WARNING (cont.)

After the diagnosis of pseudomembraneous colitis has been established, therapeutic measures should be initiated. Mild cases of pseudomembranous colitis usually respond to drug discontinuation alone. In moderate to severe cases, consideration should be given to management with fluids and electrolytes, protein supplementation, and treatment with an antibacterial drug clinically effective against *C. difficile* colitis.

Diarrhea, colitis and pseudomembranous colitis have been obsered to begin up to several weeks following cessation of therapy with lincomycin.

Indications

➤*Serious infections:* Treatment of serious infections due to susceptible strains of streptococci, pneumococci, and staphylococci. Its use should be reserved for penicillin-allergic patients or other patients for whom, in the judgment of the physician, a penicillin is inappropriate. Because of the risk of antibiotic-associated pseudomembranous collitis, as described in the Warning box, before selecting lincomycin the physician should consider the nature of the infection and the suitability of less toxic alternatives (eg, erythromycin).

Lincomycin has been demonstrated to be effective in the treatment of staphylococcal infections resistant to other antibiotics and susceptible to lincomycin. Staphylococcal strains resistant to lincomycin have been recov-

LINCOMYCIN — ORAL

ered; culture and susceptibility studies should be done in conjunction with therapy with lincomycin. In the case of macrolides, partial but not complete cross resistance may occur (see Microbiology). The drug may be administered concomitantly with other antimicrobial agents when indicated.

Administration and Dosage

➤*Approved by the FDA:* April 21, 1991.

If significant diarrhea occurs during therapy, this antibiotic should be discontinued (see Warning box).

➤*Adults:*

Serious infections – 500 mg 3 times per day (500 mg approximately every 8 hours).

More severe infections – 500 mg or more 4 times per day (500 mg or more approximately every 6 hours).

➤*Children (older than 1 month of age):*

Serious infections – 30 mg/kg/day (15 mg/lb/day) divided into 3 or 4 equal doses.

More severe infections – 60 mg/kg/day (30 mg/lb/day) divided into 3 or 4 equal doses.

With β-hemolytic streptococcal infections, treatment should continue for at least 10 days to diminish the likelihood of subsequent rheumatic fever or glomerulonephritis.

➤*Administration:* For optimal absorption it is recommended that nothing be given by mouth except water for a period of one to two hours before and after oral administration of lincomycin preparations.

➤*Renal function impairment:* When therapy with lincomycin is required in individuals with severe impairment of renal function, an appropriate dose is 25% to 30% of that recommended for patients with normally functioning kidneys.

➤*Storage/Stability:* Store at controlled room temperature 20° to 25° (68° to 77°F) [see USP].

LINCOMYCIN — INJECTION

For complete and comparartive prescribing information, refer to the Lincosamides group monograph.

WARNING

Pseudomembranous colitis has been reported with nearly all antibacterial agents, including lincomycin, and may range in severity from mild to life-threatening. Therefore, it is important to consider this diagnosis in patients who present with diarrhea subsequent to the administration of antibacterial agents.

Because lincomycin therapy has been associated with severe colitis which may end fatally, it should be reserved for serious infections where less toxic antimicrobial agents are inappropriate, as described in Indications. It should not be used in patients with nonbacterial infections such as most upper respiratory tract infections. Treatment with antibacterial agents alters the normal flora of the colon and may permit overgrowth of clostridia. Studies indicate that a toxin produced by *Clostridium difficile* is one primary cause of "antibiotic-associated colitis."

After the diagnosis of pseudomembranous colitis has been established, therapeutic measures should be initiated. Mild cases of pseudomembranous colitis usually respond to drug discontinuation alone. In moderate to severe cases, consideration should be given to management with fluids and electrolytes, protein supplementation, and treatment with an antibacterial drug clinically effective against *C. difficile* colitis.

Diarrhea, colitis and pseudomembranous colitis have been observed to begin up to several weeks following cessation of therapy with lincomycin.

Indications

➤*Serious infections:* Treatment of serious infections due to susceptible strains of streptococci, pneumococci, and staphylococci. Its use should be reserved for penicillin-allergic patients or other patients for whom, in the judgment of the physician, a penicillin is inappropriate. Because of the risk of antibiotic-associated pseudomembranous colitis, as described in the Warning box, before selecting lincomycin the physician should consider the nature of the infection and the suitability of less toxic alternatives (eg, erythromycin).

Lincomycin has been demonstrated to be effective in the treatment of staphylococcal infections resistant to other antibiotics and susceptible to lincomycin. Staphylococcal strains resistant to lincomycin have been recovered; culture and susceptibility studies should be done in conjunction with therapy with lincomycin. In the case of macrolides, partial but not complete cross resistance may occur (see Microbiology). The drug may be administered concomitantly with other antimicrobial agents when indicated.

Administration and Dosage

➤*Approved by the FDA:* April 21, 1991.

If significant diarrhea occurs during therapy, this antibiotic should be discontinued (see Warning box).

➤*Intramuscular Injection:*

Adults –

Serious infections: 600 mg (2 mL) intramuscularly every 24 hours.

More severe infections: 600 mg (2 mL) intramuscularly every 12 hours or more often.

Children (older than 1 month of age) –

Serious infections: One intramuscular injection of 10 mg/kg (5 mg/lb) every 24 hours.

More severe infections: One intramuscular injection of 10 mg/kg (5 mg/lb) every 12 hours or more often.

➤*Intravenous injection:*

Adults – The intravenous dose will be determined by the severity of the infection. For serious infections doses of 600 mg of lincomycin (2 mL of lincomycin) to 1 g are given every 8 to 12 hours. For more severe infections these doses may have to be increased. In life-threatening situations daily intravenous doses of as much as 8 g have been given. Intravenous doses are given on the basis of 1 g of lincomycin diluted in not less than 100 mL of appropriate solution and infused over a period of not less than 1 hour.

Lincomycin Infusion Rates

Dose	Volume diluent	Time
600 mg	100 mL	1 h
1 g	100 mL	1 h
2 g	200 mL	2 h
3 g	300 mL	3 h
4 g	400 mL	4 h

These doses may be repeated as often as required to the limit of the maximum recommended daily dose of 8 g of lincomycin.

Children (older than 1 month of age) – 10 to 20 mg/kg/day (5 to 10 mg/lb/day) depending on the severity of the infection may be infused in divided doses as described above for adults.

Infusion-related reactions – Severe cardiopulmonary reactions have occurred when this drug has been given at greater than the recommended concentration and rate.

➤*Subconjunctival injection:* 0.25 mL (75 mg) injected subconjunctivally will result in ocular fluid levels of antibiotic (lasting for at least 5 hours) with MICs sufficient for most susceptible pathogens.

➤*Patients with diminished renal function:* When therapy with lincomycin is required in individuals with severe impairment of renal function, an appropriate dose is 25% to 30% of that recommended for patients with normally functioning kidneys.

➤*Compatible IV solutions:* Infusion solutions which may be used for preparing intravenous lincomycin include 5% Dextrose Injection, 10% Dextrose Injection, 5% Dextrose and 0.9% Sodium Chloride Injection, 10% Dextrose and 0.9% Sodium Chloride Injection, Ringer's Injection, 1/6 M Sodium Lactate Injection, Travert 10%-Electrolyte No. 1, and Dextran in Saline 6% w/v.

➤*Storage/Stability:* Store at controlled room temperature 20° to 25° (68° to 77°F) [see USP].

CLINDAMYCIN

Rx	**Clindamycin hydrochloride** (Various, eg, Danbury)	**Capsules**: 75 mg (as hydrochloride)	In 100s.
Rx	**Cleocin** (Upjohn)		(CLEOCIN 75 mg). Tartrazine, lactose. Green. In 100s.
Rx	**Clindamycin hydrochloride** (Various, eg, Compumed, Zenith-Goldline)	**Capsules**: 150 mg (as hydrochloride)	In 100s.
Rx	**Cleocin** (Upjohn)		(CLEOCIN 150 mg). Tartrazine, lactose. Light blue and green. In 16s, 100s, and UD 100s.
Rx	**Clindamycin hydrochloride** (Ranbaxy)	**Capsules**: 300 mg (as hydrochloride)	Lactose. In 16s and 100s.
Rx	**Cleocin** (Upjohn)		(CLEOCIN 300 mg). Lactose. Light blue. In 16s, 100s, and UD 100s.
Rx	**Cleocin Pediatric** (Upjohn)	**Granules for Oral Solution**: 75 mg/5 mL (as palmitate)	Sucrose, parabens. In 100 mL.

CLINDAMYCIN

Rx	**Clindamycin Phosphate** (Various, eg, Hospira)	**Injection**: 150 mg (as phosphate) per mL	In 2, 4, 6, 60, and 100 mL vials.
Rx	**Cleocin Phosphate** (Upjohn)		In 2, 4, and 6 mL vials[a] and 4 and 6 mL *ADD-Vantage* vials[a], 50 mL *Galaxy* plastic containers, and 60 mL pharmacy bulk package.

[a] With benzyl alcohol and EDTA.

CLINDAMYCIN HYDROCHLORIDE — ORAL

For complete and comparative prescribing information, refer to the Lincosamides group monograph.

WARNING

Pseudomembranous colitis has been reported with nearly all antibacterial agents, including clindamycin, and may range in severity from mild to life-threatening. Therefore, it is important to consider this diagnosis in patients who present with diarrhea subsequent to the administration of antibacterial agents.

Because clindamycin therapy has been associated with severe colitis, which may end fatally, it should be reserved for serious infections where less toxic antimicrobial agents are inappropriate, as described in Indications. It should not be used in patients with nonbacterial infections such as most upper respiratory tract infections. Treatment with antibacterial agents alters the normal flora of the colon and may permit overgrowth of clostridia. Studies indicate that a toxin produced by *Clostridium difficile* is one primary cause of "antibiotic-associated colitis".

After the diagnosis of pseudomembranous colitis has been established, therapeutic measures should be initiated. Mild cases of pseudomembranous colitis usually respond to drug discontinuation alone. In moderate to severe cases, consideration should be given to management with fluids and electrolytes, protein supplementation, and treatment with an antibacterial drug clinically effective against *C. difficile* colitis.

Diarrhea, colitis, and pseudomembranous colitis have been observed to begin up to several weeks following cessation of therapy with clindamycin.

Indications

➤*Anaerobes:* Serious respiratory tract infections such as empyema, anaerobic pneumonitis, and lung abscess; serious skin and soft tissue infections; septicemia; intra-abdominal infections such as peritonitis and intra-abdominal abscess (typically resulting from anaerobic organisms resident in the normal gastrointestinal tract); infections of the female pelvis and genital tract such as endometritis, nongonococcal tubo-ovarian abscess, pelvic cellulitis, and postsurgical vaginal cuff infection.

➤*Streptococci:* Serious respiratory tract infections; serious skin and soft tissue infections.

➤*Staphylococci:* Serious respiratory tract infections; serious skin and soft tissue infections.

➤*Pneumococci:* Serious respiratory tract infections.

➤*Unlabeled uses:* Clindamycin (1,200 to 2,400 mg/day) may be beneficial as an alternative to sulfonamides in combination with pyrimethamine in the acute treatment of CNS toxoplasmosis in AIDS patients.

Clindamycin is effective in the treatment of *Chlamydia trachomatis* infections in women.

Clindamycin 300 mg twice daily for 7 days is effective in bacterial vaginosis due to *Gardnerella vaginalis* and may be an alternative to metronidazole.

Administration and Dosage

➤*Approved by the FDA:* April 14, 1988.

If significant diarrhea occurs during therapy, this antibiotic should be discontinued (see Warning Box).

➤*Adults:*

Serious infections – 150 to 300 mg every 6 hours.

More severe infections – 300 to 450 mg every 6 hours.

➤*Children:*

Serious infections – 8 to 16 mg/kg/day (4 to 8 mg/lb/day) divided into 3 or 4 equal doses.

More severe infections – 16 to 20 mg/kg/day (8 to 10 mg/lb/day) divided into 3 or 4 equal doses.

To avoid the possibility of esophageal irritation, clindamycin hydrochloride capsules should be taken with a full glass of water.

➤*Streptococcal infections:* In cases of β-hemolytic streptococcal infections, treatment should continue for at least 10 days.

➤*Storage/Stability:* Store at controlled room temperature 20° to 25°C (68° to 77°F) [see USP].

CLINDAMYCIN PALMITATE HYDROCHLORIDE — ORAL SOLUTION

For complete and comparative prescribing information, refer to the Lincosamides group monograph.

WARNING

Pseudomembranous colitis has been reported with nearly all antibacterial agents, including clindamycin, and may range in severity from mild to life-threatening. Therefore, it is important to consider this diagnosis in patients who present with diarrhea subsequent to the administration of antibacterial agents.

Because clindamycin therapy has been associated with severe colitis, which may end fatally, it should be reserved for serious infections where less toxic antimicrobial agents are inappropriate, as described in Indications. It should not be used in patients with nonbacterial infections such as most upper respiratory tract infections. Treatment with antibacterial agents alters the normal flora of the colon and may permit overgrowth of clostridia. Studies indicate that a toxin produced by *Clostridium difficile* is one primary cause of "antibiotic-associated colitis".

After the diagnosis of pseudomembranous colitis has been established, therapeutic measures should be initiated. Mild cases of pseudomembranous colitis usually respond to drug discontinuation alone. In moderate to severe cases, consideration should be given to management with fluids and electrolytes, protein supplementation, and treatment with an antibacterial drug clinically effective against *C. difficile* colitis.

Diarrhea, colitis, and pseudomembranous colitis have been observed to begin up to several weeks following cessation of therapy with clindamycin.

Indications

➤*Anaerobes:* Serious respiratory tract infections such as empyema, anaerobic pneumonitis, and lung abscess; serious skin and soft tissue infections; septicemia; intra-abdominal infections such as peritonitis and intra-abdominal abscess (typically resulting from anaerobic organisms resident in the normal GI tract); infections of the female pelvis and genital tract such as endometritis, nongonococcal tubo-ovarian abscess, pelvic cellulitis, and postsurgical vaginal cuff infection.

➤*Streptococci:* Serious respiratory tract infections; serious skin and soft tissue infections.

➤*Staphylococci:* Serious respiratory tract infections; serious skin and soft tissue infections.

➤*Pneumococci:* Serious respiratory tract infections.

Administration and Dosage

➤*Approved by the FDA:* April 7, 1986.

If significant diarrhea occurs during therapy, this antibiotic should be discontinued (see Warning Box).

Concomitant administration of food does not adversely affect the absorption of clindamycin palmitate hydrochloride contained in clindamycin palmitate hydrochloride flavored granules for pediatric use (see Drug Interactions).

➤*Serious infections:* 8 to 12 mg/kg/day (4 to 6 mg/lb/day) divided into 3 or 4 equal doses.

➤*Severe infections:* 13 to 16 mg/kg/day (6.5 to 8 mg/lb/day) divided into 3 or 4 equal doses.

➤*More severe infections:* 17 to 25 mg/kg/day (8.5 to 12.5 mg/lb/day) divided into 3 or 4 equal doses.

➤*Children:* In pediatric patients weighing ≤ 10 kg, ½ teaspoon (37.5 mg) 3 times a day should be considered the minimum recommended dose.

➤*Streptococcal infections:* In cases of β-hemolytic streptococcal infections, treatment should be continued for at least 10 days.

➤*Reconstitution instructions:* When reconstituted with water as follows, each 5 mL (teaspoon) of solution contains clindamycin palmitate hydrochloride equivalent to 75 mg clindamycin.

Reconstitute bottles of 100 mL with 75 mL of water. Add a large portion of the water and shake vigorously; add the remainder of the water and shake until the solution is uniform.

➤*Storage conditions:* Store at controlled room temperature 20° to 25°C (68° to 77°F) [see USP].

Do not refrigerate the reconstituted solution; when chilled, the solution may thicken and be difficult to pour. The solution is stable for 2 weeks at room temperature.

CLINDAMYCIN PHOSPHATE — INJECTION

For complete and comparative prescribing information, refer to the Lincosamides group monograph.

WARNING

Pseudomembranous colitis has been reported with nearly all antibacterial agents, including clindamycin phosphate, and may range in severity from mild to life-threatening. Therefore, it is important to consider this diagnosis in patients who present with diarrhea subsequent to the administration of antibacterial agents.

Because clindamycin phosphate therapy has been associated with severe colitis that may end fatally, it should be reserved for serious infections where less toxic antimicrobial agents are inappropriate, as described in Indications. It should not be used in patients with nonbacterial infections, such as most upper respiratory tract infections. Treatment with antibacterial agents alters the normal flora of the colon and may permit overgrowth of clostridia. Studies indicate that a toxin produced by *Clostridium difficile* is one primary cause of "antibiotic-associated colitis".

After the diagnosis of pseudomembranous colitis has been established, therapeutic measures should be initiated. Mild cases of pseudomembranous colitis usually respond to drug discontinuation alone. In moderate to severe cases, consideration should be given to management with fluids and electrolytes, protein supplementation, and treatment with an antibacterial drug clinically effective against *C. difficile* colitis.

Diarrhea, colitis, and pseudomembranous colitis have been observed to begin up to several weeks following cessation of therapy with clindamycin phosphate.

Indications

➤*Lower respiratory tract infections:* Lower respiratory tract infections including pneumonia, empyema, and lung abscess caused by anaerobes, *Streptococcus pneumoniae*, other streptococci (except *E. faecalis*), and *Staphylococcus aureus*.

➤*Skin and skin structure infections:* Caused by *Streptococcus pyogenes*, *Staphylococcus aureus*, and anaerobes.

➤*Gynecological infections:* Gynecological infections including endometritis, nongonococcal tubo-ovarian abscess, pelvic cellulitis, and postsurgical vaginal cuff infection caused by susceptible anaerobes.

➤*Intra-abdominal infections:* Intra-abdominal infections including peritonitis and intra-abdominal abscess caused by susceptible anaerobic organisms.

➤*Septicemia:* Caused by *Staphylococcus aureus*, streptococci (except *Enterococcus faecalis*), and susceptible anaerobes.

➤*Bone and joint infections:* Bone and joint infections including acute hematogenous osteomyelitis caused by *Staphylococcus aureus* and as adjunctive therapy in the surgical treatment of chronic bone and joint infections due to susceptible organisms.

➤*Unlabeled uses:* Clindamycin (1,200 to 2,400 mg/day) may be beneficial as an alternative to sulfonamides in combination with pyrimethamine in acute treatment of CNS toxoplasmosis in AIDS patients.

Administration and Dosage

➤*Approved by the FDA:* July 24, 1987.

If diarrhea occurs during therapy, this antibiotic should be discontinued (see Warning Box).

➤*Adults:*

Parenteral (IM or IV administration) – Serious infections due to aerobic gram-positive cocci and the more susceptible anaerobes (not generally including *Bacteroides fragilis, Peptococcus* species and *Clostridium* species other than *Clostridium perfringens*):

600 to 1,200 mg/day in 2, 3, or 4 equal doses.

More severe infections (particularly those due to proven or suspected Bacteroides fragilis, Peptococcus species, or Clostridium species other than Clostridium perfringens): 1,200 to 2,700 mg/day in 2, 3, or 4 equal doses.

• *Life-threatening situations* – For more severe infections, these doses may have to be increased. In life-threatening situations due to aerobes or anaerobes, these doses may be increased. Doses of as much as 4800 mg daily have been given intravenously to adults (see Dilution and infusion rates).

• *Administration* – Single IM injections of more than 600 mg are not recommended.

Alternatively, drug may be administered in the form of a single rapid infusion of the first dose followed by continuous IV infusion as follows:

Administration		
To maintain serum clindamycin levels	Rapid infusion rate	Maintenance infusion rate
> 4 mcg/mL	10 mg/min for 30 minutes	0.75 mg/min
> 5 mcg/mL	15 mg/min for 30 minutes	1 mg/min
> 6 mcg/mL	20 mg/min for 30 minutes	1.25 mg/min

➤*Children (1 month to 16 years of age):*

Parenteral (IM or IV administration) – 20 to 40 mg/kg/day in 3 or 4 equal doses. The higher doses would be used for more severe infections. As an alternative to dosing on a body weight basis, children may be dosed on the basis of square meters body surface: 350 mg/m²/day for serious infections and 450 mg/m²/day for more severe infections.

IV to oral conversion – Parenteral therapy may be changed to clindamycin palmitate hydrochloride for oral solution or clindamycin hydrochloride capsules when the condition warrants and at the discretion of the physician.

Streptococcal infections – In cases of β-hemolytic streptococcal infections, treatment should be continued for at least 10 days.

Neonates (younger than 1 month of age) – 15 to 20 mg/kg/day in 3 to 4 equal doses. The lower dosage may be adequate for small prematures.

➤*Dilution and infusion rates:* Clindamycin phosphate must be diluted prior to IV administration. The concentration of clindamycin in diluent for infusion should not exceed 18 mg/mL. Infusion rates should not exceed 30 mg/min. The usual infusion dilutions and rates are as follows:

Clindamycin Infusion Rates		
Dose	Diluent	Time
300 mg	50 mL	10 min
600 mg	50 mL	20 min
900 mg	50 to 100 mL	30 min
1,200 mg	100 mL	40 min

Administration of more than 1,200 mg in a single 1-hour infusion is not recommended.

➤*Compatibilities/Incompatibilities:* Physical and biological compatibility studies monitored for 24 hours at room temperature have demonstrated no inactivation or incompatibility with the use of clindamycin phosphate injection, USP, sterile solution in IV solutions containing sodium chloride, glucose, calcium or potassium, and solutions containing vitamin B complex in concentrations usually used clinically. No incompatibility has been demonstrated with the antibiotics cephalothin, kanamycin, gentamicin, penicillin, or carbenicillin.

The following drugs are physically incompatible with clindamycin phosphate: Ampicillin sodium, phenytoin sodium, barbiturates, aminophylline, calcium gluconate, and magnesium sulfate.

The compatibility and duration of stability of drug admixtures will vary depending on concentration and other conditions.

➤*Storage/Stability:* Store at controlled room temperature 20° to 25°C (68° to 77°F) [see USP].

Exposure of pharmaceutical products to heat should be minimized. It is recommended that *Galaxy* plastic containers be stored at room temperature (25°C; 77°F). Avoid temperatures above 30°C (86°F).

WARNING

Toxicity – Aminoglycosides are associated with significant nephrotoxicity or ototoxicity. These agents are excreted primarily by glomerular filtration; thus, the serum half-life will be prolonged and significant accumulation will occur in patients with impaired renal function. Toxicity may develop even with conventional doses, particularly in patients with prerenal azotemia or impaired renal function.

Ototoxicity – Neurotoxicity, manifested as auditory (cochlear) and vestibular ototoxicity, can occur with any of these agents. Auditory changes are irreversible, usually bilateral and may be partial or total. Risk of hearing loss increases with the degree of exposure to high peak or high trough serum concentrations and continues to progress after drug withdrawal. The risk is higher in patients with renal function impairment and with preexisting hearing loss. High frequency deafness usually occurs first and can be detected by audiometric testing. When feasible, obtain serial audiograms. There may be no clinical symptoms to warn of developing cochlear damage. Tinnitus or vertigo may occur, and are evidence of vestibular injury. Other manifestations of neurotoxicity may include numbness, skin tingling, muscle twitching, and convulsions. Total or partial irreversible bilateral deafness may occur after drug discontinuation. Aminoglycoside-induced ototoxicity usually is irreversible. Vestibular toxicity is more predominant with gentamicin and streptomycin; auditory toxicity is more common with kanamycin and amikacin. Tobramycin affects both functions equally. Relative ototoxicity is streptomycin = kanamycin > amikacin = gentamicin = tobramycin. Kanamycin, amikacin, and streptomycin appear in this relative comparison based on high-dose (kanamycin, amikacin) and antituberculosis (streptomycin) therapy.

Renal toxicity – This may be characterized by decreased creatinine clearance (Ccr), cells or casts in the urine, decreased urine specific gravity, oliguria, proteinuria, or evidence of nitrogen retention (increasing blood urea nitrogen [BUN], nonprotein nitrogen [NPN], or serum creatinine). Renal damage usually is reversible. The relative nephrotoxicity of these agents is estimated to be kanamycin = amikacin = gentamicin > tobramycin > streptomycin.

Monitoring – Closely observe all patients treated with aminoglycosides. Monitoring renal and eighth cranial nerve function at onset of therapy is essential for patients with known or suspected renal function impairment and in those whose renal function initially is normal, but who develop signs of renal dysfunction. Evidence of renal function impairment or ototoxicity requires drug discontinuation or appropriate dosage adjustments. When feasible, monitor drug serum concentrations. Avoid concomitant use with other ototoxic, neurotoxic, or nephrotoxic drugs. Other factors that may increase risk of toxicity are dehydration and advanced age.

Indications

The indications for specific agents are listed in individual drug monographs on the following pages. Reserve these drugs for treatment of infections caused by organisms not sensitive to less toxic agents. Safety for treatment periods longer than 14 days has not been established.

➤*Unlabeled uses:* In cystic fibrosis patients, the use of inhaled aminoglycosides may be beneficial in certain populations (eg, younger patients). Clinical outcome is not improved but deterioration of pulmonary function tests may be slowed or prevented.

Administration and Dosage

➤*Synergism:* In vitro studies indicate that aminoglycosides combined with penicillins or cephalosporins act synergistically against some strains of gram-negative organisms and enterococci (*Streptococcus faecalis*). Aminoglycosides may exhibit a synergistic effect when combined with carbenicillin or ticarcillin for *Pseudomonas* infections. Tests for antibiotic synergy are necessary. See also Admixture Incompatibility and Drug Interactions.

➤*Admixture incompatibility:* Beta-lactam antibiotics (eg, cephalosporins, penicillins) may inactivate aminoglycosides when admixed. Ticarcillin and carbenicillin are the worst β-lactam offenders; tobramycin and gentamicin are more susceptible than amikacin. This is most likely to occur: When the agents are mixed in the same container; during the aminoglycoside assay procedure; and in poor renal function. Concomitant cephalosporins also may falsely elevate creatinine determinations.

Ticarcillin and carbenicillin also may decrease aminoglycoside serum levels (see Overdosage).

Inactivation of tobramycin has not occurred in patients with normal renal function if they are given the drugs by separate routes. Kanamycin and methicillin inactivate each other in vitro, but this has not been seen in patients who receive them by different routes.

Guard against in vitro inactivation of aminoglycosides by β-lactam antibiotics in patients on combination therapy: 1) Place sample on ice immediately after drawing the specimen; test immediately. If testing is delayed, freeze serum as soon as possible; 2) draw the aminoglycoside level when the β-lactam antibiotic is at its trough level; 3) inactivation can still occur when the specimen is frozen (eg, ampicillin, kanamycin). If samples are to be frozen for a long period of time, inactivate the penicillin with penicillinase prior to freezing.

➤*Dosing interval:* Although further studies are needed, preliminary evidence indicates that aminoglycosides may be administered on a once daily basis without compromising efficacy and without increasing the potential for nephrotoxicity and ototoxicity. It is possible that the incidence of nephrotoxicity may be decreased.

Actions

➤*Pharmacology:* Aminoglycosides are bactericidal antibiotics used primarily in the treatment of gram-negative infections. They irreversibly bind to the 30S subunit of bacterial ribosomes, blocking the recognition step in protein synthesis and causing misreading of the genetic code. The ribosomes separate from messenger RNA; cell death ensues.

➤*Pharmacokinetics:*

Absorption – Absorption from the GI tract is poor. Aminoglycosides are occasionally used orally for enteric infections (see Aminoglycosides, Oral monograph). Absorption from IM injection is rapid, with peak blood levels achieved within 1 hour.

Distribution – Aminoglycosides are widely distributed in extracellular fluids; peak serum concentrations may be lower than usual in patients whose extracellular fluid volume is expanded (eg, patients with edema or ascites). These drugs cross the placental barrier. Concentrations are found in bile, tissues, sputum, bronchial secretions and synovial, interstitial, peritoneal, abscess, and pleural fluids. Concentrations in renal cortex are several times higher than usual serum levels. Aminoglycosides exhibit low protein binding, except for streptomycin. They do not achieve significant cerebrospinal fluid (CSF) levels in healthy patients. Although penetration is enhanced in the presence of inflamed meninges, only low levels are achieved. When intrathecal gentamicin is given with systemic gentamicin, CSF levels are substantially increased, depending on location of injection. Peak CSF concentrations following intralumbar administration generally occur 1 to 6 hours after injection.

Newborn infants, postpartum women, and patients with ascites, spinal cord injury, and cystic fibrosis may have an enlarged apparent volume of distribution. Obesity will artificially contract the apparent volume of distribution because adipose tissue contains less water than lean body mass of equal weight.

Excretion – Done by glomerular filtration, largely as unchanged drug; thus, high urine levels are attained. Probenecid does not affect renal tubular transport. The serum half-lives of all the agents are between 2 to 3 hours in patients with normal renal function. Approximately 53% to 98% of a single IV dose is excreted in the urine in 24 hours. However, when renal function is impaired, significant accumulation and subsequent toxicity may occur rapidly if dosage is not adjusted. The serum half-life is longer in young infants, as the immature renal system is unable to excrete these drugs rapidly; during the first days of life, the half-life may exceed 5 to 6 hours. Prolonged half-life also may be noted in the elderly. In severely burned patients, the half-life may be significantly decreased and result in serum concentrations lower than anticipated. Febrile and anemic states may be associated with a shorter serum half-life; dosage adjustment is usually not necessary. Aminoglycosides are removed by hemodialysis (4 to 6 hours removes approximately 50%) and peritoneal dialysis (range, removal of 23% in 8 hours to only 4% in 22 hours).

Serum levels – Because of the narrow range between therapeutic and toxic serum levels, careful attention to dosage calculations is essential, especially in patients with renal function impairment, women and elderly patients, those requiring high peak serum levels, patients on prolonged (longer than 10 days) therapy, patients with unstable renal function or those undergoing dialysis, those with abnormal extracellular fluid volume, or with prior exposure to ototoxic or nephrotoxic drugs. Age markedly affects peak concentration in children; generally, it is lower in young children and infants. Monitor drug serum levels. Peak levels indicate therapeutic levels. Trough serum level determinations (just before next dose) best indicate drug accumulation. Obtain serum levels within 48 hours of start of therapy and every 3 to 4 days assuming stable renal function; also, levels are indicated when dose is changed or in changing renal function. Generally, to measure peak levels, draw a serum sample about 30 minutes after IV infusion or 1 hour after an IM dose. For trough levels, obtain serum samples at 8 hours or just prior to the next dose.

Various Pharmacokinetic Parameters of the Aminoglycosides

Aminoglycoside	Half-life (h)		Therapeutic serum levels (peak) (mcg/mL)	Toxic serum levels (mcg/mL)		Dose (mg/kg/day) (normal Ccr)
	Normal	ESRD		Peak[a]	Trough[b]	
Amikacin	2 to 3	24 to 60	16 to 32	> 35	> 10	15
Gentamicin	2	24 to 60	4 to 8	> 12	> 2	3 to 5
Kanamycin	2 to 3	24 to 60	15 to 40	> 35	> 10	15
Streptomycin	2.5	100	20 to 30	> 50	—	15
Tobramycin	2 to 2.5	24 to 60	4 to 8	> 12	> 2	3 to 5

[a] Measured 1 hour after IM administration.
[b] Measured immediately prior to next dose.

➤*Microbiology:* The bactericidal activity of aminoglycosides is through inhibition of bacterial protein synthesis. One-way cross resistance is frequently noted. The following 3 mechanisms for the development of bacterial resistance to aminoglycosides have been identified: alteration of the drug target site (the bacterial ribosome); reduction or elimination of transport of the drug into the bacterial cell; inactivation of the drug by enzymatic modification (aminoglycoside inactivating enzymes; most significant).

Perform culture and sensitivity testing. Treat susceptible organisms with less toxic agents, especially if renal function is compromised. Resistance develops slowly, except with streptomycin. Development of streptomycin resistance may be a single-step process and may occur rapidly. Most streptococci species (particularly group D), including *S. pneumoniae*, anaerobic organisms (including *Bacteroides* sp. and *Clostridia* sp.), and anaerobic cocci are resistant to aminoglycosides.

Organisms Generally Susceptible to Aminoglycosides						
	Organisms	Amikacin	Gentamicin	Kanamycin	Streptomycin	Tobramycin
Gram-positive	*Mycobacterium tuberculosis*	✓[a]			✓[b]	
	Staphylococci	✓[c]	✓[c]			✓
	S. aureus	✓	✓	✓[c]		✓
	S. epidermidis	✓		✓		
	Streptococci				✓[b]	
	S. faecalis		✓[b]		✓[b]	✓[b]
Gram-negative	*Acinetobacter* sp.	✓		✓		
	Brucella sp.				✓	
	Citrobacter sp.	✓	✓	✓	✓	✓
	Enterobacter sp.	✓	✓	✓	✓	✓
	Escherichia coli	✓	✓	✓	✓	✓
	Hemophilus influenzae	✓		✓	✓[b]	
	Hemophilus ducreyi				✓	
	Klebsiella sp.	✓	✓	✓	✓[b]	✓
	Morganella morganii					✓
	Neisseria sp.	✓		✓	✓	
	Proteus sp.	✓[d]	✓[d]	✓[d]	✓	✓[d]
	Providencia sp.	✓	✓	✓	✓	✓
	Pseudomonas sp.	✓				
	P. aeruginosa	✓	✓[b]		✓	✓
	Salmonella sp.	✓	✓	✓	✓	✓
	Serratia sp.	✓	✓	✓	✓	✓
	Shigella sp.	✓	✓	✓	✓	✓
	Yersinia (Pasteurella) pestis	✓	✓	✓	✓	✓

[a] ✓ = generally susceptible.
[b] Usually used concomitantly with other anti-infectives.
[c] Penicillinase-producing and nonpenicillinase-producing.
[d] Indole-positive and indole-negative.

Contraindications

Previous reactions to these agents. With the exception of the use of streptomycin in tuberculosis, these agents are generally not indicated in long-term therapy because of the ototoxic and nephrotoxic hazards of extended administration.

Warnings

➤*Burn patients:* In patients with extensive burns, altered pharmacokinetics may result in reduced serum concentrations of aminoglycosides. In such patients, measurement of serum concentration is especially important for dosage determination.

➤*Hypomagnesemia:* This may occur in more than one third of patients whose oral diet is restricted or who are eating poorly.

➤*Neuromuscular blockade:* Neurotoxicity can occur after intrapleural and interperitoneal installation of large doses of an aminoglycoside; however, the reaction has followed IV, IM, and oral administration. Aminoglycosides may aggravate muscle weakness because of a potential curare-like effect on the neuromuscular junction. Use with caution in patients with neuromuscular disorders (eg, infant botulism, myasthenia gravis, parkinsonism).

Neuromuscular blockade resulting in respiratory paralysis has occurred with aminoglycosides, especially if given with or soon after anesthesia or muscle relaxants (see Drug Interactions).

During or following gentamicin therapy, paresthesias, tetany, positive Chvostek and Trousseau signs, and mental confusion have been described in patients with hypomagnesemia, hypocalcemia, and hypokalemia. When this occurred in infants, tetany and muscle weakness occurred. Adults and infants required appropriate corrective electrolyte therapy.

Use caution in newborns of mothers on magnesium sulfate; these hypermagnesemic infants may experience respiratory arrest after receiving aminoglycosides.

➤*Nephrotoxicity:* This may occur. Risk factors include the elderly, patients with a history of renal function impairment who are treated for longer periods or with higher doses than those recommended, a recent course of aminoglycosides (within 6 weeks), concurrent use of other nephrotoxic agents, frequent dosing, potassium depletion, and decreased intravascular volume. Adverse renal effects can occur in patients with initially normal renal function. Of patients receiving an aminoglycoside for several days or more, approximately 8% to 26% will develop mild renal function impairment that is generally reversible.

Because renal function may alter appreciably during therapy, test renal function daily or more frequently. Examine urine for increased excretion of protein and for presence of cells and casts, keeping in mind the effects of the primary illness on these tests. Obtain 1 or more of the following laboratory measurements at the onset of therapy, frequently during therapy and at, or shortly after, the end of therapy: Ccr rate (carefully measured or estimated from published nomograms or equations based on patient's age, sex, body weight, and serial creatinine concentrations; preferred over BUN); serum creatinine concentration (preferred over BUN); BUN. More frequent testing is desirable if renal function is changing. If signs of renal irritation appear, such as casts, white or red cells, and albumin, increase hydration; a dosage reduction may be desirable (see Administration and Dosage for individual agents). These signs usually disappear when treatment is completed. However, if azotemia or a progressive decrease of urine output occurs, stop treatment. Reduce dosage if other evidence of renal dysfunction occurs (decreased Ccr or urine-specific gravity, or increased BUN, creatinine, or oliguria).

The risk of toxic reactions is low in well-hydrated patients with normal renal function who do not receive **gentamicin** or **kanamycin** injections at higher doses or for longer periods of time than recommended.

Hydration – These drugs reach high concentrations in the renal system; keep patients well hydrated to minimize chemical irritation of tubules. Well-hydrated patients with normal renal function have low risk of nephrotoxic reactions if recommended dosage is not exceeded.

Streptomycin, given to patients with preexisting renal insufficiency, calls for extreme caution. In severely uremic patients, a single dose may produce high blood levels for several days, and the cumulative effect may produce ototoxic sequelae. Alkalinize the urine to minimize or prevent renal irritation.

➤*Elderly:* These patients may have reduced renal function that is not evident in the results of routine screening tests, such as BUN or serum creatinine. A Ccr determination may be more useful. Monitoring of renal function and drug levels during treatment is particularly important in such patients.

➤*Pregnancy: Category D* (amikacin, gentamicin, kanamycin, tobramycin). Aminoglycosides can cause fetal harm when given to pregnant women. These agents cross the placenta. Fetal serum levels may reach 16% to 50% of maternal levels. There are reports of total irreversible bilateral congenital deafness in children whose mothers received **streptomycin** during pregnancy. Prolonged use of **gentamicin** during pregnancy may result in otological damage to the fetus. Serious side effects to the mother, fetus, or newborn have not been reported with other aminoglycosides, but the potential for harm exists. Although there is no clearly defined risk, such experience cannot exclude the possibility of infrequent or subtle damage to the fetus. If these drugs are used during pregnancy, or if the patient becomes pregnant while taking these drugs, apprise her of the potential hazards to the fetus.

➤*Lactation:* Small amounts of **streptomycin** and **kanamycin** are excreted in breast milk. Decide whether to discontinue breast-feeding or discontinue the drug, taking into account the importance of the drug to the mother.

➤*Children:* Use with caution in premature infants and neonates because of their renal immaturity and the resulting prolongation of serum half-life of these drugs.

A syndrome of apparent CNS depression, characterized by stupor and flaccidity to coma and deep respiratory depression, has been reported in very young infants given **streptomycin** in doses higher than those recommended. Do not exceed recommended doses in infants.

Precautions

➤*Monitoring:* Collect urine specimens for examination during therapy (see Nephrotoxicity). Monitor peak and trough serum concentrations periodically to assure adequate levels and to avoid potentially toxic levels. Also monitor serum calcium, magnesium, and sodium (see Adverse Reactions).

Eighth cranial nerve function testing – Serial audiometric tests are suggested, particularly when renal function is impaired or prolonged aminoglycoside therapy is required; also repeat such tests periodically after treatment if there is evidence of a hearing deficit or vestibular abnormality before or during therapy, or when consecutive or concomitant use of other potentially ototoxic drugs is unavoidable. Discontinue therapy if tinnitus or subjective hearing loss develops, or if follow-up audiograms show loss of high frequency perception. Aminoglycoside-induced ototoxicity is usually irreversible.

Factors that may increase risk of aminoglycoside-induced ototoxicity include renal function impairment (especially if dialysis is required), excessive dosage, dehydration, coadministration of ethacrynic acid or furosemide, or previous use of other ototoxic drugs.

Cochlear damage usually is manifested initially by small changes in audiometric test results at the high frequencies and may not be associated with subjective hearing loss; vestibular dysfunction is usually manifested by nystagmus, vertigo, nausea, vomiting, or acute Meniere syndrome.

➤*Intrathecal gentamicin:* A patient with multiple sclerosis for 7 years was given intra-lumbar gentamicin; disseminated microscopic brainstem lesions were found at autopsy. Tissue rarefaction and marked swelling of axis cylinders with occasional calcification, loss of oligodendroglia and astroglia, and poor inflammatory response were seen. Use of excessive (40 to 160 mg) doses of intrathecal gentamicin has produced neuromuscular disturbances (eg, ataxia, incontinence, paresis).

➤*Cross-allergenicity:* Occurrence among the aminoglycosides has been demonstrated and depends largely on inactivation by bacterial enzymes.

➤*Syphilis:* In the treatment of sexually transmitted disease, if concomitant syphilis is suspected, perform a darkfield examination before treatment is started. Perform monthly serologic tests for at least 4 months.

➤*Topical use:* Aminoglycosides are quickly and almost totally absorbed when applied topically in association with surgical procedures, except to the urinary bladder. Irreversible deafness, renal failure, and death because of neuromuscular blockade have occurred following irrigation of small and large surgical fields with an aminoglycoside preparation. Consider potential toxicity.

➤*Benzyl alcohol:* This is contained in some of these products as a preservative and has been associated with a fatal "gasping syndrome" in premature infants.

➤*Superinfection:* Use of antibiotics (especially prolonged or repeated therapy) may result in bacterial or fungal overgrowth of nonsusceptible organisms. Such overgrowth may lead to a secondary infection. Take appropriate measures if this occurs.

➤*Sulfite sensitivity:* Some products contain sulfites that may cause allergic-type reactions, including anaphylactic symptoms and life-threatening/less severe asthmatic episodes in susceptible people. Overall prevalence in general population is unknown and probably low. It is more frequent in asthmatics or atopic nonasthmatics.

Drug Interactions

Aminoglycoside Drug Interactions

Precipitant drug	Object drug[a]		Description
Cephalosporins Enflurane Methoxyflurane Vancomycin	Aminoglycosides	↑	Risk of nephrotoxicity may increase above that with aminoglycoside alone. Monitor patients. With cephalosporins, bactericidal activity against certain pathogens may be enhanced (see Administration).
Indomethacin IV	Aminoglycosides	↑	In preterm infants, the use of indomethacin for closure of patent ductus arteriosus resulted in aminoglycoside accumulation in 1 study.
Loop diuretics	Aminoglycosides	↑	Auditory toxicity appears to increase during concomitant use. Hearing loss of varying degrees may occur; it may be irreversible. Monitor patients.
Penicillins	Aminoglycosides	↑	Synergism of these agents is well documented; however, certain penicillins may inactivate certain aminoglycosides. The problem may be highest in vitro (see Administration).
Aminoglycosides	Neuromuscular blockers, depolarizing and nondepolarizing	↑	The neuromuscular blocking effects are enhanced by aminoglycosides. Prolonged respiratory depression may occur.
Aminoglycosides	Polypeptide antibiotics	↑	Concurrent use of these agents may increase the risk of respiratory paralysis and renal dysfunction.

[a] ↑ = Object drug increased.

Adverse Reactions

Aminoglycoside Adverse Reactions (%)

	Adverse reaction	Amikacin	Gentamicin	Kanamycin	Streptomycin	Tobramycin
CNS	Confusion		✓			✓
	Convulsions		✓			
	Disorientation					✓
	Dizziness		✓			✓
	Encephalopathy		✓			
	Fever		✓		✓	✓
	Headache	rare	✓[a]	rare		✓
	Lethargy		✓			✓
	Muscle twitching		✓			
	Myasthenia gravis-like syndrome		✓			
	Neuromuscular blockade[b]	✓		✓	✓	
	Numbness		✓			
	Paresthesia	rare		rare		
	Peripheral neuropathy		✓			
	Skin tingling		✓			
GI	Diarrhea			rare		✓
	Nausea	rare	✓	rare	✓	✓
	Vomiting	rare	✓	rare	✓	✓

Aminoglycoside Adverse Reactions (%)

	Adverse reaction	Amikacin	Gentamicin	Kanamycin	Streptomycin	Tobramycin
Hematologic	Anemia	rare	✓			✓
	Eosinophilia	rare	✓		✓	✓
	Granulocytopenia		✓		✓	✓
	Leukopenia		✓		✓	✓
	Thrombocytopenia		✓		✓	✓
Hypersensitivity	Anaphylaxis/Anaphylactoid reaction		✓		✓	
	Itching		✓			✓
	Rash	rare	✓	rare	✓	✓
	Urticaria		✓		✓	✓
Lab test abnormalities	Increased AST/ALT		✓			✓
	Increased bilirubin		✓			✓
	Increased serum LDH		✓			✓
Renal	Azotemia	✓		✓	✓	
	Casts	✓	✓			
	Decreasing Ccr			✓		
	Oliguria	✓	✓	✓		✓
	Proteinuria	✓	✓	✓		✓
	Red and white cells in urine	✓		✓		
	Rising BUN[b]		✓	✓		✓
	Rising NPN[b]		✓			✓
	Rising serum creatinine[b]	✓	✓	✓		✓
Special senses	Hearing loss/deafness	✓	✓	✓[c]	✓	✓
	Loss of balance	✓		✓[c]		
	Roaring in ears		✓			✓
	Tinnitus		✓			✓
	Vertigo		✓		✓	✓
	Visual disturbances/blurred vision		✓			
Miscellaneous	Acute muscular paralysis	✓		✓		
	Apnea	✓	✓	✓	✓	✓
	Decreased serum Ca, Na, K, Mg[b]		✓			✓
	Drug fever	rare		rare		
	Hypotension	rare	✓			
	Pain/Irritation at injection site		✓	✓		✓

[a] ✓ = Reported; no incidence given.
[b] See Warnings.
[c] Partially reversible to irreversible bilateral hearing loss.

➤*Renal:*

Renal function changes – These are usually reversible upon discontinuation. See Warnings.

➤*Amikacin:*

Miscellaneous – Arthralgia, tremor (rare).

➤*Gentamicin:*

CNS – Acute organic brain syndrome; depression; pseudotumor cerebri; respiratory depression.

GI – Decreased appetite; hypersalivation; stomatitis; weight loss.

Hematologic – Increased and decreased reticulocyte count; transient agranulocytosis.

Hypersensitivity – Generalized burning; laryngeal edema; purpura.

Miscellaneous – Alopecia; arachnoiditis or burning at injection site after intrathecal administration (see Warnings); Fanconi-like syndrome, with aminoaciduria and metabolic acidosis; hypertension; increased CSF protein; joint pain; leg cramps; pulmonary fibrosis; splenomegaly; subcutaneous atrophy or fat necrosis (rare); transient hepatomegaly.

➤*Kanamycin:*

Miscellaneous – Granular casts; "malabsorption syndrome" characterized by an increase in fecal fat, decrease in serum carotene, and fall in xylose absorption (prolonged therapy).

➤*Streptomycin:*

CNS – Facial, circumoral or peripheral paresthesia; muscular weakness.

Hypersensitivity – Angioneurotic edema; exfoliative dermatitis.

Miscellaneous – Amblyopia; hemolytic anemia; hepatic necrosis; myocarditis; pancytopenia; serum sickness; toxic epidermal necrolysis.

➤*Tobramycin:*

Miscellaneous – Cylindruria; delirium; leukocytosis.

Overdosage

➤*Symptoms:* The severity of the signs and symptoms following overdose are dependent on the dose administered, patient's renal function, state of hydration and age, and whether or not other medications with similar toxicities are being administered concurrently. Toxicity may occur in patients treated longer than 10 days or in patients with reduced renal function where dose has not been appropriately adjusted.

Nephrotoxicity following the parenteral administration of an aminoglycoside is most closely related to the area under the curve. Nephrotoxicity is more likely if trough concentrations fail to fall below the intended concentration. Patients who are elderly, have abnormal renal function, are receiving other nephrotoxic drugs, or are volume depleted are at higher risk for developing acute tubular necrosis. Auditory and vestibular toxicities have been associated with aminoglycoside overdose. These toxicities occur in patients treated longer than 10 days, in patients with abnormal renal function, in dehydrated patients, or in patients receiving medications with additive auditory toxicities. These patients may not have signs or symptoms, or may experience dizziness, tinnitus, vertigo, and a loss of high-tone acuity as ototoxicity progresses. Ototoxic signs and symptoms may not begin to occur until long after the drug has been discontinued.

Neuromuscular blockade or respiratory paralysis may occur following aminoglycoside administration. Neuromuscular blockade, respiratory failure, and prolonged respiratory paralysis may occur more commonly in patients with myasthenia gravis or Parkinson disease. Prolonged respiratory paralysis also may occur in patients receiving neuromuscular blockers. If neuromuscular blockade occurs, it may be reversed by the administration of calcium salts but mechanical assistance may be necessary.

If an aminoglycoside were ingested, toxicity would be less likely because they are poorly absorbed from an intact GI tract.

➤*Treatment:* The initial intervention is to establish an airway and ensure oxygenation and ventilation. Initiate resuscitative measures promptly if respiratory paralysis occurs. Adequately hydrate patients and carefully monitor fluid balance, Ccr, and plasma levels.

Peritoneal dialysis or hemodialysis will aid in removal from the blood. This is especially important if renal function is, or becomes, compromised. Hemodialysis is preferable because it is more efficient in reducing serum levels. Complexation with ticarcillin or carbenicillin (12 to 30 g/day) appears as effective as hemodialysis in lowering excessive aminoglycoside serum concentrations. In newborns, consider exchange transfusions.

Range of Aminoglycoside Half-Lives (Hours) During Dialysis[a]

Aminoglycosides	Interdialysis	Hemodialysis	Peritoneal dialysis
Kanamycin	40 to 96	5	12
Gentamicin	21 to 59	6 to 11	5 to 29
Tobramycin	27 to 70	3 to 10	10 to 37
Amikacin	28 to 87	4 to 7	18 to 29

[a] Patient renal function Ccr ≤ 5 mL/min.

STREPTOMYCIN SULFATE

Rx	**Streptomycin Sulfate** (Pfizer)	**Injection:** 400 mg/ml	In 2.5 ml amps.
Rx	**Streptomycin Sulfate** (Pharma-Tek)	**Lyophilized Cake/Powder for Injection:** 200 mg/ml	In 1 g vials.

STREPTOMYCIN SULFATE — INJECTION

For complete and comparative prescribing information, refer to the Aminoglycosides group monograph.

WARNING

The risk of severe neurotoxic reactions is sharply increased in patients with impaired renal function or prerenal azotemia. These include disturbances of vestibular and cochlear function, optic nerve dysfunction, peripheral neuritis, arachnoiditis, and encephalopathy. The incidence of clinically detectable, irreversible vestibular damage is particularly high in patients treated with streptomycin.

Renal function should be monitored carefully; patients with renal impairment and/or nitrogen retention should receive reduced doses. The peak serum concentration in individuals with kidney damage should not exceed 20 to 25 mcg/mL.

The concurrent or sequential use of other neurotoxic and/or nephrotoxic drugs with streptomycin sulfate, including neomycin, kanamycin, gentamicin, cephaloridine, paromomycin, viomycin, polymyxin B, colistin, tobramycin, and cyclosporine should be avoided.

The neurotoxicity of streptomycin can result in respiratory paralysis from neuromuscular blockage, especially when the drug is given soon after the use of anesthesia or muscle relaxants.

The administration of streptomycin in parenteral form should be reserved for patients where adequate laboratory and audiometric testing facilities are available during therapy.

Indications

➤*Mycobacterium tuberculosis:* The Advisory Council for the Elimination of Tuberculosis, the American Thoracic Society, and the Centers for Disease Control and Prevention recommend that either streptomycin or ethambutol be added as a fourth drug in a regimen containing isoniazid (INH), rifampin, and pyrazinamide for initial treatment of tuberculosis unless the likelihood of INH or rifampin resistance is very low. The need for a fourth drug should be reassessed when the results of susceptibility testing are known. In the past when the national rate of primary drug resistance to isoniazid was known to be < 4% and was either stable or declining, therapy with 2 and 3 drug regimens was considered adequate. If community rates of INH resistance are currently < 4%, an initial treatment regimen with < 4 drugs may be considered.

Streptomycin is also indicated for therapy of tuberculosis when one or more of the above drugs is contraindicated because of toxicity or intolerance. The management of tuberculosis has become more complex as a consequence of increasing rates of drug resistance and concomitant HIV infection. Additional consultation from experts in the treatment of tuberculosis may be desirable in those settings.

➤*Nontuberculosis infections:* The use of streptomycin should be limited to the treatment of infections caused by bacteria that have been shown to be susceptible to the antibacterial effects of streptomycin and that are not amenable to therapy with less potentially toxic agents. Organisms usually include sensitive *Pasteurella pestis* (plague); *Francisella tularensis* (tularemia); *Brucella*; *Calymmatobacterium granulomatis* (donovanosis, granuloma inguinale); *H. ducreyi* (chancroid); *H. influenzae* (in respiratory, endocardial, and meningeal infections, concomitantly with another antibacterial agent); *K. pneumoniae* pneumonia (concomitantly with another antibacterial agent); *E. coli*, *Proteus*, *A. aerogenes*, *K. pneumoniae*, and *Enterococcus faecalis* in urinary tract infections; *Streptococcus viridans*; *Enterococcus faecalis* (in endocardial infections, concomitantly with penicillin); gram-negative bacillary bacteremia (concomitantly with another antibacterial agent).

➤*Unlabeled uses:* Streptomycin 11 to 13 mg/kg/24 hrs IV or 15 mg/kg/day IM may be used as part of a multiple-drug regimen (generally 3 to 5 agents) for *Mycobacterium avium* complex, a common infection in AIDS patients.

Administration and Dosage

➤*Approved by the FDA:* June 30, 1998.

➤*Method of administration:* IM route only.

The preferred site is the upper outer quadrant of the buttock (ie, gluteus maximus) or the mid-lateral thigh.

It is recommended that IM injections be given preferably in the mid-lateral muscles of the thigh. In infants and small children the periphery of the upper outer quadrant of the gluteal region should be used only when necessary, such as in burn patients, in order to minimize the possibility of damage to the sciatic nerve.

The deltoid area should be used only if well developed such as in certain adults and older children, and then only with caution to avoid radial nerve injury. IM injections should not be made into the lower and mid-third of the upper arm. As with all IM injections, aspiration is necessary to help avoid inadvertent injection into a blood vessel.

Injection sites should be alternated. As higher doses or more prolonged therapy with streptomycin may be indicated for more severe or fulminating infections (endocarditis, meningitis), the physician should always take adequate measures to be immediately aware of any toxic signs or symptoms occurring in the patient as a result of streptomycin therapy.

➤*Tuberculosis:* The standard regimen for the treatment of drug susceptible tuberculosis has been 2 months of INH, rifampin, and pyrazinamide followed by 4 months of INH and rifampin (patients with concomitant infection with tuberculosis and HIV may require treatment for a longer period). When streptomycin is added to this regimen because of suspected or proven drug resistance (see Indications), the recommended dosing for streptomycin is as follows:

Streptomycin Dosage in Tuberculosis

	Daily	Twice daily	Thrice weekly
Children	20 to 40 mg/kg	25 to 30 mg/kg	25 to 30 mg/kg
	Max 1 g	Max 1.5 g	Max 1.5 g
Adults	15 mg/kg	25 to 30 mg/kg	25 to 30 mg/kg
	Max 1 g	Max 1.5 g	Max 1.5 g

Streptomycin is usually administered daily as a single IM injection. A total dose of not more than 120 g over the course of therapy should be given unless there are no other therapeutic options. In patients > 60 years of age the drug should be used at a reduced dosage due to the risk of increased toxicity (see Warning Box).

Therapy with streptomycin may be terminated when toxic symptoms have appeared, when impending toxicity is feared, when organisms become resistant, or when full treatment effect has been obtained. The total period of drug treatment of tuberculosis is a minimum of 1 year; however, indications for terminating therapy with streptomycin may occur at any time as noted above.

➤*Tularemia:* 1 to 2 g daily in divided doses for 7 to 14 days until the patient is afebrile for 5 to 7 days.

➤*Plague:* 2 g of streptomycin daily in 2 divided doses should be administered intramuscularly. A minimum of 10 days of therapy is recommended.

STREPTOMYCIN SULFATE — INJECTION

➤*Bacterial endocarditis:*

Streptococcal endocarditis – In penicillin-sensitive alpha and nonhemolytic streptococcal endocarditis (penicillin MIC ≤ 0.1 mcg/mL), streptomycin may be used for 2-week treatment concomitantly with penicillin. The streptomycin regimen is 1 g twice daily for the first week, and 500 mg twice daily for the second week. If the patient is > 60 years of age, the dosage should be 500 mg twice daily for the entire 2-week period.

Enterococcal endocarditis – Streptomycin in doses of 1 g twice daily for 2 weeks and 500 mg twice daily for an additional 4 weeks is given in combination with penicillin. Ototoxicity may require termination of the streptomycin prior to completion of the 6-week course of treatment.

➤*Concomitant (agents):* For concomitant use with other agents to which the infecting organism is also sensitive, streptomycin is considered a second-line agent for the treatment of gram-negative bacillary bacteremia, meningitis, and pneumonia; brucellosis; granuloma inguinale; chancroid, and urinary tract infection.

Adults – 1 to 2 g in divided doses every 6 to 12 hours for moderate to severe infections. Doses should generally not exceed 2 g/day.

Children – 20 to 40 mg/kg/day (8 to 20 mg/lb/day) in divided doses every 6 to 12 hours. Particular care should be taken to avoid excessive dosage in children.

➤*Storage / Stability:* Store dry powder under controlled room temperature 15° to 30°C (59° to 86°F).

Sterile reconstituted solutions should be protected from light and may be stored at room temperature for 1 week without significant loss of potency.

KANAMYCIN SULFATE

Rx	**Kanamycin Sulfate** (Various, eg, Smith & Nephew)	**Injection**: 500 mg	In 2 ml vials.[a]
Rx	**Kantrex** (Apothecon)		In 2 ml vials.[b]
Rx	**Kanamycin Sulfate** (Various, eg, Smith & Nephew)	**Injection**: 1 g	In 2 ml vials.[a]
Rx	**Kantrex** (Apothecon)		In 3 ml vials.[b]
Rx	**Kanamycin Sulfate** (Various, eg, Smith & Nephew)	**Pediatric Injection**: 75 mg	In 2 ml vials.[a]
Rx	**Kantrex** (Apothecon)		In 2 ml vials.[b]

[a] May contain sulfites.
[b] With sodium bisulfite.

KANAMYCIN SULFATE — INJECTION

For complete and comparative prescribing information, refer to the Aminoglycosides group monograph.

WARNING

Ototoxicity – Patients treated with aminoglycosides by any route should be under close clinical observation because of the potential toxicity associated with their use. As with other aminoglycosides, the major toxic effects of kanamycin sulfate are its action on the auditory and vestibular branches of the eighth nerve and the renal tubules. Neurotoxicity is manifested by bilateral auditory toxicity which often is permanent and, sometimes, by vestibular ototoxicity. Loss of high frequency perception usually occurs before there is noticeable clinical hearing loss and can be detected by audiometric testing. There may not be clinical symptoms to warn of developing cochlear damage. Vertigo may occur and may be evidence of vestibular injury. Other manifestations of neurotoxicity may include numbness, skin tingling, muscle twitching, and convulsions. The risk of hearing loss increases with the degree of exposure to either high peak or high trough serum concentrations and continues to progress after drug withdrawal.

Renal toxicity – Renal impairment may be characterized by decreased creatinine clearance, the presence of cells or casts, oliguria, proteinuria, decreased urine specific gravity, or evidence of increasing nitrogen retention (increasing blood urea nitrogen [BUN], nonprotein nitrogen [NPN], or serum creatinine).

The risks of severe ototoxic and nephrotoxic reactions are sharply increased in patients with impaired renal function and in those with normal renal function who receive high doses or prolonged therapy.

Monitoring – Renal and eighth nerve function should be closely monitored, especially in patients with known or suspected reduced renal function at the onset of therapy, and also in those whose renal function is initially normal but who develop signs of renal dysfunction during therapy. Serum concentrations of parenterally administered aminoglycosides should be monitored when feasible to assure adequate levels and to avoid potentially toxic levels. Urine should be examined for decreased specific gravity, increased excretion of protein, and the presence of cells or casts. BUN, serum creatinine, or creatinine clearance should be measured periodically. Serial audiograms should be obtained when feasible in patients old enough to be tested, particularly high risk patients. Evidence of ototoxicity (dizziness, vertigo, tinnitus, roaring in the ears, and hearing loss) or nephrotoxicity requires dosage adjustment or discontinuance of the drug.

Neuromuscular blockade – Neuromuscular blockade with respiratory paralysis may occur when kanamycin sulfate is instilled intraperitoneally concomitantly with anesthesia and muscle-relaxing drugs. Neuromuscular blockade has been reported following parenteral injection and the oral use of aminoglycosides. The possibility of the occurrence of neuromuscular blockade and respiratory paralysis should be considered if aminoglycosides are administered by any route, especially in patients receiving anesthetics, neuromuscular-blocking agents such as tubocurarine, succinylcholine, decamethonium, or in patients receiving massive transfusions of citrate-anticoagulated blood. If blockage occurs, calcium salts may reduce these phenomena but mechanical respiratory assistance may be necessary.

Concurrent therapy – The concurrent or sequential systemic, oral, or topical use of kanamycin and other potentially nephrotoxic, or neurotoxic drugs, particularly polymyxin B, bacitracin, colistin, amphotericin B, cisplatin, vancomycin, and all other aminoglycosides (including paromomycin) should be avoided because the toxicity may be additive. Other factors which may increase patient risk of toxicity are advanced age and dehydration.

WARNING (cont.)

Kanamycin sulfate should not be given concurrently with potent diuretics (ethacrynic acid, furosemide, meralluride sodium, sodium mercaptomerin, or mannitol). Some diuretics themselves cause ototoxicity, and IV administered diuretics may enhance aminoglycoside toxicity by altering antibiotic concentrations in serum and tissue.

Indications

➤*Initial therapy:*

Known pathogens – Kanamycin may be considered as initial therapy in the treatment of infections where one or more of the following are the known or suspected pathogens: *E. coli*, *Proteus* species (both indole-positive and indole-negative), *Enterobacter aerogenes*, *Klebsiella pneumoniae*, *Serratia marcescens*, *Acinetobacter* species. The decision to continue therapy with the drug should be based on results of the susceptibility tests, the response of the infection to therapy, and the important additional concepts contained in the Warning box.

Unknown pathogens – In serious infections when the causative organisms are unknown, kanamycin may be administered as initial therapy in conjunction with a penicillin- or cephalosporin-type drug before obtaining results of susceptibility testing. If anaerobic organisms are suspected, consideration should be given to using other suitable antimicrobial therapy in conjunction with kanamycin.

➤*Staphylococcal infections:* Although kanamycin is not the drug of choice for staphylococcal infections, it may be indicated under certain conditions for the treatment of known or suspected staphylococcal disease. These situations include the initial therapy of severe infections where the organism is thought to be either a gram-negative bacterium or a *Staphylococcus*, infections due to susceptible strains of staphylococci in patients allergic to other antibiotics, and mixed staphylococcal/gram-negative infections.

➤*Unlabeled uses:* Kanamycin 11 to 13 mg/kg/24 hours IV or 15 mg/kg/day IM may be used as part of a multiple-drug regimen (generally 3 to 5 agents) for *Mycobacterium avium* complex, a common infection in AIDS patients.

Administration and Dosage

Kanamycin injection may be given by IM or IV. The patient's pretreatment body weight should be obtained for calculation of the correct dosage. The dosage of an aminoglycoside in obese patients should be based on an estimate of the lean body mass. The status of renal function should be determined by measurement of serum creatinine concentration or calculation of the endogenous creatinine clearance rate. The BUN level is much less reliable for this purpose. Renal function should be reassessed frequently during therapy.

➤*Therapeutic concentrations:* It is desirable to measure both peak and trough serum concentrations intermittently during therapy because both concentrations are used to determine the adequacy and safety of the dose and to adjust the dosage during treatment. Peak serum concentrations (30 to 90 minutes after injection) above 35 mcg per mL and trough concentrations (just prior to the next dose) above 10 mcg per mL should be avoided.

➤*IM:* Inject deeply into the upper outer quadrant of the gluteal muscle. The recommended dose for adults or children is 15 mg/kg/day in two equally divided dosages administered at equally divided intervals (ie, 7.5 mg/kg every 12 hours). If continuously high blood levels are desired, the daily dose of 15 mg/kg may be given in equally divided doses every 6 or 8 hours. Treatment of patients in the heavier weight classes, ie, 100 kg, should not exceed 1.5 g/day.

➤*Renal function impairment:* In patients with impaired renal function, it is desirable to follow therapy by appropriate serum assays. If this is not feasible, a suggested method is to reduce the frequency of administration in patients with renal dysfunction. The interval between doses may be calculated with the following formula:

KANAMYCIN SULFATE — INJECTION

Serum creatinine (mg/100 mL) × 9 = dosage interval (in hours); eg, if the serum creatinine is 2 mg, the recommended dose (7.5 mg/kg) should be administered every 18 hours. Changes in creatinine concentration during therapy would, of course, necessitate changes in the dosage frequency.

➤*Duration:* It is desirable to limit the duration of treatment with kanamycin to short term. The usual duration of treatment is 7 to 10 days. Total daily dose by all routes of administration should not exceed 1.5 g/day. If longer therapy is required, measurement of kanamycin peak and trough serum concentrations is particularly important as a basis for determining the adequacy and safety of the dose. These patients should be carefully monitored for changes in renal, auditory, and vestibular function. Dosage should be adjusted as needed. The risks of toxicity multiply as the length of treatment increases.

At the recommended dosage level, uncomplicated infections due to kanamycin-susceptible organisms should respond to therapy in 24 to 48 hours. If definite clinical response does not occur within 3 to 5 days, therapy should be stopped and the antibiotic susceptibility pattern of the invading organism should be rechecked. Failure of the infection to respond may be due to resistance of the organism or to the presence of septic foci requiring surgical drainage.

➤*IV:*

Adults – The dose should not exceed 15 mg/kg per day and must be administered slowly. The solution for intravenous use is prepared by adding the contents of a 500 mg vial to 100 to 200 mL of sterile diluent such as normal saline or 5% dextrose in water, or the contents of a 1 g vial to 200 to 400 mL of sterile diluent. The appropriate dose is administered over a 30- to 60-minute period. The total daily dose should be divided into 2 or 3 equally divided doses.

Children – In pediatric patients the amount of diluent used should be sufficient to infuse the kanamycin sulfate over a 30- to 60-minute period.

➤*Admixture incompatibility:* Kanamycin sulfate injection, USP should not be physically mixed with other antibacterial agents but each should be administered separately in accordance with its recommended route of administration and dosage schedule.

➤*Intraperitoneal use:* Following exploration for established peritonitis or after peritoneal contamination due to fecal spill during surgery.

Adults – 500 mg diluted in 20 mL sterile distilled water may be instilled through a polyethylene catheter sutured into the wound at closure. If possible, installation should be postponed until the patient has fully recovered from the effects of anesthesia and muscle-relaxing drugs (see duration of treatment statement above and Warning box). Serum levels should be carefully monitored during treatment.

➤*Aerosol treatment:* 250 mg 2 to 4 times a day. Withdraw 250 mg (1 mL) from a 500 mg vial and dilute it with 3 mL physiological saline and nebulize. Serum levels should be carefully monitored during treatment.

➤*Other routes of administration:* Kanamycin injection in concentrations of 0.25% (2.5 mg/mL) has been used as an irrigating solution in abscess cavities, pleural space, peritoneal and ventricular cavities. Possible absorption of kanamycin by such routes must be taken into account and dosage adjustments should be arranged so that a maximum total dose of 1.5 g/day by all routes of administration is not exceeded. Serum levels should be carefully monitored during treatment.

➤*Storage/Stability:* Occasionally, some vials may darken during the shelf-life of the product, but this does not indicate a loss of potency.

GENTAMICIN

Rx	**Gentamicin Sulfate** (Various, eg, Fujisawa, Major, Moore, Taylor)	**Injection:** 40 mg/mL (as sulfate)	In 2 and 20 mL vials and 1.5 and 2 mL cartridge-needle units.
Rx	**Gentamicin Sulfate** (Hospira)	**Injection:** 10 mg/mL (as sulfate)	In *ADD-Vantage* 60, 80, and 100 mg vials.
Rx	**Pediatric Gentamicin Sulfate** (Fujisawa)		In 2 mL vials.
Rx	**Gentamicin Sulfate in 0.9% Sodium Chloride** (Hospira)	**Injection:** 0.8 mg/mL (as gentamicin base)	In 100 mL single-dose flexible containers.
		0.9 mg/mL (as gentamicin base)	In 100 mL single-dose flexible containers.
		1 mg/mL (as gentamicin base)	In 100 mL single-dose flexible containers.
		1.2 mg/mL (as gentamicin base)	In 50 mL single-dose flexible containers.
		1.4 mg/mL (as gentamicin base)	In 50 mL single-dose flexible containers.
		1.6 mg/mL (as gentamicin base)	In 50 mL single-dose flexible containers.

GENTAMICIN SULFATE — INJECTION

For complete and comparative prescribing information, refer to the Aminoglycosides, Parenteral group monograph.

WARNING

Patients treated with aminoglycosides should be under close clinical observation because of the potential toxicity associated with their use.

As with other aminoglycosides, gentamicin sulfate injectable is potentially nephrotoxic. The risk of nephrotoxicity is greater in patients with impaired renal function and in those who receive high dosage or prolonged therapy.

Neurotoxicity manifested by ototoxicity, both vestibular and auditory, can occur in patients treated with gentamicin sulfate injectable, primarily in those with preexisting renal damage and in patients with healthy renal function treated with higher doses and/or for longer periods than recommended. Aminoglycoside-induced ototoxicity is usually irreversible. Other manifestations of neurotoxicity may include numbness, skin tingling, muscle twitching, and convulsions.

Renal and eighth cranial nerve functions should be closely monitored, especially in patients with known or suspected reduced renal function at onset of therapy, and also in those whose renal function is initially healthy but who develop signs of renal dysfunction during therapy. Urine should be examined for decreased specific gravity, increased excretion of protein, and the presence of cells or casts. Blood urea nitrogen, serum creatine, or creatine clearance should be determined periodically. When feasible, it is recommended that serial audiograms be obtained in patients old enough to be tested, particularly high-risk patients. Evidence of ototoxicity (dizziness, vertigo, ataxia, tinnitus, roaring in the ears, or hearing loss) or nephrotoxicity requires dosage adjustment or discontinuance of the drug. As with the other aminoglycosides, on rare occasions changes in renal and eighth cranial nerve function may not become manifest until soon after completion of therapy.

Serum concentrations of aminoglycosides should be monitored when feasible to ensure adequate levels and to avoid potentially toxic levels. When monitoring gentamicin peak concentrations, dosage should be adjusted so that prolonged levels above 12 mcg/mL are avoided. When monitoring gentamicin trough concentrations, dosage should be adjusted so that levels above 2 mcg/mL are avoided. Excessive peak or trough serum concentrations of aminoglycosides may increase the risk of renal and eighth cranial nerve toxicity. In the event of overdose or toxic reactions, hemodialysis may aid in the removal of gentamicin from the blood, especially if renal function is, or becomes, compromised. The rate of removal of gentamicin is considerably less by peritoneal dialysis than by hemodialysis.

WARNING (cont.)

Concurrent and/or sequential systemic or topical use of other potentially neurotoxic and/or nephrotoxic drugs, such as cisplatin, cephaloridine, kanamycin, amikacin, neomycin, polymyxin B, colistin, paromomycin, streptomycin, tobramycin, vancomycin, and viomycin, should be avoided. Other factors which may increase patient risk of toxicity are advanced age and dehydration.

The concurrent use of gentamicin with potent diuretics, such as ethacrynic acid or furosemide, should be avoided, because certain diuretics by themselves may cause ototoxicity. In addition, when administered intravenously, diuretics may enhance aminoglycoside toxicity by altering the antibiotic concentration in serum and tissue.

Indications

➤*Serious infections:* In the treatment of serious infections caused by susceptible strains of the following microorganisms: *Pseudomonas aeruginosa*, *Proteus* species (indole-positive and indole-negative), *Escherichia coli*, *Klebsiella-Enterobacter-Serratia* species, *Citrobacter* species, and *Staphylococcus* species (coagulase-positive and coagulase-negative).

Clinical studies have shown gentamicin sulfate injectable to be effective in bacterial neonatal sepsis; bacterial septicemia; and serious bacterial infections of the central nervous system (meningitis), urinary tract, respiratory tract, gastrointestinal tract (including peritonitis), skin, bone, and soft tissue (including burns). Aminoglycosides, including gentamicin, are not indicated in uncomplicated initial episodes of urinary tract infections unless the causative organisms are susceptible to these antibiotics and are not susceptible to antibiotics having less potential for toxicity.

Specimens for bacterial culture should be obtained to isolate and identify causative organisms and to determine their susceptibility to gentamicin.

➤*Gram-negative infections:* As initial therapy in suspected or confirmed gram-negative infections, and therapy may be instituted before obtaining results of susceptibility testing. The decision to continue therapy with this drug should be based on the results of susceptibility tests, the severity of the infection, and the important additional concepts contained in the warning box. If the causative organisms are resistant to gentamicin, other appropriate therapy should be instituted.

➤*Unknown pathogens:* In serious infections when the causative organisms are unknown, gentamicin sulfate injectable may be administered as initial therapy in conjunction with a penicillin-type or cephalosporin-type drug before obtaining results of susceptibility testing. If anaerobic organisms are suspected as etiologic agents, consideration should be given to using other suitable antimicrobial therapy in conjunction with gentamicin.

GENTAMICIN SULFATE — INJECTION

Following identification of the organism and its susceptibility, appropriate antibiotic therapy should then be continued.

➤*Combination therapy:* In combination with carbenicillin for the treatment of life-threatening infections caused by *Pseudomonas aeruginosa*. It has also been found effective when used in conjunction with a penicillin-type drug for the treatment of endocarditis caused by group D streptococci.

➤*Staphylococcal infections:* Treatment of serious staphylococcal infections. While not the antibiotic of first choice, gentamicin sulfate injectable may be considered when penicillins or other less potentially toxic drugs are contraindicated and bacterial susceptibility tests and clinical judgment indicate its use. It may also be considered in mixed infections caused by susceptible strains of staphylococci and gram-negative organisms.

In the neonate with suspected bacterial sepsis or staphylococcal pneumonia, a penicillin-type drug is also usually indicated as concomitant therapy with gentamicin.

➤*Unlabeled uses:* An alternative regimen for pelvic inflammatory disease is gentamicin 2 mg/kg IV followed by 1.5 mg/kg 3 times daily (healthy renal function) plus clindamycin 600 mg IV 4 times daily. Continue for at least 4 days and at least 48 hours after patient improves; then continue clindamycin 450 mg orally 4 times daily for 10 to 14 days total therapy.

Administration and Dosage

Gentamicin sulfate injectable may be given intramuscularly or intravenously. The patient's pretreatment body weight should be obtained for calculation of correct dosage. The dosage of aminoglycosides in obese patients should be based on an estimate of the lean body mass. It is desirable to limit the duration of treatment with aminoglycosides to short term.

Parenteral drug products should be inspected visually for particulate matter and discoloration prior to administration, whenever solution and container permit.

➤*Dosage for patients with healthy renal function:*

Children – 6 to 7.5 mg/kg/day. (2 to 2.5 mg/kg administered every 8 hours.)

Infants and neonates – 7.5 mg/kg/day. (2.5 mg/kg administered every 8 hours.)

Premature or full-term neonates 1 week of age or less – 5 mg/kg/day. (2.5 mg/kg administered every 12 hours.) It is desirable to measure periodically both peak and trough serum concentrations of gentamicin when feasible during therapy to assure adequate but not excessive drug levels. For example, the peak concentration (at 30 to 60 minutes after intramuscular injection) is expected to be in the range of 4 to 6 mcg/mL. When monitoring peak concentrations after intramuscular or intravenous administration, dosage should be adjusted so that prolonged levels above 12 mcg/mL are avoided. When monitoring trough concentrations (just prior to the next dose), dosage should be adjusted so that levels above 2 mcg/mL are avoided. Determination of the adequacy of a serum level for a particular patient must take into consideration the susceptibility of the causative organism, the severity of the infection, and the status of the patient's host-defense mechanisms.

In patients with extensive burns, altered pharmacokinetics may result in reduced serum concentrations of aminoglycosides. In such patients treated with gentamicin, measurement of serum concentrations is recommended as a basis for dosage adjustment.

The usual duration of treatment for all patients is 7 to 10 days. In difficult and complicated infections, a longer course of therapy may be necessary. In such cases, monitoring of renal, auditory, and vestibular functions is recommended, because toxicity is more apt to occur with treatment extended for more than 10 days. Dosage should be reduced if clinically indicated. A regimen of either 2.5 mg/kg every 18 hours or 3 mg/kg every 24 hours may also provide satisfactory peak and trough levels in preterm infants less than 32 weeks gestational age.

Adults – The recommended dosage of gentamicin sulfate injectable for patients with serious infections and healthy renal function is 3 mg/kg/day, administered in 3 equal doses every 8 hours (see table below).

For patients with life-threatening infections, dosages up to 5 mg/kg/day may be administered in 3 or 4 equal doses. This dosage should be reduced to 3 mg/kg/day as soon as clinically indicated (see table below).

Dosage Schedule Guide for Adults with Healthy Renal Function (Dosage at 8-Hour Intervals), 40 mg per mL

Patient's weight[a]		Usual dose for serious infections 1 mg/kg every 8 hours (3 mg/kg/day)		Dose for life-threatening infections (reduce as soon as clinically indicated) 1.7 mg/kg every 8 hours[b] (5 mg/kg/day)	
kg	lb	mg/dose	mL/dose	mg/dose	mL/dose
40	88	40	1	66	1.6
45	99	45	1.1	75	1.9
50	110	50	1.25	83	2.1
55	121	55	1.4	91	2.25
60	132	60	1.5	100	2.5
65	143	65	1.6	108	2.7
70	154	70	1.75	116	2.9
75	165	75	1.9	125	3.1
80	176	80	2	133	3.3
85	187	85	2.1	141	3.5
90	198	90	2.25	150	3.75
95	209	95	2.4	158	4
100	220	100	2.5	166	4.2

[a] The dosage of aminoglycosides in obese patients should be based on an estimate of lean body mass.
[b] For every-6-hour schedules, dosage should be recalculated.

Dosing interval – Although further studies are needed, preliminary evidence indicates that aminoglycosides may be administered on a once daily basis without compromising efficacy and without increasing the potential for nephrotoxicity and ototoxicity. It is possible that the incidence of nephrotoxicity may even be decreased.

➤*For intravenous administration:* The intravenous administration of gentamicin may be particularly useful for treating patients with bacterial septicemia or those in shock. It may also be the preferred route of administration for some patients with congestive heart failure, hematologic disorders, severe burns, or those with reduced muscle mass. For intermittent intravenous administration in adults, a single dose of gentamicin sulfate injectable may be diluted in 50 to 200 mL of sterile isotonic saline solution or in a sterile solution of dextrose 5% in water. For intermittent intravenous administration, a single dose of gentamicin sulfate pediatric injectable may be diluted in sterile isotonic saline solution or in a sterile solution of dextrose 5% in water.

The recommended dosage for intravenous and intramuscular administration is identical.

Gentamicin sulfate injectable should not be physically premixed with other drugs, but should be administered separately in accordance with the recommended route of administration and dosage schedule.

➤*Dosage for patients with impaired renal function:* Dosage must be adjusted in patients with impaired renal function to ensure therapeutically adequate, but not excessive, blood levels. Whenever possible, serum concentrations of gentamicin should be monitored. One method of dosage adjustment is to increase the interval between administration of the usual doses. Because the serum creatinine concentration has a high correlation with the serum half-life of gentamicin, this laboratory test may provide guidance for adjustment of the interval between doses. In adults, the interval between doses (in hours) may be approximated by multiplying the serum creatinine level (mg/100 mL) by 8. For example, a patient weighing 60 kg with a serum creatinine level of 2 mg/100 mL could be given 60 mg (1 mg/kg) every 16 hours (2×8). These guidelines may be considered when treating infants and children with serious renal impairment.

In patients with serious systemic infections and renal impairment, it may be desirable to administer the antibiotic more frequently but in reduced dosage. In such patients, serum concentrations of gentamicin should be measured so that adequate but not excessive levels result. A peak and trough concentration measured intermittently during therapy will provide optimal guidance for adjusting dosage. After the usual initial dose, a rough guide for determining reduced dosage at 8-hour intervals is to divide the normally recommended dose by the serum creatinine level (see table below). For example, after an initial dose of 60 mg (1 mg/kg), a patient weighing 60 kg with a serum creatinine level of 2 mg/100 mL could be given 30 mg every 8 hours (60 divided by 2). After an initial dose of 20 mg (2 mg/kg), a child weighing 10 kg with a serum creatinine level of 2 mg/100 mL could be given 10 mg every 8 hours (20 divided by 2). It should be noted that the status of renal function may be changing over the course of the infectious process.

It is important to recognize that deteriorating renal function may require a greater reduction in dosage than that specified in the above guidelines for patients with stable renal impairment.

Dosage Adjustment Guide for Patients with Renal Impairment (Dosage at 8-Hour Intervals After the Usual Initial Dose)

Serum creatinine (mg %)	Approximate creatinine clearance rate (mL/min/1.73 m^2)	Percent of usual doses shown above
≤ 1	> 100	100
1.1 to 1.3	70 to 100	80
1.4 to 1.6	55 to 70	65
1.7 to 1.9	45 to 55	55
2 to 2.2	40 to 45	50
2.3 to 2.5	35 to 40	40
2.6 to 3	30 to 35	35
3.1 to 3.5	25 to 30	30
3.6 to 4	20 to 25	25

GENTAMICIN SULFATE — INJECTION

Dosage Adjustment Guide for Patients with Renal Impairment (Dosage at 8-Hour Intervals After the Usual Initial Dose)		
Serum creatinine (mg %)	Approximate creatinine clearance rate (mL/min/1.73 m^2)	Percent of usual doses shown above
4.1 to 5.1	15 to 20	20
5.2 to 6.6	10 to 15	15
6.7 to 8	< 10	10

In adults with renal failure undergoing hemodialysis, the amount of gentamicin removed from the blood may vary depending upon several factors including the dialysis method used. An 8-hour hemodialysis may reduce serum concentrations of gentamicin by approximately 50%. The recommended dosage at the end of each dialysis period is 1 to 1.7 mg/kg depending upon the severity of infection. In children, a dose of 2 mg/kg may be administered. In children the recommended dose at the end of each dialysis period is 2 to 2.5 mg/kg depending upon the severity of infection.

The above dosage schedules are not intended as rigid recommendations but are provided as guides to dosage when the measurement of gentamicin serum levels is not feasible.

A variety of methods are available to measure gentamicin concentrations in body fluids; these include microbiologic, enzymatic and radioimmunoassay techniques.

➤*Storage/Stability:* Store at controlled room temperature 15° to 30°C (59° to 86°F).

TOBRAMYCIN

Rx	**Tobramycin in 0.9% Sodium Chloride** (Hospira)	**Injection:** 0.8 mg/mL (as sulfate)	In 100 mL single-dose flexible containers.
		1.2 mg/mL (as sulfate)	In 50 mL single-dose flexible containers.
Rx	**Tobramycin Sulfate Pediatric** (Various, eg, Hospira, Apothecon)	**Solution for Injection:** 10 mg/ml	In 2 ml vials.
		40 mg/ml	In 1.5 and 2 ml syringes and 2 and 30 ml vials.
Rx	**Tobramycin Sulfate** (American Pharmaceutical Partners)	**Powder for injection:** 1.2 g (40 mg/mL after reconstitution)	Preservative free. In 50 mL pharmacy bulk package vial.
Rx	**TOBI** (PathoGenesis)	**Nebulizer solution:** 300 mg/5 ml	In 5 ml ampules.[a]

[a] With sodium chloride, sulfuric acid and sodium hydroxide.

TOBRAMYCIN — INJECTION

Information beginning in the Aminoglycoside group monograph must be considered when using these products.

WARNING

Keep patients treated with tobramycin injection and other aminoglycosides under close clinical observation because these drugs have an inherent potential for causing ototoxicity and nephrotoxicity.

Ototoxicity – Neurotoxicity, manifested as both auditory and vestibular ototoxicity, can occur. The auditory changes are irreversible, are usually bilateral, and may be partial or total. Eighth nerve impairment and nephrotoxicity may develop, primarily in patients having preexisting renal damage and in those with healthy renal function to whom aminoglycosides are administered for longer periods or in higher doses than those recommended. Other manifestations of neurotoxicity may include numbness, skin tingling, muscle twitching, and convulsions. The risk of aminoglycoside-induced hearing loss increases with the degree of exposure to either high peak or high trough serum concentrations. Patients who develop cochlear damage may not have symptoms during therapy to warn them of eighth-nerve toxicity, and partial or total irreversible bilateral deafness may continue to develop after the drug has been discontinued. Rarely, nephrotoxicity may not become apparent until the first few days after cessation of therapy. Aminoglycoside-induced nephrotoxicity usually is reversible.

Monitoring – Closely monitor renal and eighth nerve function in patients with known or suspected renal impairment and also in those whose renal function is initially normal but who develop signs of renal dysfunction during therapy. Periodically monitor peak and trough serum concentrations of aminoglycosides during therapy to assure adequate levels and to avoid potentially toxic levels. Prolonged serum concentrations above 12 mcg/mL should be avoided. Rising trough levels (above 2 mcg/mL) may indicate tissue accumulation. Such accumulation, excessive peak concentrations, advanced age, and cumulative dose may contribute to ototoxicity and nephrotoxicity. Examine urine for decreased specific gravity and increased excretion of protein, cells, and casts. Periodically measure serum urea nitrogen (BUN), serum creatinine, and creatinine clearance. When feasible, it is recommended that serial audiograms be obtained in patients old enough to be tested, particularly high-risk patients. Evidence of impairment of renal, vestibular, or auditory function requires discontinuation of the drug or dosage adjustment.

Use tobramycin injection with caution in premature and neonatal infants because of their renal immaturity and the resulting prolongation of serum half-life of the drug.

Concurrent therapy – Avoid concurrent and sequential use of other neurotoxic or nephrotoxic antibiotics, particularly other aminoglycosides (eg, amikacin, streptomycin, neomycin, kanamycin, gentamicin, paromomycin), cephaloridine, viomycin, polymyxin B, colistin, cisplatin, and vancomycin. Other factors that may increase patient risk are advanced age and dehydration.

Do not give aminoglycosides concurrently with potent diuretics, such as ethacrynic acid and furosemide. Some diuretics themselves cause ototoxicity, and intravenously (IV) administered diuretics enhance aminoglycoside toxicity by altering antibiotic concentrations in serum and tissue.

Pregnancy – Aminoglycosides can cause fetal harm when administered to a pregnant woman.

Indications

➤*Septicemia:* Septicemia in the pediatric patient and adult caused by *Pseudomonas aeruginosa*, *Escherichia coli*, and *Klebsiella* sp.

➤*Lower respiratory tract infections:* Lower respiratory tract infections caused by *P. aeruginosa*, *Klebsiella* sp., *Enterobacter* sp., *Serratia* sp., *E. coli*, and *Staphylococcus aureus* (penicillinase- and non-penicillinase-producing strains).

➤*Serious CNS infections (meningitis):* Serious CNS infections (meningitis) caused by susceptible organisms.

➤*Intra-abdominal infections:* Intra-abdominal infections, including peritonitis, caused by *E. coli*, *Klebsiella* sp., and *Enterobacter* sp.

➤*Skin, bone, and skin structure infections:* Skin, bone, and skin structure infections caused by *P. aeruginosa*, *Proteus* sp., *E. coli*, *Klebsiella* sp., *Enterobacter* sp., and *S. aureus*.

➤*Complicated and recurrent urinary tract infections:* Complicated and recurrent urinary tract infections caused by *P. aeruginosa*, *Proteus* sp. (indole-positive and indole-negative), *E. coli*, *Klebsiella* sp., *Enterobacter* sp., *Serratia* sp., *S. aureus*, *Providencia* sp., and *Citrobacter* sp.

Aminoglycosides, including tobramycin injection, are not indicated in uncomplicated initial episodes of urinary tract infections unless the causative organisms are not susceptible to antibiotics having less potential toxicity. Tobramycin injection may be considered in serious staphylococcal infections when penicillin or other potentially less toxic drugs are contraindicated, and when bacterial susceptibility testing and clinical judgment indicate its use.

Administration and Dosage

➤*Approved by the FDA:* April 9, 1989.

Tobramycin injection may be given intramuscularly (IM) or IV. Recommended dosages are the same for both routes. Obtain the patient's pretreatment body weight for calculation of correct dosage. It is desirable to measure both peak and trough serum concentrations.

➤*Dosage:*

Adults with serious infections – 3 mg/kg/day in 3 equal doses every 8 hours.

Adults with life-threatening infections – Up to 5 mg/kg/day may be administered in 3 or 4 equal doses (see dosage guidelines in the following table). The dosage should be reduced to 3 mg/kg/day as soon as clinically indicated. To prevent increased toxicity due to excessive blood levels, dosage should not exceed 5 mg/kg/day unless serum levels are monitored.

Children (older than 1 week of age) – 6 to 7.5 mg/kg/day in 3 or 4 equally divided doses (2 to 2.5 mg/kg every 8 hours or 1.5 to 1.89 mg/kg every 6 hours).

Premature or full-term neonates 1 week of age or younger – Up to 4 mg/kg/day may be administered in 2 equal doses every 12 hours.

Cystic fibrosis – In patients with cystic fibrosis, altered pharmacokinetics may result in reduced serum concentrations of aminoglycosides. Measurement of tobramycin serum concentration during treatment is especially important as a basis for determining appropriate dose. In patients with severe cystic fibrosis, an initial dosing regimen of 10 mg/kg/day in 4 equally divided doses is recommended. This dosing regimen is suggested only as a guide. Measure the serum levels of tobramycin directly during treatment due to wide interpatient variability.

➤*Duration:* It is desirable to limit treatment to a short term. The usual duration of treatment is 7 to 10 days. A longer course of therapy may be necessary in difficult and complicated infections. In such cases, monitoring of renal, auditory, and vestibular functions is advised because neurotoxicity is more likely to occur when treatment is extended longer than 10 days.

➤*Renal function impairment:* Whenever possible, monitor serum tobramycin concentrations during therapy.

TOBRAMYCIN — INJECTION

Following a loading dose of 1 mg/kg, subsequent dosage in these patients must be adjusted, either with reduced doses administered at 8-hour intervals or with normal doses given at prolonged intervals. Both of these methods are suggested as guides to be used when serum levels of tobramycin cannot be measured directly. They are based on either the creatinine clearance level or the serum creatinine level of the patient because these values correlate with the half-life of tobramycin. Use the dosage schedule derived from either method in conjunction with careful clinical and laboratory observations of the patient and modify as necessary. Do not use either method when dialysis is being performed.

Reduced dosage at 8-hour intervals – When the creatinine clearance rate (Ccr) is less than or equal to 70 mL/min, or when the serum creatinine value is known, the amount of the reduced dose can be determined by multiplying the normal dose from the dosage guidelines for adults with healthy renal function by the percent of normal dose from the accompanying nomogram.

An alternate rough guide for determining reduced dosage at 8-hour intervals (for patients whose steady-state serum creatinine values are known) is to divide the normally recommended dose by the patient's serum creatinine.

Normal dosage at prolonged intervals – If the Ccr is not available, and the patient's condition is stable, a dosage frequency in hours for the dosage given in the dosage guidelines for adults with normal renal function can be determined by multiplying the patient's serum creatinine by 6.

➤*Dosage in obese patients:* The appropriate dose may be calculated by using the patient's estimated lean body weight plus 40% of the excess as the basic weight on which to figure mg/kg.

➤*IM administration:* Tobramycin injection may be administered by withdrawing the appropriate dose directly from a vial or by using a prefilled syringe. The pharmacy bulk package and tobramycin in 0.9% sodium chloride is not intended for IM administration.

➤*IV administration:* For IV administration, the usual volume of diluent (0.9% sodium chloride injection or 5% dextrose injection) is 50 to 100 mL for adult doses. For pediatric patients, the volume of diluent should be proportionately less than that for adults. The diluted solution usually should be infused over a period of 20 to 60 minutes. Infusion periods of less than 20 minutes are not recommended because peak serum levels may exceed 12 mcg/mL and should be avoided. Such accumulation, excessive peak concentrations, advanced age, and cumulative dose may contribute to ototoxicity and nephrotoxicity.

➤*Admixture incompatibility:* Do not physically premix tobramycin injection with other drugs, but administer separately according to the recommended dose and route.

➤*Storage/Stability:* Store at controlled room temperature 20° to 25°C (68° to 77°F).

TOBRAMYCIN — SOLUTION FOR INHALATION

Information beginning in the Aminoglycoside group monograph must be considered when using these products.

Indications

➤*Cystic fibrosis:* For the management of cystic fibrosis patients with *P. aeruginosa*.

Safety and efficacy have not been demonstrated in patients under the age of 6 years, patients with $FEV_1 < 25\%$ or greater than 75% predicted, or patients colonized with *Burkholderia cepacia*.

Administration and Dosage

➤*Approved by the FDA:* December 22, 1997.

➤*Dosage:* The recommended dosage for both adults and pediatric patients at least 6 years of age is 1 single-use ampule (300 mg) administered twice daily for 28 days. Dosage is not adjusted by weight. All patients should be administered 300 mg twice daily. The doses should be taken as close to 12 hours apart as possible; they should not be taken less than 6 hours apart.

➤*Administration:* Tobramycin solution for inhalation is administered by inhalation over a 10- to 15-minute period, using a handheld reusable nebulizer with a compressor.

Tobramycin solution for inhalation is inhaled while the patient is sitting or standing upright and breathing normally through the mouthpiece of the nebulizer. Nose clips may help the patient breathe through the mouth.

Tobramycin solution for inhalation is administered twice daily in alternating periods of 28 days. After 28 days of therapy, patients should stop tobramycin solution for inhalation therapy for the next 28 days, and then resume therapy for the next 28 day on/28 day off cycle.

Tobramycin solution for inhalation is supplied as a single-use ampule and is administered by inhalation, using a handheld reusable nebulizer with a compressor (use only those supplied). Tobramycin solution for inhalation is not for SC, IV or intrathecal administration.

➤*Admixture incompatibility:* You should not mix tobramycin solution for inhalation with dornase alfa in the nebulizer.

➤*Concurrent therapy:* During clinical studies, patients on multiple therapies were instructed to take them first, followed by tobramycin solution for inhalation.

The recommended order is as follows: Bronchodilator first, followed by chest physiotherapy, then other inhaled medications and, finally, tobramycin solution for inhalation.

➤*Storage/Stability:* Tobramycin solution for inhalation should be stored under refrigeration at (2° to 8°C; 36° to 46°F). Upon removal from the refrigerator, or if refrigeration is unavailable, tobramycin solution for inhalation pouches (opened or unopened) may be stored at room temperature (up to 25°C; 77°F) for up to 28 days. Tobramycin solution for inhalation should not be used beyond the expiration date stamped on the ampule when stored under refrigeration (2° to 8°C; 36° to 46°F) or beyond 28 days when stored at room temperature (25°C; 77°F).

Tobramycin solution for inhalation ampules should not be exposed to intense light. The solution in the ampule is slightly yellow, but may darken with age if not stored in the refrigerator; however, the color change does not indicate any change in the quality of the product as long as it is stored within the recommended storage conditions.

You should not use tobramycin solution for inhalation if it is cloudy, if there are particles in the solution, or if it has been stored at room temperature for > 28 days.

AMIKACIN SULFATE

Rx	**Amikacin** (Various, eg, Bedford Labs, Elkins-Sinn)	**Injection**: 250 mg/ml	In 2 and 4 ml vials.[a]
Rx	**Amikin** (Apothecon)		In 2 and 4 ml vials[b] and 2 ml disp syringes.[b]
	Amikacin (Various, eg, Gensia)	**Pediatric Injection**: 50 mg/ml	0.13% sodium metabisulfite, 0.5% sodium citrate dihydrate. In 2 and 4 ml vials.
Rx	**Amikin** (Apothecon)		In 2 ml vials.[b]

[a] May contain sodium metabisulfite, sodium citrate dihydrate or sulfuric acid.

[b] With sodium bisulfite and sulfuric acid.

AMIKACIN — INJECTION

Information beginning in the Aminoglycosides group monograph must be considered when using these products.

WARNING

Patients treated with parenteral aminoglycosides should be under close clinical observation because of the potential ototoxicity and nephrotoxicity associated with their use. Safety for treatment periods which are longer than 14 days has not been established.

Ototoxicity – Neurotoxicity, manifested as vestibular and permanent bilateral auditory ototoxicity, can occur in patients with preexisting renal damage and in patients with normal renal function treated at higher doses and/or periods longer than those recommended. The risk of aminoglycoside-induced ototoxicity is greater in patients with renal damage. High frequency deafness usually occurs first and can be detected only by audiometric testing. Vertigo may occur and may be evidence of vestibular injury. Other manifestations of neurotoxicity may include numbness, skin tingling, muscle twitching, and convulsions. The risk of hearing loss due to aminoglycosides increases with the degree of exposure to either high peak or high trough serum concentrations. Patients developing cochlear damage may not have symptoms during therapy to warn them of developing eighth-nerve toxicity, and total or partial irreversible bilateral deafness may occur after the drug has been discontinued. Aminoglycoside-induced ototoxicity is usually irreversible.

WARNING (cont.)

Nephrotoxicity – Aminoglycosides are potentially nephrotoxic. The risk of nephrotoxicity is greater in patients with impaired renal function and in those who receive high doses or prolonged therapy.

Neuromuscular blockade – Neuromuscular blockade and respiratory paralysis have been reported following parenteral injection, topical instillation (as in orthopedic and abdominal irrigation or in local treatment of empyema), and following oral use of aminoglyosides. The possibility of these phenomena should be considered if aminoglycosides are administered by any route, especially in patients receiving anesthetics, neuromuscular blocking agents such as tubocurarine, succinylcholine, decamethonium, or in patients receiving massive transfusions of citrate-anticoagulated blood. If blockage occurs, calcium salts may reverse these phenomena, but mechanical respiratory assistance may be necessary.

AMIKACIN — INJECTION

WARNING (cont.)

Monitoring – Renal and eighth-nerve function should be closely monitored especially in patients with known or suspected renal impairment at the onset of therapy and also in those whose renal function is initially normal but who develop signs of renal dysfunction during therapy. Serum concentrations of amikacin should be monitored when feasible to assure adequate levels and to avoid potentially toxic levels and prolonged peak concentrations above 35 mcg/mL. Urine should be examined for decreased specific gravity, increased excretion of proteins, and the presence of cells or casts. Blood urea nitrogen, serum creatinine, or creatinine clearance should be measured periodically. Serial audiograms should be obtained where feasible in patients old enough to be tested, particularly high-risk patients. Evidence of ototoxicity (dizziness, vertigo, tinnitus, roaring in the ears, and hearing loss) or nephrotoxicity requires discontinuation of the drug or dosage adjustment.

Concurrent therapy – Concurrent and/or sequential systemic, oral, or topical use of other neurotoxic or nephrotoxic products, particularly bacitracin, cisplatin, amphotericin B, cephaloridine, paromomycin, viomycin, polymyxin B, colistin, vancomycin, or other aminoglycosides should be avoided. Other factors that may increase risk of toxicity are advanced age and dehydration.

The concurrent use of amikacin with potent diuretics (ethacrynic acid, or furosemide) should be avoided because diuretics by themselves may cause ototoxicity. In addition, when administered intravenously, diuretics may enhance aminoglycoside toxicity by altering antibiotic concentrations in serum and tissue.

Indications

➤*Gram-negative infections:* In the short-term treatment of serious infections due to susceptible strains of gram-negative bacteria including *Pseudomonas* species, *Escherichia coli*, species of indole-positive and indole-negative *Proteus*, *Providencia* species, *Klebsiella-Enterobacter-Serratia* species, and *Acinetobacter* (Mima-Herellea) species.

➤*Serious infections:* Clinical studies have shown amikacin to be effective in bacterial septicemia (including neonatal sepsis); in serious infections of the respiratory tract, bones and joints, central nervous system (including meningitis) and skin and soft tissue; intra-abdominal infections (including peritonitis); and in burns and postoperative infections (including post-vascular surgery). Clinical studies have shown amikacin also to be effective in serious complicated and recurrent urinary tract infections due to these organisms. Aminoglycosides, including amikacin injectable, are not indicated in uncomplicated initial episodes of urinary tract infections unless the causative organisms are not susceptible to antibiotics having less potential toxicity.

➤*Suspected gram-negative infections:* Bacteriologic studies should be performed to identify causative organisms and their susceptibilities to amikacin. Amikacin may be considered as initial therapy in suspected gram-negative infections and therapy may be instituted before obtaining the results of susceptibility testing. Clinical trials demonstrated that amikacin was effective in infections caused by gentamicin and/or tobramycin-resistant strains of gram-negative organisms, particularly *Proteus rettgeri*, *Providencia stuartii*, *Serratia marcescens*, and *Pseudomonas aeruginosa*. The decision to continue therapy with the drug should be based on results of the susceptibility tests, the severity of the infection, the response of the patient and the important additional considerations contained in the Warning Box.

➤*Staphylococcal infections:* Amikacin has also been shown to be effective in staphylococcal infections and may be considered as initial therapy under certain conditions in the treatment of known or suspected staphylococcal disease such as, severe infections where the causative organism may be either a gram-negative bacterium or a staphylococcus, infections due to susceptible strains of staphylococci in patients allergic to other antibiotics, and in mixed staphylococcal/gram-negative infections. In certain severe infections such as neonatal sepsis, concomitant therapy with a penicillin-type drug may be indicated because of the possibility of infections due to gram-positive organisms such as streptococci or pneumococci.

➤*Unlabeled uses:* Intrathecal/intraventricular administration has been suggested at 8 mg/24 hours.

Amikacin 15 mg/day IV in divided doses every 8 to 12 hours may be used as a part of a multiple-drug regimen (generally 3 to 5 agents) for *Mycobacterium avium* complex, a common infection in AIDS patients.

In cystic fibrosis patients, the use of inhaled aminoglycosides may be beneficial in certain populations (eg, younger patients). Clinical outcome is not improved, but deterioration of pulmonary function tests may be slowed or prevented.

Administration and Dosage

➤*Approved by the FDA:* May 18, 1992.

The patient's pretreatment body weight should be obtained for calculation of correct dosage. Amikacin may be given intramuscularly or intravenously.

➤*Monitoring:* The status of renal function should be estimated by measurement of the serum creatinine concentration or calculation of the endogenous creatinine clearance rate. The blood urea nitrogen (BUN) is much less reliable for this purpose. Reassessment of renal function should be made periodically during therapy.

Whenever possible, amikacin concentrations in serum should be measured to ensure adequate but not excessive levels. It is desirable to measure both peak and trough serum concentrations intermittently during therapy. Peak concentrations (30 to 90 minutes after injection) above 35 mcg/mL and trough concentrations (just prior to the next dose) above 10 mcg per mL should be avoided. Dosage should be adjusted as indicated.

➤*IM:* The recommended dosage for adults, children and older infants with normal renal function is 15 mg/kg/day divided into 2 or 3 equal doses administered at equally divided intervals (ie, 7.5 mg/kg every 12 hours or 5 mg/kg every 8 hours). Treatment of patients in the heavier weight classes should not exceed 1.5 g/day.

➤*Neonates:* When amikacin is indicated in newborns, it is recommended that a loading dose of 10 mg/kg be administered initially to be followed with 7.5 mg/kg every 12 hours.

➤*Duration:* The usual duration of treatment is 7 to 10 days. It is desirable to limit the duration of treatment to short term whenever feasible. The total daily dose by all routes of administration should not exceed 15 mg/kg/day. In difficult and complicated infections where treatment beyond 10 days is considered, the use of amikacin should be reevaluated. If continued, amikacin serum levels, and renal, auditory, and vestibular functions should be monitored. At the recommended dosage level, uncomplicated infections due to amikacin-sensitive organisms should respond in 24 to 48 hours. If definite clinical response does not occur within 3 to 5 days, therapy should be stopped and the antibiotic susceptibility pattern of the invading organism should be rechecked. Failure of the infection to respond may be due to resistance of the organism or to the presence of septic foci requiring surgical drainage.

➤*Urinary tract infections:* When amikacin is indicated in uncomplicated urinary tract infections, a dose of 250 mg twice daily may be used.

➤*Renal function impairment:* Whenever possible, serum amikacin concentrations should be monitored by appropriate assay procedures. Doses may be adjusted in patients with impaired renal function either by administering normal doses at prolonged intervals or by administering reduced doses at a fixed interval.

Both methods are based on the patient's creatinine clearance or serum creatinine values because these have been found to correlate with aminoglycoside half-lives in patients with diminished renal function. These dosage schedules must be used in conjunction with careful clinical and laboratory observations of the patient and should be modified as necessary. Neither method should be used when dialysis is being performed.

These methods of dosage calculation may be misleading in patients who have undergone severe wasting and in the elderly.

Normal dosage at prolonged intervals – If the creatinine clearance rate is not available and the patient's condition is stable, a dosage interval in hours for the normal dose can be calculated by multiplying the patient's serum creatinine by 9 (eg, if the serum creatinine concentration is 2 mg/100 mL) the recommended single dose (7.5 mg/kg) should be administered every 18 hours.

Reduced dosage at fixed time intervals – When renal function is impaired and it is desirable to administer amikacin at a fixed time interval, dosage must be reduced. In these patients, serum amikacin concentrations should be measured to assure accurate administration of amikacin and to avoid concentrations above 35 mcg/mL. If serum assay determinations are not available and the patients's condition is stable, serum creatinine and creatinine clearance values are the most readily available indicators of the degree of renal impairment to use as a guide for dosage.

First, initiate therapy by administering a normal dose, 7.5 mg/kg, as a loading dose. This loading dose is the same as the normally recommended dose which would be calculated for a patient with normal renal function as described above.

To determine the size of maintenance doses administered every 12 hours, the loading dose should be reduced in proportion to the reduction in the patient's creatinine clearance rate:

$$\text{Maintenance dose every 12 hours} = \frac{\text{observed Ccr (mL/min)}}{\text{normal Ccr (mL/min)}} \times \text{calculated loading dose (mg)}$$

An alternate rough guide for determining reduced dosage at 12-hours intervals (for patients whose steady state serum creatinine values are known) is to divide the normally recommended dose by the patient's serum creatinine.

The above dosage schedules are not intended to be rigid recommendations but are provided as guides to dosage when the measurement of amikacin serum levels is not feasible.

Several predictive methods and published monograms have been compared for gentamicin, none of which performed as well as individualized pharmacokinetic dosing with serum levels. This would probably also be true for amikacin.

Dialysis: Approximately half the normal mg/kg dose can be given after hemodialysis; in peritoneal dialysis, a parenteral dose of 7.5 mg/kg is given, and then amikacin is instilled in peritoneal dialysate at a concentration desired in serum.

➤*IV:*

Adults – The individual dose, the total daily dose, and the total cumulative dose of amikacin are identical to the dose recommended for intramuscular administration. The solution for intravenous use is prepared by adding the contents of a 500 mg vial to 100 or 200 mL of sterile diluent such as 0.9% sodium chloride injection or 5% dextrose injection or any of the compatible solutions listed below.

Single doses of 500 mg (7.5 mg/kg), administered as an infusion over a period of 30 minutes, produced a mean peak serum concentration over a period of 30 minutes, produced a mean peak serum concentration of 38 mcg/mL at the end of the infusion, and levels of 24, 18, and 0.75 mcg/mL

AMIKACIN — INJECTION

at 30 minutes, 1 hour, and 10 hours post-infusion, respectively. Repeat infusions of 7.5 mg/kg every 12 hours were well tolerated and caused no drug accumulation.

The solution is administered to adults over a 30– to 60–minute period. The total daily dose should not exceed 15 mg/kg/day and may be divided into either 2 or 3 equally divided doses at equally divided intervals.

Children – In pediatric patients the amount of fluid used will depend on the amount of amikacin ordered for the patient. It should be a sufficient amount to infuse the amikacin over a 30– to 60–minute period. Infants should receive a 1– to 2–hour infusion.

➤*Compatible IV fluids:* Amikacin is stable for 24 hours at room temperature at concentrations of 0.25 and 5 mg/mL in the following solutions:

- 5% Dextrose Injection
- 5% Dextrose and 0.2% Sodium Chloride Injection
- 5% Dextrose and 0.45% Sodium Chloride Injection
- 0.9% Sodium Chloride Injection
- Lactated Ringer's Injection
- *Normosol M* in 5% Dextrose Injection (or *Plasma-Lyte 56* Injection in 5% Dextrose in Water)
- *Normosol R* in 5% Dextrose Injection (or *Plasma-Lyte 148* Injection in 5% Dextrose in Water)

➤*Admixture incompatibility:* Aminoglycosides administered by any of the above routes should not be physically premixed with other drugs but should be administered separately.

➤*Storage/Stability:* Store at controlled room temperature 15° to 30°C (59° to 86°F).

In the above solutions with amikacin concentrations of 0.25 and 5 mg/mL, solutions aged for 60 days at 4°C (39.2°F) and then stored at 25°C (77°F) had utility times of 24 hours.

At the same concentrations, solutions frozen and aged for 30 days at -15°C (+5°F), thawed, and stored at 25°C (77°F) had utility times of 24 hours.

AMINOGLYCOSIDES, ORAL

For more complete information on aminoglycosides, refer to the Aminoglycosides, Parenteral group monograph. SPECIAL NOTE: See Warning Box in Aminoglycosides, Parenteral group monograph concerning toxicity.

Indications

Suppression of intestinal bacteria.

Hepatic coma.

See individual monographs for specific information.

Actions

➤*Pharmacokinetics:* Oral aminoglycosides are poorly absorbed; therefore use only for suppression of GI bacterial flora. The small absorbed fraction is rapidly excreted with normal kidney function. The unabsorbed drug is eliminated unchanged in the feces. Most intestinal bacteria are rapidly eliminated with bacterial suppression persisting for 48 to 72 hours. Nonpathogenic yeasts and occasionally resistant strains of *Enterobacter aerogenes* replace the intestinal bacteria.

Contraindications

Presence of intestinal obstruction; hypersensitivity to aminoglycosides.

Warnings

➤*Increased absorption:* Although negligible amounts are absorbed through intact mucosa, consider the possibility of increased absorption from ulcerated or denuded areas.

➤*Nephrotoxicity/Ototoxicity:* Because of reported cases of deafness and potential nephrotoxic effects, closely observe patients. Perform urine and blood examinations and audiometric tests prior to and during extended therapy, especially in those with hepatic or renal disease. If renal insufficiency develops, reduce dosage or discontinue the drug. Refer to the Warning Box in the Aminoglycosides, Parenteral monograph concerning aminoglycoside toxicity.

➤*Pregnancy:* Safety for use during pregnancy has not been established. Use only when clearly needed and when the potential benefits outweigh the potential hazards.

Neomycin – Category D. Aminoglycosides can cause fetal harm when administered to a pregnant woman. Aminoglycosides cross the placenta. Although serious side effects to fetus or newborn have not been reported in the treatment of pregnant women, the potential for harm exists. If neomycin is used during pregnancy, or if the patient becomes pregnant while taking this drug, apprise the patient of the potential hazard to the fetus.

➤*Lactation:* Neomycin is excreted in cow milk following a single IM injection. It is not known whether neomycin is excreted in human breast milk. Other aminoglycosides are excreted in human breast milk. Because of the potential for serious adverse reactions from the aminoglycosides in nursing infants, decide whether to discontinue nursing or to discontinue the drug, taking into account the importance of the drug to the mother.

➤*Children:* The safety and efficacy of oral neomycin in patients < 18 years of age have not been established. If treatment is necessary, use with caution; do not exceed a treatment period of 3 weeks because of absorption from the GI tract.

Precautions

➤*Muscular disorders:* Use with caution in patients with muscular disorders such as myasthenia gravis or parkinsonism; these drugs may aggravate muscle weakness because of their potential curare-like effect on neuromuscular junction.

➤*GI effects:*

Neomycin – Orally administered neomycin increases fecal bile acid excretion and reduces intestinal lactase activity.

Paromomycin – Use with caution in individuals with ulcerative lesions of the bowel to avoid renal toxicity through inadvertent absorption.

➤*Superinfection:* Use of antibiotics (especially prolonged or repeated therapy) may result in bacterial or fungal overgrowth of nonsusceptible organisms. Such overgrowth may lead to a secondary infection. Take appropriate measures if superinfection occurs.

Drug Interactions

Oral Aminoglycoside Drug Interactions

Precipitant drug	Object drug*		Description
Aminoglycosides	Anticoagulants	↑	A small rise in warfarin-induced hypoprothrombinemia may occur, possibly due to interference in absorption of dietary vitamin K by aminoglycosides.
Aminoglycosides	Digoxin	↓	Rate and extent of digoxin absorption may be reduced; however, in a small number of patients (< 10%), this may be offset by a reduction in digoxin's metabolism.
Aminoglycosides	Methotrexate	↓	Methotrexate's absorption and bioavailability may be decreased.
Aminoglycosides	Neuromuscular blockers - Depolarizing and nondepolarizing	↑	The actions of the neuromuscular blockers may be enhanced; prolonged respiratory depression may occur.
Aminoglycosides	Polypeptide antibiotics	↑	Concurrent use may increase the risk of respiratory paralysis and renal dysfunction.
Aminoglycosides	Vitamin A	↓	Serum retinol and plasma carotene levels may be decreased.

* ↑ = Object drug increased. ↓ = Object drug decreased.

Adverse Reactions

Nausea, vomiting and diarrhea are most common. The "malabsorption syndrome" characterized by increased fecal fat, decreased serum carotene and fall in xylose absorption has occurred with prolonged therapy. *Clostridium difficile*-associated colitis has occurred following neomycin therapy. Nephrotoxicity and ototoxicity have occurred following prolonged and high dosage therapy in hepatic coma.

Overdosage

Because of low absorption, it is unlikely that acute overdosage would occur with oral neomycin sulfate. However, prolonged administration could result in sufficient systemic drug levels to produce neurotoxicity, ototoxicity or nephrotoxicity. Hemodialysis will remove neomycin sulfate from the blood.

Patient Information

Complete full course of therapy; take until gone. May cause nausea, vomiting or diarrhea.

Notify physician if ringing in the ears, hearing impairment or rash, problems urinating or dizziness occurs.

Drink plenty of fluids.

➤*Neomycin:* Before administering the drug, inform patients or members of their families of possible toxic effects on the eighth cranial nerve. The possibility of acute toxicity increases in premature infants and neonates.

KANAMYCIN SULFATE

Rx	**Kantrex** (Apothecon)	**Capsules:** 500 mg (as sulfate)	Lactose. In 20s & 100s.

KANAMYCIN SULFATE — ORAL

For complete and comparative prescribing information, refer to the Aminoglycosides, Oral group monograph.

Indications

➤*Suppression of intestinal bacteria:* When suppression of the normal bacterial flora of the bowel is desirable for short-term adjunctive therapy.

➤*Hepatic coma:* Prolonged administration has been shown to be effective adjunctive therapy in hepatic coma by reduction of the ammonia-forming bacteria in the intestinal tract. The subsequent reduction in blood ammonia has resulted in neurologic improvement.

Administration and Dosage

➤*Hepatic coma:* As an adjunct in therapy of hepatic coma for extended therapy: 8 to 12 g per day in divided doses.

➤*Suppression of intestinal bacteris:* As an adjunct to mechanical cleansing of the large bowel in short-term therapy: 1g (2 capsules) every hour for 4 hours followed by 1g (2 capsules) every 6 hours for 36 to 72 hours.

➤*Storage/Stability:* Store at room temperature 15° to 30°C (59° to 86°F). Dispense in tight containers.

NEOMYCIN SULFATE

Rx	**Neomycin Sulfate** (Various, eg, Goldline)	**Tablets:** 500 mg	In 100s.
Rx	**Neo-fradin** (Pharma-Tek)	**Oral solution:** 125 mg per 5 ml	Parabens. In 480 ml.

NEOMYCIN SULFATE — ORAL

Refer to the general discussion of these products in the Aminoglycosides, Oral group monograph.

WARNING

Toxicity – Systemic absorption of neomycin occurs following oral administration, and toxic reactions may occur. Patients treated with neomycin should be under close clinical observation because of the potential toxicity associated with the use of neomycin. Neurotoxicity (including ototoxicity) and nephrotoxicity following the oral use of neomycin sulfate have been reported, even when used in recommended doses. The potential for nephrotoxicity, permanent bilateral auditory ototoxicity, and sometimes vestibular toxicity, is present in patients with healthy renal function when treated with higher doses of neomycin or for longer periods than recommended. Serial, vestibular and audiometric tests, as well as tests of renal function, should be performed (especially in high-risk patients). The risk of nephrotoxicity and ototoxicity is greater in patients with impaired renal function. Ototoxicity is often delayed in onset, and patients developing cochlear damage will not have symptoms during therapy to warn them of developing eighth nerve destruction, and total or partial deafness may occur long after neomycin has been discontinued.

Other factors which increase the risk of toxicity are advanced age and dehydration.

Neuromuscular blockage – Neuromuscular blockage and respiratory paralysis have been reported following the oral use of neomycin. The possibility of the occurrence of neuromuscular blockage and respiratory paralysis should be considered if neomycin is administered, especially to patients receiving anesthetics; neuromuscular-blocking agents such as tubocurarine, succinylcholine, decamethonium; or massive transfusions of citrate anticoagulated blood. If blockage occurs, calcium salts may reverse these phenomena, but mechanical respiratory assistance may be necessary.

Concurrent therapy – Concurrent or sequential systemic, oral or topical use of other aminoglycosides, including paromomycin and other potentially nephrotoxic or neurotoxic drugs such as bacitracin, cisplatin, vancomycin, amphotericin B, polymyxin B, colistin and viomycin, should be avoided because the toxicity may be additive.

The concurrent use of neomycin with potent diuretics such as ethacrynic acid or furosemide should be avoided, since certain diuretics by themselves may cause ototoxicity. In addition, when administered IV, diuretics may enhance neomycin toxicity by altering the antibiotic concentration in serum and tissue.

Indications

➤*Suppression of intestinal bacteria (tablets only):* Adjunctive therapy as part of a regimen for the suppression of the normal bacterial flora of the bowel (eg, preoperative preparation of the bowel). It is given concomitantly with erythromycin enteric-coated base (see Administration and Dosage).

➤*Hepatic coma (portal-systemic encephalopathy) (tablets and oral solution):* Neomycin sulfate oral preparations have been shown to be effective adjunctive therapy in hepatic coma by reduction of the ammonia-forming bacteria in the intestinal tract. The subsequent reduction in blood ammonia has resulted in neurologic improvement.

Administration and Dosage

➤*Hepatic coma (tablets and oral solution):* To minimize the risk of toxicity, use the lowest possible dose and the shortest possible treatment period to control the condition. Treatment for periods greater than 2 weeks is not recommended.

Dosage – For use as an adjunct in the management of hepatic coma. Withdraw protein from diet. Avoid use of diuretic agents. Give supportive therapy, including blood products, as indicated. The recommended dose is 4 to 12 g/day given in the following regimen:

Give neomycin sulfate tablets in doses of 4 to 12 g of neomycin sulfate per day (8 to 24 tablets) in divided doses. Treatment should be continued over a period of 5 to 6 days, during which time protein should be returned incrementally to the diet.

If less potentially toxic drugs cannot be used for chronic hepatic insufficiency, neomycin in doses of up to 4 g daily (8 tablets/day) may be necessary. The risk for the development of neomycin-induced toxicity progressively increases when treatment must be extended to preserve the life of a patient with hepatic encephalopathy who has failed to fully respond. Frequent periodic monitoring of these patients to ascertain the presence of drug toxicity is mandatory (see Precautions). Also, neomycin serum concentrations should be monitored to avoid potentially toxic levels. The benefits to the patient should be weighed against the risks of nephrotoxicity, permanent ototoxicity and neuromuscular blockade following the accumulation of neomycin in the tissues.

➤*Suppression of intestinal bacteria (tablets):*

Preoperative prophylaxis for elective colorectal surgery – Listed below is an example of a recommended bowel preparation regimen. A proposed surgery time of 8 am has been used.

Preoperative day 3: Minimum residue or clear liquid diet. Bisacodyl, 1 tablet orally at 6 pm.

Preoperative day 2: Minimum residue or clear liquid diet. Magnesium sulfate, 30 mL, 50% solution (15 g) orally at 10 am, 2 pm, and 6 pm. Enema at 7 pm and 8 pm.

Preoperative day 1: Clear liquid diet. Supplemental (IV) fluids as needed. Magnesium sulfate, 30 mL, 50% solution (15 g) orally at 10 am and 2 pm. Neomycin sulfate (1 g) and erythromycin base (1 g) orally at 1 pm, 2 pm and 11 pm. No enema.

Day of operation: Patient evacuates rectum at 6:30 am for scheduled operation at 8 am.

➤*Storage/Stability:* Store at controlled room temperature 15° to 30°C (59° to 86°F). Dispense in tight containers.

PAROMOMYCIN SULFATE

Rx	**Humatin** (Parke-Davis)	**Capsules:** 250 mg paromomycin (as sulfate)	In 16s.

PAROMOMYCIN SULFATE — ORAL

Refer to the general discussion of these products in the Aminoglycosides, Oral group monograph.

Indications

➤*Intestinal amebiasis:* Acute and chronic intestinal amebiasis.

It is not effective in extraintestinal amebiasis because it is not absorbed.

➤*Hepatic coma:* Management of hepatic coma as adjunctive therapy.

➤*Unlabeled uses:* Has been recommended for other parasitic infections, including *Dientamoeba fragilis* (25 to 30 mg/kg/day in 3 doses for 7 days); *Diphyllobothrium latum, Taenia saginata, T. solium, Dipylidium caninum* (for adults, 1 g every 15 minutes for 4 doses; for pediatric patients, 11 mg/kg every 15 minutes for 4 doses); *Hymenolepsis nana* (45 mg/kg/day for 5 to 7 days).

Administration and Dosage

➤*Approved by the FDA:* June 30, 1997.

➤*Intestinal amebiasis:*

Adults and pediatric patients –

Usual dose: 25 to 35 mg/kg body weight daily, administered in 3 divided doses with meals, for 5 to 10 days.

➤*Management of hepatic coma:*

Adults –

Usual dose: 4 g daily in divided doses, given at regular intervals for 5 to 6 days.

➤*Storage/Stability:* Store at controlled room temperature 15° to 30°C (59° to 86°F). Protect from moisture.

COLISTIMETHATE SODIUM

Rx	Colistimethate Sodium (Paddock)	Lyophilized cake for injection: 150 mg colistin base[a]	In vials.
Rx	Coly-Mycin M (Parke-Davis)		In vials.

[a] As colistimethate sodium or pentasodium colistinmethane sulfonate.

COLISTIMETHATE SODIUM — INJECTION

Indications

➤*Gram-negative infections:* Treatment of acute or chronic infections due to sensitive strains of certain gram-negative bacilli. Particularly indicated when the infection is caused by sensitive strains of *P. aeruginosa*. Clinically effective in treatment of infections due to the following gram-negative organisms: *E. aerogenes*, *E. coli*, *K. pneumoniae* and *P. aeruginosa*. Pending results of bacteriologic cultures and sensitivity tests, colistimethate may be used to initiate therapy in serious infections that are suspected to be due to gram-negative organisms.

➤*Unlabeled uses:* Aerosolized colistin has been shown to be beneficial in the treatment of sensitive *Pseudomonas* infections in patients with cystic fibrosis. In addition, early aggressive use of the drug as adjunctive therapy may play a role in reducing chronic infections in this population.

Administration and Dosage

For IM or IV use.

➤*Adults and children:* 2.5 to 5 mg/kg/day in 2 to 4 divided doses for patients with normal renal function, depending upon the severity of the infection.

➤*Renal function impairment:* Reduce the daily dose in the presence of any renal impairment.

Suggested Modification of Colistimethate Dosage Schedules for Adults with Impaired Renal Function

	Renal function		Dosage			
Degree of impairment	Plasma creatinine (mg/dl)	Urea clearance % (of normal)	Dose[1] (mg)	Frequency (times per day)	Total daily dose (mg)	Approx. daily dose (mg/kg)
Normal	0.7 - 1.2	80 - 100	100 - 150	4 to 2	300	5
Mild	1.3 - 1.5	40 - 70	75 - 115	2	150 - 230	2.5 - 3.8
Moderate	1.6 - 2.5	25 - 40	66 - 150	2 or 1	133 - 150	2.5
Severe	2.6 - 4	10 - 25	100 - 150	q 36 h	100	1.5

[1] Suggested unit dose is 2.5 to 5 mg/kg; increase time interval between injections in presence of impaired renal function.

➤*IV administration:*

Direct intermittent administration – Inject one-half the total daily dose over a period of 3 to 5 minutes every 12 hours.

Continuous infusion – Slowly inject one-half the daily dose over 3 to 5 minutes. Add the remaining half of the total daily dose of colistimethate to one of the following: 0.9% Sodium Chloride; 5% Dextrose in Water; 5% Dextrose with 0.9% Sodium Chloride; 5% Dextrose with 0.45% Sodium Chloride; 5% Dextrose with 0.225% Sodium Chloride; Lactated Ringer's solution. Swirl gently to avoid frothing. Administer by slow IV infusion starting 1 to 2 hours after the initial dose over the next 22 to 23 hours in the presence of normal renal function. In the presence of impaired renal function, reduce infusion rate. Choice of IV solution and volume to be employed are dictated by requirements of fluid and electrolyte management.

➤*Storage/Stability:* Freshly prepare any infusion solution containing colistimethate and use for no longer than 24 hours.

Actions

➤*Pharmacokinetics:* Higher initial blood levels are obtained following IV administration. Blood levels peak at between 5 and 10 mcg/ml between 2 and 3 hours after IM administration. Serum half-life is 2 to 3 hours.

Average urinary levels range from about 270 mcg/ml at 2 hours to about 15 mcg/ml at 8 hours after IV administration and from about 200 to 25 mcg/ml during a similar period following IM administration.

➤*Microbiology:* Colistimethate has bactericidal activity against the following gram-negative bacilli: *Enterobacter aerogenes*, *Escherichia coli*, *Klebsiella pneumoniae* and *Pseudomonas aeruginosa*.

Contraindications

Hypersensitivity to colistimethate sodium; infections due to *Proteus* or *Neisseria* species.

Warnings

➤*Maximum dosage:* Do not exceed 5 mg/kg/day in patients with normal renal function.

➤*Neurologic effects:* May occur transiently. These include circumoral paresthesias or numbness, tingling or formication of the extremities, generalized pruritus, vertigo, dizziness and slurring of speech. Warn patients not to drive vehicles or use hazardous machinery while on therapy. Dosage reduction may alleviate symptoms. Therapy need not be discontinued, but observe such patients carefully. Overdosage can result in renal insufficiency, muscle weakness and apnea.

➤*Renal function impairment:* Since colistimethate is eliminated mainly by renal excretion, use with caution when the possibility of impaired renal function exists. Consider the decline in renal function with advanced age.

When actual renal impairment is present, use colistimethate with extreme caution; reduce the dosage in proportion to the extent of the impairment. Administration of amounts in excess of renal excretory capacity will lead to high serum levels. This can result in further impairment of renal function, initiating a cycle which, if not recognized, can lead to acute renal insufficiency, renal shutdown and further concentration of the antibiotic to toxic levels in the body. Interference with nerve transmission at neuromuscular junctions may occur and result in muscle weakness and apnea.

Signs indicating the development of impaired renal function are diminishing urine output and rising BUN or serum creatinine. If present, discontinue therapy immediately. If a life-threatening situation exists, reinstate therapy at a lower dosage after blood levels have fallen.

➤*Pregnancy: Category C.* Colistimethate sodium is transferred across the placental barrier, and blood levels of about 1 mcg/ml are obtained in the fetus following IV administration to the mother. Safety for use during pregnancy has not been established. Use only when clearly needed and when the potential benefits outweigh the potential hazards.

Precautions

➤*Respiratory effects:* Respiratory arrest has occurred following IM administration. Impaired renal function increases the possibility of apnea and neuromuscular blockade, generally because of failure to follow recommended guidelines, overdosage, failure to reduce dose commensurate with degree of renal impairment or concomitant use of other antibiotics or drugs with neuromuscular blocking potential. If apnea occurs, treat with assisted respiration, oxygen and calcium chloride injections.

➤*Nephrotoxicity:* A decrease in urine output or increase in BUN or serum creatinine can be signs of nephrotoxicity, which is probably a dose-dependent effect. These manifestations are reversible following discontinuation. Increases of BUN have occurred at dose levels of 1.6 to 5 mg/kg/day. Values returned to normal following cessation.

Drug Interactions

Colistimethate Drug Interactions

Precipitant drug	Object drug*		Description
Aminoglycosides	Colistimethate	↑	Concurrent use may increase the risk of respiratory paralysis and renal dysfunction.
Cephalothin	Colistimethate	↑	Concurrent use may increase the risk of renal dysfunction.
Colistimethate	Nondepolaizing muscle relaxants	↑	Neuromuscular blockade may be enhanced.

* ↑ = Object drug increased.

Adverse Reactions

Respiratory arrest (see Precautions); decreased urine output or increased BUN or serum creatinine (see Precautions); paresthesia; tingling of the extremities or the tongue; generalized itching or urticaria; drug fever; GI upset; vertigo; slurring of speech. The subjective symptoms reported by the adult may not be manifest in infants or young children, thus requiring close attention to renal function.

POLYMYXIN B SULFATE

Rx	**Polymyxin B Sulfate** (Bedford)	**Injection:** 500,000 units	In vials.

POLYMYXIN B — INJECTION

WARNING

When this drug is given IM or intrathecally, it should be given only to hospitalized patients, so as to provide constant supervision by a physician.

Nephrotoxicity – Renal function should be carefully determined, and patients with renal damage and nitrogen retention should have reduced dosage. Patients with nephrotoxicity due to polymyxin B sulfate usually show albuminuria, cellular casts, and azotemia. Diminishing urine output and a rising blood urea nitrogen (BUN) are indications for discontinuing therapy with this drug.

Neurotoxicity – Neurotoxic reactions may be manifested by irritability, weakness, drowsiness, ataxia, perioral paresthesia, numbness of the extremities, and blurring of vision. These are usually associated with high serum levels found in patients with impaired renal function or nephrotoxicity.

Concurrent therapy – The concurrent or sequential use of other neurotoxic or nephrotoxic drugs with polymyxin B sulfate, particularly bacitracin, streptomycin, neomycin, kanamycin, gentamicin, tobramycin, amikacin, cephaloridine, paromomycin, viomycin, and colistin should be avoided.

Neuromuscular blockade – The neurotoxicity of polymyxin B sulfate can result in respiratory paralysis from neuromuscular blockade, especially when the drug is given soon after anesthesia or muscle relaxants.

Use in pregnancy – The safety of this drug in human pregnancy has not been established.

Indications

➤*Pseudomonal infections :* Polymyxin B sulfate is a drug of choice in the treatment of infections of the urinary tract, meninges, and bloodstream caused by susceptible strains of *Pseudomonas aeruginosa*.

➤*Serious infections:* It may be indicated in serious infections caused by susceptible strains of the following organisms, when less potentially toxic drugs are ineffective or contraindicated: *H. influenzae*, specifically meningeal infections; *Escherichia coli*, specifically urinary tract infections; *Aerobacter aerogenes*, specifically bacteremia; *Klebsiella pneumoniae*, specifically bacteremia.

In meningeal infections, polymyxin B sulfate should be administered only by the intrathecal route.

Administration and Dosage

➤*IV:* Dissolve 500,000 polymyxin B units in 300 to 500 mL solutions for parenteral dextrose injection 5% for continuous drip.

Adults and children – Fifteen thousand (15,000) to 25,000 units/kg body weight/day in individuals with healthy kidney function. This amount should be reduced from 15,000 units/kg downward for individuals with kidney impairment. Infusions may be given every 12 hours; however, the total daily dose must not exceed 25,000 units/kg/day.

Infants – Infants with healthy kidney function may receive up to 40,000 units/kg/day without adverse reactions.

➤*IM:* IM administration is not recommended routinely because of severe pain at injection sites, particularly in infants and children. Dissolve 500,000 polymyxin B units in 2 mL sterile water for injection or sodium chloride injection or procaine HCl injection 1%.

Adults and children – Twenty-five thousand (25,000) to 30,000 units/kg/day. This should be reduced in the presence of renal impairment. The dosage may be divided and given at either 4- or 6-hour intervals.

Infants – Infants with healthy kidney function may receive up to 40,000 units/kg/day without adverse reactions.

Doses as high as 45,000 units/kg/day have been used in limited clinical studies in treating prematures and newborn infants for sepsis caused by *Pseudomonas aeruginosa*.

➤*Intrathecal:* A treatment of choice for *Pseudomonas aeruginosa* meningitis. Dissolve 500,000 polymyxin B units in 10 mL sodium chloride injection USP for 50,000 units/mL dosage unit.

Adults and children over 2 years of age – Dosage is 50,000 units once daily intrathecally for 3 to 4 days, then 50,000 units once every other day for at least 2 weeks after cultures of the cerebrospinal fluid are negative and sugar content has returned to normal.

Children under 2 years of age – Twenty thousand (20,000) units once daily, intrathecally for 3 to 4 days or 25,000 units once every other day. Continue with a dose of 25,000 units once every other day for at least 2 weeks after cultures of the cerebrospinal fluid are negative and sugar content has returned to normal.

Avoid total systemic instillation over 25,000 units/kg/day.

➤*Storage / Stability:*

Before reconstitution – Store at controlled room temperature 15° to 30°C (59° to 86°F).

Protect from light. Retain in carton until time of use.

After reconstitution – Product must be stored under refrigeration, between 2° to 8°C (36° to 46°F) and any unused portion should be discarded after 72 hours.

Actions

➤*Pharmacology:* Polymyxin B sulfate has a bactericidal action against almost all gram-negative bacilli except the *Proteus* group. Polymyxins increase the permeability of bacterial cell wall membranes.

➤*Pharmacokinetics:*

Absorption / Distribution – Polymyxin B sulfate is not absorbed from the normal alimentary tract. Since the drug loses 50% of its activity in the presence of serum, active blood levels are low. Repeated injections may give a cumulative effect. Levels tend to be higher in infants and children. Tissue diffusion is poor and the drug does not pass the blood-brain barrier into the cerebrospinal fluid.

Excretion – The drug is excreted slowly by the kidneys. In therapeutic dosage, polymyxin B sulfate causes some nephrotoxicity with tubule damage to a slight degree.

➤*Microbiology:* All gram-positive bacteria, fungi, and the gram-negative cocci, *N. gonorrhoeae* and *N. meningitidis*, are resistant.

Contraindications

Hypersensitivity reactions to polymyxins.

Precautions

➤*Monitoring:* Baseline renal function should be done prior to therapy, with frequent monitoring of renal function and blood levels of the drug during parenteral therapy. Renal function should be carefully determined, and patients with renal damage and nitrogen retention should have reduced dosage. Patients with nephrotoxicity due to polymyxin B sulfate usually show albuminuria, cellular casts, and azotemia. Diminishing urine output and a rising blood urea nitrogen (BUN) are indications for discontinuing therapy with this drug.

➤*Superinfection:* As with other antibiotics, use of this drug may result in overgrowth of nonsusceptible organisms, including fungi. If superinfection occurs, appropriate therapy should be instituted.

Drug Interactions

➤*Neurotoxic drugs:* Avoid concurrent use of a curariform muscle relaxant and other neurotoxic drugs (eg, ether, tubocurarine, succinylcholine, gallamine, decamethonium, sodium citrate) which may precipitate respiratory depression. If signs of respiratory paralysis appear, respiration should be assisted as required, and the drug discontinued.

Polymyxin B Drug Interactions

Precipitant drug	Object drug*		Description
Aminoglycosides	Polymyxin B	⬆	Concurrent use may increase the risk of respiratory paralysis and renal dysfunction.
Polymyxin B	Nondepolarizing muscle relaxants	⬆	Neuromuscular blockade may be enhanced.

* ⬆ = Object drug increased.

Adverse Reactions

➤*CNS:*

Neurotoxic reactions – Facial flushing, dizziness progressing to ataxia, drowsiness, peripheral paresthesias (circumoral and stocking glove), apnea due to concurrent use of curariform muscle relaxants, other neurotoxic drugs or inadvertent overdosage, and signs of meningeal irritation with intrathecal administration (eg, fever, headache, stiff neck, increased cell count and protein cerebrospinal fluid).

➤*Renal:*

Nephrotoxic reactions – Albuminuria, cylinduria, azotemia, and rising blood levels without any increase in dosage.

➤*Miscellaneous:* Other reactions occasionally reported include the following: Drug fever, urticarial rash, pain (severe) at IM injection sites, and thrombophlebitis at IV injection sites.

BACITRACIN

Rx	**Bacitracin USP** (Various, eg, Upjohn)	**Powder for Injection:** 50,000 units	In vials.
Rx	**Baci-IM** (Pharma-Tek)		In vials.

BACITRACIN — INJECTION

WARNING

Nephrotoxicity – Bacitracin in parenteral (IM) therapy may cause renal failure due to tubular and glomerular necrosis. Its use should be restricted to infants with staphylococcal pneumonia and empyema when due to organisms shown to be susceptible to bacitracin. It should be used only where adequate laboratory facilities are available and when constant supervision of the patient is possible.

Renal function should be carefully determined prior to and daily during therapy. The recommended daily dose should not be exceeded, and fluid intake and urinary output should be maintained at proper levels to avoid kidney toxicity. If renal toxicity occurs the drug should be discontinued. The concurrent use of other nephrotoxic drugs, particularly streptomycin, kanamycin, polymyxin B, polymyxin E (colistin), and neomycin should be avoided.

Indications

➤*Pneumonia / Empyema:* The use of IM bacitracin is limited to the treatment of infants with pneumonia and empyema caused by staphylococci shown to be susceptible to the drug.

See the Warning box for more information..

➤*Unlabeled uses:* Oral use in antibiotic-associated colitis has been successful.

Administration and Dosage

This medication is to be administered IM only.

IM injections of the solution should be given in the upper outer quadrant of the buttocks, alternating right and left and avoiding multiple injections in the same region because of the transient pain following injection.

➤*Infant dose:*

For infants under 2500 g – Administer 900 units/kg/24 hours in 2 or 3 divided doses.

For infants over 2500 g – Administer 1000 units/kg/24 hours, in 2 or 3 divided doses.

➤*Preparation of solutions:* Solutions should be dissolved in sodium chloride injection containing 2% procaine HCl. The concentration of the antibiotic in the solution should not be less than 5000 units/mL nor more than 10,000 units/mL.

Diluents containing parabens should not be used to reconstitute bacitracin; cloudy solutions and precipitate formation have occurred.

Reconstitution of the 50,000 unit vial with 9.8 mL of diluent will result in a concentration of 5000 units/mL.

➤*Storage / Stability:* Store the unreconstituted product in a refrigerator 2° to 8°C (36° to 46°F).

Solutions are stable for 1 week when stored in a refrigerator at 2° to 8°C (36° to 46°F).

Actions

➤*Pharmacology:* Bacitracin exerts pronounced antibacterial action in vitro against a variety of gram-positive and a few gram-negative organisms. However, among systemic diseases, only staphylococcal infections qualify for consideration of bacitracin therapy. Bacitracin is assayed against a standard and its activity is expressed in units, 1 mg having a potency of not less than 50 units.

➤*Pharmacokinetics:*

Absorption – Absorption of bacitracin following IM injection is rapid and complete. A dose of 200 or 300 units/kg every 6 hours gives serum levels of 0.2 to 2 mcg/mL in individuals with healthy renal function.

Distribution – Bacitracin injection is widely distributed in all body organs and is demonstrable in ascitic and pleural fluids after IM injection.

Excretion – Bacitracin injection is excreted slowly by glomerular filtration.

Contraindications

Hypersensitivity or toxic reaction to the drug.

Warnings

➤*Nephrotoxicity:* Bacitracin in parenteral (IM) therapy may cause renal failure due to tubular and glomerular necrosis. Its use should be restricted to infants with staphylococcal pneumonia and empyema when due to organisms shown to be susceptible to bacitracin. It should be used only where adequate laboratory facilities are available and when constant supervision of the patient is possible.

Precautions

➤*Monitoring:* Renal function should be carefully determined prior to and daily during therapy. The recommended daily dose should not be exceeded, and fluid intake and urinary output should be maintained at proper levels to avoid kidney toxicity. If renal toxicity occurs, the drug should be discontinued.

➤*Hydration:* Adequate fluid intake should be maintained orally, or if necessary, by parenteral method.

➤*Superinfection:* As with other antibiotics, use of this drug may result in overgrowth of nonsusceptible organisms, including fungi. If superinfection occurs, appropriate therapy should be instituted.

Drug Interactions

Bacitracin Drug Interactions

Precipitant drug	Object drug*		Description
Aminoglycosides	Bacitracin	⬆	Concurrent use may increase risk of respiratory paralysis and renal dysfunction.
Bacitracin	Nondepolarizing muscle relaxants	⬆	Neuromuscular blockade may be enhanced.

* ⬆ = Object drug increased

➤*Other nephrotoxic drugs:* The concurrent use of other nephrotoxic drugs, particularly streptomycin, kanamycin, polymyxin B, polymyxin E (colistin), and neomycin should be avoided.

Adverse Reactions

➤*Dermatologic:* Skin rashes.

➤*GI:* Nausea and vomiting.

➤*Local:* Pain at site of injection.

➤*Renal:* Albuminuria, cylindruria, azotemia. Rising blood levels without any increase in dosage.

RIFAXIMIN

RIFAXIMIN

Rx	**Xifaxan** (Salix)	**Tablets:** 200 mg	EDTA. (Sx). Pink, biconvex. Film-coated. In 30s.

RIFAXIMIN — ORAL

Indications

➤*Traveler's diarrhea:* Rifaximin tablets are indicated for the treatment of patients (greater than or equal to 12 years of age) with travelers' diarrhea caused by noninvasive strains of *Escherichia coli*.

Do not use rifaximin tablets in patients with diarrhea complicated by fever or blood in the stool or diarrhea due to pathogens other than *Escherichia coli*.

Administration and Dosage

➤*Approved by the FDA:* May 25, 2004.

Rifaximin tablets can be administered orally with or without food. For travelers' diarrhea, the recommended dose is one 200 mg tablet taken 3 times a day for 3 days.

➤*Storage / Stability:* Store rifaximin tablets at 20° to 25°C (68° to 77°F); excursions permitted to 15° to 30°C (59° to 86°F).

Actions

➤*Pharmacokinetics:*

Absorption – The mean pharmacokinetic parameters of rifaximin in 14 healthy subjects after a single oral 400 mg dose given as 2 × 200 mg doses under fed and fasting conditions are summarized in the following table.

Effect of Food on the Mean ± SD Pharmacokinetic Parameters Following a Single 400 mg Dose of Rifaximin (n = 14)

Parameter	Fasting	Fed
C_{max} (ng/mL)	3.8 ± 1.32	9.63 ± 5.93
T_{max} (hours)	1.21 ± 0.47	1.9 ± 1.52
Half-life (hours)	5.85 ± 4.34	5.95 ± 1.88
AUC (ng•hr/mL)	18.35 ± 9.48	34.7 ± 9.23
% excreted in urine	0.023 ± 0.009	0.051 ± 0.017

Rifaximin can be administered with or without food. Systemic absorption of rifaximin was low in both the fasting state and when administered within 30 minutes of a high-fat breakfast.

^{14}C-Rifaximin was administered as a single dose to 4 healthy male subjects. The mean overall recovery of radioactivity in the urine and feces of 3 subjects during the 168 hours after administration was 96.94% ± 5.64% of the dose. Radioactivity was excreted almost exclusively in the feces (96.62% ± 5.67% of the dose), with only a small proportion of the dose (mean 0.32% of the dose) excreted in urine. Analysis of fecal extracts indicated that rifaximin was being excreted as unchanged drug. The amount of radioactivity in urine (less than 0.4% of the dose) suggests that rifaximin is poorly absorbed from the gastrointestinal tract and is almost exclusively and completely excreted in feces as unchanged drug. Mean rifaximin pharmacokinetic

RIFAXIMIN — ORAL

parameters were C_{max} 4.3 ± 2.8 ng/mL and AUC_t 19.5 ± 16.5 ng•hr/mL with a median T_{max} of 1.25 hours.

Systemic absorption of rifaximin (200 mg 3 times daily) was also evaluated in 13 subjects with shigellosis on days 1 and 3 of a 3-day course of treatment. Rifaximin concentrations and exposures were low and variable. There was no evidence of accumulation of rifaximin following repeated administration for 3 days (9 doses). Peak plasma rifaximin concentrations after 3 and 9 consecutive doses ranged from 0.81 to 3.4 ng/mL on day 1 and 0.68 to 2.26 ng/mL on day 3. Similarly, $AUC_{0\text{-last}}$ estimates were 6.95 ± 5.15 ng•hr/mL on day 1 and 7.83 ± 4.94 ng•hr/mL on day 3. Rifaximin is not suitable for treating systemic bacterial infections because less than 0.4% of the drug is absorbed after oral administration.

Distribution – Animal pharmacokinetic studies have demonstrated that 80% to 90% of oral rifaximin is concentrated in the gut, with less than 0.2% in the liver and kidney and less than 0.01% in other tissues. In adults with infectious diarrhea treated with rifaximin 800 mg daily for 3 days, concentrations of rifaximin in stools averaged approximately 8,000 mcg/g the day after treatment ended.

Metabolism – In vitro drug interactions studies have shown that rifaximin, at concentrations ranging from 2 to 200 ng/mL, did not inhibit human hepatic cytochrome P450 isoenzymes: 1A2, 2A6, 2B6, 2C9, 2C19, 2D6, 2E1, and 3A4. In an in vitro hepatocyte induction model, rifaximin was shown to induce cytochrome P450 3A4 (CYP3A4), an isoenzyme which rifampin is known to induce. Two clinical drug-drug interaction studies using midazolam and an oral contraceptive containing ethinyl estradiol and norgestimate demonstrated that rifaximin did not alter the pharmacokinetics of these drugs.

Excretion – Rifaximin is excreted primarily in the feces. After oral administration of 400 mg ^{14}C-rifaximin to healthy volunteers, approximately 97% of the dose was recovered in feces, almost entirely as unchanged drug, and 0.32% was recovered in the urine.

➤*Microbiology:* Rifaximin acts by binding to the beta-subunit of bacterial DNA-dependent RNA polymerase resulting in inhibition of bacterial RNA synthesis.

Escherichia coli has been shown to develop resistance to rifaximin in vitro. However, the clinical significance of such an effect has not been studied.

Rifaximin has been shown to be active against the following pathogen in clinical studies of infectious diarrhea: *Escherichia coli* (enterotoxigenic and enteroaggregative strains).

Contraindications

Hypersensitivities to rifaximin, any of the rifamycin antimicrobial agents, or any of the components in rifaximin tablets.

Warnings

➤*Diarrhea:* Rifaximin tablets were not found to be effective in patients with diarrhea complicated by fever or blood in the stool or diarrhea due to pathogens other than *Escherichia coli*. Rifaximin tablets are not effective in cases of travelers' diarrhea due to *Campylobacter jejuni*. The effectiveness of rifaximin tablets in travelers' diarrhea caused by *Shigella* spp. and *Salmonella* spp. has not been proven. Rifaximin tablets should not be used in patients where *Campylobacter jejuni*, *Shigella* spp., or *Salmonella* spp. may be suspected as causative pathogens.

Discontinue rifaximin tablets if diarrhea symptoms get worse or persist more than 24 to 48 hours, and consider alternative antibiotic therapy.

➤*Pseudomembranous colitis:* Pseudomembranous colitis has been reported with nearly all antibacterial agents and may range in severity from mild to life-threatening. Therefore, it is important to consider this diagnosis in patients who present with diarrhea subsequent to the administration of antibacterial agents.

Treatment with antibacterial agents alters the normal flora of the colon and may permit overgrowth of clostridia. Studies indicate that a toxin produced by *Clostridium difficile* is the primary cause of "antibiotic-associated colitis."

After the diagnosis of pseudomembranous colitis has been established, initiate therapeutic measures. Mild cases of pseudomembranous colitis usually respond to drug discontinuation alone. In moderate to severe cases, consider management with fluids and electrolytes, protein supplementation, and treatment with an antibacterial drug clinically effective against *Clostridium difficile*.

➤*Pregnancy: Category C.* Rifaximin was teratogenic in rats at doses of 150 to 300 mg/kg (approximately 2.5 to 5 times the clinical dose, adjusted for body surface area) and in rabbits at doses of 62.5 to 1,000 mg/kg (approximately 2 to 33 times the clinical dose, adjusted for body surface area). These effects include cleft palate, agnatha, jaw shortening, hemorrhage, eye partially open, small eyes, brachygnathia, incomplete ossification, and increased thoracolumbar vertebrae. There are no adequate and well-controlled studies in pregnant women. Use during pregnancy only if the potential benefit outweighs the potential risk to the fetus.

➤*Lactation:* It is not known whether rifaximin is excreted in human milk. Because many drugs are excreted in human milk and because of the potential for adverse reactions in nursing infants from rifaximin tablets, a decision should be made whether to discontinue nursing or to discontinue the drug, taking into account the importance of the drug to the mother.

➤*Children:* The safety and efficacy of rifaximin tablets in pediatric patients less than 12 years of age have not been established.

Precautions

➤*Hazardous tasks:* Patients should be careful about driving or operating machinery if they feel dizzy while taking rifaximin.

➤*Superinfection:* The use of antibiotics may promote the overgrowth of nonsusceptible organisms. Should superinfection occur during therapy, take appropriate measures.

Drug Interactions

➤*Cytochrome P-450 system:* Although in vitro studies demonstrated the potential of rifaximin to interact with cytochrome P450 3A4 (CYP3A4), a clinical drug-drug interaction study demonstrated that rifaximin did not significantly affect the pharmacokinetics of midazolam either presystemically or systemically. An additional clinical drug-drug interaction study showed no effect of rifaximin on the presystemic metabolism of an oral contraceptive containing ethinyl estradiol and norgestimate. Therefore, clinical interactions with drugs metabolized by human cytochrome P450 isoenzymes are not expected.

Adverse Reactions

All Adverse Events with an Incidence ≥ 2% Among Patients Receiving Rifaximin Tablets, 600 mg/day, in Placebo-controlled Studies

MedDRA preferred term	Number (%) of patients: Rifaximin tablets, 600 mg/day (n = 320)	Placebo (n = 228)
Abdominal pain NOS	23 (7.2%)	23 (10.1%)
Constipation	12 (3.8%)	8 (3.5%)
Defecation urgency	19 (5.9%)	21 (9.2%)
Flatulence	36 (11.3%)	45 (19.7%)
Headache	31 (9.7%)	21 (9.2%)
Nausea	17 (5.3%)	19 (8.3%)
Pyrexia	10 (3.1%)	10 (4.4%)
Rectal tenesmus	23 (7.2%)	20 (8.8%)
Vomiting NOS	7 (2.2%)	4 (1.8%)

The following adverse events, presented by body system, have also been reported in less than 2% of patients taking rifaximin tablets in the 2 placebo-controlled clinical trials where the 200 mg taken 3 times a day dose was used. The following includes adverse events regardless of causal relationship to drug exposure:

➤*Cardiovascular:* Chest pain; hot flashes NOS.

➤*CNS:* Abnormal dreams, dizziness, migraine NOS, syncope.

➤*Dermatologic:* Clamminess, increased sweating, rash NOS, sunburn.

➤*GI:* Abdominal distension, blood in stool, diarrhea NOS, dry lips, dry throat, dysentery NOS, fecal abnormality NOS, gingival disorder NOS, inguinal hernia NOS, stomach discomfort.

➤*GU:* Blood in urine, choluria, dysuria, hematuria, polyuria, proteinuria, urinary frequency.

➤*Hematologic/Lymphatic:* Lymphocytosis, monocytosis, neutropenia.

➤*Hepatic:* Increased aspartate aminotransferase.

➤*Metabolic/Nutritional:* Anorexia, dehydration, decreased weight.

➤*Musculoskeletal:* Arthralgia, muscle spasms, myalgia, neck pain.

➤*Psychiatric:* Insomnia.

➤*Respiratory:* Dyspnea NOS, nasal passage irritation, nasopharyngitis, pharyngitis, pharyngolaryngeal pain, respiratory tract infection NOS, rhinitis NOS, rhinorrhea, upper respiratory tract infection NOS.

➤*Special senses:* Ear pain, loss of taste, motion sickness, tinnitus.

➤*Miscellaneous:* Fatigue, malaise, pain NOS, weakness.

➤*Postmarketing:*

Hypersensitivity – These events (hypersensitivity reactions, including allergic dermatitis, rash, angioneurotic edema, urticaria, and pruritus) have been identified during foreign postapproval use of rifaximin tablets. Because these events are reported voluntarily from a population of uncertain size, it is not always possible to estimate their frequency or establish a causal relationship to drug exposure.

Overdosage

➤*Symptoms:* No specific information is available on the treatment of overdosage with rifaximin tablets. In clinical studies at doses higher than the recommended dose (greater than 600 mg/day), adverse events were similar to the recommended dose (200 mg taken 3 times a day) and to placebo.

➤*Treatment:* In the case of overdosage, discontinue rifaximin tablets, treat symptomatically, and institute supportive measures as required.

METRONIDAZOLE

Rx	**Metronidazole** (Various, eg, Mutual, Teva, UDL)	**Tablets**: 250 mg	In 25s, 100s, 250s, and 500s.
Rx	**Flagyl** (Pharmacia)		(SEARLE 1831 FLAGYL 250). Blue. Film-coated. In 50s, 100s, and 2500s.
Rx	**Metronidazole** (Various, eg, Mutual, Teva, UDL)	**Tablets**: 500 mg	In 25s, 50s, 100s, and 500s.
Rx	**Flagyl** (Pharmacia)		(FLAGYL 500). Blue, oblong. Film-coated. In 50s, 100s, and 500s.
Rx	**Metronidazole** (Able)	**Tablets, extended-release**: 750 mg	Lactose, polydextrose. (A352). Yellow, oval. Film coated. In 30s, 100s, 500s, and 1000s.
Rx	**Flagyl ER** (Pharmacia)		Lactose. (SEARLE 1961 FLAGYL ER). Blue, oval. Film-coated. In 30s.
Rx	**Metronidazole** (Able)	**Capsules**: 375 mg	(A 353). Yellow and grey. In 30s, 50s, 100s, 500s, and 1000s.
Rx	**Flagyl 375** (Pharmacia)		(375 mg Flagyl). Iron gray/lt. green. In 50s and UD 100s.
Rx	**Flagyl IV** (Pharmacia)	**Powder for Injection, lyophilized**: 500 mg	In single-dose vials.[1]
Rx	**Metronidazole** (B. Braun)	**Injection**: 5 mg/mL	In 100 mL vials.

[1] 415 mg mannitol per vial.

METRONIDAZOLE — ORAL

Metronidazole is also available for topical and intravaginal use. For further information refer to the individual monographs in the Dermatologicals chapter and Renal and Genitourinary chapter.

WARNING

Metronidazole has been shown to be carcinogenic in mice and rats. Unnecessary use of the drug should be avoided. Its use should be reserved for the conditions for which this drug is indicated.

Indications

➤*Tablets and capsules:*

Symptomatic trichomoniasis – For the treatment of symptomatic trichomoniasis in females and males when the presence of the trichomonad has been confirmed by appropriate laboratory procedures (wet smears or cultures).

Asymptomatic trichomoniasis – In the treatment of asymptomatic females when the organism is associated with endocervicitis, cervicitis, or cervical erosion. Since there is evidence that presence of the trichomonad can interfere with accurate assessment of abnormal cytological smears, additional smears should be performed after eradication of the parasite.

Treatment of asymptomatic consorts – *T. vaginalis* infection is a venereal disease. Therefore, asymptomatic sexual partners of treated patients should be treated simultaneously if the organism has been found to be present, in order to prevent reinfection of the partner. The decision as to whether to treat an asymptomatic male partner who has a negative culture or one for whom no culture has been attempted is an individual one. In making this decision, it should be noted that there is evidence that a woman may become reinfected if her partner is not treated. Also, since there can be considerable difficulty in isolating the organism from the asymptomatic male carrier, negative smears and cultures cannot be relied upon in this regard. In any event, the partner should be treated with metronidazole in cases of reinfection.

Amebiasis – In the treatment of acute intestinal amebiasis (amebic dysentery) and amebic liver abscess.

In amebic liver abscess, metronidazole therapy does not obviate the need for aspiration or drainage of pus.

Anaerobic bacterial infections – In the treatment of serious infections caused by susceptible anaerobic bacteria. Indicated surgical procedures should be performed in conjunction with metronidazole therapy. In a mixed aerobic and anaerobic infection, antimicrobials appropriate for the treatment of the aerobic infection should be used in addition to metronidazole.

Intra-abdominal infections – Peritonitis, intra-abdominal abscess, and liver abscess, caused by *Bacteroides* species including the *B. fragilis* group (*B. fragilis, B. distasonis, B. ovatus, B. thetaiotaomicron, B. vulgatus*), *Clostridium* species, *Eubacterium* species, *Peptococcus niger*, and *Peptostreptococcus* species.

Skin and skin structure infections – Caused by *Bacteroides* species including the *B. fragilis* group, *Clostridium* species, *Peptococcus niger*, *Peptostreptococcus* species, and *Fusobacterium* species.

Gynecologic infections – Including endometritis, endomyometritis, tubo-ovarian abscess, and postsurgical vaginal cuff infection, caused by *Bacteroides* species including the *B. fragilis* group, *Clostridium* species, *Peptococcus niger*, and *Peptostreptococcus* species.

Bacterial septicemia – Caused by *Bacteroides* species including the *B. fragilis* group, and *Clostridium* species.

Bone and joint infections – As adjunctive therapy, caused by *Bacteroides* species including the *B. fragilis* group.

CNS infections – Including meningitis and brain abscess, caused by *Bacteroides* species including the *B. fragilis* group.

Lower respiratory tract infections – Including pneumonia, empyema, and lung abscess, caused by *Bacteroides* species including the *B. fragilis* group.

Endocarditis – Caused by *Bacteroides* species including the *B. fragilis* group.

➤*Extended-release tablets:*

Bacterial vaginosis – In the treatment of women with bacterial vaginosis.

➤*Unlabeled uses:*

Hepatic encephalopathy – Metronidazole (800 mg/day) for 1 week has comparable efficacy to neomycin.

Crohn's disease – Metronidazole (250 mg 4 times/day) plus ciprofloxacin (500 mg twice/day) has been useful for patients with active acute-phase Crohn's disease.

Diarrhea associated with Clostridium difficile – Metronidazole (500 mg 3 times/day or 250 mg 4 times/day) has similar rates of efficacy compared with vancomycin.

Helicobacter pylori – Metronidazole is useful in eradicating *H. pylori* but should be used in combination therapy.

Recurrent and persistent urethritis – The CDC recommends metronidazole 2 g orally in a single dose plus erythromycin for 7 days.

Bacterial vaginosis – Per CDC recommendations, metronidazole 500 mg twice/day for 7 days or 2 g orally in a single dose. *Flagyl ER* is approved for this use.

Pelvic inflammatory disease – For oral therapy, metronidazole 500 mg twice/day is given with ofloxacin for 14 days.

Prophylaxis after sexual assault – CDC guidelines recommend metronidazole 2 g orally in a single dose plus ceftriaxone and either azithromycin or doxycycline.

Gardnerella vaginalis and giardiasis – The CDC has recommended the use of oral metronidazole for *Gardnerella vaginalis* (500 mg twice daily for 7 days) and for giardiasis (250 mg 3 times daily for 7 days).

Administration and Dosage

➤*Hepatic function impairment:* Patients with severe hepatic disease metabolize metronidazole slowly, with resultant accumulation of metronidazole and its metabolites in the plasma. Accordingly, for such patients, doses below those usually recommended should be administered cautiously. Close monitoring of plasma metronidazole levels and toxicity is recommended.

➤*Renal function impairment:* The dose of metronidazole should not be specifically reduced in anuric patients because accumulated metabolites may be rapidly removed by dialysis.

➤*Elderly:* In elderly patients, the pharmacokinetics of metronidazole may be altered and therefore, monitoring of serum levels may be necessary to adjust the metronidazole dosage accordingly.

➤*Pregnancy:* Pregnant patients should not be treated during the first trimester.

In pregnant patients in whom alternative treatment has been inadequate, the 1-day course of therapy should not be used, as it results in higher serum levels that can reach the fetal circulation.

➤*Tablets:*

Trichomoniasis in the female – For 1-day treatment, take 2 g of metronidazole, given either as a single dose or in 2 divided doses of 1 g each given in the same day.

For a 7-day course of treatment, take 250 mg 3 times daily for 7 consecutive days. There is some indication from controlled comparative studies that cure rates as determined by vaginal smears, signs, and symptoms may be higher after a 7-day course of treatment than after a 1-day treatment regimen.

The dosage regimen should be individualized. Single-dose treatment can assure compliance, especially if administered under supervision, in those patients who cannot be relied on to continue the 7-day regimen. A 7-day course of treatment may minimize reinfection by protecting the patient long enough for the sexual contacts to obtain appropriate treatment. Further, some patients may tolerate one treatment regimen better than the other.

METRONIDAZOLE — ORAL

Capsules – Seven-day course of treatment 375 mg capsules 2 times daily for 7 consecutive days.

A 7-day course of treatment may minimize reinfection by protecting the patient long enough for the sexual contacts to obtain treatment. When repeat courses of the drug are required, it is recommended that an interval of 4 to 6 weeks elapse between courses and that the presence of the trichomonad be reconfirmed by appropriate laboratory measures. Total and differential leukocyte counts should be made before and after retreatment.

Trichomoniasis in the male – In the male, treatment should be individualized as for the female.

➤*Amebiasis:*

Adults – For acute intestinal amebiasis (acute amebic dysentery), take 750 mg orally 3 times daily for 5 to 10 days.

For amebic liver abscess – 500 mg or 750 mg orally 3 times daily for 5 to 10 days.

Children – 35 to 50 mg/kg/24 hours, divided into 3 doses orally for 10 days.

Extended-release tablets –

Bacterial vaginosis: For a 7-day course of treatment, take 750 mg once daily by mouth for 7 consecutive days.

Metronidazole extended-release tablets should be taken under fasting conditions, at least 1 hour before or 2 hours after meals. The optimum extended-release characteristics of metronidazole extended-release are obtained when the drug is taken under fasting conditions.

➤*Anaerobic bacterial infections:* In the treatment of most serious anaerobic infections, metronidazole IV is usually administered initially.

The usual adult oral dosage is 7.5 mg/kg every 6 hours (approximately 500 mg for a 70 kg adult). A maximum of 4 g should not be exceeded during a 24-hour period.

➤*Duration:* The usual duration of therapy is 7 to 10 days; however, infections of the bone and joint, lower respiratory tract, and endocardium may require longer treatment.

➤*Storage/Stability:*

Tablets – Store below 25°C (77°F) and protect from light.

Capsules – Store at controlled room temperature 15° to 25°C (59° to 77°F). Dispense in a well-closed container with a child-resistant closure.

Extended-release tablets – Store at controlled room temperature, in a dry place, between 15° to 30°C (59° to 86°F). Dispense in a well-closed container with a child-resistant closure. Protect from light.

Actions

➤*Pharmacology:* Metronidazole exerts an antimicrobial effect in an anaerobic environment by the following possible mechanism: Once metronidazole enters the organism, the drug is reduced by intracellular electron transport proteins. Because of this alteration to the metronidazole molecule, a concentration gradient is maintained, which promotes the drug's intracellular transport. Presumably, free radicals are formed, which in turn react with cellular components resulting in death of the microorganism.

➤*Pharmacokinetics:*

Absorption –

Tablets: Following oral administration, metronidazole is well absorbed with peak plasma concentrations occurring between 1 and 2 hours after administration. Plasma concentrations of metronidazole are proportional to the administered dose. Oral administration of 250, 500, or 2000 mg produced peak plasma concentrations of 6 mcg/mL, 12 mcg/mL, and 40 mcg/mL, respectively. Studies reveal no significant bioavailability differences between males and females; however, because of weight differences, the resulting plasma levels in males are generally lower.

Capsules: Metronidazole 375 mg capsules have been shown to have a rate and extent of absorption similar to metronidazole tablets and were bioequivalent at an equal single dose of 750 mg. In a study conducted with 23 adult, healthy, female volunteers, oral administration of two 375 mg metronidazole capsules under fasting conditions produced a mean (± 1 SD) peak plasma concentration (C_{max}) of 21.4 (± 2.8) mcg/mL with a mean t_{max} of 1.6 (± 0.7) hours and a mean area under the plasma concentration-time curve (AUC) of 223 (± 44) mcg•hr/mL. In the same study, three 250 mg metronidazole tablets produced a mean C_{max} of 20.4 (± 3.8) mcg/mL with a mean t_{max} of 1.4 (± 0.4) hours and a mean AUC of 218 (± 50) mcg•hr/mL.

Administration of metronidazole 375 mg capsules with food does not affect the extent of absorption of metronidazole; however, the presence of food results in a lower C_{max} and a delayed t_{max} compared to fasted conditions. In a study of 14 healthy, adult, female volunteers, administration of metronidazole 375 mg capsules under fasting conditions produced a mean C_{max} of 10.9 (± 1.5) mcg/mL, a mean t_{max} of 1.5 (± 1.4) hours, and a mean AUC of 110 (± 34) mcg•hr/mL compared to a mean C_{max} of 8.6 (± 1.6) mcg/mL, a mean t_{max} of 4.2 (± 1.7) hours, and a mean AUC of 99 (± 14) mcg•hr/mL under fed conditions.

Extended-release tablets: Relative to the fasting state, the rate of metronidazole absorption from the extended-release tablet is increased in the fed state resulting in alteration of the extended-release characteristics.

Distribution – Metronidazole appears in cerebrospinal fluid, saliva, and human milk in concentrations similar to those found in plasma. Bactericidal concentrations of metronidazole have also been detected in pus from hepatic abscesses.

Metabolism – Metronidazole is the major component appearing in the plasma, with lesser quantities of the 2-hydroxymethyl metabolite also being present. Less than 20% of the circulating metronidazole is bound to plasma proteins. Both the parent compound and the metabolite possess in vitro bactericidal activity against most strains of anaerobic bacteria and in vitro trichomonacidal activity.

Excretion – Disposition of metronidazole in the body is similar for both oral and IV dosage forms, with an average elimination half-life of 8 hours in healthy humans.

The major route of elimination of metronidazole and its metabolites is via the urine (60% to 80% of the dose), with fecal excretion accounting for 6% to 15% of the dose. The metabolites that appear in the urine result primarily from side-chain oxidation [1-(β-hydroxyethyl)-2-hydroxymethyl-5-nitroimidazole and 2-methyl-5-nitroimidazole-1-yl-acetic acid] and glucuronide conjugation, with unchanged metronidazole accounting for approximately 20% of the total. Renal clearance of metronidazole is approximately 10 mL/min/1.73 m^2.

Hepatic/Renal function impairment – Decreased renal function does not alter the single-dose pharmacokinetics of metronidazole. However, plasma clearance of metronidazole is decreased in patients with decreased liver function.

➤*Microbiology:*

Metronidazole has been shown to have in vitro and clinical activity against the following organisms –

Anaerobic gram-negative bacilli, including: Bacteroides species including the *Bacteroides fragilis* group (*B. fragilis, B. distasonis, B. ovatus, B. thetaiotaomicron, B. vulgatus*) and *Fusobacterium* species.

Anaerobic gram-positive bacilli: Clostridium species and susceptible strains of *Eubacterium*.

Anaerobic gram-positive cocci: Peptococcus niger and *Peptostreptococcus* species.

Protozoal parasites: Entamoeba histolytica and *Trichomonas vaginalis*.

Contraindications

A history of hypersensitivity to metronidazole or other nitroimidazole derivatives; during the first trimester of pregnancy.

Warnings

➤*Neurologic effects:* Convulsive seizures and peripheral neuropathy, the latter characterized mainly by numbness or paresthesia of an extremity, have been reported in patients treated with metronidazole. The appearance of abnormal neurologic signs demands the prompt discontinuation of metronidazole therapy. Metronidazole should be administered with caution to patients with CNS diseases.

➤*Hepatic function impairment:* See Administration and Dosage for more information.

➤*Carcinogenesis:* Metronidazole has shown evidence of carcinogenic activity in a number of studies involving chronic, oral administration in mice and rats, but similar studies in the hamster gave negative results.

Prominent among the effects in the mouse was the promotion of pulmonary tumorigenesis. This has been observed in all 6 reported studies in that species, including one study in which the animals were dosed on an intermittent schedule (administration during every fourth week only). When taken at very high dose levels (approximately 1500 mg/m^2, which is approximately 3 times the most frequently recommended human dose for a 50 kg adult based on mg/m^2) there was a statistically significant increase in the incidence of malignant liver tumors in males. In addition, when high dose levels (approximately 500 mg/kg/day which is approximately 33 times the most frequently recommended human dose for a 50 kg adult based on mg/kg body weight) were administered, there was a statistically significant increase in the incidence of malignant liver tumors in males. Also, the published results of one of the mouse studies indicate an increase in the incidence of malignant lymphomas and pulmonary neoplasms associated with lifetime feeding of the drug. All these effects are statistically significant.

Several long-term, oral-dosing studies in the rat have been completed. There were statistically significant increases in the incidence of various neoplasms, particularly in mammary and hepatic tumors, among female rats administered metronidazole over those noted in the concurrent female control groups.

➤*Elderly:* No overall differences have been reported in safety and effectiveness between younger and older individuals, but greater sensitivity of some older individuals cannot be ruled out. Systemic exposure to the active metabolite, 2-hydroxymethyl metronidazole, is higher in the elderly. Metronidazole is known to be substantially excreted by the kidney, and the risk of toxic reactions to this drug may be greater in patients with impaired renal function. Although decreased renal function does not alter the single dose pharmacokinetics of metronidazole, because elderly patients are more likely to have decreased liver function, care should be taken in dose selection, and it may be useful to monitor renal function.

Plasma clearance of metronidazole is decreased in patients with decreased liver function. Therefore, in elderly patients, monitoring of serum levels may be necessary to adjust the metronidazole dosage accordingly.

➤*Pregnancy: Category B.* Metronidazole crosses the placental barrier and enters the fetal circulation rapidly. Reproduction studies have been performed in rats at doses up to 5 times the human dose and have revealed no evidence of impaired fertility or harm to the fetus due to metronidazole. No fetotoxicity was observed when metronidazole was administered orally to pregnant mice at 20 mg/kg/day, approximately 1.5 times the most frequently recommended human dose (750 mg/day) based on mg/kg body weight. No fetotoxicity was observed when metronidazole was administered orally to pregnant mice at 60 mg/m^2/day, which is approximately 10% of the human dose when expressed as mg/m^2. However in a single small study where the drug was administered intraperitoneally, some intrauterine deaths were observed. The relationship of these findings to the drug is unknown. There are, however, no adequate and well-controlled studies in pregnant women.

METRONIDAZOLE — ORAL

Because animal reproduction studies are not always predictive of human response, and because metronidazole is a carcinogen in rodents, this drug should be used during pregnancy only if clearly needed.

Use of metronidazole in the second and third trimesters of pregnancy or for trichomoniasis during pregnancy should be restricted to those in whom alternative treatment has been inadequate. Use of metronidazole in the first trimester or for trichomoniasis in pregnancy should be carefully evaluated because metronidazole crosses the placental barrier and its effects on the human fetal organogenesis are not known (see above).

➤*Lactation:* Because of the potential for tumorigenicity, shown for metronidazole in mouse and rat studies, a decision should be made whether to discontinue nursing or to discontinue the drug, taking into account the importance of the drug to the mother. Metronidazole is secreted in human milk in concentrations similar to those found in plasma.

➤*Children:* Safety and efficacy in children have not been established, except for the treatment of amebiasis (tablets and capsules only).

Precautions

➤*Monitoring:* Monitoring of serum levels in elderly patients may be necessary to adjust the metronidazole dosage accordingly.

➤*Candidiasis:* Known or previously unrecognized candidiasis may present more prominent symptoms during therapy with metronidazole and requires treatment with a candidacidal agent.

➤*Hematologic effects:* Metronidazole is a nitroimidazole and should be used with caution in patients with evidence of or history of blood dyscrasia. A mild leukopenia has been observed during its administration; however, no persistent hematologic abnormalities attributable to metronidazole have been observed in clinical studies. Total and differential leukocyte counts are recommended before and after therapy for trichomoniasis and amebiasis, especially if a second course of therapy is necessary, and before and after therapy for anaerobic infections.

Drug Interactions

Metronidazole Drug Interactions

Precipitant drug	Object drug*		Description
Barbiturates Phenytoin	Metronidazole	⬇	Coadministration may accelerate the elimination of metronidazole, resulting in reduced plasma levels.
Cimetidine	Metronidazole	⬆	Decreased metronidazole clearance and increased serum levels may occur; however, data conflict.
Metronidazole	Anticoagulants	⬆	The anticoagulant effect of warfarin may be enhanced.
Metronidazole	Disulfiram	⬆	Concurrent use may result in an acute psychosis or confusional state. Do not give metronidazole to patients who have taken disulfiram within the last 2 weeks.
Metronidazole	Ethanol	⬆	A disulfiram-like reaction including symptoms of flushing, palpitations, tachycardia, nausea, vomiting, etc, may occur with concurrent use. Although the risk for most patients may be slight, caution is advised. Do not consume alcohol during therapy and for ≥ 1 to 3 days afterward.
Metronidazole	Hydantoins	⬆	The total clearance of phenytoin may be decreased and its elimination half-life prolonged.
Metronidazole	Lithium	⬆	In patients stabilized on relatively high lithium doses, short-term metronidazole has been associated with increased lithium levels and toxicity in some cases.

* ⬆ = Object drug increased. ⬇ = Object drug decreased.

➤*Drug/Lab test interactions:* Metronidazole may interfere with certain types of determinations of serum chemistry values, such AST, ALT, LDH, triglycerides, and hexokinase glucose. Values of zero may be observed. All of the assays in which interference has been reported involve enzymatic coupling of the assay to oxidation-reduction of nicotinamide adenine dinucleotide ($NAD^+ \rightleftarrows NADH$). Interference is due to the similarity in absorbance peaks of NADH (340 nm) and metronidazole (322 nm) at pH 7.

Adverse Reactions

➤*Extended-release tablets:* Most adverse events were described as being of mild or moderate severity. Among patients taking metronidazole extended-release who reported headaches, 10% considered them severe, and less than 2% of reported episodes of nausea were considered severe. Metallic taste was reported by 9% of patients taking metronidazole extended-release.

Adverse events (≥ 2% incidence rate) irrespective of treatment causality

	Metronidazole extended release tablets 7 days (n = 267)	Vaginal preparation (n = 285)
Headache	48 (18%)	44 (15%)
Vaginitis	39 (15%)	32 (12%)
Nausea	28 (10%)	8 (3%)
Taste perversion (metallic taste)	23 (9%)	1 (0%)
Infection bacterial	19 (7%)	17 (6%)
Influenza-like symptoms	17 (6%)	20 (7%)
Pruritus genital	14 (5%)	25 (9%)
Abdominal pain	10 (4%)	13 (5%)
Dizziness	11 (4%)	3 (1%)
Diarrhea	11 (4%)	3 (1%)
Upper respiratory tract infection	11 (4%)	10 (4%)
Rhinitis	12 (4%)	10 (4%)
Sinusitis	7 (3%)	6 (2%)
Urine abnormal	7 (3%)	4 (1%)
Pharyngitis	8 (3%)	4 (1%)
Dysmenorrhea	9 (3%)	7 (2%)
Moniliasis	9 (3%)	8 (3%)
Mouth dry	5 (2%)	2 (1%)
Urinary tract infection	6 (2%)	16 (6%)

➤*Adverse reactions reported during treatment with metronidazole:* The following reactions have also been reported during treatment with metronidazole:

Cardiovascular – Flattening of the T-wave may be seen in electrocardiographic tracings.

CNS – Two serious adverse reactions reported in patients treated with metronidazole have been convulsive seizures and peripheral neuropathy, the latter characterized mainly by numbness or paresthesia of an extremity. Since persistent peripheral neuropathy has been reported in some patients receiving prolonged administration of metronidazole, patients should be specifically warned about these reactions and should be told to stop the drug and report immediately to their physicians if any neurologic symptoms occur. In addition, patients have reported dizziness, vertigo, incoordination, ataxia, confusion, irritability, depression, weakness, and insomnia.

GI – The most common adverse reactions reported have been referable to the GI tract, particularly nausea reported by approximately 12% of patients, sometimes accompanied by headache, anorexia, and occasionally vomiting, diarrhea, epigastric distress, and abdominal cramping. Constipation has also been reported.

Hematologic – Reversible neutropenia (leukopenia); rarely, reversible thrombocytopenia.

Hypersensitivity – Urticaria, erythematous rash, flushing, nasal congestion, dryness of the mouth (or vagina or vulva), and fever.

Renal – Dysuria, cystitis, polyuria, incontinence, and a sense of pelvic pressure. Instances of darkened urine have been reported by approximately 1 patient in 100,000. Although the pigment, which is probably responsible for this phenomenon, has not been positively identified, it is almost certainly a metabolite of metronidazole and seems to have no clinical significance.

Special senses – A sharp, unpleasant metallic taste is not unusual. Furry tongue, glossitis, and stomatitis have occurred; these may be associated with a sudden overgrowth of *Candida*, which may occur during therapy.

Miscellaneous – Proliferation of *Candida* in the vagina, dyspareunia, decrease of libido, proctitis, and fleeting joint pains sometimes resembling "serum sickness." If patients receiving metronidazole drink alcoholic beverages, they may experience abdominal distress, nausea, vomiting, flushing, or headache. A modification of the taste of alcoholic beverages has also been reported. Rare cases of pancreatitis, which generally abated on withdrawal of the drug, have been reported.

Crohn disease – Crohn's disease patients are known to have an increased incidence of GI and certain extraintestinal cancers. There have been some reports in the medical literature of breast and colon cancer in Crohn's disease patients who have been treated with metronidazole at high doses for extended periods of time. A cause and effect relationship has not been established. Crohn's disease is not an approved indication for oral metronidazole.

Overdosage

➤*Symptoms:* Single oral doses of metronidazole up to 15 g have been reported in suicide attempts and accidental overdoses. Symptoms reported include nausea, vomiting, and ataxia.

METRONIDAZOLE — ORAL

Oral metronidazole has been studied as a radiation sensitizer in the treatment of malignant tumors. Neurotoxic effects, including seizures and peripheral neuropathy, have been reported after 5 to 7 days of doses of 6 to 10.4 g every other day.

➤*Treatment:* There is no specific antidote for metronidazole overdose; therefore, management of the patient should consist of symptomatic and supportive therapy.

Patient Information

Alcoholic beverages should be avoided while taking metronidazole and for at least 1 day (metronidazole) or 3 days (metronidazole after discontinuing.

METRONIDAZOLE — INJECTION

Metronidazole is also available for topical and intravaginal use. For further information refer to the individual monographs in the Dermatologicals chapter and Renal and Genitourinary chapter.

WARNING

Metronidazole has been shown to be carcinogenic in mice and rats. Its use, therefore, should be reserved for the conditions for which it is indicated.

Indications

➤*Anaerobic infections:* In the treatment of serious infections caused by susceptible anaerobic bacteria. Indicated surgical procedures should be performed in conjunction with metronidazole injection therapy. In a mixed aerobic and anaerobic infection, antibiotics appropriate for the treatment of the aerobic infection should be used in addition to metronidazole injection.

Effective in *Bacteroides fragilis* infections resistant to clindamycin, chloramphenicol, and penicillin.

Intra-abdominal infections – Intra-abdominal infections including peritonitis, intra-abdominal abscess, and liver abscess, caused by *Bacteroides* species including the *B. fragilis* group (*B. fragilis*, *B. distasonis*, *B. ovatus*, *B. thetaiotaomicron*, *B. vulgatus*), *Clostridium* species, *Eubacterium* species, *Peptococcus* species, and *Peptostreptococcus* species.

Skin and skin structure infections – Caused by *Bacteroides* species including the *B. fragilis* group, *Clostridium* species, *Peptococcus* species, *Peptostreptococcus* species, and *Fusobacterium* species.

Gynecologic infections – Including endometritis, endomyometritis, tubo-ovarian abscess, and postsurgical vaginal cuff infection, caused by *Bacteroides* species including the *B. fragilis* group, *Clostridium* species, *Peptococcus* species, and *Peptostreptococcus* species.

Bacterial septicemia – Caused by *Bacteroides* species including the *B. fragilis* group, and *Clostridium* species.

Bone and joint infections – As adjunctive therapy, caused by *Bacteroides* species including the *B. fragilis* group.

Central nervous system (CNS) infections – Including meningitis and brain abscess, caused by *Bacteroides* species including the *B. fragilis* group.

Lower respiratory tract infections – Including pneumonia, empyema, and lung abscess, caused by *Bacteroides* species including the *B. fragilis* group.

Endocarditis – Caused by *Bacteroides* species including the *B. fragilis* group.

➤*Prophylaxis:* The prophylactic administration of metronidazole injection preoperatively, intraoperatively, and postoperatively may reduce the incidence of postoperative infection in patients undergoing elective colorectal surgery which is classified as contaminated or potentially contaminated.

Prophylactic use of metronidazole injection should be discontinued within 12 hours after surgery. If there are signs of infection, specimens for cultures should be obtained for the identification of the causative organism(s) so that appropriate therapy may be given.

➤*Unlabeled uses:*

Pelvic inflammatory disease – As an alternative parenteral regimen, the CDC recommends metronidazole 500 mg IV every 8 hours combined with ofloxacin alone or ciprofloxacin plus doxycycline.

Administration and Dosage

➤*Elderly:* In elderly patients the pharmacokinetics of metronidazole may be altered and therefore monitoring of serum levels may be necessary to adjust the metronidazole dosage accordingly.

➤*Anaerobic infections:* The recommended dosage schedule for adults is:

Loading dose – 15 mg/kg infused over 1 hour (approximately 1 g for a 70 kg adult).

Maintenance dose – 7.5 mg/kg infused over 1 hour every 6 hours (approximately 500 mg for a 70 kg adult). The first maintenance dose should be instituted 6 hours following the initiation of the loading dose.

➤*IV to oral conversion:* Parenteral therapy may be changed to oral metronidazole when conditions warrant, based upon the severity of the disease and the response of the patient to metronidazole injection treatment. The usual adult oral dosage is 7.5 mg/kg every 6 hours.

A maximum of 4 g should not be exceeded during a 24-hour period.

➤*Hepatic function impairment:* Patients with severe hepatic disease metabolize metronidazole slowly, with resultant accumulation of metronidazole and its metabolites in the plasma. Accordingly, for such patients, doses below those usually recommended should be administered cautiously. Close monitoring of plasma metronidazole levels and toxicity is recommended.

➤*Nasogastric aspiration:* In patients receiving metronidazole injection in whom gastric secretions are continuously removed by nasogastric aspiration, sufficient metronidazole may be removed in the aspirate to cause a reduction in serum levels.

➤*Renal function impairment:* The dose of metronidazole injection should not be specifically reduced in anuric patients since accumulated metabolites may be rapidly removed by dialysis.

➤*Duration:* The usual duration of therapy is 7 to 10 days; however, infections of the bone and joint, lower respiratory tract, and endocardium may require longer treatment.

➤*Prophylaxis:* For surgical prophylactic use, to prevent postoperative infection in contaminated or potentially contaminated colorectal surgery, the recommended dosage schedule for adults is 15 mg/kg infused over 30 to 60 minutes and completed approximately 1 hour before surgery; followed by 7.5 mg/kg infused over 30 to 60 minutes at 6 and 12 hours after the initial dose.

It is important that administration of the initial preoperative dose be completed approximately 1 hour before surgery so that adequate drug levels are present in the serum and tissues at the time of initial incision. Metronidazole injection be administered, if necessary, at 6-hour intervals to maintain effective drug levels.

Prophylactic use of metronidazole injection should be limited to the day of surgery only, following the above guidelines.

➤*IV:* Metronidazole injection is to be administered by slow IV drip infusion only, either as a continuous or intermittent infusion. IV admixtures containing metronidazole and other drugs should be avoided. Additives should not be introduced into this solution. If used with a primary IV fluid system, the primary solution should be discontinued during metronidazole infusion. Do not use equipment containing aluminum (eg, needles, cannulae) that would come in contact with the drug solution.

➤*Single-dose lyophilized vials:* Metronidazole HCl cannot be given by direct IV injection (IV bolus) because of the low pH (0.5 to 2) of the reconstituted product. Metronidazole HCl must be further diluted and neutralized for IV infusion.

Metronidazole HCl is prepared for use in 2 steps:

Order of mixing is important.

1.) Reconstitution.
2.) Dilution in IV solution followed by pH neutralization with sodium bicarbonate injection into the dilution.

Reconstitution – To prepare the solution, add 4.4 mL of one of the following diluents and mix thoroughly: Sterile Water for Injection, Bacteriostatic Water for Injection, 0.9% Sodium Chloride Injection, or Bacteriostatic 0.9% Sodium Chloride Injection. The resultant approximate withdrawal volume is 5 mL with an approximate concentration of 100 mg/mL.

The pH of the reconstituted product will be in the range of 0.5 to 2. Reconstituted metronidazole HCl is clear, and pale yellow to yellow-green in color.

Dilution in IV solutions – Properly reconstituted metronidazole HCl may be added to a glass or plastic IV container not to exceed a concentration of 8 mg/mL. Any of the following IV solutions may be used: 0.9% Sodium Chloride Injection, 5% Dextrose Injection, or Lactated Ringer's Injection. Neutralization is required prior to administration. The final product should be mixed thoroughly and used within 24 hours.

Neutralization for IV infusion – Neutralize the IV solution containing metronidazole HCl with approximately 5 mEq of sodium bicarbonate injection for each 500 mg of metronidazole HCl used. Mix thoroughly. The pH of the neutralized IV solution will be approximately 6 to 7. Carbon dioxide gas will be generated with neutralization. It may be necessary to relieve gas pressure within the container.

When the contents of 1 vial (500 mg) are diluted and neutralized to 100 mL, the resultant concentration is 5 mg/mL. Do not exceed an 8 mg/mL concentration of metronidazole HCl in the neutralized IV solution, since neutralization will decrease the aqueous solubility and precipitation may occur. Do not refrigerate neutralized solutions; otherwise, precipitation may occur.

➤*Single-dose flexible containers:* Metronidazole injection is a ready-to-use isotonic solution. No dilution or buffering is required. Do not refrigerate. Each container of metronidazole injection contains 14 mEq of sodium.

Do not use flexible container in series connections. Such use could result in air embolism due to residual air being drawn from the primary container before administration of the fluid from the secondary container is complete.

➤*Storage/Stability:* Parenteral drug products should be inspected visually for particulate matter and discoloration prior to administration, whenever solution and container permit. Do not use if cloudy or precipitated or if the seal is not intact.

Use sterile equipment. It is recommended that the IV administration apparatus be replaced at least once every 24 hours.

Single-dose lyophilized vials – Reconstituted vials of IV metronidazole HCl are chemically stable for 96 hours when stored below 30°C (86°F) in room light.

METRONIDAZOLE — INJECTION

Use diluted and neutralized IV solutions containing metronidazole HCl within 24 hours of mixing.

Single-dose flexible containers – Metronidazole injection should be stored at controlled room temperature 15° to 30°C (59° to 86°F) and protected from light during storage.

Actions

➤*Pharmacology:* Metronidazole is a synthetic antibacterial compound. Disposition of metronidazole in the body is similar for both oral and IV dosage forms, with an average elimination half-life in healthy humans of 8 hours.

➤*Pharmacokinetics:*

Absorption/Distribution – Metronidazole appears in cerebrospinal fluid, saliva, and breast milk in concentrations similar to those found in plasma. Bactericidal concentrations of metronidazole have also been detected in pus from hepatic abscesses.

Plasma concentrations of metronidazole are proportional to the administered dose. An 8-hour IV infusion of 100 to 4000 mg of metronidazole in healthy subjects showed a linear relationship between dose and peak plasma concentration.

In patients treated with metronidazole, using a dosage regimen of 15 mg/kg loading dose followed 6 hours later by 7.5 mg/kg every 6 hours, peak steady-state plasma concentrations of metronidazole averaged 25 mcg/mL with trough (minimum) concentrations averaging 18 mcg/mL.

Metronidazole is the major component appearing in the plasma, with lesser quantities of the 2-hydroxymethyl metabolite also being present. Less than 20% of the circulating metronidazole is bound to plasma proteins. Both the parent compound and the metabolite possess in vitro bactericidal activity against most strains of anaerobic bacteria.

Metabolism/Excretion – The major route of elimination of metronidazole and its metabolites is via the urine (60% to 80% of the dose), with fecal excretion accounting for 6% to 15% of the dose. The metabolites that appear in the urine result primarily from side-chain oxidation [1-(β-hydroxyethyl)-2-hydroxymethyl-5-nitroimidazole and 2-methyl-5-nitroimidazole-1-yl-acetic acid] and glucuronide conjugation, with unchanged metronidazole accounting for approximately 20% of the total. Renal clearance of metronidazole is approximately 10 mL/min/1.73 m^2.

Hepatic function impairment: Decreased renal function does not alter the single-dose pharmacokinetics of metronidazole. However, plasma clearance of metronidazole is decreased in patients with decreased liver function.

Children: In 1 study, newborn infants appeared to demonstrate diminished capacity to eliminate metronidazole. The elimination half-life, measured during the first 3 days of life, was inversely related to gestational age. In infants whose gestational ages were between 28 and 40 weeks, the corresponding elimination half-lives ranged from 109 to 22.5 hours.

➤*Microbiology:* Metronidazole is active in vitro against most obligate anaerobes, but does not appear to possess any clinically relevant activity against facultative anaerobes or obligate aerobes. Against susceptible organisms, metronidazole is generally bactericidal at concentrations equal to or slightly higher than the minimal inhibitory concentrations. Metronidazole has been shown to have in vitro and clinical activity against the following organisms:

Anaerobic gram-negative bacilli, including:
- *Bacteroides* species, including the *Bacteroides fragilis* group (*B. fragilis, B. distasonis, B. ovatus, B. thetaiotaomicron, B. vulgatus*).
- *Fusobacterium* species.

Anaerobic gram-positive bacilli, including:
- *Clostridium*species.
- Susceptible strains of *Eubacterium*.

Anaerobic gram-positive cocci, including:
- *Peptococcus* species.
- *Peptostreptococcus* species.

Contraindications

Hypersensitivity to metronidazole or other nitroimidazole derivatives.

Warnings

➤*Neurologic effects:* Convulsive seizures and peripheral neuropathy, the latter characterized mainly by numbness or paresthesia of an extremity, have been reported in patients treated with metronidazole. The appearance of abnormal neurologic signs demands the prompt evaluation of the benefit/risk ratio of the continuation of therapy.

➤*Hepatic function impairment:* Patients with severe hepatic disease metabolize metronidazole slowly, with resultant accumulation of metronidazole and its metabolites in the plasma. Accordingly, for such patients, doses below those usually recommended should be administered cautiously.

➤*Carcinogenesis:* Metronidazole has shown evidence of carcinogenic activity in studies involving chronic, oral administration in mice and rats, but similar studies in the hamster gave negative results.

➤*Pregnancy: Category B.* Metronidazole crosses the placental barrier and enters the fetal circulation rapidly. Reproduction studies have been performed in rats at doses up to 5 times the human dose and have revealed no evidence of impaired fertility or harm to the fetus due to metronidazole. Metronidazole administered intraperitoneally to pregnant mice at approximately the human dose caused fetotoxicity; administered orally to pregnant mice, no fetotoxicity was observed. There are, however, no adequate and well controlled studies in pregnant women. Because animal reproduction studies are not always predictive of human response, and because metronidazole is a carcinogen in rodents, these drugs should be used during pregnancy only if clearly needed.

➤*Lactation:* Because of the potential for tumorigenicity shown for metronidazole in mouse and rat studies, a decision should be made whether to discontinue nursing or to discontinue the drug, taking into account the importance of the drug to the mother. Metronidazole is secreted in breast milk in concentrations similar to those found in plasma.

➤*Children:* Safety and efficacy in children have not been established.

Precautions

➤*Sodium content:* Administration of solutions containing sodium ions may result in sodium retention.

➤*Candidiasis:* Known or previously unrecognized candidiasis may present more prominent symptoms during therapy with metronidazole injection and requires treatment with a candidacidal agent.

➤*Hematologic effects:* Metronidazole is a nitroimidazole, and metronidazole injection should be used with care in patients with evidence of or history of blood dyscrasia. A mild leukopenia has been observed during its administration; however, no persistent hematologic abnormalities attributable to metronidazole have been observed in clinical studies. Total and differential leukocyte counts are recommended before and after therapy.

➤*Special risk:* Care should be taken when administering metronidazole injection to patients receiving corticosteroids or to patients predisposed to edema.

Drug Interactions

Metronidazole Drug Interactions

Precipitant drug	Object drug*		Description
Barbiturates Phenytoin	Metronidazole	⬇	Coadministration may accelerate the elimination of metronidazole, resulting in reduced plasma levels.
Cimetidine	Metronidazole	⬆	Decreased metronidazole clearance and increased serum levels may occur; however, data conflict.
Metronidazole	Anticoagulants	⬆	The anticoagulant effect of warfarin may be enhanced.
Metronidazole	Disulfiram	⬆	Concurrent use may result in an acute psychosis or confusional state. Do not give metronidazole to patients who have taken disulfiram within the last 2 weeks.
Metronidazole	Ethanol	⬆	A disulfiram-like reaction including symptoms of flushing, palpitations, tachycardia, nausea, vomiting, etc, may occur with concurrent use. Although the risk for most patients may be slight, caution is advised. Do not consume alcohol during therapy and for ≥ 1 to 3 days afterward.
Metronidazole	Hydantoins	⬆	The total clearance of phenytoin may be decreased and its elimination half-life prolonged.
Metronidazole	Lithium	⬆	In patients stabilized on relatively high lithium doses, short-term metronidazole has been associated with increased lithium levels and toxicity in some cases.

* ⬆ = Object drug increased. ⬇ = Object drug decreased.

➤*Drug/Lab test interactions:* Metronidazole may interfere with certain types of determinations of serum chemistry values, such as aspartate aminotransferase (AST), alanine aminotransferase (ALT), lactate dehydrogenase (LDH), triglycerides, and hexokinase glucose. Values of zero may be observed. All of the assays in which interference has been reported involve enzymatic coupling of the assay to oxidation-reduction of nicotine adenine dinucleotide ($NAD^+ \rightleftarrows NADH$). Interference is due to the similarity in absorbance peaks of NADH (340 nm) and metronidazole (322 nm) at pH 7.

Adverse Reactions

The 2 most serious adverse reactions reported in patients treated with metronidazole injection have been convulsive seizures and peripheral neuropathy, the latter characterized mainly by numbness or paresthesia of an extremity. Since persistent peripheral neuropathy has been reported in some patients receiving prolonged oral administration of metronidazole, patients should be observed carefully if neurologic symptoms occur and a prompt evaluation made of the benefit/risk ratio of the continuation of therapy.

The following reactions have also been reported during treatment with metronidazole injection:

➤*CNS:* Headache, dizziness, syncope, ataxia, and confusion.

➤*Dermatologic:* Erythematous rash and pruritus.

METRONIDAZOLE — INJECTION

➤*GI:* Nausea, vomiting, abdominal discomfort, diarrhea, and an unpleasant metallic taste.

➤*Hematologic:* Reversible neutropenia (leukopenia).

➤*Local:* Thrombophlebitis after IV infusion. This reaction can be minimized or avoided by avoiding prolonged use of indwelling IV catheters.

➤*Miscellaneous:* Fever. Instances of a darkened urine have also been reported, and this manifestation has been the subject of a special investigation. Although the pigment which is probably responsible for this phenomenon has not been positively identified, it is almost certainly a metabolite of metronidazole and seems to have no clinical significance.

➤*Crohn disease:* Crohn's disease patients are known to have an increased incidence of GI and certain extraintestinal cancers. There have been some reports in the medical literature of breast and colon cancer in Crohn's disease patients who have been treated with metronidazole at high doses for extended periods of time. A cause-and-effect relationship has not been established. Crohn's disease is not an approved indication for metronidazole injection.

Overdosage

➤*Symptoms:* Use of dosages of metronidazole injection higher than those recommended has been reported. These include the use of 27 mg/kg 3 times a day for 20 days, and the use of 75 mg/kg as a single loading dose followed by 7.5 mg/kg maintenance doses. No adverse reactions were reported in either of the 2 cases. Single oral doses of metronidazole, up to 15 g, have been reported in suicide attempts and accidental overdoses. Symptoms reported include nausea, vomiting, and ataxia.

➤*Treatment:* There is no specific antidote for overdose; therefore, management of the patient should consist of symptomatic and supportive therapy.

SULFONAMIDES

In addition to the sulfonamides listed on the following pages, other preparations that contain sulfonamides include: Ophthalmic; vaginal; burn preparations (eg, mafenide, silver sulfadiazine). Sulfasalazine is indicated for ulcerative colitis and rheumatoid arthritis and is described in other sections. See individual monographs or sections.

Indications

Sulfonamide Indications

Indications	Sulfadiazine	Sulfisoxazole
Chancroid	✓	✓
Inclusion conjunctivitis	✓	✓
Malaria[1]	✓	✓
Meningitis, *Haemophilus influenzae*	✓	✓
Meningitis, meningococcal[2]	✓	✓
Nocardiosis	✓	✓
Otitis media, acute[3]	✓	✓
Rheumatic fever	✓	
Toxoplasmosis[4]	✓	✓
Trachoma	✓	✓
Urinary tract infections[5] (pyelonephritis, cystitis)	✓	✓

[1] As adjunctive therapy because of chloroquine-resistant strains of *Plasmodium falciparum*.
[2] When the organism is susceptible and for prophylaxis when sulfonamide-sensitive group A strains prevail.
[3] Caused by *H. influenzae* when used with penicillin.
[4] As adjunctive therapy with pyrimethamine.
[5] In the absence of obstructive uropathy or foreign bodies when caused by *Escherichia coli, Klebsiella-Enterobacter, Staphylococcus aureus, Proteus mirabilis,* and *P. vulgaris.*

Administration and Dosage

See individual products for specific guidelines based on indication.

➤*CDC recommended treatment schedules for sexually transmitted diseases†:*

Lymphogranuloma venereum – As an alternative regimen to doxycycline, sulfisoxazole 500 mg 4 times/day for 21 days or equivalent sulfonamide course.

Chlamydia trachomatic infections – As an alternative regimen to doxycycline or azithromycin (or if erythromycin is not tolerated), sulfisoxazole 500 mg 4 times/day for 10 days or equivalent sulfonamide course.

Actions

➤*Pharmacology:* Sulfonamides exert their bacteriostatic action by competitive antagonism of para-aminobenzoic acid (PABA), an essential component in folic acid synthesis. Microorganisms that require exogenous folic acid and do not synthesize folic acid are not susceptible to the action of sulfonamides.

➤*Pharmacokinetics:*

Absorption/Distribution – The oral sulfonamides are readily absorbed from the GI tract. Approximately 70% to 100% of an oral dose is absorbed. These agents are distributed throughout all body tissues and readily enter the cerebrospinal fluid, pleura, synovial fluids, the eye, the placenta, and the fetus. Sulfonamides are bound to plasma proteins in varying degrees. "Free" sulfonamide serum levels of 5 to 15 mg/dL may be therapeutically effective for most infections. Avoid levels > 20 mg/dL.

Metabolism – Metabolism occurs in the liver by conjugation and acetylation to inactive metabolites. Individuals who are slow acetylators have an increased risk of toxicity from sulfonamide accumulation.

Excretion – Renal excretion is mainly by glomerular filtration. Some of the acetylated metabolites are less soluble and may contribute to crystalluria and renal complications. To prevent the possibility of crystalluria, alkalinization of the urine and adequate fluid intake are recommended when using the less soluble sulfonamides (eg, sulfadiazine). Small amounts are eliminated in the feces, and in bile, breast milk, and other secretions.

➤*Microbiology:* Sulfonamides have a broad antibacterial spectrum that includes both gram-positive and gram-negative organisms.

Resistance – Organisms that produce excessive amounts of PABA develop resistance. The increasing frequency of resistant organisms is a limitation to the usefulness of the sulfonamides alone, especially in the treatment of chronic and recurrent urinary tract infections. Cross-resistance between sulfonamides is common once resistance develops. Minimize resistance by initiating treatment promptly with adequate doses and continuing for a sufficient period. In vitro sensitivity tests are not always reliable; carefully coordinate the test with bacteriologic and clinical response.

Contraindications

Hypersensitivity to sulfonamides or chemically related drugs (eg, sulfonylureas, thiazide and loop diuretics, carbonic anhydrase inhibitors, sunscreens with PABA, local anesthetics); pregnancy at term, lactation (see Warnings); infants < 2 months of age (except in congenital toxoplasmosis as adjunct with pyrimethamine).

Warnings

➤*Deaths:* Those associated with the administration of sulfonamides have been reported from hypersensitivity reactions, hepatocellular necrosis, agranulocytosis, aplastic anemia, and other blood dyscrasias. Sore throat, fever, pallor, purpura, or jaundice may be early indications of serious blood disorders. Perform complete blood counts.

➤*Group A beta-hemolytic streptococcal infections:* Do not use for treatment of these infections. In an established infection, they will not eradicate the streptococcus and will not prevent sequelae, such as rheumatic fever and glomerulonephritis.

➤*Hypersensitivity reactions:* May cause cholestatic jaundice.

➤*Renal function impairment:* Use with caution. The frequency of renal complications is considerably lower in patients receiving the more soluble sulfonamides (sulfisoxazole). Maintain adequate fluid intake (2 to 3 L/day) to prevent crystalluria and stone formation.

➤*Hepatic function impairment:* Cholestatic jaundice occurs in 0.5% to 1% of patients because of hypersensitivity or idiosyncrasy.

➤*Pregnancy: Category C.* Safety for use during pregnancy is not established. Sulfonamides cross the placenta; fetal levels average 70% to 90% of maternal serum levels. Significant levels may persist in the neonate if these drugs are given near term; jaundice, hemolytic anemia and kernicterus may occur. Teratogenicity (eg, tracheoesophageal fistula, cataracts) has occurred in some animal species. Do not use at term.

➤*Lactation:* Sulfonamides are excreted in breast milk in low concentrations. Milk:plasma ratios for sulfonamides are as low as 0.5 to 0.6. According to the American Academy of Pediatrics, breastfeeding and sulfonamide use

† *Morbidity and Mortality Weekly Report* 1993 Sep 24;42 (No. RR-14):i-102.

are compatible because sulfonamide excretion into breast milk does not pose a significant risk to the healthy full-term neonate. However, do not nurse premature infants or those with hyperbilirubinemia or G-6-PD deficiency.

➤*Children:* Do not use in infants < 2 months of age (except for congenital toxoplasmosis as adjunctive therapy with pyrimethamine).

Precautions

➤*Monitoring:* Monitor blood counts frequently, especially during prolonged administration. Perform microscopic urinalyses once a week when a patient is treated for > 2 weeks. Use urine cultures to confirm eradication of bacteriuria.

➤*Allergy or asthma:* Give with caution to patients with severe allergy or bronchial asthma.

➤*Hemolytic anemia:* Frequently dose-related, this may occur in G-6-PD deficient individuals.

➤*Photosensitivity:* Photosensitization (photoallergy or phototoxicity) may occur; therefore, caution patients to take protective measures (eg, sunscreens, protective clothing) against exposure to ultraviolet light or sunlight until tolerance is determined.

Drug Interactions

Sulfonamide Drug Interactions

Precipitant Drug	Object Drug*		Description
Sulfonamides	Anticoagulants, oral	↑	Warfarin's anticoagulation action may be enhanced. Hemorrhage could occur.
Sulfisoxazole	Barbiturate anesthetics	↑	The anesthetic effects of thiopental may be enhanced.
Sulfonamides	Cyclosporine	↓	Cyclosporine concentrations are decreased, and the risk of nephrotoxicity may be increased.
Sulfonamides	Hydantoins	↑	Serum hydantoin levels may be increased.
Sulfonamides	Methotrexate	↑	The risk of methotrexate-induced bone marrow suppression may be enhanced.
Sulfonamides	Sulfonylureas	↑	Increased sulfonylurea half-lives and hypoglycemia may occur.
Sulfonamides	Tolbutamide	↑	The half-life of tolbutamide may be prolonged when administered with sulfamethizole.
Sulfonamides	Uricosuric agents	↑	Potentiation of uricosuric action may be noted.
Diuretics (eg, thiazide)	Sulfonamides	↑	Coadministration may cause an increased incidence of thrombocytopenia with purpura.
Indomethacin	Sulfonamides	↑	Sulfonamides may be displaced from plasma albumin resulting in increased free-drug concentrations.
Methenamine	Sulfonamides	↑	An insoluble precipitate may form in acidic urine when sulfamethizole is used concomitantly with methenamine mandelate.
Probenecid	Sulfonamides	↑	Sulfonamides may be displaced from plasma albumin resulting in increased free-drug concentrations.
Salicylates	Sulfonamides	↑	Sulfonamides may be displaced from plasma albumin resulting in increased free-drug concentrations.

* ↑ = Object drug increased. ↓ = Object drug decreased.

Adverse Reactions

➤*CNS:* Headache; peripheral neuropathy; mental depression; convulsions; ataxia; hallucinations; tinnitus; vertigo; insomnia; apathy; drowsiness; polyneuritis; neuritis; optic neuritis; transient myopia.

➤*GI:* Nausea; emesis; abdominal pains; diarrhea; anorexia; pancreatitis; stomatitis; hepatitis; hepatocellular necrosis; pseudomembranous enterocolitis; glossitis.

➤*Hematologic:* Agranulocytosis; aplastic anemia; thrombocytopenia; leukopenia; hemolytic anemia; purpura; hypoprothrombinemia; neutropenia; eosinophilia; methemoglobinemia.

➤*Hypersensitivity:* Stevens-Johnson type erythema multiforme; generalized skin eruptions; allergic myocarditis; epidermal necrolysis; urticaria; periarteritis nodosum; serum sickness; pruritus; exfoliative dermatitis; anaphylactoid reactions; periorbital edema; conjunctival, scleral injection; photosensitization; arthralgia; allergic myocarditis; transient pulmonary changes with eosinophilia and decreased pulmonary function.

➤*Renal:* Crystalluria; elevated creatinine; toxic nephrosis with oliguria and anuria.

➤*Miscellaneous:* Drug fever; chills; pyrexia; L.E. phenomenon. Reports of adverse effects in breastfeeding infants are rare.

The sulfonamides bear chemical similarities to some goitrogens, diuretics (acetazolamide and thiazides) and oral hypoglycemic agents. Goiter production, diuresis and hypoglycemia have occurred rarely in patients receiving sulfonamides. Cross-sensitivity may exist with these agents (see Contraindications).

Overdosage

➤*Symptoms:*

GI – Anorexia; colic; nausea; vomiting.

CNS – Dizziness; headache; drowsiness; unconsciousness; vertigo. Pyrexia, hematuria and crystalluria have been reported. Blood dyscrasias and jaundice are late manifestations of overdosage.

➤*Treatment:* Discontinue the drug immediately. Within 1 or 2 days after discontinuation, the less serious symptoms disappear; grave symptoms require 1 to 3 weeks for remission. Empty the stomach if large doses have been ingested. Alkalinize the urine to enhance solubility and excretion. Force fluids if kidney function is normal, up to 4 L/day, to increase excretion. Monitor renal function with appropriate blood chemistries including electrolytes closely and in the acute period. Follow hematologic parameters over the next 10 days to 2 weeks after the overdose ingestion. Methemoglobinuria can be acutely reversed with IV 1% methylene blue.

Patient Information

Complete full course of therapy.

Take with a full glass of water (2 to 3 L/day).

Avoid prolonged exposure to sunlight; photosensitivity may occur. If outside, wear protective clothing and apply sunscreen to exposed areas.

Notify physician if any of the following occurs: Blood in urine, rash, ringing in ears, difficulty in breathing, fever, sore throat or chills.

SULFADIAZINE

Rx	**Sulfadiazine** (Various, eg, Eon, Major, Rugby, UDL, Zenith-Goldline)	**Tablets:** 500 mg	In 100s, 1000s and UD 100s.

SULFADIAZINE — ORAL

For complete and comparative prescribing information, refer to the Sulfonamides group monograph.

Administration and Dosage

Systemic sulfonamides are contraindicated in infants under 2 months of age except as adjunctive therapy with pyrimethamine in the treatment of congenital toxoplasmosis.

➤*Infants over 2 months of age and children:*

Initially – One-half the 24-hour dose.

Maintenance – 150 mg/kg or 4 g/m^2, divided into 4 to 6 doses, every 24 hours, with a maximum of 6 g every 24 hours.

Rheumatic fever prophylaxis – Under 30 kg (66 lbs), 500 mg every 24 hours; over 30 kg (66 lbs), 1 g every 24 hours.

➤*Adults:*

Initially – 2 to 4 g.

Maintenance – 2 to 4 g, divided into 3 to 6 doses, every 24 hours.

➤*Storage/Stability:* Store at controlled room temperature 15° to 30°C (59° to 86°F).

Dispense in a tight, light-resistant container as defined in the USP.

SULFISOXAZOLE

Rx	**Sulfisoxazole** (Various, eg, Geneva, Moore, Rugby)	**Tablets:** 500 mg	In 100s and 1000s.
Rx	**Gantrisin Pediatric** (Roche)	**Suspension:** 500 mg/5 ml	0.3% alcohol, parabens, sugar, sucrose. Raspberry flavor. In 480 ml.

SULFISOXAZOLE — ORAL

For complete and comparative prescribing information, refer to the Sulfonamides group monograph.

Administration and Dosage

Systemic sulfonamides are contraindicated in infants under 2 months of age, except in the treatment of congenital toxoplasmosis as adjunctive therapy with pyrimethamine.

➤*Infants over 2 months of age and children:*

Initial dose – 75 mg/kg or 2 g/m^2.

Maintenance dose – 150 mg/kg per 24 hours or 4 g/M^2 per 24 hours (dose to be divided into 4 to 6 doses per 24 hours). The maximum dose should not exceed 6 g per 24 hours.

➤*Adults:*

Initial dose – 2 to 4 g.

Maintenance dose – 4 to 8 g per 24 hours, divided in 4 to 6 doses per 24 hours.

➤*Storage/Stability:* Store at controlled room temperature 15° to 30°C (59° to 86°F).

NITROFURANS

NITROFURANTOIN

Rx	**Macrodantin** (Procter & Gamble)	**Capsules:** 25 mg (as macrocrystals)	Lactose, talc. (MACRODANTIN 25 mg 0149-0007). Opaque, white. In 100s.
Rx	**Nitrofurantoin** (Various, eg, Ivax, Mylan, Watson)	**Capsules:** 50 mg (as macrocrystals)	In 100s, 500s, and 1,000s.
Rx	**Macrodantin** (Procter & Gamble)		Lactose, talc. (MACRODANTIN 50 mg 0149-0008). Opaque, yellow/white. In 100s and 1,000s.
Rx	**Nitrofurantoin** (Various, eg, Ivax, Mylan, Watson)	**Capsules:** 100 mg (as macrocrystals)	In 100s, 500s, and 1,000s.
Rx	**Macrodantin** (Procter & Gamble)		Lactose, talc. (MACRODANTIN 100 mg 0149-0009). Opaque, yellow. In 100s and 1,000s.
Rx	**Nitrofurantoin** (Various, eg, Mylan, Watson)	**Capsules:** 100 mg (as monohydrate/macrocrystals)	In 100s and 500s.
Rx	**Macrobid** (Procter & Gamble)		Lactose, talc. (Macrobid Norwich Eaton). Opaque, black/yellow. In 100s.
Rx	**Furadantin** (First Horizon)	**Oral suspension:** 25 mg per 5 mL	Glycerin, parabens, saccharin, sorbitol. In 60 and 470 mL.

NITROFURANTOIN

Indications

➤*Urinary tract infections (UTIs):* For the treatment of UTIs when caused by susceptible strains of *Escherichia coli*, enterococci, *Staphylococcus aureus*, and certain susceptible strains of *Klebsiella* and *Enterobacter* species.

Acute cystitis – Nitrofurantoin monohydrate/macrocrystals is indicated only for the treatment of acute uncomplicated UTIs (acute cystitis) caused by susceptible strains of *E. coli* or *Staphylococcus saprophyticus* in patients 12 years of age and older.

Nitrofurantoin is not indicated for the treatment of pyelonephritis or perinephric abscesses.

Administration and Dosage

➤*Approved by the FDA:* February 6, 1953.

Give nitrofurantoin with food to improve drug absorption and, in some patients, tolerance.

➤*Adults:* 50 to 100 mg 4 times a day (the lower dosage level is recommended for uncomplicated UTIs); 100 mg every 12 hours for 7 days for adults and children older than 12 years of age (monohydrate/macrocrystals only).

For long-term suppressive therapy in adults, a dosage reduction to 50 to 100 mg at bedtime may be adequate.

➤*Children (1 month of age and older):* 5 to 7 mg/kg of body weight per 24 hours, given in 4 divided doses (contraindicated in infants younger than 1 month of age).

Continue therapy for 1 week or for at least 3 days after sterility of the urine is obtained. Continued infection indicates the need for reevaluation.

For long-term suppressive therapy in pediatric patients, doses as low as 1 mg/kg per 24 hours, given in a single dose or in 2 divided doses, may be adequate.

Oral suspension – The following table is based on an average weight in each range receiving 5 to 6 mg/kg of body weight per 24 hours, given in 4 divided doses. It can be used to calculate an average dose of nitrofurantoin oral suspension (25 mg per 5 mL) for pediatric patients.

Nitrofurantoin Dosage in Children Based on Body Weight		
Body weight		Dosage amount
Pounds	Kilograms	4 times daily
15 to 26	7 to 11	2.5 mL
27 to 46	12 to 21	5 mL
47 to 68	22 to 30	7.5 mL
69 to 91	31 to 41	10 mL

➤*Storage/Stability:*

Oral suspension – Avoid exposure to strong light, which may darken the drug. It is stable when stored between 20° to 25°C (68° to 77°F). Protect from freezing. Dispense in glass amber bottles.

Capsules – Store at controlled room temperature 15° to 30°C (59° to 86°F). Dispense in a tight container using a child-resistant closure.

Actions

➤*Pharmacology:* Nitrofurantoin is bactericidal in urine at therapeutic doses. The mechanism of the antimicrobial action of nitrofurantoin is unusual among antibacterials. Nitrofurantoin is reduced by bacterial flavoproteins to reactive intermediates that inactivate or alter bacterial ribosomal proteins and other macromolecules. As a result of such inactivations, the vital biochemical processes of protein synthesis, aerobic energy metabolism, DNA synthesis, RNA synthesis, and cell wall synthesis are inhibited. The broad-based nature of this mode of action may explain the lack of acquired bacterial resistance to nitrofurantoin, as the necessary multiple and simultaneous mutations of the target macromolecules would likely be lethal to the bacteria. Development of resistance to nitrofurantoin has not been a significant problem since its introduction in 1953. Cross-resistance with antibiotics and sulfonamides has not been observed, and transferable resistance is, at most, a very rare phenomenon.

➤*Pharmacokinetics:*

Absorption – Blood concentrations at therapeutic dosage are usually low.

Oral suspension: Oral nitrofurantoin is readily absorbed.

Macrocrystals: Nitrofurantoin macrocrystals are a larger, crystal form of nitrofurantoin. The absorption of nitrofurantoin macrocrystals is slower when compared with nitrofurantoin oral suspension.

Monohydrate/macrocrystals: Each monohydrate/macrocrystals capsule contains 2 forms of nitrofurantoin. Twenty-five percent is macrocrystalline nitrofurantoin, which has slower dissolution and absorption than nitrofurantoin monohydrate. The remaining 75% is nitrofurantoin monohydrate contained in the powder blend that, upon exposure to gastric and intestinal fluids, forms a gel matrix that releases nitrofurantoin over time.

Plasma nitrofurantoin concentrations after a single oral dose of the monohydrate/macrocrystals 100 mg capsule are low, with peak levels usually less than 1 mcg/mL.

Distribution – Unlike many drugs, the presence of food or agents delaying gastric emptying can increase the bioavailability of nitrofurantoin, presumably by allowing better dissolution in gastric juices.

When monohydrate/macrocrystals is administered with food, the bioavailability of nitrofurantoin is increased by approximately 40%.

Excretion – It is highly soluble in urine, to which it may impart a brown color.

Oral suspension: Nitrofurantoin oral suspension is rapidly excreted in urine. Following a dose regimen of 100 mg 4 times daily for 7 days, average urinary drug recoveries (0 to 24 hours) on day 1 and day 7 were 42.7% and 43.6%, respectively.

Macrocrystals: Excretion for nitrofurantoin macrocrystals is somewhat less when compared with nitrofurantoin oral suspension. Following a dose regimen of 100 mg 4 times daily for 7 days, average urinary drug recoveries (0 to 24 hours) on day 1 and day 7 were 37.9% and 35%, respectively.

Monohydrate/macrocrystals: Based on urinary pharmacokinetic data, the extent and rate of urinary excretion of nitrofurantoin from the monohydrate/macrocrystals 100 mg capsule are similar to those of the macrocrystals 50 or 100 mg capsule. Approximately 20% to 25% of a single dose of nitrofurantoin is recovered from the urine unchanged over 24 hours.

➤*Microbiology:* The minimal inhibitory concentration (MIC) in urine for most susceptible organisms is 32 mcg/mL or less. Resistant species generally have an MIC of at least 100 mcg/mL. Most gram-negative bacilli and gram-positive cocci associated with UTIs are susceptible, including: *E. coli*,

NITROFURANTOIN

Klebsiella and *Enterobacter* species, enterococci (eg, *Enterococcus faecalis*), *S. aureus*, and *S. saprophyticus*. Some strains of *Enterobacter* and *Klebsiella* species are resistant. Most strains of *Proteus* and *Serratia* species are resistant. It has no activity against *Pseudomonas* species. Susceptible bacteria do not readily develop resistance to nitrofurantoin during therapy. However, plasmid-mediated, transferable resistance has been demonstrated. Although in vitro susceptibility of *Salmonella*, *Shigella*, *Neisseria*, *Streptococcus pyogenes*, *S. pneumoniae*, *Corynebacterium*, and many anaerobes has been demonstrated, nitrofurantoin is of little clinical importance for infections caused by these organisms.

Contraindications

Anuria, oliguria, or significant impairment of renal function (creatinine clearance [Ccr] less than 60 mL/min or clinically significant elevated serum creatinine); hypersensitivity to nitrofurantoin.

Because of the possibility of hemolytic anemia caused by immature erythrocyte enzyme systems (glutathione instability), the drug is contraindicated in pregnant patients at term (38 to 42 weeks gestation), during labor and delivery, or when the onset of labor is imminent; also contraindicated in neonates younger than 1 month of age.

Warnings

➤*Pulmonary reactions:* Acute, subacute, or chronic pulmonary reactions have been observed in patients treated with nitrofurantoin. If these reactions occur, discontinue nitrofurantoin and take appropriate measures. Reports have cited pulmonary reactions as a contributing cause of death. Close monitoring of the pulmonary condition of patients receiving long-term therapy is warranted and requires that the benefits of therapy be weighed against potential risks.

Acute – Acute pulmonary reactions are commonly manifested by fever, chills, cough, chest pain, dyspnea, pulmonary infiltration with consolidation or pleural effusion on x-ray, and eosinophilia. Acute reactions usually occur within the first week of treatment and are reversible with cessation of therapy. Resolution often is dramatic.

Subacute – In subacute pulmonary reactions, fever and eosinophilia occur less often than in the acute form. Upon cessation of therapy, recovery may require several months. If the symptoms are not recognized as being drug-related and nitrofurantoin therapy is not stopped, the symptoms may become more severe.

Chronic – Chronic pulmonary reactions generally occur in patients who have received continuous treatment for 6 months or longer. Malaise, dyspnea on exertion, cough, and altered pulmonary function are common manifestations that can occur insidiously. Radiologic and histologic findings of diffuse interstitial pneumonitis or fibrosis, or both, also are common manifestations of the chronic pulmonary reaction. Fever is rarely prominent.

The severity of chronic pulmonary reactions and their degree of resolution appear to be related to the duration of therapy after the first clinical signs appear. Pulmonary function may be impaired permanently, even after cessation of therapy. The risk is greater when chronic pulmonary reactions are not recognized early.

➤*Peripheral neuropathy:* Peripheral neuropathy, which may become severe or irreversible, has occurred. Fatalities have been reported. Conditions such as renal impairment (Ccr less than 60 mL/min or clinically significant elevated serum creatinine), anemia, diabetes mellitus, electrolyte imbalance, vitamin B deficiency, and debilitating disease may enhance the occurrence of peripheral neuropathy. Periodically monitor patients receiving long-term therapy for changes in renal function.

➤*Optic neuritis:* Optic neuritis has been reported rarely in postmarketing experience with nitrofurantoin formulations.

➤*Hematologic effects:* Cases of hemolytic anemia of the primaquine-sensitivity type have been induced by nitrofurantoin. Hemolysis appears to be linked to a glucose-6-phosphate dehydrogenase deficiency in the red blood cells of the affected patients. This deficiency is found in 10% of black patients and a small percentage of ethnic groups of Mediterranean and Near-Eastern origin. Hemolysis is an indication for discontinuing nitrofurantoin; hemolysis ceases when the drug is withdrawn.

➤*Pseudomembranous colitis:* Pseudomembranous colitis has been reported with nearly all antibacterial agents, including nitrofurantoin, and may range from mild to life-threatening. Therefore, it is important to consider this diagnosis in patients with diarrhea subsequent to the administration of antibacterial agents.

Treatment with antibacterial agents alters the healthy flora of the colon and may permit overgrowth of clostridia. Studies indicate that a toxin produced by *Clostridium difficile* is one primary cause of antibiotic-associated colitis.

After the diagnosis of pseudomembranous colitis has been established, initiate appropriate therapeutic measures. Mild cases of pseudomembranous colitis usually respond to drug discontinuation alone. In moderate to severe cases, give consideration to management with fluids and electrolytes, protein supplementation, and treatment with an antibacterial drug clinically effective against *C. difficile* colitis.

➤*Hepatic reactions:* Hepatic reactions, including hepatitis, cholestatic jaundice, chronic active hepatitis, and hepatic necrosis, occur rarely. Fatalities have been reported. The onset of chronic active hepatitis may be insidious; periodically monitor patients for changes in biochemical tests that would indicate liver injury. If hepatitis occurs, withdraw the drug immediately and take appropriate measures.

➤*Carcinogenesis:* Evidence of carcinogenic activity in female mice was as shown by increased incidences of tubular adenomas, benign mixed tumors, and granulosa cell tumors of the ovary. In male rats, there were increased incidences of uncommon kidney tubular cell neoplasms, osteosarcomas of the bone, and neoplasms of the subcutaneous tissue. In 1 study involving subcutaneous administration of nitrofurantoin 75 mg/kg to pregnant female mice, lung papillary adenomas of unknown significance were observed in the F1 generation.

➤*Mutagenesis:* Nitrofurantoin has been shown to induce point mutations in certain strains of *Salmonella typhimurium* and forward mutations in mouse lymphoma cells. Nitrofurantoin induced increased numbers of sister chromatid exchanges and chromosomal aberrations in Chinese hamster ovary cells but not in human cells in culture.

➤*Fertility impairment:* The administration of high doses of nitrofurantoin to rats causes temporary spermatogenic arrest; this is reversible on discontinuing the drug. Dosages of 10 mg/kg/day or greater in healthy men may, in certain unpredictable instances, produce a slight to moderate spermatogenic arrest with a decrease in sperm count.

➤*Elderly:* Spontaneous reports suggest a higher proportion of pulmonary reactions, including fatalities, in elderly patients; these differences appear to be related to the higher proportion of elderly patients receiving long-term nitrofurantoin therapy. As in younger patients, chronic pulmonary reactions generally are observed in patients receiving therapy for 6 months or longer. Spontaneous reports also suggest an increased proportion of severe hepatic reactions, including fatalities, in elderly patients.

In general, consider the greater frequency of decreased hepatic, renal, or cardiac function, and of concomitant disease or other drug therapy when prescribing nitrofurantoin. This drug is known to be substantially excreted by the kidney, and the risk of toxic reactions to this drug may be greater in patients with impaired renal function. Anuria, oliguria, or significant impairment of renal function (Ccr less than 60 mL/min or clinically significant elevated serum creatinine) are contraindications. Because elderly patients are more likely to have decreased renal function, take care in dose selection; it may be useful to monitor renal function.

➤*Pregnancy: Category B.* Because of the possibility of hemolytic anemia caused by immature erythrocyte enzyme systems (glutathione instability), the drug is contraindicated in pregnant patients at term (38 to 42 weeks gestation). In a single published study conducted in mice at 68 times the human dose (based on mg/kg administered to the dam), growth retardation and a low incidence of minor and common malformations were observed. However, at 25 times the human dose, fetal malformations were not observed; the relevance of these findings to humans is uncertain. There are, however, no adequate and well-controlled studies in pregnant women. Because animal reproduction studies are not always predictive of human response, use this drug during pregnancy only if clearly needed.

Nitrofurantoin has been shown in one published transplacental carcinogenicity study to induce lung papillary adenomas in the F1 generation mice at doses 19 times the human dose on a mg/kg basis. Because of the uncertainty regarding the human implications of these animal data, use this drug during pregnancy only if clearly needed.

Labor and delivery – Because of the possibility of hemolytic anemia caused by immature erythrocyte enzyme systems (glutathione instability), the drug is contraindicated in pregnant patients at term (38 to 42 weeks gestation), during labor and delivery, or when the onset of labor is imminent.

➤*Lactation:* Nitrofurantoin has been detected in human breast milk in trace amounts. Because of the potential for serious adverse reactions from nitrofurantoin in nursing infants younger than 1 month of age, decide whether to discontinue breast-feeding or to discontinue the drug, taking into account the importance of the drug to the mother.

➤*Children:* Nitrofurantoin is contraindicated in infants younger than 1 month of age.

Safety and efficacy of nitrofurantoin monohydrate/macrocrystals in pediatric patients younger than 12 years of age have not been established.

Precautions

➤*Monitoring:* Periodically monitor patients receiving long-term therapy for changes in renal and pulmonary function.

➤*Drug resistance:* To reduce the development of drug-resistant bacteria and maintain the efficacy of nitrofurantoin and other antibacterial drugs, only use nitrofurantoin to treat or prevent infections that are proven or strongly suspected to be caused by bacteria. Prescribing nitrofurantoin in the absence of a proven or strongly suspected bacterial infection or a prophylactic indication is unlikely to provide benefit to the patient and increases the risk of the development of drug-resistant bacteria.

➤*Superinfection:* As with other antimicrobial agents, superinfections caused by resistant organisms (eg, *Pseudomonas* or *Candida* species) can occur. There are sporadic reports of *C. difficile* superinfections, or pseudomembranous colitis, with the use of nitrofurantoin.

Drug Interactions

Nitrofurantoin Drug Interactions

Precipitant drug	Object drug*		Description
Anticholinergics	Nitrofurantoin	⬆	Anticholinergic drugs increase nitrofurantoin bioavailability by delaying gastric emptying and increasing absorption.
Magnesium salts	Nitrofurantoin	⬇	Magnesium salts may delay or decrease the absorption of nitrofurantoin.

NITROFURANTOIN

Nitrofurantoin Drug Interactions			
Precipitant drug	Object drug*		Description
Uricosurics	Nitrofurantoin	↑	Administration of high doses of probenecid with nitrofurantoin decreases renal clearance and increases serum levels of nitrofurantoin. The result could be increased toxic effects.

* ↑ = Object drug increased. ↓ = Object drug decreased.

➤*Drug/Lab test interactions:* As a result of the presence of nitrofurantoin, a false-positive reaction for glucose in the urine may occur. This has been observed with Benedict and Fehling solutions but not with the glucose enzymatic test.

Adverse Reactions

➤*Cardiovascular:* Benign intracranial hypertension (pseudotumor cerebri) has been reported rarely. Bulging fontanels, as a sign of benign intracranial hypertension in infants, have been reported rarely. Changes in electrocardiogram (eg, nonspecific ST/T wave changes, bundle branch block) have been reported in association with pulmonary reactions.

➤*CNS:* Asthenia, confusion, depression, dizziness, drowsiness, headache, nystagmus, peripheral neuropathy (see Warnings), psychotic reactions, vertigo.

➤*Dermatologic:* Erythema multiforme (including Stevens-Johnson syndrome), exfoliative dermatitis (rare); transient alopecia.

➤*GI:* Abdominal pain, anorexia, diarrhea, emesis, nausea, pancreatitis, pseudomembranous colitis, sialadenitis.

➤*Hepatic:* Cholestatic jaundice, chronic active hepatitis, hepatic necrosis, hepatic reactions, hepatitis (rare).

➤*Hypersensitivity:* Anaphylaxis; angioedema; arthralgia; chills; drug fever; eczematous, erythematous, or maculopapular eruptions; lupus-like syndrome associated with pulmonary reactions; myalgia; pruritus; urticaria.

➤*Lab test abnormalities:* Agranulocytosis, decreased hemoglobin, eosinophilia, glucose-6-phosphate dehydrogenase deficiency anemia, granulocytopenia, hemolytic anemia, increased ALT, increased AST, increased serum phosphorus, leukopenia, megaloblastic anemia, thrombocytopenia. In most cases, these hematologic abnormalities resolved following cessation of therapy. Aplastic anemia (rare).

➤*Respiratory:* Chronic, subacute, or acute pulmonary hypersensitivity reactions may occur (see Warnings); cyanosis (rare).

➤*Miscellaneous:* Optic neuritis, superinfections caused by resistant organisms.

➤*Monohydrate/macrocrystals:* In clinical trials of monohydrate/macrocrystals, the most frequent adverse reactions that were reported as possibly or probably drug-related were nausea (8%), headache (6%), and flatulence (1.5%). Additional clinical adverse reactions reported as possibly or probably drug-related occurred in less than 1% of patients studied and are listed below:

CNS – Amblyopia, dizziness, drowsiness.

Dermatologic – Alopecia.

GI – Abdominal pain, constipation, diarrhea, dyspepsia, emesis.

Hypersensitivity – Pruritus, urticaria.

Respiratory – Acute pulmonary hypersensitivity reaction.

Miscellaneous – Chills, fever, malaise.

Overdosage

➤*Symptoms:* Occasional incidents of acute overdosage of nitrofurantoin have not resulted in any specific symptoms other than vomiting.

➤*Treatment:* There is no specific antidote, but a high fluid intake should be maintained to promote urinary excretion of the drug. It is dialyzable.

Patient Information

May cause brown discoloration of the urine.

Advise patients to take nitrofurantoin with food to further enhance tolerance and improve drug absorption. Instruct patients to complete the full course of therapy; however, advise them to contact their doctors if any unusual symptoms occur during therapy.

Many patients who cannot tolerate microcrystalline nitrofurantoin are able to take nitrofurantoin macrocrystals without nausea.

Advise patients not to use antacid preparations containing magnesium trisilicate while taking nitrofurantoin.

Counsel patients that antibacterial drugs, including nitrofurantoin, should only be used to treat bacterial infections. They do not treat viral infections (eg, the common cold). When nitrofurantoin is prescribed to treat a bacterial infection, tell patients that although it is common to feel better early in the course of therapy, the medication should be taken exactly as directed. Skipping doses or not completing the full course of therapy may (1) decrease the effectiveness of the immediate treatment, and (2) increase the likelihood that bacteria will develop resistance and will not be treatable by nitrofurantoin or other antibacterial drugs in the future.

METHENAMINES

Indications

➤*Urinary tract infections:* Prophylaxis or suppression/elimination of frequently recurring urinary tract infections when long-term therapy is considered necessary. Use only after eradication of the infection by other appropriate antimicrobial agents.

Actions

➤*Pharmacology:* In acid urine, methenamine is hydrolyzed to ammonia and formaldehyde, which is bactericidal. Methenamine does not liberate formaldehyde in the serum. The acid salts (mandelate and hippurate) help maintain a low urine pH.

➤*Pharmacokinetics:*

Absorption – Methenamine is readily absorbed following oral administration; 10% to 30% of the drug will be hydrolyzed by the gastric juices unless it is protected by an enteric coating.

Metabolism/Excretion – Approximately 10% to 25% of methenamine is metabolized in the liver and has a half-life of 3 to 6 hours. Generation of formaldehyde depends upon urinary pH, the concentration of methenamine and the duration that the urine is retained in the bladder. Peak concentrations of formaldehyde occur at a urine pH of ≤ 5.5 and are seen approximately 2 hours after a dose of methenamine hippurate and 3 to 8 hours after a dose of methenamine mandelate. A urinary formaldehyde concentration of > 25 mcg/ml is necessary for antimicrobial activity. Steady-state urinary formaldehyde concentrations are achieved in 2 to 3 days. Formaldehyde levels range from 1 to 85 mcg/ml, and decrease with increasing pH, urinary volume or flow rate.

In some instances, supplementary urine acidification may be desirable, especially in infections caused by urea-splitting organisms (which raise the urine pH). Ingestion of acidifying agents (eg, mandelic acid, hippuric acid, ammonium chloride, monobasic sodium phosphate) or acid-producing foods (eg, cranberries, plums, prunes) aid in maintaining an acid urine; however, effects may be negligible. Ammonium chloride 8 to 12 g/day, methionine 8 to 15 g/day and cranberry juice 1200 to 4000 ml/day, have all been recommended, but with marginal results. There is no reliable oral urinary acidifier at present. Monitor urine pH.

Excretion occurs via glomerular filtration and tubular secretion. Approximately 90% of the methenamine moiety is excreted in the urine within 24 hours. The influence of renal dysfunction on the pharmacology of methenamine is unknown.

➤*Microbiology:* The nonspecific antibacterial action of formaldehyde is effective against gram-positive and gram-negative organisms and fungi. *Escherichia coli*, enterococci and staphylococci are usually susceptible. *Enterobacter aerogenes* and *Proteus vulgaris* are generally resistant. Urea-splitting organisms (eg, *Proteus*, *Pseudomonas*) may be resistant since they raise the pH of the urine inhibiting the release of formaldehyde. An effective urine concentration of formaldehyde must persist for a minimum of 2 hours.

Methenamine is effective clinically against most common urinary tract pathogens since most bacteria are sensitive to free formaldehyde concentrations of 20 mcg/ml.

Methenamine is particularly suited for therapy of chronic infections, since bacteria and fungi do not develop resistance to formaldehyde.

Contraindications

Renal insufficiency; severe dehydration; severe hepatic insufficiency (because it facilitates ammonia production in the intestine); use alone for acute infections with parenchymal involvement causing systemic symptoms; hypersensitivity to the drug; concurrent sulfonamides since an insoluble precipitate may form with formaldehyde in the urine.

Warnings

➤*Pregnancy:* *Category C.* Safe use of methenamine in early pregnancy has not been established. Safety in the last trimester is suggested, but not proven. Methenamine passes into the fetus, but there is no evidence that methenamine salts cause fetal abnormalities. It is not known whether the drug can cause fetal harm when administered to a pregnant woman or can affect reproduction capacity. Give to pregnant women only if clearly needed.

➤*Lactation:* Methenamine passes into breast milk, levels are about equivalent to maternal serum and peak in 1 hour. One estimate revealed that an infant would receive about 0.15 to 0.4 mg methenamine/feeding. No adverse effects on the nursing infant have been reported.

Precautions

➤*Large doses:* (8 g daily for 3 to 4 weeks). These have caused bladder irritation, painful and frequent micturition, proteinuria and gross hematuria.

➤*Acid urine pH:* This should be maintained, especially when treating infections due to urea-splitting organisms such as *Proteus* and strains of *Pseudomonas*. When acidification is contraindicated or unattainable (as with some urea-splitting bacteria) the drug is not recommended.

➤*Serum transaminases:* These have elevated mildly during treatment in a few instances and returned to normal while patients were still receiving methenamine hippurate. Perform liver function studies periodically on patients receiving methenamine hippurate, especially those with liver dysfunction.

➤*Gout:* Methenamine salts may cause precipitation of urate crystals in the urine.

➤*Tartrazine sensitivity:* Some of these products contain tartrazine, which may cause allergic-type reactions (including bronchial asthma) in certain susceptible individuals. Although the overall incidence of tartrazine sensitivity in the general population is low, it is frequently seen in patients who also have aspirin hypersensitivity. Specific products containing tartrazine are identified in the product listings.

Drug Interactions

Methenamine Drug Interactions			
Precipitant drug	Object drug*		Description
Sulfonamides	Methenamine	⬇	An insoluble precipitate between the sulfonamide and formaldehyde may form in the urine.
Urinary alkalinizers	Methenamine	⬇	Alkalinizing agents may decrease the efficacy of methenamine by inhibiting its conversion to formaldehyde.

* ⬇ = Object drug decreased.

➤*Drug/Lab test interactions:* Methenamine may interfere with laboratory urine determinations of **17-hydroxycorticosteroids, catecholamines** and **vanillylmandelic acid** (false increases); and **5-hydroxyindoleacetic acid** (false decrease).

Methenamine taken during pregnancy can interfere with laboratory tests of **urine estriol** (resulting in unmeasurably low values) when an acid hydrolysis procedure is used. This is due to the presence in the urine of methenamine or formaldehyde. Use enzymatic hydrolysis in place of acid hydrolysis.

Adverse Reactions

➤*Overall incidence:* Approximately 1% to 7%.

➤*Dermatologic:* Pruritus (rare) ; urticaria; erythematous eruptions; rash.

➤*GI:* Nausea; vomiting; cramps; stomatitis; anorexia.

➤*GU:* Bladder irritation, dysuria, proteinuria, hematuria, urinary frequency/urgency, crystalluria (large doses).

➤*Miscellaneous:* Headache, dyspnea, lipoid pneumonitis, generalized edema (rare).

Overdosage

➤*Treatment:* Immediately after ingestion of an overdose, further absorption of the drug may be minimized by inducing vomiting or by gastric lavage, followed by administration of activated charcoal. Force fluids, either oral or parenteral, to tolerance.

Patient Information

It may be necessary to attempt to acidify the urine (eg, ascorbic acid, cranberry juice).

Take with food to minimize GI upset.

Drink sufficient fluids to ensure adequate urine flow.

Avoid excessive intake of alkalinizing foods (milk products) or medication (bicarbonate, acetazolamide).

Complete full course of therapy; take until gone.

Notify physician if skin rash, painful urination or intolerable GI upset occurs.

METHENAMINE HIPPURATE

Rx	**Hiprex** (Hoechst Marion Roussel)	**Tablets**: 1 g	Tartrazine, saccharin. (Merrell 277). Yellow, scored. In 100s.
Rx	**Urex** (3M Pharm)		Saccharin. (3M Urex). White, scored. In 100s.

METHENAMINE HIPPURATE — ORAL

Complete prescribing and comparative information for these products begins in the Methenamine monograph.

Indications

➤*Urinary tract infections:* For prophylactic or suppressive treatment of frequently recurring urinary tract infections when long-term therapy is considered necessary. This drug should only be used after eradication of the infection by other appropriate antimicrobial agents.

Administration and Dosage

➤*Adults and children older than 12 years of age:* One tablet (1 g) twice daily (morning and night).

➤*Children 6 to 12 years of age:* One-half to 1 tablet (0.5 g to 1 g) twice daily (morning and night).

The antibacterial activity of methenamine hippurate is greater in acid urine. Therefore, restriction of alkalinizing foods and medications is desirable. If necessary, as indicated by urinary pH and clinical response, supplemental acidification of the urine may be instituted. The efficacy of therapy should be monitored by repeated urine cultures.

➤*Storage/Stability:* Store at controlled room temperature 15° to 30°C (59° to 86°F). Dispense in well-closed, light-resistant containers with child-resistant closures.

METHENAMINE MANDELATE

Rx	**Mandelamine** (Warner Chilcott)	**Tablets**: 0.5 g	(166). Brown. Film coated. In 100s.
Rx	**Mandelamine** (Warner Chilcott)	**Tablets**: 1 g	(167). Purple. Film coated. In 100s.
Rx	**Methenamine Mandelate** (Various, eg, Major)	**Tablets, enteric coated**: 0.5 g	In 100s and 1000s.
Rx	**Methenamine Mandelate** (Various, eg, Rugby)	**Tablets, enteric coated**: 1 g	In 100s and 1000s.
Rx	**Methenamine Mandelate** (Various, eg, Barre-National)	**Suspension**: 0.5 g/5 ml	In 480 ml.

METHENAMINE MANDELATE — ORAL

Complete prescribing and comparative information for these products begins in the Methenamine monograph.

Indications

➤*Urinary tract infections:* Suppression or elimination of bacteriuria associated with pyelonephritis, cystitis, and other chronic urinary tract infections; also for infected residual urine sometimes accompanying neurologic diseases. When used as recommended, methenamine is particularly suitable for long-term therapy because of its safety and because resistance to the nonspecific bactericidal action of formaldehyde does not develop. Pathogens resistant to other antibacterial agents may respond to methenamine because of the nonspecific effect of formaldehyde formed in an acid urine.

Administration and Dosage

➤*Adults:* 4 g daily given as 1 g after each meal and at bedtime.

➤*Children:* Children 6 to 12 years of age should receive half the adult dose, and children under 6 years of age should receive 250 mg per 30 lbs of body weight, 4 times daily.

Since an acidic urine is essential for antibacterial activity, with maximum efficacy occurring at pH 5.5 or below, restriction of alkalinizing foods and medication is thus desirable. If testing of urine pH reveals the need, supplemental acidification should be given.

➤*Storage/Stability:* Store at controlled room temperature between 15° to 30°C (59° to 86°F).

METHENAMINE COMBINATIONS

Rx	**Uretron D/S** (A. G. Marin)[1]	**Tablets**: 120 mg methenamine, 36.2 mg phenyl salicylate, 0.12 mg hyoscyamine sulfate, 10.8 mg methylene blue, 40.8 mg sodium biphosphate*Dose*: *Adults* - 1 qid followed by liberal fluid intake; *older children* - individualize dosing	Parabens, sucrose. (URETRON D/S). Purple. Sugar-coated. In 100s.
Rx	**Urelle** (Pharmelle[2])	**Tablets**: 81 mg methenamine, 32.4 mg phenyl salicylate, 10.8 mg methylene blue, 40.8 mg sodium phosphate monobasic, 0.12 mg hyoscyamine sulfate *Dose*: *Adults* - 1 qid followed by liberal fluid intake; *older children* - individualize dosing	Sugar, mineral oil. (P-002). Blue. Sugar-coated. In 90s.
Rx	**Prosed/DS** (Star)	**Tablets**: 81.6 mg methenamine, 36.2 mg phenyl salicylate, 10.8 mg methylene blue, 9 mg benzoic acid, 0.06 mg atropine sulfate, 0.06 mg hyoscyamine sulfate *Dose*: 1 tablet 4 times daily	Parabens, sugar. (Prosed/DS). Dark blue. Sugar coated. In 100s and 1000s.
Rx	**Uritact DS** (Cypress)	**Tablets**: 81.6 mg methenamine, 36.2 mg phenyl salicylate, 10.8 mg methylene blue, 9 mg benzoic acid, 0.06 mg atropine sulfate, 0.06 mg hyoscyamine sulfate *Dose*: 1 tablet 4 times daily with liquid	Alcohol-free. (CYP 516). Light blue, capsule shape. In 100s.

METHENAMINE COMBINATIONS

Rx	**Uro Blue** (R. A. McNeil[3])	**Tablets**: 120 mg methenamine, 40.8 mg sodium phosphate monobasic, 36.2 mg phenyl salicylate, 10.8 mg methylene blue, 0.12 mg hyoscyamine sulfate *Dose*: 1 tablet 4 times daily followed by liberal fluid intake	Sugar. (HMP). Purple. Sugar-coated. In 100s.
Rx	**Urogesic Blue** (Edwards)	**Tablets**: 81.6 mg methenamine, 40.8 mg sodium biphosphate, 36.2 mg phenyl salicylate, 10.8 mg methylene blue, 0.12 mg hyoscyamine sulfate *Dose*: 1 tablet 4 times daily followed by liberal fluid intake	Sucrose, parabens. (MD-20). Purple. Oval. Sugar coated. In 100s.
Rx	**Urimax** (Integrity)	**Tablets, delayed release**: 81.6 mg methenamine, 40.8 mg sodium biphosphate, 36.2 mg phenyl salicylate, 10.8 mg methylene blue, 0.12 mg hyoscyamine sulfate *Dose*: 1 tablet 4 times daily	(Urimax). Magenta. Film coated. In 100s.
Rx	**Urimar-T** (Marnel)	**Tablets**: 120 mg methenamine, 40.8 mg sodium phosphate monobasic, 36.2 mg phenyl salicylate, 10.8 mg methylene blue, 0.12 mg hyoscyamine sulfate *Dose*: 1 tablet 4 times daily followed by liberal fluid intake; not recommended for children ≤ 6 years of age.	Sugar coated. (HMP). Purple. In 4s and 100s.
Rx	**Uroquid-Acid No. 2** (Beach)	**Tablets**: 500 mg methenamine mandelate, 500 mg sodium acid phosphate monohydrate *Dose*: Initial - 2 tablets 4 times daily Maintenance - 2 to 4 tablets daily in divided doses	(Beach 1114). Yellow. Film coated. Capsule shape. In 100s.
Rx	**Urisedamine** (PolyMedica)	**Tablets**: 500 mg methenamine mandelate, 0.15 mg hyoscyamine *Dose*: 2 tablets 4 times daily Children (≥ 6 years) – Reduce dosage in proportion to age and weight	Sucrose. (W2210). Light blue. Capsule shape. In 100s.
Rx	**Atrosept** (Geneva)	**Tablets**: 40.8 mg methenamine, 18.1 mg phenyl salicylate, 0.03 mg atropine sulfate, 0.03 mg hyoscyamine (as sulfate), 4.5 mg benzoic acid, 5.4 mg methylene blue *Dose*: Adults – 2 tablets 4 times daily Children (≥ 6 years) – Reduce dosage in proportion to age and weight	(220). Deep blue. Sugar coated. In 100s and 1000s.
Rx	**Dolsed** (American Urologicals)		(Dolsed). Deep blue. Sugar coated. In 100s and 1000s.
Rx	**UAA** (Econo Med)		(UAA). Blue. Sugar coated. In 100s and 1000s.
Rx	**Uridon Modified** (Rugby)		Blue. Sugar coated. In 100s and 1000s.
Rx	**Urinary Antiseptic No. 2** (Various)		In 100s and 1000s.
Rx	**Urised** (PolyMedica)		(W 2183). Purple. Sugar coated. In 100s and 500s.
Rx	**Uritin** (Various, eg, Goldline)		In 1000s.
Rx	**MHP-A** (Cypress)	**Tablets**: 40.8 mg methenamine, 18.1 mg phenyl salicylate, 0.03 mg atropine sulfate, 0.03 mg hyoscyamine sulfate, 4.5 mg benzoic acid, 5.4 mg methylene blue *Dose*: Adults – 2 qid Children (≥ 6 years) – Dosage must be individualized by physician.	(CYP515). Green. In 100s.
Rx	**Uriseptic** (SDA Labs)[4]	**Tablets**: 40.8 mg methenamine, 18.1 mg phenyl salicylate, 0.03 mg atropine sulfate, 0.03 mg hyoscyamine sulfate, 4.5 mg benzoic acid, 5.4 mg methylene blue *Dose*: Adults – 2 qid followed by liberal fluid intake Children (≥ 6 years) – Individualize dosage	Dk. blue. Film-coated. In 100s.
otc	**Cystex** (Numark)	**Tablets**: 162 mg methenamine, 162.5 mg sodium salicylate, 32 mg benzoic acid *Dose*: Adults and children > 16 years old – 2 tablets 4 times daily with meals and at bedtime	In 40s and 100s.
Rx	**UriSym** (Vindex)	**Capsules**: 100 mg methenamine, 40 mg phenyl salicylate, 40.8 mg sodium biphosphate, 10.8 mg methylene blue, 0.12 mg hyoscyamine sulfate *Dose*: Adults – 1 capsule 4 times daily followed by liberal fluid intake Children at least 7 years of age — Dosage must be individualized by physician	(VX 531). Light blue. In 100s.

[1] A. G. Marin Pharmaceuticals, 1730 N.W. 79th Avenue, Miami, FL 33126; 305-593-5333, fax 305-593-8333.
[2] Pharmelle L.L.C., 890 N. Lafayette, Florissant, MO 63031; 314-830-4950, 877-577-2577.
[3] R. A. McNeil Company, 1210 E. Dallas Road, Chattanooga, TN 37405; 423-265-8240, 800-755-3038; fax 423-265-7373.
[4] SDA Laboratories, 280 Railroad Avenue, Greenwich, CT 06830; 203-861-0005, fax 203-861-0006.

FOLATE ANTAGONISTS

TRIMETHOPRIM (TMP)

Rx	**Trimethoprim** (Various, eg, Biocraft, Moore, Parmed, Rugby, Schein)	**Tablets**: 100 mg	In 14s, 30s, 100s and UD 100s.
Rx	**Proloprim** (GlaxoWellcome)		(Proloprim 09A). White, scored. In 100s.
Rx	**Trimethoprim** (Various, eg, Biocraft, Moore, Rugby)	**Tablets**: 200 mg	In 100s.
Rx	**Proloprim** (GlaxoWellcome)		(Proloprim 200). Yellow, scored. In 100s.
Rx	**Primsol** (Ascent Pediatrics)	**Solution, oral**: 50 mg/5 ml	Parabens, sorbitol. Alcohol free. Bubble gum flavor. In 473 ml.

TRIMETHOPRIM TABLETS

Indications

➤*Urinary tract infections:* For the treatment of initial episodes of uncomplicated urinary tract infections due to susceptible strains of the following organisms: *Escherichia coli*, *Proteus mirabilis*, *Klebsiella pneumoniae*, *Enterobacter* species and coagulase-negative *Staphylococcus* species, including *S. saprophyticus*.

Administration and Dosage

➤*Approved by the FDA:* March 30, 1980.

➤*Adults:* 100 mg every 12 hours or 200 mg every 24 hours, each for 10 days.

➤*Renal function impairment:* The use of trimethoprim in patients with a creatinine clearance of less than 15 mL/min is not recommended. For patients with a creatinine clearance of 15 to 30 mL/min, the dose should be 50 mg every 12 hours.

➤*Storage/Stability:* Store at 15° to 25°C (59° to 77°F) in a dry place and protect from light.

Actions

➤*Pharmacokinetics:*

Absorption/Distribution – Trimethoprim is rapidly absorbed following oral administration. It exists in the blood as unbound, protein-bound and metabolized forms. The free form is considered to be the therapeutically active form. Approximately 44% of trimethoprim is bound to plasma proteins.

TRIMETHOPRIM TABLETS

Mean peak serum concentrations of approximately 1 mcg/mL occur 1 to 4 hours after oral administration of a single 100 mg dose. A single 200 mg dose will result in serum levels approximately twice as high. The half-life of trimethoprim ranges from 8 to 10 hours. However, patients with severely impaired renal function exhibit an increase in the half-life of trimethoprim, which requires either dosage regimen adjustment or not using the drug in such patients. During a 13-week study of trimethoprim administered at a daily dosage of 200 mg (50 mg 4 times a day), the mean minimum steady-state concentration of the drug was 1.1 mcg/mL. Steady-state concentrations were achieved within 2 to 3 days of chronic administration and were maintained throughout the experimental period.

Since normal vaginal and fecal flora are the source of most pathogens causing urinary tract infections, it is relevant to consider the distribution of trimethoprim into these sites. Concentrations of trimethoprim in vaginal secretions are consistently greater than those found simultaneously in the serum, being typically 1.6 times the concentrations of simultaneously obtained serum samples. Sufficient trimethoprim is excreted in the feces to markedly reduce or eliminate trimethoprim-susceptible organisms from the fecal flora.

Trimethoprim also passes the placental barrier and is excreted in human milk.

Metabolism – Ten percent to 20% of trimethoprim is metabolized, primarily in the liver; the remainder is excreted unchanged in the urine. The principal metabolites of trimethoprim are the 1- and 3-oxides and the 3′- and 4′-hydroxy derivatives.

Excretion – Excretion of trimethoprim is primarily by the kidneys through glomerular filtration and tubular secretion. Urine concentrations of trimethoprim are considerably higher than are the concentrations in the blood. After a single oral dose of 100 mg, urine concentrations of trimethoprim ranged from 30 to 160 mcg/mL during the 0- to 4-hour period and declined to approximately 18 to 91 mcg/mL during the 8- to 24-hour period. A 200 mg single oral dose will result in trimethoprim urine concentrations approximately twice as high. After oral administration, 50% to 60% of trimethoprim is excreted in urine within 24 hours, approximately 80% of this being unmetabolized trimethoprim.

➤*Microbiology:* Trimethoprim blocks the production of tetrahydrofolic acid from dihydrofolic acid by binding to and reversibly inhibiting the required enzyme, dihydrofolate reductase. This binding is very much stronger for the bacterial enzyme than for the corresponding mammalian enzyme. Thus, trimethoprim selectively interferes with bacterial biosynthesis of nucleic acids and proteins.

Trimethoprim has been shown to be active against most strains of the following microorganisms, both in vitro and in clinical infections.

Aerobic gram-positive microorganisms – *Staphylococcus* species (coagulase-negative strains, including *S. saprophyticus*).

Aerobic gram-negative microorganisms –
- *Enterobacter* species.
- *Escherichia coli.*
- *Klebsiella pneumoniae.*
- *Proteus mirabilis.*

Contraindications

Hypersensitivity to trimethoprim and in those with documented megaloblastic anemia due to folate deficiency.

Warnings

➤*Hematologic effects:* Trimethoprim has been reported rarely to interfere with hematopoiesis, especially when administered in large doses or for prolonged periods.

The presence of clinical signs such as sore throat, fever, pallor or purpura may be early indications of serious blood disorders.

Obtain complete blood counts if any of these signs are noted in a patient receiving trimethoprim and discontinue the drug if a significant reduction in the count of any formed blood element is found.

➤*Hypersensitivity reactions:* Serious hypersensitivity reactions have been reported rarely in patients on trimethoprim therapy.

➤*Renal/Hepatic function impairment:* Give trimethoprim with caution to patients with impaired renal or hepatic function.

➤*Elderly:* Case reports of hyperkalemia in elderly patients receiving trimethoprim-sulfamethoxazole have been published. Trimethoprim is known to be substantially excreted by the kidney, and the risk of toxic reactions to this drug may be greater in patients with impaired renal function. Because elderly patients are more likely to have decreased renal function, care should be taken in dose selection, and it may be useful to monitor potassium concentrations and to monitor renal function by calculating creatinine clearance.

➤*Pregnancy: Category C.* Trimethoprim has been shown to be teratogenic in the rat when given in doses 40 times the human dose. In some rabbit studies, the overall increase in fetal loss (dead and resorbed and malformed conceptuses) was associated with doses 6 times the human therapeutic dose.

While there are no large well-controlled studies on the use of trimethoprim in pregnant women, Brumfitt and Pursell (Brumfitt W., Pursell, R. Trimethoprim-sulfamethoxazole in the treatment of bacteriuria in women, *J Infect Dis*, 1973; 128 (suppl): S657 to S663) in a retrospective study, reported the outcome of 186 pregnancies during which the mother received either placebo or trimethoprim in combination with sulfamethoxazole. The incidence of congenital abnormalities was 4.5% (3 of 66) in those who received placebo and 3.3% (4 of 120) in those receiving trimethoprim plus sulfamethoxazole. There were no abnormalities in the 10 children whose mothers received the drug during the first trimester. In a separate survey, Brumfitt and Pursell also found no congenital abnormalities in 35 children whose mothers had received trimethoprim plus sulfamethoxazole at the time of conception or shortly thereafter.

Because trimethoprim may interfere with folic acid metabolism, use trimethoprim during pregnancy only if the potential benefit justifies the potential risk to the fetus.

➤*Lactation:* Trimethoprim is excreted in human milk. Because trimethoprim may interfere with folic acid metabolism, exercise caution when trimethoprim is administered to a nursing woman.

➤*Children:* Safety and efficacy in pediatric patients below the age of 2 months have not been established. The effectiveness of trimethoprim has not been established in pediatric patients under 12 years of age.

Precautions

➤*Monitoring:* If any clinical signs of a blood disorder are noted in a patient receiving trimethoprim, obtain a complete blood count and discontinue the drug if a significant reduction in the count of any formed blood element is found.

➤*Folate deficiency:* Give trimethoprim with caution to patients with possible folate deficiency. Folates may be administered concomitantly without interfering with the antibacterial action of trimethoprim.

Drug Interactions

➤*Phenytoin:* Trimethoprim may inhibit the hepatic metabolism of phenytoin. Trimethoprim, given at a common clinical dosage, increased the phenytoin half-life by 51% and decreased the phenytoin metabolic clearance rate by 30%. When administering these drugs concurrently, one should be alert for possible excessive phenytoin effect.

➤*Drug/Lab test interactions:* Trimethoprim can interfere with a serum methotrexate assay as determined by the competitive binding protein technique (CBPA) when a bacterial dihydrofolate reductase is used as the binding protein. No interference occurs, however, if methotrexate is measured by a radioimmunoassay (RIA).

The presence of trimethoprim may also interfere with the Jaffé alkaline picrate reaction assay for creatinine, resulting in overestimations of about 10% in the range of normal values.

Adverse Reactions

The adverse effects encountered most often with trimethoprim were rash and pruritus.

➤*CNS:* Aseptic meningitis has been rarely reported.

➤*Dermatologic:* Rash, pruritus and phototoxic skin eruptions. At the recommended dosage regimens of 100 mg twice daily or 200 mg daily, each for 10 days, the incidence of rash is 2.9% to 6.7%. In clinical studies which employed high doses of trimethoprim, an elevated incidence of rash was noted. These rashes were maculopapular, morbilliform, pruritic and generally mild to moderate, appearing 7 to 14 days after the initiation of therapy.

➤*GI:* Epigastric distress, glossitis, nausea, and vomiting.

➤*Hematologic:* Leukopenia, megaloblastic anemia, methemoglobinemia, neutropenia, and thrombocytopenia.

➤*Hepatic:* Cholestatic jaundice has been rarely reported. Elevation of serum transaminase and bilirubin has been noted, but the significance of this finding is unknown.

➤*Hypersensitivity:* Rare reports of anaphylaxis, erythema multiforme, exfoliative dermatitis, Stevens-Johnson syndrome, and toxic epidermal necrolysis (Lyell syndrome) have been received.

➤*Metabolic:* Hyperkalemia, hyponatremia.

➤*Miscellaneous:* Fever, increases in blood urea nitrogen (BUN) and serum creatinine levels.

Overdosage

➤*Acute:*

Symptoms – Signs of acute overdosage with trimethoprim may appear following ingestion of 1 g or more of the drug and include nausea, vomiting, dizziness, headaches, mental depression, confusion and bone marrow depression (see Chronic overdosage).

Treatment – Treatment consists of gastric lavage and general supportive measures. Acidification of the urine will increase renal elimination of trimethoprim. Peritoneal dialysis is not effective and hemodialysis is only moderately effective in eliminating the drug.

➤*Chronic:*

Symptoms – Use of trimethoprim at high doses or for extended periods of time may cause bone marrow depression manifested as thrombocytopenia, leukopenia or megaloblastic anemia.

Treatment – If signs of bone marrow depression occur, trimethoprim should be discontinued and the patient should be given leucovorin; 5 to 15 mg leucovorin daily has been recommended by some investigators.

TRIMETHOPRIM HYDROCHLORIDE — ORAL SOLUTION

Indications

➤*Adults:*

Urinary tract infections – For the treatment of initial episodes of uncomplicated urinary tract infections due to susceptible strains of the following organisms: *Escherichia coli, Proteus mirabilis, Klebsiella pneumoniae, Enterobacter* species and coagulase-negative *Staphylococcus* species, including *S. saprophyticus.*

➤*Children:*

Acute otitis media – For the treatment of acute otitis media due to susceptible strains of *Streptococcus pneumoniae* and *Haemophilus influenzae. Moraxella catarrhalis* isolates were found consistently resistant to trimethoprim in vitro. Therefore, when infection with *Moraxella catarrhalis* is suspected, consider the use of alternative antimicrobial agents. Trimethoprim is not indicated for prophylactic or prolonged administration in otitis media at any age.

Administration and Dosage

➤*Approved by the FDA:* May 30, 1980.

➤*Uncomplicated urinary tract infections:* 100 mg (10 mL) every 12 hours or 200 mg (20 mL) every 24 hours, each for 10 days.

➤*Renal function impairment:* The use of trimethoprim in patients with a creatinine clearance of less than 15 mL/min is not recommended. Give patients with a creatinine clearance of 15 to 30 mL/min half the dose recommended for patients of the same age with normal renal function.

➤*Acute otitis media:* The recommended dose for pediatric patients with acute otitis media is 10 mg/kg trimethoprim per 24 hours, given in divided doses every 12 hours for 10 days.

➤*Storage/Stability:* Store between 15° to 25°C (59° to 77°F). Dispense in tight, light-resistant glass or PET plastic containers.

Actions

➤*Pharmacology:* Trimethoprim blocks the production of tetrahydrofolic acid from dihydrofolic acid by binding to and reversibly inhibiting the required enzyme, dihydrofolate reductase. This binding is very much stronger for the bacterial enzyme than for the corresponding mammalian enzyme. Thus, trimethoprim selectively interferes with bacterial biosynthesis of nucleic acids and proteins.

➤*Pharmacokinetics:*

Absorption/Distribution – Trimethoprim is rapidly absorbed following oral administration. It exists in the blood as unbound, protein-bound and metabolized forms. Approximately 44% of trimethoprim is bound to plasma proteins.

Mean peak plasma concentrations of approximately 1 mcg/mL occur 1 to 4 hours after oral administration of a single 100 mg dose. A single 200 mg dose will result in plasma concentrations approximately twice as high. The mean half-life of trimethoprim is approximately 9 hours (range, 8 to 10 hours). However, patients with severely impaired renal function exhibit an increase in the half-life of trimethoprim, which requires either dosage regimen adjustment or not using the drug in such patients. During a 13-week study of trimethoprim tablets administered at a dosage of 50 mg 4 times daily, the mean minimum steady-state concentration of the drug was 1.1 mcg/mL. Steady-state concentrations were achieved within 2 to 3 days of chronic administration and were maintained throughout the experimental period.

Trimethoprim also passes the placental barrier and is excreted in breast milk.

Since normal vaginal and fecal flora are the source of most pathogens causing urinary tract infections, it is relevant to consider the distribution of trimethoprim into these sites. Concentrations of trimethoprim in vaginal secretions are consistently greater than those found simultaneously in the serum, being typically 1.6 times the concentrations of simultaneously obtained serum samples. Sufficient trimethoprim is excreted in the feces to markedly reduce or eliminate trimethoprim-susceptible organisms from the fecal flora. The dominant non-Enterobacteriaceae fecal organisms, *Bacteroides* spp. and *Lactobacillus* spp, are not susceptible to trimethoprim concentrations obtained with the recommended dosage.

Trimethoprim also concentrates into middle ear fluid (MEF) very efficiently. In a study in children aged 1 to 12 years, administration of a single 4 mg/kg dose resulted in a mean peak MEF concentration of 2 mcg/mL.

Metabolism – Ten percent to 20% of trimethoprim is metabolized, primarily in the liver; the remainder is excreted unchanged in the urine. The principal metabolites of trimethoprim are the 1- and 3-oxides and the 3′- and 4′-hydroxy derivatives. The free form is considered to be the therapeutically active form.

Excretion – Excretion of trimethoprim is primarily by the kidneys through glomerular filtration and tubular secretion. Urine concentrations of trimethoprim are considerably higher than are the concentrations in the blood. After a single oral dose of 100 mg, urine concentrations of trimethoprim ranged from 30 to 160 mcg/mL during the 0- to 4-hour period and declined to approximately 18 to 91 mcg/mL during the 8- to 24-hour period. A 200 mg single oral dose will result in trimethoprim urine concentrations approximately twice as high. After oral administration, 50% to 60% of trimethoprim is excreted in the urine within 24 hours, approximately 80% of this being unmetabolized trimethoprim.

➤*Microbiology:* Trimethoprim has been shown to be active against most strains of the following microorganisms, both in vitro and in clinical infections.

Aerobic gram-positive microorganisms –
- *Staphylococcus* species (coagulase-negative strains, including *S. saprophyticus*).
- *Streptococcus pneumoniae* (penicillin-susceptible strains).

Aerobic gram-negative microorganisms –
- *Enterobacter* species.
- *Escherichia coli.*
- *Haemophilus influenzae* (excluding beta-lactamase-negative, ampicillin-resistant strains).
- *Klebsiella pneumoniae.*
- *Proteus mirabilis.*

Moraxella catarrhalis isolates were found consistently resistant to trimethoprim.

Contraindications

Hypersensitivity to trimethoprim and in those with documented megaloblastic anemia due to folate deficiency.

Warnings

➤*Hematologic effects:* Experience with trimethoprim alone is limited, but it has been reported rarely to interfere with hematopoiesis, especially when administered in large doses or for prolonged periods.

If any clinical signs of a blood disorder are noted in a patient receiving trimethoprim, obtain a complete blood count and discontinue the drug if a significant reduction in the count of any formed blood element is found.

The presence of clinical signs such as sore throat, fever, pallor, or purpura may be early indications of serious blood disorders.

➤*Renal/Hepatic function impairment:* Give with caution to patients with impaired renal or hepatic function.

➤*Pregnancy: Category C.* Trimethoprim has been shown to be teratogenic in the rat when given in doses 40 times the human dose. In some rabbit studies, the overall increase in fetal loss (dead and resorbed and malformed conceptuses) was associated with doses 6 times the human therapeutic dose.

While there are no large well-controlled studies on the use of trimethoprim in pregnant women, Brumfitt and Pursell, in a retrospective study, reported the outcome of 186 pregnancies during which the mother received either placebo or trimethoprim in combination with sulfamethoxazole. The incidence of congenital abnormalities was 4.5% (3 of 66) in those who received placebo and 3.3% (4 of 120) in those receiving trimethoprim plus sulfamethoxazole. There were no abnormalities in the 10 children whose mothers received the drug during the first trimester. In a separate survey, Brumfitt and Pursell also found no congenital abnormalities in 35 children whose mothers had received trimethoprim plus sulfamethoxazole at the time of conception or shortly thereafter.

Because trimethoprim may interfere with folic acid metabolism, use during pregnancy only if the potential benefit justifies the potential risk to the fetus.

➤*Lactation:* Trimethoprim is excreted in human milk. Because trimethoprim may interfere with folic acid metabolism, exercise caution when trimethoprim is administered to a nursing woman.

➤*Children:* The safety of trimethoprim has not been established in pediatric patients below the age of 2 months.

The effectiveness of trimethoprim solution in the treatment of acute otitis media has not been established in patients below the age of 6 months.

Precautions

Give with caution to patients with possible folate deficiency. Folates may be administered concomitantly without interfering with the antibacterial action of trimethoprim.

Drug Interactions

➤*Phenytoin:* Trimethoprim oral solution may inhibit the hepatic metabolism of phenytoin. Trimethoprim, given at a common clinical dosage, increased the phenytoin half-life by 51% and decreased the phenytoin metabolic clearance rate by 30%. When administering these drugs concurrently, one should be alert for possible excessive phenytoin effect.

➤*Drug/Lab test interactions:* Trimethoprim can interfere with a serum methotrexate assay as determined by the competitive binding protein technique (CBPA) when a bacterial dihydrofolate reductase is used as the bind ing protein. No interference occurs, however, if methotrexate is measured by a radioimmunoassay (RIA).

The presence of trimethoprim may also interfere with the Jaffé alkaline picrate reaction assay for creatinine resulting in overestimations of about 10% in the range of normal values.

Adverse Reactions

➤*Children (oral solution):*

Drug-related Adverse Event	Percent of Pediatric Patients: Trimethoprim oral solution (n = 310)	Percent of Pediatric Patients: Sulfamethoxazole + trimethoprim oral solution (n = 197)
Dermatologic		
Rash	1.3%	6.1%

TRIMETHOPRIM HYDROCHLORIDE — ORAL SOLUTION

Drug-related Adverse Event	Percent of Pediatric Patients: Trimethoprim oral solution (n = 310)	Percent of Pediatric Patients: Sulfamethoxazole + trimethoprim oral solution (n = 197)
GI		
Diarrhea	4.2%	4.6%
Vomiting	1.6%	1.5%
Miscellaneous		
Abdominal pain	< 1%	2.5%

Hematologic – An increase in lymphocytes and eosinophils was noted in some pediatric patients following treatment with trimethoprim oral solution or sulfamethoxazole and trimethoprim oral suspension.

➤*Other adverse reactions reported for trimethoprim:* In addition to the adverse events listed above which have been observed in pediatric patients receiving trimethoprim oral solution, the following adverse reactions and altered laboratory tests have been previously reported for trimethoprim and, therefore, may occur with trimethoprim therapy:

Dermatologic – Pruritus and exfoliative dermatitis. At the recommended adult dosage regimens of 100 mg twice daily or 200 mg daily, each for 10 days, the incidence of rash is 2.9% to 6.7%. In clinical studies which employed high doses of trimethoprim in adults, an elevated incidence of rash was noted. These rashes were maculopapular, morbilliform, pruritic, and generally mild to moderate, appearing 7 to 14 days after the initiation of therapy.

GI – Epigastric distress, glossitis, and nausea.

Hematologic – Leukopenia, megaloblastic anemia, methemoglobinemia, neutropenia, and thrombocytopenia.

Metabolic – Hyperkalemia, hyponatremia.

Miscellaneous – Elevation of serum transaminase and bilirubin, fever, and increases in blood urea nitrogen (BUN) and serum creatinine levels.

Overdosage

➤*Acute:*

Symptoms – Signs of acute overdosage with trimethoprim may appear following ingestion of 1 g or more of the drug and include bone marrow depression, confusion, dizziness, headaches, mental depression, nausea, and vomiting.

Treatment – Treatment consists of gastric lavage and general supportive measures. Acidification of the urine will increase renal elimination of trimethoprim. Peritoneal dialysis is not effective, and hemodialysis is only moderately effective in eliminating the drug.

➤*Chronic:*

Symptoms – Use of trimethoprim at high doses or for extended periods of time may cause bone marrow depression manifested as thrombocytopenia, leukopenia or megaloblastic anemia.

Treatment – If signs of bone marrow depression occur, discontinue trimethoprim, and give the patient leucovorin, 3 to 6 mg IM daily for 3 days, or as required to restore normal hematopoiesis.

TRIMETREXATE GLUCURONATE

Rx	**Neutrexin** (US Bioscience)	**Powder for Injection, lyophilized:** 25 mg trimetrexate	In 5 ml vials with or without 50 mg leucovorin.

TRIMETREXATE GLUCURONATE — INJECTION

WARNING

Trimetrexate glucuronate for injection must be used with concurrent leucovorin (leucovorin protection) to avoid potentially serious or life-threatening toxicities.

Indications

➤*Pneumocystis carinii pneumonia (PCP):* Trimetrexate glucuronate for injection with concurrent leucovorin administration (leucovorin protection) is indicated as an alternative therapy for the treatment of moderate-to-severe PCP in immunocompromised patients, including patients with the acquired immunodeficiency syndrome (AIDS), who are intolerant of, or are refractory to, trimethoprim-sulfamethoxazole therapy or for whom trimethoprim-sulfamethoxazole is contraindicated.

➤*Unlabeled uses:* Trimetrexate is being investigated for treatment of non-small cell lung, prostate, and colorectal cancer.

Administration and Dosage

➤*Approved by the FDA:* December 17, 1993.

➤*Concurrent leucovorin therapy:* Trimetrexate glucuronate for injection must be administered with concurrent leucovorin (leucovorin protection) to avoid potentially serious or life-threatening toxicities. Leucovorin (LV) therapy must extend for 72 hours past the last dose of trimetrexate glucuronate.

➤*Dosage:* 45 mg/m^2 once daily by IV infusion over 60 minutes. Leucovorin must be administered daily during treatment with trimetrexate glucuronate and for 72 hours past the last dose of trimetrexate glucuronate. Leucovorin may be administered intravenously at a dose of 20 mg/m^2 over 5 to 10 minutes every 6 hours for a total daily dose of 80 mg/m^2, or orally as 4 doses of 20 mg/m^2 spaced equally throughout the day. The oral dose should be rounded up to the next higher 25 mg increment. The recommended course of therapy is 21 days of trimetrexate glucuronate and 24 days of leucovorin.

➤*Alternate dosing:* Trimetrexate glucuronate and leucovorin may alternatively be dosed on a mg/kg basis, depending on the patient's body weight, using the conversion factors shown in the following table:

Body weight (kg)	Trimetrexate glucuronate dose (mg/kg/day)	Leucovorin dose (mg/kg/4 times a day)
< 50	1.5	0.6
50 to 80	1.2	0.5
> 80	1	0.5

➤*Dosage modifications:*

Hematologic toxicity – Trimetrexate glucuronate for injection and leucovorin doses should be modified based on the worst hematologic toxicity according to the following information. If leucovorin is given orally, doses should be rounded up to the next higher 25 mg increment.

Dose Modifications for Hematologic Toxicity

Toxicity grade	Neutrophils (polys and bands)	Platelets	Recommended dosages: Trimetrexate glucuronate	Recommended dosages: Leucovorin
1	> 1000/mm^3	> 75,000/mm^3	45 mg/m^2 once daily	20 mg/m^2 every 6 hours
2	750 to 1000/mm^3	50,000 to 75,000/mm^3	45 mg/m^2 once daily	40 mg/m^2 every 6 hours
3	500 to 749/mm^3	25,000 to 49,999/mm^3	22 mg/m^2 once daily	40 mg/m^2 every 6 hours
4	< 500/mm^3	< 25,000/mm^3	Day 1 to 9, discontinue; Day 10 to 21, interrupt up to 96 hours[a]	40 mg/m^2 every 6 hours

[a] If grade 4 hematologic toxicity occurs prior to day 10, trimetrexate glucuronate should be discontinued. Leucovorin (40 mg/m^2, every 6 hours) should be administered for an additional 72 hours. If grade 4 hematologic toxicity occurs at day 10 or later, trimetrexate glucuronate may be held up to 96 hours to allow counts to recover. If counts recover to grade 3 within 96 hours, trimetrexate glucuronate should be administered at a dose of 22 mg/mm^2 and leucovorin maintained at 40 mg/m^2, every 6 hours. When counts recover to grade 2 toxicity, trimetrexate glucuronate dose may be increased to 45 mg/m^2, but the leucovorin dose should be maintained at 40 mg/m^2 for the duration of treatment. If counts do not improve to grade 3 toxicity or less within 96 hours, trimetrexate glucuronate should be discontinued. Leucovorin at a dose of 40 mg/m^2, every 6 hours should be administered for 72 hours following the last dose of trimetrexate glucuronate.

Hepatic toxicity – Transient elevations of transaminases and alkaline phosphatase have been observed in patients treated with trimetrexate glucuronate. Interruption of treatment is advisable if transaminase levels or alkaline phosphatase levels increase to greater than 5 times the upper limit of normal range.

Renal toxicity – Interruption of trimetrexate glucuronate is advisable if serum creatinine levels increase to greater than 2.5 mg/dL and the elevation is considered to be secondary to trimetrexate glucuronate.

Other toxicities – Interruption of treatment is advisable in patients who experience severe mucosal toxicity that interferes with oral intake. Treatment should be discontinued for fever (oral temperature greater than or equal to 40.5°C [105°F]) that cannot be controlled with antipyretics. Leucovorin therapy must extend for 72 hours past the last dose of trimetrexate glucuronate.

➤*Reconstitution and dilution:* Each vial of trimetrexate glucuronate for injection should be reconstituted in accordance with labeled instructions with either 5% Dextrose Injection, USP, or Sterile Water for Injection, USP, to yield a concentration of 12.5 mg of trimetrexate per mL (complete dissolution should occur within 30 seconds). The reconstituted product will appear as a pale greenish yellow solution and must be inspected visually prior to dilution. Do not use if cloudiness or precipitate is observed. Trimetrexate glucuronate should not be reconstituted with solutions containing either chloride ion or leucovorin, since precipitation occurs instantly.

TRIMETREXATE GLUCURONATE — INJECTION

Prior to administration, the reconstituted solution should be further diluted with 5% Dextrose Injection, USP, to yield a final concentration of 0.25 to 2 mg of trimetrexate per mL. The diluted solution should be administered by intravenous infusion over 60 minutes. Trimetrexate glucuronate should not be mixed with solutions containing either chloride ion or leucovorin, since precipitation occurs instantly. The diluted solution is stable under refrigeration or at room temperature for up to 24 hours. Do not freeze. Discard any unused portion after 24 hours. The intravenous line must be flushed thoroughly with at least 10 mL of 5% Dextrose Injection, USP, before and after administering trimetrexate glucuronate.

Leucovorin protection may be administered prior to or following trimetrexate glucuronate. In either case, the intravenous line must be flushed thoroughly with at least 10 mL of 5% Dextrose Injection, USP. Leucovorin calcium for injection should be diluted according to the instructions in the leucovorin monograph, and administered over 5 to 10 minutes every 6 hours.

Parenteral products should be inspected visually for particulate matter and discoloration prior to administration, whenever solution and container permit. Trimetrexate glucuronate forms a precipitate instantly upon contact with chloride ion or leucovorin; therefore it should not be added to solutions containing sodium chloride or other anions. Trimetrexate glucuronate and leucovorin solutions must be administered separately. Intravenous lines should be flushed with at least 10 mL of 5% Dextrose Injection, USP between trimetrexate glucuronate and leucovorin infusions.

➤*Handling and disposal:* If trimetrexate glucuronate contacts the skin or mucosa, immediately wash thoroughly with soap and water. Procedures for proper disposal of cytotoxic drugs should be considered. Several guidelines on this subject have been published.

➤*Storage/Stability:* Store at controlled room temperature 20° to 25°C (68° to 77°F). Protect from exposure to light.

After reconstitution, the solution should be used immediately; however, the solution is stable for 6 hours at room temperature (20° to 25°C; 68° to 77°F), or 24 hours under refrigeration (2° to 8°C; 35.6° to 46.4°F).

Actions

➤*Pharmacology:* In vitro studies have shown that trimetrexate is a competitive inhibitor of dihydrofolate reductase (DHFR) from bacterial, protozoan, and mammalian sources. DHFR catalyzes the reduction of intracellular dihydrofolate to the active coenzyme tetrahydrofolate. Inhibition of DHFR results in the depletion of this coenzyme, leading directly to interference with thymidylate biosynthesis, as well as inhibition of folate-dependent formyltransferases, and indirectly to inhibition of purine biosynthesis. The end result is disruption of DNA, RNA, and protein synthesis, with consequent cell death.

Leucovorin (folinic acid) is readily transported into mammalian cells by an active, carrier-mediated process and can be assimilated into cellular folate pools following its metabolism. In vitro studies have shown that leucovorin provides a source of reduced folates necessary for normal cellular biosynthetic processes. Because the *Pneumocystis carinii* organism lacks the reduced folate carrier-mediated transport system, leucovorin is prevented from entering the organism. Therefore, at concentrations achieved with therapeutic doses of trimetrexate plus leucovorin, the selective transport of trimetrexate, but not leucovorin, into the *Pneumocystis carinii* organism allows the concurrent administration of leucovorin to protect normal host cells from the cytotoxicity of trimetrexate without inhibiting the antifolate's inhibition of *Pneumocystis carinii*. It is not known if considerably higher doses of leucovorin would affect trimetrexate's effect on *Pneumocystis carinii*.

➤*Pharmacokinetics:*

Absorption/Distribution – There have been inconsistencies in the reporting of trimetrexate protein binding. The in vitro plasma protein binding of trimetrexate using ultrafiltration is approximately 95% over the concentration range of 18.75 to 1000 ng/mL. There is a suggestion of capacity limited binding (saturable binding) at concentrations greater than about 1000 ng/mL, with free fraction progressively increasing to about 9.3% as concentration is increased to 15 mcg/mL. Other reports have declared trimetrexate to be greater than 98% bound at concentrations of 0.1 to 10 mcg/mL; however, specific free fractions were not stated. The free fraction of trimetrexate also has been reported to be about 15% to 16% at a concentration of 60 ng/mL, increasing to about 20% at a trimetrexate concentration of 6 mcg/mL.

Metabolism/Excretion – Trimetrexate metabolism in man has not been characterized. Preclinical data strongly suggest that the major metabolic pathway is oxidative O-demethylation, followed by conjugation to either glucuronide or the sulfate. N-demethylation and oxidation is a related minor pathway. Preliminary findings in humans indicate the presence of a glucuronide conjugate with DHFR inhibition and a demethylated metabolite in urine.

The presence of metabolite(s) in human plasma following the administration of trimetrexate is suggested by the differences seen in trimetrexate plasma concentrations when measured by HPLC and a nonspecific DHFR inhibition assay. The profiles are similar initially, but diverge with time; concentrations determined by DHFR being higher than those determined by HPLC. This suggests the presence of one or more metabolites with DHFR inhibition activity. After IV administration of trimetrexate to humans, urinary recovery averaged about 40%, using a DHFR assay, in comparison to 10% urinary recovery as determined by HPLC, suggesting the presence of one or more metabolites that retain inhibitory activity against DHFR. Fecal recovery of trimetrexate over 48 hours after IV administration ranged from 0.09% to 7.6% of the dose as determined by DHFR inhibition and 0.02% to 5.2% of the dose as determined by HPLC.

➤*Microbiology:* Trimetrexate inhibits, in a dose-related manner, in vitro growth of the trophozoite stage of rat *Pneumocystis carinii* cultured on human embryonic lung fibroblast cells. Trimetrexate concentrations between 3 and 54.1 mcM were shown to inhibit the growth of trophozoites. Leucovorin alone at a concentration of 10 mcM did not alter either the growth of the trophozoites or the antipneumocystis activity of trimetrexate. Resistance to trimetrexate's antimicrobial activity against *Pneumocystis carinii* has not been studied.

Contraindications

Clinically significant sensitivity to trimetrexate, leucovorin, or methotrexate.

Warnings

➤*Concurrent leucovorin therapy:* Trimetrexate glucuronate for injection must be used with concurrent leucovorin to avoid potentially serious or life-threatening complications including bone marrow suppression, oral and gastrointestinal mucosal ulceration, and renal and hepatic dysfunction. Leucovorin therapy must extend for 72 hours past the last dose of trimetrexate glucuronate. Patients should be informed that failure to take the recommended dose and duration of leucovorin can lead to fatal toxicity. Patients should be closely monitored for the development of serious hematologic adverse reactions. Blood tests to assess absolute neutrophil counts and platelets should be performed at least twice a week during therapy.

Trimetrexate glucuronate-associated myelosuppression, stomatitis, and GI toxicities generally can be ameliorated by adjusting the dose of leucovorin.

➤*Hypersensitivity reactions:* Hypersensitivity/allergic type reactions including but not limited to rash, chills/rigors, fever, diaphoresis and dyspnea, have occurred with trimetrexate primarily when it is administered as a bolus infusion or at doses higher than those recommended for PCP, and most frequently in combination with 5-FU and leucovorin. In rare cases, anaphylactoid reactions, including acute hypotension and loss of consciousness have occurred.

➤*Fertility impairment:* No studies have been conducted to evaluate the potential of trimetrexate to impair fertility. However, during standard toxicity studies conducted in mice and rats, degeneration of the testes and spermatocytes including the arrest of spermatogenesis was observed.

➤*Pregnancy: Category D.*

Teratogenic – Trimetrexate glucuronate can cause fetal harm when administered to a pregnant woman. Trimetrexate has been shown to be fetotoxic and teratogenic in rats and rabbits. Rats administered 1.5 and 2.5 mg/kg/day intravenously on gestational days 6 to 15 showed substantial postimplantation loss and severe inhibition of maternal weight gain. Trimetrexate administered intravenously to rats at 0.5 and 1 mg/kg/day on gestational days 6 to 15 retarded normal fetal development and was teratogenic. Rabbits administered trimetrexate intravenously at daily doses of 2.5 and 5 mg/kg/day on gestational days 6 to 18 resulted in significant maternal and fetal toxicity. In rabbits, trimetrexate at 0.1 mg/kg/day was teratogenic in the absence of significant maternal toxicity. These effects were observed using doses $\frac{1}{20}$ to $\frac{1}{2}$ the equivalent human therapeutic dose based on a mg/m^2 basis. Teratogenic effects included skeletal, visceral, ocular, and cardiovascular abnormalities. If trimetrexate glucuronate is used during pregnancy, or if the patient becomes pregnant while taking this drug, the patient should be apprised of the potential hazard to the fetus. Women of childbearing potential should be advised to avoid becoming pregnant.

➤*Lactation:* It is not known if trimetrexate is excreted in human milk. Because many drugs are excreted in human milk and because of the potential for serious adverse reactions in nursing infants from trimetrexate, it is recommended that breastfeeding be discontinued if the mother is treated with trimetrexate glucuronate.

➤*Children:* The safety and effectiveness of trimetrexate glucuronate for the treatment of histologically confirmed PCP has not been established for patients under 18 years of age. Two children, ages 15 months and 9 months, were treated with trimetrexate and leucovorin using a dose of 45 mg/m^2 of trimetrexate per day for 21 days and 20 mg/m^2 of leucovorin every 6 hours for 24 days. There were no serious or unexpected adverse effects.

Precautions

➤*Monitoring:* Patients receiving trimetrexate glucuronate with leucovorin protection should be seen frequently by a physician. Blood tests to assess the following parameters should be performed at least twice a week during therapy: Hematology (absolute neutrophil counts [ANC], platelets), renal function (serum creatinine, BUN), and hepatic function (AST, ALT, alkaline phosphatase).

➤*Pulmonary conditions:* Trimetrexate glucuronate has not been evaluated clinically for the treatment of concurrent pulmonary conditions such as bacterial, viral, or fungal pneumonia or mycobacterial diseases. In vitro activity has been observed against *Toxoplasma gondii*, *Mycobacterium avium* complex, gram-positive cocci, and gram-negative rods. If clinical deterioration is observed in patients, they should be carefully evaluated for other possible causes of pulmonary disease and treated with additional agents as appropriate.

➤*Seizures:* Seizures have been reported rarely (less than 1%) in AIDS patients receiving trimetrexate glucuronate; however, a causal relationship has not been established. Trimetrexate is a known inhibitor of histamine metabolism.

➤*Special risk:* Patients receiving trimetrexate glucuronate for injection may experience severe hematologic, hepatic, renal, and GI toxicities. Caution should be used in treating patients with impaired hematologic, renal, or hepatic function. Patients who require concomitant therapy with nephrotoxic, myelosuppressive, or hepatotoxic drugs should be treated with trimetrexate glucuronate at the discretion of the physician and monitored

TRIMETREXATE GLUCURONATE — INJECTION

carefully. To allow for full therapeutic doses of trimetrexate glucuronate, treatment with zidovudine should be discontinued during trimetrexate glucuronate therapy.

➤*Lab test abnormalities:* Mild elevations in transaminases and alkaline phosphatase have been observed with trimetrexate glucuronate administration and are usually not cause for modification of trimetrexate glucuronate therapy. Interruption of treatment is advisable if transaminase levels or alkaline phosphatase levels increase to greater than 5 times the upper limit of normal range.

Drug Interactions

Since trimetrexate is metabolized by a P450 enzyme system, drugs that induce or inhibit this drug metabolizing enzyme system may elicit important drug-drug interactions that may alter trimetrexate plasma concentrations. Agents that might be coadministered with trimetrexate in AIDS patients for other indications that could elicit this activity include erythromycin, rifampin, rifabutin, ketoconazole, and fluconazole. In vitro perfusion of isolated rat liver has shown that cimetidine caused a significant reduction in trimetrexate metabolism and that acetaminophen altered the relative concentration of trimetrexate metabolites possibly by competing for sulfate metabolites. Based on an in vitro rat liver model, nitrogen substituted imidazole drugs (clotrimazole, ketoconazole, miconazole) were potent, noncompetitive inhibitors of trimetrexate metabolism. Patients medicated with these drugs and trimetrexate should be carefully monitored.

Adverse Reactions

Trimetrexate Glucuronate Comparative Trial
Comparison of adverse reactions reported for ≥ 1% of patients

Adverse reactions	Number and percent (%) of patients with adverse reactions			
	TMTX/LV (n = 109)		TMP-SMZ (n = 111)	
Nonlaboratory adverse reactions				
Fever	9	(8.3%)	14	(12.6%)
Rash/Pruritus	6	(5.5%)	14	(12.6%)
Nausea/Vomiting	5	(4.6%)[a]	15	(13.5%)[a]
Confusion	3	(2.8%)	3	(2.7%)
Fatigue	2	(1.8%)	0	(0%)
Hematologic toxicity				
Neutropenia (≤ 1000/mm^3)	33	(30.3%)	37	(33.3%)
Thrombocytopenia (≤ 75,000/mm^3)	11	(10.1%)	17	(15.3%)
Anemia (Hgb < 8 g/dL)	8	(7.3%)	10	(9%)
Hepatotoxicity				
Increased AST (> 5 × ULN)[b]	15	(13.8%)	10	(9%)
Increased ALT (> 5 × ULN)	12	(11%)	13	(11.7%)
Increased alkaline phosphatase (> 5 × ULN)	5	(4.6%)	3	(2.7%)
Increased bilirubin (2.5 × ULN)	2	(1.8%)	1	(0.9%)
Renal				
Increased serum creatinine (> 3 × ULN)	1	(0.9%)	2	(1.8%)
Electrolyte imbalance				
Hyponatremia	5	(4.6%)	10	(9%)
Hypocalcemia	2	(1.8%)	0	(0%)
No. of patients with at least one adverse reaction[c]	58	(53.2%)	60	(54.1%)

[a] Statistically significant difference between treatment groups (Chi-square: $P = 0.022$).
[b] ULN = Upper limit of normal range.
[c] Patients could have reported more than 1 adverse reaction; therefore, the sum of adverse reactions exceeds the number of patients.

➤*Laboratory toxicities:* Laboratory toxicities were generally manageable with dose modification of trimetrexate/leucovorin.

The following table lists the adverse reactions resulting in discontinuation of study therapy in the trimetrexate glucuronate comparative study with TMP-SMZ. Twenty-nine percent (29%) of the patients on the TMP-SMZ arm discontinued therapy due to adverse reactions compared to 10% of the patients treated with TMTX/LV ($P < 0.001$).

Trimetrexate Glucuronate Comparative Trial
Adverse reactions resulting in discontinuation of therapy

Adverse reactions	Number and percent (%) of patients discontinued for adverse reactions[b]			
	TMTX/LV (n = 109)		TMP-SMZ (n = 111)	
Nonlaboratory adverse reactions				
Rash/Pruritus	3	(2.8%)	5	(4.5%)
Fever	2	(1.8%)	4	(3.6%)
Nausea/Vomiting	1	(0.9%)	8	(7.2%)
Neurologic toxicity	1	(0.9%)[c]	2	(1.8%)
Hematologic toxicity				
Neutropenia (≤ 1000/mm^3)	4	(3.7%)	6	(5.4%)
Thrombocytopenia (≤ 75,000/mm^3)	0	(0%)	4	(3.6%)
Anemia (Hgb < 8 g/dL)	0	(0%)	4	(3.6%)
Hepatotoxicity				
Increased AST (> 5 × ULN[a])	3	(2.8%)	9	(8.1%)
Increased ALT (> 5 × ULN)	1	(0.9%)	4	(3.6%)
Increased alkaline phosphatase (> 5 × ULN)	0	(0%)	1	(0.9%)
Electrolyte imbalance				
Hyponatremia	0	(0%)	3	(2.7%)
No. of patients discontinuing therapy due to an adverse reaction[b]	11	(10.1%)[d]	32	(28.8%)[d]

[a] ULN = Upper limit of normal range.
[b] Patients could discontinue therapy due to more than 1 toxicity; therefore the sum exceeds number of patients who discontinued due to toxicity.
[c] Patient discontinued TMTX/LV due to seizure, though causal relationship could not be established.
[d] Statistically significant difference between treatment groups (Chi-square: $P < 0.001$).

Hematologic toxicity was the principal dose-limiting side effect.

Overdosage

➤*Symptoms:* Trimetrexate glucuronate for injection administered without concurrent leucovorin can cause lethal complications. There has been no extensive experience in humans receiving single IV doses of trimetrexate greater than 90 mg/m^2/day with concurrent leucovorin. The toxicities seen at this dose were primarily hematologic.

➤*Treatment:* In the event of overdose, trimetrexate glucuronate should be stopped and leucovorin should be administered at a dose of 40 mg/m^2 every 6 hours for 3 days. The LD_{50} of IV trimetrexate in mice is 62 mg/kg (186 mg/m^2).

MISCELLANEOUS ANTI-INFECTIVES/ANTISEPTICS

METHYLENE BLUE

For complete and comparative prescribing information, see the Methylene blue oral monograph in the Endocrine and Metabolic Agents chapter.

FOSFOMYCIN TROMETHAMINE

Rx	**Monurol** (Forest)	**Granules:** 3 g	In single-dose packets.

FOSFOMYCIN TROMETHAMINE — ORAL

Indications

➤*Uncomplicated urinary tract infections:* For the treatment of uncomplicated urinary tract infections (acute cystitis) in women due to susceptible strains of *Escherichia coli* and *Enterococcus faecalis*. Fosfomycin tromethamine is not indicated for the treatment of pyelonephritis or perinephric abscess.

If persistence or reappearance of bacteriuria occurs after treatment with fosfomycin, other therapeutic agents should be selected.

Administration and Dosage

➤*Approved by the FDA:* December 19, 1996.

➤*Women (18 years of age and older):* 1 sachet of fosfomycin tromethamine. Fosfomycin may be taken with or without food.

Fosfomycin should not be taken in its dry form. Always mix fosfomycin with water before ingesting.

FOSFOMYCIN TROMETHAMINE — ORAL

➤*Preparation:* Fosfomycin should be taken orally. Pour the entire contents of a single-dose sachet of fosfomycin into 90 to 120 mL of water (½ cup) and stir to dissolve. Do not use hot water. Fosfomycin should be taken immediately after dissolving in water.

➤*Storage/Stability:* Store at controlled room temperature 15° to 30°C (59° to 86°F).

Keep this and all drugs out of the reach of children.

Actions

➤*Pharmacokinetics:*

Absorption – Fosfomycin tromethamine is rapidly absorbed following oral administration and converted to the free acid, fosfomycin. Absolute oral bioavailability under fasting conditions is 37%. After a single 3 g dose of fosfomycin tromethamine, the mean (± 1 SD) maximum serum concentration (C_{max}) achieved was 26.1 (± 9.1) mcg/mL within 2 hours. The oral bioavailability of fosfomycin is reduced to 30% under fed conditions. Following a single 3 g oral dose of fosfomycin tromethamine with a high-fat meal, the mean C_{max} achieved was 17.6 (± 4.4) mcg/mL within 4 hours. Cimetidine does not affect the pharmacokinetics of fosfomycin when coadministered with fosfomycin tromethamine. Metoclopramide lowers the serum concentrations and urinary excretion of fosfomycin when coadministered with fosfomycin.

Distribution – The mean apparent steady-state volume of distribution (Vss) is 136.1 (± 44.1) L following oral administration of fosfomycin tromethamine. Fosfomycin is not bound to plasma proteins. Fosfomycin is distributed to the kidneys, bladder wall, prostate, and seminal vesicles. Following a 50 mg/kg dose of fosfomycin to patients undergoing urological surgery for bladder carcinoma, the mean concentration of fosfomycin in the bladder, taken at a distance from the neoplastic site, was 18 mcg/g of tissue at 3 hours after dosing. Fosfomycin has been shown to cross the placental barrier in animals and man.

Excretion – Fosfomycin is excreted unchanged in both urine and feces. Following oral administration of fosfomycin tromethamine, the mean total body clearance (CL_{TB}) and mean renal clearance (CL_R) of fosfomycin were 16.9 (± 3.5) L/hr and 6.3 (± 1.7) L/hr, respectively. Approximately 38% of a 3 g dose of fosfomycin tromethamine is recovered from urine, and 18% is recovered from feces. Following intravenous administration, the mean CL_{TB} and mean CL_R of fosfomycin were 6.1 (± 1) L/hr and 5.5 (± 1.2) L/hr, respectively.

A mean urine fosfomycin concentration of 706 (± 466) mcg/mL was attained within 2 to 4 hours after a single oral 3 g dose of fosfomycin tromethamine under fasting conditions. The mean urinary concentration of fosfomycin was 10 mcg/mL in samples collected 72 to 84 hours following a single oral dose of fosfomycin tromethamine.

Following a 3 g dose of fosfomycin tromethamine administered with a high-fat meal, a mean urine fosfomycin concentration of 537 (± 252) mcg/mL was attained within 6 to 8 hours. Although the rate of urinary excretion of fosfomycin was reduced under fed conditions, the cumulative amount of fosfomycin excreted in the urine was the same, 1118 (± 201) mg (fed) vs 1140 (± 238) mg (fasting). Further, urinary concentrations greater than or equal to 100 mcg/mL were maintained for the same duration, 26 hours, indicating that fosfomycin tromethamine can be taken without regard to food.

Following oral administration of fosfomycin tromethamine, the mean half-life for elimination (t½) is 5.7 (± 2.8) hours.

Special populations –

Renal function impairment: In 5 anuric patients undergoing hemodialysis, the t½ of fosfomycin during hemodialysis was 40 hours. In patients with varying degrees of renal impairment (creatinine clearances varying from 54 mL/min to 7 mL/min), the t½ of fosfomycin increased from 11 hours to 50 hours. The percent of fosfomycin recovered in urine decreased from 32% to 11% indicating that renal impairment significantly decreases the excretion of fosfomycin.

➤*Microbiology:* Fosfomycin (the active component of fosfomycin tromethamine) has in vitro activity against a broad range of gram-positive and gram-negative aerobic microorganisms that are associated with uncomplicated urinary tract infections. Fosfomycin is bactericidal in urine at therapeutic doses. The bactericidal action of fosfomycin is due to its inactivation of the enzyme enolpyruvyl transferase, thereby irreversibly blocking the condensation of uridine diphosphate-N-acetylglucosamine with p-enolpyruvate, one of the first steps in bacterial cell wall synthesis. It also reduces adherence of bacteria to uroepithelial cells.

Fosfomycin has been shown to be active against most strains of the following microorganisms, both in vitro and in clinical infections.

Aerobic gram-positive microorganisms – *Enterococcus faecalis.*

Aerobic gram-negative microorganisms – *Escherichia coli.*

Contraindications

Hypersensitivity to the drug.

Warnings

➤*Elderly:* In general, dose selection for an elderly patient should be cautious, starting at the low end of the dosing range, reflecting the greater frequency of decreased hepatic, renal, or cardiac function, and of concomitant disease or other drug therapy.

➤*Pregnancy: Category B.* When administered intramuscularly as the sodium salt at a dose of 1 g to pregnant women, fosfomycin crosses the placental barrier. Fosfomycin crosses the placental barrier of rats; it does not produce teratogenic effects in pregnant rats at dosages as high as 1000 mg/kg/day (approximately 9 and 1.4 times the human dose based on body weight and mg/m², respectively). When administered to pregnant female rabbits at dosages as high as 1000 mg/kg/day (approximately 9 and 2.7 times the human dose based on body weight and mg/m², respectively), fetotoxicities were observed. However, these toxicities were seen at maternally toxic doses and were considered to be due to the sensitivity of the rabbit to changes in the intestinal microflora resulting from the antibiotic administration. There are, however, no adequate and well-controlled studies in pregnant women. Because animal reproduction studies are not always predictive of human response, this drug should be used during pregnancy only if clearly needed.

➤*Lactation:* It is not known whether fosfomycin tromethamine is excreted in human milk. Because many drugs are excreted in human milk and because of the potential for serious adverse reactions in nursing infants from fosfomycin, a decision should be made whether to discontinue nursing or the drug, taking into account the importance of the drug to the mother.

➤*Children:* Safety and efficacy in children age 12 years and under have not been established in adequate and well-controlled studies.

Precautions

➤*Monitoring:* Urine specimens for culture and susceptibility testing should be obtained before and after completion of therapy.

➤*Acute cystitis:* Do not use more than 1 single dose of fosfomycin tromethamine to treat a single episode of acute cystitis. Repeated daily doses of fosfomycin tromethamine did not improve the clinical success or microbiological eradication rates compared to single dose therapy, but did increase the incidence of adverse events.

➤*Lab test abnormalities:* Significant laboratory changes reported in US clinical trials of fosfomycin tromethamine without regard to drug relationship include increased eosinophil count, increased or decreased WBC count, increased bilirubin, increased ALT, increased AST, increased alkaline phosphatase, decreased hematocrit, decreased hemoglobin, increased and decreased platelet count. The changes were generally transient and were not clinically significant.

Drug Interactions

➤*Metoclopramide:* When coadministered with fosfomycin, metoclopramide, a drug that increases gastrointestinal motility, lowers the serum concentration and urinary excretion of fosfomycin. Other drugs that increase gastrointestinal motility may produce similar effects.

➤*Cimetidine:* Cimetidine does not affect the pharmacokinetics of fosfomycin when coadministered with fosfomycin tromethamine.

Adverse Reactions

➤*Adverse reactions from clinical trials:*

Drug-Related Adverse Reactions (%) In Fosfomycin and Comparator Populations (> 1%)

Adverse reactions	Fosfomycin (n = 1233)	Nitrofurantoin (n = 374)	Trimethoprim/ sulfamethoxazole (n = 428)	Ciprofloxacin (n = 445)
Diarrhea	9%	6.4%	2.3%	3.1%
Vaginitis	5.5%	5.3%	4.7%	6.3%
Nausea	4.1%	7.2%	8.6%	3.4%
Headache	3.9%	5.9%	5.4%	3.4%
Dizziness	1.3%	1.9%	2.3%	2.2%
Asthenia	1.1%	0.3%	0.5%	0%
Dyspepsia	1.1%	2.1%	0.7%	1.1%

➤*Adverse events in the study population:* In clinical trials, the following adverse events occurring in the study population regardless of drug relationship:

CNS – Headache (10.3%); nervousness, somnolence, paresthesia, insomnia, migraine (less than 1%).

Dermatologic – Rash (1.4%); skin disorder, pruritus (less than 1%).

GI – Diarrhea (10.4%); nausea (5.2%); dyspepsia (1.8%); abnormal stools, dry mouth, flatulence, anorexia, constipation, vomiting (less than 1%).

GU – Vaginitis (7.6%); dysmenorrhea (2.6%); hematuria, menstrual disorder, dysuria (less than 1%).

Respiratory – Rhinitis (4.5%); pharyngitis (2.5%).

Miscellaneous – Back pain (3%); dizziness (2.3%); abdominal pain (2.2%); pain (2.2%); asthenia (1.7%); myalgia, ear disorder, fever, flu syndrome, infection, lymphadenopathy, AST increase (less than 1%). One patient developed unilateral optic neuritis, an event considered possibly related to fosfomycin therapy.

➤*Postmarketing:* Serious adverse events from the marketing experience with fosfomycin tromethamine outside of the United States have been rarely reported and include angioedema, aplastic anemia, asthma (exacerbation), cholestatic jaundice, hepatic necrosis, and toxic megacolon.

Overdosage

➤*Symptoms:* In acute toxicology studies, oral administration of high doses of fosfomycin tromethamine up to 5 g/kg were well-tolerated in mice and rats, produced transient and minor incidences of watery stool in rabbits, and produced diarrhea with anorexia in dogs occurring 2 to 3 days after single dose administration. These doses represent 50 to 125 times the human therapeutic dose.

FOSFOMYCIN TROMETHAMINE — ORAL

➤*Treatment:* There have been no reported cases of overdosage. In the event of overdosage, treatment should be symptomatic and supportive.

Patient Information

Fosfomycin tromethamine can be taken with or without food. Symptoms should improve in 2 to 3 days after taking fosfomycin; if not improved, the patient should contact her healthcare provider.

ANTIBIOTIC COMBINATIONS

TRIMETHOPRIM AND SULFAMETHOXAZOLE (Co-Trimoxazole; TMP-SMZ)

Rx	**Trimethoprim and Sulfamethoxazole** (Various, eg, Geneva, Goldline, Lemmon, Moore, Rugby, Schein, URL)	**Tablets**: 80 mg trimethoprim and 400 mg sulfamethoxazole	In 100s and 500s.
Rx	**Bactrim** (Roche)		(Bactrim-Roche). Lt. green, scored. Capsule shape. In 100s.
Rx	**Trimethoprim and Sulfamethoxazole DS** (Various, eg, Goldline, Geneva, Lemmon, Moore, Rugby, Schein, URL)	**Tablets, Double Strength**: 160 mg trimethoprim and 800 mg sulfamethoxazole	In 100s and 500s.
Rx	**Bactrim DS** (Roche)		(Bactrim-DS Roche). White. Capsule shape. In 100s, 250s and 500s.
Rx	**Septra DS** (Monarch)		(Septra DS O2C). Pink, scored. Oval. In 100s, 250s and UD 100s.
Rx	**Trimethoprim and Sulfamethoxazole** (Various, eg, Goldline, Lemmon, Moore, Rugby)	**Oral Suspension**: 40 mg trimethoprim and 200 mg sulfamethoxazole per 5 ml	In 150, 200 and 480 ml.
Rx	**Cotrim Pediatric** (Lemmon)		Cherry flavor. In 473 ml.[2]
Rx	**Septra** (Monarch)		Cherry flavor in 20, 100, 150, 200 and 473 ml.[3] Grape flavor in 473 ml.[3]
Rx	**Sulfatrim** (Various, eg, URL)		In 473 ml.
Rx	**Trimethoprim and Sulfamethoxazole** (Various, eg, Sanofi)	**Injection**: 80 mg/ml sulfamethoxazole, 16 mg/ml trimethoprim per 5 ml	In 5 ml *Carpuject*.
Rx	**Bactrim IV** (Roche)	**Injection**: 80 mg trimethoprim and 400 mg sulfamethoxazole per 5 ml	In 10 and 30 ml multiple-dose vials.[4]
Rx	**Septra IV** (Monarch)		In 5 ml vials and 10 and 20 ml multiple-dose vials.[4]

[1] With 0.3% alcohol, saccharin, sorbitol, sucrose, parabens, EDTA.
[2] With ≤ 0.5% alcohol, saccharin, sorbitol.
[3] With 0.26% alcohol, 0.1% methylparaben, 0.1% sodium benzoate, saccharin, sorbitol.
[4] With 40% propylene glycol, 10% ethyl alcohol, 0.3% diethanolamine, 0.1% sodium metabisulfite and 1% benzyl alcohol.

TRIMETHOPRIM AND SULFAMETHOXAZOLE (Co-Trimoxazole; TMP-SMZ) — INJECTION

See also individual monographs for trimethoprim and sulfonamides.

Indications

➤*Oral and parenteral:*

Urinary tract infections (UTIs) due to susceptible strains of E. coli, Klebsiella and Enterobacter species, M. morganii, P. mirabilis and P. vulgaris – Treat initial uncomplicated UTIs with a single antibacterial agent.

Parenteral therapy is indicated in severe or complicated infections when oral therapy is not feasible.

Shigellosis enteritis – Caused by susceptible strains of *S. flexneri* and *S. sonnei* in children and adults.

Pneumocystis carinii pneumonia (PCP) – Treatment of PCP in children and adults.

➤*Oral:*

Pneumocystis carinii pneumonia prophylaxis – Prophylaxis against PCP in individuals who are immunosuppressed and considered to be at increased risk.

Acute otitis media in children – Due to susceptible strains of *H. influenzae* or *S. pneumoniae*. There are limited data on the safety of repeated use in children < 2 years of age. Not indicated for prophylactic use or prolonged administration.

Acute exacerbations of chronic bronchitis in adults – Due to susceptible strains of *H. influenzae* and *S. pneumoniae*.

Travelers' diarrhea in adults – Due to susceptible strains of enterotoxigenic *E. coli*.

➤*Unlabeled uses:* Treatment of cholera and salmonella-type infections and nocardiosis.

TMP 40 mg and SMZ 200 mg daily at bedtime, a minimum of 3 times weekly or postcoitally has been used to prevent recurrent UTIs in females.

Low-dose TMP–SMZ has been studied in the prophylaxis of neutropenic patients with *P. carinii* infections or leukemia patients to reduce the incidence of gram- negative rod bacteremia.

Prophylaxis with TMP-SMZ (320/1600 mg/day) appears beneficial in reducing the incidence of bacterial infection (especially of the urinary tract and blood) following renal transplantation, and may provide protection against *P. carinii* pneumonia.

Treatment of acute and chronic prostatitis – 160 mg TMP/800 mg SMZ twice daily has been used for chronic bacterial prostatitis for up to 12 weeks.

Administration and Dosage

Administration and Dosage of TMP-SMZ

Organisms/Infections	Dosage	
Urinary tract infections, shigellosis and acute otitis media:		
Adults:	160 mg TMP/800 mg SMZ every 12 hours for 10 to 14 days (5 days for shigellosis).	
Children (≥ 2 months of age):	8 mg/kg TMP/40 mg/kg SMZ per day given in 2 divided doses every 12 hours for 10 days (5 days for shigellosis).	
Guideline for proper dosage:	Dose every 12 hours:	
Weight (kg)	Teaspoonfuls	Tablets
10	1 (5 ml)	-
20	2 (10 ml)	1
30	3 (15 ml)	1½
40	4 (20 ml)	2 (or 1 double strength tablet)
Patients with impaired renal function Ccr (ml/min):	Recommended dosage regimen:	
> 30	Usual regimen	
15-30	½ usual regimen	
< 15	Not recommended	
IV: Adults and children > 2 months with normal renal function for severe UTIs and shigellosis.	8 to 10 mg/kg/day (based on TMP) in 2 to 4 divided doses every 6, 8 or 12 hours for up to 14 days for severe UTIs and 5 days for shigellosis.	
Travelers' diarrhea in adults:	160 mg TMP/800 mg SMZ every 12 hrs for 5 days.	
Acute exacerbations of chronic bronchitis in adults:	160 mg TMP/800 mg SMZ every 12 hrs for 14 days.	
Pneumocystis carinii pneumonia:	15 to 20 mg/kg TMP/100 mg/kg SMZ per day in divided doses every 6 hours for 14 to 21 days.	
Guideline for proper dosage in children	Dose every 6 hours:	
Weight (kg)	Teaspoonfuls	Tablets
8	1 (5 ml)	-
16	2 (10 ml)	1
24	3 (15 ml)	1½
32	4 (20 ml)	2 (or 1 double strength tablet)

TRIMETHOPRIM AND SULFAMETHOXAZOLE (Co-Trimoxazole; TMP-SMZ) — INJECTION

Administration and Dosage of TMP-SMZ			
Organisms/Infections	Dosage		
IV for adults and children > 2 months:	15 to 20 mg/kg/day (based on TMP) in 3 or 4 divided doses every 6 to 8 hours for up to 14 days.		
Prophylaxis:			
Adults:	160 mg TMP/800 mg SMZ given orally every 24 hours.		
Children:	150 mg/m² TMP/ 750 mg/m² SMZ per day given orally in equally divided doses twice a day, on 3 consecutive days per week. The total daily dose should not exceed 320 mg TMP/1600 mg SMZ.		
Guideline for proper dosage in children	Dose every 12 hours		
Body surface area (m²)	Teaspoonfuls	Tablets	
0.26	½ (2.5 ml)	-	
0.53	1 (5 ml)	½	
1.06	2 (10 ml)	1	

[1] Also recommended by the Public Service Task Force on Antipneumocystis Prophylaxis. CDC 1993 Sexually Transmitted Diseases Treatment Guidelines. *Morbidity and Mortality Weekly Report* 1993 Sep 24;42 (No. RR-14):1–102.

➤*Parenteral:*

IV – Administer over 60 to 90 minutes. Avoid rapid infusion or bolus injection. Do not give IM. When administered by an infusion device, thoroughly flush all lines used to remove any residual TMP-SMZ. The following infusion systems have been tested and found satisfactory: Unit-dose glass containers; unit-dose polyvinyl chloride; polyolefin containers.

Preparation of solution – Infusion must be diluted; add the contents of each 5 ml amp to 125 ml of 5% Dextrose in Water. Do not mix with other drugs or solutions. Do not refrigerate and use within 6 hours. If a dilution of 5 ml per 100 ml D5W is desired, use within 4 hours. When fluid restriction is desirable, add each 5 ml amp to 75 ml of D5W. Mix solution just prior to use and administer within 2 hours. If solution is cloudy or precipitates after mixing, discard and prepare fresh solution.

➤*Storage / Stability:* Store infusion at room temperature (15° to 30°C; 59° to 86°F). Do not refrigerate. Protect from light. After initial entry into the multi-dose vials, use the remaining contents within 48 hours.

Actions

➤*Pharmacology:* Sulfamethoxazole (SMZ) inhibits bacterial synthesis of dihydrofolic acid by competing with para-aminobenzoic acid. Trimethoprim (TMP) blocks the production of tetrahydrofolic acid by inhibiting the enzyme dihydrofolate reductase. Thus, this combination blocks two consecutive steps in the bacterial biosynthesis of essential nucleic acids and proteins. In vitro, bacterial resistance develops more slowly with this combination than with either drug alone.

➤*Pharmacokinetics:*

Absorption / Distribution – TMP-SMZ is rapidly and completely absorbed following oral administration. Peak plasma levels occur in 1 to 4 hours following oral administration and 1 to 1.5 hours after IV infusion. The 1:5 ratio of TMP to SMZ achieves an approximate 1:20 ratio of peak serum concentrations. Detectable amounts of TMP–SMZ are present in the blood 24 hours after administration. During 3 days of administration of 160 mg TMP/ 800 mg SMZ twice daily, the mean steady-state plasma TMP concentration was 1.72 mcg/ml. The steady-state mean plasma levels of free and total SMZ were 57.4 mcg/ml and 68 mcg/ml, respectively. Approximately 44% of TMP and 70% of SMZ are protein bound. Both distribute to sputum, vaginal fluid and middle ear fluid, pass the placental barrier, and are excreted in breast milk; TMP also distributes to bronchial secretion. Two to three times the serum concentration of TMP is achieved in prostatic fluid. Therapeutic concentrations are achieved in vaginal secretions, cerebrospinal fluid, pulmonary tissue, pleural effusion, bile, sputa and aqueous humor. It is also detectable in breast milk, amniotic fluid and fetal serum. Following oral administration, the half-lives of TMP (8 to 11 hours) and SMZ (10 to 12 hours) are similar. Following IV administration, the mean plasma half-life was 11.3 ± 0.7 hours for TMP and 12.8 ± 1.8 hours for SMZ. Patients with severely impaired renal function exhibit an increase in the half-lives of both components, requiring dosage regimen adjustment.

Metabolism / Excretion – TMP is metabolized to a relatively small extent; SMZ undergoes biotransformation to inactive compounds. The metabolism of SMZ occurs predominantly by N_4-acetylation, although the glucuronide conjugate has been identified. The principal metabolites of TMP are the 1- and 3-oxides and the 3'- and 4'-hydroxy derivatives. The free forms are the therapeutically active forms.

Excretion is chiefly by the kidneys through both glomerular filtration and tubular secretion. Urine concentrations are considerably higher than serum concentrations. Concurrent administration does not affect the excretion pattern of either drug. The average percentage of the dose recovered in urine from 0 to 72 hours after a single oral dose is 84.5% for total sulfonamide and 66.8% for free TMP. Of the total sulfonamide, 30% is excreted as free SMZ, with the remaining as N_4-acetylated metabolite.

➤*Microbiology:* The antibacterial activity of TMP–SMZ includes the common urinary tract pathogens except *Pseudomonas aeruginosa*. The following are usually susceptible: *Escherichia coli*, *Klebsiella* and *Enterobacter* sp., *Morganella morganii*, *Proteus mirabilis* and indole-positive *Proteus* sp. including *P. vulgaris*. The following pathogens isolated from middle ear exudate and bronchial secretions are usually susceptible: *Haemophilus influenzae* (including ampicillin-resistant strains), *Streptococcus pneumoniae*, *Shigella flexneri* and *S. sonnei*.

Contraindications

Hypersensitivity to trimethoprim or sulfonamides; megaloblastic anemia due to folate deficiency; pregnancy at term and lactation (see Warnings); infants < 2 months old.

The sulfonamides are chemically similar to some goitrogens, diuretics (acetazolamide and the thiazides) and oral hypoglycemic agents. Goiter production, diuresis and hypoglycemia occur rarely in patients receiving sulfonamides. Cross-sensitivity may exist with these agents.

Warnings

➤*Streptococcal pharyngitis:* Do not use to treat streptococcal pharyngitis. Patients with group A β-hemolytic streptococcal tonsillopharyngitis have a greater incidence of bacteriologic failure with this combination than with penicillin.

➤*Adverse reactions:* Sulfonamide-associated deaths, although rare, have occurred from hypersensitivity of the respiratory tract, Stevens-Johnson syndrome, toxic epidermal necrolysis, fulminant hepatic necrosis, agranulocytosis, aplastic anemia and other blood dyscrasias. Both TMP and SMZ can interfere with hematopoiesis. In elderly patients receiving diuretics (primarily thiazides), an increased incidence of thrombocytopenia with purpura occurred. Discontinue the drug at the first appearance of skin rash or any sign of adverse reaction. Rash, sore throat, fever, arthralgia, cough, shortness of breath, pallor, purpura or jaundice may be early indications of serious reactions. Obtain complete blood counts frequently. If significant reduction in the count of any formed blood element is noted, discontinue therapy.

IV use at high doses or for extended periods of time may cause bone marrow depression manifested as thrombocytopenia, leukopenia or megaloblastic anemia. If signs of bone marrow depression occur, give leucovorin as needed to restore normal hematopoiesis. Oral leucovorin, 5 to 15 mg/day has been recommended.

➤*Pneumocystis carinii pneumonitis in patients with AIDS:* Because of their unique immune dysfunction, AIDS patients may not tolerate or respond to TMP–SMZ. The incidence of side effects, particularly rash, fever, leukopenia, elevated aminotransferase values, hyperkalemia and hyponatremia in these patients is greatly increased compared with non-AIDS patients.

Adverse effects are generally less severe in patients receiving TMP-SMZ for prophylaxis. A history of mild intolerance to TMP-SMZ in AIDS patients does not appear to predict intolerance of subsequent secondary prophylaxis. However, if a patient develops skin rash or any sign of adverse reaction, re-evaluate therapy.

➤*Renal / Hepatic function impairment:* Use with caution. Maintain adequate fluid intake to prevent crystalluria and stone formation. Perform urinalyses and renal function tests during therapy, particularly in impaired renal function.

➤*Elderly:* There may be an increased risk of severe adverse reactions, particularly when complicating conditions exist (eg, impaired kidney or liver function, concomitant use of other drugs). Severe skin reactions, generalized bone marrow suppression or a decrease in platelets (with or without purpura) are the most frequently reported severe adverse reactions. In those concurrently receiving certain diuretics, primarily thiazides, an increased incidence of thrombocytopenia with purpura has occurred. Make appropriate dosage adjustments for impaired kidney function.

➤*Pregnancy: Category C.* Do not use at term. Sulfonamides readily cross the placenta. Fetal levels average 70% to 90% of maternal levels. Toxicities observed in the neonate include jaundice, hemolytic anemia and kernicterus. Trimethoprim crosses the placenta, producing similar levels in fetal and maternal serum. There are no large, well controlled studies; however, in one study of 186 pregnancies where the mother received either placebo or oral TMP–SMZ, the incidence of congenital abnormalities was 4.5% (3 of 66) in those who received placebo and 3.3% (4 of 120) in those receiving TMP–SMZ. There were no abnormalities in 10 children whose mothers received the drug during the first trimester or in 35 children whose mothers had taken the drug at conception or shortly thereafter.

Because TMP-SMZ may interfere with folic acid metabolism, use during pregnancy only if the potential benefits outweigh the potential hazards to the fetus.

➤*Lactation:* TMP–SMZ is not recommended in the nursing period because sulfonamides are excreted in breast milk and may cause kernicterus. Premature infants and infants with hyperbilirubinemia or G–6–PD deficiency are also at risk for adverse effects.

➤*Children:* Not recommended for infants < 2 months old. See Indications.

Precautions

➤*Extravascular infiltration:* If local irritation and inflammation due to extravascular infiltration of the infusion occurs, discontinue the infusion and restart at another site.

➤*Benzyl alcohol:* This is contained in some of these products as a preservative and has been associated with a fatal "gasping syndrome" in premature infants.

➤*Special risk:* Use with caution in patients with possible folate deficiency (eg, elderly patients, chronic alcoholics, anticonvulsant therapy, malabsorp-

TRIMETHOPRIM AND SULFAMETHOXAZOLE (Co-Trimoxazole; TMP-SMZ) — INJECTION

tion syndrome, patients in malnutrition states), severe allergy or bronchial asthma. In G-6-PD deficient individuals, hemolysis may occur; it is frequently dose-related.

➤*Superinfection:* Use of antibiotics (especially prolonged or repeated therapy) may result in bacterial or fungal overgrowth of nonsusceptible organisms. Such overgrowth may lead to a secondary infection. Take appropriate measures if this occurs.

➤*Sulfite sensitivity:* Sulfites may cause allergic-type reactions (eg, hives, itching, wheezing, anaphylaxis) in susceptible persons. Although the prevalence of sulfite sensitivity in the general population is probably low, it is more frequent in asthmatics or atopic nonasthmatic persons. Products containing sulfites are identified in the product listings.

Drug Interactions

TMP-SMZ Drug Interactions

Precipitant drug	Object drug*		Description
TMP-SMZ	Anticoagulants	↑	The prothrombin time of warfarin may be prolonged. Monitor coagulation tests and adjust dosage as required.
TMP-SMZ	Cyclosporine	↓	A decrease in the therapeutic effect of cyclosporine and an increased risk of nephrotoxicity have occurred.
TMP-SMZ	Dapsone	↑	Increased serum levels of both dapsone and TMP may occur.
Dapsone	TMP-SMZ	↑	
TMP-SMZ	Diuretics	↑	In elderly patients, concomitant use has increased incidence of thrombocytopenia with purpura.
TMP-SMZ	Hydantoins	↑	Phenytoin's hepatic clearance may be decreased and the half-life prolonged.
TMP-SMZ	Methotrexate	↑	Sulfonamides can displace methotrexate (MTX) from plasma protein binding sites, thus increasing free MTX concentrations; bone marrow depressant effects may be potentiated.
TMP-SMZ	Sulfonylureas	↑	The hypoglycemic response may be increased.
TMP-SMZ	Zidovudine	↑	The serum levels of zidovudine may be increased due to a decreased renal clearance.

* ↑ = Object drug increased. ↓ = Object drug decreased.

➤*Drug/Lab test interactions:* Trimethoprim can interfere with a serum methotrexate assay as determined by the competitive binding protein technique (CBPA) when a bacterial dihydrofolate reductase is used as the binding protein. No interference occurs if methotrexate is measured by a radioimmunoassay.

TMP-SMZ may interfere with the Jaffe alkaline picrate reaction assay for creatinine, resulting in overestimations of about 10% in the range of normal values.

Adverse Reactions

➤*Parenteral therapy:* Local reaction, pain and slight irritation on IV administration (infrequent); thrombophlebitis (rare).

➤*Most common:* GI disturbances (nausea, vomiting, anorexia); allergic skin reactions (eg, rash, urticaria).

➤*CNS:* Headache; mental depression; convulsions; ataxia; hallucinations; tinnitus; vertigo; insomnia; apathy; fatigue; weakness; nervousness; aseptic meningitis; peripheral neuritis.

➤*GI:* Glossitis; anorexia; stomatitis; nausea; emesis; abdominal pain; diarrhea; pseudomembranous enterocolitis; hepatitis (including cholestatic jaundice and hepatic necrosis); pancreatitis; elevation of serum transaminase and bilirubin.

➤*GU:* Renal failure; interstitial nephritis; BUN and serum creatinine elevation; toxic nephrosis with oliguria and anuria; crystalluria.

➤*Hematologic:* Agranulocytosis; aplastic, hemolytic or megaloblastic anemia; thrombocytopenia; leukopenia; neutropenia; hypoprothrombinemia; eosinophilia; methemoglobinemia; hyperkalemia; hyponatremia.

➤*Hypersensitivity:* Erythema multiforme; Stevens-Johnson syndrome; generalized skin eruptions; rash; toxic epidermal necrolysis; urticaria; serum sickness-like syndrome; pruritus; exfoliative dermatitis; anaphylactoid reactions; conjunctival and scleral injection; photosensitization; allergic myocarditis; angioedema; drug fever; chills; Henoch-Schoenlein purpura; systemic lupus erythematosus; generalized allergic reactions; periarteritis nodosa.

➤*Musculoskeletal:* Arthralgia; myalgia.

➤*Respiratory:* Pulmonary infiltrates.

Overdosage

➤*Symptoms:*

Acute – Signs and symptoms observed with either TMP or SMZ alone include: Anorexia; colic; nausea; vomiting; dizziness; headache; drowsiness; unconsciousness; pyrexia; hematuria; crystalluria; depression; confusion; blood dyscrasias and jaundice (late manifestations).

Chronic – High doses or use for extended periods may cause bone marrow depression manifested as thrombocytopenia, leukopenia or megaloblastic anemia. Give leucovorin; 5 to 15 mg/day has been recommended.

➤*Treatment:* Treatment includes usual supportive measures. Refer to General Management of Acute Overdosage. Perform gastric lavage or emesis, force oral fluids and administer IV fluids if urine output is low and renal function is normal. Acidifying urine will increase renal elimination of TMP. Monitor patient with blood counts and appropriate blood chemistries, including electrolytes. If significant blood dyscrasia or jaundice occurs, institute specific therapy for these complications. Peritoneal dialysis is not effective and hemodialysis is only moderately effective in eliminating TMP and SMZ.

Patient Information

Complete full course of therapy. Take each oral dose with a full glass of water.

Maintain adequate fluid intake.

Notify physician immediately if sore throat, fever, chills, pale skin, yellowing of skin or eyes, rash or unusual bleeding or bruising occurs.

ERYTHROMYCIN ETHYLSUCCINATE AND SULFISOXAZOLE

Rx	**Erythromycin and Sulfisoxasole** (Various, eg, Barr, Goldline, Harber, Lederle, Moore, Rugby, URL)	**Granules for Oral Suspension:** Erythromycin ethylsuccinate (equivalent to 200 mg erythromycin activity) and sulfisoxazole acetyl (equivalent to 600 mg sulfisoxazole) per 5 ml when reconstituted	In 100, 150 and 200 ml.
Rx	**Eryzole** (Alra)		Sucrose. Strawberry flavor. In 100, 150 and 200 ml.
Rx	**Pediazole** (Ross)		Sucrose. Strawberry-banana flavor. In 100, 150, 200 and 250 ml.

ERYTHROMYCIN ETHYLSUCCINATE AND SULFISOXAZOLE — ORAL

For complete and comparative information on each of the components, refer to Erythromycin and Sulfisoxazole individual monographs.

Indications

➤*Acute otitis media in children:* Acute otitis media caused by susceptible strains of *Haemophilus influenzae*.

Administration and Dosage

Do not administer to infants < 2 months old; systemic sulfonamides are contraindicated in this age group.

➤*Acute otitis media:* 50 mg/kg/day erythromycin and 150 mg/kg/day (to a maximum of 6 g/day), sulfisoxazole. Give in equally divided doses 4 times daily for 10 days. Administer without regard to meals.

Erythromycin/Sulfisoxazole Dosage Based on Weight

Weight		
kg	lb	Dose (every 6 hours)
< 8	< 18	Adjust dosage by body weight
8	18	2.5 ml
16	35	5 ml
24	53	7.5 ml
> 45	> 100	10 ml

ANTIFUNGAL AGENTS

FLUCYTOSINE (5-FC; 5-Fluorocytosine)

Rx	**Ancobon** (ICN)	**Capsules:** 250 mg	Talc, lactose, and parabens. (Ancobon 250 ICN). Green and gray. In 100s.
		500 mg	Talc, lactose, and parabens. (Ancobon 500 ICN). White and gray. In 100s.

FLUCYTOSINE (5-FC; 5-Fluorocytosine) — ORAL

WARNING

Use with extreme caution in patients with renal impairment. Close monitoring of hematologic, renal, and hepatic status of all patients is essential.

Indications

With the exception of urinary tract infection (UTI), use flucytosine in combination with amphotericin B for the treatment of systemic candidiasis and cryptococcosis because of rapid emergence of resistance to flucytosine in *Candida* and *Cryptococcus* isolates in patients receiving flucytosine alone.

➤*Candida:* Septicemia, endocarditis, and UTIs have been effectively treated. Limited trials in pulmonary infections justify the use of flucytosine.

➤*Cryptococcus:* For the treatment of meningitis and pulmonary infections. Good responses in septicemias and UTIs have occurred although studies are limited.

Administration and Dosage

The usual dosage is 50 to 150 mg/kg/day in divided doses at 6-hour intervals. To reduce or avoid nausea or vomiting, take capsules a few at a time over a 15-minute period.

➤*Renal function impairment:* Use a lower initial dose if BUN or serum creatinine is elevated, or if there are other signs of renal impairment (see Warnings).

➤*Storage/Stability:* Store at 25°C (77°F); excursions permitted to 15° to 30°C (59° to 86°F).

Actions

➤*Pharmacology:* Flucytosine has in vitro and in vivo activity against *Candida* and *Cryptococcus*. Although the exact mechanism is unknown, it has been reported that flucytosine acts directly on fungal organisms by competitive inhibition of purine and pyrimidine uptake and indirectly by intracellular metabolism to 5-fluorouracil. The 5-fluorouracil is extensively incorporated into fungal RNA and inhibits synthesis of DNA and RNA. The result is unbalanced growth and death of the fungal organism. It is rarely used alone; generally, it is used in combination with amphotericin B for synergistic antifungal activity (see Drug Interactions).

➤*Pharmacokinetics:*

Absorption/Distribution – Flucytosine is well absorbed after oral use with peak blood levels of 30 to 40 mcg/mL reached within 2 hours. After 5 days of continuous therapy, median peak levels in infants were 19.6, 27.7, and 83.9 mcg/mL at doses of 25, 50, and 100 mg/kg, respectively. Mean time to peak serum levels were approximately 2.5 hours, similar to that observed in adult patients. It is well distributed into aqueous humor and other body fluids and tissues; CSF concentrations are approximately 65% to 90% of serum levels. Bioavailability is 78% to 89%. Plasma protein binding is minimal. Toxicity occurs at blood levels higher than 100 mcg/mL.

Metabolism/Excretion – More than 90% of the dose is excreted unchanged in the urine by glomerular filtration; a small portion is found unchanged in the feces. Serum half-life is 2.4 and 4.8 hours in patients with normal renal function; half-life increases significantly, up to an average of 85 hours, in patients with renal failure. The median half-life observed in infants was 7.4 hours, approximately double that seen in adults. The drug is removed rapidly by hemodialysis.

➤*Microbiology:*

Fungal resistance –

Cryptococcus: Any isolate with an MIC greater than 12.5 mcg/mL is considered resistant. In vitro resistance has developed in originally susceptible strains during therapy. It is recommended that clinical cultures for susceptibility testing be taken initially and at weekly intervals during therapy. Reserve the initial culture as a reference in susceptibility testing of subsequent isolates.

Candida: As high as 40% to 50% of the pretreatment clinical isolates of *Candida* have been reported to be resistant to flucytosine. It is recommended that susceptibility studies be performed as early as possible and be repeated during therapy. An MIC value greater than 100 mcg/mL is considered resistant.

Contraindications

Hypersensitivity to flucytosine.

Warnings

➤*Bone marrow depression:* Give with extreme caution to patients with bone marrow depression. Patients may be more prone to bone marrow depression if they have a hematologic disease, are being treated with radiation or marrow-suppressant drugs, or have a history of treatment with such drugs or radiation. Bone marrow toxicity can be irreversible and may lead to death in immunosuppressed patients. Frequently monitor hepatic function and the hematopoietic system during therapy.

➤*Renal function impairment:* Give with extreme caution; drug accumulation may occur. Monitor blood levels to determine the adequacy of renal excretion in such patients. Adjust dosage to prevent progressive accumulation of the drug and to maintain the blood levels at less than 100 mcg/mL.

➤*Pregnancy: Category C.* Flucytosine is teratogenic in rats at 40 mg/kg/day. At higher doses (700 mg/kg/day) cleft lip and palate and micrognathia were reported. There are no adequate and well-controlled studies in pregnant women. Use only if the potential benefit justifies the potential risk to the fetus.

➤*Lactation:* It is not known whether this drug is excreted in breast milk. Because of potential serious adverse reactions in nursing infants, decide whether to discontinue nursing or the drug, taking into account the importance of the drug to mother.

➤*Children:* Safety and efficacy in children have not been established. Hypokalemia and acidemia were reported in one patient who received flucytosine in combination with amphotericin B, and anemia was observed in a second patient who received flucytosine alone. Transient thrombocytopenia was noted in 2 additional patients, one of whom also received amphotericin B.

Precautions

➤*Monitoring:* Before therapy is initiated, determine electrolytes and hematological and renal status of the patient (see Warnings). Because renal impairment can cause accumulation of the drug, monitor blood concentrations and renal function during therapy. Monitor hematologic status (WBC and platelet count) and liver function (alkaline phosphatase, ALT, and AST) at frequent intervals during treatment.

Drug Interactions

Drugs that impair glomerular filtration may prolong the half-life of flucytosine.

➤*Amphotericin B:* Amphotericin B may increase the therapeutic action and toxicity of flucytosine.

➤*Cytosine:* Cytosine may inactivate the antifungal activity of flucytosine.

➤*Drug/Lab test interactions:* Determine measurement of serum creatinine levels by the Jaffe reaction, because flucytosine does not interfere with the determination of creatinine values by this method.

Adverse Reactions

➤*Cardiovascular:* Cardiac arrest; myocardial toxicity; ventricular dysfunction.

➤*CNS:* Ataxia; confusion; convulsions; fatigue; hallucinations; headache; hearing loss; paresthesia; parkinsonism; peripheral neuropathy; psychosis; pyrexia; sedation; vertigo; weakness.

➤*Dermatologic:* Photosensitivity; pruritus; rash; urticaria.

➤*GI:* Abdominal pain; anorexia; bilirubin elevation; diarrhea; dry mouth; duodenal ulcer; emesis; GI hemorrhage; hepatic dysfunction; elevation of hepatic enzymes; acute hepatic injury with possible fatal outcome in debilitated patients; jaundice; nausea; ulcerative colitis.

➤*GU:* Azotemia; creatinine and BUN elevation; crystalluria; renal failure.

➤*Hematologic:* Agranulocytosis; aplastic anemia; anemia; eosinophilia; leukopenia; pancytopenia; thrombocytopenia.

➤*Respiratory:* Chest pain; dyspnea; respiratory arrest.

➤*Miscellaneous:* Allergic reactions; hypoglycemia; hypokalemia; Lyell syndrome.

Overdosage

➤*Symptoms:* There is no experience with intentional overdosage. It is reasonable to expect pronounced manifestations of known clinical adverse reactions. Prolonged serum concentration in excess of 100 mcg/mL may be associated with an increased incidence of toxicity, especially GI (diarrhea, nausea, vomiting), hematologic (leukopenia, thrombocytopenia), and hepatic (hepatitis).

➤*Treatment:* Prompt gastric lavage or emetic use is recommended. Maintain adequate fluid intake by IV route if necessary, because flucytosine is excreted unchanged in the renal tract. Hemodialysis rapidly reduced serum concentrations in anuric patients. Monitor hematologic parameters frequently, and monitor liver and kidney function. If any abnormalities appear in any of these parameters, institute appropriate therapeutic measures. Refer to General Management of Acute Overdosage.

Patient Information

May cause GI upset (eg, nausea, vomiting, diarrhea). Inform patient that this can be reduced or avoided by taking capsules a few at a time over a 15-minute period. Instruct patient to notify physician if effects become intolerable.

Inform patients that lab tests will be required while taking this medication and to be sure to keep appointments.

Advise patients that this drug may cause photosensitivity (sensitivity to sunlight). Advise them to avoid prolonged exposure to the sun and other ultraviolet light (eg, tanning beds) and to use sunscreens and wear protective clothing until tolerance is determined.

Indications

➤*Ringworm infections:* Treatment of ringworm infections of the skin, hair, and nails, namely the following: Tinea corporis, tinea pedis, tinea cruris, tinea barbae, tinea capitis, tinea unguium (onychomycosis) when caused by ≥ 1 of the following fungi: *Trichophyton rubrum, T. tonsurans, T. mentagrophytes, T. interdigitalis, T. verrucosum, T. megninii, T. gallinae, T. crateriform, T. sulphureum, T. schoenleinii, Microsporum audouinii, M. canis, M. gypseum,* and *Epidermophyton floccosum*.

➤*Note:* Prior to therapy, identify the types of fungi responsible for the infection. Use of this drug is not justified in minor or trivial infections that will respond to topical agents alone.

Griseofulvin is NOT effective in bacterial infections; candidiasis (moniliasis); histoplasmosis; actinomycosis; sporotrichosis; chromoblastomycosis; coccidioidomycosis; North American blastomycosis; cryptococcosis (torulosis); tinea versicolor; nocardiosis.

Administration and Dosage

Accurate diagnosis of the infecting organism is essential.

➤*Duration of therapy:* Continue medication until the infecting organism is completely eradicated, as indicated by appropriate clinical or laboratory examination. Representative treatment periods are as follows: Tinea capitis, 4 to 6 weeks; tinea corporis, 2 to 4 weeks; tinea pedis, 4 to 8 weeks; tinea unguium (depending on rate of growth) – fingernails, ≥ 4 months; toenails, ≥ 6 months.

➤*Hygiene:* Observe good hygiene to control sources of infection or reinfection. Concomitant use of appropriate topical agents is usually required, particularly in treatment of tinea pedis. In some forms of athlete's foot, yeasts and bacteria may be involved, as well as fungi. Griseofulvin will not eradicate the bacterial or monilial infection.

➤*Adults:*

Tinea corporis, tinea cruris, tinea capitis – A single or divided daily dose of 330 to 375 mg ultramicrosize will give a satisfactory response in most patients.

Tinea pedis, tinea unguium – 660 to 750 mg ultramicrosize per day in divided doses.

➤*Children:* Approximately 7.3 mg ultramicrosize/kg/day (3.3 mg/lb/day) is an effective dose for most children. The following dosage schedule is suggested:

Griseofulvin Dosage for Children Based on Weight

Weight		Daily dose (mg)
lb	kg	ultramicrosize
30 to 50	13.6 to 22.6	82.5 to 165
> 50	> 22.6	165 to 330

Clinical experience indicates that a single daily dose is effective in children with tinea capitis.

Children (≤ 2 years of age) – Dosage not established.

➤*Storage / Stability:*

Tablets – Store between 2° and 30°C (36° and 86°F).

Capsules – Store at room temperature, ≈ 25°C (77°F). Dispense in a well-closed container.

Oral suspension – Store at room temperature in a tight, light-resistant container.

Actions

➤*Pharmacology:* Griseofulvin, an antibiotic derived from a species of *Penicillium*, is deposited in the keratin precursor cells, which are gradually exfoliated and replaced by noninfected tissue; it has a greater affinity for diseased tissue. The drug is tightly bound to the new keratin, which becomes highly resistant to fungal invasions.

➤*Pharmacokinetics:* The peak serum level found in fasting adults given 0.5 g griseofulvin microsize occurred at ≈ 4 hours and ranged between 0.5 to 1.5 mcg/ml. Some individuals are consistently "poor absorbers" and tend to attain lower blood levels at all times. The serum level may be increased by giving the drug with a high-fat meal. GI absorption varies considerably among individuals because of insolubility of the drug in aqueous media of the upper GI tract. The efficiency of GI absorption of the ultramicrocrystalline formulation is ≈ 1.5 times that of conventional microsized griseofulvin. This factor permits the oral intake of ⅔ as much ultramicrocrystalline griseofulvin as the microsized form; however, there is no evidence this confers any significant clinical differences in regard to safety and efficacy.

➤*Microbiology:* Griseofulvin is fungistatic with in vitro activity against species of *Microsporum, Epidermophyton,* and *Trichophyton*. It has no effect on bacteria or other fungi.

Contraindications

Hypersensitivity to griseofulvin; porphyria; hepatocellular failure.

Warnings

➤*Prophylaxis:* Safety and efficacy for prophylaxis of fungal infections have not been established.

➤*Hypersensitivity reactions:* Hypersensitivity reactions (eg, skin rashes, urticaria, angioneurotic edema, erythema multiforme-like reactions) may occur and necessitate withdrawal of therapy. Institute appropriate countermeasures; refer to Management of Acute Hypersensitivity Reactions.

➤*Carcinogenesis:* Chronic feeding of griseofulvin to mice at levels ranging from 0.5% to 2.5% of the diet resulted in the development of liver tumors. Smaller particle sizes resulted in an enhanced effect. Thyroid tumors developed in male rats receiving griseofulvin at levels of 2%, 1%, and 0.2% of the diet.

In subacute toxicity studies, griseofulvin produced hepatocellular necrosis in mice, but not in other species. Griseofulvin produced disturbances in porphyrin metabolism, a colchicine-like effect on mitosis and cocarcinogenicity with methylcholanthrene in cutaneous tumor induction in laboratory animals.

➤*Fertility impairment:* Because griseofulvin has demonstrated harmful effects in vitro on the genotype bacteria, plants, and fungi, males should wait ≥ 6 months after completing therapy before fathering a child. Females should avoid risk of pregnancy while receiving griseofulvin.

➤*Pregnancy: Category C.* Griseofulvin was embryotoxic and teratogenic in rats. Rare cases of conjoined twins have been reported in patients taking griseofulvin during the first trimester of pregnancy. Do not give to pregnant women or women contemplating pregnancy.

Precautions

➤*Prolonged therapy:* Closely observe patients on prolonged therapy. Periodically monitor renal, hepatic, and hematopoietic function.

➤*Penicillin cross-sensitivity:* This is possible because griseofulvin is derived from species of *Penicillium*; however, known penicillin-sensitive patients have been treated without difficulty.

➤*Lupus erythematosus:* Lupus-like syndromes or exacerbation of lupus erythematosus have occurred in patients receiving griseofulvin.

➤*Photosensitivity:* Caution patients to take protective measures (eg, sunscreens, protective clothing) against exposure to ultraviolet light or sunlight.

Photosensitivity reactions may aggravate lupus erythematosus.

Drug Interactions

Griseofulvin Drug Interactions

Precipitant drug	Object drug*		Description
Griseofulvin	Anticoagulants	⬇	Griseofulvin may decrease the hypoprothrombinemic activity of warfarin; patients may require anticoagulant dosage adjustment.
Griseofulvin	Contraceptives, oral	⬇	Loss of contraceptive effectiveness may occur, possibly leading to breakthrough bleeding, amenorrhea, or unintended pregnancy.
Griseofulvin	Cyclosporine	⬇	Cyclosporine levels may be reduced, resulting in a decrease in pharmacologic effects.
Griseofulvin	Salicylates	⬇	Serum salicylate concentrations may be decreased.
Barbiturates	Griseofulvin	⬇	Serum griseofulvin levels may be decreased.

* ⬇ = Object drug decreased.

Adverse Reactions

➤*Most common:* Hypersensitivity reactions such as skin rashes and urticaria (see Warnings).

➤*Occasional:* Oral thrush; nausea; vomiting; epigastric distress; diarrhea; headache; fatigue; dizziness; insomnia; mental confusion; impairment of performance of routine activities.

➤*Rare:* Angioneurotic edema and erythema multiforme-like drug reactions may occur.

Griseofulvin interferes with porphyrin metabolism. Proteinuria; nephrosis; leukopenia; hepatic toxicity; GI bleeding; menstrual irregularities; paresthesias of the hands and feet after extended therapy have occurred. Discontinue administration if granulocytopenia occurs.

Rarely, serious reactions occur with griseofulvin. They are usually associated with high dosages, long periods of therapy, or both.

Patient Information

Beneficial effects may not be noticeable for some time; continue taking medication for entire course of therapy.

Photosensitivity reactions may occur; avoid prolonged exposure to sunlight or sunlamps.

Notify physician if fever, sore throat, or skin rash occurs.

Griseofulvin

GRISEOFULVIN MICROSIZE

Rx	**Grifulvin V** (Ortho)	**Tablets:** 500 mg	(ORTHO 214). White, scored. In 100s and 500s.
Rx	**Griseofulvin Microsize** (Glades)	**Oral suspension:** 125 mL per 5 mL	Orange-cream flavors. In 120 mL.[a]
Rx	**Grifulvin V** (Ortho)		In 120 mL.[a]

[a] With alcohol 0.2%, menthol, parabens, saccharin, sucrose.

GRISEOFULVIN MICROSIZE — ORAL

For complete and comparative prescribing information refer to the griseofulvin group monograph.

GRISEOFULVIN ULTRAMICROSIZE

Rx	**Gris-PEG** (Pedinol)	**Tablets:** 125 mg	Lactose, parabens. (Gris-PEG 125). White, elliptical, scored. Film-coated. In 100s.
		250 mg	Parabens. (Gris-PEG 250). White, capsule shape, scored. Film-coated. In 100s and 500s.

GRISEOFULVIN ULTRAMICROSIZE — ORAL

For complete and comparative prescribing information refer to the griseofulvin group monograph.

Polyene Antifungals

AMPHOTERICIN B DESOXYCHOLATE

Rx	**Amphotericin B** (Pharma-Tek)	**Powder for Injection:** 50 mg (as desoxycholate)	In vials.
Rx	**Amphocin** (Gensia Sicor)		In vials.
Rx	**Fungizone Intravenous** (Apothecon)		In vials.

AMPHOTERICIN B DESOXYCHOLATE — INJECTION

WARNING

This drug should be used primarily for treatment of patients with progressive and potentially life-threatening fungal infections; it should not be used to treat noninvasive forms of fungal disease such as oral thrush, vaginal candidiasis, and esophageal candidiasis in patients with normal neutrophil counts.

Exercise caution to prevent inadvertent overdose with amphotericin B. Verify the product name and dosage if dose exceeds 1.5 mg/kg.

Indications

➤*Life-threatening fungal infections:* Amphotericin B for injection, USP should be administered primarily to patients with progressive, potentially life-threatening fungal infections. This potent drug should not be used to treat noninvasive fungal infections, such as oral thrush, vaginal candidiasis and esophageal candidiasis in patients with normal neutrophil counts.

Amphotericin B for injection is specifically intended to treat potentially life-threatening fungal infections: Aspergillosis, cryptococcosis (torulosis), North American blastomycosis, systemic candidiasis, coccidioidomycosis, histoplasmosis, zygomycosis including mucormycosis due to susceptible species of the genera *Absidia*, *Mucor* and *Rhizopus*, and infections due to related susceptible species of *Conidiobolus* and *Basidiobolus*, and sporotrichosis.

➤*Leishmaniasis:* Amphotericin B may be useful in the treatment of American mucocutaneous leishmaniasis, but it is not the drug of choice as primary therapy.

➤*Unlabeled uses:* Prophylaxis of fungal infection in patients with bone marrow transplantation (0.1 mg/kg/day); for the treatment of primary amoebic meningoencephalitis caused by *Naegleria fowleri*; subconjunctival or intravitreal injection in ocular aspergillosis; as a bladder irrigation for candidal cystitis; as chemoprophylaxis by low-dose IV, intranasal, or nebulized administration in immunocompromised patients at risk of *aspergillosis*; intrathecally for patients with severe meningitis unresponsive to IV therapy; intra-articularly or IM for coccidioidal arthritis.

Administration and Dosage

➤*Approved by the FDA:* April 29, 1992.

➤*Maximum dose:* Under no circumstances should a total daily dose of 1.5 mg/kg be exceeded. Amphotericin B overdoses can result in cardiorespiratory arrest (see Overdosage).

➤*IV:* Amphotericin B for injection should be administered by slow IV infusion. IV infusion should be given over a period of ≈ 2 to 6 hours (depending on the dose) observing the usual precautions for IV therapy (see Precautions). The recommended concentration for IV infusion is 0.1 mg/mL (1 mg/10 mL).

Since patient tolerance varies greatly, the dosage of amphotericin B must be individualized and adjusted according to the patient's clinical status (eg, site and severity of infection, etiologic agent, cardio-renal function).

➤*Test dose:* A single IV test dose (1 mg in 20 mL of 5% dextrose solution) administered over 20 to 30 minutes may be preferred. The patient's temperature, pulse, respiration, and blood pressure should be recorded every 30 minutes for 2 to 4 hours.

➤*Dosage:* In patients with good cardio-renal function and a well-tolerated test dose, therapy is usually initiated with a daily dose of 0.25 mg/kg of body weight. However, in those patients having severe and rapidly progressive fungal infection, therapy may be initiated with a daily dose of 0.3 mg/kg of body weight. In patients with impaired cardio-renal function or a severe reaction to the test dose, therapy should be initiated with smaller daily doses (ie, 5 to 10 mg).

Depending on the patient's cardio-renal status (see Precautions), doses may gradually be increased by 5 to 10 mg/day to final daily dosage of 0.5 to 0.7 mg/kg.

There are insufficient data presently available to define total dosage requirements and duration of treatment necessary for eradication of specific mycoses. The optimal dose is unknown. Total daily dosage may range up to 1 mg/kg/day or up to 1.5 mg/kg when given on alternate days.

➤*Sporotrichosis:* Therapy with IV amphotericin B for sporotrichosis has ranged up to 9 months with a total dose up to 2.5 g.

➤*Aspergillosis:* Aspergillosis has been treated with amphotericin B intravenously for a period up to 11 months with a total dose up to 3.6 g.

➤*Rhinocerebral phycomycosis:* This fulminating disease, generally occurs in association with diabetic ketoacidosis. It is, therefore, imperative that diabetic control be restored in order for treatment with amphotericin B for injection to be successful. In contradistinction, pulmonary phycomycosis, which is more common in association with hematologic malignancies, is often an incidental finding at autopsy. A cumulative dose of at least 3 g of amphotericin B is recommended to treat rhinocerebral phycomycosis. Although a total dose of 3 to 4 g will infrequently cause lasting renal impairment, this would seem a reasonable minimum where there is clinical evidence of invasion of deep tissue. Since rhinocerebral phycomycosis usually follows a rapidly fatal course, the therapeutic approach must necessarily be more aggressive than that used in more indolent mycoses.

➤*Preparation of solutions:* Reconstitute as follows: An initial concentrate of 5 mg amphotericin B per mL is first prepared by rapidly expressing 10 mL Sterile Water for Injection, USP without a bacteriostatic agent directly into the lyophilized cake, using a sterile needle (minimum diameter, 20 gauge) and syringe. Shake the vial immediately until the colloidal solution is clear. The infusion solution, providing 0.1 mg amphotericin B per mL, is then obtained by further dilution (1:50) with 5% Dextrose Injection, USP of pH > 4.2. The pH of each container of Dextrose Injection should be ascertained before use. Commercial dextrose injection usually has a pH > 4.2; however, if it is < 4.2, then 1 or 2 mL of buffer should be added to the dextrose injection before it is used to dilute the concentrated solution of amphotericin B. The recommended buffer has the following composition:

- Dibasic sodium phosphate (anhydrous) equals 1.59 g
- Monobasic sodium phosphate (anhydrous) equals 0.96 g
- Water for Injection, USP equals qs 100 mL
- The buffer should be sterilized before it is added to the Dextrose Injection, either by filtration through a bacterial retentive stone, mat, or membrane, or by autoclaving for 30 minutes at 15 lb pressure (≈ 121°C; 249.8°F).

Do not use the initial concentrate or the infusion solution if there is any evidence of precipitation or foreign matter in either one.

An inline membrane filter may be used for IV infusion of amphotericin B; however, the mean pore diameter of the filter should not be less than 1 micron in order to ensure passage of the antibiotic dispersion.

➤*Storage/Stability:* Prior to reconstitution, amphotericin B for injection should be stored in the refrigerator, protected against exposure to light. The concentrate (5 mg amphotericin B per mL after reconstitution with 10 mL Sterile Water for Injection, USP) may be stored in the dark, at room temperature for 24 hours, or at refrigerator temperatures for 1 week with minimal loss of potency and clarity. Any unused material should then be discarded. Solutions prepared for IV infusion (≤ 0.1 mg amphotericin B per

AMPHOTERICIN B DESOXYCHOLATE — INJECTION

mL) should be used promptly after preparation and should be protected from light during administration.

Actions

➤*Pharmacology:* Amphotericin B is fungistatic or fungicidal depending on the concentration obtained in body fluids and the susceptibility of the fungus. The drug acts by binding to sterols in the cell membrane of susceptible fungi with a resultant change in membrane permeability allowing leakage of intracellular components. Mammalian cell membranes also contain sterols and it has been suggested that the damage to human cells and fungal cells may share common mechanisms.

➤*Pharmacokinetics:* An initial IV infusion of 1 to 5 mg of amphotericin B per day, gradually increased to 0.4 to 0.6 mg/kg/day, produces peak plasma concentrations ranging from ≈ 0.5 to 2 mcg/mL. Following a rapid initial fall, plasma concentrations plateau at ≈ 0.5 mcg/mL. An elimination half-life of ≈ 15 days follows an initial plasma half-life of ≈ 24 hours. Amphotericin B circulating in plasma is highly bound (> 90%) to plasma proteins and is poorly dialyzable. Approximately two-thirds of concurrent plasma concentrations have been detected in fluids from inflamed pleura, peritoneum, synovium, and aqueous humor. Concentrations in the cerebrospinal fluid seldom exceed 2.5% of those in the plasma. Little amphotericin B penetrates into vitreous humor or normal amniotic fluid. Complete details of tissue distribution are not known.

Amphotericin B is excreted very slowly (over weeks to months) by the kidneys with 2% to 5% of a given dose being excreted in the biologically active form. Details of possible metabolic pathways are not known. After treatment is discontinued, the drug can be detected in the urine for at least 7 weeks due to the slow disappearance of the drug. The cumulative urinary output over a 7-day period amounts to ≈ 40% of the amount of drug infused.

➤*Microbiology:* Amphotericin B shows a high order of in vitro activity against many species of fungi. *Histoplasma capsulatum*, *Coccidioides immitis*, *Candida* species, *Blastomyces dermatitidis*, *Rhodotorula*, *Cryptococcus neoformans*, *Sporothrix schenckii*, *Mucor mucedo*, and *Aspergillus fumigatus* are all inhibited by concentrations of amphotericin B ranging from 0.03 to 1 mcg/mL in vitro. While *Candida albicans* is generally quite susceptible to amphotericin B, non*albicans* species may be less susceptible. *Pseudallescheria boydii* and *Fusarium* sp. are often resistant to amphotericin B. The antibiotic is without effect on bacteria, rickettsiae, and viruses.

Contraindications

This product is contraindicated in patients who have shown hypersensitivity to amphotericin B or any other component in the formulation unless, in the opinion of the physician, the condition requiring treatment is life-threatening and amenable only to amphotericin B therapy.

Warnings

➤*Life-threatening fungal disease:* Amphotericin B is frequently the only effective treatment available for potentially life-threatening fungal disease. In each case, its possible lifesaving benefit must be balanced against its untoward and dangerous side effects.

➤*Renal function impairment:* Amphotericin B should be used with care in patients with reduced renal function; frequent monitoring of renal function is recommended (see Precautions and Adverse Reactions). In some patients, hydration and sodium repletion prior to amphotericin B administration may reduce the risk of developing nephrotoxicity. Supplemental alkali medication may decrease renal tubular acidosis complications.

➤*Pregnancy: Category B.*

Reproduction studies in animals have revealed no evidence of harm to the fetus due to amphotericin B for injection. Systemic fungal infections have been successfully treated in pregnant women with amphotericin B for injection without obvious effects to the fetus, but the number of cases reported has been small. Because animal reproduction studies are not always predictive of human response, and adequate and well-controlled studies have not been conducted in pregnant women, this drug should be used during pregnancy only if clearly indicated.

➤*Lactation:* It is not known whether amphotericin B is excreted in human milk. Because many drugs are excreted in human milk and considering the potential toxicity of amphotericin B, it is prudent to advise a nursing mother to discontinue nursing.

➤*Children:* Safety and efficacy in children have not been established through adequate and well-controlled studies. Systemic fungal infections have been successfully treated in children without reports of unusual side effects. Amphotericin B for injection, when administered to children, should be limited to the smallest dose compatible with an effective therapeutic regimen.

Precautions

➤*Monitoring:* Renal function should be monitored frequently during amphotericin B therapy (see Warnings and Adverse Reactions). It is also advisable to monitor on a regular basis liver function, serum electrolytes (particularly magnesium and potassium), blood counts, and hemoglobin concentrations. Laboratory test results should be used as a guide to subsequent dosage adjustments.

➤*Administration:* Administer IV under close clinical observation by medically trained personnel. It should be reserved for treatment of patients with progressive, potentially life-threatening fungal infections due to susceptible organisms (see Indications).

➤*Infusion reactions:* Acute reactions including fever, shaking chills, hypotension, anorexia, nausea, vomiting, headache, and tachypnea are common 1 to 3 hours after starting an IV infusion. These reactions are usually more severe with the first few doses of amphotericin B and usually diminish with subsequent doses.

Rapid IV infusion has been associated with hypotension, hypokalemia, arrhythmias, and shock and should, therefore, be avoided (see Administration and Dosage).

➤*Leukocyte transfusions:* Since acute pulmonary reactions have been reported in patients given amphotericin B during or shortly after leukocyte transfusions, it is advisable to temporarily separate these infusions as far as possible and to monitor pulmonary function (see Drug Interactions).

➤*Leukoencephalopathy:* Leukoencephalopathy has been reported following use of amphotericin B. Literature reports have suggested that total body irradiation may be a predisposition.

➤*Therapy interruption:* Whenever medication is interrupted for a period of > 7 days, therapy should be resumed by starting with the lowest dosage level (eg, 0.25 mg/kg of body weight) and increased gradually as outlined under Administration and Dosage.

➤*Lab test abnormalities:* Serum electrolytes, liver function tests, renal function tests, and other test abnormalities have been reported including the following: Hypomagnesemia, hypo- and hyperkalemia, hypocalcemia; elevations of AST, ALT, GGT, bilirubin, and alkaline phosphatase; elevations of BUN and serum creatinine.

Drug Interactions

Amphotericin B Drug Interactions

Precipitant drug	Object drug*		Description
Antineoplastic agents	Amphotericin B	↑	Concurrent administration may enhance the potential for renal toxicity, bronchospasm, and hypotension.
Azole antifungals	Amphotericin B	↓	In vitro animal studies suggest that imidazoles may induce fungal resistance to amphotericin B. Administer with caution, especially in immunocompromised patients.
Corticosteroids and corticotropin	Amphotericin B	↑	Concurrent administration may potentiate hypokalemia and predispose patients to cardiac dysfunction. Do not give unless necessary to control adverse reactions.
Zidovudine	Amphotericin B	↑	Increases in myelotoxicity and nephrotoxicity were observed in dogs administered zidovudine concomitantly with amphotericin B desoxycholate.
Amphotericin B	Cyclosporine	↑	The risk of renal toxicity is increased with concomitant administration. Severe muscle tremors were reported in 1 patient.
Cyclosporine	Amphotericin B		
Amphotericin B	Digitalis glycosides	↑	Concurrent administration may induce hypokalemia and may potentiate digitalis toxicity.
Amphotericin B	Flucytosine	↑	A synergistic relationship with amphotericin B has been reported. Flucytosine toxicity may be increased by increasing its cellular uptake or impairing renal excretion.
Amphotericin B	Nephrotoxic agents	↑	Concomitant administration may enhance risk of drug-induced renal toxicity. Use caution when administering concomitantly. Monitor renal function intensively.
Nephrotoxic agents	Amphotericin B		
Amphotericin B	Skeletal muscle relaxants	↑	Amphotericin B-induced hypokalemia may enhance the curariform effect of skeletal muscle relaxants. Monitor serum potassium levels closely.
Amphotericin B	Thiazides	↑	Electrolyte depletion may be intensified, particularly hypokalemia. Monitor potassium levels.

* ↑ = Object drug increased. ↓ = Object drug decreased.

Adverse Reactions

➤*Prevention of adverse reactions:* Although some patients may tolerate full IV doses of amphotericin B without difficulty, most will exhibit some intolerance, often at less than the full therapeutic dose.

Tolerance may be improved by treatment with aspirin, antipyretics (eg, acetaminophen), antihistamines, or antiemetics. Meperidine (25 to 50 mg IV)

AMPHOTERICIN B DESOXYCHOLATE — INJECTION

has been shown in some patients to decrease the duration of shaking chills, and fever that may accompany the infusion of amphotericin B.

Administration of amphotericin B on alternate days may decrease anorexia and phlebitis.

IV administration of small doses of adrenal corticosteroids just prior to or during the amphotericin B infusion may help decrease febrile reactions. Dosage and duration of such corticosteroid therapy should be kept to a minimum (see Drug Interactions).

Addition of heparin (1000 units per infusion) and the use of pediatric scalp-vein needle may lessen the incidence of thrombophlebitis. Extravasation may cause chemical irritation.

➤*Most common adverse reactions:*

CNS – Headache.

GI – Anorexia; nausea; vomiting; diarrhea; dyspepsia; cramping; epigastric pain.

Hematologic – Normochromic; normocytic anemia.

Local – Pain at the injection site with or without phlebitis or thrombophlebitis.

Musculoskeletal – Generalized pain, including muscle and joint pains.

Pulmonary – Hypotension; tachypnea.

Renal – Decreased renal function and renal function abnormalities including azotemia, hypokalemia, hyposthenuria, renal tubular acidosis, and nephrocalcinosis. These usually improve with interruption of therapy. However, some permanent impairment often occurs, especially in those patients receiving large amounts (> 5 g) of amphotericin B or receiving other nephrotoxic agents. In some patients hydration and sodium repletion prior to amphotericin B administration may reduce the risk of developing nephrotoxicity. Supplemental alkali medication may decrease renal tubular acidosis.

Miscellaneous – Fever (sometimes accompanied by shaking chills usually occurring within 15 to 20 minutes after initiation of treatment); malaise; weight loss.

➤*Other adverse reactions:*

Allergic – Anaphylactoid and other allergic reactions; bronchospasm; wheezing.

CNS – Convulsions; hearing loss; tinnitus; transient vertigo; visual impairment; diplopia; peripheral neuropathy; encephalopathy (see Precautions); other neurologic symptoms.

Dermatologic – Rash, in particular maculopapular; pruritus.

GI – Acute liver failure; hepatitis; jaundice; hemorrhagic gastroenteritis; melena.

Hematologic – Agranulocytosis; coagulation defects; thrombocytopenia; leukopenia; eosinophilia; leukocytosis.

Lab test abnormalities –

Serum electrolytes: Hypomagnesemia; hypo- and hyperkalemia; hypocalcemia.

Liver function tests: Elevations of AST, ALT, GGT, bilirubin, and alkaline phosphatase.

Renal function tests: Elevations of BUN and serum creatinine.

Cardiopulmonary – Cardiac arrest; shock; cardiac failure; pulmonary edema; hypersensitivity pneumonitis; arrhythmias, including ventricular fibrillation; dyspnea; hypertension.

Renal – Acute renal failure; anuria; oliguria.

Miscellaneous – Flushing.

Overdosage

➤*Symptoms:* Amphotericin B overdoses can result in cardiorespiratory arrest.

➤*Treatment:* If an overdose is suspected, discontinue therapy and monitor the patient's clinical status (eg, cardiorespiratory, renal, and liver function, hematologic status, serum electrolytes) and administer supportive therapy, as required. Amphotericin B is not hemodialyzable.

Prior to reinstituting therapy, the patient's condition should be stabilized (including correction of electrolyte deficiencies).

AMPHOTERICIN B, LIPID-BASED

Rx	**Abelcet** (Enzon)	**Suspension for Injection**: 100 mg/20 ml (as lipid complex)	In 10 and 20 ml single-use vials with 5-micron filter needles.
Rx	**Amphotec** (Sequus Pharmaceuticals)	**Powder for Injection**: 50 mg (as cholesteryl)	In 20 ml single-use vials.
		100 mg (as cholesteryl)	In 50 ml single-use vials.
Rx	**AmBisome** (Fujisawa)	**Powder for Injection**: 50 mg (as liposomal)	Sucrose. In single-dose vials with 5-micron filter.

AMPHOTERICIN B LIPID COMPLEX — INJECTION

WARNING

Use primarily for treatment of patients with progressive and potentially fatal fungal infections. Do not use to treat noninvasive forms of fungal disease such as oral thrush, vaginal candidiasis, and esophageal candidiasis in patients with normal neutrophil counts.

Indications

➤*Fungal infections, systemic:* For use in patients refractory to conventional amphotericin B desoxycholate therapy or when renal impairment or unacceptable toxicity precludes the use of the desoxycholate formulation for the treatment of invasive fungal infections (lipid complex); for the treatment of invasive aspergillosis (cholesteryl); for the treatment of infections caused by *Aspergillus*, *Candida*, or *Cryptococcus* sp. (liposomal).

➤*Fungal infections, empirical:* For empirical treatment in febrile, neutropenic patients with presumed fungal infection (*AmBisome* only).

➤*Cryptococcal meningitis in HIV:* Treatment of cryptococcal meningitis in HIV-infected patients (*AmBisome* only).

➤*Leishmaniasis:* For treatment of visceral leishmaniasis (*AmBisome* only).

➤*Unlabeled uses:* Prophylaxis of fungal infection in patients with bone marrow transplantation (0.1 mg/kg/day); for the treatment of primary amoebic meningoencephalitis caused by *Naegleria fowleri*; subconjunctival or intravitreal injection in ocular aspergillosis; as a bladder irrigation for candidal cystitis ; as chemoprophylaxis by low-dose IV, intranasal, or nebulized administration in immunocompromised patients at risk of aspergillosis; intra-articularly or IM for coccidioidal arthritis.

Administration and Dosage

Individualize and adjust dosage based on patient's clinical status (eg, cardiorenal function, reaction to test dose, site, and severity of infection). If administered through an existing IV line, flush with 5% Dextrose for Injection prior to and following infusion; otherwise administer via a separate line.

➤*Fungal infection, empirical:* Administer 3 mg/kg/day of liposomal amphotericin B for empirical fungal infections using a controlled infusion device over ≈ 120 minutes; infusion time may be reduced to 60 minutes if well tolerated or increased if patient experiences discomfort.

➤*Fungal infection, systemic:*

Abelcet – The recommended dose is 5 mg/kg/day prepared as a 1 mg/ml infusion and delivered at a rate of 2.5 mg/kg/hour. For pediatric patients and patients with cardiovascular disease, the drug may be diluted to a final concentration of 2 mg/ml. If the infusion exceeds 2 hours, mix the contents by shaking the infusion bag every 2 hours. Do not use an in-line filter.

Amphotec – A test dose is advisable (eg, 10 ml of final preparation containing 1.6 to 8.3 mg infused over 15 to 30 min). The recommended dose is 3 to 4 mg/kg/day prepared as a 0.6 mg/ml (range, 0.16 to 0.83 mg/ml) infusion delivered at a rate of 1 mg/kg/hr. Do not filter or use an in-line filter.

AmBisome – The recommended dose is 3 to 5 mg/kg/day prepared as a 1 to 2 mg/ml infusion delivered initially over 120 minutes; infusion time may be reduced to 60 minutes if well tolerated or increased if patient experiences discomfort. Lower infusion concentrations of 0.2 to 0.5 mg/ml may be appropriate for infants and small children to provide sufficient volume for infusion. An in-line membrane filter of ≥ 1 micron mean pore diameter may be used.

➤*Cryptococcal meningitis in HIV:*

AmBisome – Administer 6 mg/kg/day using a controlled infusion device over ≈ 120 minutes; infusion time may be reduced to 60 minutes if well tolerated or increased if patient experiences discomfort.

➤*Leishmaniasis:*

AmBisome – Administer 3 mg/kg/day on days 1 through 5, 14, and 21 to immunocompetent patients; a repeat course of therapy may be useful if parasitic clearance is not achieved. Administer 4 mg/kg/day on days 1 through 5, 10, 17, 24, 31, and 38 to immunosuppressed patients; seek expert advice regarding further therapy if parasitic clearance is not achieved.

➤*Unlabeled uses:*

Cystitis, candidal – Irrigate bladder with a 50 mcg/ml solution, instilled periodically or continuously for 5 to 10 days.

Paracoccidioidomycosis – Administer 0.4 to 0.5 mg/kg/day slow IV infusion; treat for 4 to 12 weeks.

➤*Preparation of infusion solutions:* Do not dilute or reconstitute with saline solutions or mix with other drugs or electrolytes. The use of any solution other than those recommended or the presence of a bacteriostatic agent (eg, benzyl alcohol) may cause precipitation of amphotericin B.

Abelcet – Shake the vial gently until there is no yellow sediment at the bottom. Withdraw the appropriate dose from the required number of vials into ≥ 1 sterile 20 ml syringes using an 18-gauge needle. Remove the needle from each syringe and replace with a 5-micron filter needle. Each filter needle may be used to filter the content of up to 4 vials. Insert the filter needle of the syringe into an IV bag containing 5% Dextrose for Injection, and empty the contents of the syringe into the bag for a final concentration of 1 mg/ml (2 mg/ml for pediatric and cardiovascular patients).

AMPHOTERICIN B LIPID COMPLEX — INJECTION

Amphotec – Reconstitute with Sterile Water for Injection. Do not use saline or dextrose for reconstitution. Using a sterile syringe and a 20-gauge needle, rapidly add the following volumes to the vial to provide a liquid containing 5 mg/ml. Shake gently by hand, rotating the vial until all solids have dissolved. Note that the fluid may be opalescent or clear. For 50 mg/vial add 10 ml Sterile Water for Injection; for the 100 mg/vial add 20 ml Sterile Water for Injection.

For infusion, further dilute the reconstituted liquid to a final concentration of ≈ 0.6 mg/ml (range, 0.16 to 0.83 mg/ml).

AmBisome – Add 12 ml of Sterile Water for Injection to each vial to yield 4 mg/ml. Immediately shake the vial vigorously for 30 seconds to completely disperse the drug until a yellow, translucent suspension is formed. Calculate total dose needed, withdraw appropriate amount of reconstituted solution into sterile syringe, attach the 5-micron filter provided, and inject contents of syringe through filter needle into an appropriate volume of 5% Dextrose (use only 1 filter needle per vial) to yield a final concentration of 1 to 2 mg/ml. Concentrations of 0.2 to 0.5 mg/ml may be more appropriate for infants and small children.

➤*Admixture incompatibility:* Do not dilute or reconstitute with saline solutions or mix with other drugs or electrolytes. The use of any solution other than those recommended or the presence of a bacteriostatic agent (eg, benzyl alcohol) may cause precipitation of amphotericin B. If administered through an existing IV line, flush with 5% Dextrose for Injection prior to and following infusion; otherwise administer via a separate line.

➤*Storage / Stability:*

Abelcet – Prior to admixture, store at 2° to 8°C (36° to 46°F). Protect from exposure to light. Do not freeze. Retain in the carton until time of use. The admixture may be stored for ≤ 48 hours at 2° to 8°C (36° to 46°F) and an additional 6 hours at room temperature.

Amphotec – Store unopened vials at 15° to 30°C (59° to 86°F). After reconstitution, refrigerate at 2° to 8°C (36° to 46°F), and use within 24 hours. Do not freeze. After further dilution with 5% Dextrose for Injection, refrigerate (2° to 8°C; 36° to 46°F), and use within 24 hours.

AmBisome – Refrigerate unopened vials at 2° to 8°C (36° to 46°F). Store reconstituted product concentrate at 2° to 8°C for ≤ 24 hours. Do not freeze. Use within 6 hours of dilution with 5% Dextrose.

Actions

➤*Pharmacology:* Amphotericin B is a polyene antibiotic produced by a strain of *Streptomyces nodosus* that is fungistatic or fungicidal, depending on the concentration obtained in body fluids and on the susceptibility of the fungus. It acts by binding to sterols (primarily ergosterol) in the fungal cell membrane with a resultant change in membrane permeability, allowing leakage of a variety of intracellular components. It can also bind to the cholesterol component of the mammalian cell, leading to cytotoxicity.

Liposomal encapsulation or incorporation in a lipid complex can substantially affect a drug's functional properties relative to those of the unencapsulated or nonlipid-associated drug. Lipid-based formulations increase the circulation time and alter the biodistribution of the associated amphotericin. Because drugs complexed with lipid vehicles have a longer residence time in the vasculature, they are able to localize and reach greater concentrations in regions with increased capillary permeability (eg, solid tumors, infection, inflammation) compared with regions of normal tissue, which are essentially impermeable to lipid-complexed drugs. This opportunistic method of increasing the localization of drugs to diseased sites is referred to as passive targeting and allows drug levels to be increased several times higher than those allowable with the free drug. Increasing drug levels at the site of action and reducing levels in normal tissues offers 2 distinct clinical advantages: An increased therapeutic index and an altered toxicity profile relative to the free drug.

In addition, different lipid-based formulations with a common active ingredient may vary from one another in the chemical composition (eg, phospholipid and cholesterol content) and physical form of the lipid component (eg, sphere, disc, ribbon). Such differences may affect functional properties of these drug products.

➤*Pharmacokinetics:*

Lipid-based formulations – The pharmacokinetics of lipid-based amphotericin B products are nonlinear. Steady-state volume of distribution (Vss) and total plasma clearance (CL) increase with escalating doses, resulting in less than proportional increases in plasma concentration over a given dose range.

The increased volume of distribution probably reflects uptake by tissues. The long terminal elimination half-life for the cholesteryl (*Amphotec*), lipid complex (*Abelcet*), and liposomal (*AmBisome*) formulations probably reflects a slow redistribution from tissues. Mean trough levels for each of these formulations remain relatively constant with repeated dosing, indicating little accumulation in plasma. The following table presents pharmacokinetic parameters at steady state for lipid-based formulations of amphotericin B; the assay used to measure serum levels did not distinguish between free and complexed amphotericin B.

Pharmacokinetic Parameters of Lipid-Based Amphotericin B Formulations[1]

Parameter	*AmBisome* 1 mg/kg/day (n = 7)	*AmBisome* 2.5 mg/kg/day (n = 7)	*AmBisome* 5 mg/kg/day (n = 9)	*Amphotec* 3 mg/kg/day (predicted)[2]	*Amphotec* 4 mg/kg/day (predicted)[2]	*Abelcet* 5 mg/kg/day (n = varied)[3]
C_{max} (mcg/ml)	≈ 12.2	≈ 31.4	≈ 83	2.6	2.9	≈ 1.7
AUC (mcg/ml•hr)	≈ 60	≈ 197	≈ 555	29	36	≈ 14
$t_{1/2}$ (hours)	≈ 7	≈ 6.3	≈ 6.8	27.5 (100 to 153)[4]	28.2 (100 to 153)[4]	≈ 173.4
Vss (L/kg)	≈ 0.14	≈ 0.16	≈ 0.1	3.8	4.1	≈ 131
CL (ml/hr/kg)	≈ 17	≈ 22	≈ 11	105	112	≈ 436

[1] Data are pooled from separate studies and are not necessarily comparable.
[2] Values based on the population model developed from 51 bone marrow transplant patients with systemic fungal infections given *Amphotec* 0.5 to 8 mg/kg/day.
[3] Data obtained from various studies in patients with mucocutaneous leishmaniasis or cancer with presumed or proven fungal infections.
[4] Based on total amphotericin B levels measured within a 24-hour dosing interval (for up to 49 days after dosing).

Following a 1 mg/kg/hour infusion, ≈ 25% of the total amphotericin B concentration measured in plasma was in the amphotericin B cholesteryl complex, dropping to ≈ 9.3% at 1 hour and ≈ 7.5% at 24 hours after the end of the infusion.

Children – In a small study of 12 children 4 months to 14 years of age infused with 0.25 to 1.5 mg/kg/day of amphotericin B, plasma levels ranged from 0.78 to 10.02 mcg/ml and were independent of dose. The mean elimination half-life was 18.1 hours. An inverse relationship between age and total clearance was observed indicating that children > 9 years of age may require lower doses.

➤*Microbiology: Abelcet* is active in animal models against *Aspergillus fumigatus, Candida albicans, C. guillermondi, C. stellatoideae , C. tropicalis, Cryptococcus* sp., *Coccidioidomyces* sp., *Histoplasma* sp., and *Blastomyces* sp.

Amphotec is active in vitro against *Aspergillus, Candida* sp., and other fungi. In animal models, it has shown additional activity against *Coccidioides immitis, Cryptococcus neoformans,* and *Leishmania* sp.

AmBisome has shown in vitro activity against *Aspergillus* sp. (*A. fumigatus , A. flavus*), *Candida* sp. (*C. albicans, C. krusei, C. lusitaniae, C. parapsilosis, C. tropicalis*), *Cryptococcus neoformans*, and *Blastomyces dermatitidis*. In animal models, it has shown additional activity against *Coccidioides immitis, Histoplasma capsulatum, Paracoccidioides brasiliensis, Leishmania donovani*, and *Leishmania infantum*.

Contraindications

Hypersensitivity to amphotericin B or any other component of the formulation unless the condition requiring treatment is life-threatening and amenable only to amphotericin B therapy.

Warnings

➤*Fatal fungal diseases:* Amphotericin B is frequently the only effective treatment for potentially fatal fungal diseases. Balance its possible lifesaving effect against its dangerous side effects.

➤*Nephrotoxicity:* Lipid formulations of amphotericin B reduced the severe kidney toxicity of amphotericin B and are indicated in patients with renal impairment or when unacceptable toxicity precludes use of amphotericin B desoxycholate in effective doses.

In a randomized, double-blind study of amphotericin B cholesteryl (*Amphotec* 4 mg/kg/day) and amphotericin B desoxycholate (0.8 mg/kg/day) as empiric treatment in febrile neutropenic patients, it was demonstrated that in patients with normal baseline renal function the incidence of nephrotoxicity was significantly lower with amphotericin B cholesteryl than with amphotericin B desoxycholate.

In a randomized, double-blind study of amphotericin B liposomal (*AmBisome*) in neutropenic patients, the incidence of nephrotoxicity is summarized in the following table.

Nephrotoxicity in Neutropenic Patients Taking *AmBisome* (%)

	AmBisome			Amphotericin B lipid complex
	3 mg/kg/day	5 mg/kg/day	Both	5 mg/kg/day
Total patients	85	81	166	78
Patients with nephrotoxicity 1.5 × baseline serum creatinine value	29.4	25.9	27.7	62.8

AMPHOTERICIN B LIPID COMPLEX — INJECTION

Nephrotoxicity in Neutropenic Patients Taking *AmBisome* (%)				
	AmBisome			Amphotericin B lipid complex
	3 mg/kg/day	5 mg/kg/day	Both	5 mg/kg/day
2 × baseline serum creatinine value	14.1	14.8	14.5	42.3

➤*Infusion reactions:* Acute reactions including fever, shaking chills, hypotension, anorexia, vomiting, nausea, headache, and tachypnea are common 1 to 3 hours after starting an IV infusion. These reactions are usually more severe with the first few doses of amphotericin B and usually diminish with subsequent doses. Acute infusion-related reactions can be managed by pretreatment with antihistamines and corticosteroids or by reducing the rate of infusion and by prompt administration of antihistamines and corticosteroids. Avoid rapid IV infusion because it has been associated with hypotension, hypokalemia, arrhythmias, bronchospasm, and shock.

➤*Leukoencephalopathy:* Leukoencephalopathy has been reported following use of amphotericin B; total body irradiation may be a predisposition.

➤*Hypersensitivity reactions:* Anaphylaxis has been reported with amphotericin B. If severe respiratory distress occurs, discontinue the infusion immediately. Do not give further infusions. Have cardiopulmonary resuscitation facilities available during administration.

➤*Renal function impairment:* Use amphotericin B with care in patients with reduced renal function; frequent monitoring is recommended (see Precautions). Lipid formulations have been reported to overcome most problems of chronic nephrotoxicity, even in patients with impaired renal function following previous treatment with amphotericin B desoxycholate.

➤*Elderly:* A total of 188 patients > 65 years of age have been treated with lipid-based formulations of amphotericin B with no reports of unexpected adverse events.

➤*Pregnancy: Category B.* Systemic fungal infections have been successfully treated in pregnant women with amphotericin B without obvious effects to the fetus, but the number of cases reported has been small. Adequate and well-controlled studies have not been conducted; therefore, use during pregnancy only if clearly needed.

➤*Lactation:* It is not known whether amphotericin B is excreted in breast milk. Because of the potential for serious adverse reactions in nursing infants, decide whether to discontinue breastfeeding or discontinue treatment, taking into account the importance of the drug to the mother.

➤*Children:* Pediatric patients < 16 years of age (n = 97) with systemic fungal infections have been treated with amphotericin B cholesteryl (*Amphotec*) at daily mg/kg doses similar to those given adults and had significantly less renal toxicity than the desoxycholate formulation (12% vs 52%); 273 pediatric patients age 1 month to 16 years of age with presumed fungal infections, confirmed systemic fungal infections, or with visceral leishmaniasis have been successfully treated with liposomal amphotericin B (*AmBisome*); 111 children < 16 years of age, including 11 patients < 1 year of age, have been treated with amphotericin B lipid complex (*Abelcet*) at 5 mg/kg/day and 5 children with hepatosplenic candidiasis were effectively treated with 2.5 mg/kg/day. Safety and efficacy in patients < 1 month of age have not been established.

Precautions

➤*Monitoring:* Monitor renal function frequently during amphotericin B therapy. Monitor liver function, serum electrolytes (particularly magnesium and potassium), blood counts, and hemoglobin concentrations on a regular basis. Use laboratory test results as a guide to subsequent dose adjustments. Monitor complete blood count and prothrombin time as medically indicated.

Testing dose – Record the patient's temperature, pulse, respiration, and blood pressure every 30 minutes for 2 to 4 hours after administration.

➤*Resistance:* Variants with reduced susceptibility to amphotericin B have been isolated from several fungal species after serial passage in cell culture media containing the drug and from some patients receiving prolonged therapy with amphotericin B desoxycholate. The relevance of drug resistance to clinical outcome has not been established.

➤*Pulmonary reactions:* Pulmonary reactions characterized by acute dyspnea, hypoxemia, and interstitial infiltrates have been observed in neutropenic patients receiving amphotericin B and leukocyte transfusions. Although pulmonary toxicity has occurred in association with either agent used alone, it was more frequent when amphotericin B was given after or during initiation of leukocyte transfusions. Administer amphotericin B cautiously in patients receiving leukocyte transfusions and separate the infusion as far as possible from the time of leukocyte transfusion.

➤*Lab test abnormalities:* Serum electrolyte, liver function, renal function, and other test abnormalities have been reported, including the following: Hypomagnesemia, hyperkalemia, hypokalemia, hypercalcemia, hypocalcemia, hypophosphatemia; increased AST, ALT, GGT, bilirubin, alkaline phosphatase, LDH, BUN, and serum creatinine; acidosis, hyperamylasemia, hypoglycemia, hyperglycemia, and hyperuricemia.

Drug Interactions

Amphotericin B Drug Interactions			
Precipitant drug	Object drug*		Description
Antineoplastic agents	Amphotericin B	↑	Concurrent administration may enhance the potential for renal toxicity, bronchospasm, and hypotension.
Corticosteroids and corticotropin	Amphotericin B	↑	Concurrent administration may potentiate hypokalemia and predispose patient to cardiac dysfunction. Do not give unless necessary to control adverse reactions.
Zidovudine	Amphotericin B	↑	Increases in myelotoxicity and nephrotoxicity were observed in dogs administered zidovudine concomitantly with amphotericin B desoxycholate or lipid complex.
Amphotericin B	Cyclosporine	↑	The risk of renal toxicity is increased with concomitant administration. Severe muscle tremors were reported in 1 patient.
Cyclosporine	Amphotericin B		
Amphotericin B	Digitalis glycosides	↑	Concurrent administration may induce hypokalemia and may potentiate digitalis toxicity.
Amphotericin B	Flucytosine	↑	A synergistic relationship with amphotericin B has been reported. Flucytosine toxicity may be increased by increasing its cellular uptake or impairing renal excretion.
Azole antifungals	Amphotericin B	↓	In vitro animal studies suggest that imidazoles may induce fungal resistance to amphotericin B. Administer with caution, especially in immunocompromised patients.
Nephrotoxic agents	Amphotericin B	↑	Concomitant administration may enhance risk of drug-induced renal toxicity. Use caution when administering concomitantly. Monitor renal function intensively.
Amphotericin B	Nephrotoxic agents		
Amphotericin B	Skeletal muscle relaxants	↑	Amphotericin B-induced hypokalemia may enhance the curariform effect of skeletal muscle relaxants. Monitor serum potassium levels closely.
Amphotericin B	Thiazides	↑	Electrolyte depletion may be intensified, particularly hypokalemia. Monitor potassium levels.

* ↑ = Object drug increased. ↓ = Object drug decreased.

Adverse Reactions

➤*Prevention of adverse reactions:* Most patients will exhibit some intolerance, often at less than full therapeutic dosage. Severe reactions may be lessened by giving aspirin, antipyretics (eg, acetaminophen), antihistamines, and antiemetics before the infusion and by maintaining sodium balance. Administration on alternate days may decrease anorexia and phlebitis. Small doses of IV adrenal corticosteroids given prior to or during the infusion may decrease febrile reactions. Keep the dosage and duration of such corticosteroid therapy to a minimum (see Drug Interactions). In 3 patients, dantrolene was a successful adjunctive agent for the prophylaxis (50 mg oral) and treatment (50 mg IV) of amphotericin B-induced rigors. Adding a small amount of heparin to the infusion (500 to 2000 units), removal of needle after infusion, rotation of infusion sites, administration through a large central vein, and using a pediatric scalp-vein needle may lessen the incidence of thrombophlebitis. Extravasation may cause chemical irritation. In some patients meperidine (25 to 50 mg IV) has been shown to decrease the duration of shaking chills and fever that may accompany infusion of amphotericin B.

AMPHOTERICIN B LIPID COMPLEX — INJECTION

Amphotericin B, Lipid-Based Adverse Reactions (%)[1]			
Adverse reaction	Abelcet (5 mg/kg/day)	Amphotec (3 to 6 mg/kg/day)	AmBisome[2]
Cardiovascular			
Hypotension	8	10-12	14.3
Cardiac arrest	6	1-5	2-10
Hypertension	5	7	7.9
Chest pain	3	≥ 5	12
Tachycardia	—	9-10	13.4
CNS			
Headache	6	4-5	19.8
Anxiety	—	1-5	13.7
Confusion	—	1-5	11.4
Insomnia	—	≥ 5	17.2
Dermatologic			
Rash	4	≥ 5	24.8
Pruritus	✓	≥ 5	10.8
Sweating	—	≥ 5	7
GI			
Nausea	9	7-8	39.7
Vomiting	8	6-11	31.8
Diarrhea	6	≥ 5	30.3
Abdominal pain	4	≥ 5	19.8
GI hemorrhage	4	1-5	9.9
Nausea/Vomiting	3	4-7	—
Hematologic			
Thrombocytopenia	5	1-6	2-10
Anemia	4	≥ 5	2-10
Leukopenia	4	1-5	—
Bilirubinemia	4	—	—
Metabolic/Nutritional			
Creatine, increased	11	12-21[3]	22.4
BUN, increased	5	1-5	21
Hyperbilirubinemia	—	3-19	18.1
Alkaline phosphatase, increased	✓	3-7	22.2
ALT, increased	✓	1-5	14.6
AST, increased	✓	1-5	12.8
Liver function test abnormality	—	4-11	2-10
Hypokalemia	5	8-26	42.9
Hypomagnesemia	✓	4-6	20.4
Hyperglycemia	✓	1-6	23
Hypernatremia	—	1-5	4.1
Hypocalcemia	✓	≥ 5	18.4
Hypervolemia	—	1-5	12.2
Peripheral edema	—	≥ 5	14.6
Edema	—	≥ 5	14.3
Respiratory			
Respiratory failure	8	—	2-10
Dyspnea	7	5-9	23
Respiratory disorder	4	1-5	2-10
Hypoxia	—	5-9	7.6
Cough increased	—	≥ 5	17.8
Epistaxis	—	≥ 5	14.9
Lung disorder	—	≥ 5	17.8
Pleural effusion	—	1-5	12.5
Rhinitis	—	≥ 5	11.1
Miscellaneous			
Chills	18	50-77	47.5
Fever	14	33-55	—
Multiple organ failure	11	—	—
Sepsis	7	≥ 5	14
Infection	5	1-5	11.1
Pain	5	≥ 5	14
Kidney failure	5	1-5	2-10
Chills and fever	—	3-7	—
Asthenia	—	1-5	13.1
Back pain	—	≥ 5	12
Blood product transfusion reaction	—	—	18.4
Hematuria	—	≥ 5	14

[1] Data are pooled from separate studies and are not necessarily comparable.
[2] Incidence of ≥ 10%.
[3] Includes patients with "abnormal kidney function," which was associated with an increase in creatinine.
* ✓ = occurred, no incidence figure reported.

➤*Abelcet:* The following adverse reactions have also been reported in patients using *Abelcet*, but the causal association between these adverse reactions and *Abelcet* is uncertain.

Cardiovascular – Cardiac failure, MI, cardiomyopathy, arrhythmias including ventricular fibrillation.

CNS – Convulsions, peripheral neuropathy, transient vertigo, encephalopathy, cerebrovascular accident, extrapyramidal syndrome and other neurologic symptoms.

Dermatologic – Maculopapular rash, exfoliative dermatitis, erythema multiforme.

GI – Melena, dyspepsia, cramping, epigastric pain.

GU – Oliguria, decreased renal function, anuria, renal tubular acidosis, impotence, dysuria.

Hematologic – Coagulation defects, leukocytosis, blood dyscrasias including eosinophilia.

Hepatic – Acute liver failure, hepatitis, jaundice, venoocclusive liver disease, hepatomegaly, cholangitis, cholecystitis.

Lab test abnormalities – Hyperkalemia, hypercalcemia, increased LDH, increased BUN, hyperamylasemia, hypoglycemia, hyperuricemia, hypophosphatemia.

Musculoskeletal – Myasthenia, bone pain, muscle pain, joint pain.

Respiratory – Bronchospasm, wheezing, asthma, pulmonary edema, hemoptysis, pulmonary embolus, tachypnea, pleural effusion.

Special senses – Deafness, tinnitus, visual impairment, hearing loss, diplopia.

Miscellaneous – Malaise, weight loss, injection site reactions including inflammation, anaphylactoid and other allergic reactions, shock, thrombophlebitis, anorexia, acidosis.

➤*Amphotec:* The following adverse events also occurred in *Amphotec* patients, but the causal relationship is uncertain.

Cardiovascular – Hemorrhage, postural hypotension (≥ 5%); arrhythmia, atrial fibrillation, bradycardia, CHF, phlebitis, shock, supraventricular tachycardia, syncope, vasodilation, venoocclusive liver disease, ventricular extrasystoles (1% to < 5%).

CNS – Dizziness, somnolence, abnormal thinking, tremor (≥ 5%); agitation, convulsion, depression, hallucinations, hypertonia, nervousness, neuropathy, paresthesia, psychosis, speech disorder, stupor (1% to < 5%).

Dermatologic – Maculopapular rash (≥ 5%); acne, alopecia, petechial rash, skin discoloration, skin disorder, skin nodule, skin ulcer, urticaria, vesiculobullous rash (1% to < 5%).

GI – Dry mouth, hematemesis, jaundice, stomatitis (≥ 5%); anorexia, bloody diarrhea, constipation, dyspepsia, fecal incontinence, gamma glutamyl transpeptidase increase, GI disorder, gingivitis, glossitis, hepatic failure, melena, mouth ulceration, oral moniliasis, rectal disorder (1% to < 5%).

GU – Albuminuria, dysuria, glycosuria, oliguria, urinary incontinence, urinary retention, urinary tract disorder (1% to < 5%).

Hematologic / Lymphatic – Coagulation disorder, prothrombin decreased (≥ 5%); ecchymosis, increased fibrinogen, hypochromic anemia, leukocytosis, petechia, decreased thromboplastin (1% to < 5%).

Metabolic / Nutritional – Hypophosphatemia, peripheral edema, weight gain (≥ 5%); acidosis, dehydration, hyponatremia, hyperkalemia, hyperlipemia, hypoglycemia, hypoproteinemia, lactic dehydrogenase increased, weight loss (1% to < 5%).

Musculoskeletal – Arthralgia, myalgia (1% to < 5%).

Respiratory – Apnea, asthma, hyperventilation (≥ 5%); hemoptysis, lung edema, pharyngitis, sinusitis (1% to < 5%).

Special senses – Eye hemorrhage (≥ 5%); amblyopia, deafness, ear disorder, tinnitus (1% to < 5%).

Miscellaneous – Abdomen enlarged, face edema, injection site inflammation, mucous membrane disorder (≥ 5%); accidental injury, allergic reaction, death, hypothermia, immune system disorder, injection site pain, injection site reaction, neck pain (1% to < 5%).

➤*AmBisome:* The following adverse reactions occurred in 2% to 10% of *AmBisome* patients receiving chemotherapy or bone marrow transplantation.

Cardiovascular – Arrhythmia, atrial fibrillation, bradycardia, cardiomegaly, hemorrhage, postural hypertension, valvular heart disease, vascular disorder, flushing.

CNS – Agitation, coma, convulsions, cough, depression, dysesthesia, dizziness, hallucinations, nervousness, paresthesia, somnolence, thinking abnormality, tremor.

Dermatologic – Alopecia, dry skin, herpes simplex, injection site inflammation, purpura, skin discoloration, skin disorder, skin ulcer, urticaria, vesiculobullous rash.

GI – Anorexia, constipation, dry mouth, dry nose, dyspepsia, dysphagia, eructation, fecal incontinence, flatulence, GI hemorrhage, hemorrhoids, gum or oral hemorrhage, hematemesis, hepatocellular damage, hepatomegaly, mucositis, rectal disorder, stomatitis, ulcerative stomatitis, venoocclusive disease.

GU – Abnormal renal function, acute renal failure, dysuria, toxic nephropathy, urinary incontinence, vaginal hemorrhage.

Hematologic / Lymphatic – Coagulation disorder, ecchymosis, fluid overload, petechia, decreased prothrombin, increased prothrombin.

Metabolic / Nutritional – Acidosis, increased amylase, hyperchloremia, hyperkalemia, hypermagnesemia, hyperphosphatemia, hyponatremia,

AMPHOTERICIN B LIPID COMPLEX — INJECTION

hypophosphatemia, hypoproteinemia, increased lactate dehydrogenase, increased nonprotein nitrogen, respiratory alkalosis.

Musculoskeletal – Arthralgia, bone pain, dystonia, myalgia, rigors.

Respiratory – Asthma, atelectasis, hemoptysis, hiccough, hyperventilation, influenza-like symptoms, lung edema, pharyngitis, pneumonia, sinusitis.

Special senses – Conjunctivitis, dry eyes, eye hemorrhage.

Miscellaneous – Abdomen enlarged, allergic reaction, cellulitis, cell-mediated immunological reaction, face edema, graft-vs-host disease, malaise, neck pain.

Postmarketing – The following have been reported during postmarketing surveillance: Angioedema, erythema, urticaria, cyanosis/hypoventilation, pulmonary edema, agranulocytosis, hemorrhagic cystitis.

Overdosage

➤*Symptoms:* Amphotericin B overdose has been reported to cause cardiorespiratory arrest. Amphotericin B lipid complex at doses of 7 to 13 mg/kg and repeated daily doses of liposomal amphotericin B up to 7.5 mg/kg have been administered without serious adverse reactions.

➤*Treatment:* If overdose is suspected, discontinue therapy, monitor clinical status, and administer supportive therapy. Refer to General Management of Acute Overdosage. Amphotericin B lipid complex and cholesteryl are not hemodialyzable.

NYSTATIN

Rx	**Nystatin** (Various, eg, Major, Teva)	**Tablets**: 500,000 units	In 100s.
Rx	**Mycostatin** (Bristol-Myers Squibb)		Lactose. (Squibb 580). Light brown, biconvex. Film-coated. In 100s.
Rx	**Nystatin** (Various, eg, Geneva, NMC, Parmed)	**Oral suspension**: 100,000 units/mL	In 5, 60 and 480 mL.
Rx	**Nilstat** (Lederle)		Cherry flavor. In 60 and 473 mL.
Rx	**Mycostatin Pastilles** (Bristol-Myers Oncology)	**Troches**: 200,000 units	In 30s.
Rx	**Nystatin** (Paddock)	**Bulk Powder**: 50 million units	
Rx	**Nilstat** (Lederle)	**Bulk Powder**: 150 million units	
Rx	**Nystatin** (Paddock)		
Rx	**Nystatin** (Paddock)	**Bulk Powder**: 500 million units	
Rx	**Nilstat** (Lederle)	**Bulk Powder**: 1 billion units	
Rx	**Nystatin** (Paddock)		
Rx	**Nilstat** (Lederle)	**Bulk Powder**: 2 billion units	
Rx	**Nystatin** (Paddock)		
Rx	**Nystatin** (Paddock)	**Bulk Powder**: 5 billion units	

NYSTATIN — ORAL

Indications

➤*Tablets:* Nystatin tablets are intended for the treatment of nonesophageal mucous membrane GI candidiasis.

➤*Lozenges / Troches, oral suspension:* For the treatment of candidiasis in the oral cavity.

➤*Powder for extemporaneous preparation of oral suspension:* Nystatin powder for oral suspension is indicated for the treatment of intestinal and oral cavity infections caused by *Candida (Monilia) albicans*.

Administration and Dosage

➤*Approved by the FDA:* December 22, 1983 (tablets); April 9, 1987 (lozenges); July 14, 1982 (oral suspension).

➤*Tablets:* The usual therapeutic dosage is 1 to 2 tablets (500,000 to 1,000,000 units nystatin) 3 times daily. Treatment should generally be continued for at least 48 hours after clinical cure to prevent relapse.

➤*Lozenges / Troches:*

Pediatric patients and adults – The recommended dose is 1 or 2 nystatin lozenges (200,000 or 400,000 units nystatin) 4 or 5 times daily for as long as 14 days if necessary. Continue the dosage regimen for at least 48 hours after disappearance of oral symptoms.

Discontinue dosage if symptoms persist after the initial 14-day period of treatment.

Administration – Allow lozenges to dissolve slowly in the mouth. Do not chew or swallow whole.

➤*Oral suspension:*

Adults and children – 400,000 to 600,000 units 4 times daily (one half of dose in each side of mouth, retaining the drug as long as possible before swallowing).

Infants – 200,000 units 4 times daily (100,000 units in each side of the mouth).

Premature and low birth weight infants – Limited clinical studies indicate that 100,000 units 4 times daily is effective.

➤*Powder for extemporaneous preparation of oral suspension:*

Adults and older children – Add ⅛ teaspoonful (approximately 500,000 units) of nystatin to about ½ cup of water and stir well. One-eighth teaspoonful of nystatin is equivalent to the recommended dose for adults and children of nystatin oral suspension (4 to 6 mL, or 400,000 to 600,000 units). This product contains no preservatives. Therefore, use immediately after mixing and do not store. It is designed for extemporaneous preparation of a single dose at a time.

Infections of the oral cavity caused by Candida (Monilia) albicans –
Infants: 200,000 units 4 times daily.
Children and adults: 400,000 to 600,000 units 4 times daily (one-half dose in each side of the mouth).

Note: Limited clinical studies in premature and low-birth-weight infants indicate that 100,000 units 4 times daily is effective. Continue local treatment at least 48 hours after perioral symptoms have disappeared and cultures have returned to normal.

Retain the drug in the mouth as long as possible before swallowing.

Intestinal candidiasis (moniliasis) –
Usual dosage: 500,000 to 1 million units (approximately ⅛ to ¼ teaspoonful) 3 times daily. Treatment should generally be continued for at least 48 hours after clinical cure to prevent relapse.

Examples for determining dosing – Determine the number of units for the entire course of treatment (eg, for thrush, 500,000 units per dose, 4 doses per day [2 million units/day], 14-day course of treatment = 28 million units.

At 500,000 units/dose, 4 doses/day [2 million units/day], 21-day course of treatment = 42 million units.

➤*Storage / Stability:*

Tablets – Store at controlled room temperature 15° to 30°C (59° to 86°F). Dispense in tight, light-resistant container.

Lozenges – Refrigerate between 2° and 8°C (36° and 46°F).

Powder for extemporaneous preparation of oral suspension – Store in a refrigerator, 2° to 8°C (36° to 46°F). Protect from light. Dispense in a tight, light-resistant container.
Note: The potency of this product cannot be ensured for longer than 90 days after the container is first opened.

Actions

➤*Pharmacology:* Nystatin acts by binding to sterols in the cell membrane of susceptible fungi, with a resultant change in membrane permeability, allowing leakage of intracellular components. Nystatin exhibits no appreciable activity against bacteria, protozoa, or viruses.

➤*Pharmacokinetics:*

Absorption – GI absorption of nystatin is insignificant. Most oral nystatin is passed unchanged in the stool. In patients with renal insufficiency receiving oral therapy with conventional dosage forms, significant plasma concentrations of nystatin may occasionally occur.

Lozenges: Mean nystatin concentrations in excess of those required in vitro to inhibit growth of clinically significant *Candida* persisted in saliva for approximately 2 hours after the start of oral dissolution of 2 nystatin lozenges (400,000 units nystatin) administered simultaneously to 12 healthy volunteers.

➤*Microbiology:* Nystatin is both fungistatic and fungicidal in vitro against a wide variety of yeasts and yeast-like fungi. *Candida albicans* demonstrates no significant resistance to nystatin in vitro on repeated subculture in increasing levels of nystatin; other *Candida* species become quite resistant. Generally, resistance does not develop in vivo.

Polyene Antifungals

NYSTATIN — ORAL

Contraindications

Nystatin tablets, lozenges, and oral suspension are contraindicated in patients with histories of hypersensitivity to any of the components.

Warnings

➤*Hypersensitivity reactions:* If irritation or hypersensitivity develops with nystatin, discontinue treatment and institute appropriate therapy.

➤*Pregnancy:* Category C.

Teratogenic – Animal reproduction studies have not been conducted with nystatin. It is also not known whether nystatin can cause fetal harm when administered to a pregnant woman or can affect reproduction capacity. Give nystatin to a pregnant woman only if clearly needed.

➤*Lactation:* It is not known whether nystatin is excreted in human milk. Although GI absorption is insignificant, because many drugs are excreted in human milk, exercise caution when nystatin is administered to a nursing woman.

➤*Children:*

Lozenges – The use of nystatin lozenges has not been systematically studied in pediatric patients.

Precautions

➤*Systemic mycoses:* Do not use these medications for the treatment of systemic mycoses. Discontinue treatment if sensitization or irritation is reported during use.

➤*Lozenges:* In order to achieve maximum effect from the medication, nystatin lozenges must be allowed to dissolve slowly in the mouth; therefore, patients for whom the nystatin lozenge is prescribed, including pediatric patients and the elderly, must be competent to utilize the dosage form as intended.

➤*Lab test abnormalities:*

Lack of therapeutic response – If there is a lack of therapeutic response, repeat appropriate microbiological studies (eg, KOH smears or cultures) to confirm the diagnosis of candidiasis and rule out other pathogens before instituting another course of therapy.

Adverse Reactions

Nystatin is generally well tolerated, even with prolonged therapy. Oral irritation and sensitization have been reported. Nausea has been reported occasionally during therapy.

➤*Dermatologic:* Rash, including urticaria, has been reported rarely. Stevens-Johnson syndrome has been reported very rarely.

➤*GI:* Diarrhea (including 1 case of bloody diarrhea), nausea, vomiting, GI upset disturbances.

Large oral doses of nystatin have occasionally produced irritation of the stomach that may result in nausea and vomiting.

➤*Miscellaneous:* Tachycardia, bronchospasm, facial swelling, and nonspecific myalgia have also been rarely reported.

Overdosage

➤*Symptoms:* Oral doses of nystatin in excess of 5 million units daily have caused nausea and GI upset. There have been no reports of serious toxic effects or superinfections.

Patient Information

Retain the drug in the mouth as long as possible. Continue use at least 2 days after symptoms have subsided.

➤*Lozenges:* Patients taking this medication should receive the following information and instructions:

- Use as directed; the medication is not for any disorder other than that for which it was prescribed.
- Allow the nystatin lozenge to dissolve slowly in the mouth; do not chew or swallow the lozenge.
- You should be advised regarding replacement of any missed doses.
- There should be no interruption or discontinuation of medication until the prescribed course of treatment is completed, even though symptomatic relief may occur within a few days.
- If symptoms of local irritation develop, notify the physician promptly.
- Good oral hygiene, including proper care of dentures, is particularly important for denture wearers.

Imidazole Antifungal

KETOCONAZOLE

Rx	**Ketoconazole** (Various, eg, Mutual, Mylan, Novopharm, Taro, Teva)	**Tablets:** 200 mg	In 30s, 50s, 100s, 250s, 500s, 1000s, blister packs of 10, and UD 30s, 50s, and 100s.
Rx	**Nizoral** (Janssen)		(Janssen/Nizoral). White, scored. In 100s.

KETOCONAZOLE — ORAL

For information on topical ketoconazole, refer to the individual monograph in the Dermatological Anti-infectives section.

WARNING

Hepatotoxicity – When used orally, ketoconazole has been associated with hepatic toxicity, including some fatalities. Patients receiving this drug should be informed by the physician of the risk and should be closely monitored (see Warnings).

Drug interactions –

Terfenadine: Coadministration of terfenadine with ketoconazole tablets is contraindicated. Rare cases of serious cardiovascular adverse events, including death, ventricular tachycardia and torsades de pointes have been observed in patients taking ketoconazole tablets concomitantly with terfenadine, due to increased terfenadine concentrations induced by ketoconazole tablets (see Contraindications, Warnings, and Drug Interactions).

Astemizole: Pharmacokinetic data indicate that oral ketoconazole inhibits the metabolism of astemizole, resulting in elevated plasma levels of astemizole and its active metabolite desmethylastemizole which may prolong QT intervals. Coadministration of astemizole with ketoconazole tablets is therefore contraindicated (see Contraindications, Warnings, and Drug Interactions).

Cisapride: Coadministration of cisapride with ketoconazole is contraindicated. Serious cardiovascular adverse events including ventricular tachycardia, ventricular fibrillation and torsades de pointes have occurred in patients taking ketoconazole concomitantly with cisapride (see Contraindications, Warnings, and Drug Interactions).

Indications

➤*Fungal infections:* Treatment of the following systemic fungal infections: Candidiasis, chronic mucocutaneous candidiasis, oral thrush, candiduria, blastomycosis, coccidioidomycosis, histoplasmosis, chromomycosis, and paracoccidioidomycosis. Ketoconazole should not be used for fungal meningitis because it penetrates poorly into the cerebrospinal fluid.

➤*Severe recalcitrant cutaneous dermatophyte infections:* Treatment of patients with severe recalcitrant cutaneous dermatophyte infections who have not responded to topical therapy or oral griseofulvin, or who are unable to take griseofulvin.

➤*Unlabeled uses:* Ketoconazole has been used successfully in the treatment of onychomycosis (caused by *Trichophyton* and *Candida* sp); pityriasis versicolor (tinea versicolor); tinea pedis, corporis, and cruris (200 to 400 mg/day); tinea capitis (3.3 to 6.6 mg/kg/day); and vaginal candidiasis.

High-dose (800 to 1200 mg/day) ketoconazole has shown some success in treating CNS fungal infections.

Ketoconazole in doses of 400 mg every 8 hours has been used in the treatment of advanced prostate cancer (see Warnings).

Ketoconazole 800 to 1200 mg/day has been used to effectively treat Cushing's syndrome because of its ability to inhibit adrenal steroidogenesis.

Treatment of refractory depression (with or without psychotic component); hypercortisolemia-related refractory depression.

Administration and Dosage

➤*Approved by the FDA:* December 31, 1985.

➤*Adults:* The recommended starting dose of ketoconazole is a single daily administration of 200 mg (1 tablet). In very serious infections or if clinical responsiveness is insufficient within the expected time, the dose of ketoconazole may be increased to 400 mg (2 tablets) once daily.

➤*Children:* In small numbers of children older than 2 years of age, a single daily dose of 3.3 to 6.6 mg/kg has been used. Ketoconazole has not been studied in children younger than 2 years of age.

➤*Duration:* There should be laboratory as well as clinical documentation of infection prior to starting ketoconazole therapy. Treatment should be continued until tests indicate that active fungal infection has subsided. Inadequate periods of treatment may yield poor response and lead to early recurrence of clinical symptoms. Minimum treatment for candidiasis is 1 or 2 weeks. Patients with chronic mucocutaneous candidiasis usually require maintenance therapy. Minimum treatment for the other indicated systemic mycoses is 6 months.

Minimum treatment for recalcitrant dermatophyte infections is 4 weeks in cases involving glabrous skin. Palmar and plantar infections may respond more slowly. Apparent cures may subsequently recur after discontinuation of therapy in some cases.

➤*Storage/Stability:* Store at controlled room temperature 15° to 25°C (59° to 77°F). Protect from moisture.

Actions

➤*Pharmacology:* In vitro studies suggest that ketoconazole impairs the synthesis of ergosterol, which is a vital component of fungal cell membranes. This allows impaired permeability and leakage of cellular components.

KETOCONAZOLE — ORAL

➤*Pharmacokinetics:*

Absorption / Distribution – Mean peak plasma levels of ≈ 3.5 mcg/mL are reached within 1 to 2 hours, following oral administration of a single 200 mg dose taken with a meal. In vitro, the plasma protein binding is ≈ 99% mainly to the albumin fraction. Only a negligible proportion of ketoconazole reaches the cerebrospinal fluid. Ketoconazole is a weak dibasic agent and thus requires acidity for dissolution and absorption.

Metabolism – Following absorption from the GI tract, ketoconazole is converted into several inactive metabolites. The major identified metabolic pathways are oxidation and degradation of the imidazole and piperazine rings, oxidative O-dealkylation and aromatic hydroxylation.

Excretion – About 13% of the dose is excreted in the urine, of which 2% to 4% is unchanged drug. The major route of excretion is through the bile into the intestinal tract.

Plasma elimination is biphasic with a half-life of 2 hours during the first 10 hours and 8 hours thereafter.

➤*Microbiology:* Ketoconazole is active against clinical infections with *Blastomyces dermatitidis*, *Candida* sp, *Coccidioides immitis*, *Histoplasma capsulatum*, *Paracoccidioides brasiliensis*, and *Phialophora*sp. Ketoconazole is also active against *Trichophyton* sp, *Epidermophyton* sp, and *Microsporum* sp. Ketoconazole is also active in vitro against a variety of fungi and yeast. In animal models, activity has been demonstrated against *Candida* sp, *Blastomyces dermatitidis*, *Histoplasma capsulatum*, *Malassezia furfur*, *Coccidioides immitis*, and *Cryptococcus neoformans*.

Contraindications

Coadministration with terfenadine, astemizole, cisapride, or oral triazolam (see Warning Box, Warnings, and Drug Interactions); hypersensitivity to the drug.

Warnings

➤*Cardiac dysrhythmias:* See the Warning box for more information.

➤*Prostate cancer:* In European clinical trials involving 350 patients with metastatic prostatic cancer, 11 deaths were reported within 2 weeks of starting treatment with high doses of ketoconazole tablets (1200 mg/day). It is not possible to ascertain from the information available whether death was related to ketoconazole therapy in these patients with serious underlying disease. However, high doses of ketoconazole are known to suppress adrenal corticosteroid secretion.

➤*Hepatotoxicity:* Hepatotoxicity, primarily of the hepatocellular type, has been associated with the use of ketoconazole, including rare fatalities. The reported incidence of hepatotoxicity has been about 1:10,000 exposed patients, but this probably represents some degree of underreporting, as is the case for most reported adverse reactions to drugs. The median duration of ketoconazole therapy in patients who developed symptomatic hepatotoxicity was ≈ 28 days, although the range extended to as low as 3 days. The hepatic injury has usually, but not always, been reversible upon discontinuation of ketoconazole treatment. Several cases of hepatitis have been reported in children.

Prompt recognition of liver injury is essential. Liver function tests (such as alkaline phosphatase, ALT, AST and bilirubin) should be measured before starting treatment and at frequent intervals during treatment. Patients receiving ketoconazole concurrently with other potentially hepatotoxic drugs should be carefully monitored, particularly those patients requiring prolonged therapy or those who have had a history of liver disease.

Most of the reported cases of hepatic toxicity have to date been in patients treated for onychomycosis. Of 180 patients worldwide developing idiosyncratic liver dysfunction during ketoconazole therapy, 61.3% had onychomycosis and 16.8% had chronic recalcitrant dermatophytoses.

Transient minor elevations in liver enzymes have occurred during treatment with ketoconazole. The drug should be discontinued if these persist, if the abnormalities worsen, or if the abnormalities become accompanied by symptoms of possible liver injury.

➤*Hypersensitivity reactions:* In rare cases anaphylaxis has been reported after the first dose. Several cases of hypersensitivity reactions including urticaria have also been reported.

➤*Pregnancy: Category C.* Ketoconazole has been shown to be teratogenic (syndactylia and oligodactylia) in the rat when given in the diet at 80 mg/kg/day (10 times the maximum recommended human dose). However, these effects may be related to maternal toxicity, evidence of which also was seen at this and higher dose levels.

There are no adequate and well-controlled studies in pregnant women. Ketoconazole tablets should be used during pregnancy only if the potential benefit justifies the potential risk to the fetus.

➤*Lactation:* Since ketoconazole is probably excreted in the milk, mothers who are under treatment should not breastfeed.

➤*Children:* Ketoconazole have not been systematically studied in children of any age, and essentially no information is available on children younger than 2 years. Ketoconazole should not be used in pediatric patients unless the potential benefit outweighs the risks.

Precautions

➤*Hormone levels:* Ketoconazole has been demonstrated to lower serum testosterone. Once therapy with ketoconazole has been discontinued, serum testosterone levels return to baseline values. Testosterone levels are impaired with doses of 800 mg/ day and abolished by 1600 mg per day. Ketoconazole also decrease ACTH-induced corticosteroid serum levels at similar high doses. The recommended dose of 200 mg to 400 mg daily should be followed closely.

➤*Gastric acidity:* In 4 subjects with drug-induced achlorhydria, a marked reduction in ketoconazole absorption was observed. Ketoconazole requires acidity for dissolution. If concomitant antacids, anticholinergics, and H_2-blockers are needed, they should be given at least 2 hours after administration of ketoconazole. In cases of achlorhydria, the patients should be instructed to dissolve each tablet in 4 mL aqueous solution of 0.2 N HCl. For ingesting the resulting mixture, they should use a drinking straw so as to avoid contact with the teeth. This administration should be followed with a cup of tap water.

Drug Interactions

Ketoconazole Drug Interactions

Precipitant drug	Object drug*		Description
Antacids	Ketoconazole	↓	Increased gastric pH may inhibit ketoconazole absorption. Consider giving antacids ≥ 2 hours after ketoconazole.
Didanosine	Ketoconazole	↓	The therapeutic effects of ketoconazole may be decreased. The buffers in didanosine chewable tablets decrease the absorption of ketoconazole.
Ketoconazole	Protease inhibitors Indinavir Ritonavir Saquinavir	↑	Plasma protease inhibitors concentrations may be elevated, increasing the risk of toxicity. Ketoconazole may inhibit the hepatic metabolism of protease inhibitors.
Ketoconazole	Tricyclic antidepressants	↑	Serum tricyclic antidepressant concentrations may be elevated, resulting in an increase in therapeutic and adverse effects.
Ketoconazole	Carbamazepine	↑	Plasma concentrations of carbamazepine may be elevated, increasing clinical and adverse effects. Ketoconazole may inhibit the metabolism of carbamazepine.
Sucralfate	Ketoconazole	↓	The therapeutic effects of ketoconazole may be reduced. The mechanism of action is unknown but likely because of a decrease in ketoconazole bioavailability. When clinical situation permits, administer ketoconazole ≥ 2 hours before sucralfate.
Proton pump inhibitors	Ketoconazole	↓	The effects of ketoconazole may be decreased. The bioavailability of ketoconazole may be decreased because of a possible reduction in tablet dissolution in the presence of a high gastric pH.
Ketoconazole	Quinidine	↑	Serum quinidine levels may be elevated, increasing therapeutic and toxic effects. Ketoconazole may inhibit quinidine metabolism.
Ketoconazole	Sulfonylureas	↑	Serum sulfonylurea concentrations may be elevated increasing the hypoglycemic effect.
Ketoconazole	Benzodiazepines	↑	Increased and prolonged serum levels, CNS depression, and psychomotor impairment with certain benzodiazepines are possible for several days after stopping ketoconazole. Concomitant administration of ketoconazole with oral triazolam is contraindicated.
Ketoconazole	Buspirone	↑	Plasma buspirone concentrations may be elevated, increasing pharmacologic and adverse effects.
Ketoconazole	Contraceptives, oral	↔	The therapeutic efficacy of oral contraceptives may be reduced. In addition, elevated ethinyl estradiol blood levels may occur. The mechanism of action is unknown. Inform women of the possible increased risk of oral contraceptive failure. Consider an alternative method of contraception.
Ketoconazole	Donepezil	↑	Donepezil plasma concentration and side effects may be increased.
Ketoconazole	HMG-CoA Reductase Inhibitors	↑	Increased plasma levels and side effects of HMG-CoA reductase inhibitors may occur. Rhabdomyolysis has been reported. If concurrent administration cannot be avoided, consider reducing the HMG-CoA reductase inhibitor dose.
Ketoconazole	Nisoldipine	↑	Nisoldipine concentrations may be elevated, increasing pharmacologic and adverse effects.
Ketoconazole	Tacrolimus	↑	Plasma concentrations may be elevated, increasing the risk of toxicity because of inhibition of tacrolimus gut metabolism.
Ketoconazole	Vinca alkaloids	↑	Increased risk of vinca alkaloid toxicity has occurred because of inhibition of vinca alkaloid metabolism (CYP3A4) by ketoconazole.
Ketoconazole	Zolpidem	↑	Plasma concentrations and the therapeutic effects of zolpidem may be increased.

KETOCONAZOLE — ORAL

Ketoconazole Drug Interactions

Precipitant drug	Object drug*		Description
Histamine H_2 antagonists	Ketoconazole	⬇	Increased gastric pH may inhibit ketoconazole absorption.
Isoniazid	Ketoconazole	⬇	Bioavailability of ketoconazole may be decreased.
Rifampin	Ketoconazole	⬇	Decreased serum levels of either drug may occur. Avoid concurrent use if possible.
Ketoconazole	Warfarin	⬆	The anticoagulant response may be enhanced secondary to inhibition of warfarin metabolism.
Ketoconazole	Corticosteroids	⬆	Corticosteroid bioavailability may be increased and clearance may be decreased, possibly resulting in toxicity.
Ketoconazole	Cyclosporine	⬆	Increased cyclosporine concentrations may occur because of inhibition of metabolism, resulting in toxicity. Because the effect on cyclosporine levels is consistent and predictable, this interaction has been used beneficially to decrease cyclosporine dosage in some patients.
Ketoconazole	Theophyllines	⬇	Decreased absorption of theophylline may occur, resulting in decreased theophylline serum levels.

* ⬆ = Object drug increased ⬇ = Object drug decreased
⟷ = Undetermined clinical effect

➤*Cytochrome P-450 3A4:* Ketoconazole is a potent inhibitor of the cytochrome P-450 3A4 enzyme system. Coadministration of ketoconazole and drugs primarily metabolized by the cytochrome P-450 3A4 enzyme system may result in increased plasma concentrations of the drugs that could increase or prolong both therapeutic and adverse effects. Therefore, unless otherwise specified, appropriate dosage adjustments may be necessary. The following drug interactions have been identified involving ketoconazole and other drugs metabolized by the cytochrome P-450 3A4 enzyme system:

➤*Terfenadine:* Ketoconazole tablets inhibit the metabolism of terfenadine, resulting in an increased plasma concentration of terfenadine and a delay in the elimination of its acid metabolite. The increased plasma concentration of terfenadine or its metabolite may result in prolonged QT intervals (see Warning Box, Contraindications, and Warnings).

➤*Astemizole:* Pharmacokinetic data indicates that oral ketoconazole inhibits the metabolism of astemizole, resulting in elevated plasma levels of astemizole and its active metabolite desmethylastemizole which may prolong QT intervals. Coadministration of astemizole with ketoconazole tablets is therefore contraindicated (see Warning Box, Contraindications, and Warnings).

➤*Cisapride:* Human pharmacokinetics data indicate that oral ketoconazole potently inhibits the metabolism of cisapride resulting in a mean 8-fold increase in the area under the plasma concentration-time curve (AUC) of cisapride. Data suggests that coadministration of oral ketoconazole and cisapride can result in prolongation of the QT interval on the ECG. Therefore concomitant administration of ketoconazole tablets with cisapride is contraindicated (see Warning Box, Contraindications, and Warnings).

➤*Cyclosporine, tacrolimus, methylprednisolone:* Ketoconazole may alter the metabolism of cyclosporine, tacrolimus, and methylprednisolone, resulting in elevated plasma concentrations of the latter drugs. Dosage adjustment may be required if cyclosporine, tacrolimus, or methylprednisolone are given concomitantly with ketoconazole.

➤*Midazolam, triazolam:* Coadministration of ketoconazole with midazolam or triazolam has resulted in elevated plasma concentrations of the latter 2 drugs. This may potentiate and prolong hypnotic and sedative effects, especially with repeated dosing or chronic administration of these agents. These agents should not be used in patients treated with ketoconazole. If midazolam is administered parenterally, special precaution is required since the sedative effect may be prolonged.

➤*Digoxin:* Rare cases of elevated plasma concentrations of digoxin have been reported. It is not clear whether this was due to the combination of therapy. It is, therefore, advisable to monitor digoxin concentrations in patients receiving ketoconazole.

➤*Hypoglycemic agents:* Because severe hypoglycemia has been reported in patients concomitantly receiving oral miconazole (an imidazole) and oral hypoglycemic agents, such a potential interaction involving the latter agents when used concomitantly with ketoconazole tablets (an imidazole) can not be ruled out.

➤*Phenytoin:* Concomitant administration of ketoconazole with phenytoin may alter the metabolism of one or both of the drugs. It is suggested to monitor both ketoconazole and phenytoin.

➤*Loratadine:* After the coadministration of 200 mg oral ketoconazole twice daily and one 20 mg dose of loratadine to 11 subjects, the AUC and C_{max} of loratadine averaged 302% (± 142 S.D.) and 251% (± 68 S.D.), respectively, of those obtained after cotreatment with placebo. The AUC and C_{max} of descarboethoxyloratadine, an active metabolite, averaged 155% (± 27 S.D.) and 141% (± 35 S.D.), respectively. However, no related changes were noted in the QTc on ECG taken at 2, 6, and 24 hours after the coadministration. Also, there were no clinically significant differences in adverse events when loratadine was administered with or without ketoconazole.

➤*Alcohol:* Rare cases of a disulfiram-like reaction to alcohol have been reported. These experiences have been characterized by flushing, rash, peripheral edema, nausea, and headache. Symptoms resolved within a few hours.

Adverse Reactions

In rare cases, anaphylaxis has been reported after the first dose. Several cases of hypersensitivity reactions including urticaria have also been reported. However, the most frequent adverse reactions were nausea or vomiting in ≈ 3%, abdominal pain in 1.2%, pruritus in 1.5%, and the following in less than 1% of the patients: Headache, dizziness, somnolence, fever and chills, photophobia, diarrhea, gynecomastia, impotence, thrombocytopenia, leukopenia, hemolytic anemia, and bulging fontanelles. Oligospermia has been reported in investigational studies with the drug at dosages above those currently approved. Oligospermia has not been reported at dosages up to 400 mg daily; however, sperm counts have been obtained infrequently in patients treated with these dosages. Most of these reactions were mild and transient and rarely required discontinuation of ketoconazole. In contrast, the rare occurrences of hepatic dysfunction require special attention (see Warnings).

In worldwide postmarketing experience with ketoconazole there have been rare reports of alopecia, paresthesia, and signs of increased intracranial pressure including bulging fontanelles and papilledema. Hypertriglyceridemia has also been reported but a causal association with ketoconazole is uncertain.

➤*Cardiovascular:* Ventricular dysrhythmias (prolonged QT intervals) have occurred with the concomitant use of terfenadine with ketoconazole tablets (see Warning Box, Contraindications, and Warnings). Data suggest that coadministration of ketoconazole tablets and cisapride can result in prolongation of the QT interval and has rarely been associated with ventricular arrhythmias (see Contraindications, Warnings, and Drug Interactions).

➤*Psychiatric:* Neuropsychiatric disturbances, including suicidal tendencies and severe depression, have occurred rarely in patients using ketoconazole tablets.

Overdosage

➤*Treatment:* In the event of accidental overdosage, supportive measures, including gastric lavage with sodium bicarbonate, should be employed.

Patient Information

Patients should not take ketoconazole with antacids; this may cause dizziness.

Patients should be instructed to report any signs and symptoms which may suggest liver dysfunction so that appropriate biochemical testing can be done. Such signs and symptoms may include unusual fatigue, anorexia, nausea or vomiting, jaundice, dark urine or pale stools (see Warnings).

VORICONAZOLE

Rx	**Vfend** (Roerig)	**Tablets:** 50 mg	Lactose. (Pfizer VOR50). White. Film-coated. In 30s.
		200 mg	Lactose. (Pfizer VOR200). White, capsule shape. Film-coated. In 30s.
		Powder for injection, lyophilized:[a] 200 mg	Preservative-free. In single-use vials.
		Powder for oral suspension: 45 g (40 mg/mL after reconstitution)	Sucrose. Orange flavor. In 100 mL high density polyethylene bottles w/ a 5 mL oral dispenser and a press-in bottle adaptor.

[a] Contains IV vehicle of 3200 mg sulfobutyl ether beta-cyclodextrin sodium (SBECD).

VORICONAZOLE — ORAL

Indications

➤*Candidemia:* For the treatment of Candidemia in nonneutropenic patients and the following *Candida* infections: disseminated infections in skin and infections in abdomen, bladder wall, kidney, and wounds.

➤*Esophageal candidiasis:* For the treatment of esophageal candidiasis.

➤*Invasive aspergillosis:* For the treatment of invasive aspergillosis. In clinical trials, the majority of isolates recovered were *Aspergillus fumigatus*. There was a small number of cases of culture-proven disease caused by species of *Aspergillus* other than *A. fumigatus* (eg, *Aspergillus flavus, Aspergillus niger, Aspergillus terreus*).

➤*Serious fungal infections:* For the treatment of serious fungal infections caused by *Scedosporium apiospermum* (asexual form of *Pseudallesch-*

VORICONAZOLE — ORAL

eria boydii) and *Fusarium* spp., including *Fusarium solani*, in patients intolerant of, or refractory to, other therapy.

Administration and Dosage

➤*Approved by the FDA:* May 24, 2002.

➤*Administration:* Voriconazole tablets or oral suspension should be taken at least 1 hour before or 1 hour after a meal.

Electrolyte disturbances such as hypocalcemia, hypokalemia, and hypomagnesemia should be corrected prior to initiation of voriconazole therapy.

➤*Dosage:*

Adults –

Candidemia in nonneutropenic patients and other deep tissue Candida infections: See the following table. Patients should be treated for a minimum of 14 days after resolution of symptoms, or following last positive culture, whichever is longer.

Esophageal candidiasis: See the following table. Patients should be treated for a minimum of 14 days and for at least 7 days following resolution of symptoms.

Invasive aspergillosis and serious fungal infections caused by Fusarium spp. and S. apiospermum: For the treatment of adults with invasive aspergillosis and infections caused by *Fusarium* spp. and *S. apiospermum*, therapy must be initiated with the specified loading dose regimen of intravenous (IV) voriconazole to achieve plasma concentrations on day 1 that are close to steady state. On the basis of high oral bioavailability, switching between IV and oral administration is appropriate when clinically indicated. Once the patient can tolerate medication given by mouth, the oral tablet form or oral suspension form of voriconazole may be utilized (see the following table).

The recommended dosing regimen of voriconazole is as follows:

Voriconazole Recommended Dosing Regimen

Infection	Loading dosage IV	Maintenance dosage IV	Maintenance dosage Oral[a]
Candidemia in nonneutropenic patients and other deep tissue *Candida* infections	6 mg/kg every 12 hours for the first 24 hours	3 to 4 mg/kg every 12 hours[b]	200 mg every 12 hours
Esophageal candidiasis	[c]	[c]	200 mg every 12 hours
Invasive aspergillosis	6 mg/kg every 12 hours for the first 24 hours	4 mg/kg every 12 hours	200 mg every 12 hours
Scedosporiosis and fusariosis	6 mg/kg every 12 hours for the first 24 hours	4 mg/kg every 12 hours	200 mg every 12 hours

[a] Patients who weigh 40 kg or more should receive an oral maintenance dosage of voriconazole 200 mg every 12 hours. Adult patients who weigh less than 40 kg should receive an oral maintenance dosage of 100 mg every 12 hours.
[b] In clinical trials, patients with candidemia received 3 mg/kg every 12 hours as primary therapy, while patients with other deep tissue *Candida* infections received 4 mg/kg as salvage therapy. Base appropriate dose on the severity and nature of the infection.
[c] Not evaluated in patients with esophageal candidiasis.

Dosage adjustment: If patient response is inadequate, the oral maintenance dosage may be increased from 200 mg every 12 hours to 300 mg every 12 hours. For adult patients weighing 40 kg or less, the oral maintenance dosage may be increased from 100 mg every 12 hours to 150 mg every 12 hours. If patients are unable to tolerate 300 mg orally every 12 hours, reduce the oral maintenance dosage by 50 mg steps to a minimum of 200 mg every 12 hours (or to 100 mg every 12 hours for adult patients weighing 40 kg or less).

• *Coadministration with phenytoin –* Phenytoin may be coadministered with voriconazole if the oral maintenance dosage is increased from 200 to 400 mg every 12 hours (100 to 200 mg every 12 hours in adult patients weighing 40 kg or less).

➤*Hepatic function impairment:* In the clinical program, patients were included who had baseline liver function tests (LFTs) (ALT, AST) up to 5 times the upper limit of normal (ULN). No dosage adjustment is necessary in patients with this degree of abnormal liver function, but continued monitoring of LFTs for further elevations is recommended. Patient management should include laboratory evaluation of hepatic function (particularly LFTs and bilirubin).

It is recommended that the standard loading-dose regimens be used, but that the maintenance dose be halved in patients with mild to moderate hepatic cirrhosis (Child-Pugh class A and B, respectively).

Voriconazole has not been studied in patients with severe hepatic cirrhosis (Child-Pugh class C) or in patients with chronic hepatitis B or chronic hepatitis C disease. Voriconazole has been associated with elevations in LFTs and clinical signs of liver damage, such as jaundice, and should only be used in patients with severe hepatic function impairment if the benefit outweighs the potential risk. Patients with hepatic function impairment must be carefully monitored for drug toxicity.

➤*Voriconazole for oral suspension:*

Reconstitution – Tap the bottle to release the powder. Add 46 mL of water to the bottle. Shake the closed bottle vigorously for about 1 minute. Remove child-resistant cap and push bottle adaptor into the neck of the bottle. Replace the cap. Write the date of expiration of the reconstituted suspension on the bottle label (the shelf-life of the reconstituted suspension is 14 days at controlled room temperature (15° to 30°C [59° to 86°F]).

Instructions for use – Shake the closed bottle of reconstituted suspension for approximately 10 seconds before each use. Only administer the reconstituted oral suspension using the oral dispenser supplied with each pack.

Incompatibilities – Voriconazole for oral suspension and the 40 mg/mL reconstituted oral suspension should not be mixed with any other medication or additional flavoring agent. The suspension should not be diluted further with water or other vehicles.

➤*Storage/Stability:* Store voriconazole tablets at controlled room temperature (15° to 30°C [59° to 86°F]).

Store voriconazole powder for oral suspension in a refrigerator at 2° to 8°C (37° to 46°F) before reconstitution. The shelf-life of the powder for oral suspension is 18 months. Store the reconstituted suspension at 15° to 30°C (59° to 86°F). Do not refrigerate or freeze. Keep the container tightly closed. The shelf-life of the reconstituted suspension is 14 days. Discard any remaining suspension 14 days after reconstitution.

Actions

➤*Pharmacology:* Voriconazole is a triazole antifungal agent. The primary mode of action of voriconazole is the inhibition of fungal cytochrome P-450–mediated 14 alpha-lanosterol demethylation, an essential step in fungal ergosterol biosynthesis. The accumulation of 14 alpha-methyl sterols correlates with the subsequent loss of ergosterol in the fungal cell wall and may be responsible for the antifungal activity of voriconazole. Voriconazole has been shown to be more selective for fungal cytochrome P-450 enzymes than for various mammalian cytochrome P-450 enzyme systems.

➤*Pharmacokinetics:*

Absorption – The pharmacokinetic properties of voriconazole are similar following administration by the IV and oral routes. Based on a population pharmacokinetic analysis of pooled data in healthy subjects (n = 207), the oral bioavailability of voriconazole is estimated to be 96% (coefficient of variation [CV] 13%). Bioequivalence was established between the 200 mg tablet and the 40 mg/mL oral suspension when administered as a 400 mg every-12-hour loading dosage followed by a 200 mg every-12-hour maintenance dosage.

C_{max} is achieved 1 to 2 hours after dosing. When multiple doses of voriconazole are administered with high-fat meals, the mean C_{max} and AUC to last time point (AUC_τ) are reduced by 34% and 24%, respectively, when administered as a tablet, and by 58% and 37%, respectively, when administered as the oral suspension.

Distribution – The volume of distribution at steady state for voriconazole is estimated to be 4.6 L/kg, suggesting extensive distribution into tissues. Plasma protein binding is estimated to be 58% and was shown to be independent of plasma concentrations achieved after single and multiple oral doses of 200 or 300 mg (approximate range is 0.9 to 15 mcg/mL). Varying degrees of hepatic and renal function impairment do not affect the protein binding of voriconazole.

Metabolism – In vitro studies showed that voriconazole is metabolized by the human hepatic cytochrome P-450 enzymes, CYP2C19, CYP2C9, and CYP3A4.

The major metabolite of voriconazole is the N-oxide, which accounts for 72% of the circulating radiolabeled metabolites in plasma. Because this metabolite has minimal antifungal activity, it does not contribute to the overall efficacy of voriconazole.

Excretion – Voriconazole is eliminated via hepatic metabolism, with less than 2% of the dose excreted unchanged in the urine. After administration of a single radiolabeled dose of oral or IV voriconazole, preceded by multiple oral or IV dosing, approximately 80% to 83% of the radioactivity is recovered in the urine. The majority (more than 94%) of the total radioactivity is excreted in the first 96 hours after oral dosing.

As a result of nonlinear pharmacokinetics, the terminal half-life of voriconazole is dose dependent and therefore not useful in predicting the accumulation or elimination of voriconazole.

Special populations –

Renal function impairment: A pharmacokinetic study in subjects with renal failure undergoing hemodialysis showed that voriconazole is dialyzed with clearance of 121 mL/min. The IV vehicle, sulfobutylether 7- beta-cyclodextrin (SBECD), is hemodialyzed with clearance of 55 mL/min. A 4-hour hemodialysis session does not remove a sufficient amount of voriconazole to warrant dosage adjustment.

Hepatic function impairment: After a single oral dose of voriconazole 200 mg in 8 subjects with mild (Child-Pugh class A) and 4 patients with moderate (Child-Pugh class B) hepatic function impairment, the mean AUC was 3.2-fold higher than in age- and weight-matched controls with healthy hepatic function. There was no difference in mean C_{max} between the groups. When only the patients with mild (Child-Pugh class A) hepatic function impairment were compared with controls, there still was a 2.3-fold increase in the mean AUC in the group with hepatic function impairment compared with controls.

In an oral, multiple-dose study, AUC_τ was similar in 6 subjects with moderate hepatic function impairment (Child-Pugh class B) given a lower maintenance dose of 100 mg twice daily, compared with 6 subjects with healthy hepatic function given the standard 200 mg twice daily maintenance dose. The mean C_{max} was 20% lower in the hepatically impaired group.

See Administration and Dosage for more information.

Gender: In a multiple, oral-dose study, the mean C_{max} and AUC_τ for healthy young women were 83% and 113% higher, respectively, than in healthy young men (18 to 45 years of age) after tablet dosing. In the same study, no signifi-

VORICONAZOLE — ORAL

cant differences in the mean C_{max} and AUC_τ were observed between healthy elderly men and healthy elderly women (65 years of age and older). In a similar study, after dosing with the oral suspension, the mean AUC for healthy young women was 45% higher than in healthy young men, whereas the mean C_{max} was comparable between genders. The steady-state trough voriconazole concentrations (C_{min}) in women were 100% and 91% higher than in men receiving the tablet and the oral suspension, respectively.

➤*Microbiology:*

Activity in vitro and in vivo – Voriconazole has demonstrated in vitro activity against *Aspergillus* species (*A. fumigatus, A. flavus, A. niger* and *A. terreus*), *Candida* species (*Candida albicans, Candida glabrata, Candida krusei, Candida parapsilosis,* and *Candida tropicalis*), *S. apiospermum* and *Fusarium* spp., including *Fusarium solani*.

Drug resistance – Fungal isolates exhibiting reduced susceptibility to fluconazole or itraconazole also may show reduced susceptibility to voriconazole, suggesting cross-resistance can occur among these azoles. The relevance of cross-resistance and clinical outcome has not been fully characterized. Clinical cases where azole cross-resistance is demonstrated may require alternative antifungal therapy.

Contraindications

Hypersensitivity to voriconazole or its excipients. There is no information regarding cross-sensitivity between voriconazole and other azole antifungal agents. Use caution when prescribing voriconazole to patients with hypersensitivity to other azoles.

Coadministration with CYP3A4 substrates, terfenadine, astemizole, cisapride, pimozide, quinidine, sirolimus, rifampin, ritonavir (400 mg every 12 hours), efavirenz, rifabutin, and ergot alkaloids (ergotamine and dihydroergotamine) (see Drug Interactions for more information).

Warnings

➤*Visual disturbances:* The effect of voriconazole on visual function is not known if treatment continues beyond 28 days. If treatment continues beyond 28 days, monitor visual function, including visual acuity, visual field, and color perception.

➤*Hepatic toxicity:* In clinical trials, there have been uncommon cases of serious hepatic reactions during treatment with voriconazole (including clinical hepatitis, cholestasis, and fulminant hepatic failure, including fatalities). Instances of hepatic reactions were noted to occur primarily in patients with serious underlying medical conditions (predominantly hematological malignancy). Hepatic reactions, including hepatitis and jaundice, have occurred among patients with no other identifiable risk factors. Liver dysfunction usually has been reversible on discontinuation of therapy.

See Precautions for more information.

➤*Galactose intolerance:* Voriconazole tablets contain lactose; do not give to patients with rare hereditary problems of galactose intolerance, Lapp-lactase deficiency, or glucose-galactose malabsorption.

➤*Renal function impairment:* In patients with moderate to severe renal dysfunction (creatinine clearance [Ccr] less than 50 mL/min), accumulation of the IV vehicle SBECD occurs. Administer oral voriconazole to these patients, unless an assessment of the benefit/risk to the patient justifies the use of voriconazole IV. Closely monitor serum creatinine levels in these patients, and, if increases occur, consider changing to oral voriconazole therapy.

➤*Hepatic function impairment:* See Administration and Dosage for more information.

➤*Carcinogenesis:* Two-year carcinogenicity studies were conducted in rats and mice. Rats were given oral doses of voriconazole 6, 18, or 50 mg/kg , or 0.2, 0.6, or 1.6 times the recommended maintenance dose (RMD) on a mg/m^2 basis. Hepatocellular adenomas were detected in females at 50 mg/kg and hepatocellular carcinomas were found in males at 6 and 50 mg/kg. Mice were given oral doses of voriconazole 10, 30, or 100 mg/kg, or 0.1, 0.4, or 1.4 times the RMD on a mg/m^2 basis. In mice, hepatocellular adenomas were detected in males and females and hepatocellular carcinomas were detected in males at 1.4 times the RMD of voriconazole.

➤*Mutagenesis:* Voriconazole demonstrated clastogenic activity (mostly chromosome breaks) in human lymphocyte cultures in vitro. Voriconazole was not genotoxic in the Ames assay, Chinese hamster ovary (CHO) assay, mouse micronucleus assay or deoxyribonucleic acid (DNA) repair test (unscheduled DNA synthesis assay).

➤*Fertility impairment:* Voriconazole produced a reduction in the pregnancy rates of rats dosed at 50 mg/kg, or 1.6 times the RMD. This was statistically significant only in the preliminary study and not in a larger fertility study.

➤*Elderly:* See Actions for more information.

➤*Pregnancy: Category D.* Voriconazole can cause fetal harm when administered to a pregnant woman.

If this drug is used during pregnancy, or if the patient becomes pregnant while taking this drug, apprise the patient of the potential hazard to the fetus.

Voriconazole was teratogenic in rats (cleft palates, hydronephrosis/hydroureter) from 10 mg/kg (0.3 times the RMD on a mg/m^2 basis) and embryotoxic in rabbits at 100 mg/kg (6 times the RMD). Other effects in rats included reduced ossification of sacral and caudal vertebrae, skull, pubic and hyoid bone, supernumerary ribs, anomalies of the sternebrae, and dilatation of the ureter/renal pelvis. Plasma estradiol in pregnant rats was reduced at all dose levels. Voriconazole treatment in rats produced increased gestational length and dystocia, which were associated with increased perinatal pup mortality at the 10 mg/kg dose. The effects seen in rabbits were an increased embryomortality; reduced fetal weight; and increased incidences of skeletal variations, cervical ribs, and extrasternebral ossification sites.

Women of childbearing potential should use effective contraception during treatment.

➤*Lactation:* The excretion of voriconazole in breast milk has not been investigated. Breast-feeding mothers should not use voriconazole unless the benefit clearly outweighs the risk.

➤*Children:* Safety and efficacy in children younger than 12 years of age have not been established.

Precautions

➤*Monitoring:* Correct electrolyte disturbances such as hypocalcemia, hypokalemia, and hypomagnesemia, prior to initiation of voriconazole therapy.

Patient management should include laboratory evaluation of renal (particularly serum creatinine) and hepatic function (particularly LFTs and bilirubin).

Evaluate LFTs at the start of and during the course of voriconazole therapy. Monitor patients who develop abnormal LFTs during voriconazole therapy for the development of more severe hepatic injury. Patient management should include laboratory evaluation of hepatic function (particularly LFTs and bilirubin). Voriconazole has been associated with elevations in LFTs and clinical signs of liver damage, such as jaundice; use only in patients with severe hepatic insufficiency if the benefit outweighs the potential risk. Patients with hepatic insufficiency must be carefully monitored for drug toxicity. Discontinuation of voriconazole must be considered if clinical signs and symptoms consistent with liver disease develop that may be attributable to voriconazole.

If treatment continues beyond 28 days, monitor visual function, including visual acuity, visual field, and color perception.

Monitor patients for the development of abnormal renal function. This should include laboratory evaluation, particularly serum creatinine.

➤*Renal toxicity:* Acute renal failure has been observed in severely ill patients undergoing treatment with voriconazole. Patients being treated with voriconazole are likely to be treated concomitantly with nephrotoxic medications and have concurrent conditions that may result in decreased renal function.

➤*Dermatological reactions:* See Adverse Reactions for more information.

➤*Arrhythmias and QT prolongation:* Some azoles, including voriconazole, have been associated with prolongation of the QT interval on the ECG. During clinical development and postmarketing surveillance, there have been rare cases of arrhythmias (including ventricular arrhythmias such as torsade de pointes), cardiac arrests, and sudden deaths in patients taking voriconazole. These cases usually involved seriously ill patients with multiple confounding risk factors, such as histories of cardiotoxic chemotherapy, cardiomyopathy, hypokalemia, and concomitant medications that may have been contributory.

Administer voriconazole with caution to patients with these potentially proarrhythmic conditions.

➤*Hazardous tasks:* Advise patients to avoid potentially hazardous tasks, such as driving or operating machinery, if they perceive any change in vision.

➤*Photosensitivity:* Voriconazole has been infrequently associated with photosensitivity skin reaction, especially during long-term therapy. It is recommended that patients avoid strong, direct sunlight during voriconazole therapy.

Drug Interactions

Voriconazole Drug Interactions

Precipitant drug	Object drug[a]		Description
Barbiturates, long acting (eg, mephobarbital, phenobarbital), carbamazepine	Voriconazole	⬇	Coadministration may decrease voriconazole plasma concentrations. Coadministration is contraindicated.
Cimetidine	Voriconazole	⬆	Cimetidine increased voriconazole C_{max} and AUC by an average of 18% and 23%, respectively. No dosage adjustment is required.
NNRTIs eg, delavirdine, nevirapine)	Voriconazole	⬆⬇	Coadministration may induce or inhibit the metabolism of voriconazole. Monitor for toxicity and effectiveness of voriconazole. Voriconazole also may inhibit the metabolism of an NNRTI. Monitor for drug toxicity. Coadministration with efavirenz is contraindicated.
Voriconazole	NNRTIs (eg, delavirdine, efavirenz)	⬆	
Phenytoin	Voriconazole	⬇	Phenytoin may decrease the C_{max} and AUC of voriconazole by 50% and 70%, respectively. Voriconazole may increase the C_{max} and AUC of phenytoin up to 2 times. Monitor for adverse reactions and phenytoin plasma concentrations.
Voriconazole	Phenytoin	⬆	

VORICONAZOLE — ORAL

Voriconazole Drug Interactions

Precipitant drug	Object drug[a]		Description
Protease inhibitors (eg, amprenavir, ritonavir, saquinavir)	Voriconazole	↑↓	Voriconazole may inhibit the metabolism of certain protease inhibitors, and the metabolism of voriconazole may be inhibited or induced by certain protease inhibitors. Monitor closely for toxicity. Coadministration with indinavir showed no significant effects on voriconazole or indinavir exposure. Ritonavir (400 mg every 12 hours) decreased voriconazole AUC and C_{max} by approximately 82% and 66%, respectively. Coadministration with ritonavir (400 mg every 12 hours) is contraindicated.
Voriconazole	Protease inhibitors (eg, amprenavir, nelfinavir, ritonavir, saquinavir)	↑	
Proton pump inhibitors (eg, omeprazole)	Voriconazole	↑	Omeprazole may increase the C_{max} and AUC of voriconazole by an average of 15% and 40%, respectively. No dosage adjustment of voriconazole is recommended. Voriconazole may increase the C_{max} and AUC of omeprazole by an average of 2 and 4 times, respectively. When initiating voriconazole in patients already receiving omeprazole doses of 40 mg or more, reduce the dose of omeprazole by 50%. Voriconazole also may inhibit the metabolism of other proton pump inhibitors that are CYP2C19 substrates.
Voriconazole	Proton pump inhibitors (eg, omeprazole)		
Rifampin, Rifabutin	Voriconazole	↓	Voriconazole plasma concentrations are significantly reduced during coadministration. Voriconazole may increase the C_{max} and AUC of rifabutin by an average of 3 and 4 times, respectively. Coadministration is contraindicated.
Voriconazole	Rifabutin	↑	
Voriconazole	Astemizole, cisapride, pimozide, quinidine, terfenadine	↑	Voriconazole may inhibit the metabolism of these drugs. Increased plasma concentration may lead to QT prolongation and rare occurrences of torsades de pointes. Coadministration is contraindicated.
Voriconazole	Benzodiazepines (eg, alprazolam, midazolam, triazolam)	↑	Voriconazole may increase the plasma concentrations of benzodiazepines that are metabolized by CYP3A4 (eg, alprazolam, midazolam, triazolam). Adjust benzodiazepine dose if needed.
Voriconazole	Calcium channel blockers	↑	Voriconazole may increase plasma concentrations of calcium channel blockers that are metabolized by CYP3A4 (eg, felodipine). Adjust calcium channel blocker dose if needed.
Voriconazole	Coumarin anticoagulants (eg, warfarin)	↑	Coadministration may significantly increase PT. Closely monitor coagulation tests and adjust warfarin dose accordingly. Voriconazole also may increase the PT in patients receiving other coumarin anticoagulants.
Voriconazole	Cyclosporine	↑	Coadministration of oral voriconazole increased cyclosporine C_{max} and AUC an average of 1.1 and 1.7 times, respectively. When initiating voriconazole therapy in patients already receiving cyclosporine, reduce the dose of cyclosporine to 50% of the original dose. Frequently monitor cyclosporine levels during coadministration and when voriconazole is discontinued.
Voriconazole	Ergot alkaloids	↑	Voriconazole may increase the plasma concentrations of ergot alkaloids (eg, dihydroergotamine, ergotamine) and lead to ergotism. Coadministration is contraindicated.
Voriconazole	HMG-CoA-reductase inhibitors (eg, lovastatin)	↑	Voriconazole has been shown to inhibit lovastatin metabolism. Voriconazole may increase the plasma concentrations of statins that are metabolized by CYP3A4. Consider dosage adjustment of the statin during coadministration.
Voriconazole	Methadone	↑	Voriconazole may increase plasma concentrations of methadone. Increased concentrations of methadone may cause QT prolongation. Dose reduction of methadone may be needed.
Voriconazole	Prednisolone	↑	Voriconazole may increase the C_{max} and AUC of prednisolone by an average 11% and 34%, respectively. No dosage adjustment is recommended.
Voriconazole	Sirolimus	↑	Voriconazole can significantly increase the C_{max} and AUC of sirolimus an average of 7- and 11-fold, respectively. Coadministration is contraindicated.
Voriconazole	Sulfonylureas	↑	Voriconazole may increase plasma concentrations of sulfonylureas. Monitor for hypoglycemia. Dose adjustment of the sulfonylurea is recommended.
Voriconazole	Tacrolimus	↑	Voriconazole can significantly increase the C_{max} and AUC of tacrolimus by an average of 2- and 3-fold, respectively. When initiating voriconazole therapy in patients already receiving tacrolimus, reduce the dose of tacrolimus to 33% of the original dose. Frequently monitor tacrolimus levels during coadministration and when voriconazole is discontinued.
Voriconazole	Vinca alkaloids (eg, vincristine, vinblastine)	↑	Coadministration may increase the plasma concentrations of the vinca alkaloids and lead to neurotoxicity. Consider adjusting the dose of the vinca alkaloid and monitor for toxicity.

[a] ↓ = Object drug decreased. ↑ = Object drug increased.

➤*Drug/Food interactions:* See Actions for more information.

Adverse Reactions

➤*Overview:* The most frequently reported adverse reactions (all causalities) in the therapeutic trials were abdominal pain, diarrhea, fever, headache, nausea, peripheral edema, rash, respiratory disorder, sepsis, visual disturbances, and vomiting. The treatment-related adverse reactions that most often led to discontinuation of voriconazole therapy were elevated LFTs, rash, and visual disturbances.

➤*Less common adverse reactions:* The following adverse reactions occurred in less than 2% of all voriconazole-treated patients in all therapeutic studies (n = 1,655). This listing includes reactions where a causal relationship to voriconazole cannot be ruled out or those that may help the health care provider in managing the risks to the patients. The list does not include reactions included in the preceding table and does not include every reaction reported in the voriconazole clinical program.

Cardiovascular – Atrial arrhythmia, atrial fibrillation, AV block complete, bigeminy, bradycardia, bundle branch block, cardiomegaly, cardiomyopathy, cerebral hemorrhage, cerebral ischemia, cerebrovascular accident, congestive heart failure, deep thrombophlebitis, endocarditis, extrasystoles, heart arrest, hypertension, hypotension, myocardial infarction, nodal arrhythmia, palpitation, phlebitis, postural hypotension, pulmonary embolus, QT interval prolonged, supraventricular extrasystoles, supraventricular tachycardia, syncope, thrombophlebitis, vasodilatation, ventricular arrhythmia, ventricular fibrillation, ventricular tachycardia (including torsade de pointes).

CNS – Abnormal dreams, acute brain syndrome, agitation, akathisia, amnesia, anxiety, ataxia, brain edema, coma, confusion, convulsion, delirium, dementia, depersonalization, depression, diplopia, dizziness,

VORICONAZOLE — ORAL

encephalitis, encephalopathy, euphoria, extrapyramidal syndrome, generalized tonic-clonic seizure, Guillain-Barré syndrome, hypertonia, hypesthesia, insomnia, intracranial hypertension, libido decreased, neuralgia, neuropathy, nystagmus, oculogyric crisis, paresthesia, psychosis, somnolence, suicidal ideation, tremor, vertigo.

Dermatologic – Alopecia, angioedema, contact dermatitis, discoid lupus erythematosis, eczema, erythema multiforme, exfoliative dermatitis, fixed drug eruption, furunculosis, herpes simplex, maculopapular rash, melanosis, photosensitivity skin reaction, pruritus, psoriasis, skin discoloration, skin disorder, skin dry, Stevens-Johnson syndrome, sweating, toxic epidermal necrolysis, urticaria.

Endocrine – Adrenal cortex insufficiency, diabetes insipidus, hyperthyroidism, hypothyroidism.

GI – Abdomen enlarged, abdominal pain, anorexia, cheilitis, cholecystitis, cholelithiasis, constipation, diarrhea, duodenal ulcer perforation, duodenitis, dyspepsia, dysphagia, dry mouth, enlarged liver, esophageal ulcer, esophagitis, flatulence, gastroenteritis, gamma-glutamyl-transferase (GGT)/lactic dehydrogenase (LDH) elevated, GI hemorrhage, gingivitis, glossitis, gum hemorrhage, gum hyperplasia, hematemesis, hepatic coma, hepatic failure, hepatitis, intestinal perforation, intestinal ulcer, jaundice, melena, mouth ulceration, pancreatitis, parotid gland enlargement, periodontitis, proctitis, pseudomembranous colitis, rectal disorder, rectal hemorrhage, stomach ulcer, stomatitis, tongue edema.

GU – Anuria, blighted ovum, Ccr decreased, dysmenorrhea, dysuria, epididymitis, glycosuria, hemorrhagic cystitis, hematuria, hydronephrosis, impotence, kidney pain, kidney tubular necrosis, metrorrhagia, nephritis, nephrosis, oliguria, scrotal edema, urinary incontinence, urinary retention, urinary tract infection, uterine hemorrhage, vaginal hemorrhage.

Hematologic/Lymphatic – Agranulocytosis, anemia (macrocytic, megaloblastic, microcytic, normocytic), aplastic anemia, hemolytic anemia, bleeding time increased, cyanosis, disseminated intravascular coagulation (DIC), ecchymosis, enlarged spleen, eosinophilia, hypervolemia, leukopenia, lymphadenopathy, lymphangitis, marrow depression, pancytopenia, petechia, purpura, thrombocytopenia, thrombotic thrombocytopenic purpura.

Metabolic/Nutritional – Albuminuria, creatine phosphokinase increased, edema, glucose tolerance decreased, hypercalcemia, hypercholesteremia, hyperglycemia, hyperkalemia, hypermagnesemia, hypernatremia, hyperuricemia, hypocalcemia, hypoglycemia, hypomagnesemia, hyponatremia, hypophosphatemia, peripheral edema, serum urea nitrogen (BUN) increased, uremia.

Musculoskeletal – Arthralgia, arthritis, bone necrosis, bone pain, leg cramps, myalgia, myasthenia, myopathy, osteomalacia, osteoporosis.

Respiratory – Cough increased, dyspnea, epistaxis, hemoptysis, hypoxia, lung edema, pharyngitis, pleural effusion, pneumonia, respiratory disorder, respiratory distress syndrome, respiratory tract infection, rhinitis, sinusitis, voice alteration.

Special senses – Abnormality of accommodation, blepharitis, color blindness, conjunctivitis, corneal opacity, deafness, dry eyes, ear pain, eye hemorrhage, eye pain, hypoacusis, keratitis, keratoconjunctivitis, mydriasis, night blindness, optic atrophy, optic neuritis, otitis externa, papilledema, retinal hemorrhage, retinitis, scleritis, taste loss, taste perversion, tinnitus, uveitis, visual field defect.

Miscellaneous – Allergic reaction, anaphylactoid reaction, ascites, asthenia, back pain, bacterial infection, cellulitis, chest pain, edema, face edema, flank pain, flu syndrome, fungal infection, graft versus host reaction, granuloma, infection, mucous membrane disorder, multiorgan failure, pain, pelvic pain, peritonitis, sepsis, substernal chest pain.

➤*Lab test abnormalities:* The overall incidence of clinically significant transaminase abnormalities in all therapeutic studies was 12.4% (206 of 1,655) of patients treated with voriconazole. Increased incidence of LFT abnormalities may be associated with higher plasma concentrations and/or doses. The majority of abnormal LFTs resolved during treatment without dose adjustment or after dose adjustment, including discontinuation of therapy.

Voriconazole Lab Test Abnormalities (Study 305)			
	Criteria [a]	Voriconazole n/N [b]	Fluconazole n/N
Total bilirubin	> 1.5 × ULN	8/185 (4.3%)	7/186 (3.8%)
AST	> 3 × ULN	38/187 (20.3%)	15/186 (8.1%)
ALT	> 3 × ULN	20/187 (10.7%)	12/186 (6.5%)
Alkaline phosphatase	> 3 × ULN	19/187 (10.2%)	14/186 (7.5%)

[a] Without regard to baseline value.
[b] n = number of patients with a clinically significant abnormality while on study therapy; N = total number of patients with at least 1 observation of the given lab test while on study therapy.

Voriconazole Lab Test Abnormalities (Study 307/602)			
	Criteria [a]	Voriconazole n/N [c]	Amphotericin B [b] n/N
Total bilirubin	> 1.5 × ULN	35/180 (19.4%)	46/173 (26.6%)
AST	> 3 × ULN	21/180 (11.7%)	18/174 (10.3%)
ALT	> 3 × ULN	34/180 (18.9%)	40/173 (23.1%)
Alkaline phosphatase	> 3 × ULN	29/181 (16%)	38/173 (22%)
Creatinine	> 1.3× ULN	39/182 (21.4%)	102/177 (57.6%)
Potassium	< 0.9 × LLN [d]	30/181 (16.6%)	70/178 (39.3%)

[a] Without regard to baseline value.
[b] Amphotericin B followed by other licensed antifungal therapy.
[c] n = number of patients with a clinically significant abnormality while on study therapy; N = total number of patients with at least 1 observation of the given lab test while on study therapy.
[d] LLN = lower limit of normal.

Voriconazole Lab Test Abnormalities (Study 608)			
	Criteria[a]	Voriconazole n/N[b]	Amphotericin B followed by fluconazole (n/N)
Total bilirubin	> 1.5 × ULN	50/261 (19.2%)	31/115 (27%)
AST	> 3 × ULN	40/261 (15.3%)	16/116 (13.8%)
ALT	> 3 × ULN	22/261 (8.4%)	15/116 (12.9%)
Alkaline phosphatase	> 3 × ULN	59/261 (22.6%)	26/115 (22.6%)
Creatinine	> 1.3 × ULN	39/260 (15%)	32/118 (27.1%)
Potassium	< 0.9 × LLN	43/258 (16.7%)	35/118 (29.7%)

[a] Without regard to baseline value.
[b] n = number of patients with a clinically significant abnormality while on study therapy; N = total number of patients with at least 1 observation of the given lab test while on study therapy.

Overdosage

➤*Symptoms:* In clinical trials, there were 3 cases of accidental overdose. All occurred in pediatric patients who received up to 5 times the recommended IV dose of voriconazole. A single adverse reaction of photophobia of 10 minutes' duration was reported.

The minimum lethal oral dose in mice and rats was 300 mg/kg (equivalent to 4 and 7 times the RMD, based on body surface area). At this dose, clinical signs observed in both mice and rats included depressed behavior, dyspnea, mydriasis, partially closed eyes, prostration, salivation, and titubation (loss of balance while moving). Other signs in mice were convulsions, corneal opacification, and swollen abdomen.

➤*Treatment:* There is no known antidote to voriconazole.

Voriconazole is hemodialyzed with clearance of 121 mL/min. The IV vehicle, SBECD, is hemodialyzed with clearance of 55 mL/min. In an overdose, hemodialysis may assist in the removal of voriconazole and SBECD from the body.

Patient Information

Advise patients to take voriconazole tablets or oral suspension at least 1 hour before or 1 hour after a meal.

Advise patients not to drive at night while taking voriconazole. Voriconazole may cause changes to vision, including blurring and/or photophobia.

Advise patients to avoid potentially hazardous tasks, such as driving or operating machinery if they perceive any change in vision.

Advise patients to avoid strong, direct sunlight during voriconazole therapy.

Advise of childbearing potential to use effective contraception during treatment.

Voriconazole for oral suspension contains sucrose and is not recommended for patients with rare hereditary problems of fructose intolerance, sucrase-isomaltase deficiency, or glucose-galactose malabsorption.

VORICONAZOLE — INJECTION

Indications

➤*Candidemia:* For the treatment of candidemia in nonneutropenic patients and the following *Candida* infections: disseminated infections in skin and infections in abdomen, kidney, bladder wall, and wounds.

➤*Esophageal candidiasis:* For the treatment of esophageal candidiasis.

➤*Invasive aspergillosis:* For the treatment of invasive aspergillosis. In clinical trials, the majority of isolates recovered were *Aspergillus fumigatus*. There was a small number of cases of culture-proven disease caused by species of *Aspergillus* other than *Aspergillus fumigatus* (eg, *A. flavus, Aspergillus niger, Aspergillus terreus*).

➤*Serious fungal infections:* For the treatment of serious fungal infections caused by *Scedosporium apiospermum* (asexual form of *Pseudallescheria boydii*) and *Fusarium* spp., including *Fusarium solani*, in patients intolerant of, or refractory to, other therapy.

Administration and Dosage

➤*Approved by the FDA:* May 24, 2002.

Not for IV bolus injection.

Electrolyte disturbances, such as hypokalemia, hypomagnesemia, and hypocalcemia, should be corrected prior to initiation of voriconazole therapy.

VORICONAZOLE — INJECTION

➤*Dosage:*

Adults –

Candidemia in nonneutropenic patients and other deep tissue Candida infections: See the following table. Patients should be treated for at least 14 days following resolution of symptoms or following last positive culture, whichever is longer.

Esophageal candidiasis: See the following table. Patients should be treated for a minimum of 14 days and for at least 7 days following resolution of symptoms.

Invasive aspergillosis and serious fungal infections caused by Fusarium spp. and S. apiospermum: For the treatment of adults with invasive aspergillosis and infections caused by *Fusarium* spp. and *S. apiospermum*, therapy must be initiated with the specified loading dose regimen of IV voriconazole to achieve plasma concentrations on day 1 that are close to steady state. On the basis of high oral bioavailability, switching between IV and oral administration is appropriate when clinically indicated. Once the patient can tolerate medication given by mouth, the oral tablet form or oral suspension form of voriconazole may be utilized.

The recommended dosing regimen of voriconazole is as follows:

Voriconazole Recommended Dosing Regimen		
	Loading dosage	Maintenance dosage
Infection	IV	IV
Candidemia in nonneutropenic patients and other deep tissue *Candida* infections	6 mg/kg every 12 h for the first 24 h	3 to 4 mg/kg every 12 h[a]
Esophageal candidiasis	[b]	[b]
Invasive aspergillosis	6 mg/kg every 12 h for the first 24 h	4 mg/kg every 12 h
Scedosporiosis and fusariosis	6 mg/kg every 12 h for the first 24 h	4 mg/kg every 12 h

[a] In clinical trials, patients with candidemia received 3 mg/kg every 12 hours as primary therapy, while patients with other deep tissue *Candida* infections received 4 mg/kg as salvage therapy. Base appropriate dosage on the severity and nature of the infection.
[b] Not evaluated in patients with esophageal candidiasis.

Dosage adjustment: If patients are unable to tolerate 4 mg/kg IV, reduce the IV maintenance dosage to 3 mg/kg every 12 hours.

• *Coadministration with phenytoin* – Phenytoin may be coadministered with voriconazole if the IV maintenance dosage of voriconazole is increased to 5 mg/kg every 12 hours.

➤*Hepatic function impairment:* In the clinical program, patients were included who had baseline liver function tests (ALT, AST) up to 5 times the upper limit of normal (ULN). No dose adjustment is necessary in patients with this degree of abnormal liver function, but continued monitoring of liver function tests for further elevations is recommended. Patient management should include laboratory evaluation of hepatic function (particularly liver function tests and bilirubin).

It is recommended that the standard loading-dose regimens be used, but that the maintenance dose be halved in patients with mild to moderate hepatic cirrhosis (Child-Pugh class A and B, respectively.).

Voriconazole has not been studied in patients with severe hepatic cirrhosis (Child-Pugh class C) or in patients with chronic hepatitis B or chronic hepatitis C disease. Voriconazole has been associated with elevations in liver function tests and clinical signs of liver damage, such as jaundice, and should only be used in patients with severe hepatic function impairment if the benefit outweighs the potential risk. Patients with hepatic function impairment must be carefully monitored for drug toxicity.

➤*Renal function impairment:* In patients with moderate or severe renal function impairment (creatinine clearance [Ccr] less than 50 mL/min), accumulation of the IV vehicle, sulfobutylether 7-beta-cyclodextrin (SBECD), occurs. Oral voriconazole should be administered to these patients, unless an assessment of the benefit/risk to the patient justifies the use of IV voriconazole. Serum creatinine levels should be monitored closely in these patients, and, if increases occur, consideration should be given to changing to oral voriconazole therapy.

➤*IV administration:*

Reconstitution – The powder is reconstituted with 19 mL of water for injection to obtain an extractable volume of 20 mL of clear concentrate containing 10 mg/mL of voriconazole. It is recommended that a standard 20 mL (nonautomated) syringe be used to ensure that the exact amount (19 mL) of water for injection is dispensed. Discard the vial if a vacuum does not pull the diluent into the vial. Shake the vial until all the powder is dissolved.

Dilution – Voriconazole must be infused over 1 to 2 hours at a concentration of 5 mg/mL or less. Therefore, the required volume of the voriconazole 10 mg/mL concentrate should be further diluted as follows:

1.) Calculate the volume of voriconazole 10 mg/mL concentrate required based on the patient's weight (see the following table).
2.) In order to allow the required volume of voriconazole concentrate to be added, withdraw and discard at least an equal volume of diluent from the infusion bag or bottle to be used. The volume of diluent remaining in the bag or bottle should be such that when the voriconazole 10 mg/mL concentrate is added, the final concentration is not less than 0.5 mg/mL nor greater than 5 mg/mL.
3.) Using a suitable size syringe and aseptic technique, withdraw the required volume of voriconazole concentrate from the appropriate number of vials and add to the infusion bag or bottle. Discard partially used vials.

The final voriconazole solution must be infused over 1 to 2 hours at a maximum rate of 3 mg/kg/h.

Required Volumes of Voriconazole 10 mg/mL Concentrate			
	Volume of voriconazole concentrate (10 mg/mL) required for:		
Body weight (kg)	3 mg/kg dose (number of vials)	4 mg/kg dose (number of vials)	6 mg/kg dose (number of vials)
30	9 mL (1)	12 mL (1)	18 mL (1)
35	10.5 mL (1)	14 mL (1)	21 mL (2)
40	12 mL (1)	16 mL (1)	24 mL (2)
45	13.5 mL (1)	18 mL (1)	27 mL (2)
50	15 mL (1)	20 mL (1)	30 mL (2)
55	16.5 mL (1)	22 mL (2)	33 mL (2)
60	18 mL (1)	24 mL (2)	36 mL (2)
65	19.5 mL (1)	26 mL (2)	39 mL (2)
70	21 mL (2)	28 mL (2)	42 mL (3)
75	22.5 mL (2)	30 mL (2)	45 mL (3)
80	24 mL (2)	32 mL (2)	48 mL (3)
85	25.5 mL (2)	34 mL (2)	51 mL (3)
90	27 mL (2)	36 mL (2)	54 mL (3)
95	28.5 mL (2)	38 mL (2)	57 mL (3)
100	30 mL (2)	40 mL (2)	60 mL (3)

The reconstituted solution can be diluted with the following: 9 mg/mL (0.9%) sodium chloride; Ringer's lactate; 5% dextrose and Ringer's lactate; 5% dextrose and 0.45% sodium chloride; 5% dextrose; 5% dextrose and 20 meq potassium chloride; 0.45% sodium chloride; 5% dextrose and 0.9% sodium chloride.

Admixture incompatibilities – Voriconazole IV must not be infused into the same line or cannula concomitantly with other drug infusions, including parenteral nutrition (eg, *Aminofusin 10% Plus*). *Aminofusin 10% Plus* is physically incompatible, with an increase in subvisible particulate matter after 24 hours storage at 4°C (39.2°F).

Infusions of blood products must not occur simultaneously with voriconazole IV.

Infusions of total parenteral nutrition can occur simultaneously with voriconazole IV.

Voriconazole IV must not be diluted with 4.2% sodium bicarbonate infusion. The mildly alkaline nature of this diluent caused slight degradation of voriconazole after 24 hours storage at room temperature. Although refrigerated storage is recommended following reconstitution, use of this diluent is not recommended as a precautionary measure. Compatibility with other concentrations is unknown.

➤*Storage/Stability:* Store unreconstituted vials at controlled room temperature 15° to 30°C (59° to 86°F). Voriconazole is a single-dose, unpreserved, sterile lyophile. From a microbiological point of view, following reconstitution of the lyophile with water for injection, use the reconstituted solution immediately. If not used immediately, in-use storage times and conditions prior to use are the responsibility of the user and should not be longer than 24 hours at 2° to 8°C (36° to 46°F). Chemical and physical in-use stability has been demonstrated for 24 hours at 2° to 8°C (36° to 46°F). This medicinal product is for single use only; discard any unused solution. Only use clear solutions without particles.

Actions

➤*Pharmacology:* Voriconazole is a triazole antifungal agent. The primary mode of action of voriconazole is the inhibition of fungal cytochrome P-450–mediated 14 alpha-lanosterol demethylation, an essential step in fungal ergosterol biosynthesis. The accumulation of 14 alpha-methyl sterols correlates with the subsequent loss of ergosterol in the fungal cell wall and may be responsible for the antifungal activity of voriconazole. Voriconazole has been shown to be more selective for fungal cytochrome P-450 enzymes than for various mammalian cytochrome P-450 enzyme systems.

➤*Pharmacokinetics:*

Absorption – The pharmacokinetic properties of voriconazole are similar following administration by the IV and oral routes.

Maximum plasma concentrations (C_{max}) are achieved 1 to 2 hours after dosing.

Distribution – The volume of distribution at steady state for voriconazole is estimated to be 4.6 L/kg, suggesting extensive distribution into tissues. Plasma protein binding is estimated to be 58%. Varying degrees of hepatic and renal function impairment do not affect the protein binding of voriconazole.

Metabolism – In vitro studies showed that voriconazole is metabolized by the human hepatic cytochrome P-450 enzymes, CYP2C19, CYP2C9, and CYP3A4. Results of in vitro metabolism studies indicate that the affinity of voriconazole is highest for CYP2C19, followed by CYP2C9, and is appreciably lower for CYP3A4. Inhibitors or inducers of these 3 enzymes may increase or decrease voriconazole systemic exposure (plasma concentrations), respectively.

The major metabolite of voriconazole is the N-oxide, which accounts for 72% of the circulating radiolabeled metabolites in plasma. Because this metabolite has minimal antifungal activity, it does not contribute to the overall efficacy of voriconazole.

VORICONAZOLE — INJECTION

Excretion – Voriconazole is eliminated via hepatic metabolism with less than 2% of the dose excreted unchanged in the urine. After administration of a single radiolabeled dose of either oral or IV voriconazole, preceded by multiple oral or IV dosing, approximately 80% to 83% of the radioactivity is recovered in the urine. The majority (greater than 94%) of the total radioactivity is excreted in the first 96 hours after both oral and IV dosing.

As a result of nonlinear pharmacokinetics, the terminal half-life of voriconazole is dose dependent and, therefore, not useful in predicting the accumulation or elimination of voriconazole.

Special populations –

Renal function impairment: In patients with moderate renal dysfunction (Ccr 30 to 50 mL/min), accumulation of the IV vehicle, SBECD, occurs. The AUC and C_{max} of SBECD were increased by 4-fold and almost 50%, respectively, in the moderately impaired group compared with the healthy control group.

Avoid IV voriconazole in patients with moderate or severe renal function impairment (Ccr less than 50 mL/min), unless an assessment of the benefit/risk to the patient justifies the use of IV voriconazole.

A pharmacokinetic study in subjects with renal failure undergoing hemodialysis showed that voriconazole is dialyzed with clearance of 121 mL/min. The IV vehicle, SBECD, is hemodialyzed with clearance of 55 mL/min. A 4-hour hemodialysis session does not remove a sufficient amount of voriconazole to warrant dosage adjustment.

Hepatic function impairment: See Administration and Dosage for more information.

Elderly: In the clinical program, no dosage adjustment was made on the basis of age. An analysis of pharmacokinetic data obtained from 552 patients from 10 voriconazole clinical trials showed that the median voriconazole plasma concentrations in the elderly patients (65 years of age and older) were approximately 80% to 90% higher than those in the younger patients (65 years of age and younger) after either IV or oral administration. However, the safety profile of voriconazole in younger and elderly subjects was similar and, therefore, no dosage adjustment is necessary for the elderly.

Children:

➤*Microbiology:* Voriconazole has demonstrated in vitro activity against *Aspergillus* species (*A. fumigatus*, *A. flavus*, *A. niger* and *A. terreus*), *Candida* species (*Candida albicans*, *Candida glabrata*, *Candida krusei*, *Candida parapsilosis*, and *Candida tropicalis*), *S. apiospermum*, and *Fusarium* spp., including *Fusarium solani*.

Drug resistance –

Fungal isolates exhibiting reduced susceptibility to fluconazole or itraconazole may also show reduced susceptibility to voriconazole, suggesting cross-resistance can occur among these azoles. The relevance of cross-resistance and clinical outcome has not been fully characterized. Clinical cases where azole cross-resistance is demonstrated may require alternative antifungal therapy.

Contraindications

Hypersensitivity to voriconazole or its excipients. There is no information regarding cross-sensitivity between voriconazole and other azole antifungal agents. Use caution when prescribing voriconazole to patients with hypersensitivity to other azoles.

Coadministration with CYP3A4 substrates, terfenadine, astemizole, cisapride, pimozide, quinidine, sirolimus, rifampin, ritonavir (400 mg every 12 hours), efavirenz, rifabutin, and ergot alkaloids (ergotamine and dihydroergotamine) (see Drug Interactions for more information).

Warnings

➤*Visual disturbances:* The effect of voriconazole on visual function is not known if treatment continues beyond 28 days. If treatment continues beyond 28 days, monitor visual function, including visual acuity, visual field, and color perception.

➤*Hepatic toxicity:* In clinical trials, there have been uncommon cases of serious hepatic reactions during treatment with voriconazole (including clinical hepatitis, cholestasis, and fulminant hepatic failure, including fatalities). Instances of hepatic reactions were noted to occur primarily in patients with serious underlying medical conditions (predominantly hematological malignancy). Hepatic reactions, including hepatitis and jaundice, have occurred among patients with no other identifiable risk factors. Liver dysfunction has usually been reversible on discontinuation of therapy.

See Precautions for more information.

➤*Renal function impairment:* See Administration and Dosage for more information.

➤*Hepatic function impairment:* See Administration and Dosage for more information.

➤*Carcinogenesis:* Two-year carcinogenicity studies were conducted in rats and mice. Rats were given oral doses of voriconazole 6, 18, or 50 mg/kg , or 0.2, 0.6, or 1.6 times the recommended maintenance dose (RMD) on a mg/m^2 basis. Hepatocellular adenomas were detected in females at 50 mg/kg, and hepatocellular carcinomas were found in males at 6 and 50 mg/kg. Mice were given oral doses of 10, 30, or 100 mg/kg voriconazole, or 0.1, 0.4, or 1.4 times the RMD on a mg/m^2 basis. In mice, hepatocellular adenomas were detected in males and females and hepatocellular carcinomas were detected in males at 1.4 times the RMD of voriconazole.

➤*Mutagenesis:* Voriconazole demonstrated clastogenic activity (mostly chromosome breaks) in human lymphocyte cultures in vitro. Voriconazole was not genotoxic in the Ames assay, Chinese hamster ovary (CHO) assay, mouse micronucleus assay, or deoxyribonucleic acid (DNA) repair test (unscheduled DNA synthesis assay).

➤*Fertility impairment:* Voriconazole produced a reduction in the pregnancy rates of rats dosed at 50 mg/kg, or 1.6 times the RMD. This was statistically significant only in the preliminary study and not in a larger fertility study.

➤*Elderly:* See Actions for more information.

➤*Pregnancy: Category D.* Voriconazole can cause fetal harm when administered to a pregnant woman.

If this drug is used during pregnancy or if the patient becomes pregnant while taking this drug, apprise the patient of the potential hazard to the fetus.

Voriconazole was teratogenic in rats (cleft palates, hydronephrosis/hydroureter) from 10 mg/kg (0.3 times the RMD on a mg/m^2 basis) and embryotoxic in rabbits at 100 mg/kg (6 times the RMD). Other effects in rats included reduced ossification of sacral and caudal vertebrae, skull, pubic and hyoid bone, supernumerary ribs, anomalies of the sternebrae, and dilatation of the ureter/renal pelvis. Plasma estradiol in pregnant rats was reduced at all dose levels. Voriconazole treatment in rats produced increased gestational length and dystocia, which were associated with increased perinatal pup mortality at the 10 mg/kg dose. The effects seen in rabbits were an increased embryomortality, reduced fetal weight, and increased incidences of skeletal variations, cervical ribs, and extrasternebral ossification sites.

Women of childbearing potential should use effective contraception during treatment.

➤*Lactation:* The excretion of voriconazole in breast milk has not been investigated. Breast-feeding mothers should not use voriconazole unless the benefit clearly outweighs the risk.

➤*Children:* Safety and efficacy in children younger than 12 years of age have not been established.

Precautions

➤*Monitoring:* Correct electrolyte disturbances such as hypokalemia, hypomagnesemia, and hypocalcemia prior to initiation of voriconazole therapy.

Patient management should include laboratory evaluation of renal (particularly serum creatinine) and hepatic function (particularly liver function tests and bilirubin).

Monitor patients for the development of abnormal renal function. This should include laboratory evaluation, particularly serum creatinine.

Evaluate liver function tests at the start of and during the course of voriconazole therapy. Monitor patients who develop abnormal liver function tests during voriconazole therapy for the development of more severe hepatic injury. Patient management should include laboratory evaluation of hepatic function (particularly liver function tests and bilirubin). Voriconazole has been associated with elevations in liver function tests and clinical signs of liver damage, such as jaundice; use only in patients with severe hepatic function impairment if the benefit outweighs the potential risk. Patients with hepatic function impairment must be carefully monitored for drug toxicity. Discontinuation of voriconazole must be considered if clinical signs and symptoms consistent with liver disease develop that may be attributable to voriconazole.

If treatment continues beyond 28 days, monitor visual function, including visual acuity, visual field and color perception.

➤*Renal toxicity:* Acute renal failure has been observed in severely ill patients undergoing treatment with voriconazole. Patients being treated with voriconazole are likely to be treated concomitantly with nephrotoxic medications and have concurrent conditions that may result in decreased renal function.

➤*Dermatological reactions:* Patients have rarely developed serious cutaneous reactions (eg, Stevens-Johnson syndrome) during treatment with voriconazole. If patients develop a rash, monitor them closely and consider discontinuation of voriconazole. Voriconazole has been infrequently associated with photosensitivity skin reaction, especially during long-term therapy. It is recommended that patients avoid strong, direct sunlight during voriconazole therapy.

➤*Infusion-related reactions:* During infusion of the IV formulation of voriconazole in healthy subjects, anaphylactoid-type reactions, including flushing, fever, sweating, tachycardia, chest tightness, dyspnea, faintness, nausea, pruritus, and rash, have occurred uncommonly. Symptoms appeared immediately upon initiating the infusion. Consider stopping the infusion if these reactions occur.

➤*Arrhythmias and QT prolongation:* Some azoles, including voriconazole, have been associated with prolongation of the QT interval on the electrocardiogram. During clinical development and postmarketing surveillance, there have been rare cases of arrhythmias (including ventricular arrhythmias such as torsade de pointes), cardiac arrests, and sudden deaths in patients taking voriconazole. These cases usually involved seriously ill patients with multiple confounding risk factors, such as histories of cardiotoxic chemotherapy, cardiomyopathy, hypokalemia, and concomitant medications that may have been contributory.

Administer voriconazole with caution to patients with these potentially proarrhythmic conditions.

➤*Hazardous tasks:* Advise patients to avoid potentially hazardous tasks, such as driving or operating machinery, if they perceive any change in vision.

VORICONAZOLE — INJECTION

➤*Photosensitivity:* Voriconazole has been infrequently associated with photosensitivity skin reaction, especially during long-term therapy. It is recommended that patients avoid strong, direct sunlight during voriconazole therapy.

Drug Interactions

Voriconazole Drug Interactions

Precipitant drug	Object drug[a]		Description
Barbiturates, long acting (eg, mephobarbital, phenobarbital), carbamazepine	Voriconazole	↓	Coadministration may decrease voriconazole plasma concentrations. Coadministration is contraindicated.
Cimetidine	Voriconazole	↑	Cimetidine increased voriconazole C_{max} and AUC an average of 18% and 23%, respectively. No dosage adjustment is required.
Nonnucleoside reverse transcriptase inhibitors (NNRTIs) (eg, delavirdine, nevirapine)	Voriconazole	↑↓	Coadministration may induce or inhibit the metabolism of voriconazole. Monitor for toxicity and effectiveness of voriconazole. Voriconazole also may inhibit the metabolism of an NNRTI. Monitor for drug toxicity. Coadministration with efavirenz is contraindicated.
Voriconazole	NNRTIs (eg, delavirdine, efavirenz)	↑	
Phenytoin	Voriconazole	↓	Phenytoin may decrease the C_{max} and AUC of voriconazole 50% and 70%, respectively. Voriconazole may increase the C_{max} and AUC of phenytoin up to 2 times. Monitor for adverse reactions and phenytoin plasma concentrations.
Voriconazole	Phenytoin	↑	
Protease inhibitors (eg, amprenavir, ritonavir, saquinavir)	Voriconazole	↑↓	Voriconazole may inhibit the metabolism of certain protease inhibitors, and the metabolism of voriconazole may be inhibited or induced by certain protease inhibitors. Monitor closely for toxicity. Coadministration with indinavir showed no significant effects on voriconazole or indinavir exposure. Ritonavir (400 mg every 12 hours) decreased voriconazole AUC and C_{max} approximately 82% and 66%, respectively. Coadministration with ritonavir (400 mg every 12 hours) is contraindicated.
Voriconazole	Protease inhibitors (eg, ritonavir, saquinavir, amprenavir, nelfinavir)	↑	
Proton pump inhibitors (eg, omeprazole)	Voriconazole	↑	Omeprazole may increase the C_{max} and AUC of voriconazole an average of 15% and 40%, respectively. No dosage adjustment of voriconazole is recommended. Voriconazole may increase the C_{max} and AUC of omeprazole by an average of 2 and 4 times, respectively. When initiating voriconazole in patients already receiving omeprazole doses of 40 mg or greater, reduce the dose of omeprazole by 50%. Voriconazole also may inhibit the metabolism of other proton pump inhibitors that are CYP2C19 substrates.
Voriconazole	Proton pump inhibitors (eg, omeprazole)		
Rifampin, rifabutin	Voriconazole	↓	Voriconazole plasma concentrations are significantly reduced during coadministration. Voriconazole may increase the C_{max} and AUC of rifabutin by an average of 3 and 4 times, respectively. Coadministration is contraindicated.
Voriconazole	Rifabutin	↑	
Voriconazole	Astemizole, cisapride, pimozide, quinidine, terfenadine	↑	Voriconazole may inhibit the metabolism of these drugs. Increased plasma concentration may lead to QT prolongation and rare occurrences of torsades de pointes. Coadministration is contraindicated.
Voriconazole	Benzodiazepines (eg, midazolam, triazolam, alprazolam)	↑	Voriconazole may increase the plasma concentrations of benzodiazepines that are metabolized by CYP3A4 (eg, alprazolam, midazolam, triazolam). Adjust benzodiazepine dose if needed.
Voriconazole	Calcium channel blockers	↑	Voriconazole may increase plasma concentrations of calcium channel blockers that are metabolized by CYP3A4 (eg, felodipine). Adjust calcium channel blocker dosage if needed.
Voriconazole	Coumarin anticoagulants (eg, warfarin)	↑	Coadministration may significantly increase PT. Closely monitor coagulation tests and adjust warfarin dose accordingly. Voriconazole also may increase the PT in patients receiving other coumarin anticoagulants.
Voriconazole	Cyclosporine	↑	Coadministration of oral voriconazole increased cyclosporine C_{max} and AUC an average of 1.1 and 1.7 times, respectively. When initiating voriconazole therapy in patients already receiving cyclosporine, reduce the dose of cyclosporine to 50% of the original dose. Frequently monitor cyclosporine levels during coadministration and when voriconazole is discontinued.
Voriconazole	Ergot alkaloids	↑	Voriconazole may increase the plasma concentrations of ergot alkaloids (eg, ergotamine, dihydroergotamine) and lead to ergotism. Coadministration is contraindicated.
Voriconazole	HMG-CoA-reductase inhibitors (eg, lovastatin)	↑	Voriconazole has been shown to inhibit lovastatin metabolism. Voriconazole may increase the plasma concentrations of statins that are metabolized by CYP3A4. Consider dosage adjustment of the statin during coadministration.
Voriconazole	Methadone	↑	Voriconazole may increase plasma concentrations of methadone. Increased concentrations of methadone may cause QT prolongation. Dose reduction of methadone may be needed.
Voriconazole	Prednisolone	↑	Voriconazole may increase the C_{max} and AUC of prednisolone by an average 11% and 34%, respectively. No dosage adjustment recommended.
Voriconazole	Sirolimus	↑	Voriconazole can significantly increase the C_{max} and AUC of sirolimus an average of 7- and 11-fold, respectively. Coadministration is contraindicated.
Voriconazole	Sulfonylureas	↑	Voriconazole may increase plasma concentrations of sulfonylureas. Monitor for hypoglycemia. Dose adjustment of the sulfonylurea is recommended.

VORICONAZOLE — INJECTION

Voriconazole Drug Interactions			
Precipitant drug	Object drug[a]		Description
Voriconazole	Tacrolimus	↑	Voriconazole can significantly increase the C_{max} and AUC of tacrolimus by an average of 2- and 3-fold, respectively. When initiating voriconazole therapy in patients already receiving tacrolimus, reduce the dose of tacrolimus to 33% of the original dose. Frequently monitor tacrolimus levels during coadministration and when voriconazole is discontinued.
Voriconazole	Vinca alkaloids (eg, vincristine, vinblastine)	↑	Coadministration may increase the plasma concentrations of the vinca alkaloids and lead to neurotoxicity. Consider adjusting the dose of the vinca alkaloid and monitor for toxicity.

[a] ↓ = Object drug decreased. ↑ = Object drug increased.

Adverse Reactions

The most frequently reported adverse reactions (all causalities) in the therapeutic trials were abdominal pain, diarrhea, fever, headache, nausea, peripheral edema, rash, respiratory disorder, sepsis, visual disturbances, and vomiting. The treatment-related adverse reactions which most often led to discontinuation of voriconazole therapy were elevated liver function tests, rash, and visual disturbances.

➤*Discussion of adverse reactions:*

Voriconazole Adverse Reactions

Rate ≥ 2% on Voriconazole or Adverse Reactions of Concern in All Therapeutic Studies Population, Studies 307/602-608 Combined, or Study 305. Possibly Related to Therapy or Causality Unknown[a]

	All studies	Studies 307/602 and 608 (IV/oral therapy)			Study 305	
Adverse reaction	Voriconazole (n = 1,655)	Voriconazole (n = 468)	Amphotericin B[b] (n = 185)	Amphotericin B followed by fluconazole (n = 131)	Voriconazole (n = 200)	Fluconazole (n = 191)
Cardiovascular						
Tachycardia	39 (2.4%)	6 (1.3%)	5 (2.7%)	0	0	0
CNS						
Hallucinations	39 (2.4%)	13 (2.8%)	1 (0.5%)	0	0	0
Headache	49 (3%)	9 (1.9%)	8 (4.3%)	1 (0.8%)	0	1 (0.5%)
Dermatologic						
Rash	88 (5.3%)	20 (4.3%)	7 (3.8%)	1 (0.8%)	3 (1.5%)	1 (0.5%)
GI						
Nausea	89 (5.4%)	18 (3.8%)	29 (15.7%)	2 (1.5%)	2 (1%)	3 (1.6%)
Vomiting	72 (4.4%)	15 (3.2%)	18 (9.7%)	1 (0.8%)	2 (1%)	1 (0.5%)
Hepatic						
Cholestatic jaundice	17 (1%)	8 (1.7%)	0	1 (0.8%)	3 (1.5%)	0
Liver function tests abnormal	45 (2.7%)	15 (3.2%)	4 (2.2%)	1 (0.8%)	6 (3%)	2 (1%)
Metabolic/Nutritional						
Alkaline phosphatase increased	59 (3.6%)	19 (4.1%)	4 (2.2%)	3 (2.3%)	10 (5%)	3 (1.6%)
ALT increased	29 (1.8%)	9 (1.9%)	1 (0.5%)	2 (1.5%)	6 (3%)	2 (1%)
AST increased	31 (1.9%)	9 (1.9%)	0	1 (0.8%)	8 (4%)	2 (1%)
Bilirubinemia	15 (0.9%)	5 (1.1%)	3 (1.6%)	2 (1.5%)	1 (0.5%)	0
Creatinine increased	4 (0.2%)	0	59 (31.9%)	10 (7.6%)	1 (0.5%)	0
Hepatic enzymes increased	30 (1.8%)	11 (2.4%)	5 (2.7%)	1 (0.8%)	3 (1.5%)	0
Hypokalemia	26 (1.6%)	3 (0.6%)	36 (19.5%)	16 (12.2%)	0	0
Renal						
Acute kidney failure	7 (0.4%)	2 (0.4%)	11 (5.9%)	7 (5.3%)	0	0
Kidney function abnormal	10 (0.6%)	6 (1.3%)	40 (21.6%)	9 (6.9%)	1 (0.5%)	1 (0.5%)
Special senses[c]						
Abnormal vision	310 (18.7%)	63 (13.5%)	1 (0.5%)	0	31 (15.5%)	8 (4.2%)
Chromatopsia	20 (1.2%)	2 (0.4%)	0	0	2 (1%)	0
Photophobia	37 (2.2%)	8 (1.7%)	0	0	5 (2.5%)	2 (1%)
Miscellaneous						
Chills	61 (3.7%)	1 (0.2%)	36 (19.5%)	8 (6.1%)	1 (0.5%)	0
Fever	94 (5.7%)	8 (1.7%)	25 (13.5%)	5 (3.8%)	0	0

[a] Study 307/602: invasive aspergillosis; study 608: candidemia; study 305: esophageal candidiasis.
[b] Amphotericin B followed by other licensed antifungal therapy.
[c] See Warnings and Patient Information.

Dermatologic – See Precautions for more information.

Ophthalmic – Voriconazole treatment-related visual disturbances are common. In therapeutic trials, approximately 21% of patients experienced abnormal vision, color vision change, and/or photophobia. The visual disturbances were generally mild and rarely resulted in discontinuation. Visual disturbances may be associated with higher plasma concentrations and/or doses.

The mechanism of action of the visual disturbance is unknown, although the site of action is most likely to be within the retina. In a study in healthy volunteers investigating the effect of 28-day treatment with voriconazole on retinal function, voriconazole caused a decrease in the electroretinogram (ERG) waveform amplitude, a decrease in the visual field, and an alteration in color perception. The ERG measures electrical currents in the retina. The effects were noted early in administration of voriconazole and continued through the course of study drug dosing.

Fourteen days after end of dosing, ERG, visual fields, and color perception returned to normal. Advise patients not to drive at night while taking voriconazole.

➤*Less common adverse reactions:* The following adverse reactions occurred in less than 2% of all voriconazole-treated patients in all therapeutic studies (n = 1,655). This listing includes reactions where a causal relationship to voriconazole cannot be ruled out or those that may help the health care provider in managing the risks to the patients. The list does not include events included in the preceding table and does not include every reaction reported in the voriconazole clinical program.

Cardiovascular – Atrial arrhythmia, atrial fibrillation, AV block complete, bigeminy, bradycardia, bundle branch block, cardiomegaly, cardiomyopathy, cerebral hemorrhage, cerebral ischemia, cerebrovascular accident, congestive heart failure, deep thrombophlebitis, endocarditis, extrasystoles, heart arrest, hypertension, hypotension, myocardial infarction, nodal arrhythmia, palpitation, phlebitis, postural hypotension, pulmonary embolus, QT interval prolonged, supraventricular extrasystoles, supraventricular tachycardia, syncope, thrombophlebitis, vasodilatation, ventricular arrhythmia, ventricular fibrillation, ventricular tachycardia (including torsades de pointes).

CNS – Abnormal dreams, acute brain syndrome, agitation, akathisia, amnesia, anxiety, ataxia, brain edema, coma, confusion, convulsion, delirium, dementia, depersonalization, depression, diplopia, dizziness, encephalitis, encephalopathy, euphoria, extrapyramidal syndrome, generalized tonic-clonic seizure, Guillain-Barré syndrome, hypertonia, hypesthesia, insomnia, intracranial hypertension, libido decreased, neuralgia, neuropathy, nystagmus, oculogyric crisis, paresthesia, psychosis, somnolence, suicidal ideation, tremor, vertigo.

VORICONAZOLE — INJECTION

Dermatologic – Alopecia, angioedema, contact dermatitis, discoid lupus erythematosis, eczema, erythema multiforme, exfoliative dermatitis, fixed drug eruption, furunculosis, herpes simplex, maculopapular rash, melanosis, photosensitivity skin reaction, pruritus, psoriasis, skin discoloration, skin disorder, skin dry, Stevens-Johnson syndrome, sweating, toxic epidermal necrolysis, urticaria.

Endocrine – Adrenal cortex insufficiency, diabetes insipidus, hyperthyroidism, hypothyroidism.

GI – Abdomen enlarged, abdominal pain, anorexia, cheilitis, cholecystitis, cholelithiasis, constipation, diarrhea, duodenal ulcer perforation, duodenitis, dyspepsia, dysphagia, dry mouth, enlarged liver, esophageal ulcer, esophagitis, flatulence, gastroenteritis, gamma-glutamyl-transferase (GGT)/lactic dehydrogenase (LDH) elevated, GI hemorrhage, gingivitis, glossitis, gum hemorrhage, gum hyperplasia, hematemesis, hepatic coma, hepatic failure, hepatitis, intestinal perforation, intestinal ulcer, jaundice, melena, mouth ulceration, pancreatitis, parotid gland enlargement, periodontitis, proctitis, pseudomembranous colitis, rectal disorder, rectal hemorrhage, stomach ulcer, stomatitis, tongue edema.

GU – Anuria, blighted ovum, Ccr decreased, dysmenorrhea, dysuria, epididymitis, glycosuria, hemorrhagic cystitis, hematuria, hydronephrosis, impotence, kidney pain, kidney tubular necrosis, metrorrhagia, nephritis, nephrosis, oliguria, scrotal edema, urinary incontinence, urinary retention, urinary tract infection, uterine hemorrhage, vaginal hemorrhage.

Hematologic/Lymphatic – Agranulocytosis, anemia (macrocytic, megaloblastic, microcytic, normocytic), aplastic anemia, hemolytic anemia, bleeding time increased, cyanosis, disseminated intravascular coagulation (DIC), ecchymosis, enlarged spleen, eosinophilia, hypervolemia, leukopenia, lymphadenopathy, lymphangitis, marrow depression, pancytopenia, petechia, purpura, thrombocytopenia, thrombotic thrombocytopenic purpura.

Metabolic/Nutritional – Albuminuria, creatine phosphokinase increased, edema, glucose tolerance decreased, hypercalcemia, hypercholesteremia, hyperglycemia, hyperkalemia, hypermagnesemia, hypernatremia, hyperuricemia, hypocalcemia, hypoglycemia, hypomagnesemia, hyponatremia, hypophosphatemia, peripheral edema, serum urea nitrogen (BUN) increased, uremia.

Musculoskeletal – Arthralgia, arthritis, bone necrosis, bone pain, leg cramps, myalgia, myasthenia, myopathy, osteomalacia, osteoporosis.

Respiratory – Cough increased, dyspnea, epistaxis, hemoptysis, hypoxia, lung edema, pharyngitis, pleural effusion, pneumonia, respiratory disorder, respiratory distress syndrome, respiratory tract infection, rhinitis, sinusitis, voice alteration.

Special senses – Abnormality of accommodation, blepharitis, color blindness, conjunctivitis, corneal opacity, deafness, dry eyes, ear pain, eye hemorrhage, eye pain, hypoacusis, keratitis, keratoconjunctivitis, mydriasis, night blindness, optic atrophy, optic neuritis, otitis externa, papilledema, retinal hemorrhage, retinitis, scleritis, taste loss, taste perversion, tinnitus, uveitis, visual field defect.

Miscellaneous – Allergic reaction, anaphylactoid reaction (including flushing, fever, sweating, tachycardia, chest tightness, dyspnea, faintness, nausea, pruritus and rash), ascites, asthenia, back pain, bacterial infection, cellulitis, chest pain, edema, face edema, flank pain, flu syndrome, fungal infection, graft versus host reaction, granuloma, infection, injection-site pain, injection-site infection/inflammation, mucous membrane disorder, multiorgan failure, pain, pelvic pain, peritonitis, sepsis, substernal chest pain.

➤*Lab test abnormalities:* The overall incidence of clinically significant transaminase abnormalities in all therapeutic studies was 12.4% (206 of 1,655) of patients treated with voriconazole. Increased incidence of liver function test abnormalities may be associated with higher plasma concentrations and/or doses. The majority of abnormal liver function tests either resolved during treatment without dosage adjustment or following dose adjustment, including discontinuation of therapy.

Voriconazole Lab Test Abnormalities (Study 305)

	Criteria [a]	Voriconazole n/N [b]	Fluconazole n/N
Total bilirubin	> 1.5 × ULN	8/185 (4.3%)	7/186 (3.8%)
AST	> 3 × ULN	38/187 (20.3%)	15/186 (8.1%)
ALT	> 3 × ULN	20/187 (10.7%)	12/186 (6.5%)
Alkaline phosphatase	> 3 × ULN	19/187 (10.2%)	14/186 (7.5%)

[a] Without regard to baseline value.
[b] n = number of patients with a clinically significant abnormality while on study therapy; N = total number of patients with at least 1 observation of the given lab test while on study therapy.

Voriconazole Lab Test Abnormalities (Study 307/602)

	Criteria [a]	Voriconazole n/N [c]	Amphotericin B [b] n/N
Total bilirubin	> 1.5 × ULN	35/180 (19.4%)	46/173 (26.6%)
AST	> 3 × ULN	21/180 (11.7%)	18/174 (10.3%)
ALT	> 3 × ULN	34/180 (18.9%)	40/173 (23.1%)
Alkaline phosphatase	> 3 × ULN	29/181 (16%)	38/173 (22%)
Creatinine	> 1.3 × ULN	39/182 (21.4%)	102/177 (57.6%)
Potassium	< 0.9 × LLN [d]	30/181 (16.6%)	70/178 (39.3%)

[a] Without regard to baseline value.
[b] Amphotericin B followed by other licensed antifungal therapy.
[c] n = number of patients with a clinically significant abnormality while on study therapy; N = total number of patients with at least 1 observation of the given lab test while on study therapy.
[d] LLN = lower limit of normal.

Voriconazole Lab Test Abnormalities (Study 608)

	Criteria[a]	Voriconazole n/N [b]	Amphotericin B followed by fluconazole n/N (%)
Total bilirubin	> 1.5 × ULN	50/261 (19.2%)	31/115 (27%)
AST	> 3 × ULN	40/261 (15.3%)	16/116 (13.8%)
ALT	> 3 × ULN	22/261 (8.4%)	15/116 (12.9%)
Alkaline phosphatase	> 3 × ULN	59/261 (22.6%)	26/115 (22.6%)
Creatinine	> 1.3 × ULN	39/260 (15%)	32/118 (27.1%)
Potassium	< 0.9 × LLN	43/258 (16.7%)	35/118 (29.7%)

[a] Without regard to baseline value.
[b] n = number of patients with a clinically significant abnormality while on study therapy; N = total number of patients with at least 1 observation of the given lab test while on study therapy.

Overdosage

➤*Symptoms:* In clinical trials, there were 3 cases of accidental overdose. All occurred in children who received up to 5 times the recommended IV dose of voriconazole. A single adverse reaction of photophobia of 10 minutes' duration was reported.

The minimum lethal oral dose in mice and rats was 300 mg/kg (equivalent to 4 and 7 times the RMD, based on body surface area). At this dose, clinical signs observed in both mice and rats included salivation, mydriasis, titubation (loss of balance while moving), depressed behavior, prostration, partially closed eyes, and dyspnea. Other signs in mice were convulsions, corneal opacification, and swollen abdomen.

➤*Treatment:* There is no known antidote to voriconazole.

Voriconazole is hemodialyzed with clearance of 121 mL/min. The IV vehicle, SBECD, is hemodialyzed with clearance of 55 mL/min. In an overdose, hemodialysis may assist in the removal of voriconazole and SBECD from the body.

Patient Information

Advise patients not to drive at night while taking voriconazole. Voriconazole may cause changes to vision, including blurring and/or photophobia.

Advise patients to avoid potentially hazardous tasks, such as driving or operating machinery, if they perceive any change in vision.

Advise patients to avoid strong, direct sunlight during voriconazole therapy.

FLUCONAZOLE

Rx	**Fluconazole** (Various, eg, Greenstone, Ivax, Ranbaxy, Sandoz, Teva)	**Tablets:** 50 mg	In 30s, 100s, 500s, and UD 100s.
Rx	**Diflucan** (Pfizer)		(Diflucan 50 Roerig). Pink, trapezoid shape. In 30s.
Rx	**Fluconazole** (Various, eg, Greenstone, Ivax, Ranbaxy, Sandoz, Teva)	**Tablets:** 100 mg	In 30s, 100s, 500s, and UD 100s.
Rx	**Diflucan** (Pfizer)		(Diflucan 100 Roerig). Pink, trapezoid shape. In 30s and UD 100s.

FLUCONAZOLE

Rx	**Fluconazole** (Various, eg, Greenstone, Ivax, Ranbaxy, Sandoz, Teva)	**Tablets:** 150 mg	In UD 1s and 12s.
Rx	**Diflucan** (Pfizer)		(Diflucan 150 Roerig). Pink, oval. In UD 1s.
Rx	**Fluconazole** (Various, eg, Greenstone, Ivax, Ranbaxy, Sandoz, Teva)	**Tablets:** 200 mg	In 30s, 100s, 500s, and UD 100s.
Rx	**Diflucan** (Pfizer)		(Diflucan 200 Roerig). Pink, trapezoid shape. In 30s and UD 100s.
Rx	**Fluconazole** (Various, eg, Greenstone, Ranbaxy)	**Powder for oral suspension:** 10 mg/mL when reconstituted	May contain sucrose. In 35 mL.
Rx	**Diflucan** (Pfizer)		Sucrose. Orange flavor. In 35 mL.
Rx	**Fluconazole** (Various, eg, Greenstone, Ranbaxy)	**Powder for oral suspension:** 40 mg/mL when reconstituted	May contain sucrose. In 35 mL.
Rx	**Diflucan** (Pfizer)		Sucrose. Orange flavor. In 35 mL.
Rx	**Fluconazole** (Various, eg, Greenstone, Hospira, Mayne, West-Ward Pharmaceutical Corp.)	**Injection:** 2 mg/mL	In 100 and 200 mL.
Rx	**Diflucan** (Pfizer)		In 100 or 200 mL bottles or *Viaflex Plus* (available with NaCl[1] or dextrose diluents).[2]

[1] Contains 9 mg/mL NaCl.
[2] Contains 56 mg/mL dextrose, hydrous.

FLUCONAZOLE — ORAL

Indications

➤*Vaginal Candidiasis:* Vaginal yeast infections due to *Candida*.

➤*Oropharyngeal and esophageal candidiasis:* In open noncomparative studies of relatively small numbers of patients, fluconazole was also effective for the treatment of *Candida* urinary tract infections, peritonitis, and systemic *Candida* infections including candidemia, disseminated candidiasis, and pneumonia.

➤*Cryptococcal meningitis:* Treatment of cryptococcal meningitis.

➤*Prophylaxis:* Fluconazole is also indicated to decrease the incidence of candidiasis in patients undergoing bone marrow transplantation who receive cytotoxic chemotherapy or radiation therapy.

Administration and Dosage

➤*Approved by the FDA:* January 29, 1990.

➤*Adults:*

Multiple dose – Since oral absorption is rapid and almost complete, the daily dose of fluconazole is the same for oral (tablets and suspension) and intravenous administration. In general, a loading dose of twice the daily dose is recommended on the first day of therapy to result in plasma concentrations close to steady-state by the second day of therapy.

The daily dose of fluconazole for the treatment of infections other than vaginal candidiasis should be based on the infecting organism and the patient's response to therapy. Treatment should be continued until clinical parameters or laboratory tests indicate that active fungal infection has subsided. An inadequate period of treatment may lead to recurrence of active infection. Patients with AIDS and cryptococcal meningitis or recurrent oropharyngeal candidiasis usually require maintenance therapy to prevent relapse.

Oropharyngeal candidiasis: 200 mg on the first day, followed by 100 mg once daily. Clinical evidence of oropharyngeal candidiasis generally resolves within several days, but treatment should be continued for at least 2 weeks to decrease the likelihood of relapse.

Esophageal candidiasis: 200 mg on the first day, followed by 100 mg once daily. Doses up to 400 mg/day may be used, based on medical judgment of the patient's response to therapy. Patients with esophageal candidiasis should be treated for a minimum of 3 weeks and for at least 2 weeks following resolution of symptoms.

Systemic Candida infections: For systemic *Candida* infections including candidemia, disseminated candidiasis, and pneumonia, optimal therapeutic dosage and duration of therapy have not been established. In open, noncomparative studies of small numbers of patients, doses of up to 400 mg daily have been used.

Urinary tract infections and peritonitis: For the treatment of *Candida* urinary tract infections and peritonitis, daily doses of 50 to 200 mg have been used in open, noncomparative studies of small numbers of patients.

Cryptococcal meningitis: The recommended dosage for treatment of acute cryptococcal meningitis is 400 mg on the first day, followed by 200 mg once daily. A dosage of 400 mg once daily may be used, based on medical judgment of the patient's response to therapy. The recommended duration of treatment for initial therapy of cryptococcal meningitis is 10 to 12 weeks after the cerebrospinal fluid becomes culture negative. The recommended dosage of fluconazole for suppression of relapse of cryptococcal meningitis in patients with AIDS is 200 mg once daily.

Prophylaxis in patients undergoing bone marrow transplantation: The recommended fluconazole daily dosage for the prevention of candidiasis of patients undergoing bone marrow transplantation is 400 mg, once daily. Patients who are anticipated to have severe granulocytopenia (less than 500 neutrophils per cu mm) should start fluconazole prophylaxis several days before the anticipated onset of neutropenia, and continue for 7 days after the neutrophil count rises above 1000 cells per cu mm.

➤*Children:* The following dose equivalency scheme should generally provide equivalent exposure in pediatric and adult patients:

Pediatric patients	Adults
3 mg/kg	100 mg
6 mg/kg	200 mg
12* mg/kg	400 mg

* Some older children may have clearances similar to that of older adults. Absolute doses exceeding 600 mg/day are not recommended.

Neonates – Experience with fluconazole in neonates is limited to pharmacokinetic studies in premature newborns (see Pharmacokinetics). Based on the prolonged half-life seen in premature newborns (gestational age 26 to 29 weeks), these children, in the first 2 weeks of life, should receive the same dosage (mg/kg) as in older children, but administered every 72 hours. After the first 2 weeks, these children should be dosed once daily. No information regarding fluconazole pharmacokinetics in full-term newborns is available.

Oropharyngeal candidiasis – 6 mg/kg on the first day, followed by 3 mg/kg once daily. Treatment should be administered for at least 2 weeks to decrease the likelihood of relapse.

Esophageal candidiasis – 6 mg/kg on the first day, followed by 3 mg/kg once daily. Doses up to 12 mg/kg/day may be used based on medical judgment of the patient's response to therapy. Patients with esophageal candidiasis should be treated for a minimum of 3 weeks and for at least 2 weeks following the resolution of symptoms.

Systemic Candida infections – For the treatment of candidemia and disseminated *Candida* infections, daily doses of 6 to 12 mg/kg/day have been used in an open, noncomparative study of a small number of children.

Cryptococcal meningitis – For the treatment of acute cryptococcal meningitis, the recommended dosage is 12 mg/kg on the first day, followed by 6 mg/kg once daily. A dosage of 12 mg/kg once daily may be used, based on medical judgment of the patient's response to therapy. The recommended duration of treatment for initial therapy of cryptococcal meningitis is 10 to 12 weeks after the cerebrospinal fluid becomes culture negative. For suppression of relapse of cryptococcal meningitis in children with AIDS, the recommended dose of fluconazole is 6 mg/kg once daily.

➤*Renal function impairment:* Fluconazole is cleared primarily by renal excretion as unchanged drug. There is no need to adjust single dose therapy for vaginal candidiasis because of impaired renal function. In patients with impaired renal function who will receive multiple doses of fluconazole, an initial loading dose of 50 to 400 mg should be given. After the loading dose, the daily dose (according to indication) should be based on the following table:

Creatinine clearance (mL/min)	Percent of recommended dose
> 50	100%
≤ 50 (no dialysis)	50%
Regular dialysis	100% after each dialysis

These are suggested dose adjustments based on pharmacokinetics following administration of multiple doses. Further adjustment may be needed depending upon clinical condition.

Although the pharmacokinetics of fluconazole has not been studied in children with renal insufficiency, dosage reduction in children with renal insufficiency should parallel that recommended for adults. The following formula may be used to estimate creatinine clearance in children:

K × linear length or height (cm) / serum creatinine (mg/100 mL). (Where K = 0.55 for children older than 1 year and 0.45 for infants).

FLUCONAZOLE — ORAL

➤*Directions for mixing the oral suspension:* Prepare a suspension at time of dispensing as follows: Tap bottle until all the powder flows freely. To reconstitute, add 24 mL of distilled water or Purified Water (USP) to fluconazole bottle and shake vigorously to suspend powder. Each bottle will deliver 35 mL of suspension. The concentrations of the reconstituted suspensions are as follows:

Fluconazole content per bottle	Concentration of reconstituted suspension
350 mg	10 mg/mL
1400 mg	40 mg/mL

➤*Storage/Stability:* Store tablets below 30°C (86°F). Store dry powder below 30°C (86°F). Store reconstituted suspension between 30°C (86°F) and 5°C (41°F) and discard unused portion after two weeks. Protect from freezing.

Actions

➤*Pharmacology:* Fluconazole is a highly selective inhibitor of fungal cytochrome P-450 sterol C-14 alpha-demethylation. Mammalian cell demethylation is much less sensitive to fluconazole inhibition. The subsequent loss of normal sterols correlates with the accumulation of 14 alpha-methyl sterols in fungi and may be responsible for the fungistatic activity of fluconazole.

➤*Pharmacokinetics:*

Absorption/Distribution – The pharmacokinetic properties of fluconazole are similar following administration by the intravenous or oral routes. In healthy volunteers, the bioavailability of orally administered fluconazole is greater than 90% compared with intravenous administration. Bioequivalence was established between the 100 mg tablet and both suspension strengths when administered as a single 200 mg dose.

Peak plasma concentrations (C_{max}) in fasted healthy volunteers occur between 1 and 2 hours with a terminal plasma elimination half-life of ≈ 30 hours (range, 20 to 50 hours) after oral administration. In fasted healthy volunteers, administration of a single oral 400 mg dose of fluconazole leads to a mean C_{max} of 6.72 mcg/mL (range, 4.12 to 8.08 mcg/mL) and after single oral doses of 50 to 400 mg, fluconazole plasma concentrations and AUC (area under the plasma concentration-time curve) are dose proportional.

Administration of a single oral 150 mg tablet of fluconazole to 10 lactating women resulted in a mean C_{max} of 2.61 mcg/mL (range, 1.57 to 3.65 mcg/mL).

Steady state concentrations are reached within 5 to 10 days following oral doses of 50 to 400 mg given once daily. Administration of a loading dose (on day 1) of twice the usual daily dose results in plasma concentrations close to steady-state by the second day. The apparent volume of distribution of fluconazole approximates that of total body water. Plasma protein binding is low (11% to 12%). Following either single- or multiple-oral doses for up to 14 days, fluconazole penetrates into all body fluids studied. In healthy volunteers, saliva concentrations of fluconazole were equal to or slightly greater than plasma concentrations regardless of dose, route, or duration of dosing. In patients with bronchiectasis, sputum concentrations of fluconazole following a single 150 mg oral dose were equal to plasma concentrations at both 4 and 24 hours post dose. In patients with fungal meningitis, fluconazole concentrations in the CSF are ≈ 80% of the corresponding plasma concentrations.

Metabolism/Excretion – In healthy volunteers, fluconazole is cleared primarily by renal excretion, with ≈ 80% of the administered dose appearing in the urine as unchanged drug. About 11% of the dose is excreted in the urine as metabolites.

Renal function impairment: The pharmacokinetics of fluconazole are markedly affected by reduction in renal function. There is an inverse relationship between the elimination half-life and creatinine clearance. The dose of fluconazole may need to be reduced in patients with impaired renal function (see Administration and Dosage). A 3-hour hemodialysis session decreases plasma concentrations by ≈ 50%.

➤*Microbiology:* Fluconazole exhibits in vitro activity against *Cryptococcus neoformans* and *Candida* spp. Fungistatic activity has also been demonstrated in normal and immunocompromised animal models for systemic and intracranial fungal infections due to *Cryptococcus neoformans* and for systemic infections due to *Candida albicans*.

In common with other azole antifungal agents, most fungi show a higher apparent sensitivity to fluconazole in vivo than in vitro. Fluconazole administered orally or intravenously was active in a variety of animal models of fungal infection using standard laboratory strains of fungi. Activity has been demonstrated against fungal infections caused by *Aspergillus flavus*and *Aspergillus fumigatus* in normal mice. Fluconazole has also been shown to be active in animal models of endemic mycoses, including one model of *Blastomyces dermatitidis* pulmonary infections in normal mice; one model of *Coccidioides immitis* intracranial infections in normal mice; and several models of *Histoplasma capsulatum* pulmonary infection in normal and immunosuppressed mice. The clinical significance of results obtained in these studies is unknown.

Contraindications

Hypersensitivity to fluconazole or to any of its excipients. There is no information regarding cross-hypersensitivity between fluconazole and other azole antifungal agents. Caution should be used in prescribing fluconazole to patients with hypersensitivity to other azoles. Coadministration with terfenadine or cisapride (see Drug Interactions).

Warnings

➤*Hepatic injury:* Fluconazole has been associated with rare cases of serious hepatic toxicity, including fatalities primarily in patients with serious underlying medical conditions. In cases of fluconazole-associated hepatotoxicity, no obvious relationship to total daily dose, duration of therapy, sex or age of the patient has been observed. Fluconazole hepatotoxicity has usually, but not always, been reversible on discontinuation of therapy. Patients who develop abnormal liver function tests during fluconazole therapy should be monitored for the development of more severe hepatic injury. Fluconazole should be discontinued if clinical signs and symptoms consistent with liver disease develop that may be attributable to fluconazole.

➤*Dermatologic disorders:* Patients have rarely developed exfoliative skin disorders during treatment with fluconazole. In patients with serious underlying diseases (predominantly AIDS and malignancy), these have rarely resulted in a fatal outcome. Patients who develop rashes during treatment with fluconazole should be monitored closely and the drug discontinued if lesions progress.

➤*Hypersensitivity reactions:* In rare cases, anaphylaxis has been reported.

➤*Carcinogenesis:* Fluconazole showed no evidence of carcinogenic potential in mice and rats treated orally for 24 months at doses of 2.5, 5, or 10 mg/kg/day (≈ 2 to 7 times the recommended human dose). Male rats treated with 5 and 10 mg/kg/day had an increased incidence of hepatocellular adenomas.

➤*Fertility impairment:* Fluconazole did not affect the fertility of male or female rats treated orally with daily doses of 5, 10, or 20 mg/kg or with parenteral doses of 5, 25, or 75 mg/kg, although the onset of parturition was slightly delayed at 20 mg/kg by mouth. In an intravenous perinatal study in rats at 5, 20, and 40 mg/kg, dystocia and prolongation of parturition were observed in a few dams at 20 mg/kg (≈ 5 to 15 times the recommended human dose) and 40 mg/kg, but not at 5 mg/kg. The disturbances in parturition were reflected by a slight increase in the number of still born pups and decrease of neonatal survival at these dose levels. The effects on parturition in rats are consistent with the species specific estrogen-lowering property produced by high doses of fluconazole. Such a hormone change has not been observed in women treated with fluconazole.

➤*Pregnancy: Category C.* Fluconazole was administered orally to pregnant rabbits during organogenesis in 2 studies, at 5, 10, and 20 mg/kg and at 5, 25, and 75 mg/kg, respectively. Maternal weight gain was impaired at all dose levels, and abortions occurred at 75 mg/kg (≈ 20 to 60 times the recommended human dose); no adverse fetal effects were detected. In several studies in which pregnant rats were treated orally with fluconazole during organogenesis, maternal weight gain was impaired and placental weights were increased at 25 mg/kg. There were no fetal effects at 5 or 10 mg/kg; increases in fetal anatomical variants (supernumerary ribs, renal pelvis dilation) and delays in ossification were observed at 25 and 50 mg/kg and higher doses. At doses ranging from 80 mg/kg (≈ 20 to 60 times the recommended human dose) to 320 mg/kg embryolethality in rats was increased and fetal abnormalities included wavy ribs, cleft palate, and abnormal cranio-facial ossification. These effects are consistent with the inhibition of estrogen synthesis in rats and may be a result of known effects of lowered estrogen on pregnancy, organogenesis, and parturition.

There are no adequate and well-controlled studies in pregnant women. There have been reports of multiple congenital abnormalities in infants whose mothers were being treated for 3 or more months with high dose (400 to 800 mg/day) fluconazole therapy for coccidioidomycosis (an unindicated use). The relationship between fluconazole use and these events is unclear. Fluconazole should be used in pregnancy only if the potential benefit justifies the possible risk to the fetus.

➤*Lactation:* Fluconazole is secreted in human milk at concentrations similar to plasma. Therefore, the use of fluconazole in nursing mothers is not recommended.

➤*Children:* An open-label, randomized, controlled trial has shown fluconazole to be effective in the treatment of oropharyngeal candidiasis in children 6 months to 13 years of age.

The use of fluconazole in children with cryptococcal meningitis, *Candida* esophagitis, or systemic *Candida* infections is supported by the efficacy shown for these indications in adults and by the results from several small noncomparative pediatric clinical studies. In addition, pharmacokinetic studies in children (see Pharmacokinetics) have established a dose proportionality between children and adults (see Administration and Dosage).

Efficacy of fluconazole has not been established in infants younger than 6 months of age. A small number of patients (29) ranging in age from 1 day to 6 months have been treated safely with fluconazole.

Precautions

➤*Vaginal candidiasis:* The convenience and efficacy of the single dose oral tablet of fluconazole regimen for the treatment of vaginal yeast infections should be weighed against the acceptability of a higher incidence of drug-related adverse events with fluconazole (26%) versus intravaginal agents (16%) in US comparative clinical studies (see Drug interactions, and Adverse reactions).

FLUCONAZOLE — ORAL

Drug Interactions

Fluconazole Drug Interactions

Precipitant drug	Object drug*		Description
Cimetidine	Fluconazole	↓	Cimetidine resulted in a reduction in fluconazole AUC and C_{max}.
Hydrochlorothiazide	Fluconazole	↑	Concomitant use resulted in a significant increase in fluconazole C_{max} and AUC, which can be attributed to reduced renal clearance.
Rifampin	Fluconazole	↓	Rifampin enhances the metabolism of concurrently administered fluconazole. Depending on the clinical circumstances, give consideration when increasing the dose of fluconazole when administered with rifampin.
Fluconazole	Alfentanil	↑	The pharmacologic and adverse effects of alfentanil may be increased. Possible inhibition of alfentanil metabolism (CYP3A4) by fluconazole may occur. Monitor for prolonged or recurrent respiratory depression. It may be necessary to administer a lower dose of alfentanil.
Fluconazole	Benzodiazepines	↑	Increased and prolonged serum levels, CNS depression, and psychomotor impairment with certain benzodiazepines may occur, possibly lasting for several days after stopping fluconazole.
Fluconazole	Buspirone	↑	Plasma buspirone concentrations may be elevated because of inhibition of buspirone metabolism. The pharmacologic and adverse effects of buspirone may be increased. Adjust the dose of buspirone as needed.
Fluconazole	Carbamazepine	↑	Plasma concentrations of carbamazepine may be elevated, increasing clinical and adverse effects because of possible inhibition of carbamazepine metabolism (CYP3A4) by fluconazole. Monitor carbamazepine concentrations.
Fluconazole	Cisapride	↑	Concurrent use may increase cisapride concentrations and cardiotoxicity may occur. Coadministration is contraindicated.
Fluconazole	Contraceptives, oral	↔	Concurrent use with an OC containing ethinyl estradiol/levonorgestrel produced an overall mean increase in the levels of the OC components; however, in some cases there were decreases ≤ 47% and 33% of ethinyl estradiol and levonorgestrel levels, respectively.
Fluconazole	Corticosteroids	↑	The effects of corticosteroids may be enhanced, resulting in increased toxicity because of inhibition of corticosteroid metabolism. Adjust corticosteroid dose as needed.
Fluconazole	Cyclosporine	↑	Significant increases in cyclosporine C_{max}, C_{min}, and AUC values and a significant decrease in oral clearance occurred following fluconazole use.
Fluconazole	Haloperidol	↑	Concurrent use may increase haloperidol plasma concentrations, increasing the risk of side effects. Adjust haloperidol dose as needed.
Fluconazole	HMG-CoA reductase inhibitors	↑	Coadministration causes increased plasma levels of the HMG-CoA reductase inhibitors. Rhabdomyolysis has been reported. If concurrent use can not be avoided, consider reducing the dose of the HMG-CoA reductase inhibitor. Pravastatin levels appear to be the least affected by concurrent use.
Fluconazole	Losartan	↑	The antihypertensive and adverse effects of losartan may be increased because of possible inhibition of metabolism (CYP2D9) of losartan by fluconazole. Monitor blood pressure.
Fluconazole	Nisoldipine	↑	Serum nisoldipine concentrations may be elevated, increasing pharmacologic and adverse effects. Fluconazole, especially > 200 mg/day, may inhibit CYP3A4.
Fluconazole	Phenytoin	↑	Coadministration resulted in an increase of phenytoin AUC values. Monitor phenytoin levels and adjust dose as needed.
Fluconazole	Protease inhibitors	↑	Concurrent use may elevate protease inhibitor levels, increasing the risk of toxicity. Adjust protease inhibitor dose as needed.
Fluconazole	Rifabutin	↑	Coadministration may increase rifabutin levels. Cases of uveitis have been reported in patients receiving both drugs. Monitor closely.
Fluconazole	Sirolimus	↑	Plasma sirolimus concentrations may be elevated because of an inhibition of sirolimus gut metabolism.
Fluconazole	Sulfonylureas	↑	Fluconazole reduces the metabolism of sulfonylureas and increases the plasma concentrations of these agents. Carefully monitor blood glucose concentrations and adjust the sulfonylurea dose as necessary when these agents are coadministered.
Fluconazole	Tacrolimus	↑	There have been reports of nephrotoxicity in patients when these agents were coadministered. Carefully monitor.
Fluconazole	Theophylline	↑	Theophylline AUC, C_{max}, and half-life were significantly increased, and clearance was decreased.
Fluconazole	Tolterodine	↑	Concurrent use may increase tolterodine plasma levels. Adjust tolterodine dose as needed. Do not give more than 1 mg of tolterodine twice daily when coadministered with azole antifungals.
Fluconazole	Tricyclic antidepressants (ie, amitriptyline, nortriptyline)	↑	Serum tricyclic antidepressant (TCA) concentrations may be elevated, resulting in an increase in therapeutic and adverse effects including cardiac arrhythmia. Inhibition of TCA metabolism is suspected (CYP2C9 by fluconazole). Adjust the TCA dose as needed.
Fluconazole	Vinca alkaloids (eg, vincristine)	↑	The risk of vinca alkaloid toxicity (eg, constipation, myalgia, neutropenia) may be increased. Avoid coadministration of these agents whenever possible.
Fluconazole	Warfarin	↑	The anticoagulant effect of warfarin may be increased. A single warfarin dose after 14 days of fluconazole resulted in an increase in the PT response. Monitor PT and INR frequently.

FLUCONAZOLE — ORAL

Fluconazole Drug Interactions			
Precipitant drug	Object drug*		Description
Fluconazole	Zidovudine	↑	There was a significant increase in zidovudine AUC following fluconazole administration.
Fluconazole	Zolpidem	↑	Plasma concentrations and therapeutic effects of zolpidem may be increased. The dose of zolpidem may need to be decreased during coadministration of azole antifungal agents.

* ↑ = Object drug increased. ↓ = Object drug decreased.
↔ = Undetermined clinical effect.

Adverse Reactions

➤*Patients receiving multiple doses for other infections:* Sixteen percent of over 4000 patients treated with fluconazole in clinical trials of 7 days or more experienced adverse reactions. Treatment was discontinued in 1.5% of patients due to adverse clinical events and in 1.3% of patients due to laboratory test abnormalities.

Clinical adverse events were reported more frequently in HIV infected patients (21%) than in non-HIV infected patients (13%); however, the patterns in HIV infected and non-HIV infected patients were similar. The proportions of patients discontinuing therapy due to clinical adverse events were similar in the 2 groups (1.5%).

The following treatment-related clinical adverse events occurred at an incidence of 1% or greater in 4048 patients receiving fluconazole for 7 or more days in clinical trials: Nausea 3.7%, headache 1.9%, skin rash 1.8%, vomiting 1.7%, abdominal pain 1.7%, diarrhea 1.5%.

The following adverse events have occurred under conditions where a causal association is probable.

Allergic – In rare cases, anaphylaxis has been reported.

Hepatic – In combined clinical trials and marketing experience, there have been rare cases of serious hepatic reactions during treatment with fluconazole (see Warnings). The spectrum of these hepatic reactions has ranged from mild transient elevations in transaminases to clinical hepatitis, cholestasis, and fulminant hepatic failure, including fatalities. Instances of fatal hepatic reactions were noted to occur primarily in patients with serious underlying medical conditions (predominantly AIDS or malignancy) and often while taking multiple concomitant medications. Transient hepatic reactions, including hepatitis and jaundice, have occurred among patients with no other identifiable risk factors. In each of these cases, liver function returned to baseline on discontinuation of fluconazole.

➤*Adverse reactions with an unknown relationship to fluconazole:* The following adverse events have occurred under conditions where a causal association is uncertain.

CNS – Seizures.

Dermatologic – Exfoliative skin disorders including Stevens-Johnson syndrome and toxic epidermal necrolysis (see Warnings), alopecia.

Hematologic/Lymphatic – Leukopenia, including neutropenia and agranulocytosis, thrombocytopenia.

Metabolic – Hypercholesterolemia, hypertriglyceridemia, hypokalemia.

➤*Children:* In Phase II/III clinical trials conducted in the United States and in Europe, 577 pediatric patients, ages 1 day to 17 years were treated with fluconazole at doses up to 15 mg/kg/day for up to 1616 days. Thirteen percent of children experienced treatment related adverse events. The most commonly reported events were vomiting (5%), abdominal pain (3%), nausea (2%), and diarrhea (2%). Treatment was discontinued in 2.3% of patients due to adverse clinical events and in 1.4% of patients due to laboratory test abnormalities. The majority of treatment-related laboratory abnormalities were elevations of transaminases or alkaline phosphatase.

Adverse reaction	Percentage of patients with treatment-related side effects fluconazole (n = 577)	Comparative agents (n = 451)
With any side effect	13%	9.3%
Vomiting	5.4%	5.1%
Abdominal pain	2.8%	1.6%
Nausea	2.3%	1.6%
Diarrhea	2.1%	2.2%

Overdosage

➤*Symptoms:* There has been 1 reported case of overdosage with fluconazole. A 42-year-old patient infected with human immunodeficiency virus developed hallucinations and exhibited paranoid behavior after reportedly ingesting 8200 mg of fluconazole. The patient was admitted to the hospital, and his condition resolved within 48 hours.

➤*Treatment:* In the event of overdose, symptomatic treatment (with supportive measures and gastric lavage if clinically indicated) should be instituted.

Fluconazole is largely excreted in urine. A 3-hour hemodialysis session decreases plasma levels by ≈ 50%.

In mice and rats receiving very high doses of fluconazole, clinical effects in both species included decreased motility and respiration, ptosis, lacrimation, salivation, urinary incontinence, loss of righting reflex, and cyanosis; death was sometimes preceded by clonic convulsions.

FLUCONAZOLE FOR — INJECTION

Indications

➤*Vaginal candidiasis:* Vaginal yeast infections due to *Candida*.

➤*Oropharyngeal and esophageal candidiasis:* In open noncomparative studies of relatively small numbers of patients, fluconazole was also effective for the treatment of *Candida* urinary tract infections, peritonitis, and systemic *Candida* infections including candidemia, disseminated candidiasis, and pneumonia.

➤*Cryptococcal meningitis:* Treatment of cryptococcal meningitis.

➤*Prophylaxis:* Fluconazole is also indicated to decrease the incidence of candidiasis in patients undergoing bone marrow transplantation who receive cytotoxic chemotherapy or radiation therapy.

Administration and Dosage

➤*Approved by the FDA:* January 29, 1990.

➤*Adults:*

Single dose (vaginal candidiasis) – 150 mg as a single dose.

Multiple dose – Since oral absorption is rapid and almost complete, the daily dose of fluconazole is the same for oral (tablets and suspension) and intravenous administration. In general, a loading dose of twice the daily dose is recommended on the first day of therapy to result in plasma concentrations close to steady-state by the second day of therapy.

The daily dose of fluconazole for the treatment of infections other than vaginal candidiasis should be based on the infecting organism and the patient's response to therapy. Treatment should be continued until clinical parameters or laboratory tests indicate that active fungal infection has subsided. An inadequate period of treatment may lead to recurrence of active infection. Patients with AIDS and cryptococcal meningitis or recurrent oropharyngeal candidiasis usually require maintenance therapy to prevent relapse.

Oropharyngeal candidiasis: 200 mg on the first day, followed by 100 mg once daily. Clinical evidence of oropharyngeal candidiasis generally resolves within several days, but treatment should be continued for at least 2 weeks to decrease the likelihood of relapse.

Esophageal candidiasis: 200 mg on the first day, followed by 100 mg once daily. Doses up to 400 mg/day may be used, based on medical judgment of the patient's response to therapy. Patients with esophageal candidiasis should be treated for a minimum of 3 weeks and for at least 2 weeks following resolution of symptoms.

Systemic Candida infections: For systemic *Candida* infections including candidemia, disseminated candidiasis, and pneumonia, optimal therapeutic dosage and duration of therapy have not been established. In open, noncomparative studies of small numbers of patients, doses of up to 400 mg daily have been used.

Urinary tract infections and peritonitis: For the treatment of *Candida* urinary tract infections and peritonitis, daily doses of 50 to 200 mg have been used in open, noncomparative studies of small numbers of patients.

Cryptococcal meningitis: The recommended dosage for treatment of acute cryptococcal meningitis is 400 mg on the first day, followed by 200 mg once daily. A dosage of 400 mg once daily may be used, based on medical judgment of the patient's response to therapy. The recommended duration of treatment for initial therapy of cryptococcal meningitis is 10 to 12 weeks after the cerebrospinal fluid becomes culture negative. The recommended dosage of fluconazole for suppression of relapse of cryptococcal meningitis in patients with AIDS is 200 mg once daily.

Prophylaxis in patients undergoing bone marrow transplantation: The recommended fluconazole daily dosage for the prevention of candidiasis of patients undergoing bone marrow transplantation is 400 mg, once daily. Patients who are anticipated to have severe granulocytopenia (less than 500 neutrophils per cu mm) should start fluconazole prophylaxis several days before the anticipated onset of neutropenia, and continue for seven days after the neutrophil count rises above 1000 cells per cu mm.

➤*Children:* The following dose equivalency scheme should generally provide equivalent exposure in pediatric and adult patients:

Pediatric patients	Adults
3 mg/kg	100 mg
6 mg/kg	200 mg
12[a] mg/kg	400 mg

[a] Some older children may have clearances similar to that of older adults. Absolute doses exceeding 600 mg/day are not recommended.

Neonates – Experience with fluconazole in neonates is limited to pharmacokinetic studies in premature newborns (see Pharmacokinetics). Based on the prolonged half-life seen in premature newborns (gestational age 26 to 29 weeks), these children, in the first 2 weeks of life, should receive the same dosage (mg/kg) as in older children, but administered every 72 hours. After the first 2 weeks, these children should be dosed once daily. No information regarding fluconazole pharmacokinetics in full-term newborns is available.

FLUCONAZOLE FOR — INJECTION

Oropharyngeal candidiasis – The recommended dosage of fluconazole for oropharyngeal candidiasis in children is 6 mg/kg on the first day, followed by 3 mg/kg once daily. Treatment should be administered for at least 2 weeks to decrease the likelihood of relapse.

Esophageal candidiasis – For the treatment of esophageal candidiasis, the recommended dosage of fluconazole in children is 6 mg/kg on the first day, followed by 3 mg/kg once daily. Doses up to 12 mg/kg/day may be used based on medical judgment of the patient's response to therapy. Patients with esophageal candidiasis should be treated for a minimum of 3 weeks and for at least 2 weeks following the resolution of symptoms.

Systemic Candida infections – For the treatment of candidemia and disseminated *Candida* infections, daily doses of 6 to 12 mg/kg/day have been used in an open, noncomparative study of a small number of children.

Cryptococcal meningitis – For the treatment of acute cryptococcal meningitis, the recommended dosage is 12 mg/kg on the first day, followed by 6 mg/kg once daily. A dosage of 12 mg/kg once daily may be used, based on medical judgment of the patient's response to therapy. The recommended duration of treatment for initial therapy of cryptococcal meningitis is 10 to 12 weeks after the cerebrospinal fluid becomes culture negative. For suppression of relapse of cryptococcal meningitis in children with AIDS, the recommended dose of fluconazole is 6 mg/kg once daily.

➤*Renal function impairment:* Fluconazole is cleared primarily by renal excretion as unchanged drug. There is no need to adjust single dose therapy for vaginal candidiasis because of impaired renal function. In patients with impaired renal function who will receive multiple doses of fluconazole, an initial loading dose of 50 to 400 mg should be given. After the loading dose, the daily dose (according to indication) should be based on the following table:

Creatinine clearance (mL/min)	Percent of recommended dose
> 50	100%
≤ 50 (no dialysis)	50%
Regular dialysis	100% after each dialysis

Suggested dose adjustments based on pharmacokinetics following administration of multiple doses – These are suggested dose adjustments based on pharmacokinetics following administration of multiple doses. Further adjustment may be needed depending upon clinical condition.

Although the pharmacokinetics of fluconazole has not been studied in children with renal insufficiency, dosage reduction in children with renal insufficiency should parallel that recommended for adults. The following formula may be used to estimate creatinine clearance in children:

$$K\dagger \times \frac{\text{linear length or height (cm)}}{\text{serum creatinine (mg/100 mL)}}$$

➤*Administration:* Fluconazole may be administered either orally or by intravenous infusion. Fluconazole injection has been used safely for up to 14 days of intravenous therapy. The intravenous infusion of fluconazole should be administered at a maximum rate of ≈ 200 mg/hour, given as a continuous infusion.

Fluconazole injections in glass and *Viaflex Plus* plastic containers are intended only for intravenous administration using sterile equipment.

Do not use if the solution is cloudy or precipitated or if the seal is not intact.

Directions for IV use of fluconazole in Viaflex Plus plastic containers – Do not remove unit from overwrap until ready for use. The overwrap is a moisture barrier. The inner bag maintains the sterility of the product.

Caution – Do not use plastic containers in series connections. Such use could result in air embolism due to residual air being drawn from the primary container before administration of the fluid from the secondary container is completed.

Preparation for administration – Suspend container from eyelet support. Remove plastic protector from outlet port at bottom of container. Attach administration set. Refer to complete directions accompanying set.

➤*Storage/Stability:* Store fluconazole injections in glass bottles between 30°C (86°F) and 5°C (41°F). Protect from freezing.

Store fluconazole injections in *Viaflex Plus* plastic containers between 25°C (77°F) and 5°C (41°F). Brief exposure up to 40°C (104°F) does not adversely affect the product. Protect from freezing.

Actions

➤*Pharmacology:* Fluconazole is a highly selective inhibitor of fungal cytochrome P-450 sterol C-14 alpha-demethylation. Mammalian cell demethylation is much less sensitive to fluconazole inhibition. The subsequent loss of normal sterols correlates with the accumulation of 14 alpha-methyl sterols in fungi and may be responsible for the fungistatic activity of fluconazole.

➤*Pharmacokinetics:*

Absorption/Distribution – The pharmacokinetic properties of fluconazole are similar following administration by the intravenous or oral routes. In healthy volunteers, the bioavailability of orally administered fluconazole is greater than 90% compared with intravenous administration. Bioequivalence was established between the 100 mg tablet and both suspension strengths when administered as a single 200 mg dose.

† (Where K = 0.55 for children older than 1 year and 0.45 for infants).

Peak plasma concentrations (C_{max}) in fasted healthy volunteers occur between 1 and 2 hours with a terminal plasma elimination half-life of ≈ 30 hours (range, 20 to 50 hours) after oral administration. In fasted healthy volunteers, administration of a single oral 400 mg dose of fluconazole leads to a mean C_{max} of 6.72 mcg/mL (range, 4.12 to 8.08 mcg/mL) and after single oral doses of 50 to 400 mg, fluconazole plasma concentrations and AUC (area under the plasma concentration-time curve) are dose proportional.

Administration of a single oral 150 mg tablet of fluconazole to 10 lactating women resulted in a mean C_{max} of 2.61 mcg/mL (range, 1.57 to 3.65 mcg/mL).

Steady state concentrations are reached within 5 to 10 days following oral doses of 50 to 400 mg given once daily. Administration of a loading dose (on day 1) of twice the usual daily dose results in plasma concentrations close to steady-state by the second day. The apparent volume of distribution of fluconazole approximates that of total body water. Plasma protein binding is low (11% to 12%). Following either single- or multiple-oral doses for up to 14 days, fluconazole penetrates into all body fluids studied. In healthy volunteers, saliva concentrations of fluconazole were equal to or slightly greater than plasma concentrations regardless of dose, route, or duration of dosing. In patients with bronchiectasis, sputum concentrations of fluconazole following a single 150 mg oral dose were equal to plasma concentrations at both 4 and 24 hours post dose. In patients with fungal meningitis, fluconazole concentrations in the CSF are ≈ 80% of the corresponding plasma concentrations.

Metabolism/Excretion – In healthy volunteers, fluconazole is cleared primarily by renal excretion, with ≈ 80% of the administered dose appearing in the urine as unchanged drug. About 11% of the dose is excreted in the urine as metabolites.

Renal function impairment: The pharmacokinetics of fluconazole are markedly affected by reduction in renal function. There is an inverse relationship between the elimination half-life and creatinine clearance. The dose of fluconazole may need to be reduced in patients with impaired renal function (see Administration and Dosage). A 3-hour hemodialysis session decreases plasma concentrations by ≈ 50%.

➤*Microbiology:* Fluconazole exhibits in vitro activity against *Cryptococcus neoformans* and *Candida* spp. Fungistatic activity has also been demonstrated in normal and immunocompromised animal models for systemic and intracranial fungal infections due to *Cryptococcus neoformans* and for systemic infections due to *Candida albicans*.

In common with other azole antifungal agents, most fungi show a higher apparent sensitivity to fluconazole in vivo than in vitro. Fluconazole administered orally or intravenously was active in a variety of animal models of fungal infection using standard laboratory strains of fungi. Activity has been demonstrated against fungal infections caused by *Aspergillus flavus* and *Aspergillus fumigatus* in normal mice. Fluconazole has also been shown to be active in animal models of endemic mycoses, including one model of *Blastomyces dermatitidis* pulmonary infections in normal mice; one model of *Coccidioides immitis* intracranial infections in normal mice; and several models of *Histoplasma capsulatum* pulmonary infection in normal and immunosuppressed mice. The clinical significance of results obtained in these studies is unknown.

Contraindications

Fluconazole is contraindicated in patients who have shown hypersensitivity to fluconazole or to any of its excipients. There is no information regarding cross-hypersensitivity between fluconazole and other azole antifungal agents. Caution should be used in prescribing fluconazole to patients with hypersensitivity to other azoles. Coadministration of terfenadine is contraindicated in patients receiving fluconazole at multiple doses of 400 mg or higher based upon results of a multiple dose interaction study. Coadministration of cisapride is contraindicated in patients receiving fluconazole (see Drug Interactions).

Warnings

➤*Hepatic injury:* Fluconazole has been associated with rare cases of serious hepatic toxicity, including fatalities primarily in patients with serious underlying medical conditions. In cases of fluconazole-associated hepatotoxicity, no obvious relationship to total daily dose, duration of therapy, sex or age of the patient has been observed. Fluconazole hepatotoxicity has usually, but not always, been reversible on discontinuation of therapy. Patients who develop abnormal liver function tests during fluconazole therapy should be monitored for the development of more severe hepatic injury. Fluconazole should be discontinued if clinical signs and symptoms consistent with liver disease develop that may be attributable to fluconazole.

➤*Dermatologic:* Patients have rarely developed exfoliative skin disorders during treatment with fluconazole. In patients with serious underlying diseases (predominantly AIDS and malignancy), these have rarely resulted in a fatal outcome. Patients who develop rashes during treatment with fluconazole should be monitored closely and the drug discontinued if lesions progress.

➤*Hypersensitivity reactions:* In rare cases, anaphylaxis has been reported.

➤*Carcinogenesis:* Fluconazole showed no evidence of carcinogenic potential in mice and rats treated orally for 24 months at doses of 2.5, 5, or 10 mg/kg/day (≈ 2 to 7 times the recommended human dose). Male rats treated with 5 and 10 mg/kg/day had an increased incidence of hepatocellular adenomas.

➤*Fertility impairment:* Fluconazole did not affect the fertility of male or female rats treated orally with daily doses of 5, 10, or 20 mg/kg or with parenteral doses of 5, 25, or 75 mg/kg, although the onset of parturition was slightly delayed at 20 mg/kg by mouth. In an intravenous perinatal study in

FLUCONAZOLE FOR — INJECTION

rats at 5, 20, and 40 mg/kg, dystocia and prolongation of parturition were observed in a few dams at 20 mg/kg (≈ 5 to 15 times the recommended human dose) and 40 mg/kg, but not at 5 mg/kg. The disturbances in parturition were reflected by a slight increase in the number of still-born pups and decrease of neonatal survival at these dose levels. The effects on parturition in rats are consistent with the species specific estrogen-lowering property produced by high doses of fluconazole. Such a hormone change has not been observed in women treated with fluconazole.

➤*Pregnancy: Category C.* Fluconazole was administered orally to pregnant rabbits during organogenesis in 2 studies, at 5, 10, and 20 mg/kg and at 5, 25, and 75 mg/kg, respectively. Maternal weight gain was impaired at all dose levels, and abortions occurred at 75 mg/kg (≈ 20 to 60 times the recommended human dose); no adverse fetal effects were detected. In several studies in which pregnant rats were treated orally with fluconazole during organogenesis, maternal weight gain was impaired and placental weights were increased at 25 mg/kg. There were no fetal effects at 5 or 10 mg/kg; increases in fetal anatomical variants (supernumerary ribs, renal pelvis dilation) and delays in ossification were observed at 25 and 50 mg/kg and higher doses. At doses ranging from 80 mg/kg (≈ 20 to 60 times the recommended human dose) to 320 mg/kg embryolethality in rats was increased and fetal abnormalities included wavy ribs, cleft palate, and abnormal cranio-facial ossification. These effects are consistent with the inhibition of estrogen synthesis in rats and may be a result of known effects of lowered estrogen on pregnancy, organogenesis, and parturition.

There are no adequate and well-controlled studies in pregnant women. There have been reports of multiple congenital abnormalities in infants whose mothers were being treated for 3 or more months with high dose (400 to 800 mg/day) fluconazole therapy for coccidioidomycosis (an unindicated use). The relationship between fluconazole use and these events is unclear. Fluconazole should be used in pregnancy only if the potential benefit justifies the possible risk to the fetus.

➤*Lactation:* Fluconazole is secreted in human milk at concentrations similar to plasma. Therefore, the use of fluconazole in nursing mothers is not recommended.

➤*Children:* An open-label, randomized, controlled trial has shown fluconazole to be effective in the treatment of oropharyngeal candidiasis in children 6 months to 13 years of age.

The use of fluconazole in children with cryptococcal meningitis, *Candida* esophagitis, or systemic *Candida* infections is supported by the efficacy shown for these indications in adults and by the results from several small noncomparative pediatric clinical studies. In addition, pharmacokinetic studies in children (see Pharmacokinetics) have established a dose proportionality between children and adults (see Administration and Dosage).

Efficacy of fluconazole has not been established in infants younger than 6 months of age. A small number of patients (29) ranging in age from 1 day to 6 months have been treated safely with fluconazole.

Drug Interactions

Fluconazole Drug Interactions

Precipitant drug	Object drug*		Description
Cimetidine	Fluconazole	↓	Cimetidine resulted in a reduction in fluconazole AUC and C_{max}.
Hydrochlorothiazide	Fluconazole	↑	Concomitant use resulted in a significant increase in fluconazole C_{max} and AUC, which can be attributed to reduced renal clearance.
Rifampin	Fluconazole	↓	Rifampin enhances the metabolism of concurrently administered fluconazole. Depending on the clinical circumstances, give consideration when increasing the dose of fluconazole when administered with rifampin.
Fluconazole	Alfentanil	↑	The pharmacologic and adverse effects of alfentanil may be increased. Possible inhibition of alfentanil metabolism (CYP3A4) by fluconazole may occur. Monitor for prolonged or recurrent respiratory depression. It may be necessary to administer a lower dose of alfentanil.
Fluconazole	Benzodiazepines	↑	Increased and prolonged serum levels, CNS depression, and psychomotor impairment with certain benzodiazepines may occur, possibly lasting for several days after stopping fluconazole.
Fluconazole	Buspirone	↑	Plasma buspirone concentrations may be elevated because of inhibition of buspirone metabolism. The pharmacologic and adverse effects of buspirone may be increased. Adjust the dose of buspirone as needed.
Fluconazole	Carbamazepine	↑	Plasma concentrations of carbamazepine may be elevated, increasing clinical and adverse effects because of possible inhibition of carbamazepine metabolism (CYP3A4) by fluconazole. Monitor carbamazepine concentrations.
Fluconazole	Cisapride	↑	Concurrent use may increase cisapride concentrations and cardiotoxicity may occur. Coadministration is contraindicated.
Fluconazole	Contraceptives, oral	↔	Concurrent use with an OC containing ethinyl estradiol/levonorgestrel produced an overall mean increase in the levels of the OC components; however, in some cases there were decreases ≤ 47% and 33% of ethinyl estradiol and levonorgestrel levels, respectively.
Fluconazole	Corticosteroids	↑	The effects of corticosteroids may be enhanced, resulting in increased toxicity because of inhibition of corticosteroid metabolism. Adjust corticosteroid dose as needed.
Fluconazole	Cyclosporine	↑	Significant increases in cyclosporine C_{max}, C_{min}, and AUC values and a significant decrease in oral clearance occurred following fluconazole use.
Fluconazole	Haloperidol	↑	Concurrent use may increase haloperidol plasma concentrations, increasing the risk of side effects. Adjust haloperidol dose as needed.
Fluconazole	HMG-CoA reductase inhibitors	↑	Coadministration causes increased plasma levels of the HMG-CoA reductase inhibitors. Rhabdomyolysis has been reported. If concurrent use can not be avoided, consider reducing the dose of the HMG-CoA reductase inhibitor. Pravastatin levels appear to be the least affected by concurrent use.
Fluconazole	Losartan	↑	The antihypertensive and adverse effects of losartan may be increased because of possible inhibition of metabolism (CYP2D9) of losartan by fluconazole. Monitor blood pressure.
Fluconazole	Nisoldipine	↑	Serum nisoldipine concentrations may be elevated, increasing pharmacologic and adverse effects. Fluconazole, especially > 200 mg/day, may inhibit CYP3A4.
Fluconazole	Phenytoin	↑	Coadministration resulted in an increase of phenytoin AUC values. Monitor phenytoin levels and adjust dose as needed.
Fluconazole	Protease inhibitors	↑	Concurrent use may elevate protease inhibitor levels, increasing the risk of toxicity. Adjust protease inhibitor dose as needed.
Fluconazole	Rifabutin	↑	Coadministration may increase rifabutin levels. Cases of uveitis have been reported in patients receiving both drugs. Monitor closely.

FLUCONAZOLE FOR — INJECTION

Fluconazole Drug Interactions

Precipitant drug	Object drug*		Description
Fluconazole	Sirolimus	↑	Plasma sirolimus concentrations may be elevated because of an inhibition of sirolimus gut metabolism.
Fluconazole	Sulfonylureas	↑	Fluconazole reduces the metabolism of sulfonylureas and increases the plasma concentrations of these agents. Carefully monitor blood glucose concentrations and adjust the sulfonylurea dose as necessary when these agents are coadministered.
Fluconazole	Tacrolimus	↑	There have been reports of nephrotoxicity in patients when these agents were coadministered. Carefully monitor.
Fluconazole	Theophylline	↑	Theophylline AUC, C_{max}, and half-life were significantly increased, and clearance was decreased.
Fluconazole	Tolterodine	↑	Concurrent use may increase tolterodine plasma levels. Adjust tolterodine dose as needed. Do not give more than 1 mg of tolterodine twice daily when coadministered with azole antifungals.
Fluconazole	Tricyclic antidepressants (ie, amitriptyline, nortriptyline)	↑	Serum tricyclic antidepressant (TCA) concentrations may be elevated, resulting in an increase in therapeutic and adverse effects including cardiac arrhythmia. Inhibition of TCA metabolism is suspected (CYP2C9 by fluconazole). Adjust the TCA dose as needed.
Fluconazole	Vinca alkaloids (eg, vincristine)	↑	The risk of vinca alkaloid toxicity (eg, constipation, myalgia, neutropenia) may be increased. Avoid coadministration of these agents whenever possible.
Fluconazole	Warfarin	↑	The anticoagulant effect of warfarin may be increased. A single warfarin dose after 14 days of fluconazole resulted in an increase in the PT response. Monitor PT and INR frequently.
Fluconazole	Zidovudine	↑	There was a significant increase in zidovudine AUC following fluconazole administration.
Fluconazole	Zolpidem	↑	Plasma concentrations and therapeutic effects of zolpidem may be increased. The dose of zolpidem may need to be decreased during coadministration of azole antifungal agents.

* ↑ = Object drug increased. ↓ = Object drug decreased.
↔ = Undetermined clinical effect.

Adverse Reactions

➤*Patients receiving multiple doses for other infections:* Sixteen percent of over 4000 patients treated with fluconazole in clinical trials of 7 days or more experienced adverse events. Treatment was discontinued in 1.5% of patients due to adverse clinical events and in 1.3% of patients due to laboratory test abnormalities.

Clinical adverse events were reported more frequently in HIV infected patients (21%) than in non-HIV infected patients (13%); however, the patterns in HIV infected and non-HIV infected patients were similar. The proportions of patients discontinuing therapy due to clinical adverse events were similar in the 2 groups (1.5%).

The following treatment-related clinical adverse events occurred at an incidence of 1% or greater in 4048 patients receiving fluconazole for 7 or more days in clinical trials: Nausea (3.7%), headache (1.9%), skin rash (1.8%), vomiting (1.7%), abdominal pain (1.7%), diarrhea (1.5%).

The following adverse events have occurred under conditions where a causal association is probable.

Allergic – In rare cases, anaphylaxis has been reported.

Hepatic – In combined clinical trials and marketing experience, there have been rare cases of serious hepatic reactions during treatment with fluconazole (see Warnings). The spectrum of these hepatic reactions has ranged from mild transient elevations in transaminases to clinical hepatitis, cholestasis, and fulminant hepatic failure, including fatalities. Instances of fatal hepatic reactions were noted to occur primarily in patients with serious underlying medical conditions (predominantly AIDS or malignancy) and often while taking multiple concomitant medications. Transient hepatic reactions, including hepatitis and jaundice, have occurred among patients with no other identifiable risk factors. In each of these cases, liver function returned to baseline on discontinuation of fluconazole.

➤*Adverse reactions of uncertain causal association with fluconazole:* The following adverse reactions have occurred under conditions where a causal association is uncertain.

CNS – Seizures.

Dermatologic – Exfoliative skin disorders including Stevens-Johnson syndrome and toxic epidermal necrolysis (see Warnings), alopecia.

Hematologic/Lymphatic – Leukopenia, including neutropenia and agranulocytosis, thrombocytopenia.

Metabolic – Hypercholesterolemia, hypertriglyceridemia, hypokalemia.

➤*Children:* In Phase II/III clinical trials conducted in the United States and in Europe, 577 pediatric patients, ages 1 day to 17 years were treated with fluconazole at doses up to 15 mg/kg/day for up to 1616 days.

Adverse reactions	Percentage of patients with treatment-related side effects fluconazole (n = 577)	Comparative agents (n = 451)
With any side effect	13%	9.3%
Vomiting	5.4%	5.1%
Abdominal pain	2.8%	1.6%
Nausea	2.3%	1.6%
Diarrhea	2.1%	2.2%

Overdosage

➤*Symptoms:* There has been 1 reported case of overdosage with fluconazole. A 42-year-old patient infected with human immunodeficiency virus developed hallucinations and exhibited paranoid behavior after reportedly ingesting 8200 mg of fluconazole. The patient was admitted to the hospital, and his condition resolved within 48 hours.

➤*Treatment:* In the event of overdose, symptomatic treatment (with supportive measures and gastric lavage if clinically indicated) should be instituted.

Fluconazole is largely excreted in urine. A 3-hour hemodialysis session decreases plasma levels by ≈ 50%.

Animal toxicology – In mice and rats receiving very high doses of fluconazole, clinical effects in both species included decreased motility and respiration, ptosis, lacrimation, salivation, urinary incontinence, loss of righting reflex, and cyanosis; death was sometimes preceded by clonic convulsions.

ITRACONAZOLE

Rx	**Itraconazole** (Various, eg, Eon)	**Capsules:** 100 mg	In 28s, 30s, 100s, 500s, and UD 28s and 30s.
Rx	**Sporanox** (Janssen)		Sucrose, sugar. (Janssen Sporanox 100). Blue/pink. In 30s, UD 30s, and *PulsePak* 28s.
Rx	**Sporanox** (Ortho Biotech)	**Injection:** 10 mg/mL	Kit: 25 mL amp, 50 mL bag of 0.9% NaCl injection, and 1 filtered infusion set.
		Oral solution: 10 mg/mL	Saccharin, sorbitol. Cherry/caramel flavor. In 150 mL.

ITRACONAZOLE — ORAL

WARNING

Congestive heart failure (CHF) – If signs or symptoms of CHF occur during administration of itraconazole, reassess continued itraconazole use.

Do not administer itraconazole capsules for the treatment of onychomycosis in patients with evidence of ventricular dysfunction such as CHF or a history of CHF. If signs or symptoms of CHF occur during administration of itraconazole capsules, discontinue administration. When itraconazole was administered intravenously (IV) to dogs and healthy human volunteers, negative inotropic effects were seen.

Drug Interactions – Coadministration of cisapride, pimozide, quinidine, or dofetilide with itraconazole is contraindicated. Itraconazole, a potent cytochrome P450 3A4 isoenzyme system (CYP3A4) inhibitor, may increase plasma concentrations of drugs metabolized by this pathway. Serious cardiovascular events, including QT prolongation, torsades de pointes, ventricular tachycardia, cardiac arrest, and/or sudden death have occurred in patients using cisapride, pimozide, or quinidine concomitantly with itraconazole and/or other CYP3A4 inhibitors.

Indications

➤*Aspergillosis (capsules):* Treatment of pulmonary and extrapulmonary aspergillosis in immunocompromised and nonimmunocompromised patients who are intolerant of or who are refractory to amphotericin B therapy.

➤*Blastomycosis (capsules):* Treatment of pulmonary and extrapulmonary blastomycosis in immunocompromised and nonimmunocompromised patients.

➤*Febrile neutropenia, empiric (oral solution):* For empiric therapy of febrile neutropenic (ETFN) patients with suspected fungal infections. Note: In a comparative trial, the overall response rate for itraconazole-treated subjects was higher than for amphotericin B-treated subjects. However, compared with amphotericin B-treated subjects, a larger number of itraconazole-treated subjects discontinued treatment because of persistent fever and a change in antifungal medication because of fever. Whereas a larger number of amphotericin B-treated subjects discontinued because of drug intolerance.

➤*Histoplasmosis (capsules):* Treatment of histoplasmosis, including chronic cavitary pulmonary disease and disseminated, nonmeningeal histoplasmosis in immunocompromised and nonimmunocompromised patients.

➤*Onychomycosis (capsules):* Treatment of onychomycosis of the toenail, with or without fingernail involvement, caused by dermatophytes (*tinea unguium*) and onychomycosis of the fingernail caused by dermatophytes (*tinea unguium*) in nonimmunocompromised patients.

Prior to initiating treatment, obtain appropriate nail specimens for laboratory testing (potassium hydroxide [KOH] preparation, fungal culture, or nail biopsy) to confirm the diagnosis of onychomycosis.

➤*Oropharyngeal/esophageal candidiasis (oral solution):* Treatment of oropharyngeal and esophageal candidiasis.

➤*Unlabeled uses:* Itraconazole solution (200 mg/day) is recommended as an alternative to fluconazole as secondary prevention of oropharyngeal, vaginal, or esophageal candidiasis in HIV-infected patients who have severe or frequent recurrences; itraconazole capsules (200 mg/day) have been used as an alternative to fluconazole for primary prevention of cryptococcosis in adults with advanced HIV disease (CD4 counts less than 50 cells/mcL) and are recommended as an alternate to fluconazole for lifelong secondary prevention of cryptococcal disease in HIV-infected adults; itraconazole capsules (200 mg/day) are recommended as first-line agent in the primary prevention of histoplasmosis in adults with advanced HIV disease (CD4 counts less than 100 cells/mcL) and live in endemic areas (rate greater than or equal to 10 cases per 100 patient-years) and also as first-line agent for lifelong secondary prophylaxis (200 mg twice daily); itraconazole capsules (200 mg twice daily) are recommended as an alternate agent to fluconazole for lifelong secondary prevention of coccidioidomycosis in HIV-infected adults; oral itraconazole also is recommended for secondary prevention of histoplasmosis (first line; 2 to 5 mg/kg every 12 to 48 hours), cryptococcal disease (alternate therapy; 2 to 5 mg/kg every 12 to 24 hours), and coccidioidomycosis (alternate therapy; 2 to 5 mg/kg every 12 to 48 hours) in children with HIV; oral itraconazole (2 to 5 mg/kg every 12 to 24 hours) is recommended for primary prevention of histoplasmosis (first-line agent) and cryptococcal disease (alternate therapy) in children with HIV, severe immunosuppression, and live in endemic areas (histoplasmosis).

Administration and Dosage

➤*Approved by the FDA:* September 11, 1992.

The itraconazole capsule is a different preparation than itraconazole oral solution and should not be used interchangeably. Only the oral solution has been demonstrated effective for oral and/or esophageal candidiasis.

➤*Capsules:* Take itraconazole capsules with a full meal to ensure maximal absorption.

Blastomycosis and histoplasmosis – The recommended dosage is 200 mg once daily (2 capsules). If there is no obvious improvement, or there is evidence of progressive fungal disease, increase the dose in 100 mg increments to a maximum of 400 mg daily. Give doses above 200 mg/day in 2 divided doses.

Aspergillosis – A daily dose of 200 to 400 mg is recommended.

Life-threatening situations – In life-threatening situations, use a loading dose whether given as oral capsules or intravenously. Although clinical studies did not provide for a loading dose, it is recommended, based on pharmacokinetic data, that a loading dose of 200 mg (2 capsules) 3 times daily (600 mg/day) be given for the first 3 days of treatment.

Continue treatment for a minimum of 3 months and until clinical parameters and laboratory tests indicate that the active fungal infection has subsided. An inadequate period of treatment may lead to recurrence of active infection.

Onychomycosis –

Toenails with or without fingernail involvement: 200 mg (2 capsules) once daily for 12 consecutive weeks.

Fingernails only: 2 treatment pulses, each consisting of 200 mg (2 capsules) twice daily (400 mg/day) for 1 week. The pulses are separated by a 3-week period without itraconazole.

➤*Oral solution:* Itraconazole oral solution should be taken without food, if possible.

Febrile neutropenia, empiric – 200 mg IV twice daily for 4 doses, followed by 200 mg once daily for up to 14 days. Infuse each IV dose over 1 hour. Continue treatment with itraconazole oral solution 200 mg (20 mL) twice daily until resolution of clinically significant neutropenia. The safety and efficacy of itraconazole use exceeding 28 days in ETFN is not known.

Oropharyngeal candidiasis – 200 mg (20 mL) daily for 1 to 2 weeks. Vigorously swish the solution in the mouth (10 mL at a time) for several seconds and swallow. Clinical signs and symptoms of oropharyngeal candidiasis generally resolve within several days.

For patients with oropharyngeal candidiasis unresponsive/refractory to treatment with fluconazole tablets, the recommended dose is 100 mg (10 mL) twice daily. For patients responding to therapy, clinical response will be seen in 2 to 4 weeks. Patients may relapse shortly after discontinuing therapy. Limited data on the safety of long-term use (greater than 6 months) of itraconazole oral solution are available at this time.

Esophageal candidiasis – 100 mg (10 mL) daily for a minimum treatment of 3 weeks. Vigorously swish the solution in the mouth (10 mL at a time) for several seconds and swallow. Continue treatment for 2 weeks following resolution of symptoms. Doses up to 200 mg (20 mL) per day may be used based on medical judgement of the patient's response to therapy.

➤*Storage/Stability:*

Capsules – Store at controlled room temperature 15° to 25°C (59° to 77°F). Protect from light and moisture.

Oral solution – Store at or below 25°C (77°F). Do not freeze.

Actions

➤*Pharmacology:* Itraconazole is a systemic triazole antifungal agent. In vitro, itraconazole inhibits the cytochrome P450-dependent synthesis of ergosterol, which is a vital component of fungal membranes.

➤*Pharmacokinetics:*

Absorption/Distribution –

The plasma protein binding of itraconazole is 99.8% and that of hydroxyitraconazole is 99.5%. Following IV administration, the volume of distribution of itraconazole averaged 796 ± 185 L.

The pharmacokinetics of itraconazole after IV administration and its absolute oral bioavailability from an oral solution were studied in a randomized crossover study in 6 healthy men. The observed absolute oral bioavailability of itraconazole was 55%.

Capsules: The oral bioavailability of itraconazole is maximal when itraconazole capsules are taken with a full meal. The pharmacokinetics of itraconazole were studied in 6 healthy men who received, in a crossover design, single doses of itraconazole 100 mg as a polyethylene glycol capsule, with or without a full meal. The same 6 volunteers also received 50 or 200 mg with a full meal in a crossover design. In this study, only itraconazole plasma concentrations were measured.

Pharmacokinetics of Various Dosages of Itraconazole Capsules (N = 6)

	50 mg (fed)	100 mg (fed)	100 mg (fasted)	200 mg (fed)
C_{max} (ng/mL)	45 ± 16[a]	132 ± 67	38 ± 20	289 ± 100
t_{max} (hours)	3.2 ± 1.3	4 ± 1.1	3.3 ± 1	4.7 ± 1.4
$AUC_{0-\infty}$ (ng•h/mL)	567 ± 264	1899 ± 838	722 ± 289	5211 ± 2116

[a] Mean ± standard deviation.

Doubling the itraconazole dose results in approximately a 3-fold increase in the itraconazole plasma concentrations.

Values given in the following table represent data from a crossover pharmacokinetics study in which 27 healthy male volunteers each took a single dose of itraconazole capsules 200 mg with or without a full meal:

Pharmacokinetics of a Single Itraconazole Capsule 200 mg (N = 27)

	Itraconazole		Hydroxyitraconazole	
	Fed	Fasted	Fed	Fasted
C_{max} (ng/mL)	239 ± 85[a]	140 ± 65	397 ± 103	286 ± 101
t_{max} (hours)	4.5 ± 1.1	3.9 ± 1	5.1 ± 1.6	4.5 ± 1.1
$AUC_{0-\infty}$ (ng•h/mL)	3423 ± 1154	2094 ± 905	7978 ± 2648	5191 ± 2489
$t_{½}$ (hours)	21 ± 5	21 ± 7	12 ± 3	12 ± 3

[a] Mean ± standard deviation.

Absorption of itraconazole under fasted conditions in individuals with relative or absolute achlorhydria, such as patients with AIDS or volunteers taking gastric acid secretion suppressors (eg, H_2 receptor antagonists), was increased when itraconazole capsules were administered with a cola beverage. Eighteen men with AIDS received single doses of itraconazole capsules

ITRACONAZOLE — ORAL

200 mg under fasted conditions with 240 mL of water or 240 mL of a cola beverage in a crossover design. The absorption of itraconazole was increased when itraconazole capsules were coadministered with a cola beverage, with AUC_{0-24} and C_{max} increasing 75% ± 121% and 95% ± 128%, respectively.

Steady-state concentrations were reached within 15 days following oral doses of 50 to 400 mg daily. Values given in the information below are data at steady-state from a pharmacokinetics study in which 27 healthy male volunteers took itraconazole capsules 200 mg twice daily (with a full meal) for 15 days:

Steady-State Pharmacokinetics of Itraconazole Capsules

	Itraconazole	Hydroxyitraconazole
C_{max} (ng/mL)	2282 ± 514[a]	3488 ± 742
C_{min} (ng/mL)	1855 ± 535	3349 ± 761
t_{max} (hours)	4.6 ± 1.8	3.4 ± 3.4
$AUC_{0-12\,hr}$ (ng•h/mL)	22569 ± 5375	38572 ± 8450
t½ (hours)	64 ± 32	56 ± 24

[a] Mean ± standard deviation.

Oral solution: The absolute bioavailability of itraconazole administered as a nonmarketed solution formulation under fed conditions was 55% in 6 healthy men. However, the bioavailability of itraconazole oral solution is increased under fasted conditions reaching higher maximum plasma concentrations (C_{max}) in a shorter period of time. In 27 healthy men, the steady-state area under the plasma concentration versus time curve (AUC_{0-24hr}) of itraconazole (itraconazole oral solution, 200 mg daily for 15 days) under fasted conditions was 131 ± 30% of that obtained under fed conditions. Therefore, unlike itraconazole capsules, it is recommended that itraconazole oral solution be administered without food. Presented in the table below are the steady-state (day 15) pharmacokinetic parameters for itraconazole and hydroxyitraconazole (itraconazole oral solution) under fasted and fed conditions:

Steady-State Pharmacokinetic Parameters for Itraconazole Oral Solution

	Itraconazole		Hydroxy-itraconazole	
	Fasted	Fed	Fasted	Fed
C_{max} (ng/mL)	1963 ± 601[a]	1435 ± 477	2055 ± 487	1781 ± 397
t_{max} (hours)	2.5 ± 0.8	4.4 ± 0.7	5.3 ± 4.3	4.3 ± 1.2
$AUC_{0-24\,h}$ (ng•h/mL)	29271 ± 10285	22815 ± 7098	45184 ± 10981	38823 ± 8907
t½ (hours)	39.7 ± 13	37.4 ± 13	27.3 ± 13	26.1 ± 10

[a] Mean ± standard deviation.

The bioavailability of itraconazole oral solution relative to itraconazole capsules was studied in 30 healthy men who received itraconazole 200 mg as the oral solution and capsules under fed conditions. The $AUC_{0-\infty}$ from itraconazole oral solution was 149 ± 68% of that obtained from itraconazole capsules; a similar increase was observed for hydroxyitraconazole. In addition, a cross study comparison of itraconazole and hydroxyitraconazole pharmacokinetics following the administration of single doses of itraconazole oral solution 200 mg (under fasted conditions) or itraconazole capsules (under fed conditions) indicates that when these 2 formulations are administered under conditions which optimize their systemic absorption, the bioavailability of the solution relative to capsules is expected to be increased further. Therefore, it is recommended that itraconazole oral solution and itraconazole capsules not be used interchangeably. The following table contains pharmacokinetic parameters for itraconazole and hydroxyitraconazole following single doses of itraconazole oral solution 200 mg (n = 27) or itraconazole capsules (n = 30) administered to healthy men under fasted and fed conditions, respectively:

Pharmacokinetic Parameters for Itraconazole Capsules (N = 30) vs Oral Solution (N = 27)

	Itraconazole		Hydroxy-itraconazole	
	Oral solution fasted	Capsules fed	Oral solution fasted	Capsules fed
C_{max} (ng/mL)	544 ± 213[a]	302 ± 119	622 ± 116	504 ± 132
t_{max} (hours)	2.2 ± 0.8	5 ± 0.8	3.5 ± 1.2	5 ± 1
$AUC_{0-24\,hr}$ (ng•h/mL)	4505 ± 1670	2682 ± 1084	9552 ± 1835	7293 ± 2144

[a] Mean ± standard deviation.

Metabolism/Excretion – Itraconazole is metabolized predominately by the cytochrome P450 3A4 isoenzyme system (CYP3A4), resulting in the formation of several metabolites, including hydroxyitraconazole, the major metabolite. Results of a pharmacokinetics study suggest that itraconazole may undergo saturable metabolism with multiple dosing. Fecal excretion of the parent drug varies between 3% to 18% of the dose. Renal excretion of the parent drug is less than 0.03% of the dose. About 40% of the dose is excreted as inactive metabolites in the urine. No single excreted metabolite represents more than 5% of a dose. Itraconazole total plasma clearance averaged 381 ± 95 mL/minute following IV administration.

Special populations –

Children:

• *Oral solution* – The pharmacokinetics of itraconazole oral solution were studied in 26 pediatric patients requiring systemic antifungal therapy. Patients were stratified by age: 6 months to 2 years of age (n = 8), 2 to 5 years of age (n = 7) and 5 to 12 years of age (n = 11), and received itraconazole oral solution 5 mg/kg once daily for 14 days. Pharmacokinetic parameters at steady-state (day 14) were not significantly different among the age strata and are summarized in the table below for all 26 patients:

Pharmacokinetics of Itraconazole Oral Solution in Pediatric Patients (N = 26)

	Itraconazole	Hydroxyitraconazole
C_{max} (ng/mL)	582.5 ± 382.4[a]	692.4 ± 355
C_{min} (ng/mL)	187.5 ± 161.4	403.8 ± 336.1
$AUC_{0-24\,h}$ (ng•h/mL)	7706.7 ± 5245.2	13356.4 ± 8942.4
t½ (hours)	35.8 ± 35.6	17.7 ± 13

[a] Mean ± standard deviation.

Renal function impairment: A pharmacokinetic study using a single dose of itraconazole 200 mg (four 50 mg capsules) was conducted in 3 groups of patients with renal impairment (uremia [n = 7]; hemodialysis [n = 7]; and continuous ambulatory peritoneal dialysis [n = 5]). In uremic subjects with a mean creatinine clearance of 13 mL/min × 1.73 m^2, the bioavailability was slightly reduced compared with healthy population parameters. This study did not demonstrate any significant effect of hemodialysis or continuous ambulatory peritoneal dialysis on the pharmacokinetics of itraconazole (t_{max}, C_{max}, and AUC_{0-8}). Plasma concentration-versus-time profiles showed wide intersubject variation in all 3 groups.

Hepatic function impairment: Carefully monitor patients with impaired hepatic function when taking itraconazole. Consider the prolonged elimination half-life of itraconazole observed in cirrhotic patients when deciding to initiate therapy with other medications metabolized by CYP3A4, such as lovastatin, simvastatin, cisapride, pimozide, quinidine, dofetilide, triazolam, and oral midazolam. Itraconazole has been associated with rare cases of hepatotoxicity, including liver failure and death. If clinical signs or symptoms develop that are consistent with liver disease, discontinue treatment.

• *Capsules* – A pharmacokinetic study using a single dose of itraconazole 100 mg (one 100 mg capsule) was conducted in 6 healthy and 12 cirrhotic subjects. No statistically significant differences in AUC were seen between these 2 groups. A statistically significant reduction in mean C_{max} (47%) and a 2-fold increase in the elimination half-life (37 ± 17 hours) of itraconazole were noted in cirrhotic subjects compared with healthy subjects.

Decreased cardiac contractility: When itraconazole was administered IV to anesthetized dogs, a dose-related negative inotropic effect was documented. In a healthy volunteer study of itraconazole injection (IV infusion), transient, asymptomatic decreases in left ventricular ejection fraction were observed using gated SPECT imaging; these resolved before the next infusion, 12 hours later.

• *Capsules* – If signs or symptoms of CHF appear during administration of itraconazole capsules, discontinue itraconazole.

• *Oral solution* – If signs or symptoms of CHF appear during administration of itraconazole oral solution, monitor carefully and consider other treatment alternatives which may include discontinuation of itraconazole oral solution administration.

Cystic fibrosis – Seventeen cystic fibrosis patients, 7 to 28 years of age, were administered itraconazole oral solution 2.5 mg/kg twice daily for 14 days in a pharmacokinetic study. Sixteen patients completed the study. Steady state trough concentrations more than 250 ng/mL were achieved in 6 out of 11 patients 16 years of age and older, but none of the 5 patients younger than 16 years of age. Large variability was observed in the pharmacokinetic data (%CV for trough concentrations = 98% and 70% for 16 years of age and older and less than 16 years of age, respectively; %CV for AUC = 75% and 58% for 16 years of age and older and less than 16 years of age, respectively). If a patient with cystic fibrosis does not respond to itraconazole oral solution, consider switching to alternative therapy.

➤*Microbiology:* In vitro studies have demonstrated that itraconazole inhibits the cytochrome P-450–dependent synthesis of ergosterol, which is a vital component of fungal cell membranes.

Activity in vitro and in vivo – Itraconazole exhibits in vitro activity against *Blastomyces dermatitidis*, *Histoplasma capsulatum*, *Histoplasma duboisii*, *Aspergillus flavus*, *Aspergillus fumigatus*, *Candida albicans*, and *Cryptococcus neoformans*. Itraconazole also exhibits varying in vitro activity against *Sporothrix schenckii*, *Trichophyton* species, *Candida krusei*, and other *Candida* species. The bioactive metabolite, hydroxyitraconazole, has not been evaluated against *Histoplasma capsulatum* and *Blastomyces dermatitidis*. Correlation between minimum inhibitory concentration (MIC) results in vitro and clinical outcome has yet to be established for azole antifungal agents.

Resistance –

Several in vitro studies have reported that some fungal clinical isolates, including *Candida* species, with reduced susceptibility to 1 azole antifungal agent may also be less susceptible to other azole derivatives. The finding of cross-resistance is dependent on a number of factors, including the species evaluated, its clinical history, the particular azole compounds compared, and the type of susceptibility test that is performed. The relevance of these in vitro susceptibility data to clinical outcome remains to be elucidated.

Contraindications

Do not administer itraconazole capsules for the treatment of onychomycosis in patients with evidence of ventricular dysfunction such as CHF or a history of CHF.

ITRACONAZOLE — ORAL

Coadministration with certain drugs metabolized by the cytochrome P-450 3A4 isoenzyme system (CYP3A4), cisapride, oral midazolam, pimozide, quinidine, dofetilide, triazolam, HMG-CoA reductase inhibitors metabolized by CYP3A4, such as lovastatin and simvastatin, and ergot alkaloids metabolized by CYP3A4, such as dihydroergotamine, ergotamine, ergonovine, and methylergonovine (see Drug interactions).

Itraconazole is contraindicated for patients who have shown hypersensitivity to itraconazole or its excipients. There is no information regarding cross-hypersensitivity between itraconazole and other azole antifungal agents. Use caution when prescribing itraconazole to patients with hypersensitivity to other azoles.

Warnings

➤*Interchangeability:* Do not use itraconazole capsules and itraconazole oral solution interchangeably. This is because drug exposure is greater with the oral solution than with the capsules when the same dose of drug is given. In addition, the topical effects of mucosal exposure may be different between the 2 formulations. Only the oral solution has been demonstrated effective for oral and/or esophageal candidiasis.

➤*Cardiac dysrhythmias:* Life-threatening cardiac dysrhythmias and/or sudden death have occurred in patients using cisapride, pimozide, or quinidine concomitantly with itraconazole and/or other CYP3A4 inhibitors. Concomitant administration of these drugs with itraconazole is contraindicated.

➤*Cardiac disease:* For patients with risk factors for CHF, carefully review the risks and benefits of itraconazole therapy. These risk factors include cardiac disease such as ischemic and valvular disease; significant pulmonary disease such as chronic obstructive pulmonary disease; and renal failure and other edematous disorders. Inform such patients of the signs and symptoms of CHF, treat with caution, and monitor for signs and symptoms of CHF during treatment. If signs or symptoms of CHF appear during administration of itraconazole capsules, discontinue administration.

See Actions for more information.

Cases of CHF, peripheral edema, and pulmonary edema have been reported in the postmarketing period among patients being treated for onychomycosis and/or systemic fungal infections.

Capsules – Do not administer itraconazole capsules for the treatment of onychomycosis in patients with evidence of ventricular dysfunction such as CHF or a history of CHF. Do not use itraconazole capsules for other indications in patients with evidence of ventricular dysfunction unless the benefit clearly outweighs the risk.

Oral solution – Do not use itraconazole oral solution in patients with evidence of ventricular dysfunction unless the benefit clearly outweighs the risk. If signs or symptoms of CHF appear during administration of itraconazole oral solution, monitor carefully and consider other treatment alternatives which may include discontinuation of itraconazole oral solution administration.

➤*Cystic fibrosis:* If a patient with cystic fibrosis does not respond to itraconazole oral solution, consider switching to alternative therapy.

➤*Severely neutropenic patients:* Itraconazole oral solution as treatment for oropharyngeal and/or esophageal candidiasis was not investigated in severely neutropenic patients. Because of its pharmacokinetic properties, itraconazole oral solution is not recommended for initiation of treatment in patients at immediate risk of systemic candidiasis.

➤*Hepatotoxicity:* Itraconazole has been associated with rare cases of serious hepatotoxicity, including liver failure and death. Some of these cases had neither preexisting liver disease nor a serious underlying medical condition and some of these cases developed within the first week of treatment. If clinical signs or symptoms develop that are consistent with liver disease, discontinue treatment and perform liver function testing. Continued itraconazole use or reinstitution of treatment with itraconazole is strongly discouraged unless there is a serious or life-threatening situation where the expected benefit exceeds the risk.

In patients with elevated or abnormal liver enzymes or active liver disease, or who have experienced liver toxicity with other drugs, treatment with itraconazole is strongly discouraged unless there is a serious or life-threatening situation where the expected benefit exceeds the risk.

➤*Carcinogenesis:* Itraconazole showed no evidence of carcinogenicity potential in mice treated orally for 23 months at dosage levels up to 80 mg/kg/day (approximately 10 times the maximum recommended human dose [MRHD]). Male rats treated with 25 mg/kg/day (3.1 times MRHD) had a slightly increased incidence of soft tissue sarcoma. These sarcomas may have been a consequence of hypercholesterolemia, which is a response of rats, but not dogs or humans, to chronic itraconazole administration. Female rats treated with 50 mg/kg/day (6.25 times MRHD) had an increased incidence of squamous cell carcinoma of the lung (2/50) as compared with the untreated group. Although the occurrence of squamous cell carcinoma in the lung is extremely uncommon in untreated rats, the increase in this study was not statistically significant.

Oral solution: Hydroxypropyl-β-cyclodextrin (HP-β-CD), the solubilizing excipient used in itraconazole oral solution, was found to produce pancreatic exocrine hyperplasia and neoplasia when administered orally to rats at doses of 500, 2,000, or 5,000 mg/kg/day for 25 months. Adenocarcinomas of the exocrine pancreas produced in the treated animals were not seen in the untreated group and are not reported in the historical controls. Development of these tumors may be related to a mitogenic action of cholecystokinin. This finding was not observed in the mouse carcinogenicity study at doses of 500, 2,000, or 5,000 mg/kg/day for 22 to 23 months; however, the clinical relevance of these findings is unknown. Based on body surface area comparisons, the exposure to humans of HP-β-CD at the recommended clinical dose of itraconazole oral solution, is approximately equivalent to 1.7 times the exposure at the lowest dose in the rat study.

➤*Fertility impairment:* Itraconazole did not affect the fertility of male or female rats treated orally with dosage levels of up to 40 mg/kg/day (5 times MRHD), even though parental toxicity was present at this dosage level. More severe signs of parental toxicity, including death, were present in the next higher dosage level, 160 mg/kg/day (20 times MRHD).

➤*Pregnancy: Category C.*

There are no studies in pregnant women. Use itraconazole for the treatment of systemic fungal infections in pregnancy only if the benefit outweighs the potential risk. Do not administer itraconazole for the treatment of onychomycosis to pregnant patients or to women contemplating pregnancy.

Itraconazole was found to cause a dose-related increase in maternal toxicity, embryotoxicity, and teratogenicity in rats at dosage levels of approximately 40 to 160 mg/kg/day (5 to 20 times MRHD), and in mice at dosage levels of approximately 80 mg/kg/day (10 times MRHD). In rats, the teratogenicity consisted of major skeletal defects; in mice, it consisted of encephaloceles and/or macroglossia.

During postmarketing experience, cases of congenital abnormalities have been reported.

Women of childbearing potential – Do not administer itraconazole to women of childbearing potential for the treatment of onychomycosis unless they are using effective measures to prevent pregnancy and they begin therapy on the second or third day following the onset of menses. Continue effective contraception throughout itraconazole therapy and for 2 months following the end of treatment.

➤*Lactation:* Itraconazole is excreted in human milk; therefore, weigh the expected benefits of itraconazole therapy for the mother against the potential risk from exposure of itraconazole to the infant. The US Public Health Service Centers for Disease Control and Prevention advises HIV-infected women not to breast feed to avoid potential transmission of HIV to uninfected infants.

➤*Children:* The efficacy and safety of itraconazole have not been established in pediatric patients.

The long-term effects of itraconazole on bone growth in children are unknown. In 3 toxicology studies using rats, itraconazole induced bone defects at dosage levels as low as 20 mg/kg/day (2.5 times MRHD). The induced defects included reduced bone plate activity, thinning of the zona compacta of the large bones, and increased bone fragility. At a dosage level of 80 mg/kg/day (10 times MRHD) over 1 year or 160 mg/kg/day (20 times MRHD) for 6 months, itraconazole induced small tooth pulp with hypocellular appearance in some rats. No such bone toxicity has been reported in adult patients.

Precautions

➤*Monitoring:* Monitor liver function in patients with preexisting hepatic function abnormalities or those who have experienced liver toxicity with other medications, and consider monitoring liver function in all patients receiving itraconazole. Stop treatment immediately and conduct liver function testing in patients who develop signs and symptoms suggestive of liver dysfunction.

➤*Neuropathy:* If neuropathy occurs that may be attributable to itraconazole, discontinue the treatment.

➤*Decreased gastric acidity:*

Capsules – Administer itraconazole capsules after a full meal. The oral bioavailability of itraconazole is maximal when itraconazole capsules are taken with a full meal.

Under fasted conditions, itraconazole absorption was decreased in the presence of decreased gastric acidity. The absorption of itraconazole may be decreased with the concomitant administration of antacids or gastric acid secretion suppressors. Studies conducted under fasted conditions demonstrated that administration with 240 mL of a cola beverage resulted in increased absorption of itraconazole in AIDS patients with relative or absolute achlorhydria. This increase relative to the effects of a full meal is unknown.

Because hypochlorhydria has been reported in HIV-infected individuals, the absorption of itraconazole in these patients may be decreased.

Drug Interactions

➤*Cytochrome P450 system:* Concomitant administration of itraconazole and certain drugs metabolized by the cytochrome P450 3A4 isoenzyme system (CYP3A4) may result in increased plasma concentrations of those drugs, leading to potentially serious and/or life-threatening adverse events. Cisapride, oral midazolam, pimozide, quinidine, dofetilide, and triazolam are contraindicated with itraconazole. HMG-CoA reductase inhibitors metabolized by CYP3A4, such as lovastatin and simvastatin, are also contraindicated with itraconazole. Ergot alkaloids metabolized by CYP3A4 such as dihydroergotamine, ergonovine, and methylergonovine are contraindicated with itraconazole. Use cilostazol and eletriptan (CYP3A4 metabolized drugs) with caution when coadministered with itraconazole.

Itraconazole and its major metabolite, hydroxyitraconazole, are inhibitors of CYP3A4.

Itraconazole may decrease the elimination of drugs metabolized by CYP3A4, resulting in increased plasma concentrations of these drugs when they are administered with itraconazole. These elevated plasma concentrations may increase or prolong both therapeutic and adverse effects of these drugs. Whenever possible, monitor plasma concentrations of these drugs, and make dosage adjustments after concomitant itraconazole therapy is initiated. When appropriate, clinical monitoring for signs or symptoms of increased or

ITRACONAZOLE — ORAL

prolonged pharmacologic effects is advised. Upon discontinuation, depending on the dose and duration of treatment, itraconazole plasma concentrations decline gradually (especially in patients with hepatic cirrhosis or in those receiving CYP3A4 inhibitors). This is particularly important when initiating therapy with drugs whose metabolism is affected by itraconazole.

Inducers of CYP3A4 may decrease the plasma concentrations of itraconazole. Itraconazole may not be effective in patients concomitantly taking itraconazole and 1 of these drugs. Therefore, administration of these drugs with itraconazole is not recommended.

Other inhibitors of CYP3A4 may increase the plasma concentrations of itraconazole. Monitor patients who must take itraconazole concomitantly with 1 of these drugs for signs or symptoms of increased or prolonged pharmacologic effects of itraconazole.

Itraconazole Drug Interactions

Precipitant drug	Object drug*		Description
Antacids Proton pump inhibitors H_2-antagonists	Itraconazole	↓	Absorption of itraconazole capsules is impaired when gastric acidity is decreased. Administer at least 1 hour before or 2 hours after itraconazole capsules. Administer itraconazole with a cola beverage when coadministering with H_2-antagonists or other gastric acid suppressors.
Didanosine (buffered formulation only)	Itraconazole	↓	The therapeutic effects of itraconazole may be decreased. Administer itraconazole ≥ 2 hours before didanosine (buffered formulation only).
Macrolide antibiotics Erythromycin Clarithromycin	Itraconazole	↑	Macrolide antibiotics may increase plasma itraconazole concentrations through inhibition of CYP3A4.
Nevirapine	Itraconazole	↓	Coadministration may lead to decreased itraconazole plasma levels and, therefore, is not recommended.
Phenobarbital	Itraconazole	↓	The plasma concentration of itraconazole may be decreased.
Itraconazole	Alfentanil	↑	Pharmacologic and adverse effects may be increased. Use caution when administering concurrently. Lower the alfentanil dose as needed.
Itraconazole	Amphotericin B	↓	Studies suggest that amphotericin B activity may be suppressed by prior azole antifungal therapy. Clinical significance is unknown.
Itraconazole	Aripiprazole	↑	Aripiprazole plasma concentrations may be elevated, increasing the pharmacologic and adverse effects. Reduce the aripiprazole dose 50% of the normal dose when coadministering with itraconazole.
Itraconazole	Benzodiazepines Triazolam Midazolam Alprazolam Diazepam	↑	Increased and prolonged serum levels, CNS depression, and psychomotor impairment with certain benzodiazepines may occur, possibly several days after stopping itraconazole. Concurrent use of triazolam and oral midazolam is contraindicated.
Itraconazole	Buspirone	↑	Plasma buspirone concentrations may be elevated, increasing the pharmacologic and adverse effects. In patients receiving itraconazole when buspirone is started, it may be prudent to start with a conservative dose. Monitor closely when an antifungal agent is stopped, started, or changed in dose in patients on buspirone therapy. Adjust the dose of buspirone as needed.
Itraconazole	Busulfan	↑	Itraconazole may elevate busulfan plasma levels, increasing the risk of toxicity (eg, pancytopenia). Monitor patients for increased toxicity and adjust the busulfan dose as needed.

Itraconazole Drug Interactions

Precipitant drug	Object drug*		Description
Itraconazole	Calcium channel blockers	↑	Concomitant administration may increase negative inotropic effects. Edema has also been reported with concomitant therapy. Itraconazole may inhibit the metabolism of calcium channel blockers such as dihydropyridines (eg, felodipine, nisoldipine, nifedipine) and verapamil. Coadminister with caution and adjust the dose of calcium channel blockers accordingly.
Itraconazole	Carbamazepine	↑	Plasma concentrations of carbamazepine may be elevated, increasing clinical and adverse effects. Monitor serum levels.
Carbamazepine	Itraconazole	↓	Decreased itraconazole plasma concentrations may occur with coadministration.
Itraconazole	Cilostazol	↑	Cilostazol plasma concentrations may be elevated, increasing the pharmacologic and adverse effects. Use caution with coadministration.
Itraconazole	Cisapride	↑	Increased cisapride concentrations with cardiotoxicity may occur. Itraconazole is contraindicated in patients receiving cisapride.
Itraconazole	Corticosteroids Budesonide Dexamethasone Methylprednisolone	↑	Itraconazole may inhibit the metabolism of certain corticosteroids, enhancing the effects and possibly resulting in increased toxicity. Monitor patients for adverse effects and adjust corticosteroids dose accordingly.
Itraconazole	Cyclosporine	↑	Increased cyclosporine levels may occur. Monitor cyclosporine levels and serum creatinine when itraconazole is added or discontinued.
Itraconazole	Digoxin	↑	Serum digoxin concentrations may be increased, enhancing its pharmacologic and adverse effects. Monitor plasma digoxin concentrations and observe the patient for signs of digoxin toxicity. Adjust digoxin dose accordingly.
Itraconazole	Disopyramide	↑	Serum disopyramide concentrations may be elevated. A high plasma concentration has the potential to increase the QT interval.
Itraconazole	Docetaxel	↑	Itraconazole may inhibit docetaxel metabolism.
Itraconazole	Dofetilide	↑	Elevated dofetilide plasma concentrations may occur with increased risk of ventricular arrhythmias, including torsades de pointes. Administration with itraconazole is contraindicated.
Itraconazole	Eletriptan Almotriptan	↑	Plasma concentrations of eletriptan may be elevated, increasing the pharmacologic and adverse effects. Eletriptan should not be taken within 72 hours of itraconazole.
Itraconazole	Eplerenone	↑	Elevated eplerenone plasma concentrations may occur, increasing the risk of hyperkalemia and associated serious arrhythmias. Coadministration is contraindicated.

ITRACONAZOLE — ORAL

Itraconazole Drug Interactions			
Precipitant drug	Object drug*		Description
Itraconazole	Ergot alkaloids Dihydroergotamine Ergonovine Ergotamine Methylergonovine	↑	The risk of ergot toxicity (eg, peripheral vasospasm, ischemia of the extremities and/or cerebral ischemia) may be increased. Concomitant administration is contraindicated.
Itraconazole	Halofantrine	↑	Halofantrine plasma concentrations may be elevated, increasing the potential of prolonging the QT interval. Use caution with coadministration.
Itraconazole	Haloperidol	↑	Haloperidol concentrations may be elevated, increasing the risk of side effects. Adjust dose as needed.
Itraconazole	HMG-CoA reductase inhibitors Atorvastatin Simvastatin Lovastatin	↑	Increased plasma levels and side effects of certain HMG-CoA reductase inhibitors may occur. If concurrent administration of these agents cannot be avoided, consider reducing the HMG-CoA reductase inhibitor dose. Coadministration with lovastatin and simvastatin is contraindicated.
Itraconazole	Hydantoins (eg, phenytoin)	↑	The plasma concentrations and pharmacologic effects of itraconazole may be decreased while those of hydantoins may be increased. Avoid concomitant use if possible.
Hydantoins (eg, phenytoin)	Itraconazole	↓	
Itraconazole	Oral hypoglycemic agents	↑	Severe hypoglycemia has been reported in those receiving concomitant therapy. Monitor blood glucose levels carefully.
Itraconazole	Phosphodiesterase Type 5 Inhibitors Sildenafil Tadalafil Vardenafil	↑	Phosphodiesterase Type 5 (PDE5) inhibitor plasma levels may be elevated, increasing the risk of side effects. Give PDE5 inhibitors with caution and in reduced doses to patients.
Itraconazole	Pimozide	↑	Concomitant use may increase pimozide plasma concentrations, resulting in serious cardiac effects. Administration with itraconazole is contraindicated.
Itraconazole	Protease inhibitors	↑	Plasma concentrations of protease inhibitors metabolized by CYP3A4 (eg, indinavir, ritonavir, saquinavir) may be elevated, increasing the risk of toxicity. Consider reducing the dose of the protease inhibitor during concurrent administration with itraconazole. Plasma concentrations of itraconazole may be increased by indinavir and ritonavir.
Protease inhibitors Indinavir Ritonavir	Itraconazole		
Itraconazole	Quinidine	↑	Quinidine concentrations may be elevated, increasing the risk of serious cardiovascular events. Coadministration is contraindicated.
Itraconazole	Rifamycins Rifabutin Rifampin Rifapentine Isoniazid	↑	Itraconazole levels may be decreased. Itraconazole may increase rifabutin plasma levels and toxicity. Anticipate similar effects with isoniazid. Coadministration is not recommended. If coadministration cannot be avoided, monitor antimicrobial activity and adjust dosage.
Rifamycins Rifabutin Rifampin Rifapentine Isoniazid	Itraconazole	↓	
Itraconazole	Sirolimus	↑	Coadministration may lead to increased sirolimus plasma levels. Monitor sirolimus plasma concentrations and observe patient for toxicity when starting or stopping itraconazole. Adjust sirolimus dose accordingly.
Itraconazole	Tacrolimus	↑	Tacrolimus concentrations may be elevated, increasing the toxicity risk.
Itraconazole	Tolterodine	↑	Tolterodine plasma concentrations may be elevated, increasing the pharmacologic and adverse effects. Patients receiving itraconazole should not receive more than 1 mg tolterodine twice daily.
Itraconazole	Trimetrexate	↑	Itraconazole may inhibit trimetrexate metabolism.
Itraconazole	Vinca alkaloids Vincristine Vinblastine	↑	Vinca alkaloid toxicity (constipation, myalgia, neutropenia) may be increased. Avoid concurrent administration of these agents if possible.
Itraconazole	Warfarin	↑	The anticoagulant effect of warfarin may be increased. Monitor prothrombin time (PT) and international normalized ratio (INR) values frequently when adding or discontinuing itraconazole. Adjust warfarin dose accordingly.
Itraconazole	Zolpidem	↑	Plasma concentrations and therapeutic effects of zolpidem may be increased. Monitor the clinical response of the patient. The dose of zolpidem may need to be decreased.

* ↑ = Object drug increased. ↓ = Object drug decreased.

➤*Drug/Food interactions:* The oral bioavailability of itraconazole is maximal when itraconazole capsules are taken with a full meal. The absorption of itraconazole was increased when itraconazole capsules were coadministered with a cola beverage. The bioavailability of itraconazole oral solution is increased under fasted conditions reaching higher maximum plasma concentrations (C_{max}) in a shorter period of time. Therefore, unlike itraconazole capsules, it is recommended that itraconazole oral solution be administered without food.

Adverse Reactions

Itraconazole has been associated with rare cases of serious hepatotoxicity, including liver failure and death. Some of these cases had neither preexisting liver disease nor a serious underlying medical condition. If clinical signs or symptoms develop that are consistent with liver disease, discontinue treatment and perform liver function testing. Reassess the risks and benefits of itraconazole use.

➤*Capsules:*

Adverse events in the treatment of systemic fungal infections – Adverse event data were derived from 602 patients treated for systemic fungal disease in US clinical trials who were immunocompromised or receiving multiple concomitant medications. Treatment was discontinued in 10.5% of patients because of adverse events. The median duration before discontinuation of therapy was 81 days (range, 2 to 776 days).

Itraconazole Capsules Adverse Events During Clinical Trials of Systemic Fungal Infections ≥ 1%	
Adverse reaction	Incidence (%) (n = 602)
CNS	
Dizziness	2%
Fatigue	3%
Headache	4%
Libido decreased	1%
Malaise	1%
Somnolence	1%
Dermatologic	
Pruritus	3%
Rash[a]	9%
GI	
Abdominal pain	2%
Anorexia	1%

ITRACONAZOLE — ORAL

Itraconazole Capsules Adverse Events During Clinical Trials of Systemic Fungal Infections ≥ 1%	
Adverse reaction	Incidence (%) (n = 602)
Diarrhea	3%
Nausea	11%
Vomiting	5%
Miscellaneous	
Albuminuria	1%
Edema	4%
Fever	3%
Hepatic function abnormal	3%
Hypertension	3%
Hypokalemia	2%
Impotence	1%

[a] Rash tends to occur more frequently in immunocompromised patients receiving immunosuppressive medications.

Adverse events infrequently reported in all studies included adrenal insufficiency, constipation, depression, gastritis, gynecomastia, insomnia, male breast pain, menstrual disorder, and tinnitus.

Adverse events reported in toenail onychomycosis clinical trials – Patients in these trials were on a continuous dosing regimen of 200 mg once daily for 12 consecutive weeks.

Patients Temporarily or Permanently Discontinuing Itraconazole Treatment of Onychomycosis of the Toenail Because of Adverse Events (%)	
Adverse reaction	Itraconazole (n = 112)
Elevated liver enzymes (greater than twice the upper limit of normal)	4%
GI disorders	4%
Headache	1%
Hypertension	2%
Malaise	1%
Myalgia	1%
Orthostatic hypotension	1%
Rash	3%
Vasculitis	1%
Vertigo	1%

The following adverse events occurred with an incidence of greater than or equal to 1% (n = 112): headache (10%); rhinitis (9%); upper respiratory tract infection (8%); injury, sinusitis (7%); abdominal pain, diarrhea, dizziness, dyspepsia, flatulence, rash (4%); cystitis, liver function abnormality, myalgia, nausea, urinary tract infection (3%); abnormal dreaming, appetite increased, asthenia, constipation, fever, gastritis, gastroenteritis, herpes zoster, pain, pharyngitis, tremor (2%).

Adverse events reported in fingernail onychomycosis clinical trials – Patients in these trials were on a pulse regimen consisting of two 1-week treatment periods of 200 mg twice daily, separated by a 3-week period without drug.

Patients Temporarily or Permanently Discontinuing Itraconazole Treatment of Onychomycosis of the Fingernail Because of Adverse Events (%)	
Adverse reaction	Itraconazole (n = 37)
Hypertriglyceridemia	3%
Rash/pruritus	3%

The following adverse events occurred with an incidence of greater than or equal to 1% (n = 37): headache (8%); nausea, pruritus, rhinitis (5%); abdominal pain, anxiety, bursitis, constipation, depression, dyspepsia, fatigue, gingivitis, hypertriglyceridemia, injury, malaise, pain, rash, sinusitis, ulcerative stomatitis (3%).

Itraconazole Capsules Adverse Events in Clinical Trials of Onychomycosis of the Toenail (≥ 1%)	
Adverse reaction	Incidence (n = 112)
CNS	
Abnormal dreaming	2%
Asthenia	4%
Dizziness	2%
Headache	10%
Tremor	2%
GI	
Abdominal pain	4%
Appetite increased	2%
Constipation	2%
Diarrhea	4%
Dyspepsia	4%
Flatulence	4%
Gastritis	2%
Gastroenteritis	2%
Nausea	3%
GU	
Cystitis	3%
Urinary tract infection	3%
Respiratory	
Pharyngitis	2%
Rhinitis	9%
Sinusitis	7%
Upper respiratory tract infection	8%
Miscellaneous	
Fever	2%
Herpes zoster	2%
Injury	7%
Liver function abnormality	3%
Myalgia	3%
Pain	2%
Rash	4%

Itraconazole Capsules Adverse Events in Clinical Trials of Onychomycosis of the Fingernail (≥ 1%)	
Adverse reaction	Incidence (n = 37)
CNS	
Anxiety	3%
Depression	3%
Fatigue	3%
Headache	8%
Malaise	3%
Dermatologic	
Pruritus	5%
Rash	3%
GI	
Abdominal pain	3%
Constipation	3%
Dyspepsia	3%
Gingivitis	3%
Nausea	5%
Ulcerative stomatitis	3%
Respiratory	
Rhinitis	5%
Sinusitis	3%
Miscellaneous	
Bursitis	3%
Hypertriglyceridemia	3%
Injury	3%
Pain	3%

➤*Oral solution:*

Adverse events reported in empiric therapy in febrile neutropenic (ETFN) patients – Adverse events considered at least possibly drug related in a clinical trial of empiric therapy in 384 febrile, neutropenic patients (192 treated with itraconazole and 192 with amphotericin B) with suspected fungal infections are listed in the table below. Patients received a regimen of itraconazole injection followed by itraconazole oral solution. The dose of itraconazole injection was 200 mg twice daily for the first 2 days followed by a single daily dose of 200 mg for the remainder of the intravenous treatment period. The majority of patients received between 7 and 14 days of itraconazole injection. The dose of itraconazole oral solution was 200 mg (20 mL) twice daily for the remainder of therapy.

ITRACONAZOLE — ORAL

Itraconazole Oral Solution Adverse Events in a Clinical Trial of Empiric Therapy in Febrile Neutropenic Patients (≥ 2%)		
Adverse reaction	Itraconazole (n = 192)	Amphotericin B (n = 192)
Cardiovascular		
Hypertension	0%	2%
Hypotension	1%	3%
Tachycardia	1%	3%
Dermatologic		
Rash	5%	3%
Sweating increased	2%	1%
GI		
Abdominal pain	3%	3%
Diarrhea	10%	9%
Nausea	11%	15%
Vomiting	7%	10%
Hepatic		
ALT increased	3%	1%
AST increased	2%	1%
Bilirubinemia	6%	3%
Hepatic function abnormal	3%	2%
Jaundice	2%	1%
Metabolic		
Alkaline phosphatase increased	2%	2%
Blood urea nitrogen increased	1%	6%
Fluid overload	1%	3%
Hypocalcemia	1%	2%
Hypokalemia	9%	28%
Hypomagnesemia	2%	4%
LDH increased	2%	0%
Serum creatinine increased	3%	25%
Miscellaneous		
Dyspnea	1%	3%
Edema	2%	2%
Fever	0%	7%
Headache	2%	2 %
Renal function abnormal	1%	12%
Rigors	1%	34%

The following additional adverse events considered at least possibly related occurred in between 1% and 2% of patients who received itraconazole injection and oral solution: constipation, dizziness, erythematous rash, GGT increased, hypophosphatemia, pruritus, pulmonary infiltration, and tremor.

Adverse events reported in oropharyngeal or esophageal candidiasis trials – US adverse experience data are derived from 350 immunocompromised patients (332 HIV seropositive/AIDS) treated for oropharyngeal or esophageal candidiasis. The table below lists adverse events reported by at least 2% of patients treated with itraconazole oral solution in US clinical trials. Data on patients receiving comparator agents in these trials are included for comparison.

Itraconazole Oral Solution Adverse Events in Clinical Trials of Oropharyngeal Candidiasis (≥ 2%)				
	Itraconazole			
Adverse reaction	Total (n = 350[a])	All controlled studies (n = 272)	Fluconazole (n = 125[b])	Clotrimazole (n = 81[c])
CNS				
Depression	2%	1%	0%	1%
Dizziness	2%	2%	4%	1%
Headache	4%	4%	6%	6%
Dermatologic				
Increased sweating	3%	4%	6%	1%
Rash	4%	5%	4%	6%
Skin disorder, unspecified	2%	2%	2%	1%
GI				
Abdominal pain	6%	4%	7%	7%
Constipation	2%	2%	1%	0%
Diarrhea	11%	10%	10%	4%
Nausea	11%	10%	11%	5%
Vomiting	7%	6%	8%	1%
Respiratory				
Coughing	4%	4%	10%	0%
Dyspnea	2%	3%	5%	1%
Pneumonia	2%	2%	0%	0%
Sinusitis	2%	2%	4%	0%
Sputum increased	2%	3%	3%	1%
Miscellaneous				
Chest pain	3%	3%	2%	0%
Fatigue	2%	1%	2%	0%
Fever	7%	6%	8%	5%
Pain	2%	2%	4%	0%
Pneumocystis carinii infection	2%	2%	2%	0%

[a] Of the 350 patients, 209 were treated for oropharyngeal candidiasis in controlled studies, 63 were treated for esophageal candidiasis in controlled studies and 78 were treated for oropharyngeal candidiasis in an open study.
[b] Of the 125 patients, 62 were treated for oropharyngeal candidiasis and 63 were treated for esophageal candidiasis.
[c] All 81 patients were treated for oropharyngeal candidiasis.

Adverse events reported by less than 2% of patients in US clinical trials with itraconazole included: adrenal insufficiency, asthenia, back pain, dehydration, dyspepsia, dysphagia, flatulence, gynecomastia, hematuria, hemorrhoids, hot flushes, implantation complication, infection unspecified, injury, insomnia, male breast pain, myalgia, pharyngitis, pruritus, rhinitis, rigors, stomatitis ulcerative, taste perversion, tinnitus, upper respiratory tract infection, vision abnormal, and weight decrease. Edema, hypokalemia, and menstrual disorders have been reported in clinical trials with itraconazole capsules.

➤*Postmarketing:* Worldwide postmarketing experiences with the use of itraconazole include adverse events of GI origin, such as abdominal pain, constipation, diarrhea, dyspepsia, nausea, and vomiting. Other reported adverse events include allergic reactions (eg, pruritus, rash, urticaria, angioedema, anaphylaxis), alopecia, anaphylactic, anaphylactoid, and allergic reaction, CHF and pulmonary edema, dizziness, headache, hepatitis, hypertriglyceridemia, hypokalemia, liver failure, menstrual disorders, neutropenia, peripheral edema, peripheral neuropathy, photosensitivity, reversible increases in hepatic enzymes, and Stevens-Johnson syndrome.

Congenital abnormalities – There is limited information on the use of itraconazole during pregnancy. Cases of congenital abnormalities, including skeletal, genitourinary tract, cardiovascular, and ophthalmic malformations, as well as chromosomal and multiple malformations have been reported during postmarketing experience. A causal relationship with itraconazole has not been established.

Overdosage

➤*Symptoms:* Limited data exist on the outcomes of patients ingesting high doses of itraconazole. In patients taking either itraconazole oral solution 1,000 mg or itraconazole capsules up to 3,000 mg, the adverse event profile was similar to that observed at recommended doses.

➤*Treatment:* Itraconazole is not removed by dialysis. In the event of accidental overdosage, employ supportive measures, including gastric lavage with sodium bicarbonate.

Patient Information

➤*Capsules:* The topical effects of mucosal exposure may be different between the itraconazole capsules and oral solution. Only the oral solution has been demonstrated effective for oral and/or esophageal candidiasis. Do not use itraconazole capsules interchangeably with itraconazole oral solution.

Instruct patients to take itraconazole capsules with a full meal.

Instruct patients about the signs and symptoms of CHF, and if these signs or symptoms occur during itraconazole administration, to discontinue itraconazole and contact their healthcare provider immediately.

Instruct patients to stop itraconazole treatment immediately and contact their healthcare provider if any signs and symptoms suggestive of liver dysfunction develop. Such signs and symptoms may include unusual anorexia, dark urine, fatigue, jaundice, nausea and/or vomiting, or pale stools.

ITRACONAZOLE — ORAL

Instruct patients to contact their physician before taking any concomitant medications with itraconazole to ensure there are no potential drug interactions.

➤*Oral solution:* Only itraconazole oral solution has been demonstrated effective for oral and/or esophageal candidiasis. Itraconazole oral solution contains the excipient hydroxypropyl-β-cyclodextrin which produced pancreatic adenocarcinomas in a rat carcinogenicity study. These findings were not observed in a similar mouse carcinogenicity study. The clinical relevance of these findings is unknown.

Taking itraconazole oral solution under fasted conditions improves the systemic availability of itraconazole. Instruct patients to take itraconazole oral solution without food, if possible.

Do not use itraconazole oral solution interchangeably with itraconazole capsules.

Patients taking itraconazole oral solution for the treatment of oropharyngeal and esophageal candidiasis should be instructed to vigorously swish in the mouth (10 mL at a time) for several seconds and swallowed.

ITRACONAZOLE — INJECTION

WARNING

Congestive heart failure (CHF) – When itraconazole was administered intravenously (IV) to dogs and healthy human volunteers, negative inotropic effects were seen. If signs or symptoms of CHF occur during administration of itraconazole injection, reassess continued itraconazole use.

Drug interactions – Coadministration of cisapride, pimozide, quinidine, or dofetilide with itraconazole is contraindicated. Itraconazole, a potent cytochrome P450 3A4 isoenzyme system (CYP3A4) inhibitor, may increase plasma concentrations of drugs metabolized by this pathway. Serious cardiovascular events, including QT prolongation, torsades de pointes, ventricular tachycardia, cardiac arrest, and/or sudden death have occurred in patients using cisapride, pimozide, or quinidine concomitantly with itraconazole and/or other CYP3A4 inhibitors. HMG-CoA reductase inhibitors metabolized by CYP3A4, such as lovastatin and simvastatin, are also contraindicated with itraconazole.

Indications

➤*Aspergillosis:* Treatment of pulmonary and extrapulmonary aspergillosis in nonimmunocompromised or immunocompromised patients who are intolerant of or who are refractory to amphotericin B therapy.

➤*Blastomycosis:* Treatment of pulmonary and extrapulmonary blastomycosis in nonimmunocompromised or immunocompromised patients.

➤*Febrile neutropenia, empiric:* For empiric therapy of febrile neutropenic (ETFN) patients with suspected fungal infections. Note: In a comparative trial, the overall response rate for itraconazole-treated subjects was higher than for amphotericin B-treated subjects. However, compared with amphotericin B-treated subjects, a larger number of itraconazole-treated subjects discontinued treatment because of persistent fever and a change in antifungal medication because of fever. Whereas a larger number of amphotericin B-treated subjects discontinued because of drug intolerance.

➤*Histoplasmosis:* Treatment of histoplasmosis, including chronic cavitary pulmonary disease and disseminated, nonmeningeal histoplasmosis in nonimmunocompromised or immunocompromised patients.

Administration and Dosage

➤*Approved by the FDA:* September 11, 1992.

Use only the components (itraconazole injection ampule, 0.9% sodium chloride injection [normal saline] bag and filtered infusion set) provided in the kit. Do not substitute.

➤*Febrile neutropenia, empiric:* The recommended dosage of itraconazole injection is 200 mg IV twice daily for 4 doses, followed by 200 mg once daily for up to 14 days. Infuse each IV dose over 1 hour. Continue treatment with itraconazole oral solution 200 mg (20 mL) twice daily until resolution of clinically significant neutropenia. The safety and efficacy of itraconazole use exceeding 28 days are ETFN is not known.

➤*Blastomycosis, histoplasmosis, and aspergillosis:* The recommended IV dosage is 200 mg twice daily for 4 doses, followed by 200 mg once daily. Infuse each IV dose over 1 hour.

For the treatment of blastomycosis, histoplasmosis, and aspergillosis, itraconazole can be given as oral capsules or IV. The safety and efficacy of itraconazole injection administered for greater than 14 days are not known.

➤*Duration:* Continue total itraconazole therapy (itraconazole injection followed by itraconazole capsules) for a minimum of 3 months and until clinical parameters and laboratory tests indicate that the active fungal infection has subsided. An inadequate period of treatment may lead to recurrence of active infection.

➤*Renal function impairment:* Do not use itraconazole injection in patients with creatinine clearance less than 30 mL/min.

➤*Admixture incompatibility:* Itraconazole injection should not be diluted with 5% dextrose injection or with lactated Ringer's injection alone or in combination with any other diluent. The compatibility of itraconazole injection with diluents other than 0.9% sodium chloride injection is not known. Not for IV bolus injection.

➤*Preparation/Administration:* Use only a dedicated infusion line for administration of itraconazole injection. Do not introduce concomitant medication into the same bag nor through the same line as itraconazole injection. Other medications may be administered after flushing the line/catheter with 0.9% sodium chloride injection as described below, and removing and replacing the entire infusion line. Alternatively, utilize another lumen, in the case of a multilumen catheter.

Correct preparation and administration of itraconazole injection are necessary to ensure maximal efficacy and safety. A precise mixing ratio is required in order to obtain a stable admixture. It is critical to maintain a 3.33 mg/mL itraconazole:diluent ratio. Failure to maintain this concentration will lead to the formation of a precipitate.

Add the full contents (25 mL) of the itraconazole injection ampule into the infusion bag provided, which contains 50 mL of 0.9% sodium chloride injection. Mix gently after the solution is completely transferred. Withdraw and discard 15 mL of the solution before administering to the patient. Using a flow control device, infuse 60 mL of the dilute solution (3.33 mg/mL = 200 mg itraconazole, pH approximately 4.8) IV over 60 minutes, using an extension line and the infusion set provided. After administration, flush the infusion set with 15 to 20 mL of 0.9% sodium chloride injection over 30 seconds to 15 minutes, via the 2-way stopcock. Do not use bacteriostatic sodium chloride injection. The compatibility of itraconazole injection with flush solutions other than 0.9% sodium chloride injection is not known. Discard the entire infusion line.

➤*Storage/Stability:* Store at or below 25°C (77°F). Protect from light and freezing. Note: After reconstitution, the diluted itraconazole injection may be stored refrigerated (2° to 8°C; 35.6° to 46.4°F) or at room temperature (15° to 25°C; 59° to 77°F) for up to 48 hours, when protected from direct light. During administration, exposure to normal room light is acceptable.

Actions

➤*Pharmacology:* Itraconazole is a systemic triazole antifungal agent. In vitro, itraconazole inhibits the cytochrome P450-dependent synthesis of ergosterol, which is a vital component of fungal membranes.

➤*Pharmacokinetics:*

Absorption –

The pharmacokinetics of itraconazole injection (200 mg twice daily for 2 days, then 200 mg once daily for 5 days) followed by oral dosing of itraconazole capsules were studied in patients with advanced HIV infection. Steady-state plasma concentrations were reached after the fourth dose for itraconazole and by the seventh dose for hydroxyitraconazole. Steady-state plasma concentrations were maintained by administration of itraconazole capsules, 200 mg twice daily.

Itraconazole Pharmacokinetics (Mean ± Standard Deviation)				
	Injection day 7 (n = 29)		Capsule, 200 mg twice daily day 36 (n = 12)	
Parameter	Itraconazole	Hydroxy-itraconazole	Itraconazole	Hydroxy-itraconazole
C_{max} (ng/mL)	2,856 ± 866[a]	1,906 ± 612	2,010 ± 1,420	2,614 ± 1,703
t_{max} (h)	1.08 ± 0.14	8.53 ± 6.36	3.92 ± 1.83	5.92 ± 6.14
$AUC_{0-12\ h}$ (ng•h/mL)	-	-	18,768 ± 13,933	28,516 ± 19,149
$AUC_{0-24\ h}$ (ng•h/mL)	30,605 ± 8,961	42,445 ± 13,282	-	-

[a] Mean ± standard deviation (SD).

Distribution – The plasma protein binding of itraconazole is 99.8% and that of hydroxyitraconazole is 99.5%. Following IV administration, the volume of distribution of itraconazole averaged 796 ± 185 L.

Metabolism – Itraconazole is metabolized predominately by the cytochrome P450 3A4 isoenzyme system (CYP3A4), resulting in the formation of several metabolites, including hydroxyitraconazole, the major metabolite. Results of a pharmacokinetics study suggest that itraconazole may undergo saturable metabolism with multiple dosing.

Excretion – The estimated mean ± SD half-life at steady state of itraconazole after IV infusion was 35.4 ± 29.4 hours. Approximately 93% to 101% of hydroxypropyl-β-cyclodextrin was excreted unchanged in the urine within 12 hours after dosing.

Fecal excretion of the parent drug varies between 3% to 18% of the dose. Renal excretion of the parent drug is less than 0.03% of the dose. About 40% of the dose is excreted as inactive metabolites in the urine. No single excreted metabolite represents more than 5% of a dose. Itraconazole total plasma clearance averaged 381 ± 95 mL/min following IV administration. Approximately 80% to 90% of hydroxypropyl-β-cyclodextrin is eliminated through the kidneys.

Special populations –

Renal function impairment: Plasma concentrations of itraconazole in patients with mild to moderate renal insufficiency were comparable with those obtained in healthy subjects. The majority of the 8 g dose of hydroxypropyl-β-cyclodextrin was eliminated in the urine during the 120-hour collection period in healthy subjects and in patients with mild to severe

ITRACONAZOLE — INJECTION

renal insufficiency. Following a single IV dose of 200 mg to subjects with severe renal impairment (creatinine clearance less than or equal to 19 mL/min), clearance of hydroxypropyl-β-cyclodextrin was reduced 6-fold compared with subjects with normal renal function. Do not use itraconazole injection in patients with creatinine clearance less than 30 mL/min.

In patients with mild to moderate renal impairment, use itraconazole injection with caution. Closely monitor serum creatinine levels and, if renal toxicity is suspected, consider changing to itraconazole capsules.

Hepatic function impairment: Carefully monitor patients with impaired hepatic function when taking itraconazole. Consider the prolonged elimination half-life of itraconazole observed in a clinical trial with itraconazole capsules in cirrhotic patients when deciding to initiate therapy with other medications metabolized by CYP3A4. Itraconazole has been associated with rare cases of serious hepatotoxicity, including liver failure and death. If signs or symptoms consistent with liver disease develop, discontinue treatment.

Decreased cardiac contractility: When itraconazole was administered IV to anesthetized dogs, a dose-related negative inotropic effect was documented. In a healthy volunteer study of itraconazole injection (IV infusion), transient, asymptomatic decreases in left ventricular ejection fraction were observed using gated SPECT imaging; these resolved before the next infusion, 12 hours later. If signs or symptoms of CHF appear during administration of itraconazole injection, monitor carefully and consider other treatment alternatives, which may include discontinuation of itraconazole injection administration. In patients with risk factors for CHF, carefully review the risks and benefits of itraconazole therapy.

➤*Microbiology:* In vitro studies have demonstrated that itraconazole inhibits the cytochrome P450-dependent synthesis of ergosterol, which is a vital component of fungal cell membranes.

Itraconazole exhibits in vitro activity against *Blastomyces dermatitidis, Histoplasma capsulatum, Histoplasma duboisii, Aspergillus flavus, Aspergillus fumigatus, Candida albicans,* and *Cryptococcus neoformans.* Itraconazole also exhibits varying in vitro activity against *Sporothrix schenckii, Trichophyton* species, *Candida krusei,* and other *Candida* species. The bioactive metabolite, hydroxyitraconazole, has not been evaluated against *Histoplasma capsulatum* and *Blastomyces dermatitidis.* Correlation between minimum inhibitory concentration (MIC) results in vitro and clinical outcome has yet to be established for azole antifungal agents.

Resistance – Several in vitro studies have reported that some fungal clinical isolates, including *Candida* species, with reduced susceptibility to one azole antifungal agent may also be less susceptible to other azole derivatives. The finding of cross-resistance is dependent on a number of factors, including the species evaluated, its clinical history, the particular azole compounds compared, and the type of susceptibility test that is performed. The relevance of these in vitro susceptibility data to clinical outcome remains to be elucidated.

Contraindications

Hypersensitivity to itraconazole or its excipients. There is no information regarding cross-hypersensitivity between itraconazole and other azole antifungal agents. Use caution when prescribing itraconazole to patients with hypersensitivity to other azoles.

Coadministration with certain drugs metabolized by the cytochrome P-450 3A4 isoenzyme system (CYP3A4), cisapride, oral midazolam, pimozide, quinidine, dofetilide, triazolam, HMG-CoA reductase inhibitors metabolized by CYP3A4, such as lovastatin and simvastatin, and ergot alkaloids metabolized by CYP3A4, such as dihydroergotamine, ergotamine, ergonovine, and methylergonovine (see Drug interactions).

Warnings

➤*Cardiac dysrhythmias:* Itraconazole, a potent cytochrome P450 3A4 isoenzyme system (CYP3A4) inhibitor, may increase plasma concentrations of drugs metabolized by this pathway. Serious cardiovascular events, including QT prolongation, torsades de pointes, ventricular tachycardia, cardiac arrest, and/or sudden death have occurred in patients using cisapride, pimozide, or quinidine concomitantly with itraconazole and/or other CYP3A4 inhibitors. Concomitant administration of these drugs with itraconazole is contraindicated.

➤*Cardiac disease:* Do not use itraconazole injection in patients with evidence of ventricular dysfunction unless the benefit clearly outweighs the risk. For patients with risk factors for CHF, carefully review the risks and benefits of itraconazole therapy. These risk factors include cardiac disease such as ischemic and valvular disease; significant pulmonary disease such as chronic obstructive pulmonary disease; and renal failure and other edematous disorders. Inform such patients of the signs and symptoms of CHF, treat with caution, and monitor for signs and symptoms of CHF during treatment. If signs or symptoms of CHF appear during administration of itraconazole injection, monitor carefully and consider other treatment alternatives, which may include discontinuation of itraconazole injection administration.

See Actions for more information.

Cases of CHF, peripheral edema, and pulmonary edema have been reported in the postmarketing period among patients being treated for onychomycosis and/or systemic fungal infections. A dose-related negative inotropic effect has been documented in IV itraconazole. Concomitant administration of digoxin and itraconazole has led to increased plasma concentrations of digoxin.

Calcium channel blockers can have a negative inotropic effect that may be additive to those of itraconazole; itraconazole can inhibit the metabolism of calcium channel blockers such as dihydropyridines (eg, nifedipine and felodipine) and verapamil. Therefore, use caution when coadministering itraconazole and calcium channel blockers.

➤*Hepatotoxicity:* Itraconazole has been associated with rare cases of serious hepatotoxicity, including liver failure and death. Some of these cases had neither preexisting liver disease nor a serious underlying medical condition and some of these cases developed within the first week of treatment. If clinical signs or symptoms develop that are consistent with liver disease, discontinue treatment and perform liver function testing. Continued itraconazole use or reinstitution of treatment with itraconazole is strongly discouraged unless there is a serious or life-threatening situation where the expected benefit exceeds the risk.

In patients with elevated or abnormal liver enzymes or active liver disease, or who have experienced liver toxicity with other drugs, treatment with itraconazole is strongly discouraged unless there is a serious or life-threatening situation where the expected benefit exceeds the risk.

➤*Renal function impairment:* Because severe renal impairment prolongs the elimination rate of hydroxypropyl-β-cyclodextrin, do not use itraconazole injection in patients with severe renal dysfunction (creatinine clearance less than 30 mL/min).

See Actions for more information.

➤*Carcinogenesis:* Itraconazole showed no evidence of carcinogenicity potential in mice treated orally for 23 months at dosage levels up to 80 mg/kg/day (approximately 10 times the maximum recommended human dose [MRHD]). Male rats treated with 25 mg/kg/day (3.1 times MRHD) had a slightly increased incidence of soft tissue sarcoma. These sarcomas may have been a consequence of hypercholesterolemia, which is a response of rats, but not dogs or humans, to chronic itraconazole administration. Female rats treated with 50 mg/kg/day (6.25 times MRHD) had an increased incidence of squamous cell carcinoma of the lung (2/50) as compared with the untreated group. Although the occurrence of squamous cell carcinoma in the lung is extremely uncommon in untreated rats, the increase in this study was not statistically significant.

Hydroxypropyl-β-cyclodextrin (HP-β-CD), the solubilizing excipient used in itraconazole injection, was found to produce pancreatic exocrine hyperplasia and neoplasia when administered orally to rats at doses of 500, 2,000, or 5,000 mg/kg/day for 25 months. Adenocarcinomas of the exocrine pancreas produced in the treated animals were not seen in the untreated group and are not reported in the historical controls. Development of these tumors may be related to a mitogenic action of cholecystokinin. This finding was not observed in the mouse carcinogenicity study at doses of 500, 2,000, or 5,000 mg/kg/day for 22 to 23 months; however, the clinical relevance of these findings is unknown. The relevance of the findings with orally administered HP-β-CD to potential carcinogenic effects for itraconazole injection is uncertain.

➤*Fertility impairment:* Itraconazole did not affect the fertility of male or female rats treated orally with dosage levels of up to 40 mg/kg/day (5 times MRHD), even though parental toxicity was present at this dosage level. More severe signs of parental toxicity, including death, were present in the next higher dosage level, 160 mg/kg/day (20 times MRHD).

➤*Elderly:* Clinical studies of itraconazole injection did not include sufficient numbers of subjects 65 years of age and older to determine whether they respond differently from younger subjects. Other reported clinical experience has not identified differences in responses between the elderly and younger patients. In general, dose selection for an elderly patient should be cautious, reflecting the greater frequency of decreased hepatic, renal, or cardiac function, and of concomitant disease or other drug therapy.

➤*Pregnancy: Category C.*

There are no studies in pregnant women. Use itraconazole for the treatment of systemic fungal infections in pregnancy only if the benefit outweighs the potential risk. Itraconazole was found to cause a dose-related increase in maternal toxicity, embryotoxicity, and teratogenicity in rats at dosage levels of approximately 40 to 160 mg/kg/day (5 to 20 times MRHD), and in mice at dosage levels of approximately 80 mg/kg/day (10 times MRHD). In rats, the teratogenicity consisted of major skeletal defects; in mice, it consisted of encephaloceles and/or macroglossia.

During postmarketing experiences, cases of congenital abnormalities have been reported.

➤*Lactation:* Itraconazole is excreted in human milk; therefore, the expected benefits of itraconazole therapy for the mother should be weighed against the potential risk from exposure of itraconazole to the infant. The US Public Health Service Centers for Disease Control and Prevention advises HIV-infected women not to breast-feed to avoid potential transmission of HIV to uninfected infants.

➤*Children:* The efficacy and safety of itraconazole have not been established in pediatric patients. No pharmacokinetic data on itraconazole injection are available in children. A small number of patients 3 to 16 years of age have been treated with 100 mg/day of itraconazole capsules for systemic fungal infections, and no serious unexpected adverse effects have been reported. Itraconazole oral solution (5 mg/kg/day) has been administered to pediatric patients (n = 26, 6 months to 12 years of age) for 2 weeks, and no serious unexpected adverse events were reported.

The long-term effects of itraconazole on bone growth in children are unknown. In 3 toxicology studies using rats, itraconazole induced bone defects at dosage levels as low as 20 mg/kg/day (2.5 times MRHD). The induced defects included reduced bone plate activity, thinning of the zona compacta of the large bones, and increased bone fragility. At a dosage level of 80 mg/kg/day (10 times MRHD) over 1 year or 160 mg/kg/day (20 times MRHD) for 6 months, itraconazole induced small tooth pulp with hypocellular appearance in some rats. No such bone toxicity has been reported in adult patients.

ITRACONAZOLE — INJECTION

Precautions

➤*Monitoring:* Monitor liver function in patients with preexisting hepatic function abnormalities or those who have experienced liver toxicity with other medications; consider monitoring in all patients. Stop treatment immediately and conduct liver function testing in patients who develop signs and symptoms suggestive of liver dysfunction.

➤*Neuropathy:* If neuropathy occurs that may be attributable to itraconazole injection, discontinue the treatment.

Drug Interactions

➤*Cytochrome P450 system:* Concomitant administration of itraconazole and certain drugs metabolized by the cytochrome P450 3A4 isoenzyme system (CYP3A4) may result in increased plasma concentrations of those drugs, leading to potentially serious and/or life-threatening adverse events. Cisapride, oral midazolam, pimozide, quinidine, dofetilide, and triazolam are contraindicated with itraconazole. HMG-CoA reductase inhibitors metabolized by CYP3A4, such as lovastatin and simvastatin, are also contraindicated with itraconazole. Cilostazol and eletriptan are CYP3A4 metabolized drugs that should be used with caution when coadministered with itraconazole. Ergot alkaloids metabolized by CYP3A4, such as dihydroergotamine, ergotamine, ergonovine, and methylergonovine, are contraindicated with itraconazole.

Itraconazole and its major metabolite, hydroxyitraconazole, are inhibitors of CYP3A4.

1.) Itraconazole may decrease the elimination of drugs metabolized by CYP3A4, resulting in increased plasma concentrations of these drugs when they are administered with itraconazole. These elevated plasma concentrations may increase or prolong both therapeutic and adverse effects of these drugs. Whenever possible, monitor plasma concentrations of these drugs, and make dosage adjustments after concomitant itraconazole therapy is initiated. When appropriate, clinical monitoring for signs or symptoms of increased or prolonged pharmacologic effects is advised. Upon discontinuation, depending on the dose and duration of treatment, itraconazole plasma concentrations decline gradually (especially in patients with hepatic cirrhosis or in those receiving CYP3A4 inhibitors). This is particularly important when initiating therapy with drugs whose metabolism is affected by itraconazole.
2.) Inducers of CYP3A4 may decrease the plasma concentrations of itraconazole. Itraconazole may not be effective in patients concomitantly taking itraconazole and 1 of these drugs. Therefore, administration of these drugs with itraconazole is not recommended.
3.) Other inhibitors of CYP3A4 may increase the plasma concentrations of itraconazole. Monitor patients who must take itraconazole concomitantly with 1 of these drugs closely for signs or symptoms of increased or prolonged pharmacologic effects of itraconazole.

Itraconazole Drug Interactions

Precipitant drug	Object drug*		Description
Macrolide antibiotics Erythromycin Clarithromycin	Itraconazole	↑	Macrolide antibiotics may increase plasma itraconazole concentrations through inhibition of CYP3A4.
Nevirapine	Itraconazole	↓	Coadministration may lead to decreased itraconazole plasma levels and, therefore, is not recommended.
Phenobarbital	Itraconazole	↓	Decreased itraconazole plasma concentrations may occur with coadministration.
Itraconazole	Alfentanil	↑	Pharmacologic and adverse effects may be increased. Use caution when administering concurrently. Lower the alfentanil dose as needed.
Itraconazole	Amphotericin B	↓	Studies suggest that amphotericin B activity may be suppressed by prior azole antifungal therapy. Clinical significance is unknown.
Itraconazole	Aripiprazole	↑	Aripiprazole plasma concentrations may be elevated, increasing the pharmacologic and adverse effects. Reduce the aripiprazole dose 50% of the normal dose when coadministering with itraconazole.
Itraconazole	Benzodiazepines Triazolam Midazolam Alprazolam Diazepam	↑	Increased and prolonged serum levels, CNS depression, and psychomotor impairment with certain benzodiazepines may occur, possibly several days after stopping itraconazole. Concurrent use of triazolam and oral midazolam is contraindicated.
Itraconazole	Buspirone	↑	Plasma buspirone concentrations may be elevated, increasing the pharmacologic and adverse effects. In patients receiving itraconazole when buspirone is started, it may be prudent to start with a conservative dose. Monitor closely when an antifungal agent is stopped, started, or changed in dose in patients on buspirone therapy. Adjust the dose of buspirone as needed.
Itraconazole	Busulfan	↑	Itraconazole may elevate busulfan plasma levels, increasing the risk of toxicity (eg, pancytopenia). Monitor patients for increased toxicity and adjust the busulfan dose as needed.
Itraconazole	Calcium channel blockers	↑	Concomitant administration may increase negative inotropic effects. Edema has also been reported with concomitant therapy. Itraconazole may inhibit the metabolism of calcium channel blockers such as dihydropyridines (eg, felodipine, nisoldipine, nifedipine) and verapamil. Coadminister with caution and adjust the dose of calcium channel blockers accordingly.
Itraconazole	Carbamazepine	↑	Plasma concentrations of carbamazepine may be elevated, increasing clinical and adverse effects. Monitor serum levels.
Carbamazepine	Itraconazole	↓	Decreased itraconazole plasma concentrations may occur with coadministration.
Itraconazole	Cilostazol	↑	Cilostazol plasma concentrations may be elevated, increasing the pharmacologic and adverse effects. Use caution with coadministration.
Itraconazole	Cisapride	↑	Increased cisapride concentrations with cardiotoxicity may occur. Itraconazole is contraindicated in patients receiving cisapride.
Itraconazole	Corticosteroids Budesonide Dexamethasone Methylprednisolone	↑	Itraconazole may inhibit the metabolism of certain corticosteroids, enhancing the effects and possibly resulting in increased toxicity. Monitor patients for adverse effects and adjust corticosteroids dose accordingly.
Itraconazole	Cyclosporine	↑	Increased cyclosporine levels may occur. Monitor cyclosporine levels and serum creatinine when itraconazole is added or discontinued.
Itraconazole	Digoxin	↑	Serum digoxin concentrations may be increased, enhancing its pharmacologic and adverse effects. Monitor plasma digoxin concentrations and observe the patient for signs of digoxin toxicity. Adjust digoxin dose accordingly.
Itraconazole	Disopyramide	↑	Serum disopyramide concentrations may be elevated. A high plasma concentration has the potential to increase the QT interval.
Itraconazole	Docetaxel	↑	Itraconazole may inhibit docetaxel metabolism.

ITRACONAZOLE — INJECTION

Itraconazole Drug Interactions

Precipitant drug	Object drug*		Description
Itraconazole	Dofetilide	↑	Elevated dofetilide plasma concentrations may occur with increased risk of ventricular arrhythmias, including torsades de pointes. Administration with itraconazole is contraindicated.
Itraconazole	Eletriptan Almotriptan	↑	Plasma concentrations of eletriptan may be elevated, increasing the pharmacologic and adverse effects. Eletriptan should not be taken within 72 hours of itraconazole.
Itraconazole	Eplerenone	↑	Elevated eplerenone plasma concentrations may occur, increasing the risk of hyperkalemia and associated serious arrhythmias. Coadministration is contraindicated.
Itraconazole	Ergot alkaloids Dihydroergotamine Ergonovine Ergotamine Methylergonovine	↑	The risk of ergot toxicity (eg, peripheral vasospasm, ischemia of the extremities and/or cerebral ischemia) may be increased. Concomitant administration is contraindicated.
Itraconazole	Halofantrine	↑	Halofantrine plasma concentrations may be elevated, increasing the potential of prolonging the QT interval. Use caution with coadministration.
Itraconazole	Haloperidol	↑	Haloperidol concentrations may be elevated, increasing the risk of side effects. Adjust dose as needed.
Itraconazole	HMG-CoA reductase inhibitors Atorvastatin Simvastatin Lovastatin	↑	Increased plasma levels and side effects of certain HMG-CoA reductase inhibitors may occur. If concurrent administration of these agents cannot be avoided, consider reducing the HMG-CoA reductase inhibitor dose. Coadministration with lovastatin and simvastatin is contraindicated.
Itraconazole	Hydantoins (eg, phenytoin)	↑	The plasma concentrations and pharmacologic effects of itraconazole may be decreased, while those of hydantoins may be increased. Avoid concomitant use if possible.
Hydantoins (eg, phenytoin)	Itraconazole	↓	
Itraconazole	Oral hypoglycemic agents	↑	Severe hypoglycemia has been reported in those receiving concomitant therapy. Monitor blood glucose levels carefully.
Itraconazole	Phosphodiesterase type 5 Inhibitors Sildenafil Tadalafil Vardenafil	↑	Phosphodiesterase type 5 (PDE5) inhibitor plasma levels may be elevated, increasing the risk of side effects. Give PDE5 inhibitors with caution and in reduced doses to patients.
Itraconazole	Pimozide	↑	Concomitant use may increase pimozide plasma concentrations, resulting in serious cardiac effects. Administration with itraconazole is contraindicated.
Itraconazole	Protease inhibitors	↑	Plasma concentrations of protease inhibitors metabolized by CYP3A4 (eg, indinavir, ritonavir, saquinavir) may be elevated, increasing the risk of toxicity. Consider reducing the dose of the protease inhibitor during concurrent administration with itraconazole. Plasma concentrations of itraconazole may be increased by indinavir and ritonavir.
Protease inhibitors Indinavir Ritonavir	Itraconazole		
Itraconazole	Quinidine	↑	Quinidine concentrations may be elevated, increasing the risk of serious cardiovascular events. Coadministration is contraindicated.
Itraconazole	Rifamycins Rifabutin Rifampin Rifapentine Isoniazid	↑	Itraconazole levels may be decreased. Itraconazole may increase rifabutin plasma levels and toxicity. Similar effects should be anticipated with isoniazid. Coadministration is not recommended. If coadministration cannot be avoided, monitor antimicrobial activity and adjust dosage.
Rifamycins Rifabutin Rifampin Rifapentine Isoniazid	Itraconazole	↓	
Itraconazole	Sirolimus	↑	Coadministration may lead to increased sirolimus plasma levels. Monitor sirolimus plasma concentrations and observe patient for toxicity when starting or stopping itraconazole. Adjust sirolimus dose accordingly.
Itraconazole	Tacrolimus	↑	Tacrolimus concentrations may be elevated, increasing the toxicity risk.
Itraconazole	Tolterodine	↑	Tolterodine plasma concentrations may be elevated, increasing the pharmacologic and adverse effects. Patients receiving itraconazole should not receive more than tolterodine 1 mg twice daily.
Itraconazole	Trimetrexate	↑	Itraconazole may inhibit trimetrexate metabolism.
Itraconazole	Vinca alkaloids Vincristine Vinblastine	↑	Vinca alkaloid toxicity (eg, constipation, myalgia, neutropenia) may be increased. Avoid concurrent administration of these agents if possible.
Itraconazole	Warfarin	↑	The anticoagulant effect of warfarin may be increased. Monitor prothrombin time (PT) and international normalized ratio (INR) values frequently when adding or discontinuing itraconazole. Adjust warfarin dose accordingly.
Itraconazole	Zolpidem	↑	Plasma concentrations and therapeutic effects of zolpidem may be increased. Monitor the clinical response of the patient. The dose of zolpidem may need to be decreased.

* ↑ = Object drug increased. ↓ = Object drug decreased.

Adverse Reactions

Itraconazole has been associated with rare cases of serious hepatotoxicity, including liver failure and death. Some of these cases had neither preexisting liver disease nor a serious underlying medical condition. If clinical signs or symptoms develop that are consistent with liver disease, discontinue treatment and perform liver function testing. Reassess the risks and benefits of itraconazole use.

Adverse events considered at least possibly drug related are shown in the table below and are based on the experience of 360 patients treated with itraconazole injection in 4 pharmacokinetic, 1 uncontrolled and 4 active controlled studies where the control was amphotericin B or fluconazole. Nearly all patients were neutropenic or were otherwise immunocompromised and were treated empirically for febrile episodes, for documented systemic fungal infections, or in trials to determine pharmacokinetics. The dose of itraconazole injection was 200 mg twice daily for the first 2 days followed by a single daily dose of 200 mg for the remainder of the IV treatment period. The majority of patients received between 7 and 14 days of itraconazole injection.

Itraconazole Injection Adverse Reactions (≥ 2%)

Adverse reaction	Total itraconazole injection (n = 360) %	Comparative studies		
		Itraconazole injection (n = 234) %	IV fluconazole (n = 32) %	IV amphotericin B (n = 202) %
Cardiovascular				
Hypertension	0%	0%	0%	2%
Hypotension	0%	0%	0%	3%

ITRACONAZOLE — INJECTION

Itraconazole Injection Adverse Reactions (≥ 2%)				
Adverse reaction	Total itraconazole injection (n = 360) %	Comparative studies		
		Itraconazole injection (n = 234) %	IV fluconazole (n = 32) %	IV amphoteri in B (n = 202) %
Tachycardia	0%	1%	0%	3%
CNS				
Dizziness	1%	2%	0%	1%
Headache	2%	2%	0%	3%
Dermatologic				
Rash	3%	3%	3%	3%
Sweating increased	1%	2%	0%	0%
GI				
Abdominal pain	2%	2%	0%	3%
Constipation	0%	1%	3%	0%
Diarrhea	6%	6%	3%	9%
Nausea	8%	9%	0%	15%
Vomiting	4%	6%	0%	10%
Hepatic				
ALT increased	2%	3%	3%	1%
AST increased	1%	2%	0%	0%
Bilirubinemia	4%	6%	9%	3%
Hepatic function abnormal	1%	2%	0%	2%
Jaundice	1%	2%	0%	0%
Metabolic				
Alkaline phosphatase increased	1%	2%	3%	2%
Blood urea nitrogen increased	0%	1%	0%	7%
Fluid overload	0%	0%	0%	3%
Hypocalcemia	0%	0%	0%	3%
Hypokalemia	5%	8%	0%	29%
Hypomagnesemia	1%	1%	0%	5%
Serum creatinine increased	2%	2%	3%	26%
Miscellaneous				
Application-site reaction	4%	0%	0%	0%
Dyspnea	0%	0%	0%	3%
Fever	0%	0%	0%	6%
Pain	1%	2%	0%	0%
Renal function abnormal	1%	1%	0%	11%
Rigors	0%	0%	0%	34%
Vein disorder	3%	0%	0%	0 %

The following adverse events occurred in less than 2% of patients in clinical trials of itraconazole injection: albuminuria, edema, hepatitis, hyperglycemia, and LDH increased.

➤*Postmarketing:* Worldwide postmarketing experiences with the use of itraconazole include adverse events of gastrointestinal origin, such as dyspepsia, nausea, vomiting, diarrhea, abdominal pain, and constipation. Other reported adverse events include peripheral edema, CHF, and pulmonary edema, headache, dizziness, peripheral neuropathy, menstrual disorders, reversible increases in hepatic enzymes, hepatitis, liver failure, hypokalemia, hypertriglyceridemia, alopecia, allergic reactions (eg, pruritus, rash, urticaria, angioedema, anaphylaxis), Stevens-Johnson syndrome, anaphylactic, anaphylactoid, and allergic reactions, photosensitivity, and neutropenia. There is limited information on the use of itraconazole during pregnancy.

Congenital abnormalities – Cases of congenital abnormalities, including skeletal, genitourinary tract, cardiovascular, and ophthalmic malformations, as well as chromosomal and multiple malformations have been reported during postmarketing experience. A causal relationship with itraconazole has not been established.

Overdosage

➤*Symptoms:* There are limited data on the outcomes of patients ingesting high doses of itraconazole. In patients taking either itraconazole oral solution 1,000 mg or up to itraconazole capsules 3,000 mg, or twice daily dosing for 4 days with itraconazole injection, the adverse event profile was similar to that observed at recommended doses.

➤*Treatment:* Itraconazole is not removed by dialysis.

Patient Information

Itraconazole injection contains the excipient hydroxypropyl-β-cyclodextrin which produced pancreatic adenocarcinomas in a rat carcinogenicity study. These findings were not observed in a similar mouse carcinogenicity study. The clinical relevance of these findings is unknown.

TERBINAFINE HYDROCHLORIDE

Rx	**Lamisil** (Novartis)	**Tablet:** 250 mg	(Lamisil 250). White to yellow-tinged white, biconvex. In 30s and 100s.

TERBINAFINE HYDROCHLORIDE — ORAL

WARNING

Rare cases of hepatic failure, some leading to death or liver transplant, have occurred with the use of terbinafine for the treatment of onychomycosis in individuals with and without preexisting liver disease. In the majority of liver cases reported in association with terbinafine use, the patients had serious underlying systemic conditions and an uncertain causal relationship with terbinafine. Terbinafine is not recommended for patients with chronic or active liver disease. Before prescribing terbinafine, assess preexisting liver disease. Hepatotoxicity may occur in patients with and without pre-existing liver disease. Pretreatment serum transaminase (ALT and AST) tests are advised for all patients before taking terbinafine.

Indications

➤*Onychomycosis:* Terbinafine HCl tablets are indicated for the treatment of onychomycosis of the toenail or fingernail due to dermatophytes (*Tinea unguium*). The optimal clinical effect is seen some months after mycological cure and cessation of treatment. This is related to the period required for outgrowth of healthy nail.

Prior to initiating treatment, appropriate nail specimens for laboratory testing (KOH preparation, fungal culture, or nail biopsy) should be obtained to confirm the diagnosis of onychomycosis.

Administration and Dosage

➤*Approved by the FDA:* May 10, 1996.

➤*Onychomycosis:* Terbinafine HCl tablets, one 250 mg tablet, should be taken once daily for 6 weeks by patients with fingernail onychomycosis. Terbinafine HCl, one 250 mg tablet, should be taken once daily for 12 weeks by patients with toenail onychomycosis. The optimal clinical effect is seen some months after mycological cure and cessation of treatment. This is related to the period required for outgrowth of healthy nail.

➤*Storage/Stability:* Store tablets below 25°C (77°F); in a tight container. Protect from light.

Actions

➤*Pharmacokinetics:*

Absorption/Distribution – Following oral administration, terbinafine is well absorbed (greater than 70%) and the bioavailability as a result of first-pass metabolism is approximately 40%. Peak plasma concentrations of 1 mcg/mL appear within 2 hour after a single 250 mg dose; the AUC (area under the curve) is approximately 4.56 mcg•hr/mL. An increase in the AUC of terbinafine of less than 20% is observed when terbinafine HCl is administered with food. No clinically relevant age-dependent changes in steady-state plasma concentrations of terbinafine have been reported. In plasma, terbinafine is greater than 99% bound to plasma proteins and there are no specific binding sites. At steady-state, in comparison to a single dose, the peak concentration of terbinafine is 25% higher and plasma AUC increases by a factor of 2.5; the increase in plasma AUC is consistent with an effective half-life of approximately 36 hours. Terbinafine is distributed to the sebum and skin. A terminal half-life of 200 to 400 hours may represent the slow elimination of terbinafine from tissues such as skin and adipose.

TERBINAFINE HYDROCHLORIDE — ORAL

Metabolism/Excretion – Prior to excretion, terbinafine is extensively metabolized. No metabolites have been identified that have antifungal activity similar to terbinafine. Approximately 70% of the administered dose is eliminated in the urine.

Special populations –

Renal and hepatic function impairment: In patients with renal impairment (creatinine clearance less than or equal to 50 mL/min) or hepatic cirrhosis, the clearance of terbinafine is decreased by approximately 50% compared with healthy volunteers.

➤*Microbiology:* Terbinafine HCl is a synthetic allylamine derivative. Terbinafine HCl is hypothesized to act by inhibiting squalene epoxidase, thus blocking the biosynthesis of ergosterol, an essential component of fungal cell membranes. In vitro, mammalian squalene epoxidase is only inhibited at higher (4000-fold) concentrations than is needed for inhibition of the dermatophyte enzyme. Depending on the concentration of the drug and the fungal species test in vitro, terbinafine HCl may be fungicidal. However, the clinical significance of in vitro data is unknown.

Terbinafine has been shown to be active against most strains of the following microorganisms both in vitro and in clinical infections: *Trichophyton mentagrophytes* and *Trichophyton rubrum*.

Contraindications

Hypersensitivity to terbinafine or to any other ingredients of the formulation.

Warnings

➤*Dermatologic effects:* There have been isolated reports of serious skin reactions (eg, Stevens-Johnson syndrome and toxic epidermal necrolysis). If progressive skin rash occurs, treatment with terbinafine HCl should be discontinued.

➤*Hepatic failure:* See the Warning box for more information.

➤*Renal function impairment:* In patients with renal impairment (creatinine clearance less than or equal to 50 mL/ min), the use of terbinafine HCl has not been adequately studied, and therefore, is not recommended.

➤*Hepatic function impairment:* Terbinafine HCl is not recommended for patients with chronic or active liver disease. Before prescribing terbinafine HCl tablets, preexisting liver disease should be assessed. Hepatotoxicity may occur in patients with and without preexisting liver disease. Pretreatment serum transaminase (ALT and AST) tests are advised for all patients before taking terbinafine HCl tablets. Patients prescribed terbinafine HCl tablets should be warned to report immediately to their physician any symptoms of persistent nausea, anorexia, fatigue, vomiting, right upper abdominal pain or jaundice, dark urine or pale stools. Patients with these symptoms should discontinue taking oral terbinafine, and the patient's liver function should be immediately evaluated.

➤*Carcinogenesis:* In a 28-month oral carcinogenicity study in rats, an increase in the incidence of liver tumors was observed in males at the highest dose tested, 69 mg/kg/day [2 times the maximum recommended human dose (MRHD) based on AUC comparisons of the parent terbinafine]; however, even though dose-limiting toxicity was not achieved at the highest tested dose, higher doses were not tested.

➤*Pregnancy: Category B.* Oral reproduction studies have been performed in rabbits and rats at doses up to 300 mg/kg/day (12 times to 23 times the MRHD, in rabbits and rats, respectively, based on BSA) and have revealed no evidence of impaired fertility or harm to the fetus due to terbinafine. There are, however, no adequate and well-controlled studies in pregnant women. Because animal reproduction studies are not always predictive of human response, and because treatment of onychomycosis can be postponed until after pregnancy is completed, it is recommended that terbinafine HCl not be initiated during pregnancy.

➤*Lactation:* After oral administration, terbinafine is present in breast milk of nursing mothers. The ratio of terbinafine in milk to plasma is 7:1. Treatment with terbinafine HCl is not recommended in nursing mothers.

➤*Children:* The safety and efficacy of terbinafine HCl have not been established in pediatric patients.

Precautions

➤*Monitoring:* Transient decreases in absolute lymphocyte counts (ALC) have been observed in controlled clinical trials. In placebo-controlled trials, 8 out of 465 of terbinafine HCl-treated patients (1.7%) and 3 out of 137 of placebo-treated patients (2.2%) had decreases in ALC to below 1000/mm^3 on 2 or more occasions. The clinical significance of this observation is unknown. However, in patients with known or suspected immunodeficiency, physicians should consider monitoring complete blood counts in individuals using terbinafine HCl therapy for greater than 6 weeks.

➤*Visual changes:* Changes in the ocular lens and retina have been reported following the use of terbinafine HCl tablets in controlled trials. The clinical significance of these changes is unknown.

➤*Neutropenia:* Isolated cases of severe neutropenia have been reported. These were reversible upon discontinuation of terbinafine HCl, with or without supportive therapy. If clinical signs and symptoms suggestive of secondary infection occur, a complete blood count should be obtained. If the neutrophil count is less than or equal to 1000 cells/mm^3, terbinafine HCl should be discontinued and supportive management started.

Drug Interactions

➤*Cytochrome P450 2D6 system:* In vitro studies with human liver microsomes showed that terbinafine does not inhibit the metabolism of tolbutamide, ethinylestradiol, ethoxycoumarin, and cyclosporine. In vitro studies have also shown that terbinafine inhibits CYP2D6-mediated metabolism. This may be of clinical relevance for compounds predominantly metabolized by this enzyme, such as tricyclic antidepressants, β-blockers, selective serotonin reuptake inhibitors (SSRIs), and monoamine oxidase inhibitors (MAOIs) type B, if they have a narrow therapeutic window.

➤*Warfarin:* There have been spontaneous reports of increase or decrease in prothrombin times in patients concomitantly taking oral terbinafine and warfarin, however, a causal relationship between terbinafine tablets and these changes has not been established.

Terbinafine Drug Interactions

Precipitant drug	Object drug*		Description
Cimetidine	Terbinafine	↑	Terbinafine clearance is decreased 33% by cimetidine.
Rifampin	Terbinafine	↓	Terbinafine clearance is increased 100% by rifampin.
Terbinafine	Caffeine	↑	Terbinafine decreases the clearance of caffeine by 19%.
Terbinafine	Cyclosporine	↓	Terbinafine increases the clearance of cyclosporine by 15%.
Terbinafine	Dextromethorphan	↑	Plasma dextromethorphan concentrations may be elevated, increasing the pharmacologic and adverse effects. Terbinafine inhibits dextromethorphan metabolism via the cytochrome P450 2D6 enzyme.

* ↑ = Object drug increased. ↓ = Object drug decreased.

Adverse Reactions

➤*Most frequently reported adverse reactions:*

Terbinafine Adverse Reactions

	Adverse reaction		Discontinuation	
	Terbinafine hydrochloride (%) (n = 465)	Placebo (%) (n = 137)	Terbinafine hydrochloride (%) (n = 465)	Placebo (%) (n = 137)
CNS				
Headache	12.9%	9.5%	0.2%	0%
GI				
Diarrhea	5.6%	2.9%	0.6%	0%
Dyspepsia	4.3%	2.9%	0.4%	0%
Abdominal pain	2.4%	1.5%	0.4%	0%
Nausea	2.6%	2.9%	0.2%	0%
Flatulence	2.2%	2.2%	0%	0%
Dermatologic				
Rash	5.6%	2.2%	0.9%	0.7%
Pruritus	2.8%	1.5%	0.2%	0%
Urticaria	1.1%	0%	0%	0%
Hepatic				
Liver enzyme abnormalities*	3.3%	1.4%	0.2%	0%
Special senses				
Taste disturbance	2.8%	0.7%	0.2%	0%
Visual disturbance	1.1%	1.5%	0.9%	0%

* Liver enzyme abnormalities greater than or equal to 2 times the upper limit of normal range.

➤*Rare adverse reactions:* Rare adverse reactions, based on worldwide experience with terbinafine HCl tablets use, include the following:

Hepatic – Idiosyncratic and symptomatic hepatic injury and more rarely, cases of liver failure, some leading to death or liver transplant.

Special senses – Uncommonly, terbinafine HCl may cause taste disturbance (including taste loss) which usually recovers within several weeks after discontinuation of the drug. There have been isolated reports of prolonged (greater than 1 year) taste disturbances. Rarely, taste disturbances associated with oral terbinafine have been reported to be severe enough to result in decreased food intake leading to significant and unwanted weight loss.

Miscellaneous – Serious skin reactions (eg, Stevens-Johnson syndrome and toxic epidermal necrolysis), severe neutropenia, thrombocytopenia and allergic reactions (including anaphylaxis).

➤*Other adverse reactions:*

Miscellaneous – Malaise, fatigue, vomiting, arthralgia, myalgia, and hair loss.

Allylamine Antifungal

TERBINAFINE HYDROCHLORIDE — ORAL

➤*Postmarketing:*

Hematologic – Clinical adverse reactions reported spontaneously since the drug was marketed include altered prothrombin time (prolongation and reduction) in patients concomitantly treated with warfarin and terbinafine HCl tablets and agranulocytosis (very rare).

Overdosage

➤*Symptoms:* Clinical experience regarding overdose with terbinafine HCl tablets is limited. Doses up to 5 g (20 times the therapeutic daily dose) have been taken without inducing serious adverse reactions. The symptoms of overdose included nausea, vomiting, abdominal pain, dizziness, rash, frequent urination, and headache.

Echinocandins

CASPOFUNGIN ACETATE

Rx	**Cancidas** (Merck)	**Powder for injection, lyophilized:** 50 mg	In single-use vials.
		70 mg	In single-use vials.

CASPOFUNGIN — INJECTION

Indications

➤*Candidemia and other Candida infections:* Treatment of candidemia and the following *Candida* infections: intra-abdominal abscesses, peritonitis, and pleural space infections. Caspofungin has not been studied in endocarditis, osteomyelitis, or meningitis caused by *Candida*.

➤*Esophageal candidiasis:* Treatment of esophageal candidiasis.

➤*Fungal infections, empirical:* Empirical therapy for presumed fungal infections in febrile, neutropenic patients.

➤*Invasive aspergillosis:* Treatment of invasive aspergillosis in patients who are refractory to or intolerant of other therapies (ie, amphotericin B, lipid formulations of amphotericin B, itraconazole). Caspofungin has not been studied as initial therapy for invasive aspergillosis.

Administration and Dosage

➤*Approved by the FDA:* January 29, 2001.

Administer caspofungin by slow intravenous (IV) infusion over approximately 1 hour.

➤*Candidemia and other Candida infections:* Administer a single 70 mg loading dose on day 1, followed by 50 mg daily thereafter. The patient's clinical and microbiological response should dictate duration of treatment. In general, continue antifungal therapy for at least 14 days after the last positive culture. Patients who remain persistently neutropenic may warrant a longer course of therapy pending resolution of the neutropenia.

➤*Esophageal candidiasis:* 50 mg daily. Because of the risk of relapse of oropharyngeal candidiasis in patients with HIV infections, suppressive oral therapy may be considered. A 70 mg loading dose has not been studied with this indication.

➤*Fungal infections, empirical:* Administer a single 70 mg loading dose on day 1, followed by 50 mg daily thereafter. Base duration of treatment on the patient's clinical response. Continue empirical therapy until resolution of neutropenia. Treat patients found to have a fungal infection for a minimum of 14 days; continue treatment for at least 7 days after both neutropenia and clinical symptoms are resolved. If the 50 mg dose is well tolerated but does not provide an adequate clinical response, the daily dose can be increased to 70 mg. Although an increase in efficacy with 70 mg daily has not been demonstrated, limited safety data suggest that an increase in dose to 70 mg daily is well tolerated.

➤*Invasive aspergillosis:* Administer a single 70 mg loading dose on day 1, followed by 50 mg daily thereafter. Base duration of treatment upon the severity of the patient's underlying disease, recovery from immunosuppression, and clinical response. The efficacy of a 70 mg dose regimen in patients who are not responding clinically to the 50 mg daily dose is not known. Limited safety data suggest that an increase in dosage to 70 mg daily is well tolerated. The safety and efficacy of doses above 70 mg have not been studied adequately.

➤*Hepatic function impairment:* Patients with mild hepatic impairment (Child-Pugh score, 5 to 6) do not need a dosage adjustment. For patients with moderate hepatic impairment (Child-Pugh score, 7 to 9), caspofungin 35 mg daily is recommended. However, where recommended, still administer a 70 mg loading dose on day 1. There is no clinical experience in patients with severe hepatic impairment (Child-Pugh score, greater than 9).

➤*Concomitant medication with inducers of drug clearance:* Patients on rifampin should receive caspofungin 70 mg daily. Patients on nevirapine, efavirenz, carbamazepine, dexamethasone, or phenytoin may require an increase in dosage to caspofungin 70 mg daily.

➤*Admixture incompatibilities:* Do not mix or coinfuse caspofungin with other medications, because there are no data available on the compatibility of caspofungin with other IV substances, additives, or medications. Do not use diluents containing dextrose (α-d-glucose), because caspofungin is not stable in diluents containing dextrose.

➤*Preparation of the 70 mg infusion:*

1.) Equilibrate the refrigerated vial of caspofungin to room temperature.
2.) Aseptically add 10.5 mL of 0.9% sodium chloride injection, sterile water for injection, bacteriostatic water for injection with methylparaben and propylparaben, or bacteriostatic water for injection with 0.9% benzyl alcohol to the vial.† This reconstituted solution may be stored for up to 1 hour at 25°C or below (77°F or below).†
3.) Aseptically transfer 10 mL of reconstituted caspofungin† to an IV bag (or bottle) containing 250 mL 0.9%, 0.45%, or 0.225% sodium chloride injection, or Ringer's lactate injection. This infusion solution must be used within 24 hours if stored at less than or equal to 25°C or below (77°F or below) or within 48 hours if stored refrigerated at 2° to 8°C (36° to 46°F). (If a 70 mg vial is unavailable, see Alternative infusion preparation methods: Preparation of 70 mg dose from two 50 mg vials.)

➤*Preparation of the daily 50 mg infusion:*

1.) Equilibrate the refrigerated vial of caspofungin to room temperature.
2.) Aseptically add 10.5 mL of 0.9% sodium chloride injection, sterile water for injection, bacteriostatic water for injection with methylparaben and propylparaben, or bacteriostatic water for injection with 0.9% benzyl alcohol to the vial.† This reconstituted solution may be stored for up to 1 hour at 25°C or below (77°F or below).†
3.) Aseptically transfer 10 mL of reconstituted caspofungin † to an IV bag (or bottle) containing 250 mL 0.9%, 0.45%, or 0.225% sodium chloride injection, or Ringer's lactate injection. This infusion solution must be used within 24 hours if stored at 25°C or below (77°F or below) or within 48 hours if stored refrigerated at 2° to 8°C (36° to 46°F). (If a reduced infusion volume is medically necessary, see Alternative infusion preparation methods: Preparation of 50 mg daily doses at reduced volume.)

➤*Alternative infusion preparation methods:*

Preparation of 70 mg dose from two 50 mg vials – Reconstitute two 50 mg vials with 10.5 mL of diluent each (see Preparation of the daily 50 mg infusion). Aseptically transfer a total of 14 mL of the reconstituted caspofungin from the 2 vials to 250 mL of 0.9%, 0.45%, or 0.225% sodium chloride injection, or Ringer's lactate injection.

Preparation of 50 mg daily doses at reduced volume – When medically necessary, the 50 mg daily doses can be prepared by adding 10 mL of reconstituted caspofungin to 100 mL of 0.9%, 0.45%, or 0.225% sodium chloride injection, or Ringer's lactate injection (see Preparation of the daily 50 mg infusion).

Preparation of a 35 mg daily dose for patients with moderate hepatic function impairment – Reconstitute one 50 mg vial (see Preparation of the daily 50 mg infusion). Aseptically transfer 7 mL of the reconstituted caspofungin from the vial to 250 mL or, if medically necessary, to 100 mL of 0.9%, 0.45%, or 0.225% sodium chloride injection or Ringer's lactate injection.

Caspofungin Concentrations

Dose	Reconstituted solution concentration	Infusion volume	Infusion solution concentration
70 mg initial dose	7.2 mg/mL	260 mL	0.28 mg/mL
50 mg daily dose	5.2 mg/mL	260 mL	0.2 mg/mL
70 mg initial dose[a] (from two 50 mg vials)	5.2 mg/mL	264 mL	0.28 mg/mL
50 mg daily dose[a] (reduced volume)	5.2 mg/mL	110 mL	0.47 mg/mL
35 mg daily dose[a] (from one 50 mg vial) for moderate hepatic impairment	5.2 mg/mL	257 or 107 mL	0.14 or 0.34 mg/mL

[a] See preceding text for these special situations.

➤*Storage/Stability:*

Vials – Store the lyophilized vials refrigerated at 2° to 8°C (36° to 46°F).

Reconstituted concentrate – Reconstituted caspofungin may be stored at 25°C or below (77°F or below) for 1 hour prior to the preparation of the patient infusion solution.

† Visually inspect the reconstituted solution for particulate matter or discoloration during reconstitution and prior to infusion. Do not use if the solution is cloudy or has precipitated.

CASPOFUNGIN — INJECTION

Diluted product – The final patient infusion solution in the IV bag or bottle can be stored at 25°C or below (77°F or below) for 24 hours or at 2° to 8°C (36° to 46°F) for 48 hours.

Actions

➤*Pharmacology:* Caspofungin inhibits the synthesis of β (1,3)-D-glucan, an essential component of the cell wall of susceptible *Aspergillus* and *Candida* species. Beta (1,3)-D-glucan is not present in mammalian cells. Caspofungin has shown activity against *Candida* species and in regions of active cell growth of the hyphae of *Aspergillus fumigatus*.

➤*Pharmacokinetics:*

Distribution – Plasma concentrations of caspofungin decline in a polyphasic manner following single 1-hour IV infusions. A short α-phase occurs immediately postinfusion, followed by a β-phase (half-life, 9 to 11 hours) that characterizes much of the profile and exhibits clear log-linear behavior from 6 to 48 hours postdose during which the plasma concentration decreases 10-fold. An additional, longer half-life phase, γ-phase (half-life, 40 to 50 hours) also occurs. Distribution, rather than excretion or biotransformation, is the dominant mechanism influencing plasma clearance. Caspofungin is bound extensively to albumin (approximately 97%), and distribution into red blood cells is minimal. Mass balance results showed that approximately 92% of the administered radioactivity was distributed to tissues by 36 to 48 hours after a single 70 mg dose of [^{3}H] caspofungin. There is little excretion or biotransformation of caspofungin during the first 30 hours after administration.

Metabolism – Caspofungin is metabolized slowly by hydrolysis and N-acetylation. Caspofungin also undergoes spontaneous chemical degradation to an open-ring peptide compound, L-747969. At later time points (greater than or equal to 5 days postdose), there is a low level (less than or equal to 7 picomoles/mg protein, or less than or equal to 1.3% of administered dose) of covalent binding of radiolabel in plasma following single-dose administration of [^{3}H] caspofungin, which may be due to 2 reactive intermediates formed during the chemical degradation of caspofungin to L-747969. Additional metabolism involves hydrolysis into constitutive amino acids and their degradates, including dihydroxyhomotyrosine and N-acetyl-dihydroxyhomotyrosine. These 2 tyrosine derivatives are found only in urine, suggesting rapid clearance of these derivatives by the kidneys.

Excretion – Two single-dose radiolabeled pharmacokinetic studies were conducted. In 1 study, plasma, urine, and feces were collected over 27 days, and in the second study plasma was collected over 6 months. Plasma concentrations of radioactivity and of caspofungin were similar during the first 24 to 48 hours postdose; thereafter drug levels fell more rapidly. In plasma, caspofungin concentrations fell below the limit of quantitation after 6 to 8 days postdose, while radiolabel fell below the limit of quantitation at 22.3 weeks postdose. After single IV administration of [^{3}H] caspofungin, excretion of caspofungin and its metabolites in humans was 35% of dose in feces and 41% of dose in urine. A small amount of caspofungin is excreted unchanged in urine (approximately 1.4% of dose). Renal clearance of parent drug is low (approximately 0.15 mL/min), and total clearance of caspofungin is 12 mL/min.

Special populations –

Renal function impairment: In a clinical study of single 70 mg doses, caspofungin pharmacokinetics were similar in volunteers with mild renal insufficiency (creatinine clearance [Ccr] 50 to 80 mL/min) and control subjects. Moderate (Ccr 31 to 49 mL/min), advanced (Ccr 5 to 30 mL/min), and end-stage (creatinine clearance less than 10 mL/min and dialysis dependent) renal insufficiency moderately increased caspofungin plasma concentrations after single-dose administration (range 30% to 49% for AUC). However, in patients with invasive aspergillosis, candidemia, or other *Candida* infections (intra-abdominal abscesses, peritonitis, or pleural space infections) who received multiple daily doses of caspofungin 50 mg, there was no significant effect of mild to end-stage renal impairment on caspofungin concentrations. No dosage adjustment is necessary for patients with renal impairment. Caspofungin is not dialyzable, thus supplementary dosing is not required following hemodialysis.

Hepatic function impairment: Plasma concentrations of caspofungin after a single 70 mg dose in patients with mild hepatic insufficiency (Child-Pugh score 5 to 6) were increased by approximately 55% in the AUC compared with healthy control subjects. In a 14-day multiple-dose study (70 mg on day 1 followed by 50 mg daily thereafter), plasma concentrations in patients with mild hepatic insufficiency were increased modestly (19% to 25% in the AUC) on days 7 and 14 relative to healthy control subjects. No dosage adjustment is recommended for patients with mild hepatic insufficiency. Patients with moderate hepatic insufficiency (Child-Pugh score, 7 to 9) who received a single 70 mg dose of caspofungin had an average plasma caspofungin increase of 76% in the AUC compared with control subjects. A dosage reduction is recommended for patients with moderate hepatic insufficiency. There is no clinical experience in patients with severe hepatic insufficiency (Child-Pugh score, greater than 9).

Age: Plasma concentrations of caspofungin in healthy older men and women (65 years of age and older) were increased slightly (approximately 28% in the AUC) compared with young healthy men after a single 70 mg dose of caspofungin. In patients who were treated empirically or who had candidemia or other *Candida* infections (intra-abdominal abscesses, peritonitis, or pleural space infections), a similar modest effect of age was seen in older patients relative to younger patients. No dosage adjustment is necessary for the elderly.

➤*Microbiology:*

Activity in vitro – Caspofungin exhibits in vitro activity against *Aspergillus* species (*A. fumigatus, Aspergillus flavus,* and *Aspergillus terreus*) and *Candida* species (*Candida albicans, Candida glabrata, Candida guilliermondii, Candida krusei, Candida parapsilosis,* and *Candida tropicalis*). Susceptibility testing was performed according to the National Committee for Clinical Laboratory Standards (NCCLS) method M38-A (for *Aspergillus* species) and M27-A (for *Candida* species). Standardized susceptibility testing methods for echinocandins have not been established for yeasts and filamentous fungi, and results of susceptibility studies do not correlate with clinical outcome.

Drug resistance – Mutants of *Candida* with reduced susceptibility to caspofungin have been identified in some patients during treatment. Similar observations were made in a study in mice infected with *C. albicans* and treated with orally administered doses of caspofungin. Do not use mean inhibitory concentration (MIC) values for caspofungin to predict clinical outcome, since a correlation between MIC values and clinical outcome has not been established. The incidence of drug resistance by various clinical isolates of *Candida* and *Aspergillus* species is unknown.

Contraindications

Hypersensitivity to any component of this product.

Warnings

➤*Concomitant use with cyclosporine:* Limit concomitant use of caspofungin injection with cyclosporine to patients for whom the potential benefit outweighs the potential risk. In 1 clinical study, 3 of 4 healthy subjects who received caspofungin 70 mg on days 1 through 10, and also received two cyclosporine 3 mg/kg doses 12 hours apart on day 10, developed transient elevations of ALT on day 11 that were 2 to 3 times the upper limit of normal (ULN). In a separate panel of subjects in the same study, 2 of 8 who received caspofungin 35 mg daily for 3 days and cyclosporine (two 3 mg/kg doses administered 12 hours apart) on day 1 had small increases in ALT (slightly above the ULN) on day 2. In both groups, elevations in AST paralleled ALT elevations, but were of lesser magnitude.

Given the limitations of these data, only use caspofungin and cyclosporine concomitantly in those patients for whom the potential benefit outweighs the potential risk. Monitor patients who develop abnormal liver function tests during concomitant therapy with cyclosporine, and evaluate the risk/benefit of continuing therapy.

➤*Hepatic function impairment:* See Administration and Dosage for more information.

➤*Elderly:* Clinical studies of caspofungin did not include sufficient numbers of patients 65 years of age and older to determine whether they respond differently from younger patients. Although the number of elderly patients was not large enough for a statistical analysis, no overall differences in safety or efficacy were observed between these and younger patients. Plasma concentrations of caspofungin in healthy older men and women (65 years of age and older) were increased slightly (approximately 28% in the AUC) compared with young healthy men. No dose adjustment is recommended for the elderly; however, greater sensitivity of some older individuals cannot be ruled out.

➤*Pregnancy: Category C.* Caspofungin was shown to be embryotoxic in rats and rabbits. Findings included incomplete ossification of the skull and torso and an increased incidence of cervical rib in rats. An increased incidence of incomplete ossifications of the talus/calcaneus was seen in rabbits. Caspofungin also produced increases in resorptions in rats and rabbits and periimplantation losses in rats. These findings were observed at doses that produced exposures similar to those seen in patients treated with a 70 mg dose. Caspofungin crossed the placental barrier in rats and rabbits and was detected in the plasma of fetuses of pregnant animals dosed with caspofungin. There are no adequate and well-controlled studies in pregnant women. Use caspofungin during pregnancy only if the potential benefit justifies the potential risk to the fetus.

➤*Lactation:* Caspofungin was found in the milk of lactating, drug-treated rats. It is not known whether caspofungin is excreted in human milk. Because many drugs are excreted in human milk, exercise caution when caspofungin is administered to a breast-feeding woman.

➤*Children:* Safety and efficacy in pediatric patients have not been established.

Precautions

➤*Monitoring:* Monitor patients who develop abnormal liver function tests during concomitant therapy with cyclosporine, and evaluate the risk/benefit of continuing therapy.

Monitor patients who develop abnormal liver function tests during caspofungin therapy for evidence of worsening hepatic function and evaluate them for risk/benefit of continuing caspofungin therapy.

➤*Administration:* The efficacy of a 70 mg dose regimen in patients with invasive aspergillosis who are not clinically responding to the 50 mg daily dose is not known. Limited safety data suggest that an increase in dosage to 70 mg daily is well tolerated. The safety and efficacy of doses above 70 mg have not been studied adequately in patients with *Candida* infections. However, caspofungin was generally well tolerated at a dosage of 100 mg once daily for 21 days when administered to 15 healthy subjects.

The safety information on treatment durations longer than 4 weeks is limited; however, available data suggest that caspofungin continues to be well tolerated with longer courses of therapy (up to 162 days).

➤*Hepatic effects:* Laboratory abnormalities in liver function tests have been seen in healthy volunteers and patients treated with caspofungin. In some patients with serious underlying conditions who were receiving multiple concomitant medications along with caspofungin, clinical hepatic abnormalities have also occurred. Isolated cases of significant hepatic dysfunction, hepatitis, or worsening hepatic failure have been reported in

CASPOFUNGIN — INJECTION

patients; a causal relationship to caspofungin has not been established. Monitor patients who develop abnormal liver function tests during caspofungin therapy for evidence of worsening hepatic function and evaluate them for risk/benefit of continuing caspofungin therapy.

Drug Interactions

Caspofungin Drug Interactions

Precipitant drug	Object drug[a]		Description
Cyclosporine	Caspofungin	⬆	Cyclosporine increased the AUC of caspofungin by approximately 35%. Concurrent use also produced transient elevations in ALT and AST.
Inducers of drug clearance or mixed inducer/ inhibitors (eg, efavirenz, nevirapine, phenytoin, rifampin, dexamethasone, carbamazepine)	Caspofungin	⬇	Coadministration may result in clinically meaningful reductions in caspofungin concentrations. Rifampin decreased caspofungin trough concentrations by 30%. Patients on rifampin should receive 70 mg of caspofungin daily. When coadministering caspofungin with the other drugs listed, consider an increase in the daily dose of caspofungin to 70 mg in patients who are not clinically responding.
Caspofungin	Tacrolimus	⬇	Concomitant administration produced a decrease in the AUC of tacrolimus by approximately 20%, C_{max} by 16%, and 12-hour blood concentration by 26%. Monitor tacrolimus blood concentrations and adjust dose accordingly.

[a] ⬇ = Object drug decreased. ⬆ = Object drug increased.

Adverse Reactions

Possible histamine-mediated symptoms have been reported, including reports of rash, facial swelling, pruritus, sensation of warmth, or bronchospasm. Anaphylaxis has been reported during administration of caspofungin.

➤*Clinical adverse reactions:* The overall safety of caspofungin was assessed in 1,440 individuals who received single or multiple doses of caspofungin: 564 febrile, neutropenic patients (empirical therapy study); 125 patients with candidemia and/or intra-abdominal abscesses, peritonitis, or pleural space infections (including 4 patients with chronic disseminated candidiasis); 285 patients with esophageal and/or oropharyngeal candidiasis; 72 patients with invasive aspergillosis; and 394 individuals in phase 1 studies. In the empirical-therapy study, patients had undergone hematopoietic stem-cell transplantation or chemotherapy. In the studies involving patients with documented *Candida* infections, the majority of the patients had serious underlying medical conditions (eg, hematologic or other malignancy, recent major surgery, HIV) requiring multiple concomitant medications. Patients in the noncomparative *Aspergillus* study often had serious predisposing medical conditions (eg, bone marrow or peripheral stem cell transplants, hematologic malignancy, solid tumors, organ transplants) requiring multiple concomitant medications.

➤*Empirical therapy:*

Drug-Related[a] Clinical Adverse Reactions Among Patients with Persistent Fever and Neutropenia Incidence ≥ 2% for at Least 1 Treatment Group by Body System

	Caspofungin[b] n = 564	Amphotericin B liposome for injection[c] n = 547
Cardiovascular		
Hypertension	1.1%	2%
Tachycardia	1.4%	2.4%
CNS		
Headache	4.3%	5.7%
Dermatologic		
Rash	6.2%	5.3%
GI		
Abdominal pain	1.4%	2.4%
Diarrhea	2.7%	2.4%
Nausea	3.5%	11.3%
Vomiting	3.5%	8.6%
Metabolic/Nutritional		
Hypokalemia	3.7%	4.2%
Musculoskeletal		
Back pain	0.7%	2.7%
Respiratory		
Dyspnea	2%	4.2%
Tachypnea	0.4%	2%
Miscellaneous		
Chills	13.8%	24.7%
Fever	17%	19.4%
Flushing	1.8%	4.2%
Perspiration/ Diaphoresis	2.8%	2.2%

[a] Determined by the investigator to be possibly, probably, or definitely drug related.
[b] 70 mg on day 1, then 50 mg daily for the remainder of treatment; daily dose was increased to 70 mg for 73 patients.
[c] 3 mg/kg/day; daily dose was increased to 5 mg/kg for 74 patients.

Drug-Related[a] Laboratory Adverse Reactions Among Patients with Persistent Fever and Neutropenia Incidence ≥ 2% for At Least 1 Treatment Group by Laboratory Test Category

	Caspofungin[b] n = 564	Amphotericin B liposome injection[c] n = 547
Hematologic		
Blood chemistry		
Alkaline phosphatase increased	7%	12%
ALT increased	8.7%	8.9%
AST increased	7%	7.6%
Direct serum bilirubin increased	2.6%	5.2%
Hypokalemia	7.3%	11.8%
Hypomagnesemia	2.3%	2.6%
Serum creatinine increased	1.2%	5.5%
Total serum bilirubin increased	3%	5.2%

[a] Determined by the investigator to be possibly, probably, or definitely drug related.
[b] 70 mg on day 1, then 50 mg daily for the remainder of treatment; daily dose was increased to 70 mg for 73 patients.
[c] 3 mg/kg/day; daily dose was increased to 5 mg/kg for 74 patients.

➤*Candidemia and other Candida infections:*

Drug-Related[a] Clinical Adverse Reactions Among Patients with Candidemia or other *Candida* Infections[b] Incidence ≥ 2% for at least 1 treatment group by body system

	Caspofungin 50 mg[c] n = 114	Amphotericin B n = 125
Cardiovascular		
Hypertension	1.8%	6.4%
Hypotension	0.9%	2.4%
Phlebitis/ Thrombophlebitis	3.5%	4.8%
Tachycardia	1.8%	10.4%
CNS		
Tremor	1.8%	2.4%
Dermatologic		
Erythema	0%	2.4%
Rash	0.9%	3.2%
Sweating	0.9%	3.2%
GI		
Diarrhea	2.6%	0.8%
Jaundice	0.9%	3.2%
Nausea	1.8%	5.6%
Vomiting	3.5%	8%
GU		
Renal insufficiency	0.9%	5.6%
Renal insufficiency, acute	0%	5.6%
Metabolic/Nutritional		
Hypokalemia	0.9%	5.6%

CASPOFUNGIN — INJECTION

Drug-Related[a] Clinical Adverse Reactions Among Patients with Candidemia or other *Candida* Infections[b]		
Incidence ≥ 2% for at least 1 treatment group by body system		
	Caspofungin 50 mg[c] n = 114	Amphotericin B n = 125
Respiratory		
Tachypnea	0%	10.4%
Miscellaneous		
Chills	5.3%	26.4%
Fever	7%	23.2%

[a] Determined by the investigator to be possibly, probably, or definitely drug related.
[b] Intra-abdominal abscesses, peritonitis, and pleural space infections
[c] Patients received caspofungin 70 mg on day 1, then 50 mg daily for the remainder of their treatment.

The incidence of drug-related clinical adverse reactions was significantly lower among patients treated with caspofungin (28.9%) than among patients treated with amphotericin B (58.4%). Also, the proportion of patients who experienced an infusion-related adverse reaction was significantly lower in the group treated with caspofungin (20.2%) than in the group treated with amphotericin B (48.8%).

Drug-Related[a] Laboratory Adverse Reactions Among Patients with Candidemia or other *Candida* Infections[b]		
Incidence ≥ 2% for at least 1 treatment group by laboratory test category		
	Caspofungin 50 mg[a] n = 114	Amphotericin B n = 125
Blood chemistry		
ALT increased	3.7%	8.1%
AST increased	1.9%	9%
Direct serum bilirubin increased	3.8%	8.4%
Serum alkaline phosphatase increased	8.3%	15.6%
Serum bicarbonate decreased	0%	3.6%
Serum creatinine increased	3.7%	22.6%
Serum phosphate increased	0%	2.7%
Serum potassium decreased	9.9%	23.4%
Serum potassium increased	0.9%	2.4%
Serum urea increased	1.9%	15.8%
Total serum bilirubin increased	2.8%	8.9%
Hematology		
Hematocrit decreased	0.9%	7.3%
Hemoglobin decreased	0.9%	10.5%
Urinalysis		
Urine protein increased	0%	3.7%

[a] Determined by the investigator to be possibly, probably, or definitely drug related.
[b] Intra-abdominal abscesses, peritonitis, and pleural space infections.
[c] Patients received caspofungin 70 mg on day 1, then 50 mg daily for the remainder of their treatment.

➤*Esophageal candidiasis and oropharyngeal candidiasis:*

Drug-Related Clinical Adverse Reactions Among Patients with Esophageal and/or Oropharyngeal Candidiasis[a]					
Incidence ≥ 2% for at least 1 treatment dose (per comparison) by body system					
	Caspofungin 50 mg[b] n = 83	Fluconazole IV 200 mg[b] n = 94	Caspofungin 50 mg[c] n = 80	Caspofungin 70 mg[c] n = 65	Amphotericin B 0.5 mg/kg[c] n = 89
Cardiovascular					
Infused vein complication	12%	8.5%	2.5%	1.5%	0%
Phlebitis/ Thrombophlebitis	15.7%	8.5%	11.3%	13.8%	22.5%
Tachycardia	0%	0%	1.3%	0%	4.5%
Vasculitis	0%	0%	0%	0%	3.4%
CNS					
Dizziness	0%	2.1%	0%	1.5%	1.1%
Headache	6%	1.1%	11.3%	7.7%	19.1%
Insomnia	1.2%	0%	0%	0%	2.2%
Paresthesia	0%	0%	1.3%	3.1%	1.1%
Tremor	0%	0%	0%	0%	7.9%
Dermatologic					
Erythema	1.2%	0%	1.3%	1.5%	7.9%
Induration	0%	0%	0%	3.1%	6.7%
Pruritus	1.2%	0%	2.5%	1.5%	0%
Rash	0%	0%	1.3%	4.6%	3.4%
Sweating	0%	0%	1.3%	0%	3.4%
GI					
Abdominal pain	3.6%	2.1%	2.5%	0%	9%
Anorexia	0%	0%	1.3%	0%	3.4%
Diarrhea	3.6%	2.1%	1.3%	3.1%	11.2%
Gastritis	0%	2.1%	0%	0%	0%
Nausea	6%	6.4%	2.5%	3.1%	21.3%
Vomiting	1.2%	3.2%	1.3%	3.1%	13.5%
Hematologic					
Anemia	0%	0%	3.8%	0%	9%
Metabolic					
Edema, facial	0%	0%	0%	3.1%	0%
Edema/ Swelling	0%	0%	0%	0%	5.6%
Musculoskeletal					
Back pain	0%	0%	0%	0%	2.2%
Musculoskeletal pain	0%	0%	1.3%	0%	4.5%
Myalgia	1.2%	0%	0%	3.1%	2.2%
Respiratory					
Tachypnea	0%	0%	1.3%	0%	4.5%
Miscellaneous					
Anaphylaxis	0%	0%	0%	0%	2.2%
Asthenia/ Fatigue	0%	0%	0%	0%	6.7%
Chills	0%	0%	2.5%	1.5%	75.3%
Fever	3.6%	1.1%	21.3%	26.2%	69.7%
Flu-like illness	0%	0%	0%	3.1%	0%
Malaise	0%	0%	0%	0%	5.6%
Pain	0%	0%	1.3%	4.6%	5.6%
Warm sensation	0%	0%	0%	1.5%	4.5%

[a] Relationship to drug was determined by the investigator to be possibly, probably, or definitely drug related.
[b] Derived from a phase 3, comparator-controlled clinical study.
[c] Derived from phase 2, comparator-controlled clinical studies. Laboratory abnormalities occurring in 2% or more of patients with esophageal and/or oropharyngeal candidiasis are presented in the following table.

Drug-Related Laboratory Abnormalities Reported Among Patients with Esophageal and/or Oropharyngeal Candidiasis[a]				
Incidence ≥ 2% (for at least 1 treatment dose) by laboratory test category				
	Caspofungin 50 mg[b] n = 163	Caspofungin 70 mg[c] n = 65	Fluconazole IV 200 mg[b] n = 94	Amphotericin B 0.5 mg/kg[c] n = 89
Blood chemistry				
ALT increased	10.6%	10.8%	11.8%	22.7%
AST increased	13%	10.8%	12.9%	22.7%
Direct serum bilirubin increased	0.6%	0%	3.3%	2.5%
Serum albumin decreased	8.6%	4.6%	5.4%	14.9%
Serum alkaline phosphatase increased	10.5%	7.7%	11.8%	19.3%

CASPOFUNGIN – INJECTION

Drug-Related Laboratory Abnormalities Reported Among Patients with Esophageal and/or Oropharyngeal Candidiasis[a]				
Incidence ≥ 2% (for at least 1 treatment dose) by laboratory test category				
	Caspofungin 50 mg[b] n = 163	Caspofungin 70 mg[c] n = 65	Fluconazole IV 200 mg[b] n = 94	Amphotericin B 0.5 mg/kg[c] n = 89
Serum bicarbonate decreased	0.9%	0%	0%	6.6%
Serum calcium decreased	1.9%	0%	3.2%	1.1%
Serum creatinine increased	0%	1.5%	2.2%	28.1%
Serum potassium decreased	3.7%	10.8%	4.3%	31.5%
Serum potassium increased	0.6%	0%	2.2%	1.1%
Serum sodium decreased	1.9%	1.5%	3.2%	1.1%
Serum urea increased	0%	0%	1.2%	10.3%
Serum uric acid increased	0.6%	0%	0%	3.4%
Total serum bilirubin increased	0%	0%	3.2%	4.5%
Total serum protein decreased	3.1%	0	3.2%	3.4%
Hematology				
Eosinophils increased	3.1%	3.1%	1.1%	1.1%
Hematocrit decreased	11.1%	1.5%	5.4%	32.6%
Hemoglobin decreased	12.3%	3.1%	5.4%	37.1%
Lymphocyte increased	0%	1.6%	2.2%	0%
Neutrophils decreased	1.9%	3.1%	3.2%	1.1%
Platelet count decreased	3.1%	1.5%	2.2%	3.4%
Prothrombin time increased	1.3%	1.5%	0%	2.3%
White blood cell (WBC) count decreased	6.2%	4.6%	8.6%	7.9%
Urinalysis				
Urine blood increased	0%	0%	0%	4%
Urine casts increased	0%	0%	0%	8%
Urine pH increased	0.8%	0%	0%	3.6%
Urine protein increased	1.2%	0%	3.3%	4.5%
Urine red blood cell (RBC) count increased	1.1%	3.8%	5.1%	12%
Urine WBC count increased	0%	7.7%	0%	24%

[a] Relationship to drug was determined by the investigator to be possibly, probably, or definitely drug related.
[b] Derived from phase 2 and 3 comparator-controlled clinical studies.
[c] Derived from phase 2, comparator-controlled clinical studies.

➤*Invasive aspergillosis:* In the open-label, noncomparative aspergillosis study, in which 69 patients received caspofungin (70 mg loading dose on day 1 followed by 50 mg daily), the following drug-related clinical adverse reactions were observed with an incidence of greater than or equal to 2%: fever, flushing, infused-vein complications, nausea, vomiting (2.9%).

Also reported infrequently in this patient population were pulmonary edema, adult respiratory distress syndrome (ARDS), and radiographic infiltrates.

Drug-related laboratory abnormalities reported with an incidence greater than or equal to 2% in patients treated with caspofungin in the noncomparative aspergillosis study were as follows: urine protein increased (4.9%), eosinophils increased (3.2%), serum alkaline phosphatase increased and serum potassium decreased (2.9%), and urine red blood cells increased (2.2%).

➤*Postmarketing:*

Hepatic – Rare cases of clinically significant hepatic dysfunction.

Metabolic – Hypercalcemia, peripheral edema, and swelling.

➤*Concomitant therapy:* In 1 clinical study, 3 of 4 subjects who received caspofungin 70 mg daily on days 1 through 10 and also received 2 cyclosporine 3 mg/kg doses 12 hours apart on day 10 developed transient elevations of ALT on day 11 that were 2 to 3 times the ULN. In a separate panel of subjects in the same study, 2 of 8 subjects who received caspofungin 35 mg daily for 3 days and cyclosporine (two 3 mg/kg doses administered 12 hours apart) on day 1 had small increases in ALT (slightly above the ULN) on day 2. In another clinical study, 2 of 8 healthy men developed transient ALT elevations of less than 2 times ULN. In this study, cyclosporine (4 mg/kg) was administered on days 1 and 12, and caspofungin 70 mg was administered daily on days 3 through 13. In 1 subject, the ALT elevation occurred on days 7 and 9 and, in the other subject, the ALT elevation occurred on day 19. These elevations returned to normal by day 27. In all groups, elevations in AST paralleled ALT elevations but were of lesser magnitude. In these clinical studies, cyclosporine (one 4 mg/kg dose or two 3 mg/kg doses) increased the AUC of caspofungin by approximately 35%.

Overdosage

In clinical studies the highest dose was 210 mg, administered as a single dose to 6 healthy subjects. This dose was generally well tolerated. In addition, 100 mg once daily for 21 days has been administered to 15 healthy subjects and was generally well tolerated. Caspofungin is not dialyzable. The minimum lethal dose of caspofungin in rats was 50 mg/kg, a dose which is equivalent to 10 times the recommended daily dose based on relative body surface area comparison.

MICAFUNGIN

Rx	**Mycamine** (Astellas Pharma, Inc.)	**Powder for injection:** 50 mg[a]	In single-use vials.

[a] Micafungin must be diluted with 0.9% sodium chloride injection or 5% dextrose injection.

MICAFUNGIN — INJECTION

Indications

➤*Esophageal candidiasis:* For the treatment of patients with esophageal candidiasis.

➤*Prophylaxis of Candida infections:* For prophylaxis of *Candida* infections in patients undergoing hematopoietic stem cell transplantation (HSCT).

Administration and Dosage

Micafungin Dosage	
Indication	Recommended dosage
Treatment of esophageal candidiasis[a]	150 mg/day
Prophylaxis of *Candida* infections in HSCT recipients[b]	50 mg/day

[a] In patients treated successfully for esophageal candidiasis, the mean duration of treatment was 15 days (range, 10 to 30 days).
[b] In HSCT recipients who experienced success of prophylactic therapy, the mean duration of prophylaxis was 19 days (range, 6 to 51 days).

➤*Administration:* Administer micafungin by intravenous (IV) infusion over the period of 1 hour. More rapid infusions may result in more frequent histamine-mediated reactions.

Flush an existing IV line with 0.9% sodium chloride injection prior to infusion of micafungin.

➤*Admixture incompatibility:* Do not mix or coinfuse micafungin with other medications. Micafungin has been shown to precipitate when mixed directly with a number of other commonly used medications.

➤*Preparation for administration:* Please read this entire section care fully before beginning reconstitution.

The diluent to be used for reconstitution and dilution is 0.9% sodium chloride injection (without a bacteriostatic agent). Alternatively, 5% dextrose injection may be used for reconstitution and dilution of micafungin.

Solutions for Infusion – Infusion are prepared as follows:

Reconstitution: Aseptically add 5 mL of 0.9% sodium chloride injection (without a bacteriostatic agent) to each 50 mg vial to yield a preparation containing approximately micafungin 10 mg/mL.

Dissolution: To minimize excessive foaming, gently dissolve the micafungin powder by swirling the vial. Do not vigorously shake the vial. Visually inspect the vial for particulate matter.

Dilution: Protect the diluted solution from light. It is not necessary to cover the infusion drip chamber or the tubing.

For prophylaxis of *Candida* infections: Add micafungin 50 mg reconstituted in sodium chloride 5 mL injection into 100 mL of 0.9% sodium chloride injection.

For treatment of esophageal candidiasis: Add micafungin 150 mg (from 3 micafungin 50 mg vials) reconstituted in sodium chloride 15 mL injection into 100 mL of 0.9% sodium chloride injection.

Micafungin is preservative free. Discard partially used vials.

➤*Storage / Stability:* The reconstituted product may be stored in the original vial for up to 24 hours at room temperature (25° C [77° F]).

Protect the diluted infusion from light. It may be stored for up to 24 hours at room temperature (25° C [77° F]).

Actions

➤*Pharmacology:* Micafungin inhibits the synthesis of 1,3-β-D-glucan, an essential component of fungal cell walls, which is not present in mammalian cells.

➤*Pharmacokinetics:*

Absorption / Distribution –

The relationship of area under the concentration-time curve (AUC) to micafungin dose was linear over the daily dose range of 50 to 150 mg and 3 to 8 mg/kg body weight.

Steady-state pharmacokinetic parameters in relevant patient populations after repeated daily administration are presented in the following table.

Pharmacokinetic Parameters of Micafungin in Adult Patients						
			Pharmacokinetic Parameters (Mean ± SD[a])			
Population	n	Dose	C_{max} (mcg/mL)	AUC_{0-24} (mcg•h/mL)	t½ (h)	Cl (mL/min/kg)
HIV-Positive Patients with EC[b] (Day 14 or 21)	20	50 mg	5.1 ± 1	54 ± 13	15.6 ± 2.8	0.3 ± 0.063
	20	100 mg	10.1 ± 2.6	115 ± 25	16.9 ± 4.4	0.301 ± 0.086
	14	150 mg	16.4 ± 6.5	167 ± 40	15.2 ± 2.2	0.297 ± 0.081
HSCT[c] Recipients (Day 7)	8	3 mg/kg	21.1 ± 2.84	234 ± 34	14 ± 1.4	0.214 ± 0.031
	10	4 mg/kg	29.2 ± 6.2	339 ± 72	14.2 ± 3.2	0.204 ± 0.036
	8	6 mg/kg	38.4 ± 6.9	479 ± 157	14.9 ± 2.6	0.224 ± 0.064
	8	8 mg/kg	60.8 ± 26.9	663 ± 212	17.2 ± 2.3	0.223 ± 0.081

[a] SD = standard deviation.
[b] EC = esophageal candidiasis.
[c] HSCT = hematopoietic stem cell transplant.

The mean ± SD volume of distribution of micafungin at terminal phase was 0.39 ± 0.11 L/kg body weight when determined in adult patients with esophageal candidiasis at the dose range of 50 to 150 mg.

Micafungin is highly (more than 99%) protein bound in vitro, independent of plasma concentrations over the range of 10 to 100 mcg/mL. The primary binding protein is albumin; however, micafungin, at therapeutically relevant concentrations, does not competitively displace bilirubin binding to albumin. Micafungin also binds to a lesser extent to α_1-acid-glycoprotein.

Metabolism – Micafungin is metabolized to M-1 (catechol form) by arylsulfatase, with further metabolism to M-2 (methoxy form) by catechol-O-methyltransferase. M-5 is formed by hydroxylation at the side chain (ω-1 position) of micafungin catalyzed by cytochrome P-450 (CYP) isozymes. Even though micafungin is a substrate for, and a weak inhibitor of, CYP3A in vitro, hydroxylation by CYP3A is not a major pathway for micafungin metabolism in vivo. Micafungin is neither a P-glycoprotein substrate nor inhibitor in vitro.

In 4 healthy volunteer studies, the ratio of metabolite to parent exposure (AUC) at a dosage of 150 mg/day was 6% for M-1, 1% for M-2, and 6% for M-5. In patients with esophageal candidiasis, the ratio of metabolite to parent exposure (AUC) at a dosage of 150 mg/day was 11% for M-1, 2% for M-2, and 12% for M-5.

Excretion – The excretion of radioactivity following a single IV dose of ^{14}C-micafungin for injection (25 mg) was evaluated in healthy volunteers. At 28 days after administration, mean urinary and fecal recovery of total radioactivity accounted for 82.5% (76.4 to 87.9%) of the administered dose. Fecal excretion is the major route of elimination (total radioactivity at 28 days was 71% of the administered dose).

Special populations –

Hepatic function impairment: A single 1-hour infusion of micafungin 100 mg was administered to 8 subjects with moderate hepatic dysfunction (Child-Pugh score, 7 to 9) and 8 age-, gender-, and weight-matched subjects with healthy hepatic function. The C_{max} and AUC values of micafungin were lower by approximately 22% in subjects with moderate hepatic insufficiency. This difference in micafungin exposure does not require dose adjustment of micafungin in patients with moderate hepatic impairment. The pharmacokinetics of micafungin have not been studied in patients with severe hepatic insufficiency.

➤*Microbiology:*

Activity in vitro – Micafungin exhibited in vitro activity against *Candida albicans, Candida glabrata, Candida krusei, Candida parapsilosis,* and *Candida tropicalis.* Standardized susceptibility testing methods for 1,3-β-D-glucan synthesis inhibitors have not been established, and the results of susceptibility studies do not correlate with clinical outcome.

Contraindications

Hypersensitivity to any component of this product.

Warnings

➤*Hypersensitivity reactions:* Isolated cases of serious hypersensitivity (anaphylaxis and anaphylactoid) reactions (including shock) have been reported in patients receiving micafungin. If these reactions occur, discontinue micafungin infusion and administer appropriate treatment.

➤*Fertility impairment:* Male rats treated IV with micafungin for 9 weeks showed vacuolation of the epididymal ductal epithelial cells at or above 10 mg/kg (about 0.6 times the recommended clinical dose for esophageal candidiasis, based on body surface area comparisons). Higher doses (about twice the recommended clinical dose, based on body surface area comparisons) resulted in higher epididymis weights and reduced numbers of sperm cells. In a 39-week IV study in dogs, seminiferous tubular atrophy and decreased sperm in the epididymis were observed at 10 and 32 mg/kg, doses equal to about 2 and 7 times the recommended clinical dose, based on body surface area comparisons. There was no impairment of fertility in animal studies with micafungin.

➤*Pregnancy: Category C.* Micafungin administration to pregnant rabbits (IV dosing on days 6 to 18 of gestation) resulted in visceral abnormalities and abortion at 32 mg/kg, a dose equivalent to about 4 times the recommended dose based on body surface area comparisons. Visceral abnormalities included abnormal lobation of the lung, levocardia, retrocaval ureter, anomalous right subclavian artery, and dilatation of the ureter.

However, adequate, well-controlled studies were not conducted in pregnant women. Animal studies are not always predictive of human response; therefore, use micafungin during pregnancy only if clearly needed.

➤*Lactation:* Micafungin was found in the milk of lactating, drug-treated rats. It is not known whether micafungin is excreted in human milk. Exercise caution when micafungin is administered to a breast-feeding woman.

➤*Children:* The safety and efficacy of micafungin in pediatric patients has not been established in clinical studies.

Precautions

➤*Hematological effects:* Acute intravascular hemolysis and hemoglobinuria was seen in a healthy volunteer during infusion of micafungin (200 mg) and oral prednisolone (20 mg). This event was transient, and the subject did not develop significant anemia. Isolated cases of significant hemolysis and hemolytic anemia have also been reported in patients treated with micafungin. Closely monitor patients who develop clinical or laboratory evidence of hemolysis or hemolytic anemia during micafungin therapy for evidence of worsening of these conditions, and evaluate them for the risk/benefit of continuing micafungin therapy.

MICAFUNGIN — INJECTION

➤*Hepatic effects:* Laboratory abnormalities in liver function tests have been seen in healthy volunteers and patients treated with micafungin. In some patients with serious underlying conditions who were receiving micafungin along with multiple concomitant medications, clinical hepatic abnormalities have occurred, and isolated cases of significant hepatic dysfunction, hepatitis, or worsening hepatic failure have been reported. Monitor patients who develop abnormal liver function tests during micafungin therapy for evidence of worsening hepatic function, and evaluate them for the risk/benefit of continuing micafungin therapy.

➤*Renal effects:* Elevations in serum urea nitrogen (BUN) and creatinine, and isolated cases of significant renal dysfunction or acute renal failure have been reported in patients who received micafungin. In controlled trials, the incidence of drug-related renal adverse reactions was 0.4% for micafungin-treated patients and 0.5% for fluconazole-treated patients. Monitor patients who develop abnormal renal function tests during micafungin therapy for evidence of worsening renal function.

Drug Interactions

➤*Sirolimus or nifedipine:* Sirolimus AUC was increased by 21% with no effect on C_{max} in the presence of steady-state micafungin compared with sirolimus alone. Nifedipine AUC and C_{max} were increased by 18% and 42%, respectively, in the presence of steady-state micafungin compared with nifedipine alone. Monitor patients receiving sirolimus or nifedipine in combination with micafungin for sirolimus or nifedipine toxicity, and reduce sirolimus or nifedipine dosage if necessary.

Adverse Reactions

➤*Hypersensitivity:* Possible histamine-mediated symptoms have been reported with micafungin, including rash, pruritus, facial swelling, and vasodilatation.

➤*Local:* Injection site reactions, including phlebitis and thrombophlebitis, have been reported at micafungin dosages of 50 to 150 mg/day. These reactions tended to occur more often in patients receiving micafungin via peripheral IV administration.

➤*Esophageal candidiasis:* In a phase 3, randomized, double-blind study for treatment of esophageal candidiasis, a total of 202/260 (77.7%) patients who received micafungin 150 mg/day and 186/258 (72.1%) patients who received fluconazole 200 mg/day IV experienced an adverse reaction. Adverse reactions considered to be drug-related occurred in 72 (27.7%) and 55 (21.3%) patients in the micafungin and fluconazole treatment groups, respectively. Drug-related adverse reactions resulting in discontinuation were reported in 6 (2.3%) micafungin-treated patients, and in 2 (0.8%) fluconazole-treated patients. Rash and delirium were the most common drug-related adverse reactions resulting in micafungin discontinuation. Drug-related adverse reactions occurring in at least 0.5% of the patients in either treatment group are shown in the following table.

Common Micafungin Adverse Reactions[a] Among Patients with Esophageal Candidiasis[b]

Adverse reactions[c]	Micafungin 150 mg/day (n = 260)	Fluconazole 200 mg/day (n = 258)
CNS		
Delirium	2 (0.8%)	2 (0.8%)
Dizziness	1 (0.4%)	2 (0.8%)
Headache	7 (2.7%)	3 (1.2%)
Somnolence	1 (0.4%)	7 (2.7%)
Dermatologic		
Pruritus	3 (1.2%)	3 (1.2%)
Rash	8 (3.1%)	5 (1.9%)
GI		
Abdominal pain	5 (1.9%)	4 (1.6%)
Nausea	6 (2.3%)	7 (2.7%)
Vomiting	3 (1.2%)	4 (1.6%)
Hematologic/Lymphatic		
Anemia	3 (1.2%)	4 (1.6%)
Eosinophilia	0 (0%)	2 (0.8%)
Leukopenia	7 (2.7%)	2 (0.8%)
Lymphopenia	2 (0.8%)	1 (0.4%)
Neutropenia	3 (1.2%)	1 (0.4%)
Thrombocytopenia	3 (1.2%)	4 (1.6%)
Lab test abnormalities		
ALT increased	1 (0.4%)	5 (1.9%)
AST increased	2 (0.8%)	4 (1.6%)
Blood alkaline phosphatase increased	4 (1.5%)	4 (1.6%)
Blood lactate dehydrogenase increased	2 (0.8%)	3 (1.2%)
Transaminases increased	2 (0.8%)	1 (0.4%)
Metabolic/Nutritional		
Hypomagnesemia	0 (0%)	3 (1.2%)
Miscellaneous		
Infusion site inflammation	4 (1.5%)	3 (1.2%)
Phlebitis	11 (4.2%)	6 (2.3%)
Pyrexia	5 (1.9%)	1 (0.4%)
Rigors	6 (2.3%)	0 (0%)

[a] Relationship to drug was determined by the investigator to be possibly, probably, or definitely drug-related.
[b] Patient base: all randomized patients who received at least 1 dose of trial drug. Common: at least 0.5% in either treatment arm.
[c] Within a system organ class, patients may experience more than 1 adverse reaction.

➤*Prophylaxis of Candida infections in HSCT recipients:* All patients who received micafungin (425) and all patients who received fluconazole (457) experienced at least 1 adverse reaction during the study. Drug-related adverse reactions occurred in 64/425 (15.1%) and 77/457 (16.8%) patients in the micafungin and fluconazole treatment groups, respectively. Drug-related adverse reactions resulting in micafungin discontinuation were reported in 11 (2.6%) patients; while those resulting in fluconazole discontinuation were reported in 16 (3.5%). Drug-related adverse reactions occurring in at least 0.5% of the patients in either treatment group are shown in the following table.

Common Micafungin Adverse Reactions[a] in Clinical Study of Prophylaxis of *Candida* Infection in HSCT Recipients[b]

Adverse reactions[c]	Micafungin 50 mg/day (n = 425)	Fluconazole 400 mg/day (n = 457)
Cardiovascular		
Flushing	1 (0.2%)	6 (1.3%)
Hypotension	1 (0.2%)	4 (0.9%)
CNS		
Dizziness	0 (0%)	5 (1.1%)
Headache	4 (0.9%)	4 (0.9%)
Dermatologic		
Pruritus	4 (0.9%)	3 (0.7%)
Rash	6 (1.4%)	4 (0.9%)
GI		
Abdominal pain	4 (0.9%)	3 (0.7%)
Abdominal pain upper	0 (0%)	3 (0.7%)
Constipation	1 (0.2%)	3 (0.7%)
Diarrhea	9 (2.1%)	14 (3.1%)
Dysgeusia	3 (0.7%)	1 (0.2%)
Dyspepsia	3 (0.7%)	1 (0.2%)
Hiccups	1 (0.2%)	3 (0.7%)
Nausea	10 (2.4%)	12 (2.6%)
Vomiting	7 (1.6%)	5 (1.1%)
Hematologic/Lymphatic		
Anemia	4 (0.9%)	3 (0.7%)
Febrile neutropenia	4 (0.9%)	1 (0.2%)
Leukopenia	4 (0.9%)	2 (0.4%)
Neutropenia	5 (1.2%)	4 (0.9%)
Thrombocytopenia	4 (0.9%)	5 (1.1%)
Lab test abnormalities		
ALT increased	4 (0.9%)	9 (2%)
AST increased	3 (0.7%)	9 (2%)
Blood creatinine increased	1 (0.2%)	3 (0.7%)
Drug level increased	1 (0.2%)	3 (0.7%)
Hyperbilirubinemia	12 (2.8%)	11 (2.4%)
Liver function tests abnormal	3 (0.7%)	6 (1.3%)
Transaminases increased	1 (0.2%)	4 (0.9%)
Metabolic/Nutritional		
Appetite decreased	3 (0.7%)	0 (0%)
Hypocalcemia	4 (0.9%)	4 (0.9%)
Hypokalemia	8 (1.9%)	8 (1.8%)
Hypomagnesemia	5 (1.2%)	6 (1.3%)

MICAFUNGIN — INJECTION

Common Micafungin Adverse Reactions[a] in Clinical Study of Prophylaxis of *Candida* Infection in HSCT Recipients[b]		
Adverse reactions[c]	Micafungin 50 mg/day (n = 425)	Fluconazole 400 mg/day (n = 457)
Hypophosphatemia	6 (1.4%)	4 (0.9%)
Miscellaneous		
Fatigue	0 (0%)	5 (1.1%)
Mycosal inflammation	1 (0.2%)	3 (0.7%)
Pyrexia	4 (0.9%)	5 (1.1%)
Rigors	1 (0.2%)	5 (1.1%)

[a] Relationship to drug was determined by the investigator to be possibly, probably, or definitely drug-related.
[b] Patient base: all randomized patients who received at least 1 dose of trial drug. Common: at least 0.5% in either treatment arm.
[c] Within a system organ class, patients may experience more than 1 adverse reaction.

➤*Overall safety experience:* The overall safety of micafungin was assessed in 1,980 patients and 422 volunteers in 32 clinical studies, including the esophageal candidiasis and prophylaxis studies, who received single or multiple doses of micafungin, ranging from 12.5 to 150 mg or more per day. A total of 606 subjects (patients and volunteers) received at least micafungin 150 mg/day for a minimum of 10 days. Overall, 2,028/2,402 (84.4%) subjects who received micafungin experienced an adverse reaction. Adverse reactions considered to be drug-related were reported in 717 (29.9%) subjects. Drug-related adverse reactions, which occurred in at least 0.5% of all subjects who received micafungin in these trials are shown in the following table.

Common Micafungin Adverse Reactions[a,b,c]	
Adverse reactions[d]	Micafungin (n = 2,402)
Cardiovascular	
Flushing	12 (0.5%)
Hypertension	14 (0.6%)
Phlebitis	39 (1.6%)
CNS	
Dizziness	16 (0.7%)
Headache	57 (2.4%)
Somnolence	12 (0.5%)
Dermatologic	
Pruritus	18 (0.7%)
Rash	38 (1.6%)
GI	
Abdominal pain	23 (1%)
Abdominal pain upper	11 (0.5)
Diarrhea	38 (1.6%)
Nausea	67 (2.8%)
Vomiting	58 (2.4%)
Hematologic/Lymphatic	
Anemia	19 (0.8%)
Leukopenia	38 (1.6%)
Neutropenia	29 (1.2%)
Thrombocytopenia	20 (0.8%)
Lab test abnormalities	
ALT increased	62 (2.6%)
AST increased	64 (2.7%)
Blood alkaline phosphatase increased	48 (2%)
Blood creatinine increased	14 (0.6%)
Blood lactate dehydrogenase increased	11 (0.5%)
Blood urea increased	12 (0.5%)
Hyperbilirubinemia	25 (1%)
Liver function tests abnormal	36 (1.5%)
Metabolic/Nutritional	
Hypocalcemia	27 (1.1%)
Hypokalemia	28 (1.2%)
Hypomagnesemia	27 (1.1%)
Miscellaneous	
Injection site pain	21 (0.9%)
Pyrexia	37 (1.5%)
Rigors	23 (1%)

[a] Relationship to drug was determined by the investigator to be possibly, probably, or definitely drug-related.
[b] Subjects included patients and volunteers.
[c] Patient base: all randomized patients who received at least 1 dose of trial drug. Common: incidence of adverse reaction at least 0.5%.
[d] Within a system organ class, patients may experience more than 1 adverse reaction.

Other clinically significant adverse reactions, regardless of causality, that occurred in these trials follow:

➤*Cardiovascular:* Arrhythmia, cardiac arrest, cyanosis, deep venous thrombosis, hypertension, myocardial infarction, tachycardia.

➤*CNS:* Convulsions, delirium, encephalopathy, intracranial hemorrhage.

➤*Dermatologic:* Erythema multiforme, skin necrosis, urticaria.

➤*Hematologic/Lymphatic:* Coagulopathy, hemolysis, hemolytic anemia, pancytopenia, thrombotic thrombocytopenic purpura.

➤*Hepatic:* Hepatic failure, hepatocellular damage, hepatomegaly, jaundice.

➤*Metabolic/Nutritional:* Acidosis, anorexia, hyponatremia.

➤*Musculoskeletal:* Arthralgia.

➤*Renal:* Anuria, hemoglobinuria, oliguria, renal failure acute, renal tubular necrosis.

➤*Respiratory:* Apnea, dyspnea, hypoxia, pneumonia, pulmonary embolism.

➤*Miscellaneous:* Infection, injection site thrombosis, sepsis.

➤*Postmarketing:* The following adverse reactions have been identified during the postapproval use of micafungin for injection in Japan. Because these reactions are reported voluntarily from a population of uncertain size, it is not always possible to reliably estimate their frequency. A causal relationship to micafungin for injection could not be excluded for these adverse reactions, which included:

CNS – Shock.

Hematologic/Lymphatic – Hemolytic anemia, white blood cell count decreased.

Hepatic – Hepatic disorder, hepatic function abnormal, hepatocellular damage, hyperbilirubinemia.

Renal – Acute renal failure and renal impairment.

Overdosage

Micafungin is highly protein bound and, therefore, is not dialyzable. No cases of micafungin overdosage have been reported. Repeated daily doses up to 8 mg/kg (maximum total dose, 896 mg) in adult patients have been administered in clinical trials with no reported dose-limiting toxicity. The minimum lethal dose of micafungin is 125 mg/kg in rats, equivalent to 8.1 times the recommended human clinical dose for esophageal candidiasis based on body surface area comparisons.

ANIDULAFUNGIN

Rx	**Eraxis** (Roerig)	**Powder for injection, lyophilized:** 50 mg	Preservative free. In single-use vial with diluent.

ANIDULAFUNGIN — INJECTION

Indications

➤*Candidemia and other Candida infections:* For the treatment of candidemia and other forms of *Candida* infections (intra-abdominal abscess and peritonitis). Anidulafungin has not been studied in endocarditis, osteomyelitis, and meningitis caused by *Candida*, and it has not been studied in sufficient numbers of neutropenic patients to determine efficacy in this group.

➤*Esophageal candidiasis:* For the treatment of esophageal candidiasis.

Administration and Dosage

➤*Approved by the FDA:* February 17, 2006.

➤*Prior to therapy:* Obtain specimens for fungal culture and other relevant laboratory studies (including histopathology) prior to therapy to isolate and identify causative organism(s). Therapy may be instituted before the results of the cultures and other laboratory studies are known. However, once these results become available, adjust antifungal therapy accordingly.

➤*Candidemia and other Candida infections:* The recommended dosage is a single 200 mg loading dose on day 1, followed by 100 mg/day thereafter. Duration of treatment should be based on the patient's clinical response. In general, continue antifungal therapy for at least 14 days after the last positive culture.

➤*Esophageal candidiasis:* The recommended dosage is a single 100 mg loading dose on day 1, followed by 50 mg/day thereafter. Treat patients for a minimum of 14 days and for at least 7 days following resolution of symptoms. Duration of treatment should be based on the patient's clinical response. Because of the risk of relapse of esophageal candidiasis in patients with HIV infection, suppressive antifungal therapy may be considered after a course of treatment.

ANIDULAFUNGIN — INJECTION

➤*Preparation for administration:* Reconstitute with the companion diluent (20% [w/w] dehydrated alcohol in water for injection) and subsequently diluted with only 5% dextrose injection or 0.9% sodium chloride injection (normal saline). The compatibility of reconstituted anidulafungin with intravenous (IV) substances, additives, or medications other than 5% dextrose injection or 0.9% sodium chloride injection (normal saline) has not been established.

Reconstitution – Aseptically reconstitute each 50-mg vial with 15 mL of the companion diluent (20% [w/w] dehydrated alcohol in water for injection) to provide a concentration of 3.33 mg/mL. The reconstituted solution must be further diluted and administered within 24 hours.

Dilution – Aseptically transfer the contents of the reconstituted vial(s) into an IV bag (or bottle) containing 5% dextrose injection or 0.9% sodium chloride injection (normal saline) to provide an infusion solution concentration of 0.5 mg/mL. The following table provides the number of vials and volumes required for each dose.

Dilution Requirements for Anidulafungin Administration

Dose	Number of 50-mg vials	Total reconstituted volume	Diluent volume required	Total infusion volume
50 mg	1	15 mL	85 mL	100 mL
100 mg	2	30 mL	170 mL	200 mL
200 mg	4	60 mL	340 mL	400 mL

Administration – The rate of infusion should not exceed 1.1 mg/min.

Compatibilities / Incompatibilities – Prior to administration, anidulafungin for injection requires reconstitution with the companion diluent (20% (w/w) dehydrated alcohol in water for injection) and subsequent dilution with 5% dextrose injection or 0.9% sodium chloride injection (normal saline). Do not dilute with other solutions or co-infuse with other medications or electrolytes.

➤*Storage / Stability:* Store unreconstituted vials, reconstituted vials, and companion diluent vials at 25°C (77°F); excursions are permitted to 15° to 30°C (59° to 86°F). Do not freeze. The reconstituted vials must be further diluted and administered within 24 hours.

Actions

➤*Pharmacology:* Anidulafungin is a semi-synthetic echinocandin with antifungal activity. Anidulafungin inhibits glucan synthase, an enzyme present in fungal, but not mammalian cells. This results in inhibition of the formation of 1,3-β-D-glucan, an essential component of the fungal cell wall.

➤*Pharmacokinetics:*

Absorption –

Systemic exposures of anidulafungin are dose-proportional and have low intersubject variability (coefficient of variation less than 25%), as shown in the following table. The steady state was achieved on the first day after a loading dose (twice the daily maintenance dose), and the estimated plasma accumulation factor at steady state is approximately 2.

Distribution – The pharmacokinetics of anidulafungin following IV administration are characterized by a short distribution half-life (0.5 to 1 hour) and a volume of distribution of 30 to 50 L that is similar to total body fluid volume. Anidulafungin is moderately bound to plasma proteins in humans (84%).

Metabolism – Anidulafungin undergoes slow chemical degradation at physiologic temperature and pH to a ring-opened peptide that lacks antifungal activity. The in vitro degradation half-life of anidulafungin under physiologic conditions is about 24 hours. In vivo, the ring-opened product is subsequently converted to peptidic degradants and eliminated.

Excretion – The clearance of anidulafungin is about 1 L/hour and anidulafungin has a terminal half-life of 40 to 50 hours.

In a single-dose clinical study, radiolabeled (^{14}C) anidulafungin was administered to healthy subjects. Approximately 30% of the administered radioactive dose was eliminated in the feces over 9 days, of which less than 10% was intact drug. Less than 1% of the administered radioactive dose was excreted in the urine. Anidulafungin concentrations fell below the lower limits of quantitation 6 days postdose. Negligible amounts of drug-derived radioactivity were recovered in blood, urine, and feces 8 weeks postdose.

Mean (% CV[a]) Steady-State Pharmacokinetic Parameters of Anidulafungin Following IV Administration of Anidulafungin Once Daily for 10 Days in Adults

Pharmacokinetic parameter[b]	Anidulafungin IV dosing regimen (LD/MD, mg)[c] 70/35[d,e] (N = 6)	200/100 (N = 10)	260/130[e,f] (N = 10)
$C_{max, ss}$ [mg/L]	3.55 (13.2)	8.6 (16.2)	10.9 (11.7)
AUC_{ss} [mg•h/L]	42.3 (14.5)	111.8 (24.9)	168.9 (10.8)
CL [L/h]	0.84 (13.5)	0.94 (24)	0.78 (11.3)
t½ [h]	43.2 (17.7)	52 (11.7)	50.3 (9.7)

[a] Coefficient of variation.
[b] Parameters were obtained from separate studies.
[c] LD/MD: loading dose/maintenance dose once daily.
[d] Data were collected on day 7.
[e] Safety and efficacy of these doses have not been established.
[f] See overdosage.

➤*Microbiology:*

Activity in vitro – Anidulafungin is active in vitro against *Candida albicans*, *Candida glabrata*, *Candida parapsilosis*, and *Candida tropicalis*.

Minimum inhibitory concentrations (MICs) were determined according to the Clinical and Laboratory Standards Institute's approved standard reference method M27 for susceptibility testing of yeasts. However, no correlation between in vitro activity (MIC) as determined by this method and clinical outcome has been established.

Activity in vivo – Parenterally administered anidulafungin was effective against *C. albicans* in immunocompetent and immunosuppressed mice and rabbits with disseminated infection as measured by prolonged survival and reduction in mycological burden. Anidulafungin also reduced the mycological burden of fluconazole-resistant *C. albicans* in an oropharyngeal/esophageal infection model in immunosuppressed rabbits.

Drug resistance – Emergence of resistance to anidulafungin has not been studied.

Anidulafungin was active against *C. albicans* resistant to fluconazole. Cross resistance with other echinocandins has not been studied.

Contraindications

Known hypersensitivity to anidulafungin, any component of anidulafungin, or other echinocandins.

Warnings

➤*Pregnancy:* Category C. Embryo-fetal development studies were conducted with doses up to 20 mg/kg/day in rats and rabbits (equivalent to 2 and 4 times, respectively, the proposed therapeutic maintenance dose of 100 mg/day on the basis of relative body surface area). Anidulafungin administration resulted in skeletal changes in rat fetuses, including incomplete ossification of various bones and wavy, misaligned, or misshapen ribs. These changes were not dose-related and were within the range of the laboratory's historical control database. Developmental effects observed in rabbits (slightly reduced fetal weights) occurred in the high-dose group, a dose that also produced maternal toxicity. Anidulafungin crossed the placental barrier in rats and was detected in fetal plasma.

There are no adequate and well-controlled studies in pregnant women. Because animal reproduction studies are not always predictive of human response, only use anidulafungin during pregnancy if the potential benefit justifies the risk to the fetus.

➤*Lactation:* Administer to breast-feeding mothers only if the potential benefit justifies the risk. Anidulafungin was found in the milk of lactating rats. It is not known whether anidulafungin is excreted in human milk.

➤*Children:* Safety and efficacy of anidulafungin in children have not been established.

Precautions

➤*Monitoring:* Monitor patients who develop abnormal liver function tests (LFTs) during andidulafungin therapy for evidence of worsening hepatic failure.

➤*Hepatic effects:* Laboratory abnormalities in LFTs have been seen in healthy volunteers and patients treated with anidulafungin. In some patients with serious underlying medical conditions who were receiving multiple concomitant medications along with anidulafungin, clinically significant hepatic abnormalities have occurred. Isolated cases of significant hepatic dysfunction, hepatitis, or worsening hepatic failure have been reported in patients; a causal relationship to anidulafungin has not been established. Monitor patients who develop abnormal LFTs during anidulafungin therapy for evidence of worsening hepatic function and evaluate for risk/benefit of continuing anidulafungin therapy.

Drug Interactions

In vitro studies showed that anidulafungin is not metabolized by human cytochrome P-450 or by isolated human hepatocytes, and does not significantly inhibit the activities of clinically important human CYP isoforms (1A2, 2C9, 2D6, 3A4). No clinically relevant drug-drug interactions were observed with drugs likely to be coadministered with anidulafungin.

➤*Cyclosporine:* In a study in which 12 healthy adult subjects received a maintenance dose of anidulafungin 100 mg/day following a 200 mg loading dose (on days 1 to 8) and in combination with oral cyclosporine 1.25 mg/kg twice daily (on days 5 to 8), the steady state C_{max} of anidulafungin was not significantly altered by cyclosporine; the steady-state AUC of anidulafungin was increased 22%. A separate in vitro study showed that anidulafungin has no effect on the metabolism of cyclosporine. No dosage adjustment of either drug is warranted when coadministered.

Adverse Reactions

➤*Hypersensitivity:* Possible histamine-mediated symptoms have been reported with anidulafungin, including dyspnea, flushing, hypotension, pruritus, rash, and urticaria. These reactions are infrequent when the rate of anidulafungin infusion does not exceed 1.1 mg/minute.

ANIDULAFUNGIN — INJECTION

➤*Candidemia/other Candida infections:*

Anidulafungin Adverse Reactions[a] for Candidemia/Other *Candida* Infections (≥ 2%)	Anidulafungin 100 mg[b] N = 131	Fluconazole 400 mg[b] N = 125
Adverse reaction	32 (24.4%)	33 (26.4%)
Cardiovascular		
Deep vein thrombosis	1 (0.8%)	3 (2.4%)
GI		
Diarrhea	4 (3.1%)	2 (1.6%)
Hepatic		
Alkaline phosphatase increased	2 (1.5%)	5 (4%)
ALT increased	3 (2.3%)	4 (3.2%)
AST increased	1 (0.8%)	3 (2.4%)
Hepatic enzyme increased	2 (1.5%)	9 (7.2%)
Metabolic/Nutritional		
Hypokalemia	4 (3.1%)	3 (2.4%)

[a] Treatment-related adverse reactions are defined as those that are possibly or probably related to study treatment, as determined by the investigator.
[b] Maintenance dose.

➤*Esophageal candidiasis:*

Anidulafungin Adverse Reactions[a] Reported in Therapy for Esophageal Candidiasis (≥ 1%)	Anidulafungin 50 mg[b] N = 300	Fluconazole 100 mg[b] N = 301
Subjects with at least 1 treatment-related adverse reaction	43 (14.3%)	50 (16.6%)
CNS		
Headache	4 (1.3%)	3 (1%)
Dermatologic		
Rash	3 (1%)	2 (0.7%)
GI		
Dyspepsia aggravated	1 (0.3%)	3 (1%)
Nausea	3 (1%)	3 (1%)
Vomiting NOS[c]	2 (0.7%)	3 (1%)
Hematologic		
Leukopenia	2 (0.7%)	4 (1.3%)
Neutropenia	3 (1%)	-
Hepatic		
ALT increased	-	3 (1%)
AST increased	1 (0.3%)	7 (2.3)
Gamma-glutamyl transferase increased	4 (1.3%)	4 (1.3%)
Miscellaneous		
Phlebitis NOS	2 (0.7%)	4 (1.3%)
Pyrexia	2 (0.7%)	3 (1%)

[a] Treatment-related adverse reactions include those that are of possible, probable, or unknown relationship to study treatment, as determined by the investigator.
[b] Maintenance dose.
[c] NOS = Not otherwise specified.

The following reactions occurred in less than 2% of patients treated for candidemia/other *Candida* infections or in less than 1% of patients treated for esophageal candidiasis and were judged by investigators to be at least possibly related to anidulafungin.

➤*Cardiovascular:* Atrial fibrillation, bundle branch block (right), hypertension, hypotension, sinus arrhythmia, thrombophlebitis superficial, ventricular extrasystoles.

➤*CNS:* Convulsion, dizziness, headache.

➤*Dermatologic:* Angioneurotic edema, erythema, pruritis, pruritis generalized, sweating increased, urticaria, urticaria NOS.

➤*GI:* Abdominal pain upper, constipation, diarrhea NOS, dyspepsia, fecal incontinence, nausea, vomiting.

➤*Hepatic:* Abnormal LFTs NOS, cholestasis, hepatic necrosis.

➤*Hematologic/Lymphatic:* Coagulopathy, thrombocytopenia.

➤*Lab test abnormalities:* Amylase increased, bilirubin increased, creatine phosphokinase (CPK) increased, creatinine increased, electrocardiogram QT prolonged, electrocardiogram early transition, gamma-glutamyl transferase increased, lipase increased, magnesium decreased, platelet count decreased, platelet count increased, potassium decreased, prothrombin time prolonged, transferase increased, urea increased.

➤*Metabolic/Nutritional:* Hypercalcemia, hyperglycemia, hyperkalemia, hypernatremia, hypomagnesemia.

➤*Musculoskeletal:* Back pain, rigors.

➤*Ophthalmic:* Eye pain, vision blurred, visual disturbance.

➤*Respiratory:* Cough.

➤*Miscellaneous:* Candidiasis, clostridial infection, flushing, fungemia, hot flushes, infusion-related reaction, oral candidiasis, peripheral edema.

Overdosage

➤*Symptoms:* During clinical trials, a single dose of anidulafungin 400 mg was inadvertently administered as a loading dose. No clinical adverse reactions were reported. In a study of 10 healthy subjects administered a loading dose of 260 mg followed by 130 mg daily, anidulafungin was generally well tolerated; 3 of the 10 subjects experienced transient, asymptomatic transaminase elevations (3 or less × upper limit of normal).

In 3-month studies, liver toxicity, including single-cell hepatocellular necrosis, hepatocellular hypertrophy, and increased liver weights, were observed in monkeys and rats at doses equivalent to 5 to 6 times the human exposure. For both species, hepatocellular hypertrophy was still noted 1 month after the end of dosing.

QUININE SULFATE

Rx	**Quinine Sulfate** (Various, eg, Moore)	**Capsules:** 200 mg	In 100s, 500s, and 1000s.
		260 mg	In 100s, 500s, and 1000s.
		325 mg	In 100s, 500s, and 1000s.
Rx	**Quinine Sulfate** (Various, eg, Moore, Zenith Goldline)	**Tablets:** 260 mg	In 100s, 500s, and 1000s.

QUININE SULFATE — ORAL

Indications

➤*Malaria:* Either alone, with pyrimethamine and a sulfonamide, or with a tetracycline. Alternative therapy for chloroquine-sensitive strains of *P. falciparum*, *P. malariae*, *P. ovale*, and *P. vivax*. Mefloquine and clindamycin may also be used with quinine depending on where the malaria was acquired (eg, Southeast Asia, Bangladesh, East Africa).

➤*Unlabeled uses:* Nocturnal recumbency leg cramps, prevention, and treatment. Dose: 260 to 300 mg at bedtime.

Administration and Dosage

➤*Approved by the FDA:* September 30, 1976.

➤*Adults:* 1 to 3 tablets or capsules 3 times a day for 6 to 12 days.

➤*Children:* Only as directed by a physician.

➤*Storage/Stability:* Store at controlled room temperature 15° to 30°C (59° to 86°F). Dispense in a tight, light-resistant container.

Actions

➤*Pharmacology:* Quinine, a cinchona alkaloid, acts on skeletal muscle by 3 mechanisms: It increases the refractory period by direct action on the muscle fiber; it decreases the excitability of the motor end-plate, an action similar to that of curare; and it affects the distribution of calcium within the muscle fiber.

➤*Pharmacokinetics:*

Absorption/Distribution – Quinine is readily absorbed when given orally. Absorption occurs mainly from the upper part of the small intestine, and is almost complete even in patients with marked diarrhea.

Peak plasma concentrations of cinchona alkaloids occur within 1 to 3 hours after a single oral dose. The half-life is 4 to 5 hours. After chronic administration of total daily doses of 1 g of drug, the average plasma quinine con-

QUININE SULFATE — ORAL

centration is approximately 7 mcg/mL. After termination of quinine therapy, the plasma level falls rapidly and only a negligible concentration is detectable after 24 hours.

A large fraction (approximately 70%) of the plasma quinine is bound to proteins. This explains in part why the concentration of the alkaloid in cerebrospinal fluid is only 2% to 5% of that in plasma. However, it can traverse the placental membrane and readily reach fetal tissues.

Tinnitus and impairment of hearing should rarely occur at plasma concentrations of less than 10 mcg/mL. An occasional patient may have some evidence of cinchonism on this product, such as tinnitus.

Metabolism/Excretion – The cinchona alkaloids in large measure are metabolically degraded in the body, especially in the liver; less than 5% of an administered dose is excreted unaltered in the urine. It is reported that there is no accumulation of the drug in the body on continued administration. The metabolic degradation products are excreted in the urine where many of them have been identified as hydroxy derivatives, but small amounts also appear in the feces, gastric juice, bile, and saliva. Renal excretion of quinine is twice as rapid when the urine is acidic as when it is alkaline, due to the greater tubular reabsorption of the alkaloidal base that occurs in an alkaline medium. Excretion is also limited by the binding of a large fraction of cinchona alkaloids to plasma proteins.

Contraindications

➤*Pregnancy:* Because of the quinine content, quinine sulfate is contraindicated in patients with known quinine hypersensitivity, in patients with glucose-6-phosphate dehydrogenase (G-6-PD) deficiency, and pregnancy.

See Warnings for more information.

Since thrombocytopenic purpura may follow the administration of quinine in highly sensitive patients, a history of this occurrence associated with previous quinine ingestion contraindicates its further use. Recovery usually occurs following withdrawal of the medication and appropriate therapy. This drug should not be used in patients with tinnitus or optic neuritis or in patients with a history of blackwater fever.

Warnings

➤*Cinchonism:* Repeated doses or overdosage of quinine in some individuals may precipitate a cluster of symptoms referred to as cinchonism. Such symptoms, in the mildest form, include ringing in the ears, headache, nausea, and slightly disturbed vision; however, when medication is continued or after large single doses, symptoms also involve the GI tract, the nervous and cardiovascular systems, and the skin.

➤*Hemolysis:* Hemolysis (with the potential for hemolytic anemia) has been associated with a G-6-PD deficiency in patients taking quinine. Quinine sulfate should be stopped immediately if evidence of hemolysis appears.

If symptoms occur, the drug should be discontinued and supportive measures instituted.

➤*Tinnitus and impaired hearing:* These may occur at plasm quinine concentrations greater than 10 mcg/mL, a level not normally attained with quinine 260 to 520 mg/day. In a hypersensitive patient, as little as 300 mg may produce tinnitus.

➤*Hypersensitivity reactions:* Quinine sulfate tablets should be discontinued if there is any evidence of hypersensitivity. (See Contraindications.) Cutaneous flushing, pruritus, skin rashes, fever, gastric distress, dyspnea, ringing in the ears, and visual impairment are the usual expressions of hypersensitivity, particularly if only small doses of quinine have been taken. Extreme flushing of the skin accompanied by intense, generalized pruritus is the most common form. Hemoglobinuria and asthma from quinine are rare types of idiosyncrasy.

➤*Mutagenesis:* Mutation studies of quinine hydrochloride, 100 mg/kg, administered orally, in Chinese hamsters showed no genotoxic activity in the sister chromatid exchange (SCE) test, micronucleus test, or chromosome aberration test. In mice given quinine hydrochloride, 100 mg/kg, administered orally, the micronucleus test and chromosome aberration test were negative; the SCE test exhibited an increase of SCEs/cell. Tests were repeated in 2 inbred strains of mice using 55, 75, and 110 mg/kg administered orally. The effect was more pronounced in these mice and the increase in SCEs/cell demonstrated a linear dose relationship. One of the inbred strains had positive micronucleus test findings. The chromosome aberration test also revealed an increase in chromatid breaks. The Ames test system results were negative for point mutation.

➤*Pregnancy: Category X.* Quinine sulfate may cause fetal harm when administered to a pregnant woman. Congenital malformations in the human have been reported with the use of quinine, primarily with large doses (up to 30 g) for attempted abortion. In about half of these reports, the malformation was deafness related to auditory nerve hypoplasia. Among the other abnormalities reported were limb anomalies, visceral defects, and visual changes. In animal tests, teratogenic effects were found in rabbits and guinea pigs and were absent in mice, rats, dogs, and monkeys. Quinine sulfate is contraindicated in women who are or may become pregnant. If this drug is used during pregnancy, or if the patient becomes pregnant while taking this drug, the patient should be apprised of the potential hazard to the fetus.

Because quinine crosses the placenta in humans, the potential for fetal effects is present. Stillbirths in mothers taking quinine have been reported in which no obvious cause for the fetal deaths was shown. Quinine in toxic amounts has been associated with abortion. Whether this action is always due to direct effect on the uterus is questionable.

➤*Lactation:* Caution should be exercised when quinine sulfate is given to nursing women because quinine is excreted in breast milk (in small amounts).

Precautions

➤*Cardiac disease:* In patients with atrial fibrillation, the administration of quinine requires the same precautions as those for quinidine.

➤*Lab test abnormalities:* Quinine may produce an elevated value for urinary 17-ketogenic steroids when the Zimmerman method is used.

Drug Interactions

Quinine Drug Interactions

Precipitant drug	Object drug*		Description
Antacids, aluminum-containing	Quinine	⬇	Aluminum-containing antacids may delay or decrease absorption of concurrent quinine.
Cimetidine	Quinine	⬆	Cimetidine may reduce quinine's oral clearance and increase its elimination half-life.
Mefloquine	Quinine	⬆	Do not use concurrently with quinine. If these agents are to be used in the initial treatment of severe malaria, delay mefloquine administration ≥ 12 hours after the last dose of quinine. ECG abnormalities or cardiac arrest may occur. The risk of convulsions may also be increased with coadministration.
Rifamycins (rifabutin, rifampin)	Quinine	⬇	Rifamycins, potent inducers of hepatic microsomal enzymes, increased the hepatic clearance of quinine. Enzyme induction can persist for several days following discontinuation of the rifamycin.
Urinary alkalinizers (eg, acetazolamide, sodium bicarbonate)	Quinine	⬆	Urinary alkalinizers administered concurrently with quinine may increase quinine blood levels with potential for toxicity.
Quinine	Anticoagulants, oral	⬆	Quinine may depress the hepatic enzyme system that synthesizes the vitamin K-dependent clotting factors and thus may enhance the action of warfarin and other oral anticoagulants.
Quinine	Digoxin	⬆	Digoxin serum concentrations may be increased by concurrent quinine. Monitor digoxin levels periodically.
Quinine	Neuromuscular blocking agents (depolarizing and nondepolarizing)	⬆	The neuromuscular blockade of these agents may be potentiated by quinine, and may result in respiratory difficulties.
Quinine	Succinylcholine	⬆	Quinidine may produce a decrease in plasma cholinesterase activity, resulting in a slowed metabolic rate for succinylcholine.

* ⬆ = Object drug increased. ⬇ = Object drug decreased.

Adverse Reactions

➤*Cardiovascular:* Anginal symptoms.

➤*CNS:* Visual disturbances, including blurred vision with scotomata, photophobia, diplopia, diminished visual fields and disturbed color vision; tinnitus, deafness, and vertigo; headache, nausea, vomiting, fever, apprehension, restlessness, confusion, and syncope.

➤*GI:* Nausea and vomiting (may be CNS-related), epigastric pain.

➤*Hematologic:* Acute hemolysis, thrombocytopenic purpura, agranulocytosis, hypoprothrombinemia.

➤*Hepatic:* Hepatitis.

➤*Hypersensitivity:* Cutaneous rashes (urticarial, the most frequent type of allergic reaction, papular, or scarlatina), pruritus, flushing of the skin, sweating, occasional edema of the face.

➤*Respiratory:* Asthmatic symptoms.

Overdosage

Fatalities with quinine have been reported from single oral doses of 2 g to 8 g; a single fatality reported with a dose of 1.5 g may reflect an idiosyncratic effect. Several cases of blindness following large overdoses of quinine, with partial recovery of vision in each instance, have been reported. Tinnitus and impaired hearing may occur at plasma concentrations over 10 mcg/mL. This level would not normally be obtained with the use of quinine sulfate daily, but in hypersensitive patients as little as 0.3 g of quinine may produce tinnitus.

➤*Symptoms:* The more common signs and symptoms of overdosage are tinnitus, dizziness, skin rash, and GI disturbance (intestinal cramping). With higher doses, cardiovascular and CNS effects may occur, including headache, fever, vomiting, apprehension, confusion, and convulsions.

➤*Treatment:* Treatment for overdosage should initially include efforts to remove any residual quinine sulfate from the stomach by gastric lavage or by emesis induced with syrup of ipecac. The blood pressure should be sup-

QUININE SULFATE — ORAL

ported and measures used to maintain renal function. Artificial respiration may be needed. Sedatives, oxygen, and other supportive measures should be used as necessary.

Fluid and electrolyte balance with intravenous fluids should be maintained. Acidification of the urine will promote renal excretion of quinine. In the presence of hemoglobinuria, however, acidification of the urine may augment renal blockade. Quinine should be readily dialyzable by hemodialysis or hemoperfusion procedures.

Evidence of angioedema or asthma may require the use of epinephrine, corticosteroids, and antihistamines. In the acute phase of toxic amaurosis caused by quinine, vasodilators administered intravenously may have a salutary effect. Stellate block has also been used effectively for quinine-associated blindness. Residual visual impairment occasionally yields to vasodilators.

Patient Information

Take with food or after meals to minimize GI irritation.

Quinine sulfate may cause diarrhea, nausea, stomach cramps or pain, vomiting, or ringing in the ears; notify physician if these become pronounced.

Quinine sulfate may produce blurred vision, vertigo, restlessness, confusion, or dizziness; patients should observe caution while driving or performing other tasks requiring alertness.

Stop the drug if there is any evidence of allergy such as flushing, itching, rash, fever, stomach pain, difficult breathing, ringing in the ears, or vision problems.

MEFLOQUINE HYDROCHLORIDE

Rx	**Mefloquine HCl** (Geneva)	**Tablets:** 250 mg	(GP 118). White, scored. In 25s.
Rx	**Lariam** (Roche)		Lactose. (LARIAM 250 ROCHE). White, scored. In UD 25s.

MEFLOQUINE HYDROCHLORIDE — ORAL

Indications

➤*Acute malaria infections:* For the treatment of mild-to-moderate acute malaria caused by mefloquine-susceptible strains of *P. falciparum* (both chloroquine-susceptible and resistant strains) or by *Plasmodium vivax*. There are insufficient clinical data to document the effect of mefloquine in malaria caused by *P. ovale* or *P. malariae*.

➤*Prevention of malaria:* For the prophylaxis of *P. falciparum* and *P. vivax* malaria infections, including prophylaxis of chloroquine-resistant strains of *P. falciparum*.

Administration and Dosage

➤*Approved by the FDA:* May 2, 1989.

➤*Adult patients:*

Treatment of mild-to-moderate malaria caused by P. vivax or mefloquine-susceptible strains of P. falciparum – 5 tablets (1,250 mg) given as a single oral dose. The drug should not be taken on an empty stomach and should be administered with at least 240 mL of water.

If a full treatment course with mefloquine HCl does not lead to improvement within 48 to 72 hours, mefloquine HCl should not be used for retreatment. An alternative treatment should be used. Similarly, if previous prophylaxis with mefloquine has failed, mefloquine HCl should not be used for curative treatment.

Malaria prophylaxis – One 250 mg mefloquine HCl tablet once weekly.

Prophylactic drug administration should begin 1 week before arrival in an endemic area. Subsequent weekly doses should be taken regularly, always on the same day of each week preferably after the main meal. To reduce the risk of malaria after leaving an endemic area, prophylaxis must be continued for 4 additional weeks to ensure suppressive blood levels of the drug when merozoites emerge from the liver. Tablets should not be taken on an empty stomach and should be administered with at least 240 mL of water.

Concurrent medications – In certain cases (eg, when a traveler is taking other medication), it may be desirable to start prophylaxis 2 to 3 weeks prior to departure, in order to ensure that the combination of drugs is well tolerated (see Drug Interactions).

➤*Children:*

Treatment of mild-to-moderate malaria caused by mefloquine-susceptible strains of P. falciparum – 20 to 25 mg/kg. Splitting the total therapeutic dose into 2 doses taken 6 to 8 hours apart may reduce the occurrence or severity of adverse reactions. Experience with mefloquine HCl in infants younger than 3 months of age or weighing less than 5 kg is limited. The drug should not be taken on an empty stomach and should be administered with ample water. For very young patients, the dose may be crushed and suspended in a small amount of water, milk or other beverage for administration to small children and other persons unable to swallow them whole.

If a full treatment course with mefloquine HCl does not lead to improvement within 48 to 72 hours, mefloquine HCl should not be used for retreatment. Alternative therapy should be given. Similarly, if previous prophylaxis with mefloquine has failed, mefloquine HCl should not be used for curative treatment.

In pediatric patients, the administration of mefloquine HCl for the treatment of malaria has been associated with early vomiting. In some cases, early vomiting has been cited as a possible cause of treatment failure. If a significant loss of drug product is observed or suspected because of vomiting, a second full dose of mefloquine HCl should be administered to patients who vomit less than 30 minutes after receiving the drug. If vomiting occurs 30 to 60 minutes after a dose, an additional half-dose should be given. If vomiting recurs, the patient should be monitored closely and alternative malaria treatment considered if improvement is not observed within a reasonable period of time.

The safety and efficacy of mefloquine HCl to treat malaria in pediatric patients below the age of 6 months have not been established.

Experience with mefloquine HCl in infants younger than 3 months of age or weighing less than 5 kg is limited.

Malaria prophylaxis – The following doses have been extrapolated from the recommended adult dose. Neither the pharmacokinetics, nor the clinical efficacy of these doses have been determined in children, owing to the difficulty of acquiring this information in pediatric subjects. The recommended prophylactic dose of mefloquine HCl is 5 mg/kg body weight once weekly. One 250 mg mefloquine HCl tablet should be taken once weekly in pediatric patients weighting greater than 45 kg. In pediatric patients weighing less than 45 kg, the weekly dose decreases in proportion to body weight: 31 to 45 kg, ¾ tablet; 21 to 30 kg, ½ tablet; 11 to 20 kg, ¼ tablet; 5 to 10 kg, ⅛ tablet (approximate tablet fraction based on a dosage of 5 mg/kg body weight. Exact doses for children weighing less than 10 kg may best be prepared and dispensed by pharmacists.

➤*Storage/Stability:* Tablets should be stored at 25°C (77°F); excursions permitted to 15° to 30°C (59° to 86°F).

Actions

➤*Pharmacology:* Mefloquine HCl is an antimalarial agent which acts as a blood schizonticide. Its exact mechanism of action is not known.

➤*Pharmacokinetics:*

Absorption – The absolute oral bioavailability of mefloquine has not been determined since an intravenous formulation is not available. The bioavailability of the tablet formation compared with an oral solution was over 85%. The presence of food significantly enhances the rate and extent of absorption, leading to about a 40% increase in bioavailability. In healthy volunteers, plasma concentrations peak 6 to 24 hours (median, about 17 hours) after a single dose of mefloquine HCl. In a similar group of volunteers, maximum plasma concentrations in mcg/L are roughly equivalent to the dose in milligrams (for example, a single 1000 mg dose produces a maximum concentration of about 1000 mcg/L).

In healthy volunteers, a dose of 250 mg once weekly, produces maximum steady-state plasma concentrations of 1000 to 2000 mcg/L, which are reached after 7 to 10 weeks.

Distribution – In healthy adults, the apparent volume of distribution, approximately 20 L/kg, indicates extensive tissue distribution. Mefloquine HCl may accumulate in parasitized erythrocytes. Experiments conducted in vitro with human blood using concentrations between 50 and 1000 mg/mL showed a relatively constant erythrocyte-to-plasma concentration ratio of about 2 to 1. The equilibrium reached in less than 30 minutes, was found to be reversible. Protein binding is about 98%.

Mefloquine crosses the placenta. Excretion into breast milk appears to be minimal (see Warnings).

Metabolism – Two metabolites have been identified in humans. The main metabolite, 2,8-bis-trifluoromethyl-4-quinoline carboxylic acid, is inactive in Plasmodium falciparum. In a study in healthy volunteers, the carboxylic acid metabolite appeared in plasma 2 to 4 hours after a single oral dose. Maximum plasma concentrations, which were about 50% higher than those of mefloquine, were reached after 2 weeks. Thereafter, plasma levels of the main metabolite and mefloquine declined at a similar rate. The area under the plasma concentration-time curve (AUC) of the main metabolite was 3 to 5 times larger than that of the parent drug. The other metabolite, an alcohol, was present in minute quantities only.

Excretion – In several studies in healthy adults, the mean elimination half-life of mefloquine varied between 2 and 4 weeks, with an average of about 3 weeks. The total clearance of the drug, which is essentially all hepatic, is approximately 30 mL/min. There is evidence that mefloquine is excreted mainly in the bile and feces. In volunteers, urinary excretion of unchanged mefloquine and its main metabolite under steady-state condition accounted for about 9% and 4% of the dose, respectively. Concentrations of other metabolites could not be measured in the urine.

➤*Microbiology:*

Activity in vitro and in vivo – Mefloquine is active against the erythrocytic stages of *Plasmodium* species (see Indications). However, the drug has no effect against the exoerythrocytic (hepatic) stages of the parasite. Mefloquine is effective against malaria parasites resistant to chloroquine (see Indications).

Drug resistance – Strains of *P. falciparum* with decreased susceptibility to mefloquine can be selected in vitro or in vivo. Resistance of *P. falciparum* to mefloquine have been reported in areas of multi-drug resistance in South East Asia. Increased incidences of resistance have also been reported in other parts of the world.

MEFLOQUINE HYDROCHLORIDE — ORAL

Contraindications

Hypersensitivity to mefloquine or related compounds (eg, quinine, quinidine) or to any of the excipients contained in the formulation. Mefloquine HCl should not be prescribed for prophylaxis in patients with active depression, generalized anxiety disorder, a recent history of depression, psychosis, or schizophrenia or other major psychiatric disorders, or with a history of convulsions.

Warnings

➤*Life-threatening P. falciparum infections:* In case of life-threatening, serious or overwhelming malaria infections due to *P. falciparum*, patients should be treated with an IV antimalarial drug. Following completion of IV treatment, mefloquine HCl may be given to complete the course of therapy.

➤*Psychiatric disturbances:* Mefloquine HCl may cause psychiatric symptoms in a number of patients, ranging from anxiety, paranoia, and depression to hallucinations and psychotic behavior. On occasions, these symptoms have been reported to continue long after mefloquine has been stopped. Rare cases of suicidal ideation and suicide have been reported; though no relationship to drug administration has been confirmed. To minimize the chances of these adverse events, mefloquine should not be taken for prophylaxis in patients with active depression or with a recent history of depression, generalized anxiety disorder, psychosis, or schizophrenia or other major psychiatric disorders. Mefloquine HCl should be used with caution in patients with a history of depression.

During prophylactic use, if psychiatric symptoms such as acute anxiety, depression, restlessness or confusion occur, these may be considered prodromal to a more serious event. In these cases, the drug must be discontinued, and an alternative medication should be substituted.

➤*Hypersensitivity reactions:* Hypersensitivity reactions ranging from mild cutaneous events to anaphylaxis cannot be predicted.

➤*Hepatic function impairment:* In patients with impaired liver function, the elimination of mefloquine may be prolonged, leading to higher plasma levels.

➤*Fertility impairment:* Fertility studies in rats at doses of 5, 20, and 50 mg/kg/day of mefloquine have demonstrated adverse reactions on fertility in the male at the high dose of 50 mg/kg/day, and in the female at doses of 20 and 50 mg/kg/day. Histopathological lesions were noted in the epididymides from male rats at doses of 20 and 50 mg/kg/day. Administration of 250 mg/week of mefloquine (base) in adult males for 22 weeks failed to reveal any deleterious effects on human spermatozoa.

➤*Pregnancy: Category C.*

Teratogenic – Mefloquine has been demonstrated to be teratogenic in rats and mice at a dose of 100 mg/kg/day. In rabbits, a high dose of 160 mg/kg/day was embryotoxic and teratogenic, and a dose of 80 mg/kg/day was teratogenic but not embryotoxic. There are no adequate and well-controlled studies in pregnant women. However, clinical experience with mefloquine HCl has not revealed an embryotoxic or teratogenic effect. Mefloquine should be used during pregnancy only if the potential benefit justifies the potential risk to the fetus. Women of childbearing potential who are traveling to areas where malaria is endemic should be warned against becoming pregnant. Women of childbearing potential should also be advised to practice contraception during malaria prophylaxis with mefloquine HCl and for up to 3 months thereafter. However, in the case of unplanned pregnancy, malaria chemoprophylaxis with mefloquine HCl is not considered an indication for pregnancy termination.

➤*Lactation:* Mefloquine is excreted in human milk in small amounts, the activity of which is unknown. Based on a study in a few subjects, low concentrations (3% to 4%) of mefloquine were excreted in human milk following a dose equivalent to 250 mg of the free base. Because of the potential for serious adverse reactions in nursing infants from mefloquine, a decision should be made whether to discontinue the drug, taking into account the importance of the drug to the mother.

➤*Children:* Use of mefloquine HCl to treat acute, uncomplicated *P. falciparum* malaria in pediatric patients is supported by evidence from adequate and well-controlled studies of mefloquine HCl in adults with additional data from published open-label and comparative trials using mefloquine HCl to treat malaria caused by *P. falciparum* in patients younger than 16 years of age. The safety and efficacy of mefloquine HCl for the treatment of malaria in pediatric patients below the age of 6 months have not been established.

Early vomiting – See Administration and Dosage for more information.

Precautions

➤*Monitoring:* This drug has been administered for greater than 1 year. If the drug is to be administered for a prolonged period, periodic evaluations, including liver function tests, should be performed.

➤*Ocular lesions:* Although retinal abnormalities seen in humans with long-term chloroquine use have not been observed with mefloquine use, long-term feeding of mefloquine to rats resulted in dose-related ocular lesions. All surviving rats given 30 mg/kg/day had ocular lesions in both eyes characterized by retinal degeneration, opacity of the lens, and retinal edema. Similar but less severe lesions were observed in 80% of female and 22% of male rats fed 12.5 mg/kg/day for 2 years. At doses of 5 mg/kg/day, only corneal lesions were observed. They occurred in 9% of rats studied. Therefore, periodic ophthalmic examinations are recommended.

➤*Cardiac effects:* Parenteral studies in animals show that mefloquine, a myocardial depressant, possesses 20% of the antifibrillatory action of quinidine and produces 50% of the increase in the PR interval reported with quinine. The effect of mefloquine on the compromised cardiovascular system has not been evaluated. However, transitory and clinically silent ECG alterations have been reported during the use of mefloquine. Alterations included sinus bradycardia, sinus arrhythmia, first-degree AV block, prolongation of the QTc interval and abnormal T-waves. The benefits of mefloquine HCl therapy should be weighed against the possibility of adverse effects in patients with cardiac disease.

➤*Epilepsy:* In patients with epilepsy, mefloquine HCl may increase the risk of convulsions. The drug should therefore be prescribed only for curative treatment in such patients and only if there are compelling medical reasons for its use.

➤*Special risk:* Mefloquine HCl should be used with caution in patients with psychiatric disturbances because mefloquine use has been associated with emotional disturbances.

➤*Hazardous tasks:* Caution should be exercised with regard to activities requiring alertness and fine motor coordination such as driving, piloting aircraft and operating machinery, and deep-sea diving, as dizziness, a loss of balance, or other disorders of the central or peripheral nervous system have been reported during and following the use of mefloquine HCl. These effects may occur after therapy is discontinued due to the long half-life of the drug.

Drug Interactions

Mefloquine Drug Interactions

Precipitant drug	Object drug*		Description
Beta-adrenergic blockers (propranolol)	Mefloquine	↑	There is one report of cardiopulmonary arrest with full recovery in a patient taking propranolol.
Chloroquine	Mefloquine	↑	The risk of convulsions may be increased with concomitant mefloquine.
Halofantrine	Mefloquine	↑	Do not give halofantrine with or subsequently to mefloquine because of the danger of a potentially fatal prolongation of the QT_c interval.
Mefloquine	Bacterial vaccines, live attenuated (ie, oral live typhoid vaccines)	↓	When mefloquine is taken concurrently with oral live typhoid vaccines, attenuation of immunization cannot be excluded. Vaccinations with attenuated live bacteria should therefore be completed at least 3 days before the first dose of mefloquine.
Mefloquine	Quinine or Quinidine	↑	Coadministration may produce ECG abnormalities. If these agents are to be used in the initial treatment of severe malaria, delay mefloquine administration at least 12 hours after the last dose of quinine or quinidine. The risk of convulsions also may be increased with concurrent mefloquine and quinine.
Mefloquine	Anticonvulsants (eg, valproic acid, carbamazepine, phenobarbital, phenytoin)	↓	Monitor anticonvulsant blood levels and adjust the dosage as necessary. Coadministration may reduce seizure control by lowering the plasma levels of the anticonvulsant.

* ↑ = Object drug increased. ↓ = Object drug decreased.

Theoretically, coadministration of other drugs known to alter cardiac conduction (eg, antiarrhythmic or beta-adrenergic-blocking agents, calcium channel blockers, antihistamines or H_1-blocking agents, tricyclic antidepressants, phenothiazines) might also contribute to a prolongation of the QTc interval. There are no data that conclusively establish whether the concomitant administration of mefloquine and the above listed agents has an effect on cardiac function.

Adverse Reactions

At the doses used for treatment of acute malaria infections, the symptoms possibly attributable to drug administration cannot be distinguished from those symptoms usually attributable to the disease itself.

➤*Prophylaxis of malaria:* Among subjects who received mefloquine for prophylaxis of malaria, the most frequently observed adverse experience was vomiting (3%). Dizziness, syncope, extrasystoles and other complaints affecting less than 1% were also reported.

➤*Treatment of malaria:* Among subjects who received mefloquine for treatment, the most frequently observed adverse experiences included the following: Dizziness, myalgia, nausea, fever, headache, vomiting, chills, diarrhea, skin rash, abdominal pain, fatigue, loss of appetite, and tinnitus. Those side effects occurring in less than 1% included bradycardia, hair loss, emotional problems, pruritus, asthenia, transient emotional disturbances and telogen effluvium (loss of resting hair). Seizures have also been reported.

Two serious adverse reactions were cardiopulmonary arrest in 1 patient shortly after ingesting a single prophylactic dose of mefloquine while con-

MEFLOQUINE HYDROCHLORIDE — ORAL

comitantly using propranolol (see Precautions), and encephalopathy of unknown etiology during prophylactic mefloquine administration. The relationship of encephalopathy to drug administration could not be clearly established.

➤*Postmarketing:* Postmarketing surveillance indicates that the same adverse experiences are reported during prophylaxis, as well as acute treatment.

The most frequently reported adverse events are nausea, vomiting, loose stools or diarrhea, abdominal pain, dizziness or vertigo, loss of balance, and neuropsychiatric events such as headache, somnolence, and sleep disorders (insomnia, abnormal dreams). These are usually mild and may decrease despite continued use.

Psychiatric – Occasionally, more severe neuropsychiatric disorders have been reported such as the following: Sensory and motor neuropathies (including paresthesia, tremor and ataxia), convulsions, agitation or restlessness, anxiety, depression, mood changes, panic attacks, forgetfulness, confusion, hallucinations, aggression, psychotic or paranoid reactions and encephalopathy. Rare cases of suicidal ideation and suicide have been reported, though no relationship to drug administration has been confirmed.

Other infrequent adverse reactions include:

Cardiovascular – Circulatory disturbances (hypotension, hypertension, flushing, syncope), chest pain, tachycardia or palpitation, bradycardia, irregular pulse, extrasystoles, AV block and other transient cardiac conduction alterations.

Dermatologic – Rash, exanthema, erythema, urticaria, pruritus, hair loss, erythema multiforme and Stevens-Johnson syndrome.

Lab test abnormalities – The most frequently observed laboratory alterations which could be possibly attributable to drug administration were decreased hematocrit, transient elevation of transaminases, leukopenia and thrombocytopenia. These alterations were observed in patients with acute malaria who received treatment doses of the drug and were attributed to the disease itself.

During prophylactic administration of mefloquine to indigenous populations in malaria-endemic areas, the following occasional alterations in laboratory values were observed: Transient elevation of transaminases, leukocytosis or thrombocytopenia.

Because of the long half-life of mefloquine, adverse reactions to mefloquine HCl may occur or persist up to several weeks after the last dose.

Musculoskeletal – Muscle weakness, muscle cramps, myalgia, arthralgia.

Miscellaneous – Visual disturbances, vestibular disorders (including tinnitus and hearing impairment), dyspnea, asthenia, malaise, fatigue, fever, sweating, chills, dyspepsia, and loss of appetite.

Overdosage

➤*Symptoms:* In cases of overdosage with mefloquine HCl, the adverse reactions may be more pronounced.

➤*Treatment:* The following procedure is recommended in case of overdosage: Induce vomiting or perform gastric lavage, as appropriate. Monitor cardiac function (if possible by ECG) and neurologic and psychiatric status for at least 24 hours. Provide symptomatic and intensive supportive treatment as required, particularly for cardiovascular disturbances. Treat vomiting or diarrhea with standard fluid therapy.

Patient Information

As required by law, a mefloquine HCl medication guide is supplied to patients when mefloquine HCl is dispensed. Patients should be instructed to read the *MedGuide* when mefloquine HCl is received.

Malaria can be a life-threatening infection in the traveler.

In a small percentage of cases, patients are unable to take this medication because of side effects, and it may be necessary to change medications.

When used as prophylaxis, the first dose of mefloquine HCl should be taken 1 week prior to arrival in an endemic area

If the patients experience psychiatric symptoms such as acute anxiety, depression, restlessness or confusion, these may be considered prodromal to a more serious event. In these cases, the drug must be discontinued, and an alternative medication should be substituted.

No chemoprophylactic regimen is 100% effective, and protective clothing, insect repellents, and bednets are important components of malaria prophylaxis.

Seek medical attention for any febrile illness that occurs after return from a malarious area and inform their physician that they may have been exposed to malaria.

DOXYCYCLINE

Refer to the Tetracyclines group monograph and the individual doxycycline monograph for more information.

4-Aminoquinoline Compounds

Indications

➤*Malaria:* Prophylaxis and treatment of acute attacks of malaria caused by *Plasmodium vivax*, *P. malariae*, *P. ovale*, and susceptible strains of *P. falciparum*. Chloroquine phosphate is the drug of choice in this situation. Chloroquine HCl is used when oral therapy is not feasible. For radical cure of *P. vivax* and *P. malariae* malaria, concomitant primaquine therapy is required.

➤*Unlabeled uses:* Chloroquine has been used to suppress rheumatoid arthritis and in the treatment of systemic and discoid lupus erythematosus, scleroderma, pemphigus, lichen planus, polymyositis, sarcoidosis, and porphyria cutanea tarda.

For other uses, refer to individual product monographs.

Actions

➤*Pharmacology:* Chloroquine's exact mechanism of action is not known, but several mechanisms have been suggested. It concentrates in parasite acid vesicles and raises internal pH. The "non-weak base effect" inhibits parasite growth at extracellular drug concentrations; this may occur due to active chloroquine-concentrating mechanism in parasite acid vesicles. Another mechanism may involve ferriprotoporphyrin IX aggregates, which are released by parasitized erythrocytes during hemoglobin degradation and serve as chloroquine receptors, causing membrane damage with lysis of parasites or erythrocytes. Chloroquine also may influence hemoglobin digestion or interfere with parasite/nucleoprotein synthesis.

➤*Pharmacokinetics:*

Absorption/Distribution – Absorbed readily from GI tract, peak plasma levels are reached in 1 to 6 hours. Plasma protein binding is 55%. Drug concentrates in liver, spleen, kidney and brain and is strongly bound in melanin-containing cells such as in eyes and skin.

Metabolism/Excretion – Chloroquine is eliminated very slowly and may persist in tissues for a prolonged period. Up to 70% of a dose may be excreted unchanged in urine and up to 25% as a metabolite. Renal excretion is enhanced by urinary acidification.

➤*Microbiology:* Active against the erythrocytic forms of *P. vivax* and *malariae* and most strains of *P. falciparum* (but not the gametocytes of *P. falciparum*).

These drugs do not prevent relapses or infection of *P. vivax* or *malariae* malaria; not effective against exoerythrocytic parasite forms. Highly effective in suppressing *P. vivax* or *malariae* malaria, terminating acute attacks and significantly lengthening interval between treatment and relapse. In *P. falciparum* malaria, they abolish acute attack and completely cure infection unless due to resistant strain. Hydroxychloroquine is not effective against chloroquine-resistant *P. falciparum* strains.

Contraindications

Retinal or visual field changes; hypersensitivity; long-term therapy in children (hydroxychloroquine). Consider an exception in acute malarial attacks caused by *Plasmodia* strains susceptible only to 4-aminoquinolines.

Warnings

➤*Resistance:* Certain strains of *P. falciparum* are resistant to 4-aminoquinoline compounds; normally adequate doses fail to prevent or cure malaria or parasitemia.

➤*Retinopathy:* Irreversible retinal damage has occurred with long-term or high dosages. Retinopathy may be dose-related. During prolonged therapy, perform baseline and periodic ophthalmologic exams. If there is any indication of abnormality in visual acuity/field or retinal macular areas or any visual symptoms not explainable by difficulties of accommodation or corneal opacities, stop drug immediately; observe for possible progression. Retinal changes/visual disturbances may progress after therapy cessation.

➤*Glucose-6-phosphate dehydrogenase (G-6-PD) deficiency:* Use with caution in patients with G-6-PD deficiencies.

➤*Muscular weakness:* Periodically question and examine patients who are on long-term therapy; test knee and ankle reflexes to detect muscular weakness. If weakness occurs, discontinue therapy.

➤*Psoriasis or porphyria:* Use of these drugs may exacerbate these conditions. Do not use in these conditions unless the benefit outweighs the possible hazard.

➤*Hepatic function impairment:* These drugs concentrate in liver; use with caution in hepatic disease or alcoholism, or in conjunction with hepatotoxic drugs.

➤*Pregnancy:* Use only when clearly needed and when potential benefits outweigh potential hazards to the fetus.

➤*Lactation:* Safety for use has not been established; these agents are excreted in breast milk. A nursing infant may consume ≈ 0.55% of a 300 mg maternal dose over 24 hours. One study determined the milk: blood ratio of the nursing mother to be 0.358.

➤*Children:* Children are especially sensitive to the 4-aminoquinoline compounds. Fatalities following accidental ingestion of relatively small doses and sudden deaths from parenteral chloroquine have been recorded. Do not exceed a single dose of 5 mg base/kg of chloroquine HCl in infants or children.

Precautions

➤*Monitoring:* Perform periodic CBCs during prolonged therapy. If any severe blood disorder not attributable to the disease appears, consider discontinuing therapy. Measure G-6-PD in susceptible individuals prior to initiating therapy. Although probably safe when given in normal therapeutic doses, these compounds may induce hemolysis in G-6-PD deficient individuals in the presence of infection or stressful conditions. An acute drop in hematocrit, hemoglobin, and red blood cell count may occur.

Drug Interactions

4-Aminoquinoline Drug Interactions			
Precipitant drug	Object drug*		Description
Cimetidine	Chloroquine	↑	Cimetidine may reduce the oral clearance rate and metabolism of chloroquine
Chloroquine	Kaolin or magnesium trisilicate	↓	GI absorption of chloroquine may be decreased by coadministration of these agents.

* ↑ = Object drug increased. ↓ = Object drug decreased.

Adverse Reactions

➤*Cardiovascular:* Hypotension; ECG changes (particularly inversion or depression of the T wave, widening of QRS complex); cardiomyopathy (rare).

➤*CNS:* Mild, transient headache; psychic stimulation; psychotic episodes, convulsions (rare).

➤*GI:* Anorexia; nausea; vomiting; diarrhea; abdominal cramps.

➤*Ophthalmic:* Irreversible retinal damage (see Warnings); visual disturbances (blurred vision, difficulty of focusing or accommodation); nyctalopia; scotomatous vision with field defects of paracentral, pericentral ring types and typically temporal scotomas (eg, difficulty reading with words tending to disappear, seeing half an object, misty vision, fog before eyes).

➤*Miscellaneous:* Agranulocytosis; hair loss; pruritus; neuromyopathy, blood dyscrasias, lichen planus-like eruptions, skin/mucosal pigment changes, pleomorphic skin eruptions. A few cases of a nerve-type deafness have occurred after prolonged high doses.

Overdosage

➤*Symptoms:* Symptoms may occur within 30 minutes in overdosage (or rarely with lower doses in hypersensitive patients) and consist of headache, drowsiness, visual disturbances, nausea, vomiting, cardiovascular collapse, and convulsions followed by sudden and early respiratory and cardiac arrest. Respiratory depression, cardiovascular collapse, shock, convulsions, and death have occurred with overdose of parenteral chloroquine HCl, especially in infants and children. The ECG may reveal atrial standstill, nodal rhythm, prolonged intraventricular conduction and bradycardia progressing to ventricular fibrillation or arrest. In a retrospective study, it was determined that ingestion of more than 5 g of chloroquine was an accurate predictor of fatal outcome in adults.

➤*Treatment:* Treatment is symptomatic; the stomach must be immediately evacuated by emesis or gastric lavage until the stomach is completely emptied. After lavage, activated charcoal (a dose not less than 5 times estimated dose ingested) may inhibit further absorption if given within 30 minutes of ingestion.

Control convulsions before attempting gastric lavage. If due to cerebral stimulation, cautious administration of a short-acting barbiturate may be tried. Treat anoxia-induced convulsions by oxygen, mechanical ventilation or, in shock with hypotension, by vasopressor therapy. Tracheal intubation or tracheostomy may be necessary. Peritoneal dialysis and exchange transfusions have been suggested.

For at least 6 hours, closely observe an asymptomatic patient who survives the acute phase. Force fluids and acidify the urine with 8 g ammonium chloride in divided doses (for adults) to help promote excretion.

In 1 study, 10 of 11 patients who ingested more than 5 g of chloroquine survived after treatment with diazepam and epinephrine for several days along with mechanical ventilation. The use of diazepam has also been successful in other reports.

Patient Information

May cause GI upset; take with food. Complete full course of therapy.

Report visual disturbances or difficulty in hearing or ringing in ears to physician.

Keep out of reach of children; overdosage is especially dangerous in children.

Medication may cause diarrhea, loss of appetite, nausea, stomach pain or vomiting, muscle weakness, or rash. Notify physician if pronounced or bothersome.

CHLOROQUINE PHOSPHATE

Rx **Chloroquine Phosphate** (Various, eg, CMC, Gallipot)	**Tablets:** 250 mg (equiv. to 150 mg base)	In 100s and 1000s.
Rx **Aralen Phosphate** (Sanofi Synthelabo)	**Tablets:** 500 mg (equiv. to 300 mg base)	(W/A77). Pink. Film coated. In 25s.

CHLOROQUINE PHOSPHATE — ORAL

WARNING

Physicians should completely familiarize themselves with the complete contents of this monograph before prescribing chloroquine phosphate.

Indications

➤*Malaria:* For the suppressive treatment and for acute attacks of malaria due to *P. vivax*, *P. malariae P. ovale*, and susceptible strains of *P. falciparum*.

➤*Extraintestinal amebiasis:* For the treatment of extraintestinal amebiasis.

Administration and Dosage

➤*Approved by the FDA:* January 13, 1982.

The dosage of chloroquine phosphate is often expressed or calculated in terms of equivalent chloroquine base. Each 250 mg tablet of chloroquine phosphate is equivalent to 150 mg base and each 500 mg tablet of chloroquine phosphate is equivalent to 300 mg base. In infants and children the dosage is preferably calculated on the body weight.

➤*Malaria:*

Prophylaxis –

Adults: 500 mg (300 mg base) on exactly the same day of each week.

Children: The weekly suppressive dosage is 5 mg calculated as base, per kg of body weight, but should not exceed the adult dose regardless of weight.

If circumstances permit, suppressive therapy should begin 2 weeks prior to exposure. However, failing this in adults, an initial double (loading) dose of 1 g (600 mg base), or in children 10 mg base/kg may be taken in 2 divided doses, 6 hours apart. The suppressive therapy should be continued for 8 weeks after leaving the endemic area.

➤*Treatment of acute attack:*

Adults – An initial dose of 1 g (600 mg base) followed by an additional 500 mg (300 mg base) after 6 to 8 hours and a single dose of 500 mg (300 mg base) on each of 2 consecutive days. This represents a total dose of 2.5 g chloroquine phosphate or 1.5 g base in 3 days.

Children – The dosage for adults may also be calculated on the basis of body weight; this method is preferred for infants and children. A total dose representing 25 mg of base per kg of body weight is administered in 3 days, as follows:

First dose: Take 10 mg base per kg (but not exceeding a single dose of 600 mg base).

Second dose: Take 5 mg base per kg (but not exceeding a single dose of 300 mg base) 6 hours after first dose.

Third dose: Take 5 mg base per kg 18 hours after second dose.

Fourth dose: Take 5 mg base per kg 24 hours after third dose.

For radical cure of vivax and malariae malaria concomitant therapy with an 8-aminoquinoline compound is necessary.

➤*Extraintestinal amebiasis:*

Adults – One gram (600 mg base) daily for 2 days, followed by 500 mg (300 mg base) daily for at least 2 to 3 weeks. Treatment is usually combined with an effective intestinal amebicide.

➤*CDC recommended schedule for chloroquine as an alternative to mefloquine:* Travelers to areas of risk where chloroquine-resistant *P. falciparum* is endemic and for whom mefloquine is contraindicated may elect to use an alternative regimen. Chloroquine alone taken weekly is recommended for travelers who cannot use mefloquine or doxycycline, especially pregnant women and children less than 15 kg. In addition, give these travelers a single treatment dose of sulfadoxine/pyrimethamine to keep during travel and to take promptly in the event of a febrile illness during their travel when professional medical care is not readily available. Continue weekly chloroquine prophylaxis after presumptive treatment with sulfadoxine/pyrimethamine.

➤*Storage / Stability:* Dispense in a tight, light-resistant container using a child-resistant closure.

Store at controlled room temperature 15° to 30°C (59° to 86°F). Protect from light and moisture.

CHLOROQUINE HYDROCHLORIDE

Rx **Aralen HCl** (Sanofi Winthrop)	**Injection:** 50 mg (equiv. to 40 mg base)/ml	In 5 ml amps.

4-Aminoquinoline Compounds

CHLOROQUINE HYDROCHLORIDE — INJECTION

WARNING

Physicians should completely familiarize themselves with the complete contents of this leaflet before prescribing chloroquine HCl.

Indications

➤*Extraintestinal amebiasis:* For the treatment of extraintestinal amebiasis.

➤*Malaria:* For treatment of acute attacks of malaria due to *P. vivax*, *P. malariae*, *P. ovale*, and susceptible strains of *P. falciparum* when oral therapy is not feasible.

➤*Unlabeled uses:* To suppress rheumatoid arthritis and in the treatment of systemic and discoid lupus erythematosus, scleroderma, pemphigus, lichen planus, polymyositis, sarcoidosis, and porphyria cutanea tarda.

Administration and Dosage

➤*Malaria:*

Adults – An initial dose of 4 mL or 5 mL (160 mg to 200 mg chloroquine base) may be injected IM and repeated in 6 hours if necessary. The total parenteral dosage in the first 24 hours should not exceed 800 mg chloroquine base. Treatment by mouth should be started as soon as practicable and continued until a course of approximately 1.5 g of base in 3 days is completed.

Children: Infants and children are extremely susceptible to overdosage of parenteral chloroquine HCl. Severe reactions and deaths have occurred. In the pediatric age range, parenteral chloroquine HCl dosage should be calculated in proportion to the adult dose based upon body weight. The recommended single dose in infants and children is 5 mg base per kg. This dose may be repeated in 6 hours; however, the total dose in any 24-hour period should not exceed 10 mg base per kg of body weight. Parenteral administration should be terminated and oral therapy instituted as soon as possible.

➤*Extraintestinal amebiasis:* In adult patients not able to tolerate oral therapy, from 4 to 5 mL (160 to 200 mg chloroquine base) may be injected daily for 10 to 12 days. Oral administration should be substituted or resumed as soon as possible.

➤*Storage/Stability:* Store at room temperature up to 30°C (86°F).

8-Aminoquinoline Compound

PRIMAQUINE PHOSPHATE

Rx	**Primaquine Phosphate** (Various, eg, Quality Care, Sanofi Winthrop)	**Tablets:** 26.3 mg (equivalent to 15 mg base)	Lactose. In 20s and 100s.

PRIMAQUINE PHOSPHATE — ORAL

WARNING

Physicians should completely familiarize themselves with the complete contents of this monograph before prescribing primaquine phosphate.

Indications

➤*Plasmodium vivax malaria:* For the radical cure (prevention of relapse) of vivax malaria.

Recommended only for the radical cure of vivax malaria, the prevention of relapse in vivax malaria, or following the termination of chloroquine phosphate suppressive therapy in an area where vivax malaria is endemic.

Administration and Dosage

Patients suffering from an attack of vivax malaria or having parasitized red blood cells should receive a course of chloroquine phosphate, which quickly destroys the erythrocytic parasites and terminates the paroxysm. Primaquine phosphate should be administered concurrently in order to eradicate the exoerythrocytic parasites in a dosage of 1 tablet (equivalent to 15 mg base) daily for 14 days.

➤*Storage/Stability:* Store at 25°C (77°F); excursions permitted to 15° to 30°C (59° to 86°F) [see USP Controlled Room Temperature].

Actions

➤*Pharmacology:* Primaquine phosphate is an 8-amino-quinoline compound which eliminates tissue (exoerythrocytic) infection. Thereby, it prevents the development of the blood (erythrocytic) forms of the parasite which are responsible for relapses in vivax malaria. Primaquine phosphate is also active against gametocytes of *Plasmodium falciparum*.

Contraindications

In acutely ill patients suffering from systemic disease manifested by tendency to granulocytopenia, such as rheumatoid arthritis and lupus erythematosus. In patients receiving concurrently other potentially hemolytic drugs or depressants of myeloid elements of the bone marrow; coadministration with quinacrine.

Warnings

➤*Hemolytic anemia:* Discontinue the use of primaquine phosphate promptly if signs suggestive of hemolytic anemia occur (eg, darkening of the urine, marked fall of hemoglobin or erythrocytic count).

Hemolytic reactions (moderate to severe) may occur in glucose-6-phosphate dehydrogenase (G-6-PD) deficient white patients (particularly in Sardinians and in individuals with a family or personal history of favism). Dark-skinned persons have a great tendency to develop hemolytic anemia (due to congenital deficiency of erythrocytic glucose-6-phosphate dehydrogenase) while receiving primaquine and related drugs.

If primaquine phosphate is prescribed for an individual who has shown a previous idiosyncrasy to primaquine phosphate (as manifested by hemolytic anemia, methemoglobinemia, or leukopenia), an individual with a family or personal history of favism, or an individual with erythrocytic glucose-6-phosphate dehydrogenase (G-6-PD) deficiency or nicotinamide adenine dinucleotide (NADH) methemoglobin reductase deficiency, the person should be observed closely for tolerance. The drug should be discontinued immediately if marked darkening of the urine or sudden decrease in hemoglobin concentration or leukocyte count occurs.

➤*Pregnancy:* Safe use of this preparation in pregnancy has not been established. Therefore, use of it during pregnancy should be avoided except when in the judgment of the physician the benefit outweighs the possible hazard.

Precautions

➤*Monitoring:* Since anemia, methemoglobinemia, and leukopenia have been observed following administration of large doses of primaquine, the adult dosage of 1 tablet (= 15 mg base) daily for 14 days should not be exceeded. It is also advisable to make routine blood examinations (particularly blood cell counts and hemoglobin determinations) during therapy.

Drug Interactions

➤*Quinacrine:* Because quinacrine hydrochloride appears to potentiate the toxicity of antimalarial compounds which are structurally related to primaquine, the use of quinacrine in patients receiving primaquine is contraindicated. Similarly, primaquine should not be administered to patients who have received quinacrine recently, as toxicity is increased.

Adverse Reactions

➤*GI:* Nausea, vomiting, epigastric distress, and abdominal cramps.

➤*Hematologic:* Leukopenia, hemolytic anemia in glucose-6-phosphate dehydrogenase (G-6-PD) deficient individuals, and methemoglobinemia in nicotinamide adenine dinucleotide (NADH) methemoglobin reductase-deficient individuals.

Overdosage

➤*Symptoms:* Symptoms of overdosage of primaquine phosphate are similar to those seen after overdosage of pamaquine. They include abdominal cramps, vomiting, burning epigastric distress, central nervous system and cardiovascular disturbances, cyanosis, methemoglobinemia, moderate leukocytosis or leukopenia, and anemia. The most striking symptoms are granulocytopenia and acute hemolytic anemia in sensitive persons. Acute homolysis occurs, but patients recover completely if the dosage is discontinued.

Folic Acid Antagonist

PYRIMETHAMINE

Rx	**Daraprim** (GlaxoSmithKline)	**Tablets:** 25 mg	Lactose. (Daraprim A3A). White, scored. In 100s.

PYRIMETHAMINE — ORAL

Indications

➤*Chemoprophylaxis of malaria:* In susceptible strains of plasmodia only. It is not suitable as a prophylactic agent for travelers to most areas because of prevalent resistance worldwide.

➤*Toxoplasmosis:* Use with a sulfonamide; synergism exists with this combination.

➤*Acute malaria:* In conjunction with a sulfonamide (eg, sulfadoxine) to initiate transmission control and suppression for susceptible strains of plasmodia. Fast-acting schizonticides (chloroquine, quinine) are preferable for the treatment of acute malaria.

Administration and Dosage

Administer with food to minimize vomiting.

➤*Chemoprophylaxis of malaria:* Do not exceed recommended dosage.

Adults and children (older than 10 years of age) – 25 mg once weekly.

Children (4 to 10 years of age) – 12.5 mg once weekly.

PYRIMETHAMINE — ORAL

Infants and children (younger than 4 years of age) – 6.25 mg once weekly.

➤*Treatment of acute malaria:* Recommended in areas where only susceptible plasmodia exist. Not recommended for use alone to treat acute malaria. Fast-acting schizonticides (chloroquine, quinine) are indicated for treatment of acute malaria. However, concomitant pyrimethamine, 25 mg daily for 2 days, with a sulfonamide will initiate transmission control and suppression of nonfalciparum malaria.

If pyrimethamine must be used alone in semi-immune people, dose as follows:

Adults and children (older than 10 years of age) – 50 mg daily for 2 days.

Children (4 to 10 years of age) – 25 mg daily for 2 days.

Follow with once weekly regimen described in the chemoprophylaxis regimen above. Extend regimens to include suppression through any characteristic periods of early recrudescence and late relapse for at least 10 weeks in each case.

➤*Toxoplasmosis:* At the dosage required, there is marked variation in tolerance. Young patients may tolerate higher doses than older patients. Coadministration of folinic acid (leucovorin) is strongly recommended in all patients. The dosage of pyrimethamine required for the treatment of toxoplasmosis is 10 to 20 times the recommended antimalaria dosage and approaches the toxic level (see Warnings).

Adults – Initial dose is 50 to 75 mg daily with 1 to 4 g of a sulfonamide of the sulfapyrimidine type (eg, sulfadoxine). Continue for 1 to 3 weeks, depending on response and tolerance. Dosage for each drug may then be reduced by one half and continued for an additional 4 or 5 weeks.

Children – Dosage is 1 mg/kg/day divided into 2 equal daily doses; after 2 to 4 days, reduce to one half and continue for approximately 1 month. The usual pediatric sulfonamide dosage is used in conjunction with pyrimethamine.

Convulsive disorders – Use lower initial dose to avoid potential CNS toxicity.

➤*Storage/Stability:* Store at 15° to 25°C (59° to 77°F) in a dry place and protect from light.

Actions

➤*Pharmacology:* Pyrimethamine is a folic acid antagonist; its therapeutic action is based on differential requirement between host and parasite for nucleic acid precursors involved in growth as it selectively inhibits plasmodial dihydrofolate reductase. Pyrimethamine inhibits the enzyme dihydrofolate reductase, which catalyzes the reduction of dihydrofolate to tetrahydrofolate. This activity is highly selective against plasmodia and *Toxoplasma gondii*. It does not destroy gametocytes but arrests sporogony in the mosquito. Pyrimethamine possesses blood schizonticidal and some tissue schizonticidal activity against human malaria parasites. The action of pyrimethamine against *T. gondii* is greatly enhanced when used in conjunction with sulfonamides.

➤*Pharmacokinetics:* Pyrimethamine is well absorbed after oral use. Peak plasma concentrations occur in 2 to 6 hours. Plasma half-life is approximately 4 days; suppressive concentrations are maintained for approximately 2 weeks (but lower in malaria patients). It is approximately 87% plasma protein-bound. Several metabolites appear in the urine.

Contraindications

Hypersensitivity to the drug or any components of the formulation; megaloblastic anemia caused by folate deficiency.

Warnings

➤*Folic acid deficiency:* The dosage of pyrimethamine required for the treatment of toxoplasmosis is 10 to 20 times the recommended antimalaria dosage and approaches the toxic level. If signs of folate deficiency develop, reduce dosage or discontinue drug according to patient response. Folinic acid (leucovorin) may be given in a dosage of 5 to 15 mg/day (oral, IM, or IV) until normal hematopoiesis is restored. Use with caution in possible folate deficiency (eg, malabsorption syndrome, alcoholism, pregnancy, phenytoin usage).

➤*Accidental ingestion:* Keep pyrimethamine out of the reach of infants and children as they are extremely susceptible to adverse effects from an overdose. Deaths in pediatric patients have been reported after accidental ingestion.

➤*Hypersensitivity reactions:* Occasionally severe hypersensitivity reactions (eg, Stevens-Johnson syndrome, toxic epidermal necrolysis, erythema multiforme, and anaphylaxis) have occurred, particularly if given with a sulfonamide (see Adverse Reactions). Refer to Management of Acute Hypersensitivity Reactions.

➤*Renal/Hepatic function impairment:* Use with caution.

➤*Carcinogenesis:* Data in 2 humans indicate that pyrimethamine may be carcinogenic: A 51-year-old female who developed chronic granulocytic leukemia after taking pyrimethamine for 2 years for toxoplasmosis, and a 56-year-old patient who developed reticulum cell sarcoma after 14 months of pyrimethamine for toxoplasmosis. Pyrimethamine has been reported to produce a significant increase in the number of lung tumors in mice when given intraperitoneally at doses of 25 mg/kg.

➤*Mutagenesis:* Pyrimethamine has been shown to be mutagenic in the L5178Y/TK +/- mouse lymphoma assay in the absence of exogenous metabolic activation. Human blood lymphocytes cultured in vitro had structural chromosome aberrations induced by pyrimethamine.

➤*Elderly:* Dose selection for an elderly patient should be cautious, usually starting at the low end of the dosing range, reflecting the greater frequency of decreased hepatic, renal, or cardiac function, and of concomitant disease or other drug therapy.

➤*Pregnancy: Category C.* Pyrimethamine has been shown to be teratogenic in rats when given in oral doses 7 times the human dose for chemoprophylaxis of malaria or 2.5 times the human dose for treatment of toxoplasmosis. At these doses in rats, there was a significant increase in abnormalities such as cleft palate, brachygnathia, oligodactyly, and microphthalmia. Pyrimethamine also has been shown to produce terata such as meningocele in hamsters and cleft palate in miniature pigs when given in oral doses 170 and 5 times the human dose, respectively, for chemoprophylaxis of malaria or for treatment of toxoplasmosis. There are no adequate and well-controlled studies in pregnant women. Use pyrimethamine during pregnancy only if the potential benefit justifies the potential risk to the fetus. Coadministration of folinic acid is strongly recommended when treating toxoplasmosis during pregnancy.

➤*Lactation:* Pyrimethamine is excreted in breast milk. Because of the potential for serious adverse reactions in nursing infants from pyrimethamine and from concurrent use of a sulfonamide with pyrimethamine for treatment of some patients with toxoplasmosis, decide whether to discontinue nursing or discontinue the drug, taking into account the importance of the drug to the mother.

➤*Children:* See Administration and Dosage.

Precautions

➤*Monitoring:* For toxoplasmosis, perform semiweekly blood counts, including platelet counts. Because of the long half-life of pyrimethamine, daily monitoring of peripheral blood counts is recommended for up to several weeks after an overdose until normal hematological values are restored.

➤*G-6-PD:* Large doses of pyrimethamine may precipitate hemolytic anemia in patients with glucose-6-phosphate dehydrogenase deficiency.

Drug Interactions

➤*Antifolate drugs or agents associated with myelosuppression (eg, proguanil, zidovudine, cytostatic agents [eg, methotrexate], sulfonamides, trimethoprim-sulfamethoxazole):* Concurrent use of antifolic acids and pyrimethamine may increase the risk of bone marrow suppression. Discontinue pyrimethamine if signs of folate deficiency develop. Administer folinic acid (leucovorin) until normal hematopoiesis is restored (see Warnings).

➤*Lorazepam:* Mild hepatotoxicity has been reported when lorazepam and pyrimethamine were coadministered.

Adverse Reactions

➤*GI:* Anorexia, vomiting (large doses); atrophic glossitis. Vomiting may be minimized by giving with meals; it usually disappears promptly upon dosage reduction.

➤*Hematologic:* Megaloblastic anemia, leukopenia, thrombocytopenia, pancytopenia, hematuria.

➤*Hypersensitivity:* Hypersensitivity reactions, occasionally severe (eg, Stevens-Johnson syndrome, toxic epidermal necrolysis, erythema multiforme, anaphylaxis), and hyperphenylalaninemia have occurred particularly when coadministered with a sulfonamide.

➤*Miscellaneous:* Rhythm disorders; pulmonary eosinophilia (rare).

Overdosage

➤*Symptoms:* Following the ingestion of 300 mg or more of pyrimethamine, GI and/or CNS signs may be present, including convulsions. Initial GI symptoms include abdominal pain, nausea, and severe and repeated vomiting possibly including hematemesis. CNS toxicity is manifested by initial excitability; generalized and prolonged convulsions, which may be followed by respiratory depression; circulatory collapse; and death within a few hours. Neurological symptoms appear rapidly (30 minutes to 2 hours after drug ingestion), suggesting that in gross overdosage, pyrimethamine has a direct toxic effect on the CNS.

Fatal dose is variable; the smallest reported fatal single dose is 375 mg. There are reports of children who have recovered after taking 375 to 625 mg.

➤*Treatment:* There is no specific antidote for pyrimethamine. Gastric lavage is effective. Use parenteral diazepam to control convulsions. Administer folinic acid (leucovorin) within 2 hours of ingestion to counteract effects on the hematopoietic system. Because of the long half-life of pyrimethamine, daily monitoring of peripheral blood counts is recommended for up to several weeks after the overdose until normal hematological values are restored. Treatment includes usual supportive measures. Refer to General Management of Acute Overdosage.

Patient Information

May cause anorexia or vomiting; inform patients to take with food or meals.

At first appearance of a skin rash, inform patients to discontinue the drug and immediately seek medical attention.

Warn patients that the appearance of sore throat, pallor, purpura, or glossitis may be early indications of serious disorders that require seeking medical treatment.

Warn women of childbearing potential against becoming pregnant.

Advise patients to keep medication out of the reach of children.

Advise patients not to exceed recommended doses.

Coadministration of folinic acid (leucovorin) is strongly recommended in all patients when used for the treatment of toxoplasmosis.

SULFADOXINE AND PYRIMETHAMINE

Rx	**Fansidar** (Roche)	**Tablets:** 500 mg sulfadoxine and 25 mg pyrimethamine	Lactose, talc. (FANSIDAR ROCHE). Scored. In UD 25s.

SULFADOXINE AND PYRIMETHAMINE — ORAL

WARNING

Fatalities associated with the administration of sulfadoxine and pyrimethamine have occurred because of severe reactions, including Stevens-Johnson syndrome and toxic epidermal necrolysis. Discontinue sulfadoxine and pyrimethamine prophylaxis at the first appearance of skin rash, if a significant reduction in the count of any formed blood elements is noted, or upon the occurrence of active bacterial or fungal infections.

Indications

➤*Malaria:* For the treatment of *Plasmodium falciparum* malaria for those patients in whom chloroquine resistance is suspected.

➤*Malaria prophylaxis:* For travelers to areas where chloroquine-resistant *P. falciparum* malaria is endemic (strains of *P. falciparum* may be encountered that have developed resistance to sulfadoxine and pyrimethamine therapy).

➤*Unlabeled uses:* Sulfadoxine and pyrimethamine combination has been used in the prophylaxis of *Pneumocystis carinii* infection .

Administration and Dosage

➤*Acute attack of malaria:* A single dose of the following number of sulfadoxine and pyrimethamine tablets is used in sequence with quinine or alone:

Sulfadoxine and Pyrimethamine Dosing for an Acute Malaria Attack

Age	Dosing
Adults	2 to 3 tablets
9 to 14 years of age	2 tablets
4 to 8 years of age	1 tablet
less than 4 years of age	½ tablet

➤*Malaria prophylaxis:* Take the first dose of sulfadoxine and pyrimethamine 1 or 2 days before departure to an endemic area; continue administration during the stay and for 4 to 6 weeks after return.

Sulfadoxine and Pyrimethamine Dosing for Malaria Prophylaxis

Age	Once weekly	Once every 2 weeks
Adults	1 tablet	2 tablets
9 to 14 years of age	¾ tablet	1½ tablets
4 to 8 years of age	½ tablet	1 tablet
less than 4 years of age	¼ tablet	½ tablet

Actions

➤*Pharmacology:* Sulfadoxine and pyrimethamine combination is an antimalarial agent that acts by reciprocal potentiation of its 2 components, achieved by a sequential blockade of 2 enzymes involved in the biosynthesis of folinic acid within the parasites. It is effective against certain strains of *P. falciparum* that are resistant to chloroquine.

➤*Pharmacokinetics:*

Absorption/Distribution – Both sulfadoxine and pyrimethamine are absorbed orally. Following a single tablet administration, sulfadoxine peak plasma concentrations of 51 to 76 mcg/mL were achieved in 2.5 to 6 hours, and the pyrimethamine peak plasma concentrations of 0.13 to 0.4 mcg/mL were achieved in 1.5 to 8 hours. Both drugs appear in the breast milk of nursing mothers.

Metabolism/Excretion – Both sulfadoxine and pyrimethamine are excreted mainly by the kidney. The apparent elimination half-life of sulfadoxine ranged from 100 to 231 hours (mean, 169 hours), whereas pyrimethamine half-lives ranged from 54 to 148 hours (mean, 111 hours).

Contraindications

Prophylactic use in patients with severe renal insufficiency, marked liver parenchymal damage, or blood dyscrasias; hypersensitivity to pyrimethamine or sulfonamides; patients with documented megaloblastic anemia caused by folate deficiency; infants younger than 2 months of age; pregnancy at term and during the nursing period.

Warnings

➤*Death:* Fatalities associated with the administration of sulfonamides, although rare, have occurred caused by severe reactions, including fulminant hepatic necrosis, agranulocytosis, aplastic anemia, and other blood dyscrasias (see Warning Box).

➤*Leukopenia:* Sulfadoxine and pyrimethamine prophylactic regimen has been reported to cause leukopenia during a treatment of 2 months or longer. This leukopenia is generally mild and reversible.

➤*Renal/Hepatic function impairment:* Administer with caution to patients with impaired renal or hepatic function. Perform a urinalysis with microscopic examination and renal function tests during therapy for patients who have impaired renal function.

➤*Mutagenesis:* Pyrimethamine was found to be mutagenic in laboratory animals and also in human bone marrow following 3 or 4 consecutive daily doses totaling 200 to 300 mg. Testicular changes have been observed in rats treated with 105 mg/kg/day of sulfadoxine and pyrimethamine and with 15 mg/kg/day of pyrimethamine alone.

➤*Fertility impairment:* The pregnancy rate of female rats was not affected following their treatment with 10.5 mg/kg/day, but was significantly reduced at dosages of 31.5 mg/kg/day or higher, a dosage approximately 30 times or more the weekly human prophylactic dose.

➤*Elderly:* Dose selection for an elderly patient should be cautious, usually starting at the low end of the dosing range, reflecting the greater frequency of decreased hepatic, renal, or cardiac function, and of concomitant disease or other drug therapy. This drug is known to be substantially excreted by the kidney, and the risk of toxic reactions to this drug may be greater in patients with impaired renal function. Because elderly patients are more likely to have decreased renal function, use caution in dose selection and monitor renal function.

➤*Pregnancy: Category C.* Sulfadoxine and pyrimethamine therapy is contraindicated during pregnancy at term. It has been shown to be teratogenic in rats when given in weekly doses approximately 12 times the weekly human prophylactic dose. Teratogenicity studies with pyrimethamine plus sulfadoxine (1:20) in rats showed the minimum oral teratogenic dose to be approximately 0.9 mg/kg pyrimethamine plus 18 mg/kg sulfadoxine. In rabbits, no teratogenic effects were noted at oral doses as high as 20 mg/kg pyrimethamine plus 400 mg/kg sulfadoxine.

There are no adequate and well-controlled studies in pregnant women. However, because of the teratogenic effect shown in animals and because pyrimethamine plus sulfadoxine may interfere with folic acid metabolism, use during pregnancy only if the potential benefit justifies the potential risk to the fetus. Warn women of childbearing potential who are traveling to areas where malaria is endemic against becoming pregnant.

➤*Lactation:* Sulfadoxine and pyrimethamine therapy is contraindicated in the nursing period because sulfonamides cross the placenta and are excreted in breast milk, which may result in kernicterus.

➤*Children:* Do not give to infants younger than 2 months of age because of inadequate development of the glucuronide-forming enzyme system.

Precautions

➤*Monitoring:* Periodic blood counts and analysis of urine for crystalluria are desirable during prolonged prophylaxis.

➤*Folic acid deficiency:* Discontinue therapy if signs of folic acid deficiency develop. Folinic acid (leucovorin) may be administered in doses of 5 to 15 mg/day IM, for 3 days or longer for depressed platelet or white blood cell counts in patients with drug-induced folic acid deficiency when recovery is too slow.

➤*Special risk:* Administer with caution to patients with possible folate deficiency and to those with severe allergy or bronchial asthma. As with some sulfonamide drugs, in glucose-6-phosphate dehydrogenase-deficient individuals, hemolysis may occur.

Drug Interactions

➤*Chloroquine:* There have been reports that may indicate an increase in incidence and severity of adverse reactions when chloroquine is used with sulfadoxine and pyrimethamine tablets as compared with the use of the sulfadoxine and pyrimethamine tablets alone.

➤*Antifolic drugs:* Do not use antifolic drugs (eg, sulfonamides or trimethoprim-sulfamethoxazole combinations) while the patient is receiving sulfadoxine and pyrimethamine tablets for antimalarial prophylaxis.

➤*Goitrogens, diuretics, hypoglycemic agents:* The sulfonamides bear certain chemical similarities to some goitrogens, diuretics (acetazolamide and the thiazides), and oral hypoglycemic agents. Diuresis and hypoglycemia have occurred rarely in patients receiving sulfonamides. Cross-sensitivity may exist with these agents.

Adverse Reactions

➤*CNS:* Headache; peripheral neuritis; mental depression; convulsions; ataxia; hallucinations; tinnitus; vertigo; insomnia; apathy; fatigue; muscle weakness; nervousness.

➤*GI:* Glossitis; stomatitis; nausea; emesis; abdominal pains; hepatitis; hepatocellular necrosis; diarrhea; pancreatitis.

➤*Hematologic:* Agranulocytosis; aplastic anemia; megaloblastic anemia; thrombopenia; leukopenia; hemolytic anemia; purpura; hypoprothrombinemia; methemoglobinemia; eosinophilia.

➤*Hypersensitivity:* Erythema multiforme; Stevens-Johnson syndrome; generalized skin eruptions; toxic epidermal necrolysis; urticaria; serum sickness; pruritus; exfoliative dermatitis; anaphylactoid reactions; periorbital edema; conjunctival and scleral injection; photosensitization; arthralgia; allergic myocarditis.

➤*Miscellaneous:* Pulmonary infiltrates; drug fever; chills; toxic nephrosis with oliguria and anuria; periarteritis nodosa; LE phenomenon.

Overdosage

➤*Symptoms:* Acute intoxication may be manifested by anorexia, vomiting, and CNS stimulation (including convulsions), followed by megaloblastic anemia, leukopenia, thrombocytopenia, glossitis, and crystalluria.

SULFADOXINE AND PYRIMETHAMINE — ORAL

➤*Treatment:* In acute intoxication, emesis and gastric lavage followed by purges may be of benefit. Adequately hydrate the patient to prevent renal damage. Monitor the renal and hematopoietic systems for at least 1 month after overdosage. If the patient is having convulsions, the use of a parenteral barbiturate is indicated. Administer folinic acid (leucovorin) 5 to 15 mg/day IM for 3 days or longer for depressed platelet or white blood cell counts.

Patient Information

Advise the patient to immediately seek medical attention and discontinue therapy at first appearance of rash. Adequate fluid intake must be maintained in order to prevent crystalluria and stone formation.

Instruct the patient to seek medical attention and discontinue prophylactic therapy if sore throat, fever, arthralgia, cough, shortness of breath, pallor, purpura, jaundice, or glossitis develop.

Caution women against becoming pregnant and not to breastfeed their infants during therapy or prophylactic treatment.

ATOVAQUONE AND PROGUANIL HYDROCHLORIDE

Rx	**Malarone** (GlaxoSmithKline)	**Tablets**: atovaquone 250 mg/ proguanil hydrochloride 100 mg	(GX CM3). Pink, biconvex. Film-coated. In 100s and UD 24s.
Rx	**Malarone Pediatric** (GlaxoSmithKline)	**Tablets**: atovaquone 62.5 mg/ proguanil hydrochloride 25 mg	(GX CG7). Pink, biconvex. Film-coated. In 100s.

ATOVAQUONE AND PROGUANIL HYDROCHLORIDE — ORAL

Indications

➤*Malaria prevention:* Prophylaxis of *Plasmodium falciparum* malaria, including areas where chloroquine resistance has been reported.

➤*Malaria treatment:* Treatment of acute, uncomplicated *P. falciparum* malaria. Atovaquone and proguanil have been shown to be effective in regions where the drugs chloroquine, halofantrine, mefloquine, and amodiaquine may have unacceptable failure rates, presumably because of drug resistance.

Administration and Dosage

➤*Approved by the FDA:* July 14, 2000.

Advise patients to take the daily dose at the same time each day with food or milk. In the event of vomiting within 1 hour after dosing, instruct patient to repeat dose. Tablets may be crushed and mixed with condensed milk just prior to administration for children who may have difficulty swallowing tablets.

➤*Malaria prevention:* Start prophylactic treatment 1 or 2 days before entering a malaria-endemic area and continue daily during the stay and for 7 days after return.

Adults – 1 tablet (adult strength = atovaquone 250 mg/proguanil 100 mg) per day.

Children – The dosage for prevention of malaria in pediatric patients is based upon body weight (see table below).

Dosage of Atovaquone/Proguanil for Prevention of Malaria in Pediatric Patients

Weight (kg)	Atovaquone/ Proguanil total daily dose	Dosage regimen
11 to 20	62.5 mg/25 mg	1 pediatric tablet daily
21 to 30	125 mg/50 mg	2 pediatric tablets as a single daily dose
31 to 40	187.5 mg/75 mg	3 pediatric tablets as a single daily dose
more than 40	250 mg/100 mg	1 tablet (adult strength) as a single daily dose

➤*Malaria treatment:*

Adults – 4 tablets (adult strength; total daily dose atovaquone 1 g/proguanil 400 mg) as a single daily dose for 3 consecutive days.

Children – The dosage for treatment of acute malaria in pediatric patients is based upon body weight (see table below).

Dosage of Atovaquone/Proguanil for Treatment of Acute Malaria in Pediatric Patients

Weight (kg)	Atovaquone/ Proguanil total daily dose	Dosage regimen
5 to 8	125 mg/50 mg	2 tablets (pediatric strength) daily for 3 consecutive days
9 to 10	187.5 mg/75 mg	3 tablets (pediatric strength) daily for 3 consecutive days
11 to 20	250 mg/100 mg	1 tablet (adult strength) daily for 3 consecutive days
21 to 30	500 mg/200 mg	2 tablets (adult strength) as a single daily dose for 3 consecutive days
31 to 40	750 mg/300 mg	3 tablets (adult strength) as a single daily dose for 3 consecutive days
more than 40	1 g/400 mg	4 tablets (adult strength) as a single daily dose for 3 consecutive days

➤*Storage/Stability:* Store at 25°C (77°F); excursions permitted to 15° to 30°C (59° to 86°F).

Actions

➤*Pharmacology:* Atovaquone/proguanil is a fixed-dose combination. The constituents of the combination interfere with 2 different pathways involved in the biosynthesis of pyrimidines required for nucleic acid replication. Atovaquone is a selective inhibitor of parasite mitochondrial electron transport. Proguanil primarily exerts its effect by means of the metabolite cycloguanil, a dihydrofolate reductase inhibitor. Inhibition of dihydrofolate reductase in the malaria parasite disrupts deoxythymidylate synthesis.

Atovaquone and cycloguanil (an active metabolite of proguanil) are active against the erythrocytic and exoerythrocytic stages of *Plasmodium* spp. Enhanced efficacy of the combination compared with either atovaquone or proguanil alone was demonstrated in clinical studies in immune and nonimmune patients.

Drug resistance – Strains of *P. falciparum* with decreased susceptibility to atovaquone or proguanil/cycloguanil alone can be selected in vitro or in vivo. The combination of atovaquone and proguanil may not be effective for treatment of recrudescent malaria that develops after prior therapy with the combination.

➤*Pharmacokinetics:*

Absorption – Atovaquone is a highly lipophilic compound with low aqueous solubility. The bioavailability of atovaquone shows considerable interindividual variability.

See Drug Interactions for more information.

Distribution – Atovaquone is highly protein bound (more than 99%) over the concentration range of 1 to 90 mcg/mL. The apparent volume of distribution of atovaquone in adults and children after oral administration is approximately 8.8 L/kg.

Proguanil is 75% protein bound. The apparent volume of distribution of proguanil in adults and children older than 15 years of age with body weights from 31 to 110 kg ranged from 1,617 to 2,502 L. In children 15 years of age and younger with body weights from 11 to 56 kg, the apparent volume of distribution of proguanil ranged from 462 to 966 L. In human plasma, the binding of atovaquone and proguanil was unaffected by the presence of the other.

Metabolism – There is indirect evidence that atovaquone may undergo limited metabolism; however, a specific metabolite has not been identified. Proguanil is metabolized to cycloguanil (primarily via CYP2C19) and 4-chlorophenylbiguanide. The main routes of elimination are hepatic biotransformation and renal excretion.

Excretion – In a study where atovaquone was administered to healthy volunteers, greater than 94% of the dose was recovered unchanged in the feces over 21 days. There was little or no excretion of atovaquone in the urine (less than 0.6%). Between 40% to 60% of proguanil is excreted by the kidneys. The elimination half-life of atovaquone is approximately 2 to 3 days in adult patients. The mean oral clearance of proguanil is 3.22 L/h/kg. The elimination half-life of proguanil is 12 to 21 hours in adult and pediatric patients but may be longer in individuals who are slow metabolizers.

Special populations –

Renal function impairment: In patients with moderate renal impairment (Ccr 30 to 50 mL/min), mean oral clearance for proguanil was reduced by approximately 35% compared with patients with normal renal function (Ccr greater than 80 mL/min) and the oral clearance of atovaquone was comparable between patients with normal renal function and mild renal impairment. In patients with severe renal impairment (Ccr less than 30 mL/min), atovaquone C_{max} and AUC are reduced, but the elimination half-lives for proguanil and cycloguanil are prolonged, with corresponding increases in AUC, resulting in the potential of drug accumulation and toxicity with repeated dosing.

Hepatic function impairment: In patients with moderate hepatic impairment, the elimination half-life of atovaquone was increased (point estimate = 1.28, 90% CI = 1 to 1.63). Proguanil AUC, C_{max}, and half-life increased in subjects with mild hepatic impairment when compared with healthy subjects. The proguanil AUC and half-life increased in patients with moderate hepatic impairment when compared with healthy subjects. Consistent with the increase in proguanil AUC, there were marked decreases in the systemic exposure of cycloguanil (C_{max} and AUC) and an increase in its elimination half-life in subjects with mild hepatic impairment when compared with healthy volunteers.

Elderly: In elderly subjects, the extent of systemic exposure (AUC) of cycloguanil was increased (point estimate = 2.36, CI = 1.7, 3.28). T_{max} was longer in elderly subjects (median, 8 hours) compared with younger subjects (median, 4 hours) and average elimination half-life was longer in elderly subjects (mean, 14.9 hours) compared with younger subjects (mean, 8.3 hours).

Children: The pharmacokinetics of proguanil and cycloguanil are similar in adult and pediatric patients. However, the elimination half-life of atovaquone is shorter in pediatric patients (1 to 2 days) than in adult patients (2 to 3 days).

ATOVAQUONE AND PROGUANIL HYDROCHLORIDE — ORAL

Contraindications

Hypersensitivity to atovaquone, proguanil, or any component of the formulation.

For prophylaxis of *P. falciparum* malaria in patients with severe renal impairment (Ccr less than 30 mL/min).

Warnings

➤*Renal function impairment:* Do not use for malaria prophylaxis in patients with severe renal impairment (Ccr less than 30 mL/min). Use with caution for the treatment of malaria in patients with severe renal impairment (Ccr less than 30 mL/min) only if the benefits of the 3-day treatment regimen outweigh the potential risks associated with increased drug exposure. Administer with caution to patients with severe pre-existing renal failure because proguanil is eliminated by renal excretion.

➤*Carcinogenesis:* Atovaquone 24-month studies in mice showed treatment-related increases in incidence of hepatocellular adenoma and hepatocellular carcinoma at all doses tested, which ranged from approximately 5 to 8 times the average steady-state plasma concentrations in humans during prophylaxis of malaria.

➤*Mutagenesis:* Cycloguanil, the active metabolite of proguanil, was negative in the Ames test, but was positive in the mouse lymphoma assay and the mouse micronucleus assay. These positive effects with cycloguanil, a dihydrofolate reductase inhibitor, were significantly reduced or abolished with folinic acid supplementation.

➤*Pregnancy: Category C.* Falciparum malaria carries a higher risk of morbidity and mortality in pregnant women than in the general population. Maternal death and fetal loss are known complications of falciparum malaria in pregnancy. In pregnant women who must travel to malaria-endemic areas, personal protection against mosquito bites should always be employed (see Patient Information) in addition to antimalarials.

In rabbits, atovaquone caused maternal toxicity at plasma concentrations that were approximately 0.6 to 1.3 times the estimated human exposure during treatment of malaria. Adverse fetal effects in rabbits, including decreased fetal body lengths and increased early resorption and postimplantation losses, were observed only in the presence of maternal toxicity. Concentrations of atovaquone in rabbit fetuses averaged 30% of the concurrent maternal plasma concentrations.

While there are no adequate and well-controlled studies of atovaquone or proguanil in pregnant women; the combination may be used if the potential benefit justifies the potential risk to the fetus. The proguanil component acts by inhibiting the parasitic dihydrofolate reductase (see Pharmacology). However, there are no clinical data indicating that folate supplementation diminishes drug efficacy, and for women of childbearing age receiving folate supplements to prevent neural tube birth defects, such supplements may be continued while taking the atovaquone/proguanil combination.

➤*Lactation:* It is not known whether atovaquone is excreted in breast milk. In a rat study, atovaquone concentrations in the milk were 30% of the concurrent atovaquone concentrations in the maternal plasma. Proguanil is excreted in breast milk in small quantities. Exercise caution when the atovaquone/proguanil combination is administered to a nursing woman.

➤*Children:* The safety and efficacy of atovaquone/proguanil for the treatment of malaria have been established in controlled studies involving pediatric patients weighing 5 kg or more. Safety and efficacy have not been established in pediatric patients who weigh less than 5 kg.

The safety and efficacy of atovaquone/proguanil have been established for the prophylaxis of malaria in controlled studies involving children weighing 11 kg or more. Safety and efficacy have not been established in children who weigh less than 11 kg.

Precautions

➤*Cerebral malaria:* Atovaquone/proguanil combination has not been evaluated for the treatment of cerebral malaria or other severe manifestations of complicated malaria, including hyperparasitemia, pulmonary edema, or renal failure. Patients with severe malaria are not candidates for oral therapy.

➤*Diarrhea/vomiting:* Absorption of atovaquone may be reduced in patients with diarrhea or vomiting. If atovaquone/proguanil combination is used in patients who are vomiting (see Administration and Dosage), closely monitor parasitemia and consider the use of an antiemetic. Vomiting occurred in 19% or less of pediatric patients given treatment doses. In controlled clinical trials, 15.3% of adults who were treated with atovaquone/proguanil received an antiemetic. Of these patients, 98.3% were successfully treated. In patients with severe or persistent diarrhea or vomiting, alternative antimalarial therapy may be required.

➤*Relapse:* Parasite relapse occurred commonly when *Plasmodium vivax* malaria was treated with atovaquone/proguanil alone. In the event of recrudescent *P. falciparum* infections after treatment with or failure of chemoprophylaxis with atovaquone/proguanil, treat patients with a different blood schizonticide.

Drug Interactions

Atovaquone is highly protein bound (more than 99%) but does not displace other highly protein-bound drugs in vitro. Proguanil is metabolized primarily by CYP2C19. Potential pharmacokinetic interactions with other substrates or inhibitors of this pathway are unknown.

Atovaquone/Proguanil Drug Interactions

Precipitant drug	Object drug*		Description
Metoclopramide	Atovaquone	⬇	Concomitant treatment with metoclopramide has been associated with decreased bioavailability of atovaquone. Use only if other antiemetics are not available.
Rifampin Rifabutin	Atovaquone	⬇	Concomitant administration of rifampin or rifabutin is known to reduce atovaquone levels by approximately 50% and 34% respectively. The concomitant administration of these agents is not recommended. The mechanism of this interaction is unknown.
Tetracycline	Atovaquone	⬇	Concomitant treatment with tetracycline has been associated with ≈ 40% reduction in plasma concentrations of atovaquone. Closely monitor parasitemia in patients receiving tetracycline.
Atovaquone	Zidovudine	⬆	Zidovudine concentrations may be elevated, increasing the risk of zidovudine toxicity.

* ⬇ = Object drug decreased. ⬆ = Object drug increased.

➤*Drug/Food interactions:* Dietary fat taken with atovaquone increases the rate and extent of absorption, increasing AUC 2 to 3 times and C_{max} 5 times over fasting. The absolute bioavailability of the tablet formulation of atovaquone when taken with food is 23%. Atovaquone/proguanil tablets should be taken with food or a milky drink. Proguanil is extensively absorbed regardless of food intake.

Adverse Reactions

Malaria prevention – Among subjects who received atovaquone/proguanil for prophylaxis of malaria, adverse reactions occurred in similar proportions of subjects receiving the combination or placebo. The most commonly reported adverse experiences possibly attributable to atovaquone/proguanil or placebo were headache and abdominal pain. Prophylaxis was discontinued prematurely because of treatment-related adverse experiences in 3 of 381 adults and 0 of 125 pediatric patients.

In an additional placebo-controlled study of malaria prophylaxis with atovaquone/proguanil involving 330 pediatric patients, the most common treatment-emergent adverse events with atovaquone/proguanil were abdominal pain and headache (13%) and cough (10%). Abdominal pain (13% vs 8%) and vomiting (5% vs 3%) were reported more often with atovaquone/proguanil than with placebo, while fever (5% vs 12%) and diarrhea (1% vs 5%) were more common with placebo.

Malaria treatment – Among adults who received atovaquone/proguanil for malaria treatment, attributable adverse experiences that occurred in 5% or more of patients were abdominal pain (17%); nausea, vomiting (12%); headache (10%); diarrhea, asthenia (8%); anorexia, dizziness (5%). Treatment was discontinued prematurely because of an adverse experience in 4 of 436 adults.

Among children (weighing 11 to 40 kg) who received atovaquone/proguanil for malaria treatment, attributable adverse experiences that occurred in 5% or more of patients were vomiting (10%) and pruritus (6%). Vomiting occurred in 43 of 319 (13%) pediatric patients who did not have symptomatic malaria but were given treatment doses of atovaquone/proguanil for 3 days in a clinical trial. The design of this clinical trial required that any patient who vomited be withdrawn from the trial. Among pediatric patients with symptomatic malaria treated with the combination, treatment was discontinued prematurely because of an adverse experience in 1 of 116 (0.9%).

In a study of 100 pediatric patients (5 to less than 11 kg body weight) who received atovaquone/proguanil for the treatment of uncomplicated *P. falciparum* malaria, only diarrhea (6%) occurred in 5% or more of patients as an adverse experience attributable to atovaquone/proguanil. In 3 patients (3%), treatment was discontinued prematurely because of an adverse experience.

➤*Lab test abnormalities:* Abnormalities in laboratory tests reported in clinical trials were limited to elevations of transaminases in malaria patients being treated with atovaquone/proguanil. The frequency of these abnormalities varied substantially across studies of treatment and were not observed in the randomized portions of the prophylaxis trials.

In one phase 3 trial of malaria treatment in Thai adults, early elevations of AST and ALT were observed to occur more frequently in patients treated with atovaquone/proguanil compared with patients treated with an active control drug. Rates for patients who had normal baseline levels of these clinical laboratory parameters were: day 7 – ALT 26.7% vs 15.6%; AST 16.9% vs 8.6%. By day 14 of this 28-day study, the frequency of transaminase elevations equalized across the 2 groups.

In this and other studies in which transaminase elevations occurred, they were noted to persist for 4 weeks or less following treatment with atovaquone/proguanil for malaria. None were associated with untoward clinical events.

ATOVAQUONE AND PROGUANIL HYDROCHLORIDE — ORAL

Adverse Reactions of Atovaquone/Proguanil Combination for Prophylaxis of Malaria (%)

	Adults			Children and adolescents	
	Placebo (n = 206)	Atovaquone/ Proguanil[a] (n = 206)	Atovaquone/ Proguanil[b] (n = 381)	Placebo (n = 140)	Atovaquone/ Proguanil (n = 125)
Any adverse event	32%	17%	17%	41%	42%
GI					
Abdominal pain	5%	4%	3%	29	31%
Diarrhea	3%	2%	1%	1%	0%
Dyspepsia	4%	2%	1%	0%	0%
Gastritis	2%	3%	2%	0%	0%
Vomiting	less than 1%	less than 1%	less than 1%	6%	7%
Respiratory					
Cough	less than 1%	less than 1%	1%	0%	0%
Upper respiratory tract infection	0%	0%	0%	0%	0%
Miscellaneous					
Back pain	0%	0%	0%	0%	0%
Fever	1%	0%	0%	less than 1%	0%
Flu syndrome	0%	0%	0%	0%	0%
Headache	7%	3%	5%	14%	14%
Myalgia	0%	0%	0%	0%	0%

[a] Subjects receiving the recommended dose of atovaquone and proguanil in placebo-controlled trials.
[b] Subjects receiving the recommended dose of atovaquone and proguanil in any trial.

➤*Postmarketing:*

CNS – Rare cases of seizures and psychotic events (eg, hallucinations); however, a causal relationship has not been established.

Dermatologic – Cutaneous reactions ranging from rash, photosensitivity, and urticaria to rare cases of erythema multiforme and Stevens-Johnson syndrome.

Overdosage

There have been no reports of overdosage of atovaquone/proguanil combination tablets substantially higher than the doses recommended for treatment.

➤*Symptoms:*

Atovaquone – Overdoses with 31,500 mg or less of atovaquone have been reported. In one such patient who also took an unspecified dose of dapsone, methemoglobinemia occurred. Rash also has been reported after overdose.

Proguanil – Overdoses of proguanil as large as 1,500 mg have been followed by complete recovery, and doses as high as 700 mg twice daily have been taken for more than 2 weeks without serious toxicity. Adverse events occasionally associated with proguanil doses of 100 to 200 mg/day, such as epigastric discomfort and vomiting, would be likely to occur with overdose. There also are reports of reversible hair loss and scaling of the skin on the palms or soles, reversible aphthous ulceration, and hematologic side effects.

➤*Treatment:*

Atovaquone – There is no known antidote for atovaquone, and it is currently unknown if atovaquone is dialyzable. The median lethal dose is higher than the maximum oral dose tested in mice and rats (1,825 mg/kg/day).

Patient Information

Instruct patients to do the following:

- Take atovaquone/proguanil combination tablets at the same time each day with food or a milky drink.
- Take a repeat dose of the combination if vomiting occurs within 1 hour after dosing.
- Consult a health care professional regarding alternative forms of prophylaxis if prophylaxis with atovaquone/proguanil is prematurely discontinued for any reason.
- Include protective clothing, insect repellants, and bed nets as important components of malaria prophylaxis.
- No chemoprophylactic regimen is 100% effective; therefore, patients should seek medical attention for any febrile illness that occurs during or after return from a malaria-endemic area and inform their health care professional that they may have been exposed to malaria.
- *Falciparum* malaria carries a higher risk of death and serious complications in pregnant women than in the general population. Pregnant women anticipating travel to malarious areas should discuss the risks and benefits of such travel with their physicians (see Pregnancy section).
- If a dose is missed, take it as soon as possible, then return to the normal schedule. If a dose is skipped, do not double the next dose.

ANTITUBERCULOSIS AGENTS

Antituberculosis drugs have been described in terms of the following 3 areas of activity: Bactericidal activity, sterilizing activity, and drug resistance prevention. Isoniazid is the most potent bactericidal antituberculosis agent, although rifampin and streptomycin have some bactericidal activity. Rifampin and pyrazinamide are the most potent sterilizing drugs for tuberculosis. Drugs that eliminate all bacterial populations and do not allow the emergence of resistant organisms prevent drug resistance.

Standard treatment regimens are divided into the following 2 phases: An initial phase, during which agents are used to kill rapidly multiplying populations of *Mycobacterium tuberculosis* and to prevent the emergence of drug resistance, followed by a continuation phase, during which sterilizing drugs kill the intermittently dividing populations.

The initial phase of the regimen must contain ≥ 3 of the following drugs: Isoniazid, rifampin, and pyrazinamide, along with either ethambutol or streptomycin if the local resistance pattern to isoniazid is not documented or is more than 4%.

➤*Directly observed therapy (DOT):* Adherence to the treatment regimen can be achieved by DOT, the "gold standard." The health care provider watches the patient swallow each dose of medication. This allows for monitoring the number of doses that an individual has taken.

DOT may be given intermittently (2 to 3 times/week) or daily. Intermittent therapy was introduced when it was shown in controlled clinical trials that therapeutic serum levels of the various antituberculosis drugs were maintained even when medications were given only 2 or 3 times/week. Intermittent regimens do not have more toxic effects than daily regimens; allow drug administration to be adapted to local conditions. All intermittent regimens must involve DOT.

Recommended Drugs for the Treatment of Tuberculosis in Children and Adults[1]

Drug	Daily dose[2]		Maximum daily dose in children and adults	Twice weekly dose		3 times/week dose	
	Children	Adults		Children	Adults	Children	Adults
Initial treatment							
Isoniazid	10 to 20 mg/kg PO or IM	5 mg/kg PO or IM	300 mg	20 to 40 mg/kg max 900 mg	15 mg/kg max 900 mg	20 to 40 mg/kg max 900 mg	15 mg/kg max 900 mg
Rifampin	10 to 20 mg/kg PO	10 mg/kg PO	600 mg	10 to 20 mg/kg max 600 mg	10 mg/kg max 600 mg	10 to 20 mg/kg max 600 mg	10 mg/kg max 600 mg
Pyrazinamide	15 to 30 mg/kg PO	15 to 30 mg/kg PO	2 g	50 to 70 mg/kg max 4 g	50 to 70 mg/kg max 4 g	50 to 70 mg/kg max 3 g	50 to 70 mg/kg max 3 g
Streptomycin	20 to 40 mg/kg IM	15 mg/kg IM	1 g[3]	25 to 30 mg/kg IM max 1.5 g	25 to 30 mg/kg IM max 1.5 g	25 to 30 mg/kg max 1.5 g	25 to 30 mg/kg max 1.5 g
Ethambutol	15 to 25 mg/kg PO	15 to 25 mg/kg PO	—	50 mg/kg	50 mg/kg	25 to 30 mg/kg	25 to 30 mg/kg
Rifapentine	—	—	—	—	600 mg PO	—	—
Second-line treatment							
Cycloserine	15 to 20 mg/kg PO	15 to 20 mg/kg PO	1 g	—	—	—	—
Ethionamide	15 to 20 mg/kg PO	15 to 20 mg/kg PO	1 g	—	—	—	—

Recommended Drugs for the Treatment of Tuberculosis in Children and Adults[1]							
	Daily dose[2]		Maximum daily dose in children and adults	Twice weekly dose		3 times/week dose	
Drug	Children	Adults		Children	Adults	Children	Adults
Capreomycin	15 to 30 mg/kg IM	15 to 30 mg/kg IM	1 g	—	—	—	—
Kanamycin	15 to 30 mg/kg IM or IV	15 to 30 mg/kg IM or IV	1 g	—	—	—	—
Ciprofloxacin	—	1000 to 1500 mg PO	1500 mg	—	—	—	—
Ofloxacin		800 mg PO	800 mg	—	—	—	—
Levofloxacin	—	500 to 750 mg PO	750 mg	—	—	—	—
Sparfloxacin	—	200 mg PO	200 mg	—	—	—	—
P-aminosalicylic acid	150 mg/kg PO	150 mg/kg PO	12 g	—	—	—	—
Rifabutin	—	300 to 450 mg PO	—	—	—	—	—

[1] For detailed dosing information and frequency, see individual monographs.
[2] Doses based on weight. Adjust as weight changes.
[3] In people ≥ 60 years of age, limit the daily dose of streptomycin to 0.5 g IM.

➤*Treatment regimens:* Treatment for tuberculosis is a long-term process. Begin treatment as soon as possible after diagnosis. Combination therapy is required. The CDC recommends at least a 3-drug regimen with rifampin, isoniazid, and pyrazinamide for a minimum of 2 months, followed by rifampin and isoniazid for 4 months in areas with a low incidence of tuberculosis. Administer streptomycin or ethambutol for the first 2 months in areas with a high incidence of tuberculosis.

➤*Retreatment:* Retreatment is necessary when treatment fails because of noncompliance or inadequate drug treatment. Retreatment regimens include ≥ 4 drugs; however, depending on disease progression and the bacteriostatic or bactericidal activity of the drug, ≤ 7 drugs can be used. Retreatment drug regimens most commonly include the second-line agents of ethionamide, aminosalicylic acid, cycloserine, and capreomycin, as well as ofloxacin and ciprofloxacin.

Therapy includes 2 or 3 agents not given previously when current susceptibility data are unavailable. Add to the initial 4-drug regimen of isoniazid, rifampin, pyrazinamide, and ethambutol or streptomycin, ≥ 2 drugs to which the organism is susceptible on the basis of local resistance patterns. The ineffective agents may be discontinued once susceptibility test results are available.

Individualize treatment on the basis of the susceptibility pattern of the infecting organism when re-treating patients known to be infected with drug-resistant isolates. Include in this regimen ≥ 3 new drugs to which the organism is susceptible. Continue therapy until sputum cultures convert to negative and then continue therapy for an additional 12 months with 2 drugs. Treatment may be continued for 24 months after sputum culture conversion.

➤*HIV:* The initial phase of a 6-month tuberculosis regimen consists of isoniazid, rifabutin, pyrazinamide, and ethambutol for patients receiving therapy with protease inhibitors or nonnucleoside reverse transcriptase inhibitors. These drugs are administered a) daily for at least the first 2 weeks, followed by twice weekly dosing for 6 weeks or b) daily for 8 weeks to complete the 2-month induction phase. The second phase of treatment consists of rifabutin and isoniazid administered twice weekly or daily for 4 months.

Patients for whom the use of rifamycins is limited or contraindicated for any reason (eg, patient/clinician decision not to combine antiretroviral therapy with rifabutin, intolerance to rifamycins), the initial phase of a 9-month tuberculosis regimen consists of isoniazid, streptomycin, pyrazinamide, and ethambutol administered a) daily for at least the first 2 weeks, followed by twice weekly dosing for 6 weeks or b) daily for 8 weeks to complete the 2-month induction phase. The second phase of treatment consists of isoniazid, streptomycin, and pyrazinamide administered 2 to 3 times/week for 7 months.

The preferred option for patients who are not candidates for antiretroviral therapy or for whom a decision is made not to combine the initiation of tuberculosis therapy with antiretroviral therapy is to administer a 6-month regimen of isoniazid, rifampin, pyrazinamide, and ethambutol or streptomycin. These drugs are administered a) daily for at least the first 2 weeks, followed by 2 or 3 times/week dosing for 6 weeks or b) daily for 8 weeks to complete the 2-month induction phase. The second phase of treatment consists of isoniazid and rifampin administered daily or 2 to 3 times/week for 4 months. Isoniazid, rifampin, pyrazinamide, and ethambutol or streptomycin can be administered 3 times/week for 6 months.

Do not use tuberculosis regimens consisting of isoniazid, ethambutol, and pyrazinamide (ie, 3-drug regimens that do not contain a rifamycin, an aminoglycoside [eg, streptomycin, amikacin, kanamycin], or capreomycin) for the treatment of patients with HIV-related tuberculosis. The minimum duration of therapy is 18 months (or 12 months after documented culture conversion) if these regimens are used for the treatment of tuberculosis.

Administer pyridoxine (vitamin B_6) 25 to 50 mg daily or 50 to 100 mg twice weekly to all HIV-infected patients who are undergoing tuberculosis treatment with isoniazid to reduce the occurrence of isoniazid-induced side effects in the central and peripheral nervous system.

Because the MMWR's most recent recommendations for the use of antiretroviral therapy strongly advise against interruptions of therapy, and because alternative tuberculosis treatments that do not contain rifampin are available, previous antituberculosis therapy options that involved stopping protease inhibitor therapy to allow the use of rifampin are no longer recommended.

➤*Pregnancy:* Do not delay treatment for suspected or confirmed tuberculosis during pregnancy. The best therapeutic choices with the least danger to the fetus appear to be combinations of isoniazid, ethambutol, and rifampin. Pyrazinamide and streptomycin are not recommended during pregnancy because of possible teratogenic effects. Administer pyridoxine to all pregnant women receiving tuberculosis treatment to prevent peripheral neuropathy as a result of taking isoniazid. In pregnant women, delay prophylaxis until after delivery.

➤*Multidrug resistance:* The most recent cultures should undergo susceptibility testing to all antituberculosis drugs if cultures remain positive after 3 to 4 months of treatment. The patient may continue to receive the most recent treatment regimen, if his or her condition is clinically stable, while awaiting results of drug susceptibility testing. Alternatively, add ≥ 2 new drugs to the original medications if the patient is acutely ill. Administer an aminoglycoside or capreomycin as one of the medications, because these drugs lead to earlier sputum conversion.

➤*Chemoprophylaxis:* Administer isoniazid to adults in a daily dose of 300 mg for 1 year. Administer 10 mg/kg to a maximum daily dose of 300 mg for 1 year to children. Consider prophylactic therapy for the following: Those exposed to tuberculosis but who have no evidence of infection; those with infection (positive tuberculin test: greater than 5 mm [HIV infected] or 10 mm [not immunocompromised] of induration to 5 units purified protein derivative [PPD]) and no apparent disease; those with a history of tuberculosis but in whom the disease is presently "inactive;" and anergic people from populations at risk for tuberculosis. Prophylaxis with isoniazid is contraindicated for patients who have had reactions to the drug or have active hepatic disease. There are insufficient data on the advisability of prophylaxis with alternative drugs such as rifampin.

ISONIAZID (Isonicotinic acid hydrazide; INH)

Rx	**Isoniazid** (Various, eg, Barr, Eon, Paddock, UDL)	**Tablets:** 100 mg	In 30s, 100s, and 1000s.
Rx	**Isoniazid** (Various, eg, Barr, Eon, Major, UDL)	**Tablets:** 300 mg	In 30s, 60s, 100s, 200s, and 1000s.
Rx	**Isoniazid** (Carolina Medical)	**Syrup:** 50 mg/5 ml	Sorbitol. Orange flavor. In pt.
Rx	**Nydrazid** (Apothecon)	**Injection:** 100 mg/ml	In 10 ml vials.[1]

[1] With 0.25% chlorobutanol.

ISONIAZID — ORAL

WARNING

Hepatitis – Severe and sometimes fatal hepatitis associated with isoniazid therapy has been reported and may occur or may develop even after many months of treatment. The risk of developing hepatitis is age related. Approximate case rates by age are as follows: less than 1 per 1,000 for persons younger than 20 years of age, 3 per 1,000 for persons in the 20- to 34-years of age group, 12 per 1,000 for persons in the 35- to 49-years of age group, 23 per 1,000 for persons in the 50- to 64-years of age group, and 8 per 1,000 for persons older than 65 years of age. The risk of hepatitis is increased with daily consumption of alcohol. Precise data to provide a fatality rate for isoniazid-related hepatitis is not available; however, in a US public health service surveillance study of 13,838 persons taking isoniazid, there were 8 deaths among 174 cases of hepatitis.

Therefore, carefully monitor patients given isoniazid and interview patients at monthly intervals. For persons older than 35 years of age, in addition to monthly symptom reviews, measure hepatic enzymes (specifically, AST and ALT) prior to starting isoniazid therapy and periodically throughout treatment. Isoniazid-associated hepatitis usually occurs during the first 3 months of treatment. Usually, enzyme levels return to normal despite continuance of drug, but, in some cases, progressive liver dysfunction occurs. Other factors associated with an increased risk of hepatitis include daily use of alcohol, chronic liver disease, and injection drug use. A recent report suggests an increased risk of fatal hepatitis associated with isoniazid among women, particularly black and Hispanic women. The risk may also be increased during the postpartum period. Consider more careful monitoring in these groups, possibly including more frequent laboratory monitoring. If abnormalities of liver function exceed 3 to 5 times the upper limit of normal (ULN), strongly consider discontinuation of isoniazid. Liver function tests are not a substitute for a clinical evaluation at monthly intervals or for the prompt assessment of signs or symptoms of adverse reactions occurring between regularly scheduled evaluations. Instruct patients to immediately report signs or symptoms consistent with liver damage or other adverse reactions. These include any of the following: unexplained anorexia, nausea, vomiting, dark urine, icterus, rash, persistent paresthesias of the hands and feet, persistent fatigue, weakness or fever of greater than 3-day duration or abdominal tenderness, especially right-upper-quadrant discomfort. If these symptoms appear or if signs suggestive of hepatic damage are detected, promptly discontinue isoniazid, because continued use of the drug in these cases has been reported to cause a more severe form of liver damage.

Give patients with tuberculosis who have hepatitis attributed to isoniazid appropriate treatment with alternative drugs. If isoniazid must be reinstituted, do so only after symptoms and laboratory abnormalities have cleared. Restart the drug in very small and gradually increasing doses and withdraw immediately if there is any indication of recurrent liver involvement.

Defer preventive treatment in persons with acute hepatic diseases.

Indications

➤*Tuberculosis treatment:* For all forms of tuberculosis in which organisms are susceptible. However, active tuberculosis must be treated with multiple, concomitant antituberculosis medications to prevent the emergence of drug resistance. Single-drug treatment of active tuberculosis with isoniazid, or any other medication, is inadequate therapy.

➤*Prophylaxis:* Isoniazid is recommended as preventive therapy for the following groups, regardless of age. (Note: The criterion for a positive reaction to a skin test [in millimeters (mm) of induration] for each group is given in parenthesis).

HIV – Persons with HIV infection (greater than or equal to 5 mm) and persons with risk factors for HIV infection whose HIV infection status is unknown but who are suspected of having HIV infection. Preventive therapy may be considered for HIV-infected persons who are tuberculin negative but belong to groups in which the prevalence of tuberculosis is high. Candidates for preventive therapy who have HIV infection should have a minimum of 12 months of therapy.

Close contacts of people with infectious tuberculosis – Close contacts of persons with newly diagnosed infectious tuberculosis (greater than or equal to 5 mm). In addition, tuberculin-negative (less than 5 mm) children and adolescents who have been close contacts of infectious persons within the past 3 months are candidates for preventive therapy until a repeat tuberculin skin test is done 12 weeks after the infectious source. If the repeat skin test is positive (greater than 5 mm), continue therapy.

Recent converters – Recent converters, as indicated by a tuberculin skin test (greater than or equal to 10 mm increase within a 2-year period for those younger than 35 years old; greater than or equal to 15 mm increase for those 35 years of age and older). All infants and children younger than 4 years of age with a greater than 10 mm skin test are included in this category.

Abnormal chest radiographs – Persons with abnormal chest radiographs that show fibrotic lesions likely to represent old healed tuberculosis (greater than or equal to 5 mm). Candidates for preventive therapy who have fibrotic pulmonary lesions consistent with healed tuberculosis or who have pulmonary silicosis should have 12 months of isoniazid or 4 months of rifampin, concomitantly.

IV drug users – Intravenous (IV) drug users known to be HIV-seronegative (greater than 10 mm).

Increased risk of tuberculosis – Persons with the following medical conditions that have been reported to increase the risk of tuberculosis (greater than or equal to 10 mm); silicosis; diabetes mellitus; prolonged therapy with adrenocorticosteroids; immunosuppressive therapy; some hematologic and reticuloendothelial diseases, such as leukemia or Hodgkin disease; end-stage renal disease; clinical situations associated with substantial rapid weight loss or chronic undernutrition (including the following: intestinal bypass surgery for obesity, the postgastrectomy state with or without weight loss, chronic peptic ulcer disease, chronic malabsorption syndromes, and carcinomas of the oropharynx and upper GI tract that prevent adequate nutritional intake). Candidates for preventive therapy who have fibrotic pulmonary lesions consistent with healed tuberculosis pulmonary silicosis should have 12 months of isoniazid or 4 months of isoniazid and rifampin, concomitantly.

Adults younger than 35 years of age with tuberculin skin test reaction of greater than or equal to 10 mm – Additionally, in the absence of any of the above risk factors, persons younger than 35 years of age with a tuberculin skin test reaction of greater than or equal to 10 mm are also appropriate candidates for preventive therapy if they are a member of any of the following high-incidence groups.

- Foreign-born persons from high-prevalence countries who never received BCG vaccine.
- Medically underserved low-income populations, including high-risk racial or ethnic minority populations, especially blacks, Hispanics, and Native Americans.
- Residents of facilities for long-term care (eg, correctional institutions, nursing homes, mental institutions).

Children younger than 4 years of age – Children who are younger than 4 years old are candidates for isoniazid-preventive therapy if they have greater than 10 mm induration from a purified protein derivative (PPD) Mantoux tuberculin skin test.

Adults younger than 35 years of age with tuberculin skin test reaction of greater than or equal to 15 mm – Finally, persons younger than 35 years of age who: have none of the above risk factors, belong to none of the high-incidence groups, and have tuberculin skin test reactions of 15 mm or more, are appropriate candidates for preventive therapy.

The risk of hepatitis must be weighed against the risk of tuberculosis in positive tuberculin reactors older than 35 of age. However, the use of isoniazid is for those with the additional risk factors listed above and on an individual basis in situations where there is likelihood of serious consequences to contacts who may become infected.

Administration and Dosage

Do not administer isoniazid with food. Studies have shown that the bioavailability of isoniazid is reduced significantly when administered with food.

➤*Treatment of tuberculosis:* Isoniazid is used in conjunction with other effective antituberculosis agents. Perform drug susceptibility testing on the organisms initially isolated from all patients with newly diagnosed tuberculosis. If the bacilli becomes resistant, therapy must be changed to agents which the bacilli are susceptible.

Usual oral dosage (depending on the regimen used) –

Adults: 5 mg/kg up to 300 mg/day in a single dose or 15 mg/kg up to 900 mg/day, 2 or 3 times/week.

Children: 10 to 15 mg/kg up to 300 mg/day in a single dose or 20 to 40 mg/kg up to 900 mg/day, 2 or 3 times/week.

Pulmonary tuberculosis without HIV infection – There are 3 regimen options for the initial treatment of tuberculosis in children and adults:

Option 1: Daily isoniazid, rifampin, and pyrazinamide for 8 weeks followed by 16 weeks of isoniazid and rifampin daily or 2 to 3 times weekly. Add ethambutol or streptomycin to the initial regimen until sensitivity to isoniazid and rifampin is demonstrated. The addition of a fourth drug is optional if the relative prevalence of isoniazid-resistant *Mycobacterium tuberculosis* isolates in the community is less than or equal to 4%.

Option 2: Daily isoniazid, rifampin, pyrazinamide, and streptomycin or ethambutol for 2 weeks followed by twice-weekly administration of the same drugs for 6 weeks, subsequently twice-weekly isoniazid and rifampin for 16 weeks.

Option 3: Three times weekly with isoniazid, rifampin, pyrazinamide, and ethambutol or streptomycin for 6 months.

Administer all regimens given twice weekly or 3 times weekly by directly observed therapy. See Directly observed therapy (DOT).

The above treatment guidelines apply only when the disease is caused by organisms that are susceptible to the standard antituberculous agents. Because of the impact of resistance to isoniazid and rifampin on the response to therapy, it is essential that health care providers initiating therapy for tuberculosis be familiar with the prevalence of drug resistance in their communities. It is suggested that ethambutol not be used in children whose visual acuity cannot be monitored.

Pulmonary tuberculosis and HIV infection – The response of the immunologically impaired host to treatment may not be as satisfactory as that of a person with normal host responsiveness. For this reason, therapeutic decisions for the impaired host must be individualized. Since patients coinfected with HIV may have problems with malabsorption, screening of antimycobacterial drug levels, especially in patients with advanced HIV disease, may be necessary to prevent the emergence of multidrug-resistant tuberculosis (MDRTB).

Extra pulmonary tuberculosis – The basic principles that underlie the treatment of pulmonary tuberculosis also apply to extra pulmonary forms of the disease. Although there have not been the same kinds of carefully conducted controlled trials of treatment of extra pulmonary tuberculosis as for pulmonary disease, increasing clinical experience indicates that a 6- to 9-month short-course regimen is effective. Because of the insufficient data,

ISONIAZID — ORAL

military tuberculosis, bone/joint tuberculosis, and tuberculous meningitis in infants and children should receive 12-month therapy.

Bacteriologic evaluation of extra pulmonary tuberculosis may be limited by the relative inaccessibility of the sites of disease. Thus, response to treatment often must be judged on the basis of clinical and radiographic findings.

The use of adjunctive therapies such as surgery and corticosteroids is more commonly required in extra pulmonary tuberculosis than in pulmonary disease. Surgery may be necessary to obtain specimens for diagnosis and to treat such processes as constrictive pericarditis and spinal cord compression from Pott disease. Corticosteroids have been shown to be of benefit in preventing cardiac constriction from tuberculous pericarditis and in decreasing the neurologic sequelae of all stages of tuberculosis meningitis, especially when administered early in the course of the disease.

Pregnant women with tuberculosis – The treatment options previously listed must be adjusted for the pregnant patient. Streptomycin interferes with in utero development of the ear and may cause congenital deafness. Routine use of pyrazinamide is also not recommended in pregnancy because of inadequate teratogenicity data. The initial treatment regimen should consist of isoniazid and rifampin. Include ethambutol unless primary isoniazid resistance is unlikely (isoniazid resistance rate documented to be less than 4%).

MDRTB – MDRTB (ie, resistance to at least isoniazid and rifampin) presents difficult treatment problems. Treatment must be individualized and based on susceptibility studies. In such cases, consultation with an expert in tuberculosis is recommended.

➤*For preventive therapy of tuberculosis:* Before isoniazid preventive therapy is initiated, bacteriologically positive or radiographically progressive tuberculosis must be excluded. Perform appropriate evaluations if extra pulmonary tuberculosis is suspected.

Adults over 30 kg – 300 mg/day in a single dose.

Infants and children – 10 mg/kg (up to 300 mg daily) in a single dose. In situations where adherence with daily preventive therapy cannot be ensured, 20 to 30 mg/kg (not to exceed 900 mg) twice weekly under the direct observation of a health care provider at the time of administration.

Continuous administration of isoniazid for a sufficient period is an essential part of the regimen because relapse rates are higher if chemotherapy is stopped prematurely. In the treatment of tuberculosis, resistant organisms may multiply and the emergence of resistant organisms during the treatment may necessitate a change in the regimen.

Directly observed therapy (DOT) – A major cause of drug-resistant tuberculosis is patient noncompliance with treatment. The use of directly observed therapy can help ensure patient compliance with drug therapy. Directly observed therapy is the observation of the patient by a healthcare provider or other responsible person as the patient ingests antituberculosis medications. Directly observed therapy can be achieved with daily, twice-weekly, or thrice-weekly regimens and is recommended for all patients.

For following patient compliance – The Potts-Cozart test, a simple colorimetric method of checking for isoniazid in the urine is a useful tool for ensuring patient compliance, which is essential for effective tuberculosis control. Additionally, isoniazid test strips are also available to check patient compliance.

Concomitant pyridoxine therapy – Administration of pyridoxine (B_6) is recommended in malnourished and in those predisposed to neuropathy (eg, alcoholics, diabetics).

➤*Storage/Stability:* Store at controlled room temperature, 15° to 30°C (59° to 86°F). Protect from moisture and light. Dispense in a well-closed and light-resistant container with a child-resistant closure.

Actions

➤*Pharmacology:* Isoniazid inhibits the synthesis of mycoloic acids, an essential component of the bacterial cell wall. At therapeutic levels isoniazid is bacteriocidal against activity growing intracellular and extracellular *M. tuberculosis* organisms.

Isoniazid-resistant *Mycobacterium tuberculosis* bacilli develop rapidly when isoniazid monotherapy is administered.

➤*Pharmacokinetics:*

Absorption/Distribution – Within 1 to 2 hours after oral administration, isoniazid produces peak blood levels that decline to 50% or less within 6 hours. It diffuses readily into all body fluids (cerebrospinal, pleural, and ascitic fluids), tissues, organs, and excreta (saliva, sputum, and feces). The drug also passes through the placental barrier and into milk in concentrations comparable with those in the plasma.

Metabolism – Isoniazid is metabolized primarily by acetylation and dehydrazination. The rate of acetylation is genetically determined. Approximately 50% of black patients and white patients are "slow inactivators" and the rest are "rapid inactivators"; the majority of Eskimo and Asian patients are "rapid inactivators."

Excretion – From 50% to 70% of a dose of isoniazid is excreted in the urine within 24 hours. The rate of acetylation does not significantly alter the efficacy of isoniazid. However, slow acetylation may lead to higher blood levels of the drug and, thus, to an increase in toxic reactions.

Pyridoxine (vitamin B_6) deficiency is sometimes observed in adults with high doses of isoniazid and is considered probably due to its competition with pyridoxal phosphate for the enzyme apotryptophanase.

Contraindications

Severe hypersensitivity reactions, including drug-induced hepatitis; previous isoniazid-associated severe adverse reactions to isoniazid such as drug fever, chills, or arthritis; and acute liver disease of any etiology.

Warnings

➤*Hepatitis:* See the Warning box for more information.

➤*Hypersensitivity reactions:* All drugs should be stopped and an evaluation made at the first sign of a hypersensitivity reaction. If isoniazid therapy must be reinstituted, give the drug only after symptoms have cleared. Restart the drug in very small and gradually increasing doses and withdraw immediately if there is any indication of a recurrent hypersensitivity reaction.

➤*Carcinogenesis:* Isoniazid has been shown to induce pulmonary tumors in a number of strains of mice. Isoniazid has not been shown to be carcinogenic in humans. (Note: A diagnosis of mesothelioma in a child with prenatal exposure to isoniazid and no other apparent risk factors has been reported).

➤*Pregnancy: Category C.* Isoniazid has been shown to have an embryocidal effect in rats and rabbits when given orally during pregnancy. Isoniazid was not teratogenic in reproduction studies in mice, rats and rabbits. There are no adequate and well-controlled studies in pregnant women. Use isoniazid as a treatment for active tuberculosis during pregnancy because the benefit justifies the potential risk to the fetus. Weigh the benefit of preventive therapy against a possible risk to the fetus. Generally, start preventive therapy after delivery to prevent putting the fetus at risk of exposure; the low levels of isoniazid in breast milk do not threaten the neonate. Since isoniazid is known to cross the placental barrier, carefully observe neonates of isoniazid-treated mothers for any evidence of adverse effects.

➤*Lactation:* The small concentrations of isoniazid in breast milk do not produce toxicity in the breast-feeding newborn; therefore, do not discourage breast-feeding. However, because levels of isoniazid are so low in breast milk, they can not be relied upon for prophylaxis or therapy of breast-feeding infants.

Precautions

➤*Monitoring:* Carefully monitor use of isoniazid in the following: Daily users of alcohol (daily ingestion of alcohol may be associated with a higher incidence of isoniazid hepatitis); patients with active chronic liver disease or severe renal dysfunction; older than 35 years of age; concurrent use of any chronically administered medication; history of previous discontinuation of isoniazid; existence of peripheral neuropathy or conditions predisposing to neuropathy; pregnancy; injection drug use; women belonging to minority groups, particularly in the postpartum period; HIV-seropositive patients.

➤*Special risk:* Because there is a higher frequency of isoniazid-associated hepatitis among certain patient groups, including those older than 35 years of age, daily users of alcohol, chronic liver disease, drug use, and women belonging to minority groups, particularly in the postpartum period, obtain transaminase measurements prior to starting and monthly during preventive therapy, or more frequently as needed. If any of the values exceed 3 to 5 times the ULN, temporarily discontinue isoniazid and consider restarting therapy.

Drug Interactions

Isoniazid Drug Interactions

Precipitant drug	Object drug*		Description
Rifampin	Isoniazid	↑	Hepatotoxicity may occur at a rate higher than either agent alone. If alterations in liver function tests occur, consider discontinuation of one or both of these agents.
Isoniazid	Acetaminophen	↑	Hepatotoxicity has been reported due to inhibition of acetaminophen metabolism. Monitor patient for acetaminophen toxicity.
Isoniazid	Carbamazepine	↑	Isoniazid hepatotoxicity may result due to carbamazepine increasing isoniazid degradation to hepatotoxic metabolites. Carbamazepine toxicity may result due to inhibition of carbamazepine metabolism by isoniazid. Monitor serum carbamazepine concentrations, monitor liver function, and adjust doses as necessary.
Carbamazepine	Isoniazid	↑	
Isoniazid	Chlorzoxazone	↑	Plasma concentrations of chlorzoxazone may be elevated, increasing therapeutic and adverse effects. Adjust the dose of chlorzoxazone as appropriate.
Isoniazid	Disulfiram	↑	The coadministration of disulfiram and isoniazid may result in acute behavioral and coordination changes. The mechanism is unknown; possible excess dopaminergic activity may occur. If acute behavioral or coordination changes develop during concurrent administration of disulfiram and isoniazid, the disulfiram dose may need to be decreased or the drug discontinued.

ISONIAZID — ORAL

Isoniazid Drug Interactions

Precipitant drug	Object drug*		Description
Isoniazid	Enflurane	↑	In rapid isoniazid acetylators, high output renal failure may occur due to nephrotoxic concentrations of inorganic fluoride. Monitor renal function in patients receiving this combination, particularly those who are rapid acetylators.
Isoniazid	Hydantoins (eg, phenytoin)	↑	Serum hydantoin levels may be increased, producing an increase in the pharmacologic and toxic effects of hydantoins. In usual therapeutic doses, phenytoin toxicity appears to be most significant in patients who are slow acetylators of isoniazid. Monitor serum hydantoin levels and observe for toxicity.
Isoniazid	Ketoconazole	↓	The therapeutic benefit of ketoconazole may be attenuated. Avoid concomitant use if possible. Monitoring of ketoconazole serum levels or antifungal activity may be necessary.
Isoniazid	Valproate	↑	A recent case study has shown a possible increase in the plasma level of valproate when coadministered with isoniazid. Monitor plasma valproate concentration when isoniazid and valproate are coadministered and make appropriate dosage adjustments of valproate.
Isoniazid	Theophylline	↑	Isoniazid may increase theophylline plasma levels. Also a slight decrease in isoniazid elimination has been noted. Monitor and adjust the dose as necessary.
Theophylline	Isoniazid	↑	

* ↑ = Object drug increased. ↓ = Object drug decreased.

➤*Drug/Food interactions:* Do not administer isoniazid with food. Studies have shown that the bioavailability of isoniazid is reduced significantly when administered with food.

Adverse Reactions

The most frequent reactions are those affecting the nervous system and the liver.

➤*CNS:* Peripheral neuropathy is the most common toxic effect. It is dose related, occurs most often in the malnourished and in those predisposed to neuritis (eg, alcoholics, diabetics), and is usually preceded by paresthesias of the feet and hands. The incidence is higher in "slow inactivators".

Other neurotoxic effects, which are uncommon with conventional doses, are convulsions, toxic encephalopathy, optic neuritis and atrophy, memory impairment, and toxic psychosis.

➤*GI:* Nausea, vomiting, epigastric distress.

➤*Hematologic:* Agranulocytosis; hemolytic, sideroblastic, or aplastic anemia; thrombocytopenia; eosinophilia.

➤*Hepatic:* Elevated serum transaminase (AST, ALT), bilirubinemia, bilirubinuria, jaundice, and occasionally severe and sometimes fatal hepatitis. The common prodromal symptoms of hepatitis are anorexia, nausea, vomiting, fatigue, malaise, and weakness. Mild hepatic dysfunction, evidenced by mild and transient elevation of serum transaminase levels occurs in 10% to 20% of patients taking isoniazid.

See the Warning box for more information.

➤*Hypersensitivity:* Fever, skin eruptions (morbilliform, maculopapular, purpuric, or exfoliative), lymphadenopathy, vasculitis.

➤*Metabolic/Nutritional:* Pyridoxine deficiency, pellagra, hyperglycemia, metabolic acidosis, gynecomastia.

➤*Miscellaneous:* Rheumatic syndrome, systemic lupus erythematosus-like syndrome.

Overdosage

➤*Symptoms:* Isoniazid overdosage produces signs and symptoms within 30 minutes to 3 hours after ingestion. Nausea, vomiting, dizziness, slurring of speech, blurring of vision, and visual hallucinations (including bright colors and strange designs) are among the early manifestations. With marked overdosage, respiratory distress and CNS depression, progressing rapidly from stupor to profound coma, are to be expected, along with severe, intractable seizures. Severe metabolic acidosis, acetonuria, and hyperglycemia are typical laboratory findings.

➤*Treatment:*

For the asymptomatic patient – Absorption of drugs from the GI tract may be decreased by giving activated charcoal. Employ gastric emptying in the asymptomatic patient. Safeguard the patient's airway when employing these procedures. Patients who acutely ingest greater than 80 mg/kg should be treated with pyridoxine IV on a gram per gram (g) basis equal to the isoniazid dose. If an unknown amount of isoniazid is ingested, consider an initial dose of 5 g of pyridoxine given over 30 to 60 minutes in adults, 80 mg/kg of pyridoxine in children.

For the symptomatic patient – Ensure adequate ventilation, support cardiac output, and protect the airway while treating seizures and attempting to limit absorption. If the dose of isoniazid is known, initially treat the patient with a slow IV bolus of pyridoxine, over 3 to 5 minutes, on a gram per gram basis, equal to the isoniazid dose. If the quantity of isoniazid ingestion is unknown, then consider an initial IV bolus of pyridoxine of 5 g in the adult or 80 mg/kg in the child. If seizures continue, the dosage of pyridoxine may be repeated. It would be rare that greater than 10 g of pyridoxine would need to be given. The maximum safe dose for pyridoxine in isoniazid intoxication is not known. If the patient does not respond to pyridoxine, diazepam may be administered. Use phenytoin cautiously because isoniazid interferes with the metabolism of phenytoin.

General – Obtain blood samples for immediate determination of gases, electrolytes, serum urea nitrogen (BUN), glucose; type and cross-match blood in preparation for possible hemodialysis.

Rapid control of metabolic acidosis – Patients with this degree of isoniazid intoxication are likely to have hypoventilation. The administration of sodium bicarbonate under these circumstances can cause exacerbation of hypercarbia. Ventilation must be monitored carefully, by measuring blood carbon dioxide levels, and supported mechanically, if there is respiratory impairment.

Dialysis – Both peritoneal and hemodialysis have been used in the management of isoniazid overdosage. These procedures are probably not required if control of seizures and acidosis is achieved with pyridoxine, diazepam, and bicarbonate.

Along with measures based on initial and repeated determination of blood gases and other laboratory tests as needed, utilize meticulous respiratory and other intensive care to protect against hypoxia, hypotension, aspiration, and pneumonitis.

ISONIAZID — INJECTION

WARNING

Hepatitis – Severe and sometimes fatal hepatitis associated with isoniazid therapy has been reported and may occur or may develop even after many months of treatment. The risk of developing hepatitis is age related. Approximate case rates by age are as follows: Less than 1/1000 for persons younger than 20 years of age, 3/1000 for persons in the 20- to 34-year age group, 12/1000 for persons in the 35- to 49-year age group, 23/1000 for persons in the 50- to 64-year age group, and 8/1000 for persons older than 65 years of age. The risk of hepatitis is increased with daily consumption of alcohol. Precise data to provide a fatality rate for isoniazid-related hepatitis are not available; however, in a US Public Health Service surveillance study of 13,838 persons taking isoniazid, there were 8 deaths among 174 cases of hepatitis.

WARNING (cont.)

Therefore, patients given isoniazid should be carefully monitored and interviewed at monthly intervals. For persons 35 years of age and older, in addition to monthly symptom reviews, hepatic enzymes (specifically, AST and ALT) should be measured prior to starting isoniazid therapy and periodically throughout treatment. Isoniazid-associated hepatitis usually occurs during the first 3 months of treatment. Usually, enzyme levels return to normal despite continuance of drug, but in some cases progressive liver dysfunction occurs. Other factors associated with an increased risk of hepatitis include daily use of alcohol, chronic liver disease and injection drug use. A report suggests an increased risk of fatal hepatitis associated with isoniazid among women, particularly black and Hispanic women. The risk may also be increased during the postpartum period. More careful monitoring should be considered in these groups, possibly including more frequent laboratory monitoring. If abnormalities of liver function exceed 3 to 5 times the upper limit of normal, discontinuation of isoniazid should be strongly considered. Liver function tests

ISONIAZID — INJECTION

WARNING (cont.)

are not a substitute for a clinical evaluation at monthly intervals or for the prompt assessment of signs or symptoms of adverse reactions occurring between regularly scheduled evaluations. Patients should be instructed to immediately report signs or symptoms consistent with liver damage or other adverse effects. These include any of the following: Unexplained anorexia, nausea, vomiting, dark urine, icterus, rash, persistent paresthesias of the hands and feet, persistent fatigue, weakness or fever of more than 3-day duration or abdominal tenderness, especially right upper quadrant discomfort. If these symptoms appear, or if signs suggestive of hepatic damage are detected, isoniazid should be discontinued promptly, since continued use of the drug in these cases has been reported to cause a more severe form of liver damage.

Patients with tuberculosis who have hepatitis attributed to isoniazid should be given appropriate treatment with alternative drugs. If isoniazid must be reinstituted, it should be reinstituted only after symptoms and laboratory abnormalities have cleared. The drug should be restarted in very small and gradually increasing doses and should be withdrawn immediately if there is any indication of recurrent liver involvement.

Preventive treatment should be deferred in persons with acute hepatic diseases.

Indications

➤*Tuberculosis treatment:* For all forms of tuberculosis in which organisms are susceptible.

However, active tuberculosis must be treated with multiple concomitant antituberculosis medications to prevent the emergence of drug resistance. Single-drug treatment of active tuberculosis with isoniazid, or any other medication, is inadequate therapy.

➤*Preventive therapy:* Isoniazid is recommended as preventive therapy for the following groups, regardless of age (the criterion for a positive reaction to a skin test [in mm of induration] for each group is given in parenthesis).

HIV – Persons with human immunodeficiency virus (HIV) infection (greater than or equal to 5 mm) and persons with risk factors for HIV infection whose HIV infection status is unknown but who are suspected of having HIV infection. Preventive therapy may be considered for HIV-infected persons who are tuberculin-negative but belong to groups in which the prevalence of tuberculosis infection is high. Candidates for preventive therapy who have HIV infection should have a minimum of 12 months of therapy.

Close contacts of people with infectious tuberculosis – Close contacts of persons with newly diagnosed infectious tuberculosis (greater than or equal to 5 mm). In addition, tuberculin-negative (less than 5 mm) children, and adolescents who have been close contacts of infectious persons within the past 3 months, are candidates for preventive therapy until a repeat tuberculin skin test is done 12 weeks after contact with the infectious source. If the repeat skin test is positive (greater than 5 mm), therapy should be continued.

Recent converters – Recent converters, as indicated by a tuberculin skin test (greater than or equal to 10 mm increase within a 2-year period for those younger than 35 years old; greater than or equal to 15 mm increase for those 35 years of age and older). All infants and children younger than 4 years of age with a greater than 10 mm skin test are included in this category.

Abnormal chest radiographs – Persons with abnormal chest radiographs that show fibrotic lesions likely to represent old healed tuberculosis (greater than or equal to 5 mm). Candidates for preventive therapy who have fibrotic pulmonary lesions consistent with healed tuberculosis or who have pulmonary silicosis should have 12 months of isoniazid or 4 months of isoniazid and rifampin, concomitantly.

IV drug users – IV drug users known to be HIV-seronegative (greater than 10 mm).

Increased risk of tuberculosis – Persons with the following medical conditions that have been reported to increase the risk of tuberculosis (greater than or equal to 10 mm): Silicosis; diabetes mellitus; prolonged therapy with adrenocorticosteroids; immunosuppressive therapy; some hematologic and reticuloendothelial diseases such as leukemia or Hodgkin's disease; end-stage renal disease; clinical situations associated with substantial rapid weight loss or chronic undernutrition (eg, intestinal bypass surgery for obesity, the postgastrectomy state with or without weight loss, chronic peptic ulcer disease, chronic malabsorption syndromes, and carcinomas of the oropharynx and upper GI tract that prevent adequate nutritional intake). Candidates for preventive therapy who have fibrotic pulmonary lesions consistent with healed tuberculosis or who have pulmonary silicosis should have 12 months of isoniazid or 4 months of isoniazid and rifampin, concomitantly.

Adults younger than 35 years of age with tuberculin skin test reaction of greater than or equal to 10 mm – Additionally, in the absence of any of the above risk factors, persons younger than 35 years of age with a tuberculin skin test reaction of greater than or equal to 10 mm are also appropriate candidates for preventive therapy if they are a member of any of the following high-incidence groups: Foreign-born persons from high-prevalence countries who never received BCG vaccine; medically underserved low-income populations, including high-risk racial or ethnic minority populations, especially black patients, Hispanic patients, and Native Americans; residents of facilities for long-term care (eg, correctional institutions, nursing homes, and mental institutions).

Children less than 4 years of age – Children who are younger than 4 years old are candidates for isoniazid preventive therapy if they have greater than 10 mm induration from a PPD Mantoux tuberculin skin test.

Adults less than 35 years of age – Persons younger than 35 years of age who have none of the above risk factors, belong to none of the high-incidence groups, and have a tuberculin skin test reaction of greater than or equal to 15 mm, are appropriate candidates for preventive therapy.

The risk of hepatitis must be weighed against the risk of tuberculosis in positive tuberculin reactors older than 35 years of age. However, the use of isoniazid is recommended for those with the additional risk factors listed above and on an individual basis in situations where there is likelihood of serious consequences to contacts who may become infected.

Administration and Dosage

Isoniazid injection is used in conjunction with other effective antituberculous agents.

➤*For treatment of tuberculosis:*

Usual parenteral dosage (depending on the regimen used) –

Adults: 5 mg/kg up to 300 mg daily in a single dose or 15 mg/kg up to 900 mg/day, 2 or 3 times/week.

Children: 10 to 15 mg/kg up to 300 mg daily in a single dose or 20 to 40 mg/kg up to 900 mg/day, 2 or 3 times/week.

Pulmonary tuberculosis without HIV infection: There are 3 regimen options for the initial treatment of tuberculosis in children and adults:

- *Option 1* – Daily isoniazid, rifampin, and pyrazinamide for 8 weeks followed by 16 weeks of isoniazid and rifampin daily or 2 to 3 times weekly. Ethambutol or streptomycin should be added to the initial regimen until sensitivity to isoniazid and rifampin is demonstrated. The addition of a fourth drug is optional if the relative prevalence of isoniazid-resistant *Mycobacterium tuberculosis* isolates in the community is ≤ 4%.
- *Option 2* – Daily isoniazid, rifampin, pyrazinamide and streptomycin or ethambutol for 2 weeks, followed by twice-weekly administration of the same drugs for 6 weeks, subsequently twice-weekly administration of isoniazid and rifampin for 16 weeks.
- *Option 3* – Three times weekly with isoniazid, rifampin, pyrazinamide and ethambutol or streptomycin for 6 months.

All regimens given twice weekly or 3 times weekly should be administered by directly observed therapy (see also Directly observed therapy).

Pulmonary tuberculosis and HIV infection – The response of the immunologically impaired host to treatment may not be satisfactory as that of a person with healthy host responsiveness. For this reason, therapeutic decisions for the impaired host must be individualized. Since patients coinfected with HIV may have problems with malabsorption, screening of antimycobacterial drug levels, especially in patients with advanced HIV disease, may be necessary to prevent the emergence of multidrug-resistant tuberculosis (MDRTB).

Extrapulmonary tuberculosis – The basic principles that underlie the treatment of pulmonary tuberculosis also apply to extrapulmonary forms of the disease. Although there have not been the same kinds of carefully conducted controlled trials of treatment of extrapulmonary tuberculosis as for pulmonary disease, increasing clinical experience indicates that 6- to 9-month short-course regimens are effective. Because of the insufficient data, miliary tuberculosis, bone/joint tuberculosis, and tuberculosis meningitis in infants and children should receive 12-month therapy.

Bacteriologic evaluation of extra pulmonary tuberculosis may be limited by the relative inaccessibility of the sites of disease. Thus, response to treatment often must be judged on the basis of clinical and radiographic findings.

The use of adjunctive therapies such as surgery and corticosteroids is more commonly required in extra pulmonary tuberculosis than in pulmonary disease. Surgery may be necessary to obtain specimens for diagnosis and to treat such processes as constrictive pericarditis and spinal cord compression from Pott's disease. Corticosteroids have been shown to be of benefit in preventing cardiac constriction from tuberculous pericarditis and in decreasing the neurologic sequelae of all stages of tuberculosis meningitis, especially when administered early in the course of the disease.

Pregnant women with tuberculosis – The options listed above must be adjusted for the pregnant patient. Streptomycin interferes with in utero development of the ear and may cause congenital deafness. Routine use of pyrazinamide is also not recommended in pregnancy because of inadequate teratogenicity data. The initial treatment regimen should consist of isoniazid and rifampin. Ethambutol should be included unless primary isoniazid resistance is unlikely (isoniazid resistance rate documented to be less than 4%).

MDRTB – Multiple-drug resistant tuberculosis (ie, resistance to at least isoniazid and rifampin) presents difficult treatment problems. Treatment must be individualized and based on susceptibility studies. In such cases, consultation with an expert in tuberculosis is recommended.

➤*Prophylaxis:* Before isoniazid preventive therapy is initiated, bacteriologically positive or radiographically progressive tuberculosis must be excluded. Appropriate evaluations should be performed if extrapulmonary tuberculosis is suspected.

Adults (heavier than 30 kg) – 300 mg/day in a single dose.

Infants and children – 10 mg/kg (up to 300 mg daily) in a single dose.

In situations where adherence with daily preventive therapy cannot be assured, 20 to 30 mg/kg (not to exceed 900 mg) twice weekly under the direct observation of a healthcare worker at the time of administration is recommended.

Continuous administration of isoniazid for a sufficient period of time is an essential part of the regimen because relapse rates are higher if chemotherapy is stopped prematurely. In the treatment of tuberculosis, resistant

ISONIAZID — INJECTION

organisms may multiply and the emergence during the treatment may necessitate a change in the regimen.

Directly observed therapy (DOT) – A major cause of drug-resistant tuberculosis is patient noncompliance with treatment. The use of DOT can help ensure patient compliance with drug therapy. DOT is the observation of the patient by a healthcare provider or other responsible person as the patient ingests antituberculosis medications. DOT can be achieved with daily, twice-weekly or 3-times-a-week regimens, and is recommended for all patients.

Patient compliance – The Potts-Cozart test, a simple colorimetric method of checking for isoniazid in the urine, is a useful tool for assuring patient compliance, which is essential for effective tuberculosis control. Additionally, isoniazid test strips are also available to check patient compliance.

Concomitant pyridoxine therapy – Concomitant administration of pyridoxine (B_6) is recommended in the malnourished and in those predisposed to neuropathy (eg, alcoholics, diabetics).

➤*Storage/Stability:* Store at controlled room temperature 15° to 30°C (59° to 86°F). Protect from light.

Isoniazid injection may crystallize at low temperatures. If this occurs, warm the vial to room temperature before use to redissolve the crystals.

Actions

➤*Pharmacology:* Pyridoxine (B_6) deficiency is sometimes observed in adults with high doses of isoniazid and is considered probably due to its competition with pyridoxal phosphate for the enzyme apotryptophanase.

Isoniazid inhibits the synthesis of mycoloic acids, an essential component of the bacterial cell wall. At therapeutic levels isoniazid is bacteriocidal against actively growing intracellular and extracellular *Mycobacterium tuberculosis* organisms.

➤*Pharmacokinetics:*

Absorption/Distribution – Within 1 to 2 hours after oral administration, isoniazid produces peak blood levels which decline to ≤ 50% within 6 hours. The medicine diffuses readily into all body fluids (cerebrospinal, pleural, and ascitic), tissues, organs, and excreta (saliva, sputum, and feces). The drug also passes through the placental barrier and into milk in concentrations comparable to those in the plasma.

Metabolism – Isoniazid is metabolized primarily by acetylation and dehydrazination. The rate of acetylation is genetically determined. Approximately 50% of black patients and white patients are "slow acetylators" and the rest are "rapid acetylators"; the majority of Eskimos and Asian patients are "rapid acetylators."

The rate of acetylation does not significantly alter the effectiveness of isoniazid therapy when dosage is administered daily. However, slow acetylation may lead to higher blood levels of the drug and thus an increase in toxic reactions.

Excretion – From 50% to 70% of a dose of isoniazid is excreted in the urine in 24 hours.

➤*Microbiology:* Isoniazid-resistant *Mycobacterium tuberculosis* bacilli develop rapidly when isoniazid monotherapy is administered.

Contraindications

Severe hypersensitivity reactions, including the following: Drug-induced hepatitis; previous isoniazid-associated hepatic injury; severe adverse reactions to isoniazid such as drug fever, chills, arthritis; acute liver disease of any etiology.

Warnings

➤*Hepatitis:* See Warning Box.

➤*Hypersensitivity reactions:* All drugs should be stopped and an evaluation made at the first sign of a hypersensitivity reaction. If isoniazid therapy must be reinstituted, the drug should be given only after symptoms have cleared. The drug should be restarted in very small and gradually increasing doses and should be withdrawn immediately if there is any indication of recurrent hypersensitivity reaction.

➤*Carcinogenesis:* Isoniazid has been shown to induce pulmonary tumors in a number of strains of mice. Isoniazid has not been shown to be carcinogenic in humans (a diagnosis of mesothelioma in a child with prenatal exposure to isoniazid and no other apparent risk factors has been reported).

➤*Pregnancy: Category C.*

Isoniazid has been shown to have an embryocidal effect in rats and rabbits when given orally during pregnancy. There are no adequate and well-controlled studies in pregnant women. Isoniazid should be used as a treatment for active tuberculosis during pregnancy because the benefit justifies the potential risk to the fetus. The benefit of preventive therapy also should be weighed against a possible risk to the fetus. Preventive therapy generally should be started after delivery to prevent putting the fetus at risk of exposure; the low levels of isoniazid in breast milk do not threaten the neonate.

Since isoniazid is known to cross the placental barrier, neonates of isoniazid-treated mothers should be carefully observed for any evidence of adverse effects.

➤*Lactation:* The small concentrations of isoniazid in breast milk do not produce toxicity in the nursing newborn; therefore, breastfeeding should not be discouraged. However, because levels of isoniazid are so low in breast milk, they can not be relied upon for prophylaxis or therapy of nursing infants.

Precautions

➤*Monitoring:* Periodic ophthalmologic examinations during isoniazid therapy are recommended when visual symptoms occur.

Because there is a higher frequency of isoniazid-associated hepatitis among certain patient groups, including those older than 35 years of age, daily users of alcohol, those with chronic liver disease, patients with injection drug use and women belonging to minority groups (particularly in the post-partum period), transaminase measurements should be obtained prior to starting, and monthly during, preventive therapy, or more frequently as needed. If any of the values exceed 3 to 5 times the upper limit of normal, isoniazid should be temporarily discontinued and consideration given to restarting therapy.

➤*Special risk:* Use of isoniazid should be carefully monitored in the following: Daily users of alcohol (daily ingestion of alcohol may be associated with a higher incidence of + isoniazid hepatitis); patients with active chronic liver disease or severe renal dysfunction; patients older than 35 years of age; patients with concurrent use of any chronically administered medication; patients with a history of previous discontinuation of isoniazid; patients with the existence of peripheral neuropathy or conditions predisposing to neuropathy; pregnant patients; patients with injection drug use; women belonging to minority groups, particularly in the postpartum period; HIV-seropositive patients.

Drug Interactions

Isoniazid Drug Interactions

Precipitant drug	Object drug*		Description
Rifampin	Isoniazid	↑	Hepatotoxicity may occur at a rate higher than either agent alone. If alterations in liver function tests occur, consider discontinuation of one or both of these agents.
Isoniazid	Acetaminophen	↑	Hepatotoxicity has been reported due to inhibition of acetaminophen metabolism. Monitor patient for acetaminophen toxicity.
Isoniazid	Carbamazepine	↑	Isoniazid hepatotoxicity may result due to carbamazepine increasing isoniazid degradation to hepatotoxic metabolites. Carbamazepine toxicity may result due to inhibition of carbamazepine metabolism by isoniazid. Monitor serum carbamazepine concentrations, monitor liver function, and adjust doses as necessary.
Carbamazepine	Isoniazid	↑	
Isoniazid	Chlorzoxazone	↑	Plasma concentrations of chlorzoxazone may be elevated, increasing therapeutic and adverse effects. Adjust the dose of chlorzoxazone as appropriate.
Isoniazid	Disulfiram	↑	The coadministration of disulfiram and isoniazid may result in acute behavioral and coordination changes. The mechanism is unknown; possible excess dopaminergic activity may occur. If acute behavioral or coordination changes develop during concurrent administration of disulfiram and isoniazid, the disulfiram dose may need to be decreased or the drug discontinued.
Isoniazid	Enflurane	↑	In rapid isoniazid acetylators, high output renal failure may occur due to nephrotoxic concentrations of inorganic fluoride. Monitor renal function in patients receiving this combination, particularly those who are rapid acetylators.
Isoniazid	Hydantoins (eg, phenytoin)	↑	Serum hydantoin levels may be increased, producing an increase in the pharmacologic and toxic effects of hydantoins. In usual therapeutic doses, phenytoin toxicity appears to be most significant in patients who are slow acetylators of isoniazid. Monitor serum hydantoin levels and observe for toxicity.
Isoniazid	Ketoconazole	↓	The therapeutic benefit of ketoconazole may be attenuated. Avoid concomitant use if possible. Monitoring of ketoconazole serum levels or antifungal activity may be necessary.

ISONIAZID — INJECTION

Isoniazid Drug Interactions			
Precipitant drug	Object drug*		Description
Isoniazid	Valproate	⬆	A recent case study has shown a possible increase in the plasma level of valproate when coadministered with isoniazid. Plasma valproate concentration should be monitored when isoniazid and valproate are coadministered, and appropriate dosage adjustments of valproate should be made.
Isoniazid	Theophylline	⬆	Isoniazid may increase theophylline plasma levels. Also a slight decrease in isoniazid elimination has been noted. Monitor and adjust the dose as necessary.
Theophylline	Isoniazid	⬆	

* ⬆ = Object drug increased. ⬇ = Object drug decreased.

Adverse Reactions

The most frequent reactions are those affecting the nervous system and the liver.

➤*CNS:* Peripheral neuropathy is the most common toxic effect. It is dose related, occurs most often in the malnourished and in those predisposed to neuritis (eg, alcoholics, diabetics), and is usually preceded by paresthesias of the feet and hands. The incidence is higher in "slow acetylators."

Other neurotoxic effects which are uncommon with conventional doses are convulsions, toxic encephalopathy, optic neuritis and atrophy, memory impairment, and toxic psychosis.

➤*GI:* Nausea, vomiting, and epigastric distress.

➤*Hematologic:* Agranulocytosis; hemolytic, sideroblastic, or aplastic anemia; thrombocytopenia; eosinophilia.

➤*Hepatic:* See Warning Box. Elevated serum transaminases (AST; ALT), bilirubinemia, bilirubinuria, jaundice, and occasionally severe and sometimes fatal hepatitis. The common prodromal symptoms of hepatitis are anorexia, nausea, vomiting, fatigue, malaise, and weakness. Mild hepatic dysfunction, evidenced by mild and transient elevation of serum transaminase levels occurs in 10% to 20% of patients taking isoniazid.

See the Warning box for more information.

➤*Hypersensitivity:* Fever, skin eruptions (morbilliform, maculopapular, purpuric, or exfoliative), lymphadenopathy, and vasculitis.

➤*Local:* Local irritation has been observed at the site of IM injection.

➤*Metabolic/Nutritional:* Pyridoxine deficiency, pellagra, hyperglycemia, metabolic acidosis, and gynecomastia.

➤*Miscellaneous:* Rheumatic syndrome and systemic lupus erythematosus-like syndrome.

Overdosage

➤*Symptoms:* Isoniazid overdosage produces signs and symptoms within 30 minutes to 3 hours after ingestion. Nausea, vomiting, dizziness, slurring of speech, blurring of vision, and visual hallucinations (including bright colors and strange designs) are among the early manifestations. With marked overdosage, respiratory distress and CNS depression, progressing rapidly from stupor to profound coma, are to be expected, along with severe, intractable seizures. Severe metabolic acidosis, acetonuria, and hyperglycemia are typical laboratory findings.

➤*Treatment:* Untreated or inadequately treated cases of gross isoniazid overdosage, 80 mg/kg to 150 mg/kg, can cause neurotoxicity and terminate fatally, but good response has been reported in most patients brought under adequate treatment within the first few hours after drug ingestion.

For the asymptomatic patient – Absorption of drugs from the GI tract may be decreased by giving activated charcoal. Gastric emptying should also be employed in the asymptomatic patient. Safeguard the patient's airway when employing these procedures. Patients who acutely ingest more than 80 mg/kg should be treated with IV pyridoxine on a gram per gram basis equal to the isoniazid dose. If an unknown amount if isoniazid is ingested, consider an initial dose of 5 g of pyridoxine given over 30 to 60 minutes in adults, or 80 mg/kg of pyridoxine in children.

For the symptomatic patient – Ensure adequate ventilation, support cardiac output, and protect the airway while treating seizures and attempting to limit absorption. If the dose of isoniazid is known, the patient should be treated initially with a slow IV bolus of pyridoxine, over 3 to 5 minutes, on a gram per gram basis, equal to the isoniazid dose. If the quantity of isoniazid ingestion is unknown, then consider an initial IV bolus of pyridoxine of 5 g in the adult or 80 mg/kg in the child. If seizures continue, the dosage of pyridoxine may be repeated. It would be rare that more than 10 g of pyridoxine would need to be given. The maximum safe dose of pyridoxine in isoniazid intoxication is not known. If the patient does not respond to pyridoxine, diazepam may be administered. Phenytoin should be used cautiously, because isoniazid interferes with the metabolism of phenytoin.

Obtain blood samples for immediate determination of gases, electrolytes, BUN, glucose; type and cross-match blood in preparation for possible hemodialysis.

Rapid control of metabolic acidosis – Patients with this degree of INH intoxication are likely to have hypoventilation. The administration of sodium bicarbonate under these circumstances can cause exacerbation of hypercarbia. Ventilation must be monitored carefully, by measuring blood carbon dioxide levels, and supported mechanically, if there is respiratory insufficiency.

Dialysis – Both peritoneal and hemodialysis have been used in the management of isoniazid overdosage. These procedures are probably not required if control of seizures and acidosis is achieved with pyridoxine, diazepam and bicarbonate.

Patient Information

Use as directed. Do not discontinue except on the advice of a physician.

Avoid certain foods (eg, fish [skipjack, tuna], and perhaps tyramine-containing products).

Notify physician of weakness, fatigue, loss of appetite, nausea and vomiting, yellowing of skin or eyes, darkening of urine, or numbness or tingling in hands and feet.

ISONIAZID COMBINATIONS

Rx	**Rifater** (Aventis)	**Tablets:** 120 mg rifampin, 50 mg isoniazid, 300 mg pyrazinamide	(Rifater). Sugar-coated. Light beige. In 60s.
Rx	**IsonaRif** (VersaPharm)	**Capsules:** 300 mg rifampin and 150 mg isoniazid	Lactose. (West-ward 3238). Scarlet opaque. In 60s.
Rx	**Rifamate** (Aventis)		(RIFAMATE). Red. In 60s.

ISONIAZID COMBINATIONS — ORAL

Refer to the general discussion in the Antituberculosal Agents Introduction.

Indications

➤*ISONIAZID:* Bacteriocidal against *Mycobacterium tuberculosis*. See individual monograph.

➤*PYRAZINAMIDE:* Acts against *M. tuberculosis*. See individual monograph.

➤*RIFAMPIN:* Bactericidal against *M. tuberculosis*. See individual monograph.

RIFAMPIN

Rx	**Rifampin** (Various, eg, Eon)	**Capsules:** 150 mg	In 30s and 100s.
Rx	**Rifadin** (Aventis)		(Rifadin 150). Maroon and scarlet. In 30s.
Rx	**Rifampin** (Various, eg, Eon, UDL)	**Capsules:** 300 mg	In 30s, 60s, 100s, and 500s.
Rx	**Rifadin** (Aventis)		(Rifadin 300). Maroon and scarlet. In 30s, 60s, and 100s.
Rx	**Rimactane** (Novartis)		(Ciba 154). Scarlet and caramel. In 30s, 60s, and 100s.
Rx	**Rifadin** (Aventis)	**Powder for Injection:** 600 mg	In vials.

RIFAMPIN

Refer to the general discussion in the Antituberculosal Agents Introduction.

Indications

➤*Tuberculosis:*

Oral – For all forms of tuberculosis. A 3-drug regimen consisting of rifampin, isoniazid, and pyrazinamide is recommended in the initial phase of short-course therapy that is usually continued for 2 months. The Advisory Council for the Elimination or Tuberculosis, the American Thoracic Society, and Centers for Disease Control and Prevention recommend that either streptomycin or ethambutol be added as a fourth drug in a regimen containing isoniazid (INH), rifampin, and pyrazinamide for initial treatment of tuberculosis unless the likelihood of INH resistance is very low. Reassess the need for a fourth drug when the results of susceptibility testing are known. If community rates of INH resistance are currently less than 4%, an initial treatment regimen with fewer than 4 drugs may be considered.

Following the initial phase, continue treatment with rifampin and isoniazid for greater than or equal to 4 months. Continue treatment for longer if the patient is still sputum- or culture-positive, if resistant organisms are present, or if the patient is HIV positive.

IV – For initial treatment and retreatment of tuberculosis when the drug cannot be taken by mouth.

➤*Neisseria meningitidis carriers:* For treatment of asymptomatic carriers of *N. meningitidis* to eliminate meningococci from the nasopharynx. Not indicated for the treatment of meningococcal infection.

➤*Unlabeled uses:* Rifampin has a broad antibacterial spectrum. Use in monotherapy is limited to *Haemophilus influenzae* type B. Rifampin, in combination with other effective agents, has been used in combination for the following: To clear pharyngeal carriage of group A beta-hemolytic streptococcus; eradicate pharyngeal carriage of group b streptococci (GBS) in infants who have had recurrent GBS sepsis; treat manifestations of cat scratch disease caused by *Bartonella henselae*; treat resistant *Streptococcus pneumoniae meningitis*; treat severe staphylococcal bone and joint infections; treat prosthetic valve endocarditis due to coagulase-negative staphylococci; treat Aspergillus; treat Leprosy. Rifampin, in combination with other agents, has also shown activity against *S. pneumoniae, Staphylococcus aureus, Staphylococcus epidermidis, C. jeikeium, L. monocytogenes, N. gonorrhoeae, M. catarrhalis, F. tularensis, Brucella* sp, *N. meningitides*, and *Chlamydia trachomatis*. Rifampin has been used for prophylaxis in high-risk, close contacts of patients infected with *Neisseria meningitidis*. Dosage in adults is 600 mg every 12 hours for 2 days; dosage in children older than 1 month is 10 mg/kg (maximum dose 600 mg) every 12 hours for 2 days; dosage in infants ≤ 1 month is 5 mg/kg every 12 hours for 2 days.

Administration and Dosage

Rifampin can be administered by the oral route or by IV infusion. IV doses are the same as oral.

➤*Oral:* Administer once daily, either 1 hour before or 2 hours after meals with a full glass of water.

Data is not available to determine dosage for children younger than 5 years of age (*Rimactane*).

For pediatric and adult patients in whom capsule swallowing is difficult or when lower doses are needed, a rifampin suspension can be prepared (see Preparation of extemporaneous oral suspension).

➤ *IV:* For IV infusion only. Must not be administered by IM or SC route. Avoid extravasation during injection; local irritation and inflammation because of extravascular infiltration of the infusion have been observed. If these occur, discontinue the infusion and restart at another site.

➤*Oral and IV:*

Tuberculosis –

Adults: 10 mg/kg in a single daily administration not to exceed 600 mg once daily.

Children: 10 to 20 mg/kg, not to exceed 600 mg/day.

Use with at least one other antituberculous agent. In general, continue therapy until bacterial conversion and maximal improvement have occurred. This information is best explained by the regimens that follow.

➤*The 2-month regimen:* According to the MMWR, the 2-month daily regimen of rifampin and pyrazinamide is recommended on the basis of a prospective randomized trial of treatment of latent tuberculosis infection (LTBI) in HIV-infected people that demonstrated the 2-month regimen to be similar in safety and efficacy to a 12-month regimen of isoniazid. Although this regimen has not been evaluated in HIV-uninfected people with LTBI, the efficacy is not expected to differ significantly. However, the drug toxicities may be increased. Two randomized prospective trials of intermittent dosing of rifampin and pyrazinamide for 2 and 3 months respectively, have been reported in HIV-infected people; in neither case was the sample size adequate to conclude with certainty that efficacy was equivalent to daily dosing.

➤*The 4-month regimen:* According to the MMWR, rifampin given daily for 3 months has resulted in better protection than placebo in treatment of LTBI in non-HIV patients with silicosis in a randomized prospective trial. However, because the patients receiving rifampin had a high rate of active tuberculosis (4%), experts have concluded that a 4-month regimen would be more prudent when using rifampin alone. This option may be useful for patients who cannot tolerate isoniazid or pyrazinamide.

➤*The 6-month regimen:* Ordinarily this consists of an initial 2-month phase of rifampin, isoniazid, and pyrazinamide and, if clinically indicated, streptomycin or ethambutol, followed by 4 months of rifampin and isoniazid. Reassess the need for a fourth drug when the results of susceptibility testing are known. If community rates of INH resistance are currently less than 4%, an initial treatment regimen with fewer than 4 drugs may be considered. Continue treatment for more than 6 months if the patient is still sputum- or culture-positive, if resistant organisms are present, or if the patient is HIV positive.

➤*Meningococcal carriers:* Once daily for 4 consecutive days in the following doses:

Adults – 600 mg (two 300 mg capsules) in a single daily administration.

Children – 10 to 20 mg/kg, not to exceed 600 mg/day.

The following dosage has also been recommended:

Adults – 600 mg every 12 hours for 2 days.

Children (1 month of age or older) – 10 mg/kg (not to exceed 600 mg/dose) every 12 hours for 2 days.

Children (younger than 1 month of age) – 5 mg/kg every 12 hours for 2 days.

➤*Preparation/Stability of solution for IV infusion:* Reconstitute the lyophilized powder by transferring 10 ml of Sterile Water for Injection to a vial containing 600 mg of rifampin for injection. Swirl vial gently to completely dissolve the antibiotic. The resultant solution contains rifampin 60 mg/ml and is stable at room temperature for 24 hours. Withdraw a volume equivalent to the amount of rifampin calculated to be administered and add to 500 ml of infusion medium. Mix well and infuse at a rate allowing for complete infusion in 3 hours. In some cases, the amount of rifampin calculated to be administered may be added to 100 ml of infusion medium and infused in 30 minutes. Dilutions in Dextrose 5% for Injection are stable at room temperature for up to 4 hours and should be prepared and used within this time. Precipitation of rifampin from the infusion solution may occur beyond this time. Dilutions in normal saline are stable at room temperature for up to 24 hours and should be prepared and used within this time. Other infusion solutions are not recommended.

➤*Incompatibilities:* Physical incompatibility (precipitate) was observed with undiluted (5 mg/ml) and diluted (1 mg/ml in normal saline) diltiazem HCl and rifampin (6 mg/ml in normal saline) during simulated Y-site administration.

➤*Preparation of extemporaneous oral suspension:* Preparation of suspension (to contain rifampin 10 mg/ml) – 1) Empty the contents of 4 rifampin 300 mg (or 8 rifampin 150 mg) capsules into a 4 oz amber glass bottle. 2) Add 20 ml of simple syrup (*Syrup NF*, Humco Laboratories), *Syrpalta syrup* (Emerson Laboratories), or *Raspberry syrup* (Humco Laboratories). Shake vigorously. 3) Add 100 ml of simple syrup. Shake again.

➤*Storage/Stability:* The extemporaneously prepared oral suspension is stable for 4 weeks when stored at room temperature or in a refrigerator (2° to 8°C; 36° to 46°F).

Actions

➤*Pharmacology:* Rifampin inhibits DNA-dependent RNA polymerase activity in susceptible cells. Specifically, it interacts with bacterial RNA polymerase but does not inhibit the mammalian enzyme. Cross-resistance has only been shown with other rifamycins. Rifampin at therapeutic levels has demonstrated bactericidal activity against intracellular and extracellular *Mycobacterium tuberculosis* organisms.

➤*Pharmacokinetics:*

Absorption/Distribution – Rifampin, 600 mg administered orally, is almost completely absorbed and achieves mean peak plasma levels within 1 to 4 hours. The peak level averages at 7 mcg/ml but may vary from 4 to 32 mcg/ml. In children, mean peak serum levels range from 3.5 to 15 mcg/ml. Absorption of rifampin is reduced by approximately 30% when the drug is ingested with food.

Metabolism – Rifampin is metabolized in the liver by deacetylation; the metabolite is still active against *M. tuberculosis*. It undergoes enterohepatic circulation; however, the deacetylated metabolite is poorly absorbed. The half-life is approximately 3 hours after a 600 mg oral dose, up to 5.1 hours after a 900 mg oral dose. With repeated administration, the half-life decreases and averages approximately 2 to 3 hours.

Excretion – Elimination occurs mainly through the bile and, to a much lesser extent, the urine. Dosage adjustment is not necessary in renal failure, but is with hepatic dysfunction. Rifampin is not significantly removed by hemodialysis.

IV – Following administration of a 300 or 600 mg IV dose in 12 volunteers, mean peak plasma concentrations were 9 and 17 mcg/ml, respectively. The average plasma concentrations remained detectable for 8 and 12 hours, respectively. The elimination of the larger dose was not as rapid. Volumes of distribution at steady state were approximately 0.66 and approximately 0.64 L/kg for the 300 and 600 mg IV doses, respectively. After repeated once daily infusions of 600 mg in 5 patients for 7 days, concentrations decreased from 5.8 mcg/ml 8 hours after the infusion on day 1 to 2.6 mcg/ml 8 hours after the infusion on day 7.

Special populations –

Children:

• *Oral* – In 1 study, pediatric patients 6 to 58 months of age were given rifampin suspended in simple syrup or as dry powder mixed with applesauce at a dose of 10 mg/kg body weight. Peak serum concentrations of approximately 10.7 and approximately 11.5 mcg/ml were obtained 1 hour after preprandial ingestion of the drug suspension and the applesauce mixture, respectively. After the administration of either preparation, the half-life of rifampin averaged 2.9 hours. It should be noted that in other studies in pediatric populations, at doses of 10 mg/kg body weight, mean peak serum concentrations of 3.5 to 15 mcg/ml have been reported.

RIFAMPIN

• *IV* – In children 0.25 to 12.8 years of age (n = 12), the mean peak serum concentration was 26 mcg/ml following a 300 mg/m^2 infusion, 11.7 to 41.5 mcg/ml 1 to 4 days after initiation of therapy, and 13.6 to 37.4 mcg/ml 5 to 14 days after initiation of therapy. The half-life was 1.17 to 3.19 hours.

Contraindications

Hypersensitivity to any rifamycin.

Warnings

➤*Hepatotoxicity:* There have been fatalities associated with jaundice in patients with liver disease or patients receiving rifampin concomitantly with other hepatotoxic agents. Since an increased risk may exist for individuals with liver disease, weigh benefits against risk of further liver damage. Carefully monitor liver function, especially AST and ALT, prior to therapy and then every 2 to 4 weeks during therapy. Withdraw rifampin if signs of hepatocellular damage occur.

➤*Hyperbilirubinemia:* This results from competition between rifampin and bilirubin for excretory pathways of the liver at the cell level can occur in the early days of treatment. An isolated report showing a moderate rise in bilirubin or transaminase level is not in itself an indication to interrupt treatment. Make the decision based on repeat tests and the patient's clinical condition.

➤*Porphyria:* Isolated reports have associated porphyria exacerbation with rifampin administration.

➤*Meningococci resistance:* The possibility of rapid emergence of resistant meningococci restricts use to short-term treatment of asymptomatic carrier state. Rifampin is not to be used for treatment of meningococcal disease.

➤*Hypersensitivity reactions:* These reactions have occurred during intermittent therapy or when treatment was resumed following accidental or intentional interruption and were reversible with rifampin discontinuation and appropriate therapy. Refer to Management of Acute Hypersensitivity Reactions (see Adverse Reactions).

➤*Carcinogenesis:* A few cases of accelerated growth of lung carcinoma have occurred in humans, but a causal relationship has not been established. An increase in the incidence of hepatomas in female mice (of a strain known to be particularly susceptible to the spontaneous development of hepatomas) was observed when rifampin was administered in doses of 2 to 10 times the average daily human dose for 60 weeks. Rifampin possesses immunosuppressive potential in animals and humans. Antitumor activity in vitro has also occurred.

➤*Pregnancy: Category C.* The effect of rifampin (alone or in combination with other antituberculous drugs) on the human fetus is not known. Rifampin crosses the placental barrier and appears in cord blood. It is teratogenic in rodents given oral doses of 15 to 25 times the human dose. An increase in congenital malformations, primarily spina bifida and cleft palate, has occurred in the offspring of rodents given oral doses of 150 to 250 mg/kg/day. Imperfect osteogenesis and embryotoxicity occurred in rabbits given doses up to 20 times the usual human daily dose. When administered during the last few weeks of pregnancy, rifampin can cause postnatal hemorrhages in the mother and infant for which treatment with vitamin K may be indicated. Carefully weigh possible teratogenic potential in women capable of bearing children against benefits of therapy (also see Antituberculosal Drugs introduction).

Carefully observe neonates of rifampin-treated mothers for any adverse effects.

➤*Lactation:* Rifampin is excreted in breast milk. Decide whether to discontinue nursing or discontinue the drug, taking into account the importance of the drug to the mother.

➤*Children:* Safety and efficacy in pediatric patients have not been established.

Precautions

➤*Monitoring:* Perform baseline measurements of hepatic enzymes, bilirubin, serum creatinine, a complete blood count, and a platelet count (or estimate) in adults treated for tuberculosis with rifampin. Baseline tests are unnecessary in pediatric patients unless a complicating condition is known or clinically suspected.

➤*Intermittent therapy:* May be used if the patient cannot or will not self-administer drugs on a daily basis. Closely monitor patients on intermittent therapy for compliance, and caution against intentional or accidental interruption of prescribed therapy because of increased risk of serious adverse reactions.

➤*Red discoloration of body fluids:* Urine, sputum, sweat, and tears may be red-orange colored. Soft contact lenses may be permanently stained. Advise patients of these possibilities.

➤*Thrombocytopenia:* This reaction has occurred, primarily with high dose intermittent therapy, but has also been noted after resumption of interrupted treatment. It rarely occurs during well-supervised daily therapy. This effect is reversible if the drug is discontinued as soon as purpura occurs. Cerebral hemorrhage and fatalities have occurred when rifampin administration has continued or resumed after appearance of purpura.

Drug Interactions

Rifampin Drug Interactions

Precipitant drug	Object drug*		Description
Aminosalicylic acid, oral	Rifampin	⬇	Aminosalicylic acid decreases the effect of rifampin. Give the combination of these 2 agents at an interval of 8 to 12 hours apart.
Halothane	Rifampin	⬆	Hepatotoxicity and hepatic encephalopathy have been reported.
Rifampin	Antiarrhythmics (eg, amiodarone, disopyramide, mexiletine, propafenone, quinidine, tocainide)	⬇	Serum concentrations of antiarrhythmics may be decreased because of CYP3A4 induction by rifampin. Closely monitor serum concentrations when starting or stopping rifampin.
Rifampin	ACE inhibitors (eg, enalapril)	⬇	The pharmacologic effects of enalapril may be decreased, resulting in a decrease in antihypertensive control. The mechanism by which this occurs is unknown. Monitor the patient's blood pressure; consider an alternative antihypertensive if blood pressure remains uncontrolled.
Rifampin	Anticoagulants	⬇	Rifampin decreases the anticoagulation activity of warfarin because of increased hepatic microsomal enzyme metabolism. Increased dosage of anticoagulants may be needed. Monitor coagulation parameters closely when rifampin is discontinued.
Rifampin	Azole antifungals (eg, fluconazole, itraconazole, ketoconazole)	⬇	Rifampin may induce the metabolism of azole antifungal agents. Ketoconazole may interfere with rifampin absorption decreasing serum rifampin levels. If concurrent use cannot be avoided, monitor and adjust the dosages as needed.
Azole antifungals (eg, fluconazole, itraconazole, ketoconazole)	Rifampin	⬇	
Rifampin	Barbiturates	⬇	Rifampin may stimulate liver microsomal enzymes resulting in more rapid degradation of barbiturates. When rifampin is added to the regimen of a patient receiving a barbiturate, monitor the patient for changes in clinical status and plasma barbiturate levels. The barbiturate dosage may need to be raised.
Rifampin	Benzodiazepines (eg, diazepam, midazolam, triazolam)	⬇	The pharmacologic effects of diazepam, midazolam, and triazolam may be decreased because of increased metabolism of benzodiazepines. Monitor the clinical response to the benzodiazepine when starting or stopping rifampin.
Rifampin	Beta blockers (eg, bisoprolol, metoprolol, propranolol)	⬇	The pharmacologic effects of certain beta blockers (eg, bisoprolol, metoprolol, propranolol) may be reduced possibly because of increased hepatic metabolism from enzyme induction by rifampin. A 3- to 4-week washout period may be necessary for the enzyme induction effect to diminish. Close monitoring of therapeutic response is essential.
Rifampin	Buspirone	⬇	Buspirone plasma concentrations and pharmacologic effects may be decreased because of induction of first-pass metabolism (CYP3A4) by rifampin. Escalation of buspirone dose may be necessary.
Rifampin	Chloramphenicol	⬇	Chloramphenicol metabolism may be increased because of induction of hepatic microsomal enzymes by rifampin.
Rifampin	Contraceptives, oral	⬇	Reduced oral contraceptive efficacy and an increased incidence of menstrual abnormalities may occur. Advise patients to use an additional form of birth control while receiving rifampin therapy.

RIFAMPIN

Rifampin Drug Interactions

Precipitant drug	Object drug*		Description
Rifampin	Corticosteroids	⬇	The pharmacologic effects of corticosteroids may be decreased. Lack of effect may occur within a few days of adding rifampin and reverse 2 to 3 weeks following discontinuation. Avoid coadministration.
Rifampin	Cyclosporine	⬇	The immunosuppressive effects of cyclosporine may be reduced 2 days following the initiation of rifampin and persist for 1 to 3 weeks after discontinuation. Cyclosporine bioavailability is decreased because of induction of intestinal cytochrome P450 enzymes. Increased doses may be necessary; avoid this combination if possible.
Rifampin	Delavirdine	⬇	Rifampin may increase the metabolism of delavirdine by enzyme induction thereby decreasing the plasma concentrations. Avoid concurrent use.
Rifampin	Digoxin	⬇	Rifampin coadministration may decrease the serum concentration of digoxin. An increased digoxin dosage may be necessary.
Rifampin	Doxycycline	⬇	Rifampin may decrease the serum concentration and half-life of doxycycline, possibly reducing the therapeutic effect. Monitor the clinical response.
Rifampin	Estrogens	⬇	Rifampin may impair the effectiveness of estrogens by inducing drug metabolism, decreasing AUC, and half-life. Consider alternate methods of contraception.
Rifampin	Fluoroquinolones	⬇	Rifampin may accelerate the metabolism of fluoroquinolones. It may be necessary to adjust the dosage of a fluoroquinolone.
Rifampin	Haloperidol	⬇	Rifampin may decrease the plasma concentration and clinical effectiveness of haloperidol. When adding or discontinuing rifamycin therapy, carefully monitor the clinical response of the patient. Adjust the haloperidol dose as indicated.
Rifampin	Hydantoins	⬇	Serum hydantoin levels may be decreased because of rifampin increasing hepatic enzyme metabolism. Monitor serum hydantoin levels and observe the patient.
Rifampin	Isoniazid	⬆	Hepatotoxicity may occur at a rate higher than with either agent alone. If alterations in liver function tests occur, consider discontinuation of one or both agents.
Isoniazid	Rifampin	⬆	
Rifampin	Losartan	⬇	Rifampin may increase the metabolism of losartan. Observe the clinical response of the patient when starting or stopping rifampin.
Rifamycins	Macrolide antibiotics (eg, clarithromycin)	⬇	The metabolism of rifampin may be inhibited, while the metabolism of the macrolide antibiotic may be increased. Monitor for increased side effects and a decrease in the response to the macrolide antibiotic.
Macrolide antibiotics (eg, clarithromycin)	Rifamycins	⬆	
Rifampin	Narcotic analgesics (eg, methadone, morphine)	⬇	Patients may experience withdrawal symptoms. Rifampin primarily appears to stimulate the hepatic metabolism of methadone. A higher dose of narcotic analgesics may be required during concurrent administration of rifampin.
Rifampin	Nifedipine	⬇	The therapeutic effects of nifedipine may be reduced. Monitor blood pressure and angina symptoms. Adjust the nifedipine dose accordingly or consider a different antihypertensive medication.
Rifampin	Ondansetron	⬇	Plasma concentrations of ondansetron may be reduced. Consider use of an alternative antiemetic.
Rifampin	Progestins	⬇	Rifampin may increase the elimination rate of progestin-containing oral contraceptives. Avoid coadministration.
Rifampin	Protease inhibitors (eg, indinavir, nelfinavir, ritonavir)	⬇	Rifampin may increase the metabolism of protease inhibitors while protease inhibitors may decrease rifampin metabolism. Avoid concomitant use.
Protease inhibitors (eg, indinavir, nelfinavir, ritonavir)	Rifampin	⬆	
Rifampin	Quinine derivatives	⬇	Rifampin increases the hepatic clearance of quinine derivatives. Enzyme induction can persist for several days following discontinuation of rifampin. Addition of rifampin to stable quinine derivative regimens may require increased doses of quinine derivatives to maintain the desired therapeutic effect. Withdrawal of rifampin may result in quinine derivative dose-related toxicity. Monitor quinine derivative serum levels and the ECG.
Rifampin	Sulfapyridine	⬇	Plasma concentrations of sulfapyridine may be reduced following the concomitant administration of sulfasalazine and rifampin. This finding may be the result of alteration in the colonic bacteria responsible for the reduction of sulfasalazine to sulfapyridine and mesalamine.
Rifampin	Sulfones	⬇	The pharmacologic effect of dapsone may be decreased because of increased metabolism of dapsone. Higher doses of dapsone may be necessary.
Rifampin	Sulfonylureas	⬇	Rifampin may decrease the half-life and serum levels while increasing the clearance of tolbutamide and chlorpropamide, possibly resulting in hyperglycemia. Closely monitor blood glucose and possibly increase the sulfonylurea dose.
Rifampin	Tacrolimus	⬇	The immunosuppressive effects of tacrolimus may be reduced as early as 2 days following the initiation of rifampin. Closely monitor tacrolimus whole blood concentrations when starting or stopping rifampin.
Rifampin	Theophylline	⬇	The addition of rifampin may result in decreased theophylline levels and exacerbation of pulmonary symptoms. Monitor theophylline levels.
Rifampin	Thyroid hormones	⬇	Thyroid stimulating hormone (TSH) levels may be increased, resulting in hypothyroidism. Monitor thyroid status in patients receiving both drugs.
Rifampin	Tricyclic antidepressants (TCAs)	⬇	TCA levels may decrease because of increased hepatic metabolism of TCAs. Consider monitoring TCA concentrations when starting, stopping, or altering the rifampin dose.
Rifampin	Verapamil	⬇	There is an increase in first-pass hepatic metabolism resulting in a lowered bioavailability of oral verapamil. Use IV verapamil or substitute another agent for either verapamil or rifampin.
Rifampin	Zidovudine	⬇	The pharmacologic effects of zidovudine may be decreased possibly because of increased hepatic metabolism.
Rifampin	Zolpidem	⬇	Plasma concentrations and therapeutic effects of zolpidem may be reduced. Monitor the clinical response of the patient.

* ⬇ = Object drug decreased. ⬆ = Object drug increased.

RIFAMPIN

➤*Cytochrome P450:* Rifampin is known to induce certain cytochrome P450 enzymes. Administration of rifampin with drugs that undergo biotransformation through these metabolic pathways may accelerate elimination of coadministered drugs. To maintain optimum therapeutic blood levels, dosages of drugs metabolized by these enzymes may require adjustment when starting or stopping concomitantly administered rifampin.

➤*Drug/Lab test interactions:* Therapeutic levels of rifampin inhibit standard assays for serum folate and vitamin B_{12}. Consider alternative methods when determining folate and vitamin B_{12} concentrations in the presence of rifampin.

Hepatitis or shock-like syndrome with hepatic involvement and abnormal liver function tests have been reported.

Transient abnormalities in liver function tests (eg, elevation in serum bilirubin, alkaline phosphatase, and serum transaminases), and reduced biliary excretion of contrast media used for visualization of the gallbladder have also been observed. Therefore, perform these tests before the morning dose of rifampin.

➤*Drug/Food interactions:* Food interferes with the absorption of rifampin, possibly resulting in increased peak plasma concentrations. Take on an empty stomach, either 1 hour before or 2 hours after a meal, with a full glass of water.

Adverse Reactions

High doses of rifampin (more than 600 mg) given once or twice weekly have resulted in a high incidence of adverse reactions including: The "flu-like" syndrome (eg, fever, chills, malaise); hematopoietic reactions (eg, leukopenia, thrombocytopenia, acute hemolytic anemia); cutaneous, GI and hepatic reactions; shortness of breath; shock; renal failure. Recent studies indicate that regimens using twice-weekly doses of rifampin 600 mg plus isoniazid 15 mg/kg are much better tolerated.

➤*CNS:* Headache; ataxia; drowsiness; fatigue; dizziness; inability to concentrate; mental confusion; psychoses; generalized numbness; behavioral changes (rare).

➤*Dermatologic:* Rash; flushing; itching (with or without rash).

➤*GI:* Heartburn; epigastric distress; anorexia; nausea; vomiting; gas; cramps; diarrhea; jaundice; pseudomembranous colitis.

➤*Hematologic:* Transient leukopenia; hemolytic anemia; decreased hemoglobin; hemolysis; disseminated intravascular coagulation; thrombocytopenia (see Precautions).

➤*Hepatic:* Hepatitis or shock-like syndrome with hepatic involvement (rare); abnormal liver function tests; transient abnormalities in liver function tests (elevations in serum bilirubin, BSP, alkaline phosphatase, serum transaminases). Perform BSP test prior to the morning dose of rifampin to avoid false-positive results.

➤*Hypersensitivity:* Pruritus; urticaria; pemphigoid reaction; erythema multiforme including Stevens-Johnson syndrome; toxic epidermal necrolysis; vasculitis; eosinophilia; sore mouth; sore tongue; conjunctivitis. Rarely hemolysis, hemoglobinuria, hematuria, renal insufficiency, or acute renal failure have occurred.

➤*Musculoskeletal:* Ataxia; muscular weakness; pain in extremities; myopathy.

➤*Renal:* Interstitial nephritis; acute tubular necrosis.

➤*Miscellaneous:* Visual disturbances; menstrual disturbances; fever; elevations in BUN and serum uric acid; adrenal insufficiency in patients with compromised adrenal function; edema of face and extremities; shortness of breath; wheezing; decrease in blood pressure; shock; flu syndrome (eg, fever, chills, headache, dizziness, bone pain).

Overdosage

➤*Symptoms:* The minimum acute lethal or toxic dose is not well established. However, nonfatal acute overdoses in adults have been reported with doses ranging from 9 to 12 g rifampin. Fatal acute overdoses in adults have been reported with doses ranging from 14 to 60 g. Alcohol or a history of alcohol abuse was involved in some of the fatal and nonfatal reports. Nonfatal overdoses in pediatric patients ages 1 to 4 years of age or 100 mg/kg for 1 to 2 doses has been reported.

Nausea, vomiting, abdominal pain, pruritus, headache, and increasing lethargy will probably occur shortly after ingestion; unconsciousness may occur with severe hepatic disease. Transient increases in liver enzymes or bilirubin may occur. Brownish-red or orange discoloration of skin, urine, sweat, saliva, tears, and feces is proportional to amount ingested. Facial or periorbital edema has also been reported in pediatric patients. Hypotension, sinus tachycardia, ventricular arrhythmias, seizures, and cardiac arrest were reported in some fatal cases. Liver enlargement, possibly with tenderness, can develop within a few hours after severe overdosage, and jaundice may develop rapidly. Hepatic involvement may be more marked in patients with prior impairment of hepatic function. Other physical findings remain essentially normal.

Direct and total bilirubin levels may increase rapidly with severe overdosage; hepatic enzyme levels may be affected, especially with prior impairment of hepatic function. A direct effect on the hematopoietic system, electrolyte levels, or acid-base balance is unlikely.

➤*Treatment:* Nausea and vomiting are likely to be present. Gastric lavage is probably preferable to inducing emesis. Instill activated charcoal slurry into stomach after evacuation of gastric contents to help absorb any remaining drug in GI tract. Antiemetic medication may be required to control severe nausea or vomiting.

Forced diuresis (with measured intake and output) will promote excretion of the drug. Hemodialysis may be of value in some patients. Bile drainage may be indicated in the presence of serious impairment of hepatic function lasting more than 24 to 48 hours; extracorporeal hemodialysis may be required. In patients with previously adequate hepatic function, reversal of liver enlargement, and impaired hepatic excretory function probably will be noted within 72 hours, with rapid return toward normal thereafter.

Patient Information

Take on an empty stomach, greater than or equal to 1 hour before or 2 hours after meals, with a full glass of water.

Take medication on a regular basis; avoid missing doses. Do not discontinue therapy except on advice of physician.

Advise patient that the reliability of oral or other systemic hormonal contraceptive may be affected; give consideration to using alternative contraceptive measures.

Medication may cause a reddish-orange discoloration of urine, stools, saliva, tears, sweat, and sputum. This is to be expected and is not harmful. It may also permanently discolor soft contact lenses.

Notify physician if fever, loss of appetite, malaise, nausea, vomiting, darkened urine, or yellowish discoloration of skin or eyes occurs.

RIFABUTIN

Rx	**Mycobutin** (Pharmacia & Upjohn)	**Capsules:** 150 mg	(MYCOBUTIN/PHARMACIA & UPJOHN). Red/brown. In 100s.

RIFABUTIN — ORAL

Refer to the general discussion in the Antituberculosal Agents Introduction.

Indications

➤*Mycobacterium avium complex:* For the prevention of disseminated *Mycobacterium avium* complex (MAC) disease in patients with advanced human immunodeficiency virus (HIV) infection.

Administration and Dosage

➤*Approved by the FDA:* December 23, 1992.

➤*Dosage:* 300 mg once daily. For those patients with propensity to nausea, vomiting, or other gastrointestinal upset, administration of rifabutin at doses of 150 mg twice daily taken with food may be useful.

Renal function impairment – For patients with severe renal impairment (creatinine clearance less than 30 mL/min), the dose of rifabutin should be reduced by 50%. No dosage adjustment is required for patients with mild to moderate renal impairment.

Concomitant drugs – Reduction of the dose of rifabutin may also be needed for patients receiving concomitant treatment with certain other drugs (see Drug Interactions).

➤*Storage/Stability:* Keep tightly closed and dispense in a tight container as defined in the USP. Store at 25°C (77°F); excursions permitted to 15° to 30°C (59° to 86°F) (see USP Controlled Room Temperature).

Actions

➤*Pharmacology:* Rifabutin inhibits DNA-dependent RNA polymerase in susceptible strains of *Escherichia coli* and *Bacillus subtilis* but not in mammalian cells. In resistant strains of *E. coli*, rifabutin, like rifampin, did not inhibit this enzyme. It is not known whether rifabutin inhibits DNA-dependent RNA polymerase in *Mycobacterium avium* or in *M. intracellulare* which comprise *M. avium* complex (MAC).

➤*Pharmacokinetics:*

Absorption – Following a single oral dose of 300 mg to nine healthy adult volunteers, rifabutin was readily absorbed from the gastrointestinal tract with mean (± SD) peak plasma levels (C_{max}) of 375 (± 267) ng/mL (range: 141 to 1033 ng/mL) attained in 3.3 (± 0.9) hours (T_{max} range: 2 to 4 hours). Absolute bioavailability assessed in 5 HIV-positive patients, who received both oral and intravenous doses, averaged 20%. Total recovery of radioactivity in the urine indicates that at least 53% of the orally administered rifabutin dose is absorbed from the gastrointestinal tract. The bioavailability of rifabutin from the capsule dosage form, relative to an oral solution, was 85% in 12 healthy adult volunteers. High-fat meals slow the rate without influencing the extent of absorption from the capsule dosage form. Plasma concentrations post-C_{max} declined in an apparent biphasic manner. Pharmacokinetic dose-proportionality was established over the 300 to 600 mg dose range in 9 healthy adult volunteers (crossover design) and in 16 early symptomatic HIV-positive patients over a 300 to 900 mg dose range.

Distribution – Due to its high lipophilicity, rifabutin demonstrates a high propensity for distribution and intracellular tissue uptake. Following intravenous dosing, estimates of apparent steady-state distribution volume (9.3 ± 1.5 L/kg) In 5 HIV-positive patients exceeded total body water by approximately 15-fold. Substantially higher intracellular tissue levels than those seen in plasma have been observed in both rat and man. The lung-to-plasma concentration ratio, obtained at 12 hours, was approximately 6.5 in 4 surgical patients who received an oral dose. Mean rifabutin steady-state trough levels ($C_{p,min}^{ss}$; 24-hour post-dose) ranged from 50 to 65 ng/mL in HIV-positive patients and in healthy adult volunteers. About 85% of the drug is bound in a concentration-independent manner to plasma proteins over a concentration range of 0.05 to 1 mcg/mL. Binding does not appear to be

RIFABUTIN — ORAL

influenced by renal or hepatic dysfunction. Rifabutin was slowly eliminated from plasma in 7 healthy adult volunteers, presumably because of distribution-limited elimination, with a mean terminal half-life of 45 (±17) hours (range: 16 to 69 hours). Although the systemic levels of rifabutin following multiple dosing decreased by 38%. Its terminal half-life remained unchanged.

Metabolism – Of the 5 metabolites that have been identified, 25-O-desacetyl and 31-hydroxy are the most predominant, and show a plasma metabolite: Parent area under the curve ratio of 0.1 and 0.07, respectively. The former has an activity equal to the parent drug and contributes up to 10% to the total antimicrobial activity.

Excretion – A mass-balance study in 3 healthy adult volunteers with ^{14}C-labeled rifabutin showed that 53% of the oral dose was excreted in the urine, primarily as metabolites. About 30% of the dose is excreted in the feces. Mean systemic clearance (CL_s/F) in healthy adult volunteers following a single oral dose was 0.69 (± 0.32) L/hr/kg (range: 0.46 to 1.34 L/hr/kg). Renal and biliary clearance of unchanged drug each contribute approximately 5% to CL_s/F.

Special populations –

Renal function impairment: The disposition of rifabutin (300 mg) was studied in 18 patients with varying degrees of renal function. Area under plasma concentration time curve (AUC) increased by about 71% in patients with severe renal insufficiency (creatinine clearance below 30 mL/min) compared to patients with creatinine clearance (Ccr) between 61 to 74 mL/min. In patients with mild to moderate renal insufficiency (Ccr between 30 to 61 mL/min), the AUC increased by about 41%. A reduction in the dosage of rifabutin is recommended for patients with Ccr less than 30 mL/min (see Administration and Dosage).

Contraindications

Clinically significant hypersensitivity to rifabutin or to any other rifamycins.

Warnings

➤*Active tuberculosis:* Rifabutin capsules must not be administered for MAC prophylaxis to patients with active tuberculosis. Tuberculosis in HIV-positive patients is common and may present with atypical or extrapulmonary findings. Patients are likely to have a nonreactive purified protein derivative (PPD) despite active disease. In addition to chest X-ray and sputum culture, the following studies may be useful in the diagnosis of tuberculosis in the HIV-positive patient: Blood culture, urine culture, or biopsy of a suspicious lymph node.

Patients who develop complaints consistent with active tuberculosis while on prophylaxis with rifabutin should be evaluated immediately, so that those with active disease may be given an effective combination regimen of antituberculosis medications. Administration of rifabutin as a single agent to patients with active tuberculosis is likely to lead to the development of tuberculosis that is resistant both to rifabutin and to rifampin.

There is no evidence that rifabutin is effective prophylaxis against *M. tuberculosis*. Patients requiring prophylaxis against both *M. tuberculosis* and *Mycobacterium avium* complex may be given isoniazid and rifabutin concurrently.

➤*Fertility impairment:* Fertility was impaired in male rats given 160 mg/kg (32 times the recommended human daily dose).

➤*Pregnancy: Category B.*

In rats, given 200 mg/kg/day, there was a decrease in fetal viability. In rats, at 40 mg/kg/day (8 times the recommended human daily dose), rifabutin caused an increase in fetal skeletal variants. In rabbits, at 80 mg/kg/day (16 times the recommended human daily dose), rifabutin caused maternotoxicity and increase in fetal skeletal anomalies. There are no adequate and well-controlled studies in pregnant women. Because animal reproduction studies are not always predictive of human response, rifabutin should be used in pregnant women only if the potential benefit justifies the potential risk to the fetus.

➤*Lactation:* It is not known whether rifabutin is excreted in human milk. Because many drugs are excreted in human milk and because of the potential for serious adverse reactions in nursing infants, a decision should be made whether to discontinue nursing or discontinue the drug, taking into account the importance of the drug to the mother.

➤*Children:* Safety and effectiveness of rifabutin for prophylaxis of MAC in children have not been established. Limited safety data are available from treatment use in 22 HIV-positive children with MAC who received rifabutin in combination with at least two other antimycobacterials for periods from 1 to 183 weeks. Mean doses (mg/kg) for these children were: 18.5 (range 15 to 25) for infants 1 year of age; 8.6 (range 4.4 to 18.8) for children 2 to 10 years of age; and 4 (range 2.8 to 5.4) for adolescents 14 to 16 years of age. There is no evidence that doses greater than 5 mg/kg daily are useful. Adverse experiences were similar to those observed in the adult population, and included leukopenia, neutropenia and rash. In addition, corneal deposits have been observed in some patients during routine ophthalmologic surveillance of HIV-positive pediatric patients receiving rifabutin as part of a multiple-drug regimen for MAC prophylaxis. These are tiny, almost transparent, asymptomatic peripheral and central corneal deposits which do not impair vision. Doses of rifabutin may be administered mixed with foods such as applesauce.

Precautions

➤*Monitoring:* Because treatment with rifabutin capsules may be associated with neutropenia, and more rarely thrombocytopenia, physicians should consider obtaining hematologic studies periodically in patients receiving prophylaxis with rifabutin.

Drug Interactions

Rifabutin Drug Interactions

Precipitant drug	Object drug[1]		Description
Rifamycins	Anticoagulants	⬇	Rifampin decreases the anticoagulation action of warfarin. Increased doses of anticoagulants may be needed when rifamycins are administered concomitantly.
Rifamycins	Azole antifungal agents (eg, ketoconazole, itraconazole, fluconazole)	⬇	Plasma levels of azole antifungal agents may be decreased, reducing antifungal activity. Ketoconazole may decrease serum rifamycin levels. Itraconazole may increase rifabutin plasma levels and toxicity. If concurrent use cannot be avoided, monitor antimicrobial activity, and adjust doses as needed.
Azole antifungal agents (eg, ketoconazole, itraconazole)	Rifamycins	⬌	
Rifamycins	Benzodiazepines	⬇	The pharmacologic effects of certain benzodiazepines may be decreased. Monitor the clinical response to the benzodiazepines when starting or stopping the rifamycin.
Rifamycins	Beta blockers	⬇	The pharmacologic effects of certain beta blockers may be reduced by rifampin. May need a 3- to 4-week wash-out period for the enzyme induction effect to disappear. Closely monitor therapeutic response (eg, blood pressure).
Rifamycins	Buspirone	⬇	Buspirone plasma concentrations and pharmacologic effects may be decreased. Escalation of buspirone dose may be necessary. Buspirone concentrations may increase following discontinuation of concomitantly administered rifamycins.
Rifamycins	Corticosteroids	⬇	The pharmacologic effects of corticosteroids may be markedly decreased with initiation of rifampin therapy. This appears to occur within a few days of adding rifampin and to reverse 2 to 3 weeks following its administration. Double corticosteroid dosage after the addition of rifampin 300 mg/day.
Rifamycins	Cyclosporine	⬇	Immunosuppressive effects of cyclosporine may be reduced as early as 2 days following rifamycin initiation. Avoid this combination if possible; otherwise, frequently monitor.
Rifamycins	Dapsone	⬇	Rifabutin (300 mg/day) decreased the AUC of dapsone (50 mg/day) in HIV-infected patients (n = 16) by about 27% to 40%.
Rifamycins	Delavirdine	⬇	Rifamycins decrease delavirdine plasma concentrations. Avoid concurrent use if possible.
Rifamycins	Didanosine	⬌	In 12 HIV-infected patients, coadministration of rifabutin (300 or 600 mg/day) and didanosine (167 to 375 mg twice daily) did not alter the pharmacokinetics of either drug.
Rifamycins	Doxycycline	⬇	Rifamycins may decrease the serum concentration of doxycycline. Monitor the clinical response. Streptomycin does not appear to decrease doxycycline concentrations.
Rifamycins	Hydantoins	⬇	Serum hydantoin levels may be decreased, resulting in a decreased pharmacologic hydantoin effect. Monitor hydantoin levels.

RIFABUTIN — ORAL

Rifabutin Drug Interactions

Precipitant drug	Object drug[1]		Description
Rifamycins	Indinavir	↓	Rifamycins may decrease indinavir serum concentrations. In addition, indinavir may elevate serum rifabutin concentrations, increasing the risk of rifabutin toxicity. It is recommended to reduce the rifabutin dose by 50% when administered with indinavir.
Indinavir	Rifamycins	↑	
Rifamycins	Losartan	↓	Losartan plasma concentrations may be reduced, decreasing antihypertensive effects. Observe the clinical response when rifamycin is started or stopped and adjust therapy as needed.
Rifamycins	Macrolide antibiotics (eg, clarithromycin, erythromycin)	↓	The antimicrobial effects of macrolide antibiotics may be decreased. The frequency of GI adverse reactions may be increased.
Rifamycins	Methadone	↓	The actions of methadone may be reduced, requiring higher doses of methadone during rifampin administration. Patients receiving methadone treatment may experience withdrawal symptoms.
Rifamycins	Morphine	↓	The analgesic effects of morphine may be decreased.
Rifamycins	Nelfinavir	↓	Rifamycins may decrease nelfinavir serum concentrations, decreasing the pharmacologic effects. Avoid concomitant rifampin and nelfinavir administration.
Rifamycins	Oral contraceptives	↓	In 22 healthy female volunteers receiving an oral contraceptive (35 mcg ethinyl estradiol (EE) and 1 mg norethindrone (NE) daily for 21 days, rifabutin decreased EE (AUC) and C_{max} by 35% and 20%, respectively, and NE AUC by 46%.
Rifamycins	Quinine, Quinidine	↓	Addition of rifamycins to stable quinine derivative regimens may require increased doses of quinine derivative to maintain the desired therapeutic effect. Monitor quinine derivative serum levels and the ECG.
Rifamycins	Saquinavir	↓	In 12 HIV-infected patients, rifabutin (300 mg/day) decreased the AUC of saquinavir (600 mg 3 times daily) by about 40%.
Rifamycins	Sulfamethoxazole-trimethoprim	↓	Coadministration of rifabutin (300 mg/day) and sulfamethoxazole-trimethoprim (double strength) in 12 HIV-infected patients decreased the AUC of sulfamethoxazole-trimethoprim by about 15% to 20%. When trimethoprim was given alone, the AUC of trimethoprim was decreased by 14% and the C_{max} by 6%. Sulfamethoxazole-trimethoprim did not alter the pharmacokinetics of rifabutin.
Rifamycins	Theophylline, Aminophylline	↓	The addition of rifamycin may cause decreased theophylline levels and exacerbation of pulmonary symptoms. Monitor theophylline levels and the patient's response.
Rifamycins	Tricyclic antidepressants	↓	Tricyclic antidepressant (TCA) levels may be decreased, resulting in a decrease in pharmacologic effects. Consider monitoring the TCA concentrations when starting, discontinuing, or altering the rifamycin dose.
Rifamycins	Zidovudine	↓	In 16 HIV-infected patients on zidovudine (100 or 200 mg every 4 hours), rifabutin (300 or 450 mg/day) lowered the C_{max} and AUC of zidovudine by about 48% and 32%, respectively. However, zidovudine levels remained within the therapeutic range during coadministration of rifabutin. Zidovudine did not affect the pharmacokinetics of rifabutin.
Rifamycins	Zolpidem	↓	Plasma concentrations and therapeutic effects of zolpidem may be reduced. Monitor the clinical response, possibly increasing the dose of zolpidem during concomitant administration of rifamycins.
Ritonavir	Rifabutin	↑	Coadministration of ritonavir (500 mg every 12 hours) and rifabutin (150 mg/day) increased the AUC and C_{max} of rifabutin by more than 400% and 250%, respectively.

[1] ↓ = Object drug decreased. ↑ = Object drug increased. ↔ = Undetermined clinical effect.

➤*Cytochrome P450 system:* Rifabutin induces the enzymes of the cytochrome P450 3A subfamily (CYP3A) and therefore may reduce the plasma concentrations of drugs that are principally metabolized by those enzymes. Rifabutin is also metabolized by CYP3A. Thus, some drugs that inhibit CYP3A may significantly increase plasma concentrations of rifabutin.

Adverse Reactions

Rifabutin capsules were generally well tolerated in the controlled clinical trials. Discontinuation of therapy due to an adverse event was required in 16% of patients receiving rifabutin compared to 8% of patients receiving placebo in these trials. Primary reasons for discontinuation of rifabutin were rash (4% of treated patients), gastrointestinal intolerance (3%), and neutropenia (2%).

The following table enumerates adverse experiences that occurred at a frequency of 1% or greater, among the patients treated with rifabutin in studies 023 and 027.

Clinical adverse experiences reported in ≥ 1% of patients treated with rifabutin

Adverse reaction	Rifabutin (n = 566)	Placebo (n = 580)
CNS		
Insomnia	1%	1%
Dermatologic		
Rash	11%	8%
GI		
Anorexia	2%	2%
Diarrhea	3%	3%
Dyspepsia	3%	1%
Eructation	3%	1%
Flatulence	2%	1%
Nausea	6%	5%
Nausea and vomiting	3%	2%
Vomiting	1%	1%
GU		
Discolored urine	30%	6%
Musculoskeletal		
Myalgia	2%	1%
Special senses		
Taste perversion	3%	1%
Miscellaneous		
Abdominal pain	4%	3%
Asthenia	1%	1%
Chest pain	1%	1%
Fever	2%	1%
Headache	3%	5%
Pain	1%	2 %

➤*Additional (less than 1%):* Considering data from the 023 and 027 pivotal trials, and from other clinical studies, rifabutin appears to be a likely cause of the following adverse events which occurred in less than 1% of treated patients: Flu-like syndrome, hepatitis, hemolysis, arthralgia, myositis, chest pressure or pain with dyspnea, and skin discoloration.

The following adverse events have occurred in more than one patient receiving rifabutin, but an etiologic role has not been established: Seizure, paresthesia, aphasia, confusion, and nonspecific T wave changes on electrocardiogram.

When rifabutin was administered at doses from 1050 mg/day to 2400 mg/day, generalized arthralgia and uveitis were reported. These adverse experiences abated when rifabutin was discontinued.

➤*Lab test abnormalities:* The following table enumerates the changes in laboratory values that were considered as laboratory abnormalities in studies 023 and 027.

RIFABUTIN — ORAL

Percentage of patients with laboratory abnormalities		
Laboratory abnormalities	Rifabutin (n = 566)	Placebo (n = 580)
Chemistry		
Increased alkaline phosphatase[1]	less than 1%	3%
Increased AST[2]	7%	12%
Increased ALT[2]	9%	11%
Hematology		
Anemia[3]	6%	7%
Eosinophilia	1%	1%
Leukopenia[4]	17%	16%
Neutropenia[5]	25%	20%
Thrombocytopenia[6]	5%	4%

[1] Includes grade 3 or 4 toxicities as specified: 1 all values greater than 450 U/L
[2] 2 all values greater than 150 U/L
[3] 3 all hemoglobin values less than 8 g/dL
[4] 4 all WBC values less than 1500/mm[3]
[5] 5 all ANC values less than 750/mm[3]
[6] 6 all platelet count values less than 50,000/mm[3]

➤*Neutropenia:* The incidence of neutropenia in patients treated with rifabutin was significantly greater than in patients treated with placebo (P = 0.03). Although thrombocytopenia was not significantly more common among patients treated with rifabutin in these trials, rifabutin has been clearly linked to thrombocytopenia in rare cases. One patient in study 023 developed thrombotic thrombocytopenic purpura, which was attributed to rifabutin.

➤*Uveitis:* Uveitis is rare when rifabutin is used as a single agent at 300 mg/day for prophylaxis of MAC in HIV-infected persons, even with the concomitant use of fluconazole and/or macrolide antibiotics. However, if higher doses of rifabutin are administered in combination with these agents, the incidence of uveitis is higher.

Patients who developed uveitis had mild to severe symptoms that resolved after treatment with corticosteroids and/or mydriatic eye drops; in some severe cases, however, resolution of symptoms occurred after several weeks.

When uveitis occurs, temporary discontinuance of rifabutin and ophthalmologic evaluation are recommended. In most mild cases, rifabutin may be restarted; however, if signs or symptoms recur, use of rifabutin should be discontinued.

Overdosage

➤*Treatment:* While there is no experience in the treatment of overdose with rifabutin, clinical experience with rifamycins suggest that gastric lavage to evacuate gastric contents (within a few hours of overdose), followed by instillation of an activated charcoal slurry into the stomach, may help absorb any remaining drug from the gastrointestinal tract.

Rifabutin is 85% protein bound and distributed extensively into tissues (V_{ss}: 8 to 9 L/kg). It is not primarily excreted via the urinary route (less than 10% as unchanged drug), therefore, neither hemodialysis nor forced diuresis is expected to enhance the systemic elimination of unchanged rifabutin from the body in a patient with an overdose of rifabutin.

Patient Information

Patients should be advised of the signs and symptoms of both MAC and tuberculosis, and should be instructed to consult their physicians if they develop new complaints consistent with either of these diseases. In addition, since rifabutin may rarely be associated with myositis and uveitis, patients should be advised to notify their physicians if they develop signs or symptoms suggesting either of these disorders.

Urine, feces, saliva, sputum, perspiration, tears, and skin may be colored brown-orange with rifabutin and some of its metabolites. Soft contact lenses may be permanently stained. Patients to be treated with rifabutin should be made aware of these possibilities.

Advise patients using oral contraceptives to consider changing to nonhormonal methods of birth control because rifabutin, like rifampin, may decrease their efficacy.

ETHAMBUTOL HYDROCHLORIDE

Rx	**Myambutol** (X-Gen)	**Tablets:** 100 mg	(M6). White, film coated. In 100s.
		400 mg	(M7). White, scored, film coated. In 100s, 1000s, and UD 10s.

ETHAMBUTOL HYDROCHLORIDE — ORAL

Refer to the general discussion in the Antituberculosal Agents Introduction.

Indications

➤*Pulmonary tuberculosis:* For the treatment of pulmonary tuberculosis. It should not be used as the sole antituberculous drug, but should be used in conjunction with at least one other antituberculous drug. Selection of the companion drug should be based on clinical experience, considerations of comparative safety and appropriate in vitro susceptibility studies. In patients who have not received previous antituberculous therapy (ie, initial treatment) the most frequently used regimens have been ethambutol plus isoniazid and ethambutol plus isoniazid plus streptomycin.

In patients who have received previous antituberculous therapy, mycobacterial resistance to other drugs used in initial therapy is frequent. Consequently, in such retreatment patients, combine ethambutol with at least 1 of the second line drugs not previously administered to the patient and to which bacterial susceptibility has been indicated by appropriate in vitro studies. Antituberculous drugs used with ethambutol have included cycloserine, ethionamide, pyrazinamide, viomycin, and other drugs. Isoniazid, aminosalicylic acid, and streptomycin have also been used in multiple drug regimens. Alternating drug regimens have also been utilized.

Administration and Dosage

Ethambutol should not be used alone, in initial treatment or in retreatment. Please consult the CDC for the most current recommendations regarding treatment of tuberculosis. Administer ethambutol on a once every 24-hour basis only. Absorption is not significantly altered by administration with food. In general, continue therapy until bacteriological conversion has become permanent and maximal clinical improvement has occurred.

➤*Children:* Ethambutol is not recommended for use in pediatric patients under 13 years of age since safe conditions for use have not been established.

➤*Initial treatment:* In patients who have not received previous antituberculous therapy, administer ethambutol 15 mg/kg (7 mg/lb) of body weight, as a single oral dose once every 24 hours. In the more recent studies, isoniazid has been administered concurrently in a single, daily, oral dose.

➤*Retreatment:* In patients who have received previous antituberculous therapy, administer ethambutol 25 mg/kg (11 mg/lb) of body weight, as a single oral dose once every 24 hours. Concurrently administer at least one other antituberculous drug to which the organisms have been demonstrated to be susceptible by appropriate in vitro tests. Suitable drugs usually consist of those not previously used in the treatment of the patient. After 60 days of ethambutol administration, decrease the dose to 15 mg/kg (7 mg/lb) of body weight, and administer as a single oral dose once every 24 hours.

During the period when a patient is on a daily dose of 25 mg/kg, monthly eye examinations are advised.

Ethambutol Weight-Dose Table		
Weight range		Daily dose
Pounds	Kilograms	In mg
15 mg/kg (7 mg/lb) schedule		
Under 85 lbs	Under 37 kg	500
85 to 94.5	37 to 43	600
95 to 109.5	43 to 50	700
110 to 124.5	50 to 57	800
125 to 139.5	57 to 64	900
140 to 154.5	64 to 71	1,000
155 to 169.5	71 to 79	1,100
170 to 184.5	79 to 84	1,200
185 to 199.5	84 to 90	1,300
200 to 214.5	90 to 97	1,400
215 and over	Over 97	1,500
25 mg/kg (11 mg/lb) schedule		
less than 85 lbs	less than 38 kg	900
85 to 92.5	38 to 42	1,000
93 to 101.5	42 to 45.5	1,100
102 to 109.5	45.5 to 50	1,200
110 to 118.5	50 to 54	1,300
119 to 128.5	54 to 58	1,400
129 to 136.5	58 to 62	1,500
137 to 146.5	62 to 67	1,600
147 to 155.5	67 to 71	1,700
156 to 164.5	71 to 75	1,800
165 to 173.5	75 to 79	1,900
174 to 182.5	79 to 83	2,000
183 to 191.5	83 to 87	2,100
192 to 199.5	87 to 91	2,200
200 to 209.5	91 to 95	2,300
210 to 218.5	95 to 99	2,400
≥ 219	over 99	2,500

ETHAMBUTOL HYDROCHLORIDE — ORAL

➤*Storage/Stability:* Store at controlled room temperature 20° to 25°C (68° to 77°F).

Actions

➤*Pharmacology:* Ethambutol diffuses into actively growing mycobacterium cells such as tubercle bacilli. Ethambutol appears to inhibit the synthesis of 1 or more metabolites, thus causing impairment of cell metabolism, arrest of multiplication, and cell death. No cross-resistance with other available antimycobacterial agents has been demonstrated.

➤*Pharmacokinetics:*

Absorption/Distribution – Ethambutol following a single oral dose of 25 mg/kg of body weight, attains a peak of 2 to 5 mcg/mL in serum 2 to 4 hours after administration. When the drug is administered daily for longer periods of time at this dose, serum levels are similar. The serum level of ethambutol falls to undetectable levels by 24 hours after the last dose except in some patients with abnormal renal function. The intracellular concentrations of erythrocytes reach peak values approximately twice those of plasma and maintain this ratio throughout the 24 hours.

Metabolism/Excretion – During the 24-hour period following oral administration of ethambutol, approximately 50% of the initial dose is excreted unchanged in the urine, while an additional 8% to 15% appears in the form of metabolites. The main path of metabolism appears to be an initial oxidation of the alcohol to an aldehydic intermediate, followed by conversion to a dicarboxylic acid. From 20% to 22% of the initial dose is excreted in the feces as unchanged drug. No drug accumulation has been observed with consecutive single daily doses of 25 mg/kg in patients with healthy kidney function, although marked accumulation has been demonstrated in patients with renal insufficiency.

Contraindications

Hypersensitive to ethambutol; optic neuritis unless clinical judgement determines that it may be used; in patients who are unable to appreciate and report visual side effects or changes in vision (eg, young children, unconscious patients).

Warnings

➤*Visual disturbances:* See Adverse Reactions for more information.

➤*Hepatic effects:* Liver toxicities including fatalities have been reported.

➤*Renal function impairment:* Patients with decreased renal function need the dosage reduced as determined by serum levels of ethambutol, since the main path of excretion of this drug is by the kidneys.

➤*Pregnancy: Category C.* There are no adequate and well-controlled studies in pregnant women. There are reports of ophthalmic abnormalities occurring in infants born to women on antituberculous therapy that included ethambutol. Use ethambutol during pregnancy only if the benefit justifies the potential risk to the fetus.

Ethambutol has been shown to be teratogenic in pregnant mice and rabbits when given in high doses. When pregnant mice or rabbits were treated with high doses of ethambutol, fetal mortality was slightly but not significantly (*P* greater than 0.05) increased. Female rats treated with ethambutol displayed slight but insignificant (*P* greater than 0.05) decreases in fertility and litter size.

In fetuses born of mice treated with high doses of ethambutol during pregnancy, a low incidence of cleft palate, exencephaly, and abnormality of the vertebral column were observed. Minor abnormalities of the cervical vertebra were seen in the newborn of rats treated with high doses of ethambutol during pregnancy. Rabbits receiving high doses of ethambutol during pregnancy gave birth to 2 fetuses with monophthalmia, 1 with a shortened right forearm accompanied by bilateral wrist-joint contracture, and 1 with hare lip and cleft palate.

➤*Lactation:* Ethambutol is excreted into breast milk. Consider the use of ethambutol only if the expected benefit to the mother outweighs the potential risk to the infant.

➤*Children:* See Administration and Dosage for more information.

Precautions

➤*Monitoring:* As with any potent drug, perform baseline and periodic assessments of organ system functions, including renal, hepatic, and hematopoietic.

Because this drug may have adverse effects on vision, physical examination should include ophthalmoscopy, finger perimetry, and testing of color discrimination. In patients with visual defects such as cataracts, recurrent inflammatory conditions of the eye, optic neuritis, and diabetic retinopathy, the evaluation of changes in visual acuity is more difficult. Take care to be sure the variations in vision are not due to the underlying disease conditions. In such patients, give consideration to the relationship between benefits expected and possible visual deterioration because evaluation of visual changes is difficult.

Drug Interactions

➤*Aluminum-containing antacids:* The results of a study of coadministration of ethambutol (50 mg/kg) with an aluminum hydroxide containing antacid to 13 patients with tuberculosis showed a reduction of mean serum concentrations and urinary excretion of ethambutol of approximately 20% and 13%, respectively, suggesting that the oral absorption of ethambutol may be reduced by these antacid products. It is recommended to avoid concurrent administration of ethambutol with aluminum hydroxide containing antacids for at least 4 hours following ethambutol administration.

Adverse Reactions

➤*Ophthalmic:* Ethambutol may produce decreases in visual acuity, including irreversible blindness, which appear to be due to optic neuritis. Optic neuropathy including optic neuritis or retrobulbar neuritis occurring in association with ethambutol therapy may be characterized by 1 or more of the following events: decreased visual acuity, scotoma, color blindness, and/or visual defect. These events have also been reported in the absence of a diagnosis of optic or retrobulbar neuritis.

Advise patients to report promptly to their physicians any change of visual acuity.

Recovery of visual acuity generally occurs over a period of weeks to months after the drug has been discontinued. Patients have then received ethambutol again without recurrence of loss of visual acuity.

➤*Hypersensitivity:* Hypersensitivity syndrome consisting of cutaneous reaction (such as rash or exfoliative dermatitis), eosinophilia, and 1 or more of the following: Hepatitis, pneumonitis, nephritis, myocarditis, pericarditis. Fever and lymphadenopathy may be present.

➤*Miscellaneous:* Other adverse reactions reported include hypersensitivity, anaphylactoid reactions, dermatitis, pruritus and joint pain, anorexia, nausea, vomiting, gastrointestinal upset, abdominal pain, fever, malaise, headache, and dizziness, mental confusion, disorientation and possible hallucinations, thrombocytopenia, leukopenia, and neutropenia. Numbness and tingling of the extremities due to peripheral neuritis have been reported infrequently.

Elevated serum uric acid levels occur and precipitation of acute gout has been reported. Pulmonary infiltrates and eosinophilia also have been reported during ethambutol therapy. Liver toxicities, including fatalities, have been reported. Since ethambutol is recommended for therapy in conjunction with one or more other antituberculous drugs, these changes may be related to the concurrent therapy.

PYRAZINAMIDE

Rx	**Pyrazinamide** (UDL & ESI)	**Tablets:** 500 mg	(P36 LL). White, scored. In UD 100s.

PYRAZINAMIDE — ORAL

Refer to the general discussion in the Antituberculosal Agents Introduction.

Indications

➤*Tuberculosis:* Initial treatment of active tuberculosis in adults and children when combined with other antituberculous agents.

The current CDC recommendation for drug-susceptible initial treatment of active tuberculosis disease is a 6-month regimen consisting of isoniazid, rifampin, and pyrazinamide given for 2 months, followed by isoniazid and rifampin for 4 months.

Administration and Dosage

Administer pyrazinamide with other effective antituberculous drugs for the initial 2 months of a ≥ 6-month treatment regimen for drug-susceptible patients. Treat patients who are known or suspected to have drug-resistant disease with regimens individualized to their situation.

➤*HIV infection:* Patients with concomitant HIV infection may require longer courses of therapy. Be alert to any revised recommendations from the CDC for this group of patients.

➤*Usual dose:* 15 to 30 mg/kg orally once daily. Do not exceed 2 g/day when given as a daily regimen.

➤*Alternative dosing:* Alternatively, a twice weekly dosing regimen (50 to 70 mg/kg twice weekly based on lean body weight) has been developed to promote patient compliance on an outpatient basis. In studies evaluating the twice weekly regimen, doses of pyrazinamide in excess of 3 g twice weekly have been administered without an increased incidence of adverse reactions.

Actions

➤*Pharmacology:* Pyrazinamide, the pyrazine analog of nicotinamide, is an antituberculous agent. Pyrazinamide may be bacteriostatic or bactericidal against *Mycobacterium tuberculosis* depending on the concentration of the drug attained at the site of infection. The mechanism of action is unknown.

➤*Pharmacokinetics:*

Absorption/Distribution – Pyrazinamide is well absorbed from the GI tract and attains peak plasma concentrations within 2 hours. Plasma concentrations generally range from 30 to 50 mcg/ml with doses of 20 to 25 mg/kg. It is widely distributed in body tissues and fluids including the liver, lungs, and cerebrospinal fluid. Pyrazinamide is ≈ 10% bound to plasma proteins.

Metabolism/Excretion – The half-life is 9 to 10 hours; it may be prolonged in patients with impaired renal or hepatic function. Pyrazinamide is hydrolyzed in the liver to its major active metabolite, pyrazinoic acid. Pyrazinoic acid is hydroxylated to the main excretory product, 5-hydroxypyrazinoic acid.

PYRAZINAMIDE — ORAL

Approximately 70% of an oral dose is excreted in urine, mainly by glomerular filtration, within 24 hours. Pyrazinamide is significantly dialyzed and should be dosed after hemodialysis.

Contraindications

Severe hepatic damage; hypersensitivity; acute gout.

Warnings

➤*Combination therapy:* Use only in conjunction with other effective antituberculous agents. Individualize regimens to treat patients with drug-resistant disease.

➤*Hyperuricemia:* Pyrazinamide inhibits renal excretion of urates, frequently resulting in hyperuricemia, which is usually asymptomatic. Patients started on pyrazinamide should have baseline serum uric acid determinations. Discontinue the drug and do not resume if signs of hyperuricemia accompanied by acute gouty arthritis appear.

➤*Renal function impairment:* It may be prudent to select doses at the low end of the dosing range.

➤*Hepatic function impairment:* Patients started on pyrazinamide should have baseline liver function determinations. Closely follow patients with preexisting liver disease or those at an increased risk for drug-related hepatitis (eg, alcohol abusers). Discontinue pyrazinamide and do not resume if signs of hepatocellular damage appear.

➤*Elderly:* In general, use caution when selecting a dose for an elderly patient. Start at the low end of the dosing range to reflect the greater frequency of decreased hepatic or renal function and of concomitant disease or other drug therapy.

➤*Pregnancy: Category C.* It is not known whether pyrazinamide can cause fetal harm when administered to a pregnant woman or can affect reproduction capacity. Give to a pregnant woman only if clearly needed.

➤*Lactation:* Pyrazinamide has been found in small amounts in breast milk. Therefore, it is advised that pyrazinamide be used with caution in nursing mothers, taking into account the risk-benefit of this therapy.

➤*Children:* Pyrazinamide regimens employed in adults are probably equally effective in children. Pyrazinamide appears to be well tolerated in children.

Precautions

➤*Monitoring:* Determine baseline liver function studies (especially ALT and AST) and uric acid levels prior to therapy. Perform appropriate laboratory testing at periodic intervals and if any clinical signs or symptoms occur during therapy.

➤*HIV infection:* In patients with concomitant HIV infection, be aware of current CDC recommendations. It is possible these patients may require a longer course of treatment.

➤*Diabetes mellitus:* Use with caution in patients with a history of diabetes mellitus, as management may be more difficult.

➤*Primary resistance of M. tuberculosis:* Primary resistance to pyrazinamide is uncommon. In cases with known or suspected drug resistance, perform in vitro susceptibility tests with recent cultures of *M. tuberculosis* against pyrazinamide and the usual primary drugs. There are few reliable in vitro tests for pyrazinamide resistance. A reference laboratory capable of performing these studies must be employed.

Drug Interactions

➤*Drug/Lab test interactions:* Pyrazinamide has been reported to interfere with *Acetest* and *Ketostix* urine tests to produce a pink-brown color.

Adverse Reactions

➤*GI:* Nausea; vomiting; anorexia.

➤*Hematologic/Lymphatic:* Thrombocytopenia and sideroblastic anemia with erythroid hyperplasia, vacuolation of erythrocytes, increased serum iron concentration and adverse effects on blood clotting mechanisms (rare).

➤*Hepatic:* The principal adverse effect is a hepatic reaction (see Warnings). Hepatotoxicity appears to be dose-related, and may appear at any time during therapy.

➤*Miscellaneous:* Mild arthralgia and myalgia (frequent); hypersensitivity reactions including rashes, urticaria, pruritus; fever, acne, photosensitivity, porphyria, dysuria, interstitial nephritis (rare); gout (see Warnings).

Overdosage

➤*Symptoms:* Overdosage experience is limited. In 1 case report of overdose, abnormal liver function tests developed. These spontaneously reverted to normal when the drug was stopped.

➤*Treatment:* Employ clinical monitoring and supportive therapy. Pyrazinamide is dialyzable. Refer to General Management of Acute Overdosage.

Patient Information

Instruct patients to notify their physician promptly if they experience any of the following: Fever, loss of appetite, malaise, nausea and vomiting, darkened urine, yellowish discoloration of the skin and eyes, pain or swelling of the joints.

Compliance with the full course of therapy must be emphasized; stress the importance of not missing any doses.

ETHIONAMIDE

Rx	**Trecator-SC** (Wyeth-Ayerst)	**Tablets:** 250 mg	(Wyeth 4130). Reddish-orange. Sugar coated. In 100s.

ETHIONAMIDE — ORAL

Refer to the general discussion in the Antituberculosal Agents Introduction.

Indications

➤*Tuberculosis:* Ethionamide is primarily indicated for the treatment of active tuberculosis in patients with *Mycobacterium tuberculosis* resistant to isoniazid or rifampin, or when there is intolerance on the part of the patient to other drugs. Its use alone in the treatment of tuberculosis results in the rapid development of resistance. It is essential, therefore, to give a suitable companion drug or drugs, the choice being based on the results of susceptibility tests. If the susceptibility tests indicate that the patient's organism is resistant to one of the first-line antituberculosis drugs (ie, isoniazid or rifampin) yet susceptible to ethionamide, ethionamide should be accompanied by at least one drug to which the *M. tuberculosis* isolate is known to be susceptible. If the tuberculosis is resistant to both isoniazid and rifampin, yet susceptible to ethionamide, ethionamide should be accompanied by at least two other drugs to which the *M. tuberculosis* isolate is known to be susceptible.

Drugs which have been used as companion agents are rifampin, ethambutol, pyrazinamide, cycloserine, kanamycin, streptomycin, and isoniazid. The usual warnings, precautions, and dosage regimens for these companion drugs should be observed.

Administration and Dosage

➤*Adults:* Ethionamide is administered orally. The usual adult dose is 15 to 20 mg/kg/day, administered once daily or, if patient exhibits poor gastrointestinal tolerance, in divided doses, with a maximum daily dosage of 1 g. Thus far, there is insufficient evidence to indicate the lowest effective dosage levels. Therefore, in order to minimize the risk of resistance developing to the drug or to the companion drug, the principle of giving the highest tolerated dose (based on gastrointestinal intolerance) has been followed. In the adult this would seem to be between 0.5 and 1 g daily, with an average of 0.75 g daily.

➤*Children:* The optimum dosage for pediatric patients has not been established. However, pediatric dosages of 10 to 20 mg/kg orally daily in 2 or 3 divided doses given after meals or 15 mg/kg/24 hrs as a single daily dose have been recommended. As with adults, ethionamide may be administered to pediatric patients once daily. It should be noted that in patients with concomitant tuberculosis and HIV infection, malabsorption syndrome may be present. Drug malabsorption should be suspected in patients who adhere to therapy, but who fail to respond appropriately. In such cases, consideration should be given to therapeutic drug monitoring (see Pharmacokinetics).

➤*Alternative dosing:* Initiation of therapy at a dose of 250 mg daily, with gradual titration to optimal doses as tolerated by the patient, also may be beneficial. A regimen of 250 mg daily for 1 or 2 days, followed by 250 mg twice daily for 1 or 2 days with a subsequent increase to 1 g in 3 or 4 divided doses has been reported.

➤*Concomitant pyridoxine therapy:* Concomitant administration of pyridoxine is recommended.

➤*Duration:* Duration of treatment should be based on individual clinical response. In general, continue therapy until bacteriological conversion has become permanent and maximal clinical improvement has occurred.

➤*Storage/Stability:* Store at room temperature ≈ 25°C (77°F). Dispense in a tight container.

Actions

➤*Pharmacology:* Ethionamide may be bacteriostatic or bactericidal in action, depending on the concentration of the drug attained at the site of infection and the susceptibility of the infecting organism. The exact mechanism of action of ethionamide has not been fully elucidated, but the drug appears to inhibit peptide synthesis in susceptible organisms.

➤*Pharmacokinetics:*

Absorption/Distribution – Ethionamide is essentially completely absorbed following oral administration and is not subjected to any appreciable first pass metabolism. Following a single 250 mg oral dose of ethionamide in healthy volunteers, peak plasma concentrations of about 2 mcg/mL were attained at 2 hours in most cases. Normal serum concentrations of 1 to 5 mcg/mL are usually seen 2 hours following doses of 250 mg to 500 mg. These concentrations approximate the therapeutic range for this drug when the therapeutic range is defined by those serum concentrations associated with a high probability of success and a low probability of dose-related toxicity. The drug is ≈ 30% bound to plasma proteins. Ethionamide is rapidly and widely distributed into body tissues and fluids, with concentrations in plasma and various organs being approximately equal. Significant concentrations also are present in cerebrospinal fluid.

Metabolism/Excretion – Ethionamide is extensively metabolized to active and inactive metabolites with less than 1% excreted as the free form in urine. Metabolism is presumed to occur in the liver and thus far 6 metabolites have been isolated: 2-ethylisonicotinamide, carbamoyldihydropyridine, thiocarbamoyl-dihydropyridine, S-oxocarbamoyl dihydropyridine, 2-ethylthioiso-nicotinamide, and ethionamide sulphoxide. The sulphoxide metabolite has been demonstrated to have antimicrobial activity against *Mycobacterium tuberculosis*. Ethionamide has a plasma elimination half-life of ≈ 2 hours after oral dosing.

ETHIONAMIDE — ORAL

Contraindications

In patients with severe hepatic impairment and in patients who are hypersensitive to the drug.

Warnings

➤*Resistance:* The use of ethionamide alone in the treatment of tuberculosis results in rapid development of resistance. It is essential, therefore, to give a suitable companion drug or drugs, the choice being based on the results of susceptibility testing.

However, therapy may be initiated prior to receiving the results of susceptibility tests as deemed appropriate by the physician. Ethionamide should be administered with at least one, sometimes two, other drugs to which the organism is known to be susceptible (see Indications).

➤*Compliance:* Patient compliance is essential to the success of the antituberculosis therapy and to prevent the emergence of drug-resistant organisms. Therefore, patients should adhere to the drug regimen for the full duration of treatment. It is recommended that directly observed therapy be practiced when patients are receiving antituberculous medication. Additional consultation from experts in the treatment of drug-resistant tuberculosis is recommended when patients develop drug-resistant organisms.

➤*Pregnancy: Category C.* Animal studies conducted with ethionamide indicate that the drug has teratogenic potential in rabbits and rats. The doses used in these studies on a mg/kg basis were considerably in excess of those recommended in humans. There are no adequate and well-controlled studies in pregnant women. Because of these animal studies, however, it must be recommended that ethionamide be withheld from women who are pregnant, or who are likely to become pregnant while under therapy, unless the prescribing physician considers it to be an essential part of the treatment.

➤*Lactation:* Because no information is available on the excretion of ethionamide in human milk, ethionamide should be administered to nursing mothers only if the benefits outweigh the risks. Newborns who are breastfed by mothers who are taking ethionamide should be monitored for adverse effects.

➤*Children:* Due to the fact that pulmonary tuberculosis resistant to primary therapy is rarely found in neonates, infants, and children, investigations have been limited in these age groups. At present, the drug should not be used in pediatric patients under 12 years of age except when the organisms are definitely resistant to primary therapy and systemic dissemination of the disease, or other life-threatening complications of tuberculosis, is judged to be imminent.

Precautions

➤*Monitoring:* Determination of serum transaminases (AST/ALT) should be made prior to initiation of therapy and should be monitored monthly. If serum transaminases become elevated during therapy, ethionamide and the companion antituberculosis drug or drugs may be discontinued temporarily until the laboratory abnormalities have resolved. Ethionamide and the companion antituberculosis medication(s) then should be reintroduced sequentially to determine which drug (or drugs) is (are) responsible for the hepatotoxicity.

Blood glucose determinations should be made prior to and periodically throughout therapy with ethionamide. Diabetic patients should be particularly alert for episodes of hypoglycemia.

Periodic monitoring of thyroid function tests is recommended as hypothyroidism, with or without goiter, has been reported with ethionamide therapy.

Ophthalmologic examinations (including ophthalmoscopy) should be performed before and periodically during therapy with ethionamide.

Drug Interactions

➤*Antituberculous agents:* Ethionamide has been found to temporarily raise serum concentrations of isoniazid. Ethionamide may potentiate the adverse effects of other antituberculous drugs administered concomitantly. In particular, convulsions have been reported when ethionamide is administered with cycloserine and special care should be taken when the treatment regimen includes both of these drugs.

➤*Ethanol:* Excessive ethanol ingestion should be avoided because a psychotic reaction has been reported.

Adverse Reactions

➤*CNS:* Psychotic disturbances (including mental depression), drowsiness, dizziness, restlessness, headache, and postural hypotension have been reported with ethionamide. Rare reports of peripheral neuritis, optic neuritis, diplopia, blurred vision, and a pellagra-like syndrome also have been reported. Concurrent administration of pyridoxine has been recommended to prevent or relieve neurotoxic effects.

➤*GI:* The most common side effects of ethionamide are gastrointestinal disturbances including nausea, vomiting, diarrhea, abdominal pain, excessive salivation, metallic taste, stomatitis, anorexia and weight loss. Adverse gastrointestinal effects appear to be dose related, with ≈ 50% of patients unable to tolerate 1 g as a single dose. Gastrointestinal effects may be minimized by decreasing dosage, by changing the time of drug administration, or by the concurrent administration of an antiemetic agent.

➤*Hepatic:* Transient increases in serum bilirubin, AST, ALT; hepatitis (with or without jaundice).

➤*Hypersensitivity:* Hypersensitivity reactions including rash, photosensitivity, thrombocytopenia and purpura have been reported rarely.

➤*Miscellaneous:* Hypoglycemia, gynecomastia, impotence, and acne also have occurred. The management of patients with diabetes mellitus may become more difficult in those receiving ethionamide.

Overdosage

➤*Treatment:* No specific information is available on the treatment of overdosage with ethionamide. If it should occur, standard procedures to evacuate gastric contents and to support vital functions should be employed.

Patient Information

Patients should be advised to consult their physician should blurred vision or any loss of vision, with or without eye pain, occur during treatment.

Excessive ethanol ingestion should be avoided because a psychotic reaction has been reported.

AMINOSALICYLIC ACID (p-aminosalicylic acid; 4-aminosalicylic acid)

Rx	**Paser** (Jacobus Pharm)	**Granules, delayed-release:** 4 g	In packets.

AMINOSALICYLIC ACID — ORAL

Refer to the general discussion in the Antituberculosal Agents Introduction.

Indications

➤*Tuberculosis:* For the treatment of tuberculosis in combination with other active agents. It is most commonly used in patients with multi-drug resistant TB (MDR-TB) or in situations when therapy with isoniazid and rifampin is not possible due to a combination of resistance or intolerance. When aminosalicylic acid is added to the treatment regimen in patients with proven or suspected drug resistance, it should be accompanied by at least 1 and preferably 2 other new agents to which the patient's organism is known or expected to be susceptible.

Administration and Dosage

Aminosalicylic acid granules should be administered with other drugs to which the organism is known or expected to be susceptible. It is most commonly administered to patients with MDR-TB or in other situations in which therapy with isoniazid or rifampin is not possible due to a combination of resistance or intolerance.

➤*Tuberculosis:* The adult dosage of 4 g (1 packet) 3 times per day or correspondingly smaller doses in children should be given by sprinkling on apple sauce or yogurt or by swirling in the glass to suspend the granules in an acidic drink such as tomato or orange juice.

Do not use if packet is swollen or the granules have lost their tan color, turning dark brown or purple.

➤*Storage/Stability:* Store below 15°C (59°F) (in a refrigerator or freezer).

Patients are urged to store aminosalicylic acid in a refrigerator or freezer. Aminosalicylic acid packets may be stored at room temperature for short periods of time.

Avoid excessive heat. Do not use if packet is swollen or the granules have lost their tan color, turning dark brown or purple.

Actions

➤*Pharmacology:* Aminosalicylic acid is bacteriostatic against *Mycobacterium tuberculosis.* It inhibits the onset of bacterial resistance to streptomycin and isoniazid. The mechanism of action has been postulated to be inhibition of folic acid synthesis (but without potentiation with antifolic compounds) or inhibition of synthesis of the cell wall component, mycobactin, thus reducing iron uptake by *M. tuberculosis.*

Enteric coating –

After 2 hours in simulated gastric fluid, 10% of unprotected aminosalicylic acid is decarboxylated to form meta-aminophenol, a known hepatotoxin. The acid-resistant coating of the aminosalicylic acid granules protects against degradation in the stomach.

The small granules are designed to escape the usual restriction on gastric emptying of large particles. Under neutral conditions such as are found in the small intestine or in neutral foods, the acid-resistant coating is dissolved within 1 minute. Care must be taken in the administration of these granules to protect the acid-resistant coating by maintaining the granules in an acidic food during dosage administration. Patients who have neutralized gastric acid with antacids will not need to protect the acid resistant coating with an acidic food since no acid is present to spoil the drug. Antacids may influence the absorption of other medications and are not necessary for aminosalicylic acid consumed with an acidic food.

Because aminosalicylic acid granules are protected by an enteric coating, absorption does not commence until they leave the stomach. The soft skeletons of the granules remain and may be seen in the stool.

➤*Pharmacokinetics:*

Absorption/Distribution – In a single 4 g pharmacokinetic study with food in healthy volunteers the initial time to a 2 mcg/mL serum level of aminosalicylic acid was 2 hours with a range of 45 minutes to 24 hours; the median time to peak was 6 hours with a range of 1.5 to 24 hours. The mean peak level was 20 mcg/mL with a range of 9 to 35 mcg/mL; a level of 2 mcg/mL was maintained for an average of 7.9 hours with a range of 5 to 9;

AMINOSALICYLIC ACID — ORAL

a level of 1 mcg/mL was maintained for an average of 8.8 hours with a range of 6 to 11.5 hours. The recommended schedule is 4 g every 8 hours.

Penetration into the cerebrospinal fluid occurs only if the meninges are inflamed.

Approximately 50% to 60% of aminosalicylic acid is protein bound; binding is reported to be reduced 50% in kwashiorkor.

Excretion – Eighty percent (80%) of aminosalicylic acid is excreted in the urine, with 50% or more of the dosage excreted in acetylated form. The acetylation process is not genetically determined as is the case for isoniazid. Aminosalicylic acid is excreted by glomerular filtration; although previously reported otherwise, probenecid, a tubular blocking agent, does not enhance plasma concentration. In a 1954 study thyroxine synthesis but not iodide uptake was reported reduced about 40% when the sodium salt (not aminosalicylic acid granules) of aminosalicylic acid was administered 1 hour before radioiodine; the sodium salt typically produces a serum level over 120 mcg/mL at 1 hour lasting 1 hour. Occasional goiter development can be prevented by the administration of thyroxine but not iodide.

Contraindications

Hypersensitivity to any component of this medication; severe renal disease.

Warnings

➤*Hepatitis:* In 1 retrospective study of 7492 patients on rapidly absorbed aminosalicylic acid preparations, drug-induced hepatitis occurred in 38 patients (0.5%): In these 38, the first symptom usually appeared within 3 months of the start of therapy with a rash as the most common event followed by fever and much less frequently by GI disturbances of anorexia, nausea or diarrhea. Only 1 patient was diagnosed on routine biochemistry.

➤*Hypersensitivity reactions:* All drugs should be stopped at the first sign suggesting a hypersensitivity reaction. They may be restarted one at a time in very small but gradually increasing doses to determine whether the manifestations are drug-induced and, if so, which drug is responsible.

Desensitization has been accomplished successfully in 15 of 17 patients starting with 10 mg aminosalicylic acid given as a single dose. The dosage is doubled every 2 days until reaching a total of 1 g after which the dosage is divided to follow the regular schedule of administration. If a mild temperature rise or skin reaction develops, the increment is to be dropped back 1 level or the progression held for 1 cycle.

Reactions are rare after a total dosage of 1.5 g.

➤*Renal function impairment:* Patients with severe renal disease will accumulate aminosalicylic acid and its acetyl metabolite but will continue to acetylate, thus leading exclusively to the inactive acetylated form; deacetylation, if any, is not significant.

➤*Mutagenesis:* Patients on isoniazid and aminosalicylic acid have been reported to have an increased number of chromosomal aberrations as compared to controls.

➤*Pregnancy: Category C.* Aminosalicylic acid has been reported to produce occipital malformations in rats when given at doses within the human dose range. Although there probably is a dose response, the frequency of abnormalities was comparable to controls at the highest level tested (2 times the human dosage). When administered to rabbits at 5 mg/kg, throughout all 3 trimesters, no teratologic or embryocidal effects were seen. Literature reports on aminosalicylic acid in pregnant women always report coadministration of other medications. Because there are no adequate and well controlled studies of aminosalicylic acid in humans, aminosalicylic acid granules should be given to a pregnant woman only if clearly needed.

➤*Lactation:* After administration of a different preparation of aminosalicylic acid to 1 patient, the maximum concentration in the milk was 1 mcg/mL at 3 hours with a half-life of 2.5 hours; the maximum maternal plasma concentration was 70 mcg/mL at 2 hours.

Precautions

➤*Malabsorption syndrome:* A malabsorption syndrome can develop in patients on aminosalicylic acid but is usually not complete. The complete syndrome includes steatorrhea, an abnormal small bowel pattern on x-ray, villus atrophy, depressed cholesterol, reduced D-xylose, and iron absorption. Triglyceride absorption always is normal.

Drug Interactions

Aminosalicylic Acid Drug Interactions

Precipitant	Object drug*		Description
Aminosalicylic acid	Isoniazid	↑	Aminosalicylic acid at a dose of 12 g in a rapidly available form has been reported to produce a 20% decrease in the acetylation of INH, especially in fast acetylators. The effect is dose related and, while it has not been studied with the current delayed-release formulation, the lower serum levels with this preparation will result in a reduced effect on the acetylation of INH. Special precautions are not deemed necessary.
Aminosalicylic acid	Digoxin	↓	Oral absorption of digoxin may be reduced when given concomitantly with aminosalicylic acid. Monitor serum digoxin levels.
Aminosalicylic acid	Vitamin B_{12}	↓	Aminosalicylic acid impairs the absorption of vitamin B_{12}. Consider vitamin B_{12} therapy for patients on aminosalicylic acid therapy more than 1 month.

* ↑ = Object drug increased. ↓ = Object drug decreased.

➤*Drug/Lab test interactions:* Aminosalicylic acid has been reported to interfere technically with the serum determinations of albumin by dye-binding, AST by the azoene dye method and with qualitative urine tests for ketones, bilirubin, urobilinogen, or porphobilinogen.

Adverse Reactions

➤*GI:* The most common side effect is gastrointestinal intolerance manifested by nausea, vomiting, diarrhea, and abdominal pain.

➤*Miscellaneous:* Fever, skin eruptions of various types, including exfoliative dermatitis, infectious mononucleosis-like, or lymphoma-like syndrome, leucopenia, agranulocytosis, thrombocytopenia, Coombs' positive hemolytic anemia, jaundice, hepatitis, pericarditis, hypoglycemia, optic neuritis, encephalopathy, Leoffler's syndrome, vasculitis, and a reduction in prothrombin.

Crystalluria may be prevented by the maintenance of urine at a neutral or an alkaline pH.

Patient Information

The patient should be advised that the first signs of hypersensitivity include a rash, often followed by fever, and much less frequently, GI disturbances of anorexia, nausea, or diarrhea. If such symptoms develop, the patient should immediately cease taking the medication and arrange for a prompt clinical visit.

Patients should be advised that poor compliance in taking anti-TB medication often leads to treatment failure, and, not infrequently, to the development of resistance of the organisms in the individual patient.

Patients should be advised that the skeleton of the granules may be seen in the stool.

The coating to protect the aminosalicylic acid granules dissolves promptly under neutral conditions; the granules therefore should be administered by sprinkling on acidic foods such as apple sauce or yogurt or by suspension in a fruit drink which will protect the coating, but the granules sink and will have to be swirled. The coating will last at least 2 hours in either system. All juices tested to date have been satisfactory; tested are: Tomato, orange, grapefruit, grape, cranberry, apple, "fruit punch".

Patients should be advised to store aminosalicylic acid in a refrigerator or freezer. Aminosalicylic acid packets may be stored at room temperature for short periods of time.

Patients should be advised not to use if the packets are swollen or the granules have lost their tan color and are dark brown or purple. The patient should inform the pharmacist or physician immediately and return the medication.

CYCLOSERINE

Rx	**Seromycin Pulvules** (Dura)	**Capsules:** 250 mg	(51479 019). Red/gray. In 40s.

CYCLOSERINE — ORAL

Refer to the general discussion in the Antituberculosal Agents Introduction.

Indications

➤*Active pulmonary and extrapulmonary tuberculosis:* Treatment of active pulmonary and extrapulmonary tuberculosis (including renal disease) when the causative organisms are susceptible to this drug and when treatment with the primary medications (streptomycin, isoniazid, rifampin, and ethambutol) has proved inadequate. Like all antituberculosis drugs, cycloserine should be administered in conjunction with other effective chemotherapy and not as the sole therapeutic agent.

➤*Acute urinary tract infections:* Treatment of acute urinary tract infections caused by susceptible strains of gram-positive and gram-negative bacteria, especially *Enterobacter* sp. and *Escherichia coli*. It is generally no more and is usually less effective than other antimicrobial agents in the treatment of urinary tract infections caused by bacteria other than mycobacteria. Use of cycloserine in these infections should be considered only when more conventional therapy has failed and when the organism has been demonstrated to be susceptible to the drug.

Administration and Dosage

➤*Adults:* 500 mg to 1 g daily in divided doses monitored by blood levels. The initial adult dosage most frequently given is 250 mg twice daily at 12-hour intervals for the first 2 weeks. A daily dosage of 1 g should not be exceeded.

CYCLOSERINE — ORAL

➤*Storage/Stability:* Store at controlled room temperature, 15° to 30°C (59° to 86°F).

Actions

➤*Pharmacology:* Cycloserine inhibits cell-wall synthesis in susceptible strains of gram-positive and gram-negative bacteria and in *Mycobacterium* tuberculosis.

➤*Pharmacokinetics:*

Absorption – After oral administration, cycloserine is readily absorbed from the GI tract, with peak blood levels occurring in 4 to 8 hours.

Distribution – Blood levels of 25 to 30 mcg/mL can generally be maintained with the usual dosage of 250 mg twice a day, although the relationship of plasma levels to dosage is not always consistent. Concentrations in the cerebrospinal fluid, pleural fluid, fetal blood, and mother's milk approach those found in the serum. Detectable amounts are found in ascitic fluid, bile, sputum, amniotic fluid, and lung and lymph tissues.

Metabolism/Excretion – The remaining 35% is apparently metabolized to unknown substances.

Approximately 65% of a single dose of cycloserine can be recovered in the urine within 72 hours after oral administration. The maximum excretion rate occurs 2 to 6 hours after administration, with 50% of the drug eliminated in 12 hours.

Contraindications

Hypersensitivity to cycloserine; epilepsy; depression, severe anxiety, or psychosis; severe renal insufficiency; excessive concurrent use of alcohol.

Warnings

➤*CNS toxicity:* Administration of cycloserine should be discontinued or the dosage reduced if the patient develops symptoms of CNS toxicity, such as convulsions, psychosis, somnolence, depression, confusion, hyperreflexia, headache, tremor, vertigo, paresis, or dysarthria.

The risk of convulsions is increased in chronic alcoholics.

➤*Allergic dermatitis:* Administration should be discontinued or the dosage reduced if the patient develops allergic dermatitis.

➤*Toxicity:* The toxicity of cycloserine is closely related to excessive blood levels (above 30 mcg/mL), as determined by high dosage or inadequate renal clearance. The ratio of toxic dose to effective dose in tuberculosis is small.

➤*Pregnancy: Category C.*

It is not known whether cycloserine can cause fetal harm when administered to a pregnant woman or can affect reproduction capacity. Cycloserine should be given to a pregnant woman only if clearly needed.

➤*Lactation:* Because of the potential for serious adverse reactions in nursing infants from cycloserine, a decision should be made whether to discontinue nursing or to discontinue the drug, taking into account the importance of the drug to the mother.

➤*Children:* Safety and effectiveness in pediatric patients have not been established.

Precautions

➤*Monitoring:* Patients should be monitored by hematologic, renal excretion, blood level, and liver function studies.

Blood levels should be determined at least weekly for patients with reduced renal function, for individuals receiving a daily dosage of more than 500 mg, and for those showing signs and symptoms suggestive of toxicity. The dosage should be adjusted to keep the blood level below 30 mcg/mL.

➤*Anticonvulsants or sedatives:* Anticonvulsant drugs or sedatives may be effective in controlling symptoms of CNS toxicity, such as convulsions, anxiety, and tremor. Patients receiving more than 500 mg of cycloserine daily should be closely observed for such symptoms. The value of pyridoxine in preventing CNS toxicity from cycloserine has not been proved.

➤*Anemia:* Administration of cycloserine and other antituberculosis drugs has been associated in a few instances with vitamin B_{12} or folic-acid deficiency, megaloblastic anemia, and sideroblastic anemia. If evidence of anemia develops during treatment, appropriate studies and therapy should be instituted.

Drug Interactions

➤*Ethionamide:* Concurrent administration of ethionamide has been reported to potentiate neurotoxic side effects.

➤*Alcohol:* Alcohol and cycloserine are incompatible, especially during a regimen calling for large doses of the latter. Alcohol increases the possibility and risk of epileptic episodes.

➤*Isoniazid:* Concurrent administration of isoniazid may result in increased incidence of CNS effects, such as dizziness or drowsiness. Dosage adjustments may be necessary and patients should be monitored closely for signs of CNS toxicity.

Adverse Reactions

Most adverse reactions occurring during therapy with cycloserine involve the nervous system or are manifestations of drug hypersensitivity. The following side effects have been observed in patients receiving cycloserine:

➤*Allergic:* Allergy apparently not related to dosage.

➤*Cardiovascular:* Sudden development of congestive heart failure in patients receiving 1 to 1.5 g of cycloserine daily has been reported.

➤*CNS:* Nervous system symptoms that appear to be related to higher dosages of the drug, ie, greater than 500 mg daily, are convulsions, drowsiness and somnolence, headache, tremor, dysarthria, vertigo, confusion and disorientation with loss of memory, psychoses, possibly with suicidal tendencies, character changes, hyperirritability, aggression, paresis, hyperreflexia, paresthesia, major and minor (localized) clonic seizures, coma.

➤*Dermatologic:* Skin rash.

➤*Miscellaneous:* Elevated serum transaminase, especially in patients with preexisting liver disease.

Overdosage

➤*Symptoms:* Acute toxicity from cycloserine can occur if more than 1 g is ingested by an adult. Chronic toxicity from cycloserine is dose related and can occur if more than 500 mg is administered daily. Patients with renal impairment will accumulate cycloserine and may develop toxicity if the dosing regimen is not modified. Patients with severe renal impairment should not receive the drug. The central nervous system is the most common organ system involved with toxicity. Toxic effects may include headache, vertigo, confusion, drowsiness, hyperirritability, paresthesias, dysarthria, and psychosis. Following larger ingestions, paresis, convulsions, and coma often occur. Ethyl alcohol may increase the risk of seizures in patients receiving cycloserine.

The oral median lethal dose in mice is 5290 mg/kg.

➤*Treatment:* Overdoses of cycloserine have been reported rarely. The following is provided to serve as a guide should such an overdose be encountered.

Protect the patient's airway and support ventilation and perfusion. Meticulously monitor and maintain, within acceptable limits, the patient's vital signs, blood gases, serum electrolytes, etc. Absorption of drugs from the GI tract may be decreased by giving activated charcoal, which, in many cases, is more effective than emesis or lavage; consider charcoal instead of or in addition to gastric emptying. Repeated doses of charcoal over time may hasten elimination of some drugs that have been absorbed. Safeguard the patient's airway when employing gastric emptying or charcoal.

In adults, many of the neurotoxic effects of cycloserine can be both treated and prevented with the administration of 200 to 300 mg of pyridoxine daily.

The use of hemodialysis has been shown to remove cycloserine from the bloodstream. This procedure should be reserved for patients with life-threatening toxicity that is unresponsive to less invasive therapy.

STREPTOMYCIN SULFATE

Refer to the streptomycin sulfate monograph in the Aminoglycosides, Parenteral section.

CAPREOMYCIN

Rx	**Capastat Sulfate** (Dura)	**Powder for Injection:** 1 g (as sulfate)/vial.	In 10 mL vials.

CAPREOMYCIN — INJECTION

Refer to the general discussion in the Antituberculosal Agents Introduction.

WARNING

The use of capreomycin for injection, USP in patients with renal insufficiency or preexisting auditory impairment must be undertaken with great caution, and the risk of additional cranial nerve VIII impairment or renal injury should be weighed against the benefits derived from therapy.

Since other parenteral antituberculosis agents (streptomycin, viomycin) also have similar and sometimes irreversible toxic effect, particularly on cranial nerve VIII and renal function, simultaneous administration of these agents with capreomycin is not recommended. Use with nonantituberculosis drugs (polymyxin A sulfate, colistin sulfate, amikacin, gentamicin, tobramycin, vancomycin, kanamycin, and neomycin) having ototoxic or nephrotoxic potential should be undertaken only with great caution.

WARNING

Pregnancy – The safety of the use capreomycin in pregnancy has not been determined.

Children – Safety and effectiveness in pediatric patients have not been established.

Indications

➤*Tuberculosis:* Pulmonary infections caused by capreomycin-susceptible strains of *M. tuberculosis* when the primary agents (isoniazid, rifampin, ethambutol, aminosalicylic acid, and streptomycin) have been ineffective or cannot be used because of toxicity or the presence of resistant tubercle bacilli.

Susceptibility studies should be performed to determine the presence of a capreomycin-susceptible strain of *M. tuberculosis*.

CAPREOMYCIN — INJECTION

Administration and Dosage

➤*Preparation/Administration:* Capreomycin may be administered intramuscularly or intravenously following reconstitution. Reconstitution is achieved by dissolving the vial contents (1 g) in 2 mL of 0.9% Sodium Chloride Injection or Sterile Water for Injection. Two to 3 minutes should be allowed for complete dissolution.

Intravenously – For intravenous infusion, reconstituted capreomycin should be diluted in 100 mL of 0.9% Sodium Chloride Injection and administered over 60 minutes.

Intramuscularly – Reconstituted capreomycin should be given by deep intramuscular injection into a large muscle mass, since superficial injection may be associated with increased pain and the development of sterile abscesses.

For administration of a 1 g dose, the entire contents of the vial should be given. For doses lower than 1 g, the following dilution table may be used.

Capreomycin Dilution Table

Diluent added to 1 g, 10 mL vial	Volume of capreomycin for injection solution	Concentration (approximate)
2.15 mL	2.85 mL	350 mg*/mL
2.63 mL	3.33 mL	300 mg*/mL
3.3 mL	4 mL	250 mg*/mL
4.3 mL	5 mL	200 mg*/mL

* Equivalent to capreomycin activity.

➤*Dosage:* Capreomycin is always administered in combination with at least 1 other antituberculosis agent to which the patient's strain of tubercle bacilli is susceptible. The usual dose is 1 g daily (not to exceed 20 mg/kg/day) given intramuscularly or intravenously for 60 to 120 days, followed by 1 g by either route 2 or 3 times weekly. (Note-Therapy for tuberculosis should be maintained for 12 to 24 months. If facilities for administering injectable medication are not available, a change to appropriate oral therapy is indicated on the patient's release from the hospital.)

➤*Renal function impairment:* Patients with reduced renal function should have dosage reduction based on creatinine clearance using the guidelines included below. These dosages are designed to achieve a mean steady-state capreomycin level of 10 mcg/mL.

Estimated Dosages to Attain Mean Steady-State Serum Capreomycin Concentration of 10 mcg/mL (Based on Creatinine Clearance)

Ccr (mL/min)	Capreomycin clearance (L/g/hr × 10^{-2})	Half-life (hours)	Dose[a] (mg/kg) for the following dosing intervals: 24 hours	48 hours	72 hours
0	0.54	55.5	1.29	2.58	3.87
10	1.01	29.4	2.43	4.87	7.3
20	1.49	20	3.58	7.16	10.7
30	1.97	15.1	4.72	9.45	14.2
40	2.45	12.2	5.87	11.7	
50	2.92	10.2	7.01	14	
60	3.4	8.8	8.16		
80	4.35	6.8	10.4[b]		
100	5.31	5.6	12.7[b]		
110	5.78	5.2	13.9[b]		

[a] For patients with renal impairment, initial maintenance dose estimates are given for optional dosing intervals; longer dosing intervals are expected to provide greater peak and lower trough serum capreomycin levels than shorter dosing intervals.

[b] The usual dosage for patients with normal renal function is 1000 mg daily, not to exceed 20 mg/kg/day, for 60 to 120 days, then 1000 mg 2 to 3 times weekly.

➤*Storage/Stability:* Store at controlled room temperature 15° to 30°C (59° to 86°F) prior to reconstitution.

The solution may acquire a pale straw color and darken with time, but this is not associated with loss of potency or the development of toxicity. After reconstitution, all solutions of capreomycin may be stored for up to 24 hours under refrigeration.

Actions

➤*Pharmacology:* Capreomycin is a polypeptide antibiotic isolated from *Streptomyces capreolus*.

➤*Pharmacokinetics:* Capreomycin is not absorbed in significant quantities from the gastrointestinal tract and must be administered parenterally. In 2 studies of 10 patients each, peak serum concentrations following 1 g of capreomycin given intramuscularly were achieved 1 to 2 hours after administration, and average peak levels reached were 28 and 32 mcg/mL respectively (range, 20 to 47 mcg/mL). Low serum concentrations were present at 24 hours. However, 1 g of capreomycin daily for 30 days or more produced no significant accumulation in subjects with healthy renal function. Two patients with marked reduction of renal function had high serum concentrations 24 hours after administration of the drug. When a 1 g dose of capreomycin was given intramuscularly to healthy volunteers, 52% was excreted in the urine within 12 hours.

Lehmann, et al, examined the pharmacokinetics of single dose capreomycin (1 g) administered intramuscularly and by intravenous infusion (1 hour) in 6 healthy volunteers. The area under the serum concentration vs. time curve was similar for the 2 routes of administration. Capreomycin peak concentrations after intravenous infusion were 30 ± 47% higher than after intramuscular administration.

Paper chromatographic studies indicated that capreomycin is excreted essentially unaltered. Urine concentrations averaged 1.68 mcg/mL (average urine volume, 228 mL) during the 6 hours following a 1 g dose.

Contraindications

Hypersensitivity to capreomycin.

Warnings

➤*Hypersensitivity reactions:* Caution should be exercised in the administration of antibiotics, including capreomycin, to any patient who has demonstrated some form of allergy, particularly to drugs.

➤*Renal function impairment:* Regular tests of renal function should be made throughout the period of treatment, and reduced dosage should be employed in patients with known or suspected renal impairment.

➤*Pregnancy: Category C.* Capreomycin has been shown to be teratogenic in rats when given in doses 3 ½ times the human dose. There are no adequate and well-controlled studies in pregnant women. Capreomycin should be used during pregnancy only if the potential benefit justifies the potential risk to the fetus (see Warning Box and Animal Pharmacology).

➤*Lactation:* It is not known whether this drug is excreted in human milk. Because many drugs are excreted in human milk, caution should be exercised when capreomycin is administered to a nursing woman.

➤*Children:* Safety and effectiveness in pediatric patients have not been established (see Warning Box).

Precautions

➤*Monitoring:* Renal function studies should be made both before therapy with capreomycin is started and on a weekly basis during treatment.

➤*Hypokalemia:* Since hypokalemia may occur during therapy, serum potassium levels should be determined frequently.

➤*Ototoxicity:* Audiometric measurements and assessment of vestibular function should be performed prior to initiation of therapy with capreomycin and at regular intervals during treatment.

➤*Nephrotoxicity:* Renal injury, with tubular necrosis, elevation of the blood urea nitrogen (BUN) or serum creatinine, and abnormal urinary sediment, has been noted. Slight elevation of the BUN and serum creatinine has been observed in a significant number of patients receiving prolonged therapy. The appearance of casts, red cells, and white cells in the urine has been noted in a high percentage of these cases. Elevation of the BUN above 30 mg/100 mL or any other evidence of decreasing renal function with or without a rise in BUN levels calls for careful evaluation of the patient, and the dosage should be reduced or the drug completely withdrawn. The clinical significance of abnormal urine sediment and slight elevation in the BUN (or serum creatinine) observed during long-term therapy with capreomycin has not been established.

➤*Neuromuscular blockade:* The peripheral neuromuscular blocking action that has been attributed to other polypeptide antibiotics (colistin sulfate, polymyxin A sulfate, paromomycin, and viomycin) and to aminoglycoside antibiotics (streptomycin, dihydrostreptomycin, neomycin, and kanamycin) has been studied with capreomycin. A partial neuromuscular blockade was demonstrated after large intravenous doses of capreomycin. This action was enhanced by ether anesthesia (as has been reported for neomycin) and was antagonized by neostigmine.

Drug Interactions

For neuromuscular blocking action of this drug, see Precautions.

Adverse Reactions

➤*Hematologic:* Leukocytosis and leukopenia have been observed. The majority of patients treated have had eosinophilia exceeding 5% while receiving daily injections of capreomycin. This has subsided with reduction of the capreomycin dosage to 2 or 3 g weekly.

Pain and induration at the injection site have been observed. Excessive bleeding at the injection site has been reported. Sterile abscesses have been noted. Rare cases of thrombocytopenia have been reported.

➤*Hepatic:* Serial tests of liver function have demonstrated a decrease in BSP excretion without change in SGOT or SGPT in the presence of preexisting liver disease. Abnormal results in liver function tests have occurred in many persons receiving capreomycin in combination with other antituberculosis agents that also are known to cause changes in hepatic function. The role of capreomycin in producing these abnormalities is not clear; however, periodic determinations of liver function are recommended.

➤*Hypersensitivity:* Urticaria and maculopapular skin rashes associated in some cases with febrile reactions have been reported when capreomycin and other antituberculosis drugs were given concomitantly.

➤*Renal:* In 36% of 722 patients treated with capreomycin, elevation of the BUN above 20 mg/100 mL has been observed. In many instances, there was also depression of PSP excretion and abnormal urine sediment. In 10% of this series, the BUN elevation exceeded 30 mg/100 mL.

Toxic nephritis was reported in 1 patient with tuberculosis and portal cirrhosis who was treated with capreomycin (1 g) and aminosalicylic acid daily for 1 month. This patient developed renal insufficiency and oliguria and died. Autopsy showed subsiding acute tubular necrosis.

CAPREOMYCIN — INJECTION

Electrolyte disturbances resembling Bartter's syndrome have been reported in 1 patient.

➤*Special senses:* Subclinical auditory loss was noted in ≈ 11% of 722 patients undergoing treatment with capreomycin. This was a 5- to 10-decibel loss in the 4000- to 8000-CPS range. Clinically apparent hearing loss occurred in 3% of the 722 subjects. Some audiometric changes were reversible. Other cases with permanent loss were not progressive following withdrawal of capreomycin.

Tinnitus and vertigo have occurred.

Overdosage

➤*Symptoms:* Nephrotoxicity following the parenteral administration of capreomycin is most closely related to the area under the curve of the serum concentration vs time graph. The elderly patient, patients with abnormal renal function or dehydration, and patients receiving other nephrotoxic drugs are at much greater risk for developing acute tubular necrosis.

Damage to the auditory and vestibular divisions of cranial nerve VIII has been associated with capreomycin given to patients with abnormal renal function or dehydration and in those receiving medications with additive auditory toxicities. These patients often experience dizziness, tinnitus, vertigo, and a loss of high-tone acuity.

Neuromuscular blockage or respiratory paralysis may occur following rapid intravenous infusion.

If capreomycin is ingested, toxicity would be unlikely because it is poorly absorbed (less than 1%) from an intact gastrointestinal system.

Hypokalemia, hypocalcemia, hypomagnesemia, and an electrolyte disturbance resembling Bartter's syndrome have been reported to occur in patients with capreomycin toxicity.

The subcutaneous median lethal dose in mice was 514 mg/kg.

➤*Treatment:* Protect the patient's airway and support ventilation and perfusion. Meticulously monitor and maintain, within acceptable limits, the patient's vital signs, blood gases, serum electrolytes, etc. Absorption of drugs from the gastrointestinal tract may be decreased by giving activated charcoal, which, in many cases, is more effective than emesis or lavage; consider charcoal instead of or in addition to gastric emptying. Repeated doses of charcoal over time may hasten elimination of some drugs that have been absorbed. Safeguard the patient's airway when employing gastric emptying or charcoal.

Patients who have received an overdose of capreomycin and have normal renal function should be carefully hydrated to maintain a urine output of 3 to 5 mL/kg/hr. Fluid balance, electrolytes, and creatinine clearance should be carefully monitored.

Hemodialysis may be effectively used to remove capreomycin in patients with significant renal disease.

RIFAPENTINE

Rx	**Priftin** (Aventis)	**Tablets:** 150 mg	EDTA, polyethylene glycol. (Priftin 150). Dark pink. Film coated. In 32s.

RIFAPENTINE — ORAL

Refer to the general discussion in the Antituberculosis Agents Introduction.

Indications

➤*Pulmonary tuberculosis:* For the treatment of pulmonary tuberculosis. Rifapentine oral must always be used in conjunction with at least one other antituberculosis drug to which the isolate is susceptible. In the intensive phase of the short-course treatment of pulmonary tuberculosis, rifapentine oral should be administered twice weekly for 2 months, with an interval of no less than 3 days (72 hours) between doses, as part of an appropriate regimen which includes daily companion drugs. It may also be necessary to add either streptomycin or ethambutol until the results of susceptibility testing are known. Compliance with all drugs in the intensive phase (ie, rifapentine oral, isoniazid, pyrazinamide, ethambutol or streptomycin) is imperative to ensure early sputum conversion and protection against relapse. Following the intensive phase, continuation phase treatment should be continued with rifapentine oral for 4 months. During this phase, rifapentine oral should be administered on a once-weekly basis in combination with an appropriate antituberculous agent for susceptible organisms.

Administration and Dosage

➤*Approved by the FDA:* June 22, 1998.

➤*Intensive phase:* Rifapentine oral should not be used alone, in initial treatment or in retreatment of pulmonary tuberculosis. In the intensive phase of short-course therapy which is to continue for 2 months, 600 mg (four 150 mg tablets) of rifapentine oral should be given twice weekly with an interval of not less than 3 days (72 hours) between doses. For those patients with propensity to nausea, vomiting or gastrointestinal upset, administration of rifapentine oral with food may be useful. In the intensive phase, rifapentine oral must be administered in combination as part of an appropriate regimen which includes daily companion drugs. Compliance with all drugs in the intensive phase (ie, rifapentine oral, isoniazid, pyrazinamide, ethambutol, or streptomycin), especially on days when rifapentine is not administered, is imperative to assure early sputum conversion and protection against relapse. The Advisory Council for the Elimination of Tuberculosis, the American Thoracic Society and the Centers for Disease Control and Prevention also recommend that either streptomycin or ethambutol be added to the regimen unless the likelihood of isoniazid resistance is very low. The need for streptomycin or ethambutol should be reassessed when the results of susceptibility testing are known. An initial treatment regimen with less than 4 drugs may be considered if there is little possibility of drug resistance (that is, less than 4% primary resistance to isoniazid in the community, and the patient has had no previous treatment with antituberculosis medications, is not from a country with a high prevalence of drug resistance, and has no known exposure to a drug-resistant case).

➤*Continuation phase:* Following the intensive phase, treatment should be continued with rifapentine oral once weekly for 4 months in combination with isoniazid or an appropriate agent for susceptible organisms. If the patient is still sputum smear or culture positive, if resistant organisms are present, or if the patient is HIV positive, follow the ATS/CDC treatment guidelines.

➤*Concomitant pyridoxine therapy:* Concomitant administration of pyridoxine (vitamin B_6) is recommended in the malnourished, in those predisposed to neuropathy (eg, alcoholics and diabetics), and in adolescents.

➤*Storage/Stability:* Store at 25°C (77°F); excursions permitted 15° to 30°C (59° to 86°F). Protect from excessive heat and humidity.

Actions

➤*Pharmacology:* Rifapentine, a cyclopentyl rifamycin, inhibits DNA-dependent RNA polymerase in susceptible strains of *Mycobacterium tuberculosis* but not in mammalian cells. At therapeutic levels, rifapentine exhibits bactericidal activity against both intracellular and extracellular *M. tuberculosis* organisms. Both rifapentine and the 25-desacetyl metabolite accumulate in human monocyte-derived macrophages with intracellular/extracellular ratios of approximately 24 to 1 and 7 to 1, respectively.

➤*Pharmacokinetics:*

Absorption – The absolute bioavailability of rifapentine has not been determined. The relative bioavailability (with an oral solution as a reference) of rifapentine after a single 600 mg dose to healthy adult volunteers was 70%. The maximum concentrations were achieved from 5 to 6 hours after administration of the 600 mg rifapentine dose. Food (850 total calories: 33 g protein, 55 g fat and 58 g carbohydrate) increased $AUC_{(0-\infty)}$ and C_{max} by 43% and 44%, respectively, over that observed when administered under fasting conditions. When oral doses of rifapentine were administered once daily or once every 72 hours to healthy volunteers for 10 days, single dose $AUC_{(0-\infty)}$ value of rifapentine was similar to its steady-state $AUC_{SS\ (0\text{-}24\ hr)}$ or $AUC_{SS\ (0\text{-}72\ hr)}$ values, suggesting no significant auto-induction effect on steady-state pharmacokinetics of rifapentine. Steady-state conditions were achieved by day 10 following daily administration of rifapentine 600 mg. The pharmacokinetic characteristics of rifapentine and 25-desacetyl rifapentine (active metabolite) on day 10 following oral administration of 600 mg rifapentine every 72 hours to healthy volunteers are discussed below.

Select Pharmacokinetic Parameters of Rifapentine

Pharmacokinetic parameter	Rifapentine[1] (n = 12)	25-desacetyl rifapentine[1] (n = 12)
C_{max} (mcg/ml)	≈ 15.05	≈ 6.26
AUC (0-72 hr) (mcg•hr/ml)	≈ 319.54	≈ 215.88
t½ (hr)	≈ 13.19	≈ 13.35
T_{max} (hr)	≈ 4.83	≈ 11.25
Cl_{po} (L/hr)	≈ 2.03	–

[1] Mean values, day 10.

Distribution – In a population pharmacokinetic analysis in 351 tuberculosis patients who received 600 mg rifapentine in combination with isoniazid, pyrazinamide and ethambutol, the estimated apparent volume of distribution was 70.2 ± 9.1 L. In healthy volunteers, rifapentine and 25-desacetyl rifapentine were 97.7% and 93.2% bound to plasma proteins, respectively. Rifapentine was mainly bound to albumin. Similar extent of protein binding was observed in healthy volunteers, asymptomatic HIV-infected subjects and hepatically impaired subjects.

Metabolism/Excretion – Following a single 600 mg oral dose of radiolabelled rifapentine to healthy volunteers (n = 4), 87% of the total ^{14}C rifapentine was recovered in the urine (17%) and feces (70%). Greater than 80% of the total ^{14}C rifapentine dose was excreted from the body within 7 days. Rifapentine was hydrolyzed by an esterase enzyme to form a microbiologically active 25-desacetyl rifapentine. Rifapentine and 25-desacetyl rifapentine accounted for 99% of the total radioactivity in plasma. Plasma $AUC_{(0-\infty)}$ and C_{max} values of the 25-desacetyl rifapentine metabolite were one-half and one-third those of the rifapentine, respectively. Based upon relative in vitro activities and $AUC_{(0-\infty)}$ values, rifapentine and 25-desacetyl rifapentine potentially contributes 62% and 38% to the clinical activities against *M. tuberculosis*, respectively.

Special populations –

Asymptomatic HIV-infected volunteers: Following oral administration of a single 600 mg dose of rifapentine to asymptomatic HIV-infected volunteers (n = 15) under fasting conditions, mean C_{max} and $AUC_{(0-\infty)}$ of rifapentine were lower (20 to 32%) than that observed in other studies in healthy volunteers (n = 55). In a cross-study comparison, mean C_{max} and AUC values of the 25-desacetyl metabolite of rifapentine, when compared to healthy volunteers were higher (6 to 21%) in one study (n = 20), but lower (15 to 16%) in

RIFAPENTINE — ORAL

a different study (n = 40). The clinical significance of this observation is not known. Food (850 total calories: 33 g protein, 55 g fat, and 58 g carbohydrate) increases the mean AUC and C_{max} of rifapentine observed under fasting conditions in asymptomatic HIV-infected volunteers by about 51% and 53%, respectively.

Contraindications

Hypersensitivity to any of the rifamycins (eg, rifampin, rifabutin).

Warnings

➤*Compliance:* Poor compliance with the dosage regimen, particularly the daily administered non-rifamycin drugs in the Intensive Phase, was associated with late sputum conversion and a high relapse rate in the rifapentine arm of Clinical Study 008. Therefore, compliance with the full course of therapy must be emphasized, and the importance of not missing any doses must be stressed.

➤*Hyperbilirubinemia:* Hyperbilirubinemia resulting from competition for excretory pathways between rifapentine and bilirubin cannot be excluded since competition between the related drug rifampin and bilirubin can occur. An isolated report showing a moderate rise in bilirubin and/or transaminase level is not in itself an indication for interrupting treatment; rather, the decision should be made after repeating the tests, noting trends in the levels and considering them in conjunction with the patient's clinical condition.

➤*Pseudomembranous colitis:* Pseudomembranous colitis has been reported to occur with various antibiotics, including other rifamycins. Diarrhea, particularly if severe and/or persistent, occurring during treatment or in the initial weeks following treatment may be symptomatic of *Clostridium difficile*-associated disease, the most severe form of which is pseudomembranous colitis. If pseudomembranous colitis is suspected, rifapentine should be stopped immediately and the patient should be treated with supportive and specific treatment without delay (eg, oral vancomycin). Products inhibiting peristalsis are contraindicated in this clinical situation.

➤*HIV-infected patients:* Experience in HIV-infected patients is limited. In an ongoing CDC TB trial, 5 out of 30 HIV-infected patients randomized to once weekly rifapentine (plus INH) in the Continuation Phase who completed treatment, relapsed. Four of these patients developed rifampin monoresistant (RMR) TB. Each RMR patient had late-stage HIV infection, low CD4 counts and extrapulmonary disease, and documented coadministration of antifungal azoles. These findings are consistent with the literature in which an emergence of RMR TB in HIV-infected TB patients has been reported in recent years. Further study in this sub-population is warranted. As with other antituberculous treatments, when rifapentine is used in HIV-infected patients, a more aggressive regimen should be employed (eg, more frequent dosing). Based on results to date of the CDC trial (see above), once weekly dosing during the continuation phase of treatment is not recommended at this time.

➤*Hepatic function impairment:* Since antituberculous multidrug treatments, including the rifamycin class, are associated with serious hepatic events, patients with abnormal liver tests and/or liver disease should only be given rifapentine in cases of necessity and then with caution and under strict medical supervision. In these patients, careful monitoring of liver tests (especially serum transaminases) should be carried out prior to therapy and then every 2 to 4 weeks during therapy. If signs of liver disease occur or worsen, rifapentine should be discontinued. Hepatotoxicity of other antituberculosis drugs (eg, isoniazid, pyrazinamide) used in combination with rifapentine should also be taken into account.

➤*Mutagenesis:* The 25–desacetyl metabolite of rifapentine did induce chromosomal aberrations in an in vitro chromosomal aberration assay.

➤*Elderly:* In general, dose selection for an elderly patient should be cautious, usually starting at the low end of the dosing range, reflecting the greater frequency of decreased hepatic, renal, or cardiac function and of concomitant disease or other drug therapy.

➤*Pregnancy: Category C.* Rifapentine has been shown to be teratogenic in rats and rabbits. In rats, when given in doses 0.6 times the human dose (based on body surface area comparisons) during the period of organogenesis, pups showed cleft palates, right aortic arch and increased incidence of delayed ossification and increased number of ribs. Rabbits treated with drug at doses between 0.3 and 1.3 times the human dose (based on body surface area comparison) displayed major malformations including ovarian agenesis, pes varus, arhinia, microphthalmia and irregularities of the ossified facial tissues (4 of 321 examined fetuses).

In rats, rifapentine administration was associated with increased resorption rate and post implantation loss, decreased mean fetus weight, increased number of stillborn pups and slightly increased mortality during lactation. Rabbits given 1.3 times the human dose (based on body surface area comparisons) showed higher postimplantation losses and an increased incidence of stillborn pups.

When rifapentine was administered at 0.3 times the human dose (based on body surface area comparisons) to mated female rats late in gestation (from day 15 of gestation to day 21 postpartum), pup weights and gestational survival (live pups born/pups born) were reduced compared to controls.

There are no adequate and well-controlled studies in pregnant women. In Clinical Study 008, 6 patients randomized to rifapentine became pregnant; 2 had normal deliveries; 2 had first trimester spontaneous abortions, 1 had an elective abortion and 1 patient was lost to follow-up. Of the 2 patients who spontaneously aborted, co-morbid conditions of ethanol abuse in 1 and HIV infection in the other were noted.

When administered during the last few weeks of pregnancy, rifampin can cause postnatal hemorrhages in the mother and infant for which treatment with vitamin K may be indicated. Thus, patients and infants who receive rifapentine during the last few weeks of pregnancy should have appropriate clotting parameters evaluated.

Rifapentine should be used during pregnancy only if the potential benefit justifies the potential risk to the fetus.

➤*Lactation:* It is not known whether rifapentine is excreted in human milk. Because many drugs are excreted in human milk and because of the potential for serious adverse reactions in nursing infants, a decision should be made whether to discontinue nursing or discontinue the drug, taking into account the importance of the drug to the mother. Since rifapentine may produce a red-orange discoloration of body fluids, there is a potential for discoloration of breast milk.

➤*Children:* The safety and effectiveness of rifapentine in pediatric patients under the age of 12 have not been established. A pharmacokinetic study was conducted in 12- to 15-year-old healthy volunteers. The pharmacokinetics of rifapentine were similar to those observed in healthy adults.

Precautions

➤*Monitoring:* Adults treated for tuberculosis with rifapentine should have baseline measurements of hepatic enzymes, bilirubin, a complete blood count, and a platelet count (or estimate).

Patients should be seen at least monthly during therapy and should be specifically questioned concerning symptoms associated with adverse reactions. All patients with abnormalities should have follow-up, including laboratory testing, if necessary. Routine laboratory monitoring for toxicity in people with normal baseline measurements is generally not necessary.

➤*Red discoloration of body fluids:* Rifapentine may produce a predominately red-orange discoloration of body tissues and/or fluids (eg, skin, teeth, tongue, urine, feces, saliva, sputum, tears, sweat, and cerebrospinal fluid).

Contact lenses or dentures may become permanently stained.

➤*Porphyria:* Rifapentine should not be used in patients with porphyria. Rifampin has enzyme-inducing properties, including induction of delta amino levulinic acid synthetase. Isolated reports have associated porphyria exacerbation with rifampin administration. Based on these isolated reports with rifampin, it may be assumed that rifapentine has a similar effect.

Drug Interactions

➤*Indinavir:* In a study in which 600 mg rifapentine was administered twice weekly for 14 days followed by rifapentine twice weekly plus 800 mg indinavir 3 times a day for an additional 14 days, indinavir C_{max} decreased by 55% while AUC reduced by 70%. Clearance of indinavir increased by 3-fold in the presence of rifapentine while half-life did not change. But when indinavir was administered for 14 days followed by coadministration with rifapentine for an additional 14 days, indinavir did not affect the pharmacokinetics of rifapentine. Rifapentine should be used with extreme caution, if at all, in patients who are also taking protease inhibitors.

➤*Cytochrome P450 system:* Rifapentine is an inducer of cytochromes P450 3A4 and P450 2C8/9. Therefore, rifapentine may increase the metabolism of other coadministered drugs that are metabolized by these enzymes. Induction of enzyme activities by rifapentine occurred within 4 days after the first dose. Enzyme activities returned to baseline levels 14 days after discontinuing rifapentine. In addition, the magnitude of enzyme induction by rifapentine was dose and dosing frequency dependent; less enzyme induction occurred when 600 mg oral doses of rifapentine were given once every 72 hours versus daily. In vitro and in vivo enzyme induction studies have suggested rifapentine induction potential may be less than rifampin but more potent than rifabutin. Rifampin has been reported to accelerate the metabolism and may reduce the activity of the following drugs; hence, rifapentine may also increase the metabolism and decrease the activity of these drugs.

Dosage adjustments of the following drugs or of drugs metabolized by cytochrome P450 3A4 or P450 2C8/9 may be necessary if they are given concurrently with rifapentine. Patients using oral or other systemic hormonal contraceptives should be advised to change to nonhormonal methods of birth control.

Drugs That May Require Dosage Adjustment When Given Concurrently with Rifapentine	
Anticonvulsants (eg, phenytoin)	Haloperidol
Antiarrhythmics (eg, disopyramide, mexiletine, quinidine, tocainide	HIV protease inhibitors (eg, indinavir, ritonavir, nelfinavir, saquinavir; see indinavir interaction above)
Antibiotics (eg, chloramphenicol, clarithromycin, dapsone, doxycycline, fluoroquinolones such as ciprofloxacin)	Oral hypoglycemic agents (eg, sulfonylureas).
Anticoagulants, oral (eg, warfarin)	Immunosuppressants (eg, cyclosporine, tacrolimus)
Antifungals (eg, fluconazole, itraconazole, ketoconazole)	Levothyroxine
Barbiturates	Narcotic analgesics (eg, methadone)
Benzodiazepines (eg, diazepam)	Progestins
Beta blockers, calcium channel blockers (eg, diltiazem, nifedipine, verapamil)	Quinine
	Reverse transcriptase inhibitors (eg, delavirdine, zidovudine)
Corticosteroids	
Cardiac glycoside preparations	Sildenafil
Clofibrate	Theophylline
Oral or other systemic hormonal contraceptives	Tricyclic antidepressants (eg, amitriptyline, nortriptyline)

Esterase enzyme – The conversion of rifapentine to 25-desacetyl rifapentine is mediated by an esterase enzyme. There is minimal potential for rifapentine metabolism to be inhibited or induced by another drug, or for rifapentine to inhibit the metabolism of another drug based upon the characteristics of the esterase enzymes. Rifapentine does not induce its own

RIFAPENTINE — ORAL

metabolism. Since rifapentine is highly bound to albumin, drug displacement interactions may also occur.

Antacids – In Clinical study 008, patients were advised to take rifapentine at least 1 hour before or 2 hours after ingestion of antacids.

➤*Drug/Lab test interactions:* Therapeutic concentrations of rifampin have been shown to inhibit standard microbiological assays for serum folate and Vitamin B_{12}. Similar drug-laboratory interactions should be considered for rifapentine; thus, alternative assay methods should be considered.

Adverse Reactions

A patient may have experienced the same adverse event more than once during the course of the study, therefore, patient counts across the columns may not equal the patient counts in the total column. "Greater than or equal to 1%" refers to rifapentine in the total column.

Treatment-Related Adverse Events Occurring in ≥ 1% of the Patients in Study 008

	Intensive phase[1]		Continuation phase[2]		Total	
Preferred term	Rifapentine combination (n = 361) n (%)	Rifampin combination (n = 361) n (%)	Rifapentine combination (n = 321) n (%)	Rifampin combination (n = 307) n (%)	Rifapentine combination (n = 361) n (%)	Rifampin combination (n = 361) n (%)
Hyperuricemia	78 (21.6%)	55 (15.2%)	0	0	78 (21.6%)	55 (15.%2)
ALT increased	12 (3.3%)	17 (4.7%)	6 (1.9%)	7 (2.3%)	18 (5%)	24 (6.6%)
AST increased	11 (3%)	16 (4.4%)	5 (1.6%)	7 (2.3%)	15 (4.2%)	23 (6.4%)
Neutropenia	7 (1.9%)	9 (2.5%)	12 (3.7%)	9 (2.9%)	18 (5%)	18 (5%)
Pyuria	11 (3%)	10 (2.8%)	6 (1.9%)	3 (1%)	14 (3.9%)	12 (3.3%)
Proteinuria	15 (4.2%)	10 (2.8%)	2 (0.6%)	1 (0.3%)	17 (4.7%)	11 (3%)
Hematuria	10 (2.8%)	12 (3.3%)	4 (1.2%)	4 (1.3%)	13 (3.6%)	15 (4.2%)
Lymphopenia	14 (3.9%)	13 (3.6%)	3 (0.9%)	1 (0.3%)	16 (4.4%)	14 (3.9%)
Urinary casts	11 (3%)	3 (0.8%)	4 (1.2%)	0	14 (3.9%)	3 (0.8%)
Rash	9 (2.5%)	19 (5.3%)	4 (1.2%)	3 (1%)	13 (3.6%)	21 (5.8%)
Pruritus	8 (2.2%)	15 (4.2%)	1 (0.3%)	1 (0.3%)	9 (2.5%)	16 (4.4%)
Acne	5 (1.4%)	3 (0.8%)	2 (0.6%)	1 (0.3%)	7 (1.9%)	4 (1.1%)
Anorexia	6 (1.7%)	8 (2.2%)	3 (0.9%)	4 (1.3%)	8 (2.2%)	10 (2.8%)
Anemia	7 (1.9%)	9 (2.5%)	2 (0.6%)	1 (0.%3)	9 (2.5%)	10 (2.8%)
Leukopenia	4 (1.1%)	4 (1.1%)	3 (0.9%)	5 (1.6%)	7 (1.9%)	8 (2.2%)
Arthralgia	9 (2.5%)	7 (1.9%)	0	0	9 (2.5%)	7 (1.9%)
Pain	7 (1.9%)	5 (1.4%)	0	1 (0.3%)	7 (1.9%)	6 (1.7%)
Nausea	7 (1.9%)	2 (0.6%)	0	1 (0.3%)	7 (1.9%)	3 (0.8%)
Vomiting	4 (1.1%)	6 (1.7%)	1 (0.3%)	1 (0.3%)	5 (1.4%)	7 (1.9%)
Headache	3 (0.8%)	4 (1.1%)	1 (0.3%)	3 (1%)	4 (1.1%)	7 (1.9%)
Dyspepsia	3 (0.8%)	5 (1.4%)	2 (0.6%)	3 (1%)	4 (1.1%)	8 (2.2%)
Hypertension	3 (0.8%)	0 (0.0%)	1 (0.3%)	1 (0.3%)	4 (1.1%)	1 (0.3%)
Dizziness	4 (1.1%)	0	0	1 (0.3%)	4 (1.1%)	1 (0.3%)
Thrombocytosis	4 (1.1%)	2 (0.6%)	0	0	4 (1.1%)	2 (0.6%)
Diarrhea	4 (1.1%)	0	0	0	4 (1.1%)	0
Rash maculopapular	4 (1.1%)	3 (0.8%)	0	0	4 (1.1%)	3 (0.8%)
Hemoptysis	2 (0.6%)	0	2 (0.6%)	0	4 (1.1%)	0

[1] Intensive phase consisted of therapy with either rifapentine or rifampin combined with isoniazid, pyrazinamide, and ethambutol administered daily (rifapentine twice weekly) for 60 days.

[2] Continuation phase consisted of therapy with either rifapentine or rifampin combined with isoniazid for 120 days. Rifapentine patients were dosed once weekly; rifampin patients were dosed twice weekly. Events recorded in this phase includes those reported up to 3 months after continuation phase therapy was completed.

Treatment-related adverse events of moderate or severe intensity in less than 1% of the rifapentine combination therapy patients in Study 008 are presented below.

➤*Dermatologic:* Urticaria, skin discoloration.

➤*GI:* Constipation, esophagitis, gastritis, pancreatitis.

➤*Hematologic:* Thrombocytopenia, neutrophilia, leukocytosis, purpura, hematoma.

➤*Hepatic:* Bilirubinemia, hepatitis.

➤*Metabolic/Nutritional:* Hyperkalemia, hypovolemia, alkaline phosphatase increased, LDH increased.

➤*Musculoskeletal:* Gout, arthrosis.

➤*Miscellaneous:* Aggressive reaction, peripheral edema, fatigue. Three (3) patients (2 rifampin combination therapy patients and 1 rifapentine combination therapy patient) were discontinued in the Intensive Phase as a result of hepatitis with increased liver function tests (ALT, AST, LDH, and bilirubin). Concomitant medications for all 3 patients included isoniazid, pyrazinamide, ethambutol, and pyridoxine. The 2 rifampin patients and 1 rifapentine patient recovered without sequelae.

Twenty-two (22) deaths occurred in Study 008 (11 in the rifampin combination therapy group and 11 in the rifapentine combination therapy group). None of the deaths were attributed to study medication. In the study, 18/361 (5%) rifampin combination therapy patients discontinued the study due to an adverse event compared to 11/361 (3%) rifapentine combination therapy patients.

The overall occurrence rate of treatment-related adverse events was higher in males with the rifapentine combination regimen (50%) versus the rifampin combination regimen (43%), while in females the overall rate was greater in the rifampin combination group (68%) compared to the rifapentine combination group (59%). However, there were higher frequencies of treatment-related hematuria and ALT increases for female patients in both treatment groups compared to those for male patients.

Adverse events associated with rifampin may occur with rifapentine: Effects of enzyme induction to increase metabolism resulting in decreased concentration of endogenous substrates, including adrenal hormones, thyroid hormones, and vitamin D.

Overdosage

There is no experience with the treatment of acute overdose with rifapentine at doses exceeding 1200 mg per dose.

In a pharmacokinetic study involving healthy volunteers (n = 9), single oral doses up to 1200 mg have been administered without serious adverse reactions. The only adverse reactions reported with the 1200 mg dose were heartburn (3/8), headache (2/8) and increased urinary frequency (1/8). In clinical trials, tuberculosis patients ranging in age from 20 to 74 years accidentally received continuous daily doses of rifapentine 600 mg. Some patients received continuous daily dosing for up to 20 days without evidence of serious adverse effects. One patient experienced a transient elevation in AST and glucose (the latter attributed to pre-existing diabetes); a second patient experienced slight pruritus. While there is no experience with the treatment of acute overdose with rifapentine, clinical experience with rifamycins suggests that gastric lavage to evacuate gastric contents (within a few hours of overdose), followed by instillation of an activated charcoal slurry into the stomach, may help absorb any remaining drug from the gastrointestinal tract.

Rifapentine and 25-desacetyl rifapentine are 97.7% and 93.2% plasma protein bound, respectively. Rifapentine and related compounds excreted in urine account for only 17% of the administered dose; therefore, neither hemodialysis nor forced diuresis is expected to enhance the systemic elimination of unchanged rifapentine from the body of a patient with a rifapentine overdose.

Patient Information

The patient should be told that rifapentine may produce a reddish coloration of the urine, sweat, sputum, tears, and breast milk and the patient should be forewarned that contact lenses or dentures may be permanently stained. The patient should be advised that the reliability of oral or other systemic hormonal contraceptives may be affected; consideration should be given to using alternative contraceptive measures. For those patients with a propensity to nausea, vomiting, or gastrointestinal upset, administration of rifapentine with food may be useful. Patients should be instructed to notify their physician promptly if they experience any of the following: Fever, loss of appetite, malaise, nausea and vomiting, darkened urine, yellowish discoloration of the skin and eyes, and pain or swelling of the joints.

RIFAPENTINE — ORAL

Compliance with the full course of therapy must be emphasized, and the importance of not missing any doses of the daily administered companion medications in the intensive phase must be stressed.

AMEBICIDES

The agents listed in this group are recommended for the following disorders (see individual monographs):

Intestinal amebiasis:	*Extraintestinal amebiasis:*	*Intestinal amebiasis:*	*Extraintestinal amebiasis:*
Paromomycin	Metronidazole	Metronidazole	Chloroquine
Iodoquinol	Emetine HCl	Emetine HCl	

PAROMOMYCIN

For paromomycin sulfate prescribing information, see the Paromomycin Sulfate monograph in the Oral Aminoglycosides section.

IODOQUINOL (Diiodohydroxyquin)

Rx	**Yodoxin** (Glenwood)	**Tablets:** 210 mg	In 100s and 1,000s.
		650 mg	In 100s and 1,000s.
		Powder	In 25 g.

IODOQUINOL — ORAL

Indications

➤*Intestinal amebiasis:* Treatment of intestinal amebiasis.

Administration and Dosage

➤*Adults:* 650 mg 3 times per day after meals for 20 days.

➤*Children:* 10 to 13.3 mg/kg 3 times per day (not to exceed 1.95 g in 24 hours) for 20 days.

➤*Storage/Stability:* Store at controlled room temperature, 15° to 30°C (59° to 86°F).

Actions

➤*Pharmacology:* Iodoquinol is amebicidal against *Entamoeba histolytica* and is considered effective against the trophozoite and cyst forms.

Contraindications

Hypersensitivity to iodine and 8-hydroxyquinolines; hepatic damage.

Warnings

➤*CNS and ophthalmic effects:* Optic neuritis, optic atrophy, and peripheral neuropathy have been reported following prolonged high dosage therapy with halogenated 8-hydroxyquinolines.

➤*Pregnancy: Category C.* Safety for use during pregnancy has not been established.

➤*Lactation:* Safety for use during lactation has not been established.

Precautions

➤*Thyroid disease:* Use iodoquinol with caution in patients with thyroid disease.

Drug Interactions

➤*Drug/Lab test interactions:* Protein-bound serum iodine levels may be increased during treatment with iodoquinol and therefore interfere with certain thyroid function tests. These effects may persist for as long as 6 months after discontinuation of therapy.

Adverse Reactions

➤*CNS:* Chills, headache, vertigo; peripheral neuropathy (associated with prolonged high-dosage 8-hydroxyquinoline therapy).

➤*Dermatologic:* Various forms of skin eruptions (acneiform papular and pustular bullae; vegetating or tuberous iododerma), urticaria, pruritus.

➤*GI:* Abdominal cramps, diarrhea, nausea, pruritus ani, and vomiting.

➤*Ophthalmic:* Optic neuritis and optic atrophy (associated with prolonged high-dosage 8-hydroxyquinoline therapy).

➤*Miscellaneous:* Fever, enlargement of thyroid.

METRONIDAZOLE

For metronidazole prescribing information, see the Metronidazole monograph.

CHLOROQUINE PHOSPHATE

For chloroquine phosphate prescribing information, see the Chloroquine phosphate monograph in the 4–Aminoquinoline Compounds section.

CHLOROQUINE HYDROCHLORIDE

For chloroquine phosphate prescribing information, see the Chloroquine Hydrochloride monograph in the 4–Aminoquinoline Compounds section.

ANTIVIRAL AGENTS

FOSCARNET SODIUM (Phosphonoformic acid; PFA)

Rx	**Foscarnet Sodium** (Hospira)	**Injection:** 24 mg/mL	Preservative-free. In 250 and 500 mL.
Rx	**Foscavir** (Astra)		Preservative-free. In 250 and 500 mL.

FOSCARNET SODIUM — INJECTION

WARNING

Renal impairment is the major toxicity of foscarnet sodium. Frequent monitoring of serum creatinine, with dose adjustment for changes in renal function, and adequate hydration with administration of foscarnet sodium, is imperative (see Administration and Dosage, Hydration).

Seizures, related to alterations in plasma minerals and electrolytes, have been associated with foscarnet sodium treatment. Therefore, patients must be carefully monitored for such changes and their potential sequelae. Mineral and electrolyte supplementation may be required.

Foscarnet sodium is indicated for use only in immunocompromised patients with cytomegalovirus (CMV) retinitis and mucocutaneous acyclovir resistant herpes simplex virus (HSV) infections (see Indications).

Indications

➤*CMV retinitis:* For the treatment of CMV retinitis in patients with acquired immunodeficiency syndrome (AIDS). Combination therapy with foscarnet sodium and ganciclovir is indicated for patients who have relapsed after monotherapy with either drug. Safety and efficacy of foscarnet sodium have not been established for treatment of other CMV infections (eg, pneumonitis, gastroenteritis); congenital or neonatal CMV disease; or nonimmunocompromised individuals.

➤*Mucocutaneous acyclovir-resistant HSV infections:* For the treatment of acyclovir-resistant mucocutaneous HSV infections in immunocompromised patients. Safety and efficacy of foscarnet sodium have not been established for treatment of other HSV infections (eg, retinitis, encephalitis); congenital or neonatal HSV disease; or HSV in nonimmunocompromised individuals.

Administration and Dosage

➤*Approved by the FDA:* September 27, 1991.

➤*IV infusion:* Do not administer foscarnet sodium by rapid or bolus intravenous injection. The toxicity of foscarnet sodium may be increased as a result of excessive plasma levels. Care should be taken to avoid unintentional overdose by carefully controlling the rate of infusion. Therefore, an infusion pump must be used. In spite of the use of an infusion pump, overdoses have occurred.

Foscarnet sodium is administered by controlled intravenous infusion, either by using a central venous line or by using a peripheral vein. The standard 24 mg/mL solution may be used with or without dilution when using a central venous catheter for infusion. When a peripheral vein catheter is used, the 24 mg/mL must be diluted to 12 mg/mL with 5% dextrose in water or with a normal saline solution prior to administration to avoid local irritation of peripheral veins. Since the dose of foscarnet sodium is calculated on the basis of body weight, it may be desirable to remove and discard any unneeded quantity from the bottle before starting with the infusion to avoid overdosage. Dilutions or removal of excess quantities should be accomplished under aseptic conditions. Solutions thus prepared should be used within 24 hours of first entry into a sealed bottle. To reduce the risk of nephrotoxicity, creatinine clearance (mL/min/kg) should be calculated even if serum creatinine is within the healthy range, and doses should be adjusted accordingly.

➤*Hydration:* Hydration may reduce the risk of nephrotoxicity. It is recommended that 750 to 1000 mL of normal saline or 5% dextrose solution should be given prior to the first infusion of foscarnet sodium to establish diuresis. With subsequent infusions, 750 to 1000 mL of hydration fluid should be given with 90 to 120 mg/kg of foscarnet sodium, and 500 mL with 40 to 60 mg/kg of foscarnet sodium. Hydration fluid may need to be decreased if clinically warranted.

After the first dose, the hydration fluid should be administered concurrently with each infusion of foscarnet sodium.

➤*Admixture compatibility:* Other drugs and supplements can be administered to a patient receiving foscarnet sodium. However, care must be taken to ensure the foscarnet sodium is only administered with normal saline or 5% dextrose solution and that no other drug or supplement is administered concurrently via the same catheter. Foscarnet has been reported to be chemically incompatible with 30% dextrose, amphotericin B, and solutions containing calcium such as Ringer's Lactate and TPN. Physical incompatibility with other IV drugs has also been reported including acyclovir sodium, ganciclovir, trimetrexate glucuronate, pentamidine isethionate, vancomycin, trimethoprim/sulfamethoxazole, diazepam, midazolam, digoxin, phenytoin, leucovorin, and prochlorperazine. Because of foscarnet's chelating properties, a precipitate can potentially occur when divalent cations are administered concurrently in the same catheter.

➤*Accidental exposure:* Accidental skin and eye contact with foscarnet sodium solution may cause local irritation and burning sensation. If accidental contact occurs, the exposed area should be flushed with water.

➤*Dosage:* The recommended dosage, frequency, or infusion rates should not be exceeded. All doses must be individualized for patient's renal function.

➤*Induction treatment:* The recommended initial dose of foscarnet sodium for patients with healthy renal function is:

CMV retinitis – For CMV retinitis patients, either 90 mg/kg (1½ to 2 hour infusion) every 12 hours or 60 mg/kg (minimum 1 hour infusion) every 8 hours over 2 to 3 weeks depending on clinical response.

HSV infections – For acyclovir-resistant HSV patients, 40 mg/kg (minimum 1 hour infusion) either every 8 or 12 hours for 2 to 3 weeks or until healed.

An infusion pump must be used to control the rate of infusion. Adequate hydration is recommended to establish a diuresis (see Hydration for recommendation), both prior to and during treatment to minimize renal toxicity (see Warnings), provided there are no clinical contraindications.

➤*Maintenance treatment:* Following induction treatment the recommended maintenance dose of foscarnet sodium for CMV retinitis is 90 mg/kg/day to 120 mg/kg/day (individualized for renal function) given as an intravenous infusion over 2 hours. Because the superiority of the 120 mg/kg/day has not been established in controlled trials, and given the likely relationship of higher plasma foscarnet levels to toxicity, it is recommended that most patients be started on maintenance treatment with a dose of 90 mg/kg/day. Escalation to 120 mg/kg/day may be considered should early reinduction be required because of retinitis progression. Some patients who show excellent tolerance to foscarnet sodium may benefit from initiation of maintenance treatment at 120 mg/kg/day earlier in their treatment.

Patients who experience progression of retinitis while receiving foscarnet sodium maintenance therapy may be retreated with the induction and maintenance regimens given above or with a combination of foscarnet sodium and ganciclovir (see Clinical Trials section). Because of physical incompatibility, foscarnet sodium and ganciclovir must not be mixed.

➤*Renal function impairment:* Foscarnet sodium should be used with caution in patients with abnormal renal function because reduced plasma clearance of foscarnet will result in elevated plasma levels (see Pharmacokinetics). In addition, foscarnet sodium has the potential to further impair renal function (see Warnings). Safety and efficacy data for patients with baseline serum creatinine levels > 2.8 mg/dL or measured 24-hour creatinine clearances < 50 mL/min are limited.

Renal function must be monitored carefully at baseline and during induction and maintenance therapy with appropriate dose adjustments for foscarnet sodium as outlined below (see Dose Adjustment and Patient Monitoring). During foscarnet sodium therapy if creatinine clearance falls below the limits of the dosing nomograms (0.4 mL/min/kg), foscarnet sodium should be discontinued, the patient hydrated, and the patient monitored daily until resolution of renal impairment is ensured.

➤*Dose adjustment:* Foscarnet sodium dosing must be individualized according to the patient's renal function status. Refer below for recommended doses and adjust the dose as indicated. Even patients with serum creatinine in the healthy range may require dose adjustment; therefore, the dose should be calculated at baseline and frequently thereafter.

To use this dosing guide, actual 24-hour creatinine clearance (mL/min) must be divided by body weight (kg), or the estimated creatinine clearance in mL/min/kg can be calculated from serum creatinine (mg/dL) using the following formula (modified Cockcroft and Gault equation):

For males: $\frac{140\text{-age}}{\text{serum creatinine} \times 72}$ (0.85 for females) = mL/min/kg.

Foscarnet sodium dosing guide

Induction				
	HSV equivalent to		CMV equivalent to	
	80 mg/kg/day total	120 mg/kg/day total	180 mg/kg/day total	
C_{cr} (mL/min/kg)	(40 mg/kg every 12 hours)	(40 mg/kg every 8 hours)	(60 mg/kg every 8 hours)	(90 mg/kg every 12 hours)
> 1.4	40 mg every k12 hours	40 mg every 8 hours	60 mg every 8 hours	90 mg every 12 hours)
> 1 to 1.4	30 mg every 12 hours	30 mg every 8 hours	45 mg every 8 hours	70 mg every 12 hours
> 0.8 to 1	20 mg every 12 hours	35 mg every 12 hours	50 mg every 12 hours	50 mg every 12 hours
> 0.6 to 0.8	35 mg every 24 hours	25 mg every 12 hours	40 mg every 12 hours	80 mg every 24 hours
> 0.5 to 0.6	25 mg every 24 hours	40 mg every 24 hours	60 mg every 24 hours	60 mg every 24 hours
≥ 0.4 to 0.5	20 mg every 24 hours	35 mg every 24 hours	50 mg every 24 hours	50 mg every 24 hours
< 0.4	Not recommended	Not recommended	Not recommended	Not recommended

Maintenance		
	CMV: equivalent to	
C_{cr} (mL/min/kg)	90 mg/kg/day (once daily)	120 mg/kg/day (once daily)
> 1.4	90 mg every 24 hours	120 mg every 24 hours
> 1 to 1.4	70 mg every 24 hours	90 mg every 24 hours
> 0.8 to 1	50 mg every 24 hours	65 mg every 24 hours
> 0.6 to 0.8	80 mg every 48 hours	105 mg every 48 hours
> 0.5 to 0.6	60 mg every 48 hours	80 mg every 48 hours
≥ 0.4 to 0.5	50 mg every 48 hours	65 mg every 48 hours
< 0.4	Not recommended	Not recommended

➤*Storage/Stability:* Foscarnet sodium injection should be stored at controlled room temperature, 15° to 30°C (59° to 86°F), and should be protected from excessive heat (above 40°C; 104°F) and from freezing. Foscarnet

FOSCARNET SODIUM — INJECTION

sodium injection should be used only if the bottle and seal are intact, a vacuum is present, and the solution is clear and colorless.

Actions

➤*Pharmacology:* Foscarnet sodium is an organic analogue of inorganic pyrophosphate that inhibits replication of herpes viruses in vitro including CMV and HSV types 1 and 2 (HSV-1 and HSV-2).

Foscarnet sodium exerts its antiviral activity by a selective inhibition at the pyrophosphate binding site on virus-specific DNA polymerases at concentrations that do not affect cellular DNA polymerases. Foscarnet sodium does not require activation (phosphorylation) by thymidine kinase or other kinases and therefore is active in vitro against HSV TK deficient mutants and CMV UL97 mutants. Thus, HSV strains resistant to acyclovir or CMV strains resistant to ganciclovir may be sensitive to foscarnet sodium. However, acyclovir— or ganciclovir—resistant mutants with alterations in the viral DNA polymerase may be resistant to foscarnet sodium and may not respond to therapy with foscarnet sodium. The combination of foscarnet sodium and ganciclovir has been shown to have enhanced activity in vitro.

➤*Pharmacokinetics:*

Absorption/Distribution – In vitro studies have shown that 14% to 17% of foscarnet is protein bound at plasma drug concentrations of 1 to 1000 mcM.

The pharmacokinetics of foscarnet have been determined after administration as an intermittent intravenous infusion during induction therapy in AIDS patients with CMV retinitis. Observed plasma foscarnet concentrations in 4 studies (FOS-01, ACTG-015, FP48PK, FP49PK) are summarized in the following table:

Foscarnet sodium pharmacokinetic characteristics*		
Parameter	60 mg/kg every 8 hours	90 mg/kg every 12 hours
C_{max} at steady state (mcM)	589 ± 192 (24)	623 ± 132 (19)
C_{trough} at steady state (mcM)	114 ± 91 (24)	63 ± 57 (17)
Volume of distribution (L/kg)	0.41 ± 0.13 (12)	0.52 ± 0.2 (18)
Plasma half-life (hours)	4 ± 2 (n = 24)	3.3 ± 1.4 (18)
Systemic clearance (L/hr)	6.2 ± 2.1 (24)	7.1 ± 2.7 (18)
Renal clearance (L/hr)	5.6 ± 1.9 (5)	6.4 ± 2.5 (13)
CSF:plasma ratio	0.69 ± 0.19 (9)[1]	0.66 ± 0.11 (5)[2]

* Values expressed as mean ± SD (number of subjects studied) for each parameter.
[1] 50 mg/kg every 8 hours for 28 days, samples taken 3 hours after end of 1 hour infusion (Astra Report 815–04 AC025–1).
[2] 90 mg/kg every 12 hours for 28 days, samples taken 1 hour after end of 2-hour infusion.

Metabolism/Excretion – The foscarnet terminal half-life determined by urinary excretion was 87.5 ± 41.8 hours, possibly due to release of foscarnet from bone. Postmortem data on several patients in European clinical trials provide evidence that foscarnet does accumulate in bone in humans; however, the extent to which this occurs has not been determined. In animal studies (mice), 40% of an intravenous dose of foscarnet sodium was deposited in bone in young animals and 7% was deposited in adult animals.

Special populations –

Renal function impairment: The pharmacokinetic properties of foscarnet have been determined in a small group of adult subjects with healthy and impaired renal function, as summarized in the following table:

Pharmacokinetic parameters (mean ± SD) after a single 60 mg/kg dose of foscarnet sodium in 4 groups* of adults with varying degrees of renal function				
Parameter	Group 1 (n = 6)	Group 2 (n = 6)	Group 3 (n = 6)	Group 4 (n = 4)
Creatinine clearance (mL/min)	108 ± 16	68 ± 8	34 ± 9	20 ± 4
Foscarnet CL (mL/min/kg)	2.13 ± 0.71	1.33 ± 0.43	0.46 ± 0.14	0.43 ± 0.26
Foscarnet half-life (hours)	1.93 ± 0.12	3.35 ± 0.87	13 ± 4.05	25.3 ± 18.7

* Group 1 patients had healthy renal function defined as a creatinine clearance (C_{cr} of greater than 80 mL/min. Group 2 C_{cr} was 50 to 80 mL min. Group 3 C_{cr} was 25 to 49 mL/min and Group 4 C_{cr} was 10 to 24 mL/min.

Total systemic clearance of foscarnet decreased and half-life increased with diminishing renal function (as expressed by creatinine clearance). Based on these observations, it is necessary to modify the dosage of foscarnet in patients with renal impairment (see Administration and Dosage).

Contraindications

Clinically significant hypersensitivity to foscarnet sodium.

Warnings

➤*Mineral and electrolyte abnormalities:* Foscarnet sodium has been associated with changes in serum electrolytes including hypocalcemia, hypophosphatemia, hyperphosphatemia, hypomagnesemia, and hypokalemia (see Adverse Reactions). Foscarnet sodium may also be associated with a dose-related decrease in ionized serum calcium which may not be reflected in total serum calcium. This effect is likely to be related to chelation of divalent metal ions such as calcium by foscarnet. Patients should be advised to report symptoms of low ionized calcium such as perioral tingling, numbness in the extremities and paresthesias. Particular caution and careful management of serum electrolytes is advised in patients with altered calcium or other electrolyte levels before treatment and especially in those with neurologic or cardiac abnormalities and those receiving other drugs known to influence minerals and electrolytes (see Administration and Dosage, Patient monitoring and Drug Interactions). Physicians should be prepared to treat these abnormalities and their sequelae such as tetany, seizures or cardiac disturbances. The rate of foscarnet sodium infusion may also affect the decrease in ionized calcium. Therefore, an infusion pump must be used for administration to prevent rapid intravenous infusion (see Administration and Dosage). Slowing the infusion rate may decrease or prevent symptoms.

➤*Seizures:* Seizures related to mineral and electrolyte abnormalities have been associated with foscarnet sodium treatment (see Warnings; Mineral and electrolyte abnormalities). Several cases of seizures were associated with death. Risk factors associated with seizures included impaired baseline renal function, low total serum calcium, and underlying CNS conditions.

➤*Nephrotoxicity:* The major toxicity of foscarnet sodium is renal impairment (see Adverse Reactions). Renal impairment is most likely to become clinically evident during the second week of induction therapy, but may occur at any time during foscarnet sodium treatment. Renal function should be monitored carefully during both induction and maintenance therapy (see Administration and Dosage, Patient monitoring). Elevations in serum creatinine are usually, but not always, reversible following discontinuation or dose adjustment of foscarnet sodium. Safety and efficacy data for patients with baseline serum creatinine levels > 2.8 mg/dL or measured 24-hour creatinine clearances < 50 mL/min are limited.

Because of foscarnet sodium's potential to cause renal impairment, dose adjustment based on serum creatinine is necessary.

➤*Hydration:* See Administration and Dosage for more information.

➤*Mutagenesis:* Foscarnet sodium showed genotoxic effects in the BALB/3T3 in vitro transformation assay at concentrations > 0.5 mcg/mL and an increased frequency of chromosome aberrations in the sister chromatid exchange assay at 1000 mcg/mL. A high dose of foscarnet (350 mg/kg) caused an increase in micronucleated polychromatic erythrocytes in vivo in mice at doses that produced exposures (area under curve) comparable to that anticipated clinically.

➤*Elderly:* No studies of the efficacy or safety of foscarnet sodium in persons over age 65 have been conducted. Since these individuals frequently have reduced glomerular filtration, particular attention should be paid to assessing renal function before and during foscarnet sodium administration (see Administration and Dosage).

➤*Pregnancy: Category C.* Daily subcutaneous doses up to 75 mg/kg administered to female rats prior to and during mating, during gestation, and 21 days post-partum caused a slight increase (< 5%) in the number of skeletal anomalies compared with the control group. Daily subcutaneous doses up to 75 mg/kg administered to rabbits and 150 mg/kg administered to rats during gestation caused an increase in the frequency of skeletal anomalies/variations. On the basis of estimated drug exposure (as measured by AUC), the 150 mg/kg dose in rats and 75 mg/kg dose in rabbits were approximately one-eighth (rat) and one-third (rabbit) the estimated maximal daily human exposure.

These studies are inadequate to define the potential teratogenicity at levels to which women will be exposed. There are no adequate and well-controlled studies in pregnant women. Because animal reproductive studies are not always predictive of human response, foscarnet sodium should be used during pregnancy only if clearly needed.

➤*Lactation:* It is not known whether foscarnet sodium is excreted in human milk; however, in lactating rats administered 75 mg/kg, foscarnet sodium was excreted in maternal milk at concentrations three times higher than peak maternal blood concentrations.

➤*Children:* The safety and effectiveness of foscarnet sodium in pediatric patients have not been established. Foscarnet sodium is deposited in teeth and bone and deposition is greater in young and growing animals. Foscarnet sodium has been demonstrated to adversely affect development of tooth enamel in mice and rats. The effects of this deposition on skeletal development have not been studied. Since deposition in human bone has also been shown to occur, it is likely that it does so to a greater degree in developing bone in pediatric patients. Administration to pediatric patients should be undertaken only after careful evaluation and only if the potential benefits for treatment outweigh the risks.

Precautions

➤*Monitoring:* The majority of patients will experience some decrease in renal function due to foscarnet sodium administration. Therefore it is recommended that creatinine clearance, either measured or estimated using the modified Cockcroft and Gault equation based on serum creatinine, be determined at baseline, 2 to 3 times per week during induction therapy and at least every 1 to 2 weeks during maintenance therapy, with foscarnet sodium dose adjusted accordingly (see Dose Adjustment). More frequent monitoring may be required for some patients. It is also recommended that a 24-hour creatinine clearance be determined at baseline and periodically thereafter to ensure correct dosing (assuming verification of an adequate collection using creatinine index). Foscarnet sodium should be discontinued if creatinine clearance drops below 0.4 mL/min/kg.

Due to foscarnet sodium's propensity to chelate divalent metal ions and alter levels of serum electrolytes, patients must be monitored closely for such changes. It is recommended that a schedule similar to that recommended for serum creatinine (see above) be used to monitor serum calcium, magnesium, potassium and phosphorus. Particular caution is advised in patients with decreased total serum calcium or other electrolyte levels before treatment, as well as in patients with neurologic or cardiac abnormalities, and in

FOSCARNET SODIUM — INJECTION

patients receiving other drugs known to influence serum calcium levels. Any clinically significant metabolic changes should be corrected. Also, patients who experience mild (eg, perioral numbness or paresthesias) or severe (eg, seizures) symptoms of electrolyte abnormalities should have serum electrolyte and mineral levels assessed as close in time to the event as possible.

Careful monitoring and appropriate management of electrolytes, calcium, magnesium, and creatinine are of particular importance in patients with conditions that may predispose them to seizures (see Warnings).

➤*Local irritation:* Care must be taken to infuse solutions containing foscarnet sodium only into veins with adequate blood flow to permit rapid dilution and distribution to avoid local irritation (see Administration and Dosage). Local irritation and ulcerations of penile epithelium have been reported in male patients receiving foscarnet sodium, possibly related to the presence of drug in the urine. One case of vulvovaginal ulcerations in a female receiving foscarnet sodium has been reported. Adequate hydration with close attention to personal hygiene may minimize the occurrence of such events.

➤*Hemopoietic system:* Anemia has been reported in 33% of patients receiving foscarnet sodium in controlled studies. Granulocytopenia has been reported in 17% of patients receiving foscarnet sodium in controlled studies; however, only 1% (2/189) were terminated from these studies because of neutropenia.

Drug Interactions

Foscarnet Drug Interactions

Precipitant drug	Object drug*		Description
Nephrotoxic drugs (eg, aminoglycosides, amphotericin B, IV pentamidine)	Foscarnet	↑	Because of foscarnet's tendency to cause renal impairment, avoid the use of foscarnet in combination with potentially nephrotoxic drugs unless the potential benefits outweigh the risks to the patient.
Ritonavir/Saquinavir	Foscarnet	↑	Abnormal renal function has occurred with concomitant use.
Foscarnet	Calcium	↓	Foscarnet decreases serum concentrations of ionized calcium. Avoid concurrent use.
Foscarnet	Pentamidine	↑	Concomitant treatment of four patients with foscarnet and IV pentamidine may have caused hypocalcemia; one patient died with severe hypocalcemia. Toxicity associated with concomitant use of aerosolized pentamidine has not been reported.

* ↑ = Object drug increased.

Adverse Reactions

➤*Electrolyte disturbance:* Foscarnet sodium has been associated with changes in serum electrolytes including hypocalcemia (15% to 30%), hypophosphatemia (8% to 26%) and hyperphosphatemia (6%), hypomagnesemia (15% to 30%), and hypokalemia (16% to 48%) (see Warnings). The higher percentages were derived from those patients receiving hydration.

➤*Renal:* The major toxicity of foscarnet sodium is renal impairment (see Warnings). Approximately 33% of 189 patients with AIDS and CMV retinitis who received foscarnet sodium (60 mg/kg 3 times daily), without adequate hydration, developed significant impairment of renal function (serum creatinine ≥ 2 mg/dL). The incidence of renal impairment in subsequent clinical trials in which 1000 mL of normal saline or 5% dextrose solution was given with each infusion of foscarnet sodium was 12% (34/280).

➤*Seizures:* Foscarnet sodium treatment was associated with seizures in 18/189 (10%) AIDS patients in the initial 5 controlled studies (see Warnings). Risk factors associated with seizures included impaired baseline renal function, low total serum calcium, and underlying CNS conditions predisposing the patient to seizures. The rate of seizures did not increase with duration of treatment. Three cases were associated with overdoses of foscarnet sodium (see Overdosage). In five controlled US clinical trials the most frequently reported adverse events in patients with AIDS and CMV retinitis are shown in the table below. These figures were calculated without reference to drug relationship or severity.

Adverse events reported in 5 controlled US clinical trials

Adverse event	n = 189
Fever	65%
Nausea	47%
Anemia	33%
Diarrhea	30%
Abnormal renal function	27%
Vomiting	26%
Headache	26%
Seizures	10%

From these same controlled trials, adverse events categorized by investigator as "severe" are shown in the table below. Although death was specifically attributed to foscarnet in only 1 case, other complications of foscarnet (ie, renal impairment, electrolyte abnormalities, and seizures) may have contributed to patient deaths (see Warnings).

Severe adverse events

Event	n = 189
Death	14%
Abnormal renal function	14%
Marrow suppression	10%
Anemia	9%
Seizures	7%

➤*Incidence ≥ 5%:* From the 5 initial US controlled trials of foscarnet sodium, the following list of adverse events has been compiled regardless of causal relationship to foscarnet sodium. Evaluation of these reports was difficult because of the diverse manifestations of the underlying disease and because most patients received numerous concomitant medications.

CNS – Headache, paresthesia, dizziness, involuntary muscle contractions, hypoesthesia, neuropathy, seizures including grand mal seizures (see Warnings).

Dermatologic – Rash, increased sweating.

GI – Anorexia, nausea, diarrhea, vomiting, abdominal pain.

GU – Alterations in renal function included increased serum creatinine, decreased creatinine clearance, and abnormal renal function (see Warnings).

Hematologic – Anemia, granulocytopenia, leukopenia (see Precautions).

Metabolic/Nutritional – Mineral and electrolyte imbalances (see Warnings) including hypokalemia, hypocalcemia, hypomagnesemia, hypophosphatemia, hyperphosphatemia.

Psychiatric – Depression, confusion, anxiety.

Respiratory – Coughing, dyspnea.

Special senses – Vision abnormalities.

Miscellaneous – Fever, fatigue, rigors, asthenia, malaise, pain, infection, sepsis, death.

➤*Incidence 1% to < 5%:*

Cardiovascular – Hypertension, palpitations, ECG abnormalities including sinus tachycardia, first degree AV block and non-specific ST-T segment changes, hypotension, flushing, cerebrovascular disorder (see Warnings).

CNS – Tremor, ataxia, dementia, stupor, generalized spasms, sensory disturbances, meningitis, aphasia, abnormal coordination, leg cramps, EEG abnormalities (see Warnings).

Dermatologic – Pruritus, skin ulceration, seborrhea, erythematous rash, maculopapular rash, skin discoloration.

GI – Constipation, dysphagia, dyspepsia, rectal hemorrhage, dry mouth, melena, flatulence, ulcerative stomatitis, pancreatitis.

GU – Albuminuria, dysuria, polyuria, urethral disorder, urinary retention, urinary tract infections, acute renal failure, nocturia, facial edema.

Hematologic – Thrombocytopenia, platelet abnormalities, thrombosis, white blood cell abnormalities, lymphadenopathy.

Hepatic – Abnormal A-G ratio, abnormal hepatic function, increased ALT, increased AST.

Metabolic/Nutritional – Hyponatremia, decreased weight, increased alkaline phosphatase, increased LDH, increased BUN, acidosis, cachexia, thirst, hypercalcemia (see Warnings).

Musculoskeletal – Arthralgia, myalgia.

Psychiatric – Insomnia, somnolence, nervousness, amnesia, agitation, aggressive reaction, hallucination.

Respiratory – Pneumonia, sinusitis, pharyngitis, rhinitis, respiratory disorders, respiratory insufficiency, pulmonary infiltration, stridor, pneumothorax, hemoptysis, bronchospasm.

Special senses – Taste perversions, eye abnormalities, eye pain, conjunctivitis.

Miscellaneous – Back pain, chest pain, edema, influenza-like symptoms, bacterial infections, moniliasis, fungal infections, abscess.
Application Site: Injection site pain, injection site inflammation.
Neoplasms: Lymphoma-like disorder, sarcoma.

➤*Incidence < 1%:* Selected adverse events occurring at a rate of less than 1% in the five initial US controlled clinical trials of foscarnet sodium include: syndrome of inappropriate antidiuretic hormone secretion, pancytopenia, hematuria, dehydration, hypoproteinemia, increases in amylase and creatinine phosphokinase, cardiac arrest, coma, and other cardiovascular and neurologic complications. Selected adverse event data from the Foscarnet vs Ganciclovir CMV Retinitis Trial (FGCRT), performed by the Studies of the Ocular Complications of AIDS (SOCA) Research Group are shown in the table below.

FOSCARNET SODIUM — INJECTION

FGCRT: Selected adverse events[1]						
	Ganciclovir			Foscarnet		
Event	No. of events	No. of patients	Rates[3]	No. of events	No. of patients	Rates[3]
Absolute neutrophil count decreasing < 0.50•10^9 per liter	63	41	1.3	31	17	0.72
Serum creatinine increasing to > 260 mcmol per liter (> 2.9 mg/dL)	6	4	0.12	13	9	0.3
Seizure[2]	21	13	0.37	19	13	0.37
Catheterization-related infection	49	27	1.26	51	28	1.46
Hospitalization	209	91	4.74	202	75	5.03

[1] Values for the treatment groups refer only to patients who completed at least 1 follow-up visit (ie, 113 to 119 patients in the ganciclovir group and 93 to 100 in the foscarnet group. "Events" denotes all events observed and "patients" the number of patients with 1 or more of the indicated events.
[2] Final frozen SOCA 1 database dated October 1991.
[3] Per person-year at risk.

Selected adverse events from ACTG Study 228 (CRRT) comparing combination therapy with foscarnet sodium or ganciclovir monotherapy are shown in the table below. The most common reason for a treatment change in patients assigned to either foscarnet sodium or ganciclovir was retinitis progression. The most frequent reason for a treatment change in the combination treatment group was toxicity.

CRRT: Selected adverse events									
	Foscarnet (n = 88)			Ganciclovir (n = 93)			Combination (n = 93)		
Adverse event	No. events	No. patients[1]	Rate[2]	No. events	No. patients[1]	Rate[2]	No. events	No. patients[1]	Rate[2]
Anemia (Hgb < 70 g/L)	11	7	0.20	9	7	0.14	19	15	0.33
Neutropenia[3]									
ANC < 0.75•10^9 cells/L	86	32	1.53	95	41	1.51	107	51	1.91
ANC < 0.50•10^9 cells/L	50	25	0.91	49	28	0.8	50	28	0.85
Thrombocytopenia									
Platelets < 50•10^9/L	28	14	0.5	19	8	0.43	40	15	0.56
Platelets < 20•10^9/L	1	1	0.01	6	2	0.05	7	6	0.18
Nephrotoxicity									
Creatinine > 260 mcmol/L (> 2.9 mg/dL)	9	7	0.15	10	7	0.17	11	10	0.2
Seizures	6	6	0.17	7	6	0.15	10	5	0.18
Hospitalizations	86	53	1.86	111	59	2.36	118	64	2.36

[1] Patients with event.
[2] Rate = events/person/year.
[3] ANC = absolute neutrophil count.

Postmarketing – Adverse events that have been reported in postmarketing surveillance include: Ventricular arrhythmia, prolongation of QT interval, diabetes insipidus (usually nephrogenic), renal calculus, and muscle disorders including myopathy, myositis, muscle weakness and rare cases of rhabdomyolysis. Cases of vesiculobullous eruptions including erythema multiforme, toxic epidermal necrolysis, and Stevens-Johnson syndrome have been reported. In most cases, patients were taking other medications that have been associated with toxic epidermal necrolysis or Stevens-Johnson syndrome.

Overdosage

➤*Symptoms:* In controlled clinical trials performed in the United States, overdosage with foscarnet sodium was reported in 10 out of 189 patients. All 10 patients experienced adverse events and all except 1 made a complete recovery. One patient died after receiving a total daily dose of 12.5 g for 3 days instead of the intended 10.9 g. The patient suffered a grand mal seizure and became comatose. Three days later the patient expired with the cause of death listed as respiratory/cardiac arrest. The other 9 patients received doses ranging from 1.14 times to 8 times their recommended doses with an average of 4 times their recommended doses. Overall, 3 patients had seizures, 3 patients had renal function impairment, 4 patients had paresthesias either in limbs or perioraliy, and 5 patients had documented electrolyte disturbances primarily involving calcium and phosphate.

➤*Treatment:* There is no specific antidote for foscarnet sodium overdose. Hemodialysis and hydration may be of benefit in reducing drug plasma levels in patients who receive an overdosage of foscarnet sodium, but the effectiveness of these interventions has not been evaluated. The patient should be observed for signs and symptoms of renal impairment and electrolyte imbalance. Medical treatment should be instituted if clinically warranted.

Patient Information

➤*CMV retinitis:* Patients should be advised that foscarnet sodium is not a cure for CMV retinitis, and that they may continue to experience progression of retinitis during or following treatment. They should be advised to have regular ophthalmologic examinations.

➤*Mucocutaneous acyclovir-resistant HSV infections:* Patients should be advised that foscarnet sodium is not a cure for HSV infections. While complete healing is possible, relapse occurs in most patients. Because relapse may be due to acyclovir-sensitive HSV, sensitivity testing of the viral isolate is advised. In addition, repeated treatment with foscarnet sodium has led to the development of resistance associated with poorer response. In the case of poor therapeutic response, sensitivity testing of the viral isolate also is advised.

➤*General:* Patients should be informed that the major toxicities of foscarnet are renal impairment, electrolyte disturbances, and seizures, and that dose modifications and possibly discontinuation may be required. The importance of close monitoring while on therapy must be emphasized. Patients should be advised of the importance of reporting to their physicians symptoms of perioral tingling, numbness in the extremities or paresthesias during or after infusion as possible symptoms of electrolyte abnormalities. Should such symptoms occur, the infusion of foscarnet sodium should be stopped, appropriate laboratory samples for assessment of electrolyte concentrations obtained, and a physician consulted before resuming treatment. The rate of infusion must be no more than 1 mg/kg/minute. The potential for renal impairment may be minimized by accompanying foscarnet sodium administration with hydration adequate to establish and maintain a diuresis during dosing.

GANCICLOVIR (DHPG)

Rx	**Ganciclovir** (Ranbaxy)	**Capsules:** 250 mg	(RX 636). Green. In 180s.
Rx	**Cytovene** (Roche)		(Roche Cytovene 250 mg). Green. In 180s.
Rx	**Ganciclovir** (Ranbaxy)	**Capsules:** 500 mg	(RX 637). Yellow/Green. In 180s.
Rx	**Cytovene** (Roche)		(Roche Cytovene 500 mg). Yellow/green. In 180s.
Rx	**Cytovene** (Roche)	**Powder for injection, lyophilized:** 500 mg/vial ganciclovir (as sodium)	46 mg sodium. In 10 mL vials.

GANCICLOVIR — ORAL

WARNING

The clinical toxicity of ganciclovir includes granulocytopenia, anemia and thrombocytopenia. In animal studies ganciclovir was carcinogenic, teratogenic and caused aspermatogenesis.

Ganciclovir capsules are indicated only for prevention of cytomegalovirus (CMV) disease in patients with advanced HIV infection at risk for CMV disease, for maintenance treatment of CMV retinitis in immunocompromised patients, and for prevention of CMV disease in solid organ transplant recipients.

Because ganciclovir capsules are associated with a risk of more rapid rate of CMV retinitis progression, they should be used as maintenance treatment only in those patients for whom this risk is balanced by the benefit associated with avoiding daily intravenous infusions.

Indications

➤*CMV disease:* For the prevention of cytomegalovirus (CMV) disease in solid organ transplant recipients and in individuals with advanced HIV infection at risk for developing CMV disease.

➤*CMV retinitis:* An alternative to the intravenous formulation for maintenance treatment of CMV retinitis in immunocompromised patients, including patients with AIDS, in whom retinitis is stable following appropriate induction therapy and for whom the risk of more rapid progression is balanced by the benefit associated with avoiding daily IV infusions.

Safety and efficacy of ganciclovir has not been established for congenital or neonatal CMV disease; nor for the treatment of established CMV disease other than retinitis; nor for use in nonimmunocompromised individuals. The safety and efficacy of ganciclovir capsules have not been established for treating any manifestation of CMV disease other than maintenance treatment of CMV retinitis.

Administration and Dosage

➤*Approved by the FDA:* December 12, 1997.

➤*Dosage:* The recommended dose for ganciclovir capsules should not be exceeded.

➤*CMV retinitis:*

Induction treatment – Ganciclovir capsules should not be used for induction treatment.

GANCICLOVIR — ORAL

Maintenance treatment –

Ganciclovir capsules: Following induction treatment, the recommended maintenance dosage of ganciclovir capsules is 1000 mg 3 times a day with food. Alternatively, the dosing regimen of 500 mg 6 times daily every 3 hours with food, during waking hours, may be used. For patients who experience progression of CMV retinitis while receiving maintenance treatment with either formulation of ganciclovir, reinduction treatment is recommended.

➤*CMV disease in patients with advanced HIV infection:* The recommended prophylactic dose of ganciclovir capsules is 1000 mg 3 times a day with food.

➤*CMV disease in transplant recipients:* The recommended prophylactic dosage of ganciclovir capsules is 1000 mg 3 times a day with food.

➤*Renal function impairment:* In patients with renal impairment, the dose of ganciclovir capsules should be modified as shown below.

Creatinine clearance* (mL/min)	Ganciclovir capsule doses
≥ 70	1000 mg 3 times daily or 500 mg every 3 hours, 6 × day
50 to 69	1500 mg once daily or 500 mg 3 times daily
25 to 49	1000 mg once daily or 500 mg twice daily
10 to 24	500 mg once daily
< 10	500 mg 3 times per week, following hemodialysis

* Creatinine clearance can be related to serum creatinine by the following formulas:

➤*Dosage adjustments:* Dosage reductions in renally impaired patients should be considered for ganciclovir capsules. Dosage reductions should also be considered for those with neutropenia, anemia and/or thrombocytopenia. Ganciclovir should not be administered in patients with severe neutropenia (ANC less than 500/mcL) or severe thrombocytopenia (platelets less than 25,000/mcL).

➤*Handling and disposal:* Caution should be exercised in the handling of ganciclovir capsules. Avoid direct contact with the skin or mucous membranes of the powder contained in ganciclovir capsules. If such contact occurs, wash thoroughly with soap and water; rinse eyes thoroughly with plain water. Ganciclovir capsules should not be opened or crushed.

Because ganciclovir shares some of the properties of antitumor agents (ie, carcinogenicity and mutagenicity), consideration should be given to handling and disposal according to guidelines issued for antineoplastic drugs. Several guidelines on this subject have been published.

➤*Storage/Stability:* Store at controlled room temperature, 20° to 25°C (68° to 77°F); excursions permitted between 15° and 30°C (59° to 86°F).

Actions

➤*Pharmacology:* Ganciclovir is an acyclic nucleoside analogue of 2′-deoxyguanosine that inhibits replication of herpes viruses. Ganciclovir has been shown to be active against cytomegalovirus (CMV) and herpes simplex virus (HSV) in human clinical studies.

To achieve anti-CMV activity, ganciclovir is phosphorylated first to the monophosphate form by a CMV-encoded (UL97 gene) protein kinase homologue, then to the di- and triphosphate forms by cellular kinases. Ganciclovir triphosphate concentrations may be 100-fold greater in CMV-infected than in uninfected cells, indicating preferential phosphorylation in infected cells. Ganciclovir triphosphate, once formed, persists for days in the CMV-infected cell. Ganciclovir triphosphate is believed to inhibit viral DNA synthesis by competitive inhibition of viral DNA polymerases; and incorporation into viral DNA, resulting in eventual termination of viral DNA elongation.

➤*Pharmacokinetics:*

Absorption – The absolute bioavailability of oral ganciclovir under fasting conditions was approximately 5% (n = 6) and following food was 6% to 9% (n = 32). When ganciclovir was administered orally with food at a total daily dosage of 3 g/day (500 mg every 3 hours, 6 times daily and 1000 mg 3 times a day), the steady-state absorption as measured by area under the serum concentration vs time curve (AUC) over 24 hours and maximum serum concentrations (C_{max}) were similar following both regimens with an $AUC_{0\text{-}24}$ of 15.9 ± 4.2 (mean ± SD) and 15.4 ± 4.3 mcg•hr/mL and C_{max} of 1.02 ± 0.24 and 1.18 ± 0.36 mcg/mL, respectively (n = 16).

When ganciclovir capsules were given with a meal containing 602 calories and 46.5% fat at a dosage of 1000 mg every 8 hours to 20 HIV-positive subjects, the steady-state AUC increased by 22% ± 22% (range, −6% to 68%) and there was a significant prolongation of time to peak serum concentrations (t_{max}) from 1.8 ± 0.8 to 3 ± 0.6 hours and a higher C_{max} (0.85 ± 0.25 vs 0.96 ± 0.27 mcg/mL) (n = 20).

Distribution – For ganciclovir capsules, no correlation was observed between AUC and reciprocal weight (range, 55 to 128 kg); oral dosing according to weight is not required. Binding to plasma proteins was 1% to 2% over ganciclovir concentrations of 0.5 and 51 mcg/mL.

Metabolism – Following oral administration of a single 1000 mg dose of ^{14}C-labeled ganciclovir, 86% ± 3% of the administered dose was recovered in the feces and 5% ± 1% was recovered in the urine (n = 4). No metabolite accounted for more than 1% to 2% of the radioactivity recovered in urine or feces.

Excretion – When administered orally, it exhibits linear kinetics up to a total daily dose of 4 g/day. Renal excretion of unchanged drug by glomerular filtration and active tubular secretion is the major route of elimination of ganciclovir. After oral administration of ganciclovir, steady-state is achieved within 24 hours. Renal clearance following oral administration was 3.1 ± 1.2 mL/min/kg (n = 22). Half-life was 4.8 ± 0.9 hours (n = 39) following oral administration.

Special populations –

Renal function impairment: The pharmacokinetics of ganciclovir following oral administration of ganciclovir capsules were evaluated in 44 patients, who were either solid organ transplant recipients or HIV positive. Apparent oral clearance of ganciclovir decreased and $AUC_{0\text{-}24\,hr}$ increased with diminishing renal function (as expressed by creatinine clearance). Based on these observations, it is necessary to modify the dosage of ganciclovir in patients with renal impairment.

Hemodialysis: See Administration and Dosage for more information.

Contraindications

Hypersensitivity to ganciclovir or acyclovir.

Warnings

➤*Hematologic:* Ganciclovir should not be administered if the absolute neutrophil count is less than 500 cells/mcL or the platelet count is less than 25,000 cells/mcL. Granulocytopenia (neutropenia), anemia and thrombocytopenia have been observed in patients treated with ganciclovir. The frequency and severity of these events vary widely in different patient populations.

Ganciclovir should, therefore, be used with caution in patients with preexisting cytopenias or with a history of cytopenic reactions to other drugs, chemicals or irradiation. Granulocytopenia usually occurs during the first or second week of treatment but may occur at any time during treatment. Cell counts usually begin to recover within 3 to 7 days of discontinuing drug.

➤*Renal function impairment:* Ganciclovir should be used with caution in patients with impaired renal function because the half-life and plasma/serum concentrations of ganciclovir will be increased due to reduced renal clearance.

Hemodialysis has been shown to reduce plasma levels of ganciclovir by approximately 50%.

Since ganciclovir is excreted by the kidneys, normal clearance depends on adequate renal function. If renal function is impaired, dosage adjustments are required for ganciclovir IV and should be considered for ganciclovir capsules. Such adjustments should be based on measured or estimated creatinine clearance values.

➤*Carcinogenesis:* Ganciclovir was carcinogenic in the mouse at oral doses of 20 and 1000 mg/kg/day (approximately 0.1× and 1.4×, respectively, the mean drug exposure in humans following the recommended intravenous dose of 5 mg/kg, based on area under the plasma concentration curve [AUC] comparisons). At the dose of 1000 mg/kg/day there was a significant increase in the incidence of tumors of the preputial gland in males, forestomach (nonglandular mucosa) in males and females, and reproductive tissues (ovaries, uterus, mammary gland, clitoral gland and vagina) and liver in females. At the dose of 20 mg/kg/day, a slightly increased incidence of tumors was noted in the preputial and harderian glands in males, forestomach in males and females, and liver in females. No carcinogenic effect was observed in mice administered ganciclovir at 1 mg/kg/day (estimated as 0.01× the human dose based on AUC comparison). Except for histiocytic sarcoma of the liver, ganciclovir-induced tumors were generally of epithelial or vascular origin. Although the preputial and clitoral glands, forestomach and harderian glands of mice do not have human counterparts, ganciclovir should be considered a potential carcinogen in humans.

Compared with the single 5 mg/kg intravenous infusion, human exposure is doubled during the intravenous induction phase (5 mg/kg 2 times a day) and approximately halved during maintenance treatment with ganciclovir capsules (1000 mg 3 times a day). The cross-species dosage treatment should be multiplied by 2 for ganciclovir capsules.

➤*Mutagenesis:* Ganciclovir increased mutations in mouse lymphoma cells and DNA damage in human lymphocytes in vitro at concentrations between 50 to 500 and 250 to 2000 mcg/mL, respectively. Ganciclovir was not mutagenic in the Ames *Salmonella* assay at concentrations of 500 to 5000 mcg/mL.

➤*Fertility impairment:* Animal data indicate that administration of ganciclovir causes inhibition of spermatogenesis and subsequent infertility. These effects were reversible at lower doses and irreversible at higher doses. Although data in humans have not been obtained regarding this effect, it is considered probable that ganciclovir at the recommended doses causes temporary or permanent inhibition of spermatogenesis. Animal data also indicate that suppression of fertility in females may occur.

➤*Elderly:* Clinical studies of ganciclovir did not include sufficient numbers of subjects aged 65 years and over to determine whether they respond differently from younger subjects. In general, dose selection for an elderly patient should be cautious, reflecting the greater frequency of decreased hepatic, renal, or cardiac function, and of concomitant disease or other drug therapy. Ganciclovir capsules are known to be substantially excreted by the kidney, and the risk of toxic reactions to this drug may be greater in patients with impaired renal function. Because elderly patients are more likely to have decreased renal function, care should be taken in dose selection. In addition, renal function should be monitored and dosage adjustments should be made accordingly.

➤*Pregnancy: Category C.* Because of the mutagenic and teratogenic potential of ganciclovir, women of childbearing potential should be advised to use effective contraception during treatment. Similarly, men should be advised to practice barrier contraception during and for at least 90 days following treatment with ganciclovir.

Ganciclovir has been shown to be embryotoxic in rabbits and mice following intravenous administration and teratogenic in rabbits. Fetal resorptions were present in at least 85% of rabbits and mice administered 60 mg/kg/day

GANCICLOVIR — ORAL

and 108 mg/kg/day (2× the human exposure based on AUC comparisons), respectively. Effects observed in rabbits included fetal growth retardation, embryolethality, teratogenicity or maternal toxicity. Teratogenic changes included cleft palate, anophthalmia/microphthalmia, aplastic organs (kidney and pancreas), hydrocephaly, and brachygnathia. In mice, effects observed were maternal/fetal toxicity and embryolethality.

Ganciclovir may be teratogenic or embryotoxic at dose levels recommended for human use. There are no adequate and well-controlled studies in pregnant women. Ganciclovir should be used during pregnancy only if the potential benefits justify the potential risk to the fetus.

➤*Lactation:* It is not known whether ganciclovir is excreted in human milk. However, many drugs are excreted in human milk and, because carcinogenic and teratogenic effects occurred in animals treated with ganciclovir, the possibility of serious adverse reactions from ganciclovir in nursing infants is considered likely. Mothers should be instructed to discontinue nursing if they are receiving ganciclovir. The minimum interval before nursing can safely be resumed after the last dose of ganciclovir is unknown.

➤*Children:* Ganciclovir capsules have not been studied in pediatric patients under age 13 years.

Safety and efficacy of ganciclovir in pediatric patients have not been established. The use of ganciclovir in the pediatric population warrants extreme caution due to the probability of long-term carcinogenicity and reproductive toxicity. Administration to pediatric patients should be undertaken only after careful evaluation and only if the potential benefits of treatment outweigh the risks.

Precautions

➤*Monitoring:* Due to the frequency of neutropenia, anemia, and thrombocytopenia in patients receiving ganciclovir, it is recommended that complete blood counts and platelet counts be performed frequently, especially in patients in whom ganciclovir or other nucleoside analogues have previously resulted in leukopenia, or in whom neutrophil counts are less than 1000 cells/mcL at the beginning of treatment. Increased serum creatinine levels have been observed in trials evaluating both ganciclovir. Patients should have serum creatinine or creatinine clearance values monitored carefully to allow for dosage adjustments in renally impaired patients.

HIV-positive patients with CMV retinitis – Ganciclovir is not a cure for CMV retinitis, and immunocompromised patients may continue to experience progression of retinitis during or following treatment. Patients should be advised to have ophthalmologic follow-up examinations at a minimum of every 4 to 6 weeks while being treated with ganciclovir capsules. Some patients will require more frequent follow-up.

Drug Interactions

Ganciclovir Drug Interactions

Precipitant drug	Object drug*		Description
Ganciclovir	Cytotoxic drugs	↑	Cytotoxic drugs that inhibit replication of rapidly dividing cell populations such as bone marrow, spermatogonia, and germinal layers of skin and GI mucosa may have additive toxicity when administered concomitantly with ganciclovir. Therefore, consider the concomitant use of drugs such as dapsone, pentamidine, flucytosine, vincristine, vinblastine, adriamycin, amphotericin B, trimethoprim/sulfamethoxazole combinations, or other nucleoside analogs only if potential benefits outweigh the risks.
Imipenem-cilastatin	Ganciclovir	↑	Generalized seizures occurred in patients who received ganciclovir and imipenem-cilastatin. Do not use these drugs concomitantly unless the potential benefits outweigh the risks.
Nephrotoxic drugs	Ganciclovir	↑	Increases in serum creatinine were observed following concurrent use of ganciclovir and either cyclosporine or amphotericin B.
Probenecid	Ganciclovir	↑	Ganciclovir AUC increased 53% (range, -14% to 299%) in the presence of probenecid. Renal clearance of ganciclovir decreased 22% (range, -54% to -4%), which is consistent with an interaction involving competition for renal tubular secretion.

Ganciclovir Drug Interactions

Precipitant drug	Object drug*		Description
Ganciclovir	Didanosine	↑	Steady-state didanosine AUC increased 111% (range, 10% to 493%) when didanosine was administered either 2 hours prior to or simultaneously with ganciclovir. A decrease in steady-state ganciclovir AUC of 21% (range, -44% to 5%) was observed when didanosine was administered 2 hours prior to administration of ganciclovir, but ganciclovir AUC was not affected by the presence of didanosine when the 2 drugs were administered simultaneously.
Didanosine	Ganciclovir	↓	
Ganciclovir	Zidovudine	↑	Mean steady-state ganciclovir AUC decreased 17% (range, -52% to 23%) in the presence of zidovudine (100 mg every 4 hours [n = 12]). Steady-state zidovudine AUC increased 19% (range, -11% to 74%) in the presence of ganciclovir. Because both drugs can cause neutropenia and anemia, some patients will not tolerate combination therapy at full dosage.
Zidovudine	Ganciclovir	↓	

* ↑ = Object drug increased. ↓ = Object drug decreased.

Adverse Reactions

Adverse events that occurred during clinical trials of ganciclovir capsules are summarized below, according to the participating study subject population.

➤*AIDS patients:* Three controlled, randomized, phase 3 trials comparing ganciclovir IV and ganciclovir capsules for maintenance treatment of CMV retinitis have been completed. During these trials, ganciclovir IV or ganciclovir capsules were prematurely discontinued in 9% of subjects because of adverse events. In a placebo-controlled, randomized, phase 3 trial of ganciclovir capsules for prevention of CMV disease in AIDS, treatment was prematurely discontinued because of adverse events, new or worsening intercurrent illness, or laboratory abnormalities in 19.5% of subjects treated with ganciclovir capsules and 16% of subjects receiving placebo.

➤*Lab test abnormalities:* Laboratory data and adverse events reported during the conduct of these controlled trials are summarized below.

Selected laboratory abnormalities in trials for treatment of CMV retinitis and prevention of CMV disease

	CMV retinitis treatment[1]		CMV disease preventions[4]	
Treatment	Ganciclovir capsules[2] 3000 mg/day	Ganciclovir IV[3] 5 mg/kg/day	Ganciclovir capsules[5] 3000 mg/day	Placebo[6]
Subjects, number	320	175	478	234
Neutropenia				
< 500 ANC/mcL	18%	25%	10%	6%
500 to < 749 ANC/mcL	17%	14%	16%	7%
750 to < 1000 ANC/mcL	19%	26%	22%	16%
Anemia				
Hemoglobin				
< 6.5 g/dL	2%	5%	1%	< 1%
6.5 to < 8 g/dL	10%	16%	5%	3%
8 to < 9.5 g/dL	25%	26%	15%	16%
Maximum serum creatinine				
≥ 2.5 mg/dL	1%	2%	1%	2%
≥ 1.5 to < 2.5 mg/dL	12%	14%	19%	11%

[1] Pooled data from treatment studies, ICM 1653, study ICM 1774, and study AVI 034.
[2] Mean time on therapy = 91 days, including allowed reinduction treatment periods.
[3] Mean time on therapy = 103 days, including allowed reinduction treatment periods.
[4] Data from prevention study, ICM 1654.
[5] Mean time on ganciclovir = 269 days.
[6] Mean time on placebo = 240 days.

GANCICLOVIR — ORAL

➤*Adverse events reported in 5% or more of the subjects:*

Selected adverse events reported in ≥ 5% of subjects in 3 randomized phase 3 studies comparing ganciclovir capsules to ganciclovir IV solution for maintenance treatment of CMV retinitis and in 1 phase 3 randomized study comparing ganciclovir capsules to placebo for prevention of CMV disease					
		Maintenance treatment		Prevention study	
Body system	Adverse event	Capsules (n = 326)	IV (n = 179)	Capsules (n = 478)	Placebo (n = 234)
Miscellaneous	Fever	38%	48%	35%	33%
	Infection	9%	13%	8%	4%
	Chills	7%	10%	7%	4%
	Sepsis	4%	15%	3%	2%
GI	Diarrhea	41%	44%	48%	42%
	Anorexia	15%	14%	19%	16%
	Vomiting	13%	13%	14%	11%
Hemic and lymphatic	Leukopenia	29%	41%	17%	9%
	Anemia	19%	25%	9%	7%
	Thrombocytopenia	6%	6%	3%	1%
CNS	Neuropathy	8%	9%	21%	15%
Other	Sweating	11%	12%	14%	12%
	Pruritus	6%	5%	10%	9%
Catheter related*	Total catheter events	6%	22%	-	-
	Catheter infection	4%	9%	-	-
	Catheter sepsis	1%	8%	-	-

* Some of these events also appear under other body systems.

➤*The following events were frequently observed in clinical trials but occurred with equal or greater frequency in placebo-treated subjects:* Abdominal pain, nausea, flatulence, pneumonia, paresthesia, rash.

➤*Retinal detachment:* Retinal detachment has been observed in subjects with CMV retinitis both before and after initiation of therapy with ganciclovir. Its relationship to therapy with ganciclovir is unknown.

Retinal detachment occurred in 11% of patients treated with ganciclovir IV solution and in 8% of patients treated with ganciclovir capsules. Patients with CMV retinitis should have frequent ophthalmologic evaluations to monitor the status of their retinitis and to detect any other retinal pathology.

➤*Transplant recipients:* There has been 1 controlled clinical trial of ganciclovir capsules for the prevention of CMV disease in transplant recipients. Laboratory data and adverse events reported during this trial is summarized below.

Laboratory data – The following table shows the frequency of granulocytopenia (neutropenia) and thrombocytopenia observed:

	Ganciclovir capsules	
	Liver allograft*	
	Ganciclovir capsules (n = 150)	Placebo (n = 154)
Neutropenia		
Minimum ANC < 500/mcL	3%	1%
Minimum ANC 500 to 1000/mcL	3%	2%
Total ANC ≤ 1000/mcL	6%	3%
Thrombocytopenia		
Platelet count < 25,000/mcL	0%	3%
Platelet count 25,000 to 50,000/mcL	5%	3%
Total platelet ≤ 50,000/mcL	5%	6%

* Study GAN040. Mean duration of ganciclovir treatment = 82 days.

The following table shows the frequency of elevated serum creatinine values in these controlled clinical trials.

	Ganciclovir capsules	
	Liver allograft	
	Study 040	
Maximum serum creatinine levels	Ganciclovir capsules (n = 150)	Placebo (n = 154)
Serum creatinine ≥ 2.5 mg/dL	16%	10%
Serum creatinine ≥ 1.5 to < 2.5 mg/dL	39%	42%

In 3 out of 4 trials, patients receiving either ganciclovir IV solution or ganciclovir capsules had elevated serum creatinine levels when compared to those receiving placebo. Most patients in these studies also received cyclosporine. The mechanism of impairment of renal function is not known. However, careful monitoring of renal function during therapy with ganciclovir capsules is essential, especially for those patients receiving concomitant agents that may cause nephrotoxicity.

➤*"Probably" or "possibly" related to ganciclovir IV solution or ganciclovir capsules:* Other adverse events that were thought to be in controlled clinical studies in either subjects with AIDS or transplant recipients are listed below. These events all occurred in at least 3 subjects.

Cardiovascular – Hypertension, phlebitis, vasodilatation.

CNS – Abnormal dreams, anxiety, confusion, depression, dizziness, dry mouth, insomnia, seizures, somnolence, thinking abnormal, tremor.

Dermatologic – Alopecia, dry skin.

GI – Abnormal liver function test, aphthous stomatitis, constipation, dyspepsia, eructation.

GU – Creatinine clearance decreased, kidney failure, kidney function abnormal, urinary frequency.

Hematologic/Lymphatic – Pancytopenia.

Metabolic/Nutritional – Creatinine increased, AST increased, ALT increased, weight loss.

Musculoskeletal – Arthralgia, leg cramps, myalgia, myasthenia.

Respiratory – Cough increased, dyspnea.

Special senses – Abnormal vision, taste perversion, tinnitus, vitreous disorder.

Miscellaneous – Abdomen enlarged, asthenia, chest pain, edema, headache, injection site inflammation, malaise, pain.

Fatal adverse events – The following adverse events reported in patients receiving ganciclovir may be potentially fatal: Gastrointestinal perforation, multiple organ failure, pancreatitis and sepsis.

➤*Postmarketing:* The following events have been identified during postapproval use of the drug. Because they are reported voluntarily from a population of unknown size, estimates of frequency cannot be made. These events have been chosen for inclusion due to either the seriousness, frequency of reporting, the apparent causal connection or a combination of these factors:

Acidosis, allergic reaction, anaphylactic reaction, arthritis, bronchospasm, cardiac arrest, cardiac conduction abnormality, cataracts, cholelithiasis, cholestasis, congenital anomaly, dry eyes, dysesthesia, dysphasia, elevated triglyceride levels, encephalopathy, exfoliative dermatitis, extrapyramidal reaction, facial palsy, hallucinations, hemolytic anemia, hemolytic uremic syndrome, hepatic failure, hepatitis, hypercalcemia, hyponatremia, inappropriate serum ADH, infertility, intestinal ulceration, intracranial hypertension, irritability, loss of memory, loss of sense of smell, myelopathy, oculomotor nerve paralysis, peripheral ischemia, pulmonary fibrosis, renal tubular disorder, rhabdomyolysis, Stevens-Johnson syndrome, stroke, testicular hypotrophy, torsades de pointes, vasculitis, and ventricular tachycardia.

Overdosage

➤*Symptoms:* There have been no reports of overdosage with ganciclovir capsules. Doses as high as 6000 mg/day, given either as 1000 mg 6 times daily or as 2000 mg 3 times a day, did not result in overt toxicity other than transient neutropenia. Daily doses of more than 6000 mg have not been studied.

➤*Treatment:* Since ganciclovir is dialyzable, dialysis may be useful in reducing serum concentrations. Adequate hydration should be maintained. The use of hematopoietic growth factors should be considered.

Patient Information

All patients should be informed that the major toxicities of ganciclovir are granulocytopenia (neutropenia), anemia, and thrombocytopenia and that dose modifications may be required, including discontinuation. The importance of close monitoring of blood counts while on therapy should be emphasized. Patients should be informed that ganciclovir has been associated with elevations in serum creatinine.

Patients should be instructed to take ganciclovir capsules with food to maximize bioavailability.

Patients should be advised that ganciclovir has caused decreased sperm production in animals and may cause infertility in humans. Women of childbearing potential should be advised that ganciclovir causes birth defects in animals and should not be used during pregnancy and to use effective contraception during treatment with ganciclovir capsules. Similarly, men should be advised to practice barrier contraception during and for at least 90 days following treatment with ganciclovir capsules.

Patients should be advised that ganciclovir causes tumors in animals. Although there is no information from human studies, ganciclovir should be considered a potential carcinogen.

➤*All HIV-positive patients:* These patients may be receiving zidovudine. Patients should be counseled that treatment with both ganciclovir and zidovudine simultaneously may not be tolerated by some patients and may result in severe granulocytopenia (neutropenia). Patients with AIDS may be receiving didanosine. Patients should be counseled that concomitant treatment with both ganciclovir and didanosine can cause didanosine serum concentrations to be significantly increased.

➤*HIV-positive patients with CMV retinitis:* Ganciclovir is not a cure for CMV retinitis, and immunocompromised patients may continue to experience progression of retinitis during or following treatment. Patients should be advised to have ophthalmologic follow-up examinations at a minimum of every 4 to 6 weeks while being treated with ganciclovir capsules. Some patients will require more frequent follow-up.

GANCICLOVIR SODIUM — INJECTION

WARNING

The clinical toxicity of ganciclovir IV includes granulocytopenia, anemia and thrombocytopenia. In animal studies ganciclovir was carcinogenic, teratogenic and caused aspermatogenesis.

Ganciclovir IV is indicated for use only in the treatment of cytomegalovirus (CMV) retinitis in immunocompromised patients and for the prevention of CMV disease in transplant patients at risk for CMV disease.

Indications

➤*CMV retinitis:* Treatment of CMV retinitis in immunocompromised patients, including patients with acquired immunodeficiency syndrome (AIDS).

➤*CMV disease prevention:* Prevention of CMV disease in transplant recipients at risk for CMV disease.

Safety and efficacy of ganciclovir IV has not been established for congenital or neonatal CMV disease; nor for the treatment of established CMV disease other than retinitis; nor for use in non-immunocompromised individuals.

➤*Unlabeled uses:* Ganciclovir may be beneficial in CMV pneumonia in organ transplant patients.

Administration and Dosage

➤*Approved by the FDA:* June 23, 1989.

➤*IV infusion:* Do not administer ganciclovir IV solution by rapid or bolus intravenous injection. The toxicity of ganciclovir IV may be increased as a result of excessive plasma levels.

Intramuscular or subcutaneous injection or reconstituted ganciclovir IV solution may result in severe tissue irritation due to the high pH of 11.

➤*Dosage:* The recommended dose and infusion rate for ganciclovir IV solution should not be exceeded.

➤*CMV retinitis:*

Induction treatment – The recommended initial dosage for patients with healthy renal function is 5 mg/kg (given intravenously at a constant rate over 1 hour) every 12 hours for 14 to 21 days. Capsules should not be used for induction.

Maintenance treatment – Following induction treatment, the recommended maintenance dosage of ganciclovir IV solution is 5 mg/kg given as a constant-rate intravenous infusion over 1 hour once daily, 7 days per week, or 6 mg/kg once daily, 5 days per week.

For patients who experience progression of CMV retinitis while receiving maintenance treatment with either formulation of ganciclovir, reinduction treatment is recommended.

➤*Prevention of CMV disease in transplant recipients:* The recommended initial dosage of ganciclovir IV solution for patients with healthy renal function is 5 mg/kg (given intravenously at a constant rate over 1 hour) every 12 hours for 7 to 14 days, followed by 5 mg/kg once daily, 7 days per week or 6 mg/kg once daily, 5 days per week.

The duration of treatment with ganciclovir IV solution in transplant recipients is dependent upon the duration and degree of immunosuppression. In controlled clinical trials in bone marrow allograft recipients, treatment with ganciclovir IV was continued until day 100 to 120 post-transplantation. CMV disease occurred in several patients who discontinued treatment with ganciclovir IV solution prematurely. In heart allograft recipients, the onset of newly diagnosed CMV disease occurred after treatment with ganciclovir IV was stopped at day 28 posttransplant, suggesting that continued dosing may be necessary to prevent late occurrence of CMV disease in this patient population. In a controlled clinical trial of liver allograft recipients, treatment with ganciclovir capsules was continued through week 14 posttransplantation (see Indications).

➤*Renal function impairment:* For patients with impairment of renal function, refer to the table below for recommended doses of ganciclovir IV solution and adjust the dosing interval as indicated:

Creatinine clearance* (mL/min)	Ganciclovir IV induction dose (mg/kg)	Dosing interval (hours)	Ganciclovir IV maintenance dose (mg/kg)	Dosing interval (hours)
≥ 70	5	12	5	24
50 to 69	2.5	12	2.5	24
25 to 49	2.5	24	1.25	24
10 to 24	1.25	24	0.625	24
< 10	1.25	3 times per week, following hemodialysis	0.625	3 times per week, following hemodialysis

* Creatinine clearance can be related to serum creatinine by the formulas given below.

Hemodialysis – Dosing for patients undergoing hemodialysis should not exceed 1.25 mg/kg 3 times per week, following each hemodialysis session. Ganciclovir IV should be given shortly after completion of the hemodialysis session, since hemodialysis has been shown to reduce plasma levels by approximately 50%.

➤*Dosage adjustment:* Dosage reductions in renally impaired patients are required for ganciclovir IV and should be considered for ganciclovir capsules (see Renal impairment). Dosage reductions should also be considered for those with neutropenia, anemia or thrombocytopenia (see Adverse Reactions). Ganciclovir should not be administered in patients with severe neutropenia (ANC less than 500/mcL) or severe thrombocytopenia (platelets less than 25,000/mcL).

➤*Preparation of ganciclovir IV solution:* Each 10 mL clear glass vial contains ganciclovir sodium equivalent to 500 mg of ganciclovir and 46 mg of sodium. The contents of the vial should be prepared for administration in the following manner:

Reconstituted solution –

1.) Reconstitute lyophilized ganciclovir IV by injecting 10 mL of Sterile Water for Injection, USP, into the vial. Do not use bacteriostatic water for injection containing parabens. It is incompatible with ganciclovir IV and may cause precipitation.
2.) Shake the vial to dissolve the drug.
3.) Visually inspect the reconstituted solution for particulate matter and discoloration prior to proceeding with infusion solution. Discard the vial if particulate matter or discoloration is observed.
4.) Reconstituted solution in the vial is stable at room temperature for 12 hours. It should not be refrigerated.

Infusion solution – Based on patient weight, the appropriate volume of the reconstituted solution (ganciclovir concentration 50 mg/mL) should be removed from the vial and added to an acceptable (see below) infusion fluid (typically 100 mL) for delivery over the course of 1 hour. Infusion concentrations > 10 mg/mL are not recommended. The following infusion fluids have been determined to be chemically and physically compatible with ganciclovir IV solution: 0.9% Sodium Chloride, 5% Dextrose, Ringer's Injection and Lactated Ringer's Injection, USP.

Ganciclovir IV, when reconstituted with sterile water for injection, further diluted with 0.9% sodium chloride injection, and stored refrigerated at 5°C (41°F) in polyvinyl chloride (PVC) bags, remains physically and chemically stable for 14 days.

However, because ganciclovir IV is reconstituted with nonbacteriostatic sterile water, it is recommended that the infusion solution be used within 24 hours of dilution to reduce the risk of bacterial contamination. The infusion should be refrigerated. Freezing is not recommended.

➤*Handling and disposal:* Caution should be exercised in the handling and preparation of solutions of ganciclovir IV. Solutions of ganciclovir IV are alkaline (pH 11). Avoid direct contact with the skin or mucous membranes of the powder contained in ganciclovir capsules or of ganciclovir IV solutions. If such contact occurs, wash thoroughly with soap and water; rinse eyes thoroughly with plain water.

Because ganciclovir shares some of the properties of antitumor agents (ie, carcinogenicity and mutagenicity), consideration should be given to handling and disposal according to guidelines issued for antineoplastic drugs. Several guidelines on this subject have been published.

➤*Storage/Stability:* Store vials at temperatures below 40°C (104°F).

Reconstituted solution – Reconstituted solution in the vial is stable at room temperature for 12 hours. It should not be refrigerated.

Ganciclovir IV, when reconstituted with sterile water for injection, further diluted with 0.9% sodium chloride injection, and stored refrigerated at 5°C (41°F) in polyvinyl chloride (PVC) bags, remains physically and chemically stable for 14 days.

However, because ganciclovir IV is reconstituted with nonbacteriostatic sterile water, it is recommended that the infusion solution be used within 24 hours of dilution to reduce the risk of bacterial contamination. The infusion should be refrigerated. Freezing is not recommended.

Actions

➤*Pharmacology:* Ganciclovir is an acyclic nucleoside analogue of 2′-deoxyguanosine that inhibits replication of herpes viruses. Ganciclovir has been shown to be active against cytomegalovirus (CMV) and herpes simplex virus (HSV) in human clinical studies.

To achieve anti-CMV activity, ganciclovir is phosphorylated first to the monophosphate form by a CMV-encoded (UL97 gene) protein kinase homologue, then to the di- and triphosphate forms by cellular kinases. Ganciclovir triphosphate concentrations may be 100-fold greater in CMV-infected than in uninfected cells, indicating preferential phosphorylation in infected cells. Ganciclovir triphosphate, once formed, persists for days in the CMV-infected cell. Ganciclovir triphosphate is believed to inhibit viral DNA synthesis by competitive inhibition of viral DNA polymerases; and incorporation into viral DNA, resulting in eventual termination of viral DNA elongation.

➤*Pharmacokinetics:*

Absorption – The absolute bioavailability of oral ganciclovir under fasting conditions was approximately 5% (n = 6) and following food was 6% to 9% (n = 32). When ganciclovir was administered orally with food at a total daily dosage of 3 g/day (500 mg every 3 hours, 6 times daily and 1000 mg 3 times a day), the steady-state absorption as measured by area under the serum concentration vs time curve (AUC) over 24 hours and maximum serum concentrations (C_{max}) were similar following both regimens with an $AUC_{0\text{-}24}$ of 15.9 ± 4.2 (mean ± SD) and 15.4 ± 4.3 mcg•hr/mL and C_{max} of 1.02 ± 0.24 and 1.18 ± 0.36 mcg/mL, respectively (n = 16).

When ganciclovir capsules were given with a meal containing 602 calories and 46.5% fat at a dosage of 1000 mg every 8 hours to 20 HIV-positive subjects, the steady-state AUC increased by 22 ± 22% (range, −6% to 68%) and there was a significant prolongation of time to peak serum concentrations (T_{max}) from 1.8 ± 0.8 to 3 ± 0.6 hours and a higher C_{max} (0.85 ± 0.25 vs 0.96 ± 0.27 mcg/mL) (n = 20).

Distribution – The steady-state volume of distribution of ganciclovir after intravenous administration was 0.74 ± 0.15 L/kg (n = 98). For ganciclovir

GANCICLOVIR SODIUM — INJECTION

capsules, no correlation was observed between AUC and reciprocal weight (range, 55 to 128 kg); oral dosing according to weight is not required. Cerebrospinal fluid concentrations obtained 0.25 to 5.67 hours postdose in 3 patients who received 2.5 mg/kg ganciclovir intravenously every 8 hours or every 12 hours ranged from 0.31 to 0.68 mcg/mL representing 24% to 70% of the respective plasma concentrations. Binding to plasma proteins was 1% to 2% over ganciclovir concentrations of 0.5 and 51 mcg/mL.

Metabolism – Following oral administration of a single 1000 mg dose of ^{14}C-labeled ganciclovir, 86% ± 3% of the administered dose was recovered in the feces and 5% ± 1% was recovered in the urine (n = 4). No metabolite accounted for more than 1% to 2% of the radioactivity recovered in urine or feces.

Excretion – When administered intravenously, ganciclovir exhibits linear pharmacokinetics over the range of 1.6 to 5 mg/kg and when administered orally, it exhibits linear kinetics up to a total daily dose of 4 g/day. Renal excretion of unchanged drug by glomerular filtration and active tubular secretion is the major route of elimination of ganciclovir. In patients with healthy renal function, 91.3% ± 5% (n = 4) of intravenously administered ganciclovir was recovered unmetabolized in the urine. Systemic clearance of intravenously administered ganciclovir was 3.52 ± 0.8 mL/min/kg (n = 98) while renal clearance was 3.20 ± 0.8 mL/min/kg (n = 47), accounting for 91% ± 11% of the systemic clearance (n = 47). After oral administration of ganciclovir, steady-state is achieved within 24 hours. Renal clearance following oral administration was 3.1 ± 1.2 mL/min/kg (n = 22). Half-life was 3.5 ± 0.9 hours (n = 98) following IV administration and 4.8 ± 0.9 hours (n = 39) following oral administration.

Special populations –

Renal function impairment: The pharmacokinetics following intravenous administration of ganciclovir IV solution were evaluated in 10 immunocompromised patients with renal impairment who received doses ranging from 1.25 to 5 mg/kg.

Estimated creatinine clearance (mL/min)	n	Dose	Clearance (mL/min) Mean ± SD	Half life (hours) Mean ± SD
50 to 79	4	3.2 to 5 mg/kg	128 ± 63	4.6 ± 1.4
25 to 49	3	3 to 5 mg/kg	57 ± 8	4.4 ± 0.4
< 25	3	1.25 to 5 mg/kg	30 ± 13	10.7 ± 5.7

• *Hemodialysis* – See Administration and Dosage for more information.

Contraindications

Hypersensitivity to ganciclovir or acyclovir.

Warnings

➤*Hematologic:* Ganciclovir IV should not be administered if the absolute neutrophil count is less than 500 cells/mcL or the platelet count is less than 25,000 cells/mcL. Granulocytopenia (neutropenia), anemia and thrombocytopenia have been observed in patients treated with ganciclovir IV and ganciclovir. The frequency and severity of these events vary widely in different patient populations (see Adverse Reactions).

Ganciclovir IV should, therefore, be used with caution in patients with preexisting cytopenias or with a history of cytopenic reactions to other drugs, chemicals or irradiation. Granulocytopenia usually occurs during the first or second week of treatment but may occur at any time during treatment. Cell counts usually begin to recover within 3 to 7 days of discontinuing drug. Colony-stimulating factors have been shown to increase neutrophil and white blood cell counts in patients receiving ganciclovir IV solution for treatment of CMV retinitis.

➤*Renal function impairment:* Ganciclovir IV should be used with caution in patients with impaired renal function because the half-life and plasma/serum concentrations of ganciclovir will be increased due to reduced renal clearance (see Administration and Dosage and Adverse Reactions, Renal).

Hemodialysis has been shown to reduce plasma levels of ganciclovir by approximately 50%.

Since ganciclovir is excreted by the kidneys, normal clearance depends on adequate renal function. If renal function is impaired, dosage adjustments are required for ganciclovir IV. Such adjustments should be based on measured or estimated creatinine clearance values (see Administration and Dosage).

➤*Carcinogenesis:* Ganciclovir was carcinogenic in the mouse at oral doses of 20 and 1000 mg/kg/day (≈ 0.1× and 1.4×, respectively, the mean drug exposure in humans following the recommended intravenous dose of 5 mg/kg, based on area under the plasma concentration curve [AUC] comparisons). At the dose of 1000 mg/kg/day there was a significant increase in the incidence of tumors of the preputial gland in males, forestomach (nonglandular mucosa) in males and females, and reproductive tissues (ovaries, uterus, mammary gland, clitoral gland and vagina) and liver in females. At the dose of 20 mg/kg/day, a slightly increased incidence of tumors was noted in the preputial and harderian glands in males, forestomach in males and females, and liver in females. No carcinogenic effect was observed in mice administered ganciclovir at 1 mg/kg/day (estimated as 0.01× the human dose based on AUC comparison). Except for histiocytic sarcoma of the liver, ganciclovir-induced tumors were generally of epithelial or vascular origin. Although the preputial and clitoral glands, forestomach and harderian glands of mice do not have human counterparts, ganciclovir should be considered a potential carcinogen in humans.†

➤*Mutagenesis:* Ganciclovir increased mutations in mouse lymphoma cells and DNA damage in human lymphocytes in vitro at concentrations between 50 to 500 and 250 to 2000 mcg/mL, respectively. In the mouse micronucleus assay, ganciclovir was clastogenic at doses of 150 and 500 mg/kg (IV) (2.8 to 10× human exposure based on AUC) but not 50 mg/kg (exposure approximately comparable to the human based on AUC). Ganciclovir was not mutagenic in the Ames *Salmonella* assay at concentrations of 500 to 5000 mcg/mL.†

➤*Fertility impairment:* Ganciclovir caused decreased mating behavior, decreased fertility, and an increased incidence of embryolethality in female mice following intravenous doses of 90 mg/kg/day (≈ 1.7× the mean drug exposure in humans following the dose of 5 mg/kg, based on AUC comparisons). Ganciclovir caused decreased fertility in male mice and hypospermatogenesis in mice and dogs following daily oral or intravenous administration of doses ranging from 0.2 to 10 mg/kg. Systemic drug exposure (AUC) at the lowest dose showing toxicity in each species ranged from 0.03 to 0.1 times the AUC of the recommended human intravenous dose.

Animal data indicate that administration of ganciclovir causes inhibition of spermatogenesis and subsequent infertility. These effects were reversible at lower doses and irreversible at higher doses. Although data in humans have not been obtained regarding this effect, it is considered probable that ganciclovir at the recommended doses causes temporary or permanent inhibition of spermatogenesis. Animal data also indicate that suppression of fertility in females may occur.†

➤*Elderly:* Clinical studies of ganciclovir IV did not include sufficient numbers of subjects aged 65 and over to determine whether they respond differently from younger subjects. In general, dose selection for an elderly patient should be cautious, reflecting the greater frequency of decreased hepatic, renal, or cardiac function, and of concomitant disease or other drug therapy. Ganciclovir IV is known to be substantially excreted by the kidney, and the risk of toxic reactions to this drug may be greater in patients with impaired renal function. Because elderly patients are more likely to have decreased renal function, care should be taken in dose selection. In addition, renal function should be monitored and dosage adjustments should be made accordingly (see Warnings, Renal impairment and Administration and Dosage).

➤*Pregnancy: Category C*†. Ganciclovir has been shown to be embryotoxic in rabbits and mice following intravenous administration and teratogenic in rabbits. Fetal resorptions were present in at least 85% of rabbits and mice administered 60 mg/kg/day and 108 mg/kg/day (2× the human exposure based on AUC comparisons), respectively. Effects observed in rabbits included fetal growth retardation, embryolethality, teratogenicity or maternal toxicity. Teratogenic changes included cleft palate, anophthalmia/microphthalmia, aplastic organs (kidney and pancreas), hydrocephaly and brachygnathia. In mice, effects observed were maternal/fetal toxicity and embryolethality.

Ganciclovir may be teratogenic or embryotoxic at dose levels recommended for human use. There are no adequate and well-controlled studies in pregnant women. Ganciclovir IV should be used during pregnancy only if the potential benefits justify the potential risk to the fetus.

Because of the mutagenic and teratogenic potential of ganciclovir, women of childbearing potential should be advised to use effective contraception during treatment. Similarly, men should be advised to practice barrier contraception during and for at least 90 days following treatment with ganciclovir IV.

➤*Lactation:* It is not known whether ganciclovir is excreted in human milk. However, many drugs are excreted in human milk and, because carcinogenic and teratogenic effects occurred in animals treated with ganciclovir, the possibility of serious adverse reactions from ganciclovir in nursing infants is considered likely (see Pregnancy). Mothers should be instructed to discontinue nursing if they are receiving ganciclovir IV. The minimum interval before nursing can safely be resumed after the last dose of ganciclovir IV is unknown.

➤*Children:* Safety and efficacy of ganciclovir IV in pediatric patients have not been established. The use of ganciclovir IV in the pediatric population warrants extreme caution due to the probability of long-term carcinogenicity and reproductive toxicity. Administration to pediatric patients should be undertaken only after careful evaluation and only if the potential benefits of treatment outweigh the risks.

The spectrum of adverse events reported in 120 immunocompromised pediatric clinical trial participants with serious CMV infections receiving ganciclovir IV solution were similar to those reported in adults. Granulocytopenia (17%) and thrombocytopenia (10%) were the most common adverse events reported.

Precautions

➤*Monitoring:* Due to the frequency of neutropenia, anemia, and thrombocytopenia in patients receiving ganciclovir IV (see Adverse Events), it is recommended that complete blood counts and platelet counts be performed frequently, especially in patients in whom ganciclovir or other nucleoside analogues have previously resulted in leukopenia, or in whom neutrophil

† All dose comparisons presented in the Carcinogenesis, Mutagenesis, Impairment of fertility, and Pregnancy subsections are based on the human AUC following administration of a single 5 mg/kg intravenous infusion of ganciclovir IV as used during the maintenance phase of treatment. Compared with the single 5 mg/kg intravenous infusion, human exposure is doubled during the intravenous induction phase (5 mg/kg 2 times a day) and approximately halved during maintenance treatment with ganciclovir capsules (1000 mg 3 times a day). The cross-species dose comparisons should be divided by 2 for intravenous induction treatment with ganciclovir IV.

GANCICLOVIR SODIUM — INJECTION

counts are less than 1000 cells/mcL at the beginning of treatment. Increased serum creatinine levels have been observed in trials evaluating ganciclovir IV. Patients should have serum creatinine or creatinine clearance values monitored carefully to allow for dosage adjustments in renally impaired patients (see Administration and Dosage).

➤*Large doses/Rapid infusion:* In clinical studies with ganciclovir IV, the maximum single dose administered was 6 mg/kg by intravenous infusion over 1 hour. Larger doses have resulted in increased toxicity. It is likely that more rapid infusions would also result in increased toxicity (see Overdosage). Administration of ganciclovir IV solution should be accompanied by adequate hydration.

➤*Phlebitis/Pain at injection site:* Initially reconstituted solutions of ganciclovir IV have a high pH (pH 11). Despite further dilution in intravenous fluids, phlebitis or pain may occur at the site of intravenous infusion. Care must be taken to infuse solutions containing ganciclovir IV only into veins with adequate blood flow to permit rapid dilution and distribution (see Administration and Dosage).

Drug Interactions

Ganciclovir Drug Interactions

Precipitant drug	Object drug*		Description
Ganciclovir	Cytotoxic drugs	↑	Cytotoxic drugs that inhibit replication of rapidly dividing cell populations such as bone marrow, spermatogonia, and germinal layers of skin and GI mucosa may have additive toxicity when administered concomitantly with ganciclovir. Therefore, consider the concomitant use of drugs such as dapsone, pentamidine, flucytosine, vincristine, vinblastine, adriamycin, amphotericin B, trimethoprim/sulfamethoxazole combinations, or other nucleoside analogs only if potential benefits outweigh the risks.
Imipenem-cilastatin	Ganciclovir	↑	Generalized seizures occurred in patients who received ganciclovir and imipenem-cilastatin. Do not use these drugs concomitantly unless the potential benefits outweigh the risks.
Nephrotoxic drugs	Ganciclovir	↑	Increases in serum creatinine were observed following concurrent use of ganciclovir and either cyclosporine or amphotericin B.
Probenecid	Ganciclovir	↑	Ganciclovir AUC increased 53% (range, -14% to 299%) in the presence of probenecid. Renal clearance of ganciclovir decreased 22% (range, -54% to -4%), which is consistent with an interaction involving competition for renal tubular secretion.
Ganciclovir	Didanosine	↑	Steady-state didanosine AUC increased 111% (range, 10% to 493%) when didanosine was administered either 2 hours prior to or simultaneously with ganciclovir. A decrease in steady-state ganciclovir AUC of 21% (range, -44% to 5%) was observed when didanosine was administered 2 hours prior to administration of ganciclovir, but ganciclovir AUC was not affected by the presence of didanosine when the 2 drugs were administered simultaneously.
Didanosine	Ganciclovir	↓	
Ganciclovir	Zidovudine	↑	Mean steady-state ganciclovir AUC decreased 17% (range, -52% to 23%) in the presence of zidovudine (100 mg every 4 hours [n = 12]). Steady-state zidovudine AUC increased 19% (range, -11% to 74%) in the presence of ganciclovir. Because both drugs can cause neutropenia and anemia, some patients will not tolerate combination therapy at full dosage.
Zidovudine	Ganciclovir	↓	

* ↑ = Object drug increased. ↓ = Object drug decreased.

Adverse Reactions

Adverse events that occurred during clinical trials of ganciclovir IV solution and ganciclovir capsules are summarized below, according to the participating study subject population.

➤*AIDS patients:* Three controlled, randomized, phase 3 trials comparing ganciclovir IV and ganciclovir capsules for maintenance treatment of CMV retinitis have been completed. During these trials, ganciclovir IV or ganciclovir capsules were prematurely discontinued in 9% of subjects because of adverse events. In a placebo-controlled, randomized, phase 3 trial of ganciclovir capsules for prevention of CMV disease in AIDS, treatment was prematurely discontinued because of adverse events, new or worsening intercurrent illness, or laboratory abnormalities in 19.5% of subjects treated with ganciclovir capsules and 16% of subjects receiving placebo. Laboratory data and adverse events reported during the conduct of these controlled trials are summarized below.

➤*Lab test abnormalities:*

	CMV retinitis treatment[1]		CMV disease prevention[4]	
Treatment	Ganciclovir capsules 3000 mg/day[2]	Ganciclovir IV 5 mg/kg/day[3]	Ganciclovir capsules 3000 mg/day[5]	Placebo[6]
Subjects, number	320	175	478	234
Neutropenia:				
< 500 ANC/mcL	18%	25%	10%	6%
500 to < 749 ANC/mcL	17%	14%	16%	7%
750 to < 1000 ANC/mcL	19%	26%	22%	16%
Anemia: Hemoglobin:				
< 6.5 g/dL	2%	5%	1%	< 1%
6.5 to < 8 g/dL	10%	16%	5%	3%
8 to < 9.5 g/dL	25%	26%	15%	16%
Maximum serum creatinine:				
≥ 2.5 mg/dL	1%	2%	1%	2%
≥ 1.5 to < 2.5 mg/dL	12%	14%	19%	11%

[1] Pooled data from treatment studies, ICM 1653, study ICM 1774, and study AVI 034.
[2] Mean time on therapy = 91 days, including allowed reinduction treatment periods.
[3] Mean time on therapy = 103 days, including allowed reinduction treatment periods.
[4] Data from prevention study, ICM 1654.
[5] Mean time on ganciclovir = 269 days.
[6] Mean time on placebo = 240 days.

➤*Adverse events reported in 5% or more of the subjects:*

		Maintenance treatment studies		Prevention study	
Body system	Adverse event	Capsules (n = 326)	IV (n = 179)	Capsules (n = 478)	Placebo (n = 234)
Miscellaneous	Fever	38%	48%	35%	33%
	Infection	9%	13%	8%	4%
	Chills	7%	10%	7%	4%
	Sepsis	4%	15%	3%	2%
GI	Diarrhea	41%	44%	48%	42%
	Anorexia	15%	14%	19%	16%
	Vomiting	13%	13%	14%	11%
Hemic and lymphatic system	Leukopenia	29%	41%	17%	9%
	Anemia	19%	25%	9%	7%
	Thrombocytopenia	6%	6%	3%	1%
Nervous system	Neuropathy	8%	9%	21%	15%
Other	Sweating	11%	12%	14%	12%
	Pruritus	6%	5%	10%	9%
Catheter related*	Total catheter events	6%	22%		
	Catheter infection	4%	9%		
	Catheter sepsis	1%	8%		

* Some of these events also appear under other body systems.

➤*The following events were frequently observed in clinical trials but occurred with equal or greater frequency in placebo-treated subjects:* Abdominal pain, nausea, flatulence, pneumonia, paresthesia, rash.

➤*Retinal detachment:* Retinal detachment has been observed in subjects with CMV retinitis both before and after initiation of therapy with ganciclovir. Its relationship to therapy with ganciclovir is unknown.

Ophthalmic – Retinal detachment occurred in 11% of patients treated with ganciclovir IV solution and in 8% of patients treated with ganciclovir capsules. Patients with CMV retinitis should have frequent ophthalmologic evaluations to monitor the status of their retinitis and to detect any other retinal pathology.

GANCICLOVIR SODIUM — INJECTION

➤*Transplant recipients:* There have been 3 controlled clinical trials of ganciclovir IV solution and 1 controlled clinical trial of ganciclovir capsules for the prevention of CMV disease in transplant recipients. Laboratory data and adverse events reported during these trials are summarized below.

Laboratory data – The following table shows the frequency of granulocytopenia (neutropenia) and thrombocytopenia observed.

Controlled trials - transplant recipients						
	Ganciclovir IV				Ganciclovir capsules	
	Heart allograft[1]		Bone marrow allograft[2]		Liver allograft[3]	
	Ganciclovir IV (n = 76)	Placebo (n = 73)	Ganciclovir IV (n = 57)	Control (n = 55)	Ganciclovir capsules (n = 150)	Placebo (n = 154)
Neutropenia						
Minimum ANC < 500/mcL	4%	3%	12%	6%	3%	1%
Minimum ANC 500 to 1000/mcL	3%	8%	29%	17%	3%	2%
Total ANC ≤ 1000/mcL	7%	11%	41%	23%	6%	3%
Thrombocytopenia						
Platelet count < 25,000/mcL	3%	1%	32%	28%	0%	3%
Platelet count 25,000 to 50,000/mcL	5%	3%	25%	37%	5%	3%
Total platelet ≤ 50,000/mcL	8%	4%	57%	65%	5%	6%

[1] Study ICM 1496. Mean duration of treatment = 28 days.
[2] Study ICM 1570 and ICM 1689. Mean duration of treatment = 45 days.
[3] Study GAN040. Mean duration of ganciclovir treatment = 82 days.

Frequency of elevated serum creatinine values in clinical trials – The following table shows the frequency of elevated serum creatinine values in these controlled clinical trials.

Controlled trials - transplant recipients								
	Ganciclovir IV						Ganciclovir capsules	
	Heart allograft ICM 1496		Bone marrow allograft ICM 1570		Bone marrow allograft ICM 1689		Liver allograft study 040	
Maximum serum creatinine levels	Ganciclovir IV (n = 76)	Placebo (n = 73)	Ganciclovir IV (n = 20)	Control (n = 20)	Ganciclovir IV (n = 37)	Placebo (n = 35)	Ganciclovir capsules (n = 150)	Placebo (n = 154)
Serum creatinine ≥ 2.5 mg/dL	18%	4%	20%	0%	0%	0%	16%	10%
Serum creatinine ≥ 1.5 to < 2.5 mg/dL	58%	69%	50%	35%	43%	44%	39%	42%

In 3 out of 4 trials, patients receiving either ganciclovir IV solution or ganciclovir capsules had elevated serum creatinine levels when compared to those receiving placebo. Most patients in these studies also received cyclosporine. The mechanism of impairment of renal function is not known. However, careful monitoring of renal function during therapy with ganciclovir IV solution or ganciclovir capsules is essential, especially for those patients receiving concomitant agents that may cause nephrotoxicity.

➤*Other adverse events:* Other adverse events that were thought to be "probably" or "possibly" related to ganciclovir IV solution or ganciclovir capsules in controlled clinical studies in either subjects with AIDS or transplant recipients are listed below. These events all occurred in at least 3 subjects.

Cardiovascular – Hypertension, phlebitis, vasodilatation.

CNS – Abnormal dreams, anxiety, confusion, depression, dizziness, dry mouth, insomnia, seizures, somnolence, thinking abnormal, tremor.

Dermatologic – Alopecia, dry skin.

GI – Abnormal liver function test, aphthous stomatitis, constipation, dyspepsia, eructation.

GU – Creatinine clearance decreased, kidney failure, kidney function abnormal, urinary frequency.

Hematologic / Lymphatic – Pancytopenia.

Metabolic / Nutritional – Creatinine increased, SGOT increased, SGPT increased, weight loss.

Musculoskeletal – Arthralgia, leg cramps, myalgia, myasthenia.

Respiratory – Cough increased, dyspnea.

Special senses – Abnormal vision, taste perversion, tinnitus, vitreous disorder.

Miscellaneous – Abdomen enlarged, asthenia, chest pain, edema, headache, injection site inflammation, malaise, pain.

Fatal adverse events: The following adverse events reported in patients receiving ganciclovir may be potentially fatal: Gastrointestinal perforation, multiple organ failure, pancreatitis and sepsis.

➤*Postmarketing:* The following events have been identified during post-approval use of the drug. Because they are reported voluntarily from a population of unknown size, estimates of frequency cannot be made. These events have been chosen for inclusion due to either the seriousness, frequency of reporting, the apparent causal connection or a combination of these factors:

Miscellaneous – Acidosis, allergic reaction, anaphylactic reaction, arthritis, bronchospasm, cardiac arrest, cardiac conduction abnormality, cataracts, cholelithiasis, cholestasis, congenital anomaly, dry eyes, dysesthesia, dysphasia, elevated triglyceride levels, encephalopathy, exfoliative dermatitis, extrapyramidal reaction, facial palsy, hallucinations, hemolytic anemia, hemolytic uremic syndrome, hepatic failure, hepatitis, hypercalcemia, hyponatremia, inappropriate serum ADH, infertility, intestinal ulceration, intracranial hypertension, irritability, loss of memory, loss of sense of smell, myelopathy, oculomotor nerve paralysis, peripheral ischemia, pulmonary fibrosis, renal tubular disorder, rhabdomyolysis, Stevens-Johnson syndrome, stroke, testicular hypotrophy, torsades de pointes, vasculitis, ventricular tachycardia.

Overdosage

➤*Symptoms:* Overdosage with ganciclovir IV has been reported in 17 patients (13 adults and 4 children under 2 years of age). Five patients experienced no adverse events following overdosage at the following doses: 7 doses of 11 mg/kg over a 3-day period (adult), single dose of 3500 mg (adult), single dose of 500 mg (72.5 mg/kg) followed by 48 hours of peritoneal dialysis (4-month-old), single dose of ≈ 60 mg/kg followed by exchange transfusion (18-month-old), 2 doses of 500 mg instead of 31 mg (21-month-old).

Irreversible pancytopenia developed in 1 adult with AIDS and CMV colitis after receiving 3000 mg of ganciclovir IV solution on each of 2 consecutive days. He experienced worsening GI symptoms and acute renal failure that required short-term dialysis. Pancytopenia developed and persisted until his death from a malignancy several months later. Other adverse events reported following overdosage included: persistent bone marrow suppression (1 adult with neutropenia and thrombocytopenia after a single dose of 6000 mg), reversible neutropenia or granulocytopenia (4 adults, overdoses ranging from 8 mg/kg daily for 4 days to a single dose of 25 mg/kg), hepatitis (1 adult receiving 10 mg/kg daily, and one 2 kg infant after a single 40 mg dose), renal toxicity (1 adult with transient worsening of hematuria after a single 500 mg dose, and 1 adult with elevated creatinine (5.2 mg/dL) after a single 5000 to 7000 mg dose), and seizure (1 adult with known seizure disorder after 3 days of 9 mg/kg). In addition, 1 adult received 0.4 mL (instead of 0.1 mL) ganciclovir IV solution by intravitreal injection, and experienced temporary loss of vision and central retinal artery occlusion secondary to increased intraocular pressure related to the injected fluid volume.

➤*Treatment:* Since ganciclovir is dialyzable, dialysis may be useful in reducing serum concentrations. Adequate hydration should be maintained. The use of hematopoietic growth factors should be considered.

Patient Information

All patients should be informed that the major toxicities of ganciclovir are granulocytopenia (neutropenia), anemia and thrombocytopenia and that dose modifications may be required, including discontinuation. The importance of close monitoring of blood counts while on therapy should be emphasized. Patients should be informed that ganciclovir has been associated with elevations in serum creatinine.

Patients should be advised that ganciclovir has caused decreased sperm production in animals and may cause infertility in humans. Women of childbearing potential should be advised that ganciclovir causes birth defects in animals and should not be used during pregnancy and to use effective contraception during treatment with ganciclovir IV. Similarly, men should be advised to practice barrier contraception during and for at least 90 days following treatment with ganciclovir IV.

Patients should be advised that ganciclovir causes tumors in animals. Although there is no information from human studies, ganciclovir should be considered a potential carcinogen.

➤*All HIV positive patients:* These patients may be receiving zidovudine. Patients should be counseled that treatment with both ganciclovir and zidovudine simultaneously may not be tolerated by some patients and may result in severe granulocytopenia (neutropenia). Patients with AIDS may be receiving didanosine. Patients should be counseled that concomitant treatment with both ganciclovir and didanosine can cause didanosine serum concentrations to be significantly increased.

➤*HIV positive patients with CMV retinitis:* Ganciclovir is not a cure for CMV retinitis, and immunocompromised patients may continue to experience progression of retinitis during or following treatment. Patients should be advised to have ophthalmologic follow-up examinations at a minimum of every 4 to 6 weeks while being treated with ganciclovir IV. Some patients will require more frequent follow-up.

➤*Transplant recipients:* Transplant recipients should be counseled regarding the high frequency of impaired renal function in transplant recipients who received ganciclovir IV solution in controlled clinical trials, particularly in patients receiving concomitant administration of nephrotoxic agents such as cyclosporine and amphotericin B. Although the specific mechanism of this toxicity, which in most cases was reversible, has not been determined, the higher rate of renal impairment in patients receiving ganciclovir IV solution compared with those who received placebo in the same trials may indicate that ganciclovir IV played a significant role.

VALGANCICLOVIR HYDROCHLORIDE

Rx	Valcyte (Roche)	Tablets: 450 mg (as base)	(VGC 450). Pink. In 60s.

VALGANCICLOVIR HYDROCHLORIDE — ORAL

WARNING

The clinical toxicity of valganciclovir hydrochloride, which is metabolized to ganciclovir, includes granulocytopenia, anemia and thrombocytopenia. In animal studies ganciclovir was carcinogenic, teratogenic and caused aspermatogenesis.

Indications

➤*CMV retinitis:* For the treatment of cytomegalovirus (CMV) retinitis in patients with acquired immunodeficiency syndrome (AIDS).

➤*CMV disease:* For the prevention of CMV disease in kidney, heart, and kidney-pancreas transplant patients at high risk (Donor CMV seropositive/ Recipient CMV seronegative [(D+/R−)]).

➤*Liver transplant patients:* See Warnings for more information.

Administration and Dosage

➤*Approved by the FDA:* March 29, 2001.

Strict adherence to dosage recommendations is essential to avoid overdose. Valganciclovir hydrochloride tablets cannot be substituted for gancyclovir capsules on a 1-to-1 basis.

Valganciclovir hydrochloride tablets are administered orally, and should be taken with food. After oral administration, valganciclovir is rapidly and extensively converted into ganciclovir. The bioavailability of ganciclovir from valganciclovir hydrochloride tablets is significantly higher than from ganciclovir capsules. Therefore, the dosage and administration of valganciclovir hydrochloride tablets as described below should be closely followed.

➤*CMV retinitis:*

Induction – For patients with active CMV retinitis, the recommended dosage is 900 mg (two 450 mg tablets) twice a day for 21 days with food.

Maintenance – Following induction treatment, or in patients with inactive CMV retinitis, the recommended dosage is 900 mg (two 450 mg tablets) once daily with food.

➤*Prevention of CMV disease in heart, kidney, and kidney-pancreas transplantation:* For patients who have received a kidney, heart, or kidney-pancreas transplant, the recommended dose is 900 mg (two 450 mg tablets) once daily with food starting within 10 days of transplantation until 100 days posttransplantation.

➤*Renal function impairment:* Serum creatinine or creatinine clearance levels should be monitored carefully. Dosage adjustment is required according to creatinine clearance as shown in the table below. Increased monitoring for cytopenias may be warranted in patients with renal impairment.

Dose modifications for patients with impaired renal function

Ccr* (mL/min)	Induction dose	Maintenance prevention dose
≥ 60	900 mg twice daily	900 mg once daily
40 to 59	450 mg twice daily	450 mg once daily
25 to 39	450 mg once daily	450 mg every 2 days
10 to 24	450 mg every 2 days	450 mg twice weekly

* An estimated creatinine clearance can be related to serum creatinine by the following formulas:

For males = (140 − age [years]) × (body weight [kg])÷(72) × (serum creatinine [mg/dL]).

For females = 0.85 × male value.

➤*Hemodialysis patients:* Should not be prescribed to patients receiving hemodialysis.

For patients on hemodialysis (Ccr less than 10 mL/min) a dose recommendation cannot be given.

➤*Handling and disposal:* Caution should be exercised in the handling of valganciclovir hydrochloride tablets. Tablets should not be broken or crushed. Since valganciclovir is considered a potential teratogen and carcinogen in humans, caution should be observed in handling broken tablets. Avoid direct contact of broken or crushed tablets with skin or mucous membranes. If such contact occurs, wash thoroughly with soap and water, and rinse eyes thoroughly with plain water.

Because ganciclovir shares some of the properties of antitumor agents (ie, carcinogenicity and mutagenicity), consideration should be given to handling and disposal according to guidelines issued for antineoplastic drugs.

➤*Storage / Stability:* Store at 25°C (77°F); excursions permitted to 15° to 30°C (59° to 86°F).

Actions

➤*Pharmacology:* Valganciclovir is an L-valyl ester (prodrug) of ganciclovir that exists as a mixture of 2 diastereomers. After oral administration, both diastereomers are rapidly converted to ganciclovir by intestinal and hepatic esterases. Ganciclovir is a synthetic analogue of 2′-deoxyguanosine, which inhibits replication of human cytomegalovirus in vitro and in vivo.

In CMV-infected cells ganciclovir is initially phosphorylated to ganciclovir monophosphate by the viral protein kinase, pUL97. Further phosphorylation occurs by cellular kinases to produce ganciclovir triphosphate, which is then slowly metabolized intracellularly (half-life 18 hours). As the phosphorylation is largely dependent on the viral kinase, phosphorylation of ganciclovir occurs preferentially in virus-infected cells. The virustatic activity of ganciclovir is due to inhibition of viral DNA synthesis by ganciclovir triphosphate.

Viral resistance – Viruses resistant to ganciclovir can arise after prolonged treatment with valganciclovir by selection of mutations in either the viral protein kinase gene (UL97) responsible for ganciclovir monophosphorylation or in the viral polymerase gene (UL54). Virus with mutations in the UL97 gene is resistant to ganciclovir alone, whereas virus with mutations in the UL54 gene may show cross-resistance to other antivirals that target the same sites on viral DNA polymerase.

The current working definition of CMV resistance to ganciclovir in in vitro assays is IC_{50} greater than or equal to 1.5 mcg/mL (greater than or equal to 6 mcM). CMV resistance to ganciclovir has been observed in individuals with AIDS and CMV retinitis who have never received ganciclovir therapy. Viral resistance has also been observed in patients receiving prolonged treatment for CMV retinitis with ganciclovir. The possibility of viral resistance should be considered in patients who show poor clinical response or experience persistent viral excretion during therapy.

➤*Pharmacokinetics:*

Absorption – Valganciclovir, a prodrug of ganciclovir, is well absorbed from the gastrointestinal tract and rapidly metabolized in the intestinal wall and liver to ganciclovir. The absolute bioavailability of ganciclovir from valganciclovir hydrochloride tablets following administration with food was approximately 60% (3 studies, n = 18; n = 16; n = 28). Ganciclovir median t_{max} following administration of 450 mg to 2,625 mg valganciclovir tablets ranged from 1 to 3 hours. Dose proportionality with respect to ganciclovir AUC following administration of valganciclovir tablets was demonstrated only under fed conditions. Systemic exposure to the prodrug, valganciclovir, is transient and low, and the AUC_{24} and C_{max} values are approximately 1% and 3% of those of ganciclovir, respectively.

When valganciclovir tablets were administered with a high fat meal containing approximately 600 total calories (31.1 g fat, 51.6 g carbohydrates, and 22.2 g protein) at a dose of 875 mg once daily to 16 HIV-positive subjects, the steady-state ganciclovir AUC increased by 30% (95% CI: 12% to 51%), and the C_{max} increased by 14% (95% CI: −5% to 36%), without any prolongation in time to peak plasma concentrations (t_{max}). Valganciclovir hydrochloride tablets should be administered with food.

Distribution – Due to the rapid conversion of valganciclovir to ganciclovir, plasma protein binding of valganciclovir was not determined. Plasma protein binding of ganciclovir is 1% to 2% over concentrations of 0.5 and 51 mcg/mL. When ganciclovir was administered intravenously, the steady state volume of distribution of ganciclovir was 0.703 ± 0.134 L/kg (n = 69).

Metabolism – Valganciclovir is rapidly hydrolyzed to ganciclovir; no other metabolites have been detected. No metabolite of orally administered radiolabeled ganciclovir (1,000 mg single dose) accounted for more than 1% to 2% of the radioactivity recovered in the feces or urine.

Excretion – Because the major elimination pathway for ganciclovir is renal, dosage reductions according to creatinine clearance are required for valganciclovir hydrochloride tablets.

The major route of elimination of valganciclovir is by renal excretion as ganciclovir through glomerular filtration and active tubular secretion. Systemic clearance of intravenously administered ganciclovir was 3.07 ± 0.64 mL/min/kg (n = 68) while renal clearance was 2.99± 0.67 mL/min/kg (n = 16).

The terminal half-life ($t_{1/2}$) of ganciclovir following oral administration of valganciclovir tablets to either healthy or HIV-positive/CMV-positive subjects was 4.08 ± 0.76 hours (n =73), and that following administration of intravenous ganciclovir was 3.81 ± 0.71 hours (n = 69). In heart, kidney, kidney-pancreas, and liver transplant patients, the terminal elimination half-life of ganciclovir following oral administration of valganciclovir was 6.48 ± 1.38 hours, and following oral administration of ganciclovir was 8.56 ± 3.62.

Special populations –

Renal function impairment:

Pharmacokinetics of ganciclovir from a single oral dose of 900 mg valganciclovir tablets

Estimated creatinine clearance (mL/min)	N	Apparent clearance (mL/min) Mean ± SD	AUC_{last} (mcg•hr/mL) Mean ± SD	Half-life (hours) Mean ± SD
51 to 70	6	249 ± 99	49.5 ± 22.4	4.85 ± 1.4
21 to 50	6	136 ± 64	91.9 ± 43.9	10.2 ± 4.4
11 to 20	6	45 ± 11	223 ± 46	21.8 ± 5.2
≤ 10	6	12.8 ± 8	366 ± 66	67.5 ± 34

Decreased renal function results in decreased clearance of ganciclovir from valganciclovir, and a corresponding increase in terminal half-life. Therefore, dosage adjustment is required for patients with impaired renal function.

Hemodialysis: Hemodialysis reduces plasma concentrations of ganciclovir by about 50% following valganciclovir administration. Patients receiving hemodialysis (Ccr less than 10 mL/min) cannot use valganciclovir hydro-

VALGANCICLOVIR HYDROCHLORIDE — ORAL

chloride tablets because the daily dose of valganciclovir hydrochloride tablets required for these patients is less than 450 mg. The pharmacokinetic properties of valganciclovir have been evaluated in HIV- and CMV-seropositive patients, patients with AIDS and CMV retinitis and in solid organ transplant patients.

Mean ganciclovir pharmacokinetic* measures in healthy volunteers and HIV-positive/CMV-positive adults at maintenance dosage			
Formulation	Valganciclovir tablets	Ganciclovir IV	Ganciclovir capsules
Dosage	900 mg once daily with food	5 mg/kg once daily	1,000 mg 3 times daily with food
$AUC_{0\text{-}24hr}$ (mcg•hr/mL)	29.1 ± 9.7 (3 studies, n = 57)	26.5 ± 5.9 (4 studies, n = 68)	Range of means 12.3 to 19.2 (6 studies, n = 94)
C_{max} (mg/mL)	5.61 ± 1.52 (3 studies, n = 58)	9.46 ± 2.02 (4 studies, n = 68)	Range of means 0.955 to 1.4 (6 studies, n = 94)
Absolute oral bioavailability (%)	59.4 ± 6.1 (2 studies, n = 32)	Not applicable	Range of means 6.22 ± 1.29 to 8.53 ± 1.53 (2 studies, n = 32)
Elimination half-life (hr)	4.08 ± 0.76 (4 studies, n = 73)	3.81 ± 0.71 (4 studies, n = 69)	Range of means 3.86 to 5.03 (4 studies, n = 61)
Renal clearance (mL/min/kg)	3.21 ± 0.75 (1 study, n = 20)	2.99 ± 0.67 (1 study, n = 16)	Range of means 2.67 to 3.98 (3 studies, n = 30)

* Data were obtained from single- and multiple-dose studies in healthy volunteers, HIV-positive patients, and HIV-positive/CMV-positive patients with and without retinitis. Patients with CMV retinitis tended to have higher ganciclovir plasma concentrations than patients without CMV retinitis.

In solid organ transplant recipients, the mean systemic exposure to ganciclovir was 1.7 times higher following administration of 900 mg valganciclovir tablets once daily versus 1,000 mg ganciclovir capsules 3 times daily, when both drugs were administered according to their renal function dosing algorithms. The systemic ganciclovir exposures attained were comparable across kidney, heart and liver transplant recipients based on a population pharmacokinetics evaluation (see table below).

Mean ganciclovir pharmacokinetic measures by organ type (study PV16000)		
Parameter	Ganciclovir capsules	Valganciclovir tablets
Dosage	1,000 mg 3 times daily with food	900 mg once daily with food
Heart transplant recipients	(n = 13)	(n = 17)
$AUC_{0\text{-}24\,hr}$ (mcg•hr/mL)	26.6 ± 11.6	40.2 ± 11.8
C_{max} (mcg/mL)	1.4 ± 0.5	4.9 ± 1.1
Elimination half-life (hr)	8.47 ± 2.84	6.58 ± 1.5
Liver transplant recipients	(n = 33)	(n = 75)
$AUC_{0\text{-}24\,hr}$ (mcg•hr/mL)	24.9 ± 10.2	46 ± 16.1
C_{max} (mcg/mL)	1.3 ± 0.4	5.4 ± 1.5
Elimination half-life (hr)	7.68 ± 2.74	6.18 ± 1.42
Kidney transplant recipients*	(n = 36)	(n = 68)
$AUC_{0\text{-}24\,hr}$ (mcg•hr/mL)	31.3 ± 10.3	48.2 ± 14.6
C_{max} (mcg/mL)	1.5 ± 0.5	5.3 ± 1.5
Elimination half-life (hr)	9.44 ± 4.37	6.77 ± 1.25

* Includes kidney-pancreas.

Contraindications

Hypersensitivity to valganciclovir or ganciclovir.

Warnings

➤*Toxicity:* The clinical toxicity of valganciclovir hydrochloride, which is metabolized to ganciclovir, includes granulocytopenia, anemia and thrombocytopenia. In animal studies ganciclovir was carcinogenic, teratogenic and caused aspermatogenesis.

➤*Hematologic:* Valganciclovir hydrochloride tablets should not be administered if the absolute neutrophil count is less than 500 cells/mcL, the platelet count is less than 25,000/mcL, or the hemoglobin is less than 8 g/dL.

Severe leukopenia, neutropenia, anemia, thrombocytopenia, pancytopenia, bone marrow depression and aplastic anemia have been observed in patients treated with valganciclovir hydrochloride tablets (and ganciclovir). Valganciclovir hydrochloride tablets should, therefore, be used with caution in patients with preexisting cytopenias, or who have received or who are receiving myelosuppressive drugs or irradiation. Cytopenia may occur at any time during treatment and may increase with continued dosing. Cell counts usually begin to recover within 3 to 7 days of discontinuing drug.

➤*Liver transplant patients:*

Tissue invasive CMV disease in liver transplant patients – In liver transplant patients, there was a significantly higher incidence of tissue-invasive CMV disease in the valganciclovir-treated group compared with the oral ganciclovir group. Valganciclovir is not indicated for use in liver transplant patients.

➤*Renal function impairment:* Since ganciclovir is excreted by the kidneys, normal clearance depends on adequate renal function. If renal function is impaired, dosage adjustments are required for valganciclovir hydrochloride tablets. Such adjustments should be based on measured or estimated creatinine clearance values.

For patients on hemodialysis (Ccr less than 10 mL/min) it is recommended that ganciclovir be used (in accordance with the dose-reduction algorithm cited in the ganciclovir IV and ganciclovir capsules drug monographs in Administration and Dosage) rather than valganciclovir hydrochloride tablets.

➤*Carcinogenesis:* No long-term carcinogenicity studies have been conducted with valganciclovir. However, upon oral administration, valganciclovir is rapidly and extensively converted to ganciclovir. Therefore, like ganciclovir, valganciclovir is a potential carcinogen.

Ganciclovir was carcinogenic in the mouse at oral doses that produced exposures approximately 0.1 times and 1.4 times, respectively, the mean drug exposure in humans following the recommended intravenous dose of 5 mg/kg, based on area under the plasma concentration curve [AUC] comparisons. At the higher dose of 1,000 mg/kg/day there was a significant increase in the incidence of tumors of the preputial gland in males, forestomach (nonglandular mucosa) in males and females, and reproductive tissues (ovaries, uterus, mammary gland, clitoral gland and vagina) and liver in females. At the lower dose, a slightly increased incidence of tumors was noted in the preputial and barderian glands in males, forestomach in males and females, and liver in females. Ganciclovir should be considered a potential carcinogen in humans.

➤*Mutagenesis:* Valganciclovir increases mutations in mouse lymphoma cells. In the mouse micronucleus assay, valganciclovir was clastogenic. Valganciclovir was not mutagenic in the Ames *Salmonella* assay. Ganciclovir increased mutations in mouse lymphoma cells and DNA damage in human lymphocytes in vitro. In the mouse micronucleus assay, ganciclovir was clastogenic. Ganciclovir was not mutagenic in the Ames *Salmonella* assay.

➤*Fertility impairment:* Valganciclovir is converted to ganciclovir and therefore is expected to have similar reproductive toxicity effects as ganciclovir. Ganciclovir caused decreased mating behavior, decreased fertility, and an increased incidence of embryolethality in female mice following intravenous doses that produced an exposure approximately 1.7 times the mean drug exposure in humans following the dose of 5 mg/kg, based on AUC comparisons. Ganciclovir caused decreased fertility in male mice and hypospermatogenesis in mice and dogs following daily oral or intravenous administration. Systemic drug exposure (AUC) at the lowest dose showing toxicity in each species ranged from 0.03 to 0.1 times the AUC of the recommended human intravenous dose. Valganciclovir caused similar effects on spermatogenesis in mice, rats, and dogs. It is considered likely that ganciclovir (and valganciclovir) could cause inhibition of human spermatogenesis.

Animal data indicate that administration of ganciclovir causes inhibition of spermatogenesis and subsequent infertility. These effects were reversible at lower doses and irreversible at higher doses. It is considered probable that in humans, valganciclovir at the recommended doses may cause temporary or permanent inhibition of spermatogenesis. Animal data also indicate that suppression of fertility in females may occur.

➤*Elderly:* Clinical studies of valganciclovir hydrochloride did not include sufficient numbers of subjects aged 65 years and over to determine whether they respond differently from younger subjects. In general, dose selection for an elderly patient should be cautious, reflecting the greater frequency of decreased hepatic, renal, or cardiac function, and of concomitant disease or other drug therapy. Valganciclovir hydrochloride is known to be substantially excreted by the kidney, and the risk of toxic reactions to this drug may be greater in patients with impaired renal function. Because elderly patients are more likely to have decreased renal function, care should be taken in dose selection. In addition, renal function should be monitored and dosage adjustments should be made accordingly.

➤*Pregnancy: Category C.* Valganciclovir is converted to ganciclovir and therefore is expected to have reproductive toxicity effects similar to ganciclovir. Ganciclovir has been shown to be embryotoxic in rabbits and mice following intravenous administration, and teratogenic in rabbits. Fetal resorptions were present in at least 85% of rabbits and mice doses that produced 2 times the human exposure based on AUC comparisons. Effects observed in rabbits included: Fetal growth retardation, embryolethality, teratogenicity or maternal toxicity. Teratogenic changes included cleft palate, anophthalmia/microphthalmia, aplastic organs (kidney and pancreas), hydrocephaly and brachygnathia. In mice, effects observed were maternal/fetal toxicity and embryolethality.

Daily intravenous doses administered to female mice prior to mating, during gestation, and during lactation caused hypoplasia of the testes and seminal vesicles in the month-old male offspring, as well as pathologic changes in the nonglandular region of the stomach. The drug exposure in mice as estimated by the AUC was approximately 1.7 times the human AUC.

Data obtained using an ex vivo human placental model show that ganciclovir crosses the placenta and that simple diffusion is the most likely mecha-

VALGANCICLOVIR HYDROCHLORIDE — ORAL

nism of transfer. The transfer was not saturable over a concentration range of 1 to 10 mg/mL and occurred by passive diffusion.

Valganciclovir may be teratogenic or embryotoxic at dose levels recommended for human use. There are no adequate and well-controlled studies in pregnant women. Valganciclovir hydrochloride tablets should be used during pregnancy only if the potential benefit justifies the potential risk to the fetus.

Because of the mutagenic and teratogenic potential of ganciclovir, women of childbearing potential should be advised to use effective contraception during treatment. Similarly, men should be advised to practice barrier contraception during, and for at least 90 days following, treatment with valganciclovir tablets.

In animal studies, ganciclovir was found to be mutagenic and carcinogenic. Valganciclovir should, therefore, be considered a potential teratogen and carcinogen in humans with the potential to cause birth defects and cancers.

➤*Lactation:* It is not known whether ganciclovir or valganciclovir is excreted in human milk. Because valganciclovir caused granulocytopenia, anemia and thrombocytopenia in clinical trials and ganciclovir was mutagenic and carcinogenic in animal studies, the possibility of serious adverse events from ganciclovir in nursing infants is possible. Because of potential for serious adverse events in nursing infants, mothers should be instructed not to breastfeed if they are receiving valganciclovir hydrochloride tablets. In addition, the Centers for Disease Control and Prevention recommend that HIV-infected mothers not breastfeed their infants to avoid risking postnatal transmission of HIV.

➤*Children:* Safety and effectiveness of valganciclovir hydrochloride tablets in pediatric patients have not been established.

Precautions

➤*Monitoring:* Due to the frequency of neutropenia, anemia, and thrombocytopenia in patients receiving valganciclovir hydrochloride tablets, it is recommended that complete blood counts and platelet counts be performed frequently, especially in patients in whom ganciclovir or other nucleoside analogues have previously resulted in leukopenia, or in whom neutrophil counts are less than 1000 cells/mcL at the beginning of treatment. Increased monitoring for cytopenias may be warranted if therapy with oral ganciclovir is changed to oral valganciclovir, because of increased plasma concentrations of ganciclovir after valganciclovir administration.

Increased serum creatinine levels have been observed in trials evaluating valganciclovir hydrochloride tablets. Patients should have serum creatinine or creatinine clearance values monitored carefully to allow for dosage adjustments in renally impaired patients. The mechanism of impairment of renal function is not known.

Strict adherence to dosage recommendations is essential to avoid overdose.

➤*Switching from ganciclovir:* The bioavailability of ganciclovir from valganciclovir hydrochloride tablets is significantly higher than from ganciclovir capsules. Patients switching from ganciclovir capsules should be advised of the risk of overdosage if they take more than the prescribed number of valganciclovir hydrochloride tablets. Valganciclovir hydrochloride tablets cannot be substituted for ganciclovir capsules on a 1-to-1 basis.

Drug Interactions

➤*Drug interaction studies conducted with valganciclovir:* No in vivo drug-drug interaction studies were conducted with valganciclovir. However, because valganciclovir is rapidly and extensively converted to ganciclovir, interactions associated with ganciclovir will be expected for valganciclovir hydrochloride tablets.

Ganciclovir Drug Interactions

Precipitant drug	Object drug*		Description
Didanosine	Ganciclovir	⬇	Steady-state didanosine AUC increased 111% (range, 10% to 493%) when didanosine was administered either 2 hours prior to or simultaneously with ganciclovir. Closely monitor for didanosine toxicity. A decrease in steady-state ganciclovir AUC of 21% (range, -44% to 5%) was observed when didanosine was administered 2 hours prior to administration of ganciclovir, but ganciclovir AUC was not affected by the presence of didanosine when the 2 drugs were administered simultaneously.
Ganciclovir	Didanosine	⬆	
Imipenem-cilastatin	Ganciclovir	⬆	Generalized seizures occurred in patients who received ganciclovir and imipenem-cilastatin. Do not administer these drugs concomitantly unless the potential benefits outweigh the risks.
Nephrotoxic drugs	Ganciclovir	⬆	Increases in serum creatinine were observed following concurrent use of ganciclovir and either cyclosporine or amphotericin B.

Ganciclovir Drug Interactions

Precipitant drug	Object drug*		Description
Probenecid	Ganciclovir	⬆	Ganciclovir AUC increased 53% (range, -14% to 299%) in the presence of probenecid. Renal clearance of ganciclovir decreased 22% (range, -54% to -4%), which is consistent with an interaction involving competition for renal tubular secretion. Monitor for ganciclovir toxicity.
Trimethoprim	Ganciclovir	⬆	Coadministration resulted in decreased ganciclovir renal clearance and increased $t_{1/2}$.
Zalcitabine	Ganciclovir	⬆	Zalcitabine 0.75 mg administered 2 hours before ganciclovir resulted in an increase in ganciclovir AUC by 13%.
Zidovudine	Ganciclovir	⬇	Mean steady-state ganciclovir AUC decreased 17% (range, -52% to 23%) in the presence of zidovudine. Zidovudine AUC increased 19% (range, -11% to 74%) in the presence of ganciclovir. Because both drugs can cause neutropenia and anemia, many patients will not tolerate combination therapy at full dosage.
Ganciclovir	Zidovudine	⬆	
Ganciclovir	Cytotoxic drugs	⬆	Cytotoxic drugs that inhibit replication of rapidly dividing cell populations such as bone marrow, spermatogonia, and germinal layers of skin and GI mucosa may have additive toxicity when administered concomitantly with ganciclovir. Therefore, consider the concomitant use of drugs such as dapsone, pentamidine, flucytosine, vincristine, vinblastine, adriamycin, amphotericin B, trimethoprim/sulfamethoxazole combinations, or other nucleoside analogs only if potential benefits outweigh the risks.

* ⬆ = Object drug increased. ⬇ = Object drug decreased.

➤*Drug/Food interactions:* When valganciclovir tablets were administered with a high-fat meal containing approximately 600 total calories (31.1 g fat, 51.6 g carbohydrates, and 22.2 g protein) at a dose of 875 mg once daily to 16 HIV-positive subjects, the steady-state ganciclovir AUC increased by 30% (95% CI 12% to 51%), and the C_{max} increased by 14% (95% CI −5% to 36%), without any prolongation in time to peak plasma concentrations (T_{max}). Administer valganciclovir tablets with food.

Adverse Reactions

Valganciclovir, a prodrug of ganciclovir, is rapidly converted to ganciclovir after oral administration. Adverse events known to be associated with ganciclovir usage can therefore be expected to occur with valganciclovir hydrochloride tablets.

➤*Treatment of CMV retinitis in AIDS patients:* As shown in the table below, the safety profiles of valganciclovir hydrochloride tablets and intravenous ganciclovir during 28 days of randomized therapy (21 days induction dose and 7 days maintenance dose) in 158 patients were comparable, with the exception of catheter-related infection, which occurred with greater frequency in patients randomized to receive IV ganciclovir.

Percentage of selected adverse events occurring during the randomized phase of Study WV15376

Adverse event	Valganciclovir arm (n = 79)	Intravenous ganciclovir arm (n = 79)
Diarrhea	16%	10%
Neutropenia	11%	13%
Nausea	8%	14%
Headache	9%	5%
Anemia	8%	8%
Catheter-related infection	3%	11%

The following tables show the pooled adverse event data and abnormal laboratory values from 2 single arm, open-label clinical trials, WV15376 and WV15705. A total of 370 patients received maintenance therapy with valganciclovir tablets 900 mg once daily. Approximately 252 (68%) of these patients received valganciclovir hydrochloride tablets for more than 9 months (maximum duration was 36 months).

VALGANCICLOVIR HYDROCHLORIDE — ORAL

Pooled selected adverse events reported in ≥ 5% of patients in 2 clinical studies in CMV retinitis	
	Patients with CMV retinitis (studies WV15376 and WV15705)
Adverse events according to body system	Valganciclovir (n = 370) %
GI	
Diarrhea	41%
Nausea	30%
Vomiting	21%
Abdominal pain	15%
Miscellaneous	
Pyrexia	31%
Headache	22%
Hemic and lymphatic	
Neutropenia	27%
Anemia	26%
Thrombocytopenia	6%
CNS	
Insomnia	16%
Peripheral neuropathy	9%
Paresthesia	8%
Special senses	
Retinal detachment	15%

Pooled laboratory abnormalities reported in 2 clinical studies in the treatment of CMV retinitis	
	CMV retinitis patients (studies WV15376 and WV15705)
Laboratory abnormalities	Valganciclovir (n = 370) %
Neutropenia: ANC/mcL	
< 500	19%
500 to < 750	17%
750 to < 1,000	17%
Anemia: Hemoglobin g/dL	
< 6.5	7%
6.5 to < 8	13%
8 to < 9.5	16%
Thrombocytopenia: Platelets/mcL	
< 25,000	4%
25,000 to < 50,000	6%
50,000 to < 100,000	22%
Serum creatinine: mg/dL	
> 2.5	3%
> 1.5 to 2.5	12%

➤*Prevention of CMV disease in selected solid organ transplantation:* The table below shows selected adverse events regardless of severity and drug relationship with an incidence of greater than or equal to 5% from a clinical trial, PV16000 (up to 28 days after study treatment) where heart, kidney, kidney-pancreas and liver transplant patients received valganciclovir (n = 244) or oral ganciclovir (n = 126). The majority of the adverse events were of mild or moderate intensity.

Percentage of selected grades 1 to 4 adverse events reported in ≥ 5% of selected solid organ transplant patients in Study PV16000		
Adverse event	Valganciclovir (n = 244) %	Oral ganciclovir (n = 126) %
Diarrhea	30%	29%
Tremors	28%	25%
Graft rejection	24%	30%
Nausea	23%	23%
Headache	22%	27%
Insomnia	20%	16%
Hypertension	18%	15%
Vomiting	16%	14%
Leukopenia	14%	7%
Pyrexia	13%	14%

Laboratory adverse events are those reported by investigators.

Adverse events not included in the table above, which either occurred at a frequency of greater than or equal to 5% in clinical study PV16000, or were selected serious adverse events reported in studies WV15376, WV15705, or PV16000 with a frequency of less than 5% are listed below.

Allergic – Valganciclovir hypersensitivity.

Cardiovascular – Hypotension.

CNS – Paresthesia, dizziness (excluding vertigo), convulsion.

Dermatologic – Dermatitis, pruritus, acne.

GI – Abdominal pain, constipation, dyspepsia, abdominal distention, ascites.

Hematologic – Potentially life-threatening bleeding associated with thrombocytopenia.

Anemia, neutropenia, thrombocytopenia, pancytopenia, bone marrow depression, aplastic anemia.

Hepatic – Abnormal hepatic function.

Metabolic/Nutritional – Hyperkalemia, hypokalemia, hypomagnesemia, hyperglycemia, appetite decreased, dehydration, hypophosphatemia, hypocalcemia.

Musculoskeletal – Back pain, arthralgia, muscle cramps, limb pain.

Psychiatric – Depression, psychosis, hallucinations, confusion, agitation.

Renal – Renal impairment, dysuria, decreased creatinine clearance.

Respiratory – Cough, dyspnea, rhinorrhea, pleural effusion.

Miscellaneous – Fatigue, pain, edema, peripheral edema, weakness.
Infections and infestations: Pharyngitis/nasopharyngitis, upper respiratory tract infection, urinary tract infection, local and systemic infections and sepsis, postoperative wound infection.
Injury, poisoning and procedural complications: Postoperative complications, postoperative pain, increased wound drainage, wound dehiscence.

Lab test abnormalities – Laboratory abnormalities reported with valganciclovir tablets in one study in solid organ transplant patients are listed in the table below.

Laboratory abnormalities reported in selected solid organ transplant patients in Study PV16000		
Laboratory abnormalities	Valganciclovir (n = 244) %	Oral ganciclovir (n = 126) %
Neutropenia: ANC/mcL		
< 500	5%	3%
500 to < 750	3%	2%
750 to < 1,000	5%	2%
Anemia: Hemoglobin g/dL		
< 6.5	1%	2%
6.5 to < 8	5%	7%
8 to < 9.5	31%	25%
Thrombocytopenia: Platelets/mcL		
< 25,000	0%	2%
25,000 to < 50,000	1%	3%
50,000 to < 100,000	18%	21%
Serum creatinine: mg/dL		
> 2.5	14%	21%
> 1.5 to 2.5	45%	47%

Overdosage

➤*Symptoms:*

Overdose experience with valganciclovir hydrochloride tablets – One adult developed fatal bone marrow depression (medullary aplasia) after several days of dosing that was at least 10-fold greater than recommended for the patient's estimated degree of renal impairment.

It is expected that an overdose of valganciclovir hydrochloride tablets could also possibly result in increased renal toxicity.

Overdose experience with intravenous ganciclovir – Reports of overdoses with intravenous ganciclovir have been received from clinical trials and during postmarketing experience. The majority of patients experienced one or more of the following adverse events:
Hematological toxicity: Pancytopenia, bone marrow depression, medullary aplasia, leukopenia, neutropenia, granulocytopenia.
Hepatotoxicity: Hepatitis, liver function disorder.
Renal toxicity: Worsening of hematuria in a patient with preexisting renal impairment, acute renal failure, elevated creatinine.
Gastrointestinal toxicity: Abdominal pain, diarrhea, vomiting.
Neurotoxicity: Generalized tremor, convulsion.

➤*Treatment:* Since ganciclovir is dialyzable, dialysis may be useful in reducing serum concentrations in patients who have received an overdose of valganciclovir hydrochloride tablets. Adequate hydration should be maintained. The use of hematopoietic growth factors should be considered.

Patient Information

Valganciclovir hydrochloride tablets cannot be substituted for ganciclovir capsules on a 1-to-1 basis. Patients switching from ganciclovir capsules should be advised of the risk of overdosage if they take more than the prescribed number of valganciclovir hydrochloride tablets.

VALGANCICLOVIR HYDROCHLORIDE — ORAL

Valganciclovir hydrochloride is changed to ganciclovir once it is absorbed into the body. All patients should be informed that the major toxicities of ganciclovir include granulocytopenia (neutropenia), anemia and thrombocytopenia and that dose modifications may be required, including discontinuation. The importance of close monitoring of blood counts while on therapy should be emphasized. Patients should be informed that ganciclovir has been associated with elevations in serum creatinine.

Patients should be instructed to take valganciclovir hydrochloride tablets with food to maximize bioavailability.

Patients should be advised that ganciclovir has caused decreased sperm production in animals and may cause decreased fertility in humans. Women of childbearing potential should be advised that ganciclovir causes birth defects in animals and should not be used during pregnancy. Because of the potential for serious adverse events in nursing infants, mothers should be instructed not to breastfeed if they are receiving valganciclovir hydrochloride tablets. Women of childbearing potential should be advised to use effective contraception during treatment with valganciclovir hydrochloride tablets. Similarly, men should be advised to practice barrier contraception during and for at least 90 days following treatment with valganciclovir hydrochloride tablets.

Although there is no information from human studies, patients should be advised that ganciclovir should be considered a potential carcinogen.

Convulsions, sedation, dizziness, ataxia or confusion have been reported with the use of valganciclovir hydrochloride tablets or ganciclovir. If they occur, such effects may affect tasks requiring alertness including the patient's ability to drive and operate machinery.

Patients should be told that ganciclovir is not a cure for CMV retinitis, and that they may continue to experience progression of retinitis during or following treatment. Patients should be advised to have ophthalmologic follow-up examinations at a minimum of every 4 to 6 weeks while being treated with valganciclovir hydrochloride tablets. Some patients will require more frequent follow-up.

Antiherpes Virus Agents

ACYCLOVIR (Acycloguanosine)

Rx	**Acyclovir** (Various, eg, Dixon-Shane, Mylan, PAR, Purepac, Teva, Zenith-Goldline)	**Tablets**: 400 mg	In 100s, 500s, and 1000s.
Rx	**Zovirax** (GlaxoWellcome)		(Zovirax). White, shield shape. In 100s.
Rx	**Acyclovir** (Various, eg, Dixon-Shane, Mylan, PAR, Purepac, Teva, Zenith-Goldline)	**Tablets**: 800 mg	In 100s and 500s.
Rx	**Zovirax** (GlaxoWellcome)		(Zovirax 800 mg). Blue, oval. In 100s and UD 100s.
Rx	**Acyclovir** (Various, eg, Dixon-Shane, Mylan, PAR, Purepac, Teva, Zenith-Goldline)	**Capsules**: 200 mg	In 100s.
Rx	**Zovirax** (GlaxoWellcome)		Lactose. (Wellcome Zovirax 200). Blue. In 100s and UD 100s.[1]
Rx	**Acyclovir** (Various, eg, Alpharma, Xactdose)	**Suspension**: 200 mg/5 mL	In 473 mL.
Rx	**Zovirax** (GlaxoWellcome)		Banana flavor. In 473 mL.[2]
Rx	**Acyclovir** (Various, eg, Bertek, APP)	**Injection**: 50 mg/mL (as sodium)	In cartons of 10.
Rx	**Acyclovir** (Various, eg, Abbott, Bedford, Gensia Sicor, Novaplus)	**Powder for injection**: 500 mg/vial (as sodium)	In 10 mL vials.
		1000 mg/vial (as sodium)	In 20 mL vials.
Rx	**Zovirax** (GlaxoWellcome)	**Powder for injection, lyophilized**: 500 mg/vial (as sodium)[3]	In 10 mL vials.

[1] May contain parabens. [2] With 0.1% methylparaben, 0.02% propylparaben, and sorbitol. [3] Contains 49 mg of sodium.

ACYCLOVIR — ORAL

Indications

➤*Herpes zoster infections:* Acyclovir is indicated for the acute treatment of herpes zoster (shingles).

➤*Genital herpes:* Acyclovir is indicated for the treatment of initial episodes and the management of recurrent episodes of genital herpes.

➤*Chickenpox:* Acyclovir is indicated for the treatment of chickenpox (varicella).

➤*Unlabeled uses:* Cytomegalovirus and herpes simplex virus (HSV) infection following bone marrow or renal transplantation; disseminated primary eczema herpeticum; herpes simplex-associated erythema multiforme; herpes simplex labialis; varicella pneumonia; herpes simplex ocular infections; herpes simplex proctitis; herpes simplex whitlow; herpes zoster encephalitis; infectious mononucleosis.

Administration and Dosage

➤*Approved by the FDA:* March 29, 1982.

➤*Acute treatment of herpes zoster:* 800 mg every 4 hours orally, 5 times daily for 7 to 10 days.

➤*Genital herpes:*

Treatment of initial genital herpes – 200 mg every 4 hours, 5 times daily for 10 days.

Chronic suppressive therapy for recurrent disease: 400 mg 2 times daily for up to 12 months, followed by re-evaluation. Alternative regimens have included doses ranging from 200 mg 3 times daily to 200 mg 5 times daily.

Intermittent therapy: 200 mg every 4 hours, 5 times daily for 5 days. Therapy should be initiated at the earliest sign or symptom (prodrome) of recurrence.

➤*Treatment of chickenpox:*

Children (2 years of age and older) – 20 mg/kg per dose orally 4 times daily (80 mg/kg per day) for 5 days. Children over 40 kg should receive the adult dose for chickenpox.

Adults and children over 40 kg – 800 mg 4 times daily for 5 days.

➤*Renal function impairment:* In patients with renal impairment, the dose of acyclovir capsules, tablets, or suspension should be modified as shown in the table below:

Dosage modification for renal impairment

Normal dosage regimen	Creatinine clearance (mL/min/1.73 m²)	Adjusted dosage regimen	
		Dose (mg)	Dosing interval
200 mg every 4 hours	> 10	200	every 4 hours,k 5 times daily
	0 to 10	200	every 12 hours
400 mg every 12 hours	> 10	400	every 12 hours
	0 to 10	200	every 12 hours
800 mg every 4 hours	> 25	800	every 4 hours, 5 times daily
	10 to 25	800	every 8 hours
	0 to 10	800	every 12 hours

➤*Hemodialysis:* For patients who require hemodialysis, the mean plasma half-life of acyclovir during hemodialysis is approximately 5 hours. This results in a 60% decrease in plasma concentrations following a 6-hour dialysis period. Therefore, the patient's dosing schedule should be adjusted so that an additional dose is administered after each dialysis.

➤*Peritoneal dialysis:* No supplemental dose appears to be necessary after adjustment of the dosing interval.

➤*Bioequivalence of dosage forms:* Acyclovir suspension was shown to be bioequivalent to acyclovir capsules (n = 20) and 1 acyclovir 800 mg tablet was shown to be bioequivalent to 4 acyclovir 200 mg capsules (n = 24).

➤*Storage/Stability:* Store at 15° to 25°C (59° to 77°F) and protect from moisture.

Actions

➤*Pharmacology:* Acyclovir is a synthetic purine nucleoside analogue with in vitro and in vivo inhibitory activity against herpes simplex virus types 1 (HSV-1), 2 (HSV-2), and varicella-zoster virus (VZV). In cell culture, acyclovir's highest antiviral activity is against HSV-1, followed in decreasing order of potency against HSV-2 and VZV.

The inhibitory activity of acyclovir is highly selective due to its affinity for the enzyme thymidine kinase (TK) encoded by HSV and VZV. This viral enzyme converts acyclovir into acyclovir monophosphate, a nucleotide analogue. The monophosphate is further converted into diphosphate by cellular guanylate kinase and into triphosphate by a number of cellular enzymes. In vitro, acyclovir triphosphate stops replication of herpes viral DNA. This is accomplished in three ways: Competitive inhibition of viral DNA polymerase; incorporation into and termination of the growing viral DNA chain; and inactivation of the viral DNA polymerase. The greater antiviral activity of

ACYCLOVIR — ORAL

acyclovir against HSV compared to VZV is due to its more efficient phosphorylation by the viral TK.

➤*Pharmacokinetics:*

Absorption/Distribution – The pharmacokinetics of acyclovir after oral administration have been evaluated in healthy volunteers and in immunocompromised patients with herpes simplex or varicella-zoster virus infection. Acyclovir pharmacokinetic parameters are summarized in the table below.

Acyclovir pharmacokinetic characteristics (range)	
Parameter	Range
Plasma protein binding	9% to 33%
Plasma elimination half-life	2.5 to 3.3 hours
Average oral bioavailability	10% to 20%*

* Bioavailability decreases with increasing dose.

In one multiple-dose, cross-over study in healthy subjects (n = 23), it was shown that increases in plasma acyclovir concentrations were less than dose proportional with increasing dose, as shown in the table below. The decrease in bioavailability is a function of the dose and not the dosage form.

Acyclovir peak and trough concentrations at steady-state			
Parameter	200 mg	400 mg	800 mg
Css_{max}	0.83 mcg/mL	1.21 mcg/mL	1.61 mcg/mL
Css_{trough}	0.46 mcg/mL	0.63 mcg/mL	0.83 mcg/mL

There was no effect of food on the absorption of acyclovir (n = 6); therefore, acyclovir capsules, tablets, and suspension may be administered with or without food.

Metabolism – The only known urinary metabolite is 9-]guanine.

Special populations –

Renal function impairment: The half-life and total body clearance of acyclovir are dependent on renal function. A dosage adjustment is recommended for patients with reduced renal function.

Elderly: Acyclovir plasma concentrations are higher in geriatric patients compared to younger adults, in part due to age-related changes in renal function. Dosage reduction may be required in geriatric patients with underlying renal impairment.

Contraindications

Hypersensitivity to acyclovir or valacyclovir.

Warnings

➤*Oral use:* Acyclovir capsules, tablets, and suspension are intended for oral ingestion only.

➤*Thrombotic thrombocytopenic purpura/hemolytic uremic syndrome (TTP/HUS):* TTP/HUS, which has resulted in death, has occurred in immunocompromised patients receiving acyclovir therapy.

➤*Renal effects:* Renal failure, in some cases resulting in death, has been observed with acyclovir therapy.

➤*Renal function impairment:* Dosage adjustment is recommended when administering acyclovir to patients with renal impairment. Caution should also be exercised when administering acyclovir to patients receiving potentially nephrotoxic agents since this may increase the risk of renal dysfunction and/or the risk of reversible central nervous system symptoms such as those that have been reported in patients treated with intravenous acyclovir.

➤*Carcinogenesis:* The data presented below include references to peak steady-state plasma acyclovir concentrations observed in humans treated with 800 mg given orally 5 times a day (dosing appropriate for treatment of herpes zoster) or 200 mg given orally 5 times a day (dosing appropriate for treatment of genital herpes). Plasma drug concentrations in animal studies are expressed as multiples of human exposure to acyclovir at the higher and lower dosing schedules.

➤*Mutagenesis:* Acyclovir was tested in 16 in vitro and in vivo genetic toxicity assays. Acyclovir was positive in 5 of the assays.

➤*Fertility impairment:* Acyclovir did not impair fertility or reproduction in mice (450 mg/kg/day orally) or in rats (25 mg/kg/day SC). In the mouse study, plasma levels were 9 to 18 times human levels, while in the rat study, they were 8 to 15 times human levels. At higher doses (50 mg/kg/day SC) in rats and rabbits (11 to 22 and 16 to 31 times human levels, respectively) implantation efficacy, but not litter size, was decreased. In a rat peri and postnatal study at 50 mg/kg/day SC, there was a statistically significant decrease in group mean numbers of corpora lutea, total implantation sites, and live fetuses.

No testicular abnormalities were seen in dogs given 50 mg/kg/day IV for 1 month (21 to 41 times human levels) or in dogs given 60 mg/kg/day orally for 1 year (6 to 12 times human levels). Testicular atrophy and aspermatogenesis were observed in rats and dogs at higher dose levels.

➤*Elderly:* Of 376 subjects who received acyclovir in a clinical study of herpes zoster treatment in immunocompetent subjects 50 years of age and older, 244 were 65 years of age and older while 111 were 75 years of age and older. No overall differences in effectiveness for time to cessation of new lesion formation or time to healing were reported between geriatric subjects and younger adult subjects. The duration of pain after healing was longer in patients 65 years of age and older. Nausea, vomiting, and dizziness were reported more frequently in elderly subjects. Elderly patients are more likely to have reduced renal function and require dose reduction. Elderly patients are also more likely to have renal or CNS adverse events. With respect to CNS adverse events observed during clinical practice, somnolence, hallucinations, confusion, and coma were reported more frequently in elderly patients.

➤*Pregnancy: Category B.* There are no adequate and well-controlled studies in pregnant women. A prospective epidemiologic registry of acyclovir use during pregnancy was established in 1984 and completed in April 1999. There were 749 pregnancies followed in women exposed to systemic acyclovir during the first trimester of pregnancy resulting in 756 outcomes. The occurrence rate of birth defects approximates that found in the general population. However, the small size of the registry is insufficient to evaluate the risk for less common defects or to permit reliable or definitive conclusions regarding the safety of acyclovir in pregnant women and their developing fetuses. Acyclovir should be used during pregnancy only if the potential benefit justifies the potential risk to the fetus.

➤*Lactation:* Acyclovir concentrations have been documented in breast milk in 2 women following oral administration of acyclovir and ranged from 0.6 to 4.1 times corresponding plasma levels. These concentrations would potentially expose the nursing infant to a dose of acyclovir as high as 0.3 mg/kg/day. Acyclovir should be administered to a nursing mother with caution and only when indicated.

➤*Children:* Safety and effectiveness in pediatric patients younger than 2 years of age have not been established.

Precautions

➤*Herpes zoster:* There are no data on treatment initiated more than 72 hours after onset of the zoster rash. Patients should be advised to initiate treatment as soon as possible after a diagnosis of herpes zoster.

➤*Genital herpes infections:* Patients should be informed that acyclovir is not a cure for genital herpes. There are no data evaluating whether acyclovir will prevent transmission of infection to others. Because genital herpes is a sexually transmitted disease, patients should avoid contact with lesions or intercourse when lesions and/or symptoms are present to avoid infecting partners. Genital herpes can also be transmitted in the absence of symptoms through asymptomatic viral shedding. If medical management of a genital herpes recurrence is indicated, patients should be advised to initiate therapy at the first sign or symptom of an episode.

➤*Chickenpox:* Chickenpox in otherwise healthy children is usually a self-limited disease of mild to moderate severity. Adolescents and adults tend to have more severe disease. Treatment was initiated within 24 hours of the typical chickenpox rash in the controlled studies, and there is no information regarding the effects of treatment begun later in the disease course.

Drug Interactions

Acyclovir Drug Interactions			
Precipitant drug	Object drug*		Description
Probenecid	Acyclovir	↑	Acyclovir bioavailability and terminal plasma half-life may be increased, and renal clearance may be decreased.
Acyclovir	Theophyllines	↑	Coadministration may result in increased theophylline plasma concentrations; monitor plasma levels and side effects. Adjust theophylline dose as necessary.
Acyclovir	Hydantoins Valproic acid	↓	Plasma levels of hydantoins and valproic acid may be decreased with coadministration of acyclovir.

* ↑ = Object drug increased. ↓ = Object drug decreased.

Adverse Reactions

Herpes simplex –

Short-term administration: The most frequent adverse events reported during clinical trials of treatment of genital herpes with acyclovir 200 mg administered orally 5 times daily every 4 hours for 10 days were nausea or vomiting in 8 of 298 patient treatments (2.7%). Nausea or vomiting occurred in 2 of 287 (0.7%) patients who received placebo.

Long-term administration: The most frequent adverse events reported in a clinical trial for the prevention of recurrences with continuous administration of 400 mg (two 200 mg capsules) 2 times daily for 1 year in 586 patients treated with acyclovir were nausea (4.8%) and diarrhea (2.4%).

The 589 control patients receiving intermittent treatment of recurrences with acyclovir for 1 year reported diarrhea (2.7%), nausea (2.4%), and headache (2.2%).

Herpes zoster – The most frequent adverse event reported during 3 clinical trials of treatment of herpes zoster (shingles) with 800 mg of oral acyclovir 5 times daily for 7 to 10 days in 323 patients was malaise (11.5%). The 323 placebo recipients reported malaise (11.1%).

Chickenpox – The most frequent adverse event reported during 3 clinical trials of treatment of chickenpox with oral acyclovir at doses of 10 to 20 mg/kg 4 times daily for 5 to 7 days or 800 mg 4 times daily for 5 days in 495 patients was diarrhea (3.2%). The 498 patients receiving placebo reported diarrhea (2.2%).

➤*Postmarketing:* In addition to adverse events reported from clinical trials, the following events have been identified during postapproval use of

ACYCLOVIR — ORAL

acyclovir. Because they are reported voluntarily from a population of unknown size, estimates of frequency cannot be made. These events have been chosen for inclusion due to a combination of their seriousness, frequency of reporting, or potential causal connection to acyclovir, or a combination of these factors.

CNS – Aggressive behavior, agitation, ataxia, coma, confusion, decreased consciousness, delirium, dizziness, dysarthria, encephalopathy, hallucinations, paresthesia, psychosis, seizure, somnolence, tremors. These symptoms may be marked, particularly in older adults or in patients with renal impairment.

Dermatologic – Alopecia, erythema multiforme, photosensitive rash, pruritus, rash, Stevens-Johnson syndrome, toxic epidermal necrolysis, urticaria.

GI – Diarrhea; gastrointestinal distress; nausea.

GU – Renal failure, elevated blood urea nitrogen, elevated creatinine, hematuria.

Hematologic/Lymphatic – Anemia, leukocytoclastic vasculitis, leukopenia, lymphadenopathy, thrombocytopenia.

Hepatic – Elevated liver function tests, hepatitis, hyperbilirubinemia, jaundice.

Musculoskeletal – Myalgia.

Special senses – Visual abnormalities.

Miscellaneous – Anaphylaxis, fever, angioedema, headache, pain, peripheral edema.

Overdosage

➤*Symptoms:* Overdoses involving ingestion of up to 100 capsules (20 g) have been reported. Adverse events that have been reported in association with overdosage include agitation, coma, seizures, and lethargy. Precipitation of acyclovir in renal tubules may occur when the solubility (2.5 mg/mL) is exceeded in the intratubular fluid. Overdosage has been reported following bolus injections or inappropriately high doses and in patients whose fluid and electrolyte balance were not properly monitored. This has resulted in elevated BUN and serum creatinine and subsequent renal failure.

➤*Treatment:* In the event of acute renal failure and anuria, the patient may benefit from hemodialysis until renal function is restored.

Patient Information

Patients are instructed to consult with their physicians if they experience severe or troublesome adverse reactions, they become pregnant or intend to become pregnant, they intend to breastfeed while taking orally administered acyclovir, or they have any other questions.

There are no data on treatment initiated more than 72 hours after onset of the zoster rash. Patients should be advised to initiate treatment as soon as possible after a diagnosis of herpes zoster.

Patients should be informed that acyclovir is not a cure for genital herpes. There are no data evaluating whether acyclovir will prevent transmission of infection to others. Because genital herpes is a sexually transmitted disease, patients should avoid contact with lesions or intercourse when lesions and/or symptoms are present to avoid infecting partners. Genital herpes can also be transmitted in the absence of symptoms through asymptomatic viral shedding. If medical management of a genital herpes recurrence is indicated, patients should be advised to initiate therapy at the first sign or symptom of an episode.

Chickenpox in otherwise healthy children is usually a self-limited disease of mild to moderate severity. Adolescents and adults tend to have more severe disease. Treatment was initiated within 24 hours of the typical chickenpox rash in the controlled studies, and there is no information regarding the effects of treatment begun later in the disease course.

ACYCLOVIR — INJECTION

Indications

➤*Herpes simplex infections in immunocompromised patients:* Acyclovir for injection is indicated for the treatment of initial and recurrent mucosal and cutaneous herpes simplex (HSV-1 and HSV-2) in immunocompromised patients.

➤*Initial episodes of herpes genitalis:* Treatment of severe initial clinical episodes of herpes genitalis in immunocompetent patients.

➤*Herpes simplex encephalitis:* Treatment of herpes simplex encephalitis.

➤*Neonatal herpes simplex virus infection:* Treatment of neonatal herpes infections.

➤*Varicella-zoster infections in immunocompromised patients:* Treatment of varicella-zoster (shingles) infections in immunocompromised patients.

➤*Unlabeled uses:* Prophylaxis of mucocutaneous HSV infection in immunosuppressed HSV-seropositive patients (oral and IV); high-dose IV acyclovir may reduce the risk of CMV infection in CMV-seropositive patients undergoing bone-marrow transplantation.

Administration and Dosage

➤*Approved by the FDA:* October 22, 1982.

Initiate therapy as early as possible following onset of signs and symptoms of herpes infections.

Do not exceed a maximum dose equivalent to 20 mg/kg every 8 hours for any patient.

➤*Caution:* Rapid or bolus intravenous (IV) injection must be avoided.

Intramuscular (IM) or subcutaneous injection must be avoided.

➤*Dosage:*

Herpes simplex infections –

Mucosal and cutaneous herpes simplex (HSV-1 and HSV-2) infections in immunocompromised patients:

• *Adults and adolescents (12 years of age and older)* – 5 mg/kg infused at a constant rate over 1 hour, every 8 hours for 7 days.

• *Pediatrics (younger than 12 years of age)* – 10 mg/kg infused at a constant rate over 1 hour, every 8 hours for 7 days.

Severe initial clinical episodes of herpes genitalis:

• *Adults and adolescents (12 years of age and older)* – 5 mg/kg infused at a constant rate over 1 hour, every 8 hours for 5 days.

Herpes simplex encephalitis:

• *Adults and adolescents (12 years of age and older)* – 10 mg/kg infused at a constant rate over 1 hour, every 8 hours for 10 days.

• *Pediatrics (3 months to 12 years of age)* – 20 mg/kg infused at a constant rate over 1 hour, every 8 hours for 10 days.

Neonatal herpes simplex virus infections (birth to 3 months of age): 10 mg/kg infused at a constant rate over 1 hour, every 8 hours for 10 days. In neonatal herpes simplex infections, doses of 15 mg/kg or 20 mg/kg (infused at a constant rate over 1 hour every 8 hours) have been used; the safety and efficacy of these doses are not known.

Varicella zoster infections –

Zoster in immunocompromised patients:

• *Adults and adolescents (12 years of age and older)* – 10 mg/kg infused at a constant rate over 1 hour, every 8 hours for 7 days.

• *Pediatrics (younger than 12 years of age)* – 20 mg/kg infused at a constant rate over 1 hour, every 8 hours for 7 days.

• *Obese patients* – Administer the recommended adult dose using ideal body weight.

Renal function impairment – See the preceding recommended doses, and adjust the dosing interval as indicated in the following table.

Dosage Adjustments for Patients with Renal Impairment		
Creatinine clearance (mL/min per 1.73 m^2)	Percent of recommended dose	Dosing interval (hours)
> 50	100%	8
25 to 50	100%	12
10 to 25	100%	24
0 to 10	50%	24

Hemodialysis – For patients who require dialysis, the mean plasma half-life of acyclovir during hemodialysis is approximately 5 hours. This results in a 60% decrease in plasma concentrations following a 6-hour dialysis period. Therefore, adjust the patient's dosing schedule so that an additional dose is administered after each dialysis.

➤*Method of preparation:* Each 10 mL vial contains acyclovir sodium equivalent to 500 mg of acyclovir. Each 20 mL vial contains acyclovir sodium equivalent to 1,000 mg of acyclovir. The contents of the vial should be dissolved in sterile water for injection as follows:

Contents of Vial	Amount of Diluent
500 mg	10 mL
1,000 mg	20 mL

The resulting solution in each case contains acyclovir 50 mg/mL (pH approximately 11). Shake the vial well to ensure complete dissolution before measuring and transferring each individual dose.

Do not use bacteriostatic water for injection containing benzyl alcohol or parabens.

➤*Administration:* Remove and add the calculated dose to any appropriate IV solution at a volume selected for administration during each 1-hour infusion. Infusion concentrations of approximately 7 mg/mL or lower are recommended. In clinical studies, the average 70 kg adult received between 60 and 150 mL of fluid per dose. Higher concentrations (eg, 10 mg/mL) may produce phlebitis or inflammation at the injection site upon inadvertent extravasation. Standard, commercially available electrolyte and glucose solutions are suitable for IV administration; biologic or colloidal fluids (eg, blood products, protein solutions) are not recommended.

Once diluted for administration, use each dose within 24 hours.

➤*Storage/Stability:* Store at 15° to 25°C (59° to 77°F).

The reconstituted solution should be used within 12 hours. Refrigeration of reconstituted solution may result in the formation of a precipitate that will redissolve at room temperature.

Actions

➤*Pharmacology:* Acyclovir is a synthetic purine nucleoside analogue with in vitro and in vivo inhibitory activity against HSV-1, HSV-2, and varicella-zoster virus (VZV). In cell culture, acyclovir's highest antiviral activity is against HSV-1, followed in decreasing order of potency against HSV-2 and VZV.

The inhibitory activity of acyclovir is highly selective due to its affinity for the enzyme thymidine kinase (TK) encoded by HSV and VZV. This viral

ACYCLOVIR — INJECTION

enzyme converts acyclovir into acyclovir monophosphate, a nucleoside analogue. The monophosphate is further converted into diphosphate by cellular guanylate kinase and into triphosphate by a number of cellular enzymes. In vitro, acyclovir triphosphate stops replication of herpes viral DNA. This is accomplished in three ways: Competitive inhibition of viral DNA polymerase, incorporation into and termination of the growing viral DNA chain, and inactivation of the viral DNA polymerase. The greater antiviral activity of acyclovir against HSV compared with VZV is due to its more efficient phosphorylation by the viral TK.

➤*Pharmacokinetics:*

Absorption/Distribution – The pharmacokinetics of acyclovir after IV administration have been evaluated in adult patients with normal renal function during Phase 1 and 2 studies after single doses ranging from 0.5 to 15 mg/kg and after multiple doses ranging from 2.5 to 15 mg/kg every 8 hours. Proportionality between dose and plasma levels is seen after single doses or at steady-state after multiple dosing.

Average steady-state peak and trough concentrations from 1-hour infusions administered every 8 hours are given in the following table.

Acyclovir Peak and Trough Concentrations at Steady-State		
Dosage regimen	Css_{max}	Css_{trough}
5 mg/kg every 8 hours (n = 8)	9.8 mcg/mL	0.7 mcg/mL
	range: 5.5 to 13.8	range: 0.2 to 1
10 mg/kg every 8 hours (n = 7)	22.9 mcg/mL	1.9 mcg/mL
	range: 14.1 to 44.1	range: 0.5 to 2.9

Concentrations achieved in the cerebrospinal fluid are approximately 50% of plasma values. Plasma protein binding is relatively low (9% to 33%) and drug interactions involving binding site displacement are not anticipated.

Metabolism/Excretion – Renal excretion of unchanged drug is the major route of acyclovir elimination accounting for 62% to 91% of the dose. The only major urinary metabolite detected is 9-carboxymethoxymethylguanine, accounting for up to 14.1% of the dose in patients with healthy renal function.

The half-life and total body clearance of acyclovir are dependent on renal function as shown in the following table.

Acyclovir Half-Life and Total Body Clearance			
Creatinine clearance (mL/min per 1.73 m^2)	Half-life (h)	Total body clearance (mL/min per 1.73 m^2)	Total body clearance (mL/min/kg)
> 80	2.5	327	5.1
50 to 80	3	248	3.9
15 to 50	3.5	190	3.4
0 (anuric)	19.5	29	0.5

Special populations –
Renal function impairment: Acyclovir was administered at a dose of 2.5 mg/kg to 6 adult patients with severe renal failure. The peak and trough plasma levels during the 47 hours preceding hemodialysis were 8.5 mcg/mL and 0.7 mcg/mL, respectively.
Elderly: Acyclovir plasma concentrations are higher in geriatric patients compared with younger adults, in part due to age-related changes in renal function. Dosage reduction may be required in geriatric patients with underlying renal impairment.

Contraindications

Hypersensitivity to acyclovir or valacyclovir.

Warnings

➤*Administration:* Reconstituted acyclovir IV has a pH of approximately 11 and should not be administered by mouth.

Acyclovir for injection is intended for IV infusion only; do not administer topically, IM, orally, subcutaneously, or in the eye. IV infusions must be given over a period of at least 1 hour to reduce the risk of renal tubular damage.

➤*Thrombotic thrombocytopenic purpura/hemolytic uremic syndrome (TTP/HUS):* TTP/HUS, which has resulted in death, has occurred in immunocompromised patients receiving acyclovir therapy.

➤*Renal function impairment:* The dose of acyclovir must be adjusted in patients with impaired renal function in order to avoid accumulation of acyclovir in the body.

In patients receiving acyclovir at higher doses, (eg, for herpes encephalitis), take specific care regarding renal function, particularly when patients are dehydrated or have any renal impairment.

Renal failure, in some cases resulting in death, has been observed with acyclovir therapy.

➤*Mutagenesis:* Acyclovir was tested in 16 in vitro and in vivo genetic toxicity assays. Acyclovir was positive in 5 of the assays.

➤*Fertility impairment:* Acyclovir did not impair fertility or reproduction in mice (450 mg/kg/day, administered orally) or in rats (25 mg/kg/day, subcutaneously). In the mouse study, plasma levels were the same as human levels, while in the rat study, they were 1 to 2 times human levels. At higher doses (50 mg/kg/day, subcutaneously) in rats and rabbits (1 to 2 and 1 to 3 times human levels, respectively) implantation efficacy, but not litter size, was decreased. In a rat peri- and postnatal study at 50 mg/kg/day, subcutaneously, there was a statistically significant decrease in group mean numbers of corpora lutea, total implantation sites, and live fetuses.

No testicular abnormalities were seen in dogs given 50 mg/kg/day IV for 1 month (1 to 3 times human levels) or in dogs given 60 mg/kg/day orally for 1 year (the same as human levels). Testicular atrophy and aspermatogenesis were observed in rats and dogs at higher dose levels.

➤*Elderly:* Clinical studies of acyclovir for injection did not include sufficient numbers of patients 65 years of age and older to determine whether they respond differently from younger patients. Other reported clinical experience has identified differences in the severity of CNS adverse reactions between elderly and younger patients. In general, dose selection for an elderly patient should be cautious, reflecting the greater frequency of decreased renal function, and of concomitant disease or other drug therapy. This drug is known to be substantially excreted by the kidney, and the risk of toxic reactions to this drug may be greater in patients with impaired renal function. Because elderly patients are more likely to have decreased renal function, take care in dose selection, and it may be useful to monitor renal function.

➤*Pregnancy: Category B.* There are no adequate and well-controlled studies in pregnant women. A prospective epidemiologic registry of acyclovir use during pregnancy was established in 1984 and completed in April 1999. There were 749 pregnancies followed in women exposed to systemic acyclovir during the first trimester of pregnancy resulting in 756 outcomes. The occurrence rate of birth defects approximates that found in the general population. However, the small size of the registry is insufficient to evaluate the risk for less common defects or to permit reliable or definitive conclusions regarding the safety of acyclovir in pregnant women and their developing fetuses. Use acyclovir during pregnancy only if the potential benefit justifies the potential risk to the fetus.

➤*Lactation:* Acyclovir concentrations have been documented in breast milk in 2 women following oral administration of acyclovir and ranged from 0.6 to 4.1 times corresponding plasma levels. These concentrations would potentially expose the nursing infant to a dose of acyclovir up to 0.3 mg/kg/day. Administer acyclovir to a breast-feeding mother with caution and only when indicated.

➤*Children:* See Administration and Dosage for more information.

Precautions

➤*Aseptic conditions:* Acyclovir IV contains no antimicrobial preservative. Reconstitution and dilution should be carried out under full aseptic conditions immediately before use and any unused solution discarded. Do not refrigerate the reconstituted or diluted solutions.

➤*Renal effects:* Precipitation of acyclovir crystals in renal tubules can occur if the maximum solubility of free acyclovir (2.5 mg/mL at 37°C [98.6°F] in water) is exceeded or if the drug is administered by bolus injection. Ensuing renal tubular damage can produce acute renal failure.

Abnormal renal function (decreased creatinine clearance) can occur as a result of acyclovir administration and depends on the state of the patient's hydration, other treatments, and the rate of drug administration. Concomitant use of other nephrotoxic drugs, preexisting renal disease, and dehydration make further renal impairment with acyclovir more likely.

When dosage adjustments are required, they should be based on estimated creatinine clearance.

➤*Hydration:* Administration of acyclovir by IV infusion must be accompanied by adequate hydration.

➤*Encephalopathic changes:* Approximately 1% of patients receiving IV acyclovir have manifested encephalopathic changes characterized by either lethargy, obtundation, tremors, confusion, hallucinations, agitation, seizures, or coma. Use acyclovir with caution in those patients who have underlying neurologic abnormalities and those with serious renal, hepatic, or electrolyte abnormalities, or significant hypoxia.

Drug Interactions

Acyclovir Drug Interactions			
Precipitant drug	Object drug*		Description
Probenecid	Acyclovir	↑	Acyclovir bioavailability and terminal plasma half-life may be increased, and renal clearance may be decreased.
Acyclovir	Theophyllines	↑	Coadministration may result in increased theophylline plasma concentrations; monitor plasma levels and side effects. Adjust theophylline dose as necessary.
Acyclovir	Hydantoins Valproic acid	↓	Plasma levels of hydantoins and valproic acid may be decreased with coadministration of acyclovir.

* ↑ = Object drug increased. ↓ = Object drug decreased.

Adverse Reactions

The most frequent adverse reactions reported during administration of acyclovir were inflammation or phlebitis at the injection site in approximately 9% of the patients, and transient elevations of serum creatinine or blood urea nitrogen in 5% to 10% (the higher incidence occurred usually following rapid [less than 10 minutes] IV infusion). Nausea or vomiting occurred in approximately 7% of the patients (the majority occurring in non-

ACYCLOVIR — INJECTION

hospitalized patients who received 10 mg/kg). Itching, rash, or hives occurred in approximately 2% of patients. Elevation of transaminases occurred in 1% to 2% of patients.

The following hematologic abnormalities occurred at a frequency of less than 1%: Anemia, neutropenia, thrombocytopenia, thrombocytosis, leukocytosis, and neutrophilia. In addition, anorexia and hematuria were observed.

➤*Postmarketing:* In addition to adverse reactions reported from clinical trials, the following reactions have been identified during post-approval use of acyclovir for injection in clinical practice. Because they are reported voluntarily from a population of unknown size, estimates of frequency cannot be made. These reactions have been chosen for inclusion due to either their seriousness, frequency of reporting, potential causal connection to acyclovir, or a combination of these factors.

Cardiovascular – Hypotension.

CNS – Aggressive behavior, agitation, ataxia, coma, confusion, delirium, dizziness, dysarthria, encephalopathy, hallucinations, obtundation, paresthesia, psychosis, seizure, somnolence, tremor. These symptoms may be marked, particularly in older adults.

Dermatologic – Alopecia, erythema multiforme, photosensitive rash, pruritus, rash, Stevens-Johnson syndrome, toxic epidermal necrolysis, urticaria. Severe local inflammatory reactions, including tissue necrosis, have occurred following infusion of acyclovir into extravascular tissues.

GI – Abdominal pain, diarrhea, GI distress, nausea.

GU – Renal failure, elevated blood urea nitrogen, elevated creatinine.

Hematologic/Lymphatic – Disseminated intravascular coagulation, hemolysis, leukocytoclastic vasculitis, leukopenia, lymphadenopathy.

Hepatic – Elevated liver function tests, hepatitis, hyperbilirubinemia, jaundice.

Musculoskeletal – Myalgia.

Special senses – Visual abnormalities.

Miscellaneous – Anaphylaxis, angioedema, fatigue, fever, headache, pain, peripheral edema.

Overdosage

➤*Symptoms:* Overdoses involving ingestions of up to 20 g have been reported. Adverse reactions that have been reported in association with overdosage include agitation, coma, seizures, and lethargy. Precipitation of acyclovir in renal tubules may occur when the solubility (2.5 mg/mL) is exceeded in the intratubular fluid. Overdosage has been reported following bolus injections or inappropriately high doses, and in patients whose fluid and electrolyte balance were not properly monitored. This has resulted in elevated blood urea nitrogen and serum creatinine, and subsequent renal failure.

➤*Treatment:* In the event of acute renal failure and anuria, the patient may benefit from hemodialysis until renal function is restored.

FAMCICLOVIR

Rx	**Famvir** (Novartis)	**Tablets:** 125 mg	Lactose. (Famvir 125). White. Film coated. In 30s.
		250 mg	Lactose. (Famvir 250). White. Film coated. In 30s.
		500 mg	Lactose. (Famvir 500). White, oval. Film coated. In 30s and UD 50s.

FAMCICLOVIR — ORAL

Indications

➤*Herpes zoster:* Treatment of acute herpes zoster (shingles).

➤*Genital herpes:* Treatment or suppression of recurrent genital herpes in immunocompetent patients.

➤*Herpes simplex:* Treatment of recurrent mucocutaneous herpes simplex infections in HIV-infected patients.

➤*Unlabeled uses:* Management of initial episodes of herpes genitalis (250 mg 3 times/day for 7 to 10 days).

Administration and Dosage

➤*Approved by the FDA:* June 29, 1994 (1S Classification)

➤*Herpes zoster:* The recommended dosage is 500 mg every 8 hours for 7 days. Therapy should be initiated promptly as soon as herpes zoster is diagnosed. No data are available on efficacy of treatment started greater than 72 hours after rash onset.

➤*Herpes simplex infections:*

Recurrent genital herpes – The recommended dosage is 125 mg twice daily for 5 days. Initiate therapy at the first sign or symptom if medical management of a genital herpes recurrence is indicated. The efficacy of famciclovir has not been established when treatment is initiated more than 6 hours after onset of symptoms or lesions.

Suppression of recurrent genital herpes – The recommended dosage is 250 mg twice daily for up to 1 year. The safety and efficacy of famciclovir therapy beyond 1 year of treatment have not been established.

➤*HIV-infected patients:* For recurrent orolabial or genital herpes simplex infection, the recommended dosage is 500 mg twice daily for 7 days.

➤*Renal function impairment:* In patients with reduced renal function, dosage reduction is recommended (see Precautions).

Indication and normal dosage regimen	Creatinine clearance (mL/min)	Adjusted dosage regimen dose (mg)	Dosing interval
Herpes zoster 500 mg every 8 hours	> 60	500	every 8 hours
	40 to 59	500	every 12 hours
	20 to 39	500	every 24 hours
	< 20	250	every 24 hours
	HD*	250	following each dialysis
Recurrent genital herpes 125 mg every 12 hours	≥ 40	125	every 12 hours
	20 to 39	125	every 24 hours
	< 20	125	every 24 hours
	HD*	125	following each dialysis

Indication and normal dosage regimen	Creatinine clearance (mL/min)	Adjusted dosage regimen dose (mg)	Dosing interval
Suppression of recurrent genital herpes 250 mg every 12 hours	≥ 40	250	every 12 hours
	20 to 39	125	every 12 hours
	< 20	125	every 24 hours
	HD*	125	following each dialysis
Recurrent orolabial and genital herpes simplex infection in HIV-infected patients 500 mg every 12 hours	≥ 40	500	every 12 hours
	20 to 39	500	every 24 hours
	< 20	250	every 24 hours
	HD*	250	following each dialysis

* Hemodialysis.

➤*Storage/Stability:* Store between 15° and 30°C (59° and 86°F).

Actions

➤*Pharmacokinetics:*

Absorption – Famciclovir is the diacetyl 6-deoxy analog of the active antiviral compound penciclovir. Following oral administration, little or no famciclovir is detected in plasma or urine.

The absolute bioavailability of famciclovir is 77% ± 8% as determined following the administration of a 500 mg famciclovir oral dose and a 400 mg penciclovir intravenous dose to 12 healthy male subjects.

Penciclovir concentrations increased in proportion to dose over a famciclovir dose range of 125 mg to 750 mg administered as a single dose. Single oral dose administration of 125 mg, 250 mg or 500 mg famciclovir to healthy male volunteers across 17 studies gave the following pharmacokinetic parameters:

Dose	AUC (0-inf)[1] (mcg•hr/mL)	C_{max}[2] (mcg/mL)	t_{max}[3] (hours)
125 mg	2.24	0.8	0.9
250 mg	4.48	1.6	0.9
500 mg	8.95	3.3	0.9

[1] AUC (0-inf) (mcg•hr/mL) = area under the plasma concentration-time profile extrapolated to infinity.
[2] C_{max} (mcg/mL) = maximum observed plasma concentration.
[3] t_{max} (hours) = time to C_{max}.

Following single oral-dose administration of 500 mg famciclovir to 7 patients with herpes zoster, the mean ± SD AUC, C_{max}, and T_{max} were 12.1 ± 1.7 mcg•hr/mL, 4 ± 0.7 mcg/mL, and 0.7 ± 0.2 hours, respectively. The AUC of penciclovir was approximately 35% greater in patients with herpes zoster

FAMCICLOVIR — ORAL

as compared to healthy volunteers. Some of this difference may be due to differences in renal function between the 2 groups.

There is no accumulation of penciclovir after the administration of 500 mg famciclovir 3 times a day for 7 days.

Penciclovir C_{max} decreased approximately 50% and T_{max} was delayed by 1.5 hours when a capsule formulation of famciclovir was administered with food (nutritional content was ≈ 910 Kcal and 26% fat). There was no effect on the extent of availability (AUC) of penciclovir. There was an 18% decrease in C_{max} and a delay in t_{max} of about 1 hour when famciclovir was given 2 hours after a meal as compared to its administration 2 hours before a meal. Because there was no effect on the extent of systemic availability of penciclovir, it appears that famciclovir can be taken without regard to meals.

Distribution – The volume of distribution ($Vd_β$) was 1.08 ± 0.17 L/kg in 12 healthy male subjects following a single intravenous dose of penciclovir at 400 mg administered as a 1-hour intravenous infusion.

Penciclovir is < 20% bound to plasma proteins over the concentration range of 0.1 to 20 mcg/mL. The blood/plasma ratio of penciclovir is ≈ 1.

Metabolism – Following oral administration, famciclovir is deacetylated and oxidized to form penciclovir. Metabolites that are inactive include 6-deoxy penciclovir, monoacetylated penciclovir, and 6-deoxy monoacetylated penciclovir (5%, < 0.5% and < 0.5% of the dose in the urine, respectively). Little or no famciclovir is detected in plasma or urine.

An in vitro study using human liver microsomes demonstrated that cytochrome P450 does not play an important role in famciclovir metabolism. The conversion of 6-deoxy penciclovir to penciclovir is catalyzed by aldehyde oxidase.

Excretion – Approximately 94% of administered radioactivity was recovered in urine over 24 hours (83% of the dose was excreted in the first 6 hours) after the administration of 5 mg/kg radiolabeled penciclovir as a 1-hour infusion to 3 healthy male volunteers. Penciclovir accounted for 91% of the radioactivity excreted in the urine.

Following the oral administration of a single 500 mg dose of radiolabeled famciclovir to 3 healthy male volunteers, 73% and 27% of administered radioactivity were recovered in urine and feces over 72 hours, respectively. Penciclovir accounted for 82% and 6-deoxy penciclovir accounted for 7% of the radioactivity excreted in the urine. Approximately 60% of the administered radiolabeled dose was collected in urine in the first 6 hours.

After intravenous administration of penciclovir in 48 healthy male volunteers, mean ± SD total plasma clearance of penciclovir was 36.6 ± 6.3 L/hr (0.48 ± 0.09 L/hr/kg). Penciclovir renal clearance accounted for 74.5 ± 8.8% of total plasma clearance.

Renal clearance of penciclovir following the oral administration of a single 500 mg dose of famciclovir to 109 healthy male volunteers was 27.7 ± 7.6 L/hr.

The plasma elimination half-life of penciclovir was 2 ± 0.3 hours after intravenous administration of penciclovir to 48 healthy male volunteers and 2.3 ± 0.4 hours after oral administration of 500 mg famciclovir to 124 healthy male volunteers. The half-life in 7 patients with herpes zoster was 3 ± 1.1 hours.

Special populations –

Renal function impairment: Apparent plasma clearance, renal clearance, and the plasma-elimination rate constant of penciclovir decreased linearly with reductions in renal function. After the administration of a single 500 mg famciclovir oral dose (n = 27) to healthy volunteers and to volunteers with varying degrees of renal insufficiency (C_{cr} ranged from 6.4 to 138.8 mL/min), the following results were obtained.

Parameter (mean ± SD)	C_{cr}[1] ≥ 60 (mL/m in)	C_{cr} 40 to 59 (mL/min)	C_{cr} 20 to 39 (mL/min)	C_{cr} < 20 (mL/min)
C_{cr} (mL/min)	88.1 ± 20.6	49.3 ± 5.9	26.5 ± 5.3	12.7 ± 5.9
CL_R (L/hr)	30.1 ± 10.6	13 ± 1.3[2]	4.2 ± 0.9	1.6 ± 1
CL/F[3] (L/hr)	66.9 ± 27.5	27.3 ± 2.8	12.8 ± 1.3	5.8 ± 2.8
Half-life (hours)	2.3 ± 0.5	3.4 ± 0.7	6.2 ± 1.6	13.4 ± 10.2
n	15	5	4	3

[1] C_{cr} is measured creatinine clearance.
[2] n = 4.
[3] CL/F consists of bioavailability factor and famciclovir to penciclovir conversion factor.

A dosage adjustment is recommended for patients with renal insufficiency (see Administration and Dosage).

Hepatic function impairment: Well-compensated chronic liver disease (chronic hepatitis [n = 6], chronic ethanol abuse [n = 8], or primary biliary cirrhosis [n = 1]) had no effect on the extent of availability (AUC) of penciclovir following a single dose of 500 mg famciclovir. However, there was a 44% decrease in penciclovir mean maximum plasma concentration and the time to maximum plasma concentration was increased by 0.75 hours in patients with hepatic insufficiency compared to healthy volunteers. No dosage adjustment is recommended for patients with well-compensated hepatic impairment. The pharmacokinetics of penciclovir have not been evaluated in patients with severe uncompensated hepatic impairment.

Elderly: Based on cross-study comparisons, mean penciclovir AUC was 40% larger and penciclovir renal clearance was 22% lower after the oral administration of famciclovir in elderly volunteers (n = 18, age 65 to 79 years) compared to younger volunteers. Some of this difference may be due to differences in renal function between the 2 groups.

➤*Microbiology:* Famciclovir undergoes rapid biotransformation to the active antiviral compound penciclovir, which has inhibitory activity against herpes simplex virus types 1 (HSV-1) and 2 (HSV-2) and varicella zoster virus (VZV). In cells infected with HSV-1, HSV-2 or VZV, viral thymidine kinase phosphorylates penciclovir to a monophosphate form that, in turn, is converted to penciclovir triphosphate by cellular kinases. In vitro studies demonstrate that penciclovir triphosphate inhibits HSV-2 DNA polymerase competitively with deoxyguanosine triphosphate. Consequently, herpes viral DNA synthesis and, therefore, replication are selectively inhibited.

Contraindications

Hypersensitivity to the product, its components, and penciclovir cream.

Warnings

➤*Renal function impairment:* Dosage adjustment is recommended when administering famciclovir to patients with creatinine clearance values < 60 mL/min (see Administration and Dosage). In patients with underlying renal disease who have received inappropriately high doses of famciclovir for their level of renal function, acute renal failure has been reported.

➤*Carcinogenesis:* Two-year dietary carcinogenicity studies with famciclovir were conducted in rats and mice. Famciclovir was administered orally unless otherwise stated. An increase in the incidence of mammary adenocarcinoma (a common tumor in animals of this strain) was seen in female rats receiving the high dose of 600 mg/kg/day (1.5 to 9 times the human systemic exposure at the recommended daily oral doses of 500 mg 3 times a day, 250 mg 2 times a day, or 125 mg 2 times a day, based on area under the plasma concentration curve comparisons [24 hour AUC] for penciclovir). No increases in tumor incidence were reported in male rats treated at doses up to 240 mg/kg/day (0.9 to 5.4 times the human AUC), or in male and female mice at doses up to 600 mg/kg/day (0.4 to 2.4 times the human AUC).

➤*Mutagenesis:* Famciclovir and penciclovir (the active metabolite of famciclovir) were tested for genotoxic potential in a battery of in vitro and in vivo assays. Famciclovir and penciclovir were negative in in vitro tests for gene mutations in bacteria (*Salmonella typhimurium* and *Escherichia coli*) and unscheduled DNA synthesis in mammalian HeLa 83 cells (at doses up to 10,000 and 5000 mcg/plate, respectively). Famciclovir was also negative in the L5178Y mouse lymphoma assay (5000 mcg/mL), the in vivo mouse micronucleus test (4800 mg/kg), and rat dominant lethal study (5000 mg/kg). Famciclovir induced increases in polyploidy in human lymphocytes in vitro in the absence of chromosomal damage (1200 mcg/mL). Penciclovir was positive in the L5178Y mouse lymphoma assay for gene mutation/chromosomal aberrations, with and without metabolic activation (1000 mcg/mL). In human lymphocytes, penciclovir caused chromosomal aberrations in the absence of metabolic activation (250 mcg/mL). Penciclovir caused an increased incidence of micronuclei in mouse bone marrow in vivo when administered intravenously at doses highly toxic to bone marrow (500 mg/kg), but not when administered orally.

➤*Fertility impairment:* Testicular toxicity was observed in rats, mice, and dogs following repeated administration of famciclovir or penciclovir. Famciclovir was administered orally unless otherwise stated. Testicular changes included atrophy of the seminiferous tubules, reduction in sperm count, or increased incidence of sperm with abnormal morphology or reduced motility. The degree of toxicity to male reproduction was related to dose and duration of exposure. In male rats, decreased fertility was observed after 10 weeks of dosing at 500 mg/kg/day (1.9 to 11.4 times the human AUC). The no observable effect level for sperm and testicular toxicity in rats following chronic administration (26 weeks) was 50 mg/kg/day (0.2 to 1.2 times the human systemic exposure based on AUC comparisons). Testicular toxicity was observed following chronic administration to mice (104 weeks) and dogs (26 weeks) at doses of 600 mg/kg/day (0.4 to 2.4 times the human AUC) and 150 mg/kg/day (1.7 to 10.2 times the human AUC), respectively. Famciclovir had no effect on general reproductive performance or fertility in female rats at doses up to 1000 mg/kg/day (3.6 to 21.6 times the human AUC). Two placebo-controlled studies in a total of 130 otherwise healthy men with a normal sperm profile over an 8-week baseline period and recurrent genital herpes receiving oral famciclovir (250 mg 2 times a day) (n = 66) or placebo (n = 64) therapy for 18 weeks showed no evidence of significant effects on sperm count, motility or morphology during treatment or during an 8-week follow-up.

➤*Pregnancy: Category B.* There are no adequate and well-controlled studies in pregnant women. Because animal reproduction studies are not always predictive of human response, famciclovir should be used during pregnancy only if the benefit to the patient clearly exceeds the potential risk to the fetus.

➤*Lactation:* Following oral administration of famciclovir to lactating rats, penciclovir was excreted in breast milk at concentrations higher than those seen in the plasma. It is not known whether it is excreted in human milk. There are no data on the safety of famciclovir in infants.

➤*Children:* Safety and efficacy in children under the age of 18 years have not been established.

Precautions

➤*Initial episodes:* The efficacy of famciclovir has not been established for initial episode genital herpes infection, ophthalmic zoster, disseminated zoster or in immunocompromised patients with herpes zoster.

➤*Lab test abnormalities:* The percentage of patients with selected laboratory abnormalities (increased or decreased from baseline and outside of specified ranges) while receiving famciclovir vs placebo in genital herpes

FAMCICLOVIR — ORAL

suppression studies are listed below. At least 660 famciclovir treated patients and 210 placebo recipients were assessed for each of the listed laboratory parameters.

- Anemia (< 0.8 x normal range low [NRL]; 0.1% vs 0)
- Leukopenia (< 0.75 x NRL; 1.3% vs 0.9%)
- Neutropenia (< 0.8 x NRL; 3.1% vs 1.5%)
- AST (SGOT) (> 2 x normal range high [NRH]; 2.3% vs 1.2%)
- ALT (SGPT) (> 2 x NRH); 3.2% vs 1.5%)
- Total bilirubin (> 1.5 x NRH; 1.9% vs 1.2%)
- Serum creatinine (> 1.5 x NRH; 0.2% vs 0.3%)
- Amylase (> 1.5 x NRH; 1.5% vs 1.9%)
- Lipase (> 1.5 x NRH; 4.9% vs 4.7%)

Drug Interactions

➤*Aldehyde oxidase:* The conversion of 6-deoxy penciclovir to penciclovir is catalyzed by aldehyde oxidase. Interactions with other drugs metabolized by this enzyme could potentially occur.

➤*Probenecid:* Concurrent use with probenecid or other drugs significantly eliminated by active renal tubular secretion may result in increased plasma concentrations of penciclovir.

Adverse Reactions

➤*Immunocompetent patients:* The safety of famciclovir has been evaluated in clinical studies involving 816 famciclovir-treated patients with herpes zoster (famciclovir, 250 mg 3 times a day to 750 mg 3 times a day); 528 famciclovir-treated patients with recurrent genital herpes (famciclovir, 125 mg 2 times a day to 500 mg 3 times a day); and 1197 patients with recurrent genital herpes treated with famciclovir as suppressive therapy (125 mg once daily to 250 mg 3 times a day) of which 570 patients received famciclovir (open-labeled or double-blind) for at least 10 months. The table below lists selected adverse reactions.

Selected adverse reactions reported by ≥ 2% of patients in placebo-controlled famciclovir trials*

	Incidence					
	Herpes zoster		Recurrent genital herpes		Genital herpes-suppression	
Adverse reaction	Famciclovir (n = 273) %	Placebo (n = 146) %	Famciclovir (n = 640) %	Placebo (n = 225) %	Famciclovir (n = 458) %	Placebo (n = 63) %
CNS						
Headache	22.7%	17.8%	23.6%	16.4%	39.3%	42.9%
Paresthesia	2.6%	0%	1.3%	0%	0.9%	0%
Migraine	0.7%	0.7%	1.3%	0.4%	3.1%	0%
GI						
Nausea	12.5%	11.6%	10%	8%	7.2%	9.5%
Diarrhea	7.7%	4.8%	4.5%	7.6%	9%	9.5%
Vomiting	4.8%	3.4%	1.3%	0.9%	3.1%	1.6%
Flatulence	1.5%	0.7%	1.9%	2.2%	4.8%	1.6%
Abdominal pain	1.1%	3.4%	3.9%	5.8%	7.9%	7.9%
Miscellaneous						
Fatigue	4.4%	3.4%	6.3%	4.4%	4.8%	3.2%
Dermatologic						
Pruritus	3.7%	2.7%	0.9%	0%	2.2%	0%
Rash	0.4%	0.7%	0.6%	0.4%	3.3%	1.6%
GU (female reproduction)						
Dysmenorrhea	0%	0.7%	2.2%	1.3%	7.6%	6.3%

* Patients may have entered into more than 1 clinical trial.

➤*Postmarketing:* The following adverse events have been reported during postapproval use of famciclovir: Urticaria, hallucinations and confusion (including delirium, disorientation, confusional state, occurring predominantly in the elderly). Because these adverse events are reported voluntarily from a population of unknown size, estimates of frequency cannot be made.

Selected laboratory abnormalities in genital herpes suppression studies[1]

Parameter	Famciclovir (n = 660)[2] %	Placebo (n = 210)[2] %
Anemia (< 0.8•NRL)	0.1%	0%
Leukopenia (< 0.75•NRL)	1.3%	0.9%
Neutropenia (< 0.8•NRL)	3.2%	1.5%
AST (> 2•NRH)	2.3%	1.2%
ALT (> 2•NRH)	3.2%	1.5%
Total bilirubin (> 1.5•NRH)	1.9%	1.2%
Serum creatinine (> 1.5•NRH)	0.2%	0.3%
Amylase (> 1.5•NRH)	1.5%	1.9%
Lipase (> 1.5•NRH)	4.9%	4.7%

[1] Percentage of patients with laboratory abnormalities that were increased or decreased from baseline and were outside of specified ranges.
[2] N values represent the minimum number of patients assessed for each laboratory parameter.
NRH = normal range high.
NRL = normal range low.

➤*HIV-infected patients:* In HIV-infected patients, the most frequently reported adverse events for famciclovir (500 mg twice daily; n = 150) and acyclovir (400 mg, 5 times a day; n = 143), respectively, were headache (16 vs 15.4%), nausea (10.7 vs 12.6%), diarrhea (6.7 vs 10.5%), vomiting (4.7 vs 3.5%), fatigue (4 vs 2.1%), and abdominal pain (3.3 vs 5.6%).

Overdosage

➤*Treatment:* Appropriate symptomatic and supportive therapy should be given. Penciclovir is removed by hemodialysis.

Patient Information

Patients should be informed that famciclovir is not a cure for genital herpes. There are no data evaluating whether famciclovir will prevent transmission of infection to others. As genital herpes is a sexually transmitted disease, patients should avoid contact with lesions or intercourse when lesions or symptoms are present to avoid infecting partners. Genital herpes can also be transmitted in the absence of symptoms through asymptomatic viral shedding. If medical management of recurrent episodes is indicated, patients should be advised to initiate therapy at the first sign or symptom (eg, pain, tenderness, burning, itching, tingling, vesicles, ulcers, or crusts).

May be taken without regard to meals.

VALACYCLOVIR HYDROCHLORIDE

Rx	**Valtrex** (GlaxoSmithKline)	**Tablets:** 500 mg (as base)	(VALTREX 500 mg). Blue, capsule shape. Film-coated. In 30s and UD 100s.
		1 g (as base)	(VALTREX 1 gram). Blue, capsule shape. Film-coated. In 21s.

VALACYCLOVIR HYDROCHLORIDE — ORAL

Indications

➤*Herpes zoster:* For the treatment of herpes zoster (shingles).

➤*Genital herpes:* For the treatment or suppression of genital herpes in immunocompetent individuals and for the suppression of recurrent genital herpes in HIV-infected individuals.

When valacyclovir is used as suppressive therapy in immunocompetent individuals with genital herpes, the risk of heterosexual transmission to susceptible partners is reduced. Use safer sex practices with suppressive therapy (see current Centers for Disease Control and Prevention [CDC] *Sexually Transmitted Diseases Treatment Guidelines*).

➤*Cold sores (herpes labialis):* For the treatment of cold sores (herpes labialis).

➤*Unlabeled uses:* For the prophylaxis of cytomegalovirus (CMV) disease in patients who have undergone renal transplantation; however, its use in patients with AIDS for CMV prophylaxis is not recommended because of a trend of increasing deaths associated with its use in this population. Valacyclovir use in patients who have undergone hematopoietic stem cell transplant is also not recommended because it is presumed to be less effective than ganciclovir.

Administration and Dosage

➤*Approved by the FDA:* June 23, 1995.

Valacyclovir may be given without regard to meals.

➤*Herpes zoster:* 1 g orally 3 times daily for 7 days. Therapy should be initiated at the earliest sign or symptom of herpes zoster and is most effective when started within 48 hours of the onset of zoster rash. No data are available on efficacy of treatment started more than 72 hours after rash onset.

➤*Genital herpes:*

Initial episodes – 1 g twice daily for 10 days. There are no data on the efficacy of treatment with valacyclovir when initiated more than 72 hours after the onset of signs and symptoms. Therapy was most effective when administered within 48 hours of the onset of signs and symptoms.

Recurrent episodes: 500 mg twice daily for 3 days.

If medical management of a genital herpes recurrence is indicated, patients should be advised to initiate therapy at the first sign or symptom of an episode. There are no data on the efficacy of treatment with valacyclovir when initiated more than 24 hours after the onset of signs or symptoms.

Suppressive therapy: 1 g once daily in patients with healthy immune function. In patients with a history of 9 or fewer recurrences per year, an alter-

VALACYCLOVIR HYDROCHLORIDE — ORAL

native dosage is 500 mg once daily. The safety and efficacy of therapy with valacyclovir beyond 1 year have not been established.

• *HIV-infected patients* – In HIV-infected patients with CD4 cell count at least 100 cells/mm^3, the recommended dosage of valacyclovir for chronic suppressive therapy of recurrent genital herpes is 500 mg twice daily. The safety and efficacy of therapy with valacyclovir beyond 6 months in patients with HIV infection have not been established.

Reduction of transmission: The recommended dosage of valacyclovir for reduction of transmission of genital herpes in patients with a history of 9 or fewer recurrences per year is 500 mg once daily for the source partner. Counsel patients to use safer sex practices in combination with suppressive therapy with valacyclovir. The efficacy of reducing transmission beyond 8 months in discordant couples has not been established.

➤*Cold sores (herpes labialis):* 2 g twice daily for 1 day, taken about 12 hours apart. Therapy should be initiated at the earliest symptom of a cold sore (eg, tingling, itching, burning). There are no data on the efficacy of treatment initiated after the development of clinical signs of a cold sore (eg, papule, vesicle, ulcer).

➤*Renal function impairment:* In patients with reduced renal function, reduction in dosage is recommended (see the following table).

Valacyclovir Dosage Adjustments for Renal Function Impairment

Indications	Normal dosage regimen (creatinine clearance ≥ 50)	Creatinine clearance (mL/min) 30 to 49	10 to 29	< 10
Herpes zoster	1 g every 8 h	1 g every 12 h	1 g every 24 h	500 mg every 24 h
Genital herpes				
Initial treatment	1 g every 12 h	No reduction	1 g every 24 h	500 mg every 24 h
Recurrent episodes	500 mg every 12 h	No reduction	500 mg every 24 h	500 mg every 24 h
Suppressive therapy	1 g every 24 h	No reduction	500 mg every 24 h	500 mg every 24 h
Suppressive therapy	500 mg every 24 h	No reduction	500 mg every 48 h	500 mg every 48 h
Suppressive therapy in HIV-infected patients	500 mg every 12 h	No reduction	500 mg every 24 h	500 mg every 24 h
Herpes labialis (cold sores) Do not exceed 1 day of treatment.	Two 2 g doses taken about 12 h apart	Two 1 g doses taken about 12 h apart	Two 500 mg doses taken about 12 h apart	500 mg single dose

Hemodialysis – During hemodialysis, the half-life of acyclovir after administration of valacyclovir is approximately 4 hours. About one-third of acyclovir in the body is removed by dialysis during a 4-hour hemodialysis session. Patients requiring hemodialysis should receive the recommended dose of valacyclovir after hemodialysis.

Peritoneal dialysis – There is no information specific to administration of valacyclovir in patients receiving peritoneal dialysis. The effect of chronic ambulatory peritoneal dialysis (CAPD) and continuous arteriovenous hemofiltration/dialysis (CAVHD) on acyclovir pharmacokinetics has been studied. The removal of acyclovir after CAPD and CAVHD is less pronounced than with hemodialysis, and the pharmacokinetic parameters closely resemble those observed in patients with end-stage renal disease (ESRD) not receiving hemodialysis. Therefore, supplemental doses of valacyclovir should not be required following CAPD or CAVHD.

➤*Storage / Stability:* Store at 15° to 25°C (59° to 77°F).

Actions

➤*Pharmacology:* Valacyclovir is rapidly converted to acyclovir, which has demonstrated antiviral activity against herpes simplex virus types 1 (HSV-1) and 2 (HSV-2) and varicella-zoster virus (VZV) both in vitro and in vivo.

The inhibitory activity of acyclovir is highly selective because of its affinity for the enzyme thymidine kinase (TK) encoded by HSV and VZV. This viral enzyme converts acyclovir into acyclovir monophosphate, a nucleotide analogue. The monophosphate is further converted into diphosphate by cellular guanylate kinase and into triphosphate by a number of cellular enzymes. In vitro, acyclovir triphosphate stops replication of herpes viral deoxyribonucleic acid (DNA). This is accomplished in the following 3 ways: competitive inhibition of viral DNA polymerase, incorporation and termination of the growing viral DNA chain, and inactivation of the viral DNA polymerase. The greater antiviral activity of acyclovir against HSV compared with VZV is due to its more efficient phosphorylation by the viral TK.

➤*Pharmacokinetics:*

Absorption – The pharmacokinetics of valacyclovir and acyclovir after oral administration of valacyclovir have been investigated in 14 volunteer studies involving 283 adults. The absolute bioavailability of acyclovir after administration of valacyclovir is 54.5% ± 9.1%, as determined following an oral dose of valacyclovir 1 g and an intravenous (IV) dose of acyclovir 350 mg to 12 healthy volunteers. Acyclovir bioavailability from the administration of valacyclovir is not altered by administration with food (30 minutes after an 873 kcal breakfast, which included 51 g of fat).

There was a lack of dose proportionality in acyclovir maximum concentration (C_{max}) and area under the acyclovir concentration-time curve (AUC) after single-dose administration of 100 mg, 250 mg, 500 mg, 750 mg, and 1 g of valacyclovir to 8 healthy volunteers. The mean C_{max} (± standard deviation [SD]) was 0.83 (± 0.14), 2.15 (± 0.5), 3.28 (± 0.83), 4.17 (± 1.14), and 5.65 (± 2.37) mcg/mL, respectively, and the mean AUC (± SD) was 2.28 (± 0.4), 5.76 (± 0.6), 11.59 (± 1.79), 14.11 (± 3.54), and 19.52 (± 6.04) mcg•h/mL, respectively.

There was also a lack of dose proportionality in acyclovir C_{max} and AUC after the multiple-dose administration of 250 mg, 500 mg, and 1 g of valacyclovir administered 4 times daily for 11 days in parallel groups of 8 healthy volunteers. The mean C_{max} (± SD) was 2.11 (± 0.33), 3.69 (± 0.87), and 4.96 (± 0.64) mcg/mL, respectively, and the mean AUC (±SD) was 5.66 (± 1.09), 9.88 (± 2.01), and 15.7 (± 2.27) mcg/mL•h, respectively.

There is no accumulation of acyclovir after the administration of valacyclovir at the recommended dosage regimens to healthy volunteers with healthy renal function.

Distribution – The binding of valacyclovir to human plasma proteins ranged from 13.5% to 17.9%.

Metabolism – After oral administration, valacyclovir is rapidly absorbed from the GI tract. Valacyclovir is converted to acyclovir and L-valine by first-pass intestinal and/or hepatic metabolism. Acyclovir is converted to a small extent to inactive metabolites by aldehyde oxidase and by alcohol and aldehyde dehydrogenase. Neither valacyclovir nor acyclovir is metabolized by cytochrome P-450 enzymes. Plasma concentrations of unconverted valacyclovir are low and transient, generally becoming nonquantifiable by 3 hours after administration. Peak plasma valacyclovir concentrations are generally less than 0.5 mcg/mL at all doses. After single-dose administration of valacyclovir 1 g, average plasma valacyclovir concentrations observed were 0.5, 0.4, and 0.8 mcg/mL in patients with hepatic function impairment, those with renal function impairment, and in healthy volunteers who received concomitant cimetidine and probenecid, respectively.

Excretion – The pharmacokinetic disposition of acyclovir delivered by valacyclovir is consistent with previous experience from IV and oral acyclovir. Following the oral administration of a single 1 g dose of radiolabeled valacyclovir to 4 healthy subjects, 45.6% and 47.12% of administered radioactivity was recovered in urine and feces over 96 hours, respectively. Acyclovir accounted for 88.6% of the radioactivity excreted in the urine. Renal clearance of acyclovir following the administration of a single 1 g dose of valacyclovir to 12 healthy volunteers was approximately 255 ± 86 mL/min, which represents 41.9% of total acyclovir apparent plasma clearance.

The plasma elimination half-life of acyclovir typically averaged 2.5 to 3.3 hours in all studies of valacyclovir in volunteers with healthy renal function.

Special populations –

Renal function impairment: Following administration of valacyclovir to volunteers with ESRD, the average acyclovir half-life is approximately 14 hours. During hemodialysis, the acyclovir half-life is approximately 4 hours. Approximately one-third of acyclovir in the body is removed by dialysis during a 4-hour hemodialysis session. Apparent plasma clearance of acyclovir in dialysis patients was 86.3 ± 21.3 mL/min/1.73 m^2, compared with 679.16 ± 162.76 mL/min/1.73 m^2 in healthy volunteers.

Reduction in dosage is recommended in patients with renal function impairment.

Hepatic function impairment: Administration of valacyclovir to patients with moderate (biopsy-proven cirrhosis) or severe (with and without ascites and biopsy-proven cirrhosis) liver disease indicated that the rate but not the extent of conversion of valacyclovir to acyclovir is reduced, and the acyclovir half-life is not affected. Dosage modification is not recommended for patients with cirrhosis.

Elderly: After single-dose administration of valacyclovir 1 g in healthy elderly volunteers, the half-life of acyclovir was 3.11 ± 0.51 hours, compared with 2.91 ± 0.63 hours in healthy volunteers. The pharmacokinetics of acyclovir after a single dose of valacyclovir 1 g was unchanged by coadministration of digoxin (2 doses of 0.75 mg). The pharmacokinetics of acyclovir following single- and multiple-dose oral administration of valacyclovir in elderly volunteers varied with renal function. Dose reduction may be required in elderly patients, depending on the underlying renal status of the patient.

➤*Microbiology:*

Antiviral activities – The quantitative relationship between the in vitro susceptibility of herpes viruses to antivirals and the clinical response to therapy has not been established in humans, and virus-sensitivity testing has not been standardized. Sensitivity testing results, expressed as the concentration of drug required to inhibit by 50% the growth of virus in cell culture (inhibitory concentration [IC_{50}]), vary greatly depending upon a number of factors. Using plaque-reduction assays, the IC_{50} against HSV isolates ranges from 0.02 to 13.5 mcg/mL for HSV-1 and from 0.01 to 9.9 mcg/mL for HSV-2. The IC_{50} for acyclovir against most laboratory strains and clinical isolates of VZV ranges from 0.12 to 10.8 mcg/mL. Acyclovir also demonstrates activity against the Oka vaccine strain of VZV with a mean IC_{50} of 1.35 mcg/mL.

Drug resistance – Resistance of HSV and VZV to acyclovir can result from qualitative or quantitative changes in the viral TK and/or DNA polymerase. Clinical isolates of VZV with reduced susceptibility to acyclovir have been recovered from patients with AIDS. In these cases, TK-deficient mutants of VZV have been recovered.

Resistance of HSV and VZV to acyclovir occurs by the same mechanisms. While most of the acyclovir-resistant mutants isolated thus far from

VALACYCLOVIR HYDROCHLORIDE — ORAL

immunocompromised patients have been found to be TK-deficient mutants, other mutants involving the viral TK gene (TK partial and TK altered) and DNA polymerase have also been isolated. TK-negative mutants may cause severe disease in immunocompromised patients. Consider the possibility of viral resistance to valacyclovir (and, therefore, to acyclovir) in patients who show poor clinical response during therapy.

Contraindications

Known hypersensitivity or intolerance to valacyclovir, acyclovir, or any component of the formulation.

Warnings

➤*Thrombotic thrombocytopenic purpura/hemolytic uremic syndrome (TTP/HUS):* TTP/HUS, in some cases resulting in death, has occurred in patients with advanced HIV disease and also in allogeneic bone marrow transplant– and renal transplant–recipients participating in clinical trials of valacyclovir at doses of 8 g/day.

➤*Renal function impairment:* Dose reduction is recommended when administering valacyclovir to patients with renal function impairment. Acute renal failure and CNS symptoms (agitation, hallucinations, confusion, delirium, and encephalopathy) have been reported in patients with underlying renal disease who have received inappropriately high doses of valacyclovir for their level of renal function. Exercise similar caution when administering valacyclovir to elderly patients and patients receiving potentially nephrotoxic agents.

Precipitation of acyclovir in renal tubules may occur when the solubility (2.5 mg/mL) is exceeded in the intratubular fluid. Maintain adequate hydration. In the event of acute renal failure and anuria, the patient may benefit from hemodialysis until renal function is restored.

➤*Mutagenesis:* In the mouse lymphoma assay, valacyclovir was not mutagenic in the absence of metabolic activation. In the presence of metabolic activation (76% to 88% conversion to acyclovir), valacyclovir was mutagenic. Valacyclovir was mutagenic in a mouse micronucleus assay.

➤*Elderly:* Of the total number of patients included in clinical studies of valacyclovir, 906 were 65 years of age or older, and 352 were 75 years of age or older. In a clinical study of herpes zoster, the duration of pain after healing (postherpetic neuralgia) was longer in patients 65 years of age and older, compared with younger adults. Elderly patients are more likely to have reduced renal function and to require dose reduction. Elderly patients are more likely to have renal or CNS adverse reactions. With respect to CNS adverse reactions observed during clinical practice, agitation, hallucinations, confusion, delirium, and encephalopathy were reported more frequently in elderly patients.

➤*Pregnancy: Category B.*

Teratogenic –

There are no adequate and well-controlled studies of valacyclovir or acyclovir in pregnant women. A prospective epidemiologic registry of acyclovir use during pregnancy was established in 1984 and completed in April 1999. There were 749 pregnancies followed in women exposed to systemic acyclovir during the first trimester of pregnancy, resulting in 756 outcomes. The occurrence rate of birth defects approximates that found in the general population. However, the small size of the registry is insufficient to evaluate the risk for less common defects or to permit reliable or definitive conclusions regarding the safety of acyclovir in pregnant women and their developing fetuses. Use valacyclovir during pregnancy only if the potential benefit justifies the potential risk to the fetus.

➤*Lactation:* Following oral administration of a dose of valacyclovir 500 mg to 5 breast-feeding mothers, peak acyclovir concentrations (C_{max}) in breast milk ranged from 0.5 to 2.3 times (median, 1.4) the corresponding maternal acyclovir serum concentrations. The acyclovir breast milk AUC ranged from 1.4 to 2.6 (median, 2.2) maternal serum AUC. A maternal dosage of valacyclovir 500 mg twice daily would provide a breast-feeding infant with an oral acyclovir dosage of approximately 0.6 mg/kg/day. This would result in less than 2% of the exposure obtained after administration of a standard neonatal dose of 30 mg/kg/day of IV acyclovir to the breast-feeding infant. Unchanged valacyclovir was not detected in maternal serum, breast milk, or infant urine. Administer valacyclovir to a breast-feeding mother with caution and only when indicated.

➤*Children:* Safety and efficacy of valacyclovir in prepubertal children have not been established.

Precautions

➤*Immunocompromised patients:* The safety and efficacy of valacyclovir have not been established in immunocompromised patients, other than for the suppression of genital herpes in HIV-infected patients. The safety and efficacy of valacyclovir for suppression of recurrent genital herpes in patients with advanced HIV disease (CD4 cell count less than 100 cells/mm³) have not been established. The efficacy of valacyclovir for the treatment of genital herpes in HIV-infected patients has not been established. The safety and efficacy of valacyclovir have not been established for the treatment of disseminated herpes zoster.

➤*Transmission of genital herpes:* The efficacy of valacyclovir for reducing transmission of genital herpes has not been established in individuals with multiple partners and nonheterosexual couples.

➤*Cold sore treatment:* Given the dosage recommendations for treatment of cold sores, pay special attention when prescribing valacyclovir for cold sores in patients who are elderly or who have impaired renal function. Treatment should not exceed 1 day (2 doses of 2 g in 24 hours). Therapy beyond 1 day does not provide additional clinical benefit.

Adverse Reactions

Frequently reported adverse reactions in clinical trials of valacyclovir in healthy patients are listed in the following table:

Valacyclovir Adverse Reactions

Adverse reaction	Herpes zoster: Valacyclovir 1 g 3 times daily (n = 967)	Herpes zoster: Placebo (n = 195)	Genital herpes treatment: Valacyclovir 1 g twice daily (n = 1,194)	Genital herpes treatment: Valacyclovir 500 mg twice daily (n = 1,159)	Genital herpes treatment: Placebo (n = 439)	Genital herpes suppression: Valacyclovir 1 g once daily (n = 269)	Genital herpes suppression: Valacyclovir 500 mg once daily (n = 266)	Genital herpes suppression: Placebo (n = 134)
CNS								
Depression	NA[a]	NA	1%	0%	< 1%	7%	5%	5%
Dizziness	3%	2%	3%	2%	3%	4%	2%	1%
Headache	14%	12%	16%	15%	14%	35%	38%	34%
GI								
Abdominal pain	3%	2%	2%	1%	3%	11%	9%	6%
Nausea	15%	8%	6%	5%	8%	11%	11%	8%
Vomiting	6%	3%	1%	< 1%	< 1%	3%	3%	2%
Lab test abnormalities								
AST (2 × ULN[b])	1%	0%	1%	—[c]	0.5%	4.1%	3.8%	3%
Hemoglobin (< 0.8 × LLN[d])	0.8%	0%	0.3%	0.2%	0%	0%	0.8%	0.8%
Platelet count (< 100,000/mm³)	1%	1.2%	0.3%	0.1%	0.7%	0.4%	1.1%	1.5%
Serum creatinine (> 1.5 × ULN)	0.2%	0%	0.7%	0%	0%	0%	0%	0%
White blood cells (< 0.75 × LLN)	1.3%	0.6%	0.7%	0.6%	0.2%	0.7%	0.8%	1.5%
Miscellaneous								
Arthralgia	NA	NA	< 1%	< 1%	< 1%	6%	5%	4%
Dysmenorrhea	NA	NA	< 1%	< 1%	1%	8%	5%	4%

[a] NA = not applicable.
[b] ULN = upper limit of normal.
[c] Data were not collected prospectively.
[d] LLN = lower limit of normal.

VALACYCLOVIR HYDROCHLORIDE — ORAL

Suppression of genital herpes in HIV-infected patients – In HIV-infected patients, frequently reported adverse reactions for valacyclovir (500 mg twice daily; n = 194; median days on therapy, 172) and placebo (n = 99; median days on therapy, 59) included headache (13% vs 8%, respectively), fatigue (8% vs 5%, respectively), and rash (8% vs 1%, respectively). Post randomization laboratory abnormalities that were reported more frequently in valacyclovir subjects vs placebo included elevated alkaline phosphatase (4% vs 2%), elevated ALT (14% vs 10%), elevated AST (16% vs 11%), decreased neutrophil counts (18% vs 10%), and decreased platelet counts (3% vs 0%).

Reduction of transmission – In a clinical study for the reduction of transmission of genital herpes, the adverse reactions reported by patients receiving valacyclovir 500 mg once daily (n = 743) or placebo once daily (n = 741) included headache (valacyclovir, 29%; placebo, 26%), nasopharyngitis (valacyclovir, 16%; placebo, 15%), and upper respiratory tract infection (valacyclovir, 9%; placebo, 10%). In this 8-month study, there were no clinically significant changes from baseline laboratory parameters in subjects receiving valacyclovir compared with placebo.

➤*Cold sores (herpes labialis):* In clinical studies for the treatment of cold sores, the adverse reactions reported by patients receiving valacyclovir (n = 609) or placebo (n = 609) included headache (valacyclovir, 14%; placebo, 10%) and dizziness (valacyclovir, 2%; placebo, 1%). The frequencies of abnormal ALT (greater than 2 times the ULN) were 1.8% for patients receiving valacyclovir, compared with 0.8% for placebo. Other laboratory abnormalities (hemoglobin, white blood cells, alkaline phosphatase, and serum creatinine) occurred with similar frequencies in the 2 groups.

➤*Postmarketing:* The following events have been identified during post-approval use of valacyclovir in clinical practice. Because they are reported voluntarily from a population of unknown size, estimates of frequency cannot be made. These events have been chosen for inclusion because of their seriousness, frequency of reporting, or causal connection to valacyclovir, or a combination of these factors.

Cardiovascular – Hypertension, tachycardia.

CNS – Aggressive behavior; agitation; ataxia; coma; confusion; decreased consciousness; dysarthria; encephalopathy; mania; psychosis, including auditory and visual hallucinations; seizures; tremors.

Dermatologic – Alopecia; erythema multiforme; rashes, including photosensitivity.

GI – Diarrhea.

Hematologic – Aplastic anemia, leukocytoclastic vasculitis, thrombocytopenia, TTP/HUS.

Hepatic – Hepatitis, liver enzyme abnormalities.

Hypersensitivity – Acute hypersensitivity reactions, including anaphylaxis, angioedema, dyspnea, pruritus, rash, and urticaria.

Ophthalmic – Visual abnormalities.

Renal – Elevated creatinine, renal failure.

Renal failure and CNS symptoms have been reported in patients with renal function impairment who received valacyclovir or acyclovir at greater than the recommended dose. Dosage reduction is recommended in this patient population.

Miscellaneous – Facial edema.

Overdosage

Exercise caution to prevent inadvertent overdose.

➤*Symptoms:* Precipitation of acyclovir in renal tubules may occur when the solubility (2.5 mg/mL) is exceeded in the intratubular fluid.

➤*Treatment:* In the event of acute renal failure and anuria, the patient may benefit from hemodialysis until renal function is restored.

Patient Information

Advise patients to maintain adequate hydration.

➤*Herpes zoster:* There are no data on treatment initiated greater than 72 hours after onset of the zoster rash. Advise patients to initiate treatment as soon as possible after a diagnosis of herpes zoster.

➤*Genital herpes:* Inform patients that valacyclovir is not a cure for genital herpes. Because genital herpes is a sexually transmitted disease, patients should avoid contact with lesions or intercourse when lesions and/or symptoms are present to avoid infecting partners. Genital herpes is frequently transmitted in the absence of symptoms through asymptomatic viral shedding. Therefore, counsel patients to use safer sex practices in combination with suppressive therapy with valacyclovir. Advise sex partners of infected persons that they might be infected even if they have no symptoms. Type-specific serologic testing of asymptomatic partners of persons with genital herpes can determine whether risk of HSV-2 acquisition exists.

Valacyclovir has not been shown to reduce transmission of sexually transmitted infections other than HSV-2.

If medical management of a genital herpes recurrence is indicated, advise patients to initiate therapy at the first sign or symptom of an episode.

There are no data on the efficacy of treatment initiated greater than 72 hours after the onset of signs and symptoms of a first episode of genital herpes or more than 24 hours after the onset of signs and symptoms of a recurrent episode.

There are no data on the safety or efficacy of chronic suppressive therapy of greater than 1 year's duration in otherwise healthy patients. There are no data on the safety or efficacy of chronic suppressive therapy of more than 6 months' duration in HIV-infected patients.

➤*Cold sores (herpes labialis):* Advise patients to initiate treatment at the earliest symptom of a cold sore (eg, tingling, itching, burning). There are no data on the efficacy of treatment initiated after the development of clinical signs of a cold sore (eg, papule, vesicle, ulcer). Instruct patients that treatment for cold sores should not exceed 1 day (2 doses) and that their doses should be taken about 12 hours apart. Inform patients that valacyclovir is not a cure for cold sores.

AMANTADINE HYDROCHLORIDE

Rx	**Amantadine Hydrochloride** (Upsher-Smith)	**Tablets:** 100 mg	(832 AMT). Peach. In 100s and 500s.
Rx	**Symmetrel** (Endo)		(SYMMETREL). Orange, triangular. In 100s and 500s.
Rx	**Amantadine HCl** (Various, eg, Banner, Geneva, Major, Martec, UDL, URL)	**Capsules:** 100 mg	In 100s, 500s, and UD 100s.
Rx	**Amantadine HCl** (Various, eg, Alpharma, Endo, Morton Grove)	**Syrup:** 50 mg per 5 mL	May contain sorbitol and parabens. In 480 mL.
Rx	**Symmetrel** (Endo)		Sorbitol and parabens. In 480 mL.

AMANTADINE HYDROCHLORIDE — ORAL

Indications

➤*Influenza A prophylaxis:* For chemoprophylaxis against signs and symptoms of influenza A virus infection when early vaccination is not feasible or when the vaccine is contraindicated or not available. In the prophylaxis of influenza, early vaccination on an annual basis as recommended by the Centers for Disease Control's Immunization Practices Advisory Committee is the method of choice. Because amantadine hydrochloride does not completely prevent the host immune response to influenza A infection, individuals who take this drug may still develop immune responses to natural disease or vaccination and may be protected when later exposed to antigenically related viruses. Following vaccination during an influenza A outbreak, amantadine hydrochloride prophylaxis should be considered for the 2- to 4-week time period required to develop an antibody response.

➤*Influenza A treatment:* Treatment of uncomplicated respiratory tract illness caused by influenza A virus strains especially when administered early in the course of illness. There are no well-controlled clinical studies demonstrating that treatment with amantadine hydrochloride will avoid the development of influenza A virus pneumonitis or other complications in high-risk patients.

➤*Parkinson disease:* Treatment of idiopathic Parkinson's disease (paralysis agitans), postencephalitic parkinsonism, and symptomatic parkinsonism which may follow injury to the nervous system by carbon monoxide intoxication. It is indicated in those elderly patients believed to develop parkinsonism in association with cerebral arteriosclerosis. In the treatment of Parkinson's disease, amantadine hydrochloride is less effective than levodopa, (-)-3-(3,4-dihydroxyphenyl)-L-alanine, and its efficacy in comparison with the anticholinergic antiparkinson drugs has not yet been established.

➤*Drug-induced extrapyramidal reactions:* In the treatment of drug-induced extrapyramidal reactions. Although anticholinergic-type side effects have been noted with amantadine hydrochloride when used in patients with drug-induced extrapyramidal reactions, there is a lower incidence of these side effects than that observed with the anticholinergic antiparkinson drugs.

Administration and Dosage

➤*Approved by the FDA:* August 5, 1986.

➤*Special risk:* The dose of amantadine hydrochloride may need reduction in patients with congestive heart failure, peripheral edema, orthostatic hypotension, or impaired renal function (see Dosage for impaired renal function).

➤*Prophylaxis and treatment of uncomplicated influenza A virus illness:*

Adults – 200 mg; two (2) 100 mg capsules or tablets or 4 teaspoonfuls of syrup as a single daily dose. The daily dosage may be split into 100 mg (2 teaspoonfuls of syrup) twice a day. If central nervous system effects develop in once-a-day dosage, a split dosage schedule may reduce such complaints. In persons 65 years of age or older, the daily dosage of amantadine hydrochloride is 100 mg.

Alternative dosing – A 100 mg daily dose has also been shown in experimental challenge studies to be effective as prophylaxis in healthy adults who are not at high risk for influenza-related complications. However, it has not been demonstrated that a 100 mg daily dose is as effective as a 200 mg daily dose for prophylaxis, nor has the 100 mg daily dose been studied in the treatment of acute influenza illness. In recent clinical trials, the incidence of central nervous system (CNS) side effects associated with the 100 mg daily dose was at or near the level of placebo. The 100 mg dose is recommended for persons who have demonstrated intolerance to 200 mg of amantadine hydrochloride daily because of CNS or other toxicities.

Children –

1 to 9 years of age: The total daily dose should be calculated on the basis of 2 to 4 mg/lb/day (4.4 to 8.8 mg/kg/day), but not to exceed 150 mg per day.

9 to 12 years of age: The total daily dose is 200 mg given as 1 capsule or tablet of 100 mg (2 teaspoonfuls of syrup) twice a day. The 100 mg daily dose has not been studied in children. Therefore, there are no data which demonstrate that this dose is as effective as or is safer than the 200 mg daily dose in this patient population. Prophylactic dosing should be started in anticipation of an influenza A outbreak and before or after contact with individuals with influenza A virus respiratory tract illness.

Amantadine hydrochloride should be continued daily for at least 10 days following a known exposure. If amantadine hydrochloride is used chemoprophylactically in conjunction with inactivated influenza A virus vaccine until protective antibody responses develop, then it should be administered for 2 to 4 weeks after the vaccine has been given. When inactivated influenza A virus vaccine is unavailable or contraindicated, amantadine hydrochloride should be administered for the duration of known influenza A in the community because of repeated and unknown exposure.

Treatment of influenza A virus illness should be started as soon as possible, preferably within 24 to 48 hours after onset of signs and symptoms, and should be continued for 24 to 48 hours after the disappearance of signs and symptoms.

➤*Parkinsonism:*

Adults – 100 mg twice a day when used alone. Amantadine hydrochloride has an onset of action usually within 48 hours.

The initial dose of amantadine hydrochloride is 100 mg daily for patients with serious associated medical illnesses or who are receiving high doses of other antiparkinson drugs. After 1 to several weeks at 100 mg once daily, the dose may be increased to 100 mg twice daily, if necessary.

Occasionally, patients whose responses are not optimal with amantadine hydrochloride at 200 mg daily may benefit from an increase up to 400 mg daily in divided doses. However, such patients should be supervised closely by their physicians.

Patients initially deriving benefit from amantadine hydrochloride not uncommonly experience a fall-off of effectiveness after a few months. Benefit may be regained by increasing the dose to 300 mg daily. Alternatively, temporary discontinuation of amantadine hydrochloride for several weeks, followed by reinitiation of the drug, may result in regaining benefit in some patients. A decision to use other antiparkinson drugs may be necessary.

➤*Dosage for concomitant therapy:* Some patients who do not respond to anticholinergic antiparkinson drugs may respond to amantadine hydrochloride. When amantadine hydrochloride or anticholinergic antiparkinson drugs are each used with marginal benefit, concomitant use may produce additional benefit.

When amantadine hydrochloride and levodopa are initiated concurrently, the patient can exhibit rapid therapeutic benefits. Amantadine hydrochloride should be held constant at 100 mg daily or twice daily while the daily dose of levodopa is gradually increased to optimal benefit.

When amantadine hydrochloride is added to optimal well-tolerated doses of levodopa, additional benefit may result, including smoothing out the fluctuations in improvement which sometimes occur in patients on levodopa alone. Patients who require a reduction in their usual dose of levodopa because of development of side effects may possibly regain lost benefit with the addition of amantadine hydrochloride.

➤*Drug-induced extrapyramidal reactions:*

Adult – 100 mg twice a day. Occasionally, patients whose responses are not optimal with amantadine hydrochloride at 200 mg daily may benefit from an increase up to 300 mg daily in divided doses.

➤*Renal function impairment:*

Amantadine HCl Impaired Renal Function Dosage	
Ccr (mL/min/1.73 m^2)	Amantadine HCl I dosage
30 to 50	200 mg first day and 100 mg each day thereafter
15 to 29	200 mg first day followed by 100 mg on alternate days
< 15	200 mg every 7 days

The recommended dosage for patients on hemodialysis is 200 mg every 7 days.

➤*Storage/Stability:* Store at controlled room temperature 25°C (77°F), excursions permitted to 15° to 30°C (59° to 86°F).

Dispense in a tight container as defined in the USP, with a child-resistant closure (as required). Protect from moisture.

Actions

➤*Pharmacology:*

Parkinson's disease – The mechanism of action of amantadine in the treatment of Parkinson's disease and drug-induced extrapyramidal reactions is not known. Data from animal studies have either shown or suggested amantadine hydrochloride to enhance extracellular concentrations of dopamine by increasing dopamine release or decreasing reuptake of dopamine into presynaptic neurons; to stimulate the dopamine receptor itself; or drive the postsynaptic dopaminergic system to a more dopamine sensitive status.

However, doses employed in the animal studies were often of a magnitude greater than the clinically therapeutic doses. More recent work using doses in the low clinically therapeutic range (low mcM) showed amantadine to inhibit the N-methyl-D-aspartic acid (NMDA) receptor-mediated stimulation of acetylcholine release from rat stratum, most likely at the MK-801 site. Although amantadine does not possess anticholinergic activity in dogs at doses of 31.5 mg/kg, equivalent to an approximate human dose of 15.8 mg/kg (based on body surface area conversions), clinically, it exhibits anticholinergic-like side effects such as dry mouth, urinary retention, and constipation.

Antiviral – The mechanism by which amantadine exerts its antiviral activity is not clearly understood. It appears to mainly prevent the release of infectious viral nucleic acid into the host cell by interfering with the function of the transmembrane domain of the viral M2 protein. In certain cases,

AMANTADINE HYDROCHLORIDE — ORAL

amantadine is also known to prevent virus assembly during virus replication. It does not appear to interfere with the immunogenicity of inactivated influenza A virus vaccine.

➤*Pharmacokinetics:* Amantadine hydrochloride is well absorbed orally. Maximum plasma concentrations are directly related to dose for doses up to 200 mg/day. Doses above 200 mg/day may result in a greater than proportional increase in maximum plasma concentrations. It is primarily excreted unchanged in the urine by glomerular filtration and tubular secretion. Eight metabolites of amantadine have been identified in human urine. One metabolite, an N-acetylated compound, was quantified in human urine and accounted for 5% to 15% of the administered dose. Plasma acetylamantadine accounted for up to 80% of the concurrent amantadine plasma concentration in 5 of 12 healthy volunteers following the ingestion of a 200 mg dose of amantadine. Acetylamantadine was not detected in the plasma of the remaining 7 volunteers. The contribution of this metabolite to efficacy or toxicity is not known.

Amantadine pharmacokinetics were determined in 24 healthy adult male volunteers after the oral administration of a single amantadine hydrochloride 100 mg capsule. The mean ± SD maximum plasma concentration was 0.22 ± 0.03 mcg/mL (range, 0.18 to 0.32 mcg/mL). The time to peak concentration was 3.3 ± 1.5 hours (range, 1.5 to 8 hours). The apparent oral clearance was 0.28 ± 0.11 L/hr/kg (range, 0.14 to 0.62 L/hr/kg). The half-life was 17 ± 4 hours (range, 10 to 25 hours). Across other studies, amantadine plasma half-life has averaged 16 ± 6 hours (range, 9 to 31 hours) in 19 healthy volunteers.

Plasma amantadine clearance ranged from 0.2 to 0.3 L/kg/hr after the administration of 5 mg to 25 mg intravenous doses of amantadine to 15 healthy volunteers.

In 6 healthy volunteers, the ratio of amantadine renal clearance to apparent oral plasma clearance was 0.79 ± 0.17 (mean ± SD).

The volume of distribution determined after the intravenous administration of amantadine to 15 healthy subjects was 3 to 8 L/kg, suggesting tissue binding. Amantadine, after single oral 200 mg doses to 6 healthy young subjects and to 6 healthy elderly subjects has been found in nasal mucus at mean ± SD concentrations of 0.15 ± 0.16, 0.28 ± 0.26, and 0.39 ± 0.34 mcg/g at 1, 4, and 8 hours after dosing, respectively. These concentrations represented 31 ± 33%, 59 ± 61%, and 95 ± 86% of the corresponding plasma amantadine concentrations. Amantadine is approximately 67% bound to plasma proteins over a concentration range of 0.1 to 2 mcg/mL. Following the administration of amantadine 100 mg as a single dose, the mean ± SD red blood cell to plasma ratio ranged from 2.7 ± 0.5 in 6 healthy subjects to 1.4 ± 0.2 in 8 patients with renal insufficiency.

Elderly – The apparent oral plasma clearance of amantadine is reduced and the plasma half-life and plasma concentrations are increased in healthy elderly individuals age 60 and older. After single dose administration of 25 to 75 mg to 7 healthy, elderly male volunteers, the apparent plasma clearance of amantadine was 0.1 ± 0.04 L/hr/kg (range 0.06 to 0.17 L/hr/kg) and the half-life was 29 ± 7 hours (range 20 to 41 hours). Whether these changes are due to decline in renal function or other age related factors is not known.

Renal function impairment – Compared with otherwise healthy adult individuals, the clearance of amantadine is significantly reduced in adult patients with renal insufficiency. The elimination half-life increases 2- to 3-fold or greater when creatinine clearance is less than 40 mL/min/1.73 m^2 and averages 8 days in patients on chronic maintenance hemodialysis. Amantadine is removed in negligible amounts by hemodialysis.

Drug interactions – The pH of the urine has been reported to influence the excretion rate of amantadine hydrochloride. Since the excretion rate of amantadine hydrochloride increases rapidly when the urine is acidic, the administration of urine acidifying drugs may increase the elimination of the drug from the body.

Contraindications

Hypersensitivity to amantadine hydrochloride.

Warnings

➤*Deaths:* Deaths have been reported from overdose with amantadine hydrochloride. The lowest reported acute lethal dose was 1 g. Acute toxicity may be attributable to the anticholinergic effects of amantadine. Drug overdose has resulted in cardiac, respiratory, renal or central nervous system toxicity. Cardiac dysfunction includes arrhythmia, tachycardia and hypertension (see Overdosage).

➤*Suicide attempts:* Suicide attempts, some of which have been fatal, have been reported in patients treated with amantadine hydrochloride, many of whom received short courses for influenza treatment or prophylaxis. The incidence of suicide attempts is not known and the pathophysiologic mechanism is not understood. Suicide attempts and suicidal ideation have been reported in patients with and without history of psychiatric illness. Amantadine hydrochloride can exacerbate mental problems in patients with a history of psychiatric disorders or substance abuse. Patients who attempt suicide may exhibit abnormal mental states which include disorientation, confusion, depression, personality changes, agitation, aggressive behavior, hallucinations, paranoia, other psychotic reactions, and somnolence or insomnia. Because of the possibility of serious adverse effects, caution should be observed when prescribing amantadine hydrochloride to patients being treated with drugs having CNS effects, or for whom the potential risks outweigh the benefit of treatment. Because some patients have attempted suicide by overdosing with amantadine, prescriptions should be written for the smallest quantity consistent with good patient management.

➤*CNS effects:* Patients with a history of epilepsy or other "seizures" should be observed closely for possible increased seizure activity.

Patients receiving amantadine hydrochloride who note central nervous system effects or blurring of vision should be cautioned against driving or working in situations where alertness and adequate motor coordination are important.

➤*CHF or peripheral edema:* Patients with a history of congestive heart failure or peripheral edema should be followed closely as there are patients who developed congestive heart failure while receiving amantadine hydrochloride.

Because amantadine hydrochloride has anticholinergic effects and may cause mydriasis, it should not be given to patients with untreated angle closure glaucoma.

➤*Parkinson disease:* Patients with Parkinson's disease improving on amantadine hydrochloride should resume normal activities gradually and cautiously, consistent with other medical considerations, such as the presence of osteoporosis or phlebothrombosis.

➤*Renal function impairment:* Because amantadine hydrochloride is mainly excreted in the urine, it accumulates in the plasma and in the body when renal function declines. Thus, the dose of amantadine hydrochloride should be reduced in patients with renal impairment and in individuals who are greater than or equal to 65 years of age. Hemodialysis does not remove significant amounts of amantadine hydrochloride; in patients with renal failure, a 4-hour hemodialysis removed 7 to 15 mg after a single 300 mg oral dose.

➤*Hepatic function impairment:* Care should be exercised when administering amantadine hydrochloride to patients with liver disease. Rare instances of reversible elevation of liver enzymes have been reported in patients receiving amantadine hydrochloride, though a specific relationship between the drug and such changes has not been established.

➤*Fertility impairment:* Failed fertility has been reported during human in vitro fertilization (IVF) when the sperm donor ingested amantadine 2 weeks prior to, and during the IVF cycle.

➤*Elderly:* Because amantadine hydrochloride is primarily excreted in the urine, it accumulates in the plasma and in the body when renal function declines. Thus, the dose of amantadine hydrochloride should be reduced in patients with renal impairment and in individuals who are greater than or equal to 65 years of age. The dose of amantadine hydrochloride may need reduction in patients with congestive heart failure, peripheral edema, or orthostatic hypotension.

➤*Pregnancy:* *Category C.*

Amantadine hydrochloride has been shown to be teratogenic in rats at 50 mg/kg/day and embryotoxic at 100 mg/kg/day (estimated human equivalent dose of 7.1 mg/kg/day and 14.2 mg/kg/day, respectively, based on body surface area conversion). There are no adequate and well-controlled studies in pregnant women. Human data regarding teratogenicity after maternal use of amantadine is scarce. Teratology of Fallot and tibial hemimelia (normal karyotype) occurred in an infant exposed to amantadine during the first trimester of pregnancy (100 mg by mouth for 7 days during the sixth and seventh week of gestation). Cardiovascular maldevelopment (single ventricle with pulmonary atresia) was associated with maternal exposure to amantadine (100 mg/day) administered during the first 2 weeks of pregnancy. Amantadine hydrochloride should be used during pregnancy only if the potential benefit justifies the potential risk to the embryo or fetus.

➤*Lactation:* Amantadine hydrochloride is excreted in human milk. Use is not recommended in nursing mothers.

➤*Children:* The safety and efficacy of amantadine hydrochloride in newborn infants and infants below the age of 1 year have not been established.

Precautions

➤*Abrupt withdrawal:* Amantadine hydrochloride should not be discontinued abruptly in patients with Parkinson's disease since a few patients have experienced a parkinsonian crisis (ie, a sudden marked clinical deterioration) when this medication was suddenly stopped. The dose of anticholinergic drugs or of amantadine hydrochloride should be reduced if atropine-like effects appear when these drugs are used concurrently. Abrupt discontinuation may also precipitate delirium, agitation, delusions, hallucinations, paranoid reaction, stupor, anxiety, depression and slurred speech.

➤*Neuroleptic malignant syndrome (NMS):* Sporadic cases of possible neuroleptic malignant syndrome (NMS) have been reported in association with dose reduction or withdrawal of amantadine hydrochloride therapy. Therefore, patients should be observed carefully when the dosage of amantadine hydrochloride is reduced abruptly or discontinued, especially if the patient is receiving neuroleptics.

➤*Bacterial infections:* Serious bacterial infections may begin with influenza-like symptoms or may coexist with or occur as complications during the course of influenza. Amantadine hydrochloride has not been shown to prevent such complications.

➤*Special risk:* The dose of amantadine hydrochloride may need careful adjustment in patients with congestive heart failure, peripheral edema, or orthostatic hypotension. Care should be exercised when administering amantadine hydrochloride to patients with a history of recurrent eczematoid rash, or to patients with psychosis or severe psychoneurosis not controlled by chemotherapeutic agents.

➤*Hazardous tasks:* See Warnings for more information.

AMANTADINE HYDROCHLORIDE — ORAL

Drug Interactions

Amantadine Drug Interactions			
Precipitant drug	Object drug*		Description
Anticholinergic agents	Amantadine	↑	Concurrent administration may potentiate the anticholinergic-like side effects of amantadine. Consider reducing the dose of the anticholinergic agent if atropine-like effects appear.
Quinidine Quinine	Amantadine	↑	Coadministration was shown to reduce renal clearance of amantadine.
Triamterene Thiazide diuretics	Amantadine	↑	Coadministration resulted in a higher plasma amantadine concentration.
Trimethoprim/ sulfamethoxazole	Amantadine	↑	Coadministration may impair renal clearance of amantadine, resulting in higher plasma concentrations.
Amantadine	CNS stimulants	↑	Careful observation is required during concomitant administration.
Thioridazine	Amantadine	↑	Coadministration of thioridazine has been reported to worsen the tremor in elderly patients with Parkinson's disease; however, it is not known if other phenothiazines produce a similar response.

* ↑ = Object drug increased.

Adverse Reactions

The adverse reactions reported most frequently at the recommended dose of amantadine hydrochloride (5% to 10%) are nausea, dizziness (lightheadedness), and insomnia.

Less frequently (1% to 5%) reported adverse reactions are the following: Depression, anxiety and irritability, hallucinations, confusion, anorexia, dry mouth, constipation, ataxia, livedo reticularis, peripheral edema, orthostatic hypotension, headache, somnolence, nervousness, dream abnormality, agitation, dry nose, diarrhea, and fatigue.

Infrequently (0.1% to 1%) occurring adverse reactions are as follows: Congestive heart failure, psychosis, urinary retention, dyspnea, fatigue, skin rash, vomiting, weakness, slurred speech, euphoria, confusion, thinking abnormality, amnesia, hyperkinesia, hypertension, decreased libido, and visual disturbance, including punctate subepithelial or other corneal opacity, corneal edema, decreased visual acuity, sensitivity to light, and optic nerve palsy.

Rare (less than 0.1%) occurring adverse reactions are the following: Instances of convulsion, leukopenia, neutropenia, eczematoid dermatitis, oculogyric episodes, suicidal attempt, suicide, and suicidal ideation.

➤*Postmarketing:*

Cardiovascular – Cardiac arrest, arrhythmias including malignant arrhythmias, hypotension, and tachycardia.

CNS – Coma, stupor, delirium, hypokinesia, hypertonia, delusions, aggressive behavior, paranoid reaction, manic reaction, involuntary muscle contractions, gait abnormalities, paresthesia, EEG changes, and tremor. Abrupt discontinuation may also precipitate delirium, agitation, delusions, hallucinations, paranoid reaction, stupor, anxiety, depression and slurred speech.

Dermatologic – Pruritus and diaphoresis.

GI – Dysphagia.

Hematologic – Leukocytosis.

Lab test abnormalities – Elevated CPK, BUN, serum creatine, alkaline phosphatase, LDH, bilirubin, GGT, AST, and ALT.

Respiratory – Acute respiratory failure, pulmonary edema, and tachypnea.

Special senses – Keratitis and mydriasis.

Miscellaneous – Neuroleptic malignant syndrome (see Warnings), allergic reactions including anaphylactic reactions, edema, and fever.

Overdosage

➤*Symptoms:* Deaths have been reported from overdose with amantadine hydrochloride. The lowest reported acute lethal dose was 1 g. Because some patients have attempted suicide by overdosing with amantadine, prescriptions should be written for the smallest quantity consistent with good patient management.

Acute toxicity may be attributable to the anticholinergic effects of amantadine. Drug overdose has resulted in cardiac, respiratory, renal or central nervous system toxicity. Cardiac dysfunction includes arrhythmia, tachycardia and hypertension. Pulmonary edema and respiratory distress (including adult respiratory distress syndrome [ARDS]) have been reported; renal dysfunction including increased BUN, decreased creatinine clearance and renal insufficiency can occur. Central nervous system effects that have been reported include insomnia, anxiety, aggressive behavior, hypertonia, hyperkinesia, tremor, confusion, disorientation, depersonalization, fear, delirium, hallucinations, psychotic reactions, lethargy, somnolence and coma. Seizures may be exacerbated in patients with history of seizure disorders. Hyperthermia has also been observed in cases where a drug overdose has occurred.

➤*Treatment:* There is no specific antidote for an overdose of amantadine hydrochloride. However, slowly administered intravenous physostigmine in 1 and 2 mg doses in an adult at 1- to 2-hour intervals and 0.5 mg doses in a child at 5- to 10-minute intervals up to a maximum of 2 mg/hr have been reported to be effective in the control of central nervous system toxicity caused by amantadine hydrochloride. For acute overdosing, general supportive measures should be employed along with immediate gastric lavage or induction of emesis. Fluids should be forced, and if necessary, given intravenously. Hemodialysis does not remove significant amounts of amantadine hydrochloride; in patients with renal failure, a 4-hour hemodialysis removed 7 to 15 mg after a single 300 mg oral dose. The pH of the urine has been reported to influence the excretion rate of amantadine hydrochloride. Since the excretion rate of amantadine hydrochloride increases rapidly when the urine is acidic, the administration of urine acidifying drugs may increase the elimination of the drug from the body. The blood pressure, pulse, respiration and temperature should be monitored. The patient should be observed for hyperactivity and convulsions; if required, sedation, and anticonvulsant therapy should be administered. The patient should be observed for the possible development of arrhythmias and hypotension; if required, appropriate antiarrhythmic and antihypotensive therapy should be given. The blood electrolytes, urine pH and urinary output should be monitored. If there is no record of recent voiding, catheterization should be done.

Care should be exercised when administering adrenergic agents, such as isoproterenol, to patients with a amantadine hydrochloride overdose, since the dopaminergic activity of amantadine hydrochloride has been reported to induce malignant arrhythmias.

Patient Information

Patients should be advised of the following information:

Blurry vision and/or impaired mental acuity may occur.

Gradually increase physical activity as the symptoms of Parkinson's disease improve.

Avoid excessive alcohol usage, because it may increase the potential for CNS effects such as dizziness, confusion, lightheadedness, and orthostatic hypotension.

Avoid getting up suddenly from a sitting or lying position. If dizziness or lightheadedness occurs, notify physician.

Notify physician if mood/mental changes, swelling of extremities, difficulty urinating, or shortness of breath occurs.

Do not take more medication than prescribed because of the risk of overdose. If there is no improvement in a few days, or if medication appears less effective after a few weeks, discuss with a physician.

Consult physician before discontinuing medication.

Seek medical attention immediately if it is suspected that an overdose of medication has been taken.

CIDOFOVIR

Rx	**Vistide** (Gilead Sciences)	**Injection:** 75 mg/mL	Preservative free. In 5 mL single-use vials.

CIDOFOVIR — INJECTION

WARNING

Renal impairment is the major toxicity of cidofovir. Cases of acute renal failure resulting in dialysis or contributing to death have occurred with as few as 1 or 2 doses of cidofovir. To reduce possible nephrotoxicity, IV prehydration with normal saline and administration of probenecid must be used with each cidofovir infusion. Renal function (serum creatinine and urine protein) must be monitored within 48 hours prior to each dose of cidofovir and the dose of cidofovir modified for changes in renal function as appropriate (see Administration and Dosage). Cidofovir is contraindicated in patients who are receiving other nephrotoxic agents.

WARNING (cont.)

Neutropenia has been observed in association with cidofovir treatment. Therefore, neutrophil counts should be monitored during cidofovir therapy.

Cidofovir is indicated only for the treatment of cytomegalovirus (CMV) retinitis in patients with acquired immunodeficiency syndrome (AIDS).

In animal studies, cidofovir was carcinogenic, teratogenic and caused hypospermia (see Warnings, Carcinogenesis, Mutagenesis, and Fertility impairment).

Indications

➤*CMV retinitis:* Treatment of cytomegalovirus (CMV) retinitis in patients with AIDS. The safety and efficacy of cidofovir have not been established for

CIDOFOVIR — INJECTION

treatment of other CMV infections (such as pneumonitis or gastroenteritis), congenital or neonatal CMV disease, or CMV disease in non-HIV-infected individuals.

Administration and Dosage

➤*Approved by the FDA:* June 26, 1996.

Cidofovir must not be administered by intraocular injection.

➤*Dosage:* The recommended dosage, frequency, or infusion rate must not be exceeded. Cidofovir must be diluted in 100 mL 0.9% (normal) saline prior to administration. To minimize potential nephrotoxicity, probenecid, and IV saline prehydration must be administered with each cidofovir infusion.

➤*Induction treatment:* The recommended induction dose of cidofovir for patients with a serum creatinine of ≤ 1.5 mg/dL, a calculated creatinine clearance > 55 mL/min, and a urine protein < 100 mg/dL (equivalent to < 2+ proteinuria) is 5 mg/kg body weight (given as an IV infusion at a constant rate over 1 hour) administered once weekly for 2 consecutive weeks. Because serum creatinine in patients with advanced AIDS and CMV retinitis may not provide a complete picture of the patient's underlying renal status, it is important to utilize the Cockcroft-Gault formula to more precisely estimate creatinine clearance (Ccr). As creatinine clearance is dependent on serum creatinine and patient weight, it is necessary to calculate clearance prior to initiation of cidofovir. Ccr (mL/min) should be calculated according to the following formula:

$$\text{Ccr}_{\text{males}} = \frac{[140 \text{ - age (in years)}] \times [\text{body weight (in kg)}]}{72 \times [\text{serum creatinine (mg/dL)}]}.$$

$$\text{Ccr}_{\text{females}} = \frac{0.85 \times [140 \text{ - age (in years)}] \times [\text{body weight (in kg)}]}{72 \times [\text{serum creatinine (mg/dL)}]}.$$

➤*Maintenance treatment:* The recommended maintenance dose of cidofovir is 5 mg/kg body weight (given as an IV infusion at a constant rate over 1 hour), administered once every 2 weeks.

➤*Dose adjustment:*

Changes in renal function during cidofovir therapy – The maintenance dose of cidofovir must be reduced from 5 mg/kg to 3 mg/kg for an increase in serum creatinine of 0.3 to 0.4 mg/dL above baseline. Cidofovir therapy must be discontinued for an increase in serum creatinine of ≥ 0.5 mg/dL above baseline or development of ≥ 3+ proteinuria.

Renal function impairment – Cidofovir is contraindicated in patients with a serum creatinine concentration> 1.5 mg/dL, a calculated creatinine clearance ≤ 55 mL/min, or a urine protein ≥ 100 mg/dL (equivalent to ≥ 2+ proteinuria).

Probenecid – Probenecid must be administered orally with each cidofovir dose. Two grams must be administered 3 hours prior to the cidofovir dose and 1 g administered at 2 and again at 8 hours after completion of the 1 hour cidofovir infusion (for a total of 4 g).

Ingestion of food prior to each dose of probenecid may reduce drug-related nausea and vomiting. Administration of an antiemetic may reduce the potential for nausea associated with probenecid ingestion. In patients who develop allergic or hypersensitivity symptoms to probenecid, the use of an appropriate prophylactic or therapeutic antihistamine or acetaminophen should be considered (see Contraindications).

Hydration – Patients must receive at least 1 L of 0.9% (normal) saline solution IV with each infusion of cidofovir. The saline solution should be infused over a 1- to 2-hour period immediately before the cidofovir infusion. Patients who can tolerate the additional fluid load should receive a second liter. If administered, the second liter of saline should be initiated either at the start of the cidofovir infusion or immediately afterwards, and infused over a 1- to 3-hour period.

➤*Preparation and administration:* Inspect vials visually for particulate matter and discoloration prior to administration. If particulate matter or discoloration is observed, the vial should not be used. With a syringe, extract the appropriate volume of cidofovir from the vial and transfer the dose to an infusion bag containing 100 ml 0.9% (normal) saline solution. Infuse the entire volume IV into the patient at a constant rate over a 1-hour period. Use of a standard infusion pump for administration is recommended.

➤*Admixture incompatibility:* The chemical stability of cidofovir admixtures was demonstrated in polyvinyl chloride composition and ethylene/propylene copolymer composition commercial infusion bags, and in glass bottles. No data are available to support the addition of other drugs or supplements to the cidofovir admixture for concurrent administration.

Cidofovir is supplied in single-use vials. Partially used vials should be discarded.

➤*Handling and disposal:* Due to the mutagenic properties of cidofovir, adequate precautions including the use of appropriate safety equipment are recommended for the preparation, administration, and disposal of cidofovir. The National Institutes of Health presently recommends that such agents be prepared in a class II laminar flow biological safety cabinet and that personnel preparing drugs of this class wear surgical gloves and a closed front surgical-type gown with knit cuffs. If cidofovir contacts the skin, wash membranes, and flush thoroughly with water. Excess cidofovir and all other materials used in the admixture preparation and administration should be placed in a leak-proof, puncture-proof container. The recommended method of disposal is high temperature incineration.

➤*Storage/Stability:* Cidofovir should be stored at controlled room temperature (20° to 25°C; 68° to 77°F).

It is recommended that cidofovir infusion admixtures be administered within 24 hours of preparation and that refrigerator or freezer storage not be used to extend this 24-hour limit.

If admixtures are not intended for immediate use, they may be stored under refrigeration (2° to 8°C; 35.6° to 46.4°F) for no more than 24 hours. Refrigerated admixtures should be allowed to equilibrate to room temperature prior to use.

Actions

➤*Pharmacokinetics:*

Absorption/Distribution – Cidofovir must be administered with probenecid. The pharmacokinetics of cidofovir, administered both without and with probenecid, are described below.

In vitro, cidofovir was < 6% bound to plasma or serum proteins over the cidofovir concentration range 0.25 to 25 mcg/mL. Cerebrospinal fluid (CSF) concentrations of cidofovir following IV infusion of cidofovir 5 mg/kg with concomitant probenecid and IV hydration were undetectable (< 0.1 mcg/mL, assay detection threshold) at 15 minutes after the end of a 1-hour infusion in one patient whose corresponding serum concentration was 8.7 mcg/mL.

The pharmacokinetics of cidofovir without probenecid were evaluated in 27 HIV-infected patients with or without asymptomatic CMV infection. Dose-independent pharmacokinetics were demonstrated after 1-hour infusions of 1 (n = 5), 3 (n = 10), 5 (n = 2) and 10 (n = 8) mg/kg. There was no evidence of cidofovir accumulation after 4 weeks of repeated administration of 3 mg/kg/week (n = 5) without probenecid. In patients with healthy renal function, ≈ 80% to 100% of the cidofovir dose was recovered unchanged in urine within 24 hours (n = 27). The renal clearance of cidofovir was greater than creatinine clearance, indicating renal tubular secretion contributes to the elimination of cidofovir.

Cidofovir pharmacokinetic parameters following 3 and 5 mg/kg infusions without and with probenecid*

Parameters	Cidofovir injection administered without probenecid		Cidofovir for injection administered with probenecid	
	3 mg/kg (n = 10)	5 mg/kg (n = 2)	3 mg/kg (n = 12)	5 mg/kg (n = 6)
AUC (mcg•hr/mL)	20 ± 2.3	28.3	25.7 ± 8.5	40.8 ± 9
C_{max} (end of infusion) (mcg/mL)	7.3 ± 1.4	11.5	9.8 ± 3.7	19.6 ± 7.2
V_{dss} (mL/kg)	537 ± 126 (n = 12)		410 ± 102 (n = 18)	
Clearance (mL/min/1.73 m^2)	179 ± 23.1 (n = 12)		148 ± 38.8 (n = 18)	
Renal clearance (mL/min/1.73 m^2)	150 ± 26.9 (n = 12)		98.6 ± 27.9 (n = 11)	

* See Administration and Dosage.

Special populations –

Renal function impairment: Pharmacokinetic data collected from subjects with creatinine clearance values as low as 11 mL/min indicate that cidofovir clearance decreases proportionally with creatinine clearance.

High-flux hemodialysis has been shown to reduce the serum levels of cidofovir by ≈ 75%.

Initiation of therapy with cidofovir is contraindicated in patients with serum creatinine >1.5 mg/dL, a calculated creatinine clearance ≤ 55 mL/min, or a urine protein ≥ 100 mg/dL (equivalent to ≥ 2+ proteinuria) (see Contraindications).

Contraindications

Initiation of therapy in patients with a serum creatinine > 1.5 mg/dL, a calculated creatinine clearance ≤ 55 mL/min, or a urine protein ≥ 100 mg/dL (equivalent to ≥ 2+ proteinuria); in patients receiving agents with nephrotoxic potential (such agents must be discontinued at least 7 days prior to starting therapy with cidofovir); hypersensitivity to cidofovir or a history of clinically severe hypersensitivity to probenecid or other sulfa-containing medications; direct intraocular injection; direct injection of cidofovir has been associated with iritis, ocular hypotony, and permanent impairment of vision.

Warnings

➤*Hematological toxicity:* Neutropenia may occur during cidofovir therapy. Neutrophil count should be monitored while receiving cidofovir therapy.

➤*Decreased IOP/ocular hypotony:* Decreased intraocular pressure (IOP) may occur during cidofovir therapy, and in some instances has been associated with decreased visual acuity. IOP should be monitored during cidofovir therapy. Among the subset of patients monitored for intraocular pressure changes, a ≥ 50% decrease from baseline intraocular pressure was reported in 17 of 70 (24%) patients at the 5 mg/kg maintenance dose. Severe hypotony (intraocular pressure of 0 to 1 mm Hg) has been reported in 3 patients. Risk of ocular hypotony may be increased in patients with preexisting diabetes mellitus.

➤*Metabolic acidosis:* Decreased serum bicarbonate associated with proximal tubule injury and renal wasting syndrome (including Fanconi's syndrome) have been reported in patients receiving cidofovir (see Adverse Reactions). Mucormycosis, aspergillus, disseminated mycobacterial infection, cases of metabolic acidosis in association with liver dysfunction and pancreatitis resulting in death have been reported in patients receiving cidofovir.

➤*Nephrotoxicity:* Dose-dependent nephrotoxicity is the major dose-limiting toxicity related to cidofovir administration. Cases of acute renal failure resulting in dialysis or contributing to death have occurred with as few as 1 or 2 doses of cidofovir. Renal function (serum creatinine and urine protein) must be monitored within 48 hours prior to each dose of cidofovir.

CIDOFOVIR — INJECTION

Dose adjustment or discontinuation is required for changes in renal function (serum creatinine or urine protein) while on therapy. Proteinuria, as measured by urinalysis in a clinical laboratory, may be an early indicator of cidofovir-related nephrotoxicity. Continued administration of cidofovir may lead to additional proximal tubular cell injury, which may result in glycosuria, decreases in serum phosphate, uric acid, and bicarbonate, elevations in serum creatinine, or acute renal failure, in some cases, resulting in the need for dialysis. Patients with these adverse events occurring concurrently and meeting a criteria of Fanconi's syndrome have been reported. Renal function that did not return to baseline after drug discontinuation has been observed in clinical studies of cidofovir.

➤*Renal function impairment:* See Administration and Dosage for more information.

➤*Carcinogenesis:* In animal studies cidofovir was carcinogenic, teratogenic, and caused hypospermia.

Chronic, 2-year carcinogenicity studies in rats and mice have not been carried out to evaluate the carcinogenic potential of cidofovir. However, a 26-week toxicology study evaluating once weekly subscapular SC injections of cidofovir in rats was terminated at 19 weeks because of the induction, in females, of palpable masses, the first of which was detected after 6 doses. The masses were diagnosed as mammary adenocarcinomas which developed at doses as low as 0.6 mg/kg/week, equivalent to 0.04 times the human systemic exposure at the recommended IV cidofovir dose based on AUC comparisons.

In a 26-week IV toxicology study in which rats received 0.6, 3, or 15 mg/kg cidofovir once weekly, a significant increase in mammary adenocarcinomas in female rats as well as a significant incidence of Zymbal's gland carcinomas in male and female rats were seen at the high dose but not at the lower 2 doses. The high dose was equivalent to 1.1 times the human systemic exposure at the recommended dose of cidofovir, based on comparisons of AUC measurements. In light of the results of these studies, cidofovir should be considered to be a carcinogen in rats as well as a potential carcinogen in humans.

➤*Mutagenesis:* An increase in micronucleated polychromatic erythrocytes in vivo was seen in mice receiving ≥ 2000 mg/kg, a dosage ≈ 65-fold higher than the maximum recommended clinical IV cidofovir dose based on body surface area estimations. Cidofovir induced chromosomal aberrations in human peripheral blood lymphocytes in vitro without metabolic activation. At the 4 cidofovir levels tested, the percentage of damaged metaphases and number of aberrations per cell increased in a concentration-dependent manner.

➤*Fertility impairment:* Studies showed that cidofovir caused inhibition of spermatogenesis in rats and monkeys. However, no adverse effects on fertility or reproduction were seen following once-weekly IV injections of cidofovir in male rats for 13 consecutive weeks at doses up to 15 mg/kg/week (equivalent to 1.1 times the recommended human dose based on AUC comparisons). Female rats dosed IV once weekly at 1.2 mg/kg/week (equivalent to 0.09 times the recommended human dose based on AUC) or higher, for up to 6 weeks prior to mating and for 2 weeks post mating had decreased litter sizes and live births per litter and increased early resorptions per litter. Peri- and post-natal development studies in which female rats received SC injections of cidofovir once daily at doses up to 1 mg/kg/day from day 7 of gestation through day 21 postpartum (≈ 5 weeks) resulted in no adverse effects on viability, growth, behavior, sexual maturation or reproductive capacity in the offspring.

➤*Elderly:* No studies of the safety or efficacy of cidofovir in patients over the age of 60 have been conducted. Since elderly individuals frequently have reduced glomerular filtration, particular attention should be paid to assessing renal function before and during cidofovir administration (see Administration and Dosage).

➤*Pregnancy: Category C.* Cidofovir was embryotoxic (reduced fetal body weights) in rats at 1.5 mg/kg/day and in rabbits at 1 mg/kg/day, doses which were also maternally toxic, following daily IV dosing during the period of organogenesis. The no-observable-effect levels for embryotoxicity in rats (0.5 mg/kg/day) and in rabbits (0.25 mg/kg/day) were ≈ 0.04 and 0.05 times the clinical dose (5 mg/kg every other week) based on AUC, respectively. An increased incidence of fetal external, soft tissue, and skeletal anomalies (meningocele, short snout, and short maxillary bones) occurred in rabbits at the high dose (1 mg/kg/day) which was also maternally toxic. There are no adequate and well-controlled studies in pregnant women. Cidofovir should be used during pregnancy only if the potential benefit justifies the potential risk to the fetus.

➤*Lactation:* It is not known whether cidofovir is excreted in human milk. Since many drugs are excreted in human milk and because of the potential for adverse reactions as well as the potential for tumorigenicity shown for cidofovir in animal studies, cidofovir should not be administered to nursing mothers. The US Public Health Service Centers for Disease Control and Prevention advises HIV-infected women not to breastfeed to avoid postnatal transmission of HIV to a child who may not yet be infected.

➤*Children:* Safety and efficacy in children have not been studied. The use of cidofovir in children with AIDS warrants extreme caution due to the risk of long-term carcinogenicity and reproductive toxicity. Administration of cidofovir to children should be undertaken only after careful evaluation and only if the potential benefits of treatment outweigh the risks.

Precautions

➤*Monitoring:* Serum creatinine and urine protein must be monitored within 48 hours prior to each dose. White blood cell counts with differential should be monitored prior to each dose. In patients with proteinuria, IV hydration should be administered and the test repeated. Intraocular pressure, visual acuity, and ocular symptoms should be monitored periodically.

➤*IV infusion only:* Cidofovir is formulated for IV infusion only and must not be administered by intraocular injection. Administration of cidofovir by infusion must be accompanied by oral probenecid and IV saline prehydration (see Administration and Dosage).

➤*Uveitis/iritis:* Uveitis or iritis was reported in clinical trials and during postmarketing in patients receiving cidofovir therapy. Treatment with topical corticosteroids with or without topical cycloplegic agents should be considered. Patients should be monitored for signs and symptoms of uveitis/iritis during cidofovir therapy.

Drug Interactions

➤*Nephrotoxic agents:* Concomitant administration of cidofovir and agents with nephrotoxic potential (eg, IV aminoglycosides [eg, tobramycin, gentamicin, and amikacin], amphotericin B, foscarnet, IV pentamidine, vancomycin, and nonsteroidal anti-inflammatory agents) is contraindicated. Such agents must be discontinued at least 7 days prior to starting therapy with cidofovir.

Adverse Reactions

➤*Nephrotoxicity:* Renal toxicity, as manifested by ≥ 2+ proteinuria, serum creatinine elevations of ≥ 0.4 mg/dL, or decreased creatinine clearance ≤ 55 mL/min, occurred in 79 of 135 (59%) patients receiving cidofovir at a maintenance dose of 5 mg/kg every other week. Maintenance dose reductions from 5 mg/kg to 3 mg/kg due to proteinuria or serum creatinine elevations were made in 12 of 41 (29%) patients who had not received prior therapy for CMV retinitis (Study 106) and in 19 of 74 (26%) patients who had received prior therapy for CMV retinitis (Study 107). Prior foscarnet use has been associated with an increased risk of nephrotoxicity; therefore, such patients must be monitored closely (see Contraindications, Warnings, Administration and Dosage).

➤*Neutropenia:* In clinical trials, at the 5 mg/kg maintenance dose, a decrease in absolute neutrophil count to ≤ 500 cells/mm^3 occurred in 24% of patients. Granulocyte colony-stimulating factor (G-CSF) was used in 39% of patients.

➤*Decreased IOP/ocular hypotony:* Among the subset of patients monitored for IOP changes, a ≥ 50% decrease from baseline IOP was reported in 17 of 70 (24%) patients at the 5 mg/kg maintenance dose. Severe hypotony (intraocular pressure of 0 to 1 mmHg) has been reported in 3 patients. Risk of ocular hypotony may be increased in patients with preexisting diabetes mellitus.

➤*Anterior uveitis/iritis:* Uveitis or iritis has been reported in clinical trials and during postmarketing in patients receiving cidofovir therapy. Uveitis or iritis was reported in 15 of 135 (11%) patients receiving 5 mg/kg maintenance dosing. Treatment with topical corticosteroids with or without topical cycloplegic agents may be considered. Patients should be monitored for signs and symptoms of uveitis/iritis during cidofovir therapy.

➤*Metabolic acidosis:* A diagnosis of Fanconi's syndrome, as manifested by multiple abnormalities of proximal renal tubular function, was reported in 1% of patients. Decreases in serum bicarbonate to ≤ 16 mEq/L occurred in 16% of cidofovir-treated patients. Cases of metabolic acidosis in association with liver dysfunction and pancreatitis resulting in death have been reported in patients receiving cidofovir.

Lab test abnormalities – In clinical trials, cidofovir was withdrawn due to adverse events in 39% of patients treated with 5 mg/kg every other week as maintenance therapy.

The incidence of adverse reactions reported as serious in 3 controlled clinical studies in patients with CMV retinitis, regardless of presumed relationship to drug, is listed in the table below.

Serious clinical adverse reactions or laboratory abnormalities occurring in > 5% of patients	
	n = 135 [a] # of patients (%)
Proteinuria (≥ 100 mg/dL)	68 (50%)
Neutropenia (≤ 500 cells/mm^3)	33 (24%)
Decreased intraocular pressure [b]	17 (24%)
Decreased serum bicarbonate (≤ 16 mEq/L)	21 (16%)
Fever	19 (14%)
Infection	16 (12%)
Creatinine elevation (≥ 2 mg/dL)	16 (12%)
Pneumonia	12 (9%)
Dyspnea	11 (8%)
Nausea/vomiting	10 (7%)

[a] Patients receiving 5 mg/kg maintenance regimen in studies 105, 106 and 107.
[b] Defined as decreased IOP to ≤ 50% that at baseline. Based on 70 patients receiving 5 mg/kg maintenance dosing (studies 105, 106 and 107) for whom baseline and follow-up IOP determinations were recorded.

➤*Observed adverse reactions/intercurrent illnesses in clinical trials (causal relationship unknown):* The following adverse reactions/intercurrent illnesses have been observed in clinical studies of cidofovir and are listed below regardless of causal relationship to cidofovir. Evaluation of these reports was difficult because of the diverse manifestations of the underlying disease and because most patients received numerous concomitant medicines.

Cardiovascular – Cardiomyopathy, cardiovascular disorder, congestive heart failure, hypertension, hypotension, migraine, pallor, peripheral vascu-

CIDOFOVIR — INJECTION

lar disorder, phlebitis, postural hypotension, shock, syncope, tachycardia, vascular disorder, and edema.

CNS – Abnormal dreams, abnormal gait, acute brain syndrome, agitation, amnesia, anxiety, ataxia, cerebrovascular disorder, confusion, convulsion, delirium, dementia, depression, dizziness, drug dependence, dry mouth, encephalopathy, facial paralysis, hallucinations, headache, hemiplegia, hyperesthesia, hypertonia, hypotony, incoordination, increased libido, insomnia, myoclonus, nervousness, neuropathy, paresthesia, personality disorder, somnolence, speech disorder, tremor, twitching, vasodilatation, and vertigo.

Dermatologic – Acne, alopecia, angioedema, dry skin, eczema, exfoliative dermatitis, furunculosis, herpes simplex, nail disorder, pruritus, rash, seborrhea, skin discoloration, skin disorder, skin hypertrophy, skin ulcer, sweating, and urticaria.

Endocrine – Adrenal cortex insufficiency.

GI – Anorexia, abdominal pain, cholangitis, colitis, constipation, esophagitis, diarrhea, dry mouth, dyspepsia, dysphagia, fecal incontinence, flatulence, gastritis, GI hemorrhage, gingivitis, hepatitis, hepatomegaly, hepatosplenomegaly, jaundice, abnormal liver function, liver damage, liver necrosis, melena, oral candidiasis, pancreatitis, proctitis, rectal disorder, stomatitis, aphthous stomatitis, tongue discoloration, mouth ulceration, and tooth caries.

GU – Decreased creatinine clearance, dysuria, glycosuria, hematuria, kidney stone, mastitis, metorrhagia, nocturia, polyuria, prostatic disorder, toxic nephrophathy, urethritis, urinary casts, urinary incontinence, urinary retention, and urinary tract infection.

Hematologic/Lymphatic – Hypochromic anemia, leukocytosis, leukopenia, lymphadenopathy, lymphoma like reaction, pancytopenia, splenic disorder, splenomegaly, thrombocytopenia, and thrombocytopenic purpura.

Metabolic/Nutritional – Cachexia, dehydration, edema, hypercalcemia, hyperglycemia, hyperkalemia, hyperlipemia, hypocalcemia, hypoglycemia, hypoglycemic reaction, hypokalemia, hypomagnesemia, hyponatremia, hypophosphatemia, hypoproteinemia, increased alkaline phosphatase, increased BUN, increased lactic dehydrogenase, increased AST, increased ALT, peripheral edema, respiratory alkalosis, thirst, weight loss, and weight gain.

Musculoskeletal – Arthralgia, arthrosis, bone necrosis, bone pain, joint disorder, leg cramps, myalgia, myasthenia, and pathological fracture.

Respiratory – Asthma, bronchitis, coughing, epistaxis, hemoptysis, hiccup, hyperventilation, hypoxia, increased sputum, larynx edema, lung disorder, pharyngitis, pneumothorax, rhinitis, and sinusitis.

Special senses – Abnormal vision, amblyopia, blindness, cataract, conjunctivitis, corneal lesion, corneal opacity, diplopia, dry eyes, ear disorder, ear pain, eye disorder, eye pain, hypotony, hyperacusis, iritis, keratitis, miosis, otitis externa, otitis media, refraction disorder, retinal detachment, retinal disorder, taste perversion, tinnitus, uveitis, visual field defect, and hearing loss.

Miscellaneous – Abdominal pain, accidental injury, AIDS, allergic reaction, back pain, catheter blocked, cellulitis, chest pain, chills and fever, cryptococcosis, cyst, death, face edema, flu-like syndrome, hypothermia, injection site reaction, malaise, mucous membrane disorder, neck pain, overdose, photosensitivity reaction, sarcoma, and sepsis.

➤*Most frequently reported adverse reactions, regardless of relationship to study drugs or severity:* The most frequently reported adverse events regardless of relationship to study drugs (cidofovir or probenecid) or severity are shown in the table below.

All clinical adverse reactions, laboratory abnormalities or intercurrent illnesses regardless of severity occurring in > 15% of patients	n = 115 [a] # of patients (%)
Any adverse reaction	115 (100%)
Proteinuria (≥ 30 mg/dL)	101 (88%)
Nausea with or without vomiting	79 (69%)
Fever	67 (58%)
Neutropenia (< 750 cells/mm^3)	50 (43%)
Asthenia	50 (43%)
Headache	34 (30%)
Rash	34 (30%)
Infection	32 (28%)
Alopecia	31 (27%)
Diarrhea	30 (26%)
Pain	29 (25%)
Creatinine elevation (> 1.5 mg/dL)	28 (24%)
Anemia	28 (24%)
Anorexia	26 (23%)
Dyspnea	26 (23%)
Chills	25 (22%)
Increased cough	22 (19%)
Oral moniliasis	21 (18%)

[a] Patients receiving 5 mg/kg maintenance regimen in studies 106 and 107.

➤*Reporting of adverse reactions:* Malignancies or serious adverse reactions that occur in patients who have received cidofovir should be reported to patients' healthcare providers.

Overdosage

➤*Symptoms:* Two cases of cidofovir overdose have been reported. These patients received single doses of cidofovir at 16.3 mg/kg and 17.4 mg/kg, respectively, with concomitant oral probenecid and IV hydration. Significant changes in renal function were not observed in either patient.

➤*Treatment:* In both cases, the patients were hospitalized and received oral probenecid (1 g 3 times daily) and vigorous IV hydration with normal saline for 3 to 5 days.

Patient Information

Patients should be advised that cidofovir is not a cure for CMV retinitis, and that they may continue to experience progression of retinitis during and following treatment. Patients receiving cidofovir should be advised to have regular follow-up ophthalmologic examinations. Patients may also experience other manifestations of CMV disease despite cidofovir therapy.

HIV-infected patients may continue taking antiretroviral therapy, but those taking zidovudine should be advised to temporarily discontinue zidovudine administration or decrease their zidovudine dose by 50%, on days of cidofovir administration only, because probenecid reduces metabolic clearance of zidovudine.

Patients should be informed of the major toxicity of cidofovir, namely renal impairment, and that dose modification, including reduction, interruption, and possibly discontinuation, may be required. Close monitoring of renal function (routine urinalysis and serum creatinine) while on therapy should be emphasized.

The importance of completing a full course of probenecid with each cidofovir dose should be emphasized. Patients should be warned of potential adverse events caused by probenecid (eg, headache, nausea, vomiting, hypersensitivity reactions). Hypersensitivity/allergic reactions may include rash, fever, chills, and anaphylaxis. Administration of probenecid after a meal or use of antiemetics may decrease the nausea. Prophylactic or therapeutic antihistamines or acetaminophen can be used to ameliorate hypersensitivity reactions.

Patients should be advised that cidofovir causes tumors, primarily mammary adenocarcinomas, in rats. Cidofovir should be considered a potential carcinogen in humans (see Warnings). Women should be advised of the limited enrollment of women in clinical trials of cidofovir.

Patients should be advised that cidofovir caused reduced testes weight and hypospermia in animals. Such changes may occur in humans and cause infertility. Women of childbearing potential should be advised that cidofovir is embryotoxic in animals and should not be used during pregnancy. Women of childbearing potential should be advised to use effective contraception during and for 1 month following treatment with cidofovir. Men should be advised to practice barrier contraceptive methods during and for 3 months after treatment with cidofovir.

RIBAVIRIN

Rx	**Ribavirin** (Various, eg, Par, Teva)	**Tablets**: 200 mg	In 168s.
Rx	**Copegus** (Roche)		(RIB 200 ROCHE). Lt. pink to pink, oval. Film-coated. In 168s.
Rx	**Ribaspheres** (Three Rivers)		Lactose. (200 3RP). Lt. blue, capsule shape. Film-coated. In 168s and 500s.
Rx	**Ribaspheres** (Three Rivers)	**Tablets**: 400 mg	Lactose. (400 3RP). Medium blue, capsule shape. Film-coated. In 56s and 500s.
Rx	**Ribatab** (PRX Pharmaceuticals)		Lactose. (400 3RP). Medium blue, capsule shape. Film-coated. In UD 14s.
Rx	**Ribaspheres** (Three Rivers)	**Tablets**: 600 mg	Lactose. (600 3RP). Dk. blue, capsule shape. Film-coated. In 56s and 250s.
Rx	**Ribatab** (PRX Pharmaceuticals)		Lactose. (600 3RP). Dk. blue, capsule shape. Film-coated. In UD 14s.[a]

RIBAVIRIN

Rx	**Ribavirin** (Various, eg, Sandoz, Teva)	**Capsules:** 200 mg	In 42s, 56s, 70s, 84s, and 100s.
Rx	**Rebetol** (Schering)		Lactose. (REBETOL 200 mg). White. In 42s, 56s, 70s, and 84s.
Rx	**Ribaspheres** (Three Rivers)		Pellet filled. Lactose. (riba 200). Opaque white. In 42s, 56s, 70s, and 84s.
Rx	**Rebetol** (Schering)	**Oral solution:** 40 mg/mL	Sucrose, sorbitol. Bubble gum flavor. In 100 mL.
Rx	**Virazole** (ICN)	**Lyophilized powder for aerosol reconstitution:** 6 g ribavirin/ 100 mL vial. Contains 20 mg/mL when reconstituted with 300 mL sterile water.	In vials.

[a] Also available in a 400 mg and 600 mg combination package (1,000 mg/day).

RIBAVIRIN — ORAL

WARNING

Capsules/Tablets/Oral solution – Ribavirin monotherapy is not effective for the treatment of chronic hepatitis C virus (HCV) infection and should not be used alone for this indication.

The primary toxicity of ribavirin is hemolytic anemia that may result in worsening of cardiac disease and lead to fatal and nonfatal myocardial infarctions (MIs). Do not treat patients with a history of significant or unstable cardiac disease with ribavirin.

Significant teratogenic and/or embryocidal effects have been demonstrated in all animal species exposed to ribavirin. In addition, ribavirin has a multiple-dose half-life of 12 days, and it may persist in nonplasma compartments for as long as 6 months. Therefore, ribavirin therapy is contraindicated in women who are pregnant and in the male partners of women who are pregnant. Extreme care must be taken to avoid pregnancy during therapy and for 6 months after completion of treatment in these individuals. At least 2 reliable forms of effective contraception must be used during treatment and during the 6-month posttreatment follow-up period.

Indications

➤*Tablets:*

Chronic HCV – In combination with peginterferon alfa-2a for the treatment of adults with chronic HCV infection who have compensated liver disease and have not been previously treated with interferon alpha. Patients in whom efficacy was demonstrated included patients with compensated liver disease and histological evidence of cirrhosis (Child-Pugh class A).

➤*Capsules/Oral solution:*

Chronic HCV – In combination with interferon alfa-2b injection for the treatment of chronic HCV in patients 3 years of age (oral solution) or 5 years of age (capsules) and older with compensated liver disease previously untreated with alpha interferon or in patients who have relapsed following alpha interferon therapy. Note: *Ribasphere* is only indicated in combination with interferon alfa-2b in patients 18 years of age and older.

In combination with peginterferon alfa-2b injection for the treatment of chronic HCV in patients with compensated liver disease who have not been previously treated with interferon alpha and are at least 18 years of age.

The safety and efficacy of ribavirin capsules or oral solution with interferons other than interferon alfa-2b or peginterferon alfa-2b products have not been established.

Children – Consider evidence of disease progression, such as hepatic inflammation and fibrosis, as well as prognostic factors for response, HCV genotype, and viral load, when deciding to treat a pediatric patient. Weigh the benefits of treatment against the safety findings observed for pediatric patients in clinical trials.

➤*Unlabeled uses:* Treatment of viral hemorrhagic fevers such as Lassa fever or hemorrhagic fever with renal syndrome.

Administration and Dosage

➤*Tablets:* The daily dose of ribavirin tablets is 800 to 1,200 mg administered orally in 2 divided doses with food. Individualize the dose depending on baseline disease characteristics (eg, genotype), response to therapy, and tolerability of the regimen.

Peginterferon Alfa-2a and Ribavirin Tablet Dosing Recommendations

Genotype[a]	Peginterferon alfa-2a dose	Ribavirin tablet dose	Duration
Genotype 1, 4	180 mcg	< 75 kg = 1,000 mg	48 wk
		≥ 75 kg = 1,200 mg	48 wk
Genotype 2, 3	180 mcg	800 mg	24 wk

[a] Genotypes non-1 showed no increased response to treatment beyond 24 weeks. Data on genotypes 5 and 6 are insufficient for dosing recommendations.

Duration – The recommended duration of treatment for patients previously untreated with ribavirin and interferon is 24 to 48 weeks.

Dose modifications – If severe adverse reactions or laboratory abnormalities develop during combination ribavirin tablets/peginterferon alfa-2a therapy, modify or discontinue the dose, if appropriate, until the adverse reactions abate. If intolerance persists after dose adjustment, discontinue ribavirin tablet/peginterferon alfa-2a therapy.

Ribavirin Tablet Dosage Modification Guidelines

Laboratory values	Reduce ribavirin tablet dose to 600 mg/day[a] if:	Discontinue ribavirin tablets if:
Hemoglobin in patients with no cardiac disease	< 10 g/dL	< 8.5 g/dL
Hemoglobin in patients with history of stable cardiac disease	≥ 2 g/dL decrease in hemoglobin during any 4-wk treatment period	< 12 g/dL despite 4 wk at reduced dose

[a] One 200 mg tablet in the morning and either two 200 mg tablets or one 400 mg tablet in the evening.

Once ribavirin tablets have been withheld because of a laboratory abnormality or clinical manifestation, an attempt may be made to restart ribavirin tablets at 600 mg/day and further increase the dose to 800 mg/day depending upon the health care provider's judgement. However, it is not recommended that ribavirin tablets be increased to the original assigned dose (1,000 to 1,200 mg).

Renal function impairment – Do not use ribavirin tablets in patients with creatinine clearance (Ccr) less than 50 mL/min.

Special populations – Administer ribavirin tablets with caution to patients with preexisting cardiac disease. Assess patients before commencement of therapy and appropriately monitor them during therapy. If there is any deterioration of cardiovascular status, stop therapy.

➤*Capsules/Oral solution:* Clinical studies with ribavirin/interferon alfa-2b were conducted without instructions with respect to food consumption. When given with interferon alfa-2b, ribavirin may be given without regard to food, but should be administered in a consistent manner with respect to food intake. During clinical studies with ribavirin/peginterferon alfa-2b, all subjects were instructed to take ribavirin capsules with food. When given in combination with peginterferon alfa-2b, it is recommended that ribavirin be administered in the evening with food.

Do not open, crush, or break capsules.

Ribavirin/Interferon alfa-2b combination –

Adults: The recommended dosing of ribavirin capsules depends on the patient's body weight and is provided in the table below:

Recommended Adult Dosing for Ribavirin Capsules

Body weight	Ribavirin capsules
≤ 75 kg	2 × 200 mg capsules AM, 3 × 200 mg capsules PM daily by mouth
> 75 kg	3 × 200 mg capsules AM, 3 × 200 mg capsules PM daily by mouth

Children: The recommended dose is 15 mg/kg/day orally (divided dose AM and PM). For children weighing 25 kg or less or who cannot swallow capsules, ribavirin oral solution is supplied in a concentration of 40 mg/mL. For children weighing more than 25 kg, administer either the oral solution or 200 mg capsule.

Pediatric Dosing for Interferon Alfa-2b and Ribavirin

Body weight	Ribavirin capsules	Interferon alfa-2b injection
25 to 36 kg	1 × 200 mg capsules AM, 1 × 200 mg capsules PM daily by mouth	3 million units/m² 3 times weekly subcutaneously
37 to 49 kg	1 × 200 mg capsules AM, 2 × 200 mg capsules PM daily by mouth	3 million units/m² 3 times weekly subcutaneously
50 to 61 kg	2 × 200 mg capsules AM, 2 × 200 mg capsules PM daily by mouth	3 million units/m² 3 times weekly subcutaneously
> 61 kg	Refer to adult dosing table	Refer to adult dosing table

Ribavirin/Peginterferon alfa-2b combination (adults) – The recommended dose of ribavirin capsules is 800 mg/day in 2 divided doses: 2 capsules (400 mg) in the morning with food and 2 capsules (400 mg) in the evening with food.

Dose modifications – If severe adverse reactions or laboratory abnormalities develop during combination therapy, modify or discontinue the dose, if

RIBAVIRIN — ORAL

appropriate, until the adverse reactions abate. If intolerance persists after dose adjustment, discontinue combination therapy.

A permanent dose reduction is required for patients with a history of stable cardiovascular disease if the hemoglobin decreases by 2 g/dL or more during any 4-week period. In addition, discontinue combination therapy in patients with a cardiac history if the hemoglobin remains less than 12 g/dL after 4 weeks on a reduced dose.

It is recommended that patients whose hemoglobin level falls below 10 g/dL have their ribavirin dose reduced to 600 mg/day (1 × 200 mg capsule AM, 2 × 200 mg capsules PM) for adults and 7.5 mg/kg/day (divided dose AM and PM) for pediatric patients. Permanently discontinue ribavirin therapy in patients whose hemoglobin level falls below 8.5 g/dL.

Ribavirin Guidelines for Dose Modifications and Discontinuation for Anemia Based on Hemoglobin Levels

Laboratory values	Dose reduction of ribavirin capsules 600 mg/day for adults and 7.5 mg/kg/day for pediatrics	Permanent discontinuation of ribavirin treatment
Hemoglobin in patients with no cardiac history	< 10 g/dL	< 8.5 g/dL
Hemoglobin in patients with a cardiac history	≥ 2 g/dL decrease during any 4-wk period during treatment	< 12 g/dL after 4 wk of dose reduction

Renal function impairment: Do not use ribavirin in patients with Ccr less than 50 mL/min.

Duration – The recommended duration of treatment for patients previously untreated with interferon is 24 to 48 weeks. Individualize the duration of the patient's treatment depending on baseline disease characteristics, response to therapy, and tolerability of the regimen. Assess virologic response after 24 weeks of treatment. Consider treatment discontinuation in any patient who has not achieved an HCV RNA below the limit of detection of the assay by 24 weeks. The recommended duration of treatment is 48 weeks for pediatric patients with genotype 1 and 24 weeks for genotype 2/3. There are no safety and efficacy data on treatment for longer than 48 weeks in the previously untreated patient population.

Therapy relapse – In patients who relapse following interferon therapy, the recommended duration of treatment is 24 weeks. There are no safety and efficacy data on treatment for longer than 24 weeks in the relapsed patient population.

➤*Storage/Stability:*

Capsules/Tablets – Store at 25°C (77°F); excursions are permitted between 15° and 30°C (59° and 86°F). Keep bottle tightly closed.

Oral solution – Store at 2° to 8°C (36° to 46°F) or at 77°F; excursions are permitted between 15° and 30°C (59° and 86°F).

Actions

➤*Pharmacology:* Ribavirin is a synthetic nucleoside analog. The mechanism by which the combination of ribavirin and an interferon product exerts its effect against HCV has not been fully established.

➤*Pharmacokinetics:*

Absorption –

Tablets: After administration of 1,200 mg/day with food for 12 weeks, the $AUC_{0-12\ h}$ was 25,361 ng•h/mL and C_{max} was 2,748 ng/mL. The average time to reach C_{max} was 2 hours. There is extensive accumulation after multiple dosing (twice daily) such that the C_{max} at steady state was 4-fold higher than that of a single dose.

Capsules: Ribavirin was rapidly and extensively absorbed following oral administration. However, because of first-pass metabolism, the absolute bioavailability averaged 64%.

Distribution –

Capsules: Upon multiple oral dosing, based on $AUC_{12\ h}$, a 6-fold accumulation of ribavirin was observed in plasma. Following oral dosing with 600 mg twice daily, steady-state was reached by about 4 weeks, with mean steady-state plasma concentrations of 2,200 ng/mL.

Metabolism –

Capsules: Ribavirin has 2 pathways of metabolism: (1) a reversible phosphorylation pathway in nucleated cells and (2) a degradative pathway involving deribosylation and amide hydrolysis to yield a triazole carboxylic acid metabolite.

Excretion –

Tablets: The terminal half-life following a single dose administration is approximately 120 to 170 hours. The total apparent clearance is about 26 L/hour.

Capsules: Ribavirin and its triazole carboxamide and triazole carboxylic acid metabolites are excreted renally. After oral administration of 600 mg ribavirin, about 61% and 12% was eliminated in the urine and feces, respectively, in 336 hours. Unchanged ribavirin accounted for 17% of the administered dose. Upon discontinuation of dosing, the mean half-life was 298 hours, which probably reflects slow elimination from nonplasma compartments.

Special populations –

Renal function impairment:

• *Capsules/Oral solution* – The pharmacokinetics of ribavirin were assessed after administration of a single oral dose (400 mg) of ribavirin to non–HCV-infected subjects with varying degrees of renal dysfunction. The mean AUC value was 3-fold greater in subjects with Ccr values between 10 to 30 mL/min when compared with control subjects (Ccr more than 90 mL/min). In subjects with Ccr values between 30 to 60 mL/min, AUC was 2-fold greater when compared with control subjects. The increased AUC appears to be because of reduction of renal and nonrenal clearance in these patients. Phase 3 efficacy trials included subjects with Ccr values more than 50 mL/min. The multiple-dose pharmacokinetics of ribavirin cannot be accurately predicted in patients with renal dysfunction. Ribavirin is not effectively removed by hemodialysis. Do not treat patients with Ccr less than 50 mL/min with ribavirin.

Hepatic function impairment:

• *Capsules/Oral solution* – The mean C_{max} values increased with severity of hepatic dysfunction and was 2-fold greater in subjects with severe hepatic dysfunction when compared with control subjects.

Contraindications

➤*Tablets/Capsules/Oral solution:* Hypersensitivity to the drug or its components; patients with hemoglobinopathies (eg, thalassemia major, sickle-cell anemia).

Ribavirin may cause birth defects and/or death of the exposed fetus. Ribavirin capsules are contraindicated in women who are pregnant or in men whose female partners are pregnant (see Warnings).

Ribavirin tablets/Peginterferon alfa-2a – Ribavirin tablets/peginterferon alfa-2a combination therapy is contraindicated in patients with autoimmune hepatitis and hepatic decompensation (Child-Pugh class B and C) before or during treatment.

Ribavirin capsules/oral solution/interferon alfa-2b – Patients with autoimmune hepatitis must not be treated with combination ribavirin capsules/interferon alfa-2b therapy because using these medicines can make the hepatitis worse.

Warnings

➤*Monotherapy (capsules/tablets/oral solution):* Based on results of clinical trials, ribavirin monotherapy is not effective for the treatment of chronic HCV infection. Therefore, ribavirin must not be used alone. The safety and efficacy of ribavirin capsules and oral solution have been established only when used with interferon alfa-2b as interferon alfa-2b/ribavirin combination therapy or with peginterferon alfa-2b injection. The safety and efficacy of ribavirin tablets have been established only when used with pegylated interferon alfa-2a.

➤*Combination therapy adverse events (capsules/tablets/oral solution):* There are significant adverse events caused by ribavirin capsules/interferon alfa-2b or peginterferon alfa-2b therapy and by ribavirin tablets/peginterferon alfa-2a therapy, including severe depression and suicidal ideation, hemolytic anemia, suppression of bone marrow function, autoimmune and infectious disorders, pulmonary dysfunction, pancreatitis, and diabetes. Review the interferon alfa-2b/ribavirin capsule combination therapy, peginterferon alfa-2b, and peginterferon alfa-2a package inserts in their entirety prior to initiation of combination treatment for additional safety information.

➤*Pancreatitis (capsules/tablets/oral solution):* Suspend ribavirin, interferon alfa-2b, peginterferon alfa-2b, or peginterferon alfa-2a therapy in patients with signs and symptoms of pancreatitis and discontinue in patients with confirmed pancreatitis.

➤*Renal function impairment (capsules/tablets/oral solution):* See Administration and Dosage for more information.

➤*Suicidal ideation (capsules/oral solution):* Severe psychiatric adverse events including depression, psychoses, aggressive behavior, hallucinations, violent behavior (suicidal ideation, suicidal attempts, suicides) and rare instances of homicidal ideation have occurred during combination ribavirin capsules/*Intron A* therapy, both in patients with and without a previous psychiatric disorder. Use ribavirin capsules/*Intron A* therapy with extreme caution in patients with a history of preexisting psychiatric disorders, and carefully monitor all patients for evidence of depression and other psychiatric symptoms. Consider suspending ribavirin capsules/*Intron A* therapy if psychiatric intervention and/or dose reduction is unsuccessful in controlling psychiatric symptoms. In severe cases, immediately stop therapy and seek psychiatric intervention.

➤*Pulmonary effects:* Pulmonary symptoms, including dyspnea, pulmonary infiltrates, pneumonitis, and pneumonia have been reported during therapy with ribavirin and interferon. Occasional cases of fatal pneumonia have occurred. In addition, sarcoidosis or the exacerbation of sarcoidosis has been reported. If there is evidence of pulmonary infiltrates or pulmonary function impairment, closely monitor the patient and, if appropriate, discontinue treatment.

➤*Hemolytic anemia:* The primary toxicity of ribavirin is hemolytic anemia (hemoglobin less than 10 g/dL), which was observed in about 10% of ribavirin capsules/interferon alfa-2b-treated patients and about 13% in ribavirin tablets/peginterferon alfa-2a-treated patients in clinical trials (see Adverse Reactions). The anemia associated with ribavirin occurs within 1 to 2 weeks of initiation of therapy. Because the initial drop in hemoglobin may be significant, it is advised that hemoglobin or hematocrit be obtained pretreatment and at weeks 2 and 4 of therapy, or more frequently if clinically indicated. Then follow patients as clinically appropriate.

➤*Cardiovascular effects:* Fatal and nonfatal MIs have been reported in patients with anemia caused by ribavirin. Assess patients for underlying cardiac disease before initiation of ribavirin therapy and appropriately monitor them during therapy. If there is any deterioration of cardiovascular status, suspend or discontinue therapy (see Administration and Dosage). Because cardiac disease may be worsened by drug-induced anemia, patients with a history of significant or unstable cardiac disease should not use ribavirin.

RIBAVIRIN — ORAL

➤*Carcinogenesis:* Ribavirin has produced positive findings in multiple in vitro and animal in vivo genotoxicity assays, and should be considered a potential carcinogen.

➤*Mutagenesis:*
Tablets: The in vitro mouse lymphoma assay demonstrated mutagenic activity. Results from studies showed clastogenic activity in the in vivo mouse micronucleus assay at oral doses up to 2,000 mg/kg.
Capsules/Oral solution: Ribavirin demonstrated increased incidences of mutation and cell transformation in multiple genotoxicity assays. Mutagenic activity was observed in the mouse lymphoma assay and at doses of 20 to 200 mg/kg (estimated human equivalent of 1.67 to 16.7 mg/kg, based on body surface area adjustment for a 60 kg adult; 0.1 to 1 times the maximum recommended human 24-hour dose of ribavirin) in a mouse micronucleus assay.

➤*Fertility impairment:* Use ribavirin with caution in fertile men. In studies in mice to evaluate the time course and reversibility of ribavirin-induced testicular degeneration at doses of 15 to 150 mg/kg/day (estimated human equivalent of 1.25 to 12.5 mg/kg/day, based on body surface area adjustment for a 60 kg adult; 0.1 to 0.8 times the maximum human 24-hour dose of ribavirin) administered for 3 or 6 months, abnormalities in sperm occurred. Upon cessation of treatment, essentially total recovery from ribavirin-induced testicular toxicity was apparent within 1 or 2 spermatogenesis cycles.

➤*Elderly:*
Capsules/Oral solution – In clinical trials, elderly subjects had a higher frequency of anemia (67%) than did younger patients (28%) (see Warnings).

In general, cautiously administer ribavirin to elderly patients, starting at the lower end of the dosing range, reflecting the greater frequency of decreased hepatic or cardiac function and of concomitant disease or other drug therapy.

Take care in dose selection because elderly patients often have decreased renal function. Monitor renal function and make dosage adjustments accordingly. Do not use ribavirin in elderly patients with Ccr less than 50 mL/min.

➤*Pregnancy: Category X.* Ribavirin has demonstrated significant teratogenic effects (ie, malformation of skull, palate, eye, jaw, limbs, skeleton, GI tract) and/or embryocidal potential in all animal species in which adequate studies have been conducted. The incidence and severity of teratogenic effects increased with escalation of the drug dose. Although clinical studies have not been performed, ribavirin may cause fetal harm in humans.

Ribavirin may cause birth defects or death of the exposed fetus. Extreme care must be taken to avoid pregnancy in female patients and in female partners of male patients. Ribavirin has demonstrated significant teratogenic and/or embryocidal effects in all animal species in which adequate studies have been conducted. These effects occurred at doses as low as one-twentieth of the recommended human dose of ribavirin. Do not start ribavirin therapy until a report of a negative pregnancy test has been obtained immediately prior to planned initiation of therapy. Instruct male and female patients to use at least 2 forms of effective contraception during treatment and during the 6-month period after treatment has been stopped based on a multiple-dose half-life of ribavirin of 12 days. Pregnancy testing should occur monthly during ribavirin therapy and for 6 months after therapy has stopped.

Patients or partners of patients should immediately report any pregnancy that occurs during treatment or within 6 months after treatment cessation to their health care provider. Health care providers should report such cases for ribavirin capsules and oral solution by calling (800) 727-7064.

Ribavirin Pregnancy Registry – A Ribavirin Pregnancy Registry has been established to monitor maternal-fetal outcomes of pregnancies of female patients and female partners of male patients exposed to ribavirin during treatment and for 6 months following cessation of treatment. Health care providers and patients are encouraged to report such cases by calling (800) 593-2214.

➤*Lactation:* It is not known if ribavirin is excreted in human milk. Because of the potential for serious adverse reactions from the drug in nursing infants, decide whether to discontinue nursing or to delay or discontinue ribavirin.

➤*Children:* Safety and efficacy of ribavirin tablets have not been established in pediatric patients younger than 18 years of age.

Suicidal ideation or attempts occurred more frequently among pediatric patients, primarily adolescents, compared with adult patients (2.4% vs 1%) during treatment and off-therapy follow-up. Safety and efficacy of ribavirin in combination with peginterferon alfa-2b has not been established in pediatric patients.

During a 48-week course of therapy there was a decrease in the rate of linear growth (mean percentile assignment decrease of 9%) and a decrease in the rate of weight gain (mean percentile assignment decrease of 13%). A general reversal of these trends was noted during the 24-week posttreatment period.

Precautions

➤*Monitoring:* Assess patients for underlying cardiac disease before initiation of ribavirin therapy and appropriately monitor them during therapy. The following laboratory tests are recommended for all patients treated with ribavirin prior to beginning treatment and periodically thereafter:

- Standard hematologic tests: Including hemoglobin (pretreatment, week 2, and week 4 of therapy, and as clinically appropriate) (see Warnings), complete and differential white blood cell counts, and platelet count.
- Blood chemistries: Liver function tests and TSH.
- Pregnancy: Including monthly monitoring for women of childbearing potential and for 6 months after discontinuing therapy.
- ECG.

Consider acceptable baseline values for initiation of ribavirin tablets and peginterferon alfa-2a therapy: Platelet count 90,000 cell/mm^3 or more; absolute neutrophil count (ANC) 1,500 cells/mm^3 or more; TSH and T_4 within normal limits or adequately controlled thyroid function; ECG.

➤*HIV or HBV coinfection:* The safety and efficacy of ribavirin and interferon alfa-2b or peginterferon alfa-2a combination therapy for the treatment of HCV have not been established in patients coinfected with HIV or HBV.

➤*Hepatitis C:* The safety and efficacy of ribavirin and interferon alfa-2b or peginterferon alfa-2a combination therapy for the treatment of HCV in patients who have received liver or other organ transplants have not been established.

➤*Other infections:* The safety and efficacy of ribavirin and peginterferon alfa-2a, interferon alfa-2b, and peginterferon alfa-2b combination therapy for the treatment of HIV infection, adenovirus RSV, parainfluenza, or influenza infections have not been established. Do not use ribavirin for these indications.

Drug Interactions

➤*Antacids:* Coadministration with an antacid containing magnesium, aluminum, and simethicone (*Mylanta*) resulted in a 14% decrease in mean ribavirin AUC. The clinical relevance of results from this single-dose study is unknown.

➤*Nucleoside analogs (eg, didanosine, stavudine, zidovudine):* Ribavirin has shown in vitro to inhibit phosphorylation of zidovudine and stavudine, which could lead to decreased antiretroviral activity. Exposure to didanosine and its metabolites is increased when coadministered with ribavirin. Avoid concomitant use.

➤*Drug/Food interactions:* Both AUC and C_{max} increased 70% when ribavirin capsules were administered with a high-fat meal. For ribavirin tablets, the absorption was slowed (T_{max} was doubled) and the AUC and C_{max} increased 42% and 66%, respectively, when taken with a high-fat meal. There are insufficient data to address the clinical relevance of these results.

Adverse Reactions

➤*Tablets:*
Ribavirin tablets/Peginterferon alfa-2a combination therapy – The most common life-threatening or fatal events induced or aggravated by ribavirin tablets/peginterferon alfa-2a combination therapy were depression, suicide, relapse of drug abuse/overdose, and bacterial infections; each occurred at a frequency of less than 1%.

The most commonly reported adverse reactions were psychiatric reactions, including anxiety; depression; flu-like symptoms such as fatigue, headache, myalgia, pyrexia, and rigors; and irritability.

The most common reasons for discontinuation of therapy were dermatologic, GI disorders, flu-like syndrome (eg, lethargy, fatigue, headache), and psychiatric.

The most common reason for dose modification in patients receiving combination therapy was for laboratory abnormalities; neutropenia (20%) and thrombocytopenia (4%) for peginterferon alfa-2a and anemia (22%) for ribavirin tablets.

Peginterferon alfa-2a dose was reduced in 12% of patients receiving 1,000 to 1,200 mg ribavirin tablets for 48 weeks and in 7% of patients receiving 800 mg ribavirin tablets for 24 weeks. Ribavirin tablet dose was reduced in 21% of patients receiving 1,000 to 1,200 mg for 48 weeks and 12% in patients receiving 800 mg for 24 weeks.

Adverse Reactions Occurring in Patients in Hepatitis C Clinical Trials (≥ 5%)

Adverse reaction	Peginterferon alfa-2a 180 mcg + 1,000 or 1,200 mg ribavirin tablet 48 wk (N = 451)	Interferon alfa-2b + 1,000 or 1,200 mg ribavirin capsules 48 wk (N = 443)
CNS		
Concentration impairment	10%	13%
Depression	20%	28%
Dizziness (excluding vertigo)	14%	14%
Fatigue/Asthenia	65%	68%
Headache	43%	49%
Insomnia	30%	37%
Irritability/Anxiety/Nervousness	33%	38%
Memory impairment	6%	5%
Mood alteration	5%	6%
Rigors	25%	37%
Dermatologic		
Alopecia	28%	33%
Dermatitis	16%	13%
Dry skin	10%	13%
Eczema	5%	4%
Injection site reaction	23%	16%
Pruritus	19%	18%

RIBAVIRIN — ORAL

Adverse Reactions Occurring in Patients in Hepatitis C Clinical Trials (≥ 5%)		
Adverse reaction	Peginterferon alfa-2a 180 mcg + 1,000 or 1,200 mg ribavirin tablet 48 wk (N = 451)	Interferon alfa-2b + 1,000 or 1,200 mg ribavirin capsules 48 wk (N = 443)
Rash	8%	5%
Sweating increased	6%	5%
GI		
Abdominal pain	8%	9%
Anorexia	24%	26%
Diarrhea	11%	10%
Dry mouth	4%	7%
Dyspepsia	6%	5%
Nausea/Vomiting	25%	29%
Weight decrease	10%	10%
Hematologic		
Anemia	11%	11%
Lymphopenia	14%	12%
Neutropenia	27%	8%
Thrombocytopenia	5%	< 1%
Musculoskeletal		
Arthralgia	22%	23%
Back pain	5%	5%
Myalgia	40%	49%
Respiratory		
Cough	10%	7%
Dyspnea	13%	14%
Dyspnea, exertional	4%	7%
Miscellaneous		
Hypothyroidism	4%	5%
Overall resistance mechanism disorders	12%	10%
Pain	10%	9%
Pyrexia	41%	55%
Vision blurred	5%	2%

The most common serious adverse event (3%) was bacterial infection (eg, endocarditis, osteomyelitis, pneumonia, pyelonephritis, sepsis). Others that occurred at a frequency of less than 1% included the following: aggression, angina, anxiety, aplastic anemia, arrhythmia, autoimmune phenomena (eg, hyperthyroidism, hypothyroidism, sarcoidosis, systemic lupus erythematous, rheumatoid arthritis), cerebral hemorrhage, cholangitis, colitis, coma, corneal ulcer, diabetes mellitus, drug abuse and drug overdose, fatty liver, GI bleeding, hepatic dysfunction, myositis, pancreatitis, peptic ulcer, peripheral neuropathy, psychosis, pulmonary embolism, suicidal ideation, suicide.

➤*Capsules / Oral solution:* The primary toxicity of ribavirin is hemolytic anemia. Reductions in hemoglobin levels occurred within the first 1 to 2 weeks of oral therapy. Cardiac and pulmonary events associated with anemia occurred in about 10% of patients (see Warnings).

Combination therapy – In clinical trials, 19% and 6% of previously untreated and relapse patients, respectively, discontinued therapy because of adverse events in the combination arms compared with 13% and 3% in the interferon arms. Selected treatment-emergent adverse events that occurred in the US studies with 5% or more incidence are provided in the table below by treatment group. In general, the selected treatment-emergent adverse events were reported with lower incidence in the international studies as compared with the US studies with the exception of asthenia, influenza-like symptoms, nervousness, and pruritus. In clinical trials for pediatric patients 3 to 16 years of age, 6% discontinued therapy because of adverse events. Dose modifications were required in 30% of patients, most commonly for anemia and neutropenia. In general, the adverse event profile in the pediatric population was similar to that observed in adults. Injection site disorders, fever, anorexia, vomiting, and emotional lability occurred more frequently in pediatric patients compared with adult patients.

Selected Adverse Events: Previously Untreated and Relapse Patients							
	US previously untreated study				US relapse study		Pediatric Patients
	24 wk of treatment		48 wk of treatment		24 wk of treatment		48 wk of treatment
Adverse reaction[a]	Interferon alfa-2b + ribavirin capsules (N = 228)	Interferon alfa-2b + placebo (N = 231)	Interferon alfa-2b + ribavirin capsules (N = 228)	Interferon alfa-2b + placebo (N = 225)	Interferon alfa-2b + ribavirin capsules (N = 77)	Interferon alfa-2b + placebo (N = 76)	Interferon alfa-2b + ribavirin capsules (N = 118)
CNS							
Asthenia	9%	4%	9%	9%	10%	4%	5%
Dizziness	17%	15%	23%	19%	26%	21%	20%
Fatigue	68%	62%	70%	72%	60%	53%	58%
Headache	63%	63%	66%	67%	66%	68%	69%
Rigors	40%	32%	42%	39%	43%	37%	25%
Dermatologic							
Alopecia	28%	27%	32%	28%	27%	26%	23%
Injection site inflammation	13%	10%	12%	14%	6%	8%	14%
Injection site reaction	7%	9%	8%	9%	5%	3%	19%
Pruritus	21%	9%	19%	8%	13%	4%	12%
Rash	20%	9%	28%	8%	21%	5%	17%
GI							
Anorexia	27%	16%	25%	19%	21%	14%	51%
Dyspepsia	14%	6%	16%	9%	16%	9%	< 1%
Nausea	38%	35%	46%	33%	47%	33%	33%
Vomiting	11%	10%	9%	13%	12%	8%	42%
Musculoskeletal							
Arthralgia	30%	27%	33%	36%	29%	29%	15%
Musculoskeletal pain	20%	26%	28%	32%	22%	28%	21%
Myalgia	61%	57%	64%	63%	61%	58%	32%
Psychiatric							
Depression	32%	25%	36%	37%	23%	14%	13%
Emotional lability	7%	6%	11%	8%	12%	8%	16%
Impaired concentration	11%	14%	14%	14%	10%	12%	5%
Insomnia	39%	27%	39%	30%	26%	25%	14%
Irritability	23%	19%	32%	27%	25%	20%	10%
Nervousness	4%	2%	4%	4%	5%	4%	3%
Respiratory							
Dyspnea	19%	9%	18%	10%	17%	12%	5%
Sinusitis	9%	7%	10%	14%	12%	7%	< 1%
Miscellaneous							
Chest pain	5%	4%	9%	8%	6%	7%	5%
Fever	37%	35%	41%	40%	32%	36%	61%
Influenza-like symptoms	14%	18%	18%	20%	13%	13%	31%
Taste perversion	7%	4%	8%	4%	6%	5%	< 1%

[a] Patients reporting 1 or more adverse event. A patient may have reported more than 1 adverse event within a body system/organ class category.

In addition, the following spontaneous adverse events have been reported during the marketing surveillance of ribavirin capsules/interferon alfa-2b therapy: Hearing disorder and vertigo.

Ribavirin capsules / Peginterferon alfa-2b combination therapy: Overall in clinical trials, 14% of patients receiving ribavirin capsules/peginterferon alfa-2b combination therapy discontinued therapy compared with 13% treated with the ribavirin capsules in combination with interferon alfa-2b. The most common reasons for discontinuation of therapy were related to psychiatric, systemic (eg, fatigue, headache), or GI adverse events. Adverse events that occurred in clinical trials at more than 5% incidence are provided below. Safety and effectiveness of ribavirin in combination with peginterferon alfa-2b have not been established in pediatric patients.

Adverse Events with Ribavirin Capsules and Peginterferon Alfa-2b Combination Therapy Compared with Ribavirin Capsules and Interferon Alfa-2b Combination Therapy (> 5%)		
Adverse reaction[a]	Peginterferon alfa-2b + ribavirin capsules (N = 511)	Interferon alfa-2b + ribavirin capsules (N = 505)
CNS		
Agitation	8%	5%
Anxiety/Emotional lability/Irritability	47%	47%
Concentration impaired	17%	21%
Depression	31%	34%
Dizziness	21%	17%
Fatigue/Asthenia	66%	63%
Headache	62%	58%
Insomnia	40%	41%
Nervousness	6%	6%
Rigors	48%	41%

RIBAVIRIN — ORAL

Adverse Events with Ribavirin Capsules and Peginterferon Alfa-2b Combination Therapy Compared with Ribavirin Capsules and Interferon Alfa-2b Combination Therapy (> 5%)		
Adverse reaction[a]	Peginterferon alfa-2b + ribavirin capsules (N = 511)	Interferon alfa-2b + ribavirin capsules (N = 505)
Dermatologic		
Alopecia	36%	32%
Flushing	4%	3%
Pruritus	29%	28%
Rash	24%	23%
Skin dry	24%	23%
Sweating increased	11%	7%
GI		
Abdominal pain	13%	13%
Anorexia	32%	27%
Constipation	5%	5%
Diarrhea	22%	17%
Dyspepsia	9%	8%
Mouth dry	12%	8%
Nausea	43%	33%
Vomiting	14%	12%
Hematologic		
Anemia	12%	17%
Leukopenia	6%	5%
Neutropenia	26%	14%
Thrombocytopenia	5%	2%
Musculoskeletal		
Arthralgia	34%	28%
Musculoskeletal pain	21%	19%
Myalgia	56%	50%
Resistance mechanism		
Infection, fungal	6%	1%
Infection, viral	12%	12%
Respiratory		
Coughing	23%	16%
Dyspnea	26%	24%
Pharyngitis	12%	13%
Rhinitis	8%	6%
Sinusitis	6%	5%
Special senses		
Conjunctivitis	4%	5%
Taste perversion	9%	4%
Vision blurred	5%	6%
Miscellaneous		
Chest pain	8%	7%
Fever	46%	33%
Hepatomegaly	4%	4%
Hypothyroidism	5%	4%
Injection site inflammation	25%	18%
Injection site reaction	58%	36%
Malaise	4%	6%
Menstrual disorder	7%	6%
Right upper quadrant pain	12%	6%
Weight decrease	29%	20%

[a] Patients reporting 1 or more adverse events. A patient may have reported more than 1 adverse event within a body system/organ class category.

➤*Laboratory values:*

Hemoglobin – Hemoglobin decreases among patients receiving ribavirin therapy began at week 1, with stabilization by week 4. Hemoglobin values returned to pretreatment levels within 4 to 8 weeks of cessation of therapy in most patients.

Ribavirin capsules induced a decrease in hemoglobin levels in approximately two-thirds of patients. Hemoglobin levels decreased to less than 11 g/dL in about 30% of patients. Severe anemia (less than 8 g/dL) occurred in less than 1% of patients. Dose modification was required in 9% and 13% of patients in the peginterferon alfa-2b/ribavirin capsules and interferon alfa-2b/ribavirin capsules groups.

Hemoglobin less than 10 g/dL was observed in 13% of ribavirin tablets and peginterferon alfa-2a combination-treated patients in clinical trials. The maximum drop in hemoglobin occurred during the first 8 weeks of initiation of ribavirin therapy (see Warnings).

Bilirubin and uric acid – Increases in bilirubin and uric acid, associated with hemolysis, were noted in clinical trials. Most were moderate biochemical changes and were reversed within 4 weeks after treatment discontinuation. This observation occurs most frequently in patients with a previous diagnosis of Gilbert syndrome.

In the peginterferon alfa-2b/ribavirin capsule combination trial, 10% to 14% of patients developed hyperbilirubinemia and 33% to 38% developed hyperuricemia in association with hemolysis. Six patients developed mild to moderate gout.

Selected Hematologic Values During Treatment with Ribavirin Capsules Plus Interferon Alfa-2b: Previously Untreated and Relapse Patients							
	US previously untreated study				US relapse study		Pediatric Patients
	24 wk of treatment		48 wk of treatment		24 wk of treatment		48 wk of treatment
	Interferon alfa-2b + ribavirin capsules (N = 228)	Interferon alfa-2b + placebo (N = 231)	Interferon alfa-2b + ribavirin capsules (N = 228)	Interferon alfa-2b + placebo (N = 225)	Interferon alfa-2b + ribavirin capsules (N = 77)	Interferon alfa-2b + placebo (N = 76)	Interferon alfa-2b + ribavirin capsules (N = 118)
Hemoglobin (g/dL)							
9.5 to 10.9	24%	1%	32%	1%	21%	3%	24%
8 to 9.4	5%	0%	4%	0%	4%	0%	3%
6.5 to 7.9	0%	0%	0%	0.4%	0%	0%	0%
< 6.5	0%	0%	0%	0%	0%	0%	0%
Leukocytes (× 10^9/L)							
2 to 2.9	40%	20%	38%	23%	45%	26%	35%
1.5 to 1.9	4%	1%	9%	2%	5%	3%	8%
1 to 1.4	0.9%	0%	2%	0%	0%	0%	0%
< 1	0%	0%	0%	0%	0%	0%	0%
Neutrophils (× 10^9/L)							
1 to 1.49	30%	32%	31%	44%	42%	34%	37%
0.75 to 0.99	14%	15%	14%	11%	16%	18%	15%
0.5 to 0.74	9%	9%	14%	7%	8%	4%	16%
< 0.5	11%	8%	11%	5%	5%	8%	3%
Platelets (× 10^9/L)							
70 to 99	9%	11%	11%	14%	6%	12%	0.8%
50 to 69	2%	3%	2%	3%	0%	5%	2%
30 to 49	0%	0.4%	0%	0.4%	0%	0%	0%
< 30	0.9%	0%	1%	0.9%	0%	0%	0%
Total bilirubin (mg/dL)							
1.5 to 3	27%	13%	32%	13%	21%	7%	2%
3.1 to 6	0.9%	0.4%	2%	0%	3%	0%	0%
6.1 to 12	0%	0%	0.4%	0%	0%	0%	0%
> 12	0%	0%	0%	0%	0%	0%	0%

Selected Hematologic Values During Treatment with Ribavirin Capsules Plus Peginterferon Alfa-2b	
	Ribavirin capsules + peginterferon alfa-2b (N = 511)
ALT	
2 × baseline	0.6%
2.1 to 5 × baseline	3%
5.1 to 10 × baseline	0%
> 10 × baseline	0%
Hemoglobin (g/dL)	
9.5 to 10.9	26%
8 to 9.4	3%
6.5 to 7.9	0.2%
< 6.5	0%
Leukocytes (× 10^9/L)	
2 to 2.9	46%
1.5 to 1.9	24%
1 to 1.4	5%
< 1	0%
Neutrophils (× 10^9/L)	
1 to 1.49	33%
0.75 to 0.99	25%
0.5 to 0.74	18%
< 0.5	4%
Platelets (× 10^9/L)	
70 to 99	15%
50 to 69	3%
30 to 49	0.2%
< 30	0%
Total bilirubin (mg/dL)	
1.5 to 3	10%
3.1 to 6	0.6%
6.1 to 12	0%
> 12	0%

Overdosage

➤*Symptoms:*

Capsules/Oral solution – Acute ingestion of up to 20 g ribavirin, ingestion of interferon alfa-2b up to 120 million units, and subcutaneous doses of up to 10 times the recommended dose have been reported. Primary effects observed were increased severity of adverse effects. However, hepatic enzyme abnormalities, renal failure, hemorrhage, and MI were observed with doses exceeding recommended single subcutaneous doses of interferon alfa-2b.

RIBAVIRIN — ORAL

➤*Treatment:*

Capsules/Oral solution – There is no specific antidote known for interferon alfa-2b and ribavirin overdose, nor is hemodialysis and peritoneal dialysis effective.

Patient Information

Ribavirin may cause birth defects or death of the exposed fetus. Ribavirin must not be used by women who are pregnant or by men whose female partners are pregnant. Extreme care must be taken to avoid pregnancy in these individuals. Do not initiate ribavirin until a report of a negative pregnancy test has been obtained immediately prior to initiation of therapy. Patients must perform a pregnancy test monthly during therapy and for 6 months posttherapy. Women of childbearing potential must be counseled about use of effective contraception (2 reliable forms) prior to initiating therapy. Patients (male and female) must be advised of the teratogenic/embryocidal risks and must be instructed to practice effective contraception during ribavirin therapy and for 6 months posttherapy. Advise patients (male and female) to notify their doctor immediately in the event of a pregnancy (see Contraindications and Warnings). Doctor should report such cases by calling (800) 727-7064 for ribavirin capsules and oral solution. A Ribavirin Pregnancy Registry has been established to monitor maternal-fetal outcomes of pregnancies of female patients and female partners of male patients exposed to ribavirin during treatment and for 6 months following cessation of treatment. Health care providers and patients are encouraged to report such cases by calling (800) 593-2214.

Inform patients receiving ribavirin of the benefits and risks associated with treatment, directed in its appropriate use, and referred to the patient medication guide. Inform patients that the effect of treatment of HCV infection on transmission is not known, and that they should take appropriate precautions to prevent transmission of HCV.

Advise the patient that laboratory evaluations are required prior to starting therapy and periodically thereafter (see Precautions). Advise patients to be well hydrated, especially during the initial stages of treatment.

Caution patients who develop dizziness, confusion, somnolence, and fatigue to avoid driving or operating machinery. Advise patients to take ribavirin tablets with food. Do not open, crush, or break capsules.

RIBAVIRIN — SOLUTION FOR INHALATION

WARNING

Use of aerosolized ribavirin in patients requiring mechanical ventilator assistance should be undertaken only by physicians and support staff familiar with this mode of administration and the specific ventilator being used. Strict attention must be paid to procedures that have been shown to minimize the accumulation of drug precipitate, which can result in mechanical ventilator dysfunction and associated increased pulmonary pressures (see Warnings).

Sudden deterioration of respiratory function has been associated with initiation of aerosolized ribavirin use in infants. Respiratory function should be carefully monitored during treatment. If initiation of aerosolized ribavirin treatment appears to produce sudden deterioration of respiratory function, treatment should be stopped and reinstituted only with extreme caution, continuous monitoring, and consideration of concomitant administration of bronchodilators (see Precautions).

Ribavirin is not indicated for use in adults. Physicians and patients should be aware that ribavirin has been shown to produce testicular lesions in rodents and to be teratogenic in all animal species in which adequate studies have been conducted (rodents and rabbits); (see Contraindications and Warnings).

Indications

➤*Severe lower respiratory tract infections:* For the treatment of hospitalized infants and young children with severe lower respiratory tract infections due to respiratory syncytial virus (RSV). Treatment early in the course of severe lower respiratory tract infection may be necessary to achieve efficacy.

Only severe RSV lower respiratory tract infection should be treated with ribavirin. The vast majority of infants and children with RSV infection have disease that is mild, self-limited, and does not require hospitalization or antiviral treatment. Many children with mild lower respiratory tract involvement will require shorter hospitalization than would be required for a full course of ribavirin aerosol (3 to 7 days) and should not be treated with the drug. Thus the decision to treat with ribavirin should be based on the severity of the RSV infection. The presence of an underlying condition such as prematurity, immunosuppression, or cardiopulmonary disease may increase the severity of clinical manifestations and complications of RSV infection.

Use of aerosolized ribavirin in patients requiring mechanical ventilator assistance should be undertaken only by physicians and support staff familiar with this mode of administration and the specific ventilator being used (see Warnings).

➤*Diagnosis:* RSV infection should be documented by a rapid diagnostic method such as demonstration of viral antigen in respiratory tract secretions by immunofluorescence or ELISA before or during the first 24 hours of treatment. Treatment may be initiated while awaiting rapid diagnostic test results. However, treatment should not be continued without documentation of RSV infection. Nonculture antigen detection techniques may have false positive or false negative results. Assessment of the clinical situation, the time of year and other parameters may warrant reevaluation of the laboratory diagnosis.

➤*Unlabeled uses:* Aerosol ribavirin has shown some success against influenza A and B.

Administration and Dosage

Before use, read thoroughly the ICN small particle aerosol generator (SPAG-2) operator's manual for small particle aerosol generator operating instructions. Aerosolized ribavirin should not be administered with any other aerosol generating device.

➤*Dosage:* 20 mg/mL ribavirin as the starting solution in the drug reservoir of the SPAG-2 unit, with continuous aerosol administration for 12 to 18 hours per day for 3 to 7 days. Using the recommended drug concentration of 20 mg/mL the average aerosol concentration for a 12 hour delivery period would be 190 mcg/L of air. Aerosolized ribavirin should not be administered in a mixture for combined aerosolization or simultaneously with other aerosolized medications.

➤*Non-mechanically ventilated infants:* Ribavirin should be delivered to an infant oxygen hood from the SPAG-2 aerosol generator. Administration by face mask or oxygen tent may be necessary if a hood cannot be employed (see SPAG-2 manual). However, the volume and condensation area are larger in a tent and this may alter delivery dynamics of the drug.

➤*Mechanically ventilated infants:* The recommended dose and administration schedule for infants who require mechanical ventilations is the same as for those who do not. Either a pressure or volume cycle ventilator may be used in conjunction with the SPAG-2. In either case, patients should have their endotracheal tubes suctioned every 1 to 2 hours, and their pulmonary pressures monitored frequently (every 2 to 4 hours). For both pressure and volume ventilators, heated wire connective tubing and bacteria filters in series in the expiratory limb of the system (which must be changed frequently, ie, every 4 hours) must be used to minimize the risk of ribavirin precipitation in the system and the subsequent risk of ventilator dysfunction. Water column pressure release valves should be used in the ventilator circuit for pressure cycled ventilators, and may be utilized with volume cycled ventilators (see SPAG-2 manual for detailed instructions).

➤*Method of preparation:* Ribavirin brand of ribavirin is supplied as 6 grams of lyophilized powder per 100 mL vial to aerosol administration only. By sterile technique, reconstitute drug with a minimum of 75 mL of sterile USP water for injection or inhalation in the original 100 mL glass vial. Shake well. Transfer to the clean, sterilized 500 mL SPAG-2 reservoir and further dilute to a final volume of 300 mL with Sterile Water for Injection, USP, or Inhalation. The final concentration should be 20 mg/mL.

Important – This water should not have had any antimicrobial agent or other substance added. The solution should be inspected visually for particulate matter and discoloration prior to administration. Solutions that have been placed in the SPAG-2 unit should be discarded at least every 24 hours and when the liquid level is low before adding newly reconstituted solution.

➤*Storage/Stability:*

Aerosol – Store lyophilized drug powder at 15° to 25°C (59° to 78°F) in a dry place. Reconstituted solutions may be stored under sterile conditions at room temperature (20° to 30°C, 68° to 86°F) for 24 hours. Discard solutions that have been placed in the SPAG-2 unit at least every 24 hours.

Actions

➤*Pharmacology:* In cell cultures the inhibitory activity of ribavirin for respiratory syncytial virus (RSV) is selective. The mechanism of action is unknown. Reversal of the in vitro antiviral activity by guanosine or xanthosine suggests ribavirin may act as an analogue of these cellular metabolites.

➤*Pharmacokinetics:*

Absorption – Ribavirin, when administered by aerosol, is absorbed systemically. Four children inhaling ribavirin aerosol administered by face mask for 2.5 hours each day for 3 days had plasma concentrations ranging from 0.44 to 1.55 mcM, with a mean concentration of 0.76 mcM. The plasma half-life was reported to be 9.5 hours. Three children inhaling aerosolized ribavirin administered by face mask or mist tent for 20 hours each day for 5 days had plasma concentrations ranging from 1.5 to 14.3 mcM, with a mean concentration of 6.8 mcM.

Distribution – The bioavailability of aerosolized ribavirin is unknown and may depend on the mode of aerosol delivery. After aerosol treatment, peak plasma concentrations of ribavirin are 85% to 98% less than the concentration that reduced RSV plaque formation in tissue culture. After aerosol treatment, respiratory tract secretions are likely to contain ribavirin in concentrations many fold higher than those required to reduce plaque formation. However, RSV is an intracellular virus and it is unknown whether plasma concentrations or respiratory secretion concentrations of the drug better reflect intracellular concentrations in the respiratory tract.

In man, rats, and rhesus monkeys, accumulation of ribavirin and/or metabolites in the red blood cells has been noted, plateauing in red cells in man in about 4 days and gradually declining with an apparent half-life of 40 days (the half-life of erythrocytes). The extent of accumulation of ribavirin following inhalation therapy is not well defined.

Immunologic effects – Neutralizing antibody responses to RSV were decreased in aerosolized ribavirin treated infants compared to placebo-treated infants. One study also showed that RSV-specific IgE antibody in bronchial secretions was decreased in patients treated with aerosolized ribavirin. In rats, ribavirin administration resulted in lymphoid atrophy of the thymus, spleen, and lymph nodes. Humoral immunity was reduced in guinea pigs and ferrets. Cellular immunity was also mildly depressed in animal studies. The clinical significance of these observations is unknown.

RIBAVIRIN — SOLUTION FOR INHALATION

Contraindications

Hypersensitivity to the drug or its components, and in women who are or may become pregnant during exposure to the drug. Ribavirin has demonstrated significant teratogenic and/or embryocidal potential in all animal species in which adequate studies have been conducted (rodents and rabbits). Therefore, although clinical studies have not been performed, it should be assumed that ribavirin may cause fetal harm in humans. Studies in which the drug has been administered systemically demonstrate that ribavirin is concentrated in the red blood cells and persists for the life of the erythrocyte.

Warnings

➤*Use with mechanical ventilators:* Use of aerosolized ribavirin in patients requiring mechanical ventilator assistance should be undertaken only by physicians and support staff familiar with this mode of administration and the specific ventilator being used. Strict attention must be paid to procedures that have been shown to minimize the accumulation of drug precipitate, which can result in mechanical ventilator dysfunction and associated increased pulmonary pressure. These procedures include the use of bacteria filters in series in the expiratory limb of the ventilator circuit with frequent changes (every 4 hours). Water column pressure release valves to indicate elevated ventilator pressure, frequent monitoring of these devices and verification that ribavirin crystals have not accumulated within the ventilator circuitry and frequent suctioning and monitoring of the patient (see Clinical Trials).

Those administering aerosolized ribavirin in conjunction with mechanical ventilator use should be thoroughly familiar with detailed descriptions of these procedures as outlined in the SPAG-2 manual.

➤*Deaths:* Deaths during or shortly after treatment with aerosolized ribavirin have been reported in 20 cases of patients treated with ribavirin (12 of these patients were being treated for RSV infections). Several cases have been characterized as possibly related to ribavirin by the treating physician; these were in infants who experienced worsening respiratory status related to bronchospasm while being treated with the drug. Several other cases have been attributed to mechanical ventilator malfunction in which ribavirin precipitation within the ventilator apparatus led to excessively high pulmonary pressures and diminished oxygenation. In these cases the monitoring procedures described in the current package insert were not employed (see Description of Studies, Precautions, and Administration and Dosage).

➤*Pulmonary effects:* Pulmonary function significantly deteriorated during aerosolized ribavirin treatment in 6 of 6 adults with chronic obstructive lung disease and in 4 of 6 asthmatic adults. Dyspnea and chest soreness were also reported in the latter group. Minor abnormalities in pulmonary function were also seen in healthy adult volunteers. In the original study population of ≈ 200 infants who received aerosolized ribavirin, several serious adverse events occurred in severely ill infants with life-threatening underlying diseases, many of whom required assisted ventilation. The role of ribavirin in these events is indeterminate. Since the drug's approval in 1986, additional reports of similar serious, though nonfatal, events have been filed infrequently. (See Adverse Reactions for events associated with aerosolized ribavirin.)

➤*Hematologic:* Although anemia was not reported with the use of aerosolized ribavirin in controlled clinical trials, most infants treated with the aerosol have not been evaluated 1 to 2 weeks post-treatment when anemia is likely to occur. Anemia has been shown to occur frequently with experimental IV ribavirin in humans. Also, cases of anemia (type unspecified), reticulocytosis and hemolytic anemia associated with aerosolized ribavirin use have been reported through postmarketing reporting systems. All have been reversible with discontinuation of the drug.

➤*Carcinogenesis:* In vivo carcinogenicity studies with ribavirin are incomplete. However, results of a chronic feeding study with ribavirin in rats, at doses of 16 to 100 mg/kg/day (estimated human equivalent of 2.3 to 14.3 mg/kg/day, based on body surface area adjustment for the adult) suggest that ribavirin may induce benign mammary, pancreatic, pituitary and adrenal tumors. Preliminary results of 2 oral gavage oncogenicity studies in the mouse and rat (18 to 24 months; doses of 20 to 75 and 10 to 40 mg/kg/day, respectively [estimated human equivalent of 1.67 to 6.25 and 1.43 to 5.71 mg/kg/day, respectively, based on body surface area adjustment for the adult]) are inconclusive as to the carcinogenic potential of ribavirin (see Pharmacokinetics). However, these studies have demonstrated a relationship between chronic ribavirin exposure and increased incidences of vascular lesions (microscopic hemorrhages in mice) and retinal degeneration (in rats).

➤*Mutagenesis:* Ribavirin increased the incidence of cell transformations and mutations in mouse Balb/c 3T3 (fibroblasts) and L5178Y (lymphoma) cells at concentrations of 0.015 and 0.03 to 5 mg/mL, respectively (without metabolic activation). Modest increases in mutation rates (3 to 4 times) were observed at concentrations between 3.75 to 10 mg/mL in L5178Y cells in vitro with the addition of a metabolic activation fraction. In the mouse micronucleus assay ribavirin was clastogenic at IV doses of 20 to 200 mg/kg (estimated human equivalent of 1.67 to 16.7 mg/kg based on body surface area adjustment for a 60 kg adult). Ribavirin was not mutagenic in a dominant lethal assay in rats at intraperitoneal doses between 50 to 200 mg/kg when administered for 5 days (estimated human equivalent of 7.14 to 28.6 mg/kg, based on body surface area adjustment; see Pharmacokinetics).

➤*Fertility impairment:* The fertility of ribavirin-treated animals (male or female) has not been fully investigated. However, in the mouse, administration of ribavirin at doses between 35 to 150 mg/kg/day (estimated human equivalent of 2.92 to 12.5 mg/kg/day, based on body surface area adjustment for the adult) resulted in significant seminiferous tubule atrophy, decreased sperm concentrations, and increased numbers of sperm with abnormal morphology. Partial recovery of sperm production was apparent 3 to 6 months following dose cessation. In several additional toxicology studies, ribavirin has been shown to cause testicular lesions (tubular atrophy) in adult rats at oral dose levels as low as 16 mg/kg/day (estimated human equivalent of 2.29 mg/kg/day, based on body surface area adjustment; see Pharmacokinetics). Lower doses were not tested. The reproductive capacity of treated male animals has not been studied.

➤*Pregnancy: Category X.* Ribavirin has demonstrated significant teratogenic and/or embryocidal potential in all animal species in which adequate studies have been conducted.

Teratogenic effects were evident after single oral doses of ≥ 2.5 mg/kg in the hamster, and after daily oral doses of 0.3 and 1 mg/kg in the rabbit and rat, respectively (estimated human equivalent doses of 0.12 and 0.14 mg/kg. Based on body surface area adjustment for the adult). Malformations of the skull, palate, eye, jaw, limbs, skeleton, and GI tract were noted. The incidence and severity of teratogenic effects increased with escalation of the drug dose. Survival of fetuses and offspring was reduced. Ribavirin caused embryolethality in the rabbit at daily oral dose levels as low as 1 mg/kg. No teratogenic effects were evident in the rabbit and rat administered daily oral doses of 0.1 and 0.3 mg/kg respectively with estimated human equivalent doses of 0.01 and 0.04 mg/kg based on body surface area adjustment (see Pharmacokinetics). These doses are considered to define the No Observable Teratogenic Effects Level (NOTEL) for ribavirin in the rabbit and rat.

Following oral administration of ribavirin in the pregnant rat (1 mg/kg) and rabbit (0.3 mg/kg), mean plasma level of drug ranged from 0.1 to 0.2 M (0.024 to 0.049 g/mL) at 1 hour after dosing to undetectable levels at 24 hours. At 1 hour following the administration of 0.3 or 0.1 mg/kg in the rat and rabbit (NOTEL), respectively, mean plasma levels of drug in both species were near or below the limit of detection (0.05M; see Pharmacokinetics).

Although clinical studies have not been performed, ribavirin may cause fetal harm in humans. As noted previously, ribavirin is concentrated in red blood cells and persists for the life of the cell. Thus the terminal half-life for the systemic elimination of ribavirin is essentially that of the half-life of circulating erythrocytes. The minimum interval following exposure to ribavirin before pregnancy may be safety initiated is unknown (see Contraindications, Warnings, Precautions, and Information for Health Care Personnel).

➤*Lactation:* Ribavirin has been shown to be toxic to lactating animals and their offspring. It is not known if ribavirin is excreted in human milk.

Precautions

➤*Monitoring:* Sudden deterioration of respiratory function has been associated with initiation of aerosolized ribavirin use in infants. Respiratory function should be carefully monitored during treatment. If initiation of aerosolized ribavirin treatment appears to produce sudden deterioration of respiratory function, treatment should be stopped and reinstituted only with extreme caution, continuous monitoring, and consideration of concomitant administration of bronchodilators.

Patients with severe lower respiratory tract infection due to respiratory syncytial virus require optimum monitoring and attention to respiratory and fluid status (see SPAG-2 manual).

➤*Health care personnel information:* Health care workers directly providing care to patients receiving aerosolized ribavirin should be aware that ribavirin has been shown to be teratogenic in all animal species in which adequate studies have been conducted (rodents and rabbits). Although no reports of teratogenesis in offspring of mothers who were exposed to aerosolized ribavirin during pregnancy have been confirmed, no controlled studies have been conducted in pregnant women. Studies of environmental exposure in treatment settings have shown that the drug can disperse into the immediate bedside area during routine patient care activities with highest ambient levels closest to the patient and extremely low levels outside of the immediate bedside area. Adverse reactions resulting from actual occupational exposure in adults are described below (see Adverse Reactions, Adverse Events in Health Care Workers). Some studies have documented ambient drug concentrations at the bedside that could potentially lead to systemic exposures above those considered safe for exposure during pregnancy (1/1000 of the NOTEL dose in the most sensitive animal species).

A 1992 study conducted by the National Institute of Occupational Safety and Health (NIOSH) demonstrated measurable urine levels of ribavirin in health workers exposed to aerosol in the course of direct patient care. Levels were lowest in workers caring for infants receiving aerosolized ribavirin with mechanical ventilation and highest in those caring for patients being administered the drug via an oxygen tent or hood. This study employed a more sensitive assay to evaluate ribavirin levels in urine than was available for several previous studies of environmental exposure that failed to detect measurable ribavirin levels in exposed workers. Creatinine adjusted urine levels in the NIOSH study ranged from < 0.001 to 0.140 mcM of ribavirin per gram of creatinine in exposed workers, plasma levels in animal studies, and the specific risk of teratogenesis in exposed pregnant women is unknown.

It is good practice to avoid unnecessary occupational exposure to chemicals wherever possible. Hospitals are encouraged to conduct training programs to minimize potential occupational exposure to ribavirin. Health care workers who are pregnant should consider avoiding direct care of patients receiving aerosolized ribavirin. If close patient contact cannot be avoided, precautions to limit exposure should be taken. These include administration of ribavirin in negative pressure rooms: adequate room ventilation (≥ 6 air exchanges per hour); the use of ribavirin aerosol scavenging devices; turning off the SPAG-2 device for 5 to 10 minutes prior to prolonged patient contact; and wearing appropriately fitted respirator masks. Surgical masks do not provide adequate filtration of ribavirin particles. Further information is available from NIOSH's Hazard Evaluation and Technical Assistance Branch and additional recommendations have been published in an Aerosol

RIBAVIRIN — SOLUTION FOR INHALATION

Consensus Statement by the American Respiratory Care Foundation and the American Association for Respiratory Care.

Adverse Reactions

Some subjects requiring assisted ventilation experienced serious difficulties, due to inadequate ventilation and gas exchange. Precipitation of drug within the ventilatory apparatus, including the endotracheal tube, has resulted in increased positive and expiratory pressure and increase positive inspiratory pressure. Accumulation of fluid in tubing (rain out) has also been noted. Measures to avoid these complications should be followed carefully (see Administration and Dosage).

➤*Cardiovascular:* Cardiac arrest; hypotension; bradycardia; digitalis toxicity. Bigeminy, bradycardia and tachycardia have been described in patients with underlying congenital heart disease.

➤*Pulmonary:* Worsening of respiratory status; bronchospasm; pulmonary edema; hypoventilation; cyanosis; dyspnea; bacterial pneumonia; pneumothorax; apnea; atelectasis; ventilator dependence.

➤*Miscellaneous:* Rash and conjunctivitis have been associated with the use of aerosolized ribavirin. These usually resolve within hours of discontinuing therapy. Seizures and asthenia associated with experimental IV ribavirin therapy have also been reported.

Adverse events in health care workers – Studies of environmental exposure to aerosolized ribavirin in health care workers administering care to patients receiving the drug have not detected adverse signs or symptoms related to exposure. However, 152 health care workers have reported experiencing adverse events through postmarketing surveillance. Nearly all were in individuals providing direct care to infants receiving aerosolized ribavirin. Of 358 events from these 152 individual health care worker reports, the most common signs and symptoms were headache (51% of reports), conjunctivitis (32%), and rhinitis, nausea, rash, dizziness, pharyngitis, or lacrimation (10% to 20% each). Several cases of bronchospasm and/or chest pain were also reported, usually in individuals with known underlying reactive airway disease. Several case reports of damage to contact lenses after prolonged close exposure to aerosolized ribavirin have also been reported. Most signs and symptoms reported as having occurred in exposed health care workers resolved within minutes to hours of discontinuing close exposure to aerosolized ribavirin (also see Precautions and Information for Health Care Personnel).

Overdosage

➤*Symptoms:* No overdosage with ribavirin by aerosol administration has been reported in humans. The LD_{50} in mice is 2 g orally and is associated with hypoactivity and GI symptoms (estimated human equivalent dose of 0.17 g/kg based on body surface area conversion). This mean plasma half-life after administration of aerosolized ribavirin for children is 9.5 hours. Ribavirin is concentrated and persists in red blood cells for the life of the erythrocyte (see Pharmacokinetics).

RIMANTADINE HYDROCHLORIDE

Rx	**Flumadine** (Forest)	**Tablets:** 100 mg	(FLUMADINE 100 FOREST). Orange, oval. Film-coated. In 100s.
		Syrup: 50 mg/5 mL	Saccharin, sorbitol, parabens. Raspberry flavor. In 240 mL.

RIMANTADINE HYDROCHLORIDE — ORAL

Indications

➤*Adults:* For the prophylaxis and treatment of illness caused by various strains of influenza A virus in adults.

➤*Children:* For prophylaxis against influenza A virus in children.

Administration and Dosage

➤*Approved by the FDA:* September 17, 1993.

➤*Prophylaxis:*

Adults – 100 mg twice a day.

Children – In children less than 10 years of age, rimantadine HCl should be administered once a day, at a dose of 5 mg/kg but not exceeding 150 mg. For children greater than or equal to 10 years of age, use the adult dose.

➤*Treatment (adults only):* 100 mg twice a day.

Rimantadine HCl therapy should be initiated as soon as possible, preferably within 48 hours after onset of signs and symptoms of influenza A infection. Therapy should be continued for approximately 7 days from the initial onset of symptoms.

➤*Renal / Hepatic function impairment / Elderly (treatment and prophylaxis):* In patients with severe hepatic dysfunction, renal failure (Ccr less than or equal to 10 mL/min) and elderly nursing home patients, a dose reduction to 100 mg daily is recommended. There are currently no data available regarding the safety of rimantadine during multiple dosing in subjects with renal or hepatic impairment. Because of the potential for accumulation of rimantadine metabolites during multiple dosing, patients with any degree of renal insufficiency should be monitored for adverse effects, with dosage adjustments being made as necessary.

➤*Storage / Stability:* Tablets and syrup should be stored at 15° to 30°C (59° to 86°F).

Actions

➤*Pharmacology:* The mechanism of action of rimantadine is not fully understood. Rimantadine appears to exert its inhibitory effect early in the viral replicative cycle, possibly inhibiting the uncoating of the virus. Genetic studies suggest that a virus protein specified by the virion M_2 gene plays an important role in the susceptibility of influenza A virus to inhibition by rimantadine.

➤*Pharmacokinetics:*

Absorption / Distribution – The tablet and syrup formulations of rimantadine HCl are equally absorbed after oral administration. The mean ± SD peak plasma concentration after a single 100 mg dose of rimantadine HCl was 74 ± 22 ng/mL (range, 45 to 138 ng/mL). The time to peak concentration was 6 ± 1 hours in healthy adults (age 20 to 44 years).

After the administration of rimantadine 100 mg twice daily to healthy volunteers (age 18 to 70 years) for 10 days, area under the curve (AUC) values were approximately 30% greater than predicted from a single dose. Plasma trough levels at steady state ranged between 118 and 468 ng/mL. In these patients no age-related differences in pharmacokinetics were detected. However, in a comparison of three groups of healthy older subjects (age 50 to 60, 61 to 70, and 71 to 79 years), the 71- to 79-year-old group had average AUC values, peak concentrations and elimination half-life values at steady state that were 20% to 30% higher than the other 2 groups. Steady-state concentrations in elderly nursing home patients (age 68 to 102 years) were 2- to 4-fold higher than those seen in healthy young and elderly adults.

The in vitro human plasma protein binding of rimantadine is about 40% over typical plasma concentrations. Albumin is the major binding protein.

Metabolism – Following oral administration, rimantadine is extensively metabolized in the liver with less than 25% of the dose excreted in the urine as unchanged drug. Three hydroxylated metabolites have been found in plasma. These metabolites, an additional conjugated metabolite and parent drug, account for 74 ± 10% (n = 4) of a single 200 mg dose of rimantadine excreted in urine over 72 hours.

Excretion – The single dose elimination half-life in this population was 25.4 ± 6.3 hours (range, 13 to 65 hours). The single dose elimination half-life in a group of healthy 71- to 79-year-old subjects was 32 ± 16 hours (range, 20 to 65 hours).

Special populations –

Renal function impairment: Studies of the effects of renal insufficiency on the pharmacokinetics of rimantadine have given inconsistent results. Following administration of a single 200 mg oral dose of rimantadine to 8 patients with a creatinine clearance (Ccr) of 31 to 50 mL/min and 6 patients with a Ccr of 11 to 30 mL/min, the apparent clearance was 37% and 16% lower, respectively, and plasma metabolite concentrations were higher when compared to weight-, age-, and sex-matched healthy subjects (n = 9, Ccr greater than 50 mL/min). After a single 200 mg oral dose of rimantadine was given to 8 hemodialysis patients (Ccr 0 to 10 mL/min), there was a 1.6-fold increase in the elimination half-life and a 40% decrease in apparent clearance compared to age-matched healthy subjects. Hemodialysis did not contribute to the clearance of rimantadine.

Hepatic function impairment: In a group (n = 14) of patients with chronic liver disease, the majority of whom were stabilized cirrhotics, the pharmacokinetics of rimantadine were not appreciably altered following a single 200 mg oral dose compared to 6 healthy subjects who were sex, age and weight matched to 6 of the patients with liver disease. After administration of a single 200 mg dose to patients (n = 10) with severe hepatic dysfunction, AUC was approximately 3-fold larger, elimination half-life was approximately 2-fold longer and apparent clearance was about 50% lower when compared to historic data from healthy subjects.

Children: The pharmacokinetic profile of rimantadine in children has not been established. In a group (n = 10) of children 4 to 8 years old who were given a single dose (6.6 mg/kg) of rimantadine HCl syrup, plasma concentrations of rimantadine ranged from 446 to 988 ng/mL at 5 to 6 hours and from 170 to 424 ng/mL at 24 hours. In some children, drug was detected in plasma 72 hours after the last dose.

Contraindications

Hypersensitivity to drugs of the adamantane class including rimantadine and amantadine.

Warnings

➤*Renal / Hepatic function impairment:* Because of the potential for accumulation of rimantadine and its metabolites in plasma, caution should be exercised when patients with renal or hepatic insufficiency are treated with rimantadine.

See Actions for more information.

➤*Pregnancy:* *Category C.* There are no adequate and well-controlled studies in pregnant women. Rimantadine is reported to cross the placenta in mice. Rimantadine has been shown to be embryotoxic in rats when given at a dose of 200 mg/kg/day (11 times the recommended human dose based on body surface area comparisons). At this dose the embryotoxic effect consisted of increased fetal resorption in rats; this dose also produced a variety of maternal effects including ataxia, tremors, convulsions and significantly reduced weight gain. No embryotoxicity was observed when rabbits were given doses up to 50 mg/kg/day (5 times the recommended human dose based on body surface area comparisons). However, there was evidence of a developmental abnormality in the form of a change in the ratio of fetuses

RIMANTADINE HYDROCHLORIDE — ORAL

with 12 or 13 ribs. This ratio is normally about 50:50 in a litter but was 80:20 after rimantadine treatment.

Rimantadine was administered to pregnant rats in a peri- and postnatal reproduction toxicity study at doses of 30, 60 and 120 mg/kg/day (1.7, 3.4 and 6.8 times the recommended human dose based on body surface area comparisons). Maternal toxicity during gestation was noted at the 2 higher doses of rimantadine, and at the highest dose, 120 mg/kg/day, there was an increase in pup mortality during the first 2 to 4 days postpartum. Decreased fertility of the F1 generation was also noted for the 2 higher doses.

For these reasons, rimantadine HCl should be used during pregnancy only if the potential benefit justifies the risk to the fetus.

➤*Lactation:* Rimantadine HCl should not be administered to nursing mothers because of the adverse effects noted in offspring of rats treated with rimantadine during the nursing period. Rimantadine is concentrated in rat milk in a dose-related manner: 2 to 3 hours following administration of rimantadine, rat breast milk levels were approximately twice those observed in the serum.

➤*Children:* In children, rimantadine HCl is recommended for the prophylaxis of influenza A. The safety and effectiveness of rimantadine HCl in the treatment of symptomatic influenza infection in children have not been established. Prophylaxis studies with rimantadine HCl have not been performed in children less than 1 year.

Precautions

➤*Epilepsy:* An increased incidence of seizures has been reported in patients with a history of epilepsy who received the related drug amantadine. In clinical trials of rimantadine HCl, the occurrence of seizure-like activity was observed in a small number of patients with a history of seizures who were not receiving anticonvulsant medication while taking rimantadine HCl. If seizures develop, rimantadine HCl should be discontinued.

➤*Resistant strains:* Transmission of rimantadine resistant virus should be considered when treating patients whose contacts are at high risk for influenza A illness. Influenza A virus strains resistant to rimantadine can emerge during treatment and such resistant strains have been shown to be transmissible and to cause typical influenza illness. Although the frequency, rapidity and clinical significance of the emergence of drug-resistant virus are not yet established, several small studies have demonstrated that 10% to 30% of patients with initially sensitive virus, upon treatment with rimantadine, shed rimantadine-resistant virus.

Drug Interactions

Rimantadine Drug Interactions

Precipitant drug	Object drug*		Description
Acetaminophen	Rimantadine	⬇	Coadministration with acetaminophen reduced the peak concentration and AUC values for rimantadine by ≈ 11%.
Aspirin	Rimantadine	⬇	Peak plasma and AUC of rimantadine were reduced ≈ 10% when coadministered with aspirin.
Cimetidine	Rimantadine	⬆	When a single 100 mg dose of rimantadine was administered 1 hour after cimetidine (300 mg 4 times/day) in healthy adults, the apparent total rimantadine clearance was reduced by 18%.

* ⬆ = Object drug increased. ⬇ = Object drug decreased.

Adverse Reactions

➤*Incidence in > 1%:* Adverse events reported most frequently (1% to 3%) at the recommended dose in controlled clinical trials are shown below.

	Rimantadine (n = 1027)	Control (n = 986)
CNS		
Insomnia	2.1%	0.9%
Dizziness	1.9%	1.1%
Headache	1.4%	1.3%
Nervousness	1.3%	0.6%
Fatigue	1%	0.9%
Miscellaneous		
Asthenia	1.4%	0.5%
GI		
Nausea	2.8%	1.6%
Vomiting	1.7%	0.6%
Anorexia	1.6%	0.8%
Dry mouth	1.5%	0.6%
Abdominal pain	1.4%	0.8%

➤*Less frequent adverse events (0.3% to 1%):*

CNS – Impairment of concentration, ataxia, somnolence, agitation, depression.

Dermatologic – Rash.

GI – Diarrhea, dyspepsia.

Respiratory – Dyspnea.

Special senses – Tinnitus.

➤*Additional adverse events (less than 0.3%):*

Cardiovascular – Pallor, palpitation, hypertension, cerebrovascular disorder, cardiac failure, pedal edema, heart block, tachycardia, syncope.

CNS – Gait abnormality, euphoria, hyperkinesia, tremor, hallucination, confusion, convulsions.

Endocrine – Non-puerperal lactation.

Respiratory – Bronchospasm, cough.

Special senses – Taste loss/change, parosmia.

➤*Other adverse events:* Rates of adverse events, particularly those involving the gastrointestinal and nervous systems, increased significantly in controlled studies using higher than recommended doses of rimantadine HCl. In most cases, symptoms resolved rapidly with discontinuation of treatment. In addition to the adverse events reported above, the following were also reported at higher than recommended doses:

Miscellaneous – Increased lacrimation, increased micturition frequency, fever, rigors, agitation, constipation, diaphoresis, dysphagia, stomatitis, hypesthesia, and eye pain.

➤*Adverse reactions in trials of rimantadine and amantadine:* In a 6-week prophylaxis study of 436 healthy adults comparing rimantadine with amantadine and placebo, the following adverse reactions were reported with an incidence greater than 1%.

	Rimantadine 200 mg/day (n = 145)	Placebo (n = 143)	Amantadine 200 mg/day (n = 148)
CNS			
Insomnia	3.4%	0.7%	7%
Nervousness	2.1%	0.7%	2.8%
Impaired concentration	2.1%	1.4%	2.1%
Dizziness	0.7%	0%	2.1%
Depression	0.7%	0.7%	3.5%
Total % of subjects with adverse reactions	6.9%	4.1%	14.7%
Total % of subjects withdrawn due to adverse reactions	6.9%	3.4%	14%

➤*Elderly:* Approximately 200 patients over the age of 64 were evaluated for safety in controlled clinical trials with rimantadine hydrochloride. Geriatric subjects who received either 200 mg or 400 mg of rimantadine daily for 1 to 50 days experienced considerably more CNS and GI adverse events than comparable geriatric subjects receiving placebo. Central nervous system events including dizziness, headache, anxiety, asthenia, and fatigue, occurred up to 2 times more often in subjects treated with rimantadine than in those treated with placebo. Gastrointestinal symptoms, particularly nausea, vomiting, and abdominal pain occurred at least twice as frequently in subjects receiving rimantadine than in those receiving placebo. The gastrointestinal symptoms appeared to be dose related. In patients over 64 years of age, the recommended dose is 100 mg daily.

Overdosage

➤*Symptoms:* Overdoses of a related drug, amantadine, have been reported with adverse reactions consisting of agitation, hallucinations, cardiac arrhythmia and death.

➤*Treatment:* The administration of IV physostigmine (a cholinergic agent) at doses of 1 to 2 mg in adults and 0.5 mg in children repeated as needed as long as the dose did not exceed 2 mg/hr has been reported anecdotally to be beneficial in patients with CNS effects from overdoses of amantadine. As with any overdose, supportive therapy should be administered as indicated.

ZANAMIVIR

Rx	**Relenza** (GlaxoSmithKline)	**Blisters of powder for inhalation:** 5 mg	20 mg lactose. In 4 blisters with 5 *Rotadisks* and 1 *Diskhaler.*

ZANAMIVIR — INHALATIONAL

Indications

➤*Treatment of influenza:* For treatment of uncomplicated acute illness due to influenza A and B virus in adults and children greater than or equal to 7 years of age who have been symptomatic for no more than 2 days.

➤*Prophylaxis of influenza:* In adults and children 5 years of age and older for prophylaxis of influenza.

Zanamivir is not recommended for treatment or prophylaxis of influenza of patients with underlying airways disease (such as asthma or chronic obstructive pulmonary disease) due to risk of serious bronchospasm.

Administration and Dosage

➤*Approved by the FDA:* July 27, 1999.

Zanamivir is for administration to the respiratory tract by oral inhalation only, using the *Diskhaler* device provided. Patients should be instructed in the use of the delivery system. Instructions should include a demonstration whenever possible. If zanamivir is prescribed for children, it should be used only under adult supervision and instruction, and the supervising adult should first be instructed by a healthcare professional.

Patients scheduled to use an inhaled bronchodilator at the same time as zanamivir should use their bronchodilator before taking zanamivir.

➤*Treatment:* Two inhalations (one 5 mg blister per inhalation for a total dose of 10 mg) twice daily (approximately 12 hours apart) for 5 days. Two doses should be taken on the first day of treatment whenever possible provided there is at least 2 hours between doses. On subsequent days, doses should be about 12 hours apart (eg, morning and evening) at approximately the same time each day. There are no data on the effectiveness of treatment with zanamivir when initiated more than 2 days after the onset of signs or symptoms.

➤*Prophylaxis:*

Household setting – 10 mg once daily for 10 days. The 10-mg dose is provided by 2 inhalations (one 5-mg blister per inhalation). Administer the dose at approximately the same time each day. There are no data on the effectiveness of prophylaxis in a household setting when initiated more than 1.5 days after the onset of signs or symptoms in the index case.

Community outbreaks – 10 mg once daily for 28 days. The 10-mg dose is provided by 2 inhalations (one 5-mg blister per inhalation). Administer the dose at approximately the same time each day. There are no data on the effectiveness of prophylaxis in a community outbreak when initiated more than 5 days after the outbreak was identified in the community. The safety and effectiveness of prophylaxis have not been evaluated for longer than 28 days duration.

➤*Storage / Stability:* Store at 25°C (77°F); excursions permitted to 15° to 30°C (59° to 86°F). Keep out of reach of children. Do not puncture any zanamivir *Rotadisk* blister until taking a dose using the *Diskhaler*.

Actions

➤*Pharmacology:* The proposed mechanism of action of zanamivir is via inhibition of influenza virus neuraminidase with the possibility of alteration of virus particle aggregation and release.

➤*Pharmacokinetics:*

Absorption – Pharmacokinetic studies of orally inhaled zanamivir indicate that approximately 4% to 17% of the inhaled dose is systemically absorbed. The peak serum concentrations ranged from 17 to 142 ng/mL within 1 to 2 hours following a 10 mg dose. The area under the serum concentration versus time curve (AUC_∞) ranged from 111 to 1364 ng•hr/mL.

Distribution – Zanamivir has limited plasma protein binding (less than 10%).

Metabolism – Zanamivir is renally excreted as unchanged drug. No metabolites have been detected in humans.

Excretion – The serum half-life of zanamivir following administration by oral inhalation ranges from 2.5 to 5.1 hours. It is excreted unchanged in the urine with excretion of a single dose completed within 24 hours. Total clearance ranges from 2.5 to 10.9 L/hr. Unabsorbed drug is excreted in the feces.

Special populations –

Renal function impairment: Systemic exposure is limited after inhalation. After a single intravenous dose of 4 mg or 2 mg of zanamivir in volunteers with mild/moderate or severe renal impairment, respectively, significant decreases in renal clearance (and hence total clearance: Normal 5.3 L/hr, mild/moderate 2.7 L/hr, and severe 0.8 L/hr; median values) and significant increases in half-life (normal 3.1 hr, mild/moderate 4.7 hr, and severe 18.5 hr; median values) and systemic exposure were observed. Safety and efficacy have not been documented in the presence of severe renal insufficiency.

Children: The pharmacokinetics of zanamivir were evaluated in pediatric patients with signs and symptoms of respiratory illness. Sixteen patients, 6 to 12 years of age, received a single dose of 10-mg zanamivir dry powder via *Diskhaler*. Five patients had either undetectable zanamivir serum concentrations or had low drug concentrations (8.32 to 10.38 ng/mL) that were not detectable after 1.5 hours. Eleven patients had C_{max} median values of 43 ng/mL (range, 15 to 74) and AUC_∞ median values of 167 ng•hr/mL (range, 58 to 279). Low or undetectable serum concentrations were related to lack of measurable PIFR in individual patients.

➤*Microbiology:*

Antiviral activity in vitro – The antiviral activity of zanamivir against laboratory and clinical isolates of influenza virus was determined in cell culture assays. The concentrations of zanamivir required for inhibition of influenza virus were highly variable depending on the assay method used and virus isolate tested. The 50% and 90% inhibitory concentrations (IC_{50} and IC_{90}) of zanamivir were in the range of 0.005 to 16 mcM and 0.05 to greater than 100 mcM, respectively (1 mcM = 0.33 mcg/mL). The relationship between the in vitro inhibition of influenza virus by zanamivir and the inhibition of influenza virus replication in humans has not been established.

Drug resistance – Influenza viruses with reduced susceptibility to zanamivir have been recovered in vitro by passage of the virus in the presence of increasing concentrations of the drug. Genetic analysis of these viruses showed that the reduced susceptibility in vitro to zanamivir is associated with mutations that result in amino acid changes in the viral neuraminidase or viral hemagglutinin or both.

In an immunocompromised patient infected with influenza B virus, a variant virus emerged after treatment with an investigational nebulized solution of zanamivir for 2 weeks. Analysis of this variant showed a hemagglutinin mutation (Thr 198 Ile) which resulted in a reduced affinity for human cell receptors, and a mutation in the neuraminidase active site (Arg 152 Lys) which reduced the enzyme's activity to zanamivir by 1000-fold.

Insufficient information is available to characterize the risk of emergence of zanamivir resistance in clinical use.

Cross-resistance – Cross-resistance has been observed between zanamivir-resistant and oseltamivir-resistant influenza virus mutants generated in vitro. No studies have been performed to assess risk of emergence of cross-resistance during clinical use.

Contraindications

Hypersensitivity to any component of the formulation.

Warnings

➤*Bronchospasm and decline in lung function:* Bronchospasm and decline in lung function have been reported in some patients receiving zanamivir. Many but not all of these patients had underlying airways disease such as asthma or chronic obstructive pulmonary disease. Because of the risk of serious adverse events and because efficacy has not been demonstrated in this population, zanamivir is not generally recommended for treatment of patients with underlying airways disease. Some patients with serious adverse events during treatment with zanamivir have had fatal outcomes, although causality was difficult to assess.

Zanamivir should be discontinued in any patient who develops bronchospasm or decline in respiratory function; immediate treatment and hospitalization may be required. Some patients without prior pulmonary disease may also have respiratory abnormalities from acute respiratory infection that could resemble adverse drug reactions or increase patient vulnerability to adverse drug reactions.

➤*Elderly:* Of the total number of patients in 6 clinical treatment studies of zanamivir, 59 were 65 years and over, while 24 were 75 years and over. No overall differences in safety or effectiveness were observed between these subjects and younger patients, and other reported clinical experience has not identified differences in responses between the elderly and younger patients, but greater sensitivity of some older individuals cannot be ruled out.

➤*Pregnancy: Category C.* Embryo/fetal development studies were conducted in rats (dosed from days 6 to 15 of pregnancy) and rabbits (dosed from days 7 to 19 of pregnancy) using the same IV doses. Pre- and postnatal developmental studies were performed in rats (dosed from day 16 of pregnancy until litter day 21 to 23). In all studies, intravenous (1, 9, and 90 mg/kg/day) instead of the inhalational route of drug administration was used. No malformations, maternal toxicity, or embryotoxicity were observed in pregnant rats or rabbits and their fetuses. Because of insufficient blood sampling timepoints in both rat and rabbit reproductive toxicity studies, AUC values were not available. However, in a subchronic study in rats at the 90 mg/kg/day IV dose, the AUC values were greater than 300 times the human exposure at the proposed clinical dose.

An additional embryo/fetal study, in a different strain of rat, was conducted using subcutaneous administration of zanamivir, 3 times daily, at doses of 1, 9, or 80 mg/kg during days 7 to 17 of pregnancy. There was an increase in the incidence rates of a variety of minor skeleton alterations and variants in the exposed offspring in this study. Based on AUC measurements, the high dose in the study produced an exposure greater than 1000 times the human exposure at the proposed clinical dose. However, the individual incidence rate of each skeletal alteration or variant, in most instances, remained within the background rates of the historical occurrence in the strain studied.

Zanamivir has been shown to cross the placenta in rats and rabbits. In these animals, fetal blood concentrations of zanamivir were significantly lower than zanamivir concentrations in the maternal blood.

There are no adequate and well-controlled studies of zanamivir in pregnant women. Zanamivir should be used during pregnancy only if the potential benefit justifies the potential risk to the fetus.

➤*Lactation:* Studies in rats have demonstrated that zanamivir is excreted in milk. However, nursing mothers should be instructed that it is not known

ZANAMIVIR — INHALATIONAL

whether zanamivir is excreted in human milk. Because many drugs are excreted in human milk, caution should be exercised when zanamivir is administered to a nursing mother.

➤*Children:* Safety and effectiveness of zanamivir have not been established in pediatric patients less than 7 years of age.

The safety and effectiveness of zanamivir have been studied in a phase 3 treatment study in pediatric patients, where 471 children 5 to 12 years of age received zanamivir or placebo. In a phase 1 study of 16 children ages 6 to 12 years with signs and symptoms of respiratory disease, 4 did not produce a measurable PIFR through the *Diskhaler* (3 with no adequate inhalation on request, 1 with missing data), 9 had measurable PIFR on each of 2 inhalations, and 3 achieved measurable PIFR on only 1 of 2 inhalations. Neither of two 6-year-olds and 1 of two 7-year-olds produced measurable PIFR. Overall, 8 of the 16 children (including all those less than 8 years old) either did not produce measurable inspiratory flow through the *Diskhaler* or produced peak inspiratory flow rates below the 60 L/min considered optimal for the device under standardized in vitro testing; lack of measurable flow rate was related to low or undetectable serum concentrations. Prescribers should carefully evaluate the ability of young children to use the delivery system if prescription of zanamivir is considered. When zanamivir is prescribed for children, it should be used only under adult supervision and with attention to proper use of the delivery system.

Adolescents were included in the 3 principal phase 3 adult treatment studies. In these studies, 67 patients were 12 to 16 years of age. No definite differences in safety and efficacy were observed between these adolescent patients and young adults.

Precautions

➤*Other illness:* There is no evidence for efficacy of zanamivir in any illness caused by agents other than influenza virus A and B. Data on treatment of influenza B are limited.

➤*Start of treatment:* No data are available to support safety or efficacy in patients who begin treatment after 48 hours of symptoms.

➤*Repeated courses:* Safety and efficacy of repeated treatment courses have not been studied.

➤*Allergic reactions:* Allergic-like reactions, including oropharyngeal edema and serious skin rashes, have been reported in postmarketing experience with zanamivir. Zanamivir should be stopped and appropriate treatment instituted if an allergic reaction occurs or is suspected.

➤*Bacterial infections:* Serious bacterial infections may begin with influenza-like symptoms or may coexist with or occur as complications during the course of influenza. Zanamivir has not been shown to prevent such complications.

➤*Prevention of influenza:* Use of zanamivir should not affect the evaluation of individuals for annual influenza vaccination in accordance with guidelines of the Centers for Disease Control and Prevention Advisory Committee on Immunization Practices. Safety and efficacy of zanamivir have not been established for prophylactic use of zanamivir to prevent influenza.

➤*Chronic pulmonary disease:* Safety and efficacy have not been demonstrated in patients with underlying chronic pulmonary disease. In particular, this product has not been shown to be effective in patients with severe or decompensated chronic obstructive pulmonary disease or asthma, and serious adverse events have been reported in such patients. Therefore, zanamivir is not generally recommended for treatment of patients with underlying airways disease such as asthma or chronic obstructive pulmonary disease.

Bronchospasm was documented following administration of zanamivir in 1 of 13 patients with mild or moderate asthma (but without acute influenza-like illness) in a phase 1 study. In interim results from an ongoing treatment study in patients with acute influenza-like illness superimposed on underlying asthma or chronic obstructive pulmonary disease, more patients on zanamivir than on placebo experienced greater than 20% decline in FEV_1 or peak expiratory flow rate.

If treatment with zanamivir is considered for a patient with underlying airways disease, the potential risks and benefits should be carefully weighed. If a decision is made to prescribe zanamivir for such a patient, this should be done only under conditions of careful monitoring of respiratory function, close observation, and appropriate supportive care including availability of fast-acting bronchodilators.

➤*High-risk patients:* Safety and efficacy have not been demonstrated in patients with high-risk underlying medical conditions. No information is available regarding treatment of influenza in patients with any medical condition sufficiently severe or unstable to be considered at imminent risk of requiring inpatient management.

Drug Interactions

No clinically significant pharmacokinetic drug interactions are predicted based on data from in vitro studies.

Adverse Reactions

Bronchospasm and decline in lung function have been reported in some patients receiving zanamivir. Many but not all of these patients had underlying airways disease such as asthma or chronic obstructive pulmonary disease. Because of the risk of serious adverse events and because efficacy has not been demonstrated in this population, zanamivir is not generally recommended for treatment of patients with underlying airways disease. Some patients with serious adverse events during treatment with zanamivir have had fatal outcomes, although causality was difficult to assess.

Zanamivir should be discontinued in any patient who develops bronchospasm or decline in respiratory function; immediate treatment and hospitalization may be required. Some patients without prior pulmonary disease may also have respiratory abnormalities from acute respiratory infection that could resemble adverse drug reactions or increase patient vulnerability to adverse drug reactions.

Allergic-like reactions, including oropharyngeal edema and serious skin rashes, have been reported in postmarketing experience with zanamivir. Zanamivir should be stopped and appropriate treatment instituted if an allergic reaction occurs or is suspected.

➤*Summary of adverse reaction in greater than or equal to 1.5%:* Adverse reactions that occurred with an incidence greater than or equal to 1.5% in treatment studies are listed below. This table shows adverse reactions occurring in patients greater than or equal to 12 years of age receiving zanamivir 10 mg inhaled twice daily, zanamivir in all inhalation regimens, and placebo inhaled twice daily (where placebo consisted of the same lactose vehicle used in zanamivir).

Zanamivir Adverse Reactions in Adults and Adolescents (≥ 1.5%)

Adverse reaction	10 mg twice-daily inhaled (n = 1132)	All dosing regimens (n = 2289)	Placebo (lactose vehicle[1]) (n = 1520)
CNS			
Dizziness	2%	1%	< 1%
Headaches	2%	2%	3%
GI			
Diarrhea	3%	3%	4%
Nausea	3%	3%	3%
Vomiting	1%	1%	2%
Respiratory			
Nasal signs and symptoms	2%	3%	3%
Bronchitis	2%	2%	3%
Cough	2%	2%	3%
Sinusitis	3%	2%	2%
Ear, nose, and throat infections	2%	1%	2%

* Includes studies where zanamivir was administered intranasally (6.4 mg 2 to 4 times per day in addition to inhaled preparation) or inhaled more frequently (4 times a day) than the currently recommended dose.

[1] Because the placebo consisted of inhaled lactose powder that is also the vehicle for the active drug, some adverse reactions occurring at similar frequencies in different treatment groups could be related to lactose vehicle inhalation.

➤*Additional adverse reaction in less than 1.5%:* Additional adverse reactions occurring in less than 1.5% of patients receiving zanamivir included malaise, fatigue, fever, abdominal pain, myalgia, arthralgia, and urticaria.

The most frequent laboratory abnormalities in phase 3 treatment studies included elevations of liver enzymes and CPK, lymphopenia, and neutropenia. These were reported in similar proportions of zanamivir and lactose vehicle placebo recipients with acute influenza-like illness.

➤*Clinical trials in children:* Adverse reactions that occurred with an incidence greater than or equal to 1.5% in children receiving treatment doses of zanamivir in 2 phase 3 studies are listed in the table below. This table shows adverse reactions occurring in pediatric patients 5 to 12 years old receiving zanamivir 10 mg inhaled twice daily, and placebo inhaled twice daily (where placebo consisted of the same lactose vehicle used in zanamivir).

Zanamivir adverse reactions in children (≥ 1.5%)*

Adverse reaction	Zanamivir 10 mg twice-daily inhaled (n = 291)	Placebo (lactose vehicle[1]) (n = 318)
Respiratory		
Ear, nose, and throat infections	5%	5%
Ear, nose, and throat hemorrhage	< 1%	2%
Asthma	< 1%	2%
Cough	< 1%	2%
GI		
Vomiting	2%	3%
Diarrhea	2%	2%
Nausea	< 1%	2%

* Includes a subset of patients receiving zanamivir for treatment of influenza in a prophylaxis study.

[1] Because the placebo consisted of inhaled lactose powder, which is also the vehicle for the active drug, some adverse reactions occurring at similar frequencies in different treatment groups could be related to lactose vehicle inhalation.

In 1 of the 2 studies described in the table above, some additional information is available from children (5 to 12 years old) without acute influenza-like illness who received an investigational prophylaxis regimen of zanamivir; 132 children received zanamivir and 145 children received placebo. Among these children, nasal signs and symptoms (zanamivir 20%, placebo 9%), cough (zanamivir 16%, placebo 8%) and throat/tonsil/discomfort and pain (zanamivir 11%, placebo 6%) were reported more frequently with zanamivir than placebo. In a subset with chronic respiratory disease, lower respiratory tract adverse reactions (described as asthma, cough, or viral res-

ZANAMIVIR — INHALATIONAL

piratory infections that could include influenza-like symptoms) were reported in 7 of 7 zanamivir recipients and 5 of 12 placebo recipients.

➤*Observed during clinical practice:* In addition to adverse reactions reported from clinical trials, the following reactions have been identified during postmarketing use of zanamivir. Because they are reported voluntarily from a population of unknown size, estimates of frequency cannot be made. These reactions have been chosen for inclusion due to a combination of their seriousness, frequency of reporting, or potential causal connection to zanamivir.

Cardiovascular – Arrhythmias, syncope.

CNS – Seizures.

Dermatologic – Facial edema; rash, including serious cutaneous reactions.

Respiratory – Bronchospasm, dyspnea.

Miscellaneous – Allergic or allergic-like reaction, including oropharyngeal edema.

Overdosage

There have been no reports of overdosage from administration of zanamivir. Doses of zanamivir up to 64 mg/day have been administered by nebulizer. Additionally, doses of up to 1200 mg/day for 5 days have been administered intravenously. Adverse reactions were similar to those seen in clinical studies at the recommended dose.

Patient Information

Patients should be instructed in use of the delivery system. Instructions should include a demonstration whenever possible.

For the proper use of zanamivir, the patient should read and follow carefully this section. Effective and safe use of zanamivir requires proper use of the *Diskhaler* to inhale the drug.

Patients should be advised to finish the entire 5-day course of treatment even if they start to feel better sooner.

Patients should be advised that the use of zanamivir for treatment of influenza has not been shown to reduce the risk of transmission of influenza to others.

Patients should be advised of the risk of bronchospasm, especially in the setting of underlying airways disease, and should stop zanamivir and contact their physician if they experience increased respiratory symptoms during treatment such as worsening wheezing, shortness of breath, or other signs or symptoms of bronchospasm. If a decision is made to prescribe zanamivir for a patient with asthma or chronic obstructive pulmonary disease, the patient should be made aware of the risks and should have a fast-acting bronchodilator available. Patients scheduled to take inhaled bronchodilators at the same times as zanamivir should be advised to use their bronchodilators before taking zanamivir.

OSELTAMIVIR PHOSPHATE

Rx	**Tamiflu** (Roche)	**Capsules:** 75 mg (as base)	Talc. (ROCHE 75 mg). Grey/yellow. In blister pack 10s.
		Powder for oral suspension: 12 mg/mL after reconstitution (as base)	Sorbitol, saccharin. Tutti-frutti flavor. In 25 mL with bottle adapter and oral dispenser.

OSELTAMIVIR PHOSPHATE — ORAL

Indications

➤*Treatment of influenza:* Treatment of uncomplicated acute illness due to influenza infection in patients greater than 1 year of age who have been symptomatic for no more than 2 days.

➤*Prophylaxis of influenza:* Prophylaxis of influenza in adult patients and adolescents greater than or equal to 13 years of age.

Oseltamivir phosphate is not a substitute for early vaccination on an annual basis as recommended by the Centers for Disease Control's Immunization Practices Advisory Committee (ACIP).

Administration and Dosage

➤*Approved by the FDA:* October 27, 1999.

Oseltamivir phosphate may be taken with or without food. However, when taken with food, tolerability may be enhanced in some patients.

Note: Shake the oseltamivir phosphate oral suspension well before each use.

The constituted oral suspension should be used within 10 days of preparation.

See Actions for more information.

➤*Treatment of influenza:*

Adults and adolescents – The recommended oral dose of oseltamivir phosphate for treatment of influenza in adults and adolescents greater than or equal to 13 years of age is 75 mg twice daily for 5 days. Treatment should begin within 2 days of onset of symptoms of influenza.

Children – The recommended oral dose of oseltamivir phosphate oral suspension for children greater than or equal to 1 year of age or adult patients who cannot swallow a capsule is as follows:

Body weight in kg	Body weight in lbs	Recommended dose for 5 days	Number of bottles needed to obtain the recommended dose
≤ 15 kg	≤ 33 lbs	30 mg twice daily	1
> 15 kg to 23 kg	> 33 lbs to 51 lbs	45 mg twice daily	2
> 23 kg to 40 kg	> 51 lbs to 88 lbs	60 mg twice daily	2
> 40 kg	> 88 lbs	75 mg twice daily	3

An oral dosing dispenser with 30, 45, and 60 mg graduations is provided with the oral suspension; the 75 mg dose can be measured using a combination of 30 mg and 45 mg. It is recommended that patients use this dispenser. In the event that the dispenser provided is lost or damaged, another dosing syringe or other device may be used to deliver the following volumes: 2.5 mL (½ tsp) for children less than or equal to 15 kg; 3.8 mL (¾ tsp) for greater than 15 to less than or equal to 23 kg; 5 mL (1 tsp) for greater than 23 to less than or equal to 40 kg; and 6.2 mL (1¼ tsp) for greater than 40 kg.

➤*Prophylaxis of influenza:* The recommended oral dose of oseltamivir phosphate for prophylaxis of influenza in adults and adolescents greater than or equal to 13 years of age following close contact with an infected individual is 75 mg once daily for at least 7 days. Therapy should begin within 2 days of exposure. The recommended dose for prophylaxis during a community outbreak of influenza is 75 mg once daily. Safety and efficacy have been demonstrated for up to 6 weeks. The duration of protection lasts for as long as dosing is continued.

➤*Renal function impairment:* For plasma concentrations of oseltamivir carboxylate predicted to occur following various dosing schedules in patients with renal impairment. Administration of 100 mg of oseltamivir phosphate twice daily for 5 days to patients with various degrees of renal impairment showed that exposure to oseltamivir carboxylate is inversely proportional to declining renal function.

Treatment of influenza – Dose adjustment is recommended for patients with creatinine clearance between 10 and 30 mL/min receiving oseltamivir phosphate for the treatment of influenza. In these patients, it is recommended that the dose be reduced to 75 mg of oseltamivir phosphate once daily for 5 days. No recommended dosing regimens are available for patients undergoing routine hemodialysis and continuous peritoneal dialysis treatment with end-stage renal disease.

Prophylaxis of influenza – For the prophylaxis of influenza, dose adjustment is recommended for patients with creatinine clearance between 10 and 30 mL/min receiving oseltamivir phosphate. In these patients, it is recommended that the dose be reduced to 75 mg of oseltamivir phosphate every other day or 30 mg of oseltamivir phosphate oral suspension every day. No recommended dosing regimens are available for patients undergoing routine hemodialysis and continuous peritoneal dialysis treatment with end-stage renal disease.

➤*Storage/Stability:* Store at 25°C (77°F); excursions permitted to 15° to 30°C (59° to 86°F). [See USP controlled room temperature.]

Store constituted suspension under refrigeration at 2° to 8°C (36° to 46°F). Do not freeze. The constituted oral suspension should be used within 10 days of preparation.

Actions

➤*Pharmacology:* Oseltamivir is an ethyl ester prodrug requiring ester hydrolysis for conversion to the active form, oseltamivir carboxylate. The proposed mechanism of action of oseltamivir is via inhibition of influenza virus neuraminidase, with the possibility of alteration of virus particle aggregation and release.

➤*Pharmacokinetics:*

Absorption – Oseltamivir is readily absorbed from the GI tract after oral administration of oseltamivir phosphate and is extensively converted, predominantly by hepatic esterases, to oseltamivir carboxylate. At least 75% of an oral dose reaches the systemic circulation as oseltamivir carboxylate. Exposure to oseltamivir is less than 5% of the total exposure after oral dosing (see the following table).

Mean (% CV) pharmacokinetic parameters of oseltamivir and oseltamivir carboxylate after a multiple 75 mg capsule twice-daily oral dose (n = 20)		
Parameter	Oseltamivir	Oseltamivir carboxylate
C_{max} (ng/mL)	65.2 (26% CV)	348 (18% CV)
$AUC_{0\text{-}12\ h}$ (ng•hr/mL)	112 (25% CV)	2719 (20% CV)

Plasma concentrations of oseltamivir carboxylate are proportional to doses less than or equal to 500 mg given twice daily.

Coadministration with food has no significant effect on the peak plasma concentration (551 ng/mL under fasted conditions and 441 ng/mL under fed conditions) and the area under the plasma concentration time curve (6218 ng•hr/mL under fasted conditions and 6069 ng•hr/mL under fed conditions) of oseltamivir carboxylate.

Distribution – The volume of distribution (V_{ss}) of oseltamivir carboxylate, following IV administration in 24 subjects, ranged between 23 and 26 L.

OSELTAMIVIR PHOSPHATE — ORAL

The binding of oseltamivir carboxylate to human plasma protein is low (3%). The binding of oseltamivir to human plasma protein is 42%, which is insufficient to cause significant displacement-based drug interactions.

Metabolism – Oseltamivir is extensively converted to oseltamivir carboxylate by esterases located predominantly in the liver. Neither oseltamivir nor oseltamivir carboxylate is a substrate for, or inhibitor of, cytochrome P450 isoforms.

Excretion – Absorbed oseltamivir is primarily (greater than 90%) eliminated by conversion to oseltamivir carboxylate. Plasma concentrations of oseltamivir declined with a half-life of 1 to 3 hours in most subjects after oral administration. Oseltamivir carboxylate is not further metabolized and is eliminated in the urine. Plasma concentrations of oseltamivir carboxylate declined with a half-life of 6 to 10 hours in most subjects after oral administration. Oseltamivir carboxylate is eliminated entirely (greater than 99%) by renal excretion. Renal clearance (18.8 L/hr) exceeds glomerular filtration rate (7.5 L/hr) indicating that tubular secretion occurs, in addition to glomerular filtration. Less than 20% of an oral radiolabeled dose is eliminated in feces.

Special populations –

Renal function impairment: Administration of 100 mg of oseltamivir phosphate twice daily for 5 days to patients with various degrees of renal impairment showed that exposure to oseltamivir carboxylate is inversely proportional to declining renal function. Oseltamivir carboxylate exposures in patients with healthy and abnormal renal function administered various dose regimens of oseltamivir are described below.

In the following table, AUC is normalized to 48 hours.

Oseltamivir carboxylate exposures in patients with normal and reduced serum creatinine clearance								
	Normal renal function			Impaired renal function				
				Creatinine clearance < 10 mL/min		Creatinine clearance > 10 and < 30 mL/min		
				CAPD	Hemodialysis			
Parameter	75 mg every day	75 mg twice daily	150 mg twice daily	30 mg weekly	30 mg alternate HD cycle	75 mg daily	75 mg alternate days	30 mg daily
C_{max}	259*	348*	705*	766	850	1638	1175	655
C_{min}	39*	138*	288*	62	48	864	209	346
AUC_{48}	7476*	10,876*	21,864*	17,381	12,429	62,636	21,999	25,054

* Observed values. All other values are predicted.

Elderly: Exposure to oseltamivir carboxylate at steady state was 25% to 35% higher in elderly patients (age range 65 to 78 years) compared to younger adults given comparable doses of oseltamivir. Half-lives observed in the elderly patients were similar to those seen in younger adults. Based on drug exposure and tolerability, dose adjustments are not required for elderly patients (for either treatment or prophylaxis; see Administration and Dosage).

Children: The pharmacokinetics of oseltamivir and oseltamivir carboxylate have been evaluated in a single-dose pharmacokinetic study in children aged 5 to 16 years (n = 18) and in a small number of children aged 3 to 12 years (n = 5) enrolled in a clinical trial. Younger children cleared both the prodrug and the active metabolite faster than adult patients resulting in a lower exposure for a given mg/kg dose. For oseltamivir carboxylate, apparent total clearance decreases linearly with increasing age (up to 12 years). The pharmacokinetics of oseltamivir in children older than 12 years of age are similar to those in adult patients.

Contraindications

Hypersensitivity to any of the components of the product.

Warnings

➤*Renal function impairment:* Dose adjustment is recommended for patients with a serum creatinine clearance less than 30 mL/min.

Treatment of influenza – See Administration and Dosage for more information.

Prophylaxis of influenza – See Administration and Dosage for more information.

➤*Pregnancy: Category C.* There are insufficient human data upon which to base an evaluation of risk of oseltamivir phosphate to the pregnant woman or developing fetus. Studies for effects on embryofetal development were conducted in rats (50, 250, and 1500 mg/kg/day) and rabbits (50, 150, and 500 mg/kg/day) by the oral route. Relative exposures at these doses were, respectively, 2, 13, and 100 times human exposure in the rat and 4, 8, and 50 times human exposure in the rabbit. Pharmacokinetic studies indicated that fetal exposure was seen in both species. In the rat study, minimal maternal toxicity was reported in the 1500 mg/kg/day group. In the rabbit study, slight and marked maternal toxicities were observed, respectively, in the 150 and 500 mg/kg/day groups. There was a dose-dependent increase in the incidence rates of a variety of minor skeletal abnormalities and variants in the exposed offspring in these studies. However, the individual incidence rate of each skeletal abnormality or variant remained within the background rates of occurrence in the species studied.

Because animal reproductive studies may not be predictive of human response, and there are no adequate and well-controlled studies in pregnant women, oseltamivir phosphate should be used during pregnancy only if the potential benefit justifies the potential risk to the fetus.

➤*Lactation:* In lactating rats, oseltamivir and oseltamivir carboxylate are excreted in the milk. It is not known whether oseltamivir or oseltamivir carboxylate is excreted in human milk. Oseltamivir phosphate should, therefore, be used only if the potential benefit for the lactating mother justifies the potential risk to the breastfed infant.

➤*Children:* The safety and efficacy of oseltamivir phosphate in children (less than 1 year of age) have not been established.

Precautions

➤*Influenza vaccination:* Use of oseltamivir phosphate should not affect the evaluation of individuals for annual influenza vaccination in accordance with guidelines of the CDC Advisory Committee on Immunization Practices.

➤*Treatment initiation:* Efficacy of oseltamivir phosphate in patients who begin treatment after 40 hours of symptoms has not been established.

➤*Bacterial infections:* Serious bacterial infections may begin with influenza-like symptoms or may coexist with or occur as complications during the course of influenza. Oseltamivir phosphate has not been shown to prevent such complications.

Drug Interactions

➤*Drug/Food interactions:* Oseltamivir phosphate may be taken with or without food. However, when taken with food, tolerability may be enhanced in some patients.

Adverse Reactions

➤*Adults:* A total of 1171 patients who participated in adult phase 3 controlled clinical trials for the treatment of influenza were treated with oseltamivir phosphate. The most frequently reported adverse reactions in these studies were nausea and vomiting. These reactions were generally of mild-to-moderate degree and usually occurred on the first 2 days of administration. Less than 1% of subjects discontinued prematurely from clinical trials due to nausea and vomiting.

Adverse reactions that occurred with an incidence of greater than or equal to 1% in 1440 patients taking placebo or oseltamivir phosphate 75 mg twice daily in adult, phase 3 treatment studies are shown in the following table. This summary includes 945 healthy young adults and 495 at risk patients (elderly patients and patients with chronic cardiac or respiratory disease). Those reactions reported numerically more frequently in patients taking oseltamivir phosphate compared with placebo were nausea, vomiting, bronchitis, insomnia, and vertigo.

Most frequent adverse reactions in studies in naturally acquired influenza				
	Treatment		Prophylaxis	
Adverse reaction	Placebo (n = 716)	Oseltamivir 75 mg twice daily (n = 724)	Placebo (n = 1434)	Oseltamivir 75 mg daily (n = 1480)
Nausea (without vomiting)	40 (5.6%)	72 (9.9%)	56 (3.9%)	104 (7%)
Vomiting	21 (2.9%)	68 (9.4%)	15 (1%)	31 (2.1%)
Diarrhea	70 (9.8%)	48 (6.6%)	38 (2.6%)	48 (3.2%)
Bronchitis	15 (2.1%)	17 (2.3%)	17 (1.2%)	11 (0.7%)
Abdominal pain	16 (2.2%)	16 (2.2%)	23 (1.6%)	30 (2%)
Dizziness	25 (3.5%)	15 (2.1%)	21 (1.5%)	24 (1.6%)
Headache	14 (2%)	13 (1.8%)	251 (17.5%)	298 (20.1%)
Cough	12 (1.7%)	9 (1.2%)	86 (6%)	83 (5.6%)
Insomnia	6 (0.8%)	8 (1.1%)	14 (1%)	18 (1.2%)
Vertigo	4 (0.6%)	7 (1%)	3 (0.2%)	4 (0.3%)
Fatigue	7 (1%)	7 (1%)	107 (7.5%)	117 (7.9%)

Additional adverse reactions occurring in less than 1% of patients receiving oseltamivir phosphate included unstable angina, anemia, pseudomembranous colitis, humerus fracture, pneumonia, pyrexia, and peritonsillar abscess.

Prophylaxis studies: A total of 3434 subjects (adolescents, healthy adults and elderly) participated in phase 3 prophylaxis studies, of whom 1480 received the recommended dose of 75 mg once daily for up to 6 weeks. Adverse reactions were qualitatively very similar to those seen in the treatment studies, despite a longer duration of dosing (see information above). Events reported more frequently in subjects receiving oseltamivir phosphate compared to subjects receiving placebo in prophylaxis studies, and more commonly than in treatment studies, were aches and pains, rhinorrhea, dyspepsia, and upper respiratory tract infections. However, the difference in incidence between oseltamivir phosphate and placebo for these reactions was less than 1%. There were no clinically relevant differences in the safety profile of the 942 elderly subjects who received oseltamivir phosphate or placebo, compared with the younger population.

➤*Children:* A total of 1032 children aged 1 to 12 years (including 698 otherwise healthy children aged 1 to 12 years and 334 asthmatic children aged 6 to 12 years) participated in phase 3 studies of oseltamivir phosphate given for the treatment of influenza. A total of 515 children received treatment with oseltamivir phosphate oral suspension. Adverse reactions occurring in greater than 1% of children receiving oseltamivir phosphate treatment are listed in the following table. The most frequently reported adverse reaction was vomiting. Other reactions reported more frequently by children treated with oseltamivir phosphate included abdominal pain, epistaxis, ear disorder, and conjunctivitis. These reactions generally occurred once and resolved despite continued dosing. They did not cause discontinuation of drug in the vast majority of cases.

OSELTAMIVIR PHOSPHATE — ORAL

The adverse reaction profile in adolescents is similar to that described for adult patients and children aged 1 to 12 years.

Adverse reactions occurring on treatment in > 1% of children enrolled in phase 3 trials of oseltamivir phosphate treatment of naturally acquired influenza

Adverse reaction	Placebo (n = 517)	Oseltamivir phosphate 2 mg/kg twice daily (n = 515)
Vomiting	48 (9.3%)	77 (15%)
Diarrhea	55 (10.6%)	49 (9.5%)
Otitis media	58 (11.2%)	45 (8.7%)
Abdominal pain	20 (3.9%)	24 (4.7%)
Asthma (including aggravated)	19 (3.7%)	18 (3.5%)
Nausea	22 (4.3%)	17 (3.3%)
Epistaxis	13 (2.5%)	16 (3.1%)
Pneumonia	17 (3.3%)	10 (1.9%)
Ear disorder	6 (1.2%)	9 (1.7%)
Sinusitis	13 (2.5%)	9 (1.7%)
Bronchitis	11 (2.1%)	8 (1.6%)
Conjunctivitis	2 (0.4%)	5 (1%)
Dermatitis	10 (1.9%)	5 (1%)
Lymphadenopathy	8 (1.5%)	5 (1%)
Tympanic membrane disorder	6 (1.2%)	5 (1%)

➤*Postmarketing:*

Allergic – Rash; swelling of the face or tongue; toxic epidermal necrolysis.

Cardiovascular – Arrhythmia.

CNS – Seizure; confusion.

Hepatic – Hepatitis; abnormal liver function tests.

Metabolic – Aggravation of diabetes.

Overdosage

➤*Symptoms:* At present, there has been no experience with overdose. Single doses less than or equal to 1000 mg of oseltamivir phosphate have been associated with nausea or vomiting.

Patient Information

Patients should be instructed to begin treatment with oseltamivir phosphate as soon as possible from the first appearance of flu symptoms. Similarly, prevention should begin as soon as possible after exposure, at the recommendation of a physician.

Patients should be instructed to take any missed doses as soon as they remember, except if it is near the next scheduled dose (within 2 hours), and then continue to take oseltamivir phosphate at the usual times.

Oseltamivir phosphate is not a substitute for a flu vaccination. Patients should continue receiving an annual flu shot according to guidelines on immunization practices.

ADEFOVIR DIPIVOXIL

Rx	**Hepsera** (Gilead Sciences)	**Tablets:** 10 mg	Lactose. (10 GILEAD). White. In 30s.

ADEFOVIR DIPIVOXIL — ORAL

WARNING

Severe acute exacerbations of hepatitis have been reported in patients who have discontinued anti–hepatitis B therapy, including therapy with adefovir dipivoxil. Closely monitor hepatic function with both clinical and laboratory follow-up for at least several months in patients who discontinue anti–hepatitis B therapy. If appropriate, resumption of anti–hepatitis B therapy may be warranted.

In patients at risk of or having underlying renal dysfunction, chronic administration of adefovir dipivoxil may result in nephrotoxicity. Closely monitor these patients for renal function; they may require dose adjustment. Carefully evaluate the risks and benefits of adefovir dipivoxil treatment prior to discontinuing adefovir dipivoxil in a patient with treatment-emergent nephrotoxicity.

Prior to initiating adefovir dipivoxil therapy, offer HIV antibody testing to all patients. HIV resistance may emerge in chronic hepatitis B patients with unrecognized or untreated HIV infection treated with anti–hepatitis B therapies, such as therapy with adefovir dipivoxil, that may have activity against HIV. Adefovir dipivoxil has not been shown to suppress HIV ribonucleic acid (RNA) in patients; however, there are limited data on the use of adefovir dipivoxil to treat patients with chronic hepatitis B coinfected with HIV.

Lactic acidosis and severe hepatomegaly with steatosis, including fatal cases, have been reported with the use of nucleoside analogs alone or in combination with other antiretrovirals.

Indications

➤*Chronic hepatitis B:* For the treatment of chronic hepatitis B in adults with evidence of active viral replication and either evidence of persistent elevations in serum aminotransferases (ALT or AST) or histologically active disease.

Administration and Dosage

➤*Approved by the FDA:* September 20, 2002.

The recommended dosage of adefovir dipivoxil in chronic hepatitis B patients with adequate renal function is 10 mg once daily, taken orally, without regard to food. The optimal duration of treatment is unknown.

➤*Renal function impairment:* Significantly increased drug exposures were seen when adefovir dipivoxil was administered to patients with renal impairment. Therefore, adjust the dosing interval of adefovir dipivoxil in patients with baseline creatinine clearance less than 50 mL/min using the following suggested guidelines. The safety and efficacy of these dosing interval adjustment guidelines have not been clinically evaluated.

Additionally, it is important to note that these guidelines were derived from data in patients with preexisting renal impairment at baseline. They may not be appropriate for patients in whom renal insufficiency evolves during treatment with adefovir dipivoxil. Therefore, closely monitor clinical response to treatment and renal function in these patients.

Dosing Interval Adjustment of Adefovir Dipivoxil in Patients with Renal Impairment

	Creatinine clearance (mL/min)[a]			
	≥ 50	20 to 49	10 to 19	Hemodialysis patients
Recommended dose and dosing interval	10 mg every 24 hours	10 mg every 48 hours	10 mg every 72 hours	10 mg every 7 days following dialysis

[a] Creatinine clearance calculated by Cockroft-Gault method using lean or ideal body weight.

The pharmacokinetics of adefovir have not been evaluated in nonhemodialysis patients with creatinine clearance less than 10 mL/min; therefore, no dosing recommendation is available for these patients.

➤*Storage/Stability:* Store in original container at 25°C (77°F), excursions permitted to 15° to 30°C (59° to 86°F).

Actions

➤*Pharmacology:* Adefovir is an acyclic nucleotide analog of adenosine monophosphate, which is phosphorylated to the active metabolite adefovir diphosphate by cellular kinases. Adefovir diphosphate inhibits HBV deoxyribonucleic acid (DNA) polymerase (reverse transcriptase) by competing with the natural substrate deoxyadenosine triphosphate and by causing DNA chain termination after its incorporation into viral DNA. The inhibition constant (K_i) for adefovir diphosphate for HBV DNA polymerase was 0.1 mcM. Adefovir diphosphate is a weak inhibitor of human DNA polymerases α and γ with K_i values of 1.18 and 0.97 mcM, respectively.

➤*Pharmacokinetics:*

Absorption – Adefovir dipivoxil is a diester prodrug of the active moiety adefovir. Based on a cross study comparison, the approximate oral bioavailability of adefovir from adefovir dipivoxil is 59%.

Following oral administration of a 10 mg single dose of adefovir dipivoxil to chronic hepatitis B patients (n = 14), the peak adefovir plasma concentration (C_{max}) was 18.4 ± 6.26 ng/mL (mean ± SD) and occurred between 0.58 and 4 hours (median, 1.75 hours) postdose. The adefovir area under the plasma concentration-time curve ($AUC_{0-\infty}$) was 220 ± 70 ng•h/mL. Plasma adefovir concentrations declined in a biexponential manner.

Adefovir exposure was unaffected when a 10 mg single dose of adefovir dipivoxil was administered with food (an approximately 1,000 kcal high-fat meal). Adefovir dipivoxil may be taken without regard to food.

Distribution – In vitro binding of adefovir to human plasma or human serum proteins is less than or equal to 4% over the adefovir concentration range of 0.1 to 25 mcg/mL. The volume of distribution at steady state following intravenous (IV) administration of 1 or 3 mg/kg/day is 392 ± 75 and 352 ± 9 mL/kg, respectively.

Metabolism/Excretion – Terminal elimination half-life is 7.48 ± 1.65 hours. Following oral administration, adefovir dipivoxil is rapidly converted to adefovir. Forty-five percent of the dose is recovered as adefovir in the urine over 24 hours at steady state following oral doses of adefovir dip-

ADEFOVIR DIPIVOXIL — ORAL

ivoxil 10 mg. Adefovir is renally excreted by a combination of glomerular filtration and active tubular secretion. Apart from lamivudine, trimethoprim/sulfamethoxazole, and acetaminophen, the effects of coadministration of adefovir dipivoxil with drugs that are excreted renally, or other drugs known to affect renal function, have not been evaluated.

Special populations –

Renal function impairment: In subjects with moderately or severely impaired renal function or with end-stage renal disease (ESRD) requiring hemodialysis, C_{max}, AUC, and half-life ($t_{½}$) were increased compared with subjects with normal renal function. It is recommended that the dosing interval of adefovir dipivoxil be modified in these patients.

The pharmacokinetics of adefovir in nonchronic hepatitis B patients with varying degrees of renal impairment are described in the following table. In this study, subjects received a single dose of adefovir dipivoxil 10 mg.

Pharmacokinetic Parameters (mean ± SD) of Adefovir Dipivoxil in Patients with Varying Degrees of Renal Function

Renal function group	Unimpaired	Mild	Moderate	Severe
Baseline creatinine clearance (mL/min)	> 80 (n = 7)	50 to 80 (n = 8)	30 to 49 (n = 7)	10 to 29 (n = 10)
C_{max} (ng/mL)	17.8 ± 3.22	22.4 ± 4.04	28.5 ± 8.57	51.6 ± 10.3
$AUC_{0-\infty}$ (ng•h/mL)	201 ± 40.8	266 ± 55.7	455 ± 176	1240 ±629
CL/F (mL/min)	469 ± 99	356 ± 85.6	237 ± 118	91.7 ± 51.3
CL_{renal} (mL/min)	231 ± 48.9	148 ± 39.3	83.9 ± 27.5	37 ± 18.4

A 4-hour period of hemodialysis removed approximately 35% of the adefovir dose. The effect of peritoneal dialysis on adefovir removal has not been evaluated.

See Administration and Dosage for more information.

Contraindications

Hypersensitivity to any of the components of the product.

Warnings

➤*Exacerbations of hepatitis after discontinuation of treatment:* In clinical trials of adefovir dipivoxil, exacerbations of hepatitis (ALT elevations 10 times the ULN or greater) occurred in up to 25% of patients after discontinuation of adefovir dipivoxil. These events were identified in studies GS-98–437 and GS-98–438 (n = 492). Most of these events occurred within 12 weeks of drug discontinuation. These exacerbations generally occurred in the absence of HBeAg seroconversion, and presented as serum ALT elevations in addition to reemergence of viral replication. In the HBeAg-positive and HBeAg-negative studies in patients with compensated liver function, the exacerbations were not generally accompanied by hepatic decompensation. However, patients with advanced liver disease or cirrhosis may be at higher risk for hepatic decompensation. Although most events appear to have been self-limited or resolved with reinitiation of treatment, severe hepatitis exacerbations, including fatalities, have been reported. Therefore, closely monitor patients after stopping treatment.

See Adverse Reactions for more information.

➤*Nephrotoxicity:* It is important to monitor renal function for all patients during treatment with adefovir dipivoxil, particularly for those with preexisting or other risks for renal impairment. Patients with renal insufficiency at baseline or during treatment may require dose adjustment. Carefully evaluate the risks and benefits of adefovir dipivoxil treatment prior to discontinuing adefovir dipivoxil in a patient with treatment-emergent nephrotoxicity.

See Adverse Reactions for more information.

➤*HIV resistance:* Prior to initiating adefovir dipivoxil therapy, offer HIV antibody testing to all patients. Treatment with anti–hepatitis B therapies, such as adefovir dipivoxil, that have activity against HIV in a chronic hepatitis B patient with unrecognized or untreated HIV infection may result in emergence of HIV resistance. Adefovir dipivoxil has not been shown to suppress HIV RNA in patients; however, there are limited data on the use of adefovir dipivoxil to treat patients with chronic hepatitis B coinfected with HIV.

➤*Lactic acidosis / Severe hepatomegaly with steatosis:* See Adverse Reactions for more information.

➤*Elderly:* Clinical studies of adefovir dipivoxil did not include sufficient numbers of patients 65 years of age and older to determine whether they respond differently from younger patients. In general, exercise caution when prescribing to elderly patients because they have greater frequency of decreased renal or cardiac function caused by concomitant disease or other drug therapy.

➤*Pregnancy: Category C.* When adefovir was administered intravenously (IV) to pregnant rats at doses associated with notable maternal toxicity (systemic exposure 38 times that in the human), embryotoxicity, and an increased incidence of fetal malformations (eg, anasarca, depressed eye bulge, umbilical hernia, kinked tail) were observed. No adverse effects on development were seen with adefovir administered IV to pregnant rats at a systemic exposure 12 times that in humans.

There are no adequate and well-controlled studies in pregnant women. Because animal reproduction studies are not always predictive of human response, use adefovir dipivoxil during pregnancy only if clearly needed and after careful consideration of the risks and benefits.

Pregnancy registry – To monitor fetal outcomes of pregnant women exposed to adefovir dipivoxil, a pregnancy registry has been established. Health care providers are encouraged to register patients by calling 1-800-258-4263.

Labor and delivery – There are no studies in pregnant women and no data on the effect of adefovir dipivoxil on transmission of HBV from mother to infant. Therefore, use appropriate infant immunizations to prevent neonatal acquisition of HBV.

➤*Lactation:* It is not known whether adefovir is excreted in human milk. Instruct mothers not to breast-feed if they are taking adefovir dipivoxil.

➤*Children:* Safety and efficacy in pediatric patients have not been established.

Precautions

➤*Monitoring:* Closely monitor patients for adverse reactions when adefovir dipivoxil is coadministered with drugs that are excreted renally or with other drugs known to affect renal function.

Monitor patients who discontinue adefovir dipivoxil at repeated intervals over a period of time for hepatic function.

➤*Duration of treatment:* The optimal duration of adefovir dipivoxil treatment and the relationship between treatment response and long-term outcomes, such as hepatocellular carcinoma or decompensated cirrhosis, are not known.

Drug Interactions

➤*Renally eliminated drugs:* Because adefovir is eliminated by the kidney, coadministration of adefovir dipivoxil with drugs that reduce renal function or compete for active tubular secretion may increase serum concentrations of either adefovir and/or these coadministered drugs. The clinical significance of this increase in adefovir exposure is unknown.

Adverse Reactions

➤*Hepatitis exacerbations:* Severe acute exacerbation of hepatitis has been reported in patients who have discontinued anti–hepatitis B therapy, including therapy with adefovir dipivoxil. Monitor patients who discontinue adefovir dipivoxil at repeated intervals over a period of time for hepatic function. If appropriate, resumption of anti–hepatitis B therapy may be warranted.

➤*Nephrotoxicity:* Nephrotoxicity, characterized by a delayed onset of gradual increases in serum creatinine and decreases in serum phosphorus, was historically shown to be the treatment-limiting toxicity of adefovir dipivoxil therapy at substantially higher dosages in HIV-infected patients (60 and 120 mg daily) and in chronic hepatitis B patients (30 mg daily). Chronic administration of adefovir dipivoxil (10 mg once daily) may result in nephrotoxicity. The overall risk of nephrotoxicity in patients with adequate renal function is low. However, this is of special importance in patients at risk of, or having, underlying renal dysfunction and patients taking concomitant nephrotoxic agents such as cyclosporine, tacrolimus, aminoglycosides, vancomycin, and NSAIDs.

➤*HIV-resistance:* Treatment with anti–hepatitis B therapies, such as adefovir dipivoxil, that have activity against HIV in a chronic hepatitis B patient with unrecognized or untreated HIV infection may result in emergence of HIV resistance.

➤*Lactic acidosis / Severe hepatomegaly:* Lactic acidosis and severe hepatomegaly with steatosis, including fatal cases, have been reported with the use of nucleoside analogs alone or in combination with antiretrovirals.

A majority of these cases have been in women. Obesity and prolonged nucleoside exposure may be risk factors. Exercise particular caution when administering nucleoside analogs to any patient with known risk factors for liver disease; however, cases also have been reported in patients with no known risk factors. Suspend treatment with adefovir dipivoxil in any patient who develops clinical or laboratory findings suggestive of lactic acidosis or pronounced hepatotoxicity (which may include hepatomegaly and steatosis even in the absence of marked transaminase elevations).

Treatment-Related Adverse Reactions (Grades 1 to 4) Reported in ≥ 3% of All Adefovir Dipivoxil–Treated Patients in the Pooled 437 and 438 Studies (0 to 48 Weeks)

	Adefovir dipivoxil 10 mg (n = 294)	Placebo (n = 228)
CNS		
Headache	9%	10%
GI		
Abdominal pain	9%	11%
Diarrhea	3%	4%
Dyspepsia	3%	2%
Flatulence	4%	4%
Nausea	5%	8%
Miscellaneous		
Asthenia	13%	14%

ADEFOVIR DIPIVOXIL — ORAL

➤*Lab test abnormalities:*

Grade 3 to 4 Laboratory Abnormalities Reported in ≥ 1% of All Adefovir Dipivoxil–Treated Patients in the Pooled 437 and 438 Studies (0 to 48 Weeks)		
	Adefovir dipivoxil 10 mg (n = 294)	Placebo (n = 228)
ALT (> 5 × ULN)	20%	41%
Amylase (> 2 × ULN)	4%	4%
AST (> 5 × ULN)	8%	23%
Creatine kinase (> 4 × ULN)	7%	7%
Glycosuria (≥ 3+)	1%	3%
Hematuria (≥ 3+)	11%	10%

In patients with adequate renal function, increases in serum creatinine greater than or equal to 0.3 mg/dL from baseline were observed in 4% of patients treated with adefovir dipivoxil 10 mg/day compared with 2% of patients in the placebo group at week 48. No patients developed a serum creatinine increase greater than or equal to 0.5 mg/dL from baseline by week 48. By week 96, 10% and 2% of adefovir dipivoxil–treated patients, by Kaplan-Meier estimate, had increases in serum creatinine greater than or equal to 0.3 mg/dL and greater than or equal to 0.5 mg/dL from baseline, respectively (no placebo-controlled results were available for comparison beyond week 48). Of the 29 of 492 patients with elevations in serum creatinine greater than or equal to 0.3 mg/dL from baseline, 20 resolved on continued treatment (less than or equal to 0.2 mg/dL from baseline), 8 remained unchanged, and 1 resolved on discontinuing treatment.

➤*Special risk patients:* The most common treatment-related adverse reactions reported in pre– and post–liver transplantation patients treated with adefovir dipivoxil with a 2% frequency or higher include the following:

Dermatologic – Pruritus, rash.

GI – Abdominal pain, diarrhea, flatulence, nausea, vomiting.

GU – Increases in creatinine, renal failure, renal insufficiency.

Hepatic – Abnormal liver function, hepatic failure, increases in ALT and AST.

Respiratory – Increased cough, pharyngitis, sinusitis.

Miscellaneous – Asthenia, fever, headache.

Overdosage

➤*Symptoms:* Dosages of adefovir dipivoxil 500 mg/day for 2 weeks and 250 mg/day for 12 weeks have been associated with GI adverse reactions.

➤*Treatment:* If overdose occurs, monitor the patient for evidence of toxicity and apply standard supportive treatment as necessary. Following a single dose of adefovir dipivoxil 10 mg, a 4-hour hemodialysis session removed approximately 35% of the adefovir dose.

ENTECAVIR

Rx	**Baraclude** (Bristol-Myers Squibb Company)	**Tablets:** 0.5 mg	Lactose. (BMS 1611). White to off-white, triangular. Film-coated. In 30s and 90s.
		1 mg	Lactose. (BMS 1612). Pink, triangular. Film-coated. In 30s.
		Oral Solution: 0.05 mg/mL	Parabens. Orange flavor. In 210 mL.

ENTECAVIR — ORAL

WARNING

Lactic acidosis and severe hepatomegaly with steatosis, including fatal cases, have been reported with the use of nucleoside analog alone or in combination with antiretrovirals.

Severe acute exacerbations of hepatitis B have been reported in patients who have discontinued anti-hepatitis B therapy, including entecavir. Closely monitor hepatic function closely with clinical and laboratory follow-up for at least several months in patients who discontinue anti-hepatitis B therapy. If appropriate, initiation of anti-hepatitis B therapy may be warranted.

Indications

➤*Chronic hepatitis B:* For the treatment of chronic hepatitis B virus (HBV) infection in adults with evidence of active viral replication and either evidence of persistent elevations in serum aminotransferases (ALT or AST) or histologically active disease.

Administration and Dosage

➤*Approved by the FDA:* March 29, 2005.

Administer entecavir on an empty stomach (at least 2 hours after a meal and 2 hours before the next meal).

➤*Nucleoside-treatment-naive patients:* The recommended dosage of entecavir for chronic HBV infection in nucleoside-treatment-naive adults and adolescents 16 years of age and older is 0.5 mg once daily.

➤*Coadministration with lamivudine or lamivudine-resistant patients:* The recommended dosage of entecavir in adults and adolescents 16 years of age and older with a history of hepatitis B viremia while receiving lamivudine or known lamivudine resistance mutations is 1 mg once daily.

➤*Renal function impairment:* In patients with renal impairment, the apparent oral clearance of entecavir decreased as creatinine clearance (Ccr) decreased. Dosage adjustment is recommended for patients with Ccr less than 50 mL/minute, including patients on hemodialysis or continuous ambulatory peritoneal dialysis (CAPD) (see the following table).

Recommended Dosage of Entecavir in Patients with Renal Function Impairment		
Ccr (mL/min)	Usual dose (0.5 mg) (nucleoside-naive)	Lamivudine-refractory (1 mg)
≥ 50	0.5 mg once daily	1 mg once daily
30 to < 50	0.25 mg once daily	0.5 mg once daily
10 to < 30	0.15 mg once daily	0.3 mg once daily
< 10; hemodialysis[a] or CAPD	0.05 mg once daily	0.1 mg once daily

[a] Administer after hemodialysis.

➤*Duration of therapy:* The optimal duration of treatment with entecavir for patients with chronic HBV infection and the relationship between treatment and long-term outcomes such as cirrhosis and hepatocellular carcinoma are unknown.

➤*Storage/Stability:*

Tablets – Store entecavir tablets in a tightly closed container at 25°C (77°F); excursions permitted between 15° to 30°C (59° to 86°F).

Oral solution – Store entecavir oral solution in the outer carton at 25°C (77°F); excursions permitted between 15° to 30°C (59° to 86°F). Protect from light. After opening, the oral solution may be used up to the expiration date on the bottle. Discard the bottle and its contents after the expiration date.

Actions

➤*Pharmacology:* Entecavir, a guanosine nucleoside analog with activity against HBV polymerase, is efficiently phosphorylated to the active triphosphate form, which has an intracellular half-life of 15 hours. By competing with the natural substrate deoxyguanosine triphosphate, entecavir triphosphate functionally inhibits all 3 activities of the HBV polymerase (reverse transcriptase, rt): base priming, reverse transcription of the negative strand from the pregenomic messenger RNA, and synthesis of the positive strand of HBV DNA. Entecavir triphosphate has an inhibition constant (K_i) for HBV DNA polymerase of 0.0012 mcM. Entecavir triphosphate is a weak inhibitor of cellular DNA polymerases alpha, beta, and delta and mitochondrial DNA polymerase gamma with K_i values ranging from 18 to more than 160 mcM.

➤*Pharmacokinetics:*

Absorption – Following oral administration in healthy subjects, entecavir peak plasma concentrations occurred between 0.5 and 1.5 hours. Following multiple daily doses ranging from 0.1 to 1 mg, C_{max} and area under the concentration-time curve (AUC) at steady state increased in proportion to dose. Steady state was achieved after 6 to 10 days of once-daily administration with approximately 2-fold accumulation. For a 0.5 mg oral dose, C_{max} at steady state was 4.2 ng/mL and trough plasma concentration (C_{trough}) was 0.3 ng/mL. For a 1 mg oral dose, C_{max} was 8.2 ng/mL and C_{trough} was 0.5 ng/mL.

In healthy subjects, the bioavailability of the tablet was 100% relative to the oral solution. The oral solution and tablet may be used interchangeably.

Distribution – Based on the pharmacokinetic profile of entecavir after oral dosing, the estimated apparent volume of distribution is in excess of total body water, suggesting that entecavir is extensively distributed into tissues.

Binding of entecavir to human serum proteins in vitro was approximately 13%.

Metabolism/Excretion – Following administration of ^{14}C-entecavir in humans and rats, no oxidative or acetylated metabolites were observed. Minor amounts of phase 2 metabolites (glucuronide and sulfate conjugates) were observed. Entecavir is not a substrate, inhibitor, or inducer of the cytochrome P-450 (CYP450) enzyme system.

After reaching peak concentration, entecavir plasma concentrations decreased in a bi-exponential manner with a terminal elimination half-life of approximately 128 to 149 hours. The observed drug accumulation index is approximately 2-fold with once-daily dosing, suggesting an effective accumulation half-life of approximately 24 hours.

Entecavir is predominantly eliminated by the kidney with urinary recovery of unchanged drug at steady state ranging from 62% to 73% of the administered dose. Renal clearance is independent of dose and ranges from 360 to 471 mL/minute, suggesting that entecavir undergoes both glomerular filtration and net tubular secretion.

Special populations –

Renal function impairment: The pharmacokinetics of entecavir following a single 1 mg dose were studied in patients (without chronic HBV infection) with selected degrees of renal impairment, including patients whose renal impairment was managed by hemodialysis or CAPD. Results are shown in the following table.

ENTECAVIR — ORAL

Pharmacokinetic Parameters in Subjects with Selected Degrees of Renal Function Impairment

Pharmacokinetic parameters	Renal function group / Baseline Ccr (mL/min): Unimpaired > 80 (n = 6)	Mild > 50 to ≤ 80 (n = 6)	Moderate 30 to 50 (n = 6)	Severe < 30 (n = 6)	Severe managed with hemo-dialysis[a] (n = 6)	Severe managed with CAPD (n = 4)
C_{max} (ng/mL) (CV%)	8.1 (30.7)	10.4 (37.2)	10.5 (22.7)	15.3 (33.8)	15.4 (56.4)	16.6 (29.7)
AUC (zero to T) (ng•hr/mL) (CV)	27.9 25.6)	51.5 (22.8)	69.5 (22.7)	145.7 (31.5)	233.9 (28.4)	221.8 (11.6)
CLR[b] (mL/min) (SD)	383.2 (101.8)	197.9 (78.1)	135.6 (31.6)	40.3 (10.1)	NA	NA
CLT/F[c] (mL/min)	588.1 (153.7)	309.2 (62.6)	226.3 (60.1)	100.6 (29.1)	50.6 (16.5)	35.7 (19.6)

[a] Dosed immediately following hemodialysis.
[b] CLR = renal clearance.
[c] CLT/F = apparent oral clearance.

• *Dialysis* – Dosage adjustment is recommended for patients with a Ccr less than 50 mL/min, including patients on hemodialysis or CAPD.

Following a single dose of entecavir 1 mg administered 2 hours before the hemodialysis session, hemodialysis removed approximately 13% of the entecavir dose over 4 hours. CAPD removed approximately 0.3% of the dose during 7 days. Administer entecavir after hemodialysis.

Elderly: The effect of age on the pharmacokinetics of entecavir was evaluated following administration of a single 1 mg oral dose in healthy younger and elderly volunteers. Entecavir AUC was 29.3% greater in elderly subjects compared to younger subjects. The disparity in exposure between elderly and younger subjects most likely was attributable to differences in renal function. Base dosage adjustment of entecavir on the renal function of the patient, rather than age.

After liver transplant: In a small pilot study of entecavir use in HBV-infected liver transplant recipients on a stable dose of cyclosporine (n = 5) or tacrolimus (n = 4), entecavir exposure was approximately 2-fold the exposure in healthy subjects with normal renal function. Altered renal function contributed to the increase in entecavir exposure in these patients. Monitor renal function carefully before and during treatment with entecavir in liver transplant recipients who have received or are receiving an immunosuppressant that may affect renal function, such as cyclosporine or tacrolimus.

Contraindications

Hypersensitivity to entecavir or any component of the product.

Warnings

➤*Lactic acidosis/hepatomegaly:* Lactic acidosis and severe hepatomegaly with steatosis, including fatal cases, have been reported with the use of nucleoside analog alone or in combination with antiretrovirals.

➤*Posttreatment exacerbations of hepatitis:* Severe acute exacerbations of hepatitis B have been reported in patients who have discontinued anti-hepatitis B therapy, including entecavir. Monitor hepatic function closely with both clinical and laboratory follow-up for at least several months in patients who discontinue anti-hepatitis B therapy. If appropriate, initiation of anti-hepatitis B therapy may be warranted.

➤*Renal function impairment:* Dosage adjustment of entecavir is recommended for patients with a Ccr less than 50 mL/ min, including patients on hemodialysis or CAPD.

➤*Carcinogenesis:* Long-term oral carcinogenicity studies of entecavir in mice and rats were conducted at exposures up to approximately 42 times (mice) and 35 times (rats) those observed in humans at the highest recommended dose of 1 mg/day. In mouse and rat studies, entecavir was positive for carcinogenic findings. In mice, lung adenomas were increased in males and females at exposures 3 and 40 times those in humans. Lung carcinomas in male and female mice were increased at exposures 40 times those in humans. Combined lung adenomas and carcinomas were increased in male mice at exposures 3 times, and in female mice at exposures 40 times those in humans. Tumor development was preceded by pneumocyte proliferation in the lung, which was not observed in rats, dogs, or monkeys administered entecavir, supporting the conclusion that lung tumors in mice may be a species-specific event. Hepatocellular carcinomas were increased in males, and combined liver adenomas and carcinomas also were increased at exposures 42 times those in humans. Vascular tumors in female mice (hemangiomas of ovaries and uterus and hemangiosarcomas of spleen) were increased at exposures 40 times those in humans. In rats, hepatocellular adenomas were increased in females at exposures 24 times those in humans; combined adenomas and carcinomas were also increased in females at exposures 24 times those in humans. Brain gliomas were induced in both males and females at exposures 35 and 24 times those in humans. Skin fibromas were induced in females at exposures 4 times those in humans. It is not known how predictive the results of rodent carcinogenicity studies may be for humans.

➤*Mutagenesis:* Entecavir was clastogenic to human lymphocyte cultures.

➤*Fertility impairment:* In rodent and dog toxicology studies, seminiferous tubular degeneration was observed at exposures greater than or equal to 35 times those achieved in humans.

➤*Elderly:* Clinical studies of entecavir did not include sufficient numbers of subjects 65 years of age and older to determine whether they respond differently from younger subjects. Entecavir is substantially excreted by the kidney, and the risk of toxic reactions to this drug may be greater in patients with impaired renal function. Because elderly patients are more likely to have decreased renal function, take care in dose selection, and monitor renal function.

➤*Pregnancy: Category C.* Reproduction studies have been performed in rats and rabbits in oral doses up to 200 and 16 mg/kg/day and showed no embryotoxicity or maternal toxicity at systemic exposures approximately 28 and 212 times those achieved at the highest recommended dose of 1 mg/day in humans. In rats, maternal toxicity, embryo-fetal toxicity (resorptions), lower fetal body weights, tail and vertebral malformations, reduced ossification (vertebrae, sternebrae, and phalanges), and extra lumbar vertebrae and ribs were observed at exposures 3,100 times those in humans. In rabbits, embryo-fetal toxicity (resorptions), reduced ossification (hyoid), and an increased incidence of 13th rib were observed at exposures 883 times those in humans. In a peri-postnatal study, no adverse effects on offspring were seen with entecavir administered orally to rats at exposures more than 94 times those in humans. There are no adequate and well-controlled studies in pregnant women. Because animal reproduction studies are not always predictive of human response, only use entecavir during pregnancy if clearly needed and after careful consideration of the risks and benefits.

There are no studies in pregnant women and no data on the effect of entecavir on transmission of HBV from mother to infant. Therefore, use appropriate interventions to prevent neonatal acquisition of HBV.

Pregnancy registry – To monitor fetal outcomes of pregnant women exposed to entecavir, a pregnancy registry has been established. Health care providers are encouraged to register patients by calling 1-800-258-4263.

➤*Lactation:* Entecavir is excreted in the milk of rats. It is not known whether this drug is excreted in human milk. Instruct mothers not to breast-feed if they are taking entecavir.

➤*Children:* Safety and effectiveness of entecavir in pediatric patients younger than 16 years of age have not been established.

Precautions

➤*Monitoring:* Periodic monitoring of hepatic function is recommended during treatment and for at least several months after treatment in patients who discontinue anti-hepatitis B therapy. Monitor patients closely for adverse events when entecavir is coadministered with drugs that are renally eliminated or known to affect renal function.

Liver transplant recipients – The safety and efficacy of entecavir in liver transplant recipients are unknown. If entecavir treatment is necessary for a liver transplant recipient who has received or is receiving an immunosuppressant that may affect renal function, such as cyclosporine or tacrolimus, renal function must be carefully monitored before and during treatment with entecavir.

Drug Interactions

➤*Drugs affected by renal function impairment:* Because entecavir primarily is eliminated by the kidneys, coadministration of entecavir with drugs that reduce renal function or compete for active tubular secretion may increase serum concentrations of either entecavir or the coadministered drug. Coadministration of entecavir with lamivudine, adefovir dipivoxil, or tenofovir disoproxil fumarate did not result in significant drug interactions. The effects of coadministration of entecavir with other drugs that are renally eliminated or are known to affect renal function have not been evaluated. Monitor patients closely for adverse events when entecavir is coadministered with such drugs.

➤*Drug/Food interactions:* Oral administration of entecavir 0.5 mg with a standard high-fat meal (945 kcal, 54.6 g fat) or a light meal (379 kcal, 8.2 g fat) resulted in a delay in absorption (1 to 1.5 hours fed vs 0.75 hours fasted), a decrease in C_{max} of 44% to 46%, and a decrease in AUC of 18% to 20%. Therefore, administer entecavir on an empty stomach (at least 2 hours after a meal and 2 hours before the next meal).

Adverse Reactions

➤*Most common adverse reactions:* The most common adverse events of any severity with at least a possible relation to study drug for entecavir-treated patients were headache, fatigue, dizziness, and nausea. The most common adverse events among lamivudine-treated patients were headache, fatigue, and dizziness.

➤*Discontinuation of treatment:* One percent of entecavir-treated patients in these 4 studies compared with 4% of lamivudine-treated patients discontinued for adverse events or abnormal laboratory test results. Selected clinical adverse events of moderate-severe intensity and considered at least possibly related to treatment occurring during therapy in 4 clinical studies in which entecavir was compared with lamivudine are presented in the following table.

ENTECAVIR — ORAL

Selected Adverse Reactions[a] of Entecavir (Moderate to Severe Intensity)				
	Nucleoside-naive[b]		Lamivudine-refractory[c]	
Adverse reaction	Entecavir 0.5 mg (n = 679)	Lamivudine 100 mg (n = 668)	Entecavir 1 mg (n = 183)	Lamivudine 100 mg (n = 190)
CNS				
Dizziness	< 1%	< 1%	0	1%
Fatigue	1%	1%	3%	3%
Headache	2%	2%	4%	1%
Insomnia	< 1%	< 1%	0	< 1%
Somnolence	< 1%	< 1%	0	0
GI				
Diarrhea	< 1%	0	1%	0
Dyspepsia	< 1%	< 1%	1%	0
Nausea	< 1%	< 1%	< 1%	2%
Vomiting	< 1%	< 1%	< 1%	0

[a] Includes events of possible, probable, certain, or unknown relationship to treatment regimen.
[b] Studies AI463022 and AI463027.
[c] Includes study AI463026 and the entecavir 1 mg and lamivudine treatment arms of study AI463014, a phase 2 multinational, randomized, double-blind study of 3 doses of entecavir (0.1, 0.5, and 1 mg) once daily vs continued lamivudine 100 mg once daily for up to 52 weeks in patients who experienced recurrent viremia on lamivudine therapy.

➤*Lab test abnormalities:*

Selected[a] Laboratory Test Abnormalities of Entecavir				
	Nucleoside-naive[b]		Lamivudine-refractory[c]	
Test	Entecavir 0.5 mg (n = 679)	Lamivudine 100 mg (n = 668)	Entecavir 1 mg (n = 183)	Lamivudine 100 mg (n = 190)
ALT > 10 ×ULN and > 2 × baseline	2%	4%	2%	11%
ALT > 5 × ULN	11%	16%	12%	24%
AST > 5 × ULN	5%	8%	5%	17%
Albumin < 2.5 g/dL	< 1%	< 1%	0	2%
Total bilirubin > 2.5 g/dL	2%	2%	3%	2%
Amylase > 2 × ULN	2%	2%	3%	3%
Lipase > 2 × ULN	7%	6%	8%	7%
Creatinine > 3 × ULN	0	0	0	0
Confirmed creatinine increase ≥ 0.5 mg/dL	1%	1%	2%	1%
Hyperglycemia, fasting > 250 mg/dL	2%	1%	2%	1%
Glycosuria[d]	4%	3%	4%	6%
Hematuria[d]	9%	10%	9%	6%
Platelets < 50,000/mm³	< 1%	< 1%	< 1%	< 1%

[a] On-treatment value worsened from baseline to grade 3 or grade 4 for all parameters except albumin (any on-treatment value less than 2.5 g/dL), confirmed creatinine increase greater than or equal to 0.5 mg/dL, and ALT greater than 10 × ULN and greater than 2 × baseline.
[b] Studies AI463022 and AI463027.
[c] Includes Study AI463026 and the entecavir 1 mg and lamivudine treatment arms of Study AI463014, a phase 2 multinational, randomized, double-blind study of 3 doses of entecavir (0.1, 0.5, and 1 mg) once daily versus continued lamivudine 100 mg once daily for up to 52 weeks in patients who experienced recurrent viremia on lamivudine therapy.
[d] Grade 3 equals 3+, large (also 500, 1,000, more than 1,000 and at least 1,000 for glycosuria); grade 4 equals 4+, 5+, marked, severe (also ++++, 4+:MANY for hematuria).

Among entecavir-treated patients in these studies, on-treatment ALT elevations more than 10 × ULN and more than 2 × baseline generally resolved with continued treatment. A majority of these exacerbations were associated with at least a 2 $\log_{10}$/mL reduction in viral load that preceded or coincided with the ALT elevation. Periodic monitoring of hepatic function is recommended during treatment.

➤*Posttreatment exacerbations of hepatitis (ALT elevations):* In the phase 3 studies, a subset of patients was allowed to discontinue treatment at 52 weeks if they achieved a protocol-defined response to therapy. An exacerbation of hepatitis or ALT flare was defined as ALT more than 10 × ULN and more than 2 × the patients baseline level. As demonstrated in the following table, a proportion of patients in the nucleoside-naive studies experienced posttreatment ALT flares. The number of lamivudine-refractory patients eligible to discontinue treatment was small, and the rates of post-treatment flares in this population could not be determined. If entecavir is discontinued without regard to treatment response, the rate of posttreatment flares could be higher.

Post-treatment Exacerbations of Hepatitis (ALT elevations) in Nucleoside-Naive Patients		
	Patients with ALT Elevations > 10 × ULN and > 2 × Baseline	
	Entecavir	Lamivudine
Nucleoside-naive	25/431 (6%)	38/392 (10%)
HBeAg-positive[a]	2/134 (1%)	9/129 (7%)
HBeAg-negative[b]	23/297 (8%)	29/263 (11%)

[a] Median time to off-treatment exacerbation was 23 weeks for entecavir-treated patients and 12 weeks for lamivudine-treated patients.
[b] Median time to off-treatment exacerbation was 24 weeks for entecavir-treated patients and 9 weeks for lamivudine-treated patients.

Overdosage

➤*Symptoms:* There is no experience of entecavir overdosage reported in patients. Healthy subjects who received single entecavir doses up to 40 mg or multiple doses up to 20 mg/day for up to 14 days had no increase in or unexpected adverse events.

➤*Treatment:* Following a single dose of entecavir 1 mg, a 4-hour hemodialysis session removed approximately 13% of the entecavir dose. If overdose occurs, the patient must be monitored for evidence of toxicity, and standard supportive treatment applied as necessary.

Patient Information

A patient package insert (PPI) for entecavir is available for patient information.

Keep patients in the care of a physician while taking entecavir. They should discuss any new symptoms or concurrent medications with their physician.

Advise patients to take entecavir on an empty stomach (at least 2 hours after a meal and 2 hours before the next meal).

Inform patients that deterioration of liver disease may occur in some cases if treatment is discontinued, and that they should discuss any change in regimen with their physician.

Advise patients that treatment with entecavir has not been shown to reduce the risk of transmission of HBV to others through sexual contact or blood contamination.

ANTIRETROVIRAL AGENTS

Protease Inhibitors

SAQUINAVIR

Rx	**Invirase** (Roche)	**Tablets:** 500 mg (as mesylate)	Lactose. (ROCHE SQV 500). Lt. orange to greyish or brownish orange. Oval, cylindrical. In 120s.
		Capsules: 200 mg (as mesylate)	Lactose. (ROCHE 0245). Lt. brown/green. In 270s.

SAQUINAVIR — ORAL

WARNING

Saquinavir soft gelatin capsules and saquinavir mesylate capsules are not bioequivalent and cannot be used interchangeably when used as the sole protease inhibitor. Only use saquinavir soft gelatin capsules for the initiation of therapy that includes saquinavir as a sole protease inhibitor because saquinavir soft gelatin capsules provide greater bioavailability and efficacy than saquinavir mesylate capsules.

Product identification in this monograph includes: Saquinavir mesylate capsules, saquinavir soft gel formulation, and saquinavir in reference to the active base.

Indications

➤*HIV infection:* For the treatment of HIV infection. This indication is based on studies that showed increased saquinavir concentrations and improved antiviral activity for saquinavir 1,200 mg 3 times daily compared to saquinavir mesylate 600 mg 3 times daily.

Administration and Dosage

➤*Approved by the FDA:* November 7, 1997.

➤*Adults (over the age of 16 years):*

Saquinavir administered without ritonavir – Saquinavir 1,200 mg 3 times daily (6 × 200 mg capsules). Take saquinavir with a meal or up to 2 hours after a meal.

Saquinavir administered with ritonavir – Saquinavir 1,000 mg twice daily (5 × 200 mg capsules) in combination with ritonavir 100 mg twice daily. Take ritonavir at the same time as saquinavir. Take saquinavir and ritonavir within 2 hours after a meal. When used in combination with nucleoside analogues, the dosage of saquinavir should not be reduced as this will lead to greater than dose proportional decreases in saquinavir plasma levels.

➤*Monitoring of patients:* See Precautions for more information.

➤*Dose adjustment for combination therapy with saquinavir:* For serious toxicities that may be associated with saquinavir, the drug should be interrupted. For recipients of combination therapy with saquinavir and other antiretroviral agents, base dose adjustment of the other antiretroviral agents on the known toxicity profile of the individual drug. Saquinavir dose adjustments may be required with some other antiretroviral agents. Refer to the complete monographs for these drugs for comprehensive dose adjustment recommendations and drug-associated adverse reactions.

➤*Storage/Stability:* Refrigerate capsules at 2° to 8°C (36° to 46°F) in tightly closed bottles until dispensed.

For patient use, refrigerated (2° to 8°C [36° to 46°F]) saquinavir soft gelatin capsules remain stable until the expiration date printed on the label. Once brought to room temperature (at or below 25°C [77°F]), use capsules within 3 months.

Actions

➤*Pharmacology:* Saquinavir is an inhibitor of HIV protease. HIV protease is an enzyme required for the proteolytic cleavage of viral polyprotein precursors into individual functional proteins found in infectious HIV. Saquinavir is a peptide-like substrate analogue that binds to the protease active site and inhibits the activity of the enzyme. Saquinavir inhibition prevents cleavage of the viral polyproteins resulting in the formation of immature noninfectious virus particles.

➤*Pharmacokinetics:*

Absorption – The pharmacokinetic properties of saquinavir when administered as saquinavir soft gelatin capsules have been evaluated in healthy volunteers (n = 207) and HIV-infected patients (n = 91) after single oral doses (range, 300 mg to 1,200 mg) and multiple oral doses (range, 400 mg to 1,200 mg 3 times daily). The disposition properties of saquinavir have been studied in healthy volunteers after IV doses of 6, 12, 36 or 72 mg (n = 21).

HIV-infected patients administered saquinavir (1,200 mg 3 times daily) had AUC and maximum plasma concentration (C_{max}) values approximately twice those observed in healthy volunteers receiving the same treatment regimen. The mean AUC values at week 1 were 4,159 (CV 88%) and 8,839 (CV 82%) ng•hr/mL, and C_{max} values were 1,420 (CV 81%) and 2477 (CV 76%) ng/mL for healthy volunteers and HIV-infected patients, respectively.

The absolute bioavailability of saquinavir administered as the free base has not been assessed. However, following single 600 mg doses, the relative bioavailability of saquinavir as the free base compared to saquinavir administered as saquinavir mesylate was estimated as 331% (95% CI: 207% to 530%). The absolute bioavailability of saquinavir administered as saquinavir mesylate averaged 4% (CV 73%; range, 1% to 9%) in 8 healthy volunteers who received a single 600 mg dose of saquinavir mesylate following a high-fat breakfast (48 g protein, 60 g carbohydrate, 57 g fat; 1,006 kcal). In healthy volunteers receiving single doses of saquinavir (300 mg to 1,200 mg) and in HIV-infected patients receiving multiple doses of saquinavir (400 mg to 1,200 mg 3 times daily), a greater than dose-proportional increase in saquinavir plasma concentrations has been observed.

Comparison of pharmacokinetic parameters between single- and multiple-dose studies shows that following multiple dosing of saquinavir (1,200 mg 3 times daily) in healthy male volunteers (n = 18), the steady-state AUC was 80% (95% CI: 22% to 176%) higher than that observed after a single 1,200 mg dose (n = 30).

When administered as the sole protease inhibitor, it has been shown that saquinavir 1,200 mg 3 times daily provides an 8-fold increase in AUC compared with saquinavir mesylate 600 mg 3 times daily.

Saquinavir in combination with ritonavir at doses of 400/400 mg twice daily, or 1,000/100 mg twice daily provide saquinavir systemic exposures over a 24-hour period similar to or greater than those achieved with saquinavir 1,200 mg 3 times daily.

Pharmacokinetic Parameters of Saquinavir at Steady-State After Administration of Different Regimens in HIV-Infected Patients

Dosing regimen	n	$AUC_{0-\tau}$* (ng•hr/mL)	AUC_{0-24h} (ng•hr/mL)	C_{min} (ng/mL)
Saquinavir 1,200 mg 3 times daily (arithmetic mean)	31	7,249	21,747	216
Saquinavir mesylate 400 mg twice daily + ritonavir 400 mg twice daily (arithmetic mean ± SD)	7	16,000 ± 8,000	32,000	480 ± 360
Saquinavir mesylate 1,000 mg twice daily + ritonavir 100 mg twice daily (geometric mean and 95% CI)	24	14,607 (10,218 to 20,882)	29,214	371 (245 to 561)
Saquinavir 1,000 mg twice daily + ritonavir 100 mg twice daily (geometric mean and 95% CI)	24	19,085 (13,943 to 26,124)	38,170	433 (301 to 622)

* τ is the dosing interval (ie, 8 hours if 3 times daily and 12 hours if twice daily).

The mean 12-hour AUC after a single 800 mg oral dose of saquinavir in healthy volunteers (n = 12) was increased from 167 ng•hr/mL (CV 45%), under fasting conditions, to 1,120 ng•hr/mL (CV 54%) when saquinavir was given following a high-fat breakfast (45 g protein, 76 g carbohydrate, 55 g fat; 961 kcal). The effect of food with saquinavir mesylate has been shown to persist for up to 2 hours. The mean 12-hour AUC after a single 1,200 mg oral dose of saquinavir in healthy volunteers (n = 12) was increased from 952 ng•hr/mL, following a light meal (21 g protein, 50 g carbohydrate, 28 g fat; 524 kcal) to 1,388 ng•hr/mL when saquinavir was given following a high-fat breakfast (45 g protein, 76 g carbohydrate, 55 g fat; 961 kcal).

Distribution – The mean steady-state volume of distribution following intravenous administration of a 12 mg dose of saquinavir (n = 8) was 700 L (CV 39%), suggesting saquinavir partitions into tissues. It has been shown that saquinavir, up to 30 mcg/mL, is approximately 97% bound to plasma proteins.

Metabolism/Excretion – In vitro studies using human liver microsomes have shown that the metabolism of saquinavir is cytochrome P450-mediated with the specific isoenzyme, CYP3A4, responsible for more than 90% of the hepatic metabolism. Based on in vitro studies, saquinavir is rapidly metabolized to a range of mono- and di-hydroxylated inactive compounds. In a mass balance study using 600 mg ^{14}C-saquinavir mesylate (n = 8), 88% and 1% of the oral radioactivity was recovered in feces and urine, respectively, within 5 days of dosing. In an additional 4 subjects administered 10.5 mg ^{14}C-saquinavir IV, 81% and 3% of the IV radioactivity was recovered in feces and urine, respectively, within 5 days of dosing. In mass balance studies, 13% of circulating radioactivity in plasma was attributed to unchanged drug after oral administration and the remainder attributed to saquinavir metabolites. Following IV administration, 66% of circulating radioactivity was attributed to unchanged drug and the remainder attributed to saquinavir metabolites, suggesting that saquinavir undergoes extensive first-pass metabolism.

Systemic clearance of saquinavir was rapid, 1.14 L/hr/kg (CV 12%) after IV doses of 6, 36, and 72 mg. The mean residence time of saquinavir was 7 hours (n = 8).

Special populations –

Children: The pharmacokinetics of saquinavir in pediatric patients differs significantly from that in adults. Children have a markedly higher apparent clearance than adults and administration of saquinavir alone will not give consistently therapeutic plasma levels. The pharmacokinetics of saquinavir when coadministered with ritonavir to pediatric patients is under investigation.

➤*Microbiology:*

Antiviral activity – In vitro antiviral activity of saquinavir was assessed in lymphoblastoid and monocytic cell lines and in peripheral blood lymphocytes. Saquinavir inhibited HIV activity in both acutely and chronically infected cells. IC_{50} and IC_{90} values (50% and 90% inhibitory concentrations) were in the range of 1 to 30 nM and 5 to 80 nM, respectively. In the presence of 40% human serum, the mean IC_{50} of saquinavir against laboratory strain HIV-1 RF in MT4 cells was 37.7 ± 5 nM, representing a 4-fold increase in IC_{50} value. In cell culture saquinavir demonstrated additive to synergistic effects against HIV-1 in combination with reverse transcriptase inhibitors zidovudine, zalcitabine, didanosine, lamivudine, stavudine and nevirapine, without enhanced cytotoxicity. Saquinavir in combination with the protease inhibitors amprenavir, atazanavir, or lopinavir resulted in synergistic antiviral activity.

Drug resistance – HIV-1 mutants with reduced susceptibility to saquinavir have been selected during in vitro passage. Genotypic analyses of these isolates showed several substitutions in the HIV protease gene. Only the

SAQUINAVIR — ORAL

G48V and L90M substitutions were associated with reduced susceptibility to saquinavir, and conferred an increase in the IC_{50} value of 8- and 3-fold, respectively.

Cross-resistance – Among protease inhibitors, variable cross-resistance has been observed. In 1 clinical study, 22 HIV-1 isolates with reduced susceptibility (greater than 4-fold increase in the IC_{50} value) to saquinavir following therapy with saquinavir mesylate were evaluated for cross-resistance to amprenavir, indinavir, nelfinavir and ritonavir. Six of the 22 isolates (27%) remained susceptible to all 4 protease inhibitors, 12 of the 22 isolates (55%) retained susceptibility to at least 1 of the PIs and 4 out of the 22 isolates (18%) displayed broad cross-resistance to all PIs.

Sixteen (73%) and 11 (50%) of the 22 isolates remained susceptible (less than 4-fold) to amprenavir and indinavir, respectively. Four of 16 (25%) and 9 of 21 (43%) with available data remained susceptible to nelfinavir and ritonavir, respectively.

After treatment failure with amprenavir, cross-resistance to saquinavir was evaluated. HIV-1 isolates from 22 of 22 patients failing treatment with amprenavir and containing 1 or more mutations at M46L/I, I50V, I54L, V32I, 147V, and 184V were susceptible to saquinavir.

Contraindications

Clinically significant hypersensitivity to saquinavir or to any of the components contained in the capsule; coadministration with cisapride, pimozide, triazolam, midazolam, or ergot derivatives, because competition for CYP3A by saquinavir could result in inhibition of the metabolism of these drugs and create the potential for serious or life-threatening reactions, such as cardiac arrhythmias or prolonged sedation; severe hepatic impairment.

Drugs that are Contraindicated with Saquinavir	
Drug class	Drugs within class that are contraindicated with saquinavir
Antiarrhythmics	Amiodarone, flecainide, propafenone, quinidine
Ergot derivatives	Dihydroergotamine, ergonovine, ergotamine, methylergonovine
Antimycobacterial agents	Rifampin
GI motility agent	Cisapride
Neuroleptics	Pimozide
Sedative/Hypnotics	Triazolam, midazolam

If saquinavir is coadministered with ritonavir, the ritonavir monograph should be reviewed for additional contraindicated drugs.

Warnings

➤*Diabetes mellitus and hyperglycemia:* New onset diabetes mellitus, exacerbation of preexisting diabetes mellitus and hyperglycemia have been reported during postmarketing surveillance in HIV-infected patients receiving protease inhibitor therapy. Some patients required either initiation or dose adjustments of insulin or oral hypoglycemic agents for the treatment of these events. In some cases diabetic ketoacidosis has occurred. In those patients who discontinued protease inhibitor therapy, hyperglycemia persisted in some cases. Because these events have been reported voluntarily during clinical practice, estimates of frequency cannot be made and a causal relationship between protease inhibitor therapy and these events has not been established.

➤*Renal function impairment:* Renal clearance is only a minor elimination pathway; the principal route of metabolism and excretion for saquinavir is by the liver. Therefore, no dose adjustment is necessary for patients with renal impairment. However, patients with severe renal impairment have not been studied and caution should be exercised when prescribing saquinavir in this population.

➤*Hepatic function impairment:* The use of saquinavir by patients with hepatic impairment has not been studied. In the absence of such studies, caution should be exercised, as increases in saquinavir levels or increases in liver enzymes may occur. In patients with underlying hepatitis B or C, cirrhosis, chronic alcoholism, or other underlying liver abnormalities, there have been reports of worsening liver disease.

➤*Elderly:* Clinical studies of saquinavir did not include sufficient numbers of subjects aged 65 years and over to determine whether they respond differently from younger subjects. In general, caution should be taken when dosing saquinavir in elderly patients due to the greater frequency of decreased hepatic, renal, or cardiac function, and of concomitant disease or other drug therapy.

➤*Pregnancy: Category B.* Clinical experience in pregnant women is limited. Only use saquinavir during pregnancy if the potential benefit justifies the potential risk to the fetus.

Antiretroviral pregnancy registry – To monitor maternal-fetal outcomes of pregnant women exposed to antiretroviral medications, including saquinavir, an antiretroviral pregnancy registry has been established. Register patients by calling 1-800-258-4263.

➤*Lactation:* The Centers for Disease Control and Prevention recommend that HIV-infected women not breastfeed their infants to avoid risking postnatal transmission of HIV. It is not known whether saquinavir is excreted in human milk. Because of both the potential for HIV transmission and the potential for serious adverse reactions in nursing infants, instruct mothers not to breastfeed if they are receiving antiretroviral medications, including saquinavir.

➤*Children:* Do not administer saquinavir as a sole protease inhibitor to pediatric patients 16 years of age and younger due to the risk of reduced saquinavir plasma concentrations compared to adults.

Safety and effectiveness of saquinavir when coadministered with ritonavir to pediatric patients are under investigation.

Precautions

➤*Monitoring:* Perform clinical chemistry tests, viral load, and CD_4 count prior to initiating saquinavir therapy and at appropriate intervals thereafter. Elevated nonfasting triglyceride levels have been observed in patients in saquinavir trials. Periodically monitor triglyceride levels during therapy. For comprehensive information concerning laboratory test alterations associated with the use of other antiretroviral therapies, refer to the complete monographs for these drugs.

➤*Hyperlipidemia:* Elevated cholesterol and/or triglyceride levels have been observed in some patients taking saquinavir in combination with ritonavir. Marked elevation in triglyceride levels is a risk factor for development of pancreatitis. Monitor cholesterol and triglyceride levels prior to initiating combination dosing regimen of saquinavir or saquinavir mesylate with ritonavir, and at periodic intervals while on such therapy. In these patients, manage lipid disorders as clinically appropriate.

➤*Bioequivalency:* See the Warning box for more information.

➤*Toxicity:* If a serious or severe toxicity occurs during treatment with saquinavir, interrupt saquinavir until the etiology of the event is identified or the toxicity resolves. At that time, consider resumption of treatment with full-dose saquinavir. For antiretroviral agents used in combination with saquinavir, refer to the complete monographs for these drugs for dose adjustment recommendations and for information regarding drug-associated adverse reactions.

➤*Hemophilia:* There have been reports of spontaneous bleeding in patients with hemophilia A and B treated with protease inhibitors. In some patients additional Factor VIII was required. In the majority of reported cases treatment with protease inhibitors was continued or restarted. A causal relationship between protease-inhibitor therapy and these episodes has not been established.

➤*Fat redistribution:* Redistribution/accumulation of body fat including central obesity, dorsocervical fat enlargement (buffalo hump), peripheral wasting, breast enlargement and "cushingoid appearance" have been observed in patients receiving antiretroviral therapy. A causal relationship between protease inhibitor therapy and these events has not been established and the long-term consequences are currently unknown.

➤*Resistance / cross-resistance:* Varying degrees of cross-resistance among protease inhibitors have been observed. Continued administration of saquinavir therapy following loss of viral suppression may increase the likelihood of cross-resistance to other protease inhibitors.

Drug Interactions

The metabolism of saquinavir is mediated by cytochrome P450, with the specific isoenzyme CYP3A4 responsible for 90% of the hepatic metabolism. Additionally, saquinavir is a substrate for P-Glycoprotein (Pgp). Therefore, drugs that affect CYP3A4 and/or Pgp, may modify the pharmacokinetics of saquinavir. Similarly, saquinavir might also modify the pharmacokinetics of other drugs that are substrates for CYP3A4 or Pgp.

See Contraindications for more information.

➤*Drugs that are mainly metabolized by CYP3A4:* Although specific studies have not been performed, coadministration with drugs that are mainly metabolized by CYP3A4 (eg, calcium channel blockers, dapsone, disopyramide, quinine, amiodarone, quinidine, warfarin, tacrolimus, cyclosporine, ergot derivatives, pimozide, carbamazepine, fentanyl, alfentanyl, alprazolam, nefazodone and triazolam) may have elevated plasma concentrations when coadministered with saquinavir; therefore, use these combinations with caution. If saquinavir is coadministered with ritonavir, review the ritonavir label for additional drugs that should not be coadministered.

➤*Inducers of CYP3A4:* Coadministration with compounds that are potent inducers of CYP3A4 (eg, phenobarbital, phenytoin, dexamethasone, carbamazepine) may result in decreased plasma levels of saquinavir.

➤*Additional drug interactions:*

Saquinavir Drug Interactions			
Precipitant drug	Object drug		Description
Aldesleukin	Saquinavir	↑	Saquinavir concentrations may be elevated, increasing risk of toxicity.
Anticonvulsants (ie, carbamazepine, phenobarbital, phenytoin)	Saquinavir	↓	Saquinavir may be less effective due to decreased plasma concentrations. Use with caution.
Azole antifungals (eg, itraconazole, ketoconazole)	Saquinavir	↑	Azole antifungals may inhibit the metabolism of saquinavir resulting in an increase in plasma concentrations.

SAQUINAVIR — ORAL

Saquinavir Drug Interactions

Precipitant drug	Object drug		Description
Clarithromycin	Saquinavir	↑	Concurrent use increased saquinavir and clarithromycin concentrations but decreased concentrations of the active metabolite 14-OH clarithromycin.
Saquinavir	Clarithromycin	↑↓	
Delavirdine	Saquinavir	↑	Coadministration may increase saquinavir concentrations.
Dexamethasone	Saquinavir	↓	Dexamethasone may decrease saquinavir levels. Use with caution.
Efavirenz	Saquinavir	↓	Coadministration may decrease saquinavir and efavirenz plasma levels.
Saquinavir	Efavirenz	↓	
Garlic capsules	Saquinavir	↓	Do not use garlic capsules while taking saquinavir as the sole protease inhibitor due to the risk of decreased saquinavir plasma concentrations. No data are available for the coadministration of saquinavir/ritonavir and garlic capsules.
Indinavir	Saquinavir	↑	Saquinavir concentrations significantly increased when given with indinavir.
Nelfinavir	Saquinavir	↑	Concurrent use significantly increased saquinavir plasma concentration and increased nelfinavir AUC by 18%.
Saquinavir	Nelfinavir		
Nevirapine	Saquinavir	↓	Saquinavir plasma levels and clinical efficacy may be reduced.
Rifamycins (eg, rifampin)	Saquinavir	↓	Coadministration is contraindicated. Rifamycins may decrease saquinavir serum concentrations. In addition, saquinavir was shown to increase serum rifabutin concentrations.
Saquinavir	Rifamycins (eg, rifabutin)	↑	
Ritonavir, lopinavir/ritonavir	Saquinavir	↑	Saquinavir plasma concentrations were significantly elevated when given with ritonavir or lopinavir/ritonavir.
St. John's wort	Saquinavir	↓	Coadministration may lead to loss of virologic response and possible resistance to saquinavir or to the class of protease inhibitors. Concomitant use is not recommended.
Saquinavir	Antiarrhythmics (ie, amiodarone, flecainide, propafenone, quinidine, lidocaine)	↑	Use lidocaine cautiously with saquinavir. Coadministration with the other antiarrhythmics is contraindicated due to the potential for serious and/or life-threatening reactions.
Saquinavir	Benzodiazepines (eg, midazolam, triazolam)	↑	Saquinavir may inhibit the CYP3A4 metabolism of certain benzodiazepines. Midazolam and triazolam are contraindicated with saquinavir due to the potential for serious and/or life-threatening reactions.
Saquinavir	Calcium channel blockers (eg, diltiazem, felodipine, verapamil)	↑	The concentration of the calcium channel blocker may be increased when given with saquinavir. Use with caution and monitor closely.
Saquinavir	Cisapride	↑	Coadministration is contraindicated due to potential for serious and/or life-threatening reactions such as cardiac arrhythmias.
Saquinavir	Ergot derivatives (ie, dihydroergotamine, ergonovine, ergotamine, methylergonovine)	↑	Coadministration is contraindicated due to the potential for serious and/or life-threatening reactions such as acute ergot toxicity characterized by peripheral vasospasm and ischemia of the extremities and other tissues.

Saquinavir Drug Interactions

Precipitant drug	Object drug		Description
Saquinavir	Fentanyl	↑	Concurrent use may increase fentanyl plasma concentrations and prolong the half-life, increasing the risk of adverse effects (eg, respiratory depression).
Saquinavir	HMG-CoA reductase inhibitors (ie, atorvastatin, lovastatin, simvastatin)	↑	Concentrations of certain HMG-CoA reductase inhibitors may be elevated, increasing the risk of side effects such as myopathy including rhabdomyolysis. Avoid coadministration of saquinavir with lovastatin or simvastatin. Use the lowest dose of atorvastatin or use pravastatin or rosuvastatin.
Saquinavir	Immunosuppressants (ie, cyclosporine, tacrolimus)	↑	Coadministration may increase the concentrations of the immunosuppressant. Monitor levels.
Saquinavir	Methadone	↓	Methadone levels may decrease. Adjust methadone dose as needed.
Saquinavir	Oral contraceptives	↓	Concurrent use may decrease ethinyl estradiol concentrations. Use alternative or additional contraceptive measures when estrogen-based oral contraceptives are taken with saquinavir.
Saquinavir	PDE5 inhibitors (sildenafil, tadalafil, vardenafil)	↑	Concurrent use may increase the PDE5 inhibitor concentration, resulting in severe and potentially fatal hypotension. Reduce the dose and increase the dosing interval of the PDE5 inhibitor.
Saquinavir	Pimozide	↑	Coadministration is contraindicated due to the potential for serious and/or life-threatening reactions.
Saquinavir	Pravastatin	↓	Pravastatin plasma levels may be reduced, decreasing efficacy.
Saquinavir	Trazodone	↑	Trazodone concentrations may be elevated.
Saquinavir	Tricyclic antidepressants (ie, amitriptyline, imipramine)	↑	Tricyclic antidepressant concentrations may increase when coadministered with saquinavir.

➤*Drug/Food interactions:* Saquinavir levels may be elevated due to inhibition of saquinavir metabolism (CYP3A4). Avoid coadministration of saquinavir and grapefruit products.

Adverse Reactions

The safety of saquinavir was studied in more than 500 patients who received the drug either alone or in combination with other antiretroviral agents. The majority of treatment-related adverse events were of mild intensity. The most frequently reported treatment-emergent adverse events among patients receiving saquinavir in combination with other antiretroviral agents were diarrhea, nausea, abdominal discomfort, and dyspepsia.

Rare occurrences of the following serious adverse reactions have been reported during clinical trials of saquinavir or saquinavir mesylate and were considered at least possibly related to use of study drugs: Confusion, ataxia and weakness; seizures; headache; acute myeloblastic leukemia; hemolytic anemia; thrombocytopenia; thrombocytopenia and intracranial hemorrhage leading to death; attempted suicide; Stevens-Johnson syndrome; bullous skin eruption and polyarthritis; severe cutaneous reaction associated with increased liver function tests; isolated elevation of transaminases; exacerbation of chronic liver disease with grade 4 elevated liver function tests, jaundice, ascites, and right and left upper quadrant abdominal pain; pancreatitis leading to death; intestinal obstruction; portal hypertension; thrombophlebitis; peripheral vasoconstriction; drug fever; nephrolithiasis; and acute renal insufficiency.

Saquinavir Adverse Reactions (≥ 2%)[a]

	NV15182 (48 weeks) (n = 442)	NV15355 (48 weeks) Naive patients (n = 90)
Adverse event	Saquinavir + TOC[b]	Saquinavir + 2 RTIs[c]
CNS		
Headaches	5%	5.6%
Dermatologic		

SAQUINAVIR — ORAL

Saquinavir Adverse Reactions (≥ 2%)[a]

Adverse event	NV15182 (48 weeks) (n = 442) Saquinavir + TOC[b]	NV15355 (48 weeks) Naive patients (n = 90) Saquinavir + 2 RTIs[c]
Eczema	-	-
Rash	-	-
Verruca	-	2.2%
GI		
Abdominal discom-fort	8.6%	10%
Abdominal pain	2.3%	4.4%
Constipation	-	3.3%
Diarrhea	19.9%	15.6%
Dyspepsia	8.4%	7.8%
Flatulence	5.7%	10%
Nausea	10.6%	13.3%
Vomiting	2.9%	4.4%
Musculoskeletal		
Pain	-	3.3%
Psychiatric		
Anxiety	-	2.2%
Depression	2.7%	-
Insomnia	-	5.6%
Libido disorder	-	3.3%
Special senses		
Taste alteration	-	4.4%
Miscellaneous		
Appetite decreased	-	2.2%
Chest pain	-	2.2%
Fatigue	4.8%	8.9%

[a] Includes adverse events at least possibly related to study drug or of unknown intensity or relationship to treatment (corresponding to ACTG Grade 2, 3, and 4).
[b] Antiretroviral Treatment of Choice.
[c] Reverse Transcriptase Inhibitor.

➤*Concomitant therapy with ritonavir:*

Saquinavir Adverse Reactions(≥ 2%)[a]

Adverse reaction	Saquinavir 1,000 mg plus ritonavir 100 mg twice daily (48 weeks) n = 148 n (% = n/N)
Dermatologic	
Dry lips/skin	3 (2%)
Eczema	3 (2%)
Pruritus	5 (3.4%)
Rash	5 (3.4%)
Endocrine	
Diabetes mellitus/hyperglycemia	4 (2.7%)
Lipodystrophy	8 (5.4%)
GI	
Abdominal pain	9 (6.1%)
Constipation	3 (2%)
Diarrhea	12 (8.1%)
Nausea	16 (10.8%)
Vomiting	11 (7.4%)
Musculoskeletal	
Back pain	3 (2%)
Respiratory	
Bronchitis	4 (2.7%)
Influenza	4 (2.7%)
Pneumonia	8 (5.4%)
Sinusitis	4 (2.7%)
Miscellaneous	
Fatigue	9 (6.1%)
Fever	5 (3.4%)

[a] Includes events with unknown relationship to study drug.

➤*Lab test abnormalities:* In the MaxC$_{min}$ 1 study, Grade 3 and 4 thrombocytopenia (2% of patients) and anemia (2%) were observed with saquinavir in combination with ritonavir. At 48 weeks, other lab abnormalities included increased ALT, increased AST, increased GGT, hyperglycemia, hypertriglyceridemia, increased TSH, neutropenia, raised amylase, and increased LDH.

In the safety study (NV15182), 27% to 33% of subjects experienced greater than or equal to 1 grade shifts in ALT and AST during the 48-week study period. In 46% of such events, there was a single abnormal transaminase level with no evidence of persistently elevated enzyme values during the course of study. Only 3% to 4% of patients had greater than or equal to 3 grade shifts in transaminase levels and less than 0.5% of patients had to discontinue the study for increased liver function test values.

Marked Laboratory Abnormalities[a] with Saquinavir

Biochemistry	Limit	NV 15182 (48 weeks) Saquinavir + TOC[b] (n = 442)	NV15355 (48 weeks) Saquinavir + 2 RTIs[c] (n = 90)
Alkaline phosphate (high)	> 5 × ULN[d]	0.5	0
Calcium (high)	> 12.5 mg/dL	0.2	0
Creatine kinase (high)	> 4 × ULN[d]	7.8	6
Gamma GT (high)	> 5 × ULN[d]	5.7	5
Glucose (low)	< 40 mg/dL	6.4	3.5
Glucose (high)	> 250 mg/dL	1.4	0
Phosphate (low)	< 1.5 mg/dL	0.5	1
Potassium (high)	> 6.5 mEq/L	2.7	3.5
Serum amylase (high)	> 2 × ULN[d]	1.9	ND[e]
AST (high)	> 5 × ULN[d]	4.1	0
ALT (high)	> 5 × ULN[d]	5.7	1
Sodium (high)	> 157 mEq/L	0.7	0
Sodium (low)	< 123 mEq/L	0	1
Total bilirubin (high)	> 2.5 × ULN[d]	1.6	0
Triglycerides (high)	> 750 mg/dL	0	2
Hematology			
Hemoglobin (low)	< 7 gm/dL	0.7	1
Absolute neutrophil count (low)	< 750 mm^3	2.9	1
Platelets (low)	< 50,000 mm^3	0.9	0

[a] ACTG grade 3 or above.
[b] Antiretroviral Treatment of Choice.
[c] Reverse Transcriptase Inhibitor.
[d] ULN = Upper limit of normal range.
[e] ND = not done.

Additional marked lab abnormalities have been observed with saquinavir mesylate. These include the following: Calcium (low), phosphate (low), potassium (low), sodium (low).

➤*Monotherapy and combination studies:* Other clinical adverse reactions of any intensity, at least remotely related to saquinavir and saquinavir mesylate, including those in less than 2% of patients, are listed below by body system.

Cardiovascular – Cyanosis, heart murmur, heart rate disorder, heart valve disorder, hypertension, hypotension, stroke, syncope, vein distended.

CNS – Ataxia, cerebral hemorrhage, confusion, convulsions, dizziness, dry mouth, dysarthria, dysesthesia, face numbness, hyperesthesia, hyperreflexia, hyporeflexia, increased sweating, lightheaded feeling, myelopolyradiculoneuritis, neuropathy, night sweats, numbness of extremities, paresis, paresthesia, peripheral neuropathy, poliomyelitis, prickly sensation, progressive multifocal leukoencephalopathy, spasms, tremor, unconsciousness.

Dermatologic – Acne, alopecia, chalazion, dermatitis, erythema, folliculitis, furunculosis, hair changes, hot flushes, maculopapular rash, nail disorder, papillomatosis, papular rash, parasites external, photosensitivity reaction, pruritus, psoriasis, pruritic rash, red face, seborrheic dermatitis, skin disorder, skin pigment changes, skin nodule, skin syndrome, skin ulceration, urticaria, verruca, xeroderma.

GI – Abdominal colic, abdominal distention, anorexia, appetite decreased, appetite disturbances, bloodstained feces, buccal mucosa ulceration, cheilitis, discolored feces, dysphagia, esophageal ulceration, eructation, esophagi-

SAQUINAVIR — ORAL

tis, fecal incontinence, frequent bowel movements, gastritis, gastralgia, gastroesophageal reflux, gastrointestinal ulcer, GI inflammation, gingivitis, glossitis, hemorrhage of rectum, hemorrhoids, infectious diarrhea, melena, oral canker sores, painful defecation, parotid disorder, pruritus ani, pyrosis, salivary glands disorder, stomach upset, stomatitis, toothache, tooth disorder, unpleasant taste.

GU – Epididymitis, erectile impotence, impotence, menstrual disorder, menstrual irregularity, micturition disorder, nocturia, renal calculus, renal colic, penis disorder, prostate enlarged, urinary tract bleeding, urinary tract infection, vaginal discharge.

Hematologic – Anemia, dermal bleeding, hemorrhage, microhemorrhages, neutropenia, pancytopenia, splenomegaly, thrombocytopenia.

Hepatic – Cholelithiasis, hepatitis, hepatomegaly, hepatosplenomegaly, jaundice, liver enzyme disorder, pancreatitis, sclerosing cholangitis.

Metabolic – Dehydration, diabetes mellitus, hyperglycemia, hypoglycemia, hypothyroidism, thirst, triglyceride increase, weight increase.

Musculoskeletal – Arthralgia, arthritis, back pain, facial pain, jaw pain, leg cramps, leg pain, lumbago, muscle cramps, musculoskeletal disorders, musculoskeletal pain, myalgia, myopathy, stiffness, tissue changes.

Psychiatric – Agitation, amnesia, anxiety attack, behavior disturbances, euphoria, excessive dreaming, hallucination, irritability, lethargy, overdose effect, psychic disorder, psychosis, reduced intellectual ability, somnolence, speech disorder.

Respiratory – Allergic atopic rhinitis, bronchial asthma, bronchitis, cough, dyspnea, epistaxis, hemoptysis, laryngitis, pharyngitis, pneumonia, pulmonary disease, respiratory disorder, rhinitis, sinusitis, upper respiratory tract infection.

Special senses – Blepharitis, conjunctivitis, cytomegalovirus retinitis, dry eye syndrome, earache, ear pressure, eye irritation, hearing decreased, otitis, tinnitus, unpleasant taste, visual disturbance, xerophthalmia.

Miscellaneous – Allergic reaction, asthenia, body pain, chest pain, edema, fever, intoxication, malaise, olfactory disorder, pelvic pain, redistribution/accumulation of body fat, retrosternal pain, shivering, trauma, wasting syndrome, weakness generalized, weight decrease.

Neoplasm: Kaposi's sarcoma, tumor.

Resistance mechanism: Abscess, angina tonsillaris, candidiasis, cellulitis, herpes simplex, herpes zoster, infection bacterial, infection mycotic, infection staphylococcal, infestation parasitic, influenza, lymphadenopathy, molluscum contagiosum, moniliasis.

➤*Postmarketing:* Additional adverse events that have been observed during the postmarketing period are similar to those seen in clinical trials with saquinavir mesylate and saquinavir and administration of saquinavir mesylate and saquinavir in combination with ritonavir.

Overdosage

Two cases of saquinavir overdosage have been received (1 case with unknown amount of saquinavir, the second case with 3.6 to 4 g at once). No adverse events have been reported in both cases.

There were 2 patients who had overdoses with saquinavir mesylate. No acute toxicities or sequelae were noted in the first patient after ingesting 8 g of saquinavir mesylate as a single dose. The patient was treated with induction of emesis within 2 to 4 hours after ingestion. The second patient ingested 2.4 g of saquinavir mesylate in combination with 600 mg of ritonavir and experienced pain in the throat that lasted for 6 hours and then resolved.

Patient Information

Advise patients that saquinavir, like other protease inhibitors, is recommended for use in combination with active antiretroviral therapy. Greater activity has been observed when new antiretroviral therapies are begun at the same time as saquinavir. As with all protease inhibitors, adherence to the prescribed regimen is strongly recommended. Base concomitant therapy on a patient's prior drug exposure.

Inform patients that any change from saquinavir mesylate to saquinavir or saquinavir to saquinavir mesylate coadministered with ritonavir should be made only under the supervision of a physician.

Saquinavir may interact with some drugs; therefore, advise patients to report to their physicians the use of any other prescription, nonprescription medication, or herbal products, particularly St. John's wort.

Inform patients that saquinavir is not a cure for HIV infection and that they may continue to contract illnesses associated with advanced HIV infection, including opportunistic infections. Advise patients that saquinavir should be used only in combination with other active antiretroviral medications.

Inform patients that redistribution or accumulation of body fat may occur in patients receiving protease inhibitors and that the cause and long-term health effects of these conditions are not known at this time.

Tell patients that the long-term effects of saquinavir are unknown at this time. Inform them that saquinavir therapy has not been shown to reduce the risk of transmitting HIV to others through sexual contact or blood contamination.

Advise patients that saquinavir should be taken within 2 hours after a full meal. When saquinavir is coadministered with ritonavir, a light meal is sufficient. Advise patients of the importance of taking their medication every day, as prescribed, to achieve maximum benefit. Patients should not alter the dose or discontinue therapy without consulting their physicians. If a dose is missed, patients should take the next dose as soon as possible. However, the patient should not double the next dose.

Inform patients that refrigerated (2° to 8°C; 36° to 46°F) capsules of saquinavir remain stable until the expiration date printed on the label. Once brought to room temperature (at or below 25°C [77°F]), use capsules within 3 months.

SAQUINAVIR MESYLATE — ORAL

WARNING

Saquinavir mesylate capsules and tablets and saquinavir soft gelatin capsules are not bioequivalent and cannot be used interchangeably. Use saquinavir mesylate only if it is combined with ritonavir, which significantly inhibits saquinavir's metabolism to provide plasma saquinavir levels at least equal to those achieved with saquinavir soft gelatin capsules. When using saquinavir as the sole protease inhibitor (PI) in an antiviral regimen, saquinavir soft gelatin capsules are the recommended formulation.

Product identification in this document includes the following: saquinavir mesylate (capsules and tablets), saquinavir soft gelatin formulation, and saquinavir in reference to the active base.

Indications

➤*HIV infection:* Saquinavir mesylate in combination with ritonavir and other antiretroviral agents is indicated for the treatment of HIV infection. The twice-daily administration of saquinavir mesylate in combination with ritonavir is supported by safety data from the MaxCmin 1 study and pharmacokinetic data. The efficacy of saquinavir mesylate with ritonavir or saquinavir soft gelatin capsules (with or without ritonavir coadministration) has not been compared against the efficacy of antiretroviral regimens currently considered standard of care.

Administration and Dosage

➤*Approved by the FDA:* December 6, 1995.

➤*Adults (over the age of 16 years):* 1,000 mg twice daily (5 × 200 mg capsules or 2 × 500 mg tablets) in combination with ritonavir 100 mg twice daily. Give ritonavir at the same time as saquinavir mesylate. Give saquinavir mesylate and ritonavir within 2 hours after a meal.

➤*Dose adjustment for combination therapy with saquinavir mesylate:* For serious toxicities that may be associated with saquinavir mesylate, the drug should be interrupted. Saquinavir mesylate at doses less than 1,000 mg with ritonavir 100 mg twice daily are not recommended since lower doses have not shown antiviral activity. For recipients of combination therapy with saquinavir mesylate and ritonavir, dose adjustments may be necessary. These adjustments should be based on the known toxicity profile of the individual agent and the pharmacokinetic interaction between saquinavir and the coadministered drug. Health care providers should refer the complete monographs for these drugs for comprehensive dose adjustment recommendations and drug-associated adverse reactions of nucleoside analogues.

➤*Storage/Stability:* Store capsules and tablets at 15° to 30°C (59° to 86°F) in tightly closed bottles.

Actions

➤*Pharmacology:* Saquinavir is an inhibitor of HIV protease. HIV protease is an enzyme required for the proteolytic cleavage of viral polyprotein precursors into individual functional proteins found in infectious HIV. Saquinavir is a peptide-like substrate analogue that binds to the protease active site and inhibits the activity of the enzyme. Saquinavir inhibition prevents cleavage of the viral polyproteins resulting in the formation of immature noninfectious virus particles.

➤*Pharmacokinetics:*

Absorption – HIV-infected patients administered saquinavir mesylate (600 mg 3 times daily) had area under the curve (AUC) and maximum plasma concentration (C_{max}) values approximately 2 to 2.5 times those observed in healthy volunteers receiving the same treatment regimen.

Absolute bioavailability of saquinavir administered as saquinavir mesylate averaged 4% (CV 73%; range, 1% to 9%) in 8 healthy volunteers who received a single 600 mg dose (3 × 200 mg) of saquinavir mesylate following a high-fat breakfast (48 g protein, 60 g carbohydrate, 57 g fat; 1,006 kcal). The low bioavailability is thought to be due to a combination of incomplete absorption and extensive first-pass metabolism. Following single 600 mg doses, the relative bioavailability of saquinavir as saquinavir soft gelatin capsules compared with saquinavir administered as saquinavir mesylate was estimated at 331% (95% CI, 207% to 530%).

Pharmacokinetic Parameters of Saquinavir at Steady-State After Administration of Different Regimens in HIV-Infected Patients

Dosing regimen	N	AUC_{τ}[a] (ng•h/mL)	AUC_{24hr} (ng•h/mL)	C_{min} (ng/mL)
Saquinavir mesylate 600 mg 3 times daily (arithmetic mean, %CV)	10	866 (62)	2,598	79

SAQUINAVIR MESYLATE — ORAL

Pharmacokinetic Parameters of Saquinavir at Steady-State After Administration of Different Regimens in HIV-Infected Patients

Dosing regimen	N	AUC_{τ}[a] (ng•h/mL)	AUC_{24hr} (ng•h/mL)	C_{min} (ng/mL)
Saquinavir 1,200 mg soft gelatin capsules 3 times daily (arithmetic mean)	31	7,249	21,747	216
Saquinavir mesylate 400 mg twice daily + ritonavir 400 mg twice daily (arithmetic mean ± SD)[b]	7	16,000 ± 8,000	32,000	480 ± 360
Saquinavir mesylate 1,000 mg twice daily + ritonavir 100 mg twice daily (geometric mean and 95% CI)	24	14,607 (10,218 to 20,882)	29,214	371 (245 to 561)
Saquinavir 1,000 mg soft gelatin capsules twice daily + ritonavir 100 mg twice daily (geometric mean and 95% CI)	24	19,085 (13,943 to 26,124)	38,170	433 (301 to 622)

[a] τ is the dosing interval (ie, 8 hours if 3 times daily and 12 hours if twice daily).
[b] SD = standard deviation.

The mean 24-hour AUC after a single 600 mg oral dose (6 × 100 mg) in healthy volunteers (n = 6) was increased from 24 ng•h/mL (CV 33%), under fasting conditions, to 161 ng•h/mL (CV 35%) when saquinavir mesylate was given following a high-fat breakfast (48 g protein, 60 g carbohydrate, 57 g fat; 1,006 kcal). Saquinavir 24-hour AUC and C_{max} (n = 6) following the administration of a higher-calorie meal (943 kcal, 54 g fat) were on average 2 times higher than after a lower-calorie, lower-fat meal (355 kcal, 8 g fat). The effect of food has been shown to persist for up to 2 hours.

Saquinavir exposure was similar when saquinavir soft gelatin capsules plus ritonavir (1,000 mg/100 mg twice daily) were administered following a high-fat (45 g fat) or moderate-fat (20 g fat) breakfast.No food effect data are available for saquinavir mesylate in combination with ritonavir.

Distribution – The mean steady-state volume of distribution following intravenous (IV) administration of a 12 mg dose of saquinavir (n = 8) was 700 L (CV 39%), suggesting saquinavir partitions into tissues. Saquinavir was approximately 98% bound to plasma proteins over a concentration range of 15 to 700 ng/mL. In 2 patients receiving saquinavir mesylate 600 mg 3 times daily, cerebrospinal fluid concentrations were negligible when compared with concentrations from matching plasma samples.

Metabolism/Excretion – In vitro studies using human liver microsomes have shown that the metabolism of saquinavir is cytochrome P-450-mediated with the specific isoenzyme CYP3A4 responsible for more than 90% of the hepatic metabolism. Based on in vitro studies, saquinavir is rapidly metabolized to a range of mono- and di-hydroxylated inactive compounds. In a mass balance study using 600 mg of ^{14}C-saquinavir (n = 8), 88% and 1% of the oral radioactivity was recovered in feces and urine, respectively, within 5 days of dosing. In an additional 4 subjects administered 10.5 mg of ^{14}C-saquinavir IV, 81% and 3% of the IV radioactivity was recovered in feces and urine, respectively, within 5 days of dosing. In mass balance studies, 13% of circulating radioactivity in plasma was attributed to unchanged drug after oral administration and the remainder attributed to saquinavir metabolites. Following IV administration, 66% of circulating radioactivity was attributed to unchanged drug and the remainder attributed to saquinavir metabolites, suggesting that saquinavir undergoes extensive first-pass metabolism.

Systemic clearance of saquinavir was rapid, 1.14 L/h/kg (CV 12%) after IV doses of 6, 36, and 72 mg. The mean residence time of saquinavir was 7 hours (n = 8).

The pharmacokinetic properties of saquinavir mesylate have been evaluated in healthy volunteers (n = 351) and HIV-infected patients (n = 270) after single and multiple oral doses of 25, 75, 200, and 600 mg 3 times daily and in healthy volunteers after IV doses of 6, 12, 36 or 72 mg (n = 21). The pharmacokinetics of saquinavir mesylate/ritonavir 400/400 mg twice daily and saquinavir mesylate/ritonavir 1,000/100 mg twice daily have also been evaluated in HIV-infected patients.

Special populations –

Gender and age: A gender difference was observed with women, showing higher saquinavir exposure than men (mean AUC increase of 56%, mean C_{max} increase of 26%), in the relative bioavailability study comparing saquinavir mesylate 500 mg film-coated tablets with the saquinavir mesylate 200 mg capsules in combination with ritonavir. There was no evidence that age and body weight explained the gender difference in this study. A clinically significant difference in safety and efficacy between men and women has not been reported with the approved dosage regimen (saquinavir mesylate 1,000 mg/ritonavir 100 mg twice daily).

➤*Microbiology:*

Drug resistance – HIV-1 mutants with reduced susceptibility to saquinavir have been selected during in vitro passage. Genotypic analyses of these isolates showed several substitutions in the HIV protease gene. Only the G48V and L90M substitutions were associated with reduced susceptibility to saquinavir, and conferred an increase in the IC_{50} value of 8- and 3-fold, respectively.

Cross-resistance – Among protease inhibitors, variable cross-resistance has been observed. In one clinical study, 22 HIV-1 isolates with reduced susceptibility (greater than 4-fold increase in the IC_{50} value) to saquinavir following therapy with saquinavir mesylate were evaluated for cross-resistance to amprenavir, indinavir, nelfinavir, and ritonavir. Six of the 22 isolates (27%) remained susceptible to all 4 protease inhibitors, 12 of the 22 isolates (55%) retained susceptibility to at least one of the protease inhibitors, and 4 out of the 22 isolates (18%) displayed broad cross-resistance to all protease inhibitors. Sixteen (73%) and 11 (50%) of the 22 isolates remained susceptible (less than 4-fold) to amprenavir and indinavir, respectively. Four of 16 (25%) and nine of 21 (43%) with available data remained susceptible to nelfinavir and ritonavir, respectively.

After treatment failure with amprenavir, cross-resistance to saquinavir was evaluated. HIV-1 isolates from 22 of 22 patients failing treatment with amprenavir and containing 1 or more mutations M46L/I, I50V, I54L, V32I, I47V, and I84V were susceptible to saquinavir.

Contraindications

Hypersensitivity to saquinavir or to any of the components contained in the capsule.

Saquinavir mesylate when administered with ritonavir is contraindicated in patients with severe hepatic impairment.

Saquinavir mesylate may be used only if it is combined with ritonavir, which significantly inhibits saquinavir's metabolism and provides plasma saquinavir levels at least equal to those achieved with saquinavir soft gelatin capsules.

Do not administer saquinavir mesylate concurrently with drugs listed in the following table. Inhibition of CYP3A4 by saquinavir could result in elevated plasma concentrations of these drugs, potentially causing serious or life-threatening reactions such as cardiac arrhythmias or prolonged sedation.

Drugs That are Contraindicated with Saquinavir Mesylate/Ritonavir

Drug class	Drugs within class that are contraindicated with saquinavir mesylate
Antiarrhythmics	Amiodarone, flecainide, propafenone, quinidine
Ergot derivatives	Dihydoergotamine, ergonovine, ergotamine, methylergonovine
Antimycobacterial agents	Rifampin[a]
GI motility agent	Cisapride
Neuroleptics	Pimozide
Sedative/Hypnotics	Triazolam, midazolam

[a] Saquinavir mesylate used as a sole protease inhibitor.

Warnings

➤*Diabetes mellitus, new onset:* New onset diabetes mellitus, exacerbation of preexisting diabetes mellitus, and hyperglycemia have been reported during postmarketing surveillance in HIV-infected patients receiving protease inhibitor therapy. Some patients required either initiation or dose adjustments of insulin or oral hypoglycemic agents for the treatment of these events. In some cases, diabetic ketoacidosis has occurred. In those patients who discontinued protease inhibitor therapy, hyperglycemia persisted in some cases. Because these events have been reported voluntarily during clinical practice, estimates of frequency cannot be made and a causal relationship between protease inhibitor therapy and these events has not been established.

➤*Renal function impairment:* Renal clearance is only a minor elimination pathway; the principal route of metabolism and excretion for saquinavir is by the liver. Therefore, no initial dose adjustment is necessary for patients with renal impairment. However, patients with severe renal impairment have not been studied; exercise caution when prescribing saquinavir in this population.

➤*Hepatic function impairment:* The use of saquinavir mesylate (in combination with ritonavir) in patients with hepatic impairment has not been studied. In the absence of such studies, exercise caution, as increases in saquinavir levels and/or increases in liver enzymes may occur. In patients with underlying hepatitis B or C, cirrhosis, chronic alcoholism, and/or other underlying liver abnormalities, there have been reports of worsening liver disease. Saquinavir mesylate is contraindicated in patients with severe hepatic impairment.

➤*Elderly:* Clinical studies of saquinavir mesylate did not include sufficient numbers of subjects 65 years of age and older to determine whether they respond differently from younger subjects. In general, use caution when dosing saquinavir mesylate in elderly patients because of the greater frequency of decreased hepatic, renal, or cardiac function, and of concomitant disease or other drug therapy.

SAQUINAVIR MESYLATE — ORAL

➤*Pregnancy: Category B.* Clinical experience in pregnant women is limited. Use saquinavir during pregnancy only if the potential benefit justifies the potential risk to the fetus.

Antiretroviral pregnancy registry – To monitor maternal-fetal outcomes of pregnant women exposed to antiretroviral medications, including saquinavir mesylate, an antiretroviral pregnancy registry has been established. Health care providers are encouraged to register patients by calling 1-800-258-4263.

➤*Lactation:* The Centers for Disease Control and Prevention recommend that HIV-infected mothers not breast-feed their infants to avoid risking postnatal transmission of HIV. It is not known whether saquinavir is excreted in human milk. Because of both the potential for HIV transmission and the potential for serious adverse reactions in breast-feeding infants, instruct mothers not to breast-feed if they are receiving antiretroviral medications, including saquinavir mesylate.

➤*Children:* Safety and efficacy of saquinavir mesylate in HIV-infected pediatric patients younger than 16 years of age have not been established.

Precautions

➤*Monitoring:* Perform clinical chemistry tests, viral load, and CD4 count prior to initiating saquinavir mesylate therapy and at appropriate intervals thereafter. Elevated cholesterol and/or triglyceride levels have been observed in patients in saquinavir trials. Monitor cholesterol and triglyceride levels prior to initiating the combination dosing regimen and at periodic intervals during therapy.

➤*Bioequivalency:* See the Warning box for more information.

➤*Toxicity:* If a serious or severe toxicity occurs during treatment with saquinavir mesylate, interrupt saquinavir mesylate until the etiology of the event is identified or the toxicity resolves. At that time, resumption of treatment with full-dose saquinavir mesylate may be considered. For antiretroviral agents used in combination with saquinavir mesylate, health care providers should refer to the monographs for these drugs for dose adjustment recommendations and for information regarding drug-associated adverse reactions.

➤*Hemophilia:* There have been reports of spontaneous bleeding in patients with hemophilia A and B treated with protease inhibitors. In some patients, additional factor VIII was required. In the majority of reported cases, treatment with protease inhibitors was continued or restarted. A causal relationship between protease inhibitor therapy and these episodes has not been established.

➤*Hyperlipidemia:* Elevated cholesterol and/or triglyceride levels have been observed in some patients taking saquinavir in combination with ritonavir. Marked elevation in triglyceride levels is a risk factor for development of pancreatitis. Monitor cholesterol and triglyceride levels prior to initiating the combination dosing regimen of saquinavir soft gelatin capsules or saquinavir mesylate with ritonavir, and at periodic intervals while on such therapy. In these patients, manage lipid disorders as clinically appropriate.

➤*Lactose intolerance:* Each capsule contains lactose (anhydrous) 63.3 mg. This quantity should not induce specific symptoms of intolerance.

➤*Fat redistribution:* Redistribution/accumulation of body fat including central obesity, dorsocervical fat enlargement (buffalo hump), peripheral wasting, breast enlargement, facial wasting, and "cushingoid appearance" have been observed in patients receiving antiretroviral therapy. A causal relationship between protease inhibitor therapy and these events has not been established and the long-term consequences are currently unknown.

➤*Resistance/cross-resistance:* Varying degrees of cross-resistance among protease inhibitors have been observed. Continued administration of saquinavir mesylate therapy following loss of viral suppression may increase the likelihood of cross-resistance to other protease inhibitors.

Drug Interactions

➤*Cytochrome P-450/P-Glycoprotein system:* The metabolism of saquinavir is mediated by cytochrome P-450, with the specific isoenzyme CYP3A4 responsible for 90% of the hepatic metabolism. Additionally, saquinavir is a substrate for P-Glycoprotein (Pgp). Therefore, drugs that affect CYP3A4 and/or Pgp may modify the pharmacokinetics of saquinavir. Similarly, saquinavir might also modify the pharmacokinetics of other drugs that are substrates for CYP3A4 or Pgp.

➤*Drugs that are mainly metabolized by CYP3A4:* Although specific studies have not been performed, coadministration with drugs that are mainly metabolized by CYP3A4 (eg, calcium channel blockers, dapsone, disopyramide, quinine, amiodarone, quinidine, warfarin, tacrolimus, cyclosporine, ergot derivatives, pimozide, carbamazepine, fentanyl, alfentanyl, alprazolam, triazolam) may have elevated plasma concentrations when coadministered with saquinavir; therefore, use these combinations with caution. Since saquinavir mesylate is coadministered with ritonavir, review the ritonavir label for additional drugs that should not be coadministered.

➤*Additional drug interactions:*

Saquinavir Drug Interactions

Precipitant drug	Object drug[a]		Description
Aldesleukin	Saquinavir	↑	Saquinavir concentrations may be elevated, increasing risk of toxicity.
Anticonvulsants (eg, carbamazepine, phenobarbital, phenytoin)	Saquinavir	↓	Saquinavir may be less effective because of decreased plasma concentrations. Use with caution.
Azole antifungals (eg, itraconazole, ketoconazole)	Saquinavir	↑	Azole antifungals may inhibit the metabolism of saquinavir resulting in an increase in plasma concentrations.
Cimetidine	Saquinavir	↑	Saquinavir plasma concentrations may be elevated, increasing the therapeutic and adverse effects.
Clarithromycin	Saquinavir	↑	Concurrent use increased saquinavir and clarithromycin concentrations but decreased concentrations of the active metabolite 14-OH clarithromycin.
Saquinavir	Clarithromycin	↑↓	
Delavirdine	Saquinavir	↑	Coadministration may increase saquinavir concentrations.
Dexamethasone	Saquinavir	↓	Dexamethasone may decrease saquinavir levels. Use with caution.
Efavirenz	Saquinavir	↓	Coadministration may decrease saquinavir and efavirenz plasma levels.
Saquinavir	Efavirenz	↓	
Garlic capsules	Saquinavir	↓	Garlic capsules should not be used while taking saquinavir as the sole protease inhibitor because of the risk of decreased saquinavir plasma concentrations. No data are available for the coadministration of saquinavir/ritonavir and garlic capsules.
Grapefruit juice	Saquinavir	↑	Saquinavir plasma levels and pharmacologic and adverse effects may be increased.
Indinavir	Saquinavir	↑	Saquinavir concentrations significantly increased when given with indinavir.
Nelfinavir	Saquinavir	↑	Concurrent use significantly increased saquinavir plasma concentration and increased nelfinavir AUC by 18%.
Saquinavir	Nelfinavir		
Nevirapine	Saquinavir	↓	Saquinavir plasma levels and clinical efficacy may be reduced.
Rifamycins (eg, rifampin)	Saquinavir	↓	Coadministration is contraindicated. Rifamycins may decrease saquinavir serum concentrations. In addition, saquinavir was shown to increase serum rifabutin concentrations.
Saquinavir	Rifamycins (eg, rifabutin)	↑	
Ritonavir, lopinavir/ritonavir	Saquinavir	↑	Saquinavir plasma concentrations were significantly elevated when given with ritonavir or lopinavir/ritonavir.
St. John's wort	Saquinavir	↓	Coadministration may lead to loss of virologic response and possible resistance to saquinavir or to the class of protease inhibitors. Concomitant use is not recommended.
Saquinavir	Antiarrhythmics (eg, amiodarone, bepridil, flecainide, propafenone, quinidine, lidocaine)	↑	Use lidocaine cautiously with saquinavir. Coadministration with the other antiarrhythmics is contraindicated because of the potential for serious and/or life-threatening reactions.
Saquinavir	Benzodiazepines (eg, midazolam, triazolam)	↑	Saquinavir may inhibit the CYP3A4 metabolism of certain benzodiazepines. Midazolam and triazolam are contraindicated with saquinavir because of the potential for serious and/or life-threatening reactions.

SAQUINAVIR MESYLATE — ORAL

Saquinavir Drug Interactions			
Precipitant drug	Object drug[a]		Description
Saquinavir	Calcium channel blockers (eg, diltiazem, felodipine, verapamil)	↑	The concentration of the calcium channel blocker may be increased when given with saquinavir. Use with caution and monitor closely.
Saquinavir	Cisapride	↑	Coadministration is contraindicated because of potential for serious and/or life-threatening reactions such as cardiac arrhythmias.
Saquinavir	Ergot derivatives (eg, dihydroergotamine, ergonovine, ergotamine, methylergonovine)	↑	Coadministration is contraindicated because of the potential for serious and/or life-threatening reactions such as acute ergot toxicity characterized by peripheral vasospasm and ischemia of the extremities and other tissues.
Saquinavir	Fentanyl	↑	Concurrent use may increase fentanyl plasma concentrations and prolong the half-life, increasing the risk of adverse effects (eg, respiratory depression).
Saquinavir	HMG-CoA reductase inhibitors (eg, atorvastatin, lovastatin, simvastatin)	↑	Concentrations of certain HMG-CoA reductase inhibitors may be elevated, increasing the risk of side effects such as myopathy, including rhabdomyolysis. Avoid coadministration of saquinavir with lovastatin or simvastatin. Use the lowest dose of atorvastatin or use pravastatin or rosuvastatin.
Saquinavir	Immunosuppressants (eg, cyclosporine, tacrolimus)	↑	Coadministration may increase the concentrations of the immunosuppressant. Monitor levels.
Saquinavir	Levothyroxine	↑	Thyroxine serum concentrations may be increased, resulting in hyperthyroidism.
Saquinavir	Methadone	↓	Methadone levels may decrease. Adjust methadone dose as needed.
Saquinavir	Oral contraceptives	↓	Concurrent use may decrease ethinyl estradiol concentrations. Alternative or additional contraceptive measures should be used when estrogen-based oral contraceptives are taken with saquinavir.
Saquinavir	PDE5 inhibitors (sildenafil, tadalafil, vardenafil)	↑	Concurrent use may increase the PDE5 inhibitor concentration, resulting in severe and potentially fatal hypotension. Reduce the dose and increase the dosing interval of the PDE5 inhibitor.
Saquinavir	Pimozide	↑	Coadministration is contraindicated because of the potential for serious and/or life-threatening reactions.
Saquinavir	Pravastatin	↓	Pravastatin plasma levels may be reduced, decreasing efficacy.
Saquinavir	Risperidone	↑	Risperidone plasma concentrations may be elevated, increasing the risk of side effects.
Saquinavir	Trazodone	↑	Trazodone concentrations may be elevated.
Saquinavir	Tricyclic antidepressants (eg, amitriptyline, imipramine)	↑	Tricyclic antidepressant concentrations may increase when coadministered with saquinavir.
Saquinavir	Warfarin	↓	The anticoagulant effect of warfarin may be decreased.

[a] ↑ = Object drug increased. ↓ = Object drug decreased.

➤*Drug/Food interactions:* See Actions for more information.

Adverse Reactions

The following grade 2 to grade 4 adverse reactions (considered at least possibly related to study drug or of unknown relationship) occurred in greater than or equal to 2% of patients receiving saquinavir mesylate 600 mg 3 times daily alone or in combination with zidovudine and/or zalcitabine: abdominal discomfort, abdominal pain, appetite disturbances, asthenia, buccal mucosa ulceration, diarrhea, dizziness, dyspepsia, extremity numbness, headache, mucosa damage, musculoskeletal pain, myalgia, nausea, paresthesia, peripheral neuropathy, pruritus, and rash.

➤*Saquinavir alone or in combination with zidovudine or zalcitabine:* The safety of saquinavir mesylate was studied in patients who received the drug either alone or in combination with zidovudine or zalcitabine. The majority of adverse reactions were of mild intensity. The most frequently reported adverse reactions among patients receiving saquinavir mesylate in clinical trials (excluding those toxicities known to be associated with zidovudine and zalcitabine when used in combinations) were diarrhea, abdominal discomfort, and nausea.

➤*Serious adverse reactions (rare):* Rare occurrences of the following serious adverse reactions have been reported during clinical trials of saquinavir mesylate and were considered at least possibly related to use of study drugs: confusion, ataxia, and weakness; acute myeloblastic leukemia; hemolytic anemia; attempted suicide; Stevens-Johnson syndrome; seizures; severe cutaneous reaction associated with increased liver function tests; isolated elevation of transaminases; thrombophlebitis; headache; thrombocytopenia; exacerbation of chronic liver disease with grade 4 elevated liver function tests, jaundice, ascites, and right and left upper quadrant abdominal pain; drug fever; bullous skin eruption and polyarthritis; pancreatitis leading to death; nephrolithiasis; thrombocytopenia and intracranial hemorrhage leading to death; peripheral vasoconstriction; portal hypertension; intestinal obstruction. These reactions were reported from a database of greater than 6,000 patients. Over 100 patients on saquinavir mesylate therapy have been followed for greater than 2 years.

➤*Concomitant therapy with ritonavir:*

Saquinavir Adverse Reactions ≥ 2%[a]	
Adverse reaction	Saquinavir 1,000 mg soft gelatin capsules plus ritonavir 100 mg twice daily (48 weeks) (N = 148) n (% = n/N)
Dermatological	
Dry lips/skin	3 (2%)
Eczema	3 (2%)
Pruritus	5 (3.4%)
Rash	5 (3.4%)
GI	
Abdominal pain	9 (6.1%)
Constipation	3 (2%)
Diarrhea	12 (8.1%)
Nausea	16 (10.8%)
Vomiting	11 (7.4%)
Metabolic	
Diabetes mellitus/hyperglycemia	4 (2.7%)
Lipodystrophy	8 (5.4%)
Musculoskeletal	
Back pain	3 (2%)
Respiratory	
Bronchitis	4 (2.7%)
Influenza	4 (2.7%)
Pneumonia	8 (5.4%)
Sinusitis	4 (2.7%)
Miscellaneous	
Fatigue	9 (6.1%)
Fever	5 (3.4%)

[a] Includes events with unknown relationship to study drug.

Additionally, adverse reactions that occurred in clinical trials with saquinavir soft gelatin capsules, which are not listed above, are listed for completeness. However, due to the higher bioavailability of saquinavir soft gelatin capsules, these adverse reactions might not be predictive of the safety profile of saquinavir mesylate.

➤*Experience from clinical trials with saquinavir soft gelatin capsules:* The safety of saquinavir soft gelatin capsules was studied in more than 500 patients who received the drug either alone or in combination with other antiretroviral agents. The most frequently reported adverse reactions among patients receiving saquinavir soft gelatin capsules in combination with other antiretroviral agents were diarrhea, nausea, abdominal discomfort, and dyspepsia. Clinical adverse reactions of at least moderate intensity, which occurred in greater than or equal to 2% of patients in 2 studies with saquinavir soft gelatin capsules, which are not listed above, are listed below by body system.

CNS – Anxiety, depression, insomnia, libido disorder.

SAQUINAVIR MESYLATE — ORAL

Dermatologic – Eczema, verruca.

GI – Constipation, flatulence, vomiting.

Miscellaneous – Appetite decreased, chest pain, fatigue, taste alteration.

➤*Lab test abnormalities with saquinavir mesylate:* Grade 3 and 4 lab abnormalities have been observed with saquinavir soft gelatin capsules in combination with ritonavir. At 48 weeks, lab abnormalities included increased ALT, anemia, increased AST, increased gamma-glutamyltranspeptidase (GGT), hyperglycemia, hypertriglyceridemia, increased thyroid-stimulating hormones, neutropenia, raised amylase, raised lactate dehydrogenase, and thrombocytopenia.

In studies NV14255/ACTG 229 and NV14256, the following grade 3 or grade 4 abnormalities in laboratory tests were reported among patients receiving saquinavir mesylate 600 mg 3 times daily alone or in combination with zidovudine and/or zalcitabine:

Biochemistry –
- Incidence between less than 1% and 4%: hypoglycemia, hyper- or hypocalcemia, hypophosphatemia, hyper- or hypokalemia, hyper- or hyponatremia, raised serum amylase grade 3 or 4 elevations in transaminases (AST, ALT), hyperbilirubinemia.
- Incidence of less than or equal to 5%: hyperglycemia.
- Incidence of between 7% and 12%: elevated creatine phosphokinase.

Hematology –
- Incidence of less than or equal to 2%: thrombocytopenia and anemia.
- Incidence between 1% and 8%: leukopenia. Additional marked lab abnormalities have been observed with saquinavir soft gelatin capsules. These include alkaline phosphatase (high), GGT (high), and triglycerides (high).

➤*Monotherapy and combination studies:* Other clinical adverse reactions of any intensity, at least remotely related to saquinavir mesylate, including those in less than 2% of patients on arms containing saquinavir mesylate in studies NV14255/ACTG229 and NV14256, and those in smaller clinical trials, are listed below by body system.

Cardiovascular – Cyanosis, heart murmur, heart rate disorder, heart valve disorder, hypertension, hypotension, syncope, vein distended.

CNS – Ataxia, confusion, convulsions, dysarthria, dysesthesia, face numbness, hyperesthesia, hyperreflexia, hyporeflexia, light-headed feeling, myelopolyradiculoneuritis, paresis, poliomyelitis, prickly sensation, progressive multifocal leukoencephalopathy, spasms, tremor, unconsciousness.

Dermatologic – Acne, alopecia, chalazion, dermatitis, eczema, erythema, folliculitis, furunculosis, hair changes, hot flushes, maculopapular rash, nail disorder, papillomatosis, photosensitivity reaction, seborrheic dermatitis, skin disorder, skin nodule, skin pigment changes, skin ulceration, sweating increased, urticaria, verruca, xeroderma.

GI – Bloodstained feces, bowel movements frequent, cheilitis, colic abdominal, constipation, discolored feces, dry mouth, dyspepsia, dysphagia, esophagitis, eructation, flatulence, gastralgia, gastritis, gastrointestinal inflammation, gingivitis, glossitis, hemorrhage rectum, hemorrhoids, infectious diarrhea, melena, pain pelvic, painful defecation, pancreatitis, parotid disorder, salivary glands disorder, stomach upset, stomatitis, toothache, tooth disorder, vomiting.

GU – Impotence, prostate enlarged, vaginal discharge.

Micturition disorder, renal calculus, urinary tract bleeding, urinary tract infection.

Hematologic – Anemia, bleeding dermal, microhemorrhages, neutropenia, pancytopenia, splenomegaly, thrombocytopenia.

Hepatic – Hepatitis, hepatomegaly, hepatosplenomegaly, jaundice, liver enzyme disorder.

Metabolic – Dehydration, diabetes mellitus, hyperglycemia, weight decrease, weight increase.

Musculoskeletal – Arthralgia, arthritis, back pain, cramps leg, creatine phosphokinase increased, facial pain, generalized weakness, muscle cramps, musculoskeletal disorders, stiffness, tissue changes, trauma.

Psychiatric – Agitation, amnesia, anxiety, anxiety attack, depression, dreaming excessive, euphoria, hallucination, insomnia, intellectual ability reduced, irritability, lethargy, libido disorder, overdose effect, psychic disorder, psychosis, somnolence, speech disorder, suicide attempt.

Respiratory – Bronchitis, cough, dyspnea, epistaxis, hemoptysis, laryngitis, pharyngitis, pneumonia, pulmonary disease, respiratory disorder, rhinitis, sinusitis, upper respiratory tract infection.

Special senses – Blepharitis, decreased hearing, dry eye syndrome, earache, ear pressure, eye irritation, otitis, taste alteration, tinnitus, visual disturbance, xerophthalmia.

Miscellaneous – Allergic reaction, anorexia, chest pain, edema, external parasites, fatigue, fever, intoxication, night sweats, redistribution/accumulation of body fat, retrosternal pain, shivering, wasting syndrome.

Resistance mechanism: Abscess, angina tonsillaris, candidiasis, cellulitis, herpes simplex, herpes zoster, infection bacterial, infection mycotic, infection staphylococcal, influenza, lymphadenopathy, moniliasis, tumor.

➤*Postmarketing:* Additional adverse events that have been observed during the postmarketing period are similar to those seen in clinical trials with saquinavir mesylate and saquinavir soft gelatin capsules and administration of saquinavir mesylate and saquinavir soft gelatin capsules in combination with ritonavir.

Overdosage

No acute toxicities or sequelae were noted in 1 patient who ingested saquinavir mesylate 8 g as a single dose. The patient was treated with induction of emesis within 2 to 4 hours after ingestion. A second patient ingested saquinavir mesylate 2.4 g in combination with ritonavir 600 mg and experienced pain in the throat that lasted for 6 hours and then resolved. In an exploratory phase 2 study of oral dosing with saquinavir mesylate at 7,200 mg/day (1,200 mg every 4 hours), there were no serious toxicities reported through the first 25 weeks of treatment.

Patient Information

Inform patients that any change from saquinavir mesylate to saquinavir soft gelatin capsules or saquinavir soft gelatin capsules to saquinavir mesylate coadministered with a drug which inhibits its metabolism, such as ritonavir, should be made only under the supervision of a health care provider.

Saquinavir mesylate may interact with some drugs; therefore, advise patients to report to their doctors the use of any other prescription, nonprescription medication, or herbal products, particularly St. John's wort.

Inform patients that saquinavir mesylate is not a cure for HIV infection and that they may continue to acquire illnesses associated with advanced HIV infection, including opportunistic infections. Advise patients that saquinavir mesylate may be used only if it is combined with ritonavir, which significantly inhibits saquinavir's metabolism to provide plasma saquinavir levels at least equal to those achieved with saquinavir soft gelatin capsules.

Inform patients that redistribution or accumulation of body fat may occur in patients receiving protease inhibitors and that the cause and long-term health effects of these conditions are not known at this time.

Tell patients that the long-term effects of saquinavir mesylate are unknown at this time. Inform them that saquinavir mesylate therapy has not been shown to reduce the risk of transmitting HIV to others through sexual contact or blood contamination.

Advise patients that saquinavir mesylate should be taken within 2 hours after a full meal. When saquinavir mesylate is taken without food, concentrations of saquinavir in the blood are substantially reduced and may result in no antiviral activity. Advise patients of the importance of taking their medication every day, as prescribed, to achieve maximum benefit. Patients should not alter the dose or discontinue therapy without consulting their health care providers. If a dose is missed, patients should take the next dose as soon as possible. However, the patient should not double the next dose.

INDINAVIR SULFATE

Rx	**Crixivan** (Merck)	**Capsules:** 100 mg[a]	Lactose. (CRIXIVAN 100 mg). White. In unit-of-use 180s.
		200 mg[a]	Lactose. (CRIXIVAN 200 mg). White. In unit-of-use 360s.
		333 mg[a]	Lactose. (CRIXIVAN 333 mg). White. In unit-of-use 135s.
		400 mg[a]	Lactose. (CRIXIVAN 400 mg). White. In unit dose 42s, and unit-of-use 18s, 90s, 120s, and 180s.

[a] Corresponding to 125, 250, 416.3, and 500 mg of indinavir sulfate, respectively.

INDINAVIR SULFATE — ORAL

Indications

➤*HIV Infection:* Indinavir with antiretroviral agents is indicated for the treatment of HIV infection.

Administration and Dosage

➤*Approved by the FDA:* March 13, 1995.

The recommended dosage of indinavir is 800 mg (usually two 400 mg capsules) orally every 8 hours.

Indinavir must be taken at intervals of 8 hours. For optimal absorption, indinavir should be administered without food but with water 1 hour before or 2 hours after a meal. Alternatively, indinavir may be administered with other liquids such as skim milk, juice, coffee, or tea, or with a light meal (eg, dry toast with jelly, juice, and coffee with skim milk and sugar; or corn flakes, skim milk, and sugar).

To ensure adequate hydration, it is recommended that the patient drink at least 1.5 L (approximately 48 ounces) of liquids during the course of 24 hours.

➤*Concomitant therapy:*

Delavirdine – Dose reduction of indinavir to 600 mg every 8 hours should be considered when administering delavirdine 400 mg 3 times a day.

Didanosine – If indinavir and didanosine are coadministered, they should be administered at least 1 hour apart on an empty stomach.

INDINAVIR SULFATE — ORAL

Itraconazole – Dosage reduction of indinavir to 600 mg every 8 hours is recommended when administering itraconazole 200 mg twice daily concurrently.

Ketoconazole – Dosage reduction of indinavir to 600 mg every 8 hours is recommended when administering ketoconazole concurrently.

Rifabutin – Dose reduction of rifabutin to half the standard dose and a dosage increase of indinavir to 1,000 mg (three 333 mg capsules) every 8 hours are recommended when rifabutin and indinavir are coadministered.

➤*Hepatic function impairment:* The dosage of indinavir should be reduced to 600 mg every 8 hours in patients with mild to moderate hepatic insufficiency caused by cirrhosis.

➤*Nephrolithiasis/Urolithiasis:* In addition to adequate hydration, medical management in patients who experience nephrolithiasis/urolithiasis may include temporary interruption (eg, 1 to 3 days) or discontinuation of therapy.

➤*Storage/Stability:* Store in a tightly closed container at room temperature (15° to 30°C; 59° to 86°F). Protect from moisture.

Indinavir capsules are sensitive to moisture. Dispense and store indinavir in the original container. The desiccant should remain in the original bottle.

Actions

➤*Pharmacology:* HIV-1 protease is an enzyme required for the proteolytic cleavage of the viral polyprotein precursors into the individual functional proteins found in infectious HIV-1. Indinavir binds to the protease active site and inhibits the activity of the enzyme. This inhibition prevents cleavage of the viral polyproteins, resulting in the formation of immature noninfectious viral particles.

Drug resistance – Isolates of HIV-1 with reduced susceptibility to the drug have been recovered from some patients treated with indinavir. Viral resistance was correlated with the accumulation of mutations that resulted in the expression of amino acid substitutions in the viral protease. Eleven amino acid residue positions (L10I/V/R, K20I/M/R, L24I, M46I/L, I54A/V, L63P, I64V, A71T/V, V82A/F/T, I84V, and L90M), at which substitutions are associated with resistance, have been identified. Resistance was mediated by the coexpression of multiple and variable substitutions at these positions. No single substitution was either necessary or sufficient for measurable resistance (at least 4-fold increase in IC_{95}). In general, higher levels of resistance were associated with the coexpression of greater numbers of substitutions, although their individual effects varied and were not additive. At least 3 amino acid substitutions must be present for phenotypic resistance to indinavir to reach measurable levels. In addition, mutations in the p7/p1 and p1/p6 gag cleavage sites were observed in some indinavir-resistant HIV-1 isolates.

Cross-resistance to other antiviral agents – Varying degrees of HIV-1 cross-resistance have been observed between indinavir and other HIV-1 protease inhibitors. In studies with ritonavir, saquinavir, and amprenavir, the extent and spectrum of cross-resistance varied with the specific mutational patterns observed. In general, the degree of cross-resistance increased with the accumulation of resistance-associated amino acid substitutions. Within a panel of 29 viral isolates from indinavir-treated patients that exhibited measurable (at least 4-fold) phenotypic resistance to indinavir, all were resistant to ritonavir. Of the indinavir resistant HIV-1 isolates, 63% showed resistance to saquinavir and 81% to amprenavir.

➤*Pharmacokinetics:*

Absorption – Indinavir was rapidly absorbed in the fasted state with a time to peak plasma concentration (T_{max}) of 0.8 ± 0.3 hours (mean ± SD; n = 11). A greater than dose-proportional increase in indinavir plasma concentrations was observed over the 200 to 1,000 mg dose range. At a dosing regimen of 800 mg every 8 hours, steady-state area under the plasma concentration time curve (AUC) was 30,691 ± 11,407 nM•h (n = 16), peak plasma concentration (C_{max}) was 12,617 ± 4,037 nM (n = 16), and plasma concentration 8 hours post dose (trough) was 251 ± 178 nM (n = 16).

Administration of indinavir with a meal high in calories, fat, and protein (784 kcal, 48.6 g fat, 31.3 g protein) resulted in a 77% ± 8% reduction in AUC and an 84% ± 7% reduction in C_{max} (n = 10). Administration with lighter meals (eg, a meal of dry toast with jelly, apple juice, and coffee with skim milk and sugar or a meal of corn flakes, skim milk and sugar) resulted in little or no change in AUC, C_{max}, or trough concentration.

Distribution – Indinavir was approximately 60% bound to human plasma proteins over a concentration range of 81 to 16,300 nM.

Metabolism – Following a 400 mg dose of ^{14}C-indinavir, 83 ± 1% (n = 4) and 19 ± 3% (n = 6) of the total radioactivity was recovered in feces and urine, respectively; radioactivity caused by parent drug in feces and urine was 19.1% and 9.4%, respectively. Seven metabolites have been identified, 1 glucuronide conjugate and 6 oxidative metabolites. In vitro studies indicate that cytochrome P-450 3A4 (CYP3A4) is the major enzyme responsible for formation of the oxidative metabolites.

Excretion – Less than 20% of indinavir is excreted unchanged in the urine. Mean urinary excretion of unchanged drug was 10.4 ± 4.9% (n = 10) and 12 ± 4.9% (n = 10) following a single 700 mg and 1,000 mg dose, respectively. Indinavir was rapidly eliminated with a half-life of 1.8 ± 0.4 hours (n = 10). Significant accumulation was not observed after multiple dosing at 800 mg every 8 hours.

Special populations –

Hepatic function impairment: Patients with mild to moderate hepatic insufficiency and clinical evidence of cirrhosis had evidence of decreased metabolism of indinavir resulting in approximately 60% higher mean AUC following a single 400 mg dose (n = 12). The half-life of indinavir increased to 2.8 ± 0.5 hours. Indinavir pharmacokinetics have not been studied in patients with severe hepatic insufficiency. Reduce the dosage of indinavir to 600 mg every 8 hours in patients with mild to moderate hepatic insufficiency caused by cirrhosis.

Children: The optimal dosing regimen for use of indinavir in pediatric patients has not been established. In HIV-infected pediatric patients (4 to 15 years of age), a dosage regimen of indinavir 500 mg/m² capsules every 8 hours produced $AUC_{0\text{-}8h}$ of 38,742 ± 24,098 nM•h (n = 34), C_{max} of 17,181 ± 9,809 nM (n = 34), and trough concentrations of 134 ± 91 nM (n = 28). The pharmacokinetic profiles of indinavir in pediatric patients were not comparable to profiles previously observed in HIV-infected adults receiving the recommended dose of 800 mg every 8 hours. The AUC and C_{max} values were slightly higher and the trough concentrations were considerably lower in pediatric patients. Approximately 50% of the pediatric patients had trough values below 100 nM; whereas, approximately 10% of adult patients had trough levels below 100 nM. The relationship between specific trough values and inhibition of HIV replication has not been established.

Pregnant patients: See Warnings for more information.

Contraindications

Clinically significant hypersensitivity to any of its components. Inhibition of CYP3A4 by indinavir could result in elevated plasma concentrations of the following drugs, potentially causing serious or life-threatening reactions.

Contraindicated Drugs with Indinavir

Drug class	Drugs within class that are contraindicated with indinavir
Antiarrhythmics	Amiodarone
Ergot derivatives	Dihydroergotamine, ergonovine, ergotamine, methylergonovine
Sedative/Hypnotics	Midazolam, triazolam
GI motility agents	Cisapride
Neuroleptics	Pimozide

Warnings

➤*Nephrolithiasis/Urolithiasis:* Nephrolithiasis/urolithiasis has occurred with indinavir therapy. The cumulative frequency of nephrolithiasis is substantially higher in pediatric patients (29%) than in adult patients (12.4%; range across individual trials, 4.7% to 34.4%). The cumulative frequency of nephrolithiasis events increases with increasing exposure to indinavir; however, the risk over time remains relatively constant. In some cases, nephrolithiasis/urolithiasis has been associated with renal insufficiency or acute renal failure, and/or pyelonephritis with or without bacteremia. If signs or symptoms of nephrolithiasis/urolithiasis (including flank pain with or without hematuria or microscopic hematuria) occur, consider temporary interruption (eg, 1 to 3 days) or discontinuation of therapy. Adequate hydration is recommended in all patients treated with indinavir.

➤*Hemolytic anemia:* Acute hemolytic anemia, including cases resulting in death, has been reported in patients treated with indinavir. Once a diagnosis is apparent, institute appropriate measures for the treatment of hemolytic anemia, including discontinuation of indinavir.

➤*Hepatitis:* Hepatitis, including cases resulting in hepatic failure and death, has been reported in patients treated with indinavir. Because the majority of these patients had confounding medical conditions and/or were receiving concomitant therapy(ies), a causal relationship between indinavir and these events has not been established.

➤*Hyperglycemia:* New onset diabetes mellitus, exacerbation of preexisting diabetes mellitus, and hyperglycemia have been reported during postmarketing surveillance in HIV-infected patients receiving protease inhibitor therapy. Some patients required either initiation or dose adjustments of insulin or oral hypoglycemic agents for treatment of these events. In some cases, diabetic ketoacidosis has occurred. In those patients who discontinued protease inhibitor therapy, hyperglycemia persisted. Because these events have been reported voluntarily during clinical practice, estimates of frequency cannot be made and a causal relationship between protease inhibitor therapy and these events has not been established.

➤*Hepatic function impairment:* In these patients, lower the dosage of indinavir because of decreased metabolism of indinavir. Reduce the dosage of indinavir to 600 mg every 8 hours in patients with mild to moderate hepatic insufficiency caused by cirrhosis.

➤*Carcinogenesis:* Carcinogenicity studies were conducted in mice and rats. In mice, no increased incidence of any tumor type was observed. The highest dosage tested in rats was 640 mg/kg/day; at this dose a statistically significant increased incidence of thyroid adenomas was seen only in male rats. At that dose, daily systemic exposure in rats was approximately 1.3 times higher than daily systemic exposure in humans.

➤*Elderly:* Clinical studies of indinavir did not include sufficient numbers of subjects 65 years of age and older to determine whether they respond differently from younger subjects. In general, exercise caution in dose selection for an elderly patient, reflecting the greater frequency of decreased hepatic, renal, or cardiac function and of concomitant disease or other drug therapy.

➤*Pregnancy: Category C.* Developmental toxicity studies were performed in rabbits (at dosages up to 240 mg/kg/day), dogs (at dosages up to 80 mg/kg/day), and rats (at dosages up to 640 mg/kg/day). Treatment-related increases over controls in the incidence of supernumerary ribs (at exposures at or below those in humans) and of cervical ribs (at exposures comparable with or slightly greater than those in humans) were seen in rats. In all 3 species, no treatment-related effects on embryonic/fetal survival or fetal weights were observed.

Indinavir was administered to rhesus monkeys during the third trimester of pregnancy (at dosages up to 160 mg/kg twice daily) and to neonatal rhesus monkeys (at dosages up to 160 mg/kg twice daily). When administered to neonates, indinavir caused an exacerbation of the transient physiologic hyperbilirubinemia seen in this species after birth; serum bilirubin values were approximately 4-fold above controls at 160 mg/kg twice daily. A similar exacerbation did not occur in neonates after in utero exposure to indinavir during the third trimester of pregnancy. In rhesus monkeys, fetal plasma drug levels were approximately 1% to 2% of maternal plasma drug levels approximately 1 hour after maternal dosing at 40, 80, or 160 mg/kg twice daily.

There are no adequate and well-controlled studies in pregnant women. Use during pregnancy only if the potential benefit justifies the potential risk to the fetus.

A dose of indinavir 800 mg every 8 hours with zidovudine 200 mg every 8 hours and lamivudine 150 mg twice daily has been studied in 16 HIV-infected pregnant patients at 14 to 28 weeks of gestation at enrollment (Study PACTG 358). Given the substantially lower antepartum exposures observed and the limited data in this patient population, indinavir use is not recommended in HIV-infected pregnant patients.

Antiviral pregnancy registry – To monitor maternal-fetal outcomes of pregnant women exposed to indinavir, an Antiretroviral Pregnancy Registry has been established. Health care providers are encouraged to register patients by calling 1-800-258-4263.

Hyperbilirubinemia – See Precautions for more information.

➤*Lactation:* Studies in lactating rats have demonstrated that indinavir is excreted in milk. Although it is not known whether indinavir is excreted in human milk, there exists the potential for adverse reactions from indinavir in breast-feeding infants. Instruct mothers to discontinue breast-feeding if they are receiving indinavir. This is consistent with the recommendation by the US Public Health Service Centers for Disease Control and Prevention that HIV-infected mothers not breast-feed their infants to avoid risking postnatal transmission of HIV.

➤*Children:* The optimal dosing regimen for use of indinavir in pediatric patients has not been established. A dosage of 500 mg/m^2 every 8 hours has been studied in uncontrolled studies of 70 children 3 to 18 years of age. The pharmacokinetic profiles of indinavir at this dose were not comparable with profiles previously observed in adults receiving the recommended dose. The AUC and C_{max} values were slightly higher and the trough concentrations were considerably lower in pediatric patients. Approximately 50% of the pediatric patients had trough values below 100 nM, whereas, approximately 10% of adult patients had trough levels below 100 nM. The relationship between specific trough values and inhibition of HIV replication has not been established. Although viral suppression was observed in some of the 32 children who were followed on this regimen through 24 weeks, a substantially higher rate of nephrolithiasis was reported when compared with adult historical data. Health care providers considering the use of indinavir in pediatric patients without other protease inhibitor options should be aware of the limited data available in this population and the increased risk of nephrolithiasis.

Precautions

➤*Hyperbilirubinemia:* Indirect hyperbilirubinemia has occurred frequently during treatment with indinavir and has infrequently been associated with increases in serum transaminases. Asymptomatic hyperbilirubinemia (total bilirubin greater than or equal to 2.5 mg/dL), reported predominantly as elevated indirect bilirubin, has occurred in approximately 14% of patients treated with indinavir. In less than 1%, this was associated with elevations in ALT or AST. It is not known whether indinavir will exacerbate the physiologic hyperbilirubinemia seen in neonates.

➤*Immune reconstitution syndrome:* Immune reconstitution syndrome has been reported in patients treated with combination antiretroviral therapy (CART), including indinavir. During the initial phase of treatment, patients responding to antiretroviral therapy whose immune system responds to CART may develop an inflammatory response to indolent or residual opportunistic infections (eg, *Mycobacterium avium*, cytomegalovirus, *Pneumocystis carinii*, pneumonia, tuberculosis [TB]), which may necessitate further evaluation and treatment.

➤*Tubulointerstitial nephritis:* Reports of tubulointerstitial nephritis with medullary calcification and cortical atrophy have been observed in patients with asymptomatic severe leukocyturia (greater than 100 cells/high power field). Closely follow patients with asymptomatic severe leukocyturia, and frequently monitor with urinalysis. Further diagnostic evaluation may be warranted; consider discontinuation of indinavir in all patients with severe leukocyturia.

➤*Hemophilia:* There have been reports of spontaneous bleeding in patients with hemophilia A and B treated with protease inhibitors. In some patients, additional factor VIII was required. In many of the reported cases, treatment with protease inhibitors was continued or restarted. A causal relationship between protease inhibitor therapy and these episodes has not been established.

➤*Fat redistribution:* Redistribution/accumulation of body fat, including central obesity, dorsocervical fat enlargement (buffalo hump), peripheral wasting, facial wasting, breast enlargement, and "cushingoid appearance", have been observed in patients receiving antiretroviral therapy. The mechanism and long-term consequences of these events are currently unknown. A causal relationship has not been established.

Drug Interactions

➤*Cytochrome P-450 3A4:* Indinavir is an inhibitor of the cytochrome P-450 isoform CYP3A4. Coadministration of indinavir and drugs primarily metabolized by CYP3A4 may result in increased plasma concentrations of the other drug, which could increase or prolong its therapeutic and adverse effects.

Indinavir is metabolized by CYP3A4. Drugs that induce CYP 3A4 activity would be expected to increase the clearance of indinavir, resulting in lowered plasma concentrations of indinavir. Coadministration of indinavir and other drugs that inhibit CYP3A4 may decrease the clearance of indinavir and may result in increased plasma concentrations of indinavir.

Indinavir Drug Interactions

Precipitant drug	Object drug[a]		Description
Anticonvulsants (carbamazepine, phenobarbital, phenytoin)	Indinavir	↓	Use with caution. Indinavir may not be effective because of decreased indinavir concentrations in patients taking these agents concomitantly.
Azole antifungals (itraconazole, ketoconazole)	Indinavir	↑	Plasma indinavir concentrations may be elevated, increasing the toxicity. Dose reduction of indinavir to 600 mg every 8 hours is recommended when administering concurrently.
Delavirdine	Indinavir	↑	Indinavir plasma concentrations may be elevated, increasing the pharmacologic and adverse effects. Reduce dose of indinavir to 600 mg every 8 hours when administering delavirdine 400 mg 3 times daily.
Didanosine	Indinavir	↓	The therapeutic effect of indinavir may be decreased. Administer indinavir and buffered didanosine formulations at least 1 hour apart on an empty stomach.
Efavirenz	Indinavir	↓	The optimal dose of indinavir, when given in combination with efavirenz, is not known. Increasing the indinavir dose to 1,000 mg every 8 hours does not compensate for the increased indinavir metabolism caused by efavirenz.
Interleukins	Indinavir	↑	Indinavir concentrations may be elevated, increasing the risk of toxicity. Adjust dose of indinavir as needed when interleukins are started or stopped.
Nelfinavir	Indinavir	↑	Indinavir concentrations may be elevated, increasing the risk of toxicity.
Nevirapine	Indinavir	↓	Indinavir concentrations may be decreased in the presence of nevirapine. Monitor indinavir levels, and adjust dose of indinavir as needed.
Protease inhibitors (atazanavir)	Indinavir	↔	Both indinavir and atazanavir are associated with indirect (unconjugated) hyperbilirubinemia. Combinations of these drugs have not been studied and coadministration of indinavir and atazanavir is not recommended.
Rifabutin	Indinavir	↓	Dose reduction of rifabutin to half the standard dose and a dose increase of indinavir to 100 mg (three 333 mg capsules) every 8 hours are recommended when rifabutin and indinavir are coadministered.
Indinavir	Rifabutin	↑	

INDINAVIR SULFATE — ORAL

Indinavir Drug Interactions			
Precipitant drug	Object drug[a]		Description
Rifampin	Indinavir	↓	Rifampin decreases indinavir serum concentrations which may lead to loss of virologic response and possible resistance to indinavir or to the class protease inhibitors. Concurrent administration is not recommended. Indinavir may elevate serum rifampin concentrations, increasing the risk of toxicity.
Indinavir	Rifampin	↑	
Ritonavir	Indinavir	↑	Ritonavir and indinavir concentrations may be elevated, increasing the pharmacologic and adverse effects.
Indinavir	Ritonavir	↑	
St. John's wort (*Hypericum perforatum*)	Indinavir	↓	Coadministration substantially decreases indinavir concentrations which may lead to loss of virologic response and possible resistance to indinavir or to the class of protease inhibitors. Coadministration not recommended.
Indinavir	Amiodarone	↑	Increases in serum amiodarone concentrations may occur, increasing the risk of serious and/or life-threatening reactions such as cardiac arrhythmias. Concurrent use of indinavir with amiodarone is contraindicated.
Indinavir	Antiarrhythmics (bepridil, lidocaine [systemic], quinidine)	↑	Caution is warranted and therapeutic concentration monitoring is recommended for antiarrhythmics when coadministered with indinavir.
Indinavir	Benzodiazepines (midazolam, triazolam)	↑	Serum concentrations of benzodiazepines may be elevated, resulting in prolonged or increased sedation or respiratory depression. Midazolam and triazolam are contraindicated in patients taking indinavir.
Indinavir	Clarithromycin	↑	Concentrations of clarithromycin and indinavir may be elevated, increasing the pharmacologic and adverse effects.
Clarithromycin	Indinavir	↑	
Indinavir	Cisapride	↑	Increased cisapride plasma concentrations with cardiotoxicity may occur. Coadministration is contraindicated.
Indinavir	Dihydropyridine calcium channel blockers (felodipine, nicardipine, nifedipine)	↑	Caution is warranted and clinical monitoring of patients is recommended.
Indinavir	Ergot derivatives (dihydroergotamine, ergonovine, ergotamine, methylergonovine)	↑	The risk of ergot toxicity (peripheral vasospasm, ischemia of the extremities) may be increased. Coadministration is contraindicated.
Indinavir	Fentanyl	↑	Plasma concentrations may be increased and the half-life prolonged, increasing the risk of adverse reactions (eg, respiratory depression).
Indinavir	HMG-CoA reductase inhibitors (atorvastatin, lovastatin, simvastatin)	↑	Coadministration may result in elevated plasma levels, increasing the risk of myopathy including rhabdomyolysis. Lovastatin and simvastatin are not recommended for concomitant use with indinavir. Use the lowest possible dose of atorvastatin and monitor for side effects or consider drugs not metabolized by CYP3A4, such as pravastatin, fluvastatin, or rosuvastatin.

Indinavir Drug Interactions			
Precipitant drug	Object drug[a]		Description
Indinavir	Immunosuppressant agents (sirolimus, tacrolimus)	↑	Plasma concentrations of immunosuppressants may be increased by indinavir.
Indinavir	Neuroleptic (pimozide)	↑	Inhibition of CYP3A4 by indinavir can result in elevated plasma concentrations of pimozide, potentially causing serious or life-threatening reactions. Coadministration is contraindicated.
Indinavir	Phosphodiesterase type 5 inhibitors (sildenafil, tadalafil, vardenafil)	↑	Elevated plasma concentrations of sildenafil, tadalafil, and vardenafil may occur, resulting in an increase in adverse reactions, including hypotension, visual changes, and priapism. Sildenafil dose should not exceed a maximum of 25 mg in a 48 h period in patients receiving concomitant indinavir therapy. Tadalafil dose should not exceed a maximum of 10 mg in a 72 h period in patients on concomitant therapy. Vardenafil dose should not exceed a maximum of 2.5 mg in a 24 h period in patients receiving concomitant therapy.
Indinavir	Saquinavir	↑	Saquinavir concentrations may be elevated, increasing the pharmacologic and adverse effects.
Indinavir	Trazodone	↑	Trazodone plasma concentrations may be elevated, increasing the pharmacologic and adverse effects. Monitor patient and adjust the dose of trazodone as needed.

[a] ↑ = Object drug increased. ↓ = Object drug decreased. ↔ = Undetermined clinical effect.

➤*Drug/Food interactions:* See Actions for more information.

Adverse Reactions

Adverse Reactions (≥ 2%)					
	Indinavir	Indinavir plus zidovudine	Zidovudine	Indinavir plus zidovudine plus lamivudine	Zidovudine plus lamivudine
Adverse reaction	% (n = 332)	% (n = 332)	% (n = 332)	% (n = 571)	% (n = 575)
CNS					
Dizziness	3%	3.9%	0.9%	0.5%	0.7%
Headache	5.4%	9.6%	6%	2.4%	2.8%
Somnolence	2.4%	3.3%	3.3%	0	0
Dermatologic					
Pruritus	4.2%	2.4%	1.8%	0.5%	0
Rash	1.2%	0.6%	2.4%	1.1%	0.5%
GI					
Abdominal pain	16.6%	16%	12%	1.9%	0.7%
Acid regurgitation	2.7%	5.4%	1.8%	0.4%	0
Anorexia	2.7%	5.4%	3%	0.5%	0.2%
Appetite increase	2.1%	1.5%	1.2%	0	0
Diarrhea	3.3%	3%	2.4%	0.9%	1.2%
Dyspepsia	1.5%	2.7%	0.9%	0	0
Jaundice	1.5%	2.1%	0.3%	0	0
Nausea	11.7%	31.9%	19.6%	2.8%	1.4%
Vomiting	8.4%	17.8%	9%	1.4%	1.4%
GU					
Dysuria	1.5%	2.4%	0.3%	0.4%	0.2%
Nephrolithiasis/ Urolithiasis[a]	8.7%	7.8%	2.1%	2.6%	0.3%
Respiratory					
Cough	1.5%	0.3%	0.6%	1.6%	1%
Difficulty breathing/ Dyspnea/Shortness of breath	0	0.6%	0.3%	1.8%	1%

INDINAVIR SULFATE — ORAL

Adverse Reactions (≥ 2%)					
Adverse reaction	Indinavir % (n = 332)	Indinavir plus zidovudine % (n = 332)	Zidovudine % (n = 332)	Indinavir plus zidovudine plus lamivudine % (n = 571)	Zidovudine plus lamivudine % (n = 575)
Miscellaneous					
Anemia	0.6%	1.2%	2.1%	2.4%	3.5%
Asthenia/Fatigue	2.1%	4.2%	3.6%	2.4%	4.5%
Back pain	8.4%	4.5%	1.5%	0.9%	0.7%
Fever	1.5%	1.5%	2.1%	3.8%	3%
Malaise	2.1%	2.7%	1.8%	0	0
Taste perversion	2.7%	8.4%	1.2%	0.2%	0

[a] Including renal colic, and flank pain with and without hematuria.

➤*Hyperbilirubinemia:* See Warnings for more information.

Hyperbilirubinemia and nephrolithiasis/urolithiasis occurred more frequently at doses exceeding 2.4 g/day compared to doses less than or equal to 2.4 g/day.

➤*Nephrolithiasis / Urolithiasis:* Nephrolithiasis/urolithiasis, including flank pain with or without hematuria (including microscopic hematuria), has been reported in approximately 12.4% (301 of 2,429; range across individual trials: 4.7% to 34.4%) of patients receiving indinavir at the recommended dosage in clinical trials with a mean follow-up of 47 weeks (range: 1 day to 242 weeks; 2,238 patient-years follow-up). The cumulative frequency of nephrolithiasis events increases with duration of exposure to indinavir; however, the risk over time remains relatively constant. Of the patients treated with indinavir who developed nephrolithiasis/urolithiasis in clinical trials during the double-blind phase, 2.8% (7 of 246) were reported to develop hydronephrosis and 4.5% (11 of 246) underwent stent placement. Following the acute episode, 4.9% (12 of 246) of patients discontinued therapy.

➤*Miscellaneous:* In phase 1 and 2 controlled trials, the following adverse reactions were reported significantly more frequently by those randomized to the arms containing indinavir than by those randomized to nucleoside analogues: rash, upper respiratory tract infection, dry skin, pharyngitis, taste perversion.

➤*Lab test abnormalities:*

Selected Laboratory Abnormalities					
Lab test abnormalities	Indinavir % (n = 329)	Indinavir plus zidovudine % (n = 320)	Zidovudine % (n = 330)	Indinavir plus zidovudine plus lamivudine % (n = 571)	Zidovudine plus lamivudine % (n = 575)
Blood chemistry					
Increased ALT > 500% ULN[a]	4.9%	4.1%	3%	2.6%	2.6%
Increased AST > 500% ULN	3.7%	2.8%	2.7%	3.3%	2.8%
Total serum bilirubin > 250% ULN	11.9%	9.7%	0.6%	6.1%	1.4%
Increased serum amylase > 200% ULN	2.1%	1.9%	1.8%	0.9%	0.3%
Increased glucose > 250 mg/dL	0.9%	0.9%	0.6%	1.6%	1.9%
Increased creatinine > 300% ULN	0%	0%	0.6%	0.2%	0%
Hematology					
Decreased hemoglobin < 7 g/dL	0.6%	0.9%	3.3%	2.4%	3.5%
Decreased platelet count < 50 THS/mm^3	0.9%	0.9%	1.8%	0.2%	0.9%
Decreased neutrophils < 0.75 THS/mm^3	2.4%	2.2%	6.7%	5.1%	14.6%

[a] Upper limit of the normal range.

➤*Postmarketing:*

Cardiovascular – Cardiovascular disorders, including myocardial infarction and angina pectoris, cerebrovascular disorder.

CNS – Oral paresthesia, depression.

Dermatologic – Rash, including erythema multiforme and Stevens-Johnson syndrome; hyperpigmentation; alopecia; ingrown toenails or paronychia; pruritus.

Endocrine – New onset diabetes mellitus, exacerbation of preexisting diabetes mellitus, hyperglycemia.

GI – Pancreatitis; abdominal distention; dyspepsia.

GU – Nephrolithiasis/urolithiasis, in some cases resulting in renal insufficiency or acute renal failure; pyelonephritis with or without bacteremia; interstitial nephritis, sometimes with indinavir crystal deposits (in some patients, the interstitial nephritis did not resolve following discontinuation of indinavir); leukocyturia; crystalluria; dysuria.

Hematologic – Increased spontaneous bleeding in patients with hemophilia; acute hemolytic anemia.

Hepatic – Liver function abnormalities; hepatitis, including reports of hepatic failure; jaundice.

Hypersensitivity – Anaphylactoid reactions, urticaria, vasculitis.

Lab test abnormalities – Increased serum triglycerides, increased serum cholesterol.

Miscellaneous – Redistribution/accumulation of body fat; arthralgia.

Overdosage

There have been more than 60 reports of acute or chronic human overdosage (up to 23 times the recommended total daily dose of 2,400 mg) with indinavir. The most commonly reported symptoms were renal (eg, nephrolithiasis/urolithiasis, flank pain, hematuria) and GI (eg, nausea, vomiting, diarrhea).

It is not known whether indinavir is dialyzable by peritoneal or hemodialysis.

Patient Information

Indinavir is not a cure for HIV infection and patients may continue to develop opportunistic infections and other complications associated with HIV disease. The long-term effects of indinavir are unknown at this time. Indinavir has not been shown to reduce the risk of transmission of HIV to others through sexual contact or blood contamination.

Advise patients to remain under the care of a doctor when using indinavir and not to modify or discontinue treatment without first consulting the doctor. Therefore, if a dose is missed, advise patients to take the next dose at the regularly scheduled time and to not double this dose. Initiate and maintain therapy with indinavir at the recommended dosage.

Indinavir may interact with some drugs; therefore, advise patients to report to their doctor the use of any other prescription medication, nonprescription medication, or herbal products, particularly St. John's wort.

For optimal absorption, administer indinavir without food but with water 1 hour before or 2 hours after a meal. Alternatively, indinavir may be administered with other liquids such as skim milk, juice, coffee, or tea, or with a light meal (eg, dry toast with jelly, juice, and coffee with skim milk and sugar; or corn flakes, skim milk, and sugar). Ingestion of indinavir with a meal high in calories, fat, and protein reduces the absorption of indinavir.

Advise patients receiving a phosphodiesterase type 5 (PDE5) inhibitor (sildenafil, tadalafil, vardenafil) that they may be at an increased risk of PDE5-associated adverse reactions, including hypotension, visual changes, and priapism, and to promptly report any symptoms to their doctors.

Inform patients that redistribution or accumulation of body fat may occur in patients receiving protease inhibitors and that the cause and long-term health effects of these conditions are not known at this time.

Indinavir capsules are sensitive to moisture. Inform patients to store and use indinavir in the original container and to leave the desiccant in the bottle.

TIPRANAVIR ORAL

Rx	**Aptivus** (Boehringer Ingelheim)	**Capsules:** 250 mg	7% w/w dehydrated alcohol, polyoxyl 35 castor oil. (TPV 250). Pink, oblong. In 120s.

TIPRANAVIR — ORAL

WARNING

Tipranavir coadministered with ritonavir 200 mg has been associated with reports of both fatal and nonfatal intracranial hemorrhage.

Tipranavir coadministered with ritonavir 200 mg has been associated with reports of clinical hepatitis and hepatic decompensation, including some fatalities. Extra vigilance is warranted in patients with chronic hepatitis B or C coinfection, as these patients have an increased risk of hepatotoxicity.

Indications

➤*HIV infection:* Tipranavir, coadministered with ritonavir 200 mg, is indicated for combination antiretroviral treatment of HIV-1 infected adult patients with evidence of viral replication, who are highly treatment-experienced or have HIV-1 strains resistant to multiple protease inhibitors (PIs).

This indication is based on analyses of plasma HIV-1 RNA levels in 2 controlled studies of tipranavir/ritonavir of 24 weeks' duration. Both studies were conducted in clinically advanced, 3-class antiretroviral (nucleoside reverse transcriptase inhibitor [NRTI], nonnucleoside reverse transcriptase inhibitor [NNRTI], PI) treatment–experienced adults with evidence of HIV-1 replication despite ongoing antiretroviral therapy.

Consider the following points when initiating therapy with tipanavir/ritonavir:

- The use of other active agents with tipranavir/ritonavir is associated with a greater likelihood of treatment response.
- Genotypic or phenotypic testing and/or treatment history should guide the use of tipranavir/ritonavir. The number of baseline primary PI mutations affects the virologic response to tipranavir/ritonavir.
- Use caution when prescribing tipranavir/ritonavir in patients who may be at risk of increased bleeding or who are receiving medications known to increase the risk of bleeding.
- Perform liver function tests at initiation of therapy with tipranavir/ritonavir and monitor them frequently throughout the duration of treatment.
- Use caution when prescribing tipranavir/ritonavir to patients with elevated transaminases, hepatitis B or C coinfection, or other underlying hepatic function impairment.
- The extensive drug-drug interaction potential of tipranavir/ritonavir when coadministered with multiple classes of drugs must be considered prior to and during tipranavir/ritonavir use.
- The risk-benefit of tipranavir/ritonavir has not been established in treatment-naive adult or pediatric patients.

There are no study results demonstrating the effect of tipranavir/ritonavir on clinical progression of HIV-1.

Administration and Dosage

➤*Approved by the FDA:* June 22, 2005.

Tipranavir, coadministered with ritonavir 200 mg, should be taken with food. Bioavailability is increased with a high-fat meal. Swallow the capsules whole.

➤*Dosage:* The recommended dosage of tipranavir is 500 mg (two 250 mg capsules) coadministered with ritonavir 200 mg, twice daily.

➤*Storage / Stability:* Store tipranavir in a refrigerator, 2° to 8°C (36° to 46°F), prior to opening the bottle. After opening the bottle, the capsules may be stored at 25°C (77°F); excursions permitted to 15° to 30°C (59° to 86°F), and must be used within 60 days.

Actions

➤*Pharmacology:* Tipranavir is a nonpeptidic HIV-1 PI that inhibits the virus-specific processing of the viral Gag and Gag-Pol polyproteins in HIV-1–infected cells, thus preventing formation of mature virions.

➤*Pharmacokinetics:*

Absorption – Absorption of tipranavir in humans is limited, although no absolute quantification of absorption is available. Tipranavir is a P-glycoprotein (P-gp) substrate, a weak P-gp inhibitor, and appears to be a potent P-gp inducer as well. In vivo data suggest that the net effect of tipranavir/ritonavir at the proposed dose regimen (500 mg/200 mg) is P-gp induction at steady state, although ritonavir is a P-gp inhibitor. Tipranavir trough concentrations at steady state are approximately 70% lower than those on day 1, presumably because of intestinal P-gp induction. Steady state is attained in most subjects after 7 to 10 days of dosing.

Dosing with tipranavir 500 mg concomitant with ritonavir 200 mg twice daily for longer than 2 weeks and without meal restriction produced the following pharmacokinetic parameters for female and male HIV-positive patients (see the following table).

Pharmacokinetic Parameters[a] of Tipranavir 500 mg/Ritonavir 200 mg for HIV-Positive Patients by Gender

Parameter	Women (n = 14)	Men (n = 106)
Cp_{trough} (mcM)	41.6 ± 24.3	35.6 ± 16.7
C_{max} (mcM)	94.8 ± 22.8	77.6 ± 16.6
T_{max} (h)	2.9	3

Pharmacokinetic Parameters[a] of Tipranavir 500 mg/Ritonavir 200 mg for HIV-Positive Patients by Gender

Parameter	Women (n = 14)	Men (n = 106)
$AUC_{0\text{-}12h}$ (mcM•h)	851 ± 309	710 ± 207
CL (L/h)	1.15	1.27
V (L)	7.7	10.2
$t_{1/2}$ (h)	5.5	6

[a] Population pharmacokinetic parameters reported as mean ± standard deviation.

Tipranavir capsules coadministered with ritonavir should be taken with food. Bioavailability is increased with a high-fat meal. Tipranavir capsules, administered under high-fat meal conditions or with a light snack of toast and skimmed milk, were tested in a multiple-dose study. High-fat meals (868 kcal, 53% derived from fat, 31% derived from carbohydrates) enhanced the extent of bioavailability (AUC point estimate 1.31; confidence interval [CI], 1.23 to 1.39), but had minimal effect on peak tipranavir concentrations (C_{max} point estimate 1.16; CI, 1.09 to 1.24).

When tipranavir, coadministered with low-dose ritonavir, was coadministered with 20 mL of an aluminum- and magnesium-based liquid antacid, tipranavir AUC_{12h}, C_{max}, and C_{12h} were reduced by 25% to 29%. Give consideration to separating tipranavir/ritonavir dosing from antacid administration to prevent reduced absorption of tipranavir.

Distribution – Tipranavir is extensively bound to plasma proteins (more than 99.9%). It binds to both human serum albumin and α_1-acid glycoprotein. The mean fraction of tipranavir (dosed without ritonavir) unbound in plasma was similar in clinical samples from healthy volunteers (0.015% ± 0.006%) and HIV-positive patients (0.019% ± 0.076%). Total plasma tipranavir concentrations for these samples ranged from 9 to 82 mcM. The unbound fraction of tipranavir appeared to be independent of total drug concentration over this concentration range.

Metabolism – In vitro metabolism studies with human liver microsomes indicated that CYP3A4 is the predominant CYP enzyme involved in tipranavir metabolism.

The oral clearance of tipranavir decreased after the addition of ritonavir, which may represent diminished first-pass clearance of the drug at the GI tract as well as the liver.

The metabolism of tipranavir in the presence of ritonavir 200 mg is minimal. Administration of ^{14}C-tipranavir to subjects that received tipranavir 500 mg/ritonavir 200 mg dosed to steady state demonstrated that unchanged tipranavir accounted for 98.4% or greater of the total plasma radioactivity circulating at 3, 8, or 12 hours after dosing. Only a few metabolites were found in plasma, and all were at trace levels (0.2% or less of the plasma radioactivity). In feces, unchanged tipranavir represented the majority of fecal radioactivity (79.9% of fecal radioactivity). The most abundant fecal metabolite, at 4.9% of fecal radioactivity (3.2% of dose), was a hydroxyl metabolite of tipranavir. In urine, unchanged tipranavir was found in trace amounts (0.5% of urine radioactivity). The most abundant urinary metabolite, at 11% of urine radioactivity (0.5% of dose), was a glucuronide conjugate of tipranavir.

Excretion – Administration of ^{14}C-tipranavir to subjects (n = 8) that received tipranavir 500 mg/ritonavir 200 mg dosed to steady state demonstrated that most radioactivity (median, 82.3%) was excreted in feces, while only a median of 4.4% of the radioactive dose administered was recovered in urine. In addition, most radioactivity (56%) was excreted between 24 and 96 hours after dosing. The effective mean elimination half-life of tipranavir/ritonavir in healthy volunteers (n = 67) and HIV-infected adult patients (n = 120) was approximately 4.8 and 6 hours, respectively, at steady state following a dosage of 500 mg/200 mg twice daily with a light meal.

Special populations –

Gender: Evaluation of steady-state plasma tipranavir trough concentrations at 10 to 14 hours after dosing from studies 1182.12 and 1182.48 demonstrated that women generally had higher tipranavir concentrations than men. After 4 weeks of tipranavir 500 mg/ritonavir 200 mg twice daily, the median plasma trough concentration of tipranavir was 43.9 mcM for women and 31.1 mcM for men. The difference in concentrations does not warrant a dose adjustment.

➤*Microbiology:* Tipranavir inhibits the replication of laboratory strains of HIV-1 and clinical isolates in acute models of T-cell infection, with 50% effective concentrations (EC_{50}) ranging from 0.03 to 0.07 mcM (18 to 42 ng/mL). Tipranavir demonstrates antiviral activity in vitro against a broad panel of HIV-1 group M non-clade B isolates (A, C, D, F, G, H, CRF01 AE, CRF02 AG, CRF12 BF). Group O and HIV-2 isolates have reduced susceptibility in vitro to tipranavir with EC_{50} values ranging from 0.164 to 1 mcM and 0.233 to 0.522 mcM, respectively. Protein binding studies have shown that the antiviral activity of tipranavir decreases on average 3.75-fold in conditions where human serum is present. When used with other antiretroviral agents in vitro, the combination of tipranavir was additive to antagonistic with other PIs (amprenavir, atazanavir, indinavir, lopinavir, nelfinavir, ritonavir, and saquinavir) and generally additive with the NNRTIs (delavirdine, efavirenz, and nevirapine) and the NRTIs (abacavir, didanosine, emtricitabine, lamivudine, stavudine, tenofovir, and zidovudine). Tipranavir was synergistic with the HIV fusion inhibitor enfuvirtide. There was no antagonism of the in vitro combinations of tipranavir with either adefovir or ribavirin, used in the treatment of viral hepatitis.

Resistance –

Clinical studies of treatment-experienced patients: In phase 3 studies 1182.12 and 1182.48, multiple PI-resistant HIV-1 isolates from 59 highly

TIPRANAVIR — ORAL

treatment-experienced patients who received tipranavir/ritonavir and experienced virologic rebound developed amino acid substitutions that were associated with resistance to tipranavir. The most common amino acid substitutions that developed on tipranavir 500 mg/ritonavir 200 mg in greater than 20% of tipranavir/ritonavir virologic failure isolates were L33V/I/F, V82T, and I84V. Other substitutions that developed in 10% to 20% of tipranavir/ritonavir virologic failure isolates included L10V/I/S, I13V, E35D/G/N, I47V, K55R, V82L, and L89V/M. Tipranavir resistance was detected at virologic rebound after an average of 38 weeks of tipranavir/ritonavir treatment with a median 14-fold decrease in tipranavir susceptibility. The resistance profile in treatment-naive subjects has not been characterized.

Cross-resistance – Cross-resistance among PIs has been observed. Tipranavir had less than 4-fold decreased susceptibility against 90% (94 of 105) of HIV-1 isolates resistant to amprenavir, atazanavir, indinavir, lopinavir, nelfinavir, ritonavir, or saquinavir. Tipranavir-resistant viruses that emerged in vitro had decreased susceptibility to the PIs amprenavir, atazanavir, indinavir, lopinavir, nelfinavir, and ritonavir but remained sensitive to saquinavir.

Contraindications

Hypersensitivity to any of the ingredients of the product; moderate to severe (Child-Pugh class B and C, respectively) hepatic insufficiency.

Coadministration of tipranavir and ritonavir 200 mg with drugs that are highly dependent on CYP3A for clearance and for which elevated plasma concentrations are associated with serious and/or life-threatening events is contraindicated. These drugs are listed in the following table.

Drugs that are Contraindicated with Tipranavir Coadministered with Ritonavir 200 mg

Drug class	Drugs within class that are contraindicated with tipranavir coadministered with ritonavir 200 mg
Antiarrhythmics	Amiodarone, bepridil, flecainide, propafenone, quinidine
Antihistamines	Astemizole, terfenadine
Ergot derivatives	Dihydroergotamine, ergonovine, ergotamine, methylergonovine
GI motility agent	Cisapride
Neuroleptic	Pimozide
Sedatives/Hypnotics	Midazolam, triazolam

Because of the required coadministration of tipranavir with ritonavir 200 mg, refer to the ritonavir monograph for a description of ritonavir contraindications.

Warnings

➤*Coadministration with ritonavir:* Tipranavir must be coadministered with ritonavir 200 mg to exert its therapeutic effect. Failure to correctly coadminister tipranavir with ritonavir will result in reduced plasma levels of tipranavir that will be insufficient to achieve the desired antiviral effect and will alter some drug interactions (effect of tipranavir and ritonavir on other drugs).

Refer to the ritonavir monograph for additional information on precautionary measures.

➤*Diabetes mellitus/Hyperglycemia:* New-onset diabetes mellitus, exacerbation of preexisting diabetes mellitus, and hyperglycemia have been reported during postmarketing surveillance in HIV-1–infected patients receiving PI therapy. Some patients required either initiation or dose adjustments of insulin or oral hypoglycemic agents for treatment of these events. In some cases, diabetic ketoacidosis has occurred. In those patients who discontinued PI therapy, hyperglycemia persisted in some cases. Because these events have been reported voluntarily during clinical practice, estimates of frequency cannot be made and a causal relationship between PI therapy and these events has not been established.

➤*Hepatic toxicity:* Tipranavir coadministered with ritonavir 200 mg has been associated with reports of clinical hepatitis and hepatic decompensation, including some fatalities. These have generally occurred in patients with advanced HIV disease taking multiple concomitant medications. A causal relationship to tipranavir/ritonavir could not be established. Closely follow all patients with clinical and laboratory monitoring, especially those with chronic hepatitis B or C coinfection because these patients have an increased risk of hepatotoxicity. Perform liver function tests prior to initiating therapy with tipranavir/ritonavir, and frequently throughout the duration of treatment.

Health care providers and patients should be vigilant for the appearance of signs or symptoms of hepatitis, such as fatigue, malaise, anorexia, nausea, jaundice, bilirubinuria, acholic stools, liver tenderness, or hepatomegaly. Patients with signs or symptoms of clinical hepatitis should discontinue tipranavir/ritonavir treatment and seek medical evaluation.

➤*Hepatic function impairment:* Patients with chronic hepatitis B or hepatitis C coinfection or elevations in transaminases are at an approximately 2.5-fold risk for developing further transaminase elevations or hepatic decompensation. Additionally, grade 3 and 4 increases in hepatic transaminases were observed in 6% of healthy volunteers in phase 1 studies and 6% of subjects receiving tipranavir/ritonavir in phase 3 studies.

Tipranavir is principally metabolized by the liver. Therefore, exercise caution when administering tipranavir/ritonavir to patients with hepatic impairment because tipranavir concentrations may be increased. Tipranavir/ritonavir is contraindicated in patients with moderate to severe (Child-Pugh class B and C, respectively) hepatic insufficiency.

➤*Elderly:* Clinical studies of tipranavir did not include sufficient numbers of subjects 65 years of age and older to determine whether they respond differently from younger subjects. In general, exercise caution in the administration and monitoring of tipranavir in elderly patients, reflecting the greater frequency of decreased hepatic, renal, or cardiac function, and of concomitant disease or other drug therapy.

➤*Pregnancy: Category C.* At 400 mg/kg/day and above in rats, fetal toxicity (decreased sternebrae ossification and body weights) was observed, corresponding to an AUC of 1,310 mcM•h or approximately 0.8-fold human exposure at the recommended dose.

In pre- and postdevelopment studies in rats, tipranavir showed no adverse effects at 40 mg/kg/day (approximately 0.2-fold human exposure), but caused growth inhibition in pups and maternal toxicity at dose levels of 400 mg/kg/day (approximately 0.8-fold human exposure). No postweaning functions were affected at any dose level.

There are no adequate and well-controlled studies in pregnant women for the treatment of HIV-1 infection. Use tipranavir during pregnancy only if the potential benefit justifies the potential risk to the fetus.

Antiretroviral pregnancy registry – To monitor maternal-fetal outcomes of pregnant women exposed to tipranavir, an antiretroviral pregnancy registry has been established. Health care providers are encouraged to register patients by calling 1-800-258-4263.

➤*Lactation:* The Centers for Disease Control and Prevention recommend that HIV-infected mothers not breast-feed their infants to avoid risking postnatal transmission of HIV. Because of the potential for HIV transmission and possible adverse reactions of tipranavir, instruct mothers not to breast-feed if they are receiving tipranavir.

➤*Children:* Safety and efficacy in pediatric patients have not been established.

Precautions

➤*Monitoring:* Perform liver function tests prior to initiating therapy with tipranavir/ritonavir, and frequently throughout the duration of treatment.

Perform triglyceride and cholesterol testing prior to initiating tipranavir/ritonavir therapy and at periodic intervals during therapy. Manage lipid disorders as clinically appropriate.

➤*Sulfa allergy:* Use tipranavir with caution in patients with a known sulfonamide allergy. Tipranavir contains a sulfonamide moiety. The potential for cross-sensitivity between drugs in the sulfonamide class and tipranavir is unknown.

➤*Rash:* Mild to moderate rashes including urticarial rash, maculopapular rash, and possible photosensitivity have been reported in subjects receiving tipranavir/ritonavir. In phase 2 and 3 trials, rash was observed in 14% of women and in 8% to 10% of men receiving tipranavir/ritonavir. Additionally, in 1 drug interaction trial in healthy female volunteers administered a single dose of ethinyl estradiol followed by tipranavir/ritonavir, 33% of subjects developed a rash. Rash accompanied by joint pain or stiffness, throat tightness, or generalized pruritus has been reported in both men and women receiving tipranavir/ritonavir.

➤*Hemophilia:* There have been reports of increased bleeding, including spontaneous skin hematomas and hemarthrosis in patients with hemophilia type A and B treated with PIs. In some patients, additional Factor VIII was given. In more than half of the reported cases, treatment with PIs was continued or reintroduced if treatment had been discontinued. A causal relationship between PIs and these events has not been established.

➤*Lipid elevations:* Treatment with tipranavir coadministered with ritonavir 200 mg has resulted in large increases in the concentration of total cholesterol and triglycerides. Perform triglyceride and cholesterol testing prior to initiating tipranavir/ritonavir therapy and at periodic intervals during therapy. Manage lipid disorders as clinically appropriate.

➤*Fat redistribution:* Redistribution/accumulation of body fat, including central obesity, dorsocervical fat enlargement (buffalo hump), peripheral wasting, facial wasting, breast enlargement, and "cushingoid appearance," have been observed in patients receiving antiretroviral therapy. The mechanism and long-term consequences of these events are currently unknown. A causal relationship has not been established.

➤*Immune reconstitution syndrome:* Immune reconstitution syndrome has been reported in patients treated with combination antiretroviral therapy, including tipranavir. During the initial phase of combination antiretroviral treatment, patients whose immune system responds may develop an inflammatory response to indolent or residual opportunistic infections (eg, *Mycobacterium avium* infection, cytomegalovirus, *Pneumocystis jeroveci* pneumonia, tuberculosis, reactivation of herpes simplex and herpes zoster), which may necessitate further evaluation and treatment.

Drug Interactions

Tipranavir is a CYP3A substrate and a P-gp substrate. Coadministration of tipranavir/ritonavir and drugs that induce CYP3A and/or P-gp may decrease tipranavir plasma concentrations. Coadministration of tipranavir/ritonavir and drugs that inhibit P-gp may increase tipranavir plasma concentrations.

Coadministration of tipranavir/ritonavir with drugs that inhibit CYP3A may not further increase tipranavir plasma concentrations, because the level of

TIPRANAVIR — ORAL

metabolites is low following steady-state administration of tipranavir 500 mg/ritonavir 200 mg twice daily.

Tipranavir Drug Interactions

Precipitant drug	Object drug[a]		Description
Aluminum- and magnesium-based antacids	Tipranavir	↓	Aluminum- and magnesium-based antacids may decrease tipranavir absorption. Consider separating tipranavir/ritonavir dosing from antacid administration.
Azole antifungals (ie, fluconazole)	Tipranavir	↑	Fluconazole may increase tipranavir concentrations. Dosage adjustment is not needed. High doses (> 200 mg) of fluconazole, itraconazole, and ketoconazole are not recommended. Studies have not been done with itraconazole, ketoconazole, or voriconazole.
Tipranavir	Azole antifungals (ie, fluconazole, itraconazole, ketoconazole, voriconazole)	↔	
Clarithromycin	Tipranavir	↑	Concurrent use may increase tipranavir and clarithromycin levels. Dosage adjustment is not needed in patients with normal renal function. For patients with Ccr 30 to 60 mL/min, decrease clarithromycin dose by 50%. For patients with Ccr < 30 mL/min, decrease the clarithromycin dose by 75%.
Tipranavir	Clarithromycin		
Efavirenz	Tipranavir	↓	Efavirenz coadministered with tipranavir/ritonavir (500 mg/100 mg twice daily) cause tipranavir concentrations to decrease. Higher doses of tipranavir/ritonavir did not cause significant changes in tipranavir pharmacokinetics.
Loperamide	Tipranavir	↓	Coadministration may decrease the concentrations of both tipranavir and loperamide.
Tipranavir	Loperamide		
NRTIs (ie, didanosine, zidovudine)	Tipranavir	↓	Didanosine and zidovudine may decrease tipranavir concentrations. Plasma levels of NRTIs may be decreased. Clinical relevance is currently unknown. Separate didanosine dosing from tipranavir/ritonavir by at least 2 hours.
Tipranavir	NRTIs (ie, abacavir, didanosine, zidovudine)		
Rifamycins (ie, rifampin)	Tipranavir	↓	Coadministration of tipranavir with rifampin may lead to loss of virologic response and possible resistance to tipranavir. Concurrent use is not recommended.
Tipranavir	Rifamycins (ie, rifabutin)	↑	Coadministration of tipranavir with rifabutin may increase rifabutin (and its metabolite) concentrations. Reduce rifabutin dose by 75% (eg, 150 mg every other day) and increase monitoring.
St. John's wort	Tipranavir	↓	Coadministration may lead to loss of virologic response and possible resistance to tipranavir. Concurrent use is not recommended.
Tenofovir	Tipranavir	↓	Coadministration may decrease the concentrations of both tipranavir and tenofovir.
Tipranavir	Tenofovir		
Tipranavir	Antiarrhythmic agents (ie, amiodarone, bepridil, flecainide, propafenone, quinidine)	↑	Coadministration is contraindicated because of the potential for cardiac arrhythmias secondary to increases in plasma concentrations of antiarrhythmics.
Tipranavir	Antihistamines (ie, astemizole, terfenadine)	↑	Coadministration is contraindicated because of the potential for serious and/or life-threatening reactions such as cardiac arrhythmias.
Tipranavir	Benzodiazepines (ie, midazolam, triazolam)	↑	Coadministration is contraindicated because of the risk of prolonged or increased sedation or respiratory depression.

Tipranavir Drug Interactions

Precipitant drug	Object drug[a]		Description
Tipranavir	Calcium channel blockers (ie, diltiazem, felodipine, nicardipine, nisoldipine, verapamil)	↔	Although not studied, caution is warranted and clinical monitoring is recommended.
Tipranavir	Cisapride	↑	Coadministration is contraindicated because of the risk of cardiac arrhythmias.
Tipranavir	Contraceptives, oral (estrogen-containing)	↓	Concurrent use may decrease ethinyl estradiol by 50%. Use alternative methods of nonhormonal contraception. Monitor patients taking estrogen-based hormone replacement therapy for signs of estrogen deficiency. Patients also may have an increased risk of rash.
Tipranavir	Desipramine	↑	Although not studied, increased desipramine levels are suspected. Dosage reduction and concentration monitoring of desipramine are recommended.
Tipranavir	Disulfiram, Metronidazole	↑	Tipranavir capsules contain alcohol that can produce disulfiram-like reactions when coadministered with disulfiram or other drugs that can produce this reaction (eg, metronidazole).
Tipranavir	Ergot derivatives	↑	The risk of ergot toxicity is increased. Coadministration is contraindicated.
Tipranavir	HMG-CoA reductase inhibitors (ie, lovastatin, simvastatin, atorvastatin)	↑	Concurrent use increases the risk of myopathy, including rhabdomyolysis. Concurrent use of tipranavir with lovastatin or simvastatin is not recommended. If using atorvastatin, start with the lowest possible dose with careful monitoring.
Tipranavir	Hypoglycemic agents (ie, glimepiride, glipizide, glyburide, tolbutamide, pioglitazone, repaglinide)	↔	Although not studied, careful glucose monitoring is recommended.
Tipranavir	Immunosuppressants (ie, cyclosporine, sirolimus, tacrolimus)	↔	Although not studied, careful drug concentration monitoring is recommended.
Tipranavir	Opioid analgesics (ie, meperidine, methadone)	↑↓	Although not studied, the levels of meperidine and methadone may be decreased. However, the levels of the metabolite normeperidine may be increased and thus increase the risk for seizures. Increased dosage and long-term use of meperidine are not recommended. Methadone dosage may need to be increased.
Tipranavir	PDE5 inhibitors (ie, sildenafil, tadalafil, vardenafil)	↑	Although not studied, use concomitantly with caution. The PDE5 inhibitor dose should not exceed the following: sildenafil 25 mg within 48 hours; tadalafil 10 mg every 72 hours; vardenafil 2.5 mg every 72 hours.
Tipranavir	Pimozide	↑	Coadministration is contraindicated because of the potential for cardiac arrhythmias.
Tipranavir	Protease inhibitors (ie, amprenavir, lopinavir, saquinavir)	↓	Protease inhibitor concentrations may be decreased. Coadministration is not recommended.

TIPRANAVIR — ORAL

Tipranavir Drug Interactions			
Precipitant drug	Object drug[a]		Description
Tipranavir	SSRIs (ie, fluoxetine, paroxetine, sertraline)	↑	Although not studied, SSRI dose may need to be adjusted.
Tipranavir	Warfarin	↔	Although not studied, monitor the international normalized ratio frequently upon initiation of tipranavir/ritonavir.

[a] ↑ = Object drug increased. ↓ = Object drug decreased. ↔ = Undetermined clinical effect.

➤*Drug/Food interactions:* See Actions for more information.

Adverse Reactions

In 1182.12 and 1182.48 in the tipranavir/ritonavir arm, the most frequent adverse reactions were diarrhea, fatigue, headache, nausea, and vomiting. Adverse reactions leading to discontinuation were reported by 7.8% of the tipranavir-treated patients and 4.9% of the comparator arm patients.

Because of the need for coadministration of tipranavir with ritonavir 200 mg, refer to the ritonavir monograph for ritonavir-associated adverse reactions.

Tipranavir Treatment-Emergent Adverse Reactions of at Least Moderate Intensity (Grades 2 to 4) in ≥ 2% of Patients in Either Treatment Group[a]		
	Phase 3 studies 1182.12 and 1182.48 (24 weeks)	
Adverse reaction	Tipranavir/Ritonavir (500 mg/200 mg twice daily) + OBR (n = 746)	Comparator PI/Ritonavir[b] + OBR (n = 737)
CNS		
Depression	2%	3%
Headache	3.1%	3.1%
Insomnia	1.2%	2.6%
Dermatologic		
Rash	2%	2%
GI		
Abdominal pain[c]	2.8%	3.7%
Diarrhea	10.9%	9.4%
Nausea	6.7%	4.6%
Vomiting	3.4%	3%
Respiratory		
Bronchitis	2.9%	1.1%
Cough	0.8%	2.2%
Miscellaneous		
Asthenia	1.5%	2.3%
Fatigue	4%	3.9%
Pyrexia	4.6%	4.3%

[a] Excludes laboratory abnormalities that were adverse reactions.
[b] Comparator PI/ritonavir: lopinavir 400 mg/ritonavir 100 mg twice daily, indinavir 800 mg/ritonavir 100 mg twice daily, saquinavir 1,000 mg/ritonavir 100 mg twice daily, amprenavir 600 mg/ritonavir 100 mg twice daily.
[c] Abdominal pain includes preferred terms "abdominal pain" and "abdominal pain, upper."

Clinically meaningful adverse reactions in less than 2% of adult patients (n = 1,397) treated with tipranavir 500 mg/ritonavir 200 mg in phase 2 and 3 trials are listed by body system:

➤*CNS:* Dizziness, insomnia, peripheral neuropathy, sleep disorder, somnolence.

➤*Dermatologic:* Acquired lipodystrophy, exanthem, lipoatrophy, lipohypertrophy, pruritus.

➤*GI:* Abdominal distension, anorexia, dyspepsia, flatulence, gastroesophageal reflux disease, pancreatitis.

➤*Hematologic/Lymphatic:* Anemia, neutropenia, thrombocytopenia.

➤*Hepatic:* Hepatic failure, hepatitis.

➤*Lab test abnormalities:* Hepatic enzymes increased, lipase increased, liver function test abnormal.

➤*Metabolic/Nutritional:* Decreased appetite, dehydration, diabetes mellitus, facial wasting, hyperamylasemia, hypercholesterolemia, hyperglycemia.

➤*Musculoskeletal:* Muscle cramp, myalgia.

➤*Renal:* Renal insufficiency.

➤*Respiratory:* Dyspnea.

➤*Miscellaneous:* Hypersensitivity, influenza-like illness, malaise, pyrexia, reactivation of herpes simplex and varicella zoster, weight decreased.

➤*Lab test abnormalities:*

Tipranavir Treatment-Emergent Laboratory Abnormalities Reported in ≥ 2% of Adult Patients			
		Studies 1182.12 and 1182.48 (24 weeks)	
	Limit	Tipranavir/Ritonavir (500 mg/200 mg twice daily) + OBR (n = 732)	Comparator PI/Ritonavir + OBR[a] (n = 726)
Hematology			
White blood cell count decrease (grade 3 to 4)	< 2 × 10³/mcL	3.6%	5.4%
Chemistry			
Amylase (grade 3 to 4)	> 2 × ULN[b]	2.9%	4.8%
ALT			
Grade 2	> 2.5 to 5 × ULN[b]	10.7%	5.4%
Grade 3	> 5 to 10 × ULN[b]	3.1%	1.4%
Grade 4	> 10 × ULN[b]	2.7%	0.4%
AST			
Grade 2	> 2.5 to 5 × ULN[b]	6%	5.8%
Grade 3	> 5 to 10 × ULN[b]	3.3%	1%
Grade 4	> 10 × ULN[b]	0.7%	0.4%
ALT and/or AST (grade 2 to 4)	> 2.5 × ULN[b]	17.5%	9.9%
Cholesterol			
Grade 2	> 300 to 400 mg/dL	11.3%	4.3%
Grade 3	> 400 to 500 mg/dL	2.5%	0.3%
Grade 4	> 500 mg/dL	0.8%	0%
Triglycerides			
Grade 2	400 to 750 mg/dL	26.2%	14.7%
Grade 3	> 750 to 1,200 mg/dL	12.8%	5.6%
Grade 4	> 1,200 mg/dL	6.1%	3.4%

[a] Comparator PI/ritonavir: lopinavir 400 mg/ritonavir 100 mg twice daily, indinavir 800 mg/ritonavir 100 mg twice daily, saquinavir 1,000 mg/ritonavir 100 mg twice daily, amprenavir 600 mg/ritonavir 100 mg twice daily.
[b] ULN = upper limit of normal. In clinical trials extending up to 48 weeks, the proportion of patients who developed grade 2 to 4 ALT and/or AST elevations increased to 24.4% with tipranavir/ritonavir and to 12.8% with comparator PI/ritonavir.

Overdosage

➤*Treatment:* There is no known antidote for tipranavir overdose. Treatment of overdose should consist of general supportive measures, including monitoring of vital signs and observation of the patient's clinical status. If indicated, elimination of unabsorbed tipranavir should be achieved by gastric lavage. Administration of activated charcoal also may be used to aid in removal of unabsorbed drug. Because tipranavir is highly protein bound, dialysis is unlikely to be beneficial in significant removal of this medicine.

Patient Information

Inform patients that tipranavir coadministered with ritonavir 200 mg has been associated with severe liver disease, including some deaths. Instruct patients with signs or symptoms of clinical hepatitis to discontinue tipranavir/ritonavir treatment and seek medical evaluation. Symptoms of hepatitis include fatigue, malaise, anorexia, nausea, jaundice, bilirubinuria, acholic stools, liver tenderness, or hepatomegaly. Extra vigilance is needed for patients with chronic hepatitis B or C coinfection because these patients have an increased risk of hepatotoxicity.

Advise patients that liver function tests will be performed prior to initiating therapy with tipranavir and ritonavir 200 mg, and frequently throughout the duration of treatment. Patients with chronic hepatitis B or C coinfection or elevations in liver enzymes prior to treatment are at increased risk (approximately 2.5-fold) for developing further liver enzyme elevations or severe liver disease. Exercise caution when administering tipranavir/ritonavir to patients with liver enzyme abnormalities or history of chronic liver disease. Increased liver function testing is warranted in these patients. Do not give tipranavir to patients with moderate to severe liver disease.

Mild to moderate rash has been reported in HIV-infected men and women receiving tipranavir/ritonavir.

Instruct women receiving estrogen-based hormonal contraceptives to use additional or alternative contraceptive measures during therapy with

TIPRANAVIR — ORAL

tipranavir/ritonavir. There may be an increased risk of rash when tipranavir is given with hormonal contraceptives.

Inform patients that redistribution or accumulation of body fat may occur in patients receiving antiretroviral therapy and that the cause and long-term health effects of these conditions are not known at this time.

Inform patients that tipranavir must be coadministered with ritonavir 200 mg to ensure its therapeutic effect. Failure to correctly coadminister tipranavir with ritonavir will result in reduced plasma levels of tipranavir that may be insufficient to achieve the desired antiviral effect.

Tell patients that sustained decreases in plasma HIV-1 RNA have been associated with a reduced risk of progression to AIDS and death. Instruct patients to remain under the care of a health care provider while using tipranavir. Advise patients to take tipranavir and other concomitant antiretroviral therapy every day as prescribed. Tipranavir, coadministered with ritonavir, must be given in combination with other antiretroviral drugs. Instruct patients not to alter the dose or discontinue therapy without consulting their health care provider. If a dose of tipranavir is missed, instruct patients to take the dose as soon as possible and then return to their normal schedule. However, if a dose is skipped, the patient should not double the next dose.

Inform patients that tipranavir is not a cure for HIV-1 infection and that they may continue to develop opportunistic infections and other complications associated with HIV disease. The long-term effects of tipranavir are unknown at this time. Tell patients that there are currently no data demonstrating that therapy with tipranavir can reduce the risk of transmitting HIV to others through sexual contact.

Tipranavir may interact with some drugs; therefore, advise patients to report to their health care provider the use of any other prescription or nonprescription medications or herbal products, particularly St. John's wort.

Instruct patients to take tipranavir with food to enhance absorption.

DARUNAVIR ETHANOLATE

Rx	**Prezista** (Ortho Biotech)	**Tablets:** 300 mg (as base)	(300 TMC114). Orange, oval. Film coated. In 120s.

DARUNAVIR ETHANOLATE — ORAL

Indications

➤*HIV:* Darunavir, coadministered with 100 mg ritonavir and with other antiretroviral agents, is indicated for the treatment of human immunodeficiency virus (HIV) infection in antiretroviral treatment-experienced adult patients, such as those with HIV-1 strains resistant to more than 1 protease inhibitor.

Administration and Dosage

➤*Approved by the FDA:* June 23, 2006.

➤*Adults:* 600 mg (two 300 mg tablets) twice daily taken with ritonavir 100 mg twice daily and with food. The type of food does not affect exposure to darunavir.

➤*Hepatic function impairment:* There are no data regarding the use of darunavir/ritonavir when coadministered to patients with varying degrees of hepatic function impairment; therefore, specific dosage recommendations cannot be made. Darunavir/Ritonavir should be used with caution in patients with hepatic function impairment.

➤*Storage/Stability:* Store at 25°C (77°F); excursions permitted to 15° to 30°C (59° to 86°F).

NELFINAVIR MESYLATE

Rx	**Viracept** (Agouron)	**Tablets:** 250 mg (as base)	(Viracept 250 mg). Lt. blue, capsule shape. In 270s and 300s.
		625 mg (as base)	(V 625). White, oval. In 120s.
		Powder: 50 mg/g (as base)	Aspartame,[1] sucrose. In multiple-dose bottles containing 144 g powder with 1 g scoop.

[1] 11.2 mg/g phenylalanine

NELFINAVIR MESYLATE — ORAL

Indications

➤*HIV infection:* In combination with other antiretroviral agents, for the treatment of HIV infection.

➤*Unlabeled uses:* Used as part of a 3-drug regimen for occupational HIV postexposure prophylaxis in cases where there is an increased risk for transmission; for HIV infection in neonates; twice daily dosing for HIV infection in children older than 6 years of age.

Administration and Dosage

➤*Approved by the FDA:* March 14, 1997.

➤*Adults:* 1,250 mg (five 250 mg tablets or two 625 mg tablets) twice daily or 750 mg (three 250 mg tablets) 3 times daily. Take with a meal. Patients unable to swallow the 250 or 625 mg tablets may dissolve the tablets in a small amount of water. Once dissolved, mix the cloudy liquid well, and consume it immediately. Rinse the glass with water and swallow the rinse to ensure the entire dose is consumed.

➤*Children (2 to 13 years):* 45 to 55 mg/kg twice daily or 25 to 35 mg/kg 3 times daily. Take all doses with a meal. Doses higher than the adult maximum dose of 2,500 mg per day have not been studied in children. For children unable to take tablets, nelfinavir mesylate oral powder may be administered.

Assess appropriate formulation and dosage for each patient. Crushed 250 mg tablets can be used in lieu of powder.

Dosing Table for Children ≥ 2 Years of Age (Tablets)

Body weight		Twice daily 45 to 55 mg/kg ≥ 2 years	3 times daily 25 to 35 mg/kg ≥ 2 years
Kg	Lbs	No. of tablets (250 mg)	No. of tablets (250 mg)
10 to 12	22 to 26.4	2	1
13 to 18	28.6 to 39.6	3	2
19 to 20	41.8 to 44	4	2
≥ 21	≥ 46.2	4 to 5[a]	3[b]

[a] For twice-daily dosing, the maximum dose per day is 5 tablets twice daily.
[b] For 3-times-a-day dosing, the maximum dose per day is 3 tablets 3 times a day.

Dosing Table for Children ≥ 2 Years of Age (Powder)

Body weight		Twice daily 45 to 55 mg/kg		3 times daily 25 to 35 mg/kg	
kg	lbs	Scoops of powder (50 mg/g)	Teaspoons[a] of powder	Scoops of powder (50 mg/g)	Teaspoons[a] of powder
9 to < 10.5	20 to < 23	10	2 ½	6	1 ½
10.5 to < 12	23 to < 26.5	11	2 ¾	7	1 ¾
12 to < 14	26.5 to < 31	13	3 ¼	8	2
14 to < 16	31 to < 35	15	3 ¾	9	2 ¼
16 to < 18	35 to < 39.5	Not recommended[b]	Not recommended[b]	10	2 ½
18 to < 23	39.5 to < 50.5	Not recommended[b]	Not recommended[b]	12	3
≥ 23	≥ 50.5	Not recommended[b]	Not recommended[b]	15	3 ¾

[a] If a teaspoon is used to measure nelfinavir oral powder, 1 level teaspoon contains 200 mg of nelfinavir (4 level scoops equals 1 level teaspoon).
[b] Use nelfinavir 250 mg tablet.

Oral powder – The oral powder may be mixed with a small amount of water, milk, formula, soy formula, soy milk, or dietary supplements; once mixed, consume the entire contents in order to obtain the full dose. If the mixture is not consumed immediately, store it under refrigeration, but storage must not exceed 6 hours. Acidic food or juice (eg, orange juice, apple juice, or applesauce) are not recommended to be used in combination with nelfinavir mesylate, because the combination may result in a bitter taste. Do not reconstitute oral powder with water in its original container.

➤*Storage/Stability:* Keep container tightly closed. Dispense in original container. Store at 15° to 30°C (59° to 86°F).

NELFINAVIR MESYLATE — ORAL

Actions

➤*Pharmacology:* Nelfinavir is an inhibitor of the HIV-1 protease. Inhibition of the viral protease prevents cleavage of the gag and gag-pol polyprotein resulting in the production of immature, noninfectious virus.

➤*Pharmacokinetics:*

Absorption – The pharmacokinetic properties of nelfinavir were evaluated in healthy volunteers and HIV-infected patients; no substantial differences were observed between the 2 groups.

Summary of a Pharmacokinetic Study in HIV-Positive Patients with Multiple Dosing of 1,250 mg Twice a Day for 28 Days and 750 mg 3 Times a Day for 28 Days

Regimen	AUC_{24} mg•hr/L	C_{max} mg/L	C_{trough} morning mg/L	C_{trough} afternoon or evening mg/L
1,250 mg twice a day	52.8 ± 15.7	4 ± 0.8	2.2 ± 1.3	0.7 ± 0.4
750 mg 3 times a day	43.6 ± 17.8	3 ± 1.6	1.4 ± 0.6	1 ± 0.5

Data are mean ± SD.

The difference between morning and afternoon or evening trough concentrations for the 3-times-a-day and 2-times-a-day regimens was also observed in healthy volunteers who were dosed at precisely 8- or 12-hour intervals.

In healthy volunteers receiving a single 1,250 mg dose, the 625 mg tablet was not bioequivalent to the 250 mg tablet formulation. Under fasted conditions (n = 27), the AUC and C_{max} were 34% and 24% higher, respectively, for the 625 mg tablets. In a relative bioavailability assessment under fed conditions (n = 28), the AUC was 24% higher for the 625 mg tablet; the C_{max} was comparable for both formulations.

Food increases nelfinavir exposure and decreases nelfinavir pharmacokinetic variability relative to the fasted state. In one study, healthy volunteers received a single dose of 1,250 mg of nelfinavir 250 mg tablets (5 tablets) under fasted or fed conditions (3 different meals). In a second study, healthy volunteers received single doses of 1,250 mg nelfinavir (5 × 250 mg tablets) under fasted or fed conditions (2 different fat content meals).

Increase in AUC, C_{max} and t_{max} for Nelfinavir in Fed State Relative to Fasted State Following 1,250 mg Nelfinavir (5 × 250 mg Tablets)

Number of Kcal	% fat	Number of subjects	AUC fold increase	C_{max} fold increase	Increase in t_{max} (hr)
125	20	n = 21	2.2	2	1
500	20	n = 22	3.1	2.3	2
1,000	50	n = 23	5.2	3.3	2

Increase in Nelfinavir AUC, C_{max} and t_{max} in Fed Low-Fat (20%) vs High-Fat (50%) State Relative to Fasted State Following 1,250 mg Nelfinavir (5 × 250 mg Tablets)

Number of Kcal	% fat	Number of subjects	AUC fold increase	C_{max} fold increase	Increase in t_{max} (hr)
500	20	n = 22	3.1	2.5	1.8
500	50	n = 22	5.1	3.8	2.1

Nelfinavir exposure can be increased by increasing the calorie or fat content in meals taken with nelfinavir.

Distribution – The apparent volume of distribution following oral administration of nelfinavir was 2 to 7 L/kg. Nelfinavir in serum is extensively protein bound (greater than 98%).

Metabolism – Unchanged nelfinavir comprised 82% to 86% of the total plasma radioactivity after a single oral 750 mg dose of ^{14}C-nelfinavir. In vitro, multiple cytochrome P450 enzymes including CYP3A and CYP2C19 are responsible for metabolism of nelfinavir. One major and several minor oxidative metabolites were found in plasma. The major oxidative metabolite has in vitro antiviral activity comparable to the parent drug.

Excretion – The terminal half-life in plasma was typically 3.5 to 5 hours. The majority (87%) of an oral 750 mg dose containing ^{14}C-nelfinavir was recovered in the feces; fecal radioactivity consisted of numerous oxidative metabolites (78%) and unchanged nelfinavir (22%). Only 1% to 2% of the dose was recovered in urine, of which unchanged nelfinavir was the major component.

Special populations –

Children: The pharmacokinetics of nelfinavir have been investigated in 5 studies in pediatric patients from birth to 13 years of age either receiving nelfinavir 3 times or twice daily.

Summary of Steady-State AUC_{24} of Nelfinavir in Pediatric Studies

Protocol no.	Dosing regimen[a]	N[b]	Age	AUC_{24} (mg•hr/L) arithmetic mean ± SD
AG1343-524	20 (19 to 28) mg/kg 3 times daily	14	2 to 13 years	56.1 ± 29.8
PACTG 725	55 (48 to 60) mg/kg twice daily	6	3 to 11 years	101.8 ± 56.1
PENTA 7	40 (34 to 43) mg/kg 3 times daily	4	2 to 9 months	33.8 ± 8.9
PENTA 7	75 (55 to 83) mg/kg twice daily	12	2 to 9 months	37.2 ± 19.2
PACTG 353	40 (14 to 56) mg/kg twice daily	10	6 weeks	44.1 ± 27.4
			1 week	45.8 ± 32.1

[a] Protocol specified dose (actual dose range).
[b] N: Number of subjects with evaluable pharmacokinetic results C_{trough} values are not presented in the table because they are not available for all studies.

Overall, use of nelfinavir in the pediatric population is associated with highly variable drug exposure. The high variability may be due to inconsistent food intake in pediatric patients.

➤*Microbiology:*

Antiviral activity in vitro – The antiviral activity of nelfinavir in vitro has been demonstrated in both acute or chronic HIV infections in lymphoblastoid cell lines, peripheral blood lymphocytes, and monocytes/macrophages. Nelfinavir was found to be active against several laboratory strains of HIV-1 and several clinical isolates of HIV-1 and the HIV-2 strain ROD. The EC_{95} (95% effective concentration) of nelfinavir ranged from 7 to 196 nM. Drug combination studies with protease inhibitors showed nelfinavir had antagonistic interactions with indinavir, additive interactions with ritonavir or saquinavir, and synergistic interactions with amprenavir and lopinavir. Minimal to no cellular cytotoxicity was observed with any of these protease inhibitors alone or in combination with nelfinavir. In combination with reverse transcriptase inhibitors, nelfinavir demonstrated additive (didanosine or stavudine) to synergistic (abacavir, delavirdine, efavirenz, lamivudine, nevirapine, tenofovir, zalcitabine, or zidovudine) antiviral activity in vitro without enhanced cytotoxicity.

Drug resistance – HIV-1 isolates with reduced susceptibility to nelfinavir have been selected in vitro. HIV isolates from selected patients treated with nelfinavir alone or in combination with reverse transcriptase inhibitors were monitored for phenotypic (n = 19) and genotypic (n = 195, 157 of which were evaluable) changes in clinical trials over a period of 2 to 82 weeks. One or more virus protease mutations at amino acid positions 30, 35, 36, 46, 71, 77, and 88 were detected in the HIV-1 of greater than 10% of patients with evaluable isolates. The overall incidence of the D30N mutation in the virus protease of evaluable patients (n = 157) receiving nelfinavir monotherapy or nelfinavir in combination with zidovudine and lamivudine or stavudine was 54.8%. The overall incidence of other mutations associated with primary protease inhibitor resistance was 9.6% for the L90M substitution whereas substitutions at 48, 82, or 84 were not observed. Of 19 clinical isolates for which both phenotypic and genotypic analyses were performed on clinical isolates, 9 showed reduced susceptibility (5- to 93-fold) to nelfinavir in vitro. All 9 patients possessed 1 or more mutations in the virus protease gene. Amino acid position 30 appeared to be the most frequent mutation site.

Cross-resistance –

Nonclinical studies: Patient-derived recombinant HIV isolates containing the D30N mutation (n = 4) and demonstrating high-level (greater than 10-fold) NFV-resistance remained susceptible (less than 2.5-fold resistance) to amprenavir, indinavir, lopinavir, and saquinavir, in vitro. Patient-derived recombinant HIV isolates containing the L90M mutation (n = 8) demonstrated moderate-to high-level resistance to NFV and had varying levels of susceptibility to amprenavir, indinavir, lopinavir, and saquinavir, in vitro. Most patient-derived recombinant isolates with phenotypic and genotypic evidence of reduced susceptibility (greater than 2.5-fold) to amprenavir, indinavir, lopinavir, or saquinavir demonstrated high-level cross-resistance to nelfinavir, in vitro. Mutations associated with resistance to other PIs (eg, G48V, V82A/F/T, I84V, L90M) appeared to confer high-level cross-resistance to NFV Following ritonavir therapy, 6 of 7 clinical isolates with decreased ritonavir susceptibility (8- to 113-fold) in vitro compared to baseline also exhibited decreased susceptibility to nelfinavir in vitro (5- to 40-fold). Cross-resistance between nelfinavir and reverse transcriptase inhibitors is unlikely because different enzyme targets are involved. Clinical isolates (n = 5) with decreased susceptibility to zidovudine, lamivudine, or nevirapine remain fully susceptible to nelfinavir in vitro.

Contraindications

Hypersensitivity to any of its components.

Coadministration of nelfinavir is contraindicated with drugs that are highly dependent on CYP3A for clearance and for which elevated plasma concentrations are associated with serious or life-threatening events.

Drugs That are Contraindicated with Nelfinavir

Drug class	Drugs within class that are contraindicated with nelfinavir
Antiarrhythmics	Amiodarone, quinidine
Ergot derivatives	Dihydroergotamine, ergonovine, ergotamine, methylergonovine
Neuroleptic	Pimozide
Sedative/hypnotics	Midazolam, triazolam

NELFINAVIR MESYLATE — ORAL

Warnings

➤*Phenylketonurics:* Nelfinavir mesylate oral powder contains 11.2 mg phenylalanine per g of powder.

➤*Diabetes mellitus / hyperglycemia:* New onset diabetes mellitus, exacerbation of preexisting diabetes mellitus, and hyperglycemia have been reported during postmarketing surveillance in HIV-infected patients receiving protease inhibitor therapy. Some patients required either initiation or dose adjustments of insulin or oral hypoglycemic agents for treatment of these events. In some cases, diabetic ketoacidosis has occurred. In those patients who discontinued protease inhibitor therapy, hyperglycemia persisted in some cases. Because these events have been reported voluntarily during clinical practice, estimates of frequency cannot be made and a causal relationship between protease inhibitor therapy and these events has not been established.

➤*Hepatic function impairment:* Nelfinavir is principally metabolized by the liver. Therefore, exercise caution when administering this drug to patients with hepatic impairment.

➤*Carcinogenesis:* Carcinogenicity studies in mice and rats were conducted with nelfinavir at oral doses up to 1,000 mg/kg/day. No evidence of a tumorigenic effect was noted in mice at systemic exposures (C_{max}) up to 9-fold those measured in humans at the recommended therapeutic dose (750 mg 3 times daily or 1,250 mg twice daily). In rats, thyroid follicular cell adenomas and carcinomas were increased in males at 300 mg/kg/day and higher and in females at 1,000 mg/kg/day. Systemic exposures (C_{max}) at 300 and 1,000 mg/kg/day were 1- to 3-fold, respectively, those measured in humans at the recommended therapeutic dose. Repeated administration of nelfinavir to rats produced effects consistent with hepatic microsomal enzyme induction and increased thyroid hormone disposition; these effects predispose rats, but not humans, to thyroid follicular cell neoplasms.

➤*Pregnancy: Category B.* There are no adequate and well-controlled studies in pregnant women. Because animal reproduction studies are not always predictive of human response, use nelfinavir mesylate during pregnancy only if clearly needed.

Antiretroviral pregnancy registry (APR) – To monitor maternal-fetal outcomes of pregnant women exposed to nelfinavir mesylate and other antiretroviral agents, an Antiretroviral Pregnancy Registry has been established. Register patients by calling (800) 258-4263.

➤*Lactation:* The Centers for Disease Control and Prevention advises HIV-infected women not to breastfeed to avoid postnatal transmission of HIV to a child who may not yet be infected. Studies in lactating rats have demonstrated that nelfinavir is excreted in milk. Because of both the potential for HIV transmission and the potential for serious adverse reactions in nursing infants, instruct mothers not to breastfeed if they are receiving nelfinavir.

➤*Children:* The safety and effectiveness of nelfinavir have been established in patients from 2 to 13 years of age. The use of nelfinavir in these age groups is supported by evidence from adequate and well-controlled studies of nelfinavir in adults and pharmacokinetic studies and studies supporting activity in pediatric patients. In patients less than 2 years of age, nelfinavir was found to be safe at the doses studied but a reliably effective dose could not be established.

Precautions

➤*Resistance / cross-resistance:* HIV cross-resistance between protease inhibitors has been observed.

➤*Hemophilia:* There have been reports of increased bleeding, including spontaneous skin hematomas and hemarthrosis, in patients with hemophilia type A and B treated with protease inhibitors. In some patients, additional Factor VIII was given. In more than half of the reported cases, treatment with protease inhibitors was continued or reintroduced. A causal relationship has not been established.

➤*Redistribution / accumulation of body fat:* Redistribution/accumulation of body fat including central obesity, dorsocervical fat enlargement (buffalo hump), peripheral wasting, breast enlargement, and "cushingoid appearance" have been observed in patients receiving antiretroviral therapy. The mechanism and long-term consequences of these events are currently unknown. A causal relationship has not been established.

Drug Interactions

CYP3A and CYP2C19 appear to be the predominant enzymes that metabolize nelfinavir in humans. The potential ability of nelfinavir to inhibit the major human cytochrome P450 isoforms (CYP3A, CYP2C19, CYP2D6, CYP2C9, CYP1A2 and CYP2E1) has been investigated in vitro. Only CYP3A was inhibited at concentrations in the therapeutic range.

Nelfinavir Drug Interactions

Precipitant drug	Object drug*		Description
Anticonvulsants (ie, carbamazepine, phenobarbital)	Nelfinavir	↓	Concurrent use may decrease nelfinavir plasma concentrations.
Azithromycin	Nelfinavir	↓	Coadministration resulted in a decrease in the AUC and C_{max} of nelfinavir by 15% and 10%, respectively.
Nelfinavir	Azithromycin	↑	Coadministration resulted in an increase in the AUC of 112% and C_{max} of 136% of azithromycin. Dose adjustment is not recommended; closely monitor for liver enzyme abnormalities and hearing impairment.
Azole antifungals	Nelfinavir	↑	May inhibit the metabolism of protease inhibitors. Ketoconazole increased nelfinavir AUC and C_{max} by 35% and 25%, respectively. Monitor for protease inhibitor toxicity and adjust dose as needed.
Efavirenz Delavirdine	Nelfinavir	↑	Coadministration resulted in an increase in the AUC and C_{max} of nelfinavir, 107% and 88% with delavirdine, and 20% and 21% with efavirenz, respectively.
Nelfinavir	Efavirenz Delavirdine	↓	Coadministration caused a decrease in the AUC and C_{max} of efavirenz of 12% and 12%, respectively, and delavirdine of 31% and 27%, respectively.
Indinavir	Nelfinavir	↑	Coadministration resulted in an 83% increase in nelfinavir AUC and a 51% increase in indinavir AUC.
Nelfinavir	Indinavir		
Interleukins	Nelfinavir	↑	May inhibit protease inhibitor metabolism. May be necessary to adjust protease inhibitor dose.
Nevirapine	Nelfinavir	↓	Increased hepatic metabolism of the protease inhibitor is suspected. Monitor protease inhibitor blood levels and adjust dose as necessary.
Rifabutin	Nelfinavir	↓	Coadministration resulted in a 32% decrease in nelfinavir AUC and a 207% increase in rifabutin AUC. It is recommended that the dose of rifabutin be reduced to one half the usual dose when administered with nelfinavir.
Nelfinavir	Rifabutin	↑	
Rifampin	Nelfinavir	↓	Coadministration resulted in an 83% decrease in nelfinavir AUC. Do not coadminister nelfinavir with rifampin.
Ritonavir	Nelfinavir	↑	Coadministration resulted in a 152% increase in nelfinavir AUC and very little change in ritonavir AUC.
Saquinavir	Nelfinavir	↑	Coadministration resulted in an 18% increase in nelfinavir AUC and a 392% increase in saquinavir AUC. If used in combination, no dose adjustments are needed.
Nelfinavir	Saquinavir		
St. John's wort	Nelfinavir	↓	Increased metabolism of the protease inhibitor is suspected and may lead to loss of virologic response and possible resistance to nelfinavir. Avoid coadministration.
Nelfinavir	Didanosine	↔	It is recommended that didanosine be administered on an empty stomach; administer nelfinavir (with food) 1 hour after or > 2 hours before didanosine.
Nelfinavir	HMG-CoA reductase inhibitors (atorvastatin, lovastatin, simvastatin)	↑	Coadministration resulted in an increase in the C_{max} and AUC of simvastatin (517% and 505%) and atorvastatin (122% and 74%). Concomitant administration with nelfinavir is contraindicated due to potential for serious reactions such as risk of myopathy including rhabdomyolysis.

NELFINAVIR MESYLATE — ORAL

Nelfinavir Drug Interactions

Precipitant drug	Object drug*		Description
Nelfinavir	Lamivudine	↑	Coadministration resulted in an increase in lamivudine's AUC and C_{max} by 10% and 31%, respectively.
Nelfinavir	Oral contraceptives	↓	Coadministration resulted in a 47% decrease in ethinyl estradiol and an 18% decrease in norethindrone plasma levels. Use alternate or additional contraceptive measures during nelfinavir therapy.
Nelfinavir	Phenytoin	↓	Coadministration resulted in a decrease in the AUC and C_{max} of phenytoin, 29% and 21%, respectively. Monitor phenytoin plasma levels and adjust dose as necessary.
Nelfinavir	Pimozide	↑	Coadministration is contraindicated due to potential for serious or life-threatening reactions such as cardiac arrhythmias.
Nelfinavir	Zidovudine	↓	Coadministration of zidovudine with nelfinavir resulted in a 35% decrease in zidovudine AUC.
Nelfinavir	Antiarrhythmics (amiodarone, quinidine)	↑	Protease inhibitors may inhibit the metabolism via cytochrome P450 3A4 isoenzyme. Coadministration with nelfinavir is contraindicated.
Nelfinavir	Benzodiazepines	↑	Possibly severe sedation and respiratory depression caused by the inhibition of the metabolism of benzodiazepines that undergo oxidation. Midazolam and triazolam are contraindicated in patients receiving nelfinavir.
Nelfinavir	Cisapride	↑	Protease inhibitors may inhibit the metabolism of cisapride via cytochrome P450 3A4 isoenzyme.
Nelfinavir	Ergot alkaloids	↑	Protease inhibitors may inhibit the metabolism of ergot alkaloids via cytochrome P450 3A4 isoenzyme. Coadministration with nelfinavir is contraindicated due to potential for serious or life-threatening reactions, such as acute ergot toxicity characterized by peripheral vasospasm and ischemia of the extremities and other tissues.
Nelfinavir	Fentanyl	↑	Possible inhibition of metabolism of fentanyl. Closely monitor respiratory function if coadministered. A reduction in the fentanyl dose may be necessary.
Nelfinavir	Methadone	↓	Increased metabolism of methadone is suspected. Coadministration resulted in a decrease of the AUC and C_{max} of methadone, 47% and 46%, respectively. Monitor for withdrawal symptoms and adjust dose as necessary.
Nelfinavir	Sildenafil	↑	Inhibition of sildenafil metabolism. Coadminister with extreme caution; sildenafil should not exceed a maximum single dose of 25 mg/48 hours when used concomitantly.
Nelfinavir	Tacrolimus Sirolimus	↑	Plasma concentrations of the immunosuppressants may be increased with concomitant administration. Carefully monitor renal function and immunosuppressant concentrations when starting, stopping, or changing the dose of a protease inhibitor and adjust the dose of the immunosuppressant as necessary.

Nelfinavir is an inhibitor of CYP3A enzyme. Coadministration of nelfinavir mesylate and drugs primarily metabolized by CYP3A (eg, dihydropyridine calcium channel blockers, HMG-CoA reductase inhibitors, immunosuppressants, sildenafil) may result in increased plasma concentrations of the other drug that could increase or prolong both its therapeutic and adverse effects. Exercise caution when inhibitors of CYP3A, including nelfinavir, are coadministered with drugs that are metabolized by CYP3A and that prolong the QT interval. Nelfinavir is metabolized by CYP3A and CYP2C19. Coadministration of nelfinavir mesylate and drugs that induce CYP3A or CYP2C19, such as rifampin, may decrease nelfinavir plasma concentrations and reduce its therapeutic effect. Coadministration of nelfinavir mesylate and drugs that inhibit CYP3A or CYP2C19 may increase nelfinavir plasma concentrations.

Adverse Reactions

The safety of nelfinavir mesylate was studied in over 5,000 patients who received drug either alone or in combination with nucleoside analogues. The majority of adverse events were of mild intensity. The most frequently reported adverse event among patients receiving nelfinavir mesylate was diarrhea, which was generally of mild to moderate intensity. The frequency of nelfinavir-associated diarrhea may be increased in patients receiving the 625 mg tablet because of the increased bioavailability of this formulation.

Percentage of Patients with Treatment-Emergent[a] Adverse Reactions of Moderate or Severe Intensity Reported in ≥ 2% of Patients

	Study 511; 24 weeks			Study 542; 48 weeks	
Adverse events	Placebo + zidovudine/ lamivudine (n = 101)	500 mg 3 times daily nelfinavir mesylate + zidovudine/ lamivudine (n = 97)	750 mg 3 times daily nelfinavir mesylate + zidovudine/ lamivudine (n = 100)	1,250 mg twice daily nelfinavir mesylate + stavudine/ lamivudine (n = 344)	750 mg 3 times daily nelfinavir mesylate + stavudine/ lamivudine (n = 210)
Dermatologic					
Rash	1%	1%	3%	2%	1%
GI system					
Diarrhea	3%	14%	20%	20%	15%
Flatulence	0%	5%	2%	1%	1%
Nausea	4%	3%	7%	3%	3%

[a] Includes those adverse events at least possibly related to study drug or of unknown relationship and excludes concurrent HIV conditions.

Adverse events occurring in less than 2% of patients receiving nelfinavir mesylate in all phase 2/3 clinical trials and considered at least possibly related or of unknown relationship to treatment and of at least moderate severity are listed below.

➤*CNS:* Anxiety, depression, dizziness, emotional lability, hyperkinesia, insomnia, migraine, paresthesia, seizures, sleep disorder, somnolence, and suicidal ideation.

➤*Dermatologic:* Dermatitis, folliculitis, fungal dermatitis, maculopapular rash, pruritus, sweating, and urticaria.

➤*GI:* Anorexia, dyspepsia, epigastric pain, GI bleeding, hepatitis, mouth ulceration, pancreatitis, vomiting, and abdominal pain.

➤*GU:* Kidney calculus, sexual dysfunction, and urine abnormality.

➤*Hematologic/Lymphatic:* Anemia, leukopenia, and thrombocytopenia.

➤*Metabolic/Nutritional:* Increases in alkaline phosphate, amylase, creatine phosphokinase, lactic dehydrogenase, ALT, AST and gamma glutamyl transpeptidase; hyperlipemia, hyperuricemia, hyperglycemia, hypoglycemia, dehydration, and abnormal liver function tests.

➤*Musculoskeletal:* Arthralgia, arthritis, cramps, myalgia, myasthenia, and myopathy.

➤*Respiratory:* Dyspnea, pharyngitis, rhinitis, and sinusitis.

➤*Special senses:* Acute iritis and eye disorder.

➤*Miscellaneous:* Accidental injury, allergic reaction, back pain, fever, headache, malaise, pain and redistribution/accumulation of body fat including central obesity, dorsocervical fat enlargement (buffalo hump), peripheral wasting, breast enlargement, and "cushingoid appearance".

➤*Postmarketing:* The following additional adverse experiences have been reported from postmarketing surveillance as at least possibly related or of unknown relationship to nelfinavir mesylate:

Cardiovascular – QTc prolongation, torsades de pointes.

GI – Jaundice.

Metabolic/Nutritional – Bilirubinemia, metabolic acidosis.

Miscellaneous – Hypersensitivity reactions (including bronchospasm, moderate to severe rash, fever, and edema).

➤*Lab test abnormalities:* The percentage of patients with marked laboratory abnormalities in studies 542 and 511 are presented below. Marked laboratory abnormalities are defined as a Grade 3 or 4 abnormality in a patient with a normal baseline value or a Grade 4 abnormality in a patient with a Grade 1 abnormality at baseline.

NELFINAVIR MESYLATE — ORAL

Percentage of Patients by Treatment Group with Marked Laboratory Abnormalities in> 2% of Patients					
		Study 511		Study 542	
	Placebo + zidovudine/ lamivudine (n = 101)	500 mg 3 times daily nelfinavir mesylate + zidovudine/ lamivudine (n = 97)	750 mg 3 times daily nelfinavir mesylate + zidovudine/ lamivudine (n = 100)	1,250 mg twice daily nelfinavir mesylate + stavudine/ lamivudine (n = 344)	750 mg 3 times daily nelfinavir mesylate + stavudine/ lamivudine (n = 210)
Chemistry					
ALT	6%	1%	1%	2%	1%
AST	4%	1%	0%	2%	1%
Creatine kinase	7%	2%	2%	N/A	N/A
Hematology					
Hemoglobin	6%	3%	2%	0%	0%
Lymphocytes	1%	6%	1%	1%	0%
Neutrophils	4%	3%	5%	2%	1%

[a] Marked laboratory abnormalities are defined as a shift from Grade 0 at baseline to at least Grade 3 or from Grade 1 to Grade 4.

Children – The most commonly reported drug-related, treatment-emergent adverse events reported in the pediatric studies included diarrhea, leukopenia/neutropenia, rash, anorexia, and abdominal pain. Diarrhea, regardless of assigned relationship to study drug, was reported in 39% to 47% of pediatric patients receiving nelfinavir in 2 of the larger treatment trials. Leukopenia/neutropenia was the laboratory abnormality most commonly reported as a significant event across the pediatric studies.

Overdosage

➤*Treatment:* Human experience of acute overdose with nelfinavir mesylate is limited. There is no specific antidote for overdose with nelfinavir mesylate. If indicated, achieve elimination of unabsorbed drug by emesis or gastric lavage. Administration of activated charcoal may also be used to aid removal of unabsorbed drug. Since nelfinavir is highly protein bound, dialysis is unlikely to significantly remove drug from blood.

Patient Information

For optimal absorption, advise patients to take nelfinavir mesylate with food. Maximum plasma concentrations and area under the plasma concentration-time curve (AUC) were 2 – to 3-fold higher under fed conditions compared to fasting. The effect of food on nelfinavir absorption was evaluated in 2 studies (n = 14, total). The meals evaluated contained 517 to 759 Kcal, with 153 to 313 Kcal derived from fat.

Inform patients that nelfinavir mesylate is not a cure for HIV infection and that they may continue to acquire illnesses associated with advanced HIV infection, including opportunistic infections.

Tell patients that there is currently no data demonstrating that nelfinavir mesylate therapy can reduce the risk of transmitting HIV to others through sexual contact or blood contamination.

Tell patients that sustained decreases in plasma HIV RNA have been associated with a reduced risk of progression to AIDS and death. Advise patients to take nelfinavir mesylate and other concomitant antiretroviral therapy every day as prescribed. Patients should not alter the dose or discontinue therapy without consulting with their doctor. If a dose of nelfinavir mesylate is missed, patients should take the dose as soon as possible and then return to their normal schedule. However, if a dose is skipped, the patient should not double the next dose.

Inform patients that nelfinavir tablets are film-coated and that this film-coating is intended to make the tablets easier to swallow.

The most frequent adverse event associated with nelfinavir mesylate is diarrhea, which can usually be controlled with nonprescription drugs, such as loperamide, which slow GI motility.

Inform patients that redistribution or accumulation of body fat may occur in patients receiving antiretroviral therapy including protease inhibitors and that the cause and long-term health effects of these conditions are not known at this time.

Nelfinavir may interact with some drugs; therefore, advise patients to report to their doctor the use of any other prescription, nonprescription medication, or herbal products, particularly St. John's wort.

Instruct patients receiving oral contraceptives to use alternate or additional contraceptive measures during therapy with nelfinavir mesylate.

Advise patients receiving sildenafil and nelfinavir that they may be at an increased risk of sildenafil-associated adverse events including hypotension, visual changes, and prolonged penile erection, and should promptly report any symptoms to their doctor.

FOSAMPRENAVIR CALCIUM

Rx	**Lexiva** (GlaxoSmithKline)	**Tablets:** 700 mg (equivalent to 600 mg amprenavir)	(GX LL7). Pink, capsule shape. Film-coated. In 60s.

FOSAMPRENAVIR CALCIUM — ORAL

Indications

➤*HIV infection:* In combination with other antiretroviral agents for the treatment of human immunodeficiency virus (HIV) infection in adults.

Administration and Dosage

➤*Approved by the FDA:* October 21, 2003.

Fosamprenavir may be taken with or without food. Consult the full monograph for ritonavir when using this agent in combination with fosamprenavir.

➤*Therapy-naive patients:* The recommended oral dose of fosamprenavir alone or in combination with ritonavir is as follows: Fosamprenavir 1400 mg twice daily (without ritonavir); fosamprenavir 1400 mg once daily plus ritonavir 200 mg once daily; fosamprenavir 700 mg twice daily plus ritonavir 100 mg twice daily.

➤*Protease inhibitor (PI)-experienced patients:* The recommended oral dose is fosamprenavir 700 mg twice daily plus ritonavir 100 mg twice daily. Once-daily administration of fosamprenavir plus ritonavir is not recommended in PI-experienced patients.

➤*Adjustment of ritonavir dose when fosamprenavir plus ritonavir are administered with efavirenz:* An additional 100 mg/day (300 mg total) of ritonavir is recommended when efavirenz is administered with fosamprenavir plus ritonavir once daily.

➤*Hepatic function impairment:* Use fosamprenavir with caution, at a reduced dosage of 700 mg twice daily, in patients with mild or moderate hepatic impairment (Child-Pugh score ranging from 5 to 8) receiving fosamprenavir without concurrent ritonavir. Do not use fosamprenavir in patients with severe hepatic impairment (Child-Pugh score ranging from 9 to 12) because the dose cannot be reduced below 700 mg. There are no data on the use of fosamprenavir in combination with ritonavir in patients with any degree of hepatic impairment.

➤*Storage/Stability:* Store at controlled room temperature of 25°C (77°F); excursions permitted to 15° to 30°C (59° to 86°F). Keep container tightly closed.

Actions

➤*Pharmacology:* Fosamprenavir is a prodrug of amprenavir, an inhibitor of HIV protease. Fosamprenavir is rapidly converted to amprenavir by cellular phosphatases in vivo. Amprenavir is an inhibitor of HIV-1 protease. Amprenavir binds to the active site of HIV-1 protease and thereby prevents the processing of viral Gag and Gag-Pol polyprotein precursors, resulting in the formation of immature noninfectious viral particles.

➤*Pharmacokinetics:*

Absorption – Fosamprenavir is a prodrug that is rapidly hydrolyzed to amprenavir by enzymes in the gut epithelium as it is absorbed. After administration of a single dose of fosamprenavir to HIV-1-infected patients, the time to peak amprenavir concentration (T_{max}) occurred between 1.5 and 4 hours (median 2.5 hours). The absolute oral bioavailability of amprenavir after administration of fosamprenavir in humans has not been established.

Administration of a single 1400 mg dose of fosamprenavir in the fed state compared with the fasted state was associated with no significant changes in amprenavir C_{max}, T_{max}, or $AUC_{0-\infty}$.

The pharmacokinetic parameters of amprenavir after administration of fosamprenavir (with and without concomitant ritonavir) are shown in the table below.

Mean Steady-State Plasma Amprenavir Pharmacokinetic Parameters				
Regimen	C_{max} (mcg/mL)	T_{max} (hours)[1]	AUC_{24} (mcg•h/mL)	C_{min} (mcg/mL)
Fosamprenavir 1400 mg bid	4.82	1.3	33	0.35
Fosamprenavir 1400 mg qd plus ritonavir 200 mg qd	7.24	2.1	69.4	1.45
Fosamprenavir 700 mg bid plus ritonavir 100 mg bid	6.08	1.5	79.2	2.12

[1] Data shown are median (range).

Distribution – In vitro, amprenavir is approximately 90% bound to plasma proteins, primarily to alpha$_1$-acid glycoprotein. In vitro, concentration-dependent binding was observed over the concentration range of 1 to 10 mcg/mL, with decreased binding at higher concentrations. The partitioning of amprenavir into erythrocytes is low but increases as amprenavir concentrations increase, reflecting the higher amount of unbound drug at higher concentrations.

Metabolism – After oral administration, fosamprenavir is rapidly and almost completely hydrolyzed to amprenavir and inorganic phosphate prior

FOSAMPRENAVIR CALCIUM — ORAL

to reaching the systemic circulation. This occurs in the gut epithelium during absorption. Amprenavir is metabolized in the liver by the cytochrome P450 3A4 (CYP3A4) enzyme system. The 2 major metabolites result from oxidation of the tetrahydrofuran and aniline moieties. Glucuronide conjugates of oxidized metabolites have been identified as minor metabolites in urine and feces.

Excretion – Excretion of unchanged amprenavir in urine and feces is minimal. Approximately 14% and 75% of an administered single dose of ^{14}C-amprenavir can be accounted for as metabolites in urine and feces, respectively. Two metabolites accounted for more than 90% of the radiocarbon in fecal samples. The plasma elimination half-life of amprenavir is approximately 7.7 hours.

Special populations –

Hepatic function impairment: The pharmacokinetics of amprenavir after administration of fosamprenavir have not been studied in patients with hepatic insufficiency. Based on amprenavir capsule data (see amprenavir monograph for further information), patients with impaired hepatic function receiving fosamprenavir without concurrent ritonavir may require dosage reduction. There are no data on the use of fosamprenavir in combination with ritonavir in patients with any degree of hepatic impairment (see Warnings and Administration and Dosage).

➤*Microbiology:*

Antiviral activity in vitro – Fosamprenavir has little or no antiviral activity in vitro. The in vitro antiviral activity observed with fosamprenavir is not measurable because of trace amounts of amprenavir (see amprenavir monograph for further information).

Resistance – HIV-1 isolates with a decreased susceptibility to amprenavir have been selected in vitro and obtained from patients treated with fosamprenavir. Genotypic analysis of isolates from amprenavir-treated patients showed mutations in the HIV-1 protease gene, resulting in amino acid substitutions primarily at positions V32I, M46I/L, I47V, I50V, I54L/M, and I84V, as well as mutations in the p7/p1 and p1/p6 Gag and Gag-Pol polyprotein precursor cleavage sites. Some of these amprenavir resistance-associated mutations also have been detected in HIV-1 isolates from antiretroviral-naive patients treated with fosamprenavir. Of the 488 antiretroviral-naive patients treated with fosamprenavir or fosamprenavir/ritonavir, 61 patients (29 receiving fosamprenavir and 32 receiving fosamprenavir/ritonavir) with virologic failure (plasma HIV-1 RNA greater than 1000 copies/mL on 2 occasions on or after week 12) were genotyped. Five of the 29 antiretroviral-naive patients (17%) receiving fosamprenavir without ritonavir had evidence of genotypic resistance to amprenavir: I54L/M (n = 2), I54L + L33F (n = 1), V32I + I47V (n = 1), and M46I + I47V (n = 1). No amprenavir-associated mutations were detected in antiretroviral-naive patients treated with fosamprenavir/ritonavir.

Cross-resistance – Varying degrees of cross-resistance among HIV-1 PI have been observed. An association between virologic response at 48 weeks (HIV-1 RNA level less than 400 copies/mL) and PI-resistance mutations detected in baseline HIV-1 isolates from PI-experienced patients receiving fosamprenavir/ritonavir twice daily (n = 88) or lopinavir/ritonavir twice daily (n = 85) in study APV30003 is shown in the table below. The majority of subjects had previously received either 1 (47%) or 2 (36%) PIs, most commonly nelfinavir (57%) and indinavir (53%). Of the 102 subjects with baseline phenotypes receiving twice-daily fosamprenavir/ritonavir, 54% (55) had resistance to at least 1 PI with 98% (54) of those having resistance to nelfinavir. Of 97 subjects with baseline phenotypes in the lopinavir/ritonavir arm, 60% (58) had resistance to at least 1 PI with 97% (56) of those having resistance to nelfinavir.

Responders at Week 48 by Presence of Baseline PI Resistance-Associated Mutations (%)[1]

PI-mutations[2]	Fosamprenavir/ ritonavir bid (n = 88)	Lopinavir/ ritonavir bid (n = 85)
D30N	95	89
N88D/S	91	100
L90M	52	59
M46I/L	50	50
V82A/F/T/S	22	35
I54V	18	55
I84V	17	40

[1] Interpret results with caution because the subgroups were small.
[2] Most patients had more than 1 PI resistance-associated mutation at baseline.

The virologic response based upon baseline phenotype was assessed. Baseline isolates from PI-experienced patients responding to fosamprenavir/ritonavir twice daily had a median shift in susceptibility to amprenavir relative to a standard wild-type reference strain of 0.7 (range, 0.1 to 5.4, n = 62), and baseline isolates from individuals failing therapy had a median shift in susceptibility of 1.9 (range, 0.2 to 14, n = 29). Because this was a select patient population, these data do not constitute definitive clinical susceptibility break points. Additional data are needed to determine clinically relevant break points for fosamprenavir.

Isolates from 15 of the 20 patients receiving twice-daily fosamprenavir/ritonavir and experiencing virologic failure/ongoing replication were subjected to genotypic analysis. The following amprenavir resistance-associated mutations were found either alone or in combination: V32I, M46I/L, I47V, I50V, I54L/M, and I84V.

Contraindications

Previously demonstrated clinically significant hypersensitivity to any of the components of this product or to amprenavir; coadministration with dihydroergotamine, ergonovine, ergotamine, methylergonovine, cisapride, pimozide, midazolam, or triazolam.

If fosamprenavir is coadministered with ritonavir, the antiarrhythmic agents flecainide and propafenone also are contraindicated.

Warnings

➤*Drug interactions:* Serious and/or life-threatening drug interactions could occur between fosamprenavir and amiodarone, lidocaine (systemic), tricyclic antidepressants, and quinidine. Concentration monitoring of these agents is recommended if these agents are used concomitantly with fosamprenavir (see Contraindications and Drug Interactions).

➤*Skin reactions:* Severe or life-threatening skin reactions, including 1 case of Stevens-Johnson syndrome among 700 patients treated with fosamprenavir, were reported in less than 1% of patients treated with fosamprenavir in the clinical studies. Discontinue treatment with fosamprenavir for severe or life-threatening rashes and moderate rashes accompanied by systemic symptoms.

Skin rash (without regard to causality) occurred in approximately 19% of patients treated with fosamprenavir in the pivotal efficacy studies. Rashes usually were maculopapular and of mild or moderate intensity, some with pruritus. Rash had a median onset of 11 days after initiation of fosamprenavir and had a median duration of 13 days. Skin rash led to discontinuation of fosamprenavir in less than 1% of patients. In some patients with mild or moderate rash, dosing with fosamprenavir was often continued without interruption; if interrupted, reintroduction of fosamprenavir generally did not result in rash recurrence.

➤*Hemolytic anemia:* Acute hemolytic anemia has been reported in a patient treated with amprenavir.

➤*Diabetes mellitus / hyperglycemia:* New-onset diabetes mellitus, exacerbation of preexisting diabetes mellitus, and hyperglycemia have been reported during postmarketing surveillance in HIV-infected patients receiving PI therapy. Some patients required either initiation or dose adjustments of insulin or oral hypoglycemic agents for treatment of these events. In some cases, diabetic ketoacidosis has occurred. In those patients who discontinued PI therapy, hyperglycemia persisted in some cases. Because these events have been voluntarily reported during clinical practice, estimates of frequency cannot be made and causal relationships between PI therapy and these events have not been established.

➤*Hepatic function impairment:* Fosamprenavir is principally metabolized by the liver; therefore, exercise caution when administering fosamprenavir to patients with hepatic impairment because amprenavir concentrations may be increased (see Actions). Patients with impaired hepatic function receiving fosamprenavir without concurrent ritonavir may require dose reduction (see Administration and Dosage). There are no data on the use of fosamprenavir in combination with ritonavir in patients with any degree of hepatic impairment.

Patients with underlying hepatitis B or C or marked elevations in transaminases prior to treatment may be at increased risk for developing transaminase elevations. Conduct appropriate laboratory testing prior to initiating therapy with fosamprenavir and closely monitor patients during treatment.

➤*Carcinogenesis:* Carcinogenicity studies of fosamprenavir in rats and mice are in progress; however, results are available from carcinogenicity studies with amprenavir. Amprenavir was evaluated for carcinogenic potential by oral gavage administration to mice and rats for up to 104 weeks. Results showed an increase in the incidence of benign hepatocellular adenomas and an increase in the combined incidence of hepatocellular adenomas plus carcinoma in males of both species at the highest doses tested. Female mice and rats were not affected. These observations were made at systemic exposures equivalent to approximately 2 (mice) and 4 (rats) times the human exposure (based on $AUC_{0\text{-}24\,h}$ measurement) at the recommended dose of 1200 mg twice daily.

➤*Elderly:* In general, dose selection for an elderly patient should be cautious, reflecting the greater frequency of decreased hepatic, renal, or cardiac function, and of concomitant disease or other drug therapy.

➤*Pregnancy: Category C.* Administration of fosamprenavir to pregnant rats and rabbits produced no major effects on embryo-fetal development; however, the incidence of abortion was increased in rabbits. Systemic exposures ($AUC_{0\text{-}24\,h}$) to amprenavir at these dosages were 0.8 (rabbits) to 2 (rats) times the exposures in humans following administration of the maximum recommended human dose (MRHD) of fosamprenavir alone or 0.3 (rabbits) to 0.7 (rats) times the exposures in humans following administration of the MRHD of fosamprenavir in combination with ritonavir. In contrast, administration of amprenavir was associated with abortions and an increased incidence of minor skeletal variations resulting from deficient ossification of the femur, humerus, and trochlea in pregnant rabbits at the tested dose; approximately one-twentieth the exposure seen at the recommended human dose.

The mating and fertility of the F_1 generation born to female rats given fosamprenavir was not different from control animals; however, fosamprenavir did cause a reduction in both pup survival and body weights. Surviving F_1 female rats showed an increased time to successful mating, an increased length of gestation, a reduced number of uterine implantation sites per litter, and reduced gestational body weights compared with control animals. Systemic exposure ($AUC_{0\text{-}24\,h}$) to amprenavir in the F_0 pregnant rats was approximately 2 times higher than exposures in humans following the administration of the MRHD of fosamprenavir alone or approximately the

FOSAMPRENAVIR CALCIUM — ORAL

same as those seen in humans following administration of the MRHD of fosamprenavir in combination with ritonavir.

There are no adequate and well-controlled studies in pregnant women. Use fosamprenavir during pregnancy only if the potential benefit justifies the potential risk to the fetus.

Antiretroviral pregnancy registry – To monitor maternal-fetal outcomes of pregnant women exposed to fosamprenavir, an Antiretroviral Pregnancy Registry has been established. Physicians are encouraged to register patients by calling 1-800-258-4263.

➤*Lactation:* The Centers for Disease Control and Prevention recommend that HIV-infected mothers not breastfeed their infants to avoid risking postnatal transmission of HIV. Although it is not known if amprenavir is excreted in human milk, amprenavir is secreted into the milk of lactating rats. Because of both the potential for HIV transmission and the potential for serious adverse reactions in nursing infants, instruct mothers not to breastfeed if they are receiving fosamprenavir.

➤*Children:* The safety and efficacy of fosamprenavir have not been established in pediatric patients.

Precautions

➤*Sulfa sensitivity:* Use fosamprenavir with caution in patients with a known sulfonamide allergy. Fosamprenavir contains a sulfonamide moiety. The potential for cross-sensitivity between drugs in the sulfonamide class and fosamprenavir is unknown. In a clinical study of fosamprenavir used as the sole PI, rash occurred in 2 of 10 patients (20%) with a history of sulfonamide allergy compared with 42 of 126 patients (33%) with no history of sulfonamide allergy. In 2 clinical studies of fosamprenavir plus low-dose ritonavir, rash occurred in 8 of 50 patients (16%) with a history of sulfonamide allergy compared with 50 of 412 patients (12%) with no history of sulfonamide allergy.

➤*Hemophilia:* There have been reports of spontaneous bleeding in patients with hemophilia A and B treated with PI. In some patients, additional factor VIII was required. In many of the reported cases, treatment with PI was continued or restarted. A causal relationship between PI therapy and these episodes has not been established.

➤*Opportunistic infections:* During the initial phase of treatment, patients responding to antiretroviral therapy may develop an inflammatory response to indolent or residual opportunistic infections such as *Mycobacterium avium* complex, cytomegalovirus, *Pneumocystis carinii*, and tuberculosis that may necessitate further evaluation and treatment.

➤*Fat redistribution:* Redistribution/accumulation of body fat including central obesity, dorsocervical fat enlargement (buffalo hump), peripheral wasting, facial wasting, breast enlargement, and "cushingoid appearance" have been observed in patients receiving antiretroviral therapy, including fosamprenavir. The mechanism and long-term consequences of these events are currently unknown. A causal relationship has not been established.

➤*Lipid elevations:* Treatment with fosamprenavir plus ritonavir has resulted in increases in the concentration of triglycerides. Perform triglyceride and cholesterol testing prior to initiating therapy with fosamprenavir and at periodic intervals during therapy. Manage lipid disorders as clinically appropriate.

➤*Resistance/Cross-resistance:* Because the potential for HIV cross-resistance among PI has not been fully explored, it is unknown what effect therapy with fosamprenavir will have on the activity of subsequently administered PI. Fosamprenavir has been studied in patients who have experienced treatment failure with PI.

Drug Interactions

Because amprenavir is the active metabolite of fosamprenavir, please refer to the amprenavir monograph for other possible drug interactions. Amprenavir is metabolized by CYP3A4 and is an inhibitor (and possibly an inducer) of CYP3A4. Coadministration of fosamprenavir and drugs that induce CYP3A4, such as rifampin, may decrease amprenavir concentrations and reduce its therapeutic effect. Coadministration of fosamprenavir and drugs that inhibit CYP3A4 may increase amprenavir concentrations and increase the incidence of adverse effects.

➤*CYP450 system:* The potential for drug interactions with fosamprenavir changes when fosamprenavir is coadministered with the potent CYP3A4 inhibitor ritonavir. Because ritonavir is a CYP2D6 inhibitor, clinically significant interactions with drugs metabolized by CYP2D6 are possible when coadministered with fosamprenavir plus ritonavir.

Fosamprenavir Drug Interactions

Precipitant drug	Object drug*		Description
Fosamprenavir	Amiodarone Lidocaine (systemic) Quinidine	↑	Coadminister with caution because of potential serious and/or life-threatening reactions. Monitor concentrations if available.
Fosamprenavir	Amitriptyline Imipramine	↑	Therapeutic concentration monitoring is recommended for the tricyclic antidepressants when coadministered.
Fosamprenavir	Benzodiazepines	↑	Coadministration with midazolam or triazolam is contraindicated because of serious and/or life-threatening reactions such as prolonged or increased sedation or respiratory depression. Alprazolam, clorazepate, diazepam, and flurazepam may have increased serum concentrations, which could increase their activity.
Fosamprenavir	Calcium channel blockers	↑	Concurrent use may increase bepridil concentrations, possibly causing life-threatening reactions such as cardiac arrhythmias. Use with caution. The concentrations of other calcium channel blockers may be increased when given with fosamprenavir.
Fosamprenavir	Cisapride Pimozide	↑	Coadministration is contraindicated because of potential for serious and/or life-threatening reactions such as cardiac arrhythmias.
Fosamprenavir	Contraceptives, oral	↓	Coadministration of fosamprenavir with ethinyl estradiol/norethindrone may alter the hormonal levels. Alternative nonhormonal methods of contraception are recommended.
Fosamprenavir	Cyclosporine Tacrolimus	↑	Therapeutic concentration monitoring of immunosuppressants is recommended with coadministration.
Fosamprenavir	Ergot derivatives	↑	Coadministration is contraindicated because of potential for serious and/or life-threatening reactions such as acute ergot toxicity (peripheral vasospasm and ischemia of the extremities and other tissues).
Fosamprenavir	HMG-CoA reductase inhibitors	↑	Fosamprenavir may increase serum concentrations of atorvastatin, lovastatin, and simvastatin, which could increase their toxicity such as myopathy including rhabdomyolysis. Avoid administration with lovastatin or simvastatin, use ≤ 20 mg/day of atorvastatin with careful monitoring, or use fluvastatin, pravastatin, or rosuvastatin. Administration of atorvastatin with fosamprenavir produced a decrease in amprenavir C_{max} and AUC.
HMG-CoA reductase inhibitors Atorvastatin	Fosamprenavir	↓	
Fosamprenavir	Ketoconazole Itraconazole	↑	Coadministration may lead to increase in ketoconazole or itraconazole adverse events. Dose reduction of ketoconazole or itraconazole may be necessary in patients who are receiving more than 400 mg/day of ketoconazole or itraconazole.
Fosamprenavir	Methadone	↓	Dosage of methadone may need to be increased with coadministration.
Fosamprenavir	Rifabutin	↑	Monitor for neutropenia weekly when coadministered. When coadministered, a dosage reduction of rifabutin by at least half the usual dose is recommended. When coadministered with fosamprenavir plus ritonavir, a dosage reduction of rifabutin by at least 75% of the usual dose is recommended (max dose of 150 mg every other day or 3 times/week).

FOSAMPRENAVIR CALCIUM — ORAL

Fosamprenavir Drug Interactions			
Precipitant drug	Object drug*		Description
Fosamprenavir	Sildenafil Vardenafil	↑	Use with caution. When coadministered, decreased doses of sildenafil (25 mg every 48 hours) and vardenafil (2.5 mg every 24 hours) are recommended with increased monitoring for adverse events. When vardenafil is coadministered with fosamprenavir plus ritonavir, decrease vardenafil dose to no more than 2.5 mg every 72 hours.
Fosamprenavir	Warfarin	↔	Concentrations of warfarin may be affected. Monitor INR.
Fosamprenavir plus ritonavir	Flecainide Propafenone	↑	Coadministration may increase the plasma concentrations of the antiarrhythmics and cause serious and/or life-threatening reactions such as cardiac arrhythmias. Coadministration is contraindicated.
Antacids	Fosamprenavir	↓	Coadministration resulted in a decrease in the amprenavir C_{max} and AUC by 35% and 18%, respectively.
Efavirenz	Fosamprenavir with or without ritonavir	↓	Coadministration led to decreases in fosamprenavir concentrations. An additional 100 mg/day of ritonavir is recommended when efavirenz is administered with fosamprenavir plus ritonavir once daily. No change in dose is necessary when efavirenz is administered with fosamprenavir plus ritonavir twice daily.
Efavirenz plus ritonavir	Fosamprenavir plus ritonavir	↑	Coadministration led to increases in amprenavir C_{max} and AUC by 18% and 11%, respectively.
Indinavir Nelfinavir	Fosamprenavir	↑	Coadministration has led to increases in amprenavir concentrations.
Lopinavir plus ritonavir	Fosamprenavir plus ritonavir	↓	Coadministration decreased amprenavir C_{max} and AUC but increased lopinavir C_{max} and AUC.
Fosamprenavir plus ritonavir	Lopinavir plus ritonavir	↑	
Nevirapine Saquinavir	Fosamprenavir	↓	Coadministration has led to decreases in amprenavir concentrations.
Ranitidine	Fosamprenavir	↓	Coadministration led to decreases in amprenavir C_{max} and AUC by 51% and 30%, respectively.
Rifampin St. John's wort Delavirdine Carbamazepine Phenobarbital Phenytoin Dexamethasone Histamine H_2- receptor antagonists Proton pump inhibitors	Fosamprenavir	↓	Coadministration may result in loss of virologic response and possible resistance to fosamprenavir and/or other PI. Rifampin decreases plasma levels of amprenavir by approximately 90% after coadministration. Avoid administration with rifampin, St. John's wort, and delavirdine.

* ↑ = Object drug increased. ↓ = Object drug decreased. ↔ = Undetermined clinical effect.

Adverse Reactions

Fosamprenavir was studied in 700 patients in phase 3 controlled clinical studies. The most common treatment-emergent adverse events in clinical studies of fosamprenavir were diarrhea, nausea, vomiting, headache, and rash (see Warnings) and were generally mild to moderate in severity. Treatment discontinuation because of adverse events occurred in 6.4% of patients receiving fosamprenavir and in 5.9% of patients receiving comparator treatments.

➤*Antiretroviral-naive patients:*

Adverse Reactions in Antiretroviral-Naive Patients (%)								
	Fosamprenavir 1400 mg bid[1] (n = 166)		Nelfinavir 1250 mg bid[1] (n = 83)		Fosamprenavir 1400 mg qd/ ritonavir 200 mg qd[1] (n = 322)		Nelfinavir 1250 mg bid[1] (n = 327)	
Adverse reaction	Moderate/severe drug-related	All grades[2]	Moderate/severe drug-related	All grades[2]	Moderate/severe drug-related	All grades[2]	Moderate/severe drug-related	All grades[2]
CNS								
Headache	2	19	4	20	3	21	3	27
Fatigue	2	10	1	7	4	18	2	13
Depressive/mood disorders	1	8	0	8	< 1	8	0	6
Paresthesia, oral	0	2	0	0	< 1	10	0	< 1
Dermatologic								
Rash	8	35	2	19	3	17	2	21
Pruritus	0	7	0	11	< 1	7	1	9
GI								
Nausea	7	39	4	24	7	37	5	27
Diarrhea	5	34	18	63	10	52	18	72
Vomiting	2	16	4	17	6	20	4	13
Abdominal pain	1	5	0	8	2	11	2	11

[1] All patients also received abacavir and lamivudine twice daily.
[2] Includes adverse events of all grades regardless of causality reported in more than 5% of patients.

Laboratory abnormalities –

Grade 3/4 Laboratory Abnormalities Reported in ≥ 2% of Antiretroviral-Naive Adult Patients[1]				
Laboratory abnormality	Fosamprenavir 1400 mg bid[2] (n = 166)	Nelfinavir 1250 mg bid[2] (n = 83)	Fosamprenavir 1400 mg qd/ ritonavir 200 mg qd[2] (n = 322)	Nelfinavir 1250 mg bid[2] (n = 327)
Serum lipase (> 2 × ULN)	8	4	6	4
AST (> 5 × ULN)	6	6	6	7
ALT (> 5 × ULN)	6	5	8	8
Hypertriglyceridemia[3] (> 750 mg/dL)	0	1	6	2
Neutropenia (< 750 cells/mm³)	3	6	3	4

[1] The incidence of grade 3 or 4 hyperglycemia in antiretroviral-naive patients who received fosamprenavir in the pivotal studies was less than 1%.
[2] All patients also received abacavir and lamivudine twice daily.
[3] Fasting specimens.
ULN = Upper limit of normal.

➤*Protease inhibitor-experienced patients:*

Fosamprenavir Adverse Reactions Reported in Protease Inhibitor-Experienced Patients (%)				
	Fosamprenavir 700 mg bid/ ritonavir 100 mg bid[1] (n = 106)		Lopinavir 400 mg bid/ ritonavir 100 mg bid[1] (n = 103)	
Adverse reaction	Moderate/severe drug-related	All grades[2]	Moderate/severe drug-related	All grades[2]
CNS				
Headache	4	27	2	20
Depressive/ mood disorders	< 1	11	< 1	10
Fatigue	< 1	9	< 1	14
Paresthesia, oral	0	< 1	0	0
Dermatologic				
Rash	3	9	0	22
Pruritus	< 1	8	0	3
GI				
Diarrhea	13	38	11	47
Nausea	3	20	9	31
Vomiting	3	10	5	17
Abdominal pain	< 1	11	2	9

[1] All patients also received 2 reverse transcriptase inhibitors.
[2] Includes adverse events of all grades regardless of causality reported in more than 5% of patients.

FOSAMPRENAVIR CALCIUM — ORAL

Laboratory abnormalities –

Grade 3/4 Laboratory Abnormalities Reported in ≥ 2% of Protease Inhibitor-Experienced Adult Patients		
Laboratory abnormality	Fosamprenavir 700 mg bid/ ritonavir 100 mg bid[1] (n = 104)	Lopinavir 400 mg bid/ ritonavir 100 mg bid[1] (n = 103)
Hypertriglyceridemia[2] (> 750 mg/dL)	11[3]	6[3]
Serum lipase (> 2 × ULN)	5	12
ALT (> 5 × ULN)	4	4
AST (> 5 × ULN)	4	2
Hyperglycemia (> 251 mg/dL)	2[3]	2[3]

[1] All patients also received 2 reverse transcriptase inhibitors.
[2] Fasting specimens.
[3] n = 100 for fosamprenavir/ritonavir, n = 98 for lopinavir/ritonavir.
ULN = Upper limit of normal.

Overdosage

There is no known antidote for fosamprenavir. It is not known whether amprenavir can be removed by peritoneal dialysis or hemodialysis. If overdosage occurs, monitor the patient for evidence of toxicity and apply standard supportive treatment as necessary.

Patient Information

A patient information sheet for fosamprenavir is available for patient information.

Inform patients that fosamprenavir is not a cure for HIV infection and that they may continue to develop opportunistic infections and other complications associated with HIV disease. The long-term effects of fosamprenavir are unknown at this time. Inform patients that there are currently no data demonstrating that therapy with fosamprenavir can reduce the risk of transmitting HIV to others.

Inform patients that sustained decreases in plasma HIV-1 RNA have been associated with a reduced risk of progression to AIDS and death. Advise patients to remain under the care of a physician while using fosamprenavir and to take fosamprenavir every day as prescribed. Fosamprenavir must always be used in combination with other antiretroviral drugs.

Instruct patients not to alter the dose or discontinue therapy without consulting their physician. If a dose is missed, advise patients to take the dose as soon as possible and then return to their normal schedule. However, if a dose is skipped, instruct patients not to double the next dose.

Advise patients to inform their health care provider if they have a sulfa allergy. The potential for cross-sensitivity between drugs in the sulfonamide class and fosamprenavir is unknown.

Fosamprenavir may interact with many drugs; therefore, advise patients to report to their health care provider the use of any other prescription or nonprescription medication or herbal products, particularly St. John's wort.

Advise patients receiving phosphodiesterase type 5 (PDE5) inhibitors that they may be at an increased risk of PDE5 inhibitor-associated adverse events, including hypotension, visual changes, and priapism, and to promptly report any symptoms to their health care provider.

Instruct patients receiving hormonal contraceptives to use alternative contraceptive measures during therapy with fosamprenavir because hormonal levels may be altered.

Inform patients that redistribution or accumulation of body fat may occur in patients receiving antiretroviral therapy, including fosamprenavir, and that the cause and long-term health effects of these conditions are not known at this time.

AMPRENAVIR

Rx	**Agenerase** (GlaxoSmithKline)	**Capsules:** 50 mg[a]	(GX CC1). Off-white to cream. Oblong. In 480s.
		Solution, oral: 15 mg/mL[b,c]	Grape/bubblegum/peppermint flavor. In 240 mL.

[a] With D-sorbitol, d-alpha tocopheryl polyethylene glycol 1,000 succinate (TPGS), propylene glycol 19 mg.
[b] With acesulfame potassium, saccharin, propylene glycol 550 mg.
[c] Each mL of amprenavir oral solution contains 46 units vitamin E in the form of TPGS.

AMPRENAVIR — ORAL

WARNING

Oral solution – Because of the potential risk of toxicity from the large amount of the excipient, propylene glycol, amprenavir oral solution is contraindicated in infants and children below 4 years of age, pregnant women, patients with hepatic or renal failure, and patients treated with disulfiram or metronidazole. Disulfiram and metronidazole are contraindicated due to potential risk of toxicity from the large amount of the excipient, propylene glycol, in amprenavir oral solution.

Amprenavir oral solution should be used only when amprenavir capsules or other protease inhibitor formulations are not therapeutic options.

Indications

➤*HIV infection:* In combination with other antiretroviral agents for the treatment of HIV-1 infection.

➤*Oral solution:* Use only when amprenavir capsules or other protease inhibitor formulations are not therapeutic options.

Administration and Dosage

➤*Approved by the FDA:* April 16, 1999.

Amprenavir may be taken with or without food; however, a high-fat meal decreases the absorption of amprenavir and should be avoided. Adult and pediatric patients should be advised not to take supplemental vitamin E since the vitamin E content of amprenavir capsules and oral solution exceeds the reference daily intake (adults 30 IU, pediatrics approximately 10 IU).

➤*Bioequivalency:* Amprenavir capsules and amprenavir oral solution are not interchangeable on a milligram-per-milligram basis. Amprenavir oral solution was 14% less bioavailable compared to the capsules.

➤*Capsules:*

Adults – 1,200 mg (eight 150 mg capsules) twice daily in combination with other antiretroviral agents.

Children –

Patients 4 to 12 years of age, or patients 13 to 16 years of age who weigh less than 50 kg: 20 mg/kg twice daily or 15 mg/kg 3 times daily (to a maximum daily dose of 2,400 mg) in combination with other antiretroviral agents. The recommended dose of amprenavir for use in combination with ritonavir has not been established in pediatric patients.

Patients 13 to 16 years of age: 1,200 mg (eight 150 mg capsules) twice daily in combination with other antiretroviral agents.

➤*Oral solution:* The recommended dose of amprenavir oral solution based on body weight and age is shown in the following table. Consideration should be given to switching patients from amprenavir oral solution to amprenavir capsules as soon as they are able to take the capsule formulation.

Recommended dosages of amprenavir oral solution		
	Dose	
Age/Weight criteria	Twice daily	3 times daily
4 to 12 years, or 13 to 16 years and < 50 kg	22.5 mg/kg (1.5 mL/kg) (maximum dose 2,800 mg per day)	17 mg/kg (1.1 mL/kg) (maximum dose 2,800 mg per day)
13 to 16 years and ≥ 50 kg or > 16 years	1,400 mg	NA

➤*Concomitant therapy:*

Capsules – If amprenavir and ritonavir are used in combination, the recommended dosage regimens are the following: Amprenavir 1,200 mg with ritonavir 200 mg once daily or amprenavir 600 mg with ritonavir 100 mg twice daily.

Oral solution – Concurrent use of amprenavir oral solution and ritonavir oral solution is not recommended because the large amount of propylene glycol in amprenavir oral solution and ethanol in ritonavir oral solution may compete for the same metabolic pathway for elimination.

➤*Hepatic function impairment:*

Capsules – Amprenavir capsules should be used with caution in patients with moderate or severe hepatic impairment. Patients with a Child-Pugh score ranging from 5 to 8 should receive a reduced dose of amprenavir capsules of 450 mg twice daily, and patients with a Child-Pugh score ranging from 9 to 12 should receive reduced doses of amprenavir capsules of 300 mg twice daily.

Oral solution – Amprenavir oral solution is contraindicated in patients with hepatic failure.

Patients with hepatic impairment are at increased risk of propylene glycol-associated adverse events. Amprenavir oral solution should be used with caution in patients with hepatic impairment. Based on a study with amprenavir capsules, adult patients with a Child-Pugh score ranging from 5 to 8 should receive a reduced dose of amprenavir oral solution of 513 mg (34 mL) twice daily, and adult patients with a Child-Pugh score ranging from 9 to 12 should receive a reduced dose of amprenavir oral solution of 342 mg (23 mL) twice daily.

➤*Renal function impairment:*

Oral solution – Amprenavir oral solution is contraindicated in patients with renal failure.

Patients with renal impairment are at increased risk of propylene glycol-associated adverse events. Amprenavir oral solution should be used with caution in patients with renal impairment.

AMPRENAVIR — ORAL

➤*Storage/Stability:* Store at controlled room temperature of 25°C (77°F).

Actions

➤*Pharmacokinetics:*

Absorption –

Amprenavir was rapidly absorbed after oral administration in HIV-1-infected patients with a time to peak concentration (t_{max}) typically between 1 and 2 hours after a single oral dose. The absolute oral bioavailability of amprenavir in humans has not been established.

Increases in the area under the plasma concentration versus time curve (AUC) after single oral doses between 150 and 1,200 mg were slightly greater than dose proportional. Increases in AUC were dose proportional after 3 weeks of dosing with doses from 300 to 1,200 mg twice daily. The pharmacokinetic parameters after administration of amprenavir 1,200 mg twice daily for 3 weeks to HIV-infected subjects are shown in the following table:

Average (% CV) pharmacokinetic parameters after 1,200 mg twice daily of amprenavir capsules (n = 54)					
C_{max} (mcg/mL)	t_{max} (hours)	AUC_{0-12} (mcg•hr/mL)	C_{avg} (mcg/mL)	C_{min} (mcg/mL)	CL/F (mL/min/kg)
7.66 (54%)	1 (42%)	17.7 (47%)	1.48 (47%)	0.32 (77%)	19.5 (46%)

The relative bioavailability of amprenavir capsules and oral solution was assessed in healthy adults. Amprenavir oral solution was 14% less bioavailable compared to the capsules; therefore, amprenavir capsules and amprenavir oral solution are not interchangeable on a milligram-per-milligram basis.

Effects of food on oral absorption: The relative bioavailability of amprenavir capsules was assessed in the fasting and fed states in healthy volunteers (standardized high-fat meal: 967 kcal, 67 grams fat, 33 grams protein, 58 grams carbohydrate). Administration of a single 1,200 mg dose of amprenavir in the fed state compared to the fasted state was associated with changes in C_{max} (fed: 6.18 ± 2.92 mcg/mL, fasted: 9.72 ± 2.75 mcg/mL), t_{max} (fed: 1.51 ± 0.68, fasted: 1.05 ± 0.63), and $AUC_{0-\infty}$ (fed: 22.06 ± 11.6 mcg•hr/mL, fasted: 28.05 ± 10.1 mcg•hr/mL). Amprenavir may be taken with or without food, but should not be taken with a high-fat meal.

Distribution – The apparent volume of distribution (V_z/F) is approximately 430 L in healthy adult subjects. In vitro binding is approximately 90% to plasma proteins. The high affinity binding protein for amprenavir is alpha-1-acid glycoprotein (AAG). The partitioning of amprenavir into erythrocytes is low, but increases as amprenavir concentrations increase, reflecting the higher amount of unbound drug at higher concentrations.

Metabolism – Amprenavir is metabolized in the liver by the cytochrome P450 3A4 (CYP3A4) enzyme system. The 2 major metabolites result from oxidation of the tetrahydrofuran and aniline moieties. Glucuronide conjugates of oxidized metabolites have been identified as minor metabolites in urine and feces.

Oral solution: Amprenavir oral solution contains a large amount of propylene glycol, which is hepatically metabolized by the alcohol and aldehyde dehydrogenase enzyme pathway. Alcohol dehydrogenase (ADH) is present in the human fetal liver at 2 months of gestational age, but at only 3% of adult activity. Although the data are limited, it appears that by 12 to 30 months of postnatal age, ADH activity is equal to or greater than that observed in adults. Additionally, certain patient groups (female, Asian, Eskimo, Native American) may be at increased risk of propylene glycol-associated adverse events due to diminished ability to metabolize propylene glycol.

Excretion – Excretion of unchanged amprenavir in urine and feces is minimal. Approximately 14% and 75% of an administered single dose of ^{14}C-amprenavir can be accounted for as radiocarbon in urine and feces, respectively. Two metabolites accounted for greater than 90% of the radiocarbon in fecal samples. The plasma elimination half-life of amprenavir ranged from 7.1 to 10.6 hours.

Special populations –

Renal function impairment: The impact of renal impairment on amprenavir elimination in adult patients has not been studied. The renal elimination of unchanged amprenavir represents less than 3% of the administered dose.

• *Oral solution* – Amprenavir oral solution is contraindicated in patients with renal failure.

Patients with renal impairment are at increased risk of propylene glycol-associated adverse events. Additionally, because metabolites of the excipient, propylene glycol, in amprenavir oral solution may alter acid-base balance, patients with renal impairment should be monitored for potential adverse events. Amprenavir oral solution should therefore be used with caution in patients with renal impairment. The impact of renal impairment on amprenavir elimination has not been studied. The renal elimination of unchanged amprenavir represents less than 3% of the administered dose.

Hepatic function impairment: Amprenavir oral solution is contraindicated in patients with hepatic failure.

Amprenavir has been studied in adult patients with impaired hepatic function using a single 600 mg oral dose. The $AUC_{0-\infty}$ was significantly greater in patients with moderate cirrhosis (25.76 ± 14.68 mcg•hr/mL) compared with healthy volunteers (12 ± 4.38 mcg•hr/mL). The $AUC_{0-\infty}$ and C_{max} were significantly greater in patients with severe cirrhosis ($AUC_{0-\infty}$: 38.66 ± 16.08 mcg•hr/mL; C_{max}: 9.43 ± 2.61 mcg/mL) compared with healthy volunteers ($AUC_{0-\infty}$: 12 ± 4.38 mcg•hr/mL; C_{max}: 4.9 ± 1.39 mcg/mL). Patients with impaired hepatic function require dosage adjustment.

Amprenavir capsules should be used with caution in patients with moderate or severe hepatic impairment. Patients with a Child-Pugh score ranging from 5 to 8 should receive a reduced dose of amprenavir capsules of 450 mg twice daily, and patients with a Child-Pugh score ranging from 9 to 12 should receive a reduced dose of amprenavir capsules of 300 mg twice daily.

• *Oral solution* – Amprenavir oral solution is contraindicated in patients with hepatic failure.

Patients with hepatic impairment are at increased risk of propylene glycol-associated adverse events. Amprenavir oral solution should be used with caution in patients with hepatic impairment.

Children: The pharmacokinetics of amprenavir have been studied after either single or repeat doses of amprenavir capsules or oral solution in 84 pediatric patients. Twenty HIV-1-infected children ranging in age from 4 to 12 years received single doses from 5 mg/kg to 20 mg/kg using 25 mg or 150 mg capsules. The C_{max} of amprenavir increased less than proportionally with dose. The $AUC_{0-\infty}$ increased proportionally at doses between 5 and 20 mg/kg.

Amprenavir is 14% less bioavailable from the liquid formulation than from the capsules; therefore, amprenavir capsules and oral solution are not interchangeable on a milligram-per-milligram basis.

Amprenavir oral solution is contraindicated in infants and children below the age of 4 years due to the potential risk of toxicity from the large amount of the excipient, propylene glycol.

• *Oral solution* – Amprenavir oral solution is contraindicated in infants and children below 4 years of age.

Average (% CV) pharmacokinetic parameters in children ages 4 to 12 years receiving 20 mg/kg twice daily or 15 mg/kg 3 times daily of amprenavir oral solution							
Dose	n	C_{max} (mcg/mL)	t_{max} (hours)	AUC_{ss}* (mcg•hr/mL)	C_{avg} (mcg/mL)	C_{min} (mcg/mL)	CL/F (mL/min/kg)
20 mg/kg twice daily	20	6.77 (51%)	1.1 (21%)	15.46 (59%)	1.29 (59%)	0.24 (98%)	29 (58%)
15 mg/kg 3 times daily	17	3.99 (37%)	1.4 (90%)	8.73 (36%)	1.09 (36%)	0.27 (95%)	32 (34%)

* AUC is 0 to 12 hours for twice daily and 0 to 8 hours for 3 times daily; therefore the C_{avg} is a better comparison of the exposures.

Gender:

• *Oral solution* – Females may have a lower amount of alcohol dehydrogenase compared with males and may be at increased risk of propylene glycol-associated adverse events; no data are available on propylene glycol metabolism in females.

Race:

• *Oral solution* – Certain ethnic populations (Asian patients, Eskimo patients, and Native American patients) may be at increased risk of propylene glycol-associated adverse events because of alcohol dehydrogenase polymorphisms; no data are available on propylene glycol metabolism in these groups.

➤*Microbiology:* Amprenavir is an inhibitor of HIV-1 protease. Amprenavir binds to the active site of HIV-1 protease and thereby prevents the processing of viral gag and gag-pol polyprotein precursors, resulting in the formation of immature noninfectious viral particles.

Antiviral activity in vitro – The in vitro antiviral activity of amprenavir was evaluated against HIV-1 IIIB in both acutely and chronically infected lymphoblastic cell lines (MT-4, CEM-CCRF, H9) and in peripheral blood lymphocytes. The 50% inhibitory concentration (IC_{50}) of amprenavir ranged from 0.012 to 0.08 mcM in acutely infected cells and was 0.41 mcM in chronically infected cells (1 mcM = 0.5 mcg/mL). Amprenavir exhibited synergistic anti-HIV-1 activity in combination with abacavir, zidovudine, didanosine, or saquinavir, and additive anti-HIV-1 activity in combination with indinavir, nelfinavir, and ritonavir in vitro. These drug combinations have not been adequately studied in humans. The relationship between in vitro anti-HIV-1 activity of amprenavir and the inhibition of HIV-1 replication in humans has not been defined.

Resistance – HIV-1 isolates with a decreased susceptibility to amprenavir have been selected in vitro and obtained from patients treated with amprenavir. Genotypic analysis of isolates from amprenavir-treated patients showed mutations in the HIV-1 protease gene resulting in amino acid substitutions primarily at positions V32I, M46I/L, I47V, I50V, I54L/M, and I84V as well as mutations in the p7/p1 and p1/p6 gag cleavage sites. Phenotypic analysis of HIV-1 isolates from 21 NRTI-experienced, protease inhibitor-naive patients treated with amprenavir in combination with NRTIs for 16 to 48 weeks identified isolates from 15 patients who exhibited a 4- to 17-fold decrease in susceptibility to amprenavir in vitro compared to wild-type virus. Clinical isolates that exhibited a decrease in amprenavir susceptibility harbored one or more amprenavir-associated mutations. The clinical relevance of the genotypic and phenotypic changes associated with amprenavir therapy is under evaluation.

Cross-resistance – Varying degrees of HIV-1 cross-resistance among protease inhibitors have been observed. Five of 15 amprenavir-resistant isolates exhibited a 4- to 8-fold decrease in susceptibility to ritonavir. However, amprenavir-resistant isolates were susceptible to either indinavir or saquinavir.

Contraindications

Coadministration of amprenavir is contraindicated with drugs that are highly dependent on CYP3A4 for clearance and for which elevated plasma

AMPRENAVIR — ORAL

concentrations are associated with serious or life-threatening events. These drugs are listed in the following table:

Drugs that are Contraindicated with Amprenavir	
Drug class	Drugs within class that are contraindicated with amprenavir
Alcohol-dependence treatment	Disulfiram (oral solution only)
Antibiotic	Metronidazole (oral solution only)
Ergot derivatives	Dihydroergotamine, ergonovine, ergotamine, methylergonovine
GI motility agent	Cisapride
Neuroleptic	Pimozide
Sedatives/hypnotics	Midazolam, triazolam

If amprenavir is coadministered with ritonavir, the antiarrhythmic agents flecainide and propafenone are also contraindicated.

Amprenavir is contraindicated in patients with previously demonstrated clinically significant hypersensitivity to any of the components of this product.

➤*Propylene glycol:* See the Warning box for more information.

Warnings

➤*Propylene glycol:* Because of the possible toxicity associated with the large amount of propylene glycol and the lack of information on chronic exposure to large amounts of propylene glycol, amprenavir oral solution should be used only when amprenavir capsules or other protease inhibitor formulations are not therapeutic options. Certain ethnic populations (Asian patients, Eskimo patients, Native American patients) and women may be at increased risk of propylene glycol-associated adverse events due to diminished abilities to metabolize propylene glycol; no data are available on propylene glycol metabolism in these groups.

If patients require treatment with amprenavir oral solution, they should be monitored closely for propylene glycol-associated adverse events, including seizures, stupor, tachycardia, hyperosmolality, lactic acidosis, renal toxicity, and hemolysis. Patients should be switched from amprenavir oral solution or amprenavir capsules as soon as they are able to take the capsule formulation.

Concurrent use of amprenavir oral solution and ritonavir oral solution is not recommended because the large amount of propylene glycol in amprenavir oral solution and ethanol in ritonavir oral solution may compete for the same metabolic pathway for elimination.

Use of alcoholic beverages is not recommended in patients treated with amprenavir oral solution.

See the Warning box for more information.

➤*Skin reactions:* See Adverse Reactions for more information.

➤*Hemolytic anemia:* Acute hemolytic anemia has been reported in a patient treated with amprenavir.

➤*Diabetes mellitus / Hyperglycemia:* New onset diabetes mellitus, exacerbation of preexisting diabetes mellitus, and hyperglycemia have been reported during postmarketing surveillance in HIV-infected patients receiving protease inhibitor therapy. Some patients required either initiation or dose adjustments of insulin or oral hypoglycemic agents for treatment of these events. In some cases, diabetic ketoacidosis has occurred. In those patients who discontinued protease inhibitor therapy, hyperglycemia persisted in some cases. Because these events have been reported voluntarily during clinical practice, estimates of frequency cannot be made, and causal relationships between protease inhibitor therapy and these events have not been established.

➤*Hepatic function impairment:* Amprenavir is principally metabolized by the liver. Amprenavir, when used alone and in combination with low-dose ritonavir, has been associated with elevations of AST and ALT in some patients. Caution should be exercised when administering amprenavir to patients with hepatic impairment.

Appropriate laboratory testing should be conducted prior to initiating therapy with amprenavir and at periodic intervals during treatment.

Capsules – See Administration and Dosage for more information.

Oral solution – See Administration and Dosage for more information.

➤*Carcinogenesis:* Amprenavir was evaluated for carcinogenic potential by oral gavage administration to mice and rats for up to 104 weeks. Daily doses of 50, 275 to 300, and 500 to 600 mg/kg/day were administered to mice and doses of 50, 190, and 750 mg/kg/day were administered to rats. Results showed an increase in the incidence of benign hepatocellular adenomas and an increase in the combined incidence of hepatocellular adenomas plus carcinoma in males of both species at the highest doses tested. Female mice and rats were not affected. These observations were made at systemic exposures equivalent to approximately 2 times (mice) and 4 times (rats) the human exposure (based on $AUC_{0\text{-}24\,hr}$ measurement) at the recommended dose of 1,200 mg twice daily. Administration of amprenavir did not cause a statistically significant increase in the incidence of any other benign or malignant neoplasm in mice or rats. It is not known how predictive the results of rodent carcinogenicity studies may be for humans.

➤*Elderly:* Clinical studies of amprenavir did not include sufficient numbers of patients aged 65 and over to determine whether they respond differently from younger adults. In general, dose selection for an elderly patient should be cautious, reflecting the greater frequency of decreased hepatic, renal, or cardiac function, and of concomitant disease or other drug therapy.

➤*Pregnancy: Category C.*

Embryo/fetal development studies were conducted in rats (dosed from 15 days before pairing to day 17 of gestation) and rabbits (dosed from day 8 to day 20 of gestation). In pregnant rabbits, amprenavir administration was associated with abortions and an increased incidence of 3 minor skeletal variations resulting from deficient ossification of the femur, humerus trochlea, and humerus. Systemic exposure at the highest tested dose was approximately one-twentieth of the exposure seen at the recommended human dose. In rat fetuses, thymic elongation and incomplete ossification of bones were attributed to amprenavir. Both findings were seen at systemic exposures that were one half of that associated with the recommended human dose.

Pre- and postnatal development studies were performed in rats dosed from day 7 of gestation to day 22 of lactation. Reduced body weights (10% to 20%) were observed in the offspring. The systemic exposure associated with this finding was approximately twice the exposure in humans following administration of the recommended human dose. The subsequent development of these offspring, including fertility and reproductive performance, was not affected by the maternal administration of amprenavir.

There are no adequate and well-controlled studies in pregnant women. Amprenavir should be used during pregnancy only if the potential benefit justifies the potential risk to the fetus.

Amprenavir oral solution is contraindicated during pregnancy due to the potential risk of toxicity to the fetus from the high propylene glycol content. Therefore, if amprenavir is used in pregnant women, the amprenavir capsule formulation should be used.

Antiretroviral pregnancy registry – To monitor maternal-fetus outcomes of pregnant women exposed to amprenavir, an antiretroviral pregnancy registry has been established. Physicians are encouraged to register patients by calling 1-800-258-4263.

➤*Lactation:* The Centers for Disease Control and Prevention recommended that HIV-infected mothers not breastfeed their infants to avoid risking postnatal transmission of HIV. Although it is not known if amprenavir is excreted in human milk, amprenavir is secreted into the milk of lactating rats. Because of both the potential for HIV transmission and the potential for serious adverse reactions in nursing infants, mothers should be instructed not to breastfeed if they are receiving amprenavir.

➤*Children:* Amprenavir capsules have not been evaluated in pediatric patients below 4 years of age.

Amprenavir oral solution is contraindicated in infants and children below the age of 4 years due to the potential risk of toxicity from the excipient, propylene glycol. Alcohol dehydrogenase (ADH), which metabolizes propylene glycol, is present in the human fetal liver at 2 months of gestational age, but at only 3% of adult activity. Although the data are limited, it appears that by 12 to 30 months of postnatal age, ADH activity is equal to or greater than that observed in adults.

Precautions

➤*Monitoring:* Amprenavir is principally metabolized by the liver. Amprenavir, when used alone and in combination with low-dose ritonavir, has been associated with elevations of AST and ALT in some patients. Caution should be exercised when administering amprenavir to patients with hepatic impairment. Appropriate laboratory testing should be conducted prior to initiating therapy with amprenavir and at periodic intervals during treatment.

If patients require treatment with amprenavir oral solution, they should be monitored closely for propylene glycol-associated adverse events, including seizures, stupor, tachycardia, hyperosmolality, lactic acidosis, renal toxicity, and hemolysis. Patients should be switched from amprenavir oral solution to amprenavir capsules as soon as they are able to take the capsule formulation.

The combination of amprenavir and low-dose ritonavir has been associated with elevations of cholesterol and triglycerides, AST, and ALT in some patients. Appropriate laboratory testing should be considered prior to initiating combination therapy with amprenavir and ritonavir and at periodic intervals or if any clinical signs or symptoms of hyperlipidemia or elevated liver function tests occur during therapy. For comprehensive information concerning laboratory test alterations associated with ritonavir, refer to the complete monograph for ritonavir.

➤*Doseform interchangeability:* Amprenavir capsules and amprenavir oral solution are not interchangeable on a milligram-per-milligram basis. Amprenavir oral solution was 14% less bioavailable compared to the capsules.

➤*Vitamin E:* Formulations of amprenavir provide high daily doses of vitamin E. The effects of long-term, high-dose vitamin E administration in humans is not well characterized and has not been specifically studied in HIV-infected individuals. High vitamin E doses may exacerbate the blood coagulation defect of vitamin K deficiency caused by anticoagulant therapy or malabsorption.

➤*Hemophilics:* There have been reports of spontaneous bleeding in patients with hemophilia A and B treated with protease inhibitors. In some patients, additional factor VIII was required. In many of the reported cases, treatment with protease inhibitors was continued or restarted. A causal relationship between protease inhibitor therapy and these episodes has not been established.

➤*Fat redistribution:* Redistribution/accumulation of body fat, including central obesity, dorsocervical fat enlargement (buffalo hump), peripheral wasting, facial wasting, breast enlargement, and "cushingoid appearance," have been observed in patients receiving antiretroviral therapy. The mechanism and long-term consequences of these events are currently unknown. A causal relationship has not been established.

AMPRENAVIR — ORAL

➤*Lipid elevations:* Treatment with amprenavir alone or in combination with ritonavir has resulted in increases in the concentration of total cholesterol and triglycerides. Triglyceride and cholesterol testing should be performed prior to initiation of therapy with amprenavir and at periodic intervals during treatment. Lipid disorders should be managed as clinically appropriate.

➤*Resistance/cross-resistance:* Because the potential for HIV cross-resistance among protease inhibitors has not been fully explored, it is unknown what effect amprenavir therapy will have on the activity of subsequently administered protease inhibitors. It is also unknown what effect previous treatment with other protease inhibitors will have on the activity of amprenavir.

➤*Sulfite sensitivity:* Amprenavir is a sulfonamide. The potential for cross-sensitivity between drugs in the sulfonamide class and amprenavir is unknown. Amprenavir should be used with caution in patients with a known sulfonamide allergy.

Drug Interactions

Amprenavir Drug Interactions

Precipitant drug	Object drug[a]		Description
Abacavir	Amprenavir	↑	Concurrent use may increase amprenavir's C_{max}, AUC, and C_{min}.
Aldesleukin	Amprenavir	↑	Amprenavir concentration may be elevated.
Antacids	Amprenavir	↓	It is advisable that antacids not be taken at the same time as amprenavir because of potential interference with absorption. Take amprenavir at least 1 hour before or after antacids.
Anticonvulsants Carbamazepine Phenobarbital Phenytoin	Amprenavir	↓	Carbamazepine, phenobarbital, and phenytoin induce CYP3A4 and may decrease amprenavir concentrations. Amprenavir may increase carbamazepine plasma concentrations.
Amprenavir	Anticonvulsants Carbamazepine	↑	
Azole antifungals Fluconazole Itraconazole Ketoconazole	Amprenavir	↑↓	Itraconazole may increase amprenavir serum concentrations, and ketoconazole may increase amprenavir's AUC and decrease its C_{max}. Amprenavir may increase ketoconazole's C_{max} and AUC. Dose reduction of ketoconazole or itraconazole may be needed for patients receiving more than 400 mg of ketoconazole or itraconazole per day.
Amprenavir	Azole antifungals Ketoconazole	↑	
Clarithromycin	Amprenavir	↑	Clarithromycin may increase amprenavir's C_{max}, AUC, and C_{min}. Concurrent use may slightly decrease clarithromycin's C_{max}.
Amprenavir	Clarithromycin	↓	
Contraceptives, oral	Amprenavir	↓	Concurrent use of amprenavir with ethinyl estradiol/norethindrone may decrease amprenavir's AUC and C_{min} and also increase the AUC and C_{min} of the oral contraceptive. Alternative methods of nonhormonal contraception are recommended.
Amprenavir	Contraceptives, oral	↑	
Cyclosporine Tacrolimus	Amprenavir	↑	The concentration of the immunosuppressant may be increased. Monitor therapeutic concentration. Protease inhibitor concentrations also may be increased. Monitor the clinical response to the protease inhibitor.
Amprenavir	Cyclosporine		
Dexamethasone	Amprenavir	↓	Use with caution. Amprenavir concentrations may be decreased.
Didanosine (buffered formulation only)	Amprenavir	↓	Coadministration may decrease amprenavir concentrations. Take amprenavir at least 1 hour before or after the buffered formulation of didanosine.
Disulfiram Metronidazole	Amprenavir (oral solution)	↑	Coadministration is contraindicated because of the potential risk for toxicity from the large amount of the excipient, propylene glycol, in the amprenavir oral solution.
Ethanol	Amprenavir (oral solution)	↑	Concurrent use is not recommended because the large amount of propylene glycol and ethanol may compete for the same metabolic pathway for elimination.
Indinavir	Amprenavir	↑	Concurrent use may increase amprenavir's C_{max}, AUC, and C_{min}, and decrease indinavir's C_{max}, AUC, and C_{min}.
Amprenavir	Indinavir	↓	
Methadone	Amprenavir	↓	Amprenavir plasma concentrations may be decreased; consider alternate antiretroviral therapy. Methadone plasma concentrations may be decreased; therefore, the dosage of methadone may need to be increased.
Amprenavir	Methadone		
Nelfinavir	Amprenavir	↔	Concurrent use may decrease amprenavir's C_{max} and increase its C_{min}, and nelfinavir's C_{max}, AUC, and C_{min} may be increased.
Amprenavir	Nelfinavir	↑	
NNRTIs Delavirdine Efavirenz Nevirapine	Amprenavir	↑↓	NNRTIs have the potential to increase (delavirdine) or decrease (efavirenz, nevirapine) amprenavir serum concentrations. Delavirdine serum concentrations may be decreased when given with amprenavir. Do not coadminister delavirdine with amprenavir.
Amprenavir	NNRTIs Delavirdine	↓	
Rifamycins Rifampin Rifabutin	Amprenavir	↓	Coadministration with rifabutin results in a 15% decrease in amprenavir AUC and a 193% increase in rifabutin AUC. A dose reduction of rifabutin to at least half the recommended dose is required during concurrent use. Perform a weekly complete blood count and as clinically indicated to monitor for neutropenia. Do not coadminister rifampin because it reduces amprenavir C_{max} 70% and AUC 82%.
Amprenavir	Rifamycins Rifabutin	↑	
Ritonavir	Amprenavir	↑	Concurrent use may increase amprenavir's AUC and C_{min} and decrease ritonavir's C_{max}, AUC, and C_{min}. Reduce the amprenavir capsule dose when given with ritonavir capsules (see Administration and Dosage). Concurrent use of amprenavir oral solution and ritonavir oral solution is not recommended (see Warnings).
Amprenavir	Ritonavir	↓	
Saquinavir	Amprenavir	↓	Concurrent use may decrease amprenavir's C_{max}, AUC, and C_{min}, and increase saquinavir's C_{max} and decrease its AUC and C_{min}.
Amprenavir	Saquinavir	↑↓	
St. John's wort	Amprenavir	↓	St. John's wort may increase the metabolism (CYP3A4) of amprenavir, thus decreasing the concentration and clinical efficacy of amprenavir. Concurrent use is not recommended.
Zidovudine	Amprenavir	↑	Concurrent use may increase amprenavir's AUC and zidovudine's C_{max} and AUC.
Amprenavir	Zidovudine		
Amprenavir	Antiarrhythmics Amiodarone Lidocaine (systemic) Quinidine	↑	Serious and/or life-threatening interactions can occur between amprenavir and amiodarone, lidocaine, or quinidine. Concentration monitoring is recommended.

AMPRENAVIR — ORAL

Amprenavir Drug Interactions			
Precipitant drug	Object drug[a]		Description
Amprenavir	Benzodiazepines	↑	Do not use amprenavir and midazolam or triazolam concurrently. Coadministration may result in competitive inhibition of these benzodiazepines and cause serious and/or life-threatening adverse reactions. Alprazolam, clorazepate, diazepam, and flurazepam may have increased serum concentrations, which could increase their activity.
Amprenavir	Calcium channel blockers	↑	The concentrations of amlodipine, diltiazem, felodipine, isradipine, nifedipine, nicardipine, nimodipine, nisoldipine, or verapamil may be increased when given with amprenavir.
Amprenavir	Cisapride	↑	Do not use concurrently. Coadministration may result in increased cisapride concentrations and cause serious and/or life-threatening adverse reactions, such as cardiac arrhythmias.
Amprenavir	Ergot alkaloids	↑	Contraindicated because of potential for serious and/or life-threatening reactions such as acute ergot toxicity characterized by peripheral vasospasm and ischemia of the extremities and other tissues.
Amprenavir	Fentanyl	↑	Fentanyl plasma concentrations may be increased and the half-life prolonged. Monitor closely; dosage reduction may be needed.
Amprenavir	HMG-CoA reductase inhibitors Atorvastatin Lovastatin Simvastatin	↑	Amprenavir may increase serum concentrations of atorvastatin, lovastatin, and simvastatin, which could increase their toxicity, such as myopathy, including rhabdomyolysis. Use the lowest possible dose of atorvastatin with careful monitoring. Do not coadminister lovastatin and simvastatin with amprenavir.
Amprenavir	Pimozide	↑	Contraindicated because of potential for serious and/or life-threatening reactions such as cardiac arrhythmias.
Amprenavir	Phosphodiesterase type 5 inhibitors Sildenafil Tadalafil Vardenafil	↑	Amprenavir may inhibit sildenafil's metabolism (CYP3A4), increasing the concentration of sildenafil and possibly resulting in severe and potentially fatal hypotension. Use sildenafil with caution at reduced doses of 25 mg every 48 hours with increased monitoring. Similar effects are expected with tadalafil and vardenafil, and dosage modifications are needed.
Amprenavir	Trazodone	↑	Trazodone plasma concentrations may be elevated. Monitor closely and adjust trazodone dosage as needed.
Amprenavir	Tricyclic antidepressants Amitriptyline Imipramine	↑	Concentrations of the tricyclic antidepressant may be increased. Therapeutic concentration monitoring is recommended.
Amprenavir	Warfarin	↔	Plasma warfarin concentrations may be affected. Coadministration requires monitoring of international normalized ratio (INR).

[a] ↑ = Object drug increased. ↓ = Object drug decreased.
↔ = Undetermined clinical effect.

Amprenavir is an inhibitor of cytochrome P450 3A4 metabolism and therefore should not be administered concurrently with medications with narrow therapeutic windows that are substrates of CYP3A4. There are other agents that may result in serious or life-threatening drug interactions.

Adverse Reactions

In clinical studies, adverse reactions leading to amprenavir discontinuation occurred primarily during the first 12 weeks of therapy, and were mostly due to GI events (nausea, vomiting, diarrhea, and abdominal pain/discomfort), which were mild to moderate in severity.

➤*Dermatologic:* Skin rash occurred in 22% of patients treated with amprenavir in studies PROAB3001 and PROAB3006. Rashes were usually maculopapular and of mild or moderate intensity, some with pruritus. Rashes had a median onset of 11 days after amprenavir initiation and a median duration of 10 days. Skin rashes led to amprenavir discontinuation in approximately 3% of patients. In some patients with mild or moderate rash, amprenavir dosing was often continued without interruption; if interrupted, reintroduction of amprenavir generally did not result in rash recurrence.

Severe or life-threatening rash (grade 3 or 4), including cases of Stevens-Johnson syndrome, occurred in approximately 1% of recipients of amprenavir. Amprenavir therapy should be discontinued for severe or life-threatening rashes and for moderate rashes accompanied by systemic symptoms.

Selected clinical adverse events of all grades reported in > 5% of adult patients				
	PROAB3001 therapy-naive patients		PROAB3006 NRTI-experienced patients	
Adverse reaction	Amprenavir*/ lamivudine/ zidovudine (n = 113)	Lamivudine/ zidovudine (n = 109)	Amprenavir*/ NRTI (n = 245)	Indinavir/ NRTI (n = 241)
GI				
Nausea	74%	50%	43%	35%
Vomiting	34%	17%	24%	20%
Diarrhea or loose stools	39%	35%	60%	41%
Taste disorders	10%	6%	2%	8%
Dermatologic				
Rash	27%	6%	20%	15%
CNS				
Paresthesia, oral/ erioral	26%	6%	31%	2%
Paresthesia, peripheral	10%	4%	14%	10%
Psychiatric				
Depressive or mood disorders	16%	4%	9%	13%

* Amprenavir capsules.

➤*Miscellaneous:* Among amprenavir-treated patients in phase 3 studies, 2 patients developed de novo diabetes mellitus, 1 patient developed a dorsocervical fat enlargement (buffalo hump), and 9 patients developed fat redistribution.

➤*Children:* An adverse event profile similar to that seen in adults was seen in pediatric patients.

➤*Concomitant therapy with ritonavir:* The following tables present adverse clinical events and laboratory abnormalities observed in subjects who received amprenavir plus ritonavir. Since the trials were small, open-label, of varying duration, and often included different patient populations, direct comparison to the frequency of events with amprenavir capsules alone cannot be made.

Selected clinical adverse events of all grades reported in adult patients in open-label clinical trials of amprenavir capsules in combination with ritonavir		
Adverse event	Amprenavir 1,200 mg plus ritonavir 200 mg daily* (n = 101)	Amprenavir 600 mg plus ritonavir 100 mg twice daily[1] (n = 239)
Nausea	31%	23%
Diarrhea/loose stools	30%	28%
Headache	16%	12%
Abdominal symptoms	14%	14%
Vomiting	11%	9%
Rash	10%	9%
Paresthesias	9%	11%
Fatigue	7%	14%
Depressive and mood disorders	4%	9%

* Data from 2 open-label studies in treatment-naive patients also receiving abacavir/ lamivudine.
[1] Data from 3 open-label studies in treatment-naive patients and treatment-experienced patients receiving combination antiretroviral therapy.

AMPRENAVIR — ORAL

➤*Lab test abnormalities:*

Grade 3/4 laboratory abnormalities reported in ≥ 2% of adult patients in open-label clinical trials of amprenavir capsules in combination with ritonavir		
Laboratory abnormality (non-fasting specimens)	Amprenavir 1,200 mg plus ritonavir 200 mg daily* (n = 101)	Amprenavir 600 mg plus ritonavir 100 mg twice daily[1] (n = 239)
Hypertriglyceridemia (> 750 mg/dL)	8%	13%
Hyperglycemia (> 251 mg/dL)	2%	3%
AST (> 5 × ULN)	3%	5%
ALT (> 5 × ULN)	4%	4%
Amylase (> 2 × ULN)	4%	3%

* Data from 2 open-label studies in treatment-naive patients also receiving abacavir/lamivudine.
[1] Data from 3 open-label studies in treatment-naive and treatment-experienced patients receiving combination antiretroviral therapy.

Overdosage

➤*Treatment:* There is no known antidote for amprenavir. It is not known whether amprenavir can be removed by peritoneal dialysis or hemodialysis. If overdosage occurs, the patient should be monitored for evidence of toxicity and standard supportive treatment should be applied as necessary.

Amprenavir oral solution contains large amounts of propylene glycol. In the event of overdosage, monitoring and management of acid-base abnormalities is recommended. Propylene glycol can be removed by hemodialysis.

Patient Information

➤*Alert:* Find out about medicines that should not be taken with amprenavir.

Patients treated with amprenavir capsules should be cautioned against switching to amprenavir oral solution because of the increased risk of adverse events from the large amount of propylene glycol in amprenavir oral solution.

Patients should be informed that amprenavir is not a cure for HIV infection and that they may continue to develop opportunistic infections and other complications associated with HIV disease. The long-term effects of amprenavir are unknown at this time. Patients should be told that there are currently no data demonstrating that therapy with amprenavir can reduce the risk of transmitting HIV to others through sexual contact.

Patients should remain under the care of their physicians while using amprenavir. Patients should be advised to take amprenavir every day as prescribed. Amprenavir must always be used in combination with other antiretroviral drugs.

Patients should not alter their doses or discontinue therapy without consulting their physicians. If a dose is missed, the patient should take the dose as soon as possible and then return to his normal schedule. However, if a dose is skipped, the patient should not double the next dose.

Patients should inform their doctors if they have sulfa allergies. The potential for cross-sensitivity between drugs in the sulfonamide class and amprenavir is unknown.

Amprenavir may interact with many drugs; therefore, patients should be advised to report to their doctors the use of any other prescription or nonprescription medication or herbal products, particularly St. John's wort.

Patients taking antacids (or the buffered formulation of didanosine) should take amprenavir at least 1 hour before or after antacid (or the buffered formulation of didanosine) use.

Patients receiving sildenafil should be advised that they may be at an increased risk of sildenafil-associated adverse events, including hypotension, visual changes, and priapism, and should promptly report any symptoms to their doctors.

Patients taking amprenavir should be instructed not to use hormonal contraceptives because some birth control pills (those containing ethinyl estradiol/norethindrone) have been found to decrease the concentration of amprenavir. Therefore, patients receiving hormonal contraceptives should be instructed to use alternate contraceptive measures during therapy with amprenavir.

High-fat meals may decrease the absorption of amprenavir and should be avoided. Amprenavir may be taken with meals of normal fat content.

Patients should be informed that redistribution or accumulation of body fat may occur in patients receiving antiretroviral therapy and that the cause and long-term health effects of these conditions are not known at this time.

Adult and pediatric patients should be advised not to take supplemental vitamin E since the vitamin E content of amprenavir capsules and oral solution exceeds the Reference Daily Intake (adults 30 IU, pediatrics approximately 10 IU).

➤*Oral solution:* Amprenavir oral solution is contraindicated in infants and children below the age of 4 years, pregnant women, patients with hepatic or renal failure, and patients treated with disulfiram or metronidazole. Amprenavir oral solution should be used only when amprenavir capsules or other protease inhibitor formulations are not therapeutic options.

Women, Asian patients, Eskimo patients, or Native American patients, as well as patients who have hepatic or renal insufficiency, should be informed that they may be at increased risk of adverse events from the large amount of propylene glycol in amprenavir oral solution.

Patients should be informed that amprenavir is not a cure for HIV infection and that they may continue to develop opportunistic infections and other complications associated with HIV disease. The long-term effects of amprenavir are unknown at this time. Patients should be told that there are currently no data demonstrating that therapy with amprenavir can reduce the risk of transmitting HIV to others through sexual contact.

Patients should be advised that drinking alcoholic beverages is not recommended while taking amprenavir oral solution.

ATAZANAVIR SULFATE

Rx	**Reyataz** (Bristol-Myers Squibb)	**Capsules:** 100 mg (as base)	Lactose, alcohols, simethicone. (BMS 100 mg 3623). Blue/White. In 60s.
		150 mg (as base)	Lactose, alcohols, simethicone. (BMS 150 mg 3624). Blue/Powder blue. In 60s.
		200 mg (as base)	Lactose, alcohols, simethicone. (BMS 200 mg 3631). Blue. In 60s.

ATAZANAVIR SULFATE — ORAL

Indications

➤*HIV infection:* In combination with other antiretroviral agents for the treatment of HIV-1 infection.

Administration and Dosage

➤*Approved by the FDA:* June 20, 2003.

Atazanavir capsules must be taken with food.

➤*Therapy-naive patients:* Atazanavir 400 mg (two 200 mg capsules) once daily taken with food.

➤*Therapy-experienced patients:* Atazanavir 300 mg (two 150 mg capsules) once daily plus ritonavir 100 mg once daily taken with food.

Atazanavir without ritonavir is not recommended for treatment-experienced patients with prior virologic failure.

Safety and efficacy of atazanavir with ritonavir in doses greater than 100 mg once daily have not been established. The use of higher ritonavir doses might alter the safety profile of atazanavir (eg, cardiac effects, hyperbilirubinemia) and, therefore, is not recommended. Prescribers should consult the complete monograph for ritonavir when using this agent.

➤*Concomitant therapy:*

– Important dosing information: Efavirenz. In treatment-naive patients who receive efavirenz and atazanavir, the recommended dose is atazanavir 300 mg with ritonavir 100 mg and efavirenz 600 mg (all once daily). Dosing recommendations for efavirenz and atazanavir in treatment-experienced patients have not been established.

Didanosine – When coadministered with didanosine-buffered formulations, give atazanavir (with food) 2 hours before or 1 hour after didanosine.

Tenofovir disoproxil fumarate – When coadministered with tenofovir, it is recommended that atazanavir 300 mg be given with ritonavir 100 mg and tenofovir 300 mg (all as a single daily dose with food). Atazanavir without ritonavir should not be coadministered with tenofovir.

Indinavir – Both atazanavir and indinavir are associated with indirect (unconjugated) indinavir hyperbilirubinemia. Coadministration of atazanavir and indinavir is not recommended.

Nevirapine – Nevirapine is expected to decrease atazanavir exposure. Coadministration is not recommended.

Ritonavir – If atazanavir is coadministered with ritonavir, it is recommended that atazanavir 300 mg once daily be given with ritonavir 100 mg once daily with food.

Other protease inhibitors – The coadministration of atazanavir/ritonavir and other protease inhibitors would be expected to increase exposure to the other protease inhibitor. Such coadministration is not recommended.

➤*Hepatic function impairment:* Use atazanavir with caution in patients with mild to moderate hepatic impairment. For patients with moderate hepatic impairment (Child-Pugh class B) who have not experienced prior virologic failure, consider a dose reduction to 300 mg once daily. Do not use atazanavir in patients with severe hepatic impairment (Child-Pugh class C). Atazanavir/ritonavir has not been studied in subjects with hepatic impairment and is not recommended.

➤*Storage/Stability:* Store atazanavir capsules at 25°C (77°F); excursions permitted to 15° to 30°C (59° to 86°F).

ATAZANAVIR SULFATE — ORAL

Actions

➤*Pharmacology:* Atazanavir is an azapeptide HIV-1 protease inhibitor. The compound selectively inhibits the virus-specific processing of viral Gag and Gag-Pol polyproteins in HIV-1 infected cells, thus preventing formation of mature virions.

➤*Pharmacokinetics:*

Absorption – Atazanavir is rapidly absorbed with a T_{max} of approximately 2.5 hours. Atazanavir demonstrates nonlinear pharmacokinetics with greater than dose-proportional increases in AUC and C_{max} values over the dose range of 200 to 800 mg once daily. Steady state is achieved between days 4 and 8, with an accumulation of approximately 2.3 fold.

Administration of atazanavir with food enhances bioavailability and reduces pharmacokinetic variability. Administration of a single atazanavir 400 mg dose with a light meal (357 kcal, 8.2 g fat, 10.6 g protein) resulted in a 70% increase in AUC and 57% increase in C_{max} relative to the fasting state. Administration of a single atazanavir 400 mg dose with a high-fat meal (721 kcal, 37.3 g fat, 29.4 g protein) resulted in a mean increase in AUC of 35% with no change in C_{max} relative to the fasting state. Administration of atazanavir with either a light meal or high-fat meal decreased the coefficient of variation of AUC and C_{max} by approximately one half compared with the fasting state.

Distribution – Atazanavir is 86% bound to human serum proteins, and protein binding is independent of concentration. Atazanavir binds to both alpha-1-acid glycoprotein (AAG) and albumin to a similar extent (89% and 86%, respectively). In a multiple-dose study in HIV-infected patients dosed with atazanavir 400 mg once daily with a light meal for 12 weeks, atazanavir was detected in the cerebrospinal fluid and semen. The cerebrospinal fluid/plasma ratio for atazanavir (n = 4) ranged between 0.0021 and 0.0226 and seminal fluid/plasma ratio (n = 5) ranged between 0.11 and 4.42.

Metabolism – Atazanavir is extensively metabolized in humans. The major biotransformation pathways of atazanavir in humans consisted of monooxygenation and dioxygenation. Other minor biotransformation pathways for atazanavir or its metabolites consisted of glucuronidation, N-dealkylation, hydrolysis, and oxygenation with dehydrogenation. Two minor metabolites of atazanavir in plasma have been characterized. Neither metabolite demonstrated in vitro antiviral activity. In vitro studies using human liver microsomes suggested that atazanavir is metabolized by CYP3A.

Excretion – Following a single 400 mg dose of ^{14}C-atazanavir, 79% and 13% of the total radioactivity was recovered in the feces and urine, respectively. Unchanged drug accounted for approximately 20% and 7% of the administered dose in the feces and urine, respectively. The mean elimination half-life of atazanavir in healthy volunteers (n = 214) and HIV-infected adult patients (n = 13) was approximately 7 hours at steady state following a dose of 400 mg daily with a light meal.

Steady-State Pharmacokinetics of Atazanavir in Healthy Subjects or HIV-Infected Patients in the Fed State

Parameter	400 mg once daily		300 mg with 100 mg ritonavir once daily	
	Healthy subjects (n = 14)	HIV-infected patients (n = 13)	Healthy subjects (n = 28)	HIV-infected patients (n = 10)
C_{max} (ng/mL)				
Geometric mean (CV%)	5,199 (26%)	2,298 (71%)	6,129 (31%)	4,422 (58%)
Mean (SD)	5,358 (1,371)	3,152 (2,231)	6,450 (2,031)	5,233 (3,033)
T_{max} (h)				
Median	2.5	2	2.7	3
AUC (ng•h/mL)				
Geometric mean (CV%)	28,132 (28%)	14,874 (91%)	57,039 (37%)	46,073 (66%)
Mean (SD)	29,303 (8,263)	22,262 (20,159)	61,435 (22,911)	53,761 (35,294)
$t_{½}$ (h)				
Mean (SD)	7.9 (2.9)	6.5 (2.6)	18.1 (6.2)[a]	8.6 (2.3)
C_{min} (ng/mL)				
Geometric mean (CV%)	159 (88%)	120 (109%)	1,227 (53%)	636 (97%)
Mean (SD)	218 (191)	273 (298)[b]	1,441 (757)	862 (838)

[a] (n = 26). [b] (n = 12).

Special populations –

Hepatic function impairment: Atazanavir is metabolized and eliminated primarily by the liver. Atazanavir has been studied in adult subjects with moderate to severe hepatic impairment (14 Child-Pugh B and 2 Child-Pugh C subjects) after a single 400 mg dose. The mean $AUC_{(0-\infty)}$ was 42% greater in subjects with impaired hepatic function than in healthy volunteers. The mean half-life of atazanavir in hepatically impaired subjects was 12.1 hours compared with 6.4 hours in healthy volunteers. Increased concentrations of atazanavir are expected in patients with moderately or severely impaired hepatic function. The pharmacokinetics of atazanavir in combination with ritonavir have not been studied in subjects with hepatic impairment.

Electrocardiogram (EKG) – Concentration- and dose-dependent prolongation of the PR interval in the EKG has been observed in healthy volunteers receiving atazanavir. In a placebo-controlled study (AI424-076), the mean (± SD) maximum change in PR interval from the predose value was 24 (± 15) msec following oral dosing with atazanavir 400 mg (n = 65) compared with 13 (± 11) msec following dosing with placebo (n = 67). The PR interval prolongations in this study were asymptomatic. There is limited information on the potential for a pharmacodynamic interaction in humans between atazanavir and other drugs that prolong the PR interval of the EKG.

➤*Microbiology:*

Antiviral activity in vitro – Atazanavir exhibits anti-HIV-1 activity with a mean 50% inhibitory concentration (IC_{50}) in the absence of human serum of 2 to 5 nM against a variety of laboratory and clinical HIV-1 isolates grown in peripheral blood mononuclear cells, macrophages, CEM-SS cells, and MT-2 cells. Two-drug combination studies with atazanavir showed additive to antagonistic antiviral activity in vitro with abacavir and the NNRTIs (delavirdine, efavirenz, and nevirapine) and additive antiviral activity in vitro with the protease inhibitors (amprenavir, indinavir, lopinavir, nelfinavir, ritonavir, and saquinavir), NRTIs (didanosine, emtricitabine, lamivudine, stavudine, tenofovir, zalcitabine, and zidovudine), the HIV-1 fusion inhibitor enfuvirtide, and 2 compounds used in the treatment of viral hepatitis, adefovir and ribavirin, without enhanced cytotoxicity.

Resistance –

In vitro: HIV-1 isolates with a decreased susceptibility to atazanavir have been selected in vitro and obtained from patients treated with atazanavir or atazanavir/ritonavir. HIV-1 isolates that were 93- to 183-fold resistant to atazanavir from 3 different viral strains were selected in vitro by 5 months. The mutations in these HIV-1 viruses that contributed to atazanavir resistance included I50L, N88S, I84V, A71V, and M46I. Changes were also observed at the protease cleavage sites following drug selection. Recombinant viruses containing the I50L mutation were growth impaired and displayed increased in vitro susceptibility to other protease inhibitors (amprenavir, indinavir, lopinavir, nelfinavir, ritonavir, and saquinavir). The I50L and I50V substitutions yielded selective resistance to atazanavir and amprenavir, respectively, and did not appear to be cross-resistant.

Clinical studies of treatment-experienced patients: In contrast, from studies of treatment-experienced patients treated with atazanavir or atazanavir/ritonavir, most atazanavir-resistant isolates from patients who experienced virologic failure developed mutations that were associated with resistance to multiple protease inhibitors and displayed decreased susceptibility to multiple protease inhibitors. The most common protease mutations to develop in the viral isolates of patients who failed treatment with atazanavir 300 mg once daily and ritonavir 100 mg once daily (together with tenofovir and an NRTI) included V32I, L33F/V/I, E35D/G, M46I/L, I50L, F53L/V, I54V, A71V/T/I, G73S/T/C, V82A/T/L, I85V, and L89V/Q/M/T. Other mutations that developed on atazanavir/ritonavir treatment including E34K/A/Q, G48V, I84V, N88S/D/T, and L90M occurred in less than 10% of patient isolates. Generally, if multiple protease inhibitor resistance mutations were present in the HIV-1 of the patient at baseline, atazanavir resistance developed through mutations associated with resistance to other protease inhibitors and could include the development of the I50L mutation.

Cross-resistance – Cross-resistance among protease inhibitors has been observed. Baseline phenotypic and genotypic analyses of clinical isolates from atazanavir clinical trials of protease inhibitor-experienced subjects showed that isolates cross-resistant to multiple protease inhibitors were cross-resistant to atazanavir. Greater than 90% of the isolates with mutations that included I84V or G48V were resistant to atazanavir. Greater than 60% of isolates containing L90M, G73S/T/C, A71V/T, I54V, M46I/L, or a change at V82 were resistant to atazanavir, and 38% of isolates containing a D30N mutation in addition to other changes were resistant to atazanavir. Isolates resistant to atazanavir were also cross-resistant to other protease inhibitors with greater than 90% of the isolates resistant to indinavir, lopinavir, nelfinavir, ritonavir, and saquinavir, and 80% resistant to amprenavir. In treatment-experienced patients, protease inhibitor-resistant viral isolates that developed the I50L mutation in addition to other protease inhibitor resistance-associated mutations were also cross-resistant to other protease inhibitors.

Contraindications

Hypersensitivity to any ingredients, including atazanavir.

Coadministration of atazanavir is contraindicated with the following drugs that are highly dependent on CYP3A for clearance and for which elevated plasma concentrations are associated with serious and/or life-threatening events. These drugs are listed in the table below:

Drugs that are Contraindicated with Atazanavir Due to Potential P450-Mediated Interactions

Drug class	Drugs within class that are contraindicated with atazanavir
Benzodiazepines	Midazolam, triazolam
Ergot derivatives	Dihydroergotamine, ergotamine, ergonovine, methylergonovine
GI motility agent	Cisapride
Neuroleptic	Pimozide

ATAZANAVIR SULFATE — ORAL

Warnings

➤*PR interval prolongation:* Atazanavir has been shown to prolong the PR interval of the EKG in some patients. In healthy volunteers and in patients, abnormalities in atrioventricular (AV) conduction were asymptomatic and generally limited to first-degree AV block. There have been rare reports of second-degree AV block and other conduction abnormalities and no reports of third-degree AV block. In clinical trials, asymptomatic first-degree AV block was observed in 5.9% of atazanavir-treated patients (n = 920), 5.2% of lopinavir/ritonavir-treated patients (n = 252), 10.4% of nelfinavir-treated patients (n = 48), and 3% of efavirenz-treated patients (n = 329). In Study AI424-045, asymptomatic first-degree AV block was observed in 5% (6/118) of atazanavir/ritonavir-treated patients and 5% (6/116) of lopinavir/ritonavir-treated patients who had on-study EKG measurements. Because of limited clinical experience, use atazanavir with caution in patients with preexisting conduction system disease (eg, marked first-degree AV block or second- or third-degree AV block).

See Drug Interactions for more information.

➤*Diabetes mellitus/Hyperglycemia:* New-onset diabetes mellitus, exacerbation of preexisting diabetes mellitus, and hyperglycemia have been reported during postmarketing surveillance in HIV-infected patients receiving protease inhibitor therapy. Some patients required either initiation or dose adjustments of insulin or oral hypoglycemic agents for treatment of these events. In some cases, diabetic ketoacidosis has occurred. In those patients who discontinued protease inhibitor therapy, hyperglycemia persisted in some cases. Because these events have been reported voluntarily during clinical practice, estimates of frequency cannot be made and a causal relationship between protease inhibitor therapy and these events has not been established.

➤*Hepatic function impairment:* Atazanavir is principally metabolized by the liver; exercise caution when administering this drug to patients with hepatic impairment because atazanavir concentrations may be increased. Patients with underlying hepatitis B or C viral infections or marked elevations in transaminases prior to treatment may be at increased risk for developing further transaminase elevations or hepatic decompensation. There are no clinical trial data on the use of atazanavir/ritonavir in patients with any degree of hepatic impairment.

➤*Carcinogenesis:* Long-term carcinogenicity studies of atazanavir in animals have not been completed. Atazanavir tested positive in an in vitro clastogenicity test using primary human lymphocytes, in the absence and presence of metabolic activation.

➤*Elderly:* In general, exercise appropriate caution in the administration and monitoring of atazanavir in elderly patients reflecting the greater frequency of decreased hepatic, renal, or cardiac function, and of concomitant disease or other drug therapy.

➤*Pregnancy: Category B.* At maternal doses producing the systemic drug exposure levels equal to (in rabbits) or 2 times (in rats) those at the human clinical dose (400 mg once daily), atazanavir did not produce teratogenic effects. In the pre- and post-natal development assessment in rats, atazanavir, at maternally toxic drug exposure levels 2 times those at the human clinical dose, caused body weight loss or weight gain suppression in the offspring. Offspring were unaffected at a lower dose that produced maternal exposure equivalent to that observed in humans given 400 mg once daily.

Hyperbilirubinemia occurred frequently during treatment with atazanavir. It is not known whether atazanavir administered to the mother during pregnancy will exacerbate physiological hyperbilirubinemia and lead to kernicterus in neonates and young infants. In the prepartum period, consider additional monitoring and alternative therapy to atazanavir.

There are no adequate and well-controlled studies in pregnant women. Cases of lactic acidosis syndrome, sometimes fatal, and symptomatic hyperlactatemia have been reported in patients (including pregnant women) receiving atazanavir in combination with nucleoside analogues, which are known to be associated with increased risk of lactic acidosis syndrome. Only use atazanavir during pregnancy if the potential benefit justifies the potential risk to the fetus.

Antiretroviral pregnancy registry – To monitor maternal-fetal outcomes of pregnant women exposed to atazanavir, an antiretroviral pregnancy registry has been established. Physicians are encouraged to register patients by calling 1-800-258-4263.

➤*Lactation:* The Centers for Disease Control and Prevention recommend that HIV-infected mothers not breastfeed their infants to avoid risking postnatal transmission of HIV. It is not known whether atazanavir is secreted in human milk. A study in lactating rats has demonstrated that atazanavir is secreted in milk. Because of both the potential for HIV transmission and the potential for serious adverse reactions in nursing infants, instruct mothers not to breastfeed if they are receiving atazanavir.

➤*Children:* The optimal dosing regimen for use of atazanavir in pediatric patients has not been established. Do not administer atazanavir to pediatric patients younger than 3 months of age due to the risk of kernicterus.

Precautions

➤*Hyperbilirubinemia:* Most patients taking atazanavir experience asymptomatic elevations in indirect (unconjugated) bilirubin related to inhibition of UDP-glucuronosyl transferase (UGT). This hyperbilirubinemia is reversible upon discontinuation of atazanavir. Evaluate hepatic transaminase elevations that occur with hyperbilirubinemia for alternative etiologies. No long-term safety data are available for patients experiencing persistent elevations in total bilirubin greater than 5 times the upper limit of normal (ULN). Alternative antiretroviral therapy to atazanavir may be considered if jaundice or scleral icterus associated with bilirubin elevations presents cosmetic concerns for patients. Dose reduction of atazanavir is not recommended since long-term efficacy of reduced doses has not been established.

➤*Rash:* In controlled clinical trials (n = 1,597), rash (all grades, regardless of causality) occurred in 21% of patients treated with atazanavir. The median time to onset of rash was 8 weeks after initiation of atazanavir and the median duration of rash was 1.3 weeks. Rashes were generally mild to moderate maculopapular skin eruptions. Dosing with atazanavir was often continued without interruption in patients who developed rash. The discontinuation rate for rash in clinical trials was 0.4%. Discontinue atazanavir if severe rash develops. Cases of Stevens-Johnson syndrome and erythema multiforme have been reported in patients receiving atazanavir.

➤*Resistance/cross-resistance:* Various degrees of cross-resistance among protease inhibitors have been observed. Resistance to atazanavir may not preclude the subsequent use of other protease inhibitors.

➤*Hemophilia:* There have been reports of increased bleeding, including spontaneous skin hematomas and hemarthrosis, in patients with hemophilia type A and B treated with protease inhibitors. In some patients, additional factor VIII was given. In more than half of the reported cases, treatment with protease inhibitors was continued or reintroduced. A causal relationship between protease inhibitor therapy and these events has not been established.

➤*Fat redistribution:* Redistribution/accumulation of body fat including central obesity, dorsocervical fat enlargement (buffalo hump), peripheral wasting, facial wasting, breast enlargement, and "cushingoid appearance" have been observed in patients receiving antiretroviral therapy. The mechanism and long-term consequences of these events are currently unknown. A causal relationship has not been established.

➤*Immune reconstitution syndrome:* Immune reconstitution syndrome has been reported in patients treated with combination antiretroviral therapy, including atazanavir. During the initial phase of combination antiretroviral treatment, patients whose immune system responds may develop an inflammatory response to indolent or residual opportunistic infections (such as *Mycobacterium avium* infection, cytomegalovirus, *Pneumocystis carinii* pneumonia, or tuberculosis), which may necessitate further evaluation and treatment.

Drug Interactions

Atazanavir is an inhibitor of CYP3A and UGT1A1. Coadministration of atazanavir and drugs primarily metabolized by CYP3A (eg, calcium channel blockers, HMG-CoA reductase inhibitors, immunosuppressants, and PDE5 inhibitors) or UGT1A1 (eg, irinotecan) may result in increased plasma concentrations of the other drug that could increase or prolong both its therapeutic and adverse effects (see tables below). Atazanavir is metabolized in the liver by the cytochrome P450 enzyme system. Coadministration of atazanavir and drugs that induce CYP3A, such as rifampin, may decrease atazanavir plasma concentrations and reduce its therapeutic effect. Coadministration of atazanavir and drugs that inhibit CYP3A may increase atazanavir plasma concentrations.

Atazanavir Drug Interactions

Precipitant drug	Object drug*		Description
Antacids and buffered medications	Atazanavir	↓	Reduced plasma concentrations of atazanavir are expected if antacids, including buffered medications, are administered with atazanavir. Administer atazanavir 2 h before or 1 h after these medications.
Antifungals Itraconazole Ketoconazole	Atazanavir/ Ritonavir	↑	Coadministration of ketoconazole has only been studied with atazanavir without ritonavir (negligible increase in atazanavir AUC and C_{max}). Because of the effect of ritonavir on ketoconazole, high doses of ketoconazole and itraconazole (> 200 mg/day) should be used cautiously with atazanavir/ritonavir.
Atazanavir/ Ritonavir	Antifungals Itraconazole Ketoconazole		
Clarithromycin	Atazanavir	↑	Increased concentrations of clarithromycin may cause QTc prolongations; therefore, consider a 50% dose reduction of clarithromycin when it is administered with atazanavir. In addition, concentrations of the active metabolite 14-OH clarithromycin are significantly reduced; consider alternative therapy for indications other than infections because of *M. avium* complex.
Atazanavir	Clarithromycin	↑↓	

ATAZANAVIR SULFATE — ORAL

Atazanavir Drug Interactions

Precipitant drug	Object drug*		Description
Didanosine (buffered formulation only)	Atazanavir	↓	Coadministration may decrease atazanavir concentrations. Take atazanavir (with food) 2 h before or 1 h after the buffered formulation of didanosine. Because didanosine enteric-coated capsules are to be given on an empty stomach and atazanavir is to be given with food, administer at different times.
Efavirenz	Atazanavir	↓	If atazanavir is to be coadministered with efavirenz, which decreases atazanavir exposure, it is recommended that atazanavir 300 mg with ritonavir 100 mg be coadministered with efavirenz 600 mg (all as a single daily dose with food). Atazanavir without ritonavir should not be coadministered with efavirenz.
H_2-receptor antagonists	Atazanavir	↓	Reduced plasma concentrations of atazanavir are expected if coadministered with H_2-receptor antagonists. This may result in loss of therapeutic effect and development of resistance. Administer atazanavir 12 h apart (or as far apart as possible) from H_2-receptor antagonists.
Nevirapine	Atazanavir	↓	Nevirapine, a CYP3A inducer, is expected to decrease atazanavir exposure. Coadministration is not recommended.
Proton pump inhibitors	Atazanavir	↓	Coadministration is not recommended because of expected substantial decreases in atazanavir concentrations and decreased therapeutic effect.
Rifampin	Atazanavir	↓	Rifampin decreases plasma concentrations and AUC of most protease inhibitors by ≈ 90%, possibly resulting in loss of therapeutic effect and development of resistance. Coadministration is not recommended.
Ritonavir	Atazanavir	↑	If atazanavir is coadministered with ritonavir, it is recommended that atazanavir 300 mg once daily be given with ritonavir 100 mg once daily with food.
St. John's wort	Atazanavir	↓	Concurrent use may be expected to reduce plasma concentrations of atazanavir. This may result in loss of therapeutic effect and development of resistance. Concurrent use is not recommended.
Tenofovir disoproxil fumarate	Atazanavir	↓	Tenofovir may decrease the AUC and C_{min} of atazanavir. When coadministered with tenofovir, it is recommended that atazanavir 300 mg be given with ritonavir 100 mg and tenofovir 300 mg (all as a single daily dose with food). Atazanavir without ritonavir should not be coadministered with tenofovir. Also, atazanavir may increase tenofovir concentrations. Monitor patients receiving atazanavir and tenofovir for tenofovir-associated adverse reactions.
Atazanavir	Tenofovir disoproxil fumarate		
Voriconazole	Atazanavir/ Ritonavir	↑	Until data are available, do not coadminister voriconazole with atazanavir/ritonavir.
Atazanavir/ Ritonavir	Voriconazole	↔	

Atazanavir Drug Interactions

Precipitant drug	Object drug*		Description
Atazanavir	Antiarrhythmics (eg, amiodarone, systemic lidocaine, quinidine)	↑	Concurrent use of atazanavir with antiarrhythmics have the potential to produce serious and/or life-threatening adverse reactions. Concentration monitoring of the antiarrhythmic agent is recommended if they are used concomitantly.
Atazanavir	Atenolol	↑	Atazanavir has the potential to prolong the PR interval in some patients. Use with caution when coadministering with atenolol.
Atazanavir	Benzodiazepines (eg, midazolam, triazolam)	↑	Contraindicated because of potential for serious and/or life-threatening events such as prolonged or increased sedation or respiratory depression.
Atazanavir	Calcium channel blockers (eg, diltiazem, felodipine, nicardipine, nifedepine, verapamil)	↑	Atazanavir has the potential to prolong the PR interval in some patients. Caution is warranted. Consider a dose reduction of diltiazem by 50% and consider dose titration of other calcium channel blockers. ECG monitoring is recommended.
Atazanavir	Cisapride	↑	Contraindicated because of potential for serious and/or life-threatening events such as cardiac arrhythmias.
Atazanavir	Contraceptives, oral (ethinyl estradiol and norethindrone)	↑	Mean concentrations of ethinyl estradiol and norethindrone are increased when administered with atazanavir. Exercise caution and use the lowest effective dose of each oral contraceptive component or use an alternate nonhormonal contraceptive.
Atazanavir	Ergot derivatives (dihydroergotamine, ergotamine)	↑	Contraindicated because of potential for serious and/or life-threatening events such as acute ergot toxicity.
Atazanavir	HMG-CoA reductase inhibitors (eg, lovastatin, simvastatin, atorvastatin)	↑	Atazanavir may increase serum concentrations of HMG-CoA reductase inhibitors, which could increase their toxicity, including rhabdomyolysis. Do not coadminister with simvastatin or lovastatin.
Atazanavir	Immunosuppressants (cyclosporine, sirolimus, tacrolimus)	↑	Coadministration may result in increased plasma concentrations of the immunosuppressant. Therapeutic concentration monitoring is recommended for the immunosuppressant agents when coadministered with atazanavir.
Atazanavir	Indinavir	↑	Both atazanavir and indinavir are associated with indirect (unconjugated) hyperbilirubinemia. Coadministration is not recommended.
Indinavir	Atazanavir		
Atazanavir	Irinotecan	↑	Atazanavir inhibits UGT and may interfere with the metabolism of irinotecan, resulting in increased irinotecan toxicities. Coadministration is not recommended.
Atazanavir	PDE5 inhibitors (sildenafil, tadalafil, vardenafil)	↑	Coadministration may result in an increase in sildenafil-associated adverse reactions, including hypotension, visual changes, and priapism. Use with caution at reduced doses: sildenafil 25 mg every 48 hours, tadalafil 10 mg every 72 hours, or vardenafil up to 2.5 mg every 72 hours. Monitor for adverse reactions.
Atazanavir	Pimozide	↑	Contraindicated because of increased serum pimozide concentrations and increased toxicity such as cardiac arrhythmias.

ATAZANAVIR SULFATE — ORAL

Atazanavir Drug Interactions

Precipitant drug	Object drug*		Description
Atazanavir	Rifabutin	↑	Concentrations of rifabutin may be increased. A rifabutin dose reduction of up to 75% (eg, 150 mg every other day or 3 times/wk) is recommended.
Atazanavir	Saquinavir	↑	Appropriate dosing recommendations for this combination, with respect to efficacy and safety, have not been established.
Atazanavir	Tricyclic antidepressants	↑	Concentrations of the tricyclic antidepressant may be increased. Concentration monitoring of the tricyclic antidepressant is recommended.
Atazanavir	Warfarin	↑	Coadministration has the potential to produce serious and/or life-threatening bleeding and has not been studied. It is recommended that INR be monitored.

* ↑ = Object drug increased. ↓ = Object drug decreased.
↔ = Undetermined clinical effect.

Adverse Reactions

➤*Adult patients:*
Treatment-naive patients –

Atazanavir Adverse Reactions[a] of Moderate or Severe Intensity Reported in Adult Treatment-Naive Patients[b]

Adverse reaction	Phase 3 study AI424-034		Phase 2 studies AI424-007, -008	
	64 weeks[c] atazanavir 400 mg once daily + lamivudine + zidovudine[e] (n = 404)	64 weeks[c] efavirenz 600 mg once daily + lamivudine + zidovudine[e] (n = 401)	120 weeks[c,d] atazanavir 400 mg once daily + stavudine + lamivudine or + stavudine + didanosine (n = 279)	73 weeks[c,d] nelfinavir 750 mg 3 times daily or 1,250 mg twice daily + stavudine + lamivudine or + stavudine + didanosine (n = 191)
CNS				
Dizziness	2%	7%	< 1%	—
Headache	6%	6%	1%	2%
Insomnia	3%	3%	< 1%	—
Peripheral neurologic symptoms	< 1%	1%	4%	3%
Dermatologic				
Rash	7%	10%	5%	1%
GI				
Abdominal pain	4%	4%	4%	2%
Diarrhea	1%	2%	3%	16%
Jaundice/Scleral icterus	7%	—	7%	—
Nausea	14%	12%	6%	4%
Vomiting	4%	7%	3%	3%

[a] Includes events of possible, probably, certain, or unknown relationship to treatment regimen.
[b] Based on regimens containing atazanavir.
[c] Median time on therapy.
[d] Includes long-term follow-up.
[e] As a fixed-dose combination: 150 mg lamivudine, 300 mg zidovudine twice daily.

Treatment-experienced patients –

Atazanavir Treatment-Emergent Adverse Reactions[a] of Moderate or Severe Intensity Reported in ≥ 2% of Adult Treatment-Experienced Patients[b], Study AI424-045

Adverse reaction	48 weeks[c] Atazanavir/ritonavir 300/100 mg once daily + tenofovir + NRTI (n = 119)	48 weeks[c] Lopinavir/ritonavir 400/100 mg twice daily[d] + tenofovir + NRTI (n = 118)
CNS		
Depression	2%	< 1%
GI		
Diarrhea	3%	11%
Jaundice/Scleral icterus	9%	—
Nausea	3%	2%
Musculoskeletal		
Myalgia	4%	—
Miscellaneous		
Fever	2%	—

[a] Includes event of possible, probable, certain, or unknown relationship to treatment regimen.
[b] Based on the regimen containing atazanavir.
[c] Median time on therapy.
[d] As a fixed-dose combination.

➤*Lab test abnormalities:*
Treatment-naive patients –

Grade 3 and 4 Laboratory Abnormalities Reported in ≥ 2% of Adult Treatment-Naive Patients[a]

Variable	Limit	Phase 3 study AI424-034		Phase 2 studies AI424-007, -008	
		64 weeks[b] atazanavir 400 mg once daily + lamivudine + zidovudine (n = 404)	64 weeks[b] efavirenz 600 mg once daily + lamivudine + zidovudine (n = 401)	120 weeks[b,c] atazanavir 400 mg once daily + stavudine + lamivudine or + stavudine + didanosine (n = 279)	73 weeks[b,c] nelfinavir 750 mg 3 times daily or 1,250 mg twice daily + stavudine + lamivudine or + stavudine + didanosine (n = 191)
Chemistry	High				
ALT	≥ 5.1 × ULN	4%	3%	9%	7%
Amylase	≥ 2.1 ×ULN	—	—	14%	10%
AST	≥ 5.1 × ULN	2%	2%	7%	5%
Creatine kinase	≥ 5.1 × ULN	6%	6%	11%	9%
Lipase	≥ 2.1 × ULN	< 1%	1%	4%	5%
Total bilirubin	≥ 2.6 × ULN	35%	< 1%	47%	3%
Total cholesterol	≥ 240 mg/dL	6%	24%	19%	48%
Triglycerides	≥ 751 mg/dL	< 1%	3%	4%	2%
Hematology	Low				
Hemoglobin	< 8 g/dL	5%	3%	< 1%	4%
Neutrophils	< 750 cells/mm^3	7%	9%	3%	7%

[a] Based on regimen(s) containing atazanavir.
[b] Median time on therapy.
[c] Includes long-term follow-up.
[e] As a fixed-dose combination: 150 mg lamivudine, 300 mg zidovudine twice daily.
[f] None reported in this treatment arm.

Lipids, change from baseline – For Study AI424-034, changes from baseline in fasting LDL-cholesterol, HDL-cholesterol, total cholesterol, and fasting triglycerides are shown in the table below:

Lipid Values, Mean Change from Baseline, Study AI424-034

	Atazanavir[a,b]			Efavirenz[b,c]		
	Baseline	Week 48		Baseline	Week 48	
	mg/dL (n = 383[e])	mg/dL (n = 283[e])	Change[d] (n = 272[e])	mg/dL (n = 378[e])	mg/dL (n = 264[e])	Change[d] (n = 253[e])
HDL cholesterol	39	43	+13%	38	46	+24%
LDL cholesterol[f]	98	98	+1%	98	114	+18%
Total cholesterol	164	168	+2%	162	195	+21%
Triglycerides[f]	138	124	−9%	129	168	+23%

[a] Atazanavir 400 mg once daily with the fixed-dose combination: 150 mg lamivudine, 300 mg zidovudine twice daily.
[b] Values obtained after initiation of serum lipid-reducing agents were not included in these analyses. Use of serum lipid-reducing agents was more common in the efavirenz treatment arm (3%) than in the atazanavir arm (1%).
[c] Efavirenz 600 mg once daily with the fixed-dose combination: 150 mg lamivudine, 300 mg zidovudine twice daily.
[d] The change from baseline is the mean of within-patient changes from baseline for patients with both baseline and week-48 values and is not a simple difference of the baseline and week-48 mean values.
[e] Number of patients with LDL-cholesterol measured.
[f] Fasting.

ATAZANAVIR SULFATE — ORAL

Treatment-experienced patients –

Grade 3 to 4 Laboratory Abnormalities Reported in ≥ 2% of Adult Treatment-Experienced Patients, Study AI424-045[a]			
Variable	Limit	48 weeks[b] atazanavir/ritonavir 300/100 mg once daily + tenofovir + NRTI (n = 119)	48 weeks[b] lopinavir/ritonavir 400/100 mg twice daily[c] + tenofovir + NRTI (n = 118)
Chemistry	High		
ALT	≥ 5.1 × ULN	4%	3%
AST	≥ 5.1 × ULN	3%	3%
Creatine kinase	≥ 5.1 × ULN	8%	8%
Glucose	≥ 251 mg/dL	5%	< 1%
Lipase	≥ 2.1 × ULN	5%	6%
Total bilirubin	≥ 2.6 × ULN	49%	< 1%
Total cholesterol	≥ 240 mg/dL	25%	26%
Triglycerides	≥ 751 mg/dL	8%	12%
Hematology	Low		
Platelets	< 50,000 cells/mm^3	2%	3%
Neutrophils	< 750 cells/mm^3	7%	8%

[a] Based on regimen(s) containing atazanavir.
[b] Median time on therapy.
[c] ULN = Upper limit of normal.
[d] As a fixed-dose combination.

Lipids, change from baseline – For Study AI424-045, changes from baseline in fasting LDL-cholesterol, HDL-cholesterol, total cholesterol, and fasting triglycerides are shown in the table below. The observed magnitude of dyslipidemia was less with atazanavir/ritonavir than with lopinavir/ritonavir. However, the clinical impact of such findings has not been demonstrated.

Lipid Values, Mean Change from Baseline, Study AI424-045						
	Atazanavir/ritonavir[a,b]			Lopinavir/ritonavir[b,c]		
	Baseline	Week 48		Baseline	Change[d]	
	mg/dL (n = 111[e])	mg/dL (n = 75[e])	Change[d] (n = 74[e])	mg/dL (n = 108[e])	mg/dL (n = 76[e])	Change[d] (n = 73[e])
HDL cholesterol	40	39	−7%	39	41	+2%
LDL cholesterol[f]	108	98	−10%	104	103	+1%
Total cholesterol	188	170	−8%	181	187	+6%
Triglycerides[f]	215	161	−4%	196	224	+30%

[a] Atazanavir 300 mg once daily plus ritonavir plus tenofovir plus 1 NRTI.
[b] Values obtained after initiation of serum lipid-reducing agents were not included in these analyses. Use of serum lipid-reducing agents was more common in the lopinavir/ritonavir treatment arm (19%) than in the atazanavir/ritonavir arm (8%).
[c] Lopinavir/ritonavir (400/100 mg) twice daily plus tenofovir plus 1 NRTI.
[d] The change from baseline is the mean of within-patient changes from baseline for patients with both baseline and Week 48 values and is not a simple difference of the baseline and Week 48 mean values.
[e] Number of patients with LDL cholesterol measured.
[f] Fasting.

Patients co-infected with hepatitis B and/or hepatitis C virus – Monitor liver function tests in patients with a history of hepatitis B or C. In studies AI424-008 and AI424-034, 74 patients treated with 400 mg of atazanavir once daily, 58 who received efavirenz, and 12 who received nelfinavir were seropositive for hepatitis B and/or C at study entry. ALT levels greater than 5 times the upper limit of normal (ULN) developed in 15% of the atazanavir-treated patients, 14% of the efavirenz-treated patients, and 17% of the nelfinavir-treated patients. AST levels greater than 5 times ULN developed in 9% of the atazanavir-treated patients, 5% of the efavirenz-treated patients, and 17% of the nelfinavir-treated patients. Within atazanavir and control regimens, no difference in frequency of bilirubin elevations was noted between seropositive and seronegative patients.

In study AI424-045, 20 patients treated with atazanavir/ritonavir 300 mg/100 mg once daily and 18 patients treated with lopinavir/ritonavir 400 mg/100 mg twice daily were seropositive for hepatitis B and/or C at study entry. ALT levels greater than 5 times ULN developed in 25% (5/20) of the atazanavir/ritonavir-treated patients and 6% (1/18) of the lopinavir/ritonavir-treated patients. AST levels greater than 5 times ULN developed in 10% (2/20) of the atazanavir/ritonavir-treated patients and 6% (1/18) of the lopinavir/ritonavir-treated patients.

Overdosage

➤*Symptoms:* Human experience of acute overdose with atazanavir is limited. Single doses up to 1,200 mg have been taken by healthy volunteers without symptomatic untoward effects. A single self-administered overdose of atazanavir 29.2 g in an HIV-infected patient (73 times the 400 mg recommended dose) was associated with asymptomatic bifascicular block and PR interval prolongation. These events resolved spontaneously. At high doses that lead to high drug exposures, jaundice due to indirect (unconjugated) hyperbilirubinemia (without associated liver function test changes) or PR interval prolongation may be observed.

➤*Treatment:* Treatment of overdosage with atazanavir should consist of general supportive measures, including monitoring of vital signs and EKG, and observations of the patient's clinical status. If indicated, achieve elimination of unabsorbed atazanavir by emesis or gastric lavage. Administration of activated charcoal may also be used to aid removal of unabsorbed drug. There is no specific antidote for overdose with atazanavir. Since atazanavir is extensively metabolized by the liver and is highly protein bound, dialysis is unlikely to be beneficial in significant removal of this medicine.

Patient Information

Inform patients that sustained decreases in plasma HIV RNA have been associated with a reduced risk of progression to AIDS and death. Patients should remain under the care of a physician while using atazanavir. Advise patients to take atazanavir with food every day and take other concomitant antiretroviral therapy as prescribed. Atazanavir must always be used in combination with other antiretroviral drugs. Advise patients not to alter the dose or discontinue therapy without consulting their doctor. If a dose of atazanavir is missed, patients should take the dose as soon as possible and then return to their normal schedule. However, if a dose is skipped, the patient should not double the next dose.

Inform patients that atazanavir is not a cure for HIV infection and that they may continue to develop opportunistic infections and other complications associated with HIV disease. Tell patients that there are currently no data demonstrating that therapy with atazanavir can reduce the risk of transmitting HIV to others through sexual contact.

Atazanavir may interact with some drugs; therefore, advise patients to report to their doctors the use of any other prescription, nonprescription medication, or herbal products, particularly St. John's wort.

Advise patients receiving a PDE5 inhibitor and atazanavir that they may be at an increased risk of PDE5 inhibitor-associated adverse events including hypotension, visual changes, and prolonged penile erection, and that they should promptly report any symptoms to their doctors.

Inform patients that atazanavir may produce changes in the EKG (PR prolongation). Patients should consult their physicians if they are experiencing symptoms such as dizziness or lightheadedness.

Tell patients to take atazanavir with food to enhance absorption.

Inform patients that asymptomatic elevations in indirect bilirubin have occurred in patients receiving atazanavir. This may be accompanied by yellowing of the skin or whites of the eyes and alternative antiretroviral therapy may be considered if the patient has cosmetic concerns.

Inform patients that redistribution or accumulation of body fat may occur in patients receiving antiretroviral therapy including protease inhibitors and that the cause and long-term health effects of these conditions are not known at this time. It is unknown whether long-term use of atazanavir will result in a lower incidence of lipodystrophy than with other protease inhibitors.

RITONAVIR

Rx	**Norvir** (Abbott)	**Capsules, soft gelatin:** 100 mg	Ethanol. (100 DS). White. In 120s.
		Oral solution: 80 mg/mL	Saccharin, ethanol. Peppermint and caramel flavor. In 240 mL.

RITONAVIR — ORAL

WARNING

Coadministration of ritonavir with certain nonsedating antihistamines, sedative hypnotics, antiarrhythmics, or ergot alkaloid preparations may result in potentially serious and/or life-threatening adverse reactions due to possible effects of ritonavir on the hepatic metabolism of certain drugs (see Contraindications).

Indications

➤*HIV infection:* Ritonavir is indicated in combination with other antiretroviral agents for the treatment of HIV infection.

Administration and Dosage

➤*Approved by the FDA:* March 1, 1996.

➤*Adults:*

Recommended dosage – The recommended dosage of ritonavir is 600 mg twice daily by mouth. Use of a dose titration schedule may help to reduce treatment-emergent adverse reactions while maintaining appropriate ritonavir plasma levels. Ritonavir should be started at no less than 300 mg twice daily and increased at 2- to 3-day intervals by 100 mg twice daily.

Concomitant therapy – If saquinavir and ritonavir are used in combination, the dosage of saquinavir should be reduced to 400 mg twice daily. The optimum dosage of ritonavir (400 or 600 mg twice daily), in combination with saquinavir, has not been determined; however, the combination regimen was better tolerated in patients who received ritonavir 400 mg twice daily.

➤*Children:* Ritonavir should be used in combination with other antiretroviral agents. The recommended dosage of ritonavir is 400 mg/m^2 twice daily by mouth and should not exceed 600 mg twice daily. Ritonavir should be

RITONAVIR — ORAL

started at 250 mg/m^2 and increased at 2- to 3-day intervals by 50 mg/m^2 twice daily. If patients do not tolerate 400 mg/m^2 twice daily because of adverse reactions, the highest tolerated dose may be used for maintenance therapy in combination with other antiretroviral agents; however, alternative therapy should be considered. When possible, dose should be administered using a calibrated dosing syringe.

Pediatric Dosage Guidelines

Body surface area[a] (m^2)	Twice daily dose 250 mg/m^2	Twice daily dose 300 mg/m^2	Twice daily dose 350 mg/m^2	Twice daily dose 400 mg/m^2
0.25	0.8 mL (62.5 mg)	0.9 mL (75 mg)	1.1 mL (87.5 mg)	1.25 mL (100 mg)
0.5	1.6 mL (125 mg)	1.9 mL (150 mg)	2.2 mL (175 mg)	2.5 mL (200 mg)
1	3.1 mL (250 mg)	3.75 mL (300 mg)	4.4 mL (350 mg)	5 mL (400 mg)
1.25	3.9 mL (312.5 mg)	4.7 mL (375 mg)	5.5 mL (437.5 mg)	6.25 mL (500 mg)
1.5	4.7 mL (375 mg)	5.6 mL (450 mg)	6.6 mL (525 mg)	7.5 mL (600 mg)

[a] Body surface area (m^2) can be calculated with the following equation: Take the square root of a patient's height in centimeters multiplied by the patient's weight in kilograms divided by 3,600.

➤*Dosing guidelines:* Patients should be aware that frequently observed adverse reactions, such as mild to moderate GI disturbances and paresthesias, may diminish as therapy is continued. In addition, patients initiating combination regimens with ritonavir and nucleosides may improve GI tolerance by initiating ritonavir alone and subsequently adding nucleosides before completing 2 weeks of ritonavir monotherapy.

Ritonavir is administered orally. It is recommended that ritonavir be taken with meals if possible. Patients may improve the taste of ritonavir oral solution by mixing with chocolate milk or enteral nutritional therapy liquids (eg, *Ensure* or *Advera*) within 1 hour of dosing. The effects of antacids on the absorption of ritonavir have not been studied.

➤*Storage/Stability:*

Capsules – Store soft gelatin capsules in the refrigerator between 2° to 8°C (36° to 46°F) until dispensed. Refrigeration of ritonavir soft gelatin capsules by the patient is recommended, but not required if used within 30 days and stored below 25°C (77°F). Protect from light. Avoid exposure to excessive heat.

Oral solution – Store ritonavir oral solution at room temperature 20° to 25°C (68° to 77°F). Do not refrigerate. Shake well before each use. Use by product expiration date. Store and dispense in its original container. Avoid exposure to excessive heat. Keep cap tightly closed.

Actions

➤*Pharmacology:* Ritonavir is a peptidomimetic inhibitor of both the HIV-1 and HIV-2 proteases. Inhibition of HIV protease renders the enzyme incapable of processing the gag-pol polyprotein precursor that leads to production of noninfectious immature HIV particles.

➤*Pharmacokinetics:*

Absorption –

The absolute bioavailability of ritonavir has not been determined. After a 600 mg dose of oral solution, peak concentrations of ritonavir were achieved approximately 2 and 4 hours after dosing under fasting and nonfasting (514 KCal; 9% fat, 12% protein, and 79% carbohydrate) conditions, respectively.

Effect of food on oral absorption: When the oral solution was given under nonfasting conditions, peak ritonavir concentrations decreased 23% and the extent of absorption decreased 7% relative to fasting conditions. Dilution of the oral solution, within 1 hour of administration, with 240 mL of chocolate milk or enteral nutritional therapy liquids (eg, *Ensure* or *Advera*) did not significantly affect the extent and rate of ritonavir absorption. After a single 600 mg dose under nonfasting conditions in 2 separate studies, the soft gelatin capsule (n = 57) and oral solution (n = 18) formulations yielded mean ± SD areas under the plasma concentration-time curve (AUCs) of 121.7 ± 53.8 and 129 ± 39.3 mcg•h/mL, respectively. Relative to fasting conditions, the extent of absorption of ritonavir from the soft gelatin capsule formulation was 13% higher when administered with a meal (615 KCal; 14.5% fat, 9% protein, and 76% carbohydrate).

Metabolism – Nearly all of the plasma radioactivity after a single oral dose of ^{14}C-ritonavir 600 mg oral solution (n = 5) was attributed to unchanged ritonavir. Five ritonavir metabolites have been identified in human urine and feces. The isopropylthiazole oxidation metabolite (M-2) is the major metabolite and has antiviral activity similar to that of parent drug; however, the concentrations of this metabolite in plasma are low. In vitro studies utilizing human liver microsomes have demonstrated that cytochrome P-450 3A (CYP3A) is the major isoform involved in ritonavir metabolism, although CYP2D6 also contributes to the formation of M-2.

Excretion – In a study of 5 subjects receiving a dose of ^{14}C-ritonavir 600 mg oral solution, 11.3% ± 2.8% of the dose was excreted into the urine, with 3.5% ± 1.8% of the dose excreted as unchanged parent drug. In that study, 86.4% ± 2.9% of the dose was excreted in the feces with 33.8% ± 10.8% of the dose excreted as unchanged parent drug. Upon multiple dosing, ritonavir accumulation is less than predicted from a single dose possibly because of a time- and dose-related increase in clearance.

Ritonavir Pharmacokinetic Characteristics

Parameter	n	Values (mean ± SD)
C_{max} SS[a]	10	11.2 ± 3.6 mcg/mL
C_{trough} SS[a]	10	3.7 ± 2.6 mcg/mL
V_{β}/F[b]	91	0.41 ± 0.25 L/kg
$t_{½}$		3 to 5 hours
CL/F SS[a]	10	8.8 ± 3.2 L/h
CL/F[b]	91	4.6 ± 1.6 L/h
CL_R	62	< 0.1 L/h
RBC/plasma ratio		0.14
Percent bound[c]		98% to 99%

[a] SS = steady state; patients taking ritonavir 600 mg every 12 hours.
[b] Single ritonavir 600 mg dose.
[c] Primarily bound to human serum albumin and alpha$_1$ acid glycoprotein over the ritonavir concentration range of 0.01 to 30 mcg/mL.

Special populations –

Hepatic function impairment: Dose-normalized steady-state ritonavir exposures in subjects with moderate hepatic impairment (400 mg twice daily, n = 6) were about 40% lower than those in subjects with normal hepatic function (500 mg twice daily, n = 6).

No dose adjustment is recommended in patients with mild or moderate hepatic impairment. However, health care providers should be aware of the potential for lower ritonavir concentrations in patients with moderate hepatic impairment and should monitor patient response carefully. Ritonavir has not been studied in patients with severe hepatic impairment.

Children: The pharmacokinetic profile of ritonavir in pediatric patients younger than 2 years of age has not been established. Steady-state pharmacokinetics were evaluated in 37 HIV-infected patients ages 2 to 14 years of age receiving doses ranging from 250 to 400 mg/m^2 twice daily. Across dose groups, ritonavir steady-state oral clearance (CL/F/m^2) was approximately 1.5 times faster in pediatric patients than in adult subjects. Ritonavir concentrations obtained after 350 to 400 mg/m^2 twice daily in pediatric patients were comparable to those obtained in adults receiving 600 mg (approximately 330 mg/m^2) twice daily.

Contraindications

Hypersensitivity to ritonavir or any of its ingredients.

Coadministration of ritonavir is contraindicated with the drugs listed in the table below because competition for primarily CYP3A by ritonavir could result in inhibition of the metabolism of these drugs and create the potential for serious and/or life-threatening reactions such as cardiac arrhythmias, prolonged or increased sedation, and respiratory depression.

Drugs That are Contraindicated with Ritonavir

Drug class	Drugs within class that are contraindicated with ritonavir
Alpha$_1$-adrenoreceptor antagonist	Alfuzosin hydrochloride
Antiarrhythmics	Amiodarone, bepridil, flecainide, propafenone, quinidine
Antihistamines	Astemizole, terfenadine
Ergot derivatives	Dihydroergotamine, ergonovine, ergotamine, methylergonovine
GI motility agent	Cisapride
Neuroleptic	Pimozide
Sedative/Hypnotics	Midazolam, triazolam

Warnings

➤*Pancreatitis:* Pancreatitis has been observed in patients receiving ritonavir therapy, including those who developed hypertriglyceridemia. In some cases fatalities have been observed. Patients with advanced HIV disease may be at increased risk of elevated triglycerides and pancreatitis.

Consider pancreatitis if clinical symptoms (eg, nausea, vomiting, abdominal pain) or abnormalities in laboratory values (eg, increased serum lipase or amylase values) suggestive of pancreatitis occur. Evaluate patients who exhibit these signs or symptoms and discontinue ritonavir therapy if a diagnosis of pancreatitis is made.

➤*Diabetes mellitus/Hyperglycemia:* New onset diabetes mellitus, exacerbation of preexisting diabetes mellitus, and hyperglycemia have been reported during postmarketing surveillance in HIV-infected patients receiving protease inhibitor therapy. Some patients required either initiation or dose adjustments of insulin or oral hypoglycemic agents for treatment of these events. In some cases, diabetic ketoacidosis has occurred. In those patients who discontinued protease inhibitor therapy, hyperglycemia persisted in some cases. Because these events have been reported voluntarily during clinical practice, estimates of frequency cannot be made and a causal relationship between protease inhibitor therapy and these events has not been established.

➤*Hypersensitivity reactions:* Allergic reactions including urticaria, mild skin eruptions, bronchospasm, and angioedema have been reported. Rare cases of anaphylaxis and Stevens-Johnson syndrome have also been reported.

RITONAVIR — ORAL

➤*Hepatic function impairment:* Hepatic transaminase elevations exceeding 5 times the upper limit of normal, clinical hepatitis, and jaundice have occurred in patients receiving ritonavir alone or in combination with other antiretroviral drugs. There may be an increased risk for transaminase elevations in patients with underlying hepatitis B or C. Therefore, exercise caution when administering ritonavir to patients with preexisting liver diseases, liver enzyme abnormalities, or hepatitis. Consider increased AST/ALT monitoring in these patients, especially during the first 3 months of ritonavir treatment.

There have been postmarketing reports of hepatic dysfunction, including some fatalities. These have generally occurred in patients taking multiple concomitant medications and/or with advanced AIDS.

Ritonavir is principally metabolized by the liver. Therefore, exercise caution when administering this drug to patients with impaired hepatic function.

➤*Carcinogenesis:* Carcinogenicity studies in mice and rats have been carried out on ritonavir. In male mice, at levels of 50, 100, or 200 mg/kg/day, there was a dose-dependent increase in the incidence of both adenomas and combined adenomas and carcinomas in the liver. Based on AUC measurements, the exposure at the high dose was approximately 0.3-fold for males that of the exposure in humans with the recommended therapeutic dose (600 mg twice daily).

➤*Elderly:*

In general, dose selection for an elderly patient should be cautious, usually starting at the low end of the dosing range, reflecting the greater frequency of decreased hepatic, renal, or cardiac function, and of concomitant disease or other drug therapy.

➤*Pregnancy: Category B.*

Developmental toxicity observed in rats (eg, early resorptions, decreased fetal body weight and ossification delays and developmental variations) occurred at a maternally toxic dosage at an exposure equivalent to approximately 30% of that achieved with the proposed therapeutic dose. A slight increase in the incidence of cryptorchidism was also noted in rats at an exposure approximately 22% of that achieved with the proposed therapeutic dose. Developmental toxicity observed in rabbits (eg, resorptions, decreased litter size and decreased fetal weights) also occurred at a maternally toxic dosage equivalent to 1.8 times the proposed therapeutic dose.

There are no adequate and well-controlled studies in pregnant women. Because animal reproduction studies are not always predictive of human response, only use this drug during pregnancy if clearly needed.

Antiretroviral pregnancy registry – To monitor maternal-fetal outcomes of pregnant women exposed to ritonavir, an antiretroviral pregnancy registry has been established. Health care providers are encouraged to register patients by calling 1-800-258-4263.

➤*Lactation:* The Centers for Disease Control and Prevention recommend that HIV-infected mothers not breast-feed their infants to avoid risking postnatal transmission of HIV. It is not known whether ritonavir is secreted in human milk. Because of both the potential for HIV transmission and the potential for serious adverse reactions in breast-feeding infants, instruct mothers not to breast-feed if they are receiving ritonavir.

➤*Children:* The safety and pharmacokinetic profile of ritonavir in pediatric patients younger than 2 years of age have not been established. In HIV-infected patients 2 to 16 years of age, the adverse reaction profile seen during a clinical trial and postmarketing experience was similar to that for adult patients. The evaluation of the antiviral activity of ritonavir in pediatric patients in clinical trials is ongoing.

Precautions

➤*Monitoring:* There may be an increased risk for transaminase elevations in patients with underlying hepatitis B or C. Consider increased AST/ALT monitoring in these patients, especially during the first 3 months of ritonavir treatment.

Ritonavir has been shown to increase triglycerides, cholesterol, AST, ALT, GGT, CPK, and uric acid. Perform appropriate laboratory testing prior to initiating ritonavir therapy and at periodic intervals or if any clinical signs or symptoms occur during therapy.

➤*Resistance / Cross-resistance:* Varying degrees of cross-resistance among protease inhibitors have been observed. Continued administration of ritonavir therapy following loss of viral suppression may increase the likelihood of cross-resistance to other protease inhibitors.

➤*Hemophilia:* There have been reports of increased bleeding, including spontaneous skin hematomas and hemarthrosis, in patients with hemophilia type A and B treated with protease inhibitors. In some patients, additional factor VIII was given. In more than half of the reported cases, treatment with protease inhibitors was continued or reintroduced. A causal relationship has not been established.

➤*Fat redistribution:* Redistribution/accumulation of body fat including central obesity, dorsocervical fat enlargement (buffalo hump), peripheral wasting, facial wasting, breast enlargement, and "cushingoid appearance" have been observed in patients receiving antiretroviral therapy. The mechanism and long-term consequences of these events are currently unknown. A causal relationship has not been established.

➤*Lipid disorders:* Treatment with ritonavir therapy alone or in combination with saquinavir has resulted in substantial increases in the concentration of total triglycerides and cholesterol. Perform triglyceride and cholesterol testing prior to initiating ritonavir therapy and at periodic intervals during therapy. Manage lipid disorders as clinically appropriate.

➤*Lab test abnormalities:* Ritonavir has been shown to increase triglycerides, cholesterol, AST, ALT, GGT, CPK, and uric acid. Perform appropriate laboratory testing prior to initiating ritonavir therapy and at periodic intervals or if any clinical signs or symptoms occur during therapy.

Drug Interactions

Ritonavir Drug Interactions

Precipitant drug	Object drug[a]		Description
Azole antifungals (ie, fluconazole, ketoconazole)	Ritonavir	↑↓	Ritonavir plasma concentrations may be elevated, increasing the risk of toxicity. Ketoconazole AUC was shown to increase 3.4-fold and the C_{max} increased by 55%. High doses of ketoconazole (> 200 mg/day) are not recommended. Itraconazole levels may be increased. Voriconazole levels may be decreased when coadministered with ritonavir. Therefore, voriconazole coadministered with ritonavir is contraindicated.
Ritonavir	Azole antifungals (ie, ketoconazole, itraconazole, voriconazole)		
Clarithromycin	Ritonavir	↑	Concurrent use may increase ritonavir and clarithromycin levels. Dosage adjustment is not needed in patients with normal renal function. For patients with Ccr 30 to 60 mL/min, decrease clarithromycin dose by 50%. For patients with Ccr < 30 mL/min, decrease the clarithromycin dose by 75%.
Ritonavir	Clarithromycin		
Didanosine	Ritonavir	↔	Coadministration for 4 days decreased the didanosine AUC by 13% and the C_{max} by 16%. Separate dosing of didanosine and ritonavir by 2.5 hours to avoid formulation incompatibility.
Ritonavir	Didanosine	↓	
Nevirapine	Ritonavir	↓	Ritonavir plasma levels and clinical efficacy may be decreased.
Rifamycins (ie, rifampin)	Ritonavir	↓	Coadministration of ritonavir with rifampin may lead to loss of virologic response to ritonavir. Consider alternate antimycobacterial agents (eg, rifabutin). Coadministration of ritonavir with rifabutin may increase rifabutin (and its metabolite) concentrations. Reduce rifabutin dose by at least 75% (eg, 150 mg every other day or 3 times weekly). Further dosage reduction may be necessary.
Ritonavir	Rifamycins (ie, rifabutin)	↑	
SSRIs (ie, fluoxetine)	Ritonavir	↑	Fluoxetine may increase ritonavir levels. SSRI levels may be increased. Monitor closely.
Ritonavir	SSRIs		
St. John's wort	Ritonavir	↓	Coadministration may lead to loss of virologic response and possible resistance to ritonavir. Concurrent use is not recommended.
Ritonavir	Antiarrhythmic agents (eg, amiodarone, bepridil, flecainide, propafenone, quinidine)	↑	Coadministration of ritonavir with amiodarone, bepridil, flecainide, propafenone, or quinidine is contraindicated because of the potential for cardiac arrhythmias secondary to increases in plasma concentrations of antiarrhythmics. Coadministration of ritonavir with other antiarrhythmics (disopyramide, lidocaine, mexiletine) may also cause an increase in the antiarrhythmic concentration.
Ritonavir	Antihistamines (ie, astemizole, terfenadine)	↑	Coadministration is contraindicated because of the potential for serious and/or life-threatening reactions such as cardiac arrhythmias.
Ritonavir	Atovaquone	↓	Atovaquone levels may be decreased.

RITONAVIR — ORAL

Ritonavir Drug Interactions

Precipitant drug	Object drug[a]		Description
Ritonavir	Benzodiazepines (eg, midazolam, triazolam, clonazepam, clorazepate, diazepam, estazolam, fluraxepam)	↑	Coadministration of ritonavir with midazolam or triazolam is contraindicated because of the risk of prolonged or increased sedation or respiratory depression. Plasma levels of the other benzodiazepines may be increased.
Ritonavir	Beta-blockers (ie, metoprolol, timolol)	↑	Metoprolol and timolol concentrations may be increased.
Ritonavir	Bupropion	↑	Increased serum bupropion concentrations may occur, increasing bupropion toxicity.
Ritonavir	Calcium channel blockers (ie, diltiazem, nifedipine verapamil)	↑	Calcium channel blocker levels may be increased.
Ritonavir	Carbamazepine	↑	Carbamazepine levels may be increased.
Ritonavir	Cisapride	↑	Coadministration is contraindicated due to the risk of cardiac arrhythmias.
Ritonavir	Clozapine	↑	Increases in serum concentrations may occur, possibly increasing clozapine toxicity.
Ritonavir	Contraceptives, oral (estrogen-containing)	↓	Coadministration decreased the ethinyl estradiol AUC by 40% and the C_{max} by 32%. Consider dosage increase or alternate contraceptive measures.
Ritonavir	Desipramine	↑	Concurrent use increased the desipramine AUC by 145% and the C_{max} by 22%. Dosage reduction and concentration monitoring of desipramine is recommended.
Ritonavir	Digoxin	↑	Digoxin levels may be elevated, increasing the risk of toxicity. Monitor digoxin levels closely and adjust dosage as needed.
Ritonavir	Disulfiram Metronidazole	↑	Ritonavir formulations contain alcohol, which can produce disulfiram-like reactions when coadministered with disulfiram or other drugs that produce this reaction (eg, metronidazole).
Ritonavir	Divalproex	↓	Divalproex levels may be decreased.
Ritonavir	Dronabinol	↑	Dronabinol levels may be increased.
Ritonavir	Eplerenone	↑	Eplerenone levels may be elevated, increasing the risk for hyperkalemia and associated arrhythmias. Coadministration is contraindicated.
Ritonavir	Ergot derivatives	↑	The risk of ergot toxicity may be increased. Coadministration is contraindicated.
Ritonavir	Ethosuximide	↑	Ethosuximide levels may be increased.
Ritonavir	HMG-CoA reductase inhibitors (ie, lovastatin, simvastatin, atorvastatin)	↑	Concurrent use increases the risk of myopathy including rhabdomyolysis. Concurrent use of ritonavir with lovastatin or simvastatin is not recommended. If using atorvastatin, start with the lowest possible dose with careful monitoring.
Ritonavir	Immunosuppressants (ie, cyclosporine, sirolimus, tacrolimus)	↑	Immunosuppressant levels may be increased.
Ritonavir	Indinavir	↑	Indinavir plasma concentrations may be elevated. Appropriate doses for this combination have not been established.
Ritonavir	Lamotrigine	↓	Lamotrigine levels may be decreased.
Ritonavir	Loperamide	↑	Loperamide levels may be increased.
Ritonavir	Methamphetamine	↑	Methamphetamine levels may be increased.
Ritonavir	Nefazodone	↑	Nefazodone levels may be increased.
Ritonavir	Olanzapine	↓	Olanzapine levels may be decreased.
Ritonavir	Opioid analgesics (eg, fentanyl, meperidine, methadone propoxyphene, tramadol)	↑↓	Plasma concentrations of fentanyl, propoxyphene, and tramadol may be increased, possibly causing toxicity. Methadone concentration may be decreased; therefore, consider dosage increase of methadone. Meperidine levels may decrease, possibly decreasing efficacy. However, the levels of the metabolite normeperidine may be increased and increase neurologic toxicity. Dosage increase and long-term use of meperidine with ritonavir are not recommended.
Ritonavir	PDE5 inhibitors (ie, sildenafil, tadalafil, vardenafil)	↑	Use concomitantly with caution; the PDE5 inhibitor dose should not exceed the following: sildenafil 25 mg within 48 hours; tadalafil 10 mg every 72 hours; vardenafil 2.5 mg every 72 hours.
Ritonavir	Phenothiazines (ie, perphenazine, thioridazine)	↑	Phenothiazine levels may be increased.
Ritonavir	Phenytoin	↓	Phenytoin levels may be decreased.
Ritonavir	Pimozide	↑	Coadministration is contraindicated because of the potential for cardiac arrhythmias.
Ritonavir	Quinine	↑	Quinine levels may be increased.
Ritonavir	Risperidone	↑	Risperidone levels may be increased.
Ritonavir	Saquinavir	↑	Coadministration may increase saquinavir plasma concentrations.
Ritonavir	Steroids (ie, fluticasone, dexamethasone, prednisone)	↑	Steroid levels may be increased. Coadministration of ritonavir with fluticasone (nasal spray) increased fluticasone AUC by 350-fold and C_{max} by 25-fold and caused a significant decrease (86%) in plasma cortisol AUC. Coadministration of ritonavir with fluticasone is not recommended unless the potential benefits outweigh the risks.
Ritonavir	Sulfamethoxazole	↓	Coadministration of ritonavir with sulfamethoxazole/trimethoprim decreased sulfamethoxazole AUC by 20%.
Ritonavir	Theophylline	↓	Coadministration decreased the theophylline AUC by 43% and the C_{max} by 32%. Consider monitoring of theophylline levels and increased dosage.
Ritonavir	Trazodone	↑	Concurrent use with ritonavir may cause elevated trazodone plasma concentrations and therefore increase adverse effects. Use with caution and consider a lower dose of trazodone.

RITONAVIR — ORAL

Ritonavir Drug Interactions			
Precipitant drug	Object drug[a]		Description
Ritonavir	Trimethoprim	↑	Coadministration of ritonavir with sulfamethoxazole/trimethoprim increased trimethoprim AUC by 20%.
Ritonavir	Tricyclic antidepressants	↑	Tricyclic antidepressant levels may be increased.
Ritonavir	Warfarin	↑↓	Initial frequent monitoring of INR is indicated.
Ritonavir	Zidovudine	↓	Coadministration may decrease zidovudine plasma concentrations.
Ritonavir	Zolpidem	↑	Zolpidem levels may be increased.

[a] ↑ = Object drug increased. ↓ = Object drug decreased. ↔ = Undetermined effect.

➤*Drug/Food interactions:* When the oral solution was given under nonfasting conditions, peak ritonavir concentrations decreased 23% and extent of absorption decreased 7% relative to fasting conditions. Extent of absorption or ritonavir from the capsule was 13% higher when given with a meal relative to fasting conditions. Take ritonavir with meals, if possible.

Adverse Reactions

The most frequently reported clinical adverse reactions, other than asthenia, among patients receiving ritonavir were GI and neurological disturbances including nausea, diarrhea, vomiting, anorexia, abdominal pain, taste perversion, and circumoral and peripheral paresthesias.

Ritonavir Adverse Reactions[a] (≥ 2%)						
	Study 245 naive patients[b]			Study 247 advanced patients[c]		Study 462 PI-naive patients[d]
Adverse reactions	Ritonavir + zidovudine (n = 116)	Ritonavir (n = 117)	Zidovudine (n = 119)	Ritonavir (n = 541)	Placebo (n = 545)	Ritonavir + saquinavir (n = 141)
Cardiovascular						
Syncope	0.9%	1.7%	0.8%	0.6%	0%	2.1%
Vasodilation	3.4%	1.7%	0.8%	1.7%	0%	3.5%
CNS						
Anxiety	0.9%	0%	0.8%	1.7%	0.9%	2.1%
Circumoral paresthesia	5.2%	3.4%	0%	6.7%	0.4%	6.4%
Confusion	0%	0.9%	0%	0.6%	0.6%	2.1%
Depression	1.7%	1.7%	2.5%	1.7%	0.7%	7.1%
Dizziness	5.2%	2.6%	3.4%	3.9%	1.1%	8.5%
Headache	7.8%	6%	6.7%	6.5%	5.7%	4.3%
Insomnia	3.4%	2.6%	0.8%	2%	1.8%	2.8%
Paresthesia	5.2%	2.6%	0%	3%	0.4%	2.1%
Peripheral paresthesia	0%	6%	0.8%	5%	1.1%	5.7%
Somnolence	2.6%	2.6%	0%	2.4%	0.2%	0%
Thinking abnormal	2.6%	0%	0.8%	0.9%	0.4%	0.7%
Dermatologic						
Rash	0.9%	0%	0.8%	3.5%	1.5%	0.7%
Sweating	3.4%	2.6%	1.7%	1.7%	1.1%	2.8%
GI						
Anorexia	8.6%	1.7%	4.2%	7.8%	4.2%	4.3%
Constipation	3.4%	0%	0.8%	0.2%	0.4%	1.4%
Diarrhea	25%	15.4%	2.5%	23.3%	7.9%	22.7%
Dyspepsia	2.6%	0%	1.7%	5.9%	1.5%	0.7%
Fecal incontinence	0%	0%	0%	0%	0%	2.8%
Flatulence	2.6%	0.9%	1.7%	1.7%	0.7%	3.5%
Local throat irritation	0.9%	1.7%	0.8%	2.8%	0.4%	1.4%
Nausea	46.6%	25.6%	26.1%	29.8%	8.4%	18.4%
Vomiting	23.3%	13.7%	12.6%	17.4%	4.4%	7.1%
GU						
Nocturia	0%	0%	0%	0.2%	0%	2.8%
Metabolic/Nutritional						
Weight loss	0%	0%	0%	2.4%	1.7%	0%
Musculoskeletal						
Arthralgia	0%	0%	0%	1.7%	0.7%	2.1%
Myalgia	1.7%	1.7%	0.8%	2.4%	1.1%	2.1%
Respiratory						
Pharyngitis	0.9%	2.6%	0%	0.4%	0.4%	1.4%
Special senses						
Taste perversion	17.2%	11.1%	8.4%	7%	2.2%	5%
Miscellaneous						
Abdominal pain	5.2%	6%	5.9%	8.3%	5.1%	2.1%
Asthenia	28.4%	10.3%	11.8%	15.3%	6.4%	16.3%
Fever	1.7%	0.9%	1.7%	5%	2.4%	0.7%
Malaise	5.2%	1.7%	3.4%	0.7%	0.2%	2.8%
Pain (unspecified)	0.9%	1.7%	0.8%	2.2%	1.8%	4.3%

[a] Includes those adverse reactions at least possibly related to study drug or of unknown relationship and excludes concurrent HIV conditions.
[b] The median duration of treatment for patients randomized to regimens containing ritonavir in study 245 was 9.1 months.
[c] The median duration of treatment for patients randomized to regimens containing ritonavir in study 247 was 9.4 months.
[d] The median duration of treatment for patients in ongoing study 462 was 48 weeks.

➤*Adverse reactions occurring in less than 2% of patients:*

Cardiovascular – Cardiovascular disorder, cerebral ischemia, cerebral venous thrombosis, hypertension, hypotension, myocardial infarct, palpitation, peripheral vascular disorder, phlebitis, postural hypotension, tachycardia, vasospasm.

CNS – Abnormal dreams, abnormal gait, agitation, amnesia, aphasia, ataxia, coma, convulsion, dementia, depersonalization, diplopia, emotional lability, euphoria, grand mal convulsion, hallucinations, hyperesthesia, hyperkinesia, hypesthesia, incoordination, libido decreased, manic reaction, migraine, nervousness, neuralgia, neuropathy, paralysis, peripheral neuropathic pain, peripheral neuropathy, peripheral sensory neuropathy, personality disorder, sleep disorder, speech disorder, stupor, subdural hematoma, tremor, vertigo, vestibular disorder.

Dermatologic – Acne, contact dermatitis, dry skin, eczema, erythema multiforme, exfoliative dermatitis, folliculitis, fungal dermatitis, furunculosis, maculopapular rash, molluscum contagiosum, onychomycosis, pruritus, psoriasis, pustular rash, seborrhea, skin discoloration, skin disorder, skin hypertrophy, skin melanoma, urticaria, vesiculobullous rash.

Endocrine – Adrenal cortex insufficiency, diabetes mellitus.

RITONAVIR — ORAL

GI – Abnormal stools, bloody diarrhea, cheilitis, cholestatic jaundice, colitis, dry mouth, dysphagia, eructation, esophageal ulcer, esophagitis, gastritis, gastroenteritis, GI disorder, GI hemorrhage, gingivitis, melena, mouth ulcer, pancreatitis, pseudomembranous colitis, rectal disorder, rectal hemorrhage, sialadenitis, stomatitis, tenesmus, thirst, tongue edema, ulcerative colitis.

GU – Acute kidney failure, breast pain, cystitis, dysuria, hematuria, impotence, kidney calculus, kidney failure, kidney function abnormal, kidney pain, menorrhagia, penis disorder, polyuria, urethritis, urinary frequency, urinary retention, urinary tract infection, vaginitis.

Hematologic/Lymphatic – Acute myeloblastic leukemia, anemia, ecchymosis, leukopenia, lymphadenopathy, lymphocytosis, myeloproliferative disorder, thrombocytopenia.

Hepatic – Hepatic coma, hepatitis, hepatomegaly, hepatosplenomegaly, ileus, liver damage.

Metabolic/Nutritional – Albuminuria, alcohol intolerance, avitaminosis, blood urea nitrogen (BUN) increased, cachexia, dehydration, edema, enzymatic abnormality, glycosuria, gout, hypercholesteremia, peripheral edema, xanthomatosis.

Musculoskeletal – Arthritis, arthrosis, bone disorder, bone pain, extraocular palsy, joint disorder, leg cramps, muscle cramps, muscle weakness, myositis, twitching.

Respiratory – Asthma, bronchitis, dyspnea, epistaxis, hiccup, hypoventilation, increased cough, interstitial pneumonia, larynx edema, lung disorder, rhinitis, sinusitis.

Special senses – Abnormal electro-oculogram, abnormal electroretinogram, abnormal vision, amblyopia/blurred vision, blepharitis, conjunctivitis, ear pain, eye disorder, eye pain, hearing impairment, increased cerumen, iritis, parosmia, photophobia, taste loss, tinnitus, uveitis, visual field defect, vitreous disorder.

Miscellaneous – Abdomen enlarged, accidental injury, allergic reaction, back pain, chest pain, chills, facial edema, facial pain, flu syndrome, hormone level altered, hypothermia, neck pain, neck rigidity, pelvic pain, photosensitivity reaction, substernal chest pain.

➤*Postmarketing:* The following adverse reactions have been reported during postmarketing use of ritonavir. Because these reactions are reported voluntarily from a population of unknown size, it is not possible to reliably estimate their frequency or establish a causal relationship to ritonavir exposure.

Cardiac and neurologic events have been reported when ritonavir has been coadministered with disopyramide, mexiletine, nefazodone, fluoxetine, and beta-blockers. The possibility of drug interactions cannot be excluded.

CNS – There have been postmarketing reports of seizure. Also, see Cardiovascular system effects.

Endocrine – Cushing syndrome and adrenal suppression have been reported when ritonavir, primarily at higher doses, has been coadministered with fluticasone propionate.

Hematologic/Lymphatic – There have been reports of increased bleeding in patients with hemophilia A or B.

Dehydration, usually associated with GI symptoms, and sometimes resulting in hypotension, syncope, or renal insufficiency has been reported. Syncope, orthostatic hypotension, and renal insufficiency have also been reported without known dehydration.

Coadministration of ritonavir with ergotamine or dihydroergotamine has been associated with acute ergot toxicity characterized by vasospasm and ischemia of the extremities and other tissues including the CNS.

Redistribution/accumulation of body fat, including central obesity, dorsocervical fat enlargement (buffalo hump), peripheral wasting, facial wasting, breast enlargement, and "cushingoid appearance" have been observed in patients receiving antiretroviral therapy. The mechanism and long-term consequences of these events are currently unknown. A causal relationship has not been established.

➤*Lab test abnormalities:*

Laboratory Abnormalities with Ritonavir Therapy (> 3%)

		Naive patients			Advanced patients		Protease inhibitor-naive patients
Variable	Limit	Ritonavir + zidovudine	Ritonavir	Zidovudine	Ritonavir	Placebo	Ritonavir + saquinavir
Chemistry values	High						
Cholesterol	> 240 mg/dL	30.7%	44.8%	9.3%	36.5%	8%	65.2%
CPK	> 1,000 units/L	9.6%	12.1%	11%	9.1%	6.3%	9.9%
GGT	> 300 units/L	1.8%	5.2%	1.7%	19.6%	11.3%	9.2%
AST	> 180 units/L	5.3%	9.5%	2.5%	6.4%	7%	7.8%
ALT	> 215 units/L	5.3%	7.8%	3.4%	8.5%	4.4%	9.2%
Triglycerides	> 800 mg/dL	9.6%	17.2%	3.4%	33.6%	9.4%	23.4%
Triglycerides	> 1,500 mg/dL	1.8%	2.6%	—[a]	12.6%	0.4%	11.3%
Triglycerides fasting	> 1,500 mg/dL	1.5%	1.3%	—	9.9%	0.3%	—
Uric acid	> 12 mg/dL	—	—	—	3.8%	0.2%	1.4%
Hematology values	Low						
Hematocrit	< 30%	2.6%	—	0.8%	17.3%	22%	0.7%
Hemoglobin	< 8 g/dL	0.9%	—	—	3.8%	3.9%	—
Neutrophils	≤ 0.5×10^9/L	—	—	—	6%	8.3%	—
RBC	< 3×10^{12}/L	1.8%	—	5.9%	18.6%	24.4%	—
WBC	< 2.5×10^9/L	—	0.9%	6.8%	36.9%	59.4%	3.5%

[a] Indicates no events reported.

Overdosage

➤*Symptoms:* Human experience of acute overdose with ritonavir is limited. One patient in clinical trials took ritonavir 1,500 mg/day for 2 days. The patient reported paresthesias that resolved after the dose was decreased. A postmarketing case of renal failure with eosinophilia has been reported with ritonavir overdose.

The approximate lethal dose was found to be greater than 20 times the related human dose in rats and 10 times the related human dose in mice.

➤*Treatment:* Ritonavir oral solution contains 43% alcohol by volume. Accidental ingestion of the product by a young child could result in significant alcohol-related toxicity and could approach the potential lethal dose of alcohol.

Treatment of overdose with ritonavir consists of general supportive measures including monitoring of vital signs and observation of the clinical status of the patient. There is no specific antidote for overdose with ritonavir. If indicated, achieve elimination of unabsorbed drug by gastric lavage; observe usual precautions to maintain the airway. Administration of activated charcoal may also be used to aid in removal of unabsorbed drug. Because ritonavir is extensively metabolized by the liver and is highly protein bound, dialysis is unlikely to be beneficial in significant removal of the drug. A certified poison control center should be consulted for up-to-date information on the management of overdose with ritonavir.

Patient Information

Inform patients that ritonavir is not a cure for HIV infection and that they may continue to acquire illnesses associated with advanced HIV infection, including opportunistic infections.

Tell patients that the long-term effects of ritonavir are unknown at this time. Inform them that ritonavir therapy has not been shown to reduce the risk of transmitting HIV to others through sexual contact or blood contamination.

Advise patients to take ritonavir with food, if possible.

Inform patients to take ritonavir every day as prescribed. Inform patients not to alter the dose or discontinue ritonavir without consulting their health care provider. If a dose is missed, instruct patients to take the next dose as soon as possible. However, if a dose is skipped, advise the patient not to double the next dose.

Inform patients that redistribution or accumulation of body fat may occur in patients receiving antiretroviral therapy and that the cause and long-term health effects of these conditions are not known at this time.

Ritonavir may interact with some drugs; therefore, advise patients to report to their doctor the use of any other prescription, nonprescription medications or herbal products, particularly St. John's wort.

LOPINAVIR/RITONAVIR

Rx	**Kaletra** (Abbott)	**Tablets:** 200 mg lopinavir/50 mg ritonavir	(KA). Yellow, oval. Film coated. In 120s.
		Capsules, soft gelatin: 133.3 mg lopinavir/ 33.3 mg ritonavir	Sorbitol. (PK). Orange. In 180s.
		Solution, oral: 80 mg lopinavir/20 mg ritonavir per mL	42.4% alcohol, menthol, corn syrup, saccharin, peppermint oil. Cotton candy or vanilla flavors. In 160 mL bottles with dosing cup.

LOPINAVIR/RITONAVIR — ORAL

Indications

➤*HIV infection:* In combination with other antiretroviral agents for the treatment of HIV infection. This indication is based on analyses of plasma HIV RNA levels and CD4 cell counts in a controlled study of lopinavir/ritonavir combination of 48 weeks duration and in smaller uncontrolled dose-ranging studies of 144 to 204 weeks duration. At present, there are no results from controlled trials evaluating the effect on clinical progression of HIV.

Administration and Dosage

➤*Approved by the FDA:* September 15, 2000.

➤*Adults:*

Therapy-naive patients – The recommended dosage is 400/100 mg of lopinavir/ritonavir (3 capsules or 5 mL taken with food, or 2 tablets taken with or without food) twice daily or 800/200 mg of lopinavir/ritonavir (6 capsules or 10 mL taken with food, or 4 tablets with or without food) once daily.

Therapy-experienced patients – The recommended dosage is 400/100 mg (3 capsules or 5 mL taken with food, or 2 tablets taken with or without food) twice daily. Once daily administration of lopinavir/ritonavir is not recommended in therapy-experienced patients.

Concomitant therapy with efavirenz, nevirapine, fosamprenavir, or nelfinavir – Consider a dose increase to 533/133 mg lopinavir/ritonavir (4 capsules or 6.5 mL) twice daily taken with food when used in combination with efavirenz, nevirapine, amprenavir, or nelfinavir, or 600/150 mg (3 tablets) twice daily with or without food when used in combination with efavirenz, nevirapine, fosamprenavir without ritonavir, or nelfinavir in treatment-experienced patients where decreased susceptibility to lopinavir is clinically suspected (by treatment history or laboratory evidence).

➤*Children (6 months to 12 years of age):* The recommended dosage of lopinavir/ritonavir oral solution is 12/3 mg/kg for those weighing 7 to less than 15 kg and 10/2.5 mg/kg for those 15 to 40 kg (approximately equivalent to 230/57.5 mg/m^2) twice daily with food, up to a maximum dose of 400/100 mg in children greater than 40 kg (5 mL or 3 capsules, or 2 tablets) twice daily. It is preferred that the prescriber calculate the appropriate milligram dose for each individual child 12 years of age and younger and determine the corresponding volume of solution or number of capsules or tablets.

Lopinavir/Ritonavir Pediatric Dosage Without Efavirenz, Nevirapine, or Amprenavir

Weight (kg)[1]	Dose (mg/kg)[2]	Volume of oral solution BID (80 mg lopinavir/20 mg ritonavir per mL)
7 to < 15	12 mg/kg BID	
7 to 10		1.25 mL
> 10 to < 15		1.75 mL
15 to 40	10 mg/kg BID	
15 to 20		2.25 mL
> 20 to 25		2.75 mL
> 25 to 30		3.5 mL
> 30 to 35		4 mL
> 35 to 40		4.75 mL
> 40	Adult dose	5 mL (or 3 capsules or 2 tablets)

[1] Note: Use adult dosage recommendation for children above 12 years of age.
[2] Dosing based on the lopinavir component of lopinavir/ritonavir solution (80 mg/20 mg per mL).

Concomitant therapy with efavirenz, nevirapine, or amprenavir – Consider a dose increase of lopinavir/ritonavir oral solution to 13/3.25 mg/kg for those weighing 7 to less than 15 kg and 11/2.75 mg/kg for those 15 to 45 kg (approximately equivalent to 300/75 mg/m^2) twice daily with food, up to a maximum dose of 533/133 mg in children over 45 kg twice daily when used in combination with efavirenz, nevirapine, or amprenavir in children 6 months to 12 years of age.

Lopinavir/Ritonavir Pediatric Dosage with Efavirenz, Nevirapine, or Amprenavir

Weight (kg)[1]	Dose (mg/kg)[2]	Volume of oral solution BID (80 mg lopinavir/20 mg ritonavir per mL)
7 to < 15	13 mg/kg BID	
7 to 10		1.5 mL
> 10 to < 15		2 mL
15 to 45	11 mg/kg BID	
15 to 20		2.5 mL
> 20 to 25		3.25 mL
> 25 to 30		4 mL
> 30 to 35		4.5 mL
> 35 to 40		5 mL (or 3 capsules)

Lopinavir/Ritonavir Pediatric Dosage with Efavirenz, Nevirapine, or Amprenavir

Weight (kg)[1]	Dose (mg/kg)[2]	Volume of oral solution BID (80 mg lopinavir/20 mg ritonavir per mL)
> 40 to 45	Adult dose	5.75 mL (or 2 tablets)
> 45	Adult dose	6.5 mL (or 4 capsules or 2 tablets)

[1] Note: Use adult dosage recommendation for children over 12 years of age.
[2] Dosing based on the lopinavir component of lopinavir/ritonavir solution (80 mg/20 mg per mL).

➤*Administration:* Lopinavir/ritonavir tablets may be taken with or without food; capsules and oral solution must be taken with food. Tablets should be swallowed whole and not chewed, broken, or crushed.

➤*Storage/Stability:*

Capsules and oral solution – Store capsules and oral solution at 2° to 8°C (36° to 46°F) until dispensed. Avoid exposure to excessive heat. Under refrigeration, the capsules and solution remain stable until the expiration date printed on the label. If stored at room temperature up to 25°C (77°F), use within 2 months.

Tablets – Store at 20° to 25°C (68° to 77°F); excursions permitted to 15° to 30°C (59° to 86°F). Dispense in original container. Exposure to high humidity outside the original container for longer than 2 weeks is not recommended.

Actions

➤*Pharmacology:* Lopinavir, an HIV protease inhibitor, prevents cleavage of the Gag-Pol polyprotein, resulting in the production of immature, noninfectious viral particles. As coformulated in the lopinavir/ritonavir combination, ritonavir inhibits the CYP3A-mediated metabolism of lopinavir, providing increased lopinavir plasma levels.

➤*Pharmacokinetics:*

Absorption – Administration of a single 400/100 mg dose of lopinavir/ritonavir with a moderate-fat meal was associated with a mean increase of 48% and 23% in lopinavir AUC and C_{max}, respectively, relative to fasting. For lopinavir/ritonavir oral solution, the corresponding increases in lopinavir AUC and C_{max} were 80% and 54%, respectively. Relative to fasting, administration of lopinavir/ritonavir with a high-fat meal increased lopinavir AUC and C_{max} by 97% and 43%, respectively, for capsules, and 130% and 56%, respectively, for oral solution. To enhance bioavailability and minimize pharmacokinetic variability, take lopinavir/ritonavir with food.

Distribution – At steady state, lopinavir is approximately 98% to 99% bound to plasma proteins. Lopinavir binds to alpha-1-acid glycoprotein (AAG) and albumin, but has a higher affinity for AAG. At steady state, lopinavir protein binding remains constant over the range of observed concentrations after 400/100 mg lopinavir/ritonavir twice daily, and is similar between healthy volunteers and HIV-positive patients.

Metabolism – In vitro experiments with human hepatic microsomes indicate that lopinavir primarily undergoes oxidative metabolism. Lopinavir is extensively metabolized by the hepatic cytochrome P450 system, almost exclusively by the CYP3A isozyme. Ritonavir is a potent CYP3A inhibitor that inhibits the metabolism of lopinavir, and therefore increases plasma levels of lopinavir. At least 13 lopinavir oxidative metabolites have been identified in man. Ritonavir has been shown to induce metabolic enzymes, resulting in the induction of its own metabolism. Pre-dose lopinavir concentrations decline with time during multiple dosing, stabilizing after approximately 10 to 16 days.

Across studies, administration of lopinavir/ritonavir 400/100 mg twice daily yields mean steady-state lopinavir plasma concentrations 15- to 20-fold higher than those of ritonavir in HIV-infected patients. The plasma levels of ritonavir are less than 7% of those obtained after the ritonavir dose of 600 mg twice daily. The in vitro antiviral 50% effective concentration (EC_{50}) of lopinavir is approximately 10-fold lower than that of ritonavir. Therefore, the antiviral activity of lopinavir/ritonavir combination is due to lopinavir.

Excretion – Following a 400/100 mg ^{14}C-lopinavir/ritonavir dose, approximately 10.4% and approximately 82.6% of an administered dose of ^{14}C-lopinavir can be accounted for in urine and feces, respectively, after 8 days. Unchanged lopinavir accounted for approximately 2.2% and 19.8% of the administered dose in urine and feces, respectively. After multiple dosing, less than 3% of the lopinavir dose is excreted unchanged in the urine. The half-life of lopinavir over a 12-hour dosing interval averaged 5 to 6 hours, and the apparent oral clearance (CL/F) of lopinavir is 6 to 7 L/h.

➤*Microbiology:*

Antiviral activity in vitro – The in vitro antiviral activity of lopinavir against laboratory HIV strains and clinical HIV isolates was evaluated in acutely infected lymphoblastic cell lines and peripheral blood lymphocytes, respectively. In the absence of human serum, the mean EC_{50} of lopinavir against 5 different HIV-1 laboratory strains ranged from 10 to 27 nM (0.006 to 0.017 mcg/mL, 1 mcg/mL = 1.6 mcM) and ranged from 4 to 11 nM (0.003 to

LOPINAVIR/RITONAVIR — ORAL

0.007 mcg/mL) against several HIV-1 clinical isolates (n = 6). In the presence of 50% human serum, the mean EC_{50} of lopinavir against these 5 laboratory strains ranged from 65 to 289 nM (0.04 to 0.18 mcg/mL), representing a 7- to 11-fold attenuation. Combination drug activity studies with lopinavir and other protease inhibitors or reverse transcriptase inhibitors have not been completed.

Resistance – HIV-1 isolates with reduced susceptibility to lopinavir have been selected in vitro. The presence of ritonavir does not appear to influence the selection of lopinavir-resistant viruses in vitro.

The selection of resistance to lopinavir/ritonavir in antiretroviral treatment-naive patients has not yet been characterized. In a Phase III study of 653 antiretroviral treatment-naive patients, plasma viral isolates from each patient on treatment with plasma HIV greater than 400 copies/mL at week 24, 32, 40, and/or 48 were analyzed. No evidence of resistance to lopinavir/ritonavir was observed in 37 evaluable lopinavir/ritonavir-treated patients. Evidence of genotypic resistance to nelfinavir, defined as the presence of the D30N and/or L90M mutation in HIV protease, was observed in 25/76 (33%) of evaluable nelfinavir-treated patients. The selection of resistance to lopinavir/ritonavir in antiretroviral treatment-naive pediatric patients appears to be consistent with that seen in adult patients.

Resistance to lopinavir/ritonavir has been noted to emerge in patients treated with other protease inhibitors prior to lopinavir/ritonavir therapy. In Phase II studies of 227 antiretroviral treatment-naive and protease inhibitor-experienced patients, isolates from 4 of 23 patients with quantifiable (greater than 400 copies/mL) viral RNA following treatment for 12 to 100 weeks displayed significantly reduced susceptibility to lopinavir compared with the corresponding baseline viral isolates. Three of these patients previously had received treatment with a single protease inhibitor (nelfinavir, indinavir, or saquinavir) and 1 patient had received treatment with multiple protease inhibitors (indinavir, saquinavir, and ritonavir). All 4 of these patients had at least 4 mutations associated with protease inhibitor resistance immediately prior to lopinavir/ritonavir therapy. Following viral rebound, isolates from these patients all contained additional mutations, some of which are recognized to be associated with protease inhibitor resistance. However, there are insufficient data at this time to identify lopinavir-associated mutational patterns in isolates from patients on lopinavir/ritonavir therapy. The assessment of these mutational patterns is under study.

Cross-resistance (preclinical studies) – Varying degrees of cross-resistance have been observed among protease inhibitors. Little information is available on the cross-resistance of viruses that developed decreased susceptibility to lopinavir during therapy.

The in vitro activity of lopinavir against clinical isolates from patients previously treated with a single protease inhibitor was determined. Isolates that displayed greater than 4-fold reduced susceptibiltiy to nelfinavir (n = 13) and saquinavir (n = 4) displayed less than 4-fold reduced susceptibility to lopinavir. Isolates with greater than 4-fold reduced susceptibility to indinavir (n = 16) and ritonavir (n = 3) displayed a mean of 5.7- and 8.3-fold reduced susceptibility to lopinavir, respectively. Isolates from patients previously treated with 2 or more protease inhibitors showed greater reductions in susceptibility to lopinavir.

Contraindications

Hypersensitivity to any of its ingredients, including ritonavir.

Coadministration of lopinavir/ritonavir is contraindicated with drugs that are highly dependent on CYP3A or CYP2D6 for clearance and for which elevated plasma concentrations are associated with serious and/or life-threatening events (see Drug Interactions). These drugs include the following: Flecainide, propafenone, dihydroergotamine, ergonovine, ergotamine, methylergonovine, pimozide, midazolam, cisapride, triazolam.

Warnings

➤*Hepatic function impairment:* Lopinavir/ritonavir is principally metabolized by the liver; therefore, exercise caution when administering this drug to patients with hepatic impairment because lopinavir concentrations may be increased. Patients with underlying hepatitis B or C or marked elevations in transaminases prior to treatment may be at increased risk for developing further transaminase elevations or hepatic decompensation. There have been postmarketing reports of hepatic dysfunction, including some fatalities. These have generally occurred in patients with advanced HIV disease taking multiple concomitant medications in the setting of underlying chronic hepatitis or cirrhosis. A causal relationship with lopinavir/ritonavir therapy has not been established. Consider increased AST/ALT monitoring in these patients, especially during the first several months of lopinavir/ritonavir treatment.

➤*Carcinogenesis:* In male mice, at levels of 50, 100, or 200 mg/kg/day of ritonavir, there was a dose-dependent increase in the incidence of both adenomas and combined adenomas and carcinomas in the liver. Based on AUC measurements, the exposure for males at the high dose was approximately 4-fold that of the exposure in humans with the recommended therapeutic dose (400/100 mg lopinavir/ritonavir twice daily). There were no carcinogenic effects seen in females at the dosages tested. The exposure for females at the high dose was approximately 9-fold that of the exposure in humans. In rats dosed at levels of 7, 15, or 30 mg/kg/day, there were no carcinogenic effects. In this study, the exposure at the high dose was approximately 0.7-fold that of the exposure in humans with 400/100 mg lopinavir/ritonavir twice-daily regimen. Based on the exposures achieved in the animal studies, the significance of the observed effects is not known.

➤*Elderly:* Exercise appropriate caution in the administration and monitoring of lopinavir/ritonavir in elderly patients, reflecting the greater frequency of decreased hepatic, renal, or cardiac function and of concomitant disease or other drug therapy.

➤*Pregnancy: Category C.* There are no adequate and well-controlled studies in pregnant women. Use lopinavir/ritonavir during pregnancy only if the potential benefit justifies the potential risk to the fetus. To monitor maternal-fetal outcomes of pregnant women exposed to lopinavir/ritonavir, an antiretroviral pregnancy registry has been established. Physicians are encouraged to register patients by calling (800) 258-4263.

➤*Lactation:* The Centers for Disease Control and Prevention recommend that HIV-infected mothers not breastfeed their infants to avoid risking post-natal transmission of HIV. Studies in rats have demonstrated that lopinavir is secreted in breast milk. It is not known whether lopinavir is secreted in human milk. Because of both the potential for HIV transmission and the potential for serious adverse reactions in nursing infants, instruct mothers not to breastfeed if they are receiving lopinavir/ritonavir.

➤*Children:* The safety and pharmacokinetic profiles of lopinavir/ritonavir in children under 6 months of age have not been established. In HIV-infected patients 6 months to 12 years of age, the adverse event profile seen during a clinical trial was similar to that for adult patients. The evaluation of the antiviral activity of lopinavir/ritonavir in pediatric patients in clinical trials is ongoing.

Precautions

➤*Pancreatitis:* Pancreatitis has been observed in patients receiving lopinavir/ritonavir therapy, including those who developed marked triglyceride elevations. Fatalities have been observed. Although a causal relationship to lopinavir/ritonavir has not been established, marked triglyceride elevation is a risk factor for development of pancreatitis. Patients with advanced HIV disease may be at increased risk of elevated triglycerides and pancreatitis, and patients with a history of pancreatitis may be at increased risk for recurrence during therapy.

Consider pancreatitis if clinical symptoms (nausea, vomiting, abdominal pain) or abnormalities in laboratory values (eg, increased serum lipase, amylase values) suggestive of pancreatitis should occur. Evaluate patients who exhibit these signs or symptoms and suspend lopinavir/ritonavir or other antiretroviral therapy as clinically appropriate.

➤*Diabetes mellitus/hyperglycemia:* New-onset diabetes mellitus, exacerbation of pre-existing diabetes mellitus, and hyperglycemia have been reported during postmarketing surveillance in HIV-infected patients receiving protease inhibitor therapy. Some patients required initiation or dose adjustments of insulin or oral hypoglycemic agents for treatment of these events. In some cases, diabetic ketoacidosis has occurred. In those patients who discontinued protease inhibitor therapy, hyperglycemia persisted in some cases. Because these events have been reported voluntarily during clinical practice, estimates of frequency cannot be made. A causal relationship between protease inhibitor therapy and these events has not been established.

➤*Resistance/Cross-resistance:* Various degrees of cross-resistance among protease inhibitors have been observed. The effect of lopinavir/ritonavir therapy on the efficacy of subsequently administered protease inhibitors is under investigation.

➤*Hemophilia:* There have been reports of increased bleeding, including spontaneous skin hematomas and hemarthrosis, in patients with hemophilia type A and B treated with protease inhibitors. In some patients, additional factor VIII was given. In more than 50% of the reported cases, treatment with protease inhibitors was continued or reintroduced. A causal relationship between protease inhibitor therapy and these events has not been established.

➤*Fat redistribution:* Redistribution/accumulation of body fat including central obesity, dorsocervical fat enlargement (buffalo hump), peripheral wasting, facial wasting, breast enlargement, and "cushingoid appearance" have been observed in patients receiving antiretroviral therapy. The mechanism and long-term consequences of these events are currently unknown. A causal relationship has not been established.

➤*Lipid elevations:* Treatment with lopinavir/ritonavir has resulted in large increases in the concentration of total cholesterol and triglycerides. Perform triglyceride and cholesterol testing prior to initiating therapy and at periodic intervals during therapy. Manage lipid disorders as clinically appropriate.

Drug Interactions

➤*CYP 450:* Lopinavir/ritonavir is an inhibitor of the P450 isoform CYP3A in vitro. Coadministration of the combination and drugs primarily metabolized by CYP3A may result in increased plasma concentrations of the other drug, which could increase or prolong its therapeutic and adverse effects.

Lopinavir/ritonavir inhibits CYP2D6 in vitro, but to a lesser extent than CYP3A. Clinically significant drug interactions with drugs metabolized by CYP2D6 are possible with the combination at the recommended dose, but the magnitude is not known. Lopinavir/ritonavir does not inhibit CYP2C9, CYP2C19, CYP2E1, CYP2B6, or CYP1A2 at clinically relevant concentrations.

Lopinavir/ritonavir has been shown in vivo to induce its own metabolism and to increase the biotransformation of some drugs metabolized by cytochrome P450 enzymes and by glucuronidation.

Lopinavir/ritonavir is metabolized by CYP3A. Drugs that induce CYP3A activity would be expected to increase the clearance of lopinavir, resulting in lowered plasma concentrations of lopinavir. Although not noted with concurrent ketoconazole, coadministration of lopinavir/ritonavir and other drugs that inhibit CYP3A may increase lopinavir plasma concentrations.

LOPINAVIR/RITONAVIR — ORAL

Lopinavir and Ritonavir Drug Interactions			
Precipitant drug	Object drug*		Description
Anticonvulsants (eg, carbamazepine, phenobarbital, phenytoin)	Lopinavir	↓	Use with caution. Lopinavir/Ritonavir may be less effective because of decreased lopinavir plasma concentrations in patients taking these agents concomitantly.
Azole antifungals	Ritonavir	↑	Plasma ritonavir concentrations may be elevated, increasing the risk of toxicity.
Corticosteroids (eg, dexamethasone)	Lopinavir	↓	Use with caution. Lopinavir/Ritonavir may be less effective because of decreased lopinavir plasma concentrations in patients taking these agents concomitantly.
Delavirdine	Lopinavir	↔	Appropriate doses of the combination with respect to safety and efficacy have not been established.
Efavirenz Nevirapine	Lopinavir Ritonavir	↓	Plasma levels and clinical efficacy may be reduced. Consider a dose increase of lopinavir/ritonavir to 533/133 mg (4 capsules or 6.5 mL) twice daily taken with food when used in combination with efavirenz or nevirapine in patients where reduced susceptibility to lopinavir is clinically suspected (by treatment history or laboratory evidence) (see Administration and Dosage). Note: Efavirenz and nevirapine induce the activity of CYP3A and thus have the potential to decrease plasma concentrations of other protease inhibitors when used in combination with lopinavir/ritonavir.
Rifabutin	Ritonavir	↓	Rifamycins may decrease ritonavir serum concentrations.
Rifampin	Lopinavir Ritonavir	↓	May lead to loss of virologic response and possible resistance to lopinavir/ritonavir or to the protease inhibitors class or other coadministered antiretroviral agents when administered with rifampin. Avoid coadministration.
St. John's wort (*Hypericum perforatum*)	Lopinavir Ritonavir	↓	Concomitant use of lopinavir/ritonavir and St. John's wort or products containing St. John's wort, is not recommended. Coadministration of protease inhibitors, including lopinavir/ritonavir with St. John's wort, is expected to substantially decrease protease inhibitor concentrations and may result in suboptimal levels of lopinavir and lead to loss of virologic response and possible resistance to lopinavir or to the protease inhibitors class.
Lopinavir	Atovaquone	↔	Clinical significance is unknown; however, increase in atovaquone doses may be needed.
Lopinavir	Calcium channel blockers, dihydropyridine (eg, felodipine, nifedipine, nicardipine)	↑	Caution is warranted and clinical monitoring of patients is recommended.
Lopinavir	HMG-CoA reductase inhibitors (eg, atorvastatin, lovastatin, simvastatin)	↑	Use lowest possible dose of atorvastatin with careful monitoring, or consider other HMG-CoA reductase inhibitors such as pravastatin or fluvastatin in combination with lopinavir/ritonavir. Avoid coadministration because of potential for serious reactions, such as risk of myopathy including rhabdomyolysis.
Lopinavir	Ketoconazole Itraconazole	↑	High doses of ketoconazole or itraconazole (> 200 mg/day) are not recommended.
Lopinavir	Pimozide	↑	Contraindicated because of potential serious and/or life-threatening reactions (eg, cardiac arrhythmias).
Lopinavir Ritonavir	Antiarrhythmics (eg, flecainide, propafenone, amiodarone, bepridil, lidocaine [systemic], quinidine)	↑	Amiodarone, flecainide, and propafenone are contraindicated because of the potential for serious and/or life-threatening reactions such as cardiac arrhythmia. Caution is warranted and therapeutic concentration monitoring is recommended for antiarrhythmics when coadministered with lopinavir/ritonavir, if available.
Lopinavir Ritonavir	Cisapride	↑	Contraindicated because of potential for serious and/or life-threatening reactions such as cardiac arrhythmias.
Lopinavir Ritonavir	Clarithromycin	↑	Clarithromycin AUC increased by 77% and C_{max} by 31% with coadministration of ritonavir. For patients with renal impairment, consider the following dosage adjustments: For patients with Ccr 30 to 60 mL/min, reduce the dose of clarithromycin by 50%. For patients with Ccr < 30 mL/min, reduce the dose of clarithromycin by 75%. No dose adjustment for patients with normal renal function is necessary.
Lopinavir Ritonavir	Disulfiram Metronidazole	↑	Lopinavir/Ritonavir oral solution contains alcohol, which can produce disulfiram-like reactions when coadministered with disulfiram or other drugs that produce this reaction (eg, metronidazole).
Lopinavir Ritonavir	Ergot derivatives (eg, dihydroergotamine, ergonovine, ergotamine, methylergonovine)	↑	Contraindicated because of potential for serious and/or life-threatening reactions, such as acute ergot toxicity characterized by peripheral vasospasm and ischemia of the extremities and other tissues.
Lopinavir Ritonavir	HIV protease inhibitors (amprenavir, indinavir, saquinavir)	↔	Amprenavir 750 mg BID and indinavir 600 mg BID, when coadministered with lopinavir/ritonavir 400/100 mg BID, may produce a similar AUC, lower C_{max}, and higher C_{min} compared with their respective established clinical dosing regimens. Saquinavir 800 mg BID, when coadministered with lopinavir/ritonavir 400/100 mg BID, may produce a similar AUC and higher C_{min} to its respective established clinical dosing regimen (no comparative information regarding C_{max}). The clinical significance of the lower C_{max} and higher C_{min} is unknown. Appropriate doses of amprenavir, indinavir, and saquinavir in combination with lopinavir/ritonavir with respect to safety and efficacy have not been established.
Lopinavir Ritonavir	Immunosuppressants (eg, cyclosporine, tacrolimus, rapamycin)	↑	Therapeutic concentration monitoring is recommended for immunosuppressant agents when co-administered with lopinavir/ritonavir.
Lopinavir Ritonavir	Midazolam Triazolam	↑	Contraindicated because of potential serious and/or life-threatening reactions such as prolonged or increased sedation or respiratory depression.
Lopinavir Ritonavir	Narcotic analgesics (eg, propoxyphene, methadone, fentanyl, meperidine)	↓	Dosage of methadone may need to be increased when coadministered with lopinavir/ritonavir. Plasma concentrations of propoxyphene and fentanyl may be increased possibly, causing toxicity. Meperidine levels may decrease, possibly decreasing efficacy but increasing neurologic toxicity. Concurrent use of propoxyphene or meperidine is contraindicated with ritonavir.
Lopinavir Ritonavir	Oral contraceptives (eg, ethinyl estradiol)	↓	Use alternative or additional contraceptive measures when estrogen-based oral contraceptives and lopinavir/ritonavir are coadministered.

LOPINAVIR/RITONAVIR — ORAL

Lopinavir and Ritonavir Drug Interactions			
Precipitant drug	Object drug*		Description
Lopinavir Ritonavir	Rifabutin and rifabutin metabolite	↑	Dosage reduction of rifabutin by at least 75% of the usual dose of 300 mg/day is recommended (ie, a maximum dose of 150 mg every other day or 3 times/week). Increased monitoring for adverse events is warranted in patients receiving the combination. Further dosage reduction of rifabutin may be necessary.
Lopinavir Ritonavir	Sildenafil	↑	Use with caution at reduced doses of 25 mg sildenafil every 48 hours with increased monitoring for adverse events.
Lopinavir Ritonavir	Warfarin	↓	The anticoagulant effect of warfarin may be decreased. Carefully monitor the international normalized ratio when starting or stopping a protease inhibitor.
Ritonavir	Bupropion	↑	Increased serum bupropion concentrations may occur, increasing bupropion toxicity. Ritonavir is contraindicated in patients taking bupropion.
Ritonavir	Clozapine	↑	Increases of serum concentrations may occur, possibly increasing clozapine toxicity.
Ritonavir	Desipramine	↑	Concurrent use increased the desipramine AUC by 145% and the C_{max} by 22%. Dosage reduction and concentration monitoring of desipramine is recommended.
Ritonavir	Piroxicam	↑	Large increases in serum piroxicam concentrations may occur, increasing piroxicam toxicity. Concomitant use is contraindicated.
Ritonavir	Quinidine	↑	Large increases in serum quinidine concentrations may occur, increasing the risk of quinidine toxicity. Concurrent use is contraindicated.
Ritonavir	Theophylline	↓	Coadministration decreased the theophylline AUC by 43% and the C_{max} by 27%.
Ritonavir	Zolpidem	↓	Possibly severe sedation and respiratory depression may occur. Coadministration is contraindicated.

* ↑ = Object drug increased. ↓ = Object drug decreased. ↔ = Undetermined clinical effect.

➤*Drug/Food interactions:*

Didanosine – It is recommended that didanosine be administered on an empty stomach; therefore, give didanosine 1 hour before or 2 hours after lopinavir/ritonavir (give with food).

Adverse Reactions

The most common adverse event associated with lopinavir/ritonavir therapy was diarrhea (generally of mild to moderate severity).

Lopinavir/Ritonavir Adverse Reactions of Moderate or Severe Intensity in Adult Patients (≥ 2%)				
	Antiretroviral-naive patients			Protease inhibitor-experienced patients
Adverse reaction	Lopinavir/Ritonavir 400/100 mg BID + d4T* + 3TC* (N = 326)[1]	Nelfinavir 750 mg TID + d4T* + 3TC* (N = 327)[1]	Lopinavir/Ritonavir BID[2] + d4T* + 3TC* (N = 84)[3]	Lopinavir/Ritonavir BID[4] + NNRTI + NRTIs* (N = 186)
CNS				
Headache	2.5	1.8	7.1	1.6
Insomnia	1.5	1.2	2.4	1.1
GI				
Abdominal pain	4	3.1	4.8	1.6
Abnormal stools	0	0.3	6	1.6
Diarrhea	15.6	17.1	23.8	15.6
Dyspepsia	2.1	0.3	1.2	0.5
Nausea	6.7	4.6	15.5	2.7
Vomiting	2.5	2.4	4.8	1.6
Miscellaneous				
Asthenia	4	3.4	7.1	5.4
Pain	0.6	0	2.4	1.6
Rash	0.6	1.5	3.6	2

* d4T = stavudine; 3TC = lamivudine; NRTIs = nucleoside reverse transcriptase inhibitors; NNRTI = nonnucleoside reverse transcriptase inhibitor

[1] Study performed over the course of 48 weeks.

[2] Includes adverse event data from dose group I (400/100 mg BID only [N = 16]) and dose group II (400/100 mg BID [N = 35] and 400/200 mg BID [N = 33]). Within dosing groups, moderate to severe nausea of probable/possible relationship to lopinavir/ritonavir occurred at a higher rate in the 400/200 mg dose arm compared with the 400/100 mg dose arm in group II.

[3] Study performed over the course of 72 weeks.

[4] Includes adverse event data from patients receiving 400/100 mg BID, 400/200 mg BID, and 533/133 mg BID for 16 to 72 weeks. All 186 patients received lopinavir/ritonavir in combination with NRTIs and either nevirapine or efavirenz.

Adverse events occurring in less than 2% of adult patients receiving lopinavir/ritonavir are as follows:

➤*Cardiovascular:* Deep vein thrombosis; hypertension; palpitation; thrombophlebitis; vasculitis.

➤*CNS:* Abnormal dreams; agitation; amnesia; anxiety; ataxia; confusion; depression; dizziness; dyskinesia; emotional lability; encephalopathy; hypertonia; libido decreased; nervousness; neuropathy; paresthesia; peripheral neuritis; somnolence; abnormal thinking; tremor; migraine; facial paralysis.

➤*Dermatologic:* Acne; alopecia; dry skin; exfoliative dermatitis; furunculosis; maculopapular rash; nail disorder; pruritus; skin benign neoplasm; skin discoloration; sweating; eczema; seborrhea; skin ulcer.

➤*Endocrine:* Cushing syndrome; hypothyroidism; diabetes mellitus.

➤*GI:* Anorexia; cholecystitis; constipation; dry mouth; dyspepsia; dysphagia; enterocolitis; eructation; esophagitis; fecal incontinence; flatulence; gastritis; gastroenteritis; GI disorder; hemorrhagic colitis; increased appetite; pancreatitis; sialadenitis; stomatitis; ulcerative stomatitis; enlarged abdomen; mouth ulceration.

➤*GU:* Abnormal ejaculation; gynecomastia; hypogonadism (male); kidney calculus; urine abnormality.

➤*Hematologic/Lymphatic:* Anemia; leukopenia; lymphadenopathy.

➤*Lab test abnormalities:*

Grade 3 to 4 Lopinavir/Ritonavir Lab Test Abnormalities in Adult Patients (≥ 2%)					
		Antiretroviral-naive patients			Antiretroviral-experienced patients
Variable	Limit[1]	Lopinavir/Ritonavir 400/100 mg BID + d4T* + 3TC* (N = 326)[2]	Nelfinavir 750 mg TID + d4T* + 3TC* (N = 327)[2]	Lopinavir/Ritonavir BID[3] + d4T* + 3TC* (N = 84)[4]	Lopinavir/Ritonavir BID[5] + NNRTI* + NRTIs* (N = 186)
Glucose	> 250 mg/dL	2.2	1.6	2.4	4.4
Uric acid	> 12 mg/dL	2.2	1.6	3.6	0.5
AST	> 180 U/L	2.2	4.1	9.5	5.5

LOPINAVIR/RITONAVIR — ORAL

Grade 3 to 4 Lopinavir/Ritonavir Lab Test Abnormalities in Adult Patients (≥ 2%)					
		Antiretroviral-naive patients			Antiretroviral-experienced patients
Variable	Limit[1]	Lopinavir/Ritonavir 400/100 mg BID + d4T* + 3TC* (N = 326)[2]	Nelfinavir 750 mg TID + d4T* + 3TC* (N = 327)[2]	Lopinavir/Ritonavir BID[3] + d4T* + 3TC* (N = 84)[4]	Lopinavir/Ritonavir BID[5] + NNRTI* + NRTIs* (N = 186)
ALT	> 215 U/L	3.8	3.8	8.3	7.1
GGT	> 300 U/L	N/A	N/A	3.6	24.6[6]
Total cholesterol	> 300 mg/dL	9	5	14.3	28.4
Triglycerides	> 750 mg/dL	9.3	1.3	10.7	28.4
Amylase	> 2 × ULN	3.2	2.2	4.8	4.9
Inorganic phosphorus	< 1.5 mg/dL	0	0	0	2.2
Neutrophils	0.75 × 10⁹/L	0.6	2.5	2.4	2.7

* d4T = stavudine; 3TC = lamivudine; NRTIs = nucleoside reverse transcriptase inhibitors; NNRTI = nonnucleoside reverse transcriptase inhibitor; N/A = not applicable
[1] ULN = upper limit of normal range.
[2] Study performed over the course of 48 weeks.
[3] Includes clinical laboratory data from dose group I (400/100 mg BID only [N = 16]) and dose group II (400/100 mg BID [N = 35] and 400/200 mg BID [N = 33]).
[4] Study performed over the course of 72 weeks.
[5] Includes clinical laboratory data from patients receiving 400/100 mg BID, 400/200 mg BID, and 533/133 mg BID for 16 to 72 weeks. All 186 patients received lopinavir/ritonavir in combination with NRTIs and either nevirapine or efavirenz.
[6] GGT was only measured in 69 patients receiving 400/100 mg BID or 400/200 mg BID in combination with nevirapine.

➤*Metabolic/Nutritional:* Avitaminosis; dehydration; edema; glucose tolerance, decreased; lactic acidosis; obesity; peripheral edema; weight loss; weight gain.

➤*Musculoskeletal:* Arthralgia; arthrosis; myalgia.

➤*Respiratory:* Bronchitis; dyspnea; lung edema; sinusitis; rhinitis.

➤*Special senses:* Abnormal vision; eye disorder; otitis media; taste perversion; tinnitus.

➤*Miscellaneous:* Back pain; chest pain; substernal chest pain; chills; drug interaction; drug level increased; face edema; fever; flu syndrome; malaise; viral infection; cyst; hypertrophy; bacterial infection; varicose vein.

➤*Postmarketing:* Redistribution/Accumulation of body fat has been reported (see Precautions).

➤*Children:* The adverse event profile seen during a clinical trial was similar to that for adults. Rash (3%) was the only drug-related clinical adverse event of moderate or severe intensity in 2% or more of pediatric patients enrolled.

Grade 3 to 4 Lopinavir/Ritonavir Lab Test Abnormalities in Children (≥ 2%)		
Variable	Limit[1]	Lopinavir/Ritonavir BID + RTIs* (N = 100)
Sodium, high	> 149 mEq/L	3
Total bilirubin	≥ 3 × ULN	3
AST	> 180 U/L	8
ALT	> 215 U/L	7
Total cholesterol	> 300 mg/dL	3
Amylase	> 2.5 × ULN	7[2]
Sodium, low	< 130 mEq/L	3
Platelet count	< 50 × 10⁹/L	4
Neutrophils	< 0.4 × 10⁹/L	2

* RTIs = reverse transcriptase inhibitors
[1] ULN = upper limit of normal range.
[2] Subjects with Grade 3 to 4 amylase confirmed by elevations in pancreatic amylase.

Overdosage

Lopinavir/ritonavir oral solution contains 42.4% alcohol (v/v). Accidental ingestion of the product by a young child could result in significant alcohol-related toxicity and could approach the potential lethal dose of alcohol.

➤*Treatment:* Treatment of overdose with lopinavir/ritonavir should consist of general supportive measures, including monitoring of vital signs and observation of the clinical status of the patient. There is no specific antidote for overdose with lopinavir/ritonavir. If indicated, elimination of unabsorbed drug should be achieved by emesis or gastric lavage. Administration of activated charcoal also may be used to aid in removal of unabsorbed drug. Because lopinavir/ritonavir is highly protein bound, dialysis is unlikely to be beneficial in significant removal of the drug. Refer to Management of Acute Overdosage.

Patient Information

A patient package insert for lopinavir/ritonavir is available for patient information.

Inform patients that sustained decreases in plasma HIV RNA have been associated with a reduced risk of progression to AIDS and death. Patients should remain under the care of a physician while using lopinavir/ritonavir. Advise patients to take lopinavir/ritonavir and other concomitant antiretroviral therapy every day as prescribed. It must always be used in combination with other antiretroviral drugs. Patients should not alter the dose or discontinue therapy without consulting their doctor. If a dose is missed, patients should take the dose as soon as possible and then return to their normal schedule. However, if a dose is skipped, the patient should not double the next dose.

Inform patients that lopinavir/ritonavir is not a cure for HIV infection and that they may continue to develop opportunistic infections and other complications associated with HIV disease. The long-term effects of lopinavir/ritonavir are unknown at this time. There are currently no data demonstrating that therapy with lopinavir/ritonavir can reduce the risk of transmitting HIV to others through sexual contact.

Lopinavir/ritonavir may interact with some drugs; therefore, advise patients to report to their doctor the use of any other prescription or nonprescription medication or herbal product, particularly St. John's wort.

Patients taking didanosine should take didanosine 1 hour before or 2 hours after lopinavir/ritonavir.

Advise patients receiving sildenafil that they may be at an increased risk of sildenafil-associated adverse events, including hypotension, visual changes, and sustained erection, and to promptly report any symptoms to their doctor.

Instruct patients receiving estrogen-based hormonal contraceptives to use additional or alternate contraceptive measures during therapy.

Take with food to enhance absorption.

Inform patients that redistribution or accumulation of body fat may occur in patients receiving antiretroviral therapy, including protease inhibitors, and that the cause and long-term health effects of these conditions are not known at this time.

TENOFOVIR DISOPROXIL FUMARATE (PMPA)

Rx	**Viread** (Gilead Sciences)	**Tablets:** 300 mg (equivalent to tenofovir disoproxil 245 mg)	Lactose. (GILEAD 4331 300). Light blue, almond shape. Film-coated. In 30s.

TENOFOVIR DISOPROXIL FUMARATE — ORAL

WARNING

Lactic acidosis and severe hepatomegaly with steatosis, including fatal cases, have been reported with the use of nucleoside analogs alone or in combination with other antiretrovirals (see Warnings).

Tenofovir is not indicated for the treatment of chronic hepatitis B virus (HBV) infection, and the safety and efficacy of tenofovir have not been established in patients coinfected with HBV and human immunodeficiency virus (HIV). Severe acute exacerbations of hepatitis B have been reported in patients who are coinfected with HBV and HIV and have discontinued tenofovir. Closely monitor hepatic function with both clinical and laboratory follow-up for at least several months in patients who discontinue tenofovir and are coinfected with HBV and HIV. If appropriate, initiation of anti-hepatitis B therapy may be warranted.

Indications

➤*HIV infection:* In combination with other antiretroviral agents for the treatment of HIV-1 infection.

Administration and Dosage

➤*Approved by the FDA:* October 26, 2001.

➤*Dosage:* 300 mg once daily taken orally without regard to food.

➤*Renal function impairment:* Significantly increased drug exposures occurred when tenofovir was administered to patients with moderate to severe renal impairment. Adjust the dosing interval of tenofovir in patients with baseline creatinine clearance (Ccr) less than 50 mL/min using the recommendations in the following table. The safety and effectiveness of these dosing interval adjustment recommendations have not been clinically evaluated, therefore, closely monitor clinical response to treatment and renal function in these patients.

Tenofovir Dosage Adjustment for Patients with Altered Ccr

	Ccr (mL/min)[a]			Hemodialysis patients
	≥ 50	30 to 49	10 to 29	
Recommended 300 mg dosing interval	Every 24 hours	Every 48 hours	Twice a week	Every 7 days or after a total of ≈ 12 hours of dialysis[b]

[a] Calculated using ideal (lean) body weight.
[b] Generally once weekly assuming 3 hemodialysis sessions/week of approximately 4-hours duration. Administer tenofovir following completion of dialysis.

The pharmacokinetics of tenofovir have not been evaluated in nonhemodialysis patients with Ccr less than 10 mL/min; therefore, no dosing recommendation is available for these patients.

➤*Storage/Stability:* Store at 25°C (77°F); excursions permitted to 15° to 30°C (59° to 86°F).

Actions

➤*Pharmacology:* Tenofovir disoproxil fumarate is an acyclic nucleoside phosphonate diester analog of adenosine monophosphate. Tenofovir disoproxil fumarate requires initial diester hydrolysis for conversion to tenofovir and subsequent phosphorylations by cellular enzymes to form tenofovir diphosphate. Tenofovir diphosphate inhibits the activity of HIV-1 reverse transcriptase by competing with the natural substrate deoxyadenosine 5′-triphosphate and, after incorporation into DNA, by DNA chain termination.

➤*Pharmacokinetics:*

Absorption – The oral bioavailability of tenofovir in fasted patients is approximately 25%. Following oral administration of a single dose of tenofovir disoproxil 300 mg to HIV-1 infected patients in the fasted state, maximum serum concentrations (C_{max}) are achieved in approximately 1 hour. C_{max} and AUC values are approximately 296 ng/mL and approximately 2287 ng•h/mL, respectively.

Administration of tenofovir disoproxil following a high-fat meal increases the oral bioavailability with an increase in tenofovir $AUC_{0-\infty}$ of approximately 40% and an increase in C_{max} of approximately 14%. Food delays the time to C_{max} by approximately 1 hour. C_{max} and AUC of tenofovir are approximately 326 ng/mL and approximately 3324 ng•h/mL following multiple doses of tenofovir 300 mg/day in the fed state.

Distribution – In vitro binding of tenofovir to human plasma or serum proteins is less than 0.7% and 7.2%, respectively, over the tenofovir concentration range of 0.01 to 25 mcg/mL. The volume of distribution at steady state is approximately 1.3 L/kg and 1.2 L/kg following IV administration of tenofovir 1 and 3 mg/kg, respectively.

Metabolism/Excretion – In vitro studies indicate that neither tenofovir disoproxil nor tenofovir are substrates of CYP450 enzymes. Following IV administration of tenofovir, approximately 70% to 80% of the dose is recovered in the urine as unchanged tenofovir within 72 hours of dosing. Following a single oral dose of tenofovir, the terminal elimination half-life is approximately 17 hours. After multiple oral doses of tenofovir 300 mg/day (under fed conditions), approximately 32% of the administered dose is recovered in urine over 24 hours. Tenofovir is eliminated by a combination of glomerular filtration and active tubular secretion. There may be competition for elimination with other compounds that are also renally eliminated.

Special populations –

Renal function impairment: In patients with Ccr less than 50 mL/min or with end-stage renal disease requiring dialysis, C_{max} and AUC of tenofovir were increased (see the following table). It is recommended that the dosing interval be modified in these patients.

Pharmacokinetic Parameters (Mean ± SD) of Tenofovir[a] in Patients with Varying Degrees of Renal Function

Baseline Ccr (mL/min)	> 80 (n = 3)	50 to 80 (n = 10)	30 to 49 (n = 8)	12 to 29 (n = 11)
C_{max} (ng/mL)	335.4 ± 31.8	330.4 ± 61	372.1 ± 156.1	601.6 ± 185.3
$AUC_{0-\infty}$ (ng•h/mL)	2,184.5 ± 257.4	3,063.8 ± 927	6,008.5 ± 2,504.7	15,984.7 ± 7,223
CL/F (mL/min)	1,043.7 ± 15.4	807.7 ± 279.2	444.4 ± 209.8	177 ± 97.1
CL_{renal} (mL/min)	243.5 ± 33.3	168.6 ± 27.5	100.6 ± 27.5	43 ± 31.2

[a] Single dose of tenofovir 300 mg.

Tenofovir is efficiently removed by hemodialysis with an extraction coefficient of approximately 54%. Following a single 300 mg dose, a 4-hour hemodialysis session removed approximately 10% of the administered tenofovir dose (see Administration and Dosage).

➤*Microbiology:*

Antiviral activity in vitro – In drug combination studies of tenofovir with nucleoside and non-nucleoside reverse transcriptase inhibitors, and protease inhibitors, additive to synergistic effects were observed.

Drug resistance – HIV-1 isolates with reduced susceptibility to tenofovir have been selected in vitro. These viruses expressed a K65R mutation in reverse transcriptase and showed a 3- to 4-fold reduction in susceptibility to tenofovir.

Tenofovir-resistant isolates of HIV-1 have also been recovered from some patients treated with tenofovir in combination with certain antiretroviral agents. In treatment-naive patients treated with tenofovir + lamivudine + efavirenz, viral isolates from 24% of patients with virologic failure showed reduced susceptibility to tenofovir. In treatment-experienced patients, 4.6% of the tenofovir-treated patients with virologic failure showed reduced susceptibility to tenofovir. Genotypic analysis of the resistant isolates showed a mutation in the HIV-1 reverse transcriptase gene resulting in the K65R amino acid substitution.

Cross-resistance – Cross-resistance among certain reverse transcriptase inhibitors has been recognized. The K65R mutation selected by tenofovir also is selected in some HIV-1 infected subjects treated with abacavir, didanosine, or zalcitabine. HIV isolates with this mutation also show reduced susceptibility to emtricitabine and lamivudine. Therefore, cross-resistance among these drugs may occur in patients whose virus harbors the K65R mutation. HIV-1 isolates from patients (n = 20) whose HIV-1 expressed a mean of 3 zidovudine-associated reverse transcriptase mutations (M41L, D67N, K70R, L210W, T215Y/F, or K219Q/E/N), showed a 3.1-fold decrease in the susceptibility to tenofovir. Multinucleoside resistant HIV-1 with a T69S double insertion mutation in the reverse transcriptase showed reduced susceptibility to tenofovir.

Contraindications

Previously demonstrated hypersensitivity to any of the components of the product.

Warnings

➤*HIV and hepatitis B coinfection:* It is recommended that all patients with HIV be tested for the presence of HBV before initiating antiretroviral therapy. Tenofovir is not indicated for the treatment of chronic HBV infection and the safety and efficacy of tenofovir have not been established in patients coinfected with HBV and HIV. Severe acute exacerbations of hepatitis B have been reported in patients who are coinfected with HBV and HIV, and have discontinued tenofovir. Closely monitor patients coinfected with HBV and HIV who discontinue tenofovir with both clinical and laboratory follow-up for at least several months. If appropriate, initiation of anti-hepatitis B therapy may be warranted.

➤*Lactic acidosis/severe hepatomegaly with steatosis:* Lactic acidosis and severe hepatomegaly with steatosis, including fatal cases, have been reported with the use of nucleoside analogs alone or in combination with other antiretrovirals. A majority of these cases have been in women. Obesity and prolonged nucleoside exposure may be risk factors. Exercise particular caution when administering nucleoside analogs to any patient with known risk factors for liver disease. Cases also have been reported in patients with no known risk factors. Suspend treatment with tenofovir in any patient who develops clinical or laboratory findings suggestive of lactic acidosis or pronounced hepatotoxicity, which may include hepatomegaly and steatosis even in the absence of marked transaminase elevations (see Warning Box).

➤*Virologic failure:* A high rate of early virologic failure and emergence of nucleoside reverse transcriptase inhibitor (NRTI) resistance mutations have been observed in a study of HIV-infected treatment-naive patients receiving a once-daily 3-drug combination including enteric-coated didanosine, lamivudine, and tenofovir. These new data are consistent with the high rates of virologic failure observed in several recent clinical studies that have evaluated the use of triple NRTI regimens. Based on these results, tenofovir in combination with didanosine and lamivudine is not recommended when considering a new treatment regimen for therapy-naive or experienced patients with HIV infection. Consider patients currently on this regimen for treat-

TENOFOVIR DISOPROXIL FUMARATE — ORAL

ment modification. Early virologic failure and high rates of resistance also have been reported with abacavir, lamivudine, and tenofovir.

➤*Renal function impairment:* Tenofovir is principally eliminated by the kidney. Dosing interval adjustment is recommended in all patients with Ccr less than 50 mL/min (see Administration and Dosage). No safety data are available in patients with renal dysfunction who received tenofovir using these dosing guidelines.

Renal impairment, including cases of acute renal failure and Fanconi syndrome (renal tubular injury with severe hypophosphatemia), has been reported in association with the use of tenofovir (see Adverse Reactions, Postmarketing). The majority of these cases occurred in patients with underlying systemic or renal disease or in patients taking nephrotoxic agents; however, some cases occurred in patients without identified risk factors.

Avoid tenofovir with concurrent or recent use of a nephrotoxic agent. Carefully monitor patients at risk for, or with a history of, renal dysfunction and patients receiving concomitant nephrotoxic agents for changes in serum creatinine and phosphorus.

➤*Carcinogenesis:* Long-term oral carcinogenicity studies of tenofovir in mice and rats were carried out at exposures up to approximately 16 times (mice) and 5 times (rats) those observed in humans at the therapeutic dose for HIV infection. At the high dose in female mice, liver adenomas were increased at exposures 16 times that in humans.

➤*Mutagenesis:* Tenofovir was mutagenic in the in vitro mouse lymphoma assay.

➤*Fertility impairment:* There was an alteration of the estrous cycle in female rats at a dose equivalent to 10 times the human dose based on body surface area.

➤*Elderly:* In general, be cautious with dose selection for the elderly patient, keeping in mind the greater frequency of decreased hepatic, renal, or cardiac function, and of concomitant disease or other drug therapy.

➤*Pregnancy: Category B.* There are no adequate and well-controlled studies in pregnant women. Use during pregnancy only if clearly needed.

Antiretroviral Pregnancy Registry – To monitor fetal outcomes of pregnant women exposed to tenofovir, an Antiretroviral Pregnancy Registry has been established. Health care providers are encouraged to register patients by calling (800) 258-4263.

➤*Lactation:* The Centers for Disease Control and Prevention recommend that HIV-infected mothers not breastfeed their infants to avoid risking postnatal transmission of HIV. Studies in rats have demonstrated that tenofovir is secreted in milk. It is not known whether tenofovir is excreted in human milk. Because of the potential for HIV transmission and the potential for serious adverse reactions, instruct mothers not to breastfeed if they are receiving tenofovir.

➤*Children:* Safety and efficacy in pediatric patients have not been established.

Precautions

➤*Monitoring:* Closely monitor patients coinfected with HBV and HIV who discontinue tenofovir with both clinical and laboratory follow-up for at least several months. Monitor patients at risk for, or with a history of, renal dysfunction and patients receiving concomitant nephrotoxic agents for changes in serum creatinine and phosphorus. Consider bone monitoring for HIV infected patients who have a history of pathologic bone fracture or are at substantial risk for osteopenia.

➤*Bone toxicity:* In a 48-week, active-controlled study, percent decreases in bone mineral density (BMD) from mean baseline were greater in patients receiving tenofovir plus lamivudine plus efavirenz (spine, approximately −3.3%; hip, approximately −3.2%) compared with patients receiving stavudine plus lamivudine plus efavirenz (spine, approximately −2%; hip, approximately −1.8%). The proportion of patients who met a protocol defined value of BMD loss (5% decrease in spine or 7% decrease in hip) was higher in the tenofovir group than the stavudine group. In addition, there were significant increases in levels of 4 biochemical markers of bone metabolism in the tenofovir group relative to the stavudine group, suggesting increased bone turnover. Serum parathyroid hormone levels also were higher in the tenofovir group. Except for bone specific alkaline phosphatase, these changes resulted in values that remained within the normal range. There was 1 bone fracture reported in the tenofovir group, compared with 4 in the stavudine group. The clinical significance of the changes in BMD and biochemical markers is unknown and follow-up is continuing to assess long-term impact.

Consider bone monitoring for HIV-infected patients who have a history of pathologic bone fracture or are at substantial risk for osteopenia. Supplementation with calcium and vitamin D may be considered for HIV-associated osteopenia or osteoporosis. If bone abnormalities are suspected, obtain appropriate consultation.

➤*Fat redistribution:* Redistribution and accumulation of body fat including central obesity, dorsocervical fat enlargement (buffalo hump), peripheral wasting, facial wasting, breast enlargement, and "cushingoid appearance" have been observed in patients receiving antiretroviral therapy. The mechanism and long-term consequences of these events are currently unknown. A causal relationship has not been established.

Drug Interactions

➤*Drugs eliminated by the kidneys:* Because tenofovir is eliminated primarily by the kidneys, coadministration of tenofovir with drugs that reduce renal function or compete for active tubular secretion may increase serum concentrations of tenofovir or increase the concentrations of other renally eliminated drugs. Some examples include, but are not limited to, adefovir dipivoxil, cidofovir, acyclovir, valacyclovir, ganciclovir, and valganciclovir.

Higher tenofovir concentrations could potentiate tenofovir-associated adverse reactions, including renal disorders.

Tenofovir Drug Interactions

Precipitant drug	Object drug[a]		Description
Atazanavir	Tenofovir	↑	Concurrent use increased tenofovir AUC 22% and C_{max} 14%. Monitor closely. Coadministration of tenofovir and unboosted atazanavir resulted in decreased concentrations of atazanavir, which may lead to loss or lack of response and possible resistance.
Tenofovir	Atazanavir	↓	
Indinavir	Tenofovir	↑	Coadministration increased tenofovir C_{max} approximately 14% but AUC remained unchanged. The C_{max} of indinavir decreased ≈ 11% but AUC remained unchanged.
Tenofovir	Indinavir	↓	
Lopinavir/ Ritonavir	Tenofovir	↑	Concurrent use increased tenofovir AUC 32%. Monitor closely.
Tenofovir	Abacavir	↑	Concurrent use increased abacavir C_{max} 12% but AUC remained unchanged.
Tenofovir	Didanosine (buffered or enteric coated)	↑	The C_{max} and AUC of didanosine (buffered formulation or enteric coated) increased when given with tenofovir. Increases in didanosine concentrations could potentiate adverse events, including pancreatitis and neuropathy. In adults weighing > 60 kg, reduce the didanosine dose to 250 mg when administered with tenofovir.
Tenofovir	Lamivudine	↓	Concurrent use decreased lamivudine C_{max} 24% but AUC remained unchanged.

[a] ↑= Object drug increased. ↓= Object drug decreased.

Adverse Reactions

➤*Treatment-experienced patients:* The most common adverse events that occurred in patients receiving tenofovir with other antiretroviral agents in clinical trials were mild to moderate GI events such as nausea, diarrhea, vomiting, and flatulence. Less than 1% discontinued participation in the clinical studies because of GI adverse events.

Tenofovir Adverse Events (Grades 2 to 4) (≥ 3%)

Adverse reaction	Tenofovir (n = 368) (week 0 to 24)	Placebo (n = 182) (week 0 to 24)	Tenofovir (n = 368) (week 0 to 48)	Placebo crossover to tenofovir (n = 170) (week 24 to 48)
CNS				
Asthenia	7	6	11	1
Depression	4	3	8	4
Dizziness	1	3	3	1
Headache	5	5	8	2
Insomnia	3	2	4	4
Peripheral neuropathy[a]	3	3	5	2
GI				
Abdominal pain	4	3	7	6
Anorexia	3	2	4	1
Diarrhea	11	10	16	11
Dyspepsia	3	2	4	2
Flatulence	3	1	4	1
Nausea	8	5	11	7
Vomiting	4	1	7	5
Skin and appendages				
Rash event[b]	5	4	7	1
Sweating	3	2	3	1
Miscellaneous				
Back pain	3	3	4	2
Chest pain	3	1	3	2
Fever	2	2	4	2
Myalgia	3	3	4	1
Pain	7	7	12	4
Pneumonia	2	0	3	2
Weight loss	2	1	4	2

[a] Peripheral neuropathy includes peripheral neuritis and neuropathy.
[b] Rash event includes rash, pruritus, maculopapular rash, urticaria, vesiculobullous rash, and pustular rash.

Nucleotide Analog Reverse Transcriptase Inhibitor

TENOFOVIR DISOPROXIL FUMARATE — ORAL

Lab test abnormalities –

Tenofovir Grade 3/4 Laboratory Abnormalities (≥ 1%)

Lab abnormality	Tenofovir (n = 368) (week 0 to 24)	Placebo (n = 182) (week 0 to 24)	Tenofovir (n = 368) (week 0 to 48)	Placebo crossover to tenofovir (n = 170) (week 24 to 48)
Any ≥ grade 3 laboratory abnormality	25	38	35	34
Triglycerides (> 750 mg/dL)	8	13	11	9
Creatine kinase (M: > 990 units/L) (F:> 845 units/L)	7	14	12	12
Serum amylase (> 175 units/L)	6	7	7	6
Urine glucose (≥ 3+)	3	3	3	2
AST (M: > 180 units/L) (F: > 170 units/L)	3	3	4	5
ALT (M: > 215 units/L) (F: > 170 units/L)	2	2	4	5
Serum glucose (> 250 units/L)	2	4	3	3
Neutrophils (< 750 mg/dL)	1	1	2	1

➤*Treatment-naive patients:* Adverse reactions seen in treatment-naive patients were generally consistent, with the addition of dizziness, with those seen in treatment-experienced patients. Mild adverse events (grade 1) were common and included dizziness, diarrhea, and nausea.

Tenofovir Adverse Events (Grades 2 to 4) (≥ 3%)

Adverse reaction	Tenofovir plus lamivudine plus efavirenz (n = 299)	Stavudine plus lamivudine plus efavirenz (n = 301)
CNS		
Abnormal dreams	3	3
Depression	7	5
Dizziness	3	5
Headache	10	11
Insomnia	4	6
Paresthesia	2	3
Peripheral neuropathy[a]	1	4
GI		
Abdominal pain	4	8
Diarrhea	6	6
Dyspepsia	3	2
Nausea	5	6
Vomiting	3	6
Miscellaneous		
Arthralgia	2	4
Asthenia	3	5
Back pain	4	3
Fever	5	6
Pain	7	6
Pneumonia	3	3
Rash event[b]	15	11

[a] Peripheral neuropathy includes peripheral neuritis and neuropathy.
[b] Rash event includes rash, pruritus, maculopapular rash, urticaria, vesiculobullous rash, and pustular rash.

Lab test abnormalities –

Tenofovir Grade 3/4 Laboratory Abnormalities (≥ 1%)

Lab abnormality	Tenofovir plus lamivudine plus efavirenz (n = 299)	Stavudine plus lamivudine plus efavirenz (n = 301)
Any ≥ grade 3 laboratory abnormality	28	31
Creatine kinase (M: > 990 units/L) (F:> 845 units/L)	8	9
Serum amylase (> 175 units/L)	7	6
AST (M: > 180 units/L) (F: > 170 units/L)	4	5
ALT (M: > 215 units/L) (F: > 170 units/L)	4	4
Hematuria (> 100 RBC/HPF)	4	4
Neutrophil (< 750/mm³)	3	1
Triglyceride (> 750 mg/dL)	2	8

➤*Postmarketing:* In addition to adverse reactions reported from clinical trials, the following reactions have been identified during postapproval use of tenofovir. Because they are reported voluntarily from a population of unknown size, estimates of frequency cannot be made. These events have been chosen for inclusion because of a combination of their seriousness, frequency of reporting, or potential causal connection to tenofovir.

GI – Abdominal pain, pancreatitis.

GU – Acute renal failure, acute tubular necrosis, Fanconi syndrome, increased creatinine, proteinuria, proximal tubulopathy, renal failure, renal impairment.

Metabolic/Nutritional – Hypophosphatemia, lactic acidosis.

Respiratory – Dyspnea.

Miscellaneous – Allergic reaction.

Overdosage

➤*Symptoms:* Limited clinical experience at doses higher than the therapeutic dose of tenofovir 300 mg is available. In a study, tenofovir disoproxil fumarate 600 mg was administered to 8 patients orally for 28 days. No severe adverse reactions were reported. The effects of higher doses are not known.

➤*Treatment:* If overdose occurs, monitor the patient for evidence of toxicity and apply standard supportive treatment as necessary. Tenofovir is efficiently removed by hemodialysis with an extraction coefficient of approximately 54%. Following a single dose of tenofovir 300 mg, a 4-hour hemodialysis session removed approximately 10% of the administered tenofovir dose.

Patient Information

Tenofovir does not cure HIV infection or AIDS. The long-term effects of tenofovir are not known at this time. People taking tenofovir may still get opportunistic infections or other conditions that happen with HIV infection.

Tenofovir does not reduce the risk of passing HIV to others through sexual contact or blood contamination. Instruct the patient to continue to practice safe sex and to not use or share dirty needles.

Instruct patients not to breastfeed if they are taking tenofovir.

Instruct the patient to take tenofovir with or without a meal.

The most common side effects of tenofovir are diarrhea, nausea, vomiting, and flatulence.

Changes in body fat have been seen in some patients taking anti-HIV medicine.

Nucleoside Reverse Transcriptase Inhibitors

DIDANOSINE (ddI; dideoxyinosine)

Rx	**Videx** (Bristol-Myers Squibb)	**Tablets, buffered, chewable/dispersible**[1]: 25 mg	(VIDEX 25). Off-white to light orange/yellow, mottled. Orange flavor. In 60s.
		50 mg	(VIDEX 50). Off-white to light orange/yellow, mottled. Orange flavor. In 60s.
		100 mg	(VIDEX 100). Off-white to light orange/yellow, mottled. Orange flavor. In 60s.
		200 mg	(VIDEX 200). Off-white to light orange/yellow, mottled. Orange flavor. In 60s.
Rx	**Videx EC** (Bristol-Myers Squibb)	**Capsules, delayed-release (with enteric-coated beadlets)**: 125 mg	(BMS 125 mg 6671). White. In 30s and 60s.

DIDANOSINE (ddI; dideoxyinosine)

Rx	**Didanosine** (Barr Labs)	**Capsules, delayed-release (with enteric-coated beadlets):** 200 mg	Dextrose, talc. (barr 588). Opaque green and white. In UD 30s.
Rx	**Videx EC** (Bristol-Myers Squibb)		(BMS 200 mg 6672). White. In 30s and 60s.
Rx	**Didanosine** (Barr Labs)	**Capsules, delayed-release (with enteric-coated beadlets):** 250 mg	Dextrose, talc. (barr 589). Opaque blue and white. In UD 30s.
Rx	**Videx EC** (Bristol-Myers Squibb)		(BMS 250 mg 6673). White. In 30s and 60s.
Rx	**Didanosine** (Barr Labs)	**Capsules, delayed-release (with enteric-coated beadlets):** 400 mg	Dextrose, talc. (barr 590). Opaque red and white. In UD 30s.
Rx	**Videx EC** (Bristol-Myers Squibb)		(BMS 400 mg 6674). White. In 30s and 60s.
Rx	**Videx** (Bristol-Myers Squibb)	**Powder for oral solution, buffered**[2]**:** 100 mg	In single-dose packets.
		250 mg	In single-dose packets.
		Powder for oral solution, pediatric: 2 g	In 4 oz bottles.
		4 g	In 8 oz bottles.

[1] Buffered with calcium carbonate and magnesium hydroxide. With aspartame, sorbitol, magnesium stearate, and phenylalanine (see Precautions).

[2] Buffered with dibasic sodium phosphate, sodium citrate, and citric acid. Total sodium content 1380 mg/packet. With sucrose.

DIDANOSINE — ORAL

WARNING

Fatal and nonfatal pancreatitis has occurred during therapy with didanosine used alone or in combination regimens in both treatment-naive and treatment-experienced patients, regardless of degree of immunosuppression. Didanosine should be suspended in patients with suspected pancreatitis and discontinued in patients with confirmed pancreatitis (see Warnings).

Lactic acidosis and severe hepatomegaly with steatosis, including fatal cases, have been reported with the use of nucleoside analogues alone or in combination, including didanosine and other antiretrovirals (see Warnings). Fatal lactic acidosis has been reported in pregnant women who received the combination of didanosine and stavudine with other antiretroviral agents. The combination of didanosine and stavudine should be used with caution during pregnancy and is recommended only if the potential benefits clearly outweighs the potential risk (see Warnings, Pregnancy).

Indications

➤*HIV infection:* The treatment of HIV-1 infection in combination with other antiretroviral agents.

Administration and Dosage

➤*Approved by the FDA:* October 1991.

All didanosine formulations should be administered on an empty stomach, at least 30 minutes before or 2 hours after eating. For either a once-daily or twice-daily regimen, patients must take at least 2 of the appropriate strength tablets at each dose to provide adequate buffering and prevent gastric acid degradation of didanosine. Because of the need for adequate buffering, the 200 mg strength tablet should only be used as a component of a once-daily regimen. To reduce the risk of GI side effects, patients should take no more than 4 tablets at each dose.

➤*Adults:* The preferred dosing frequency of didanosine is twice daily because there is more evidence to support the effectiveness of this dosing regimen. Once-daily dosing should be considered only for adult patients whose management requires once-daily dosing of didanosine. The daily dose in adult patients is dependent on weight as outlined in the table below.

Adult dosing		
Patient weight	Didanosine tablets[a]	Didanosine buffered powder[b]
Preferred dosing		
≥ 60 kg	200 mg twice daily	250 mg twice daily
< 60 kg	125 mg twice daily	167 twice daily
Dosing for patients whose management requires once-daily frequency		
≥ 60 kg	400 mg once daily	[b]
< 60 kg	250 mg once daily	[b]

[a] The 200 mg strength tablet should only be used as a component of a once-daily regimen.
[b] Not suitable for once-daily dosing except for patients with renal impairment. See table below (recommended dosage of didanosine in renal impairment).

➤*Children:* The recommended dose of didanosine in pediatric patients is 120 mg/m² twice a day. There are no data on once-daily dosing of didanosine in pediatric patients.

➤*Didanosine delayed-release capsules:* Didanosine delayed-release capsules should be administered on an empty stomach; the capsules should be swallowed intact. The recommended daily dose is dependent on body weight and is administered as one capsule given on a once-daily schedule as follows.

Dosing of didanosine delayed-release capsules	
Patient weight	Dosage
≥ 60 kg	400 mg once daily
< 60 kg	250 mg once daily

➤*Dose adjustment:* Clinical and laboratory signs suggestive of pancreatitis should prompt dose suspension and careful evaluation of the possibility of pancreatitis. Didanosine use should be discontinued in patients with confirmed pancreatitis (see Warnings).

Patients with symptoms of peripheral neuropathy may tolerate a reduced dose of didanosine after resolution of the symptoms of peripheral neuropathy upon drug discontinuation. If neuropathy recurs after resumption of didanosine, permanent discontinuation of didanosine should be considered.

Renal function impairment – In adult patients with impaired renal function, the dose of didanosine should be adjusted to compensate for the slower rate of elimination. The recommended doses and dosing intervals of didanosine in adult patients with renal insufficiency are presented in the table below.

Recommended dosage of didanosine in renal impairment				
Creatinine clearance (mL/min)	≥ 60 kg		< 60 kg	
	Tablet[a] (mg)	Buffered powder[b] (mg)	Tablet[a] (mg)	Buffered powder [b](mg)
≥ 60	200 twice daily[c]	250 twice daily[c]	125 twice daily[c]	167 twice daily
30 to 59	200 once daily or 100 twice daily	100 twice daily	150 once daily or 75 twice daily	100 twice daily
10 to 29	150 once daily	167 once daily	100 once daily	100 once daily
< 10	100 once daily	100 once daily	75 once daily	100 once daily

[a] Didanosine chewable/dispersible buffered tablet. Two didanosine tablets must be taken with each dose; different strengths of tablets may be combined to yield the recommended dose.
[b] Didanosine buffered powder for oral solution.
[c] 400 mg once daily (greater than or equal to 60 kg) or 250 mg once daily (less than 60 kg) for patients whose management requires once-daily frequency of administration.

Patients requiring continuous ambulatory peritoneal dialysis (CAPD) or hemodialysis: It is recommended that one-fourth of the total daily dose of didanosine be administered once a day. It is not necessary to administer a supplemental dose of didanosine following hemodialysis.

Recommended dosage of didanosine delayed-release capsules in renal impairment by body weight:

Recommended dosage of didanosine in renal impairment in body weight[a]		
	Dosage (mg)	
Creatinine clearance (mL/min)	≥ 60 kg	< 60 kg
≥ 60	400 once daily	250 once daily
30 to 59	200 once daily	125 once daily
10 to 29	125 once daily	125 once daily
< 10	125 once daily	[b]

[a] Based on studies using a buffered formulation of didanosine.
[b] Not suitable for use in patients less than 60 kg with Ccr less than 10 mL/min. An alternate formulation of didanosine should be used.

Urinary excretion is also a major route of elimination of didanosine in pediatric patients; therefore, the clearance of didanosine may be altered in children with renal impairment. Although there are insufficient data to recommend a specific dose adjustment of didanosine in this patient population, a reduction in the dose or an increase in the interval between doses should be considered.

➤*Method of preparation:*

Chewable/dispersible buffered tablets (Adult dosing) – To provide adequate buffering, at least 2 of the appropriate strength tablets, but no more than 4 tablets, should be thoroughly chewed or dispersed in at least 1 ounce of water prior to consumption (see Patient Information). To disperse tablets, add 2 tablets to at least 1 ounce of drinking water. Stir until a uniform dispersion forms, and drink the entire dispersion immediately. If additional flavoring is desired, the dispersion may be diluted with one ounce of clear apple juice. Stir the further diluted dispersion just prior to consumption. The dispersion with clear apple juice is stable at room temperature, 17° to 23°C (62° to 73°F), for up to 1 hour.

DIDANOSINE — ORAL

Buffered powder for oral solution –

1.) Open packet carefully and pour contents into a container with ≈ 120 mL of drinking water. Do not mix with fruit juice or other acid-containing liquid.
2.) Stir until the powder completely dissolves (≈ 2 to 3 minutes).
3.) Drink the entire solution immediately.

Pediatric powder for oral solution – Prior to dispensing, the pharmacist must constitute dry powder with purified water, USP, to an initial concentration of 20 mg/mL and immediately mix the resulting solution with antacid to a final concentration of 10 mg/mL as follows:

20 mg/mL initial solution: Constitute the product to 20 mg/mL by adding 100 mL or 200 mL of purified water, USP, to the 2 g or 4 g of didanosine powder, respectively, in the product bottle.

10 mg/mL final admixture:

1.) Immediately mix one part of the 20 mg/mL initial solution with one part of either aluminum hydroxide, magnesium hydroxide and simethicone suspension or aluminum hydroxide and magnesium hydroxide suspension for a final dispensing concentration of 10 mg didanosine per mL. For patient home use, the admixture should be dispensed in appropriately sized, flint-glass or plastic (HDPE, PET, or PETG) bottles with child-resistant closures. This admixture is stable for 30 days under refrigeration, 2° to 8°C (36° to 46°F).
2.) Instruct the patient to shake the admixture thoroughly prior to use and to store the tightly closed container in the refrigerator, 2° to 8°C (36° to 46°F), up to 30 days.

➤*Storage/Stability:* The bottles of powder should be stored at 15° to 30°C (59° to 86°F). The didanosine admixture may be stored up to 30 days in a refrigerator, 2° to 8°C (36° to 46°F). Discard any unused portion after 30 days.

Actions

➤*Pharmacokinetics:*

Absorption/Distribution – Didanosine is rapidly absorbed, with peak plasma concentrations generally observed from 0.25 to 1.5 hours following oral dosing. Increases in plasma didanosine concentrations were dose proportional over the range of 50 to 400 mg. Steady-state pharmacokinetic parameters did not differ significantly from values obtained after a single dose. Binding of didanosine to plasma proteins in vitro was low (< 5%). Based on data from in vitro and animal studies, it is presumed that the metabolism of didanosine in man occurs by the same pathways responsible for the elimination of endogenous purines.

Mean ± SD pharmacokinetic parameters for didanosine in adult and pediatric patients

Parameter	Adult patients[a]	n	Pediatric patients[b]: 8 months to 19 years	n	Pediatric patients[b]: 2 weeks to 4 months	n
Oral bioavailability (%)	42 ± 12	6	25 ± 20	46	ND**	
Apparent volume of distribution[c] (L/m²)	43.7 ± 8.9	6	28 ± 15	49	ND	
CSF*-plasma ratio[d]	21 ± 0.03%[e]	5	46% (range, 12% to 85%)	7	ND	
Systemic clearance[c] (mL/min/m²)	526 ± 64.7	6	516 ± 184	49	ND	
Renal clearance[f] (mL/min/m²)	223 ± 85	6	240 ± 90	15	ND	
Apparent oral clearance[g] (mL/min/m²)	1252 ± 154	6	2064 ± 736	48	1353 ± 759	41
Elimination half-life[f] (hr)	1.5 ± 0.4	6	0.8 ± 0.3	60	1.2 ± 0.3	21
Urinary recovery of didanosine[f] (%)	18 ± 8	6	18 ± 10	15	ND	

* CSF = Cerebrospinal fluid.
** ND = Not determined.
[a] Parameter units for adults were converted to the same units in pediatric patients to facilitate comparisons among populations: Mean adult body weight = 70 kg and mean adult body surface area = 1.73 m².
[b] In 1-day old infants (n = 10), the mean ± SD apparent oral clearance was 1523 ± 1176 mL/min/m² and half-life was 2 ± 0.7 hr.
[c] Following IV administration.
[d] Following IV administration in adults and IV or oral administration in pediatric patients.
[e] Mean ± SE.
[f] Following oral administration.
[g] Apparent oral clearance estimate was determined as the ratio of the mean systemic clearance and the mean oral bioavailability estimate.

Comparison of didanosine formulations: In didanosine delayed-release capsules, the active ingredient, didanosine, is protected against degradation by stomach acid by the use of an enteric coating on the beadlets in the capsule. The enteric coating dissolves when the beadlets empty into the small intestine, the site of drug absorption. With buffered formulations of didanosine, administration with antacid provides protection from degradation by stomach acid.

In healthy volunteers, as well as subjects infected with HIV, the area under the plasma concentration time curve (AUC) is equivalent for didanosine administered as the didanosine delayed-release capsule formulation relative to a buffered tablet formulation. The peak plasma concentration (C_{max}) of didanosine, administered as didanosine delayed-release capsules, is reduced ≈ 40% relative to didanosine buffered tablets. The time to the peak concentration (T_{max}) increases from ≈ 0.67 hours for dianosine buffered tablets to 2 hours for didanosine delayed-release capsules.

Effect of food on absorption of didanosine: Didanosine peak plasma concentrations (C_{max}) and area under the plasma concentration time curve (AUC) were decreased by ≈ 55% when didanosine tablets were administered up to 2 hours after a meal. Administration of didanosine tablets up to 30 minutes before a meal did not result in any significant changes in bioavailability. Didanosine should be taken on an empty stomach, at least 30 minutes before or 2 hours after eating. In the presence of food, the C_{max} and AUC for didanosine delayed-release capsules were reduced by ≈ 46% and 19%, respectively, compared to the fasting state. Didanosine delayed-release capsules should be taken on an empty stomach (see Administration and Dosage).

Special populations –

Renal function impairment: It is recommended that the didanosine dose be modified in patients with reduced creatinine clearance and in patients receiving maintenance hemodialysis (see Administration and Dosage). Data from 2 studies indicated that the apparent oral clearance of didanosine decreased and the terminal elimination half-life increased as creatinine clearance decreased. Following oral administration, didanosine was not detectable in peritoneal dialysate fluid (n = 6); recovery in hemodialysate (n = 5) ranged from 0.6% to 7.4% of the dose over a 3- to 4-hour dialysis period. The absolute bioavailability of didanosine was not affected in patients requiring dialysis.

Mean ± SD pharmacokinetic parameters for didanosine following a single oral dose of a buffered formulation*

Parameter	Creatinine clearance (mL/min): ≥ 90 (n = 12)	60 to 90 (n = 6)	30 to 59 (n = 6)	10 to 29 (n = 3)	Dialysis patients (n = 11)
Ccr (mL/min)	112 ± 22	68 ± 8	46 ± 8	13 ± 5	ND
CL/F (mL/min)	2164 ± 638	1566 ± 833	1023 ± 378	628 ± 104	543 ± 174
CL_R (mL/min)	458 ± 164	247 ± 153	100 ± 44	20 ± 8	< 10
t½ (hr)	1.42 ± 0.33	1.59 ± 0.13	1.75 ± 0.43	2 ± 0.3	4.1 ± 1.2

* ND = not determined due to anuria; Ccr = creatinine clearance; CL/F = apparent oral clearance; CL_R = renal clearance.

Children: The pharmacokinetics of didanosine have been evaluated in HIV-infected pediatric patients from 0.7 to 18.9 years of age. Overall, the pharmacokinetics of didanosine in pediatric patients > 0.7 years of age are similar to those of didanosine in adults. Didanosine plasma concentrations increased in proportion to oral doses ranging from 80 to 180 mg/m². The pharmacokinetics of didanosine administered as delayed release capsules have not been studied in pediatric patients.

➤*Microbiology:* Didanosine is a synthetic nucleoside analogue of the naturally occurring nucleoside deoxyadenosine in which the 3'-hydroxyl group is replaced by hydrogen. Intracellularly, didanosine is converted by cellular enzymes to the active metabolite, dideoxyadenosine 5'-triphosphate. Dideoxyadenosine 5'-triphosphate inhibits the activity of HIV-1 reverse transcriptase both by competing with the natural substrate, deoxyadenosine 5'-triphosphate, and by its incorporation into viral DNA causing termination of viral DNA chain elongation.

Drug resistance – HIV-1 isolates with reduced sensitivity to didanosine have been selected in vitro and were also obtained from patients treated with didanosine. Genetic analysis of isolates from didanosine-treated patients showed mutations in the reverse transcriptase gene that resulted in the amino acid substitutions K65R, L74V, and M184V. The L74V mutation was most frequently observed in clinical isolates. Phenotypic analysis of HIV-1 isolates from 60 patients (some with prior zidovudine treatment) receiving 6 to 24 months of didanosine monotherapy showed that isolates from 10 of 60 patients exhibited an average of a 10-fold decrease in susceptibility to didanosine in vitro compared to baseline isolates. Clinical isolates that exhibited a decrease in didanosine susceptibility harbored one or more didanosine-associated mutations. The clinical relevance of genotypic and phenotypic changes associated with didanosine therapy has not been established.

Cross-resistance – HIV-1 isolates from 2 of 39 patients receiving combination therapy for up to 2 years with zidovudine and didanosine exhibited decreased susceptibility to zidovudine, didanosine, zalcitabine, stavudine, and lamivudine in vitro. These isolates harbored 5 mutations (A62V, V751, F77L, F116Y, and Q151M) in the reverse transcriptase gene. The clinical relevance of these observations has not been established.

Contraindications

Clinically significant hypersensitivity to any of the components of the formulations.

Warnings

➤*Pancreatitis:* See the Warning box for more information.

When treatment with life-sustaining drugs known to cause pancreatic toxicity is required, suspension of didanosine therapy is recommended. In patients with risk factors for pancreatitis, didanosine should be used with extreme caution and only if clearly indicated. Patients with advanced HIV infection, especially the elderly, are at increased risk of pancreatitis and

DIDANOSINE — ORAL

should be followed closely. Patients with renal impairment may be at greater risk for pancreatitis if treated without dose adjustment.

The frequency of pancreatitis is dose related. In phase 3 studies, incidence ranged from 1% to 10% with doses higher than are currently recommended and 1% to 7% with recommended dose.

In pediatric studies, pancreatitis occurred in 3% (2/60) of patients treated at entry doses below 300 mg/m^2/day and in 13% (5/38) of patients treated at higher doses. Didanosine use should be suspended in pediatric patients with signs or symptoms of pancreatitis and discontinued in pediatric patients with confirmed pancreatitis.

➤*Lactic acidosis/severe hepatomegaly with steatosis:* Lactic acidosis and severe hepatomegaly with steatosis, including fatal cases, have been reported with the use of nucleoside analogues alone or in combination, including didanosine and other antiretrovirals. A majority of these cases have been in women. Obesity and prolonged nucleoside exposure may be risk factors. Particular caution should be exercised when administering didanosine to any patient with known risk factors for liver disease; however, cases have also been reported in patients with no known risk factors. Treatment with didanosine should be suspended in any patient who develops clinical or laboratory findings suggestive of lactic acidosis or pronounced hepatotoxicity (which may include hepatomegaly and steatosis even in the absence of marked transaminase elevations).

➤*Retinal changes and optic neuritis:* Retinal changes and optic neuritis have been reported in adult and pediatric patients. Periodic retinal examinations should be considered for patients receiving didanosine (see Adverse Reactions).

➤*Hyperuricemia:* Didanosine has been associated with asymptomatic hyperuricemia; treatment suspension may be necessary if clinical measures aimed at reducing uric acid levels fail.

➤*Renal function impairment:* Patients with renal impairment (creatinine clearance < 60 mL/min) may be at greater risk of toxicity from didanosine due to decreased drug clearance (see Pharmacokinetics). A dose reduction is recommended in these patients (see Administration and Dosage). The magnesium content of each buffered tablet of didanosine is 8.6 mEq. This may present an excessive load of magnesium to patients with significant renal impairment, particularly after prolonged dosing.

➤*Hepatic function impairment:* It is unknown if hepatic impairment significantly affects didanosine pharmacokinetics. Therefore, these patients should be monitored closely for evidence of didanosine toxicity.

➤*Mutagenesis:* Didanosine was positive in the following genetic toxicology assays: The *Escherichia coli* tester strain WP2 uvrA bacterial mutagenicity assay; the L5178Y/TK+/−mouse lymphoma mammalian cell gene mutation assay; the in vitro chromosomal aberrations assay in cultured human peripheral lymphocytes; the in vitro chromosomal aberrations assay in Chinese Hamster Lung cells; and the BALB/c 3T3 in vitro transformation assay. No evidence of mutagenicity was observed in an Ames *Salmonella* bacterial mutagenicity assay or in rat and mouse in vivo micronucleus assays.

➤*Elderly:* In an Expanded Access Program for patients with advanced HIV infection, patients aged 65 years and older had a higher frequency of pancreatitis (10%) than younger patients (5%). Clinical studies of didanosine did not include sufficient numbers of subjects aged 65 years and over to determine whether they respond differently than younger subjects. Didanosine is known to be substantially excreted by the kidney, and the risk of toxic reactions to this drug may be greater in patients with impaired renal function. Because elderly patients are more likely to have decreased renal function, care should be taken in dose selection. In addition, renal function should be monitored and dosage adjustments should be made accordingly (see Administration and Dosage, Dose adjustment).

➤*Pregnancy: Category B.* At ≈ 12 times the estimated human exposure, didanosine was slightly toxic to female rats and their pups during mid and late lactation. These rats showed reduced food intake and body weight gains but the physical and functional development of the offspring was not impaired and there were no major changes in the F2 generation. A study in rats showed that didanosine or its metabolites are transferred to the fetus through the placenta.

There are no adequate and well-controlled studies in pregnant women. Because animal reproduction studies are not always predictive of human response, this drug should be used during pregnancy only if clearly needed.

Fatal lactic acidosis has been reported in pregnant women who received the combination of didanosine and stavudine with other antiretroviral agents. It is unclear if pregnancy augments the risk of lactic acidosis/hepatic steatosis syndrome reported in non-pregnant individuals receiving nucleoside analogues (See Warnings, Lactic acidosis/Severe hepatomegaly with steatosis). The combination of didanosine and stavudine should be used with caution during pregnancy and is recommended only if the potential benefit clearly outweighs the potential risk. Health care providers caring for HIV-infected pregnant women receiving didanosine should be alert for early diagnosis of lactic acidosis/hepatic steatosis syndrome.

Antiretroviral pregnancy registry – To monitor maternal-fetal outcomes of pregnant women exposed to didanosine and other antiretroviral agents, an Antiretroviral Pregnancy Registry has been established. Physicians are encouraged to register patients by calling 1-800-258-4263.

➤*Lactation:* The Centers for Disease Control And Prevention recommend that HIV-infected mothers not breastfeed their infants to avoid risking postnatal transmission of HIV. A study in rats showed that following oral administration, didanosine or its metabolites were excreted into the milk of lactating rats. It is not known if didanosine is excreted in human milk. Because of both the potential for HIV transmission and the potential for serious adverse reactions in nursing infants, mothers should be instructed not to breast-feed if they are receiving didanosine.

➤*Children:* The safety and efficacy of didanosine delayed-release capsules in pediatric patients have not been established.

Precautions

➤*Peripheral neuropathy:* Peripheral neuropathy, manifested by numbness, tingling, or pain in the hands or feet, has been reported in patients receiving didanosine therapy. Peripheral neuropathy has occurred more frequently in patients with advanced HIV disease, in patients with a history of neuropathy, or in patients being treated with neurotoxic drug therapy, including stavudine (see Adverse Reactions).

➤*Phenylketonuria:* Didanosine chewable/dispersible buffered tablets contain 73 mg phenylalanine per 2-tablet dose (36.5 mg phenylalanine per tablet).

➤*Sodium-restricted diets:* Didanosine buffered powder for oral solution: Each single-dose packet of didanosine buffered powder for oral solution contains 1380 mg sodium.

Drug Interactions

Coadministration of didanosine with drugs that are known to cause pancreatitis may increase the risk of this toxicity (see Warnings). Because didanosine formulations either contain buffers or are mixed with antacids before administration, interactions may be anticipated with drugs whose absorption can be affected by the level of acidity in the stomach and with drugs that have been demonstrated to interact with antacids containing magnesium, calcium, or aluminum. Predicted drug interactions with didanosine are listed in the table below.

Didanosine Drug Interactions

Precipitant drug	Object drug*		Description
Allopurinol	Didanosine	↑	The AUC of didanosine was increased ≈ 4-fold when 300 mg/day allopurinol was coadministered with a single 200 mg dose of didanosine to 2 patients with renal impairment. Coadministration of these 2 drugs is not recommended.
Ganciclovir	Didanosine	↑	Administration of didanosine 2 hours prior to or concurrent with oral ganciclovir was associated with an increase in the steady-state AUC of didanosine. A decrease in the steady-state AUC of ganciclovir was observed when didanosine was administered 2 hours prior to ganciclovir, but not when the 2 drugs were administered simultaneously.
Didanosine	Ganciclovir	↓	
Methadone	Didanosine	↓	Administration of a single 200 mg dose of didanosine with chronic methadone dosing decreased the AUC and C_{max} of didanosine by 41% and 59%, respectively.
Didanosine	Antacids	↑	Concomitant administration of antacids containing magnesium or aluminum with didanosine chewable/dispersible tablets and pediatric powder may potentiate adverse events associated with the antacid components.
Didanosine	Antifungal agents	↓	The therapeutic effects of azole antifungal agents may be decreased. The buffers in didanosine chewable tablets appear to decrease the absorption of azole antifungal agents. Administer the azole antifungal drugs ≥ 2 hours before chewable tablets.

DIDANOSINE — ORAL

Didanosine Drug Interactions

Precipitant drug	Object drug*		Description
Didanosine	Antiretroviral drugs	⬇	Significant decreases in the AUC of delavirdine and indinavir occurred following simultaneous administration of these agents with didanosine. To avoid this interaction, give delavirdine or indinavir 1 hour prior to dosing with didanosine. The pharmacokinetics of nelfinavir are not altered to a clinically significant degree when it is administered with a light meal 1 hour after didanosine.
Didanosine	Fluoroquinolones	⬇	Plasma concentrations of some quinolone antibiotics are decreased when administered with antacids containing magnesium, calcium, or aluminum. Therefore, if concurrent use cannot be avoided, give the quinolone ≥ 2 hours before or 6 hours after didanosine.
Didanosine	Stavudine	⬆	Combination therapy of didanosine, stavudine, and other antiretrovirals has caused fatal lactic acidosis in women. Peripheral neuropathy has occurred more frequently in patients treated with neurotoxic drugs, including stavudine.

* ⬆ = Object drug increased. ⬇ = Object drug decreased.
⬌ = Undetermined clinical effect.

Predicted drug interactions with didanosine*

Drug or drug class	Effect	Clinical comment
Use with caution or not recommended, risk of adverse reactions may be increased		
Drugs that may cause pancreatic toxicity	⬆ Risk of pancreatitis	Use only with extreme caution.[a]
Neurotoxic drugs	⬆ Risk of neuropathy	Use with caution.[b]
Antacids containing magnesium or aluminum	⬆ Side effects associated with antacid components	Use caution with didanosine chewable/dispersable buffered tablets and pediatric powder for oral solution.
Ribavirin	⬆ Risk of toxicity	Ribavirin has been shown in vitro to increase intracellular triphosphate levels of didanosine. Coadministration is not recommended (see below).
Use with caution; plasma concentrations may be decreased by coadministration with didanosine		
Drug class	**Effect**	**Clinical comment**
Azole antifungals	⬇ Ketoconazole or itraconazole concentration	Administer drugs such as ketoconazole or itraconazole at least 2 hours before didanosine.
Quinolone antibiotics (see also ciprofloxacin in table above)	⬇ Quinolone concentration	Consult monograph for the quinolone
Tetracycline antibiotics	⬇ Antibiotic concentration	Consult monograph of the tetracycline.

* ⬆ = indicates increase; ⬇ = indicates decrease.
[a] Only if other drugs are not available and if clearly indicated. If treatment with life-sustaining drugs that cause pancreatic toxicity is required, suspension of didanosine is recommended (see Warnings, Pancreatitis).
[b] See Precautions: Peripheral Neuropathy.

Adverse Reactions

A serious toxicity of didanosine is pancreatitis, which may be fatal. Other important toxicities include lactic acidosis/severe hepatomegaly with steatosis; retinal changes and optic neuritis; and peripheral neuropathy.

When didanosine is used in combination with other agents with similar toxicities, the incidence of these toxicities may be higher than when didanosine is used alone. Thus, patients treated with didanosine in combination with stavudine, with or without hydroxyurea, may be at increased risk for pancreatitis and liver function abnormalities (see Warnings). Patients treated with didanosine in combination with stavudine may also be at increased risk for peripheral neuropathy (see Precautions).

➤*Adults:*

Selected clinical adverse events from monotherapy studies

	Percent of patients			
	ACTG 116A		ACTG 116B/117	
Adverse events	Didanosine (n = 197)	Zidovudine (n = 212)	Didanosine (n = 298)	Zidovudine (n = 304)
Diarrhea	19	15	28	21
Peripheral neurologic symptoms/neuropathy	17	14	20	12
Rash/pruritus	7	8	9	5
Abdominal pain	13	8	7	8
Pancreatitis	7	3	6	2

Selected clinical adverse events from combination studies

	Percent of patients[a]			
	AI454-148[b]		Start 2[b]	
Adverse events	Didanosine + stavudine + nelfinavir (n = 482)	Zidovudine + lamivudine + nelfinavir (n = 248)	Didanosine + stavudine + indinavir (n = 102)	Zidovudine + lamivudine + indinavir (n = 103)
Diarrhea	70	60	45	39
Nausea	28	40	53	67
Headache	21	30	46	37
Peripheral neurologic symptoms/neuropathy	26	6	21	10
Rash	13	16	30	18
Vomiting	12	14	30	35
Pancreatitis (see below)	1	*	< 1	*

[a] Percentages based on treated subjects.
[b] Median duration of treatment 48 weeks.
* This event was not observed in this study arm.

Pancreatitis – Pancreatitis resulting in death was observed in one patient who received didanosine plus stavudine plus nelfinavir in Study AI454-148 and in one patient who received didanosine plus stavudine plus indinavir in the Start 2 study. In addition, pancreatitis resulting in death was observed in 2 of 68 patients who received didanosine plus stavudine plus indinavir plus hydroxyurea in an ACTG clinical trial (see Warnings).

➤*Lab test abnormalities:*

Selected laboratory abnormalities from monotherapy studies*

	Percent of patients			
	ACTG 116A		ACTG 116B/117	
Parameter	Didanosine (n = 197)	Zidovudine (n = 212)	Didanosine (n = 298)	Zidovudine (n = 304)
AST (> 5•ULN)	9	4	7	6
ALT (> 5•ULN)	9	6	6	6
Alkaline phosphatase (> 5•ULN)	4	1	1	1
Amylase (≥ 1.4•ULN)	17	12	15	5
Uric acid (> 12 mg/dL)	3	1	2	1

* ULN = upper limit of normal.

Selected laboratory abnormalities from combinations studies (Grades 3 to 4)*

	Percent of patients[a]			
	AI454-148[b]		Start 2[b]	
Parameter	Didanosine + stavudine + nelfinavir (n = 482)	Zidovudine + lamivudine + nelfinavir (n = 248)	Didanosine + stavudine + indinavir (n = 102)	Zidovudine + lamivudine + indinavir (n = 103)
Bilirubin (> 2.6•ULN)	< 1	< 1	16	8
AST (> 5•ULN)	3	2	7	7
ALT (> 5•ULN)	3	3	8	5
GGT (> 5•ULN)	NC	NC	5	2

DIDANOSINE — ORAL

Selected laboratory abnormalities from combinations studies (Grades 3 to 4)*				
	Percent of patients[a]			
	AI454-148[b]		Start 2[b]	
Parameter	Didanosine + stavudine + nelfinavir (n = 482)	Zidovudine + lamivudine + nelfinavir (n = 248)	Didanosine + stavudine + indinavir (n = 102)	Zidovudine + lamivudine + indinavir (n = 103)
Lipase (> 2•ULN)	7	2	5	5
Amylase (> 2•ULN)	NC	NC	8	2

* ULN = upper limit of normal.NC = not collected.
[a] Percentages based on treated subjects.
[b] Median duration of treatment 48 weeks.

Selected laboratory abnormalties from combination studies (all grades)*				
	Percent of patients[a]			
	AI454-148[b]		Start 2[b]	
Parameter	Didanosine + stavudine + nelfinavir (n = 482)	Zidovudine + lamivudine + nelfinavir (n = 248)	Didanosine + stavudine + indinavir (n = 102)	Zidovudine + lamivudine + indinavir (n = 103)
Bilirubin	7	3	68	55
AST	42	23	53	20
ALT	37	24	50	18
GGT	NC	NC	28	12
Lipase	17	11	26	19
Amylase	NC	NC	31	17

* NC = not collected.
[a] Percentages based on treatment subjects.
[b] Median duration of treatment 48 weeks.

➤*Didanosine delayed-release capsules:*

Selected clinical adverse events from combination studies of didanosine dosed once daily				
	Percent of patients[a]			
	AI454-152[b]		AI454-148[c]	
Adverse events	Didanosine delayed-release capsule + stavudine + nelfinavir (n = 255)	Zidovudine/ lamivudine[d] + nelfinavir (n = 250)	Didanosine delayed release chewable tablet + stavudine + nelfinavir (n = 482)	Zidovudine + lamivudine + nelfinavir (n = 248)
Diarrhea	54	56	70	60
Nausea	21	35	28	40
Headache	20	16	21	30
Peripheral neurologic symptoms/neuropathy	20	8	26	6
Vomiting	13	18	12	14
Rash	10	10	13	16
Pancreatitis	< 1	[e]	1	[e]

[a] Percentages based on treatment patients.
[b] Median duration of treatment 43 weeks in the didanosine delayed-release capsule + stavudine + nelfinavir group and 39 weeks in the ziduvudine/lamivudine + nelfinavir group.
[c] Median duration of treated 48 weeks.
[d] Zidovudine/lamivudine combination tablet.
[e] This event was not observed in this study arm.

In clinical trials using a buffered formulation of didanosine, pancreatitis resulting in death was observed in 1 patient who received didanosine plus stavudine plus nelfinavir, 1 patient who received didanosine plus stavudine plus indinavir, and 2 of 68 patients who received didanosine plus stavudine plus indinavir plus hydroxyurea. In an early access program, pancreatitis resulting in death was observed in 1 patient who received didanosine delayed-release capsules plus stavudine plus hydroxyurea plus ritonavir plus indinavir plus efavirenz (see Warnings).

The frequency of pancreatitis is dose related. In phase 3 studies with buffered formulations of didanosine, incidence ranged from 1% to 10% with doses higher than are currently recommended and 1% to 7% with recommended dose.

Lab test abnormalities –

Selected laboratory abnormalities from combination studies of didanosine dosed once daily								
	Percent of patients[a]							
	AI454-152[b]				AI454-148[c]			
	Didanosine delayed-release capsules + stavudine + nelfinavir (n = 255)		Zidovudine/ lamivudine[d] + nelfinavir (n = 250)		Didanosine chewable tablet + stavudine + nelfinavir (n = 482)		Zidovudine + lamivudine + nelfinavir (n = 248)	
Parameter	Grades 3 to 4[e]	All grades	Grades 3 to 4[e]	All grades	Grades 3 to 4[e]	All grades	Grades 3 to 4[e]	ll grades
AST	4	40	4	17	3	42	2	23
ALT	4	39	4	20	3	37	3	24
Lipase	3	18	< 1	8	7	17	2	11
Bilirubin	< 1	7	< 1	3	< 1	7	< 1	3

[a] Percentages based on treated patients.
[b] Median duration of treatment 43 weeks in didanosine delayed-release + stavudine + nelfinavir group and 39 weeks in the zidovudine/lamivudine + nelfinavir group.
[c] Median duration of treatment 48 weeks.
[d] Zidovudine/lamivudine combination tablet.
[e] > 5•ULN for AST and ALT, ≥ 2.1•ULN for lipase, and ≥ 2.6•ULN for bilirubin (ULN = upper limit of normal).

➤*Postmarketing:* The following events have been identified during post-approval use of didanosine. Because they are reported voluntarily from a population of unknown size, estimates of frequency cannot be made. These events have been chosen for inclusion due to their seriousness, frequency of reporting, causal connection to didanosine, or a combination of these factors.

Endocrine – Pancreatitis (including fatal cases) (see Warnings), sialoadenitis, parotid gland enlargement, dry mouth, and dry eyes.

Hematologic – Anemia, leukopenia, and thrombocytopenia.

Hepatic – Lactic acidosis and hepatic steatosis (see Warnings); hepatitis and liver failure.

Metabolic – Diabetes mellitus, elevated serum alkaline phosphatase level, elevated serum amylase level, elevated serum gamma-glutamyltransferase level, elevated serum uric acid level, hypoglycemia, and hyperglycemia.

Musculoskeletal – Myalgia (with or without increases in creatinine phosphokinase), rhabdomyolysis including acute renal failure and hemodialysis, arthralgia, and myopathy.

Ophthalmic – Retinal depigmentation and optic neuritis (see Warnings).

Systemic – Anorexia, dyspepsia, and flatulence.

Miscellaneous – Abdominal pain, alopecia, anaphylactoid reaction, asthenia, chills/fever, and pain.

➤*Children:* In pediatric phase 1 studies, pancreatitis occurred in 2 of 60 (3%) patients treated at entry doses below 300 mg/m²/day and in 5 of 38 (13%) patients treated at higher doses.

Retinal changes and optic neuritis have been reported in pediatric patients.

Overdosage

➤*Symptoms:* In phase 1 studies, in which didanosine was initially administered at doses ten times the currently recommended dose, toxicities included: pancreatitis, peripheral neuropathy, diarrhea, hyperuricemia, and hepatic dysfunction.

➤*Treatment:* There is no known antidote for didanosine overdosage. Didanosine is not dialyzable by peritoneal dialysis, although there is some clearance by hemodialysis (see Pharmacokinetics).

Patient Information

Inform patients that pancreatitis, a serious toxicity of didanosine when used alone and in combination regimens, has been fatal.

Advise patients that peripheral neuropathy, manifested by numbness, tingling, or pain in the hands or feet, may develop during therapy with didanosine. Counsel patients that peripheral neuropathy occurs with greatest frequency in patients with advanced HIV disease or a history of peripheral neuropathy, and that dose modification or discontinuation of didanosine may be required if toxicity develops.

Inform patients that when didanosine is used in combination with other agents with similar toxicities, the incidence of adverse events may be higher than when didanosine is used alone. Follow these patients closely.

Caution patients about the use of medications or other substances, including alcohol, that may exacerbate didanosine toxicities.

Didanosine is not a cure for HIV infection, and patients may continue to develop HIV-associated illnesses, including opportunistic infections. There-

DIDANOSINE — ORAL

fore, counsel patients to remain under the care of a physician when using didanosine. Advise patients that didanosine therapy has not been shown to reduce the risk of HIV transmission to others through sexual contact or blood contamination. Inform patients that the long-term effects of didanosine are unknown at this time.

Inform patients that the preferred dosing frequency of didanosine is twice daily because there is more evidence to support the effectiveness of this dosing frequency. Consider once-daily dosing only for adult patients whose management requires once-daily dosing of didanosine.

Advise patients that to ensure proper acid neutralization in the stomach they must take ≥ 2 of the appropriate strength didanosine buffered tablets at each dose. To reduce the risk of GI side effects from excess antacid, patients should take no more than 4 didanosine buffered tablets at each dose.

LAMIVUDINE (3TC)

Rx	**Epivir-HBV** (GlaxoSmithKline)	**Tablets:** 100 mg	(GX CG5). Butterscotch color, capsule shape. Film-coated. In 60s.
Rx	**Epivir** (GlaxoSmithKline)	**Tablets:** 150 mg	(GX CJ7 150). White, diamond shape. Film-coated. In 60s.
		300 mg	(GX EJ7). Gray, diamond shape. Film-coated. In 30s.
Rx	**Epivir-HBV** (GlaxoSmithKline)	**Oral solution:** 5 mg/mL	Parabens, sucrose. Strawberry-banana flavor. In 240 mL.
Rx	**Epivir** (GlaxoSmithKline)	**Oral solution:** 10 mg/mL	Parabens, sucrose. Strawberry-banana flavor. In 240 mL.

LAMIVUDINE — ORAL

WARNING

Lactic acidosis and severe hepatomegaly with steatosis, including fatal cases, have been reported with the use of nucleoside analogues alone or in combination, including lamivudine and other antiretrovirals. A majority of these cases have been in women. Obesity and prolonged nucleoside exposure may be risk factors. Most of these reports have described patients receiving nucleoside analogues for treatment of HIV infection, but there have been reports of lactic acidosis in patients receiving lamivudine for hepatitis B. Particular caution should be exercised when administering lamivudine to any patient with known risk factors for liver disease; however, cases have also been reported in patients with no known risk factors. Treatment with lamivudine or lamivudine-HBV should be suspended in any patient who develops clinical or laboratory findings suggestive of lactic acidosis or pronounced hepatotoxicity (which may include hepatomegaly and steatosis even in the absence of marked transaminase elevations).

Lamivudine tablets and oral solution (used to treat HIV infection) contain a higher dose of the active ingredient (lamivudine) than lamivudine-HBV tablets and oral solution (used to treat chronic hepatitis B). Patients with HIV infection should receive only dosing forms appropriate for treatment of HIV. Lamivudine-HBV tablets and oral solution contain a lower dose of the same active ingredient (lamivudine) as lamivudine tablets and oral solution, lamivudine/zidovudine combination tablets, and abacavir, lamivudine, and zidovudine combination tablets used to treat HIV infection. The formulation and dosage of lamivudine in lamivudine-HBV are not appropriate for patients dually infected with HBV and HIV. Lamivudine has not been adequately studied for treatment of chronic hepatitis B in patients dually infected with HIV and HBV.

Lamivudine-HBV – Human immunodeficiency virus (HIV) counseling and testing should be offered to all patients before beginning lamivudine-HBV and periodically during treatment, because lamivudine-HBV tablets and oral solution contain a lower dose of the same active ingredient (lamivudine) as lamivudine tablets and oral solution used to treat HIV infection. If treatment with lamivudine-HBV is prescribed for chronic hepatitis B for a patient with unrecognized or untreated HIV infection, rapid emergence of HIV resistance is likely because of subtherapeutic dose and inappropriate monotherapy.

Indications

➤*HIV infection (Epivir):* In combination with other antiretroviral agents, for the treatment of HIV infection.

➤*Chronic hepatitis B:* Lamivudine-HBV for hepatitis B virus (HBV) is indicated for the treatment of chronic hepatitis B associated with evidence of hepatitis B viral replication and active liver inflammation.

Administration and Dosage

➤*Approved by the FDA:* November 17, 1995 (lamivudine oral solution and tablets); December 8, 1998 (lamivudine-HBV oral solution and tablets).

➤*Lamivudine:*

Adults – 300 mg daily, administered as either 150 mg twice daily or 300 mg once daily, in combination with other antiretroviral agents.

Children –

Infants/children/adolescents: The recommended oral dose of lamivudine for HIV-infected pediatric patients 3 months up to 16 years of age is 4 mg/kg twice daily (up to a maximum of 150 mg twice a day), administered in combination with other antiretroviral agents.

Renal function impairment – See Actions for more information.

Adjustment of dosage of lamivudine in adults and adolescents in accordance with creatinine clearance

Creatinine clearance (mL/min)	Recommended dosage of lamivudine
≥ 50	150 mg twice daily or 300 mg once daily
30 to 49	150 mg once daily
15 to 29	150 mg first dose, then 100 mg once daily
5 to 14	150 mg first dose, then 50 mg daily
< 5	50 mg first dose, then 25 mg once daily

Insufficient data are available to recommend a dosage of lamivudine in patients undergoing dialysis. Although there are insufficient data to recommend a specific dose adjustment of lamivudine in pediatric patients with renal impairment, a reduction in the dose or an increase in the dosing interval should be considered.

➤*Lamivudine-HBV:*

Adults – 100 mg once daily. Safety and efficacy of treatment beyond 1 year have not been established, and the optimum duration of treatment is not known.

Monitoring: See Precautions for more information.

HIV coinfection – The formulation and dosage of lamivudine in lamivudine-HBV are not appropriate for patients dually infected with HBV and HIV. If lamivudine is administered to such patients, the higher dosage indicated for HIV therapy should be used as part of an appropriate combination regimen, and the information for lamivudine, as well as for lamivudine-HBV, should be consulted.

Children – The recommended oral dose of lamivudine-HBV for pediatric patients 2 to 17 years of age with chronic hepatitis B is 3 mg/kg once daily up to a maximum daily dose of 100 mg. Safety and efficacy of treatment beyond 1 year have not been established, and the optimum duration of treatment is not known (see above).

Dose adjustment – It is recommended that doses of lamivudine-HBV be adjusted in accordance with renal function.

Adjustment of adult dosage of lamivudine-HBV in accordance with creatinine clearance

Creatinine clearance (mL/min)	Recommended dosage of lamivudine-HBV
≥ 50	100 mg once daily
30 to 49	100 mg first dose, then 50 mg once daily
15 to 29	100 mg first dose, then 25 mg once daily
5 to 14	35 mg first dose, then 15 mg once daily
< 5	35 mg first dose, then 10 mg once daily

Although there are insufficient data to recommend a specific dose adjustment of lamivudine-HBV in pediatric patients with renal impairment, a dose reduction should be considered.

No additional dosing of lamivudine-HBV is required after routine (4-hour) hemodialysis. Insufficient data are available to recommend a dosage of lamivudine-HBV in patients undergoing peritoneal dialysis.

➤*Storage/Stability:*

Lamivudine tablets – Store at 25°C (77°F); excursions permitted to 15° to 30°C (59° to 86°F).

Lamivudine oral solution – Store in tightly closed bottles at 25°C (77°F).

Lamivudine-HBV tablets – Store at 25°C (77°F); excursions permitted to 15° to 30°C (59° to 86°F).

Lamivudine-HBV oral solution – Store at controlled room temperature of 20° to 25°C (68° to 77°F) in tightly closed bottles.

LAMIVUDINE — ORAL

Actions

➤*Pharmacology:* Lamivudine is a synthetic nucleoside analogue. Intracellularly, lamivudine is phosphorylated to its active 5-triphosphate metabolite, lamivudine triphosphate (L-TP). The principal mode of action of L-TP is the inhibition of HIV-1 reverse transcriptase (RT) via DNA chain termination after incorporation of the nucleoside analogue. L-TP is a weak inhibitor of mammalian DNA polymerases alpha and beta, and mitochondrial DNA polymerase.

Lamivudine-HBV – Lamivudine is a synthetic nucleoside analogue. Lamivudine is phosphorylated intracellularly to lamivudine triphosphate, L-TP. Incorporation of the monophosphate form into viral DNA by hepatitis B virus (HBV) polymerase results in DNA chain termination. L-TP also inhibits the RNA- and DNA-dependent DNA polymerase activities of HIV-1 reverse transcriptase (RT). L-TP is a weak inhibitor of mammalian alpha-, beta-, and gamma-DNA polymerases.

➤*Pharmacokinetics:*

Absorption –

Lamivudine: Lamivudine was rapidly absorbed after oral administration in HIV-infected patients. Absolute bioavailability in 12 adult patients was 86% ± 16% (mean ± SD) for the 150 mg tablet and 87% ± 13% for the 10 mg/mL oral solution. After oral administration of 2 mg/kg twice a day to 9 adults with HIV, the peak serum lamivudine concentration (C_{max}) was 1.5 ± 0.5 mcg/mL (mean ± SD). The area under the plasma concentration vs time curve (AUC) and C_{max} increased in proportion to oral dose over the range from 0.25 to 10 mg/kg.

An investigational, 25 mg dosage form of lamivudine was administered orally to 12 asymptomatic, HIV-infected patients on 2 occasions, once in the fasted state and once with food (1099 kcal; 75 g fat, 34 g protein, 72 g carbohydrate). Absorption of lamivudine was slower in the fed state (t_{max}, 3.2 ± 1.3 hours) compared with the fasted state (t_{max}, 0.9 ± 0.3 hours); C_{max} in the fed state was 40% ± 23% (mean ± SD) lower than in the fasted state. There was no significant difference in systemic exposure (AUC_{∞}) in the fed and fasted states; therefore, lamivudine tablets and oral solution may be administered with or without food.

Lamivudine-HBV: Lamivudine was rapidly absorbed after oral administration in HBV-infected patients and in healthy subjects. Following single oral doses of 100 mg, the peak serum lamivudine concentration (C_{max}) in HBV-infected patients (steady state) and healthy subjects (single dose) was 1.28 ± 0.56 mcg/mL and 1.05 ± 0.32 mcg/mL (mean ± SD), respectively, which occurred between 0.5 and 2 hours after administration. The area under the plasma concentration vs time curve ($AUC_{0\text{-}24\ hr}$) following 100 mg lamivudine oral single and repeated daily doses to steady state was 4.3 ± 1.4 (mean ± SD) and 4.7 ± 1.7 mcg•hr/mL, respectively. The relative bioavailability of the tablet and solution was then demonstrated in healthy subjects. Although the solution demonstrated a slightly higher peak serum concentration (C_{max}), there was no significant difference in systemic exposure (AUC_{∞}) between the solution and the tablet. Therefore, the solution and the tablet may be used interchangeably.

After oral administration of lamivudine once daily to HBV-infected adults, the AUC and peak serum levels (C_{max}) increased in proportion to dose over the range from 5 mg to 600 mg once daily.

The 100 mg tablet was administered orally to 24 healthy subjects on 2 occasions, once in the fasted state and once with food (standard meal: 967 kcal; 67 g fat, 33 g protein, 58 g carbohydrate). There was no significant difference in systemic exposure (AUC_{∞}) in the fed and fasted states; therefore, lamivudine-HBV tablets and oral solution may be administered with or without food.

Distribution – The apparent volume of distribution after IV administration of lamivudine to 20 asymptomatic, HIV-infected patients was 1.3 ± 0.4 L/kg, suggesting that lamivudine distributes into extravascular spaces. Volume of distribution was independent of dose and did not correlate with body weight.

Binding of lamivudine to human plasma proteins is low (less than 36%). In vitro studies showed that, over the concentration range of 0.1 to 100 mcg/mL, the amount of lamivudine associated with erythrocytes ranged from 53% to 57% and was independent of concentration.

Metabolism – Metabolism of lamivudine is a minor route of elimination. In man, the only known metabolite of lamivudine is the trans-sulfoxide metabolite.

Lamivudine: Within 12 hours after a single oral dose of lamivudine in 6 HIV-infected adults, 5.2% ± 1.4% (mean ± SD) of the dose was excreted as the trans-sulfoxide metabolite in the urine. Serum concentrations of the trans-sulfoxide metabolite have not been determined.

Lamivudine-HBV: In 9 healthy subjects receiving 300 mg of lamivudine as single oral doses, a total of 4.2% (range, 1.5% to 7.5%) of the dose was excreted as the trans-sulfoxide metabolite in the urine, the majority of which was excreted in the first 12 hours. Serum concentrations of the trans-sulfoxide metabolite have not been determined.

Excretion – The majority of lamivudine is eliminated unchanged in urine by active organic cationic secretion. In 9 healthy subjects given a single 300 mg oral dose of lamivudine, renal clearance was 199.7 ± 56.9 mL/min (mean ± SD). In 20 HIV-infected patients given a single IV dose, renal clearance was 280.4 ± 75.2 mL/min (mean ± SD), representing 71% ± 16% (mean ± SD) of total clearance of lamivudine.

In most single-dose studies in HIV-infected patients, HBV-infected patients, or healthy subjects with serum sampling for 24 hours after dosing, the observed mean elimination half-life ($t_{1/2}$) ranged from 5 to 7 hours. In HIV-infected patients, total clearance was 398.5 ± 69.1 mL/min (mean ± SD). Oral clearance and elimination half-life were independent of dose and body weight over an oral dosing range from 0.25 to 10 mg/kg.

Special populations –

Renal function impairment: Exposure (AUC_{∞}), C_{max}, and half-life increased with diminishing renal function (as expressed by creatinine clearance). Apparent total oral clearance (Cl/F) of lamivudine decreased as creatinine clearance decreased. Time to maximum plasma concentration (t_{max}) was not significantly affected by renal function. Based on these observations, it is recommended that the dosage of lamivudine be modified in patients with renal impairment.

• *Lamivudine* –

Pharmacokinetic parameters (mean ± SD) after a single 300 mg oral dose of lamivudine in 3 groups of adults with varying degrees of renal function

Parameter	Creatinine clearance criterion (number of subjects)		
	> 60 mL/min (n = 6)	10 to 30 mL/min (n = 4)	< 10 mL/min (n = 6)
Creatinine clearance (mL/min)	111 ± 14	28 ± 8	6 ± 2
C_{max} (mcg/mL)	2.6 ± 0.5	3.6 ± 0.8	5.8 ± 1.2
AUC_{∞} (mcg•hr/mL)	11 ± 1.7	48 ± 19	157 ± 74
Cl/F (mL/min)	464 ± 76	114 ± 34	36 ± 11

• *Lamivudine-HBV* –

Pharmacokinetic parameters (mean ± SD) dose normalized to a single 100 mg oral dose of lamivudine in patients with varying degrees of renal function

Parameter	Creatinine clearance criterion (number of subjects)		
	≥ 80 mL/min (n = 9)	20 to 59 mL/min (n = 8)	< 20 mL/min (n = 6)
Creatinine clearance (mL/min)	97 (range 82 to 117)	39 (range 25 to 49)	15 (range 13 to 19)
C_{max} (mcg/mL)	1.31 ± 0.35	1.85 ± 0.4	1.55 ± 0.31
AUC_{∞} (mcg•hr/mL)	5.28 ± 1.01	14.67 ± 3.74	27.33 ± 6.56
Cl/F (mL/min)	326.4 ± 63.8	120.1 ± 29.5	64.5 ± 18.3

Hemodialysis increases lamivudine clearance from a mean of 64 to 88 mL/min; however, the length of time of hemodialysis (4 hours) was insufficient to significantly alter mean lamivudine exposure after a single-dose administration. Therefore, it is recommended, following correction of dose for creatinine clearance, that no additional dose modification be made after routine hemodialysis.

It is not known whether lamivudine can be removed by peritoneal dialysis or continuous (24-hour) hemodialysis.

Children:

• *Lamivudine* – Systemic clearance decreased with increasing age in pediatric patients.

After oral administration of lamivudine 4 mg/kg twice daily to 11 pediatric patients ranging from 4 months to 14 years of age, C_{max} was 1.1 ± 0.6 mcg/mL, and half-life was 2 ± 0.6 hours. In adults with similar blood sampling, the half-life was 3.7 ± 1 hours. Total exposure to lamivudine, as reflected by mean AUC values, was comparable between pediatric patients receiving an 8 mg/kg/day dose and adults receiving a 4 mg/kg/day dose.

• *Lamivudine-HBV* – Lamivudine pharmacokinetics were evaluated in a 28-day, dose-ranging study in 53 pediatric patients with chronic hepatitis B. Patients aged 2 to 12 years of age were randomized to receive lamivudine 0.35 mg/kg twice daily, 3 mg/kg once daily, 1.5 mg/kg twice daily, or 4 mg/kg twice daily. Patients aged 13 to 17 years of age received lamivudine 100 mg once daily. Lamivudine was rapidly absorbed (t_{max} 0.5 to 1 hour). In general, both C_{max} and exposure (AUC) showed dose proportionality in the dosing range studied. Weight-corrected oral clearance was highest at age 2 and declined from 2 to 12 years, where values were then similar to those seen in adults. A dose of 3 mg/kg given once daily produced a steady-state lamivudine AUC (mean 5953 ng•hr/mL ± 1562 SD) similar to that associated with a dose of 100 mg/day in adults.

➤*Microbiology:*

Antiviral activity in vitro –

Lamivudine: In HIV-1-infected MT-4 cells, lamivudine in combination with zidovudine at various ratios exhibited synergistic antiretroviral activity. The relationship between in vitro susceptibility of HIV to lamivudine and the inhibition of HIV replication in humans has not been established.

Drug resistance –

Lamivudine: Lamivudine-resistant variants of HIV-1 have been selected in vitro. Genotypic analysis showed that the resistance was due to a specific amino acid substitution in the HIV-1 reverse transcriptase at codon 184 changing the methionine residue to either isoleucine or valine.

HIV-1 strains resistant to both lamivudine and zidovudine have been isolated from patients. Susceptibility of clinical isolates to lamivudine and zidovudine was monitored in controlled clinical trials. In patients receiving lamivudine monotherapy or combination therapy with lamivudine plus zidovudine, HIV-1 isolates from most patients became phenotypically and genotypically resistant to lamivudine within 12 weeks. In some patients harboring zidovudine-resistant virus at baseline, phenotypic sensitivity to zidovudine was restored by 12 weeks of treatment with lamivudine and zidovudine. Combination therapy with lamivudine plus zidovudine delayed the emergence of mutations conferring resistance to zidovudine.

LAMIVUDINE — ORAL

Lamivudine-HBV – Mutations in the HBV polymerase YMDD motif have been associated with reduced susceptibility of HBV to lamivudine in vitro. In studies of non-HIV-infected patients with chronic hepatitis B, HBV isolates with YMDD mutations were detected in some patients who received lamivudine daily for 6 months or more, and were associated with evidence of diminished treatment response; similar HBV mutants have been reported in HIV-infected patients who received lamivudine-containing antiretroviral regimens in the presence of concurrent infection with hepatitis B virus.

Mutant viruses were associated with evidence of diminished treatment response at 52 weeks relative to lamivudine-treated patients without evidence of YMDD mutations in both adult and pediatric studies. These mutations can be detected by a research assay and have been associated with reduced susceptibility to lamivudine in vitro. Lamivudine-treated patients (adult and pediatric) with YMDD-mutant HBV at 52 weeks showed diminished treatment responses in comparison to lamivudine-treated patients without evidence of YMDD mutations, including lower rates of HBeAg seroconversion and HBeAg loss (no greater than placebo recipients), more frequent return of positive HBV DNA by solution hybridization or branched-chain DNA assay, and more frequent ALT elevations. In the controlled trials, when patients developed YMDD-mutant HBV, they had a rise in HBV DNA and ALT from their own previous on-treatment levels. Progression of hepatitis B, including death, has been reported in some patients with YMDD-mutant HBV, including patients from the liver transplant setting and from other clinical trials. The long-term clinical significance of YMDD-mutant HBV is not known. Increased clinical and laboratory monitoring may aid in treatment decisions if emergence of viral mutants is suspected.

Lamivudine –

Cross-resistance: Lamivudine-resistant HIV-1 mutants were cross-resistant to didanosine (ddI) and zalcitabine (ddC). In some patients treated with zidovudine plus didanosine or zalcitabine, isolates resistant to multiple reverse transcriptase inhibitors, including lamivudine, have emerged.

Contraindications

Previously demonstrated clinically significant hypersensitivity to any of the components of the products.

Warnings

➤*Pancreatitis:* Pancreatitis has been reported in patients receiving lamivudine, particularly in HIV-infected pediatric patients with prior nucleoside exposure.

In pediatric patients with a history of antiretroviral nucleoside exposure, a history of pancreatitis, or other significant risk factors for the development of pancreatitis, lamivudine should be used with caution. Treatment with lamivudine should be stopped immediately if clinical signs, symptoms, or laboratory abnormalities suggestive of pancreatitis occur. In early, open-label studies of lamivudine in children with HIV, pancreatitis was observed in 14% to 15% of patients.

➤*Lactic acidosis / severe hepatomegaly with steatosis:* See the Warning box for more information.

➤*Important differences among lamivudine-containing products:*

Differences between lamivudine-containing products, HIV testing, and risk of emergence of resistant HIV – Lamivudine-HBV tablets and oral solution contain a lower dose of the same active ingredient (lamivudine) as lamivudine tablets and oral solution, lamivudine/zidovudine combination tablets, and abacavir, lamivudine, and zidovudine combination tablets used to treat HIV infection. The formulation and dosage of lamivudine in lamivudine-HBV are not appropriate for patients dually infected with HBV and HIV. Lamivudine has not been adequately studied for treatment of chronic hepatitis B in patients dually infected with HIV and HBV.

If treatment with lamivudine-HBV is prescribed for chronic hepatitis B for a patient with unrecognized or untreated HIV infection, rapid emergence of HIV resistance is likely to result because of the subtherapeutic dose and the inappropriateness of monotherapy HIV treatment. If a decision is made to administer lamivudine to such patients, the higher dosage indicated for HIV therapy should be used as part of an appropriate combination regimen, and the prescribing information for lamivudine, lamivudine/zidovudine, or abacavir, lamivudine, and zidovudine, as well as for lamivudine-HBV should be consulted.

➤*Posttreatment exacerbations of hepatitis:* In clinical trials in non-HIV-infected patients treated with lamivudine for chronic hepatitis B, clinical and laboratory evidence of exacerbations of hepatitis have occurred after discontinuation of lamivudine or lamivudine-HBV. These exacerbations have been detected primarily by serum ALT elevations in addition to reemergence of HBV DNA commonly observed after stopping treatment. Although most events appear to have been self-limited, fatalities have been reported in some cases. Similar events have been reported from postmarketing experience after changes from lamivudine-containing HIV treatment regimens to non-lamivudine-containing regimens in patients infected with both HIV and HBV. The causal relationship to discontinuation of lamivudine treatment is unknown. Patients should be closely monitored with both clinical and laboratory followup for at least several months after stopping treatment. There is insufficient evidence to determine whether reinitiation of lamivudine alters the course of posttreatment exacerbations of hepatitis.

➤*Renal function impairment:* See Actions for more information.

➤*Elderly:* Clinical studies of lamivudine did not include sufficient numbers of subjects aged 65 and over to determine whether they respond differently from younger subjects. In general, dose selection for an elderly patient should be cautious, reflecting the greater frequency of decreased hepatic, renal, or cardiac function, and of concomitant disease or other drug therapy. In particular, because lamivudine is substantially excreted by the kidney and elderly patients are more likely to have decreased renal function, renal function should be monitored and dosage adjustments should be made accordingly.

➤*Pregnancy: Category C.* Evidence of early embryolethality was seen in the rabbit at exposure levels similar to those observed in humans, but there was no indication of this effect in the rat at exposure levels up to 35 times that in humans (up to 60 times that in humans for HBV). Studies in pregnant rats and rabbits showed that lamivudine is transferred to the fetus through the placenta.

In a subset of subjects from whom amniotic fluid specimens were obtained following natural rupture of membranes, amniotic fluid concentrations of lamivudine ranged from 1.2 to 2.5 mcg/mL (150 mg twice daily) and 2.1 to 5.2 mcg/mL (300 mg twice daily) and were typically greater than 2 times the maternal serum levels. Lamivudine should be used during pregnancy only if the potential benefits outweigh the risks.

Lamivudine-HBV – Lamivudine has not been shown to affect the transmission of HBV from mother to infant, and appropriate infant immunizations should be used to prevent neonatal acquisition of HBV.

Antiretroviral pregnancy registry – To monitor maternal-fetal outcomes of pregnant women exposed to lamivudine, a pregnancy registry has been established. Physicians are encouraged to register patients by calling the toll-free number.

➤*Lactation:* The Centers for Disease Control and Prevention recommend that HIV-infected mothers not breastfeed their infants to avoid risking postnatal transmission of HIV infection.

A study in lactating rats administered 45 mg/kg of lamivudine showed that lamivudine concentrations in milk were slightly greater than those in plasma. Lamivudine is also excreted in human milk. Samples of breast milk obtained from 20 mothers receiving lamivudine monotherapy (300 mg twice daily) or combination therapy (150 mg lamivudine twice daily and 300 mg zidovudine twice daily) had measurable concentrations of lamivudine.

Because of both the potential for HIV transmission and the potential for serious adverse reactions in nursing infants, mothers should be instructed not to breastfeed if they are receiving lamivudine.

➤*Children:*

Lamivudine – Limited, uncontrolled pharmacokinetic and safety data are available from administration of lamivudine (and zidovudine) to 36 infants up to 1 week of age in 2 studies in South Africa. In these studies, lamivudine clearance was substantially reduced in 1-week-old neonates relative to pediatric patients (greater than 3 months of age) studied previously. There is insufficient information to establish the time course of changes in clearance between the immediate neonatal period and the age ranges greater than 3 months old.

See Actions for more information.

Lamivudine-HBV – Safety and efficacy in pediatric patients younger than 2 years of age have not been established.

See Actions for more information.

Precautions

➤*Monitoring:* Patients should be monitored regularly during treatment by a physician experienced in the management of chronic hepatitis B. The safety and effectiveness of treatment with lamivudine-HBV beyond 1 year have not been established. During treatment, combinations of such events such as return of persistently elevated ALT, increasing levels of HBV DNA over time after an initial decline below assay limit, progression of clinical signs or symptoms of hepatic disease, or worsening of hepatic necroinflammatory findings may be considered as potentially reflecting loss of therapeutic response. Such observations should be taken into consideration when determining the advisability of continuing therapy with lamivudine-HBV.

The optimal duration of treatment, the durability of HBeAg seroconversions occurring during treatment, and the relationship between treatment response and long-term outcomes such as hepatocellular carcinoma or decompensated cirrhosis are not known.

➤*Patients with HIV and hepatitis B virus coinfection:* Safety and efficacy of lamivudine have not been established for treatment of chronic hepatitis B in patients dually infected with HIV and HBV. In non-HIV-infected patients treated with lamivudine for chronic hepatitis B, emergence of lamivudine-resistant HBV has been detected and has been associated with diminished treatment response. Emergence of hepatitis B virus variants associated with resistance to lamivudine has also been reported in HIV-infected patients who have received lamivudine-containing antiretroviral regimens in the presence of concurrent infection with hepatitis B virus.

➤*Differences between dosing regimens:* Trough levels of lamivudine in plasma and of intracellular lamivudine triphosphate were lower with once-daily dosing than with twice-daily dosing. The clinical significance of this observation is not known.

➤*Fat redistribution:* Redistribution/accumulation of body fat including central obesity, dorsocervical fat enlargement (buffalo hump), peripheral wasting, facial wasting, breast enlargement, and "cushingoid appearance" have been observed in patients receiving antiretroviral therapy. The mechanism and long-term consequences of these events are currently unknown. A causal relationship has not been established.

➤*Emergence of resistance-associated HBV mutations:* See Actions for more information.

➤*Special risk:* Safety and efficacy of lamivudine-HBV have not been established in patients with decompensated liver disease or organ transplants;

LAMIVUDINE — ORAL

pediatric patients less than 2 years of age; patients dually infected with HBV and HCV, hepatitis delta, or HIV; or other populations not included in the principal phase III controlled studies. There are no studies in pregnant women and no data regarding effect on vertical transmission, and appropriate infant immunizations should be used to prevent neonatal acquisition of HBV.

Drug Interactions

➤*Trimethoprim/sulfamethoxazole:* Trimethoprim (TMP) 160 mg and sulfamethoxazole (SMZ) 800 mg once daily has been shown to increase lamivudine exposure (AUC) by 44%. No change in dose of either drug is recommended. There is no information regarding the effect on lamivudine pharmacokinetics of higher doses of TMP/SMZ such as those used to treat *Pneumocystis carinii* pneumonia. No data are available regarding interactions with other drugs that have renal clearance mechanisms similar to that of lamivudine.

➤*Zalcitabine:* Lamivudine and zalcitabine may inhibit the intracellular phosphorylation of one another. Therefore, use of lamivudine in combination with zalcitabine is not recommended.

➤*Zidovudine:* Lamivudine and zidovudine were coadministered to 12 asymptomatic HIV-positive adult patients in a single-center, open-label, randomized, crossover study. No significant differences were observed in AUC_∞ or total clearance for lamivudine or zidovudine when the 2 drugs were administered together. Coadministration of lamivudine with zidovudine resulted in an increase of 39% ± 62% (mean ± SD) in C_{max} of zidovudine.

Adverse Reactions

➤*HIV infection:*

Adults –

Selected clinical adverse reactions (≥ 5% frequency) in 4 controlled clinical trials (A3001, A3002, B3001, B3002)		
Adverse reaction	Lamivudine 150 mg twice daily plus zidovudine (n = 251)	Zidovudine (n = 230)
Miscellaneous		
Headache	35%	27%
Malaise/fatigue	27%	23%
Fever or chills	10%	12%
GI		
Nausea	33%	29%
Diarrhea	18%	22%
Nausea/vomiting	13%	12%
Anorexia or decreased appetite	10%	7%
Abdominal pain	9%	11%
Abdominal cramps	6%	3%
Dyspepsia	5%	5%
CNS		
Neuropathy	12%	10%
Insomnia and other sleep disorders	11%	7%
Dizziness	10%	4%
Depressive disorders	9%	4%
Respiratory		
Nasal signs/symptoms	20%	11%
Cough	18%	13%
Dermatologic		
Skin rashes	9%	6%
Musculoskeletal		
Musculoskeletal pain	12%	10%
Myalgia	8%	6%
Arthralgia	5%	5%

The types and frequencies of clinical adverse reactions reported in patients receiving lamivudine 300 mg once daily or lamivudine 150 mg twice daily (in 3-drug combination regimens in EPV 20001 and EPV 40001) were similar. The most common adverse reactions in both treatment groups were nausea, dizziness, fatigue or malaise, headache, dreams, insomnia and other sleep disorders, and skin rash.

Pancreatitis was observed in 9 of the 2613 adult patients (0.3%) who received lamivudine in the controlled clinical trials EPV20001, NUCA3001, NUCB3001, NUCA3002, NUCB3002, and B3007.

Lab test abnormalities:

Frequencies of selected laboratory abnormalities in adults in four 24-week surrogate endpoint studies (A3001, A3002, B3001, B3002) and a clinical endpoint study (B3007)				
	24-week surrogate endpoint studies		Clinical endpoint study *	
Test (threshold level)	Lamivudine plus zidovudine	Zidovudine	Lamivudine plus current therapy	Placebo plus current therapy **
Absolute neutrophil count (ANC < 750/mm³)	7.2%	5.4%	15%	13%
Hemoglobin (< 8 g/dL)	2.9%	1.8%	2.2%	3.4%
Thrombocytopenia (platelets < 50,000/mm³)	0.4%	1.3%	2.8%	3.8%
ALT (> 5 × ULN [a])	3.7%	3.6%	3.8%	1.9%
AST (> 5 × ULN)	1.7%	1.8%	4%	2.1%
Bilirubin (> 2.5 × ULN)	0.8%	0.4%	ND [b]	ND
Amylase (> 2 × ULN)	4.2%	1.5%	2.2%	1.1%

* The median duration on study was 12 months.
** Current therapy was either zidovudine, zidovudine plus didanosine, or zidovudine plus zalcitabine.
[a] ULN – Upper limit of normal.
[b] ND = Not done.

Miscellaneous: In small, uncontrolled studies in which pregnant women were given lamivudine alone or in combination with zidovudine beginning in the last few weeks of pregnancy, reported adverse reactions included anemia, urinary tract infections, and complications of labor and delivery. In postmarketing experience, liver function abnormalities and pancreatitis have been reported in women who received lamivudine in combination with other antiretroviral drugs during pregnancy. It is not known whether risks of adverse reactions associated with lamivudine are altered in pregnant women compared to other HIV-infected patients.

Children –

Selected clinical adverse reactions and physical findings (≥ 5% frequency) in pediatric patients in Study ACTG300		
Adverse reaction	Lamivudine plus zidovudine (n = 236)	Didanosine (n = 235)
Miscellaneous		
Fever	25%	32%
Lymphadenopathy	9%	11%
GI		
Hepatomegaly	11%	11%
Nausea/vomiting	8%	7%
Diarrhea	8%	6%
Stomatitis	6%	12%
Splenomegaly	5%	8%
Respiratory		
Cough	15%	18%
Abnormal breath sounds/ wheezing	7%	9%
Ear, nose, and throat		
Signs or symptoms of ears *	7%	6%
Nasal discharge or congestion	8%	11%
Dermatologic		
Skin rashes	12%	14%

* Includes pain, discharge, erythema, or swelling of an ear.

Lab test abnormalities:

Frequencies of selected laboratory abnormalities in pediatric patients in Study ACTG300		
Test (abnormal level)	Lamivudine plus zidovudine	Didanosine
ANC [a]< 400/mm³	8%	3%
Hgb < 7 g/dL	4%	2%
Platelets < 50,000/mm³	1%	3%
ALT (> 10 × ULN [b])	1%	3%
AST (> 10 × ULN)	2%	4%

LAMIVUDINE — ORAL

Frequencies of selected laboratory abnormalities in pediatric patients in Study ACTG300		
Test (abnormal level)	Lamivudine plus zidovudine	Didanosine
Lipase (> 2.5 × ULN)	3%	3%
Total amylase (> 2.5 × ULN)	3%	3%

[a] ANC = Absolute neutrophil count.
[b] ULN = Upper limit of normal.

Pancreatitis: Pancreatitis, which has been fatal in some cases, has been observed in antiretroviral nucleoside-experienced pediatric patients receiving lamivudine alone or in combination with other antiretroviral agents. In an open-label dose-escalation study (A2002), 14 patients (14%) developed pancreatitis while receiving monotherapy with lamivudine. Three of these patients died of complications of pancreatitis. In a second open-label study (A2005), 12 patients (18%) developed pancreatitis. In Study ACTG300, pancreatitis was not observed in 236 patients randomized to lamivudine plus zidovudine. Pancreatitis was observed in 1 patient in this study who received open-label lamivudine in combination with zidovudine and ritonavir following discontinuation of didanosine monotherapy.

CNS: Paresthesias and peripheral neuropathies were reported in 15 patients (15%) in Study A2002, 6 patients (9%) in Study A2005, and 2 patients (less than 1%) in Study ACTG300.

Miscellaneous: Limited short-term safety information is available from 2 small, uncontrolled studies in South Africa in neonates receiving lamivudine with or without zidovudine for the first week of life following maternal treatment starting at week 38 or 36 of gestation. Adverse reactions reported in these neonates included increased liver function tests, anemia, diarrhea, electrolyte disturbances, hypoglycemia, jaundice and hepatomegaly, rash, respiratory infections, sepsis, and syphilis; 3 neonates died (1 from gastroenteritis with acidosis and convulsions, 1 from traumatic injury, and 1 from unknown causes). Two other nonfatal gastroenteritis or diarrhea cases were reported, including 1 with convulsions; 1 infant had transient renal insufficiency associated with dehydration. The absence of control groups further limits assessments of causality, but it should be assumed that perinatally exposed infants may be at risk for adverse reactions comparable to those reported in pediatric and adult HIV-infected patients treated with lamivudine-containing combination regimens. Long-term effects of in utero and infant lamivudine exposure are not known.

➤*Clinical trials in HBV (lamivudine-HBV):* Several serious adverse reactions reported with lamivudine (lactic acidosis and severe hepatomegaly with steatosis, posttreatment exacerbations of hepatitis B, pancreatitis, and emergence of viral mutants associated with reduced drug susceptibility and diminished treatment response) have occurred.

Adults –

Selected clinical adverse reactions (≥ 5% frequency in 3 placebo-controlled clinical trials in adults during treatment*) (studies 1 to 3)		
Adverse reaction	Lamivudine-HBV (n = 332)	Placebo (n = 200)
Non-site specific		
Malaise and fatigue	24%	28%
Fever or chills	7%	9%
Ear, nose, and throat		
Ear, nose, and throat infections	25%	21%
Sore throat	13%	8%
GI		
Nausea/vomiting	15%	17%
Abdominal discomfort and pain	16%	17%
Diarrhea	14%	12%
Musculoskeletal		
Myalgia	14%	17%
Arthralgia	7%	5%
CNS		
Headache	21%	21%
Dermatologic		
Skin rashes	5%	5%

* Includes patients treated for 52 to 68 weeks.

Lab test abnormalities: Frequencies of specified laboratory abnormalities during therapy with lamivudine-HBV compared with placebo are listed in the following table:

Frequencies of specified laboratory abnormalities in 3 placebo-controlled trials in adults during treatment* (studies 1 to 3)		
	Patients with abnormality/ patients with observations	
Test (abnormal level)	Lamivudine-HBV	Placebo
ALT > 3 × baseline [1]	37/331 (11%)	26/199 (13%)
Albumin < 2.5 g/dL	0/331 (0%)	2/199 (1%)
Amylase > 3 × baseline	2/259 (< 1%)	4/167 (2%)
Serum lipase ≥ 2.5 × the upper limit of normal (ULN)[2]	19/189 (10%)	9/127 (7%)
CPK ≥ 7 × baseline	31/329 (9%)	9/198 (5%)
Neutrophils < 750/mm^3	0/331 (0%)	1/199 (< 1%)
Platelets < 50,000/mm^3	10/272 (4%)	5/168 (3%)

* Includes patients treated for 52 to 68 weeks.
[1] See the following table for posttreatment ALT values.
[2] Includes observations during and after treatment in the 2 placebo-controlled trials that collected this information.

In patients followed for up to 16 weeks after discontinuation of treatment, posttreatment ALT elevations were observed more frequently in patients who had received lamivudine-HBV than in patients who had received placebo. A comparison of ALT elevations between weeks 52 and 68 in patients who discontinued lamivudine-HBV at week 52 and patients in the same studies who received placebo throughout the treatment course is shown in the following table:

Posttreatment ALT elevations in 2 placebo-controlled studies in adults with no-active-treatment follow-up (studies 1 and 3)		
	Patients with ALT elevation/ patients with observations *	
Abnormal value	Lamivudine-HBV	Placebo
ALT ≥ 2 × baseline value	37/137 (27%)	22/116 (19%)
ALT ≥ 3 × baseline value **	29/137 (21%)	9/116 (8%)
ALT ≥ 2 × baseline value and absolute ALT> 500 IU/L	21/137 (15%)	8/116 (7%)
ALT ≥ 2 × baseline value; and bilirubin> 2 × the upper limit of normal (ULN) and ≥ 2 × baseline value	1/137 (0.7%)	1/116 (0.9%)

* Each patient may be represented in 1 or more category.
** Comparable to a grade 3 toxicity in accordance with modified WHO criteria.

Lamivudine (HIV) vs lamivudine-HBV: In HIV-infected patients, safety information reflects a higher dose of lamivudine (150 mg twice daily) than the dose used to treat chronic hepatitis B in HIV-negative patients. In clinical trials using lamivudine as part of a combination regimen for treatment of HIV infection, several clinical adverse reactions occurred more often in lamivudine-containing treatment arms than in comparator arms. These included nasal signs and symptoms (20% vs 11%), dizziness (10% vs 4%), and depressive disorders (9% vs 4%). Pancreatitis was observed in 9 of 2613 adult patients (less than 0.5%) who received lamivudine in controlled clinical trials. Laboratory abnormalities reported more often in lamivudine-containing arms included neutropenia and elevations of liver function tests (also more frequent in lamivudine-containing arms for a retrospective analysis of HIV/HBV dually infected patients in one study), and amylase elevations.

Children with hepatitis B: Most commonly observed adverse reactions in the pediatric trials were similar to those in adult trials; in addition, respiratory symptoms (cough, bronchitis, and viral respiratory tract infections) were reported in both lamivudine and placebo recipients. Posttreatment transaminase elevations were observed in some patients followed after cessation of lamivudine.

➤*Postmarketing:*

CNS – Paresthesia, peripheral neuropathy.

Dermatologic – Alopecia, rash, pruritus.

Endocrine – Hyperglycemia.

GI – Stomatitis.

Hematologic/Lymphatic – Anemia (including pure red cell aplasia and severe anemias progressing on therapy), lymphadenopathy, splenomegaly.

Hepatic – Lactic acidosis and hepatic steatosis, pancreatitis, posttreatment exacerbation of hepatitis B.

Hypersensitivity – Anaphylaxis, urticaria.

Musculoskeletal – Muscle weakness, CPK elevation, rhabdomyolysis.

Respiratory – Abnormal breath sounds/wheezing.

Miscellaneous – Redistribution/accumulation of body fat, weakness.

Overdosage

➤*Symptoms:* One case of an adult ingesting 6 g of lamivudine was reported; there were no clinical signs or symptoms noted, and hematologic tests remained normal. Two cases of pediatric overdose were reported in ACTG300. One case was a single dose of 7 mg/kg of lamivudine; the second

LAMIVUDINE — ORAL

case involved use of 5 mg/kg of lamivudine twice daily for 30 days. There were no clinical signs or symptoms noted in either case.

➤*Treatment:* There is no known antidote for lamivudine. It is not known whether lamivudine can be removed by peritoneal dialysis or hemodialysis. If overdose occurs, the patient should be monitored, and standard supportive treatment applied as required.

Patient Information

➤*Lamivudine:* Lamivudine is not a cure for HIV infection and patients may continue to experience illnesses associated with HIV infection, including opportunistic infections. Patients should remain under the care of a physician when using lamivudine. Patients should be advised that the use of lamivudine has not been shown to reduce the risk of transmission of HIV to others through sexual contact or blood contamination.

Patients should be advised that lamivudine tablets and oral solution contain a higher dose of the same active ingredient (lamivudine) as lamivudine-HBV tablets and oral solution. If a decision is made to include lamivudine in the HIV treatment regimen of a patient dually infected with HIV and HBV, the formulation and dosage of lamivudine in lamivudine (not lamivudine-HBV) should be used.

Patients should be advised that the long-term effects of lamivudine are unknown at this time.

Lamivudine tablets and oral solution are for oral ingestion only.

Patients should be advised of the importance of taking lamivudine with combination therapy on a regular dosing schedule and to avoid missing doses.

Patients should be advised of the importance of taking lamivudine exactly as it is prescribed.

Parents or guardians should be advised to monitor pediatric patients for signs and symptoms of pancreatitis.

Patients should be informed that redistribution or accumulation of body fat may occur in patients receiving antiretroviral therapy and that the cause and long-term effects of these conditions are not known at this time.

Diabetic patients should be advised that each 15 mL dose of lamivudine oral solution contains 3 g of sucrose.

➤*Lamivudine-HBV:* Patients should remain under the care of a physician while taking lamivudine-HBV. They should discuss any new symptoms or concurrent medications with their physicians.

Patients should be advised that lamivudine-HBV is not a cure for hepatitis B, that the long-term treatment benefits of lamivudine-HBV are unknown at this time, and, in particular, that the relationship of initial treatment response to outcomes such as hepatocellular carcinoma and decompensated cirrhosis is unknown. Patients should be informed that deterioration of liver disease has occurred in some cases if treatment was discontinued, and that they should discuss any change in regimen with their physicians. Patients should be informed that emergence of resistant hepatitis B virus and worsening of disease can occur during treatment, and they should promptly report any new symptoms to their physicians.

Patients should be counseled on the importance of testing for HIV to avoid inappropriate therapy and development of resistant HIV, and HIV counseling and testing should be offered before starting lamivudine-HBV and periodically during therapy. Patients should be advised that lamivudine-HBV tablets and lamivudine-HBV oral solution contain a lower dose of the same active ingredient (lamivudine) as lamivudine tablets, lamivudine oral solution, lamivudine/zidovudine tablets, and abacavir sulfate/lamivudine/zidovudine tablets. Lamivudine-HBV should not be taken concurrently with lamivudine, lamivudine/zidovudine, or abacavir sulfate/lamivudine/zidovudine. Patients infected with both HBV and HIV who are planning to change their HIV treatment regimen to a regimen that does not include lamivudine, lamivudine/zidovudine, or abacavir sulfate/lamivudine/zidovudine should discuss continued therapy for hepatitis B with their physician.

Patients should be advised that treatment with lamivudine-HBV has not been shown to reduce the risk of transmission of HBV to others through sexual contact or blood contamination.

Diabetic patients should be advised that each 20 mL dose of lamivudine-HBV oral solution contains 4 g of sucrose.

STAVUDINE (d4T)

Rx	**Zerit** (BMS Virology)	**Capsules:** 15 mg	Lactose. (BMS 1964 15). Lt. yellow/dark red. In 60s.
		20 mg	Lactose. (BMS 1965 20). Lt. brown. In 60s.
		30 mg	Lactose. (BMS 1966 30). Lt. orange/dk. orange. In 60s.
		40 mg	Lactose. (BMS 1967 40). Dk. orange. In 60s.
		Powder for oral solution: 1 mg/mL when reconstituted	Sucrose, parabens. Dye-free. Fruit flavor. In 200 mL.

STAVUDINE — ORAL

WARNING

Lactic acidosis and severe hepatomegaly with steatosis, including fatal cases, have been reported with the use of nucleoside analogues alone or in combination, including stavudine and other antiretrovirals. Fatal lactic acidosis has been reported in pregnant women who received the combination of stavudine and didanosine with other antiretroviral agents. The combination of stavudine and didanosine should be used with caution during pregnancy and is recommended only if the potential benefit clearly outweighs the potential risk.

Fatal and nonfatal pancreatitis have occurred during therapy when stavudine was part of a combination regimen that included didanosine, with or without hydroxyurea, in both treatment-naïve and treatment-experienced patients, regardless of degree of immunosuppression.

Indications

➤*HIV infection:* For the treatment of HIV-1 infection in combination with other antiretroviral agents.

Administration and Dosage

➤*Approved by the FDA:* June 24, 1994.

➤*Capsules and oral solution:* The interval between doses of stavudine should be 12 hours. Stavudine may be taken without regard to meals.

Adults – The recommended dose based on body weight is as follows:
40 mg twice daily for patients greater than or equal to 60 kg.
30 mg twice daily for patients less than 60 kg.

Children – The recommended dose for newborns from birth to 13 days old is 0.5 mg/kg/dose given every 12 hours. The recommended dose for pediatric patients at least 14 days old and weighing less than 30 kg is 1 mg/kg/dose, given every 12 hours. Pediatric patients weighing 30 kg or greater should receive the recommended adult dosage.

Renal function impairment –

Recommended dosage adjustment for renal impairment

Creatinine clearance (mL/min)	Recommended stavudine dose by patient weight: ≥ 60 kg	< 60 kg
> 50	40 mg every 12 hours	30 mg every 12 hours
26 to 50	20 mg every 12 hours	15 mg every 12 hours
10 to 25	20 mg every 24 hours	15 mg every 24 hours

Since urinary excretion is also a major route of elimination of stavudine in pediatric patients, the clearance of stavudine may be altered in children with renal impairment. Although there are insufficient data to recommend a specific dose adjustment of stavudine in this patient population, a reduction in the dose or an increase in the interval between doses should be considered.

Hemodialysis patients – The recommended dose is 20 mg every 24 hours (greater than or equal to 60 kg) or 15 mg every 24 hours (less than 60 kg), administered after the completion of hemodialysis and at the same time of day on non-dialysis days.

Method of preparation for oral solution – Prior to dispensing, the pharmacist must constitute the dry powder with purified water to a concentration of 1 mg stavudine per mL of solution, as follows:

1.) Add 202 mL of purified water to the container.
2.) Shake container vigorously until the powder dissolves completely. Constitution in this way produces 200 mL (deliverable volume) of 1 mg/mL stavudine solution. The solution may appear slightly hazy.
3.) Dispense solution in original container with measuring cup provided. Instruct patient to shake the container vigorously prior to measuring each dose and to store the tightly closed container in a refrigerator, 2° to 8°C (36° to 46°F). Discard any unused portion after 30 days.

➤*Extended-release capsules:* Stavudine extended-release may be taken with or without food.

Stavudine extended-release is based on body weight and is administered in a once-daily schedule as follows:
100 mg once daily for patients greater than or equal to 60 kg.
75 mg once daily for patients less than or equal to 60 kg.

For patients who have difficulty swallowing intact capsules, the capsule can be carefully opened and the contents mixed with 2 tablespoons of yogurt or applesauce. Patients should be cautioned not to chew or crush the beads while swallowing.

Children – Stavudine extended-release has not been studied in pediatric patients.

STAVUDINE — ORAL

Renal function impairment – Stavudine extended-release has not been studied in patients with renal impairment.

➤*Dosage adjustment:* Patients should be monitored for the development of peripheral neuropathy, which is usually manifested by numbness, tingling, or pain in the feet or hands. These symptoms may be difficult to detect in young children. Peripheral neuropathy has occurred more frequently in patients with advanced HIV disease, a history of neuropathy, or concurrent neurotoxic drug therapy, including didanosine. If these symptoms develop during treatment, stavudine therapy should be interrupted. Symptoms may resolve if therapy is withdrawn promptly, although in some cases, symptoms may worsen temporarily following discontinuation of therapy. Switching the patient to an alternate treatment regimen should be considered. If switching to an alternate regimen is not suitable and if symptoms resolve satisfactorily after temporary withdrawal, treatment with stavudine extended-release may be resumed at 50% of the recommended dosage.

Immediate-release –
Patients greater than or equal to 60 kg: 20 mg twice daily.
Patients less than 60 kg: 15 mg twice daily .

Extended-release –
Patients greater than or equal to 60 kg: 50 mg once daily.
Patients less than 60 kg: 37.5 mg once daily.

If peripheral neuropathy recurs, permanent discontinuation of stavudine extended-release should be considered.

➤*Storage / Stability:*

Capsules – Store in tightly closed containers at controlled room temperature, 15° to 30°C (59° to 86°F).

Oral solution – Protect from excessive moisture and store in tightly closed containers at controlled room temperature, 15° to 30°C (59° to 86°F). After constitution, store tightly closed containers in a refrigerator, 2° to 8°C (36° to 46°F). Discard any unused portion after 30 days.

Extended-release capsules – Store in tightly closed containers at 25°C (77°F). Excursions between 15° and 30°C (59° and 86°F) are permitted.

Actions

➤*Pharmacology:* Stavudine, a nucleoside analogue of thymidine, inhibits the replication of HIV in human cells in vitro. Stavudine is phosphorylated by cellular kinases to the active metabolite stavudine triphosphate. Stavudine triphosphate inhibits the activity of HIV-1 reverse transcriptase (RT) by competing with the natural substrate thymidine tri-phosphate (K_i = 0.0083 to 0.032 mcM) and by causing DNA chain termination following its incorporation into viral DNA. Stavudine triphosphate inhibits cellular DNA polymerases beta and gamma, and markedly reduces the synthesis of mitochondrial DNA.

➤*Pharmacokinetics:*

Absorption –
Capsules and oral solution: Following oral administration, stavudine is rapidly absorbed, with peak plasma concentrations occurring within 1 hour after dosing. The systemic exposure to stavudine is the same following administration as capsules or solution.
Extended-release capsules: In a crossover study in healthy volunteers, equivalent values for stavudine AUC (total daily exposure) were observed for the extended-release and immediate-release formulations. AUC increased proportionally with dose in the oral dose range of 37.5 to 100 mg.

In parallel groups of HIV-infected patients, stavudine exposure was on average 23% lower following administration of 100 mg once daily of the extended-release formulation compared with 40 mg twice daily of the immediate-release formulation. The maximum plasma concentration (C_{max}) for the extended-release capsule is 43% of the value for the immediate-release capsule, and the time to reach C_{max} (t_{max}) is approximately 3 hours for the extended-release capsule compared with 1 hour for the immediate-release capsule. No significant accumulation of stavudine was observed after repeated administration of the extended-release capsule every 24 hours.

Compared to the fasted condition, the administration of stavudine extended-release capsules with a high-fat meal (945 kcal), a light meal (373 kcal), yogurt (26 kcal, 2 tablespoons), or applesauce (32 kcal, 2 tablespoons) did not significantly alter the stavudine AUC and C_{max}.

Distribution – Binding of stavudine to serum proteins was negligible over the concentration range of 0.01 to 11.4 mcg/mL. Stavudine distributes equally between red blood cells and plasma.

Metabolism – The metabolic fate of stavudine has not been elucidated in humans.

Excretion – Renal elimination accounted for about 40% of the overall clearance regardless of the route of administration.

The mean renal clearance is about twice the average endogenous creatinine clearance, indicating active tubular secretion in addition to glomerular filtration. The remaining 60% of the drug is presumably eliminated by endogenous pathways. The elimination half-life of stavudine is 1.6 hours.

Special populations –
Renal function impairment:
• *Capsules and oral solution* – Data from 2 studies indicated that the apparent oral clearance of stavudine decreased and the terminal elimination half-life increased as creatinine clearance decreased (see table below). C_{max} and t_{max} were not significantly altered by renal insufficiency. The mean ± SD hemodialysis clearance value of stavudine was 120 ± 18 mL/min (n = 12); the mean ± SD percentage of the stavudine dose recovered in the dialysate, timed to occur between 2 to 6 hours post-dose, was 31 ± 5%. Based on these observations, it is recommended that stavudine dosage be modified in patients with reduced creatinine clearance and in patients receiving maintenance hemodialysis.

Mean ± SD pharmacokinetic parameter values single 40 mg oral dose of stavudine[1]

	Creatinine clearance			Hemodialysis patients* (n = 11)
	> 50 mL/min (n = 10)	26 to 50 mL/min (n = 5)	9 to 25 mL/min (n = 5)	
Ccr (mL/min)	104 ± 28	41 ± 5	17 ± 3	NA
CL/F (mL/min)	335 ± 57	191 ± 39	116 ± 25	105 ± 17
CL_R (mL/min)	167 ± 65	73 ± 18	17 ± 3	NA
$t_{½}$ (hr)	1.7 ± 0.4	3.5 ± 2.5	4.6 ± 0.9	5.4 ± 1.4

* Determined while patients were off dialysis.
[1] Ccr = creatinine clearance; CL/F = apparent oral clearance; CL_R = renal clearance; $t_{½}$ = terminal elimination half-life; NA = not applicable.

• *Extended-release capsules* – The extended-release formulation of stavudine should not be used in patients with creatinine clearance less than or equal to 50 mL/min.

The effects of renal dysfunction on the pharmacokinetics of the extended-release capsule have not been investigated. With an immediate-release formulation of stavudine indicated that the apparent oral clearance of stavudine decreased and the terminal elimination half-life increased as creatinine clearance decreased. The applicability of the results from the immediate-release formulation to the extended-release formulation needs to be further investigated.

Children:
• *Capsules and oral solution* – For pharmacokinetic properties of stavudine in pediatric patients, see the table below.

Pharmacokinetic parameters (mean ± SD) of stavudine in HIV-exposed or HIV-infected pediatric patients

Parameter	Ages 5 weeks to 15 years	n	Ages 14 to 28 days	n	Day of birth	n
Oral bioavailability (%)	76.9 ± 31.7	20	ND*		ND*	
Volume of distribution[a] (L/kg)	0.73 ± 0.32	21	ND*		ND*	
Ratio of CSF:plasma concentrations (as %)[b]	59 ± 35	8	ND*		ND*	
Total body clearance[a] (mL/min/kg)	9.75 ± 3.76	21	ND*		ND*	
Apparent oral clearance[c] (mL/min/kg)	13.75 ± 4.29	20	11.52 ± 5.93	30	5.08 ± 2.8	17
Elimination half-life, IV dose[a] (hr)	1.11 ± 0.28	21	ND*		ND*	
Elimination half-life oral dose[c] (hr)	0.96 ± 0.26	20	1.59 ± 0.29	30	5.27 ± 2.01	17
Urinary recovery of stavudine (% of dose)[c]	34 ± 16	19	ND*		ND*	

[a] Following 1-hour IV infusion.
[b] Following multiple oral doses.
[c] Following single oral doses.
* ND = not determined.

Capsules and oral solution –
Pharmacokinetics in adults: The pharmacokinetics of stavudine have been evaluated in HIV-infected adult and pediatric patients (see tables below). Peak plasma concentrations (C_{max}) and area under the plasma concentration-time curve (AUC) increased in proportion to dose after both single and multiple doses ranging from 0.03 to 4 mg/kg. There was no significant accumulation of stavudine with repeated administration every 6, 8, or 12 hours.

Pharmacokinetic parameters of stavudine in adult HIV-infected patients

Parameter	Mean ± SD	n
Oral bioavailability	86.4 ± 18.2%	25
Volume of distribution[a]	58 ± 21 L	44
Apparent oral volume of distribution[b]	66 ± 22 L	71
Total body clearance[a]	8.3 ± 2.3 mL/min/kg	44
Apparent oral clearance[b]	8 ± 2.6 mL/min/kg	113
Elimination half-life, IV dose[a]	1.15 ± 0.35 hr	44
Elimination half-life, oral dose[b]	1.44 ± 0.3 hr	115
Urinary recovery of stavudine (% of dose)[b]	39 ± 23%	88

[a] Following 1-hour IV infusion.
[b] Following single oral dose.

STAVUDINE — ORAL

Steady-state pharmacokinetic parameters of stavudine extended-release in HIV-infected adults are compared with those of the immediate-release formulation in the table below.

Pharmacokinetic parameters of stavudine in HIV-infected adults, stavudine extended-release versus stavudine immediate-release: Absorption*		
Parameter	Stavudine extended-release 100 mg once daily	Stavudine immediate-release 40 mg twice daily
	Mean ± SD (n = 19[a])	Mean ± SD (n = 8[a])
AUC (ng•hr/mL)	1966 ± 629	2568 ± 454
C_{max} (ng/mL)	228 ± 62	536 ± 146
C_{min} (ng/mL)	24 ± 17	8 ± 9

[a] Parallel groups for extended-release and immediate-release formulations in HIV-infected adults.
* AUC = area under the curve over 24 hours. C_{max} = maximum plasma concentration. C_{min} = trough or minimum plasma concentration.

Extended-release capsules –
Pharmacokinetics in adults: The pharmacokinetic properties of stavudine administered as an extended-release capsule have been evaluated in healthy adult volunteers and HIV-infected adults. The slow release of stavudine from the extended-release capsule maintains measurable plasma concentrations for 24 hours after once-daily dosing. With once-daily dosing of the extended-release capsule, there is approximately 50% lower fluctuation of plasma concentration than observed with twice-daily dosing of the immediate-release formulation of stavudine.

➤*Microbiology:*

In vitro HIV susceptibility – The in vitro antiviral activity of stavudine was measured in peripheral blood mononuclear cells, monocytic cells, and lymphoblastoid cell lines. The concentration of drug necessary to inhibit viral replication by 50% (ED_{50}) ranged from 0.009 to 4 mcM against laboratory and clinical isolates of HIV-1. Stavudine had additive and synergistic activity in combination with didanosine and zalcitabine, respectively, in vitro. Stavudine combined with zidovudine had additive or antagonistic activity in vitro depending upon the molar ratios of the agents tested. The relationship between in vitro susceptibility of HIV to stavudine and the inhibition of HIV replication in humans has not been established.

Drug resistance –
Capsules and oral solution: HIV isolates with reduced susceptibility to stavudine have been selected in vitro and were also obtained from patients treated with stavudine. Phenotypic analysis of HIV isolates from stavudine-treated patients revealed, in 3 of 20 paired isolates, a 4- to 12-fold decrease in susceptibility to stavudine in vitro. The genetic basis for these susceptibility changes has not been identified. The clinical relevance of changes in stavudine susceptibility has not been established.
Extended-release capsules: HIV-1 isolates with reduced susceptibility to stavudine have been selected in vitro (strain-specific) and were also obtained from patients treated with stavudine. Phenotypic analysis of HIV-1 isolates from 61 patients receiving prolonged (6 to 29 months) stavudine monotherapy showed that post-therapy isolates from 4 patients exhibited IC_{50} values more than 4-fold (range 7- to 16-fold) higher than the average pretreatment susceptibility of baseline isolates. Of these, HIV-1 isolates from 1 patient contained the zidovudine-resistance-associated mutations T215Y and K219E, and isolates from another patient contained the multiple-nucleoside-resistance-associated mutation Q151M. Mutations in the RT gene of HIV-1 isolates from the other 2 patients were not detected. The genetic basis for stavudine susceptibility changes has not been identified.

Cross-resistance –
Capsules and oral solution: Five of 11 stavudine post-treatment isolates developed moderate resistance to zidovudine (9- to 176-fold) and 3 of those 11 isolates developed moderate resistance to didanosine (7- to 29-fold). The clinical relevance of these findings is unknown.
Extended-release capsules: Several studies have demonstrated that prolonged stavudine treatment can select or maintain mutations associated with zidovudine resistance. HIV-1 isolates with 1 or more zidovudine-resistance-associated mutations (M41L, D67N, K7OR, L210W, T215Y/F, K219Q/E) exhibited reduced susceptibility to stavudine in vitro.

Contraindications

Clinically significant hypersensitivity to stavudine or to any of the components contained in the formulation.

Warnings

➤*Lactic acidosis/severe hepatomegaly with steatosis/hepatic failure:* Lactic acidosis and severe hepatomegaly with steatosis, including fatal cases, have been reported with the use of nucleoside analogues alone or in combination, including stavudine and other antiretrovirals. Although relative rates of lactic acidosis have not been assessed in prospective well-controlled trials, longitudinal cohort and retrospective studies suggest that this infrequent event may be more often associated with antiretroviral combinations containing stavudine. Female gender, obesity, and prolonged nucleoside exposure may be risk factors. Fatal lactic acidosis has been reported in pregnant women who received the combination of stavudine and didanosine with other antiretroviral agents. The combination of stavudine and didanosine should be used with caution during pregnancy and is recommended only if the potential benefit clearly outweighs the potential risk.

Particular caution should be exercised when administering stavudine to any patient with known risk factors for liver disease; however, cases of lactic acidosis have also been reported in patients with no known risk factors. Generalized fatigue, digestive symptoms (nausea, vomiting, abdominal pain, and sudden unexplained weight loss); respiratory symptoms (tachypnea and dyspnea); or neurologic symptoms (including motor weakness, see Neurologic symptoms) might be indicative of lactic acidosis syndrome or the development of symptomatic hyperlactatemia.

Treatment with stavudine should be suspended in any patient who develops clinical or laboratory findings suggestive of lactic acidosis or pronounced hepatotoxicity (which may include hepatomegaly and steatosis even in the absence of marked transaminase elevations).

An increased risk of hepatotoxicity may occur in patients treated with stavudine in combination with didanosine and hydroxyurea compared to when stavudine is used alone. Deaths attributed to hepatotoxicity have occurred in patients receiving this combination. Patients treated with this combination should be closely monitored for signs of liver toxicity.

➤*Neurologic symptoms:* Motor weakness has been reported rarely in patients receiving combination antiretroviral therapy including stavudine. Most of these cases occurred in the setting of lactic acidosis. The evolution of motor weakness may mimic the clinical presentation of Guillain-Barré syndrome (including respiratory failure). Symptoms may continue or worsen following discontinuation of therapy.

Peripheral neuropathy, manifested by numbness, tingling, or pain in the hands or feet, has been reported in patients receiving stavudine therapy. Peripheral neuropathy has occurred more frequently in patients with advanced HIV disease, a history of neuropathy, or concurrent neurotoxic drug therapy, including didanosine.

See Administration and Dosage for more information.

➤*Pancreatitis:* Fatal and nonfatal pancreatitis have occurred during therapy when stavudine was part of a combination regimen that included didanosine, with or without hydroxyurea, in both treatment-naive and treatment-experienced patients, regardless of degree of immunosuppression. The combination of stavudine and didanosine (with or without hydroxyurea) and any other agents that are toxic to the pancreas should be suspended in patients with suspected pancreatitis. Reinstitution of stavudine after a confirmed diagnosis of pancreatitis should be undertaken with particular caution and close patient monitoring. The new regimen should contain neither didanosine nor hydroxyurea.

➤*Carcinogenesis:* In 2-year carcinogenicity studies in mice and rats, stavudine was noncarcinogenic at doses which produced exposures (AUC) 39 and 168 times, respectively, human exposure at the recommended clinical dose. Benign and malignant liver tumors in mice and rats and malignant urinary bladder tumors in male rats occurred at levels of exposure 250 (mice) and 732 (rats) times human exposure at the recommended clinical dose.

➤*Mutagenesis:* Stavudine was not mutagenic in the Ames, *E. coli* reverse mutation, or the CHO/HGPRT mammalian cell forward gene mutation assays, with and without metabolic activation. Stavudine produced positive results in the in vitro human lymphocyte clastogenesis and mouse fibroblast assays, and in the in vivo mouse micronucleus test. In the in vitro assays, stavudine elevated the frequency of chromosome aberrations in human lymphocytes (concentrations of 25 to 250 mcg/mL, without metabolic activation) and increased the frequency of transformed foci in mouse fibroblast cells (concentrations of 25 to 2500 mcg/mL, with and without metabolic activation). In the in vivo micronucleus assay, stavudine was clastogenic in bone marrow cells following oral stavudine administration to mice at dosages of 600 to 2000 mg/kg/day for 3 days.

➤*Elderly:* In a monotherapy Expanded Access Program in which patients with advanced HIV infection were treated with stavudine immediate-release, peripheral neuropathy or peripheral neuropathic symptoms were observed in 15 of 40 (38%) elderly patients receiving 40 mg twice daily and 8 of 51 (16%) elderly patients receiving 20 mg twice daily. Of the approximately 12,000 patients enrolled in the Expanded Access Program, peripheral neuropathy or peripheral neuropathic symptoms developed in 30% of patients receiving 40 mg twice daily and 25% of patients receiving 20 mg twice daily. Elderly patients should be closely monitored for signs and symptoms of peripheral neuropathy.

Stavudine is known to be substantially excreted by the kidney, and the risk of toxic reactions to this drug may be greater in patients with impaired renal function. Because elderly patients are more likely to have decreased renal function, it may be useful to monitor renal function. Stavudine immediate-release, with dose adjustment, is recommended for patients with creatinine clearance less than or equal to 50 mL/min.

➤*Pregnancy: Category C.* Reproduction studies have been performed in rats and rabbits with exposures (based on C_{max}) up to 399 and 183 times, respectively, of that seen at a clinical dosage of 1 mg/kg/day and have revealed no evidence of teratogenicity. The incidence in fetuses of a common skeletal variation, unossified or incomplete ossification of sternebra, was increased in rats at 399 times human exposure, while no effect was observed at 216 times human exposure. A slight post-implantation loss was noted at 216 times the human exposure with no effect noted at approximately 135 times the human exposure. An increase in early rat neonatal mortality (birth to 4 days of age) occurred at 399 times the human exposure, while survival of neonates was unaffected at approximately 135 times the human exposure. A study in rats showed that stavudine is transferred to the fetus through the placenta. The concentration in fetal tissue was approximately one-half the concentration in maternal plasma. Animal reproduction studies are not always predictive of human response. There are no adequate and well-controlled studies of stavudine in pregnant women. Stavudine should be used during pregnancy only if the potential benefit justifies the potential risk. Fatal lactic acidosis has been reported in pregnant women who received the combination of stavudine and didanosine with other antiretroviral agents. It is unclear if pregnancy augments the risk of lactic acidosis/hepatic steatosis syndrome reported in non-pregnant individuals receiving nucleoside analogues (see Lactic acidosis/severe hepatomegaly with steatosis). The combination of stavudine and didanosine should be used with caution during pregnancy and is recommended only if the potential benefit clearly outweighs the potential risk. Healthcare providers caring for HIV-infected pregnant women receiving stavudine should be alert for early diagnosis of lactic acidosis/hepatic steatosis syndrome.

Antiretroviral pregnancy registry – To monitor maternal-fetal outcomes of pregnant women exposed to stavudine and other antiretroviral agents, an Antiretroviral Pregnancy Registry has been established. Physicians are encouraged to register patients by calling (800) 258-4263.

➤*Lactation:* The Centers for Disease Control and Prevention recommend that HIV-infected mothers not breastfeed their infants to avoid risking postnatal transmission of HIV. Studies in lactating rats demonstrated that stavudine is excreted in milk. Although it is not known whether stavudine is excreted in human milk, there exists the potential for adverse effects from stavudine in nursing infants. Because of both the potential for HIV transmission and the potential for serious adverse reactions in nursing infants, mothers should be instructed not to breastfeed if they are receiving stavudine.

➤*Children:*

Capsules and oral solution – Use of stavudine in pediatric patients from birth through adolescence, is supported by evidence from adequate and well-controlled studies of stavudine in adults with additional pharmacokinetic and safety data in pediatric patients.

Extended-release capsules – The safety and efficacy of stavudine extended-release in pediatric patients have not been established.

Precautions

➤*Fat redistribution:* Redistribution/accumulation of body fat including central obesity, dorsocervical fat enlargement (buffalo hump), peripheral wasting, facial wasting, breast enlargement, and "cushingoid appearance" have been observed in patients receiving antiretroviral therapy. The mechanism and long-term consequences of these events are currently unknown. A causal relationship has not been established.

Drug Interactions

Stavudine Drug Interactions

Precipitant drug	Object drug*		Description
Didanosine Hydroxyurea	Stavudine	↑	Coadministration may increase the risk for lactic acidosis, hepatotoxicity, pancreatitis, or peripheral neuropathy (see Warnings).
Doxorubicin Ribavirin	Stavudine	↓	Phosphorylation of stavudine is inhibited at relevant concentrations by doxorubicin and ribavirin. Coadministration should be undertaken with caution.
Methadone	Stavudine	↓	Coadministration produced a 25% decrease in AUC and a 44% decrease in peak drug concentration of stavudine.
Zidovudine	Stavudine	↓	Zidovudine may competitively inhibit the intracellular phosphorylation of stavudine. Coadministration is not recommended.

Drug interaction studies have demonstrated that there are no clinically significant interaction between stavudine and the following: Didanosine, lamivudine, or nelfinavir.

Adverse Reactions

➤*Adults:* Fatal lactic acidosis has occurred in patients treated with stavudine in combination with other antiretroviral agents. Patients with suspected lactic acidosis should immediately suspend therapy with stavudine. Permanent discontinuation of stavudine should be considered for patients with confirmed lactic acidosis.

Stavudine therapy has rarely been associated with motor weakness, occurring predominantly in the setting of lactic acidosis. If motor weakness develops, stavudine should be discontinued.

Stavudine therapy has also been associated with peripheral sensory neuropathy, which can be severe, is dose related, and occurs more frequently in patients being treated with neurotoxic drug therapy, including didanosine, in patients with advanced HIV infection, or in patients who have previously experienced peripheral neuropathy.

Neuropathy: See Administration and Dosage for more information.

When stavudine is used in combination with other agents with similar toxicities, the incidence of adverse reactions may be higher than when stavudine is used alone. Pancreatitis, peripheral neuropathy, and liver function abnormalities occur more frequently in patients treated with the combination of stavudine and didanosine, with or without hydroxyurea. Fatal pancreatitis and hepatotoxicity may occur more frequently in patients treated with stavudine in combination with didanosine and hydroxyurea.

Selected clinical adverse reactions in Study AI455-019[a] (monotherapy)

Adverse reactions	Stavudine (40 mg twice daily) (n = 412)	Zidovudine (200 mg 3 times daily) (n = 402)
Headache	54%	49%
Diarrhea	50%	44%
Peripheral neurologic symptoms/neuropathy	52%	39%
Rash	40%	35%
Nausea/vomiting	39%	44%

[a] Median duration of stavudine therapy = 79 weeks; median duration of zidovudine therapy = 53 weeks.

Pancreatitis was observed in 3 of the 412 adult patients who received stavudine in a controlled monotherapy study.

Selected clinical adverse reactions that occurred in antiretroviral naive adult patients receiving stavudine from 2 controlled combination studies are provided in the following data:

Stavudine Adverse Reactions in START 1 and START 2 Studies[1] (%)

	START 1		START 2	
Adverse reaction	Stavudine + lamivudine + indinavir (n = 100)[2]	Zidovudine + lamivudine + indinavir (n = 102)	Stavudine + didanosine + indinavir (n = 102)[2]	Zidovudine + lamivudine + indinavir (n = 103)
Nausea	43	63	53	67
Diarrhea	34	16	45	39
Headache	25	26	46	37
Rash	18	13	30	18
Vomiting	18	33	30	35
Peripheral neurologic symptoms/ neuropathy	8	7	21	10

[a] START 2 compared 2 triple-combination regimens in 205 treatment-naive patients. Patients received either stavudine (40 mg twice daily) plus didanosine plus indinavir or zidovudine plus lamivudine plus indinavir.
[b] Duration of stavudine therapy = 48 weeks.

Pancreatitis resulting in death has been observed in patients treated with stavudine plus didanosine, with or without hydroxyurea, in controlled clinical studies and in postmarketing reports.

Lab test abnormalities – Selected laboratory abnormalities reported in a controlled monotherapy study (Study AI455-019) are provided in the following data.

Selected adult laboratory abnormalities in Study AI455-019[a,b]

	(%)	
Parameter	Stavudine (40 mg twice daily) (n = 412)	Zidovudine (200 mg 3 times daily) (n = 402)
AST (> 5 x ULN[c])	11%	10%
ALT (> 5 x ULN)	13%	11%
Amylase (≥ 1.4 x ULN)	14%	13%

[a] Data presented for patients for whom laboratory evaluations were performed.
[b] Median duration of stavudine therapy = 79 weeks; median duration of zidovudine therapy = 53 weeks.
[c] ULN = upper limit of normal.

Selected laboratory abnormalities reported in 2 controlled combination studies are provided in the following data.

Selected Stavudine Lab Test Abnormalities in START 1 and START 2 (Grades 3 to 4) (%)

	START 1		START 2	
Parameter	Stavudine + lamivudine + indinavir (n = 100)	Zidovudine + lamivudine + indinavir (n = 102)	Stavudine + didanosine + indinavir (n = 102)	Zidovudine + lamivudine + indinavir (n = 103)
Bilirubin (> 2.6 x ULN)	7	6	16	8
AST (> 5 x ULN)	5	2	7	7
ALT (> 5 x ULN)	6	2	8	5
GGT (> 5 x ULN)	2	2	5	2
Lipase (> 2 x ULN)	6	3	5	5
Amylase (> 2 x ULN)	4	< 1	8	2

[a] ULN = upper limit of normal.

STAVUDINE — ORAL

Stavudine Lab Test Abnormalities in START 1 and START 2 Studies (All Grades) (%)

Parameter	START 1		START 2	
	Stavudine + lamivudine + indinavir (n = 100)	Zidovudine + lamivudine + indinavir (n = 102)	Stavudine + didanosine + indinavir (n = 102)	Zidovudine + lamivudine + indinavir (n = 103)
Total bilirubin	65	60	68	55
AST	42	20	53	20
ALT	40	20	50	18
GGT	15	8	28	12
Lipase	27	12	26	19
Amylase	21	19	31	17

➤*Extended-release capsules:*

Peripheral neuropathy – See Administration and Dosage for more information. In clinical trials, less than 1% of 466 patients treated with stavudine extended-release for a median duration of 56 weeks (ranging up to 120 weeks) discontinued therapy because of peripheral neuropathy.

In the pooled database from trials AI455-099 and AI455-096 and an ongoing long-term follow-up study for patients completing these 2 trials (median duration of therapy 56 weeks, ranging up to 120 weeks), the rates of discontinuation of therapy due to adverse reactions were 5% for the stavudine extended-release regimen and 7% for the stavudine immediate-release regimen.

Selected Clinical Adverse Events[a] of Any Severity from Combination Studies of Stavudine Extended-Release (Pooled Data) (%)[b]

Adverse reactions	Stavudine extended-release + lamivudine + efavirenz (n = 466)	Stavudine immediate-release + lamivudine + efavirenz (n = 467)
Miscellaneous		
Headache	12%	8%
Fatigue	6%	4%
GI		
Diarrhea	10%	10%
Nausea	10%	9%
Dyspepsia	4%	3%
Vomiting	3%	4%
Metabolic/nutritional		
Lipodystrophy	3%	4%
CNS		
Dizziness	30%	30%
PNS[c]/neuropathy	16%	19%
Abnormal dreams	13%	14%
Somnolence	8%	8%
Insomnia	8%	6%
Abnormal thinking	3%	2%
Depression	2%	1%
Dermatologic		
Rash	16%	12%
Pruritus	4%	4%

[a] Considered by the investigator to be of possible, probable, or unknown relationship to any component of the drug regimen.
[b] Patients received either stavudine extended-release 100 mg once daily or stavudine immediate release 40 mg twice daily each in combination with lamivudine 150 mg twice daily and efavirenz 600 mg once daily. Median duration of treatment was 56 weeks (ranging up to 120 weeks).
[c] PNS = Peripheral neurologic symptoms (includes neuropathy, paresthesia, and peripheral neuritis).

In clinical trials, lactic acidosis syndrome/symptomatic hyperlactatemia (LAS/SHL), sometimes fatal, was reported. LAS/SHL occurred in 3 of 466 patients treated with stavudine extended-release (stavudine) and in 6 of 467 patients treated with stavudine immediate release. The overall incidence of LAS/SHL for these trials was 8.8/1000 patient years.

Elevations in liver function tests or progression of liver disease, sometimes fatal, that resulted in discontinuation of study drug were observed in 3 of 466 patients in the stavudine extended-release arm and 3 of 467 patients in the stavudine immediate-release arm of clinical trials. All 6 patients were co-infected with hepatitis B or C.

Pancreatitis was observed in 1 of 466 patients treated with stavudine extended-release and 4 of 467 patients treated with stavudine immediate release in clinical trials. Pancreatitis resulting in death was observed in patients treated with stavudine plus didanosine, with or without hydroxyurea, in controlled clinical studies and in postmarketing reports.

Selected laboratory abnormalities from combination studies of stavudine extended-release (pooled data)[a]

Parameter	Stavudine extended-release + lamivudine + efavirenz (n = 466)	Stavudine immediate-release + lamivudine + efavirenz (n = 467)
AST (> 5 × ULN)	2%	3%
ALT (> 5 × ULN)	3%	3%
Lipase (≥ 2.1 × ULN)	4%	3%
Total bilirubin (≥ 2.6 × ULN)	< 1%	0
Neutropenia (ANC[b] < 750/mm³)	5%	5%
Anemia (hemoglobin < 8 g/dL)	< 1%	< 1%
Thrombocytopenia (platelets < 50,000/mm³)	1%	2%

[a] Patients received either stavudine extended-release 100 mg once daily or stavudine immediate release 40 mg twice daily each in combination with lamivudine 150 mg twice daily and efavirenz 600 mg once daily. Median duration of treatment was 56 weeks (ranging up to 120 weeks).
[b] ANC = Absolute neutrophil count.

➤*Postmarketing:*

CNS – Insomnia, severe motor weakness (most often reported in the setting of lactic acidosis.

GI – Anorexia.

Hematologic – Anemia, leukopenia, and thrombocytopenia.

Hepatic – Symptomatic hyperlactatemia/lactic acidosis and hepatic steatosis, hepatitis and liver failure.

Musculoskeletal – Myalgia.

Systemic – Abdominal pain, allergic reaction, chills/fever, and redistribution/accumulation of body fat.

Miscellaneous – Pancreatitis, including fatal cases.

Children – Adverse reactions and serious laboratory abnormalities in pediatric patients from birth through adolescence were similar in type and frequency to those seen in adult patients.

Overdosage

➤*Symptoms:* Experience with adults treated with 12 to 24 times the recommended daily dosage of the immediate-release formulation revealed no acute toxicity. Complications of chronic overdosage include peripheral neuropathy and hepatic toxicity.

➤*Treatment:* Stavudine can be removed by hemodialysis; the mean ± SD hemodialysis clearance of stavudine is 120 ± 18 mL/min. Whether stavudine is eliminated by peritoneal dialysis has not been studied.

Patient Information

Patients should be informed of the importance of early recognition of symptoms of symptomatic hyperlactatemia or lactic acidosis syndrome, which include abdominal discomfort, nausea, vomiting, fatigue, dyspnea, and motor weakness. Patients in whom these symptoms develop should seek medical attention immediately. Discontinuation of stavudine therapy may be required.

Patients should be informed that an important toxicity of stavudine is peripheral neuropathy. Patients should be aware that peripheral neuropathy is manifested by numbness, tingling, or pain in hands or feet, and that these symptoms should be reported to their physicians. Patients should be counseled that peripheral neuropathy occurs with greatest frequency in patients who have advanced HIV disease or a history of peripheral neuropathy, and that dose modification or discontinuation of stavudine may be required if toxicity develops.

Caregivers of young children receiving stavudine therapy should be instructed regarding detection and reporting of peripheral neuropathy.

Patients should be informed that when stavudine is used in combination with other agents with similar toxicities, the incidence of adverse reactions may be higher than when stavudine is used alone. An increased risk of pancreatitis, which may be fatal, may occur in patients treated with the combination of stavudine and didanosine, with or without hydroxyurea. Patients treated with this combination should be closely monitored for symptoms of pancreatitis. An increased risk of hepatotoxicity, which may be fatal, may occur in patients treated with stavudine in combination with didanosine and hydroxyurea. Patients treated with this combination should be closely monitored for signs of liver toxicity.

Patients should be informed that stavudine is not a cure for HIV infection, and that they may continue to acquire illnesses associated with HIV infection, including opportunistic infections. Patients should be advised to remain under the care of a physician when using stavudine. They should be advised that stavudine therapy has not been shown to reduce the risk of transmission of HIV to others through sexual contact or blood contamination. Patients should be informed that the long-term effects of stavudine are unknown at this time.

STAVUDINE — ORAL

Patients should be informed that the Centers for Disease Control and Prevention (CDC) recommend that HIV-infected mothers not nurse newborn infants to reduce the risk of postnatal transmission of HIV infection.

Patients should be informed that redistribution or accumulation of body fat may occur in patients receiving antiretroviral therapy and that the cause and long-term health effects of these conditions are not known at this time.

Patients should be advised of the importance of adherence to any antiretroviral regimen, including those that contain stavudine immediate release or extended-release.

ZALCITABINE (Dideoxycytidine; ddC)

Rx	**Hivid** (Roche)	**Tablets:** 0.375 mg	Lactose. (Hivid 0.375 Roche). Beige, oval. Film-coated. In 100s.
		0.75 mg	Lactose. (Hivid 0.750 Roche). Gray, oval. Film-coated. In 100s.

ZALCITABINE — ORAL

WARNING

The use of zalcitabine has been associated with significant clinical adverse reactions, some of which are potentially fatal. Zalcitabine can cause severe peripheral neuropathy and because of this should be used with extreme caution in patients with preexisting neuropathy. Zalcitabine may also rarely cause pancreatitis and patients who develop any symptoms suggestive of pancreatitis while using zalcitabine should have therapy suspended immediately until this diagnosis is excluded.

Lactic acidosis and severe hepatomegaly with steatosis, including fatal cases, have been reported with the use of antiretroviral nucleoside analogues alone or in combination, including zalcitabine. A majority of these cases have been in women. Obesity and prolonged exposure to antiretroviral nucleoside analogues may be risk factors. Particular caution should be exercised when administering zalcitabine to any patient with known risk factors for liver disease; however, cases have also been reported in patients with no known risk factors. Treatment with zalcitabine should be suspended in any patient who develops clinical or laboratory findings suggestive of lactic acidosis or pronounced hepatotoxicity.

In addition, rare cases of hepatic failure and death considered possibly related to underlying hepatitis B and zalcitabine have been reported. Treatment with zalcitabine in patients with preexisting liver disease, liver enzyme abnormalities, a history of ethanol abuse, or hepatitis should be approached with caution. Treatment with zalcitabine should be suspended in any patient who develops clinical or laboratory findings suggestive of pronounced hepatotoxicity. In clinical trials, drug interruption was recommended if liver function tests exceeded greater than 5 times the upper limit of normal.

Indications

➤*HIV infection:* For the treatment of HIV infection in combination with antiretroviral agents.

Administration and Dosage

➤*Approved by the FDA:* June 19, 1992.

Patients should be advised that zalcitabine is recommended for use in combination with active antiretroviral therapy. Greater activity has been observed when new antiretroviral therapies are begun at the same time as zalcitabine. Concomitant therapy should be based on a patient's prior drug exposure. The recommended regimen is one 0.75 mg tablet of zalcitabine orally every 8 hours (2.25 mg zalcitabine total daily dose) in combination with other antiretroviral agents.

➤*Renal function impairment:* Based on preliminary data, the recommended zalcitabine dosage reduction for patients with impaired renal function is the following:

Ccr 10 to 40 mL/min – 0.75 mg of zalcitabine every 12 hours.

Ccr less than 10 mL/min – 0.75 mg of zalcitabine every 24 hours.

➤*Monitoring:* Complete blood counts and clinical chemistry tests should be performed prior to initiating zalcitabine therapy and at appropriate intervals thereafter. Serum amylase levels should be monitored in those individuals who have a history of elevated amylase, pancreatitis, ethanol abuse, who are on parenteral nutrition or who are otherwise at high risk of pancreatitis. Careful monitoring for signs or symptoms suggestive of peripheral neuropathy is recommended, particularly in individuals with a low CD_4 cell count or who are at a greater risk of developing peripheral neuropathy while on therapy. The major clinical toxicity of zalcitabine is peripheral neuropathy, which may occur in up to one-third of patients with advanced disease treated with zalcitabine. The incidence in patients with less-advanced disease is lower.

➤*Dose adjustment:* For toxicities that are likely to be associated with zalcitabine (eg, peripheral neuropathy, severe oral ulcers, pancreatitis, elevated liver function tests especially in patients with chronic hepatitis B), zalcitabine should be interrupted or dose reduced. For severe toxicities or those persisting after dose reduction, zalcitabine should be interrupted. For recipients of combination therapy with zalcitabine and other antiretroviral agents, dose adjustments or interruption for each drug should be based on the known toxicity profile of the individual drugs. See information for each drug used in combination for a description of known drug-associated adverse reactions.

Peripheral neuropathy – Patients developing moderate discomfort with signs or symptoms of peripheral neuropathy should stop zalcitabine. Zalcitabine-associated peripheral neuropathy may continue to worsen despite interruption of zalcitabine. Zalcitabine should be reintroduced at 50% dose, 0.375 mg every 8 hours only if all findings related to peripheral neuropathy have improved to mild symptoms. Zalcitabine should be permanently discontinued if patients experience severe discomfort related to peripheral neuropathy or moderate discomfort that progresses. If other moderate-to-severe clinical adverse reactions or laboratory abnormalities (such as increased liver function tests) occur, then zalcitabine or the other potential causative agent(s) should be interrupted until the adverse reaction abates. Zalcitabine or the other potential causative agent(s) should then be carefully reintroduced at lower doses if appropriate. If adverse reactions recur at the reduced dose, therapy should be discontinued. The minimum effective dose of zalcitabine in combination with zidovudine for the treatment of adult patients with advanced HIV infection has not been established.

Hematologic toxicities – In patients with poor bone marrow reserve, particularly those patients with advanced symptomatic HIV disease, frequent monitoring of hematologic indices is recommended to detect serious anemia or granulocytopenia. Significant toxicities, such as anemia (hemoglobin of less than 7.5 g/dL or reduction of greater than 25% of baseline) or granulocytopenia (granulocyte count of less than 750 cells/mm^3 or reduction of greater than 50% from baseline), may require a treatment interruption of zalcitabine and zidovudine until evidence of marrow recovery is observed. For less severe anemia or granulocytopenia, a reduction in daily dose of zidovudine in those patients receiving combination therapy may be adequate. In patients who experience hematologic toxicity, reduction in hemoglobin may occur as early as 2 to 4 weeks after initiation of therapy, and granulocytopenia usually occurs after 6 to 8 weeks of therapy. In patients who develop significant anemia, dose modification does not necessarily eliminate the need for transfusion. If marrow recovery occurs following dose modification, gradual increases in dose may be appropriate depending on hematologic indices and patient tolerance. For more details, refer to the complete monograph for zidovudine.

➤*Storage/Stability:* Store in tightly closed bottles at 15° to 30°C (59° to 86°F).

Actions

➤*Pharmacokinetics:*

Absorption – Following oral administration to HIV-infected patients, the mean absolute bioavailability of zalcitabine was greater than 80% (30% CV; range, 23% to 124%; n = 19). The absorption rate of a 1.5 mg oral dose of zalcitabine (n = 20) was reduced when administered with food. This resulted in a 39% decrease in mean maximum plasma concentrations (C_{max}) from 25.2 ng/mL (35% CV; range, 11.6 to 37.5 ng/mL) to 15.5 ng/mL (24% CV; range, 9.1 to 23.7 ng/mL), and a 2-fold increase in time to achieve maximum plasma concentrations from a mean of 0.8 hours under fasting conditions to 1.6 hours when the drug was given with food. The extent of absorption (as reflected by AUC) was decreased by 14%, from 72 ng•hr/mL (28% CV; range, 43 to 119 ng•hr/mL) to 62 ng•hr/mL (23% CV; range, 42 to 91 ng•hr/mL). The clinical relevance of these decreases is unknown. Absorption of zalcitabine does not appear to be reduced in patients with diarrhea not caused by an identified pathogen.

Distribution – The steady-state volume of distribution following intravenous administration of a 1.5 mg dose of zalcitabine averaged 0.534 (±0.127) L/kg (24% CV; range, 0.304 to 0.734 L/kg; n = 20). Cerebrospinal fluid obtained from 9 patients at 2 to 3.5 hours following 0.06 mg/kg or 0.09 mg/kg intravenous infusion showed measurable concentrations of zalcitabine. The CSF:plasma concentration ratio ranged from 9% to 37% (mean, 20%), demonstrating penetration of the drug through the blood-brain barrier. The clinical relevance of these ratios has not been evaluated.

Metabolism/Excretion – Zalcitabine is phosphorylated intracellularly to zalcitabine triphosphate, the active substrate for HIV-reverse transcriptase. Concentrations of zalcitabine triphosphate are too low for quantitation following administration of therapeutic doses to humans.

Zalcitabine does not undergo a significant degree of metabolism by the liver. The primary metabolite of zalcitabine that has been identified is dideoxyuridine (ddU), which accounts for less than 15% of an oral dose in both urine and feces (n = 4). Approximately 10% of an orally administered radiolabeled dose of zalcitabine appears in the feces (n = 10), comprised primarily of unchanged drug and ddU. Renal excretion of unchanged drug appears to be the primary route of elimination, accounting for approximately 80% of an intravenous dose and 60% of an orally administered dose within 24 hours after dosing (n = 19). The mean elimination half-life is 2 hours and generally ranges from 1 to 3 hours in individual patients. Total clearance following an intravenous dose averaged 285 mL/min (29% CV; range, 165 to 447 mL/min; n = 20). Renal clearance averaged approximately 235 mL/min or about 80% of total clearance (30% CV; range, 129 to 348 mL/min; n = 20). Renal clear-

ZALCITABINE — ORAL

ance exceeds glomerular filtration rate suggesting renal tubular secretion contributes to the elimination of zalcitabine by the kidneys.

Special populations –
Renal function impairment: In patients with impaired kidney function, prolonged elimination of zalcitabine may be expected. Preliminary results from 7 patients with renal impairment (estimated Ccr less than 55 mL/min) indicate that the half-life was prolonged (up to 8.5 hours) in these patients compared to those with normal renal function. Maximum plasma concentrations were higher in some patients after a single dose.

Children: Limited pharmacokinetic data have been reported for 5 HIV-positive pediatric patients using doses of 0.03 and 0.04 mg/kg zalcitabine administered orally every 6 hours. The mean bioavailability of zalcitabine in these pediatric patients was 54% and mean apparent systemic clearance was 150 mL/min/m^2. Due to the small number of subjects and different analytical techniques, it is difficult to make comparisons between pediatric and adult data.

➤*Microbiology:* Zalcitabine is a synthetic nucleoside analogue of the naturally occurring nucleoside deoxycytidine, in which the 3′-hydroxyl group is replaced by hydrogen. Within cells, zalcitabine is converted to the active metabolite, dideoxycytidine 5′-triphosphate (ddCTP), by the sequential action of cellular enzymes. Dideoxycytidine 5′-triphosphate inhibits the activity of the HIV-reverse transcriptase both by competing for utilization of the natural substrate, deoxycytidine 5′-triphosphate (dCTP), and by its incorporation into viral DNA. The lack of a 3′-OH group in the incorporated nucleoside analogue prevents the formation of the 5′ to 3′ phosphodiester linkage essential for DNA chain elongation and, therefore, the viral DNA growth is terminated. The active metabolite, ddCTP, is also an inhibitor of cellular DNA polymerase-beta and mitochondrial DNA polymerase-gamma and has been reported to be incorporated into the DNA of cells in culture.

In vitro HIV susceptibility – In drug combination studies with zidovudine (ZDV) or saquinavir, zalcitabine showed additive to synergistic activity in cell culture. The relationship between the in vitro susceptibility of HIV to reverse-transcriptase inhibitors and the inhibition of HIV replication in humans has not been established.

Drug resistance – HIV isolates with a reduction in sensitivity to zalcitabine (ddC) have been isolated from a small number of patients treated with zalcitabine by 1 year of therapy. Genetic analysis of these isolates showed point mutations (Lys 65 Arg or Asn, Thr 69 Asp, Leu 74 Val, Val 75 Thr or Ala, Met 184 Val or Tyr 215 Cys) in the pol gene that encodes for the reverse transcriptase. Combination therapy with zalcitabine and zidovudine (ZDV) does not appear to prevent the emergence of zidovudine-resistant isolates.

Contraindications

Clinically significant hypersensitivity to zalcitabine or to any of the excipients contained in the tablets.

Warnings

➤*Significant adverse reactions:* Significant clinical adverse reactions, some of which are potentially fatal, have been reported with zalcitabine. Patients with decreased CD_4 cell counts appear to have an increased incidence of adverse events.

➤*Peripheral neuropathy:* The major clinical toxicity of zalcitabine is peripheral neuropathy, which may occur in up to one-third of patients with advanced disease treated with zalcitabine. The incidence in patients with less-advanced disease is lower.

Zalcitabine-related peripheral neuropathy is a sensorimotor neuropathy characterized initially by numbness and burning dysesthesia involving the distal extremities. These symptoms may be followed by sharp shooting pains or severe continuous burning pain if the drug is not withdrawn. The neuropathy may progress to severe pain requiring narcotic analgesics and is potentially irreversible. In some patients, symptoms of neuropathy may initially progress despite discontinuation of zalcitabine. With prompt discontinuation of zalcitabine, the neuropathy is usually slowly reversible.

There are no data regarding the use of zalcitabine in patients with preexisting peripheral neuropathy since these patients were excluded from clinical trials; therefore, zalcitabine should be used with extreme caution in these patients. Individuals with moderate or severe peripheral neuropathy, as evidenced by symptoms accompanied by objective findings, are advised to avoid zalcitabine.

Zalcitabine should be used with caution in patients with a risk of developing peripheral neuropathy: Patients with low CD_4 cell counts (CD_4 less than 50 cells/mm^3), diabetes, weight loss, or patients receiving zalcitabine concomitantly with drugs that have the potential to cause peripheral neuropathy. Drugs that have been associated with peripheral neuropathy include antiretroviral nucleoside analogues, chloramphenicol, cisplatin, dapsone, disulfiram, ethionamide, glutethimide, gold, hydralazine, iodoquinol, isoniazid, metronidazole, nitrofurantoin, phenytoin, ribavirin, and vincristine. Concomitant use of zalcitabine with didanosine is not recommended. Careful monitoring is strongly recommended for these individuals.

Zalcitabine should be stopped promptly if signs or symptoms of peripheral neuropathy occur, such as when moderate discomfort from numbness, tingling, burning or pain of the extremities progresses, or any related symptoms occur that are accompanied by an objective finding.

➤*Pancreatitis:* Pancreatitis, which has been fatal in some cases, has been observed with the administration of zalcitabine. Pancreatitis is an uncommon complication of zalcitabine occurring in up to 1.1% of patients.

Patients with a history of pancreatitis or known risk factors for the development of pancreatitis should be followed more closely while on zalcitabine therapy. Of 528 zalcitabine-treated patients enrolled in an expanded-access safety study (N3544), who had a history of pancreatitis or increased amylase, 28 (5.3%) developed pancreatitis, and an additional 23 (4.4%) developed asymptomatic elevated serum amylase.

Treatment with zalcitabine should be stopped immediately if clinical signs or symptoms (nausea, vomiting, abdominal pain) or if abnormalities in laboratory values (hyperamylasemia associated with dysglycemia, rising triglyceride level, decreasing serum calcium) suggestive of pancreatitis should occur. If clinical pancreatitis develops during zalcitabine administration, it is recommended that zalcitabine be permanently discontinued. Treatment with zalcitabine should also be interrupted if treatment with another drug known to cause pancreatitis (eg, intravenous pentamidine) is required. Death due to fulminant pancreatitis possibly related to intravenous pentamidine and zalcitabine has been reported.

➤*Lactic acidosis/severe hepatomegaly with steatosis and hepatic toxicity:* See the Warning box for more information.

➤*Oral ulcers:* Severe oral ulcers occurred in up to 3% of patients receiving zalcitabine in CPCRA 002 and ACTG 175; less severe oral ulcerations have occurred at higher frequencies in other clinical trials.

➤*Esophageal ulcers:* Infrequent cases of esophageal ulcers have also been attributed to zalcitabine therapy. Interruption of zalcitabine should be considered in patients who develop esophageal ulcers that do not respond to specific treatment for opportunistic pathogens in order to assess a possible relationship to zalcitabine.

➤*Cardiomyopathy/congestive heart failure:* Cardiomyopathy and congestive heart failure in patients with AIDS have been associated with the use of nucleoside analogues. Infrequent cases have been reported in patients receiving zalcitabine. Treatment with zalcitabine in patients with baseline cardiomyopathy or history of congestive heart failure should be approached with caution.

➤*Hypersensitivity reactions:* An anaphylactoid reaction was reported in a patient receiving both zalcitabine and zidovudine. In addition, there have been several reports of hypersensitivity reactions (including anaphylactic reaction or urticaria without other signs of anaphylaxis).

➤*Renal function impairment:* Patients with renal impairment (estimated creatinine clearance less than 55 mL/min) may be at a greater risk of toxicity from zalcitabine due to decreased drug clearance. Dosage adjustment is recommended in these patients.

See Administration and Dosage for more information.

➤*Carcinogenesis:* A significant increase in thymic lymphoma in all zalcitabine dose groups and Harderian gland (a gland of the eye of rodents) adenoma in the 2 highest dose groups was observed in female CD-1 mice after 2 years of dosing. No increase in tumor incidence was observed in rats or male mice treated with zalcitabine. In an independent study, administration of zalcitabine to $B_6C_3F_1$ mice at a dose of 1000 mg/kg/day for 3 months induced an increased incidence of thymic lymphoma. A high rate of spontaneous lymphoreticular neoplasms have previously been noted in this strain of mice.

➤*Mutagenesis:* Zalcitabine was positive in a cell transformation assay and induced chromosomal aberrations in vitro in human peripheral blood lymphocytes. Oral doses of zalcitabine at 2500 and 4500 mg/kg were clastogenic in the mouse micronucleus assay. Zalcitabine showed no evidence of mutagenicity in Ames tests, Chinese hamster lung cell assays and the mouse lymphoma assay. An unscheduled DNA synthesis assay in rat hepatocytes showed that zalcitabine had no effect on DNA repair.

➤*Fertility impairment:* Fertility and reproductive performance were assessed in rats at plasma concentrations up to 2142 times those achieved with the maximum recommended human dose (MRHD) based on AUC measurements. No adverse effects on rate of conception or general reproductive performance were observed. The highest dose was associated with embryolethality and evidence of teratogenicity. The next lower dose studied (plasma concentrations equivalent to 485 times the MRHD) was associated with a lower frequency of embryotoxicity but no teratogenicity. The fertility of F_1 males was significantly reduced at a calculated dose of 2142 (but not 485) times the MRHD (based on AUC measurements) in a teratology study in which rat mothers were dosed on gestation days 7 to 15. No adverse effects were observed on the fertility of parents or F_1 generation in the study of fertility and general reproductive performance or in the perinatal and postnatal reproduction study.

➤*Elderly:* Clinical studies of zalcitabine did not include sufficient numbers of subjects greater than or equal to 65 years of age to determine whether they respond differently than younger subjects. In general, dose selection for an elderly patient should be cautious, reflecting the greater frequency of decreased hepatic, renal, or cardiac function, and of concomitant disease or other drug therapy. Zalcitabine is known to be substantially excreted by the kidney, and the risk of toxic reactions to this drug may be greater in patients with impaired renal function. Because elderly patients are more likely to have decreased renal function, care should be taken in dose selection. In addition, renal function should be monitored and dosage adjustments should be made accordingly (see Renal impairment).

➤*Pregnancy: Category C.* Zalcitabine has been shown to be teratogenic in mice at calculated exposure levels of 1365 and 2730 times that of the MRHD (based on AUC measurements). In rats, zalcitabine was teratogenic at a calculated exposure level of 2142 times the MRHD but not at an exposure level of 485 times the MRHD. In a perinatal and postnatal study in the rat, a high incidence of hydrocephalus was observed in the F_1 offspring derived from litters of dams treated with 1071 (but not 485) times the MRHD (based on AUC measurements). There are no adequate and well-controlled studies of zalcitabine in pregnant women. Zalcitabine should be used during pregnancy only if the potential benefit justifies the potential risk to the fetus.

ZALCITABINE — ORAL

Fertile women should not receive zalcitabine unless they are using effective contraception during therapy. If pregnancy occurs, physicians are encouraged to report such cases by calling (800) 526-6367.

Increased embryolethality was observed in pregnant mice at doses 2730 times the MRHD and in pregnant rats above 485 (but not 98) times the MRHD (based on AUC measurements). Average fetal body weight was significantly decreased in mice at doses of 1365 times the MRHD and in rats at 2142 times the MRHD (based on AUC measurements). In a perinatal and postnatal study, the learning and memory of a significant number of F_1 offspring were impaired, and they tended to stay hyperactive for a longer period of time. These effects, observed at a calculated exposure level of 1071 (but not 485) times the MRHD (based on AUC measurements), were considered to result from extensive damage to or gross underdevelopment of the brain of these F_1 offspring consistent with the finding of hydrocephalus.

Antiretroviral pregnancy registry – To monitor maternal-fetal outcomes of pregnant women exposed to antiretroviral medications, including zalcitabine, an antiretroviral pregnancy registry has been established. Physicians are encouraged to register patients by calling 1-800-258-4263.

➤*Lactation:* The Centers for Disease Control and Prevention recommend that HIV-infected mothers not breastfeed their infants to avoid risking postnatal transmission of HIV. It is not known whether zalcitabine is excreted in human milk. Because of both the potential for HIV transmission and the potential for serious adverse reactions in nursing infants, mothers should be instructed not to breastfeed if they are receiving antiretroviral medications, including zalcitabine.

➤*Children:* Safety and effectiveness of zalcitabine in HIV-infected pediatric patients younger than 13 years of age have not been established.

Precautions

➤*Monitoring:* Complete blood counts and clinical chemistry tests should be performed prior to initiating zalcitabine therapy and at appropriate intervals thereafter. Baseline testing of serum amylase and triglyceride levels should be performed in individuals with a history of pancreatitis, increased amylase, those on parenteral nutrition, or with a history of ethanol abuse.

➤*Lymphoma:* High doses of zalcitabine, administered for 3 months to $B_6C_3F_1$ mice (resulting in plasma concentrations over 1000 times those seen in patients taking the recommended doses of zalcitabine) induced an increased incidence of thymic lymphoma. Although the pathogenesis of the effect is uncertain, a predisposition to chemically induced thymic lymphoma and high rates of spontaneous lymphoreticular neoplasms have previously been noted in this strain of mice.

The incidence of lymphomas was reviewed in 13 comparative studies conducted by Roche, the NIAID and the NCI, as well as 7 Roche expanded-access studies that included zalcitabine. In 1 study, ACTG 155, a statistically significant increased rate of lymphomas was seen in patients receiving zalcitabine or combination zalcitabine and zidovudine compared to zidovudine alone (rates of 0, 1.3, and 2.3 per 100 person years for zidovudine, zalcitabine, and combination zalcitabine and zidovudine, respectively; log rank P-value = 0.01, pooling zalcitabine, and combination zalcitabine and zidovudine vs zidovudine, P-value = 0.003). Based on review of the literature, the incidence of lymphomas in HIV-infected patients with advanced disease on zidovudine monotherapy would be expected to be approximately 1 to 2 per 100 person years of follow-up.

None of the other comparative studies evaluated showed a statistically significant difference in rates of lymphomas in patients receiving zalcitabine. In a large, controlled clinical trial (ACTG 175) zalcitabine in combination with zidovudine was not associated with an increase in the incidence of lymphoma over that seen with zidovudine monotherapy (6 of 615 and 9 of 619, respectively).

Lymphoma has been identified as a consequence of HIV infection. This most likely represents a consequence of prolonged immunosuppression; however, an association between the occurrence of lymphoma and antiviral therapy cannot be excluded.

➤*Fat redistribution:* Redistribution/accumulation of body fat including central obesity, dorsocervical fat enlargement (buffalo hump), peripheral wasting, facial wasting, breast enlargement, and "cushingoid appearance" have been observed in patients receiving antiretroviral therapy. The mechanism and long-term consequences of these events are currently unknown. A causal relationship has not been established.

➤*Development of opportunistic infections:* Patients receiving zalcitabine or any other antiretroviral therapy may continue to develop opportunistic infections and other complications of HIV infections, and therefore should remain under close clinical observation by physicians experienced in the treatment of patients with associated HIV diseases.

➤*Clinical benefit from antiretroviral therapy:* The duration of clinical benefit from antiretroviral therapy may be limited. Alterations in antiretroviral therapy should be considered in cases of disease progression, either clinical or as demonstrated by viral rebound (increase in HIV RNA after initial decline).

Drug Interactions

Zalcitabine Drug Interactions

Precipitant drug	Object drug*		Description
Amphotericin, foscarnet, aminoglycosides	Zalcitabine	↑	These drugs may increase the risk of developing peripheral neuropathy or other zalcitabine-associated adverse events by interfering with the renal clearance of zalcitabine (and thereby raising systemic exposure). Patients who require the use of 1 of these drugs with zalcitabine should have frequent clinical and laboratory monitoring with dosage adjustment for any significant change in renal function.
Antacids (aluminum and magnesium-containing)	Zalcitabine	↓	Zalcitabine absorption is moderately reduced (≈ 25%) when coadministered with magnesium/aluminum-containing antacids. Do not ingest simultaneously.
Antiretroviral nucleoside analogs Chloramphenicol Cisplatin Dapsone Didanosine Disulfiram Ethionamide Glutethimide Gold Hydralazine Iodoquinol Isoniazid Metronidazole Nitrofurantoin Phenytoin Ribavirin Vincristine	Zalcitabine	↑	These drugs have been associated with peripheral neuropathy. Avoid concomitant use when possible. Concomitant use of zalcitabine with didanosine is not recommended.
Cimetidine	Zalcitabine	↑	Concomitant use decreases zalcitabine elimination, most likely by inhibition of renal tubular secretion. Monitor for signs of toxicity and reduce zalcitabine dose if warranted.
Doxorubicin	Zalcitabine	↓	Doxorubicin caused a decrease in zalcitabine phosphorylation (> 50% inhibition of total phosphate formation) in U937/Molt 4 cells. Although there may be decreased zalcitabine activity because of lessened active metabolite formation, the clinical relevance of these in vitro results are not known.
Metoclopramide	Zalcitabine	↓	Zalcitabine bioavailability is mildly reduced (≈ 10%).
Pentamidine (and other agents that have potential to cause pancreatitis)	Zalcitabine	↑	Interrupt treatment when the use of a drug that has the potential to cause pancreatitis is required. Death because of fulminant pancreatitis possibly related to zalcitabine and IV pentamidine was reported. If IV pentamidine is required to treat *Pneumocystis carinii* pneumonia, interrupt treatment with zalcitabine.
Probenecid	Zalcitabine	↑	Concomitant use decreases zalcitabine elimination, most likely by inhibition of renal tubular secretion. Monitor for signs of toxicity and reduce the zalcitabine dose if warranted.

* ↑ = Object drug increased. ↓ = Object drug decreased.

➤*Lamivudine:* In vitro studies in peripheral blood mononuclear cells, U937 and Molt-4 cells revealed that lamivudine significantly inhibited zalcitabine phosphorylation in a dose-dependent manner. Effects were already seen with doses corresponding to relevant plasma levels in humans, and the intracellular phosphorylation of zalcitabine to its 3 metabolites (including the active zalcitabine triphosphate metabolite) was significantly inhibited. Zalcitabine inhibited lamivudine phophorylation at high concentration

ZALCITABINE — ORAL

ratios (10 and 100); however, it is considered to be unlikely that this decrease of phosphorylated lamivudine concentration is of clinical significance, as lamivudine is a more efficient substrate for deoxycytidine kinase than zalcitabine. These in vitro studies suggest that concomitant administration of zalcitabine and lamivudine in humans may result in subtherapeutic concentrations of active phosphorylated zalcitabine, which may lead to a decreased antiretroviral effect of zalcitabine. It is unknown how the effect seen in these in vitro studies translates into clinical consequences. Concomitant use of zalcitabine and lamivudine is not recommended.

Adverse Reactions

Percentage of patients with clinical adverse reactions ≥ Grade 3[1] in ≥ 1% of patients receiving zalcitabine

	CPCRA 002[1] ZDV intolerant or failure		ACTG 175[2] ZDV naive/experienced	
Body system/ adverse reaction	Zalcitabine 0.75 mg every 8 hours (n = 237)	Didanosine (ddl) 250 mg every 12 hours (n = 230)	Zidovudine (ZDV) 200 mg every 8 hours (n = 619)	Zalcitabine + zidovudine (ZDV) 0.75 mg every 8 hours + 200 mg every 8 hours (n = 615)
Miscellaneous				
Fatigue	3.8%	2.6%	2.7%	2.3%
Headache	2.1%	1.3%	2.4%	2.6%
Fever	1.7%	0.4%	2.7%	2.9%
GI				
Abdominal pain	3%	7%	2.3%	1.8%
Oral lesions/ stomatitis[3]	3%	0%	0.6%	1.5%
Vomiting/ nausea[3]	3.4%	7%	4.9%	2.1%
Diarrhea/ constipation[3]	2.5%	17.4%	2.9%	1%
Hepatic				
Abnormal hepatic function	8.9%	7%	[4]	[4]
Neurologic				
Convulsions	1.3%	2.2%		
Peripheral neuropathy[5]	28.3%	13%	3.1%	3.3%
Dermatologic				
Rash/pruritus/ urticaria	3.4%	3.9%	1.8%	1.6%
Metabolic/nutritional				
Pancreatitis	0%	1.7%	0.2%	0.5%
Psychological				
Depression	0.4%	0%	1.1%	1.8%
Musculoskeletal				
Painful/ swollen joints	0.4%	0%	0.3%	1%

[1] Grade 2 adverse events possibly or probably related to treatment or unassessable were included if study drug dosage was changed or interrupted. Grade 3 severity: Event causing marked limitation in activity, requiring medical care and possible hospitalization. Grade 4 severity: Completely disabling, unable to care for self, requiring active medical intervention, probable hospitalization or hospice care.
[2] All relationships.
[3] See table below.
[4] Adverse reactions were combined to form this category.
[5] CPCRA 002 included patients who were dose-adjusted for grade 2 reactions; ACTG 175 required dose adjustment for grade 2 peripheral neuropathy but recorded only grade 3 reactions.

Percentage of patients with laboratory abnormalities (protocol grade 3/4)

	CPCRA 002* zidovudine (ZDV) intolerant or failure		ACTG 175## zidovudine (ZDV) naive/experienced	
Lab abnormality	Zalcitabine 0.75 mg every 8 hours (n = 237)	Didanosine (ddl) 250 mg every 12 hours (n = 230)	Zidovudine 200 mg every 8 hours (n = 619)	Zalcitabine + zidovudine (ZDV) 0.75 mg every 8 hours + 200 mg every 8 hours (n = 615)
Anemia (< 7.5 g/dL)	0.4%	7.4%	1.8%	3.1%
Leukopenia (< 1500 cells/mm³)	13.1%	9.6%	N/A=	N/A=
Eosinophilia (> 1000 cells/mm³ or 25%)	2.5%	1.7%	N/A=	N/A=
Neutropenia (< 750 cells/mm³)	16.9%	11.7%	1.9%	4.2%
Thrombocytopenia (< 50,000 cells/mm³)	1.3%	4.8%	1.1%	1.8%
CPK elevation* (> 4 x ULN)	0.8%	0%	5.8%	5.7%
ALT (> 5 x ULN)	N/A=	N/A=	3.6%	5%
AST (> 5 x ULN)	7.6%	5.7%	2.9%	4.1%
Bilirubin (> 2.5 x ULN)	0.8%	0.9%	0.5%	1%
GGT (> 5 x ULN)	N/A=	N/A=	0.5%	1%
Amylase (> 2 x ULN)	5.1%	3.9%	1%	1.5%
Hyperglycemia* (> 250 mg/dL)	0%	1.7%	0.8%	2%

* Grade 3 of higher reported for CPCRA 002.
All relationships.
= N/A = not available.

➤*Additional clinical adverse reactions:* Adverse reactions associated with zalcitabine that occurred in less than 1% of patients in CPCRA 002 (at least possibly related, grade 3 or higher), ACTG 175 (any relationship, grade 3/4) or in other clinical studies are listed below by body system. Several of these reactions occurred in slightly higher rates in other studies. The incidence of adverse reactions varied in different studies, generally being lower in patients with less-advanced disease.

Cardiovascular – Abnormal cardiac movement, arrhythmia, atrial fibrillation, cardiac failure, cardiac dysrhythmias, cardiomyopathy, heart racing, hypertension, palpitation, subarachnoid hemorrhage, syncope, tachycardia, ventricular ectopy.

CNS – Abnormal coordination, aphasia, ataxia, Bell's palsy, confusion, decreased concentration, decreased neurological function, disequilibrium, dizziness, dysphonia, facial nerve palsy, focal motor seizures, grand mal seizure, hyperkinesia, hypertonia, hypokinesia, memory loss, migraine, neuralgia, neuritis, paralysis, seizures, speech disorder, status epilepticus, stupor, tremor, twitch, vertigo.

Dermatologic – Acne, alopecia, bullous eruptions, carbuncle/furuncle, cellulitis, cold sore, dermatitis, dry skin, dry rash desquamation, erythematous rash, exfoliative dermatitis, finger inflammation, follicular rash, impetigo, infection, itchy rash, lip blisters/lesions, macular/papular rash, maculopapular rash, moniliasis, mucocutaneous/skin disorder, nail disorder, photosensitivity reaction, pruritic disorder, pruritus, skin disorder, skin lesions, skin fissure, skin ulcer, urticaria.

Endocrine – Altered serum glucose, diabetes mellitus.

GI – Abdominal bloating or cramps, acute pancreatitis, anal/rectal pain, anorexia, bleeding gums, bloody or black stools, colitis, dental abscess, dry mouth, dyspepsia, dysphagia, enlarged abdomen, epigastric pain, eructation, esophageal pain, esophageal ulcers, esophagitis, flatulence, gagging with pills, gastritis, gastrointestinal hemorrhage, gingivitis, glossitis, gum disorder, heartburn, hemorrhagic pancreatitis, hemorrhoids, increased saliva, left quadrant pain, melena, mouth lesion, odynophagia, painful sore gums, painful swallowing, pancreatitis, rectal hemorrhage, rectal mass, rectal ulcers, salivary gland enlargement, sore tongue, sore throat, tongue disorder, tongue ulcer, toothache, unformed/loose stools, vomiting.

GU – Abnormal renal function, acute renal failure, albuminuria, bladder pain, dysuria, frequent urination, genital lesion/ulcer, increased blood urea nitrogen, increased creatinine, micturition frequency, nocturia, painful penis sore, pain on urination, penile edema, polyuria, renal cyst, renal calculus, testicular swelling, toxic nephropathy, urinary retention, vaginal itch, vaginal ulcer, vaginal pain, vaginal/cervical disorder, vaginal discharge.

Hematologic – Absolute neutrophil count alteration, anemia, epistaxis, decreased hematocrit, granulocytosis, hemoglobinemia, leukopenia, neutrophilia, platelet alteration, purpura, thrombus, unspecified hematologic toxicity, white blood cell alteration.

Hepatic – Abnormal lactate dehydrogenase, bilirubinemia, cholecystitis, decreased alkaline phosphatase, hepatitis, hepatocellular damage, hepatomegaly, increased alkaline phosphatase, jaundice.

ZALCITABINE — ORAL

Metabolic – Abnormal triglycerides, abnormal lipase, altered glucose, decreased bicarbonate, diabetes mellitus, glycosuria, gout, hot flushes, hypercalcemia, hyperkalemia, hyperlipemia, hypernatremia, hyperuricemia, hypocalcemia, hypoglycemia, hypokalemia, hypomagnesemia, hyponatremia, hypophosphatemia, increased nonprotein nitrogen, lactic acidosis.

Musculoskeletal – Arthralgia, arthritis, arthropathy, arthrosis, back pain, backache, bone pains/aches, bursitis, cold extremities, extremity pain, joint inflammation, leg cramps, muscle aches, muscle weakness, muscle disorder, muscle stiffness, muscle cramps, myalgia, myopathy, myositis, neck pain, rib pain, stiff neck.

Psychiatric – Acute psychotic disorder, acute stress reaction, agitation, amnesia, anxiety, confusion, decreased motivation, decreased sexual desire, depersonalization, emotional lability, euphoria, hallucination, impaired concentration, insomnia, manic reaction, mood swings, nervousness, paranoid state, somnolence, suicide attempt, dementia.

Respiratory – Acute nasopharyngitis, chest congestion, coughing, cyanosis, difficulty breathing, dry nasal mucosa, dyspnea, flu-like symptoms, hemoptysis, nasal discharge, pharyngitis, rales/rhonchi, respiratory distress, sinus congestion, sinus pain, sinusitis, wheezing.

Special senses – Abnormal vision, blurred vision, burning eyes, decreased taste, decreased vision, ear pain/problem, ear blockage, eye abnormality, eye inflammation, eye itching, eye pain, eye irritation, eye redness, eye hemorrhage, fluid in ears, hearing loss, increased tears, loss of taste, mucopurulent conjunctivitis, parosmia, photophobia, smell dysfunction, taste perversion, tinnitus, unequal-sized pupils, xerophthalmia, yellow sclera.

Miscellaneous – Abnormal weight loss, asthenia, cachexia, chest tightness or pain, chills, cutaneous/allergic reaction, debilitation, difficulty moving, dry eyes/mouth, edema, facial pain or swelling, flank pain, flushing, increased sweating, lymphadenopathy, hypersensitivity reactions (including anaphylactic reaction or urticaria without other signs of anaphylaxis), malaise, night sweats, pain, pelvic/groin pain, rigors, redistribution/accumulation of body fat.

Overdosage

➤*Acute overdosage:* Inadvertent pediatric overdoses have occurred with doses up to 1.5 mg/kg zalcitabine. Pediatric patients had prompt gastric lavage and treatment with activated charcoal and had no sequelae. Mixed overdoses including zalcitabine and other drugs have led to drowsiness and vomiting (with zalcitabine or placebo, zidovudine and trimethoprim/sulfamethoxazole [TMP-SMZ]), or increased GGT (with 18.75 mg zalcitabine with zidovudine and lormetazepam) or increased creatine phosphokinase (with zalcitabine or placebo, zidovudine, fluconazole, dapsone, and wine). There is no experience with acute zalcitabine overdosage at higher doses and sequelae are unknown. There is no known antidote for zalcitabine overdosage. It is not known whether zalcitabine is dialyzable by peritoneal dialysis or hemodialysis.

➤*Chronic overdosage:* In an initial dose-finding study in which zalcitabine was administered at doses 25 times (0.25 mg/kg every 8 hours) the currently recommended dose, 1 patient discontinued zalcitabine after one and a half weeks of treatment subsequent to the development of a rash and fever. In the early phase 1 studies, all patients receiving zalcitabine at approximately 6 times the current total daily recommended dose experienced peripheral neuropathy by week 10. Eighty percent (80%) of patients who received approximately 2 times the current total daily recommended dose experienced peripheral neuropathy by week 12.

Patient Information

Patients should be informed that zalcitabine is not a cure for HIV infection and that they may continue to acquire illnesses associated with advanced HIV infection, including opportunistic infections.

Patients should be told that there is currently no data demonstrating that zalcitabine therapy can reduce the risk of transmitting HIV to others through sexual contact or blood contamination.

Patients should be advised to take zalcitabine every day as prescribed. Patients should not alter the dose or discontinue therapy without consulting with their doctor. If a dose is missed, patients should take the dose as soon as possible and then return to their normal schedule. However, if a dose is skipped, the patient should not double the next dose.

Patients should be instructed that the major toxicity of zalcitabine is peripheral neuropathy. Pancreatitis and hepatic toxicity are other serious potentially life-threatening toxicities that have been reported in patients treated with zalcitabine. Patients should be advised of the early symptoms of these conditions and instructed to promptly report them to their physician. Since the development of peripheral neuropathy appears to be dose-related to zalcitabine, patients should be advised to follow their physicians' instructions regarding the prescribed dose.

Patients should be informed that redistribution or accumulation of body fat may occur in patients receiving antiretroviral therapy and that the cause and long-term health effects of these conditions are not known at this time.

ZIDOVUDINE (Azidothymidine; AZT; Compound S)

Rx	**Zidovudine** (Various, eg, Roxane, Teva)	**Tablets:** 300 mg	In 60s.
Rx	**Retrovir** (GlaxoSmithKline)		(GX CW3 300). White. Film-coated. In 60s.
Rx	**Retrovir** (GlaxoSmithKline)	**Capsules:** 100 mg	(Wellcome Y9C 100). White with blue band. In 100s and UD 100s.
		Syrup: 50 mg/5 mL	0.2% sodium benzoate, sucrose. Strawberry flavor. In 240 mL.
		Injection: 10 mg/mL	In 20 mL single-use vial.

ZIDOVUDINE — ORAL

WARNING

Zidovudine has been associated with hematologic toxicity, including neutropenia and severe anemia, particularly in patients with advanced HIV disease. Prolonged use of zidovudine has been associated with symptomatic myopathy.

Lactic acidosis and severe hepatomegaly with steatosis, including fatal cases, have been reported with the use of nucleoside analogues alone or in combination, including zidovudine and other antiretrovirals.

Indications

➤*HIV infection:* For the treatment of HIV infection in combination with other antiretroviral agents.

➤*Maternal-fetal HIV transmission:* For the prevention of maternal-fetal HIV transmission as part of a regimen that includes oral zidovudine beginning between 14 and 34 weeks of gestation, intravenous zidovudine during labor, and administration of zidovudine syrup to the neonate after birth. The efficacy of this regimen for preventing HIV transmission in women who have received zidovudine for a prolonged period before pregnancy has not been evaluated. The safety of zidovudine for the mother or fetus during the first trimester of pregnancy has not been assessed.

Administration and Dosage

➤*Approved by the FDA:* March 19, 1987.

➤*Adults:* 600 mg/day in divided doses in combination with other antiretroviral agents. The effectiveness of this dose compared to higher dosing regimens in improving the neurologic dysfunction associated with HIV disease is unknown.

➤*Children:* The recommended dose in pediatric patients 6 weeks to 12 years of age is 160 mg/m^2 every 8 hours (480 mg/m^2/day up to a maximum of 200 mg every 8 hours) in combination with other antiretroviral agents.

➤*Maternal-fetal HIV transmission:* The recommended dosing regimen for administration to pregnant women (greater than 14 weeks of pregnancy) and their neonates is as follows:

Maternal dosing – 100 mg orally 5 times/day until the start of labor. During labor and delivery, intravenous zidovudine should be administered at 2 mg/kg (total body weight) over 1 hour, followed by a continuous intravenous infusion of 1 mg/kg/hr (total body weight) until clamping of the umbilical cord.

Neonatal dosing – 2 mg/kg orally every 6 hours starting within 12 hours after birth and continuing through 6 weeks of age. Neonates unable to receive oral dosing may be administered zidovudine intravenously at 1.5 mg/kg infused over 30 minutes every 6 hours.

➤*Dose adjustment:*

Anemia – Significant anemia (hemoglobin of less than 7.5 g/dL or reduction of greater than 25% of baseline) or significant neutropenia (granulocyte count of less than 750 cells/mm^3 or reduction of greater than 50% from baseline) may require a dose interruption until evidence of marrow recovery is observed (see Warnings). In patients who develop significant anemia, dose interruption does not necessarily eliminate the need for transfusion. If marrow recovery occurs following dose interruption, resumption in dose may be appropriate using adjunctive measures such as epoetin alfa at recommended doses, depending on hematologic indices such as serum erythropoietin level and patient tolerance.

For patients experiencing pronounced anemia while receiving chronic coadministration of zidovudine and some of the drugs (eg, fluconazole, valproic acid) listed in the information above, zidovudine dose reduction may be considered.

Renal function impairment – In patients maintained on hemodialysis or peritoneal dialysis, the recommended dosing is 100 mg every 6 to 8 hours.

See Actions for more information.

Hepatic function impairment – There are insufficient data to recommend dose adjustment of zidovudine in patients with mild-to-moderate impaired hepatic function or liver cirrhosis. Since zidovudine is primarily eliminated by hepatic metabolism, a reduction in the daily dose may be necessary in these patients. Frequent monitoring for hematologic toxicities is advised.

ZIDOVUDINE — ORAL

➤*Storage/Stability:* Store at 15° to 25°C (59° to 77°F). Protect from moisture.

Actions

➤*Pharmacokinetics:*

Special populations –

Renal function impairment:

• *Adults with impaired renal function –* Zidovudine clearance was decreased resulting in increased zidovudine and GZDV half-life and AUC in patients with impaired renal function (n = 14) following a single 200-mg oral dose (see table below). Plasma concentrations of AMT were not determined. A dose adjustment should not be necessary for patients with creatinine clearance (Ccr) of 15 mL/min or greater.

Zidovudine pharmacokinetic parameters in patients with severe renal impairment*		
Parameter	Control subjects (healthy renal function) (n = 6)	Patients with renal impairment (n = 14)
Ccr (mL/min)	120 ± 8	18 ± 2
Zidovudine AUC (ng•hr/mL)	1,400 ± 200	3,100 ± 300
Zidovudine half-life (hr)	1 ± 0.2	1.4 ± 0.1

* Data are expressed as mean ± standard deviation.

Hepatic function impairment:

• *Adults with impaired hepatic function –* Data describing the effect of hepatic impairment on the pharmacokinetics of zidovudine are limited. However, because zidovudine is eliminated primarily by hepatic metabolism, it is expected that zidovudine clearance would be decreased and plasma concentrations would be increased following administration of the recommended adult doses to patients with hepatic impairment.

Children:

• *Patients less than 3 months of age –* Zidovudine pharmacokinetics have been evaluated in pediatric patients from birth to 3 months of life. Zidovudine elimination was determined immediately following birth in 8 neonates who were exposed to zidovudine in utero. The half-life was 13 ± 5.8 hours. In neonates less than or equal to 14 days old, bioavailability was greater, total body clearance was slower, and half-life was longer than in pediatric patients greater than 14 days old.

Zidovudine pharmacokinetic parameters in pediatric patients*			
Parameter	Birth to 14 days of age	14 days to 3 months of age	3 months to 12 years of age
Oral bioavailability (%)	89 ± 19 (n = 15)	61 ± 19 (n = 17)	65 ± 24 (n = 18)
CSF:plasma ratio	no data	no data	0.68 [0.03 to 3.25]** (n = 38)
CL (L/hr/kg)	0.65 ± 0.29 (n = 18)	1.14 ± 0.24 (n = 16)	1.85 ± 0.47 (n = 20)
Elimination half-life (hr)	3.1 ± 1.2 (n = 21)	1.9 ± 0.7 (n = 18)	1.5 ± 0.7 (n = 21)

* Data presented as mean ± standard deviation except where noted.
** Median [range].

Adults – Following oral administration, zidovudine is rapidly absorbed and extensively distributed, with peak serum concentrations occurring within 0.5 to 1.5 hours. Binding to plasma protein is low. Zidovudine is primarily eliminated by hepatic metabolism. The major metabolite of zidovudine is 3'-azido-3'-deoxy-5'-O-β-D-glucopyranuronosylthymidine (GZDV). GZDV area under the curve (AUC) is about 3-fold greater than the zidovudine AUC. Urinary recovery of zidovudine and GZDV accounts for 14% and 74%, respectively, of the dose following oral administration. A second metabolite, 3'-amino-3'-deoxythymidine (AMT), has been identified in the plasma following single-dose intravenous (IV) administration of zidovudine. The AMT AUC was one-fifth of the zidovudine AUC. Pharmacokinetics of zidovudine were dose independent at oral dosing regimens ranging from 2 mg/kg every 8 hours to 10 mg/kg every 4 hours.

The extent of absorption (AUC) was equivalent when zidovudine was administered as zidovudine tablets or syrup compared to zidovudine capsules.

Zidovudine pharmacokinetic parameters in fasting adult patients	
Parameter	Mean ± SD (except where noted)
Oral bioavailability (%)	64 ± 10 (n = 5)
Apparent volume of distribution (L/kg)	1.6 ± 0.6 (n = 8)
Plasma protein binding (%)	< 38
CSF:plasma ratio*	0.6 [0.04 to 2.62] (n = 39)
Systemic clearance (L/hr/kg)	1.6 ± 0.6 (n = 6)
Renal clearance (L/hr/kg)	0.34 ± 0.05 (n = 9)
Elimination half-life (hr)**	0.5 to 3 (n = 19)

* Median [range].
** Approximate range.

Effect of food on absorption – Zidovudine may be administered with or without food. The extent of zidovudine absorption (AUC) was similar when a single dose of zidovudine was administered with food.

➤*Microbiology:* Zidovudine is a synthetic nucleoside analogue of the naturally occurring nucleoside, thymidine, in which the 3'-hydroxy (−OH) group is replaced by an azido ($-N_3$) group. Within cells, zidovudine is converted to the active metabolite, zidovudine 5'-triphosphate (AztTP), by the sequential action of the cellular enzymes. Zidovudine 5'-triphosphate inhibits the activity of the HIV reverse transcriptase both by competing for utilization with the natural substrate, deoxythymidine 5'-triphosphate (dTTP), and by its incorporation into viral DNA. The lack of a 3'−OH group in the incorporated nucleoside analogue prevents the formation of the 5' to 3' phosphodiester linkage essential for DNA chain elongation and, therefore, the viral DNA growth is terminated. The active metabolite AztTP is also a weak inhibitor of the cellular DNA polymerase-alpha and mitochondrial polymerase gamma and has been reported to be incorporated into the DNA of cells in culture.

In vitro HIV susceptibility – The in vitro anti-HIV activity of zidovudine was assessed by infecting cell lines of lymphoblastic and monocytic origin and peripheral blood lymphocytes with laboratory and clinical isolates of HIV. The IC_{50} and IC_{90} values (50% and 90% inhibitory concentrations) were 0.003 to 0.013 and 0.03 to 0.13 mcg/mL, respectively (1 nM = 0.27 ng/mL). The IC_{50} and IC_{90} values of HIV isolates recovered from 18 untreated AIDS/ARC patients were in the range of 0.003 to 0.013 mcg/mL and 0.03 to 0.3 mcg/mL, respectively. Zidovudine showed antiviral activity in all acutely infected cell lines; however, activity was substantially less in chronically infected cell lines. In drug combination studies with zalcitabine, didanosine, lamivudine, saquinavir, indinavir, ritonavir, nevirapine, delavirdine, or interferon alpha, zidovudine showed additive to synergistic activity in cell culture. The relationship between the in vitro susceptibility of HIV to reverse transcriptase inhibitors and the inhibition of HIV replication in humans has not been established.

Drug resistance – HIV isolates with reduced sensitivity to zidovudine have been selected in vitro and were also recovered from patients treated with zidovudine. Genetic analysis of the isolates showed mutations which result in 5 amino acid substitutions (Met41→Leu, A67→Asn, Lys70→Arg, Thr215→Tyr or Phe, and Lys219→Gln) in the viral reverse transcriptase. In general, higher levels of resistance were associated with greater number of mutations with 215 mutation being the most significant.

Cross-resistance – The potential for cross-resistance between HIV reverse transcriptase inhibitors and protease inhibitors is low because of the different enzyme targets involved. Combination therapy with zidovudine plus zalcitabine or didanosine does not appear to prevent the emergence of zidovudine-resistant isolates. Combination therapy with zidovudine plus lamivudine delayed the emergence of mutations conferring resistance to zidovudine. In some patients harboring zidovudine-resistant virus, combination therapy with zidovudine plus lamivudine restored phenotypic sensitivity to zidovudine by 12 weeks of treatment. HIV isolates with multidrug resistance to zidovudine, didanosine, zalcitabine, stavudine, and lamivudine were recovered from a small number of patients treated for greater than or equal to 1 year with the combination of zidovudine and didanosine or zalcitabine. The pattern of resistant mutations in the combination therapy was different (Ala62→Val, Val75→Ile, Phe77→116Tyr, and Gln→151Met) from monotherapy, with mutation 151 being most significant for multidrug resistance. Site-directed mutagenesis studies showed that these mutations could also result in resistance to zalcitabine, lamivudine, and stavudine.

Contraindications

For patients who have potentially life-threatening allergic reactions to any of the components of the formulations.

Warnings

➤*Combination products:* Lamivudine plus zidovudine (*Combivir*) and abacavir sulfate plus lamivudine plus zidovudine (*Trizivir*) are combination product tablets that contain zidovudine as one of their components. Zidovudine should not be administered concomitantly with these combinations.

➤*Bone marrow suppression:* Zidovudine should be used with caution in patients who have bone marrow compromise evidenced by granulocyte count less than 1000 cells/mm^3 or hemoglobin less than 9.5 g/dL. In patients with advanced symptomatic HIV disease, anemia and neutropenia were the most significant adverse reactions observed. There have been reports of pancytopenia associated with the use of zidovudine, which was reversible in most instances after discontinuance of the drug. However, significant anemia, in many cases requiring dose adjustment, discontinuation of zidovudine, or blood transfusions has occurred during treatment with zidovudine alone or in combination with other antiretrovirals.

Frequent blood counts are strongly recommended in patients with advanced HIV disease who are treated with zidovudine. For HIV-infected individuals and patients with asymptomatic or early HIV disease, periodic blood counts are recommended. If anemia or neutropenia develops, dosage adjustments may be necessary.

➤*Myopathy:* Myopathy and myositis with pathological changes, similar to that produced by HIV disease, have been associated with prolonged use of zidovudine.

➤*Lactic acidosis/severe hepatomegaly with steatosis:* Lactic acidosis and severe hepatomegaly with steatosis, including fatal cases, have been reported with the use of nucleoside analogues alone or in combination, including zidovudine and other antiretrovirals. A majority of these cases have been in women. Obesity and prolonged exposure to antiretroviral nucleoside analogues may be risk factors. Particular caution should be exercised when administering zidovudine to any patient with known risk factors

ZIDOVUDINE — ORAL

for liver disease; however, cases have also been reported in patients with no known risk factors. Treatment with zidovudine should be suspended in any patient who develops clinical or laboratory findings suggestive of lactic acidosis or pronounced hepatotoxicity (which may include hepatomegaly and steatosis even in the absence of marked transaminase elevations).

➤*Renal/Hepatic function impairment:* Zidovudine is eliminated from the body primarily by renal excretion following metabolism in the liver (glucuronidation). In patients with severely impaired renal function (Ccr less than 15 mL/min), dosage reduction is recommended. Although the data are limited, zidovudine concentrations appear to be increased in patients with severely impaired hepatic function that may increase the risk of hematologic toxicity (see Administration and Dosage and Pharmacokinetics).

➤*Carcinogenesis:* In mice, 7 late-appearing (after 19 months) vaginal neoplasms (5 nonmetastasizing squamous cell carcinomas, 1 squamous cell papilloma, and 1 squamous polyp) occurred in animals given the highest dose. One late-appearing squamous cell papilloma occurred in the vagina of a middle-dose animal. No vaginal tumors were found at the lowest dose.

In rats, 2 late-appearing (after 20 months), nonmetastasizing vaginal squamous cell carcinomas occurred in animals given the highest dose. No vaginal tumors occurred at the low or middle dose in rats. No other drug-related tumors were observed in either sex of either species.

Two transplacental carcinogenicity studies were conducted in mice. One study administered zidovudine at doses of 20 mg/kg/day or 40 mg/kg/day from gestation day 10 through parturition and lactation with dosing continuing in offspring for 24 months postnatally. The doses of zidovudine employed in this study produced zidovudine exposures approximately 3 times the estimated human exposure at recommended doses. After 24 months, an increase in incidence of vaginal tumors was noted with no increase in tumors in the liver or lung or any other organ in either gender. These findings are consistent with results of the standard oral carcinogenicity study in mice, as described earlier. A second study administered zidovudine at maximum tolerated doses of 12.5 mg/day or 25 mg/day (approximately 1000 mg/kg nonpregnant body weight or approximately 450 mg/kg of term body weight) to pregnant mice from days 12 through 18 of gestation. There was an increase in the number of tumors in the lung, liver, and female reproductive tracts in the offspring of mice receiving the higher dose level of zidovudine.

➤*Mutagenesis:* Zidovudine was mutagenic in a 5178Y/TK$^{+/-}$ mouse lymphoma assay, positive in an in vitro cell transformation assay, clastogenic in a cytogenetic assay using cultured human lymphocytes, and positive in mouse and rat micronucleus tests after repeated doses. It was negative in a cytogenetic study in rats given a single dose.

➤*Elderly:* In general, dose selection for an elderly patient should be cautious, reflecting the greater frequency of decreased hepatic, renal, or cardiac function, and of concomitant disease or other drug therapy.

➤*Pregnancy: Category C.* Oral teratology studies in the rat and in the rabbit at doses up to 500 mg/kg/day revealed no evidence of teratogenicity with zidovudine. Zidovudine treatment resulted in embryo/fetal toxicity as evidenced by an increase in the incidence of fetal resorptions in rats given 150 or 450 mg/kg/day and rabbits given 500 mg/kg/day. The doses used in the teratology studies resulted in peak zidovudine plasma concentrations (after one half of the daily dose) in rats 66 to 226 times, and in rabbits 12 to 87 times, mean steady-state peak human plasma concentrations (after one sixth of the daily dose) achieved with the recommended daily dose (100 mg every 4 hours). In an in vitro experiment with fertilized mouse oocytes, zidovudine exposure resulted in a dose-dependent reduction in blastocyst formation. In an additional teratology study in rats, a dose of 3000 mg/kg/day (very near the oral median lethal dose in rats of 3683 mg/kg) caused marked maternal toxicity and an increase in the incidence of fetal malformations. This dose resulted in peak zidovudine plasma concentrations 350 times peak human plasma concentrations. (Estimated area-under-the-curve [AUC] in rats at this dose level was 300 times the daily AUC in humans given 600 mg/day.) No evidence of teratogenicity was seen in this experiment at doses of 600 mg/kg/day or less.

A randomized, double-blind, placebo-controlled trial was conducted in HIV-infected pregnant women to determine the utility of zidovudine for the prevention of maternal-fetal HIV-transmission. Congenital abnormalities occurred with similar frequency between neonates born to mothers who received zidovudine and neonates born to mothers who received placebo. Abnormalities were either problems in embryogenesis (prior to 14 weeks) or were recognized on ultrasound before or immediately after initiation of study drug.

Antiretroviral pregnancy registry – To monitor maternal-fetal outcomes of pregnant women exposed to zidovudine, an Antiretroviral Pregnancy Registry has been established. Physicians are encouraged to register patients by calling 1-800-258-4263.

➤*Lactation:* The CDC recommend that HIV-infected mothers not breastfeed their infants to avoid risking postnatal transmission of HIV. Zidovudine is excreted in human milk. Because of both the potential for HIV transmission and the potential for serious adverse reactions in nursing infants, mothers should be instructed not to breastfeed if they are receiving zidovudine.

➤*Children:* Zidovudine has been studied in HIV-infected pediatric patients greater than 3 months of age who have HIV-related symptoms or who are asymptomatic with abnormal laboratory values indicating significant HIV-related immunosuppression. Zidovudine has also been studied in neonates perinatally exposed to HIV.

Precautions

➤*Monitoring:* The incidence of adverse reactions appears to increase with disease progression, and patients should be monitored carefully, especially as disease progression occurs.

Hematologic toxicities appear to be related to pretreatment bone marrow reserve and to dose and duration of therapy. In patients with poor bone marrow reserve, particularly in patients with advanced symptomatic HIV disease, frequent monitoring of hematologic indices is recommended to detect serious anemia or neutropenia. In patients who experience hematologic toxicity, reduction in hemoglobin may occur as early as 2 to 4 weeks, and neutropenia usually occurs after 6 to 8 weeks.

➤*Fat redistribution:* Redistribution/accumulation of body fat, including central obesity, dorsocervical fat enlargement (buffalo hump), peripheral wasting, facial wasting, breast enlargement and "cushingoid appearance", have been observed in patients receiving antiretroviral therapy. The mechanism and long-term consequences of these events are currently unknown. A causal relationship has not been established.

Drug Interactions

Zidovudine Drug Interactions

Precipitant drug	Object drug*		Description
Acetaminophen	Zidovudine	⬇	Acetaminophen may decrease the AUC of zidovudine.
Atovaquone	Zidovudine	⬆	Atovaquone appears to inhibit glucuronidation of zidovudine, thus increasing zidovudine concentrations and decreasing clearance.
Bone marrow suppressive/ cytotoxic agents (eg, interferon-alpha, interferon-beta-1b)	Zidovudine	⬆	Coadministration may increase the hematologic toxicity of zidovudine.
Clarithromycin	Zidovudine	⬌	Peak serum zidovudine concentrations may be increased or decreased.
Doxorubicin	Zidovudine	⬇	Avoid coadministration. An antagonistic relationship has been demonstrated.
Fluconazole	Zidovudine	⬆	Concurrent use may increase the zidovudine AUC.
Ganciclovir	Zidovudine	⬆	Concomitant use may increase zidovudine plasma levels and AUC, thus increasing risk of life-threatening hematologic toxicities.
Methadone	Zidovudine	⬆	Zidovudine serum concentrations and AUC may be elevated, increasing the risk of side effects.
Nelfinavir/ Ritonavir	Zidovudine	⬇	Zidovudine AUC is decreased.
Probenecid	Zidovudine	⬆	Probenecid may increase zidovudine AUC by inhibiting glucuronidation or reducing renal excretion. Some patients have developed symptoms consisting of myalgia, malaise or fever, and maculopapular rash.
Rifamycins	Zidovudine	⬇	The AUC of zidovudine may be decreased.
Stavudine, ribavirin	Zidovudine	⬇	Avoid concomitant use because some nucleoside analogs affect viral replication and may antagonize antiviral activity of zidovudine against HIV.
Trimethoprim	Zidovudine	⬆	Serum levels of zidovudine and its metabolite may be increased, especially in patients with impaired hepatic glucuronidation from liver disease or drug inhibition.
Valproic acid	Zidovudine	⬆	Concurrent use may inhibit glucuronide metabolism, thus increasing zidovudine AUC.

ZIDOVUDINE — ORAL

Zidovudine Drug Interactions			
Precipitant drug	Object drug*		Description
Zidovudine	Phenytoin	↔	Phenytoin levels have been reported to increase, decrease or not change with concurrent use. In addition, zidovudine clearance was decreased by phenytoin.
Phenytoin	Zidovudine	↑	

* ↑ = Object drug increased. ↓ = Object drug decreased.
↔ = Undetermined clinical effect.

Adverse Reactions

➤*Adults:* The frequency and severity of adverse reactions associated with the use of zidovudine are greater in patients with more advanced infection at the time of initiation of therapy. The table below summarizes reactions reported at a statistically significant greater incidence for patients receiving zidovudine in a monotherapy study:

Percentage (%) of patients with adverse reactions* in asymptomatic HIV infection (ACTG019)		
Adverse reaction	Zidovudine 500 mg/day (n = 453)	Placebo (n = 428)
Miscellaneous		
Asthenia	8.6%[1]	5.8%
Headache	62.5%	52.6%
Malaise	53.2%	44.9%
GI		
Anorexia	20.1%	10.5%
Constipation	6.4%[1]	3.5%
Nausea	51.4%	29.9%
Vomiting	17.2%	9.8%

* Reported in greater than or equal to 5% of study population.
[1] Not statistically significant versus placebo.

Other adverse reactions observed in clinical studies were the following: Abdominal cramps, abdominal pain, arthralgia, chills, dyspepsia, fatigue, hyperbilirubinemia, insomnia, musculoskeletal pain, myalgia, and neuropathy. Selected laboratory abnormalities observed during a clinical study of monotherapy with zidovudine are shown in the table below.

Frequencies of selected (grade 3/4) laboratory abnormalities in patients with asymptomatic HIV infection (ACTG019)		
Adverse reaction	Zidovudine 500 mg/day (n = 453)	Placebo (n = 428)
Anemia (Hgb < 8 g/dL)	1.1%	0.2%
Granulocytopenia (< 750 cells/mm³)	1.8%	1.6%
Thrombocytopenia (platelets < 50,000/mm³)	0%	0.5%
ALT (> 5 × ULN)[1]	3.1%	2.6%
AST (> 5 × ULN)[1]	0.9%	1.6%
Alkaline phosphatase (> 5 × ULN)[1]	0%	0%

[1] ULN = Upper limit of normal.

➤*Children:* Selected clinical adverse reactions and physical findings with a greater than or equal to 5% frequency during therapy with lamivudine 4 mg/kg twice daily plus zidovudine 160 mg/m² 3 times daily compared with didanosine in therapy-naive (less than or equal to 56 days of antiretroviral therapy) pediatric patients are listed in the table below.

Selected clinical adverse reactions and physical findings (≥ 5% frequency) in pediatric patients in Study ACTG300		
Adverse reaction	Lamivudine plus zidovudine (n = 236)	Didanosine (n = 235)
Miscellaneous		
Fever	25%	32%
Skin rashes	12%	14%
Lymphadenopathy	9%	11%
GI		
Hepatomegaly	11%	11%
Nausea/vomiting	8%	7%
Diarrhea	8%	6%
Stomatitis	6%	12%
Splenomegaly	5%	8%
Respiratory		
Cough	15%	18%
Abnormal breath sounds/wheezing	7%	9%
Ear, nose, and throat		
Signs or symptoms of ears*	7%	6%
Nasal discharge or congestion	8%	11%

* Includes pain, discharge, erythema, or swelling of an ear.

Lab test abnormalities – Selected laboratory abnormalities experienced by therapy-naive (less than or equal to 56 days of antiretroviral therapy) pediatric patients are listed in the table below.

Frequencies of selected (grade 3/4) laboratory abnormalities in pediatric patients in Study ACTG300		
Test (abnormal level)	Lamivudine plus zidovudine	Didanosine
Neutropenia (ANC < 400 cells/mm³)[1]	8%	3%
Anemia (Hgb < 7 g/dL)	4%	2%
Thrombocytopenia (platelets < 50,000/mm³)	1%	3%
ALT (> 10 × ULN)[2]	1%	3%
AST (> 10 × ULN)[2]	2%	4%
Lipase (> 2.5 × ULN)[2]	3%	3%
Total amylase (> 2.5 × ULN)[2]	3%	3%

[1] ANC = Absolute neutrophil count.
[2] ULN = Upper limit of normal.

Additional adverse reactions reported in open-label studies in pediatric patients receiving zidovudine 180 mg/m² every 6 hours were the following: Congestive heart failure, decreased reflexes, ECG abnormality, edema, hematuria, left ventricular dilation, macrocytosis, nervousness/irritability, and weight loss.

The clinical adverse reactions reported among adult recipients of zidovudine may also occur in pediatric patients.

➤*Use for the prevention of maternal-fetal transmission of HIV:* In a randomized, double-blind, placebo-controlled trial in HIV-infected women and their neonates conducted to determine the utility of zidovudine for the prevention of maternal-fetal HIV transmission, zidovudine syrup at 2 mg/kg was administered every 6 hours for 6 weeks to neonates beginning within 12 hours following birth. The most commonly reported adverse reactions were anemia (hemoglobin less than 9 g/dL) and neutropenia (less than 1000 cells/mm³). Anemia occurred in 22% of the neonates who received zidovudine and in 12% of the neonates who received placebo. The mean difference in hemoglobin values was less than 1 g/dL for neonates receiving zidovudine compared to neonates receiving placebo. No neonates with anemia required transfusion and all hemoglobin values spontaneously returned to normal within 6 weeks after completion of therapy with zidovudine. Neutropenia was reported with similar frequency in the group that received zidovudine (21%) and in the group that received placebo (27%). The long-term consequences of in utero and infant exposure to zidovudine are unknown.

➤*Postmarketing:*

Cardiovascular – Cardiomyopathy, syncope.

CNS – Anxiety, confusion, depression, dizziness, loss of mental acuity, mania, paresthesia, seizures, somnolence, vertigo.

Dermatologic – Changes in skin and nail pigmentation, pruritus, rash, Stevens-Johnson syndrome, toxic epidermal necrolysis, sweat, urticaria.

Endocrine – Gynecomastia.

GI – Constipation, dysphagia, flatulence, oral mucosa pigmentation, mouth ulcer.

GU – Urinary frequency, urinary hesitancy.

Hematologic/Lymphatic – Aplastic anemia, hemolytic anemia, leukopenia, lymphadenopathy, pancytopenia with marrow hypoplasia, pure red cell aplasia.

Hepatic – Hepatitis, hepatomegaly with steatosis, jaundice, lactic acidosis, pancreatitis.

Musculoskeletal – Increased CPK, increased LDH, muscle spasm, myopathy and myositis with pathological changes (similar to that produced by HIV disease), rhabdomyolysis, tremor.

Ophthalmic – Macular edema.

Respiratory – Cough, dyspnea, rhinitis, sinusitis.

Special senses – Amblyopia, hearing loss, photophobia, taste perversion.

Miscellaneous – Back pain, chest pain, flu-like syndrome, generalized pain, sensitization reactions including anaphylaxis and angioedema, vasculitis. Redistribution/accumulation of body fat, including central obesity, dor-

ZIDOVUDINE — ORAL

socervical fat enlargement (buffalo hump), peripheral wasting, facial wasting, breast enlargement and "cushingoid appearance", have been observed in patients receiving antiretroviral therapy.

Overdosage

➤*Symptoms:* Acute overdoses of zidovudine have been reported in pediatric patients and adults. These involved exposures up to 50 g. No specific symptoms or signs have been identified following acute overdosage with zidovudine apart from those listed as adverse reactions (eg, fatigue, headache, vomiting, and occasional reports of hematological disturbances). All patients recovered without permanent sequelae.

➤*Treatment:* Hemodialysis and peritoneal dialysis appear to have a negligible effect on the removal of zidovudine while elimination of its primary metabolite, GZDV, is enhanced.

Patient Information

Zidovudine is not a cure for HIV infection, and patients may continue to acquire illnesses associated with HIV infection, including opportunistic infections. Therefore, patients should be advised to seek medical care for any significant change in their health status.

The safety and efficacy of zidovudine in women, intravenous drug users, and racial minorities is not significantly different than that observed in white males.

Patients should be informed that the major toxicities of zidovudine are neutropenia or anemia. The frequency and severity of these toxicities are greater in patients with more advanced disease and in those who initiate therapy later in the course of their infection. They should be told that if toxicity develops, they may require transfusions or dose modifications including possible drug discontinuation. They should be told of the extreme importance of having their blood counts followed closely while on therapy, especially for patients with advanced symptomatic HIV disease. They should be cautioned about the use of other medications, including ganciclovir and interferon alpha, that may exacerbate the toxicity of zidovudine. Patients should be informed that other adverse effects of zidovudine include nausea and vomiting. Patients should also be encouraged to contact their physicians if they experience muscle weakness, shortness of breath, symptoms of hepatitis or pancreatitis, or any other unexpected adverse reactions while being treated with zidovudine.

Zidovudine tablets, capsules, and syrup are for oral ingestion only. Patients should be told of the importance of taking zidovudine exactly as prescribed. They should be told not to share medication and not to exceed the recommended dose. Patients should be told that the long-term effects of zidovudine are unknown at this time.

Pregnant women considering the use of zidovudine during pregnancy for prevention of HIV-transmission to their infants should be advised that transmission may still occur in some cases despite therapy. The long-term consequences of in utero and infant exposure to zidovudine are unknown, including the possible risk of cancer.

HIV-infected pregnant women should be advised not to breastfeed to avoid postnatal transmission of HIV to a child who may not yet be infected.

Patients should be advised that therapy with zidovudine has not been shown to reduce the risk of transmission of HIV to others through sexual contact or blood contamination.

Patients should be informed that redistribution or accumulation of body fat may occur in patients receiving antiretroviral therapy and that the cause and long-term health effects of these conditions are not known at this time.

ZIDOVUDINE — INJECTION

WARNING

Zidovudine has been associated with hematologic toxicity, including neutropenia and severe anemia, particularly in patients with advanced HIV disease. Prolonged use of zidovudine has been associated with symptomatic myopathy.

Lactic acidosis and severe hepatomegaly with steatosis, including fatal cases, have been reported with the use of nucleoside analogues alone or in combination, including zidovudine and other antiretrovirals.

Indications

➤*HIV infection:* For the treatment of HIV infection in combination with other antiretroviral agents.

➤*Maternal-fetal HIV transmission:* For the prevention of maternal-fetal HIV transmission as part of a regimen that includes oral zidovudine beginning between 14 and 34 weeks of gestation, intravenous zidovudine during labor, and administration of zidovudine syrup to the neonate after birth. The efficacy of this regimen for preventing HIV transmission in women who have received zidovudine for a prolonged period before pregnancy has not been evaluated. The safety of zidovudine for the mother or fetus during the first trimester of pregnancy has not been assessed.

Administration and Dosage

➤*Approved by the FDA:* March 19, 1987.

➤*Adults:* The recommended intravenous dose is 1 mg/kg infused over 1 hour. This dose should be administered 5 to 6 times daily (5 to 6 mg/kg daily). The effectiveness of this dose compared to higher dosing regimens in improving the neurologic dysfunction associated with HIV disease is unknown. A small randomized study found a greater effect of higher doses of zidovudine on improvement of neurological symptoms in patients with pre-existing neurological disease.

Patients should receive zidovudine IV infusion only until oral therapy can be administered. The intravenous dosing regimen equivalent to the oral administration of 100 mg every 4 hours is approximately 1 mg/kg intravenously every 4 hours.

➤*Maternal-fetal HIV transmission:* The recommended dosing regimen for administration to pregnant women (greater than 14 weeks of pregnancy) and their neonates is as follows:

Maternal dosing – 100 mg orally 5 times per day until the start of labor. During labor and delivery, intravenous zidovudine should be administered at 2 mg/kg (total body weight) over 1 hour followed by a continuous intravenous infusion of 1 mg/kg/hour (total body weight) until clamping of the umbilical cord.

Neonatal dosing – 2 mg/kg orally every 6 hours starting within 12 hours after birth and continuing through 6 weeks of age. Neonates unable to receive oral dosing may be administered zidovudine intravenously at 1.5 mg/kg, infused over 30 minutes, every 6 hours.

➤*Monitoring:* Hematologic toxicities appear to be related to pretreatment bone marrow reserve and to dose and duration of therapy. In patients with poor bone marrow reserve, particularly in patients with advanced symptomatic HIV disease, frequent monitoring of hematologic indices is recommended to detect serious anemia or neutropenia. In patients who experience hematologic toxicity, reduction in hemoglobin may occur as early as 2 to 4 weeks, and neutropenia usually occurs after 6 to 8 weeks.

➤*Dose adjustment:*

Anemia – Significant anemia (hemoglobin of less than 7.5 g/dL or reduction of greater than 25% of baseline) or significant neutropenia (granulocyte count of less than 750 cells/mm^3 or reduction of greater than 50% from baseline) may require a dose interruption until evidence of marrow recovery is observed. In patients who develop significant anemia, dose interruption does not necessarily eliminate the need for transfusion. If marrow recovery occurs following dose interruption, resumption in dose may be appropriate using adjunctive measures such as epoetin alfa at recommended doses, depending on hematologic indices such as serum erythropoetin level and patient tolerance.

For patients experiencing pronounced anemia while receiving chronic coadministration of zidovudine and certain drugs (eg, atovaquone, fluconazole, methadone, nelfinavir, probenecid, ritonavir, valproic acid), zidovudine dose reduction may be considered.

Renal function impairment – In patients with severely impaired renal function (Ccr less than 15 mL/min), dosage reduction is recommended.

In patients maintained on hemodialysis or peritoneal dialysis (Ccr less than 15 mL/min), recommended dosing is 1 mg/kg every 6 to 8 hours.

Hepatic function impairment – Although the data are limited, zidovudine concentrations appear to be increased in patients with severely impaired hepatic function, which may increase the risk of hematologic toxicity.

There are insufficient data to recommend dose adjustment of zidovudine in patients with mild to moderate impaired hepatic function or liver cirrhosis. Since zidovudine is primarily eliminated by hepatic metabolism, a reduction in the daily dose may be necessary in these patients. Frequent monitoring of hematologic toxicities is advised.

➤*Method of preparation:* Zidovudine IV infusion must be diluted prior to administration. The calculated dose should be removed from the 20 mL vial and added to 5% Dextrose Injection solution to achieve a concentration no greater than 4 mg/mL. Admixture in biologic or colloidal fluids (eg, blood products, protein solutions) is not recommended.

➤*Administration:* Zidovudine IV infusion is administered intravenously at a constant rate over 1 hour. Rapid infusion or bolus injection should be avoided. Zidovudine IV infusion should not be given intramuscularly.

➤*Storage/Stability:* Store vials at 15° to 25°C (59° to 77°F) and protect from light.

After dilution, the solution is physically and chemically stable for 24 hours at room temperature and 48 hours if refrigerated at 2° to 8°C (36° to 46°F). Care should be taken during admixture to prevent inadvertent contamination. As an additional precaution, the diluted solution should be administered within 8 hours if stored at 25°C (77°F) or 24 hours if refrigerated at 2° to 8°C to minimize potential administration of a microbially contaminated solution.

Actions

➤*Pharmacology:* Zidovudine is a synthetic nucleoside analogue of the naturally occurring nucleoside, thymidine, in which the 3'-hydroxy (-OH) group is replaced by an azido (-N_3) group. Within cells, zidovudine is converted to the active metabolite, zidovudine 5'-triphosphate (AztTP), by the sequential action of the cellular enzymes. Zidovudine 5'-triphosphate inhibits the activity of the HIV reverse transcriptase both by competing for utilization with the natural substrate, deoxythymidine 5'-triphosphate (dTTP), and by its incorporation into viral DNA. The lack of a 3'-OH group in the incorporated nucleoside analogue prevents the formation of the 5' to 3' phosphodiester linkage essential for DNA chain elongation and, therefore, the viral DNA growth is terminated. The active metabolite AztTP is also a weak

ZIDOVUDINE — INJECTION

inhibitor of the cellular DNA polymerase-alpha and mitochondrial polymerase-gamma and has been reported to be incorporated into the DNA of cells in culture.

➤*Pharmacokinetics:*

Absorption/Distribution – The pharmacokinetics of zidovudine have been evaluated in 22 adult HIV-infected patients in a Phase 1 dose-escalation study. Following IV dosing, dose-independent kinetics was observed over the range of 1 to 5 mg/kg.

The mean steady-state peak and trough concentrations of zidovudine at 2.5 mg/kg every 4 hours were 1.06 and 0.12 mcg/mL, respectively. The apparent volume of distribution of zidovudine was 1.6 ± 0.6 L/kg. Plasma protein binding of zidovudine was less than 38%.

The zidovudine cerebrospinal fluid (CSF)/plasma concentration ratio was determined in 39 patients receiving chronic therapy with zidovudine. The median ratio measured in 50 paired samples drawn 1 to 8 hours after the last dose of zidovudine was 0.6. (0.04 to 2.62).

Metabolism – The major metabolite of zidovudine is 3'-azido-3'-deoxy-5'-O-β-D-glucopyranuronosylthymidine (GZDV). GZDV area under the curve (AUC) is about 3-fold greater than the zidovudine AUC. Urinary recovery of zidovudine and GZDV accounts for 18% and 60%, respectively, following IV dosing. A second metabolite, 3'-amino-3'-deoxythymidine (AMT), has been identified in the plasma following single-dose IV administration of zidovudine. The AMT AUC was one fifth of the zidovudine AUC.

Excretion – The elimination half-life of zidovudine was 1.1 hours (0.5 to 2.9 hours) and systemic clearance of zidovudine was 1.6 L/hr/kg (0.8 to 2.7 L/hr/kg).

Renal clearance rate of zidovudine following IV administration in HIV-infected patients was 0.34 ± 0.05 L/hr/kg. Urinary recovery of zidovudine and GZDV accounts for 18% and 60%, respectively, following IV dosing.

Special populations –

Renal function impairment: Zidovudine clearance was decreased resulting in increased zidovudine and GZDV half-life and AUC in patients with impaired renal function (n = 14) following a single 200 mg oral dose (see table below). Plasma concentrations of AMT were not determined. A dose adjustment should not be necessary for patients with creatinine clearance (Ccr) greater than or equal to 15 mL/min.

Zidovudine pharmacokinetic parameters in patients with severe renal impairment*

Parameter	Control subjects (healthy renal function) (n = 6)	Patients with renal impairment (n = 14)
Ccr (mL/min)	120 ± 8	18 ± 2
Zidovudine AUC (ng•hr/mL)	1,400 ± 200	3,100 ± 300
Zidovudine half-life (hr)	1 ± 0.2	1.4 ± 0.1

* Data are expressed as mean ± standard deviation.

Hepatic function impairment: Data describing the effect of hepatic impairment on the pharmacokinetics of zidovudine are limited. However, because zidovudine is eliminated primarily by hepatic metabolism, it is expected that zidovudine clearance would be decreased and plasma concentrations would be increased following administration of the recommended adult doses to patients with hepatic impairment.

Children:

• *Patients younger than 3 months of age* – Zidovudine pharmacokinetics have been evaluated in pediatric patients from birth to 3 months of life. Zidovudine elimination was determined immediately following birth in 8 neonates who were exposed to zidovudine in utero. The half-life was 13.0 ± 5.8 hours. In neonates less than or equal to 14 days old, bioavailability was greater, total body clearance was slower, and half-life was longer than in pediatric patients greater than 14 days old.

Zidovudine pharmacokinetic parameters in pediatric patients*

Parameter	Birth to 14 days of age	14 days to 3 months of age	3 months to 12 years of age
Oral bioavailability (%)	89 ± 19 (n = 15)	61 ± 19 (n = 17)	65 ± 24 (n = 18)
CSF:plasma ratio	no data	no data	0.26 ± 0.17** (n = 28)
CL (L/hr/kg)	0.65 ± 0.29 (n = 18)	1.14 ± 0.24 (n = 16)	1.85 ± 0.47 (n = 20)
Elimination half-life (hr)	3.1 ± 1.2 (n = 21)	1.9 ± 0.7 (n = 18)	1.5 ± 0.7 (n = 21)

* Data presented as mean ± standard deviation except where noted.
** CSF ratio determined at steady-state on constant IV infusion.

Pharmacokinetic parameters in adults –

Zidovudine pharmacokinetic parameters following IV administration in HIV-infected patients

Parameter	Mean ± SD (except where noted)
Apparent volume of distribution (L/kg)	1.6 ± 0.6 (n = 11)
Plasma protein binding (%)	< 38
CSF:plasma ratio*	0.6 [0.04 to 2.62] (n = 39)
Systemic clearance (L/hr/kg)	1.6 (0.8 to 2.7) (n = 18)
Renal clearance (L/hr/kg)	0.34 ± 0.05 (n = 16)
Elimination half-life (hr)**	1.1 (0.5 to 2.9) (n = 19)

* Median [range].
** Approximate range.

➤*Microbiology:*

In vitro HIV susceptibility – The in vitro anti-HIV activity of zidovudine was assessed by infecting cell lines of lymphoblastic and monocytic origin and peripheral blood lymphocytes with laboratory and clinical isolates of HIV. The IC_{50} and IC_{90} values (50% and 90% inhibitory concentrations) were 0.003 to 0.013 and 0.03 to 0.13 mcg/mL, respectively (1 nM = 0.27 ng/mL). The IC_{50} and IC_{90} values of HIV isolates recovered from 18 untreated AIDS/ARC patients were in the range of 0.003 to 0.013 mcg/mL and 0.03 to 0.3 mcg/mL, respectively. Zidovudine showed antiviral activity in all acutely infected cell lines; however, activity was substantially less in chronically infected cell lines. In drug combination studies with zalcitabine, didanosine, lamivudine, saquinavir, indinavir, ritonavir, nevirapine, delavirdine, or interferon-alpha, zidovudine showed additive to synergistic activity in cell culture. The relationship between the in vitro susceptibility of HIV to reverse transcriptase inhibitors and the inhibition of HIV replication in humans has not been established.

Drug resistance – HIV isolates with reduced sensitivity to zidovudine have been selected in vitro and were also recovered from patients treated with zidovudine. Genetic analysis of the isolates showed mutations that result in 5 amino acid substitutions (Met41→Leu, A67→Asn, Lys70→Arg, Thr215→Tyr or Phe, and Lys219→Gln) in the viral reverse transcriptase. In general, higher levels of resistance were associated with greater number of mutations, with 215 mutation being the most significant.

Cross-resistance – The potential for cross-resistance between HIV reverse transcriptase inhibitors and protease inhibitors is low because of the different enzyme targets involved. Combination therapy with zidovudine plus zalcitabine or didanosine does not appear to prevent the emergence of zidovudine-resistant isolates. Combination therapy with zidovudine plus lamivudine delayed the emergence of mutations conferring resistance to zidovudine. In some patients harboring zidovudine-resistant virus, combination therapy with zidovudine plus lamivudine restored phenotypic sensitivity to zidovudine by 12 weeks of treatment. HIV isolates with multidrug resistance to zidovudine, didanosine, zalcitabine, stavudine, and lamivudine were recovered from a small number of patients treated for greater than or equal to 1 year with the combination of zidovudine and didanosine or zalcitabine. The pattern of resistant mutations in the combination therapy was different (Ala62→Val, Val75→Ile, Phe77→116Tyr, and Gln→151Met) from monotherapy, with mutation 151 being most significant for multidrug resistance. Site-directed mutagenesis studies showed that these mutations could also result in resistance to zalcitabine, lamivudine, and stavudine.

Contraindications

In patients who have potentially life-threatening allergic reactions to any of the components of the formulation.

Warnings

➤*Combination products:* Lamivudine/zidovudine tablets and abacavir sulfate/lamivudine/zidovudine tablets are combination product tablets that contain zidovudine as one of their components. Zidovudine should not be administered concomitantly with lamivudine/zidovudine tablets or abacavir sulfate/lamivudine/zidovudine tablets.

➤*Bone marrow suppression:* Zidovudine should be used with caution in patients who have bone marrow compromise evidenced by granulocyte count less than 1000 cells/mm^3 or hemoglobin less than 9.5 g/dL. In patients with advanced symptomatic HIV disease, anemia and neutropenia were the most significant adverse reactions observed. There have been reports of pancytopenia associated with the use of zidovudine, which was reversible in most instances, after discontinuance of the drug. However, significant anemia, in many cases requiring dose adjustment, discontinuation of zidovudine, or blood transfusions, has occurred during treatment with zidovudine alone or in combination with other antiretrovirals.

See Precautions for more information.

➤*Myopathy:* Myopathy and myositis with pathological changes, similar to that produced by HIV disease, have been associated with prolonged use of zidovudine.

➤*Lactic acidosis/severe hepatomegaly with steatosis:* Lactic acidosis and severe hepatomegaly with steatosis, including fatal cases, have been reported with the use of nucleoside analogues alone or in combination, including zidovudine and other antiretrovirals. A majority of these cases have been in women. Obesity and prolonged exposure to antiretroviral nucleoside analogues may be risk factors. Particular caution should be exercised when administering zidovudine to any patient with known risk factors for liver disease; however, cases have also been reported in patients with no known risk factors. Treatment with zidovudine should be suspended in any patient who develops clinical or laboratory findings suggestive of lactic acidosis or pronounced hepatotoxicity (which may include hepatomegaly and steatosis even in the absence of marked transaminase elevations).

➤*Renal/Hepatic function impairment:* Zidovudine is eliminated from the body primarily by renal excretion following metabolism in the liver (glucuronidation).

ZIDOVUDINE — INJECTION

See Administration and Dosage for more information.

➤*Carcinogenesis:* In mice, 7 late-appearing (after 19 months) vaginal neoplasms (5 nonmetastasizing squamous cell carcinomas, 1 squamous cell papilloma, and 1 squamous polyp) occurred in animals given the highest dose. One late-appearing squamous cell papilloma occurred in the vagina of a middle-dose animal. No vaginal tumors were found at the lowest dose.

In rats, 2 late-appearing (after 20 months), nonmetastasizing vaginal squamous cell carcinomas occurred in animals given the highest dose. No vaginal tumors occurred at the low or middle dose in rats. No other drug-related tumors were observed in either sex of either species.

Two transplacental carcinogenicity studies were conducted in mice. One study administered zidovudine at doses of 20 mg/kg/day or 40 mg/kg/day from gestation day 10 through parturition and lactation with dosing continuing in offspring for 24 months postnatally. The doses of zidovudine employed in this study produced zidovudine exposures approximately 3 times the estimated human exposure at recommended doses. After 24 months, an increase in incidence of vaginal tumors was noted with no increase in tumors in the liver or lung or any other organ in either gender. These findings are consistent with results of the standard oral carcinogenicity study in mice, as described earlier. A second study administered zidovudine at maximum tolerated doses of 12.5 mg/day or 25 mg/day (approximately 1,000 mg/kg nonpregnant body weight or approximately 450 mg/kg of term body weight) to pregnant mice from days 12 through 18 of gestation. There was an increase in the number of tumors in the lung, liver, and female reproductive tracts in the offspring of mice receiving the higher dose level of zidovudine. It is not known how predictive the results of rodent carcinogenicity studies may be for humans.

➤*Mutagenesis:* Zidovudine was mutagenic in a 5178Y/TK$^{+/-}$ mouse lymphoma assay, positive in an in vitro cell transformation assay, clastogenic in a cytogenetic assay using cultured human lymphocytes, and positive in mouse and rat micronucleus tests after repeated doses. It was negative in a cytogenetic study in rats given a single dose.

➤*Elderly:* In general, dose selection for an elderly patient should be cautious, reflecting the greater frequency of decreased hepatic, renal, or cardiac function, and of concomitant disease or other drug therapy.

➤*Pregnancy: Category C.* Oral teratology studies in the rat and in the rabbit at doses up to 500 mg/kg/day revealed no evidence of teratogenicity with zidovudine. Zidovudine treatment resulted in embryo/fetal toxicity as evidenced by an increase in the incidence of fetal resorptions in rats given 150 or 450 mg/kg/day and rabbits given 500 mg/kg/day. The doses used in the teratology studies resulted in peak zidovudine plasma concentrations (after one half of the daily dose) in rats 66 to 226 times, and in rabbits 12 to 87 times, mean steady-state peak human plasma concentrations (after one sixth of the daily dose) achieved with the recommended daily dose (100 mg every 4 hours). In an in vitro experiment with fertilized mouse oocytes, zidovudine exposure resulted in a dose-dependent reduction in blastocyst formation. In an additional teratology study in rats, a dose of 3000 mg/kg/day (very near the oral median lethal dose in rats of 3683 mg/kg) caused marked maternal toxicity and an increase in the incidence of fetal malformations. This dose resulted in peak zidovudine plasma concentrations 350 times peak human plasma concentrations. (Estimated area-under-the-curve [AUC] in rats at this dose level was 300 times the daily AUC in humans given 600 mg per day.) No evidence of teratogenicity was seen in this experiment at doses of 600 mg/kg/day or less.

A randomized, double-blind, placebo-controlled trial was conducted in HIV-infected pregnant women to determine the utility of zidovudine for the prevention of maternal-fetal HIV transmission. Congenital abnormalities occurred with similar frequency between neonates born to mothers who received zidovudine and neonates born to mothers who received placebo. Abnormalities were either problems in embryogenesis (prior to 14 weeks) or were recognized on ultrasound before or immediately after initiation of study drug.

Antiretroviral pregnancy registry – To monitor maternal-fetal outcomes of pregnant women exposed to zidovudine, an antiretroviral pregnancy registry has been established. Physicians are encouraged to register patients by calling 1-800-258-4263.

➤*Lactation:* The Centers for Disease Control and Prevention recommend that HIV-infected mothers not breastfeed their infants to avoid risking postnatal transmission of HIV.

Zidovudine is excreted in human milk. Because of both the potential for HIV transmission and the potential for serious adverse reactions in nursing infants, mothers should be instructed not to breastfeed if they are receiving zidovudine.

➤*Children:* Zidovudine has been studied in HIV-infected pediatric patients over 3 months of age who had HIV-related symptoms or who were asymptomatic with abnormal laboratory values indicating significant HIV-related immunosuppression. Zidovudine has also been studied in neonates perinatally exposed to HIV.

Precautions

➤*Monitoring:* Frequent blood counts are strongly recommended in patients with advanced HIV disease who are treated with zidovudine. For HIV-infected individuals and patients with asymptomatic or early HIV disease, periodic blood counts are recommended. Significant anemia (hemoglobin of less than 7.5 g/dL or reduction of greater than 25% of baseline) or significant neutropenia (granulocyte count of less than 750 cells/mm^3 or reduction of greater than 50% from baseline) may require a dose interruption until evidence of marrow recovery is observed.

The incidence of adverse reactions appears to increase with disease progression; patients should be monitored carefully, especially as disease progression occurs.

Drug Interactions

Zidovudine Drug Interactions

Precipitant drug	Object drug*		Description
Acetaminophen	Zidovudine	⬇	Acetaminophen may decrease the AUC of zidovudine.
Atovaquone	Zidovudine	⬆	Atovaquone appears to inhibit glucuronidation of zidovudine, thus increasing zidovudine concentrations and decreasing clearance.
Bone marrow suppressive/ cytotoxic agents (eg, interferon-alpha, interferon-beta-1b)	Zidovudine	⬆	Coadministration may increase the hematologic toxicity of zidovudine.
Clarithromycin	Zidovudine	⟷	Peak serum zidovudine concentrations may be increased or decreased.
Doxorubicin	Zidovudine	⬇	Avoid coadministration. An antagonistic relationship has been demonstrated.
Fluconazole	Zidovudine	⬆	Concurrent use may increase the zidovudine AUC.
Ganciclovir	Zidovudine	⬆	Concomitant use may increase zidovudine plasma levels and AUC, thus increasing risk of life-threatening hematologic toxicities.
Methadone	Zidovudine	⬆	Zidovudine serum concentrations and AUC may be elevated, increasing the risk of side effects.
Nelfinavir/ Ritonavir	Zidovudine	⬇	Zidovudine AUC is decreased.
Probenecid	Zidovudine	⬆	Probenecid may increase zidovudine AUC by inhibiting glucuronidation or reducing renal excretion. Some patients have developed symptoms consisting of myalgia, malaise or fever, and maculopapular rash.
Rifamycins	Zidovudine	⬇	The AUC of zidovudine may be decreased.
Stavudine, ribavirin	Zidovudine	⬇	Avoid concomitant use because some nucleoside analogs affect viral replication and may antagonize antiviral activity of zidovudine against HIV.
Trimethoprim	Zidovudine	⬆	Serum levels of zidovudine and its metabolite may be increased, especially in patients with impaired hepatic glucuronidation from liver disease or drug inhibition.
Valproic acid	Zidovudine	⬆	Concurrent use may inhibit glucuronide metabolism, thus increasing zidovudine AUC.
Zidovudine	Phenytoin	⟷	Phenytoin levels have been reported to increase, decrease or not change with concurrent use. In addition, zidovudine clearance was decreased by phenytoin.
Phenytoin	Zidovudine	⬆	

* ⬆ = Object drug increased. ⬇ = Object drug decreased.
⟷ = Undetermined clinical effect.

Adverse Reactions

The adverse reactions reported during intravenous administration of zidovudine IV infusion are similar to those reported with oral administration; neutropenia and anemia were reported most frequently. Long-term intravenous administration beyond 2 to 4 weeks has not been studied in adults and may enhance hematologic adverse reactions. Local reaction, pain, and slight irritation during intravenous administration occur infrequently.

➤*Adults:* The frequency and severity of adverse reactions associated with the use of zidovudine are greater in patients with more advanced infection at the time of initiation of therapy.

ZIDOVUDINE — INJECTION

Percentage (%) of patients with adverse reactions[1] in asymptomatic HIV infection (ACTG 019)		
Adverse reaction	Zidovudine 500 mg/day (n = 453)	Placebo (n = 428)
Miscellaneous		
Asthenia	8.6%	5.8%
Headache	62.5%	52.6%
Malaise	53.2%	44.9%
GI		
Constipation	6.4%[2]	3.5%
Nausea	51.4%	29.9%
Vomiting	17.2%	9.8%
Psychiatric		
Anorexia	20.1%	10.5%

[1] Reported in greater than or equal to 5% of study population.
[2] Not statistically significant versus placebo.

In addition to the adverse reactions listed in the table above, other adverse reactions observed in clinical studies were abdominal cramps, abdominal pain, arthralgia, chills, dyspepsia, fatigue, hyperbilirubinemia, insomnia, musculoskeletal pain, myalgia, and neuropathy.

Lab test abnormalities –

Frequencies of selected (grade 3/4) laboratory abnormalities in patients with asymptomatic HIV infection (ACTG 019)		
Adverse reaction	Zidovudine 500 mg/day (n = 453)	Placebo (n = 428)
Anemia (Hgb < 8 g/dL)	1.1%	0.2%
Granulocytopenia (< 750 cells/mm^3)	1.8%	1.6%
Thrombocytopenia (platelets < 50,000/mm^3)	0%	0.5%
ALT (> 5 x ULN)[1]	3.1%	2.6%
AST (> 5 x ULN)[1]	0.9%	1.6%
Alkaline phosphate (> 5 x ULN)[1]	0%	0%

[1] ULN = Upper limit of normal.

➤*Children:* Selected clinical adverse reactions and physical findings with a greater than or equal to 5% frequency during therapy with lamivudine/zidovudine tablets 4 mg/kg twice daily plus zidovudine 160 mg/m^2 orally 3 times daily compared with didanosine in therapy-naive (less than or equal to 56 days of antiretroviral therapy) pediatric patients are listed in the table below.

Selected clinical adverse reactions and physical findings (greater than or equal to 5% frequency) in pediatric patients in study ACTG300		
Adverse reaction	Lamivudine plus zidovudine (n = 236)	Didanosine (n = 235)
Miscellaneous		
Fever	25%	32%
Lymphadenopathy	9%	11%
GI		
Hepatomegaly	11%	11%
Nausea and vomiting	8%	7%
Diarrhea	8%	6%
Stomatitis	6%	12%
Splenomegaly	5%	8%
Respiratory		
Cough	15%	18%
Abnormal breathing sounds/wheezing	7%	9%
Nasal discharge or congestion	8%	11%
Special senses		
Signs or symptoms of ears*	7%	6%
Dermatologic		
Skin rashes	12%	14%

* Includes pain, discharge, erythema, or swelling of an ear.

Lab test abnormalities –

Frequencies of selected (grade 3/4) laboratory abnormalities in pediatric patients in study ACTG300		
Test (abnormal level)	Lamivudine plus zidovudine	Didanosine
Neutropenia (ANC < 400 cells/mm^3)[1]	8%	3%
Anemia (Hgb < 7.0 g/dL)	4%	2%
Thrombocytopenia (platelets < 50,000/mm^3)	1%	3%
ALT (> 10 x ULN)[2]	1%	3%
AST (> 10 x ULN)[2]	2%	4%
Lipase (> 2.5 x ULN)[2]	3%	3%
Total amylase (> 2.5 x ULN)[2]	3%	3%

[1] ANC = Absolute neutrophil count
[2] ULN = Upper limit of normal

Additional adverse reactions reported in open-label studies in pediatric patients receiving zidovudine 180 mg/m^2 every 6 hours were congestive heart failure, decreased reflexes, ECG abnormality, edema, hematuria, left ventricular dilation, macrocytosis, nervousness/irritability, and weight loss.

The clinical adverse reactions reported among adult recipients of zidovudine may also occur in pediatric patients.

➤*Use for the prevention of maternal-fetal transmission of HIV:* In a randomized, double-blind, placebo-controlled trial in HIV-infected women and their neonates conducted to determine the utility of zidovudine for the prevention of maternal-fetal HIV transmission, zidovudine syrup at 2 mg/kg was administered every 6 hours for 6 weeks to neonates beginning within 12 hours following birth. The most commonly reported adverse reactions were anemia (hemoglobin less than 9 g/dL) and neutropenia (less than 1000 cells/mm^3). Anemia occurred in 22% of the neonates who received zidovudine and in 12% of the neonates who received placebo. The mean difference in hemoglobin values was less than 1 g/dL for neonates receiving zidovudine compared to neonates receiving placebo. No neonates with anemia required transfusion and all hemoglobin values spontaneously returned to normal within 6 weeks after completion of therapy with zidovudine. Neutropenia was reported with similar frequency in the group that received zidovudine (21%) and in the group that received placebo (27%). The long-term consequences of in utero and infant exposure to zidovudine are unknown.

➤*Postmarketing:*

Cardiovascular – Cardiomyopathy, syncope.

CNS – Anxiety, confusion, depression, dizziness, loss of mental acuity, mania, paresthesia, seizures, somnolence, vertigo.

Dermatologic – Changes in skin and nail pigmentation, pruritus, rash, Stevens-Johnson syndrome, toxic epidermal necrolysis, sweat, urticaria.

Endocrine – Gynecomastia.

GI – Constipation, dysphagia, flatulence, oral mucosal pigmentation, mouth ulcer.

GU – Urinary frequency, urinary hesitancy.

Hematologic/Lymphatic – Aplastic anemia, hemolytic anemia, leukopenia, lymphadenopathy, pancytopenia with marrow hypoplasia, pure red cell aplasia.

Hepatic – Hepatitis, hepatomegaly with steatosis, jaundice, lactic acidosis, pancreatitis.

Hypersensitivity – Sensitization reactions including anaphylaxis and angioedema.

Musculoskeletal – Increased CPK, increased LDH, muscle spasm, myopathy and myositis with pathological changes (similar to that produced by HIV disease), rhabdomyolysis, tremor.

Respiratory – Cough, dyspnea, rhinitis, sinusitis.

Special senses – Macular edema, amblyopia, hearing loss, photophobia, taste perversion.

Miscellaneous – Back pain, chest pain, flu-like syndrome, generalized pain, vasculitis.

Overdosage

Acute overdoses of zidovudine have been reported in pediatric patients and adults. These involved exposures up to 50 g.

➤*Symptoms:* No specific symptoms or signs have been identified following acute overdosage with zidovudine apart from those listed as adverse reactions such as fatigue, headache, vomiting, and occasional reports of hematological disturbances. All patients recovered without permanent sequelae.

➤*Treatment:* Hemodialysis and peritoneal dialysis appear to have a negligible effect on the removal of zidovudine, while elimination of its primary metabolite, GZDV, is enhanced.

Patient Information

Zidovudine is not a cure for HIV infection, and patients may continue to acquire illnesses associated with HIV infection, including opportunistic infections. Therefore, patients should be advised to seek medical care for any significant change in their health status.

ZIDOVUDINE — INJECTION

The safety and efficacy of zidovudine in treating women, intravenous drug users, and racial minorities is not significantly different than that observed in white males.

Patients should be informed that the major toxicities of zidovudine are neutropenia and anemia. The frequency and severity of these toxicities are greater in patients with more advanced disease and in those who initiate therapy later in the course of their infection. They should be told that if toxicity develops, they may require transfusions or drug discontinuation. They should be told of the extreme importance of having their blood counts followed closely while on therapy, especially for patients with advanced symptomatic HIV disease. They should be cautioned about the use of other medications, including ganciclovir and interferon-alpha, which may exacerbate the toxicity of zidovudine. Patients should be informed that other adverse effects of zidovudine include nausea and vomiting. Patients should also be encouraged to contact their physicians if they experience muscle weakness, shortness of breath, symptoms of hepatitis or pancreatitis, or any other unexpected adverse reactions while being treated with zidovudine.

Pregnant women considering the use of zidovudine during pregnancy for prevention of HIV transmission to their infants should be advised that transmission may still occur in some cases despite therapy. The long-term consequences of in utero and neonatal exposure to zidovudine are unknown, including the possible risk of cancer.

HIV-infected pregnant women should be advised not to breastfeed to avoid postnatal transmission of HIV to a child who may not yet be infected.

Patients should be advised that therapy with zidovudine has not been shown to reduce the risk of transmission of HIV to others through sexual contact or blood contamination.

ABACAVIR SULFATE

Rx	**Ziagen** (GlaxoSmithKline)	**Tablets:** 300 mg	(GX 623). Yellow, capsule shape. Film-coated. In 60s and UD blister packs of 60s.
		Oral solution: 20 mg/mL	Parabens, saccharin, sorbitol. Strawberry-banana flavor. In 240 mL.

ABACAVIR SULFATE — ORAL

WARNING

Hypersensitivity reactions – Serious and sometimes fatal hypersensitivity reactions have been associated with abacavir therapy. Hypersensitivity to abacavir is a multi-organ clinical syndrome usually characterized by a sign or symptom in 2 or more of the following groups:

- constitutional, including achiness, fatigue, or generalized malaise;
- fever;
- GI, including abdominal pain, diarrhea, nausea, or vomiting;
- rash;
- respiratory, including cough, dyspnea, or pharyngitis.

Discontinue abacavir as soon as a hypersensitivity reaction is suspected. Permanently discontinue abacavir if hypersensitivity cannot be ruled out, even when other diagnoses are possible.

Following a hypersensitivity reaction to abacavir, never restart abacavir or any abacavir-containing product because more severe symptoms can occur within hours and may include life-threatening hypotension and death.

Reintroduction of abacavir or any other abacavir-containing product, even in patients who have no identified history or unrecognized symptoms of hypersensitivity to abacavir therapy, can result in serious or fatal hypersensitivity reactions. Such reactions can occur within hours.

Lactic acidosis and severe hepatomegaly – Lactic acidosis and severe hepatomegaly with steatosis, including fatal cases, have been reported with the use of nucleoside analogs alone or in combination, including abacavir and other antiretrovirals.

Indications

➤*HIV infection:* In combination with other antiretroviral agents, for the treatment of HIV-1 infection.

Administration and Dosage

➤*Approved by the FDA:* December 17, 1998.

Abacavir should always be used in combination with other antiretroviral agents. Abacavir should not be added as a single agent when antiretroviral regimens are changed because of loss of virologic response.

A *Medication Guide* and warning card that provide information about recognition of hypersensitivity reactions should be dispensed with each new prescription and refill. To facilitate reporting of hypersensitivity reactions and collection of information on each case, an abacavir hypersensitivity registry has been established. Physicians should register patients by calling 1-800-270-0425.

➤*Adults:* 600 mg daily, administered as 300 mg twice daily or 600 mg once daily, in combination with other antiretroviral agents.

➤*Children (3 months to 16 years of age):* 8 mg/kg twice daily (up to a maximum of 300 mg twice daily) in combination with other antiretroviral agents.

➤*Hepatic function impairment:* The recommended dose of abacavir in patients with mild hepatic function impairment (Child-Pugh score 5 to 6) is 200 mg twice daily. To enable dose reduction, abacavir oral solution (10 mL twice daily) should be used for the treatment of these patients. The safety, efficacy, and pharmacokinetic properties of abacavir have not been established in patients with moderate to severe hepatic function impairment, therefore abacavir is contraindicated in these patients.

➤*Storage / Stability:*

Tablets – Store at controlled room temperature of 20° to 25°C (68° to 77°F).

Oral solution – Store at controlled room temperature of 20° to 25°C (68° to 77°F). Do not freeze. May be refrigerated.

Actions

➤*Pharmacology:* Abacavir is a carbocyclic synthetic nucleoside analog. Abacavir is converted intracellularly by cellular enzymes to the active metabolite carbovir triphosphate, an analog of deoxyguanosine-5'-triphosphate (dGTP). Carbovir triphosphate inhibits the activity of HIV-1 reverse transcriptase (RT) by competing with the natural substrate dGTP and by its incorporation into viral DNA. The lack of a 3'-OH group in the incorporated nucleoside analog prevents the formation of the 5' to 3' phosphodiester linkage essential for DNA chain elongation, and therefore, the viral DNA growth is terminated. Abacavir is a weak inhibitor of cellular DNA polymerases α, β, and γ.

➤*Pharmacokinetics:*

Absorption – The pharmacokinetic properties of abacavir have been studied in asymptomatic, HIV-infected adult patients after administration of a single IV dose of 150 mg and after single and multiple oral doses. The pharmacokinetic properties of abacavir were independent of dose over the range of 300 to 1,200 mg/day.

Abacavir was rapidly and extensively absorbed after oral administration. The geometric mean absolute bioavailability of the tablet was 83%. After oral administration of 300 mg twice daily in 20 patients, the steady-state peak serum abacavir concentration (C_{max}) was 3 ± 0.89 mcg/mL (mean ± SD) and $AUC_{(0\ to\ 12\ h)}$ was 6.02 ± 1.73 mcg•h/mL. After oral administration of a single dose of abacavir 600 mg in 20 patients, C_{max} was 4.26 ± 1.19 mcg/mL (mean ± SD) and AUC_{∞} was 11.95 ± 2.51 mcg•h/mL. Bioavailability of abacavir tablets was assessed in the fasting and fed states. There was no significant difference in systemic exposure (AUC_{∞}) in the fed and fasting states; therefore, abacavir tablets may be administered with or without food. Systemic exposure to abacavir was comparable after administration of abacavir oral solution and abacavir tablets. Therefore, these products may be used interchangeably.

Distribution – The apparent volume of distribution after IV administration of abacavir was 0.86 ± 0.15 L/kg, suggesting that abacavir distributes into extravascular space. In 3 subjects, the CSF $AUC_{(0\ to\ 6\ h)}$ to plasma abacavir $AUC_{(0\ to\ 6\ h)}$ ratio ranged from 27% to 33%.

Binding of abacavir to human plasma proteins is approximately 50%. Binding of abacavir to plasma proteins was independent of concentration. Total blood and plasma drug-related radioactivity concentrations are identical, demonstrating that abacavir readily distributes into erythrocytes.

Metabolism – In humans, abacavir is not significantly metabolized by cytochrome P-450 enzymes. The primary routes of elimination of abacavir are metabolism by alcohol dehydrogenase (to form the 5'-carboxylic acid) and glucuronyl transferase (to form the 5'-glucuronide). The metabolites do not have antiviral activity. In vitro experiments reveal that abacavir does not inhibit human CYP3A4, CYP2D6, or CYP2C9 activity at clinically relevant concentrations.

Excretion – Elimination of abacavir was quantified in a mass-balance study following administration of ^{14}C-abacavir 600 mg was as follows: 99% of the radioactivity was recovered, 1.2% was excreted in the urine as abacavir, 30% as the 5'-carboxylic acid metabolite, 36% as the 5'-glucuronide metabolite, and 15% as unidentified minor metabolites in the urine. Fecal elimination accounted for 16% of the dose.

In single-dose studies, the observed elimination half-life ($t_{1/2}$) was 1.54 ± 0.63 hours. After IV administration, total clearance was 0.8 ± 0.24 L/h/kg (mean ± SD).

Special populations –

Hepatic function impairment: The pharmacokinetics of abacavir have been studied in patients with mild hepatic function impairment (Child-Pugh score 5 to 6). Results show that there was a mean increase of 89% in the abacavir AUC, and an increase of 58% in the $t_{1/2}$ of abacavir after a single dose of abacavir 600 mg. The AUCs of the metabolites were not modified by mild liver disease; however, the rates of formation and elimination of the metabolites were decreased. A dose of 200 mg (provided by 10 mL of abacavir oral solution) administered twice daily is recommended for patients with mild liver disease. The safety, efficacy, and pharmacokinetics of abacavir have not been studied in patients with moderate or severe hepatic function impairment, therefore abacavir is contraindicated in these patients.

Children: The pharmacokinetics of abacavir have been studied after either single or repeat doses of abacavir in 68 children. Following multiple-dose administration of abacavir 8 mg/kg twice daily, steady-state $AUC_{(0\ to\ 12\ h)}$ and C_{max} were 9.8 ± 4.56 mcg•h/mL and 3.71 ± 1.36 mcg/mL (mean ± SD), respectively. The safety and efficacy of abacavir have been established in pediatric patients 3 months to 13 years of age.

ABACAVIR SULFATE — ORAL

➤*Microbiology:*

Antiviral activity in vitro – The in vitro, anti-HIV-1 activity of abacavir was evaluated against a T-cell tropic laboratory strain HIV-1_{IIIB} in lymphoblastic cell lines, a monocyte/macrophage tropic laboratory strain HIV-1_{BaL} in primary monocytes/macrophages, and clinical isolates in peripheral blood mononuclear cells. The concentration of drug necessary to inhibit viral replication by 50% (IC_{50}) ranged from 3.7 to 5.8 mcM (1 mcM = 0.28 mcg/mL) and 0.07 to 1 mcM against HIV-1_{IIIB} and HIV-1_{BaL}, respectively, and was 0.26 ± 0.18 mcM against 8 clinical isolates. The IC_{50} values of abacavir against different HIV-1 clades (A-E) ranged from 0.0015 to 1 mcM, and against HIV-2 isolates, from 0.024 to 0.49 mcM. Abacavir had synergistic activity in vitro in combination with amprenavir, nevirapine, and zidovudine, and additive activity in combination with didanosine, lamivudine, stavudine, tenofovir, and zalcitabine. Ribavirin had no effect on the in vitro anti-HIV-1 activity of abacavir.

Contraindications

Hypersensitivity to abacavir or any other component of the products; moderate or severe hepatic function impairment (Child-Pugh score higher than 6). See the Warning box for more information.

Warnings

➤*Lactic acidosis/severe hepatomegaly with steatosis:* Lactic acidosis and severe hepatomegaly with steatosis, including fatal cases, have been reported with the use of nucleoside analogs alone or in combination, including abacavir and other antiretrovirals. A majority of these cases have been in women. Obesity and prolonged nucleoside exposure may be risk factors. Exercise particular caution when administering abacavir to any patient with known risk factors for liver disease; however, cases also have been reported in patients with no known risk factors. Suspend treatment with abacavir in any patient who develops clinical or laboratory findings suggestive of lactic acidosis or pronounced hepatotoxicity (which may include hepatomegaly and steatosis even in the absence of marked transaminase elevations).

➤*Hypersensitivity reactions:* Serious and sometimes fatal hypersensitivity reactions have been associated with abacavir and other abacavir-containing products. To minimize the risk of a life-threatening hypersensitivity reaction, permanently discontinue abacavir sulfate if hypersensitivity cannot be ruled out, even when other diagnoses are possible.

See the Warning box for more information.

Hypersensitivity to abacavir following the presentation of a single sign or symptom has been reported infrequently. Hypersensitivity to abacavir was reported in approximately 8% of 2,670 patients (n = 206) in 9 clinical trials (range, 2% to 9%) with enrollment from November 1999 to February 2002. Data on time to onset and symptoms of suspected hypersensitivity were collected on a detailed data collection module. Symptoms usually appeared within the first 6 weeks of treatment with abacavir, although the reaction may occur at any time during therapy. Median time to onset was 9 days; 89% appeared within the first 6 weeks; 95% of patients reported symptoms from 2 or more of the 5 groups listed previously.

Other less common signs and symptoms of hypersensitivity include abnormal chest x-ray findings (predominantly infiltrates, which can be localized), edema, lethargy, myolysis, and paresthesia. Adult respiratory distress syndrome, anaphylaxis, death, hypotension, liver failure, renal failure, and respiratory failure have occurred in association with hypersensitivity reactions. In one study, 4 patients (11%) receiving abacavir 600 mg once daily experienced hypotension with a hypersensitivity reaction compared with 0 patients receiving abacavir 300 mg twice daily.

Physical findings associated with hypersensitivity to abacavir in some patients include lymphadenopathy, mucous membrane lesions (conjunctivitis and mouth ulcerations), and rash. The rash usually appears maculopapular or urticarial, but may be variable in appearance. There have been reports of erythema multiforme. Hypersensitivity reactions have occurred without rash.

Laboratory abnormalities associated with hypersensitivity to abacavir in some patients include elevated liver function tests, elevated creatinine phosphokinase, elevated creatinine, and lymphopenia.

Clinical management of hypersensitivity – Discontinue abacavir as soon as a hypersensitivity reaction is suspected. To minimize the risk of a life-threatening hypersensitivity reaction, permanently discontinue abacavir if hypersensitivity cannot be ruled out, even when other diagnoses are possible (eg, acute onset respiratory diseases such as bronchitis, influenza, pharyngitis, or pneumonia; gastroenteritis; reactions to other medications). Following a hypersensitivity reaction to abacavir, do not restart abacavir or any other abacavir-containing product because more severe symptoms can occur within hours and may include life-threatening hypotension and death.

When therapy with abacavir has been discontinued for reasons other than symptoms of a hypersensitivity reaction and if reinitiation of abacavir or any other abacavir-containing product is under consideration, carefully evaluate the reason for discontinuation of abacavir to ensure that the patient did not have symptoms of a hypersensitivity reaction. If hypersensitivity cannot be ruled out, do not reintroduce abacavir or any other abacavir-containing product. If symptoms consistent with hypersensitivity are not identified, reintroduction can be undertaken with continued monitoring for symptoms of a hypersensitivity reaction. Inform patients that a hypersensitivity reaction may occur with reintroduction of abacavir or any other abacavir-containing product and that reintroduction of abacavir or any other abacavir-containing product needs to be undertaken only if medical care can be readily accessed by the patient or others.

Hypersensitivity reaction registry – To facilitate reporting of hypersensitivity reactions and collection of information on each case, an abacavir hypersensitivity registry has been established. Physicians should register patients by calling 1-800-270-0425.

➤*Hepatic function impairment:* The safety, efficacy, and pharmacokinetics of abacavir have not been studied in patients with moderate or severe hepatic function impairment, therefore abacavir is contraindicated in these patients.

➤*Carcinogenesis:* Abacavir was administered orally at 3 dosage levels to separate groups of mice and rats in 2-year carcinogenicity studies. Results showed an increase in the incidence of malignant and nonmalignant tumors. Malignant tumors occurred in the preputial gland of males, the clitoral gland of females of both species, and in the liver of female rats. In addition, nonmalignant tumors also occurred in the liver and thyroid gland of female rats. These observations were made at systemic exposures in the range of 6 to 32 times the human exposure at the recommended dose (300 mg twice daily). It is not known how predictive the results of rodent carcinogenicity studies may be for humans.

➤*Mutagenesis:* Abacavir-induced chromosomal aberrations in the presence and absence of metabolic activation in an in vitro cytogenetic study in human lymphocytes. Abacavir was mutagenic in the absence of metabolic activation, although it was not mutagenic in the presence of metabolic activation in an L5178Y mouse lymphoma assay. Abacavir was clastogenic in males and not clastogenic in females in an in vivo mouse bone marrow micronucleus assay. Abacavir was not mutagenic in bacterial mutagenicity assays in the presence and absence of metabolic activation.

➤*Pregnancy: Category C.* Studies in pregnant rats showed that abacavir is transferred to the fetus through the placenta. Fetal malformations (increased incidences of fetal anasarca and skeletal malformations) and developmental toxicity (depressed fetal body weight and reduced crown-rump length) were observed in rats at a dose that produced 35 times the human exposure, based on AUC. Embryonic and fetal toxicities (increased resorptions, decreased fetal body weights) and toxicities to the offspring (increased incidence of stillbirth and lower body weights) occurred at half of the above-mentioned dose in separate fertility studies conducted in rats. In the rabbit, no developmental toxicity and no increases in fetal malformations occurred at doses that produced 8.5 times the human exposure at the recommended dose based on AUC.

There are no adequate and well-controlled studies in pregnant women. Use abacavir during pregnancy only if the potential benefits outweigh the risk.

Antiretroviral pregnancy registry – To monitor maternal-fetal outcomes of pregnant women exposed to abacavir, an antiretroviral pregnancy registry has been established. Physicians are encouraged to register patients by calling 1-800-258-4263.

➤*Lactation:* The Centers for Disease Control and Prevention recommend that HIV-infected mothers not breast-feed their infants to avoid risking postnatal transmission of HIV infection.

Although it is not known if abacavir is excreted in human milk, abacavir is secreted into the milk of lactating rats. Because of both the potential for HIV transmission and the potential for serious adverse reactions in nursing infants, instruct mothers not to breast-feed if they are receiving abacavir.

➤*Children:* The safety and efficacy of abacavir have been established in children 3 months to 13 years of age. Use of abacavir in these age groups is supported by pharmacokinetic studies and evidence from adequate and well-controlled studies of abacavir in adults and children.

Precautions

➤*Cross-resistance:* In clinical trials, patients with prolonged prior NRTI exposure or who had HIV-1 isolates that contained multiple mutations conferring resistance to NRTIs had limited response to abacavir. Consider the potential for cross-resistance between abacavir and other NRTIs when choosing new therapeutic regimens in therapy-experienced patients. Recombinant laboratory strains of HIV-1 (HXB_2) containing multiple reverse transcriptase mutations conferring abacavir resistance exhibited cross-resistance to lamivudine, didanosine, and zalcitabine in vitro.

➤*Fat redistribution:* See Adverse Reactions for more information.

Drug Interactions

➤*Ethanol:* Because of the common metabolic pathways via alcohol dehydrogenase, the pharmacokinetic interaction between abacavir and ethanol was studied in 24 HIV-infected men. Each patient received the following treatments on separate occasions: single dose of abacavir 600 mg, ethanol 0.7 g/kg (equivalent to 5 alcoholic drinks), and abacavir 600 mg plus ethanol 0.7 g/kg. Coadministration of ethanol and abacavir resulted in a 41% increase in abacavir AUC_∞ and a 26% increase in abacavir $t_{½}$. In men, abacavir had no effect on the pharmacokinetic properties of ethanol, so no clinically significant interaction is expected in men. This interaction has not been studied in women.

➤*Methadone:* The addition of methadone has no clinically significant effect on the pharmacokinetic properties of abacavir. In a study of 11 HIV-infected subjects receiving methadone-maintenance therapy (40 and 90 mg daily), with abacavir 600 mg twice daily (twice the current recommended dose), oral methadone clearance increased 22% (90% CI: 6% to 42%). This alteration will not result in a methadone dose modification in the majority of patients; however, an increased methadone dose may be required in a small number of patients.

ABACAVIR SULFATE — ORAL

Adverse Reactions

➤*Hypersensitivity:* Serious and sometimes fatal hypersensitivity reactions have been associated with abacavir. In one study, once-daily dosing of abacavir was associated with more severe hypersensitivity reactions.

Therapy-naive adults –
Study CNA30024:

Abacavir Adverse Reactions in Therapy-Naive Adults (CNA30024) (≥ 5%)		
Adverse reaction	Abacavir plus lamivudine plus efavirenz (n = 324)	Zidovudine plus lamivudine plus efavirenz (n = 325)
CNS		
Depressive disorders	6%	6%
Dizziness	6%	6%
Dreams/Sleep disorders	10%	10%
Fatigue/Malaise	7%	10%
Headaches/Migraine	7%	11%
Dermatologic		
Rashes	6%	12%
GI		
Abdominal pain/ Gastritis/ GI signs and symptoms	6%	8%
Diarrhea	7%	6%
Nausea	7%	11%
Vomiting	2%	9%
Musculoskeletal		
Musculoskeletal pain	6%	5%
Respiratory		
Bronchitis	4%	5%
Miscellaneous		
Drug hypersensitivity	9%	< 1%[b]

[a] This study used double-blind ascertainment of suspected hypersensitivity reactions. During the blinded portion of the study, suspected hypersensitivity to abacavir was reported by investigators in 9% of 324 patients in the abacavir group and 3% of 325 patients in the zidovudine group.
[b] Ten (3%) cases of suspected drug hypersensitivity were reclassified as not being caused by abacavir following unblinding.

Study CNA3005:

Abacavir Adverse Reactions in Therapy-Naive Adults (CNA3005) (≥ 5%)		
Adverse reaction	Abacavir sulfate plus lamivudine/zidovudine n = 262)	Indinavir plus lamivudine/zidovudine (n = 264)
CNS		
Anxiety	5%	3%
Depressive disorders	6%	4%
Headache	13%	9%
Malaise and fatigue	12%	12%
Dermatologic		
Skin rashes	5%	4%
GI		
Diarrhea	7%	5%
Nausea	19%	17%
Nausea and vomiting	10%	10%
Musculoskeletal		
Musculoskeletal pain	5%	7%
Miscellaneous		
Ear/Nose/Throat infections	5%	4%
Fever and/or chills	6%	3%
Pain (nonsite-specific)	< 1%	5%
Renal sign/Symptoms	< 1%	5%
Viral respiratory infections	5%	5%

Five patients receiving abacavir sulfate in study CNA3005 experienced worsening of pre-existing depression compared with none in the indinavir arm. The background rates of pre-existing depression were similar in the 2 treatment arms.

➤*Therapy-experienced children:*
Children –

Abacavir Adverse Reactions in Therapy-experienced Children (≥ 5%)		
Adverse reaction	Abacavir plus lamivudine plus zidovudine (n = 102)	Lamivudine plus zidovudine (n = 103)
CNS		
Headache	1%	5%
Dermatologic		
Skin rashes	7%	1%
GI		
Nausea and vomiting	9%	2%
Miscellaneous		
Ear/nose/throat infections	5%	1%
Fever and/or chills	9%	7%
Pneumonia	4%	5%

➤*Miscellaneous:* In addition to adverse reactions in the previous tables, other adverse reactions observed in the expanded access program were pancreatitis and increased gamma-glutamyl-transferase (GGT).

➤*Lab test abnormalities:*

Abacavir Laboratory Abnormalities in Therapy-Naive Adults (CNA30024)		
Grade 3/4 laboratory abnormalities	Abacavir plus lamivudine plus efavirenz (n = 324)	Zidovudine plus lamivudine plus efavirenz (n = 325)
Elevated CPK (> 4 × ULN)	8%	8%
Elevated ALT (> 5 × ULN)	6%	6%
Elevated AST (> 5 × ULN)	6%	5%
Hypertriglyceridemia (> 750 mg/dL)	6%	5%
Hyperamylasemia (> 2 × ULN)	4%	5%
Neutropenia (ANC < 750/mm^3)	2%	4%
Anemia (Hgb ≤ 6.9 gm/dL0	< 1%	2%
Thrombocytopenia (P1t < 50,000/mm^3)	1%	< 1%
Leukopenia (WBC ≤ 1,500/mm^3)	< 1%	2%

➤*Postmarketing:*
Dermatologic – Suspected Stevens-Johnson syndrome (SJS) and toxic epidermal necrolysis (TEN) have been reported in patients receiving abacavir primarily in combination with medications known to be associated with SJS and TEN, respectively. Because of the overlap of clinical signs and symptoms between hypersensitivity to abacavir and SJS and TEN, and the possibility of multiple drug sensitivities in some patients, discontinue abacavir and do not restart in such cases.

There also have been reports of erythema multiforme with abacavir use.

Hepatic – Hepatic steatosis and lactic acidosis.

Fat redistibution – Redistribution/accumulation of body fat, including breast enlargement, central obesity, "cushingoid appearance", dorsocervical fat enlargement (buffalo hump), facial wasting, and peripheral wasting have been observed in patients receiving antiretroviral therapy. The mechanism and long-term consequences of these reactions are currently unknown. A causal relationship has not been established.

Overdosage

➤*Treatment:* There is no known antidote for abacavir sulfate. It is not known whether abacavir can be removed by peritoneal dialysis or hemodialysis.

Patient Information

Inform patients that some HIV medicines, including abacavir, may cause a rare but serious condition called lactic acidosis with liver enlargement (hepatomegaly).

Abacavir is not a cure for HIV infection, and patients may continue to experience illnesses associated with HIV infection, including opportunistic infections. Patients should remain under the care of a physician when using abacavir. Advise patients that the use of abacavir has not been shown to reduce the risk of transmission of HIV to others through sexual contact or blood contamination.

Inform patients that redistribution or accumulation of body fat may occur in patients receiving antiretroviral therapy, and the cause and long-term health effects of these conditions are not known at this time.

EMTRICITABINE

Rx	**Emtriva** (Gilead Sciences)	**Capsules:** 200 mg	(200 mg GILEAD). Blue/White. In 30s.
		Oral solution: 10 mg/mL	Xylitol, parabens. Cotton candy flavor. In 170 mL with dosing cup.

EMTRICITABINE — ORAL

WARNING

Lactic acidosis and severe hepatomegaly with steatosis, including fatal cases, have been reported with the use of nucleoside analogs alone or in combination with other antiretrovirals.

Emtricitabine is not indicated for the treatment of chronic hepatitis B virus (HBV) infection, and the safety and efficacy of emtricitabine have not been established in patients coinfected with HBV and HIV. Severe acute exacerbations of hepatitis B have been reported in patients after the discontinuation of emtricitabine. Closely monitor hepatic function with clinical and laboratory follow-up for at least several months in patients who discontinue emtricitabine and are coinfected with HIV and HBV. If appropriate, initiation of anti-HBV therapy may be warranted.

Indications

➤*HIV infection:* In combination with other antiretroviral agents, for the treatment of HIV-1 infection in patients older than 3 months of age.

In antiretroviral treatment–experienced patients, the use of emtricitabine may be considered for patients with HIV strains that are expected to be susceptible to emtricitabine as assessed by genotypic or phenotypic testing.

➤*Unlabeled uses:* HBV treatment.

Administration and Dosage

➤*Approved by the FDA:* July 2, 2003.

May be taken without regard to food.

➤*Adults (18 years of age and older):*

Capsules – 200 mg administered once daily orally.

Oral solution – 240 mg (24 mL) administered once daily orally.

➤*Children (3 months through 17 years of age):*

Capsules – For children weighing more than 33 kg who can swallow an intact capsule, one 200 mg capsule administered once daily orally.

Oral solution – 6 mg/kg up to a maximum of 240 mg (24 mL) administered once daily orally.

➤*Renal function impairment:* Significantly increased drug exposures were seen when emtricitabine was administered to patients with renal impairment. Therefore, the dosing interval of emtricitabine should be adjusted in patients with baseline creatinine clearance (Ccr) less than 50 mL/min using the following guidelines. The safety and efficacy of these dose adjustment guidelines have not been clinically evaluated. Therefore, clinical response to treatment and renal function should be closely monitored in these patients.

Emtricitabine Dosage Adjustment in Adult Patients with Renal Function Impairment

	Ccr			
Formulation	≥ 50 mL/min	30 to 49 mL/min	15 to 29 mL/min	< 15 mL/min or on hemodialysis[a]
Capsule (200 mg)	200 mg every 24 hours	200 mg every 48 hours	200 mg every 72 hours	200 mg every 96 hours
Oral solution (10 mg/mL)	240 mg every 24 hours (24 mL)	120 mg every 24 hours (12 mL)	80 mg every 24 hours (8 mL)	60 mg every 24 hours (6 mL)

[a] Hemodialysis patients: If dosing on day of dialysis, administer after dialysis.

Although there are insufficient data to recommend a specific dose adjustment of emtricitabine in pediatric patients with renal impairment, a reduction in the dose and/or an increase in the dosing interval similar to adjustments for adults should be considered.

➤*Storage / Stability:*

Capsules – Store at 25°C (77°F); excursions are permitted to 15° to 30°C (59° to 86°F).

Oral solution – Refrigerate at 2° to 8°C (36° to 46°F). Use within 3 months if stored at 25°C (77°F); excursions are permitted to 15° to 30°C (59° to 86°F).

Actions

➤*Pharmacology:* Emtricitabine, a synthetic nucleoside analog of cytosine, is phosphorylated by cellular enzymes to form emtricitabine 5'-triphosphate. Emtricitabine 5'-triphosphate inhibits the activity of the HIV-1 reverse transcriptase by competing with the natural substrate deoxycytidine 5'-triphosphate and by being incorporated into nascent viral deoxyribonucleic acid (DNA), which results in chain termination. Emtricitabine 5'-triphosphate is a weak inhibitor of mammalian DNA polymerase α, β, ε, and mitochondrial DNA polymerase γ.

Pharmacodynamics – The in vivo activity of emtricitabine was evaluated in 2 clinical trials in which 101 patients were administered 25 to 400 mg a day of emtricitabine as monotherapy for 10 to 14 days. A dose-related antiviral effect was observed, with a median decrease from baseline in plasma HIV-1 ribonucleic acid (RNA) of 1.3 log_{10} at a dosage of 25 mg once daily and 1.7 log_{10} to 1.9 log_{10} at a dosage of 200 mg once daily or twice daily.

➤*Pharmacokinetics:*

Absorption – Emtricitabine is rapidly and extensively absorbed following oral administration with peak plasma concentrations occurring at 1 to 2 hours postdose. Following multiple dose oral administration of emtricitabine capsules to 20 HIV-infected subjects, the (mean ± standard deviation [SD]) steady-state plasma emtricitabine peak concentration (C_{max}) was 1.8 ± 0.7 mcg/mL and the area under the plasma concentration-time curve (AUC) over a 24-hour dosing interval was 10 ± 3.1 mcg•h/mL. The mean steady-state plasma trough concentration at 24 hours postdose was 0.09 mcg/mL. The mean absolute bioavailability of emtricitabine capsules was 93% while the mean absolute bioavailability of emtricitabine oral solution was 75%. The relative bioavailability of emtricitabine oral solution was approximately 80% of emtricitabine capsules.

The multiple-dose pharmacokinetics of emtricitabine are dose proportional over a dose range of 25 to 200 mg.

Effects of food: Emtricitabine capsules and oral solution may be taken with or without food. Emtricitabine systemic exposure (AUC) was unaffected while C_{max} decreased by 29% when emtricitabine capsules were administered with food (an approximately 1,000 kcal high-fat meal). Emtricitabine systemic exposure (AUC) and C_{max} were unaffected when emtricitabine 200 mg oral solution was administered with either a high- or low-fat meal.

Distribution – In vitro binding of emtricitabine to human plasma proteins was less than 4% and independent of concentration over the range of 0.02 to 200 mcg/mL. At peak plasma concentration, the mean plasma to blood drug concentration ratio was approximately 1 and the mean semen to plasma drug concentration ratio was approximately 4.

Metabolism – In vitro studies indicate that emtricitabine is not an inhibitor of human CYP-450 enzymes. Following administration of ^{14}C-emtricitabine, complete recovery of the dose was achieved in urine (approximately 86%) and feces (approximately 14%). Thirteen percent of the dose was recovered in urine as 3 putative metabolites. The biotransformation of emtricitabine includes oxidation of the thiol moiety to form the 3'-sulfoxide diastereomers (approximately 9% of dose) and conjugation with glucuronic acid to form 2'-O-glucuronide (approximately 4% of dose). No other metabolites were identifiable.

Excretion – The plasma emtricitabine half-life is approximately 10 hours. The renal clearance of emtricitabine is greater than the estimated Ccr, suggesting elimination by glomerular filtration and active tubular secretion. There may be competition for elimination with other compounds that also are renally eliminated.

Special populations –

Renal function impairment: The pharmacokinetics of emtricitabine are altered in patients with renal impairment. In adult patients with Ccr less than 50 mL/min or with end-stage renal disease (ESRD) requiring dialysis, C_{max} and AUC of emtricitabine were increased because of a reduction in renal clearance (see the following table). It is recommended that the dosing interval for emtricitabine be modified in adult patients with Ccr less than 50 mL/min or in adult patients with ESRD who require dialysis. The effects of renal impairment on emtricitabine pharmacokinetics in pediatric patients are not known.

Emtricitabine Mean Pharmacokinetic Parameters in Adults With Renal Function Impairment

Ccr (mL/min)	> 80 (n = 6)	50 to 80 (n = 6)	30 to 49 (n = 6)	< 30 (n = 5)	ESRD[a] < 30 (n = 5)
Baseline Ccr (mL/min)	107 ± 21	59.8 ± 6.5	40.9 ± 5.1	22.9 ± 5.3	8.8 ± 1.4
C_{max} (mcg/mL)	2.2 ± 0.6	3.8 ± 0.9	3.2 ± 0.6	2.8 ± 0.7	2.8 ± 0.5
AUC (h•mcg/mL)	11.8 ± 2.9	19.9 ± 1.2	25.1 ± 5.7	33.7 ± 2.1	53.2 ± 9.9
CL/F[b] (mL/min)	302 ± 94	168 ± 10	138 ± 28	99 ± 6	64 ± 12
CLr[c] (mL/min)	213 ± 89	121 ± 39	69 ± 32	30 ± 11	NA[d]

[a] End stage renal disease patients requiring dialysis.
[b] CL/F = apparent oral clearance.
[c] CLr = apparent renal clearance.
[d] NA = not applicable.

Children: The pharmacokinetics of emtricitabine at steady state were determined in 77 HIV-infected children, and the pharmacokinetic profile was characterized in 4 age groups. The emtricitabine exposure achieved in

EMTRICITABINE — ORAL

children receiving a daily dose of 6 mg/kg up to a maximum of 240 mg oral solution or a 200 mg capsule is similar to exposures achieved in adults receiving a once-daily dose of 200 mg.

Emtricitabine Mean Pharmacokinetic Parameters in Children				
Age	3 to 24 months (n = 14)	25 months to 6 years (n = 19)	7 to 12 years (n = 17)	13 to 17 years (n = 27)
Formulation				
Capsules (n)	0	0	10	26
Oral solution (n)	14	19	7	1
Dose (mg/kg)[a]	6.1 (5.5 to 6.8)	6.1 (5.6 to 6.7)	5.6 (3.1 to 6.6)	4.4 (1.8 to 7)
C_{max} (mcg/mL)	1.9 ± 0.6	1.9 ± 0.7	2.7 ± 0.8	2.7 ± 0.9
AUC (h•mcg/mL)	8.7 ± 3.2	9 ± 3	12.6 ± 3.5	12.6 ± 5.4
$t_{½}$[b] (h)	8.9 ± 3.2	11.3 ± 6.4	8.2 ± 3.2	8.9 ± 3.3

[a] Mean (range).
[b] $t_{½}$ = terminal half-life.

Hemodialysis – See Overdosage for more information.

➤*Microbiology:*

Antiviral activity in vitro – The in vitro antiviral activity of emtricitabine against laboratory and clinical isolates of HIV was assessed in lymphoblastoid cell lines, the multinuclear-activation-of-galactosidase-indicator-CCR5 cell line, and peripheral blood mononuclear cells. The 50% inhibitory concentration (IC_{50}) value for emtricitabine was in the range of 0.0013 to 0.64 mcM (0.0003 to 0.158 mcg/mL). In drug combination studies of emtricitabine with nucleoside reverse transcriptase inhibitors (abacavir, lamivudine, stavudine, tenofovir, zalcitabine, zidovudine), nonnucleoside reverse transcriptase inhibitors (NNRTIs; delavirdine, efavirenz, nevirapine), and protease inhibitors (amprenavir, nelfinavir, ritonavir, saquinavir), additive to synergistic effects were observed. Most of these drug combinations have not been studied in humans. Emtricitabine displayed antiviral activity in vitro against HIV-1 clades A, C, D, E, F, and G (IC_{50} values ranged from 0.007 to 0.075 mcM) and showed strain specific activity against HIV-2 (IC_{50} values ranged from 0.007 to 1.5 mcM).

Drug resistance – Emtricitabine-resistant isolates of HIV have been selected in vitro. Genotypic analysis of these isolates showed that the reduced susceptibility to emtricitabine was associated with a mutation in the HIV reverse transcriptase gene at codon 184, which resulted in an amino acid substitution of methionine by valine or isoleucine (M184V/I).

Emtricitabine-resistant isolates of HIV have been recovered from some patients treated with emtricitabine alone or in combination with other antiretroviral agents. In a clinical study, viral isolates from 37.5% of treatment-naïve patients with virologic failure showed reduced susceptibility to emtricitabine. Genotypic analysis of these isolates showed that the resistance was because of M184V/I mutations in the HIV reverse transcriptase gene.

Cross-resistance – Cross-resistance among certain nucleoside analog reverse transcriptase inhibitors has been recognized. Emtricitabine-resistant isolates (M184V/I) were cross-resistant to lamivudine and zalcitabine but retained sensitivity to abacavir, didanosine, stavudine, tenofovir, zidovudine, and NNRTIs (delavirdine, efavirenz, and nevirapine). HIV-1 isolates containing the K65R mutation, selected in vivo by abacavir, didanosine, tenofovir, and zalcitabine, demonstrated reduced susceptibility to inhibition by emtricitabine. Viruses harboring mutations conferring reduced susceptibility to stavudine and zidovudine (M41L, D67N, K70R, L210W, T215Y/F, K219Q/E) or didanosine (L74V) remained sensitive to emtricitabine. HIV-1 containing the K103N mutation associated with resistance to NNRTIs was susceptible to emtricitabine.

Contraindications

Previously demonstrated hypersensitivity to any of the components of the products.

Warnings

➤*Lactic acidosis / Severe hepatomegaly with steatosis:* Lactic acidosis and severe hepatomegaly with steatosis, including fatal cases, have been reported with the use of nucleoside analogs alone or in combination, including emtricitabine and other antiretrovirals. A majority of these cases have been in women. Obesity and prolonged nucleoside exposure may be risk factors. However, cases have also been reported in patients with no known risk factors. Suspend treatment with emtricitabine in any patient who develops clinical or laboratory findings suggestive of lactic acidosis or pronounced hepatotoxicity (which may include hepatomegaly and steatosis even in the absence of marked transaminase elevations).

➤*Coinfection with HIV and HBV:* It is recommended that all patients with HIV be tested for the presence of chronic HBV before initiating antiretroviral therapy.

See the Warning box for more information.

➤*Renal function impairment:* See Administration and Dosage for more information.

➤*Elderly:* Clinical studies of emtricitabine did not contain sufficient numbers of subjects 65 years of age and older to determine whether they respond differently from younger subjects. In general, exercise caution in dose selection for the elderly patient, keeping in mind the greater frequency of decreased hepatic, renal, or cardiac function, and of concomitant disease or other drug therapy.

➤*Pregnancy:* *Category B.* The incidence of fetal variations and malformations was not increased in embryofetal toxicity studies performed with emtricitabine in mice at exposures (AUC) approximately 60-fold higher and in rabbits at approximately 120-fold higher than human exposures at the recommended daily dose. There are, however, no adequate and well-controlled studies in pregnant women. Because animal reproduction studies are not always predictive of human response, use emtricitabine during pregnancy only if clearly needed.

Antiretroviral pregnancy registry – To monitor fetal outcomes of pregnant women exposed to emtricitabine, an antiretroviral pregnancy registry has been established. Doctors are encouraged to register patients by calling 1-800-258-4263.

➤*Lactation:* The Centers for Disease Control and Prevention recommends that HIV-infected mothers not breast-feed their infants to avoid risking postnatal transmission of HIV. It is not known whether emtricitabine is secreted into human milk. Because of the potential for HIV transmission and for serious adverse reactions in breast-feeding infants, instruct mothers not to breast-feed if they are receiving emtricitabine.

➤*Children:* Safety and efficacy in children younger than 3 months of age have not been established.

Precautions

➤*Monitoring:* Closely monitor hepatic function with clinical and laboratory follow-up for at least several months in patients who discontinue emtricitabine and are coinfected with HIV and HBV. HBV testing is recommended prior to initiation of therapy.

➤*Fat redistribution:* Redistribution/accumulation of body fat, including central obesity, dorsocervical fat enlargement ("buffalo hump"), peripheral wasting, facial wasting, breast enlargement, and cushingoid appearance, have been observed in patients receiving antiretroviral therapy. The mechanism and long-term consequences of these reactions are unknown. A causal relationship has not been established.

➤*Immune reconstitution syndrome:* Immune reconstitution syndrome has been reported in patients treated with combination antiretroviral therapy including emtricitabine. During the initial phase of combination antiretroviral treatment, patients whose immune system responds may develop an inflammatory response to indolent or residual opportunistic infections (eg, *Mycobacterium avium* infection, cytomegalovirus, *Pneumocystis jirovecii* pneumonia, tuberculosis), which may necessitate further evaluation and treatment.

Drug Interactions

None known.

Adverse Reactions

➤*Adults:* The most common adverse reactions that occurred in patients receiving emtricitabine with other antiretroviral agents in clinical trials were headache, diarrhea, nausea, and rash, which were generally of mild to moderate severity. Approximately 1% of patients discontinued participation in the clinical studies because of these reactions. All adverse reactions were reported with similar frequency in emtricitabine and control treatment groups with the exception of skin discoloration, which was reported with higher frequency in the emtricitabine-treated group.

Skin discoloration, manifested by hyperpigmentation on the palms and/or soles, was generally mild and asymptomatic. The mechanism and clinical significance are unknown.

Emtricitabine Adverse Reactions (≥ 3%)				
	Study 303		Study 301A	
Adverse reaction	Emtricitabine + zidovudine or stavudine + NNRTI or protease inhibitor (n = 294)	Lamivudine + zidovudine or stavudine + NNRTI or protease inhibitor (n = 146)	Emtricitabine + didanosine + efavirenz (n = 286)	Stavudine + didanosine + efavirenz (n = 285)
CNS				
Abnormal dreams	2%	< 1%	11%	19%
Asthenia	16%	10%	12%	17%
Depressive disorders	6%	10%	9%	13%
Dizziness	4%	5%	25%	26%
Headache	13%	6%	22%	25%
Insomnia	7%	3%	16%	21%
Neuropathy/ Peripheral neuritis	4%	3%	4%	13%
Paresthesia	5%	7%	6%	12%

EMTRICITABINE — ORAL

Emtricitabine Adverse Reactions (≥ 3%)

Adverse reaction	Study 303		Study 301A	
	Emtricitabine + zidovudine or stavudine + NNRTI or protease inhibitor (n = 294)	Lamivudine + zidovudine or stavudine + NNRTI or protease inhibitor (n = 146)	Emtricitabine + didanosine + efavirenz (n = 286)	Stavudine + didanosine + efavirenz (n = 285)
Dermatologic				
Rash event[a]	17%	14%	30%	33%
GI				
Abdominal pain	8%	11%	14%	17%
Diarrhea	23%	18%	23%	32%
Dyspepsia	4%	5%	8%	12%
Nausea	18%	12%	13%	23%
Vomiting	9%	7%	9%	12%
Lab test abnormalities				
Percentage with grade 3 or 4 laboratory abnormality	31%	28%	34%	38%
ALT (> 5 × ULN[b])	2%	1%	5%	6%
AST (> 5 × ULN)	3%	< 1%	6%	9%
Bilirubin (> 2.5 × ULN)	1%	2%	< 1%	< 1%
Creatine kinase (> 4 × ULN)	11%	14%	12%	11%
Neutrophils (< 750 mm^3)	5%	3%	5%	7%
Pancreatic amylase (> 2 × ULN)	2%	2%	< 1%	1%
Serum amylase (> 2 × ULN)	2%	2%	5%	10%
Serum glucose (< 40 or > 250 mg/dL)	3%	3%	2%	3%
Serum lipase (> 2 × ULN)	< 1%	< 1%	1%	2%
Triglycerides (> 750 mg/dL)	10%	8%	9%	6%
Musculoskeletal				
Arthralgia	3%	4%	5%	6%
Myalgia	4%	4%	6%	3%
Respiratory				
Increased cough	14%	11%	14%	8%
Rhinitis	18%	12%	12%	10%

[a] Rash event includes rash, pruritus, maculopapular rash, urticaria, vesiculobullous rash, and allergic reaction.
[b] ULN = upper limit of normal.

➤*Children:* Assessment of adverse reactions is based on data from 169 HIV-infected pediatric patients who received emtricitabine through week 48. The adverse reaction profile in pediatric patients was generally comparable with that observed in clinical studies of emtricitabine in adult patients.

Selected treatment-emergent adverse reactions, regardless of causality, reported in patients during 48 weeks of treatment were the following: infection (44%), hyperpigmentation (32%), increased cough (28%), vomiting (23%), otitis media (23%), rash (21%), rhinitis (20%), diarrhea (20%), fever (18%), pneumonia (15%), gastroenteritis (11%), abdominal pain (10%), and anemia (7%).

Lab test abnormalities: Treatment-emergent grade 3/4 laboratory abnormalities were experienced by 9% of pediatric patients, including amylase greater than 2 times the ULN (n = 4), neutrophils less than 750/mm^3 (n = 3), ALT greater than 5 times the ULN (n = 2), elevated creatine phosphokinase (greater than 4 times the ULN) (n = 2) and 1 patient each with elevated bilirubin (greater than 3 times the ULN), elevated gamma-glutamyltransferase (greater than 10 times the ULN), elevated lipase (greater than 2.5 times the ULN), decreased hemoglobin (less than 7 g/dL), and decreased glucose (less than 40 mg/dL).

Overdosage

➤*Symptoms:* Limited clinical experience is available at doses higher than the therapeutic dose of emtricitabine. The effects of higher doses are not known. In one clinical pharmacology study, single doses of emtricitabine 1,200 mg were administered to 11 patients. No severe adverse reactions were reported.

➤*Treatment:* There is no known antidote for emtricitabine. If overdose occurs, monitor the patient for signs of toxicity and apply standard supportive treatment as necessary.

Hemodialysis treatment removes approximately 30% of the emtricitabine dose over a 3-hour dialysis period starting within 1.5 hours of emtricitabine dosing (blood flow rate of 400 mL/min and a dialysate flow rate of 600 mL/min). It is not known whether emtricitabine can be removed by peritoneal dialysis.

Patient Information

Emtricitabine is not a cure for HIV infection and patients may continue to experience illnesses associated with HIV infection, including opportunistic infections. Advise patients to remain under the care of a doctor when using this medicine.

Patients should be advised that:

- the use of emtricitabine has not been shown to reduce the risk of transmission of HIV to others through sexual contact or blood contamination.
- the long-term effects of emtricitabine are unknown.
- emtricitabine capsules are for oral ingestion only.
- it is important to take emtricitabine with combination therapy on a regular dosing schedule to avoid missing doses.
- redistribution or accumulation of body fat may occur in patients receiving antiretroviral therapy and the cause and long-term health effects of these conditions are not known.

Nucleoside Analog Reverse Transcriptase Inhibitor Combination

LAMIVUDINE/ZIDOVUDINE (3TC/ZDV, 3TC/AZT)

Rx	**Combivir** (GlaxoSmithKline)	**Tablets:** 150 mg lamivudine/300 mg zidovudine	(GXFC3). White, capsule shape. Film-coated. In 60s and UD 120s.

LAMIVUDINE/ZIDOVUDINE (3TC/ZDV, 3TC/AZT) — ORAL

Consult the complete prescribing information for each agent, lamivudine and zidovudine, prior to administration of lamivudine/zidovudine combination tablets.

WARNING

Zidovudine has been associated with hematologic toxicity, including neutropenia and severe anemia, particularly in patients with advanced HIV disease. Prolonged use of zidovudine has been associated with symptomatic myopathy.

Lactic acidosis and severe hepatomegaly with steatosis, including fatal cases, have been reported with use of nucleoside analogs alone or in combination, including lamivudine, zidovudine, and other antiretrovirals.

Severe acute exacerbations of hepatitis B have been reported in patients who are coinfected with hepatitis B virus (HBV) and HIV and have discontinued lamivudine. Monitor hepatic function closely with both clinical and laboratory follow-up for at least several months in patients who discontinue lamivudine/zidovudine and are coinfected with HIV and HBV. If appropriate, initiation of hepatitis B therapy may be warranted.

Indications

➤*HIV infection:* In combination with other antiretrovirals for the treatment of HIV-1 infection.

Administration and Dosage

➤*Approved by the FDA:* September 26, 1997.

➤*Dosage:* The recommended oral dosage for adults and adolescents (at least 12 years of age) is 1 tablet (containing 150 mg of lamivudine and 300 mg of zidovudine) twice daily.

➤*Renal function impairment:* Because it is a fixed-dose combination, lamivudine/zidovudine should not be prescribed for patients requiring dosage adjustment, such as those with reduced renal function (creatinine clearance [Ccr] less than 50 mL/min) or patients experiencing dose-limiting adverse reactions.

➤*Hepatic function impairment:* A reduction in the daily dose of zidovudine may be necessary in patients with mild to moderate impaired hepatic function impairment or liver cirrhosis. Because lamivudine/zidovudine is a fixed-dose combination that cannot be adjusted for this patient population, it is not recommended for patients with impaired hepatic function.

➤*Storage/Stability:* Store between 2° and 30°C (36° and 86°F).

Actions

➤*Pharmacology:*

Lamivudine – Lamivudine is a synthetic nucleoside analogue. Intracellularly, lamivudine is phosphorylated to its active 5'-triphosphate metabolite, lamivudine triphosphate (3TC-TP). The principal mode of action of 3TC-TP is inhibition of reverse transcriptase (RT) via deoxyribonucleic acid (DNA) chain termination after incorporation of the nucleotide analogue. 3TC-TP is a weak inhibitor of cellular DNA polymerases α, β, and γ.

Zidovudine – Zidovudine is a synthetic nucleoside analogue. Intracellularly, zidovudine is phosphorylated to its active 5'-triphosphate metabolite, zidovudine triphosphate (ZDV-TP). The principal mode of action of ZDV-TP is inhibition of RT via DNA chain termination after incorporation of the nucleotide analogue. ZDV-TP is a weak inhibitor of the cellular DNA polymerases α and γ, and has been reported to be incorporated into the DNA of cells in culture.

➤*Pharmacokinetics:*

Absorption/Distribution – Following oral administration, lamivudine and zidovudine are rapidly absorbed and extensively distributed. Binding to plasma protein is low.

Bioequivalence: One lamivudine/zidovudine tablet was bioequivalent to 1 lamivudine tablet (150 mg) plus 1 zidovudine tablet (300 mg) following single-dose administration to fasting healthy subjects (n = 24).

Effects of food: Lamivudine/zidovudine may be administered with or without food. The extent of lamivudine and zidovudine absorption (area under the curve [AUC]) following administration of lamivudine/zidovudine with food was similar when compared with fasting healthy subjects (n = 24).

Metabolism/Excretion –

Lamivudine: Approximately 70% of an intravenous dose of lamivudine is recovered as unchanged drug in the urine. Metabolism of lamivudine is a minor route of elimination. In humans, the only known metabolite is the trans-sulfoxide metabolite (approximately 5% of an oral dose after 12 hours).

Zidovudine: Zidovudine is eliminated primarily by hepatic metabolism. The major metabolite of zidovudine is 3'-azido-3'-deoxy-5'-*O*-β-*D*- glucopyranuronosylthymidine (GZDV). GZDV AUC is about 3-fold greater than the zidovudine AUC. Urinary recovery of zidovudine and GZDV accounts for 14% and 74%, respectively, of the dose following oral administration. A second metabolite, 3'-amino- 3'-deoxythymidine (AMT), has been identified in plasma. The AMT AUC was ⅕ of the zidovudine AUC.

Special populations –

Renal function impairment: See Administration and Dosage for more information.

Hepatic function impairment: See Administration and Dosage for more information.

Children:

• *Lamivudine/Zidovudine* – Do not administer lamivudine/zidovudine to pediatric patients younger than 12 years of age because it is a fixed-dose combination that cannot be adjusted for this patient population.

Pharmacokinetic parameters – The pharmacokinetic parameters of lamivudine and zidovudine in fasting patients are summarized in the following table:

Pharmacokinetic Parameters[a] for Lamivudine and Zidovudine in Adults				
Parameter	Lamivudine		Zidovudine	
Oral bioavailability (%)	86 ± 16	n = 12	64 ± 10	n = 5
Apparent volume of distribution (L/kg)	1.3 ± 0.4	n = 20	1.6 ± 0.6	n = 8
Plasma protein binding (%)	< 36		< 38	
CSF:plasma ratio[b]	0.12 (0.04 to 0.47)	n = 38[c]	0.6 (0.04 to 2.62)	n = 39[d]
Systemic clearance (L/h/kg)	0.33 ± 0.06	n = 20	1.6 ± 0.6	n = 6
Renal clearance (L/h/kg)	0.22 ± 0.06	n = 20	0.34 ± 0.05	n = 9
Elimination half-life (h)[e]	5 to 7		0.5 to 3	

[a] Data presented as mean ± standard deviation except where noted.
[b] Median (range).
[c] Children.
[d] Adults.
[e] Approximate range.

Contraindications

Previously demonstrated clinically significant hypersensitivity to any of the components of this product.

Warnings

➤*Fixed-dose combination:* Lamivudine/zidovudine is a fixed-dose combination. Ordinarily, do not coadminister lamivudine/zidovudine with lamivudine, zidovudine, a fixed-dose combination of abacavir and lamivudine, or a fixed-dose combination of abacavir, lamivudine, and zidovudine.

Consult the complete monographs for all agents being considered for use with lamivudine/zidovudine before combination therapy with lamivudine/zidovudine is initiated.

➤*Bone marrow suppression:* Use lamivudine/zidovudine with caution in patients who have bone marrow compromise evidenced by granulocyte count less than 1,000 cells/mm^3 or hemoglobin less than 9.5 g/dL. Frequent blood cell counts are strongly recommended in patients with advanced HIV disease who are treated with lamivudine/zidovudine. For HIV-infected individuals and patients with asymptomatic or early HIV disease, periodic blood cell counts are recommended.

➤*Lactic acidosis/severe hepatomegaly with steatosis:* Lactic acidosis and severe hepatomegaly with steatosis, including fatal cases, have been reported with the use of nucleoside analogues alone or in combination, including lamivudine, zidovudine, and other antiretrovirals. A majority of these cases have been in women. Obesity and prolonged nucleoside exposure may be risk factors. Exercise particular caution when administering lamivudine/zidovudine to any patient with known risk factors for liver disease; however, cases have also been reported in patients with no known risk factors. Suspend treatment with lamivudine/zidovudine in any patient who develops clinical or laboratory findings suggestive of lactic acidosis or pronounced hepatotoxicity (which may include hepatomegaly and steatosis even in the absence of marked transaminase elevations).

➤*Myopathy:* Myopathy and myositis, with pathological changes similar to that produced by HIV disease, have been associated with prolonged use of zidovudine, and, therefore, may occur with therapy with lamivudine/zidovudine.

➤*Posttreatment exacerbations of hepatitis:* In clinical trials in non-HIV–infected patients treated with lamivudine for chronic HBV, clinical and laboratory evidence of exacerbations of hepatitis have occurred after discontinuation of lamivudine. These exacerbations have been detected primarily by serum ALT elevations in addition to reemergence of HBV DNA. Although most events appear to have been self-limited, fatalities have been reported in some cases. Similar events have been reported from postmarketing experience after changes from lamivudine-containing HIV treatment regimens to non-lamivudine–containing regimens in patients infected with both HIV and HBV. The causal relationship to discontinuation of lamivudine treatment is unknown. Closely monitor patients with both clinical and laboratory follow-up for at least several months after stopping treatment. There is insufficient evidence to determine whether reinitiation of lamivudine alters the course of posttreatment exacerbations of hepatitis.

➤*Use with interferon- and ribavirin-based regimens:* In vitro studies have shown ribavirin can reduce the phosphorylation of pyrimidine nucleoside analogues such as lamivudine and zidovudine. Although no evidence of a pharmacokinetic or pharmacodynamic interaction (eg, loss of HIV/hepatitis C virus [HCV] virologic suppression) was seen when ribavirin was coadministered with lamivudine/zidovudine in HIV/HCV coinfected patients, hepatic decompensation (some fatal) has occurred in HIV/HCV coinfected patients receiving combination antiretroviral therapy for HIV and interferon alfa and ribavirin. Closely monitor patients receiving interferon alfa with or without ribavirin and lamivudine/zidovudine for

LAMIVUDINE/ZIDOVUDINE (3TC/ZDV, 3TC/AZT) — ORAL

treatment-associated toxicities, especially hepatic decompensation, neutropenia, and anemia. Consider discontinuation of lamivudine/zidovudine as medically appropriate. Consider dose reduction or discontinuation of interferon alfa, ribavirin, or both if worsening clinical toxicities are observed, including hepatic decompensation (eg, Child-Pugh greater than 6) (see the complete monographs for interferon and ribavirin).

➤*Renal function impairment:* See Administration and Dosage for more information.

➤*Hepatic function impairment:* See Administration and Dosage for more information.

➤*Carcinogenesis:*

Zidovudine: Zidovudine was administered orally at 3 dosage levels to separate groups of mice and rats (60 females and 60 males in each group). Initial single daily doses were 30, 60, and 120 mg/kg/day in mice and 80, 220, and 600 mg/kg/day in rats. The dosages in mice were reduced to 20, 30, and 40 mg/kg/day after day 90 because of treatment-related anemia, whereas in rats only the high dosage was reduced to 450 mg/kg/day on day 91 and then to 300 mg/kg/day on day 279.

In mice, 7 late-appearing (after 19 months) vaginal neoplasms (5 nonmetastasizing squamous cell carcinomas, 1 squamous cell papilloma, and 1 squamous polyp) occurred in animals given the highest dose. One late-appearing squamous cell papilloma occurred in the vagina of a middle-dose animal. No vaginal tumors were found at the lowest dose.

In rats, 2 late-appearing (after 20 months), nonmetastasizing vaginal squamous cell carcinomas occurred in animals given the highest dose. No vaginal tumors occurred at the low or middle dose in rats. No other drug-related tumors were observed in either sex of either species.

At doses that produced tumors in mice and rats, the estimated drug exposure (as measured by AUC) was approximately 3 times (mouse) and 24 times (rat) the estimated human exposure at the recommended therapeutic dose of 100 mg every 4 hours.

Two transplacental carcinogenicity studies were conducted in mice. One study administered zidovudine at dosages of 20 or 40 mg/kg/day from gestation day 10 through parturition and lactation with dosing continuing in offspring for 24 months postnatally. The doses of zidovudine employed in this study produced zidovudine exposures approximately 3 times the estimated human exposure at recommended doses. After 24 months at the highest dose, an increase in incidence of vaginal tumors was noted with no increase in tumors in the liver or lung or any other organ in either gender. These findings are consistent with results of the standard oral carcinogenicity study in mice, as described earlier. A second study administered zidovudine at maximum tolerated dosages of 12.5 or 25 mg/day (approximately 1,000 mg/kg nonpregnant body weight or approximately 450 mg/kg of term body weight) to pregnant mice from days 12 through 18 of gestation. There was an increase in the number of tumors in the lung, liver, and female reproductive tracts in the offspring of mice receiving the higher dose level of zidovudine.

It is not known how predictive the results of rodent carcinogenicity studies may be for humans.

➤*Mutagenesis:*

Lamivudine: Lamivudine was mutagenic in an L5178Y/TK$^{\pm}$ mouse lymphoma assay and clastogenic in a cytogenetic assay using cultured human lymphocytes. Lamivudine was negative in a microbial mutagenicity assay, in an in vitro cell transformation assay, in a rat micronucleus test, in a rat bone marrow cytogenetic assay, and in an assay for unscheduled DNA synthesis in rat liver.

Zidovudine: Zidovudine was mutagenic in an L5178Y/TK$^{\pm}$ mouse lymphoma assay, positive in an in vitro cell transformation assay, clastogenic in a cytogenetic assay using cultured human lymphocytes, and positive in mouse and rat micronucleus tests after repeated doses. It was negative in a cytogenetic study in rats given a single dose.

➤*Pregnancy: Category C.*

Lamivudine/Zidovudine – There are no adequate and well-controlled studies of lamivudine/zidovudine in pregnant women. Reproduction studies with lamivudine and zidovudine have been performed in animals. Only use lamivudine/zidovudine during pregnancy if the potential benefits outweigh the risks.

Lamivudine – Studies in pregnant rats and rabbits showed that lamivudine is transferred to the fetus through the placenta. Reproduction studies with orally administered lamivudine have been performed in rats and rabbits at dosages up to 4,000 and 1,000 mg/kg/day, respectively, producing plasma levels up to approximately 35 times that for the adult HIV dose. No evidence of teratogenicity due to lamivudine was observed. Evidence of early embryolethality was seen in the rabbit at exposure levels similar to those observed in humans, but there was no indication of this effect in the rat at exposure levels up to 35 times those in humans.

Zidovudine – Reproduction studies with orally administered zidovudine in the rat and in the rabbit at dosages up to 500 mg/kg/day revealed no evidence of teratogenicity with zidovudine. Zidovudine treatment resulted in embryo/fetal toxicity as evidenced by an increase in the incidence of fetal resorptions in rats given 150 or 450 mg/kg/day and rabbits given 500 mg/kg/day. The doses used in the teratology studies resulted in peak zidovudine plasma concentrations (after one half of the daily dose) in rats 66 to 226 times, and in rabbits 12 to 87 times, mean steady-state peak human plasma concentrations (after one sixth of the daily dose) achieved with the recommended daily dose (100 mg every 4 hours). In an additional teratology study in rats, a dosage of 3,000 mg/kg/day (very near the oral median lethal dose in rats of 3,683 mg/kg) caused marked maternal toxicity and an increase in the incidence of fetal malformations. This dose resulted in peak zidovudine plasma concentrations 350 times peak human plasma concentrations. No evidence of teratogenicity was seen in this experiment at dosages of 600 mg/kg/day or less. Two rodent carcinogenicity studies were conducted (see Carcinogenesis).

Antiretroviral pregnancy registry – To monitor maternal-fetal outcomes of pregnant women exposed to lamivudine/zidovudine and other antiretroviral agents, an antiretroviral pregnancy registry has been established. Register patients by calling 1-800-258-4263.

➤*Lactation:* The Centers for Disease Control and Prevention recommend that HIV-infected mothers not breast-feed their infants to avoid risking postnatal transmission of HIV infection. No specific studies of lamivudine and zidovudine excretion in breast milk after dosing with lamivudine/zidovudine have been performed. Lamivudine and zidovudine are excreted in human breast milk. A study in lactating rats administered 45 mg/kg of lamivudine showed that lamivudine concentrations in milk were slightly greater than those in plasma. Because of both the potential for HIV transmission and the potential for serious adverse reactions in breast-feeding infants, instruct mothers not to breast-feed if they are receiving lamivudine/zidovudine.

➤*Children:* Lamivudine/zidovudine should not be administered to pediatric patients younger than 12 years of age because it is a fixed-dose combination that cannot be adjusted for this patient population.

Precautions

➤*Monitoring:* Blood cell counts are recommended frequently for patients with advanced HIV disease and periodically for patients with asymptomatic or early HIV disease.

Monitor hepatic function closely with both clinical and laboratory follow-up for at least several months in patients who discontinue lamivudine/zidovudine and are coinfected with HIV and HBV.

➤*Patients with HIV and HBV coinfection:* See the Warning box for more information.

➤*Immune reconstitution syndrome:* Immune reconstitution syndrome has been reported in patients treated with combination antiretroviral therapy, including lamivudine/zidovudine. During the initial phase of combination antiretroviral treatment, patients whose immune system responds may develop an inflammatory response to indolent or residual opportunistic infections (eg, *Mycobacterium avium* infection, cytomegalovirus, *Pneumocystis jirovecii* pneumonia, tuberculosis), which may necessitate further evaluation and treatment.

➤*Fat redistribution:* Redistribution/accumulation of body fat, including central obesity, dorsocervical fat enlargement (buffalo hump), peripheral wasting, facial wasting, breast enlargement, and cushingoid appearance, has been observed in patients receiving antiretroviral therapy. The mechanism and long-term consequences of these events are currently unknown. A causal relationship has not been established.

Drug Interactions

Lamivudine/Zidovudine Drug Interactions

Precipitant Drug	Object Drug[a]		Description
Acetaminophen	Zidovudine	↓	Acetaminophen may decrease the AUC of zidovudine.
Atovaquone	Zidovudine	↑	Atovaquone appears to inhibit glucuronidation of zidovudine, thus increasing zidovudine concentrations and decreasing clearance.
Bone marrow suppressive/ cytotoxic agents (eg, ganciclovir, interferon alfa)	Zidovudine	↑	Coadministration may increase the hematologic toxicity of zidovudine.
Clarithromycin	Zidovudine	↑↓	Peak serum zidovudine concentrations may be increased or decreased.
Doxorubicin	Zidovudine	↓	Avoid coadministration. An antagonistic relationship has been demonstrated.
Fluconazole	Zidovudine	↑	Concurrent use may increase the zidovudine AUC.
Methadone	Zidovudine	↑	Zidovudine serum concentrations and AUC may be elevated, increasing the risk of side effects.
Nelfinavir Ritonavir	Zidovudine	↓	Zidovudine AUC is decreased.
Nelfinavir	Lamivudine	↑	Lamivudine AUC is increased.

LAMIVUDINE/ZIDOVUDINE (3TC/ZDV, 3TC/AZT) — ORAL

Lamivudine/Zidovudine Drug Interactions

Precipitant Drug	Object Drug[a]		Description
Probenecid	Zidovudine	↑	Probenecid may increase zidovudine AUC by inhibiting glucuronidation or reducing renal excretion. Some patients have developed symptoms consisting of myalgia, malaise or fever, and maculopapular rash.
Ribavirin/ Interferon	Zidovudine	↑	Coadministration of zidovudine, in combination with pegylated interferon and ribavirin, may increase the hematologic toxicity of zidovudine.
Rifamycins	Zidovudine	↓	The AUC of zidovudine may be decreased.
Stavudine	Zidovudine	↓	Avoid coadministration. An antagonistic relationship has been demonstrated.
Trimethoprim Trimethoprim/ Sulfamethox-azole	Lamivudine/ Zidovudine	↑	Plasma lamivudine concentrations may be increased. Trimethoprim appears to inhibit the renal secretion of lamivudine. Serum levels of zidovudine and its metabolite may be increased, especially in patients with impaired hepatic glucuronidation from liver disease or drug inhibition.
Valproic acid	Zidovudine	↑	Concurrent use may inhibit glucuronide metabolism, thus increasing zidovudine AUC.
Zalcitabine	Lamivudine	↓	Lamivudine and zalcitabine may inhibit the intracellular phosphorylation of one another.
Lamivudine	Zalcitabine		
Zidovudine	Didanosine	↓	The AUC of didanosine may be decreased, while the plasma concentration of zidovudine may be increased.
Didanosine	Zidovudine	↑	

[a] ↑ = Object drug increased. ↓ = Object drug decreased.

Adverse Reactions

➤*Lamivudine plus zidovudine administered as separate formulations:* In 4 randomized, controlled trials of lamivudine 300 mg per day plus zidovudine 600 mg per day, the following selected clinical and laboratory adverse reactions were observed (see the following tables).

Lamivudine/Zidovudine Adverse Reactions (≥ 5%)

Adverse Reaction	Lamivudine plus Zidovudine (n = 251)
CNS	
Depressive disorders	9%
Dizziness	10%
Headache	35%
Insomnia and other sleep disorders	11%
Malaise and fatigue	27%
Neuropathy	12%
Dermatologic	
Nasal signs and symptoms	20%
Skin rashes	9%
GI	
Abdominal cramps	6%
Abdominal pain	9%
Anorexia and/or decreased appetite	10%
Diarrhea	18%
Dyspepsia	5%
Nausea	33%
Nausea and vomiting	13%
Lab test abnormalities[a,b]	
ALT (> 5 × ULN[c])	3.7% (241)
Amylase (> 2 × ULN)	4.2% (72)
Anemia (hemoglobin < 8 g/dL)	2.9% (241)
AST (> 5 × ULN)	1.7% (241)
Bilirubin (> 2.5 × ULN)	0.8% (241)
Neutropenia (ANC < 750/mm³)	7.2% (237)

Lamivudine/Zidovudine Adverse Reactions (≥ 5%)

Adverse Reaction	Lamivudine plus Zidovudine (n = 251)
Thrombocytopenia (platelets < 50,000/mm³)	0.4% (240)
Musculoskeletal	
Arthralgia	5%
Musculoskeletal pain	12%
Myalgia	8%
Respiratory	
Cough	18%
Miscellaneous	
Fever or chills	10%

[a] Frequencies of these laboratory abnormalities were higher in patients with mild laboratory abnormalities at baseline.
[b] (n) = number of patients assessed.
[c] ULN = upper limit of normal.

Pancreatitis was observed in 3 of the 656 adult patients (less than 0.5%) who received lamivudine in controlled clinical trials.

➤*Postmarketing:* In addition to adverse reactions reported from clinical trials, the following reactions have been identified during post-approval use of lamivudine, zidovudine, and/or lamivudine/zidovudine. Because they are reported voluntarily from a population of unknown size, estimates of frequency cannot be made. These reactions have been chosen for inclusion because of a combination of their seriousness, frequency of reporting, or potential causal connection to lamivudine, zidovudine, and/or lamivudine/zidovudine.

Cardiovascular – Cardiomyopathy.

CNS – Paresthesia, peripheral neuropathy, seizures, weakness.

Dermatologic – Alopecia, erythema multiforme, Stevens-Johnson syndrome.

GI – Oral mucosal pigmentation, stomatitis.

Hematologic / Lymphatic – Anemia (including pure red cell aplasia and severe anemias progressing on therapy), lymphadenopathy, splenomegaly.

Hepatic – Lactic acidosis and hepatic steatosis, pancreatitis, posttreatment exacerbation of hepatitis B.

Hypersensitivity – Sensitization reactions (including anaphylaxis), urticaria.

Metabolic – Gynecomastia, hyperglycemia.

Musculoskeletal – Creatine phosphokinase elevation, muscle weakness, rhabdomyolysis.

Respiratory – Abnormal breath sounds/wheezing.

Miscellaneous – Redistribution/accumulation of body fat, vasculitis.

Overdosage

➤*Lamivudine / Zidovudine:* There is no known antidote for lamivudine/zidovudine.

➤*Lamivudine:* One case of an adult ingesting 6 g of lamivudine was reported; there were no clinical signs or symptoms noted and hematologic tests remained normal. Because a negligible amount of lamivudine was removed via (4-hour) hemodialysis, continuous ambulatory peritoneal dialysis, and automated peritoneal dialysis, it is not known if continuous hemodialysis would provide clinical benefit in a lamivudine overdose event.

➤*Zidovudine:* Acute overdoses of zidovudine have been reported in pediatric patients and adults. These involved exposures up to 50 g. The only consistent findings were nausea and vomiting. Other reported occurrences included headache, dizziness, drowsiness, lethargy, confusion, and 1 report of a grand mal seizure. Hematologic changes were transient. All patients recovered. Hemodialysis and peritoneal dialysis appear to have a negligible effect on the removal of zidovudine, while elimination of its primary metabolite, GZDV, is enhanced.

Patient Information

Lamivudine/zidovudine is not a cure for HIV infection and patients may continue to experience illnesses associated with HIV infection, including opportunistic infections. Advise patients that the use of lamivudine/zidovudine has not been shown to reduce the risk of transmission of HIV to others through sexual contact or blood contamination. Advise patients of the importance of taking lamivudine/zidovudine exactly as it is prescribed.

Inform patients that redistribution or accumulation of body fat may occur in patients receiving antiretroviral therapy and that the cause and long-term health effects of these conditions are not known at this time.

➤*Lamivudine:* Inform patients coinfected with HIV and HBV that deterioration of liver disease has occurred in some cases when treatment with lamivudine was discontinued. Advise patients to discuss any changes in regimen with their health care provider.

➤*Zidovudine:* Inform patients that the important toxicities associated with zidovudine are neutropenia and/or anemia. Tell patients about the extreme importance of having their blood cell counts followed closely while on therapy, especially patients with advanced HIV disease.

Nucleoside Analog Reverse Transcriptase Inhibitor Combination

ABACAVIR SULFATE/LAMIVUDINE/ZIDOVUDINE

Rx	**Trizivir** (GlaxoSmithKline)	**Tablets:** 300 mg abacavir sulfate/150 mg lamivudine/ 300 mg zidovudine	(GX LL1). Blue-green, capsule shape. Film-coated. In 60s.

ABACAVIR SULFATE/LAMIVUDINE/ZIDOVUDINE — ORAL

Consult the complete prescribing information for each agent (ie, abacavir, lamivudine, zidovudine), prior to administration of abacavir/lamivudine/zidovudine combination tablets.

WARNING

This product contains 3 nucleoside analogs (ie, abacavir sulfate, lamivudine, zidovudine) and is intended only for patients whose regimen would otherwise include these 3 components.

Hypersensitivity reactions – Serious and sometimes fatal hypersensitivity reactions have been associated with abacavir sulfate, a component of abacavir/lamivudine/zidovudine. Hypersensitivity to abacavir is a multi-organ clinical syndrome usually characterized by a sign or symptom in 2 or more of the following groups:

1.) fever
2.) rash
3.) gastrointestinal (eg, abdominal pain, diarrhea, nausea, vomiting)
4.) constitutional (eg, achiness, fatigue, generalized malaise)
5.) respiratory (eg, cough, dyspnea, pharyngitis).

Discontinue abacavir/lamivudine/zidovudine as soon as a hypersensitivity reaction is suspected. Permanently discontinue abacavir/lamivudine/zidovudine if hypersensitivity cannot be ruled out, even when other diagnoses are possible.

Following a hypersensitivity reaction to abacavir, never restart abacavir/lamivudine/zidovudine or any other abacavir-containing product because more severe symptoms can occur within hours and may include life-threatening hypotension and death.

Reintroduction of abacavir/lamivudine/zidovudine or any other abacavir-containing product, even in patients who have no identified history or unrecognized symptoms of hypersensitivity to abacavir therapy, can result in serious or fatal hypersensitivity reactions. Such reactions can occur within hours (see Warnings).

Hematologic toxicity – Zidovudine has been associated with hematologic toxicity including neutropenia and severe anemia, particularly in patients with advanced HIV disease (see Warnings). Prolonged use of zidovudine has been associated with symptomatic myopathy.

Lactic acidosis and severe hepatomegaly – Lactic acidosis and severe hepatomegaly with steatosis, including fatal cases, have been reported with the use of nucleoside analogs alone or in combination, including abacavir, lamivudine, zidovudine, and other antiretrovirals (see Warnings).

Exacerbations of hepatitis B – Severe acute exacerbations of hepatitis B have been reported in patients who are co-infected with hepatitis B virus (HBV) and HIV and have discontinued lamivudine, which is one component of abacavir/lamivudine/zidovudine. Hepatic function should be monitored closely with both clinical and laboratory follow-up for at least several months in patients who discontinue abacavir/lamivudine/zidovudine and are co-infected with HIV and HBV. If appropriate, initiation of anti-HBV therapy may be warranted (see Warnings).

Indications

➤*HIV infection:* In combination with other antiretrovirals or alone for the treatment of HIV-1 infection.

Administration and Dosage

➤*Approved by the FDA:* November 14, 2000.

➤*Dosage (adults and adolescents 40 kg or more):* 1 tablet twice daily. Abacavir/lamivudine/zidovudine is not recommended in adolescents who weigh less than 40 kg because it is a fixed-dose tablet.

➤*Dose adjustment:* Because it is a fixed-dose tablet, abacavir/lamivudine/zidovudine should not be prescribed for patients requiring dosage adjustment such as those with creatinine clearance (Ccr) less than 50 mL/min, patients with hepatic impairment, or patients experiencing dose-limiting adverse reactions.

➤*Medication Guide / Warning card:* A medication guide and warning card that provide information about recognition of hypersensitivity reactions should be dispensed with each new prescription and refill. To facilitate reporting of hypersensitivity reactions and collection of information on each case, an Abacavir Hypersensitivity Registry has been established. Physicians should register patients by calling 1-800-270-0425.

➤*Storage / Stability:* Store at 25°C (77°F); excursions permitted to 15° to 30°C (59° to 86°F).

Actions

➤*Pharmacology:*

Abacavir – Abacavir is a carbocyclic synthetic nucleoside analog. Abacavir is converted by cellular enzymes to the active metabolite, carbovir triphosphate (CBV-TP), an analog of deoxyguanosine-5'-triphosphate (dGTP). CBV-TP inhibits the activity of HIV-1 reverse transcriptase (RT) both by competing with the natural substrate dGTP and by its incorporation into viral DNA. The lack of a 3'-OH group in the incorporated nucleotide analog prevents the formation of the 5' to 3' phosphodiester linkage essential for DNA chain elongation, and therefore, the viral DNA growth is terminated. CBV-TP is a weak inhibitor of cellular DNA polymerases α, β, and γ.

Lamivudine – Lamivudine is a synthetic nucleoside analog. Intracellularly, lamivudine is phosphorylated to its active 5'-triphosphate metabolite, lamivudine triphosphate (3TC-TP). The principal mode of action of 3TC-TP is inhibition of RT via DNA chain termination after incorporation of the nucleotide analog. 3TC-TP is a weak inhibitor of cellular DNA polymerases α, β, and γ.

Zidovudine – Zidovudine is a synthetic nucleoside analog. Intracellularly, zidovudine is phosphorylated to its active 5'-triphosphate metabolite, zidovudine triphosphate (ZDV-TP). The principal mode of action of ZDV-TP is inhibition of RT via DNA chain termination after incorporation of the nucleotide analog. ZDV-TP is a weak inhibitor of the cellular DNA polymerases α and γ and has been reported to be incorporated into the DNA of cells in culture.

➤*Pharmacokinetics:*

Absorption / Distribution – In a single-dose, 3-way crossover bioavailability study of 1 abacavir/lamivudine/zidovudine tablet versus 1 abacavir 300 mg tablet, 1 lamivudine 150 mg tablet, plus 1 zidovudine 300 mg tablet administered simultaneously in healthy subjects (n = 24), there was no difference in the extent of absorption, as measured by the area under the plasma concentration-time curve (AUC) and maximal peak concentration (C_{max}) of all 3 components. One abacavir/lamivudine/zidovudine tablet was bioequivalent to 1 abacavir 300 mg tablet, 1 lamivudine 150 mg tablet, plus 1 zidovudine 300 mg tablet following single-dose administration to fasting healthy subjects (n = 24).

Abacavir: Following oral administration, abacavir is rapidly absorbed and extensively distributed. Binding of abacavir to human plasma proteins is approximately 50%. Binding of abacavir to plasma proteins was independent of concentration. Total blood and plasma drug-related radioactivity concentrations are identical, demonstrating that abacavir readily distributes into erythrocytes.

Lamivudine, zidovudine: Following oral administration, lamivudine and zidovudine are rapidly absorbed and extensively distributed. Binding to plasma protein is low.

Food effects: Abacavir/lamivudine/zidovudine may be administered with or without food. Administration with food in a single-dose bioavailability study resulted in lower C_{max}, similar to results observed previously for the reference formulations. The average (90% CI) decrease in abacavir, lamivudine, and zidovudine C_{max} was 32% (24% to 38%), 18% (10% to 25%), and 28% (13% to 40%), respectively, when administered with a high-fat meal, compared to administration under fasted conditions. Administration of abacavir/lamivudine/zidovudine with food did not alter the extent of abacavir, lamivudine, and zidovudine absorption (AUC), as compared with administration under fasted conditions (n = 24).

Metabolism / Excretion –

Abacavir: The primary routes of elimination of abacavir are metabolism by alcohol dehydrogenase to form the 5′-carboxylic acid and glucuronyl transferase to form the 5′-glucuronide.

Lamivudine: Approximately 70% of an intravenous dose of lamivudine is recovered as unchanged drug in the urine. Metabolism of lamivudine is a minor route of elimination. In humans, the only known metabolite is the trans-sulfoxide metabolite (approximately 5% of an oral dose after 12 hours).

Zidovudine: Zidovudine is eliminated primarily by hepatic metabolism. The major metabolite of zidovudine is 3′-azido-3′-deoxy-5′-*O*-β-*D*-glucopyranuronosylthymidine (GZDV). GZDV AUC is about 3-fold greater than the zidovudine AUC. Urinary recovery of zidovudine and GZDV accounts for 14% and 74% of the dose following oral administration, respectively. A second metabolite, 3'-amino- 3'-deoxythymidine (AMT), has been identified in plasma. The AMT AUC was one fifth of the zidovudine AUC. In humans, abacavir, lamivudine, and zidovudine are not significantly metabolized by CYP450 enzymes.

The pharmacokinetic properties of abacavir, lamivudine, and zidovudine in fasting patients are summarized in the following table.

Pharmacokinetic Parameters for Abacavir, Lamivudine, and Zidovudine in Adults

Parameter	Abacavir	Lamivudine	Zidovudine
Oral bioavailability (%)	≈ 86	≈ 86	≈ 64
Apparent volume of distribution (L/kg)	≈ 0.86	≈ 1.3	≈ 1.6
Systemic clearance (L/h/kg)	≈ 0.8	≈ 0.33	≈ 1.6
Renal clearance (L/h/kg)	≈ 0.007	≈ 0.22	≈ 0.34
Elimination half-life (h)[a]	≈ 1.45	5 to 7	0.5 to 3

[a] Approximate range.

Special populations –

Renal function impairment: Because lamivudine and zidovudine require dose adjustment in the presence of renal insufficiency, abacavir/lamivudine/zidovudine is not recommended for use in patients with Ccr less than 50 mL/min.

Hepatic function impairment: A reduction in the daily dose of zidovudine may be necessary in patients with mild to moderate hepatic function impairment or liver cirrhosis. Abacavir is contraindicated in patients with moder-

ABACAVIR SULFATE/LAMIVUDINE/ZIDOVUDINE — ORAL

ate to severe hepatic impairment, and dose reduction is required in patients with mild hepatic impairment. Because abacavir/lamivudine/zidovudine is a fixed-dose combination that cannot be adjusted for this patient population, abacavir/lamivudine/zidovudine is contraindicated for patients with hepatic function impairment.

Children: Abacavir/lamivudine/zidovudine is not intended for use in pediatric patients. Abacavir/lamivudine/zidovudine should not be administered to adolescents who weigh less than 40 kg because it is a fixed-dose tablet that cannot be dose adjusted for this patient population.

➤*Microbiology:*

Antiviral Activity –

Abacavir: The in vitro anti-HIV-1 activity of abacavir was evaluated against a T-cell tropic laboratory strain HIV-1_{IIIB} in lymphoblastic cell lines, a monocyte/macrophage tropic laboratory strain HIV-1_{BaL} in primary monocytes/macrophages, and clinical isolates in peripheral blood mononuclear cells. The concentration of drug necessary to inhibit viral replication by 50% (IC_{50}) ranged from 3.7 to 5.8 mcM (1 mcM = 0.28 mcg/mL) and 0.07 to 1.0 mcM against HIV-1_{IIIB} and HIV-1_{BaL}, respectively, and was 0.26 ± 0.18 mcM against 8 clinical isolates. The IC_{50} values of abacavir against different HIV-1 clades (A-G) ranged from 0.0015 to 1.05 mcM, and against HIV-2 isolates, from 0.024 to 0.49 mcM. Abacavir had synergistic activity in vitro in combination with the nucleoside reverse transcriptase inhibitor (NRTI) zidovudine, the non-nucleoside reverse transcriptase inhibitor (NNRTI) nevirapine, and the protease inhibitor (PI) amprenavir; and additive activity in combination with the NRTIs didanosine, emtricitabine, lamivudine, stavudine, tenofovir, and zalcitabine. Ribavirin (50 mcM) had no effect on the in vitro anti-HIV-1 activity of abacavir.

Lamivudine: The in vitro activity of lamivudine against HIV-1 was assessed in a number of cell lines (including monocytes and fresh human peripheral blood lymphocytes) using standard susceptibility assays. IC_{50} values (50% inhibitory concentrations) were in the range of 0.003 to 15 mcM (1 mcM = 0.23 mcg/mL). The IC_{50} values of lamivudine against different HIV-1 clades (A- G) ranged from 0.001 to 0.120 mcM and against HIV-2 isolates from 0.003 to 0.120 mcM. In HIV-1 infected MT-4 cells, lamivudine in combination with zidovudine at various ratios exhibited synergistic antiretroviral activity. Ribavirin (50 mcM) decreased the anti-HIV-1 activity of lamivudine by 3.5 fold.

Zidovudine: In vitro activity of zidovudine against HIV-1 was assessed in a number of cell lines (including monocytes and fresh human peripheral blood lymphocytes). The IC_{50} and IC_{90} values for zidovudine were 0.01 to 0.49 mcM (1 mcM = 0.27 mcg/mL) and 0.1 to 9 mcM, respectively. Zidovudine had anti-HIV-1 activity in all acute virus-cell infections tested. However, zidovudine activity was substantially less in chronically infected cell lines. The IC_{50} values of zidovudine against different HIV-1 clades (A-G) ranged from 0.00018 to 0.02 mcM, and against HIV-2 isolates from 0.00049 to 0.004 mcM. In cell culture drug combination studies, zidovudine demonstrated synergistic activity with the NRTIs abacavir, didanosine, lamivudine, and zalcitabine; the NNRTIs delavirdine and nevirapine; and the PIs indinavir, nelfinavir, ritonavir, and saquinavir; and additive activity with interferon-alfa. Ribavirin has been found to inhibit the phosphorylation of zidovudine in vitro.

Resistance – HIV-1 isolates with reduced sensitivity to abacavir, lamivudine, or zidovudine have been selected in vitro and were also obtained from patients treated with abacavir, lamivudine, and zidovudine, or the combination of lamivudine and zidovudine.

Abacavir: Genotypic analysis of isolates selected in vitro and recovered from abacavir-treated patients demonstrated that amino acid substitutions K65R, L74V, Y115F, and M184V/I in RT contributed to abacavir resistance. In a study of subjects receiving abacavir once or twice daily in combination with lamivudine and efavirenz once daily, 39% of the isolates from patients who experienced virologic failure in the abacavir once-daily arm had a more than 2.5-fold decrease in abacavir susceptibility with a median-fold decrease of 1.3 (range 0.5 to 11) compared with 29% of the failure isolates in the twice-daily arm with a median-fold decrease of 0.92 (range 0.7 to 13).

Lamivudine: Genotypic analysis of isolates selected in vitro and recovered from lamivudine-treated patients showed that the resistance was due to a specific amino acid substitution in the HIV-1 reverse transcriptase at codon 184 changing the methionine to either isoleucine or valine.

Zidovudine: Genotypic analyses of the isolates selected in vitro and recovered from zidovudine-treated patients showed mutations in the HIV-1 RT gene resulting in 6 amino acid substitutions (M41L, D67N, K70R, L210W, T215Y or F, and K219Q) that confer zidovudine resistance. In general, higher levels of resistance were associated with a greater number of mutations. In some patients harboring zidovudine-resistant virus at baseline, phenotypic sensitivity to zidovudine was restored by 12 weeks of treatment with lamivudine and zidovudine. Combination therapy with lamivudine plus zidovudine delayed the emergence of mutations conferring resistance to zidovudine.

Cross-resistance –

Abacavir: Isolates containing abacavir resistance-associated mutations, namely, K65R, L74V, Y115F, and M184V, exhibited cross-resistance to didanosine, emtricitabine, lamivudine, tenofovir, and zalcitabine in vitro and in patients. The K65R mutation can confer resistance to abacavir, didanosine, emtricitabine, lamivudine, stavudine, tenofovir, and zalcitabine; the L74V mutation can confer resistance to abacavir, didanosine, and zalcitabine; and the M184V mutation can confer resistance to abacavir, didanosine, emtricitabine, lamivudine, and zalcitabine. An increasing number of thymidine analog mutations (TAMs: M41L, D67N, K70R, L210W, T215Y/F, K219E/R/H/Q/N) is associated with a progressive reduction in abacavir susceptibility.

Lamivudine: Cross-resistance to abacavir, didanosine, tenofovir, and zalcitabine has been observed in some patients harboring lamivudine-resistant HIV-1 isolates. In some patients treated with zidovudine plus didanosine or zalcitabine, isolates resistant to multiple drugs, including lamivudine, have emerged (see Zidovudine below). Cross-resistance between lamivudine and zidovudine has not been reported.

Zidovudine: In a study of 167 HIV-infected patients, isolates (n = 2) with multidrug resistance to didanosine, lamivudine, stavudine, zalcitabine, and zidovudine were recovered from patients treated for at least 1 year with zidovudine plus didanosine or zidovudine plus zalcitabine. The pattern of resistance-associated mutations with such combination therapies was different (A62V, V75I, F77L, F116Y, Q151M) from the pattern with zidovudine monotherapy, with the Q151M mutation being most commonly associated with multidrug resistance. The mutation at codon 151 in combination with mutations at 62, 75, 77, and 116 results in a virus with reduced susceptibility to didanosine, lamivudine, stavudine, zalcitabine, and zidovudine. TAMs are selected by zidovudine and confer cross-resistance to abacavir, didanosine, stavudine, tenofovir, and zalcitabine.

Contraindications

Previously demonstrated hypersensitivity to abacavir or to any other component of the product; hepatic impairment.

See the Warning box for more information.

Warnings

➤*Hypersensitivity reactions:* Serious and sometimes fatal hypersensitivity reactions have been associated with abacavir/lamivudine/zidovudine and other abacavir-containing products. To minimize the risk of a life-threatening hypersensitivity reaction, permanently discontinue abacavir/lamivudine/zidovudine if hypersensitivity cannot be ruled out, even when other diagnoses are possible. Important information on signs and symptoms of hypersensitivity, as well as clinical management, is presented below.

Abacavir hypersensitivity reaction registry – To facilitate reporting of hypersensitivity reactions and collection of information on each case, an Abacavir Hypersensitivity Registry has been established. Register patients by calling 1-800-270-0425.

➤*Lactic acidosis / severe hepatomegaly with steatosis:* Lactic acidosis and severe hepatomegaly with steatosis, including fatal cases, have been reported with the use of nucleoside analogs alone or in combination, including abacavir, lamivudine, zidovudine, and other antiretrovirals. A majority of these cases have been in women. Obesity and prolonged nucleoside exposure may be risk factors. Exercise particular caution when administering abacavir/lamivudine/zidovudine to any patient with known risk factors for liver disease; however, cases have also been reported in patients with no known risk factors. Suspend treatment in any patient who develops clinical or laboratory findings suggestive of lactic acidosis or pronounced hepatotoxicity (which may include hepatomegaly and steatosis even in the absence of marked transaminase elevations).

➤*Bone marrow suppression:* Because abacavir/lamivudine/zidovudine contains zidovudine, use abacavir/lamivudine/zidovudine with caution in patients who have bone marrow compromise evidenced by granulocyte count less than 1,000 cells/mm^3 or hemoglobin less than 9.5 g/dL. Frequent blood counts are strongly recommended in patients with advanced HIV disease who are treated with abacavir/lamivudine/zidovudine. For HIV-infected individuals and patients with asymptomatic or early HIV disease, periodic blood counts are recommended.

➤*Myopathy:* Myopathy and myositis, with pathological changes similar to that produced by HIV disease, have been associated with prolonged use of zidovudine, and therefore may occur with therapy with abacavir/lamivudine/zidovudine.

➤*Posttreatment exacerbations of hepatitis:* In clinical trials in non-HIV-infected patients treated with lamivudine for chronic HBV, clinical and laboratory evidence of exacerbations of hepatitis have occurred after discontinuation of lamivudine. These exacerbations have been detected primarily by serum ALT elevations in addition to re-emergence of HBV DNA. Although most events appear to have been self-limited, fatalities have been reported in some cases. Similar events have been reported from postmarketing experience after changes from lamivudine-containing HIV treatment regimens to nonlamivudine-containing regimens in patients infected with both HIV and HBV. The causal relationship to discontinuation of lamivudine treatment is unknown. Closely monitor patients with clinical and laboratory follow-up for at least several months after stopping treatment. There is insufficient evidence to determine whether re-initiation of lamivudine alters the course of posttreatment exacerbations of hepatitis.

➤*Fixed-dose combination:* Abacavir/lamivudine/zidovudine contains fixed doses of 3 nucleoside analogs: abacavir, lamivudine, and zidovudine and should not be administered concomitantly with abacavir, lamivudine, emtricitabine, or zidovudine. Do not administer abacavir/lamivudine/zidovudine concomitantly with the fixed-dose combination drugs: lamivudine/zidovudine, abacavir and lamivudine, or emtricitabine and tenofovir.

Because abacavir/lamivudine/zidovudine is a fixed-dose tablet, it should not be prescribed for adolescents who weigh less than 40 kg or other patients requiring dosage adjustment.

➤*Renal function impairment:* Because abacavir/lamivudine/zidovudine is a fixed-dose tablet and the dosage of the individual components cannot be altered, patients with Ccr less than 50 mL/min should not receive abacavir/lamivudine/zidovudine.

➤*Hepatic function impairment:* Abacavir/lamivudine/zidovudine is contraindicated in patients with hepatic impairment since it is a fixed-dose tablet and the dosage of the individual components cannot be altered.

ABACAVIR SULFATE/LAMIVUDINE/ZIDOVUDINE — ORAL

➤*Carcinogenesis:*

Abacavir: Abacavir was administered orally at 3 dosage levels to separate groups of mice and rats in 2-year carcinogenicity studies. Results showed an increase in the incidence of malignant and nonmalignant tumors. Malignant tumors occurred in the preputial gland of males and the clitoral gland of females of both species, and in the liver of female rats. In addition, nonmalignant tumors also occurred in the liver and thyroid gland of female rats.

Zidovudine: Zidovudine was administered orally at 3 dosage levels to separate groups of mice and rats (60 females and 60 males in each group). Initial single daily doses were 30, 60, and 120 mg/kg/day in mice and 80, 220, and 600 mg/kg/day in rats. The doses in mice were reduced to 20, 30, and 40 mg/kg/day after day 90 because of treatment-related anemia, whereas in rats only the high dose was reduced to 450 mg/kg per day on day 91 and then to 300 mg/kg/day on day 279.

In mice, 7 late-appearing (after 19 months) vaginal neoplasms (5 nonmetastasizing squamous cell carcinomas, 1 squamous cell papilloma, and 1 squamous polyp) occurred in animals given the highest dose. One late-appearing squamous cell papilloma occurred in the vagina of a middle-dose animal. No vaginal tumors were found at the lowest dose.

In rats, 2 late-appearing (after 20 months), nonmetastasizing vaginal squamous cell carcinomas occurred in animals given the highest dose. No vaginal tumors occurred at the low or middle dose in rats. No other drug-related tumors were observed in either sex of either species.

At doses that produced tumors in mice and rats, the estimated drug exposure (as measured by AUC) was approximately 3 times (mouse) and 24 times (rat) the estimated human exposure at the recommended therapeutic dose of 100 mg every 4 hours.

Two transplacental carcinogenicity studies were conducted in mice. One study administered zidovudine at doses of 20 mg/kg/day or 40 mg/kg/day from gestation day 10 through parturition and lactation with dosing continuing in offspring for 24 months postnatally. At these doses, exposures were approximately 3 times the estimated human exposure at the recommended doses. After 24 months at the 40 mg/kg/day dose, an increase in incidence of vaginal tumors was noted with no increase in tumors in the liver or lung or any other organ in either gender. These findings are consistent with results of the standard oral carcinogenicity study in mice, as described earlier. A second study administered zidovudine at maximum tolerated doses of 12.5 mg/day or 25 mg/day (approximately 1,000 mg/kg nonpregnant body weight or approximately 450 mg/kg of term body weight) to pregnant mice from days 12 through 18 of gestation. There was an increase in the number of tumors in the lung, liver, and female reproductive tracts in the offspring of mice receiving the higher dose level of zidovudine.

➤*Mutagenesis:*

Abacavir: Abacavir induced chromosomal aberrations both in the presence and absence of metabolic activation in an in vitro cytogenetic study in human lymphocytes. Abacavir was mutagenic in the absence of metabolic activation, although it was not mutagenic in the presence of metabolic activation in an L5178Y/TK$^{\pm}$ mouse lymphoma assay. Abacavir was clastogenic in males and not clastogenic in females in an in vivo mouse bone marrow micronucleus assay. Abacavir was not mutagenic in bacterial mutagenicity assays in the presence and absence of metabolic activation.

Lamivudine: Lamivudine was mutagenic in an L5178Y/TK$^{\pm}$ mouse lymphoma assay and clastogenic in a cytogenetic assay using cultured human lymphocytes. Lamivudine was negative in a microbial mutagenicity assay, in an in vitro cell transformation assay, in a rat micronucleus test, in a rat bone marrow cytogenetic assay, and in an assay for unscheduled DNA synthesis in rat liver.

Zidovudine: Zidovudine was mutagenic in an L5178Y/TK$^{\pm}$ mouse lymphoma assay, positive in an in vitro cell transformation assay, clastogenic in a cytogenetic assay using cultured human lymphocytes, and positive in mouse and rat micronucleus tests after repeated doses. It was negative in a cytogenetic study in rats given a single dose.

➤*Elderly:* Clinical studies of abacavir, lamivudine, and zidovudine did not include sufficient numbers of patients 65 years of age and older to determine whether they respond differently from younger patients. In general, dose selection for an elderly patient should be cautious, reflecting the greater frequency of decreased hepatic, renal, or cardiac function, and of concomitant disease or other drug therapy. Abacavir/lamivudine/zidovudine is not recommended for patients with impaired renal function (ie, Ccr less than 50 mL/min).

➤*Pregnancy:* *Category C.* There are no adequate and well-controlled studies of abacavir/lamivudine/zidovudine in pregnant women. Reproduction studies with abacavir, lamivudine, and zidovudine have been performed in animals (see Abacavir, Lamivudine, and Zidovudine sections below). Only use abacavir/lamivudine/zidovudine during pregnancy if the potential benefits outweigh the risks.

Abacavir – Studies in pregnant rats showed that abacavir is transferred to the fetus through the placenta. Fetal malformations (increased incidences of fetal anasarca and skeletal malformations) and developmental toxicity (depressed fetal body weight and reduced crown-rump length) were observed in rats at a dose which produced 35 times the human exposure, based on AUC. Embryonic and fetal toxicities (increased resorptions, decreased fetal body weights) and toxicities to the offspring (increased incidence of stillbirth and lower body weights) occurred at half of the above-mentioned dose in separate fertility studies conducted in rats. In the rabbit, no developmental toxicity and no increases in fetal malformations occurred at doses that produced 8.5 times the human exposure at the recommended dose based on AUC.

Lamivudine – Studies in pregnant rats and rabbits showed that lamivudine is transferred to the fetus through the placenta. Reproduction studies with orally administered lamivudine have been performed in rats and rabbits at doses up to 4,000 mg/kg/day and 1,000 mg/kg/day, respectively, producing plasma levels up to approximately 35 times that for the adult HIV dose. No evidence of teratogenicity due to lamivudine was observed. Evidence of early embryolethality was seen in the rabbit at exposure levels similar to those observed in humans, but there was no indication of this effect in the rat at exposure levels up to 35 times that in humans.

Zidovudine – Reproduction studies with orally administered zidovudine in rats and rabbits at doses up to 500 mg/kg/day revealed no evidence of teratogenicity with zidovudine. Zidovudine treatment resulted in embryo/fetal toxicity as evidenced by an increase in the incidence of fetal resorptions in rats given 150 or 450 mg/kg/day and rabbits given 500 mg/kg/day. The doses used in the teratology studies resulted in peak zidovudine plasma concentrations (after one half of the daily dose) in rats 66 to 226 times, and in rabbits 12 to 87 times, mean steady-state peak human plasma concentrations (after one sixth of the daily dose) achieved with the recommended daily dose (100 mg every 4 hours). In an additional teratology study in rats, a dose of 3,000 mg/kg/day (very near the oral median lethal dose in rats of approximately 3,700 mg/kg) caused marked maternal toxicity and an increase in the incidence of fetal malformations. This dose resulted in peak zidovudine plasma concentrations 350 times peak human plasma concentrations. No evidence of teratogenicity was seen in this experiment at doses of 600 mg/kg/day or less. Two rodent carcinogenicity studies were conducted (see Carcinogenesis, Mutagenesis, and Impairment of Fertility).

Antiretroviral pregnancy registry – To monitor maternal-fetal outcomes of pregnant women exposed to abacavir/lamivudine/zidovudine or other antiretroviral agents, an Antiretroviral Pregnancy Registry has been established. Physicians are encouraged to register patients by calling 1-800-258-4263.

➤*Lactation:* The Centers for Disease Control and Prevention recommend that HIV-infected mothers not breast-feed their infants to avoid risking postnatal transmission of HIV infection.

Lamivudine and zidovudine are excreted in human breast milk; abacavir and lamivudine are secreted into the milk of lactating rats.

Because of both the potential for HIV transmission and the potential for serious adverse reactions in nursing infants, instruct mothers not to breast-feed if they are receiving abacavir/lamivudine/zidovudine.

➤*Children:* Abacavir/lamivudine/zidovudine is not intended for use in pediatric patients. Abacavir/lamivudine/zidovudine should not be administered to adolescents who weigh less than 40 kg because it is a fixed-dose tablet that cannot be adjusted for this patient population.

Therapy-experienced pediatric patients – A randomized, double-blind study, CNA3006, compared abacavir plus lamivudine and zidovudine versus lamivudine and zidovudine in pediatric patients, most of whom were extensively pretreated with nucleoside analog antiretroviral agents. Patients in this study had a limited response to abacavir.

Precautions

➤*Therapy-experienced patients:* In clinical trials, patients with prolonged prior NRTI exposure or who had HIV-1 isolates that contained multiple mutations conferring resistance to NRTIs had limited response to abacavir. Consider the potential for cross-resistance between abacavir and other NRTIs when choosing new therapeutic regimens in therapy-experienced patients (see Microbiology: Cross-Resistance).

➤*HIV and HBV coinfection:* Safety and efficacy of lamivudine have not been established for treatment of chronic hepatitis B in patients dually infected with HIV and HBV. In non-HIV-infected patients treated with lamivudine for chronic hepatitis B, emergence of lamivudine-resistant HBV has been detected and has been associated with diminished treatment response. Emergence of HBV variants associated with resistance to lamivudine has also been reported in HIV-infected patients who have received lamivudine-containing antiretroviral regimens in the presence of concurrent infection with HBV.

➤*Immune reconstitution syndrome:* Immune reconstitution syndrome has been reported in patients treated with combination antiretroviral therapy, including abacavir/lamivudine/zidovudine. During the initial phase of combination antiretroviral treatment, patients whose immune system responds may develop an inflammatory response to indolent or residual opportunistic infections (eg, *Mycobacterium avium* infection, cytomegalovirus, *Pneumocystis jirovecii* pneumonia, tuberculosis), which may necessitate further evaluation and treatment.

➤*Fat redistribution:* Redistribution/accumulation of body fat including central obesity, dorsocervical fat enlargement (buffalo hump), peripheral wasting, facial wasting, breast enlargement, and cushingoid appearance have been observed in patients receiving antiretroviral therapy. The mechanism and long-term consequences of these events are currently unknown. A causal relationship has not been established.

Drug Interactions

The drug interactions described are based on studies conducted with the individual nucleoside analogs. In humans, abacavir, lamivudine, and zidovudine are not significantly metabolized by CYP450 enzymes; therefore, it is unlikely that clinically significant drug interactions will occur with drugs metabolized through these pathways.

ABACAVIR SULFATE/LAMIVUDINE/ZIDOVUDINE — ORAL

Abacavir/Lamivudine/Zidovudine Drug Interactions

Precipitant drug	Object drug*		Description
Acetaminophen	Zidovudine	↓	Acetaminophen may decrease the AUC of zidovudine.
Atovaquone	Zidovudine	↑	Atovaquone appears to inhibit glucuronidation of zidovudine, thus increasing zidovudine concentrations and decreasing clearance.
Bone marrow suppressive/ cytotoxic agents (eg, interferon-alpha, interferon-beta-1b, ganciclovir)	Zidovudine	↑	Coadministration may increase the hematologic toxicity of zidovudine.
Clarithromycin	Zidovudine	↔	Peak serum zidovudine concentrations may be increased or decreased.
Doxorubicin	Zidovudine	↓	Avoid coadministration. An antagonistic relationship has been demonstrated.
Ethanol	Abacavir	↑	Ethanol decreases the elimination of abacavir, causing an increase in overall exposure because of their common metabolic pathway. Coadministration of ethanol 0.7 g/kg and abacavir 600 mg resulted in a 41% increase in abacavir AUC and a 26% increase in abacavir half-life.
Fluconazole	Zidovudine	↑	Concurrent use may increase the zidovudine AUC.
Ganciclovir	Zidovudine	↑	Concomitant use may increase zidovudine plasma levels and AUC, thus increasing risk of life-threatening hematologic toxicities.
Methadone	Zidovudine	↑	Zidovudine serum concentrations and AUC may be elevated, increasing the risk of side effects.
Nelfinavir/ Ritonavir	Zidovudine	↓	Zidovudine AUC is decreased.
Probenecid	Zidovudine	↑	Probenecid may increase zidovudine AUC by inhibiting glucuronidation or reducing renal excretion. Some patients have developed symptoms consisting of myalgia, malaise or fever, and maculopapular rash.
Rifamycins	Zidovudine	↓	The AUC of zidovudine may be decreased.
Stavudine, ribavirin	Zidovudine	↓	Avoid concomitant use because some nucleoside analogs affect viral replication and may antagonize antiviral activity of zidovudine against HIV.
Trimethoprim/ Sulfamethoxazole	Zidovudine	↑	Serum levels of zidovudine and its metabolite may be increased, especially in patients with impaired hepatic glucuronidation from liver disease or drug inhibition.
	Lamivudine		Coadministration resulted in an increase of approximately 44% in lamivudine AUC, a decrease of approximately 29% in oral clearance, and a decrease of approximately 30% in renal clearance. No change in the dose of either drug is recommended.
Valproic acid	Zidovudine	↑	Concurrent use may inhibit glucuronide metabolism, thus increasing zidovudine AUC.

Abacavir/Lamivudine/Zidovudine Drug Interactions

Precipitant drug	Object drug*		Description
Abacavir	Methadone	↓	Coadministration increased oral methadone clearance by 22% (90% CI 6% to 42%). This alteration will not result in a methadone dose modification in the majority of patients; however, an increased methadone dose may be required in a small number of patients.
Lamivudine	Zalcitabine	↑	Lamivudine and zalcitabine may inhibit the intracellular phosphorylation of one another. Therefore, use of abacavir/lamivudine/zidovudine in combination with zalcitabine is not recommended.
Zalcitabine	Lamivudine	↑	
Zidovudine	Phenytoin	↔	Phenytoin levels have been reported to increase, decrease, or not change with concurrent use. In addition, zidovudine clearance was decreased by phenytoin.
Phenytoin	Zidovudine	↑	

* ↑ = Object drug increased. ↓ = Object drug decreased. ↔ = Undetermined clinical effect.

Adverse Reactions

➤*Hypersensitivity reactions:* Serious and sometimes fatal hypersensitivity reactions have been associated with abacavir sulfate, a component of abacavir/lamivudine/zidovudine (see Warning Box and Warnings).

➤*Treatment-emergent adverse reactions:* Treatment-emergent clinical adverse reactions (rated by the investigator as moderate or severe) with a 5% or more frequency during therapy with abacavir 300 mg twice daily, lamivudine 150 mg twice daily, and zidovudine 300 mg twice daily compared with indinavir 800 mg 3 times daily, lamivudine 150 mg twice daily, and zidovudine 300 mg twice daily from CNA3005 are listed in the following table.

Treatment-Emergent Adverse Reactions of at Least Moderate Intensity (Grades 2 through 4) in Therapy-Naive Adults Through 48 Weeks of Treatment (≥ 5%)

Adverse reaction	Abacavir plus Lamivudine/Zidovudine (n = 262)	Indinavir plus Lamivudine/Zidovudine (n = 264)
CNS		
Anxiety	5%	3%
Depressive disorders	6%	4%
Headache	13%	9%
Malaise and fatigue	12%	12%
GI		
Diarrhea	7%	5%
Nausea	19%	17%
Nausea and vomiting	10%	10%
Miscellaneous		
Ear/nose/throat infections	5%	4%
Fever and/or chills	6%	3%
Hypersensitivity reaction	8%	2%
Musculoskeletal pain	5%	7%
Pain (non-site-specific)	< 1%	5%
Renal sign/symptoms	< 1%	5%
Skin rashes	5%	4%
Viral respiratory infections	5%	5%

Five patients receiving abacavir in the study above experienced worsening of pre-existing depression compared to none in the indinavir arm. The background rates of pre-existing depression were similar in the 2 treatment arms.

➤*Lab test abnormalities:*

Treatment-Emergent Laboratory Abnormalities (Grades 3 to 4)

Grade 3/4 laboratory abnormalities	Abacavir plus Lamivudine/ Zidovudine (n = 262)	Indinavir plus Lamivudine/ Zidovudine (n = 264)
Elevated CPK (> 4 x ULN[a])	7%	7%
ALT (> 5.0 x ULN)	6%	6%
Neutropenia (< 750/mm^3)	5%	5%
Hypertriglyceridemia (> 750 mg/dL)	2%	1%
Hyperamylasemia (> 2.0 x ULN)	2%	< 1%
Hyperglycemia (> 13.9 mmol/L)	< 1%	< 1%
Anemia (Hgb ≤ 6.9 g/dL)	0%	1%

[a] Upper limit of normal.

ABACAVIR SULFATE/LAMIVUDINE/ZIDOVUDINE — ORAL

➤*Other adverse reactions:* In addition, other adverse reactions observed in the expanded access program for abacavir were pancreatitis and increased gamma-glutamyltransferase.

➤*Postmarketing: abacavir, lamivudine, and/or zidovudine:*
Abacavir: Suspected Stevens-Johnson syndrome (SJS) and toxic epidermal necrolysis (TEN) have been reported in patients receiving abacavir primarily in combination with medications known to be associated with SJS and TEN, respectively. Because of the overlap of clinical signs and symptoms between hypersensitivity to abacavir and SJS and TEN, and the possibility of multiple drug sensitivities in some patients, abacavir should be discontinued and not restarted in such cases.

There have also been reports of erythema multiforme with abacavir use.

Cardiovascular – Cardiomyopathy.

CNS – Dizziness, insomnia and other sleep disorders, paresthesia, peripheral neuropathy, seizures, weakness.

Dermatologic – Alopecia, erythema multiforme, Stevens-Johnson syndrome.

Endocrine – Gynecomastia, hyperglycemia.

GI – Anorexia and/or decreased appetite, abdominal pain, dyspepsia, oral mucosal pigmentation; stomatitis.

Hematologic/Lymphatic – Aplastic anemia, anemia (including pure red cell aplasia and severe anemias progressing on therapy), lymphadenopathy, splenomegaly, thrombocytopenia.

Hepatic – Lactic acidosis and hepatic steatosis, elevated bilirubin, elevated transaminases, pancreatitis, posttreatment exacerbation of hepatitis B (see Warnings).

Hypersensitivity – Sensitization reactions (including anaphylaxis), urticaria.

Musculoskeletal – Arthralgia, myalgia, muscle weakness, CPK elevation, rhabdomyolysis.

Respiratory – Abnormal breath sounds/wheezing.

Miscellaneous – Redistribution/accumulation of body fat (see Precautions: Fat Redistribution); vasculitis.

Overdosage

➤*Abacavir:* There is no known antidote for abacavir. It is not known whether abacavir can be removed by peritoneal dialysis or hemodialysis.

Animal toxicology – Myocardial degeneration was found in mice and rats following administration of abacavir for 2 years. The systemic exposures were equivalent to 7 to 24 times the expected systemic exposure in humans. The clinical relevance of this finding has not been determined.

➤*Lamivudine:* One case of an adult ingesting 6 g of lamivudine was reported; there were no clinical signs or symptoms noted and hematologic tests remained normal. Because a negligible amount of lamivudine was removed via (4-hour) hemodialysis, continuous ambulatory peritoneal dialysis, and automated peritoneal dialysis, it is not known if continuous hemodialysis would provide clinical benefit in a lamivudine overdose event.

➤*Zidovudine:* Acute overdoses of zidovudine have been reported in pediatric patients and adults. These involved exposures up to 50 g. The only consistent findings were nausea and vomiting. Other reported occurrences included headache, dizziness, drowsiness, lethargy, and confusion. Hematologic changes were transient. All patients recovered. Hemodialysis and peritoneal dialysis appear to have a negligible effect on the removal of zidovudine, while elimination of its primary metabolite, GZDV, is enhanced.

Patient Information

➤*Abacavir hypersensitivity reaction:* Inform patients of the following:
- a *Medication Guide* and warning card summarizing the symptoms of the abacavir hypersensitivity reaction and other product information will be dispensed by the pharmacist with each new prescription and refill of abacavir/lamivudine/zidovudine, and encourage the patient to read the *Medication Guide* and warning card every time to obtain any new information that may be present about abacavir/lamivudine/zidovudine. (The complete text of the *Medication Guide* is reprinted at the end of this document.)
- to carry the warning card with them.
- how to identify a hypersensitivity reaction (see Warnings and *Medication Guide*). If they develop symptoms consistent with a hypersensitivity reaction to discontinue treatment with abacavir/lamivudine/zidovudine and seek medical evaluation immediately.
- that a hypersensitivity reaction can worsen and lead to hospitalization or death if abacavir/lamivudine/zidovudine is not immediately discontinued.
- to not restart abacavir/lamivudine/zidovudine or any other abacavir-containing product following a hypersensitivity reaction because more severe symptoms can occur within hours and may include life-threatening hypotension and death.
- that a hypersensitivity reaction is usually reversible if it is detected promptly and abacavir/lamivudine/zidovudine is stopped right away.
- that if they have interrupted abacavir/lamivudine/zidovudine for reasons other than symptoms of hypersensitivity (ie, those who have an interruption in drug supply), a serious or fatal hypersensitivity reaction may occur with reintroduction of abacavir.
- to not restart abacavir/lamivudine/zidovudine or any other abacavir-containing product without medical consultation and that restarting abacavir needs to be undertaken only if medical care can be readily accessed by the patient or others.
- abacavir/lamivudine/zidovudine should not be co-administered with lamivudine/zidovudine combination, emtricitabine, lamivudine, abacavir/lamivudine combination, zidovudine, emtricitabine/tenofovir combination, or abacavir.

➤*Lamivudine:* Inform patients co-infected with HIV and HBV that deterioration of liver disease has occurred in some cases when treatment with lamivudine was discontinued. Advise patients to discuss any changes in regimen with their physician.

➤*Zidovudine:* Inform patients that the important toxicities associated with zidovudine are neutropenia and/or anemia. Inform them of the extreme importance of having their blood counts followed closely while on therapy, especially for patients with advanced HIV disease.

➤*Abacavir/lamivudine/zidovudine:* Inform patients that some HIV medicines, including abacavir/lamivudine/zidovudine can cause a rare, but serious condition called lactic acidosis with liver enlargement (hepatomegaly).

Abacavir/lamivudine/zidovudine is not a cure for HIV infection and patients may continue to experience illnesses associated with HIV infection, including opportunistic infections. Patients should remain under the care of a physician when using abacavir/lamivudine/zidovudine. Advise patients that the use of abacavir/lamivudine/zidovudine has not been shown to reduce the risk of transmission of HIV to others through sexual contact or blood contamination.

Inform patients that redistribution or accumulation of body fat may occur in patients receiving antiretroviral therapy and that the cause and long-term health effects of these conditions are not known at this time.

Abacavir/lamivudine/zidovudine tablets are for oral ingestion only.

Advise patients of the importance of taking abacavir/lamivudine/zidovudine exactly as prescribed.

EMTRICITABINE/TENOFOVIR DISOPROXIL FUMARATE

Rx	**Truvada** (Gilead)	**Tablets:** 200 mg emtricitabine/300 mg tenofovir disoproxil fumarate (equivalent to 245 mg tenofovir disoproxil)	(GILEAD 701). Blue, capsule shape. Film-coated. In 30s.

EMTRICITABINE/TENOFOVIR DISOPROXIL FUMARATE — ORAL

Consult the complete prescribing information for each agent, emtricitabine and tenofovir disoproxil fumarate, prior to administration of emtricitabine/tenofovir disoproxil fumarate combination tablets.

WARNING

Lactic acidosis and severe hepatomegaly with steatosis, including fatal cases, have been reported with the use of nucleoside analogs alone or in combination with other antiretrovirals (see Warnings).

Emtricitabine/tenofovir disoproxil fumarate is not indicated for the treatment of chronic hepatitis B virus (HBV) infection, and the safety and efficacy of emtricitabine/tenofovir disoproxil fumarate has not been established in patients coinfected with HBV and HIV. Severe acute exacerbations of hepatitis B have been reported in patients who have discontinued emtricitabine or tenofovir disoproxil fumarate. Closely monitor hepatic function with clinical and laboratory follow-up for at least several months in patients who discontinue emtricitabine/tenofovir disoproxil fumarate and are coinfected with HIV and HBV. If appropriate, initiation of antihepatitis B therapy may be warranted (see Warnings).

Indications

➤*HIV infection:* For the treatment of HIV-1 infection in adults in combination with other antiretroviral agents (such as nonnucleoside reverse transcriptase inhibitors or protease inhibitors) .

In treatment-naïve patients, consider emtricitabine/tenofovir disoproxil fumarate as an alternative to the combination of tenofovir disoproxil fumarate plus lamivudine (3TC) for those patients who might benefit from a once-daily regimen. In treatment-experienced patients, guide the use of emtricitabine/tenofovir disoproxil fumarate by laboratory testing and treatment history.

Administration and Dosage

➤*Approved by the FDA:* August 2, 2004.

The dose of emtricitabine/tenofovir disoproxil fumarate is 1 tablet (containing 200 mg emtricitabine/300 mg tenofovir disoproxil fumarate) taken orally once daily with or without food.

EMTRICITABINE/TENOFOVIR DISOPROXIL FUMARATE — ORAL

➤*Renal function impairment:* Significantly increased drug exposures occurred when emtricitabine or tenofovir disoproxil fumarate were administered to patients with moderate to severe renal impairment. Therefore, adjust the dosing interval of emtricitabine/tenofovir disoproxil fumarate in patients with baseline creatinine clearance (Ccr) 30 to 49 mL/min using the recommendations in the table below. The safety and effectiveness of these dosing interval adjustment recommendations have not been clinically evaluated; therefore, closely monitor clinical response to treatment and renal function in these patients.

Dosage Adjustment for Patients with Altered Ccr			
Ccr (mL/min)[a]	≥ 50	30 to 49	< 30 (including patients requiring hemodialysis)
Recommended dosing interval	Every 24 hours	Every 48 hours	Not to be administered

[a] Calculated using ideal (lean) body weight.

➤*Storage/Stability:* Store at 25°C (77°F); excursions permitted to 15° to 30°C (59° to 86°F).

Actions

➤*Pharmacology:* The combination tablets contain the following 2 synthetic nucleoside analog reverse transcriptase inhibitors with activity against HIV: emtricitabine and tenofovir disoproxil fumarate. Refer to individual monographs for a complete explanation of mechanisms of action.

➤*Pharmacokinetics:* One emtricitabine/tenofovir disoproxil fumarate tablet was bioequivalent to 1 emtricitabine capsule (200 mg) plus 1 tenofovir disoproxil fumarate tablet (300 mg) following single-dose administration to fasting healthy subjects.

Single Dose Pharmacokinetic Parameters for Emtricitabine and Tenofovir in Adults	Emtricitabine	Tenofovir
Fasted oral bioavailability[a] (%)	≈ 92	≈ 25
Plasma terminal elimination half-life[a] (h)	≈ 10	≈ 17
C_{max}[b] (mcg/mL)	≈ 1.8[c]	≈ 0.30
AUC[b] (mcg•h/mL)	≈ 10[c]	≈ 2.29
CL/F[b] (mL/min)	≈ 302	≈ 1043
CL_{renal}[b] (mL/min)	≈ 213	≈ 243

[a] Median (range)
[b] Mean (≈ SD)
[c] Data presented as steady-state values.

Special populations –
Renal function impairment: The pharmacokinetics of emtricitabine/tenofovir disoproxil fumarate are altered in patients with renal impairment. In patients with Ccr less than 50 mL/min, C_{max}, and $AUC_{0\ to\ \infty}$ of emtricitabine/tenofovir disoproxil fumarate were increased. It is recommended that the dosing interval for emtricitabine/tenofovir disoproxil fumarate be modified in patients with Ccr 30 to 49 mL/min. Do not use emtricitabine/tenofovir disoproxil fumarate in patients with Ccr less than 30 mL/min and in patients with end-stage renal disease requiring dialysis.

Contraindications

Hypersensitivity to any of the components of the product.

Warnings

➤*Fixed dose combination:* This combination contains fixed doses of 2 nucleoside analogs: emtricitabine and tenofovir disoproxil fumarate. Do not administer concomitantly with emtricitabine or tenofovir disoproxil fumarate.

➤*Lactic acidosis/severe hepatomegaly with steatosis:* Lactic acidosis and severe hepatomegaly with steatosis, including fatal cases, have been reported with the use of nucleoside analogs alone or in combination with other antiretrovirals. A majority of these cases have been in women. Obesity and prolonged nucleoside exposure may be risk factors. Exercise particular caution when administering nucleoside analogs to any patient with known risk factors for liver disease; however, cases also have been reported in patients with no known risk factors. Suspend treatment with emtricitabine/tenofovir disoproxil fumarate in any patient who develops clinical or laboratory findings suggestive of lactic acidosis or pronounced hepatotoxicity (which may include hepatomegaly and steatosis even in the absence of marked transaminase elevations).

➤*Patients with HIV and hepatitis B coinfection:* It is recommended that all patients with HIV be tested for the presence of hepatitis B virus (HBV) before initiating antiretroviral therapy.

See the Warning box for more information.

➤*Renal function impairment:* See Actions for more information.

Renal effects – Renal impairment, including cases of acute renal failure and Fanconi syndrome (renal tubular injury with severe hypophosphatemia), has been reported in association with the use of tenofovir disoproxil fumarate. The majority of these cases occurred in patients with underlying systemic or renal disease, or in patients taking nephrotoxic agents; however, some cases occurred in patients without identified risk factors.

Avoid emtricitabine/tenofovir disoproxil fumarate with concurrent or recent use of a nephrotoxic agent. Carefully monitor patients at risk for or with a history of renal dysfunction and patients receiving concomitant nephrotoxic agents for changes in serum creatinine and phosphorus.

➤*Pregnancy: Category B.* There are no adequate and well-controlled studies in pregnant women. Because animal reproduction studies are not always predictive of human response, use emtricitabine/tenofovir disoproxil fumarate during pregnancy only if clearly needed.

Antiretroviral pregnancy registry – To monitor fetal outcomes of pregnant women exposed to emtricitabine/tenofovir disoproxil fumarate, an Antiretroviral Pregnancy Registry has been established. Health care providers are encouraged to register patients by calling 1-800-258-4263.

➤*Lactation:* The Centers for Disease Control and Prevention recommend that HIV-infected mothers not breastfeed their infants to avoid risking postnatal transmission of HIV. It is not known whether emtricitabine/tenofovir disoproxil fumarate is excreted in human milk. Because of the potential for HIV transmission and the potential for serious adverse reactions in nursing infants, instruct mothers not to breastfeed if they are receiving emtricitabine/tenofovir disoproxil fumarate.

ABACAVIR/LAMIVUDINE

Rx	**Epzicom** (GlaxoSmithKline)	**Tablets:** 600 mg abacavir (as sulfate)/ 300 mg lamivudine	(GS FC2). Orange. Film-coated. In 30s.

ABACAVIR/LAMIVUDINE — ORAL

Consult the complete prescribing information for each agent, Abacavir sulfate and Lamivudine, prior to administration of abacavir/lamivudine combination tablets.

WARNING

This product contains 2 nucleoside analogs (abacavir sulfate and lamivudine) and is intended only for patients whose regimen would otherwise include these 2 components.

Hypersensitivity reactions – Serious and sometimes fatal hypersensitivity reactions have been associated with abacavir, a component of *Epzicom.* Hypersensitivity to abacavir is a multiorgan clinical syndrome usually characterized by a sign or symptom in 2 or more of the following groups: fever, rash, GI (eg, nausea, vomiting, diarrhea, abdominal pain), constitutional (eg, generalized malaise, fatigue, achiness), and respiratory (eg, dyspnea, cough, pharyngitis). Discontinue abacavir/lamivudine as soon as a hypersensitivity reaction is suspected. Permanently discontinue abacavir/lamivudine if hypersensitivity cannot be ruled out, even when other diagnoses are possible.

Following a hypersensitivity reaction to abacavir, never restart abacavir/lamivudine or any other abacavir-containing product because more severe symptoms can occur within hours and may include life-threatening hypotension and death.

Reintroduction of abacavir/lamivudine or any other abacavir-containing product, even in patients who have no identified history or unrecognized symptoms of hypersensitivity to abacavir therapy, can result in serious or fatal hypersensitivity reactions. Such reactions can occur within hours.

WARNING (cont.)

Lactic acidosis and severe hepatomegaly – Lactic acidosis and severe hepatomegaly with steatosis, including fatal cases, has been reported with the use of nucleoside analogs alone or in combination, including abacavir, lamivudine, and other antiretrovirals (see Warnings sections in individual monographs).

Exacerbations of hepatitis B – Severe acute exacerbations of hepatitis B have been reported in patients who are co-infected with hepatitis B virus (HBV) and human immunodeficiency virus (HIV) and have discontinued lamivudine, which is one component of abacavir/lamivudine. Closely monitor hepatic function with clinical and laboratory follow-up for at least several months in patients who discontinued abacavir/lamivudine and are co-infected with HIV and HBV. If appropriate, initiation of anti-hepatitis B therapy may be warranted (see Warnings sections in individual monographs).

Indications

➤*HIV infection:* For use in combination with other antiretroviral agents for the treatment of HIV-1 infection.

Administration and Dosage

➤*Approved by the FDA:* August 2, 2004.

Dispense a Medication Guide and Warning Card that provide information about recognition of hypersensitivity reactions with each new prescription and refill. To facilitate reporting of hypersensitivity reactions and collection

ABACAVIR/LAMIVUDINE — ORAL

of information on each case, an Abacavir Hypersensitivity Registry has been established. Physicians should register patients by calling (800) 270-0425.

➤*Adults:* 1 tablet daily, in combination with other antiretroviral agents. May be taken without regard to food.

➤*Dose adjustment:* Because it is a fixed-dose tablet, do not prescribe abacavir/lamivudine to patients requiring dosage adjustment such as those with Ccr less than 50 mL/min, those with hepatic impairment, or those experiencing dose-limiting adverse events.

➤*Storage / Stability:* Store at 25°C (77°F); excursions permitted to 15° to 30°C (59° to 86°F).

Actions

➤*Pharmacology:* The combination tablets contain 2 synthetic nucleoside analogs, abacavir sulfate and lamivudine, with inhibitory activity against HIV. Refer to abacavir and lamivudine individual monographs for a complete explanation of mechanisms of action.

➤*Pharmacokinetics:* Following oral administration, abacavir and lamivudine are absorbed rapidly and distributed extensively. Binding of abacavir to human plasma proteins is about 50%; binding of lamivudine to plasma proteins is low.

The pharmacokinetic properties of abacavir and lamivudine in fasting patients are summarized below.

Pharmacokinetic Parameters for Abacavir and Lamivudine in Adults

Parameter	Abacavir	Lamivudine
Oral bioavailability (%)	≈ 86	≈ 86
Apparent volume of distribution (L/kg)	≈ 0.86	≈ 1.3
Systemic clearance (L/hr/kg)	≈ 0.8	≈ 0.33
Renal clearance (L/hr/kg)	≈ 0.007	≈ 0.22
Elimination half-life (hr)	≈ 1.45	5 to 7[1]

[1] Approximate range.

Special populations –

Renal function impairment: Lamivudine requires dose adjustment in the presence of renal insufficiency; abacavir/lamivudine is not recommended for use in patients with Ccr less than 50mL/min.

Liver function impairment: Abacavir is contraindicated in patients with moderate to severe hepatic impairment, and dose reduction is required in patients with mild hepatic impairment. Because abacavir/lamivudine is a fixed-dose combination and cannot be dose adjusted, abacavir/lamivudine is contraindicated for patients with hepatic impairment.

Contraindications

Abacavir sulfate has been associated with fatal hypersensitivity reactions. Do not restart abacavir following a hypersensitivity reaction to any abacavir containing product (see Warning box); hepatic impairment; previously demonstrated hypersensitivity to any of the components of the product.

Warnings

➤*Hypersensitivity reaction:* An Abacavir Hypersensitivity Registry has been established. Physicians should register patients by calling (800) 270-0425.

See the Warning box for more information.

➤*Lactic acidosis / severe hepatomegaly with steatosis:* Lactic acidosis and severe hepatomegaly with steatosis, including fatal cases, have been reported with the use of nucleoside analogs alone or in combination, including abacavir and lamivudine and other antiretrovirals. A majority of these cases have been in women. Obesity and prolonged nucleoside exposure may be risk factors. Exercise particular caution when administering abacavir/lamivudine to any patient with known risk factors for liver disease; however, cases also have been reported in patients with no known risk factors. Suspend abacavir/lamivudine treatment in any patient who develops clinical or laboratory findings suggestive of lactic acidosis or pronounced hepatotoxicity (which may include hepatomegaly and steatosis even in the absence of marked transaminase elevations).

➤*Posttreatment exacerbations of hepatitis:* In clinical trials in non-HIV-infected patients treated with lamivudine for chronic HBV, clinical and laboratory evidence of exacerbations of hepatitis have occurred after discontinuation of lamivudine. These exacerbations have been detected primarily by serum ALT elevations in addition to re-emergence of HBV DNA. Although most events appear to have been self-limited, fatalities have been reported in some cases.

➤*Fixed-dose combination:* This combination contains fixed doses of 2 nucleoside analogs, abacavir and lamivudine, and should not be administered concomitantly with other abacavir-containing and/or lamivudine-containing products.

➤*Pregnancy: Category C.* There are no adequate and well-controlled studies of abacavir/lamivudine in pregnant women. Use abacavir/lamivudine during pregnancy only if the potential benefits outweigh the risks. Refer to abacavir and lamivudine individual monographs for more information.

Antiretroviral pregnancy registry – To monitor maternal-fetal outcomes of pregnant women exposed to abacavir/lamivudine or other antiretroviral agents, an Antiretroviral Pregnancy Registry has been established. Physicians are encouraged to register patients by calling (800) 258-4263.

➤*Lactation:* Because of the potential for HIV transmission and the potential for serious adverse reactions in nursing infants, instruct mothers not to breastfeed if they are receiving abacavir/lamivudine. Lamivudine is excreted in human breast milk.

NEVIRAPINE

Rx	**Viramune** (Boehringer Ingelheim)	**Tablets:** 200 mg	Lactose. (54 193). White. Oval. In 60s, 100s, and UD 100s.
		Oral suspension: 50 mg/5 mL (as hemihydrate)	Parabens, sorbitol, sucrose. In 240 mL.

NEVIRAPINE — ORAL

WARNING

Severe, life-threatening, and in some cases fatal hepatotoxicity, including fulminant and cholestatic hepatitis, hepatic necrosis, and hepatic failure, has been reported in patients treated with nevirapine. In some cases, patients presented with nonspecific prodromal signs or symptoms of hepatitis and progressed to hepatic failure. These events are often associated with rash. Women, and patients with higher CD4 counts, are at increased risk of these hepatic events. Women with CD4 counts greater than 250 cells/mm^3, including pregnant women receiving chronic treatment for HIV infection, are at considerably higher risk of these events. Patients with signs or symptoms of hepatitis must discontinue nevirapine and seek medical evaluation immediately.

Severe, life-threatening skin reactions, including fatal cases, have occurred in patients treated with nevirapine. These have included cases of Stevens-Johnson syndrome, toxic epidermal necrolysis, and hypersensitivity reactions characterized by rash, constitutional findings, and organ dysfunction. Patients developing signs or symptoms of severe skin reactions or hypersensitivity reactions must discontinue nevirapine and seek medical evaluation immediately.

WARNING (cont.)

It is essential that patients be monitored intensively during the first 18 weeks of therapy with nevirapine to detect potentially life-threatening hepatotoxicity or skin reactions. The greatest risk of severe rash or hepatic events (often associated with rash) occurs in the first 6 weeks of therapy. However, the risk of any hepatic event, with or without rash, continues past this period and monitoring should continue at frequent intervals. In some cases, hepatic injury has progressed despite discontinuation of treatment. Nevirapine should not be restarted following severe hepatic, skin or hypersensitivity reactions. In addition, the 14-day lead-in period with nevirapine 200 mg daily dosing must be strictly followed.

Indications

➤*HIV infection:* For use in combination with other antiretroviral agents for the treatment of HIV-1 infection.

Administration and Dosage

➤*Approved by the FDA:* June 21, 1996.

➤*Adults:* One 200 mg tablet daily for the first 14 days (this lead-in period should be used because it has been found to lessen the frequency of rash), followed by one 200 mg tablet twice daily, in combination with antiretroviral agents. For concomitantly administered antiretroviral therapy, the manufacturer's recommended dosage and monitoring should be followed.

➤*Children:* The recommended oral dose of nevirapine for pediatric patients 2 months up to 8 years of age is 4 mg/kg once daily for the first 14 days followed by 7 mg/kg twice daily thereafter. For patients 8 years and older the recommended dose is 4 mg/kg once daily for 2 weeks followed by 4 mg/kg twice daily thereafter. The total daily dose should not exceed 400 mg for any patient.

NEVIRAPINE — ORAL

Suspension – Nevirapine suspension should be shaken gently prior to administration. It is important to administer the entire measured dose of suspension by using an oral dosing syringe or dosing cup. An oral dosing syringe is recommended, particularly for volumes of 5 mL or less. If a dosing cup is used, it should be thoroughly rinsed with water and the rinse should also be administered to the patient.

➤*Monitoring of patients:* See Precautions for more information.

➤*Dosage adjustment:* Nevirapine should be discontinued if patients experience severe rash or a rash accompanied by constitutional findings. Patients experiencing rash during the 14-day lead-in period of 200 mg/day (4 mg/kg/day in pediatric patients) should not have their nevirapine dose increased until the rash has resolved.

If clinical hepatitis occurs, nevirapine should be permanently discontinued and not restarted after recovery.

Missed doses – Patients who interrupt nevirapine dosing for more than 7 days should restart the recommended dosing, using one 200 mg tablet daily (4 mg/kg/day in pediatric patients) for the first 14 days (lead-in) followed by one 200 mg tablet twice daily (4 or 7 mg/kg twice daily, according to age, for pediatric patients).

Renal function impairment – An additional 200 mg dose of nevirapine following each dialysis treatment is indicated in patients requiring dialysis. Nevirapine metabolites may accumulate in patients receiving dialysis; however, the clinical significance of this accumulation is not known. Patients with Ccr greater than or equal to 20 mL/min do not require an adjustment in nevirapine dosing.

➤*Storage/Stability:* Store at 25°C (77°F); excursions permitted to 15° to 30°C (59° to 86°F). Store in a safe place out of the reach of children.

Actions

➤*Pharmacology:* Nevirapine is a non-nucleoside reverse transcriptase inhibitor (NNRTI) of HIV-1. Nevirapine binds directly to reverse transcriptase (RT) and blocks the RNA-dependent and DNA-dependent DNA polymerase activities by causing a disruption of the enzyme's catalytic site. The activity of nevirapine does not compete with template or nucleoside triphosphates. HIV-2 RT and eukaryotic DNA polymerases (such as human DNA polymerases α, β, γ, or δ) are not inhibited by nevirapine.

Microbiology –

In vitro HIV susceptibility: The in vitro antiviral activity of nevirapine was measured in peripheral blood mononuclear cells, monocyte-derived macrophages, and lymphoblastoid cell lines. IC_{50} values (50% inhibitory concentration) ranged from 10 to 100 nM against laboratory and clinical isolates of HIV-1. In cell culture, nevirapine demonstrated additive to synergistic activity against HIV in drug combination regimens with zidovudine (ZDV), didanosine (ddI), stavudine (d4T), lamivudine (3TC), saquinavir, and indinavir. The relationship between in vitro susceptibility of HIV-1 to nevirapine and the inhibition of HIV-1 replication in humans has not been established.

Resistance: HIV-1 isolates with reduced susceptibility (100- to 250-fold) to nevirapine emerge in vitro. Genotypic analysis showed mutations in the HIV-1 RT gene Y181C and/or V106A depending upon the virus strain and cell line employed. Time to emergence of nevirapine resistance in vitro was not altered when selection included nevirapine in combination with several other NNRTIs.

Phenotypic and genotypic changes in HIV-1 isolates from patients treated with either nevirapine (n = 24) or nevirapine and ZDV (n = 14) were monitored in Phase I/II trials over 1 to greater than or equal to 12 weeks. After 1 week of nevirapine monotherapy, isolates from 3/3 patients had decreased susceptibility to nevirapine in vitro; 1 or more of the RT mutations K103N, V106A, V1081, Y181C, Y188C, and G190A were detected in HIV-1 isolates from some patients as early as 2 weeks after therapy initiation. By week 8 of nevirapine monotherapy, 100% of the patients tested (n = 24) had HIV-1 isolates with a greater than 100-fold decrease in susceptibility to nevirapine in vitro compared to baseline, and had 1 or more of the nevirapine-associated RT resistance mutations; 19 of 24 patients (80%) had isolates with Y181C mutations regardless of dose. Nevirapine+ZDV combination therapy did not alter the emergence rate of nevirapine-resistant virus or the magnitude of nevirapine resistance in vitro. The clinical relevance of phenotypic and genotypic changes associated with nevirapine therapy has not been established.

Cross-resistance: Rapid emergence of HIV strains which are cross-resistant to NNRTIs has been observed in vitro. Nevirapine-resistant HIV-1 isolates were cross-resistant to the NNRTIs efavirenz and delavirdine. However, nevirapine-resistant isolates were susceptible to the nucleoside analogues ZDV and ddI. Similarly, ZDV-resistant isolates were susceptible to nevirapine in vitro.

➤*Pharmacokinetics:*

Absorption – Nevirapine is readily absorbed (greater than 90%) after oral administration in healthy volunteers and in adults with HIV-1 infection. Absolute bioavailability in 12 healthy adults following single-dose administration was 93 ± 9% (mean ± SD) for a 50 mg tablet and 91 ± 8% for an oral solution. Peak plasma nevirapine concentrations of 2 ± 0.4 mcg/mL (7.5 mcM) were attained by 4 hours following a single 200 mg dose. Following multiple doses, nevirapine peak concentrations appear to increase linearly in the dose range of 200 to 400 mg/day. Steady-state trough nevirapine concentrations of 4.5 ± 1.9 mcg/mL (17 ± 7 mcM), (n = 242) were attained at 400 mg/day. Nevirapine tablets and suspension have been shown to be comparably bioavailable and interchangeable at doses up to 200 mg. When nevirapine (200 mg) was administered to 24 healthy adults (12 female, 12 male), with either a high fat breakfast (857 kcal, 50 g fat, 53% of calories from fat) or antacid (*Maalox* 30 mL), the extent of nevirapine absorption (AUC) was comparable to that observed under fasting conditions. In a separate study in HIV-1-infected patients (n = 6), nevirapine steady-state systemic exposure (AUC_T) was not significantly altered by ddI, which is formulated with an alkaline buffering agent. Nevirapine may be administered with or without food, antacid or ddI.

Distribution – Nevirapine is highly lipophilic and is essentially nonionized at physiologic pH. Following intravenous administration to healthy adults, the apparent volume of distribution (Vdss) of nevirapine was 1.21 ± 0.09 L/kg, suggesting that nevirapine is widely distributed in humans. Nevirapine readily crosses the placenta and is found in breast milk. Nevirapine is about 60% bound to plasma proteins in the plasma concentration range of 1 to 10 mcg/mL. Nevirapine concentrations in human cerebrospinal fluid (n = 6) were 45% (± 5%) of the concentrations in plasma; this ratio is approximately equal to the fraction not bound to plasma protein.

Metabolism/Excretion – In vivo studies in humans and in vitro studies with human liver microsomes have shown that nevirapine is extensively biotransformed via cytochrome P450 (oxidative) metabolism to several hydroxylated metabolites. In vitro studies with human liver microsomes suggest that oxidative metabolism of nevirapine is mediated primarily by cytochrome P450 (CYP) isozymes from the CYP3A and CYP2B6 families, although other isozymes may have a secondary role. In a mass balance/excretion study in 8 healthy male volunteers dosed to steady state with nevirapine 200 mg given twice daily followed by a single 50 mg dose of $_{14}C$-nevirapine, approximately 91.4% ± 10.5% of the radiolabeled dose was recovered, with urine (81.3% ± 11.1%) representing the primary route of excretion compared to feces (10.1% ± 1.5%). Greater than 80% of the radioactivity in urine was made up of glucuronide conjugates of hydroxylated metabolites. Thus cytochrome P450 metabolism, glucuronide conjugation, and urinary excretion of glucuronidated metabolites represent the primary route of nevirapine biotransformation and elimination in humans. Only a small fraction (less than 5%) of the radioactivity in urine (representing less than 3% of the total dose) was made up of parent compound; therefore, renal excretion plays a minor role in elimination of the parent compound.

Nevirapine is an inducer of hepatic cytochrome P450 (CYP) metabolic enzymes 3A4 and 2B6. Nevirapine induces CYP3A4 and CYP2B6 by approximately 20% to 25%, as indicated by erythromycin breath test results and urine metabolites. Autoinduction of CYP3A4 and CYP2B6 mediated metabolism leads to an approximately 1.5- to 2-fold increase in the apparent oral clearance of nevirapine as treatment continues from a single dose to 2 to 4 weeks of dosing with 200 to 400 mg/day. Autoinduction also results in a corresponding decrease in the terminal phase half-life of nevirapine in plasma from approximately 45 hours (single dose) to approximately 25 to 30 hours following multiple dosing with 200 to 400 mg/day.

Special populations –

Renal function impairment: In subjects with renal impairment (mild, moderate or severe), there were no significant changes in the pharmacokinetics of nevirapine. However, subjects requiring dialysis exhibited a 44% reduction in nevirapine AUC over a 1-week exposure period. There was also evidence of accumulation of nevirapine hydroxy-metabolites in plasma in subjects requiring dialysis. An additional 200 mg dose following each dialysis treatment is indicated.

Hepatic function impairment: In the majority of patients with mild or moderate hepatic impairment, no significant changes were seen in the pharmacokinetics of nevirapine. However, a significant increase in the AUC of nevirapine observed in 1 patient with Child-Pugh class B and ascites suggests that patients with worsening hepatic function and ascites may be at risk of accumulating nevirapine in the systemic circulation. Because nevirapine induces its own metabolism with multiple dosing, a single dose study may not reflect the impact of hepatic impairment on multiple dose pharmacokinetics. Nevirapine should not be administered to patients with severe hepatic impairment.

Children: The pharmacokinetics of nevirapine have been studied in 2 open-label studies in children with HIV-1 infection. In 1 study (BI 853; ACTG 165), 9 HIV-1-infected children ranging in age from 9 months to 14 years were administered a single dose (7.5 mg, 30 mg, or 120 mg per m^2; n = 3 per dose) of nevirapine suspension after an overnight fast. The mean nevirapine apparent clearance adjusted for body weight was greater in children compared to adults.

In a multiple dose study (BI 882; ACTG 180), nevirapine suspension or tablets (240 or 400 mg/m^2/day) were administered as monotherapy or in combination with ZDV or ZDV+ddI to 37 HIV-1-infected pediatric patients with the following demographics: Male (54%), racial minority groups (73%), median age of 11 months (range, 2 months to 15 years). The majority of these patients received 120 mg/m^2/day of nevirapine for approximately 4 weeks followed by 120 mg/m^2/twice daily (patients older than 9 years of age) or 200 mg/m^2/twice daily (patients 9 years of age or younger). Nevirapine apparent clearance adjusted for body weight reached maximum values by age 1 to 2 years and then decreased with increasing age. Nevirapine apparent clearance adjusted for body weight was at least 2-fold greater in children younger than 8 years compared to adults. The relationship between nevirapine clearance with long-term drug administration and age is shown in the figure below. The pediatric dosing regimens were selected in order to achieve steady-state plasma concentrations in pediatric patients that approximate those in adults.

Contraindications

Hypersensitivity to any of the components contained in the tablet or the oral suspension.

Warnings

➤*Hepatotoxicity:* In addition, serious hepatotoxicity (including liver failure requiring transplantation in 1 instance) has been reported in HIV-uninfected individuals receiving multiple doses of nevirapine in the setting of post-exposure prophylaxis, an unapproved use.

NEVIRAPINE — ORAL

In general, women have a 3-fold higher risk than men for symptomatic, often rash-associated, hepatic events (5.8% vs 2.2%), and patients with higher CD4 counts at initiation of nevirapine therapy are at higher risk for symptomatic hepatic events with nevirapine. In a retrospective review, women with CD4 counts greater than 250 cells/mm^3 had a 12-fold higher risk of symptomatic hepatic adverse events compared to women with CD4 counts less than 250 cells/mm^3 (11% vs 0.9%). An increased risk was observed in men with CD4 counts greater than 400 cells/mm^3 (6.3% vs 2.3% for men with CD4 counts less than 400 cells/mm^3).

Because increased nevirapine levels and nevirapine accumulation may be observed in patients with serious liver disease, nevirapine should not be administered to patients with severe hepatic impairment.

Intensive clinical and laboratory monitoring, including liver function tests, is essential at baseline and during the first 18 weeks of treatment. Monitoring should continue at frequent intervals thereafter. Liver function tests should be performed if a patient experiences signs or symptoms suggestive of hepatitis and/or hypersensitivity reaction. Liver function tests should also be obtained for all patients who develop a rash in the first 18 weeks of treatment. Physicians and patients should be vigilant for the appearance of signs or symptoms of hepatitis, such as fatigue, malaise, anorexia, nausea, jaundice, bilirubinuria, acholic stools, liver tenderness or hepatomegaly. The diagnosis of hepatotoxicity should be considered in this setting, even if liver function tests are initially normal or alternative diagnoses are possible.

If clinical hepatitis occurs, nevirapine should be permanently discontinued and not restarted after recovery. In some cases, hepatic injury progresses despite discontinuation of treatment.

See the Warning box for more information.

➤*Hypersensitivity reactions:*

Skin reactions – If patients present with a suspected nevirapine-associated rash, liver function tests should be performed. Patients with rash-associated AST or ALT elevations should be permanently discontinued from nevirapine.

Therapy with nevirapine must be initiated with a 14-day lead-in period of 200 mg/day (4 mg/kg/day in pediatric patients), which has been shown to reduce the frequency of rash. If rash is observed during this lead-in period, dose escalation should not occur until the rash has resolved. Patients should be monitored closely if isolated rash of any severity occurs.

Women appear to be at higher risk than men of developing rash with nevirapine.

In a clinical trial, concomitant prednisone use (40 mg/day for the first 14 days of nevirapine administration) was associated with an increase in incidence and severity of rash during the first 6 weeks of nevirapine therapy. Therefore, use of prednisone to prevent nevirapine-associated rash is not recommended.

See the Warning box for more information.

➤*Renal function impairment:* Nevirapine is extensively metabolized by the liver and nevirapine metabolites are extensively eliminated by the kidney. No adjustment in nevirapine dosing is required in patients with Ccr greater than or equal to 20 mL/min. In patients undergoing chronic hemodialysis, an additional 200 mg dose following each dialysis treatment is indicated. Nevirapine metabolites may accumulate in patients receiving dialysis; however, the clinical significance of this accumulation is not known.

➤*Hepatic function impairment:* It is not clear whether a dosing adjustment is needed for patients with mild to moderate hepatic impairment, because multiple dose pharmacokinetic data are not available for this population. However, patients with moderate hepatic impairment and ascites may be at risk of accumulating nevirapine in the systemic circulation. Caution should be exercised when nevirapine is administered to patients with moderate hepatic impairment. Nevirapine should not be administered to patients with severe hepatic impairment.

➤*Carcinogenesis:* Long-term carcinogenicity studies in mice and rats were carried out with nevirapine. Mice were dosed with 0, 50, 375 or 750 mg/kg/day for 2 years. Hepatocellular adenomas and carcinomas were increased at all doses in males and at the 2 high doses in females. In studies in which rats were administered nevirapine at doses of 0, 3.5, 17.5 or 35 mg/kg/day for 2 years, an increase in hepatocellular adenomas was seen in males at all doses and in females at the high dose. The systemic exposure (based on AUCs) at all doses in the 2 animal studies were lower than that measured in humans at the 200 mg twice daily dose. The mechanism of the carcinogenic potential is unknown.

➤*Fertility impairment:* In reproductive toxicology studies, evidence of impaired fertility was seen in female rats at doses providing systemic exposure, based on AUC, approximately equivalent to that provided with the recommended clinical dose of nevirapine.

➤*Elderly:* Clinical studies of nevirapine did not include sufficient numbers of subjects aged 65 and older to determine whether elderly subjects respond differently from younger subjects. In general, dose selection for an elderly patient should be cautious, reflecting the greater frequency of decreased hepatic, renal or cardiac function, and of concomitant disease or other drug therapy.

➤*Pregnancy: Category C.* No observable teratogenicity was detected in reproductive studies performed in pregnant rats and rabbits. In rats, a significant decrease in fetal body weight occurred at doses providing systemic exposure approximately 50% higher, based on AUC, than that seen at the recommended human clinical dose.

The maternal and developmental no-observable-effect level dosages in rats and rabbits produced systemic exposures approximately equivalent to or approximately 50% higher, respectively, than those seen at the recommended daily human dose, based on AUC. There are no adequate and well-controlled studies in pregnant women. Nevirapine should be used during pregnancy only if the potential benefit justifies the potential risk to the fetus. Severe hepatic events, including fatalities, have been reported in pregnant women receiving chronic nevirapine therapy as part of combination treatment of HIV infection. It is unclear if pregnancy augments the already increased risk observed in non-pregnant women.

Antiretroviral pregnancy registry – To monitor maternal-fetal outcomes of pregnant women exposed to nevirapine, an antiretroviral pregnancy registry has been established. Physicians are encouraged to register patients by calling (800) 258-4263.

➤*Lactation:* The Centers for Disease Control and Prevention recommend that HIV-infected mothers not breastfeed their infants to avoid risking postnatal transmission of HIV. Nevirapine is excreted in breast milk. Because of both the potential for HIV transmission and the potential for serious adverse reactions in nursing infants, mothers should be instructed not to breastfeed if they are receiving nevirapine.

➤*Children:* The most frequently reported adverse events related to nevirapine in pediatric patients were similar to those observed in adults, with the exception of granulocytopenia, which was more commonly observed in children. The evaluation of the antiviral activity of nevirapine in pediatric patients is ongoing.

See Actions for more information.

Precautions

➤*Monitoring:* The first 18 weeks of therapy with nevirapine are a critical period during which intensive monitoring of patients is required to detect potentially life-threatening hepatic events and skin reactions. The optimal frequency of monitoring during this time period has not been established. Some experts recommend clinical and laboratory monitoring more often than once per month, and in particular, would include monitoring of liver function tests at baseline, prior to dose escalation and at 2 weeks post dose escalation. After the initial 18-week period, frequent clinical and laboratory monitoring should continue throughout nevirapine treatment. In addition, the 14-day lead-in period with nevirapine 200 mg daily dosing has been demonstrated to reduce the frequency of rash. In some cases, hepatic injury has progressed despite discontinuation of treatment.

➤*Opportunistic infections:* The duration of clinical benefit from antiretroviral therapy may be limited. Patients receiving nevirapine or any other antiretroviral therapy may continue to develop opportunistic infections and other complications of HIV infection, and therefore should remain under close clinical observation by physicians experienced in the treatment of patients with associated HIV diseases.

➤*Fat redistribution:* Redistribution/accumulation of body fat including central obesity, dorsocervical fat enlargement (buffalo hump), peripheral wasting, facial wasting, breast enlargement, and "cushingoid appearance" have been observed in patients receiving antiretroviral therapy. The mechanism and long-term consequences of these events are currently unknown. A causal relationship has not been established.

➤*Superinfection:* Resistant virus emerges rapidly and uniformly when nevirapine is administered as monotherapy. Therefore, nevirapine should always be administered in combination with other antiretroviral agents for the treatment of HIV-1 infection.

Drug Interactions

➤*Cytochrome P-450 system:* Nevirapine is principally metabolized by the liver via the cytochrome P450 isoenzymes, 3A4 and 2B6. Nevirapine is known to be an inducer of these enzymes. As a result, drugs that are metabolized by these enzyme systems may have lower than expected plasma levels when coadministered with nevirapine.

Nevirapine Drug Interactions

Precipitant drug	Object drug*		Description
Fluconazole	Nevirapine	↑	Nevirapine concentrations may be increased. Use with caution.
Rifamycins (eg, rifampin, rifabutin)	Nevirapine	↓	Nevirapine plasma concentrations may be reduced and, therefore, should not be used with rifampin. When treating tuberculosis, use rifabutin instead. Rifabutin and its metabolite concentrations are moderately increased when coadministered with nevirapine. Use this combination with caution. Rifampin AUC also may increase slightly.
Nevirapine	Rifamycins (eg, rifampin, rifabutin)	↑	
St. John's wort	Nevirapine	↓	Nevirapine concentrations may be reduced because of increased hepatic metabolism. Coadministration is not recommended.
Nevirapine	Clarithromycin	↑↓	Clarithromycin exposure may be decreased; however, the active metabolite concentration may be increased. Consider an alternative to clarithromycin such as azithromycin.

NEVIRAPINE — ORAL

Nevirapine Drug Interactions			
Precipitant drug	Object drug*		Description
Nevirapine	Contraceptives, oral	⬇	Reduced oral contraceptive efficacy may occur. An alternative nonhormonal or additional method of contraception is recommended.
Nevirapine	Efavirenz	⬇	Efavirenz plasma concentration may be decreased. Appropriate dose for this combination has not been established.
Nevirapine	Ketoconazole	⬇	Ketoconazole plasma concentrations may be decreased. Do not coadminister.
Nevirapine	Methadone	⬇	Methadone levels may be decreased. Adjust methadone dose as needed. Narcotic withdrawal syndrome has been reported.
Nevirapine	Protease inhibitors	⬇	Nevirapine may decrease plasma levels and clinical efficacy of protease inhibitors. An increase in indinavir and saquinavir dose may be required. A dose increase of lopinavir/ritonavir to 533/133 mg twice daily with food is recommended.
Nevirapine	Warfarin	⬇	The anticoagulant effect of warfarin may be decreased. Monitor coagulation parameters and adjust warfarin dose as needed.
Nevirapine	Zidovudine	⬇	Coadministration decreased zidovudine AUC and C_{max} 28% and 30%, respectively.

* ⬆ = Object drug increased. ⬇ = Object drug decreased.
⬌ = Undetermined clinical effect.
[a] Based on reports of narcotic withdrawal syndrome in patients treated with nevirapine and methadone concurrently, and evidence of decreased plasma concentrations of methadone.

Potential drug interactions: Use with caution, dose adjustment of coadministered drug may be needed due to possible decrease in clinical effect	
Examples of drugs in which plasma concentrations may be decreased by coadministration with nevirapine	
Drug class	Examples of drugs
Antiarrhythmics	Amiodarone, disopyramide, lidocaine
Anticonvulsants	Carbamazepine, clonazepam, ethosuximide
Antifungals	Itraconazole
Calcium channel blockers	Diltiazem, nifedipine, verapamil
Cancer chemotherapy	Cyclophosphamide
Ergot alkaloids	Ergotamine
Immunosuppressants	Cyclosporine, tacrolimus, sirolimus
Motility agents	Cisapride
Opiate agonists	Fentanyl
Examples of drugs in which plasma concentrations may be increased by coadministration with nevirapine	
Antithrombotics	Warfarin: Potential effect on anticoagulation. Monitoring of anticoagulation levels is recommended.

Adverse Reactions

➤*Adults:* Clinical practice has shown that the most serious adverse reactions associated with nevirapine are clinical hepatitis/hepatic failure, Stevens-Johnson syndrome, toxic epidermal necrolysis, and hypersensitivity reactions. Clinical hepatitis/hepatic failure may be isolated or associated with signs of hypersensitivity which may include severe rash or rash accompanied by fever, general malaise, fatigue, muscle or joint aches, blisters, oral lesions, conjunctivitis, facial edema, and/or hepatitis, eosinophilia, granulocytopenia, lymphadenopathy, and renal dysfunction.

Hepatic – Severe and life-threatening hepatotoxicity, and fatal fulminant hepatitis have been reported in patients treated with nevirapine. Hepatic adverse events have been reported to occur more frequently during the first 18 weeks of treatment, but such events may occur at any time during treatment.

In controlled clinical trials, clinical hepatic events regardless of severity occurred in 4% (range 2.5% to 11%) of patients who received nevirapine and 1.2% of patients in control groups. Transaminase elevations (ALT or AST greater than 5 × ULN) were observed in 8.8% of patients receiving nevirapine and 6.2% of patients in control groups in clinical trials. In a retrospective analysis of controlled and uncontrolled clinical trials, patients with higher CD4 counts at initiation of nevirapine therapy, particularly women, were at greater risk for acute symptomatic hepatic events, including death, especially in the firs 6 weeks of therapy. Patients with chronic hepatitis B or C infection were at higher risk for later hepatic events.

Dermatologic – The most common clinical toxicity of nevirapine is rash. Severe or life-threatening rash occurred in approximately 2% of nevirapine-treated patients, most frequently within the first 6 weeks of therapy (see table below). Rashes are usually mild to moderate, maculopapular or erythematous cutaneous eruptions, with or without pruritus, located on the trunk, face, and extremities. Women tend to be at higher risk for development of nevirapine-associated rash.

Risk of rash (%) in adult placebo controlled trials[1] regardless of causality			
Through 6 weeks of treatment[2]		Nevirapine (n = 1374) %	Placebo (n = 1331) %
Rash events of all grades[3]		14.8%	5.9%
Grade 1	Erythema, pruritus	8.5%	4.2%
Grade 2	Diffuse maculopapular rash, dry desquamation	4.8%	1.6%
Grade 3 or 4	Grade 3: Vesiculation, moist desquamation, ulceration; Grade 4: Erythema multiforme, necrolysis, necrosis requiring surgery, exfoliative dermatitis	1.5%	0.1%
Through 52 weeks of treatment[2]			
Rash events of all grades[3]		24%	14.9%
Grade 1	See above	15.5%	10.8%
Grade 2	See above	7.1%	3.9%
Grade 3 or 4	See above	1.7%	0.2%
Proportion of patients who discontinued treatment due to rash		4.3%	1.2%

[1] Trials 1037, 1038, 1046, and 1090.
[2] Percentage based on Kaplan-Meier probability estimates.
[3] NCI grading system.

Percentage of patients with moderate or severe drug related events in adult placebo controlled trials				
	Trial 1090[1]		Trials 1037, 1038, 1046[2]	
	Nevirapine (n = 1121)	Placebo (n = 1128)	Nevirapine (n = 253)	Placebo (n = 203)
Median exposure (weeks)	58	52	28	28
Any adverse event	14.5%	11.1%	31.6%	13.3%
Rash	5.1%	1.8%	6.7%	1.5%
Abnormal LFTs	1.2%	0.9%	6.7%	1.5%
Nausea	0.5%	1.1%	8.7%	3.9%
Granulocytopenia	1.8%	2.8%	0.4%	0%
Headache	0.7%	0.4%	3.6%	0.5%
Fatigue	0.2%	0.3%	4.7%	3.9%
Diarrhea	0.2%	0.8%	2%	0.5%
Abdominal pain	0.1%	0.4%	2%	0%
Myalgia	0.2%	0%	1.2%	2%

[1] Background therapy included 3TC for all patients and combinations of NRTIs and PIs. Patients had CD4+ cell counts less than 200 cells/mm^3.
[2] Background therapy included ZDV and ZDV+ddl; nevirapine monotherapy was administered in some patients. Patients had CD4+ cell counts greater than or equal to 200 cells/mm^3.

Lab test abnormalities – Liver function test abnormalities (AST, ALT) were observed more frequently in patients receiving nevirapine than in controls (see table below). Asymptomatic elevations in GGT occur frequently but are not a contraindication to continue nevirapine therapy in the absence of elevations in other liver function tests. Other laboratory abnormalities (bilirubin, anemia, neutropenia, thrombocytopenia) were observed with similar frequencies in clinical trials comparing nevirapine and control regimens (see table below).

NEVIRAPINE — ORAL

Percentage of adult patients with laboratory abnormalities				
	Trial 1090[1]		Trials 1037, 1038, 1046[2]	
Laboratory abnormality	Nevirapine (n = 1121)	Placebo (n = 1128)	Nevirapine (n = 253)	Placebo (n = 203)
Blood chemistry				
ALT > 250 U/L	5.3%	4.4%	14%	4%
AST > 250 U/L	3.7%	2.5%	7.6%	1.5%
Bilirubin > 2.5 mg/dL	1.7%	2.2%	1.7%	1.5%
Hematology				
Hemoglobin < 8 g/dL	3.2%	4.1%	0%	0%
Platelets < 50,000/mm³	1.3%	1%	0.4%	1.5%
Neutrophils < 750/mm³	13.3%	13.5%	3.6%	1%

[1] Background therapy included 3TC for all patients and combinations of NRTIs and PIs. Patients had CD4+ cell counts less than 200 cells/mm³.
[2] Background therapy included ZDV and ZDV+ddI; nevirapine monotherapy was administered in some patients. Patients had CD4+ cell counts greater than or equal to 200 cells/mm³.

Because clinical hepatitis has been reported in nevirapine-treated patients, intensive clinical and laboratory monitoring, including liver function tests, is essential at baseline and during the first 18 weeks of treatment. Monitoring should continue at frequent intervals thereafter, depending on the patient's clinical status.

➤*Postmarketing:*

CNS – Paraesthesia.

Dermatologic – Allergic reactions including anaphylaxis, angioedema, bullous eruptions, ulcerative stomatitis and urticaria have all been reported. In addition, hypersensitivity syndrome and hypersensitivity reactions with rash associated with constitutional findings such as fever, blistering, oral lesions, conjunctivitis, facial edema, muscle or joint aches, general malaise, fatigue or significant hepatic abnormalities plus 1 or more of the following: Hepatitis, eosinophilia, granulocytopenia, lymphadenopathy and/or renal dysfunction have been reported with the use of nevirapine.

GI – Vomiting.

Hematologic – Anemia, eosinophilia, neutropenia.

Hepatic – Jaundice, fulminant and cholestatic hepatitis, hepatic necrosis, hepatic failure.

Musculoskeletal – Arthralgia.

Miscellaneous – Fever, somnolence, drug withdrawal, redistribution/accumulation of body fat.

➤*Children:* Safety was assessed in trial BI 882 in which patients were followed for a mean duration of 33.9 months (range: 6.8 months to 5.3 years, including long-term follow-up in 29 of these patients in trial BI 892). The most frequently reported adverse events related to nevirapine in pediatric patients were similar to those observed in adults, with the exception of granulocytopenia, which was more commonly observed in children. Serious adverse events were assessed in ACTG 245, a double-blind, placebo-controlled trial of nevirapine (n = 305) in which pediatric patients received combination treatment with nevirapine. In this trial, 2 patients were reported to experience Stevens-Johnson syndrome or Stevens-Johnson/toxic epidermal necrolysis transition syndrome. Cases of allergic reaction, including 1 case of anaphylaxis, were also reported.

Number of pediatric patients (%) with laboratory abnormalities in trials BI 882 and BI 892 combined	
	Number (%) of patients (n = 37)
Blood chemistry	
Increased ALT (> 250 U/L)	4 (11%)
Increased AST (> 250 U/L)	5 (14%)
Increased GGT (> 450 U/L)	4 (11%)
Increased total bilirubin (> 2.5 mg/dL)	1 (3%)
Increased alkaline phosphate (> 2 × ULN)	19 (51%)
Increased amylase (> 2 × ULN)	6 (16%)
Hematology	
Decreased Hg (< 8 g/dL)	7 (19%)
Decreased platelets (< 50,000/mm³)	4 (11%)
Decreased neutrophils (< 750/mm³)	14 (38%)
Increased MCV (> 100 F/L)	13 (35%)

Overdosage

➤*Symptoms:* Cases of nevirapine overdose at doses ranging from 800 to 1800 mg per day for up to 15 days have been reported. Patients have experienced events including edema, erythema nodosum, fatigue, fever, headache, insomnia, nausea, pulmonary infiltrates, rash, vertigo, vomiting and weight decrease.

➤*Treatment:* There is no known antidote for nevirapine overdosage. All events subsided following discontinuation of nevirapine.

Patient Information

Patients should be informed of the possibility of severe liver disease or skin reactions associated with nevirapine that may result in death. Patients developing signs or symptoms of liver disease or severe skin reactions should be instructed to discontinue nevirapine and seek medical attention immediately, including performance of laboratory monitoring. Symptoms of liver disease include fatigue, malaise, anorexia, nausea, jaundice, acholic stools, liver tenderness or hepatomegaly. Symptoms of severe skin or hypersensitivity reactions include rash accompanied by fever, general malaise, fatigue, muscle or joint aches, blisters, oral lesions, conjunctivitis, facial edema and/or hepatitis.

Intensive clinical and laboratory monitoring, including liver function tests, is essential during the first 18 weeks of therapy with nevirapine to detect potentially life-threatening hepatotoxicity. However, liver disease can occur after this period, therefore monitoring should continue at frequent intervals throughout nevirapine treatment. Extra vigilance is warranted during the first 6 weeks of therapy, which is the period of greatest risk of hepatic events and skin reactions. Patients with signs and symptoms of hepatitis should discontinue nevirapine and seek medical evaluation immediately. If nevirapine is discontinued due to hepatitis, it should not be restarted. Patients should be advised that coinfection with hepatitis B or C and/or increased liver function tests at the start of antiretroviral therapy are associated with a greater risk of hepatic events with nevirapine. Patients, particularly women, with increased CD4+ cell count at initiation of nevirapine therapy (greater than 250 cells/mm³ in women and greater than 400 cells/mm³ in men) may be at substantially higher risk for development of hepatic events, often associated with rash.

The majority of rashes associated with nevirapine occur within the first 6 weeks of initiation of therapy. Patients should be instructed that if any rash occurs during the 2-week lead-in period, the nevirapine dose should not be escalated until the rash resolves. Any patient experiencing severe rash or hypersensitivity reactions should discontinue nevirapine and consult a physician. Nevirapine should be not be restarted following severe skin rash or hypersensitivity reaction. Women tend to be at higher risk for development of nevirapine-associated rash.

Oral contraceptives and other hormonal methods of birth control should not be used as a method of contraception in women taking nevirapine, since nevirapine may lower the plasma levels of these medications. Additionally, when oral contraceptives are used for hormonal regulation during nevirapine therapy, the therapeutic effect of the hormonal therapy should be monitored.

Patients should be informed that nevirapine therapy has not been shown to reduce the risk of transmission of HIV-1 to others through sexual contact or blood contamination. The long-term effects of nevirapine are unknown at this time.

Nevirapine is not a cure for HIV-1 infection; patients may continue to experience illnesses associated with advanced HIV-1 infection, including opportunistic infections. Patients should be advised to remain under the care of a physician when using nevirapine.

Patients should be informed to take nevirapine every day as prescribed. Patients should not alter the dose without consulting their doctor. If a dose is missed, patients should take the next dose as soon as possible. However, if a dose is skipped, the patient should not double the next dose. Patients should be advised to report to their doctor the use of any other medications. Based on the known metabolism of methadone, nevirapine may decrease plasma concentrations of methadone by increasing its hepatic metabolism. Narcotic withdrawal syndrome has been reported in patients treated with nevirapine and methadone concomitantly. Methadone-maintained patients beginning nevirapine therapy should be monitored for evidence of withdrawal and methadone dose should be adjusted accordingly.

Nevirapine may interact with some drugs; therefore, patients should be advised to report to their doctor the use of any other prescription, nonprescription medication or herbal products, particularly St. John's wort.

Patients should be informed that redistribution or accumulation of body fat may occur in patients receiving antiretroviral therapy and that the cause and long-term health effects of these conditions are not known at this time.

DELAVIRDINE MESYLATE

Rx	**Rescriptor** (Agouron)	**Tablets:** 100 mg	Lactose. (U 3761). White, capsule shape. In 360s.
		200 mg	Lactose. (RESCRIPTOR 200 mg). White, capsule shape. In 180s.

DELAVIRDINE MESYLATE — ORAL

WARNING

Delavirdine tablets are indicated for the treatment of HIV-1 infection in combination with appropriate antiretroviral agents when therapy is warranted. This indication is based on surrogate marker changes in clinical studies. Clinical benefit was not demonstrated for delavirdine based on survival or incidence of AIDS-defining clinical events in a completed trial comparing delavirdine plus didanosine with didanosine monotherapy.

Resistant virus emerges rapidly when delavirdine is administered as monotherapy. Therefore, always administer delavirdine in combination with appropriate antiretroviral therapy.

Indications

➤*HIV infection:* For the treatment of HIV-1 (human immunodeficiency virus type 1) infection in combination with at least 2 other active antiretroviral agents when therapy is warranted.

Administration and Dosage

➤*Approved by the FDA:* April 4, 1997.

The recommended dosage for delavirdine mesylate tablets is 400 mg (four 100 mg or two 200 mg tablets) 3 times daily. Delavirdine mesylate should be used in combination with other appropriate antiretroviral therapy.

The 100 mg delavirdine mesylate tablets may be dispersed in water prior to consumption. To prepare a dispersion, add four 100 mg delavirdine mesylate tablets to at least 3 ounces of water; allow to stand for a few minutes, and then stir until a uniform dispersion occurs (see Pharmacokinetics, Absorption). The dispersion should be consumed promptly. The glass should be rinsed with water and the rinse swallowed to insure the entire dose is consumed. The 200 mg tablets should be taken as intact tablets, because they are not readily dispersed in water.

Delavirdine mesylate tablets may be administered with or without food (see Pharmacokinetics). Patients with achlorhydria should take delavirdine mesylate with an acidic beverage (eg, orange or cranberry juice). However, the effect of an acidic beverage on the absorption of delavirdine in patients with achlorhydria has not been investigated.

➤*Concurrent antacid administration:* Patients taking both delavirdine mesylate and antacids should be advised to take them at least 1 hour apart.

➤*Storage/Stability:* Store at controlled room temperature 20° to 25°C (68° to 77°F). Keep container tightly closed. Protect from high humidity.

Actions

➤*Pharmacokinetics:*

Absorption – Delavirdine is rapidly absorbed following oral administration, with peak plasma concentrations occurring at approximately 1 hour. Following administration of delavirdine 400 mg 3 times a day (n = 67, HIV-1-infected patients), the mean ± SD steady-state peak plasma concentration (C_{max}) was 35 ± 20 mcM (range, 2 to 100 mcM), systemic exposure (AUC) was 180 ± 100 mcM•hr (range, 5 to 515 mcM•hr) and trough concentration (C_{min}) was 15 ± 10 mcM (range, 0.1 to 45 mcM). The single-dose bioavailability of delavirdine tablets relative to an oral solution was 85 ± 25% (n = 16, non-HIV-infected subjects). The single-dose bioavailability of delavirdine tablets (100 mg strength) was increased by approximately 20% when a slurry of drug was prepared by allowing delavirdine tablets to disintegrate in water before administration (n = 16, non-HIV-infected subjects). The bioavailability of the 200 mg strength delavirdine tablets has not been evaluated when administered as a slurry, because they are not readily dispersed in water (see Administration and Dosage).

Delavirdine may be administered with or without food. In a multiple-dose study, delavirdine was administered every 8 hours with food or every 8 hours, 1 hour before or 2 hours after a meal (n = 13, HIV-1-infected patients). Patients remained on their typical diet throughout the study; meal content was not standardized. When multiple doses of delavirdine were administered with food, mean C_{max} was reduced by 22% but AUC and C_{min} were not altered.

Distribution – Delavirdine is extensively bound (≈ 98%) to plasma proteins, primarily albumin. The percentage of delavirdine that is protein bound is constant over a delavirdine concentration range of 0.5 to 196 mcM. In 5 HIV-1-infected patients whose total daily dose of delavirdine ranged from 600 to 1200 mg, cerebrospinal fluid concentrations of delavirdine averaged 0.4% ± 0.07% of the corresponding plasma delavirdine concentrations; this represents about 20% of the fraction not bound to plasma proteins. Steady-state delavirdine concentrations in saliva (n = 5, HIV-1-infected patients who received delavirdine 400 mg 3 times a day) and semen (n = 5 healthy volunteers who received delavirdine 300 mg 3 times a day) were about 6% and 2%, respectively, of the corresponding plasma delavirdine concentrations collected at the end of a dosing interval.

Metabolism/Excretion – Delavirdine is extensively converted to several inactive metabolites. Delavirdine is primarily metabolized by cytochrome P450 3A (CYP3A), but in vitro data suggest that delavirdine may also be metabolized by CYP2D6. The major metabolic pathways for delavirdine are N-desalkylation and pyridine hydroxylation. Delavirdine exhibits nonlinear steady-state elimination pharmacokinetics, with apparent oral clearance decreasing by about 22-fold as the total daily dose of delavirdine increases from 60 to 1200 mg/day. In a study of ^{14}C-delavirdine in 6 healthy volunteers who received multiple doses of delavirdine tablets 300 mg 3 times a day, approximately 44% of the radiolabeled dose was recovered in feces, and approximately 51% of the dose was excreted in urine. Less than 5% of the dose was recovered unchanged in urine. The apparent plasma half-life of delavirdine increases with dose; mean half-life following 400 mg 3 times a day is 5.8 hours, with a range of 2 to 11 hours.

In vitro and in vivo studies have shown that delavirdine reduces CYP3A activity and inhibits its own metabolism. In vitro studies have also shown that delavirdine reduces CYP2C9, CYP2D6, and CYP2C19 activity. Inhibition of CYP3A by delavirdine is reversible within 1 week after discontinuation of drug.

➤*Microbiology:* Delavirdine is a non-nucleoside reverse transcriptase inhibitor (NNRTI) of HIV-1. Delavirdine binds directly to reverse transcriptase (RT) and blocks RNA-dependent and DNA-dependent DNA polymerase activities. Delavirdine does not compete with template: primer or deoxynucleoside triphosphates. HIV-2 RT and human cellular DNA polymerases α, γ, or δ are not inhibited by delavirdine. In addition, HIV-1 group O, a group of highly divergent strains that are uncommon in North America, may not be inhibited by delavirdine.

In vitro HIV-1 susceptibility – In vitro anti-HIV-1 activity of delavirdine was assessed by infecting cell lines of lymphoblastic and monocytic origin and peripheral blood lymphocytes with laboratory and clinical isolates of HIV-1. IC_{50} and IC_{90} values (50% and 90% inhibitory concentrations) for laboratory isolates (n = 5) ranged from 0.005 to 0.03 mcM and 0.04 to 0.1 mcM, respectively. Mean IC_{50} of clinical isolates (n = 74) was 0.038 mcM (range, 0.001 to 0.69 mcM); 73 of 74 clinical isolates had an $IC_{50} \le 0.18$ mcM. The IC_{90} of 24 of these clinical isolates ranged from 0.05 to 0.1 mcM. In drug combination studies of delavirdine with zidovudine, didanosine, zalcitabine, lamivudine, interferon-α, and protease inhibitors, additive to synergistic anti-HIV-1 activity was observed in cell culture. The relationship between the in vitro susceptibility of HIV-1 RT inhibitors and the inhibition of HIV replication in humans has not been established.

Drug resistance – Phenotypic analyses of isolates from patients treated with delavirdine as monotherapy showed a 50-fold to 500-fold reduction in sensitivity in 14 of 15 patients by week 8 of therapy. Genotypic analyses of HIV-1 isolates from patients receiving delavirdine plus zidovudine combination therapy (n = 79) showed resistance conferring mutations in all isolates by week 24 of therapy. In delavirdine treated patients the mutations in RT occurred predominantly at amino acid positions 103 and less frequently at positions 181 and 236. In a separate study, an average 86-fold increase in the zidovudine susceptibility of patient isolates (n = 24) was observed after 24 weeks on delavirdine and zidovudine combination therapy. The clinical relevance of the phenotypic and the genotypic changes associated with delavirdine therapy has not been determined.

Cross-resistance – Delavirdine may confer cross-resistance to other NNRTIs when used alone or in combination. Mutations at positions 103 or 181 has been found in resistant virus during treatment with delavirdine and other NNRTIs. These mutations have been associated with cross-resistance among NNRTIs in vitro.

Contraindications

Hypersensitivity to delavirdine or any of its ingredients. Coadministration of delavirdine mesylate is contraindicated with drugs that are highly dependent on CYP3A for clearance and for which elevated plasma concentrations are associated with serious or life-threatening events.

Drugs that are contraindicated with delavirdine mesylate	
Drug class	Drugs within class that are contraindicated with delavirdine mesylate
Antihistamines	Astemizole, terfenadine
Ergot derivatives	Dihydroergotamine, ergonovine, ergotamine, methylergonovine
GI motility agent	Cisapride
Neuroleptic	Pimozide
Sedative/hypnotics	Alprazolam, midazolam, triazolam

Warnings

➤*Cytochrome P-450 inhibition:* Coadministration of delavirdine mesylate with certain nonsedating antihistamines, sedative hypnotics, antiarrhythmics, calcium channel blockers, ergot alkaloid preparations, amphetamines, cisapride, and sildenafil, may result in potentially serious or life-threatening adverse events due to possible effects of delavirdine mesylate on the hepatic metabolism of certain drugs (see Drug Interactions).

➤*Hepatic function impairment:* Delavirdine is metabolized primarily by the liver. Therefore, caution should be exercised when administering delavirdine mesylate tablets to patients with impaired hepatic function.

➤*Carcinogenesis:* Lifetime carcinogenicity studies were conducted in rats at doses of 10, 32, and 100 mg/kg/day, in mice at doses of 62.5, 250, and 500 mg/kg/day for males, and 62.5, 125, and 250 mg/kg/day for females. In rats, delavirdine was noncarcinogenic at maximally tolerated doses that produced exposures (AUC) up to 12 (male rats) and 9 (female rats) times human exposure at the recommended clinical dose. In mice, delavirdine produced significant increases in the incidence of hepatocellular adenoma/adenocarcinoma in both males and females, hepatocellular adenoma in females, and mesenchymal urinary bladder tumors in males. The systemic drug exposures (AUC) in female mice were given 0.5 to 3 fold and in male mice 0.2 to 4 fold of those in humans at the recommended clinical dose. Given the lack of genotoxic activity of delavirdine, the relevance of urinary bladder and hepatocellular neoplasm in delavirdine-treated mice to humans in not known.

DELAVIRDINE MESYLATE — ORAL

➤*Elderly:* Clinical studies of delavirdine did not include sufficient numbers of subjects aged 65 and older to determine whether they respond differently from younger subjects. In general, caution should be taken when dosing delavirdine in elderly patients due to the greater frequency of decreased hepatic, renal or cardiac function and of concomitant disease or other drug therapy.

➤*Pregnancy: Category C.*

Delavirdine has been shown to be teratogenic in rats. Delavirdine caused ventricular septal defects in rats at doses of 50, 100, and 200 mg/kg/day when administered during the period of organogenesis. The lowest dose of delavirdine that caused malformations produced systemic exposures in pregnant rats equal to or lower than the expected human exposure to delavirdine mesylate (C_{min} 15 mcM) at the recommended dose. Exposure in rats approximately 5-fold higher than the expected human exposure resulted in marked maternal toxicity, embryotoxicity, fetal developmental delay, and reduced pup survival. Additionally, reduced pup survival on postpartum day 0 occurred at an exposure (mean C_{min}) approximately equal to the expected human exposure.

Delavirdine at doses of 200 and 400 mg/kg/day administered during the period of organogenesis caused maternal toxicity, embryotoxicity, and abortions in rabbits. The lowest dose of delavirdine that resulted in these toxic effects produced systemic exposures in pregnant rabbits approximately 6-fold higher than the expected human exposure to delavirdine mesylate (C_{min} 15 mcM) at the recommended dose. The no-observed-adverse-effect dose in the pregnant rabbit was 100 mg/kg/day. Various malformations were observed at this dose, but the incidence of such malformations was not statistically significantly different from those observed in the control group. Systemic exposures in pregnant rabbits at a dose of 100 mg/kg/day were lower than those expected in humans at the recommended clinical dose. Malformations were not apparent at 200 and 400 mg/kg/day; however, only a limited number of fetuses were available for examination as a result of maternal and embryo death.

No adequate and well-controlled studies in pregnant women have been conducted. Delavirdine mesylate should be used during pregnancy only if the potential benefit justifies the potential risk to the fetus. Of 9 pregnancies reported in premarketing clinical studies and postmarketing experience, a total of 10 infants were born (including 1 set of twins). Eight of the infants were born healthy. One infant was born HIV-positive but was otherwise healthy and with no congenital abnormalities detected, and 1 infant was born prematurely (34 to 35 weeks) with a small muscular ventricular septal defect that spontaneously resolved. The patient received approximately 6 weeks of treatment with delavirdine and zidovudine early in the course of the pregnancy.

Antiretroviral pregnancy registry – To monitor maternal-fetal outcomes of pregnant women exposed to delavirdine and other antiretroviral agents, an Antiretroviral Pregnancy Registry has been established. Physicians are encouraged to register patients by calling (800) 258–4263.

➤*Lactation:* Delavirdine was excreted in the milk of lactating rats at a concentration 3 to 5 times that of rat plasma.

The US public health services Centers for Disease Control and Prevention advises HIV-infected women not to breastfeed to avoid postnatal transmission of HIV. Because of both the potential for HIV transmission and any possible adverse reactions in nursing infants, mothers should be instructed not to breastfeed if they are receiving delavirdine.

➤*Children:* Safety and effectiveness of delavirdine in combination with other antiretroviral agents have not been established in HIV-1-infected individuals younger than 16 years of age.

Precautions

➤*Resistance/cross-resistance:* Non-nucleoside reverse transcriptase inhibitors, when used alone or in combination, may confer cross-resistance to other nonnucleoside reverse transcriptase inhibitors.

➤*Fat redistribution:* Redistribution/accumulation of body fat including central obesity, dorsocervical fat enlargement (buffalo hump), peripheral wasting, facial wasting, breast enlargement, and "cushingoid appearance" have been observed in patients receiving antiretroviral therapy. The mechanism and long-term consequences of these events are currently unknown. A causal relationship has not been established.

➤*Skin rash:* Severe rash including rare cases of erythema multiforme and Stevens-Johnson syndrome have been reported in patients receiving delavirdine mesylate. Erythema multiforme and Stevens-Johnson syndrome were rarely seen in clinical trials and resolved after withdrawal of delavirdine mesylate. Any patient experiencing severe rash or rash accompanied by symptoms such as fever, blistering, oral lesions, conjunctivitis, swelling, muscle or joint aches should discontinue delavirdine mesylate and consult a physician. Two cases of Stevens-Johnsons syndrome have been reported through postmarketing surveillance out of a total of 339 surveillance reports.

In studies 21 part II and 13C, rash (including maculopapular rash) was reported in more patients who were treated with delavirdine mesylate 400 mg 3 times a day (35% and 32%, respectively) than in those who were not treated with delavirdine mesylate (21% and 16%, respectively). The highest intensity of rash reported in these studies was severe (grade 3), which was observed in approximately 4% of patients treated with delavirdine in each study and in none of the patients who were not treated with delavirdine mesylate. Also in studies 21 part II and 13C, discontinuations due to rash were reported in more patients who received delavirdine mesylate 400 mg 3 times a day (3% and 4%, respectively) than in those who did not receive delavirdine mesylate (0% and 1%, respectively). In most cases, the duration of the rash was less than 2 weeks and did not require dose reduction or discontinuation of delavirdine mesylate. Most patients were able to resume therapy after rechallenge with delavirdine mesylate following a treatment interruption due to rash. The distribution of the rash was mainly on the upper body and proximal arms, with decreasing intensity of the lesions on the neck and face, and progressively less on the rest of the trunk and limbs. Occurrence of a delavirdine-associated rash after 1 month is uncommon. Symptomatic relief has been obtained using diphenhydramine hydrochloride, hydroxyzine hydrochloride, or topical corticosteroids.

Drug Interactions

➤*Serious drug interactions:* Because delavirdine may inhibit the metabolism of many different drugs (eg, antiarrhythmics, calcium channel blockers, sedative hypnotics and others), serious or life-threatening drug interactions could result from inappropriate coadministration of some drugs with delavirdine. In addition, some drugs may markedly reduce delavirdine plasma concentrations, resulting suboptimal antiviral activity and subsequent emergence of drug resistance. All prescribers should become familiar with the data available in this section and in Contraindications, Warnings, and Pharmacokinetics.

➤*Cytochrome P-450 system:* Delavirdine is an inhibitor of CYP3A isoform and other CYP isoforms to a lesser extent including CYP2C9, CYP2D6, and CYP2C19. Coadministration of delavirdine and drugs primarily metabolized by CYP3A (eg, HMG-CoA reductase inhibitors and sildenafil) may result in increased plasma concentrations of the coadministered drug that could increase or prolong both its therapeutic or adverse effects.

Delavirdine is metabolized primarily by CYP3A, but in vitro data suggest that delavirdine may also be metabolized by CYP2D6. Coadministration of delavirdine and drugs that induce CYP3A, such as rifampin, may decrease delavirdine plasma concentrations and reduce its therapeutic effect. Coadministration of delavirdine and drugs that inhibit CYP3A may increase delavirdine plasma concentrations. See the following table:

Drugs that should not be coadministered with delavirdine mesylate

Drug class: drug name	Clinical comment
Anticonvulsant agents: phenytoin, phenobarbital, and carbamazepine	May lead to loss of virologic response and possible resistance to delavirdine or to the class of nonnucleoside reverse transcriptase inhibitors.
Antihistamines: astemizole and terfenadine	Contraindicated due to potential for serious or life-threatening reactions such as cardiac arrhythmias.
Antimycobacterials: rifabutin*, rifampin*	May lead to loss of virologic response and possible resistance to delavirdine mesylate or to the class of nonnucleoside reverse transcriptase inhibitors or other coadministered antiviral agents.
Ergot derivatives: dihydroergotamine, ergonovine, ergotamine, methylergonovine	Contraindicated due to potential for serious or life-threatening reactions such as acute ergot toxicity characterized by peripheral vasospasm and ischemia of the extremities and other tissues.
GI motility agent: cisapride	Contraindicated due to potential for serious or life-threatening reactions such as cardiac arrhythmias.
Herbal products: St. John's wort (*hypericum perforatum*)	May lead to loss of virologic response and possible resistance to delavirdine mesylate or to the class of nonnucleoside reverse transcriptase inhibitors
HMG-CoA reductase inhibitors: lovastatin, simvastatin	Potential for serious reactions such as risk of myopathy including rhabdomyolysis.
Neuroleptic: pimozide	Contraindicated due to potential for serious or life-threatening reactions such as cardiac arrhythmias.
Sedative/hypnotics: alprazolam, midazolam, triazolam	Contraindicated due to potential for serious or life-threatening reactions such as prolonged or increased sedation or respiratory depression.

* See Pharmacokinetics for magnitude of interactions.

DELAVIRDINE MESYLATE — ORAL

Delavirdine Drug Interactions

Precipitant drug	Object drug*		Description
Antacids	Delavirdine	↓	Separate administration by ≥ 1 hour because antacids may reduce absorption of delavirdine.
Anticonvulsants (eg, phenytoin, phenobarbital, carbamazepine)	Delavirdine	↓	Coadministration not recommended because anticonvulsants may decrease plasma delavirdine concentrations.
Clarithromycin	Delavirdine	↑	Clarithromycin may increase plasma delavirdine concentrations.
Didanosine	Delavirdine	↓	Coadministration reduces AUC of both drugs by 20%. Separate administration times by ≥ 1 hour.
Delavirdine	Didanosine		
Fluoxetine, ketoconazole	Delavirdine	↑	These drugs may increase trough plasma delavirdine concentrations by ≈ 50%.
H_2 receptor antagonists	Delavirdine	↓	H_2 antagonists increase gastric pH and may decrease absorption of delavirdine. Although the effect on delavirdine absorption is unknown, chronic use is not recommended.
Rifabutin, rifampin	Delavirdine	↓	Coadministration not recommended because plasma delavirdine concentrations may be decreased.
Saquinavir	Delavirdine	↓	Coadministration with saquinavir may decrease delavirdine AUC. Monitor ALT/AST closely when coadministering.
Delavirdine	Amprenavir	↑	Plasma concentrations of amprenavir may be increased.
Delavirdine	Benzodiazepines (eg, alprazolam, midazolam, triazolam)	↑	Alprazolam, midazolam, and triazolam plasma concentrations may be increased.
Delavirdine	Cisapride	↑	Plasma concentrations of cisapride may be increased.
Delavirdine	Clarithromycin, dapsone, rifabutin	↑	Rifabutin, clarithromycin, or dapsone plasma concentrations of may be increased.
Delavirdine	Dihydropyridine calcium channel blockers	↑	Delavirdine may increase plasma concentrations of nifedipine and other dihydropyridine calcium channel blockers.
Delavirdine	Ergot derivatives	↑	Coadministration is not recommended because of increased risk for ergot toxicity.
Delavirdine	Indinavir	↑	Delavirdine inhibits metabolism of indinavir. When coadministered, reduce indinavir dose to 600 mg 3 times daily.
Delavirdine	Quinidine	↑	Plasma concentrations of quinidine may be increased.
Delavirdine	Saquinavir	↑	Saquinavir AUC increased 5-fold when coadministered with delavirdine. Monitor ALT/AST closely when coadministered.
Delavirdine	Sildenafil	↑	Delavirdine may increase sildenafil plasma concentration. Do not exceed a single 25 mg dose of sildenafil in a 48-hour period.
Delavirdine	Warfarin	↑	Plasma concentrations of warfarin may be increased.

[1] ↑ indicates increase.
[2] ↓ indicates decrease.
* See Pharmacokinetics for magnitude of interaction.

Adverse Reactions

Percent of patients with treatment-emergent rash in pivotal trials (Studies 21 Part II and 13C)[a]

Percent of patients with:	Description of rash grade[b]	Delavirdine mesylate 400 mg 3 times a day (n = 412)	Control group patients (n = 295)
Grade 1 rash	Erythema, pruritus	69 (16.7%)	35 (11.9%)
Grade 2 rash	Diffuse maculopapular rash, dry desquamation	59 (14.3%)	17 (5.8%)
Grade 3 rash	Vesiculation, moist desquamation, ulceration	18 (4.4%)	0 (0%)
Grade 4 rash	Erythema multiforme, Stevens-Johnson syndrome, toxic epidermal necrolysis, necrosis requiring surgery, exfoliative dermatitis	0 (0%)	0 (0%)
Rash of any grade		146 (35.4%)	52 (17.6%)
Treatment discontinuation as a result of rash		13 (3.2%)	1 (0.3%)

[a] Includes events reported regardless of causality.
[b] ACTG toxicity grading system, includes events reported as "rash", "maculopapular rash", and "urticaria".

➤*Adverse events of moderate to severe intensity:*

Treatment-emergent events, regardless of causality, of moderate to severe or life-threatening intensity reported by at least 5% of evaluable[a] patients in any treatment group

	Study 21 part II			Study 13C	
Adverse events	ZDV + 3TC (n = 123) % of patients (n)	400 mg 3 times a day delavirdine mesylate + ZDV (n = 123) % of patients (n)	400 mg 3 times a day delavirdine mesylate + ZDV + 3TC (n = 119) % of patients (n)	ZDV + ddI, ddC or 3TC (n = 172) % of patients (n)	400 mg 3 times a day delavirdine mesylate + ZDV + ddI, ddC or 3TC (n = 170) % of patients (n)
Miscellaneous					
Abdominal pain generalized	2.4% (3)	3.3% (4)	5% (6)	1.7% (3)	2.4% (4)
Asthenia/fatigue	16.3% (20)	15.4 %(19)	16% (19)	8.1% (14)	5.3% (9)
Fever	2.4% (3)	1.6% (2)	3.4% (4)	6.4 %(11)	7.1% (12)
Flu syndrome	4.9% (6)	7.3% (9)	5% (6)	5.2% (9)	2.4% (4)
Headache	14.6% (18)	12.2% (15)	16.8% (20)	12.8% (22)	11.2% (19)
Localized pain	4.9% (6)	5.7% (7)	5% (6)	2.9% (5)	1.8% (3)
GI					
Diarrhea	8.1% (10)	2.4% (3)	4.2% (5)	8.1% (14)	5.9% (10)
Nausea	17.1% (21)	20.3% (25)	16.8% (20)	9.3% (16)	14.7% (25)
Vomiting	8.9% (11)	4.9% (6)	2.5% (3)	4.1% (7)	6.5% (11)
CNS					
Anxiety	1.6% (2)	2.4% (3)	6.7% (8)	4.1% (7)	3.5% (6)
Depressive symptoms	6.5% (8)	4.9% (6)	12.6% (15)	3.5% (6)	5.9% (10)
Insomnia	4.9% (6)	4.9% (6)	5% (6)	2.9% (5)	1.2% (2)
Respiratory					
Bronchitis	4.1% (5)	6.5% (8)	6.7% (8)	3.5% (6)	3.5% (6)
Cough	9.8% (12)	4.1% (5)	5% (6)	5.2% (9)	3.5% (6)
Pharyngitis	6.5% (8)	1.6% (2)	5% (6)	4.1% (7)	3.5% (6)
Sinusitis	8.9% (11)	7.3% (9)	5% (6)	2.3% (4)	1.2% (2)
Upper respiratory tract infection	11.4% (14)	6.5% (8)	7.6% (9)	8.7% (15)	4.7% (8)
Dermatologic					
Rashes	3.3% (4)	19.5% (24)	13.4% (16)	7.6% (13)	18.8% (32)

[a] Evaluable patients in Study 21 part II were those who received at least 1 dose of study medication and returned for at least 1 clinic visit. Evaluable patients in Study 13C were those who received at least 1 dose of study medication.

DELAVIRDINE MESYLATE — ORAL

➤*Other adverse events:*

Cardiovascular – Abnormal cardiac rate and rhythm, cardiac insufficiency, cardiomyopathy, hypertension, migraine, pallor, peripheral vascular disorder, and postural hypotension.

CNS – Abnormal coordination, agitation, amnesia, change in dreams, cognitive impairment, confusion, decreased libido, disorientation, dizziness, emotional lability, euphoria, hallucination, hyperesthesia, hyperreflexia, hypertonia, hypesthesia, impaired concentration, manic symptoms, muscle cramp, nervousness, neuropathy, nystagmus, paralysis, paranoid symptoms, restlessness, sleep cycle disorder, somnolence, tingling, tremor, vertigo, and weakness.

Dermatologic – Angioedema, dermal leukocytoclastic vasculitis, dermatitis, desquamation, diaphoresis, discolored skin, dry skin, erythema, erythema multiforme, folliculitis, fungal dermatitis, hair loss, herpes zoster or simplex, nail disorder, petechiae, pruritus non-application site, seborrhea, skin hypertrophy, skin disorder, skin nodule, Stevens-Johnson syndrome, urticaria, vesiculobullous rash, and wart.

GI – Anorexia, bloody stool, colitis, constipation, decreased appetite, diarrhea (*Clostridium difficile*), diverticulitis, dry mouth, dyspepsia, dysphagia, enteritis at all levels, eructation, fecal incontinence, flatulence, gagging, gastroenteritis, gastroesophageal reflux, gastrointestinal bleeding, gastrointestinal disorder, gingivitis, gum hemorrhage, hepatomegaly, increased appetite, increased saliva, increased thirst, jaundice, mouth or tongue inflammation or ulcers, nonspecific hepatitis, oral/enteric moniliasis, pancreatitis, rectal disorder, sialadenitis, tooth abscess, and toothache.

GU – Amenorrhea, breast enlargement, calculi of the kidney, chromaturia, epididymitis, hematuria, hemospermia, urinary tract infection, impaired urination, impotence, kidney pain, metrorrhagia, nocturia, polyuria, proteinuria, testicular pain, and vaginal moniliasis.

Hematologic/Lymphatic – Adenopathy, bruising, eosinophilia, granulocytosis, leukopenia, pancytopenia, purpura, spleen disorder, and thrombocytopenia, and prolonged prothrombin time.

Metabolic/Nutritional – Alcohol intolerance, amylase increased, bilirubinemia, hyperglycemia, hyperkalemia, hypertriglyceridemia, hyperuricemia, hypocalcemia, hyponatremia, hypophosphatemia, increased AST, increased gamma glutamyl transpeptidase, increased lipase, increased serum alkaline phosphatase, increased serum creatine, and weight increase or decrease.

Musculoskeletal – Arthralgia or arthritis of single and multiple joints, bone disorder, bone pain, myalgia, tendon disorder, tenosynovitis, tetany, and vertigo.

Ophthalmic – Blepharitis, blurred vision, conjunctivitis, diplopia, dry eyes, and photophobia.

Respiratory – Chest congestion, dyspnea, epistaxis, hiccups, laryngismus, pneumonia, and rhinitis.

Special senses – Ear pain, parosmia, otitis media, taste perversion, and tinnitus.

Miscellaneous – Abdominal cramps, abdominal distention, abdominal pain (localized), abscess, allergic reaction, chills, edema (generalized or localized), epidermal cyst, fever, infection, infection viral, lip edema, malaise, *Mycobacterium tuberculosis* infection, neck rigidity, redistribution/accumulation of body fat (see Precautions, Fat redistribution, and sebaceous cyst.

➤*Postmarketing:*

Hepatic – Hepatic failure.

Hematologic/Lymphatic – Hemolytic anemia.

Musculoskeletal – Rhabdomyolysis.

Renal – Acute kidney failure.

➤*Lab test abnormalities:*

Marked laboratory abnormalities reported by ≥ 2% of patients

		Study 21 part II			Study 13C	
		ZDV + 3TC (n = 123)	400 mg 3 times a day delavirdine mesylate + ZDV (n = 123)	400 mg 3 times a day delavirdine mesylate + ZDV + 3TC (n = 119)	ZDV + ddI, ddC or 3TC (n = 172)	400 mg 3 times a day delavirdine mesylate + ZDV + ddI, ddC or 3TC (n = 170)
Adverse event	Toxicity limit	% of patients	% of patients	% of patients	% of patients	% of patients
Hematology						
Hemoglobin	< 7 mg/dL	4.1%	2.5%	0.9%	1.7%	2.9%
Neutrophils	< 750/mm^3	5.7%	4.9%	3.4%	10.4%	7.6%
PT[a]	> 1.5 x ULN	0%	0%	1.7%	2.9%	2.4%
APTT[b]	> 2.33 x ULN	0%	0.8%	0%	5.8%	2.4%
Chemistry						
ALT[c]	> 5 x ULN	2.5%	4.1%	5.1%	3.5%	4.1%
Amylase	> 2 x ULN	0.8%	2.5%	2.6%	3.5%	2.9%
AST[d]	> 5 x ULN	1.6%	2.5%	3.4%	3.5%	2.3%
Bilirubin	> 2.5 x ULN	0.8%	2.5%	1.7%	1.2%	0%
GGT[e]	> 5 x ULN	N/A	N/A	N/A	4.1%	1.8%
Glucose[f]	< 40 mg/dL > 250 mg/dL	4.1%	0.8%	1.7%	1.2%	0%

[a] Prothrombin time.
[b] Activated partial thromboplastin.
[c] Alananine aminotransferase.
[d] Aspartate aminotransferase.
[e] Gamma glutamyl transferase.
[f] Hypo/hyperglycemia.
N/A = Not applicable because no predose values were obtained for patients.

Overdosage

➤*Treatment:* Human experience of acute overdose with delavirdine mesylate is limited.

Treatment of overdosage with delavirdine mesylate should consist of general supportive measures, including monitoring of vital signs and observation of the patient's clinical status. There is no specific antidote for overdosage with delavirdine mesylate. If indicated, elimination of unabsorbed drug should be achieved by emesis or gastric lavage. Since delavirdine is extensively metabolized by the liver and is highly protein bound, dialysis is unlikely to result in significant removal of the drug.

Patient Information

Patients should be informed that delavirdine mesylate is not a cure for HIV-1 infection and that they may continue to acquire illnesses associated with HIV-1 infection, including opportunistic infections. Treatment with delavirdine mesylate has not been shown to reduce the incidence or frequency of such illnesses, and patients should be advised to remain under the care of a physician when using delavirdine mesylate.

Patients should be advised that the use of delavirdine mesylate has not been shown to reduce the risk of transmission of HIV-1.

Patients should be instructed that the major toxicity of delavirdine mesylate is rash and should be advised to promptly notify their physician should rash occur. The majority of rashes associated with delavirdine mesylate occur within 1 to 3 weeks after initiating treatment with delavirdine mesylate. The rash normally resolves in 3 to 14 days and may be treated symptomatically while therapy with delavirdine mesylate is continued. Any patient experiencing severe rash or rash accompanied by symptoms such as fever, blistering, oral lesions, conjunctivitis, swelling, muscle or joint aches should discontinue medication and consult a physician.

Patients should be informed that redistribution or accumulation of body fat may occur in patients receiving antiretroviral therapy and that the cause and long-term health effects of these conditions are not known at this time.

Patients should be informed to take delavirdine mesylate every day as prescribed. Patients should not alter the dose of delavirdine mesylate without consulting their doctor. If a dose is missed, patients should take the next dose as soon as possible. However, if a dose is skipped, the patient should not double the next dose.

Patients with achlorhydria should take delavirdine mesylate with an acidic beverage (eg, orange or cranberry juice). However, the effect of an acidic beverage on the absorption of delavirdine in patients with achlorhydria has not been investigated.

Patients taking both delavirdine mesylate and antacids should be advised to take them at least 1 hour apart.

Because delavirdine mesylate may interact with certain drugs, patients should be advised to report to their doctor the use of any prescription, nonprescription medication or herbal products, particularly St. John's wort.

DELAVIRDINE MESYLATE — ORAL

Patients receiving sildenafil and delavirdine mesylate should be advised that they may be at an increased risk of sildenafil-associated adverse events, including hypotension, visual changes, and prolonged penile erection, and should promptly report any symptoms to their doctor.

EFAVIRENZ

Rx	**Sustiva** (Bristol-Myers Squibb Oncology/Immunology)	**Capsules:** 50 mg	Lactose. (SUSTIVA 50 mg). Gold/white. In 30s.
		100 mg	Lactose. (SUSTIVA 100 mg). White. In 30s.
		200 mg	Lactose. (SUSTIVA 200 mg). Gold. In 90s.
		Tablets: 600 mg	Lactose. (SUSTIVA). Yellow, capsule shape. Film-coated. In 30s and UD blister 100s.

EFAVIRENZ — ORAL

Indications

➤*HIV infection:* In combination with other antiretroviral agents, for the treatment of HIV-1 infection.

Administration and Dosage

➤*Approved by the FDA:* September 18, 1998.

➤*Adults:* The recommended dosage of efavirenz is 600 mg orally, once daily, in combination with a protease inhibitor or NRTIs. It is recommended that efavirenz be taken on an empty stomach, preferably at bedtime. The increased efavirenz concentrations observed following administration of efavirenz with food may lead to increase in frequency of adverse reactions.

In order to improve the tolerability of nervous system side effects, bedtime dosing is recommended during the first 2 to 4 weeks of therapy and in patients who continue to experience these symptoms. Dosing at bedtime improves the tolerability of these nervous system symptoms and is recommended during the first weeks of therapy and for patients who continue to experience these symptoms.

➤*Concomitant antiretroviral therapy:* Efavirenz must be given in combination with other antiretroviral medications. Efavirenz demonstrated synergistic activity against HIV-1 in cell culture when combined with zidovudine, didanosine, or indinavir.

➤*Children:* It is recommended that efavirenz be taken on an empty stomach, preferably at bedtime. The table below describes the recommended dose of efavirenz for pediatric patients 3 years of age or older and weighing 10 to 40 kg. The recommended dosage of efavirenz for pediatric patients weighing greater than 40 kg is 600 mg, once daily.

Pediatric dose to be administered once daily		
Body weight		
kg	lb	Efavirenz dose (mg)
10 to < 15	22 to < 33	200
15 to < 20	33 to < 44	250
20 to < 25	44 to < 55	300
25 to < 32.5	55 to < 71.5	350
32.5 to < 40	71.5 to < 88	400
≥ 40	≥ 88	600

➤*Storage/Stability:* Store at 25°C (77°F); excursions permitted to 15° to 30°C (59° to 86°F).

Actions

➤*Pharmacokinetics:*

Absorption – Peak efavirenz plasma concentrations of 1.6 to 9.1 mcM were attained by 5 hours following single oral doses of 100 mg to 1,600 mg administered to uninfected volunteers. Dose-related increases in C_{max} and AUC were seen for doses up to 1600 mg; the increases were less than proportional suggesting diminished absorption at higher doses.

In HIV-infected patients at steady-state, mean C_{max}, mean C_{min}, and mean AUC were dose proportional following 200 mg, 400 mg, and 600 mg daily doses. Time-to-peak plasma concentrations were approximately 3 to 5 hours and steady-state plasma concentrations were reached in 6 to 10 days. In 35 patients receiving efavirenz 600 mg once daily, steady-state C_{max} was 12.9 ± 3.7 mcM (mean ± SD), steady-state C_{min} was 5.6 ± 3.2 mcM, and AUC was 184 ± 73 mcM•hr.

Capsules: Administration of a single 600 mg dose of efavirenz capsules with a high fat/high caloric meal (894 kcal, 54 g fat, 54% calories from fat) or a reduced fat/normal caloric meal (440 kcal, 2 g fat, 4% calories from fat) was associated with a mean increase of 22% and 17% in efavirenz AUC_∞ and a mean increase of 39% and 51% in efavirenz C_{max}, respectively, relative to the exposures achieved when given under fasted conditions.

Tablets: Administration of a single 600 mg efavirenz tablet with a high fat/high caloric mean (approximately 1,000 kcal, 500 to 600 kcal from fat) was associated with a 28% increase in mean AUC_∞ of efavirenz and a 79% increase in mean C_{max} of efavirenz relative to the exposures achieved under fasted conditions.

Distribution – Efavirenz is highly protein-bound (approximately 99.5% to 99.75%) to human plasma proteins, predominantly albumin. In HIV-1 infected patients (n = 9) who received efavirenz 200 to 600 mg once daily for at least 1 month, cerebrospinal fluid concentrations ranged from 0.26% to 1.19% (mean, 0.69%) of the corresponding plasma concentration. This proportion is approximately 3-fold higher than the nonprotein-bound (free) fraction of efavirenz in plasma.

Metabolism – Studies in humans and in vitro studies using human liver microsomes have demonstrated that efavirenz is principally metabolized by the cytochrome P450 system to hydroxylated metabolites with subsequent glucuronidation of these hydroxylated metabolites. These metabolites are essentially inactive against HIV-1. The in vitro studies suggest that CYP3A4 and CYP2B6 are the major isozymes responsible for efavirenz metabolism.

Efavirenz has been shown to induce P450 enzymes, resulting in the induction of its own metabolism. Multiple doses of 200 to 400 mg/day for 10 days resulted in a lower than predicted extent of accumulation (22% to 42% lower) and a shorter terminal half-life of 40 to 55 hours (single dose half-life 52 to 76 hours).

Excretion – Efavirenz has a terminal half-life of 52 to 76 hours after single doses and 40 to 55 hours after multiple doses. A 1-month mass balance/excretion study was conducted using 400 mg/day with a ^{14}C-labeled dose administered on day 8. Approximately 14% to 34% of the radiolabel was recovered in the urine and 16% to 61% was recovered in the feces. Nearly all of the urinary excretion of the radiolabeled drug was in the form of metabolites. Efavirenz accounted for the majority of the total radioactivity measured in feces.

Special populations –

Children: ACTG 382 is an ongoing open-label 48-week study in 57 NRTI-experienced pediatric patients to characterize the safety, pharmacokinetics, and antiviral activity of efavirenz in combination with nelfinavir (20 to 30 mg/kg 3 times a day) and NRTIs. Mean age was 8 years (range, 3 to 16). Efavirenz has not been studied in pediatric patients below 3 years of age or who weigh less than 13 kg. The type and frequency of adverse experiences was generally similar to that of adult patients with the exception of a higher incidence of rash which was reported in 46% (26 out of 57) of pediatric patients compared to 26% of adults, and a higher frequency of grade 3 or 4 rash reported in 5% (3 out of 57) of pediatric patients compared to 0.9% of adults.

➤*Microbiology:* Efavirenz is a nonnucleoside reverse transcriptase inhibitor (NNRTI) of human immunodeficiency virus type 1 (HIV-1). Efavirenz activity is mediated predominantly by noncompetitive inhibition of HIV-1 RT. HIV-2 RT and human cellular DNA polymerases alpha, beta, gamma, and delta are not inhibited by efavirenz.

In vitro HIV susceptibility – The clinical significance of in vitro susceptibility of HIV-1 to efavirenz has not been established. The in vitro antiviral activity of efavirenz was assessed in lymphoblastoid cell lines, peripheral blood mononuclear cells (PBMCs) and macrophage/monocyte cultures. The 90% to 95% inhibitory concentration (IC_{90-95}) of efavirenz for wild type laboratory adapted strains and clinical isolates ranged from 1.7 to 25 nM. Efavirenz demonstrated synergistic activity against HIV-1 in cell culture when combined with zidovudine (ZDV), didanosine, or indinavir (IDV).

Resistance – HIV-1 isolates with reduced susceptibility to efavirenz (greater than 380-fold increase in IC_{90}) compared to baseline can emerge in vitro. Phenotypic (n = 26) changes in evaluable HIV-1 isolates and genotypic (n = 104) changes in plasma virus from selected patients treated with efavirenz in combination with IDV, or with ZDV plus lamivudine were monitored. One or more RT mutations at amino acid positions 98, 100, 101, 103, 106, 108, 188, 190, and 225, were observed in 102 of 104 patients with a frequency of at least 9% compared to baseline. The mutation at RT amino acid position 103 (lysine to asparagine) was the most frequently observed (greater than or equal to 90%). A mean loss in susceptibility (IC_{90}) to efavirenz of 47-fold was observed in 26 clinical isolates. Five clinical isolates were evaluated for both genotypic and phenotypic changes from baseline. Decreases in efavirenz susceptibility (range from 9- to greater than 312-fold increase in IC_{90}) were observed for these isolates in vitro compared to baseline. All 5 isolates possessed at least 1 of the efavirenz-associated RT mutations. The clinical relevance of phenotypic and genotypic changes associated with efavirenz therapy is under evaluation.

Cross-resistance – Rapid emergence of HIV-1 strains that are cross-resistant to NNRTI has been observed in vitro. Thirteen clinical isolates previously characterized as efavirenz-resistant were also phenotypically resistant to nevirapine and delavirdine in vitro compared to baseline. Clinically derived ZDV-resistant HIV-1 isolates tested in vitro retained susceptibility to efavirenz. Cross-resistance between efavirenz and HIV protease inhibitors is unlikely because of the different enzyme targets involved.

Contraindications

Hypersensitivity to efavirenz or any of its components.

Efavirenz should not be administered concurrently with astemizole, cisapride, midazolam, triazolam, or ergot derivatives because competition for CYP3A4 by efavirenz could result in inhibition of metabolism of these drugs and create the potential for serious or life-threatening adverse reactions (eg, cardiac arrhythmias, prolonged sedation or respiratory depression).

EFAVIRENZ — ORAL

Warnings

➤*Resistance:* Efavirenz must not be used as a single agent to treat HIV or added on as a sole agent to a failing regimen. As with all other nonnucleoside reverse transcriptase inhibitors, resistant virus emerges rapidly when efavirenz is administered as monotherapy. The choice of new antiretroviral agents to be used in combination with efavirenz should take into consideration the potential for viral cross-resistance.

➤*Psychiatric symptoms:* Serious psychiatric adverse experiences have been reported in patients treated with efavirenz. In controlled trials of 1008 patients treated with regimens containing efavirenz for an average of 1.6 years and 635 patients treated with control regimens for an average of 1.3 years, the frequency of specific serious psychiatric reactions among patients who received efavirenz or control regimens, respectively, were as follows: Severe depression (1.6%, 0.6%), suicidal ideation (0.6%, 0.3%), nonfatal suicide attempts (0.4%, 0%), aggressive behavior (0.4%, 0.3%), paranoid reactions (0.4%, 0.3%), and manic reactions (0.1%, 0%). Patients with a history of psychiatric disorders appear to be at greater risk for these serious psychiatric adverse experiences, with the frequency of each of the above reactions ranging from 0.3% for manic reactions to 2% for both severe depression and suicidal ideation. There have also been occasional postmarketing reports of death by suicide, delusions and psychosis-like behavior, although a causal relationship to the use of efavirenz cannot be determined from these reports. Patients with serious psychiatric adverse experiences should seek immediate medical evaluation to assess the possibility that the symptoms may be related to the use of efavirenz, and if so, to determine whether the risks of continued therapy outweigh the benefits.

➤*Nervous system symptoms:* Fifty-three percent (53%) of patients receiving efavirenz in controlled trials reported central nervous system symptoms compared to 25% of patients receiving control regimens. These symptoms included, but were not limited to, dizziness (28.1%), insomnia (16.3%), impaired concentration (8.3%), somnolence (7%), abnormal dreams (6.2%), and hallucinations (1.2%). These symptoms were severe in 2% of patients and 2.1% of patients discontinued therapy as a result. These symptoms usually begin during the first or second day of therapy and generally resolve after the first 2 to 4 weeks of therapy. After 4 weeks of therapy, the prevalence of nervous system symptoms of at least moderate severity ranged from 5% to 9% in patients treated with regimens containing efavirenz and from 3% to 5% in patients treated with a control regimen. Patients should be informed that these common symptoms were likely to improve with continued therapy and were not predictive of subsequent onset of the less frequent psychiatric symptoms. Dosing at bedtime improves the tolerability of these nervous system symptoms and is recommended during the first weeks of therapy and for patients who continue to experience these symptoms.

Patients receiving efavirenz should be alerted to the potential for additive central nervous system effects when efavirenz is used concomitantly with alcohol or psychoactive drugs.

➤*Hepatic function impairment:* In patients with known or suspected history of hepatitis B or C infection and in patients treated with other medications associated with liver toxicity, monitoring of liver enzymes is recommended. In patients with persistent elevations of serum transaminases to greater than 5 times the upper limit of the normal range, the benefit of continued therapy with efavirenz needs to be weighed against the unknown risks of significant liver toxicity.

Because of the extensive cytochrome P450-mediated metabolism of efavirenz and limited clinical experience in patients with hepatic impairment, caution should be exercised in administering efavirenz to these patients.

➤*Carcinogenesis:* Long-term carcinogenicity studies in mice and rats were carried out with efavirenz. Mice were dosed with 0, 25, 75, 150, or 300 mg/kg/day for 2 years. Incidences of hepatocellular adenomas and carcinomas and pulmonary alveolar/bronchiolar adenomas were increased above background in females. No increases in tumor incidence above background were seen in males. In studies in which rats were administered efavirenz at doses of 0, 25, 50, or 100 mg/kg/day for 2 years, no increases in tumor incidence above background were observed. The systemic exposure (based on AUCs) in mice was approximately 1.7-fold that in humans receiving the 600 mg/day dose. The exposures in rats was lower than that in humans. The mechanism of the carcinogenic potential is unknown.

➤*Elderly:* Clinical studies of efavirenz did not include sufficient numbers of subjects aged 65 years and over to determine whether they respond differently from younger subjects. In general, dose selection for an elderly patient should be cautious, reflecting the greater frequency of decreased hepatic, renal, or cardiac function and of concomitant disease or other therapy.

➤*Pregnancy: Category C.* Pregnancy should be avoided in women receiving efavirenz. Barrier contraception should always be used in combination with other methods of contraception (eg, oral or other hormonal contraceptives). Women of childbearing potential should undergo pregnancy testing prior to initiation of efavirenz.

Malformations have been observed in 3 of 20 fetuses/infants from efavirenz-treated cynomolgus monkeys (versus 0 of 20 concomitant controls) in a developmental toxicity study. The pregnant monkeys were dosed throughout pregnancy (postcoital days 20 to 150) with efavirenz 60 mg/kg daily, a dose which resulted in plasma drug concentrations similar to those in humans given 600 mg/day of efavirenz. Anencephaly and unilateral anophthalmia were observed in 1 fetus, microophthalmia was observed in another fetus, and cleft palate was observed in a third fetus. Efavirenz crosses the placenta in cynomolgus monkeys and produces fetal blood concentrations similar to maternal blood concentrations.

Efavirenz has been shown to cross the placenta in rats and rabbits and produces fetal blood concentrations of efavirenz similar to maternal concentrations. An increase in fetal resorptions was observed in rats at efavirenz doses that produced peak plasma concentrations and AUC values in female rats equivalent to, or lower than those achieved in humans given 600 mg once daily of efavirenz. Efavirenz produced no reproductive toxicities when given to pregnant rabbits at doses that produced peak plasma concentrations similar to, and AUC values approximately half of those achieved in humans given 600 mg once daily of efavirenz.

There are no adequate and well-controlled studies in pregnant women. Efavirenz should be used during pregnancy only if the potential benefit justifies the potential risk to the fetus, such as in pregnant women without other therapeutic options. As of November 2002, the Antiretroviral Pregnancy Registry has received reports of 113 pregnancies exposed to efavirenz-containing regimens, the majority of which were first-trimester exposures (108 pregnancies). Birth defects occurred in 3 of 88 live births (first-trimester exposure) and 0 of 11 live births (second- /third-trimester exposure). In addition, there has been 1 report of multiple defects including abnormalities consistent with Dandy-Walker syndrome in a fetus from a spontaneous abortion, 1 report of a neural tube defect in a fetus from a pregnancy electively terminated in the second trimester, and 1 report of meningomyelocele in an infant. All 3 mothers were exposed to efavirenz-containing regimens in the first trimester. A causal relationship of these events to the use of efavirenz cannot be established.

Antiretroviral pregnancy registry – To monitor fetal outcomes of pregnant women exposed to efavirenz, an Antiretroviral Pregnancy Registry has been established. Physicians are encouraged to register patients by calling (800) 258-4263.

➤*Lactation:* The Centers for Disease Control and Prevention recommend that HIV-infected mothers not breastfeed their infants to avoid risking postnatal transmission of HIV infection. Although it is not known if efavirenz is secreted in human milk, efavirenz is secreted into the milk of lactating rats. Because of the potential for HIV transmission and the potential for serious adverse effects in nursing infants, mothers should be instructed not to breastfeed if they are receiving efavirenz.

➤*Children:* See Actions for more information.

Precautions

➤*Monitoring:*

Cholesterol – Monitoring of cholesterol and triglycerides should be considered in patients treated with efavirenz.

See Adverse Reactions for more information.

➤*Skin rash:* In controlled clinical trials, 26% (266 out of 1,008) of patients treated with 600 mg efavirenz experienced new onset skin rash compared with 17% (111 out of 635) of patients treated in control groups. Rash associated with blistering, moist desquamation, or ulceration occurred in 0.9% (9 out of 1,008) of patients treated with efavirenz. The incidence of grade 4 rash (eg, erythema multiforme, Stevens-Johnson syndrome) in patients treated with efavirenz in all studies and expanded access was 0.1%. The median time to onset of rash in adults was 11 days and the median duration, 16 days. The discontinuation rate for rash in clinical trials was 1.7% (17 out of 1008). Efavirenz should be discontinued in patients developing severe rash associated with blistering, desquamation, mucosal involvement or fever. Appropriate antihistamines or corticosteroids may improve the tolerability and hasten the resolution of rash.

Rash was reported in 26 of 57 pediatric patients (46%) treated with efavirenz. One pediatric patient experienced grade 3 rash (confluent rash with fever), and 1 patient had grade 4 rash (erythema multiforme). The median time to onset of rash in pediatric patients was 8 days. Prophylaxis with appropriate antihistamines prior to initiating therapy with efavirenz in pediatric patients should be considered. Efavirenz should be discontinued in patients developing severe rash associated with blistering, desquamation, mucosal involvement or fever.

➤*Fat distribution:* Redistribution/accumulation of body fat including central obesity, dorsocervical fat enlargement (buffalo hump), peripheral wasting, facial wasting, breast enlargement, and "cushingoid appearance" have been observed in patients receiving antiretroviral therapy. The mechanism and long-term consequences of these events are currently unknown. A causal relationship has not been established.

➤*Convulsions:* Convulsions have been observed infrequently in patients receiving efavirenz, generally in the presence of known medical history of seizures. Patients who are receiving concomitant anticonvulsant medications primarily metabolized by the liver, such as phenytoin, carbamazepine, and phenobarbital, may require periodic monitoring of plasma levels. Caution must be taken in any patient with a history of seizures.

➤*Hazardous tasks:* Patients who experience central nervous system symptoms such as dizziness, impaired concentration or drowsiness should avoid potentially hazardous tasks such as driving or operating machinery.

Drug Interactions

➤*Cytochrome p-450 system:* Efavirenz has been shown in vivo to induce CYP3A4. Other compounds that are substrates of CYP3A4 may have decreased plasma concentrations when coadministered with efavirenz. In vitro studies have demonstrated that efavirenz inhibits 2C9, 2C19, and 3A4 isozymes in the range of observed efavirenz plasma concentrations. Coadministration of efavirenz with drugs primarily metabolized by these isozymes may result in altered plasma concentrations of the coadministered drug. Therefore, appropriate dose adjustments may be necessary for these drugs.

EFAVIRENZ — ORAL

Drugs which induce CYP3A4 activity (eg, phenobarbital, rifampin, rifabutin) would be expected to increase the clearance of efavirenz resulting in lowered plasma concentrations. Drug interactions with efavirenz are summarized in the table below.

Drugs that should not be coadministered with efavirenz

Drug class	Drugs within class not to be coadministered with efavirenz
Antihistamines	astemizole
Benzodiazepines	midazolam, triazolam
GI motility agents	cisapride
Anti-migraine	ergot derivatives

Efavirenz Drug Interactions

Precipitant drug	Object drug*		Description
Phenytoin Phenobarbital Carbamazepine	Efavirenz	↓	Potential for reduction in anticonvulsant or efavirenz plasma levels; periodically monitor anticonvulsant plasma levels.
Efavirenz	Phenytoin Phenobarbital Carbamazepine		
Rifampin	Efavirenz	↓	Decreased efavirenz plasma concentrations may occur; the clinical significance is unknown.
Rifabutin	Efavirenz	↓	Rifabutin would be expected to increase the clearance of efavirenz caused by CYP3A4 induction. Coadministration also may decrease rifabutin concentration. Increase daily dose of rifabutin by 50%. Consider doubling the rifabutin dose when rifabutin is given 2 to 3 times/week.
Efavirenz	Rifabutin		
Ritonavir	Efavirenz	↑	With concurrent use, the concentration for each drug was increased. The combination was associated with a higher frequency of adverse clinical experiences (eg, dizziness, nausea, paresthesia) and laboratory abnormalities (elevated liver enzymes). Monitoring of liver enzymes is recommended.
Efavirenz	Ritonavir		
St. John's wort (*Hypericum perforatum*)	Efavirenz	↓	Expected to substantially decrease plasma levels of efavirenz; although, the drug combination has not been studied.
Efavirenz	Amprenavir	↓	Efavirenz has the potential to decrease serum concentrations of amprenavir.
Efavirenz	Benzodiazepines (midazolam, triazolam), cisapride, ergot derivatives	↑	Do not coadminister. Competition for CYP3A4 by efavirenz could result in serious or life-threatening adverse events (eg, cardiac arrhythmias, prolonged sedation, respiratory depression).
Efavirenz	Clarithromycin	↔	Clarithromycin plasma levels decreased while clarithromycin hydroxymetabolite levels increased. The clinical significance of these changes is unknown. No dose adjustment of efavirenz is recommended. Consider alternatives to clarithromycin, such as azithromycin. Other macrolide antibiotics have not been studied.
Efavirenz	Ethinyl estradiol	↔	The AUC of a single dose of ethinyl estradiol was increased; no significant changes were observed in C_{max}. The clinical significance is unknown. Because the interaction with oral contraceptives has not been fully characterized, use a reliable method of barrier contraception in addition to oral contraception.
Efavirenz	Indinavir	↓	Coadministration decreased indinavir AUC and C_{max}. Therefore, increase the indinavir dose from 800 to 1000 mg every 8 hours when efavirenz and indinavir are coadministered.
Efavirenz	Itraconazole Ketoconazole	↓	Although no drug interaction studies have been conducted, efavirenz has the potential to decrease plasma concentrations of itraconazole and ketoconazole.
Efavirenz	Methadone	↓	Coadministration decreased methadone AUC and C_{max}. Monitor for withdrawal symptoms and increase methadone dose as needed.
Efavirenz	Nelfinavir	↑	The AUC and C_{max} of nelfinavir are increased with coadministration. No dose adjustment is necessary.
Efavirenz	Saquinavir	↓	Coadministration decreased saquinavir AUC and C_{max} by 62% and 50%, respectively. Do not use saquinavir with efavirenz as the sole protease inhibitor.
Efavirenz	Warfarin	↔	Plasma concentrations and effects potentially increased or decreased by efavirenz.

* ↑ = Object drug increased. ↓ = Object drug decreased. ↔ = Undetermined clinical effect.

➤*Drug/Lab test interactions:* Efavirenz does not bind to cannabinoid receptors. False-positive urine cannabinoid test results have been observed in non-HIV-infected volunteers receiving efavirenz when the Microgenics *Cedia* DAU Multi-Level THC assay was used for screening. Negative results were obtained when more specific confirmatory testing was performed with gas chromatography/mass spectrometry.

Adverse Reactions

The most significant adverse reactions observed in patients treated with efavirenz are nervous system symptoms, psychiatric symptoms, and rash.

➤*CNS:* Fifty-three percent (53%) of patients receiving efavirenz reported central nervous system symptoms. The frequency of the symptoms of different degrees of severity, and discontinuation rates in clinical trials for 1 or more of the following nervous system symptoms are listed below: Dizziness, insomnia, impaired concentration, somnolence, abnormal dreaming, euphoria, confusion, agitation, amnesia, hallucinations, stupor, abnormal thinking, and depersonalization. The frequencies of specific central and peripheral nervous system symptoms are provided in the table below.

Percent of patients with 1 or more selected nervous system symptoms[1,2]

Percent of patients with:	Efavirenz 600 mg once daily (n = 1,008) %	Control groups (n = 635) %
Symptoms of any severity	52.7%	24.6%
Mild symptoms[3]	33.3%	15.6%
Moderate symptoms[4]	17.4%	7.7%
Severe symptoms[5]	2%	1.3%
Treatment discontinuation as a result of symptoms	2.1%	1.1%

[1] Includes reactions reported regardless of causality.
[2] Data from Study 006 and 3 Phase 2/3 studies.
[3] "Mild" = Symptoms which do not interfere with patient's daily activities.
[4] "Moderate" = Symptoms which may interfere with daily activities.
[5] "Severe" = Events which interrupt patient's usual daily activities.

➤*Psychiatric:* Serious psychiatric adverse reactions have been reported in patients treated with efavirenz. In controlled trials the frequency of specific serious psychiatric symptoms among patients who received efavirenz or control regimens, respectively, were severe depression (1.6%, 0.6%), suicidal ideation or attempts (0.6%, 0.3%), aggressive behavior (0.4%, 0.3%), paranoid reactions (0.2%, 0.3%), and manic reactions (0.1%, 0%). Additional psychiatric symptoms observed at a frequency of greater than 2% among patients treated with efavirenz or control regimens, respectively, in controlled clinical trials were depression (15.8%, 13.1%), anxiety (11.1%, 7.6%), and nervousness (6.3%, 2%).

➤*Dermatologic:* Rashes are usually mild-to-moderate maculopapular skin eruptions that occur within the first 2 weeks of initiating therapy with efavirenz. In most patients, rash resolves with continuing efavirenz therapy within 1 month. Efavirenz can be reinitiated in patients interrupting therapy because of rash. Use of appropriate antihistamines or corticosteroids may be considered when efavirenz is restarted. Efavirenz should be

EFAVIRENZ — ORAL

discontinued in patients developing severe rash associated with blistering, desquamation, mucosal involvement or fever. The frequency of rash by NCI grade and the discontinuation rates as a result of rash are provided below.

Percent of patients with treatment-emergent rash[1,2]				
Percent of patients with:	Description of rash grade[3]	Efavirenz 600 mg once daily adults (n = 1,008)	Efavirenz pediatric patients (n = 57)	Control groups adults (n = 635)
		%	%	%
Rash of any grade		26.3%	45.6%	17.5%
Grade 1 rash	Erythema, pruritus	10.7%	8.8%	9.8%
Grade 2 rash	Diffuse maculopapular rash, dry desquamation	14.7%	31.6%	7.4%
Grade 3 rash	Vesiculation, moist desquamation, ulceration	0.8%	1.8%	0.3%
Grade 4 rash	Erythema multiforme, Stevens-Johnson syndrome, toxic epidermal necrolysis, necrosis requiring surgery, exfoliative dermatitis	0.1%	3.5%	0%
Treatment discontinuation as a result of rash		1.7%	8.8%	0.3%

[1] Includes reactions reported regardless of causality.
[2] Data from Study 006 and 3 Phase 2/3 studies.
[3] NCI grading system.

Experience with efavirenz in patients who discontinued other antiretroviral agents of the NNRTI class is limited. Nineteen patients who discontinued nevirapine because of rash have been treated with efavirenz. Nine of these patients developed mild-to-moderate rash while receiving therapy with efavirenz, and 2 of these patients discontinued because of rash.

➤*GI:*

Pancreatitis – A few cases of pancreatitis have been described, although a causal relationship with efavirenz has not been established. Asymptomatic increases in serum amylase levels were observed in a significantly higher number of patients treated with efavirenz 600 mg than in control patients. Drug-related clinical adverse reactions of moderate or severe intensity observed in greater than or equal to 2% of patients in 2 controlled clinical trials are presented in the table below.

Percent of patients with treatment-emergent[1] adverse reactions of moderated or severe intensity reported in ≥ 2% of patients in studies 006 and ACTG 364						
	Study 006 LAM-, NNRTI, and protease inhibitor-naive patients			Study ACTG 364 NRTI-experienced NNRTI-, and protease inhibitor-naive patients		
Adverse reactions	Efavirenz[2] + ZDV/LAM[3] (n = 412)	Efavirenz[2] + indinavir (n = 415)	Indinavir + ZDV/LAM[3] (n = 401)	Efavirenz[2] + nelfinavir + NRTIs (n = 64)	Efavirenz[2] + NRTIs (n = 65)	Nelfinavir + NRTIs (n = 66)
	%	%	%	%	%	%
Miscellaneous						
Fatigue	7%	5%	8%	0%	2%	3%
Pain	1%	1%	5%	13%	6%	17%
CNS						
Dizziness	8%	8%	3%	2%	6%	6%
Headache	7%	4%	4%	5%	2%	3%
Concentration impaired	5%	2%	0%	0%	0%	0%
Insomnia	6%	7%	3%	0%	0%	2%
Abnormal dreams	3%	1%	0%	-	-	-
Somnolence	3%	2%	2%	0%	0%	0%
Anorexia	1%	0%	1%	0%	2%	2%
GI						
Nausea	12%	7%	25%	3%	2%	2%
Vomiting	7%	6%	14%	-	-	-
Diarrhea	6%	8%	6%	14%	3%	9%
Dyspepsia	3%	3%	5%	0%	0%	2%
Abdominal pain	1%	2%	4%	3%	3%	3%
Psychiatric						
Anxiety	1%	3%	0%	-	-	-
Depression	2%	1%	0%	3%	0%	5%
Nervousness	2%	2%	0%	2%	0%	2%
Dermatologic						
Rash	13%	20%	7%	9%	5%	9%
Pruritus	0%	1%	1%	9%	5%	9%
Increased sweating	2%	1%	0%	0%	0%	0%

[1] Includes adverse reactions at least possibly related to study drug of unknown relationship for Study 006. Includes all adverse reactions regardless of relationship to study drug for Study ACTG 364.
[2] Efavirenz provided as 600 mg once daily.
[3] ZDV = zidovudine, LAM = lamivudine.
\- = Not specified.

Children – In Study 006, lipodystrophy was reported in 2.3% of patients with efavirenz + IDV, 0.7% of patients treated with efavirenz + ZDV + LAM and 1% of patients treated with IDV + ZDV + LAM. Clinical adverse reactions of moderate to severe intensity observed in greater than or equal to 10% of 57 pediatric patients aged 3 to 16 years who received efavirenz, nelfinavir, and 1 or more NRTIs were the following: Rash (46%), diarrhea/loose stools (39%), fever (21%), cough (16%), headache (11%), and nausea/vomiting (12%). The incidence of nervous system symptoms was 18% (10 out of 57). One patient experienced grade 3 rash, 2 patients had grade 4 rash, and 5 patients (9%) discontinued because of rash.

➤*Postmarketing:*

Cardiovascular – Flushing; palpitations.

CNS – Abnormal coordination; ataxia; convulsions; hypoesthesia; paresthesia; neuropathy; tremor.

Dermatologic – Erythema multiforme; nail disorders; skin discoloration; Stevens-Johnson syndrome.

Endocrine – Gynecomastia.

GI – Constipation; malabsorption.

EFAVIRENZ — ORAL

Hepatic – Hepatic enzyme increase; hepatic failure; hepatitis.

Lab test abnormalities –

Hepatic enzymes: Among 1,008 patients treated with 600 mg efavirenz in controlled clinical trials, 3% developed AST levels and 3% developed ALT levels greater than 5 times the upper limit of normal. Similar elevations of AST and ALT were seen in patients treated with control regimens.

Liver function tests should be monitored in patients with a history of hepatitis B or C. In 156 patients treated with 600 mg of efavirenz who were seropositive for hepatitis B or C, 7% developed AST levels and 8% developed ALT levels greater than 5 times the upper limit of normal. In 91 patients seropositive for hepatitis B or C treated with control regimens, 5% developed AST elevations and 4% developed ALT elevations to these levels. Elevations of GGT to greater than 5 times the upper limit of the normal range were observed in 4% of all patients treated with 600 mg of efavirenz and in 10% of patients seropositive for hepatitis B or C. In patients treated with control regimens, the incidence of GGT elevations to this level was 1.5% to 2%, irrespective of hepatitis B or C serology. Isolated elevations of GGT in patients receiving efavirenz may reflect enzyme induction not associated with liver toxicity.

Lipids: Increases in total cholesterol of 10% to 20% have been observed in some uninfected volunteers receiving efavirenz. In patients treated with efavirenz + ZDV + LAM, increases in non-fasting total cholesterol and HDL of approximately 20% and 25%, respectively, were observed. In patients treated with efavirenz + IDV, increases in non-fasting cholesterol and HDL of approximately 40% and 35%, respectively, were observed. The effects of efavirenz on triglycerides and LDL were not well-characterized since samples were taken from non-fasting patients. The clinical significance of these findings is unknown.

Serum amylase: Asymptomatic elevations in serum amylase greater than 1.5 times the upper limit of normal were seen in 10% of patients treated with efavirenz and in 6% of patients treated with control regimens. The clinical significance of asymptomatic increases in serum amylase is unknown.

Metabolic/Nutritional – Hypercholesterolemia; hypertriglyceridemia.

Musculoskeletal – Arthralgia; myalgia; myopathy.

Psychiatric – Aggressive reactions; agitation; delusions; emotional lability; mania; neurosis; paranoia; psychosis; suicide.

Respiratory – Dyspnea.

Special senses – Abnormal vision; tinnitus.

Miscellaneous – Allergic reactions; asthenia; redistribution/accumulation of body fat.

Overdosage

➤*Symptoms:* Some patients accidentally taking 600 mg twice daily have reported increased nervous system symptoms. One patient experienced involuntary muscle contractions.

➤*Treatment:* Treatment of overdose with efavirenz should consist of general supportive measures, including monitoring of vital signs and observation of the patient's clinical status. Administration of activated charcoal may be used to aid removal of unabsorbed drug. There is no specific antidote for overdose with efavirenz. Since efavirenz is highly protein bound, dialysis is unlikely to significantly remove the drug from blood.

Patient Information

Patients should be informed that efavirenz is not a cure for HIV infection and that they may continue to develop opportunistic infections and other complications associated with HIV disease. (The long-term effects are unknown at this time.) Patients should be told that there are currently no data demonstrating that efavirenz therapy can reduce the risk of transmitting HIV to others through sexual contact or blood contamination.

Patients should be advised to take efavirenz every day as prescribed. Efavirenz must always be used in combination with other antiretroviral drugs. A patient should remain under the care of a physician while taking efavirenz. (Instruct patients not to alter the dose or discontinue therapy without consulting their physicians.) Patients should be informed that central nervous system symptoms including dizziness, insomnia, impaired concentration, drowsiness and abnormal dreams are commonly reported during the first weeks of therapy with efavirenz. Dosing at bedtime improves the tolerability of these symptoms and is recommended during the first weeks of therapy and in patients who continue to experience these symptoms. These symptoms are likely to improve with continued therapy. Patients should be alerted to the potential for additive central nervous system effects when efavirenz is used concomitantly with alcohol or psychoactive drugs and that they occur in approximately half the patients taking efavirenz. Patients should be instructed that if they experience these symptoms they should avoid potentially hazardous tasks such as driving or operating machinery (or other tasks requiring coordination or physical dexterity). In clinical trials, patients who develop central nervous system symptoms were not more likely to subsequently develop psychiatric symptoms.

Patients should also be informed that serious psychiatric symptoms including severe depression, suicide attempts, aggressive behavior, delusions, paranoia and psychosis-like symptoms have also been infrequently reported in patients receiving efavirenz. Patients should be informed that if they experience severe psychiatric adverse experiences they should seek immediate medical evaluation to assess the possibility that the symptoms may be related to the use of efavirenz, and if so, to determine whether discontinuation of efavirenz may be required. Patients should also inform their physicians of any history of mental illness or substance abuse.

Patients should be informed that another common side effect is rash. These rashes usually go away without any change in treatment. In a small number of patients, rash may be serious. Patients should be advised that they should contact their physicians promptly if they develop a rash.

Because malformations have been observed in fetuses from efavirenz-treated animals, instructions should be given to avoid pregnancy in women receiving efavirenz. Women should be advised to notify their physicians if they become pregnant while taking efavirenz. A reliable form of barrier contraception should always be used in combination with other methods of contraception, including oral or other hormonal contraception because the effects of efavirenz on hormonal contraceptives are not fully characterized.

Efavirenz may interact with some drugs; therefore, patients should be advised to report to their doctors the use of any other prescriptions, nonprescription medications, or herbal products, particularly St. John's wort.

Patients should be informed that redistribution or accumulation of body fat may occur in patients receiving antiretroviral therapy and that the cause and long-term health effects of these conditions are not known at this time.

Fusion Inhibitors

ENFUVIRTIDE

Rx	**Fuzeon** (Hoffman-La Roche)	**Powder for injection, lyophilized:** 108 mg (≈ 90 mg/mL when reconstituted)	Preservative-free. Convenience Kit contains: Single-use vials, syringes, diluent, and alcohol wipes.

ENFUVIRTIDE — INJECTION

Indications

➤*HIV infection:* In combination with other antiretroviral agents, for the treatment of HIV-1 infection in treatment-experienced patients with evidence of HIV-1 replication despite ongoing antiretroviral therapy.

Administration and Dosage

➤*Approved by the FDA:* March 13, 2003.

➤*Adults:* 90 mg (1 mL) twice daily injected SC into the upper arm, anterior thigh or abdomen. Each injection should be given at a site different from the preceding injection site, and only where there is no current injection site reaction from an earlier dose. Enfuvirtide should not be injected into moles, scar tissue, bruises or the navel. Additional detailed information regarding the administration of enfuvirtide is described in the enfuvirtide injection instructions.

➤*Children:* No data are available to establish a dose recommendation of enfuvirtide in pediatric patients below the age of 6 years. In pediatric patients 6 years through 16 years of age, the recommended dosage of enfuvirtide is 2 mg/kg twice daily up to a maximum dose of 90 mg twice daily injected SC into the upper arm, anterior thigh or abdomen. Each injection should be given at a site different from the preceding injection site and only where there is no current injection site reaction from an earlier dose. Enfuvirtide should not be injected into moles, scar tissue, bruises or the navel. The following table contains dosing guidelines for enfuvirtide based on body weight. Weight should be monitored periodically and the enfuvirtide dose adjusted accordingly.

Pediatric dosing guidelines

Weight		Dose per twice daily injection (mg/dose)	Injection volume (90 mg enfuvirtide per mL)
Kilograms (kg)	Pounds (lbs)		
11 to 15.5	24 to 34	27	0.3 mL
15.6 to 20	> 34 to 44	36	0.4 mL
20.1 to 24.5	> 44 to 54	45	0.5 mL
24.6 to 29	> 54 to 64	54	0.6 mL
29.1 to 33.5	> 64 to 74	63	0.7 mL
33.6 to 38	> 74 to 84	72	0.8 mL
38.1 to 42.5	> 84 to 94	81	0.9 mL
≥ 42.6	> 94	90	1 mL

➤*Preparation for administration:* Enfuvirtide must only be reconstituted with 1.1 mL of Sterile Water for Injection. After adding sterile water, the vial should be gently tapped for 10 seconds and then gently rolled between the hands to avoid foaming and to ensure all particles of drug are in contact with the liquid and no drug remains on the vial wall. The vial should then be allowed to stand until the powder goes completely into solution, which could take up to 45 minutes. Reconstitution time can be reduced by gently rolling the vial between the hands until the product is completely dis-

ENFUVIRTIDE — INJECTION

solved. Before the solution is withdrawn for administration, the vial should be inspected visually to ensure that the contents are fully dissolved in solution, and that the solution is clear, colorless and without bubbles or particulate matter. If there is evidence of particulate matter, the vial must not be used and should be returned to the pharmacy.

Enfuvirtide contains no preservatives. Once reconstituted, enfuvirtide should be injected immediately or kept refrigerated in the original vial until use. Reconstituted enfuvirtide must be used within 24 hours. The subsequent dose of enfuvirtide can be reconstituted in advance and must be stored in the refrigerator in the original vial and used within 24 hours. Refrigerated reconstituted solution should be brought to room temperature before injection and the vial should be inspected visually again to ensure that the contents are fully dissolved in solution and that the solution is clear, colorless, and without bubbles or particulate matter.

➤*Administration:* The reconstituted solution should be injected SC in the upper arm, abdomen or anterior thigh. The injection should be given at a site different from the preceding injection site and only where there is no current injection site reaction. Also, do not inject into moles, scar tissue, bruises or the navel. A vial is suitable for single use only; unused portions must be discarded.

Patients should contact their healthcare providers for any questions regarding the administration of enfuvirtide. Patients should be taught to recognize the signs and symptoms of injection-site reactions and instructed when to contact their healthcare providers about these reactions.

➤*Storage / Stability:* Store at 25°C (77°F); excursions permitted to 15° to 30°C (59° to 86°F).

Reconstituted solution should be stored under refrigeration at 2° to 8°C (36° to 46°F) and used within 24 hours.

Actions

➤*Pharmacology:* Enfuvirtide interferes with the entry of HIV-1 into cells by inhibiting fusion of viral and cellular membranes. Enfuvirtide binds to the first heptad-repeat (HR1) in the gp41 subunit of the viral envelope glycoprotein and prevents the conformational changes required for the fusion of viral and cellular membranes.

➤*Pharmacokinetics:*

Absorption – The pharmacokinetic properties of enfuvirtide were evaluated in HIV-1 infected adult and pediatric patients. Following a 90 mg single SC injection of enfuvirtide into the abdomen in 12 HIV-1 infected subjects, the mean (± SD) C_{max} was 4.59 ± 1.5 mcg/mL, the AUC was 55.8 ± 12.1 mcg•hr/mL, and the median t_{max} was 8 hours (range from 3 to 12 hours). The absolute bioavailability (using a 90 mg IV dose as a reference) was 84.3% ± 15.5%. Following 90 mg twice-daily dosing of enfuvirtide SC in combination with other antiretroviral agents in 11 HIV-1 infected subjects, the mean (±SD) steady-state C_{max} was 5 ± 1.7 mcg/mL, C_{trough} was 3.3 ± 1.6 mcg/mL, $AUC_{0\text{-}12h}$ was 48.7 ± 19.1 mcg•hr/mL, and the median t_{max} was 4 hours (ranged from 4 to 8 hours).

Absorption of the 90 mg dose was comparable when injected into the SC tissue of the abdomen, thigh or arm.

Distribution – The mean (± SD) steady-state volume of distribution after IV administration of a 90 mg dose of enfuvirtide (n = 12) was 5.5 ± 1.1 L.

Enfuvirtide is approximately 92% bound to plasma proteins in HIV-infected plasma over a concentration range of 2 to 10 mcg/mL. It is bound predominantly to albumin and to a lower extent to alpha-1-acid glycoprotein.

Metabolism / Excretion – As a peptide, enfuvirtide is expected to undergo catabolism to its constituent amino acids, with subsequent recycling of the amino acids in the body pool.

Mass-balance studies to determine elimination pathway(s) of enfuvirtide have not been performed in humans.

In vitro studies with human microsomes and hepatocytes indicate that enfuvirtide undergoes hydrolysis to form a deamidated metabolite at the C-terminal phenylalanine residue, M3. The hydrolysis reaction is not NADPH dependent. The M3 metabolite is detected in human plasma following administration of enfuvirtide, with an AUC ranging from 2.4% to 15% of the enfuvirtide AUC.

Following a 90 mg single SC dose of enfuvirtide (n = 12) the mean ± SD elimination half-life of enfuvirtide is 3.8 ± 0.6 hours and the mean ± SD apparent clearance was 24.8 ± 4.1 mL/hr/kg. Following 90 mg twice-daily dosing of enfuvirtide SC in combination with other antiretroviral agents in 11 HIV-1 infected subjects, the mean ± SD apparent clearance was 30.6 ± 10.6 mL/hr/kg.

Special populations –

Children: The pharmacokinetics of enfuvirtide have been studied in 18 pediatric subjects aged 6 through 16 years at a dose of 2 mg/kg. Enfuvirtide pharmacokinetics were determined in the presence of concomitant medications including antiretroviral agents. A dose of 2 mg/kg twice daily (maximum 90 mg twice daily) provided enfuvirtide plasma concentrations similar to those obtained in adult patients receiving 90 mg twice daily.

In the 18 pediatric subjects receiving the 2 mg/kg twice-daily dose, the mean ± SD steady-state AUC was 53.6 ± 21.4 mcg•hr/mL, C_{max} was 5.9 ± 2.2 mcg/mL, C_{trough} was 3 ± 1.5 mcg/mL, and apparent clearance was 40 ± 14 mL/hr/kg.

Gender: Analysis of plasma concentration data from subjects in clinical trials indicated that the clearance of enfuvirtide is 20% lower in females than males after adjusting for body weight.

Weight: Enfuvirtide clearance decreases with decreased body weight irrespective of gender. Relative to the clearance of a 70 kg male, a 40 kg male will have 20% lower clearance and a 110 kg male will have a 26% higher clearance. Relative to a 70 kg male, a 40 kg female will have a 36% lower clearance and a 110 kg female will have the same clearance.

No dose adjustment is recommended for weight or gender.

➤*Microbiology:*

Antiviral activity in vitro –

Enfuvirtide exhibited additive to synergistic effects in cell culture assays when combined with individual members of various antiretroviral classes, including zidovudine, lamivudine, nelfinavir, indinavir, and efavirenz.

Drug resistance –

In clinical trials, HIV-1 isolates with reduced susceptibility to enfuvirtide have been recovered from subjects treated with enfuvirtide in combination with other antiretroviral agents. Posttreatment HIV-1 virus from 185 subjects exhibited decreases in susceptibility to enfuvirtide ranging from 4- to 422-fold relative to their respective baseline virus and exhibited genotypic changes in gp41 amino acids 36 to 45. Substitutions in this region were observed with decreasing frequency at amino acid positions 38, 43, 36, 40, 42, and 45.

Cross-resistance: HIV-1 clinical isolates resistant to nucleoside analogue reverse transcriptase inhibitors (NRTI), nonnucleoside analogue reverse transcriptase inhibitors (NNRTI), and protease inhibitors (PI) were susceptible to enfuvirtide in cell culture.

Contraindications

Hypersensitivity to enfuvirtide or any of its components.

Warnings

➤*Local injection-site reactions:* The most common adverse reactions associated with enfuvirtide use are local injection site reactions. Manifestations may include pain and discomfort, induration, erythema, nodules and cysts, pruritus, and ecchymosis. Nine percent (9%) of patients had local reactions that required analgesics or limited usual activities. Reactions are often present at more than 1 injection site. Patients must be familiar with the enfuvirtide injection instructions in order to know how to inject enfuvirtide appropriately and how to monitor carefully for signs or symptoms of cellulitis or local infection.

➤*Pneumonia:* An increased rate of bacterial pneumonia was observed in subjects treated with enfuvirtide in the phase 3 clinical trials compared to the control arm. It is unclear if the increased incidence of pneumonia is related to enfuvirtide use. However, because of this finding, patients with HIV infection should be carefully monitored for signs and symptoms of pneumonia, especially if they have underlying conditions which may predispose them to pneumonia. Risk factors for pneumonia included low initial CD4 cell count, high initial viral load, IV drug use, smoking, and a history of lung disease.

➤*Hypersensitivity reactions:* Hypersensitivity reactions have been associated with enfuvirtide therapy and may recur on rechallenge. Hypersensitivity reactions have included the following, individually and in combination: Rash, fever, nausea and vomiting, chills, rigors, hypotension, and elevated serum liver transaminases. Other adverse reactions that may be immune mediated and have been reported in subjects receiving enfuvirtide include primary immune complex reaction, respiratory distress glomerulonephritis, and Guillain-Barre syndrome. Patients developing signs and symptoms suggestive of a systemic hypersensitivity reaction should discontinue enfuvirtide and should seek medical evaluation immediately. Therapy with enfuvirtide should not be restarted following systemic signs and symptoms consistent with a hypersensitivity reaction. Risk factors that may predict the occurrence or severity of hypersensitivity to enfuvirtide have not been identified.

➤*Elderly:* Clinical studies of enfuvirtide did not include sufficient numbers of subjects aged 65 years of age and over to determine whether they respond differently from younger subjects.

➤*Pregnancy: Category B.* There are no adequate and well-controlled studies in pregnant women. Because animal reproduction studies are not always predictive of human response, this drug should be used during pregnancy only if clearly needed.

Antiretroviral pregnancy registry – To monitor maternal-fetal outcomes of pregnant women exposed to enfuvirtide and other antiretroviral drugs, an antiretroviral pregnancy registry has been established.

➤*Lactation:* The Centers for Disease Control and Prevention recommends that HIV-infected mothers not breastfeed their infants to avoid the risk of postnatal transmission of HIV. It is not known whether enfuvirtide is excreted in human milk. Because of both the potential for HIV transmission and the potential for serious adverse reactions in nursing infants, mothers should be instructed not to breastfeed if they are receiving enfuvirtide.

Studies where radiolabeled ^{3}H-enfuvirtide was administered to lactating rats indicated that radioactivity was present in the milk. It is not known whether the radioactivity in the milk was from radiolabeled enfuvirtide or from radiolabeled metabolites of enfuvirtide (ie, amino acids and peptide fragments).

➤*Children:* The safety and pharmacokinetics of enfuvirtide have not been established in pediatric subjects below 6 years of age. Limited efficacy data is available in pediatric subjects 6 years of age and older.

Thirty-five HIV-1 infected pediatric subjects ages 6 through 16 years have received enfuvirtide in 2 open-label, single-arm clinical trials. Adverse experiences were similar to those observed in adult patients.

ENFUVIRTIDE — INJECTION

Precautions

➤*Hazardous tasks:* Patients should be advised that no studies have been conducted on the ability to drive or operate machinery while taking enfuvirtide. If patients experience dizziness while taking enfuvirtide, they should be advised to talk to their healthcare providers before driving or operating machinery.

Drug Interactions

➤*Drug/Lab test indteractions:* There is a theoretical risk that enfuvirtide use may lead to the production of antienfuvirtide antibodies which cross react with HIV gp41. This could result in a false-positive HIV test with an ELISA assay; a confirmatory western blot test would be expected to be negative. Enfuvirtide has not been studied in non-HIV-infected individuals.

Adverse Reactions

➤*Hypersensitivity:* Hypersensitivity reactions have been attributed to enfuvirtide (less than or equal to 1%) and in some cases have recurred upon rechallenge.

➤*Local:* Local injection-site reactions were the most frequent adverse events associated with the use of enfuvirtide. In phase 3 clinical studies (T20-301 and T20-302), 98% of subjects had at least 1 local injection site reaction (ISR). Three percent (3%) of subjects discontinued treatment with enfuvirtide because of ISRs. Eighty-six percent (86%) of subjects experienced their first ISR during the initial week of treatment. The majority of ISRs were associated with mild-to-moderate pain at the injection site, erythema, induration, and the presence of nodules or cysts. For most subjects the severity of signs and symptoms associated with ISRs did not change during the 24 weeks of treatment. In 17% of subjects an individual ISR lasted for longer than 7 days. Because of the frequency and duration of individual ISRs, 23% of subjects had 6 or more ongoing ISRs at any given time. Individual signs and symptoms characterizing local ISRs are summarized in the following table. Infection at the injection site (including abscess and cellulitis) was reported in 1% of subjects.

Summary of individual signs/symptoms characterizing local injection-site reactions to enfuvirtide in studies T20-301 and T20-302 combined (% of subjects)

	(n = 663)		
Event category	Any severity grade	% of reactions comprising grade 3 reactions	% of reactions comprising grade 4 reactions
Pain/discomfort [a]	95%	9%	0%
Induration[b]	89%	41%	16%
Erythema [c]	89%	22%	10%
Nodules and cysts[d]	76%	26%	0%
Pruritus [e]	62%	4%	NA
Ecchymosis [f]	48%	8%	5%

[a] Grade 3 = Severe pain requiring analgesics (or narcotic analgesics for less than or equal to 72 hours) or limiting usual activities.Grade 4 = Severe pain requiring hospitalization or prolongation of hospitalization, resulting in death, or persistent or significant disability/incapacity, or life-threatening, or medically significant.
[b] Grade 3 = Greater than or equal to 25 mm but less than 50 mm; grade 4 = greater than or equal to 50 mm average diameter.
[c] Grade 3 = Greater than or equal to 50 mm but less than 85 mm average diameter; grade 4 = greater than or equal to 85 mm average diameter.
[d] Grade 3 = Greater than or equal to 3 cm; grade 4 = if draining.
[e] Grade 3 = Refractory to topical treatment or requiring oral or parenteral treatment; grade 4 = not applicable.
[f] Grade 3 = Greater than 3 cm but less than or equal to 5 cm; grade 4 = greater than 5 cm.

➤*Other adverse reactions:* The reactions most frequently reported in subjects receiving enfuvirtide + background regimen, excluding injection-site reactions, were diarrhea (26.8%), nausea (20.1%), and fatigue (16.1%). These events were also commonly observed in subjects that received background regimen alone: Diarrhea (33.5%), nausea (23.7%), and fatigue (17.4%).

Percentage of patients with selected treatment-emergent adverse reactions * reported in greater than or equal to 2% of adult patients and occurring more frequently in patients treated with enfuvirtide (pooled studies T20-301/T20-302 at 24 weeks)

Adverse reaction (by system organ class)	Enfuvirtide + background regimen (n = 663)	Background regimen (n = 334)
CNS		
Peripheral neuropathy	8.9%	6.3%
Taste disturbance	2.4%	1.5%
Psychiatric		
Insomnia	11.3%	8.7%
Depression	8.6%	7.2%
Anxiety	5.7%	3%
Respiratory, thoracic, and mediastinal disorders		
Cough	7.4%	5.4%

Percentage of patients with selected treatment-emergent adverse reactions * reported in greater than or equal to 2% of adult patients and occurring more frequently in patients treated with enfuvirtide (pooled studies T20-301/T20-302 at 24 weeks)

Adverse reaction (by system organ class)	Enfuvirtide + background regimen (n = 663)	Background regimen (n = 334)
Infections		
Sinusitis	6.2%	2.1%
Herpes simplex	5%	3.9%
Skin papilloma	4.2%	1.5%
Influenza	3.9%	1.8%
Miscellaneous		
Decreased weight	6.5%	5.1%
Decreased appetite	6.3%	2.4%
Asthenia	5.7%	4.2%
Anorexia	2.6%	1.8%
Influenza-like illness	2.3%	0.9%
Dermatologic		
Pruritus not otherwise specified	5.1%	4.2%
Musculoskeletal, connective tissue, and bone disorders		
Myalgia	5%	2.4%
GI		
Constipation	3.9%	2.7%
Upper abdominal pain	3%	2.7%
Pancreatitis	2.4%	0.9%
Ophthalmic		
Conjunctivitis	2.4%	0.9%
Hematologic		
Lymphadenopathy	2.3%	0.3%

* Excludes injection-site reactions.

Respiratory – An increased rate of bacterial pneumonia was observed in subjects treated with enfuvirtide in the phase 3 clinical trials compared to the control arm (4.68 pneumonia events per 100 patient-years versus 0.61 events per 100 patient-years, respectively). Approximately half of the study subjects with pneumonia required hospitalization. One subject death in the enfuvirtide arm was attributed to pneumonia. Risk factors for pneumonia included low initial CD4 lymphocyte count, high initial viral load, IV drug use, smoking, and a history of lung disease. It is unclear if the increased incidence of pneumonia was related to enfuvirtide use. However, because of this finding patients with HIV infection should be carefully monitored for signs and symptoms of pneumonia, especially if they have underlying conditions which may predispose them to pneumonia.

➤*Less common events:* The following adverse reactions have been reported in 1 or more subjects; however, a causal relationship to enfuvirtide has not been established.

CNS – Guillain-Barre syndrome (fatal); sixth nerve palsy.

Hematologic/Lymphatic – Thrombocytopenia; neutropenia, and fever.

Hypersensitivity – Worsening abacavir hypersensitivity reaction.

Lab test abnormalities –

Percentage of treatment-emergent laboratory abnormalities that occurred in ≥ 2% of adult patients and more frequently in patients receiving enfuvirtide (pooled studies T20-301 and T20-302 at 24 weeks

Laboratory parameters	Grading	Enfuvirtide + background regimen (n = 663)	Background regimen (n = 334)
Eosinophilia			
1-2 X ULN (0.7 × 10^9/L)	0.7-1.4 × 10^9/L	8.3%	1.5%
> 2 x ULN (0.7 × 10^9/L)	> 1.4 × 10^9/L	1.8%	0.9%
Amylase (U/L)			
Gr. 3	> 2 to 5 × ULN	6.2%	3.6%
Gr. 4	> 5 × ULN or clinical pancreatitis	0.9%	0.6%
Lipase (U/L)			
Gr. 3	> 2-5 × ULN	5.9%	3.6%
Gr. 4	> 5 × ULN	2.3%	1.8%

ENFUVIRTIDE — INJECTION

Percentage of treatment-emergent laboratory abnormalities that occurred in ≥ 2% of adult patients and more frequently in patients receiving enfuvirtide (pooled studies T20-301 and T20-302 at 24 weeks)			
Laboratory parameters	Grading	Enfuvirtide + background regimen (n = 663)	Background regimen (n = 334)
Triglycerides (mmol/L)			
Gr. 3	> 1000 mg/dL	8.9%	7.2%
ALT			
Gr. 3	> 5 to 10 × ULN	3.5%	2.1%
Gr. 4	> 10 × ULN	0.9%	0.6%
AST			
Gr. 3	> 5 to 10 × ULN	3.6%	3%
Gr. 4	> 10 × ULN	1.2%	0.6%
Creatine phosphokinase (U/L)			
Gr. 3	> 5 to 10 × ULN	5.9%	3.6%
Gr. 4	> 10 × ULN	2.3%	3.6%
GGT (U/L)			
Gr. 3	> 5 to 10 × ULN	3.5%	3.3%
Gr. 4	> 10 × ULN	2.4%	1.8%
Hemoglobin (g/dL)			
Gr. 3	6.5 to 7.9 g/dL	1.5%	0.9%
Gr. 4	< 6.5 g/dL	0.6%	0.6%

Metabolic – Hyperglycemia.

Renal – Renal insufficiency (glomerulonephritis); renal failure.

Respiratory – Pneumonia.

Overdosage

➤*Symptoms:* There are no reports of human experience of acute overdose with enfuvirtide. The highest dose administered to 12 subjects in a clinical trial was 180 mg as a single dose SC.

➤*Treatment:* There is no specific antidote for overdose with enfuvirtide. Treatment of overdose should consist of general supportive measures.

Patient Information

To ensure safe and effective use of enfuvirtide, the following information and instructions should be given to patients:

Patients should be informed that injection-site reactions occur commonly. Patients must be familiar with the enfuvirtide injection instructions for instructions on how to appropriately inject enfuvirtide and how to carefully monitor for signs or symptoms of cellulitis or local infection. Patients should be instructed when to contact their healthcare provider about these reactions.

Patients should be made aware that an increased rate of bacterial pneumonia was observed in subjects treated with enfuvirtide in phase 3 clinical trials compared to the control arm. Patients should be advised to seek medical evaluation immediately if they develop signs or symptoms suggestive of pneumonia (cough with fever, rapid breathing, shortness of breath).

Patients should be advised of the possibility of a hypersensitivity reaction to enfuvirtide. Patients should be advised to discontinue therapy and immediately seek medical evaluation if they develop signs/symptoms of hypersensitivity. Hypersensitivity reactions have included the following, individually and in combination: Rash, fever, nausea and vomiting, chills, rigors, hypotension, and elevated serum liver transaminases.

Enfuvirtide is not a cure for HIV-1 infection and patients may continue to contract illnesses associated with HIV-1 infection. The long-term effects of enfuvirtide are unknown at this time. Enfuvirtide therapy has not been shown to reduce the risk of transmitting HIV-1 to others through sexual contact or blood contamination.

Enfuvirtide must be taken as part of a combination antiretroviral regimen. Use of enfuvirtide alone may lead to rapid development of virus resistant to enfuvirtide and possibly other agents of the same class.

Patients and caregivers must be instructed in the use of aseptic technique when administering enfuvirtide in order to avoid injection-site infections. Appropriate training for enfuvirtide reconstitution and self-injection must be given by a healthcare provider, including a careful review of the enfuvirtide patient prescribing information and enfuvirtide injection instructions. The first injection should be performed under the supervision of an appropriately qualified healthcare provider. It is recommended that the patient or caregiver's understanding and use of aseptic self-injection techniques and procedures be periodically reevaluated.

Patients should contact their healthcare providers for any questions regarding the administration of enfuvirtide. Patients should be told not to reuse needles or syringes, and be instructed in safe disposal procedures including the use of a puncture-resistant container for disposal of used needles and syringes. Patients must be instructed on the safe disposal of full containers as per local requirements. Caregivers who experience an accidental needlestick after patient injection should contact a healthcare provider immediately.

Patients should inform their healthcare providers if they are pregnant, plan to become pregnant or become pregnant while taking this medication.

Patients should inform their healthcare providers if they are breastfeeding.

Patients should not change the dose or dosing schedule of enfuvirtide or any antiretroviral medication without consulting their healthcare provider.

Patients should contact their healthcare providers immediately if they stop taking enfuvirtide or any other drug in their antiretroviral regimen.

Patients should be advised that no studies have been conducted on the ability to drive or operate machinery while taking enfuvirtide. If patients experience dizziness while taking enfuvirtide, they should be advised to talk to their healthcare provider before driving or operating machinery.

LEPROSTATICS

DAPSONE (DDS)

Rx	**Dapsone** (Jacobus)	**Tablets:** 25 mg	(Jacobus 25 102). White, scored. In 100s.
		100 mg	(Jacobus 100 101). White, scored. In 100s.

DAPSONE — ORAL

Indications

➤*Dermatitis herpetiformis (DH):* Treatment of DH and all forms of leprosy except for cases of proven dapsone resistance.

➤*Unlabeled uses:*

Leprosy – Unlabeled uses of dapsone include treatment of relapsing polychondritis; prophylaxis of malaria; inflammatory bowel disorders; Leishmaniasis; *Pneumocystis carinii* pneumonia; rheumatic/connective tissue disorders (eg, rheumatoid arthritis, lupus erythematosus); brown recluse spider bites. Doses used generally range from 50 to 200 mg/day.

Administration and Dosage

➤*Dermatitis herpetiformis:* The dosage should be individually titrated starting in adults with 50 mg daily and correspondingly smaller doses in children. If full control is not achieved within the range of 50 to 300 mg daily, higher doses may be tried. Dosage should be reduced to a minimum maintenance level as soon as possible. In responsive patients there is a prompt reduction in pruritus followed by clearance of skin lesions. There is no affect on the GI component of the disease.

Dapsone levels are influenced by acetylation rates. Patients with high acetylation rates, or who are receiving treatment affecting acetylation may require an adjustment in dosage.

A strict gluten-free diet is an option for the patient to elect, permitting many to reduce or eliminate the need for dapsone; the average time for dosage reduction is 8 months with a range of 4 months to 2½ years and for dosage elimination, 29 months with a range of 6 months to 9 years.

➤*Leprosy:* In order to reduce secondary dapsone resistance, the WHO Expert Committee on Leprosy and the USPHS at Carville, LA recommended that dapsone should be commenced in combination with one or more antileprosy drugs. In the multidrug program dapsone should be maintained at the full dosage of 100 mg daily without interruption (with corresponding smaller doses for children) and provided to all patients who have sensitive organisms with new or recrudescent disease or who have not yet completed a two year course of dapsone monotherapy. For advice and other drugs, the USPHS at Carville, LA (1-800-642-2477) should be contacted. Before using other drugs consult appropriate product labeling.

Bacteriologically negative tuberculoid and indeterminate disease – In bacteriologically negative tuberculoid and indeterminate disease, the recommendation is the coadministration of dapsone 100 mg daily with 6 months of rifampin 600 mg daily.

Under WHO, daily rifampin may be replaced by 600 mg rifampin monthly, if supervised. The dapsone is continued until all signs of clinical activity are controlled, usually after an additional 6 months. Then dapsone should be continued for an additional 3 years for tuberculoid and indeterminate patients and for 5 years for borderline tuberculoid patients.

DAPSONE — ORAL

Lepromatous and borderline lepromatous – In lepromatous and borderline lepromatous patients, the recommendation is the coadministration of dapsone 100 mg daily with 2 years of rifampin 600 mg daily. Under WHO daily rifampin may be replaced by 600 mg rifampin monthly, if supervised. One may elect the concurrent administration of a third anti-leprosy drug, usually either clofazamine 50 to 100 mg daily or ethionamide 250 to 500 mg daily. Dapsone 100 mg daily is continued 3 to 10 years until all signs of clinical activity are controlled with skin scrapings and biopsies negative for 1 year. Dapsone should then be continued for an additional 10 years for borderline patients and for life for lepromatous patients.

Secondary dapsone resistance should be suspected whenever a lepromatous or borderline lepromatous patient receiving dapsone treatment relapses clinically and bacteriologically, solid staining bacilli being found in the smears taken from the new active lesions. If such cases show no response to regular and supervised dapsone therapy within 3 to 6 months or good compliance for the past 3 to 6 months can be assured. Dapsone resistance should be considered confirmed clinically. Determination of drug sensitivity using the mouse footpad method is recommended and, after prior arrangement, is available without charge from the USPHS, Carville, LA. Patients with proven dapsone resistance should be treated with other drugs.

➤*Storage/Stability:* Store at controlled room temperature, 20° to 25°C (68° to 77°F).

Protect from light.

Dispense this product in a well-closed child-resistant container.

Actions

➤*Pharmacology:* The mechanism of action in dermatitis herpetiformis has not been established. By the kinetic method in mice, dapsone is bactericidal as well as bacteriostatic against *Mycobacterium leprae*.

➤*Pharmacokinetics:*

Absorption – Dapsone, when given orally, is rapidly and almost completely absorbed. Detected a few minutes after ingestion, the drug reaches peak concentration in 4 to 8 hours. Daily administration for at least 8 days is necessary to achieve a plateau level. With doses of 200 mg daily, this level averaged 2.3 mcg/mL with a range of 0.1 to 7 mcg/mL.

Excretion – The half-life in the plasma in different individuals varies from 10 to 50 hours and averages 28 hours. Repeat tests in the same individual are constant. Daily administration (50 to 100 mg) in leprosy patients will provide blood levels in excess of the usual minimum inhibitory concentration even for patients with a short dapsone half-life. Excretion of the drug is slow and a constant blood level can be maintained with the usual dosage. About 85% of the daily intake is recoverable from the urine mainly in the form of water-soluble metabolites.

Contraindications

Hypersensitivity to dapsone or its derivatives.

Warnings

➤*Hematologic effects:* The patient should be warned to respond to the presence of clinical signs such as sore throat, fever, pallor, purpura or jaundice. Deaths associated with the administration of dapsone have been reported from agranulocytosis, aplastic anemia and other blood dyscrasias. Complete blood counts should be done frequently in patients receiving dapsone. The FDA Dermatology Advisory Committee recommended that, when feasible, counts should be done weekly for the first month, monthly for 6 months and semi-annually thereafter. If a significant reduction in leucocytes, platelets or hemopoiesis is noted, dapsone should be discontinued and the patient followed intensively. Folic acid antagonists have similar effects and may increase the incidence of hematologic reactions; if co-administered with dapsone the patient should be monitored more frequently. Patients on weekly pyrimethamine and dapsone have developed agranulocytosis during the second and third month of therapy.

Severe anemia – Severe anemia should be treated prior to initiation of therapy and hemoglobin monitored. Hemolysis and methemoglobin may be poorly tolerated by patients with severe cardiopulmonary disease.

➤*Cutaneous reactions:* Cutaneous reactions, especially bullous, include exfoliative dermatitis and are probably one of the most serious, though rare, complications of sulfone therapy. They are directly due to drug sensitization. Such reactions include toxic erythema, erythema multiforme, toxic epidermal necrolysis, morbilliform and scarlatiniform reactions, urticaria and erythema nodosum. If new or toxic dermatologic reactions occur, sulfone therapy must be promptly discontinued and appropriate therapy instituted.

➤*Leprosy reactional states:* Leprosy reactional states, including cutaneous, are not hypersensitivity reactions to dapsone and do not require discontinuation (see Administration and Dosage, Leprosy reactional states).

Abrupt changes in clinical activity occur in leprosy with any effective treatment and are known as reactional states. The majority can be classified into 2 groups.

The "reversal" reaction (Type 1) may occur in borderline or tuberculoid leprosy patients often seen after chemotherapy is started. The mechanism is presumed to result from a reduction in the antigenic load: The patient is able to mount an enhanced delayed hypersensitivity response to residual infection leading to swelling ("reversal") of existing skin and nerve lesions. If severe, or if neuritis is present, large doses of steroids should always be used. If severe, the patient should be hospitalized. In general antileprosy treatment is continued and therapy to suppress the reaction is indicated such as analgesics, steroids, or surgical decompression of swollen nerve trunks. USPHS at Carville, LA should be contacted for advice in management.

Erythema nodosum leprosum (ENL) or lepromatous reaction (Type 2 reaction) occurs mainly in lepromatous patients and small numbers of borderline patients. Approximately 50% of treated patients show this reaction in the first year. The principal clinical features are fever and tender erythematous skin nodules sometimes associated with malaise, neuritis, orchitis, albuminuria, joint swelling, iritis, epistaxis or depression. Skin lesions can become pustular or ulcerate. Histologically there is a vasculitis with an intense polymorphonuclear infiltrate. Elevated circulating immune complexes are considered to be the mechanism of reaction. If severe, patients should be hospitalized. In general, anti-leprosy treatment is continued. Analgesics, steroids, and other agents available from USPHS at Carville, LA are used to suppress the reaction.

➤*Carcinogenesis:* Dapsone has been found carcinogenic (sarcomagenic) for male rats and female mice causing mesenchymal tumors in the spleen and peritoneum, and thyroid carcinoma in female rats.

➤*Pregnancy: Category C.* Animal reproduction studies have not been conducted with dapsone. Extensive, but uncontrolled experience and two published surveys on the use of dapsone in pregnant women have not shown that dapsone increases the risk of fetal abnormalities if administered during all trimesters of pregnancy or can affect reproduction capacity. Because of the lack of animal studies or controlled human experience, dapsone should be given to a pregnant woman only if clearly needed. In general, for leprosy, USPHS at Carville recommends maintenance of dapsone. Dapsone has been important for the management of some pregnant DH patients.

➤*Lactation:* Dapsone is excreted in breast milk in substantial amounts. Hemolytic reactions can occur in neonates (see Precautions). Because of the potential for tumorgenicity shown for dapsone in animal studies a decision should be made whether to discontinue nursing or discontinue the drug taking into account the importance of drug to the mother.

➤*Children:* Children are treated on the same schedule as adults but with correspondingly smaller doses. Dapsone is generally not considered to have an effect on the later growth, development and functional development of the child.

Precautions

➤*Hemolysis:* Hemolysis and Heinz body formation may be exaggerated in individuals with a glucose-6-phosphate dehydrogenase (G-6-PD) deficiency, or methemoglobin reductase deficiency, or hemoglobin M. This reaction is frequently dose-related. Dapsone should be given with caution to these patients or if the patient is exposed to other agents or conditions such as infection or diabetic ketosis capable of producing hemolysis. Drugs or chemicals which have produced significant hemolysis in G-6-PD or methemoglobin reductase-deficient patients include dapsone, sulfanilamide, nitrite, aniline, phenylhydrazine, napthalene, niridazole, nitrofurantoin and 8-aminoantimalarials such as primaquine.

➤*Hepatic effects:* Toxic hepatitis and cholestatic jaundice have been reported early in therapy. Hyperbilirubinemia may occur more often in G-6-PD-deficient patients. When feasible, baseline and subsequent monitoring of liver function is recommended: If abnormal, dapsone should be discontinued until the source of the abnormality is established.

Drug Interactions

Dapsone Drug Interactions

Precipitant drug	Object drug*		Description
Charcoal, activated	Dapsone	⬇	Activated charcoal may decrease dapsone's GI absorption and enterohepatic recycling.
Didanosine	Dapsone	⬇	Possible therapeutic failure of dapsone, leading to an increase in infection.
Folic acid antagonists	Dapsone	⬆	Folic acid antagonists such as pyrimethamine may increase the likelihood of hematologic reactions. Weekly concomitant use has caused agranulocytosis during the second and third months of therapy.
Para-aminobenzoic acid	Dapsone	⬇	Para-aminobenzoic acid may antagonize the effect of dapsone by interfering with the primary mechanism of action.
Probenecid	Dapsone	⬆	Probenecid reduces urinary excretion of dapsone metabolites, increasing plasma concentrations.
Rifampin	Dapsone	⬇	Rifampin lowers dapsone levels seven to tenfold by accelerating plasma clearance.
Trimethoprim	Dapsone	⬆	Increased serum levels of both drugs may occur, possibly increasing the pharmologic and toxic effects of each drug.
Dapsone	Trimethoprim	⬆	

* ⬆ = Object drug increased. ⬇ = Object drug decreased.

Adverse Reactions

➤*Hematologic:* Dose-related hemolysis is the most common adverse effect and is seen in patients with or without G-6-PD deficiency. Almost all patients demonstrate the inter-related changes of a loss of 1 to 2 g of hemo-

DAPSONE — ORAL

globin, an increase in the reticulocytes (2% to 12%), a shortened red cell life span and a rise in methemoglobin. G-6-PD deficient patients have greater responses.

➤*Miscellaneous:* In addition to the warnings and adverse effects reported above, additional adverse reactions include: Nausea, vomiting, abdominal pains, pancreatitis, vertigo, blurred vision, tinnitus, insomnia, fever, headache, psychosis, phototoxicity, pulmonary eosinophilia, tachycardia, albuminuria, the nephrotic syndrome, hypoalbuminemia without proteinuria, renal papillary necrosis, male infertility, drug-induced Lupus erythematosus and an infectious mononucleosis-like syndrome. In general, with the exception of the complications of severe anoxia from overdosage (eg, retinal and optic nerve damage) these adverse reactions have regressed following drug discontinuation.

Peripheral nervous system – Peripheral neuropathy is a definite but unusual complication of dapsone therapy in non-leprosy patients. Motor loss is predominant. If muscle weakness appears, dapsone should be withdrawn. Recovery on withdrawal is usually substantially complete. The mechanism of recovery is reported by axonal regeneration. Some recovered patients have tolerated retreatment at reduced dosage. In leprosy this complication may be difficult to distinguish from a leprosy reactional state.

Overdosage

➤*Symptoms:* Nausea, vomiting, and hyperexcitability can appear a few minutes up to 24 hours after ingestion of an overdosage. Methemoglobin induced depression, convulsions or severe cyanosis requires prompt treatment.

➤*Treatment:* In normal and methemoglobin reductase deficient patients, methylene blue, 1 to 2 mg/kg of body weight, given slowly intravenously is the treatment of choice. The effect is complete in 30 minutes, but may have to be repeated if methemoglobin reaccumulates. For non-emergencies, if treatment is needed, methylene blue may be given orally in doses of 3 to 5 mg/kg every 4 to 6 hours. Methylene blue reduction depends on G-6-PD and should not be given to fully expressed G-6-PD-deficient patients.

ANTIPROTOZOALS

NITAZOXANIDE

Rx	**Alinia** (Romark Laboratories)	**Tablets:** 500 mg	Sucrose, polyvinyl alcohol, talc. (ALINIA 500). Round, yellow, film-coated. In 60s and UD 6s.
		Powder for oral suspension: 100 mg per 5 mL (after reconstitution)	With sugar and sucrose 1.48 mg per 5 mL. Strawberry flavor. In 60 mL.

NITAZOXANIDE — ORAL

Indications

➤*Diarrhea caused by Giardia lamblia:* Nitazoxanide oral suspension (patients 1 year of age and older) and tablets (patients 12 years of age and older) are indicated for the treatment of diarrhea caused by *G. lamblia*.

➤*Diarrhea caused by Cryptosporidium parvum:* Nitazoxanide oral suspension is indicated for patients 1 to 11 years of age for the treatment of diarrhea caused by *C. parvum*.

Nitazoxanide oral suspension and tablets have not been shown to be superior to placebo for the treatment of diarrhea caused by *C. parvum* in HIV-infected or immunodeficient patients.

Administration and Dosage

➤*Approved by the FDA:* November 22, 2002.

Indication	Age	Dosage	Duration
Treatment of diarrhea caused by *G. lamblia*	1 to 3 years	Nitazoxanide 5 mL oral suspension (nitazoxanide 100 mg) every 12 hours with food.	3 days
	4 to 11 years	Nitazoxanide 10 mL oral suspension (nitazoxanide 200 mg) every 12 hours with food.	
	≥ 12 years	1 nitazoxanide tablet (nitazoxanide 500 mg) every 12 hours with food or 25 mL nitazoxanide oral suspension (nitazoxanide 500 mg) every 12 hours with food.	
Treatment of diarrhea caused by *C. parvum*	1 to 3 years	Nitazoxanide 5 mL oral suspension (nitazoxanide 100 mg) every 12 hours with food.	3 days
	4 to 11 years	Nitazoxanide 10 mL oral suspension (nitazoxanide 200 mg) every 12 hours with food.	

➤*Tablets:* A single nitazoxanide tablet contains a greater amount of nitazoxanide than is recommended for pediatric dosing and, therefore, should not be used in pediatric patients 11 years of age or younger.

➤*HIV-infected or immunodeficient patients:* See Warnings for more information.

➤*Reconstitution of suspension:* Prepare a suspension at time of dispensing as follows: The amount of water required for preparation of the suspension is 48 mL. Tap bottle until all powder flows freely. Add approximately ½ of the total amount of water required for reconstitution and shake vigorously to suspend powder. Add remainder of water and again shake vigorously.

Shake the suspension well before each administration.

➤*Storage/Stability:* Store the tablets, unsuspended powder, and the reconstituted oral suspension at 25°C (77°F); excursions permitted to 15° to 30°C (59° to 86°F). The suspension may be stored for 7 days, after which any unused portion must be discarded.

Actions

➤*Pharmacology:* The antiprotozoal activity of nitazoxanide is believed to be caused by interference with the pyruvate:ferredoxin oxidoreductase (PFOR) enzyme-dependent electron transfer reaction which is essential to anaerobic energy metabolism. Studies have shown that the PFOR enzyme from *G. lamblia* directly reduces nitazoxanide by transfer of electrons in the absence of ferredoxin. The DNA-derived PFOR protein sequence of *C. parvum* appears to be similar to that of *G. lamblia*. Interference with the PFOR enzyme-dependent electron transfer reaction may not be the only pathway by which nitazoxanide exhibits antiprotozoal activity.

➤*Pharmacokinetics:*

Absorption – Following oral administration of nitazoxanide tablets or oral suspension, maximum plasma concentrations of the active metabolites tizoxanide and tizoxanide glucuronide are observed within 1 to 4 hours. The parent nitazoxanide is not detected in plasma.

Mean (±SD) Plasma Pharmacokinetic Parameter Values Following Administration of a Single Dose of 1 Nitazoxanide 500 mg Tablet with Food to Subjects ≥ 12 Years of Age

	Tizoxanide			Tizoxanide glucuronide		
Age	C_{max} (mcg/mL)	T_{max} (h)[a]	$AUC_τ$ (mcg•h/mL)	C_{max} (mcg/mL)	T_{max}[a] (h)	$AUC_τ$ (mcg•h/mL)
12 to 17 years	9.1 (6.1)	4 (1 to 4)	39.5 (24.2)	7.3 (1.9)	4 (2 to 8)	46.5 (18.2)
≥ 18 years	10.6 (2)	3 (2 to 4)	41.9 (6)	10.5 (1.4)	4.5 (4 to 6)	63 (12.3)

[a] T_{max} is given as a mean (range).

Mean (± SD) Plasma Pharmacokinetic Parameter Values Following Administration of a Single Dose of Nitazoxanide for Oral Suspension with Food to Subjects 1 to 11 Years of Age

		Tizoxanide			Tizoxanide glucuronide		
Age	Dose	C_{max} (mcg/mL)	T_{max}[a] (h)	$AUC_τ$ (mcg•h/mL)	C_{max} (mcg/mL)	T_{max}[a] (h)	$AUC_τ$ (mcg•h/mL)
1 to 3 years	100 mg	3.11 (2)	3.5 (2 to 4)	11.7 (4.46)	3.64 (1.16)	4 (3 to 4)	19 (5.03)
4 to 11 years	200 mg	3 (0.99)	2 (1 to 4)	13.5 (3.3)	2.84 (0.97)	4 (2 to 4)	16.9 (5)

[a] T_{max} is given as mean (range).

Nitazoxanide oral suspension is not bioequivalent to nitazoxanide tablets. The relative bioavailability of the suspension compared with the tablet was 70%.

Nitazoxanide tablets and oral suspension were administered with food in clinical trials, and, therefore, they are recommended to be administered with food.

Distribution – In plasma, more than 99% of tizoxanide is bound to proteins.

Metabolism – Following oral administration in humans, nitazoxanide is rapidly hydrolyzed to an active metabolite, tizoxanide (desacetyl-nitazoxanide). Tizoxanide then undergoes conjugation, primarily by glucuronidation. In vitro metabolism studies have demonstrated that tizoxanide has no significant inhibitory effect on cytochrome P450 enzymes.

Excretion – Tizoxanide is excreted in the urine, bile, and feces, and tizoxanide glucuronide is excreted in urine and bile. Approximately two-thirds of the oral dose of nitazoxanide is excreted in the feces and one-third in the urine.

➤*Microbiology:* Nitazoxanide and its metabolite, tizoxanide, are active in vitro in inhibiting the growth of sporozoites and oocysts of *C. parvum* and trophozoites of *G. lamblia*.

See Indications for more information.

NITAZOXANIDE — ORAL

Contraindications

Prior hypersensitivity to nitazoxanide or any other ingredient in the formulations.

Warnings

➤*HIV-infected or immunodeficient patients:* Nitazoxanide tablets and oral suspension have not been studied for the treatment of diarrhea caused by *G. lamblia* in HIV-infected or immunodeficient patients. Nitazoxanide tablets and oral suspension have not been shown to be superior to placebo for the treatment of diarrhea caused by *C. parvum* in HIV-infected or immunodeficient patients.

➤*Renal/Hepatic function impairment:* The pharmacokinetics of nitazoxanide in patients with compromised renal or hepatic function have not been studied. Therefore, nitazoxanide must be administered with caution to patients with hepatic and biliary disease, to patients with renal disease, and to patients with combined renal and hepatic disease.

➤*Mutagenesis:* Nitazoxanide was not genotoxic in the Chinese hamster ovary (CHO) cell chromosomal aberration assay or the mouse micronucleus assay. Nitazoxanide was genotoxic in one tester strain (TA 100) in the Ames bacterial mutation assay.

➤*Elderly:* In general, consider the greater frequency of decreased hepatic, renal, or cardiac function, and of concomitant disease or other drug therapy in elderly patients when prescribing nitazoxanide tablets and oral suspension. This therapy must be administered with caution to patients with renal and/or hepatic impairment.

➤*Pregnancy: Category B.* There are no adequate and well-controlled studies in pregnant women.

➤*Lactation:* It is not known whether nitazoxanide is excreted in human milk. Because many drugs are excreted in human milk, exercise caution when nitazoxanide is administered to a nursing woman.

➤*Children:* A single nitazoxanide tablet contains a greater amount of nitazoxanide than is recommended for pediatric dosing and, therefore, should not be used in pediatric patients 11 years of age and younger. Use only nitazoxanide oral suspension for dosing nitazoxanide in pediatric patients. Safety and effectiveness of nitazoxanide for oral suspension in pediatric patients younger than 1 year of age have not been studied.

Drug Interactions

Tizoxanide is highly bound to plasma protein (greater than 99.9%). Therefore, use caution when administering nitazoxanide concurrently with other highly plasma protein-bound drugs with narrow therapeutic indices, as competition for binding sites may occur (eg, warfarin).

Adverse Reactions

In controlled and uncontrolled clinical studies of 1,628 HIV-uninfected patients 12 years of age and older who received various dosage regimens of nitazoxanide tablets, the most common adverse reactions reported regardless of causality assessment were abdominal pain (6.7%), diarrhea (4.3%), nausea (3.1%), and headache (3.1%). In placebo-controlled clinical trials using the recommended dose, the rates of occurrence of these events did not differ significantly from those of the placebo. In the placebo-controlled trials of HIV-uninfected patients 12 years of age and older who received nitazoxanide tablets for the treatment of diarrhea caused by *G. lamblia*, approximately 1% of patients discontinued therapy because of an adverse reaction.

In controlled and uncontrolled clinical studies of 613 HIV-negative pediatric patients who received nitazoxanide for oral suspension, the most frequent adverse reactions reported regardless of causality assessment were abdominal pain (7.8%), diarrhea (2.1%), vomiting (1.1%), and headache (1.1%). These were typically mild and transient in nature. In placebo-controlled clinical trials, the rates of occurrence of these reactions did not differ significantly from those of the placebo. None of the 613 pediatric patients discontinued therapy because of adverse reactions.

The adverse reactions seen in adult patients treated with nitazoxanide oral suspension were similar to those observed in adult patients treated with nitazoxanide tablets.

➤*Adverse reactions (tablets in patients 12 years of age and older, less than 1%):*

Cardiovascular – Hypertension, syncope, tachycardia.

CNS – Dizziness, hypesthesia, insomnia, somnolence, tremor.

Dermatologic – Pruritus, rash.

GI – Anorexia, constipation, dry mouth, dyspepsia, flatulence, thirst, vomiting.

GU – Amenorrhea, discolored urine, dysuria, edema labia, kidney pain, metrorrhagia.

Hematologic/Lymphatic – Anemia, leukocytosis.

Metabolic/Nutritional – Increased ALT.

Musculoskeletal – Leg cramps, myalgia, spontaneous bone fracture.

Respiratory – Epistaxis, lung disease, pharyngitis.

Special senses – Ear ache, eye discoloration.

Miscellaneous – Allergic reaction, asthenia, chills, fever, chills and fever, flu syndrome, pain, pelvic pain.

➤*Adverse reactions (oral suspension in children, less than 1%) :*

CNS – Dizziness.

Dermatologic – Pruritus, sweating.

GI – Anorexia, appetite increase, enlarged salivary glands, flatulence, nausea.

GU – Discolored urine.

Metabolic/Nutritional – Increased ALT, increased creatinine.

Respiratory – Rhinitis.

Special senses – Eye discoloration (pale yellow).

Miscellaneous – Fever, infection, malaise.

Overdosage

➤*Symptoms:* Information on nitazoxanide overdosage is not available. In acute studies in rodents and dogs, the oral LD_{50} was higher than 10,000 mg/kg. Single oral doses of up to 4,000 mg nitazoxanide in a tablet formulation have been administered to healthy adult volunteers without significant adverse effects.

➤*Treatment:* In the event of overdose, gastric lavage may be appropriate soon after oral administration. Observe patients carefully and give symptomatic and supportive treatment.

Patient Information

Take nitazoxanide tablets and oral suspension with food.

Diabetic patients and caregivers should be aware that the oral suspension contains 1.48 g of sucrose per 5 mL.

TINIDAZOLE

Rx	**Tindamax** (Presutti)	**Tablets:** 250 mg	(P L 250). Pink, scored. Film-coated. In 40s and 100s.
		500 mg	(P L 500). Pink, caplet-shaped, scored. Film-coated. In 20s and 60s.

TINIDAZOLE — ORAL

WARNING

Carcinogenicity has been seen in mice and rats treated chronically with another agent in the nitroimidazole class (metronidazole). Although such data have not been reported for tinidazole, avoid unnecessary use of tinidazole. Reserve its use for the conditions for which it is indicated.

Indications

➤*Trichomoniasis:* Treatment of trichomoniasis caused by *Trichomoniasis vaginalis* in both men and women. Identify the organism by appropriate diagnostic procedures. Because trichomoniasis is a sexually transmitted disease with potentially serious sequelae, treat partners of infected patients simultaneously in order to prevent reinfection.

➤*Giardiasis:* Treatment of giardiasis caused by *Giardiasis duodenalis* (also termed *Giardiasis lamblia*) in both adults and pediatric patients older than 3 years of age.

➤*Amebiasis:* Treatment of intestinal amebiasis and amebic liver abscess caused by *Entamoeba histolytica* in both adults and pediatric patients older than 3 years of age. It is not indicated in the treatment of asymptomatic cyst passage.

Administration and Dosage

➤*Approved by the FDA:* May 17, 2004.

Take tinidazole with food to minimize the incidence of epigastric discomfort and other GI adverse reactions. Food does not affect the oral bioavailability of tinidazole.

➤*Trichomoniasis:* A single 2 g oral dose taken with food. Since trichomoniasis is a sexually transmitted disease, treat sexual partners with the same dose and at the same time.

➤*Giardiasis:* In adults, a single 2 g dose taken with food. In pediatric patients older than 3 years of age, a single dose of 50 mg/kg (up to 2 g) with food.

➤*Amebiasis:*

Intestinal – In adults, a 2 g dose per day for 3 days taken with food. In pediatric patients older than 3 years of age, 50 mg/kg/day (up to 2 g per day) for 3 days with food.

Amebic liver abscess – In adults, a 2 g dose per day for 3 to 5 days taken with food. In pediatric patients older than 3 years of age, 50 mg/kg/day (up to 2 g per day) for 3 to 5 days with food. There are limited pediatric data on durations of therapy exceeding 3 days, although a small number of children were treated for 5 days without reported adverse reactions. Closely monitor children when treatment durations exceed 3 days.

➤*Children:* For those unable to swallow tablets, tinidazole tablets may be crushed in an artificial cherry syrup to be taken with food.

TINIDAZOLE — ORAL

Extemporaneous oral suspension (as used in pharmacokinetics studies) – Four 500 mg oral tablets were ground to a fine powder with a mortar and pestle. Approximately 10 mL of cherry syrup were added to the powder and mixed until smooth. The suspension was transferred to a graduated amber container. Several small rinses of cherry syrup were used to transfer any remaining drug in the mortar to the final suspension for a final volume of 30 mL. The suspension of crushed tablets in artificial cherry syrup (*Humco*) is stable for 7 days at room temperature. When this suspension is used, shake it well before each administration.

➤*Hemodialysis:* During hemodialysis, clearance of tinidazole is significantly increased; the half-life is reduced from 12 hours to 4.9 hours. Approximately 43% of the amount present in the body is eliminated during a 6-hour hemodialysis session. Thus, if tinidazole is administered on a day when dialysis is performed, it is recommended that an additional dose of tinidazole equivalent to one half of the recommended dose be administered after the end of the hemodialysis.

The pharmacokinetics of tinidazole in patients undergoing routine continuous peritoneal dialysis have not been investigated.

➤*Hepatic function impairment:* There are no data on tinidazole pharmacokinetics in patients with impaired hepatic function. Reduction of metabolic elimination of metronidazole, a chemically-related nitroimidazole, in patients with hepatic dysfunction has been reported in several studies. In the absence of data on tinidazole, cautiously administer usually recommended doses of tinidazole in such patients.

➤*Storage/Stability:* Store at controlled room temperature 20° to 25°C (68° to 77°F); excursions permitted to 15° to 30°C (59° to 86°F). Protect contents from light.

Actions

➤*Pharmacology:* Tinidazole is an antiprotozoal agent. The nitro group of tinidazole is reduced by cell extracts of *Trichomonas*. The free nitro radical generated as a result of this reduction may be responsible for the antiprotozoal activity. The mechanism by which tinidazole exhibits activity against *Giardia* and *Entamoeba* species is not known.

➤*Pharmacokinetics:*

Absorption – After oral administration, tinidazole is rapidly and completely absorbed. A bioavailability study of tinidazole tablets was conducted in adult healthy volunteers. All subjects received a single oral dose of 2 g (four 500 mg tablets) of tinidazole following an overnight fast. Oral administration of four 500 mg tablets of tinidazole under fasted conditions produced a mean peak plasma concentration (C_{max}) of 47.7 (± 7.5) mcg/mL with a mean time to peak concentration (T_{max}) of 1.6 (± 0.7) hours and a mean area under the plasma concentration-time curve ($AUC_{0-\infty}$) of 901.6 (± 126.5) mcg•h/mL at 72 hours. The elimination half-life ($t_{1/2}$) was 13.2 (± 1.4) hours. Mean plasma levels decreased to 14.3 mcg/mL at 24 hours, 3.8 mcg/mL at 48 hours and 0.8 mcg/mL at 72 hours following administration. Steady-state conditions are reached in 2.5 to 3 days of multi-day dosing. Administration of tinidazole tablets with food resulted in a delay in T_{max} of approximately 2 hours and a decline in C_{max} of approximately 10%, compared to fasted conditions. However, administration of tinidazole with food did not affect AUC or $t_{1/2}$ in this study.

In healthy volunteers, administration of crushed tinidazole tablets in artificial cherry syrup after an overnight fast has no effect on any pharmacokinetic parameter as compared with tablets swallowed whole under fasted conditions.

Distribution – Tinidazole is distributed into virtually all tissues and body fluids and also crosses the blood-brain barrier. The apparent volume of distribution is about 50 liters. Plasma protein binding of tinidazole is 12%.

Tinidazole crosses the placental barrier and is secreted in breast milk.

Metabolism – Tinidazole, like metronidazole, is significantly metabolized in humans prior to excretion. Tinidazole is partly metabolized by oxidation, hydroxylation, and conjugation. Tinidazole is the major drug-related constituent in plasma after human treatment, along with a small amount of the 2-hydroxymethyl metabolite.

Tinidazole is biotransformed mainly by CYP3A4. In an in vitro metabolic drug interaction study, tinidazole concentrations of up to 75 mcg/mL did not inhibit the enzyme activities of CYP1A2, CYP2B6, CYP2C9, CYP2D6, CYP2E1, and CYP3A4.

The potential of tinidazole to induce the metabolism of other drugs has not been evaluated.

Excretion – The plasma half-life of tinidazole is approximately 12 to 14 hours. Tinidazole is excreted by the liver and the kidneys. Tinidazole is excreted in the urine mainly as unchanged drug (approximately 20% to 25% of the administered dose). Approximately 12% of the drug is excreted in the feces.

Special populations –

Renal function impairment: The pharmacokinetics of tinidazole in patients with severe renal impairment (Ccr less than 22 mL/min) are not significantly different from the pharmacokinetics seen in healthy subjects. However, during hemodialysis, clearance of tinidazole is significantly increased; the half-life is reduced from 12 hours to 4.9 hours. Approximately 43% of the amount present in the body is eliminated during a 6-hour hemodialysis session. The pharmacokinetics of tinidazole in patients undergoing routine continuous peritoneal dialysis have not been investigated.

Hepatic function impairment: See Administration and Dosage for more information.

➤*Microbiology:* Tinidazole demonstrates activity both in vitro and in clinical infections against the following protozoa: *T. vaginalis*, *G. duodenalis* (also termed *G. lamblia*), and *E. histolytica*.

Tinidazole does not appear to have activity against most strains of vaginal lactobacilli.

Cross-resistance – Approximately 38% of *T. vaginalis* isolates exhibiting reduced susceptibility to metronidazole also show reduced susceptibility to tinidazole in vitro. The clinical significance of such an effect is not known.

Contraindications

Hypersensitivity to tinidazole, any component of the tablet, or other nitroimidazole derivatives; during the first trimester of pregnancy.

Warnings

➤*Neurologic effects:* Convulsive seizures and peripheral neuropathy, the latter characterized mainly by numbness or paresthesia of an extremity, have been reported in patients treated with nitroimidazole drugs, including tinidazole and metronidazole. The appearance of abnormal neurologic signs demands the prompt discontinuation of tinidazole therapy. Administer with caution to patients with CNS diseases.

➤*Hepatic function impairment:* The disposition of tinidazole in patients with hepatic impairment has not been evaluated. Patients with severe hepatic disease metabolize nitroimidazoles slowly, with resultant accumulation of parent drug in the plasma. Accordingly, for patients with hepatic dysfunction, cautiously administer usual recommended doses of tinidazole.

➤*Carcinogenesis:* Metronidazole, a chemically-related nitroimidazole, has been reported to be carcinogenic in mice and rats but not hamsters. In several studies metronidazole showed evidence of pulmonary, hepatic and lymphatic tumorigenesis in mice, and mammary and hepatic tumors in female rats. Tinidazole carcinogenicity studies in rats, mice or hamsters have not been reported.

➤*Mutagenesis:* Tinidazole was mutagenic in the TA 100, *Salmonella typhimurium* tester strain both with and without the metabolic activation system and was negative for mutagenicity in the TA 98 strain. Mutagenicity results were mixed (positive and negative) in the TA 1535, 1537 and 1538 strains. Tinidazole was also mutagenic in a tester strain of *Klebsiella pneumonia*. Tinidazole was negative for mutagenicity in a mammalian cell culture system utilizing Chinese hamster lung V79 cells (HGPRT test system) and negative for genotoxicity in the Chinese hamster ovary (CHO) sister chromatid exchange assay. Tinidazole was positive for in vivo genotoxicity in the mouse micronucleus assay.

➤*Fertility impairment:* In a 60-day fertility study, tinidazole reduced fertility and produced testicular histopathology in male rats at a 600 mg/kg/day dosage level (approximately 3-fold the highest human therapeutic dose based upon body surface area conversions). Spermatogenic effects resulted from 300 and 600 mg/kg/day dosage levels. The no observed adverse effect level for testicular and spermatogenic effects was 100 mg/kg/day (approximately 0.5-fold the highest human therapeutic dosage based upon body surface area conversions). This effect is characteristic of agents in the 5-nitroimidazole class.

➤*Elderly:* Clinical studies of tinidazole did not include sufficient numbers of subjects 65 years of age and older to determine whether they respond differently from younger subjects. In general, dose selection for an elderly patient should be cautious, reflecting the greater frequency of decreased hepatic, renal, or cardiac function, and of concomitant disease or other drug therapy.

➤*Pregnancy: Category C.*

Teratogenic – The use of tinidazole in pregnant patients has not been studied. Since tinidazole crosses the placental barrier and enters fetal circulation, do not administer to pregnant patients in the first trimester. Embryo-fetal developmental toxicity studies in pregnant mice indicated no embryo-fetal toxicity or malformations at the highest dose level of 2,500 mg/kg (approximately 6.3-fold the highest human therapeutic dose based upon body surface area conversions). In a study with pregnant rats a slightly higher incidence of fetal mortality was observed at a maternal dose of 500 mg/kg (2.5-fold the highest human therapeutic dose based upon body surface area conversions). No biologically relevant neonatal developmental effects were observed in rat neonates following maternal doses as high as 600 mg/kg (3-fold the highest human therapeutic dose based upon body surface area conversions). Because animal reproduction studies are not always predictive of human response and because there is some evidence of mutagenic potential, the use of tinidazole during pregnancy requires that the potential benefits of the drug be weighed against the possible risks to both the mother and the fetus.

➤*Lactation:* Tinidazole is excreted in breast milk in concentrations similar to those seen in serum. Tinidazole can be detected in breast milk for up to 72 hours following administration. Interruption of breast-feeding is recommended during tinidazole therapy and for 3 days following the last dose.

➤*Children:* Other than for use in the treatment of giardiasis and amebiasis in pediatric patients older than 3 years of age, safety and efficacy of tinidazole in pediatric patients have not been established.

Precautions

➤*Monitoring:* Total and differential leukocyte counts are recommended if retreatment is necessary.

➤*Candidiasis:* Known or previously unrecognized candidiasis may present more prominent symptoms during therapy with tinidazole and requires treatment with an antifungal agent.

➤*Special risk:* Tinidazole is a nitroimidazole; use with caution in patients with evidence of or history of blood dyscrasia.

TINIDAZOLE — ORAL

➤*Lab test abnormalities:* Tinidazole, like metronidazole, may produce transient leukopenia and neutropenia; however, no persistent hematological abnormalities attributable to tinidazole have been observed in clinical studies.

Drug Interactions

Although not studied specifically for tinidazole, the following drug interactions were reported for metronidazole, a chemically-related nitroimidazole. Therefore, these drug interactions may occur with tinidazole.

Tinidazole Drug Interactions

Precipitant drug	Object drug*		Description
Cholestyramine	Tinidazole	↓	Cholestyramine was shown to decrease the oral bioavailability of metronidazole. Thus, consider separating the dosing of cholestyramine and tinidazole.
CYP3A4 inducers (eg, phenobarbital, rifampin, phenytoin)	Tinidazole	↓	CYP3A4 inducers may accelerate the elimination of tinidazole.
CYP3A4 inhibitors (eg, cimetidine, ketoconazole)	Tinidazole	↑	CYP3A4 inhibitors may prolong the half-life and decrease plasma clearance of tinidazole.
Oxytetracycline	Tinidazole	↓	Oxytetracycline was reported to antagonize the therapeutic effect of metronidazole.
Tinidazole	Alcohols	↑	Avoid alcoholic beverages and preparations containing ethanol or propylene glycol during tinidazole therapy and for 3 days after discontinuation. Symptoms such as abdominal cramps, nausea, vomiting, headaches, and flushing may occur.
Tinidazole	Anticoagulants	↑	Tinidazole may enhance the effect of warfarin, resulting in a prolongation of prothrombin time. Adjust the anticoagulant dose as needed during coadministration and up to 8 days after tinidazole discontinuation.
Tinidazole	Cyclosporine Tacrolimus	↑	Several case reports suggest that metronidazole has the potential to increase the levels of cyclosporine and tacrolimus. During tinidazole coadministration, monitor for toxicities.
Tinidazole	Disulfiram	↑	Psychotic reactions have been reported in patients using metronidazole and disulfiram. Although no similar reactions have been reported with tinidazole, do not give tinidazole to patients who have taken disulfiram within the last 2 weeks.
Tinidazole	Fluorouracil	↑	Metronidazole was shown to decrease the clearance of fluorouracil, resulting in toxicities. If concomitant use of tinidazole and fluorouracil cannot be avoided, monitor for toxicities.
Tinidazole	Hydantoins (eg, fosphenytoin)	↑	Administration of oral metronidazole with IV fosphenytoin (prodrug of phenytoin) was reported to prolong the half-life and reduce the clearance of phenytoin. Orally administered phenytoin was not affected by metronidazole.
Tinidazole	Lithium	↑	Metronidazole has been reported to increase serum lithium levels. Although it is not known if tinidazole will interact with lithium, consider monitoring lithium and creatinine levels.

* ↑ = Object drug increased. ↓ = Object drug decreased.

➤*Drug/Lab test interactions:* Tinidazole, like metronidazole, may interfere with certain types of determinations of serum chemistry values, such as AST, ALT, lactate dehydrogenase (LDH), triglycerides, and hexokinase glucose. Values of zero may be observed. All of the assays in which interference has been reported involve enzymatic coupling of the assay to oxidation-reduction of nicotinamide adenine dinucleotide (NAD^+ ↔ NADH). Potential interference is due to the similarity of absorbance peaks of NADH and tinidazole.

Adverse Reactions

Among 3,669 patients treated with a single 2 g dose of tinidazole, in both controlled and uncontrolled trichomoniasis and giardiasis clinical studies, adverse reactions were reported by 11% of patients. For multi-day dosing in controlled and uncontrolled amebiasis studies, adverse reactions were reported by 13.8% of 1,765 patients. Reported adverse reactions from clinical trials have generally been mild and self-limiting.

Tinidazole Adverse Reactions

	2 g	Multi-Day Dose
CNS		
Dizziness	1.1%	0.5%
Weakness/Fatigue/Malaise	2.1%	1.1%
GI		
Anorexia	1.5%	2.5%
Constipation	0.4%	1.4%
Dyspepsia/Cramps/Epigastric discomfort	1.8%	1.4%
Metallic/Bitter taste	3.7%	6.3%
Nausea	3.2%	4.5%
Vomiting	1.5%	0.9%
Miscellaneous		
Headache	1.3%	0.7%
Total patients with adverse reactions	11% (403/3669)	13.8% (244/1765)

Other adverse reactions reported with tinidazole include:

➤*CNS:* Two serious adverse reactions reported include convulsions and transient peripheral neuropathy including numbness and paresthesia. Other CNS reports include vertigo, ataxia, giddiness, insomnia, drowsiness.

➤*GI:* Tongue discoloration, stomatitis, diarrhea.

➤*Hypersensitivity:* Urticaria, pruritis, rash, flushing, sweating, dryness of mouth, fever, burning sensation, thirst, salivation, angioedema.

➤*Renal:* Darkened urine.

➤*Cardiovascular:* Palpitations.

➤*Hematologic:* Transient neutropenia, transient leukopenia.

➤*Miscellaneous: Candida* overgrowth, increased vaginal discharge, oral candidiasis, hepatic abnormalities including raised transaminase level, arthralgias, myalgias, arthritis. Rare reported adverse reactions include bronchospasm, dyspnea, coma, confusion, depression, furry tongue, pharyngitis, and reversible thrombocytopenia.

➤*Children:* Among 6 pooled pediatric studies, 287 patients between the ages of 4 months and 11 years were evaluated. Adverse reactions reported in pediatric patients taking tinidazole were similar in nature and frequency to adult findings, including nausea, vomiting, diarrhea, taste change, anorexia, and abdominal pain.

Overdosage

There are no reported overdoses with tinidazole in humans. In acute studies with mice and rats, the LD_{50} for mice was generally greater than 3,600 mg/kg for oral administration and was greater than 2,300 mg/kg for intraperitoneal administration. In rats, the LD_{50} was greater than 2,000 mg/kg for both oral and intraperitoneal administration.

➤*Treatment:* There is no specific antidote for the treatment of overdosage with tinidazole; therefore, treatment should be symptomatic and supportive. Gastric lavage may be helpful. Hemodialysis can be considered because approximately 43% of the amount present in the body is eliminated during a 6-hour hemodialysis session.

Patient Information

Take with food.

Avoid alcoholic beverages while taking tinidazole and for 3 days afterward.

ATOVAQUONE

Rx	**Mepron** (GlaxoWellcome)	**Suspension:** 750 mg/5 ml	Benzyl alcohol, saccharin. Bright yellow. Citrus flavor. In 210 ml.

ATOVAQUONE — ORAL

Indications

➤*Pneumocystis carinii pneumonia:*

Prophylaxis – For the prevention of *P. carinii* pneumonia (PCP) in patients who are intolerant to trimethoprim-sulfamethoxazole (TMP-SMZ).

Treatment – For the acute oral treatment of mild-to-moderate PCP in patients who are intolerant to TMP-SMZ.

Administration and Dosage

➤*Approved by the FDA:* November 25, 1992.

➤*Dosage:*

Prevention of PCP –
Adults and adolescents (13 to 16 years of age): 1500 mg (10 mL) once daily administered with a meal.

Treatment of mild-to-moderate PCP –
Adults and adolescents (13 to 16 years): 750 mg (5 mL) administered with meals twice daily for 21 days (total daily dose 1500 mg). Failure to administer atovaquone suspension with meals may result in lower plasma atovaquone concentrations and may limit response to therapy.

Absorption of orally administered atovaquone is limited but can be significantly increased when the drug is taken with food. Plasma atovaquone concentrations have been shown to correlate with the likelihood of successful treatment and survival. Therefore, parenteral therapy with other agents should be considered for patients who have difficulty taking atovaquone with food. GI disorders may limit absorption of orally administered drugs. Patients with these disorders also may not achieve plasma concentrations of atovaquone associated with response to therapy in controlled trials.

➤*Storage/Stability:* Store at 15° to 25°C (59° to 77°F). Do not freeze. Dispense in tight container as defined in USP.

Actions

➤*Pharmacology:* Atovaquone is a hydroxy-1,4-naphthoquinone, an analog of ubiquinone, with antipneumocystis activity. The mechanism of action against *Pneumocystis carinii* has not been fully elucidated. In *Plasmodium* species, the site of action appears to be the cytochrome bc_1 complex (Complex III). Several metabolic enzymes are linked to the mitochondrial electron transport chain via ubiquinone. Inhibition of electron transport by atovaquone will result in indirect inhibition of these enzymes. The ultimate metabolic effects of such blockade may include inhibition of nucleic acid and ATP synthesis.

➤*Pharmacokinetics:*

Absorption – Atovaquone is a highly lipophilic compound with low aqueous solubility. The bioavailability of atovaquone is highly dependent on formulation and diet. The absolute bioavailability of a 750 mg dose of atovaquone suspension administered under fed conditions in 9 HIV-infected (CD4 greater than 100 cells/mm^3) volunteers was 47% ± 15%.

Administering atovaquone with food enhances its absorption by approximately 2-fold. In 1 study, 16 healthy volunteers received a single dose of 750 mg atovaquone suspension after an overnight fast and following a standard breakfast (23 g fat, 610 kcal). The mean (± SD) area under the concentration-time curve (AUC) values were 324 ± 115 and 801 ± 320 mcg•hr/mL under fasting and fed conditions, respectively, representing a 2.6 ± 1-fold increase. The effect of food (23 g fat, 400 kcal) on plasma atovaquone concentrations was also evaluated in a multiple-dose, randomized, crossover study in 19 HIV-infected volunteers (CD4 less than 200 cells/mm^3) receiving daily doses of 500 mg atovaquone suspension. AUC was 280 ± 114 mcg•hr/mL when atovaquone was administered with food as compared to 169 ± 77 mcg•hr/mL under fasting conditions. Maximum plasma atovaquone concentration (C_{max}) was 15.1 ± 6.1 and 8.8 ± 3.7 mcg/mL when atovaquone was administered with food and under fasting conditions, respectively.

Dose proportionality: Plasma atovaquone concentrations do not increase proportionally with dose. When atovaquone suspension was administered with food at dosage regimens of 500 mg once daily, 750 mg once daily, and 1000 mg once daily, average steady-state plasma atovaquone concentrations were 11.7 ± 4.8, 12.5 ± 5.8, and 13.5 ± 5.1 mcg/mL, respectively. The corresponding C_{max} concentrations were 15.1 ± 6.1, 15.3 ± 7.6, and 16.8 ± 6.4 mcg/mL. When atovaquone suspension was administered to 5 HIV-infected volunteers at a dose of 750 mg twice daily, the average steady-state plasma atovaquone concentration was 21.0 ± 4.9 mcg/mL, and C_{max} was 24 ± 5.7 mcg/mL. The minimum plasma atovaquone concentration (C_{min}) associated with the 750 mg twice-daily regimen was 16.7 ± 4.6 mcg/mL.

Distribution – Following the IV administration of atovaquone, the volume of distribution at steady state (Vd_{ss}) was 0.6 ± 0.17 L/kg (n = 9). Atovaquone is extensively bound to plasma proteins (99.9%) over the concentration range of 1 to 90 mcg/mL. In 3 HIV-infected children who received 750 mg atovaquone as the tablet formulation 4 times daily for 2 weeks, the cerebrospinal fluid concentrations of atovaquone were 0.04, 0.14, and 0.26 mcg/mL, representing less than 1% of the plasma concentration.

Excretion – The plasma clearance of atovaquone following IV administration in 9 HIV-infected volunteers was 10.4 ± 5.5 mL/min (0.15 ± 0.09 mL/min per kg). The half-life of atovaquone was 62.5 ± 35.3 hours after IV administration and ranged from 67 ± 33.4 to 77.6 ± 23.1 hours across studies following administration of atovaquone suspension. The half-life of atovaquone is long due to presumed enterohepatic cycling and eventual fecal elimination. In a study where ^{14}C-labeled atovaquone was administered to healthy volunteers, greater than 94% of the dose was recovered as unchanged atovaquone in the feces over 21 days. There was little or no excretion of atovaquone in the urine (less than 0.6%). There is indirect evidence that atovaquone may undergo limited metabolism; however, a specific metabolite has not been identified.

Special populations –
Children: In a study of atovaquone suspension in 27 HIV-infected, asymptomatic infants and children between 1 month and 13 years of age, the pharmacokinetics of atovaquone were age-dependent. These patients were dosed once daily with food for 12 days. The average steady-state plasma atovaquone concentrations (C_{ss}, mcg/mL) in the 24 patients with available concentration data are shown in the following information. Values are mean ± SD.

• *Average steady-state plasma atovaquone concentrations in pediatric patients* – In patients aged 1 to 3 months, atovaquone 10 mg/kg resulted in an average C_{ss} = 5.9 mcg/mL (n = 1), and atovaquone 30 mg/kg resulted in an average C_{ss} = 27.8 ± 5.8 mcg/mL (n = 4).

In patients aged greater than 3 months to 24 months, atovaquone 10 mg/kg resulted in an average C_{ss} = 5.7 ± 5.1 mcg/mL (n = 4), atovaquone 30 mg/kg resulted in an average C_{ss} = 9.8 ± 3.2 mcg/mL (n = 4), and atovaquone 45 mg/kg resulted in an average C_{ss} = 15.4 ± 6.6 mcg/mL (n = 4).

In patients greater than 2 to 13 years of age, atovaquone 10 mg/kg resulted in an average C_{ss} = 16.8 ± 6.4 mcg/mL (n = 4), and atovaquone 30 mg/kg resulted in an average C_{ss} = 37.1 ± 10.9 mcg/mL (n = 3).

➤*Microbiology:*

Drug resistance – Phenotypic resistance to atovaquone in vitro has not been demonstrated for *P. carinii*. However, in 2 patients who developed *P. carinii* pneumonia (PCP) after prophylaxis with atovaquone, DNA sequence analysis identified mutations in the predicted amino acid sequence of *P. carinii* cytochrome b (a likely target site for atovaquone). The clinical significance of this is unknown.

Contraindications

Patients who develop or have a history of potentially life-threatening allergic reactions to any of the components of the formulation.

Warnings

➤*Severe PCP:* Clinical experience with atovaquone for the treatment of PCP has been limited to patients with mild-to-moderate PCP [(A-a)DO_2 less than or equal to 45 mmHg]. Treatment of more severe episodes of PCP has not been systematically studied with this agent. Also, the efficacy of atovaquone in patients who are failing therapy with TMP-SMZ has not been systematically studied.

➤*Hepatic function impairment:* If it is necessary to treat patients with severe hepatic impairment, caution is advised, and administration should be monitored closely.

➤*Carcinogenesis:* Carcinogenicity studies in rats were negative; 24-month studies in mice showed treatment-related increases in incidence of hepatocellular adenoma and hepatocellular carcinoma at all doses tested which ranged from 1.4 to 3.6 times the average steady-state plasma concentrations in humans during acute treatment of *Pneumocystis carinii* pneumonia.

➤*Elderly:* In general, dose selection for an elderly patient should be cautious, reflecting the greater frequency of decreased hepatic, renal, or cardiac function, and of concomitant disease or other drug therapy.

➤*Pregnancy: Category C.* Atovaquone caused maternal toxicity in rabbits at plasma concentrations that were approximately one-half the estimated human exposure. Mean fetal body lengths and weights were decreased, and there were higher numbers of early resorption and postimplantation loss per dam. It is not clear whether these effects were caused by atovaquone directly or were secondary to maternal toxicity. Concentrations of atovaquone in rabbit fetuses averaged 30% of the concurrent maternal plasma concentrations. In a separate study in rats given a single ^{14}C-radiolabeled dose, concentrations of radiocarbon in rat fetuses were 18% (middle gestation) and 60% (late gestation) of concurrent maternal plasma concentrations. There are no adequate and well-controlled studies in pregnant women. Atovaquone should be used during pregnancy only if the potential benefit justifies the potential risk to the fetus.

➤*Lactation:* It is not known whether atovaquone is excreted into human milk. Because many drugs are excreted into human milk, caution should be exercised when atovaquone is administered to a nursing woman. In a rat study, atovaquone concentrations in the milk were 30% of the concurrent atovaquone concentrations in the maternal plasma.

➤*Children:* Evidence of safety and efficacy in pediatric patients has not been established. A relationship between plasma atovaquone concentrations and successful treatment of PCP has been established in adults (see the information below). In a study of atovaquone suspension in 27 HIV-infected, asymptomatic infants and children between 1 month and 13 years of age, the pharmacokinetics of atovaquone were age-dependent.

Average steady-state plasma atovaquone concentrations in pediatric patients – No drug-related, treatment-limiting adverse reactions were observed in the pharmacokinetic study.

See Actions for more information.

ATOVAQUONE — ORAL

Precautions

➤*Concurrent pulmonary infections:* Based upon the spectrum of in vitro antimicrobial activity, atovaquone is not effective therapy for concurrent pulmonary conditions such as bacterial, viral, or fungal pneumonia or mycobacterial diseases. Clinical deterioration in patients may be due to infections with other pathogens, as well as progressive PCP. All patients with acute PCP should be carefully evaluated for other possible causes of pulmonary disease and treated with additional agents as appropriate.

Drug Interactions

➤*Plasma protein-bound drugs:* Atovaquone is highly bound to plasma protein (greater than 99.9%). Therefore, caution should be used when administering atovaquone concurrently with other highly plasma protein-bound drugs with narrow therapeutic indices, as competition for binding sites may occur. The extent of plasma protein binding of atovaquone in human plasma is not affected by the presence of therapeutic concentrations of phenytoin (15 mcg/mL), nor is the binding of phenytoin affected by the presence of atovaquone.

➤*Trimethoprim/sulfamethoxazole (TMP-SMZ):* The possible interaction between atovaquone and TMP-SMZ was evaluated in 6 HIV-infected adult volunteers as part of a larger multiple-dose, dose-escalation, and chronic-dosing study of atovaquone suspension. In this crossover study, atovaquone suspension 500 mg once daily, or TMP-SMZ tablets (160 mg trimethoprim and 800 mg sulfamethoxazole) twice daily, or the combination were administered with food to achieve steady state. No difference was observed in the average steady-state plasma atovaquone concentration after coadministration with TMP-SMZ. Coadministration of atovaquone with TMP-SMZ resulted in a 17% and 8% decrease in average steady-state concentrations of trimethoprim and sulfamethoxazole in plasma, respectively. This effect is minor and would not be expected to produce clinically significant events.

Atovaquone/Proguanil Drug Interactions			
Precipitant drug	Object drug*		Description
Metoclopramide	Atovaquone	⬇	Concomitant treatment with metoclopramide has been associated with decreased bioavailability of atovaquone. Use only if other antiemetics are not available.
Rifampin Rifabutin	Atovaquone	⬇	Concomitant administration of rifampin or rifabutin is known to reduce atovaquone levels by approximately 50% and 34% respectively. The concomitant administration of these agents is not recommended. The mechanism of this interaction is unknown.
Tetracycline	Atovaquone	⬇	Concomitant treatment with tetracycline has been associated with ≈ 40% reduction in plasma concentrations of atovaquone. Closely monitor parasitemia in patients receiving tetracycline.
Atovaquone	Zidovudine	⬆	Zidovudine concentrations may be elevated, increasing the risk of zidovudine toxicity.

➤*Drug/Lab test interactions:* It is not known if atovaquone interferes with clinical laboratory test or assay results.

Adverse Reactions

Because many patients who participated in clinical trials with atovaquone had complications of advanced HIV disease, it was often difficult to distinguish adverse events caused by atovaquone from those caused by underlying medical conditions. There were no life-threatening or fatal adverse experiences caused by atovaquone.

➤*PCP prevention studies:*

Treatment-limiting adverse reactions in the dapsone comparative PCP prevention study				
	Percentage of patients with treatment-limiting adverse reactions			
	All patients		Patients not taking either drug at enrollment	
Treatment-limiting adverse reaction	Atovaquone 1,500 mg/day (n = 536)	Dapsone 100 mg/day (n = 521)	Atovaquone 1500 mg/day (n = 238)	Dapsone 100 mg/day (n = 249)
Any event	24.4%	25.9%	20.2%	43.4%
Rash	6.3%	8.8%	7.6%	16.1%
Nausea	4.1%	0.6%	2.5%	0.8%
Diarrhea	3.2%	0.2%	2.1%	0.4%
Vomiting	2.2%	0.6%	1.3%	0.8%
Allergic reaction	1.1%	2.9%	0.8%	4.8%
Fever	0.6%	2.9%	0%	5.6%
Anemia	0%	1.5%	0%	2%

Treatment-emergent adverse reactions:

Treatment-emergent adverse reactions in the aerosolized pentamidine comparative PCP prevention study			
	Percentage of patients with treatment-emergent adverse reactions		
Treatment-emergent adverse reaction	Atovaquone 1500 mg/day (n = 175)	Atovaquone 750 mg/day (n = 188)	Aerosolized pentamidine (n = 186)
Diarrhea	42%	42%	35%
Rash	39%	46%	28%
Headache	28%	31%	22%
Nausea	26%	32%	23%
Increased cough	25%	25%	31%
Fever	25%	31%	18%
Rhinitis	24%	18%	17%
Asthenia	22%	31%	31%
Infection	22%	18%	19%
Abdominal pain	20%	21%	20%
Dyspnea	15%	21%	16%
Vomiting	15%	22%	11%
Patients discontinuing therapy due to an adverse reaction	25%	16%	7%
Patients reporting at least 1 adverse reaction	98%	96%	89%

Other events: Other events occurring in greater than or equal to 10% of the patients receiving the recommended dose of atovaquone included sweating, flu syndrome, pain, sinusitis, pruritus, insomnia, depression, and myalgia. Bronchospasm occurred more frequently in patients receiving aerosolized pentamidine (11%) than in patients receiving atovaquone 1500 mg/day (4%) and atovaquone 750 mg/day (2%).

➤*PCP treatment studies:*
Clinical adverse reactions reported by greater than or equal to 5%:

Treatment-emergent adverse reactions in the TMP-SMZ comparative PCP treatment study		
	Percentage of patients with treatment-emergent adverse reactions	
Treatment-emergent adverse reaction	Atovaquone (n = 203)	TMP-SMZ (n = 205)
Rash (including maculopapular)	23%	34%
Nausea	21%	44%
Diarrhea	19%	7%
Headache	16%	22%
Vomiting	14%	35%
Fever	14%	25%
Insomnia	10%	9%
Asthenia	8%	8%
Pruritus	5%	9%
Oral monilia	5%	10%
Abdominal pain	4%	7%
Constipation	3%	17%
Dizziness	3%	8%
Patients discontinuing therapy due to an adverse reaction	9%	24%
Patients reporting at least 1 adverse reaction	63%	65%

Discontinuation of therapy: Although an equal percentage of patients receiving atovaquone and TMP-SMZ reported at least 1 adverse reaction, more patients receiving TMP-SMZ required discontinuation of therapy due to an adverse reaction. Twenty-four percent (24%) of patients receiving TMP-SMZ were prematurely discontinued from therapy due to an adverse experience vs 9% of patients receiving atovaquone. Four percent (4%) of patients receiving atovaquone had therapy discontinued due to development of rash. The majority of cases of rash among patients receiving atovaquone were mild and did not require the discontinuation of dosing. The only other clinical adverse experience that led to premature discontinuation of dosing of atovaquone by more than 1 patient was vomiting (less than 1%). The most common adverse reaction requiring discontinuation of dosing in the TMP-SMZ group was rash (8%).

Lab test abnormalities – Laboratory test abnormalities reported for greater than or equal to 5% of the study population during the treatment period are summarized in the table below. Two percent (2%) of patients treated with atovaquone and 7% of patients treated with TMP-SMZ had therapy prematurely discontinued due to elevations in ALT/AST. In general,

ATOVAQUONE — ORAL

patients treated with atovaquone developed fewer abnormalities in measures of hepatocellular function (ALT, AST, alkaline phosphatase) or amylase values than patients treated with TMP-SMZ.

Treatment-emergent laboratory test abnormalities in the TMP-SMZ comparative PCP treatment study

Laboratory test abnormality	Percentage of patients developing a laboratory test abnormality	
	Atovaquone	TMP-SMZ
Anemia (Hgb < 8 g/dL)	6%	7%
Neutropenia (ANC < 750 cells/mm^3)	3%	9%
Elevated ALT (> 5 × ULN [1])	6%	16%
Elevated AST (> 5 × ULN)	4%	14%
Elevated alkaline phosphatase (> 2.5 × ULN)	8%	6%
Elevated amylase (> 1.5 × ULN)	7%	12%
Hyponatremia (< 0.96 × LLN [2])	7%	26%

Treatment-emergent adverse reactions in the pentamidine comparative PCP treatment study (primary therapy group)

Treatment-emergent adverse reaction	Percentage of patients with treatment-emergent adverse reaction	
	Atovaquone (n = 73)	Pentamidine (n = 71)
Fever	40%	25%
Nausea	22%	37%
Rash	22%	13%
Diarrhea	21%	31%
Insomnia	19%	14%
Headache	18%	28%
Vomiting	14%	17%
Cough	14%	1%
Abdominal pain	10%	11%
Pain	10%	10%
Sweat	10%	3%
Oral monilia	10%	3%
Asthenia	8%	14%
Dizziness	8%	14%
Anxiety	7%	10%
Anorexia	7%	10%
Sinusitis	7%	6%
Dyspepsia	5%	10%
Rhinitis	5%	7%
Taste perversion	3%	13%
Hypoglycemia	1%	15%
Hypotension	1%	10%
Patients discontinuing therapy due to an adverse reaction	7%	41%
Patients reporting at least 1 adverse reaction	63%	72%

Lab test abnormalities – Laboratory test abnormalities reported in greater than or equal to 5% of patients in the pentamidine comparative study are presented in the table below. Laboratory abnormality was reported as the reason for discontinuation of treatment in 2 of 73 patients who received atovaquone. One patient (1%) had elevated creatinine and BUN levels and 1 patient (1%) had elevated amylase levels. Laboratory abnormalities were the sole or contributing factor in 14 patients who prematurely discontinued pentamidine therapy. In the 71 patients who received pentamidine, laboratory parameters most frequently reported as reasons for discontinuation were hypoglycemia (11%), elevated creatinine levels (6%), and leukopenia (4%).

Treatment-emergent laboratory test abnormalities in the pentamidine comparative PCP treatment study

Laboratory test abnormality	Percentage of patients developing a laboratory test abnormality	
	Atovaquone	Pentamidine
Anemia (Hgb < 8 g/dL)	4%	9%
Neutropenia (ANC < 750 cells/mm^3)	5%	9%
Hyponatremia (< 0.96 × LLN [1])	10%	10%
Hyperkalemia (> 1.18 × ULN [2])	0%	5%
Alkaline phosphatase (> 2.5 × ULN)	5%	2%
Hyperglycemia (> 1.8 × ULN)	9%	13%
Elevated AST (> 5 × ULN)	0%	5%
Elevated amylase (> 1.5 × ULN)	8%	4%
Elevated creatinine (> 1.5 × ULN)	0%	7%

[1] LLN = lower limit of normal range.
[2] ULN = upper limit of normal range.

➤*Postmarketing:*

Dermatologic – Allergic reactions including erythema multiforme.

GU – Acute renal impairment.

Hematologic / Lymphatic – Methemoglobinemia, thrombocytopenia.

Hepatic – Pancreatitis.

Ophthalmic – Vortex keratopathy.

Overdosage

➤*Symptoms:* The median lethal dose is higher than the maximum oral dose tested in mice and rats (1825 mg/kg/day). Overdoses up to 31,500 mg of atovaquone have been reported. In 1 such patient who also took an unspecified dose of dapsone, methemoglobinemia occurred. Rash has also been reported after overdose.

➤*Treatment:* There is no known antidote for atovaquone, and it is currently unknown if atovaquone is dialyzable.

Patient Information

The importance of taking the prescribed dose of atovaquone should be stressed. Patients should be instructed to take their daily doses of atovaquone with meals, as the presence of food will significantly improve the absorption of the drug.

PENTAMIDINE ISETHIONATE

Rx	**Pentam 300** (American Pharmaceutical Partners)	**Injection:** 300 mg	In single-dose vials.
Rx	**Pentamidine Isethionate** (Abbott)	**Powder for Injection, lyophilized:** 300 mg	In single-dose flip-top vials.
Rx	**NebuPent** (American Pharmaceutical Partners)	**Aerosol:** 300 mg	In single dose vials.

PENTAMIDINE ISETHIONATE — INJECTION

Indications

➤*Pneumocystis carinii:* For the treatment of pneumonia due to *Pneumocystis carinii.*

➤*Unlabeled uses:* Pentamidine has been used in the treatment of trypanosomiasis and visceral leishmaniasis.

Administration and Dosage

➤*Approved by the FDA:* October 16, 1984.

➤*Admixture incompatibility:* Do not use sodium chloride injection, USP for initial reconstitution because precipitation will occur.

IV solutions of pentamidine isethionate have been shown to be incompatible with fluconazole and foscarnet sodium. IV solutions of pentamidine isethionate have been shown to be compatible with IV solutions of zidovudine (AZT) and diltiazem hydrochloride.

➤*Dosage:* Pentamidine isethionate should be administered IM or IV only. The recommended regimen for adults and pediatric patients beyond 4 months of age is 4 mg/kg once a day for 14 to 21 days. Therapy for longer than 21 days with pentamidine isethionate has also been used but may be associated with increased toxicity.

PENTAMIDINE ISETHIONATE — INJECTION

➤*IM injection:* The contents of one vial (300 mg) should be dissolved in 3 mL of sterile water for injection, USP at 22° to 30°C (72° to 86°F). The calculated daily dose should then be withdrawn and administered by deep IM injection.

➤*IV injection:* The contents of one vial (300 mg) should first be dissolved in 3 to 5 mL of Sterile Water for Injection, USP, or 5% Dextrose Injection, USP at 22° to 30°C (72° to 86°F). The calculated dose of pentamidine isethionate should then be withdrawn and diluted further in 50 to 250 mL of 5% Dextrose Injection, USP.

The diluted IV solutions containing pentamidine isethionate should be infused over a period of 60 to 120 minutes.

➤*Storage/Stability:* After reconstitution with sterile water, the pentamidine isethionate solution is stable for 48 hours in the original vial at room temperature if protected from light. To avoid crystallization, store at 22° to 30°C (72° to 86°F). IV infusion solutions of pentamidine isethionate at 1 mg/mL and 2.5 mg/mL prepared in 5% Dextrose Injection, USP are stable at room temperature for up to 24 hours.

Store the dry product at controlled room temperature 15° to 30°C (59° to 86°F) and protect from light.

Preservative free; discard unused portion.

Actions

➤*Pharmacology:* Pentamidine isethionate, an aromatic diamidine, is known to have activity against *Pneumocystis carinii*. The mode of action of pentamidine is not fully understood. In vitro studies indicate that the drug interferes with protozoal nuclear metabolism by inhibition of DNA, RNA, phospholipid and protein synthesis.

➤*Pharmacokinetics:*

Absorption/Distribution – Pharmacokinetic parameters following the administration of 4 mg/kg pentamidine isethionate as a single 2-hour IV infusion or after a single IM injection to 12 patients with AIDS are presented in the following table:

Mean ± SD	C_{max} (ng/mL)	Clearance (L/hr)	Half-life (hours)	Vdss (L)	Concentration (ng/mL) 8 hour	24 hour
2-hour IV infusion 4 mg/kg (n = 6)	612 ± 371	248 ± 91	6.4 ± 1.3	821 ± 535	19.3 ± 16.9	2.9 ± 1.4
IM 4 mg/kg (n = 6)	209 ± 48	305 ± 81	9.4 ± 2	2724 ± 1066	22.9 ± 8	6.6 ± 3.5

In 7 patients treated with daily IM doses of pentamidine at 4 mg/kg for 10 to 12 days, plasma concentrations were between 300 to 500 ng/mL. The concentrations did not appreciably change with time after injection or from day to day. Higher plasma concentrations were encountered in patients with an elevated blood urea nitrogen.

Following multiple IV administration: Following multiple IV administration of pentamidine isethionate (3.7 to 4 mg/kg/day infused over 4 hours) to 6 patients with AIDS being treated for PCP, the pharmacokinetic parameters obtained on days 1, 4 and 7 are summarized in the following table:

Mean ± SD	C_{max} *(ng/mL)	C_{min}* (ng/mL)	Clearance (mL/min)	Renal clearance (mL/min/ 1.73 m²)	Creatinine clearance (mL/min/ 1.73 m²)
Day 1	175.3 ± 54	-	5737 ± 1878	269 ± 149	97 ± 12
Day 4	210.9 ± 80	17.6 ± 9.5	3350 ± 1944	214 ± 145	93 ± 17
Day 7	256.7 ± 89	40.8 ± 16.1	1989 ± 566	134 ± 60	69 ± 17

* Derived from Lidman.

Compared to the mean AUC on day 1, AUC on day 4 and day 7 were about 2- and 3-fold higher, respectively, suggesting that steady state was not achieved by day 7 of dosing.

Metabolism – In other published reports of pharmacokinetics of pentamidine following daily IV doses of 2 to 4 mg/kg/day, clearance ranged from 30 to 40 mL/min/kg, and the volume of distribution at steady state ranged from 200 to 400 L/kg. Reported values for terminal half-lives of 2.8 to 12 days is suggestive of a deep peripheral compartment. In the urine, up to 12% of the administered dose has been recovered during a dosing interval as unchanged pentamidine.

Excretion – The patients continued to excrete decreasing amounts of pentamidine in urine up to 6 to 8 weeks after cessation of the treatment.

Contraindications

History of hypersensitivity to pentamidine isethionate.

Warnings

➤*Ulceration, tissue necrosis or sloughing at the injection site:* Extravasations have been reported which, in some instances, proceeded to ulceration, tissue necrosis or sloughing at the injection site. While not common, surgical debridement and skin grafting has been necessary in some of these cases; long-term sequelae have been reported. Prevention is the most effective means of limiting the severity of extravasation. The IV needle or catheter must be properly positioned and closely observed throughout the period of pentamidine isethionate administration. If extravasation occurs, the injection should be discontinued immediately and restarted in another vein. Because there are no known local treatment measures which have proven to be useful, management of the extravasation should be symptomatic.

➤*Hypersensitivity reactions:* Fatalities due to severe hypotension, hypoglycemia, acute pancreatitis, and cardiac arrhythmias have been reported in patients treated with pentamidine isethionate, both by the IM and IV routes. Severe hypotension may result after a single IM or IV dose and is more likely with rapid IV administration (see Precautions). The administration of the drug should, therefore, be limited to the patients in whom *Pneumocystis carinii* has been demonstrated. Patients should be closely monitored for the development of serious adverse reactions (see Precautions and Adverse Reactions).

➤*Pregnancy: Category C.* Animal reproduction studies have not been conducted with pentamidine isethionate. It is also not known whether pentamidine isethionate can cause fetal harm when administered to a pregnant woman or can affect reproduction capacity. Pentamidine isethionate should not be given to a pregnant woman unless the potential benefits are judged to outweigh the unknown risks.

➤*Lactation:* It is not known whether pentamidine isethionate is excreted in human milk. Because of the potential for serious adverse reactions in nursing infants from pentamidine isethionate, a decision should be made whether to discontinue nursing or to discontinue the drug, taking into account the importance of the drug to the mother. Because many drugs are excreted in human milk, pentamidine isethionate should not be given to a nursing mother unless the potential benefits are judged to outweigh the unknown risks.

➤*Children:* IV and IM pentamidine has been described as an effective treatment for *Pneumocystis carinii* pneumonia (PCP) in immunocompromised pediatric patients beyond 4 months of age. The efficacy and safety profiles in these pediatric patients were similar to those observed in adult patients (see Administration and Dosage and Overdosage).

Precautions

➤*Monitoring:* The following tests should be carried out before, during and after therapy:

1.) Daily blood urea nitrogen and serum creatinine determinations.
2.) Daily blood glucose determinations.
3.) Complete blood count and platelet count.
4.) Liver function test, including serum bilirubin, alkaline phosphatase, AST, and ALT.
5.) Serum calcium determinations.
6.) ECGs.

➤*Hypotension:* Patients may develop sudden, severe hypotension after a single dose of pentamidine isethionate, whether given IV or IM. Therefore, patients receiving the drug should be lying down and the blood pressure should be monitored closely during administration of the drug and several times thereafter until the blood pressure is stable. Equipment for emergency resuscitation should be readily available. If pentamidine isethionate is administered IV, it should be infused over a period of 60 to 120 minutes.

➤*Hypoglycemia:* Pentamidine isethionate-induced hypoglycemia has been associated with pancreatic islet cell necrosis and inappropriately high plasma insulin concentrations. Hyperglycemia and diabetes mellitus, with or without preceding hypoglycemia, have also occurred, sometimes several months after therapy with pentamidine isethionate. Therefore, blood glucose levels should be monitored daily during therapy with pentamidine isethionate, and several times thereafter.

➤*Special risk:* Pentamidine isethionate should be used with caution in patients with hypertension, hypotension, ventricular tachycardia, hypoglycemia, hyperglycemia, hypocalcemia, pancreatitis, leukopenia, thrombocytopenia, anemia, hepatic or renal dysfunction and Stevens-Johnson syndrome.

Drug Interactions

➤*Other nephrotoxic drugs:* Because the nephrotoxic effects may be additive, the concomitant or sequential use of pentamidine isethionate and other nephrotoxic drugs such as aminoglycosides, amphotericin B, cisplatin, foscarnet, or vancomycin should be closely monitored and avoided, if possible.

Adverse Reactions

Fatalities due to severe hypotension, hypoglycemia, acute pancreatitis and cardiac arrhythmias have been reported in patients treated with pentamidine isethionate, both by the IM and IV routes. Nephrotoxic events (increased creatinine, impaired renal function, azotemia, and renal failure) are common with the parenteral administration of pentamidine isethionate. The administration of the drug should, therefore, be limited to the patients in whom *Pneumocystis carinii* has been demonstrated.

The most frequently reported spontaneous adverse events (1% to 30%) reported in clinical trials, regardless of their relation to pentamidine isethionate therapy were as follows (n = 424):

➤*Cardiovascular:* Hypotension, 5%.

➤*CNS:* Confusion/hallucinations, 1.7%.

➤*Dermatologic:* Rash, 3.3%.

➤*GI:* Anorexia/nausea, 5.9%.

➤*GU:* Azotemia, 8.5%; elevated serum creatinine, 23.6%; elevated blood urea nitrogen, 6.6%; impaired renal function, 28.8%.

➤*Hematologic:* Anemia, 1.2%; leukopenia, 10.4%; thrombocytopenia, 2.6%.

➤*Hepatic:* Elevated liver function tests, 8.7%.

➤*Local:* Sterile abscess or necrosis, pain, or induration at the site of IM injection, 11.1%.

PENTAMIDINE ISETHIONATE — INJECTION

➤*Metabolic:* Hypoglycemia, 5.9%.

➤*Special senses:* Bad taste, 1.7%.

➤*Adverse events (< 1%):* Adverse events with a frequency of less than 1% incidence were as follows (no causal relationship to treatment has been established for these adverse events):

Allergic – Allergic reaction (ie, urticaria, itching, rash), anaphylaxis.

Cardiovascular – Abnormal ST segment of ECG, cardiac arrhythmias, cerebrovascular accident, hypertension, palpitations, phlebitis, syncope, tachycardia, vasodilatation, vasculitis and ventricular tachycardia.

CNS – Anxiety, confusion, depression, dizziness, drowsiness, emotional lability, hypesthesia, insomnia, memory loss, neuropathy, nervousness, neuralgia, paranoia, paresthesia, peripheral neuropathy, seizure, tremors, unsteady gait, and vertigo.

Dermatologic – Desquamation, dry and breaking hair, dry skin, erythema, dermatitis, pruritus, rash, and urticaria.

GI – Abdominal pain, diarrhea, dry mouth, dyspepsia, hematochezia, hypersalivation, melena, pancreatitis, splenomegaly, and vomiting.

GU – Flank pain, hematuria, and incontinence.

Hematologic – Defibrination, eosinophilia, neutropenia, pancytopenia, and prolonged clotting time.

Hepatic – Hepatic dysfunction, hepatitis and hepatomegaly.

Metabolic – Hyperglycemia, hyperkalemia, hypocalcemia, and hypomagnesemia.

Ophthalmic – Blepharitis, blurred vision, conjunctivitis, contact lens discomfort, eye pain or discomfort.

Renal – Nephritis, renal dysfunction, and renal failure.

Respiratory – Asthma, bronchitis, bronchospasm, chest congestion, chest tightness, coryza, cyanosis, eosinophilic or interstitial pneumonitis, gagging, hemoptysia, hyperventilation, laryngitis, laryngospasm, non-specific lung disorder, nasal congestion, pleuritis, pneumothorax, rales, rhinitis, shortness of breath, and tachypnea.

Special senses – Loss of hearing, loss of taste, and loss of smell.

Miscellaneous – Arthralgia, chills, extrapulmonary pneumocystosis, headache, night sweats, and Stevens-Johnson syndrome.

➤*Postmarketing:* From postmarketing clinical experience with pentamidine isethionate, the following adverse events have been reported:

Miscellaneous – Cough, diabetes mellitus/ketoacidosis, dyspnea, infiltration (extravasation-see Warnings), and torsades de pointes.

Overdosage

➤*Symptoms:* A 17-month-old infant inadvertently received 1600 mg of IV pentamidine isethionate which was followed by renal and hepatic function impairment, hypotension and cardiopulmonary arrest.

➤*Treatment:* Treatment included cardiopulmonary resuscitation, epinephrine, atropine and intubation. In addition, a 4-hour course of charcoal hemoperfusion was accompanied by reduction of pentamidine serum concentration and stabilization of the patient's condition. The patient recovered from these adverse events, but later died due to an unknown cause.

PENTAMIDINE ISETHIONATE — INHALATIONAL

Indications

➤*Pneumocystis carinii pneumonia prophylaxis:* For the prevention of *Pneumocystis carinii* pneumonia (PCP) in high-risk, HIV-infected patients defined by 1 or both of the following criteria:

A history of 1 or more episodes of PCP.

A peripheral CD4+ (T4 helper/inducer) lymphocyte count less than or equal to 200/mm^3.

➤*Unlabeled uses:* Pentamidine has been used in the treatment of trypanosomiasis and visceral leishmaniasis.

Administration and Dosage

➤*Approved by the FDA:* June 15, 1989.

➤*Admixture incompatibility:* Pentamidine isethionate must be dissolved only in Sterile Water for Injection. Do not use saline solution for reconstitution because the drug will precipitate. Do not mix the pentamidine isethionate solution with any other drugs. Do not use the *Respirgard II* nebulizer to administer a bronchodilator.

➤*Reconstitution:* The contents of 1 vial (300 mg) must be dissolved in 6 mL Sterile Water for Injection. Place the entire reconstituted contents of the vial into the *Respirgard II* nebulizer reservoir for administration.

➤*Dosage:* 300 mg once every 4 weeks administered via the *Respirgard II* nebulizer.

The dose should be delivered until the nebulizer chamber is empty (approximately 30 to 45 minutes). The flow rate should be 5 to 7 L per minute from a 40 to 50 pounds per square inch (PSI) air or oxygen source. Alternatively, a 40 to 50 PSI air compressor can be used with flow limited by setting the flowmeter at 5 to 7 L per minute or by setting the pressure at 22 to 25 PSI. Low pressure (less than 20 PSI) compressors should not be used.

➤*Storage/Stability:* Store the dry product at controlled room temperature 15° to 30°C (59° to 86°F).

Protect the dry product and the reconstituted solution from light.

Freshly prepared solutions for aerosol use are recommended. After reconstitution with sterile water, the pentamidine isethionate solution is stable for 48 hours in the original vial at room temperature if protected from light.

Actions

➤*Pharmacology:* Pentamidine isethionate, an aromatic diamidine, is known to have activity against *Pneumocystis carinii*. The mode of action is not fully understood. In vitro studies indicate that the drug interferes with protozoal nuclear metabolism by inhibition of DNA, RNA, phospholipid, and protein synthesis.

➤*Pharmacokinetics:*

Absorption – In 5 AIDS patients with suspected *Pneumocystis carinii* pneumonia (PCP), the mean concentrations of pentamidine determined 18 to 24 hours after inhalation therapy were 23.2 ng/mL (range 5.1 to 43 ng/mL) in bronchoalveolar lavage fluid and 705 ng/mL (range 140 to 1336 ng/mL) in sediment after administration of a 300 mg single dose via the *Respirgard II* nebulizer. In 3 AIDS patients with suspected PCP, the mean concentrations of pentamidine determined 18 to 24 hours after a 4 mg/kg intravenous dose were 2.6 ng/mL (range 1.5 to 4 ng/mL) in bronchoalveolar lavage fluid and 9.3 ng/mL (range 6.9 to 12.8 ng/mL) in sediment. In the patients who received aerosolized pentamidine, the peak plasma levels of pentamidine were at or below the lower limit of detection of the assay (2.3 ng/mL).

Following a single 2-hour intravenous infusion of 4 mg/kg of pentamidine isethionate to 6 AIDS patients, the mean plasma C_{max}, $t_{1/2}$ and clearance were 612 ± 371 ng/mL, 6.4 ± 1.3 hr and 248 ± 91 L/hr, respectively. In another study of aerosolized pentamidine in 13 AIDS patients with acute PCP who received 4 mg/kg/day administered via the *Ultra Vent* jet nebulizer, peak plasma levels of pentamidine averaged 18.8 ± 11.9 ng/mL after the first dose. During the next 14 days of repeated dosing, the highest observed C_{max} averaged 20.5 ± 21.2 ng/mL. In a third study, following daily administration of 600 mg of inhaled pentamidine isethionate with the *Respirgard II* nebulizer for 21 days in 11 patients with acute PCP, mean plasma levels measured shortly after the 21st dose averaged 11.8 ± 10 ng/mL.

Metabolism/Excretion – Plasma concentrations after aerosol administration are substantially lower than those observed after a comparable intravenous dose. The extent of pentamidine accumulation and distribution following chronic inhalation therapy are not known.

Contraindications

History of an anaphylactic reaction to inhaled or parenteral pentamidine isethionate.

Warnings

➤*Development of acute PCP:* The potential for development of acute PCP still exists in patients receiving pentamidine isethionate prophylaxis. Therefore, any patient with symptoms suggestive of the presence of a pulmonary infection, including but not limited to dyspnea, fever, or cough, should receive a thorough medical evaluation and appropriate diagnostic tests for possible acute PCP as well as for other opportunistic and nonopportunistic pathogens. The use of pentamidine isethionate may alter the clinical and radiographic features of PCP and could result in an atypical presentation, including but not limited to mild disease or focal infection.

Prior to initiating pentamidine isethionate prophylaxis, symptomatic patients should be evaluated appropriately to exclude the presence of PCP. The recommended dose of pentamidine isethionate for the prevention of PCP is insufficient to treat acute PCP.

➤*Pregnancy: Category C.* Animal reproduction studies have not been conducted with pentamidine isethionate. It is also not known whether pentamidine isethionate inhalation can cause fetal harm when administered to a pregnant woman or can affect reproduction capacity. Pentamidine isethionate inhalation should be given to a pregnant woman only if clearly needed. Pentamidine isethionate inhalation should not be given to a pregnant woman unless the potential benefits are judged to outweigh the risks.

➤*Lactation:* It is not known whether pentamidine isethionate inhalation is excreted in human milk. Because of the potential for serious adverse reactions in nursing infants from pentamidine isethionate inhalation, a decision should be made whether to discontinue nursing or to discontinue the drug, taking into account the importance of the drug to the mother. Because many drugs are excreted in human milk, pentamidine isethionate inhalation should not be given to a nursing mother unless the potential benefits are judged to outweigh the unknown risks.

➤*Children:* The safety and efficacy of pentamidine isethionate inhalation in pediatric patients (birth to 16 years of age) have not been established.

Precautions

➤*Monitoring:* The extent and consequence of pentamidine accumulation following chronic inhalation therapy are not known. As a result, patients receiving pentamidine isethionate inhalation should be closely monitored for the development of serious adverse reactions that have occurred in patients receiving parenteral pentamidine, including hypotension, hypoglycemia, hyperglycemia, hypocalcemia, anemia, thrombocytopenia, leukopenia, hepatic or renal dysfunction, ventricular tachycardia, pancreatitis, Stevens-Johnson syndrome, hyperkalemia, and abnormal ST segment of ECG.

➤*Pulmonary:* Inhalation of pentamidine isethionate may induce bronchospasm or cough. This has been noted particularly in some patients who have a history of smoking or asthma. In clinical trials, cough and bronchospasm were the most frequently reported adverse experiences associated with pentamidine isethionate administration (38% and 15%, respectively, of patients receiving the 300 mg dose); however, less than 1% of the doses were inter-

PENTAMIDINE ISETHIONATE — INHALATIONAL

rupted or terminated due to these effects. For the majority of patients, cough and bronchospasm were controlled by administration of an aerosolized bronchodilator (only 1% of patients withdrew from the study due to treatment-associated cough or bronchospasm). In patients who experience bronchospasm or cough, administration of an inhaled bronchodilator prior to giving each pentamidine isethionate dose may minimize recurrence of the symptoms.

Extrapulmonary infection with *P. carinii* has been reported infrequently. Most, but not all, of the cases have been reported in patients who have a history of PCP. The presence of extrapulmonary pneumocystosis should be considered when evaluating patients with unexplained signs and symptoms.

➤*Pancreatitis:* Cases of acute pancreatitis have been reported in patients receiving aerosolized pentamidine. Pentamidine isethionate should be discontinued if signs or symptoms of acute pancreatitis develop.

Drug Interactions

Because the nephrotoxic effects may be additive, the concomitant or sequential use of pentamidine isethionate and other nephrotoxic drugs such as aminoglycosides, amphotericin B, cisplatin, foscarnet, or vancomycin should be closely monitored and avoided, if possible.

Adverse Reactions

➤*Most frequently reported adverse reactions (1% to 5%):* The most frequently reported unsolicited adverse events (1% to 5%) in clinical trials, regardless of their relation to pentamidine isethionate therapy were as follows (n = 931):

CNS – Headache.

GI – Diarrhea and nausea.

Hematologic – Anemia.

Respiratory – Chest pain, cough, and wheezing.

Special senses – Bad taste.

Miscellaneous – Night sweats.

Infection: Bronchitis, non-specific herpes, herpes zoster, non-specific influenza, oral *Candida*, pharyngitis, sinusitis, and upper respiratory tract infection.

➤*Adverse reactions with less than 1% incidence:* Adverse events of less than 1% incidence were as follows (no causal relationship to treatment has been established for these adverse events):

Cardiovascular – Cerebrovascular accident, hypotension, hypertension, palpitations, poor circulation, syncope, tachycardia, vasodilatation and vasculitis.

CNS – Anxiety, confusion, depression, drowsiness, emotional lability, hallucination, hypesthesia, insomnia, memory loss, neuralgia, neuropathy, nonspecific neuropathy, nervousness, paranoia, paresthesia, peripheral neuropathy, seizure, tremors, unsteady gait, and vertigo.

Dermatologic – Desquamation, dry and breaking hair, dry skin, erythema, non-specific dermatitis, pruritus, rash, and urticaria.

GI – Abdominal cramps, abdominal pain, constipation, dry mouth, dyspepsia, gastritis, gastric ulcer, gingivitis, hiatal hernia, hypersalivation, oral ulcer/abscess, splenomegaly, and vomiting.

GU – Flank pain, incontinence, nephritis, renal failure, and renal pain.

Hematologic – Eosinophilia, neutropenia, nonspecific cytopenia, pancytopenia, and thrombocytopenia.

Hepatic – Hepatitis, hepatomegaly, and hepatic dysfunction.

Metabolic – Hyperglycemia, hypoglycemia, and hypocalcemia.

Musculoskeletal – Arthralgia, gout, and myalgia.

Respiratory – Asthma, bronchitis, bronchospasm, chest congestion, chest tightness, coryza, cyanosis, eosinophilic or interstitial pneumonitis, gagging, hemoptysis, hyperventilation, laryngitis, laryngospasm, nonspecific lung disorder, nasal congestion, pleuritis, pneumothorax, rales, rhinitis, shortness of breath, nonspecific sputum, and tachypnea.

Special senses – Blepharitis, blurred vision, conjunctivitis, contact lens discomfort, eye pain or discomfort, hemianopsia, loss of taste, nonspecific odor, and smell.

Miscellaneous – Miscarriage.

Allergic reaction, non-specific allergy, body odor, facial edema, fever, leg edema, lethargy, low body temperature, and temperature abnormality.

Infection: Bacterial pneumonia, central venous line related sepsis, cryptococcal meningitis, cytomegalovirus (CMV) colitis, CMV retinitis, esophageal *Candida*, histoplasmosis, Kaposi's sarcoma, nonspecific mycoplasma, oral herpes, nonspecific otitis, nonspecific pharyngitis, pharyngeal herpes, nonspecific serious infection, tonsillitis, tuberculosis, and viral encephalitis.

➤*Postmarketing:* From postmarketing clinical experience with pentamidine isethionate the following spontaneous adverse events have been reported: Anaphylaxis, colitis, diabetes, dyspnea, esophagitis, hematochezia, increased blood urea nitrogen (BUN) and serum creatinine levels, melena, pancreatitis, syndrome of inappropriate antidiuretic hormone (SIADH), and torsade de pointes.

Overdosage

Overdosage has not been reported with pentamidine isethionate. The symptoms and signs of overdosage are not known.

A serious overdosage, to the point of producing systemic drug levels similar to those following parenteral administration, would have the potential of producing similar types of serious systemic toxicity. Patients receiving pentamidine isethionate inhalation should be closely monitored for the development of serious adverse reactions that have occurred in patients receiving parenteral pentamidine, including hypotension, hypoglycemia, hyperglycemia, hypocalcemia, anemia, thrombocytopenia, leukopenia, hepatic or renal dysfunction, ventricular tachycardia, pancreatitis, Stevens-Johnson syndrome, hyperkalemia, and abnormal ST segment of ECG.

Available clinical pharmacology data suggest that a dose up to 40 times the recommended pentamidine isethionate dosage would be required to produce systemic levels similar to a single 4 mg/kg intravenous dose.

ANTHELMINTICS

The following table lists the major parasitic infections, causative organisms and drugs of choice for treatment. For investigational antiparasitic agents available from the Centers for Disease Control, refer to the CDC Anti-Infective Agents monograph.

Major Parasite Infections			
	Infection (common name)	Organism	Drug(s) of Choice
Intestinal Nematodes	Ascariasis[1] (Roundworm)	*Ascaris lumbricoides*	Mebendazole, Pyrantel pamoate or Diethylcarbamazine
	Uncinariasis (Hookworm)	*Ancylostoma duodenale* *Necator americanus*	Mebendazole or Pyrantel pamoate[2]
	Strongyloidiasis (Threadworm)	*Strongyloides stercoralis*	Thiabendazole
	Trichuriasis (Whipworm)	*Trichuris trichiura*	Mebendazole
	Enterobiasis[3] (Pinworm)	*Enterobius vermicularis*	Mebendazole, Pyrantel pamoate or Albendazole
	Capillariasis	*Capillaria philippinensis*	Mebendazole, Thiabendazole or Albendazole
Tissue Nematodes	Trichinosis	*Trichinella spiralis*	Steroids for severe symptoms plus Thiabendazole, Albendazole, Flubendazole[6] or Mebendazole[2]
	Cutaneous larva migrans (Creeping eruption)	*Ancylostoma braziliense* and others	Thiabendazole, Albendazole or Ivermectin[4]
	Onchocerciasis (River blindness)	*Onchocerca volvulus*	Suramin[5], Diethylcarbamazine or Ivermectin[4]
	Dracontiasis (Guinea worm)	*Dracunculus medinensis*	Thiabendazole or Mebendazole
	Angiostrongyliasis (Rat lungworm)	*Angiostrongylus cantonensis*	Thiabendazole or Mebendazole
	Loiasis	*Loa loa*	Diethylcarbamazine
Cestodes	Taeniasis (Beef tapeworm)	*Taenia saginata*	Praziquantel[2] or Niclosamide[6]
	(Pork tapeworm)	*Taenia solium*	Praziquantel[2], Niclosamide[6] or Albendazole
	Diphyllobothriasis (Fish tapeworm)	*Diphyllobothrium latum*	Praziquantel[2] or Niclosamide[6]
	Dog tapeworm	*Dipylidium caninum*	Praziquantel[2]
	Hymenolepiasis (Dwarf tapeworm)	*Hymenolepis nana*	Praziquantel[2] or Niclosamide[6]
	Hydatid cysts	*Echinococcus granulosus*	Albendazole or Praziquantel

Major Parasite Infections			
	Infection (common name)	Organism	Drug(s) of Choice
Trematodes	Schistosomiasis	*Schistosoma mansoni*	Praziquantel or Oxamniquine
		Schistosoma japonicum	Praziquantel
		Schistosoma haematobium	Praziquantel
		Schistosoma mekongi	Praziquantel
	Hermaphroditic Flukes		
	Fasciolopsiasis (Intestinal fluke)	*Fasciolopsis buski*	Praziquantel
		Heterophyes heterophyes	Praziquantel
		Metagonimus yokogawai	
	Clonorchiasis (Chinese liver fluke)	*Clonorchis sinensis*	Praziquantel
	Fascioliasis (Sheep liver fluke)	*Fasciola hepatica*	Praziquantel or Bithionol[4]
	Opisthorchiasis (Liver fluke)	*Opisthorchis viverrini*	Praziquantel
	Paragonimiasis (Lung fluke)	*Paragonimus westermani*	Praziquantel or Bithionol[4] (alternate)

[1] Thiabendazole is also indicated in Ascariasis.
[2] Unlabeled use.
[3] Thiabendazole is also indicated in Enterobiasis.
[4] Available from the CDC.
[5] Available from the CDC, although generally not recommended.
[6] Not available in the US.

Benzimidazoles

MEBENDAZOLE

Rx	**Vermox** (Janssen)	**Tablets, chewable:** 100 mg	(VERMOX JANSSEN). In 12s.
Rx	**Mebendazole** (Copley)		In 12s.

MEBENDAZOLE — ORAL

Refer to the general discussion of these products in the Anthelmintics introduction.

Indications

➤*Helminths:* For the treatment of *Enterobius vermicularis* (pinworm), *Trichuris trichiura* (whipworm), *Ascaris lumbricoides* (common roundworm), *Ancylostoma duodenale* (common hookworm), and *Necator americanus* (American hookworm) in single or mixed infections.

Administration and Dosage

➤*Dosage:* The same dosage schedule applies to children and adults. The tablet may be chewed, swallowed, or crushed and mixed with food.

	Pinworm (enterobiasis)	Whipworm (trichuriasis)	Common roundworm (ascariasis)	Hookworm
Dose	1 tablet once	1 tablet morning and evening for 3 consecutive days.	1 tablet morning and evening for 3 consecutive days.	1 tablet morning and evening for 3 consecutive days.

If the patient is not cured 3 weeks after treatment, a second course of treatment is advised. No special procedures, such as fasting or purging, are required.

➤*Storage/Stability:* Store at controlled room temperature 15° to 25°C (59° to 77°F).

Actions

➤*Pharmacology:* Mebendazole inhibits the formation of the worms' microtubules and causes the worms' glucose depletion.

➤*Pharmacokinetics:*

Absorption – Following administration of 100 mg twice daily for 3 consecutive days, plasma levels of mebendazole and its primary metabolite, the 2-amine, do not exceed 0.03 mcg/mL and 0.09 mcg/mL respectively. All metabolites are devoid of anthelmintic activity.

Excretion – In man, ≈ 2% of administered mebendazole is excreted in urine and the remainder in the feces as unchanged drug or a primary metabolite.

Contraindications

Hypersensitivity to the drug.

Warnings

➤*Hydatid disease:* There is no evidence that mebendazole, even at high doses, is effective for hydatid disease. There have been rare reports of neutropenia and agranulocytosis when mebendazole was taken for prolonged periods and at dosages substantially above those recommended.

➤*Pregnancy: Category C.*

Teratogenic – Mebendazole has shown embryotoxic and teratogenic activity in pregnant rats at single oral doses as low as 10 mg/kg (approximately equal to the human dose, based on mg/m^2). In view of these findings the use of mebendazole is not recommended in pregnant women. Although there are no adequate and well-controlled studies in pregnant women, a postmarketing survey has been done of a limited number of women who inadvertently had consumed mebendazole during the first trimester of pregnancy. The incidence of spontaneous abortion and malformation did not exceed that in the general population. In 170 deliveries on term, no teratogenic risk of mebendazole was identified.

➤*Lactation:* It is not known whether mebendazole is excreted in human milk. Because many drugs are excreted in human milk, caution should be exercised when mebendazole is administered to a nursing woman.

➤*Children:* The drug has not been extensively studied in children under 2 years; therefore, in the treatment of children under 2 years the relative benefit/risk should be considered.

Precautions

➤*Monitoring:* Periodic assessment of organ system functions, including hematopoietic and hepatic, is advisable during prolonged therapy.

Drug Interactions

Preliminary evidence suggests that cimetidine inhibits mebendazole metabolism and may result in an increase in plasma concentrations of mebendazole.

Adverse Reactions

➤*CNS:* Very rare cases of convulsions have been reported.

➤*GI:* Transient symptoms of abdominal pain and diarrhea in cases of massive infection and expulsion of worms.

➤*Hematologic:* Neutropenia and agranulocytosis (see Warnings).

➤*Hepatic:* There have been liver function test elevations (AST [SGOT], ALT [SGPT], and GGT) and rare reports of hepatitis when mebendazole was taken for prolonged periods and at dosages substantially above those recommended.

➤*Hypersensitivity:* Rash, urticaria and angioedema have been observed on rare occasions.

Overdosage

➤*Symptoms:* In the event of accidental overdosage, GI complaints lasting up to a few hours may occur.

➤*Treatment:* Vomiting and purging should be induced.

Patient Information

Patients should be informed of the potential risk to the fetus in women taking mebendazole during pregnancy, especially during the first trimester (see Warnings, Pregnancy).

Patients should also be informed that cleanliness is important to prevent reinfection and transmission of the infection.

THIABENDAZOLE

Rx	**Mintezol** (Merck)	**Tablets, chewable:** 500 mg	Lactose, saccharin. (MSD 907). White, scored. Orange flavor. In 36s.
		Oral Suspension: 500 mg/5 ml	Sorbic acid, sorbitol. In 120 ml.

THIABENDAZOLE — ORAL

Refer to the general discussion of these products in the Anthelmintics introduction.

Indications

➤*Helminths:* Treatment of strongyloidiasis (threadworm), cutaneous larva migrans (creeping eruption), visceral larva migrans, and trichinosis (relief of symptoms and fever and a reduction of eosinophilia have followed the use of thiabendazole during the invasion stage of the disease).

Thiabendazole is usually inappropriate as first-line therapy for enterobiasis (pinworm). However, when enterobiasis occurs with any of the conditions listed above, additional therapy is not required for most patients.

➤*Second-line therapy:* Only use thiabendazole in the following infestations when more specific therapy is not available or cannot be used or when further therapy with a second agent is desirable: Uncinariasis (hookworm: *Necator americanus* and *Ancylostoma duodenale*); Trichuriasis (whipworm); Ascariasis (large roundworm).

Administration and Dosage

➤*Approved by the FDA:* April 7, 1967.

➤*Maximum dose:* The recommended maximum daily dose of thiabendazole is 3 g.

➤*Usual dsage:* Give thiabendazole after meals if possible. Chew thiabendazole tablets before swallowing. Dietary restriction, complementary medications, and cleansing enemas are not needed.

The usual dosage schedule for all conditions is 2 doses/day. The dosage is determined by the patient's weight.

Weight	Each dose g	Each dose mL
30 lb	0.25 g (½ tablet)	2.5 mL (½ teaspoon)
50 lb	0.5 g (1 tablet)	5 mL (1 teaspoon)
75 lb	0.75 g (1½ tablet)	7.5 mL (1½ teaspoons)
100 lb	1 g (2 tablets)	10 mL (2 teaspoons)
125 lb	1.25 g (2½ tablets)	12.5 mL (2½ teaspoons)
150 lb and over	1.5 g (3 tablets)	15 mL (3 teaspoons)

Indication	Therapeutic regimens: Regimen	Therapeutic regimens: Comments
Strongyloidiasis[a]	2 doses per day for 2 successive days	A single dose of 20 mg/lb or 50 mg/kg may be employed as an alternative schedule, but expect a higher incidence of side effects.
Cutaneous larva migrans (creeping eruption)	2 doses per day for 2 successive days	If active lesions are still present 2 days after completion of therapy, a second course is recommended.
Visceral larva migrans	2 doses per day for 7 successive days	Safety and efficacy data on the 7-day treatment course are limited.
Trichinosis[a]	2 doses per day for 2 to 4 successive days according to the response of the patient	The optimal dosage for the treatment of trichinosis has not been established.
Other indications		
Intestinal roundworms[a] (including Ascariasis, Uncinariasis, and Trichuriasis)	2 doses per day for 2 successive days	A single dose of 20 mg/lb or 50 mg/kg may be employed as an alternative schedule, but expect a higher incidence of side effects.

[a] Clinical experience with thiabendazole for treatment of each of these conditions in pediatric patients weighing less than 30 lbs has been limited.

➤*Storage/Stability:* Store in a well-closed container at controlled room temperature (15° to 30°C [59° to 86°F]). Protect the suspension from freezing.

Actions

➤*Pharmacology:* The precise mode of action of thiabendazole on the parasite is unknown, but it may inhibit the helminth-specific enzyme fumarate reductase.

Microbiology – Thiabendazole is vermicidalor vermifugal against *Ascaris lumbricoides* ("common roundworm"), *Strongyloides stercoralis* (threadworm), *Necator americanus*, and *Ancylostoma duodenale* (hookworm), *Trichuris trichiura* (whipworm), *Ancylostoma braziliense* (dog and cat hookworm), *Toxocara canis* and *Toxocara cati* (ascarids), and *Enterobius vermicularis* (pinworm).

Its effect on larvae of *Trichinella spiralis* that have migrated to muscle is questionable.

Thiabendazole also suppresses egg or larval production and may inhibit the subsequent development of those eggs or larvae which are passed in the feces.

➤*Pharmacokinetics:*

Absorption – In humans, thiabendazole is rapidly absorbed and peak plasma concentration is reached within 1 to 2 hours after the oral administration of a suspension.

Metabolism – It is metabolized almost completely to the 5-hydroxy form which appears in the urine as glucuronide or sulfate conjugates.

Excretion – In 48 hours, about 5% of the administered dose is recovered from the feces and about 90% from the urine. Most is excreted in the first 24 hours.

Contraindications

Hypersensitivity to this product. Thiabendazole is contraindicated as prophylactic treatment for pinworm infestation.

Warnings

➤*Visual effects:* Abnormal sensation in eyes, xanthopsia, blurred vision, drying of mucous membranes, and Sicca syndrome have been reported in patients treated with thiabendazole. These adverse reactions of the eye were in some cases persistent for prolonged intervals which have exceeded 1 year.

➤*Enterobiasis:* Thiabendazole should not usually be used as first-line therapy for the treatment of enterobiasis. Reserve it for use in patients who have experienced allergic reactions or resistance to other treatments.

➤*Hepatic effects:* Jaundice, cholestasis, and parenchymal liver damage have been reported in patients treated with thiabendazole. In rare cases, liver damage has been severe and has led to irreversible hepatic failure.

➤*Hypersensitivity reactions:* If hypersensitivity reactions occur, the drug should be discontinued immediately and not be resumed. Erythema multiforme has been associated with thiabendazole therapy; in severe cases (Stevens-Johnson syndrome), fatalities have occurred.

➤*Elderly:* This drug is metabolized almost completely by the liver, and the metabolites are known to be substantially excreted by the kidney; therefore, the risk of toxicity may be greater in patients with impaired renal function. Because elderly patients are more likely to have decreased renal function, take care in dose selection, and it may be useful to monitor renal function.

➤*Pregnancy: Category C.* Reproduction and teratogenic studies done in the rabbit at a dose up to 15 times the usual human dose, in the rat at a dose equivalent to the human dose, and in the mouse at a dose up to 2½ times the usual human dose, revealed no evidence of harm to the fetus. In an additional study in the mouse, no defects were observed when thiabendazole was given in aqueous suspension, at a dose 10 times the usual human dose; however, cleft palate and axial skeletal defects were observed when thiabendazole was suspended in olive oil and given at the same dose. There are no adequate and well-controlled studies in pregnant women. Only use thiabendazole during pregnancy if the potential benefit justifies the potential risk to the fetus.

➤*Lactation:* It is not known whether this drug is excreted in human milk. Because of the potential for serious adverse reactions in nursing infants from thiabendazole, a decision should be made whether to discontinue nursing or to discontinue the drug, taking into account the importance of the drug to the mother.

➤*Children:* The safety and effectiveness of thiabendazole for the treatment of Strongyloidiasis, Ascariasis, Uncinariasis, Trichuriasis, and Trichinosis in pediatric patients weighing less than 30 lbs has been limited.

Precautions

➤*Monitoring:* In the presence of hepatic or renal dysfunction, carefully monitor patients.

➤*Mixed infections with ascaris:* Thiabendazole is not suitable for the treatment of mixed infections with ascaris because it may cause these worms to migrate.

➤*Supportive therapy:* Ideally, supportive therapy is indicated for anemic, dehydrated, or malnourished patients prior to initiation of the anthelmintic therapy.

➤*Susceptible worm infestations:* Thiabendazole should be used only in patients in whom susceptible worm infestation has been diagnosed and should not be used prophylactically.

➤*Lab test abnormalities:* Rarely, a transient rise in liver function tests has occurred in patients receiving thiabendazole.

➤*Hazardous tasks:* Because CNS side effects may occur quite frequently, tell patients to avoid activities requiring mental alertness.

Drug Interactions

➤*Xanthines:* Thiabendazole may compete with other drugs, such as theophylline, for sites of metabolism in the liver, thus elevating the serum levels of such compounds to potentially toxic levels. Therefore, when concomitant use of thiabendazole and xanthine derivatives is anticipated, it may be nec-

THIABENDAZOLE — ORAL

essary to monitor blood levels or reduce the dosage of such compounds. Administer such concomitant use under careful medical supervision.

Adverse Reactions

➤*Cardiovascular:* Hypotension.

➤*CNS:* Dizziness, weariness, drowsiness, giddiness, headache, numbness, hyperirritability, convulsions, collapse, confusion, depression, floating sensation, weakness and lack of coordination.

➤*GI:* Anorexia, nausea, vomiting, diarrhea, epigastric distress, abdominal pain, jaundice, cholestasis, parenchymal liver damage and hepatic failure.

➤*GU:* Hematuria, enuresis, malodor of the urine, crystalluria.

➤*Hematologic:* Transient leukopenia.

➤*Hypersensitivity:* Pruritus, fever, facial flush, chills, conjunctival injection, angioedema, anaphylaxis, skin rashes (including perianal), erythema multiforme (including Stevens-Johnson syndrome), and lymphadenopathy.

➤*Metabolic:* Hyperglycemia.

➤*Special senses:* Tinnitus, abnormal sensation in eyes, xanthopsia, blurred vision, reduced vision, drying of mucous membranes (eg, mouth, eyes), Sicca syndrome.

➤*Miscellaneous:* Appearance of live Ascaris in the mouth and nose.

Overdosage

➤*Symptoms:* Overdosage may be associated with transient disturbances of vision and psychic alterations.

➤*Treatment:* There is no specific antidote in the event of overdosage. Therefore, employ symptomatic and supportive measures. Induce emesis or carefully perform gastric lavage.

Patient Information

Because CNS side effects may occur quite frequently, avoid activities requiring mental alertness.

ALBENDAZOLE

Rx	**Albenza** (SmithKline Beecham)	**Tablets:** 200 mg	Lactose, saccharin. (SB 5500). Biconvex. In film-coated *Tiltab.* In 112s.

ALBENDAZOLE — ORAL

Refer to the general discussion of these products in the Anthelmintics introduction.

Indications

➤*Neurocysticercosis:* For the treatment of parenchymal neurocysticercosis due to active lesions caused by larval forms of the pork tapeworm, *Taenia solium.*

➤*Hydatid disease:* For the treatment of cystic hydatid disease of the liver, lung, and peritoneum, caused by the larval form of the dog tapeworm, *Echinococcus granulosus.*

When medically feasible, surgery is considered the treatment of choice for hydatid disease. When administering albendazole in the pre- or postsurgical setting, optimal killing of cyst contents is achieved when 3 courses of therapy have been given.

The efficacy of albendazole in the therapy of alveolar hydatid disease caused by *Echinococcus multilocularis* has not been clearly demonstrated in clinical studies.

Administration and Dosage

➤*Approved by the FDA:* June 11, 1996.

Dosing of albendazole will vary, depending upon which of the following parasitic infections is being treated.

➤*Dosage:*

Indication	Patient weight	Dose	Duration
Hydatid disease	60 kg or greater	400 mg twice daily, with meals	28-day cycle followed by a 14-day albendazole-free interval, for a total of 3 cycles
	Less than 60 kg	15 mg/kg/day given in divided doses twice daily with meals (maximum total daily dose 800 mg)	
	Note: When administering albendazole in the pre- or post-surgical setting, optimal killing of cyst contents is achieved when 3 courses of therapy have been given.		
Neurocysticercosis	60 kg or greater	400 mg twice daily, with meals	8 to 30 days
	Less than 60 kg	15 mg/kg/day given in divided doses twice daily with meals (maximum total daily dose 800 mg)	

➤*Adjunct therapy:* Patients being treated for neurocysticercosis should receive appropriate steroid and anticonvulsant therapy as required. Oral or intravenous corticosteroids should be considered to prevent cerebral hypertensive episodes during the first week of treatment.

➤*Storage / Stability:* Store between 20° and 25°C (68° and 77°F).

Actions

➤*Pharmacology:* The principal mode of action for albendazole is by its inhibitory effect on tubulin polymerization which results in the loss of cytoplasmic microtubules.

In the specified treatment indications albendazole appears to be active against the larval forms of the following organisms: *Echinococcus granulosus* and *Taenia solium.*

➤*Pharmacokinetics:*

Absorption / Distribution – Albendazole is poorly absorbed from the gastrointestinal tract due to its low aqueous solubility.

Albendazole sulfoxide is 70% bound to plasma protein and is widely distributed throughout the body; it has been detected in urine, bile, liver, cyst wall, cyst fluid, and cerebrospinal fluid (CSF). Concentrations in plasma were 3- to 10-fold and 2- to 4-fold higher than those simultaneously determined in cyst fluid and CSF, respectively. Limited in vitro and clinical data suggest that albendazole sulfoxide may be eliminated from cysts at a slower rate than observed in plasma.

Albendazole concentrations are negligible or undetectable in plasma as it is rapidly converted to the sulfoxide metabolite prior to reaching the systemic circulation. The systemic anthelmintic activity has been attributed to the primary metabolite, albendazole sulfoxide. Oral bioavailability appears to be enhanced when albendazole is coadministered with a fatty meal (estimated fat content 40 g) as evidenced by higher (up to 5-fold on average) plasma concentrations of albendazole sulfoxide as compared to the fasted state.

Maximal plasma concentrations of albendazole sulfoxide are typically achieved 2 to 5 hours after dosing and are on average 1.31 mcg/mL (range, 0.46 to 1.58 mcg/mL) following oral doses of albendazole (400 mg) in 6 hydatid disease patients, when administered with a fatty meal. Plasma concentrations of albendazole sulfoxide increase in a dose-proportional manner over the therapeutic dose range following ingestion of a fatty meal (fat content 43.1 g).

Metabolism / Excretion – The mean apparent terminal elimination half-life of albendazole sulfoxide typically ranges from 8 to 12 hours in 25 healthy subjects, as well as in 14 hydatid and 8 neurocysticercosis patients.

Following 4 weeks of treatment with albendazole (200 mg 3 times daily), twelve patients' plasma concentrations of albendazole sulfoxide were approximately 20% lower than those observed during the first half of the treatment period, suggesting that albendazole may induce its own metabolism.

Albendazole is rapidly converted in the liver to the primary metabolite, albendazole sulfoxide, which is further metabolized to albendazole sulfone and other primary oxidative metabolites that have been identified in human urine. Following oral administration, albendazole has not been detected in human urine. Urinary excretion of albendazole sulfoxide is a minor elimination pathway with < 1% of the dose recovered in the urine. Biliary elimination presumably accounts for a portion of the elimination as evidenced by biliary concentrations of albendazole sulfoxide similar to those achieved in plasma.

Special populations –

Biliary effects: In patients with evidence of extrahepatic obstruction (n = 5), the systemic availability of albendazole sulfoxide was increased, as indicated by a 2-fold increase in maximum serum concentration and a 7-fold increase in area under the curve. The rate of absorption/conversion and elimination of albendazole sulfoxide appeared to be prolonged with mean T_{max} and serum elimination half-life values of 10 hours and 31.7 hours, respectively. Plasma concentrations of parent albendazole were measurable in only 1 of 5 patients.

Contraindications

Hypersensitivity to the benzimidazole class of compounds or any components of albendazole.

Warnings

➤*Hepatic function impairment:* Patients with abnormal liver function test results prior to commencing albendazole therapy should be carefully evaluated, since the drug is metabolized by the liver and has been associated with hepatotoxicity in a few patients.

ALBENDAZOLE — ORAL

➤*Elderly:* Experience in patients 65 years of age or older is limited. The number of patients treated for either hydatid disease or neurocysticercosis is limited, but no problems associated with an older population have been observed.

➤*Pregnancy: Category C.* There are no adequate and well-controlled studies of albendazole administration in pregnant women. Albendazole should be used during pregnancy only if the potential benefit justifies the potential risk to the fetus.

Albendazole should not be used in pregnant women except in clinical circumstances where no alternative management is appropriate. Patients should not become pregnant for at least 1 month following cessation of albendazole therapy. If a patient becomes pregnant while taking this drug, albendazole should be discontinued immediately. If pregnancy occurs while taking this drug, the patient should be apprised of the potential hazard to the fetus.

Teratogenic – Albendazole has been shown to be teratogenic (to cause embryotoxicity and skeletal malformations) in pregnant rats and rabbits. The teratogenic response in the rat was shown at oral doses of 10 and 30 mg/kg/day (0.10 times and 0.32 times the recommended human dose based on body surface area in mg/m^2, respectively) during gestation days 6 to 15 and in pregnant rabbits at oral doses of 30 mg/kg/day (0.60 times the recommended human dose based on body surface area in mg/m^2) administered during gestation days 7 to 19. In the rabbit study, maternal toxicity (33% mortality) was noted at 30 mg/kg/day. In mice, no teratogenic effects were observed at oral doses up to 30 mg/kg/day (0.16 times the recommended human dose based on body surface area in mg/m^2), administered during gestation days 6 to 15.

➤*Lactation:* Albendazole is excreted in animal milk. It is not known whether it is excreted in human milk. Because many drugs are excreted in human milk, caution should be exercised when albendazole is administered to a nursing woman.

➤*Children:* Experience in children under the age of 6 years is limited. In hydatid disease, infection in infants and young children is uncommon, but no problems have been encountered in those who have been treated. In neurocysticercosis, infection is more frequently encountered. In 5 published studies involving pediatric patients as young as 1 year, no significant problems were encountered, and the efficacy appeared similar to the adult population.

Precautions

➤*Hematologic effects:* Rare fatalities associated with the use of albendazole have been reported due to granulocytopenia or pancytopenia. Blood counts should be monitored at the beginning of each 28-day cycle of therapy, and every 2 weeks while on therapy with albendazole. Albendazole may be continued if the total white blood cell count and absolute neutrophil count decrease appear modest and do not progress.

Albendazole has been shown to cause occasional (< 1% of treated patients) reversible reductions in total white blood cell count. Rarely, more significant reductions may be encountered including granulocytopenia, agranulocytosis, or pancytopenia.

➤*Cysticercosis:* Cysticercosis may, in rare cases, involve the retina. Before initiating therapy for neurocysticercosis, the patient should be examined for the presence of retinal lesions. If such lesions are visualized, the need for anticysticeral therapy should be weighed against the possibility of retinal damage caused by albendazole-induced changes to the retinal lesion.

➤*Hepatic effects:* In clinical trials, treatment with albendazole has been associated with mild to moderate elevations of hepatic enzymes in approximately 16% of patients. These have returned to normal upon discontinuation of therapy.

Liver function tests (transaminases) should be performed before the start of each treatment cycle and at least every 2 weeks during treatment. If enzymes are significantly increased, albendazole therapy should be discontinued. Therapy can be reinstituted when liver enzymes have returned to pretreatment levels, but laboratory tests should be performed frequently during repeat therapy.

➤*Adjunct therapy:* See Administration and Dosage for more information.

Drug Interactions

Albendazole Drug Interactions			
Precipitant drug	Object drug*		Description
Dexamethasone	Albendazole	↑	Steady-state trough concentrations of albendazole sulfoxide were ≈ 56% higher when 8 mg dexamethasone was coadministered with each dose of albendazole (15 mg/kg/day) in eight neurocysticercosis patients.
Praziquantel	Albendazole	↑	Praziquantel (40 mg/kg) increased mean maximum plasma concentration and AUC of albendazole sulfoxide by ≈ 50% in healthy subjects.
Cimetidine	Albendazole	↑	Albendazole sulfoxide concentrations in bile and cystic fluid were increased (≈ 2-fold) in hydatid cyst patients treated with cimetidine.

* ↑ = Object drug increased.

➤*Theophylline:* Although single doses of albendazole have been shown not to inhibit theophylline metabolism, albendazole does induce cytochrome P450 1A in human hepatoma cells. Therefore, it is recommended that plasma concentrations of theophylline be monitored during and after treatment with albendazole.

Adverse Reactions

The adverse event profile of albendazole differs between hydatid disease and neurocysticercosis.

These symptoms were usually mild and resolved without treatment. Treatment discontinuations were predominantly due to leukopenia (0.7%) or hepatic abnormalities (3.8% in hydatid disease). The following incidence reflects events that were reported by investigators to be at least possibly or probably related to albendazole.

Adverse event incidence ≥ 1% in hydatid disease and neurocysticercosis		
Adverse Event	Hydatid Disease	Neurocysticercosis
Abnormal Liver Function Tests	15.6%	< 1%
Abdominal Pain	6%	0%
Nausea/Vomiting	3.7%	6.2%
Headache	1.3%	11%
Dizziness/Vertigo	1.2%	< 1%
Raised Intracranial Pressure	0%	1.5%
Meningeal Signs	0%	1%
Reversible Alopecia	1.6%	< 1%
Fever	1%	0%

➤*Adverse events less than 1%:*

Dermatologic – Rash, urticaria.

Hematologic – Leukopenia. There have been rare reports of granulocytopenia, pancytopenia, agranulocytosis, or thrombocytopenia (see Warnings).

Hypersensitivity – Allergic reactions.

Renal – Acute renal failure related to albendazole therapy has been observed.

Overdosage

➤*Symptoms:* Significant toxicity and mortality were shown in male and female mice at doses exceeding 5000 mg/kg; in rats, at estimated doses between 1300 and 2400 mg/kg; in hamsters, at doses exceeding 10,000 mg/kg; and in rabbits, at estimated doses between 500 and 1250 mg/kg. In the animals, symptoms were demonstrated in a dose-response relationship and included diarrhea, vomiting, tachycardia, and respiratory distress.

➤*Treatment:* One overdosage has been reported with albendazole in a patient who took at least 16 g over 12 hours. No untoward effects were reported. In case of overdosage, symptomatic therapy (eg, gastric lavage and activated charcoal) and general supportive measures are recommended.

Patient Information

Albendazole may cause fetal harm; therefore, women of childbearing age should begin treatment after a negative pregnancy test.

Women of childbearing age should be cautioned against becoming pregnant while on albendazole or within 1 month of completing treatment.

During albendazole therapy, because of the possibility of harm to the liver or bone marrow, routine (every 2 weeks) monitoring of blood counts and liver function tests should take place.

Albendazole should be taken with food.

DIETHYLCARBAMAZINE CITRATE

Rx	**Hetrazan**[1] (Wyeth-Ayerst)	**Tablets**: 50 mg	In 100s.

[1] Hetrazan is available from Wyeth-Ayerst Labs without charge for compassionate use only. For more information, physicians should contact: Wyeth-Ayerst Labs, P.O. Box 8299, Philadelphia, PA 19101; (610) 688-4400.

DIETHYLCARBAMAZINE CITRATE — ORAL

Refer to the general discussion of these products in the Anthelmintics introduction.

Indications

Treatment of Bancroftian filariasis, onchocerciasis, ascariasis, tropical eosinophilia, loiasis.

Administration and Dosage

➤*Bancroft's filariasis, onchocerciasis and loiasis:* Usual dose is 2 mg/kg 3 times a day immediately following meals. When the disease is in the acute stage, continue treatment for 3 to 4 weeks. Recurrences have been more frequent with smaller doses. When, as a public health measure, it is desirable to treat large numbers of patients known to harbor microfilariae, use the same dosage schedule for 3 to 5 days. Laboratory tests in randomly selected patients are helpful in assessing efficacy of therapy.

➤*Ascariasis:*

Outpatients – 13 mg/kg, given once a day for 7 days, should reduce the number of worms by 85% to 100%. No pretreatment fasting or post-treatment purging is required. Expulsion of ascarids usually begins 1 or 2 days after therapy initiation.

Children – Give 6 to 10 mg/kg 3 times daily for 7 to 10 days. In particularly obstinate cases, an additional course consisting of 10 mg/kg 3 times daily is indicated.

➤*Tropical eosinophilia:* 13 mg/kg/day for 4 to 7 days.

Actions

➤*Pharmacology:* Diethylcarbamazine does not resemble other antiparasitic compounds. It is a synthetic organic compound which is highly specific for several common parasites and does not contain any toxic metallic elements. Diethylcarbamazine has demonstrated a low order of toxicity in animals.

➤*Microbiology:* The drug is effective against the following organisms: *Wuchereria bancrofti, Onchocerca volvulus, Loa loa,* and *Ascaris lumbricoides.*

Precautions

➤*Administration:* Administer carefully to avoid or to control allergic or other untoward reactions.

Adverse Reactions

➤*Wuchereria bancrofti:* Mild reactions are transient but fairly frequent. Headache, lassitude, weakness or general malaise are most common. Nausea, vomiting and skin rash occasionally occur. These effects are not considered serious and do not usually require discontinuation of therapy. However, it may be necessary to stop therapy when severe allergic phenomena appear in conjunction with skin rash. It has not yet been determined what proportion or type of reactions result from the death of the parasites rather than from the influence of the drug.

➤*Onchocerciasis:* Facial edema and pruritus, especially of the eyes, are often encountered. Severe reactions may develop after a single dose when intense infestations are treated. In such cases, only 1 dose should be given on the first day, 2 doses the second day and 3 daily thereafter for 30 days. If very severe reactions occur, discontinue the drug and start antihistamine therapy. After 1 or 2 days, therapy may be resumed, but if severe allergic phenomena again supervene, use the drug only with extreme caution.

➤*Ascariasis:* Giddiness, nausea, vomiting and malaise may occur more frequently following treatment of ascariasis in children who are malnourished or who suffer from various debilitating diseases.

PYRANTEL

otc	**Pin-Rid** (Apothecary)	**Capsules, soft gel**: 180 mg pyrantel pamoate (equiv. to 62.5 mg pyrantel base)	In 24s.
otc	**Reese's Pinworm** (Reese)		(RC P). In 24s.
otc	**Reese's Pinworm** (Reese)	**Tablets**: 180 mg pyrantel pamoate (equiv. to 62.5 mg pyrantel base)	Capsule shaped. In 24s.
otc	**Antiminth** (Pfizer Labs)	**Oral Suspension**: 50 mg pyrantel (as pamoate) per mL	Sorbitol. Caramel-currant flavor. In 60 mL.
otc	**Reese's Pinworm** (Reese)		Glycerin, saccharin, sorbitol. Banana flavor. In 30 mL.
otc	**Pin-X** (Effcon)	**Liquid**: 50 mg pyrantel (as pamoate) per mL	Sorbitol, parabens. Caramel flavor. In 30 mL.
otc	**Reese's Pinworm** (Reese)		In 30 mL.

PYRANTEL PAMOATE — ORAL

Refer to the general discussion of these products in the Anthelmintics introduction.

Indications

➤*Helminths:* For the treatment of ascariasis (roundworm infection) and enterobiasis (pinworm infection).

➤*Unlabeled uses:* Pyrantel pamoate is also used in the treatment of hairworm.

Administration and Dosage

➤*Dosage:* 5 mg of pyrantel base per pound, or 11 mg/kg of body weight, not to exceed 1 g (16 tablets or 20 mL of suspension).

Take only according to directions and do not exceed the recommended dosage unless directed by a doctor. Medication should only be taken 1 time as a single dose. Do not repeat the treatment unless directed by a doctor. When one individual in a household has pinworms, the entire household should be treated unless otherwise advised (see Warnings). If any worms other than pinworms are present before or after treatment, consult a doctor.

Shake suspension well.

Pyrantel pamoate can be taken any time of day with or without meals. It may be taken alone or with milk or fruit juice. Use of a laxative is not necessary prior to, during, or after medication.

➤*Storage/Stability:* Store at room temperature.

Actions

➤*Pharmacology:* Pyrantel is a depolarizing neuromuscular blocking agent, resulting in spastic paralysis of the worm. It also inhibits cholinesterases. It is active against *Enterobius vermicularis* (pinworm) and *Ascaris lumbricoides* (roundworm); it is also effective against *Ancylostoma duodenale* (hookworm).

➤*Pharmacokinetics:* Pyrantel is poorly absorbed from the GI tract. Plasma levels of unchanged drug are low. Greater than 50% is excreted in feces as unchanged drug, ≤ 7% of the dose is found in the urine as parent drug and metabolites.

Contraindications

Hepatic disease; pregnancy (see Warnings); hypersensitivity to pyrantel.

Warnings

➤*Hepatic function impairment:* Patients who have hepatic disease should not take pyrantel pamoate unless directed by a physician.

➤*Pregnancy: Category C.* Patients who are pregnant should not take pyrantel pamoate unless directed by a physician.

➤*Children:* Safety and efficacy for use in children < 2 years of age have not been established.

Drug Interactions

➤*Piperazine:* In ascariasis (roundworm), pyrantel and piperazine are mutually antagonistic; therefore, concomitant use is unwise.

➤*Theophylline:* Serum levels increased in a pediatric patient following pyrantel pamoate administration. Further study is needed.

Adverse Reactions

Abdominal cramps, nausea, vomiting, diarrhea, headaches, or dizziness, sometimes occur after taking this drug. If any of these conditions persist consult a doctor.

Patient Information

As with any drug, if you are pregnant or nursing a baby, seek the advise of a health professional before using this product.

Wear tight underpants both day and night. For several days after treatment clean the bedroom floor by vacuuming or damp mopping. After treatment, wash bed linens and night clothes (don't shake them). Keep toilet seats clean.

➤*Pinworms:* Many patients who have pinworms do not have symptoms, however, many will have itching in and around the rectal opening. The itching may be very annoying and continued scratching can cause an irritation in this area. The itching may be prominent at night when sleeping. That is why restless sleep is sometimes a sign of pinworms, especially in children. Other symptoms include insomnia, GI distress, irritability, enuresis (bedwetting) and secondary infection due to localized scratching. Treat with pyrantel pamoate only after pinworms have been observed and identified.

Pinworms look like tiny white threads. The female pinworm is ≈ ½ inch long (the male pinworm is shorter); they live in the bowel. Usually, at night,

PYRANTEL PAMOATE — ORAL

the female pinworm travels to the rectal opening and lays eggs within the skin folds around the opening. This usually takes place within 1 to 2 hours after the child has been put to sleep for the night. The sticky gelatin like substance in which the eggs (they are too small to see) are deposited and the movement of the female pinworm may cause annoying itching and possibly restless sleep. By checking the rectal opening at this time, you can attempt to see the pinworm as described.

Scratching will cause pinworm eggs to stick to the fingers. Reinfection will result if the fingers are placed in the mouth. The eggs, which are too small to see, contaminate whatever they come in contact with, including bed clothes, underwear, toys, hands, and food touched by contaminated hands. Even eggs floating in the air can be swallowed and cause infection. Eggs deposited can survive for as long as 3 weeks. Pinworms are highly contagious; therefore, after treatment with pyrantel pamoate you should wash hands and fingernails with soap often during the day in order to prevent spreading to others and reinfection.

PRAZIQUANTEL

Rx	**Biltricide** (Bayer)	**Tablets:** 600 mg	(Bayer LG). White to orange-tinged, oblong, tri-scored. Film-coated. In 6s.

PRAZIQUANTEL — ORAL

Refer to the general discussion of these products in the Anthelmintics introduction.

Indications

For infections caused by the following: All species of schistosoma (eg, *Schistosoma mekongi, S. japonicum, S. mansoni,* and *S. hematobium*); liver flukes, *Clonorchis sinensis/Opisthorchis viverrini* (approval of this indication was based on studies in which the 2 species were not differentiated).

➤*Unlabeled uses:* Praziquantel has been used in the treatment of neurocysticercosis. It may also be beneficial in the treatment of other tissue flukes (eg, *Opisthorchis felineus, Paragonimus westermani,* and other species, toxemic schisto, Katayama fever), intestinal flukes (eg, *Heterophyes heterophyes, Fasciolopsis buski, Metagonimus yokogawai, Paragonimus westermani*), and intestinal cestodes (eg, *Diphyllobothrium latum, Taenia saginata* and *T. solium, Dipylidium caninum, Hymenolepis nana,* and *H. diminuta*).

Administration and Dosage

➤*Schistosomiasis:* 3 doses of 20 mg/kg as a 1 day treatment.

➤*Clonorchiasis and opisthorchiasis:* 3 doses of 25 mg/kg as a 1 day treatment.

The interval between the doses should not be < 4 and not > 6 hours.

Swallow the tablets unchewed with some liquid during meals. Keeping the tablets or the segments thereof in the mouth may reveal a bitter taste that can produce gagging or vomiting.

Segments are broken off by pressing the score (notch) with thumbnails. If ¼ of a tablet is required, this is best achieved by breaking the segment from the outer end.

Actions

➤*Pharmacology:* Praziquantel increases cell membrane permeability in susceptible worms, resulting in a loss of intracellular calcium, massive contractions, and paralysis of their musculature. The drug further results in vacuolization and disintegration of the schistosome tegument. This effect is followed by attachment of phagocytes to the parasite and death.

➤*Pharmacokinetics:* Praziquantel is rapidly absorbed (80%), reaching maximal serum concentration in 1 to 3 hours. CSF levels are ≈ 14% to 20% the total amount of drug in plasma. It undergoes significant first-pass biotransformation and the elimination half-life is 0.8 to 1.5 hours. Metabolites are excreted primarily in urine.

Contraindications

Previous hypersensitivity to praziquantel; ocular cysticercosis.

Warnings

➤*Ocular cysticercosis:* Because parasite destruction within the eyes may cause irreparable lesions, do not treat ocular cysticercosis with praziquantel.

➤*Pregnancy: Category B.* An increase in the abortion rate was found in rats at 3 times the single human therapeutic dose. There are no adequate and well-controlled studies in pregnant women. Use this drug during pregnancy only if clearly needed.

➤*Lactation:* Praziquantel appeared in breast milk at a concentration of ≈ 25% that of maternal serum. Do not nurse during treatment or the subsequent 72 hours.

➤*Children:* Safety in children < 4 years of age has not been established.

Precautions

➤*Hepatic effects:* Minimal increases in liver enzymes have occurred in some patients.

➤*Cerebral cysticercosis:* When schistosomiasis or fluke infection is found to be associated with cerebral cysticercosis, hospitalize the patient for the duration of treatment.

➤*Hazardous tasks:* May produce dizziness or drowsiness; observe caution while driving or performing other tasks requiring alertness on the day of and the day after treatment.

Drug Interactions

➤*H_2 antagonists:* Plasma concentrations of praziquantel may be elevated, increasing the effectiveness and risk of adverse reactions.

Adverse Reactions

In general, praziquantel is very well tolerated. Side effects are usually mild and transient and do not need treatment but may be more frequent or serious in patients with a heavy worm burden.

In order of severity: Malaise; headache; dizziness; abdominal discomfort (with or without nausea); rising temperature; urticaria (rare). Such symptoms can, however, also result from the infection itself. In patients with liver impairment caused by the infection, no adverse effects occurred that necessitated restriction in use.

Overdosage

➤*Treatment:* In the event of overdose, institute symptomatic treatment.

Patient Information

Take with liquids during meals. Do not chew tablets.

May cause dizziness or drowsiness; observe caution while driving or performing other tasks requiring alertness.

IVERMECTIN

Rx	**Stromectol** (Merck)	**Tablets:** 3 mg	(MSD 32) White. In UD 20s.
		6 mg	(MSD 139). White, scored. In UD 10s.

IVERMECTIN — ORAL

Indications

➤*Strongyloidiasis of the intestinal tract:* For the treatment of intestinal (ie, nondisseminated) strongyloidiasis due to the nematode parasite *Strongyloides stercoralis.*

➤*Onchocerciasis:* For the treatment of onchocerciasis due to the nematode parasite *Onchocerca volvulus.*

Ivermectin has no activity against adult *Onchocerca volvulus* parasites. The adult parasites reside in SC nodules which are infrequently palpable. Surgical excision of these nodules (nodulectomy) may be considered in the management of patients with onchocerciasis, since this procedure will eliminate the microfilariae-producing adult parasites.

➤*Unlabeled uses:* Treatment and prophylaxis of infections with Loa loa and *Wucheria bancrofti,* scabies, and human cutaneous larva migrans.

Used orally and topically in the treatment of head lice (*Pediculosis capitis*).

Administration and Dosage

➤*Approved by the FDA:* November 1996.

➤*Strongyloidiasis:* The recommended dosage is a single oral dose designed to provide approximately 200 mcg of ivermectin/kg of body weight. Patients should take tablets with water. In general, additional doses are not necessary. However, follow-up stool examinations should be performed to verify eradication of infection.

Dosage guidelines for ivermectin for strongyloidiasis

Body weight (kg)	Single oral dose: Number of 3 mg tablets	Number of 6 mg tablets
15 to 24	1 tablet	one-half tablet
25 to 35	2 tablets	1 tablet
36 to 50	3 tablets	1 and one-half tablets
51 to 65	4 tablets	2 tablets
66 to 79	5 tablets	2 and one-half tablets
≥ 80	200 mcg/kg	200 mcg/kg

➤*Onchocerciasis:* The recommended dosage is a single oral dose designed to provide approximately 150 mcg of ivermectin/kg of body weight. See the table below for dosage guidelines. Patients should take tablets with water. In mass-distribution campaigns in international treatment programs, the

IVERMECTIN — ORAL

most commonly used dose interval is 12 months. For the treatment of individual patients, retreatment may be considered at intervals as short as 3 months.

Dosage guidelines for ivermectin for onchocerciasis		
	Single oral dose	
Body weight (kg)	Number of 3 mg tablets	Number of 6 mg tablets
15 to 25	1 tablet	one-half tablet
26 to 44	2 tablets	1 tablet
45 to 64	3 tablets	1 and one-half tablets
65 to 84	4 tablets	2 tablets
≥ 85	150 mcg/kg	150 mcg/kg

➤*Storage/Stability:* Store at temperatures < 30°C (86°F).

Actions

➤*Pharmacology:* Ivermectin is a member of the avermectin class of broad-spectrum antiparasitic agents which have a unique mode of action. Compounds of the class bind selectively and with high affinity to glutamate-gated chloride ion channels which occur in invertebrate nerve and muscle cells. This leads to an increase in the permeability of the cell membrane to chloride ions with hyperpolarization of the nerve or muscle cell, resulting in paralysis and death of the parasite. Compounds of this class may also interact with other ligand-gated chloride channels, such as those gated by the neurotransmitter gamma-aminobutyric acid (GABA).

The selective activity of compounds of this class is attributable to the facts that some mammals do not have glutamate-gated chloride channels and that the avermectins have a low affinity for mammalian ligand-gated chloride channels. In addition, ivermectin does not readily cross the blood-brain barrier in humans.

Ivermectin is active against various life-cycle stages of many but not all nematodes. It is active against the tissue microfilariae of *Onchocerca volvulus* but not against the adult form. Its activity against *Strongyloides stercoralis* is limited to the intestinal stages.

➤*Pharmacokinetics:*

Absorption/Distribution – Following oral administration of ivermectin, plasma concentrations are approximately proportional to the dose. In 2 studies, after single 12 mg doses of ivermectin (2 times 6 mg) in fasting healthy volunteers (representing a mean dose of 165 mcg/kg), the mean peak plasma concentrations of the major component (H_2B_{1a}) were 46.6 (± 21.9 [range 16.4 to 101.1]) and 30.6 (± 15.6 [range 13.9 to 68.4]) ng/mL respectively at ≈ 4 hours after dosing.

Metabolism/Excretion – Ivermectin is metabolized in the liver, and ivermectin or its metabolites are excreted almost exclusively in the feces over an estimated 12 days, with < 1% of the administered dose excreted in the urine. The apparent plasma half-life of ivermectin is approximately at least 16 hours following oral administration.

Contraindications

Hypersensitivity to any component of this product.

Warnings

➤*Mazzotti reaction:* Historical data have shown that microfilaricidal drugs, such as diethylcarbamazine citrate (DEC-C), might cause cutaneous or systemic reactions of varying severity (the Mazzotti reaction) and ophthalmological reactions in patients with onchocerciasis. These reactions are probably due to allergic and inflammatory responses to the death of microfilariae. Patients treated with ivermectin for onchocerciasis may experience these reactions in addition to clinical adverse reactions possibly, probably, or definitely related to the drug itself (see Adverse Reactions).

The treatment of severe Mazzotti reactions has not been subjected to controlled clinical trials. Oral hydration, recumbency, IV normal saline, or parenteral corticosteroids have been used to treat postural hypotension. Antihistamines or aspirin have been used for most mild-to-moderate cases.

➤*Pregnancy: Category C.*

Ivermectin has been shown to be teratogenic in mice, rats, and rabbits when given in repeated doses of 0.2, 8.1, and 4.5 times the maximum recommended human dose, respectively (on a mg/m²/day basis). Teratogenicity was characterized in the 3 species tested by cleft palate; clubbed forepaws were additionally observed in rabbits. These development effects were found only at or near doses that were maternotoxic to the pregnant female. Therefore, ivermectin does not appear to be selectively fetotoxic to the developing fetus. There are, however, no adequate and well-controlled studies in pregnant women. Ivermectin should not be used during pregnancy since safety in pregnancy has not been established.

➤*Lactation:* Ivermectin is excreted in human milk in low concentrations. Treatment of mothers who intend to breastfeed should only be undertaken when the risk of delayed treatment to the mother outweighs the possible risk to the newborn.

➤*Children:* Safety and effectiveness in pediatric patients weighing < 15 kg have not been established.

Precautions

➤*Hyperreactive onchodermatitis:* After treatment with microfilaricidal drugs, patients with hyperreactive onchodermatitis (sowda) may be more likely than others to experience severe adverse reactions, especially edema and aggravation of onchodermatitis.

➤*Strongyloidiasis in immunocompromised hosts:* In immunocompromised (including HIV-infected) patients being treated for intestinal strongyloidiasis, repeated courses of therapy may be required. Adequate and well-controlled clinical studies have not been conducted in such patients to determine the optimal dosing regimen. Several treatments (ie, at 2-week intervals) may be required, and cure may not be achievable. Control of extraintestinal strongyloidiasis in these patients is difficult, and suppressive therapy (ie, once per month) may be helpful.

Adverse Reactions

➤*Strongyloidiasis:*

CNS – Dizziness (2.8%); somnolence (0.9%); vertigo (0.9%); tremor (0.9%).

Dermatologic – Pruritus (2.8%); rash (0.9%); urticaria (0.9%).

GI – Anorexia (0.9%); constipation (0.9%); diarrhea (1.8%); nausea (1.8%); vomiting (0.9%).

Lab test abnormalities – In clinical trials involving 109 patients given either 1 or 2 doses of 170 to 200 mcg/kg ivermectin, the following laboratory abnormalities were seen irrespective of drug relationship: Elevation in ALT or AST (2%), and decrease in leukocyte count (3%). Leukopenia and anemia were seen in 1 patient.

Miscellaneous – Asthenia/fatigue (0.9%) and abdominal pain (0.9%).

➤*Onchocerciasis:* In clinical trials involving 963 adult patients treated with 100 to 200 mcg/kg ivermectin, worsening of the following Mazzotti reactions during the first 4 days posttreatment were reported: Arthralgia/synovitis (9.3%); axillary lymph node enlargement and tenderness (11% and 4.4%, respectively); cervical lymph node enlargement and tenderness (5.3% and 1.2%, respectively); inguinal lymph node enlargement and tenderness (12.6% and 13.9%, respectively); other lymph node enlargement and tenderness (3% and 1.9%, respectively); pruritus (27.5%); skin involvement including edema, papular and pustular or frank urticarial rash (22.7%), and fever (22.6%) (see Warnings).

Ophthalmic – In clinical trials, ophthalmological conditions were examined in 963 adult patients before treatment, at day 3, and months 3 and 6 after treatment with 100 to 200 mcg/kg ivermectin. Changes observed were primarily deterioration from baseline 3 days posttreatment. Most changes either returned to baseline condition or improved over baseline severity at the month 3 and 6 visits. The percentages of patients with worsening of the following conditions at day 3, month 3, and 6, respectively, were as follows: Limbitis, 5.5%, 4.8%, and 3.5%, and punctate opacity, 1.8%, 1.8%, and 1.4%. The corresponding percentages for patients treated with placebo were as follows: Limbitis, 6.2%, 9.9%, and 9.4%, and punctate opacity, 2%, 6.4%, and 7.2% (see Warnings).

The following ophthalmological side effects do occur due to the disease itself but have also been reported after treatment with ivermectin: Abnormal sensation in the eyes, eyelid edema, anterior uveitis, conjunctivitis, limbitis, keratitis, and chorioretinitis or choroiditis. These have rarely been severe or associated with loss of vision and have generally resolved without corticosteroid treatment.

In clinical trials involving 963 adult patients who received 100 to 200 mcg/kg ivermectin, the following clinical adverse reactions were reported as possibly, probably, or definitely related to the drug in ≥ 1% of the patients: Facial edema (1.2%), peripheral edema (3.2%), orthostatic hypotension (1.1%), and tachycardia (3.5%).

Drug-related headache and myalgia occurred in < 1% of patients (0.2% and 0.4%, respectively). However, these were the most common adverse experiences reported overall during these trials regardless of causality (22.3% and 19.7%, respectively).

A similar safety profile was observed in an open study in pediatric patients ages 6 to 13.

Additionally, hypotension (mainly orthostatic hypotension) and worsening of bronchial asthma have been reported since the drug was registered overseas.

Lab test abnormalities – In controlled clinical trials, the following laboratory adverse experiences were reported as possibly, probably, or definitely related to the drug in ≥ 1% of the patients: Eosinophilia (3%) and hemoglobin increase (1%).

Overdosage

➤*Symptoms:* In accidental intoxication with or significant exposure to unknown quantities of veterinary formulations of ivermectin in humans, either by ingestion, inhalation, injection, or exposure to body surfaces, the following adverse effects have been reported most frequently: Rash, edema, headache, dizziness, asthenia, nausea, vomiting, and diarrhea. Other adverse effects that have been reported include seizure, ataxia, dyspnea, abdominal pain, paresthesia, and urticaria.

➤*Treatment:* In case of accidental poisoning, supportive therapy, if indicated, should include parenteral fluids and electrolytes, respiratory support (oxygen and mechanical ventilation if necessary) and pressor agents if clinically significant hypotension is present. Induction of emesis or gastric lavage as soon as possible, followed by purgatives and other routine antipoison measures, may be indicated if needed to prevent absorption of ingested material.

Patient Information

Ivermectin should be taken with water.

➤*Strongyloidiasis:* The patient should be reminded of the need for repeated stool examinations to document clearance of infection with *Strongyloides stercoralis*.

➤*Onchocerciasis:* The patient should be reminded that treatment with ivermectin does not kill the adult *Onchocerca* parasites, and therefore repeated follow-up and retreatment is usually required.

CDC ANTI-INFECTIVE AGENTS

In addition to the commercially available anti-infective agents, the Centers for Disease Control and Prevention (CDC) can supply several investigational agents upon request. These agents may be requested from the Drug Service, Division of Host Factors, Center for Infectious Disease, by calling 404-639-3670, 8:00 am to 4:30 pm EST Monday through Friday; for emergencies (evenings, weekends, or holidays), call 404-639-2888.

Indications

Available CDC Anti-Infective Agents

Generic name	Trade name	Disease/Infestation	Organism
Bithionol	*Lorothidol* *Bitin*	Paragonimiasis Fascioliasis	*Paragonimus* sp. *Fasciola hepatica*
Dehydroemetine	*Mebadin*	Extraintestinal amebiasis that fails to respond to metronidazole Amebic dysentery	*Entamoeba histolytica*
Diethylcarbamazine citrate (DEC)	*Hetrazan*	Lymphatic filariasis Tropical pulmonary eosinophilia Loiasis	*Wuchereria bancrofti* *Brugia malayi* *Brugia timori*
Melarsoprol	*Arsobal* *Mel B*	Trypanosomiasis (African sleeping sickness) with neurologic involvement and for the treatment of early African (Gambian and Rhodesian) sleeping sickness that is resistant to treatment with suramin or pentamidine	*Trypanosoma brucei gambiense* *Trypanosoma brucei rhodesiense*
Nifurtimox	*Lampit* *Bayer 2502*	Chagas' disease	*Trypanosoma cruzi*
Sodium antimony gluconate (sodium stibogluconate)	*Pentostam*	Leishmaniasis (visceral [kala azar], cutaneous [Oriental sore], or mucosal)	*Leishmania* sp.
Suramin	*Fourneau 309* *Bayer 205* *Germanin* *Moranyl* *Belganyl* *Naphuride* *Antrypol*	Trypanosomiasis (African sleeping sickness) Onchocerciasis (river blindness)	*Trypanosoma brucei rhodesiense* *Trypanosoma brucei gambiense* (second-line therapy to pentamidine) *Onchocerca volvulus*

The following general information applies to all immune sera. For specific information on individual agents, refer to specific monographs:

- Cytomegalovirus Immune Globulin, IV (CMV-IGIV)
- Hepatitis B Immune Globulin (HBIG)
- Immune Globulin, IM (IGIM)
- Immune Globulin, IV (IGIV)
- Lymphocyte Immune Globulin, Antithymocyte Globulin (Equine) (ATG equine)
- Antithymocyte Globulin (Rabbit) (ATG rabbit)
- Rabies Immune Globulin (RIG)
- Rh_o(D) Immune Globulin, IM (Rh_o[D] IGIM)
- Rh_o(D) Immune Globulin, IV (Rh_o[D] IGIV)
- Rh_o(D) Immune Globulin Micro-dose (Rh_o[D] IG Micro-dose)
- Respiratory Syncytial Virus Immune Globulin, IV (RSV-IGIV)
- Tetanus Immune Globulin (TIG)
- Varicella-Zoster Immune Globulin (VZIG)

WARNING

Immune globulin IV (human) – **IGIV** (human) products have been associated with renal dysfunction, acute renal failure, osmotic nephrosis, and death. Patients predisposed to acute renal failure include patients with any degree of pre-existing renal insufficiency, diabetes mellitus, > 65 years of age, volume depletion, sepsis, paraproteinemia, or patients receiving known nephrotoxic drugs. Especially in such patients, administer IGIV products at the minimum concentration available and the minimum rate of infusion practicable. While these reports of renal dysfunction and acute renal failure have been associated with the use of many of the licensed IGIV products, those containing sucrose as a stabilizer accounted for a disproportionate share of the total number. See Precautions and Administration and Dosage sections for important information intended to reduce the risk of acute renal failure. (*Polygam S/D*, *Gammagard S/D*, *Gamimune N*, *Venoglobulin-S*, and *Iveegam* do not contain sucrose.)

Antithymocyte globulin (equine) – Only physicians experienced in immunosuppressive therapy in the treatment of renal transplant or aplastic anemia patients should use **antithymocyte globulin** (equine).

Treat patients receiving antithymocyte globulin (equine) in facilities equipped and staffed with adequate laboratory and supportive medical resources.

Antithymocyte globulin (rabbit) – **Antithymocyte globulin** (rabbit) should only be used by physicians experienced in immunosuppressive therapy for the management of renal transplant patients.

Indications

To provide passive immunization to ≥ 1 infectious diseases. Protection derived will be of rapid onset, but of short duration (1 to 3 months). See individual monographs for specific indications.

Actions

➤*Pharmacology:*

CMV-IGIV – This product contains IgG antibodies representative of the large number of healthy people who contributed to the plasma pools from which the product was derived. The globulin contains a relatively high concentration of antibodies directed against CMV. In people who may be exposed to CMV, this product can raise the relevant antibodies to levels sufficient to attenuate or reduce the incidence of serious CMV disease.

HBIG – HBIG provides passive immunization for individuals exposed to the hepatitis B virus (HBV). The administration of the usual recommended dose of this immune globulin generally results in a detectable level of circulating anti-HBs, which persists for ≈ 2 months or longer.

IGIM – IGIM is a transient source of IgG that specifically and nonspecifically inactivates various bacteria, viruses, and fungi. IgG antibodies activate the complement system, promote opsonization, neutralize microorganisms and their toxins, and participate in antibody-dependent cytolytic reactions.

Hepatitis A: IGIM is 80% to 95% effective in preventing hepatitis A, depending on the temporal relation between administration and exposure and on the severity of exposure.

Measles: IGIM reduces the risk of clinical evidence of measles by an estimated 50%. A lower incidence of measles encephalitis also has been associated with the use of IGIM.

Varicella: IGIM reduces severity of disease, as measured by temperature and the number of pox.

IGIV – IGIV passively supplies a broad spectrum of IgG antibodies against bacterial, viral, parasitic, and mycoplasmic antigens. IGIV antibodies act through a variety of mechanisms, including antimicrobial or antitoxin neutralization. IGIV appears to work by contributing anti-idiotypic antibodies that bind and neutralize pathogenic autoantibodies. There may also be negative feedback and down-regulation of antibody production. Other mechanisms may involve binding to CD5 receptors, interleukin-1a, IL-6, tumor necrosis factor-alpha, and T-cell receptors, suppressing pathogenic cytokines and phagocytes. IGIV also interferes with pathogenic effects of products of complement activation.

ATG equine – ATG equine is a lymphocyte-selective immunosuppressant. It reduces the number of circulating, thymus-dependent lymphocytes that form rosettes with sheep erythrocytes. This antilymphocytic effect is believed to reflect an alteration of the function of the T-lymphocytes, which are responsible, in part, for cell-mediated immunity and are involved in humoral immunity. It also contains low concentrations of antibodies against other formed elements of the blood. In rhesus and cynomolgus monkeys, this drug reduces lymphocytes in the thymus-dependent areas of the spleen and lymph nodes. It also decreases the circulating sheep-erythrocyte-rosetting lymphocytes that can be detected, but ordinarily does not cause severe lymphopenia.

In general, when administered with other immunosuppressive therapy, such as antimetabolites and corticosteroids, the patient's own antibody response to horse gamma globulin is minimal.

Precise methods of determining potency have not been established; thus activity may potentially vary from lot to lot.

In general, ATG equine enables a 1 year graft survival rate of ≥ 80%. Graft and patient survival are dependent on whether the transplanted organ is harvested from a living or deceased host, the degree of antigenic matching, the combination of immunosuppressive drugs delivered, and other factors.

ATG rabbit – The mechanism of action by which polyclonal antilymphocyte preparations suppress immune responses is not fully understood. Possible mechanisms by which ATG rabbit may induce immunosuppression in vivo include: T-cell clearance from the circulation and modulation of T-cell activation, homing, and cytotoxic activities. ATG rabbit includes antibodies against T-cell markers such as CD2, CD3, CD4, CD8, CD11a, CD18, CD25, CD44, CD45, HLA-DR, HLA Class 1 heavy chains, and β2 microglobulin. In vitro, ATG rabbit (concentrations > 0.1 mg/mL) mediates T-cell suppressive effects via inhibition of proliferative responses to several mitogens. In patients, T-cell depletion is usually observed within a day from initiating ATG rabbit therapy. ATG rabbit has not been shown to be effective for treating antibody (humoral) mediated rejections.

RIG – Rabies antibody provides passive protection when given immediately to individuals exposed to rabies virus. RIG of adequate potency was used in conjunction with rabies vaccine of duck embryo origin. When a globulin dose of 20 IU/kg of rabies antibody was given simultaneously with the first dose of vaccine, levels of passive rabies antibody were detected 24 hours after injection in all individuals. There was minimal or no interference with the immune response to the initial and subsequent doses of vaccine, including booster doses. Studies of RIG given with the first of 5 doses of HDCV confirmed that passive immunization with 20 IU/kg of RIG provides maximum circulating antibody with minimum interference of active immunization by HDCV.

Rh_o(D) IGIM – Rh_o(D) IGIM acts by suppressing the immune response of Rh_o(D)-negative individuals to Rh_o(D)-positive red blood cells. The mechanism of action of the full dose is not fully understood.

Passive immunization with Rh_o(D) prevents the formation of anti-Rh_o(D) antibodies in nonsensitized Rh_o(D) antigen-negative individuals who receive Rh_o(D) antigen-positive red blood cells. Rh_o(D) antibody binds circulating antigen, thus preventing stimulation of antigen-sensitive lymphocytes and the resulting production of anti-Rh_o(D). Prevention of Rh_o(D) sensitization in turn prevents hemolytic disease of the fetus and newborn in subsequent Rh_o(D) antigen-positive children.

Rh_o(D) IGIV –

Suppression of Rh isoimmunization: Rh_o(D) IGIV is used to suppress the immune response of nonsensitized Rh_o(D)-negative individuals following Rh_o(D)-positive red blood cell exposure by fetomaternal hemorrhage during delivery of an Rh_o(D)-positive infant, abortion (spontaneous or induced), amniocentesis, abdominal trauma, or mismatched transfusion. The mechanism of action is not completely understood.

Idiopathic thrombocytopenic purpura (ITP): The mechanism of action is not completely understood, but is thought to be due to the formation of anti-Rh_o(D) (anti-D)-coated RBC complexes resulting in Fc receptor blockade, thus sparing antibody-coated platelets.

Rh_o(D) IG micro-dose – Rh_o(D) IG micro-dose is used to prevent the formation of anti-Rh_o(D) antibody in Rh_o(D)-negative women who are exposed to the Rh_o(D) antigen at the time of spontaneous or induced abortion (up to 12 weeks gestation). Rh_o(D) IG micro-dose suppresses the stimulation of active immunity by Rh_o(D)-positive fetal erythrocytes that may enter the maternal circulation at the time of termination of the pregnancy.

The amount of anti-Rh_o(D) in Rh_o(D) IG micro-dose has been shown to effectively prevent material isosensitization to the Rh_o(D) antigens following spontaneous or induced abortion occurring up to the 12th week of gestation. After the 12th week of gestation, a standard dose of Rh_o(D) IGIM full dose is indicated.

Rh_o(D) IG micro-dose acts by suppressing the immune response of Rh-negative individuals to Rh-positive red blood cells. The risk of immunization is related to the number of D-positive red blood cells received. The risk was found to be 3% when 0.1 mL of fetal red blood cells is present in the mother and 65% when 5 mL is present. In the first 12 weeks of gestation, the total volume of red blood cells in the fetus is estimated at < 2.5 mL.

RSV-IGIV – RSV-IGIV is a sterile liquid immunoglobulin G (IgG) containing neutralizing antibody to respiratory syncytial virus (RSV). The immunoglobulin is purified from pooled adult human plasma selected for high titers of neutralizing antibody against RSV. A widely utilized solvent-detergent viral inactivation process is used to decrease the possibility of transmission of bloodborne pathogens. Each milliliter contains 50 ± 10 mg immunoglobulin, primarily IgG, and trace amounts of IgA and IgM.

TIG – TIG is an antibody preparation containing antitoxin that neutralizes the free form of the powerful tetanus exotoxin. TIG does not affect toxin fixed to nerve tissue.

VZIG – VZIG is the globulin fraction of human plasma, primarily immunoglobulin G (IgG) found in routine screening of normal volunteer blood donors. When absorbed into the circulation, the antibodies persist for ≥ 1 month. The precise concentration of varicella-zoster antibodies that must be achieved or maintained in order to attenuate varicella is not known. In the clinical studies demonstrating its efficacy, VZIG was given within 96 hours of chickenpox exposure. It significantly reduces mortality and morbidity from varicella among immunodeficient children.

➤*Pharmacokinetics:* Immunoglobulins are primarily eliminated by catabolism.

CMV-IGIV – The onset of action is rapid. The mean half-life is 21 days, shorter in transplant recipients, where half-lives have been measured as 8 days immediately after transplant, or 13 to 15 days if given ≥ 60 days after transplant. The protective level is unknown.

HBIG – Antibodies appear within 1 to 6 days after IM administration and peak in 3 to 11 days. The mean half-life is 17 to 25 days (range, 6 to 35) and clinical protection typically persists for ≈ 2 months. The protective level of anti-HBs titer is ≥ 10 mIU/mL. The clearance rate was 0.433 ± 0.144 L/day, with a volume of distribution of 15.3 ± 6.2 L.

IGIM – IgG titers peak 2 to 5 days after IM injection. Mean IgG half-life in circulation of people with normal IgG levels is 23 days. Protective levels are 200 mg/100 mL of plasma as a target in immunoglobulin replacement therapy.

IGIV – The onset is rapid. In general, the mean half-life in healthy people is 18 to 25 days, although there is tremendous intersubject variability. Fever or infection may decrease antibody half-life because of increased catabolism or consumption, respectively. In idiopathic thrombocytopenic purpura (ITP), the increase in platelets usually lasts from several days to several weeks, although it may rarely persist for ≥ 1 year. In a group of burn patients, the half-life ranged from 47 to 154 days.

IV administration makes essentially 100% of the dose immediately available in the recipient's circulation. After ≈ 6 days, ≈ 50% of the body pool partitions into the extravascular space, with the balance remaining in the serum.

Expect a rapid fall in serum IgG in the first week after infusion, mainly because of equilibration of IgG between plasma and the extravascular space. The decrease averages 40% of peak level after infusion; within 24 hours, 30% of a single dose is removed from circulation to extravascular fluid, tissue, cells, and catabolism.

ATG equine – Onset is rapid. Peak plasma level of equine IgG occurs after 5 days of infusion at 10 mg/kg/day. Peak values vary depending on recipient's ability to catabolize equine IgG. In a small study, mean peak plasma value was 727 ± 310 mcg/mL. Rosette-forming cells decrease immediately after beginning therapy. Recovery to normal values after therapy cessation is dependent on recipient's catabolic rate and, in some cases, upon length of therapy. Mean half-life is ≈ 5.7 days (range, 2.7 to 8.7 days).

ATG rabbit – After an IV dose of 1.25 to 1.5 mg/kg/day (over 4 hours for 7 to 11 days) 4 to 8 hours post-infusion, ATG rabbit levels were on average 21.5 mcg/mL (10 to 40 mcg/mL) with a half-life of 2 to 3 days after the first dose, and 87 mcg/mL (23 to 170 mcg/mL) after the last dose.

RIG – Adequate levels of antibody appear in serum within 24 hours and peak within 2 to 13 days. Because rabies vaccine takes ≈ 1 week to induce active immunity, the importance of RIG cannot be overemphasized. The mean serum half-life of rabies antibody is 24 days, consistent with the 21-day half-life expected of IgG.

TIG – The efficacy is high, with a rapid onset of action and peak serum titer occurring within 2 to 3 days after IM injection. The mean half-life is 3.5 to 4.5 weeks and adequate antibody titer persists for ≈ 4 weeks. The protective level is 0.01 antitoxin units/mL; 250 units yield at least 0.01 IU/mL of tetanus antitoxin in serum for 4 weeks, an adequate response.

Rh_o(D) IGIM (human) – The onset of action is prompt. The mean half-life is 23 to 26 days, with antibody titers ≥ 1:5 by RFFIT indicative of adequate protection.

Rh_o(D) immune globulin, when administered within 72 hours of a full-term delivery of an Rh_o(D)-positive infant by an Rh_o(D)-negative mother, will reduce the incidence of Rh isoimmunization from between 12% and 13% to between 1% and 2%. The 1% to 2% range is due, for the most part, to isoimmunization during the last trimester of pregnancy. When treatment is given both antenatally at 28 weeks gestation and postpartum, the Rh immunization rate drops to ≈ 0.1%.

When 600 IU (120 mcg) of Rh_o(D) IGIV is given to pregnant women, passive anti-Rh_o(D) antibodies are not detectable in the circulation for > 6 weeks; therefore, give a dose of 1500 IU (300 mcg) for antenatal administration.

IM vs IV administration: In a clinical study involving Rh_o(D)-negative volunteers, 2 subjects were given 600 IU (120 mcg) IM and 2 subjects were given this dose IV. Peak levels (36 to 48 ng/mL) were reached within 2 hours of IV administration; for IM, peak levels (18 to 19 ng/mL) were reached at 5 to 10 days. The calculated areas under the curve were the same for both routes of administration. The half-life was ≈ 24 and 30 days following IV and IM administration, respectively.

Rh_o(D) IG micro-dose – Administration of Rh_o(D) IG micro-dose within 3 hours following abortion was 100% effective in preventing Rh immunization. Studies showed Rh_o(D) IG micro-dose to be effective when given as long as 72 hours after the infusion of Rh-positive red cells. A lesser degree of protection is afforded if the antibody is administered beyond this time period.

RSV-IGIV – The onset of action is rapid with the mean half-life of serum RSV neutralizing antibodies after RSV-IG infusion as 22 to 28 days. The protective level is not established. In one study, monthly doses of 750 mg/kg of RSV-IG attained trough geometric mean serum RSV neutralization antibody titers of 1:297 ± 38 (SE) 1 month after the first infusion, 1:477 ± 85 1 month after the second infusion, 1:490 ± 61 1 month after the third infusion, and 1:429 ± 23 1 month after the fourth infusion.

VZIG – Onset of action is prompt, but the duration of protection is unknown. The mean half-life is 21 days. The concentration of varicella-zoster antibodies that must be achieved or maintained in order to attenuate varicella is unknown.

Contraindications

History of systemic allergic reactions following administration of human immunoglobulin preparations.

Allergic response to gamma globulin or anti-immunoglobulin A (IgA) antibodies.

Allergic response to thimerosal.

People with isolated immunoglobulin A (IgA) deficiency. Such people have the potential for developing antibodies to IgA and could have anaphylactic reactions to subsequent administration of blood products that contain IgA.

➤*IGIM:* Patients who have severe thrombocytopenia or any coagulation disorder that would contraindicate IM use.

➤*ATG equine:* Severe prior systemic reaction with the administration of antithymocyte globulin (equine) or other equine immunoglobulin preparations.

➤*ATG rabbit:* In patients with a history of allergy or anaphylaxis to rabbit proteins, or who have an acute viral illness.

➤*RIG (Imogam):* Rabies immune globulin should not be administered in repeated doses once vaccine treatment has been initiated. Repeating the dose may interfere with maximum active immunity expected from the vaccine.

➤*Rh_o(D) IGIV:* Anaphylactic or severe systemic reaction to any human globulin. Rh_o(D) immune globulin contains trace amounts of IgA (≈ 5 mcg per 600 IU [120 mcg] vial). Individuals who are deficient in IgA may have the potential for developing IgA antibodies and have anaphylactic reactions. Weigh the potential benefit of treatment with Rh_o(D) immune globulin against the potential for hypersensitivity reactions.

➤*Rh_o(D) IG micro-dose (MICRhoGAM):* Must not be used for any indication with continuation of pregnancy; not recommended for any indication beyond 12 weeks gestation.

Warnings

➤*Renal risks:* IGIV (Human) products have been reported to be associated with renal dysfunction, acute renal failure, osmotic nephrosis, and death. Patients predisposed to acute renal failure include patients with any degree of pre-existing renal insufficiency, diabetes mellitus, > 65 years of age, volume depletion, sepsis, paraproteinemia, or patients receiving known nephrotoxic drugs. Especially in such patients, IGIV products should be administered at the minimum concentrations available and at the minimum rate of infusion practical. While these reports of renal dysfunction and acute renal failure have been associated with the use of many IGIV products, those containing sucrose as a stabilizer (and given at daily doses of ≥ 400 mg/kg) account for a disproportionate share of the total number. See Precautions and Administration and Dosage sections for important information intended to reduce the risk of acute renal failure.

➤*Bloodborne viral transmission:* Most of these products are made from human plasma and like other plasma products, they carry the possibility for transmission of bloodborne pathogenic agents. The risk of transmission of recognized bloodborne viruses is considered to be low because of the screening of plasma donors, and the collection and testing of plasma, through the application of viral elimination/reduction step such as alcohol fractionation, PEG/Bentonite precipitation and solvent-detergent treatment. Despite these measures, such products can still potentially transmit disease; therefore, the risk of infectious agents cannot be totally eliminated. Report all infections thought by the physician to have been possibly transmitted by these products to the manufacturer. Weigh the risks and benefits of the use of this product and discuss these with the patient.

➤*Route of administration:* Administer these agents only as indicated (eg, IM or IV). Inappropriate IV injections may cause a precipitous fall in blood pressure and a picture similar to anaphylaxis (ie, RIG). Administer IM.

➤*Rate of administration:* Except for hypersensitivity reactions, adverse reactions to IGIVs may be related to the rate of administration. Careful adherence to the infusion rate outlined under Administration and Dosage is therefore important. Have loop diuretics available for the management of patients who are at risk for fluid overload. Although systemic allergic reactions are rare (see Adverse Reactions), have epinephrine and diphenhydramine available for treatment of acute allergic symptoms.

➤*Immunoglobulin A deficiency:* People with isolated immunoglobulin A (IgA) deficiency have the potential for developing antibodies to IgA and could have anaphylactic reactions to subsequent administration of blood products that contain IgA.

➤*Aseptic meningitis syndrome (AMS):* Rare occurrences of AMS have been reported in association with IGIV treatment. AMS usually begins within several hours to 2 days following IGIV treatment and is characterized by symptoms including severe headache, drowsiness, fever, photophobia, painful eye movements, muscle rigidity, nausea, and vomiting. Cerebrospinal fluid studies generally demonstrate pleocytosis, predominately granulocytic, and elevated protein levels. Thoroughly evaluate patients exhibiting such signs and symptoms to rule out other causes of meningitis. AMS may occur more frequently in association with high-dose (2 g/kg) IGIV treatment. Discontinuation of IGIV treatment has resulted in remission of AMS within several days without sequelae.

➤*Bleeding complications:* As will all preparations administered by the IM route, bleeding complications may be encountered in patients with thrombocytopenia or other bleeding disorders.

➤*ATG equine:* Only physicians experienced in immunosuppressive therapy in the treatment of renal transplant or aplastic anemia patients should use lymphocyte immune globulin. Treat patients receiving lymphocyte immune globulin in facilities equipped and staffed with adequate laboratory and supportive medical resources.

Discontinuation – Discontinue treatment if any of the following occurs: Anaphylaxis; severe and unremitting thrombocytopenia and severe and unremitting leukopenia in renal transplant patients.

Hemolysis: Clinically significant hemolysis is rare. Treatment may include transfusion of erythrocytes; if necessary, administer IV mannitol, furosemide, sodium bicarbonate, and fluids. Severe and unremitting hemolysis may require discontinuation of therapy.

Thrombocytopenia: Thrombocytopenia is usually transient; platelet counts generally return to adequate levels without discontinuing therapy; platelet transfusions may be necessary in patients with aplastic anemia.

➤*ATG rabbit:* ATG rabbit should only be used by physicians experienced in immunosuppressive therapy for the treatment of renal transplant patients. Medical surveillance is required during ATG rabbit infusion.

Hematologic effects – Thrombocytopenia or neutropenia may result from cross-reactive antibodies and is reversible following dose adjustments.

➤*Criteria for $Rh_o(D)$ IGIV administration:* The criteria for an Rh-incompatible pregnancy requiring administration of $Rh_o(D)$ immune globulin at 28 weeks gestation and within 72 hours after delivery are the following: The mother must be $Rh_o(D)$ antigen-negative; the mother is carrying a child whose father is either $Rh_o(D)$ antigen-positive or $Rh_o(D)$ unknown; the infant is either $Rh_o(D)$ antigen-positive or $Rh_o(D)$ unknown; and the mother must not be previously sensitized to the $Rh_o(D)$ antigen.

Rh_oD-negative or splenectomized patients – Do not administer $Rh_o(D)$ immune globulin IV to $Rh_o(D)$-negative or splenectomized individuals as its efficacy in these patients has not been demonstrated.

➤*RSV-IGIV:*

Fluid overload – Infants with underlying pulmonary disease may be sensitive to the extra fluid volume. Infusion of RSV-IGIV, particularly in children with bronchopulmonary dysplasia (BPD), may precipitate symptoms of fluid overload. Overall, 8.4% of participants (1% premature and 13% BPD) received new or extra diuretics during the period 24 hours before through 48 hours after at least one of their infusions in the PREVENT trial. RSV-IGIV-related fluid overload was reported in 3 patients (1.2%) and RSV-IGIV-related respiratory distress was reported in 4 patients (1.6%); all had underlying BPD. These children were managed with diuretics or modification of the infusion rate and went on to receive subsequent infusions.

Complications related to fluid volume were recorded as a reason for incomplete or prolonged infusion in 2% of children receiving RSV-IGIV (2.5% BPD and 1.1% premature) and in 1.5% of children receiving placebo. Children with clinically apparent fluid overload should not be infused with RSV-IGIV.

➤*Anaphylactic reactions:* Anaphylactic reactions (rare) may occur following injection of human immune globulin preparations. Anaphylaxis is more likely if immune globulin is given IV; therefore, except for IGIV, these products must only be given IM. In highly allergic individuals, repeated injections may lead to anaphylactic shock.

➤*Hypersensitivity reactions:* Give with caution to patients with prior systemic allergic reactions following use of human immunoglobulin preparations. Hypersensitivity reactions are rare; the incidence may be increased by use of large IM doses or repeated injections of immune globulin. Have epinephrine available for treatment of acute allergic symptoms. Refer to Management of Acute Hypersensitivity Reactions.

Severe reactions – Severe reactions, such as anaphylaxis or angioneurotic edema, have been reported in association with IV immunoglobulins, even in patients not known to be sensitive to human immunoglobulins or blood products. If hypotension, anaphylaxis, or severe allergic reaction occurs, discontinue infusion and administer epinephrine (1:1000) as required. Administer steroids, assist respiration, and provide other resuscitative measures. If hypotension occurs, stop infusion and stabilize blood pressure with pressors if necessary. Respiratory distress may also indicate anaphylaxis. Pain in the chest, flank, or back may indicate anaphylaxis or hemolysis. Treat appropriately with an antihistamine, epinephrine, corticosteroids, or some combination of the three. Refer to Management of Acute Hypersensitivity Reactions.

Although systemic reactions to immunoglobulin preparations are rare, epinephrine should be available for treatment of acute anaphylactic symptoms.

➤*Pregnancy:* *Category C.* No studies have been conducted in pregnant patients. Clinical experience suggests no adverse effects on the fetus per se; however, it is not known whether these agents can cause fetal harm.

It should be noted again that *BayRho-D Mini-Dose* is not indicated for use during pregnancy and it should be administered only postabortion or postmiscarriage.

Intact IgG crosses the placenta significantly after 32 weeks gestation.

➤*Lactation:* Safety for use in the nursing mother has not been established. It is not known whether immune globulin is excreted in breast milk.

➤*Children:* Safety and efficacy have not been established in pediatric patients. Do not inject infants with **$Rh_o(D)$ IGIV**, **$Rh_o(D)$ IGIM**, or **$Rh_o(D)$ IG micro-dose**.

ATG equine has been administered safely to a small number of pediatric renal allograft recipients and pediatric aplastic anemia patients at dosage levels comparable to those used in adults on a mg/kg basis.

RSV-IGIV is indicated for use in children < 24 months of age. However, the safety and efficacy of RSV-IGIV in children with congenital heart disease have not been established. Although equivalent proportions of children in the RSV-IGIV and control groups in one trial had adverse events, a larger number of RSV-IGIV recipients had severe or life-threatening adverse events. These events were most frequently observed in infants with CHD with right to left shunts who underwent cardiac surgery.

IGIV – The safety and efficacy of *Gammar-P I.V.* has not been established in neonates and infants with primary defective antibody syntheses.

High-dose administration of *Panglobulin* in pediatric patients with acute or chronic immune thrombocytopenic purpura did not reveal any pediatric-specific hazard.

Venoglobulin-S:

• *Immunodeficiency* – The safety and effectiveness of *Venoglobulin-S* in the treatment of primary immunodeficiency was established in adults and a limited number of children. No infants or neonates were studied. No differences in dosing were found necessary for pediatric patients, nor were any special precautions required.

• *ITP* – The safety and effectiveness of *Venoglobulin-S* was established in both pediatric and adult populations and included all pediatric age groups except neonates. No differences in dosing were found necessary for pediatric patients, nor were any special precautions required.

• *Kawasaki disease* – The safety and efficacy of *Venoglobulin* was established in pediatric populations containing all age groups except neonates.

Sandoglobulin: High-dose administration of *Sandoglobulin* in pediatric patients with acute or chronic ITP did not reveal any pediatric-specific hazard.

Precautions

➤*Monitoring:* Assure that patients are not volume depleted prior to the initiation of therapy.

Periodic monitoring of renal function tests and urine output is particularly important in patients judged to have a potential increased risk for developing acute renal failure. Renal function, including the measurement of blood urea nitrogen (BUN) or serum creatinine should be assessed prior to the initial infusion, and again at appropriate intervals thereafter. If renal function deteriorates, discontinuation of the product should be considered.

For patients judged to be at risk for developing renal dysfunction, it may be prudent to reduce the amount of product infused per unit time (see specific product inserts for measurements).

Administer **RSV-IGIV** cautiously. During administration, monitor the patient's vital signs frequently for increases in heart rate, respiratory rate, retractions, and rales. A loop diuretic such as furosemide or bumetanide should be available for management of fluid overload.

During **ATG rabbit** therapy, monitoring the lymphocyte count (eg, total lymphocyte or T-cell subset) may help assess the degree of T-cell depletion. For safety, monitor the WBC and platelet counts.

➤*Skin testing:* Skin testing should not be performed. Intradermal injection of concentrated gamma globulin causes a localized area of inflammation that can be misinterpreted as a positive allergic reaction. It is actually localized chemical tissue irritation. Misinterpretation can cause necessary medication to be withheld from a patient not actually allergic to this material. True allergic responses to human gamma globulin given in the prescribed IM manner are extremely rare.

➤*Mercury:* Some of these products contain mercury in the form of ethyl mercury from thimerosal. While there are no definitive data on the toxicity of ethyl mercury, literature suggests that information related to methyl mercury toxicities may be applicable.

➤*Latex sensitivity:* Certain components of some of the packaging of these products contain natural rubber latex, which may cause an allergic reaction in sensitive individuals.

➤*Admixture incompatibilities:* Do not admix with other medications.

➤*$Rh_o(D)$ IGIM:*

Hemorrhage – A large fetomaternal hemorrhage late in pregnancy or following delivery may cause a weak mixed field positive D^u test result. If there is any doubt about the mother's Rh type, she should be given $Rh_o(D)$ immune globulin. A screening test to detect fetal red blood cells may be helpful in such cases.

If > 15 mL of D-positive fetal red blood cells are present in the mother's circulation, more than a single dose of $Rh_o(D)$ immune globulin full dose is required. Failure to recognize this may result in the administration of an inadequate dose.

➤*Rh_oD IGIV:* Do not administer $Rh_o(D)$ IGIV as immunoglobulin replacement therapy for immune globulin deficiency syndromes.

Treatment of ITP – Following administration of $Rh_o(D)$ IGIV, monitor $Rh_o(D)$-positive patients for signs and symptoms of intravascular hemolysis (IVH), clinically compromising anemia, and renal insufficiency. If patients are to be transfused, use $Rh_o(D)$-negative packed RBCs so as not to exacerbate ongoing IVH. Platelet products may contain up to 5 mL of RBCs, thus exercise caution if platelets from $Rh_o(D)$-positive donors are transfused.

Suppression of Rh isoimmunization – Do not administer $Rh_o(D)$ IGIV to $Rh_o(D)$-negative individuals who are Rh immunized, as evidenced by an indirect antiglobulin (Coombs') test revealing the presence of anti-$Rh_o(D)$ (anti-D) antibody.

Fetomaternal hemorrhage: A large fetomaternal hemorrhage late in pregnancy or following delivery may cause a weak mixed field positive D^u test result. Assess such an individual for a large fetomaternal hemorrhage and adjust the dose of Rh_o (D) immune globulin accordingly. Administer $Rh_o(D)$ immune globulin if there is any doubt about the mother's blood type.

Hemoglobin – If a patient has a lower than normal hemoglobin level (< 10 g/dL), give a reduced dose of 125 to 200 IU/kg to minimize the risk of increasing the severity of anemia in the patient. $Rh_o(D)$ IGIV must be used with extreme caution in patients with a hemoglobin level that is < 8 g/dL because of the risk of increasing the severity of the anemia (see Administration and Dosage).

➤*ATG equine:*

Infection – Because this agent is ordinarily given with corticosteroids and antimetabolites, monitor patients carefully for leukopenia, thrombocytopenia, or for concurrent infection. If infection occurs, institute adjunctive therapy promptly. On the basis of the clinical circumstances, decide whether therapy will continue.

Concomitant immunosuppressive therapy – Safety and efficacy have been demonstrated in renal transplant patients who received concomitant immunosuppressive therapy and in patients with aplastic anemia.

When the dose of corticosteroids and other immunosuppressants is being reduced, some previously masked reactions to the drug may appear; observe patients carefully during therapy.

Chills and fever – Chills and fever occur frequently. ATG equine may release endogenous leukocyte pyrogens. Prophylactic or therapeutic administration of antihistamines, antipyretics, or corticosteroids generally controls this reaction.

Chemical phlebitis – Chemical phlebitis can be caused by infusion through peripheral veins. Avoid by administering the solution into a high-flow vein. An SC arterialized vein produced by a Brescia fistula is also a useful administration site.

Itching and erythema – Itching and erythema probably result from the drug's effect on blood elements. Antihistamines control the symptoms.

Serum sickness-like symptoms – Serum sickness-like symptoms in aplastic anemia patients have been treated with oral or IV corticosteroids. Resolution of symptoms has generally been prompt and long-term sequelae have not been observed. Prophylactic administration of corticosteroids may decrease the frequency of this reaction.

➤*ATG rabbit:*

Chills and fever – ATG rabbit infusion may produce fever and chills. To minimize these, infuse the first dose over a minimum of 6 hours into a high-flow vein. Also premedication with corticosteroids, acetaminophen, or an antihistamine or slowing the infusion rate may reduce reaction incidence and intensity (see Administration and Dosage).

Prolonged use or overdosage – Prolonged use or overdosage of ATG rabbit in association with other immunosuppressive agents may cause over-immunosuppression resulting in severe infections and may increase the incidence of lymphoma or posttransplant lymphoproliferative disease (PTLD) or other malignancies. Appropriate antiviral, antibacterial, antiprotozoal, or antifungal prophylaxis is recommended.

➤*RSV-IGIV:*

Rate of administration – Except for hypersensitivity reactions, adverse reactions to IGIVs may be related to the rate of administration. Careful adherence to the infusion rate outlined under Administration and Dosage is therefore important. Have loop diuretics available for the management of patients who are at risk for fluid overload. Although systemic allergic reactions are rare (see Adverse Reactions), have epinephrine and diphenhydramine available for treatment of acute allergic symptoms.

Discard after use – RSV-IGIV does not contain a preservative. Enter the single-use vial only once for administration purposes and begin the infusion within 6 hours. Closely adhere to the infusion schedule (see Administration and Dosage). Do not use if the solution is turbid.

➤*Thrombotic events:* There is clinical evidence of a possible association between IGIV administration and the potential for the development of thrombotic events. The exact cause of this is unknown; therefore, exercise caution in the prescribing and infusion of IGIV in patients with a history of and predisposing factors toward cardiovascular disease or thrombotic episodes. Analysis of adverse event reports has indicated that a rapid rate of infusion may be a risk factor for vascular occlusive events.

Drug Interactions

Immune Globulin Drug Interactions

Precipitant drug	Object drug*		Description
RIG, RSV-IGIV, VZIG, IGIV	Virus vaccines, live (measles/mumps/rubella vaccine)	⬇	Antibodies present in immune globulin preparations may interfere with the immune response to live virus vaccines, such as mumps, rubella and particularly, measles. As a general rule, administer live virus vaccines 14 to 30 days before or 6 to 12 weeks after immune globulin administration. Administer live virus vaccines during this interval if corresponding antibody titers are measured 3 months after **RIG** administration. For varicella vaccine, wait 5 months. For a vaccine containing the measles virus, wait 4 months. If live vaccines are given during or within 10 months after **RSV-IGIV** infusion, reimmunization is recommended, if appropriate. Do not administer within 3 months of immune globulin administration [Rh_o(D), HBIG, CMV-IGIV, IG, RIG, TIG] because antibodies in the globulin preparation may interfere with the immune response to the live virus vaccinations (eg, measles, mumps, polio, or rubella). It may be necessary to revaccinate people who received immune globulin shortly after live virus vaccination. Live virus vaccines should be deferred until ≈ 5 months after VZIG administration. People who received VZIG within 14 days of live virus vaccination should be revaccinated with the live virus vaccine 5 months later. Use of live vaccines should be deferred for ≈ 6 months after (IGIV) administration.
Rho(D), HBIG, CMV-IGIV, IG, TIG	Inactivated vaccines (DPT, Hib, OPV)	⬇	Responses to non-live childhood vaccines (eg, DPT) do not appear to be substantially influenced by administration of IGIVs. Limited information available from infants who receive **RSV-IGIV** concurrently with one or more doses of their primary immunization series indicates that antibody responses to diphtheria, tetanus, pertussis and *Haemophilus influenzae* b may be lower in RSV-IGIV recipients than in controls. It is not known whether antibody responses to trivalent oral polio vaccine might be affected. Consider giving a booster dose of these vaccines 3 to 4 months after the last dose of RSV-IGIV in order to ensure immunity to DPT, DtaP, Hib and OPV (oral polio virus).
RIG	Rabies vaccine	⬇	Simultaneous administration may slightly delay the antibody response to rabies vaccine; follow CDC recommendations exactly and give no more than the recommended dose of **RIG**.
ATG rabbit	Immunosuppressants	⬆	Because **antithymocyte globulin (rabbit)** is administered to patients receiving a standard immunosuppressive regimen, this may predispose patients to over-immunosuppression. Many transplant centers decrease maintenance immunosuppression therapy during the period of antibody therapy. **Antithymocyte globulin (rabbit)** can stimulate the production of antibodies that cross-react with rabbit immune globulins.
ATG equine	Immunosuppressants	⬇	When dose of corticosteroids and other immunosuppressants is being reduced, some previously masked reactions to antithymocyte globulin (equine) may appear. Observe patient carefully.

* ⬇ = Object drug decreased. ⬆ = Object drug increased.

➤*Drug/Lab test interactions:*

Rh_o(D) IGIM – Babies born of women given Rh_o(D) IGIM antepartum may have a weakly positive direct antiglobulin test at birth.

Passively acquired anti-Rh_o(D) may be detected in maternal serum if antibody screening tests are performed subsequent to antepartum or postpartum administration of Rh_o(D) IGIM. This does not preclude further antepartum or postpartum prophylaxis.

Late in pregnancy or following delivery, there may be sufficient fetal red blood cells in the maternal circulation to cause a positive antiglobulin test for weak D(D^u). When there is any doubt as to the patient's Rh type, administer Rh_o(D) IGIM.

Elevated bilirubin levels have been reported in some individuals receiving multiple doses of Rh_o(D) IGIM following mismatched transfusions. This is believed to be due to a relatively rapid rate of foreign red cell destruction. About 25% of a group of 22 individuals who were given multiple doses of Rh_o(D) IGIM to treat mismatched transfusions noted fever, myalgia, and lethargy, and 1 had splenomegaly.

Rh_o(D) IGIV – The presence of passively administered anti-Rh_o(D) antibodies in maternal or fetal blood can lead to a positive direct antiglobulin (Coombs') test. If there is an uncertainty about the mother's Rh group or immune status, administer Rh_o(D) immune globulin to the mother.

In addition to anti-D, Rh_o(D) IGIV contains trace amounts of anti-A, anti-B, anti-C, and anti-E antibodies. Passively acquired anti-A, anti-B, anti-C, and anti-E blood group antibodies may be detectable in direct and indirect antiglobulin (Coombs') tests obtained following Rh_o(D) IGIV administration. Interpretation of direct and indirect antiglobulin tests must be made in the context of the patients' underlying clinical condition and supporting laboratory data.

ATG rabbit – ATG rabbit has not been shown to interfere with any routine clinical laboratory tests that do not use immunoglobulins. ATG rabbit may interfere with rabbit antibody-based immunoassays and with cross-match or panel-reactive antibody cytotoxicity assays.

VZIG – Administration of VZIG will result in false-positive tests for immunity to VZV for ≈ 2 months after receiving VZIG. Therefore, do not perform serodiagnostic tests to determine immunity to VZV should within 2 months of VZIG administration.

Adverse Reactions

There is a remote chance of an idiosyncratic or anaphylactic reaction in individuals with hypersensitivity to blood products.

➤*Local:* Tenderness, pain, muscle stiffness at injection site, urticaria, angioedema, ache, erythema, burning; may persist for several hours.

➤*Systemic:* Urticaria; angioedema; malaise, nausea, diarrhea. The most common adverse events were headache, chills, and fever. Less frequently reported reactions include the following: Emesis; chills; fever; fatigue; lightheadedness; abdominal cramping; retching; myalgia; lethargy; chest tightness; nausea. Isolated cases of angioneurotic edema and nephrotic syndrome have occurred.

Systemic reactions associated with administration are extremely rare. Discomfort at the site of injection has been reported and a small number of women have noted a slight elevation in temperature. While sensitization to repeated injections is extremely rare, it has occurred.

Potential reactions for all immune globulin IV products are often related to infusion rate and may include the following: Nausea, vomiting, abdominal cramps, chills, pyrexia, chest tightness, palpitations, tachycardia, blood pressure changes, edema, flushing, diaphoresis, rash, erythema, pruritus, cyanosis, dizziness, headache, backache, or other body aches, anxiety, wheezing (and other respiratory events), myalgia, shaking, fatigue, malaise, and arthralgia, usually beginning within 1 hour of the start of the infusion. Other reactions include feeling of faintness; chest tightness; shortness of breath; dyspnea; chills; headache; mild hemolysis; hypertension; pallor; irritability; pain (chest/hip/back/neck/legs); urticaria (hives); rash (rare).

➤*CMV-IGIV:* Minor reactions such as flushing, chills, muscle cramps, back pain, fever, nausea, vomiting, arthralgia, and wheezing were the most frequent adverse reactions observed during the clinical trials of CMV-IGIV. The incidence of these reactions during the clinical trials was < 6% of all infusions and such reactions were most often related to infusion rates. A decrease in blood pressure was observed in 1 of 1039 infusions in clinical trials. If a patient develops a minor side effect, slow the rate immediately or temporarily interrupt the infusion.

Increases in serum creatinine and BUN have been observed as soon as 1 to 2 days following IGIV infusion. Progression to oliguria or anuria requiring dialysis has been observed. Types of severe renal adverse events that have been seen following IGIV therapy include acute renal failure, acute tubular necrosis, proximal tubular nephropathy, and osmotic nephrosis.

Severe reactions such as angioneurotic edema and anaphylactic shock, although not observed during clinical trials, are a possibility. Clinical anaphylaxis may occur even when the patient is not known to be sensitized to immune globulin products. A reaction may be related to the rate of infusion; therefore, carefully adhere to the infusion rates as outlined under Administration and Dosage. If anaphylaxis or drop in blood pressure occurs, discontinue infusion and use antidote such as diphenhydramine and epinephrine. Refer to the Management of Acute Hypersensitivity Reactions.

➤*IGIV:* Increases in creatinine and BUN have been observed as soon as 1 to 2 days following infusion. Progression to oliguria and anuria requiring dialysis has been observed, although some patients have improved spontaneously following cessation of treatment. Types of severe renal adverse reactions that have been seen following IGIV therapy include the following: acute renal failure, acute tubular necrosis, proximal tubular nephropathy, and osmotic nephrosis.

➤*ATG equine:*

Renal transplantation: Fever (33%); chills, leukopenia (14%); dermatological reactions (eg, rash, pruritus, urticaria, wheal, flare) (13%); thrombocytopenia (11%); arthralgia, chest/back pain, clotted A/V fistula, diarrhea, dyspnea, headache, hypotension, nausea, vomiting, night sweats, pain at the infusion site, peripheral thrombophlebitis, stomatitis (1% to 5%); anaphylaxis, dizziness, weakness, faintness, edema, herpes simplex reactivation, hiccoughs, epigastric pain, hyperglycemia, hypertension, iliac vein obstruction, laryngospasm, localized infection, lymphadenopathy, malaise, myalgia, paresthesia, possible serum sickness, pulmonary edema, renal artery thrombosis, seizures, systemic infection, tachycardia, toxic epidermal necrosis, wound dehiscence (< 1%).

Aplastic anemia: Chills, arthralgia (50%); headache (17%); myalgia (10%); nausea, chest pain (7%); phlebitis (5%); diaphoresis, joint stiffness, periorbital edema, aches, edema, muscle ache, vomiting, agitation/lethargy, listlessness, lightheadedness, seizures, diarrhea, bradycardia, myocarditis, cardiac irregularity, hepatosplenomegaly, encephalitis or postviral encephalopathy, hypotension, CHF, hypertension, burning soles/palms, foot sole pain, lymphadenopathy, postcervical lymphadenopathy, tender lymph nodes, bilateral pleural effusion, respiratory distress, anaphylaxis, proteinuria (< 5%); abnormal tests of liver function (eg, AST, ALT, alkaline phosphatase) and renal function (eg, serum creatinine). In some trials, clinical and laboratory findings of serum sickness were seen in a majority of patients.

Postmarketing experience: Fever (51%); thrombocytopenia (30%); rashes (27%); chills (16%); leukopenia (14%); systemic infection (13%); abnormal renal function tests, serum sickness-like symptoms, dyspnea or apnea, arthralgia, chest/back/flank pain, diarrhea, nausea, vomiting (5% to 10%); hypertension, herpes simplex infection, pain, swelling or redness at the infusion site, eosinophilia, headache, myalgia, leg pains, hypotension, anaphylaxis, tachycardia, edema, localized infection, malaise, seizures, GI bleeding/perforation, deep vein thrombosis, sore mouth/throat, hyperglycemia, acute renal failure, abnormal liver function tests, confusion, disorientation, cough, neutropenia, granulocytopenia, anemia, thrombophlebitis, dizziness, epigastric/stomach pain, lymphadenopathy, pulmonary edema, CHF, abdominal pain, nosebleed, vasculitis, aplasia, pancytopenia, abnormal involuntary movement, tremor, rigidity, sweating, laryngospasm, edema, hemolysis/hemolytic anemia, viral hepatitis, faintness, enlarged/ruptured kidney, paresthesias, renal artery thrombosis (< 5%).

➤*ATG rabbit:* ATG rabbit adverse events are generally manageable or reversible. In the US Phase III controlled clinical trial (n = 163) comparing the efficacy and safety of ATG rabbit and ATG equine, there were no significant differences in clinically significant adverse events between the 2 treatment groups. Malignancies were reported in 3 patients who received ATG rabbit and in 3 patients who received ATG equine during the 1-year follow-up period. These included 2 PTLDs in the ATG rabbit group and 2 PTLDs in the ATG equine group. Infections occurring in both treatment groups during the 3-month follow-up are summarized in the following table. No significant differences were seen between the ATG rabbit and ATG equine groups for all types of infections, and the incidence of CMV infection was equivalent in both groups. (Viral prophylaxis was by the centers discretion during antibody treatment, but all centers used ganciclovir infusion during treatment.)

Antithymocyte Globulin Adverse Reactions (%)

Adverse reactions	ATG rabbit (n = 82)	ATG equine (n = 81)
Cardiovascular		
Hypertension	36.6	28.4
Tachycardia	26.8	23.5
Respiratory		
Dyspnea	28	19.8
Pneumonia	0	1.2
GI		
Abdominal pain	37.8	27.2
Diarrhea	36.6	32.1
Nausea	36.6	28.4
GI moniliasis	4.9	1.2
Oral moniliasis	3.7	2.5
Gastritis	1.2	0
GU		
Urinary tract infection	18.3	25.9
Vaginitis	0	1.2
Hematologic		
Leukopenia	57.3	29.6
Thrombocytopenia	36.6	44.4
Miscellaneous		
Fever	63.4	63
Chills	57.3	43.2
Pain	46.3	43.2
Headache	40.2	34.6
Peripheral edema	34.1	34.6
Asthenia	26.8	32.1
Hyperkalemia	26.8	18.5
Infection	30.5	23.5
Infection (other)	17.1	13.6
Infection (CMV)	13.4	11.1
Malaise	13.4	3.7
Sepsis	12.2	9.6
Dizziness	8.5	24.7
Herpes simplex	4.9	0
Infection (not specified)	0	2.5
Moniliasis	0	1.2

➤*Rh_o(D) IGIV:* Rh_o(D) IGIV is administered to Rh_o(D) positive patients with ITP. Side effects related to the destruction of Rh_o(D)-positive red cells, such as decreased hemoglobin, can be expected. At the recommended initial IV dose of 250 IU/kg, the mean maximum decrease in hemoglobin was 1.7 g/dL (range, +0.4 to -6.1 g/dL). At a reduced dose, ranging from 125 to 200 IU/kg, the mean maximum decrease in hemoglobin was 0.81 g/dL (range, +0.65 to -1.9 g/dL). Only 5 of the 137 (3.7%) patients had a maximum decrease in hemoglobin of > 4 g/dL (range, 4.2 to 6.1 g/dL).

In most cases, the RBC destruction is believed to occur in the spleen. However, signs and symptoms consistent with IVH, including back pain, shaking chills, or hemoglobinuria have been reported, occurring within 4 hours of Rh_o(D) IGIV administration.

IVH-related complications that have been reported include death (4 cases reported between May 1996 and April 1999), acute onset or exacerbation of anemia, and acute onset or exacerbation of renal insufficiency. One patient died from complications secondary to IVH-induced exacerbation of anemia after administration of Rh_o(D) IGIV for treatment of ITP. Although the primary cause of death in the other 3 ITP patients treated with Rh_o(D) IGIV was related to underlying disease, the extent to which IVH-related clinical complications exacerbated their conditions and contributed to their deaths is unknown.

In addition to the adverse reactions described above, the following have been reported infrequently in clinical trials or postmarketing experience, in patients treated for ITP or Rh isoimmunization suppression, and are thought to be temporally associated with Rh_o(D) IGIV use: Asthenia, abdominal or back pain, hypotension, pallor, diarrhea, increased LDH, arthralgia, myalgia, dizziness, hyperkinesia, somnolence, vasodilation, pruritus, rash, and sweating.

➤*RSV-IGIV:* RSV-IGIV is generally well tolerated. In the PREVENT trial of RSV-IGIV in children with BPD or prematurity, there was no difference in the proportion of children in the RSV-IGIV and placebo groups who report adverse events.

RSV-IGIV Adverse Reactions (%)		
Adverse Reaction	RSV-IGIV (n = 250)	Placebo (n = 260)
Fever/Pyrexia	6	2
Respiratory distress	2	< 1
Vomiting/Emesis	2	1
Wheezing	2	2
Diarrhea	1	< 1
Rales	1	0
Fluid overload	1	0
Tachycardia/Increased pulse rate	1	0
Rash	1	2
Hypertension	1	0
Hypoxia/Hypoxemia	1	1
Tachypnea	1	< 1
Gastroenteritis	1	< 1
Injection site inflammation	1	1
Overdose effect	1	< 1

Infrequent adverse reactions included: Edema, pallor, hypotension, heart murmur, gagging, cyanosis, sleepiness, cough, rhinorrhea, eczema, cold and clammy skin, conjunctival hemorrhage (< 1%).

Reactions similar to those reported with other IGIVs may occur with RSV-IGIV. These include: Dizziness; flushing; blood pressure changes; anxiety; palpitations; chest tightness; dyspnea; abdominal cramps; pruritus; myalgia; arthralgia. Such reactions are often related to the rate of infusion. Immediate allergic, anaphylactic, or hypersensitivity reactions may be observed (see Warnings). Rarely, aseptic meningitis syndrome (AMS) has been reported in association with IGIV treatment, particularly at high dosage (2 g/kg; see Precautions).

In the PREVENT trial, 3 children developed aseptic meningitis of unknown etiology. In the single-blind, controlled NIAID trial in children with BPD, CHD or prematurity, adverse reactions were reported in 3% of all RSV-IGIV infusions. Five of 160 children were considered to have had mild fluid overload associated with infusion. The remaining adverse reactions consisted of mild decreases in oxygen saturation (n = 8) and fever (n = 5). In the open-label study in children with BPD or prematurity (n = 6), infusion-associated adverse reactions were noted in 14 of 294 (4.8%) infusions. Six adverse events were considered related to infusion, including 4 mild and 2 moderate events. In the CARDIAC study, children with CHD with right to left shunts appeared to have an increased frequency of cardiac surgery and had a greater frequency of severe and life-threatening adverse events associated with cardiac surgery (see Warnings).

Overdosage

Although few data are available, clinical experience with other immune globulin preparations suggests that the major manifestations would be those related to fluid volume overload. Other reactions would include pain and tenderness at the injection site.

➤*ATG equine:* Because of its mode of action and because it is a biologic substance, the maximal tolerated dose of ATG equine solution would be expected to vary from patient to patient. To date, the largest single daily dose administered to a patient, a renal transplant recipient, was 7000 mg administered at a concentration of ≈ 10 mg/mL Sodium Chloride Injection, USP, ≈ 7 times the recommended total dose and infusion concentration. In this patient, administration of ATG equine was not associated with any signs of acute intoxication.

The greatest number of doses (10 to 20 mg/kg/dose) that can be administered to a single patient has not yet been determined. Some renal transplant patients have received up to 50 doses in 4 months, and others have received 28-day courses of 21 doses followed by as many as 3 more courses for the treatment of acute rejection. The incidence of toxicologic manifestations did not increase with any of these regimens.

➤*ATG rabbit:* ATG rabbit overdosage may result in leukopenia or thrombocytopenia, which can be managed with dose reduction (see Administration and Dosage).

➤*Rh_o(D) IGIV:* There are no reports of known overdoses in patients being treated for Rh isoimmunization or ITP. In clinical studies with nonpregnant Rh_o(D) positive patients with ITP (n = 141) treated with 600 to 32,500 IU (120 to 6500 mcg) of Rh_o(D) IGIV, there were no signs or symptoms that warranted medical intervention. However, these same doses were associated with a mild, transient hemolytic anemia.

Patient Information

Instruct patients to report symptoms of decreased urine output, sudden weight gain, fluid retention/edema and/or shortness of breath (which may suggest kidney damage) immediately to their physician.

Instruct patients, parents, or guardians to report any serious adverse reaction to their health care provider.

Patients, parents, or guardians should be fully informed by their health care provider of the benefits and risks of these products.

CYTOMEGALOVIRUS IMMUNE GLOBULIN INTRAVENOUS, HUMAN (CMV-IGIV)

Rx	CytoGam (MedImmune)	Solution for injection:[a] 50 ± 10 mg/mL	In 20 and 50 mL vials.

[a] Preservative free. 5% sucrose, 1% Albumin (human). Solvent/Detergent treated.

CYTOMEGALOVIRUS IMMUNE GLOBULIN INTRAVENOUS (HUMAN) — INJECTION

For complete and comparative prescribing information, refer to the Immune Globulins group monograph.

Indications

➤*Cytomegalovirus prophylaxis:* For the prophylaxis of cytomegalovirus disease associated with transplantation of kidney, lung, liver, pancreas, and heart. In transplants of these organs other than kidney from CMV seropositive donors into seronegative recipients, prophylactic CMV-IGIV should be considered in combination with ganciclovir.

➤*Unlabeled uses:* For prevention or attenuation of primary CMV disease in immunosuppressed recipients of organ transplants (eg, bone marrow, liver). Also used in immunocompromised patients with CMV pneumonia or to prevent CMV disease.

Administration and Dosage

The maximum recommended total dosage per infusion is 150 mg/kg, administered according to the following schedule:

	Type of transplant	
Within:	Kidney	Liver, pancreas, lung, heart
72 hours of transplant	150 mg/kg	150 mg/kg
2 weeks post-transplant	100 mg/kg	150 mg/kg
4 weeks post-transplant	100 mg/kg	150 mg/kg
6 weeks post-transplant	100 mg/kg	150 mg/kg
8 weeks post-transplant	100 mg/kg	150 mg/kg
12 weeks post-transplant	50 mg/kg	100 mg/kg
16 weeks post-transplant	50 mg/kg	100 mg/kg

➤*Preparation for administration:* Remove the tab portion of the vial cap and clean the rubber stopper with 70% alcohol or equivalent. Do not shake vial; avoid foaming.

➤*Infusion:* Infusion should begin within 6 hours after entering the vial and should be complete within 12 hours of entering the vial. Vital signs should be taken preinfusion, mid-way and post-infusion as well as before any rate increase. Cytomegalovirus immune globulin intravenous (human) should be administered through an intravenous line using an administration set that contains an in-line filter (pore size 15μ) and a constant infusion pump (ie, IVAC pump or equivalent). A smaller in-line filter (0.2μ) is also acceptable. Pre-dilution of cytomegalovirus immune globulin intravenous (human) before infusion is not recommended. Cytomegalovirus immune globulin intravenous (human) should be administered through a separate intravenous line. If this is not possible, cytomegalovirus immune globulin intravenous (human) may be piggybacked into a pre-existing line if that line contains either sodium chloride, injection, USP, or one of the following dextrose solutions (with or without NaCl added): 2.5% dextrose in water, 5% dextrose in water, 10% dextrose in water, 20% dextrose in water. If a pre-existing line must be used, the cytomegalovirus immune globulin intravenous (human) should not be diluted more than 1:2 with any of the above-named solutions. Admixtures of cytomegalovirus immune globulin intravenous (human) with any other solutions have not been evaluated.

➤*Initial dose:* Administer intravenously at 15 mg/kg/hr. If no adverse reactions occur after 30 minutes, the rate may be increased to 30 mg/kg/hr; if no adverse reactions occur after a subsequent 30 minutes, then the infusion may be increased to 60 mg/kg/hr (volume not to exceed 75 mL/hr). Do not exceed this rate of administration. The patient should be monitored closely during and after each rate change.

➤*Subsequent doses:* Administer at 15 mg/kg/hr for 15 minutes. If no adverse reactions occur, increase to 30 mg/kg/hr for 15 minutes and then increase to a maximum rate of 60 mg/kg/hr (volume not to exceed 75 mL/hr). Do not exceed this rate of administration. The patient should be monitored closely during each rate change.

➤*Special risk:* Cytomegalovirus immune globulin intravenous (human) should be used with caution in patients with pre-existing renal insufficiency and in patients judged to be at increased risk of developing renal insufficiency (including, but not limited to those with diabetes mellitus, age > 65, volume depletion, paraproteinemia, sepsis and patients receiving known nephrotoxic drugs). In these cases especially, it is important to assure that patients are not volume depleted prior to cytomegalovirus immune globulin intravenous (human) (CMV-IGIV) infusion. While most cases of renal insufficiency have occurred in patients receiving total doses of 400 mg/kg or greater, no prospective data are presently available to identify a maximum safe dose, concentration or rate of infusion in patients determined to be at increased risk of acute renal failure. In the absence of prospective data, recommended doses should not be exceeded and the concentration and infusion rate selected should be the minimum practicable. The product should be infused at a rate of 180 mg/kg/hr or less.

Potential adverse reactions are flushing, chills, muscle cramps, back pain, fever, nausea, vomiting, wheezing, drop in blood pressure. Minor adverse reactions have been infusion rate related - if the patient develops a minor side effect (ie, nausea, back pain, flushing), slow the rate or temporarily

CYTOMEGALOVIRUS IMMUNE GLOBULIN INTRAVENOUS (HUMAN) — INJECTION

interrupt the infusion. If anaphylaxis or drop in blood pressure occurs, discontinue infusion and use antidote such as diphenhydramine and adrenalin.

➤*Storage/Stability:* Store between 2°C and 8°C (35.6°F and 46.4°F), and used within 6 hours after entering the vial.

HEPATITIS B IMMUNE GLOBULIN (HUMAN) (HBIG)

Rx	**BayHep B** (Bayer Pharmaceutical)	**Solution for Injection:**[a] 15% to 18% protein	In 1 and 5 mL single-dose vials and 0.5 mL neonatal single-dose syringe.
Rx	**Nabi-HB** (Nabi)	**Solution for Injection:**[b] 5% ± 1% protein	In 1 and 5 mL single-dose vials.

[a] Preservative free. With 0.21 to 0.32 M glycine. Solvent/Detergent treated.
[b] Preservative free. With 0.15 M glycine. Solvent/Detergent treated.

HEPATITIS B IMMUNE GLOBULIN (HUMAN) - INJECTION

For complete and comparative prescribing information, refer to the Immune Globulins group monograph.

Indications

➤*Postexposure hepatitis B prophylaxis:*

Acute exposure to blood containing HBsAg – After either parenteral exposure (eg, by accidental "needlestick") or direct mucous membrane contact (accidental splash), or oral ingestion (pipetting accident) involving HBsAg-positive materials such as blood, plasma or serum. For inadvertent percutaneous exposure, a regimen of 2 doses of hepatitis B immune globulin (human), 1 given after exposure and 1 a month later, is about 75% effective in preventing hepatitis B in this setting.

Perinatal exposure of infants born to HBsAg-positive mothers – Infants born to HBsAg-positive mothers are at risk of being infected with hepatitis B virus and becoming chronic carriers. This risk is especially great if the mother is HBeAg-positive. Studies conducted with hepatitis B immune globulins similar to hepatitis B immune globulin (human) indicated that for an infant with perinatal exposure to an HBsAg-positive and HBeAg-positive mother, a regimen combining 1 dose of hepatitis B immune globulin (human) at birth with the hepatitis B vaccine series started soon after birth is 85% to 95% effective in preventing development of the HBV carrier state. Regimens involving either multiple doses of hepatitis B immune globulin (human) alone or the vaccine series alone have 70% to 90% efficacy, while a single dose of hepatitis B immune globulin (human) alone has only 50% efficacy.

Sexual exposure to an HBsAg-positive person – Sex partners of HBsAg-positive persons are at increased risk of acquiring HBV infection. For sexual exposure to a person with acute hepatitis B, a single dose of hepatitis B immune globulin (human) is 75% effective if administered within 2 weeks of last sexual exposure.

Household exposure to persons with acute HBV infection – Since infants have close contact with primary caregivers and they have a higher risk of becoming HBV carriers after acute HBV infection, prophylaxis of an infant less than 12 months of age with hepatitis B immune globulin (human) and hepatitis B vaccine is indicated if the mother or primary caregiver has acute HBV infection.

Administration and Dosage

➤*For IM use only:* This product is for intramuscular use only. The use of this product by the intravenous route is not indicated. Parenteral drug products should be inspected visually for particulate matter and discoloration prior to administration.

➤*Administration:* It is important to use a separate vial, sterile syringe, and needle for each individual patient, in order to prevent transmission of infectious agents from 1 person to another. Any vial of hepatitis B immune globulin (human) that has been entered should be used promptly. Do not reuse or save for future use. This product contains no preservative; therefore, partially used vials should be discarded immediately.

Hepatitis B immune globulin (human) may be administered at the same time (but at a different site), or up to 1 month preceding hepatitis B vaccination without impairing the active immune response to hepatitis B vaccine.

➤*Acute exposure to blood containing HBsAg:* The following information summarizes prophylaxis for percutaneous (needlestick, bite, sharps), ocular, or mucous membrane exposure to blood according to the source of exposure and vaccination status of the exposed person. For greatest effectiveness, passive prophylaxis with hepatitis B immune globulin (human) should be given as soon as possible after exposure (its value beyond 7 days of exposure is unclear). If hepatitis B immune globulin (human) is indicated, an injection of 0.06 mL/kg of body weight should be administered intramuscularly as soon as possible after exposure and within 24 hours, if possible. Consult hepatitis B vaccine monograph for dosage information regarding that product.

For persons who refuse hepatitis B vaccine or are known non-responders to vaccine, a second dose of hepatitis B immune globulin (human) should be given 1 month after the first dose.

Recommendations for hepatitis B prophylaxis following percutaneous or permucosal exposure

Source	Exposed person: Unvaccinated	Exposed person: Vaccinated
HBsAg-positive	1. Hepatitis B immune globulin (human) × 1 immediately*	1. Test exposed person for anti-HBs
	2. Initiate HB vaccine series+	2. If inadequate antibody++, hepatitis B immune globulin (human) × 1 immediately plus × 1 HB vaccine booster dose
Known source - high risk for HBsAg-positive	1. Initiate HB vaccine series	1. Test source for HBsAg only if exposed is vaccine non-responder. If source is HBsAg-positive, give hepatitis B immune globulin (human) × 1 immediately plus × 1 HB vaccine booster dose
	2. Test source for HBsAg. If positive, hepatitis B immune globulin (human) × 1	
Known source - low risk for HBsAg-positive	Initiate HB vaccine series	Nothing required
Unknown source	Initiate HB vaccine series	Nothing required

* Hepatitis B immune globulin (human) dose of 0.06 mL/kg IM.
\+ HB vaccine dose 20 mcg IM for adults; 10 mcg IM for infants or children under 10 years of age. First dose within 1 week; second and third doses, 1 and 6 months later.
\++ Less than 10 mIU/mL anti-HBs by radioimmunoassay, negative by enzyme immunoassay.

➤*Prophylaxis of infants born to mothers who are positive for HBsAg with or without HBeAg:* The table below contains the recommended schedule of hepatitis B prophylaxis for infants born to mothers that are either known to be positive for HBsAg or have not been screened.

Infants born to mothers known to be HBsAG-positive should receive 0.5 mL hepatitis B immune globulin (human) after psysiologic stabilization of the infant and preferably within 12 hours of birth. The hepatitis B vaccine series should be initiated simultaneously, if not contraindicated, with the first dose of the vaccine given concurrently with the hepatitis B immune globulin (human), but at a different site. Subsequent doses of the vaccine should be administered in accordance with the recommendations of the manufacturer.

Women admitted for delivery, who were not screened for HBsAg during the prenatal period, should be tested. While test results are pending, the newborn infant should receive hepatitis B vaccine within 12 hours of birth (see manufacturers' recommendations for dose). If the mother is later found to be HBsAg-positive, the infant should receive 0.5 mL hepatitis B immune globulin (human) as soon as possible and within 7 days of birth; however, the efficacy of hepatitis B immune globulin (human) administered after 48 hours of age is not known. Testing for HBsAg and anti-HBs is recommended at 12 to 15 months of age. If HBsAg is not detectable and anti-HBs is present, the child has been protected.

Recommended schedule of hepatitis B immunoprophylaxis to prevent perinatal transmission of hepatitis B virus infection

Administer	Age of infant: Infant born to mother known to be HBsAg-positive	Age of infant: Infant born to mother not screened for HBsAg
First vaccination*	Birth (within 12 hours)	Birth (within 12 hours)
Hepatitis B immune globulin (human)+	Birth (within 12 hours)	If mother is found to be HBsAg-positive, administer dose to infant as soon as possible, not later than 1 week after birth
Second vaccination*	1 month	1 to 2 months
Third vaccination*	6 months++	6 months++

* See manufacturers' recommendations for appropriate dose.
\+ 0.5 mL administered IM at a site different from that used for the vaccine.
\++ See ACIP recommendation.

➤*Sexual exposure to an HBsAg-positive person:* All susceptible persons whose sex partners have acute hepatitis B infection should receive a single dose of hepatitis B immune globulin (human) (0.06 mL/kg) and should begin the hepatitis B vaccine series, if not contraindicated, within 14 days of the last sexual contact or if sexual contact with the infected person will continue. Administering the vaccine with hepatitis B immune globulin (human) may improve the efficacy of postexposure treatment. The vaccine has the added advantage of conferring long-lasting protection.

HEPATITIS B IMMUNE GLOBULIN (HUMAN) – INJECTION

Recommendations for postexposure prophylaxis for sexual exposure to hepatitis B			
HBIG*		Vaccine	
Dose	Recommended timing	Dose	Recommended timing
0.06 mL/kg IM+	Single dose within 14 days of last sexual contact	1 mL IM+	First dose at time of HBIG* treatment$

* HBIG = hepatitis B immune globulin (human). +IM = intramuscularly.
$ The first dose can be administered the same time as the HBIG dose but at a different site; subsequent doses should be administered as recommended for specific vaccine.

➤*Household exposure to persons with acute HBV infection:* Prophylactic treatment with a 0.5 mL dose of hepatitis B immune globulin (human) and hepatitis B vaccine is indicated for infants less than 12 months of age who have been exposed to a primary caregiver who has acute hepatitis B. Prophylaxis for other household contacts of persons with acute HBV infection is not indicated unless they have had identifiable blood exposure to the index patient, such as by sharing toothbrushes or razors. Such exposures should be treated like sexual exposures. If the index patient becomes an HBV carrier, all household contacts should receive hepatitis B vaccine.

➤*Storage / Stability:* Store at 2° to 8°C (36° to 46°F). Do not freeze. Do not use after expiration date. Use within 6 hours after the vial has been entered.

IMMUNE GLOBULIN (HUMAN) (IG; IGIM; Gamma Globulin; IgG)

Rx	**BayGam** (Bayer)	**Solution for Injection:**[a] 15% to 18% protein	In 2 and 10 mL single-dose vials.

[a] Preservative-free. With 0.21 to 0.32 M glycine. Solvent/Detergent treated.

IMMUNE GLOBULIN (HUMAN) IG; IGIM; Gamma Globulin; IgG) — INJECTION

For complete and comparative prescribing information, refer to the Immune Globulins group monograph.

Indications

➤*Hepatitis A:* The prophylactic value of IGIM is greatest when given before or soon after exposure to hepatitis A. Not indicated in individuals with clinical manifestations of hepatitis A or in those exposed > 2 weeks previously.

➤*Measles (Rubeola):* For the prevention or modification of measles in susceptible contacts (one who has not been vaccinated and has not had measles previously) exposed < 6 days previously. May be especially indicated for susceptible household contacts of measles patients, particularly those < 1 year of age, for whom the risk of complications is highest. Do not give with measles vaccine. If a child > 12 months of age has received IGIM, give measles vaccine ≈ 3 months later, when the measles antibody titer will have disappeared.

If a susceptible child exposed to measles is immunocompromised, administer IGIM immediately. Do not give children who are immunocompromised the measles vaccine or any other live viral vaccine.

➤*Immunoglobulin deficiency:* IGIM therapy may prevent serious infection if circulating IgG levels of ≈ 200 mg/dL plasma are maintained. However, it may not prevent chronic infections of external secretory tissues such as the respiratory and GI tracts.

Prophylactic therapy, especially against infections due to encapsulated bacteria, is often effective in Bruton-type, sex-linked congenital agammaglobulinemia, agammaglobulinemia associated with thymoma, and acquired agammaglobulinemia.

➤*Varicella:* Passive immunization against varicella in immunosuppressed patients is best accomplished with varicella-zoster immune globulin. If unavailable, IGIM may be used.

➤*Rubella:* The routine use of IGIM for rubella prophylaxis in early pregnancy is of dubious value and cannot be justified. Some studies suggest that the use of IGIM in susceptible women exposed to rubella can lessen the likelihood of infection and fetal damage. See Administration and Dosage.

Administration and Dosage

➤*Administration:* For IM injection only, preferably in the anterolateral aspects of the upper thigh and the deltoid muscle of the upper arm. Do not use the gluteal region routinely as an injection site because of the risk of injury to the sciatic nerve. Divide and inject doses > 10 mL into several muscle sites to reduce local pain and discomfort. An individual decision as to which muscle is injected must be made for each patient based on the volume of material to be administered. If the gluteal region is used when very large volumes are to be injected or multiple doses are necessary, avoid the central region; use only the upper outer quadrant.

➤*Hepatitis A:* A dose of 0.02 mL/kg (0.01 mL/lb) is recommended for household and institutional hepatitis A case contacts. The following doses are recommended for people who plan to travel in areas where hepatitis A is common:

IG Dose for Common Hepatitis A Areas	
Length of stay	Dose (mL/kg)
< 3 months	0.02
Prolonged (> 3 months)	0.06 (repeat every 4 to 6 months)

➤*Measles (Rubeola):* To prevent or modify measles in a susceptible person exposed < 6 days previously, give 0.11 mL/lb (0.25 mL/kg). If a susceptible child who is also immunocompromised is exposed to measles, give 0.5 mL/kg (15 mL maximum) immediately.

➤*Immunoglobulin deficiency:* The usual dosage consists of an initial dose of 1.3 mL/kg followed in 3 or 4 weeks by 0.66 mL/kg (≥ 100 mg/kg) to be given every 3 to 4 weeks. Some patients may require more frequent injections.

➤*Varicella:* Give 0.6 to 1.2 mL/kg promptly, if varicella-zoster immune globulin is unavailable.

➤*Rubella:* Some studies suggest that the use of IG in exposed susceptible women can lessen the likelihood of infection and fetal damage; therefore, a dose of 0.55 mL/kg may benefit those women who do not consider a therapeutic abortion.

➤*Storage / Stability:* Store between 2° to 8°C (36° to 46°F). Do not freeze.

IMMUNE GLOBULIN INTRAVENOUS (IGIV)

Rx	**Flebogamma 5%** (Grifols)	**Injection:** 5% immune globulin (human) (50 mg/mL)[a]	In 10, 50, 100, and 200 mL vials.
Rx	**Octagam** (Octapharma)	**Injection:** 5% immune globulin (human) (50 mg/mL)[b]	In 1, 2.5, 5, and 10 g single-use bottles.
Rx	**Gammagard Liquid** (Baxter)	**Injection:** 10% immune globulin (human)	Preservative free. In 1, 2.5, 5, 10, and 20 g single-use bottles.
Rx	**Gamunex** (Talecris Biotherapeutics)	**Injection:** 10% immune globulin (human)[c]	In 10, 25, 50, 100, and 200 mL.
Rx	**Polygam S/D** (American Red Cross)	**Powder for injection (freeze-dried):** 50 mg/mL; 90% gammaglobulin[d]	In 2.5, 5, and 10 g single-use bottles with diluent, transfer device, and administration set.
Rx	**Carimune NF** (ZLB Bioplasma)	**Powder for injection, lyophilized:** 1, 3, 6, 12 g immune globulin IV[e]	In 1, 3, 6, and 12 g vials.
Rx	**Iveegam EN** (Baxter)	**Powder for Injection (freeze-dried):** 5 g immune globulin IV[f]	In 5 g bottle with diluent (contains dry natural rubber), transfer device, and infusion set with filter.

[a] 50 mg sorbitol, ≤ 6 mg/mL polyethylene glycol, preservative-free.
[b] 100 mg maltose.
[c] With 0.16 to 0.24 M glycine. Caprylate/Chromatography purified.
[d] Preservative free. With 20 mg glucose, 2 mg polyethylene glycol, 22.5 mg glycine, 1 mcg tri-n-butyl phosphate, 1 mcg octoxynol 9, 100 mcg polysorbate 80, 3 mg albumin (human) per mL. Solvent/Detergent treated.
[e] Preservative free. With 1.67 g sucrose/g protein.
[f] Preservative free. 50 mg glucose and 3 mg sodium chloride.

IMMUNE GLOBULIN INTRAVENOUS (HUMAN) — INTRAVENOUS (*FLEBOGAMMA*)

For complete and comparative prescribing information, refer to the Immune Globulins group monograph.

WARNING

Immune globulin intravenous (human) (IGIV) products have been reported to be associated with renal dysfunction, acute renal failure, osmotic nephrosis, and death. Patients predisposed to acute renal failure include patients with any degree of preexisting renal insufficiency, diabetes mellitus, volume depletion, sepsis, or paraproteinemia; patients older than 65 years of age; or patients receiving known nephrotoxic drugs. Especially in such patients, administer IGIV products at the minimum concentration available and the minimum rate of infusion practicable. While these reports of renal dysfunction and acute renal failure have been associated with the use of many of the licensed IGIV products, those containing sucrose as a stabilizer accounted for a disproportionate share of the total number. *Flebogamma* does not contain sucrose.

Indications

➤*Primary humoral immunodeficiency:* For replacement therapy in primary (inherited) humoral immunodeficiency disorders, such as common variable immunodeficiency, x-linked agammaglobulinemia, severe combined immunodeficiency, and Wiskott-Aldrich syndrome. *Flebogamma* is especially useful when rapid replacement of immunoglobulin G (IgG) or the attainment of high serum levels of IgG is desired.

➤*Unlabeled uses:* Treatment of posttransfusion purpura, Guillain-Barré syndrome, and chronic inflammatory demyelinating polyneuropathy (as an alternative to plasma exchange). IGIV is being investigated in the prevention or treatment of the following diseases: autoimmune diseases (eg, rhesus hemolytic disease, factor VIII deficiencies, bullous pemphigoid, rheumatoid arthritis, Sjogren syndrome, type 1 diabetes mellitus), IgG4 subclass deficiencies, intractable epilepsy (possibly caused by IgG2 subclass deficiency), cystic fibrosis, trauma, thermal injury (eg, severe burns), cytomegalovirus infection, neuromuscular disorders, prophylaxis of infections associated with bone marrow transplantation, and GI protection (oral administration).

Administration and Dosage

➤*Approved by the FDA:* December 15, 2003.

➤*Dosage:* The usual dosage for replacement therapy in primary humoral immunodeficiency is 300 to 600 mg/kg body weight administered every 3 to 4 weeks. Doses may be adjusted over time to achieve the desired trough IgG levels and clinical responses. No randomized controlled trial data are available to determine an optimum target trough serum IgG level.

➤*Infusion rates:* The infusion should be initiated at a rate of 0.01 mL/kg body weight/min (0.5 mg/kg/min). If during the first 30 minutes the patient does not experience any discomfort, the rate may be gradually increased to a maximum of 0.1 mL/kg/min (5 mg/kg/min).

➤*Renal function impairment:* For patients judged to be at risk for developing renal dysfunction, it may be prudent to limit the amount of product infused per unit time by infusing at a maximum rate less than 0.06 mL/kg body weight/min (3 mg/kg/min). No prospective data are available to identify a maximum safe dose, concentration, and rate of infusion in patients determined to be at increased risk of acute renal failure. In the absence of prospective data, recommended doses should not be exceeded, and the concentration and infusion rate should be the minimum level practicable. Reduction in dose, concentration, and/or rate of infusion in patients at risk of acute renal failure, which includes patients older than 65 years of age (see Warning Box), has been proposed in the literature in order to reduce the risk of acute renal failure.

➤*Administration:* *Flebogamma* should be inspected visually for particulate matter and color prior to administration. Do not use if turbid. If large doses are to be administered, several vials of *Flebogamma* may be pooled into an empty sterile IV solution container by using aseptic technique. Dilution with IV fluids is not recommended. Filters with a pore size of 15 to 20 microns may be used optionally for the infusion. Antibacterial filters (0.2 micron) also may be used, although they may slow infusions. Discard unused contents and administration devices after use.

➤*Admixture incompatibility:* Specific drug interactions and incompatibilities have not been studied. *Flebogamma* should be infused through a separate IV line. Do not add any medications or IV fluids to the *Flebogamma* infusion container. Do not mix IGIV products of different formulations or from different manufacturers.

➤*Storage/Stability:* Store at 2° to 25°C (36° to 77°F). Do not freeze.

IMMUNE GLOBULIN (HUMAN) — INTRAVENOUS 5% (*OCTAGAM*)

For complete and comparative prescribing information, refer to the Immune Globulins group monograph.

WARNING

Immune globulin intravenous (human) (IGIV) products have been reported to be associated with renal dysfunction, acute renal failure, osmotic nephrosis, and death. Patients predisposed to acute renal failure include patients with any degree of pre-existing renal insufficiency, diabetes mellitus, older than 65 years of age, volume depletion, sepsis, paraproteinemia, or patients receiving known nephrotoxic drugs. Especially in such patients, IGIV products should be administered at the minimum concentration available and the minimum rate of infusion practicable. While these reports of renal dysfunction and acute renal failure have been associated with the use of many of the licensed IGIV products, those containing sucrose as stabilizer accounted for a disproportionate share of the total number.

Indications

➤*Primary immune deficiency diseases:* For the treatment of primary immune deficient diseases, such as congenital agammaglobulinemia and hypogammaglobulinemia, common variable immunodeficiency, Wiskott-Aldrich syndrome, and severe combined immunodeficiencies.

➤*Unlabeled uses:* Posttransfusion purpura, Guillain-Barré syndrome, and chronic inflammatory demyelinating polyneuropathy (as an alternative to plasma exchange). IGIV is being investigated in the prevention or treatment of the following diseases: Autoimmune diseases (eg, rhesus hemolytic disease, Factor VIII deficiencies, bullous pemphigoid, rheumatoid arthritis, Sjogren syndrome, type 1 diabetes mellitus), IgG_4 subclass deficiencies, intractable epilepsy (possibly caused by IgG_2 subclass deficiency), cystic fibrosis, trauma, thermal injury (eg, severe burns), cytomegalovirus infection, neuromuscular disorders, prophylaxis of infections associated with bone marrow transplantation, and GI protection (ie, oral administration).

Administration and Dosage

➤*Approved by the FDA:* May 21, 2004.

➤*Primary immunodeficiency diseases:* As there are significant differences in the half-life of IgG among patients with primary immunodeficiencies, the frequency and amount of immunoglobulin therapy may vary from patient to patient. The proper amount can be determined by monitoring clinical response.

The usual dose for replacement therapy in primary immunodeficiency diseases is 300 to 600 mg/kg body weight administered every 3 to 4 weeks. Doses may be adjusted over time to achieve the desired trough levels and clinical responses.

➤*Rate of administration:* It is recommended that a 5% solution be initially infused at a rate of 30 mg/kg/hour for the first 30 minutes; if tolerated, advance to 60 mg/kg/hour for the second 30 minutes; and if further tolerated, advance to 120 mg/kg/hour for the third 30 minutes. Thereafter the infusion can be maintained at a rate up to, but not exceeding, 200 mg/kg/hour.

➤*Renal function impairment:* For patients judged to be at risk for developing renal dysfunction, it may be prudent to reduce the amount of product infused per unit time by infusing IGIV (human) 5%, *Octagam*, at a maximum rate less than 0.07 mL/kg (3.3 mg/kg)/minute (200 mg/kg/hour).

➤*Infusion rate:* Certain severe adverse drug reactions may be related to the rate of infusion. Slowing or stopping the infusion usually allows the symptoms to disappear promptly.

Rate of administration	mg/kg/hour	mL/kg/min
First 30 min	30	0.01
Next 30 min	60	0.02
Next 30 min	120	0.04
Maximum	< 200	< 0.07

➤*Admixture incompatibility:* Admixtures of IGIV (human) 5%, *Octagam*, with other drugs and intravenous solutions have not been evaluated. It is recommended that IGIV (human) 5%, *Octagam*, be administered separately from other drugs or medications that the patient may be receiving. Do not mix the product with IGIVs from other manufacturers.

➤*Lab test abnormalities:* Various passively transferred antibodies in immunoglobulin preparations can confound the results of serological testing.

IGIV (human) 5%, *Octagam*, contains maltose, which could interfere with blood and urine glucose tests.

➤*Administration:* IGIV (human) 5%, *Octagam*, should be at room temperature during administration.

Use any vial that has been entered promptly. Discard partially used vials.

➤*Storage/Stability:* IGIV (human) 5%, *Octagam*, may be stored for 24 months at 2° to 8°C (36° to 46°F) or may be stored at temperatures not to exceed 25°C (77°F) for up to 18 months from the date of manufacture.

IMMUNE GLOBULIN INTRAVENOUS (HUMAN) — INTRAVENOUS (*GAMMAGARD LIQUID*)

For complete and comparative prescribing information, refer to the Immune Globulins group monograph.

WARNING

Immune globulin intravenous (human) (IGIV) products have been reported to be associated with renal dysfunction, acute renal failure, osmotic nephrosis, and death. Patients predisposed to acute renal failure include patients with any degree of preexisting renal insufficiency, diabetes mellitus, volume depletion, sepsis, or paraproteinemia; patients older than 65 years of age; or patients receiving known nephrotoxic drugs. Especially in such patients, administer IGIV products at the minimum concentration available and the minimum rate of infusion practicable. While these reports of renal dysfunction and acute renal failure have been associated with the use of many of the licensed IGIV products, those containing sucrose as a stabilizer accounted for a disproportionate share of the total number. Glycine, an amino acid, is used as a stabilizer. *Gammagard Liquid* does not contain sucrose.

Indications

➤*Primary immunodeficiency:* For the treatment of primary immunodeficiency disorders associated with defects in humoral immunity. These include, but are not limited to, congenital X-linked agammaglobulinemia, common variable immunodeficiency, Wiskott-Aldrich syndrome, and severe combined immunodeficiencies.

➤*Unlabeled uses:* Treatment of posttransfusion purpura, Guillain-Barré syndrome, and chronic inflammatory demyelinating polyneuropathy (as an alternative to plasma exchange). IGIV is being investigated in the prevention or treatment of the following diseases: autoimmune diseases (eg, rhesus hemolytic disease, factor VIII deficiencies, bullous pemphigoid, rheumatoid arthritis, Sjogren syndrome, type 1 diabetes mellitus), immunoglobulin G4 (IgG4) subclass deficiencies, intractable epilepsy (possibly caused by IgG2 subclass deficiency), cystic fibrosis, trauma, thermal injury (eg, severe burns), cytomegalovirus infection, neuromuscular disorders, prophylaxis of infections associated with bone marrow transplantation, and GI protection (oral administration).

Administration and Dosage

➤*Approved by the FDA:* April 27, 2005.

➤*Administration: Gammagard Liquid* should be at room temperature during administration.

Parenteral drug products should be inspected visually for particulate matter and discoloration prior to administration. Do not use if particulate matter and/or discoloration is observed. Only clear or slightly opalescent and colorless or pale yellow solutions are to be administered. *Gammagard Liquid* should only be administered IV. Other routes of administration have not been evaluated. The use of an in-line filter is optional.

➤*Dosage:* For patients with primary immunodeficiency, monthly doses of approximately 300 to 600 mg/kg infused at 3- to 4-week intervals are commonly used. As there are significant differences in the half-life of IgG among patients with primary immunodeficiency, the frequency and amount of immunoglobulin therapy may vary from patient to patient. The proper amount can be determined by monitoring clinical response. The minimum serum concentration of IgG necessary for protection varies among patients and has not been established by controlled clinical studies.

➤*Infusion rates:* During the first infusion of the phase 3 clinical study, *Gammagard Liquid* was infused at an initial rate of 0.5 mL/kg/h (0.8 mg/kg/min). The rate was gradually increased every 30 minutes to a rate of 5 mL/kg/h (8.9 mg/kg/min) if it was well tolerated. However, some patients completed the infusion before the maximum rate could be obtained. During subsequent infusions the initial rate and the rate of escalation were based on their previous infusion history; however, the maximum rate attained during the first infusion was used throughout the remainder of the study. The mean rate attained by all patients was 4.3 mL/kg/h. Fifty-eight subjects (95%) achieved a maximum rate of 4 mL/kg/h or greater and of these, 16 subjects (26%) attained a rate of 5 mL/kg/h.

In general, it is recommended that patients beginning therapy with IGIV or switching from one IGIV product to another be started at the lower rates and then advanced to the maximal rate if they have tolerated several infusions at intermediate rates of infusion. It is important to individualize rates for each patient.

Special populations – Patients who have underlying renal disease or who are judged to be at risk of developing thrombotic events should not be infused rapidly with any IGIV product. Although there are no prospective studies demonstrating that any concentration or rate of infusion is completely safe, it is believed that risk is decreased at lower rates of infusion. Therefore, as a guideline, it is recommended that these patients who are judged to be at risk of renal dysfunction or thrombotic complications be gradually titrated up to a more conservative maximal rate of less than 3.3 mg IgG/kg/min (less than 2 mL/kg/h).

Adverse reactions – A rate of administration that is too rapid may cause flushing and changes in pulse rate and blood pressure. Slowing or stopping the infusion usually results in the prompt disappearance of signs. The infusion may then be resumed at a rate that is comfortable for the patient.

➤*Drug interactions:* Antibodies in IGIV products may interfere with patient responses to live vaccines, such as those for measles, mumps, and rubella. The immunizing health care provider should be informed of recent therapy with IGIV products so that appropriate precautions can be taken.

➤*Admixture incompatibilities:* Admixtures of *Gammagard Liquid* with other drugs and IV solutions have not been evaluated. It is recommended that *Gammagard Liquid* be administered separately from other drugs or medications that the patient may be receiving. The product should not be mixed with IGIV products from other manufacturers.

Normal saline should not be used as a diluent. If dilution is preferred, *Gammagard Liquid* may be diluted with 5% dextrose in water. No other drug interactions or compatibilities have been evaluated.

➤*Storage / Stability:*

Refrigeration – May be refrigerated for 36 months at 2° to 8°C (36° to 46°F). Do not freeze.

Room temperature – May be stored for 9 months at room temperature, 25°C (77°F), within the first 24 months of the date of manufacture. See prescribing information for detailed storage information. The total storage time of *Gammagard Liquid* depends on the point of time the vial is transferred to room temperature. The new expiration date must be recorded on the package when the product is transferred to room temperature.

IMMUNE GLOBULIN (HUMAN) — INTRAVENOUS (*GAMUNEX*)

For complete and comparative prescribing information, refer to the Immune Globulins group monograph.

WARNING

Immune globulin intravenous (IGIV) (human) products have been reported to be associated with renal dysfunction, acute renal failure, osmotic nephrosis, and death. Patients predisposed to acute renal failure include patients with any degree of pre-existing renal insufficiency, diabetes mellitus, patients older than 65 years of age, volume depletion, sepsis, paraproteinemia, or patients receiving known nephrotoxic drugs. Especially in such patients, administer IGIV products at the minimum concentration available and the minimum rate of infusion practicable. While these reports of renal dysfunction and acute renal failure have been associated with the use of many of the licensed IGIV products, those containing sucrose as a stabilizer accounted for a disproportionate share of the total number. *Gamunex* does not contain sucrose. Glycine, a natural amino acid, is used as a stabilizer.

Indications

➤*Primary humoral immunodeficiency (PI):* As replacement therapy of primary immunodeficiency states in which severe impairment of antibody forming capacity has been shown, such as congenital agammaglobulinemia, common variable immunodeficiency, X-linked immunodeficiency with hyper IgM, Wiskott-Aldrich syndrome, and severe combined immunodeficiencies.

➤*Idiopathic thrombocytopenic purpura (ITP):* In idiopathic thrombocytopenic purpura to rapidly raise platelet counts to prevent bleeding or to allow a patient with ITP to undergo surgery.

➤*Unlabeled uses:* Posttransfusion purpura, Guillain-Barré syndrome, and chronic inflammatory demyelinating polyneuropathy (as an alternative to plasma exchange). IGIV is being investigated in the prevention or treatment of the following diseases: Autoimmune diseases (eg, rhesus hemolytic disease, Factor VIII deficiencies, bullous pemphigoid, rheumatoid arthritis, Sjogren syndrome, type 1 diabetes mellitus), IgG_4 subclass deficiencies, intractable epilepsy (possibly caused by IgG_2 subclass deficiency), cystic fibrosis, trauma, thermal injury (eg, severe burns), cytomegalovirus infection, neuromuscular disorders, prophylaxis of infections associated with bone marrow transplantation, and GI protection (ie, oral administration).

Administration and Dosage

➤*Approved by the FDA:* August 27, 2003.

➤*Renal function impairment:* For patients judged to be at increased risk for developing renal dysfunction, it may be prudent to reduce the amount of product infused per unit time by infusing *Gamunex* at a rate less than 8 mg/kg/min (0.08 mL/kg/min). No prospective data are currently available to identify a maximum safe dose, concentration, and rate of infusion in patients determined to be at increased risk of acute renal failure. In the absence of prospective data, recommended doses should not be exceeded and the concentration and infusion rate should be the minimum level practicable. Reduction in dose, concentration, and/or rate of administration in patients at risk of acute renal failure has been proposed in the literature in order to reduce the risk of acute renal failure.

➤*PI: Gamunex* doses between 300 and 600 mg/kg (3 and 6 mL/kg), which represented the dose range for 92% of the subjects in the therapeutic equivalence trial (100175), may be used for infection prophylaxis. The dose should be individualized taking into account dosing intervals (eg, 3 or 4 weeks) and the *Gamunex* dose (between 300 and 600 mg/kg). A target serum IgG trough level (ie, prior to the next infusion) of at least 5 g/L has been proposed in the literature; however, no randomized controlled trial data are available to validate this recommendation. In a clinical trial with 73 subjects with primary immune deficiencies, treated for 9 months with *Gamunex*, the relationship of validated infections and serum IgG levels at trough are shown in the table below:

IMMUNE GLOBULIN (HUMAN) — INTRAVENOUS (*GAMUNEX*)

Average serum IgG levels (g/L) before next *Gamunex* infusion (at trough)[1]		
Average serum IgG levels (g/L)	Number of subjects with validated infections	Number of subjects with any infection (validated plus clinically defined non-validated infections of any organ system)
	Gamunex	*Gamunex*
≤ 7	3/22 (14%)	19/22 (86%)
> 7 and ≤ 9	5/33 (15%)	24/33 (73%)
> 9	1/18 (6%)	13/18 (72%)
Cochran-Armitage Trend Test	P = 0.46 (NS)	P = 0.27 (NS)

[1] NS = Non-significant.

➤*ITP:* A total dose of 2 g/kg, divided in 2 doses of 1 g/kg (10 mL/kg) given on 2 consecutive days or into 5 doses of 0.4 g/kg (4 mL/kg) given on 5 consecutive days. If after administration of the first of 2 daily 1 g/kg (10 mL/kg) doses, an adequate increase in the platelet count is observed at 24 hours, the second dose of 1 g/kg body weight may be withheld.

Forty-eight ITP subjects were treated with 2 g/kg *Gamunex*, divided in two 1 g/kg doses (10 mL/kg) given on 2 successive days. With this dose regimen, 35/39 subjects (90%) responded with a platelet count from less than or equal to 20 × 10^9/L to more than or equal to 50 × 10^9/L within 7 days after treatment.

The high dose regimen (1 g/kg × 1 to 2 days) is not recommended for individuals with expanded fluid volumes or where fluid volume may be a concern.

➤*Incompatibility: Gamunex* is not compatible with saline. If dilution is required, *Gamunex* may be diluted with 5% dextrose in water (D5/W). No other drug interactions or compatibilities have been evaluated.

➤*Needle gauge:* It is recommended that *Gamunex* should initially be infused at a rate of 0.01 mL/kg per minute (1 mg/kg per minute) for the first 30 minutes. If well tolerated, the rate may be gradually increased to a maximum of 0.08 mL/kg per minute (8 mg/kg per minute). If side effects occur, the rate may be reduced, or the infusion interrupted until symptoms subside. The infusion may then be resumed at the rate which is comfortable for the patient.

Only 18 gauge needles should be used to penetrate the stopper for dispensing product from 10 mL vial sizes; 16 gauge needles or dispensing pins should only be used with 25 mL vial sizes and larger. Needles or dispensing pins should only be inserted within the stopper area delineated by the raised ring. The stopper should be penetrated perpendicular to the plane of the stopper within the ring.

Gamunex vial size	Gauge of needle to penetrate stopper
10 mL	18 gauge
25, 50, 100, 200 mL	16 gauge

➤*Infusion bags:* Content of vials may be pooled under aseptic conditions into sterile infusion bags and infused within 8 hours after pooling.

➤*Admixture incompatibility:* It is recommended to infuse *Gamunex* using a separate line by itself, without mixing with other intravenous fluids or medications the patient might be receiving.

➤*Storage/Stability: Gamunex* may be stored for 36 months at 2° to 8°C (36° to 46°F), and product may be stored at temperatures not to exceed 25°C (77°F) for up to 5 months during the first 18 months from date of manufacture, after which the product must be immediately used or discarded. Do not freeze.

IMMUNE GLOBULIN (HUMAN) — INTRAVENOUS (*POLYGAM SD*)

For complete and comparative prescribing information, refer to the Immune Globulins group monograph.

WARNING

Immune globulin intravenous (human) products have been reported to be associated with renal dysfunction, acute renal failure, osmotic nephrosis, and death. Patients predisposed to acute renal failure include patients with any degree of preexisting renal insufficiency, diabetes mellitus, age greater than 65 years, volume depletion, sepsis, paraproteinemia, or patients receiving known nephrotoxic drugs. Especially in such patients, IGIV products should be administered at the minimum concentration available and the minimum rate of infusion practicable. While these reports of renal dysfunction and acute renal failure have been associated with the use of many of the licensed IGIV products, those containing sucrose as a stabilizer accounted for a disproportionate share of the total number. *Polygam S/D* does not contain sucrose.

This product is derived from blood collected from volunteer donors.

Indications

➤*Primary immunodeficiency diseases:* For the treatment of primary immunodeficient states, such as: Congenital agammaglobulinemia, common variable immunodeficiency, Wiskott-Aldrich syndrome, and severe combined immunodeficiencies.

Polygam S/D is especially useful when high levels or rapid elevation of circulating IgG are desired or when intramuscular injections are contraindicated (eg, small muscle mass).

➤*B-cell chronic lymphocytic leukemia (CLL):* For prevention of bacterial infections in patients with hypogammaglobulinemia and/or recurrent bacterial infections associated with B-cell chronic lymphocytic leukemia (CLL).

➤*Idiopathic thrombocytopenic purpura (ITP):* When a rapid rise in platelet count is needed to prevent and/or to control bleeding in a patient with idiopathic thrombocytopenic purpura, the administration of *Polygam S/D* should be considered.

➤*Kawasaki syndrome:* For the prevention of coronary artery aneurysms associated with Kawasaki syndrome.

➤*Unlabeled uses:* Posttransfusion purpura, Guillain-Barré syndrome, and chronic inflammatory demyelinating polyneuropathy (as an alternative to plasma exchange). IGIV is being investigated in the prevention or treatment of the following diseases: Autoimmune diseases (eg, rhesus hemolytic disease, Factor VIII deficiencies, bullous pemphigoid, rheumatoid arthritis, Sjogren syndrome, type 1 diabetes mellitus), IgG_4 subclass deficiencies, intractable epilepsy (possibly caused by IgG_2 subclass deficiency), cystic fibrosis, trauma, thermal injury (eg, severe burns), cytomegalovirus infection, neuromuscular disorders, prophylaxis of infections associated with bone marrow transplantation, and GI protection (ie, oral administration).

Administration and Dosage

➤*Primary immunodeficiency diseases:* Monthly doses of at least 100 mg/kg are recommended. Initially, patients may receive 200 to 400 mg/kg. As there are significant differences in the half-life of IgG among patients with primary immunodeficiencies, the frequency and amount of immunoglobulin therapy may vary from patient to patient. The proper amount can be determined by monitoring clinical response. The minimum serum concentration of IgG necessary for protection has not been established.

➤*B-cell CLL:* For patients with hypogammaglobulinemia and/or recurrent bacterial infections due to B-cell chronic lymphocytic leukemia, a dose of 400 mg/kg every 3 to 4 weeks is recommended.

➤*Kawasaki syndrome:* Either a single 1 g/kg dose or a dose of 400 mg/kg for 4 consecutive days beginning within 7 days of the onset of fever, administered concomitantly with appropriate aspirin therapy (80 to 100 mg/kg/day in 4 divided doses) is recommended.

➤*ITP:* 1 g/kg is recommended. The need for additional doses can be determined by clinical response and platelet count. Up to 3 separate doses may be given on alternate days if required.

No prospective data are presently available to identify a maximum safe dose, concentration, and rate of infusion in patients determined to be at increased risk of acute renal failure. In the absence of prospective data, recommended doses should not be exceeded and the concentration and infusion rate selected should be the minimum level practicable. Reduction in dose, concentration, or rate of administration in patients at risk of acute renal failure has been proposed in the literature in order to reduce the risk of acute renal failure.

➤*Reconstitution:* Use aseptic technique. When reconstitution is performed aseptically outside of a sterile laminar air flow hood, administration should begin as soon as possible, but not more than 2 hours after reconstitution.

When reconstitution is performed aseptically in a sterile laminar air flow hood, the reconstituted product may be either maintained in the original glass container or pooled into *Viaflex* bags and stored under constant refrigeration (2° to 8°C [35.6° to 46.4°F]), for up to 24 hours. (The date and time of reconstitution/pooling should be recorded.) If these conditions are not met, sterility of the reconstituted product cannot be maintained. Partially used vials should be discarded.

5% solution –

1.) Note: Reconstitute immediately before use.
2.) If refrigerated, warm the Sterile Water for Injection (diluent) and immune globulin IV (human), *Polygam S/D* (dried concentrate), to room temperature.
3.) Remove caps from concentrate and diluent bottles to expose central portion of rubber stoppers.
4.) Cleanse stoppers with germicidal solution.
5.) Remove protective covering from the spike at one end of the transfer device.
6.) Note: Invert the diluent bottle with attached transfer device rapidly into the concentrate bottle in order to avoid loss of diluent. Caution: Failure to use center of stopper may result in dislodging the stopper and loss of vacuum.
7.) The diluent will flow into the concentrate bottle quickly. When diluent transfer is complete, remove empty diluent bottle and transfer device from concentrate bottle. Discard transfer device after single use.
8.) Thoroughly wet the dried material by tilting or inverting and gently rotating the bottle. Do not shake. Avoid foaming.
9.) Repeat gentle rotation as long as undissolved product is observed.

10% solution – Follow steps 1 to 4 as previously described above. To prepare a 10% solution, reconstitute with the appropriate volume of diluent as indicated in the table below, which indicates the volume of diluent required for 5% or 10% concentration. Using aseptic technique, draw the required volume of diluent into a sterile hypodermic syringe and needle. Discard the filled syringe. Using the residual diluent in the diluent vial, follow steps 5 to 12 as previously described in A.

IMMUNE GLOBULIN (HUMAN) — INTRAVENOUS (*POLYGAM SD*)

Required diluent volume			
Concentration	2.5 g bottle	5 g bottle	10 g bottle
5%	50 mL	96 mL	192 mL
10%	25 mL	48 mL	96 mL

➤*Rate of administration:* It is recommended that initially a 5% solution be infused at a rate of 0.5 mL/kg/hr. If infusion at this rate and concentration causes the patient no distress, the administration rate may be gradually increased to a maximum rate of 4 mL/kg/hr. Patients who tolerate the 5% concentration at 4 mL/kg/hr can be infused with the 10% concentration starting at 0.5 mL/kg/hr. If no adverse effects occur, the rate can be increased gradually up to a maximum of 8 mL/kg/hr. For patients judged to be at risk for developing renal dysfunction, it may be prudent to reduce the amount of product infused per unit time by infusing immune globulin intravenous (human), *Polygam S/D*, at a rate less than 4 mL/kg/hr (less than 3.3 mg IG/kg/min) for a 5% solution or at a rate of less than 2 mL/kg/hr (less than 3.3 mg IG/kg/min) for a 10% solution.

It is recommended that antecubital veins be used especially for 10% solutions, if possible. This may reduce the likelihood of the patient experiencing discomfort at the infusion site.

A rate of administration which is too rapid may cause flushing and changes in pulse rate and blood pressure. Slowing or stopping the infusion usually allows the symptoms to disappear promptly.

➤*Admixture incompatibility:* Admixtures of immune globulin intravenous (human), *Polygam S/D*, with other drugs and intravenous solutions have not been evaluated. It is recommended that *Polygam S/D* be administered separately from other drugs or medications which the patient may be receiving. The product should not be mixed with immune globulin intravenous (human) from other manufacturers.

➤*Live vaccines:* Antibodies in immune globulin preparations may interfere with patient responses to live vaccines, such as those for measles, mumps, and rubella. The immunizing physician should be informed of recent therapy with immune globulin intravenous (human) so that appropriate precautions can be taken.

➤*Administration: Polygam S/D* should be administered as soon after reconstitution as possible, or as described above.

The reconstituted material should be at room temperature during administration.

Follow directions for use which accompany the administration set provided. If another administration set is used, ensure that the set contains a similar filter.

➤*Storage/Stability: Polygam S/D* is to be stored at a temperature not to exceed 25°C (77°F). Freezing should be avoided to prevent the diluent bottle from breaking.

IMMUNE GLOBULIN (HUMAN) — INTRAVENOUS (*CARIMUNE* AND *CARIMUNE NF*)

For complete and comparative prescribing information, refer to the Immune Globulins group monograph.

WARNING

Immune globulin intravenous (human) (IGIV) products have been reported to be associated with renal dysfunction, acute renal failure, osmotic nephrosis, and death. Patients predisposed to acute renal failure include patients with:
1.) Any degree of preexisting renal insufficiency.
2.) Diabetes mellitus.
3.) Age greater than 65 years.
4.) Volume depletion.
5.) Sepsis.
6.) Paraproteinemia.
7.) Patients receiving known nephrotoxic drugs.

In such patients, IGIV products should be administered at the minimum concentration available and the minimum rate of infusion practicable. While these reports of renal dysfunction and acute renal failure have been associated with the use of many of the licensed IGIV products, those containing sucrose as a stabilizer accounted for a disproportionate share of the total number.

Indications

➤*Immunodeficiency:* For the maintenance treatment of patients with primary immunodeficiencies (PID) (eg, common variable immunodeficiency, X-linked agammaglobulinemia, severe combined immunodeficiency). *Carimune* or *Carimune NF* is preferable to intramuscular immune globulin IV (human) preparations in treating patients who require an immediate and large increase in the intravascular immunoglobulin level, in patients with limited muscle mass, and in patients with bleeding tendencies for whom intramuscular injections are contraindicated. The infusions must be repeated at regular intervals.

➤*Immune thrombocytopenic purpura (ITP):*

Acute –

Carimune has been used with good results in the treatment of acute ITP in adult patients.

Chronic – Children and adults with chronic (defined as greater than 6 months duration) ITP have also shown an increase (sometimes temporary) in platelet counts upon administration of immune globulin IV (human) (*Carimune*). Therefore, in situations that require a rapid rise in platelet count, for example prior to surgery or to control excessive bleeding, use of *Carimune* should be considered.

➤*Unlabeled uses:* Posttransfusion purpura, Guillain-Barré syndrome, and chronic inflammatory demyelinating polyneuropathy (as an alternative to plasma exchange). IGIV is being investigated in the prevention or treatment of the following diseases: Autoimmune diseases (eg, rhesus hemolytic disease, Factor VIII deficiencies, bullous pemphigoid, rheumatoid arthritis, Sjogren syndrome, type 1 diabetes mellitus), IgG_4 subclass deficiencies, intractable epilepsy (possibly caused by IgG_2 subclass deficiency), cystic fibrosis, trauma, thermal injury (eg, severe burns), cytomegalovirus infection, neuromuscular disorders, prophylaxis of infections associated with bone marrow transplantation, and GI protection (ie, oral administration).

Administration and Dosage

➤*Admixture incompatibility:* It is generally advisable not to dilute plasma derivatives with other infusable drugs. Immune globulin IV (human) (*Carimune* or *Carimune NF*) should be given by a separate infusion line. No other medications or fluids should be mixed with *Carimune* or *Carimune NF* preparation.

➤*Renal function impairment: Carimune* or *Carimune NF* should be used with caution in patients with preexisting renal insufficiency and in patients judged to be at increased risk of developing renal insufficiency (including, but not limited to those with diabetes mellitus, age greater than 65 years, volume depletion, paraproteinemia, sepsis, and patients receiving known nephrotoxic drugs). In these cases especially it is important to assure that patients are not volume depleted prior to *Carimune* or *Carimune NF* infusion. No prospective data are presently available to identify a maximum safe dose, concentration, and rate of infusion in patients determined to be at increased risk of acute renal failure. In the absence of prospective data, recommended doses should not be exceeded and the concentration and infusion rate selected should be the minimum practicable. The product should be infused at a rate less than 2 mg/kg/min.

➤*Adult and child substitution therapy:* The usual dose of*Carimune* or *Carimune NF* in immunodeficiency syndromes is 0.2 g/kg of body weight administered once a month by IV infusion. If the clinical response is inadequate, the dose may be increased to 0.3 g/kg of body weight or the infusion may be repeated more frequently than once a month.

The first infusion of *Carimune* or *Carimune NF* in previously untreated agammaglobulinemic or hypogammaglobulinemic patients must be given as a 3% immunoglobulin solution (use the total volume of fluid provided, or see the table below, to reconstitute the lyophilized product).
1.) Start with a flow rate of 10 to 20 drops (0.5 to 1 mL) per minute.
2.) After 15 to 30 minutes the rate of infusion may be further increased to 30 to 50 drops (1.5 to 2.5 mL) per minute.
3.) After the first bottle of 3% solution is infused and the patient shows good tolerance, subsequent infusions may be administered at a higher rate or concentration. Such increases should be made gradually allowing 15 to 30 minutes before each increment.

The first infusion of *Carimune* or *Carimune NF* in previously untreated agammaglobulinemic and hypogammaglobulinemic patients may lead to systemic side effects. The nature of these effects has not been fully elucidated. Some of them may be due to the release of proinflammatory cytokines by activated macrophages in immunodeficient recipients. Subsequent administration of *Carimune* or *Carimune NF* to immunodeficient patients as well as to healthy individuals usually does not cause further untoward side effects.

➤*Therapy of idiopathic thrombocytopenic purpura (ITP):*

Induction – 0.4 g/kg of body weight on 2 to 5 consecutive days.

Acute ITP - childhood – If an initial platelet count response to the first 2 doses is adequate (30,000 to 50,000/mcL), therapy may be discontinued after the second day of the 5-day course.

Maintenance - chronic ITP – In adults and children, if after induction therapy the platelet count falls to less than 30,000/mcL and/or the patient manifests clinically significant bleeding, 0.4 g/kg of body weight may be given as a single infusion. If an adequate response does not result, the dose can be increased to 0.8 to 1 g/kg of body weight given as a single infusion.

➤*Reconstitution:*

Carimune –

For a 3% solution using the transfer set:
1.) Tear off the protective caps from the bottle containing the solvent and the immune globulin IV (human) (*Carimune*). Disinfect both rubber stoppers with alcohol.
2.) Remove the protective cover from 1 end of the transfer set and insert the needle through the rubber stopper into the bottle containing the solvent.
3.) Remove the cover from the other needle and plunge the inverted *Carimune* bottle onto it.
4.) Invert the 2 bottles so that the solvent flows into the *Carimune* bottle until the required amount has been transferred.
5.) Discard any unused solvent and the transfer set.

For a 6% solution using the transfer set:
1.) Follow steps 1 through 3, aforementioned.
2.) Invert the 2 bottles so that the solvent flows into the *Carimune* bottle. Use the appropriate amount of solvent by removing the solvent bottle with transfer needle as soon as the fluid reaches the 6% mark printed on the *Carimune* label.
3.) Discard any unused solvent and the transfer set.

IMMUNE GLOBULIN (HUMAN) — INTRAVENOUS (*CARIMUNE* AND *CARIMUNE NF*)

Carimune NF –

1.) Remove the protective plastic caps from the lyophilisate and diluent bottles and disinfect both rubber stoppers with alcohol. Remove the protective cover from one end of the transfer set and insert the exposed needle through the rubber stopper into the bottle containing the diluent.
2.) Remove the second protective cover from the other end of the transfer set. Grasp both bottles, quickly plunge the diluent bottle onto the lyophilisate bottle and bring the bottles into an upright position. Only if this is done quickly and the bottles are immediately brought into an upright position can the vacuum in the lyophilisate bottle be maintained, thus speeding up reconstitution and facilitating the transfer. Allow the diluent to flow into the lyophilisate bottle.
3.) Once the appropriate amount of diluent is transferred, lift the diluent bottle off the spike to release the vacuum. This will reduce foaming and facilitate dissolution. Remove the spike.
4.) Swirl vigorously but do not shake, otherwise a foam will form which is very slow to subside. The lyophilisate dissolves within a few minutes.
   To reconstitute *Carimune* or *Carimune NF* from the individual vial package, or when using other diluents or higher concentrations, the table below indicates the volume of sterile diluent required. Observing aseptic technique, this volume should be drawn into a sterile hypodermic syringe and needle. The diluent is then injected into the corresponding *Carimune* or *Carimune NF* vial size.

Required diluent volume*				
	1 g	3 g	6 g	12 g
Concentration	Vial	Vial	Vial	Vial
3%	33 mL	100 mL	200 mL	**
6%	16.5 mL	50 mL	100 mL	200 mL
9%	11 mL	33 mL	66 mL	132 mL
12%	8.3 mL	25 mL	50 mL	100 mL

* In patients judged to be at increased risk of developing renal insufficiency, the concentration and infusion rate of *Carimune* or *Carimune NF* should be the minimum practicable.
** Container not large enough to permit this concentration.

If large doses of *Carimune* or *Carimune NF* are to be administered, several reconstituted vials of identical concentration and diluent may be pooled in an empty sterile glass or plastic IV infusion container using aseptic technique. *Carimune* or *Carimune NF* normally dissolves within a few minutes, though in exceptional cases it may take up to 20 minutes.

Do not shake. Excessive shaking will cause foaming. Any undissolved particles should respond to careful rotation of the bottle. Avoid foaming. Parenteral drug products should be inspected visually for particulate matter and discoloration prior to administration, whenever solution and container permit. Filtering of *Carimune* or *Carimune NF* is acceptable but not required. Pore sizes of 15 microns or larger will be less likely to slow infusion, especially with higher *Carimune* or *Carimune NF* concentrations. Antibacterial filters (0.2 microns) may be used. When reconstitution of *Carimune* or *Carimune NF* occurs outside of sterile laminar air flow conditions, administration must begin promptly with partially used vials discarded. When reconstitution is carried out in a sterile laminar flow hood using aseptic technique, administration may begin within 24 hours provided the solution has been refrigerated during that time. Do not freeze *Carimune* or *Carimune NF* solution.

Proceed with infusion only if solution is clear and at approximately room temperature.

➤*Storage/Stability:* Store at room temperature not exceeding 30°C (86°F). Use promptly after reconstitution.

IMMUNE GLOBULIN (HUMAN) — INTRAVENOUS (*IVEEGAM EN*)

For complete and comparative prescribing information, refer to the Immune Globulins group monograph.

WARNING

Immune globulin intravenous (IGIV) (human) products have been reported to be associated with renal dysfunction, acute renal failure, osmotic nephrosis, and death. Patients predisposed to acute renal failure include patients with any degree of pre-existing renal insufficiency, diabetes mellitus, patients older than 65 years of age, volume depletion, sepsis, paraproteinemia, or patients receiving known nephrotoxic drugs. Especially in such patients, administer IGIV products at the minimum concentration available and the minimum rate of infusion practicable. While these reports of renal dysfunction and acute renal failure have been associated with the use of many of the licensed IGIV products, those containing sucrose as a stabilizer accounted for a disproportionate share of the total number. *Iveegam EN* does not contain sucrose.

Indications

➤*Immunodeficiency syndromes:* For replacement therapy in patients with primary immunodeficiency syndromes such as congenital agammaglobulinemia, common variable immunodeficiency, x-linked agammaglobulinemia (with or without hyper IgM) and Wiskott-Aldrich syndrome.

Patients with severe combined immunodeficiency have, in addition to a T-cell defect, an impairment of antibody production. They may benefit from replacement therapy with immune globulin intravenous (human) even through this therapy will not correct the cellular immune defect.

Immune globulin intravenous (human) is especially useful when high levels or rapid elevation of circulating antibodies are desired or when intramuscular injections are contraindicated.

➤*Kawasaki syndrome:* In the treatment of Kawasaki syndrome.

➤*Unlabeled uses:* Posttransfusion purpura, Guillain-Barre syndrome, and chronic inflammatory demyelinating polyneuropathy (as an alternative to plasma exchange). IGIV is being investigated in the prevention or treatment of the following diseases: Autoimmune diseases (eg, rhesus hemolytic disease, Factor VIII deficiencies, bullous pemphigoid, rheumatoid arthritis, Sjogren syndrome, type 1 diabetes mellitus), IgG_4 subclass deficiencies, intractable epilepsy (possibly caused by IgG_2 subclass deficiency), cystic fibrosis, trauma, thermal injury (eg, severe burns), cytomegaloviris infection, neuromuscular disorders, prophylaxis of infections associated with bone marrow transplantation, and GI protection (ie, oral administration).

Administration and Dosage

➤*Admixture compatibility/incompatibility:* Reconstitute immune globulin intravenous (human), with Sterile Water for injection only. The reconstituted product may be diluted with 5% dextrose or saline.

Interactions or incompatibilities with other drugs have not been evaluated.

Do not mix immune globulin intravenous (human) with other brands of intravenous immunoglobulins in preparing a large dose.

If administered with other preparations, always use separate infusion lines. When using primary infusion lines, rinse with saline prior to the infusion of immune globulin intravenous (human).

➤*Administration rate:* Immune globulin intravenous (human), must be administered intravenously after reconstitution. The usual rate of administration is 1 mL/min up to a maximum of 2 mL/min for the 5% solution.

➤*Renal function impairment:* For patients judged to be at risk for developing renal dysfunction, it may be prudent to reduce the amount of product infused per unit time by infusing immune globulin intravenous (human) at a rate less than 1.5 mg Ig per kg body weight per minute (0.03 mL/kg/min).

No prospective data are presently available to identify a maximum safe dose, concentration, and rate of infusion in patients determined to be at increased risk of acute renal failure. In the absence of prospective data, the recommended doses should not be exceeded and the concentration and infusion rate selected should be the minimum level practicable.

➤*Immunodeficiency syndromes:* 200 mg/kg per month is recommended for treatment of primary humoral immunodeficiency syndromes.

If the desired clinical results are not obtained, the dose may be increased up to 4-fold or intervals between infusions shortened. Doses up to 800 mg/kg body mass per month were tolerated by immunodeficient patients.

If adequate doses are given at regular intervals, pre-infusion IgG levels may be expected to rise steadily over a period of 6 to 12 months until a plateau is reached. The minimum serum concentration of IgG necessary for protection has not been established.

Dose regimens have been modified in an attempt to prevent adverse reactions in previously untreated, severe, immunodeficient patients. In a limited number of such patients, treatment has been initiated with lower doses of immune globulin intravenous (human) diluted with saline or 5% dextrose. With gradually increasing dose levels and protein concentrations (up to 5% protein) adverse reactions were not observed.

➤*Kawasaki syndrome:* Initiate within 10 days of onset of the disease. Either a dosage of 400 mg/kg body mass daily for 4 consecutive days or a single dose of 2000 mg/kg given over a 10-hour period may be used. Because all studies of this product, to date, have involved concurrent administration of aspirin, the treatment regimen should include aspirin, 100 mg/kg each day through the 14th day of illness, then 3 to 5 mg/kg each day thereafter for a period of 5 weeks.

➤*Reconstitution:* Reconstitution with Sterile Water for injection (diluent provided in each package results in a 5% solution.

1.) Remove protective caps from the concentrate and diluent bottles and disinfect rubber stoppers of both bottles.
2.) Remove protective covering from 1 end of the accompanying transfer deviceand insert the exposed spike end perpendicularly through the center of the diluent bottle stopper. Press down firmly so that the transfer device fits snugly against the diluent bottle. Caution: Failure to use center of stopper may result in dislodging the stopper.
3.) Remove protective cap from the other end of the transfer device. Do not touch the exposed spike end.
4.) Hold concentrate bottle firmly and at an angle of approximately 45 degrees. Invert the diluent bottle with the transfer device at an angle complementary to the concentrate bottle (approximately 45 degrees) and firmly insert the transfer device into the concentrate bottle through the center of the rubber stopper. Diluent will be drawn into the concentrate bottle by vacuum. Note: Invert the diluent bottle with

IMMUNE GLOBULIN (HUMAN) — INTRAVENOUS (*IVEEGAM EN*)

attached transfer device rapidly into the concentrate bottle in order to avoid loss of diluent. Caution: Failure to use center of stopper may result in dislodging the stopper and loss of vacuum.

5.) Disconnect the 2 bottles, leaving the transfer device on the diluent bottle. Accelerate reconstitution by agitating or rotating the concentrate bottle. Do not shake vigorously.

6.) Either draw up the clear solution into a syringe using the accompanying filter needle (500 mg and 1000 mg sizes) or administer the solution directly using the accompanying infusion set with filter (2500 mg and 5000 mg sizes).

➤*Storage/Stability:* Store at 2° to 8°C (35° to 46°F). Avoid freezing, which may damage the diluent bottle.

IMMUNE GLOBULIN (HUMAN) — INTRAVENOUS (*GAMMAGARD S/D*)

For complete and comparative prescribing information, refer to the Immune Globulins group monograph.

IMMUNE GLOBULIN (HUMAN) — INTRAVENOUS (*GAMMAR-PIV*)

For complete and comparative prescribing information, refer to the Immune Globulins group monograph.

IMMUNE GLOBULIN SUBCUTANEOUS (HUMAN)

Rx	**Vivaglobin** (ZLB Behring LLC)	**Injection**: 16% protein solution, (160 mg/mL)[a]	Preservative free. In 3, 10, and 20 mL single-use vials.

[a] With 2.25% glycine, 0.3% sodium chloride.

IMMUNE GLOBULIN (HUMAN) — SUBCUTANEOUS

Indications

➤*Primary immune deficiency (PID):* For the treatment of patients with PID.

Administration and Dosage

➤*Approved by the FDA:* January 9, 2006.

➤*Dosage:* All subjects who received immune globulin subcutaneous in clinical trials had previously been treated with immune globulin. It is recommended that the patient start treatment with immune globulin subcutaneous 1 week after receiving a regularly scheduled immunoglobulin intravenous (IGIV) infusion.

The initial weekly immune globulin subcutaneous dose can be calculated by multiplying the previous IGIV dose by 1.37, then dividing this dose into weekly doses based on the patient's previous IGIV treatment interval; for example, if IGIV was administered every 3 weeks, divide by 3. This dose of immune globulin subcutaneous will provide a systemic immunoglobulin G (IgG) exposure (area under the curve [AUC]) comparable with that of the previous IGIV treatment. Weekly administration of this dose will lead to stable steady-state serum IgG levels with lower IgG peak levels and higher IgG trough levels compared with monthly IGIV treatment.

The recommended weekly dose of immune globulin subcutaneous is 100 to 200 mg/kg body weight. Doses may be adjusted over time to achieve the desired clinical response and serum IgG levels. As there can be differences in the half-life of IgG among patients with primary immune deficiencies, the dose and dosing interval of immunoglobulin therapy may vary.

➤*Doses and associated IgG levels:* The minimum serum concentration of IgG necessary for protection against infections has not been established in randomized and controlled clinical trials. However, based on clinical experience, a target serum IgG trough level (ie, prior to the next infusion) of at least 500 mg/dL has been proposed in the literature for IGIV therapy.

Serum IgG levels can be sampled at any time during routine weekly treatment. Subjects on immune globulin subcutaneous therapy maintained relatively constant IgG levels, rather than the peak and trough pattern observed with monthly IGIV therapy.

➤*Administration:* Do not inject intravenously (IV). Do not inject into a blood vessel.

In the clinical study with immune globulin subcutaneous, a volume of 15 mL per injection site at a rate of 20 mL per hour per site was not exceeded. Doses over 15 mL were divided and infused into several sites using an infusion pump. Multiple simultaneous injections were enabled by administration tubing and Y-site connection tubing (*CADD-Legacy* pumps were used in the study conducted in the United States and Canada). Injection sites were at least 2 inches apart.

The following areas were used for subcutaneous injection of immune globulin subcutaneous: abdomen, thighs, upper arms, and/or lateral hip. The actual point of injection was changed with each weekly administration.

➤*Instructions for administration:* Prior to use, allow the solution to reach ambient room temperature. Immune globulin subcutaneous should be inspected visually for discoloration and particulate matter prior to administration. Do not shake. The appearance of immune globulin subcutaneous can vary from colorless to light brown. Do not use if the solution is cloudy or has particulates. Check the product expiration date on the vial. Do not use beyond the expiration date.

1.) Use aseptic technique when preparing and administering immune globulin subcutaneous for injection.
2.) Remove the protective cap from the vial to expose the central portion of the rubber stopper.
3.) Wipe the rubber stopper with alcohol and allow to dry.
4.) Using a sterile syringe and needle, prepare to withdraw immune globulin subcutaneous by first injecting air into the vial that is equivalent to the amount of immune globulin subcutaneous to be withdrawn. Then withdraw the desired volume of immune globulin subcutaneous. If multiple vials are required to achieve the desired dose, repeat this step.
5.) Follow the manufacturer's instructions for filling the pump reservoir and preparing the pump, administration tubing, and Y-site connection tubing, if needed. Be sure to prime the administration tubing to ensure that no air is left in the tubing or needle by filling the tubing/needle with immune globulin subcutaneous.
6.) Select the number and location of injection sites depending on the volume of the total dose. Note: In clinical studies with immune globulin subcutaneous, a volume of 15 mL per injection site was not exceeded.
7.) Cleanse the injection sites with antiseptic solution using a circular motion working from the center of the site and moving to the outside. Sites should be clean, dry, and at least 2 inches apart.
8.) Grasp the skin between 2 fingers and insert the needle into the subcutaneous tissue.
9.) Immune globulin subcutaneous must not be injected into a blood vessel. After each needle is inserted into the tissue, test to make sure that a blood vessel has not been accidentally accessed. This must be done prior to starting the infusion. To do this, attach a sterile syringe to the end of the primed administration tubing, gently pull back on the syringe plunger, and look to see if any blood is flowing back into the administration tubing. If you see any blood, remove and discard the needle and administration tubing. Repeat priming and needle insertion steps using a new needle, administration tubing, and infusion site. Secure the needle in place by applying sterile gauze or transparent dressing over the site.
10.) If using multiple, simultaneous injection sites, use Y-site connection tubing and secure to the administration tubing.
11.) Infuse immune globulin subcutaneous following the manufacturer's instructions for the pump.
12.) Remove the peel-off label with the product lot number and expiration date from the immune globulin subcutaneous vial and use this to complete the patient record.

After administration, discard any unused solution and administration equipment in accordance with biohazard procedures. Immune globulin subcutaneous contains no preservative; discard unused product immediately after use.

➤*Home treatment:* If home administration is appropriate, provide the patient with instructions on subcutaneous infusion for home treatment. This should include the type of equipment to be used along with its maintenance, proper infusion techniques, selection of appropriate infusion sites (eg, abdomen, thighs, upper arms, and/or lateral hip), maintenance of a treatment diary, and measures to be taken in case of adverse reactions.

➤*Admixture incompatibility:* Immune globulin subcutaneous must not be mixed with other products.

➤*Storage/Stability:* Store in the refrigerator at 2° to 8°C (36° to 46°F). Do not freeze. Keep vials in storage box until use.

LYMPHOCYTE IMMUNE GLOBULIN, ANTITHYMOCYTE GLOBULIN (EQUINE) (LIG, ATG, ATG equine)

Rx	**Atgam** (Pharmacia)	**Injection:**[a] 50 mg horse gamma globulin/ mL	In 5 mL amps.

[a] With 0.3 M glycine.

LYMPHOCYTE IMMUNE GLOBULIN — INJECTION

For complete and comparative prescribing information, refer to the Immune Globulins group monograph.

WARNING

Only physicians experienced in immunosuppressive therapy in the treatment of renal transplant or aplastic anemia patients should use lymphocyte immune globulin.

Patients receiving lymphocyte immune globulin should be treated in facilities equipped and staffed with adequate laboratory and supportive medical resources.

Indications

➤*Renal transplantation:* For the management of allograft rejection in renal transplant patients. When administered with conventional therapy at the time of rejection, it increases the frequency of resolution of the acute rejection episode. The drug has also been administered as an adjunct to other immunosuppressive therapy to delay the onset of the first rejection episode. Data accumulated to date have not consistently demonstrated improvement in functional graft survival associated with therapy to delay the onset of the first rejection episode.

➤*Aplastic anemia:* For the treatment of moderate-to-severe aplastic anemia in patients who are unsuitable for bone marrow transplantation.

When administered with a regimen of supportive care, lymphocyte immune globulin may induce partial or complete hematologic remission. In a controlled trial, patients receiving lymphocyte immune globulin showed a statistically significantly higher improvement rate compared with standard supportive care at 3 months. Improvement was defined in terms of sustained increase in peripheral blood counts and reduced transfusion needs.

➤*Unlabeled uses:* As an immunosuppressant in the course of liver, bone-marrow, heart, and other organ transplants; treatment of multiple sclerosis, myasthenia gravis, pure red cell aplasia, and scleroderma, although efficacy is not definitively established.

Administration and Dosage

➤*Skin testing:* Before the first infusion of lymphocyte immune globulin, the manufacturer strongly recommends that patients be tested with an intradermal injection of 0.1 mL of a 1:1000 dilution (5 mcg horse IgG) of lymphocyte immune globulin in sodium chloride injection, USP and a contralateral sodium chloride injection control. Use only freshly diluted lymphocyte immune globulin for skin testing. The patient, and specifically the skin test, should be observed every 15 to 20 minutes over the first hour after intradermal injection. A local reaction of ≥ 10 mm with a wheal or erythema, or both, with or without pseudopod formation and itching or a marked local swelling should be considered a positive test.

A systemic reaction such as a generalized rash, tachycardia, dyspnea, hypotension, or anaphylaxis precludes any additional administration of lymphocyte immune globulin.

Note – The predictive value of this test has not been proved clinically. Allergic reactions such as anaphylaxis have occurred in patients whose skin test is negative. In the presence of a locally positive skin test to lymphocyte immune globulin, serious consideration to alternative forms of therapy should be given. The risk to benefit ratio must be carefully weighed. If therapy with lymphocyte immune globulin is deemed appropriate following a locally positive skin test, treatment should be administered in a setting where intensive life support facilities are immediately available and with a physician familiar with the treatment of potentially life-threatening allergic reactions in attendance.

➤*Renal allograft recipients:* Adult renal allograft patients have received lymphocyte immune globulin sterile solution at the dosage of 10 to 30 mg/kg of body weight daily. The few children studied received 5 to 25 mg/kg daily. Lymphocyte immune globulin has been used to delay the onset of the first rejection episode and at the time of the first rejection episode. Most patients who received lymphocyte immune globulin for the treatment of acute rejection had not received it starting at the time of transplantation.

Usually, lymphocyte immune globulin is used concomitantly with azathioprine and corticosteroids, which are commonly used to suppress the immune response. Exercise caution during repeat courses of lymphocyte immune globulin; carefully observe patients for signs of allergic reactions.

Delaying the onset of allograft rejection – Give a fixed dose of 15 mg/kg/day for 14 days, then every other day for 14 days for a total of 21 doses in 28 days. Administer the first dose within 24 hours before or after the transplant.

Treatment of rejection – The first dose of lymphocyte immune globulin can be delayed until the diagnosis of the first rejection episode. The recommended dose is 10 to 15 mg/kg/day for 14 days. Additional alternate-day therapy up to a total of 21 doses can be given.

➤*Aplastic anemia:* 10 to 20 mg/kg/day for 8 to 14 days. Additional alternate-day therapy up to a total of 21 doses can be administered. Because thrombocytopenia can be associated with the administration of lymphocyte immune globulin, patients receiving it for the treatment of aplastic anemia may need prophylactic platelet transfusions to maintain platelets at clinically acceptable levels.

➤*Preparation of solution:* Parenteral drug products should be inspected visually for particulate matter and discoloration prior to administration whenever solution and container permit. However, because lymphocyte immune globulin is a gamma globulin product, it can be transparent to slightly opalescent, colorless to faintly pink or brown, and may develop a slight granular or flaky deposit during storage. Lymphocyte immune globulin (diluted or undiluted) should not be shaken because excessive foaming or denaturation of the protein may occur.

Dilute lymphocyte immune globulin for IV infusion in an inverted bottle of sterile vehicle so the undiluted lymphocyte immune globulin does not contact the air inside. Add the total daily dose of lymphocyte immune globulin to the sterile vehicle (see below). The concentration should not exceed 4 mg of lymphocyte immune globulin per mL. The diluted solution should be gently rotated or swirled to effect thorough mixing.

➤*Administration:* The diluted lymphocyte immune globulin should be allowed to reach room temperature before infusion. Lymphocyte immune globulin is appropriately administered into a vascular shunt, arterial venous fistula, or a high-flow central vein through an in-line filter with a pore size of 0.2 to 1 micron. The in-line filter should be used with all infusions of lymphocyte immune globulin to prevent the administration of any insoluble material that may develop in the product during storage. The use of high-flow veins will minimize the occurrence of phlebitis and thrombosis. Do not infuse a dose of lymphocyte immune globulin in < 4 hours. Always keep appropriate resuscitation equipment at the patient's bedside while lymphocyte immune globulin is being administered. Observe the patient continuously for possible allergic reactions throughout the infusions (see Adverse Reactions).

➤*Compatibility and stability:* Lymphocyte immune globulin, once diluted, has been shown to be physically and chemically stable for up to 24 hours at concentrations of up to 4 mg/mL in the following diluents: 0.9% sodium chloride injection, 5% dextrose and 0.225% sodium chloride injection, and 5% dextrose and 0.45% sodium chloride injection.

Adding lymphocyte immune globulin to dextrose injection is not recommended, as low salt concentrations can cause precipitation. Highly acidic infusion solutions can also contribute to physical instability over time. It is recommended that diluted lymphocyte immune globulin be stored in a refrigerator if it is prepared prior to the time of infusion. Even if it is stored in a refrigerator, the total time in dilution should not exceed 24 hours (including infusion time).

➤*Storage / Stability:* Store in a refrigerator at 2° to 8°C (36° to 46°F). Do not freeze.

ANTITHYMOCYTE GLOBULIN (RABBIT) (ATG Rabbit)

Rx	**Thymoglobulin** (SangStat)	**Powder for Injection, lyophilized:**[a] 25 mg	In 7 mL vials with 5 mL vial of diluent.

[a] 50 mg glycine, 50 mg mannitol, 10 mg NaCl.

ANTI-THYMOCYTE GLOBULIN — INJECTION

For complete and comparative prescribing information, refer to the Immune Globulins group monograph.

WARNING

Anti-thymocyte globulin should only be used by physicians experienced in immunosuppressive therapy for the management of renal transplant patients.

Indications

➤*Acute renal transplant rejection:* For the treatment of renal transplant acute rejection in conjunction with concomitant immunosuppression.

➤*Unlabeled uses:* Treatment of refractory aplastic anemia; prophylaxis and treatment of acute allograft rejection in renal-pancreatic, liver, cardiac, renal, and lung transplantation; treatment of refractory graft-vs-host disease (GVHD) in allogeneic bone marrow transplantation; prophylaxis of GVHD in allogeneic bone marrow transplantation; allogeneic bone marrow transplantation.

Administration and Dosage

➤*Dose:* 1.5 mg/kg of body weight administered daily for 7 to 14 days. The recommended route of administration is intravenous infusion using a high-flow vein. Anti-thymocyte globulin should be infused over a minimum of 6 hours for the first infusion and over at least 4 hours on subsequent days of therapy. Anti-thymocyte globulin should be administered through an in-line 0.22 mcm filter.

➤*Premedication:* Anti-thymocyte globulin is supplied as 2 vials: One (1) vial contains lyophilized (solid) anti-thymocyte globulin (25 mg) and the second vial contains 5 mL Sterile Water for Injection (WFI) labeled as "Diluent." For vial reconstitution, dilution in infusion solution and infusion procedure, see Preparation for administration. Investigations indicate that anti-thymocyte globulin is well tolerated and less likely to produce side effects when administered at the recommended rate. Administration of antiviral prophylactic therapy is recommended. Premedication with corticosteroids, acetaminophen, or an antihistamine 1 hour prior to the infusion is recommended and may reduce the incidence and intensity of side effects during the infusion. Medical personnel should monitor patients for adverse events during and after infusion. Monitoring T-cell counts (absolute or sub-

ANTI-THYMOCYTE GLOBULIN — INJECTION

sets) to assess the level of T-cell depletion is recommended. Total white blood cell and platelet counts should be monitored.

➤*Dose reduction/discontinuation:* Overdosage of anti-thymocyte globulin may result in leukopenia or thrombocytopenia. The anti-thymocyte globulin dose should be reduced by one-half if the WBC count is between 2000 and 3000 cells/mm^3 or if the platelet count is between 50,000 and 75,000 cells/mm^3. Stopping anti-thymocyte globulin treatment should be considered if the WBC count falls below 2000 cells/mm^3 or platelets below 50,000 cells/mm^3.

➤*Preparation for administration:*

Reconstitution – After calculating the number of vials needed, using aseptic technique, reconstitute anti-thymocyte globulin with the supplied diluent, Sterile Water for Injection (WFI), immediately before use. Anti-thymocyte globulin should be used within 4 hours after reconstitution if kept at room temperature.

1.) Allow anti-thymocyte globulin and diluent (sterile WFI) vials to reach room temperature before reconstituting the lyophilized product.
2.) Aseptically remove caps and tabs of the aluminum seals to expose rubber stoppers.
3.) Clean stoppers with germicidal or alcohol swab.
4.) Aseptically remove 5 mL of diluent (sterile WFI) using a sterile, single-use syringe and inject it slowly into the vial containing anti-thymocyte globulin lyophilized powder.
5.) Reconstitute each vial of anti-thymocyte globulin lyophilized powder with 5 mL of sterile diluent.
6.) Rotate vial gently until powder is completely dissolved. Each reconstituted vial contains 25 mg or 5 mg/mL of anti-thymocyte globulin.
7.) Inspect solution for particulate matter after reconstitution. Should some particulate matter remain, continue to gently rotate the vial until no particulate matter is visible. If particulate matter persists, discard this vial.

Dilution –

1.) Transfer the contents of the calculated number of anti-thymocyte globulin vials into the bag of infusion solution (saline or dextrose). Recommended volume: Per 1 vial of anti-thymocyte globulin use 50 mL of infusion solution (total volume usually between 50 to 500 mL).
2.) Mix the solution by inverting the bag gently only once or twice.

Infusion –

1.) Follow the manufacturer's instructions for the infusion administration set. Infuse through a 0.22-micron filter into a high-flow vein.
2.) Set the flow rate to deliver the dose over a minimum of 6 hours for the first dose and over at least 4 hours for subsequent doses.

➤*Storage/Stability:* Store in refrigerator between 2° to 8°C (36° to 46°F). Protect from light. Do not freeze. Do not use after the expiration date indicated on the label. Reconstituted vials of anti-thymocyte globulin should be used within 4 hours. Infusion solutions of anti-thymocyte globulin must be used immediately. Any unused drug remaining after infusion must be discarded.

RABIES IMMUNE GLOBULIN, HUMAN (RIG)

Rx	**BayRab**[a] (Bayer Pharmaceutical)	**Injection:** 150 IU/mL	In 2 and 10 mL single-dose vials.
Rx	**Imogam Rabies - HT**[b] (Aventis Pasteur)		In 2 and 10 mL vials.

[a] Preservative free. With 0.21 to 0.32 M glycine. Solvent/Detergent treated.

[b] Preservative free. With 0.3 M glycine. Heat treated.

RABIES IMMUNE GLOBULIN (HUMAN) — INJECTION

For complete and comparative prescribing information, refer to the general discussion for Rabies Prophylaxis in the Treatment Guidelines section of the Appendix.

Indications

➤*Rabies exposure:* For individuals suspected of exposure to rabies, particularly severe exposure, with one exception; persons who have been previously immunized with human diploid cell vaccine (HDCV) rabies vaccine in a preexposure- or postexposure-treatment series should receive only vaccine. Persons who have received rabies vaccines other than HDCV, (rabies vaccine adsorbed) RVA or PCEC (purified chick embryo cell vaccine) vaccines should have confirmed adequate rabies antibody titers if they are to receive only vaccine.

Administration and Dosage

Rabies immune globulin (human) should be injected as promptly as possible after exposure along with the first dose of vaccine. If initiation of treatment is delayed for any reason, rabies immune globulin (human) and the first dose of vaccine should still be given, regardless of the interval between exposure and treatment. *Imogam Rabies-HT* may be given up to 8 days and *BayRab* may be given up to 7 days after the first dose of vaccine is given.

➤*Imogam Rabies - HT*: Rabies immune globulin (human) should be used in conjunction with a rabies vaccine such as *Rabies Vaccine Imovax Rabies*, for IM immunization, vaccine prepared from human diploid cell cultures. The recommended dose of rabies immune globulin (human) is 20 IU/kg (0.133 mL/kg) or 9 IU/lb (0.06 mL/lb) of body weight administered at time of the first vaccine dose. The gluteal area should never be used for HDCV, RVA or PCEC injections because administration of HDCV in this area results in lower neutralizing antibody titers. If anatomically feasible, the full dose of rabies immune globulin (human) (RIG) should be thoroughly infiltrated in the area around and into the wounds. Any remaining volume should be injected IM at a site distant from vaccine administration. Because of risk of injury to the sciatic nerve, the central region of the gluteal area must be avoided; only the upper, outer quadrant should be used. Two injections would be given in the gluteal muscle if the volume is > 5 mL.

Human rabies immune globulin (HRIG) should never be administered in the same syringe or into the same anatomical site as vaccine. Because HRIG may partially suppress active production of antibody, no more than the recommended dose should be given.

➤*BayRab*: The recommended dose for *BayRab* is 20 IU/kg (0.133 mL/kg) of body weight given preferably at the time of the first vaccine dose. It may also be given through the seventh day after the first dose of vaccine is given. If anatomically feasible, up to the full dose of *BayRab* should be thoroughly infiltrated in the area around the wound and the rest should be administered IM in the gluteal area or lateral thigh muscle. Because of risk of injury to the sciatic nerve, the central region of the gluteal area must be avoided; only the upper, outer quadrant should be used. *BayRab* should never be administered in the same syringe or needle or in the same anatomical site as vaccine.

Rabies postexposure prophylaxis schedule, United States 1999*

Vaccination status	Treatment	Regimen**
Not previously vaccinated	Wound cleansing	All postexposure treatment should being with immediate thorough cleansing of all wounds with soap and water. If available, a virucidal agent such as a povidone-iodine solution should be used to irrigate the wounds.
	RIG	Administer 20 IU/kg body weight. If anatomically feasible, the full dose should be administered IM at anatomical site distant from vaccine administration. Also, RIG should not be administered in the same syringe as vaccine. Because RIG might partially suppress active production of antibody, no more than the recommended dose should be given.
	Vaccine	HDCV, RVA, or PCEC 1 mL, IM (deltoid area[1]), 1 each on days 0[2], 3, 7, 14, and 28
Previously vaccinated[3]	Wound cleansing	All postexposure treatment should being with immediate thorough cleansing of all wounds with soap and water. If available, a virucidal agent such as a povidone-iodine solution should be used to irrigate the wounds.
	RIG	RIG should not be administered.
	Vaccine	HDCV, RVA, or PCEC 1 mL, IM (deltoid area[1]), 1 each on days 0[2] and 3

* HDCV = human diploid cell vaccine; PCEC = purified chick embryo cell vaccine; RIG = rabies immune globulin; RVA = rabies vaccine adsorbed; IM = intramuscular.

** These regimens are applicable for all age groups, including children.

[1] The deltoid area is the only acceptable site of vaccination for adults and older children. For younger children, the outer aspect of the thigh may be used. Vaccine should never be administered in the gluteal area.

[2] Day 0 is the day the first dose of vaccine is administered.

[3] Any person with a history of preexposure vaccination with HDCV, RVA, or PCEC; prior postexposure prophylaxis with HDCV, RVA, or PCEC; or previous vaccination with any other type of rabies vaccine and a documented history of antibody response to the prior vaccination.

➤*Storage/Stability:* Rabies immune globulin (human) should be stored in the refrigerator between 2° and 8°C (35° and 46°F). Do not freeze. Rabies immune globulin (human) contains no preservative and unused portion must be discarded immediately.

Rh_o(D) IMMUNE GLOBULIN (Rh_o[D] IGIM)

Rx	**BayRho-D Full Dose** (Bayer Pharmaceutical)	**Solution for Injection:**[a] 15% to 18% protein	In individual and multiple-pack single-dose syringes with attached needles and vials.
Rx	**RhoGAM** (Ortho Diagnostics)	**Solution for Injection:**[b] 5% ± 1% gamma globulin	In packages with prefilled single-dose syringes, package insert, control form, and patient ID card. In 5s, 25s, and 100s.

[a] Preservative free. With 0.21 to 0.32 M glycine. Solvent/Detergent treated.

[b] Preservative free. With 2.9 mg sodium chloride, 0.01% polysorbate 80, 15 mg/mL glycine. Filtrated.

RH_o(D) IMMUNE GLOBULIN (HUMAN) — INTRAMUSCULAR

For complete and comparative prescribing information, refer to the Immune Globulins group monograph.

Indications

➤*Pregnancy and other obstetric conditions:* For the prevention of Rh hemolytic disease of the newborn by its administration to the Rh_o(D) negative mother within 72 hours after birth of an Rh_o(D) positive infant, providing the following criteria are met:

1.) The mother must be Rh_o(D) negative and must not already be sensitized to the Rh_o(D) factor.
2.) Her child must be Rh_o(D) positive, and should have a negative direct antiglobulin test (see Precautions).

If Rh_o(D) immune globulin is administered antepartum, it is essential that the mother receive another dose of Rh_o(D) immune globulin after delivery of an Rh_o(D) positive infant.

If the father can be determined to be Rh_o(D) negative, Rh_o(D) immune globulin need not be given.

Rh_o(D) immune globulin should be administered within 72 hours to all nonimmunized Rh_o(D) negative women who have undergone spontaneous or induced abortion, following ruptured tubal pregnancy, amniocentesis or abdominal trauma unless the blood group of the fetus or the father is known to be Rh_o(D) negative. If the fetal blood group cannot be determined, one must assume that it is Rh_o(D) positive, and Rh_o(D) immune globulin should be administered to the mother.

Transfusion – Rh_o(D) immune globulin may be used to prevent isoimmunization in Rh_o(D) negative individuals who have been transfused with Rh_o(D) positive red blood cells or blood components containing red blood cells.

➤*Unlabeled uses:* Although controversial, some physicians advocate administration prior to external version attempts for breech presentations (due to induced fetomaternal hemorrhage) and following tubal ligation after delivery of a Rh_o(D)-positive infant (to prevent problems should the sterilization fail or subsequent tubal reanastomoses occur.

Administration and Dosage

A full dose of Rh_o(D) immune globulin (human) has traditionally been referred to as a "300 mcg" dose and this usage is employed here for convenience in terminology. It should not be construed as the actual anti-D content. Each full dose of Rh_o(D) Immune Globulin (human) must contain at least as much anti-D as 1 mL of the US Reference Rh_o(D) Immune Globulin. Studies performed at the FDA have shown that the US Reference contains 820 international units (IU) of anti-D per mL. When the conversion factor determined for the International (WHO) Reference Preparation is used, 820 IU per mL is equivalent to 164 mcg per mL of anti-D.

➤*Pregnancy and other obstetric conditions:*

1.) For postpartum prophylaxis, administer 1 vial or syringe of Rh_o(D) immune globulin (≈ 300 mcg*), preferably within 72 hours of delivery. Although a lesser degree of protection is afforded if Rh antibody is administered beyond the 72-hour period, Rh_o(D) immune globulin may still be given. Full-term deliveries can vary in their dosage requirements depending on the magnitude of the fetomaternal hemorrhage. One 300 mcg* vial or syringe of Rh_o(D) immune globulin provides sufficient antibody to prevent Rh sensitization if the volume of red blood cells that has entered the circulation is ≤ 15 mL. In instances where a large (> 30 mL of whole blood or 15 mL red blood cells) fetomaternal hemorrhage is suspected, a fetal red cell count by an approved laboratory technique (eg, modified Kleihauer-Betke acid elution stain technique) should be performed to determine the dosage of immune globulin required. The red blood cell volume of the calculated fetomaternal hemorrhage is divided by 15 mL to obtain the number of vials or syringes of Rh_o(D) immune globulin for administration. If > 15 mL of red cells is suspected or if the dose calculation results in a fraction, administer the next higher whole number of vials or syringes (eg, if 1.4, give 2 vials or 2 syringes).
2.) For antenatal prophylaxis, one 300 mcg* vial or syringe of Rh_o(D) immune globulin is administered at ≈ 28 weeks' gestation. This must be followed by another 300 mcg* dose, preferably within 72 hours following delivery, if the infant is Rh-positive.
3.) Following threatened abortion at any stage of gestation with continuation of pregnancy, it is recommended that 300 mcg* of Rh_o(D) immune globulin be given. If > 15 mL of red cells is suspected due to fetomaternal hemorrhage, the same dose modification in the first item above applies.
4.) Following miscarriage, abortion, or termination of ectopic pregnancy at or beyond 13 weeks' gestation, it is recommended that 300 mcg* of Rh_o(D) immune globulin be given. If > 15 mL of red cells is suspected due to fetomaternal hemorrhage, the same dose modification in the first item above applies. If pregnancy is terminated prior to 13 weeks' gestation, where licensed, a single dose of Rh_o(D) immune globulin micro-dose (≈ 50 mcg*) may be used instead of Rh_o(D) immune globulin.
5.) Following amniocentesis at either 15 to 18 weeks' gestation or during the third trimester, or following abdominal trauma in the second or third trimester, it is recommended that 300 mcg* of Rh_o(D) immune globulin be administered. If there is a feto-maternal hemorrhage in excess of 15 mL of red cells, the same dose modification in No. 1 applies.

If abdominal trauma, amniocentesis, or other adverse event requires the administration of Rh_o(D) immune globulin at 13 to 18 weeks' gestation, another 300 mcg* dose should be given at 26 to 28 weeks. To maintain protection throughout pregnancy, the level of passively acquired anti-Rh_o(D) should not be allowed to fall below the level required to prevent an immune response to Rh positive red cells. The half-life of IgG is 23 to 26 days. In any case, a dose of Rh_o(D) immune globulin should be given within 72 hours after delivery if the baby is Rh positive. If delivery occurs within 3 weeks after the last dose, the postpartum dose may be withheld unless there is a fetomaternal hemorrhage in excess of 15 mL of red blood cells.

➤*Transfusion:* In the case of a transfusion of Rh_o(D) positive red cells to an Rh_o(D) negative recipient, the volume of Rh positive whole blood administered is multiplied by the hematocrit of the donor unit giving the volume of red blood cells transfused. The volume of red blood cells is divided by 15 mL, which provides the number of vials or syringes of Rh_o(D) immune globulin (human) to be administered.

If the dose calculated results in a fraction, the next higher whole number of vials or syringes should be administered (eg, if 1.4, give 2 vials or 2 syringes). Rh_o(D) immune globulin should be administered within 72 hours after an incompatible transfusion, but preferably as soon as possible.

➤*Injection procedure:* Do not inject IV. Do not inject neonate. Rh_o(D) immune globulin is administered IM, preferably in the anterolateral aspects of the upper thigh and the deltoid muscle of the upper arm. The gluteal region should not be used routinely as an injection site because of the risk of injury to the sciatic nerve. If the gluteal region is used, the central region must be avoided; only the upper, outer quadrant should be used.

➤*Single vial or syringe dose:* Inject entire contents of the vial or syringe into the individual IM.

➤*Multiple vial or syringe dose:*

1.) Calculate the number of vials or syringes of Rh_o(D) immune globulin to be given (see Administration and Dosage).
2.) The total volume of Rh_o(D) immune globulin can be given in divided doses at different sites at one time or the total dose may be divided and injected at intervals, provided the total dosage is given within 72 hours of the fetomaternal hemorrhage or transfusion. Using sterile technique, inject the entire contents of the calculated number of vials or syringes IM into the patient.

➤*Directions for syringe usage:*

1.) Remove the prefilled syringe from the package. Lift syringe by barrel, not by plunger.
2.) Twist the plunger rod clockwise until the threads are seated.
3.) With the rubber needle shield secured on the syringe tip, push the plunger rod forward a few millimeters to break any friction seal between the rubber stopper and the glass syringe barrel.
4.) Remove the needle shield and expel air bubbles.
5.) Proceed with hypodermic needle puncture.
6.) Aspirate prior to injection to confirm that the needle is not in a vein or artery.
7.) Inject the medication.
8.) Withdraw the needle and destroy it.

➤*Storage/Stability:* Store at 2° to 8°C (36° to 46°F). Do not freeze.

Rh_0(D) IMMUNE GLOBULIN INTRAVENOUS (HUMAN) (Rh_0[D] IGIV)

Rx	**Rhophylac** (ZLB Bioplasma)	**Injection:** 1,500 units (300 mcg)	Preservative-free. In 2 mL pre-filled syringes.
Rx	**WinRho SDF** (Baxter)	**Powder for injection, freeze-dried:**[a] 600 units (120 mcg)	With 2.5 mL 0.9% Sodium Chloride Injection diluent. In single-dose vials.
		1,500 units (300 mcg)	With 2.5 mL 0.9% Sodium Chloride Injection diluent. In single-dose vials.
		5,000 units (1000 mcg)	With 8.5 mL 0.9% Sodium Chloride Injection diluent. In single-dose vials.
		Liquid for IV or IM injection:[b] 600 units (120 mcg)	Preservative free. In single dose vials.
		1,500 units (300 mcg)	Preservative free. In single dose vials.
		2,500 units (500 mcg)	Preservative free. In single dose vials.
		5,000 units (1,000 mcg)	Preservative free. In single dose vials.
		15,000 units (3,000 mcg)	Preservative free. In single dose vials.

[a] Preservative free. Contains 0.1 M glycine, 0.04 M sodium chloride, 0.01% polysorbate 80. Solvent/Detergent treated.

[b] Contains 10% maltose and 0.03% polysorbate 80.

RH_0(D) IMMUNE GLOBULIN — INTRAVENOUS

For complete and comparative prescribing information, refer to the Immune Globulins group monograph.

Indications

➤*Treatment of immune thrombocytopenic purpura (ITP):* Rh_0(D) immune globulin intravenous (human), is recommended for the treatment of non-splenectomized, Rh_0(D) positive children with chronic or acute immune thrombocytopenic purpura (ITP), adults with chronic ITP, or children and adults with ITP secondary to HIV infection, in clinical situations requiring an increase in platelet count to prevent excessive hemorrhage. The safety and efficacy of RH_0(D) immune globulin intravenous have not been evaluated in clinical trials for patients with non-ITP causes of thrombocytopenia or in previously splenectomized patients or in patients who are Rh_0(D) negative.

➤*Suppression of Rh isoimmunization:*

Pregnancy and other obstetric conditions – Rh_0(D) IGIV is recommended for the suppression of Rh isoimmunization in non-sensitized, Rh_0(D) negative (D-negative) women within 72 hours after spontaneous or induced abortions, amniocentesis, chorionic villus sampling, ruptured tubal pregnancy, abdominal trauma or transplacental hemorrhage or in the normal course of pregnancy unless the blood type of the fetus or father is known to be Rh_0(D) negative. In the case of maternal bleeding due to threatened abortion, Rho(D) immune globulin intravenous should be administered as soon as possible. Suppression of Rh isoimmunization reduces the likelihood of hemolytic disease in an Rh_0(D) positive fetus in present and future pregnancies. Rh_0(D) immune globulin intravenous should not be administered to infants born to Rh incompatible mothers.

The criteria for an Rh-incompatible pregnancy requiring administration of Rh_0(D) IGIV at 28 weeks gestation and within 72 hours after delivery are:
- The mother must be Rh_0(D) negative.
- The mother is carrying a child whose father is either Rh_0(D) positive or Rh_0(D) unknown.
- The baby is either Rh_0(D) positive or Rh_0(D) unknown.
- The mother must not be previously sensitized to the Rh_0(D) factor.

➤*Transfusion:* Rh_0(D) IGIV is recommended for the suppression of Rh isoimmunization in Rh_0(D) negative female children and female adults in their childbearing years transfused with Rh_0(D) positive RBCs or blood components containing Rh_0(D) positive RBCs. Treatment should be initiated within 72 hours of exposure. Treatment should be given (without preceding exchange transfusion) only if the transfused Rh_0(D) positive blood represents less than 20% of the total circulating red cells. A 300 mcg (1500 units) dose will suppress the immunizing potential of approximately 17 mL of Rh_0(D) positive RBCs.

Rh_0(D) IGIV (human) is not indicated for use as immunoglobulin replacement therapy for immune globulin deficiency syndromes. Do not use for the treatment of ITP in Rh_0(D) negative or splenectomized individuals; efficacy in these patients has not been demonstrated.

Administration and Dosage

➤*Approved by the FDA:* March 24, 1995.

➤*Administration:* Rh_0(D) IGIV (human) may be administered either intramuscularly or intravenously.

For use in the treatment of immune thrombocytopenic purpura (ITP), Rh_0(D) IGIV must be administered intravenously.

For use in the suppression of Rh isoimmunization, Rh_0(D) IGIV may be administered either intramuscularly or intravenously.

➤*Preparation for administration:* Rh_0(D) IGIV, should be reconstituted only with the accompanying vial of 0.9% sodium chloride injection. It should not be administered concurrently with other products.

Reconstitution –

Intravenous administration: Aseptically reconstitute the product shortly before use with 2.5 mL of 0.9% sodium chloride injection for 120 mcg (600 units) and 300 mcg (1500 units) and 8.5 mL of 0.9% sodium chloride injection for 1000 mcg (5000 units). Discard unused portion of diluent. Inject the diluent slowly onto the inside wall of the vial and gently swirl until dissolved. Do not shake.

Intramuscular administration: Aseptically reconstitute the product shortly before use with 1.25 mL of 0.9% sodium chloride injection for 120 mcg (600 units) and 300 mcg (1500 units) and 8.5 mL of 0.9% sodium chloride injection for 1000 mcg (5000 units). Inject the diluent slowly onto the inside wall of the vial and gently swirl until dissolved. Do not shake.

Reconstitution of Rh_0(D) immune globulin IV

Vial size	Volume of diluent to be added to vial
IV injection	
120 mcg (600 units)	2.5 mL
300 mcg (1,500 units)	2.5 mL
1,000 mcg (5,000 units)	8.5 mL
IM injection	
120 mcg (600 units)	1.25 mL
300 mcg (1,500 units)	1.25 mL
1,000 mcg (5,000 units)	8.5 mL*

* To be administered into several sites.

Liquid – There is no reconstitution required. The following table describes the target fill volumes for each of the dosage sizes for the liquid presentation.

Vial size	Target fill volume
120 mcg (600 units)	0.5 mL
300 mcg (1,500 units)	1.3 mL
500 mcg (2,500 units)	2.2 mL
1,000 mcg (5,000 units)	4.4 mL
3,000 mcg (15,000 units)	13 mL

Note: Remove the entire contents of the vial to obtain the labeled dosage. If partial vials are required for dosage calculation, the entire contents of the vial should be withdrawn to ensure accurate calculation of the dosage requirement.

Injection – Parenteral products such as Rh_0(D) IGIV should be inspected for particulate matter and discoloration prior to administration. Use the product within 12 hours of reconstitution. Discard any unused portion.

Intravenous administration: Infuse the entire dose into a suitable vein over 3 to 5 minutes. Rh_0(D) IGIV should be administered separately from other drugs.

Intramuscular administration: Administer into the deltoid muscle of the upper arm or the anterolateral aspects of the upper thigh. Due to the risk of sciatic nerve injury, the gluteal region should not be used as a routine injection site. If the gluteal region is used, use only the upper, outer quadrant.

➤*Treatment of immune thrombocytopenic purpura:* Rh_0(D) IGIV must be given by intravenous administration for the treatment of ITP.

Initial dosing – After confirming that the patient is Rh_0(D) positive, an initial dose of 50 mcg/kg (250 units/kg) body weight, given as a single injection, is recommended for the treatment of ITP. The initial dose may be administered in 2 divided doses given on separate days, if desired. If the patient has a hemoglobin level that is less than 10 g/dL, a reduced dose of 25 to 40 mcg/kg (125 to 200 units/kg) should be given to minimize the risk of increasing the severity of anemia in the patient. All patients should be monitored to determine clinical response by assessing platelet counts, red cell counts, hemoglobin, and reticulocyte levels.

Subsequent dosing – If subsequent therapy is required to elevate platelet counts, an intravenous dose of 25 to 60 mcg/kg (125 to 300 units/kg) body weight of Rh_0(D) IGIV is recommended. The frequency and dose used in maintenance therapy should be determined by the patient's clinical response by assessing platelet counts, red cell counts, hemoglobin, and reticulocyte levels.

If patient responded to initial dose with a satisfactory increase in platelets, the maintenance therapy dosing (25 to 60 mcg/kg [125 to 300 units/kg]) is individualized based on platelet and Hgb levels.

If patient did not respond to initial dose, administer a subsequent dose based on Hgb: If Hgb between 8 to 10 g/dL, redose between 25 to 40 mcg/kg (125 to 200 units/kg). If Hgb greater than 10 g/dL, redose between 50 to 60 mcg/kg (250 to 300 units/kg). If Hgb less than 8 g/dL, use with caution.

RH_0(D) IMMUNE GLOBULIN — INTRAVENOUS

The following equations are provided to determine the dosage and number of vials needed for the treatment of ITP:

Weight in lbs/2.2083 = weight in kg

Weight in kg × selected mcg (units) dosing level = dosage

Dosage/vial size = number of vials needed

➤*Suppression of Rh isoimmunization:* Rh_0(D) IGIV may be given by intravenous or intramuscular administration for the suppression of Rh isoimmunization.

Pregnancy – The same dosage, as described below, is to be administered by either the intramuscular or intravenous routes.

A 300 mcg (1500 units) dose of Rh_0(D) IGIV should be administered at 28 weeks gestation. If Rh_0(D) IGIV is administered early in the pregnancy, it is recommended that Rh_0(D) IGIV be administered at 12-week intervals in order to maintain an adequate level of passively acquired anti-Rh.

A 120 mcg (600 units) dose should be administered as soon as possible after delivery of a confirmed Rh_0(D) positive baby and normally no later than 72 hours after delivery. In the event that the Rh status of the baby is not known at 72 hours, Rh_0(D) IGIV should be administered to the mother at 72 hours after delivery. If more than 72 hours have elapsed, Rh_0(D) IGIV should not be withheld, but administered as soon as possible up to 28 days after delivery.

Other obstetric conditions – The same dosage, as described below, is to be administered by either the intramuscular or intravenous routes.

A 120 mcg (600 units) dose of Rh_0(D) IGIV should be administered immediately after abortion, amniocentesis (after 34 weeks gestation) or any other manipulation late in pregnancy (after 34 weeks gestation) associated with increased risk of Rh isoimmunization. Administration should take place within 72 hours after the event.

A 300 mcg (1500 units) dose of Rh_0(D) IGIV should be administered immediately after amniocentesis before 34 weeks gestation or after chorionic villus sampling. This dose should be repeated every 12 weeks while the woman is pregnant. In the case of threatened abortion, Rh_0(D) IGIV should be administered as soon as possible.

Obstetric indications and recommended dose

Indication	Dose (administer IM or IV)
Pregnancy	
28 weeks gestation	300 mcg (1,500 units)
Postpartum (if newborn Rh positive)	120 mcg (600 units)
Obstetric conditions	
Threatened abortion at any time	300 mcg (1,500 units)
Amniocentesis and chorionic villus sampling before 34 weeks gestation	300 mcg (1,500 units)
Abortion, amniocentesis, or any other manipulation after 34 weeks gestation	120 mcg (600 units)

Transfusion –

Transfusion indication and recommended dose

Route of administration	Rh_o(D) immune globulin IV dose	
	If exposed to Rh_o (D) positive whole blood	If exposed to Rh_o(D) positive red blood cells
IV	9 mcg (45 units)/mL blood	18 mcg (90 units)/mL cells
IM	12 mcg (60 units)/mL blood	24 mcg (120 units)/mL cells

Intravenous administration: Administer 600 mcg (3000 units) every 8 hours via the intravenous route, until the total dose, calculated from below, is administered.

If exposed to Rh_0(D) positive whole blood, the total intravenous dose of Rh_0(D) IGIV is 9 mcg (45 units)/mL blood

If exposed to Rh_0(D) positive red blood cells, the total intravenous dose of Rh_0 (D) IGIV is 18 mcg (90 units)/mL cells. Administer 600 mcg (3000 units) every 8 hours via the intravenous route, until the total dose is administered.

Intramuscular administration – Administer 1200 mcg (6000 units) every 12 hours via the intramuscular route, until the total dose, calculated from below, is administered.

If exposed to Rh_0(D) positive whole blood, the total intramuscular dose of Rh_0(D) IGIV is 12 mcg (60 units)/mL blood.

If exposed to Rh_0(D) positive red blood cells the total intramuscular dose of Rh_0(D) IGIV is 24 mcg (120 units)/mL cells.

➤*Storage/Stability:* Store at 2° to 8°C (35° to 46°F). Do not freeze. Do not use after expiration date.

If the reconstituted product is not used immediately, store it at room temperature for no longer than 12 hours. Do not freeze the reconstituted product. Discard the product if not administered within 12 hours.

Rx only.

Actions

➤*Pharmacology:*

Treatment of immune thrombocytopenic purpura – Rh_0(D) immune globulin intravenous (human) has been shown to increase platelet counts in non-splenectomized, Rh_0(D) positive patients with ITP. Platelet counts usually rise within 1 to 2 days and peak within 7 to 14 days after initiation of therapy. The duration of response is variable; however, the average duration is approximately 30 days. The mechanism of action is not completely understood, but is thought to be due to the formation of anti-Rh_0(D) (anti-D)-coated RBC complexes resulting in Fc receptor blockade, thus sparing antibody-coated platelets.

Suppression of Rh isoimmunization – Rh_0(D) IGIV is used to suppress the immune response of non-sensitized Rh_0(D) negative individuals following exposure to Rh_0(D) positive RBCs by fetomaternal hemorrhage during delivery of an Rh_0(D) positive infant, abortion (spontaneous or induced), amniocentesis, abdominal trauma, or mismatched transfusion. The mechanism of action is not completely understood.

Rh_0(D) IGIV, when administered within 72 hours of a full-term delivery of an Rh_0(D) positive infant by an Rh_0(D) negative mother, will reduce the incidence of Rh isoimmunization from 12% to 13% to 1% to 2%. The 1% to 2% is, for the most part, due to isoimmunization during the last trimester of pregnancy. When treatment is given both antenatally at 28 weeks gestation and postpartum, the Rh immunization rate drops to about 0.1%.

When 120 mcg (600 units) of Rh_0(D) IGIV is administered to pregnant women, passive anti-Rh_0(D) antibodies are not detectable in the circulation for more than 6 weeks and therefore a dose of 300 mcg (1500 units) should be used for antenatal administration.

In a clinical study with Rh_0(D) negative volunteers (9 males and 1 female), Rh_0(D) positive red cells were completely cleared from the circulation within 8 hours of intravenous administration of Rh_0(D) IGIV. There was no indication of Rh isoimmunization of these subjects at 6 months after the clearance of the Rh_0(D) positive red cells.

➤*Pharmacokinetics:*

Intramuscular versus intravenous administration – In a clinical study involving Rh_0(D) negative volunteers, 2 subjects received 120 mcg (600 units) Rh_0(D) IGIV by intravenous administration and 2 subjects received this dose by intramuscular administration. Peak levels (36 to 48 ng/mL) were reached within 2 hours of intravenous administration and peak levels (18 to 19 ng/mL) were reached at 5 to 10 days after intramuscular administration. The calculated areas under the curve were the same for both routes of administration. The $t_{½}$ for anti-Rh_0(D) was about 24 days following intravenous administration and about 30 days following intramuscular administration.

Contraindications

➤*Treatment of immune thrombocytopenic purpura and suppression of Rh isoimmunization:* Individuals known to have had an anaphylactic or severe systemic reaction to human globulin should not receive Rh_0(D) immune globulin intravenous (human), or any other immune globulin (human). Rh_0(D) IGIV contains trace amounts of IgA (approximately 5 mcg/mL). Individuals who are deficient in IgA may have the potential for developing IgA antibodies and have anaphylactic reactions. The physician must weigh the potential benefit of treatment with Rh_0(D) IGIV against the potential for hypersensitivity reactions.

Warnings

Rh_0(D) immune globulin intravenous (human) is made from human plasma. Products made from human plasma may carry a risk of transmitting infectious agents (eg, viruses) and theoretically, the Creutzfeldt-Jakob disease (CJD) agent. The risk that such products will transmit an infectious agent has been reduced by screening plasma donors for prior exposure to certain viruses, by testing for the presence of certain current virus infections, and by inactivating or removing certain viruses. The Rh_0(D) IGIV manufacturing process includes a solvent detergent treatment step (using tri-n-butyl phosphate and *Triton X-100*) that is effective in inactivating lipid enveloped viruses such as hepatitis B, hepatitis C, and HIV. Rh_0(D) IGIV is filtered using a *Planova 35 nm Virus Filter* that is effective in reducing the level of some non-lipid enveloped viruses such as hepatitis A. These 2 processes are designed to increase product safety by reducing the risk of transmission of lipid enveloped and non-lipid enveloped viruses, respectively. Despite these measures, such products can still potentially transmit disease. There is also the possibility that unknown infectious agents may be present in such products. All infections thought by a physician possibly to have been transmitted by this product should be reported by the physician or other healthcare provider to the distributor. The physician should discuss the risks and benefits of this product with the patient.

➤*Treatment of immune thrombocytopenic purpura:* Rh_0(D) IGIV must be administered via the intravenous route for the treatment of ITP as its efficacy has not been established by the intramuscular or subcutaneous routes.

Rh_0(D) IGIV should not be administered to Rh_0(D) negative or splenectomized individuals as its efficacy in these patients has not been demonstrated.

➤*Fertility impairment:* Animal reproduction studies have not been conducted with Rh_0(D) IGIV. It is not known whether Rh_0(D) IGIV can cause fetal harm when administered to a pregnant woman or can affect reproductive capacity.

➤*Pregnancy:* Category C.

Treatment of immune thrombocytopenic purpura and suppression of Rh isoimmunization – Animal reproduction studies have not been conducted with Rh_0(D) IGIV. It is not known whether Rh_0(D) IGIV can cause fetal harm when administered to a pregnant woman or can affect reproductive capacity. Rh_0(D) IGIV should be given to a pregnant woman only if clearly needed.

➤*Children:*

Suppression of Rh isoimmunization – For the suppression of Rh isoimmunization in the mother, do not administer to the infant.

RH_0(D) IMMUNE GLOBULIN — INTRAVENOUS

Precautions

➤*Monitoring:*

Treatment of immune thrombocytopenic purpura – Following administration of Rh_0(D) IGIV, Rh_0(D) positive ITP patients should be monitored for signs or symptoms of intravascular hemolysis (IVH), clinically compromising anemia, and renal insufficiency.

If patients are to be transfused, Rh_0(D) negative red blood cells (PRBCs) should be used so as not to exacerbate ongoing IVH. Platelet products may contain up to 5 mL of RBCs, thus caution should likewise be exercised if platelets from Rh_0(D) positive donors are transfused.

If the patient has a lower than normal hemoglobin level (less than 10 g/dL), a reduced dose of 25 to 40 mcg/kg (125 to 200 units/kg) should be given to minimize the risk of increasing the severity of anemia in the patient. Rh_0(D) IGIV must be used with extreme caution in patients with a hemoglobin level that is less than 8 g/dL due to the risk of increasing the severity of the anemia.

Rh_0(D) IGIV should not be administered as immunoglobulin replacement therapy for immune globulin deficiency syndromes.

➤*Suppression of Rh isoimmunization:* Rh_0(D) IGIV should not be administered to Rh_0(D) negative individuals who are Rh immunized as evidenced by an indirect antiglobulin (Coombs') test revealing the presence of anti-Rh_0(D) (anti-D) antibody.

A large fetomaternal hemorrhage late in pregnancy or following delivery may cause a weak mixed field positive D^u test result. Such an individual should be assessed for a large fetomaternal hemorrhage and the dose of Rh_0(D) IGIV adjusted accordingly. Rh_0(D) IGIV should be administered if there is any doubt about the mother's blood type.

➤*Lab test abnormalities:* In addition to anti-D, Rh_0(D) IGIV contains trace amounts of anti-A, anti-B, anti-C and anti-E antibodies.

Treatment of immune thrombocytopenic purpura – Passively acquired anti-A, anti-B, anti-C, and anti-E blood group antibodies may be detectable in direct and indirect antiglobulin (Coombs') tests obtained following Rh_0(D) IGIV administration. Interpretation of direct and indirect antiglobulin tests must be made in the context of the patient's underlying clinical condition and supporting laboratory data.

Suppression of Rh isoimmunization – The presence of passively administered anti-Rh_0(D) in maternal or fetal blood can lead to a positive direct antiglobulin (Coombs') test. If there is an uncertainty about the mother's Rh group or immune status, Rh_0(D) IGIV should be administered to the mother.

Drug Interactions

➤*Treatment of immune thrombocytopenic purpura and suppression of Rh isoimmunization:* Administration of Rh_0(D) IGIV concomitantly with other drugs has not been evaluated. Other antibodies contained in Rh_0(D) IGIV may interfere with the response to live virus vaccines such as measles, mumps, polio or rubella. Therefore, immunization with live vaccines should not be given within 3 months after Rh_0(D) IGIV administration.

Rh_0(D) IGIV, should be reconstituted only with the accompanying vial of 0.9% sodium chloride injection. It should not be administered concurrently with other products.

Adverse Reactions

➤*Treatment of immune thrombocytopenic purpura:* In clinical trials of subjects (n = 161) with childhood acute ITP, adults and children with chronic ITP, and adults and children with ITP secondary to HIV, 60 out of 848 (7%) of infusions were associated with at least 1 adverse reaction that was considered to be related to the study medication. The most common adverse reactions were headache (19 infusions; 2%), chills (14 infusions; less than 2%), and fever (9 infusions; 1%). All are expected adverse reactions associated with infusions of immunoglobulins.

Rh_0(D) IGIV is administered to Rh_0(D) positive patients with ITP. Therefore, side effects related to the destruction of Rh_0(D) positive red blood cells, most notably a decreased hemoglobin, can be expected. In 4 clinical trials of patients treated with the recommended initial intravenous dose of 50 mcg/kg (250 units/kg), the mean maximum decrease in hemoglobin was 1.7 g/dL (range: +0.4 to −6.1 g/dL). At a reduced dose, ranging from 25 to 40 mcg/kg (125 to 200 units/kg), the mean maximum decrease in hemoglobin was 0.81 g/dL (range: +0.65 to 1.9 g/dL). Only 5/137 (3.7%) of patients had a maximum decrease in hemoglobin of greater than 4 g/dL (range 4.2 to 6.1 g/dL).

In most cases, the RBC destruction is believed to occur in the spleen. However, signs and symptoms consistent with IVH, including back pain, shaking chills, or hemoglobinuria, have been reported, occurring within 4 hours of Rh_0(D) IGIV. IVH-related complications that have been reported include death (4 cases reported between May 1996 and April 1999), acute onset or exacerbation of anemia, and acute onset or exacerbation of renal insufficiency. One patient died from complications secondary to IVH-induced exacerbation of anemia after administration of Rh_0(D) IGIV for treatment of ITP. Although the primary cause of death in the other 3 ITP patients treated with Rh_0(D) IGIV was related to underlying disease, the extent to which IVH-related clinical complications exacerbated their conditions and contributed to their deaths is unknown.

The mean maximum decrease in hemoglobin in patients who were not transfused with PRBCs was 3.7 g/dL (range: 0 to 7.6 g/dL). Transfusions for treatment-associated anemia were administered within hours to days of the onset of IVH and consisted of between 1 to 6 units of PRBCs. Acute renal insufficiency was noted within 2 to 48 hours of the onset of IVH. The mean maximum increase in serum creatinine was 3.5 mg/dL (range: 0.8 to 10.3 mg/dL) and occurred within 2 to 9 days. The renal insufficiency in all surviving patients resolved with medical management, including dialysis, within 4 to 23 days.

The etiology of IVH following Rh_0(D) IGIV administration is unknown. No known risk factors associated with this adverse event have yet been identified from among those examined, which included age, gender, pretreatment renal function, pretreatment hemoglobin, concomitantly administered PRBCs, or Rh_0(D) IGIV dose.

➤*Suppression of Rh isoimmunization:* Adverse reactions to Rh_0(D) immune globulin intravenous (human) are infrequent in Rh_0(D) negative individuals. In the clinical trial of 1186 Rh_0(D) negative pregnant women, no adverse reactions were attributed to Rh_0(D) IGIV. Discomfort and slight swelling at the site of injection and slight elevation in temperature have been reported in a small number of cases. A postmarketing survey conducted since the Canadian licensure of Rh_0(D) IGIV in 1980 for this indication included data obtained from 31,059 injections (25,068 for routine Rh prophylaxis and 5991 following abortions, amniocentesis, chorionic villus sampling, and antepartum hemorrhage). There were 9905 Rh_0(D) negative women who delivered Rh_0(D) positive infants, almost all of whom had received antenatal as well as postnatal prophylaxis. Of the patients followed in this survey, there were 26 reported treatment failures that resulted in the development of Rh_0(D) antibodies. There were no adverse reactions related to Rh_0(D) IGIV reported in this survey.

➤*Hypersensitivity:* As is the case with all drugs of this nature, there is a remote chance of an idiosyncratic or anaphylactic reaction with Rh_0(D) IGIV in individuals with hypersensitivity to blood products.

➤*Miscellaneous:* In addition to the adverse reactions described above, the following have been reported infrequently in clinical trials or postmarketing experience, in patients treated for ITP or the suppression of Rh isoimmunization, and are thought to be temporally associated with Rh_0(D) IGIV use: Asthenia, abdominal or back pain, hypotension, pallor, diarrhea, increased LDH, arthralgia, myalgia, dizziness, hyperkinesia, somnolence, vasodilation, pruritus, rash, and sweating.

Overdosage

➤*Symptoms:*

Treatment of immune thrombocytopenic purpura and suppression of Rh isoimmunization – There are no reports of known overdoses in patients being treated for Rh isoimmunization or ITP. In clinical studies with nonpregnant Rh_0(D) positive patients with ITP (n = 141) treated with 120 to 6500 mcg (600 to 32,500 units) of Rh_0(D) IGIV, there were no signs or symptoms that warranted medical intervention. However, these same doses were associated with a mild, transient hemolytic anemia.

RH_0(D) IMMUNE GLOBULIN MICRO-DOSE (Rh_0[D] IG Micro-dose)

Rx	**HyperRHO S/D Mini-Dose** (Talecris Biotherapeutics)	**Solution for Injection:** 15% to 18% protein	In single-dose syringes (10s).[a]
Rx	**MICRhoGAM** (Ortho Diagnostics)	**Solution for Injection:** 5% ± 1% gamma globulin	In packages with prefilled single-dose syringes, package insert, injection control form, and patient ID card. In 5s and 25s.[b]

[a] Preservative free. With 0.21 to 0.32 M glycine. Solvent/Detergent treated.
[b] Preservative free. With 2.9 mg/mL NaCl, 0.01% polysorbate 80, 15 mg/mL glycine. Filtrated.

RH_0(D) IMMUNE GLOBULIN (Rh_0[D] IG Micro-dose) — INTRAMUSCULAR MICRO-DOSE

For complete and comparative prescribing information, refer to the Immune Globulins group monograph.

Indications

➤*Prevention of isoimmunization:* Rh_0(D) IG micro-dose is recommended to prevent the isoimmunization of Rh_0(D)-negative women at the time of spontaneous or induced abortion of up to 12 weeks' gestation, provided the following criteria are met:

1.) The mother must be Rh_0(D)-negative and must not already be sensitized to the Rh_0(D) antigen.
2.) The father is not known to be Rh_0(D) negative.
3.) Gestation is ≤ 12 weeks at termination.

➤*Note:* Rh_0(D) immune globulin prophylaxis is not indicated if the fetus or father can be determined to be Rh negative. If the Rh status of the fetus is unknown, the fetus must be assumed to be Rh_0(D) positive, and Rh_0(D) IG micro-dose should be administered to the mother.

For abortions or miscarriages occurring after 12 weeks' gestation, a standard dose of Rh_0(D) immune globulin (human) is indicated.

Administration and Dosage

Do not give Rh_0(D) IG micro-dose IV. Inject only IM. Administer to women postabortion or postmiscarriage of ≤ 12 weeks gestation. Never administer to the neonate. One vial will suppress the immune response to 2.5 mL of Rh_0(D)-positive packed red blood cells or the equivalent (5 mL) of whole blood. One vial contains ≈ 50 mcg immunoglobulin.

$RH_o(D)$ IMMUNE GLOBULIN ($Rh_o[D]$ IG Micro-dose) — INTRAMUSCULAR MICRO-DOSE

Give 1 vial IM as soon as possible after termination of pregnancy. At or beyond 13 weeks' gestation, administer a full dose (300 mcg) $Rh_o(D)$ immune globulin.

Administer $Rh_o(D)$ IG micro-dose within 3 hours or as soon as possible after spontaneous passage or surgical removal of the products of conception. However, if $Rh_o(D)$ IG micro-dose is not given within this time period, consideration should still be given to its administration since clinical studies in male volunteers have demonstrated the effectiveness of $Rh_o(D)$ immune globulin in preventing isoimmunization as long as 72 hours after infusion of $Rh_o(D)$-positive red cells.

➤*Storage/Stability:* Store at 2° to 8°C (35° to 46°F). Do not freeze.

RESPIRATORY SYNCYTIAL VIRUS IMMUNE GLOBULIN INTRAVENOUS (HUMAN) (RSV-IGIV)

Rx	**RespiGam** (MedImmune)	**Injection:**[a] 50 ± 10 mg immunoglobulin/mL	In single-use 20 and 50 mL vials.

[a] Preservative free. Contains 5% sucrose, 1% albumin (human) and 1 to 1.5 mEq sodium per 50 mL. Solvent/Detergent treated.

RESPIRATORY SYNCYTIAL VIRUS IMMUNE GLOBULIN (HUMAN) (RSV-IGIV) — INTRAVENOUS

For complete and comparative prescribing information, refer to the Immune Globulins group monograph.

Indications

➤*Respiratory syncytial virus (RSV):* Prevention of serious lower respiratory tract infection caused by RSV in children < 24 months of age with bronchopulmonary dysplasia (BPD) or a history of premature birth (≤ 35 weeks gestation). RSV-IGIV is safe and effective in reducing the incidence and duration of RSV hospitalization and the severity of RSV illness in these high-risk infants.

➤*Unlabeled uses:* Consider using RSV-IGIV rather than IGIV during the RSV season in immunocompromised children who receive IGIV monthly.

Administration and Dosage

➤*Approved by the FDA:* January 18, 1996.

➤*Renal insufficiency:* Use IGIV products containing sucrose with caution in patients with pre-existing renal insufficiency and in patients judged to be at increased risk for developing renal insufficiency (including, but not limited to those with diabetes mellitus, > 65 years of age, volume depletion, paraproteinemia, sepsis, and patients receiving known nephrotoxic drugs). RSV-IGIV contains sucrose; therefore, it is important to assure that patients are not volume depleted prior to infusion. While most cases of renal insufficiency have occurred in patients receiving total doses of ≥ 400 mg Ig/kg of IGIV products containing sucrose, no prospective data are presently available to identify a maximum safe dose, concentration, or rate of infusion in patients determined to be at increased risk of acute renal failure. In the absence of prospective data, do not exceed recommended doses in patients at increased risk of renal failure and select the minimum practicable concentration and infusion rate.

➤*Recommended dose:* The maximum recommended total dosage per monthly infusion is 750 mg/kg, administered according to the following schedule:

RSV-IGIV Infusion Schedule	
Time after start of infusion	Rate of infusion (mL/kg of body mass per hour)
0 to 15 minutes	1.5 mL/kg/hr
15 minutes to end of infusion	3.6 mL/kg/hr

➤*Administration:* Administer RSV-IGIV intravenously at 1.5 mL/kg/hr for 15 minutes. If the clinical condition does not contraindicate a higher rate, increase the rate to 3.6 mL/kg/hr for the remainder of the infusion. *Do not exceed this rate of administration.* Monitor the patient closely during and after each rate change. In especially ill children with BPD, slower rates of infusion may be indicated.

Consider factors such as other clinical illness, how well the child has grown, and the risk of exposure from siblings or daycare when determining whether to use RSV-IGIV. Administer the first dose prior to commencement of the RSV season and subsequent doses monthly throughout the RSV season in order to maintain protection. In the Northern Hemisphere, the RSV season typically commences in November and runs through April. Infuse children from early November through April, unless RSV activity begins earlier or persists later in a community. It is recommended that RSV-IGIV be administered separately from other drugs or medications that the patient may be receiving. It is recommended that children infected with RSV continue to receive monthly doses for the duration of the RSV season.

➤*Infusion:* Begin infusion within 6 hours and complete within 12 hours after the single-use vial is entered. Assess the patient's vital signs and cardiopulmonary status prior to infusion, before each rate increase, and thereafter, at 30-minute intervals until 30 minutes following completion of the infusion. Administer RSV-IGIV through an IV line using a constant infusion pump (ie, *IVAC* pump or equivalent). Predilution of RSV-IGIV before infusion is not recommended. If possible, administer RSV-IGIV through a separate IV line, although it may be "piggy-backed" into a preexisting line if that line contains one of the following dextrose solutions (with or without sodium chloride): 2.5%, 5%, 10%, or 20% Dextrose in Water. If a preexisting line must be used, the RSV-IGIV should not be diluted more than 1:2 with any of the above-named solutions. An in-line filter with a pore size > 15 micrometers may be used for RSV-IGIV infusions.

➤*Admixture incompatibility:* It is recommended that RSV-IGIV be administered separately from other drugs or medications that the patient may be receiving.

➤*Storage/Stability:* Store between 2° and 8°C (36° and 46°F). Do not freeze. Do not shake vial; avoid foaming.

TETANUS IMMUNE GLOBULIN (HUMAN) (TIG)

Rx	**BayTet** (Bayer Pharmaceutical)	**Solution for Injection:**[a] 15% to 18% protein	In 250 unit vial and 250 unit syringe.

[a] Preservative free. With 0.21 to 0.32 M glycine. Solvent/Detergent treated.

TETANUS IMMUNE GLOBULIN (HUMAN) — INJECTION

For complete and comparative prescribing information, refer to the Immune Globulins group monograph.

Indications

➤*Tetanus prophylaxis:* For prophylaxis against tetanus following injury in patients whose immunization is incomplete or uncertain. It is also indicated, although evidence of effectiveness is limited, in the regimen of treatment of active cases of tetanus.

Guide to tetanus prophylaxis in wound management				
History of tetanus immunization (doses)	Clean, minor wounds		All other wounds*	
	Td[1]	TIG[2]	Td	TIG
Uncertain of less than 3	Yes	No	Yes	Yes
3 or more[3]	No[4]	No	No[5]	No

* Such as, but not limited to, wounds contaminated with dirt, feces, soil, and saliva; puncture wounds, avulsions, and wounds resulting from missiles, crushing, burns, and frostbite.
[1] Adult type tetanus and diphtheria toxoids. If the patient is less than 7 years old, DT or DTP is preferred to tetanus toxoid alone. For persons greater than or equal to 7 years of age, Td is preferred to tetanus toxoid alone (see Administration and Dosage).
[2] Tetanus immune globulin (human).
[3] If only 3 doses of fluid tetanus toxoid have been received, a fourth dose of toxoid, preferably an adsorbed toxoid, should be given.
[4] Yes, if more than 10 years since the last dose.
[5] Yes, if more than 5 years since the last dose (more frequent boosters are not needed and can accentuate side effects).

Administration and Dosage

➤*Routine prophylactic dosage schedule:*

Adults and children 7 years and older – Tetanus immune globulin (human), 250 units should be given by deep intramuscular injection (see Precautions). At the same time, but in a different extremity and with a separate syringe, Td should be administered according to the manufacturer's package insert. Adults with uncertain histories of a complete primary vaccination series should receive a primary series using the combined Td toxoid. To ensure continued protection, booster doses of Td should be given every 10 years.

Children < 7 years old – In small children the routine prophylactic dose of tetanus immune globulin (human) may be calculated by the body weight (4 units/kg). However, it may be advisable to administer the entire contents of the vial or syringe of tetanus immune globulin (human) (250 units) regardless of the child's size, since theoretically the same amount of toxin will be produced in the child's body by the infecting tetanus organism as it will in an adult's body. At the same time but in a different extremity and with a different syringe, DTP or DT, if pertussis vaccine is contraindicated, should be administered per the manufacturer's package insert.

The single injection of tetanus toxoid only initiates the series for producing active immunity in the recipient. The physician must impress upon the patient the need for further toxoid injections in 1 month and 1 year. Without such, the active immunization series is incomplete. If a contraindication to using tetanus toxoid-containing preparations exists for a person who has not completed a primary series of tetanus toxoid immunization and that person has a wound that is neither clean nor minor, only passive immunization should be given using tetanus immune globulin. See section regarding wound management under Indications.

TETANUS IMMUNE GLOBULIN (HUMAN) — INJECTION

Booster doses – Available evidence indicates that complete primary vaccination with tetanus toxoid provides long lasting protection ≥ 10 years for most recipients. Consequently, after complete primary tetanus vaccination, boosters even for wound management need be given only every 10 years when wounds are minor and uncontaminated. For other wounds, a booster is appropriate if the patient has not received tetanus toxoid within the preceding 5 years. Persons who have received at least 2 doses of tetanus toxoid rapidly develop antibodies. The prophylactic dosage schedule for these patients and for those with incomplete or uncertain immunity is shown in Indications.

Wound care – Since tetanus is actually a local infection, proper initial wound care is of paramount importance. The use of antitoxin is adjunctive to this procedure. However, in approximately 10% of recent tetanus cases, no wound or other breach in skin or mucous membrane could be implicated.

➤*Treatment of active cases of tetanus:* Standard therapy for the treatment of active tetanus including the use of tetanus immune globulin (human) must be implemented immediately. The dosage should be adjusted according to the severity of the infection.

Parenteral drug products should be inspected visually for particulate matter and discoloration prior to administration, whenever solution and container permit. They should not be used if particulate matter or discoloration are present.

➤*Directions for syringe usage:*

1.) Remove the prefilled syringe from the package. Lift syringe by barrel, not by plunger.
2.) Twist the plunger rod clockwise until the threads are seated.
3.) With the rubber needle shield secured on the syringe tip, push the plunger rod forward a few millimeters to break any friction seal between the rubber stopper and the glass syringe barrel.
4.) Remove the needle shield and expel air bubbles.
5.) Proceed with hypodermic needle puncture.
6.) Aspirate prior to injection to confirm that the needle is not in a vein or artery.
7.) Inject the medication.
8.) Withdraw the needle and dispose or destroy it.

➤*Storage/Stability:* Store at 2° to 8°C (36° to 46°F). Solution that has been frozen should not be used.

VARICELLA-ZOSTER IMMUNE GLOBULIN (HUMAN)

Rx	**Varicella-Zoster Immune Globulin (Human)** (American Red Cross)[a]	**Injection:**[b] A sterile 10% to 18% solution of the globulin fraction of human plasma, primarily IgG.	In single dose vials containing 125 units of varicella-zoster virus antibody in ≈ 1.25 mL and 625 units in ≈ 6.25 mL.

[a] Within MA, VZIG is distributed by the MA Public Health Biologic Laboratories. Outside Mass., distribution is arranged by the American Red Cross Blood Services – Northeast Region through other regional distribution centers. VZIG is distributed free of charge to MA residents.

[b] Preservative free. In 0.3 M glycine. Solvent/Detergent treated.

VARICELLA-ZOSTER IMMUNE GLOBULIN (HUMAN) — INJECTION

For complete and comparative prescribing information, refer to the Immune Globulins group monograph.

Indications

➤*Varicella prophylaxis:* For the passive immunization of exposed, susceptible individuals who are at greater risk of complications from varicella than healthy children. High-risk groups include immunocompromised children, newborns of mothers with varicella shortly before or after delivery, premature infants, immunocompromised adults, and normal susceptible adults, and may also include susceptible high-risk infants less than 1 year of age.

➤*Immunocompromised children:* For passive immunization of susceptible, immunocompromised children after significant exposure to chickenpox or zoster. These children include those with primary cellular immune deficiency disorders or neoplastic diseases and those currently receiving immunosuppressive treatments. Although VZIG administration has been shown to reduce the severity of disease and decrease the rate of complications, severe varicella and death may still occur in exposed immunocompromised children despite VZIG administration. Antiviral chemotherapy should be considered if significant clinical varicella develops after VZIG administration.

➤*Newborns of mothers with varicella shortly before or after delivery:* For newborns of mothers who develop chickenpox within 5 days before or within 48 hours after delivery. Despite VZIG administration some of these neonates may still develop varicella which can be severe or fatal. Antiviral chemotherapy should be considered in neonates who develop clinical varicella following VZIG administration.

➤*Premature infants:* Although the risk of postnatally acquired varicella in the premature infant is unknown, it has been judged prudent to administer varicella-zoster immune globulin (human) to exposed premature infants of 28 weeks gestation or more if their mothers have a negative or uncertain history of varicella. Premature infants of less than 28 weeks gestation or birth weight of less than 1000 g should be considered for VZIG regardless of maternal history since they may not yet have acquired transplacental maternal antibody.

➤*Full-term infants less than 1 year of age:* Mortality from varicella in the first year of life is 4 times higher than that in older children, but lower than mortality in immunocompromised children or healthy adults. The decision to administer VZIG to infants less than 1 year of age should be evaluated on an individual basis. After careful evaluation of the type of exposure, susceptibility to varicella including maternal history of varicella and zoster, and presence of underlying disease, VZIG may be administered to selected infants.

➤*Immunocompromised adults:* The complication rate for immunocompromised adults who contract varicella is likely to be substantially greater than for healthy adults. Approximately 90% of immunocompromised adults with negative or unknown histories of prior varicella are likely to be immune. After a careful evaluation, which might include the measurement of antibody to varicella-zoster virus by a reliable and sensitive assay such as fluorescent antibody to membrane antigen (FAMA), adults who are believed susceptible should receive VZIG.

➤*Healthy adults:* Chickenpox can be severe in healthy adults. The decision to administer VZIG to an adult should be evaluated on an individual basis. Approximately 90% of adults with negative or uncertain histories of varicella will be immune. The objective is to modify rather than prevent illness in hopes of inducing lifelong immunity. The clinician should consider the patient's health status, type of exposure, and likelihood of previous unrecognized varicella infection in deciding whether to administer VZIG. Adults who are older siblings of large families and adults whose children have had varicella are more likely to be immune. If reliable and sensitive tests for varicella antibody are available, they might be used to determine susceptibility, if time permits. If, after careful evaluation, a healthy adult with significant exposure to varicella is believed susceptible, VZIG may be administered.

➤*Pregnant women:* Pregnant women may be at higher risk of complications of chickenpox than healthy adults. They should be evaluated the same way as other adults. There is no evidence that administration of VZIG to a susceptible, pregnant woman will prevent viremia, fetal infection or congenital varicella syndrome. Therefore the primary indication for VZIG in pregnant women is to prevent complications of varicella in a susceptible adult patient rather than to prevent intrauterine infection. Pregnant women should be evaluated for type of exposure and history of infection as described for healthy adults.

➤*Timing of VZIG after varicella or zoster exposure:* Greatest effectiveness of treatment is to be expected when it is begun within 96 hours after exposure; treatment after 96 hours is of uncertain value. There is no evidence that established infections with varicella-zoster virus can be modified by varicella-zoster immune globulin (human). There is no indication for the prophylactic use of varicella-zoster immune globulin (human) in immunodeficient children or adults when there is a history of varicella, unless the patient has undergone bone marrow transplantation.

➤*Multiple exposures:* The duration of protection from a single dose of VZIG is not known. Therefore a second dose of VZIG should be considered when high risk patients have second exposures to varicella-zoster.

Administration and Dosage

➤*For IM use only:* Administer by deep intramuscular injection in the gluteal muscle, or in a physician-directed site if there are contraindications to the gluteal site. Never administer this material intravenously. The recommended dose is based on body weight according to the following schedule:

Weight of patients		Dose	
Kilograms	Pounds	Units	Number of vials
0 to 10	0 to 22	125	1 @ 125 units
10.1 to 20	22.1 to 44	250	2 @ 125 units
20.1 to 30	44.1 to 66	375	3 @ 125 units
30.1 to 40	66.1 to 88	500	4 @ 125 units
Over 40	Over 88	625	1 @ 625 units or 5 @ 125 units

Since VZIG does not contain a preservative administer the entire contents of each vial. Each 125 unit vial contains 125 units of antibody to varicella-zoster virus in a volume of approximately 1.25 mL and each 625 unit vial contains 625 units of antibody in a volume of approximately 6.25 mL. For patients weighing 10 kg or less, 125 units (1.25 mL) may be given in a single injection site. For patients weighing more than 10 kg, it is recommended that no more than 2.5 mL be given in a single injection site; however, some clinicians elect to give larger or smaller volumes. The number of units required to prevent pneumonia and death and to reduce the number of pox is unknown. The proposed dosage regimen was found to be effective in significantly modifying the expected severity of chickenpox and reducing the observed frequency of death, pneumonia, and encephalitis to less than 25% of the expected rate without treatment.

➤*Storage/Stability:* The product should be stored between 2° and 8°C (35.6° to 46.4°F). Do not freeze.

BOTULISM IMMUNE GLOBULIN IV (HUMAN) (BIG-IV)

Rx	**BabyBIG** (California Dept. of Health Services)	**Powder for injection, lyophilized**[a]: 100 ± 20 mg (50 mg/mL when reconstituted)	Preservative-free. In single-dose vial with 2 mL vial of diluent.

[a] Contains 5% sucrose, 1% albumin (human). Solvent/detergent treated.

BOTULISM IMMUNE GLOBULIN IV (HUMAN) (BIG-IV) — INJECTION (*BabyBIG*)

For complete and comparative prescribing information, refer to the Immune Globulins group monograph.

Indications

➤*Botulism:* For the treatment of patients below 1 year of age with infant botulism caused by toxin type A or B.

Administration and Dosage

➤*Approved by the FDA:* October 23, 2003.

➤*Recommended dose:* 1 mL/kg (50 mg/kg), given as a single intravenous infusion as soon as the clinical diagnosis of infant botulism is made. *BabyBIG* should be used with caution in patients with preexisting renal insufficiency and in patients judged to be at increased risk of developing renal insufficiency (including, but not limited to, those with diabetes mellitus, volume depletion, paraproteinemia, sepsis, or who are receiving known nephrotoxic drugs). In the absence of prospective data allowing identification of the maximum safe dose, concentration, and rate of infusion in these patients, do not exceed the dose, concentration, and rate of infusion recommended below.

➤*Preparation for administration:* Remove the tab portion of the vial cap and clean the rubber stopper with 70% alcohol or equivalent. Reconstitute the lyophilized powder with 2 mL of Sterile Water for Injection to obtain a 50 mg/mL *BabyBIG* solution. A double-ended transfer needle or large syringe is suitable for adding the water for reconstitution. When using a double-ended transfer needle, insert one end first into the vial of water. The lyophilized powder is supplied in an evacuated vial; therefore, the water should transfer by suction (the jet of water should be aimed to the side of the vial). After the water is transferred into the evacuated vial, the residual vacuum should be released to hasten the dissolution.

Rotate the container gently to wet all the powder. An approximately 30-minute interval should be allowed for dissolving the powder. Do not shake the vial, as this will cause foaming.

➤*Infusion:* Infusion should begin within 2 hours after reconstitution is complete and should be concluded within 4 hours of reconstitution. Vital signs should be monitored continuously during infusion. *BabyBIG* should be administered intravenously using low volume tubing and a constant infusion pump (ie, an IVAC pump or equivalent). Pre-dilution of *BabyBIG* before infusion is not recommended. The product should be administered through a separate intravenous line. If this is not possible, it may be "piggybacked" into a preexisting line if that line contains either Sodium Chloride Injection, or 1 of the following dextrose solutions (with or without NaCl added): 2.5% dextrose in water, 5% dextrose in water, 10% dextrose in water, or 20% dextrose in water. If a preexisting line must be used, *BabyBIG* should not be diluted more than 1:2 with any of the above-named solutions. Admixtures of *BabyBIG* with any other solutions have not been evaluated. Use of an in-line or syringe-tip sterile, disposable filter (18 mcm) is recommended for the administration of *BabyBIG*.

➤*Infusion rate:* The infusion should begin slowly. *BabyBIG* should be administered intravenously at 0.5 mL per kg body weight per hour (25 mg/kg/hr). If no untoward reactions occur after 15 minutes, the rate may be increased to 1 mL/kg/hr (50 mg/kg/hr, see table below). Do not exceed this rate of administration. The patient should be monitored closely during and after each rate change. At the recommended rates, infusion of the indicated dose should take 67.5 minutes total elapsed time.

Time	Rate of 5% solution	mg/kg/h
0 to 15 minutes	0.5 mL/kg/hr	25
15 minutes to end of infusion	1 mL/kg/hr	50

Minor adverse reactions experienced by patients treated with IGIV products have been related to the infusion rate. If the patient develops a minor side effect (ie, flushing), slow the rate of infusion or temporarily interrupt the infusion. If anaphylaxis or a significant drop in blood pressure occurs, discontinue the infusion and administer epinephrine.

➤*Storage/Stability:* The product should be stored between 2° and 8°C (35.6° to 46.4°F). Reconstituted *BabyBIG* should be used within 2 hours. *BabyBIG* should not be stored in the reconstituted state.

VACCINIA IMMUNE GLOBULIN INTRAVENOUS (VIGIV) (HUMAN)

Rx	**Vaccinia Immune Globulin Intravenous (Human)** (Dynport Vaccine Company LLC)	**Solution for injection**: 50 mg/mL (immunoglobulin 2,500 mg /vial).	With 5% sucrose and 1% albumin (human). In vials.

VACCINIA IMMUNE GLOBULIN INTRAVENOUS (VIGIV) (HUMAN) — INJECTION

WARNING

Immune globulin intravenous (human) (IGIV) products have been reported to be associated with renal dysfunction, acute renal failure, osmotic nephrosis, proximal tubular nephropathy, and death. Although the reports of renal dysfunction and acute renal failure have been associated with the use of many licensed IGIV products, those that contained sucrose as a stabilizer and were administered at daily doses of 400 mg/kg or greater have accounted for a disproportionate share of the total number. Vaccinia immune globulin intravenous (VIGIV) contains sucrose 5% as a stabilizer, and the recommended dose is 100 mg/kg. Patients predisposed to acute renal failure include the following: patients with any degree of preexisting renal insufficiency, diabetes mellitus, volume depletion, sepsis, or paraproteinemia, patients who are 65 years of age or older, or patients who are receiving known nephrotoxic drugs. In such patients, administer VIGIV at the minimum concentration available and at the minimum rate of infusion practical.

Indications

➤*Vaccinia conditions:* For the treatment and/or modification of the following conditions:

- Aberrant infections induced by vaccinia virus that include its accidental implantation in eyes (except in cases of isolated keratitis), mouth, or other areas where vaccinia infection would constitute a special hazard.
- Eczema vaccinatum
- Progressive vaccinia
- Severe generalized vaccinia, and
- Vaccinia infections in individuals who have skin conditions such as burns, impetigo, varicella-zoster, or poison ivy; or in individuals who have eczematous skin lesions because of either the activity or extensiveness of such lesions.

Perform treatment of complications that include vaccinia keratitis with VIGIV with caution because a single study in rabbits has demonstrated increased corneal scarring with intramuscular VIG administration. VIGIV is not considered to be effective in the treatment of postvaccinial encephalitis.

Administration and Dosage

➤*Approved by the FDA:* February 18, 2005.

➤*Recommended dose:* 2 mL/kg (100 mg/kg), given as an IV infusion, when the clinical diagnosis of a severe vaccinia-related complication is established. This dose may be repeated, depending on the severity of the symptoms and response to treatment.

The administration of higher doses (200 or 500 mg/kg) may be considered in the event that the patient does not respond to the initial 100 mg/kg dose.

➤*Preparation for administration:* Remove the tab portion of the vial cap and clean the rubber stopper with 70% alcohol or equivalent. Do not shake vial; avoid foaming.

➤*Infusion:* Begin IV infusion within 6 hours after entering the vial and complete within 12 hours of entering the vial. Monitor vital signs continuously. Administer VIGIV through an IV catheter with an administration set that contains an in-line filter (pore size: 0.22 mcm) and a constant infusion pump (ie, an IVAC pump or equivalent). Predilution of VIGIV before infusion is not recommended. Administer VIGIV through a dedicated IV catheter. Otherwise, VIGIV may be "piggybacked" into a preexisting catheter if the catheter contains either 0.9% sodium chloride for injection or 1 of the following dextrose solutions (with or without sodium chloride added): 2.5% dextrose in water, 5% dextrose in water, 10% dextrose in water, and 20% dextrose in water. If a preexisting access must be used, flush the line before use and do not dilute the VIGIV more than 1:2 (v/v) with any of these solutions. Admixtures of VIGIV with any other solutions have not been evaluated. It is recommended that VIGIV be administrated separately from other drugs or medications that the patient may be receiving.

➤*Infusion rate:* Infuse VIGIV at a rate of 1 mL/kg/h for the first 30 minutes, increased to 2 mL/kg/h for the next 30 minutes and then to 3 mL/kg/h for the remainder of the infusion, as tolerated. Do not exceed these rates of administration.

Monitor the patient closely during and after each infusion rate change. At the recommended rates, infusion at the indicated dose (100 mg/kg [2 mL/kg]) should take approximately 70 minutes.

Adverse reactions related to the infusion rate have been experienced by patients treated with IGIV products; most infusion rate-related adverse reactions reported for other IGIV products have been minor (including flushing, chills, muscle cramps, back pain, fever, nausea, vomiting, arthralgia, and wheezing). However, major adverse events are possible. Observe patients for increase in heart rate, respiratory rate, retractions, and rales. If the patient develops a minor adverse reaction (eg, flushing), slow the rate of infusion or temporarily interrupt the infusion. For serious adverse reactions, such as anaphylaxis or a significant drop in blood pressure, discontinue the infusion and administer epinephrine with or without diphenhydramine. A loop diuretic should be available for management of fluid overload during administration. To prevent the transmission of hepatitis viruses or other infectious agents, use sterile, disposable syringes and needles. Never reuse the syringes and needles.

VACCINIA IMMUNE GLOBULIN INTRAVENOUS (VIGIV) (HUMAN) — INJECTION

➤*Renal function impairment:* Use VIGIV with caution in patients with preexisting renal insufficiency and in patients judged to be at increased risk of developing renal insufficiency (including, but not limited to those with diabetes mellitus, age greater than 65 years, volume depletion, paraproteinemia, sepsis, and patients receiving known nephrotoxic drugs). In such patients who do not respond to the 100 mg/kg dose, the concentration and infusion selected should be the minimum practicable. Most cases of renal insufficiency have occurred in patients receiving total doses of IGIV containing 400 mg/kg of sucrose or greater. Doses of VIGIV higher than 400 mg/kg will exceed this level of sucrose and are thus not recommended in patients with potential renal problems.

➤*Storage/Stability:* Store VIGIV between 2° and 8°C (35.6° to 46.4°F). Start IV infusion within 6 hours after entering the vial.

MONOCLONAL ANTIBODY

PALIVIZUMAB

Rx	**Synagis** (MedImmune)	**Powder for Injection, lyophilized:** 50 mg	5.2 mg histidine, 0.2 mg glycine, 40.5 mg mannitol. Preservative-free. In 0.5 mL single-use vials.
		100 mg	8.7 mg histidine, 0.3 mg glycine, 67.5 mg mannitol. Preservative-free. In 1 mL single-use vials.
		Injection: 100 mg/mL	Preservative free. In 0.5[a] and 1[b] mL single-use vials.

[a] With 2.7 mg histidine and 0.08 mg glycine/mL.

[b] With 4.7 mg histidine and 0.1 mg glycine/mL.

PALIVIZUMAB — INJECTION

Indications

➤*Respiratory syncytial virus (RSV):* For the prevention of serious lower respiratory tract disease caused by RSV in pediatric patients at high risk of RSV disease. Safety and efficacy were established in infants with bronchopulmonary dysplasia (BPD), infants with a history of premature birth (35 weeks gestational age), and children with hemodynamically significant congenital heart disease (CHD).

Administration and Dosage

➤*Approved by the FDA:* June 19, 1998.

➤*Dosage:* The recommended dose of palivizumab is 15 mg/kg of body weight given intramuscularly (IM). Patients, including those who develop an RSV infection, should receive monthly doses throughout the RSV season. Administer the first dose prior to commencement of the RSV season. In the northern hemisphere, the RSV season typically commences in November and lasts through April, but it may begin earlier or persist later in certain communities.

Administer palivizumab at a dose of 15 mg/kg IM using aseptic technique, preferably in the anterolateral aspect of the thigh. Do not use the gluteal muscle routinely as an injection site because of the risk of damage to the sciatic nerve.

The dose per month = (patient weight [kg] × 15 mg/kg ÷ 100 mg/mL of palivizumab).Give injection volumes larger than 1 mL as a divided dose.

➤*Cardiopulmonary bypass procedure:* Palivizumab serum levels are decreased after cardiopulmonary bypass. Administer a dose of palivizumab to patients undergoing cardiopulmonary bypass as soon as possible after the cardiopulmonary bypass procedure (even if sooner than 1 month from the previous dose). Thereafter, administer doses monthly.

➤*Preparation for administration:*

Lyophilized powder –

1.) To reconstitute, remove the tab portion of the vial cap and clean the rubber stopper with 70% ethanol or equivalent.
2.) Both the 50 and 100 mg vials contain an overfill to allow the withdrawal of 50 or 100 mg, respectively, when reconstituted following the directions described in the following paragraphs.
3.) Slowly add 0.6 mL sterile water for injection to the 50 mg vial or add 1 mL sterile water for injection to the 100 mg vial. Tilt the vial slightly and gently rotate for 30 seconds to avoid foaming. Do not shake or vigorously agitate the vial. This is a critical step to avoid prolonged foaming.
4.) Let reconstituted palivizumab stand undisturbed at room temperature for a minimum of 20 minutes until the solution clarifies.
5.) Visually inspect reconstituted palivizumab for particulate matter or discoloration prior to administration. The reconstituted solution should appear clear or slightly opalescent (a thin layer of microbubbles on the surface is normal and will not affect the dosage). Do not use if there is particulate matter or if the solution is discolored.
6.) Reconstituted palivizumab does not contain a preservative. Administer within 6 hours of reconstitution. Administer immediately after withdrawal from the vial. Palivizumab is supplied in single-use vials. Do not reenter the vial. Discard any unused portion.

Liquid solution –

1.) Remove tab portion of the vial cap and clean the rubber stopper with 70% ethanol or equivalent.
2.) Both the 50 and 100 mg vials contain an overfill to allow the withdrawal of 50 or 100 mg.
3.) Palivizumab does not contain a preservative. Administer immediately after withdrawal from vial. Palivizumab is supplied in single-use vials. Do not reenter the vial. Discard any unused portion.

➤*Storage/Stability:* Upon receipt and until reconstitution for use, store palivizumab between 2° and 8°C (35.6° and 46.4°F) in its original container. Do not freeze. Reconstituted palivizumab does not contain a preservative; administer within 6 hours of reconstitution. Vials are for single-use only; do not reenter the vial and discard any unused portion. Do not use beyond the expiration date.

Actions

➤*Pharmacology:* Palivizumab exhibits neutralizing and fusion-inhibitory activity against RSV. These activities inhibit RSV replication in laboratory experiments. Although resistant RSV strains may be isolated in laboratory studies, a panel of 57 clinical RSV isolates were all neutralized by palivizumab. Palivizumab serum concentrations equal to 40 mcg/mL have been shown to reduce pulmonary RSV replication in the cotton rat model of RSV infection by 100-fold. The in vivo neutralizing activity of the active ingredient in palivizumab was assessed in a randomized, placebo-controlled study of 35 pediatric patients tracheally intubated because of RSV disease. In these patients, palivizumab significantly reduced the quantity of RSV in the lower respiratory tract compared with control patients.

➤*Pharmacokinetics:* In pediatric patients younger than 24 months of age without CHD, the mean half-life of palivizumab was 20 days, and monthly IM doses of 15 mg/kg achieved mean ± SD 30-day trough serum drug concentrations of 37 ± 21 mcg/mL after the first injection, 57 ± 41 mcg/mL after the second injection, 68 ± 51 mcg/mL after the third injection, and 72 ± 50 mcg/mL after the fourth injection. Trough concentrations following the first and fourth palivizumab dose were similar in children with CHD and in noncardiac patients. In pediatric patients given palivizumab for a second season, the mean ± SD serum concentrations following the first and fourth injections were 61 ± 17 mcg/mL and 86 ± 31 mcg/mL, respectively.

Cardiopulmonary bypass procedure – In 139 pediatric patients 24 months of age or younger with hemodynamically significant CHD who received palivizumab and underwent cardiopulmonary bypass for open-heart surgery, the mean ± SD serum palivizumab concentration was 98 ± 52 mcg/mL before bypass and declined to 41 ± 33 mcg/mL after bypass, a reduction of 58%. The clinical significance of this reduction is unknown.

Contraindications

Pediatric patients with a history of a severe reaction to palivizumab or other components of this product.

Warnings

➤*Hypersensitivity reactions:* Very rare cases of anaphylaxis (less than 1 case per 100,000 patients) have been reported following reexposure to palivizumab. Rare severe acute hypersensitivity reactions also have been reported on initial exposure or reexposure to palivizumab. None of the reported hypersensitivity reactions were fatal. Hypersensitivity reactions may include dyspnea, cyanosis, respiratory failure, urticaria, pruritus, angioedema, hypotonia, and unresponsiveness. The relationship between these reactions and the development of antibodies to palivizumab is unknown. If a severe hypersensitivity reaction occurs, permanently discontinue therapy with palivizumab. If milder hypersensitivity reactions occur, use caution on readministration of palivizumab. If anaphylaxis or severe allergic reactions occur, administer appropriate medications (eg, epinephrine) and provide supportive care as required.

➤*Pregnancy: Category C.* Palivizumab is not indicated for adult usage and animal reproduction studies have not been conducted. It also is not known whether palivizumab could affect reproductive capacity or cause fetal harm when administered to a pregnant woman.

➤*Children:* Palivizumab is indicated for use in pediatric patients.

Precautions

➤*Established RSV disease:* The safety and efficacy of palivizumab have not been demonstrated for treatment of established RSV disease.

➤*For IM use only:* Palivizumab is for IM use only. As with any IM injection, give palivizumab with caution to patients with thrombocytopenia or any coagulation disorder.

➤*Immunogenicity:* In trial 1, the incidence of antipalivizumab antibody following the fourth injection was 1.1% in the placebo group and 0.7% in the palivizumab group. In pediatric patients receiving palivizumab for a second season, 1 of 56 patients had transient, low-titer reactivity. This reactivity was not associated with adverse reactions or alteration in palivizumab serum concentrations. Immunogenicity was not assessed in trial 2.

These data reflect the percentage of patients whose test results were considered positive for antibodies to palivizumab in an ELISA assay, and are highly dependent on the sensitivity and specificity of the assay. Additionally,

PALIVIZUMAB — INJECTION

the observed incidence of antibody positivity in an assay may be influenced by several factors, including, sample handling, concomitant medications, and underlying disease. For these reasons, comparison of the incidence of antibodies to palivizumab with the incidence of antibodies to other products may be misleading.

Adverse Reactions

The most serious adverse reactions occurring with palivizumab treatment are anaphylaxis and other acute hypersensitivity reactions. The adverse reactions most commonly observed in palivizumab-treated patients were the following: cough, diarrhea, fever, gastroenteritis, otitis media, rash, rhinitis, upper respiratory tract infection, vomiting, and wheezing. Upper respiratory tract infection, otitis media, fever, and rhinitis occurred at a rate of 1% or greater in the palivizumab group compared with placebo (see the following table).

The data described reflect palivizumab exposure for 1,641 pediatric patients 3 days to 24.1 months of age in trials 1 and 2. Among these patients, 496 had bronchopulmonary dysplasia, 506 were premature birth infants younger than 6 months of age, and 639 had CHD. Adverse reactions observed in the 153 patient crossover study comparing the liquid and lyophilized formulations were similar between the 2 formulations, and similar to the adverse reactions observed with palivizumab in trials 1 and 2.

Palivizumab Adverse Reactions (≥ 1%)[a]

Adverse reaction	Palivizumab (n = 1,641)	Placebo (n = 1,148)
Fever	446 (27.1%)	289 (25.2%)
Hernia	68 (4.1%)	30 (2.6%)
Otitis media	597 (36.4%)	397 (34.6%)
Rhinitis	439 (26.8%)	282 (24.6%)
AST increased	49 (3%)	20 (1.7%)
Upper respiratory tract infection	830 (50.6%)	544 (47.4%)

[a] Cyanosis (palivizumab [9.1%]/placebo [6.9%] and arrythmia (palivizumab [3.1%]/placebo [1.7%]) were reported during trial 2 in CHD patients.

➤*Postmarketing:* The following adverse reactions have been identified and reported during postapproval use of palivizumab. Because the reports of these reactions are voluntary and the population is of uncertain size, it is not always possible to reliably estimate the frequency of the reaction or establish a causal relationship to drug exposure.

Hypersensitivity – Based on experience in over 400,000 patients who have received palivizumab (greater than 2 million doses), rare severe acute hypersensitivity reactions have been reported on initial or subsequent exposure. Very rare cases of anaphylaxis (less than 1 case per 100,000 patients) also have been reported, following reexposure. None of the reported hypersensitivity reactions were fatal. Hypersensitivity reactions may include the following: angioedema, cyanosis, dyspnea, hypotonia, pruritus, respiratory failure, unresponsiveness, and urticaria. The relationship between these reactions and the development of antibodies to palivizumab is unknown.

Limited information from postmarketing reports suggests that, within a single RSV season, adverse reactions after a sixth or greater dose of palivizumab are similar in character and frequency to those after the initial 5 doses.

Overdosage

➤*Symptoms:* No data from clinical studies are available on overdosage. No toxicity was observed in rabbits administered a single IM or subcutaneous injection of palivizumab at a dose of 50 mg/kg. No data are available from human subjects who have received more than 5 monthly palivizumab doses during a single RSV season.

ANTITOXINS/ANTIVENINS

ANTIVENIN (LATRODECTUS MACTANS) (Black Widow Spider Antivenin) (Equine Origin)

Rx	**Antivenin** (*Latrodectus mactans*) (Merck)	**Powder for Injection:** ≥ 6000 antivenin units/vial[a]	In single-use vials with 1 vial diluent (2.5 mL vial of sterile water for injection) and 1 mL vial of normal horse serum[a] (1:10 dilution) for sensitivity testing.

[a] With 1:10,000 thimerosal.

ANTIVENIN (LATRODECTUS MACTANS) (Black Widow Spider Antivenin) (Equine Origin) — INJECTION

Indications

➤*Envenomations:* For passive, transient protection from toxic effects of bites by the black widow (*Latrodectus mactans*) and similar spiders. Emphasize early use of this antivenin for prompt relief. The best effect occurs with antivenin administration within 4 hours after envenomation.

Administration and Dosage

➤*Sensitivity testing (horse serum):* Prior to treatment with any product prepared from horse serum, carefully review the patient's history emphasizing prior exposure to horse serum or any allergies. Serious sickness and even death could result from the use of horse serum in a sensitive patient. Perform a skin or conjunctival test prior to administration.

Skin test – Inject into (not under) the skin no more than 0.02 mL of the test material (1:10 dilution of normal horse serum in physiologic saline). Evaluate result in 10 minutes. A positive reaction is an urticarial wheal surrounded by a zone of erythema. A control test using sodium chloride injection facilitates interpretation of the results.

Conjunctival test – For adults, instill 1 drop of a 1:10 dilution of horse serum into the conjunctival sac, and for children instill 1 drop of 1:100 dilution. Itching of the eye and reddening of the conjunctiva indicate a positive reaction, usually within 10 minutes.

➤*Adults and children:* Inject 1 vial (2.5 mL) of antivenin IM, preferably in the region of the anterolateral thigh so that a tourniquet may be applied in the event of a systemic reaction. Symptoms usually subside in 1 to 3 hours. Although 1 dose is usually adequate, a second dose may be necessary.

May also be given IV in 10 to 50 mL of saline over 15 minutes. This is the preferred route in severe cases, when the patient is younger than 12 years of age, or in shock. One vial is usually adequate.

➤*Desensitization:* Attempt desensitization only when the administration of antivenin is considered necessary to save a life. Epinephrine must be available in case of untoward reaction.

If the history is positive or the results of the sensitivity tests are mildly or questionably positive, administer antivenin as follows to reduce the risk of an immediate severe allergic reaction:

1.) In separate sterile vials or syringes, prepare 1:10 or 1:100 dilutions of antivenin in sodium chloride for injection.
2.) Allow at least 15 but preferably 30 minutes between injections and only proceed with the next dose if no reactions occurred following the previous dose.
3.) Using a tuberculin syringe, inject SC 0.1, 0.2, and 0.5 mL of the 1:100 dilution at 15- or 30-minute intervals; repeat with the 1:10 dilution, and finally the undiluted antivenin.
4.) If there is a reaction after any of the injections, place a tourniquet proximal to the sites of injection and administer epinephrine 1:1000 (0.3 to 1 mL SC, 0.05 to 0.1 mL IV), proximal to the tourniquet or into another extremity. Wait at least 30 minutes before giving another injection of antivenin, the amount of which should be the same as the last one not evoking a reaction.
5.) If no reaction has occurred after 0.5 mL of undiluted antivenin has been given, it is probably safe to continue the dose at 15-minute intervals until the entire dose has been injected.

➤*Storage/Stability:* Refrigerate at 2° to 8°C (36° to 46°F). Do not freeze. Discard if frozen. Do not expose to excessive heat. When reconstituted, the color of the antivenin ranges from light (straw) to very dark (iced tea), but the color has no effect on potency.

Actions

➤*Pharmacology:* Prepared from blood serum of horses immunized against black widow spider venom. Moderately effective in pain relief and can be life-saving. IV effect is rapid; concentration peaks 2 to 3 days after IM injection. Mean half-life is less than 15 days. Symptoms begin to subside within 1 to 3 hours following administration.

Warnings

➤*Serum sickness:* Observe patients for serum sickness for an average of 8 to 12 days following administration of antivenin.

➤*Pregnancy: Category C.* It is not known whether the antivenin can cause fetal harm when administered to a pregnant woman or can affect reproduction capacity. Give to a pregnant woman only if clearly needed and when potential benefits outweigh potential hazards to the fetus.

Envenomation has produced spontaneous abortion.

➤*Lactation:* It is not known whether this drug is excreted in breast milk. Use caution when administering to a nursing woman.

➤*Children:* Controlled studies have not been conducted. However, there have been virtually no adverse effects in children receiving this product.

Adverse Reactions

➤*Hypersensitivity:* Anaphylaxis and serum sickness have been reported following use of antivenin.

Patient Information

Advise patients to contact their physician immediately if they experience any signs and symptoms of delayed allergic reactions or serum sickness (eg, rash, pruritus, urticaria, muscle aches, fever) after hospital discharge.

ANTIVENIN (CROTALIDAE) POLYVALENT (Equine Origin)

Rx	Antivenin (Crotalidae) Polyvalent (Wyeth-Ayerst)[a]	Powder for Injection, lyophilized[b]	In single-use vials with 1 vial diluent (10 mL Bacteriostatic Water for Injection, USP).[c]

[a] The manufacturer is in the process of discontinuing this product; however, it will continue to produce the product until an alternative source is identified.

[b] With 0.25% phenol and 0.005% thimerosal.

[c] With 0.001% phenylmercuric nitrate.

ANTIVENIN (CROTALIDAE) POLYVALENT (Equine Origin) – INJECTION

Indications

➤*Envenomations:* For treatment of envenomations caused by the bites of crotalids (pit vipers) native to North, Central, and South America, including rattlesnakes (*Crotalus*, *Sistrurus*); copperhead and cottonmouth (*Agkistrodon*), including *A. halys* of Korea and Japan; the Fer-de-lance and other species of Bothrops; the tropical rattler (*C. durissus* and similar species); the Cantil (*A. bilineatus*); and bushmaster (*Lachesis mutus*) of South and Central America.

Administration and Dosage

➤*Test for sensitivity to horse serum:* Test for sensitivity whenever a product containing horse serum is administered. There is a possibility of a severe immediate reaction. Constant observation for untoward reactions is mandatory. Should any systemic reaction occur, discontinue use and initiate appropriate treatment including a tourniquet, airway, oxygen, epinephrine, an injectable pressor amine, and corticosteroids. See also Management of Acute Hypersensitivity Reactions.

➤*Sensitivity testing (horse serum):* Before administration of any product prepared from horse serum, appropriate measures must be taken in an effort to detect the presence of dangerous sensitivity:

1.) A careful review of the patient's history including any report of the following:
 a.) asthma, hay fever, urticaria, or other allergic manifestations;
 b.) allergic reactions upon exposure to horses;
 c.) prior injections of horse serum.
2.) A suitable test for detection of sensitivity. Perform a skin test in every patient prior to administration, regardless of clinical history.

Skin test – Intracutaneously inject 0.02 to 0.03 mL of a 1:10 dilution of Normal Horse Serum or Antivenin. A control test on the opposite extremity, using Sodium Chloride Injection, USP, facilitates interpretation. Use of larger amounts for the skin-test dose increases the likelihood of false-positive reactions, and in the exquisitely sensitive patient, increases the risk of a systemic reaction from the skin-test dose. Use ≥ 1:100 dilution for preliminary skin testing if the history suggests sensitivity. A positive reaction to a skin test occurs within 5 to 30 minutes and is manifested by a wheal with or without pseudopodia and surrounding erythema. In general, the shorter the interval between injection and the beginning of the skin reaction, the greater the sensitivity.

If the history is negative for allergy and the result of a skin test is negative, proceed with administration of antivenin as outlined. If the history is positive, and a skin test is strongly positive, administration may be dangerous, especially if the positive sensitivity test is accompanied by systemic allergic manifestations. In such instances, the risk of administering antivenin must be weighed against the risk of withholding it, keeping in mind that severe envenomation can be fatal.

A negative allergic history and absence of reaction to a properly applied skin test do not rule out the possibility of an immediate reaction. Also, a negative skin test has no bearing on whether or not delayed serum reactions (serum sickness) will occur after administration of the full dose.

Desensitization – If the history is negative, and the skin test is mildly or questionably positive, administer as follows to reduce the risk of a severe immediate systemic reaction:

1.) Prepare, in separate sterile vials or syringes, 1:100 and 1:10 dilutions of antivenin.
2.) Allow ≥ 15 minutes between injections and proceed with the next dose if no reaction follows the previous dose.
3.) Inject SC using a tuberculin-type syringe, 0.1, 0.2, and 0.5 mL of the 1:100 dilution at 15-minute intervals; repeat with the 1:10 dilution, and finally undiluted antivenin.
4.) If a systemic reaction occurs after any injection, place a tourniquet proximal to the site of injections and administer an appropriate dose of epinephrine, 1:1000, proximal to the tourniquet or into another extremity. Wait ≥ 30 minutes before injecting another dose. The amount of the next dose should be the same as the last that did not evoke a reaction.
5.) If no reaction occurs after 0.5 mL of undiluted antivenin has been administered, switch to the IM route and continue doubling the dose at 15-minute intervals until the entire dose has been injected IM or proceed to the IV route as described in Administration and Dosage.

Obviously, if the just-described schedule is used, ≥ 3 to 5 hours would be required to administer the initial dose suggested for a moderate or severe envenomation, and time is an important factor in neutralization of venom in a critically ill patient. Wingert and Wainschel have described a procedure based on the experience of their group, which they have used in some severely envenomated patients who have positive sensitivity tests: 50 to 100 mg of diphenhydramine HCl is given IV followed by slow IV infusion of diluted antivenin for 15 to 20 minutes while carefully observing the patient for symptoms and signs of anaphylaxis; if anaphylaxis does not occur, antivenin is continued, maintaining close observation of the patient. Patients who require antivenin but develop signs of impending anaphylaxis in spite of this or the procedure described earlier, present a difficult problem; seek consultation.

➤*IV route:* IV route is preferred; if shock is present, IV use is mandatory. Administer within 4 hours of bite; it is less effective when given after 8 hours, and may be of questionable value after 12 hours. However, in severe poisonings, administer antivenin even if 24 hours have elapsed since time of bite. Maximum blood levels of antivenin may not be obtained for ≥ 8 hours following IM administration.

➤*Reconstituting dried antivenin:* Withdraw diluent and inject into the vial of antivenin. Gentle agitation will hasten complete dissolution of the lyophilized drug.

For IV drip, prepare a 1:1 to 1:10 dilution of reconstituted drug in Sodium Chloride Injection, USP, or 5% Dextrose Injection, USP. Gently swirl to avoid foaming. Infuse initial 5 to 10 mL over 3 to 5 minutes, while observing patient; if no immediate systemic reactions appear, continue infusion with delivery at the maximum safe rate for IV fluid administration. To determine dilution, type of electrolyte solution, and delivery rate, consider the patient's age, weight, and cardiac status; severity of envenomation; estimated total amount of parenteral fluids needed; and interval between bite and therapy initiation.

➤*Initial dose:* Give entire initial dose as soon as possible based on the best estimate of the severity of envenomation. The following doses are recommended:

No envenomation – No local or systemic manifestations: No dose given.

Minimal envenomation – Local swelling and other local changes; no systemic manifestations; normal laboratory findings: 20 to 40 mL (2 to 4 vials).

Moderate envenomation – Swelling progresses beyond the site of bite; ≥ 1 systemic manifestations; abnormal laboratory findings (eg, decreased hematocrit or platelets): 50 to 90 mL (5 to 9 vials).

Severe envenomation – Marked local response, severe systemic manifestations, significant alteration in laboratory findings: ≥ 100 to 150 mL (≥ 10 to 15 vials).

Base the need for additional antivenin on clinical response to initial dose and continuing assessment of severity of poisoning. If swelling progresses, systemic symptoms increase in severity, or if new manifestations appear, administer an additional 10 to 50 mL (1 to 5 vials) IV.

➤*Children:* Envenomation by large snakes in children or small adults requires larger doses of antivenin. The amount administered to a child is not based on weight (see Warnings).

➤*IM:* Administer into large muscle mass, preferably the gluteal area, taking care to avoid nerve trunks. Never inject into a finger or toe.

➤*Other treatment:* The efficacy of corticosteroids in treatment of envenomation per se or venom shock is not resolved. Do not give corticosteroids simultaneously with antivenin on a routine basis or during the acute state of envenomation; however, their use may be necessary to treat immediate allergic reactions to antivenin, and corticosteroids are the agents of choice for treating serious delayed reactions to antivenin.

Snakes' mouths do not harbor *Clostridium tetani*. However, appropriate tetanus prophylaxis is indicated, since tetanus spores may be carried into the fang puncture wounds by dirt present on skin at time of bite or by non-sterile first-aid procedures.

A broad-spectrum antibiotic in adequate dosage is indicated if local tissue damage is evident.

➤*Storage/Stability:* Store at room temperature, not exceeding 37°C (99°F). The lyophilized form can tolerate 3 freeze/thaw cycles. The product can be stored ≤ 10 days at 45°C (113°F). Use reconstituted solution within 48 hours and dilutions within 12 hours. To avoid foaming and protein degradation, mix by gently swirling rather than shaking.

Actions

➤*Pharmacology:* Concentrated serum globulins from horses immunized with the following venoms: *Crotalus adamanteus* (Eastern diamond rattlesnake), *C. atrox* (Western diamond rattlesnake), *C. durissus terrificus* (tropical rattlesnake, Cascabel), and *Bothrops atrox* (Fer-de-lance). IV effect is rapid; concentration peaks in ≥ 8 hours after IM injection. Mean half-life is < 15 days.

The location of antivenins for rare species and names and telephone numbers of experts on venomous bites can be obtained at any hour from the Arizona Poison Control Center (520-626-6016).

Warnings

➤*Pit viper bites and envenomation:* Symptoms, signs, and severity of snake venom poisoning depend on many factors including species, age, and size of the snake; number and location of bite(s); depth of venom deposit; condition of the snake's fangs and venom glands; length of time the snake "hangs on"; age, general health and size of the victim; timing, type, and efficacy of first-aid treatment rendered to remove venom. In any snake bite, the actual amount of venom introduced is unknown. The type of clothing or leg/footwear through which the snake's fangs pass may affect the amount of venom delivered. Although most North American pit vipers tend to bite and introduce venom superficially, their fangs may get hung up in SC tissues during the biting act and penetrate deeper tissues during the attempt to release the bitten part. In some bites, fangs may penetrate into muscle. In such cases, the usual local superficial manifestations of envenomation may not appear early in the course of poisoning. In bites by some species, systemic evidence of envenomation may be present in the absence of significant local manifestations. It may be difficult to determine the severity of enven-

ANTIVENIN (CROTALIDAE) POLYVALENT (Equine Origin) – INJECTION

omation during the first several hours after a pit viper bite; estimates of severity may need to be revised as poisoning progresses. Not all pit viper bites result in envenomation. In ≈ 20% of rattlesnake bites, the snake may not inject any venom.

➤*Local (fang punctures) signs and symptoms of envenomation:*

Swelling – Edema, usually seen around the bite area within 5 minutes, may progress rapidly and involve the entire extremity within an hour. Generally, edema spreads more slowly, usually over a period of ≥ 8 hours. Swelling is usually most severe following envenomation by the Eastern diamondback; less severe after bites by the Western diamondback, prairie, timber, red, Pacific, Mojave, and blacktailed rattlers, the sidewinder, and the cottonmouth; least severe after bites by copperheads, massasauga, and pygmy rattlers.

Ecchymosis and skin discoloration – These effects often appear in the bite area within a few hours. Vesicules may form in a few hours and are usually present at 24 hours. Hemorrhagic blebs and petechiae are common. Necrosis may develop, necessitating amputation.

Pain – Pain frequently begins shortly after a bite by most pit vipers. Pain may be absent after bites by Mojave rattlers.

➤*Systemic signs and symptoms of envenomation:* Weakness; faintness; nausea; sweating; numbness or tingling around the mouth, tongue, scalp, fingers, toes, bite area; muscle fasciculations; hypotension; prolonged bleeding and clotting times; hemoconcentration followed by decrease in erythrocytes; thrombocytopenia; hematuria; proteinuria; vomiting, including hematemesis; melena; hemoptysis; epistaxis.

In fatal poisoning, cause of death is frequently associated with destruction of erythrocytes and changes in capillary permeability, especially of the pulmonary vascular system, leading to pulmonary edema; hemoconcentration usually occurs early, probably as a result of plasma loss secondary to vascular permeability; hemoglobin may fall, and bleeding may occur throughout the body as early as 6 hours after the bite. Renal involvement is common. Mojave rattler venom may cause neuromuscular changes leading to respiratory failure.

Defibrination and disseminated intravascular coagulation syndromes have been associated with envenomation caused by some pit vipers native to the US, and appropriate therapy may be indicated.

➤*Supportive care:* Treat suspected envenomation as a medical emergency. Until careful observation provides clear evidence that envenomation has not occurred or is minimal, follow these procedures: Monitor vital signs frequently. Draw blood as soon as possible for baseline lab studies, including type and cross-match, CBC, hematocrit, platelet count, prothrombin time, clot retraction, bleeding and coagulation times, BUN, electrolytes, and bilirubin. During the first 4 or 5 days after a severe envenomation, perform hemoglobin, hematocrit, and platelet counts several times a day. Obtain urine samples at frequent intervals, with special attention to microscopic examination for presence of erythrocytes. Chart fluid intake and urine output. To monitor progression of edema, measure the circumference of the bitten extremity every 15 to 30 minutes, just proximal to the bite and at ≥ 1 additional points, each several inches closer to the trunk.

Have the following available for immediate use: Oxygen and resuscitation equipment including airway, epinephrine, parenteral antihistamines, and corticosteroids.

Start IV infusions: Use 1 line for supportive therapy, if needed, and the other line for administration of the antivenin and electrolytes.

Treat shock following envenomation like shock from hypovolemia of any cause, including administration of blood products or plasma expanders, as indicated.

Codeine is usually adequate for relieving pain. Sedation with phenobarbital or mild tranquilizers may be used if indicated, but not in the presence of respiratory failure.

Do not pack the bitten extremity in ice, and cryotherapy is contraindicated.

Compartment syndromes may complicate pit viper envenomations, especially those caused by bites on the lower extremities. Prompt surgical consultation is indicated whenever a closed-compartment syndrome is suspected.

➤*Hypersensitivity reactions:* The immediate reaction (eg, shock, anaphylaxis) usually occurs within 30 minutes. Symptoms and signs include the following: Apprehension; flushing; itching; urticaria; edema of the face, tongue, and throat; cough; dyspnea; cyanosis; vomiting; collapse.

Serum sickness – Serum sickness usually occurs 5 to 24 days after administration. The incubation period may be < 5 days, especially in those who have received horse-serum-containing preparations in the past. The usual symptoms and signs are malaise, fever, urticaria, lymphadenopathy, edema, arthralgia, nausea, and vomiting. Occasionally, neurological manifestations develop, such as meningismus or peripheral neuritis. Peripheral neuritis usually involves the shoulders and arms. Pain and muscle weakness are frequently present, and permanent atrophy may develop.

➤*Pregnancy: Category C.* Use only if clearly needed, with appropriate consideration of the risk-benefit ratio. It is not known if antivenin antibodies cross the placenta. Intact IgG crosses the placenta from the maternal circulation increasingly after 30 weeks gestation.

➤*Lactation:* It is not known if antivenin antibodies are excreted into breast milk. Problems in humans have not been documented.

➤*Children:* Children may require larger doses than adults, because of a child's relatively small volume of body fluid in which to dilute the venom. Do not adjust pediatric doses by the weight of the patient.

Adverse Reactions

➤*Hypersensitivity:* The immediate reaction (eg, shock, anaphylaxis) usually occurs within 30 minutes. Symptoms and signs include the following: Apprehension; flushing; itching; urticaria; edema of the face, tongue, and throat; cough; dyspnea; cyanosis; vomiting; collapse.

Serum sickness – Serum sickness usually occurs 5 to 24 days after administration. The incubation period may be < 5 days, especially in those who have received horse-serum-containing preparations in the past. The usual symptoms and signs are malaise, fever, urticaria, lymphadenopathy, edema, arthralgia, nausea, and vomiting. Occasionally, neurological manifestations develop, such as meningismus or peripheral neuritis. Peripheral neuritis usually involves the shoulders and arms. Pain and muscle weakness are frequently present, and permanent atrophy may develop.

Patient Information

Advise patients to contact their physician immediately if they experience any signs or symptoms of delayed allergic reactions or serum sickness (eg, rash, pruritus, urticaria) after hospital discharge.

CROTALIDAE POLYVALENT IMMUNE FAB (Ovine Origin)

Rx	**CroFab** (Altana)	**Powder for Injection, lyophilized**	1 g total protein and thimerosal (0.11 mg mercury)/vial. Diluent not included. In single-use vials.

CROTALIDAE POLYVALENT IMMUNE FAB (OVINE) — INJECTION

Indications

➤*Envenomation:* Crotalidae polyvalent immune fab (ovine) injection is indicated for the management of patients with minimal or moderate North American rattlesnake envenomation. Crotalidae polyvalent immune fab (ovine) injection was effective in neutralizing the venoms of 10 clinically important North American Crotalid snakes in a murine lethality model. Early use of Crotalidae polyvalent immune fab (ovine) injection (within 6 hours of snakebite) is advised to prevent clinical deterioration and the occurrence of systemic coagulation abnormalities.

Administration and Dosage

➤*Approved by the FDA:* October 2, 2000.

➤*Reconstitution:* Each vial of Crotalidae polyvalent immune fab (ovine) injection should be reconstituted with 10 mL of sterile water for injection (diluent not included) and mixed by continuous gentle swirling. The contents of the reconstituted vials should be further diluted in 250 mL of 0.9% Sodium Chloride and mixed by gently swirling. The reconstituted and diluted product should be used within 4 hours.

➤*Administration:* Administration of antivenin should be initiated as soon as possible after crotalid snakebite in patients who develop signs of progressive envenomation (eg, worsening local injury, coagulation abnormality, systemic signs of envenomation). Crotalidae polyvalent immune fab (ovine) injection was shown in the clinical studies to be effective when given within 6 hours of snakebite.

➤*Dosing schedule:* Antivenin dosage requirements are contingent upon an individual patient's response; however, based on clinical experience with Crotalidae polyvalent immune fab (ovine) injection, the recommended initial dose is 4 to 6 vials. The patient should be observed for up to 1 hour following the completion of this first dose to determine if initial control of the envenomation has been achieved (as defined by complete arrest of local manifestations and return of coagulation tests and systemic signs to normal). If initial control is not achieved by the first dose, an additional dose of 4 to 6 vials should be repeated until initial control of the envenomation syndrome has been achieved. After initial control has been established, additional 2-vial doses of Crotalidae polyvalent immune fab (ovine) injection every 6 hours for up to 18 hours (3 doses) is recommended. Optimal dosing following the 18-hour scheduled dose of Crotalidae polyvalent immune fab (ovine) injection has not been determined. Additional 2-vial doses may be administered as deemed necessary by the treating physician, based on the patient's clinical course.

➤*Infusion rate:* The initial dose of Crotalidae polyvalent immune fab (ovine) injection diluted in 250 mL of saline should be infused IV over 60 minutes. However, the infusion should proceed slowly over the first 10 minutes at a 25 to 50 mL/hr rate with careful observation for any allergic reaction. If no such reaction occurs, the infusion rate may be increased to the full 250 mL/hr rate until completion. Close patient monitoring is necessary.

➤*Additional patient care:* Supportive measures are often utilized to treat certain manifestations of crotalid snake envenomation, such as pain, swelling, hypotension, and wound infection. Poison control centers are a helpful resource for individual treatment advice.

➤*Storage / Stability:* The product should be stored at 2° to 8°C (36° to 46°F). Do not freeze. The product must be used within 4 hours after reconstitution.

Actions

➤*Pharmacology:* Crotalidae polyvalent immune fab (ovine) injection is a venom-specific fab fragment of immunoglobulin G (IgG) that works by binding and neutralizing venom toxins, facilitating their redistribution away from target tissues and their elimination from the body.

CROTALIDAE POLYVALENT IMMUNE FAB (OVINE) — INJECTION

➤*Pharmacokinetics:*

Excretion – The planned pharmacokinetic study of Crotalidae polyvalent immune fab (ovine) injection was not adequately performed. A limited number of samples were collected from 3 patients. Based on these data, estimates of elimination half-life were made. The elimination half-life for total fab ranged from approximately 12 to 23 hours. These limited pharmacokinetic estimates of half-life are augmented by data obtained with an analogous ovine fab product that was produced using a similar production process. In that study, 8 healthy subjects were given 1 mg of IV digoxin followed by an approximately equimolar neutralizing dose of 76 mg of digoxin immune fab (ovine). Total fab was shown to have a volume of distribution of 0.3 L/kg, a systemic clearance of 32 mL/min (approximately 0.4 mL/min/kg) and an elimination half-life of approximately 15 hours.

Contraindications

Crotalidae polyvalent immune fab (ovine) injection should not be administered to patients with a known history of hypersensitivity to papaya or papain, unless the benefits outweigh the risks and appropriate management for anaphylactic reactions is readily available.

Warnings

➤*Coagulopathy:* Coagulopathy is a complication noted in many victims of viper envenomation that arises due to the ability of the snake venom to interfere with the blood coagulation cascade. In clinical trials with Crotalidae polyvalent immune fab (ovine) injection, recurrent coagulopathy (the return of a coagulation abnormality after it has been successfully treated with antivenin), characterized by decreased fibrinogen, decreased platelets, and elevated prothrombin time, occurred in approximately half of patients studied. The clinical significance of these recurrent abnormalities is not known. Recurrent coagulation abnormalities were observed only in patients who experienced coagulation abnormalities during their initial hospitalizations. Optimal dosing to completely prevent recurrent coagulopathy has not been determined. Because Crotalidae polyvalent immune fab (ovine) injection has a shorter persistence in the blood than crotalid venoms that can leak from depot sites over a prolonged period of time, repeat dosing to prevent or treat such recurrence may be necessary. Additional 2-vial doses may be administered as deemed necessary by the treating physician, based on the patient's clinical course.

Recurrent coagulopathy may persist for 1 to 2 weeks or more. Patients who experience coagulopathy due to snakebite during hospitalization for initial treatment should be monitored for signs and symptoms of recurrent coagulopathy for up to 1 week or longer at the physician's discretion. During this period, the physician should carefully assess the need for retreatment with Crotalidae polyvalent immune fab (ovine) injection and use of any type of anticoagulant or antiplatelet drug.

➤*Hypersensitivity reactions:* Papain is used to cleave the whole antibody into fab and Fc fragments, and trace amounts of papain or inactivated papain residues may be present in Crotalidae polyvalent immune fab (ovine) injection. Patients with allergies to papain, chymopapain, other papaya extracts, or the pineapple enzyme bromelain may also be at risk for allergic reactions to Crotalidae polyvalent immune fab (ovine) injection. In addition, it has been noted in the literature that some dust mite allergens and some latex allergens share antigenic structures with papain, and patients with these allergies may be allergic to papain.

Crotalidae polyvalent immune fab (ovine) injection should not be administered to patients with known histories of hypersensitivity to papaya or papain, unless the benefits outweigh the risks and appropriate management for anaphylactic reactions is readily available.

Anaphylaxis, anaphylactoid reactions and allergic reactions – The possible risks and side effects that attend the administration of heterologous animal proteins in humans include anaphylactic and anaphylactoid reactions, delayed allergic reactions (late serum reaction or serum sickness) and possible febrile responses to immune complexes formed by animal antibodies and neutralized venom components. Although no patient in the clinical studies of Crotalidae polyvalent immune fab (ovine) injection has experienced a severe anaphylactic reaction, the possibility of an anaphylactic reaction should be considered. The patient should be informed of the possibility of an anaphylactic reaction, and close patient monitoring and readiness with IV therapy using epinephrine and diphenhydramine hydrochloride is recommended during the infusion of Crotalidae polyvalent immune fab (ovine) injection. If an anaphylactic reaction occurs during the infusion, Crotalidae polyvalent immune fab (ovine) injection administration should be terminated at once and appropriate treatment administered. Patients with known allergies to sheep protein would be particularly at risk for an anaphylactic reaction.

See Precautions for more information.

Infusion reactions: It has been noted in the literature with the use of other antibody therapies that reactions during the infusion, such as fever, low back pain, wheezing and nausea are often related to the rate of infusion and can be controlled by decreasing the rate of administration of the solution.

Sensitivity: Patients who receive courses of treatment with foreign proteins such as Crotalidae polyvalent immune fab (ovine) injection may become sensitized to them. Therefore, caution should be used when administering a repeat course of treatment with Crotalidae polyvalent immune fab (ovine) injection for a subsequent envenomation episode.

➤*Pregnancy: Category C.* Animal reproduction studies have not been conducted with Crotalidae polyvalent immune fab (ovine) injection. It is also not known whether Crotalidae polyvalent immune fab (ovine) injection can cause fetal harm when administered to a pregnant woman or can affect reproduction capacity. Crotalidae polyvalent immune fab (ovine) injection should be given to a pregnant woman only if clearly needed.

Crotalidae polyvalent immune fab (ovine) injection contains mercury in the form of ethyl mercury from thimerosal. The final product contains up to 104.5 mcg or approximately 0.11 mg of mercury per vial, which amounts to no more than 1.9 mg of mercury per dose (based on the maximum dose of 18 vials studied in clinical trials of Crotalidae polyvalent immune fab [ovine]injection). While there are no definitive data on the toxicity of ethyl mercury, literature suggests that information related to methyl mercury toxicities may be applicable. Developing fetuses and very young children are most susceptible and, therefore, at greater risk.

➤*Lactation:* It is not known whether Crotalidae polyvalent immune fab (ovine) injection is excreted in human breast milk. Because many drugs are excreted in human milk, caution should be exercised when Crotalidae polyvalent immune fab (ovine) injection is administered to a nursing woman.

➤*Children:* Specific studies in pediatric patients have not been conducted. The absolute venom dose following snakebite is expected to be the same in children and adults, therefore, no dosage adjustment for age should be made.

Crotalidae polyvalent immune fab (ovine) injection contains mercury in the form of ethyl mercury from thimerosal. Although there are limited toxicology data on ethyl mercury, high dose and acute exposures to methyl mercury have been associated with neurological and renal toxicities. Developing fetuses and very young children are most susceptible and, therefore, at greater risk.

Precautions

➤*Monitoring:* All patients treated with antivenin should be carefully monitored for signs and symptoms of an acute allergic reaction (eg, urticaria, pruritus, erythema, angioedema, bronchospasm with wheezing or cough, stridor, laryngeal edema, hypotension, tachycardia) and treated with appropriate emergency medical care (eg, epinephrine, IV antihistamines, albuterol). All patients should be followed up for signs and symptoms of delayed allergic reactions or serum sickness (eg, rash, fever, myalgia, arthralgia) and treated appropriately, if necessary.

➤*Mercury:* Crotalidae polyvalent immune fab (ovine) injection contains mercury in the form of ethyl mercury from thimerosal. The final product contains up to 104.5 mcg or approximately 0.11 mg of mercury per vial, which amounts to no more than 1.9 mg of mercury per dose (based on the maximum dose of 18 vials studied in clinical trials of Crotalidae polyvalent immune fab [ovine]injection). While there are no definitive data on the toxicity of ethyl mercury, literature suggests that information related to methyl mercury toxicities may be applicable.

➤*Special risk:* Because snake envenomation can cause coagulation abnormalities, the following conditions, which are also associated with coagulation defects, should be considered: Cancer, collagen disease, congestive heart failure, diarrhea, elevated temperature, hepatic disorders, hyperthyroidism, poor nutritional state, steatorrhea, vitamin K deficiency.

Adverse Reactions

The most common adverse reactions reported in the clinical studies were urticaria and rash. Adverse reactions involving the skin and appendages (primarily rash, urticaria, and pruritus) were reported in 14 of the 42 patients (see the following table).

Of the 25 patients who experienced adverse reactions, 3 patients experienced severe or serious adverse reactions. The 1 patient who experienced a serious adverse event had a recurrent coagulopathy due to envenomation, which required rehospitalization and additional antivenin administration. This patient eventually made a complete recovery. The other 2 patients that had severe adverse reactions consisted of 1 patient who developed severe hives following treatment and 1 patient who developed a severe rash and pruritus several days following treatment. Both patients recovered following treatment with antihistamines and prednisone.

One patient discontinued Crotalidae polyvalent immune fab (ovine) injection therapy due to an allergic reaction.

Incidence of clinical adverse reactions in studies of Crotalidae polyvalent immune fab (ovine) injection by body system

Adverse reactions	n = 42 *; number of reactions
Miscellaneous	
Back pain	2
Chest pain	1
Cellulitis	1
Wound infection	1
Chills	1
Allergic reaction **	1
Serum sickness	1
Dermatologic	
Urticaria	7
Rash	5
Pruritus	3
Subcutaneous nodule	1
Cardiovascular	
Hypotension	1

CROTALIDAE POLYVALENT IMMUNE FAB (OVINE) — INJECTION

Incidence of clinical adverse reactions in studies of Crotalidae polyvalent immune fab (ovine) injection by body system

Adverse reactions	n = 42 *; number of reactions
Respiratory	
Asthma	1
Cough	1
Increased sputum	1
GI	
Nausea	3
Anorexia	1
Hematologic/lymphatic	
Coagulation disorder	3
Ecchymosis	1
Musculoskeletal	
Myalgia	1
CNS	
Circumoral paresthesia	1
General paresthesia	1
Nervousness	1

* Of the 42 patients receiving Crotalidae polyvalent immune fab (ovine) injection in the clinical studies, 25 experienced an adverse reaction. A total of 40 adverse reactions was experienced by these 25 patients.
** Allergic reactions consisted of urticaria, dyspnea, and wheezing in 1 patient.

In the 42 patients treated with Crotalidae polyvalent immune fab (ovine) injection for minimal or moderate crotalid envenomations, there were 7 reactions classified as early serum reactions and 5 reactions classified as late serum reactions, and none was serious. In the clinical studies, serum reactions consisted mainly of urticaria and rash, and all patients recovered without sequelae.

Incidence of early and late serum reactions (reactions associated with Crotalidae polyvalent immune fab (ovine) injection

	n = 42 *; number of reactions
Early serum reactions	
Urticaria	5
Cough	1
Allergic reaction **	1
Late serum reactions	
Rash	2
Pruritus	1
Urticaria	1
Serum sickness ***	1

* Six of the 42 patients experienced an adverse reaction associated with an early serum reaction, and 4 experienced an adverse reaction associated with a late serum reaction. Two additional patients were considered to have a late serum reaction by the investigator, although no associated adverse reaction was reported.
** Allergic reaction consisted of urticaria, dyspnea and wheezing in 1 patient.
*** Serum sickness consisted of severe rash and pruritus in 1 patient.

Overdosage

The maximum amount of Crotalidae polyvalent immune fab (ovine) injection that can safely be administered in single or multiple doses has not been determined. Doses of up to 18 vials (approximately 13.5 g of protein) have been administered without any observed direct toxic effect.

Patient Information

Patients should be advised to contact their physicians immediately if they experience any signs and symptoms of delayed allergic reactions or serum sickness (eg, rash, pruritus, urticaria) after hospital discharge.

Patients should be advised to contact their physicians immediately if they experience unusual bruising or bleeding (eg, nosebleeds, excessive bleeding after brushing teeth, the appearance of blood in stools or urine, excessive menstrual bleeding, petechiae, excessive bruising or persistent oozing from superficial injuries) after hospital discharge, as they may need additional antivenin treatment. Such bruising or bleeding may occur for up to 1 week or longer following initial treatment, and patients should be advised to follow up with their physicians for monitoring.

ANTIVENIN (MICRURUS FULVIUS) (North American Coral Snake Antivenin) (Equine Origin)

Rx	**Antivenin** (*Micrurus fulvius*)[a] (Wyeth-Ayerst)	**Powder for Injection, lyophilized**[b]	In single-use vials with 1 vial diluent (10 mL Water for Injection).[c]

[a] The manufacturer is in the process of discontinuing this product; however, it will be producing enough antivenin to satisfy demand for several years.
[b] Prior to lyophilization, product contains 0.25% phenol and 0.005% thimerosal.
[c] With 1:100,000 phenylmercuric nitrate.

ANTIVENIN (MICRURUS FULVIUS) (North American Coral Snake Antivenin) (Equine Origin)

Indications

➤*Envenomations:* For passive, transient protection from toxic effects of venoms of *Micrurus fulvius fulvius* (Eastern coral snake). Also neutralizes venom of *M. fulvius tenere* (Texas coral snake). If indicated, the best effect results if antivenin administration begins within 4 hours of envenomation.

This antivenin partially neutralizes the venom of *M. dumerilii carinicauda* and minimally neutralizes the venom of *M. spixii*. It may also provide some protection against the venom of *M. nigrocinctus*.

Administration and Dosage

➤*Test for sensitivity to horse serum:* Whenever a product containing horse serum is administered, there is a possibility of a severe immediate reaction. Have appropriate therapeutic agents available (not corticosteroids). See also Management of Acute Hypersensitivity Reactions.

➤*Sensitivity testing (horse serum):* Before administration of any product prepared from horse serum, take appropriate measures in an effort to detect the presence of dangerous sensitivity:

1.) A careful review of the patient's history should be noted, including any report of the following:
  a.) Asthma, hay fever, urticaria, or other allergic manifestations;
  b.) allergic reactions upon exposure to horses;
  c.) prior injections of horse serum.
2.) A suitable test for detection of sensitivity. Perform a skin test in every patient prior to administration, regardless of clinical history.

Skin test – Intracutaneously inject 0.02 to 0.03 mL of a 1:10 dilution of Normal Horse Serum or Antivenin. A control test on the opposite extremity, using Sodium Chloride Injection, USP, facilitates interpretation. Use of larger amounts for the skin-test dose increases the likelihood of false-positive reactions, and in the exquisitely sensitive patient, increases the risk of a systemic reaction from the skin-test dose. A ≥ 1:100 dilution should be used for preliminary skin testing if the history suggests sensitivity. A positive reaction to a skin test occurs within 5 to 30 minutes and is manifested by a wheal with or without pseudopodia and surrounding erythema. In general, the shorter the interval between injection and the beginning of the skin reaction, the greater the sensitivity.

If the history is negative for allergy and the result of a skin test is negative, proceed with administration of antivenin as outlined. If the history is positive and a skin test is strongly positive, administration may be dangerous, especially if the positive sensitivity test is accompanied by systemic allergic manifestations. In such instances, the risk of administering antivenin must be weighed against the risk of withholding it, keeping in mind that severe envenomation can be fatal.

A negative allergic history and absence of reaction to a properly applied skin test do not rule out the possibility of an immediate reaction. Also, a negative skin test has no bearing on whether or not delayed serum reactions (serum sickness) will occur after administration of the full dose.

➤*Desensitization:* If the history is negative, and the skin test is mildly or questionably positive, administer as follows to reduce the risk of a severe immediate systemic reaction:

1.) Prepare, in separate sterile vials or syringes, 1:100 and 1:10 dilutions of antivenin.
2.) Allow ≥ 15 minutes between injections and proceed with the next dose if no reaction follows the previous dose.
3.) Inject SC using a tuberculin-type syringe, 0.1, 0.2, and 0.5 mL of the 1:100 dilution at 15-minute intervals; repeat with the 1:10 dilution, and finally undiluted antivenin.
4.) If a systemic reaction occurs after any injection, place a tourniquet proximal to the site of injections and administer an appropriate dose of epinephrine, 1:1000, proximal to the tourniquet or into another extremity. Wait ≥ 30 minutes before injecting another dose. The amount of the next dose should be the same as the last that did not evoke a reaction.
5.) If no reaction occurs after 0.5 mL of undiluted antivenin has been administered, switch to the IM route and continue doubling the dose at 15-minute intervals until the entire dose has been injected IM or proceed to the IV route as described in Administration and Dosage.

➤*Reconstituting dried antivenin:* Withdraw diluent and inject into the vial of antivenin. Gentle agitation will hasten complete dissolution of lyophilized drug. Do not shake.

➤*Antivenin therapy:* If symptoms or signs of envenomation occur or are already present at the time the patient is first seen, give IV antivenin promptly. With vigorous treatment and careful observation, patients with complete respiratory paralysis have recovered.

Start an IV drip of 250 to 500 mL of Sodium Chloride Injection, USP. If the results of appropriate tests have indicated the patient is not dangerously hypersensitive to horse serum and depending on the nature and severity of the signs and symptoms of envenomation, administer the contents of 3 to 5 vials as the initial dose IV by slow injection directly into the IV tubing or by slow IV infusion by adding to the reservoir bottle of the IV drip. In either case, give the first 1 to 2 mL of the antivenin dilution over 3 to 5 minutes and watch the patient carefully for evidence of an allergic reaction. If no signs or symptoms of anaphylaxis appear, continue the injection or infusion. Administer additional antivenin as required. Some envenomed patients may need the contents of > 10 vials.

ANTIVENIN (MICRURUS FULVIUS) (North American Coral Snake Antivenin) (Equine Origin)

Adjust the rate of delivery by the severity of signs and symptoms of envenomation and tolerance of antivenin. Nonetheless, until the contents of 3 to 5 vials of antivenin have been given, administer at the maximum safe rate for IV fluids, based on body weight and general condition of the patient. For example, 250 to 500 mL over 30 minutes may be appropriate in a healthy adult, while small children may receive the first 100 mL rapidly, followed by a rate not to exceed 4 mL/min. Response to treatment may be rapid and dramatic.

➤*Storage / Stability:* Store at 2° to 8°C (36° to 46°F). Do not expose to temperatures greater than 40°C (104°F). Do not freeze diluent. Product can tolerate 10 days in solution at room temperature. Use reconstituted solutions within 48 hours and dilutions within 12 hours. To avoid foaming and protein degradation, mix by gently swirling rather than shaking. Product shelf life expires within 60 months.

Actions

➤*Pharmacology:* Refined, concentrated, lyophilized preparation of serum globulins obtained by fractionating blood from healthy horses immunized with eastern coral snake (*Micrurus fulvius fulvius*) venom.

Two genera of coral snakes inhabit the US: *Micrurus* (including the eastern and Texas varieties), and *Micruroides* (the Arizonan or Sonoran variety). *Micrurus fulvius fulvius* inhabits an area from North Carolina south to Florida and west to the Mississippi River. *Micrurus fulvius tenere* inhabits an area west of the Mississippi River including Louisiana, Arkansas, and Texas. Several other species of coral snake inhabit much of Central and South America, including 3 genera, *Leptomicrurus*, *Micrurus*, and *Micruroides*.

Warnings

➤*Not effective:* Not effective against the venom of *Euryxanthus* (Arizonan or Sonoran coral snake), found only in southeastern Arizona, southwestern New Mexico, and portions of Mexico. Not effective in other snakes not described above.

➤*Supportive therapy:* Appropriate tetanus prophylaxis is indicated. Morphine or other narcotics that depress respiration are contraindicated. Use sedatives with extreme caution.

If practical, immobilize victim immediately and completely. If complete immobilization is not practical, splint bitten extremity to limit spread of venom.

Hemoglobinuria has occurred in animals. Therefore, continuous bladder drainage with careful attention to urinary output and blood electrolyte balance is recommended.

➤*Hypersensitivity reactions:* The immediate reaction (eg, shock, anaphylaxis) usually occurs within 30 minutes. Symptoms and signs may include apprehension; flushing; itching; urticaria; edema of the face, tongue, and throat; cough; dyspnea; cyanosis; vomiting; and collapse.

Serum sickness – See Adverse Reactions for more information.

➤*Pregnancy: Category C.* Use only if clearly needed, with appropriate consideration of the risk-benefit ratio. It is not known if antivenom antibodies cross the placenta. Intact IgG crosses the placenta from the maternal circulation increasingly after 30 weeks' gestation.

➤*Lactation:* It is not known if antivenom antibodies are excreted into breast milk. Problems in humans have not been documented.

➤*Children:* The pediatric dose is equivalent to the adult dose. Pediatric doses are not adjusted by the weight of the patient.

Adverse Reactions

➤*Hypersensitivity:* The immediate reaction (eg, shock, anaphylaxis) usually occurs within 30 minutes. Symptoms and signs may include apprehension; flushing; itching; urticaria; edema of the face, tongue, and throat; cough; dyspnea; cyanosis; vomiting; and collapse.

Serum sickness – Serum sickness usually occurs 5 to 24 days after administration. The incubation period may be < 5 days, especially in those who have received horse-serum-containing preparations on the past. The usual symptoms and signs are malaise, fever, urticaria, lymphadenopathy, edema, arthralgia, nausea, and vomiting. Occasionally, neurological manifestations develop, such as meningismus or peripheral neuritis. Peripheral neuritis usually involves the shoulders and arms. Pain and muscle weakness are frequently present, and permanent atrophy may develop.

Patient Information

Advise patients to contact their physician immediately if they experience any signs and symptoms of delayed allergic reactions or serum sickness (eg, rash, pruritus, urticaria) after hospital discharge.

In contrast to the immune serums and antitoxins, which contain exogenous antibodies to provide passive immunity, the Agents for Active Immunization include specific antigens that induce the endogenous production of antibodies. Agents that induce active immunity include vaccines and the subset of vaccines called toxoids.

Vaccines contain whole (killed or attenuated live) or partial microorganisms capable of inducing antibody formation, but which are not pathogenic. Toxoids are detoxified by-products derived from organisms that induce disease primarily through the elaboration of exotoxins. Although toxoids are not toxic, they are antigenic, and therefore, stimulate specific antibody production. Active immunization induced through administration of vaccines and toxoids provides prolonged immunity, whereas passive immunization with immune sera or antitoxins is of short duration.

Vaccination with any vaccine may not result in a protective antibody response in all individuals given the vaccine.

The following table indicates the recommended immunization schedule for infants and children. This schedule has been approved by the Advisory Committee on Immunization Practices (ACIP), the American Academy of Pediatrics (AAP), and the American Academy of Family Physicians (AAFP). This table is revised annually.

Recommended Childhood Immunization Schedule[a] — United States 2006

Vaccine	Birth	1 mo	2 mo	4 mo	6 mo	12 mo	15 mo	18 mo	24 mo	4 to 6 y	11 to 12 y	13 to 14 y	15 y	16 to 18 y
Hepatitis B (HepB)[b]	HepB	HepB[c]		HepB[b]	HepB[c]				HepB series[d]					
Diphtheria, tetanus, pertussis (DTaP)[e]			DTaP	DTaP	DTaP		DTaP[c]			DTaP	Tdap	Tdap[d]		
Haemophilus influenzae type b (Hib)[f]			Hib	Hib	Hib[f]	Hib[c]								
Inactivated poliovirus (IPV)			IPV	IPV	IPV[c]					IPV				
Measles, mumps, rubella (MMR)[g]						MMR[c]				MMR	MMR[d]			
Varicella (Var)[h]						Var[c]			Var[d]					
Meningococcal[i]											MCV4		MCV4[d]	
									MPSV4[c,j]		MCV4[c,j]			
Pneumococcal[k]			PCV	PCV	PCV	PCV[c]			PCV[d,j]					
									PPV[c,j]					
Influenza[l]					Influenza (yearly)[c]				Influenza (yearly)[c,j]					
Hepatitis A (HepA)[m]						HepA series[c]			HepA series[c,j]					

[a] This schedule indicates the recommended age for routine administration of currently licensed childhood vaccines as of December 1, 2005, for children through 18 years of age. Any dose not administered at the recommended age should be administered at any subsequent visit when indicated and feasible. Age groups that warrant special effort to administer those vaccines not previously administered are marked via table reference. Additional vaccines may be licensed and recommended during the year. Licensed combination vaccines may be used whenever any components of the combination are indicated and other components of the vaccine are not contraindicated and if approved by the Food and Drug Administration for that dose of the series. Providers should consult the respective ACIP statement for detailed recommendations. Report clinically significant adverse reactions that follow vaccination to the Vaccine Adverse Event Reporting System (VAERS). Guidance about how to obtain and complete a VAERS form is available at http://www.vaers.hhs.gov or 800-822-7967.

[b] **At birth: All newborns** should receive monovalent HepB soon after birth and before hospital discharge. **Infants born to mothers who are HBsAg-positive** should receive HepB and 0.5 mL of hepatitis B immune globulin (HBIG) within 12 hours of birth. **Infants born to mothers whose HBsAg status is unknown** should receive HepB within 12 hours of birth. The mother should have blood drawn as soon as possible to determine her HBsAg status; if HBsAg-positive, the infant should receive HBIG as soon as possible (no later than 1 week of age). **For infants born to HBsAg-negative mothers,** the birth dose can be delayed in rare circumstances but only if a health care provider's order to withhold the vaccine and a copy of the mother's original HBsAg-negative laboratory report are documented in the infant's medical record. **Following the birth dose:** The HepB series should be completed with either monovalent HepB or a combination vaccine containing HepB. The second dose should be administered at 1 to 2 months of age. The final dose should be administered at ≥ 24 weeks of age. It is permissible to administer 4 doses of HepB (eg, when combination vaccines are given after the birth dose); however, if monovalent HepB is used, a dose at 4 months of age is not needed. **Infants born to HBsAg-positive mothers** should be tested for HBsAg and antibody to HBsAg after completion of the HepB series at 9 to 18 months of age (generally at the next well-child visit after completion of the vaccine series).

[c] Range of acceptable ages for vaccination.

[d] Age range for catch-up immunization.

[e] The fourth dose of DTaP may be administered as early as 12 months of age, provided 6 months have elapsed since the third dose and the child is unlikely to return at 15 to 18 months of age. Give the final dose in the series at ≥ 4 years of age. Tetanus and diphtheria toxoids and acellular pertussis vaccine (Tdap — adolescent preparation) is recommended at 11 to 12 years of age for those who have completed the recommended childhood DTP/DTaP vaccination series and have not received a tetanus and diphtheria toxoids (Td) booster dose. Adolescents 13 to 18 years of age who missed the 11 to 12 year Td/Tdap booster dose should also receive a single dose of Tdap if they have completed the recommended childhood DTP/DTaP vaccination series. Subsequent Td are recommended every 10 years.

[f] Three Hib conjugate vaccines are licensed for infant use. If PRP-OMP (*Pedvax-HIB* or *ComVax*) is administered at 2 and 4 months of age, a dose at 6 months of age is not required. Do not use DTaP/Hib combination products for primary immunization in infants at 2, 4, or 6 months of age, but use as boosters following any Hib vaccine. Give the final dose in the series at ≥ 12 months of age.

[g] The second dose of MMR vaccine is routinely recommended at 4 to 6 years of age but may be administered during any visit provided 4 weeks or more have elapsed since the first dose and that both doses are administered at or after 12 months of age. Those who have not previously received the second dose should complete the schedule by 11 to 12 years of age.

[h] Varicella vaccine is recommended at any visit on or after 12 months of age for susceptible children (ie, those who lack a reliable history of chickenpox). Susceptible people ≥ 13 years of age should receive 2 doses given at least 4 weeks apart.

[i] Give meningococcal conjugate vaccine (MCV4) to all children at the 11 to 12 years of age as well as to unvaccinated adolescents at high school entry (15 years of age). Other adolescents who wish to decrease their risk for meningococcal disease may also be vaccinated. All college freshmen living in dormitories should also be vaccinated, preferably with MCV4, although meningococcal polysaccharide vaccine (MPSV4) is an acceptable alternative. Vaccination against invasive meningococcal disease is recommended for children and adolescents ≥ 2 years of age with terminal complement deficiencies or anatomic or functional asplenia and certain other high risk groups; use MPSV4 for children 2 to 10 years of age and MCV4 for older children, although MPSV4 is an acceptable alternative.

[j] Recommended for selected populations.

[k] The heptavalent pneumococcal conjugate vaccine (PCV) is recommended for all children 2 to 23 months of age and for certain children 24 to 59 months of age. Give the final dose in the series at ≥ 12 months of age. Pneumococcal polysaccharide vaccine (PPV) is recommended in addition to PCV for certain high-risk groups.

[l] Influenza vaccine is recommended annually for children ≥ 6 months of age with certain risk factors (including, but not limited to asthma, cardiac disease, sickle cell disease, HIV, diabetes, and conditions that can compromise respiratory function or handling of respiratory secretions or that can increase the risk for aspiration), health care workers, and other people (including household members) in close contact with people in the groups at high risk. In addition, healthy children 6 to 23 months of age and close contacts of healthy children 0 to 5 months of age are recommended to receive influenza vaccine because children in this age group are at substantially increased risk for influenza-related hospitalizations. For healthy people 5 to 49 years of age, the intranasally administered live, attenuated influenza vaccine (LAIV) is an acceptable alternative to the intramuscular trivalent inactivated influenza vaccine (TIV). Children receiving TIV should be administered a dosage appropriate for their age (0.25 mL if 6 to 35 months of age or 0.5 mL if ≥ 3 years of age). Children ≤ 8 years of age who are receiving influenza vaccine for the first time should receive 2 doses separated by at least 4 weeks for TIV and at least 6 weeks for LAIV.

[m] HepA is recommended for all children at 1 year of age (ie, 12 to 23 months). The 2 doses in the series should be administered at least 6 months apart. States, counties, and communities with existing HepA vaccination programs for children 2 to 18 years of age are encouraged to maintain these programs. In these areas, new efforts focused on routine vaccination of 1 year old children should enhance, not replace, ongoing programs directed at a broader population of children. HepA is also recommended for certain high risk groups.

Vaccine Catch-up Schedule for Children 4 Months to 6 Years of Age Who Start Late or Who Are More Than 1 Month Behind[a]

Vaccine (minimum age for dose 1)	Minimum interval between doses			
	Dose 1 to dose 2	Dose 2 to dose 3	Dose 3 to dose 4	Dose 4 to dose 5
DTaP (6 wk)	4 wk	4 wk	6 mo	6 mo[b]
IPV (6 wk)	4 wk	4 wk	4 wk[c]	
HepB[d] (birth)	4 wk	8 wk (and 16 wk after first dose)		
MMR (12 mo)	4 wk[e]			
Varicella (12 mo)				
Hib[f] (6 wk)	**4 wk:** If first dose given at < 12 mo of age **8 wk (as final dose):** If first dose given at 12 to 14 mo of age **No further doses needed:** If first dose given at ≥ 15 mo of age	**4 wk**[g]**:** If currently < 12 mo of age **8 wk (as final dose)**[g]**:** If currently ≥ 12 mo of age and dose 2 given at < 15 mo of age **No further doses needed:** If previous dose given at ≥ 15 mo of age	**8 wk (as final dose):** This dose is only necessary for children 12 mo to 5 y of age who received 3 doses before 12 mo of age	
PCV[f] (6 wk)	**4 wk:** If first dose given at < 12 mo of age and currently < 24 mo of age **8 wk (as final dose):** If first dose given at ≥ 12 mo of age or currently 24 to 59 mo of age **No further doses needed:** For healthy children if first dose given at ≥ 24 mo of age	**4 wk:** If currently < 12 mo of age **8 wk (as final dose):** If currently ≥ 12 mo of age **No further doses needed:** For healthy children if previous dose given at ≥ 24 mo of age	**8 wk (as final dose):** This dose is only necessary for children 12 mo to 5 y of age who received 3 doses before 12 mo of age	

[a] This table gives catch-up schedules and minimum intervals between doses for children who have delayed immunizations. There is no need to restart a vaccine series regardless of the time that has elapsed between doses.
[b] The fifth dose is not necessary if the fourth dose was given at ≥ 4 years of age.
[c] For children who received an all-IPV or all–oral poliovirus (OPV) series, a fourth dose is not necessary if third dose was given at ≥ 4 years of age. If both OPV and IPV were given as part of a series, give a total of 4 doses regardless of the child's current age.
[d] Administer the 3-dose series to all children and adolescents < 19 years of age if they were not previously vaccinated.
[e] The second dose of MMR is recommended routinely at 4 to 6 years of age, but may be given earlier if desired.
[f] Vaccine is not generally recommended for children ≥ 5 years of age.
[g] If currently < 12 months of age and first 2 doses were PRP-OMP (*PedvaxHIB* or *ComVax*), give the third (and final) dose at 12 to 15 months of age and at least 8 weeks after the second dose.

Vaccine Catch-up Schedule for Children 7 to 18 Years of Age Who Start Late or Who Are More Than 1 Month Behind[a]

Vaccine	Minimum interval between doses		
	Dose 1 to dose 2	Dose 2 to dose 3	Dose 3 to booster dose
Td[b]	4 wk	6 mo	6 mo: if first dose given at < 12 mo of age and currently < 11 y of age; otherwise 5 y
IPV[c]	4 wk	4 wk	IPV[c,d]
HepB	4 wk	8 wk (and 16 wk after first dose)	
MMR	4 wk		
Varicella[e]	4 wk		

[a] This table gives catch-up schedules and minimum intervals between doses for children who have delayed immunizations. There is no need to restart a vaccine series, regardless of the time that has elapsed between doses.
[b] Adolescent Tdap may be substituted for any dose in a primary catch-up series or as a booster if age appropriate for Tdap. A 5-year interval from the last Td dose is encouraged when Tdap is used as a booster dose.
[c] Vaccine is not generally recommended for patients ≥ 18 years of age.
[d] For children who received an all-IPV or all-OPV series, a fourth dose is not necessary if third dose was given at ≥ 4 years of age. If both OPV and IPV were given as part of a series, give a total of 4 doses regardless of the child's current age.
[e] Give 2-dose series to all susceptible adolescents ≥ 13 years of age.

➤*Concomitant vaccination:* Several routine pediatric vaccines may safely and effectively be administered simultaneously at separate injection sites. National authorities recommend simultaneous immunization at separate sites as indicated by age or health risk if the return of a vaccine recipient for a subsequent visit is doubtful.

➤*Immunization for other diseases:* Immunization for other diseases is recommended for people with a risk of exposure. Specific immunization requirements and recommendations for international travel may be obtained from the Centers for Disease Control and Prevention (CDC) Web site (http://www.cdc.gov), including their online publication "Health Information for International Travel." These also may be found in the following publication: Grabenstein JD. *ImmunoFacts: Vaccines & Immunologic Drugs.* St. Louis, MO: Wolters Kluwer Health, Inc.; 2006.

➤*Hypersensitivity to vaccine components:* Vaccine antigens produced in systems containing allergenic substances (eg, embryonated chicken eggs) may cause hypersensitivity reactions, including anaphylaxis. Do not give such vaccines to individuals with known hypersensitivity to these components. Influenza vaccine antigens (whole or split), although prepared in embryonated eggs, are highly purified and rarely associated with hypersensitivity reactions.

Live virus vaccines prepared by growing viruses in cell cultures are essentially devoid of allergenic substances. On very rare occasions, hypersensitivity reactions to measles vaccine have been reported in individuals with anaphylactic hypersensitivity to gelatin. However, measles vaccine may be given safely to egg-allergic individuals provided the allergies are not manifested by anaphylactic symptoms. The same precautions apply to mumps and varicella vaccines.

Some vaccines contain preservatives (eg, thimerosal) or trace amounts of antibiotics (eg, neomycin) to which patients may be hypersensitive. Such allergies are relevant only if they reflect immediate hypersensitivity (eg, the airway).

Before the injection of any biological, take all precautions known for prevention of allergic or other adverse reactions, including a review of the patient's history regarding possible sensitivity, occurrence of any adverse reaction–related symptoms or signs to determine any contraindication to immunization, and a knowledge of the recent literature pertaining to the use of the biological concerned. Have epinephrine 1:1000 available for immediate use when this product is injected. Refer to Management of Acute Hypersensitivity Reactions.

➤*Altered immunocompetence:* Microbial replication after administration of live, attenuated vaccines may be enhanced in people with immune deficiency diseases and in those with suppressed capability for immune response (eg, leukemia, lymphoma, generalized malignancy or therapy with corticosteroids, alkylating agents, antimetabolites, radiation). Do not give live, attenuated vaccines to such patients or to a member of a household in which there is a family history of congenital or hereditary immunodeficiency until the immune competence of the recipient is known.

➤*Disease transmission:* Use a separate, sterilized syringe and needle for each patient to prevent transmission of Hep B virus and other infectious agents from one patient to another.

➤*Vaccine reconstitution:* When preparing injections for reconstitution, cleanse the rubber stoppers of both vials with a suitable germicide prior to reconstitution.

➤*Aspirate:* Before delivering the intramuscular or subcutaneous dose, aspirate to help avoid inadvertent injection into a blood vessel.

➤*HIV infection:* Special immunization recommendations are appropriate for patients infected with HIV.

Live bacterial or viral vaccines – Patients infected with HIV and those who have developed AIDS are theoretically at risk of disseminated infection following immunization with a live, albeit attenuated, bacterial or viral vaccine.

Inactivated vaccines or toxoids – In general, immunization with an inactivated vaccine or toxoid poses no additional risk to patients infected with HIV and those who have developed AIDS, but these patients may be less likely to develop an adequate immune response to vaccination and may remain susceptible to the disease at issue. While HIV-infected patients and AIDS patients may develop less than optimal immunity, compared with uninfected people, immunization is often still recommended to confer at least partial protection. Optimally, complete the immunization of HIV-infected patients before they meet the criteria for AIDS.

Immunization of HIV-infected patients – In vitro studies demonstrate that proliferating CD4 cells are more susceptible to infection with HIV than nonproliferating cells, raising the possibility that immunization may be a cofactor in exacerbating the progression of HIV infection to AIDS. CDC and the World Health Organization (WHO) continue to recommend immunization of HIV-infected patients when the benefits of immunization outweigh the risks of infection.

Summary Recommendations for Routine Immunization of HIV-infected Patients in the United States

Drug	Known asymptomatic	Symptomatic
DTP/Td	yes	yes
OPV	no	no
e-IPV[a]	yes	yes
MMR	yes	yes[b]
Hib[c]	yes	yes
Pneumococcal	yes	yes
Influenza	yes[b]	yes
BCG	no	no
Cholera	yes	yes
HepA	yes	yes
HepB	yes	yes
Meningococcal	yes	yes
Rabies	yes	yes
Typhoid	yes (injection only)	yes (injection only)
Vaccinia	no	no
Varicella[d]	yes	no
Yellow fever	yes, if high risk	no

[a] For adults 18 years of age and older; use only if indicated.
[b] Consider risk and benefit.
[c] Consider for HIV-infected adults also.
[d] Consult detailed references.

➤*Severe febrile illnesses:* Generally defer immunization of individuals with severe febrile illnesses until they have recovered.

➤*Vaccination during pregnancy:* On the grounds of a theoretical risk to the developing fetus, live, attenuated virus vaccines are not generally given to pregnant women or to those likely to become pregnant within 3 months after receiving the vaccine. With some of these vaccines, particularly rubella, measles, and mumps, pregnancy is contraindicated. When the vaccine is to be given during pregnancy, waiting until the second or third trimester to minimize any concern over teratogenicity is a reasonable precaution. However, there has been no evidence of congenital rubella syndrome in infants born to susceptible mothers who received rubella vaccine during pregnancy.

Measles, mumps, rubella, or oral polio vaccines may be safely administered to children of pregnant women. Experience to date has not revealed any risks of polio vaccine virus to the fetus.

There is no convincing evidence of risk to the fetus from immunization of pregnant women using inactivated virus vaccines, bacterial vaccines, or toxoids. Give tetanus and Td to inadequately immunized pregnant women because it affords protection against neonatal tetanus. Similarly, HepB, influenza, and meningococcal vaccines may be indicated during pregnancy.

➤*Adverse reactions following immunization:* Modern vaccines are extremely safe and effective; although, adverse reactions following immunization have been reported with all vaccines. These range from frequent, minor local reactions to extremely rare, severe systemic illness, such as paralysis associated with oral polio vaccine.

Provide vaccine information required to be given with each vaccine to the patient, parent, or guardian, and inform them of the benefits and risks associated with the vaccine.

Reporting of adverse reactions – The National Vaccine Injury Compensation Program, established by the National Childhood Vaccine Injury Act of 1986, requires health care providers who administer vaccines to maintain permanent vaccination records and report occurrences of certain adverse reactions to the US Department of Health and Human Services (DHHS). Reportable reactions include those listed in the Act for each vaccine and reactions specified in the package insert as contraindications to further doses of that vaccine.

Encourage patients, parents, and guardians to report all adverse reactions occurring after vaccine administration. Adverse reactions following immunization with vaccine should be reported by the health care provider to VAERS. Reporting forms and information about reporting requirements or completion of the form can be obtained from VAERS at http://www.vaers.hhs.gov or 800-822-7967. Also report these reactions to the manufacturer.

Record the date, lot number, and manufacturer of the vaccine as part of the patient's immunization record.

Vaccines, Bacterial

BCG VACCINE

Rx	**BCG Vaccine** (Organon)	**Powder for injection, lyophilized:** TICE strain[a] (1 to 8 × 10^8 CFU equivalent to ≈ 50 mg)	In vials.[b]

[a] Developed at the University of Illinois.
[b] Preservative free.

BCG VACCINE — INJECTION

For complete and comparative prescribing information, refer to the Agents for Active Immunization introduction. TICE BCG vaccine is also indicated for carcinoma in situ of the bladder. See individual monograph in the Antineoplastics section.

Indications

➤*Tuberculosis (TB) prevention:* For the prevention of tuberculosis (TB) in people not previously infected with *Mycobacterium tuberculosis* who are at high risk for exposure. As with any vaccine, immunization with BCG vaccine may not protect 100% of susceptible individuals.

The Advisory Committee on Immunization Practices (ACIP) and the Advisory Committee for the Elimination of Tuberculosis has recommended that BCG vaccination be considered in the following circumstances.

➤*TB exposed tuberculin skin test-negative infants and children:* BCG vaccination is recommended for infants and children with negative tuberculin skin test who are at high risk of intimate and prolonged exposure to persistently untreated or ineffectively treated patients with infectious pulmonary tuberculosis and who cannot be removed from the source of exposure and cannot be placed on long-term preventive therapy, or who are continuously exposed to people with infectious pulmonary tuberculosis who have bacilli resistant to isoniazid and rifampin.

➤*TB exposed health care workers (HCW) in high risk settings:* Consider BCG vaccination of HCWs on an individual basis in settings where a high percentage of TB patients are infected with *M. tuberculosis* strains resistant to both isoniazid and rifampin, transmission of such drug resistant *M. tuberculosis* strains to HCWs and subsequent infection are likely, and comprehensive TB infection control precautions have been implemented and have not been successful. Vaccination should not be required for employment or for assignment of HCWs in specific work areas. Counsel HCWs considered for BCG vaccination regarding the risks and benefits associated with BCG vaccinations and TB preventive therapy.

➤*Exposed HCWs in low risk settings:* BCG vaccination is not recommended for HCWs in settings in which the risk for *M. tuberculosis* transmission is low.

➤*Unlabeled uses:* BCG vaccine induces antibodies that bind to *M. leprae* and may be effective in the prevention of leprosy.

Administration and Dosage

➤*Preparation:* Add 1 mL sterile water for injection at 4° to 25°C (39° to 77°F) to one vial of vaccine. Gently swirl the vial until a homogenous suspension is obtained. Avoid forceful agitation, which may cause clumping of the mycobacteria.

➤*Treatment and schedule:* Vaccination is recommended only for those who are tuberculin negative to a recent skin test with 5 tuberculin units (5TU). The vaccine is administered after fully explaining the risks and benefits to the vaccinee, parent, or guardian. After the vaccine is prepared, the immunizing dose of 0.2 to 0.3 mL is dropped on the cleansed surface of the skin and spread over a 1 × 2 inch area using the edge of the multiple puncture device. The vaccine is administered percutaneously utilizing a sterile multiple-puncture device. While holding the skin taut, press downward on the device, allowing the points to be well buried in the skin for 5 seconds. Do not "rock" the device. After successful puncture, spread vaccine as evenly as possible over the puncture area with the edge of the device. An additional 1 to 2 drops of BCG vaccine may be added to ensure a very wet vaccination site. No dressing is required; however, it is recommended that the site be kept dry for 24 hours. Advise the patient that the vaccine contains live organisms. Although the vaccine will not survive in a dry state for long, infection of others is possible.

Repeat vaccination for those who remain tuberculin-negative to 5TU of tuberculin after 2 to 3 months.

➤*Children:* In infants under 1 month of age, reduce the dosage of vaccine by 50% by using 2 mL sterile water when reconstituting. If a vaccinated infant remains tuberculin negative to 5TU on skin testing, and if indications for vaccination persist, the infant should receive a full dose after 1 year of age.

➤*Storage/Stability:* Refrigerate the intact vial at 2° to 8°C (36° to 46°F). Protect from light. Do not use after the expiration date printed on the label.

Keep reconstituted vaccine refrigerated; protect from light; use within 2 hours. Freezing of the reconstituted product is not recommended.

Actions

➤*Pharmacology:* BCG vaccine for percutaneous use is an attenuated, live culture preparation of the Bacillus of Calmette and Guerin (BCG) strain of *M. bovis*. The TICE strain was developed at the University of Illinois from a strain originated at the Pasteur Institute.

BCG VACCINE — INJECTION

Contraindications

Impaired immunologic responses because of HIV infections, congenital immunodeficiency such as chronic granulomatous disease or interferon gamma receptor deficiency, leukemia, lymphoma, or generalized malignancy; immunologic responses that have been suppressed by steroids, alkylating agents, antimetabolites, or radiation; HIV- infected or immunocompromised infants, children, or adults; hypersensitivity or history of hypersensitivity to the product; active tuberculosis. Do not use in infants, children, or adults with severe immune deficiency syndromes.

Warnings

➤*Route of administration:* Do not inject IV, SC, or intradermally. Use percutaneous administration with the multiple puncture device (see Administration and Dosage).

➤*Immune deficiency syndromes:* Administer with caution to people in groups at high risk for HIV infection. Do not vaccinate children with a family history of immune deficiency disease. If they are, consult an infectious disease specialist and administer antituberculous therapy if clinically indicated.

➤*BCG infection:* Symptoms such as fever of 103°F or greater, or acute localized inflammation persisting longer than 2 to 3 days suggest active infections, and evaluation for serious infectious complication should be considered. If a BCG infection is suspected, the physician should consult with an infectious disease expert before therapy is initiated. Treatment should be started without delay. In patients who develop persistent fever or experience an acute febrile illness consistent with BCG infection, 2 or more antimycobacterial agents should be administered while diagnostic evaluation, including cultures, is conducted. Negative cultures do not necessarily rule out infection. The most serious complication of BCG vaccination is disseminated BCG infection. BCG osteitis affecting the epiphyses of the long bones, particularly the epiphyses of the leg can occur from 4 months to 2 years after vaccination. Fatal disseminated BCG disease has occurred at a rate of 0.06 to 1.56 cases per million doses of vaccine administered; these deaths occurred primarily among immunocompromised people.

➤*Hypersensitivity reactions:* Assess the possibility of allergic reactions. Epinephrine injection (1:1000) for the control of immediate allergic reactions must be available should an acute anaphylactic reaction occur.

➤*Pregnancy: Category C.* It is not known whether BCG vaccine can cause fetal harm when administered to a pregnant woman or can affect reproduction capacity. Although no harmful effects to the fetus have been associated with BCG vaccine, its use is not recommended during pregnancy.

➤*Lactation:* It is not known whether BCG vaccine is excreted in breast milk. Because many drugs are excreted in human milk and because of the potential for serious adverse reactions in nursing infants from BCG vaccine, decide whether to discontinue nursing or not to vaccinate, taking into account the importance of tuberculosis vaccination to the mother.

➤*Children:* Take precautions with respect to infants vaccinated with BCG and exposed to individuals with active tuberculosis (see Administration and Dosage).

Precautions

➤*Biohazardous:* BCG contains live bacteria; use with aseptic technique. Handle and dispose of all equipment, supplies, and receptacles in contact with BCG vaccine as biohazardous.

➤*Normal reaction:* The intensity and duration of the local reaction depends on the depth of penetration of the multiple-puncture device and individual variations in patients' tissue reactions. The initial skin lesions usually appear within 10 to 14 days and consist of small red papules at the site. The papules reach maximum diameter (about 3 mm) after 4 to 6 weeks, after which they may scale and then slowly subside.

After vaccination, it is usually not possible to clearly distinguish between a tuberculin reaction caused by persistent postvaccination sensitivity and one caused by a virulent suprainfection. Caution is advised in attributing a positive skin test to BCG vaccination. Further investigate a sharp rise in the tuberculin reaction since the latest test (except in the immediate postvaccination period).

Drug Interactions

➤*Antimicrobial or immunosuppressive agents:* These may interfere with the development of the immune response; use only under medical supervision.

➤*Live vaccines:* Because BCG is a live vaccine, the immune response to the vaccine might be impaired if administered within 30 days of another live vaccine. However, no evidence exists for currently available vaccines to support this concern. Whenever possible, live vaccines administered on different days should be administered at least 30 days apart.

➤*Drug/Lab test interactions:* BCG vaccination results in tuberculin skin test reactivity. Tuberculin skin test reactivity as a result of BCG vaccination cannot be readily differentiated from reactivity following exposure to tuberculosis. BCG vaccination should not be administered to individuals with a positive tuberculin skin test.

Adverse Reactions

All suspected adverse reactions to BCG vaccination should be reported to Organon at (800) 842-3220 and to the Vaccine Adverse Effect Reporting System (VAERS) at (800) 822-7967. These reactions occasionally could occur more than 1 year after vaccination.

➤*Local:* Although BCG vaccination often results in local adverse effects, serious or long-term complications are rare. Reactions that can be expected after vaccination include moderate axillary or cervical lymphadenopathy and induration and subsequent pustule formation at the injection site; these reactions can persist for as long as 3 months after vaccination. More severe local reactions include ulceration at the vaccination site, regional suppurative lymphadenitis with draining sinuses, and caseous lesions or purulent drainage at the puncture site; these manifestations might occur within the 5 months after vaccination and could persist for several weeks.

➤*Systemic:* Acute, localized irritative toxicities of BCG may be accompanied by systemic manifestations, consistent with a flu-like syndrome. Systemic adverse effects of 1 to 2 days' duration such as fever, anorexia, myalgia, and neuralgia, often reflect hypersensitivity reactions.

Overdosage

➤*Symptoms:* Accidental overdosages, if treated immediately with antituberculous drugs, have not led to complications. If vaccination response is allowed to progress, it can still be treated successfully with antituberculous drugs but complications may occur (eg, regional adenitis, lupus vulgaris, SC cold abscesses, ocular lesions).

Patient Information

Keep the vaccination site clean until the local reaction has disappeared.

Following BCG vaccination, no dressing is required; however, it is recommended that the site be loosely covered and kept dry for 24 hours.

The patients should be advised that the vaccine contains live organisms. Although the vaccine will not survive in a dry state for long, infection of others is possible. Following vaccination with BCG, initial skin lesions usually appear within 10 to 14 days and consist of small red papules at the vaccination site. The papules reach a maximum diameter (about 3 mm) after 4 to 6 weeks, after which they may scale and slowly subside.

Patients may experience flu-like symptoms for 24 to 48 hours following BCG vaccination. However, the patients should consult with their physician immediately if they experience fever of 103°F or greater, or acute local reactions persisting longer than 2 to 3 days.

HAEMOPHILUS B CONJUGATE VACCINE

Rx	**HibTITER** (Wyeth-Lederle)	**Injection:** 10 mcg purified *Haemophilus* b saccharide capsular oligosaccharide and ≈ 25 mcg diphtheria CRM_{197} protein/0.5 mL	In 1 and 10 dose vials.[a]
Rx	**ActHIB** (Aventis Pasteur)	**Powder for injection, lyophilized:** 10 mcg purified *Haemophilus* b capsular polysaccharide, 24 mcg tetanus toxoid/0.5 mL	8.5% sucrose. In single-dose vials with 7.5 mL vials of diphtheria and tetanus toxoids and pertussis vaccine as diluents or with 0.6 mL vial containing 0.4% sodium chloride diluent.
Rx	**Liquid PedvaxHIB** (Merck)	**Injection:** 7.5 mcg *Haemophilus* b PRP, 125 mcg *Neisseria meningitidis* OMPC and 225 mcg aluminum (as aluminum hydroxide)/ 0.5 mL	In single-dose vials.

[a] Multidose vials contain thimerosal 1:10,000.

HAEMOPHILUS B CONJUGATE VACCINE — INJECTION

For complete and comparative prescribing information, refer to the Agents for Active Immunization introduction.

Indications

➤*HibTITER* and *Liquid PedvaxHIB*: For routine vaccination against invasive disease caused by *Haemophilus influenzae* type b in infants and children 2 to 71 months of age.

➤*ActHIB*: *ActHIB* or *ActHIB* combined with DTP vaccine by reconstitution is indicated for the active immunization of infants and children 2 through 18 months of age for the prevention of invasive disease caused by *H. influenzae* type b or diphtheria, tetanus and pertussis.

ActHIB combined with diphtheria and tetanus toxoids and acellular pertussis vaccine, absorbed (DTaP) by reconstitution is indicated for the active immunization of children 15 to 18 months of age for prevention of invasive disease caused by *H. influenzae* type b and diphtheria, tetanus and pertussis.

Administration and Dosage

➤*Administration:* The vaccines should be injected IM, preferably into the midlateral muscles of the thigh or deltoid, with care to avoid major peripheral nerve trunks. Do not inject in the gluteal area. Do not inject IV.

➤*HibTITER*: The vaccine is to be administered immediately after being drawn up into a syringe. Single dose 0.5 mL vial contains no preservative. Use 1 dose per vial; do not re-enter vial. Discard unused portions.

HAEMOPHILUS B CONJUGATE VACCINE — INJECTION

HibTITER may be administered simultaneously but at different sites from other routine pediatric vaccines (eg, diphtheria and tetanus toxoids and pertussis vaccine adsorbed "DTP], oral poliovirus vaccine "OPV], and measles-mumps-rubella vaccine "MMR]).

For infants 2 to 6 months of age, the immunizing dose is 3 separate injections of 0.5 mL given at approximately 2-month intervals. Previously unvaccinated infants from 7 through 11 months of age should receive 2 separate injections approximately 2 months apart. Children from 12 through 14 months of age who have not been vaccinated previously receive 1 injection. All vaccinated children should receive a single booster dose at 15 months of age or older, but not less than 2 months after the previous dose. Previously unvaccinated children 15 to 71 months of age should receive a single injection of *HibTITER*. Preterm infants should be vaccinated with *HibTITER* according to their chronological age from birth.

Recommended immunization schedule		
Age at first immunization (months)	Number of doses	Booster
2 to 6 months	3	Yes
7 to 11 months	2	Yes
12 to 14 months	1	Yes
15 and over	1	No

Interruption of the recommended schedules with a delay between doses does not interfere with the final immunity achieved nor does it necessitate starting the series over again, regardless of the length of time elapsed between doses.

Data support that *HibTITER* may be interchanged with other *Haemophilus influenzae* type b conjugate vaccines for the primary immunization series

➤*ActHIB*:

Reconstitution – Only whole-cell DTP, DTaP or 0.4% Sodium Chloride diluent may be used for reconstitution of lyophilized *ActHIB*. *ActHIB* combined with DTaP by reconstitution, should not be administered to infants younger than 15 months of age.

Whole-cell DTP: Cleanse both the DTP and *ActHIB* vial rubber stoppers with a suitable germicide prior to reconstitution. Thoroughly agitate the vial of DTP; then withdraw a 0.6 mL dose and inject into the vial of lyophilized *ActHIB*. After reconstitution and thorough agitation, the combined vaccines will appear whitish in color. Withdraw and administer 0.5 mL dose of the combined vaccines IM. Vaccine should be used within 24 hours after reconstitution.

DTaP: To prepare *Haemophilus* b conjugate vaccine reconstituted with DTaP, cleanse both the DTaP and *ActHIB* vial rubber stoppers with a suitable germicide prior to reconstitution. Thoroughly agitate the vial of DTaP; then withdraw a 0.6 mL dose and inject into the vial of lyophilized *ActHIB* (tetanus toxoid conjugate). After reconstitution and thorough agitation, the combined vaccines will appear whitish in color. Withdraw and administer 0.5 mL dose of the combined vaccines IM. Vaccine should be used immediately (within 30 minutes) after reconstitution.

0.4% sodium chloride: Using saline diluent (0.4% sodium chloride), cleanse the vaccine vial rubber stopper with a suitable germicide and inject the entire volume of diluent contained in the vial or syringe into the vial of lyophilized vaccine. Thorough agitation is advised to ensure complete reconstitution. The entire volume of reconstituted vaccine is then drawn back into the syringe before injecting one 0.5 mL dose IM. The vaccine will appear clear and colorless. Vaccine should be used within 24 hours after reconstitution.

Recommended immunization schedule for *ActHIB* and DTP or DTaP (for previously unvaccinated children)		
Dose	Age	Immunization
First, second, and third	At 2, 4, and 6 months	*ActHIB*, reconstituted with DTP or with saline diluent (0.4% sodium chloride)
Fourth	At 15 to 18 months	*ActHIB* reconstituted with DTP or with DTaP or with saline diluent (0.4% sodium chloride)
Fifth	At 4 to 6 years	DTP or DTaP

For previously unvaccinated children – The number of doses of *ActHIB* indicated depends on the age at which immunization is begun. A child 7 to 11 months of age should receive 2 doses of *ActHIB* at 8-week intervals and a booster dose at 15 to 18 months of age. A child 12 to 14 months of age should receive 1 dose of *ActHIB*, followed by a booster 2 months later.

Preterm infants should be vaccinated according to their chronological age from birth.

Interruption of the recommended schedule with a delay between doses should not interfere with the final immunity achieved with *ActHIB* reconstituted with DTP or *ActHIB* reconstituted with DTaP or saline diluent (0.4% Sodium Chloride). There is no need to start the series over again, regardless of the time elapsed between doses.

It is acceptable to administer a booster dose of *ActHIB* reconstituted with DTaP following a primary series of *ActHIB* and whole-cell DTP vaccines, or a primary series of a combination vaccine containing whole-cell DTP.

For *ActHIB* reconstituted with whole-cell DTP or with 0.4% sodium chloride diluent, administer vaccine within 24 hours after reconstitution.

For *ActHIB* reconstituted with DTaP, administer vaccine immediately (within 30 minutes) after reconstitution.

➤*Liquid PedvaxHIB*: If there is an interruption or delay between doses in the primary series, there is no need to repeat the series, but dosing should be continued at the next clinic visit.

2 to 14 months of age – Infants 2 to 14 months of age should receive a 0.5 mL dose of vaccine, ideally beginning at 2 months of age, followed by a 0.5 mL dose 2 months later (or as soon as possible thereafter). When the primary 2-dose regimen is completed before 12 months of age, a booster dose is required (see below and the table below). Infants born prematurely, regardless of birth weight, should be vaccinated at the same chronological age and according to the same schedule and precautions as full-term infants and children.

15 months of age and older – Children 15 months of age and older previously unvaccinated against Hib disease should receive a single 0.5 mL dose of vaccine.

Booster dose – In infants completing the primary 2-dose regimen before 12 months of age, a booster dose (0.5 mL) should be administered at 12 to 15 months of age, but not earlier than 2 months after the second dose.

Vaccination regimens for *Liquid PedvaxHIB* by age groups		
Age (months) at first dose	Primary	Age (months) at booster dose
2 to 10 months	2 doses, 2 months apart	12 to 15 months
11 to 14 months	2 doses, 2 months apart	-
15 to 71 months	1 dose	

Interchangeability – *PedvaxHIB* may be interchanged with other licensed *Haemophilus* b conjugate vaccines for the primary and booster doses.

Use with other vaccines – Results from clinical studies indicate that *Liquid PedvaxHIB* can be administered concomitantly with DTP, OPV, eIPV (enhanced inactivated poliovirus vaccine), varicella virus vaccine live, *M-M-R II* (measles, mumps, and rubella virus vaccine live) or hepatitis B vaccine (recombinant). No impairment of immune response to these individually tested vaccine antigens was demonstrated.

Administration – The vaccine should be used as supplied; no reconstitution is necessary.

Shake well before withdrawal and use. Thorough agitation is necessary to maintain suspension of the vaccine.

Inject 0.5 mL IM, preferably into the anterolateral thigh or the outer aspect of the upper arm. The buttocks should not be used for active vaccination of infants and children, because of the potential risk of injury to the sciatic nerve.

➤*Storage/Stability:*

HibTITER – Do not freeze. Store refrigerated away from freezer compartments at 2° to 8°C (36° to 46°F). Discard if the vaccine has been frozen.

ActHIB – Store lyophilized vaccine packaged with saline diluent, diphtheria and tetanus toxoids and pertussis or DTaP between 2° to 8°C (35° to 46°F). Do not freeze.

Liquid PedvaxHIB – Store vaccine at 2° to 8°C (36° to 46°F). Do not freeze.

Actions

➤*Pharmacology:*

HibTITER – The protective activity of antibody to *Haemophilus* b polysaccharide was demonstrated by passive antibody studies in animals and in children with agammaglobulinemia or with *Haemophilus* b disease and confirmed with the efficacy study of *Haemophilus* b polysaccharide (HbPs) vaccine. Data from passive antibody studies indicate that a preexisting titer of antibody to HbPs of 0.15 mcg/mL correlates with protection. Data from a Finnish field trial in children 18 to 71 months of age indicate that a titer of greater than 1 mcg/mL 3 weeks after vaccination is associated with long-term protection.

Linkage of *Haemophilus* b saccharides to a protein such as CRM^{197} converts the saccharide (HbO) to a T-dependent (HbOC) antigen, and results in an enhanced antibody response to the saccharide in young infants that primes for an anamnestic response and is predominantly of the IgG class. Laboratory evidence indicates that the native state of the CRM^{197} protein and the use of oligosaccharides in the formulation of *HibTITER* enhances its immunogenicity.

ActHIB – The response to *ActHIB* is typical of a T-dependent immune response to antigen. The prominent isotype of anticapsular PRP antibody induced by *ActHIB* is IgG. A substantial booster response has been demonstrated in children 12 months of age or older who previously received 2 or 3 doses. Bactericidal activity against *H. influenzae* type b is demonstrated in serum after immunization and statistically correlates with the anti-PRP antibody response induced by *ActHIB*.

Antibody to *H. influenzae* capsular polysaccharide (anti-PRP) titers of greater than 1 mcg/mL following vaccination with unconjugated PRP vaccine correlated with long-term protection against invasive *H. influenzae* type b disease in children older than 24 months of age. Although the relevance of this threshold to clinical protection after immunization with conjugate vaccines is not known, particularly in light of the induced, immunologic memory, this level continues to be considered as indicative of long-term protection. The immunogenicity and safety of *ActHIB* has been demonstrated in the United States and worldwide. *ActHIB* induced, on average, anti-PRP

HAEMOPHILUS B CONJUGATE VACCINE — INJECTION

levels greater than or equal to 1 mcg/mL in 90% of infants after the primary series and in more than 98% of infants after a booster dose.

Liquid PedvaxHIB – An important virulence factor of the Hib bacterium is its polysaccharide capsule (PRP). Antibody to PRP (anti-PRP) has been shown to correlate with protection against Hib disease. While the anti-PRP level associated with protection using conjugated vaccines has not yet been determined, the level of anti-PRP associated with protection in studies using bacterial polysaccharide immune globulin or nonconjugated PRP vaccines ranged from greater than 0.15 to greater than 1 mcg/mL.

Nonconjugated PRP vaccines are capable of stimulating B-lymphocytes to produce antibody without the help of T-lymphocytes (T-independent). The responses to many other antigens are augmented by helper T-lymphocytes (T-dependent). *PedvaxHIB* is a PRP-conjugate vaccine in which the PRP is covalently bound to the OMPC carrier, producing an antigen which is postulated to convert the T-independent antigen (PRP alone) into a T-dependent antigen resulting in both an enhanced antibody response and immunologic memory.

Contraindications

Hypersensitivity to any component of the vaccine or to the diluent. Persons who develop symptoms suggestive of hypersensitivity after an injection should not receive further injections of the vaccine.

➤*HibTITER*: The occurrence of an allergic or anaphylactic reaction following a prior dose of *HibTITER* is a contraindication to the use of *HibTITER*.

The decision to administer or delay vaccination because of a current or recent febrile illness depends largely on the severity of the symptoms and their etiology. Although a severe or even moderate febrile illness is sufficient reason to postpone vaccinations, minor illnesses, such as a mild respiratory tract infection with or without low-grade fever, are not generally contraindications.

➤*ActHIB*: *ActHIB* is contraindicated in children with histories of hypersensitivity to any component of the vaccine, including diphtheria toxoid or thimerosal in the multidose presentation and to any component of DTP or DTaP when combined by reconstitution with these vaccines. Any contraindication for DTP is a contraindication for *ActHIB* reconstituted with DTP. Any contraindication for DTaP is a contraindication for *ActHIB* reconstituted with DTaP.

Warnings

➤*HibTITER*: *HibTITER* will not protect against *H. influenza* other than type b strains, nor will *HibTITER* protect against other microorganisms that cause meningitis or septic disease.

As with any IM injection, *HibTITER* should be given with caution to infants or children with thrombocytopenia or any coagulation disorder, or to those receiving anticoagulant therapy.

The vial stopper contains dry natural rubber that may cause hypersensitivity reactions when handled by or when the product is injected in persons with known or possible latex sensitivity.

➤*ActHIB*: This product contains dry natural latex rubber as follows: The stopper to the diluent vial contains dry natural latex rubber. The lyophilized vaccine vial contains no rubber of any kind.

If *ActHIB* or *ActHIB* reconstituted with DTP or *ActHIB* reconstituted with DTaP is administered to immunosuppressed persons or persons receiving immunosuppressive therapy, the expected antibody responses may not be obtained. This includes patients with asymptomatic or symptomatic HIV infection, severe combined immunodeficiency, hypogammaglobulinemia, or agammaglobulinemia; altered immune states due to diseases such as leukemia, lymphoma, or generalized malignancy; or an immune system compromised by treatment with corticosteroids, alkylating drugs, antimetabolites or radiation.

➤*Elderly:* This vaccine is not recommended for use in adult populations.

➤*Pregnancy: Category C.* Animal reproduction studies have not been conducted with *Haemophilus* b conjugate vaccines or *Haemophilus* b conjugate vaccine (tetanus toxoid conjugate) reconstituted with DTP or *Haemophilus* b conjugate vaccine (tetanus toxoid conjugate) reconstituted with DTaP or saline diluent (0.4% Sodium Chloride). It is also not known whether *Haemophilus* b conjugate vaccine or *Haemophilus* b conjugate vaccine (tetanus toxoid conjugate) reconstituted with DTP or *Haemophilus* b conjugate vaccine (tetanus toxoid conjugate) reconstituted with DTaP or saline diluent (0.4% Sodium Chloride) can cause fetal harm when administered to a pregnant woman or can affect reproduction capacity. *Haemophilus* b conjugate vaccine (tetanus toxoid conjugate) reconstituted with DTP or *Haemophilus* b conjugate vaccine (tetanus toxoid conjugate) reconstituted with DTaP or saline diluent (0.4% Sodium Chloride) is not recommended for use in a pregnant woman and is not approved for use in children 5 years of age or older.

➤*Children:*

HibTITER – Safety and efficacy of *HibTITER* in infants below the age of 6 weeks have not been established.

ActHIB – Safety and efficacy of *ActHIB* reconstituted with DTaP in infants below the age of 15 months have not been established.

Safety and efficacy of *ActHIB* reconstituted with AvP DTP or saline diluent (0.4% sodium chloride) in infants below the age of 6 weeks have not been established.

Liquid PedvaxHIB – Safety and efficacy in infants below the age of 2 months and in children 6 years of age and older have not been established. In addition, *Liquid PedvaxHIB* should not be used in infants younger than 6 weeks of age because this will lead to a reduced anti-PRP response and may lead to immune tolerance (impaired ability to respond to subsequent exposure to the PRP antigen). *Liquid PedvaxHIB* is not recommended for use in individuals 6 years of age and older because they are generally not at risk of Hib disease.

Precautions

➤*Administration:* Special care should be taken to ensure that the injection does not enter a blood vessel.

➤*Allergic reaction:* Epinephrine injection (1:1000) must be immediately available should an anaphylactic or other allergic reaction occur due to any component of the vaccine.

➤*Immunosuppression:* Children with impaired immune responsiveness, whether due to the use of immunosuppressive therapy (including radiation, corticosteroids, antimetabolites, alkylating agents, and cytotoxic agents), a genetic defect, human immunodeficiency virus (HIV) infection, or other causes, may have reduced antibody response to active immunization procedures. Deferral of administration of vaccine may be considered in individuals receiving immunosuppressive therapy. Other groups should receive this vaccine according to the usual recommended schedule.

➤*HIV infection: Haemophilus* b conjugate vaccine is not contraindicated based on the presence of HIV infection.

➤*Infection:* Any acute infection or febrile illness is reason for delaying use of *Haemophilus* b conjugate vaccine, except when in the opinion of the physician, withholding the vaccine entails a greater risk. Minor illnesses such as upper respiratory infection with or without low-grade fever are not contraindications for use of *Haemophilus* b conjugate vaccine (tetanus toxoid conjugate).

➤*Active disease:* As reported with *Haemophilus* b polysaccharide vaccines, cases of *H. influenzae* type b disease may occur subsequent to vaccination and prior to the onset of protective effects of the vaccine.

➤*For IM use: Haemophilus* b conjugate vaccine should not be injected intradermally, since the safety and immunogenicity of this route have not been evaluated. The vaccine should be given IM.

➤*Disease transmission:* The evidence favors rejection of a causal relation between immunization with *Haemophilus* b conjugate vaccines and early-onset *Haemophilus* b disease.

➤*Antigenuria:* Antigenuria has been detected in some instances following receipt of *Haemophilus* b conjugate vaccines; therefore, urine antigen detection may not have definite diagnostic value in suspected *H. influenzae* type b disease within 1 week of immunization.

➤*ActHIB*: Antibody levels associated with protection may not be achieved earlier than 2 weeks following the last recommended dose.

As with any vaccine, vaccination with *ActHIB* (tetanus toxoid conjugate) reconstituted with DTP or *ActHIB* (tetanus toxoid conjugate) reconstituted with DTaP or 0.4% Sodium Chloride diluent may not protect 100% of susceptible individuals.

➤*HibTITER*: As with any vaccine, *HibTITER* may not protect 100% of individuals receiving the vaccine.

Although some antibody response to diphtheria toxin occurs, immunization with *HibTITER* does not substitute for routine diphtheria immunization.

See Warnings for more information.

➤*Liquid PedvaxHIB*: *Liquid PedvaxHIB* will not protect against disease caused by *Haemophilus influenzae* other than type b or against other microorganisms that cause invasive disease such as meningitis or sepsis.

As with any vaccine, vaccination with *Liquid PedvaxHIB* may not result in a protective antibody response in all individuals given the vaccine.

Sensitive tests (eg, Latex Agglutination Kits) may detect PRP derived from the vaccine in urine of some vaccinees for at least 30 days following vaccination with lyophilized *PedvaxHIB*; in clinical studies with lyophilized *PedvaxHIB*, such children demonstrated normal immune response to the vaccine.

Drug Interactions

➤*Anticoagulants:* As with other IM injections, use with caution in patients on anticoagulant therapy.

➤*Immunosuppressives:* Immunosuppressive therapies, including irradiation, antimetabolites, alkylating agents, cytotoxic drugs, and corticosteroids (used in greater than physiologic doses), may reduce the immune response to vaccines. Short-term (less than 2 weeks) corticosteroid therapy or intra-articular, bursal, or tendon injections with corticosteroids should not be immunosuppressive. Although no specific studies with pertussis vaccine are available, if immunosuppressive therapy will be discontinued shortly, it is reasonable to defer vaccination until the patient has been off therapy for one month; otherwise, the patient should be vaccinated while still on therapy.

If *Haemophilus* b conjugate vaccine reconstituted with DTP or *Haemophilus* b conjugate vaccine reconstituted with DTaP has been administered to persons receiving immunosuppressive therapy, a recent injection of immunoglobulin or having an immunodeficiency disorder, an adequate immunologic response may not be obtained.

➤*Vaccines:* The American Academy of Pediatrics (AAP), the Advisory Committee on Immunization Practices (ACIP) and the American Academy of Family Physicians (AAFP) encourage routine simultaneous administration of DTaP, IPV, *Haemophilus influenzae* type b vaccine, pneumococcal conjugate vaccine, measles-mumps-rubella (MMR), varicella vaccine and hepa-

HAEMOPHILUS B CONJUGATE VACCINE — INJECTION

titis B vaccine for children who are the recommended age to receive these vaccines and for whom no specific contraindications exist at the time of the visit, unless, in the judgment of the provider, complete vaccination of the child will not be compromised by administering different vaccines at different visits. Simultaneous administration is particularly important if the child might not return for subsequent vaccinations.

Adverse Reactions

➤*HibTITER*:

Number of subjects (%) manifesting side effects associated with *HibTITER* administered independently from DTP* (infants vaccinated initially at 1 to 6 months of age)

Symptoms	Dose 1 (n = 401) Same day as vacc.	Dose 1 +1 day	Dose 1 +2 days	Dose 2 (n = 383) Same day as vacc.	Dose 2 +1 day	Dose 2 +2 day	Dose 3 (n = 334) Same day as vacc.	Dose 3 +1 day	Dose 3 +2 days
Temp > 38.3°C (100.4°F)	0	2	2	2	3	2	2	6	5
	-	< 1%	< 1%	< 1%	< 1%	< 1%	< 1%	1.8%	1.5%
Redness ≥ 2 cm	1	0	0	1	6	0	5	4	0
	< 1%	-	-	< 1%	1.6%	-	1.5%	1.2%	-
Warmth ≥ 2 cm	1	1	0	2	1	0	1	6	0
	< 1%	< 1%	-	< 1%	< 1%	-	< 1%	1.8%	-
Swelling ≥ 2 cm	5	1	0	2	2	0	1	0	0
	1.2%	< 1%	-	< 1%	< 1%	-	< 1%	-	-

* DTP and *HibTITER* given 2 weeks apart, with DTP having been given first.

The following complaints were also observed after 1118 vaccinations with *HibTITER*: Irritability (133), sleepiness (91), prolonged crying [greater than or equal to 4 hours] (38), appetite loss (23), vomiting (9), diarrhea (2), and rash (1).

Selected adverse reactions* in children of 15 to 23 months of age following vaccination with HibTITER

Adverse reaction	Number of subjects	Reaction within 24 hours	% Postvaccination at 48 hours
Fever > 38.3°C (100.4°F)	354	1.4	0.6%
Erythema	354	2	-
Swelling	354	1.7	
Tenderness	354	3.7	0.3%

* The following complaints were reported after vaccination of these 354 children in the indicated number of children: Diarrhea (9), vomiting (5), prolonged crying (greater than 4 hours) (4), and rashes (2).

Postmarketing –

Injection site reactions: Injection site reactions, including hypersensitivity (including urticaria), induration, inflammation, mass, and skin discoloration.

Systemic events: Anaphylactoid/anaphylactic reactions (including shock), angioneurotic edema, convulsions, erythema multiforme, facial edema, febrile seizures, Guillain-Barré syndrome, headache, hives (urticaria), hypersensitivity reaction, lethargy, and malaise. Also reported, hypotonia or hyporesponsive-hypotonic-episodes (in many instances pertussis-containing vaccine was coadministered).

➤*ActHIB*:

Percentage of infants presenting with local or systemic reactions at 6, 24, and 48 hours of immunization with *ActHIB* administered simultaneously, at separate sites, with AvP DTP vaccine

Reaction	2 months (n = 365) 6 hours	2 months 24 hours	2 months 48 hours	4 months (n = 364) 6 hours	4 months 24 hours	4 months 48 hours	6 months (n = 365) 6 hours	6 months 24 hours	6 months 48 hours
Local[1]									
Tenderness	46.3%	11.5%	2.2%	23.4%	7.4%	1.1%	19.2%	6%	1.1%
Erythema	14.3%	4.1%	0.3%	8.8%	5.8%	0.6%	11.5%	6.9%	1.6%
Induration	22.5%	6.3%	1.9%	12.4%	4.7%	0.8%	9.6%	3.8%	1.1%
Systemic[2]									
Fever > 100.8°F[3]	20.1%	1.3%	0.6%	14.6%	6.6%	1.4%	15.7%	8.8%	0.8%
Irritability	72.6%	21.9%	12.6%	48.4%	25%	13.2%	44.1%	25.2%	10.1%
Drowsiness	57.5%	29.9%	10.4%	44.2%	18.1%	7.4%	32.6%	13.4%	2.5%
Anorexia	15.3%	5.8%	4.9%	8%	5%	3%	5.5%	4.9%	2.2%
Diarrhea	4.4%	6.6%	5.2%	5%	4.7%	4.7%	4.7%	6.3%	3.6%
Vomiting	2.7%	4.1%	2.7%	2.5%	3.3%	2.8%	2.2%	2.7%	1.9%
Persistent crying	Percentage of infants within 72 hours after immunization was 1.6% after dose one, 0.6% after dose two, and 0.3% after dose three								

[1] Local reactions were evaluated at the *ActHIB* injection site.

[2] The adverse reaction profile is defined by the concomitant use of AvP DTP vaccine.

[3] The number of individuals observed at each time point for fever varied from 357 to 363.

In general, the rates of minor systemic reactions after *ActHIB* and DTP immunization were comparable to those usually reported after DTP vaccine alone.

Percentage of infants presenting with local or systemic reactions at 6, 24, and 48 hours of immunization with *ActHIB* combined with AvP DTP vaccine by reconstitution

Reaction	2 months (n = 204) 6 hours	2 months 24 hours	2 months 48 hours	4 months (n = 199) 6 hours	4 months 24 hours	4 months 48 hours	6 months (n = 200) 6 hours	6 months 24 hours	6 months 48 hours
Local									
Tenderness	47.1%	18.6%	3.4%	33.2%	17.6%	4%	25%	17%	3.5%
Erythema > 1″	11.8%	2.5%	0%	11.6%	9.1%	2.5%	10.5%	13.5%	3.5%
Induration	31.4%	17.2%	3.9%	26.1%	20.1%	7.5%	28.5%	22.5%	10%
Systemic									
Fever > 100.4°F	24.6%	2%	0.5%	15.8%	6.1%	3.6%	13%	10.3%	3.1%
Irritability	70.6%	22.1%	12.8%	56.8%	31.2%	19.1%	40.5%	28.2%	15.9%
Drowsiness	60.3%	23.5%	11.3%	42.2%	20.6%	9.6%	30.3%	12.3%	5.6%
Anorexia	17.7%	6.4%	2.9%	10.1%	7.5%	5.5%	5.1%	4.6%	4.1%
Diarrhea	2.5%	5.4%	1.5%	3.5%	3.5%	2.5%	2.6%	4.1%	5.6%
Vomiting	2.9%	5.4%	2.9%	3%	5%	3%	3.6%	3.6%	1.5%
Persistent crying	Percentage of infants within 72 hours after immunization was 0% after dose one, 0% after dose two, and 0.005% after dose three								

In a third US trial when *ActHIB* was combined with DTP by reconstitution, approximately 1450 doses were administered to infants starting at 2 months of age. Adverse reactions observed at 6 and 24 hours, respectively, after the first immunization (n = 498) were tenderness 66.9% and 30.7%; erythema (greater than 1 inch) 8.6% and 2.2%; induration 38.2% and 21.7%; irritability 77.9% and 35.7%; drowsiness 63.7% and 34.1%; anorexia 26.1% and 12.9%; diarrhea 6.8% and 9%; and vomiting 3.4% and 3.8%. One hypotonic/hyporesponsive episode (HHE) was seen in an infant following the second dose in this trial. This is consistent with the HHE incidence rate observed with DTP vaccination alone.

Adverse reactions associated with *ActHIB* generally subsided after 24 hours and usually do not persist beyond 48 hours after immunization.

Other studies – ActHIB combined with DTaP by reconstitution, was administered to approximately 850 children, aged 15 to 20 months. All children received 3 doses of a *Haemophilus* b conjugate vaccine and 3 doses of whole-cell DTP at approximately 2, 4, and 6 months of age. Local reactions were typically mild and usually resolved within the 24- to 48-hour period after immunization. The most common local reactions were pain and tenderness at the injection site. Systemic reactions occurring were usually mild and resolved within 72 hours of immunization. The reaction rates were similar to those observed above when *ActHIB* reconstituted with DTaP was administered and when DTaP was administered alone as a booster.

In a randomized, double-blind US clinical trial, *ActHIB* was given concomitantly with DTP to more than 5,000 infants and hepatitis B vaccine was given with DTP to a similar number. In this large study, deaths due to sudden infant death syndrome (SIDS) and other causes were observed but were not different in the 2 groups. In the first 48 hours following immunization, 2 definite and 3 possible seizures were observed after *ActHIB* and DTP in comparison with none after hepatitis B vaccine and DTP. This rate of seizures following *Haemophilus* b conjugate vaccine (tetanus toxoid conjugate) and DTP was not greater than previously reported in infants receiving DTP alone. Other adverse reactions reported with administration of other *Haemophilus* b conjugate vaccines include urticaria, seizures, hives, renal failure and Guillain-Barré syndrome (GBS). A cause-and-effect relationship among any of these events and the vaccination has not been established.

However, the number of subjects studied with *ActHIB* combined with DTaP by reconstitution was inadequate to detect rare serious adverse events.

➤*PedvaxHIB*:

Liquid PedvaxHIB –

During a 3-day period following primary vaccination with *Liquid PedvaxHIB* in these infants, the most frequently reported (greater than 1%) adverse reactions, without regard to causality, excluding those shown in the table below, in decreasing order of frequency, were as follows: Irritability,

HAEMOPHILUS B CONJUGATE VACCINE — INJECTION

sleepiness, injection site pain/soreness, injection site erythema (less than or equal to 2.5 cm diameter, see also table below), injection site swelling/induration (less than or equal to 2.5 cm diameter, see also table below), unusual high-pitched crying, prolonged crying (greater than 4 hours), diarrhea, vomiting, crying, pain, otitis media, rash, and upper respiratory tract infection.

Selected objective observations reported by parents over a 48-hour period in these infants following primary vaccination with *Liquid PedvaxHIB* are summarized in the following table:

Fever or local reactions in subjects first vaccinated at 2 to 6 months of age with *Liquid PedvaxHIB*[*]

Reaction	Number of subjects evaluated	Post-dose 1 (hours)			Number of subjects evaluated	Post-dose 2 (hours)		
		6	24	48		6	24	48
		Percentage				Percentage		
Fever[**] > 38.3°C (≥ 101°F) rectal	222	18.1%	4.4%	0.5%	206	14.1%	9.4%	2.8%
Erythema > 2.5 cm diameter	674	2.2%	1%	0.5%	562	1.6%	1.1%	0.4%
Swelling > 2.5 cm diameter	674	2.5%	1.9%	0.9%	562	0.9%	0.9%	1.3%

[*] DTP and OPV were administered concomitantly to most subjects.
[**] Fever was also measured by another method or reported as normal for an additional 345 infants after dose 1 and for an additional 249 infants after dose 2; however, these data are not included in the this table.

Potential adverse reactions – The use of *Haemophilus* b polysaccharide vaccines and another *Haemophilus* b conjugate vaccine has been associated with the following additional adverse effects: Early onset Hib disease and Guillain-Barré syndrome. A cause-and-effect relationship between these side effects and the vaccination was not established.

➤*Postmarketing:*

CNS – Febrile seizures.

Dermatologic – Sterile injection site abscess.

Hematologic / Lymphatic – Lymphadenopathy.

Hypersensitivity – Rarely, angioedema.

Overdosage

There have been reports of overdose with *HibTITER*. Many cases were due to inadvertent coadministration with another *Haemophilus* b conjugate-containing vaccine. Most individuals were asymptomatic. In general, adverse events reported with overdosage have also been reported with recommended single doses.

Patient Information

The healthcare provider should inform the parent, guardian, or other responsible adult of the recommended immunization schedule for protection against *Haemophilus* b disease and of the benefits and risks of the vaccine.

Prior to administration of *Haemophilus* b conjugate vaccine or *Haemophilus* b conjugate vaccine (tetanus toxoid conjugate) reconstituted with DTP or *Haemophilus* b conjugate vaccine (tetanus toxoid conjugate) reconstituted with DTaP or saline diluent (0.4% Sodium Chloride), the parent or guardian should be asked about the recent health status of the infant or child to be immunized, previous vaccination history, and reactions to previous *Haemophilus* vaccines, if any.

The physician should inform the parent or guardian about the significant adverse reactions that have been temporally associated with the administration of *Haemophilus* b conjugate vaccine or *Haemophilus* b conjugate vaccine (tetanus toxoid conjugate) reconstituted with saline or DTP, or *Haemophilus* b conjugate vaccine (tetanus toxoid conjugate) reconstituted with DTaP. Guidance should be provided on measures to be taken should adverse events occur, such as antipyretic measures for elevated temperatures and the need to report adverse events to the healthcare provider. Parents should be provided with vaccine information pamphlets at the time of each vaccination, as stated in the National Childhood Vaccine Injury Act.

The US Department of Health and Human Services has established a new Vaccine Adverse Event Reporting System (VAERS) to accept all reports of suspected adverse events after the administration of any vaccine, including but not limited to the reporting of events required by the National Childhood Vaccine Injury Act of 1986. The toll-free number for VAERS forms and information is 1-800-822-7967.

The National Vaccine Injury Compensation Program, established by the National Childhood Vaccine Injury Act of 1986, requires physicians and other health-care providers who administer vaccines to maintain permanent vaccination records and to report occurrences of certain adverse events to the US Department of Health and Human Services. Reportable events include those listed in the Act for each vaccine and events specified in the package insert as contraindications to further doses of the vaccine.

The healthcare provider should inform the parent or guardian of the importance of completing the immunization series.

The healthcare provider should provide the Vaccine Information Materials (VIMs) which are required to be given with each immunization.

HAEMOPHILUS B CONJUGATE VACCINE WITH HEPATITIS B VACCINE

Rx	**Comvax** (Merck)	**Injection:** 7.5 mcg *Haemophilus* b PRP, 5 mcg hepatitis B surface antigen/0.5 mL[a]	In 0.5 mL single-dose vials.

[a] With 125 mcg *Neisseria meningitidis* OMPC, approximately 225 mcg aluminum (as aluminum hydroxide), and 35 mcg sodium borate (decahydrate) in 0.9% sodium chloride.

HAEMOPHILUS B CONJUGATE AND HEPATITIS B — INJECTION

For complete and comparative prescribing information, refer to the Agents for Active Immunization introduction. For complete and comparative prescribing information, refer to the Haemophilus b conjugate vaccine monograph.

Indications

➤*Haemophilus b / Hepatitis B vaccination:* For vaccination against invasive disease caused by *Haemophilus influenzae* type b and against infection caused by all known subtypes of hepatitis B virus in infants 6 weeks to 15 months of age born of HBsAg negative mothers.

See Administration and Dosage for more information.

Vaccination with haemophilus b conjugate and hepatitis B should ideally begin at approximately 2 months of age or as soon thereafter as possible. In order to complete the 3-dose regimen of haemophilus b conjugate and hepatitis B, vaccination should be initiated no later than 10 months of age. Infants in whom vaccination with a PRP-OMPC-containing product (ie, *PedvaxHIB*, haemophilus b conjugate and hepatitis B) is not initiated until 11 months of age do not require 3 doses of PRP-OMPC; however, 3 doses of an HBsAg-containing product are required for complete vaccination against hepatitis B, regardless of age. For infants and children not vaccinated according to the recommended schedule see Administration and Dosage.

Haemophilus b conjugate and hepatitis B will not protect against invasive disease caused by *Haemophilus influenzae* other than type b or against invasive disease (such as meningitis or sepsis) caused by other microorganisms. Haemophilus b conjugate and hepatitis B will not prevent hepatitis caused by other viruses known to infect the liver. Because of the long incubation period for hepatitis B, it is possible for unrecognized infection to be present at the time the vaccine is given. The vaccine may not prevent hepatitis B in such patients.

➤*Use with other vaccines:* Immunogenicity results from open-labeled studies indicate that haemophilus b conjugate and hepatitis B can be administered concomitantly with DTP (diphtheria, tetanus and whole cell pertussis vaccine), DTaP (diphtheria, tetanus and acellular pertussis vaccine), OPV (oral poliomyelitis vaccine), IPV (inactivated poliomyelitis vaccine), M-M-R II (measles, mumps, and rubella virus vaccine live), and *VARIVAX* (varicella virus vaccine live) using separate sites and syringes for injectable vaccines (see Pharmacology).

Administration and Dosage

➤*Recommended schedule:* Infants born to HBsAg negative mothers should be vaccinated with three 0.5 mL doses of haemophilus b conjugate and hepatitis B, ideally at 2, 4, and 12 to 15 months of age. If the recommended schedule cannot be followed, the interval between the first 2 doses should be at least 6 weeks and the interval between the second and third dose should be as close as possible to 8 to 11 months.

Infants born to HBsAg-positive mothers should receive hepatitis B immune globulin and hepatitis B vaccine (recombinant) at birth and should complete the hepatitis B vaccination series given according to a particular schedule (see manufacturer's circular for hepatitis B vaccine [recombinant]).

Infants born to mothers of unknown HBsAg status should receive hepatitis B vaccine (recombinant) at birth and should complete the hepatitis B vaccination series given according to a particular schedule (see manufacturer's circular for hepatitis B vaccine [recombinant]).

➤*Modified schedules:*

Children previously vaccinated with 1 or more doses of either hepatitis B vaccine or haemophilus b conjugate vaccine – Children who receive 1 dose of hepatitis B vaccine at or shortly after birth may be administered haemophilus b conjugate and hepatitis B on the schedule of 2, 4, and 12 to 15 months of age. There are no data to support the use of a 3-dose series of haemophilus b conjugate and hepatitis B in infants who have previously received more than 1 dose of hepatitis B vaccine. However, haemophilus b conjugate and hepatitis B may be administered to children otherwise scheduled to receive concurrent *RECOMBIVAX HB* and *PedvaxHIB*.

Children not vaccinated according to recommended schedule for haemophilus b conjugate and hepatitis B – Vaccination schedules for children not vaccinated according to the recommended schedule should be considered on an individual basis. The number of doses of a PRP-OMPC-containing product (ie, haemophilus b conjugate and hepatitis B, *PedvaxHIB*) depends on the age that vaccination is begun. An infant 2 to 10 months of age should receive 3 doses of a product containing PRP-OMPC. An infant 11 to 14 months of age should receive 2 doses of a product containing PRP-

HAEMOPHILUS B CONJUGATE AND HEPATITIS B — INJECTION

OMPC. A child 15 to 71 months of age should receive 1 dose of a product containing PRP-OMPC. Infants and children, regardless of age, should receive 3 doses of an HBsAg-containing product.

➤*Preparation and administration:* Haemophilus b conjugate and hepatitis B is for intramuscular injection. The anterolateral thigh is the recommended site for intramuscular injection in infants. Data suggests that injections given in the buttocks frequently are given into fatty tissue instead of into muscle. Such injections have resulted in a lower seroconversion rate (for hepatitis B vaccine) than was expected.

Injection must be accomplished with a needle long enough to ensure intramuscular deposition of the vaccine. The ACIP has recommended that for intramuscular injections, the needle should be of sufficient length to reach the muscle mass itself. In a clinical trial with haemophilus b conjugate and hepatitis B (see Pharmacology) vaccination was accomplished with a needle length of 5/8 inches in accordance with ACIP recommendations in effect at that time. ACIP currently recommends that needles of longer length (7/8 to 1 inch) be used.

The vaccine should be used as supplied; no reconstitution is necessary.

Shake well before withdrawal and use. Thorough agitation is necessary to maintain suspension of the vaccine.

➤*Storage/Stability:* Store vaccine at 2° to 8°C (36° to 46°F). Storage above or below the recommended temperature may reduce potency.

Do not freeze since freezing destroys potency.

MENINGOCOCCAL VACCINE

Rx	**Menomune-A/C/Y/W-135** (Aventis Pasteur)	**Powder for injection**: When reconstituted, each 0.5 mL contains 50 mcg "isolated product" from each of groups A, C, Y, and W-135	Freeze-dried. In single- and 10-dose vials with diluent.[a,b]
Rx	**Menactra (Groups A, C, Y, and W-135)** (Aventis Pasteur)	**Injection**: 4 mcg each of groups A, C, Y, and W-135[b]	In single-dose vials.[c]

[a] With lactose (2.5 to 5 mg per dose). Single-dose vial supplied with 0.78 mL preservative-free distilled water diluent. Ten-dose vial supplied with 6 mL diluent with 1:10,000 thimerosal.

[b] Stopper to the vial contains dry, natural latex rubber.

[c] Conjugated to approximately 48 mcg of diphtheria toxoid protein carrier.

MENINGOCOCCAL (GROUPS A, C, Y, and W-135) POLYSACCHARIDE DIPHTHERIA TOXOID CONJUGATE VACCINE — INJECTION

For complete and comparative prescribing information, refer to the Agents for Active Immunization introduction.

Indications

➤*Menomune*: Active immunization against invasive meningococcal disease caused by serogroups A, C, Y, and W-135; may be used to prevent and control outbreaks of serogroup C meningococcal disease.

Menomune is not indicated for infants and children younger than 2 years of age except as short-term protection of infants at least 3 months of age against group A. For people remaining at high risk, especially children who were first vaccinated at younger than 4 years of age, revaccination may be indicated.

May not protect 100% of individuals.

➤*Menactra*: Active immunization of adolescents and adults 11 to 55 years of age for the prevention of invasive meningococcal disease caused by *Neisseria meningitidis* serogroups A, C, Y, and W-135.

Menactra is not indicated for immunization against diphtheria.

As with any vaccine, *Menactra* may not protect 100% of individuals.

Do not use meningococcal vaccine for treatment of actual infection.

Routine vaccination is recommended for the following high-risk groups:

1.) Deficiencies in late complement components (C3, C5-C9).
2.) Functional or actual asplenia.
3.) People with laboratory or industrial exposure to *N. meningitidis* aerosols.
4.) Travelers to, and residents of, hyperendemic areas such as sub-Saharan Africa. For information concerning geographic areas for which vaccination is recommended, contact the Centers for Disease Control and Prevention (CDC) at 888-232-3299.

The American College Health Association (ACHA) and the CDC also recommend that college students consider vaccination to reduce the risk for potentially fatal meningococcal disease.

Consider vaccinations for household or institutional contacts of people with meningococcal disease and for medical and laboratory personnel at risk of exposure to meningococcal disease.

Not indicated for the prevention of meningitis caused by other microorganisms.

Routine vaccination is not recommended in the United States for the following reasons:

1.) Meningococcal disease is infrequent (about 3,000 cases/year).
2.) No vaccine exists for serogroup B, which accounts for about 50% of cases in the United States.
3.) Vaccine is not efficacious against group C disease in children younger than 2 years of age, which account for 28% of the group C cases in the United States.

The Advisory Committee on Immunization Practices (ACIP) has published recommendations for the prevention and control of meningococcal disease in the United States (refer to http://www.cdc.gov).

Administration and Dosage

Before administration, take all appropriate precautions to prevent adverse reactions. This includes a review of the patient's previous immunization history, the presence of any contraindications to immunization, the current health status, and history concerning possible sensitivity to the vaccine, similar vaccine, or to latex.

Record the date, lot number, and manufacturer of the vaccine administered as part of the patient's immunization record.

➤*Menomune*: Take special care to avoid injecting the vaccine intradermally, intramuscularly (IM), or intravenously (IV) because clinical studies have not been done to establish safety and efficacy of the vaccine using these routes of administration.

Simultaneous administration of *Menomune* can be given with other vaccines at separate sites and with separate syringes. However, because of the combined endotoxin content, do not administer the vaccine at the same time as whole-cell pertussis or whole-cell typhoid vaccines (see Drug Interactions). Do not use multiple-dose needle and syringe with jet injector.

Primary immunization – For adults and children, *Menomune* is administered subcutaneously as a single 0.5 mL dose. Protective antibody levels may be achieved within 7 to 10 days after vaccination.

Revaccination – Revaccination of a single 0.5 mL dose administered subcutaneously may be indicated for individuals at high risk of infection, particularly children who were first vaccinated when they were younger than 4 years of age; consider such children for revaccination after 2 or 3 years if they remain at high risk. Although the need for revaccination in older children and adults has not been determined, antibody levels decline rapidly over 2 to 3 years, and, if indications still exist for immunization, consider revaccination within 3 to 5 years.

Reconstitution – Reconstitute *Menomune* using only the diluent supplied for this purpose. Draw the volume of diluent shown on the diluent label into a suitable size syringe and inject into the vial containing the vaccine. Shake vial until the vaccine is dissolved. The reconstituted vaccine is a clear, colorless liquid.

➤*Menactra*: Administer *Menactra* as a single 0.5 mL injection by the IM route, preferably in the deltoid region. After insertion of the needle, aspirate to ensure that the needle has not entered a blood vessel.

Do not administer *Menactra* IV, subcutaneously, or intradermally.

The need for or timing of a booster dose of *Menactra* vaccine has not yet been determined.

Incompatibilities – Do not mix *Menactra* with any vaccine in the same syringe. Use separate injection sites and different syringes in case of coadministration.

➤*Storage/Stability:*

Menomune – Store freeze-dried vaccine and reconstituted vaccine, when not in use, between 2° and 8°C (35° to 46°F). Discard remainder of multidose vials of vaccine within 5 days after reconstitution. Use the single-dose vial within 30 minutes after reconstitution.

MENINGOCOCCAL (GROUPS A, C, Y, and W-135) POLYSACCHARIDE DIPHTHERIA TOXOID CONJUGATE VACCINE — INJECTION

Menactra – Store between 2° and 8°C (35° and 46°F). Do not freeze. Do not use product that has been exposed to freezing. Protect from light. Do not use after expiration date.

Actions

➤*Pharmacology:* The presence of bactericidal anticapsular meningococcal antibodies has been associated with protection from invasive meningococcal disease. Meningococcal polysaccharide diphtheria toxoid conjugate vaccine induces the production of bactericidal antibodies specific to the capsular polysaccharides of serogroups A, C, Y, and W-135.

The immunogenicity and clinical efficacy of serogroups A and C meningococcal vaccines have been well established. The serogroup A polysaccharide induces antibody in some children as young as 3 months of age, although a response comparable with that among adults is not achieved until 4 or 5 years of age; the serogroup C component is poorly immunogenic in recipients who are younger than 18 to 24 months of age. The serogroups A and C vaccines have demonstrated estimated clinical efficacies of 85% to 100% in older children and adults and are useful in controlling epidemics. Serogroups Y and W-135 polysaccharides are safe and immunogenic in adults and in children older than 2 years of age.

Measurable levels of antibodies against the group A and C polysaccharides decrease markedly during the first 3 years following a single dose of vaccine. This decrease in antibody occurs more rapidly in infants and young children than in adults. Similarly, although vaccine-induced clinical protection probably persists in schoolchildren and adults for at least 3 years, the efficacy of the group A vaccine in young children may decrease markedly with the passage of time. In a 3-year study, efficacy declined from more than 90% to less than 10% among children who were younger than 4 years of age at the time of vaccination, whereas among children who were 4 years of age or older when vaccinated, efficacy was 67% 3 years later.

Contraindications

➤*Menomune*: Defer use during the course of any acute illness or sensitivity to thimerosal or any other component of the vaccine. For individuals sensitive to thimerosal, administer the 1-dose package size and reconstitute with the 0.78 mL vial of diluent that contains no preservatives.

➤*Menactra*: Known hypersensitivity to any component of *Menactra*, including diphtheria toxoid, or a life-threatening reaction after previous administration of a vaccine containing similar components, are contraindications to vaccine administration.

Known hypersensitivity to dry, natural rubber latex is a contraindication to *Menactra* administration.

Warnings

➤*Latex sensitivity:* Use caution in patients with a possible history of latex sensitivity; the stopper to the vial contains natural latex rubber.

➤*Recent or acute illness:* The ACIP has published guidelines for vaccination of persons with recent or acute illness (refer to http://www.cdc.gov).

➤*Hypersensitivity reactions:* As a precautionary measure, epinephrine injection (1:1,000) and other appropriate agents and equipment must be immediately available in case of anaphylactic or serious allergic reactions.

➤*Elderly:* Safety and efficacy of *Menactra* in adults older than 55 years of age have not been established.

➤*Pregnancy: Category C.* It is not known whether meningococcal vaccine can cause fetal harm when given to a pregnant woman or can affect reproduction capacity. Give meningococcal vaccine to a pregnant woman only if clearly needed.

Health care providers are encouraged to register pregnant women who receive *Menactra* in the manufacturer's pregnancy registry by calling 1-800-822-2463.

➤*Lactation:* It is not known whether this drug is excreted in breast milk. Exercise caution when meningococcal vaccine is given to a breast-feeding woman.

➤*Children:* Safety and efficacy of *Menomune* in children younger than 2 years of age have not been established.

Safety and efficacy of *Menactra* in children younger than 11 years of age have not been established.

Precautions

➤*Immunosuppressed patients:* If *Menomune* is administered to immunosuppressed patients or patients receiving immunosuppressive therapy, an adequate immunologic response may not be obtained.

The immune response to *Menactra* administered to immunosuppressed patients has not been studied.

Drug Interactions

➤*Immunosuppressive therapy:* If meningococcal vaccine is used in people receiving immunosuppressive therapy (including irradiation, antimetabolites, alkylating agents, cytotoxic drugs, and corticosteroids [used in greater than physiologic doses]), the expected immune response may not be obtained.

➤*Other vaccines:* Do not give *Menomune* at the same time as whole-cell pertussis or whole-cell typhoid vaccines because of combined endotoxin content.

The safety and immunogenicity of coadministration of *Menactra* with vaccines other than typhoid Vi polysaccharide or tetanus and diphtheria toxoids, adsorbed (for adult use) vaccines have not been determined.

Adverse Reactions

Report adverse reactions following immunization to Vaccine Adverse Event Reporting System (VAERS). Obtain reporting forms and information about reporting requirements or completion of the form from VAERS through a toll-free number, 1-800-822-7967. Reporting forms also may be obtained at the Food and Drug Administration (FDA) Web site at http://www.vaers.org. Health care providers should also report these reactions to the manufacturer or call 1-800-822-2463.

➤*Menomune*: Adverse reactions to *Menomune* are mild and consist principally of pain and redness at the injection site for 1 to 2 days. Pain at the injection site is the most commonly reported adverse reaction, and a transient fever might develop in 2% or less of young children.

The following adverse reactions were reported by 150 adults following vaccination with *Menomune* and occurred within 3 weeks following vaccination. Local reactions resolved within 48 hours, and no significant systemic reactions were reported.

Local – Diameter (mild, less than 2 inches; moderate, 2 inches or greater), erythema (mild, 3.8%; moderate, 1.2%), induration (mild, 4.4%; moderate, 1.2%), pain (mild reaction, 2.6%; moderate reaction, 2%), tenderness (mild, 36%; moderate, 9%).

In a clinical study involving 73 children 2 to 12 years of age who received *Menomune*, local reactions consisting of erythema or tenderness were seen in approximately 40% of the children. In another clinical study involving 53 children 4 to 6 years of age who received *Menomune* , erythema was seen in 89% of the children, swelling in 92%, and tenderness in 64%. None of these reactions was considered serious or necessitated medical intervention.

Systemic – Chills (mild, 2.5%), headaches (mild, 5.2%; moderate, 1.8%), malaise (mild, 2.5%), oral temperature (mild, 2.6% [100° to 101°F]; moderate, 0.6% [greater than 101°F]).

On rare occasions, immunoglobulin A (IgA) nephropathy has occurred following vaccinations with *Menomune*; however, a cause-and-effect relationship has not been established.

➤*Menactra:*

Solicited adverse reactions in the primary safety studies – The most commonly reported solicited adverse reactions in adolescents 11 to 18 years of age (see the following table), and adults 18 to 55 years of age (see the second table that follows), were local pain, headache, and fatigue. Except for redness in adults, local reactions were more frequently reported after *Menactra* vaccination than after *Menomune* vaccination. The majority of local and systemic reactions following *Menactra* or *Menomune* were reported as mild in intensity. No important differences in rates of malaise, diarrhea, anorexia, vomiting, or rash were observed between the vaccine groups.

Meningococcal Vaccine Adverse Reactions in Patients 11 to 18 Years of Age (%)

Adverse reaction	*Menactra* vaccine			*Menomune* vaccine		
	Any	Moderate	Severe	Any	Moderate	Severe
CNS						
Headache[a]	35.6%[b]	9.6%[b]	1.1%	29.3%	6.5%	0.4%
Seizure[c]	0%	—	—	0%	—	—
Dermatologic						
Rash[c]	1.6%	—	—	1.4%	—	—
Redness[d]	10.9%[b]	1.6%[b]	0.6%[b]	5.7%	0.4%	0%
GI						
Anorexia[e]	10.7%[b]	2%	0.3%	7.7%	1.1%	0.2%
Diarrhea[f]	12%	1.6%	0.3%	10.2%	1.3%	0%
Vomiting[g]	1.9%	0.4%	0.3%	1.4%	0.5%	0.3%
Miscellaneous						
Arthralgia[a]	17.4%[b]	3.6%[b]	0.4%	10.2%	2.1%	0.1%
Chills[a]	7%[b]	1.7%[b]	0.2%	3.5%	0.4%	0.1%
Fatigue[a]	30%[b]	7.5%	1.1%[b]	25.1%	6.2%	0.2%
Fever[h]	5.1%[b]	0.6%	0%	3%	0.3%	0.1%
Induration[d]	15.7%[b]	2.5%[b]	0.3%	5.2%	0.5%	0%
Malaise[a]	21.9%[b]	5.8%[b]	1.1%	16.8%	3.4%	0.4%
Pain[i]	59.2%[b]	12.8%[b]	0.3%	28.7%	2.6%	0%
Swelling[d]	10.8%[b]	1.9%[b]	0.5%[b]	3.6%	0.3%	0%

[a] Severe: requiring bed rest.
[b] Denotes $P < 0.05$ level of significance. The *P* values were calculated for each category and severity using Chi Square test.
[c] These solicited adverse reactions were reported as present or absent only.
[d] Moderate: 1 to 2 inches; severe: greater than 2 inches.
[e] Severe: skipped 3 or more meals.
[f] Severe: 5 or more episodes.
[g] Severe: 3 or more episodes.
[h] Severe: 39.5°C (103.1°F) or higher.
[i] Moderate: interferes with normal activities; severe: disabling, unwilling to move arm.

MENINGOCOCCAL (GROUPS A, C, Y, and W-135) POLYSACCHARIDE DIPHTHERIA TOXOID CONJUGATE VACCINE — INJECTION

Meningococcal Vaccine Adverse Reactions in Patients 18 to 55 Years of Age (%)

Adverse reaction	Menactra			Menomune		
	Any	Moderate	Severe	Any	Moderate	Severe
CNS						
Headache[a]	41.4%	10.1%	1.2%	41.8%	8.9%	0.9%
Seizure[b]	0%	—	—	0%	—	—
Dermatologic						
Rash[b]	1.4%	—	—	0.8%	—	—
Redness[c]	14.4%	2.9%	1.1%[d]	16%	1.9%	0.1%
GI						
Anorexia[e]	11.8%	2.3%	0.4%	9.9%	1.6%	0.4%
Diarrhea[f]	16%	2.6%	0.4%	14%	2.9%	0.3%
Vomiting[g]	2.3%	0.4%	0.2%	1.5%	0.2%	0.4%
Miscellaneous						
Arthralgia[a]	19.8%[d]	4.7%[d]	0.3%	16%	2.6%	0.1%
Chills[a]	9.7%[d]	2.1%[d]	0.6%[d]	5.6%	1%	0%
Fatigue[a]	34.7%	8.3%	0.9%	32.3%	6.6%	0.4%
Fever[h]	1.5%[d]	0.3%	0%	0.5%	0.1%	0%
Induration[c]	17.1%[d]	3.4%[d]	0.7%[d]	11%	1%	0%
Malaise[a]	23.6%	6.6%[d]	1.1%	22.3%	4.7%	0.9%
Pain[i]	53.9%[d]	11.3%[d]	0.2%	48.1%	3.3%	0.1%
Swelling[c]	12.6%[d]	2.3%[d]	0.9%[d]	7.6%	0.7%	0%

[a] Severe: requiring bed rest.
[b] These solicited adverse reactions were reported as present or absent only.
[c] Moderate: 1 to 2 inches; severe: greater than 2 inches.
[d] Denotes $P < 0.05$ level of significance. The P values were calculated for each category and severity using Chi Square test.
[e] Severe: skipped 3 or more meals.
[f] Severe: 5 or more episodes.
[g] Severe: 3 or more episodes.
[h] Severe: 40°C (104°F) or higher.
[i] Moderate: interferes with normal activities; severe: disabling, unwilling to move arm.

Patient Information

Prior to administration of meningococcal vaccine, inform the patient, parent, guardian, or other responsible adult of the potential benefits and risks to the patient and provide vaccine information statements. Instruct patients, parents, or guardians to report any suspected adverse reactions to their doctors.

Inform women of childbearing potential that the manufacturer maintains a pregnancy registry to monitor fetal outcomes of pregnant women exposed to meningococcal vaccine. If they are pregnant or become aware they were pregnant at the time of meningococcal polysaccharide diphtheria toxoid conjugate vaccine immunization, they should contact their doctors.

PNEUMOCOCCAL VACCINE, POLYVALENT

Rx	**Pneumovax 23** (Merck)	**Injection:** 25 mcg each of 23 polysaccharide isolates per 0.5 mL dose	In 1- and 5-dose vials.[a]

[a] With 0.25% phenol.

PNEUMOCOCCAL VACCINE POLYVALENT — INJECTION

For complete and comparative information, refer to the Agents for Active Immunization introduction.

Indications

➤*Pneumococcal disease prevention:* For vaccination against pneumococcal disease caused by those pneumococcal types included in the vaccine. Effectiveness of the vaccine in the prevention of pneumococcal pneumonia and pneumococcal bacteremia has been demonstrated in controlled trials in South Africa, France and in case-control studies.

Pneumococcal vaccine polyvalent will not prevent disease caused by capsular types of pneumococcus other than those contained in the vaccine.

If it is known that a person has not received any pneumococcal vaccine or if earlier pneumococcal vaccination status is unknown, then persons in the categories listed below should be administered pneumococcal vaccine; however, if a person has received a primary dose of pneumococcal vaccine, before administering an additional dose of vaccine, please refer to the Revaccination section.

Vaccination with pneumococcal vaccine polyvalent is recommended for selected individuals as follows:

➤*Immunocompetent persons:*
- Routine vaccination for persons 50 years of age or older†
- Persons 2 years of age or older with chronic cardiovascular disease (including congestive heart failure and cardiomyopathies), chronic pulmonary disease (including chronic obstructive pulmonary disease and emphysema), or diabetes mellitus
- Persons 2 years of age or older with alcoholism, chronic liver disease (including cirrhosis) or cerebrospinal fluid leaks
- Persons 2 years of age or older with functional or anatomic asplenia (including sickle cell disease and splenectomy)
- Persons 2 years of age or older living in special environments or social settings (including Alaskan Natives and certain American Indian populations)

➤*Immunocompromised persons:* Persons aged ≥ 2 years, including those with HIV infection, leukemia, lymphoma, Hodgkin's disease, multiple myeloma, generalized malignancy, chronic renal failure or nephrotic syndrome; those receiving immunosuppressive chemotherapy (including corticosteroids); and those who have received an organ or bone marrow transplant.

➤*Timing of vaccination:* Pneumococcal vaccine should be given at least 2 weeks before elective splenectomy, if possible.

For planning cancer chemotherapy or other immunosuppressive therapy (eg, for patients with Hodgkin's disease or those who undergo organ or bone marrow transplantation), the interval between vaccination and initiation of immunosuppressive therapy should be at least 2 weeks. Vaccination during chemotherapy or radiation therapy should be avoided. Pneumococcal vaccine may be given several months following completion of chemotherapy or radiation therapy for neoplastic disease. In Hodgkin's disease, immune response to vaccination may be suboptimal for 2 years or longer after intensive chemotherapy (with or without radiation). For some patients, during the 2 years following the completion of chemotherapy or other immunosuppressive therapy (with or without radiation), significant improvement in antibody response has been observed, particularly as the interval between the end of treatment and pneumococcal vaccination increased.

Persons with asymptomatic or symptomatic HIV infection should be vaccinated as soon as possible after their diagnosis is confirmed.

➤*Use with Other Vaccines:* See Administration and Dosage for more information.

➤*Revaccination:* Early studies have indicated that local reactions (ic, arthus-type reactions) among adults receiving the second dose of 14-valent vaccine within 2 years after the first dose are more severe than those occurring after initial vaccination. However, subsequent studies have suggested that revaccination after intervals of 4 years or more is not associated with an increased incidence of adverse side effects.

Routine revaccination of immunocompetent persons previously vaccinated with 23-valent polysaccharide vaccine is not recommended. However, revaccination once is recommended for persons 2 years of age or older who are at highest risk of serious pneumococcal infection and those likely to have a rapid decline in pneumococcal antibody levels, provided that at least 5 years have passed since receipt of a first dose of pneumococcal vaccine.

The highest risk group includes persons with functional or anatomic asplenia (eg, sickle cell disease or splenectomy), HIV infection, leukemia, lymphoma, Hodgkin's disease, multiple myeloma, generalized malignancy, chronic renal failure, nephrotic syndrome, or other conditions associated with immunosuppression (eg, organ or bone marrow transplantation), and those receiving immunosuppressive chemotherapy (including long-term systemic corticosteroids).

For children 10 years of age or younger at revaccination and at highest risk of severe pneumococcal infection (eg, children with functional or anatomic asplenia, including sickle cell disease or splenectomy or conditions associated with rapid antibody decline after initial vaccination including nephrotic syndrome, renal failure or renal transplantation), the ACIP recommends that revaccination may be considered 3 years after the previous dose.

If prior vaccination status is unknown for patients in the high risk group, patients should be given pneumococcal vaccine.

All persons 65 years of age or older who have not received vaccine within 5 years (and were younger than 65 years of age at the time of vaccination) should receive another dose of vaccine.

Because data are insufficient concerning the safety of pneumococcal vaccine when administered 3 or more times, revaccination following a second dose is not routinely recommended.

Administration and Dosage

➤*Recommended dose:* Do not inject intravenously or intradermally.

For the vial, withdraw 0.5 mL from the vial using a sterile needle and syringe free of preservatives, antiseptics, and detergents.

Administer a single 0.5 mL dose of pneumococcal vaccine polyvalent subcutaneously or intramuscularly (preferably in the deltoid muscle or lateral midthigh), with appropriate precautions to avoid intravascular administration.

† The ACIP recommends routine vaccination for immunocompetent persons 65 years of age and older.

PNEUMOCOCCAL VACCINE POLYVALENT — INJECTION

➤*Use with other vaccines:* The ACIP states that pneumococcal vaccine may be administered at the same time as influenza vaccine (by separate injection in the other arm) without an increase in side effects or decreased antibody response to either vaccine. In contrast to pneumococcal vaccine, influenza vaccine is recommended annually, for appropriate populations.

➤*Storage/Stability:* Store unopened and opened vials and prefilled syringes at 2° to 8°C (36° to 46°F). The vaccine is used directly as supplied. No dilution or reconstitution is necessary. Phenol 0.25% has been added as a preservative. All vaccine must be discarded after the expiration date.

Actions

➤*Pharmacology:*

Immunogenicity – It has been established that the purified pneumococcal capsular polysaccharides induce antibody production and that such antibody is effective in preventing pneumococcal disease. Clinical studies have demonstrated the immunogenicity of each of the 23 capsular types when tested in polyvalent vaccines.

Studies with 12-, 14-, and 23-valent pneumococcal vaccines in children 2 years of age and older and in adults of all ages showed immunogenic responses. Protective capsular type-specific antibody levels generally develop by the third week following vaccination.

Bacterial capsular polysaccharides induce antibodies primarily by T-cell-independent mechanisms. Therefore, antibody response to most pneumococcal capsular types is generally poor or inconsistent in children younger than 2 years of age whose immune systems are immature.

Efficacy – The protective efficacy of pneumococcal vaccines containing 6 or 12 capsular polysaccharides was investigated in 2 controlled studies of young, healthy gold miners in South Africa, in whom there was a high attack rate for pneumococcal pneumonia and bacteremia. Capsular type-specific attack rates for pneumococcal pneumonia were observed for the period from 2 weeks through about 1 year after vaccination. Protective efficacy was 76% and 92%, respectively, in the two studies for the capsular types represented.

In similar studies carried out by Dr. R. Austrian and associates, using similar pneumococcal vaccines prepared for the National Institute of Allergy and Infectious Diseases, the reduction in pneumonia caused by the capsular types contained in the vaccines was 79%. Reduction in type-specific pneumococcal bacteremia was 82%.

A prospective study in France found pneumococcal vaccine to be 77% effective in reducing the incidence of pneumonia among nursing home residents.

Duration of Immunity – Following pneumococcal vaccination, serotype-specific antibody levels decline after 5 to 10 years. A more rapid decline in antibody levels may occur in some groups (eg, children). Limited published data suggest that antibody levels may decline in patients older than 60 years of age.

The Advisory Committee on Immunization Practices (ACIP) states that these findings indicate that revaccination may be needed to provide continued protection (see Indications, Revaccination).

The results from one epidemiologic study suggest that vaccination may provide protection for at least nine years after receipt of the initial dose. Decreasing estimates of effectiveness with increasing interval since vaccination, particularly among the very elderly (persons aged ≥ 85 years) have been reported.

Contraindications

Hypersensitivity to any component of the vaccine. Epinephrine injection (1:1000) must be immediately available should an acute anaphylactoid reaction occur due to any component of the vaccine.

Warnings

➤*Timing of vaccination:* See Indications for more information.

If the vaccine is used in persons receiving immunosuppressive therapy, the expected serum antibody response may not be obtained and potential impairment of future immune responses to pneumococcal antigens may occur (see Indications, Timing of Vaccination).

➤*Intradermal use:* Intradermal administration may cause severe local reactions.

➤*Elderly:* Because elderly individuals may not tolerate medical interventions as well as younger individuals, a higher frequency and/or a greater severity of reactions in some older individuals cannot be ruled out.

➤*Pregnancy: Category C.* Animal reproduction studies have not been conducted with pneumococcal vaccine polyvalent. It is also not known whether pneumococcal vaccine polyvalent can cause fetal harm when administered to a pregnant woman or can affect reproduction capacity. Pneumococcal vaccine polyvalent should be given to a pregnant woman only if clearly needed.

➤*Lactation:* It is not known whether this drug is excreted in human milk. Because many drugs are excreted in human milk, caution should be exercised when pneumococcal vaccine polyvalent is administered to a nursing woman.

➤*Children:* In general, children less than 2 years of age respond poorly to the capsular types of pneumococcal vaccine polyvalent that are most often the cause of pneumococcal disease in this age group (see Pharmacology, Immunogenicity). Safety and effectiveness in children below the age of 2 years have not been established. Accordingly, pneumococcal vaccine polyvalent is not recommended in this age group.

Precautions

➤*Antibiotic prophylaxis:* In patients who require penicillin (or other antibiotic) prophylaxis against pneumococcal infection, such prophylaxis should not be discontinued after vaccination with pneumococcal vaccine polyvalent.

➤*Skull fracture:* Pneumococcal vaccine polyvalent may not be effective in preventing infection resulting from basilar skull fracture or from external communication with cerebrospinal fluid.

➤*Revaccination:* Routine revaccination of immunocompetent persons previously vaccinated with a 23-valent vaccine is not recommended. However, revaccination once is recommended for persons 2 years of age or older who are at highest risk for serious pneumococcal infections and those likely to have a rapid decline in pneumococcal antibody levels (see Indications, Revaccination).

➤*Special risk:* Caution and appropriate care should be exercised in administering pneumococcal vaccine polyvalent to individuals with severely compromised cardiovascular and/or pulmonary function in whom a systemic reaction would pose a significant risk.

Any febrile respiratory illness or other active infection is reason for delaying use of pneumococcal vaccine polyvalent, except when, in the opinion of the physician, withholding the agent entails even greater risk.

Adverse Reactions

➤*Most common adverse experiences reported in clinical trials:*

Local – Local reactions at injection site including soreness, warmth, erythema, swelling and induration; fever ≤ 102°F.

➤*Other adverse experiences reported in clinical trials and in postmarketing experience:*

CNS – Headache; paresthesia; radiculoneuropathy; Guillain-Barré syndrome.

Dermatologic – Rash; urticaria.

GI – Nausea; vomiting.

Hematologic/Lymphatic – Lymphadenitis; thrombocytopenia in patients with stabilized idiopathic thrombocytopenic purpura; hemolytic anemia in patients who have had other hematologic disorders.

Hypersensitivity – Anaphylactoid reactions; serum sickness.

Musculoskeletal – Arthralgia; arthritis; myalgia.

Miscellaneous – Asthenia; malaise; fever (greater than 102°F).

Patient Information

The health care provider should inform the patient, parent or guardian of the benefits and risks associated with vaccination. For risks associated with vaccination, see Warnings, Precautions, and Adverse Reactions.

Patients, parents, and guardians should be instructed to report any serious adverse reactions to their healthcare provider who in turn should report such events to the vaccine manufacturer or the US Department of Health and Human Services through the Vaccine Adverse Event Reporting System (VAERS), 1-800-822-7967.

PNEUMOCOCCAL 7-VALENT CONJUGATE VACCINE (DIPHTHERIA CRM_{197} PROTEIN)

Rx	**Prevnar** (Wyeth Lederle Vaccines)	**Injection:** 2 mcg each of 6 polysaccharide isolates; 4 mcg of 1 polysaccharide isolate per 0.5 mL dose[a]	In 0.5 mL single-dose vials.

[a] Contains 0.125 mg aluminum per dose as aluminum phosphate adjuvant.

PNEUMOCOCCAL 7-VALENT CONJUGATE VACCINE (DIPHTHERIA CRM_{197} PROTEIN) — INJECTION

For complete and comparative prescribing information, refer to the Agents for Active Immunization introduction.

Indications

➤*Immunization against Streptococcus pneumoniae:* Active immunization of infants and toddlers against invasive disease caused by *S. pneumoniae* due to the capsular serotypes included in the vaccine (4, 6B, 9V, 14, 18C, 19F, and 23F).

➤*Immunization against otitis media:* Active immunization of infants and toddlers against otitis media caused by serotypes included in the vaccine. However, for vaccine serotypes, protection against otitis media is expected to be substantially lower than protection against invasive disease. Additionally, because otitis media is caused by many organisms other than serotypes of *S. pneumoniae* represented in the vaccine, protection against all causes of otitis media is expected to be low.

This vaccine is not intended to be used for treatment of active infection.

Administration and Dosage

➤*Approved by the FDA:* February 17, 2000.

Administer as one 0.5 mL IM injection. Do not inject IV.

The preferred sites of IM injection are the anterolateral aspect of the thigh in infants or the deltoid muscle of the upper arm in toddlers and young chil-

PNEUMOCOCCAL 7-VALENT CONJUGATE VACCINE (DIPHTHERIA CRM_{197} PROTEIN) — INJECTION

dren. Do not inject the vaccine in the gluteal area or areas where there may be a major nerve trunk or blood vessel.

➤*Vaccination schedule:* For infants, the immunization series of pneumococcal 7-valent conjugate vaccine consists of 3 doses of 0.5 mL each, at approximately 2-month intervals, followed by a fourth dose of 0.5 mL at 12 to 15 months of age. The customary age for the first dose is 2 months of age, but it can be given as young as 6 weeks of age. The recommended dosing interval is 4 to 8 weeks. Administer the fourth dose at least 2 months after the third dose.

➤*Previously unvaccinated older infants and children:* For previously unvaccinated older infants and children who are beyond the age of the routine infant schedule, the following schedule applies:

Pneumococcal Vaccine Dosage in Previously Unvaccinated Older Infants and Children	
Age at first dose	Total number of 0.5 mL doses
7 to 11 months of age	3[a]
12 to 23 months of age	2[b]
≥ 24 months through 9 years of age	1

[a] Two doses at least 4 weeks apart; third dose after the 1-year birthday, separated from the second dose by at least 2 months.
[b] Two doses at least 2 months apart.

➤*Preparation:* Because this product is a suspension containing an aluminum phosphate adjuvant, shake vigorously immediately prior to use to obtain a uniform suspension prior to withdrawing the dose. Do not use the vaccine if it cannot be resuspended. After shaking, the vaccine appears as a homogeneous, white suspension. Administer immediately after drawing the vaccine up into the syringe.

➤*Storage/Stability:* Refrigerate at 2° to 8°C (36° to 46°F). Do not freeze.

Actions

➤*Pharmacology:* Pneumococcal 7-valent conjugate vaccine is a sterile solution of saccharides of the capsular antigens of *S. pneumoniae* serotypes 4, 6B, 9V, 14, 18C, 19F, and 23F individually conjugated to diphtheria CRM_{197} protein. The polysaccharides are chemically activated to make saccharides, which are directly conjugated to the protein carrier CRM_{197} to form the glycoconjugate. This is effected by reductive amination. CRM_{197} is a nontoxic variant of diphtheria toxin isolated from cultures of *Corynebacterium diphtheriae* strain C7 (β197) grown in a casamino acids and yeast extract-base medium.

Contraindications

Hypersensitivity to any component of the vaccine, including diphtheria toxoid.

➤*Infections:* Severe or even a moderate febrile illness is sufficient reason to postpone vaccinations. Minor illnesses, such as a mild upper respiratory tract infection, with or without low-grade fever, are not generally contraindications.

Warnings

➤*Efficacy:* This vaccine will not protect against *S. pneumoniae* disease other than that caused by the 7 serotypes included in the vaccine, nor will it protect against other microorganisms that cause invasive infection such as bacteremia and meningitis or noninvasive infections such as otitis media.

Immunization with pneumococcal 7-valent conjugate vaccine does not substitute for routine diphtheria immunization.

➤*Immunosuppressed patients:* Children with impaired immune responsiveness, whether caused by the use of immunosuppressive therapy (including irradiation, corticosteroids, antimetabolites, alkylating agents, and cytotoxic agents), a genetic defect, HIV infection, or other causes, may have reduced antibody response to active immunization (see Drug Interactions).

➤*Latex sensitivity:* Use caution in patients with a possible history of latex sensitivity; the packaging contains dry natural rubber.

➤*Hypersensitivity reactions:* Epinephrine 1:1000 and other appropriate agents must be available to control immediate allergic reaction. Refer to Management of Acute Hypersensitivity Reactions.

➤*Elderly:* This vaccine is not recommended for use in adult populations. Do not use as a substitute for the pneumococcal polysaccharide vaccine in geriatric populations.

➤*Pregnancy: Category C.* It is not known whether pneumococcal 7-valent conjugate vaccine can cause fetal harm when administered to a pregnant woman or whether it can affect reproductive capacity. Pneumococcal 7-valent conjugate vaccine is not recommended for use in pregnant women.

➤*Lactation:* It is not known whether vaccine antigens or antibodies are excreted in breast milk. This vaccine is not recommended for use in nursing mothers.

➤*Children:* Pneumococcal 7-valent conjugate vaccine has been shown to be usually well-tolerated and immunogenic in infants. The safety and efficacy of pneumococcal 7-valent conjugate vaccine in children under 6 weeks of age or on or after the tenth birthday have not been established. Immune responses elicited by pneumococcal 7-valent conjugate vaccine among infants born prematurely have not been studied. See Administration and Dosage for the recommended pediatric dosage.

Precautions

➤*Route of administration:* Pneumococcal 7-valent conjugate vaccine is for IM use only. Do not administer IV under any circumstances. The safety and immunogenicity for other routes of administration (eg, SC) have not been evaluated. Take special care to prevent injection into or near a blood vessel or nerve.

➤*Postvaccination fever:* Fever and, rarely, febrile seizure have been reported in children receiving pneumococcal 7-valent conjugate vaccine. For children at higher risk of seizures than the general population, acetaminophen or other appropriate antipyretics (dosed according to respective prescribing information) may be administered around the time of vaccination to reduce the possibility of postvaccination fever.

Drug Interactions

➤*Immunosuppressive agents:* Children receiving therapy with immunosuppressive agents (large amounts of corticosteroids, antimetabolites, alkylating agents, cytotoxic agents) may not respond optimally to active immunization.

Adverse Reactions

Pneumococcal Vaccine Adverse Reactions Within 2 or 3 Days of Administration to Infants as a Primary Series at 2, 4, and 6 Months of Age (%)			
	Pneumococcal 7-valent conjugate vaccine concurrently with DTP-HbOC	Pneumococcal 7-valent conjugate vaccine concurrently with DTaP and HbOC	DTaP and HbOC only
Number of doses	9191[a]	3848[b]	538[c]
GI			
Decreased appetite	24.7	18.1	13.6
Vomiting	16.2	13.4	9.8
Diarrhea	11.4	9.8	4.4
Miscellaneous			
Irritability	69.1	52.5	45.2
Drowsiness	36.9	32.9	27.7
Fever of 38°C (100.4°F) or higher	35.6	21.1	14.2
Restless sleep	25.8	20.6	22.3
Fever of greater than 39°C (102.2°F)	3.1	1.8	0.4
Urticaria-like rash	0.9	0.6	0.3

[a] Total from which reaction data are available varies between reactions from 8874 to 9191 doses.
[b] Total from which reaction data are available varies between reactions from 3121 to 3848 doses.
[c] Total from which reaction data are available varies between reactions from 295 to 538 doses.

Pneumococcal Vaccine Adverse Reactions Within 2 or 3 Days of Administration to Toddlers as a Fourth Dose at 12 to 15 Months of Age (%)			
	Pneumococcal 7-valent conjugate vaccine concurrently with DTP-HbOC	Pneumococcal 7-valent conjugate vaccine concurrently with DTaP and HbOC	Pneumococcal 7-valent conjugate vaccine only
Number of doses	709[a]	270[b]	727[c]
GI			
Decreased appetite	33	21.1	18.3
Diarrhea	12.1	13.7	12.8
Vomiting	9.6	5.6	6.3
Miscellaneous			
Irritability	72.8	45.9	45.8
Fever of 38°C (100.4°F) or higher	41.9	19.6	13.4
Restless sleep	29.9	21.2	21.2
Drowsiness	21.3	17.5	15.9
Fever of greater than 39°C (102.2°F)	4.5	1.5	1.2
Urticaria-like rash	1.4	0.7	1.2

[a] Total from which reaction data are available varies between reactions from 706 to 709 doses.
[b] Total from which reaction data are available varies between reactions from 269 to 270 doses.
[c] Total from which reaction data are available varies between reactions from 725 to 727 doses.

➤*Local:* With vaccines in general, including pneumococcal 7-valent conjugate vaccine, it is not uncommon for patients to note within 48 to 72 hours the following minor reactions at or around the injection site: edema; pain or tenderness; redness, inflammation, or skin discoloration; mass; local hypersensitivity reaction. Such local reactions are usually self-limited and require no therapy.

As with other aluminum-containing vaccines, a nodule may occasionally be palpable at the injection site for several weeks.

➤*Postmarketing:*

Hypersensitivity – Hypersensitivity reaction including face edema, dyspnea, bronchospasm, anaphylactic/anaphylactoid reaction including shock.

Local – Injection-site dermatitis; injection-site urticaria; injection-site pruritus.

Miscellaneous – Lymphadenopathy localized to the region of the injection site; angioneurotic edema; erythema multiforme.

PNEUMOCOCCAL 7-VALENT CONJUGATE VACCINE (DIPHTHERIA CRM$_{197}$ PROTEIN) — INJECTION

Overdosage

➤*Symptoms:* There have been reports of overdose with pneumococcal 7-valent conjugate vaccine, including cases of administration of a higher than recommended dose and cases of subsequent doses administered closer than recommended to the previous dose. Most individuals were asymptomatic. In general, adverse events reported with overdose have also been reported with recommended single doses of pneumococcal 7-valent conjugate vaccine.

Patient Information

Prior to administration of this vaccine, inform the parent, guardian, or other responsible adult of the potential benefits and risks to the patient (see Adverse Reactions and Warnings) and the importance of completing the immunization series unless contraindicated. Instruct parents or guardians to report any suspected adverse reactions to their health care professional. Provide vaccine information prior to each vaccination.

TYPHOID VACCINE

Rx	**Vivotif Berna** (Berna)	**Capsules, enteric-coated:** 2 to 6 × 10^9 colony-forming units of viable *Salmonella typhi* Ty21a and 5 to 50 × 10^9 bacterial cells of nonviable *S. typhi* Ty21a[a]	Salmon/White. In blister pack 4s.
Rx	**Typhim Vi** (Aventis Pasteur)	**Injection:** 25 mcg purified Vi capsular polysaccharide/0.5 mL[b]	In 0.5 mL syringes and 20 and 50 dose vials.

[a] With 26 to 130 mg sucrose, 1 to 5 mg ascorbic acid, 1.4 to 7 mg amino acid mixture, 100 to 180 mg lactose, and 3.6 to 4.4 mg magnesium stearate.

[b] With 4.15 mg NaCl, 0.065 mg disodium phosphate, 0.023 mg monosodium phosphate, 0.5 mL sterile water for injection.

TYPHOID VACCINE

For complete and comparative prescribing information, refer to the Agents for Active Immunization introduction.

Indications

➤*Oral:* For immunization of adults and children over 6 years of age against disease caused by *Salmonella typhi*. Complete the vaccine regimen at least 1 week before potential exposure to typhoid bacteria.

➤*Parenteral:* For active immunity against typhoid fever for people 2 years of age. Complete the vaccine regimen at least 2 weeks before potential exposure to typhoid bacteria.

Routine immunization against typhoid fever is not recommended in the United States. Selective immunization against typhoid fever is recommended under the following circumstances: 1) Expected intimate exposure to a household contact with typhoid fever or a known carrier; 2) travelers to typhoid-endemic areas (especially Africa, Asia, and South and Central America), especially if prolonged exposure to potentially contaminated food and water is likely, and travelers to areas of the world with a risk of exposure to typhoid fever; and 3) workers in microbiology laboratories with expected frequent contact with *S. typhi*.

➤*Unlabeled uses:* Parenteral typhoid vaccine may offer some cross-protection against *Salmonella paratyphi* A. These bacteria share a common O antigen factor 12 with *S. typhi*.

Administration and Dosage

➤*Oral:*

Primary immunization – One capsule on alternate days (eg, days 1, 3, 5, and 7) swallowed whole about 1 hour before a meal with cold or lukewarm drink, not to exceed body temperature (37°C; 98.6°F). The vaccine capsule should not be chewed; swallow as soon as possible after placing in the mouth. A complete immunization schedule is the ingestion of 4 vaccine capsules as described above. Immunization (ingestion of all 4 doses should be completed at least 1 week prior to potential exposure to *S. typhi*). Unless a complete immunization schedule is followed, an optimum immune response may not be achieved. Not all recipients will be fully protected against typhoid fever. Travelers should take all necessary precautions to avoid contact or ingestion of potentially contaminated food or water.

Booster dose – The optimum booster schedule has not been determined. Efficacy persists for at least 5 years. Further, there is no experience with oral typhoid vaccine as a booster in people previously immunized with parenteral typhoid vaccine. It is recommended that a booster dose consisting of 4 vaccine capsules taken on alternate days be given every 5 years under conditions of repeated or continued exposure to typhoid fever.

➤*Parenteral:*

Primary immunization – For IM use only. Do not inject IV. Indicated only for individuals 2 years of age or older. Give a single 0.5 mL (25 mcg) IM dose. Inject adults in the deltoid muscle. Inject children in the deltoid or vastus lateralis. Do not inject in the gluteal area or where there may be a nerve trunk. There are no published data on safety and efficacy with administration by jet injector.

Booster doses – Give a single 0.5 mL (25 mcg) dose every 2 years under conditions of repeated or continued exposure. Booster doses do not elicit higher antibody levels than primary immunization with the polysaccharide antigen.

➤*Storage/Stability:*

Oral – The oral vaccine is not stable when exposed to ambient temperatures. Ship and store between 2° and 8°C (36° to 46°F). If frozen, thaw capsules before use. Product can tolerate 48 hours at 25°C (77°F). Each package of vaccine has an expiration date. This expiration date is valid only if the product has been maintained at these temperatures.

Parenteral – Store at 2° to 8°C (36° to 46°F). Discard frozen vaccine.

Actions

➤*Pharmacology:* Upon ingestion, virulent strains of *S. typhi* are able to pass through the stomach acid barrier, colonize the intestinal tract, penetrate the lumen, and enter the lymphatic system and blood stream, thereby causing disease.

The ability of *S. typhi* to cause disease and to induce a protective immune response is dependent upon the bacteria possessing a complete lipopolysaccharide. The *S. typhi* Ty21a vaccine strain is restricted in its ability to produce a complete lipopolysaccharide. However, a sufficient quantity of complete lipopolysaccharide is synthesized to evoke a protective immune response.

➤*Pharmacokinetics:*

Onset –

Oral: Finish the fourth capsule at least 1 week before travel.

Parenteral: Protective antibody titers develop within 2 weeks after a single dose.

Duration –

Oral: Approximately 5 years.

Parenteral: Approximately 2 years.

Contraindications

Typhoid fever or a chronic typhoid carrier.

➤*Oral:* Hypersensitivity to any component of the vaccine or the capsule. Do not administer the capsules during acute febrile illness or during an acute GI illness (eg, persistent diarrhea or vomiting).

Safety of the vaccine has not been demonstrated in people deficient in their ability to mount a humoral or cell-mediated immune response because of a congenital or acquired immunodeficient state, including treatment with immunosuppressive or antimitotic drugs. Do not administer the vaccine to these people regardless of benefit.

➤*Parenteral:* Hypersensitivity to any component of the vaccine. Defer administration in the presence of acute respiratory or other active infection, or intensive physical activity (particularly when environmental temperatures are high).

Warnings

➤*Immunodeficiency:* If administered to immunosuppressed people or those receiving immunosuppressive therapy, the expected immune response may not be obtained. This includes patients with asymptomatic or symptomatic HIV infection, severe combined immunodeficiency, hypogammaglobulinemia, or agammaglobulinemia, altered immune states because of diseases such as leukemia, lymphoma, or generalized malignancy; or an immune system compromised by treatment with corticosteroids, alkylating drugs, antimetabolites, or radiation.

➤*Hypersensitivity reactions:* Allergic reactions have been reported rarely in postmarketing experience. Epinephrine injection (1:1000) must be immediately available following immunization should anaphylactic or other allergic reactions occur because of any component of the vaccine.

➤*Pregnancy: Category C.* It is not known whether typhoid vaccine can cause fetal harm when administered to pregnant women or can affect reproduction capacity. Give to a pregnant woman only if clearly needed.

➤*Lactation:* There are no data to warrant the use of the product in nursing mothers. It is not known if the vaccine is excreted in breast milk.

➤*Children:*

Oral – Safety and efficacy have not been established for the oral vaccine in children under 6 years of age and is, therefore, not recommended for use in this age group.

Parenteral – Vaccine is not recommended for children under 2 years of age because no safety or efficacy data are available for that age group.

Precautions

➤*Protection:* Not all recipients of typhoid vaccine will be fully protected against typhoid fever. Travelers should take all necessary precautions to avoid contact with or ingestion of potentially contaminated food or water sources.

➤*Latex sensitivity:* The parenteral form of this product contains dry natural latex rubber as follows: The stopper to the vial contains no rubber of any kind. In the case of the syringe, the needle cover contains dry natural latex rubber, but the plunger for the syringe contains no rubber of any kind.

TYPHOID VACCINE

➤*Infection:* Acute infection or febrile illness may be reason for delaying use of typhoid vaccine except when in the opinion of the physician, withholding the vaccine entails a greater risk.

Drug Interactions

Typhoid Vaccine Drug Interactions			
Precipitant drug	Object drug*		Description
Immunosuppressants	Typhoid vaccine	⬇	Administration of typhoid vaccine to people receiving immunosuppressant drugs, including high-dose corticosteroids or radiation therapy may result in an insufficient response to immunization. They may remain susceptible despite immunization.
Proguanil	Typhoid vaccine (oral)	⬇	Coadministration may decrease the immune response rate. Administer proguanil only if at least 10 days have elapsed since the final dose of the oral typhoid vaccine.
Sulfonamides Antibiotics	Typhoid vaccine (oral)	⬇	Do not administer the vaccine to individuals receiving sulfonamides and antibiotics because these agents may be active against the vaccine strain and prevent a sufficient degree of multiplication to occur in order to induce a protective immune response.

* ⬇ = Object drug decreased.

Adverse Reactions

➤*Oral:* Reported adverse reactions include the following: Nausea (5.8%), abdominal pain (6.4%), headache (4.8%), fever (3.3%), diarrhea (2.9%), vomiting (1.5%), skin rash (1%), abdominal cramps, or urticaria on the trunk or extremities. One case of nonfatal anaphylactic shock, considered to be an allergic reaction, has been reported. Only the incidence of nausea occurred at a statistically higher frequency in the vaccinated group compared with placebo.

➤*Parenteral:*

Typhoid Vaccine Adverse Reactions Occurring within 48 Hours in Adults (%)			
Adverse reaction	Trial 1 Placebo (N = 54)	Trial 1 Typhoid vaccine (parenteral) (1 lot) (N = 54)	Trial 2 Typhoid vaccine (parenteral) (2 lots combined) (N = 98)
Local			
Tenderness	13	98	96.9
Pain	7.4	40.7	26.5
Induration	0	14.8	5.1
Erythema	0	3.7	5.1
Systemic			
Malaise	14.8	24	4.1
Headache	13	20.4	16.3
Diarrhea	3.7	0	3.1
Nausea	3.7	1.9	8.2
Fever ≥ 100°F	0	1.9	0
Feverish (subjective)	0	11.1	3.1
Myalgia	0	7.4	3.1
Vomiting	0	1.9	0

Patient Information

Advise vaccine recipients to take standard food and water precautions to avoid typhoid fever. Vaccine protection can be overwhelmed by swallowing a large dose of typhoid bacteria.

➤*Oral:* It is essential that all 4 doses of vaccine be taken at the prescribed alternate day interval to obtain a maximal protective immune response.

Vaccine potency is dependent upon storage under refrigeration (2° to 8°C; 36° to 46°F). Store the vaccine under refrigeration at all times. It is essential to replace unused vaccine in the refrigerator between doses.

Swallow the vaccine capsule about 1 hour before a meal with a cold or lukewarm drink, not to exceed body temperature (37°C; 98.6°F). Do not chew the vaccine capsule; swallow as soon as possible.

MEASLES VIRUS VACCINE, LIVE, ATTENUATED

Rx	**Attenuvax** (Merck)	**Powder for injection, lyophilized:** ≥ 1000 $TCID_{50}$ (tissue culture infectious doses) per 0.5 ml dose	Preservative free. With ≈ 25 mcg neomycin, 14.5 mg sorbitol, 1.9 mg sucrose, 14.5 mg hydrolyzed gelatin, 0.3 mg human albumin, < 1 ppm fetal bovine serum per dose. In single-dose vials with diluent and 50-dose vials with 30 ml diluent.

MEASLES VIRUS VACCINE LIVE — INJECTION

For information on recommended immunization schedules, refer to the Agents for Active Immunization introduction.

Indications

➤*Measles vaccination:* For vaccination against measles in persons 12 months of age or older.

Individuals first vaccinated with the measles virus vaccine at 12 months of age or older should be revaccinated with measles, mumps, and rubella virus vaccine live prior to elementary school entry. Revaccination may seroconvert primary failures or boost antibody titers of those individuals whose titers have declined. The Advisory Committee on Immunization Practices (ACIP) recommends administration of the first dose of measles, mumps, and rubella virus vaccine live at 12 to 15 months of age and administration of the second dose of measles, mumps, and rubella virus vaccine live at 4 to 6 years of age. In addition, some public health jurisdictions mandate the age for revaccination. Consult the complete text of applicable guidelines regarding routine revaccination including that of high-risk adult populations.

➤*Measles outbreak schedule:*

Infants between 6 to 12 months of age – Local health authorities may recommend measles vaccination of infants between 6 to 12 months of age in outbreak situations. This population may fail to respond to the measles component of the vaccine. The younger the infant, the lower the likelihood of seroconversion. Such infants should receive a second dose of measles, mumps, and rubella virus vaccine live between 12 to 15 months of age followed by revaccination prior to elementary school entry.

➤*Other vaccination considerations:*

Other populations – Individuals planning travel outside the United States, if not immune, can acquire measles, mumps or rubella and import these diseases into the US. Therefore, prior to international travel, individuals known to be susceptible to one or more of these diseases can receive either a monovalent vaccine (measles, mumps or rubella), or a combination vaccine as appropriate. However, measles, mumps, and rubella virus vaccine live is preferred for persons likely to be susceptible to mumps and rubella; and if monovalent measles vaccine is not readily available, travelers should receive measles, mumps, and rubella virus vaccine live regardless of their immune status to mumps or rubella.

Vaccination is recommended for susceptible individuals in high-risk groups such as college students, healthcare workers, and military personnel.

According to ACIP recommendations, most persons born in 1956 or earlier are likely to have been infected with measles naturally and generally need not be considered susceptible. All children, adolescents, and adults born after 1956 are considered susceptible and should be vaccinated, if there are no contraindications. This includes persons who may be immune to measles but who lack adequate documentation of immunity such as:

1.) Physician-diagnosed measles.
2.) Laboratory evidence of measles immunity.
3.) Adequate immunization with live measles vaccine on or after the first birthday.

The ACIP recommends that "Persons vaccinated with inactivated vaccine followed within 3 months by live vaccine should be revaccinated with 2 doses of live vaccine. Revaccination is particularly important when the risk of exposure to natural measles virus is increased, as may occur during international travel."

Postexposure vaccination – The measles virus vaccine given immediately after exposure to natural measles may provide some protection if the vaccine can be administered within 72 hours of exposure. If, however, the vaccine is given a few days before exposure, substantial protection may be provided.

Use with other vaccines – See Administration and Dosage for more information.

Administration and Dosage

➤*Recommended dosage:* Do not inject by IV. The dose for any age is 0.5 mL administered SC, preferably into the outer aspect of the upper arm.

See Indications for more information.

➤*Immune globulin:* Immune Globulin (IG) is not to be given concurrently with the measles virus vaccine.

➤*Syringe selection:* A sterile syringe free of preservatives, antiseptics, and detergents should be used for each injection or reconstitution of the vaccine because these substances may inactivate the live virus vaccine. A 25 gauge, ⅝ inch needle is recommended.

➤*Reconstitution:* To reconstitute, use only the diluent supplied, since it is free of preservatives or other antiviral substances which might inactivate the vaccine.

MEASLES VIRUS VACCINE LIVE — INJECTION

➤*Single-dose vial:* First withdraw the entire volume of diluent into the syringe to be used for reconstitution. Inject all the diluent in the syringe into the vial of lyophilized vaccine, and agitate to mix thoroughly. If the lyophilized vaccine cannot be dissolved, discard. Withdraw the entire contents into a syringe and inject the total volume of restored vaccine SC.

➤*50-dose vial (available only to government agencies/institutions):* Withdraw the entire contents (30 mL) of diluent vial into the sterile syringe to be used for reconstitution and introduce into the 50-dose vial of lyophilized vaccine. Agitate to ensure thorough mixing. If the lyophilized vaccine cannot be dissolved, discard. With full aseptic precautions, attach the vial to the sterilized multidose jet injector apparatus. Use 0.5 mL of the reconstituted vaccine for SC injection.

➤*Use with other vaccines:* The measles virus vaccine should not be given less than 1 month before or after administration of other live viral vaccines.

Routine administration of DTP (diphtheria, tetanus, pertussis) or OPV (oral poliovirus vaccine) concurrently with measles, mumps and rubella vaccines is not recommended because there are limited data relating to the simultaneous administration of these antigens.

However, other schedules have been used. The ACIP has stated, "Although data are limited concerning the simultaneous administration of the entire recommended vaccine series (ie, DTP, OPV, MMR, and Hib vaccines, with or without hepatitis B vaccine), data from numerous studies have indicated no interference between routinely recommended childhood vaccines (either live, attenuated, or killed). These findings support the simultaneous use of all vaccines as recommended."

➤*Storage/Stability:* During shipment, to ensure that there is no loss of potency, the vaccine must be maintained at a temperature of 10°C (50°F) or colder. Freezing during shipment will not affect potency.

Protect the vaccine from light at all times, since such exposure may inactivate the virus.

Before reconstitution, store the vial of lyophilized vaccine at 2° to 8°C (36° to 46°F) or colder. The diluent may be stored in the refrigerator with the lyophilized vaccine or separately at room temperature.

It is recommended that the vaccine be used as soon as possible after reconstitution. Store reconstituted vaccine in the vaccine vial in a dark place at 2° to 8°C (36° to 46°F) and discard if not used within 8 hours.

Actions

➤*Pharmacology:* Measles is a common childhood disease, caused by measles virus (paramyxovirus), that may be associated with serious complications or death. For example, pneumonia and encephalitis are caused by measles.

Contraindications

➤*Hypersensitivity:* Hypersensitivity to any component of the vaccine, including gelatin.

Anaphylactic or anaphylactoid reactions to neomycin (each dose of reconstituted vaccine contains approximately 25 mcg of neomycin).

➤*Pregnancy:* Do not give measles vaccine to pregnant females; the possible effects of the vaccine on fetal development are unknown at this time. If vaccination of postpubertal females is undertaken, pregnancy should be avoided for 3 months following vaccination (see Warnings, Pregnancy).

➤*Febrile respiratory illness or other active febrile infection:* Febrile respiratory illness or other active febrile infection. However, the ACIP has recommended that all vaccines can be administered to persons with minor illnesses such as diarrhea, mild upper respiratory infection with or without low-grade fever, or other low-grade febrile illness.

➤*Hematology issues:* Individuals with blood dyscrasias, leukemia, lymphomas of any type, or other malignant neoplasms affecting the bone marrow or lymphatic systems.

➤*Immunosuppressive or immunodeficiency states:* Patients receiving immunosuppressive therapy. This contraindication does not apply to patients who are receiving corticosteroids as replacement therapy, eg, for Addison's disease.

Primary and acquired immunodeficiency states, including patients who are immunosuppressed in association with AIDS or other clinical manifestations of infection with human immunodeficiency viruses; cellular immune deficiencies; and hypogammaglobulinemic and dysgammaglobulinemic states. Measles inclusion body encephalitis (MIBE), pneumonitis and death as a direct consequence of disseminated measles vaccine virus infection has been reported in immunocompromised individuals inadvertently vaccinated with measles-containing vaccine.

Individuals with a family history of congenital or hereditary immunodeficiency, until the immune competence of the potential vaccine recipient is demonstrated.

Warnings

➤*Thrombocytopenia:* Individuals with current thrombocytopenia may develop more severe thrombocytopenia following vaccination. In addition, individuals who experienced thrombocytopenia with the first dose of measles, mumps, and rubella virus vaccine live (or its component vaccines) may develop thrombocytopenia with repeat doses. Serologic status may be evaluated to determine whether or not additional doses of vaccine are needed. The potential risk to benefit ratio should be carefully evaluated before considering vaccination in such cases (see Adverse Reactions).

➤*Hypersensitivity reactions:* Adequate treatment provisions including epinephrine injection (1:1000), should be available for immediate use should an anaphylactic or anaphylactoid reaction occur.

Special care should be taken to ensure that the injection does not enter a blood vessel.

Eggs – The live measles vaccine is produced in chick embryo cell culture. Persons with a history of anaphylactic, anaphylactoid or other immediate reactions (eg, hives, swelling of the mouth and throat, difficulty breathing, hypotension and shock) subsequent to egg ingestion may be at an enhanced risk of immediate-type hypersensitivity reactions after receiving vaccines containing traces of chick embryo antigen. The potential risk to benefit ratio should be carefully evaluated before considering vaccination in such cases. Such individuals may be vaccinated with extreme caution, having adequate treatment on hand should a reaction occur (see Warnings).

However, the AAP has stated, "Most children with a history of anaphylactic reactions to eggs have no untoward reactions to measles or MMR vaccine. Persons are not at increased risk if they have egg allergies that are not anaphylactic, and they should be vaccinated in the usual manner. In addition, skin testing of egg-allergic children with vaccine has not been predictive of which children will have an immediate hypersensitivity reaction...Persons with allergies to chickens or chicken feathers are not at increased risk of reaction to the vaccine."

Neomycin – The AAP states, "Persons who have experienced anaphylactic reactions to topically or systemically administered neomycin should not receive measles vaccine. Most often, however, neomycin allergy manifests as a contact dermatitis, which is a delayed-type (cell-mediated) immune response rather than anaphylaxis. In such persons, an adverse reaction to neomycin in the vaccine would be an erythematous, pruritic nodule or papule, 48 to 96 hours after vaccination. A history of contact dermatitis to neomycin is not a contraindication to receiving measles vaccine."

➤*Pregnancy: Category C.* Animal reproduction studies have not been conducted with the measles virus vaccine. It is also not known whether the measles virus vaccine can cause fetal harm when administered to a pregnant woman or can affect reproduction capacity. Therefore, the vaccine should not be administered to pregnant females; furthermore, pregnancy should be avoided for 3 months following vaccination (see Contraindications).

In counseling women who are inadvertently vaccinated when pregnant or who become pregnant within 3 months of vaccination, the physician should be aware that reports have indicated that contracting natural measles during pregnancy enhances fetal risk. Increased rates of spontaneous abortion, stillbirth, congenital defects and prematurity have been observed subsequent to natural measles during pregnancy. There are no adequate studies of the attenuated (vaccine) strain of measles virus in pregnancy. However, it would be prudent to assume that the vaccine strain of virus is also capable of inducing adverse fetal effects.

➤*Lactation:* It is not known whether the measles vaccine virus is secreted in human milk. Therefore, because many drugs are excreted in human milk, caution should be exercised when the measles virus vaccine is administered to a nursing woman.

➤*Children:* Safety and effectiveness in infants younger than 6 months of age have not been established.

Children with HIV – Children and young adults who are known to be infected with HIV and are not immunosuppressed may be vaccinated. However, vaccinees who are infected with HIV should be monitored closely for vaccine-preventable diseases because immunization may be less effective than for uninfected persons (see Contraindications).

Vaccination should be deferred for 3 months or longer following blood or plasma transfusions, or administration of immune globulin (human).

Children under treatment for tuberculosis – Children under treatment for tuberculosis (TB) have not experienced exacerbation of the disease when immunized with live measles virus vaccine; no studies have been reported to date of the effect of measles virus vaccines on untreated TB children. However, individuals with active untreated TB should not be vaccinated.

Precautions

➤*Special risk:*

Cerebral injury/convulsions – Due caution should be employed in administration of the measles virus vaccine to persons with a history of cerebral injury, individual or family histories of convulsions, or any other condition in which stress due to fever should be avoided. The physician should be alert to the temperature elevation which may occur following vaccination (see Adverse Reactions).

Drug Interactions

Measles Virus Vaccine Drug Interactions

Precipitant drug	Object drug*		Description
Immunosuppressants	Measles vaccine	⬇	Administration of measles vaccine to patients receiving immunosuppressants, including corticosteroids or radiation therapy, may result in insufficient response to immunization. They may remain susceptible despite immunization.

MEASLES VIRUS VACCINE LIVE — INJECTION

Measles Virus Vaccine Drug Interactions

Precipitant drug	Object drug*		Description
Immune globulins	Measles vaccine	⬇	To avoid inactivation of the attenuated virus, administer the vaccine at least 14 to 30 days before or 6 to 8 weeks after the immune globulin. Alternately, check antibody titers or repeat the vaccine dose 3 months after immune globulin administration. Base the interval on the dose of IgG administered: 3 months for 3 to 10 mg/kg, 4 months for 20 mg/kg, 5 months for 40 mg/kg, 6 months for 60 to 100 mg/kg, 7 months for 160 mg/kg, 8 months for 300 to 400 mg/kg, 10 months for 1 g/kg, 11 months for 2 g/kg.
Interferon	Measles vaccine	⬇	Concurrent use may inhibit antibody response to the vaccine.
Vitamin A	Measles vaccine	⬇	Simultaneous administration of large doses of vitamin A impaired the response to Schwarz-strain measles vaccine in a group of Indonesian infants at 6 months of age.
Measles vaccine	Meningococcal vaccine	⬇	Reduced seroconversion rate to meningococci may occur with concurrent immunization. If possible, separate these 2 vaccinations by ≥ 1 month.
Measles vaccine	Tuberculin skin test	⬇	Measles vaccine may temporarily depress tuberculin skin sensitivity. Administer the test before or simultaneously with the vaccine.
Measles vaccine	Virus vaccines, other	⬇	To avoid the hypothetical concern over antigenic competition, give measles vaccine ≥ 1 month before or after other virus vaccines. However, several vaccines may be given simultaneously at separate injection sites (eg, DTP, OPV or e-IPV, MMR, Hib, hepatitis B, varicella, influenza).

* ⬇ = Object drug decreased.

➤*Drug/Lab test interactions:* It has been reported that attenuated measles virus vaccine live may result in a temporary depression of TB skin sensitivity. Therefore, if a tuberculin test is to be done, it should be administered either before or simultaneously with the measles virus vaccine.

Adverse Reactions

The following adverse reactions are listed in decreasing order of severity, without regard to causality, within each body system category and have been reported during clinical trials, with use of the marketed vaccine, or with use of polyvalent vaccine containing measles:

➤*Cardiovascular:* Vasculitis.

➤*CNS:* Encephalitis; encephalopathy; measles inclusion body encephalitis (MIBE) (see Contraindications); subacute sclerosing panencephalitis (SSPE); Guillain-Barré syndrome (GBS); febrile convulsions; afebrile convulsions or seizures; ataxia; ocular palsies.

There have been reports of subacute sclerosing panencephalitis (SSPE) in children who did not have a history of natural measles but did receive measles vaccine. Some of these cases may have resulted from unrecognized measles in the first year of life or possibly from the measles vaccination. Based on estimated nationwide measles vaccine distribution, the association of SSPE cases to measles vaccination is about one case per million vaccine doses distributed. This is far less than the association with natural measles, 6 to 22 cases of SSPE per million cases of measles. The results of a retrospective case-controlled study conducted by the Centers for Disease Control and Prevention suggest that the overall effect of measles vaccine has been to protect against SSPE by preventing measles with its inherent higher risk of SSPE.

➤*Dermatologic:* Stevens-Johnson syndrome; erythema multiforme; urticaria; rash.

➤*GI:* Diarrhea.

➤*Hematologic/Lymphatic:* Thrombocytopenia (see Warnings, Thrombocytopenia); purpura; lymphadenopathy; leukocytosis.

➤*Hypersensitivity:* Anaphylaxis and anaphylactoid reactions have been reported as well as related phenomena such as angioneurotic edema (including peripheral or facial edema) and bronchial spasm.

➤*Local:* Burning/stinging at injection site; wheal and flare; redness (erythema); swelling; vesiculation at injection site.

➤*Ophthalmic:* Retinitis; optic neuritis; papillitis; retrobulbar neuritis; conjunctivitis.

➤*Respiratory:* Pneumonitis (see Contraindications); cough; rhinitis.

➤*Special senses:*

Ear – Nerve deafness; otitis media.

➤*Miscellaneous:* Panniculitis; atypical measles; fever; syncope; headache; dizziness; malaise; irritability.

Patient Information

The health care provider should provide the vaccine information required to be given with each vaccination to the patient, parent or guardian.

The health care provider should inform the patient, parent or guardian of the benefits and risks associated with vaccination. For risks associated with vaccination, see Warnings, Precautions, and Adverse Reactions.

➤*Adverse reactions:* Patients, parents or guardians should be instructed to report any serious adverse reactions to their health care provider who in turn should report such events to the US Department of Health and Human Services through the Vaccine Adverse Event Reporting System (VAERS), 1-800-822-7967.

Pregnancy – See Contraindications for more information.

Immunosuppressive therapy – The immune status of patients about to undergo immunosuppressive therapy should be evaluated so that the physician can consider whether vaccination prior to the initiation of treatment is indicated (see Contraindications and Precautions).

The ACIP has stated that "Patients with leukemia in remission who have not received chemotherapy for at least 3 months may receive live-virus vaccines. Short-term (less than 2 weeks), low- to moderate-dose systemic corticosteroid therapy, topical steroid therapy (eg, nasal, skin), long-term alternate-day treatment with low to moderate doses of short-acting systemic steroid, and intra-articular, bursal, or tendon injection of corticosteroids are not immunosuppressive in their usual doses and do not contraindicate the administration of measles vaccine."

Immune globulin – Administration of immune globulins concurrently with the measles virus vaccine may interfere with the expected immune response.

RUBELLA VIRUS VACCINE, LIVE

Rx	**Meruvax** II (Merck)	**Powder for Injection:** ≥ 1000 $TCID_{50}$ (tissue culture infectious doses) of rubella per 0.5 ml dose.	With 25 mcg neomycin. In single dose vials.

RUBELLA VIRUS VACCINE LIVE — INJECTION

For information on recommended immunization schedules, refer to the Agents for Active Immunization introduction.

Indications

➤*Rubella vaccination:* For vaccination against rubella in persons 12 months of age or older.

It is not recommended for infants younger than 12 months of age because they may retain maternal rubella neutralizing antibodies that may interfere with the immune response.

Children in kindergarten and the first grades of elementary school deserve priority for vaccination because often they are epidemiologically the major source of virus dissemination in the community. A history of rubella illness is usually not reliable enough to exclude children from immunization.

Previously unimmunized children of susceptible pregnant women should receive live attenuated rubella vaccine, because an immunized child will be less likely to acquire natural rubella and introduce the virus into the household.

Individuals first vaccinated with rubella virus live at 12 months of age or older should be revaccinated with measles, mumps, and rubella virus vaccine live prior to elementary school entry. Revaccination may seroconvert primary failures or boost antibody titers of those individuals whose titers have declined. The Advisory Committee on Immunization Practices (ACIP) recommends administration of the first dose of measles, mumps, and rubella virus vaccine live at 12 to 15 months of age and administration of the second dose of measles, mumps, and rubella virus vaccine live at 4 to 6 years of age. In addition, some public health jurisdictions mandate the age for revaccination. Consult the complete text of applicable guidelines regarding routine revaccination including that of high-risk adult populations.

Unnecessary doses of a vaccine are best avoided by ensuring that written documentation of vaccination is preserved and a copy given to each vaccinee's parent or guardian.

➤*Other vaccination considerations:*

Adolescent and adult males – Vaccination of adolescent or adult males may be a useful procedure in preventing or controlling outbreaks of rubella in circumscribed population groups (eg, military bases and schools).

Non-pregnant adolescent and adult females – Immunization of susceptible non-pregnant adolescent and adult females of childbearing age with live attenuated rubella virus vaccine is indicated if certain precautions are

RUBELLA VIRUS VACCINE LIVE — INJECTION

observed (see below and Precautions). Vaccinating susceptible postpubertal females confers individual protection against subsequently acquiring rubella infection during pregnancy, which in turn prevents infection of the fetus and consequent congenital rubella injury.

Women of childbearing age should be advised not to become pregnant for 3 months after vaccination and should be informed of the reason for this precaution. The ACIP has recommended "In view of the importance of protecting this age group against rubella, reasonable practices in a rubella immunization program include asking women if they are pregnant, excluding those who say they are, explaining the concern about risk for the fetus to the others, and explaining the importance of not becoming pregnant during the 3 months following vaccination."

The ACIP has stated "If it is practical and if reliable laboratory services are available, women of childbearing age who are potential candidates for vaccination can have serologic tests to determine susceptibility to rubella. However, with the exception of premarital and prenatal screening, routinely performing serologic tests for all women of childbearing age to determine susceptibility (so that vaccine is given only to proven susceptible women) can be effective but is expensive. Also, 2 visits to the healthcare provider would be necessary one for screening and one for vaccination. Accordingly, rubella vaccination of a woman who is not known to be pregnant and has no history of vaccination is justifiable without serologic testing—and may be preferable, particularly when costs of serology are high and follow-up of identified susceptible women for vaccination is not assured."

Postpubertal females should be informed of the frequent occurrence of generally self-limited arthralgia or arthritis beginning 2 to 4 weeks after vaccination (see Adverse Reactions).

➤*Other populations:* Previously unvaccinated children in contact with susceptible pregnant women should receive live attenuated rubella vaccine (such as that contained in rubella virus live) to reduce the risk of exposure of the pregnant woman.

Individuals planning travel outside the United States, if not immune, can acquire measles, mumps or rubella and import these diseases into the United States. Therefore, prior to international travel, individuals known to be susceptible to one or more of these diseases can receive either a monovalent vaccine (measles, mumps or rubella), or a combination vaccine as appropriate. However, measles, mumps, and rubella virus vaccine live is preferred for persons likely to be susceptible to mumps and rubella; and if monovalent measles vaccine is not readily available, travelers should receive measles, mumps, and rubella virus vaccine live regardless or their immune status to mumps or rubella.

Vaccination is recommended for susceptible individuals in high-risk groups such as college students, healthcare workers, and military personnel.

➤*Postpartum women:* It has been found convenient in many instances to vaccinate rubella-susceptible women in the immediate postpartum period (see Warnings, Lactation).

➤*Postexposure vaccination:* There is no conclusive evidence that vaccination of individuals recently exposed to natural rubella will provide protection. There is, however, no contraindication to vaccinating children already exposed to natural rubella.

➤*Use with other vaccines:* See Administration and Dosage for more information.

➤*Unlabeled uses:* Intranasal administration may boost antibody titers, although this route is not confirmed as safe and effective by the FDA and is not commonly employed.

Administration and Dosage

➤*Recommended dosage:* Do not inject by IV.

The dose for any age is 0.5 mL administered SC, preferably into the outer aspect of the upper arm.

See Indications for more information.

Immune globulin – Immune Globulin (IG) is not to be given concurrently with rubella virus live .

➤*Syringe selection:* A sterile syringe free of preservatives, antiseptics, and detergents should be used for each injection or reconstitution of the vaccine because these substances may inactivate the live virus vaccine. A 25 gauge, ⅝ inch needle is recommended.

To reconstitute, use only the diluent supplied, since it is free of preservatives or other antiviral substances which might inactivate the vaccine.

➤*Single-dose vial:* First withdraw the entire volume of diluent into the syringe to be used for reconstitution. Inject all the diluent in the syringe into the vial of lyophilized vaccine, and agitate to mix thoroughly. If the lyophilized vaccine cannot be dissolved, discard. Withdraw the entire contents into a syringe and inject the total volume of restored vaccine SC.

➤*Use with other vaccines:* Rubella virus live should not be given less than 1 month before or after administration of other live viral vaccines.

Measles, mumps, and rubella virus vaccine live has been administered concurrently with varicella virus vaccine live, and *Haemophilus b* conjugate vaccine (meningococcal protein conjugate) using separate sites and syringes. No impairment of immune response to individual tested vaccine antigens was demonstrated. The type, frequency, and severity of adverse experiences observed in these studies with measles, mumps, and rubella virus vaccine live were similar to those seen when each vaccine was given alone.

Routine administration of DTP (diphtheria, tetanus, pertussis) or OPV (oral poliovirus vaccine) concurrently with measles, mumps and rubella vaccines is not recommended because there are limited data relating to the simultaneous administration of these antigens.

However, other schedules have been used. The ACIP has stated "Although data are limited concerning the simultaneous administration of the entire recommended vaccine series (ie, DTP, OPV, MMR, and Hib vaccines, with or without hepatitis B vaccine), data from numerous studies have indicated no interference between routinely recommended childhood vaccines (either live, attenuated, or killed). These findings support the simultaneous use of all vaccines as recommended."

➤*Storage / Stability:* During shipment, to ensure that there is no loss of potency, the vaccine must be maintained at a temperature of 10°C (50°F) or colder. Freezing during shipment will not affect potency.

Protect the vaccine from light at all times, since such exposure may inactivate the virus.

Before reconstitution, store the vial of lyophilized vaccine at 2° to 8°C (36° to 46°F) or colder. The diluent may be stored in the refrigerator with the lyophilized vaccine or separately at room temperature.

It is recommended that the vaccine be used as soon as possible after reconstitution. Store reconstituted vaccine in the vaccine vial in a dark place at 2° to 8°C (36° to 46°F) and discard if not used within 8 hours.

Actions

➤*Pharmacology:* Rubella is a common childhood disease, caused by rubella virus (togavirus), that may be associated with serious complications or death. For example, rubella during pregnancy may cause congenital rubella syndrome in the infants of infected mothers.

Extensive clinical trials of rubella virus vaccines, prepared using RA 27/3 strain rubella virus, have been carried out in more than 28,000 human subjects (≈ 11,000 with rubella virus live) in the USA and more than 20 additional countries. A single injection of the vaccine has been shown to induce rubella hemagglutination-inhibition (HI) antibodies in 97% or more of susceptible persons. However, a small percentage (1% to 5%) of vaccinees may fail to seroconvert after the primary dose (see also Indications, Recommended vaccination schedule).

Efficacy of rubella vaccine was established in a series of double-blind controlled field trials which demonstrated a high degree of protective efficacy. These studies also established that seroconversion in response to rubella vaccination paralleled protection from this disease.

Following vaccination, antibodies associated with protection can be measured by neutralization assays, hemagglutination-inhibition, or ELISA (enzyme linked immunosorbent assay) tests. Neutralizing and ELISA antibodies to rubella virus are still detectable in most individuals 11 to 13 years after primary vaccination. See Indications, Non-pregnant adolescents and adult females, for rubella susceptibility testing.

The RA 27/3 rubella strain elicits higher immediate post-vaccination HI, complement-fixing and neutralizing antibody levels than other strains of rubella vaccine and has been shown to induce a broader profile of circulating antibodies including anti-theta and anti-iota precipitating antibodies. The RA 27/3 rubella strain immunologically simulates natural infection more closely than other rubella vaccine viruses. The increased levels and broader profile of antibodies produced by RA 27/3 strain rubella virus vaccine appear to correlate with greater resistance to subclinical reinfection with the wild virus, and provide greater confidence for lasting immunity.

Contraindications

Hypersensitivity to any component of the vaccine, including gelatin.

Do not give rubella virus live to pregnant females; the possible effects of the vaccine on fetal development are unknown at this time. If vaccination of postpubertal females is undertaken, pregnancy should be avoided for 3 months following vaccination (see Warnings, Pregnancy).

Anaphylactic or anaphylactoid reactions to neomycin (each dose of reconstituted vaccine contains ≈ 25 mcg of neomycin).

Febrile respiratory illness or other active febrile infection. However, the ACIP has recommended that all vaccines can be administered to persons with minor illnesses such as diarrhea, mild upper respiratory infection with or without low-grade fever, or other low-grade febrile illness.

Patients receiving immunosuppressive therapy. This contraindication does not apply to patients who are receiving corticosteroids as replacement therapy, eg, for Addison's disease.

Individuals with blood dyscrasias, leukemia, lymphomas of any type, or other malignant neoplasms affecting the bone marrow or lymphatic systems.

Primary and acquired immunodeficiency states, including patients who are immunosuppressed in association with AIDS or other clinical manifestations of infection with human immunodeficiency viruses; cellular immune deficiencies; and hypogammaglobulinemic and dysgammaglobulinemic states.

Individuals with a family history of congenital or hereditary immunodeficiency, until the immune competence of the potential vaccine recipient is demonstrated.

Warnings

➤*Fever:* The physician should be alert to the temperature elevation which may occur following vaccination (see Adverse Reactions).

➤*Thrombocytopenia:* Individuals with current thrombocytopenia may develop more severe thrombocytopenia following vaccination. In addition, individuals who experienced thrombocytopenia with the first dose of measles, mumps, and rubella virus vaccine live (or its component vaccines) may develop thrombocytopenia with repeat doses. Serologic status may be evaluated to determine whether or not additional doses of vaccine are needed. The

RUBELLA VIRUS VACCINE LIVE — INJECTION

potential risk to benefit ratio should be carefully evaluated before considering vaccination in such cases (see Adverse Reactions).

➤*Hypersensitivity reactions:*

Hypersensitivity to neomycin – The AAP states, "Persons who have experienced anaphylactic reactions to topically or systemically administered neomycin should not receive measles vaccine. Most often, however, neomycin allergy manifests as a contact dermatitis, which is a delayed-type (cell-mediated) immune response rather than anaphylaxis. In such persons, an adverse reaction to neomycin in the vaccine would be an erythematous, pruritic nodule or papule, 48 to 96 hours after vaccination. A history of contact dermatitis to neomycin is not a contraindication to receiving measles vaccine."

➤*Pregnancy: Category C.* Animal reproduction studies have not been conducted with rubella virus live. It is also not known whether rubella virus live can cause fetal harm when administered to a pregnant woman or can affect reproduction capacity. There is evidence suggesting transmission of rubella vaccine viruses to products of conception. Therefore, rubella vaccine should not be administered to pregnant females (see Contraindications).

In counseling women who are inadvertently vaccinated when pregnant or who become pregnant within 3 months of vaccination, the physician should be aware of the following: In a 10-year survey involving over 700 pregnant women who received rubella vaccine within 3 months before or after conception, (of whom 189 received the Wistar RA 27/3 strain) none of the newborns had abnormalities compatible with congenital rubella syndrome.

➤*Lactation:* Recent studies have shown that lactating postpartum women immunized with live attenuated rubella vaccine may secrete the virus in breast milk and transmit it to breastfed infants. In the infants with serological evidence of rubella infection, none exhibited severe disease; however, one exhibited mild clinical illness typical of acquired rubella. Caution should be exercised when rubella virus live is administered to a nursing woman.

➤*Children:* Safety and effectiveness in infants younger than 12 months of age have not been established (see Indications, Recommended vaccination schedule).

Children and young adults who are known to be infected with HIV and are not immunosuppressed may be vaccinated. However, vaccinees who are infected with HIV should be monitored closely for vaccine-preventable diseases because immunization may be less effective than for uninfected persons (see Contraindications).

Precautions

➤*Anaphylactoid reaction:* Adequate treatment provisions including epinephrine injection (1:1000), should be available for immediate use should an anaphylactic or anaphylactoid reaction occur.

➤*Administration precaution:* Special care should be taken to ensure that the injection does not enter a blood vessel.

➤*Virus transmission:* Excretion of small amounts of the live attenuated rubella virus from the nose or throat has occurred in the majority of susceptible individuals 7 to 28 days after vaccination. There is no confirmed evidence to indicate that such virus is transmitted to susceptible persons who are in contact with the vaccinated individuals. Consequently, transmission through close personal contact, while accepted as a theoretical possibility, is not regarded as a significant risk. However, transmission of the vaccine virus to infants via breast milk has been documented (see Warnings, Lactation).

As for any vaccine, vaccination with rubella virus live may not result in protection in 100% of vaccinees.

➤*Special risk:* Vaccination should be deferred for 3 months or longer following blood or plasma transfusions, or administration of immune globulin (human). However, susceptible postpartum patients who received blood products may receive rubella virus live prior to discharge provided that a repeat HI titer is drawn 6 to 8 weeks after vaccination to ensure seroconversion. Similarly, although studies with other live rubella virus vaccines suggest that rubella virus live may be given in the immediate postpartum period to those nonimmune women who have received anti-Rho (D) globulin (human) without interfering with vaccine effectiveness, a follow-up post-vaccination HI titer should also be determined.

Tuberculosis – It has been reported that attenuated rubella virus vaccine, live, may result in a temporary depression of tuberculin skin sensitivity. Therefore, if a tuberculin test is to be done, it should be administered either before or simultaneously with rubella virus live .

Individuals with active untreated tuberculosis should not be vaccinated.

➤*Lab test abnormalities:* See Indications, Non-pregnant adolescents and adult females, for rubella susceptibility testing, and Pharmacology.

Immunosuppressive therapy – The immune status of patients about to undergo immunosuppressive therapy should be evaluated so that the physician can consider whether vaccination prior to the initiation of treatment is indicated. (see Contraindications).

The ACIP has stated that "patients with leukemia in remission who have not received chemotherapy for at least 3 months may receive live-virus vaccines. Short-term (less than 2 weeks), low- to moderate-dose systemic corticosteroid therapy, topical steroid therapy (eg, nasal, skin), long-term alternate-day treatment with low to moderate doses of short-acting systemic steroid, and intra-articular, bursal, or tendon injection of corticosteroids are not immunosuppressive in their usual doses and do not contraindicate the administration of rubella vaccine."

Immune globulin – Administration of immune globulins concurrently with rubella virus live may interfere with the expected immune response.

Drug Interactions

Rubella Virus Vaccine Drug Interactions

Precipitant drug	Object drug*		Description
Immunosuppressants	Rubella vaccine	⬇	Administration of rubella vaccine to patients receiving immunosuppressants, including corticosteroids or radiation therapy, may result in insufficient response to immunization. They may remain susceptible despite immunization.
Immune globulins	Rubella vaccine	⬇	To avoid inactivation of the attenuated virus, administer the vaccine at least 14 to 30 days before or 6 to 8 weeks after the immune globulin. Alternately, check antibody titers or repeat the vaccine dose 3 months after IgG.
Interferon	Rubella vaccine	⬇	Concurrent use may inhibit antibody response to the vaccine.
Rubella vaccine	Meningococcal vaccine	⬇	Reduced seroconversion rate to meningococci may occur with concurrent immunization.
Rubella vaccine	Virus vaccines, other	⬇	To avoid the hypothetical concern over antigenic competition, give rubella vaccine after or ≥ 1 month before other virus vaccines. However, several vaccines may be given simultaneously at separate injection sites (eg, DTP, OPV, MMR, Hib, hepatitis B).

* ⬇ = Object drug decreased.

Adverse Reactions

The following adverse reactions are listed in decreasing order of severity, without regard to causality, within each body system category and have been reported during clinical trials, with use of the marketed vaccine, or with use of polyvalent vaccine containing rubella:

➤*Cardiovascular:* Vasculitis.

➤*CNS:* Encephalitis; Guillain-Barré syndrome (GBS); polyneuritis; polyneuropathy; paresthesia.

➤*Dermatologic:* Stevens-Johnson syndrome; erythema multiforme; urticaria; rash.

➤*GI:* Diarrhea; vomiting; nausea.

➤*Hematologic/Lymphatic:* Thrombocytopenia (see Warnings, Thrombocytopenia); purpura; regional lymphadenopathy; leukocytosis.

➤*Hypersensitivity:* Anaphylaxis and anaphylactoid reactions have been reported as well as related phenomena such as angioneurotic edema (including peripheral or facial edema) and bronchial spasm.

➤*Local:* Burning/stinging at injection site; wheal and flare; redness (erythema); pain; induration.

➤*Musculoskeletal:* Arthritis; arthralgia; myalgia.

Chronic arthritis has been associated with natural rubella infection and has been related to persistent virus or viral antigen isolated from body tissues. Only rarely have vaccine recipients developed chronic joint symptoms.

Following vaccination in children, reactions in joints are uncommon and generally of brief duration. In women, incidence rates for arthritis and arthralgia are generally higher than those seen in children (children, 0% to 3%; women, 12% to 26%) and the reactions tend to be more marked and of longer duration. Symptoms may persist for a matter of months or on rare occasions for years. In adolescent girls, the reactions appear to be intermediate in incidence between those seen in children and in adult women. Even in women older than 35 years of age, these reactions are generally well tolerated and rarely interfere with normal activities. Myalgia and paresthesia have been reported rarely after administration of rubella virus live.

➤*Ophthalmic:* Optic neuritis; papillitis; retrobulbar neuritis; conjunctivitis.

➤*Respiratory:* Sore throat; cough; rhinitis.

➤*Special senses:*

Ear – Nerve deafness; otitis media.

➤*Miscellaneous:* Fever; syncope; headache; dizziness; malaise; irritability.

Patient Information

The healthcare provider should provide the vaccine information required to be given with each vaccination to the patient, parent or guardian.

The healthcare provider should inform the patient, parent or guardian of the benefits and risks associated with vaccination. For risks associated with vaccination see Warnings, Precautions, Adverse Reactions.

RUBELLA VIRUS VACCINE LIVE — INJECTION

Patients, parents or guardians should be instructed to report any serious adverse reactions to their health-care provider who in turn should report such events to the U.S. Department of Health and Human Services through the Vaccine Adverse Event Reporting System (VAERS), 1-800-822-7967.

Pregnancy should be avoided for 3 months following vaccination.

MUMPS VIRUS VACCINE, LIVE

Rx	**Mumpsvax** (Merck)	**Powder for Injection:** ≥ 20,000 $TCID_{50}$ (tissue culture infectious doses) per 0.5 ml dose.	25 mcg neomycin. In single-dose vials with vials of diluent.

MUMPS VIRUS VACCINE LIVE — INJECTION

For information on recommended immunization schedules, refer to the Agents for Active Immunization introduction.

Indications

➤*Mumps vaccination:* For vaccination against mumps in persons 12 months of age or older.

It is not recommended for infants younger than 12 months because they may retain maternal, mumps-neutralizing antibodies which may interfere with the immune response.

Individuals first vaccinated with mumps virus vaccine live at 12 months of age or older should be revaccinated with measles, mumps, and rubella virus vaccine live prior to elementary school entry. Revaccination may seroconvert primary failures or boost antibody titers of those individuals whose titers have declined. The Advisory Committee on Immunization Practices (ACIP) recommends administration of the first dose of measles, mumps, and rubella virus vaccine live at 12 to 15 months of age and administration of the second dose of measles, mumps, and rubella virus vaccine live at 4 to 6 years of age. In addition, some public health jurisdictions mandate the age for revaccination. Consult the complete text of applicable guidelines regarding routine revaccination, including that of high-risk adult populations.

Unnecessary doses of a vaccine are best avoided by ensuring that written documentation of vaccination is preserved and a copy given to each vaccinee's parent or guardian.

➤*Other vaccination considerations:*

Other populations – Individuals planning travel outside the United States, if not immune, can acquire measles, mumps or rubella and import these diseases into the United States. Therefore, prior to international travel, individuals known to be susceptible to 1 or more of these diseases can receive either a monovalent vaccine (measles, mumps or rubella), or a combination vaccine as appropriate. However, measles, mumps, and rubella virus vaccine live is preferred for persons likely to be susceptible to mumps and rubella; and if monovalent measles vaccine is not readily available, travelers should receive measles, mumps, and rubella virus vaccine live regardless of their immune status to mumps or rubella. Vaccination is recommended for susceptible individuals in high-risk groups such as college students, healthcare workers, and military personnel.

Postexposure vaccination – There is no conclusive evidence that vaccination of individuals recently exposed to natural mumps will provide protection.

Administration and Dosage

➤*Administration:* For SC administration. Do not inject IV.

The dose for any age is 0.5 mL administered SC, preferably into the outer aspect of the upper arm.

See Indications for more information.

➤*Immune globulin:* Immune globulin (IG) is not to be given concurrently with mumps virus vaccine live.

➤*Syringe selection:* A sterile syringe free of preservatives, antiseptics, and detergents should be used for each injection or reconstitution of the vaccine because these substances may inactivate the live virus vaccine. A 25-gauge, ⅝″ needle is recommended.

➤*Reconstitution:* To reconstitute, use only the diluent supplied, since it is free of preservatives or other antiviral substances which might inactivate the vaccine.

➤*Single-dose vial:* First, withdraw the entire volume of diluent into the syringe to be used for reconstitution. Inject all the diluent in the syringe into the vial of lyophilized vaccine, and agitate to mix thoroughly. If the lyophilized vaccine cannot be dissolved, discard. Withdraw the entire contents into a syringe and inject the total volume of restored vaccine SC.

➤*Use with other vaccines:* Mumps virus vaccine live should not be given less than 1 month before or after administration of other live viral vaccines.

Measles, mumps, and rubella virus vaccine live has been administered concurrently with varicella virus vaccine live and *Haemophilus B* conjugate vaccine (meningococcal protein conjugate), using separate sites and syringes. No impairment of immune response to individually tested vaccine antigens was demonstrated. The type, frequency, and severity of adverse reactions observed with measles, mumps, and rubella virus vaccine live were similar to those seen when each vaccine was given alone.

Routine administration of DTP (diphtheria, tetanus, pertussis) or OPV (oral poliovirus vaccine) concurrently with measles, mumps and rubella vaccines is not recommended because there are limited data relating to the simultaneous administration of these antigens.

However, other schedules have been used. The ACIP has stated "Although data are limited concerning the simultaneous administration of the entire recommended vaccine series (ie, DTP, OPV, MMR, and Hib vaccines, with or without hepatitis B vaccine), data from numerous studies have indicated no interference between routinely recommended childhood vaccines (either live, attenuated, or killed). These findings support the simultaneous use of all vaccines as recommended."

➤*Storage / Stability:* During shipment, to ensure that there is no loss of potency, the vaccine must be maintained at a temperature of ≤ 10°C (50°F). Freezing during shipment will not affect potency.

Protect the vaccine from light at all times, since such exposure may inactivate the virus.

Before reconstitution, store the vial of lyophilized vaccine at 2° to 8°C (36° to 46°F) or colder. The diluent may be stored in the refrigerator with the lyophilized vaccine or separately at room temperature.

It is recommended that the vaccine be used as soon as possible after reconstitution. Store reconstituted vaccine in the vaccine vial in a dark place at 2° to 8°C (36° to 46°F) and discard if not used within 8 hours.

Actions

➤*Pharmacology:* Mumps is a common childhood disease, caused by mumps virus (paramyxovirus), that may be associated with serious complications or death. For example, mumps is associated with aseptic meningitis, deafness and orchitis.

Extensive clinical trials have demonstrated that mumps virus vaccine live is highly immunogenic and well tolerated. A single injection of the vaccine has been shown to induce mumps-neutralizing antibodies in ≈ 97% of susceptible children and ≈ 93% of susceptible adults. The pattern of antibody response closely resembles that observed for natural mumps. Although the antibody level is significantly lower than that following natural infection; it is protective and long lasting. However, a small percentage (1% to 5%) of vaccinees may fail to seroconvert after the primary dose (see also Indications, Recommended Vaccination Schedule).

Efficacy of mumps vaccine was established in a series of double-blind, controlled field trials which demonstrated a high degree of protective efficacy. These studies also established that seroconversion in response to mumps vaccination paralleled protection from these diseases.

Following vaccination, antibodies associated with protection can be measured by neutralization assays, hemagglutination-inhibition (HI), or ELISA (enzyme-linked immunosorbent assay) tests. Neutralizing and ELISA antibodies to mumps virus are still detectable in most individuals 11 to 13 years after primary vaccination.

Contraindications

Hypersensitivity to any component of the vaccine, including gelatin.

Do not give mumps virus vaccine live to pregnant females; the possible effects of the vaccine on fetal development are unknown at this time. If vaccination of postpubertal females is undertaken, pregnancy should be avoided for 3 months following vaccination (see Warnings, Pregnancy).

Anaphylactic or anaphylactoid reactions to neomycin (each dose of reconstituted vaccine contains ≈ 25 mcg of neomycin).

Any febrile respiratory illness or other active febrile infection. However, the ACIP has recommended that all vaccines can be administered to persons with minor illnesses such as diarrhea, mild upper respiratory tract infection with or without low-grade fever, or other low-grade febrile illness.

Patients receiving immunosuppressive therapy. This contraindication does not apply to patients who are receiving corticosteroids as replacement therapy (eg, for Addison's disease).

Individuals with blood dyscrasias, leukemia, lymphomas of any type, or other malignant neoplasms affecting the bone marrow or lymphatic systems.

Primary and acquired immunodeficiency states, including patients who are immunosuppressed in association with AIDS or other clinical manifestations of infection with human immunodeficiency viruses; cellular immune deficiencies; and hypogammaglobulinemic and dysgammaglobulinemic states.

Individuals with a family history of congenital or hereditary immunodeficiency, until the immune competence of the potential vaccine recipient is demonstrated.

Warnings

➤*Fever:* The physician should be alert to the temperature elevation which may occur following vaccination (see Adverse Reactions).

➤*Thrombocytopenia:* Individuals with current thrombocytopenia may develop more severe thrombocytopenia following vaccination. In addition, individuals who experienced thrombocytopenia with the first dose of measles, mumps, and rubella virus vaccine live (or its component vaccines) may develop thrombocytopenia with repeat doses. Serologic status may be evaluated to determine whether or not additional doses of vaccine are needed. The potential risk to benefit ratio should be carefully evaluated before considering vaccination in such cases.

➤*Hypersensitivity reactions:*

Hypersensitivity to eggs – Live mumps vaccine is produced in chick embryo cell culture. Persons with a history of anaphylactic, anaphylactoid,

MUMPS VIRUS VACCINE LIVE — INJECTION

or other immediate reactions (eg, hives, swelling of the mouth and throat, difficulty breathing, hypotension, or shock) subsequent to egg ingestion may be at an enhanced risk of immediate-type hypersensitivity reactions after receiving vaccines containing traces of chick embryo antigen. The potential risk to benefit ratio should be carefully evaluated before considering vaccination in such cases. Such individuals may be vaccinated with extreme caution, having adequate treatment on hand should a reaction occur (see Precautions).

However, the American Academy of Pediatrics (AAP) has stated, "Most children with a history of anaphylactic reactions to eggs have no untoward reactions to measles or MMR vaccine. Persons are not at increased risk if they have egg allergies that are not anaphylactic, and they should be vaccinated in the usual manner. In addition, skin testing of egg-allergic children with vaccine has not been predictive of which children will have an immediate hypersensitivity reaction ... Persons with allergies to chickens or chicken feathers are not at increased risk of reaction to the vaccine."

Hypersensitivity to neomycin – The AAP states, "Persons who have experienced anaphylactic reactions to topically or systemically administered neomycin should not receive measles vaccine. Most often, however, neomycin allergy manifests as a contact dermatitis, which is a delayed-type (cell-mediated) immune response rather than anaphylaxis. In such persons, an adverse reaction to neomycin in the vaccine would be an erythematous, pruritic nodule or papule, 48 to 96 hours after vaccination. A history of contact dermatitis to neomycin is not a contraindication to receiving measles vaccine."

➤*Pregnancy: Category C.* Animal reproduction studies have not been conducted with mumps virus vaccine live. It is also not known whether mumps virus vaccine live can cause fetal harm when administered to a pregnant woman or can affect reproduction capacity. Therefore, mumps virus vaccine should not be given to persons known to be pregnant; furthermore, pregnancy should be avoided for 3 months following vaccination (see Contraindications).

In counseling women who are inadvertently vaccinated when pregnant or who become pregnant within 3 months of vaccination, the physician should be aware that mumps infection during the first trimester of pregnancy may increase the rate of spontaneous abortion. Although mumps vaccine virus has been shown to infect the placenta and fetus, there is no evidence that it causes congenital malformations in humans.

➤*Lactation:* It is not known whether mumps vaccine virus is secreted in human milk. Therefore, because many drugs are excreted in human milk, caution should be exercised when mumps virus vaccine live is administered to a nursing woman.

➤*Children:* See Indications for more information.

Precautions

➤*Anaphylactoid reactions:* Adequate treatment provisions including epinephrine injection (1:1000), should be available for immediate use should an anaphylactic or anaphylactoid reaction occur.

➤*Administration precautions:* Special care should be taken to ensure that the injection does not enter a blood vessel.

➤*Immunodeficiency:* Children and young adults who are known to be infected with human immunodeficiency viruses and are not immunosuppressed may be vaccinated. However, vaccinees who are infected with HIV should be monitored closely for vaccine-preventable diseases because immunization may be less effective than for uninfected persons (see Contraindications).

➤*Blood transfusions/Immune globulin:* Vaccination should be deferred for 3 months or longer following blood or plasma transfusions, or administration of immune globulin (human).

➤*Tuberculosis:* It has been reported that mumps virus vaccine live may result in a temporary depression of tuberculin skin sensitivity. Therefore, if a tuberculin test is to be done, it should be administered either before or simultaneously with mumps virus vaccine live.

Individuals with active untreated tuberculosis should not be vaccinated.

➤*Virus protection:* As for any vaccine, vaccination with mumps virus vaccine live may not result in protection in 100% of vaccinees.

Drug Interactions

See Administration and Dosage, Use with other vaccines.

Mumps Virus Vaccine Drug Interactions

Precipitant drug	Object drug*		Description
Immunosuppressants	Mumps vaccine	⬇	Administration of mumps vaccine to patients receiving immunosuppressants, including corticosteroids or radiation therapy, may result in insufficient response to immunization. They may remain susceptible despite immunization.
Immune globulins	Mumps vaccine	⬇	To avoid inactivating attenuated virus, give the vaccine at least 14 to 30 days before or 6 to 8 weeks after immune globulin. Alternately, check antibody titers or repeat the vaccine 3 months after IgG.
Interferon	Mumps vaccine	⬇	Concurrent use may inhibit antibody response to the vaccine.
Mumps vaccine	Virus vaccines, other	⬇	To avoid the hypothetical concern over antigenic competition, give mumps vaccine after or ≥ 1 month before other virus vaccines. However, several vaccines may be given simultaneously at separate injection sites (eg, DTP, OPV, MMR, Hib, hepatitis B).

* ⬇ = Object drug decreased.

Adverse Reactions

The following adverse reactions are listed in decreasing order of severity, without regard to causality, within each body system category and have been reported during clinical trials, with use of the marketed vaccine, or with use of polyvalent vaccine containing mumps:

➤*Cardiovascular:* Vasculitis.

➤*CNS:* Encephalitis; Guillain-Barré syndrome (GBS); febrile seizures; ocular palsies. Cases of aseptic meningitis have been reported to VAERS following measles, mumps, and rubella vaccination. Although a causal relationship between the Urabe strain of mumps vaccine and aseptic meningitis has been shown, there are no data to link Jeryl Lynn mumps vaccine to aseptic meningitis.

➤*Dermatologic:* Stevens-Johnson syndrome; erythema multiforme; urticaria. Local reactions including burning/stinging at injection site; wheal and flare.

➤*Endocrine:* Diabetes mellitus.

➤*GI:* Pancreatitis; diarrhea; parotitis.

➤*GU:* Orchitis.

➤*Hematologic/Lymphatic:* Thrombocytopenia; purpura; lymphadenopathy; leukocytosis.

➤*Immunologic:* Anaphylaxis and anaphylactoid reactions have been reported as well as related phenomena such as angioneurotic edema (including peripheral or facial edema) and bronchial spasm.

➤*Respiratory:* Cough; rhinitis.

➤*Special senses:*

Eye – Optic neuritis; papillitis; retrobulbar neuritis; conjunctivitis.

Ear – Nerve deafness; otitis media.

➤*Miscellaneous:* Fever; syncope; irritability. Death from various, and in some cases unknown, causes has been reported rarely following vaccination with measles, mumps, and rubella vaccines; however, a causal relationship has not been established. No deaths or permanent sequelae were reported in a published postmarketing surveillance study in Finland involving 1.5 million children and adults who were vaccinated with measles, mumps, and rubella virus vaccine live during 1982 to 1993.

Patient Information

The healthcare provider should provide the vaccine information required to be given with each vaccination to the patient, parent or guardian.

The healthcare provider should inform the patient, parent or guardian of the benefits and risks associated with vaccination. For risks associated with vaccination see Warnings, Precautions, Adverse Reactions.

Patients, parents or guardians should be instructed to report any serious adverse reactions to their healthcare provider who in turn should report such events to the US Department of Health and Human Services through the Vaccine Adverse Event Reporting System (VAERS), 1-800-822-7967.

Pregnancy should be avoided for 3 months following vaccination.

➤*Immunosuppressive therapy:* The immune status of patients about to undergo immunosuppressive therapy should be evaluated so that the physician can consider whether vaccination prior to the initiation of treatment is indicated (see Contraindications and Precautions).

The ACIP has indicated that patients with leukemia in remission who have not received chemotherapy for at least 3 months may receive live virus vaccines. Short-term (less than 2 weeks), low- to moderate-dose systemic corticosteroid therapy, topical steroid therapy (eg, nasal, skin), long-term, alternate-day treatment with low to moderate doses of short-acting systemic steroid, and intra-articular, bursal, or tendon injection of corticosteroids are not immunosuppressive in their usual doses and do not contraindicate the administration of mumps vaccine.

➤*Immune globulin:* Administration of immune globulins concurrently with mumps virus vaccine live may interfere with the expected immune response (see Precautions).

RUBELLA AND MUMPS VIRUS VACCINE, LIVE

Rx	**Biavax** II (Merck)	**Powder for Injection**: Mixture of 2 viruses: ≥ 20,000 mumps $TCID_{50}$ (tissue culture infectious doses) and ≥ 1000 rubella $TCID_{50}$ per 0.5 ml dose	25 mcg neomycin. In single-dose vials with diluent.

RUBELLA AND MUMPS VIRUS VACCINE LIVE — INJECTION

For information on recommended immunization schedules, refer to the Agents for Active Immunization introduction. Consider the prescribing information for rubella virus vaccine and for mumps virus vaccine when using this product (see individual monographs).

Indications

➤*Rubella and mumps vaccination:* For simultaneous immunization against rubella and mumps in persons 12 months of age or older. A booster is not needed.

The vaccine is not recommended for infants younger than 12 months because they may retain maternal rubella and mumps neutralizing antibodies which may interfere with the immune response.

Previously unimmunized children of susceptible pregnant women should receive live, attenuated rubella vaccine because an immunized child will be less likely to acquire natural rubella and introduce the virus into the household.

Individuals planning travel outside the United States, if not immune, can acquire measles, mumps or rubella and import these diseases to the United States. Therefore, prior to international travel, individuals known to be susceptible to one or more of these diseases can receive either a single antigen vaccine (measles, mumps, or rubella), or a combined antigen vaccine as appropriate. However, measles, mumps, and rubella virus vaccine live is preferred for persons likely to be susceptible to mumps and rubella; and if single-antigen measles vaccine is not readily available, travelers should receive measles, mumps, and rubella virus vaccine live regardless of their immune status to mumps or rubella.

➤*Nonpregnant adolescent and adult women:* Immunization of susceptible nonpregnant adolescent and adult women of childbearing age with live, attenuated rubella virus vaccine is indicated if certain precautions are observed. Vaccinating susceptible postpubertal females confers individual protection against subsequently acquiring rubella infection during pregnancy, which in turn prevents infection of the fetus and consequent congenital rubella injury.

Advise women of childbearing age not to become pregnant for 3 months after vaccination and inform them of the reasons for this precaution. The Immunization Practices Advisory Committee (ACIP) has recommended "In view of the importance of protecting this age group against rubella, reasonable precautions in a rubella immunization program include asking females if they are pregnant, excluding those who say they are, and explaining the theoretical risks to the others."

➤*Postpartum women:* It has been found convenient in many instances to vaccinate rubella-susceptible women in the immediate postpartum period.

➤*Revaccination:* Revaccinate children vaccinated when younger than 12 months of age. Based on available evidence, there is no reason to routinely revaccinate persons who were vaccinated originally when 12 months of age or older. However, persons should be revaccinated if there is evidence to suggest that initial immunization was ineffective.

➤*Use with other vaccines:* Routine administration of DTP (diphtheria, tetanus, pertussis) or OPV (oral poliovirus vaccine) concomitantly with measles, mumps and rubella vaccines is not recommended because there are insufficient data relating to the simultaneous administration of these antigens. However, the American Academy of Pediatrics has noted that in some circumstances, particularly when the patient may not return, some practitioners prefer to administer all these antigens on a single day. If done, use separate sites and syringes for DTP and rubella and mumps virus vaccine.

Do not give rubella and mumps virus vaccine less than 1 month before or after administration of other virus vaccines.

Administration and Dosage

➤*Recommended administration:* For subcutaneous administration.

Do not inject by IV.

The dosage of vaccine is the same for all persons. Inject the total volume (about 0.5 mL) of reconstituted vaccine subcutaneously, preferably into the outer aspect of upper arm. Do not give immune globulin (IG) concurrently with rubella and mumps virus vaccine.

➤*Syringe selection:* A sterile syringe free of preservatives, antiseptics, and detergents should be used for each injection of the vaccine because these substances may inactivate the live virus vaccine. A 25-gauge, ⅝ inch needle is recommended.

➤*Reconstitution:* To reconstitute, use only the diluent supplied because it is free of preservatives or other antiviral substances which might inactivate the vaccine. First, withdraw the entire volume of diluent into the syringe to be used for reconstitution. Inject all the diluent in the syringe into the vial of lyophilized vaccine, and agitate to mix thoroughly. Withdraw the entire contents into a syringe and inject the total volume of restored vaccine subcutaneously.

➤*Storage / Stability:* It is recommended that the vaccine be used as soon as possible after reconstitution. Protect the vaccine from light at all times, since such exposure may inactivate the virus. Store reconstituted vaccine in the vaccine vial in a dark place at 2° to 8°C (36° to 46°F) and discard if not used within 8 hours.

Shipping conditions – During shipment, to ensure that there is no loss of potency, the vaccine must be maintained at a temperature of 10°C (50°F) or less.

MEASLES, MUMPS, AND RUBELLA VIRUS VACCINE, LIVE

Rx	**M-M-R** II (Merck)	**Powder for injection**: Mixture of 3 viruses: ≥ 1000 measles $TCID_{50}$ (tissue culture infectious doses), ≥ 20,000 mumps $TCID_{50}$ and ≥ 1000 rubella $TCID_{50}$ per 0.5 ml dose.	With 25 mcg neomycin. In single dose vials with diluent.

MEASLES, MUMPS, AND RUBELLA VIRUS VACCINE LIVE — INJECTION

For information on recommended immunization schedules, refer to the Agents for Active Immunization introduction. Consider the prescribing information for measles (rubeola) virus vaccine, mumps virus vaccine and rubella virus vaccine when using this product (see individual monographs).

Indications

➤*Measles, mumps, and rubella vaccination:* For simultaneous vaccination against measles, mumps, and rubella in individuals at least 12 months of age.

Revaccinate individuals first vaccinated at at least 12 months of age prior to elementary school entry. Revaccination may seroconvert primary failures or boost antibody titers of previously vaccinated individuals whose titers have declined. The Advisory Committee on Immunization Practices (ACIP) recommends administration of the first dose of measles, mumps and rubella virus vaccine live at 12 to 15 months of age and administration of the second dose of measles, mumps and rubella virus vaccine live at 4 to 6 years of age. In addition, some public health jurisdictions mandate the age for revaccination. Consult the complete text of applicable guidelines regarding routine revaccination including that of high-risk adult populations.

➤*Measles outbreak schedule:*

Infants between 6 and 12 months of age – Local health authorities may recommend measles vaccination of infants between 6 and 12 months of age in outbreak situations. This population may fail to respond to the components of the vaccine. Safety and efficacy of mumps and rubella vaccine in infants younger than 12 months of age have not been established. The younger the infant, the lower the likelihood of seroconversion. Such infants should receive a second dose of measles, mumps and rubella virus vaccine live between 12 and 15 months of age, followed by revaccination at elementary school entry.

➤*Other vaccination considerations:*

Nonpregnant adolescent and adult women – Immunization of susceptible nonpregnant adolescent and adult women of childbearing age with live, attenuated rubella virus vaccine is indicated if certain precautions are observed. Vaccinating susceptible postpubertal women confers individual protection against subsequently acquiring rubella infection during pregnancy, which in turn prevents infection of the fetus and consequent congenital rubella injury.

Advise women of childbearing age not to become pregnant for 3 months after vaccination and inform them of the reasons for this precaution.†

Postpartum women – It has been found convenient in many instances to vaccinate rubella-susceptible women in the immediate postpartum period.

Other populations – Previously unvaccinated children older than 12 months who are in contact with susceptible pregnant women should receive live, attenuated rubella vaccine (such as that contained in monovalent rubella vaccine or in measles, mumps and rubella virus vaccine live) to reduce the risk of exposure of the pregnant woman.

Individuals planning travel outside the United States, if not immune, can acquire measles, mumps or rubella and import these diseases into the United States. Therefore, prior to international travel, individuals known to be susceptible to 1 or more of these diseases can receive either a monovalent vaccine (measles, mumps or rubella), or a combination vaccine as appropriate. However, measles, mumps and rubella virus vaccine live is preferred for persons likely to be susceptible to mumps and rubella; and if monovalent measles vaccine is not readily available, travelers should receive measles, mumps and rubella virus vaccine live regardless of their immune status to mumps or rubella.

Vaccination is recommended for susceptible individuals in high-risk groups such as college students, health care workers, and military personnel.

MEASLES, MUMPS, AND RUBELLA VIRUS VACCINE LIVE — INJECTION

According to ACIP recommendations, most persons born in 1956 or earlier are likely to have been infected with measles naturally and generally need not be considered susceptible. All children, adolescents, and adults born after 1956 are considered susceptible and should be vaccinated if there are no contraindications. This includes persons who may be immune to measles but who lack adequate documentation of immunity such as physician-diagnosed measles, laboratory evidence of measles immunity, or adequate immunization with live measles vaccine on or after the first birthday.

The ACIP recommends that "Persons vaccinated with inactivated vaccine followed within 3 months by live vaccine should be revaccinated with 2 doses of live vaccine. Revaccination is particularly important when the risk of exposure to natural measles virus is increased, as may occur during international travel."

➤*Postexposure vaccination:* Vaccination of individuals exposed to natural measles may provide some protection if the vaccine can be administered within 72 hours of exposure. If, however, vaccine is given a few days before exposure, substantial protection may be afforded. There is no conclusive evidence that vaccination of individuals recently exposed to natural mumps or natural rubella will provide protection.

Administration and Dosage

➤*Recommended dosage:* For subcutaneous administration. Do not inject IV.

The dose for any age is 0.5 mL administered subcutaneously, preferably into the outer aspect of the upper arm.

See Indications for more information.

➤*Immune globulin:* Immune globulin (IG) is not to be given concurrently with measles, mumps and rubella virus vaccine live.

➤*Syringe selection:* Use a sterile syringe free of preservatives, antiseptics, and detergents for each injection or reconstitution of the vaccine because these substances may inactivate the live virus vaccine. A 25-gauge, ⅝" needle is recommended.

➤*Reconstitution:* To reconstitute, use only the diluent supplied because it is free of preservatives or other antiviral substances which might inactivate the vaccine.

➤*Single-dose vial:* First, withdraw the entire volume of diluent into the syringe to be used for reconstitution. Inject all the diluent in the syringe into the vial of lyophilized vaccine, and agitate to mix thoroughly. If the lyophilized vaccine cannot be dissolved, discard. Withdraw the entire contents into a syringe and inject the total volume of restored vaccine subcutaneously. It is important to use a separate sterile syringe and needle for each individual patient to prevent transmission of hepatitis B and other infectious agents from one person to another.

➤*Use with other vaccines:* Measles, mumps and rubella virus vaccine live should be given 1 month before or after administration of other live viral vaccines.

Measles, mumps and rubella virus vaccine live has been administered concurrently with varicella virus vaccine live, and *Haemophilus* B conjugate vaccine (meningococcal protein conjugate), using separate sites and syringes. No impairment of immune response to individual tested vaccine antigens was demonstrated. The type, frequency, and severity of adverse experiences observed with measles, mumps and rubella virus vaccine live were similar to those seen when each vaccine was given alone.

Routine administration of DTP (diphtheria, tetanus, pertussis) or OPV (oral poliovirus vaccine) concurrently with measles, mumps and rubella vaccines is not recommended because there are limited data relating to the simultaneous administration of these antigens.

However, other schedules have been used. The ACIP has stated "Although data are limited concerning the simultaneous administration of the entire recommended vaccine series (ie, DTP, OPV, MMR, and Hib vaccines, with or without hepatitis B vaccine), data from numerous studies have indicated no interference between routinely recommended childhood vaccines (either live, attenuated, or killed). These findings support the simultaneous use of all vaccines as recommended."

➤*Storage/Stability:* During shipment, to ensure that there is no loss of potency, the vaccine must be maintained at a temperature of ≤ 10°C (50°F). Freezing during shipment will not affect potency.

Protect the vaccine from light at all times, since such exposure may inactivate the virus.

Before reconstitution, store the vial of lyophilized vaccine at 2° to 8°C (36° to 46°F) or colder. The diluent may be stored in the refrigerator with the lyophilized vaccine or separately at room temperature.

It is recommended that the vaccine be used as soon as possible after reconstitution. Store reconstituted vaccine in the vaccine vial in a dark place at 2° to 8°C (36° to 46°F) and discard if not used within 8 hours.

MEASLES, MUMPS, RUBELLA, AND VARICELLA VIRUS VACCINE, LIVE, ATTENUATED

Rx	**ProQuad** (Merck & Co.)	**Powder for injection, lyophilized:** Mixture of 4 viruses: ≥ 3.00 log_{10} measles $TCID_{50}$ (50% tissue culture infectious doses), 4.30 log_{10} mumps $TCID_{50}$, 3.00 log_{10} rubella $TCID_{50}$, and ≥ 3.99 log_{10} varicella PFU (plaque-forming units) per 0.5 mL dose.	Preservative free.[a] In single dose vials with diluent.

[a] Sucrose, hydrolyzed gelatin, sodium chloride, sorbitol, monosodium L-glutamate, sodium phosphate dibasic, human albumin, sodium bicarbonate, potassium phosphate monobasic, potassium chloride, potassium phosphate dibasic, residual components of MRC-5 cells including DNA and protein, neomycin, bovine calf serum.

MEASLES, MUMPS, RUBELLA, AND VARICELLA VIRUS VACCINE, LIVE, ATTENUATED — INJECTION

Indications

➤*Measles, mumps, rubella, and varicella vaccination:* Measles, mumps, rubella, and varicella virus (MMRV) vaccine live is indicated for simultaneous vaccination against measles, mumps, rubella, and varicella in children 12 months to 12 years of age. It may be used in children 12 months to 12 years of age if a second dose of measles, mumps, and rubella vaccine is to be administered.

Administration and Dosage

➤*Approved by the FDA:* September 6, 2005.

➤*Administration:* For subcutaneous administration; do not inject intravascularly. The vaccine is to be injected subcutaneously in the outer aspect of the deltoid region of the upper arm or in the higher anterolateral area of the thigh. Use a separate sterile syringe and needle for each patient to prevent transmission of infectious agents from one individual to another.

➤*Children (12 months to 12 years of age):* Individuals 12 months through 12 years of age should receive a single dose of MMRV vaccine 0.5 mL administered subcutaneously. At least 1 month should elapse between a dose of a measles-containing vaccine such as *M-M-R II* (measles, mumps, and rubella virus vaccine, live), and a dose of MMRV vaccine. If for any reason a second dose of varicella-containing vaccine is required, at least 3 months should elapse between administration of the 2 doses.

➤*Reconstitution:* Withdraw the entire volume of the supplied diluent into a syringe. Use only the diluent supplied with the vaccine because it is free of preservatives or other antiviral substances.

Preservatives, antiseptics, detergents, and other antiviral substances may inactivate the vaccine. Use only sterile syringes that are free of preservatives, antiseptics, detergents and other antiviral substances for reconstitution and injection of MMRV vaccine.

Inject the entire content of the syringe into the vial containing the powder. Gently agitate to dissolve completely.

Withdraw the entire amount of the reconstituted vaccine from the vial into the same syringe and inject the entire volume.

When reconstituted, each vial of MMRV vaccine contains a single 0.5 mL dose.

To minimize loss of potency, the vaccine should be administered immediately after reconstitution. Discard reconstituted vaccine if it is not used within 30 minutes.

➤*Concomitant vaccination:* If another vaccine is coadministered, a different injection site should be used.

➤*Storage/Stability:* During shipment, to ensure that there is no loss of potency, the vaccine must be maintained at a temperature of −20°C (−4°F) or colder.

Before reconstitution, store the lyophilized vaccine continuously in a freezer (eg, chest, frostfree) for up to 18 months, at an average temperature of −15°C (5°F) or colder. Any freezer that reliably maintains an average temperature of −15°C (5°F) or colder and has a separate sealed freezer door is acceptable for storing MMRV vaccine.

Do not store lyophilized vaccine in the refrigerator. If lyophilized vaccine is inadvertently stored in the refrigerator, discard it.

Protect the vaccine from light at all times because such exposure may inactivate the vaccine viruses. Discard reconstituted vaccine if it is not used within 30 minutes. Do not freeze reconstituted vaccine.

Store diluent separately at room temperature (20° to 25° [68° to 77° F]), or in a refrigerator (2° to 8° [36° to 46° F]).

POLIOVIRUS VACCINE, INACTIVATED (IPV)

Rx	**IPOL** (Connaught)	**Injection:** Suspension of 3 types of poliovirus (Types 1, 2 and 3) grown in monkey kidney cell cultures	In 0.5 ml single-dose syringe with integrated needle.[1]

[1] Each dose contains 0.5% 2-phenoxyethanol, a maximum of 0.02% formaldehyde and not more than 200 ng streptomycin, 25 ng polymyxin B and 5 ng neomycin.

POLIOVIRUS VACCINE, INACTIVATED (IPV) — INJECTION

For complete and comparative prescribing information, refer to the Agents for Active Immunization introduction.

Indications

➤*Poliovirus prevention:* Poliovirus vaccine, inactivated (IPV) is indicated for active immunization of infants (as young as 6 weeks of age), children and adults for the prevention of poliomyelitis caused by poliovirus types 1, 2, and 3.

➤*Infants, children, and adolescents:* It is recommended that all infants (as young as 6 weeks of age), unimmunized children, and adolescents not previously immunized be vaccinated routinely against paralytic poliomyelitis. Following the eradication of poliomyelitis caused by wild poliovirus from the Western Hemisphere (including North and South America) vaccine-associated paralytic poliomyelitis (VAPP) is the only cause of paralytic poliomyelitis in the US. The use of IPV has been suggested as a way to reduce VAPP incidence.

All children should receive 4 doses of IPV at ages 2, 4, 6 to 18 months, and 4 to 6 years. Oral poliovirus vaccine (OPV) is no longer recommended for routine immunization. In the special circumstances that OPV is acceptable, please refer to the monograph for the appropriate administration schedule and all other issues related to the use of OPV.

Children incompletely immunized – Children of all ages should have their immunization status reviewed and be considered for supplemental immunization as follows for adults. Time intervals between doses longer than those recommended for routine primary immunization do not necessitate additional doses as long as a final total of 4 doses is reached.

➤*Adults:* Routine primary poliovirus vaccination of adults (generally those 18 years of age and older) residing in the United States is not recommended. Unimmunized adults residing in a household when a child is receiving OPV or adults who have increased risk of exposure to either oral vaccine or wild poliovirus and have not been adequately immunized should receive polio vaccination in accordance with the schedule given in Administration and Dosage.

Persons with previous wild poliovirus disease, who are incompletely immunized or unimmunized, should be given additional doses of IPV if they fall into one or more categories listed previously.

The following categories of adults are at an increased risk of exposure to wild polioviruses:

- Travelers to regions or countries where poliomyelitis is endemic or epidemic.
- Healthcare workers in close contact with patients who may be excreting polioviruses.
- Laboratory workers handling specimens that may contain polioviruses.
- Members of communities or specific population groups with disease caused by wild polioviruses.
- Incompletely vaccinated or unvaccinated adults in a household (or other close contacts) with children given OPV. The adult should be informed of the risk of VAPP associated with contact of those receiving OPV.

➤*Immunodeficiency and altered immune status:* Patients with recognized immunodeficiency are at greater risk of developing paralysis when exposed to live poliovirus than persons with a healthy immune system. Under no circumstances should oral poliovirus vaccine be used in such patients or introduced into a household where such a patient resides.

IPV should be used in all patients with immunodeficiency diseases and members of such patients' households when vaccination of such persons is indicated. This includes patients with asymptomatic HIV infection, AIDS or AIDS-related complex, severe combined immunodeficiency, hypogammaglobulinemia, or agammaglobulinemia; altered immune states due to diseases such as leukemia, lymphoma, or generalized malignancy; or an immune system compromised by treatment with corticosteroids, alkylating drugs, antimetabolites, or radiation. Immunogenicity of IPV in individuals receiving immunoglobulin could be impaired and patients with an altered immune state may or may not develop a protective response against paralytic poliomyelitis after administration of IPV.

Administration and Dosage

➤*Latex allergy:* See Warnings for more information.

➤*Administration:* After preparation of the injection site, immediately administer poliovirus vaccine, inactivated intramuscularly (IM) or subcutaneously. In infants and small children, the mid-lateral aspect of the thigh is the preferred site. In older children and adults IPV should be administered IM or subcutaneously in the deltoid area.

Care should be taken to avoid administering the injection into or near blood vessels and nerves. After aspiration, if blood or any suspicious discoloration appears in the syringe, do not inject but discard contents and repeat procedures using a new dose of vaccine administered at a different site.

Do not administer vaccine intravenously.

➤*Children:* The primary series of poliovirus vaccine, inactivated consists of three 0.5 mL doses administered IM or subcutaneously, preferably 8 or more weeks apart and usually at ages 2, 4, and 6 to 18 months. Under no circumstances should the vaccine be given more frequently than 4 weeks apart. The first immunization may be administered as early as 6 weeks of age. For this series, a booster dose of IPV is administered at 4 to 6 years of age.

➤*Use with other vaccines:* From historical data on the antibody responses to diphtheria, tetanus, whole-cell or acellular pertussis, Hib, or hepatitis B vaccines used concomitantly with IPV, no interferences have been observed on the immunological end points accepted for clinical protection. If the third dose of poliovirus vaccine, inactivated is given between 12 to 18 months of age, it may be desirable to administer this dose with measles, mumps, and rubella (MMR) or other vaccines using separate syringes at separate sites, but no data on the immunological interference between IPV and these vaccines exist.

➤*Use in previously vaccinated children:* Children and adolescents with a previously incomplete series of IPV/OPV or IPV only should receive sufficient additional doses of poliovirus vaccine, inactivated to complete the series. OPV is no longer recommended for routine immunization and is recommended only in special circumstances (see Indications).

Interruption of the recommended schedule with a delay between doses does not interfere with the final immunity. There is no need to start either series over again, regardless of the time elapsed between doses.

➤*Adults:*

Unvaccinated adults – A primary series of IPV is recommended for unvaccinated adults at increased risk of exposure to poliovirus. While the responses of adults to primary series have not been studied, the recommended schedule for adults is 2 doses given at a 1- to 2-month interval and a third dose given 6 to 12 months later. If less than 3 months but greater than 2 months are available before protection is needed, 3 doses of IPV should be given at least 1 month apart. Likewise, if only 1 or 2 months are available, 2 doses of poliovirus vaccine, inactivated should be given at least 1 month apart. If less than 1 month is available, a single dose of IPV is recommended.

Incompletely vaccinated adults – Adults who are at an increased risk of exposure to poliovirus and who have had at least 1 dose of OPV, fewer than 3 doses of conventional IPV (inactivated poliovirus vaccine available in the US prior to 1988) or a combination of conventional IPV or OPV totaling fewer than 3 doses should receive at least 1 dose of poliovirus vaccine, inactivated. Additional doses needed to complete a primary series should be given if time permits.

Completely vaccinated adults – Adults who are at an increased risk of exposure to poliovirus and who have previously completed a primary series with 1 or a combination of polio vaccines can be given a dose of IPV. The preferred injection site of IPV for adults is in the tissue of the deltoid area.

➤*Storage/Stability:* The vaccine is stable if stored in the refrigerator between 2° and 8°C (35° and 46°F). The vaccine must not be frozen.

Actions

➤*Pharmacology:* Poliomyelitis is caused by poliovirus Types 1, 2, or 3. It is primarily spread by the fecal-oral route of transmission but may also be spread by the pharyngeal route.

Poliovirus vaccine, inactivated induces the production of neutralizing antibodies against each type of virus which are related to protective efficacy and induces antibody responses in most children after administering fewer doses than the vaccine available in the United States prior to 1988.

IPV is able to induce secretory antibody (IgA) produced in the pharynx and gut and reduces pharyngeal excretion of poliovirus Type 1 from 75% in children with neutralizing antibodies at levels less than 1:8 to 25% in children with neutralizing antibodies at levels more than 1:64. There is also evidence of induction of herd immunity with IPV, and that this herd immunity is sufficiently maintained in a population vaccinated only with IPV.

Paralytic polio and VAPP have not been reported in association with administration of poliovirus vaccine, inactivated. It is expected that an IPV only schedule will eliminate the risk of VAPP in both recipients and contacts compared to a schedule that included OPV.

Contraindications

Poliovirus vaccine, inactivated is contraindicated in persons with a history of hypersensitivity to any component of the vaccine, including 2-phenoxyethanol, formaldehyde, neomycin, streptomycin and polymyxin B.

No further doses should be given if anaphylaxis or anaphylactic shock occurs within 24 hours of administration of 1 dose of vaccine.

Vaccination of persons with an acute, febrile illness should be deferred until after recovery; however, minor illness, such as mild upper respiratory tract infection, with or without low grade fever, are not reasons for postponing vaccine administration.

Warnings

➤*Latex allergy:* This product contains dry, natural latex rubber as follows: The stopper to the vial contains no rubber of any kind. In the case of the syringe, the needle cover contains dry, natural latex rubber but the plunger for the syringe contains no rubber of any kind.

➤*Hypersensitivity reactions:* Neomycin, streptomycin, polymyxin B, 2-phenoxyethanol, and formaldehyde are used in the production of this vaccine. Although purification procedures eliminate measurable amounts of these substances, traces may be present (see Ingredients) and allergic reactions may occur in persons sensitive to these substances (see Contraindications).

Although no causal relationship between IPV and Guillain-Barré syndrome (GBS) has been established, GBS has been temporally related to administration of another inactivated poliovirus vaccine. Deaths have been reported in temporal association with the administration of inactivated poliovirus vaccine (see Adverse Reactions).

Epinephrine injection (1:1000) and other appropriate agents should be available to control immediate allergic reactions.

POLIOVIRUS VACCINE, INACTIVATED (IPV) — INJECTION

➤*Pregnancy:* *Category C.* Animal reproduction studies have not been conducted with poliovirus vaccine, inactivated. It is also not known whether IPV can cause fetal harm when administered to a pregnant woman or can affect reproduction capacity. Poliovirus vaccine, inactivated should be given to a pregnant woman only if clearly needed.

➤*Lactation:* It is not known whether IPV is excreted in human milk. Because many drugs are excreted in human milk, exercise caution when IPV is administered to a breast-feeding woman.

➤*Children:* See Indications for more information.

Precautions

➤*Immunodeficiency:* Immunodeficient patients or patients under immunosuppressive therapy may not develop a protective immune response against paralytic poliomyelitis after administration of IPV.

Administration of IPV is not contraindicated in individuals infected with HIV.

Drug Interactions

➤*Immunosuppressive agents:* If poliovirus vaccine, inactivated has been administered to persons receiving immunosuppressive therapy, an adequate immunologic response may not be obtained.

Adverse Reactions

In earlier studies with the vaccine grown in primary monkey kidney cells, transient local reactions at the site of injection were observed. Erythema, induration and pain occurred in 3.2%, 1%, and 13%, respectively, of vaccinees within 48 hours postvaccination. Temperatures of greater than or equal to 39°C (greater than or equal to 102°F) were reported in 38% of vaccinees. Other symptoms included irritability, sleepiness, fussiness, and crying. Because IPV was given in a different site but concurrently with diphtheria and tetanus toxoids and pertussis vaccine adsorbed (DTP), these systemic reactions could not be attributed to a specific vaccine. However, these systemic reactions were comparable in frequency and severity to that reported for DTP given alone without IPV. Although no causal relationship has been established, deaths have occurred in temporal association after vaccination of infants with IPV.

IPV Adverse Reactions (Administered Intramuscularly, Concomitantly at Separate Sites with AvP[a] Whole-Cell DTP Vaccine at 2 and 4 Months of Age and with AvP Acellular Pertussis Vaccine at 18 months of age)

	Age at immunization								
	2 months (n = 211)			4 months (n = 206)			18 months[b] (n = 74)		
Reaction	6 hours	24 hours	48 hours	6 hours	24 hours	48 hours	6 hours	24 hours	48 hours
Local, IPV alone[c]									
Erythema greater than 1 inch	0.5%	0.5%	0.5%	1%	0%	0%	1.4%	0%	0%
Swelling	11.4%	5.7%	0.9%	11.2%	4.9%	1.9%	2.7%	0%	0%
Tenderness	29.4%	8.5%	2.8%	22.8%	4.4%	1%	13.5%	4.1%	0%
Systemic[d]									
Fever greater than 39°C (102.2°F)	1%	0.5%	0.5%	2%	0.5%	0%	0%	0%	4.2%
Irritability	64.5%	24.6%	17.5%	49.5%	25.7%	11.7%	14.7%	6.7%	8%
Tiredness	60.7%	31.8%	7.1%	38.8%	18.4%	6.3%	9.3%	5.3%	4%
Anorexia	16.6%	8.1%	4.3%	6.3%	4.4%	2.4%	2.7%	1.3%	2.7%
Vomiting	1.9%	2.8%	2.8%	1.9%	1.5%	1%	1.3%	1.3%	0%
Persistent crying	Percentage of infants within 72 hours after immunization was 0% after dose 1, 1.4% after dose 2, and 0% after dose 3.								

[a] AvP (Aventis Pasteur Inc) formerly known as Connaught Laboratories, Inc.
[b] Children vaccinated with DTaP vaccine.
[c] Data are from the IPV administration site, given intramuscularly.
[d] The adverse reaction profile includes the concomitant use of AvP whole-cell DTP vaccine or DTaP (diphtheria and tetanus toxoids and acellular pertussis vaccine, adsorbed) with IPV. Rates are comparable in frequency and severity to that reported for whole-cell DTP given alone.

➤*CNS:* See Warnings for more information.

➤*GI:* Anorexia and vomiting occurred with frequencies not significantly different as reported when DTP was given alone without IPV or OPV.

Patient Information

Instruct patients, parents, or guardians to report any serious adverse reactions to their health care provider.

Inform the patient, parent, or guardian of the benefits and risks of the vaccine.

Inform the patient, parent, or guardian of the importance of completing the immunization series.

Provide the Vaccine Information Materials (VIMs) which are required to be given with each immunization.

INFLUENZA VIRUS VACCINE

Rx	**Fluarix** (GlaxoSmithKline)	**Injection (purified split-virus):** 15 mcg HA of each of A/New Caledonia/20/99 (H1N1), A/Wisconsin/67/2005 (H3N2), and B/Malaysia/2506/2004 per 0.5 mL	Preservative-free. In 0.5 mL prefilled, single-dose syringes.[a]
Rx	**Fluzone** (Sanofi Pasteur)	**Injection (purified split-virus):** 15 mcg each of A/New Caledonia/20/99 (H1N1), A/Wisconsin/67/2005 (H3N2), and B/Malaysia/2506/2004 per 0.5 mL	In preservative-free 0.25 and 0.5 mL prefilled syringes, preservative-free 0.5 mL vial, and 5 mL vials with preservative (thimerosal).[b]
Rx	**Fluvirin** (Chiron)	**Injection (purified split-virus):** 15 mcg each of A/New Caledonia/20/99 IVR–116, A/Wisconsin/67/2005 NYMC X-161, and B/Malaysia/2506/2004 per 0.5 mL	Thimerosal 0.01%. In 5 mL multidose vial.[c]
Rx	**FluMist** (MedImmune Vaccines)	**Intranasal spray:** A/New Caledonia/20/99 (H1N1), A/Wisconsin/67/2005 (H3N2), and B/Malaysia/2506/2004 per 0.5 mL	Preservative free. In 0.5 mL prefilled single-use sprayers.

[a] Thimerosal is used at the early stages of manufacture and is removed by subsequent purification steps to a trace amount (≤ 1 mcg mercury/dose). Each dose also may contain residual amounts of hydrocortisone ≤ 0.0016 mcg, gentamicin sulfate ≤ 0.15 mcg, ovalbumin ≤ 1 mcg, formaldehyde ≤ 50 mcg, and sodium deoxycholate ≤ 50 mcg from the manufacturing process.
[b] With 25 mcg mercury/dose.
[c] With 24.5 mcg mercury per 0.5 mL dose as a preservative.

INFLUENZA VIRUS VACCINE

For additional information, refer to the Agents for Active Immunization introduction.

Indications

➤*Influenza vaccination:* For active immunization against the specific influenza virus strains contained in the formulation. Influenza vaccine is strongly recommended for anyone 6 months of age or older who, because of age or underlying medical conditions, is at increased risk for complications from influenza. Vaccinate health care workers and others (including household members) in close contact with high-risk people. In addition, influenza vaccine may be given to any person 6 months of age or older who wishes to reduce the chance of becoming infected with influenza. (Note: *Fluvirin* is not indicated in children younger than 4 years of age. *FluMist* is indicated in healthy children and adolescents 5 to 17 years of age and heathy adults 18 to 49 years of age.) The following are guidelines for use of the vaccine in specific groups.

➤*Groups at increased risk of influenza-related complications:*

1.) People 65 years of age or older. Vaccination also is recommended for people 50 to 64 years of age because of increased prevalence of people with high-risk conditions.

INFLUENZA VIRUS VACCINE

2.) Residents of nursing homes and other chronic-care facilities that house people of any age with chronic medical conditions.
3.) Adults and children with chronic disorders of the pulmonary or cardiovascular systems, including asthma.
4.) Adults and children who have required regular medical follow-up or hospitalization during the preceding year because of chronic metabolic diseases (including diabetes mellitus), renal dysfunction, hemoglobinopathies, or immunosuppression (including immunosuppression caused by medications or by human immunodeficiency virus [HIV]).
5.) Adults and children who have any condition (eg, cognitive dysfunction, spinal cord injuries, seizure disorders, other neuromuscular disorders) that can compromise respiratory function or the handling of respiratory secretions or that can increase the risk for aspiration.
6.) Children and adolescents (6 months to 18 years of age) who are receiving long-term aspirin therapy and, therefore, may be at risk of developing Reye syndrome after influenza.
7.) Women who will be pregnant during the influenza season.
8.) Although not recommended by the Advisory Committee on Immunization Practices (ACIP), consider vaccination in people who smoke tobacco products because of increased risk for influenza-related complications.

➤*Groups that can transmit influenza to high-risk people:* People who are clinically or subclinically infected can transmit influenza virus to people at high risk for complications from influenza. Decreasing transmission of influenza from caregivers to people at high risk might reduce influenza-related deaths among people at high risk. Vaccination of health care workers and others in close contact with people at high risk, including household members, is recommended. Therefore, vaccinate the following groups:

1.) Physicians, nurses, and other personnel in hospital and outpatient-care settings, including emergency response workers.
2.) Employees of nursing homes and chronic-care facilities who have contact with patients or residents.
3.) Providers of home care to high-risk people (eg, visiting nurses, volunteer workers).
4.) Household members (including children) of high-risk people.
5.) Employees of assisted living and other residences for people in high-risk groups.

In addition, because children 0 to 23 months of age are at an increased risk for influenza-related hospitalization, vaccination is encouraged for their household contacts and out-of-home caretakers, particularly for contacts of children 0 to 5 months of age because influenza vaccines have not been approved by the FDA for use among children younger than 6 months of age.

➤*General population:* Any individual wishing to reduce the chance of acquiring an influenza infection. People who provide essential community service and students or other people in institutional settings may be considered for vaccination programs to minimize potential disruption of routine activities during outbreaks.

➤*Children:* Because children 6 to 23 months of age are at substantially increased risk for influenza-related hospitalizations, influenza vaccination of all children in this age group is encouraged when feasible.

➤*People infected with HIV:* Limited information exists regarding the frequency and severity of influenza illness in HIV-infected people, but reports suggest that symptoms may be prolonged and the risk of complications increased for some patients in this group. Because influenza may result in serious illness and complications, vaccination is a prudent precaution and will result in protective antibody titers in many recipients. However, the antibody response to vaccine may be low in people with advanced HIV-related illnesses; a booster dose of vaccine has not improved the immune response for these individuals.

➤*Foreign travelers:* The risk of exposure to influenza during foreign travel varies, depending on season and destination. In the tropics, influenza can occur throughout the year. People at high risk for complications of influenza who were not vaccinated with influenza vaccine during the preceding fall or winter should consider receiving influenza vaccine before travel if they plan to do any of the following:

- Travel to the tropics.
- Travel with organized tourist groups at any time of the year.
- Travel to the Southern Hemisphere from April through September.

Revaccinate people at high risk who received the previous season's vaccine before travel with the current vaccine in the following fall or winter. People 50 years of age and older and others at high risk may wish to consult with their physicians before embarking on travel during the summer to discuss the symptoms and risks of influenza and the advisability for carrying antiviral medications for prophylaxis or treatment of influenza.

Administration and Dosage

Do not use remaining 2005 to 2006 vaccine during influenza vaccination for 2006 to 2007.

➤*Fluarix:* The prefilled syringe should be shaken well before administration. Do not inject intravenously (IV).

The dose is a single 0.5 mL injection in adults. Injections should be administered intramuscularly (IM), preferably in the region of the deltoid muscle. The vaccine should not be injected in the gluteal area or areas where there may be a major nerve trunk. A needle length of at least 1 inch is preferred because needles less than 1 inch might be of insufficient length to penetrate muscle tissue in certain adults.

➤*Fluzone:* Do not inject IV. Parenteral drug products should be inspected visually for particulate matter and discoloration prior to administration. Shake well before withdrawing each dose. Give injections IM, preferably in the deltoid muscle for adults and older children. A needle length greater than or equal to 1 inch can be considered for these age groups because needles less than 1 inch might be of insufficient length to penetrate muscle tissue in certain adults and older children. Infants and young children should be vaccinated in the anterolateral aspect of the thigh. When injecting into the deltoid muscle among children with adequate deltoid muscle mass, a needle length of ⅞ to 1¼ inches is recommended. It is recommended that clinicians should use small syringes (0.5 or 1 mL) to minimize any product loss. Before immunization, the skin over the site to be injected should be cleansed with a suitable germicide. After insertion of the needle, aspirate to help avoid inadvertent injection into a blood vessel. The use of needleless injectors for administration is not recommended. Special care should be taken to prevent injection into a blood vessel.

Children younger than 9 years of age who have not previously been vaccinated should receive 2 doses of vaccine 1 month or more apart to maximize the likelihood of a satisfactory antibody response to all 3 vaccine antigens. If possible, the second dose should be administered before December.

This product is to be used for persons 6 months of age and older. It is not approved for infants younger than 6 months of age. The dosage is as follows.

Fluzone Dosage Recommendations by Age Group

Age	Dosage (mL)	Number of doses	Route[a]
6 to 35 months	0.25	1 or 2[b]	IM
3 to 8 years	0.5	1 or 2[b]	IM
≥ 9 years	0.5	1	IM

[a] For adults and older children, the recommended site of vaccination is the deltoid muscle. The preferred site for infants and young children is the anterolateral aspect of the thigh.
[b] Two doses administered at least 1 month apart are recommended for children younger than 9 years of age who are receiving influenza vaccine for the first time.

➤*Fluvirin:* For IM use only. Shake well before withdrawing each dose. Do not inject IV.

Adults and older children should be vaccinated in the deltoid muscle. A needle length of at least 1 inch can be considered for these age groups because needles shorter than 1 inch might be of insufficient length to penetrate muscle tissue in certain adults and older children.

Infants and young children should be vaccinated in the anterolateral aspect of the thigh. When injecting into the deltoid muscle among children with adequate deltoid muscle mass, a needle length of ⅞ to 1¼ inch is recommended. It is recommended that clinicians use small syringes (0.5 to 1 mL) to minimize any product loss. Before immunization, the skin over the site to be injected should be cleansed with a suitable germicide. After insertion of the needle, aspirate to help avoid inadvertent injection into a blood vessel.

Dosage recommendations vary according to age group as follows.

Fluvirin Dosing Schedule

Age group	Dose	Number of doses
< 4 years of age	Vaccine should not be used	
Children 4 through 8 years of age	0.5 mL	1 or 2 doses
9 years of age and older	0.5 mL	1 dose

Among previously unvaccinated children younger than 9 years of age, 2 doses administered at least 1 month apart are recommended for satisfactory antibody responses. If possible, the second dose should be administered before December. If a child younger than 9 years of age receiving vaccine for the first time does not receive a second dose of vaccine within the same season, only one dose of vaccine should be administered the following season. Two doses are not required at that time. Among adults, studies have indicated little or no improvement in antibody response when a second dose is administered during the same season. Because of their decreased potential for causing febrile reactions, only split-virus vaccines should be used for children younger than 13 years of age. The vaccines might be labelled as "split", "subvirion", or "purified surface antigen" vaccine. Doses of 0.25 mL should not be used.

➤*FluMist:* For nasal use only. Do not administer parenterally.

Administer according to the following schedule:

FluMist Dosing Schedule

Age group	Vaccination status	Dosage schedule
Children 5 through 8 years of age	Not previously vaccinated	2 doses (0.5 mL each, 60 days apart ± 14 days) for initial season
Children 5 through 8 years of age	Previously vaccinated with *FluMist*	1 dose (0.5 mL) per season
Children and adults 9 through 49 years of age	Not applicable	1 dose (0.5 mL) per season

For healthy children 5 through 8 years of age previously unvaccinated at anytime with *FluMist* or parenteral vaccine, the recommended dosage schedule for *FluMist* is one 0.5 mL dose followed by a second 0.5 mL dose given 6 weeks later.

For all other healthy individuals, including children 5 through 8 years of age who have previously received at least 1 dose of *FluMist*, the recommended schedule is 1 dose.

FluMist must be thawed prior to administration. *FluMist* may be thawed by holding the sprayer in the palm of the hand and supporting the plunger rod with the thumb; the vaccine must be administered immediately thereafter.

INFLUENZA VIRUS VACCINE

Alternatively, *FluMist* may be thawed in a refrigerator and stored at 2° to 8°C (36° to 46°F) for no more than 60 hours prior to use.

Approximately 0.25 mL (half of the dose from a single *FluMist* sprayer) is administered into each nostril while the recipient is in an upright position. Insert the tip of the sprayer just inside the nose and depress the plunger to spray. The dose divider clip is removed from the sprayer to administer the second half of the dose (approximately 0.25 mL) into the other nostril. Once *FluMist* has been administered, dispose of the used sprayer according to the standard procedures for biohazardous waste products.

➤*Vaccination timing (ACIP guidelines):* Beginning each September, offer influenza vaccines to people at high risk when they are seen by health care providers. Begin vaccinating children younger than 9 years of age who are receiving the vaccine for the first time in October because they need a booster dose 1 month after the initial dose. The optimal time to vaccinate is usually from October through November because influenza activity in the United States generally peaks between late December and early March. Therefore, although the timing of influenza activity can vary by region, vaccine administered after November is likely to be beneficial in most influenza seasons. Adults develop peak antibody protection against influenza infection 2 weeks after vaccination. To minimize the possibility that large organized vaccination campaigns will need to be cancelled because vaccine is unavailable, people planning substantial organized vaccination campaigns may consider scheduling these events after mid-October because the availability of vaccine in any location cannot be assured consistently in the early fall. Administering vaccine before October generally should be avoided in facilities such as nursing homes because antibody levels can begin to decline within a few months after vaccination.

➤*Storage/Stability:*

Parenteral – Store between 2° to 8°C (36° to 46°F). Freezing destroys potency; do not use vaccine if it has been frozen.

Inhalational – Store at or below −15°C (5°F). Do not refreeze after thawing. Upon receipt, immediately store *FluMist* at −15°C (5°F) or below. *FluMist* may be thawed in a refrigerator and stored at 2° to 8°C (36° to 46°F) for no more than 60 hours prior to use.

Actions

➤*Pharmacology:* Influenza A viruses are classified into subtypes on the basis of the following 2 surface antigens: hemagglutinin (H) and neuraminidase (N). A person's immunity to the surface antigens, especially hemagglutinin, reduces the likelihood of infection and severity of disease if infection occurs.

Influenza vaccines are standardized to contain the hemagglutinins of strains (typically 2 type A and 1 type B), representing the influenza viruses likely to circulate in the United States in the upcoming influenza season. The vaccine is made from highly purified, egg-grown viruses that have been made noninfectious (inactivated). Subvirion and purified surface-antigen preparations are available. Because the vaccine viruses initially are grown in embryonated hens' eggs, the vaccine might contain small amounts of residual egg protein.

The trivalent influenza vaccine prepared for the 2006 to 2007 season will include A/New Caledonia/20/99 (H1N1), A/Wisconsin/67/2005 (H3N2), and B/Malaysia/2506/2004 antigens. Manufacturers may use the antigenically equivalent A/Wisconsin/67/2005 NYMC X-161 virus for the A/Wisconsin/67/2005 (H3N2) virus, and may use the antigenically equivalent A/New Caledonia/20/99 IVR-116 virus for the A/New Caledonia/20/99 (H1N1) virus.. These viruses will be used because of their growth properties, and because they are representative of influenza viruses likely to circulate in the United States during the 2006 to 2007 influenza season.

The influenza vaccine is available as a split-virus (synonymous with subvirion or purified surface antigen) preparation. Because of their decreased potential for causing febrile reactions, only split-virus vaccines should be used for children younger than 13 years of age. The vaccines might be labelled as "split," "subviron," or "purified-surface-antigen" vaccine. Doses of 0.25 mL should not be used.

FluMist contains live attenuated influenza viruses that replicate in the nasopharynx of the recipient and are shed in respiratory secretions. Assessing the probability that these shed vaccine viruses will be transmitted from a vaccinated individual to a nonvaccinated individual was the primary objective of a prospective, randomized, double-blind, placebo-controlled trial in a daycare setting in Finland. Of *FluMist* recipients, 80% shed at least 1 vaccine strain, with a mean duration of shedding 7.6 days (range, 1 to 21 days). Assuming that a single transmission event occurred (isolation of the Type B vaccine strain), the probability of a young child acquiring vaccine virus following close contact with a single *FluMist* vaccinee in this daycare setting was 0.58%.

Contraindications

Hypersensitivity to any component of the vaccine; hypersensitivity to eggs or egg products or chicken proteins. Before being vaccinated, give a skin test to people suspected of being hypersensitive to egg protein, using the influenza virus vaccine as the antigen. Do not vaccinate people with adverse reactions to such testing. Chemoprophylaxis (with amantadine or rimantadine) may be indicated for prevention of influenza A in such people. The vaccine is also contraindicated in individuals hypersensitive to any component of the vaccine, including thimerosal (a mercury derivative).

Do not administer the influenza virus vaccine to patients with a history of Guillain-Barré syndrome (GBS). However, the ACIP recommends influenza vaccination in patients with a history of GBS who are at a high risk for severe complications from influenza.

Defer vaccination in patients with acute febrile illnesses (and/or respiratory illness for at least 72 hours [*FluMist* only]), until their symptoms have abated. Minor illnesses, with or without fever, are not contraindicated in the use of influenza virus vaccine, particularly in children with a mild upper respiratory tract infection or allergic rhinitis.

Delay immunization in patients with an active neurologic disorder characterized by changing neurological findings until stabilized. The occurrence of any neurological symptoms after vaccination is a contraindication for further use.

➤*FluMist*: Under no circumstances should *FluMist* be administered parenterally.

FluMist is contraindicated in children and adolescents 5 to 17 years of age receiving aspirin therapy or aspirin-containing therapy because of the association of Reye syndrome with aspirin and wild-type influenza infection.

As with other live virus vaccines, do not administer *FluMist* to individuals with known or suspected immune deficiency diseases such as combined immunodeficiency, agammaglobulinemia, and thymic abnormalities, and conditions such as HIV infection, malignancy, leukemia, or lymphoma. *FluMist* is also contraindicated in patients who may be immunosuppressed or have altered or compromised immune status as a consequence of treatment with systemic corticosteroids, alkylating drugs, antimetabolites, radiation, or other immunosuppressive therapies.

Warnings

➤*Postvaccination (FluMist)*: Because of the possible transmission of vaccine virus, vaccine recipients or their parents/guardians should be advised to avoid close contact (eg, within the same household) with immunocompromised individuals for at least 21 days. Healthcare workers should refrain from contact with severely immunosuppressed patients for 7 days after vaccine receipt.

➤*Asthma/Reactive airways disease:* The safety of *FluMist* in individuals with asthma or reactive airways disease has not been established. In a large safety study in children 1 to 17 years of age, children under 5 years of age who received *FluMist* were found to have an increased rate of asthma within 42 days of vaccination compared with placebo recipients. Do not administer *FluMist* to individuals with a history of asthma or reactive airways disease.

➤*Impaired immune response:* Patients with impaired immune responsiveness, whether caused by the use of immunosuppressive therapy (including irradiation, large amounts of corticosteroids, antimetabolites, alkylating agents, and cytotoxic agents), a genetic defect, HIV infection, AIDS, leukemia, lymphoma, generalized malignancy, or other causes, may have a reduced antibody response to active immunization procedures and may remain susceptible despite immunization. Chemoprophylaxis of influenza A with amantadine or rimantadine may be indicated.

The safety of *FluMist* in individuals with underlying medical conditions that may predispose them to severe disease following wild-type influenza infection has not been established. *FluMist* is not indicated for these individuals. According to the ACIP, such individuals include, but are not limited to, adults and children with chronic disorders of the cardiovascular and pulmonary systems (including asthma), pregnant women, adults and children who required regular medical follow-up or hospitalization during the preceding year because of chronic metabolic diseases (including diabetes), renal dysfunction, or hemoglobinopathies; and adults and children with congenital or acquired immunosuppression caused by underlying disease or immunosuppressive therapy. IM administered inactivated influenza vaccines are available to immunize high-risk individuals. Severely immunosuppressed persons should not administer *FluMist*.

➤*People infected with HIV:* Limited information exists regarding the frequency and severity of influenza illness or the benefits of influenza vaccination among people with HIV infection. Reports suggest influenza symptoms may be prolonged and the risk for complications increased. Vaccination will benefit many HIV-infected patients. However, in patients with advanced HIV-related illnesses, the antibody response for vaccination may be low; a booster dose has not improved the immune response for these individuals.

➤*Thrombocytopenia/Blood coagulation disorders:* Do not give influenza virus vaccine to individuals with thrombocytopenia or any coagulation disorder that would contraindicate IM injection unless, in the judgement of the health care provider, the potential benefits clearly outweigh the risk of administration.

➤*Hypersensitivity reactions:* Have epinephrine 1:1,000 immediately available. Refer to Management of Acute Hypersensitivity Reactions.

➤*Pregnancy: Category C.* It is not known whether the influenza virus vaccine can cause fetal harm when administered to a pregnant woman. Do not administer *FluMist* to pregnant women. The ACIP recommends parenteral vaccination for women who will be pregnant during influenza season.

A study of influenza vaccination of more than 2,000 pregnant women demonstrated no adverse fetal effects associated with parenteral influenza vaccine. However, more data are needed to confirm the safety of vaccination during pregnancy. Some experts prefer to administer influenza vaccine during the second trimester to avoid a coincidental association with spontaneous abortion, which is common in the first trimester, and because exposures to vaccines traditionally have been avoided during the first trimester.

➤*Lactation:*

Parenteral – Influenza vaccine does not affect the safety of breast-feeding for mothers or infants.

Inhalational – It is not known whether *FluMist* is excreted in human milk. Therefore, because some viruses are excreted in human milk and because of the possibility of vaccine virus shedding and the close proximity

INFLUENZA VIRUS VACCINE

of a breast-feeding infant and mother, exercise caution if *FluMist* is administered to breast-feeding mothers.

➤*Children:* Safety and efficacy of *Fluzone* have not been established in infants younger than 6 months of age. The safety and efficacy of *Fluvirin* in children younger than 4 years of age have not been established. The safety of *FluMist* in infants and children younger than 60 months of age has not been established.

Precautions

➤*Concurrent vaccination:* The target groups for influenza and pneumococcal vaccination overlap considerably. For people at high risk who have not previously been vaccinated with pneumococcal vaccine, health care providers should strongly consider administering pneumococcal and influenza vaccines concurrently. Both vaccines can be administered at the same time, using separate syringes, and at different sites without increasing side effects. However, influenza vaccine is administered each year, whereas pneumococcal vaccine is not. Children at high risk for influenza-related complications, including those 6 to 23 months of age, can receive influenza vaccine at the same time they receive other routine vaccinations.

➤*Seroconversion:* Vaccination may not result in seroconversion in all individuals.

➤*Latex:* Dry, natural latex rubber may be contained in vial stoppers.

➤*GBS:* During 3 of 4 influenza seasons studied from 1977 through 1991, the overall relative risk estimates for GBS after influenza vaccination were elevated slightly, but were not statistically significant in any of these studies. However, in a study of the 1992 to 1993 and 1993 to 1994 seasons, the overall relative risk for GBS was 1.7 (95% confidence intervals = 1 to 2.8; $P = 0.04$) during the 6 weeks following vaccination, representing approximately 1 additional case of GBS per million people vaccinated; the combined number of GBS cases peaked 2 weeks after vaccination. Thus, investigations to date suggest no large increase in GBS associated with influenza vaccines (other than the swine influenza vaccine of 1976) and that if influenza vaccine does pose a risk, it is probably slightly more than 1 additional case per million people vaccinated.

The incidence of GBS in the general population is low, but people with a history of GBS have a substantially greater likelihood of subsequently developing GBS than people without such a history. Thus, the likelihood of coincidentally developing GBS after influenza vaccination is expected to be greater among people with a history of GBS than among people with no history of this syndrome. Whether influenza vaccination specifically might increase the risk for recurrence of GBS is not known. The potential benefits of influenza vaccination in preventing serious illness, hospitalization, and death substantially outweigh the possible risks for developing vaccine-associated GBS. The average case-fatality ratio for GBS is 6% and increases with age. No evidence indicates that the case-fatality ratio for GBS differs among vaccinated persons and those not vaccinated.

➤*Thimerosal sensitivity:* Hypersensitivity reactions to any vaccine component can occur. Although exposure to vaccines containing thimerosal can lead to induction of hypersensitivity, most patients do not develop reactions to thimerosal when it is administered as a component of vaccines, even when patch or intradermal tests for thimerosal indicate hypersensitivity. When reported, hypersensitivity to thimerosal usually has consisted of local, delayed-type hypersensitivity reactions.

Drug Interactions

➤*Aspirin:* See Contraindications for more information.

➤*Antivirals:* The concurrent use of *FluMist* with antiviral compounds that are active against influenza A and/or B viruses has not been evaluated. However, based upon the potential for interference between such compounds and *FluMist*, it is advisable not to administer *FluMist* until 48 hours after the cessation of antiviral therapy and that antiviral agents not be administered until 2 weeks after administration of *FluMist* unless medically indicated.

➤*Other vaccines:* The safety and immunogenicity of *FluMist* when administered concurrently with other vaccines have not been determined. Therefore, *FluMist* should not be administered concurrently with other vaccines. Studies of *FluMist* in healthy individuals excluded subjects who received any live virus vaccine within 1 month of enrollment and any inactivated or subunit vaccine within 2 weeks of enrollment; therefore, health care providers should adhere to these intervals when administering *FluMist*.

➤*Drug/Lab test interactions:* Nasopharyngeal secretions or swabs collected from *FluMist* vaccinees may test positive for influenza virus for up to 3 weeks.

Adverse Reactions

➤*Parenteral:*

CNS – Neurological disorders temporally associated with influenza vaccination such as encephalopathy, unspecified neuritis, encephalitis, peripheral nerve disease, paresthesia, hypesthesia, brachial neuritis, demyelinating disease, labyrinthitis, meningitis, allergic asthma, systemic anaphylaxis, encephalopathy, optic neuritis/neuropathy, partial facial paralysis, and brachial plexus neuropathy have been reported; however, no cause-and-effect has been established. Transverse myelitis has been reported rarely. Almost all persons affected were adults, and the clinical reactions began as soon as a few hours and as late as 2 weeks after vaccination; full recovery was almost always reported.

Local – The most frequent side effect (affecting 10% to 64% of patients) was soreness at the injection site that lasted up to 2 days.

Systemic – Fever, malaise, myalgia, and other symptoms occur more often in young children and others who have had no exposure to the influenza virus antigens. These reactions begin 6 to 12 hours after vaccination and persist for 1 to 2 days.

Immediate, presumably allergic responses (eg, hives, angioedema, allergic asthma, systemic anaphylaxis) have occurred rarely, probably resulting from hypersensitivity to some vaccine component, most likely residual egg protein.

Microscopic polyangitis (vasculitis) has been reported temporally associated with influenza vaccination.

➤*FluMist:*

Children –

FluMist Adverse Reactions Observed Within 10 Days After Each Dose for Healthy Children 60 to 71 Months of Age[a]

Adverse reaction	Postdose 1 *FluMist* (n = 214)[b]	Postdose 1 Placebo (n = 95)[b]	Postdose 2 *FluMist* (n = 161)[b]	Postdose 2 Placebo (n = 75)[b]
Any reaction	65%	62.1%	66.5%	53.3%
Chills	6.1%	5.3%	2.5%	4%
Cough	25.7%	32.6%	38.5%	30.7%
Decreased activity	14%	12.6%	10.6%	13.3%
Fever[c]				
Temp 1	10.3%	9.5%	4.3%	4%
Temp 2	2.3%	2.1%	0.6%	1.3%
Temp 3	0%	0%	0%	0%
Headache	17.8%	11.6%	6.8%	16%
Irritability	17.8%	15.8%	9.9%	9.3%
Muscle aches	6.1%	4.2%	5%	4%
Runny nose/nasal congestion	48.1%	44.2%	46%	32%
Sore throat	12.6%	19.8%	9.3%	16%
Vomiting	4.7%	3.2%	5.6%	12%

[a] There were no statistically significant differences in any of these reactions (*P*-value > 0.05); Fisher's Exact method.
[b] Number of evaluable subjects (those who returned diary cards) for each reaction.
[c] Fever: Temp 1 - Oral more than 100°F, rectal or aural more than 100.6°F, or axillary more than 99.6°F; temp 2 - oral more than 102°F, rectal or aural more than 102.6°F, or axillary more than 101.6°F; temp 3 - oral more than 104°F, rectal or aural more than 104.6°F, axillary more than 103.6°F.

Among healthy children 60 to 71 months in the pediatric efficacy study, the reactions that occurred in at least 1% of *FluMist* recipients and at a higher rate compared with placebo were abdominal pain (3.7% *FluMist* vs 0% placebo), otitis media (1.4% *FluMist* vs 0% placebo), accidental injury (2.3% *FluMist* vs 2.1% placebo), diarrhea (3.7% *FluMist* vs 1.1% placebo), following dose 1 and otitis media (3.1% *FluMist* vs 1.3% placebo) following dose 2. None of these differences were statistically significant.

Adults –

FluMist Adverse Reactions Observed Within 7 Days in Healthy Adults 18 to 49 Years of Age

Adverse reaction	*FluMist* (n = 2,548)[a]	Placebo (n = 1,290)[a]
Any reaction	71.9%[b]	62.6%
Chills	8.6%[b]	6%
Cough	13.9%[b]	10.8%
Fever		
Oral temp > 100°F	1.5%	1.3%
Oral temp > 101°F	0.5%	0.7%
Oral temp > 102°F	0.1%	0.2%
Oral temp > 103°F	0%	0%
Headache	40.4%	38.4%
Muscle aches	16.7%	14.6%
Runny nose	44.5%[b]	27.1%
Sore throat	27.8%[b]	17.1%
Tiredness/weakness	25.7%[b]	21.6%

[a] Denotes statistically significant *P*-value ≤ 0.05; no adjustments for multiple comparisons; Fisher's Exact Method.
[b] Number of evaluable subjects (those who returned diary cards): 97.9% of *FluMist* recipients and 97.9% of placebo recipients.

For adults 18 to 49 years of age in the adult effectiveness study, nasal congestion (9.2% *FluMist* vs 2.2% placebo), rhinitis (6.3% *FluMist* vs 3.1% placebo), and sinusitis (4.1% *FluMist* vs 2.2% placebo) were reported significantly more often by *FluMist* recipients compared with placebo recipients.

Postmarketing – Nausea, rash, epistaxis, and hypersensitivity reactions (including anaphylaxis, facial edema, and urticaria).

INFLUENZA VIRUS VACCINE

Patient Information

Prior to administration of this vaccine, inform the parent, guardian, or adult patient of the benefits and risks of immunization against influenza.

➤*FluMist:* Inform vaccine recipients or their parents/guardians of the potential benefits and risks of *FluMist* and the need for 2 doses for the first use of *FluMist* in children 5 to 8 years of age. Because of the possible transmission of vaccine virus, advise vaccine recipients or their parents/guardians to avoid close contact (eg, within the same household) with immunocompromised individuals for at least 21 days.

Tell the vaccine recipient or the parent/guardian accompanying the vaccine recipient to report any suspected adverse reactions to their health care provider or clinic where the vaccine was administered.

JAPANESE ENCEPHALITIS VIRUS VACCINE

Rx	**JE-VAX** (Connaught)	**Powder for Injection, lyophilized**[a,b]	In single-dose vial with 1.3 ml diluent (sterile water for injection) and 10 dose vial with 11 ml diluent (sterile water for injection).

[a] Potency is determined by immunizing mice with either the test vaccine or the JE Reference Vaccine. Neutralizing antibodies are measured in a plaque-neutralization assay performed on sera from the immunized mice. The potency of the test vaccine must be no less than that of the reference vaccine.

[b] With thimerosal 0.007%. Each 1 ml dose contains ≈ 500 mcg gelatin, < 100 mcg formaldehyde and < 50 ng mouse serum protein.

JAPANESE ENCEPHALITIS VIRUS VACCINE

For complete and comparative prescribing information, refer to the Agents for Active Immunization introduction.

Indications

➤*Japanese encephalitis (JE) vaccination:* For active immunization against JE for persons one year of age and older.

➤*Patient selection:* JE vaccine should be considered for use in persons who plan to reside in or travel to areas where JE is endemic or epidemic during a transmission season. JE vaccine is not recommended for all persons traveling to or residing in Asia. The incidence of JE in the location of intended stay, the conditions of housing, nature of activities, duration of stay, and the possibility of unexpected travel to high-risk areas are factors that should be considered in the decision to administer vaccine. In general, vaccine should be considered for use in persons spending a month or longer in epidemic or endemic areas during the transmission season, especially if travel will include rural areas. Depending on the epidemic circumstances, vaccine should be considered for persons spending less than 30 days whose activities, such as extensive outdoor activities in rural areas, place them at particularly high risk for exposure.

➤*Elderly / Pregnancy:* Advanced age may be a risk factor for developing symptomatic illness after infection. JE acquired during pregnancy carries the potential for intrauterine infection and fetal death. These factors should be considered when advising elderly persons and pregnant women who plan visits to JE endemic areas.

➤*Research laboratory workers:* Laboratory-acquired JE has been reported in 22 cases. JE virus may be transmitted in a laboratory setting through needle sticks and other accidental exposures. Vaccine-derived immunity presumably protects against exposure through these percutaneous routes. Exposure to aerosolized JE virus, and particularly to high concentrations of virus, such as may occur during viral purification, potentially could lead to infection through mucous membranes and possibly directly into the central nervous system through the olfactory mucosa. It is unknown whether vaccine-derived immunity protects against such exposures, but immunization is recommended for all laboratory workers with a potential for exposure to infectious JE virus.

➤*Protection:* As with any vaccine, vaccination with JE vaccine may not result in protection in all individuals. Long-term protection, as demonstrated by persistence of neutralizing antibody for more than 2 years, has not yet been shown.

Administration and Dosage

➤*Approved by the FDA:* December 10, 1992.

➤*Recommended dose:* For persons 3 years of age and older, a single dose is 1 mL of vaccine. For children 1 year to 3 years of age, a single dose is 0.5 mL of vaccine (see Primary immunization schedule).

➤*Single-dose vial of lyophilized vaccine:* Remove plastic tab of flip-off cap. Do not remove rubber stopper. Cleanse stopper with a suitable disinfectant. Reconstitute only with the supplied 1.3 mL of diluent (sterile water for injection). Shake vial thoroughly. After reconstitution the vaccine should be stored between 2° to 8°C (35° to 46°F) and used within 8 hours. Do not freeze reconstituted vaccine.

➤*Ten-dose vial of lyophilized vaccine:* Remove plastic tab of flip-off cap. Do not remove rubber stopper. Cleanse stopper with a suitable disinfectant. Reconstitute only with the supplied 11 mL of diluent (sterile water for injection). Shake vial thoroughly. After reconstitution the vaccine should be stored between 2° to 8°C (35° to 46°F) and used within 8 hours. Do not freeze reconstituted vaccine.

➤*For subcutaneous use only:* The vaccine is to be given by subcutaneous administration only.

➤*Primary immunization schedule:* The recommended primary immunization series is three doses of 1 mL each for individuals older than 3 years of age given subcutaneously on days 0, 7, and 30. For children 1 to 3 years of age a series of 3 doses of 0.5 mL each should be given subcutaneously on days 0, 7, and 30. An abbreviated schedule of days 0, 7, and 14 can be used when the longer schedule is impractical because of time constraints. (When it is impossible to follow one of the above recommended schedules, 2 doses given a week apart will induce antibodies in ≈ 80% of vaccinees; however, this 2-dose regimen should not be used except under unusual circumstances). The last dose should be given at least 10 days before the commencement of international travel to ensure an adequate immune response and access to medical care in the event of delayed adverse reactions.

➤*Booster dose:* A booster dose of 1 mL (0.5 mL for children from 1 to 3 years of age) may be given after 2 years. In the absence of firm data on the persistence of antibody after primary immunization, a definite recommendation cannot be made on the spacing of boosters beyond 2 years.

➤*Children:* There are no data on the safety and efficacy of JE vaccine in infants under 1 year of age. Whenever possible, immunization of infants should be deferred until they are 1 year of age or older.

➤*Administration:* The skin at the site of injection first should be cleansed and disinfected. Shake vial thoroughly before each use. Cleanse top of rubber stopper of the vial with a suitable antiseptic and wipe away all excess before withdrawing vaccine.

➤*Concurrent vaccine:* When JE vaccine and any other vaccines are given concurrently, separate syringes and separate sites should be used.

➤*Storage / Stability:* The vaccine should be stored between 2° to 8°C (35° to 46°F). Do not freeze. After reconstitution the vaccine should be stored between 2° to 8°C (35° to 46°F) and used within 8 hours. Do not freeze reconstituted vaccine.

Actions

➤*Pharmacology:* Japanese encephalitis (JE), a mosquito-borne arboviral Flavivirus infection, is the leading cause of viral encephalitis in Asia.

A 3-dose vaccination schedule is recommended for US travelers and military personnel, based on the CDC experience and on a controlled immunogenicity trial performed in US military personnel. The CDC experience demonstrated that neutralizing antibody was produced in fewer than 80% of vaccinees following 2 doses of vaccine in US travelers and antibody levels declined substantially in most vaccinees within 6 months. The US Army studied the immunogenicity of JE vaccine in 538 volunteers. Two 3-dose regimens were evaluated (day 0, 7, and 14 or day 0, 7, and 30). All vaccine recipients demonstrated neutralizing antibodies at 2 months and 6 months after initiation of vaccination. The schedule of day 0, 7, and 30 produced higher antibody responses than the day 0, 7, and 14 schedule. Two hundred and seventy-three of the original study participants were tested at 12 months post-vaccination and there was no longer a statistical difference in antibody titers between the 2 vaccination regimens.

The full duration of protection is unknown. Of US Army volunteers completing a three-dose regimen, 252 agreed to receive a booster dose of vaccine 1 year after the primary series. All boosted participants still had antibody 12 months after the booster. Protective levels of neutralizing antibody persisted for 24 months (2 years) in all 21 persons who had not received a booster. Definitive recommendations cannot be given on the timing of booster doses at this time.

Contraindications

Adverse reactions to a prior dose of JE vaccine manifesting as generalized urticaria and angioedema; proven or suspected hypersensitivity to proteins of rodent or neural origin; hypersensitivity to thimerosal.

Warnings

See Precautions for more information.

➤*Hypersensitivity reactions:* Persons with a history of urticaria after hymenoptera envenomation, drugs, physical or other provocations, or of idiopathic cause appear to have a greater risk of developing reactions to JE vaccine (relative risk 9.1, 95% confidence interval 1.8 to 50.9). This history should be considered when weighing risks and benefits of the vaccine for an individual patient. When patients with such a history are offered JE vaccine, they should be alerted to their increased risk for reaction and monitored appropriately. There are no data supporting the efficacy of prophylactic antihistamines or steroids in preventing JE vaccine-related allergic reactions.

Another case control study consisting of 5 cases and 15 controls identified an increased risk of hypersensitivity reactions to JE vaccine in individuals who had unusual alcohol consumption during the 2 days following vaccination ($p = 0.005$). Recipients should be advised to avoid more than the usual alcohol intake during the 48 hours following JE vaccination.

In the same study an increased risk for hypersensitivity reactions was seen in individuals who received other vaccines within the 7-day period prior to receipt of JE vaccine. Where possible JE vaccine should be administered concurrently with other vaccines.

➤*Pregnancy: Category C.* Animal reproduction studies have not been conducted with JE vaccine. It is not known whether JE vaccine can cause fetal harm when administered to a pregnant woman or can affect reproductive capacity. Pregnant women who must travel to an area where risk of JE is

JAPANESE ENCEPHALITIS VIRUS VACCINE

high should be immunized when the theoretical risks of immunization are outweighed by the risk of infection to the mother and developing fetus. JE vaccine should be given to a pregnant woman only if clearly needed.

➤*Lactation:* It is not known whether JE vaccine is excreted in human milk. Because many drugs are excreted in human milk, caution should be exercised when JE vaccine is administered to a nursing woman.

➤*Children:* See Administration and Dosage for more information.

Precautions

➤*Monitoring:* Vaccinees should be observed for 30 minutes after vaccination and warned about the possibility of delayed generalized urticaria, often in a generalized distribution or angioedema of the extremities, face and oropharynx, especially of the lips.

➤*Anaphylactoid reaction:* Epinephrine injection (1:1000) must be immediately available should an acute anaphylactic reaction occur due to any component of the vaccine.

➤*Antibody titers:* Although substantial neutralizing antibody titers are elicited by JE vaccine in more than 90% of US travelers without history of JE immunization or of exposure to JE, the precise relationship between antibody level and efficacy has not been established even though these titers persisted for at least 2 years after immunization.

Adverse Reactions

➤*Local and systemic adverse reactions:* JE vaccine is associated with a moderate frequency of local and mild systemic adverse effects. Tenderness, redness, swelling and other local effects have been reported in about 20% of vaccinees (less than 1% to 31%). Systemic side effects, principally fever, headache, malaise, rash, and other reactions, such as chills, dizziness, myalgia, nausea, vomiting and abdominal pain have been reported in approximately 10% of vaccinees.

In a study conducted by the CDC, less than 5% of the 1756 US travelers immunized with a 3-dose regimen of the vaccine reported headache, flu-like symptoms, fever, and other systemic complaints. Hives and facial swelling were reported in 0.2% and 0.1% of vaccinees, respectively. Local soreness occurred in 5.9% and local redness in 2.9%. There was no increase in the number or severity of reactions with increasing numbers of doses.

The US Army studied 4034 personnel from 1987 to 1989. Using a 2- or 3-dose regimen of JE vaccine, arm soreness was described in 22.7%, local redness in 4.8%, headache in 15.2%, and a febrile episode in 5.5%. In another trial evaluating the safety and immunogenicity of a three-dose immunizing series (day 0, 7, and 30 or day 0, 7, and 14), performed in 538 adult volunteers in 1990, the Army determined that local soreness and redness occurred in 21% of vaccinees after the first dose, then decreased with subsequent injections ($p < 0.0001$, Chi-square for downward trend). Systemic symptoms including feverishness, headache and rash occurred in 5% of vaccinees after the first dose, then decreased with subsequent injections ($p < 0.001$, Chi-square for downward trend). Participants who received the third dose on day 14 reported more side effects than those who received the injection on day 30. Among these volunteers, 252 received a booster injection of vaccine 1 year after receiving the first dose of the primary series. Side effects reported after the booster injection included local symptoms of soreness (24.5%) and redness (6.1%) at the injection site and systemic complaints of headache (4.9%), fever (1.6%), and rash (0.8%). Less than 1% of all reported symptoms was graded as severe. No generalized urticaria or anaphylaxis was reported.

Since 1989, an apparently new pattern of adverse reactions has been reported among vaccinees in Europe, North America, and Australia. The reactions have been characterized by urticaria, often in a generalized distribution, or angioedema of the extremities, face, especially of the lips and oropharynx. Three vaccine recipients developed respiratory distress. Distress or collapse due to hypotension or other causes led to hospitalization in several cases. Most reactions were treated successfully with antihistamines or oral steroids; however some patients were hospitalized for parenteral steroid therapy. Three patients developed an erythema multiforme or erythema nodosum and some patients have had joint swelling. Some vaccinees complained of generalized itching without objective evidence of a rash.

An important feature of the reactions has been the interval between vaccination and onset of symptoms. Reactions after a first vaccine dose occurred after a median of 12 hours after immunization (88% of reactions occurred within 3 days). The interval between administration of a second dose and onset of symptoms generally was longer, (median 3 days and possibly as long as 2 weeks). Reactions have occurred after a second or third dose, when preceding doses were received uneventfully.

Between November 1991 and May 1992, the US Navy immunized 35,253 US personnel (marines, other military and dependents) with JE vaccine on Okinawa. The overall reaction rate, 62.4 per 10,000 vaccinees (95% confidence interval 54.2 to 70.6) includes persons reporting urticaria, angioedema, generalized itching and wheezing. The reaction rate per 10,000 vaccinees was 26.7 (95% confidence interval 21.3 to 32.1), 30.8 (95% confidence interval 24.6 to 37) or 12.2 (95% confidence interval 7.9 to 16.5) after the first, second or third dose, respectively. These reactions were generally mild to moderate in severity. Nine out of 35,253 persons immunized were hospitalized (2.6 per 10,000 vaccinees) primarily to allow administration of intravenous steroids for refractory urticaria. None of these reactions were considered life-threatening.

A case-control study conducted as part of the JE immunization campaign in Okinawa found that persons developing these reactions after JE vaccination were more likely to have had a history of urticaria after hymenoptera envenomation, drugs, physical or other provocations or of idiopathic origins (relative risk 9.1, 95% confidence interval 1.8 to 50.9). The vaccine constituents responsible for these adverse reactions have not been identified.

➤*Other serious adverse reactions:* Other serious adverse events reported following vaccination include (1) one case of Guillain-Barré syndrome after JE vaccination has been reported in the United States since 1984 (this patient was diagnosed as having mononucleosis 3 weeks before the onset of weakness); (2) one case of urticaria, hepatitis and respiratory failure 1 week after dose 2 (this person showed effusion and infiltrate on chest x-ray and eosinophilia); (3) one case of respiratory and renal failure 1 week after a dose (this 26-month-old male had infiltrate on chest x-ray and acid fast bacilli in sputum); and (4) one case of newly diagnosed hypertension in a young adult male presenting with a headache several hours after receiving dose 1. The relationship of JE vaccine to the etiology of these adverse events is unknown.

Optic neuritis has been reported for 1 patient. In addition to JE vaccine, this patient concurrently received a number of other vaccines.

Fatal myocarditis has been reported in a patient who had recently been given meningococcal vaccine and at least 1 dose of JE vaccine. Any causal role for the vaccines is unclear.

Sudden death occurred ≈ 60 hours after receiving the first dose of JE vaccine in a 21-year-old US military person with a history of recurrent hypersensitivity and an episode of possible anaphylaxis. This person also received the third dose of plague vaccine ≈ 12 to 15 hours prior to the death. There was no evidence of urticaria or angioedema. Cause of death was not established at autopsy.

Surveillance of JE vaccine related complications in Japan from 1965 to 1973 disclosed neurologic events (primarily encephalitis, encephalopathy, seizures, and peripheral neuropathy) in 1 to 2.3 per million vaccinees. Very rarely, deaths occurred with vaccine-associated encephalitis. Between 1987 and 1989, two cases of neurologic dysfunction were reported from Japan; one of these was a transverse myelitis, while the second included seizures, cranial nerve paresis, cerebellar ataxia, and behavior disorder. In 1992, two cases of acute disseminated encephalomyelitis were reported from Japan; one occurred 14 days after the second dose and the second occurred 17 days after a booster dose of JE vaccine. Both cases recovered. One case of Bell's palsy was reported from Thailand.

Patient Information

JE vaccine is given to provide immunization against Japanese encephalitis virus.

A 3-dose immunizing series should be completed, except in unusual circumstances (see Contraindications and Administration and Dosage).

JE vaccine should be given to a pregnant woman only if, in the opinion of a physician, withholding the vaccine entails even greater risk.

Any adverse events following JE vaccine should be reported through the Vaccine Adverse Event Reporting System (VAERS) 1-800-822-7967 after contacting the physician immediately.

If the patient has a history of urticaria (hives) (following hymenoptera envenomation, drugs, physical or other provocation or of idiopathic origin), adverse effects are more likely.

Adverse events consisting of arm soreness and local redness can occur shortly after vaccination.

Adverse events consisting of headache, rash, edema and generalized urticaria or angioedema may occur shortly after vaccination or up to 17 days (usually within 10 days) following vaccination.

International travel should not be initiated within 10 days of vaccination with JE vaccine because of the possibility of delayed adverse reactions. Patients should be instructed to seek medical attention immediately upon onset of any adverse reaction.

Personal precautions should be taken to avoid exposure to mosquito bites by the use of insect repellents, and protective clothing. Avoiding outdoor activity, especially during twilight periods and in the evening, will reduce risk even further.

ROTAVIRUS VACCINE LIVE

Rx	**RotaTeq** (Merck)	**Oral liquid:** Minimum dose levels — 2.2×10^6 infectious units rotavirus outer capsid protein G1, 2.8×10^6 infectious units rotavirus outer capsid protein G2, 2.2×10^6 infectious units rotavirus outer capsid protein G3, 2×10^6 infectious units rotavirus outer capsid protein G4, and 2.3×10^6 infectious units rotavirus attachment protein P1A per 2 mL	Preservative free. Sucrose. In 2 mL single-dose tubes (1s and 10s).

ROTAVIRUS VACCINE, LIVE — ORAL

Indications

➤*Rotavirus gastroenteritis prevention:* For the prevention of rotavirus gastroenteritis in infants and children caused by the serotypes G1, G2, G3, and G4 when administered as a 3-dose series to infants between 6 and 32 weeks of age. Administer the first dose of rotavirus vaccine when the patient is between 6 and 12 weeks of age.

Administration and Dosage

➤*Approved by the FDA:* February 3, 2006.

ROTAVIRUS VACCINE, LIVE — ORAL

➤*Vaccination schedule:* The vaccination series consists of 3 ready-to-use liquid doses of rotavirus vaccine administered orally starting when the patient is 6 to 12 weeks of age, with the subsequent doses administered at 4- to 10-week intervals. The third dose should not be given after the patient reaches 32 weeks of age.

➤*Administration:* For oral use only. Not for injection. Do not reconstitute or dilute.

There are no restrictions on the infant's consumption of food or liquid, including breast milk, either before or after vaccination with rotavirus vaccine.

Each dose is supplied in a container consisting of a squeezable plastic, latex-free dosing tube with a twist-off cap, allowing for direct oral administration. The dosing tube is contained in a pouch.

➤*Admixture incompatibility:* Do not mix the rotavirus vaccine with any other vaccines or solutions.

➤*Instructions for use:* To administer the vaccine, tear open the pouch and remove the dosing tube. Clear the fluid from the dispensing tip by holding the tube vertically and tapping the cap. Open the dosing tube in 2 easy motions (puncture the dispensing tip by screwing the cap clockwise until it becomes tight and then remove the cap by turning it counterclockwise).

Administer the dose by gently squeezing the liquid into the infant's mouth toward the inner cheek until the dosing tube is empty. (A residual drop may remain in the tip of the tube.)

If for any reason an incomplete dose is administered (eg, infant spits or regurgitates the vaccine), a replacement dose is not recommended because such dosing was not studied in the clinical trials. The infant should continue to receive any remaining doses in the recommended series.

Discard the empty tube and cap in approved biological waste containers according to local regulations.

➤*Use with other vaccines:* In clinical trials, rotavirus vaccine was routinely coadministered with diphtheria and tetanus toxoids and acellular pertussis (DTaP), inactivated poliovirus vaccine (IPV), *Haemophilus influenzae* type b conjugate vaccine (Hib), hepatitis B vaccine, and pneumococcal conjugate vaccine.

There was no evidence for reduced antibody responses to the diphtheria or tetanus toxoid components of DTaP or to the other vaccines that were coadministered with rotavirus vaccine. However, insufficient immunogenicity data are available to confirm lack of interference of immune responses when rotavirus vaccine is coadministered with childhood vaccines to prevent pertussis.

➤*Storage/Stability:* Store and transport refrigerated at 2° to 8°C (36° to 46°F). Rotavirus vaccine should be administered as soon as possible after being removed from refrigeration. Protect from light. Rotavirus vaccine should be discarded in approved biological waste containers according to local regulations. The product must be used before the expiration date. For information regarding stability under conditions other than those recommended, call 1-800-637-2590.

Actions

➤*Pharmacology:* Rotavirus is a leading cause of severe acute gastroenteritis in infants and young children, with over 95% of these children infected by 5 years of age. The most severe cases occur among infants and young children between 6 months and 24 months of age.

The exact immunologic mechanism by which rotavirus vaccine protects against rotavirus gastroenteritis is unknown. Rotavirus vaccine is a live viral vaccine that replicates in the small intestine and induces immunity.

Contraindications

History of hypersensitivity to any component of the vaccine. Do not give further doses of rotavirus vaccine to infants who develop symptoms suggestive of hypersensitivity after receiving a dose of rotavirus vaccine.

Warnings

➤*Children:* Safety and efficacy have not been established in infants younger than 6 weeks of age or older than 32 weeks of age.

Data are available from clinical studies to support the use of rotavirus vaccine in preterm infants according to their age in weeks since birth.

Data are available from clinical studies to support the use of rotavirus vaccine in infants with controlled gastroesophageal reflux disease.

Precautions

➤*Patient history:* Prior to administration of rotavirus vaccine, determine the current health status and previous vaccination history of the infant, including whether there has been a reaction to a previous dose of rotavirus vaccine or other rotavirus vaccine.

➤*Febrile illness:* Febrile illness may be reason for delaying use of rotavirus vaccine except when, in the opinion of the doctor, withholding the vaccine entails a greater risk. Low-grade fever (less than 100.5°F [38.1°C]) itself and mild upper respiratory infection do not preclude vaccination with rotavirus vaccine.

➤*Level of protection:* The level of protection provided by only 1 or 2 doses of rotavirus vaccine was not studied in clinical trials.

As with any vaccine, vaccination with rotavirus vaccine may not result in complete protection in all recipients.

➤*Postexposure:* Regarding postexposure prophylaxis, no clinical data are available for rotavirus vaccine when administered after exposure to rotavirus.

➤*Intussusception:* Following administration of a previously licensed live rhesus rotavirus-based vaccine, an increased risk of intussusception was observed. In the Rotavirus Efficacy and Safety Trial (REST) (n = 69,625), the data did not show an increased risk of intussusception for rotavirus vaccine when compared with placebo.

➤*Immunocompromised:* No safety or efficacy data are available for the administration of rotavirus vaccine to infants who are potentially immunocompromised, including the following:

- infants with blood dyscrasias, leukemia, lymphomas of any type, or other malignant neoplasms affecting the bone marrow or lymphatic system.
- infants on immunosuppressive therapy (including high-dose systemic corticosteroids). Rotavirus vaccine may be administered to infants who are being treated with topical corticosteroids or inhaled steroids.
- infants with primary and acquired immunodeficiency states, including HIV/AIDS or other clinical manifestations of infection with human immunodeficiency viruses; cellular immune deficiencies; and hypogammaglobulinemic and dysgammaglobulinemic states. There are insufficient data from the clinical trials to support administration of rotavirus vaccine to infants with indeterminate HIV status who are born to mothers with HIV/AIDS.
- infants who have received a blood transfusion or blood products, including immunoglobulins within 42 days.

GI disorders – No safety or efficacy data are available for administration of rotavirus vaccine to infants with a history of GI disorders, including infants with active acute GI illness, infants with chronic diarrhea and failure to thrive, and infants with a history of congenital abdominal disorders, abdominal surgery, and intussusception. Therefore, caution is advised when considering administration of rotavirus vaccine to these infants.

➤*Shedding and transmission:* Shedding was evaluated among a subset of subjects in REST 4 to 6 days after each dose and among all subjects who submitted a stool antigen rotavirus positive sample at any time. Rotavirus vaccine was shed in the stools of 32 of 360 (8.9%; 95% CI, 6.2%, 12.3%) vaccine recipients tested after dose 1; 0 of 249 (0%; 95% CI, 0%, 1.5%) vaccine recipients tested after dose 2; and in 1 of 385 (0.3%; 95% CI, less than 0.1%, 1.4%) vaccine recipients after dose 3. In phase 3 studies, shedding was observed as early as 1 day and as late as 15 days after a dose. Transmission was not evaluated.

Immunodeficient contacts – Caution is advised when considering whether to administer rotavirus vaccine to individuals with immunodeficient close contacts, such as individuals with malignancies or who are otherwise immunocompromised, or to individuals receiving immunosuppressive therapy.

Virus transmission – There is a theoretical risk that the live virus vaccine can be transmitted to nonvaccinated contacts. Weigh the potential risk of transmission of vaccine virus against the risk of acquiring and transmitting natural rotavirus.

Drug Interactions

➤*Immunosuppressants:* Immunosuppressive therapies, including irradiation, antimetabolites, alkylating agents, cytotoxic drugs, and corticosteroids (used in greater than physiologic doses), may reduce the immune response to vaccines.

Adverse Reactions

➤*Serious adverse reactions:* Serious adverse reactions occurred in 2.4% of recipients of rotavirus vaccine when compared with 2.6% of placebo recipients within the 42-day period of a dose in the phase 3 clinical studies of rotavirus vaccine. The most frequently reported serious adverse reactions for rotavirus vaccine compared with placebo were bronchiolitis (0.6% rotavirus vaccine vs 0.7% placebo), gastroenteritis (0.2% rotavirus vaccine vs 0.3% placebo), pneumonia (0.2% rotavirus vaccine vs 0.2% placebo), fever (0.1% rotavirus vaccine vs 0.1% placebo), and urinary tract infection (0.1% rotavirus vaccine vs 0.1% placebo).

➤*Deaths:* Across the clinical studies, 52 deaths were reported. There were 25 deaths in the rotavirus vaccine recipients compared with 27 deaths in the placebo recipients. The most commonly reported cause of death was sudden infant death syndrome (SIDS), which was observed in 8 recipients of rotavirus vaccine and 9 placebo recipients.

➤*Intussusception:* In REST, 34,837 vaccine recipients and 34,788 placebo recipients were monitored by active surveillance to identify potential cases of intussusception at 7, 14, and 42 days after each dose, and every 6 weeks thereafter for 1 year after the first dose.

For the primary safety outcome, cases of intussusception occurring within 42 days of any dose, there were 6 cases among rotavirus vaccine recipients and 5 cases among placebo recipients (see the following table). The data did not suggest an increased risk of intussusception to placebo.

Confirmed Cases of Intussusception with Rotavirus Vaccine

	Rotavirus vaccine (n = 34,837)	Placebo (n = 34,788)
Confirmed intussusception cases within 42 days of any dose	6	5
Relative risk (95% CI)[a]	1.6 (0.4, 6.4)	
Confirmed intussusception cases within 365 days of dose	13	15

ROTAVIRUS VACCINE, LIVE — ORAL

Confirmed Cases of Intussusception with Rotavirus Vaccine		
	Rotavirus vaccine (n = 34,837)	Placebo (n = 34,788)
Relative risk (95% CI)	0.9 (0.4, 1.9)	

[a] Relative risk and 95% CI based upon group sequential design stopping criteria employed in REST.

Among vaccine recipients, there were no confirmed cases of intussusception within the 42-day period after the first dose, which was the period of highest risk for the rhesus rotavirus-based product (see the following table).

Intussusception Cases by Day Range in Relation to Dose with Rotavirus Vaccine								
	Dose 1		Dose 2		Dose 3		Any Dose	
Day range	Rotavirus vaccine	Placebo	Rotavirus vaccine	Placebo	Rotavirus vaccine	Placebo	Rotavirus vaccine	Placebo
1 to 7	0	0	1	0	0	0	1	0
1 to 14	0	0	1	0	0	1	1	1
1 to 21	0	0	3	0	0	1	3	1
1 to 42	0	1	4	1	2	3	6	5

All of the children who developed intussusception recovered without sequelae with the exception of a 9-month-old male who developed intussusception 98 days after dose 3 and died of postoperative sepsis. There was a single case of intussusception among 2,470 recipients of rotavirus vaccine in a 7-month-old male in the phase 1 and 2 studies (716 placebo recipients).

➤*Seizures:* All seizures reported in the phase 3 trials of rotavirus vaccine (by vaccination group and interval after dose) are shown in the following table.

Reported Seizures with Rotavirus Vaccine			
Day range	1 to 7	1 to 14	1 to 42
Rotavirus vaccine	10	15	33
Placebo	5	8	24

Seizures reported as serious adverse reactions occurred in less than 0.1% (27/36,150) of vaccine and less than 0.1% (18/35,536) of placebo recipients (not significant). Ten febrile seizures were reported as serious adverse reactions, 5 were observed in vaccine recipients and 5 in placebo recipients.

➤*Most common adverse reactions:*

Solicited adverse reactions – Detailed safety information was collected from 11,711 infants (6,138 recipients of rotavirus vaccine), which included a subset of subjects in REST and all subjects from Studies 007 and 009 (Detailed Safety Cohort). A Vaccination Report Card was used by parents/guardians to record the child's temperature and any episodes of diarrhea and vomiting on a daily basis during the first week following each vaccination. The following table summarizes the frequencies of these adverse reactions and irritability.

Rotavirus Vaccine Adverse Reactions						
	Dose 1		Dose 2		Dose 3	
Adverse reaction	Rotavirus vaccine	Placebo	Rotavirus vaccine	Placebo	Rotavirus vaccine	Placebo
	(n = 6,130)	(n = 5,560)	(n = 5,703)	(n = 5,173)	(n = 5,496)	(n = 4,989)
CNS						
Irritability	7.1%	7.1%	6%	6.5%	4.3%	4.5%
GI						
Diarrhea	10.4%	9.1%	8.6%	6.4%	6.1%	5.4%
Vomiting	6.7%	5.4%	5%	4.4%	3.6%	3.2%
	(n = 5,616)	(n = 5,077)	(n = 5,215)	(n = 4,725)	(n = 4,865)	(n = 4,382)
Miscellaneous						
Elevated temperature[a]	17.1%	16.2%	20%	19.4%	18.2%	17.6%

[a] Temperature greater than or equal to 100.5°F (38.1°C) rectal equivalent obtained by adding 1°F to otic and oral temperatures and 2°F to axillary temperatures.

Other adverse reactions – Fever was observed at similar rates in vaccine (n = 6,138) and placebo (n = 5,573) recipients (42.6% vs 42.8%). Adverse reactions that occurred at a statistically higher incidence (ie, 2-sided P value < 0.05) within the 42 days of any dose among recipients of rotavirus vaccine as compared with placebo recipients are shown in the following table.

Rotavirus Vaccine Adverse Reactions		
Adverse reaction	Rotavirus vaccine (n = 6,138) n (%)	Placebo (n = 5,573) n (%)
GI		
Diarrhea	1,479 (24.1%)	1,186 (21.3%)
Vomiting	929 (15.2%)	758 (13.6%)
Respiratory		
Bronchospasm	66 (1.1%)	40 (0.7%)
Nasopharyngitis	422 (6.9%)	325 (5.8%)
Special senses		
Otitis media	887 (14.5%)	724 (13%)

Preterm infants – Rotavirus vaccine or placebo was administered to 2,070 preterm infants (25 to 36 weeks gestational age; median, 34 weeks) according to their age in weeks since birth in REST. All preterm infants were followed for serious adverse reactions; a subset of 308 infants was monitored for all adverse reactions. There were 4 deaths throughout the study, 2 among vaccine recipients (1 SIDS and 1 motor vehicle accident) and 2 among placebo recipients (1 SIDS and 1 unknown cause). No cases of intussusception were reported. Serious adverse reactions occurred in 5.5% of vaccine and 5.8% of placebo recipients. The most common serious adverse reaction was bronchiolitis, which occurred in 1.4% of vaccine and 2% of placebo recipients. Parents/guardians were asked to record the child's temperature and any episodes of vomiting and diarrhea daily for the first week following vaccination. The frequencies of these adverse reactions and irritability within the week after dose 1 are summarized in the following table.

Rotavirus Vaccine Adverse Reactions in Preterm Infants						
	Dose 1		Dose 2		Dose 3	
Adverse reaction	Rotavirus vaccine	Placebo	Rotavirus vaccine	Placebo	Rotavirus vaccine	Placebo
	(n = 154)	(n = 154)	(n = 137)	(n = 137)	(n = 135)	(n = 129)
CNS						
Irritability	3.9%	5.2%	2.9%	4.4%	8.1%	5.4%
GI						
Diarrhea	6.5%	5.8%	7.3%	7.3%	3.7%	3.9%
Vomiting	5.8%	7.8%	2.9%	2.2%	4.4%	4.7%
	(n = 127)	(n = 133)	(n = 124)	(n = 121)	(n = 115)	(n = 108)
Miscellaneous						
Elevated temperature[a]	18.1%	17.3%	25%	28.1%	14.8%	20.4%

[a] Temperature greater than or equal to 100.5°F (38.1°C) rectal equivalent obtained by adding 1°F to otic and oral temperatures and 2°F to axillary temperatures.

Reporting adverse reactions – Instruct parents or guardians to report any adverse reactions to their health care provider. The US Department of Health and Human Services has established a Vaccine Adverse Event Reporting System (VAERS) to accept all reports of suspected adverse reactions after the administration of any vaccine, including but not limited to the reporting of events required by the National Childhood Vaccine Injury Act of 1986. For information or a copy of the vaccine reporting form, call the VAERS toll-free number at 1-800-822-7967 or report online to http://www.vaers.hhs.gov.

Patient Information

Give parents or guardians a copy of the required vaccine information and the patient information appended to the package insert. Encourage parents and/or guardians to read the patient information that describes the benefits and risks associated with the vaccine and ask for any questions they may have during the visit.

YELLOW FEVER VACCINE

Rx	**YF-Vax**[a] (Aventis Pasteur)	**Lyophilized Powder for Injection:** Not less than 4.74 $\log_{10}$ plaque-forming units (PFU) per 0.5 mL dose when reconstituted[b]	In single-dose vials with 0.6 mL diluent, and 5-dose vials with 3 mL of diluent.

[a] Supplied only to designated Yellow Fever Vaccination Centers authorized to issue certificates of Yellow Fever Vaccination.

[b] With gelatin and sorbitol.

YELLOW FEVER VACCINE — INJECTION

Indications

As with any vaccine, vaccination with yellow fever vaccine may not protect 100% of susceptible individuals.

➤*Yellow fever vaccination:* For active immunization of persons 9 months of age and older in the following categories:

➤*Persons living in or traveling to endemic areas:* While the actual risk for contracting yellow fever during travel is probably low, variability of itineraries and behaviors and the seasonal incidence of disease make it difficult to predict the actual risk for a given individual traveling to a known endemic or epidemic area. Vaccinate persons 9 months of age and older traveling to or living in areas of South America and Africa where yellow fever infection is officially reported at the time of travel. Vaccination is also recommended for travel outside the urban areas of countries that do not officially report the disease but lie in a yellow fever endemic zone.

➤*Persons traveling internationally:* Yellow fever vaccination may be required for international travel. Some countries in Africa require evidence of vaccination from all entering travelers and some countries may waive the requirements for travelers staying less than 2 weeks that are coming from areas where there is no current evidence of significant risk for contracting yellow fever. Some countries require an individual, even if only in transit, to have a valid International Certificate of Vaccination if the individual has been in countries either known or thought to harbor yellow fever virus. The certificate becomes valid 10 days after vaccination with yellow fever vaccine.

YELLOW FEVER VACCINE — INJECTION

➤*Laboratory personnel:* Vaccinate those laboratory personnel who might be exposed to virulent yellow fever virus or concentrated preparations of the yellow fever vaccine strain by direct or indirect contact or by aerosols.

Administration and Dosage

➤*Primary vaccination:* For all eligible persons, a single subcutaneous injection of 0.5 mL of reconstituted vaccine (formulated to contain not less than 4.74 $\log_{10}$ plaque-forming units [PFU]) should be administered. Immunity develops by the 10th day after primary vaccination.

➤*Booster doses:* Re-immunization is recommended every 10 years for those at continuing risk of exposure and is required by International Health Regulations. Revaccination boosts antibody titer, although evidence from several studies suggests that yellow fever vaccine immunity persists for at least 30 to 35 years and probably for life, and epidemiologic data suggest that a single infection with wild-type yellow fever virus provides lifelong immunity against illness due to subsequent exposure.

➤*Concomitant vaccines:* Determination of whether to administer yellow fever vaccine and other immunobiologics simultaneously should be made on the basis of convenience to the traveler in completing the desired vaccinations before travel and on information regarding possible interference. Limited data are available related to administration of yellow fever vaccine with other vaccines. In those specific instances in which vaccines may be given concurrently, injections should be administered at separate sites. When there are no data to support administration of yellow fever vaccine concurrently with other vaccines, 4 weeks should elapse between sequential vaccinations.

➤*Preparation and administration:* Reconstitute the vaccine using only the diluent supplied (0.6 mL vial of sodium chloride injection for single dose vial of vaccine and 3 mL vial of sodium chloride injection for 5-dose vial of vaccine). Draw the volume of the diluent, shown on the diluent label, into a suitable size syringe and slowly inject into the vial containing the vaccine. Allow the reconstituted vaccine to sit for 1 to 2 minutes and then carefully swirl mixture until a uniform suspension is achieved. Avoid vigorous shaking as this tends to cause foaming of the suspension. Do not dilute reconstituted vaccine.

The vaccine should appear slightly opalescent and light orange in color after reconstitution. If the product contains extraneous particulate matter or is discolored, do not administer the vaccine.

Swirl vaccine well before withdrawing each dose. Administer the single immunizing dose of 0.5 mL subcutaneously using a ⅝- to ¾-inch long needle within 60 minutes of reconstituting the vial. Properly dispose of all reconstituted vaccine and containers that remain unused after 1 hour (eg, sterilized, disposed in red hazardous waste containers).

➤*Desensitization:* If immunization is imperative and the individual has a history of severe egg sensitivity and has a positive skin test to the vaccine, this desensitization procedure may be used to administer the vaccine.

Desensitization should only be performed under the direct supervision of a health care provider experienced in the management of anaphylaxis with necessary emergency equipment immediately available.

The following successive doses should be administered subcutaneously at 15- to 20-minute intervals:

- 0.05 mL of 1:10 dilution
- 0.05 mL of full strength
- 0.1 mL of full strength
- 0.15 mL of full strength
- 0.2 mL of full strength

➤*Storage/Stability:* Yellow fever vaccine is shipped frozen in a container with solid carbon dioxide; do not use unless the shipping case contains some dry ice upon arrival.

Upon receipt, lyophilized vaccine must be maintained continuously at 0° to 5°C (32° to 41°F). Do not refreeze.

Yellow fever vaccine does not contain a preservative; therefore, all reconstituted vaccine and containers that remain unused after 1 hour must be properly disposed (eg, sterilized, disposed in red hazardous waste containers).

Actions

➤*Pharmacology:* Vaccination with 17D strain viruses is predicted to elicit an immune response identical in quality to that induced by wild-type infection. This response is presumed to result from initial infection of cells in the dermis or other subcutaneous tissues near the injection site, with subsequent replication and limited spread of virus leading to the processing and presentation of viral antigens to the immune system, as would occur during infection with wild-type yellow fever virus. The humoral immune response to the viral structural proteins, as opposed to a cell-mediated response, is most important in the protective effect induced by 17D vaccines. Yellow fever antibodies with specificities that prevent or abort infection of cells are detected as neutralizing antibodies in assays that measure the ability of serum to reduce plaque formation in tissue culture cells. The titer of virus-neutralizing antibodies in sera of vaccinees is a surrogate for efficacy. A $\log_{10}$ neutralization index (LNI; measured by a plaque reduction assay) of 0.7 or greater was shown to protect 90% of monkeys from lethal intracerebral challenge. This is the definition of seroconversion adopted for clinical trials of yellow fever vaccine. The standard has also been adopted by WHO for efficacy of yellow fever vaccines in humans

Contraindications

➤*Hypersensitivity reactions:* Because the yellow fever virus used in the production of this vaccine is propagated in chicken embryos, do not administer yellow fever vaccine to anyone with a history of acute hypersensitivity to eggs or egg products; anaphylaxis may occur. Less severe or localized manifestations of allergy to eggs or feathers are not contraindications to vaccine administration and do not usually warrant vaccine skin testing. Generally, persons who are able to eat eggs or egg products may receive the vaccine.

➤*Children:* Vaccination of infants younger than 9 months of age is contraindicated because of the risk of encephalitis, and travel of such persons to rural areas in yellow fever endemic zones or to countries experiencing an epidemic should be postponed or avoided whenever possible.

➤*Immunodeficiency:* Exposure to yellow fever vaccine, which is a live virus vaccine, poses a risk of encephalitis or other serious adverse reactions to patients with illnesses that commonly result in immunosuppression (eg, AIDS or other manifestations of HIV infection, leukemia, lymphoma, thymoma, generalized malignancy) or patients whose immunologic responses are suppressed by drug therapy (eg, corticosteroids, alkylating drugs, antimetabolites) or radiation. Therefore, do not immunize immunosuppressed subjects, and such persons' travel to yellow fever endemic areas should be postponed or avoided. If travel to a yellow fever-infected zone is unavoidable, advise immunosuppressed patients of the risk, instruct them in methods for avoiding vector mosquitoes, and supply them with vaccination waiver letters by their health care providers.

Family members of immunosuppressed persons, who themselves have no contraindications, may receive yellow fever vaccine.

Warnings

➤*Viscerotropic disease:* Yellow fever vaccines must be considered as a possible, but rare, cause of vaccine-associated viscerotropic disease (previously described as multiple organ system failure), which is similar to fulminant yellow fever caused by wild-type yellow fever virus. Available evidence suggests that the occurrence of this syndrome may depend upon the presence of undefined host factors, rather than intrinsic virulence of the yellow fever strain 17D vaccine viruses isolated from subjects with vaccine-associated viscerotropic disease.

➤*Neurotropic disease:* Vaccine-associated neurotropic disease (previously described as postvaccinal encephalitis) is a known rare adverse reaction associated with yellow fever vaccination. Age younger than 9 months and immunosuppression are known risk factors for this adverse reaction.

➤*Immunodeficiency:* Exposure to yellow fever vaccine, which is a live virus vaccine, poses a risk of encephalitis or other serious adverse reactions to patients with illnesses that commonly result in immunosuppression (eg, AIDS or other manifestations of HIV infection, leukemia, lymphoma, thymoma, generalized malignancy) or patients whose immunologic responses are suppressed by drug therapy (eg, corticosteroids, alkylating drugs, antimetabolites) or radiation. Therefore, do not immunize immunosuppressed subjects, and such persons' travel to yellow fever endemic areas should be postponed or avoided. If travel to a yellow fever-infected zone is unavoidable, advise immunosuppressed patients of the risk, instruct them in methods for avoiding vector mosquitoes, and supply them with vaccination waiver letters by their health care providers.

Family members of immunosuppressed persons, who themselves have no contraindications, may receive yellow fever vaccine.

➤*Hypersensitivity reactions:* Anaphylaxis may occur following the use of yellow fever vaccine, even in individuals with no prior history of hypersensitivity to the vaccine components.

Epinephrine injection (1:1,000) should always be immediately available in case of an unexpected anaphylactic or other serious allergic reaction.

Do not administer yellow fever vaccine to an individual with a history of hypersensitivity to egg or chicken protein. Less severe or localized manifestations of allergy to eggs or feathers are not contraindications to vaccine administration and do not usually warrant vaccine skin testing. Generally, persons who are able to eat eggs or egg products may receive the vaccine. However, if a subject is suspect as being an egg-sensitive individual, the following test can be performed before the vaccine is administered:

1.) Scratch, prick, or puncture test: Place a drop of a 1:10 dilution of the vaccine in physiologic saline on a superficial scratch, prick, or puncture on the volar surface of the forearm. Also use positive (histamine) and negative (physiologic saline) controls. The test is read after 15 to 20 minutes. A positive test is a wheal 3 mm larger than that of the saline control, usually with surrounding erythema. The histamine control must be positive for valid interpretation. If the result of this test is negative, perform an intradermal (ID) test.
2.) Intradermal test: Inject a dose of 0.02 mL of a 1:100 dilution of the vaccine in physiologic saline. Perform positive and negative control skin tests concurrently. A wheal 5 mm or larger than the negative control with surrounding erythema is considered a positive reaction.

If vaccination is considered essential, despite a positive skin test, then desensitization can be considered.

➤*Elderly:* Limit vaccination of subjects older than 65 years of age to individuals who are traveling to or reside in known yellow fever endemic or epidemic areas because of the increased risk for systemic adverse reactions in this age group. When vaccination is deemed necessary, evaluate the health status of such individuals prior to vaccination. Additionally, if vaccinated, carefully monitor elderly subjects for adverse reactions for 10 days postvaccination.

YELLOW FEVER VACCINE — INJECTION

➤*Pregnancy: Category C.* Safety of yellow fever vaccine was evaluated in a study involving 101 Nigerian women, the majority of whom (88%) were in the third trimester of pregnancy. In this study, it appeared that vaccinating pregnant women with the 17D-204 strain of yellow fever vaccine was not associated with adverse reactions affecting the mother or fetus. There were no adverse reactions among 40 infants who were carefully followed up for 1 year after birth, and none of these infants tested positive for immunoglobulin M (IgM) antibodies as a criterion for transplacental infection. However, the percentage of pregnant women who seroconverted was significantly reduced compared with a nonpregnant control group (38.6% vs 81.5%).

Following a mass immunization campaign in Trinidad, during which 100 to 200 pregnant women were immunized, no adverse reactions related to pregnancy were reported. In addition, 41 cord blood samples were obtained from infants born to mothers immunized during the first trimester. One of these infants tested positive for IgM antibodies in cord blood. The infant appeared normal at delivery and no subsequent adverse sequelae of infection were reported. However, this result suggests that transplacental infection with 17D vaccine viruses can occur.

A recent case-control study of spontaneous abortion following vaccination of Brazilian women found no significant difference in the odds ratio among vaccinated women compared with a similar unvaccinated group.

Animal reproduction studies have not been conducted with yellow fever vaccine. It is also not known whether yellow fever vaccine can cause fetal harm when administered to a pregnant woman or can affect reproductive capacity. Because of the lack of large-scale controlled studies to verify its safety in pregnancy, give yellow fever vaccine to a pregnant woman only if clearly needed. The seroconversion rate to 17D vaccines is markedly reduced in pregnant women.

➤*Lactation:* It is not known whether this vaccine is excreted in human milk. There have been no reports of adverse reactions or transmission of 17D vaccine virus from breast-feeding mother to infant. However, avoid vaccination of breast-feeding mothers when possible because of the theoretical risk of the transmission of 17D virus to the breast-fed infant. When travel of breast-feeding mothers to high-risk yellow fever endemic areas cannot be avoided or postponed, such individuals may be immunized.

➤*Children:* See Contraindications for more information.

Precautions

➤*Monitoring:* Prior to an injection of any vaccine, all known precautions should be taken to prevent adverse reactions. Review the patient's previous immunization history, current health status, and medical history for previous hypersensitivity reactions and other adverse reactions related to this vaccine or similar vaccines. Monitor all vaccinees for possible adverse reactions.

➤*Latex sensitivity:* The stopper of the vial contains dry natural latex rubber, which may cause allergic reactions. In some instances in which symptoms appear soon after a vaccine is administered, differentiation between allergic reaction to the vaccine and reaction to an environmental allergen may not be possible.

➤*Revaccination:* Existing data suggest that the small percentage of immunologically healthy subjects who fail to develop an immune response to an initial vaccination may do so upon revaccination.

➤*HIV infection:* Subjects with asymptomatic HIV infection who have had recent laboratory verification of adequate immune system function and who cannot avoid potential exposure to yellow fever virus should be offered the choice of vaccination. Monitor vaccinees for possible adverse reactions. The seroconversion rate to 17D vaccines is likely to be reduced in these patients. Therefore, documentation of a protective antibody response is recommended before travel.

Adverse Reactions

➤*Reporting of adverse reactions:* The US Department of Health and Human Services (DHHS) has established a Vaccine Adverse Event Reporting System (VAERS) to accept all reports of suspected adverse reactions after the administration of any vaccine, including but not limited to the reporting of events required by the National Childhood Vaccine Injury Act of 1986. Reporting by patients, parents, or guardians of all adverse reactions occurring after vaccine administration is encouraged. Adverse reactions following immunization with vaccine should be reported by the health care provider to the US DHHS VAERS. The VAERS toll-free number for forms and information is 1-800-822-7967. Forms may also be available for downloading at the DHHS Web site http://www.hhs.gov.

Also report adverse reactions to the Pharmacovigilance Department, Aventis Pasteur Inc., Discovery Drive, Swiftwater, PA 18370, or call 1-800-822-2463. Adverse reactions to 17D yellow fever vaccine include mild headaches, myalgia, low-grade fevers, or other minor symptoms for 5 to 10 days. Local reactions, including edema, hypersensitivity, or pain or mass at the injection site, have also been reported following yellow fever vaccine administration. Immediate hypersensitivity reactions, characterized by rash, urticaria, and/or asthma, are uncommon and occur principally among persons with histories of egg allergy.

No placebo-controlled trials to assess the safety of yellow fever 17D vaccines have been performed. However, between 1953 and 1994, reactogenicity of 17D-204 vaccine was monitored in 10 uncontrolled clinical trials. The trials included a total of 3,933 adults and 264 infants older than 4 months of age residing in Europe or yellow fever endemic areas. Self-limited and mild local reactions consisting of erythema and pain at the injection site and systemic reactions consisting of headache and/or fever occurred in a minority of subjects (typically less than 5%) 5 to 7 days after immunization. In one study involving 115 infants 4 to 24 months of age, the incidence of fever was as high as 21%. Also in this study, reactogenicity of the vaccine was markedly reduced among a subset of subjects who had serological evidence of previous exposure to yellow fever virus. Only 2 of the 10 studies provided diary cards for daily reporting; this method resulted in a slightly higher incidence of local and systemic complaints.

In 2001, yellow fever vaccine was used as a control in a double-blind, randomized, comparative trial with another 17D-204 vaccine, conducted at 9 centers in the United States. Yellow fever vaccine was administered to 725 adults at least 18 years of age (mean age, 38 years). Safety data were collected by diary card for days 1 through 10 after vaccination and by interview on days 5, 11, and 31. Among subjects who received yellow fever vaccine, there were no serious adverse reactions, and 71.9% experienced nonserious adverse reactions judged to have been related to vaccination. Most of these were injection site reactions of mild to moderate severity. Four such local reactions were considered severe. Rash occurred in 3.2% and urticaria in 2 subjects. Systemic reactions (headache, myalgia, malaise, and asthenia) were usually mild and occurred in 10% to 30% of subjects during the first few days after vaccination. The incidence of nonserious adverse reactions, including headache, malaise, injection site edema, and pain, was significantly lower in subjects older than 60 years of age compared with younger subjects. Adverse reactions were less frequent in the 1.7% of vaccinated subjects who had preexisting immunity to yellow fever virus, compared with those who had not been previously exposed.

➤*Elderly:* A Centers for Disease Control (CDC) analysis of data submitted to the VAERS between 1990 and 1998 suggests that patients 65 years of age or older are at increased risk for systemic adverse reactions temporally associated with vaccination, compared with the group 25 to 44 years of age. The rate of systemic adverse reactions occurring postvaccination in patients 65 to 74 years of age was 2.5 times higher than the rate occurring in patients 25 to 44 years of age, based on incidence rates of 6.21 and 2.49 per 100,000 doses of vaccine in the 2 groups, respectively.

➤*Neurotropic disease:* Vaccine-associated neurotropic disease (previously described as postvaccinal encephalitis) is a known rare serious adverse reaction associated with 17D vaccination. Age younger than 9 months and immunosuppression are known risk factors. Twenty-one cases of vaccine-associated neurotropic disease associated with all licensed 17D vaccines have been reported between 1952 and the present, 18 in children or adolescents. Fifteen of these cases occurred prior to 1960, 13 of which occurred in infants 4 months of age or younger, and 2 of which occurred in infants 6 and 7 months of age. Six cases were reported between 1960 and 1996 worldwide. Three occurred in children, including an infant 1 month of age, a 3-year-old, and a 13-year-old. The 3-year-old died of encephalitis, and a genetic variant of the vaccine virus was isolated from the brain in this case. This is the only verified fatality due to yellow fever vaccine-associated neurotropic disease. The 3 remaining cases of vaccine-associated neurotropic disease since 1960 occurred in adults.

The incidence of vaccine-associated neurotropic disease in infants younger than 4 months of age is estimated to be between 0.5 and 4 per 1,000, based on 2 historical reports where denominators are available. No data are available for calculation of an age-specific incidence rate in the group 4 to 9 months of age. A study in Senegal described 2 fatal cases of encephalitis possibly associated with 17D-204 vaccination among 67,325 children between the ages of 6 months and 2 years, for an incidence rate of 3 per 100,000. One study conducted in Kenya in 1993 detected 4 cases of encephalitis temporally associated with vaccination, 1 in a child 2 years of age and 3 in adults, for an incidence of 5.3 cases per million vaccinees of all ages.

➤*Viscerotropic disease:* Between 1996 and 1998, four patients, 63, 67, 76, and 79 years of age, became severely ill 2 to 5 days after vaccination with yellow fever vaccine. Three of these 4 subjects died. The clinical presentations were characterized by a nonspecific febrile syndrome with fatigue, myalgia, and headache, rapidly progressing to a severe illness including respiratory failure, elevated hepatocellular enzymes, lymphocytopenia and thrombocytopenia, hyperbilirubinemia, and renal failure requiring hemodialysis. None of these subjects had vaccine-associated neurotropic disease. This severe adverse reaction is known as "vaccine-associated viscerotropic disease" (previously described as multiple organ system failure). No cause-and-effect relationship has been established between vaccination and these subsequent illnesses. In 2 cases in which vaccine virus was recovered from serum, limited nucleotide sequence analysis of the viral genome suggested that the isolates had not undergone a mutation associated with an increase in virulence. The incidence rate for these serious adverse reactions was estimated at 1 per 400,000 doses of yellow fever vaccine, based on the total number of doses administered in the US civilian population during the surveillance period.

Vaccine-associated viscerotropic disease temporally associated with yellow fever vaccination has also been reported in Australia and Brazil. One Australian citizen became ill after receiving an immunization with the 17D-204 strain of yellow fever vaccine in his home country, and 2 Brazilian citizens (5 and 22 years of age) became ill 3 to 4 days after receiving 17DD vaccine in Brazil. In the Brazilian and Australian cases, histopathologic changes in the liver included midzonal necrosis, microvesicular fatty change, and Councilman bodies, which are characteristic of wild-type yellow fever. Vaccine-type yellow fever virus was isolated from blood and autopsy material (ie, brain, liver, kidney, spleen, lung, skeletal muscle, skin) of each of these 3 persons, all of whom died 8 to 11 days after vaccination. In Brazil, an estimated 23 million vaccine doses were administered during the 15-month period during which the 2 cases of multiple organ system failure were reported.

In view of the data cited, both the 17D-204 and 17DD yellow fever vaccines may be considered as a possible, but rare, cause of vaccine-associated viscerotropic disease that is similar to fulminant yellow fever caused by wild-type yellow fever virus. All available evidence from complete nucleotide

YELLOW FEVER VACCINE — INJECTION

sequence analysis and testing in experimental animals of vaccine-type yellow fever viruses isolated from the Brazilian subjects suggests that the occurrences are due to undefined host factors, rather than to intrinsic virulence of the 17DD vaccine viruses.

Patient Information

Prior to administration of yellow fever vaccine, ask potential vaccinees or their parents or guardians about their recent health status. Fully inform all potential vaccinees or their parents or guardians of the benefits and risks of immunization and potential for adverse reactions that have been temporally associated with yellow fever vaccine administration. Instruct vaccinees or their parents or guardians to report all serious adverse reactions that occur up to 30 days postvaccination to their health care providers.

All travelers should seek information regarding vaccination requirements by consulting local health departments, the CDC, and WHO. Travel agencies, international airlines, and/or shipping lines may also have up-to-date information. Such requirements may be strictly enforced, particularly for persons traveling from Africa or South America to Asia. Consult the latest published version of Health Information for International Travel to determine requirements and regulations for vaccination.

An International Certificate of Vaccination must be completed, signed, and validated with the center's stamp where the vaccine is administered and provided to all vaccinees. The immunization record contains the date, lot number, and manufacturer of the vaccine administered. Inform subjects that US vaccination certificates are valid for a period of 10 years commencing 10 days after initial vaccination or revaccination.

HEPATITIS B VACCINE, RECOMBINANT

Rx	**Recombivax HB** (Merck)	**Injection (adult formulation):** 10 mcg hepatitis B surface antigen/mL[a]	In 1 mL single-dose vials, 3 mL multi-dose vials, and 1 mL prefilled single-dose syringes.
		Injection (pediatric/adolescent formulation): 5 mcg hepatitis B surface antigen/0.5 mL	Preservative free. In 0.5 mL single-dose vials.
		Injection (dialysis formulation): 40 mcg hepatitis B surface antigen/mL[a]	In 1 mL single-dose vials.
Rx	**Engerix-B** (GlaxoSmithKline)	**Injection (adult formulation):** 20 mcg hepatitis B surface antigen/mL[b]	Preservative free. In single-dose vials.
		Injection (pediatric/adolescent formulation): 10 mcg hepatitis B surface antigen/0.5 mL[c]	Preservative free. In single-dose vials and prefilled syringes.

[a] With thimerosal 50 mcg/mL.
[b] With thimerosal (< 1 mcg mercury).
[c] With thimerosal (< 0.5 mcg mercury).

HEPATITIS B VACCINE (RECOMBINANT) — INJECTION

For complete and comparative prescribing information, refer to the Agents for Active Immunization introduction.

Indications

➤*Hepatitis B vaccination:* For immunization against infection caused by all known subtypes of hepatitis B virus. As hepatitis D (caused by the delta virus) does not occur in the absence of hepatitis B infection, it can be expected that hepatitis D will also be prevented by hepatitis B vaccination.

Hepatitis B vaccination will not prevent hepatitis caused by other agents, such as hepatitis A, C and E viruses, or other pathogens known to infect the liver.

Immunization is recommended for persons of all ages, especially those who are, or will be, at increased risk of exposure to hepatitis B virus.

➤*Patient selection:* Vaccination with hepatitis B vaccine (recombinant) is recommended for: infants, including those born of HBsAg-positive mothers, whether HBsAg-positive or -negative; children born after November 21, 1991; adolescents.

Other persons of all ages in areas of high prevalence or those who are or may be at increased risk of infection with hepatitis B virus, such as:

➤*Healthcare personnel:* Dentists and oral surgeons; physicians and surgeons; nurses; paramedical personnel and custodial staff who may be exposed to the virus via blood or other patient specimens; dental hygienists and dental nurses; laboratory personnel handling blood, blood products, and other patient populations; dental, medical and nursing students.

➤*Selected patients and patient contacts:* Staff in hemodialysis units and hematology/oncology units; hemodialysis patients and patients with early renal failure before they require hemodialysis; patients requiring frequent or large volume blood transfusions or clotting factor concentrates (eg, persons with hemophilia, thalassemia, sickle-cell anemia, cirrhosis); individuals with hepatitis C virus infection; clients (residents) and staff of institutions for the mentally handicapped; classroom contacts of deinstitutionalized mentally handicapped persons who have persistent hepatitis B surface antigenemia and who show aggressive behavior; household and other intimate contacts of persons with persistent hepatitis B surface antigenemia.

➤*Subpopulations with a known high incidence of the disease:* Persons who may be exposed to the hepatitis B virus by travel to high-risk areas. HBV infection is highly endemic in China and Southeast Asia, most of Africa, most Pacific Islands, parts of the Middle East, and in the Amazon Basin. In these areas, most persons acquire infection at birth or during childhood, and 8% to 15% of the population are chronically infected with HBV. Police and fire department personnel who render first aid or medical assistance, and any others who, through their work or personal lifestyles, may be exposed to the hepatitis B virus; Alaskan Natives, Pacific Islanders, Indochinese immigrants, and Haitian immigrants; refugees from areas where HBV is endemic; all infants of women born in areas where the infection is highly endemic; adoptees from countries where hepatitis B virus infection is endemic; international travelers; military personnel identified as being at increased risk; morticians and embalmers; blood bank and plasma fractionation workers

➤*Persons at increased risk of the disease due to their sexual practices:* Persons who have heterosexual activity with multiple partners (greater than 1 sexual partner in a 6-month period); persons who repeatedly contract sexually transmitted diseases; homosexual and bisexual adolescent and adult men; female prostitutes; prisoners; injection drug users.

➤*Individuals with chronic hepatitis C:* Risk factors for hepatitis C are similar to those for hepatitis B. Consequently, immunization with hepatitis B vaccine is recommended for individuals with chronic hepatitis C.

➤*Indications for Recombivax HB* dialysis formulation (40 mcg/mL): Vaccination of adult predialysis (eg, patients with early renal failure before they require hemodialysis) and dialysis patients.

➤*Use with other vaccines:* The Advisory Committee on Immunization Practices (ACIP) states that, in general, simultaneous administration of certain live and inactivated pediatric vaccines has not resulted in impaired antibody responses or increased rates of adverse reactions. Separate sites and syringes should be used for simultaneous administration of injectable vaccines.

➤*Unlabeled uses:* Hepatitis B vaccination is appropriate for people expected to receive human alpha-1 proteinase inhibitor that is produced from heat-treated, pooled human plasma that may contain the causative agents of hepatitis and other viral diseases.

Administration and Dosage

➤*General guidelines:* Hepatitis B vaccine (recombinant) should be administered by IM injection. Do not inject IV or intradermally. In adults, the injection should be given in the deltoid region, but it may be preferable to inject in the anterolateral thigh in neonates and infants, who have smaller deltoid muscles. Hepatitis B vaccine (recombinant) should not be administered in the gluteal region; such injections may result in suboptimal response and a lower seroconversion rate than expected. The attending physician should determine final selection of the injection site and needle size, depending upon the patient's age and the size of the target muscle. A 1-inch, 23-gauge needle is sufficient to penetrate the anterolateral thigh in infants less than 12 months of age. A ⅝ inch, 25-gauge needle may be used to administer the vaccine in the deltoid region of toddlers and children up to and including 10 years of age. The 1-inch, 23-gauge needle is appropriate for use in older children and adults.

Hepatitis B vaccine (recombinant) may be administered SC to persons at risk of hemorrhage (eg, hemophiliacs). However, hepatitis B vaccines administered SC are known to result in lower geometric mean antibody titers (GMTs). Additionally, when other aluminum-adsorbed vaccines have been administered SC, an increased incidence of local reactions including SC nodules has been observed. Therefore, SC administration should be used only in persons who are at risk of hemorrhage with IM injections.

Dosing schedules – The usual immunization regimen consists of 3 doses of vaccine given according to the following schedule: The first dose is given on the elected date, the second dose 1 month later, and the third dose 6 months after the first dose.

➤*Engerix-B*:

Preparation for administration – Shake well before withdrawal and use. Parenteral drug products should be inspected visually for particulate matter or discoloration prior to administration. With thorough agitation, *Engerix-B* is a slightly turbid white suspension. Discard if it appears otherwise. The vaccine should be used as supplied; no dilution is necessary. The full recommended dose of the vaccine should be used. Any vaccine remaining in a single-dose vial should be discarded.

HEPATITIS B VACCINE (RECOMBINANT) — INJECTION

Recommended Dosage and Administration Schedule for *Engerix-B*		
Group	Dose	Schedules
Infants born of:		
HBsAg-negative mothers	10 mcg/0.5 mL	0, 1, 6 months
HBsAg-positive mothers	10 mcg/0.5 mL	0, 1, 6 months
Children:		
Birth through 10 years of age	10 mcg/0.5 mL	0, 1, 6 months
Adolescents:		
11 through 19 years of age	10 mcg/0.5 mL	0, 1, 6 months
Adults (> 19 years)	20 mcg/mL	0, 1, 6 months
Adult hemodialysis	40 mcg/2 mL*	0, 1, 2, 6 months

* Two × 20 mcg in 1 or 2 injections. For hemodialysis patients, in whom vaccine-induced protection is less complete and may persist only as long as antibody levels remain above 10 mIU/mL, the need for booster doses should be assessed by annual antibody testing. Forty (40) mcg (2 × 20 mcg) booster doses with *Engerix-B* should be given when antibody levels decline below 10 mIU/mL. Data show individuals given a booster with *Engerix-B* achieve high antibody titers. In a clinical trial of adults who had been on hemodialysis for a mean of 56 months (n = 43), 67% of patients were seroprotected 2 months after the last dose of 40 mcg of *Engerix-B* (2 × 20 mcg) given on a 0-, 1-, 2-, 6-month schedule; the GMT among seroconverters was 93 mIU/mL.

Alternate Dosage and Administration Schedules		
Group	Dose	Schedules
Infants born of:		
HBsAg-positive mothers	10 mcg/0.5 mL	0, 1, 2, 12 months*
Children:		
Birth through 10 years of age	10 mcg/0.5 mL	0, 1, 2, 12 months*
5 through 10 years of age	10 mcg/0.5 mL	0, 12, 24 months[1]
Adolescents:		
11 through 16 years of age	10 mcg/0.5 mL	0, 12, 24 months[1]
11 through 19 years of age	20 mcg/mL	0, 1, 6 months
11 through 19 years of age	20 mcg/mL	0, 1, 2, 12 months[1]
Adults (> 19 years)	20 mcg/mL	0, 1, 2, 12 months[1]

* This schedule is designed for certain populations (eg, neonates born of hepatitis B-infected mothers, others who have or might have been recently exposed to the virus, certain travelers to high-risk areas). On this alternate schedule, an additional dose at 12 months is recommended for prolonged maintenance of protective titers.

[1] For children and adolescents for whom an extended administration schedule is acceptable based on risk of exposure.

Booster vaccinations – Whenever administration of a booster dose is appropriate, the dose of *Engerix-B* is 10 mcg for children less than or equal to 10 years of age; 20 mcg for adolescents 11 through 19 years of age and 20 mcg for adults. Studies have demonstrated a substantial increase in antibody titers after *Engerix-B* booster vaccination following an initial course with both plasma- and yeast-derived vaccines.

Known or presumed exposure to hepatitis B virus – Unprotected individuals with known or presumed exposure to the hepatitis B virus (eg, neonates born of infected mothers, others experiencing percutaneous or permucosal exposure) should be given hepatitis B immune globulin (HBIG) in addition to *Engerix-B* in accordance with ACIP recommendations and with the monograph for HBIG. *Engerix-B* can be given on either dosing schedule.

➤***Recombivax HB***: *Recombivax HB* hepatitis B vaccine (recombinant) dialysis formulation (40 mcg/mL) (without preservative) is intended only for adult predialysis/dialysis patients.

Recombivax HB hepatitis B vaccine (recombinant) pediatric/adolescent (without preservative) and adult formulations (without preservative) are not intended for use in predialysis/dialysis patients.

2-dose regimen (adolescents, 11 to 15 years of age) – An alternate 2-dose regimen is available for routine vaccination of adolescents (11 to 15 years of age). The regimen consists of 2 doses of vaccine (10 mcg) given according to the following schedule: First injection, at elected date; second injection, 4 to 6 months later.

Dose and Formulation of *Recombivax HB* for Specific Populations, Regardless of the Risk of Infection with Hepatitis B Virus			
Group	Dose/regimen	Formulation	Color code
Infants, children, and adolescents 0 to 19 years of age	5 mcg (0.5 mL) 3 × 5 mcg	Pediatric/adolescent	Yellow
Adolescents* 11 through 15 years of age	10 mcg** (1 mL) 2 × 10 mcg	Adult	Green
Adults ≥ 20 years of age	10 mcg** (1 mL) 3 × 10 mcg	Adult	Green
Predialysis and dialysis patients[1]	40 mcg (1 mL) 3 × 40 mcg	Dialysis	Blue

* Adolescents (11 through 15 years of age) may receive either regimen: The 3 × 5 mcg (pediatric/adolescent formulation) or the 2 × 10 mcg (adult formulation).

** If the suggested formulation is not available, the appropriate dosage can be achieved from another formulation provided that the total volume of vaccine administered does not exceed 1 mL. However, the dialysis formulation may be used only for adult predialysis/dialysis patients.

[1] See also recommendations for revaccination of predialysis and dialysis patients.

The vaccine should be used as supplied; no dilution or reconstitution is necessary. The full recommended dose of the vaccine should be used.

For all formulations – Since none of the formulations contain a preservative, once the single-dose vial has been penetrated, the withdrawn vaccine should be used promptly, and the vial must be discarded.

Shake well before use. Thorough agitation at the time of administration is necessary to maintain suspension of the vaccine. Parenteral drug products should be inspected visually for particulate matter and discoloration prior to administration. After thorough agitation, the vaccine is a slightly opaque, white suspension.

Guidelines for treatment of infants born of HBsAg-positive mothers or mothers of unknown HBsAg status – Each infant should receive three 5 mcg doses of *Recombivax HB* irrespective of the mother's HBsAg status (see table above). The ACIP recommends that if the mother is determined to be HBsAg-positive within 7 days of delivery, the infant also should be given a dose of HBIG (0.5 mL) immediately. The first dose of *Recombivax HB* may be given at the same time as HBIG, but it should be administered in the opposite anterolateral thigh.

Revaccination – The duration of the protective effect of *Recombivax HB* in healthy vaccinees is unknown at present and the need for booster doses is not yet defined. However, long-term follow-up (5 to 9 years) of approximately 3000 high-risk vaccinees (infants of carrier mothers, male homosexuals, Alaskan Natives) who developed an anti-HBs titer of greater than or equal to 10 mIU/mL when given a similar plasma-derived vaccine at intervals of 0, 1, and 6 months showed that no subjects developed clinically apparent hepatitis B infection and that 5 subjects developed antigenemia, even though up to half of the subjects failed to maintain a titer at this level. Persistence of vaccine-induced immunologic memory among healthy vaccinees who responded to a primary course of plasma-derived or recombinant hepatitis B vaccine has been demonstrated by an anamnestic antibody response to a booster dose of *Recombivax HB* given 5 to 12 years later.

Booster dose – A booster dose or revaccination with *Recombivax HB Dialysis Formulation* (blue color code) may be considered in predialysis/dialysis patients if the anti-HBs level is less than 10 mIU/mL 1 to 2 months after the third dose. The ACIP recommends that the need for booster doses of vaccine should be assessed by annual antibody testing and a booster dose given when antibody levels decline to less than 10 mIU/mL.

Known or presumed exposure to HBsAg – There are no prospective studies directly testing the efficacy of a combination of HBIG and *Recombivax HB* in preventing clinical hepatitis B following percutaneous, ocular or mucous membrane exposure to hepatitis B virus. However, since most persons with such exposures (eg, healthcare workers) are candidates for *Recombivax HB*, and since combined HBIG plus vaccine is more efficacious than HBIG alone in perinatal exposures, the following guidelines are recommended for persons who have been exposed to hepatitis B virus such as through percutaneous (needlestick), ocular, mucous membrane exposure to blood known or presumed to contain HBsAg, human bites by known or presumed HBsAg carriers, that penetrate the skin, or following intimate sexual contact with known or presumed HBsAg carriers.

HBIG (0.06 mL/kg) should be given IM as soon as possible after exposure and within 24 hours if possible. *Recombivax HB* (see dosage recommendation) should be given IM at a separate site within 7 days of exposure and second and third doses given 1 and 6 months, respectively, after the first dose.

➤***Storage/Stability:*** Store between 2° and 8°C (36° and 46°F). Storage above or below the recommended temperature may reduce potency. Do not freeze; discard if product has been frozen as freezing destroys potency. Do not dilute to administer.

Actions

➤***Pharmacology:*** Hepatitis B virus is 1 of several hepatitis viruses that cause a systemic infection, with a major pathology in the liver. These include hepatitis A virus, hepatitis B virus, and hepatitis C and E viruses, previously referred to as non-A, non-B hepatitis viruses.

Reduced risk of hepatocellular carcinoma – Hepatocellular carcinoma is another serious complication of hepatitis B virus infection. Studies have

HEPATITIS B VACCINE (RECOMBINANT) — INJECTION

demonstrated the link between chronic hepatitis B infection and hepatocellular carcinoma; 80% of primary liver cancers are caused by hepatitis B virus infection. The CDC has recognized hepatitis B vaccine as the first anticancer vaccine because it can prevent primary liver cancer.

Contraindications

Hypersensitivity to yeast or any other component of the vaccine; hypersensitivity to any hepatitis B-containing vaccine. Patients experiencing hypersensitivity after a hepatitis B vaccine (recombinant) injection should not receive further injections of hepatitis B vaccine (recombinant).

Warnings

➤*Engerix-B*: The vial stopper is latex-free. The tip cap and the rubber plunger of the needleless prefilled syringes contain dry natural latex rubber that may cause allergic reactions in latex-sensitive individuals.

➤*Active infection:* Because of the long incubation period for hepatitis B, it is possible for unrecognized infection to be present at the time the vaccine is given. The vaccine may not prevent hepatitis B in such patients.

➤*Hypersensitivity reactions:* Patients who develop symptoms suggestive of hypersensitivity after an injection should not receive further injections of the vaccine.

As with any percutaneous vaccine, epinephrine (1:1000) should be available for immediate use in case of anaphylaxis or an anaphylactoid reaction.

➤*Elderly:* Clinical trials of *Recombivax HB* did not include sufficient numbers of subjects aged 65 years and over to determine whether they respond differently from younger subjects. Other reports from the clinical literature indicate that hepatitis B vaccines are less immunogenic in adults aged 65 years or older than in younger individuals. No overall differences in safety were observed between these subjects and younger subjects.

➤*Pregnancy: Category C.* Animal reproduction studies have not been conducted with hepatitis B vaccine (recombinant). It is also not known whether this vaccine can cause fetal harm when administered to a pregnant woman or can affect reproduction capacity. Hepatitis B vaccine (recombinant) should be given to a pregnant woman only if clearly needed.

➤*Lactation:* It is not known whether hepatitis B vaccine (recombinant) is excreted in human milk. Because many drugs are excreted in human milk, caution should be exercised when hepatitis B vaccine (recombinant) is administered to a nursing woman.

➤*Children:* Hepatitis B vaccine (recombinant) has been shown to be well tolerated and highly immunogenic in infants and children of all ages. Newborns also respond well; maternally transferred antibodies do not interfere with the active immune response to the vaccine. The safety and efficacy of *Recombivax HB Dialysis Formulation* in children have not been established.

Precautions

➤*Postponing vaccination:* As with other vaccines, although a moderate or severe febrile illness is sufficient reason to postpone vaccination, minor illnesses such as mild upper respiratory tract infections, with or without low-grade fever, are not contraindications.

Any serious active infection (including febrile illness) is reason for delaying use of the vaccine, except when, in the opinion of the physician, withholding the vaccine entails a greater risk.

➤*Administration precautions:* Special care should be taken to prevent injection into a blood vessel.

➤*Immunosuppressed patients:* As with any vaccine administered to immunosuppressed persons or persons receiving immunosuppressive therapy, the expected immune response may not be obtained. For individuals receiving immunosuppressive therapy, deferral of vaccination for at least 3 months after therapy may be considered.

➤*Multiple sclerosis:* Although no causal relationship has been established, rare instances of exacerbation of multiple sclerosis have been reported following administration of hepatitis B vaccines and other vaccines. In persons with multiple sclerosis, the benefit of immunization for prevention of hepatitis B infection and sequelae must be weighed against the risk of exacerbation of the disease.

➤*Special risk:* Caution and appropriate care should be exercised in administering the vaccine to individuals with severely compromised cardiopulmonary status or to others in whom a febrile or systemic reaction could pose a significant risk.

Drug Interactions

Hepatitis B Vaccine (HBV) Drug Interactions

Precipitant drug	Object drug*		Description
Immunosuppressants	HBV	⬇	Administration of HBV to people receiving immunosuppressant drugs, including high-dose corticosteroids or radiation therapy, may result in an inadequate response to immunization.
HBV	Yellow fever vaccine	⬇	In 1 study, concurrent vaccination against hepatitis B and yellow fever viruses reduced the antibody titer otherwise expected from yellow fever vaccine. Separate these vaccines by a month, if possible.
Interleukin-2	HBV	⟷	Natural interleukin 2 may boost systemic immune response to HBsAg in immunodeficient nonresponders to hepatitis B vaccination, but recombinant interleukin 2 did not augment response to hepatitis B vaccine in healthy adults in 1 study.

* ⬇ = Object drug decreased. ⟷ = Undetermined clinical effect.

Adverse Reactions

Using a symptom checklist, the most frequently reported adverse reactions were injection site soreness (22%) and fatigue (14%). Parents or guardians completed forms for children and neonates. The neonatal checklist did not include headache, fatigue or dizziness. Other reactions are listed below.

➤*Cardiovascular:*
Less than 1% – Hypotension.

➤*CNS:*
1% to 10% – Headache, dizziness.
Less than 1% – Somnolence, insomnia, irritability, agitation.

➤*Dermatologic:*
Less than 1% – Rash, urticaria, petechiae, pruritus, erythema.

➤*GI:*
Less than 1% – Nausea, anorexia, abdominal pain/cramps, vomiting, constipation, diarrhea.

➤*Local:*
1% to 10% – Induration, erythema, swelling.
Less than 1% – Pain, pruritus, ecchymosis at injection site.

➤*Lymphatic:*
Less than 1% – Lymphadenopathy.

➤*Musculoskeletal:*
Less than 1% – Pain/stiffness in arm, shoulder or neck, arthralgia, myalgia, back pain.

➤*Respiratory:*
Less than 1% – Influenza-like symptoms, upper respiratory tract illnesses.

➤*Systemic:*
1% to 10% – Fever (greater than 37.5°C [99.5°F]).
Less than 1% – Sweating, malaise, chills, weakness, flushing, tingling.

➤*Postmarketing experience with Engerix-B*: Additional adverse reactions have been reported with the commercial use of *Engerix-B*. Those listed below are to serve as alerting information to physicians.

Cardiovascular – Tachycardia/palpitations.

CNS – Migraine; syncope; paresis; neuropathy including hypoesthesia, paresthesia, Guillain-Barré syndrome and Bell's palsy, transverse myelitis; optic neuritis; multiple sclerosis; seizures.

Dermatologic – Eczema; purpura; herpes zoster; erythema nodosum; alopecia.

GI – Abnormal liver function tests, dyspepsia.

Hematologic – Thrombocytopenia.

Hypersensitivity – Anaphylaxis; erythema multiforme including Stevens-Johnson syndrome; angioedema; arthritis. An apparent hypersensitivity syndrome (serum-sickness-like) of delayed onset has been reported days to weeks after vaccination, including arthralgia/arthritis (usually transient), fever, and dermatologic reactions such as urticaria, erythema multiforme, ecchymoses and erythema nodosum.

Patients who have experienced a hypersensitivity reaction after a hepatitis B (recombinant) vaccine injection should not receive further injections of hepatitis B (recombinant) vaccine.

Respiratory – Bronchospasm including asthma-like symptoms.

Special senses – Conjunctivitis; keratitis; visual disturbances; vertigo; tinnitus; earache.

➤*Recombivax HB*: *Recombivax HB* and *Recombivax HB Dialysis Formulation* are generally well tolerated. No serious adverse reactions attributable to the vaccine have been reported during the course of clinical trials. No adverse experiences were reported during clinical trials which could be related to changes in the titers of antibodies to yeast. As with any vaccine, there is the possibility that broad use of the vaccine could reveal adverse reactions not observed in clinical trials.

HEPATITIS B VACCINE (RECOMBINANT) — INJECTION

In 3 clinical studies, 434 doses of *Recombivax HB*, 5 mcg, were administered to 147 healthy infants and children (up to 10 years of age) who were monitored for 5 days after each dose. Injection site reactions and systemic complaints were reported following 0.2% and 10.4% of the injections, respectively. The most frequently reported systemic adverse reactions (greater than 1% of injections), in decreasing order of frequency, were irritability, fever (greater than or equal to 38.3°C [101°F] oral equivalent), diarrhea, fatigue/weakness, diminished appetite, and rhinitis.

In a study that compared the 3-dose regimen (5 mcg) with the 2-dose regimen (10 mcg) of *Recombivax HB* in adolescents, the overall frequency of adverse reactions was generally similar.

In a group of studies, 3258 doses of *Recombivax HB*, 10 mcg, were administered to 1252 healthy adults who were monitored for 5 days after each dose. Injection site reactions and systemic complaints were reported following 17% and 15% of the injections, respectively. The following adverse reactions were reported:

Cardiovascular –
Less than 1%: Hypotension.

CNS –
Less than 1%: Vertigo/dizziness, and paresthesia.

Dermatologic –
Less than 1%: Pruritus, rash (nonspecified), angioedema, and urticaria.

GI –
Greater than or equal to 1%: Nausea and diarrhea.
Less than 1%: Vomiting, abdominal pains/cramps, dyspepsia, and diminished appetite.

GU –
Less than 1%: Dysuria.

Hematologic / Lymphatic –
Less than 1%: Lymphadenopathy.

Local –
Greater than or equal to 1%: Injection site reactions consisting principally of soreness, and including pain, tenderness, pruritus, erythema, ecchymosis, swelling, warmth, and nodule formation.

Musculoskeletal –
Less than 1%: Arthralgia including monoarticular, myalgia, back pain, neck pain, shoulder pain, and neck stiffness.

Psychiatric –
Less than 1%: Insomnia/disturbed sleep.

Respiratory –
Greater than or equal to 1%: Pharyngitis and upper respiratory tract infection.
Less than 1%: Rhinitis, influenza, and cough.

Special senses –
Less than 1%: Earache.

Miscellaneous –
Greater than or equal to 1%: The most frequent systemic complaints include fatigue/weakness, headache, fever (greater than or equal to 37.7°C [100°F]), and malaise.
Less than 1%: Sweating, achiness, sensation of warmth, lightheadedness, chills, and flushing.

➤*Postmarketing experience with Recombivax HB:* The following additional adverse reactions have been reported with use of the marketed vaccine. In many instances, the relationship to the vaccine was unclear.

Cardiovascular – Syncope; tachycardia.

CNS – Guillain-Barré syndrome; multiple sclerosis; exacerbation of multiple sclerosis; myelitis, including transverse myelitis; seizure; febrile seizure; peripheral neuropathy including Bell's palsy; radiculopathy; herpes zoster; migraine; muscle weakness; hypesthesia; encephalitis.

Dermatologic – Stevens-Johnson syndrome; alopecia; petechiae.

Hematologic – Increased erythrocyte sedimentation rate; thrombocytopenia.

Hypersensitivity – Anaphylaxis and symptoms of immediate hypersensitivity reactions including rash, pruritus, urticaria, edema, angioedema, dyspnea, chest discomfort, bronchial spasm, palpitation, or symptoms consistent with a hypotensive episode have been reported within the first few hours after vaccination. An apparent hypersensitivity syndrome (serum-sickness-like) of delayed onset has been reported days to weeks after vaccination, including arthralgia/arthritis (usually transient), fever, and dermatologic reactions such as urticaria, erythema multiforme, ecchymoses, and erythema nodosum.

Patients who experience a hypersensitivity reaction to hepatitis B vaccine (recombinant) should not receive further doses of hepatitis B vaccine (recombinant).

GI – Elevation of liver enzymes; constipation.

Musculoskeletal – Arthritis.

Psychiatric – Irritability; agitation; somnolence.

Special senses – Optic neuritis; tinnitus; conjunctivitis; visual disturbances.

Systemic – Systemic lupus erythematosus (SLE); lupus-like syndrome; vasculitis.

Miscellaneous – The following adverse reaction has been reported with another hepatitis B vaccine (recombinant) but not with *Recombivax HB*: Keratitis. Patients, parents and guardians should be instructed to report any serious adverse reactions to their healthcare provider.

Patient Information

The healthcare provider should provide the vaccine information required to be given with each vaccination to the patient, parent or guardian.

The healthcare provider should inform the patient, parent or guardian of the benefits and risks associated with vaccination, as well as the importance of completing the immunization series.

Patients, parents and guardians should be instructed to report any serious adverse reactions to their healthcare providers.

HEPATITIS A VACCINE, INACTIVATED

Rx	**Havrix** (GlaxoSmithKline)	**Injection (pediatric formulation)**: 720 EL.U. of viral antigen per 0.5 mL[a]	In single-dose vials and prefilled syringes.
		Injection (adult formulation): 1440 EL.U. of viral antigen per 1 mL[a]	In single-dose vials and prefilled syringes.
	Vaqta (Merck)	**Injection (pediatric/adolescent)**: 25 U hepatitis A virus antigen per 0.5 mL	In single-dose vials and prefilled syringes.
		Injection (adult): 50 U hepatitis A virus antigen per 1 mL	In single-dose vials and prefilled syringes.

[a] EL.U. = ELISA (enzyme linked immunosorbent assay) Units.

HEPATITIS A VACCINE, INACTIVATED — INJECTION

For complete and comparative prescribing information, refer to the Agents for Active Immunization introduction.

Indications

➤*Hepatitis A virus (HAV):* For active immunization of persons 12 months of age and older against disease caused by HAV. Primary immunization should be administered at least 2 weeks prior to expected exposure to HAV.

Administration and Dosage

➤*Approved by the FDA:* February 22, 1995.

➤*Preparation and administration:* Do not inject intravenously (IV), intradermally, intravascularly, or subcutaneously. Hepatitis A vaccine, inactivated is for intramuscular (IM) injection. The deltoid muscle is the preferred site for IM injection in adults. Hepatitis A vaccine, inactivated should not be administered in the gluteal region; such injections may result in suboptimal response.

The following are the Advisory Committee on Immunization Practices (ACIP) and American Academy of Family Physicians recommendations for all IM injections: For administration of hepatitis A vaccine, inactivated for children and adolescents (persons 12 months to 18 years of age), the deltoid muscle can be used if the muscle mass is adequate. The needle size can range from 22 to 25 gauge and from ⅞ to 1 ¼ inches, on the basis of the size of the muscle. For toddlers, the anterolateral thigh can be used, but the needle should be longer, usually 1 inch.

For adults (persons older than 18 years of age), the deltoid muscle is recommended for routine IM vaccinations. The anterolateral thigh can be used. The suggested needle size is 1 to 1.5 inches and 22 to 25 gauge.

A separate sterile syringe and sterile disposable needle or a sterile disposable unit should be used for each individual patient to prevent transmission of hepatitis or other infectious agents from one person to another. Needles should be disposed of properly and should not be recapped.

The vaccine should be used as supplied; no dilution or reconstitution is necessary. The full recommended dose of the vaccine should be used. After removal of the appropriate volume from a single-dose vial, any vaccine remaining in the vial should be discarded.

Shake well before withdrawal and use. Thorough agitation is necessary to maintain suspension of the vaccine. Discard if the suspension does not appear homogenous.

Parenteral drug products should be inspected visually for extraneous particulate matter and discoloration prior to administration whenever solution and container permit. After thorough agitation, hepatitis A vaccine, inactivated is a slightly opaque, white suspension. Discard if it appears otherwise.

➤*Havrix:*

Children / Adolescents – Primary immunization for children and adolescents (12 months through 18 years of age) consists of a single dose of 720 enzyme-linked immunosorbent assay (ELISA) units (EL.U.) in 0.5 mL, and a booster dose (720 EL.U. in 0.5 mL) should be administered anytime between 6 and 12 months later.

HEPATITIS A VACCINE, INACTIVATED — INJECTION

Adults – Primary immunization for adults consists of a single dose of 1,440 EL.U. in 1 mL, and a booster dose (1,440 EL.U. in 1 mL) should be administered anytime between 6 and 12 months later.

All patients: For all age groups, a booster dose should be administered anytime between 6 and 12 months after the initiation of the primary dose in order to ensure the highest antibody titers.

Clotting factor disorders: For individuals with clotting factor disorders at risk of hematoma formation following IM injection, the ACIP recommends that when any IM vaccine is indicated for such patients, that the vaccine should be administered IM if, in the opinion of a health care provider familiar with the patient's bleeding risk, the vaccine can be administered with reasonable safety by this route. If the patient receives antihemophilia or other similar therapy, IM vaccinations can be scheduled shortly after such therapy is administered. A fine needle (less than or equal to 23 gauge) should be used for the vaccination and firm pressure applied to the site, without rubbing, for at least 2 minutes. The patient or family should be instructed concerning the risk for hematoma from the injection.

Impaired immune system: In patients with an impaired immune system, adequate anti-HAV response may not be obtained after the primary immunization course. Such patients may therefore require administration of additional doses of vaccine.

➤*Vaqta*: The vaccination regimen consists of 1 primary dose and 1 booster dose for healthy children, adolescents, and adults, as follows:

Children/Adolescents – Individuals 12 months through 18 years of age should receive a single 0.5 mL (approximately 25 units) dose of vaccine at elected date and a booster dose of 0.5 mL (approximately 25 units) 6 to 18 months later.

Adults – Adults 19 years of age and older should receive a single 1 mL (approximately 50 units) dose of vaccine at elected date and a booster dose of 1 mL (approximately 50 units) 6 to 18 months later.

All patients – For all age groups, a booster dose is recommended anytime between 6 and 18 months after the administration of the primary dose in order to elicit a high antibody titer.

Interchangeability of the booster dose – A booster dose of *Vaqta* may be given at 6 to 12 months following the initial dose of other inactivated hepatitis A vaccines (eg, *Havrix*).

➤*Use with other vaccines:*

Vaqta – *Vaqta* may be given concomitantly with typhoid and yellow fever vaccines. The geometric mean titers (GMTs) for hepatitis A when *Vaqta*, typhoid, and yellow fever vaccines were coadministered were reduced when compared with *Vaqta* alone. Following receipt of the booster dose of *Vaqta*, the GMTs for hepatitis A in these 2 groups were observed to be comparable. *Vaqta* may be given concomitantly with measles, mumps, and rubella virus vaccine (*M-M-R II*). Data on concomitant use with other vaccines are limited. Separate injection sites and syringes should be used for coadministration of injectable vaccines.

Use with immune globulin:

• *Havrix* – *Havrix* may be coadministered with immune globulin, although the ultimate antibody titer obtained is likely to be lower than when the vaccine is given alone.

When coadministration of other vaccines or immune globulin is required, they should be given with different syringes and at different injection sites.

• *Vaqta* – *Vaqta* may be coadministered with immune globulin using separate sites and syringes. The vaccination regimen for *Vaqta* should be followed as stated above. Consult the manufacturer for the appropriate dosage of immune globulin. A booster dose of *Vaqta* should be administered at the appropriate time as previously outlined.

➤*Known or presumed exposure to HAV/travel to endemic areas:* For individuals requiring either postexposure prophylaxis or combined immediate and longer-term protection (eg, travelers departing on short notice to endemic areas), *Vaqta* and *Havrix* may be coadministered with immune globulin using separate sites and syringes.

➤*Storage/Stability:* Store refrigerated between 2° and 8°C (36° and 46°F).

Do not freeze because freezing destroys potency; discard if product has been frozen. Do not dilute to administer.

Contraindications

Hypersensitivity to any component of the vaccine, including neomycin; patients with previous hypersensitivity to any hepatitis A-containing vaccine or to a vaccine component.

Warnings

➤*Immunocompromised patients:* As with any vaccine, if administered to immunocompromised persons, including individuals receiving immunosuppressive therapy, the expected immune response may not be obtained.

➤*Latex sensitivity:* Certain components of the *Havrix* packaging (the tip cap and the rubber plunger of the needleless prefilled syringes) and the *Vaqta* packaging (the vial stopper and the syringe plunger stopper) contain dry natural latex rubber that may cause allergic reactions in latex-sensitive individuals.

➤*Preexisting infection/antibody development:* Hepatitis A has a relatively long incubation period (15 to 50 days). Hepatitis A vaccine may not prevent hepatitis A infection in individuals who have an unrecognized hepatitis A infection at the time of vaccination. Additionally, it may not prevent infection in individuals who do not achieve protective antibody titers (although the lowest titer needed to confer protection has not been determined).

➤*Hypersensitivity reactions:* Do not give further injections of hepatitis A vaccine, inactivated to individuals who develop symptoms suggestive of hypersensitivity after an injection the vaccine, inactivated.

There have been rare reports of anaphylaxis/anaphylactoid reactions following commercial use of the vaccine. Appropriate medical treatment and supervision should be readily available for immediate use in case of a rare anaphylactic reaction following the administration of the vaccine. Epinephrine injection (1:1,000) and other appropriate agents used for the control of immediate allergic reactions must be immediately available.

➤*Elderly:*

Havrix – Clinical studies of *Havrix* did not include sufficient numbers of subjects 65 years of age and older to determine whether they respond differently from younger subjects. Other reported clinical experience has not identified differences in overall safety between these subjects and younger adult subjects.

Vaqta – Of the total number of adults in clinical studies of *Vaqta*, conducted pre- and post-licensure, 68 were 65 years of age or older, 10 of whom were 75 years of age or older. No overall differences in safety and immunogenicity were observed between these subjects and younger subjects; however, greater sensitivity of some older individuals cannot be ruled out. In a large, postmarketing safety study in 42,110 individuals 2 years of age and older, 4,769 were 65 years of age or older, 1,073 of whom were 75 years of age or older. There were no adverse reactions judged by the investigator to be vaccine related in the geriatric study population. Other reported clinical experience has not identified differences in responses between the elderly and younger subjects.

➤*Pregnancy: Category C.* Animal reproduction studies have not been conducted with hepatitis A vaccine, inactivated. It is also not known whether hepatitis A vaccine, inactivated can cause fetal harm when administered to a pregnant woman or can affect reproduction capacity. Give hepatitis A vaccine, inactivated to a pregnant woman only if clearly needed.

➤*Lactation:* It is not known whether hepatitis A vaccine, inactivated is excreted in human milk. Because many drugs are excreted in human milk, exercise caution when hepatitis A vaccine, inactivated is administered to a woman who is breast-feeding.

➤*Children:* The safety and efficacy of hepatitis A vaccine, inactivated have not been established in subjects younger than 12 months of age.

Havrix – The safety and efficacy of *Havrix* have been evaluated in 20,436 subjects 1 year to 18 years of age.

Vaqta – The safety of *Vaqta* has been evaluated in 706 children 12 through 23 months of age and 2,615 children and adolescents 2 through 18 years of age.

Precautions

➤*Patient history:* Prior to immunization with hepatitis A vaccine, inactivated, review the patient's current health status and medical history. Review the patient's immunization history for possible vaccine sensitivity, previous vaccination-related adverse reactions, and occurrence of any adverse reaction-related symptoms and/or signs in order to determine the existence of any contraindication to immunization with hepatitis A vaccine, inactivated and to allow an assessment of benefits and risks.

➤*Administration:* Use a separate, sterile syringe and needle or a sterile disposable unit for each patient to prevent the transmission of other infectious agents from person to person. Dispose of needles properly and do not recap them.

➤*Hepatitis:* Hepatitis A vaccine, inactivated will not prevent hepatitis caused by infectious agents (eg, hepatitis B, C, or E virus) other than hepatitis A virus.

➤*Bleeding disorders:* As with other IM injections, do not give hepatitis A vaccine, inactivated to individuals with bleeding disorders such as hemophilia or thrombocytopenia or to persons on anticoagulant therapy unless the potential benefits clearly outweigh the risk of administration. If the decision is made to administer the vaccine to such persons, give it with caution and take steps to avoid the risk of hematoma following the injection.

➤*Protective response:* As with any vaccine, vaccination with hepatitis A vaccine, inactivated may not result in a protective response in all susceptible vaccinees.

➤*Acute infection/febrile illness:* An acute infection or febrile illness may be reason for delaying use of hepatitis A vaccine, inactivated except when, in the opinion of the health care provider, withholding the vaccine entails a greater risk.

Drug Interactions

➤*Anticoagulant therapy:* As with other IM injections, give hepatitis A vaccine, inactivated with caution to individuals on anticoagulant therapy.

➤*Havrix*:

Other vaccines – *Havrix* may be given concurrently with Hib conjugate vaccines in children 15 to 18 months of age. The safety of *Havrix* given concomitantly with diphtheria and tetanus toxoids and acellular pertussis vaccine, adsorbed has been evaluated. Insufficient data are available to assess the immune response of a fourth dose of diphtheria and tetanus toxoids and acellular pertussis vaccine when administered with *Havrix*. There are limited data to assess the concomitant use of *Havrix* with other vaccines.

➤*Admixture incompatibilities:* Do not mix hepatitis A vaccine, inactivated with any other vaccine in the same syringe or vial.

HEPATITIS A VACCINE, INACTIVATED — INJECTION

Adverse Reactions

➤*Havrix*: The safety of *Havrix* has been evaluated in clinical trials involving more than 31,000 individuals receiving doses ranging from 360 to 1,440 EL.U. and during postmarketing experience in Europe. As with all pharmaceuticals, however, it is possible that expanded commercial use of the vaccine could reveal rare adverse reactions not observed in clinical studies.

The frequency of solicited adverse reactions tended to decrease with successive doses of *Havrix*. Most events reported were considered by the subjects as mild and did not last for more than 24 hours.

Of solicited adverse reactions in clinical trials, the most frequently reported by volunteers was injection site soreness (56% of adults and 21% of children); however, less than 0.5% of soreness was reported as severe. Headache was reported by 14% of adults and less than 9% of children.

The following are other solicited and unsolicited reactions occurring during clinical trials:

CNS – Fatigue, malaise (1% to 10%); hypertonic episode, insomnia, photophobia, vertigo (less than 1%).

Dermatologic – Pruritus, rash, urticaria (less than 1%).

GI – Anorexia, nausea (1% to 10%); abdominal pain, diarrhea, dysgeusia, vomiting (less than 1%).

Hematologic – Lymphadenopathy (less than 1%).

Local – Induration, redness, swelling (1% to 10%); hematoma (less than 1%).

Musculoskeletal – Arthralgia, elevation of creatine phosphokinase, myalgia (less than 1%).

Respiratory – Pharyngitis, upper respiratory tract infections (less than 1%).

Miscellaneous – Fever (greater than 37.5°C [99.5°F]) (1% to 10%).

➤*Additional safety data (Havrix)*: Safety data were obtained from 2 additional sources in which large populations were vaccinated. In an outbreak setting in which 4,930 individuals were immunized with a single dose of either 720 or 1,440 EL.U. of *Havrix*, the vaccine was well tolerated and no serious adverse reactions due to vaccination were reported. Overall, less than 10% of vaccinees reported solicited general adverse reactions following the vaccine. The most common solicited local adverse reaction was pain at the injection site, reported in 22.3% of subjects at 24 hours and decreasing to 2.4% by 72 hours.

In a field efficacy trial, 19,037 children received the 360 EL.U. dose of *Havrix*. The most commonly reported adverse reactions following administration of *Havrix* were injection site pain (9.5%) and tenderness (8.1%), which were reported following first doses of *Havrix*. Other adverse reactions were infrequent and comparable with the control vaccine hepatitis B vaccine, recombinant. Additionally, no serious adverse reactions due to the vaccine were reported. The large trial further allowed for analysis of rare adverse reactions, including hospitalization and death. No significant differences were found between the cohorts.

In subjects with chronic liver disease, *Havrix* was safe and well-tolerated. Local injection-site reactions were similar among all 4 groups, and no serious adverse reactions attributed to the vaccine were reported in subjects with chronic liver disease.

Safety data for Havrix 720 EL.U. per 0.5 mL beginning at 11 months of age – In the multicenter study, parents/guardians recorded local and general symptoms on diary cards for 4 days (days 0 to 3) after vaccination. In the 3 groups of children who received *Havrix* alone, safety data were available for 723 children who received 1,396 documented doses of *Havrix*. Additional safety data were available for 181 children who received *Havrix* coadministered with diphtheria and tetanus toxoids and acellular pertussis vaccine, adsorbed and Hib conjugate vaccine (PRP-T). Most adverse reactions were mild and transient. The frequencies of solicited local and systemic reactions following receipt of *Havrix* were monitored during the 4-day observation period.

The following rates of solicited adverse reactions in children who received their first dose of *Havrix* alone between 11 and 25 months of age were observed. Among local reactions, pain was reported in 15% to 21% of subjects, redness in 16% to 21%, and swelling in 8% of subjects. Among general reactions, irritability was reported in 24% to 36% of subjects, loss of appetite in 16% to 19% of subjects, drowsiness in 15% to 17% of subjects, and fever greater than 39.5°C (103.1°F) in 1% or less of subjects.

Following the booster dose of *Havrix*, among local reactions, pain was reported in 16% to 21% of subjects, redness in 17% to 22%, and swelling in 8% to 10% of subjects. Following the booster dose of *Havrix*, among general reactions, irritability was reported in 19% to 29% of subjects, loss of appetite in 14% to 18% of subjects, drowsiness in 13% to 16% of subjects, and fever greater than 39.5°C (103.1°F) in less than or equal to 2% of subjects or less.

Drowsiness and loss of appetite occurred at statistically significantly higher rates in subjects 15 to 18 months of age who received Hib conjugate vaccine (PRP-T) and diphtheria and tetanus toxoids and acellular pertussis vaccine, adsorbed concomitantly with *Havrix* as compared with subjects 15 to 18 months of age who received Hib conjugate vaccine (PRP-T) and diphtheria and tetanus toxoids and acellular pertussis vaccine, adsorbed (drowsiness 34% and 22% and loss of appetite 29% and 19%, respectively). With the exception of fever (greater than 39.5°C [103.1°F]), the solicited general symptoms occurred at statistically significantly higher rates in subjects 15 to 18 months of age who received Hib conjugate vaccine (PRP-T) and diphtheria and tetanus toxoids and acellular pertussis vaccine, adsorbed concomitantly with *Havrix* as compared with subjects 15 to 18 months of age who received *Havrix* alone (irritability 46% and 30%, drowsiness 34% and 17%, and loss of appetite 29% and 17%, respectively).

A febrile seizure was reported in a subject 18 months of age 2 days after receiving the first dose of *Havrix*. Other serious adverse reactions reported during the course of this study included a single case each of hepatitis approximately 5 months postdose 1, insulin-dependent diabetes approximately 4 months post dose 1, and Kawasaki disease approximately 3.5 months post dose 1. The association of these events with vaccination is unknown.

➤*Postmarketing (Havrix)*: Rare voluntary reports of adverse reactions in people receiving *Havrix* that have been reported since market introduction of the vaccine include localized edema.

While no causal relationship has been established, the following rare events have been reported:

Cardiovascular – Syncope.

CNS – Convulsions, dizziness, encephalopathy, Guillain-Barré syndrome, multiple sclerosis, myelitis, neuropathy, paresthesia, somnolence.

Dermatologic – Erythema multiforme, hyperhydrosis.

Hematologic – Lymphadenopathy, thrombocytopenia.

Hepatic – Hepatitis, jaundice.

Hypersensitivity – Anaphylaxis/anaphylactoid reactions, angioedema.

Respiratory – Dyspnea.

Miscellaneous – Congenital abnormality.

➤*Vaqta*: The safety of *Vaqta* has been evaluated in over 10,000 subjects 1 to 85 years of age. Subjects were given 1 or 2 doses of the vaccine. The second (booster dose) was given 6 months or more after the first dose. As with any vaccine, there is the possibility that use of *Vaqta* in very large populations might reveal adverse reactions not observed in clinical trials.

Children (12 through 23 months of age) – In combined clinical trials involving 706 healthy children 12 through 23 months of age who received 1 or more approximately 25-unit dose, subjects were monitored for local adverse reactions and fever for 5 days after each vaccination and systemic adverse reactions for 14 days after each vaccination by diary cards. Some of these children received *Vaqta* in combination with other routinely recommended pediatric vaccines. The following information lists the complaints (with 95% CI) for all solicited events and for unsolicited events reported at 1% or more without regard to causality in decreasing order of frequency within each body system.

Hepatitis A Vaccine, Inactivated Adverse Reactions

Adverse reaction	Vaqta Dose 1	Vaqta Booster
	Adverse reaction rate (n/total n) (95% CI)	
Local		
Erythema	1.3% (9/682) (0.6%, 2.6%)	1.6% (10/622) (0.8%, 3%)
Pain/Tenderness/ Soreness	3.5% (24/682) (2.3%, 5.2%)	3.1% (19/622) (1.9%, 4.9%)
Swelling	1.6% (11/682) (0.8%, 2.9%)	1.3% (8/622) (0.6%, 2.6%)
Warmth	0.9% (6/682) (0.4%, 2%)	0.8% (5/622) (0.3%, 2%)
Miscellaneous		
Fever ≥ 100.4°F, oral	9.1% (62/678) (7.1%, 11.6%)	11.3% (69/611) (9%, 14.1%)
Fever ≥ 102°F, oral	3.8% (26/678) (2.5%, 5.6%)	3.1% (19/611) (1.9%, 4.9%)
Rash, measles-like/rubella-like	1% (7/683) (0.4%, 2%)	—
Rash, varicella-like	0.9% (6/683) (0.3%, 2%)	—

➤*Unsolicited adverse reactions of 1% or more (95% CI) (Vaqta)*:

CNS – Crying 1.8% (1%, 3.2%); irritability 10.8% (8.6%, 13.4%).

Dermatologic – Rash 4.5% (3.1%, 6.4%); viral exanthema 1% (0.4%, 2.2%).

GI – Anorexia 1.2% (0.6%, 2.4%); diarrhea 5.9% (4.3%, 8%); vomiting 4% (2.7%, 5.8%).

Local – Ecchymosis 1% (0.4%, 2.2%).

Respiratory – Cough 5.1% (3.6%, 7.1%); laryngotracheobronchitis 1.2% (0.6%, 2.4%); nasal congestion 1.2% (0.6%, 2.4%); respiratory congestion 1.6% (0.8%, 2.9%); rhinorrhea 5.7% (4.1%, 7.8%); upper respiratory tract infection 10.1% (8%, 12.7%).

Special senses – Conjunctivitis 1.3% (0.6%, 2.6%); otitis 1.8% (1%, 3.2%); otitis media 7.6% (5.8%, 9.9%).

Serious adverse reactions (Vaqta) – There were 7 children who experienced 9 seizures during the entire study period. Seizures were reported between 9 and 81 days following the administration of *Vaqta*. Some subjects had received concomitant or noncomitant immunization with measles, mumps, and rubella virus vaccine and varicella virus vaccine live. None of the events were considered to be related to *Vaqta* by the investigator. Other serious reactions that occurred during the study included bronchiolitis,

HEPATITIS A VACCINE, INACTIVATED — INJECTION

dehydration, right lower lobe pneumonia, asthma, and asthma exacerbation, which were also considered by the investigator to be unrelated to *Vaqta*. These events occurred 9 to 46 days following the administration of *Vaqta*. Some subjects received concomitant or nonconcomitant immunization with measles, mumps, and rubella virus vaccine and varicella virus vaccine live or diphtheria and tetanus toxoids and acellular pertussis vaccine, adsorbed, and/or inactivated polio vaccine.

➤*Children/Adolescents 2 through 18 years of age (safety data gathered from The Monroe Efficacy Study) (Vaqta)*: In The Monroe Efficacy study, 1,037 healthy children and adolescents, 2 through 16 years of age, received a primary dose of approximately 25 units of *Vaqta* and a booster 6, 12, or 18 months later, or placebo. Subjects were followed during a 5-day period for fever and local complaints and during a 14-day period for systemic complaints. Injection-site complaints, generally mild and transient, were the most frequently reported complaints. The following table summarizes the local and systemic complaints (1% or greater) reported in this study, without regard to causality. There were no significant differences in the rates of any complaints between vaccine and placebo recipients after dose 1.

Adverse Reactions in Children and Adolescents (≥ 1%)

Adverse reaction	*Vaqta* Dose 1[a]	*Vaqta* Booster	Placebo[a,b]
CNS			
Headache	0.4% (2/519)	0.8% (4/475)	1% (5/518)
GI			
Abdominal pain	1.2% (6/519)	1.1% (5/475)	1% (5/518)
Local			
Erythema	1.9% (10/515)	0.8% (4/475)	1.8% (9/510)
Pain	6.4% (33/515)	3.4% (16/475)	6.3% (32/510)
Swelling	1.7% (9/515)	1.5% (7/475)	1.6% (8/510)
Tenderness	4.9% (25/515)	1.7% (8/475)	6.1% (31/510)
Warmth	1.7% (9/515)	0.6% (3/475)	1.6% (8/510)
Respiratory			
Pharyngitis	1.2% (6/519)	0% (0/475)	0.8% (4/518)

[a] No statistically significant differences between the 2 groups.
[b] Second injection of placebo not administered because code for the trial was broken.

➤*Children/Adolescents (2 through 18 years of age) (combined clinical trials) (Vaqta)*: In combined clinical trials (including The Monroe Efficacy Study participants) involving 2,615 healthy children (2 years of age and older) who received 1 or more approximately 25 unit dose of *Vaqta*, subjects were followed for fever and local complaints during a 5-day period postvaccination and systemic complaints during a 14-day period postvaccination. Injection-site complaints, generally mild and transient, were the most frequently reported complaints. The following adverse reactions are the complaints reported by 1% or more of subjects, without regard to causality, in decreasing order of frequency within each body system:

CNS – Headache (2.3%).

GI – Abdominal pain (1.6%); diarrhea (1%); vomiting (1%).

Lab test abnormalities – Very few laboratory abnormalities were reported and included isolated reports of elevated liver function tests, eosinophilia, and increased urine protein.

Local – Ecchymosis (1.3%); erythema (7.5%); pain (18.7%); swelling (7.3%); tenderness (16.9%); warmth (8.6%).

Respiratory – Cough (1%); pharyngitis (1.5%); upper respiratory tract infection (1.1%).

Miscellaneous – Fever (38.8°C [102°F] or higher, oral) (3.1%).

➤*Adults (19 years of age or older) (Vaqta)*: In combined clinical trials involving 1,512 healthy adults who received 1 or more approximately 50-unit dose of *Vaqta*, subjects were followed for fever and local complaints during a 5-day period postvaccination and systemic complaints during a 14–day period postvaccination. Injection-site complaints, generally mild and transient, were the most frequently reported complaints. Listed below are the complaints reported by 1% or more of subjects, without regard to causality, in decreasing order of frequency within each body system:

CNS – Asthenia/fatigue (3.9%); headache (16%).

GI – Abdominal pain (1.3%); diarrhea (2.5%); nausea (2.3%).

GU – Menstruation disorder (1.1%).

Local – Ecchymosis (1.5%); erythema (13.1%); pain (51.1%); pain/soreness (1.2%); swelling (13.8%); tenderness (52.7%); warmth (17.4%).

Musculoskeletal – Arm pain (1.3%); back pain (1.1%); myalgia (1.9%); stiffness (1%).

Respiratory – Nasal congestion (1.1%); pharyngitis (2.7%); upper respiratory tract infection (2.7%).

Miscellaneous – Fever (2.7%).

➤*Hypersensitivity (Vaqta)*: Local and/or systemic allergic reactions that occurred in less than 1% of children/adolescents or adults in clinical trials regardless of causality included the following:

Local – Injection-site pruritus and/or rash.

Systemic – Asthma, bronchial constriction, dermatitis, edema/swelling, eye irritation/itching, generalized erythema, pruritus, rash, urticaria, wheezing.

➤*Postmarketing (Vaqta)*: The following additional adverse reactions have been reported with use of the marketed vaccine.

CNS – Very rarely, Guillain-Barré syndrome, cerebellar ataxia, and encephalitis.

Hematologic – Very rarely, thrombocytopenia. In a postmarketing short-term safety surveillance study conducted at a large health maintenance organization in the United States, a total of 42,110 individuals 2 years of age and older received 1 or 2 doses of *Vaqta* (13,735 children/adolescents and 28,375 adult subjects). Safety was passively monitored by electronic search of the automated medical records database for emergency room and outpatient visits, hospitalizations, and deaths. Medical charts were reviewed when indicated. There was no serious, vaccine-related adverse reaction identified among the 42,110 vaccine recipients in this study. Diarrhea/gastroenteritis, resulting in outpatient visits, was determined by the investigator to be the only vaccine-related, nonserious adverse reaction in the study. There was no vaccine-related adverse reaction identified that had not been reported in earlier clinical trials with *Vaqta*.

➤*Reporting of adverse reactions:* The US Department of Health and Human Services has established the Vaccine Adverse Events Reporting System (VAERS) to accept reports of suspected adverse reactions after the administration of any vaccine including, but not limited to, the reporting of events required by the National Childhood Vaccine Injury Act of 1986. The toll-free number for VAERS forms and information is 1-800-822-7967. Reporting forms may also be obtained at the VAERS Web site at http://www.vaers.org.

Patient Information

Inform vaccine recipients, parents, and guardians of the potential benefits and risks of immunization with hepatitis A vaccine, inactivated. When educating vaccine recipients and guardians regarding potential side effects, emphasize that hepatitis A vaccine, inactivated contains noninfectious killed viruses and cannot cause hepatitis A infection. It is important to question the vaccine recipient, parent, or guardian concerning the occurrence of any symptoms and/or signs of an adverse reaction after a previous dose of hepatitis A vaccine. Inform the patients, parents, or guardians about the potential for adverse reactions that have been temporally associated with administration of hepatitis A, inactivated. Instruct the patient, parent, or guardian accompanying the recipient to report severe or unusual adverse reactions to the health care provider or clinic where the vaccine was administered.

Give vaccine recipients or guardians the vaccine information statements, which are required by the National Childhood Vaccine Injury Act of 1986 to be given prior to immunization. These materials are available free of charge at the CDC Web site (http://www.cdc.gov/nip). The US Department of Health and Human Services has established a VAERS to accept all reports of suspected adverse reactions after the administration of any vaccine including, but not limited to, the reporting of events required by the National Childhood Vaccine Injury Act of 1986. The VAERS toll-free number is 1–800–822–7967. Reporting forms also may be obtained at the VAERS Web site at http://www.vaers.org.

HEPATITIS A, INACTIVATED AND HEPATITIS B, RECOMBINANT VACCINE

Rx	**Twinrix** (GlaxoSmithKline)	**Injection:** ≥ 720 EL.U.[a] inactivated hepatitis A, 20 mcg recombinant HBsAg[b] protein/mL[c]	In single-dose vials (1s and 10s).

[a] EL.U. = ELISA (enzyme linked immunosorbent assay) units.
[b] HBsAg = Hepatitis B surface antigen.
[c] With thimerosal (< 1 mcg mercury).

HEPATITIS A (INACTIVATED) AND HEPATITIS B (RECOMBINANT) VACCINE — INJECTION

For complete and comparative prescribing information, refer to the Agents for Active Immunization introduction and the individual Hepatitis A, Inactivated and Hepatitis B, Recombinant monographs.

Indications

➤*Hepatitis A and B vaccination:* For active immunization of people ≥ 18 years of age against disease caused by hepatitis A virus (HAV) and infection by all known subtypes of hepatitis B virus (HBV). As with any vaccine, vaccination with this product may not protect 100% of recipients. As hepatitis D (caused by the delta virus) does not occur in the absence of HBV infection, it can be expected that hepatitis D also will be prevented by vaccination.

➤*Patient selection:* Immunization is recommended for all susceptible people ≥ 18 years of age who are or will be at risk of exposure to hepatitis A and B viruses, including, but not limited to, the following: Travelers to areas

HEPATITIS A (INACTIVATED) AND HEPATITIS B (RECOMBINANT) VACCINE — INJECTION

of high/intermediate endemicity for HAV and HBV (see table) who are at increased risk of HBV infection because of behavioral or occupational factors.

➤*Patients with chronic liver disease:* Patients with chronic liver disease, including alcoholic cirrhosis, chronic hepatitis C, autoimmune hepatitis, and primary biliary cirrhosis.

➤*People at risk through their work:* Laboratory workers who handle live hepatitis A and hepatitis B viruses, police, and other personnel who render first-aid or medical assistance, workers who come in contact with feces or sewage.

➤*People exposed to HAV and HBV:* Health care personnel who render first-aid or emergency medical assistance; personnel employed in day care centers and correctional facilities; residents of drug and alcohol treatment centers; staff of hemodialysis units; people living in, or relocating to, areas of high/intermediate endemicity of HAV and who have risk factors for HBV; men who have sex with men; people at increased risk of disease because of their sexual practices; patients frequently receiving blood products, including people who have clotting-factor disorders (hemophiliacs and other recipients of therapeutic blood products); military recruits and other military personnel at increased risk for HBV; users of injectable illicit drugs; individuals who are at increased risk for HBV infection and who are close household contacts of patients with acute or relapsing hepatitis A; individuals who are at increased risk for HAV infection and who are close household contacts of individuals with acute or chronic hepatitis B infection.

Administration and Dosage

➤*Approved by the FDA:* May 11, 2001.

➤*Vaccination schedule:* Primary immunization for adults consists of 3 doses, given on a 0-, 1-, and 6-month schedule.

➤*Administration:* Administer by IM injection. Do not inject IV or ID. In adults, give the injection in the deltoid region. Do not administer in the gluteal region; such injections may result in a suboptimal response.

When concomitant administration of other vaccines or immunoglobulin is required, give with different syringes and at different injection sites.

➤*Preparation:* Shake vial or syringe well before withdrawal and use. Visually inspect parenteral drug products for particulate matter or discoloration prior to administration. With thorough agitation, the vaccine is a slightly turbid white suspension. Discard if it appears otherwise.

Use vaccine as supplied; no dilution or reconstitution is necessary. Use the full recommended dose of the vaccine. After removal of the appropriate volume from a single-dose vial, discard any vaccine remaining in the vial.

➤*Storage/Stability:* Store refrigerated between 2° and 8°C (36° and 46°F). Do not freeze; discard if product has been frozen. Do not dilute to administer.

HUMAN PAPILLOMAVIRUS RECOMBINANT VACCINE, QUADRIVALENT

Rx	**Gardasil** (Merck)	**Solution for injection**: 20 mcg of HPV 6 L1 protein, 40 mcg of HPV 11 L1 protein, 40 mcg of HPV 16 L1 protein, 20 mcg of HPV 18 L1 protein per 0.5 mL	Preservative free. In 0.5 mL single-dose vials.

HUMAN PAPILLOMAVIRUS RECOMBINANT VACCINE, QUADRIVALENT — INJECTION

Indications

In girls and women 9 to 26 years of age for the prevention of the following diseases caused by human papillomavirus (HPV) types 6, 11, 16, and 18:

- Cervical cancer
- Genital warts (condyloma acuminata) and the following precancerous or dysplastic lesions:
  - Cervical adenocarcinoma in situ (AIS)
  - Cervical intraepithelial neoplasia (CIN) grade 2 or grade 3
  - Vulvar intraepithelial neoplasia (VIN) grade 2 or grade 3
  - Vaginal intraepithelial neoplasia (VAIN) grade 2 or grade 3
  - CIN grade 1

Administration and Dosage

➤*Approved by the FDA:* June 8, 2006.

Quadrivalent HPV (types 6, 11, 16, 18) recombinant vaccine should be administered intramuscularly (IM) as 3 separate 0.5 mL doses according to the following schedule:

- First dose: at elected date
- Second dose: 2 months after the first dose
- Third dose: 6 months after the first dose

➤*Method of administration:* Quadrivalent HPV (types 6, 11, 16, 18) recombinant vaccine should be administered IM in the deltoid region of the upper arm or in the higher anterolateral area of the thigh.

It must not be injected intravascularly. Subcutaneous and intradermal administration have not been studied, and therefore are not recommended.

The prefilled syringe is for single use only and should not be used for more than one individual. For single-use vials, a separate sterile syringe and needle must be used for each individual.

The vaccine should be used as supplied; no dilution or reconstitution is necessary. The full recommended dose of the vaccine should be used.

Shake well before use. Thorough agitation immediately before administration is necessary to maintain suspension of the vaccine.

After thorough agitation, quadrivalent HPV (types 6, 11, 16, 18) recombinant vaccine is a white, cloudy liquid. Parenteral drug products should be inspected visually for particulate matter and discoloration prior to administration. Do not use the product if particulates are present or if it appears discolored.

➤*Single-dose vial use:* Withdraw the 0.5 mL dose of vaccine from the single-dose vial using a sterile needle and syringe free of preservatives, antiseptics, and detergents. Once the single-dose vial has been penetrated, the withdrawn vaccine should be used promptly, and the vial must be discarded.

➤*Prefilled syringe use:* Inject the entire contents of the syringe.

Use the enclosed needle for administration. If a different needle is chosen, it should fit securely on the syringe and be no longer than 1 inch to ensure proper functioning of the needle guard device. Two detachable labels are provided that can be removed after the needle is guarded.

Remove syringe tip cap. Attach luer needle. Depress both anti-rotation tabs to secure the syringe and attach the luer needle by twisting clockwise direction. The needle guard device will not activate to cover and protect the needle unless the entire dose has been given. Remove the needle sheath. Administer the injection per standard protocol as stated above. Depress the plunger while grasping the finger flange until the entire dose has been given. Remove the needle from the vaccine recipient. Release the plunger and allow the syringe to move up until the entire needle is guarded. For documentation of vaccination, remove detachable labels by pulling slowly on them. Dispose of in an approved sharps container.

➤*Storage/Stability:* Store refrigerated at 2° to 8°C (36° to 46°F). Do not freeze. Protect from light.

ZOSTER VACCINE LIVE (OKA/MERCK)

Rx	**Zostavax** (Merck)	**Injection, lyophilized**: 19,400 PFU of Oka/Merck varicella-zoster virus (live)	Sucrose. Preservative-free. In single-dose vials of 1s and 10s.

ZOSTER VACCINE LIVE (OKA/MERCK) — INJECTION

Indications

➤*Herpes zoster prevention:* For prevention of herpes zoster (shingles) in persons 60 years of age and older.

Not indicated for the treatment of zoster or postherpetic neuralgia.

Administration and Dosage

➤*Approved by the FDA:* May 25, 2006.

➤*For subcutaneous use:* For subcutaneous administration. Do not inject intravascularly.

➤*Syringe selection:* Use only sterile syringes free of preservatives, antiseptics, and detergents for each injection and/or reconstitution of zoster vaccine. Preservatives, antiseptics, and detergents may inactivate the vaccine virus.

➤*Reconstitution:* Zoster vaccine is stored frozen and should be reconstituted immediately upon removal from the freezer. Reconstitute the vaccine using only the diluent supplied. The supplied diluent is free of preservatives or other antiviral substances that might inactivate the vaccine virus. Withdraw the entire contents of the diluent vial into a syringe. Inject all of the diluent in the syringe into the vial of lyophilized vaccine and gently agitate to mix thoroughly. The vaccine should be administered immediately after reconstitution to minimize loss of potency. Discard reconstituted vaccine if it is not used within 30 minutes. Do not freeze reconstituted vaccine.

➤*Administration:* Zoster vaccine is administered as a single dose. Withdraw the entire contents into a syringe and inject the total volume of reconstituted vaccine subcutaneously, preferably in the upper arm.

➤*Storage/Stability:* During shipment, to ensure that there is no loss of potency, the vaccine must be maintained at a temperature of −20°C (−4°F) or colder.

Store frozen at an average temperature of −15°C (5°F) or colder until it is reconstituted for injection. Any freezer, including frost-free, that has a separate sealed freezer door and reliably maintains an average temperature of −15°C or colder is acceptable for storing zoster vaccine.

For information regarding stability under conditions other than those recommended, call 1-800-637-2590.

Before reconstitution, protect from light.

Store the diluent separately at room temperature (20° to 25°C; 68° to 77°F) or in the refrigerator (2° to 8°C; 36° to 46°F).

ZOSTER VACCINE LIVE (OKA/MERCK) — INJECTION

Actions

➤*Pharmacology:* The risk of developing zoster appears to be related to a decline in varicella-zoster virus–specific immunity. Zoster vaccine was shown to boost varicella-zoster virus–specific immunity, which is thought to be the mechanism by which it protects against zoster and its complications.

Contraindications

Contraindicated in persons with a history of anaphylactic/anaphylactoid reaction to gelatin, neomycin, or any other component of the vaccine; with a history of primary or acquired immunodeficiency states including leukemia, lymphomas of any type, or other malignant neoplasms affecting the bone marrow or lymphatic system, or AIDS or other clinical manifestations of infection with HIV; on immunosuppressive therapy, including high-dose corticosteroids; with active untreated tuberculosis; and who are or may become pregnant.

Warnings

➤*Immunosuppression:* Vaccination with a live attenuated vaccine, such as zoster vaccine, may result in a more extensive vaccine-associated rash or disseminated disease in patients who are immunosuppressed. Safety and efficacy of zoster vaccine have not been evaluated in patients on immunosuppressive therapy, nor in patients receiving daily topical or inhaled corticosteroids or low-dose oral corticosteroids.

➤*Neomycin allergy:* Neomycin allergy commonly manifests as a contact dermatitis, which is not a contraindication to receiving this vaccine. Do not give zoster vaccine to persons with a history of anaphylactic reaction to topically or systemically administered neomycin.

➤*Anaphylactoid reactions:* As with any vaccine, make adequate treatment provisions, including epinephrine injection (1:1,000), available for immediate use should an anaphylactic/anaphylactoid reaction occur.

➤*Varicella virus:* Zoster vaccine is not a substitute for varicella virus vaccine.

➤*Pregnancy: Category C.* Animal reproduction studies have not been conducted with zoster vaccine. It is also not known whether zoster vaccine can cause fetal harm when administered to a pregnant woman or can affect reproduction capacity. However, naturally occurring varicella-zoster virus infection is known to sometimes cause fetal harm. Therefore, do not administer zoster vaccine to a pregnant woman; furthermore, pregnancy should be avoided for 3 months following vaccination.

Pregnancy registry – Vaccinees and health care providers are encouraged to report any exposure to zoster vaccine during pregnancy by calling 1-800-986-8999.

➤*Lactation:* Some viruses are excreted in human milk; however, it is not known whether varicella-zoster virus is secreted in human milk. Therefore, because some viruses are secreted in human milk, exercise caution if zoster vaccine is administered to a breast-feeding woman.

➤*Children:* Do not administer zoster vaccine in children.

Precautions

➤*Acute illness:* Consider deferral of vaccination in acute illness, for example, in the presence of fever higher than 38.5°C (higher than 101.3°F).

➤*Duration:* The duration of protection after vaccination with zoster vaccine is unknown. In the Shingles Prevention Study (SPS), protection from zoster was demonstrated through 4 years of follow-up. The need for revaccination has not been defined.

➤*Protection:* As with any vaccine, vaccination with zoster vaccine may not result in protection of all vaccine recipients.

➤*Transmission:* In clinical trials with zoster vaccine, transmission of the vaccine virus has not been reported. However, postmarketing experience with varicella vaccines suggests that transmission of the vaccine virus may occur rarely between vaccinees who develop a varicella-like rash and susceptible contacts. Transmission of the vaccine virus from varicella vaccine recipients without a varicella-zoster virus–like rash has been reported but has not been confirmed. Weigh the risk of transmitting the attenuated vaccine virus to a susceptible person against the risk of developing natural zoster that could be transmitted to a susceptible person.

Adverse Reactions

The remainder of subjects in the SPS (n = 15,925 received zoster vaccine and n = 16,005 received placebo) were actively followed for safety outcomes through day 42 postvaccination and passively followed for safety after day 42.

Because clinical trials are conducted under conditions that may not be typical of those observed in clinical practice, the adverse reaction rates presented below may not be reflective of those observed in clinical practice.

➤*Serious adverse reactions:* The following table displays selected cardiovascular serious adverse reactions (SARs) occurring in the SPS within 42 days postvaccination.

Zoster Vaccine Cardiovascular Adverse Reactions

	Adverse Event Monitoring Substudy		Entire study cohort	
	Zoster vaccine 3,326[a]	Placebo 3,249[a]	Zoster vaccine 18,671[a]	Placebo 18,717[a]
	n[b]	n[b]	n[b]	n[b]
Overall cardiovascular reactions by body system	20 (0.6%)	12 (0.4%)	81 (0.4%)	72 (0.4%)
Coronary artery disease-related conditions[c]	10 (0.3%)	5 (0.2%)	45 (0.2%)	35 (0.2%)

[a] Number of subjects with safety follow-up.
[b] n = number of subjects reporting SARs within the category.
[c] Angina pectoris, coronary artery disease, coronary occlusion, cardiovascular disorder, myocardial ischemia, and myocardial infarction

Investigator-determined, vaccine-related serious adverse reactions were reported for 2 subjects vaccinated with zoster vaccine (asthma exacerbation and polymyalgia rheumatica) and 3 subjects who received placebo (Goodpasture syndrome, anaphylactic reaction, and polymyalgia rheumatica).

➤*Deaths:* The overall incidence of death occurring days 0 to 42 postvaccination was similar between vaccination groups during the days 0 to 42 postvaccination period; 14 deaths occurred in the group of subjects who received zoster vaccine, and 16 deaths occurred in the group of subjects who received placebo. The most common reported cause of death was cardiovascular disease (10 in the group of subjects who received zoster vaccine, 8 in the group of subjects who received placebo). The overall incidence of death occurring at any time during the study was similar between vaccination groups: 793 deaths (4.1%) occurred in subjects who received zoster vaccine and 795 deaths (4.1%) in subjects who received placebo.

➤*Most common adverse reactions:*

Zoster Vaccine Adverse Reactions (≥ 1%)

Adverse reaction	Zoster vaccine (3,345)	Placebo (3,271)
CNS		
Headache	1.4%	0.8%
Local		
Erythema[a]	33.7%	6.4%
Hematoma	1.4%	1.4%
Pain/tenderness[a]	33.4%	8.3%
Pruritus	6.6%	1%
Swelling[a]	24.9%	4.3%
Warmth	1.5%	0.3%

[a] Designates a solicited adverse reaction. Injection-site adverse reactions were solicited only from days 0 to 4 postvaccination.

The following adverse reactions in the Adverse Event Monitoring Substudy of the SPS (days 0 to 42 postvaccination) were reported at an incidence of 1% or greater in subjects who received zoster vaccine than in subjects who received placebo, respectively.

➤*CNS:* Asthenia (32 [1%] vs 14 [0.4%]).

➤*Dermatologic:* Skin disorder (35 [1.1%] vs 31 [1%])

➤*GI:* Diarrhea (51 [1.5%] vs 41 [1.3%])

➤*Respiratory:* Respiratory disorder (35 [1.1%] vs 27 [0.8%]), respiratory infection (65 [1.9%] vs 55 [1.7%]), rhinitis (46 [1.4%] vs 36 [1.1%])

➤*Miscellaneous:* Fever (59 [1.8%] vs 53 [1.6%]), flu syndrome (57 [1.7%] vs 52 [1.6%])

➤*Adverse reactions occurring after day 42 postvaccination:* Over the course of the study (4.9 years), 51 subjects (1.5%) receiving zoster vaccine were reported to have congestive heart failure (CHF) or pulmonary edema compared with 39 subjects (1.2%) receiving placebo in the Adverse Event Monitoring Substudy; 58 subjects (0.3%) receiving zoster vaccine were reported to have CHF or pulmonary edema compared with 45 (0.2%) subjects receiving placebo in the overall study.

➤*Varicella-zoster virus rashes following vaccination:* Within the 42-day postvaccination reporting period in the SPS, noninjection-site, zoster-like rashes were reported by 53 subjects (17 for zoster vaccine and 36 for placebo). Of 41 specimens that were adequate for polymerase chain reaction (PCR) testing, wild-type varicella-zoster virus was detected in 25 (5 for zoster vaccine, 20 for placebo) of these specimens. The Oka/Merck strain of varicella-zoster virus was not detected from any of these specimens.

Of reported varicella-like rashes (n = 59), 10 had specimens that were available and adequate for PCR testing. Varicella-zoster virus was not detected in any of these specimens.

ZOSTER VACCINE LIVE (OKA/MERCK) — INJECTION

In all other clinical trials in support of zoster vaccine, the reported rates of noninjection-site, zoster-like and varicella-like rashes within 42 days post-vaccination were also low in both zoster vaccine recipients and placebo recipients. Of the 17 reported varicella-like rashes and noninjection-site, zoster-like rashes, 10 specimens were available and adequate for PCR testing. The Oka/Merck strain was identified by PCR analysis from the lesion specimens of 2 subjects who reported varicella-like rashes (onset on day 8 and 17).

➤*Reporting adverse reactions:* The US Department of Health and Human Services has established a Vaccine Adverse Event Reporting System (VAERS) to accept all reports of suspected adverse reactions after the administration of any vaccine. For information or a copy of the vaccine reporting form, call the VAERS toll-free number at 1-800-822-7967 or report online to http://www.vaers.hhs.gov.

Patient Information

Question the vaccine recipient about reactions to previous vaccines. Inform the vaccine recipient of the benefits and risks of zoster vaccine. Provide a copy of the patient information sheet and an opportunity to discuss any questions or concerns.

Inform vaccinees of the theoretical risk of transmitting the vaccine virus to varicella-susceptible persons, including pregnant women who have not had chickenpox. Advise patients that pregnancy should be avoided for 3 months following vaccination.

Advise patients to report any adverse reactions to their health care provider.

VARICELLA VIRUS VACCINE

Rx	**Varivax** (Merck)	**Powder for Injection:** 1350 PFU of Oka/Merck varicella virus (live)	Sucrose. In single-dose vials of 1s and 10s.

VARICELLA VIRUS VACCINE LIVE — INJECTION

For complete and comparative prescribing information, refer to the Agents for Active Immunization introduction.

Indications

➤*Varicella vaccination:* Varicella virus vaccine live is indicated for vaccination against varicella in individuals 12 months of age and older.

➤*Revaccination:* The duration of protection of varicella virus vaccine live is unknown at present and the need for booster doses is not defined. However, a boost in antibody levels has been observed in vaccinees following exposure to natural varicella as well as following a booster dose of varicella virus vaccine live administered 4 to 6 years postvaccination.

In a highly vaccinated population, immunity for some individuals may wane due to lack of exposure to natural varicella as a result of shifting epidemiology. Postmarketing surveillance studies are ongoing to evaluate the need and timing for booster vaccination.

➤*Protection:* Vaccination with varicella virus vaccine live may not result in protection of all healthy, susceptible children, adolescents, and adults.

Administration and Dosage

➤*For subcutaneous administration:* Do not inject intravenously.

➤*Children 12 months to 12 years of age:* Children 12 months to 12 years of age should receive a single 0.5 mL dose administered subcutaneously.

➤*Adults and children 13 years of age and older:* Adolescents and adults 13 years of age and older should receive a 0.5 mL dose administered subcutaneously at elected date and a second 0.5 mL dose 4 to 8 weeks later.

➤*Administration / Reconstitution:* Varicella virus vaccine live is for subcutaneous administration. The outer aspect of the upper arm (deltoid) is the preferred site of injection. Varicella virus vaccine live should be stored frozen at an average temperature of −15°C (+5°F) or colder until it is reconstituted for injection. Any freezer (eg, chest, frost-free) that reliably maintains an average temperature of −15°C (+5°F) and has a separate sealed freezer door is acceptable for storing varicella virus vaccine live. The diluent should be stored separately at room temperature or in the refrigerator. To reconstitute the vaccine, first withdraw 0.7 mL of diluent into the syringe to be used for reconstitution. Inject all the diluent in the syringe into the vial of lyophilized vaccine and gently agitate to mix thoroughly. Withdraw the entire contents into a syringe and inject the total volume (about 0.5 mL) of reconstituted vaccine subcutaneously, preferably into the outer aspect of the upper arm (deltoid) or the anterolateral thigh. It is recommended that the vaccine be administered immediately after reconstitution, to minimize loss of potency. Discard if reconstituted vaccine is not used within 30 minutes.

➤*Caution:* A sterile syringe free of preservatives, antiseptics, and detergents should be used for each injection or reconstitution of varicella virus vaccine live because these substances may inactivate the vaccine virus.

To reconstitute the vaccine, use only the sterile diluent supplied with varicella virus vaccine live, measles, mumps, and rubella virus vaccine live, or the component vaccines of measles, mumps, and rubella virus vaccine live, since it is free of preservatives or other antiviral substances which might inactivate the vaccine virus.

Do not freeze reconstituted vaccine.

➤*Use with other vaccines:* See Drug Interactions for more information.

➤*Storage / Stability:* Varicella virus vaccine live retains a potency level of 1500 PFU or higher per dose for at least 24 months in a frost-free freezer with an average temperature of −15°C (+5°F) or colder.

Varicella virus vaccine live has a minimum potency level of approximately 1350 PFU 30 minutes after reconstitution at room temperature (20° to 25°C; 68° to 77°F).

For information regarding stability under condition other than those recommended, call 1-800-9-VARIVAX.

During shipment, to ensure that there is no loss of potency, the vaccine must be maintained at a temperature of −20°C (−4°F) or colder.

Varicella virus vaccine live may be stored at refrigerator temperature (2° to 8°C; 36° to 46°F) for up to 72 continuous hours prior to reconstitution. Vaccine stored at 2° to 8°C which is not used within 72 hours of removal from −15°C storage should be discarded.

Before reconstitution, protect from light.

Contraindications

Hypersensitivity to any component of the vaccine, including gelatin; anaphylactoid reaction to neomycin (each dose of reconstituted vaccine contains trace quantities of neomycin); blood dyscrasias, leukemia, lymphomas of any type, or other malignant neoplasms affecting the bone marrow or lymphatic systems; active untreated tuberculosis; any febrile respiratory illness or other active febrile infection.

Individuals receiving immunosuppressive therapy. Individuals who are on immunosuppressant drugs are more susceptible to infections than healthy individuals. Vaccination with live attenuated varicella vaccine can result in a more extensive vaccine-associated rash or disseminated disease in individuals on immunosuppressant doses of corticosteroids.

Individuals with primary and acquired immunodeficiency states, including those who are immunosuppressed in association with AIDS or other clinical manifestations of infection with human immunodeficiency virus; cellular immune deficiencies; and hypogammaglobulinemic and dysgammaglobulinemic states.

A family history of congenital or hereditary immunodeficiency, unless the immune competence of the potential vaccine recipient is demonstrated.

➤*Pregnancy:* The possible effects of the vaccine on fetal development are unknown at this time. However, natural varicella is known to sometimes cause fetal harm. If vaccination of postpubertal females is undertaken, pregnancy should be avoided for 3 months following vaccination.

Warnings

➤*Acute lymphoblastic leukemia:* Children and adolescents with acute lymphoblastic leukemia (ALL) in remission can receive the vaccine under an investigational protocol. More information is available by contacting the varicella virus vaccine live coordinating center, Omnicare Clinical Research, Inc., 630 Allendale Road, King of Prussia, PA 19406, (484) 679-2856.

➤*Hypersensitivity reactions:* Adequate treatment provisions, including epinephrine injection (1:1000), should be available for immediate use should an anaphylactoid reaction occur.

➤*Pregnancy: Category C.* Animal reproduction studies have not been conducted with varicella virus vaccine live. It is also not known whether varicella virus vaccine live can cause fetal harm when administered to a pregnant woman or can affect reproduction capacity. Therefore, varicella virus vaccine live should not be administered to pregnant females; furthermore, pregnancy should be avoided for 3 months following vaccination. Merck & Co, Inc. maintains a Pregnancy Registry to monitor fetal outcomes of pregnant women exposed to varicella virus vaccine live. Patients and health care providers are encouraged to report any exposure to varicella virus vaccine live during pregnancy by calling (800) 986-8999.

➤*Lactation:* It is not known whether varicella vaccine virus is secreted in human milk. Therefore, because some viruses are secreted in human milk, caution should be exercised if varicella virus vaccine live is administered to a nursing woman.

➤*Children:* No clinical data are available on safety or efficacy of varicella virus vaccine live in children less than 1 year of age and administration to infants under 12 months of age is not recommended.

Precautions

➤*Anaphylactoid reactions:* See Warnings for more information.

➤*Protection:* The duration of protection from varicella infection after vaccination with varicella virus vaccine live is unknown.

➤*Live virus:* It is not known whether varicella virus vaccine live given immediately after exposure to natural varicella virus will prevent illness.

➤*Use with other vaccines:* See Drug Interactions for more information.

➤*Immunosuppression:* The safety and efficacy of varicella virus vaccine live have not been established in children and young adults who are known to be infected with human immunodeficiency viruses with and without evidence of immunosuppression. These patients should not receive varicella virus vaccine live.

The healthcare provider should question the patient, parent, or guardian about reactions to a previous dose of varicella virus vaccine live or a similar product.

VARICELLA VIRUS VACCINE LIVE — INJECTION

➤*Administration precautions:* Varicella virus vaccine live should not be injected into a blood vessel.

➤*Congenital immunodeficiency:* Vaccination should be deferred in patients with a family history of congenital or hereditary immunodeficiency until the patient's own immune system has been evaluated.

➤*Transmission:* Postmarketing experience suggests that transmission of vaccine virus may occur rarely between healthy vaccinees who develop a varicella-like rash and healthy susceptible contacts. Transmission of vaccine virus from vaccinees without a varicella-like rash has been reported but has not been confirmed.

Therefore, vaccine recipients should attempt to avoid, whenever possible, close association with susceptible high-risk individuals for up to 6 weeks. In circumstances where contact with high-risk individuals is unavoidable, the potential risk of transmission of vaccine virus should be weighed against the risk of acquiring and transmitting natural varicella virus. Susceptible high risk individuals include:

- Immunocompromised individuals.
- Pregnant women without documented history of chickenpox or laboratory evidence of prior infection.
- Newborn infants of mothers without documented history of chickenpox or laboratory evidence of prior infection.

Drug Interactions

➤*Use with other vaccines:* Vaccination should be deferred for at least 5 months following blood or plasma transfusions, or administration of immune globulin or varicella-zoster immune globulin (VZIG).

Varicella Vaccine Drug Interactions

Precipitant drug	Object drug*		Description
Immune globulins	Varicella vaccine	⟷	Defer vaccination for at least 5 months following blood or plasma transfusions, or administration of immune globulin or varicella-zoster immune globulin (VZIG). Following administration of varicella vaccine, do not give any immune globulin, including VZIG, for 2 months thereafter unless its use outweighs the benefits of vaccination.
Immunosuppressants	Varicella vaccine	↓	Individuals who are on immunosuppressant drugs are more susceptible to infections than healthy individuals. Vaccination with live attenuated varicella vaccine can result in a more extensive vaccine-associated rash or disseminated disease in individuals on immunosuppressant doses of corticosteroids.
Salicylates	Varicella vaccine	↑	Avoid use of salicylates for 6 weeks after varicella vaccine; Reye syndrome has been reported following salicylate use during natural varicella infections.

* ↑ = Object drug increased. ↓ = Object drug decreased. ⟷ = Undetermined clinical effect.

Adverse Reactions

Children 1 to 12 years of age – In clinical trials involving healthy children monitored for up to 42 days after a single dose of varicella virus vaccine live, the frequency of fever, injection-site complaints, or rashes were reported as follows:

Fever, local reactions, or rashes (%) in children 0 to 42 days postvaccination

Reaction	N	Post dose 1	Peak occurrence in postvaccination days
Fever ≥ 39°C (102°F) oral	8827	14.7%	0 to 42
Injection-site complaints (pain/soreness, swelling or erythema, rash, pruritus, hematoma, induration, stiffness)	8916	19.3%	0 to 2
Varicella-like rash (injection site)	8916	3.4%	8 to 19
Varicella-like rash (injection site) (median number of lesions)		2	
Varicella-like rash (generalized)	8916	3.8%	5 to 26
Varicella-like rash (generalized) (median number of lesions)		5	

In addition, the most frequently (greater than or equal to 1%) reported adverse experiences, without regard to causality, are listed in decreasing order of frequency: Upper respiratory tract illness, cough, irritability/nervousness, fatigue, disturbed sleep, diarrhea, loss of appetite, vomiting, otitis, diaper rash/contact rash, headache, teething, malaise, abdominal pain, other rash, nausea, eye complaints, chills, lymphadenopathy, myalgia, lower respiratory tract illness, allergic reactions (including allergic rash, hives), stiff neck, heat rash/prickly heat, arthralgia, eczema/dry skin/dermatitis, constipation, itching.

Pneumonitis has been reported rarely (less than 1%) in children vaccinated with varicella virus vaccine live; a causal relationship has not been established.

Febrile seizures have occurred rarely (less than 0.1%) in children vaccinated with varicella virus vaccine live; a causal relationship has not been established.

Adolescents and adults 13 years of age and older – In clinical trials involving healthy adolescents and adults, the majority of whom received 2 doses of varicella virus vaccine live and were monitored for up to 42 days after any dose, the frequency of fever, injection-site complaints, or rashes were reported as follows:

Fever, local reactions, or rashes (%) in adolescents and adults 0 to 42 days postvaccination

Reaction	N	Post dose 1	Peak occurrence in postvaccination days	N	Post dose 2	Peak occurrence in postvaccination days
Fever ≥37.7°C (100°F) oral	1584	10.2%	14 to 27	956	9.5%	0 to 42
Injection-site complaints (soreness, erythema, swelling, rash, pruritus, pyrexia, hematoma, induration, numbness)	1606	24.4%	0 to 2	955	32.5%	0 to 2
Varicella-like rash (injection site)	1606	3%	6 to 20	955	1%	0 to 6
Varicella-like rash (injection site) (median number of lesions)		2			2	
Varicella-like rash (generalized)	1606	5.5%	7 to 21	955	0.9%	0 to 23
Varicella-like rash (generalized) (median number of lesions)		5			5.5	

In addition, the most frequently (greater than or equal to 1%) reported adverse experiences, without regard to causality, are listed in decreasing order of frequency: Upper respiratory tract illness, headache, fatigue, cough, myalgia, disturbed sleep, nausea, malaise, diarrhea, stiff neck, irritability/nervousness, lymphadenopathy, chills, eye complaints, abdominal pain, loss of appetite, arthralgia, otitis, itching, vomiting, other rashes, constipation, lower respiratory tract illness, allergic reactions (including allergic rash, hives), contact rash, cold/canker sore. As with any vaccine, there is the possibility that broad use of the vaccine could reveal adverse reactions not observed in clinical trials.

➤*Postmarketing reports:* The following additional adverse reactions have been reported since the vaccine has been marketed:

CNS – Encephalitis; cerebrovascular accident; non-febrile seizures; Guillain-Barré syndrome; transverse myelitis; Bell's palsy; ataxia; dizziness; paresthesia.

Dermatologic – Stevens-Johnson syndrome; erythema multiforme; Henoch-Schönlein purpura; secondary bacterial infections of skin and soft tissue, including impetigo and cellulitis; herpes zoster.

Hematologic/Lymphatic – Thrombocytopenia.

Hypersensitivity – Anaphylaxis in individuals with or without an allergic history.

Respiratory – Pharyngitis.

Patient Information

The healthcare provider should inform the patient, parent or guardian of the benefits and risks of varicella virus vaccine live.

Patients, parents, or guardians should be instructed to report any adverse reactions to their healthcare provider.

The US Department of Health and Human Services has established a Vaccine Adverse Event Reporting System (VAERS) to accept all reports of suspected adverse events after the administration of any vaccine, including but not limited to the reporting of events required by the National Childhood Vaccine Injury Act of 1986. The VAERS toll-free number for VAERS forms and information is 1-800-822-7967. Pregnancy should be avoided for 3 months following vaccination.

RABIES VACCINE

Rx	**Imovax Rabies Vaccine (Human Diploid Cell)** (Connaught)	**Powder for Injection**: Freeze-dried suspension of Wistar rabies virus strain PM-1503-3M grown in human diploid cell cultures (inactivated whole virus). Contains ≥ 2.5 IU rabies antigen per ml.	In single dose vial[a] with disposable needle and syringe containing diluent and disposable needle for administration.
Rx	**Imovax Rabies I.D. Vaccine (Human Diploid Cell)**[b] (Connaught)	**Powder for Injection**: Freeze-dried suspension of Wistar rabies virus strain PM-1503-3M grown in human diploid cell cultures. Contains 0.25 IU rabies antigen per 0.1 ml intradermal dose.	In single-dose syringe with 1 vial diluent.[c]
Rx	**RabAvert** (Chiron)	**Powder for Injection**: Freeze-dried fixed-virus strain Flury LEP grown in cultures of chicken fibroblasts. Contains ≥ 2.5 IU rabies antigen per 1 ml intramuscular dose.	Preservative-free. In single-dose vial[d] with 1 vial diluent, 1 disposable syringe, 1 longer needle for reconstitution, 1 smaller needle for injection.
Rx	**Rabies Vaccine (Adsorbed)** (Various, eg, Michigan Department of Public Health, SK-Beecham)	**Injection**: Challenge Virus Standard (CVS) Kissling/MDPH strain	In single-dose 1 ml vial.[e]

[a] With < 100 mg human albumin, < 150 mcg neomycin sulfate and 20 mcg phenol red indicator.
[b] This product is for preexposure use only by the intradermal route.
[c] With < 15 mg human albumin, < 22 mcg neomycin sulfate and 3 mcg phenol red indicator/dose.
[d] With < 3 ng ovalbumin, < 12 mg processed bovine gelatin, 1 mg potassium glutamate, 0.3 mg sodium EDTA, < 1 mcg neomycin, < 20 ng chlortetracycline and < 2 ng amphotericin B/dose.
[e] With ≤ 2 mg/ml aluminum phosphate and 0.01% thimerosal.

RABIES VACCINE — INJECTION

Refer to the general discussion in the Rabies Prophylaxis Products introduction.

Indications

➤*Rabies vaccination:*

Preexposure immunization – Vaccinate persons with greater than usual risk of exposure to rabies virus by reason of occupation or avocation, including veterinarians, certain laboratory workers, animal handlers, forest rangers, spelunkers and persons staying > 1 month in countries (eg, India) where rabies is a constant threat.

Postexposure prophylaxis – If a bite from a carrier animal is unprovoked, the animal is not apprehended and rabies is present in that species in the area, administer RIG and vaccine as indicated. Consider vaccine recipients adequately immunized if they previously completed pre- or postexposure prophylaxis with any current rabies vaccine or have a documented adequate antibody response to duck-embryo rabies vaccine (DEV).

Administration and Dosage

➤*Dosage:*

Preexposure prophylaxis – Vaccine doses on days 0, 7 and 21 to 28, and then every 2 to 5 years based on antibody titers. Give 1 ml IM (either *Imovax Rabies Vaccine* or *Rabies Vaccine Adsorbed*) or 0.1 ml ID (*Imovax Rabies ID Vaccine* only).

Postexposure prophylaxis – Do not inject postexposure vaccine intradermally. Give rabies immune globulin (20 IU/kg) as soon after exposure as possible, followed by IM vaccine doses (either manufacturer) on days 0, 3, 7, 14 and 28.

For patients who have previously received preexposure prophylaxis, give 1 ml of either vaccine IM only on days 0 and 3. Do not give RIG.

➤*Route and site:* The deltoid area is the only acceptable site for postexposure vaccination of adults and older children. For younger children, use the outer aspect of the thigh. Never administer rabies vaccine in the gluteal area.

Travelers to endemic areas may receive vaccine by the ID route if the 3-dose series can be completed ≥ 30 days before departure; otherwise give the vaccine IM.

HDCV – IM in deltoid muscle or ID. Use only the IM route for postexposure prophylaxis. ID injections given in the lateral aspect of the upper arm are less likely to result in adverse reactions, compared with ID injection in the forearm.

RVA – IM only, in deltoid muscle. Do not inject ID. Vaccinate children in the anterolateral aspect of the thigh muscle.

➤*Booster dose:* For occupational or other continuing risk, every 2 to 5 years based on antibody titers, in a single 1 ml IM or 0.1 ml ID injection.

Preexposure booster immunization – Test people who work with live rabies virus in research laboratories or in vaccine production or with diagnostic tests for serum rabies antibody titer every 6 months. Give booster vaccine doses as needed to maintain an adequate titer. Give workers (eg, veterinarians, animal control and wildlife officers in areas where animal rabies is epizootic) booster doses every 2 years or have their serum rabies antibody titer determined every 2 years. If the titer is insufficient, give a booster dose. Veterinarians and similar workers in areas of low rabies endemicity do not require routine booster doses of rabies vaccine after completion of primary preexposure immunization or postexposure prophylaxis.

➤*Missed doses:*

Preexposure prophylaxis – Prolonging the interval between doses does not interfere with immunity achieved after the concluding dose of the basic series.

Postexposure prophylaxis – Prolonging the interval between doses may seriously delay achieving protective antibody titers, with potentially fatal consequences.

➤*Storage/Stability:* Refrigerate dried vaccine at 2° to 8°C (36° to 46°F). Do not freeze. HDCV can presumably tolerate 30 days at room temperature.

Actions

➤*Pharmacology:* Rabies vaccine is available as a human diploid-cell vaccine (HDCV) and an adsorbed vaccine (RVA).

Preexposure immunization – High titer antibody responses of HDCV have been demonstrated. Seroconversion was often obtained with only one dose. With two doses 1 month apart, 100% of recipients developed specific antibody.

Postexposure immunization – Postexposure immunization efficacy was proven in conjunction with antirabies serum. Individuals severely bitten by rabid dogs and wolves received the vaccine within hours of, and up to 14 days after, the bites. All individuals were fully protected against rabies.

Contraindications

Theoretically, rabies vaccine may be contraindicated in people who have had life-threatening allergic reactions to rabies vaccine or any of its components, but carefully consider a patient's risk of developing rabies before deciding to discontinue vaccination.

Warnings

➤*Guillain-Barré syndrome:* Two cases of acute polyradiculoneuropathy (Guillain-Barré syndrome) that resolved within 12 weeks, and a focal subacute CNS disorder temporally associated with HDCV have been reported.

➤*Immune complex-like reactions:* Recently, a significant increase has been noted in "immune complex-like" reactions (6%) in people receiving booster doses of HDCV. The illness, characterized by onset at 2 to 21 days postbooster, presents with a generalized urticaria and may also include arthralgia, arthritis, angioedema, nausea, vomiting, fever and malaise. In no case were the illnesses life-threatening. This reaction occurred much less frequently in people receiving primary immunization.

➤*Hypersensitivity reactions:* May give antihistamines. Have epinephrine available to counteract anaphylactic reactions. Refer to Management of Acute Hypersensitivity Reactions.

While the concentration of antibiotics in each dose of vaccine is extremely small, people with known hypersensitivity to any of these agents could manifest an allergic reaction.

➤*Pregnancy: Category C.* Give rabies vaccine to a pregnant woman only if clearly needed. Pregnancy is not a contraindication to postexposure therapy. There have been no fetal abnormalities associated with rabies vaccination. If there is substantial risk of rabies exposure, preexposure prophylaxis may also be indicated during pregnancy.

➤*Lactation:* It is not known if rabies vaccine or corresponding antibodies are excreted in breast milk. Problems in humans have not been documented.

➤*Children:* Pediatric and adult doses are the same. Safety and efficacy are established in children. Safe and effective use of the Michigan/SKB vaccine is established for people ≥ 6 years of age.

Precautions

➤*Route of administration:*

Imovax Rabies Vaccine and Rabies Vaccine Adsorbed – Inject IM only in the deltoid area; possible vaccine failure may occur if injected in the gluteal area. Do not inject intradermally (ID).

Imovax Rabies ID Vaccine – Inject intradermally only; do not inject IM.

RABIES VACCINE — INJECTION

Drug Interactions

Rabies Vaccine Drug Interactions			
Precipitant drug	Object drug*		Description
Chloroquine	Rabies vaccine, ID	⬇	Long-term therapy with chloroquine may suppress the immune response to low-dose HDCV administered ID. Complete preexposure rabies vaccination 1 to 2 months before chloroquine administration begins. If this is not feasible, perform serologic tests several weeks after vaccination to determine the magnitude of the recipient's antibody response.
Immunosuppressants	Rabies vaccine	⬇	Like all inactivated vaccines, administration of rabies vaccine to people receiving immunosuppressants, including high-dose corticosteroids, or radiation therapy, may result in an insufficient response to immunization. They may remain susceptible despite immunization. Do not give immunosuppressives during postexposure therapy unless essential. It may be helpful to test steroid-treated patients for development of antirabies antibodies.
Rabies immune globulin	Rabies vaccine	⬇	Simultaneous administration may slightly delay the antibody response to rabies vaccine. Because of this possibility, follow CDC recommendations exactly and give no more than the recommended dose of RIG.

* ⬇ = Object drug decreased.

Adverse Reactions

HDCV – Transient pain, erythema, swelling or itching at the injection site (25%). Treat such reactions with simple analgesics.

Mild systemic reactions (20%): Headache, nausea, abdominal pain, muscle aches and dizziness. In general, ID administration results in fewer adverse reactions, except for a slight increase in transient local reactions. Serum-sickness-like reactions occur in 6% of those receiving ID booster doses 2 to 21 days after injection. These reactions may be due to albumin in the vaccine formula rendered allergenic by beta-propiolactone during the manufacturing process.

RVA – Transient pain, redness and swelling at the injection site (65% to 70%). In a few cases, these effects persist 48 hours and may be successfully treated with simple analgesics. Mild, transient constitutional reactions (8% to 10%); headache, nausea, slight fever or fatigue. Serum-sickness-like reaction (< 1%), between 7 and 14 days after booster vaccination, perhaps due to lack of albumin in the vaccine formula.

SMALLPOX VACCINE

Rx	**Dryvax**[a] (Wyeth-Ayerst)	**Powder for injection:** Dried, calf lymph type live-virus preparation of vaccinia virus.[b] The reconstituted vaccine contains ≈ 100 million infectious vaccinia viruses/mL.	In vials with 1 diluent syringe[c] (0.25 mL), 1 vented needle, 100 bifurcated needles.

[a] Licensed for restricted use and available only from the Centers for Disease Control and Prevention (CDC).

[b] Polymyxin B sulfate, dihydrostreptomycin sulfate, chlortetracycline HCl, and neomycin sulfate are added in trace amounts.

[c] With 50% glycerin and 0.25% phenol.

SMALLPOX VACCINE — INJECTION

Indications

➤*Smallpox vaccination:* Active immunization against smallpox disease.

Patient selection – The Advisory Committee on Immunization Practices (ACIP) recommends vaccination of laboratory workers who directly handle cultures or animals contaminated or infected with non-highly attenuated vaccinia virus, recombinant vaccinia viruses derived from non-highly attenuated vaccinia strains, or other Orthopoxviruses that infect humans (eg, monkeypox, cowpox, vaccinia, variola). The ACIP also recommends that vaccination be considered for health care workers who have contact with clinical specimens, contaminated materials (eg, dressings), or patients receiving vaccinia or recombinant vaccinia viruses. Laboratory and other health care personnel who work with highly attenuated poxvirus strains such as modified vaccinia Ankara (MVA), NYVAC (derived from the Copenhagen vaccinia strain), ALVAC (derived from canarypox virus), and TROVAC (derived from fowlpox virus) do not require routine vaccination.

The Armed Forces continue to recommend the use of smallpox vaccine for certain categories of personnel.

➤*Response to bioterrorism:* Recommendations for use of smallpox vaccine in response to bioterrorism are periodically updated by the CDC; the most recent recommendations can be found at http://www.cdc.gov.

Administration and Dosage

➤*Reconstitution:*

1.) Lift up tab of aluminum seal on vaccine vial. Do not break off or tear down tab.
2.) Place vaccine vial upright on a hard, flat surface. Insert a sterile 21-gauge or smaller needle into the rubber stopper to release the vacuum from the vaccine vial. The needle to release the vacuum is not included in the kit.
3.) To reduce viscosity of cold diluent, warm by holding diluent cartridge in palm of hand for a minute or so.
4.) After attaching the vented needle to the diluent syringe, aseptically insert the vented needle through the rubber stopper into the vaccine vial up to the first hub.
5.) Depress the plunger to ensure the entire volume of diluent is delivered into the vial.
6.) Withdraw diluent syringe/vented needle and discard in biohazard waste container.
7.) Allow vaccine vial to stand undisturbed for 3 to 5 minutes. Then, if necessary, swirl vial gently to effect complete reconstitution.
8.) Record date of reconstitution.

➤*Route and site:* Do not inject IM, IV, or SC. For conventional smallpox vaccination (scarification) only.

The skin over the insertion of the deltoid muscle or the posterior aspect of the arm over the triceps muscle is the preferred site for smallpox vaccination.

➤*Administration:*

1.) Remove entire aluminum seal from the vaccine vial. Then remove rubber stopper from vaccine vial and aseptically retain stopper (set aside inverted) for subsequent reuse.
2.) Carefully dip bifurcated end of needle into vaccine. Visually confirm that the needle picks up a drop of vaccine in the space between the 2 tips.
3.) Deposit the drop of vaccine onto clean, dry site previously prepared for vaccination. Do not redip needle into vaccine if needle has touched skin.
4.) With the same needle, and using multiple-puncture technique, vaccinate through drop of vaccine. Holding the bifurcated needle perpendicular to the skin, punctures are rapidly made with strokes vigorous enough to allow a trace of blood to appear after 15 to 20 seconds. Two or 3 punctures are recommended for primary vaccination; 15 punctures for revaccination. Any remaining vaccine should be wiped off with dry sterile gauze and the gauze disposed of in a biohazard waste container.
5.) If the vaccine is to be stored for subsequent use, restopper the vial with rubber stopper and store at 2° to 8°C (36° to 46°F). The vaccine may be stored for no more than 15 days after reconstitution.
6.) When next needed, remove vial from refrigerator, gently swirl suspension to ensure resuspension, and then carefully take off stopper cap.

➤*Interpretation of responses:* Inspect the vaccination site 6 to 8 days after vaccination. Two types of responses have been defined by the World Health Organization (WHO) Expert Committee on Smallpox. They are: 1) Major reaction, indicating that virus replication has taken place and vaccination was successful; or 2) equivocal reaction, indicating a possible consequence of immunity capable of suppressing viral multiplication or allergic reactions to an inactive vaccine with production of immunity.

Major reaction – Major reaction is defined as a vesicular or pustular lesion or an area of definite palpable induration or congestion surrounding a central lesion that might be a crust or an ulcer. The inoculation site becomes reddened and pruritic 3 to 4 days after vaccination. A vesicle surrounded by a red areola then forms, which becomes umbilicated and then pustular the 7th to 11th day after vaccination, and the pustule begins to dry, the redness subsides, and the lesion usually becomes crusted between the 14th and 21st days. By the end of approximately the third week, the scab falls off, leaving a permanent scar, which at first is pink in color but eventually becomes flesh-colored. Primary vaccination also may be accompanied by fever, regional lymphadenopathy, and malaise persisting for a few days. Revaccination is considered successful if a vesicular or pustular lesion is present or an area of definite palpable induration or congestion surrounding a central

SMALLPOX VACCINE — INJECTION

lesion, which may be a scar or ulcer, is present on examination 6 to 8 days after revaccination. Major reactions, especially when there has been an interval of many years since the last successful vaccination, may be accompanied by fever, regional lymphadenopathy, and malaise persisting for a few days.

Equivocal reaction – Equivocal reactions are defined as all responses other than major reactions. If an equivocal reaction is observed, check vaccination procedures and repeat vaccination with vaccine from another vial or vaccine lot, if available. If a repeat vaccination by using vaccine from another vial or vaccine lot fails to produce a major reaction, health care providers should consult the CDC or their state or local health department before giving another vaccination.

➤*Revaccination:* For those in the special-risk categories, as defined by ACIP, revaccination is recommended at appropriate intervals (every 10 years).

➤*Disposal:* The vaccine vial, its stopper, the needle to release the vacuum, the diluent syringe, the vented needle used for reconstitution, the bifurcated needle used for administration, and any gauze or cotton that came in contact with the vaccine should be burned, boiled, or autoclaved before disposal.

➤*Storage/Stability:* Store unreconstituted smallpox vaccine in the refrigerator (2° to 8°C, 36° to 46°F). Do not freeze. Reconstituted smallpox vaccine may be used for 15 days if stored at 2° to 8°C (36° to 46°F) when not in actual use. At time of reconstitution, record date. Do not use the smallpox vaccine after the expiration date regardless of whether it is in the dry or reconstituted form.

Actions

➤*Pharmacology:* Introduction of potent smallpox vaccine containing infectious vaccinia viruses into the superficial layers of the skin results in viral multiplication, immunity, and cellular hypersensitivity. With the primary vaccination, a papule appears at the site of vaccination on about the second to fifth day. This becomes a vesicle on the fifth or sixth day, which becomes pustular, umbilicated, and surrounded by erythema and induration. The maximal area of erythema is attained between the eighth and twelfth day following vaccination (usually the tenth). The erythema and swelling then subside, and a crust forms that comes off about the fourteenth to twenty-first day. At the height of the primary reaction known as the Jennerian response, there is usually regional lymphadenopathy and there may be systemic manifestations of fever and malaise.

Primary vaccination with product at a potency of 100 million pock-forming units (pfu)/mL elicits a 97% response rate by major reaction (see Administration and Dosage) and neutralizing antibody response in children. Immunity wanes after several years, and an allergic sensitization to viral proteins can persist. This allergy is manifested by the appearance of a papule and a small area of redness appearing within the first 24 hours after revaccination; this may be the maximum reaction but not infrequently vesicles appear in 24 to 48 hours with ultimate scabbing. The peak of this type of reaction is passed within 3 days following the application of fully potent vaccine with an antibody rise occurring in roughly half of those who exhibit such a reaction. As immunity wanes, revaccination with potent vaccine elicits this allergic response followed by the changes produced by propagating virus. The lesion may then go through the same course as the primary vaccination or may exhibit an accelerated development of the lesion and its attendant erythema. Viral propagation is assumed to have occurred (and an immune response evoked) when the greatest area of skin involvement (erythema) occurs after the third day following revaccination. Revaccination is considered successful if a vesicular or pustular lesion is present or an area of definite palpable induration or congestion surrounding a central lesion, which may be a scar or ulcer, is present on examination 6 to 8 days after revaccination.

Contraindications

➤*Routine nonemergency vaccine use:* Primary vaccination and revaccination with smallpox vaccine are contraindicated as follows:

1.) For any individuals who are allergic to any component of the vaccine, including polymyxin B sulfate, dihydrostreptomycin sulfate, chlortetracycline HCl, and neomycin sulfate.
2.) Infants less than 12 months of age. The ACIP advises against nonemergency use of smallpox vaccine in children less than 18 years of age.
3.) For individuals of any age with eczema or past history of eczema or for those whose household contacts have eczema, other acute, chronic, or exfoliative skin conditions (eg, atopic dermatitis, wounds, burns, impetigo, varicella zoster), and for siblings or other household contacts of such individuals.
4.) For people of any age receiving therapy with systemic corticosteroids at certain doses (eg, greater than or equal to 2 mg/kg body weight or greater than or equal to 20 mg/day of prednisone for 2 weeks or longer), immunosuppressive drugs (eg, alkylating agents, antimetabolites), or radiation. Do not vaccinate household contacts of such individuals.
5.) For individuals with congenital or acquired deficiencies of the immune system, including individuals infected with the human immunodeficiency virus (HIV). Do not vaccinate household contacts of such individuals.
6.) For individuals with immunosuppression (eg, leukemia, lymphomas of any type, generalized malignancy, solid organ transplantation, hematopoietic stem cell transplantation, cellular or humoral immunity disorders, agammaglobulinemia, other malignant neoplasms affecting the bone marrow or lymphatic systems) or household contacts of such individuals.
7.) During pregnancy, suspected pregnancy, or to household contacts of pregnant women.

➤*Smallpox emergency vaccine use:* There are no absolute contraindications regarding vaccination of a person with a high-risk exposure to smallpox. People at greatest risk for experiencing serious vaccination complications are often those at greatest risk for death from smallpox. If a relative contraindication to vaccination exists, the risk for experiencing serious vaccination complications must be weighed against the risks for experiencing a potentially fatal smallpox infection.

Warnings

➤*Elderly:* There are no published data to support the use of this vaccine in geriatric populations. This vaccine is not recommended for use in geriatric populations in nonemergency conditions. For use in emergency conditions, see Contraindications.

➤*Pregnancy: Category C.* Animal reproduction studies have not been conducted with smallpox vaccine. Do not give smallpox vaccine to pregnant women in routine, nonemergency conditions. For emergency conditions, see Contraindications and Indications. On rare occasions, almost always after primary vaccination, vaccinia virus has been reported to cause fetal infection. Fetal vaccinia usually results in stillbirth or death of the infant shortly after delivery. Vaccinia vaccine is not known to cause congenital malformations.

➤*Lactation:* It is not known whether vaccine antigens or antibodies are excreted in human milk. This vaccine is not recommended for use in a nursing mother in nonemergency conditions. For use in emergency conditions, see Contraindications.

➤*Children:* The vaccine is considered safe and effective in children. However, smallpox vaccine is not recommended for use in nonemergency situations and is contraindicated for infants less than 12 months of age in nonemergency situations.

Precautions

➤*Complications of vaccine:* The CDC can assist physicians in the diagnosis and management of patients with suspected complications of vaccinia (smallpox) vaccination. Vaccinia Immune Globulin (VIG) is indicated for certain complications of smallpox vaccination. Several antiviral compounds have been shown to have activity against vaccinia virus or other Orthopoxviruses in vitro and in animal models. However, insufficient information exists on which to base recommendations for any antiviral compound to treat postvaccination complications or Orthopoxvirus infections, including smallpox. If VIG is needed or additional information is required, physicians should contact the CDC at (404) 639-3670 or (404) 639-2888.

➤*Latex sensitivity:* The vial stopper contains dry natural rubber that may cause hypersensitivity reactions when handled by, or when the product is administered to, people with known or possible latex sensitivity.

➤*Prevention of contact transmission:* Vaccinia virus may be cultured from the site of primary vaccination beginning at the time of development of a papule (2 to 5 days after vaccination) until the scab separates from the skin lesion (14 to 21 days after vaccination). During this time, care must be taken to prevent spread of the virus to another area of the body or to another person.

Identify individuals susceptible to adverse effects of vaccinia virus (eg, those with eczema or immunodeficiency states, including HIV infection) and take measures to avoid contact with people with active vaccination lesions.

Recently vaccinated health care workers should avoid contact with patients, particularly those with immunodeficiencies, until the scab has separated from the skin at the vaccination site. However, if continued contact with patients is essential and unavoidable, they may continue to have contact with patients, including those with immunodeficiencies, as long as the vaccination site is well covered and good hand-washing technique is maintained by the vaccinee. In this setting, a more occlusive dressing may be required. Semipermeable polyurethane dressings are effective barriers to vaccinia and recombinant vaccinia viruses. However, exudate may accumulate beneath the dressing, and care must be taken to prevent viral contamination when the dressing is removed. In addition, accumulation of fluid beneath the dressing may increase the maceration of the vaccination site. Accumulation of exudate may be decreased by first covering the vaccination with dry gauze, then applying the dressing over the gauze. The dressing should also be changed at least once a day.

The most important measure to prevent inadvertent implantation and contact transmission from vaccinia vaccination is thorough hand washing after changing the bandage or after any other contact with the vaccination site.

Adverse Reactions

➤*Local:* Generalized rashes (erythematous, urticarial, nonspecific) and secondary pyogenic infections at the site of vaccine applications may occur. Bullous erythema multiforme (Stevens-Johnson syndrome) occurs rarely.

Inadvertent inoculation at other sites is the most frequent complication of vaccinia vaccination, usually resulting from autoinoculation of the vaccine virus transferred from the site of vaccination. The most common sites involved are the face, eyelid, nose, mouth, genitalia, and rectum. Accidental infection (autoinoculation) of the eye may result in blindness.

Generalized vaccinia among people without underlying illnesses is characterized by a vesicular rash of varying extent. The rash is generally self-limited and requires little or no therapy except among patients whose conditions appear to be toxic or who have serious underlying illnesses.

➤*Systemic:* A fever is common after vaccinia vaccination is administered. Up to 70% of children have 1 or more days of temperature of 38°C (100°F) or

SMALLPOX VACCINE — INJECTION

higher from 4 to 14 days after primary vaccination, and 15% to 20% have temperatures of 39°C (102°F) or higher. After revaccination, 35% of children develop temperatures of 38°C (100°F) or higher, and 5% have temperatures of 39°C (102°F) or higher. Fever is less common in adults than children after vaccination or revaccination.

More severe complications that may follow primary vaccination or revaccination include the following: Postvaccinial encephalitis, encephalomyelitis, encephalopathy, progressive vaccinia (vaccinia necrosum), eczema vaccinatum. Such complications may result in severe disability, permanent neurological sequelae, and/or death. Although a rare event, approximately 1 death per million primary vaccinations and 1 death per 4 million revaccinations have occurred after vaccinia vaccination. Death is most often the result of postvaccinial encephalitis or progressive vaccinia. Death also has been reported in unvaccinated contacts of individuals who have been vaccinated.

➤*Revaccination:* The risk of complications associated with revaccination is low. Complications have occurred, especially in patients with underlying diseases, in patients receiving therapy that impairs immunologic competence, or in subjects who have not been vaccinated for many years. Subjects who have not been vaccinated for many years may respond as primary vaccinees as regards both the local and systemic reaction to vaccine administration and risk of occurrence of the above-mentioned serious complications.

TETANUS TOXOID

For complete and comparative prescribing information, refer to the Agents for Active Immunization introduction.

WARNING

Trivalent DTP is the preferred immunizing agent for most children up to their seventh birthday. Tetanus and diphtheria toxoids (Td) for adult use is the preferred immunizing agent for most adults and older children. For information about tetanus therapy, refer to the monograph on tetanus immune globulin.

Indications

➤*Tetanus vaccination:*

Tetanus toxoid, adsorbed – Active immunization of adults and children 7 years of age or older against tetanus, wherever combined antigen preparations are not indicated.

Not recommended for immunizing children less than 7 years of age. In children older than 7 years of age, either diphtheria and tetanus toxoids and acellular pertussis vaccine adsorbed (DTaP) or diphtheria and tetanus toxoids and pertussis vaccine adsorbed (for pediatric use) is recommended. If a contraindication to pertussis immunization exists, the recommended vaccine is diphtheria and tetanus toxoids adsorbed (for pediatric use) (DT).

For the prevention of neonatal tetanus in infants born of unvaccinated pregnant women.

Tetanus infection: See Warnings for more information.

Tetanus toxoid, fluid – For booster injection against tetanus in people 7 years of age or older. Not indicated for primary immunization.

Primary immunization schedule for children younger than 7 years of age should consist of 5 doses of a vaccine containing tetanus toxoid. The initial 3 doses are given as diphtheria and tetanus toxoids and pertussis vaccine adsorbed (DTP). The fourth and fifth doses are DTaP. If the pertussis component is contraindicated, DT (for pediatric use) is recommended. For people 7 years of age or older, tetanus and diphtheria toxoids adsorbed (for adult use) (Td) is preferred to tetanus toxoid alone.

For the prevention of neonatal tetanus in infants born of unvaccinated pregnant women.

Tetanus infection: See Warnings for more information.

Administration and Dosage

➤*Administration:* Shake well. Inject in the area of the lateral mid-thigh or deltoid. Do not inject into the gluteal area or areas where there may be a major nerve trunk.

➤*Tetanus toxoid, adsorbed:* For primary immunization of people 7 years of age or older, a series of three 0.5 mL IM injections is given. The second dose of 0.5 mL IM is given 4 to 8 weeks after the first dose, and the third dose of 0.5 mL IM is given 6 to 12 months after the second dose.

For children ≥ 1 year of age in whom vaccines containing pertussis and diphtheria antigens are contraindicated, 2 doses of 0.5 mL each, 4 to 8 weeks apart, followed by a third dose of 0.5 mL, 6 to 12 months after the second dose are recommended.

For booster injections, a booster dose of 0.5 mL of Td (for adult use) vaccine or tetanus toxoid adsorbed vaccine every 10 years thereafter is recommended.

➤*Tetanus toxoid, fluid:* After the initial immunization series is completed, give a booster dose of 0.5 mL IM every 10 years to maintain adequate immunity.

➤*Tetanus prophylaxis in wound management:* Td is the preferred vaccine for active tetanus immunization in wound management of patients 7 years of age or older. This is to enhance diphtheria protection, because a large proportion of adults are susceptible. TIG is the product of choice for passive immunization. Refer to the Diphtheria and Tetanus Toxoids monograph or the Tetanus Immune Globulin monograph.

Tetanus Prophylaxis in Routine Wound Management

History of adsorbed tetanus toxoid (doses)	Clean, minor wounds		All other wounds[a]	
	Td	TIG[b]	Td	TIG
Unknown or < 3	Yes	No	Yes	Yes
≥ 3	No[c]	No	No[d]	No

[a] Such as, but not limited to, wounds contaminated with dirt, feces, soil, or saliva; puncture wounds; avulsions; and wounds resulting from missiles, crushing burns, and frostbite.
[b] TIG (human).
[c] Yes, if more than 10 years since last dose.
[d] Yes, if more than 5 years since last dose.

➤*Concomitant vaccines:* Several routine vaccines may safely and effectively be administered simultaneously at separate injection sites (eg, DTP or Td, MMR, Hib, hepatitis B). National authorities recommend simultaneous immunization at separate sites as indicated by age or health risk, if return of a vaccine recipient for a subsequent visit is doubtful.

➤*Storage / Stability:* Store at 2° to 8°C (36° to 46°F). Do not freeze. Discard frozen toxoid.

Actions

➤*Pharmacology:* Adsorbed tetanus toxoid induces specific protective antibodies against the exotoxin excreted by *Clostridium tetani*. The aluminum salt, a mineral adjuvant, prolongs and enhances the antigenic properties of tetanus toxoid by retarding the rate of absorption. Its duration is approximately 10 years.

While the rate of seroconversion and promptness of antibody response are essentially equivalent for the fluid and adsorbed forms of tetanus toxoid, adsorbed toxoids induce more persistent antitoxin titers. Therefore, adsorbed tetanus toxoid is strongly recommended for primary and booster immunizations. Use fluid tetanus toxoid to immunize the rare patient who is hypersensitive to the aluminum adjuvant. The only other rational use for fluid tetanus toxoid is in compounding dilutions of a reagent for delayed-hypersensitivity skin-testing.

Contraindications

History of systemic allergic or neurologic reactions following a previous dose or hypersensitivity to thimerosal.

Give only passive immunization, using TIG (human), if a contraindication exists in a person who has not completed a primary immunizing course of tetanus toxoid and other than a clean, minor wound is sustained.

Defer elective immunization during the course of any febrile illness or acute infection, or during an outbreak of poliomyelitis. A minor afebrile illness such as a mild upper respiratory tract infection should not preclude immunization.

Warnings

➤*Tetanus immune globulin (TIG):* Under no circumstances should tetanus toxoid be used to treat actual tetanus infections. Employ tetanus antitoxin, preferably TIG (human), in all such cases.

➤*Immunodeficiency:* People receiving immunosuppressive therapy, including radiation, corticosteroids, antimetabolites, alkylating agents, and cytotoxic drugs, or with other immunodeficiencies may have a diminished antibody response to active immunization. This is a reason to consider deferring immunization. Nonetheless, routine immunization of symptomatic and asymptomatic HIV-infected people is recommended.

➤*Hypersensitivity reactions:* Take every precaution to prevent and arrest allergic and other untoward reactions. A careful history should review possible sensitivity to the vaccine or similar vaccines, to dry natural latex rubber, or to the type of protein to be injected. Epinephrine 1:1000 and other appropriate agents should be readily available to combat unexpected allergic reactions. Refer to Management of Acute Hypersensitivity Reactions.

People who experience Arthus-type hypersensitivity reactions or temperature greater than 39.4°C (103°F) after a previous dose of tetanus toxoid usually have very high serum tetanus antitoxin levels and should not be given even emergency doses of tetanus toxoid more frequently than every 10 years, even if they have a wound that is neither clean nor minor.

➤*Elderly:* The elderly develop lower to normal antitoxin levels following tetanus immunization than younger people.

➤*Pregnancy:* *Category C.* Use only if clearly needed, although Td is preferred. Based on extensive human experience, there is no evidence that tetanus toxoid is teratogenic. Give a previously unimmunized pregnant woman who may deliver her child under nonhygienic conditions 2 doses of Td 4 to 8 weeks apart before delivery, preferably during the last 2 trimesters. Incompletely immunized pregnant women should complete their 3 dose primary series. Give those immunized more than 10 years previously a booster dose. It is not known if tetanus toxoid or corresponding antibodies cross the placenta. Generally, most IgG passage across the placenta occurs during the third trimester.

➤*Lactation:* It is not known if tetanus toxoid or corresponding antibodies are excreted in breast milk. It is unlikely that intradermal tetanus toxoid is excreted in breast milk.

➤*Children:* DTaP is the preferred immunizing agent for most children until their seventh birthday. Safety and efficacy of tetanus toxoid in infants younger than 6 weeks of age have not been established. However, tetanus toxoid is not indicated for children younger than 7 years of age.

TETANUS TOXOID

Drug Interactions

Tetanus Toxoid Drug Interactions			
Precipitant drug	Object drug*		Description
Immunosuppressants	Tetanus toxoid	⬇	Administration of tetanus toxoid to patients receiving immunosuppressants including corticosteroids or radiation therapy, may result in insufficient response to immunization. They may remain susceptible despite immunization.
Chloramphenicol	Tetanus toxoid, adsorbed	⬇	Systemic chloramphenicol may impair anamnestic response to tetanus toxoid. Avoid concurrent use.
TIG	Tetanus toxoid, adsorbed	⬇	Concurrent use may delay development of active immunity by several days; however, this interaction is not clinically significant and does not preclude concurrent use.

* ⬇ = Object drug decreased.

Adverse Reactions

➤*CNS:* Cochlear lesion; brachial plexus neuropathies; paralysis of the radial nerve; paralysis of the recurrent nerve; accommodation paresis; Guillain-Barré syndrome; EEG disturbances with encephalopathy.

➤*Dermatologic:* Urticaria; rash.

➤*Local:* Redness; warmth; edema; induration with or without tenderness; nodule; sterile abscess formation; SC atrophy.

➤*Miscellaneous:* Malaise; transient fever; chills; pain; hypotension; nausea; myalgia; arthralgia; headaches; Arthus-type hypersensitivity (characterized by severe local reactions, generally starting 2 to 8 hours after injection, particularly in patients who have received multiple prior boosters).

Rarely, anaphylactic reaction and death have been reported after receiving preparations containing tetanus and diphtheria antigens.

TETANUS TOXOID, FLUID

Rx	**Tetanus Toxoid** (Aventis Pasteur)	**Injection:** 4 Lf units tetanus per 0.5 mL dose	In 7.5 mL vials.[a]

[a] With thimerosal.

TETANUS TOXOID, FLUID

For complete and comparative prescribing information, refer to the Tetanus Toxoid group monograph.

TETANUS TOXOID, ADSORBED

Rx	**Tetanus Toxoid, Adsorbed** (Aventis Pasteur)	**Injection:** 5 Lf units tetanus per 0.5 mL dose	In 5 mL vials.[a]
Rx	**Tetanus Toxoid, Adsorbed, Purogenated** (Lederle)	**Injection:** 5 Lf units tetanus per 0.5 mL dose	In 0.5 mL disposable syringes and 5 mL vials[b]

[a] With aluminum potassium sulfate and thimerosal.
[b] With aluminum phosphate and thimerosal.

TETANUS TOXOID ALUMINUM PHOSPHATE ADSORBED

For complete and comparative prescribing information, refer to the Tetanus Toxoid group monograph.

DIPHTHERIA AND TETANUS TOXOIDS, ADSORBED

Rx	**Diphtheria & Tetanus Toxoids, Adult** (Aventis Pasteur)	**Injection:** 2 Lf units diphtheria and 5 Lf units tetanus per 0.5 mL dose	In 5 mL vials and 0.5 mL syringes.[a]
Rx	**Decavac** (Aventis Pasteur)		Preservative free. In 0.5 mL *Luer-Lok* syringe.[b]
Rx	**Diphtheria & Tetanus Toxoids, Adult** (Massachusetts Public Health Biologic Labs)	**Injection:** 2 Lf units diphtheria and 2 Lf units tetanus per 0.5 mL dose	In 5 and 10 mL vials.[c]
Rx	**Diphtheria & Tetanus Toxoids, Pediatric** (Aventis Pasteur)	**Injection:** 6.7 Lf units diphtheria and 5 Lf units tetanus per 0.5 mL dose	In 5 mL multidose vials.[a]

[a] With aluminum potassium sulfate, thimerosal.
[b] With not more than 0.28 mg of aluminum and trace thimerosal (up to 0.3 mcg mercury/dose).
[c] With aluminum phosphate, thimerosal.

DIPHTHERIA AND TETANUS TOXOIDS, ADSORBED — INJECTION

Indications

➤*Diphtheria and tetanus toxoids adsorbed for pediatric use (DT):* Diphtheria and tetanus toxoids adsorbed for pediatric use (DT) is indicated for active immunization against diphtheria and tetanus diseases in infants and children from 2 months of age up to 7 years of age (prior to their seventh birthday) for whom the use of a combined vaccine containing pertussis antigen is contraindicated (see Administration and Dosage).

Protection against diphtheria and tetanus is based on a full course of immunization.

DT is intended only for active immunization against diphtheria and tetanus and is not to be used for treatment of actual infection or in people 7 years of age or older.

Persons recovering from tetanus or diphtheria – Diphtheria or tetanus infection may not confer immunity; therefore, initiation or completion of active immunization is indicated at the time of recovery from these infections.

If a contraindication to using tetanus toxoid-containing preparations exists in a person who has not completed a primary immunizing course of tetanus toxoid, and other than a clean minor wound is sustained, only passive immunization should be given using human tetanus immune globulin (TIG). If passive immunization for diphtheria is needed, equine diphtheria antitoxin is recommended (see Administration and Dosage).

As with any vaccine, DT may not protect 100% of individuals receiving the vaccine.

➤*Tetanus and diphtheria toxoids adsorbed for adult use (Td):* Tetanus and diphtheria toxoids adsorbed for adult use (Td) is indicated for active immunization of children 7 years of age or older and adults against tetanus and diphtheria. Td is the preparation of choice for vaccination of all persons 7 years of age or older because side effects from higher doses of diphtheria toxoid are more common in this group than they are among younger children.

➤*Pregnancy:* See Warnings for more information.

➤*Active infection:* This vaccine is not to be used for the treatment of tetanus or diphtheria infection.

➤*Children:* See Warnings for more information.

➤*Protection:* As with any vaccine, vaccination with Td may not protect 100% of susceptible individuals.

➤*Passive immunization:* See Administration and Dosage for more information.

Administration and Dosage

➤*Approved by the FDA:* May 1950 (DT) and December 1954 (Td).

➤*DT for pediatric use:*

For IM injection only – The dose is 0.5 mL to be given IM.

Preparation – Since this product is a suspension containing an adjuvant, shake vigorously immediately prior to use to obtain a uniform suspension in the vaccine container. The vaccine should not be used if it cannot be resuspended.

DIPHTHERIA AND TETANUS TOXOIDS, ADSORBED — INJECTION

Administration – The vaccine should be injected IM. The preferred sites are the anterolateral aspect of the thigh or the deltoid muscle of the upper arm. The vaccine should not be injected in the gluteal area or areas where there may be a major nerve trunk or blood vessel. Before injection, the skin at the injection site should be cleansed and prepared with a suitable germicide.

After insertion of the needle, aspirate and wait to see if any blood appears in the syringe, which will help avoid inadvertent injection into a blood vessel. If blood appears, withdraw the needle and prepare for a new injection at another site.

Active immunization – It is recommended that active immunization against diphtheria and tetanus be started at 2 months of age.

Unimmunized infants and children younger than 1 year of age – Unimmunized infants and children younger than 1 year of age for whom vaccine containing pertussis antigen is contraindicated should receive 3 doses of 0.5 mL each of DT at 4-week to preferably 8-week intervals, followed by a fourth (reinforcing) dose of 0.5 mL, 6 to 12 months after the third dose, for the primary series.

Unimmunized children from 1 up to 7 years of age (prior to the seventh birthday) – Unimmunized children from 1 up to 7 years of age (prior to the seventh birthday) for whom vaccine containing pertussis antigen is contraindicated should receive 2 doses of 0.5 mL each of DT, at 4- to preferably 8-week intervals, followed by a third (reinforcing) dose 6 to 12 months later, for the primary series.

If, after beginning a DTP series, further doses of vaccine containing pertussis antigen become contraindicated, DT should be substituted for each of the remaining doses.

The reinforcing dose is an integral part of the primary immunizing series.

Interruption of doses – Interruption of the recommended schedule with a delay between doses does not interfere with the final immunity achieved, nor does it necessitate starting the series over again, regardless of the length of time elapsed between doses.

Booster doses – A booster dose of 0.5 mL is indicated at age 4 to 6 years (prior to the seventh birthday), preferably prior to entrance into kindergarten or elementary school. However, if the last dose of the primary immunizing series was administered after the fourth birthday, a booster prior to school entry is not considered necessary.

For either primary or booster immunization against tetanus and diphtheria of individuals 7 years of age or older, the use of tetanus and diphtheria toxoids adsorbed, for adult use, is recommended. The following information provides summary recommendations for routine diphtheria, tetanus, and pertussis vaccination for children younger than 7 years of age in the United States:

Dosing schedule – The customary age for the initial primary dose of diphtheria, tetanus, and pertussis vaccination is 2 months or older than 6 weeks of age. The second primary dose is administered when the child is 4 months of age and approximately 4 to 8 weeks after the first primary dose. The third primary dose is administered when the child is 6 months of age and approximately 4 to 8 weeks after the second primary dose. The fourth primary dose is administered when the child is 15 months of age and approximately 6 to 12 months after the third primary dose. A booster dose should be administered when the child is 4 to 6 years old before entering kindergarten or elementary school; though this is not necessary if the fourth primary dose was administered after the child's fourth birthday. In all cases, prolonging the dosing interval between vaccinations does not require restarting the series. Children should receive either DTaP (diphtheria, tetanus, and acellular pertussis vaccine) or DTP (diptheria, tetanus, and whole-cell pertussis vaccine) unless pertussis vaccine is contraindicated. In this case, the child should receive DT. If the child is 1 year of age or older at the time that primary dose 3 is due, a third dose 6 to 12 months after the second completes primary vaccination with DT.

Diphtheria prophylaxis for case contacts – All case contacts, household and others, who have previously received fewer than 3 doses of diphtheria toxoid should receive an immediate dose of an appropriate diphtheria toxoid-containing preparation and should complete the series according to schedule. Case contacts who previously received fewer than 3 doses, but who have not received a dose of a preparation containing diphtheria toxoid within the previous 5 years, should receive a dose of a diphtheria toxoid-containing preparation appropriate for their age. This combined preparation against both diphtheria and tetanus is designed particularly to meet the needs of children younger than 7 years of age for whom the use of a combined vaccine containing pertussis antigen is contraindicated.

Tetanus prophylaxis in wound management – The need for diphtheria and tetanus toxoids (active immunization), with or without human TIG (passive immunization) depends upon the condition of the wound and the patient's immunization history. Tetanus has rarely occurred among persons with a documented primary series of tetanus toxoid injections.

For routine wound management of children younger than 7 years of age who are not completely immunized, DT should be used instead of single-antigen tetanus toxoid (if pertussis antigen is contraindicated or individual circumstances are such that potential febrile reactions following DTP might confound the management of the patient). Completion of primary vaccination thereafter should be ensured.

If emergency tetanus prophylaxis is indicated during the period between the last primary dose and the reinforcing dose, a 0.5 mL dose of DT should be given. If given before 6 months have elapsed, it should be counted as a primary dose; if given after 6 months, it should be regarded as the reinforcing dose.

For tetanus-prone wounds in children who have had fewer than 3, or an unknown number of immunizations with a tetanus toxoid-containing product, passive immunization with human TIG is also recommended. A separate syringe and site of injection should be used.

If a contraindication to using tetanus toxoid-containing preparations exists in a person who has not completed a primary immunizing course of tetanus toxoid and other than a clean, minor wound is sustained, only passive immunization should be given using human TIG.

The following information provides a summary of recommendations for tetanus prophylaxis in routine wound management:

If there is an unknown history of tetanus toxoid administration or the patient has previously received fewer than 3 doses and the wound is clean or minor, then the patient should receive a dose of tetanus toxoid; a dose of TIG is not required. For all other wounds, such as, but not limited to, wounds contaminated with dirt, feces, soil, and saliva, puncture wounds, avulsions, and wounds resulting from missiles, crushing, burns, and frostbite, the patient should receive both tetanus toxoid and TIG.

If the patient has previously received 3 or more doses of tetanus toxoid (if only 3 doses of fluid toxoid have been received, then a fourth dose of toxoid, preferably an adsorbed toxoid, should be given) with a clean or minor wound, then the patient does not require additional tetanus toxoid unless it has been more than 10 years since the last dose. TIG is not indicated in this situation either. For all other wounds, tetanus toxoid is not required unless it has been more than 5 years since the last dose (more frequent boosters are not needed and can accentuate side effects).

➤*Td for adult use:* Shake vial well before withdrawing each dose. Discard vial of vaccine if it cannot be resuspended.

Inject 0.5 mL IM in the area of the vastus lateralis (mid-thigh laterally) or deltoid. The vaccine should not be injected into the gluteal area or areas where there may be a major nerve trunk.

The following guidelines are derived from the Advisory Committee on Immunization Practices (ACIP).

Primary immunization for children 7 years of age or older and adults – A series of 3 doses of 0.5 mL each of Td should be given IM; the second dose of 0.5 mL is given 4 to 8 weeks after the first dose; the third dose of 0.5 mL is given 6 to 12 months after the second dose. Td is the agent of choice for immunization of all individuals 7 years of age or older, because side effects from higher doses of diphtheria toxoid are more common in older children and adults.

Children who remain incompletely immunized after their seventh birthday should be counted as having prior exposure to tetanus and diphtheria toxoids (eg, a child who previously received 2 doses of DTP needs only 1 dose of Td to complete the primary series for tetanus and diphtheria).

Interruption of the recommended schedule with a delay between doses does not interfere with the final immunity achieved with Td. There is no need to start the series over again, regardless of the time elapsed between doses.

Routine recall injections – To maintain adequate protection a booster dose of 0.5 mL every 10 years thereafter is recommended.

Recall injection after injury – A thorough attempt must be made to determine whether a patient has completed primary immunization. Patients with unknown or uncertain previous immunization histories should be considered to have no previous tetanus toxoid doses. Persons who had military service since 1941 can be considered to have received at least 1 dose; although most people in the military since 1941 may have completed a primary series of tetanus toxoid and passive immunization at the time of wound cleaning and debridement (see information following).

Protection – Available evidence indicates that complete primary vaccination with tetanus toxoid provides long-lasting protection more than 10 years for most recipients. Consequently, after complete primary tetanus vaccination, boosters, even for wound management, need to be given only every 10 years when wounds are minor and uncontaminated. For other wounds, a booster is appropriate if the patient has not received tetanus toxoid within the preceding 5 years. Persons who have received at least 2 doses of tetanus toxoid rapidly develop antitoxin antibodies.

Passive immunization – If passive immunization for tetanus is needed, human TIG is the product of choice. It provides longer protection than antitoxin of animal origin and causes few adverse reactions. The currently recommended prophylactic dose of human TIG for wounds of average severity is 250 units IM. When tetanus toxoid and human TIG are given concurrently, separate syringes and separate sites should be used. The ACIP recommends the use of only adsorbed toxoid in this situation.

➤*Storage / Stability:* Do not freeze. Store refrigerated, away from freezer compartment, at 2° to 8°C (35° to 46°F).

Actions

➤*Pharmacology:* The potency of tetanus and diphtheria toxoids was determined on the basis of immunogenicity studies, with a comparison to a serological correlate of protection (0.01 antitoxin units/mL) established by the Panel on Review of Bacterial Vaccines and Toxoids.

A clinical study to evaluate the serological responses and adverse reactions was performed in 58 individuals 6 years of age or older. The results indicated protective levels of antibody were achieved in more than 90% of the study population after primary immunization with both components. Booster effects were achieved in 100% of the individuals with preexisting antibody responses.

DIPHTHERIA AND TETANUS TOXOIDS, ADSORBED — INJECTION

Contraindications

Hypersensitivity to any component of the vaccine, including thimerosal, a mercury derivative, is a contraindication.

A history of systemic allergic or neurologic reactions following a previous dose of Td is an absolute contraindication for further use.

The decision to administer or delay vaccination because of a current or recent febrile illness depends largely on the severity of symptoms and their etiology. Although a moderate or severe febrile illness is sufficient reason to postpone vaccination, minor illnesses such as a mild upper respiratory tract infection with or without low-grade fever are not contraindications.

Routine immunization should be deferred during an outbreak of poliomyelitis, provided the patient has not sustained an injury that increases the risk of tetanus and provided an outbreak of diphtheria disease does not occur simultaneously.

If a contraindication to using tetanus toxoid-containing preparations exists in a person who has not completed a primary immunizing course of tetanus toxoid and other than a clean, minor wound is sustained, only passive immunization should be given using human TIG.

Warnings

➤*DT for pediatric use:* This product is not recommended for immunizing persons on or after their seventh birthday.

For individuals 7 years of age or older, tetanus and diphtheria toxoids adsorbed, for adult use (Td), should be used instead of DT. The concentration of diphtheria toxoid in preparations intended for use in persons 7 years of age or older is approximately 80% lower than that of the pediatric formulation. The lower dosage of diphtheria toxoid is recommended for persons 7 years of age or older because adverse reactions to the diphtheria component are thought to be related to both dose and age.

➤*Td for adult use:* A routine booster should not be given more frequently than every 10 years. This guideline should not preclude wound management considerations.

➤*Both DT and Td:* DT or Td should not be given to infants, children, or adults with thrombocytopenia or any coagulation disorder that would contraindicate IM injection unless the potential benefits clearly outweigh the risk of administration. If the decision is made to administer DT or Td, it should be given with caution (see Drug Interactions).

Deaths have been reported in temporal association with the administration of preparations containing diphtheria or tetanus antigens; however, no causal relationship was proven (see Adverse Reactions).

➤*Hypersensitivity reactions:*

Both DT and Td – Persons who experience Arthus-type hypersensitivity reactions or temperatures higher than 39.4°C (103°F) after a previous dose of tetanus toxoid usually have very high serum tetanus antibody levels and should not be given even emergency doses of a tetanus toxoid-containing preparation more frequently than every 10 years, even if they have a wound that is neither clean nor minor.

➤*Elderly:*

DT for pediatric use – This vaccine is not recommended for use in adult populations.

➤*Pregnancy:*

DT for pediatric use – *Category C.* Animal reproduction studies have not been conducted with DT vaccine. It is not known whether DT vaccine can cause fetal harm when administered to a pregnant woman or can affect reproductive capacity. DT is not recommended for use in a pregnant woman. This product is not recommended for use in individuals 7 years of age or older.

Td for adult use – Animal reproduction studies have not been conducted with Td vaccine. It is also not known whether Td vaccine can cause fetal harm when administered to a pregnant woman or can affect reproduction capacity. Td vaccine should be given to a pregnant woman only if clearly needed.

Adequate immunization by routine boosters in nonpregnant women of childbearing age can obviate the need to vaccinate women during pregnancy (see Administration and Dosage).

However, the ACIP recommends the following: A previously unvaccinated pregnant woman whose child might be born under unhygienic circumstances (without sterile technique) should receive 2 doses of Td 4 to 8 weeks apart before delivery, preferably during the last 2 trimesters. Pregnant women in similar circumstances who have not had a complete vaccination series should complete the 3-dose series. Those vaccinated more than 10 years previously should have a booster dose. No evidence exists to indicate that tetanus and diphtheria toxoids administered during pregnancy are teratogenic.

It has been reported that tetanus toxoid administered to pregnant women prevents neonatal tetanus in newborns. However, the data reported on the safety of tetanus toxoid when so used is inconclusive because the incidence of neonatal deaths in New Guinea was significantly higher than in the United States. A prospective study in the US has not been done to confirm these reports.

➤*Lactation:*

DT for pediatric use – This product is not recommended for use in individuals 7 years of age or older.

➤*Children:*

DT for pediatric use – The safety and efficacy of DT for pediatric use, in children younger than 6 weeks of age have not been established (see Administration and Dosage).

Td for adult use – Safety and efficacy of Td for adult use in children younger than 7 years of age have not been established.

In children younger than 7 years of age, either diphtheria and tetanus toxoids and acellular pertussis vaccine adsorbed (DTaP) or diphtheria and tetanus toxoids and pertussis vaccine adsorbed USP (for pediatric use) (DTP) is recommended. If a contraindication to pertussis immunization exists, the recommended vaccine is DT.

Precautions

➤*Before administration:* Before the injection of any biological, the healthcare professional should take all precautions known for prevention of allergic or any other adverse reactions. These should include the following: A review of the patient's history regarding possible sensitivity and any previous adverse reactions to the vaccine or similar vaccine or to dry natural latex rubber; the ready availability of epinephrine 1:1000 (should an acute anaphylactic reaction occur due to any component of the vaccine) and other appropriate agents used for control of immediate allergic reactions; a current knowledge of the literature concerning the use of the vaccine under consideration.

➤*HIV infection:* These products (DT and Td) are not contraindicated for use in individuals with HIV infection.

➤*Administration precautions:* Special care should be taken to prevent injection into or near a blood vessel or nerve.

➤*DT for pediatric use:*

Immunodeficiency – See Drug Interactions for more information.

➤*Td for adult use:*

Immunodeficiency – Immunosuppressive therapies including radiation, corticosteroids, antimetabolites, alkylating agents, and cytotoxic drugs may reduce the immune response to vaccines. Therefore, routine vaccination should be deferred, if possible, while patients are receiving such therapy. If Td has been administered to persons receiving immunosuppressive therapy, or having an immunodeficiency disorder, an adequate antibody response may not be obtained. When possible, immunosuppressive treatment should be interrupted when immunization is required due to a tetanus-prone wound.

Wound prophylaxis – It is advisable to use Td (for adult use in those 7 years of age or older) in wound prophylaxis instead of tetanus toxoid alone in order to maintain adequate levels of diphtheria immunity.

➤*Latex allergy:* Healthcare professionals should prescribe or administer this product with caution to patients with a possible history of latex sensitivity since this packaging contains dry natural rubber.

➤*Guillain-Barre syndrome:* Healthcare professionals should administer these products with caution to patients with a history of Guillain-Barre syndrome (see Adverse Reactions).

Drug Interactions

➤*Anticoagulants:* As with other IM injections, DT or Td should be given with caution to patients on anticoagulant therapy.

➤*Human TIG/equine diphtheria antitoxin:* Human TIG or equine diphtheria antitoxin, if used, should be given in a separate site with a separate needle and syringe.

➤*DT for pediatric use:*

Immunosuppressive therapy – Infants or children receiving immunosuppressive therapy (including irradiation, systemic corticosteroids, antimetabolites, alkylating agents, and cytotoxic agents) may have a reduced response to active immunization procedures. Although no specific studies are available, if immunosuppressive therapy will be discontinued shortly, it would be reasonable to defer immunization until the patient has been off therapy for 1 month; otherwise the patient should be vaccinated while still on therapy.

➤*Passive immunization:* See Administration and Dosage for more information.

Immunosuppressants – See Precautions for more information.

Adverse Reactions

➤*DT for pediatric use:* In a prospective study that compared the reaction rates of a similar diphtheria and tetanus toxoid-containing vaccine to diphtheria and tetanus toxoids and pertussis vaccine (DTP), 781 children 0 to 6 years of age who were scheduled to receive routine DTP immunization instead received a dose of DT vaccine. Of these children, 684 and 110 were enrolled in the open-label and double-blind portions of the study, respectively. Most (98.8%) of the children received DT vaccine as a first, second, or third dose of the primary immunization series; the remainder of the immunizations were administered as a booster (fourth or fifth) dose. Local and systemic reactions that occurred within 48 hours of immunization were reported by parents through home visit, telephone call or mail-in questionnaire.

Local – Local reactions occurring within 48 hours following immunization for both the blinded and unblinded groups included redness (7.6%), swelling (7.6%), and pain (9.9%).

Systemic – Systemic symptoms included drowsiness (14.9%), fretfulness (22.6%), vomiting (2.6%), anorexia (7%), and persistent crying (0.7%). The

DIPHTHERIA AND TETANUS TOXOIDS, ADSORBED — INJECTION

incidence rates of fever 38° C (100.4°F) or higher and 39°C (102.2°F) or higher, reported in a subset of children (n = 292) three to 6 hours postimmunization, were 9.3% and 0.7%, respectively.

➤*Td for adult use:* In a clinical study involving 58 individuals 6 years of age or older, 19% of the individuals noted local reactions consisting of erythema, tenderness and induration at the injection site and 2% systemic reactions consisting of headache, malaise and temperature elevations.

Cardiovascular – Acute anaphylactic reactions may occur rarely following administration of tetanus and diphtheria antigens which may cause acute hives and cardiovascular collapse.

Adverse reactions to diphtheria toxoid in adults are minimized by the small amount of the antigen (not more than 2 Lf units per dose) contained in Td.

Epinephrine injection (1:1000) must be immediately available should an acute anaphylactic reaction occur due to any component of the vaccine.

➤*CNS:*

DT for pediatric use – Neurological complications, such as convulsions, encephalopathy, and various mono- and polyneuropathies, including Guillain-Barre syndrome (GBS), have been reported following administration of preparations containing diphtheria or tetanus antigens. A review by the Institute Of Medicine (IOM) found evidence of a causal relation between tetanus toxoid and brachial neuritis and GBS, but did not find evidence of a causal relation between DT and sudden infant death syndrome (SIDS).

Td for adult use – The following neurologic illnesses have been reported as temporally associated with vaccines containing tetanus toxoid: Neurological complications, including cochlear lesions, brachial plexus neuropathies, paralysis of the radial nerve, paralysis of the recurrent nerve, accommodation paresis, Guillain-Barre syndrome (GBS), and EEG disturbances with encephalopathy. The IOM following review of the reports of neurologic events following vaccination with tetanus toxoid, Td or DT, concluded the evidence favored acceptance of a causal relationship between tetanus toxoid and brachial neuritis and GBS.

➤*Hypersensitivity:* Allergic and hypersensitivity reactions, urticaria, erythema multiforme or other rash, arthralgias and, more rarely, a severe anaphylactic reaction (ie, urticaria with swelling of the mouth, difficulty breathing, hypotension, shock, or death) have been reported following administration of preparations containing diphtheria or tetanus antigens.

Deaths have been reported in temporal association to receipt of preparations containing tetanus and diphtheria toxoids. The IOM found inadequate evidence to accept or reject a causal relationship between tetanus toxoid-containing products and death from causes other than anaphylaxis or GBS.

See Warnings for more information.

➤*Local:* Local reactions, manifested by varying degree of erythema, warmth, edema, induration with or without tenderness, as well as urticaria and rash may occur after administration of DT or Td. With vaccines in general, it is not uncommon for patients to note within 48 to 72 hours at or around the injection site the following minor reactions: Edema; pain or tenderness; redness, inflammation or skin discoloration; mass or induration; local hypersensitivity. Such local reactions are usually self-limited and require no therapy. As with other aluminum-containing vaccines, a nodule may occasionally be palpable at the injection site for several weeks. Sterile abscess formation or subcutaneous atrophy at the injection site may also occur.

➤*Miscellaneous:* Other adverse events which have been reported in temporal association with various tetanus toxoid-containing products include the following: Warmth, swelling, cellulitis, malaise, weakness or fatigue, dizziness, irritability, aches and pains, arthralgia, flushing, tachycardia, syncope, nausea, vomiting, lymphadenopathy, phlebitis, pruritis/itching, hives, sweating, acute midbrain syndrome, EEG disturbances, accommodation pareses, paresthesia, radiculopathy, brachial plexus neuropathy, cranial nerve pareses, myelopathy, myelitis, and cochlear lesions.

Pallor, coldness, and hyporesponsiveness have been reported in a child receiving a DT vaccine.

Patient Information

Prior to the administration of these vaccines, healthcare professionals should inform the parent or guardian or adult patient of the recommended immunization schedule for protection against tetanus and diphtheria diseases and the benefits and risks of vaccination against tetanus and diphtheria diseases, and also inquire about the recent health status of the patient to be injected.

As part of the child's or adult's permanent immunization record, the date, lot number and manufacturer of the vaccine administered must be recorded.

The healthcare provider should inform the parent, guardian or adult patient about the potential for adverse reactions that have been temporally associated with the administration of these vaccines.

It is extremely important that when the parent, guardian or adult patient returns for the next dose in the series, the parent, guardian or adult patient should be questioned concerning occurrence of any symptoms or signs of an adverse reaction after the previous dose.

Guidance should be provided on measures to be taken by the parent or guardian should suspected adverse events occur, such as antipyretic measures for elevated temperatures and the need to report any suspected adverse occurrences to the healthcare professional. Parents or guardians should be provided with vaccine information statements prior to the time of vaccination, as required by the National Childhood Vaccine Injury Act (see previous information). The healthcare provider should provide the Vaccine Information Materials (VIMs) which are required to be given with each immunization.

The healthcare professional should inform the parent or guardian of the importance of completing the immunization series unless contraindicated.

DIPHTHERIA AND TETANUS TOXOIDS AND ACELLULAR PERTUSSIS VACCINE, ADSORBED (DTaP)

Rx	**Adacel** (Aventis Pasteur)	**Injection**: 2 Lf units diphtheria toxoid, 5 Lf units tetanus toxoid, 3 mcg pertactin, 5 mcg FHA,[a] 2.5 mcg detoxified pertussis toxins, 5 mcg fimbriae types 2 and 3 per 0.5 mL	In vials.[b]
Rx	**Boostrix** (GlaxoSmithKline)	**Injection**: 2.5 Lf units diphtheria toxoid, 5 Lf units tetanus toxoid, 2.5 mcg pertactin, 8 mcg FHA,[a] 8 mcg inactivated pertussis toxins per 0.5 mL	In preservative-free single-dose[c] vials and disposable prefilled *Tip-Lok* syringes.
Rx	**Tripedia** (Aventis Pasteur)	**Injection**: 6.7 Lf units diphtheria toxoid, 5 Lf units tetanus toxoid, 46.8 mcg pertussis antigens (≈ 23.4 mcg each of inactivated pertussis toxin and FHA[a]) per 0.5 mL	In preservative-free single-dose[d] and 7.5 mL multidose vials.[e]
Rx	**Daptacel** (Aventis Pasteur)	**Injection**: 15 Lf units diphtheria toxoid, 5 Lf units tetanus toxoid, 10 mcg pertussis toxoid, 5 mcg FHA,[a] 3 mcg pertactin, 5 mcg fimbriae types 2 and 3 per 0.5 mL	In single-dose vials.[f]
Rx	**Infanrix** (SmithKline Beecham)	**Injection**: 25 Lf units diphtheria toxoid, 10 Lf units tetanus toxoid, 25 mcg inactivated pertussis toxin, 25 mcg FHA,[a] 8 mcg pertactin per 0.5 mL	In single-dose vials[g] and disposable *Tip-Lok* syringes.

[a] Filamentous hemagglutinin.
[b] Each 0.5 mL dose contains 0.33 mg aluminum as the adjuvant, ≤ 5 mcg residual formaldehyde, < 50 ng residual glutaraldehyde, and 3.3 mg 2-phenoxyethanol (not as a preservative).
[c] Each 0.5 mL dose contains 4.5 mg of NaCl, aluminum adjuvant (not more than 0.39 mg aluminum by assay), ≤ 100 mcg of residual formaldehyde, and ≤ 100 mcg of polysorbate 80 (Tween 80).
[d] With thimerosal (not more than 0.3 mcg mercury/dose). Also contains gelatin.
[e] With thimerosal (25 mcg mercury/dose), not more than 0.17 mg aluminum and not more than 100 mcg of residual formaldehyde per 0.5 mL dose. Also contains gelatin and polysorbate 80.
[f] With 3.3 mg 2-phenoxyethanol, 0.33 mg of aluminum as the adjuvant, < 0.1 mg residual formaldehyde, and < 50 ng residual glutaraldehyde.
[g] With 2.5 mg 2-phenoxyethanol as a preservative, 4.5 mg sodium chloride, not more than 0.625 mg aluminum by assay, not more than 100 mcg of residual formaldehyde, and not more than 100 mcg of polysorbate 80.

DIPHTHERIA AND TETANUS TOXOIDS AND ACELLULAR PERTUSSIS VACCINE, ADSORBED (DTaP) – INJECTION

For complete and comparative prescribing information, refer to the Agents for Active Immunization introduction.

Indications

Active immunization against diphtheria, tetanus, and pertussis simultaneously in infants and children 6 weeks to 7 years of age (prior to the seventh birthday).

Children 7 years of age or older should receive diphtheria and tetanus toxoids (Td) (for adult use).

In instances where the pertussis vaccine component is contraindicated, use diphtheria and tetanus toxoids adsorbed (DT) (for pediatric use) for the remaining doses.

Adacel vaccine is indicated for active booster immunization for the prevention of tetanus, diphtheria, and pertussis as a single dose in people 11 through 64 years of age. The use of *Adacel* vaccine as a primary series, or to complete the primary series, has not been studied.

Children who have had well-documented pertussis (ie, positive culture for *Bordetella pertussis* or epidemiologic linkage to a culture-positive case) should complete the vaccination series with at least DT. Some experts recommend including the pertussis component as well (ie, administration of DTaP). Although well-documented pertussis disease is likely to confer immunity against pertussis, the duration of such immunity is unknown.

Not to be used for treatment of pertussis, diphtheria, or tetanus infections. If passive immunization is required, use tetanus immune globulin and/or diphtheria antitoxin.

Administration and Dosage

The National Childhood Vaccine Injury Act requires that the manufacturer and lot number of the vaccine administered be recorded by the health care provider in the vaccine recipient's permanent medical record, along with the

DIPHTHERIA AND TETANUS TOXOIDS AND ACELLULAR PERTUSSIS VACCINE, ADSORBED (DTaP) – INJECTION

date of administration of the vaccine and the name, address, and title of the person administering the vaccine.

Interrupting the recommended schedule or delaying subsequent doses should not interfere with the final immunity achieved with the vaccine and does not require restarting the series. Use Td, rather than DTaP, for any doses needed after a child's seventh birthday.

➤*Administration:* Shake well. Administer IM only. The anterolateral aspect of the thigh (for children under 1 year of age) or the deltoid muscle of the upper arm (for older children) is preferred. Do not inject DTaP in the gluteal area or other areas where there may be a major nerve trunk.

➤*Primary immunization:* The primary series consists of three 0.5 mL IM doses. The customary age for the first dose is 2 months of age, but it may be given as early as 6 weeks of age and up to the seventh birthday. Preterm infants should be vaccinated according to their chronological age from birth.

Vaccination Schedule for DTaP

Dose	CDC recommendations	*Daptacel*	*Infanrix* or *Tripedia*
Doses 1 to 3	2, 4, and 6 months	2, 4, and 6 months[a]	2, 4, and 6 months[b]
Dose 4	15 to 18 months[c]	17 to 20 months[d]	15 to 20 months[d]
Dose 5	4 to 6 years		4 to 6 years[e]

[a] 6- to 8-week intervals.
[b] 4- to 8-week intervals.
[c] May be administered as early 12 months, provided 6 months have elapsed since the third dose and the child is unlikely to return at age 15 to 18 months.
[d] At least 6 months between the third and fourth doses.
[e] Preferably prior to school entry. If the fourth dose was administered after the fourth birthday, a fifth dose prior to school entry is not necessary.

➤*Booster dose:* When DTaP is given for the primary series, a fourth dose is recommended. The interval between the third and fourth dose should be at least 6 months.

If a child receives whole-cell pertussis DTP for 1 or more doses, DTaP vaccines may be given to complete the series.

Infanrix may be used to complete a DTaP immunization series initiated with *Pediarix*.

➤*Adacel*: *Adacel* vaccine should be administered as a single injection of 1 dose (0.5 mL) by the intramuscular route. The preferred site is into the deltoid muscle. Five years should have elapsed since the recipient's last dose of tetanus toxoid, diphtheria toxoid, and/or pertussis containing vaccine. There are no data to support repeat administration of *Adacel* vaccine.

➤*Interchangeability of vaccines:* The manufacturers recommend that the same vaccine be given for the vaccination series. The CDC recommends that the same brand of DTaP vaccine be used for all doses of the vaccination series when feasible. However, when this is not possible, use any DTaP vaccine to continue or complete the series. Do not defer vaccination because the previously used brand is not available or is unknown.

➤*Concomitant vaccine administration:* According to the recommendations of the Advisory Committee on Immunization Practices (ACIP) and the American Academy of Family Physicians (AAFP), children aged 12 to 15 months can receive 7 or less injections (DTaP, MMR, varicella, *Haemophilus influenzae* type B [Hib], pneumococcal conjugate, inactivated polio virus [IPV], and hepatitis B vaccines) during a single visit, depending on vaccines given in the first year of life.

When concomitant administration of other vaccines is required, give with different syringes and at different injection sites.

According to the manufacturer, no immunogenicity data are available on the simultaneous administration of *Infanrix* with pneumococcal conjugate vaccine or IPV. No immunogenicity or safety date is available on the simultaneous administration of *Infanrix* with MMR or varicella vaccine.

There are no data available to the manufacturer about the simultaneous administration of *Tripedia* with varicella vaccine, IPV, or pneumococcal conjugate vaccine.

According to the manufacturer, no safety and immunogenicity data are available about the simultaneous administration of *Daptacel* with pneumococcal conjugate vaccine, MMR, and varicella vaccine, and no immunogenicity data are currently available about the simultaneous administration of IPV.

➤*Storage/Stability:* Store at 2° to 8°C (36° to 46°F). Do not freeze. Temperature extremes may adversely affect resuspendability of the vaccine. Discard if vaccine has been frozen. Do not use after expiration date.

Actions

➤*Pharmacology:* These preparations combine diphtheria and tetanus toxoids with acellular pertussis bacterial vaccine. The acellular pertussis antigens are pertussis toxin (PT), FHA, and pertactin. Adequate immunization with diphtheria and tetanus toxoids is thought to confer protection for at least 10 years. However, diphtheria toxoid does not eliminate carriage of *Corynebacterium diphtheriae* in the pharynx or nose or on the skin.

Protection against pertussis persists approximately 4 to 6 years. Serum diphtheria and tetanus antitoxin levels of 0.1 IU/mL and higher are regarded as protective. Efficacy of the pertussis component does not have a well-established correlate of protection.

Contraindications

Not recommended for use in adults or children 7 years of age or older (except for *Adacel*).

Hypersensitivity to any component of the vaccine; history of a serious allergic reaction (eg, anaphylaxis) temporally associated with a previous dose of the vaccine or with any component of the vaccine.

Encephalopathy (eg, coma, decreased level of consciousness, prolonged seizures) within 7 days of administration of a previous dose of DTP or DTaP and is not attributable to another identifiable cause.

Progressive neurologic disorders, including infantile spasms, uncontrolled epilepsy, or progressive encephalopathy. Pertussis vaccine should not be administered to individuals with such conditions until a treatment regimen has been established and the condition has stabilized.

If a contraindication to the pertussis vaccine component occurs, substitute diphtheria and tetanus toxoids for pediatric use (DT) for each of the remaining doses.

Defer elective immunization procedures during an outbreak of poliomyelitis because of the risk of provoking paralysis.

Warnings

➤*Special risk patients:* If any of the following events occurs in temporal relation with the receipt of either whole-cell pertussis DTP or DTaP, carefully consider the decision to administer subsequent doses of vaccine containing the pertussis component. Although these events were once considered contraindications to whole-cell pertussis DTP, there may be circumstances, such as high incidence of pertussis, in which the potential benefits outweigh the possible risks, particularly because the following events have not been proven to cause permanent sequelae:

1.) Temperature of at least 40.5°C (105°F) within 48 hours, not caused by another identifiable cause.
2.) Collapse or shock-like state (hypotonic-hyporesponsive episode) within 48 hours.
3.) Persistent, inconsolable crying lasting at least 3 hours, occurring within 48 hours.
4.) Convulsions, with or without fever, occurring within 3 days.

When the decision is made to withhold the pertussis component, continue immunization with DT.

The decision to administer or delay vaccination because of a current or recent febrile illness depends on the severity of symptoms and on the etiology of the disease. All vaccines can be administered to people with mild illness such as diarrhea, mild upper respiratory tract infection with or without low-grade fever, or other low grade febrile illness. However, do not immunize children with moderate or serious illnesses until recovered.

If Guillain-Barré syndrome occurs within 6 weeks of receipt of prior vaccine containing tetanus toxoid, base the decision to give subsequent doses of DTaP or any vaccine containing tetanus toxoid on careful consideration of the potential benefits and possible risks.

➤*Immunodeficiency:* People receiving immunosuppressive therapy, including irradiation, antimetabolites, alkylating agents, cytotoxic drugs, and corticosteroids (used in greater than physiologic doses), or with other immunodeficiencies may have diminished antibody response to active immunization. If immunosuppressive therapy will be discontinued shortly, it would be reasonable to defer immunization until the patient has been off therapy for more than 1 month; otherwise, vaccinate the patient while still on therapy. If DTaP vaccine has been administered to people receiving immunosuppressive therapy, a recent injection of immune globulin, or having an immunodeficiency disorder, an adequate immunological response may not be obtained. Nonetheless, routine immunization of symptomatic and asymptomatic HIV-infected people is recommended.

➤*Convulsions:* The Advisory Committee on Immunization Practices (ACIP) and the American Academy of Pediatrics (AAP) recognize cases when children with stable CNS disorders, including well-controlled seizures or satisfactorily explained single seizures, may receive acellular pertussis vaccine. The ACIP and AAP do not consider a family history of seizures to be a contraindication to pertussis vaccine. Studies suggest that when given whole-cell pertussis DTP vaccine, infants and children with a history of convulsions in first-degree family members (ie, siblings, parents) have an increased risk for neurologic events, compared with those without such histories.

For children at higher risk for seizures than the general population, an appropriate antipyretic may be administered at the time of vaccination with a vaccine containing an acellular pertussis component (including DTaP) and for the ensuing 24 hours to reduce the possibility of postvaccination fever.

➤*Latex sensitivity:* The stopper of the *Tripedia* and *Daptacel* vials and the tip cap and rubber plunger of the *Infanrix* needleless prefilled syringes contain dry natural latex rubber, which may cause allergic reactions in latex sensitive individuals.

➤*Hypersensitivity reactions:* Rarely, an anaphylactic reaction (eg, hives, swelling of the mouth, difficulty breathing, hypotension, shock) has been reported after receiving preparations containing diphtheria, tetanus, and/or pertussis antigens (see Adverse Reactions). Refer to the Management of Acute Hypersensitivity Reactions.

➤*Pregnancy: Category C.* DTaP is generally contraindicated after the seventh birthday. It is not known if DTaP antigens or corresponding antibodies cross the placenta. Most IgG passage across the placenta occurs during the third trimester. Not recommended for use in pregnant women.

DIPHTHERIA AND TETANUS TOXOIDS AND ACELLULAR PERTUSSIS VACCINE, ADSORBED (DTaP) – INJECTION

➤*Lactation:* It is not known if DTaP antigens or corresponding antibodies are excreted into breast milk.

➤*Children:* Safety and efficacy of DTaP in infants below 6 weeks of age have not been established. DTaP is not recommended for adults and children 7 years of age and older.

Precautions

➤*Adverse events:* When an infant or child returns for the next dose in the series, question the parent concerning occurrence of any symptoms or signs of adverse reactions after the previous dose (see Contraindications, Warnings, and Adverse Reactions).

Drug Interactions

➤*Immunosuppressants:* Immunosuppressive therapies, including irradiation, antimetabolites, alkylating agents, cytotoxic drugs, and corticosteroids (used in greater than physiologic doses), may reduce the immune response to vaccines. If immunosuppressive therapy will be discontinued shortly, it would be reasonable to defer immunization until the patient has been off therapy for 3 months; otherwise, vaccinate the patient while still on therapy. If DTaP is administered to a person receiving immunosuppressive therapy, or who received a recent injection of immune globulin, or who has an immunodeficiency disorder, an adequate immunologic response may not be obtained.

Adverse Reactions

The National Childhood Vaccine Injury Act requires the health care provider to report to the US Department of Health and Human Services through the Vaccine Adverse Event Reporting System (VAERS) the occurrence following immunization of any event set forth in the Vaccine Injury Table, including the following: Anaphylaxis or anaphylactic shock within 7 days; encephalopathy or encephalitis within 7 days; brachial neuritis within 28 days; any acute complication or sequelae (including death) of above events; any event that would contraindicate further doses of vaccine. The VAERS toll-free number for forms and information is (800) 822-7967.

Adverse Reactions Occurring within 72 Hours after Primary Immunization with *Tripedia, Infanrix,* and *Daptacel* (%)[a]

	Tripedia			*Infanrix*			*Daptacel*		
Adverse reaction	Dose 1 (2 mo)	Dose 2 (4 mo)	Dose 3 (6 mo)	Dose 1 (2 mo)	Dose 2 (4 mo)	Dose 3 (6 mo)	Dose 1 (2 mo)	Dose 2 (4 mo)	Dose 3 (6 mo)
Local									
Redness (any)	12.6	12.7	19.1	16.6	15.4	26.3	12.5	15.8	19.7
Swelling	8.8	8.2	10.7	12.5	15.4	21	14.3	15.4	17.8
Pain/Tenderness	8.1[b]	3.7[b]	2.3[b]	5[b]	5.1[b]	0.9[b]	30.5	19.6	15.9
GI									
Anorexia	8.1	9.7	9.9	7.5	6	9.6	26.2	14.8	17.8
Vomiting	5.2	1.5	2.3	5.8	6.8	3.5	-	-	-
Miscellaneous									
Fever[c]	0.7	1.4	3.1	0	0.9	3.5	11.9	9.9	9.9
Drowsiness	28.9	17.9	4.6	37.5	19.7	13.2	62	44.8	35.6
Irritability/Fussiness	8.1[d]	7.4[d]	7.6[d]	3.3[d]	7.7[d]	8.8[d]	72	61.2	56.2
Crying ≥ 3 hours	-	-	-	-	-	-	0.3	0	0

[a] Data are pooled from separate studies and are not necessarily comparable.
[b] Moderate or severe; cried or protested to touch or cried when limb was moved.
[c] *Tripedia*: ≥ 38.3°C, > 101°F (rectal); *Infanrix*: ≥ 38.4°C, ≥ 101.1°F (rectal); *Daptacel*: ≥ 38°C, ≥ 100.4°F (rectal).
[d] Moderate or severe; prolonged or persistent crying that could not be comforted and refusal to play.

Adverse Reactions Occurring within 72 Hours after Booster Doses with *Tripedia* and *Infanrix* (%)[a]

	Tripedia		*Infanrix*
Adverse reaction	Dose 4 (15 to 20 mo)	Dose 5 (4 to 6 yr)	Dose 4 (15 to 20 mo)
Local			
Redness (any)	17.1	33.3	39.5
Swelling	15.9	27.8	32.9
Pain	7.3[b]	11.1[b]	10.5[b]
GI			
Anorexia	8.5	0	11.8
Vomiting	2.4	0	2.6
Miscellaneous			
Fever[c]	2.4	5.6	6.6
Drowsiness	6.1	5.6	6.6
Irritability/Fussiness[d]	3.7	0	9.2

[a] Data are pooled from separate studies and are not necessarily comparable.
[b] Moderate or severe; cried or protested to touch or cried when limb was moved.
[c] *Tripedia*: ≥ 38.3°C, > 100.1°F (oral); *Infanrix*: ≥ 38.4°C, ≥ 101.1°F (rectal).
[d] Moderate or severe; prolonged or persistent crying that could not be comforted and refusal to play.

➤*CNS:* A review by the Institute of Medicine found a causal relation between tetanus toxoid and brachial neuritis and Guillain Barré syndrome. The following illnesses have been reported as temporally associated with vaccine containing tetanus toxoid: Neurological complications including cochlear lesion, brachial plexus neuropathies, paralysis of the radial nerve, paralysis of the recurrent nerve, accommodation paresis, and EEG disturbances with encephalopathy.

➤*Miscellaneous:* Rarely, an anaphylactic reaction (eg, hives, swelling of the mouth, difficulty breathing, hypotension, shock) has been reported after receiving preparations containing diphtheria, tetanus, and/or pertussis antigens.

Arthus-type hypersensitivity reactions, characterized by severe local reactions (generally starting 2 to 8 hours after an injection), may follow receipt of tetanus toxoid. A few cases of peripheral neuropathy have been reported following tetanus toxoid administration, although the evidence is inadequate to accept or reject a causal relation.

➤*Postmarketing:* Worldwide voluntary reports of adverse events for *Infanrix* since market introduction are listed below. This list includes adverse events for which 20 or more reports were received with the exception of intussusception, idiopathic thrombocytopenic purpura, thrombocytopenia, anaphylactic reaction, encephalopathy, and hypotonic-hyporesponsive episode for which fewer than 20 reports were received. These latter events are included either because of the seriousness of the event or the strength of causal connection to components of this or other vaccines or drugs.

CNS – Convulsions, crying, encephalopathy, hypotonia, hypotonic-hyporesponsive episode, irritability, somnolence.

Dermatologic – Erythema, pruritus, rash, urticaria.

GI – Diarrhea, intussusception, vomiting.

Hematologic/Lymphatic – Idiopathic thrombocytopenic purpura, lymphadenopathy, thrombocytopenia.

Miscellaneous – Anaphylactic reaction, cellulitis, cyanosis, ear pain, fever, hypersensitivity, injection site reactions, limb swelling, respiratory tract infection, Sudden Infant Death Syndrome.

Patient Information

This medicine is used to immunize children 6 weeks to 7 years of age (before the seventh birthday) against diphtheria, tetanus, and pertussis (whooping cough). It is not to be used to treat diphtheria, tetanus, or patients older than 7 years of age.

Inform the parent or guardian of the importance of completing the pertussis immunization series, unless a contraindication to further immunization exists.

Children with minor illnesses, such as a cold, may be vaccinated. Wait to vaccinate children who are moderately or severely ill until they recover.

Advise the parent or guardian to contact a health care provider at once if the child develops the following signs of encephalopathy within 7 days after receiving a vaccination: Changes in alertness; unresponsiveness; seizure activity.

Advise the parent or guardian to contact a health care provider at once if the child develops a fever of 105°F or more, faints, persistently cries for more than 3 hours within 48 hours of receiving this vaccine, or has a seizure with or without fever within 3 days of receiving this vaccine.

Inform the parent or guardian of the following adverse effects that may occur.

➤*Common mild problems that may occur:*
- Fever (up to about 1 child in 4);
- Redness or swelling where the shot was given (up to about 1 child in 4);
- Soreness or tenderness where the shot was given (up to about 1 child in 4).

These problems occur more often after the fourth and fifth doses of the DTaP series than after earlier doses. Sometimes the fourth and fifth dose of DTaP vaccine is followed by swelling of the entire arm or leg in which the shot was given, lasting 1 to 7 days (up to about 1 child in 30).

➤*Other mild problems:*
- Fussiness (up to 1 child in 3);
- Tiredness or poor appetite (up to about 1 child in 10);
- Vomiting (up to about 1 child in 50).

These problems generally occur 1 to 3 days after the shot.

Controlling fever is especially important for children who have had seizures, for any reason. It is also important if another family member has had seizures. Reduce fever and pain by giving the child an aspirin-free pain reliever when the shot is given and for the next 24 hours, following the package instructions.

DIPHTHERIA AND TETANUS TOXOIDS, ACELLULAR PERTUSSIS, AND HAEMOPHILUS INFLUENZAE TYPE B CONJUGATE VACCINES (DTaP-HIB)

Rx	**TriHIBit**[a] (Aventis Pasteur)	**Injection:** 10 mcg *Haemophilus influenzae* type b purified capsular polysaccharide conjugated to 24 mcg inactivated tetanus toxoid, 6.7 Lf diphtheria toxoid, 5 Lf tetanus toxoid, 46.8 mcg pertussis antigens per 0.5 mL	Sucrose, trace thimerosal. In vials.[b]

[a] Supplied as *ActHIB* (*Haemophilus* b conjugate vaccine [tetanus toxoid conjugate]) with *Tripedia* (diphtheria and tetanus toxoids and acellular pertussis vaccine adsorbed [DTaP]).

[b] *ActHIB* single-dose vials of dry lyophilized powder for reconstitution with 0.6 mL single-use vials of *Tripedia*.

DIPHTHERIA AND TETANUS TOXOIDS, ACELLULAR PERTUSSIS, AND HAEMOPHILUS INFLUENZAE TYPE B CONJUGATE VACCINES (DTaP-HIB) — INJECTION

For complete and comparative prescribing information, refer to the *Haemophilus* b Conjugate Vaccine and the Diphtheria and Tetanus Toxoids and Acellular Pertussis Vaccine monographs. For additional information, also refer to the Agents for Active Immunization introduction.

Indications

➤*Active immunization:* For the active immunization of children 15 to 18 months of age who previously have been immunized against diphtheria, tetanus, and pertussis with 3 doses consisting of tetanus, tetanus, tetanus, tetanus, tetanus, tetanus, tetanus, tetanus, tetanus, diphtheria and tetanus toxoids and whole cell pertussis (DTP) or DTaP vaccine and 3 doses or fewer of *ActHIB* within the first year of life for the prevention of invasive diseases caused by *Haemophilus influenzae* type b or by diphtheria, tetanus, and pertussis (refer to *ActHIB* package insert).

Do not administer *TriHIBit* to infants younger than 15 months of age.

Administration and Dosage

Do not administer IV. Administer IM in the outer aspect of the mid-thigh or deltoid. Do not inject the vaccine into the gluteal area or areas where there may be a nerve trunk.

Recommended Immunization Schedule for *ActHIB* and DTP or *Tripedia* for Previously Unvaccinated Children

Dose	Age	Immunization
First, second, and third	At 2, 4, and 6 mo	*ActHIB* reconstituted with DTP or saline diluent (0.4% sodium chloride)
Fourth	At 15 to 18 mo	*ActHIB* reconstituted with DTP or *Tripedia* (*TriHIBit*) or with saline diluent (0.4% sodium chloride)
Fifth	At 4 to 6 yr	*Tripedia* or DTP

Vaccinate preterm infants according to their chronological age from birth.

Interruption of the recommended schedule with a delay between doses should not interfere with the final immunity achieved with *ActHIB* reconstituted with DTP or *Tripedia* (*TriHIBit*) or saline diluent (0.4% sodium chloride). There is no need to start the series over again, regardless of the time elapsed between doses.

It is acceptable to administer a booster dose of *TriHIBit* following a primary series of *Haemophilus* b conjugate and whole-cell DTP vaccines or a primary series of a combination vaccine containing whole-cell DTP.

➤*Reconstitution:* To prepare *TriHIBit*, clean the *Tripedia* and *ActHIB* vial rubber stoppers with a suitable germicide prior to reconstitution. Thoroughly agitate the vial of *Tripedia*, then withdraw a 0.6 mL dose and inject into the vial of lyophilized *ActHIB*. After reconstitution and thorough agitation, the combined vaccines will appear whitish in color. Withdraw a 0.5 mL dose of the combined vaccines and administer IM. Use vaccine immediately (within 30 minutes) after reconstitution.

➤*Storage/Stability:* Store between 2° to 8°C (35° to 46°F). Do not freeze. Temperature extremes may adversely affect vaccine resuspendability. Use vaccine immediately (within 30 minutes) after reconstitution.

DIPHTHERIA AND TETANUS TOXOIDS AND ACELLULAR PERTUSSIS ADSORBED, HEPATITIS B (RECOMBINANT) AND INACTIVATED POLIOVIRUS VACCINE COMBINED

Rx	**Pediarix** (SmithKline Beecham)	**Injection:** 25 Lf diphtheria toxoid, 10 Lf tetanus toxoid, 25 mcg inactivated pertussis toxin (PT), 25 mcg filamentous hemagglutinin (FHA), 8 mcg pertactin, 10 mcg hepatitis B surface antigen (HBsAg), 40 D-antigen units (DU) Type 1 poliovirus, 8 DU Type 2 poliovirus, and 32 DU Type 3 poliovirus per 0.5 mL.[a]	Preservatives.[b] In single-dose vials and prefilled syringes.

[a] Each 0.5 mL dose also contains 2.5 mg 2-phenoxyethanol as a preservative, 4.5 mg NaCl, and aluminum adjuvant (not more than 0.85 mg aluminum by assay). Each dose also contains up to 100 mcg of residual formaldehyde and up to 100 mcg of polysorbate 80 (*Tween 80*).

[b] Thimerosal (less than 12.5 ng mercury per dose); neomycin sulfate, polymyxin B (up to 0.05 ng neomycin and up to 0.01 ng polymyxin B per dose); up to 5% yeast protein.

DIPHTHERIA AND TETANUS TOXOIDS AND ACELLULAR PERTUSSIS ADSORBED, HEPATITIS B (RECOMBINANT) AND INACTIVATED POLIOVIRUS VACCINE COMBINED — INJECTION

For complete and comparative prescribing information, refer to the Diphtheria and Tetanus Toxoids and Acellular Pertussis Vaccine, Hepatitis B Recombinant Vaccine, and Poliovirus Inactivated Vaccine monographs. For additional information, also refer to the Agents for Active Immunization introduction.

Indications

➤*Immunization:* Active immunization against diphtheria, tetanus, pertussis (whooping cough), all known subtypes of hepatitis B virus, and poliomyelitis caused by poliovirus Types 1, 2, and 3 as a 3-dose primary series in infants born of HBsAg-negative mothers, beginning as early as 6 weeks of age.

Do not administer to any infant before the age of 6 weeks or to individuals 7 years of age or older.

➤*Infants born of HBsAg-positive mothers:* Infants should receive hepatitis B immune globulin (human) (HBIG) and monovalent hepatitis B vaccine (recombinant) within 12 hours of birth and should complete the hepatitis B vaccination series according to a particular schedule (see Hepatitis B Vaccine [Recombinant] monograph).

➤*Infants born of mothers of unknown HBsAg status:* Infants should receive monovalent hepatitis B vaccine (recombinant) within 12 hours of birth and should complete the hepatitis B vaccination series according to a particular schedule (see Hepatitis B Vaccine [Recombinant] monograph).

Hepatitis D – Pediarix will not prevent hepatitis caused by other agents, such as hepatitis A, C, and E viruses, or other pathogens known to infect the liver. As hepatitis D (caused by the delta virus) does not occur in the absence of hepatitis B infection, hepatitis D also will be prevented by vaccination with *Pediarix*.

When passive protection against tetanus or diphtheria is required, administer tetanus immune globulin or diphtheria antitoxin, respectively.

Protection – Pediarix may not protect 100% of individuals receiving the vaccine and is not recommended for treatment of actual infections.

Administration and Dosage

➤*Approved by the FDA:* December 16, 2002.

➤*Administration: Pediarix* contains an adjuvant; therefore, shake vigorously to obtain a homogeneous, turbid, white suspension. Do not use if resuspension does not occur with vigorous shaking. Discard any vaccine remaining in the vial.

Administer by IM injection. The preferred sites are the anterolateral aspects of the thigh or the deltoid muscle of the upper arm. Do not inject the vaccine into the gluteal area or areas where there may be a major nerve trunk. Gluteal injections may result in suboptimal hepatitis B immune response.

Do not administer this product SC or IV.

➤*Primary immunization:* The primary immunization series for *Pediarix* is 3 doses of 0.5 mL, given IM, at 6- to 8-week intervals (preferably 8 weeks). The customary age for the first dose is 2 months of age, but it may be given starting at 6 weeks of age.

Do not administer *Pediarix* to any infant before the age of 6 weeks. Only monovalent hepatitis B vaccine can be used for the birth dose.

➤*Children previously vaccinated with 1 or more doses of hepatitis B vaccine:* Infants born of HBsAg-negative mothers and who received a dose of hepatitis B vaccine at or shortly after birth may be administered 3 doses of *Pediarix* according to the recommended schedule.

➤*Children previously vaccinated with 1 or more doses of Infanrix: Pediarix* may be used to complete the first 3 doses of the DTaP series in infants who have received 1 or 2 doses of *Infanrix* and also are scheduled to receive the other vaccine components of *Pediarix*.

➤*Children previously vaccinated with 1 or more doses of inactivated poliovirus vaccine (IPV): Pediarix* may be used to complete the first 3 doses

DIPHTHERIA AND TETANUS TOXOIDS AND ACELLULAR PERTUSSIS ADSORBED, HEPATITIS B (RECOMBINANT) AND INACTIVATED POLIOVIRUS VACCINE COMBINED — INJECTION

of the IPV series in infants who have received 1 or 2 doses of IPV and also are scheduled to receive the other vaccine components of *Pediarix*.

➤*Interchangeability of Pediarix* and licensed DTaP, IPV, or recombinant hepatitis B vaccines: It is recommended that *Pediarix* be given for all 3 doses because data are limited regarding the safety and efficacy of using acellular pertussis vaccines from different manufacturers for successive doses of the pertussis vaccination series. *Pediarix* is not recommended for completion of the first 3 doses of the DTaP vaccination series initiated with a DTaP vaccine from a different manufacturer because no data are available regarding the safety or efficacy of using such a regimen.

Pediarix may be used to complete a hepatitis B vaccination series initiated with a licensed hepatitis B vaccine (recombinant) vaccine from a different manufacturer.

Pediarix may be used to complete the first 3 doses of the IPV vaccination series initiated with IPV from a different manufacturer.

➤*Additional dosing information:* If any recommended dose of pertussis vaccine cannot be given, DT (for pediatric use), hepatitis B (recombinant), and IPV should be given as needed to complete the series.

Interruption of the recommended schedule with a delay between doses should not interfere with the final immunity achieved with *Pediarix*. There is no need to start the series over again, regardless of the time elapsed between doses.

The use of reduced volume (fractional doses) is not recommended.

Children who have received a 3-dose primary series of *Pediarix* should receive a fourth dose of IPV at 4 to 6 years of age and a fourth dose of DTaP vaccine at 15 to 18 months of age. Because the pertussis antigen components of *Infanrix* are the same as those components in *Pediarix*, these children should receive *Infanrix* as their fourth dose of DTaP.

➤*Concomitant vaccine administration:* When concomitant administration of other vaccines is required, they should be given with separate syringes and at different injection sites.

➤*Storage/Stability:* Refrigerate between 2° and 8°C (36° and 46°F). Do not freeze. Discard if the vaccine has been frozen.

Indications

Diagnosis of specific allergies, when properly diluted.

Relief of allergic symptoms (eg, hay fever, rhinitis, allergic asthma, insect-sting anaphylaxis) due to specifically identified materials by means of a graduated schedule of doses.

Administration and Dosage

Begin immunotherapy with very small doses; increase progressively until maintenance levels are reached. Dosages vary depending on the type of standardization used. Individualize dosage.

Do not inject IV. SC injection is preferable because it is less painful, allows better delineation of reaction size and slows the absorption rate, thus lowering the likelihood of an anaphylactic reaction. Although IM administration is acceptable, it is more painful and more difficult to assess the local reaction.

➤*Combining allergens:* Do not combine allergens to which the patient is extremely sensitive with allergens for which only a nominal sensitivity is shown. Distinct treatment schedules for each formula are frequently employed. (See Precautions.)

➤*Children:* Dosage is the same as for adults; divide large volume doses among several injection sites.

➤*Diagnostic testing:* Perform puncture (prick) or intradermal testing with appropriate dilutions, employing positive and negative controls. Consult manufacturer's literature for each allergen. Do not conduct test with alum-precipitated allergen extracts.

➤*Therapeutic dosing:* Typical doses are given SC every 3 to 14 days (or 7 to 14 days with alum-precipitated allergen extracts). Progress to the maximum tolerated dose or a weekly maintenance dose. Consult manufacturer's literature for each allergen.

➤*Admixtures:* Limit combinations of allergens so that each allergen will be present at a therapeutic concentration. Do not combine allergens of different standardization types. Stability varies with diluent, storage condition and concentration. Stability will be shortest in the low concentration ranges.

➤*Storage/Stability:* Store between 2° and 8°C (36° to 46°F).

Actions

➤*Pharmacology:* Allergenic extracts are derived individually from various biological sources containing antigens that possess immunologic activity. They are categorized based standardization and doseform. Standardization systems include the following: 1) Standardized by biological activity (in allergenic units, AU), 2) weight-to-volume (w/v) standardized, and 3) protein nitrogen unit (PNU) standardized. Doseforms include: 1) aqueous, 2) glycerinated and 3) alum-precipitated.

The mechanism of action is not completely defined. Specific immunoglobulin G (IgG) appears in the serum following injection of allergenic extracts. IgG competes with specific IgE for a specific antigen. Bound to receptors on mast cell membranes, IgE produces an allergenic reaction by releasing histamine and other agents upon coupling with an antigen. Serum IgE levels decrease over time. Decreased leukocyte sensitivity to allergens and increased numbers of T-suppressor cells for IgE-producing plasma cells are also noted. The histamine release response of circulating basophils to a specific allergen may be reduced in some patients by hyposensitization.

Onset/Duration – Relief of symptoms is dose-related. It is rarely achieved before maintenance dosage levels are reached, which often takes 4 to 6 months, sometimes 12 months. Serum IgG levels remain elevated for weeks to months following injection and vary markedly between individuals.

Contraindications

As initial therapy when an allergen can be environmentally avoided.

Frequent large local reactions or systemic reactions are relative contraindications for continued immunotherapy.

Foodstuff allergen extracts are diagnostic tools; efficacy for hyposensitization immunotherapy has not been demonstrated.

Warnings

➤*Cross-sensitivity:* Cross-immunoreactivity has been documented within botanical genus groups, especially among grasses. Exercise caution in prescribing since the additive effects could precipitate an allergic reaction. Markedly increased exposure to allergens in the environment may have an additive effect when coupled with an allergen extract injection. Dosage reduction may be necessary.

➤*Hypersensitivity reactions:* Anaphylactic reactions may occur with an overdose or in extremely sensitive individuals. Administer allergen extracts only where emergency facilities are immediately available. Refer to Management of Acute Hypersensitivity Reactions.

➤*Pregnancy: Category C.* Controlled studies of hyposensitization with allergen extracts throughout pregnancy failed to demonstrate any fetal or maternal risk. Because histamine can produce uterine contraction, avoid any reaction that releases significant amounts of histamine, whether from natural allergen exposure or from hyposensitization overdose. IgG crosses the placenta, especially in the third trimester. Administer during pregnancy only if clearly needed and with caution. Although pregnancy is not an indication to stop allergen extract therapy in women receiving maintenance doses without side effects, some allergists empirically decrease the maintenance dose by 50% throughout gestation.

➤*Lactation:* Minimal amounts of IgG are excreted in breast milk. No problems in humans have been documented. Various nutritional, immunologic and other advantages of breastfeeding have been described, especially in children of atopic mothers.

➤*Children:* Dosage for children is generally the same as for adults. The larger dosage volumes may produce relatively greater discomfort. To achieve the total dose required, the volume of the dose may be distributed among several injection sites.

Precautions

➤*Mixed allergens:* Mixed allergens are not to be used for skin testing. In the case of a negative reaction, a mixture fails to indicate whether one of the individual components at the full labeled concentration is capable of evoking a positive reaction. If the patient responds positively, there is no indication which component of the mixture produced the antigenic response. Treatment with nonreactive allergens can lead to sensitization and induction of IgE production.

➤*Combining allergens:* Do not combine allergens to which the patient is extremely sensitive with allergens for which only a nominal sensitivity is shown. Administer separately to individualize and better control dosage.

➤*Seasonal exposure:* Delay the start of immunotherapy until after any period of symptoms from seasonal environmental exposure. Typical allergic symptoms may follow shortly after an injection, particularly when the sum of the antigen load from the environment and from the injection exceeds the patient's antigen tolerance.

➤*Routine immunizations:* While routine immunizations may theoretically exacerbate autoimmune diseases, studies have failed to demonstrate this. Give hyposensitization cautiously to patients with autoimmune diseases and only if the risk from exposure exceeds the risk of exacerbating the underlying condition.

Drug Interactions

➤*Drug/Lab test interactions:* **Histamine H_1 antagonists** and **tricyclic antidepressants** may produce a false-negative reaction to cutaneous diagnostic testing with allergen extracts, unless a 72-hour period of antihistamine abstinence is observed. Long-acting antihistamines may interfere for weeks. **H_2 antagonists** do not decrease skin-test responsiveness alone, but may enhance suppression synergistically with H_1 antihistamines. **Topical corticosteroids** suppress dermal reactivity to allergen extracts locally.

Adverse Reactions

Most serious reactions begin within 30 minutes of an injection. Observe patients for at least 30 minutes after every injection, even once they have achieved maintenance therapy.

➤*Local:* Erythema and swelling at the injection site are common, but not significant unless they persist > 24 hours or exceed the diameter of a nickel (about 2 cm).

➤*Systemic:* Anaphylaxis, including fainting, pallor, bradycardia, hypotension, angioedema, wheezing, cough, conjunctivitis, rhinitis, generalized urticaria (see Warnings).

Patient Information

Comply with full course of therapy. To achieve efficacy, take regularly and in the proper dosage. Medication will not cure allergies, but will help control them.

Notify physician of increased environmental exposure to natural allergens; a dosage reduction may be required.

➤*Missed dose:* Depending on the amount of time elapsed, dosage reduction may be required. Do *not* double the dose to make up for the missed dose. More frequent injections may be necessary to return to maintenance doses.

Notify physician if erythema, swelling or generalized urticaria persists.

Notify physician immediately if fainting, wheezing, hypotension or bradycardia occurs.

AQUEOUS AND GLYCERINATED ALLERGENIC EXTRACTS

Rx	**Allergenic Extracts, Aqueous and Glycerinated** (Various, eg, ALK, Allergy Laboratories, Allermed, ALO, Antigen Laboratories, Center, Greer, Iatric, Meridian, Miles, Nelco)	**Injection:** Over 900 distinct allergens available in these categories: Animal products, foods, grass pollens, insect products, molds, tree pollens, weed pollens and other inhalants	Extracts supplied in various aqueous diluents or with varying concentrations of glycerin. In multidose vials of 2, 5, 10, 20, 30 and 50 ml.

For complete and comparative prescribing information, refer to the Allergenic Extracts group monograph.

ALUM-PRECIPITATED ALLERGENIC EXTRACTS

Rx	**Allpyral** (Miles)	**Injection**: Alum-precipitated extracts, prepared by pyridine extraction	In multidose vials of 10 and 30 ml at 5000, 10,000 and 20,000 PNU/ml.
Rx	**Center-Al** (Center)	**Injection**: Alum-precipitated extracts	In multidose vials of 10 and 30 ml at 10,000 and 20,000 PNU/ml.

For complete and comparative prescribing information, refer to the Allergenic Extracts group monograph.

HYMENOPTERA VENOM/VENOM PROTEIN

Rx	**Albay, Venomil** (Miles)	**Injection**: Purified venoms of honey bee, wasp, white faced hornet, yellow hornet, yellow jacket and mixed vespids (both hornets and yellow jackets)	In vials of 12, 120 and 550 mcg.
Rx	**Pharmalgen** (ALK)		In vials of 120 and 1100 mcg.

For complete and comparative prescribing information, refer to the Allergenic Extracts group monograph.

IMMUNOLOGIC AGENTS

Immunostimulants

PEGADEMASE BOVINE

Rx	**Adagen** (Enzon)	**Injection**: 250 units[a]/ml	In 1.5 ml vials.[b]

[a] One unit of activity is defined as the amount of ADA that converts 1 mcM of adenosine to inosine per minute at 25°C and pH 7.3.

[b] With 1.2 mg monobasic sodium phosphate, 5.58 mg dibasic sodium phosphate, 8.5 mg sodium chloride and water for injection.

PEGADEMASE BOVINE — INJECTION

Indications

➤*Adenosine deaminase deficiency:* For enzyme replacement therapy for adenosine deaminase (ADA) deficiency in patients with severe combined immunodeficiency disease who are not suitable candidates for or who have failed bone marrow transplantation. Pegademase bovine is recommended for use in infants from birth or in children of any age at the time of diagnosis. It is not intended as a replacement for HLA identical bone marrow transplant therapy, and it is also not intended to replace continued close medical supervision and the initiation of appropriate diagnostic tests and therapy (eg, antibiotics, nutrition, oxygen, gammaglobulin) as indicated for intercurrent illnesses.

Administration and Dosage

➤*Dose:* Administer every 7 days as an IM injection. Individualize the dosage.

First dose – 10 U/kg.

Second dose – 15 U/kg.

Third dose – 20 U/kg.

Usual maintenance dose – 20 U/kg/week. Further increases of 5 U/kg/week may be necessary, but a maximum single dose of 30 U/kg should not be exceeded.

➤*Plasma levels:* Plasma levels of ADA more than twice the upper limit of 35 mcmol/hr/ml have occurred on occasion in several patients, and have been maintained for several weeks in one patient who received twice weekly injections (20 U/kg per dose). No adverse effects have been observed at these higher levels; there is no evidence that maintaining preinjection plasma ADA > 35 mcmol/hr/ml produces any additional clinical benefits.

➤*Administration precautions:* Dose proportionality has not been established; closely monitor patients when the dosage is increased. Pegademase bovine is not recommended for IV administration.

Establish the optimal dosage and schedule of administration for each patient based on monitoring of plasma ADA activity levels (trough levels before maintenance injection), biochemical markers of ADA deficiency (primarily red cell deoxyadenosine triphosphate [dATP] content). Since improvement in immune function follows correction of metabolic abnormalities, maintenance dosage in individual patients should be aimed at achieving the following biochemical goals: 1) Maintain plasma ADA activity (trough levels before maintenance injection) in the range of 15 to 35 mcmol/hr/ml (assayed at 37°C [98.6°F]); and 2) decline in erythrocyte dATP to ≤ 0.005 to 0.015 mcmol/ml packed erythrocytes, or ≤ 1% of the total erythrocyte adenine nucleotide (ATP = dATP) content, with a normal ATP level, as measured in a preinjection sample. In addition, continued monitoring of immune function and clinical status is essential in any patient with a primary immunodeficiency disease and should be continued in patients being treated with pegademase bovine.

➤*Admixture incompatibility:* Pegademase bovine should not be diluted nor mixed with any other drug prior to administration.

➤*Storage/Stability:* Refrigerate. Store between 2°C and 8°C (36°F and 46°F). Do not freeze. Pegademase bovine should not be stored at room temperature. This product should not be used if there are any indications that it may have been frozen.

Actions

➤*Pharmacology:* Pegademase bovine is a modified enzyme used for enzyme replacement therapy for the treatment of severe combined immunodeficiency disease (SCID) associated with a deficiency of adenosine deaminase. The drug will not benefit patients with immunodeficiency due to other causes. It is a conjugate of numerous strands of monomethoxypolyethylene glycol (PEG), covalently attached to the enzyme ADA. ADA, used in the manufacture of pegademase bovine, is derived from bovine intestine.

Pegademase bovine provides specific replacement of the deficient enzyme. In the absence of the enzyme ADA, the purine substrates adenosine, 2′-deoxyadenosine and their metabolites are toxic to lymphocytes. The direct action of pegademase bovine is the correction of these metabolic abnormalities. Improvement in immune function and diminished frequency of opportunistic infections only occurs after metabolic abnormalities are corrected. There is a lag between the correction of the metabolic abnormalities and improved immune function. This period of time is variable, from a few weeks to as long as 6 months. In contrast to the natural history of combined immunodeficiency disease due to ADA deficiency, a trend toward diminished frequency of opportunistic infections and fewer complications of infections has occurred in patients receiving pegademase bovine.

SCID associated with ADA deficiency is a rare, inherited and often fatal disease. In the absence of ADA enzyme, purine substrates adenosine and 2′-deoxyadenosine accumulate, causing metabolic abnormalities that are directly toxic to lymphocytes.

The immune deficiency can be cured by bone marrow transplantation. When a suitable bone marrow donor is unavailable or when bone marrow transplantation fails, non-selective replacement of the ADA enzyme has been provided by periodic irradiated red blood cell transfusions. However, transmission of viral infections and iron overload are serious risks, and relatively few ADA-deficient patients have benefited from chronic transfusion therapy.

➤*Pharmacokinetics:* Pharmacokinetics and biochemical effects have been studied in six children ranging in age from 6 weeks to 12 years with SCID associated with ADA deficiency. After IM injection, peak plasma ADA activity levels were reached in 2 to 3 days. ADA plasma elimination half-life of was variable, even for the same child. Range was 3 to > 6 days. Following weekly injections of 15 U/kg, average trough level of ADA activity in plasma was between 20 and 25 mcmol/hr/ml.

The changes in red blood cell deoxyadenosine nucleotide (ie, dATP) and S-adenosylhomocysteine hydrolase (SAHase) have been evaluated. In patients with ADA deficiency, inadequate elimination of 2′-deoxyadenosine caused a marked elevation in dATP and a decrease in SAHase level in red blood cells. Prior to treatment with pegademase bovine, the levels of dATP in the red blood cells ranged from 0.056 to 0.899 mcmol/ml of erythrocytes. After 2 months of maintenance treatment, the levels decreased to 0.007 to 0.015 mcmol/ml. The normal value of dATP is below 0.001 mcmol/ml. In the same period of time, SAHase increased from pretreatment range of 0.09 to 0.22 nmol/hr/mg protein to 2.37 to 5.16 nmol/hr/mg protein. Normal value for SAHase is 4.18 ± 1.9 nmol/hr/mg protein.

Contraindications

There is no evidence to support the safety and efficacy of pegademase bovine as preparatory or support therapy for bone marrow transplantation. Since the drug is administered by IM injection, use with caution in patients with thrombocytopenia and do not use if thrombocytopenia is severe.

Warnings

➤*Product potency:* Product potency testing prior to distribution may not assure the initial and continuing potency of each new lot of pegademase bovine. Report any laboratory or clinical indication of a decrease in potency immediately by telephone to Enzon (732-980-4500).

➤*Pregnancy: Category C.* It is not known whether pegademase bovine can cause fetal harm when administered to a pregnant woman or can affect reproduction capacity. Give to a pregnant woman only if clearly needed.

➤*Lactation:* It is not known whether pegademase bovine is excreted in breast milk. Exercise caution when administering to a nursing woman.

Precautions

➤*Monitoring:* Monitor the treatment of SCID associated with ADA deficiency with pegademase bovine by measuring plasma ADA activity and red blood cell dATP levels.

PEGADEMASE BOVINE — INJECTION

Determine plasma ADA activity and red cell dATP prior to treatment. Once treatment has been initiated, a desirable range of plasma ADA activity (trough level before maintenance injection) should be 15 to 35 mcmol/hr/ml. This minimum trough level will ensure that plasma ADA activity from injection to injection is maintained above the level of total erythrocyte ADA activity in the blood of normal individuals.

Determine plasma ADA activity (preinjection) every 1 to 2 weeks during the first 8 to 12 weeks of treatment in order to establish an effective dose. After 2 months of maintenance treatment, red cell dATP levels should decrease to a range of ≤ 0.005 to 0.015 mcmol/ml. The normal value of dATP is below 0.001 mcmol/ml. Once the level of dATP has fallen adequately, measure 2 to 4 times during the remainder of the first year and 2 to 3 times a year thereafter, assuming no interruption in therapy.

Between 3 and 9 months, determine plasma ADA twice a month, then monthly until after 18 to 24 months of treatment. In patients who have successfully been maintained on therapy for 2 years, continue to have plasma ADA measured every 2 to 4 months and red cell dATP measured twice yearly. More frequent monitoring would be necessary if therapy were interrupted or if an enhanced rate of clearance of plasma ADA activity develops.

Once effective ADA plasma levels have been established, should a patient's plasma ADA activity level fall below 10 mcmol/hr/ml (which cannot be attributed to improper dosing, sample handling or antibody development) then all patients receiving this lot of pegademase bovine will be required to have a blood sample for plasma ADA determination taken prior to their next injection. The index patient will require retesting for determination of plasma ADA activity prior to their next injection. If this value, as well as the value from one of the other patients from a different site, is < 10 mcmol/hr/ml, then the lot in use will be recalled and replaced with a new clinical lot by Enzon.

➤*Immunodeficiency:* Maintain appropriate care to protect immunedeficient patients until improvement in immune function has been documented. The degree of immune function improvement may vary from patient to patient and, therefore, each patient will require appropriate care consistent with immunologic status.

➤*Immune function:* Immune function, including the ability to produce antibodies, generally improves after 2 to 6 months of therapy, and matures over a longer period. Compared with the natural history of combined immunodeficiency disease due to ADA deficiency, a trend toward diminished frequency of opportunistic infections and fewer complications of infections has occurred in patients receiving pegademase bovine. However, the lag between the correction of the metabolic abnormalities and improved immune function with a trend toward diminished frequency of infections and complications of infection is variable, and has ranged from a few weeks to ≈ 6 months. Improvement in the general clinical status of the patient may be gradual (as evidenced by improvement in various clinical parameters) but should be apparent by the end of the first year of therapy.

A decline in immune function, with increased risk of opportunistic infections and complications of infection, will result from failure to maintain adequate levels of plasma ADA activity (whether due to the development of antibody, improper calculation of dosage, interruption of treatment or to improper storage with subsequent loss of activity). If a persistent decline in plasma ADA activity occurs, monitor immune function and clinical status closely and take precautions to minimize the risk of infection. If antibody to ADA or pegademase bovine is found to be the cause of a persistent fall in plasma ADA activity, then adjustment in the dosage and other measures may be taken to induce tolerance and restore adequate ADA activity.

➤*Antibody:* Antibody to pegademase bovine may develop in patients and may result in more rapid clearance of the drug. Suspect antibody to pegademase bovine if a persistent fall in preinjection level of plasma ADA to < 10 mcmol/hr/ml occurs. If other causes for a decline in plasma ADA levels can be ruled out (eg, improper storage of vials [freezing or prolonged storage at temperatures> 4°C], or improper handling of plasma samples [eg, repeated freezing and thawing during transport to laboratory]), then perform a specific assay for antibody to ADA and pegademase bovine (ELISA, enzyme inhibition).

One of 12 patients showed an enhanced rate of clearance of plasma ADA activity after 5 months of therapy at 15 U/kg/week. Enhanced clearance was correlated with the appearance of an antibody that directly inhibited both unmodified ADA and pegademase bovine. Subsequently, the patient was treated with twice weekly IM injections at an increased dose of 20 U/kg, or a total weekly dose of 40 U/kg. No adverse effects were observed at the higher dose and effective levels of plasma ADA were restored. After 4 months, the patient returned to a weekly dosage schedule of 20 U/kg and effective plasma levels have been maintained.

Drug Interactions

➤*Vidarabine:* Vidarabine is a substrate for ADA and **2'-deoxycoformycin** is a potent inhibitor of ADA. Thus, the activities of these drugs and pegademase bovine could be substantially altered if they are used in combination with one another.

Adverse Reactions

Clinical experience is limited. The following adverse reactions have occurred: Headache (1 patient) and pain at the injection site (2 patients).

Overdosage

An intraperitoneal dose of 50,000 U/kg of pegademase bovine in mice resulted in weight loss up to 9%.

ALEFACEPT

Rx	**Amevive** (Biogen Idec)	**Powder for injection, lyophilized:** 15 mg	12.5 mg sucrose. Preservative-free. In dose pack 1s and 4s.[a]

[a] In single-use vials with 10 mL single-use diluent (sterile water for injection).

ALEFACEPT — INJECTION

Indications

➤*Plaque psoriasis:* Treatment of adult patients with moderate to severe chronic plaque psoriasis who are candidates for systemic therapy or phototherapy.

Administration and Dosage

➤*Approved by the FDA:* January 30, 2003.

➤*Recommended dose:* The recommended dosage of alefacept is 15 mg given once weekly as an intramuscular (IM) injection. The recommended regimen is a course of 12 weekly injections. Retreatment with an additional 12-week course may be initiated provided that CD4+ T lymphocyte counts are within the normal range, and a minimum of a 12-week interval has passed since the previous course of treatment.

See Precautions for more information.

➤*Preparation:* Do not use an alefacept dose tray beyond the date stamped on the carton, drug/diluent pack, alefacept vial label, or diluent container label.

Alefacept 15 mg lyophilized powder for IM administration should be reconstituted with 0.6 mL of the supplied diluent (sterile water for injection). 0.5 mL of the reconstituted solution contains 15 mg of alefacept.

Do not add other medications to solutions containing alefacept. Do not reconstitute alefacept with other diluents. Do not filter reconstituted solution during preparation or administration.

All procedures require the use of aseptic technique. Using the supplied syringe and 1 of the supplied needles, withdraw only 0.6 mL of the supplied diluent (sterile water for injection). Keeping the needle pointed at the sidewall of the vial, slowly inject the diluent into the vial of alefacept. Some foaming will occur, which is normal. To avoid excessive foaming, do not shake or vigorously agitate. The contents should be swirled gently during dissolution. Generally, dissolution of alefacept takes less than 2 minutes. The solution should be used as soon as possible after reconstitution.

The reconstituted solution should be clear and colorless to slightly yellow. Visually inspect the solution for particulate matter and discoloration prior to administration. The solution should not be used if discolored or cloudy, or if undissolved material remains.

Following reconstitution, the product should be used immediately or within 4 hours if stored in the vial at 2° to 8°C (36° to 46°F). Alefacept not used within 4 hours of reconstitution should be discarded.

Remove the needle used for reconstitution and attach the other supplied needle. Withdraw 0.5 mL of the alefacept solution into the syringe. Some foam or bubbles may remain in the vial.

➤*Administration:*

For IM use – Inject the full 0.5 mL of solution. Rotate injection sites so that a different site is used for each new injection. New injections should be given at least 1 inch from an old site and never into areas where the skin is tender, bruised, red, or hard.

➤*Storage/Stability:* Store the drug/diluent pack containing alefacept (lyophilized powder) in a refrigerator between 2° and 8°C (36° and 46°F). Protect from light. Retain in drug/diluent pack until time of use.

Actions

➤*Pharmacology:* Alefacept interferes with lymphocyte activation by specifically binding to the lymphocyte antigen, CD2, and inhibiting leukocyte function antigen-3 (LFA-3)/CD2 interaction. Activation of T lymphocytes involving the interaction between LFA-3 on antigen-presenting cells and CD2 on T lymphocytes plays a role in the pathophysiology of chronic plaque psoriasis. The majority of T lymphocytes in psoriatic lesions are of the memory effector phenotype characterized by the presence of the CD45RO marker, express activation markers (eg, CD25, CD69) and release inflammatory cytokines, such as interferon γ.

Alefacept also causes a reduction in subsets of CD2+ T lymphocytes (primarily CD45RO+), presumably by bridging between CD2 on target lymphocytes and immunoglobulin Fc receptors on cytotoxic cells, such as natural killer cells. Treatment with alefacept results in a reduction in circulating total

ALEFACEPT — INJECTION

CD4+ and CD8+ T lymphocyte counts. CD2 is also expressed at low levels on the surface of natural killer cells and certain bone marrow B lymphocytes. Therefore, the potential exists for alefacept to affect the activation and numbers of cells other than T lymphocytes. In clinical studies of alefacept, minor changes in the numbers of circulating cells other than T lymphocytes have been observed.

➤*Pharmacokinetics:*

Absorption – Following an IM injection, bioavailability was 63%.

Distribution – In patients with moderate to severe plaque psoriasis, following a 7.5 mg intravenous (IV) administration, the mean volume of distribution of alefacept was 94 mL/kg.

Excretion – The mean clearance was 0.25 mL/h/kg and the mean elimination half-life was approximately 270 hours.

Contraindications

Do not administer alefacept to patients infected with HIV. Alefacept reduces CD4+ T lymphocyte counts, which might accelerate disease progression or increase complications of disease in these patients. Do not administer alefacept to patients with known hypersensitivity to alefacept or any of its components.

Warnings

➤*Lymphopenia:* Alefacept induces dose-dependent reductions in circulating CD4+ and CD8+ T lymphocyte counts.

Do not initiate a course of alefacept therapy in patients with a CD4+ T lymphocyte count below normal.

See Precautions for more information.

➤*Malignancies:* Alefacept may increase the risk of malignancies. In the 24-week period constituting the first course of placebo-controlled studies, 13 malignancies were diagnosed in 11 alefacept-treated patients. The incidence of malignancies was 1.3% (11/876) for alefacept-treated patients, compared with 0.5% (2/413) in the placebo group. In preclinical studies, animals developed B cell hyperplasia, and 1 animal developed a lymphoma. Do not administer alefacept to patients with a history of systemic malignancy. Exercise caution when considering the use of alefacept in patients at high risk for malignancy. If a patient develops a malignancy, discontinue alefacept.

➤*Serious infections:* Alefacept is an immunosuppressive agent and, therefore, has the potential to increase the risk of infection and reactivate latent, chronic infections. Do not administer alefacept to patients with a clinically important infection. Exercise caution when considering the use of alefacept in patients with chronic infections or a history of recurrent infection. Monitor patients for signs and symptoms of infection during or after a course of alefacept. Closely monitor new infections. If a patient develops a serious infection, discontinue alefacept. In the 24-week period constituting the first course of placebo-controlled studies, serious infections (infections requiring hospitalization) were observed at a rate of 0.9% (8/876) in alefacept-treated patients and 0.2% (1/413) in the placebo group.

➤*Hypersensitivity reactions:* Hypersensitivity reactions (urticaria, angioedema) were associated with the administration of alefacept. If an anaphylactic reaction or other serious allergic reaction occurs, discontinue administration of alefacept immediately and initiate appropriate therapy.

➤*Carcinogenesis:* In a chronic toxicity study, cynomolgus monkeys were dosed weekly for 52 weeks with alefacept IV at 1 or 20 mg/kg/dose. One animal in the high dose group developed a B-cell lymphoma that was detected after 28 weeks of dosing. Additional animals in both dose groups developed B-cell hyperplasia of the spleen and lymph nodes. One-year posttreatment, there was no evidence of alefacept-related lymphoma or B-cell hyperplasia in any of the remaining treated monkeys.

All animals in the study were positive for an endemic primate gammaherpes virus also known as lymphocryptovirus (LCV). Latent LCV infection is generally asymptomatic, but can lead to B-cell lymphomas when animals are immune suppressed.

In a separate study, baboons given 3 doses of alefacept at 1 mg/kg every 8 weeks were found to have centroblast proliferation in B-cell dependent areas in the germinal centers of the spleen following a 116-day washout period.

The role of alefacept in the development of the lymphoid malignancy and the hyperplasia observed in nonhuman primates and the relevance to humans is unknown. Immunodeficiency-associated lymphocyte disorders (plasmacytic hyperplasia, polymorphic proliferation, and B-cell lymphomas) occur in patients who have congenital or acquired immunodeficiencies including those resulting from immunosuppressive therapy.

➤*Elderly:* Because the incidence of infections and certain malignancies is higher in the elderly population, in general, use caution in treating the elderly.

➤*Pregnancy: Category B.* Women of childbearing potential make up a considerable segment of the patient population affected by psoriasis. Because the effect of alefacept on pregnancy and fetal development, including immune system development, is not known, health care providers are encouraged to enroll patients taking alefacept who become pregnant into the manufacturer's pregnancy registry by calling 1-866-263-8483.

Animal reproduction studies, however, are not always predictive of human response and there are no adequate and well-controlled studies in pregnant women. Because the risk to the development of the fetal immune system and postnatal immune function in humans is unknown, use alefacept during pregnancy only if clearly needed. If pregnancy occurs while taking alefacept, assess continued use of the drug.

➤*Lactation:* It is not known whether alefacept is excreted in human milk. Because many drugs are excreted in human milk, and because there exists the potential for serious adverse reactions in breast-feeding infants from alefacept, decide whether to discontinue breast-feeding during drug therapy or to discontinue the use of the drug, taking into account the importance of the drug to the mother.

➤*Children:* The safety and efficacy of alefacept in children have not been studied. Alefacept is not indicated for children.

Precautions

➤*Monitoring:* Monitor CD4+ T lymphocyte counts weekly before initiating dosing and every 2 weeks throughout the 12-week dosing period and use them to guide dosing. Patients should have normal CD4+ T lymphocyte counts prior to an initial or a subsequent course of treatment with alefacept. If CD4+ T lymphocyte counts are below 250 cells/mcL, withhold alefacept dosing and institute weekly monitoring. Discontinue alefacept if CD4+ T lymphocyte counts remain below 250 cells/mcL for 1 month.

Monitor patients for signs and symptoms of infection during or after a course of alefacept. Closely monitor new infections.

➤*Phototherapy:* Patients receiving phototherapy should not receive concurrent therapy with alefacept because of the possibility of excessive immunosuppression.

➤*Hepatic injury:* In postmarketing experience, there have been reports of liver injury, including asymptomatic transaminase elevation, fatty infiltration of the liver, hepatitis, decompensation of cirrhosis with liver failure, and acute liver failure. Two cases of liver failure were reported with concomitant alcohol use. In the 24-week period constituting the first course of placebo-controlled studies, 1.7% (15/876) of alefacept-treated patients and 1.2% (5/413) of the placebo group experienced ALT and/or AST elevations of at least 3 times the upper limit of normal. While the exact relationship of these occurrences with the use of alefacept has not been established, fully evaluate patients with signs or symptoms of liver injury. Discontinue alefacept in patients who develop significant clinical signs of liver injury.

Drug Interactions

No formal interaction studies have been performed.

➤*Immunosuppressants:* Patients receiving other immunosuppressive agents should not receive concurrent therapy with alefacept because of the possibility of excessive immunosuppression.

➤*Vaccines:* The safety and efficacy of vaccines, specifically live or live-attenuated vaccines, administered to patients being treated with alefacept have not been studied. In a study of 46 patients with chronic plaque psoriasis, the ability to mount immunity to tetanus toxoid (recall antigen) and an experimental neo-antigen was preserved in those patients undergoing alefacept therapy.

Adverse Reactions

Commonly observed adverse reactions seen in the first course of placebo-controlled clinical trials with at least a 2% higher incidence in the alefacept-treated patients compared with placebo-treated patients were pharyngitis, dizziness, increased cough, nausea, pruritus, myalgia, chills, injection site pain, injection site inflammation, and accidental injury. The only adverse reaction that occurred at a 5% or higher incidence among alefacept-treated patients compared with placebo-treated patients was chills (1% placebo vs 6% alefacept), which occurred predominantly with IV administration.

The adverse reactions that most commonly resulted in clinical intervention were cardiovascular events, including coronary artery disorder in less than 1% of patients and myocardial infarct in less than 1% of patients. These reactions were not observed in any of the 413 placebo-treated patients. The total number of patients hospitalized for cardiovascular events in the alefacept-treated group was 1.2% (11/876).

The most common reactions resulting in discontinuation of treatment with alefacept were CD4+ T lymphocyte levels below 250 cells/mcgL, headache (0.2%), and nausea (0.2%).

The most serious adverse reactions were lymphopenia, malignancies, serious infections requiring hospitalization, and hypersensitivity reactions.

➤*Lymphopenia:* In the IM study (study 2), 4% of patients temporarily discontinued treatment and no patients permanently discontinued treatment due to CD4+ T lymphocyte counts below the specified threshold of 250 cells/mcL. In study 2, 10%, 28%, and 42% of patients had total lymphocyte, CD4+, and CD8+ T lymphocyte counts below normal, respectively. Twelve weeks after a course of therapy (12 weekly doses), 2%, 8%, and 21% of patients had total lymphocyte, CD4+, and CD8+ T cell counts below normal.

In the first course of the IV study (study 1), 10% of patients temporarily discontinued treatment and 2% permanently discontinued treatment due to CD4+ T lymphocyte counts below the specified threshold of 250 cells/mcL. During the first course of study 1, 22% of patients had total lymphocyte counts below normal, 48% had CD4+ T lymphocyte counts below normal and 59% had CD8+ T lymphocyte counts below normal. The maximal effect on lymphocytes was observed within 6 to 8 weeks of initiation of treatment. Twelve weeks after a course of therapy (12 weekly doses), 4% of patients had total lymphocyte counts below normal, 19% had CD4+ T lymphocyte counts below normal, and 36% had CD8+ T lymphocyte counts below normal.

For patients receiving a second course of alefacept in study 1, 17% of patients had total lymphocyte counts below normal, 44% had CD4+ T lymphocyte counts below normal, and 56% had CD8+ T lymphocyte counts below normal. Twelve weeks after completing dosing, 3% of patients had total lymphocyte counts below normal, 17% had CD4+ T lymphocyte counts below normal, and 35% had CD8+ T lymphocyte counts below normal.

ALEFACEPT — INJECTION

➤*Malignancies:* See Warnings for more information.

Among 1,869 patients who received alefacept at any dose in clinical trials, 43 patients were diagnosed with 63 treatment-emergent malignancies. The majority of the malignancies were nonmelanoma skin cancers: 46 cases (20 basal cell, 26 squamous cell carcinomas) in 27 patients. Other malignancies observed in alefacept-treated patients included melanoma (n = 3), solid organ malignancies (n = 12 in 11 patients), and lymphomas (n = 5); the latter consisted of 2 Hodgkin and 2 non-Hodgkin lymphomas, and 1 cutaneous T cell lymphoma (mycosis fungoides).

➤*Hypersensitivity:* In clinical studies, 4 of 1,869 (0.2%) patients were reported to experience angioedema: 2 of these patients were hospitalized. In the 24-week period constituting the first course of placebo-controlled studies, urticaria was reported in 6 (less than 1%) alefacept-treated patients versus 1 patient in the control group. Urticaria resulted in discontinuation of therapy in 1 of the alefacept-treated patients.

➤*Hepatic:* See Precautions for more information.

➤*Immunogenicity:* Approximately 3% (40/1,357) of patients receiving alefacept developed low-titer antibodies to alefacept. No apparent correlation of antibody development and clinical response or adverse reactions was observed. The long-term immunogenicity of alefacept is unknown.

The data reflect the percentage of patients whose test results were considered positive for antibodies to alefacept in an enzyme-linked immunosorbent assay (ELISA), and are highly dependent on the sensitivity and specificity of the assay. Additionally, the observed incidence of antibody positivity in an assay may be influenced by several factors, including sample handling, timing of sample collection, concomitant medications, and underlying disease. For these reasons, comparison of the incidence of antibodies to alefacept with the incidence of antibodies to other products may be misleading.

➤*Infections:* In the 24-week period constituting the first course of placebo-controlled studies, serious infections (infections requiring hospitalization) were seen at a rate of 0.9% (8/876) in alefacept-treated patients and 0.2% (1/413) in the placebo group. In patients receiving repeated courses of alefacept therapy, the rates of serious infections remained similar across courses of therapy. Serious infections among 1,869 alefacept-treated patients included cellulitis, abscesses, wound infections, toxic shock, pneumonia, appendicitis, cholecystitis, gastroenteritis, and herpes infections.

➤*Local:* In the IM study (study 2), 16% of alefacept-treated patients and 8% of placebo-treated patients reported injection site reactions. In patients receiving repeated courses of alefacept IM therapy, the incidence of injection site reactions remained similar across courses of therapy. Reactions at the site of injection were generally mild, typically occurred on single occasions, and included either pain (7%), inflammation (4%), bleeding (4%), edema (2%), nonspecific reaction (2%), mass (1%), or skin hypersensitivity (less than 1%). In the clinical trials, a single case of injection site reaction led to the discontinuation of alefacept.

➤*Postmarketing:* In postmarketing experience there have been reports of asymptomatic transaminase elevation, fatty infiltration of the liver, hepatitis, and severe liver failure.

Overdosage

➤*Symptoms:* The highest dose tested in humans (0.75 mg/kg IV) was associated with chills, headache, arthralgia, and sinusitis within 1 day of dosing.

➤*Treatment:* Closely monitor patients who have been inadvertently administered an excess of the recommended dose for effects on total lymphocyte count and CD4+ T lymphocyte count.

Patient Information

Inform patients of the need for regular monitoring of white blood cell (lymphocyte) counts during therapy and that alefacept must be administered under the supervision of a health care provider. Also inform patients that alefacept reduces lymphocyte counts, which could increase their chances of developing an infection or a malignancy. Advise patients to inform their health care provider promptly if they develop any signs of an infection or malignancy while undergoing a course of treatment with alefacept.

Also advise female patients to notify their health care provider if they become pregnant while taking alefacept (or within 8 weeks of discontinuing alefacept). Advise them of the existence of and encourage them to enroll in the manufacturer's pregnancy registry. Call 1-866-263-8483 to enroll into the registry.

Advise patients that serious liver injury has been reported in patients receiving alefacept. Advise patients to report to their health care provider persistent nausea, anorexia, fatigue, vomiting, abdominal pain, jaundice, easy bruising, dark urine, or pale stools.

EFALIZUMAB

Rx	**Raptiva** (Genentech)	**Powder for injection, lyophilized:** 150 mg (designed to deliver 125 mg/1.25 mL)	Preservative-free. In single-use vials.[a] With 1 single-use, prefilled diluent syringe containing 1.3 mL sterile water for injection, two 25 gauge × ⅝ inch needles, and 2 alcohol prep pads.

[a] With 123.2 mg sucrose, 6.8 mg L-histidine hydrochloride monohydrate, and 4.3 mg L-histidine.

EFALIZUMAB — INJECTION

Indications

➤*Plaque psoriasis:* For the treatment of adult patients (18 years of age or older) with chronic moderate to severe plaque psoriasis who are candidates for systemic therapy or phototherapy.

Administration and Dosage

➤*Approved by the FDA:* October 27, 2003.

➤*Recommended dose:* The recommended dose of efalizumab is a single 0.7 mg/kg SC conditioning dose followed by weekly SC doses of 1 mg/kg (maximum single dose not to exceed a total of 200 mg).

Efalizumab is intended for use under the guidance and supervision of a physician. If it is determined to be appropriate, patients may self-inject efalizumab after proper training in the preparation and injection technique and with medical follow-up.

➤*Preparation for administration:* Efalizumab should be administered using the sterile, disposable syringe and needles provided. Remove the cap from the prefilled syringe containing sterile water for injection (non-USP) and attach the needle to the syringe. Remove the plastic cap protecting the rubber stopper of the efalizumab vial and wipe the top of the rubber stopper with 1 of the provided alcohol swabs. After cleaning with the alcohol swab, do not touch the top of the vial. To prepare the efalizumab solution, using the provided prefilled diluent syringe slowly inject the 1.3 mL of sterile water for injection (non-USP) into the efalizumab vial. Swirl the vial with a gentle rotary motion to dissolve the product. Do not shake. Shaking will cause foaming of the efalizumab solution. Generally, dissolution of efalizumab takes less than 5 minutes. Efalizumab is provided as a single-use vial and contains no antibacterial preservatives. Reconstitute immediately before use and use only once. If the reconstituted efalizumab is not used immediately, store the efalizumab vial at room temperature and use within 8 hours. The reconstituted solution should be clear to pale yellow and free of particulates.

➤*Administration:* Replace the needle on the syringe with a new needle. Insert the needle into the vial containing the efalizumab solution, invert the vial, and keeping the needle below the level of the liquid, withdraw the dose to be given into the syringe.

No other medications should be added to solutions containing efalizumab, and efalizumab should not be reconstituted with other diluents.

Sites for injection include thigh, abdomen, buttocks, or upper arm. Injection sites should be rotated.

Following administration, discard any unused reconstituted efalizumab solution.

➤*Storage/Stability:* Do not use a vial beyond the expiration date stamped on the carton or vial label. Efalizumab (lyophilized powder) must be refrigerated at 2° to 8°C (36° to 46°F). Protect the vial from exposure to light. Store in original carton until time of use.

Actions

➤*Pharmacology:* Efalizumab binds to CD11a, the α subunit of leukocyte function antigen-1 (LFA-1), which is expressed on all leukocytes, and decreases cell surface expression of CD11a. Efalizumab inhibits the binding of LFA-1 to intercellular adhesion molecule-1 (ICAM-1), thereby inhibiting the adhesion of leukocytes to other cell types. Interaction between LFA-1 and ICAM-1 contributes to the initiation and maintenance of multiple processes, including activation of T lymphocytes, adhesion of T lymphocytes to endothelial cells, and migration of T lymphocytes to sites of inflammation including psoriatic skin. Lymphocyte activation and trafficking to skin play a role in the pathophysiology of chronic plaque psoriasis. In psoriatic skin, ICAM-1 cell surface expression is upregulated on endothelium and keratinocytes. CD11a is also expressed on the surface of B lymphocytes, monocytes, neutrophils, natural killer cells, and other leukocytes. Therefore, the potential exists for efalizumab to affect the activation, adhesion, migration, and numbers of cells other than T lymphocytes.

Pharmacodynamics – At a dose of 1 mg/kg/week SC, efalizumab reduced expression of CD11a on circulating T lymphocytes to approximately 15% to 25% of pre-dose values and reduced free CD11a binding sites to a mean of less than or equal to 5% of pre-dose values. These pharmacodynamic effects were seen 1 to 2 days after the first dose, and were maintained between weekly 1 mg/kg SC doses. Following discontinuation of efalizumab, CD11a expression returned to a mean of 74% of baseline at 5 weeks and stayed at comparable levels at 8 and 13 weeks. Following discontinuation of efalizumab, free CD11a binding sites returned to a mean of 86% of baseline at 8 weeks and stayed at comparable levels at 13 weeks. No assessments of CD11a expression or free CD11a binding sites were made after 13 weeks.

In clinical trials, efalizumab treatment resulted in a mean increase (relative to baseline) in white blood cell (WBC) count of 34%, a doubling of mean lymphocyte counts and an increase in eosinophil counts of 29% due to decreased leukocyte adhesion to blood vessel walls and decreased trafficking from the vascular compartment to tissues. At day 56 of 1 mg/kg/week efalizumab treatment, 32% (213/676) of patients had a shift in total WBC from low or normal baseline value to above normal, 46% (324/701) had a shift to above normal absolute lymphocyte counts, and 5% (35/675) had a shift to above normal eosinophil counts. Following discontinuation of efalizumab

EFALIZUMAB — INJECTION

treatment, the abnormal elevated lymphocyte counts took approximately 8 weeks to normalize among patients who had above normal lymphocyte counts. Plasma samples collected after first administration of 0.3 mg/kg IV efalizumab indicate that at 2 hours TNF-α and IL-6 plasma levels were elevated 9- and 90-fold, respectively, compared with baseline. Plasma samples collected after first administration of 0.7 mg/kg SC efalizumab indicate that at 2 days, IL-6 levels were elevated (10 pg/mL as compared with 5 pg/mL at baseline), whereas TNF-α was not detectable. In efalizumab-treated patients the mean levels of C-reactive protein increased from baseline by 67% and the mean levels of fibrinogen increased by 15%.

➤*Pharmacokinetics:*

Absorption – In patients with moderate to severe plaque psoriasis, following an initial SC efalizumab dose of 0.7 mg/kg followed by 11 weekly SC doses of 1 mg/kg/week, serum concentrations reached a steady-state at 4 weeks with a mean trough concentration of approximately 9 mcg/mL (n = 26). After the last dose, the mean peak concentration was approximately 12 mcg/mL (n = 25). Mean steady-state clearance was 24 mL/kg/day (range = 5 to 76 mL/kg/day, n = 25). Mean time to eliminate efalizumab after the last steady-state dose was 25 days (range = 13 to 35 days, n = 17). The mean estimated efalizumab SC bioavailability was 50%.

Excretion – In a population pharmacokinetic analysis of 1088 patients, body weight was found to be the most significant covariate affecting efalizumab clearance. In patients receiving weekly SC doses of 1 mg/kg, efalizumab exposure was similar across body weight quartiles. Efalizumab clearance was not significantly affected by gender or race.

Contraindications

Hypersensitivity to efalizumab or any of its components.

Warnings

➤*Serious infections:* Efalizumab is an immunosuppressive agent and has the potential to increase the risk of infection and reactivate latent, chronic infections. Efalizumab should not be administered to patients with clinically important infections. Caution should be exercised when considering the use of efalizumab in patients with a chronic infection or history of recurrent infections. If a patient develops a serious infection, efalizumab should be discontinued. New infections developing during efalizumab treatment should be monitored. During the first 12 weeks of controlled trials, serious infections occurred in 7 of 1620 (0.4%) efalizumab-treated patients compared with 1 of 715 (0.1%) placebo-treated patients. Serious infections requiring hospitalization included cellulitis, pneumonia, abscess, sepsis, bronchitis, gastroenteritis, aseptic meningitis, Legionnaire's disease, and vertebral osteomyelitis (note some patients had more than one infection).

➤*Malignancies:* Efalizumab is an immunosuppressive agent. Many immunosuppressive agents have the potential to increase the risk of malignancy. The role of efalizumab in the development of malignancies is not known. Caution should be exercised when considering the use of efalizumab in patients at high risk for malignancy or with a history of malignancy. If a patient develops a malignancy, efalizumab should be discontinued.

➤*Thrombocytopenia:* Platelet counts at or below 52,000 cells per mcL were observed in 8 (0.3%) efalizumab-treated patients during clinical trials compared with none among the placebo-treated patients. Five of the 8 patients received a course of systemic steroids for thrombocytopenia. Thrombocytopenia resolved in the 7 patients receiving adequate follow-up (1 patient was lost to follow-up). Physicians should follow patients closely for signs and symptoms of thrombocytopenia. Assessment of platelet counts is recommended during treatment with efalizumab and efalizumab should be discontinued if thrombocytopenia develops.

➤*Psoriasis worsening and variants:* Worsening of psoriasis can occur during or after discontinuation of efalizumab. During clinical studies, 19 of 2589 (0.7%) of efalizumab-treated patients had serious worsening of psoriasis during treatment (n = 5) or worsening past baseline after discontinuation of efalizumab (n = 14). In some patients these events took the form of psoriatic erythroderma or pustular psoriasis. Some patients required hospitalization and alternative antipsoriatic therapy to manage the psoriasis worsening. Patients, including those not responding to efalizumab treatment, should be closely observed following discontinuation of efalizumab, and appropriate psoriasis treatment instituted as necessary.

➤*Pregnancy: Category C.* Animal reproduction studies have not been conducted with efalizumab. It is also not known whether efalizumab can cause fetal harm when administered to a pregnant woman or can affect reproduction capacity. Efalizumab should be given to a pregnant woman only if clearly needed.

In a developmental toxicity study conducted in mice using an anti-mouse CD11a antibody at up to 30 times the equivalent of the recommended clinical dose of efalizumab, no evidence of maternal toxicity, embryotoxicity, or teratogenicity was observed when administered during organogenesis. No adverse effects on behavioral, reproductive, or growth parameters were observed in offspring of female mice subcutaneously treated with an anti-mouse CD11a antibody during gestation and lactation using doses 3 to 30 times the equivalent of the recommended clinical dose of efalizumab. At 11 weeks of age, the offspring of these females exhibited a significant reduction in their ability to mount an antibody response, which showed evidence of partial reversibility by 25 weeks of age. Animal studies, however, are not always predictive of human response, and there are no adequate and well-controlled studies in pregnant women.

Since the effects of efalizumab on pregnant women and fetal development, including immune system development are not known, healthcare providers are encouraged to enroll patients who become pregnant while taking efalizumab (or within 6 weeks of discontinuing efalizumab) in the efalizumab pregnancy registry.

➤*Lactation:* It is not known whether efalizumab is excreted in human milk. An anti-mouse CD11a antibody was detected in milk samples of lactating mice exposed to anti-mouse CD11a antibody and the offspring of the exposed females exhibited significant reduction in antibody responses. Since maternal immunoglobulins are known to be present in the milk of lactating mothers, and animal data suggest the potential for adverse effects in nursing infants from efalizumab, a decision should be made whether to discontinue nursing while taking the drug or to discontinue the use of the drug, taking into account the importance of the drug to the mother.

➤*Children:* The safety and efficacy of efalizumab in pediatric patients have not been studied.

Precautions

➤*Monitoring:* Assessment of platelet counts is recommended upon initiating and periodically while receiving efalizumab treatment. It is recommended that assessments be more frequent when initiating therapy (eg, monthly) and may decrease in frequency with continued treatment (eg, every 3 months). Severe thrombocytopenia has been observed.

➤*Immunosuppression:* The safety and efficacy of efalizumab in combination with other immunosuppressive agents or phototherapy have not been evaluated. Patients receiving other immunosuppressive agents should not receive concurrent therapy with efalizumab because of the possibility of increased risk of infections and malignancies.

➤*Immunizations:* See Drug Interactions for more information.

➤*First dose reactions:* First dose reactions including headache, fever, nausea, and vomiting are associated with efalizumab treatment and are dose-level related in incidence and severity. Therefore, a conditioning dose of 0.7 mg/kg is recommended to reduce the incidence and severity of reactions associated with initial dosing. One case of aseptic meningitis resulting in hospitalization has been observed in association with initial dosing.

➤*Lab test abnormalities:* Increases in lymphocyte counts related to the pharmacologic mechanism of action are frequently observed during efalizumab treatment.

Drug Interactions

➤*Immunizations:* Acellular, live and live-attenuated vaccines should not be administered during efalizumab treatment.

Adverse Reactions

➤*Common adverse reactions:* The most common adverse reactions associated with efalizumab were a first dose reaction complex that included headache, chills, fever, nausea, and myalgia within 2 days following the first 2 injections. These reactions are dose-level related in incidence and severity and were largely mild to moderate in severity when a conditioning dose of 0.7 mg/kg was used as the first dose. In placebo-controlled trials, 29% of patients treated with efalizumab 1 mg/kg developed 1 or more of these symptoms following the first dose compared with 15% of patients receiving placebo. After the third dose, 4% and 3% of patients receiving efalizumab 1 mg/kg and placebo, respectively, experienced these symptoms. Less than 1% of patients discontinued efalizumab treatment because of these adverse events.

➤*Other adverse reactions:* Other adverse events resulting in discontinuation of efalizumab treatment were psoriasis (0.6%), pain (0.4%), arthritis (0.4%), and arthralgia (0.3%).

Adverse events in placebo controlled study periods reported at a ≥ 2% higher rate in the 1 mg/kg/wk efalizumab treatment than placebo groups

Adverse reaction	Placebo (n = 715)	Efalizumab 1 mg/kg/wk (n = 1213)
Headache	159 (22%)	391 (32%)
Infection[a]	188 (26%)	350 (29%)
Chills	32 (4%)	154 (13%)
Nausea	51 (7%)	128 (11%)
Pain	38 (5%)	122 (10%)
Myalgia	35 (5%)	102 (8%)
Flu syndrome	29 (4%)	83 (7%)
Fever	24 (3%)	80 (7%)
Back pain	14 (2%)	50 (4%)
Acne	4 (1%)	45 (4%)

[a] Includes diagnosed infections and other non-specific infections. Most common non-specific infection was upper respiratory tract infection.

Adverse events occurring at a rate between 1% and 2% greater in the efalizumab group compared with placebo were arthralgia, asthenia, peripheral edema, and psoriasis.

➤*Serious adverse reactions:* The following serious adverse reactions were observed in efalizumab-treated patients:

Infections – In the first 12 weeks of placebo-controlled studies, the proportion of patients with serious infection was 0.4% (7/1620) in the efalizumab-treated group (5 of these were hospitalized, 0.3%) and 0.1% (1/715) in the placebo group. In the complete safety data from both controlled and uncontrolled studies, the overall incidence of hospitalization for infections was 1.6 per 100 patient-years for efalizumab-treated patients compared with 1.2 per

EFALIZUMAB — INJECTION

100 patient-years for placebo-treated patients. Including both controlled, uncontrolled, and follow-up study treatment periods there were 27 serious infections in 2475 efalizumab-treated patients. These infections included cellulitis, pneumonia, abscess, sepsis, sinusitis, bronchitis, gastroenteritis, aseptic meningitis, Legionnaire's disease, septic arthritis, and vertebral osteomyelitis. In controlled trials, the overall rate of infections in efalizumab-treated patients was 3% higher than in placebo-treated patients (see table above).

Malignancies – Among the 2762 psoriasis patients who received efalizumab at any dose (median duration 8 months), 31 patients were diagnosed with 37 malignancies. The overall incidence of malignancies of any kind was 1.8 per 100 patient-years for efalizumab-treated patients compared with 1.6 per 100 patient-years for placebo-treated patients. Malignancies observed in the efalizumab-treated patients included non-melanoma skin cancer, non-cutaneous solid tumors, Hodgkin's lymphoma and non-Hodgkin's lymphoma, and malignant melanoma. The incidence of non-cutaneous solid tumors (8 in 1790 patient-years) and malignant melanoma were within the range expected for the general population.

The majority of the malignancies were non-melanoma skin cancers; 26 cases (13 basal, 13 squamous) in 20 patients (0.7% of 2762 efalizumab-treated patients). The incidence was comparable for efalizumab-treated and placebo-treated patients. However, the size of the placebo group and duration of follow-up were limited and a difference in rates of non-melanoma skin cancers cannot be excluded.

Thrombocytopenia – In the combined safety database of 2762 efalizumab-treated patients, there were 8 occurrences (0.3%) of thrombocytopenia of less than 52,000 cells per mcL reported. Three of the 8 patients were hospitalized for thrombocytopenia, including 1 patient with heavy uterine bleeding; all cases were consistent with an immune mediated thrombocytopenia. Antiplatelet antibody was evaluated in 1 patient and was found to be positive. Each case resulted in discontinuation of efalizumab. Based on available platelet count measurements, the onset of platelet decline was between 8 and 12 weeks after the first dose of efalizumab in 5 of the patients. Onset was more delayed in 3 patients, occurring as late as 1 year in 1 patient. In these cases, the platelet count nadirs occurred between 12 and 72 weeks after the first dose of efalizumab.

Adverse events of psoriasis – In the combined safety database from all studies, serious psoriasis adverse events occurred in 19 efalizumab-treated patients (0.7%) including hospitalization in 17 patients. Most of these events (14/19) occurred after discontinuation of study drug and occurred in both patients responding and not responding to efalizumab treatment. Serious adverse events of psoriasis included pustular, erythrodermic, and guttate subtypes. During the first 12 weeks of treatment within placebo-controlled studies, the rate of psoriasis adverse events (serious and non-serious) was 3.2% (52/1620) in the efalizumab-treated patients and 1.4% (10/715) in the placebo-treated patients.

Hypersensitivity reactions – Symptoms associated with a hypersensitivity reaction (eg, dyspnea, asthma, urticaria, angioedema, maculopapular rash) were evaluated by treatment group. In the first 12 weeks of the controlled clinical studies, the proportion of patients reporting at least 1 hypersensitivity reaction was 8% (95/1213) in the 1 mg/kg/wk group and 7% (49/715) patients in the placebo group. Urticaria was observed in 1% of patients (16/1213) receiving efalizumab and 0.4% of patients (3/715) receiving placebo during the initial 12-week treatment period. Other observed adverse events in patients receiving efalizumab that may be indicative of hypersensitivity included laryngospasm, angioedema, erythema multiforme, asthma, and allergic drug eruption. One patient was hospitalized with a serum sickness-like reaction.

Inflammatory/immune-mediated reactions – In the entire efalizumab clinical development program of 2762 efalizumab-treated patients, inflammatory, potentially immune-mediated adverse events resulting in hospitalization included inflammatory arthritis (12 cases, 0.4% of patients) and interstitial pneumonitis (2 cases). One case each of the following serious adverse reactions was observed: Transverse myelitis, bronchiolitis obliterans, aseptic meningitis, idiopathic hepatitis, sialedenitis, and sensorineural hearing loss.

Laboratory values – In efalizumab-treated patients, a mean elevation in alkaline phosphatase (5 U/L) was observed; 4% of efalizumab-treated patients experienced a shift to above normal values compared with 0.6% of placebo-treated patients. The clinical significance of this change is unknown. Higher numbers of efalizumab-treated patients experienced elevations above normal in 2 or more liver function tests than placebo (3.1% vs 1.5%).

Other laboratory adverse reactions that were observed included thrombocytopenia, lymphocytosis (40%) (including 3 cases of transient atypical lymphocytosis), and leukocytosis (26%).

Immunogenicity – In patients evaluated for antibodies to efalizumab after efalizumab treatment ended, predominantly low-titer antibodies to efalizumab or other protein components of the efalizumab drug product were detected in 6.3% (67/1063) of patients. The long-term immunogenicity of efalizumab is unknown.

The data reflect the percentage of patients whose test results were considered positive for antibodies to efalizumab in the ELISA assay, and are highly dependent on the sensitivity and specificity of the assay. Additionally, the observed incidence of antibody positivity in an assay may be influenced by several factors including sample handling, timing of sample collection, concomitant medications, and underlying disease. For these reasons, comparison of the incidence of antibodies to efalizumab with the incidence of antibodies to other products may be misleading.

Overdosage

Doses up to 4 mg/kg/week SC for 10 weeks following a conditioning (0.7 mg/kg) first dose have been administered without an observed increase in acute toxicity. The maximum administered single dose was 10 mg/kg IV. This was administered to one patient, who subsequently was admitted to the hospital for severe vomiting. In case of overdose, it is recommended that the patient be monitored for 24 to 48 hours for any acute signs or symptoms of adverse reactions or effects and appropriate treatment instituted.

Patient Information

Patients should be informed that their physician may monitor platelet counts during therapy. Patients should be advised to seek immediate medical attention if they develop any of the signs and symptoms associated with severe thrombocytopenia, such as easy bleeding from the gums, bruising, or petechiae. Patients should also be informed that efalizumab is an immunosuppressant, and could increase their chances of developing an infection or a malignancy. Patients should be advised to promptly call the prescribing doctor's office if they develop any new signs of, or receive a new diagnosis of infection or malignancy while undergoing treatment with efalizumab.

Female patients should also be advised to notify their physicians if they become pregnant while taking efalizumab (or within 6 weeks of discontinuing efalizumab) and be advised of the existence of and encouraged to enroll in the efalizumab pregnancy registry.

If a patient or caregiver is to administer efalizumab, he/she should be instructed regarding injection techniques and how to measure the correct dose to ensure proper administration of efalizumab. Patients should be also referred to the efalizumab patient package insert. In addition, patients should have available materials for and be instructed in the proper disposal of needles and syringes to comply with state and local laws. Patients should also be cautioned against reuse of syringes and needles.

AZATHIOPRINE

Rx	**Azasan** (aaiPharma)	**Tablets:** 25 mg	Lactose. Yellow, oval, scored. In 100s.
Rx	**Azathioprine** (aaiPharma)	**Tablets:** 50 mg	In 100s.
Rx	**Imuran** (Prometheus)		(Imuran 50). Yellow to off-white, scored. In 100s and UD 100s.
Rx	**Azasan** (aaiPharma)		Lactose. Yellow, capsule shape, scored. In 100s.
Rx	**Azasan** (aaiPharma)	**Tablets:** 75 mg	Lactose. Yellow, triangular, scored. In 100s.
Rx	**Azasan** (aaiPharma)	**Tablets:** 100 mg	Lactose. Yellow, diamond shape, scored. In 100s.
Rx	**Azathioprine Sodium** (Various, eg, Bedford)	**Injection:** 100 mg (as sodium) per vial	In 20 ml vials.

AZATHIOPRINE — ORAL

WARNING

Chronic immunosuppression with this purine antimetabolite increases risk of neoplasia in humans. Physicians using this drug should be very familiar with this risk as well as with the mutagenic potential to both men and women and with possible hematologic toxicities (see Warnings).

Indications

➤*Renal homotransplantation:* Adjunct for the prevention of rejection in renal homotransplantation. Experience with > 16,000 transplants shows a 5 year patient survival of 35% to 55%, but this is dependent on donor, match for HLA antigens, anti-donor or anti-B-cell alloantigen antibody, and other variables. The effect of azathioprine on these variables has not been tested in controlled trials.

➤*Rheumatoid arthritis:* Azathioprine is indicated only in adult patients meeting criteria for classic or definite rheumatoid arthritis as specified by the American Rheumatism Association. Azathioprine should be restricted to patients with severe, active and erosive disease not responsive to conventional management including rest, aspirin, or other nonsteroidal drugs, or to agents in the class of which gold is an example. Rest, physiotherapy, and salicylates should be continued while azathioprine is given, but it may be possible to reduce the dose of corticosteroids in patients on azathioprine. The combined use of azathioprine with gold, antimalarials, or penicillamine has not been studied for either added benefit or unexpected adverse effects. The use of azathioprine with these agents cannot be recommended.

Administration and Dosage

➤*Renal homotransplantation:* The dose of azathioprine required to prevent rejection and minimize toxicity will vary with individual patients; this necessitates careful management. The initial dose is usually 3 to 5 mg/kg daily, beginning at the time of transplant. Azathioprine is usually given as a single daily dose on the day of, and in a minority of cases 1 to 3 days before, transplantation. Azathioprine is often initiated with the intravenous administration of the sodium salt, with subsequent use of tablets (at the same dose level) after the postoperative period. Intravenous administration of the sodium salt is indicated only in patients unable to tolerate oral medications. Dose reduction to maintenance levels of 1 to 3 mg/kg daily is usually possible. The dose of azathioprine should not be increased to toxic levels because of threatened rejection. Discontinuation may be necessary for severe hematologic or other toxicity, even if rejection of the homograft may be a consequence of drug withdrawal.

➤*Rheumatoid arthritis:* Azathioprine is usually given on a daily basis. The initial dose should be approximately 1 mg/kg (50 to 100 mg) given as a single dose or on a twice-daily schedule. The dose may be increased, beginning at 6 to 8 weeks and thereafter by steps at 4 week intervals, if there are no serious toxicities and if initial response is unsatisfactory. Dose increments should be 0.5 mg/kg daily, up to a maximum dose of 2.5 mg/kg per day. Therapeutic response occurs after several weeks of treatment, usually 6 to 8; an adequate trial should be a minimum of 12 weeks. Patients not improved after 12 weeks can be considered refractory. Azathioprine may be continued long-term in patients with clinical response, but patients should be monitored carefully, and gradual dosage reduction should be attempted to reduce risk of toxicities.

Maintenance therapy should be at the lowest effective dose, and the dose given can be lowered decrementally with changes of 0.5 mg/kg or approximately 25 mg daily every 4 weeks while other therapy is kept constant. The optimum duration of maintenance azathioprine has not been determined. Azathioprine can be discontinued abruptly, but delayed effects are possible.

➤*Use in renal dysfunction:* Relatively oliguric patients, especially those with tubular necrosis in the immediate postcadaveric transplant period, may have delayed clearance of azathioprine or its metabolites, may be particularly sensitive to this drug, and are usually given lower doses.

➤*Storage/Stability:* Store at 15° to 25°C (59° to 77°F) in a dry place and protect from light.

Actions

➤*Pharmacology:*

Homograft survival – Summary information from transplant centers and registries indicates relatively universal use of azathioprine with or without other immunosuppressive agents. Although the use of azathioprine for inhibition of renal homograft rejection is well established, the mechanism(s) for this action are somewhat obscure. The drug suppresses hypersensitivities of the cell-mediated type and causes variable alterations in antibody production. Suppression of T-cell effects, including ablation of T-cell suppression, is dependent on the temporal relationship to antigenic stimulus or engraftment. This agent has little effect on established graft rejections or secondary responses.

Alterations in specific immune responses or immunologic functions in transplant recipients are difficult to relate specifically to immunosuppression by azathioprine. These patients have subnormal responses to vaccines, low numbers of T-cells, and abnormal phagocytosis by peripheral blood cells, but their mitogenic responses, serum immunoglobulins, and secondary antibody responses are usually normal.

Immunoinflammatory response – Azathioprine suppresses disease manifestations as well as underlying pathology in animal models of autoimmune disease. For example, the severity of adjuvant arthritis is reduced by azathioprine.

The mechanisms whereby azathioprine affects autoimmune diseases are not known. Azathioprine is immunosuppressive, delayed hypersensitivity and cellular cytotoxicity tests being suppressed to a greater degree than are antibody responses. In the rat model of adjuvant arthritis, azathioprine has been shown to inhibit the lymph node hyperplasia, which precedes the onset of the signs of the disease. Both the immunosuppressive and therapeutic effects in animal models are dose-related. Azathioprine is considered a slow-acting drug and effects may persist after the drug has been discontinued.

➤*Pharmacokinetics:* Azathioprine is well absorbed following oral administration. Maximum serum radioactivity occurs at 1 to 2 hours after oral ^{35}S-azathioprine and decays with a half-life of 5 hours. This is not an estimate of the half-life of azathioprine itself, but is the decay rate for all ^{35}S-containing metabolites of the drug. Because of extensive metabolism, only a fraction of the radioactivity is present as azathioprine. Usual doses produce blood levels of azathioprine, and of mercaptopurine derived from it, which are low (less than 1 mcg/mL). Blood levels are of little predictive value for therapy since the magnitude and duration of clinical effects correlate with thiopurine nucleotide levels in tissues rather than with plasma drug levels. Azathioprine and mercaptopurine are moderately bound to serum proteins (30%) and are partially dialyzable.

Azathioprine is cleaved in vivo to mercaptopurine. Both compounds are rapidly eliminated from blood and are oxidized or methylated in erythrocytes and liver; no azathioprine or mercaptopurine is detectable in urine after 8 hours. Conversion to inactive 6-thiouric acid by xanthine oxidase is an important degradative pathway, and the inhibition of this pathway in patients receiving allopurinol is the basis for the azathioprine dosage reduction required in these patients. Patients receiving azathioprine and allopurinol concomitantly should have a dose reduction of azathioprine, to approximately ⅓ to ¼ the usual dose. Proportions of metabolites are different in individual patients, and this presumably accounts for variable magnitude and duration of drug effects. Renal clearance is probably not important in predicting biological effectiveness or toxicities, although dose reduction is practiced in patients with poor renal function.

Contraindications

Hypersensitivity to the drug.

Treating rheumatoid arthritis in pregnant women.

Patients with rheumatoid arthritis previously treated with alkylating agents (cyclophosphamide, chlorambucil, melphalan, or others) may have a prohibitive risk of neoplasia if treated with azathioprine.

Warnings

➤*Hematologic effects:* Severe leukopenia or thrombocytopenia may occur in patients on azathioprine. Macrocytic anemia and severe bone marrow depression may also occur. Hematologic toxicities are dose-related and may be more severe in renal transplant patients whose homograft is undergoing rejection. It is suggested that patients on azathioprine have complete blood counts, including platelet counts, weekly during the first month, twice monthly for the second and third months of treatment, then monthly or more frequently if dosage alterations or other therapy changes are necessary. Delayed hematologic suppression may occur. Prompt reduction in dosage or temporary withdrawal of the drug may be necessary if there is a rapid fall in or persistently low leukocyte count, or other evidence of bone marrow depression. Leukopenia does not correlate with therapeutic effect; therefore the dose should not be increased intentionally to lower the white blood cell count.

➤*Serious infections:* Serious infections are a constant hazard for patients receiving chronic immunosuppression, especially for homograft recipients. Fungal, viral, bacterial, and protozoal infections may be fatal and should be treated vigorously. Reduction of azathioprine dosage or use of other drugs should be considered.

➤*Carcinogenesis:* Azathioprine is carcinogenic in animals, and may increase the patient's risk of neoplasia. Renal transplant patients are known to have an increased risk of malignancy, predominantly skin cancer and reticulum cell or lymphomatous tumors. The risk of post-transplant lymphomas may be increased in patients who receive aggressive treatment with immunosuppressive drugs. The degree of immunosuppression is determined, not only by the immunosuppressive regimen, but also by a number of other patient factors. The number of immunosuppressive agents may not necessarily increase the risk of post-transplant lymphomas. However, transplant patients who receive multiple immunosuppressive agents may be at risk for over-immunosuppression; therefore, immunosuppressive drug therapy should be maintained at the lowest effective levels. Information is available on the spontaneous neoplasia risk in rheumatoid arthritis, and on neoplasia following immunosuppressive therapy of other autoimmune diseases. It has not been possible to define the precise risk of neoplasia due to azathioprine. The data suggest the risk may be elevated in patients with rheumatoid arthritis, though lower than for renal transplant patients. However, acute myelogenous leukemia as well as solid tumors have been reported in patients with rheumatoid arthritis who have received azathioprine. Data on neoplasia in patients receiving azathioprine can be found under Adverse Reactions.

➤*Fertility impairment:* Azathioprine has been reported to cause temporary depression in spermatogenesis and reduction in sperm viability and sperm count in mice at doses 10 times the human therapeutic dose; a reduced percentage of fertile matings occurred when animals received 5 mg/kg.

➤*Pregnancy:* *Category D.* Azathioprine can cause fetal harm when administered to a pregnant woman. Azathioprine should not be given during pregnancy without careful weighing of risk versus benefit. Whenever possible, use of azathioprine in pregnant patients should be avoided. This drug should not be used for treating rheumatoid arthritis in pregnant women.

AZATHIOPRINE — ORAL

Azathioprine is teratogenic in rabbits and mice when given in doses equivalent to the human dose (5 mg/kg daily). Abnormalities included skeletal malformations and visceral anomalies.

Limited immunologic and other abnormalities have occurred in a few infants born of renal allograft recipients on azathioprine, in a detailed case report, documented lymphopenia, diminished IgG and IgM levels, CMV infection, and a decreased thymic shadow were noted in an infant born to a mother receiving 150 mg azathioprine and 30 mg prednisone daily throughout pregnancy. At 10 weeks most features were normalized. DeWitte et al reported pancytoponia and severe immune deficiency in a preterm infant whose mother received 125 mg azathioprine and 12.5 mg prednisone daily. There have been 2 published reports of abnormal physical findings. Williamson and Karp described an infant born with preaxial polydactyly whose mother received azathioprine 200 mg daily and prednisone 20 mg every other day during pregnancy. Tallent et al described an infant with a large myelomeningocele in the upper lumbar region, bilateral dislocated hips, and bilateral talipes equinovarus. The father was on long-term azathioprine therapy.

Benefit versus risk must be weighed carefully before use of azathioprine in patients of reproductive potential. There are no adequate and well-controlled studies in pregnant women. If this drug is used during pregnancy or if the patient becomes pregnant while taking this drug, the patient should be apprised of the potential hazard to the fetus. Women of childbearing age should be advised to avoid becoming pregnant.

➤*Lactation:* The use of azathioprine in nursing mothers is not recommended. Azathioprine or its metabolites are transferred at low levels, both transplacentally and in breast milk. Because of the potential for tumorigenicity shown for azathioprine, a decision should be made whether to discontinue nursing or discontinue the drug, taking into account the importance of the drug to the mother.

➤*Children:* Safety and efficacy of azathioprine in children have not been established.

Precautions

➤*GI effects:* A GI hypersensitivity reaction characterized by severe nausea and vomiting has been reported. These symptoms may also be accompanied by diarrhea, rash, fever, malaise, myalgias, elevations in liver enzymes, and occasionally, hypotension. Symptoms of gastrointestinal toxicity most often develop within the first several weeks of therapy with azathioprine and are reversible upon discontinuation of the drug. The reaction can recur within hours after rechallenge with a single dose of azathioprine.

Drug Interactions

➤*Other agents affecting myeloposis:* Drugs that may affect leukocyte production, including cotrimoxazole, may lead to exaggerated leukopenia, especially in renal transplant recipients.

Azathioprine Drug Interactions

Precipitant drug	Object drug*		Description
ACE inhibitors	Azathioprine	↑	Concurrent use may induce severe leukopenia.
Allopurinol	Azathioprine	↑	Allopurinol may increase the pharmacologic and toxic effects of azathioprine. Patients receiving azathioprine and allopurinol concomitantly should have a dose reduction of azathioprine, to approximately ⅓ to ¼ the usual dose.
Methotrexate	Azathioprine	↑	Plasma levels of the 6-MP metabolite may be increased.
Azathioprine	Anticoagulants	↓	Azathioprine may decrease the action of the anticoagulants.
Azathioprine	Cyclosporine	↓	Cyclosporine plasma levels may be decreased.
Azathioprine	Nondepolarizing neuromuscular blockers	↓	Pharmacologic actions of the neuromuscular blockers may be decreased or reversed.

* ↑ = Object drug increased. ↓ = Object drug decreased.

Adverse Reactions

The principal and potentially serious toxic effects of azathioprine are hematologic and gastrointestinal. The risks of secondary infection and neoplasia are also significant (see Warnings). The frequency and severity of adverse reactions depend on the dose and duration of azathioprine as well as on the patient's underlying disease or concomitant therapies. The incidence of hematologic toxicities and neoplasia encountered in groups of renal homograft recipients is significantly higher than that in studies employing azathioprine for rheumatoid arthritis. The relative incidences in clinical studies are summarized below:

Toxicity	Renal homograft	Rheumatoid arthritis
Leukopenia (any degree)	> 50%	28%
< 2500 cells/mm^3	18%	5.3%
Infections	20%	< 1%
Neoplasia		*
Lymphoma	0.5%	
Others	2.8%	

* Data on the rate and risk of neoplasia among persons with rheumatoid arthritis are limited. The incidence of lymphoproliferative disease in patients with rheumatoid arthritis appears to be significantly higher than that in the general population. In 1 completed study, the rate of lymphoproliferative disease in RA patients receiving higher than recommended doses of azathioprine (5 mg/kg per day) was 1.8 cases per 1000 patient-years of follow-up, compared with 0.8 cases per 1000 patient-years of follow-up in those not receiving azathioprine. However, the proportion of the increased risk attributable to the azathioprine dosage or to other therapies (ie, alkylating agents) received by patients treated with azathioprine cannot be determined.

➤*GI:* Nausea and vomiting may occur within the first few months of therapy with azathioprine, and occurred in ≈12% of 676 rheumatoid arthritis patients. The frequency of gastric disturbance often can be reduced by administration of the drug in divided doses or after meals. However, in some patients, nausea and vomiting may be severe and may be accompanied by symptoms such as diarrhea, fever, malaise, and myalgias (see Precautions). Vomiting with abdominal pain may occur rarely with a hypersensitivity pancreatitis. Hepatotoxicity manifest by elevation of serum alkaline phosphatase, bilirubin, or serum transaminases is known to occur following azathioprine use, primarily in allograft recipients. Hepatotoxicity has been uncommon (< 1%) in rheumatoid arthritis patients. Hepatotoxicity following transplantation most often occurs within 5 months of transplantation and is generally reversible after interruption of azathioprine. A rare, but life-threatening hepatic veno-occlusive disease associated with chronic administration of azathioprine has been described in transplant patients and in 1 patient receiving azathioprine for panuveitis. Periodic measurement of serum transaminases, alkaline phosphatase, and bilirubin is indicated for early detection of hepatotoxicity. If hepatic veno-occlusive disease is clinically suspected, azathioprine should be permanently withdrawn.

➤*Hematologic:* Leukopenia or thrombocytopenia are dose-dependent and may occur late in the course of therapy with azathioprine. Dose reduction or temporary withdrawal allows reversal of these toxicities. Infection may occur as a secondary manifestation of bone marrow suppression or leukopenia, but the incidence of infection in renal homotransplantation is 30 to 60 times that in rheumatoid arthritis. Macrocytic anemia or bleeding have been reported.

There are rare individuals with an inherited deficiency of the enzyme thiopurine methyltransferase (TPMT) who may be unusually sensitive to the myelosuppressive effect of azathioprine and prone to developing rapid bone marrow suppression following the initiation of treatment with azathioprine.

➤*Miscellaneous:* Additional side effects of low frequency have been reported. Those include skin rashes, alopecia, fever, arthralgias, diarrhea, steatorrhea, negative nitrogen balance, and reversible interstitial pneumonitis.

Overdosage

➤*Symptoms:* The oral LD_{50}s for single doses of azathioprine in mice and rats are 2500 mg/kg and 400 mg/kg, respectively. Very large doses of this antimetabolite may lead to marrow hypoplasia, bleeding, infection, and death. About 30% of azathioprine is bound to serum proteins, but ≈ 45% is removed during an 8 hour hemodialysis. A single case has been reported of a renal transplant patient who ingested a single dose of 7500 mg azathioprine. The immediate toxic reactions were nausea, vomiting, and diarrhea, followed by mild leukopenia and mild abnormalities in liver function. The white blood cell count, AST, and bilirubin returned to normal 6 days after the overdose.

Patient Information

Patients being started on azathioprine should be informed of the necessity of periodic blood counts while they are receiving the drug and should be encouraged to report any unusual bleeding or bruising to their physician. They should be informed of the danger of infection while receiving azathioprine and asked to report signs and symptoms of infection to their physician. Careful dosage instructions should be given to the patient, especially when azathioprine is being administered in the presence of impaired renal function or concomitantly with allopurinol (see Administration and Dosage and Drug Interactions). Patients should be advised of the potential risks of the use of azathioprine during pregnancy and during the nursing period. The increased risk of neoplasia following therapy with azathioprine should be explained to the patient.

AZATHIOPRINE — INJECTION

WARNING

Chronic immunosuppression with this purine antimetabolite increases risk of neoplasia in humans. Physicians using this drug should be very familiar with this risk as well as with the mutagenic potential to both men and women and with possible hematologic toxicities. (See Warnings.)

Indications

➤*Renal homotransplantation:* Adjunct for the prevention of rejection in renal homotransplantation. Experience with over 16,000 transplants shows a 5 year patient survival of 35% to 55%, but this is dependent on donor, match for HLA antigens, anti-donor or anti-B-cell alicantigen antibody, and other variables. The effect of azathioprine on these variables has not been tested in controlled trials.

➤*Rheumatoid arthritis:* Azathioprine is indicated only in adult patients meeting criteria for classic or definite rheumatoid arthritis as specified by the American Rheumatism Association. Azathioprine should be restricted to patients with severe, active and erosive disease not responsive to conventional management including rest, aspirin, or other nonsteroidal drugs, or to agents in the class of which gold is an example. Rest, physiotherapy, and salicylates should be continued while azathioprine is given, but it may be possible to reduce the dose of corticosteroids in patients on azathioprine. The combined use of azathioprine with gold, antimalarials, or penicillamine has not been studied for either added benefit or unexpected adverse effects. The use of azathioprine with these agents cannot be recommended.

Administration and Dosage

➤*Approved by the FDA:* March 31, 1995.

➤*Renal homotransplantation:* The dose of azathioprine required to prevent rejection and minimize toxicity will vary with individual patients; this necessitates careful management. The initial dose is usually 3 to 5 mg/kg daily, beginning at the time of transplant. Azathioprine is usually given as a single daily dose on the day of, and in a minority of cases 1 to 3 days before, transplantation. Azathioprine is often initiated with the intravenous administration of the sodium salt, with subsequent use of tablets (at the same dose level) after the postoperative period. Intravenous administration of the sodium salt is indicated only in patients unable to tolerate oral medications. Dose reduction to maintenance levels of 1 to 3 mg/kg daily is usually possible. The dose of azathioprine should not be increased to toxic levels because of threatened rejection. Discontinuation may be necessary for severe hematologic or other toxicity, even if rejection of the homograft may be a consequence of drug withdrawal.

➤*Rheumatoid arthritis:* Azathioprine is usually given on a daily basis. The initial dose should be ≈ 1 mg/kg (50 to 100 mg) given as a single dose or on a twice-daily schedule. The dose may be increased, beginning at 6 to 8 weeks and thereafter by steps at 4 week intervals, if there are no serious toxicities and if initial response is unsatisfactory. Dose increments should be 0.5 mg/kg daily, up to a maximum dose of 2.5 mg/kg per day. Therapeutic response occurs after several weeks of treatment, usually 6 to 8; an adequate trial should be a minimum of 12 weeks. Patients not improved after 12 weeks can be considered refractory. Azathioprine may be continued long-term in patients with clinical response, but patients should be monitored carefully, and gradual dosage reduction should be attempted to reduce risk of toxicities.

Maintenance therapy should be at the lowest effective dose, and the dose given can be lowered decrementally with changes of 0.5 mg/kg or ≈ 25 mg daily every 4 weeks while other therapy is kept constant. The optimum duration of maintenance azathioprine has not been determined. Azathioprine can be discontinued abruptly, but delayed effects are possible.

➤*Use in renal dysfunction:* Relatively oliguric patients, especially those with tubular necrosis in the immediate postcadaveric transplant period, may have delayed clearance of azathioprine or its metabolites, may be particularly sensitive to this drug, and are usually given lower doses.

➤*Parenteral administration:* Add 10 mL of Sterile Water for Injection, and swirl until a clear solution results. This solution, equivalent to 100 mg azathioprine, is for intravenous use only; it has a pH of ≈ 9.6, and it should be used within 24 hours. Further dilution into sterile saline or dextrose is usually made for infusion; the final volume depends on time for the infusion, usually 30 to 60 minutes, but as short as 5 minutes and as long as 8 hours for the daily dose.

➤*Storage / Stability:* Store at 15°C to 25°C (59°F to 77°F) in a dry place and protect from light.

Actions

➤*Pharmacology:*

Homograft survival – Summary information from transplant centers and registries indicates relatively universal use of azathioprine with or without other immunosuppressive agents. Although the use of azathioprine for inhibition of renal homograft rejection is well established, the mechanism(s) for this action are somewhat obscure. The drug suppresses hypersensitivities of the cell-mediated type and causes variable alterations in antibody production. Suppression of T-cell effects, including ablation of T-cell suppression, is dependent on the temporal relationship to antigenic stimulus or engraftment. This agent has little effect on established graft rejections or secondary responses.

Alterations in specific immune responses or immunologic functions in transplant recipients are difficult to relate specifically to immunosuppression by azathioprine. These patients have subnormal responses to vaccines, low numbers of T-cells, and abnormal phagocytosis by peripheral blood cells, but their mitogenic responses, serum immunoglobulins, and secondary antibody responses are usually normal.

Immunoinflammatory response – Azathioprine suppresses disease manifestations as well as underlying pathology in animal models of autoimmune disease. For example, the severity of adjuvant arthritis is reduced by azathioprine.

The mechanisms whereby azathioprine affects autoimmune diseases are not known. Azathioprine is immunosuppressive, delayed hypersensitivity and cellular cytotoxicity tests being suppressed to a greater degree than are antibody responses. In the rat model of adjuvant arthritis, azathioprine has been shown to inhibit the lymph node hyperplasia which precedes the onset of the signs of the disease. Both the immunosuppressive and therapeutic effects in animal models are dose-related. Azathioprine is considered a slow-acting drug and effects may persist after the drug has been discontinued.

➤*Pharmacokinetics:*

Metabolism – Usual doses produce blood levels of azathioprine, and of mercaptopurine derived from it, which are low (< 1 mcg/mL). Blood levels are of little predictive value for therapy since the magnitude and duration of clinical effects correlate with thiopurine nucleotide levels in tissues rather than with plasma drug levels. Azathioprine and mercaptopurine are moderately bound to serum proteins (30%) and are partially dialyzable.

Azathioprine is cleaved in vivo to mercaptopurine. Both compounds are rapidly eliminated from blood and are oxidized or methylated in erythrocytes and liver; no azathioprine or mercaptopurine is detectable in urine after 8 hours. Conversion to inactive 6-thiouric acid by xanthine oxidase is an important degradative pathway, and the inhibition of this pathway in patients receiving allopurinol is the basis for the azathioprine dosage reduction required in these patients (see Drug Interactions). Proportions of metabolites are different in individual patients, and this presumably accounts for variable magnitude and duration of drug effects. Renal clearance is probably not important in predicting biological effectiveness or toxicities, although dose reduction is practiced in patients with poor renal function.

Contraindications

Hypersensitivity to the drug.

Treating rheumatoid arthritis in pregnant women.

Patients with rheumatoid arthritis previously treated with alkylating agents (cyclophosphamide, chlorambucil, melphalan, or others) may have a prohibitive risk of neoplasia if treated with azathioprine.

Warnings

➤*Hematologic effects:* Severe leukopenia or thrombocytopenia may occur in patients on azathioprine. Macrocytic anemia and severe bone marrow depression may also occur. Hematologic toxicities are dose-related and may be more severe in renal transplant patients whose homograft is undergoing rejection. It is suggested that patients on azathioprine have complete blood counts, including platelet counts, weekly during the first month, twice monthly for the second and third months of treatment, then monthly or more frequently if dosage alterations or other therapy changes are necessary. Delayed hematologic suppression may occur. Prompt reduction in dosage or temporary withdrawal of the drug may be necessary if there is a rapid fall in or persistently low leukocyte count, or other evidence of bone marrow depression. Leukopenia does not correlate with therapeutic effect; therefore the dose should not be increased intentionally to lower the white blood cell count.

➤*Serious infections:* Serious infections are a constant hazard for patients receiving chronic immunosuppression, especially for homograft recipients. Fungal viral, bacterial, and protozoal infections may be fatal and should be treated vigorously. Reduction of azathioprine dosage or use of other drugs should be considered.

➤*Carcinogenesis:* Azathioprine is carcinogenic in animals, and may increase the patient's risk of neoplasia. Renal transplant patients are known to have an increased risk of malignancy, predominantly skin cancer and reticulum cell or lymphomatous tumors. The risk of post-transplant lymphomas may be increased in patients who receive aggressive treatment with immunosuppressive drugs. The degree of immunosuppression is determined not only by the immunosuppressive regimen, but also by a number of other patient factors. The number of immunosuppressive agents may not necessarily increase the risk of post-transplant lymphomas. However, transplant patients who receive multiple immunosuppressive agents may be at risk for over-immunosuppression; therefore, immunosuppressive drug therapy should be maintained at the lowest effective levels. Information is available on the spontaneous neoplasia risk in rheumatoid arthritis, and on neoplasia following immunosuppressive therapy of other autoimmune diseases. It has not been possible to define the precise risk of neoplasia due to azathioprine. The data suggest the risk may be elevated in patients with rheumatoid arthritis, though lower than for renal transplant patients. However, acute myelogenous leukemia as well as solid tumors have been reported in patients with rheumatoid arthritis who have received azathioprine. Data on neoplasia in patients receiving azathioprine can be found under Adverse Reactions.

➤*Fertility impairment:* Azathioprine has been reported to cause temporary depression in spermatogenesis and reduction in sperm viability and sperm count in mice at doses 10 times the human therapeutic dose; a reduced percentage of fertile matings occurred when animals received 5 mg/kg.

AZATHIOPRINE — INJECTION

➤*Pregnancy: Category D.* Azathioprine can cause fetal harm when administered to a pregnant woman. Azathioprine should not be given during pregnancy without careful weighing of risk versus benefit. Whenever possible, use of azathioprine in pregnant patients should be avoided. This drug should not be used for treating rheumatoid arthritis in pregnant women.

Azathioprine is teratogenic in rabbits and mice when given in doses equivalent to the human dose (5 mg/kg daily). Abnormalities included skeletal malformations and visceral anomalies.

Limited immunologic and other abnormalities have occurred in a few infants born of renal allograft recipients on azathioprine, in a detailed case report, documented lymphopenia, diminished IgG and IgM levels, CMV infection, and a decreased thymic shadow were noted in an infant born to a mother receiving 150 mg azathioprine and 30 mg prednisone daily throughout pregnancy. At 10 weeks most features were normalized. DeWitte et al reported pancytopenia and severe immune deficiency in a preterm infant whose mother received 125 mg azathioprine and 12.5 mg prednisone daily. There have been 2 published reports of abnormal physical findings. Williamson and Karp described an infant born with preaxial polydactyly whose mother received azathioprine 200 mg daily and prednisone 20 mg every other day during pregnancy. Tallent et al described an infant with a large myelomeningocele in the upper lumbar region, bilateral dislocated hips, and bilateral talipes equinovarus. The father was on long-term azathioprine therapy.

Benefit vs risk must be weighed carefully before use of azathioprine in patients of reproductive potential. There are no adequate and well-controlled studies in pregnant women. If this drug is used during pregnancy or if the patient becomes pregnant while taking this drug, the patient should be apprised of the potential hazard to the fetus. Women of childbearing age should be advised to avoid becoming pregnant.

➤*Lactation:* The use of azathioprine in nursing mothers is not recommended. Azathioprine or its metabolites are transferred at low levels, both transplacentally and in breast milk. Because of the potential for tumorigenicity shown for azathioprine, a decision should be made whether to discontinue nursing or discontinue the drug, taking into account the importance of the drug to the mother.

➤*Children:* Safety and efficacy of azathioprine in children have not been established.

Precautions

➤*GI toxicity:* A gastrointestinal hypersensitivity reaction characterized by severe nausea and vomiting has been reported. These symptoms may also be accompanied by diarrhea, rash, fever, malaise, myalgias, elevations in liver enzymes, and occasionally, hypotension. Symptoms of GI toxicity most often develop within the first several weeks of therapy with azathioprine and are reversible upon discontinuation of the drug. The reaction can recur within hours after rechallenge with a single dose of azathioprine.

Drug Interactions

➤*Other agents affecting myeloposis:* Drugs that may affect leukocyte production, including cotrimoxazole, may lead to exaggerated leukopenia, especially in renal transplant recipients.

Azathioprine Drug Interactions

Precipitant drug	Object drug*		Description
ACE inhibitors	Azathioprine	⬆	Concurrent use may induce severe leukopenia.
Allopurinol	Azathioprine	⬆	Allopurinol may increase the pharmacologic and toxic effects of azathioprine. Patients receiving azathioprine and allopurinol concomitantly should have a dose reduction of azathioprine, to ≈ ¼ to ⅓ the usual dose.
Methotrexate	Azathioprine	⬆	Plasma levels of the 6-MP metabolite may be increased.
Azathioprine	Anticoagulants	⬇	Azathioprine may decrease the action of the anticoagulants.
Azathioprine	Cyclosporine	⬇	Cyclosporine plasma levels may be decreased.
Azathioprine	Nondepolarizing neuromuscular blockers	⬇	Pharmacologic actions of the neuromuscular blockers may be decreased or reversed.

* ⬆ = Object drug increased. ⬇ = Object drug decreased.

Adverse Reactions

The principal and potentially serious toxic effects of azathioprine are hematologic and GI. The risks of secondary infection and neoplasia are also significant (see Warnings). The frequency and severity of adverse reactions depend on the dose and duration of azathioprine and on the patient's underlying disease or concomitant therapies. The incidence of hematologic toxicities and neoplasia encountered in groups of renal homograft recipients is significantly higher than that in studies employing azathioprine for rheumatoid arthritis. The relative incidences in clinical studies are summarized below.

Toxicity	Renal homograft	Rheumatoid arthritis
Leukopenia (any degree)	> 50%	28%
< 2500/mm³	16%	5.3%
Infections	20%	< 1%
Neoplasia		*
Lymphoma	0.5%	
Others	2.8%	

* Data on the rate and risk of neoplasm among persons with rheumatoid arthritis treated with azathioprine are limited. The incidence of lymphoproliferative disease in patients with RA appears to be significantly higher than that in the general population. In one completed study, the rate of lymphoproliferative disease in RA patients receiving higher than recommended doses of azathioprine (5 mg/kg/day) was 1.8 cases per 1000 patient-years of follow-up, compared to 0.8 cases per 1000 patient-years of follow-up in those not receiving azathioprine. However, the proportion of the increased risk attributable to the azathioprine dosage or to other therapies (ie, alkylating agents) received by patients treated with azathioprine cannot be determined.

➤*GI:* Nausea and vomiting may occur within the first few months of therapy with azathioprine, and occurred in ≈ 12% of 676 rheumatoid arthritis patients. The frequency of gastric disturbance often can be reduced by administration of the drug in divided doses or after meals. However, in some patients, nausea and vomiting may be severe and may be accompanied by symptoms such as diarrhea, fever, malaise, and myalgias (see Precautions). Vomiting with abdominal pain may occur rarely with a hypersensitivity pancreatitis. Hepatotoxicity manifest by elevation of serum alkaline phosphatase, bilirubin, or serum transaminases is known to occur following azathioprine use, primarily in allograft recipients. Hepatotoxicity has been uncommon (< 1%) in rheumatoid arthritis patients. Hepatotoxicity following transplantation most often occurs within 5 months of transplantation and is generally reversible after interruption of azathioprine. A rare, but life-threatening hepatic veno-occlusive disease associated with chronic administration of azathioprine has been described in transplant patients and in one patient receiving azathioprine for panuveitis. Periodic measurement of serum transaminases, alkaline phosphatase, and bilirubin is indicated for early detection of hepatotoxicity. If hepatic veno-occlusive disease is clinically suspected, azathioprine should be permanently withdrawn.

➤*Hematologic:* Leukopenia or thrombocytopenia are dose-dependent and may occur late in the course of therapy with azathioprine. Dose reduction or temporary withdrawal allows reversal of these toxicities. Infection may occur as a secondary manifestation of bone marrow suppression or leukopenia, but the incidence of infection in renal homotransplantation is 30 to 60 times that in rheumatoid arthritis. Macrocytic anemia or bleeding have been reported.

There are rare individuals with an inherited deficiency of the enzyme thiopurine methyltransferase (TPMT) who may be unusually sensitive to the myelosuppressive effect of azathioprine and prone to developing rapid bone marrow suppression following the initiation of treatment with azathioprine.

➤*Miscellaneous:* Additional side effects of low frequency have been reported. Those include skin rashes, alopecia, fever, arthralgias, diarrhea, steatorrhea, negative nitrogen balance, and reversible interstitial pneumonitis.

Overdosage

➤*Symptoms:* The oral LD_{50}s for single doses of azathioprine in mice and rats are 2500 mg/kg and 400 mg/kg, respectively. Very large doses of this antimetabolite may lead to marrow hypoplasia, bleeding, infection, and death. About 30% of azathioprine is bound to serum proteins, but ≈ 45% is removed during an 8 hour hemodialysis. A single case has been reported of a renal transplant patient who ingested a single dose of 7500 mg azathioprine. The immediate toxic reactions were nausea, vomiting, and diarrhea, followed by mild leukopenia and mild abnormalities in liver function. The white blood cell count, AST, and bilirubin returned to normal 6 days after the overdose.

Patient Information

Patients being started on azathioprine should be informed of the necessity of periodic blood counts while they are receiving the drug and should be encouraged to report any unusual bleeding or bruising to their physician. They should be informed of the danger of infection while receiving azathioprine and asked to report signs and symptoms of infection to their physician. Careful dosage instructions should be given to the patient, especially when azathioprine is being administered in the presence of impaired renal function or concomitantly with allopurinol (see Administration and Dosage and Drug Interactions). Patients should be advised of the potential risks of the use of azathioprine during pregnancy and during the nursing period. The increased risk of neoplasia following therapy with azathioprine should be explained to the patient.

BASILIXIMAB

Rx	**Simulect** (Novartis)	**Powder for injection, lyophilized:** 20 mg	Preservative free. Sucrose, mannitol, potassium phosphate, sodium chloride. In single-use vials.

BASILIXIMAB — INJECTION

WARNING

Only physicians experienced in immunosuppression therapy and management of organ transplantation patients should prescribe basiliximab. The physician responsible for basiliximab administration should have complete information requisite for the follow-up of the patient. Patients receiving the drug should be managed in facilities equipped with adequate laboratory and supportive medical resources.

Indications

➤*Organ rejection:* For the prophylaxis of acute organ rejection in patients receiving renal transplantation when used as part of an immunosuppressive regimen that includes cyclosporine and corticosteroids.

The efficacy of basiliximab for the prophylaxis of acute rejection in recipients of other solid organ allografts has not been demonstrated.

Administration and Dosage

➤*Approved by the FDA:* May 12, 1998.

➤*Administration:* Basiliximab is used as part of an immunosuppressive regimen that includes cyclosporine (modified) and corticosteroids. Basiliximab is for central or peripheral intravenous administration only. Reconstituted basiliximab should be given either as a bolus injection or diluted to a volume of 25 mL (10 mg) vial or 50 mL (20 mg) vial with normal saline or dextrose 5% and administered as an intravenous infusion over 20 to 30 minutes. Bolus administration may be associated with nausea, vomiting, and local reactions, including pain.

➤*Re-exposure:* Basiliximab should only be administered once it has been determined that the patient will receive the graft and concomitant immunosuppression. Patients previously administered basiliximab should only be re-exposed to a subsequent course of therapy with extreme caution.

➤*Incompatibilities:* No incompatibility between basiliximab and polyvinyl chloride bags or infusion sets has been observed. No data are available on the compatibility of basiliximab with other intravenous substances. Other drug substances should not be added or infused simultaneously through the same intravenous line.

➤*Adult:* In adult patients, the recommended regimen is 2 doses of 20 mg each. The first 20 mg dose should be given within 2 hours prior to transplantation surgery. The second 20 mg dose should be given 4 days after transplantation. The second dose should be withheld if complications such as severe hypersensitivity reactions to basiliximab or graft loss occur.

➤*Children:* In pediatric patients weighing less than 35 kg, the recommended regimen is 2 doses of 10 mg each. In pediatric patients weighing 35 kg or more, the recommended regimen is 2 doses of 20 mg each. The first dose should be given within 2 hours prior to transplantation surgery. The recommended second dose should be given 4 days after transplantation. The second dose should be withheld if complications such as severe hypersensitivity reactions to basiliximab or graft loss occur.

➤*Reconstitution of 10 mg basiliximab vial:* To prepare the reconstituted solution, add 2.5 mL of Sterile Water for Injection, using aseptic technique, to the vial containing the basiliximab powder. Shake the vial gently to dissolve the powder.

The reconstituted solution is isotonic and may be given either as a bolus injection or diluted to a volume of 25 mL with normal saline or dextrose 5% for infusion. When mixing the solution, gently invert the bag in order to avoid foaming; do not shake.

➤*Reconstitution of 20 mg basiliximab vial:* To prepare the reconstituted solution, add 5 mL of Sterile Water for Injection, using aseptic technique, to the vial containing the basiliximab powder. Shake the vial gently to dissolve the powder.

The reconstituted solution is isotonic and may be given either as a bolus injection or diluted to a volume of 50 mL with normal saline or dextrose 5% for infusion. When mixing the solution, gently invert the bag in order to avoid foaming; do not shake.

➤*Storage/Stability:* Store lyophilized basiliximab under refrigerated conditions (2° to 8°C; 36° to 46°F). Do not use beyond the expiration date stamped on the vial.

Care must be taken to ensure sterility of the prepared solution because the drug product does not contain any antimicrobial preservatives or bacteriostatic agents.

It is recommended that after reconstitution, the solution should be used immediately. If not used immediately, it can be stored at 2° to 8°C (35.6° to 46.4°F) for 24 hours or at room temperature for 4 hours. Discard the reconstituted solution if not used within 24 hours.

Actions

➤*Pharmacology:* Basiliximab functions as an IL-2 receptor antagonist by binding with high affinity ($K_a = 1 \bullet 10^{10}\ M^{-1}$) to the alpha chain of the high affinity IL-2 receptor complex and inhibiting IL-2 binding. Basiliximab is specifically targeted against IL-2Rα, which is selectively expressed on the surface of activated T-lymphocytes. This specific high affinity binding of basiliximab to IL-2Rα competitively inhibits IL-2-mediated activation of lymphocytes, a critical pathway in the cellular immune response involved in allograft rejection. While in the circulation, basiliximab impairs the response of the immune system to antigenic challenges. Whether the ability to respond to repeated or ongoing challenges with those antigens returns to normal after basiliximab is cleared is unknown.

Pharmacodynamics – Complete and consistent binding to IL-2Rα in adults is maintained as long as serum basiliximab levels exceed 0.2 mcg/mL. As concentrations fall below this threshold, the IL-2Rα sites are no longer fully bound and the number of T-cells expressing unbound IL-2Rα returns to pretherapy values within 1 to 2 weeks. The relationship between serum concentration and receptor saturation was assessed in 13 pediatric patients and was similar to that characterized in adult renal transplantation patients. In vitro studies using human tissues indicate that basiliximab binds only to lymphocytes.

The duration of clinically relevant IL-2 receptor blockade after the recommended course of basiliximab is not known. When basiliximab was added to a regimen of cyclosporine (modified) and corticosteroids in adult patients, the duration of IL-2Rα saturation was 36 ± 14 days (mean ± SD), similar to that observed in pediatric patients (36 ± 14 days). When basiliximab was added to a triple therapy regimen consisting of cyclosporine (modified), corticosteroids, and azathioprine in adults, the duration was 50 ± 20 days and when added to cyclosporine (modified), corticosteroids, and mycophenolate mofetil in adults, the duration was 59 ± 17 days. No significant changes to circulating lymphocyte numbers or cell phenotypes were observed by flow cytometry.

➤*Pharmacokinetics:*

Adults – Single-dose and multiple-dose pharmacokinetic studies have been conducted in patients undergoing first kidney transplantation. Cumulative doses ranged from 15 mg up to 150 mg. Peak mean ± SD serum concentration following intravenous infusion of 20 mg over 30 minutes is 7.1 ± 5.1 mg/L. There is a dose-proportional increase in C_{max} and AUC up to the highest tested single dose of 60 mg. The volume of distribution at steady state is 8.6 ± 4.1 L. The extent and degree of distribution to various body compartments have not been fully studied. The terminal half-life is 7.2 ± 3.2 days. Total body clearance is 41 ± 19 mL/hr. No clinically relevant influence of body weight or gender on distribution volume or clearance has been observed in adult patients. Elimination half-life was not influenced by age (20 to 69 years), gender, or race.

Children – The pharmacokinetics of basiliximab have been assessed in 39 pediatric patients undergoing renal transplantation. In infants and children (1 to 11 years of age, n = 25), the distribution volume and clearance were reduced by about 50% compared to adult renal transplantation patients. The volume of distribution at steady state was 4.8 ± 2.1 L, half-life was 9.5 ± 4.5 days and clearance was 17 ± 6 mL/hr. Disposition parameters were not influenced to a clinically relevant extent by age (1 to 11 years of age), body weight (9 to 37 kg) or body surface area (0.44 to 1.2 m^2) in this age group. In adolescents (12 to 16 years of age, n = 14), disposition was similar to that in adult renal transplantation patients. The volume of distribution at steady state was 7.8 ± 5.1 L, half-life was 9.1 ± 3.9 days and clearance was 31 ± 19 mL/hr.

Contraindications

Basiliximab is contraindicated in patients with known hypersensitivity to basiliximab or any other component of the formulation.

Warnings

See the Warning box for more information.

➤*Opportunistic infections/lymphoproliferative disorders:* While neither the incidence of lymphoproliferative disorders nor of opportunistic infections was higher in basiliximab-treated patients than in placebo-treated patients, patients on immunosuppressive therapy are at increased risk for developing these complications and should be monitored accordingly.

➤*Infectious episodes:* See Adverse Reactions for more information.

➤*Immunogenicity:* Of renal transplantation patients treated with basiliximab and tested for anti-idiotype antibodies, 4 out of 339 developed an anti-idiotype antibody response, with no deleterious clinical effect upon the patient. In none of these cases was there evidence that the presence of anti-idiotype antibody accelerated basiliximab clearance or decreased the period of receptor saturation. In study 2, the incidence of human anti-murine antibody (HAMA) in renal transplantation patients treated with basiliximab was 2 out of 138 in patients not exposed to muromonab-CD3 and 4 out of 34 in patients who subsequently received muromonab-CD3. The available clinical data on the use of muromonab-CD3 in patients previously treated with basiliximab suggest that subsequent use of muromonab-CD3 or other murine anti-lymphocytic antibody preparations is not precluded.

These data reflect the percentage of patients whose test results were considered positive for antibodies to basiliximab in an ELISA assay, and are highly dependent on the sensitivity and specificity of the assay. Additionally the observed incidence of antibody positivity in an assay may be influenced by several factors including sample handling, concomitant medications, and underlying disease. For these reasons, comparison of the incidence of antibodies to basiliximab with the incidence of antibodies to other products may be misleading.

➤*Hypersensitivity reactions:* Severe acute (onset within 24 hours) hypersensitivity reactions including anaphylaxis have been observed both on initial exposure to basiliximab or following re-exposure after several months. These reactions may include hypotension, tachycardia, cardiac failure, dyspnea, wheezing, bronchospasm, pulmonary edema, respiratory failure, urticaria, rash, pruritus, or sneezing. If a severe hypersensitivity reaction occurs, therapy with basiliximab should be permanently discontinued. Medications for the treatment of severe hypersensitivity reactions including anaphylaxis should be available for immediate use. Patients previously administered basiliximab should only be re-exposed to a subsequent course

BASILIXIMAB — INJECTION

of therapy with extreme caution. The potential risks of such re-administration, specifically those associated with immunosuppression, are not known.

➤*Pregnancy: Category B.* There are no adequate and well-controlled studies in pregnant women.

Because IgG molecules are known to cross the placental barrier, because IL-2 receptor may play an important role in development of the immune system, and because animal reproduction studies are not always predictive of human response, basiliximab should only be used in pregnant women when the potential benefit justifies the potential risk to the fetus. Women of childbearing potential should use effective contraception before beginning basiliximab therapy, during therapy, and for 4 months after completion of basiliximab therapy.

➤*Lactation:* It is not known whether basiliximab is excreted in human milk. Because many drugs including human antibodies are excreted in human milk, and because of the potential for adverse reactions, a decision should be made to discontinue nursing or to discontinue the drug, taking into account the importance of the drug to the mother.

Precautions

➤*Immunogenicity:* See Warnings for more information.

Adverse Reactions

The most frequently reported adverse reactions were gastrointestinal disorders, reported in 69% of basiliximab-treated patients and 67% of placebo-treated patients.

➤*The following adverse reactions occurred in greater than or equal to 10% of basiliximab-treated patients:* The incidence and types of adverse reactions were similar in basiliximab-treated and placebo-treated patients.

Cardiovascular – Hypertension.

CNS – Headache, tremor.

Dermatologic – Acne.

GI – Constipation, nausea, abdominal pain, vomiting, diarrhea, dyspepsia.

GU – Urinary tract infection.

Hematologic – Anemia.

Metabolic/Nutritional – Hyperkalemia, hypokalemia, hyperglycemia, hypercholesterolemia, hypophosphatemia, hyperuricemia.

Psychiatric – Insomnia.

Respiratory – Dyspnea, upper respiratory tract infection.

Miscellaneous – Surgical wound complications, pain, peripheral edema, fever, viral infection.

➤*Adverse reactions, not mentioned above, reported with an incidence of greater than or equal to 3% and less than 10% in patients* : The following adverse reactions, not mentioned above, were reported with an incidence of greater than or equal to 3% and less than 10% in pooled analysis of patients treated with basiliximab in the 4 controlled clinical trials, or in an analysis of the 2 dual-therapy trials:

Cardiovascular – Arrhythmia, atrial fibrillation, tachycardia, vascular disorder, abnormal heart sounds, aggravated hypertension, angina pectoris, cardiac failure, chest pain, hypotension.

CNS – Dizziness, neuropathy, paraesthesia, hypoesthesia.

Dermatologic – Cyst, herpes simplex, herpes zoster, hypertrichosis, pruritus, rash, skin disorder, skin ulceration.

Endocrine – Increased glucocorticoids.

GI – Enlarged abdomen, esophagitis, flatulence, gastrointestinal disorder, gastroenteritis, GI hemorrhage, gum hyperplasia, melena, moniliasis, ulcerative stomatitis.

GU – Albuminuria, bladder disorder, dysuria, frequent micturition, hematuria, increased non-protein nitrogen, oliguria, abnormal renal function, renal tubular necrosis, surgery, ureteral disorder, urinary retention.
Male: Genital edema, impotence.

Hematologic – Hematoma, hemorrhage, purpura, thrombocytopenia, thrombosis. White blood cell: Leucopenia. Red blood cell: Polycythemia

Among these reactions, leukopenia and hypertriglyceridemia occurred more frequently in the 2 triple-therapy studies using azathioprine and mycophenolate mofetil than in the dual-therapy studies.

Metabolic/Nutritional – Acidosis, dehydration, diabetes mellitus, fluid overload, hypercalcemia, hyperlipemia, hypertriglyceridemia, hypocalcemia, hypoglycemia, hypomagnesemia, hypoproteinemia, weight increase.

Musculoskeletal – Arthralgia, arthropathy, back pain, bone fracture, cramps, hernia, myalgia, leg pain.

Psychiatric – Agitation, anxiety, depression.

Respiratory – Bronchitis, bronchospasm, abnormal chest sounds, coughing, pharyngitis, pneumonia, pulmonary disorder, pulmonary edema, rhinitis, sinusitis.

Special senses – Cataract, conjunctivitis, abnormal vision.

Miscellaneous – Accidental trauma, asthenia, chest pain, increased drug level, infection, face edema, fatigue, dependent edema, generalized edema, leg edema, malaise, rigors, sepsis.

➤*Malignancies:* The overall incidence of malignancies among all patients in the controlled studies was not significantly different between the basiliximab- and placebo-treatment groups. Overall, lymphoma/lymphoproliferative disease occurred in 1 out of 590 patients in the basiliximab group compared with 3 out of 594 patients in the placebo group. Other malignancies were reported among 8 out of 590 patients in the basiliximab group compared with 9 out of 594 patients in the placebo group.

➤*Infections:* The overall incidence of cytomegalovirus infection was similar in basiliximab- and placebo-treated patients (15% vs 17%) receiving a dual- or triple-immunosuppression regimen. However, in patients receiving a triple-immunosuppression regimen, the incidence of serious cytomegalovirus infection was higher in basiliximab-treated patients compared to placebo-treated patients (11% vs 5%). The rates of infections, serious infections, and infectious organisms were similar in the basiliximab- and placebo-treatment groups among dual- and triple-therapy treated patients.

➤*Postmarketing experience:* Severe acute hypersensitivity reactions including anaphylaxis characterized by hypotension, tachycardia, cardiac failure, dyspnea, wheezing, bronchospasm, pulmonary edema, respiratory failure, urticaria, rash, pruritus, or sneezing, as well as capillary leak syndrome and cytokine release syndrome, have been reported during postmarketing experience with basiliximab.

Overdosage

A maximum tolerated dose of basiliximab has not been determined in patients. During the course of clinical studies, basiliximab has been administered to adult renal transplantation patients in single doses of up to 60 mg, or in divided doses over 3 to 5 days of up to 120 mg, without any associated serious adverse reactions. There has been 1 spontaneous report of a pediatric renal transplantation patient who received a single 20 mg dose (2.3 mg/kg) without adverse reactions.

CYCLOSPORINE (Cyclosporin A)

Rx	**Gengraf** (Abbott)	**Capsules:** 25 mg	12.8% alcohol, castor oil. (25 mg OR). White, oval. In UD 30s.
		100 mg	12.8% alcohol, castor oil. (100 mg OT). White, oval. In UD 30s.
Rx	**Cyclosporine** (Apotex, Eon Labs, Pliva)	**Capsules, soft gelatin:** 25 mg	Castor oil, sorbitol, alcohol. (0932). Clear, oblong. In UD 30s.
Rx	**Neoral** (Novartis)		11.9% dehydrated alcohol. (Neoral 25 mg). Blue-gray, oval. In UD 30s.
Rx	**Sandimmune** (Novartis)		Sorbitol, ≤ 12.7% dehydrated alcohol. (78/240). Pink, oblong. In UD 30s.
Rx	**Cyclosporine** (Apotex, Eon Labs, Pliva)	100 mg	Castor oil, sorbitol, alcohol. (0933). Clear, oblong. In UD 30s.
Rx	**Neoral** (Novartis)		11.9% dehydrated alcohol. (Neoral 100 mg). Blue-gray, oblong. In UD 30s.
Rx	**Sandimmune** (Novartis)		Sorbitol, ≤ 12.7% dehydrated alcohol. (78/241). Rose, oblong. In UD 30s.
Rx	**Cyclosporine** (Pliva)	**Oral solution:** 100 mg/mL	In 50 mL.
Rx	**Gengraf** (Abbott)		Castor oil. In 50 mL with syringe.
Rx	**Neoral** (Novartis)		11.9% dehydrated alcohol. In 50 mL.
Rx	**Sandimmune** (Novartis)		12.5% alcohol. In 50 mL with syringe.
Rx	**Cyclosporine Injection** (Bedford Labs)	**Injection:** 50 mg/mL	In 5 mL single-use vials.
Rx	**Sandimmune** (Novartis)		650 mg polyoxyethylated castor oil/mL and 32.9% alcohol. In 5 mL amps.

[1] Product tables do not imply bioequivalence (see page xi). Also refer to Bioequivalency (in Administration and Dosage).

CYCLOSPORINE — ORAL

WARNING

Only physicians experienced in the management of systemic immunosuppressive therapy for the indicated disease should prescribe cyclosporine. Patients receiving the drug should be managed in facilities equipped and staffed with adequate laboratory and supportive medical resources. The physician responsible for maintenance therapy should have complete information requisite for the follow-up of the patient.

Administer *Sandimmune* with adrenal corticosteroids but not with other immunosuppressive agents. Increased susceptibility to infection and other possible development of lymphoma may result from immunosuppression.

Neoral and *Gengraf* may increase the susceptibility to infection and the development of neoplasia. In kidney, liver, and heart transplant patients, *Gengraf* and *Neoral* may be administered with other immunosuppressive agents. Increased susceptibility to infection and the possible development of lymphoma and other neoplasms may result from the increase in the degree of immunosuppression in transplant patients.

The absorption of *Sandimmune* during chronic administration was found to be erratic. It is recommended that patients taking *Sandimmune* over a period of time be monitored at repeated intervals to avoid toxicity from high levels and possible organ rejection from low absorption. This is of special importance in liver transplants.

Sandimmune capsules and oral solution have decreased bioavailability in comparison with *Neoral* capsules, *Neoral* oral solution, *Gengraf* capsules, and *Gengraf* oral solution. *Gengraf* and *Neoral* are not bioequivalent to *Sandimmune* and cannot be used interchangeably without physician supervision. For given trough concentrations, cyclosporine exposure will be greater with *Neoral* and *Gengraf* than with *Sandimmune*. If a patient receiving exceptionally high doses of *Sandimmune* is converted to *Neoral* or *Gengraf*, exercise particular caution. Monitor cyclosporine blood levels in transplant and rheumatoid arthritis (RA) patients taking *Gengraf* and *Neoral* to minimize possible organ rejection due to high concentrations. Make dose adjustments in transplant patients to minimize possible organ rejection due to low concentrations. Comparison of blood concentrations in the published literature with blood concentrations obtained using current assays must be done with detailed knowledge of the assay methods employed.

Psoriasis patients previously treated with PUVA and to a lesser extent, methotrexate or other immunosuppressive agents, UVB, coal tar, or radiation therapy, are at an increased risk of developing skin malignancies when taking *Neoral* or *Gengraf*.

Cyclosporine, in recommended doses, can cause systemic hypertension and nephrotoxicity. The risk increases with increasing dose and duration of cyclosporine therapy. Renal dysfunction, including structural kidney damage, is a potential consequence of cyclosporine, and therefore, renal function must be monitored during therapy.

Indications

➤*Allogeneic transplants:* For prophylaxis of organ rejection in kidney, liver, and heart allogeneic transplants. *Gengraf* and *Neoral* have been used in combination with azathioprine and corticosteroids. *Sandimmune* always is to be used with adrenal corticosteroids. *Sandimmune* also may be used in the treatment of chronic rejection in patients previously treated with other immunosuppressive agents. Because of the risk of anaphylaxis, reserve *Sandimmune* injection for patients who are unable to take the soft gelatin capsule or oral solution.

➤*Psoriasis: Neoral* and *Gengraf* are indicated for the treatment of adult, nonimmunocompromised patients with severe (ie, extensive and/or disabling), recalcitrant, plaque psoriasis who have failed to respond to at least 1 systemic therapy (eg, PUVA, retinoids, methotrexate) or in patients for whom other systemic therapies are contraindicated or cannot be tolerated. While rebound rarely occurs, most patients will experience relapse with *Neoral* or *Gengraf* as with other therapies upon cessation of treatment.

➤*RA: Neoral* and *Gengraf* are indicated for the treatment of patients with severe, active, RA where the disease has not adequately responded to methotrexate. *Neoral* and *Gengraf* can be used in combination with methotrexate in RA patients who do not respond adequately to methotrexate alone.

➤*Unlabeled uses:* Prevention and treatment of acute graft-versus-host disease (GVHD) following bone marrow transplantation; aplastic anemia; resistant leukemias.

Administration and Dosage

➤*Bioequivalency: Sandimmune* capsules and oral solution have decreased bioavailability in comparison with *Neoral* capsules, *Neoral* oral solution, *Gengraf* capsules, and *Gengraf* oral solution. *Gengraf* and *Neoral* are not bioequivalent to *Sandimmune* and cannot be used interchangeably without physician supervision.

Because *Sandimmune* is not bioequivalent to *Neoral* or *Gengraf*, conversion from *Neoral* or *Gengraf* to *Sandimmune* using a 1:1 ratio (mg/kg/day) may result in lower cyclosporine blood concentration. Conversion from *Neoral* or *Gengraf* to *Sandimmune* should be made with increased blood concentration monitoring to avoid the potential of underdosing.

➤*Allogenic transplants:* In children, the same dose and dosing regimen may be used as in adults; although, in several studies, children have required and tolerated higher doses than those used in adults.

➤*Sandimmune*, oral: Give the initial dose of Sandimmune 4 to 12 hours prior to transplantation as a single dose of 15 mg/kg. Although a single daily dose of 14 to 18 mg/kg was used in most clinical trials, few centers continue to use the highest dose, most favoring the lower end of the scale. There is a trend towards use of even lower initial doses for renal transplantation in the ranges of 10 to 14 mg/kg/day. The initial single daily dose is continued postoperatively for 1 to 2 weeks and then tapered by 5% per week to a maintenance dose of 5 to 10 mg/kg/day. Some centers have successfully tapered the maintenance dose to as low as 3 mg/kg/day in selected renal transplant patients without an apparent rise in rejection rate.

➤*Neoral* and *Gengraf*: Always give the daily dosage of *Neoral* and *Gengraf* in 2 divided doses (bid) on a consistent schedule with regard to time of day and relation to meals.

➤*Newly transplanted patients:* Give the initial dose of *Neoral* and *Gengraf* 4 to 12 hours prior to transplantation or postoperatively. The initial dose of *Neoral* and *Gengraf* varies depending on the transplanted organ and the other immunosuppressive agents included in the immunosuppressive protocol. In newly transplanted patients, the initial oral dose of *Neoral* and *Gengraf* are the same as the initial dose of *Sandimmune*. The mean approximate initial doses were 9 mg/kg/day for renal transplant patients, 8 mg/kg/day for liver transplant patients, and 7 mg/kg/day for heart transplant patients. Total daily doses were divided into equal daily doses. The *Neoral* and *Gengraf* dose is subsequently adjusted to achieve a predefined cyclosporine blood concentration. Using the same trough concentration target for *Neoral* and *Gengraf* as for *Sandimmune* results in greater cyclosporine exposure when *Neoral* and *Gengraf* are administered. Titrate dosing based on clinical assessments of rejection and tolerability. Lower *Neoral* and *Gengraf* doses may be sufficient as maintenance therapy.

➤*Conversion from Sandimuune*: In transplanted patients who are considered for conversion to *Neoral* or *Gengraf* from *Sandimmune*, start *Neoral* or *Gengraf* with the same daily dose as was previously used with *Sandimmune* (1:1 dose conversion). Subsequently, adjust the *Neoral* or *Gengraf* dose to attain the preconversion cyclosporine blood trough concentration. Using the same trough concentration target range for *Neoral* and *Gengraf* as for *Sandimmune* results in greater cyclosporine exposure when *Neoral* and *Gengraf* are administered. Patients with suspected poor absorption of *Sandimmune* require different dosing strategies. In some patients, the increase in blood trough concentration is more pronounced and may be of clinical significance.

Until the blood trough concentration attains the preconversion value, it is strongly recommended that the cyclosporine blood-trough concentration be monitored every 4 to 7 days after conversion to *Neoral* or *Gengraf*. In addition, monitor clinical safety parameters such as serum creatinine and blood pressure every 2 weeks during the first 2 months after conversion. If the blood trough concentrations are outside the desired range and/or if the clinical safety parameters worsen, adjust the dosage of *Neoral* or *Gengraf* accordingly.

➤*Poor Sandimmune* absorption: Patients with lower than expected cyclosporine blood trough concentrations in relation to the oral dose of *Sandimmune* may have poor or inconsistent absorption of cyclosporine from *Sandimmune*. After conversion to *Neoral* or *Gengraf*, patients tend to have higher cyclosporine concentrations. Due to the increase in bioavailability of cyclosporine following conversion to *Neoral* or *Gengraf*, the cyclosporine blood trough concentration may exceed the target range. Exercise particular caution when converting patients to *Neoral* or *Gengraf*; the cyclosporine blood trough concentration may exceed the target range. Exercise particular caution when converting patients to *Neoral* or *Gengraf* at doses greater than 10 mg/kg/day. Individually titrate the dose of *Neoral* or *Gengraf* based on cyclosporine trough concentrations, tolerability, and clinical response. In this population, measure the cyclosporine trough concentrations more frequently, at least twice a week (daily, if initial dose exceeds 10 mg/kg/day), until the concentration stabilizes within the desired range.

➤*Oral solution preparation:*

Sandimmune – To make *Sandimmune* oral solution more palatable, it may be diluted with milk, chocolate milk, or orange juice, preferably at room temperature. Instruct patients to stir well and drink at once, not allowing the solution to stand before drinking. It is best to use a glass container and rinse it with more diluent to ensure that the total dose is taken. Instruct patients to not rinse the dosage syringe with water or other cleaning agents either before or after use. If the dosage syringe requires cleaning, it must be completely dry before resuming use. Introduction of water into the product by any means will cause variation in dose. Patients should avoid switching diluents frequently. Administer *Sandimmune* soft gelatin capsules and oral solution on a consistent schedule with regard to time of day and relation to meals.

Neoral or *Gengraf* – It is recommended that *Neoral* and *Gengraf* be administered on a consistent schedule with regard to time of day and relation to meals. Grapefruit and grapefruit juice affect metabolism, increasing blood concentration of cyclosporine, and thus, should be avoided. To make *Neoral* or *Gengraf* more palatable, it should be diluted with orange or apple juice that is at room temperature. Instruct patients to not switch diluents frequently. The combination of *Neoral* or *Gengraf* solution with milk can be unpalatable. The effect of milk on the bioavailability of cyclosporine when administered as *Neoral* or *Gengraf* oral solution has not been evaluated. Instruct patients to remove the protective cover from dosing syringe supplied, and transfer the solution to a glass of orange or apple juice. Advise patients to stir well and drink at once, not allowing the diluted solution to stand before drinking. A glass container, not plastic, should be used. Tell patients to rinse the glass with more diluent to ensure that the total dose is consumed. After use, the outside of the dosing syringe should be dried with

CYCLOSPORINE — ORAL

a clean towel and the protective cover should be replaced. The dosing syringe should not be rinsed with water or other cleaning agents. If the syringe requires cleaning, it must be completely dry before resuming use.

➤*Adjunct therapy:* Adjunct therapy with adrenal corticosteroids is recommended initially. Different tapering dosage schedules of prednisone appear to achieve similar results. A representative dosage schedule based on the patient's weight started with 2 mg/kg/day for the first 4 days tapered to 1 mg/kg/day by 1 week, 0.6 mg/kg/day by 2 weeks, 0.3 mg/kg/day by 1 month, and 0.15 mg/kg/day by 2 months and thereafter as a maintenance dose. Steroid doses may be further tapered on an individualized basis depending on status of patient and function of graft. Adjustments in dosage of prednisone must be made according to the clinical situation.

➤*Psoriasis:* The initial dose of *Neoral* or *Gengraf* should be 2.5 mg/kg/day. Take *Neoral* or *Gengraf* twice daily, as a divided (1.25 mg/kg BID) oral dose. Keep patients at that dose for at least 4 weeks, barring adverse events. Increase dosage at 2-week intervals if significant clinical improvement has not occurred by that time. Based on patient response, make dose increases of approximately 0.5 mg/kg/day to a maximum of 4 mg/kg/day.

Make dose decreases by 25% to 50% at any time to control adverse events, such as hypertension, serum creatinine elevations (greater than or equal to 25% above the patient's pretreatment level), or clinically significant laboratory abnormalities. If dose reduction is not effective in controlling abnormalities, or if the adverse event or abnormality is severe, discontinue *Neoral* or *Gengraf* therapy.

Patients generally show some improvement in the clinical manifestations of psoriasis in 2 weeks. Satisfactory control and stabilization of the disease may take 12 to 16 weeks to achieve. Discontinue treatment if satisfactory response cannot be achieved after 6 weeks at 4 mg/kg/day or the patient's maximum tolerated dose. Once a patient is adequately controlled and appears stable, lower the dose of *Neoral* or *Gengraf*. Doses below 2.5 mg/kg/day may also be equally effective.

Upon stopping treatment with cyclosporine, relapse will occur in approximately 6 weeks (50% of patients) to 16 weeks (75% of patients). In the majority of patients, rebound does not occur after cessation of treatment with cyclosporine. Continuous treatment for extended periods longer than 1 year is not recommended. Consider alteration with other forms of treatment in the long-term management of patients with life-long disease.

➤*RA:* The initial dose of *Neoral* or *Gengraf* is 2.5 mg/kg/day, taken twice daily as a divided (bid) oral dose. Salicylates, NSAIDS, and oral corticosteroids may be continued. Onset of action generally occurs between 4 and 8 weeks. If sufficient clinical benefit is seen and tolerability is good (including serum creatinine less than 30% above baseline), the dose may be increased by 0.5 to 0.75 mg/kg/day after 8 weeks and again after 12 weeks to a maximum of 4 mg/kg/day. If no benefit is seen by 16 weeks of therapy, discontinue *Neoral* or *Gengraf* therapy.

Make dose decreases by 25% to 50% at any time to control adverse events, such as hypertension, serum creatinine elevations (greater than or equal to 25% above the patient's pretreatment level), or clinically significant laboratory abnormalities. If dose reduction is not effective in controlling abnormalities, or if the adverse event or abnormality is severe, discontinue *Neoral* or *Gengraf*.

Use with methotrexate – Use the same initial dose and dosage range if *Neoral* or *Gengraf* is combined with the recommended dose of methotrexate. Most patients can be treated with *Neoral* or *Gengraf* doses of 3 mg/kg/day or less when combined with methotrexate doses of up to 15 mg/week.

➤*Storage/Stability:*

Sandimmune –

Capsules: Store at 25°C (77°F); excursions permitted to 15° to 30°C (59° to 86°F).

Oral solution: Store in the original container at temperatures below 30°C (86°F). Do not store in the refrigerator. Protect from freezing. Once opened, the contents must be used within 2 months.

Neoral –

Capsules: Store in the original unit-dose container at controlled room temperature 20° to 25°C (68° to 77°F).

Oral solution: Store in the original container at controlled room temperature 20° to 25°C (68° to 77°F). Do not store in the refrigerator. Once opened, the contents must be used within 2 months. At temperatures below 20°C (68°F), the solution may gel; light flocculation or the formation of a light sediment also may occur. There is no impact on product performance or dosing using the syringe provided. Allow to warm to room temperature 25°C (77°F) to reverse these changes.

Gengraf –

Capsules: Store in the original unit-dose container at controlled room temperature 15° to 30°C (59° to 86°F).

Oral solution: Store in the original container at controlled room temperature (15° to 30°C; 59° to 86°F). Do not store in the refrigerator. Once opened, the contents must be used within 2 months. At temperatures below 20°C (68°F) the solution may gel; light flocculation or the formation of a light sediment also may occur. There is no impact on product performance or dosing using the syringe provided. Allow to warm to room temperature (15° to 30°C; 59° to 86°F) to reverse these changes.

Actions

➤*Pharmacology:* Cyclosporine is a potent immunosuppressive agent that in animals prolongs survival of allogenic transplants involving skin, kidney, liver, heart, pancreas, bone marrow, small intestine, and lung. Cyclosporine has been demonstrated to suppress some humoral immunity and to a greater extent, cell-mediated immune reactions such as allograft rejection, delayed hypersensitivity, experimental allergic encephalomyelitis, Freund's adjuvant arthritis, and graft vs host disease in many animal species for a variety of organs.

The effectiveness of cyclosporine results from specific and reversible inhibition of immunocompetent lymphocytes in the G_0 and G_1-phase of the cell cycle. T-lymphocytes are preferentially inhibited. The T-helper cell is the main target, although the T-suppressor cell also may be suppressed. Cyclosporine also inhibits lymphokine production and release including interleukin-2.

➤*Pharmacokinetics:*

Absorption –

Select Pharmacokinetic Parameters of Cyclosporine Formulations

	Absolute bioavailability (%)	T_{max} (hours)	C_{max} (ng/mL/mg of dose)	t½ (hours)
Sandimmune	30[a]	3.5	≈ 1 (2.7 to 1.4)[b]	19 (range, 10 to 27)
Neoral	Not determined in adults	1.5 to 2	40% to 106% or greater[c]	8.4 (range, 5 to 18)
Gengraf	Not determined in adults	1.5 to 2	40% to 106% or greater[c]	8.4 (range, 5 to 18)

[a] Based upon the results in 2 patients.
[b] Blood levels for low to high doses, respectively.
[c] In renal transplant patients treated with *Neoral* and *Gengraf*, peak levels were 40% to 106% greater than those following *Sandimmune* administration.

The absorption of cyclosporine from the GI tract is incomplete and variable. The extent of absorption of cyclosporine is dependent on the individual patient, the patient population, and the formulation. Very little difference in absorption was observed when patients were administered *Gengraf* or *Neoral* with and without T-tube diversion of bile. For *Sandimmune*, C_{max} and area under the plasma or blood concentration-time curve (AUC) increase with administered dose; for blood, the relationship is curvilinear (parabolic) between 0 and 1400. The relationship between administered dose and exposure AUC is linear within the therapeutic dose range for *Neoral* and *Gengraf*. The intersubject variability of cyclosporine exposure (AUC) when *Gengraf*, *Neoral*, or *Sandimmune* is administered ranges from about 20% to 50% in renal transplant patients. This intersubject variability contributes to the need for individualization of the dosing regimen for optimal therapy. Intrasubject variability of AUC in renal transplant recipients was 9% to 21% for *Gengraf* and *Neoral* and 19% to 26% for *Sandimmune*. In the same studies, intrasubject variability of trough concentrations was 17% to 30% for *Gengraf* and *Neoral* and 16% to 38% for *Sandimmune*.

The dose normalized AUC in renal transplant patients taking *Gengraf* or *Neoral* 28 days after transplantation was 50% greater than in those patients administered *Sandimmune*. The increase in AUC is accompanied by an increase in peak blood cyclosporine concentration in the range of 40% to 106% in renal transplant patients and approximately 90% in liver transplant patients. AUC and C_{max} also are increased (*Gengraf* or *Neoral* relative to *Sandimmune*) in heart transplant patients, but data are very limited. Although the AUC and C_{max} values are higher with *Gengraf* and *Neoral* relative to *Sandimmune*, the pre-dose trough concentrations (dose-normalized) are similar between the formulations.

Drug/Food interactions: See Drug Interactions for more information.

Distribution – Cyclosporine is distributed largely outside the blood volume; approximately 33% to 47% is in plasma, 4% to 9% in lymphocytes, 5% to 12% in granulocytes, and 41% to 58% in erythrocytes. At high concentrations, the binding capacity of leukocytes and erythrocytes becomes saturated. In plasma, approximately 90% is bound to proteins, primarily lipoproteins. The steady-state volume of distribution during IV dosing has been reported as 3 to 5 L/kg in solid organ transplant recipients. In blood, the distribution is concentration dependent.

Metabolism – Cyclosporine is extensively metabolized by the cytochrome P450 3A4 enzyme system in the liver and, to a lesser degree, in the GI tract and the kidney. At least 25 metabolites have been identified from human bile, feces, blood, and urine. The biological activity of the metabolites and their contributions to toxicity are considerably less than those of the parent compound. At steady-state following the oral administration of *Sandimmune*, the mean AUCs for blood concentrations of the major metabolites M1, M9, and M4N are about 70%, 21%, and 7.5% of the AUC for blood cyclosporine concentrations, respectively. Based on blood concentration data from stable renal transplant patients and bile concentration data from de novo liver transplant patients, the percentage of dose present as M1, M9, and M4N metabolites is similar when *Gengraf*, *Neoral*, or *Sandimmune* is administered.

Excretion – Only 0.1% of a dose is excreted unchanged in the urine. Excretion is primarily biliary with only 6% of the dose (parent drug and metabolites) excreted in urine. Neither dialysis nor renal failure alter cyclosporine clearance significantly.

Contraindications

Hypersensitivity to cyclosporine, or any component of the products; *Gengraf* and *Neoral* in psoriasis or RA patients with abnormal renal function, uncontrolled hypertension, or malignancies; *Gengraf* and *Neoral* concomitantly with PUVA or UVB, methotrexate or other immunosuppressive agents, coal tar or radiation therapy in psoriasis patients.

CYCLOSPORINE — ORAL

Warnings

➤*Elevated BUN and serum creatinine:* It is not unusual for serum creatinine and BUN levels to be elevated during cyclosporine therapy. These elevations in renal transplant patients do not necessarily indicate rejection, and each patient must be fully evaluated before dosage adjustment is indicated. These increases reflect a reduction in the glomerular filtration rate. Impaired renal function at any time requires close monitoring, and frequent dosage adjustments may be indicated. The frequency and severity of serum creatinine elevations increase with dose and duration of cyclosporine therapy. These elevations are likely to become more pronounced without dose reduction or discontinuation.

➤*Nephrotoxicity:* Nephrotoxicity has been noted in 25% of cases of renal transplantation, 38% of cases of cardiac transplantation, and 37% of cases of liver transplantation. Mild nephrotoxicity was generally noted 2 to 3 months after transplant and consisted of an arrest in the fall of the preoperative elevations of BUN and creatinine at a range of 35 to 45 mg/dL and 2 to 2.5 mg/dL, respectively. These elevations are often responsive to dosage reductions. More overt nephrotoxicity was seen early after transplantation and was characterized by a rapidly rising BUN and creatinine. Because these events are similar to rejection episodes, care must be taken to differentiate between them. This form of toxicity is usually responsive to cyclosporine dosage reduction.

Although specific diagnostic criteria that reliably differentiate renal graft rejection from drug toxicity have not been found, a number of parameters have been significantly associated to one or the other. However, it should be noted that up to 20% of patients may have simultaneous nephrotoxicity and rejection.

A form of a cyclosporine-associated nephrotoxicity is characterized by serial deterioration in renal function and morphologic changes in the kidneys. From 5% to 15% of transplant patients who have received cyclosporine will fail to show a reduction in rising serum creatinine despite a decrease or discontinuation of cyclosporine therapy. Renal biopsies from these patients will demonstrate one or several of the following alterations: tubular vacuolization, tubular microcalcifications, peritubular capillary congestion, arteriolopathy, and a striped form of interstitial fibrosis with tubular atrophy. Though none of these morphologic changes are entirely specific, a diagnosis of cyclosporine-associated structural nephrotoxicity requires evidence of these findings. When considering the development of cyclosporine-associated nephropathy, it is noteworthy that several authors have reported an association between the appearance of interstitial fibrosis and higher cumulative doses or persistently high circulating trough levels of cyclosporine. This is particularly true during the first 6 posttransplant months when the dosage tends to be highest and when, in kidney recipients, the organ appears to be most vulnerable to the toxic effects of cyclosporine. Among other contributing factors to the development of interstitial fibrosis in these patients are prolonged perfusion time, warm ischemia time, as well as episodes of acute toxicity, and acute and chronic rejection. The reversibility of interstitial fibrosis and its correlation to renal function have not yet been determined. Reversibility of arteriopathy has been reported after stopping cyclosporine and lowering the dosage.

Cyclosporine nephropathy was detected in renal biopsies of 6 out of 60 (10%) RA patients after the average treatment duration of 19 months. Only 1 patient out of these 6 patients was treated with a dose of approximately 4 mg/kg/day. Serum creatinine improved in all but 1 patient after discontinuation of cyclosporine. The maximal creatinine increase appears to be a factor in predicting cyclosporine nephropathy.

Kidney biopsies from 86 psoriasis patients treated for a mean duration of 23 months with 1.2 to 7.6 mg/kg/day of cyclosporine showed evidence of cyclosporine nephropathy in 18/86 (21%) of the patients. The pathology consisted of renal tubular atrophy and interstitial fibrosis. On repeat biopsy of 13 of these patients maintained on various dosages of cyclosporine for a mean of 2 additional years, the number with cyclosporine induced nephropathy rose to 26/86 (30%). The majority of patients (19/26) were on a dose of greater than or equal to 5 mg/kg/day. The patients were also on cyclosporine for greater than 15 months (18/26) and/or had a clinically significant increase for greater than 1 month (21/26). Creatinine levels returned to normal in 7 of 11 patients in whom cyclosporine therapy was discontinued.

Diagnostic Criteria Differentiating Nephrotoxicity From Rejection

Parameter	Nephrotoxicity	Rejection
History	• Donor > 50 years of age or hypotensive, • Prolonged kidney preservation, • Prolonged anastomosis time, • Concomitant nephrotoxic drugs	• Antidonor immune response, • Retransplant patient
Clinical	• Often > 6 weeks post-op, • Prolonged initial nonfunction (acute tubular necrosis)	• Often < 4 weeks post-op • Fever > 37.5°C, • Decrease in daily urine volume > 500 mL (or 50%), • Graft swelling and tenderness, • Weight gain > 0.5 kg
Laboratory	• CyA serum trough level > 200 ng/mL, • Gradual rise in Cr (< 0.15 mg/dL/day), • Cr plateau < 25% above baseline, • BUN/Cr ≥ 20	• CyA serum trough level < 150 ng/mL, • Rapid rise in Cr (> 0.3 mg/dL/day), • Cr> 25% above baseline, • BUN/Cr < 20
Biopsy	• Arteriolopathy (medial hypertrophy, hyalinosis, nodular deposits, intimal thickening, endothelial vacuolization, progressive scarring), • Tubular atrophy, isometric vacuolization, isolated calcifications, • Minimal edema, • Mild focal infiltrates, • Diffuse interstitial fibrosis, often striped form	• Endovasculitis (proliferation, intimal arteritis, necrosis, sclerosis), • Tubulitis with RBC and WBC casts, some irregular vacuolization, • Interstitial edema and hemorrhage, • Diffuse moderate to severe mononuclear infiltrates, • Glomerulitis (mononuclear cells)
Aspiration cytology	• CyA deposits in tubular and endothelial cells, • Fine isometric vacuolization of tubular cells	• Inflammatory infiltrate with mono-nuclear phagocytes, macrophages, lymphoblastoid cells, and activated T-cells, • These strongly express HLA-DR antigens
Urine cytology	• Tubular cells with vacuolization and granularization	• Degenerative tubular cells, plasmacells and lymphocyturia > 20% of sediment
Manometry	• Intracapsular pressure < 40 mm Hg	• Intracapsular pressure> 40 mm Hg
Ultrasonography	• Unchanged graft cross sectional area	• Increase in graft cross sectional area, • AP diameter ≥ transverse diameter
Magnetic resonance imagery	• Normal appearance	• Loss of distinct corticomedullary junction, swelling image intensity of parachyma approaching that of psoas, loss of hilar fat
Radionuclide scan	• Normal or generally decreased perfusion, • Decrease in tubular function, • (^{131}I-hippuran)> decrease in perfusion (^{99m}Tc DTPA)	• Patchy arterial flow, • Decrease in perfusion > decrease in tubular function, • Increased uptake of indium 111 labeled platelets or Tc-99m in colloid
Therapy	• Responds to decreased cyclosporine	• Responds to increased steroids or antilymphocyte globulin

➤*Thrombocytopenia and microangiopathic hemolytic anemia:* Occasionally patients have developed a syndrome of thrombocytopenia and microangiopathic hemolytic anemia that may result in graft failure. The vasculopathy can occur in the absence of rejection and is accompanied by avid platelet consumption within the graft. Neither the pathogenesis nor the management of this syndrome is clear. Though resolution has occurred after reduction or discontinuation of cyclosporine and 1) administration of streptokinase and heparin or 2) plasmapheresis, this appears to depend upon early detection with Indium 111 platelet scans.

➤*Hyperkalemia:* Significant hyperkalemia (sometimes associated with hyperchloremic metabolic acidosis) and hyperuricemia have been seen occasionally in individual patients.

➤*Hepatotoxicity:* Hepatotoxicity has been noted in 4% of cases of renal transplantation, 7% of cases of cardiac transplantation, and 4% of cases of liver transplantation. This was usually noted during the first month of therapy when high doses of cyclosporine were used and consisted of elevations of hepatic enzymes and bilirubin. The chemistry elevations usually decreased with a reduction in dosage.

CYCLOSPORINE — ORAL

➤*Convulsions:* Convulsions have occurred in adult and pediatric patients receiving cyclosporine, particularly in combination with high-dose methylprednisolone.

➤*Encephalopathy:* Encephalopathy has been described in postmarketing reports and in the literature. Manifestations include impaired consciousness, convulsions, visual disturbances (including blindness), loss of motor function, movement disorders, and psychiatric disturbances. In many cases, changes in the white matter have been detected using imaging techniques and pathologic specimens. Predisposing factors such as hypertension, hypomagnesemia, hypocholesterolemia, high-dose corticosteroids, high cyclosporine blood concentrations, and graft vs host disease have been noted in many but not all of the reported cases. The changes in most cases have been reversible upon discontinuation of cyclosporine, and in some cases improvement was noted after reduction of dose. It appears that patients receiving liver transplants are more susceptible to encephalopathy than those receiving kidney transplants.

➤*Bioequivalency:* See Administration and Dosage for more information.

➤*Vaccination:* During treatment with cyclosporine, vaccination may be less effective; avoid the use of live attenuated vaccines.

➤*Glomerular capillary thrombosis:* See Adverse Reactions for more information.

➤*Hypomagnesemia:* See Adverse Reactions for more information.

➤*Renal function impairment:* Renal function impairment requires close monitoring and possibly frequent dosage adjustment. In patients with persistent high elevations of BUN and creatinine unresponsive to dosage adjustments, consider switching to other immunosuppressive therapy. In the event of severe and unremitting rejection, when rescue therapy with pulse steroids and monoclonal antibodies fails to reverse the rejection episode, it is preferable to switch to alternative immunosuppressive therapy or allow the kidney transplant to be rejected and removed rather than increase the dosage to a very high level in an attempt to reverse the rejection.

➤*Carcinogenesis:* As in patients receiving other immunosuppressants, those patients receiving cyclosporine are at increased risk of development of lymphomas and other malignancies, particularly those of the skin. The increased risk appears related to the intensity and duration of immunosuppression rather than to the use of specific agents. Because of the danger of oversuppression of the immune system resulting in increased risk of infection or malignancy, use a treatment regimen containing multiple immunosuppressants with caution. Reduction or discontinuance of immunosuppression may cause the lesions to regress.

Do not treat patients for psoriasis concurrently with cyclosporine and PUVA or UVB, other radiation therapy, or other immunosuppressive agents because of the possibility of excessive immunosuppression and the subsequent risk of malignancies (see Contraindications).

Thoroughly evaluate patients before and during cyclosporine treatment for the development of malignancies. Moreover, use of cyclosporine therapy with other immunosuppressive agents may induce an excessive immunosuppression that is known to increase the risk of malignancy.

➤*Elderly:* In RA clinical trials with cyclosporine, 17.5% of patients were 65 years of age and older. These patients were more likely to develop systolic hypertension on therapy, and more likely to show serum creatinine rises greater than or equal to 50% above the baseline after 3 to 4 months of therapy. Monitor elderly patients with particular care, because decreases in renal function also occur with age. If patients are not properly monitored and dosages are not properly adjusted, cyclosporine therapy can cause structural kidney damage and persistent renal dysfunction.

➤*Pregnancy:* *Category C. Sandimmune* oral solution is embryotoxic and fetotoxic as indicated by increased pre- and postnatal mortality and reduced fetal weight together with related skeletal retardation in rats and rabbits when given in doses 2 to 5 times the human dose. There are no adequate and well-controlled studies in pregnant women. Use during pregnancy only if the potential benefit justifies the risk to the fetus.

The following data represent the reported outcomes of 116 pregnancies in women receiving cyclosporine during pregnancy, 90% of whom were transplant patients and most of whom received cyclosporine throughout the entire gestational period. The only consistent patterns of abnormality were premature birth (gestational period of 28 to 36 weeks) and low birth weight for gestational age. Sixteen fetal losses occurred. Most of the pregnancies (85 of 100) were complicated by disorders, including pre-eclampsia, eclampsia, premature labor, abruptio placentae, oligohydramnios, Rh incompatibility, and fetoplacental dysfunction. Pre-term delivery occurred in 47%. Seven malformations were reported in 5 viable infants and in 2 cases of fetal loss. Twenty-eight percent of the infants were small for gestational age. Neonatal complications occurred in 27%. Therefore, weigh the risks and benefits of using cyclosporine during pregnancy.

Because of the possible disruption of maternal-fetal interaction, carefully weigh the risk/benefit ratio of using cyclosporine in psoriasis patients during pregnancy with seriously considering discontinuing cyclosporine.

➤*Lactation:* Cyclosporine is excreted in breast milk; avoid nursing.

➤*Children:* Although no adequate and well-controlled studies have been completed in children, patients as young as 6 months of age have received *Sandimmune* with no unusual adverse effects. Transplant recipients as young as 1 year of age have received *Neoral* or *Gengraf* with no unusual adverse effects.

The safety and efficacy of *Neoral* or *Gengraf* treatment in children with juvenile RA or psoriasis younger than 18 years of age have not been established.

Precautions

➤*Monitoring:*

Blood levels – Transplant centers have found blood concentration monitoring of cyclosporine to be an essential component of patient management. Of importance to blood concentration analysis are the type of assay used, the transplanted organ, and other immunosuppressant agents being administered. While no fixed relationship has been established, blood concentration monitoring may assist in the clinical evaluation of rejection and toxicity, dose adjustments, and the assessment of compliance.

Various assays have been used to measure blood concentrations of cyclosporine. HPLC is the standard reference, but the monoclonal antibody RIAs and the monoclonal antibody FPIA offer sensitivity, reproducibility, and convenience. Most clinicians base their monitoring on trough cyclosporine concentrations. Blood concentration monitoring is not a replacement for renal function monitoring or tissue biopsies.

Laboratory tests – Assess renal and liver functions repeatedly by measurement of BUN, serum creatinine, serum bilirubin, and liver enzymes. Also monitor serum lipids, magnesium, and potassium. Routinely monitor cyclosporine blood concentrations in transplant patients and periodically in RA patients.

Special monitoring for RA patients – Before initiating treatment, perform a careful physical exam, including blood pressure measurements (on at least 2 occasions) and 2 creatinine levels to estimate baseline. Evaluate blood pressure and serum creatinine every 2 weeks during the initial 3 months and then monthly if the patient is stable. It is advisable to monitor serum creatinine and blood pressure always after an increase of the dose of NSAIDs and after initiation of new NSAID therapy during *Neoral* or *Gengraf* treatment. If coadministered with methotrexate, CBC and liver function tests are recommended to be monitored monthly.

Special monitoring for psoriasis patients – Before initiating treatment, perform a careful dermatological and physical examination, including blood pressure measurements (on at least 2 occasions). Because *Neoral* and *Gengraf* are immunosuppressive agents, evaluate patients for the presence of occult infection on their first physical examination and for the presence of tumors initially, and throughout treatment with *Neoral* or *Gengraf.* Biopsy skin lesions are not typical for psoriasis before starting *Neoral* or *Gengraf.* Treat patients with malignant or premalignant changes of the skin with *Neoral* or *Gengraf* only after appropriate treatment of such lesions and if no other treatment option exists. Baseline laboratories include serum creatinine (on 2 occasions), BUN, CBC, serum magnesium, potassium, uric acid, and lipids.

Evaluate serum creatinine and BUN every 2 weeks during the initial 3 months of therapy and then monthly if the patient is stable. If the serum creatinine is greater than or equal to 25% above the patient's pretreatment level, repeat serum creatinine within 2 weeks. If the change in serum creatinine remains greater than or equal to 25% above baseline, reduce *Neoral* or *Gengraf* by 25% to 50%. Discontinue *Neoral* or *Gengraf* if reversibility (within 25% of baseline) of serum creatinine is not achievable after 2 dosage modifications.

Evaluate blood pressure every 2 weeks during the initial 3 months of therapy and then monthly if the patient is stable, or more frequently when dosage adjustments are made. Patients without a history of previous hypertension before initiation of treatment with *Neoral* or *Gengraf* should have the drug reduced by 25% to 50% if found to have sustained hypertension. If the patient continues to be hypertensive despite multiple reductions of *Neoral* or *Gengraf*, then discontinue *Neoral* or *Gengraf.* For patients treated with hypertension, before the initiation of *Neoral* or *Gengraf* therapy, discontinue their medication if a change in hypertension management is not effective or tolerable.

Also monitor CBC, uric acid, potassium, lipids, and magnesium every 2 weeks for the first 3 months of therapy, and then monthly if the patient is stable or more frequently when dosage adjustments are made. Reduce *Neoral* or *Gengraf* dosage by 25% to 50% for any abnormality of clinical concern. In controlled trials of cyclosporine in psoriasis patients, cyclosporine blood concentrations did not correlate well with either improvement or with side effects such as renal dysfunction.

➤*Hypertension:* Mild or moderate hypertension is encountered more frequently than severe hypertension and the incidence decreases over time. In recipients of kidney, liver, and heart allografts treated with cyclosporine, antihypertensive therapy may be required. However, because cyclosporine may cause hyperkalemia, do not use potassium-sparing diuretics. While calcium antagonists can be effective agents in treating cyclosporine-associated hypertension, they can interfere with cyclosporine metabolism.

➤*Malabsorption:* Patients with malabsorption may have difficulty achieving therapeutic levels with *Sandimmune* capsules or oral solution.

Drug Interactions

➤*Nephrotoxic drugs:* Concomitant nonsteroidal anti-inflammatory drugs (NSAIDS), particularly in the setting of dehydration, may potentiate renal dysfunction. Other drugs that may potentiate renal dysfunction are antibiotics such as gentamicin, tobramycin, vancomycin, TMP-SMZ; antineoplastics such as melphalan; antifungals such as amphotericin B, ketoconazole; anti-inflammatory drugs such as diclofenac, naproxen, sulindac, colchicines; GI drugs such as cimetidine and ranitidine; and immunosuppressives such as tacrolimus.

➤*Cytochrome P450 system:* Cyclosporine is extensively metabolized by cytochrome P450 3A4. Monitoring of circulating cyclosporine concentrations and appropriate *Neoral* or *Gengraf* dosage adjustments are essential when these drugs are used concomitantly with other drugs that are inducers or

CYCLOSPORINE — ORAL

inhibitors of this isoenzyme (eg, calcium channel blockers, glucocorticoids, anticonvulsants, protease inhibitors).

Cyclosporine Drug Interactions

Precipitant Drug	Object Drug*		Description
Allopurinol	Cyclosporine	↑	Coadministration may increase cyclosporine concentrations.
Amiodarone	Cyclosporine	↑	Amiodarone may increase cyclosporine blood levels, possibly increasing the risk of nephrotoxicity.
Androgens (eg, danazol, methyltestosterone)	Cyclosporine	↑	Increased cyclosporine blood concentrations and possible nephrotoxicity.
Anticonvulsants (eg, carbamazepine, phenytoin)	Cyclosporine	↓	Cyclosporine levels may be decreased, resulting in a reduction in the pharmacologic effects.
Azole antifungals (eg, fluconazole, ketoconazole)	Cyclosporine	↑	Cyclosporine levels and toxicity may increase 1 to 3 days after starting therapy and persist more than 1 week after stopping antifungal therapy.
Beta blockers (eg, carvedilol)	Cyclosporine	↑	Elevated cyclosporine concentrations with a risk of nephrotoxicity and neurotoxicity may occur.
Bosentan	Cyclosporine	↑↓	Trough concentrations of bosentan may be elevated, increasing the risk of adverse effects, while cyclosporine plasma levels may be decreased. Coadministration is contraindicated.
Cyclosporine	Bosentan		
Bromocriptine	Cyclosporine	↑	Coadministration may increase cyclosporine concentrations.
Calcium channel blockers (eg, nicardipine, diltiazem, verapamil)	Cyclosporine	↑	Increased cyclosporine levels with possible nephrotoxicity. However, administration of verapamil before cyclosporine may be nephroprotective. The interaction is typically observed within 7 days of starting verapamil and may abate within 1 week after discontinuation.
Colchicine	Cyclosporine	↑	Severe adverse clinical symptoms including GI, hepatic, renal, and neuromuscular toxicity may occur during concurrent administration.
Contraceptives, oral	Cyclosporine	↑	Severe hepatotoxicity and raised plasma-cyclosporine trough values have resulted with coadministration in one case.
Corticosteroids	Cyclosporine	↑	Although this combination is therapeutically beneficial for organ transplants, toxicity may be enhanced.
Fluoroquinolones (eg, ciprofloxacin)	Cyclosporine	↑	Increased cyclosporine toxicity may occur.
Foscarnet	Cyclosporine	↑	The risk of renal failure may be increased.
Imipenem-cilastatin	Cyclosporine	↑	The CNS side effects of both agents may be increased.
Macrolide antibiotics	Cyclosporine	↑	Elevated cyclosporine levels, increasing the risk of nephrotoxicity and neurotoxicity, may occur.
Metoclopramide	Cyclosporine	↑	An increase in the immunosuppressive and toxic effects of cyclosporine may result with metoclopramide coadministration.
Nafcillin	Cyclosporine	↓	Coadministration may decrease cyclosporine concentrations.
Nefazodone	Cyclosporine	↑	Cyclosporine concentrations and toxicity may be increased.
Orlistat	Cyclosporine	↓	Whole blood cyclosporine concentrations may be decreased, possibly resulting in a decrease in the immunosuppressive action of cyclosporine.
Probucol	Cyclosporine	↓	Whole blood cyclosporine concentrations may be reduced, producing a decrease in clinical effect.
Rifamycins (rifampin and rifabutin)	Cyclosporine	↓	The immunosuppressive effect of cyclosporine may be reduced. This appears to occur as early as 2 days following the initiation of rifamycins and may persist for 1 to 3 weeks after their discontinuation.
Serotonin reuptake inhibitors (SSRIs) (eg, fluoxetine, sertraline)	Cyclosporine	↑	SSRIs may increase cyclosporine concentrations and toxicity.
St. John's wort	Cyclosporine	↓	Decreased cyclosporine levels and efficacy may occur with coadministration.
Sulfonamides (eg, TMP-SMZ)	Cyclosporine	↓	The action of cyclosporine may be reduced. Oral sulfonamides may increase the risk of nephrotoxicity.
Terbinafine	Cyclosporine	↓	Terbinafine may decrease cyclosporine concentrations.
Ticlopidine	Cyclosporine	↓	Cyclosporine whole blood concentrations may decrease, producing a decrease in pharmacologic effects.
Cyclosporine	Digoxin	↑	Elevated digoxin levels with toxicity may occur.
Cyclosporine	Etoposide	↑	Serum etoposide concentration may be elevated, resulting in increased toxicity.
Cyclosporine	HMG-CoA reductase inhibitors	↑	Severe myopathy or rhabdomyolysis may occur with coadministration.
Cyclosporine	Methotrexate	↑	Coadministration resulted in increased methotrexate AUC ≈ 30% and the AUC of its metabolite was decreased ≈ 80%.
Cyclosporine	Potassium-sparine diuretics	↑	Coadministration may lead to hyperkalemia. Avoid concomitant use.
Cyclosporine	Sirolimus	↑	Sirolimus plasma concentrations may be increased, resulting in increased toxicity. Administer sirolimus 4 hours after cyclosporine to prevent variations in sirolimus concentrations.

* ↑ = Object drug increased. ↓ = Object drug decreased.

➤*Drug/Food interactions:* Administration of food with *Gengraf* and *Neoral* decreases the AUC and C_{max} of cyclosporine. A high-fat meal (669 kcal, 45 g fat) consumed within 30 minutes of *Gengraf* and *Neoral* administration decreased the AUC by 13% and C_{max} by 33%. The effects of a low-fat meal (667 kcal, 15 g fat) were similar. Unless patients have been instructed by a health care provider to take cyclosporine with grapefruit juice, caution them to avoid fluctuations in the ingestion of grapefruit juice while taking cyclosporine.

Adverse Reactions

➤*Most common:* The principal adverse reactions of cyclosporine therapy are renal dysfunction, tremor, hirsutism, hypertension, and gum hyperplasia. Hypertension, which is usually mild to moderate, may occur in approximately 50% of patients following renal transplantation and in most cardiac transplant patients.

Glomerular capillary thrombosis – Glomerular capillary thrombosis has been found in patients treated with cyclosporine and may progress to graft failure. The pathologic changes resemble those seen in the hemolytic-uremic syndrome and include thrombosis of the renal microvasculature, with platelet-fibrin thrombi occluding glomerular capillaries and afferent arterioles, microangiopathic hemolytic anemia, thrombocytopenia, and decreased renal function. Similar findings have been observed when other immunosuppressives have been employed posttransplantation.

Hypomagnesemia – Hypomagnesemia has been reported in some, but not all, patients exhibiting convulsions while on cyclosporine therapy. Although magnesium-depletion studies in normal subjects suggest that hypomagnesemia is associated with neurologic disorders, multiple factors, including hypertension, high dose methylprednisolone, hypocholesterolemia, and neph-

CYCLOSPORINE — ORAL

rotoxicity associated with high plasma concentrations of cyclosporine appear to be related to the neurological manifestations of cyclosporine toxicity.

Cyclosporine (*Sandimmune*) Adverse Reactions (%)

Adverse reactions	Randomized kidney patients: *Sandimmune* (n = 227)	Randomized kidney patients: Azathioprine (n = 228)	All *Sandimmune* patients (kidney, heart, liver transplants) (n = 892)
Cardiovascular			
Flushing	< 1	0	≤ 4
Hypertension	26	18	13 - 53
CNS			
Confusion	≤ 2	—	—
Convulsions	3	1	1 - 5
Headache	2	< 1	2 - 15
Paresthesia	3	0	1 - 2
Tremor	12	0	21 - 55
Dermatologic			
Acne	6	8	1 - 2
Brittle fingernails	≤ 2	—	—
Hirsutism	21	< 1	21 - 45
GI			
Abdominal discomfort	< 1	0	≤ 7
Anorexia	≤ 2	—	—
Diarrhea	3	< 1	3 - 8
Gastritis	≤ 2	—	—
Gum hyperplasia	4	0	5 - 16
Nausea/vomiting	2	< 1	4 - 10
Peptic ulcer	≤ 2	—	—
Hematopoietic			
Anemia	≤ 2	—	—
Leukopenia	2	19	≤ 6
Lymphoma	< 1	0	1 - 6
Thrombocytopenia	≤ 2	—	—
Miscellaneous			
Allergic reaction	≤ 2	—	—
Conjunctivitis	≤ 2	—	—
Cramps	4	< 1	≤ 2
Edema	≤ 2	—	—
Fever	≤ 2	—	—
Gynecomastia	< 1	0	≤ 4
Hearing loss	≤ 2	—	—
Hepatotoxicity	< 1	< 1	4 - 7
Hiccoughs	≤ 2	—	—
Hyperglycemia	≤ 2	—	—
Muscle pain	≤ 2	—	—
Renal dysfunction	32	6	25 - 38
Sinusitis	< 1	0	3 - 7
Tinnitus	≤ 2	—	—

Rare adverse reactions: The following reactions occurred rarely: anxiety, chest pain, constipation, depression, hair breaking, hematuria, joint pain, lethargy, mouth sores, MI, night sweats, pancreatitis, pruritus, swallowing difficulty, tingling, upper GI bleeding, visual disturbance, weakness, weight loss.

Discontinuation: Among 705 kidney transplant patients treated with *Sandimmune* in clinical trials, the reason for treatment discontinuation was renal toxicity (5.4%), infection (0.9%), lack of efficacy (1.4%), acute tubular necrosis (1%), lymphoproliferative disorders (0.3%), hypertension (0.3%), and other reasons (0.7%).

Infectious Complications in Randomized Renal Transplant Patients (%)

Complication	Cyclosporine (n = 227)	Azathioprine with steroids[a] (n = 228)
Abscess	4.4	5.3
Cytomegalovirus	4.8	12.3
Local fungal infections	7.5	9.6
Pneumonia	6.2	9.2
Septicemia	5.3	4.8
Systemic fungal infections	2.2	3.9
Urinary tract infection	21.1	20.2
Viral infections	15.9	18.4
Wound and skin infections	7	10.1

[a] Some patients also received antilymphocytic globulin.

➤*Sandimmune, Neoral, Gengraf:*

RA – The principal adverse reactions associated with the use of cyclosporine in RA are renal dysfunction, hypertension, headache, GI disturbances, and hirsutism/hypertrichosis.

In RA patients treated in clinical trials within the recommended dose range, cyclosporine was discontinued in 5.3% of patients because of hypertension and in 7% of patients because of increased creatinine. These changes are usually reversible with timely dose decreases or discontinuation. The frequency and severity of serum creatinine elevations increase with dose and duration of cyclosporine therapy. These elevations are likely to become more pronounced without dose reduction or discontinuation.

Neoral/Sandimmune RA Adverse Events (≥ 3%)

Adverse event	*Sandimmune*[a] (N = 269)	*Sandimmune* (N = 155)	Methotrexate + *Sandimmune* (N = 74)	*Neoral* (N = 143)
Cardiovascular				
Arrhythmia	2	5	5	2
Chest pain	4	5	1	6
Flushing	2	2	3	5
Hypertension	8	26	16	25
CNS				
Depression	3	6	3	1
Dizziness	8	6	7	8
Headache	17	23	22	25
Insomnia	4	1	1	3
Migraine	2	3	0	3
Paresthesia	8	7	8	11
Tremor	8	7	7	13
Dermatologic				
Alopecia	3	0	1	4
Bullous eruptions	1	0	4	1
Hypertrichosis	19	17	12	15
Rash	7	12	10	8
Skin ulceration	1	1	3	0
GI				
Abdominal pain	15	15	15	15
Anorexia	3	3	1	3
Diarrhea	12	12	18	13
Dyspepsia	12	12	10	8
Flatulence	5	5	5	4
GI disorder NOS[b]	0	2	1	4
Gingivitis	4	3	0	0
Gum hyperplasia	2	4	1	4
Nausea	23	14	24	18
Rectal hemorrhage	0	3	0	1
Stomatitis	7	5	16	6
Vomiting	9	8	14	6
GU				
Dysuria	0	0	11	1
Leukorrhea	1	0	4	1
Menstrual disorder	3	2	1	1
Micturition frequency	2	4	3	2
NPN, increased	0	19	12	18
UTI	0	3	5	3
Lab test abnormalities				
Creatinine elevations ≥ 30%	43	39	55	48
Creatinine elevations ≥ 50%	24	18	26	18
Respiratory				
Bronchitis	1	3	1	1
Coughing	5	3	5	4
Dyspnea	5	1	3	1
Infection NOS	9	5	0	3
Pharyngitis	3	5	5	4
Pneumonia	1	0	4	1
Rhinitis	0	3	11	1
Sinusitis	4	4	8	3
Upper respiratory tract infection	0	14	23	13
Miscellaneous				
Accidental trauma	0	1	10	4
Edema NOS	5	14	12	10
Fatigue	6	3	8	3
Fever	2	3	0	2
Flu-like symptoms	< 1	6	1	3
Pain	6	9	10	13
Rigors	1	1	4	3
Ear disorder NOS	0	5	0	1
Purpura	3	4	1	2

[a] Includes patients in 2.5 mg/kg/day dose group only.
[b] NOS = not otherwise specified.

CYCLOSPORINE — ORAL

In addition, the following adverse events have been reported in 1% to less than 3% of the RA patients in the cyclosporine treatment group in controlled clinical trials.

Cardiovascular – Abnormal heart sounds, cardiac failure, MI, peripheral ischemia.

CNS – Anxiety, confusion, decreased libido, emotional lability, hypoesthesia, impaired concentration, increased libido, nervousness, neuropathy, paranoia, somnolence, vertigo.

Dermatologic – Abnormal pigmentation, angioedema, dermatitis, dry skin, eczema, nail disorder, pruritus, skin disorder, urticaria.

GI – Constipation, dysphagia, enanthema, eructation, esophagitis, gastric ulcer, gastritis, gastroenteritis, gingival bleeding, glossitis, peptic ulcer, salivary gland enlargement, tongue disorder, tooth disorder.

GU – Abnormal urine, breast pain, breast fibroadenosis, hematuria, increased BUN, micturition urgency, nocturia, polyuria, pyelonephritis, urinary incontinence, uterine hemorrhage.

Hematologic – Anemia, epistaxis, leucopenia, lymphadenopathy.

Metabolic/Nutritional – Diabetes mellitus, hyperkalemia, hyperuricemia, hypoglycemia, weight decrease, weight increase.

Musculoskeletal – Arthralgia, bone fracture, bursitis, joint dislocation, myalgia, stiffness, synovial cyst, tendon disorder.

Respiratory – Abnormal chest sounds, bronchospasm, tonsillitis.

Special senses – Abnormal vision, cataract, conjunctivitis, deafness, eye pain, taste perversion, tinnitus, vestibular disorder.

Miscellaneous – Abscess, allergy, asthenia, bacterial infection, bilirubinemia, carcinoma, cellulitis, dry mouth, folliculitis, fungal infection, goiter, herpes simplex, herpes zoster, hot flushes, increased sweating, malaise, moniliasis, overdose, procedure NOS, renal abscess, tumor NOS, viral infection.

Psoriasis – The principal adverse reactions associated with the use of cyclosporine in patients with psoriasis are renal dysfunction, headache, hypertension, hypertriglyceridemia, hirsutism/hypertrichosis, paresthesia or hyperesthesia, influenza-like symptoms, nausea/vomiting, diarrhea, abdominal discomfort, lethargy, and musculoskeletal or joint pain.

In psoriasis patients treated in US controlled trials within the recommended dose range, cyclosporine therapy was discontinued in 1% of patients because of hypertension and in 5.4% of patients because of increased creatinine. In the majority of cases, these changes were reversible after dose reduction or discontinuation of cyclosporine. There has been one reported death associated with the use of cyclosporine in psoriasis. A 27-year-old male developed renal deterioration and was continued on cyclosporine. He had progressive renal failure leading to death.

Frequency and severity of serum creatinine increases with dose and duration of cyclosporine therapy. These elevations are likely to become more pronounced and may result in irreversible renal damage without dose reduction or discontinuation.

Adverse Events Occurring in Psoriasis Patients (≥ 1%)

Adverse reaction	*Neoral* (n = 182)	*Sandimmune* (n = 185)
Cardiovascular		
Chest pain	1 to < 3	1 to < 3
Hypertension	27.5	25.4
CNS		
Dizziness	1 to < 3	1 to < 3
Headache	15.9	14
Insomnia	1 to < 3	1 to < 3
Nervousness	1 to < 3	1 to < 3
Paresthesia	7.1	4.8
Vertigo	1 to < 3	1 to < 3
Dermatologic		
Acne	1 to < 3	1 to < 3
Dry skin	1 to < 3	1 to < 3
Folliculitis	1 to < 3	1 to < 3
Hypertrichosis	6.6	5.4
Keratosis	1 to < 3	1 to < 3
Pruritus	1 to < 3	1 to < 3
Rash	1 to < 3	1 to < 3
GI		
Abdominal pain	2.7	6
Abdominal distention	1 to < 3	1 to < 3
Constipation	1 to < 3	1 to < 3
Diarrhea	5	5.9
Dyspepsia	2.2	3.2
Gingival bleeding	1 to < 3	1 to < 3
Gum hyperplasia	3.8	6
Nausea	5.5	5.9
GU		
Increased creatinine	19.8	15.7
Micturition frequency	1 to < 3	1 to < 3
Hematologic		
White cell and RES	4.4	2.7
Platelet, bleeding, and clotting disorders	1 to < 3	1 to < 3
Red blood cell disorders	1 to < 3	1 to < 3
Respiratory		
Bronchospasm	5	4.9
Coughing	5	4.9
Dyspnea	5	4.9
Infection (viral, other)	1 to < 3	1 to < 3
Rhinitis	5	4.9
Upper respiratory tract infections	7.7	11.3
Miscellaneous		
Abnormal vision	1 to < 3	1 to < 3
Arthralgia	6	1.1
Fever	1 to < 3	1 to < 3
Flu-like symptoms	9.9	8.1
Flushes	1 to < 3	1 to < 3
Hot flushes	1 to < 3	1 to < 3
Hyperbilirubinemia	1 to < 3	1 to < 3
Increased appetite	1 to < 3	1 to < 3
Pain	4.4	3.2
Skin malignancies (squamous cell [0.9%], basal cell [0.4%] carcinomas)	1 to < 3	1 to < 3

Mild hypomagnesemia and hyperkalemia may occur but are asymptomatic. Increases in uric acid may occur and attacks of gout have been rarely reported. A minor dose-related hyperbilirubinemia has been observed in the absence of hepatocellular damage. Cyclosporine therapy may be associated with a modest increase of serum triglycerides and cholesterol. Elevations of triglycerides (greater than 750 mg/dL) occur in about 15% of psoriasis patients; elevations of cholesterol (greater than 300 mg/dL) are observed in less than 3% of psoriasis patients. Generally these laboratory abnormalities are reversible upon dose reduction or discontinuation of cyclosporine.

Overdosage

➤*Treatment:* There is minimal experience with cyclosporine overdosage. Forced emesis can be of value up to 2 hours after administration of cyclosporine. Follow general supportive measures and symptomatic treatment in all cases of overdosage. Cyclosporine is not dialyzable to any great extent, nor is it cleared well by charcoal hemoperfusion.

Patient Information

Advise patients to take cyclosporine with food at the same time each day.

Advise patients to not eat grapefruit or drink grapefruit juice while taking this medicine.

Women who could become pregnant should use nonhormonal contraceptives (diaphragms, condoms) while taking cyclosporine.

Instruct patients to contact their health care provider if fever, sore throat, tiredness, unusual bleeding or bruising, urination, or yellow skin/eyes occurs.

An odor may be present upon opening the *Sandimmune* package. The odor will disappear shortly after opening and does not mean that there is anything wrong with the medicine.

Instruct patients to not take potassium supplements while taking cyclosporine.

Cyclosporine may increase skin cancer risk. Advise patients to avoid prolonged exposure to the sun and other UV light and to use sunscreens and wear protective clothing while taking this medicine. Patients who are being treated for psoriasis will need to have at least 2 careful skin and physical examinations, including blood pressure measurements, before starting cyclosporine.

Patients should avoid live vaccines (eg, measles, mumps, oral polio) while taking cyclosporine. The vaccination may be less effective.

Cyclosporine may increase risk of high blood pressure and abnormal kidney function.

Cyclosporine may affect blood sugar level in diabetic patients.

Instruct patients not to switch to another form of this medication without contacting a health care provider.

CYCLOSPORINE — INJECTION

WARNING

Only physicians experienced in the management of systemic immunosuppressive therapy for the indicated disease should prescribe cyclosporine. Patients receiving the drug should be managed in facilities equipped and staffed with adequate laboratory and supportive medical resources. The physician responsible for maintenance therapy should have complete information requisite for the follow-up of the patient.

Administer *Sandimmune* with adrenal corticosteroids but not with other immunosuppressive agents. Increased susceptibility to infection and other possible development of lymphoma may result from immunosuppression.

Indications

➤*Allogeneic transplants:* For prophylaxis of organ rejection in kidney, liver, and heart allogeneic transplants. *Sandimmune* always is to be used with adrenal corticosteroids. *Sandimmune* also may be used in the treatment of chronic rejection in patients previously treated with other immunosuppressive agents. Because of the risk of anaphylaxis, reserve *Sandimmune* injection for patients who are unable to take the soft gelatin capsule or oral solution.

➤*Unlabeled uses:* Prevention and treatment of acute graft-versus-host disease (GVHD) following bone marrow transplantation; aplastic anemia; resistant leukemias.

Administration and Dosage

➤*Sandimmune*, parenteral: For infusion only. *Sandimmune* injection is administered at one-third the oral dose. Give the initial dose 4 to 12 hours prior to transplantation as a single IV dose of 5 to 6 mg/kg/day. This single dose is continued postoperatively until the patient can tolerate oral therapy. Switch patients to oral therapy as soon as possible after surgery.

Immediately before use, dilute the IV concentrate 1 mL *Sandimmune* in 20 to 100 mL 0.9% sodium chloride injection or 5% dextrose injection and given in a slow IV infusion over approximately 2 to 6 hours. Discard diluted infusion solutions after 24 hours. The *Cremophor EL* (polyoxyethylated castor oil) contained in the concentrate for IV infusion can cause phthalate stripping from PVC.

➤*Adjunct therapy:* Adjunct therapy with adrenal corticosteroids is recommended initially. Different tapering dosage schedules of prednisone appear to achieve similar results. A representative dosage schedule based on the patient's weight started with 2 mg/kg/day for the first 4 days tapered to 1 mg/kg/day by 1 week, 0.6 mg/kg/day by 2 weeks, 0.3 mg/kg/day by 1 month, and 0.15 mg/kg/day by 2 months and thereafter as a maintenance dose. Steroid doses may be further tapered on an individualized basis depending on status of patient and function of graft. Adjustments in dosage of prednisone must be made according to the clinical situation.

➤*Storage / Stability:* Store at temperatures below 30°C (86°F) and protect from light.

Actions

➤*Pharmacology:* Cyclosporine is a potent immunosuppressive agent that in animals prolongs survival of allogenic transplants involving skin, kidney, liver, heart, pancreas, bone marrow, small intestine, and lung. Cyclosporine has been demonstrated to suppress some humoral immunity and to a greater extent, cell-mediated immune reactions such as allograft rejection, delayed hypersensitivity, experimental allergic encephalomyelitis, Freund's adjuvant arthritis, and graft vs host disease in many animal species for a variety of organs.

The effectiveness of cyclosporine results from specific and reversible inhibition of immunocompetent lymphocytes in the G_0 and G_1-phase of the cell cycle. T-lymphocytes are preferentially inhibited. The T-helper cell is the main target, although the T-suppressor cell also may be suppressed. Cyclosporine also inhibits lymphokine production and release including interleukin-2.

➤*Pharmacokinetics:*

Distribution – Cyclosporine is distributed largely outside the blood volume; approximately 33% to 47% is in plasma, 4% to 9% in lymphocytes, 5% to 12% in granulocytes, and 41% to 58% in erythrocytes. At high concentrations, the binding capacity of leukocytes and erythrocytes becomes saturated. In plasma, approximately 90% is bound to proteins, primarily lipoproteins. The steady-state volume of distribution during IV dosing has been reported as 3 to 5 L/kg in solid organ transplant recipients. In blood, the distribution is concentration dependent.

Metabolism – Cyclosporine is extensively metabolized by the cytochrome P450 3A4 enzyme system in the liver and, to a lesser degree, in the GI tract and the kidney. At least 25 metabolites have been identified from human bile, feces, blood, and urine. The biological activity of the metabolites and their contributions to toxicity are considerably less than those of the parent compound.

Contraindications

Hypersensitivity to polyoxyethylated castor oil (injection only; see Warnings and Administration and Dosage), cyclosporine, or any component of the products.

Warnings

➤*Elevated BUN and serum creatinine:* It is not unusual for serum creatinine and BUN levels to be elevated during cyclosporine therapy. These elevations in renal transplant patients do not necessarily indicate rejection, and each patient must be fully evaluated before dosage adjustment is indicated. These increases reflect a reduction in the glomerular filtration rate. Impaired renal function at any time requires close monitoring, and frequent dosage adjustments may be indicated. The frequency and severity of serum creatinine elevations increase with dose and duration of cyclosporine therapy. These elevations are likely to become more pronounced without dose reduction or discontinuation.

➤*Nephrotoxicity:* Nephrotoxicity has been noted in 25% of cases of renal transplantation, 38% of cases of cardiac transplantation, and 37% of cases of liver transplantation. Mild nephrotoxicity was generally noted 2 to 3 months after transplant and consisted of an arrest in the fall of the preoperative elevations of BUN and creatinine at a range of 35 to 45 mg/dL and 2 to 2.5 mg/dL, respectively. These elevations are often responsive to dosage reductions. More overt nephrotoxicity was seen early after transplantation and was characterized by a rapidly rising BUN and creatinine. Because these events are similar to rejection episodes, care must be taken to differentiate between them. This form of toxicity is usually responsive to cyclosporine dosage reduction.

Although specific diagnostic criteria that reliably differentiate renal graft rejection from drug toxicity have not been found, a number of parameters have been significantly associated to one or the other. However, it should be noted that up to 20% of patients may have simultaneous nephrotoxicity and rejection.

A form of a cyclosporine-associated nephrotoxicity is characterized by serial deterioration in renal function and morphologic changes in the kidneys. From 5% to 15% of transplant patients who have received cyclosporine will fail to show a reduction in rising serum creatinine despite a decrease or discontinuation of cyclosporine therapy. Renal biopsies from these patients will demonstrate one or several of the following alterations: tubular vascuolization, tubular microcalcifications, peritubular capillary congestion, arteriolopathy, and a striped form of interstitial fibrosis with tubular atrophy. Though none of these morphologic changes are entirely specific, a diagnosis of cyclosporine-associated structural nephrotoxicity requires evidence of these findings. When considering the development of cyclosporine-associated nephropathy, it is noteworthy that several authors have reported an association between the appearance of interstitial fibrosis and higher cumulative doses or persistently high circulating trough levels of cyclosporine. This is particularly true during the first 6 posttransplant months when the dosage tends to be highest and when, in kidney recipients, the organ appears to be most vulnerable to the toxic effects of cyclosporine. Among other contributing factors to the development of interstitial fibrosis in these patients are prolonged perfusion time, warm ischemia time, as well as episodes of acute toxicity, and acute and chronic rejection. The reversibility of interstitial fibrosis and its correlation to renal function have not yet been determined. Reversibility of arteriopathy has been reported after stopping cyclosporine and lowering the dosage.

Cyclosporine nephropathy was detected in renal biopsies of 6 out of 60 (10%) RA patients after the average treatment duration of 19 months. Only 1 patient out of these 6 patients was treated with a dose of approximately 4 mg/kg/day. Serum creatinine improved in all but 1 patient after discontinuation of cyclosporine. The maximal creatinine increase appears to be a factor in predicting cyclosporine nephropathy.

Kidney biopsies from 86 psoriasis patients treated for a mean duration of 23 months with 1.2 to 7.6 mg/kg/day of cyclosporine showed evidence of cyclosporine nephropathy in 18/86 (21%) of the patients. The pathology consisted of renal tubular atrophy and interstitial fibrosis. On repeat biopsy of 13 of these patients maintained on various dosages of cyclosporine for a mean of 2 additional years, the number with cyclosporine induced nephropathy rose to 26/86 (30%). The majority of patients (19/26) were on a dose of greater than or equal to 5 mg/kg/day. The patients were also on cyclosporine for greater than 15 months (18/26) and/or had a clinically significant increase for greater than 1 month (21/26). Creatinine levels returned to normal in 7 of 11 patients in whom cyclosporine therapy was discontinued.

CYCLOSPORINE — INJECTION

Diagnostic Criteria Differentiating Nephrotoxicity From Rejection		
Parameter	Nephrotoxicity	Rejection
History	• Donor > 50 years of age or hypotensive, • Prolonged kidney preservation, • Prolonged anastomosis time, • Concomitant nephrotoxic drugs	• Antidonor immune response, • Retransplant patient
Clinical	• Often > 6 weeks post-op, • Prolonged initial nonfunction (acute tubular necrosis)	• Often < 4 weeks post-op • Fever > 37.5°C, • Decrease in daily urine volume > 500 mL (or 50%), • Graft swelling and tenderness, • Weight gain > 0.5 kg
Laboratory	• CyA serum trough level > 200 ng/mL, • Gradual rise in Cr (< 0.15 mg/dL/day), • Cr plateau < 25% above baseline, • BUN/Cr ≥ 20	• CyA serum trough level < 150 ng/mL, • Rapid rise in Cr (> 0.3 mg/dL/day), • Cr > 25% above baseline, • BUN/Cr < 20
Biopsy	• Arteriolopathy (medial hypertrophy, hyalinosis, nodular deposits, intimal thickening, endothelial vacuolization, progressive scarring), • Tubular atrophy, isometric vacuolization, isolated calcifications, • Minimal edema, • Mild focal infiltrates, • Diffuse interstitial fibrosis, often striped form	• Endovasculitis (proliferation, intimal arteritis, necrosis, sclerosis), • Tubulitis with RBC and WBC casts, some irregular vacuolization, • Interstitial edema and hemorrhage, • Diffuse moderate to severe mononuclear infiltrates, • Glomerulitis (mononuclear cells)
Aspiration cytology	• CyA deposits in tubular and endothelial cells, • Fine isometric vacuolization of tubular cells	• Infla mmatory infiltrate with mono-nuclear phagocytes, macrophages, lymphoblastoid cells, and activated T-cells, • These strongly express HLA-DR antigens
Urine cytology	• Tubular cells with vacuolization and granularization	• Degenerative tubular cells, plasma cells and lymphocyturia > 20% of sediment
Manometry	• Intracapsular pressure < 40 mm Hg	• Intracapsular pressure > 40 mm Hg
Ultrasonography	• Unchanged graft cross sectional area	• Increase in graft cross sectional area, • AP diameter ≥ transverse diameter
Magnetic resonance imagery	• Normal appearance	• Loss of distinct corticomedullary junction, swelling image intensity of parachyma approaching that of psoas, loss of hilar fat
Radionuclide scan	• Normal or generally decreased perfusion, • Decrease in tubular function, • (^{131}I-hippuran) > decrease in perfusion (^{99m}Tc DTPA)	• Patchy arterial flow, • Decrease in perfusion > decrease in tubular function, • Increased uptake of indium 111 labeled platelets or Tc-99m in colloid
Therapy	• Responds to decreased cyclosporine	• Responds to increased steroids or antilymphocyte globulin

➤*Thrombocytopenia and microangiopathic hemolytic anemia:* Occasionally patients have developed a syndrome of thrombocytopenia and microangiopathic hemolytic anemia that may result in graft failure. The vasculopathy can occur in the absence of rejection and is accompanied by avid platelet consumption within the graft. Neither the pathogenesis nor the management of this syndrome is clear. Though resolution has occurred after reduction or discontinuation of cyclosporine and 1) administration of streptokinase and heparin or 2) plasmapheresis, this appears to depend upon early detection with Indium 111 platelet scans.

➤*Hyperkalemia:* Significant hyperkalemia (sometimes associated with hyperchloremic metabolic acidosis) and hyperuricemia have been seen occasionally in individual patients.

➤*Hepatotoxicity:* Hepatotoxicity has been noted in 4% of cases of renal transplantation, 7% of cases of cardiac transplantation, and 4% of cases of liver transplantation. This was usually noted during the first month of therapy when high doses of cyclosporine were used and consisted of elevations of hepatic enzymes and bilirubin. The chemistry elevations usually decreased with a reduction in dosage.

➤*Convulsions:* Convulsions have occurred in adult and pediatric patients receiving cyclosporine, particularly in combination with high-dose methylprednisolone.

➤*Encephalopathy:* Encephalopathy has been described in postmarketing reports and in the literature. Manifestations include impaired consciousness, convulsions, visual disturbances (including blindness), loss of motor function, movement disorders, and psychiatric disturbances. In many cases, changes in the white matter have been detected using imaging techniques and pathologic specimens. Predisposing factors such as hypertension, hypomagnesemia, hypocholesterolemia, high-dose corticosteroids, high cyclosporine blood concentrations, and graft vs host disease have been noted in many but not all of the reported cases. The changes in most cases have been reversible upon discontinuation of cyclosporine, and in some cases improvement was noted after reduction of dose. It appears that patients receiving liver transplants are more susceptible to encephalopathy than those receiving kidney transplants.

➤*Vaccination:* During treatment with cyclosporine, vaccination may be less effective; avoid the use of live attenuated vaccines.

➤*Glomerular capillary thrombosis:* See Adverse Reactions for more information.

➤*Hypomagnesemia:* See Adverse Reactions for more information.

➤*Hypersensitivity reactions:* Rarely (approximately 1 in 1000), patients receiving *Sandimmune* injection have experienced anaphylactic reactions. Although the exact cause of these reactions is unknown, it is believed to be due to the *Cremophor EL* (polyoxyethylated castor oil) used as the vehicle for the IV formulation. These reactions have consisted of flushing of the face and upper thorax, acute respiratory distress with dyspnea and wheezing, blood pressure changes, and tachycardia. One patient died after respiratory arrest and aspiration pneumonia. In some cases, the reaction subsided after the infusion stopped. Continually observe patients receiving *Sandimmune* injection for at least the first 30 minutes following the start of the infusion and at frequent intervals thereafter. If anaphylaxis occurs, stop the infusion. An aqueous solution of epinephrine 1:1000 should be available at the bedside as well as a source of oxygen. Anaphylactic reactions have not been reported with the capsules or oral solution, which lack *Cremophor EL* (polyoxyethylated castor oil). In fact, patients experiencing anaphylactic reactions have been treated subsequently with the capsules or oral solution without incident.

➤*Renal function impairment:* Renal function impairment requires close monitoring and possibly frequent dosage adjustment. In patients with persistent high elevations of BUN and creatinine unresponsive to dosage adjustments, consider switching to other immunosuppressive therapy. In the event of severe and unremitting rejection, when rescue therapy with pulse steroids and monoclonal antibodies fails to reverse the rejection episode, it is preferable to switch to alternative immunosuppressive therapy or allow the kidney transplant to be rejected and removed rather than increase the dosage to a very high level in an attempt to reverse the rejection.

➤*Carcinogenesis:* As in patients receiving other immunosuppressants, those patients receiving cyclosporine are at increased risk of development of lymphomas and other malignancies, particularly those of the skin. The increased risk appears related to the intensity and duration of immunosuppression rather than to the use of specific agents. Because of the danger of oversuppression of the immune system resulting in increased risk of infection or malignancy, use a treatment regimen containing multiple immunosuppressants with caution. Reduction or discontinuance of immunosuppression may cause the lesions to regress.

➤*Pregnancy: Category C.* There are no adequate and well-controlled studies in pregnant women. Use during pregnancy only if the potential benefit justifies the risk to the fetus.

The following data represent the reported outcomes of 116 pregnancies in women receiving cyclosporine during pregnancy, 90% of whom were transplant patients and most of whom received cyclosporine throughout the entire gestational period. The only consistent patterns of abnormality were premature birth (gestational period of 28 to 36 weeks) and low birth weight for gestational age. Sixteen fetal losses occurred. Most of the pregnancies (85 of 100) were complicated by disorders, including pre-eclampsia, eclampsia, premature labor, abruptio placentae, oligohydramnios, Rh incompatibility, and fetoplacental dysfunction. Pre-term delivery occurred in 47%. Seven malformations were reported in 5 viable infants and in 2 cases of fetal loss. Twenty-eight percent of the infants were small for gestational age. Neonatal

CYCLOSPORINE — INJECTION

complications occurred in 27%. Therefore, weigh the risks and benefits of using cyclosporine during pregnancy.

➤*Lactation:* Cyclosporine is excreted in breast milk; avoid nursing.

➤*Children:* Although no adequate and well-controlled studies have been completed in children, patients as young as 6 months of age have received *Sandimmune* with no unusual adverse effects.

Precautions

➤*Monitoring:*

Blood levels – Transplant centers have found blood concentration monitoring of cyclosporine to be an essential component of patient management. Of importance to blood concentration analysis are the type of assay used, the transplanted organ, and other immunosuppressant agents being administered. While no fixed relationship has been established, blood concentration monitoring may assist in the clinical evaluation of rejection and toxicity, dose adjustments, and the assessment of compliance.

Various assays have been used to measure blood concentrations of cyclosporine. HPLC is the standard reference, but the monoclonal antibody RIAs and the monoclonal antibody FPIA offer sensitivity, reproducibility, and convenience. Most clinicians base their monitoring on trough cyclosporine concentrations. Blood concentration monitoring is not a replacement for renal function monitoring or tissue biopsies.

Laboratory tests – Assess renal and liver functions repeatedly by measurement of BUN, serum creatinine, serum bilirubin, and liver enzymes. Also monitor serum lipids, magnesium, and potassium. Routinely monitor cyclosporine blood concentrations in transplant patients.

➤*Hypertension:* Mild or moderate hypertension is encountered more frequently than severe hypertension and the incidence decreases over time. In recipients of kidney, liver, and heart allografts treated with cyclosporine, antihypertensive therapy may be required. However, because cyclosporine may cause hyperkalemia, do not use potassium-sparing diuretics. While calcium antagonists can be effective agents in treating cyclosporine-associated hypertension, they can interfere with cyclosporine metabolism.

Drug Interactions

➤*Nephrotoxic drugs:* Concomitant nonsteroidal anti-inflammatory drugs (NSAIDS), particularly in the setting of dehydration, may potentiate renal dysfunction. Other drugs that may potentiate renal dysfunction are antibiotics such as gentamicin, tobramycin, vancomycin, TMP-SMZ; antineoplastics such as melphalan; antifungals such as amphotericin B, ketoconazole; anti-inflammatory drugs such as diclofenac, naproxen, sulindac, colchicines; GI drugs such as cimetidine and ranitidine; and immunosuppressives such as tacrolimus.

➤*Cytochrome P450 system:* Cyclosporine is extensively metabolized by cytochrome P450 3A4.

Cyclosporine Drug Interactions

Precipitant Drug	Object Drug*		Description
Allopurinol	Cyclosporine	↑	Coadministration may increase cyclosporine concentrations.
Amiodarone	Cyclosporine	↑	Amiodarone may increase cyclosporine blood levels, possibly increasing the risk of nephrotoxicity.
Androgens (eg, danazol, methyltestosterone)	Cyclosporine	↑	Increased cyclosporine blood concentrations and possible nephrotoxicity.
Anticonvulsants (eg, carbamazepine, phenytoin)	Cyclosporine	↓	Cyclosporine levels may be decreased, resulting in a reduction in the pharmacologic effects.
Azole antifungals (eg, fluconazole, ketoconazole)	Cyclosporine	↑	Cyclosporine levels and toxicity may increase 1 to 3 days after starting therapy and persist more than 1 week after stopping antifungal therapy.
Beta blockers (eg, carvedilol)	Cyclosporine	↑	Elevated cyclosporine concentrations with a risk of nephrotoxicity and neurotoxicity may occur.
Bosentan	Cyclosporine	↑↓	Trough concentrations of bosentan may be elevated, increasing the risk of adverse effects, while cyclosporine plasma levels may be decreased. Coadministration is contraindicated.
Cyclosporine	Bosentan		
Bromocriptine	Cyclosporine	↑	Coadministration may increase cyclosporine concentrations.
Calcium channel blockers (eg, nicardipine, diltiazem, verapamil)	Cyclosporine	↑	Increased cyclosporine levels with possible nephrotoxicity. However, administration of verapamil before cyclosporine may be nephroprotective. The interaction is typically observed within 7 days of starting verapamil and may abate within 1 week after discontinuation.
Colchicine	Cyclosporine	↑	Severe adverse clinical symptoms including GI, hepatic, renal, and neuromuscular toxicity may occur during concurrent administration.
Contraceptives, oral	Cyclosporine	↑	Severe hepatotoxicity and raised plasma-cyclosporine trough values have resulted with coadministration in one case.
Corticosteroids	Cyclosporine	↑	Although this combination is therapeutically beneficial for organ transplants, toxicity may be enhanced.
Fluoroquinolones (eg, ciprofloxacin)	Cyclosporine	↑	Increased cyclosporine toxicity may occur.
Foscarnet	Cyclosporine	↑	The risk of renal failure may be increased.
Imipenem-cilastatin	Cyclosporine	↑	The CNS side effects of both agents may be increased.
Macrolide antibiotics	Cyclosporine	↑	Elevated cyclosporine levels, increasing the risk of nephrotoxicity and neurotoxicity, may occur.
Metoclopramide	Cyclosporine	↑	An increase in the immunosuppressive and toxic effects of cyclosporine may result with metoclopramide coadministration.
Nafcillin	Cyclosporine	↓	Coadministration may decrease cyclosporine concentrations.
Nefazodone	Cyclosporine	↑	Cyclosporine concentrations and toxicity may be increased.
Probucol	Cyclosporine	↓	Whole blood cyclosporine concentrations may be reduced, producing a decrease in clinical effect.
Rifamycins (rifampin and rifabutin)	Cyclosporine	↓	The immunosuppressive effect of cyclosporine may be reduced. This appears to occur as early as 2 days following the initiation of rifamycins and may persist for 1 to 3 weeks after their discontinuation.
Serotonin reuptake inhibitors (SSRIs) (eg, fluoxetine, sertraline)	Cyclosporine	↑	SSRIs may increase cyclosporine concentrations and toxicity.
St. John's wort	Cyclosporine	↓	Decreased cyclosporine levels and efficacy may occur with coadministration.
Sulfonamides (eg, TMP-SMZ)	Cyclosporine	↓	The action of cyclosporine may be reduced. Oral sulfonamides may increase the risk of nephrotoxicity.
Terbinafine	Cyclosporine	↓	Terbinafine may decrease cyclosporine concentrations.
Ticlopidine	Cyclosporine	↓	Cyclosporine whole blood concentrations may decrease, producing a decrease in pharmacologic effects.
Cyclosporine	Digoxin	↑	Elevated digoxin levels with toxicity may occur.

CYCLOSPORINE — INJECTION

Cyclosporine Drug Interactions			
Precipitant Drug	Object Drug*		Description
Cyclosporine	Etoposide	↑	Serum etoposide concentration may be elevated, resulting in increased toxicity.
Cyclosporine	HMG-CoA reductase inhibitors	↑	Severe myopathy or rhabdomyolysis may occur with coadministration.
Cyclosporine	Methotrexate	↑	Coadministration resulted in increased methotrexate AUC ≈ 30% and the AUC of its metabolite was decreased ≈ 80%.
Cyclosporine	Potassium-sparine diuretics	↑	Coadministration may lead to hyperkalemia. Avoid concomitant use.
Cyclosporine	Sirolimus	↑	Sirolimus plasma concentrations may be increased, resulting in increased toxicity. Administer sirolimus 4 hours after cyclosporine to prevent variations in sirolimus concentrations.

* ↑ = Object drug increased. ↓ = Object drug decreased.

Adverse Reactions

➤*Most common:* The principal adverse reactions of cyclosporine therapy are renal dysfunction, tremor, hirsutism, hypertension, and gum hyperplasia. Hypertension, which is usually mild to moderate, may occur in approximately 50% of patients following renal transplantation and in most cardiac transplant patients.

Glomerular capillary thrombosis – Glomerular capillary thrombosis has been found in patients treated with cyclosporine and may progress to graft failure. The pathologic changes resemble those seen in the hemolytic-uremic syndrome and include thrombosis of the renal microvasculature, with platelet-fibrin thrombi occluding glomerular capillaries and afferent arterioles, microangiopathic hemolytic anemia, thrombocytopenia, and decreased renal function. Similar findings have been observed when other immunosuppressives have been employed posttransplantation.

Polyoxyethylated castor oil – *Cremophor EL* (polyoxyethylated castor oil) is known to cause hyperlipidemia and electrophoretic abnormalities of lipoproteins. These effects are reversible upon discontinuation of treatment but are usually not a reason to stop treatment.

Hypomagnesemia – Hypomagnesemia has been reported in some, but not all, patients exhibiting convulsions while on cyclosporine therapy. Although magnesium-depletion studies in normal subjects suggest that hypomagnesemia is associated with neurologic disorders, multiple factors, including hypertension, high dose methylprednisolone, hypocholesterolemia, and nephrotoxicity associated with high plasma concentrations of cyclosporine appear to be related to the neurological manifestations of cyclosporine toxicity.

Cyclosporine (*Sandimmune*) Adverse Reactions (%)			
	Randomized kidney patients		All *Sandimmune* patients (kidney, heart, liver transplants)
Adverse reactions	*Sandimmune* (n = 227)	Azathioprine (n = 228)	(n = 892)
Cardiovascular			
Flushing	< 1	0	≤ 4
Hypertension	26	18	13 - 53
CNS			
Confusion	≤ 2	—	—
Convulsions	3	1	1 - 5
Headache	2	< 1	2 - 15
Paresthesia	3	0	1 - 2
Tremor	12	0	21 - 55
Dermatologic			
Acne	6	8	1 - 2
Brittle fingernails	≤ 2	—	—
Hirsutism	21	< 1	21 - 45
GI			
Abdominal discomfort	< 1	0	≤ 7
Anorexia	≤ 2	—	—
Diarrhea	3	< 1	3 - 8
Gastritis	≤ 2	—	—
Gum hyperplasia	4	0	5 - 16
Nausea/vomiting	2	< 1	4 - 10
Peptic ulcer	≤ 2	—	—

Cyclosporine (*Sandimmune*) Adverse Reactions (%)			
	Randomized kidney patients		All *Sandimmune* patients (kidney, heart, liver transplants)
Adverse reactions	*Sandimmune* (n = 227)	Azathioprine (n = 228)	(n = 892)
Hematopoietic			
Anemia	≤ 2	—	—
Leukopenia	2	19	≤ 6
Lymphoma	< 1	0	1 - 6
Thrombocytopenia	≤ 2	—	—
Miscellaneous			
Allergic reaction	≤ 2	—	—
Conjunctivitis	≤ 2	—	—
Cramps	4	< 1	≤ 2
Edema	≤ 2	—	—
Fever	≤ 2	—	—
Gynecomastia	< 1	0	≤ 4
Hearing loss	≤ 2	—	—
Hepatotoxicity	< 1	< 1	4 - 7
Hiccoughs	≤ 2	—	—
Hyperglycemia	≤ 2	—	—
Muscle pain	≤ 2	—	—
Renal dysfunction	32	6	25 - 38
Sinusitis	< 1	0	3 - 7
Tinnitus	≤ 2	—	—

Rare adverse reactions: The following reactions occurred rarely: anxiety, chest pain, constipation, depression, hair breaking, hematuria, joint pain, lethargy, mouth sores, MI, night sweats, pancreatitis, pruritus, swallowing difficulty, tingling, upper GI bleeding, visual disturbance, weakness, weight loss.

Discontinuation: Among 705 kidney transplant patients treated with *Sandimmune* in clinical trials, the reason for treatment discontinuation was renal toxicity (5.4%), infection (0.9%), lack of efficacy (1.4%), acute tubular necrosis (1%), lymphoproliferative disorders (0.3%), hypertension (0.3%), and other reasons (0.7%).

Infectious Complications in Randomized Renal Transplant Patients (%)		
Complication	Cyclosporine (n = 227)	Azathioprine with steroids[a] (n = 228)
Abscess	4.4	5.3
Cytomegalovirus	4.8	12.3
Local fungal infections	7.5	9.6
Pneumonia	6.2	9.2
Septicemia	5.3	4.8
Systemic fungal infections	2.2	3.9
Urinary tract infections	21.1	20.2
Viral infections	15.9	18.4
Wound and skin infections	7	10.1

[a] Some patients also received antilymphocytic globulin.

Overdosage

➤*Treatment:* There is minimal experience with cyclosporine overdosage. Follow general supportive measures and symptomatic treatment in all cases of overdosage. Cyclosporine is not dialyzable to any great extent, nor is it cleared well by charcoal hemoperfusion.

Patient Information

Advise patients to not eat grapefruit or drink grapefruit juice while taking this medicine.

Women who could become pregnant should use nonhormonal contraceptives (diaphragms, condoms) while taking cyclosporine.

Instruct patients to contact their health care provider if fever, sore throat, tiredness, unusual bleeding or bruising, urination, or yellow skin/eyes occurs.

Instruct patients to not take potassium supplements while taking cyclosporine.

Cyclosporine may increase skin cancer risk. Advise patients to avoid prolonged exposure to the sun and other UV light and to use sunscreens and wear protective clothing while taking this medicine. Patients who are being treated for psoriasis will need to have at least 2 careful skin and physical examinations, including blood pressure measurements, before starting cyclosporine.

Patients should avoid live vaccines (eg, measles, mumps, oral polio) while taking cyclosporine. The vaccination may be less effective.

Cyclosporine may increase risk of high blood pressure and abnormal kidney function.

Cyclosporine may affect blood sugar level in diabetic patients.

DACLIZUMAB

Rx	**Zenapax** (Roche)	**Injection:** 25 mg/5 mL	Preservative-free. In single-use vials.

DACLIZUMAB — INJECTION

WARNING

Only physicians experienced in immunosuppressive therapy and management of organ transplant patients should prescribe daclizumab. The physician responsible for daclizumab administration should have complete information requisite for the follow-up of the patient. Daclizumab should only be administered by healthcare personnel trained in the administration of the drug who have available adequate laboratory and supportive medical resources.

Indications

➤*Renal rejection prophylaxis:* For the prophylaxis of acute organ rejection in patients receiving renal transplants. It is used as part of an immunosuppressive regimen that includes cyclosporine and corticosteroids.

Administration and Dosage

➤*Approved by the FDA:* December 10, 1997.

➤*Recommended dose:* Daclizumab is used as part of an immunosuppressive regimen that includes cyclosporine and corticosteroids. The recommended dose for daclizumab is 1 mg/kg. The calculated volume of daclizumab should be mixed with 50 mL of sterile 0.9% sodium chloride solution and administered via a peripheral or central vein over a 15-minute period.

Based on the clinical trials, the standard course of daclizumab therapy is 5 doses. The first dose should be given no more than 24 hours before transplantation. The 4 remaining doses should be given at intervals of 14 days.

➤*Instructions for administration:*

- Daclizumab is not for direct injection. The calculated volume should be diluted in 50 mL of sterile 0.9% sodium chloride solution before IV administration to patients. When mixing the solution, gently invert the bag in order to avoid foaming. Do not shake.
- Parenteral drug products should be inspected visually for particulate matter and discoloration before administration. If particulate matter is present or the solution colored, do not use.
- Care must be taken to ensure sterility of the prepared solution, since the drug product does not contain any antimicrobial preservative or bacteriostatic agents.
- Daclizumab is a colorless solution provided as a single-use vial; any unused portion of the drug should be discarded.
- Once the infusion is prepared, it should be administered IV within 4 hours. If it must be held longer, it should be refrigerated between 2° to 8°C (36° to 46°F) for up to 24 hours. After 24 hours, the prepared solution should be discarded.
- No incompatibility between daclizumab and polyvinyl chloride or polyethylene bags or infusion sets has been observed. No data are available concerning the incompatibility of daclizumab with other drug substances. However, other drug substances should not be added or infused simultaneously through the same IV line.
- Daclizumab may be administered by healthcare personnel trained in the administration of the drug who have available adequate laboratory and supportive medical resources.

➤*Storage/Stability:* Daclizumab is supplied in single-use glass vials. Vials should be stored between 2° to 8°C (36° to 46°F); do not shake or freeze. Protect undiluted solution against direct sunlight. Diluted medication is stable for 24 hours at 4°C (39.2°F) or for 4 hours at room temperature.

Actions

➤*Pharmacology:* Daclizumab functions as an IL-2 receptor antagonist that binds with high affinity to the Tac subunit of the high affinity IL-2 receptor complex and inhibits IL-2 binding. Daclizumab binding is highly specific for Tac, which is expressed on activated but not resting lymphocytes. Administration of daclizumab inhibits IL-2-mediated activation of lymphocytes, a critical pathway in the cellular immune response involved in allograft rejection.

While in the circulation, daclizumab impairs the response of the immune system to antigenic challenges. Whether the ability to respond to repeated or ongoing challenges with those antigens returns to normal after daclizumab is cleared is unknown.

Pharmacodynamics – In vitro and in vivo data suggest that serum levels of 5 to 10 mcg/mL are necessary for saturation of the Tac subunit of the IL-2 receptors to block the responses of activated T lymphocytes. At the recommended dosage regimen, daclizumab saturates the Tac subunit of the IL-2 receptor for approximately 90 and 120 days posttransplant, respectively, in pediatric and adult patients. The duration of clinically significant IL-2 receptor blockade after the recommended course of daclizumab is not known. No significant changes to circulating lymphocyte numbers or cell phenotypes were observed by flow cytometry. Cytokine release syndrome has not been observed after daclizumab administration.

➤*Pharmacokinetics:*

Adults – In clinical trials involving renal allograft patients treated with a 1 mg/kg IV dose of daclizumab every 14 days for a total of 5 doses, peak serum concentration (mean ± SD) rose between the first dose (21 ± 14 mcg/mL) and fifth dose (32 ± 22 mcg/mL). The mean trough serum concentration before the fifth dose was 7.6 ± 4 mcg/mL. In vitro and in vivo data suggest that serum levels of 5 to 10 mcg/mL are necessary for saturation of the Tac subunit of the IL-2 receptors to block the responses of activated T lymphocytes.

Population pharmacokinetic analysis of the data using a 2-compartment open model gave the following values for a reference patient (45-year-old male white patient with a body weight of 80 kg and no proteinuria): Systemic clearance = 15 mL/hour, volume of central compartment = 2.5 L, volume of peripheral compartment = 3.4 L. The estimated terminal elimination half-life for the reference patient was 20 days (480 hours), which is similar to the terminal elimination half-life for human IgG (18 to 23 days). Bayesian estimates of terminal elimination half-life ranged from 11 to 38 days for the 123 patients included in the population analysis.

The influence of body weight on systemic clearance supports the dosing of daclizumab on a mg/kg basis. For patients studied, this dosing maintained drug exposure within 30% of the reference exposure. Covariate analyses showed that no dosage adjustments based on age, race, gender, or degree of proteinuria, are required for renal allograft patients. The estimated interpatient variability (percent coefficient of variation) in systemic clearance and central volume of distribution were 15% and 27%, respectively.

Children – Pharmacokinetic parameters were evaluated in 61 pediatric patients treated with a 1 mg/kg IV dose of daclizumab every 14 days for a total of 5 doses. Peak serum concentration (mean ± SD) rose between the first dose (16 ± 12 mcg/mL) and fifth dose (21 ± 14 mcg/mL). The mean trough serum concentration before the fifth dose was 5 ± 2.7 mcg/mL. Population pharmacokinetic analysis of the data using a 2-compartment open model gave the following values for a reference patient (white patient with a body weight of 29.7 kg): Systemic clearance = 10 mL/hour, volume of central compartment = 2 L, volume of peripheral compartment = 1.4 L. The estimated terminal elimination half-life for the reference patient was 13 days (317 hours). For the patients studied, this dosing maintained drug exposure within 50% of the reference exposure. Covariate analyses suggested that disposition parameters were not influenced to a clinically relevant extent by race, gender, or degree of proteinuria. The estimated interpatient variability (percent coefficient of variation) in systemic clearance and central volume of distribution were 30% and 40%, respectively.

Contraindications

Hypersensitivity to daclizumab or to any components of this product.

Warnings

➤*Mortality:* The use of daclizumab as part of an immunosuppressive regimen including cyclosporine, mycophenolate mofetil, and corticosteroids may be associated with an increase in mortality. In a randomized, double-blind, placebo-controlled trial of daclizumab for the prevention of allograft rejection in 434 cardiac transplant recipients receiving concomitant cyclosporine, mycophenolate mofetil, and corticosteroids, mortality at 6 and 12 months was increased in those patients receiving daclizumab compared to those receiving placebo (7% vs 5%, respectively, at 6 months; 10% vs 6%, respectively, at 12 months). Some, but not all, of the increase in mortality appeared related to a higher incidence of severe infections. Concomitant use of antilymphocyte antibody therapy may also be a factor in some of the fatal infections.

See the Warning box for more information.

➤*Lymphoproliferative disorders/opportunistic infections:* While the incidence of lymphoproliferative disorders and opportunistic infections in the limited clinical trial experience was no higher in daclizumab-treated patients compared with placebo-treated patients, patients on immunosuppressive therapy are at increased risk for developing lymphoproliferative disorders and opportunistic infections and should be monitored accordingly.

➤*Hypersensitivity reactions:* Severe, acute (onset within 24 hours) hypersensitivity reactions including anaphylaxis have been observed both on initial exposure to daclizumab and following reexposure. These reactions may include hypotension, bronchospasm, wheezing, laryngeal edema, pulmonary edema, cyanosis, hypoxia, respiratory arrest, cardiac arrhythmia, cardiac arrest, peripheral edema, loss of consciousness, fever, rash, urticaria, diaphoresis, pruritus, and/or injection site reactions. If a severe hypersensitivity reaction occurs, therapy with daclizumab should be permanently discontinued. Medications for the treatment of severe hypersensitivity reactions including anaphylaxis should be available for immediate use. Patients previously administered daclizumab should only be reexposed to a subsequent course of therapy with caution. The potential risks of such readministration, specifically those associated with immunosuppression, are not known.

➤*Elderly:* Clinical studies of daclizumab did not include sufficient numbers of subjects 65 years of age and older to determine whether they respond differently from younger subjects. Caution must be used in giving immunosuppressive drugs to elderly patients.

➤*Pregnancy: Category C.* In general, IgG molecules are known to cross the placental barrier. Daclizumab should not be used in pregnant women unless the potential benefit justifies the potential risk to the fetus. Women of childbearing potential should use effective contraception before beginning daclizumab therapy, during therapy, and for 4 months after completion of daclizumab therapy.

DACLIZUMAB — INJECTION

➤*Lactation:* It is not known whether daclizumab is excreted in human milk. Because many drugs are excreted in human milk, including human antibodies, and because of the potential for adverse reactions, a decision should be made to discontinue nursing or to discontinue the drug, taking into account the importance of the drug to the mother.

➤*Children:* The safety profile of daclizumab in pediatric transplant patients was shown to be comparable with that in adult transplant patients with the exception of the following adverse reactions, which occurred more frequently in pediatric patients (greater than 15% difference in incidence): Diarrhea, postoperative pain, fever, vomiting, aggravated hypertension, pruritus, and infections of the upper respiratory tract and urinary tract.

Precautions

➤*Readministration:* Readministration of daclizumab after an initial course of therapy has not been studied in humans. The potential risks of such readministration, specifically those associated with immunosuppression and/or the occurrence of anaphylaxis/anaphylactoid reactions, are not known.

Drug Interactions

See Warnings for more information.

Adverse Reactions

➤*Mortality:* See Warnings for more information.

➤*Discontinuation:* Adverse events were reported by 95% of the patients in the placebo-treated group and 96% of the patients in the daclizumab-treated group. The proportion of patients prematurely withdrawn from the combined studies because of adverse events was 8.5% in the placebo-treated group and 8.6% in the daclizumab-treated group.

➤*Most common:* Daclizumab did not increase the number of serious adverse events observed compared with placebo. The most frequently reported adverse events were GI disorders, which were reported with equal frequency in daclizumab (67%) and placebo-treated (68%) patient groups.

The incidence and types of adverse events were similar in both placebo-treated and daclizumab-treated patients. These events included:

➤*Cardiovascular:*

Greater than or equal to 5% – Tachycardia, thrombosis.

➤*CNS:*

Greater than or equal to 5% – Tremor, headache, dizziness, hypertension, hypotension, aggravated hypertension.

Less than 5% to greater than or equal to 2% – Urinary retention, leg cramps, prickly sensation.

➤*Dermatologic:*

Greater than or equal to 5% – Impaired wound healing without infection, acne.

Less than 5% to greater than or equal to 2% – Pruritus, hirsutism, rash, night sweats, increased sweating.

➤*GI:*

Greater than or equal to 5% – Constipation, nausea, diarrhea, vomiting, abdominal pain, pyrosis, dyspepsia, abdominal distention, epigastric pain not food-related.

Less than 5% to greater than or equal to 2% – Flatulence, gastritis, hemorrhoids.

➤*GU:*

Greater than or equal to 5% – Oliguria, dysuria, renal tubular necrosis.

Less than 5% to greater than or equal to 2% – Renal damage, hydronephrosis, urinary tract bleeding, urinary tract disorder, renal insufficiency.

➤*Hematologic:*

Greater than or equal to 5% – Bleeding.

➤*Hematologic/Lymphatic:*

Greater than or equal to 5% – Lymphocele.

➤*Musculoskeletal:*

Greater than or equal to 5% – Musculoskeletal pain, back pain.

Less than 5% to greater than or equal to 2% – Arthralgia, myalgia.

➤*Metabolic/Nutritional:*

Greater than or equal to 5% – Edema extremities, edema.

Less than 5% to greater than or equal to 2% – Fluid overload, diabetes mellitus, dehydration.

➤*Ophthalmic:*

Less than 5% to greater than or equal to 2% – Vision blurred.

➤*Psychiatric:*

Greater than or equal to 5% – Insomnia.

Less than 5% to greater than or equal to 2% – Depression, anxiety.

➤*Respiratory:*

Greater than or equal to 5% – Dyspnea, pulmonary edema, coughing.

Less than 5% to greater than or equal to 2% – Atelectasis, congestion, pharyngitis, rhinitis, hypoxia, rales, abnormal breath sounds, pleural effusion.

➤*Miscellaneous:*

Greater than or equal to 5% – Posttraumatic pain, chest pain, fever, pain, fatigue.

Less than 5% to greater than or equal to 2% – Application site reaction, shivering, generalized weakness.

➤*Incidence of malignancies:* One and 3 years after treatment, the incidence of malignancies was 2.7% and 7.8%, respectively, in the placebo group compared with 1.5% and 6.4%, respectively, in the daclizumab group. Addition of daclizumab did not increase the number of posttransplant lymphomas up to 3 years posttransplant. Lymphomas occurred at a frequency of less than or equal to 1.5% in both placebo-treated and daclizumab-treated groups.

➤*Hyperglycemia:* No differences in abnormal hematologic or chemical laboratory test results were seen between placebo-treated and daclizumab-treated groups with the exception of fasting blood glucose. Fasting blood glucose was measured in a small number of placebo- and daclizumab-treated patients. A total of 16% (10 of 64 patients) of placebo-treated and 32% (28 of 88 patients) of daclizumab-treated patients had high fasting blood glucose values. Most of these high values occurred either on the first day posttransplant when patients received high doses of corticosteroids or in patients with diabetes.

➤*Incidence of infectious episodes:* The overall incidence of infectious episodes, including viral infections, fungal infections, bacteremia and septicemia, and pneumonia, was not higher in daclizumab-treated patients than in placebo-treated patients in trials of renal transplantation. In a large randomized study of daclizumab used for the prevention of allograft rejection in patients receiving cardiac allografts, more patients receiving daclizumab experienced severe or fatal infections after 12 months of therapy when compared to those receiving placebo (10% vs 7%, respectively). The risks of infection or death may be increased in patients receiving concomitant antilymphocyte antibody therapy.

The types of infections reported were similar in both the daclizumab-treated and the placebo-treated groups. Cytomegalovirus infection was reported in 16% of the patients in the placebo group and 13% of the patients in the daclizumab group. One exception was cellulitis and wound infections, which occurred in 4.1% of placebo-treated and 8.4% of daclizumab-treated patients. At 1 year posttransplant, 7 placebo patients and only 1 daclizumab-treated patient had died of an infection. At 3 years posttransplant, 8 placebo patients and 4 patients treated with daclizumab had died of an infection.

➤*Immunogenicity:* Low titers of antiidiotype antibodies to daclizumab were detected in the adult patients treated with daclizumab with an overall incidence of 14%. The incidence of antidaclizumab antibodies observed in the pediatric patients was 34%. No antibodies that affected efficacy, safety, serum daclizumab levels or any other clinically relevant parameter examined were detected. The data reflect the percentage of patients whose test results were considered positive for antibodies to daclizumab in an ELISA assay and are highly dependent on the sensitivity and specificity of the assay. Additionally, the observed incidence of antibody positivity in the assay may be influenced by several factors including sample handling, timing of sample collection, concomitant medications, and underlying disease. For these reasons, comparison of the incidence of antibodies to daclizumab with the incidence of antibodies to other products may be misleading.

➤*Postmarketing experience:* Severe acute hypersensitivity reactions including anaphylaxis characterized by hypotension, bronchospasm, wheezing, laryngeal edema, pulmonary edema, cyanosis, hypoxia, respiratory arrest, cardiac arrhythmia, cardiac arrest, peripheral edema, loss of consciousness, fever, rash, urticaria, diaphoresis, pruritus, and/or injection site reactions, as well as cytokine release syndrome, have been reported during postmarketing experience with daclizumab. The relationship between these reactions and the development of antibodies to daclizumab is unknown.

Overdosage

There have not been any reports of overdoses with daclizumab. A maximum tolerated dose has not been determined in patients. A dose of 1.5 mg/kg has been administered to bone marrow transplant recipients without any associated adverse events.

GLATIRAMER ACETATE

Rx	**Copaxone** (Teva)	**Injection, premixed:** 20 mg/mL	40 mg mannitol. Preservative free. In single-use prefilled syringes.

GLATIRAMER ACETATE — INJECTION

Indications

➤*Multiple sclerosis:* For reduction of the frequency of relapses in patients with relapsing-remitting multiple sclerosis (MS).

Administration and Dosage

➤*Approved by the FDA:* December 20, 1996.

➤*Recommended dose:* 20 mg/day injected SC.

➤*Instructions for use:* Remove 1 blister with the syringe inside from the glatiramer acetate injection pre-filled syringes package from the refrigerator. Let the pre-filled syringe package stand at room temperature for 20 minutes to allow the solution to warm up to room temperature. Store all unused syringes in the refrigerator. Inspect the reconstituted product visually and discard or return the product to the pharmacist before use if it contains particulate matter.

Sites for self-injection include arms, abdomen, hips, and thighs. The pre-filled syringe is suitable for single use only; unused portions should be discarded.

➤*Storage/Stability:* The recommended storage condition for the unreconstituted product is refrigeration (2° to 8°C; 36° to 46°F). However, excursions from recommended storage conditions to room temperature conditions (15° to 30°C; 59° to 86°F) for up to 1 week have been shown to have no adverse impact on the product. Exposure to higher temperatures or intense light should be avoided.

Glatiramer acetate injection contains no preservative. Do not use if the solution contains any particulate matter.

Actions

➤*Pharmacology:* The mechanism(s) by which glatiramer acetate exerts its effects in patients with multiple sclerosis (MS) is (are) not fully elucidated. However, it is thought to act by modifying immune processes that are currently believed to be responsible for the pathogenesis of MS. This hypothesis is supported by findings of studies that have been carried out to explore the pathogenesis of experimental allergic encephalomyelitis (EAE), a condition induced in several animal species through immunization against central nervous system-derived material containing myelin and often used as an experimental animal model of MS. Studies in animals and in vitro systems suggest that upon its administration, glatiramer acetate-specific suppressor T-cells are induced and activated in the periphery.

Because glatiramer acetate can modify immune functions, concerns exist about its potential to alter naturally occurring immune responses. Results of a limited battery of tests designed to evaluate the risk produced no finding of concern; nevertheless, there is no logical way to absolutely exclude this possibility.

➤*Pharmacokinetics:* Results obtained in pharmacokinetic studies performed in humans (healthy volunteers) and animals support the assumption that a substantial fraction of the therapeutic dose delivered to patients subcutaneously is hydrolyzed locally. Nevertheless, larger fragments of glatiramer acetate can be recognized by glatiramer acetate-reactive antibodies. Some fraction of the injected material, either intact or partially hydrolyzed, is presumed to enter the lymphatic circulation, enabling it to reach regional lymph nodes, and some may enter the systemic circulation intact.

Contraindications

Hypersensitivity to glatiramer acetate or mannitol.

Warnings

➤*For subcutaneous use:* The only recommended route of administration of glatiramer acetate injection is the SC route. Glatiramer acetate should not be administered by the IV route.

➤*Pregnancy:* Category B.

There are no adequate and well-controlled studies in pregnant women. Because animal reproduction studies are not always predictive of human response, glatiramer acetate should be used during pregnancy only if clearly needed.

➤*Lactation:* It is not known whether glatiramer acetate is excreted in human milk. Because many drugs are excreted in human milk, caution should be exercised when glatiramer acetate is administered to a nursing woman.

➤*Children:* The safety and efficacy of glatiramer acetate have not been established in individuals under 18 years of age.

Precautions

➤*Considerations regarding the use of a product capable of modifying immune response:* Because glatiramer acetate can modify immune response, it could possibly interfere with useful immune function. For example, treatment with glatiramer acetate might, in theory, interfere with the recognition of foreign antigens in a way that would undermine the body's tumor surveillance and its defenses against infection. There is no evidence that glatiramer acetate does this, but there has as yet been no systematic evaluation of the risk. Also, while glatiramer acetate is intended to minimize the autoimmune response to myelin, the possibility exists that continued alteration of cellular immunity from chronic treatment with glatiramer acetate might result in untoward effects. Because glatiramer acetate is an antigenic material it is possible that its use may lead to the induction of host responses that are untoward.

Although there is no evidence that use of glatiramer acetate induces untoward host responses in humans, systematic surveillance for these effects has not been undertaken. Studies in both the rat and monkey, however, have suggested that immune complexes are deposited in the renal glomeruli. Furthermore, in a controlled trial of 125 relapsing-remitting MS patients given glatiramer acetate, 20 mg, SC every day for 2 years, serum IgG levels reached ≈ 3 times baseline values in 80% of patients within 3 to 6 months of initiation of treatment. These values returned to about 50% greater than baseline during the remainder of treatment.

Although glatiramer acetate is intended to minimize the autoimmune response to myelin, there is the possibility that continued alteration of cellular immunity due to chronic treatment with glatiramer acetate might result in untoward effects. Anaphylaxis can be associated with the administration of almost any foreign substance. Based on the protein nature of glatiramer acetate, the risk of anaphylaxis cannot be excluded. Of the ≈ 900 patients treated in premarketing trials, none experienced anaphylactic shock.

Adverse Reactions

➤*Most common:* In controlled clinical trials the most commonly observed adverse experiences associated with the use of glatiramer acetate and not seen at an equivalent frequency among placebo-treated patients were the following: Injection site reactions, vasodilatation, chest pain, asthenia, infection, pain, nausea, arthralgia, anxiety, and hypertonia.

➤*Discontinuation:* Approximately 8% of the 893 subjects receiving glatiramer acetate discontinued treatment because of an adverse reaction. The adverse reactions most commonly associated with discontinuation were the following: Injection site reaction (6.5%), vasodilatation, unintended pregnancy, depression, dyspnea, urticaria, tachycardia, dizziness, and tremor.

➤*Immediate postinjection reaction:* Approximately 10% of MS patients exposed to glatiramer acetate in premarketing studies experienced a constellation of symptoms immediately after injection that included flushing, chest pain, palpitations, anxiety, dyspnea, constriction of the throat, and urticaria. In clinical trials, the symptoms were generally transient and self-limited and did not require specific treatment. In general, these symptoms have their onset several months after the initiation of treatment, although they may occur earlier, and a given patient may experience 1 or several episodes of these symptoms. Whether or not any of these symptoms actually represent a specific syndrome is uncertain. During the postmarketing period, there have been reports of patients with similar symptoms who received emergency medical care.

➤*Chest pain:* Approximately 26% of glatiramer acetate patients in the multicenter controlled trial (compared to 10% of placebo patients) experienced at least 1 episode of what was described as transient chest pain. While some of these episodes occurred in the context of the immediate postinjection reaction described above, many did not. The temporal relationship of this chest pain to an injection of glatiramer acetate was not always known. The pain was transient (usually lasting only a few minutes), often unassociated with other symptoms, and appeared to have no important clinical sequelae. EKG monitoring was not performed during any of these episodes. Some patients experienced more than one such episode, and episodes usually began at least 1 month after the initiation of treatment. The pathogenesis of this symptom is unknown.

Controlled trials in patients with MS (incidence of glatiramer acetate adverse reactions ≥ 2% and more frequent than placebo

	Glatiramer acetate (n = 201)		Placebo (n = 206)	
Preferred term	n	%	n	%
Miscellaneous				
Asthenia	83%	41%	78%	38%
Back pain	33%	16%	30%	15%
Bacterial infection	11%	5%	9%	4%
Chest pain	43%	21%	22%	11%
Chills	8%	4%	2%	1%
Cyst	5%	2%	1%	0%
Face edema	12%	6%	2%	1%
Fever	17%	8%	15%	7%
Flu syndrome	38%	19%	35%	17%
Infection	101%	50%	99%	48%
Injection site erythema	132%	66%	40%	19%
Injection site hemorrhage	11%	5%	6%	3%
Injection site induration	26%	13%	1%	0%
Injection site inflammation	98%	49%	22%	11%
Injection site mass	54%	27%	21%	10%
Injection site pain	147%	73%	78%	38%
Injection site pruritus	80%	40%	12%	6%
Injection site urticaria	10%	5%	0%	0%
Injection site welt	22%	11%	5%	2%
Neck pain	16%	8%	9%	4%
Pain	56%	28%	52%	25%

GLATIRAMER ACETATE — INJECTION

Controlled trials in patients with MS (incidence of glatiramer acetate adverse reactions ≥ 2% and more frequent than placebo				
	Glatiramer acetate (n = 201)		Placebo (n = 206)	
Preferred term	n	%	n	%
Cardiovascular				
Migraine	10%	5%	5%	2%
Palpitations	35%	17%	16	8%
Syncope	10%	5%	5%	2%
Tachycardia	11%	5%	8%	4%
Vasodilatation	55%	27%	21%	10%
GI				
Anorexia	17%	8%	15%	7%
Diarrhea	25%	12%	23%	11%
Gastroenteritis	6%	3%	2%	1%
Gastrointestinal disorder	10%	5%	8%	4%
Nausea	44%	22%	34%	17%
Vomiting	13%	6%	8%	4%
Hemic/lymphatic				
Ecchymosis	16%	8%	13%	6%
Lymphadenopathy	25%	12%	12%	6%
Metabolic/nutritional				
Edema	5%	3%	1%	0%
Peripheral edema	14%	7%	8%	4%
Weight gain	7%	3%	0%	0%
Musculoskeletal				
Arthralgia	49%	24%	39%	19%
CNS				
Agitation	8%	4%	4%	2%
Anxiety	46%	23%	40%	19%
Confusion	5%	2%	1%	0%
Foot drop	6%	3%	4%	2%
Hypertonia	44%	22%	37%	18%
Nervousness	4%	2%	2%	1%
Nystagmus	5%	2%	2%	1%
Speech disorder	5%	2%	3%	1%
Tremor	14%	7%	7%	3%
Vertigo	12%	6%	11%	5%
Respiratory				
Bronchitis	18%	9%	12%	6%
Dyspnea	38%	19%	15%	7%
Laryngismus	10%	5%	7%	3%
Rhinitis	29%	14%	27%	13%
Dermatologic				
Erythema	8%	4%	4%	2%
Herpes simplex	8%	4%	6%	3%
Pruritus	36%	18%	26%	13%
Rash	37%	18%	30%	15%
Skin nodule	4%	2%	1%	0%
Sweating	31%	15%	21%	10%
Urticaria	9%	4%	5%	2%
Special senses				
Ear pain	15%	7%	12%	6%
Eye disorder	8%	4%	1%	0%
GU				
Dysmenorrhea	12%	6%	10%	5%
Urinary urgency	20%	10%	17%	8%
Vaginal moniliasis	16%	8%	9%	4%

➤*Other reactions that occurred in at least 2%:* Other reactions that occurred in at least 2% of glatiramer acetate patients but were present at equal or greater rates in the placebo group included:

CNS – Dizziness, hypesthesia, paresthesia, insomnia, depression, dysesthesia, incoordination, somnolence, abnormal gait, amnesia, emotional lability, Lhermitte's sign, abnormal thinking, twitching, euphoria, and sleep disorder.

Dermatologic – Acne, alopecia, and nail disorder.

GI – Dyspepsia, constipation, dysphagia, fecal incontinence, flatulence, nausea and vomiting, gastritis, gingivitis, periodontal abscess, and dry mouth.

GU – Urinary tract infection, urinary frequency, urinary incontinence, urinary retention, dysuria, cystitis, metrorrhagia, breast pain, and vaginitis.

Lab test abnormalities – Laboratory analyses were performed on all patients participating in the clinical program for glatiramer acetate. Clinically significant laboratory values for hematology, chemistry, and urinalysis were similar for both glatiramer acetate and placebo groups in blinded clinical trials. No patient receiving glatiramer acetate withdrew from any trial because of abnormal laboratory findings.

Musculoskeletal – Myasthenia and myalgia.

Respiratory – Pharyngitis, sinusitis, increased cough and laryngitis.

Special senses – Abnormal vision, diplopia, amblyopia, eye pain, conjunctivitis, tinnitus, taste perversion, and deafness.

Miscellaneous – Headache, injection site ecchymosis, accidental injury, abdominal pain, allergic rhinitis, neck rigidity, and malaise.

Data on adverse reactions occurring in the controlled clinical trials were analyzed to evaluate differences based on sex. No clinically significant differences were identified. Ninety-two percent of patients in these clinical trials were white. This percentage reflects the racial composition of the MS population. In addition, the vast majority of patients treated with glatiramer acetate were between the ages of 18 and 45. Consequently, data are inadequate to perform an analysis of the adverse reaction incidence related to clinically relevant age subgroups.

➤*Other adverse reactions observed during clinical trials:* Reactions are further classified within body system categories and listed in order of decreasing frequency using the following definitions: Frequent adverse reactions are defined as those occurring in at least 1/100 patients; infrequent adverse reactions are those occurring in 1/100 to 1/1000 patients; rare adverse reactions are those occurring in less than 1/1000 patients.

Cardiovascular –
Frequent: Hypertension.
Infrequent: Hypotension, midsystolic click, systolic murmur, atrial fibrillation, bradycardia, fourth heart sound, postural hypotension, and varicose veins.

CNS –
Frequent: Abnormal dreams, emotional lability, and stupor.
Infrequent: Aphasia, ataxia, convulsion, circumoral paresthesia, depersonalization, hallucinations, hostility, hypokinesia, coma, concentration disorder, facial paralysis, decreased libido, manic reaction, memory impairment, myoclonus, neuralgia, paranoid reaction, paraplegia, psychotic depression, and transient stupor.

Dermatologic –
Frequent: Eczema, herpes zoster, pustular rash, skin atrophy, and warts.
Infrequent: Dry skin, skin hypertrophy, dermatitis, furunculosis, psoriasis, angioedema, contact dermatitis, erythema nodosum, fungal dermatitis, maculopapular rash, pigmentation, benign skin neoplasm, skin carcinoma, skin striae, and vesiculobullous rash.

Endocrine –
Infrequent: Goiter, hyperthyroidism, and hypothyroidism.

GI –
Frequent: Bowel urgency, oral moniliasis, salivary gland enlargement, tooth caries, and ulcerative stomatitis.
Infrequent: Dry mouth, stomatitis, burning sensation on tongue, cholecystitis, colitis, esophageal ulcer, esophagitis, gastrointestinal carcinoma, gum hemorrhage, hepatomegaly, increased appetite, melena, mouth ulceration, pancreas disorder, pancreatitis, rectal hemorrhage, tenesmus, tongue discoloration, and duodenal ulcer.

GU –
Frequent: Amenorrhea, hematuria, impotence, menorrhagia, suspicious papanicolaou smear, urinary frequency and vaginal hemorrhage.
Infrequent: Vaginitis, flank pain (kidney), abortion, breast engorgement, breast enlargement, carcinoma in situ cervix, fibrocystic breast, kidney calculus, nocturia, ovarian cyst, priapism, pyelonephritis, abnormal sexual function, and urethritis.

Hematologic / Lymphatic –
Infrequent: Leukopenia, anemia, cyanosis, eosinophilia, hematemesis, lymphedema, pancytopenia, and splenomegaly.

Metabolic / Nutritional –
Infrequent: Weight loss, alcohol intolerance, Cushing's syndrome, gout, abnormal healing, and xanthoma.

Musculoskeletal –
Infrequent: Arthritis, muscle atrophy, bone pain, bursitis, kidney pain, muscle disorder, myopathy, osteomyelitis, tendon pain, and tenosynovitis.

Ophthalmic –
Frequent: Visual field defect.
Infrequent: Dry eyes, cataract, corneal ulcer, mydriasis, photophobia, and optic neuritis.

Respiratory –
Frequent: Hyperventilation, hay-fever.
Infrequent: Asthma, pneumonia, epistaxis, hypoventilation, and voice alteration.

GLATIRAMER ACETATE — INJECTION

Special senses –
Infrequent: Otitis externa, ptosis, and taste loss.

Miscellaneous –
Frequent: Injection site edema, injection site atrophy, abscess, injection site hypersensitivity.
Infrequent: Injection site hematoma, injection site fibrosis, moon face, cellulitis, generalized edema, hernia, injection site abscess, serum sickness, suicide attempt, injection site hypertrophy, injection site melanosis, lipoma, and photosensitivity reaction.

➤*Postmarketing:* Postmarketing experience has shown an adverse event profile similar to that presented above. Reports of adverse reactions occurring under treatment with glatiramer acetate not mentioned, above that have been received since market introduction and that may have or not have causal relationship to the drug include the following:

Cardiovascular – Thrombosis; peripheral vascular disease; pericardial effusion; myocardial infarct; deep thrombophlebitis; coronary occlusion; congestive heart failure; cardiomyopathy cardiomegaly; arrythmia; angina pectoris.

CNS – Myelitis; meningitis; CNS neoplasm; cerebrovascular accident; brain edema; abnormal dreams; aphasia; convulsion; neuralgia.

GI – Tongue edema; stomach ulcer hemorrhage; liver function abnormality; liver damage; hepatitis; eructation; cirrhosis of the liver; cholelithiasis.

GU – Urogenital neoplasm; urine abnormality; ovarian carcinoma; nephrosis; kidney failure; breast carcinoma; bladder carcinoma; urinary frequency.

Hematologic / Lymphatic – Thrombocytopenia; lymphoma-like reaction; acute leukemia.

Metabolic / Nutritional – Hypercholesterolemia.

Musculoskeletal – Rheumatoid arthritis; generalized spasm.

Ophthalmic – Glaucoma; blindness; visual field defect.

Respiratory – Pulmonary embolus; pleural effusion; carcinoma of lung; hay fever.

Miscellaneous – Sepsis; LE syndrome; hydrocephalus; enlarged abdomen; injection site hypersensitivity; allergic reaction; anaphylactoid reaction.

Patient Information

Before you begin using glatiramer acetate, make sure you understand all the information in this section about its possible benefits and risks. If you do not understand some of the information, contact your doctor for help.

Glatiramer acetate is not recommended for use in pregnancy. Therefore, tell your doctor if you are pregnant, if you are planning to have a child, or if you become pregnant while you are taking this medicine.

Tell your doctor if you are nursing. We do not know if glatiramer acetate is passed through the milk to the baby.

Do not change the dose or dosing schedule without talking with your doctor.

Do not stop taking the drug without talking with your doctor.

The most common side effects of glatiramer acetate are redness, pain, swelling, itching, or a lump at the site of injection. These reactions are usually mild and seldom require professional treatment. Be sure to tell your doctor about any side effects.

Some patients report a short-term reaction right after injecting glatiramer acetate. This reaction can involve flushing (feeling of warmth or redness), chest tightness or pain with heart palpitations, anxiety, and trouble breathing. These symptoms generally appear within minutes of an injection, last about 15 minutes, and go away by themselves without further problems.

After you inject glatiramer acetate, call your doctor right away if you develop hives, skin rash with irritation, dizziness, sweating, chest pain, trouble breathing, severe pain at the injection site or other uncomfortable changes in your general health. Make no more injections until your doctor tells you to begin again.

If symptoms become severe, call 911 or the appropriate emergency phone number in your area. Make no more injections until your physician tells you to begin again.

Your prescription includes 2 types of vials (small bottles): Brown vials containing glatiramer acetate and clear vials of sterile water (diluent).

Store the brown vials of glatiramer acetate in the refrigerator as soon as you bring them home.

Store the clear vials labeled "Sterile Water for Injection" (diluent) at room temperature.

Keep glatiramer acetate out of the reach of children.

MUROMONAB-CD3

Rx	**Orthoclone OKT3** (Ortho Biotech)	**Injection:** 5 mg per 5 ml	With 1 mg polysorbate 80. In 5 ml amps.

MUROMONAB-CD3 — INJECTION

WARNING

Only physicians experienced in immunosuppressive therapy and management of renal transplant patients should use muromonab-CD3.

Anaphylactic or anaphylactoid reactions may occur following administration of any dose or course of muromonab-CD3. Serious and occasionally life-threatening systemic, cardiovascular and CNS reactions have been reported. These have included: Pulmonary edema, especially in patients with volume overload; shock; cardiovascular collapse; cardiac or respiratory arrest; seizures; coma. Hence, a patient being treated with muromonab-CD3 must be managed in a facility equipped and staffed for cardiopulmonary resuscitation.

Indications

➤*Renal allograft rejection:* Treatment of acute allograft rejection in renal transplant patients.

➤*Cardiac / Hepatic allograft rejection:* Treatment of steroid-resistant acute allograft rejection in cardiac and hepatic transplant patients.

➤*Unlabeled uses:* Prophylaxis and treatment of acute graft-versus-host disease (GVHD) in allogenic bone marrow transplantation.

Administration and Dosage

➤*Approved by the FDA:* 1986.

Administer as an IV bolus in < 1 minute. Do not give by IV infusion or in conjunction with other drug solutions.

➤*Renal allograft rejection, acute:* 5 mg/day for 10 to 14 days. Begin treatment once acute renal rejection is diagnosed.

➤*Cardiac / hepatic allograft rejection, steroid resistant:* 5 mg/day for 10 to 14 days. Begin treatment when it is determined that a rejection has not been reversed by an adequate course of corticosteroid therapy.

➤*Premedication:* Monitor patients closely for the first few doses. Methylprednisolone sodium succinate 8 mg/kg IV given 1 to 4 hours prior to muromonab-CD3 administration is strongly recommended to decrease the incidence of reactions to the first dose. Acetaminophen and antihistamines, given concomitantly, may reduce early reactions. Patient temperature should not exceed 37.8°C (100°F) prior to first administration.

➤*Other immune-suppressive drugs:* Reduce the dose of concomitant immunosuppressive drugs during muromonab-CD3 administration to the lowest level compatible with an effective therapeutic response. Resume maintenance immunosuppression ≈ 3 days prior to cessation of muromonab-CD3.

➤*Preparation of solution:* Draw solution into a syringe through a low protein-binding 0.2 or 0.22 micrometer (μm) filter.

➤*Admixture incompatibility:* Do not add or infuse other drugs simultaneously through the same IV line. If the same IV line is used for sequential infusion of several different drugs, flush with saline before and after infusion of muromonab-CD3.

➤*Storage / Stability:* Refrigerate at 2° to 8°C (36° to 46°F). Do not freeze or shake. Because this drug is a protein solution, it may develop a few fine translucent particles which do not affect its potency. Since no bacteriostatic agent is present in this product, use the amp immediately once opened and discard the unused portion.

Actions

➤*Pharmacology:* Muromonab-CD3 is a murine monoclonal antibody to the T3 (CD3) antigen of human T-cells that functions as an immunosuppressant. Muromonab-CD3 is for IV use only. The antibody is a biochemically purified IgG_{2a} immunoglobulin. It reverses graft rejection, probably by blocking the T-cell function, which plays a major role in acute allograft rejection. The drug reacts with, and blocks the function of, a molecule (CD3) in the membrane of human T-cells that is associated with the antigen recognition structure of T-cells and is essential for signal transduction. Muromonab-CD3 blocks all known T-cell functions and reacts with most peripheral T-cells in blood and in body tissues. Following termination of therapy, T-cell function usually returns to normal within 1 week.

A rapid concomitant decrease in the number of circulating CD2, CD3, CD4 and CD8 positive T-cells was observed within minutes after administration. This decrease in the number of CD3 positive T-cells results from the specific interaction between muromonab-CD3 and the CD3 antigen on the surface of all T-lymphocytes. T-cell activation results in the release of numerous cytokines/lymphokines, which are thought to be responsible for many of the acute clinical manifestations seen following muromonab-CD3 therapy (see Warnings).

Between days 2 and 7, increasing numbers of circulating CD4 and CD8 positive cells have been observed, although CD3 positive cells are not detectable. CD3 positive cells reappear rapidly and reach pretreatment levels within a week after therapy termination. Increasing numbers of CD3 positive cells have been observed in patients prior to termination of therapy, possibly caused by the development of neutralizing antibodies.

Antibodies have occurred (incidence of 21% for IgM, 86% for IgG and 29% for IgE). Mean time of appearance of IgG antibodies was 20 days. Early IgG antibodies occur towards the end of the second week of treatment in 3% of patients.

➤*Pharmacokinetics:* Serum levels are measured with an enzyme-linked immunosorbent assay (ELISA). During treatment with 5 mg/day for 14 days, mean serum trough levels rose over the first 3 days and then aver-

MUROMONAB-CD3 — INJECTION

aged 0.9 mcg/mL on days 3 to 14. Circulating serum levels ≥ 0.8 mcg/mL block the function of cytotoxic T-cells in vitro and in vivo.

Contraindications

Hypersensitivity to this or any product of murine origin; anti-mouse antibody titers ≥ 1:1000; patients in fluid overload or uncompensated heart failure, as evidenced by chest x-ray or > 3% weight gain within the week prior to treatment; history of seizures or predisposition to seizures; pregnancy, breastfeeding (see Warnings).

Warnings

➤*Cytokine release syndrome (CRS):* Temporally associated with the administration of the first few doses of muromonab-CD3 (particularly, the first two to three doses), most patients have developed an acute clinical syndrome (CRS) that has been attributed to the release of cytokines by activated lymphocytes or monocytes. This clinical syndrome has ranged from a more frequently reported mild, self-limited, "flu-like" illness to a less frequently reported severe, life-threatening shock-like reaction, which may include serious cardiovascular and CNS manifestations. The syndrome typically begins approximately 30 to 60 minutes after administration of a dose (but may occur later) and may persist for several hours. The frequency and severity of this symptom complex is usually greatest with the first dose. With each successive dose, both the frequency and severity of the CRS tend to diminish. Increasing the amount of a dose or resuming treatment after a hiatus may result in a reappearance of the CRS.

Common clinical manifestations – High fever (often spiking, up to 107°F); chills/rigors; headache; tremor; nausea/vomiting; diarrhea; abdominal pain; malaise; muscle/joint aches and pains; generalized weakness. Less frequently reported adverse experiences include minor dermatologic reactions (eg, rash, pruritus) and a spectrum of often serious, occasionally fatal, cardiorespiratory and neuro psychiatric adverse experiences.

Cardiorespiratory – Cardiorespiratory findings may include the following: Dyspnea; shortness of breath; bronchospasm/wheezing; tachypnea; respiratory arrest/failure/distress; cardiovascular collapse; cardiac arrest; angina/MI; chest pain/tightness; tachycardia (including ventricular); hypertension; hemodynamic instability; hypotension, including profound shock; heart failure; pulmonary edema (cardiogenic and non-cardiogenic); adult respiratory distress syndrome; hypoxemia; apnea; arrhythmias.

Pulmonary edema – In the initial renal rejection studies, potentially fatal, severe pulmonary edema, the most serious postdose reaction, occurred in 4.7% of the initial 107 patients. Fluid overload was present before treatment in all of these cases. However, it occurred in none of the subsequent 311 patients treated with first-dose volume/weight restrictions. In subsequent trials and in postmarketing experience, severe pulmonary edema has occurred in patients who appeared to be euvolemic. The pathogenesis of pulmonary edema may involve all or some of the following: Volume overload; increased pulmonary vascular permeability; reduced left ventricular compliance/contractility.

Serum creatinine – During the first 1 to 3 days of therapy, some patients have experienced an acute and transient decline in the glomerular filtration rate and diminished urine output with a resulting increase in the level of serum creatinine. Massive release of cytokines appears to lead to reversible renal function impairment or delayed renal allograft function. Similarly, transient elevations in hepatic transaminases have been reported following administration of the first few doses.

Fluid status – Prior to administration, assess the patient's volume (fluid) status carefully. It is imperative, especially prior to the first few doses, that there be no clinical evidence of volume overload or uncompensated heart failure, including a clear chest X-ray and weight restriction of ≤ 3% above the patient's minimum weight during the week prior to injection.

Prevention / Minimization of CRS – Manifestations of the CRS may be prevented or minimized by pretreatment with 8 mg/kg methylprednisolone (ie, high-dose steroids), given 1 to 4 hours prior to administration of the first dose of muromonab-CD3 and by closely following recommendations for dosage and treatment duration. If any of the more serious presentations of the CRS occur, intensive treatment including oxygen, IV fluids, corticosteroids, pressor amines, antihistamines, and intubation may be required.

➤*Neuropsychiatric events:* Seizures, encephalopathy, cerebral edema, aseptic meningitis, and headaches have occurred during therapy with muromonab-CD3, even following the first dose, resulting in part from T-cell activation and subsequent systemic release of cytokines.

Seizures – Seizures, some accompanied by loss of consciousness or cardiorespiratory arrest, or death, have occurred independently or in conjunction with any of the neurologic syndromes described below. Patients predisposed to seizures may include those with the following conditions: Acute tubular necrosis/uremia; fever; infection; a precipitous fall in serum calcium; fluid overload; hypertension; hypoglycemia, history of seizures and electrolyte imbalances; those who are taking a medication concomitantly that may, by itself, cause seizures. The number and regularity of seizure reports indicate that this hazard appears not to be rare. Anticipate convulsions clinically with appropriate patient monitoring.

Encephalopathy – Manifestations may include the following: Impaired cognition; confusion; obtundation; altered mental status; auditory/visual hallucinations; psychosis (delirium, paranoia); mood changes (eg, mania, agitation, combativeness); diffuse hypotonus; hyperreflexia; myoclonus; tremor; asterixis; involuntary movements; major motor seizures; lethargy/stupor/coma; diffuse weakness. Approximately one-third of patients with a diagnosis of encephalopathy may have had coexisting aseptic meningitis syndrome.

Cerebral edema – Cerebral edema and other signs of increased vascular permeability (eg, otitis media, nasal and ear stuffiness) have been seen in patients treated with muromonab-CD3 and may accompany some of the other neurologic manifestations.

Aseptic meningitis syndrome – The incidence of this syndrome was 6%. Fever (89%), headache (44%), meningismus (ie, neck stiffness; 14%) and photophobia (10%) were the most commonly reported symptoms; a combination of these 4 symptoms occurred in 5% of patients. Diagnosis is confirmed by CSF analysis demonstrating leukocytosis with pleocytosis, elevated protein and normal or decreased glucose, with negative viral, bacterial, and fungal cultures. In any immunosuppressed transplant patient with clinical findings suggesting meningitis, evaluate the possibility of infection. Approximately one-third of the patients with a diagnosis of aseptic meningitis had coexisting signs and symptoms of encephalopathy. Most patients with the aseptic meningitis syndrome had a benign course and recovered without any permanent sequelae during therapy or subsequent to its completion or discontinuation.

Headache – Headache is frequently seen after any of the first few doses and may occur in any of the aforementioned neurologic syndromes or by itself.

The following additional neurologic events have been reported occasionally: Irreversible blindness; impaired vision; quadri- or paraparesis/plegia; cerebrovascular accident (hemiparesis/-plegia); aphasia; transient ischemic attack; subarachnoid hemorrhage; palsy of the VI cranial nerve; hearing loss.

Signs or symptoms of encephalopathy, meningitis, seizures, and cerebral edema, with or without headache, have typically been reversible. Headache, aseptic meningitis, seizures, and less severe forms of encephalopathy resolved in most patients despite continued treatment. However, some events have been irreversible.

CNS adverse experiences – Patients who may be at greater risk for CNS adverse experiences include the following: Known or suspected CNS disorders (eg, history of seizure disorder); cerebrovascular disease (small or large vessel); conditions having associated neurologic problems (eg, head trauma, uremia); underlying vascular diseases; concomitant medication that may, by itself, affect the CNS.

➤*Infections:* Muromonab-CD3 is usually added to immunosuppressive therapeutic regimens, thereby augmenting the degree of immunosuppression. This increase in the total burden of immunosuppression may alter the spectrum of infections observed and increase the risk, the severity and the potential gravity (morbidity) of infectious complications. Approximately 1 to 6 months posttransplant, patients are at risk for viral infections (eg, cytomegalovirus, Epstein-Barr virus, herpes simplex virus), which produce serious systemic disease and also increase the overall state of immunosuppression. Multiple or intensive courses of any anti-T cell antibody preparation, including muromonab-CD3, which produce profound impairment of cell-mediated immunity, further increase the risk of (opportunistic) infection, especially with the herpes viruses and fungi. Anti-infective prophylaxis may reduce the morbidity associated with certain potential pathogens and should be considered for high-risk patients.

➤*Hypersensitivity reactions:* Serious and occasionally fatal, immediate (usually within 10 minutes) hypersensitivity (anaphylactic) reactions have occurred. Manifestations of anaphylaxis may appear similar to manifestations of the CRS. It may be impossible to determine the mechanism responsible for any systemic reaction(s). Reactions attributed to hypersensitivity have been reported less frequently than those attributed to cytokine release. Acute hypersensitivity reactions may be characterized by the following: Cardiovascular collapse; cardiorespiratory arrest; loss of consciousness; hypotension/shock; tachycardia; tingling; angioedema (including laryngeal, pharyngeal or facial edema); airway obstruction; bronchospasm; dyspnea; urticaria; pruritus.

Serious allergic events, including anaphylactic or anaphylactoid reactions, have been reported in patients re-exposed to muromonab-CD3 subsequent to their initial course of therapy. Pretreatment with antihistamines or steroids may not reliably prevent anaphylaxis in this setting. Weigh the possible allergic hazards of retreatment against expected therapeutic benefits and alternatives. If retreatment is employed, have epinephrine and other emergency life support equipment available, and monitor the patient closely.

If hypersensitivity is suspected, discontinue the drug immediately and do not resume therapy or re-expose the patient to muromonab-CD3. Serious acute hypersensitivity reactions may require emergency treatment with 0.3 to 0.5 mL aqueous epinephrine (1:1000 dilution) SC and other resuscitative measures. Refer to Management of Acute Hypersensitivity Reactions.

➤*Carcinogenesis:* As a result of depressed cell-mediated immunity, organ transplant patients have an increased risk of developing malignancies. This risk is evidenced almost exclusively by the occurrence of lymphoproliferative disorders (LPD), lymphomas and skin cancers. Following the initiation of muromonab-CD3 therapy, continuously monitor patients for evidence of LPD. Vigilant surveillance is advised, as early detection with subsequent reduction of total immunosuppression may result in regression of some of these lymphoproliferative disorders.

Because the potential for the development of LPD is related to the duration and extent (intensity) of total immunosuppression, it is advisable to adhere to the recommended dosage and duration of muromonab-CD3 and other anti-T lymphocyte antibody preparations administered within a short period of time. If appropriate, reduce the dosage(s) of immunosuppressive drugs used concomitantly to the lowest level compatible with an effective therapeutic response.

➤*Pregnancy: Category C.* It is not known whether muromonab-CD3 can cause fetal harm when administered to a pregnant woman or can affect

MUROMONAB-CD3 — INJECTION

reproduction capacity. However, it is an IgG antibody and may cross the placenta. If this drug is used during pregnancy, or the patient becomes pregnant while taking this drug, apprise the patient of the potential hazard to the fetus.

➤*Lactation:* It is not known whether muromonab-CD3 is excreted in breast milk. Because of the potential for serious adverse reactions/oncogenesis, decide whether to discontinue nursing or to discontinue the drug, taking into account the importance of the drug to the mother.

➤*Children:* Safety and efficacy in children have not been established. Muromonab-CD3 has been used in infants/children, beginning with a dose of ≤ 5 mg. Based on immunologic monitoring, the dosage has been adjusted accordingly. Pediatric recipients may be significantly immunosuppressed for a prolonged period of time and therefore require close monitoring post-therapy for opportunistic infection, particularly varicella (VZV), which poses an infectious complication unique to this population. GI fluid loss secondary to diarrhea or vomiting resulting from the CRS may be significant when treating small children and may require parenteral hydration. It is unknown whether there may be significant long-term sequelae (eg, neurodevelopmental language difficulties in infants < 1 year of age) related to the occurrence of seizures, high fever, CNS infections, or aseptic meningitis following muromonab-CD3 treatment. In cases where administration would be deemed medically appropriate, more vigilant and frequent monitoring is required for children than in adults.

Precautions

➤*Monitoring:* Monitor the following tests prior to and during therapy:

Renal – BUN, serum creatinine.

Hepatic – Transaminases, alkaline phosphatase, bilirubin.

Hematopoietic – WBCs and differential, platelet count.

Chest X-ray – Within 24 hours before initiating treatment, which should be free of any evidence of heart failure or fluid overload.

Monitor one of the following immunologic tests during therapy:

Plasma levels determined by an ELISA (target levels should be ≥ 800 ng/mL); or

Quantitative T-lymphocyte surface phenotyping (CD3, CD4, CD8); target CD3 positive T-cells < 25 cells/mm^3.

Testing for human-mouse antibody titers is strongly recommended; a titer ≥ 1:1000 is a contraindication for use.

➤*Intravascular thrombosis:* As with other immunosuppressive therapies, arterial, or venous thrombosis of allografts and other vascular beds (eg, heart, lungs, brain, bowel) have been reported. Consider these findings when deciding to use muromonab-CD3 in patients with a history of thrombotic events or underlying vascular disease. Consider concomitant use of prophylactic anti-thrombotic interventions (eg, minidose heparin).

➤*Special risk:* Patients at risk for more serious complications of the CRS may include those with the following conditions: Unstable angina; recent MI or symptomatic ischemic heart disease; heart failure of any etiology; pulmonary edema of any etiology; any form of chronic obstructive pulmonary disease; intravascular volume overload or depletion of any etiology (eg, excessive dialysis, recent intensive diuresis, blood loss); cerebrovascular disease; patients with advanced symptomatic vascular disease or neuropathy; history of seizures; septic shock. Make efforts to correct or stabilize background conditions prior to the initiation of therapy.

Drug Interactions

➤*Indomethacin:* Encephalopathy and other CNS effects have occurred with concurrent use.

Adverse Reactions

Cytokine release syndrome – See Warnings. In trials, the majority of patients experienced pyrexia (90%), of which 19% were ≥ 40°C (104°F), and chills (59%). Other adverse experiences occurring in ≥ 8% during the first 2 days included the following: Dyspnea (21%); nausea, vomiting (19%); chest pain, diarrhea (14%); tremor, wheezing (13%); headache (11%); tachycardia (10%); rigor, hypertension (8%).

Infections – See Warnings.

Renal rejection trial: The most common infections during the first 45 days of therapy were due to herpes simplex (27%) and cytomegalovirus (CMV; 19%). Other severe and life-threatening infections were *Staphylococcus epidermidis* (4.8%), *Pneumocystis carinii* (3.1%), *Legionella*, *Cryptococcus*, *Serratia*, and gram-negative bacteria (1.6%).

Hepatic rejection trial: The most common infections during the first 45 days of treatment were CMV (15.7%), fungal infections (14.9%) and herpes simplex (7.5%). Other severe and life-threatening infections were gram-positive (9%), gram-negative (7.5%), viral (1.5%), *Legionella* (0.7%). In another hepatic rejection trial, incidence of fungal infections was 34% and of herpes simplex virus infections was 31%.

Cardiac rejection trial: The most common infections reported during the first 45 days of treatment were herpes simplex (5%), fungal (4%), and CMV (3%).

Neoplasia – See Warnings.

Neuropsychiatric – See Warnings.

➤*Hypersensitivity:* See Warnings.

➤*Other:*

Cardiovascular – Cardiac arrest; hypotension/shock; heart failure; cardiovascular collapse; angina/MI; tachycardia; bradycardia; hemodynamic instability; hypertension; left ventricular dysfunction; arrhythmias; chest pain/tightness.

Dermatologic – Rash; Stevens-Johnson syndrome; urticaria; pruritus; erythema; flushing; diaphoresis.

GI – Diarrhea; nausea/vomiting; abdominal pain; bowel infarction; GI hemorrhage.

Hepatic – Increases in transaminases (eg, AST, ALT); hepato/splenomegaly or hepatitis, usually secondary to viral infection or lymphoma.

Musculoskeletal – Arthralgia; arthritis; myalgia; stiffness/aches/pains.

Renal – Anuria/oliguria; delayed graft function; transient and reversible increases in BUN and serum creatinine; abnormal urinary cytology, including exfoliation of damaged lymphocytes, collecting duct cells and cellular casts.

Respiratory – Respiratory arrest; adult respiratory distress syndrome (ARDS); respiratory failure; pulmonary edema (cardiogenic or noncardiogenic); apnea; dyspnea; bronchospasm; wheezing; shortness of breath; hypoxemia; tachypnea/hyperventilation; abnormal chest sounds; pneumonia/pneumonitis.

Special senses – Blindness; blurred vision; diplopia; hearing loss; otitis media; tinnitus; vertigo; VI cranial nerve palsy; photophobia; conjunctivitis; nasal/ear stuffiness.

Miscellaneous – Pancytopenia; aplastic anemia; neutropenia; leukopenia; thrombocytopenia; lymphopenia; leukocytosis; lymphadenopathy; arterial and venous thrombosis of allografts and other vascular beds (eg, heart, lung, brain, bowel); disturbances of coagulation; fever (including spiking temperatures as high as 107°F); chills/rigors; flu-like syndrome; fatigue/malaise; generalized weakness; anorexia.

Overdosage

Symptoms of overdose may include hyperthermia, severe chills, myalgia, vomiting, diarrhea, edema, oliguria, pulmonary edema, and acute renal failure. A high incidence (5%) of microangiopathic hemolytic anemia/HUS syndrome in patients receiving 10 mg/day was also reported. In the event of acute overdosage, carefully observe the patient and give symptomatic and supportive treatment.

Patient Information

Advise patients of the signs and symptoms associated with the cytokine release syndrome, including the potentially serious nature of this symptom complex (eg, systemic, cardiovascular, neuro-psychiatric events).

Advise patients to seek medical attention at the first sign of skin rash, urticaria, rapid heartbeat, difficulty in swallowing and breathing, or any swelling that may suggest angioedema or other allergic reaction.

Patients should know how they might react before operating an automobile or machinery, or engaging in activities requiring mental alertness, coordination, or physical dexterity.

MYCOPHENOLATE MOFETIL

Rx	**CellCept** (Roche)	**Capsules**: 250 mg (as mofetil)	(CellCept 250 Roche). Blue/brown. In 100s, 500s, and packages containing 12 bottles of 120s.
		Tablets: 500 mg (as mofetil)	Alcohols. (CellCept 500 Roche). Lavender. Caplet-shaped. Film-coated. In 100s and 500s.
Rx	**CellCept** (Roche)	**Powder for oral suspension**: 200 mg/mL (constituted) (as mofetil)	0.56 mg/mL phenylalanine, aspartame, methylparaben, sorbitol. Mixed fruit flavor. In 225 mL.
		Powder for injection, lyophilized: 500 mg (as mofetil)	Sodium hydroxide. Preservative free. In 20 mL vials.

MYCOPHENOLATE MOFETIL — ORAL

WARNING

Increased susceptibility to infection and the possible development of lymphoma may result from immunosuppression. Only health care providers experienced in immunosuppressive therapy and management of renal, cardiac, or hepatic transplant patients should use mycophenolate. Manage patients receiving the drug in facilities equipped and staffed with adequate laboratory and supportive medical resources. The health care provider responsible for maintenance therapy should have complete information requisite for the follow-up of the patient.

Indications

➤*Renal, cardiac, and hepatic transplant:* For the prophylaxis of organ rejection in patients receiving allogeneic renal, cardiac, or hepatic transplants. Use mycophenolate concomitantly with cyclosporine and corticosteroids.

➤*Unlabeled uses:* Refractory uveitis (2 g/day or in combination with previous corticosteroid, cyclosporine, or tacrolimus therapy); second-line therapy for Churg-Strauss syndrome; in combination with prednisolone for the treatment of diffuse proliferative lupus nephritis.

Administration and Dosage

➤*Approved by the FDA:* May 9, 1995.

➤*Renal transplantation:*

Adults – 1 g administered orally twice a day (daily dosage of 2 g). Although a dosage of 1.5 g administered twice a day (daily dosage of 3 g) was used in clinical trials and was shown to be safe and effective, no efficacy advantage could be established for renal transplant patients. Patients receiving 2 g/day of mycophenolate demonstrated an overall better safety profile than did patients receiving 3 g/day of mycophenolate.

➤*Pediatric patients:* The recommended dosage of mycophenolate oral suspension is 600 mg/m^2 administered twice a day (up to a maximum daily dosage of 2 g per 10 mL oral suspension). Patients with a body surface area of 1.25 to 1.5 m^2 may be dosed with mycophenolate capsules at a dosage of 750 mg twice a day (1.5 g daily dosage). Patients with a body surface area greater than 1.5 m^2 may be dosed with mycophenolate capsules or tablets at a dosage of 1 g twice a day (2 g daily dosage).

➤*Cardiac transplantation:* 1.5 g twice a day administered orally (daily dosage of 3 g).

➤*Hepatic transplantation:* 1.5 g twice a day administered orally (daily dosage of 3 g).

➤*Capsules, tablets, and oral suspension:* Give the initial oral dose of mycophenolate as soon as possible following renal, cardiac, or hepatic transplantation. Food has been shown to decrease mycophenolic acid C_{max} by 40%. Therefore, it is recommended that mycophenolate be administered on an empty stomach. However, in stable renal transplant patients, mycophenolate may be administered with food if necessary.

Note – If required, mycophenolate oral suspension can be administered via a nasogastric tube with a minimum size of 8 French (minimum 1.7 mm interior diameter).

➤*Preparation of oral suspension:* Mycophenolate has demonstrated teratogenic effects in rats and rabbits. There are no adequate and well-controlled studies in pregnant women. Take care to avoid inhalation or direct contact with skin or mucous membranes of the dry powder or the constituted suspension. If such contact occurs, wash thoroughly with soap and water; rinse eyes with water.

1.) Tap the closed bottle several times to loosen the powder.
2.) Measure 94 mL of water in a graduated cylinder.
3.) Add approximately half the total amount of water for constitution to the bottle and shake the closed bottle well for about 1 minute.
4.) Add the remainder of water and shake the closed bottle well for about 1 minute.
5.) Remove the child-resistant cap and push bottle adapter into neck of bottle.
6.) Close bottle with child-resistant cap tightly. This will ensure the proper seating of the bottle adapter in the bottle and child-resistant status of the cap.

Dispense with patient instruction sheet and oral dispensers. It is recommended to write the date of expiration of the constituted suspension on the bottle label. (The shelf-life of the constituted suspension is 60 days.)

➤*Dosage adjustments:* In renal transplant patients with severe chronic renal impairment (glomerular filtration rate [GFR] less than 25 mL/min per 1.73 m^2) outside the immediate posttransplant period, avoid dosages of mycophenolate greater than 1 g administered twice a day. Also carefully observe these patients. No dosage adjustments are needed in renal transplant patients experiencing delayed graft function postoperatively.

If neutropenia develops (absolute neutrophil count [ANC] less than 1.3 × 10^3/mcL), interrupt dosing or reduce the dosage of mycophenolate, perform appropriate diagnostic tests, and manage the patient appropriately.

➤*Handling and disposal:* Mycophenolate has demonstrated teratogenic effects in rats and rabbits. Do not crush mycophenolate tablets, and do not open or crush mycophenolate capsules. Avoid inhalation or direct contact with skin or mucous membranes of the powder contained in mycophenolate capsules and mycophenolate oral suspension (before or after constitution). If such contact occurs, wash thoroughly with soap and water; rinse eyes with plain water. If a spill occurs, wipe up using paper towels wetted with water to remove spilled powder or suspension.

➤*Storage/Stability:* Store at 25°C (77°F); excursions permitted to 15° to 30°C (59° to 86°F).

500 mg tablets – Dispense in light-resistant containers, such as the manufacturer's original containers.

Oral suspension – Store dry powder at 25°C (77°F); excursions permitted to 15° to 30°C (59° to 86°F). Store constituted suspension at 25°C (77°F); excursions permitted to 15° to 30°C (59° to 86°F) for up to 60 days. Storage in a refrigerator at 2° to 8°C (36° to 46°F) is acceptable. Do not freeze.

Discard any unused portion 60 days after constitution.

Actions

➤*Pharmacology:* Mycophenolate mofetil has been demonstrated in experimental animal models to prolong the survival of allogeneic transplants (kidney, heart, liver, intestine, limb, small bowel, pancreatic islets, and bone marrow).

Mycophenolate mofetil has also been shown to reverse ongoing acute rejection in the canine renal and rat cardiac allograft models. Mycophenolate mofetil also inhibited proliferative arteriopathy in experimental models of aortic and heart allografts in rats, as well as in primate cardiac xenografts. Mycophenolate mofetil was used alone or in combination with other immunosuppressive agents in these studies. Mycophenolate mofetil has been demonstrated to inhibit immunologically mediated inflammatory responses in animal models and to inhibit tumor development and prolong survival in murine tumor transplant models.

Mycophenolate mofetil is absorbed rapidly following oral administration and hydrolyzed to form mycophenolic acid, which is the active metabolite. Mycophenolic acid is a potent, selective, uncompetitive, and reversible inhibitor of inosine monophosphate dehydrogenase, and, therefore, inhibits the de novo pathway of guanosine nucleotide synthesis without incorporation into deoxyribonucleic acid (DNA). Because T- and B-lymphocytes are critically dependent for their proliferation on de novo synthesis of purines, whereas other cell types can utilize salvage pathways, mycophenolic acid has potent cytostatic effects on lymphocytes. Mycophenolic acid inhibits proliferative responses of T- and B-lymphocytes to both mitogenic and allospecific stimulation. Addition of guanosine or deoxyguanosine reverses the cytostatic effects of mycophenolic acid on lymphocytes. Mycophenolic acid also suppresses antibody formation by B-lymphocytes. mycophenolic acid prevents the glycosylation of lymphocyte and monocyte glycoproteins that are involved in intercellular adhesion to endothelial cells and may inhibit recruitment of leukocytes into sites of inflammation and graft rejection. Mycophenolate mofetil did not inhibit early events in the activation of human peripheral blood mononuclear cells (eg, the production of interleukin-1 and interleukin-2), but did block the coupling of these events to DNA synthesis and proliferation.

➤*Pharmacokinetics:*

Absorption – Mycophenolate mofetil is rapidly absorbed following oral administration and hydrolyzed to form mycophenolic acid, which is the active metabolite. Oral absorption of the drug is rapid and essentially complete. After oral administration, mycophenolate mofetil concentration is below the limit of quantitation (0.4 mcg/mL).

In 12 healthy volunteers, the mean absolute bioavailability of oral mycophenolate mofetil relative to IV mycophenolate mofetil (based on mycophenolic acid AUC) was 94%. The AUC for mycophenolic acid appears to increase in a dose-proportional fashion in renal transplant patients receiving multiple doses of mycophenolate mofetil up to a daily dosage of 3 g (see the following table).

Food (27 g fat, 650 calories) had no effect on the extent of absorption (mycophenolic acid AUC) of mycophenolate mofetil when administered at dosages of 1.5 g twice a day to renal transplant patients. However, mycophenolic acid C_{max} was decreased by 40% in the presence of food.

Distribution – The mean (± SD) apparent volume of distribution of mycophenolic acid in 12 healthy volunteers is approximately 3.6 (± 1.5) and 4 (± 1.2) L/kg following IV and oral administration, respectively. Mycophenolic acid, at clinically relevant concentrations, is 97% bound to plasma albumin. Mycophenolic acid glucuronate is 82% bound to plasma albumin at mycophenolic acid glucuronate concentration ranges that are normally seen in stable renal transplant patients; however, at higher mycophenolic acid glucuronate concentrations (observed in patients with renal impairment or delayed graft function), the binding of mycophenolic acid may be reduced as a result of competition between mycophenolic acid glucuronate and mycophenolic acid for protein binding. Mean blood-to-plasma ratio of radioactivity concentrations was approximately 0.6, indicating that mycophenolic acid and mycophenolic acid glucuronate do not distribute extensively into the cellular fractions of blood.

Metabolism – Following oral dosing, mycophenolate mofetil undergoes complete metabolism to mycophenolic acid, the active metabolite. Metabolism to mycophenolic acid occurs presystemically after oral dosing. Mycophenolic acid is metabolized principally by glucuronyl transferase to form the phenolic glucuronide of mycophenolic acid (mycophenolic acid glucuronate) which is not pharmacologically active. In vivo, mycophenolic acid glucuronate is converted to mycophenolic acid via enterohepatic recirculation. The following metabolites of the 2-hydroxyethyl-morpholino moiety are also recovered in the urine following oral administration of mycophenolate mofetil to healthy subjects: N-(2-carboxymethyl)-morpholine, N-(2-hydroxyethyl)-morpholine, and the N-oxide of N-(2-hydroxyethyl)-morpholine.

MYCOPHENOLATE MOFETIL — ORAL

Secondary peaks in the plasma mycophenolic acid concentration-time profile are usually observed 6 to 12 hours postdose. The coadministration of cholestyramine (4 g 3 times daily) resulted in approximately a 40% decrease in the mycophenolic acid AUC (largely as a consequence of lower concentrations in the terminal portion of the profile). These observations suggest that enterohepatic recirculation contributes to mycophenolic acid plasma concentrations.

Excretion – Negligible amount of drug is excreted as mycophenolic acid (less than 1% of dosage) in the urine. Oral radiolabeled mycophenolate mofetil resulted in complete recovery of the administered dose, with 93% of the administered dose recovered in the urine and 6% recovered in feces. Most (about 87%) of the administered dose is excreted in the urine as mycophenolic acid glucuronate. At clinically encountered concentrations, mycophenolic acid and mycophenolic acid glucuronate are usually not removed by hemodialysis. However, at high mycophenolic acid glucuronate plasma concentrations (greater than 100 mcg/mL), small amounts of mycophenolic acid glucuronate are removed. Bile acid sequestrants, such as cholestyramine, reduce mycophenolic acid AUC by interfering with enterohepatic circulation of the drug.

Mean (± SD) apparent half-life and plasma clearance of mycophenolic acid are 17.9 (± 6.5) hours and 193 (± 48) mL/min following oral administration.

Special populations –

Renal function impairment: Increased plasma concentrations of mycophenolate mofetil metabolites (mycophenolic acid 50% increase and mycophenolic acid glucuronate about a 3-fold to 6-fold increase) are observed in patients with renal insufficiency.

Pharmacokinetic Parameters for Mycophenolic Acid (Mean ± SD) Following Single Doses of Mycophenolate Capsules in Chronic Renal and Hepatic Impairment

Parameter	Dosage	T_{max} (h)	C_{max} (mcg/mL)	AUC (mcg•h/mL)
Renal impairment (number of patients)				
Healthy volunteers GFR > 80 mL/min per 1.73 m² (n = 6)	1 g	0.75 (± 0.27)	25.3 (± 7.99)	45 (± 22.6)[a]
Mild renal impairment GFR 50 to 80 mL/min per 1.73 m² (n = 6)	1 g	0.75 (± 0.27)	26 (± 3.82)	59.9 (± 12.9)[a]
Moderate renal impairment GFR 25 to 49 mL/min per 1.73 m² (n = 6)	1 g	0.75 (± 0.27)	19 (± 13.2)	52.9 (± 25.5)[a]
Severe renal impairment GFR < 25 mL/min per 1.73 m² (n = 7)	1 g	1 (± 0.41)	16.3 (± 10.8)	78.6 (± 46.4)[a]
Hepatic impairment (number of patients)				
Healthy volunteers (n = 6)	1 g	0.63 (± 0.14)	24.3 (± 5.73)	29 (± 5.78)[b]
Alcoholic cirrhosis (n = 18)	1 g	0.85 (± 0.58)	22.4 (± 10.1)	29.8 (± 10.7)[b]

[a] Interdosing interval $AUC_{0-96\ h}$.
[b] Interdosing interval $AUC_{0-48\ h}$.

Children:

Mean (± SD) Computed Pharmacokinetic Parameters for Mycophenolic Acid by Age and Time After Allogeneic Renal Transplantation

Age group (years)	(n)	Time	T_{max} (h)	Dose adjusted[a] C_{max} (mcg/mL)	Dosage adjusted[a] $AUC_{0-12\ h}$ (mcg•h/mL)
1 to < 2	(6)[b]	Early (day 7)	3.03 (4.7)	10.3 (5.8)	22.5 (6.66)
1 to < 6	(17)		1.63 (2.85)	13.2 (7.16)	27.4 (9.54)
6 to < 12	(16)		0.94 (0.546)	13.1 (6.3)	33.2 (12.1)
12 to 18	(21)		1.16 (0.83)	11.7 (10.7)	26.3 (9.14)[c]
1 to < 2	(4)[b]	Late (month 3)	0.725 (0.276)	23.8 (13.4)	47.4 (14.7)
1 to < 6	(15)		0.989 (0.511)	22.7 (10.1)	49.7 (18.2)
6 to < 12	(14)		1.21 (0.532)	27.8 (14.3)	61.9 (19.6)
12 to 18	(17)		0.978 (0.484)	17.9 (9.57)	53.6 (20.3)[d]
1 to < 2	(4)[b]	Late (month 9)	0.604 (0.208)	25.6 (4.25)	55.8 (11.6)
1 to < 6	(12)		0.869 (0.479)	30.4 (9.16)	61 (10.7)
6 to < 12	(11)		1.12 (0.462)	29.2 (12.6)	66.8 (21.2)
12 to 18	(14)		1.09 (0.518)	18.1 (7.29)	56.7 (14)

[a] Adjusted to a dosage of 600 mg/m².
[b] A subset of 1 to less than 6 years.
[c] n = 20.
[d] n = 16.

Pharmacokinetics in healthy volunteers, renal, cardiac, and hepatic transplant patients –

Pharmacokinetic Parameters for Mycophenolic Acid (Mean ± SD) Following Administration of Mycophenolate to Healthy Volunteers (Single Dose), Renal, Cardiac, and Hepatic Transplant Patients (Multiple Doses)

Parameter	Dose/Route	T_{max} (h)	C_{max} (mcg/mL)	AUC (mcg•h/mL)
Healthy volunteers (single dose)	1 g/oral	0.8 (± 0.36) (n = 129)	24.5 (± 9.5) (n = 129)	63.9 (±16.2) (n = 117)
Renal transplant patients (twice-daily dosing) Time after transplantation				
5 days (n = 31)	1 g/IV	1.58 (± 0.46)	12 (± 3.82)	40.8 (± 11.4)[a]
6 days (n = 31)	1 g/oral	1.33 (± 1.05)	10.7 (± 4.83)	32.9 (± 15)[a]
Early (< 40 days) (n = 25)	1 g/oral	1.31 (± 0.76)	8.16 (± 4.5)	27.3 (± 10.9)[a]
Early (< 40 days) (n = 27)	1.5 g/oral	1.21 (± 0.81)	13.5 (± 8.18)	38.4 (± 15.4)[a]
Late (> 3 months) (n = 23)	1.5 g/oral	0.9 (± 0.24)	24.1 (± 12.1)	65.3 (± 35.4)[a]
Cardiac transplant patients (twice-daily dosing) Time after transplantation				
Early (day before discharge)	1.5 g/oral	1.8 (± 1.3) (n = 11)	11.5 (± 6.8) (n = 11)	43.3 (± 20.8)[a] (n = 9)
Late (> 6 months)	1.5 g/oral	1.1 (± 0.7) (n = 52)	20 (± 9.4) (n = 52)	54.1 (± 20.4)[b] (n = 49)
Hepatic transplant patients (twice-daily dosing) Time after transplantation				
4 to 9 days (n = 22)	1 g/IV	1.5 (± 0.517)	17 (± 12.7)	34 (± 17.4)[a]
Early (5 to 8 days) (n = 20)	1.5 g/oral	1.15 (± 0.432)	13.1 (± 6.76)	29.2 (± 11.9)[a]
Late (> 6 months) (n = 6)	1.5 g/oral	1.54 (± 0.51)	19.3 (± 11.7)	49.3 (± 14.8)[a]

[a] Interdosing interval $AUC_{0-12\ h}$.
[b] $AUC_{0-12\ h}$ values quoted are extrapolated from data from samples collected over 4 hours.

Bioequivalence – Two 500 mg tablets have been shown to be bioequivalent to four 250 mg capsules. Five mL of the 200 mg/mL constituted oral suspension have been shown to be bioequivalent to four 250 mg capsules.

Contraindications

Hypersensitivity to mycophenolate, mycophenolic acid, or any component of the drug product.

Warnings

➤*Lymphomas/Malignancies:* Patients receiving immunosuppressive regimens involving combinations of drugs, including mycophenolate, as part of an immunosuppressive regimen are at increased risk of developing lymphomas and other malignancies, particularly of the skin. The risk appears to be related to the intensity and duration of immunosuppression rather than to the use of any specific agent. Oversuppression of the immune system can also increase susceptibility to infection, including opportunistic infections, fatal infections, and sepsis.

As usual for patients with increased risk for skin cancer, limit exposure to sunlight and ultraviolet (UV) light by wearing protective clothing and using a sunscreen with a high protection factor.

See Adverse Reactions for more information.

In pediatric patients, no other malignancies besides lymphoproliferative disorder (2 of 148 patients) have been observed.

➤*Infection/Sepsis:* In patients receiving mycophenolate (2 or 3 g) in controlled studies for prevention of renal, cardiac or hepatic rejection, fatal infection/sepsis occurred in approximately 2% of renal and cardiac patients and in 5% of hepatic patients.

➤*Neutropenia:* Severe neutropenia (ANC less than 0.5 × 10^3/mcL) developed in up to 2% of renal, up to 2.8% of cardiac, and up to 3.6% of hepatic transplant patients receiving mycophenolate 3 g daily. Monitor patients receiving mycophenolate for neutropenia. The development of neutropenia may be related to mycophenolate itself, concomitant medications, viral infections, or some combination of these causes. If neutropenia develops (ANC less than 1.3 × 10^3/mcL), interrupt dosing with mycophenolate or reduce the dosage, perform appropriate diagnostic tests, and manage the patient appropriately. Neutropenia has been observed most frequently in the period from 31 to 180 days posttransplant in patients treated for prevention of renal, cardiac, and hepatic rejection.

MYCOPHENOLATE MOFETIL — ORAL

➤*Renal function impairment:* Patients with severe chronic renal impairment (GFR less than 25 mL/min/1.73 m^2) who have received single doses of mycophenolate showed higher plasma mycophenolic acid and mycophenolic acid glucuronate AUCs relative to subjects with lesser degrees of renal impairment or healthy volunteers. No data are available on the safety of long-term exposure to these levels of mycophenolic acid glucuronate. Avoid dosages of mycophenolate greater than 1 g administered twice a day to renal transplant patients and carefully observe these patients.

No data are available for cardiac or hepatic transplant patients with severe chronic renal impairment. Mycophenolate may be used for cardiac or hepatic transplant patients with severe chronic renal impairment if the potential benefits outweigh the potential risks.

In patients with delayed renal graft function posttransplant, mean mycophenolic acid $AUC_{0\text{-}12\ h}$ was comparable, but mycophenolic acid glucuronate $AUC_{0\text{-}12\ h}$ was 2-fold to 3-fold higher, compared with that seen in posttransplant patients without delayed renal graft function. In the 3 controlled studies of prevention of renal rejection, there were 298 of 1,483 patients (20%) with delayed graft function. Although patients with delayed graft function have a higher incidence of certain adverse reactions (eg, anemia, thrombocytopenia, hyperkalemia) than patients without delayed graft function, these events were not more frequent in patients receiving mycophenolate than azathioprine or placebo. No dosage adjustment is recommended for these patients; however, carefully observe them.

➤*Mutagenesis:* The genotoxic potential of mycophenolate was determined in 5 assays. Mycophenolate was genotoxic in the mouse lymphoma/thymidine kinase assay and the in vivo mouse micronucleus assay. Mycophenolate was not genotoxic in the bacterial mutation assay, the yeast mitotic gene conversion assay, or the Chinese hamster ovary cell chromosomal aberration assay.

➤*Elderly:* In general, use cautious dosage selection for an elderly patient, reflecting the greater frequency of decreased hepatic, renal, or cardiac function and of concomitant or other drug therapy. Elderly patients may be at an increased risk of adverse reactions compared with younger individuals.

➤*Pregnancy: Category C.* In teratology studies in rats and rabbits, fetal resorptions and malformations occurred in rats at 6 mg/kg/day and in rabbits at 90 mg/kg/day, in the absence of maternal toxicity. These levels are equivalent to 0.03 to 0.92 times the recommended clinical dosage in renal transplant patients and 0.02 to 0.61 times the recommended clinical dosage in cardiac transplant patients on a BSA basis. In a female fertility and reproduction study conducted in rats, oral dosages of 4.5 mg/kg/day caused malformations (principally of the head and eyes) in the first generation offspring in the absence of maternal toxicity. This dosage was 0.02 times the recommended clinical dosage in renal transplant patients and 0.01 times the recommended clinical dose in cardiac transplant patients when corrected for BSA.

There are no adequate and well-controlled studies in pregnant women. Do not use mycophenolate in a pregnant woman unless the potential benefit justifies the potential risk to the fetus. Effective contraception must be used before beginning mycophenolate therapy, during therapy, and for 6 weeks after mycophenolate has been stopped.

Adverse reactions on fetal development (including malformations) occurred when pregnant rats and rabbits were dosed during organogenesis. These responses occurred at dosages lower than those associated with maternal toxicity, and at dosages below the recommended clinical dosage for renal, hepatic, or cardiac transplantation. There are no adequate and well-controlled studies in pregnant women. However, as mycophenolate has been shown to have teratogenic effects in animals, it may cause fetal harm when administered to a pregnant woman. Therefore, do not use mycophenolate in pregnant women unless the potential benefit justifies the potential risk to the fetus.

Women of childbearing potential should have a negative serum or urine pregnancy test with a sensitivity of at least 50 milliunits/mL within 1 week prior to beginning therapy. It is recommended that mycophenolate therapy not be initiated by the health care provider until a report of a negative pregnancy test has been obtained.

Effective contraception must be used before beginning mycophenolate therapy, during therapy, and for 6 weeks following discontinuation of therapy, even where there has been a history of infertility, unless due to hysterectomy. Two reliable forms of contraception must be used simultaneously unless abstinence is the chosen method. If pregnancy does occur during treatment, the health care provider and patient should discuss the desirability of continuing the pregnancy.

➤*Lactation:* Studies in rats treated with mycophenolate have shown mycophenolic acid to be excreted in milk. It is not known whether this drug is excreted in human milk. Because many drugs are excreted in human milk, and because of the potential for serious adverse reactions in breast-feeding infants from mycophenolate, decide whether to discontinue breast-feeding or the drug, taking into account the importance of the drug to the mother.

➤*Children:* Safety and efficacy in pediatric patients receiving allogeneic cardiac or hepatic transplants have not been established. See Administration and Dosage for more information.

Precautions

➤*Monitoring:* Perform complete blood counts weekly during the first month, twice monthly for the second and third months of treatment, then monthly through the first year.

➤*Infections:* In cardiac transplant patients, the overall incidence of opportunistic infections was approximately 10% higher in patients treated with mycophenolate than in those receiving azathioprine therapy, but this difference was not associated with excess mortality due to infection/sepsis among patients treated with mycophenolate.

There were more herpes virus (herpes simplex, herpes zoster, and cytomegalovirus) infections in cardiac transplant patients treated with mycophenolate compared with those treated with azathioprine.

➤*Rare hereditary deficiency:* On theoretical grounds, because mycophenolate is an IMPDH inhibitor, avoid its use in patients with rare hereditary deficiency of hypoxanthine-guanine phosphoribosyl-transferase (HGPRT) such as Lesch-Nyhan and Kelley-Seegmiller syndrome.

➤*Live, attenuated vaccines:* During treatment with mycophenolate, avoid the use of live, attenuated vaccines and advise patients that vaccinations may be less effective.

➤*Phenylketonurics:* Mycophenolate oral suspension contains aspartame, a source of phenylalanine (phenylalanine 0.56 mg/mL of suspension). Therefore, take care if mycophenolate oral suspension is administered to patients with phenylketonuria.

➤*GI effects:* GI bleeding (requiring hospitalization) has been observed in approximately 3% of renal, 1.7% of cardiac, and 5.4% of hepatic transplant patients treated with mycophenolate 3 g daily. In pediatric renal transplant patients, 5 of 148 cases of GI bleeding (requiring hospitalization) were observed.

GI perforations have been observed rarely. Most patients receiving mycophenolate were also receiving other drugs known to be associated with these complications. Patients with active peptic ulcer disease were excluded from enrollment in studies with mycophenolate. Because mycophenolate has been associated with an increased incidence of digestive system adverse reactions, including infrequent cases of GI tract ulceration, hemorrhage, and perforation, administer mycophenolate with caution in patients with active serious digestive system disease.

Drug Interactions

➤*Drugs that alter the GI flora:* Drugs that alter the GI flora may interact with mycophenolate by disrupting enterohepatic recirculation. Interference of mycophenolic acid glucuronate hydrolysis may lead to less mycophenolic acid available for absorption.

Mycophenolate Drug Interactions

Precipitant drug	Object drug[a]		Description
Acyclovir Ganciclovir	Mycophenolate	↑	Mycophenolic acid glucuronide and acyclovir plasma AUCs were increased 10.6% and 21.9%, respectively. Because mycophenolic acid glucuronide plasma concentrations are increased in the presence of renal impairment, as are acyclovir and ganciclovir concentrations, the potential exists for the 2 drugs to compete for tubular secretion, further increasing the concentrations of both drugs.
Mycophenolate	Acyclovir Ganciclovir		
Antacids	Mycophenolate	↓	Absorption of a single mycophenolate dose was decreased when coadministered with an aluminum/magnesium hydroxide antacid. The C_{max} and AUC for mycophenolic acid were 33% and 17% lower, respectively, than when mycophenolate was given alone. Avoid simultaneous administration.
Azathioprine	Mycophenolate	↔	It is recommended to avoid concomitant use because of a lack of clinical studies.
Cholestyramine	Mycophenolate	↓	Following coadministration, mycophenolic acid AUC decreased ≈ 40%. Do not give with cholestyramine or agents that may interfere with enterohepatic recirculation.
Iron	Mycophenolate	↓	Following coadministration, mycophenolate absorption and mycophenolic acid AUC were significantly decreased. Avoid concomitant administration.
Probenecid	Mycophenolate	↑	In animals, coadministration resulted in a 3-fold increase in plasma mycophenolic acid glucuronide AUC and a 2-fold increase in plasma mycophenolic acid AUC.
Salicylates	Mycophenolate	↑	Coadministration increased the free fraction of mycophenolic acid.

MYCOPHENOLATE MOFETIL — ORAL

Mycophenolate Drug Interactions

Precipitant drug	Object drug[a]		Description
Mycophenolate	Live attenuated vaccines	⬇	Coadministration may cause vaccinations to be less effective. Avoid if possible.
Mycophenolate	Oral contraceptives	⬇	Coadministration of mycophenolate and oral contraceptives containing levonorgestrel produced a significant decrease in the levonorgestrel AUC by ≈ 15%. Mean serum levels of LH, FSH, and progesterone were not significantly affected. Administer with caution and consider additional birth control methods.
Mycophenolate	Phenytoin	⬆	Mycophenolic acid decreased protein binding of phenytoin and may, therefore, increase free phenytoin levels.
Mycophenolate	Theophylline	⬆	Mycophenolic acid decreased protein binding of theophylline and may, therefore, increase free theophylline levels.

[a] ⬆ = Object drug increased. ⬇ = Object drug decreased. ⟷ = Undetermined clinical effect.

Adverse Reactions

The principal adverse reactions associated with the administration of mycophenolate include diarrhea, leukopenia, sepsis, vomiting, and there is evidence of a higher frequency of certain types of infections (eg, opportunistic infection). Adverse reactions were similar for oral and IV dosage forms.

➤*Elderly:* Elderly patients (65 years of age or older), particularly those who are receiving mycophenolate as part of a combination immunosuppressive regimen, may be at increased risk of certain infections (including cytomegalovirus [CMV] tissue-invasive disease) and possibly GI hemorrhage and pulmonary edema, compared with younger individuals.

Adverse Reactions in Controlled Studies in Prevention of Renal, Cardiac, or Hepatic Allograft Rejection (Reported in ≥ 20% of Patients in the Mycophenolate Mofetil Group)

	Renal studies			Cardiac study		Hepatic study	
Adverse reaction	Mycophenolate 2 g/day (n = 336)	Mycophenolate 3 g/day (n = 330)	Azathioprine 1 to 2 mg/kg/day or 100 to 150 mg/day (n = 326)	Mycophenolate 3 g/day (n = 289)	Azathioprine 1.5 to 3 mg/kg/day (n = 289)	Mycophenolate 3 g/day (n = 277)	Azathioprine 1 to 2 mg/kg/day (n = 287)
Cardiovascular							
Cardiovascular disorder	—	—	—	25.6%	24.2%	—	—
Hypertension	32.4%	28.2%	32.2%	77.5%	72.3%	62.1%	59.6%
Hypotension	—	—	—	32.5%	36%	—	—
Tachycardia	—	—	—	20.1%	18%	22%	15.7%
CNS							
Anxiety	—	—	—	28.4%	23.9%	—	—
Dizziness	—	—	—	28.7%	27.7%	—	—
Insomnia	—	—	—	40.8%	37.7%	52.3%	47%
Paresthesia	—	—	—	20.8%	18%	—	—
Tremor	—	—	—	24.2%	23.9%	33.9%	35.5%
Dermatologic							
Rash	—	—	—	22.1%	18%	—	—
GI							
Anorexia	—		—		—	25.3%	17.1%
Constipation	22.9%	18.5%	22.4%	41.2%	37.7%	37.9%	38.3%
Diarrhea	31%	36.1%	20.9%	45.3%	34.3%	51.3%	49.8%
Dyspepsia	—	—	—	—	—	22.4%	20.9%
Liver function tests abnormal	—	—	—	—	—	24.9%	19.2%
Nausea	19.9%	23.6%	24.5%	54%	54.3%	54.5%	51.2%
Vomiting	—	—	—	33.9%	28.4%	32.9%	33.4%
GU							
Kidney function abnormal	—	—	—	21.8%	26.3%	25.6%	28.9%
Urinary tract infection	37.2%	37%	33.7%	—	—	—	—
Hematologic/Lymphatic							
Anemia	25.6%	25.8%	23.6%	42.9%	43.9%	43%	53%
Hypochromic anemia	—	—	—	24.6%	23.5%	—	—
Leukocytosis	—	—	—	40.5%	35.6%	22.4%	21.3%
Leukopenia	23.2%	34.5%	24.8%	30.4%	39.1%	45.8%	39%
Thrombocytopenia	—	—	—	23.5%	27%	38.3%	42.2%
Metabolic/Nutritional							
Serum urea nitrogen (BUN) increased	—	—	—	34.6%	32.5%		—
Creatinine increased	—	—	—	39.4%	36%	—	—
Edema	—	—	—	26.6%	25.6%	28.2%	28.2%
Hypercholesterolemia	—	—	—	41.2%	38.4%	—	—
Hyperglycemia	—	—	—	46.7%	52.6%	43.7%	48.8%
Hyperkalomia	—	—	—	—	—	22%	23.7%
Hypocalcemia	—	—	—		—	30%	30%
Hypokalemia	—	—	—	31.8%	25.6%	37.2%	41.1%
Hypomagnesemia	—	—	—	—	—	39%	37.6%
Lactic dehydrogenase increased	—	—	—	23.2%	17%	—	—
Peripheral edema	28.6%	27%	28.2%	64%	53.3%	48.4%	47.7%
Respiratory							
Cough increased	—	—	—	31.1%	25.6%	—	—
Dyspnea	—	—	—	36.7%	36.3%	31%	30.3%
Infection	22%	23.9%	19.6%	37%	35.3%	—	—
Lung disorder	—	—	—	30.1%	29.1%	22%	18.8%
Pleural effusion	—	—	—	—	—	34.3%	35.9%

MYCOPHENOLATE MOFETIL — ORAL

Adverse Reactions in Controlled Studies in Prevention of Renal, Cardiac, or Hepatic Allograft Rejection (Reported in ≥ 20% of Patients in the Mycophenolate Mofetil Group)							
	Renal studies			Cardiac study		Hepatic study	
Adverse reaction	Mycophenolate 2 g/day (n = 336)	Mycophenolate 3 g/day (n = 330)	Azathioprine 1 to 2 mg/kg/day or 100 to 150 mg/day (n = 326)	Mycophenolate 3 g/day (n = 289)	Azathioprine 1.5 to 3 mg/kg/day (n = 289)	Mycophenolate 3 g/day (n = 277)	Azathioprine 1 to 2 mg/kg/day (n = 287)
Sinusitis	—	—	—	26%	19%	—	—
Miscellaneous							
Abdominal pain	24.7%	27.6%	23%	33.9%	33.2%	62.5%	51.2%
Ascites	—	—	—	—	—	24.2%	22.6%
Asthenia	—	—	—	43.3%	36.3%	35.4%	33.8%
Back pain	—	—	—	34.6%	28.4%	46.6%	47.4%
Chest pain	—	—	—	26.3%	26%	—	—
Fever	21.4%	23.3%	23.3%	47.4%	46.4%	52.3%	56.1%
Headache	21.1%	16.1%	21.2%	54.3%	51.9%	53.8%	49.1%
Infection	18.2%	20.9%	19.9%	25.6%	19.4%	27.1%	25.1%
Pain	33%	31.2 %	32.2%	75.8%	74.7%	74%	77.7%
Sepsis	—	—	—	—	—	27.4%	26.5%

➤*Lymphomas/Malignancies:* Lymphoproliferative disease or lymphoma developed in 0.4% to 1% of patients receiving mycophenolate (2 or 3 g daily) with other immunosuppressive agents in controlled clinical trials of renal, cardiac, and hepatic transplant patients followed for at least 1 year. Nonmelanoma skin carcinomas occurred in 1.6% to 4.2% of patients, other types of malignancy in 0.7% to 2.1% of patients. Three-year safety data in renal and cardiac transplant patients did not reveal any unexpected changes in incidence of malignancy compared with the 1-year data.

➤*Neutropenia:* See Warnings for more information.

➤*Infections:* All transplant patients are at increased risk of opportunistic infections. The risk increases with total immunosuppressive load. The following table shows the incidence of opportunistic infections that occurred in the renal, cardiac, and hepatic transplant populations in the azathioprine-controlled prevention trials:

Viral and Fungal Infections in Controlled Studies in Prevention of Renal, Cardiac, or Hepatic Transplant Rejection							
	Renal studies			Cardiac study		Hepatic study	
Infection	Mycophenolate 2 g/day (n = 336)	Mycophenolate 3 g/day (n = 330)	Azathioprine 1 to 2 mg/kg/day or 100 to 150 mg/day (n = 326)	Mycophenolate 3 g/day (n = 289)	Azathioprine 1.5 to 3 mg/kg/day (n = 289)	Mycophenolate 3 g/day (n = 277)	Azathioprine 1 to 2 mg/kg/day (n = 287)
Candida	17%	17.3%	18.1%	18.7%	17.6%	22.4%	24.4%
Mucocutaneous	15.5%	16.4%	15.3%	18%	17.3%	18.4%	17.4%
CMV							
Viremia/Syndrome	13.4%	12.4%	13.8%	12.1%	10%	14.1%	12.2%
Tissue-invasive disease	8.3%	11.5%	6.1%	11.4%	8.7%	5.8%	8%
Herpes simplex	16.7%	20%	19%	20.8%	14.5%	10.1%	5.9%
Herpes zoster	6%	7.6%	5.8%	10.7%	5.9%	4.3%	4.9%
Cutaneous disease	6%	7.3%	5.5%	10%	5.5%	4.3%	4.9%

The following other opportunistic infections occurred with an incidence of less than 4% in mycophenolate patients in the above azathioprine-controlled studies: herpes zoster, visceral disease; *Candida*, urinary tract infection, fungemia/disseminated disease, tissue-invasive disease; cryptococcosis; *Aspergillus*/Mucor; *Pneumocystis carinii*.

In patients receiving mycophenolate (2 or 3 g) in controlled studies for prevention of renal, cardiac, or hepatic rejection, fatal infection/sepsis occurred in approximately 2% of renal and cardiac patients and in 5% of hepatic patients.

See Precautions for more information.

Mycophenolate Adverse Reactions Reported in 3% to < 20% of Patients Treated with Mycophenolate in Combination with Cyclosporine and Corticosteroids	
Body system	Adverse reaction
Cardiovascular	Angina pectoris, arrhythmia, arterial thrombosis, atrial fibrillation, atrial flutter, bradycardia, cardiovascular disorder, congestive heart failure, extrasystole, heart arrest, heart failure, hypotension, pallor, palpitation, pericardial effusion, peripheral vascular disorder, postural hypotension, pulmonary hypertension, supraventricular extrasystoles, supraventricular tachycardia, syncope, tachycardia, thrombosis, vasodilatation, vasospasm, ventricular extrasystole, ventricular tachycardia, venous pressure increased.
CNS	Agitation, anxiety, confusion, convulsion, delirium, depression, dry mouth, emotional lability, hallucinations, hypertonia, hypesthesia, nervousness, neuropathy, paresthesia, psychosis, somnolence, thinking abnormal, vertigo.
Dermatologic	Acne, alopecia, fungal dermatitis, hemorrhage, hirsutism, pruritus, rash, skin benign neoplasm, skin carcinoma, skin disorder, skin hypertrophy, skin ulcer, sweating, vesiculobullous rash.
Endocrine	Cushing syndrome, diabetes mellitus, hypothyroidism, parathyroid disorder.
GI	Anorexia, cholangitis, cholestatic jaundice, dysphagia, esophagitis, flatulence, gastritis, gastroenteritis, GI disorder, GI hemorrhage, GI moniliasis, gingivitis, gum hyperplasia, hepatitis, ileus, infection, jaundice, liver damage, liver function tests abnormal, melena, mouth ulceration, nausea and vomiting, oral moniliasis, rectal disorder, stomach ulcer, stomatitis.
GU	Acute kidney failure, albuminuria, dysuria, hematuria, hydronephrosis, impotence, kidney failure, kidney tubular necrosis, nocturia, oliguria, pain, prostatic disorder, pyelonephritis, scrotal edema, urinary frequency, urinary incontinence, urinary retention, urinary tract disorder, urine abnormality.
Hemic and lymphatic	Coagulation disorder, ecchymosis, pancytopenia, petechia, polycythemia, prothrombin time increased, thromboplastin time increased.
Metabolic and nutritional	Abnormal healing, acidosis, alkaline phosphatase increased, alkalosis, ALT increased, AST increased, bilirubinemia, creatinine increased, dehydration, gamma-glutamyl transpeptidase increased, generalized edema, gout, hypercalcemia, hypercholesteremia, hyperlipemia, hyperphosphatemia, hyperuricemia, hypervolemia, hypocalcemia, hypochloremia, hypoglycemia, hyponatremia, hypophosphatemia, hypoproteinemia, hypovolemia, hypoxia, lactic dehydrogenase increased, respiratory acidosis, thirst, weight gain, weight loss.
Musculoskeletal	Arthralgia, joint disorder, leg cramps, myalgia, myasthenia, osteoporosis.

MYCOPHENOLATE MOFETIL — ORAL

Mycophenolate Adverse Reactions Reported in 3% to < 20% of Patients Treated with Mycophenolate in Combination with Cyclosporine and Corticosteroids	
Body system	Adverse reaction
Respiratory	Apnea, asthma, atelectasis, bronchitis, epistaxis, hemoptysis, hiccup, hyperventilation, lung disorder, lung edema, neoplasm, pain, pharyngitis, pleural effusion, pneumonia, pneumothorax, respiratory disorder, respiratory moniliasis, rhinitis, sinusitis, sputum increased, voice alteration.
Special senses	Abnormal vision, amblyopia, cataract (not specified), conjunctivitis, deafness, ear disorder, ear pain, eye hemorrhage, lacrimation disorder, tinnitus.
Miscellaneous	Abdomen enlarged, abscess, accidental injury, cellulitis, chills occurring with fever, cyst, face edema, flu syndrome, hemorrhage, hernia, lab test abnormal, malaise, neck pain, pelvic pain, peritonitis.

➤*Children:* The type and frequency of adverse reactions in a clinical study in 100 pediatric patients 3 months to 18 years of age dosed with mycophenolate 600 mg/m^2 oral suspension twice a day (up to 1 g twice a day) were generally similar to those observed in adult patients dosed with mycophenolate capsules at a dose of 1 g twice a day with the exception of abdominal pain, fever, infection, pain, sepsis, diarrhea, vomiting, pharyngitis, respiratory tract infection, hypertension, and anemia, which were observed in a higher proportion in pediatric patients.

➤*Postmarketing:*

GI – Colitis (sometimes caused by cytomegalovirus), pancreatitis, isolated cases of intestinal villous atrophy.

Respiratory – Interstitial lung disorders, including fatal pulmonary fibrosis, have been reported rarely and should be considered in the differential diagnosis of pulmonary symptoms ranging from dyspnea to respiratory failure in posttransplant patients receiving mycophenolate.

Resistance mechanism disorders – Serious life-threatening infections such as meningitis and infectious endocarditis have been reported occasionally and there is evidence of a higher frequency of certain types of serious infections such as tuberculosis and atypical mycobacterial infection.

Overdosage

➤*Symptoms:* There has been no reported experience of overdosage of mycophenolate in humans. The highest dosage administered to renal transplant patients in clinical trials has been 4 g/day. In limited experience with cardiac and hepatic transplant patients in clinical trials, the highest dosages used were 4 or 5 g/day. At dosages of 4 or 5 g/day, there appears to be a higher rate, compared with the use of less than or equal to 3 g/day, of GI intolerance (nausea, vomiting, or diarrhea), and occasional hematologic abnormalities, principally neutropenia, leading to a need to reduce or discontinue dosing.

In acute oral toxicity studies, no deaths occurred in adult mice at doses up to 4,000 mg/kg or in adult monkeys at doses up to 1,000 mg/kg; these were the highest doses of mycophenolate tested in these species. These doses represent 11 times the recommended clinical dose in renal transplant patients and approximately 7 times the recommended clinical dose in cardiac transplant patients when corrected for BSA. In adult rats, deaths occurred after single oral doses of 500 mg/kg of mycophenolate. The dose represents approximately 3 times the recommended clinical dosage in cardiac transplant patients when corrected for BSA.

➤*Treatment:* Mycophenolic acid and mycophenolic acid glucuronate are usually not removed by hemodialysis. However, at high mycophenolic acid glucuronate plasma concentrations (greater than 100 mcg/mL), small amounts of mycophenolic acid glucuronate are removed. By increasing excretion of the drug, mycophenolic acid can be removed by bile acid sequestrants (eg, cholestyramine).

Patient Information

Inform patients of the need for repeated appropriate laboratory tests while they are receiving mycophenolate. Give patients complete dosage instructions and inform them of the increased risk of lymphoproliferative disease and certain other malignancies. Instruct women of childbearing potential of the potential risks during pregnancy, and tell them to use effective contraception before beginning mycophenolate therapy, during therapy, and for 6 weeks after mycophenolate has been stopped.

Instruct patients receiving mycophenolate to report immediately any evidence of infection, unexpected bruising, bleeding, or any other manifestation of bone marrow depression.

➤*Phenylketonurics:* Mycophenolate oral suspension contains aspartame, a source of phenylalanine (phenylalanine 0.56 mg/mL of suspension).

MYCOPHENOLATE MOFETIL — INJECTION

WARNING

Increased susceptibility to infection and the possible development of lymphoma may result from immunosuppression. Only health care providers experienced in immunosuppressive therapy and management of renal, cardiac or hepatic transplant patients should use mycophenolate injection. Manage patients receiving the drug in facilities equipped and staffed with adequate laboratory and supportive medical resources. The health care provider responsible for maintenance therapy should have complete information requisite for the follow-up of the patient.

Indications

➤*Renal, cardiac, and hepatic transplant:* For the prophylaxis of organ rejection in patients receiving allogeneic renal, cardiac, or hepatic transplants. Use mycophenolate concomitantly with cyclosporine and corticosteroids.

Mycophenolate intravenous (IV) is an alternative dosage form to mycophenolate capsules, tablets, and oral suspension. Administer mycophenolate IV within 24 hours following transplantation. Mycophenolate IV can be administered for up to 14 days; switch patients to oral mycophenolate as soon as they can tolerate oral medication.

➤*Unlabeled uses:* Refractory uveitis (2 g/day alone or in combination with previous corticosteroid, cyclosporine, or tacrolimus therapy); second-line therapy for Churg-Strauss syndrome; in combination with prednisolone for the treatment of diffuse proliferative lupus nephritis.

Administration and Dosage

➤*Approved by the FDA:* August 12, 1998.

➤*Renal transplantation:*

Adults – 1 g administered IV (over no less than 2 hours) twice a day (daily dosage of 2 g). Although a dosage of 1.5 g administered twice a day (daily dosage of 3 g) was used in clinical trials and was shown to be safe and effective, no efficacy advantage could be established for renal transplant patients. Patients receiving 2 g/day of mycophenolate demonstrated an overall better safety profile than did patients receiving 3 g/day of mycophenolate.

➤*Cardiac transplantation:* 1.5 g twice a day administered IV (over no less than 2 hours).

➤*Hepatic transplantation:* 1 g twice a day administered IV (over no less than 2 hours).

➤*Mycophenolate IV:* Reconstitute and dilute mycophenolate IV to a concentration of 6 mg/mL using 5% dextrose injection (D5W). Mycophenolate IV is incompatible with other IV infusion solutions. Following reconstitution, administer mycophenolate IV by slow IV infusion over a period of no less than 2 hours by either peripheral or central vein.

Caution – Never administer mycophenolate IV solution by rapid or bolus IV injection.

Preparation of infusion solution (6 mg/mL) – Exercise caution in the handling and preparation of solutions of mycophenolate IV. Avoid direct contact of the prepared solution of mycophenolate IV with skin or mucous membranes. If such contact occurs, wash thoroughly with soap and water; rinse eyes with plain water.

Mycophenolate IV does not contain an antibacterial preservative; therefore, perform reconstitution and dilution of the product under aseptic conditions.

Mycophenolate IV infusion solution must be prepared in 2 steps: 1) reconstitution with 5% dextrose injection, and 2) dilution with 5% dextrose injection. Following is a detailed description of the preparation:

Step 1:

1.) Two vials of mycophenolate IV are used for preparing each 1 g dose, whereas 3 vials are needed for each 1.5 g dose. Reconstitute the contents of each vial by injecting 14 mL of 5% dextrose injection.
2.) Gently shake the vial to dissolve the drug.
3.) Inspect the resulting slightly yellow solution for particulate matter and discoloration prior to further dilution. Discard the vial if particulate matter or discoloration is observed.

Step 2:

1.) To prepare a 1 g dose, further dilute the contents of the 2 reconstituted vials (approximately 2 × 15 mL) into 140 mL of 5% dextrose injection. To prepare a 1.5 g dose, further dilute the contents of the 3 reconstituted vials (approximately 3 × 15 mL) into 210 mL of 5% dextrose injection. The final concentration of both solutions is mycophenolate 6 mg/mL.
2.) Inspect the infusion solution for particulate matter or discoloration. Discard the infusion solution if particulate matter or discoloration is observed.

If the infusion solution is not prepared immediately prior to administration, commence administration of the infusion solution within 4 hours from reconstitution and dilution of the drug product. Keep solutions at 25°C (77°F); excursions permitted to 15° to 30°C (59° to 86°F).

Do not administer mycophenolate IV or coadminister via the same infusion catheter with other IV drugs or infusion admixtures.

➤*Dosage adjustments:* In renal transplant patients with severe chronic renal impairment (glomerular filtration rate [GFR] less than 25 mL/min per 1.73 m^2) outside the immediate posttransplant period, avoid dosages of mycophenolate greater than 1 g administered twice a day. Carefully observe these patients. No dosage adjustments are needed in renal transplant patients experiencing delayed graft function postoperatively.

No data are available for cardiac or hepatic transplant patients with severe chronic renal impairment. Mycophenolate may be used for cardiac or hepatic transplant patients with severe chronic renal impairment if the potential benefits outweigh the potential risks.

MYCOPHENOLATE MOFETIL — INJECTION

If neutropenia develops (absolute neutrophil count [ANC] less than 1.3 × 10^3/mcL), interrupt dosing or reduce the dosage of mycophenolate, perform appropriate diagnostic tests, and manage the patient appropriately.

➤*Handling and disposal:* Mycophenolate has demonstrated teratogenic effects in rats and rabbits. Exercise caution in the handling and preparation of solutions of mycophenolate IV. Avoid direct contact of the prepared solution of mycophenolate IV with skin or mucous membranes. If such contact occurs, wash thoroughly with soap and water; rinse eyes with plain water.

➤*Storage / Stability:* Store powder and reconstituted/infusion solutions at 25°C (77°F); excursions permitted to 15° to 30°C (59° to 86°F).

Actions

➤*Pharmacology:* Mycophenolate has been demonstrated in experimental animal models to prolong the survival of allogeneic transplants (eg, kidney, heart, liver, intestine, limb, small bowel, pancreatic islets, bone marrow).

Mycophenolate has also been shown to reverse ongoing acute rejection in the canine renal and rat cardiac allograft models. Mycophenolate also inhibited proliferative arteriopathy in experimental models of aortic and heart allografts in rats, as well as in primate cardiac xenografts. Mycophenolate was used alone or in combination with other immunosuppressive agents in these studies. Mycophenolate has been demonstrated to inhibit immunologically mediated inflammatory responses in animal models and to inhibit tumor development and prolong survival in murine tumor transplant models.

Mycophenolate mofetil is hydrolyzed to form 2-morpholinoethyl ester of mycophenolic acid, which is the active metabolite. Mycophenolic acid is a potent, selective, uncompetitive, and reversible inhibitor of inosine monophosphate dehydrogenase, and, therefore, inhibits the de novo pathway of guanosine nucleotide synthesis without incorporation into deoxyribonucleic acid (DNA). Because T- and B-lymphocytes are critically dependent for their proliferation on de novo synthesis of purines, whereas other cell types can utilize salvage pathways, mycophenolic acid has potent cytostatic effects on lymphocytes. Mycophenolic acid inhibits proliferative responses of T- and B-lymphocytes to both mitogenic and allospecific stimulation. Addition of guanosine or deoxyguanosine reverses the cytostatic effects of mycophenolic acid on lymphocytes. Mycophenolic acid also suppresses antibody formation by B-lymphocytes. Mycophenolic acid prevents the glycosylation of lymphocyte and monocyte glycoproteins that are involved in intercellular adhesion to endothelial cells and may inhibit recruitment of leukocytes into sites of inflammation and graft rejection. Mycophenolate mofetil did not inhibit early events in the activation of human peripheral blood mononuclear cells, such as the production of interleukin-1 (IL-1) and interleukin-2 (IL-2), but did block the coupling of these events to DNA synthesis and proliferation.

➤*Pharmacokinetics:*

Absorption – Following IV administration, mycophenolate mofetil undergoes rapid and complete metabolism to mycophenolic acid, the active metabolite. Mycophenolic acid is metabolized to form the phenolic glucuronide of mycophenolic acid, which is not pharmacologically active. The parent drug, mycophenolate mofetil, can be measured systemically during the IV infusion; however, shortly (about 5 minutes) after the infusion is stopped, mycophenolate mofetil concentration is below the limit of quantitation (0.4 mcg/mL).

Distribution – The mean (± SD) apparent volume of distribution of mycophenolic acid in 12 healthy volunteers is approximately 3.6 (± 1.5) and 4 (± 1.2) L/kg following IV and oral administration, respectively. Mycophenolic acid, at clinically relevant concentrations, is 97% bound to plasma albumin. Mycophenolic acid glucuronide (phenotic glucuronide of mycophenolic acid) is 82% bound to plasma albumin at mycophenolic acid glucuronide concentration ranges that are normally seen in stable renal transplant patients; however, at higher mycophenolic acid glucuronide concentrations (observed in patients with renal impairment or delayed graft function), the binding of mycophenolic acid may be reduced as a result of competition between mycophenolic acid glucuronide and mycophenolic acid for protein binding. Mean blood-to-plasma ratio of radioactivity concentrations was approximately 0.6, indicating that mycophenolic acid and mycophenolic acid glucuronide do not distribute extensively into the cellular fractions of blood.

Metabolism – Following IV administration, mycophenolate mofetil undergoes complete metabolism to mycophenolic acid, the active metabolite. Mycophenolic acid is metabolized principally by glucuronyl transferase to form the phenolic glucuronide of mycophenolic acid (mycophenolic acid glucuronide) which is not pharmacologically active. The parent drug, mycophenolate mofetil, can be measured systemically during the IV infusion; however, shortly (about 5 minutes) after the infusion stopped or after oral administration, mycophenolate mofetil concentration is below the limit of quantitation (0.4 mcg/mL). In vivo, mycophenolic acid glucuronide is converted to mycophenolic acid via enterohepatic recirculation. The following metabolites of the 2-hydroxyethyl-morpholino moiety are also recovered in the urine following oral administration of mycophenolate mofetil to healthy subjects: N-(2-carboxymethyl)-morpholine, N-(2-hydroxyethyl)-morpholine, and the N-oxide of N-(2-hydroxyethyl)-morpholine.

Secondary peaks in the plasma mycophenolic acid concentration-time profile are usually observed 6 to 12 hours postdose. The coadministration of cholestyramine (4 g 3 times daily) resulted in approximately a 40% decrease in the mycophenolic acid AUC (largely as a consequence of lower concentrations in the terminal portion of the profile). These observations suggest that enterohepatic recirculation contributes to mycophenolic acid plasma concentrations.

Excretion – Negligible amount of drug is excreted as mycophenolic acid (less than 1% of dose) in the urine. Oral radiolabeled mycophenolate mofetil resulted in complete recovery of the administered dose, with 93% of the administered dose recovered in the urine and 6% recovered in feces. Most (about 87%) of the administered dose is excreted in the urine as mycophenolic acid glucuronide. At clinically encountered concentrations, mycophenolic acid and mycophenolic acid glucuronide are usually not removed by hemodialysis. However, at high mycophenolic acid glucuronide plasma concentrations (greater than 100 mcg/mL), small amounts of mycophenolic acid glucuronide are removed. Bile acid sequestrants, such as cholestyramine, reduce mycophenolic acid AUC by interfering with enterohepatic circulation of the drug.

Mean (± SD) apparent half-life and plasma clearance of mycophenolic acid are 16.6 (± 5.8) hours and 177 (± 31) mL/min following IV administration.

Special populations –

Renal function impairment: In a single-dose study, mycophenolate was administered as capsule or IV infusion over 40 minutes. Plasma mycophenolic acid AUC observed after oral dosing to volunteers with severe chronic renal impairment (GFR less than 25 mL/min per 1.73 m^2) was about 75% higher relative to that observed in healthy volunteers (GFR greater than 80 mL/min per 1.73 m^2). In addition, the single-dose plasma mycophenolic acid glucuronide AUC was 3-fold to 6-fold higher in volunteers with severe renal impairment than in volunteers with mild renal impairment or healthy volunteers, consistent with the known renal elimination of mycophenolic acid glucuronide. No data are available on the safety of long-term exposure to this level of mycophenolic acid glucuronide.

Plasma mycophenolic acid AUC observed after single-dose (1 g) IV dosing to volunteers (n = 4) with severe chronic renal impairment (GFR less than 25 mL/min per 1.73 m^2) was 62.4 mcg•h/mL (± 19.3). Multiple dosing of mycophenolate in patients with severe chronic renal impairment has not been studied.

See Warnings for more information.

In 8 patients with primary nonfunction of the organ following renal transplantation, plasma concentrations of mycophenolic acid glucuronide accumulated about 6-fold to 8-fold after multiple dosing for 28 days. Accumulation of mycophenolic acid was about 1-fold to 2-fold.

Hepatic function impairment: In a single dose (1 g oral) study of 18 volunteers with alcoholic cirrhosis and 6 healthy volunteers, hepatic mycophenolic acid glucuronidation processes appeared to be relatively unaffected by hepatic parenchymal disease when pharmacokinetic parameters of healthy volunteers and alcoholic cirrhosis patients within this study were compared. However, note that, for unexplained reasons, the healthy volunteers in this study had about a 50% lower AUC as compared with healthy volunteers in other studies, thus making comparisons between volunteers with alcoholic cirrhosis and healthy volunteers difficult. Effects of hepatic disease on this process probably depend on the particular disease. Hepatic disease with other etiologies, such as primary biliary cirrhosis, may show a different effect. In a single-dose (1 g) IV study of 6 volunteers with severe hepatic impairment (aminopyrine breath test less than 0.2% of dose) due to alcoholic cirrhosis, mycophenolate was rapidly converted to mycophenolic acid. Mycophenolic acid AUC was 44.1 mcg•h/mL (± 15.5).

Pharmacokinetics in healthy volunteers, renal, cardiac, and hepatic transplant patients –

Pharmacokinetic Parameters for Mycophenolic Acid (Mean ± SD) Following Administration of Mycophenolate to Healthy Volunteers (Single Dose), Renal, Cardiac, and Hepatic Transplant Patients (Multiple Doses)

Parameter	Dose/Route	T_{max} (h)	C_{max} (mcg/mL)	AUC (mcg•h/mL)
Healthy volunteers (single dose)	1 g/oral	0.8 (± 0.36) (n = 129)	24.5 (± 9.5) (n = 129)	63.9 (±16.2) (n = 117)
Renal transplant patients (twice-daily dosing) Time after transplantation				
5 days (n = 31)	1 g/IV	1.58 (± 0.46)	12 (± 3.82)	40.8 (± 11.4)[a]
6 days (n = 31)	1 g/oral	1.33 (± 1.05)	10.7 (± 4.83)	32.9 (± 15)[a]
Early (< 40 days) (n = 25)	1 g/oral	1.31 (± 0.76)	8.16 (± 4.5)	27.3 (± 10.9)[a]
Early (< 40 days) (n = 27)	1.5 g/oral	1.21 (± 0.81)	13.5 (± 8.18)	38.4 (± 15.4)[a]
Late (> 3 months) (n = 23)	1.5 g/oral	0.9 (± 0.24)	24.1 (± 12.1)	65.3 (± 35.4)[a]
Cardiac transplant patients (twice-daily dosing) Time after transplantation				
Early (day before discharge)	1.5 g/oral	1.8 (± 1.3) (n = 11)	11.5 (± 6.8) (n = 11)	43.3 (± 20.8)[a] (n = 9)
Late (> 6 months)	1.5 g/oral	1.1 (± 0.7) (n = 52)	20 (± 9.4) (n = 52)	54.1 (± 20.4)[b] (n = 49)
Hepatic transplant patients (twice-daily dosing) Time after transplantation				
4 to 9 days (n = 22)	1 g/IV	1.5 (± 0.517)	17 (± 12.7)	34 (± 17.4)[a]
Early (5 to 8 days) (n = 20)	1.5 g/oral	1.15 (± 0.432)	13.1 (± 6.76)	29.2 (± 11.9)[a]
Late (> 6 months) (n = 6)	1.5 g/oral	1.54 (± 0.51)	19.3 (± 11.7)	49.3 (± 14.8)[a]

[a] Interdosing interval $AUC_{0-12\ h}$.
[b] $AUC_{0-12\ h}$ values quoted are extrapolated from data from samples collected over 4 hours.

MYCOPHENOLATE MOFETIL — INJECTION

Contraindications

Hypersensitivity to mycophenolate, mycophenolic acid or any component of the drug product, or polysorbate 80 (Tween 80).

Warnings

➤*Lymphomas / Malignancies:* Patients receiving immunosuppressive regimens involving combinations of drugs, including mycophenolate, as part of an immunosuppressive regimen are at increased risk of developing lymphomas and other malignancies, particularly of the skin. The risk appears to be related to the intensity and duration of immunosuppression rather than to the use of any specific agent. Oversuppression of the immune system can also increase susceptibility to infection, including opportunistic infections, fatal infections, and sepsis.

As usual for patients with increased risk for skin cancer, they should limit exposure to sunlight and ultraviolet (UV) light by wearing protective clothing and using a sunscreen with a high protection factor.

Mycophenolate has been administered in combination with the following agents in clinical trials: antithymocyte globulin, muromonab-CD3, cyclosporine or modified cyclosporine, and corticosteroids. The efficacy and safety of the use of mycophenolate in combination with other immunosuppressive agents have not been determined.

See Adverse Reactions for more information.

In pediatric patients, no other malignancies besides lymphoproliferative disorder (2 of 148 patients) have been observed.

➤*Infection / Sepsis:* In patients receiving mycophenolate (2 or 3 g) in controlled studies for prevention of renal, cardiac, or hepatic rejection, fatal infection/sepsis occurred in approximately 2% of renal and cardiac patients and in 5% of hepatic patients.

Instruct patients receiving mycophenolate to report immediately any evidence of infection, unexpected bruising, bleeding, or any other manifestation of bone marrow depression.

➤*Caution:* See Administration and Dosage for more information.

➤*Renal function impairment:* See Actions for more information.

See Administration and Dosage for more information.

In patients with delayed renal graft function posttransplant, mean mycophenolic acid $AUC_{0\text{-}12h}$ was comparable, but mycophenolic acid glucuronide $AUC_{0\text{-}12h}$ was 2-fold to 3-fold higher, compared with that seen in posttransplant patients without delayed renal graft function. In the 3 controlled studies of prevention of renal rejection, there were 298 of 1,483 patients (20%) with delayed graft function. Although patients with delayed graft function have a higher incidence of certain adverse reactions (eg, anemia, thrombocytopenia, hyperkalemia) than patients without delayed graft function, these reactions were not more frequent in patients receiving mycophenolate than azathioprine or placebo. No dosage adjustment is recommended; however, carefully observe these patients.

➤*Mutagenesis:* The genotoxic potential of mycophenolate was determined in 5 assays. Mycophenolate was genotoxic in the mouse lymphoma/thymidine kinase assay and the in vivo mouse micronucleus assay. Mycophenolate was not genotoxic in the bacterial mutation assay, the yeast mitotic gene conversion assay or the Chinese hamster ovary cell chromosomal aberration assay.

➤*Elderly:* Clinical studies of mycophenolate did not include sufficient numbers of subjects 65 years of age and older to determine whether they respond differently from younger subjects. Other reported clinical experience has not identified differences in responses between the elderly and younger patients. In general, use cautious dosage selection for an elderly patient, reflecting the greater frequency of decreased hepatic, renal, or cardiac function and of concomitant or other drug therapy. Elderly patients may be at an increased risk of adverse reactions compared with younger individuals.

➤*Pregnancy: Category C.* In teratology studies in rats and rabbits, fetal resorptions and malformations occurred in rats at 6 mg/kg/day and in rabbits at 90 mg/kg/day, in the absence of maternal toxicity. These levels are equivalent to 0.03 to 0.92 times the recommended clinical dosage in renal transplant patients and 0.02 to 0.61 times the recommended clinical dosage in cardiac transplant patients on a BSA basis. In a female fertility and reproduction study conducted in rats, oral dosages of 4.5 mg/kg/day caused malformations (principally of the head and eyes) in the first generation offspring in the absence of maternal toxicity. This dosage was 0.02 times the recommended clinical dosage in renal transplant patients and 0.01 times the recommended clinical dosage in cardiac transplant patients when corrected for BSA.

There are no adequate and well-controlled studies in pregnant women. Do not use mycophenolate in a pregnant woman unless the potential benefit justifies the potential risk to the fetus. Effective contraception must be used before beginning mycophenolate therapy, during therapy, and for 6 weeks after mycophenolate has been stopped.

Adverse reactions on fetal development (including malformations) occurred when pregnant rats and rabbits were dosed during organogenesis. These responses occurred at dosages lower than those associated with maternal toxicity, and at dosages below the recommended clinical dosage for renal, cardiac, or hepatic transplantation. There are no adequate and well-controlled studies in pregnant women. However, as mycophenolate has been shown to have teratogenic effects in animals, it may cause fetal harm when administered to a pregnant woman. Therefore, do not use mycophenolate in pregnant women unless the potential benefit justifies the potential risk to the fetus.

Women of childbearing potential should have a negative serum or urine pregnancy test with a sensitivity of at least 50 milliunits/mL within 1 week prior to beginning therapy. It is recommended that mycophenolate therapy not be initiated until a report of a negative pregnancy test has been obtained.

Effective contraception must be used before beginning mycophenolate therapy, during therapy, and for 6 weeks following discontinuation of therapy, even where there has been a history of infertility, unless due to hysterectomy. Two reliable forms of contraception must be used simultaneously unless abstinence is the chosen method. If pregnancy does occur during treatment, discuss the desirability of continuing the pregnancy with the patient.

➤*Lactation:* Studies in rats treated with mycophenolate have shown mycophenolic acid to be excreted in milk. It is not known whether this drug is excreted in human milk. Because many drugs are excreted in human milk, and because of the potential for serious adverse reactions in breast-feeding infants from mycophenolate, decide whether to discontinue breast-feeding or to discontinue the drug, taking into account the importance of the drug to the mother.

➤*Children:* Safety and efficacy in pediatric patients receiving allogeneic cardiac or hepatic transplants have not been established.

Precautions

➤*Monitoring:* Perform complete blood counts weekly during the first month, twice monthly for the second and third months of treatment, then monthly through the first year.

➤*Neutropenia:* Severe neutropenia (ANC less than 0.5×10^3/mcL) developed in up to 2% of renal, up to 2.8% of cardiac, and up to 3.6% of hepatic transplant patients receiving mycophenolate 3 g daily. Monitor patients receiving mycophenolate for neutropenia. The development of neutropenia may be related to mycophenolate itself, concomitant medications, viral infections, or some combination of these causes. If neutropenia develops (ANC less than 1.3×10^3/mcL), interrupt dosing or reduce the dosage of mycophenolate, perform appropriate diagnostic tests, and manage the patient appropriately. Neutropenia has been observed most frequently in the period from 31 to 180 days posttransplant in patients treated for prevention of renal, cardiac, and hepatic rejection.

➤*Infections:* In cardiac transplant patients, the overall incidence of opportunistic infections was approximately 10% higher in patients treated with mycophenolate than in those receiving azathioprine therapy, but this difference was not associated with excess mortality due to infection/sepsis among patients treated with mycophenolate.

There were more herpes virus (herpes simplex, herpes zoster, and cytomegalovirus) infections in cardiac transplant patients treated with mycophenolate compared with those treated with azathioprine.

➤*Rare hereditary deficiency:* On theoretical grounds, because mycophenolate is an inosine monophosphate dehydrogenase inhibitor, avoid it in patients with rare hereditary deficiency of hypoxanthine-guanine phosphoribosyl-transferase (HGPRT) such as Lesch-Nyhan and Kelley-Seegmiller syndrome.

➤*Live, attenuated vaccines:* During treatment with mycophenolate, avoid the use of live, attenuated vaccines and advise patients that vaccinations may be less effective.

➤*GI effects:* GI bleeding (requiring hospitalization) has been observed in approximately 3% of renal, 1.7% of cardiac, and 5.4% of hepatic transplant patients treated with mycophenolate 3 g daily. In pediatric renal transplant patients, 5 of 148 cases of GI bleeding (requiring hospitalization) were observed.

GI perforations have been observed rarely. Most patients receiving mycophenolate were also receiving other drugs known to be associated with these complications. Patients with active peptic ulcer disease were excluded from enrollment in studies with mycophenolate. Because mycophenolate has been associated with an increased incidence of digestive system adverse reactions, including infrequent cases of GI tract ulceration, hemorrhage, and perforation, administer mycophenolate with caution in patients with active serious digestive system disease.

Drug Interactions

➤*Drugs that alter the GI flora:* Drugs that alter the GI flora may interact with mycophenolate by disrupting enterohepatic recirculation. Interference of mycophenolic acid glucuronide hydrolysis may lead to less mycophenolic acid available for absorption.

Mycophenolate Drug Interactions

Precipitant drug	Object drug[a]		Description
Acyclovir Ganciclovir	Mycophenolate	↑	Mycophenolic acid glucuronide and acyclovir plasma AUCs were increased 10.6% and 21.9%, respectively. Because mycophenolic acid glucuronide plasma concentrations are increased in the presence of renal impairment, as are acyclovir and ganciclovir concentrations, the potential exists for the 2 drugs to compete for tubular secretion, further increasing the concentrations of both drugs.
Mycophenolate	Acyclovir Ganciclovir		

MYCOPHENOLATE MOFETIL — INJECTION

Mycophenolate Drug Interactions

Precipitant drug	Object drug[a]		Description
Antacids	Mycophenolate	↓	Absorption of a single mycophenolate dose was decreased when coadministered with an aluminum/magnesium hydroxide antacid. The C_{max} and AUC for mycophenolic acid were 33% and 17% lower, respectively, than when mycophenolate was given alone. Avoid simultaneous administration.
Azathioprine	Mycophenolate	↔	It is recommended to avoid concomitant use because of a lack of clinical studies.
Cholestyramine	Mycophenolate	↓	Following coadministration, mycophenolic acid AUC decreased ≈ 40%. Do not give with cholestyramine or agents that may interfere with enterohepatic recirculation.
Iron	Mycophenolate	↓	Following coadministration, mycophenolate absorption and mycophenolic acid AUC were significantly decreased. Avoid concomitant administration.
Probenecid	Mycophenolate	↑	In animals, coadministration resulted in a 3-fold increase in plasma mycophenolic acid glucuronide AUC and a 2-fold increase in plasma mycophenolic acid AUC.
Salicylates	Mycophenolate	↑	Coadministration increased the free fraction of mycophenolic acid.
Mycophenolate	Live attenuated vaccines	↓	Coadministration may cause vaccinations to be less effective. Avoid if possible.
Mycophenolate	Oral contraceptives	↓	Coadministration of mycophenolate and oral contraceptives containing levonorgestrel produced a significant decrease in the levonorgestrel AUC by ≈ 15%. Mean serum levels of LH, FSH, and progesterone were not significantly affected. Administer with caution and consider additional birth control methods.
Mycophenolate	Phenytoin	↑	Mycophenolic acid decreased protein binding of phenytoin and may, therefore, increase free phenytoin levels.
Mycophenolate	Theophylline	↑	Mycophenolic acid decreased protein binding of theophylline and may, therefore, increase free theophylline levels.

[a] ↑ = Object drug increased. ↓ = Object drug decreased.
↔ = Undetermined clinical effect.

Adverse Reactions

➤*Principal adverse reactions:* The principal adverse reactions associated with the administration of mycophenolate include diarrhea, leukopenia, sepsis, and vomiting, and there is evidence of a higher frequency of certain types of infections (eg, opportunistic infection). The adverse reaction profile associated with the administration of mycophenolate IV has been shown to be similar to that observed after administration of oral dosage forms of mycophenolate.

➤*Elderly:* Elderly patients (65 years of age or older), particularly those who are receiving mycophenolate as part of a combination immunosuppressive regimen, may be at increased risk of certain infections (including cytomegalovirus [CMV] tissue-invasive disease) and possibly GI hemorrhage and pulmonary edema, compared with younger individuals.

➤*Mycophenolate oral:* See Mycophenolate Mofetil Oral monograph.

➤*Mycophenolate IV:* Adverse reactions attributable to peripheral venous infusion were phlebitis and thrombosis, both observed at 4% in patients treated.

➤*Postmarketing:*

GI – Colitis (sometimes caused by cytomegalovirus), pancreatitis, isolated cases of intestinal villous atrophy.

Respiratory – Interstitial lung disorders, including fatal pulmonary fibrosis, have been reported rarely; consider these in the differential diagnosis of pulmonary symptoms ranging from dyspnea to respiratory failure in post-transplant patients receiving mycophenolate.

Miscellaneous –
Resistance mechanism disorders: Serious life-threatening infections such as meningitis and infectious endocarditis have been reported occasionally, and there is evidence of a higher frequency of certain types of serious infections such as tuberculosis and atypical mycobacterial infection.

Overdosage

➤*Symptoms:* There has been no reported experience of overdosage of mycophenolate in humans. The highest dosage administered to renal transplant patients in clinical trials has been 4 g/day. In limited experience with cardiac and hepatic transplant patients in clinical trials, the highest dosages used were 4 or 5 g/day. At dosages of 4 or 5 g/day, there appears to be a higher rate, compared with the use of 3 g/day or less, of GI intolerance (eg, nausea, vomiting, diarrhea), and occasional hematologic abnormalities, principally neutropenia, leading to a need to reduce or discontinue dosing.

In acute oral toxicity studies, no deaths occurred in adult mice at doses up to 4,000 mg/kg or in adult monkeys at doses up to 1,000 mg/kg; these were the highest doses of mycophenolate tested in these species. These doses represent 11 times the recommended clinical dose in renal transplant patients and approximately 7 times the recommended clinical dose in cardiac transplant patients when corrected for BSA. In adult rats, deaths occurred after single oral doses of 500 mg/kg of mycophenolate. The dose represents approximately 3 times the recommended clinical dose in cardiac transplant patients when corrected for BSA.

➤*Treatment:* Mycophenolic acid and mycophenolic acid glucuronide are usually not removed by hemodialysis. However, at high mycophenolic acid glucuronide plasma concentrations (greater than 100 mcg/mL), small amounts of mycophenolic acid glucuronide are removed. By increasing excretion of the drug, mycophenolic acid can be removed by bile acid sequestrants, such as cholestyramine.

Patient Information

Inform patients of the need for repeated appropriate laboratory tests while they are receiving mycophenolate. Give patients complete dosage instructions and inform them of the increased risk of lymphoproliferative disease and certain other malignancies. Instruct women of childbearing potential of the potential risks during pregnancy, and that they should use effective contraception before beginning mycophenolate therapy, during therapy, and for 6 weeks after mycophenolate has been stopped.

Instruct patients receiving mycophenolate to report immediately any evidence of infection, unexpected bruising, bleeding, or any other manifestation of bone marrow depression.

MYCOPHENOLATE SODIUM

Rx	**Myfortic** (Novartis)	**Tablets, delayed-release:** 180 mg (as sodium)	Lactose. (C). Lime green. Film-coated. In 120s.
		360 mg (as sodium)	Lactose. (CT). Pale orange-red. Film-coated. In 120s.

MYCOPHENOLATE SODIUM — ORAL

WARNING

Increased susceptibility to infection and the possible development of lymphoma and other neoplasms may result from immunosuppression. Only physicians experienced in immunosuppressive therapy and management of organ transplant recipients should use mycophenolic acid. Manage patients receiving mycophenolic acid in facilities equipped and staffed with adequate laboratory and supportive medical resources. The physician responsible for maintenance therapy should have complete information requisite for the follow-up of the patient.

Indications

➤*Allogeneic renal transplant:* Prophylaxis of organ rejection in patients receiving allogeneic renal transplants, administered in combination with cyclosporine and corticosteroids.

Administration and Dosage

➤*Recommended dose:* 720 mg administered twice daily (1,440 mg total daily dose) on an empty stomach, 1 hour before or 2 hours after food intake.

➤*Interchangeability:* Mycophenolic acid delayed-release tablets and mycophenolate mofetil tablets and capsules should not be used interchangeably without physician supervision because the rate of absorption following the administration of these 2 products is not equivalent.

MYCOPHENOLATE SODIUM — ORAL

➤*Administration:* Do not crush, chew, or cut tablets prior to ingesting. Swallow the tablets whole in order to maintain the integrity of the enteric coating.

➤*Children:* Based on a pharmacokinetic study conducted in stable renal pediatric transplant patients, the recommended dose of mycophenolic acid in stable pediatric patients is 400 mg/m^2 body surface area (BSA) administered twice daily (up to a maximum dose of 720 mg administered twice daily). Patients with a BSA of 1.19 to 1.58 m^2 may be dosed either with 3 mycophenolic acid 180 mg tablets or one 180 mg tablet plus one 360 mg tablet twice daily (1,080 mg daily dose). Patients with a BSA of greater than 1.58 m^2 may be dosed either with 4 mycophenolic acid 180 mg tablets or 2 mycophenolic acid 360 mg tablets twice daily (1,440 mg daily dose). Pediatric doses for patients with BSA less than 1.19 m^2 cannot be accurately administered using currently available formulations of mycophenolic acid tablets.

➤*Elderly:* The maximum recommended dose is 720 mg administered twice daily.

➤*Storage/Stability:* Store at 25°C (77°F); excursions permitted to 15° to 30°C (59° to 86°F). Protect from moisture. Dispense in a tight container. Do not crush or cut tablets.

Actions

➤*Pharmacology:* Mycophenolic acid is an uncompetitive and reversible inhibitor of inosine monophosphate dehydrogenase (IMPDH), and therefore inhibits the de novo pathway of guanosine nucleotide synthesis without incorporation to DNA. Because T- and B-lymphocytes are critically dependent for their proliferation on de novo synthesis of purines, whereas other cell types can utilize salvage pathways, mycophenolic acid has potent cytostatic effect on lymphocytes.

➤*Pharmacokinetics:*

Absorption – In vitro studies demonstrated that the enteric-coated mycophenolic acid tablet does not release mycophenolic acid under acidic conditions (pH less than 5) as in the stomach but is highly soluble in neutral pH conditions as in the intestine. Following mycophenolic acid oral administration without food in several pharmacokinetic studies conducted in renal transplant patients, consistent with its enteric-coated formulation, the median delay (t_{lag}) in the rise of mycophenolic acid concentration ranged between 0.25 and 1.25 hours and the median time to maximum concentration (T_{max}) of mycophenolic acid ranged between 1.5 and 2.75 hours. In comparison, following the administration of mycophenolate mofetil, the median T_{max} ranged between 0.5 and 1 hours. In stable renal transplant patients on modified cyclosporine-based immunosuppression, GI absorption, and absolute bioavailability of mycophenolic acid following the administration of mycophenolic acid delayed-release tablet was 93% and 72%, respectively. Mycophenolic acid pharmacokinetics are dose proportional over the dose range of 360 to 2,160 mg.

Distribution – The mean (± SD) volume of distribution at steady state and elimination phase for mycophenolic acid is 54 (± 25) L and 112 (± 48) L, respectively. Mycophenolic acid is highly protein bound to albumin, greater than 98%. The protein binding of mycophenolic acid glucuronide is 82%. The free mycophenolic acid concentration may increase under conditions of decreased protein binding (eg, uremia, hepatic failure, hypoalbuminemia).

Metabolism – Mycophenolic acid is metabolized principally by glucuronyl transferase to glucuronidated metabolites. The phenolic glucuronide of mycophenolic acid, mycophenolic acid glucuronide, is the predominant metabolite of mycophenolic acid and does not manifest pharmacological activity. The acyl glucuronide is a minor metabolite and has comparable pharmacological activity to mycophenolic acid. In stable renal transplant patients on modified cyclosporine based immunosuppression, approximately 28% of the oral mycophenolic acid dose was converted to mycophenolic acid glucuronate by presystemic metabolism. The AUC ratio of mycophenolic acid:mycophenolic acid glucuronide is approximately 1:24:0.28 at steady state. The mean clearance of mycophenolic acid was 140 (± 30) mL/min.

Excretion – The majority of mycophenolic acid dose administered in eliminated in the urine primarily as mycophenolic acid glucuronide (greater than 60%) and approximately 3% as unchanged mycophenolic acid following mycophenolic acid administration to stable renal transplant patients. The mean renal clearance of mycophenolic acid glucuronide was 15.5 (± 5.9) mL/min. Mycophenolic acid glucuronide is also secreted in the bile and available for deconjugation by gut flora. Mycophenolic acid resulting from the deconjugation may then be reabsorbed and produce a second peak of mycophenolic acid approximately 6 to 8 hours after mycophenolic acid dosing. The mean elimination half-life of mycophenolic acid and mycophenolic acid glucuronide ranged between 8 and 16 hours, and 13 and 17 hours, respectively.

Food effect – Compared with the fasting state, administration of mycophenolic acid 720 mg with a high-fat meal (55 g fat, 1,000 calories) had no effect on the systemic exposure (AUC) of mycophenolic acid. However, there was a 33% decrease in the maximal concentration (C_{max}), a 3.5-hour delay in the t_{lag} (range, −6 to 18 hour), and a 5-hour delay in the T_{max} (range, −9 to 20 hour) of mycophenolic acid. To avoid the variability in mycophenolic acid absorption between doses, take mycophenolic acid on an empty stomach.

Pharmacokinetics in renal transplant patients –

Mean ± SD Pharmacokinetic Parameters for Mycophenolic Acid Following the Oral Administration of Mycophenolic Acid to Renal Transplant Patients on Modified Cyclosporine-Based Immunosuppression

Study patient	Mycophenolic acid dosing	n	Dose (mg)	T_{max}[a] (h)	C_{max} (mcg/mL)	$AUC_{0\text{-}12\ hour}$ (mcg•h/mL)
Adult	Single	24	720	2 (0.8 to 8)	26.1 ± 12	66.5 ± 22.6[b]
Pediatric[c]	Single	10	450/m^2	2.5 (1.5 to 24)	36.3 ± 20.9	74.3 ± 22.5[b]
Adult	Multiple × 6 days, twice daily	10	720	2 (1.5 to 3)	37 ± 13.3	67.9 ± 20.3
Adult	Multiple × 28 days, twice daily	36	720	2.5 (1.5 to 8)	31.2 ± 18.1	71.2 ± 26.3
Adult	Chronic, multiple dose, twice daily					
	2 weeks posttransplant	12	720	1.8 (1 to 5.3)	15 ± 10.7	28.6 ± 11.5
	3 months posttransplant	12	720	2 (0.5 to 2.5)	26.2 ± 12.7	52.3 ± 17.4
	6 months posttransplant	12	720	2 (0 to 3)	24.1 ± 9.6	57.2 ± 15.3
Adult	Chronic, multiple dose, twice daily	18	720	1.5 (0 to 6)	18.9 ± 7.9	57.4 ± 15

[a] Median (range).
[b] $AUC_{0-\infty}$.
[c] Age range of 5 to 16 years.

Contraindications

Hypersensitivity to mycophenolate sodium, mycophenolic acid, mycophenolate mofetil, or to any of its excipients.

Warnings

➤*Lymphomas/Malignancies:* Patients receiving immunosuppressive regimens involving combinations of drugs, including mycophenolic acid, as part of an immunosuppressive regimen are at increased risk of developing lymphomas and other malignancies, particularly of the skin. The risk appears to be related to the intensity and duration of immunosuppression rather than to the use of any specific agent. Oversuppression of the immune system can also increase susceptibility to infection, including opportunistic infections, fatal infections, and sepsis.

As usual for patients with increased risk for skin cancer, exposure to sunlight and ultraviolet (UV) light should be limited by wearing sunscreen with a high protection factor.

The rates for lymphoproliferative disease or lymphoma in mycophenolic acid-treated patients were comparable to the mycophenolate mofetil group in the de novo and maintenance studies.

➤*Fatal infections:* Fatal infections can occur in patients receiving immunosuppressive therapy.

➤*Neutropenia:* Monitor patients receiving mycophenolic acid for neutropenia. The development of neutropenia may be related to mycophenolic acid itself, concomitant medications, viral infections, or some combination of these events. If neutropenia develops (absolute neutrophil count [ANC] less than 1.3 × 10^3/mcL), interrupt dosing with mycophenolic acid or reduce the dose, use appropriate diagnostic tests, and manage the patient appropriately.

Instruct patients receiving mycophenolic acid to immediately report any evidence of infection, unexpected bruising, bleeding, or any other manifestation of bone marrow suppression.

➤*Renal function impairment:* Subjects with severe chronic renal impairment (GFR less than 25 mL/min/1.73 m^2) may present higher plasma mycophenolic acid and mycophenolic acid glucuronide AUCs relative to subjects with lesser degrees of renal impairment or healthy volunteers. No data are available on the safety of long-term exposure to these levels of mycophenolic acid glucuronide.

➤*Mutagenesis:* The genotoxic potential of mycophenolate sodium was determined in 5 assays. Mycophenolate sodium was genotoxic in the mouse lymphoma/thymidine kinase assay, the micronucleus test in V79 Chinese hamster cells, and the in vivo mouse micronucleus assay. Mycophenolate sodium was not genotoxic in the bacterial mutation assay (*Salmonella typhimurium* TA 1535, 97a, 98, 100, and 102) or the chromosomal aberration assay in human lymphocytes. Mycophenolate mofetil generated similar genotoxic activity. The genotoxic activity of mycophenolic acid is probably due to the depletion of the nucleotide pool required for DNA synthesis as a result of the pharmacodynamic mode of action of mycophenolic acid (inhibition of nucleotide synthesis).

MYCOPHENOLATE SODIUM — ORAL

➤*Elderly:* Patients 65 years of age and older may generally be at increased risk of adverse drug reactions due to immunosuppression. Clinical studies of mycophenolic acid did not include sufficient numbers of subjects 65 years of age and older to determine whether they respond differently from younger subjects. Other reported clinical experience has not identified differences in responses between the elderly and younger patients. In general, dose selection for an elderly patient should be cautious, reflecting the greater frequency of decreased hepatic, renal, or cardiac function, and of concomitant disease or other drug therapy.

➤*Pregnancy: Category C.* In a teratology study performed with mycophenolate sodium in rats, at a dose as low as 1 mg/kg, malformations in the offspring were observed, including anophthalmia, exencephaly, and umbilical hernia. The systemic exposure at this dose represents 0.05 times the clinical exposure at the dose of mycophenolic acid 1.44 g/day. In teratology studies in rabbits, fetal resorptions and malformations occurred from 80 mg/kg/day, in the absence of maternal toxicity (dose levels are equivalent to about 0.8 times the recommended clinical dose, corrected for BSA). There are no relevant qualitative or quantitative differences in the teratogenic potential of mycophenolate sodium and mycophenolate mofetil.

Do not initiate mycophenolic acid therapy until a negative pregnancy test has been obtained. Instruct patients to consult their physician immediately should pregnancy occur.

There are no adequate and well-controlled studies in pregnant women conducted with mycophenolic acid, or mycophenolate mofetil. Since mycophenolic acid may cause fetal harm when administered to a pregnant woman, do not use mycophenolic acid in pregnant women unless the potential benefit justifies the potential risk to the fetus.

Women of childbearing potential should have a negative serum or urine pregnancy test with a sensitivity of at least 50 milliunits/mL within 1 week prior to beginning therapy. Do not initiate mycophenolic acid therapy until a report of a negative pregnancy test has been obtained.

Use effective contraception before beginning mycophenolic acid therapy, during therapy, and for 6 weeks following discontinuation of therapy, even where there has been a history of infertility, unless due to hysterectomy. Use 2 reliable forms of contraception simultaneously unless abstinence is the chosen method. If pregnancy does occur during treatment, discuss the potential risk to the fetus.

➤*Lactation:* It is not known whether mycophenolic acid is excreted in human milk. Because of the potential for serious adverse reactions in breast-feeding infants from mycophenolic acid, decide whether to discontinue the drug or to discontinue breast-feeding while on treatment or within 6 weeks after stopping therapy, taking into account the importance of the drug to the mother.

➤*Children:*

De novo renal transplant – The safety and effectiveness of mycophenolic acid in de novo pediatric renal transplant patients have not been established.

Stable renal transplant – There are no pharmacokinetic data available for pediatric patients younger than 5 years of age. The safety and effectiveness of mycophenolic acid have been established in the age group 5 to 16 years in stable pediatric renal transplant patients. Use of mycophenolic acid in this age group is supported by evidence from adequate and well-controlled studies of mycophenolic acid in stable adult renal transplant patients. Limited pharmacokinetic data are available for stable pediatric renal transplant patients in the age group 5 to 16 years. Pediatric doses for patients with BSA less than 1.19 m^2 cannot be accurately administered using currently available formulations of mycophenolic acid tablets.

Precautions

➤*Monitoring:* Perform complete blood count weekly during the first month, twice monthly for the second and the third month of treatment, then monthly through the first year. If neutropenia develops (ANC less than 1.3 $\times$ 10^3/mcL), interrupt dosing with mycophenolic acid or reduce the dose, perform appropriate tests, and manage the patient accordingly.

➤*GI bleeding:* GI bleeding (requiring hospitalization) has been reported in de novo renal transplant patients (1%) and maintenance patients (1.3%) treated with mycophenolic acid (up to 12 months). Intestinal perforations, GI hemorrhage, gastric ulcers, and duodenal ulcers have rarely been observed. Most patients receiving mycophenolic acid were also receiving other drugs known to be associated with these complications. Patients with active peptic ulcer disease were excluded from enrollment in studies with mycophenolic acid. Because mycophenolic acid derivatives have been associated with an increased incidence of digestive system adverse reactions, including infrequent cases of GI tract ulceration, hemorrhage, and perforation, administer mycophenolic acid with caution in patients with active serious digestive system disease.

➤*Delayed graft function:* In the de novo study, 18.3% of mycophenolic acid patients versus 16.7% in the mycophenolate mofetil group experienced delayed graft function. Although patients with delayed graft function experienced a higher incidence of certain adverse reactions (eg, anemia, leukopenia, hyperkalemia) than patients without delayed graft function, these reactions in delayed graft function patients were not more frequent in patients receiving mycophenolic acid compared with mycophenolate mofetil. No dose adjustment is recommended for these patients; however, carefully observe such patients.

➤*Rare hereditary deficiency:* On theoretical grounds, because mycophenolic acid is an inosine monophosphate dehydrogenase inhibitor, it should be avoided in patients with rare hereditary deficiency of hypoxanthine-guanine phosphoribosyl-transferase, inosine monophosphate dehydrogenase such as Lesch-Nyhan and Kelley-Seegmiller syndrome.

➤*Live, attenuated vaccines:* See Drug Interactions for more information.

Drug Interactions

➤*Drugs that alter the GI flora:* Drugs that alter the GI flora may interact with mycophenolic acid by disrupting enterohepatic recirculation. Interference of mycophenolic acid glucuronide hydrolysis may lead to less mycophenolic acid available for absorption.

Mycophenolic Acid Drug Interactions

Precipitant drug	Object drug[a]		Description
Acyclovir Ganciclovir	Mycophenolic acid	↑	Acyclovir/ganciclovir may be taken with mycophenolic acid; however, during the treatment period, monitor blood cell counts. Both acyclovir/ganciclovir and mycophenolic acid glucuronide concentrations are increased in the presence of renal impairment; their coexistence may compete for tubular secretion and further increase the concentration of the two.
Mycophenolic acid	Acyclovir Ganciclovir		
Antacids	Mycophenolic acid	↓	Absorption of mycophenolic acid may be decreased. The C_{max} and AUC values for mycophenolic acid were 25% and 37% lower, respectively, than when mycophenolic acid was administered alone under fasting conditions. Do not administer simultaneously.
Azathioprine/ Mycophenolate mofetil	Mycophenolic acid	↔	Given that azathioprine and mycophenolate mofetil inhibit purine metabolism, do not administer mycophenolic acid concomitantly with azathioprine and/or mycophenolate mofetil.
Cholestyramine	Mycophenolic acid	↓	Cholestyramine interrupts enterohepatic recirculation and reduces mycophenolic acid exposure. Do not administer simultaneously because of the potential to reduce the efficacy of mycophenolic acid.
Mycophenolic acid	Live, attenuated vaccines	↓	Coadministration may cause vaccinations to be less effective. Avoid if possible.
Mycophenolic acid	Oral contraceptives	↓	Coadministration of mycophenolate and oral contraceptives containing levonorgestrel produced a decrease in the levonorgestrel AUC by ≈ 15%. Administer with caution and consider additional birth control methods.

[a] ↑ = Object drug increased. ↓ = Object drug decreased.
↔ = Undetermined clinical effect.

Adverse Reactions

➤*Principal adverse reactions:* The principal adverse reactions associated with the administration of mycophenolic acid include constipation, nausea, and urinary tract infection in de novo patients, and nausea, diarrhea, and nasopharyngitis in maintenance patients.

Adverse Reactions in Controlled De Novo and Maintenance Renal Studies Reported in ≥ 20% of Patients

	De novo renal study		Maintenance renal study	
Adverse reaction	Mycophenolic acid 1.44 g/day (n = 213)	Mycophenolate mofetil 2 g/day (n = 210)	Mycophenolic acid 1.44 g/day (n = 159)	Mycophenolate mofetil 2 g/day (n = 163)
CNS				
Insomnia	23.5%	23.8%	—	—
GI				
Constipation	38%	39.5%	—	—
Diarrhea	23.5%	24.8%	21.4%	24.5%
Dyspepsia	22.5%	19%	—	—
Nausea	29.1%	27.1%	24.5%	19%
Vomiting	23%	20%	—	—
GU				
Urinary tract infection	29.1%	33.3%	—	—
Hematologic/ Lymphatic				
Anemia	21.6%	21.9%	—	—
Leukopenia	19.2%	20.5%	—	—

MYCOPHENOLATE SODIUM — ORAL

Adverse Reactions in Controlled De Novo and Maintenance Renal Studies Reported in ≥ 20% of Patients

Adverse reaction	de novo renal study: Mycophenolic acid 1.44 g/day (n = 213)	de novo renal study: Mycophenolate mofetil 2 g/day (n = 210)	Maintenance renal study: Mycophenolic acid 1.44 g/day (n = 159)	Maintenance renal study: Mycophenolate mofetil 2 g/day (n = 163)
Miscellaneous				
CMV[a] infection	20.2%	18.1%	—	—
Postoperative pain	23.9%	18.6%	—	—

[a] CMV = cytomegalovirus.

➤*Infections:*

Viral and Fungal Infections Reported Over 0 to 12 Months

Infection	de novo renal study: Mycophenolic acid 1.44 g/day (n = 213)	de novo renal study: Mycophenolate mofetil 2 g/day (n = 210)	Maintenance renal study: Mycophenolic acid 1.44 g/day (n = 159)	Maintenance renal study: Mycophenolate mofetil 2 g/day (n = 163)
Any CMV	21.6%	20.5%	1.9%	1.8%
CMV disease	4.7%	4.3%	0%	0.6%
Herpes simplex	8%	6.2%	1.3%	2.5%
Herpes zoster	4.7%	3.8%	1.9%	3.1%
Any fungal infection	10.8%	11.9%	2.5%	1.8%
Candida NOS	5.6%	6.2%	0%	1.8%
Candida albicans	2.3%	3.8%	0.6%	0%

The following opportunistic infections occurred rarely in the above controlled trials: *Aspergillus* and *Cryptococcus*.

➤*Lymphomas/Malignancies:* The incidence of malignancies and lymphoma is consistent with that reported in the literature for this patient population. Lymphoma developed in 2 de novo patients (0.9%), (1 diagnosed 9 days after treatment initiation) and in 2 maintenance patients (1.3%) (1 was AIDS-related), receiving mycophenolic acid with other immunosuppressive agents in the 12-month controlled clinical trials. Nonmelanoma skin carcinoma occurred in 0.9% de novo and 1.8% maintenance patients. Other types of malignancy occurred in 0.5% de novo and 0.6% maintenance patients.

Adverse Reactions Reported in 3% to Less than 20% of Patients Treated With Mycophenolic Acid in Combination With Cyclosporine[a] and Corticosteroids

Adverse reaction	de novo renal study	Maintenance renal study
Blood and lymphatic disorders	Lymphocele, thrombocytopenia	Leukopenia, anemia
Cardiac disorder	Tachycardia	—
Eye disorder	Vision blurred	—
Endocrine disorders	Cushingoid, hirsutism	—
GI disorder	Abdominal pain upper, flatulence, abdominal distension, sore throat, abdominal pain lower, abdominal pain, gingival hyperplasia, loose stool	Vomiting, dyspepsia, abdominal pain, constipation, gastroesophageal reflux disease, loose stool, flatulence, abdominal pain upper
General disorders and administration site conditions	Edema, edema lower limb, pyrexia, pain, fatigue, edema peripheral, chest pain	Fatigue, pyrexia, edema, chest pain, peripheral edema
Infections and infestations	Nasopharyngitis, herpes simplex, upper respiratory tract infection, oral candidiasis, herpes zoster, sinusitis, wound infection, implant infection, pneumonia	Nasopharyngitis, upper respiratory tract infection, urinary tract infection, influenza, sinusitis
Injury, poisoning, and procedural complications	Drug toxicity	Post procedural pain
Investigations	Blood creatinine increased, hemoglobin decrease, blood pressure increased, liver function tests abnormal	Blood creatinine increase, weight increase
Metabolism and nutrition disorders	Hypocalcemia, hyperuricemia, hyperlipidemia, hypokalemia, hypophosphatemia, hypercholesterolemia, hyperkalemia, hypomagnesemia, diabetes mellitus, hyperphosphatemia, dehydration, fluid overload, hyperglycemia, hypercalcemia	Dehydration, hypokalemia, hypercholesterolemia
Musculoskeletal and connective tissue disorders	Back pain, arthralgia, pain in limb, muscle cramps, myalgia	Arthralgia, pain in limb, back pain, muscle cramps, peripheral swelling, myalgia
CNS disorders	Tremor, headache, dizziness (excluding vertigo)	Headache, dizziness
Psychiatric disorders	Anxiety	Insomnia, depression
Renal and urinary disorders	Renal tubular necrosis, renal impairment, dysuria, hematuria, hydronephrosis, bladder spasm, urinary retention	—
Respiratory, thoracic, and mediastinal disorders	Cough, dyspnea, dyspnea exertional	Cough, dyspnea, pharyngolaryngeal pain, sinus congestion
Skin and subcutaneous tissue disorder	Acne, pruritus	Rash, contusion
Surgical and medical procedures	Complications of transplant surgery, post operative complications, postoperative wound complication	—
Vascular disorder	Hypertension, hypertension aggravated, hypotension	Hypertension

[a] Modified.

➤*Other:*

GI – Colitis (sometimes caused by CMV), pancreatitis, esophagitis, intestinal perforation, gastrointestinal hemorrhage, gastric ulcers, duodenal ulcers, and ileus.

Immunologic – Serious life-threatening infections such as meningitis and infectious endocarditis have been reported occasionally and there is evidence of a higher frequency of certain types of serious infections such as tuberculosis and atypical mycobacterial infection.

Respiratory – Interstitial lung disorders, including fatal pulmonary fibrosis, have been reported rarely with mycophenolic acid administration and should be considered in the differential diagnosis of pulmonary symptoms ranging from dyspnea to respiratory failure in posttransplant patients receiving mycophenolic acid derivatives.

Overdosage

➤*Symptoms:* Possible signs and symptoms of acute overdose could include the following: hematological abnormalities such as leukopenia and neutropenia, and gastrointestinal symptoms such as abdominal pain, diarrhea, nausea and vomiting, and dyspepsia.

➤*Treatment:* Follow general supportive measures and symptomatic treatment in all cases of overdosage. Although dialysis may be used to remove the inactive metabolite mycophenolic acid glucuronide, it would not be expected to remove clinically significant amounts of the active moiety mycophenolic acid due to the 98% plasma protein binding of mycophenolic acid. By interfering with enterohepatic circulation of mycophenolic acid, activated charcoal or bile acid sequestrants, such as cholestyramine, may reduce the systemic mycophenolic acid exposure.

Patient Information

Administer mycophenolic acid on an empty stomach, 1 hour before or 2 hours after food intake.

In order to maintain the integrity of the enteric coating of the tablet, do not crush, chew, or cut mycophenolic acid tablets; swallow the tablets whole. Inform patients of the need for repeated appropriate laboratory tests while they are receiving mycophenolic acid. Give patients complete dosage instructions, and inform them of the increased risk of lymphoproliferative disease and certain other malignancies.

Instruct women of childbearing potential of the potential risks during pregnancy, and that they should use effective contraception before beginning mycophenolic acid therapy, during therapy, and for 6 weeks after mycophenolic acid has been stopped.

TACROLIMUS

Rx	**Prograf** (Astellas)	**Capsules:** 0.5 mg	Lactose. (f 607). Light yellow, oblong. In 100s and blister cards of 10s.
		1 mg	Lactose. (f 617). White, oblong. In 100s and blister cards of 10s.
		5 mg	Lactose. (f 657). Grayish/red, oblong. In 100s and blister cards of 10s.
		Injection: 5 mg/mL	In 1 mL amps.[a]

[a] Contains polyoxyl 60 hydrogenated castor oil (HCO-60) 200 mg/mL and 80% dehydrated alcohol.

TACROLIMUS — ORAL

Tacrolimus also is available as an ointment for use in mild to moderate atopic dermatitis. For complete and comparative prescribing information for the ointment, refer to the Dermatologics chapter.

WARNING

Increased susceptibility to infection and the possible development of lymphoma may result from immunosuppression. Only physicians experienced in immunosuppressive therapy and management of organ transplant patients should prescribe tacrolimus. Patients receiving the drug should be managed in facilities equipped and staffed with adequate laboratory and supportive medical resources. The physician responsible for maintenance therapy should have complete information requisite for the follow-up of the patient.

Indications

➤*Organ rejection prophylaxis:* For the prophylaxis of organ rejection in patients receiving allogeneic liver, kidney, or heart transplants. It is recommended that tacrolimus be used concomitantly with adrenal corticosteroids. Because of the risk of anaphylaxis, tacrolimus injection should be reserved for patients unable to take tacrolimus capsules orally. In heart transplant recipients, it is recommended that tacrolimus be used in conjunction with azathioprine or mycophenolate mofetil (MMF). The safety and efficacy of the use of tacrolimus with sirolimus has not been established.

➤*Unlabeled uses:* Prevention and treatment of acute graft-versus-host disease (GVHD) following hematopoietic stem cell transplantation.

Administration and Dosage

➤*Approved by the FDA:* April 8, 1994.

Oral Dosage Recommendations and Typical Whole Blood Trough Concentrations

Patient population	Recommended initial oral dose*	Typical whole blood trough concentrations
Adult kidney transplant patients	0.2 mg/kg/day	Month 1 through 3: 7 to 20 ng/mL Month 4 through 12: 5 to 15 ng/mL
Adult liver transplant patients	0.1 to 0.15 mg/kg/day	Month 1 through 12: 5 to 20 ng/mL
Pediatric liver transplant patients	0.15 to 0.2 mg/kg/day	Month 1 to 12: 5 to 20 ng/mL
Adult heart transplant patients	0.075 mg/kg/day	Month 1 through 3: 10 to 20 ng/mL Month 4 and after: 5 to 15 ng/mL

* Note: Two divided doses every 12 hours.

➤*Liver transplantation:* It is recommended that patients initiate oral therapy with tacrolimus capsules if possible. If IV therapy is necessary, conversion from IV to oral tacrolimus is recommended as soon as oral therapy can be tolerated. This usually occurs within 2 to 3 days. The initial dose of tacrolimus should be administered no sooner than 6 hours after transplantation. In a patient receiving an IV infusion, the first dose of oral therapy should be given 8 to 12 hours after discontinuing the IV infusion. The recommended starting oral dose of tacrolimus capsules is 0.1 to 0.15 mg/kg/day administered in 2 divided daily doses every 12 hours. Coadministered grapefruit juice has been reported to increase tacrolimus blood trough concentrations in liver transplant patients. Grapefruit juice affects CYP3A-mediated metabolism and should be avoided.

Dosing should be titrated based on clinical assessments of rejection and tolerability. Lower tacrolimus dosages may be sufficient as maintenance therapy. Adjunct therapy with adrenal corticosteroids is recommended early posttransplant.

➤*Kidney transplantation:* The recommended starting oral dose of tacrolimus is 0.2 mg/kg/day administered every 12 hours in 2 divided doses. The initial dose of tacrolimus may be administered within 24 hours of transplantation, but should be delayed until renal function has recovered (as indicated for example by a serum creatinine less than or equal to 4 mg/dL). Black patients may require higher doses to achieve comparable blood concentrations. Dosage and typical tacrolimus whole blood trough concentrations are shown in the table above; blood concentration details are described in Blood concentration monitoring: Kidney transplantation (see below).

The data in kidney transplant patients indicate that black patients required a higher dose to attain comparable trough concentrations compared to white patients.

Time after transplant	White (n = 114)		Black (n = 56)	
	Dose (mg/kg)	Trough concentrations (ng/mL)	Dose (mg/kg)	Trough concentrations (ng/mL)
Day 7	0.18	12	0.23	10.9
Month 1	0.17	12.8	0.26	12.9
Month 6	0.14	11.8	0.24	11.5
Month 12	0.13	10.1	0.19	11

➤*Heart transplantation:* The recommended starting oral dose is 0.075 mg/kg/day administered every 12 hours in two divided doses. If possible, initiating oral therapy with tacrolimus is recommended. If IV therapy is necessary, conversion from IV to oral tacrolimus is recommended as soon as oral therapy can be tolerated. This usually occurs within 2 to 3 days. The initial dose of tacrolimus should be administered no sooner than 6 hours after transplantation. In a patient receiving an IV infusion, the first dose of oral therapy should be given 8 to 12 hours after discontinuing the IV infusion.

Dosing should be titrated based on clinical assessments of rejection and tolerability. Lower tacrolimus dosages may be sufficient as maintenance therapy. Adjunct therapy with adrenal corticosteroids is recommended early posttransplant.

➤*Children:* Pediatric liver transplantation patients without preexisting renal or hepatic dysfunction have required and tolerated higher doses than adults to achieve similar blood concentrations. Therefore, it is recommended that therapy be initiated in children at a starting IV dose of 0.03 to 0.05 mg/kg/day and a starting oral dose of 0.15 to 0.2 mg/kg/day. Dose adjustments may be required. Experience in pediatric kidney and heart transplantation patients is limited.

➤*Hepatic/Renal function impairment:* Due to the reduced clearance and prolonged half-life, patients with severe hepatic impairment (Pugh score greater than or equal to 10) may require lower doses of tacrolimus. Close monitoring of blood concentrations is warranted.

Due to the potential for nephrotoxicity, patients with renal or hepatic impairment should receive doses at the lowest value of the recommended IV and oral dosing ranges. Further reductions in dose below these ranges may be required. Tacrolimus therapy usually should be delayed up to 48 hours or longer in patients with postoperative oliguria.

➤*Conversion from one immunosuppressive regimen to another:* Tacrolimus should not be used simultaneously with cyclosporine. Tacrolimus or cyclosporine should be discontinued at least 24 hours before initiating the other. In the presence of elevated tacrolimus or cyclosporine concentrations, dosing with the other drug usually should be further delayed.

➤*Blood concentration monitoring:* Monitoring of tacrolimus blood concentrations in conjunction with other laboratory and clinical parameters is considered an essential aid to patient management for the evaluation of rejection, toxicity, dose adjustments and compliance. Factors influencing frequency of monitoring include but are not limited to hepatic or renal dysfunction, the addition or discontinuation of potentially interacting drugs and the posttransplant time. Blood concentration monitoring is not a replacement for renal and liver function monitoring and tissue biopsies.

Two methods have been used for the assay of tacrolimus, a microparticle enzyme immunoassay (MEIA) and an enzyme linked immunosorbent assay (ELISA). Both methods have the same monoclonal antibody for tacrolimus. Comparison of the concentrations in published literature to patient concentrations using the current assays must be made with detailed knowledge of the assay methods and biological matrices employed. Whole blood is the matrix of choice and specimens should be collected into tubes containing ethylene diamine tetraacetic acid (EDTA) anticoagulant. Heparin anticoagulation is not recommended because of the tendency to form clots on storage. Samples that are not analyzed immediately should be stored at room temperature or in a refrigerator and assayed within 7 days; if samples are to be kept longer they should be deep frozen at −20°C (-4°F) for up to 12 months.

➤*Liver transplantation:* Although there is a lack of direct correlation between tacrolimus concentrations and drug efficacy, data from phase 2 and 3 studies of liver transplant patients have shown an increasing incidence of adverse events with increasing trough blood concentrations. Most patients are stable when trough whole blood concentrations are maintained between 5 to 20 ng/mL. Long-term posttransplant patients often are maintained at the low end of this target range.

TACROLIMUS — ORAL

Data from the US clinical trial show that tacrolimus whole blood concentrations, as measured by ELISA, were most variable during the first week posttransplantation. After this early period, the median trough blood concentrations, measured at intervals from the second week to 1 year posttransplantation, ranged from 9.8 ng/mL to 19.4 ng/mL.

➤*Kidney transplantation:* Data from the phase 3 study indicates that trough concentrations of tacrolimus in whole blood, as measured by tacrolimus-specific assay test, were most variable during the first week of dosing. During the first 3 months, 80% of the patients maintained trough concentrations between 7 to 20 ng/mL, and then between 5 to 15 ng/mL, through 1 year.

The relative risk of toxicity is increased with higher trough concentrations. Therefore, monitoring of whole blood trough concentrations is recommended to assist in the clinical evaluation of toxicity.

➤*Heart transplantation:* Data from a phase 3 study indicate that trough concentrations of tacrolimus in whole blood were most variable during the first week of dosing. From week 1 to 3 months posttransplant, approximately 80% of patients maintained trough concentrations between 8 to 20 ng/mL and, from 3 months through 18 months posttransplant, approximately 80% of patients maintained trough concentrations between 6 to 8 ng/mL.

The relative risk of toxicity; for example, nephrotoxicity and posttransplant diabetes mellitus, is increased with higher trough concentrations. Therefore, monitoring of whole blood trough concentrations is recommended to assist in the clinical evaluation of toxicity.

➤*Storage/Stability:* Store at 25°C (77°F); excursion permitted to 15° to 30°C (59° to 86°F).

Actions

➤*Pharmacology:* Tacrolimus prolongs the survival of the host and transplanted graft in animal transplant models of liver, kidney, heart, bone marrow, small bowel and pancreas, lung and trachea, skin, cornea, and limb.

In animals, tacrolimus has been demonstrated to suppress some humoral immunity and, to a greater extent, cell-mediated reactions such as allograft rejection, delayed-type hypersensitivity, collagen-induced arthritis, experimental allergic encephalomyelitis, and graft vs host disease.

Tacrolimus inhibits T-lymphocyte activation, although the exact mechanism of action is not known. Experimental evidence suggests that tacrolimus binds to an intracellular protein, FKBP-12. A complex of tacrolimus-FKBP-12, calcium, calmodulin, and calcineurin is then formed and the phosphatase activity of calcineurin inhibited. This effect may prevent the dephosphorylation and translocation of nuclear factor of activated T-cells (NF-AT), a nuclear component thought to initiate gene transcription for the formation of lymphokines (such as interleukin-2, gamma interferon). The net result is the inhibition of T-lymphocyte activation (ie, immunosuppression).

➤*Pharmacokinetics:*

Absorption – Absorption of tacrolimus from the GI tract after oral administration is incomplete and variable. The absolute bioavailability of tacrolimus was 17 ± 10% in adult kidney transplant patients (n = 26), 22 ± 6% in adult liver transplant patients (n = 17), and 18 ± 5% in healthy volunteers (n = 16).

A single dose study conducted in 32 healthy volunteers established the bioequivalence of the 1 and 5 mg capsules. Another single dose study in 32 healthy volunteers established the bioequivalence of the 0.5 mg and 1 mg capsules. Tacrolimus maximum blood concentrations (C_{max}) and area under the curve (AUC) appeared to increase in a dose-proportional fashion in 18 fasted healthy volunteers receiving a single oral dose of 3, 7, and 10 mg.

In 18 kidney transplant patients, tacrolimus trough concentrations from 3 to 30 ng/mL measured at 10 to 12 hours postdose (C_{min}) correlated well with the AUC (correlation coefficient 0.93). In 24 liver transplant patients over a concentration range of 10 to 60 ng/mL, the correlation coefficient was 0.94.

Food effects: See Drug Interactions for more information.

Distribution – The plasma protein binding of tacrolimus is approximately 99% and is independent of concentration over a range of 5 to 50 ng/mL. Tacrolimus is bound mainly to albumin and alpha-1-acid glycoprotein, and has a high level of association with erythrocytes. The distribution of tacrolimus between whole blood and plasma depends on several factors, such as hematocrit, temperature at the time of plasma separation, drug concentration, and plasma protein concentration. In a US study, the ratio of whole blood concentration to plasma concentration averaged 35 (range 12 to 67).

Metabolism – Tacrolimus is extensively metabolized by the mixed-function oxidase system, primarily the cytochrome P450 system (CYP3A). A metabolic pathway leading to the formation of 8 possible metabolites has been proposed. Demethylation and hydroxylation were identified as the primary mechanisms of biotransformation in vitro. The major metabolite identified in incubations with human liver microsomes is 13-demethyl tacrolimus. In in vitro studies, a 31-demethyl metabolite has been reported to have the same activity as tacrolimus.

Excretion – When administered orally, the mean recovery of the radiolabel was 94.9 ± 30.7%. Fecal elimination accounted for 92.6 ± 30.7%, urinary elimination accounted for 2.3 ± 1.1% and the elimination half-life based on radioactivity was 31.9 ± 10.5 hours whereas it was 48.4 ± 12.3 hours based on tacrolimus concentrations. The mean clearance of radiolabel was 0.226 ± 0.116 L/hr/kg and clearance of tacrolimus 0.172 ± 0.088 L/hr/kg.

Pharmacokinetic parameters – Tacrolimus activity is primarily due to the parent drug. The pharmacokinetic parameters (mean ± SD) of tacrolimus have been determined following IV and oral administration in healthy volunteers, liver transplant and kidney transplant patients (see table below).

Population	N	Route (dose)	Parameters					
			C_{max} (ng/mL)	t_{max} (hr)	AUC (ng•hr/mL)	t½ (hr)	Cl (L/hr/kg)	V (L/kg)
Healthy volunteers	8	IV (0.025 mg/kg/4 hr)	-	-	598* ± 125	34.2 ± 7.7	0.04 ± 0.009	1.91 ± 0.31
	16	Oral (5 mg)	29.7 ± 7.2	1.6 ± 0.7	243** ± 73	34.8 ± 11.4	0.041[1] ± 0.008	1.94[1] ± 0.53
Kidney transplant patients	26	IV (0.02 mg/kg/ 12 hr)	-	-	294*** ± 262	18.8 ± 16.7	0.083 ± 0.05	1.41 ± 0.66
		Oral (0.2 mg/kg/day)	19.2 ± 10.3	3	203*** ± 42	NA[2]	NA	NA
		Oral (0.3 mg/kg/day)	24.2 ± 15.8	1.5	288*** ± 93	NA	NA	NA
Liver transplant patients	17	IV (0.05 mg/kg/12 hr)	-	-	3300*** ± 2130	11.7 ± 3.9	0.053 ± 0.017	0.85 ± 0.3
		Oral (0.3 mg/kg/day)	68.5 ± 30	2.3 ± 1.5	519*** ± 179	NA	NA	NA

[1] Corrected for individual bioavailability.
[2] NA = not applicable.
* AUC_{0-120}.
** AUC_{0-72}.
*** $AUC_{0-\infty}$.

Due to intersubject variability in tacrolimus pharmacokinetics, individualization of dosing regimen is necessary for optimal therapy. Pharmacokinetic data indicate that whole blood concentrations rather than plasma concentrations serve as the more appropriate sampling compartment to describe tacrolimus pharmacokinetics.

Special populations –

Children: Pharmacokinetics of tacrolimus have been studied in liver transplantation patients, 0.7 to 13.2 years of age. Following oral administration to 9 patients, mean AUC and C_{max} were 337 ± 167 ng•hr/mL and 43.4 ± 27.9 ng/mL, respectively. The absolute bioavailability was 31 ± 21%.

See Indications for more information.

Renal and hepatic insufficiency: The mean pharmacokinetic parameters for tacrolimus following single administrations to patients with renal and hepatic impairment are given in the following table.

Population (number of patients)	Dose	AUC_{0-t} (ng•hr/mL)	t½ (hr)	V (L/kg)	Cl (L/hr/kg)
Renal impairment (n = 12)	0.02 mg/kg/4 hr IV	393 ± 123 (t = 60 hr)	26.3 ± 9.2	1.07 ± 0.2	0.038 ± 0.014
Mild hepatic impairment (n = 6)	0.02 mg/kg/4 hr IV	367 ± 107 (t = 72 hr)	60.6 ± 43.8 Range: 27.8 to 141	3.1 ± 1.6	0.042 ± 0.02
	7.7 mg oral	488 ± 320 (t = 72 hr)	66.1 ± 44.8 Range: 29.5 to 138	3.7 ± 4.7*	0.034 ± 0.019*
Severe hepatic impairment (n = 6, IV)	0.02 mg/kg/4 hr IV (n = 2)	762 ± 204 (t = 120 hr)	198 ± 158 Range: 81 to 436	3.9 ± 1	0.017 ± 0.013
	0.01 mg/kg/8 hr IV (n = 4)	289 ± 117 (t = 144 hr)			
Severe hepatic impairment (n = 5, oral)[1]	8 mg oral (n = 1)	658 (t = 120 hr)	119 ± 35 Range: 85 to 178	3.1 ± 3.4*	0.016 ± 0.011*
	5 mg oral (n = 4)	533 ± 156 (t = 144 hr)			
	4 mg oral (n = 1)				

* Corrected for bioavailability.
[1] One patient did not receive the oral dose.

TACROLIMUS — ORAL

• *Renal insufficiency* – Tacrolimus pharmacokinetics following a single IV administration were determined in 12 patients (7 not on dialysis and 5 on dialysis, serum creatinine of 3.9 ± 1.6 and 12 ± 2.4 mg/dL, respectively) prior to their kidney transplants. The pharmacokinetic parameters obtained were similar for both groups.

• *Hepatic insufficiency* – Tacrolimus pharmacokinetics have been determined in 6 patients with mild hepatic dysfunction (mean Pugh score: 6.2) following single IV and oral administrations. The mean clearance of tacrolimus in patients with mild hepatic dysfunction was not substantially different from that in healthy volunteers (see previous information). Tacrolimus pharmacokinetics were studied in 6 patients with severe hepatic dysfunction (mean Pugh score greater than 10). The mean clearance was substantially lower in patients with severe hepatic dysfunction, irrespective of the route of administration.

Race: A formal study to evaluate the pharmacokinetic disposition of tacrolimus in black transplant patients has not been conducted. However, a retrospective comparison of black and white kidney transplant patients indicated that black patients required higher tacrolimus doses to attain similar trough concentrations.

The data in kidney transplant patients indicate that black patients required a higher dose to attain comparable trough concentrations compared to white patients.

	White (n = 114)		Black (n = 56)	
Time after transplant	Dose (mg/kg)	Trough concentrations (ng/mL)	Dose (mg/kg)	Trough concentrations (ng/mL)
Day 7	0.18	12	0.23	10.9
Month 1	0.17	12.8	0.26	12.9
Month 6	0.14	11.8	0.24	11.5
Month 12	0.13	10.1	0.19	11

Contraindications

Tacrolimus is contraindicated in patients with a hypersensitivity to tacrolimus. Tacrolimus injection is contraindicated in patients with a hypersensitivity to HCO-60 (polyoxyl 60 hydrogenated castor oil).

Warnings

See the Warning box for more information.

➤*Insulin-dependent posttransplant diabetes mellitus:* Insulin-dependent posttransplant diabetes mellitus (PTDM) was reported in 20% of tacrolimus-treated kidney transplant patients without pretransplant history of diabetes mellitus in the phase 3 study (see tables below). The median time to onset of PTDM was 68 days. Insulin dependence was reversible in 15% of these patients at 1 year and in 50% at 2 years posttransplant. Black and Hispanic kidney transplant patients were at an increased risk of development of PTDM.

Incidence of PTDM and insulin use at 2 years in kidney transplant recipients in the phase 3 study

Status of PTDM*	Tacrolimus	CBIR[1]
Patients without pretransplant history of diabetes mellitus	151	151
New onset of PTDM*, first year	30/151 (20%)	6/151 (4%)
Still insulin dependent at 1 year in those without history of diabetes	25/151 (17%)	5/151 (3%)
New onset of PTDM* post 1 year	1	0
Patients with PTDM* at 2 years	16/151 (11%)	5/151 (3%)

* Use of insulin for 30 or more consecutive days, with less than a 5-day gap, without a history of type 1 diabetes mellitus or type 2 diabetes mellitus.
[1] Cyclosporine-based immunosuppressive regimen.

Development of PTDM by race and by treatment group during first-year post kidney transplantation in the phase 3 study

	Tacrolimus		CBIR	
Patient race	Number of patients at risk	Patients who developed PTDM*	Number of patients at risk	Patients who developed PTDM*
Black	41	15 (37%)	36	3 (8%)
Hispanic	17	5 (29%)	18	1 (6%)
White	82	10 (12%)	87	1 (1%)
Other	11	0 (0%)	10	1 (10%)
Total	151	30 (20%)	151	6 (4%)

* Use of insulin for 30 or more consecutive days, with less than a 5-day gap, without a history of type 1 diabetes mellitus or type 2 diabetes mellitus.

Insulin-dependent was reported in 18% and 11% of tacrolimus-treated liver transplant patients and was reversible in 45% and 31% of these patients at 1 year posttransplant, in the US and European randomized studies, respectively (see table below). Hyperglycemia was associated with the use of tacrolimus in 47% and 33% of liver transplant recipients in the US and European randomized studies, respectively, and may require treatment with insulin.

Incidence of posttransplant diabetes mellitus and insulin use at 1 year in liver transplant recipients

	US study		European study	
Status of PTDM*	Tacrolimus	CBIR	Tacrolimus	CBIR
Patients at risk**	239	236	239	249
New onset PTDM*	42 (18%)	30 (13%)	26 (11%)	12 (5%)
Patients still on insulin at 1 year	23 (10%)	19 (8%)	18 (8%)	6 (2%)

* Use of insulin for 30 or more consecutive days, with less than a 5-day gap, without a history of type 1 diabetes mellitus or type 2 diabetes mellitus.
** Patients without a pretransplant history of diabetes mellitus.

➤*Neurotoxicity and nephrotoxicity:* Tacrolimus can cause neurotoxicity and nephrotoxicity, particularly when used in high doses. Nephrotoxicity was reported in approximately 52% of kidney transplantation patients and in 40% and 36% of liver transplantation patients receiving tacrolimus in the US and European randomized trials, respectively. More overt nephrotoxicity is seen early after transplantation, characterized by increasing serum creatinine and a decrease in urine output. Patients with impaired renal function should be monitored closely as the dosage of tacrolimus may need to be reduced. In patients with persistent elevations of serum creatinine who are unresponsive to dosage adjustments, consideration should be given to changing to another immunosuppressive therapy. Care should be taken in using tacrolimus with other nephrotoxic drugs. In particular, to avoid excess nephrotoxicity, tacrolimus should not be used simultaneously with cyclosporine. Tacrolimus or cyclosporine should be discontinued at least 24 hours prior to initiating the other. In the presence of elevated tacrolimus or cyclosporine concentrations, dosing with the other drug usually should be further delayed.

Neurotoxicity, including tremor, headache, and other changes in motor function, mental status, and sensory function were reported in approximately 55% of liver transplant recipients in the 2 randomized studies. Tremor occurred more often in tacrolimus-treated kidney transplant patients (54%) compared to cyclosporine-treated patients. The incidence of other neurological events in kidney transplant patients was similar in the two treatment groups (headache, 44% vs 38%; insomnia, 32% vs 30%; paresthesia, 23% vs 16%; dizziness, 19% vs 16%, respectively. Tremor and headache have been associated with high whole-blood concentrations of tacrolimus and may respond to dosage adjustment. Seizures have occurred in adults and children receiving tacrolimus. Coma and delirium also have been associated with high plasma concentrations of tacrolimus.

➤*Hyperkalemia:* Mild to severe hyperkalemia was reported in 31% of kidney transplant recipients and in 45% and 13% of liver transplant recipients treated with tacrolimus in the US and European randomized trials, respectively, and may require treatment. Serum potassium levels should be monitored and potassium-sparing diuretics should not be used during tacrolimus therapy.

➤*Immunosuppressants:* As in patients receiving other immunosuppressants, patients receiving tacrolimus are at increased risk of developing lymphomas and other malignancies, particularly of the skin. The risk appears to be related to the intensity and duration of immunosuppression rather than to the use of any specific agent. A lymphoproliferative disorder (LPD) related to Epstein-Barr virus (EBV) infection has been reported in immunosuppressed organ transplant recipients. The risk of LPD appears greatest in young children who are at risk for primary EBV infection while immunosuppressed or who are switched to tacrolimus following long-term immunosuppression therapy. Because of the danger of oversuppression of the immune system, which can increase susceptibility to infection, combination immunosuppressant therapy should be used with caution.

➤*Hypersensitivity reactions:* A few patients receiving tacrolimus injection have experienced anaphylactic reactions. Although the exact cause of these reactions is not known, other drugs with castor oil derivatives in the formulation have been associated with anaphylaxis in a small percentage of patients. Because of this potential risk of anaphylaxis, tacrolimus injection should be reserved for patients who are unable to take tacrolimus capsules.

➤*Renal / Hepatic function impairment:* See Administration and Dosage for more information.

The use of tacrolimus in liver transplant recipients experiencing posttransplant hepatic impairment may be associated with increased risk of developing renal insufficiency related to high whole-blood levels of tacrolimus. These patients should be monitored closely and dosage adjustments should be considered. Some evidence suggests that lower doses should be used in these patients.

In patients who develop renal failure or clinical manifestations of ventricular dysfunction while receiving tacrolimus therapy, echocardiographic evaluation should be considered.

➤*Carcinogenesis:* An increased incidence of malignancy is a recognized complication of immunosuppression in recipients of organ transplants. The most common forms of neoplasms are non-Hodgkin's lymphomas and carcinomas of the skin. As with other immunosuppressive therapies, the risk of malignancies in tacrolimus recipients may be higher than in the healthy population. Lymphoproliferative disorders associated with Epstein-Barr virus infection have been seen. It has been reported that reduction or discontinuation of immunosuppression may cause the lesions to regress.

➤*Fertility impairment:* No impairment of fertility was demonstrated in studies of male and female rats. Tacrolimus, given orally at 1 mg/kg (0.7 to 4 times the recommended clinical dose range of 0.1 to 0.2 mg/kg/day based on body surface area corrections) to male and female rats, prior to and during mating, as well as to dams during gestation and lactation, was associ-

TACROLIMUS — ORAL

ated with embryolethality and with adverse effects on female reproduction. Effects on female reproductive function (parturition) and embryolethal effects were indicated by a higher rate of pre-implantation loss and increased numbers of undelivered and nonviable pups. When given at 3.2 mg/kg (2.3 to 4.6 times the recommended clinical dose range based on body surface area correction), tacrolimus was associated with maternal and paternal toxicity and reproductive toxicity including marked adverse effects on estrus cycles, parturition, pup viability, and pup malformations.

➤*Pregnancy: Category C.* In reproduction studies in rats and rabbits, adverse effects on the fetus were observed mainly at dose levels that were toxic to dams. Tacrolimus at oral doses of 0.32 and 1 mg/kg during organogenesis in rabbits was associated with maternal toxicity as well as an increase in incidence of abortions; these doses are equivalent to 0.5 to 1 times and 1.6 to 3.3 times the recommended clinical dose range (0.1 to 0.2 mg/kg) based on body surface area corrections. At the higher dose only, an increased incidence of malformations and developmental variations was also seen. Tacrolimus, at oral doses of 3.2 mg/kg during organogenesis in rats, was associated with maternal toxicity and caused an increase in late resorptions, decreased numbers of live births, and decreased pup weight and viability. Tacrolimus, given orally at 1 and 3.2 mg/kg (equivalent to 0.7 to 1.4 times and 2.3 to 4.6 times the recommended clinical dose range based on body surface area corrections) to pregnant rats after organogenesis and during lactation, was associated with reduced pup weights.

There are no adequate and well-controlled studies in pregnant women. Tacrolimus is transferred across the placenta. The use of tacrolimus during pregnancy has been associated with neonatal hyperkalemia and renal dysfunction. Tacrolimus should be used during pregnancy only if the potential benefit to the mother justifies potential risk to the fetus.

➤*Lactation:* Since tacrolimus is excreted in human milk, breastfeeding should be avoided.

➤*Children:* Experience with tacrolimus in pediatric kidney transplant patients is limited. Successful liver transplants have been performed in children (16 years of age or older) using tacrolimus. The 2 randomized active-controlled trials of tacrolimus in primary liver transplantation included 56 children. Thirty-one patients were randomized to tacrolimus-based and 25 to cyclosporine-based therapies. Additionally, a minimum of 122 children were studied in an uncontrolled trial of tacrolimus in living related donor liver transplantation. Children generally required higher doses of tacrolimus to maintain blood trough concentrations of tacrolimus similar to adult patients.

See Indications for more information.

Precautions

➤*Monitoring:* See Administration and Dosage for more information.

Serum creatinine, potassium, and fasting glucose should be assessed regularly. Routine monitoring of metabolic and hematologic systems should be performed as clinically warranted.

➤*Hypertension:* Hypertension is a common adverse effect of tacrolimus therapy. Mild or moderate hypertension is more frequently reported than severe hypertension. Antihypertensive therapy may be required; the control of blood pressure can be accomplished with any of the common antihypertensive agents. Since tacrolimus may cause hyperkalemia, potassium-sparing diuretics should be avoided. While calcium-channel blocking agents can be effective in treating tacrolimus-associated hypertension, care should be taken since interference with tacrolimus metabolism may require a dosage reduction.

➤*Myocardial hypertrophy:* Myocardial hypertrophy has been reported in association with the administration of tacrolimus, and is generally manifested by echocardiographically demonstrated concentric increases in left ventricular posterior wall and interventricular septum thickness. Hypertrophy has been observed in infants, children and adults. This condition appears reversible in most cases following dose reduction or discontinuance of therapy. In a group of 20 patients with pre- and posttreatment echocardiograms who showed evidence of myocardial hypertrophy, mean tacrolimus whole blood concentrations during the period prior to diagnosis of myocardial hypertrophy ranged from 11 to 53 ng/mL in infants (n = 10, age 0.4 to 2 years), 4 to 46 ng/mL in children (n = 7, age 2 to 15 years) and 11 to 24 ng/mL in adults (n = 3, age 37 to 53 years).

If myocardial hypertrophy is diagnosed, dosage reduction or discontinuation of tacrolimus should be considered.

Drug Interactions

➤*Drugs that may alter tacrolimus concentrations:* Since tacrolimus is metabolized mainly by the CYP3A enzyme systems, substances known to inhibit these enzymes may decrease the metabolism of tacrolimus with resultant increases in whole blood or plasma concentrations. Drugs known to induce these enzyme systems may result in an increased metabolism of tacrolimus and decreased whole blood or plasma concentrations. Monitoring of blood concentrations and appropriate dosage adjustments are essential when such drugs are used concomitantly.

Drugs that may increase tacrolimus blood concentrations*

Calcium channel blockers	Antifungal agents	Macrolide antibiotics	GI prokinetic agents	Other drugs
Diltiazem	Clotrimazole	Clarithromycin	Cisapride	Bromocriptine
Nicardipine	Fluconazole	Erythromycin	Metoclopramide	Cimetidine
Nifedipine	Itraconazole	Troleandomycin		Cyclosporine
Verapamil	Ketoconazole			Danazol
				Ethinyl estradiol
				Methylprednisolone
				Omeprazole
				Protease inhibitors
				Nefazodone

* This table is not all inclusive.

Drugs that may decrease tacrolimus blood concentrations*

Anticonvulsants	Antibiotics	Herbal preparations
Carbamazepine	Rifabutin	St. John's wort
Phenobarbital	Rifampin	
Phenytoin		

* This table is not all inclusive.

Interaction studies with drugs used in HIV therapy have not been conducted. However, care should be exercised when drugs that are nephrotoxic (eg, ganciclovir) or that are metabolized by CYP3A (eg, ritonavir) are administered concomitantly with tacrolimus.

➤*Other drug interactions:* Tacrolimus may affect the pharmacokinetics of other drugs (eg, phenytoin) and increase their concentration. Immunosuppressants may affect vaccination. Therefore, during treatment with tacrolimus, vaccination may be less effective. The use of live vaccines should be avoided; live vaccines may include, but are not limited to measles, mumps, rubella, oral polio, BCG, yellow fever, and TY21a typhoid.

Tacrolimus Drug Interactions

Precipitant drug	Object drug*		Description
Nephrotoxic agents (eg, aminoglycosides, amphotericin B, cisplatin, cyclosporine)	Tacrolimus	↑	Because of the potential for additive or synergistic impairment of renal function, take care when administering tacrolimus with drugs that may be associated with renal dysfunction. Coadministration with cyclosporine resulted in additive/synergistic nephrotoxicity; tacrolimus blood levels also may be increased. Give the first tacrolimus dose no sooner than 24 hours after the last cyclosporine dose.
Bromocriptine, Cimetidine, Cisapride, Chloramphenicol, Danazol, Ethinyl estradiol, Methylprednisolone, Metoclopramide, Metronidazole, Nefazodone, Omeprazole, Protease inhibitors, Macrolide antibiotics, (eg, clarithromycin, erythromycin, troleandomycin), Calcium channel blockers (eg, diltiazem, nicardepine, nifedipine, verapamil), Antifungal Agents (eg, clotrimazole, fluconazole, itraconazole, ketoconazole, miconazole)	Tacrolimus	↑	These agents may increase tacrolimus blood levels, increasing risk of toxicity.
Carbamazepine, Fosphenytoin, Phenobarbital, Phenytoin, Antibiotics eg, rifabutin, rifampin, rifapentine)	Tacrolimus	↓	These agents may decrease tacrolimus blood levels.
St. John's wort	Tacrolimus	↓	St. John's wort induces CYP3A4 and P-glycoprotein. Because tacrolimus is a substrate for CYP3A4, tacrolimus blood levels may decrease.
Tacrolimus	Mycophenolate mofetil	↑	Mycophenolate trough plasma concentrations may be elevated, increasing risk of side effects.

TACROLIMUS — ORAL

Tacrolimus Drug Interactions			
Precipitant drug	Object drug*		Description
Tacrolimus	Vaccines	⬇	Immunosuppressants may affect vaccination. Therefore, during treatment with tacrolimus, vaccination may be less effective. Avoid the use of live vaccines (eg, measles, mumps, rubella, oral polio, BCG, yellow fever, TY 21a typhoid).

* ⬆ = Object drug increased. ⬇ = Object drug decreased.

➤*Drug/Food interactions:* The rate and extent of tacrolimus absorption were greatest under fasted conditions. The presence and composition of food decreased both the rate and extent of tacrolimus absorption when administered to 15 healthy volunteers. Coadministered grapefruit juice has been reported to increase tacrolimus blood trough concentrations in liver transplant patients. Grapefruit juice affects CYP3A-mediated metabolism and should be avoided.

The effect was most pronounced with a high-fat meal (848 kcal, 46% fat): Mean AUC and C_{max} were decreased 37% and 77%, respectively; t_{max} was lengthened 5-fold. A high-carbohydrate meal (668 kcal, 85% carbohydrate) decreased mean AUC and mean C_{max} by 28% and 65%, respectively.

In healthy volunteers (n = 16), the time of the meal also affected tacrolimus bioavailability. When given immediately following the meal, mean C_{max} was reduced 71%, and mean AUC was reduced 39%, relative to the fasted condition. When administered 1.5 hours following the meal, mean C_{max} was reduced 63%, and mean AUC was reduced 39%, relative to the fasted condition.

In 11 liver transplant patients, tacrolimus administered 15 minutes after a high fat (400 kcal, 34% fat) breakfast, resulted in decreased AUC (27 ± 18%) and C_{max} (50 ± 19%), as compared to a fasted state.

Adverse Reactions

➤*Liver transplantation:* The principal adverse reactions of tacrolimus are tremor, headache, diarrhea, hypertension, nausea, and renal dysfunction. These occur with oral and IV administration of tacrolimus and may respond to a reduction in dosing. Diarrhea was sometimes associated with other GI complaints such as nausea and vomiting.

Hyperkalemia and hypomagnesemia have occurred in patients receiving tacrolimus therapy. Hyperglycemia has been noted in many patients; some may require insulin therapy. Serum potassium levels should be monitored and potassium-sparing diuretics should not be used during tacrolimus therapy.

Liver transplantation: Adverse events occurring in ≥ 15% of tacrolimus-treated patients				
	US study (%)		European study (%)	
	Tacrolimus (n = 250)	CBIR (n = 250)	Tacrolimus (n = 264)	CBIR (n = 265)
CNS				
Headache	64%	60%	37%	26%
Tremor	56%	46%	48%	32%
Insomnia	64%	68%	32%	23%
Paresthesia	40%	30%	17%	17%
GI				
Diarrhea	72%	47%	37%	27%
Nausea	46%	37%	32%	27%
Constipation	24%	27%	23%	21%
LFT Abnormal	36%	30%	6%	5%
Anorexia	34%	24%	7%	5%
Vomiting	27%	15%	14%	11%
Cardiovascular				
Hypertension	47%	56%	38%	43%
GU				
Kidney function abnormal	40%	27%	36%	23%
Creatinine increased	39%	25%	24%	19%
BUN increased	30%	22%	12%	9%
Urinary tract infection	16%	18%	21%	19%
Oliguria	18%	15%	19%	12%
Metabolic and nutritional				
Hyperkalemia	45%	26%	13%	9%
Hypokalemia	29%	34%	13%	16%
Hyperglycemia	47%	38%	33%	22%
Hypomagnesemia	48%	45%	16%	9%

Liver transplantation: Adverse events occurring in ≥ 15% of tacrolimus-treated patients				
	US study (%)		European study (%)	
	Tacrolimus (n = 250)	CBIR (n = 250)	Tacrolimus (n = 264)	CBIR (n = 265)
Hemic and lymphatic				
Anemia	47%	38%	5%	1%
Leukocytosis	32%	26%	8%	8%
Thrombocytopenia	24%	20%	14%	19%
Miscellaneous				
Abdominal pain	59%	54%	29%	22%
Pain	63%	57%	24%	22%
Fever	48%	56%	19%	22%
Asthenia	52%	48%	11%	7%
Back pain	30%	29%	17%	17%
Ascites	27%	22%	7%	8%
Peripheral edema	26%	26%	12%	14%
Respiratory				
Pleural effusion	30%	32%	36%	35%
Atelectasis	28%	30%	5%	4%
Dyspnea	29%	23%	5%	4%
Dermatologic				
Pruritus	36%	20%	15%	7%
Rash	24%	19%	10%	4%

Less frequently observed adverse reactions in both liver transplantation and kidney transplantation patients are described under the subsection Less frequently reported adverse reactions below.

➤*Kidney transplantation:* The most common adverse reactions reported were infection, tremor, hypertension, decreased renal function, constipation, diarrhea, headache, abdominal pain, and insomnia.

Adverse events that occurred in greater than or equal to 15% of tacrolimus-treated kidney transplant patients are presented below:

Kidney transplantation: Adverse events occurring in ≥ 15% of tacrolimus-treated patients		
	Tacrolimus (n = 205)	CBIR (n = 207)
CNS		
Tremor	54%	34%
Headache	44%	38%
Insomnia	32%	30%
Paresthesia	23%	16%
Dizziness	19%	16%
GI		
Diarrhea	44%	41%
Nausea	38%	36%
Constipation	35%	43%
Vomiting	29%	23%
Dyspepsia	28%	20%
Cardiovascular		
Hypertension	50%	52%
Chest pain	19%	13%
GU		
Creatinine increased	45%	42%
Urinary tract infection	34%	35%
Metabolic and nutritional		
Hypophosphatemia	49%	53%
Hypomagnesemia	34%	17%
Hyperlipemia	31%	38%
Hyperkalemia	31%	32%
Diabetes mellitus	24%	9%
Hypokalemia	22%	25%
Hyperglycemia	22%	16%
Edema	18%	19%
Hemic and lymphatic		
Anemia	30%	24%
Leukopenia	15%	17%

TACROLIMUS — ORAL

Kidney transplantation: Adverse events occurring in ≥ 15% of tacrolimus-treated patients		
	Tacrolimus (n = 205)	CBIR (n = 207)
Miscellaneous		
Infection	45%	49%
Peripheral edema	36%	48%
Asthenia	34%	30%
Abdominal pain	33%	31%
Pain	32%	30%
Fever	29%	29%
Back pain	24%	20%
Respiratory		
Dyspnea	22%	18%
Cough increased	18%	15%
Musculoskeletal		
Arthralgia	25%	24%
Dermatologic		
Rash	17%	12%
Pruritus	15%	7%

Less frequently observed adverse reactions in both liver transplantation and kidney transplantation patients are described below.

➤*Less frequently reported adverse reactions:* The following adverse events were reported in the range of 3% to less than 15% incidence in either liver or kidney transplant recipients who were treated with tacrolimus in the phase 3 comparative trials.

Cardiovascular – Angina pectoris; chest pain; deep thrombophlebitis; abnormal ECG; hemorrhage; hypotension; postural hypotension; peripheral vascular disorder; phlebitis; tachycardia; thrombosis; vasodilatation.

CNS – Abnormal dreams; agitation; amnesia; anxiety; confusion; convulsion; depression; dizziness; emotional lability; encephalopathy; hallucinations; hypertonia; incoordination; myoclonus; nervousness; neuropathy; psychosis; somnolence; thinking abnormal. Neurotoxicity, including tremor, headache, and other changes in motor function, mental status, and sensory function were reported in approximately 55% of liver transplant recipients in the 2 randomized studies. Tremor occurred more often in tacrolimus-treated kidney transplant patients (54%) compared to cyclosporine-treated patients.

Dermatologic – Acne; alopecia; exfoliative dermatitis; fungal dermatitis; herpes simplex; hirsutism; skin discoloration; skin disorder; skin ulcer; sweating.

Endocrine – PTDM; Cushing's syndrome; diabetes mellitus.

GI – Anorexia; cholangitis; cholestatic jaundice; dyspepsia; dysphagia; esophagitis; flatulence; gastritis; GI hemorrhage; GGT increase; GI perforation; hepatitis; ileus; increased appetite; jaundice; liver damage; liver function test abnormal; oral moniliasis; rectal disorder; stomatitis.

GU – Albuminuria; cystitis; dysuria; hematuria; hydronephrosis; kidney failure; kidney tubular necrosis; nocturia; pyuria; toxic nephropathy; oliguria; urinary frequency; urinary incontinence; vaginitis.

Hematologic/Lymphatic – Coagulation disorder; ecchymosis; hypochromic anemia; leukocytosis; leukopenia; polycythemia; prothrombin decreased; serum iron decreased; thrombocytopenia.

Metabolic/Nutritional – Acidosis; alkaline phosphatase increased; alkalosis; ALT increased; AST increased; bicarbonate decreased; bilirubinemia; BUN increased; dehydration; GGT increased; healing abnormal; hypercalcemia; hypercholesterolemia; hyperlipemia; hyperphosphatemia; hyperuricemia; hypervolemia; hypocalcemia; hypoglycemia; hyponatremia; hypophosphatemia; hypoproteinemia; lactic dehydrogenase increase; weight gain.

Musculoskeletal – Arthralgia; cramps; generalized spasm; joint disorder; leg cramps; myalgia; myasthenia; osteoporosis.

Respiratory – Asthma; bronchitis; cough increased; lung disorder; pneumothorax; pulmonary edema; pharyngitis; pneumonia; respiratory disorder; rhinitis; sinusitis; voice alteration.

Special senses – Abnormal vision; amblyopia; ear pain; otitis media; tinnitus.

Miscellaneous – Abdomen enlarged; abscess; accidental injury; allergic reaction; cellulitis; chills; flu syndrome; generalized edema; hernia; peritonitis; photosensitivity reaction; sepsis.

There have been rare spontaneous reports of myocardial hypertrophy associated with clinically manifested ventricular dysfunction in patients receiving tacrolimus therapy. Myocardial hypertrophy has been reported in association with the administration of tacrolimus, and is generally manifested by echocardiographically demonstrated concentric increases in left ventricular posterior wall and interventricular septum thickness. Hypertrophy has been observed in infants, children and adults. This condition appears reversible in most cases following dose reduction or discontinuance of therapy. In a group of 20 patients with pre- and posttreatment echocardiograms who showed evidence of myocardial hypertrophy, mean tacrolimus whole blood concentrations during the period prior to diagnosis of myocardial hypertrophy ranged from 11 to 53 ng/mL in infants (n = 10, age 0.4 to 2 years), 4 to 46 ng/mL in children (n = 7, age 2 to 15 years) and 11 to 24 ng/mL in adults (n = 3, age 37 to 53 years). If myocardial hypertrophy is diagnosed, dosage reduction or discontinuation of tacrolimus should be considered.

➤*Postmarketing:* The following have been reported: Increased amylase including pancreatitis, hearing loss including deafness, leukoencephalopathy, thrombocytopenic purpura, hemolytic-uremia syndrome, acute renal failure, Stevens-Johnson syndrome, stomach ulcer, glycosuria, cardiac arrythmia, and gastroenteritis.

Overdosage

➤*Symptoms:* Limited overdosage experience is available. Acute overdosages of up to 30 times the intended dose have been reported. Almost all cases have been asymptomatic and all patients recovered with no sequelae. Occasionally, acute overdosage has been followed by tacrolimus adverse reactions except in 1 case where transient urticaria and lethargy were observed.

In acute oral and IV toxicity studies, mortalities were seen at or above the following doses: In adult rats, 52 times the recommended human oral dose; in immature rats, 16 times the recommended oral dose; and in adult rats, 16 times the recommended human IV dose (all based on body surface area corrections).

➤*Treatment:* Based on the poor aqueous solubility and extensive erythrocyte and plasma protein binding, it is anticipated that tacrolimus is not dialyzable to any significant extent; there is no experience with charcoal hemoperfusion. The oral use of activated charcoal has been reported in treating acute overdoses, but experience has not been sufficient to warrant recommending its use. General supportive measures and treatment of specific symptoms should be followed in all cases of overdosage.

Patient Information

Patients should be informed of the need for repeated appropriate laboratory tests while they are receiving tacrolimus. They should be given complete dosage instructions, advised of the potential risks during pregnancy, and informed of the increased risk of neoplasia. Patients should be informed that changes in dosage should not be undertaken without first consulting their physicians.

Patients should be informed that tacrolimus can cause diabetes mellitus and should be advised of the need to see their physicians if they develop frequent urination, increased thirst or hunger.

TACROLIMUS — INJECTION

Tacrolimus also is available as an ointment for use in mild to moderate atopic dermatitis. For complete and comparative prescribing information for the ointment, refer to the Dermatologics chapter.

WARNING

Increased susceptibility to infection and the possible development of lymphoma may result from immunosuppression. Only health care providers experienced in immunosuppressive therapy and management of organ transplant patients should prescribe tacrolimus. Manage patients receiving the drug in facilities equipped and staffed with adequate laboratory and supportive medical resources. The health care provider responsible for maintenance therapy should have complete information necessary for the follow-up of the patient.

Indications

➤*Organ rejection prophylaxis:* For the prophylaxis of organ rejection in patients receiving allogeneic liver, kidney, or heart transplants. It is recommended that tacrolimus be used concomitantly with adrenal corticosteroids. Because of the risk of anaphylaxis, tacrolimus injection should be reserved for patients unable to take tacrolimus capsules orally. In heart transplant recipients, it is recommended that tacrolimus be used in conjunction with azathioprine or mycophenolate mofetil. The safety and efficacy of the use of tacrolimus with sirolimus has not been established.

➤*Unlabeled uses:* Tacrolimus is being investigated for bone marrow, pancreas, pancreatic island cell, small bowel, and lung transplantation. It may be beneficial for the treatment of autoimmune disease (ie, rheumatoid arthritis, inflammatory bowel disease) and severe recalcitrant psoriasis.

Prevention and treatment of acute graft-versus-host disease following hematopoietic stem cell transplantation.

Administration and Dosage

➤*Approved by the FDA:* April 8, 1994 (1P,E classification).

➤*Injection:* Anaphylactic reactions have occurred with injectables containing castor oil derivatives. See Warnings.

For intravenous (IV) infusion only.

In patients unable to take the capsules, therapy may be initiated with the injection. Administer the initial dose no sooner than 6 hours after transplantation. The recommended starting dose is 0.01 mg/kg/day (heart) or 0.03 to 0.05 mg/kg/day (liver, kidney) as a continuous IV infusion. Give adult patients doses at the lower end of the dosing range. Concomitant adrenal

TACROLIMUS — INJECTION

corticosteroid therapy is recommended early posttransplantation. Continue continuous IV infusion only until the patient can tolerate oral administration.

Preparation for administration – Tacrolimus must be diluted with 0.9% sodium chloride injection or 5% dextrose injection to a concentration between 0.004 and 0.02 mg/mL prior to use. In situations in which more dilute solutions are utilized (eg, pediatric dosing), polyvinyl chloride (PVC)-free tubing should likewise be used to minimize the potential for significant drug adsorption onto the tubing. Parenteral drug products should be inspected visually for particulate matter and discoloration prior to administration, whenever solution and container permit.

➤*Admixture incompatibilities:* Because of the chemical instability of tacrolimus in alkaline media, tacrolimus injection should not be mixed or co-infused with solutions of pH 9 or greater (eg, ganciclovir, acyclovir).

➤*Liver transplantation:* Convert patients from IV to oral therapy as soon as oral therapy can be tolerated. This usually occurs within 2 to 3 days. Administer the initial dose no sooner than 6 hours after transplantation. Give the first dose of oral therapy 8 to 12 hours after discontinuing the IV infusion. The recommended starting oral dose is 0.1 to 0.15 mg/kg/day administered in 2 divided daily doses every 12 hours. Coadministered grapefruit juice has been reported to increase tacrolimus blood trough concentrations in liver transplant patients.

Titrate dosing based on clinical assessments of rejection and tolerability. Lower dosages may be sufficient as maintenance therapy. Adjunct therapy with adrenal corticosteroids is recommended early posttransplant.

➤*Kidney transplantation:* See the previous information and the tacrolimus oral dosing information.

➤*Heart transplantation:* The recommended starting oral dose is 0.075 mg/kg/day administered every 12 hours in 2 divided doses. If possible, initiating oral therapy with tacrolimus capsules is recommended. If IV therapy is necessary, conversion from IV to oral tacrolimus is recommended as soon as oral therapy can be tolerated. This usually occurs within 2 to 3 days. The initial dose of tacrolimus should be administered no sooner than 6 hours after transplantation. In a patient receiving an IV infusion, the first dose of oral therapy should be given 8 to 12 hours after discontinuing the IV infusion.

Dosing should be titrated based on clinical assessments of rejection and tolerability. Lower tacrolimus dosages may be sufficient as maintenance therapy. Adjunct therapy with adrenal corticosteroids is recommended early posttransplant.

➤*Children:* Pediatric liver transplantation patients without preexisting renal or hepatic dysfunction have required and tolerated higher doses than adults to achieve similar blood concentrations. Therefore, it is recommended that therapy be initiated in pediatric patients in the IV and oral dosing ranges of 0.03 to 0.05 mg/kg/day IV and 0.15 to 0.2 mg/kg/day oral. Dose adjustments may be required. Experience in pediatric kidney and heart transplantation patients is limited.

➤*Hepatic/Renal function impairment:* Because of the reduced clearance and prolonged half-life, patients with severe hepatic impairment (Child-Pugh score of 10 or more) may require lower doses of tacrolimus. Close monitoring of blood concentrations is warranted.

Because of the potential for nephrotoxicity, give patients with renal or hepatic function impairment doses at the lowest value of the recommended IV and oral dosing ranges. Further reductions in dose below these ranges may be required. Therapy may need to be delayed by up to 48 hours or longer in patients with postoperative oliguria.

➤*Conversion from one immunosuppressive regimen to another:* Do not use tacrolimus simultaneously with cyclosporine. Discontinue either agent at least 24 hours before initiating the other. In the presence of elevated tacrolimus or cyclosporine concentrations, dosing with the other drug usually should be further delayed.

➤*Blood concentration monitoring:* Monitoring of tacrolimus blood concentrations in conjunction with other laboratory and clinical parameters is considered an essential aid to patient management for the evaluation of rejection, toxicity, dose adjustments, and compliance. Factors influencing frequency of monitoring include but are not limited to hepatic or renal dysfunction, the addition or discontinuation of potentially interacting drugs, and the posttransplant time. Blood concentration monitoring is not a replacement for renal and hepatic function monitoring and tissue biopsies.

Two methods have been used for the assay of tacrolimus, a microparticle enzyme immunoassay and an enzyme-linked immunosorbent assay (ELISA). Both methods have the same monoclonal antibody for tacrolimus. Comparison of the concentrations in published literature with patient concentrations using the current assays must be made with detailed knowledge of the assay methods and biological matrices employed. Whole blood is the matrix of choice and specimens should be collected into tubes containing ethylenediaminetetraacetic acid (EDTA) anticoagulant. Heparin anticoagulation is not recommended because of the tendency to form clots on storage. Samples that are not analyzed immediately should be stored at room temperature or in a refrigerator and assayed within 7 days; if samples are to be kept longer they should be deep frozen at −20°C (−4°F) for up to 12 months.

Liver transplantation – Although there is a lack of direct correlation between tacrolimus concentrations and drug efficacy, data from phase 2 and 3 studies of liver transplant patients have shown an increasing incidence of adverse reactions with increasing trough blood concentrations. Most patients are stable when trough whole blood concentrations are maintained between 5 to 20 ng/mL. Long-term posttransplant patients often are maintained at the low end of this target range.

Data from the US clinical trial show that tacrolimus whole blood concentrations, as measured by ELISA, were most variable during the first week post-transplantation. After this early period, the median trough blood concentrations, measured at intervals from the second week to 1-year post-transplantation, ranged from 9.8 to 19.4 ng/mL.

Kidney transplantation – Data from the phase 3 study indicate that trough concentrations of tacrolimus in whole blood were most variable during the first week of dosing. During the first 3 months, 80% of the patients maintained trough concentrations between 7 to 20 ng/mL, and then between 5 to 15 ng/mL, through 1 year.

The relative risk of toxicity is increased with higher trough concentrations. Therefore, monitoring of whole blood trough concentrations is recommended to assist in the clinical evaluation of toxicity.

Heart transplantation – Data from a phase 3 study indicate that trough concentrations of tacrolimus in whole blood were most variable during the first week of dosing. From 1 week to 3 months posttransplant, approximately 80% of patients maintained trough concentrations between 8 to 20 ng/mL and, from 3 through 18 months posttransplant, approximately 80% of patients maintained trough concentrations between 8 to 16 ng/mL.

The relative risk of toxicity (eg, nephrotoxicity, posttransplant diabetes mellitus) is increased with higher trough concentrations. Therefore, monitoring of whole blood trough concentrations is recommended to assist in the clinical evaluation of toxicity.

➤*Storage/Stability:* Store between 5° and 25°C (41° and 77°F). Store diluted infusion solution in glass or polyethylene containers and discard after 24 hours. Do not store the diluted infusion solution in a PVC container because of decreased stability and the potential for extraction of phthalates.

Actions

➤*Pharmacology:* Tacrolimus, previously known as FK506, is a macrolide immunosuppressant produced by *Streptomyces tsukubaensis*. Tacrolimus prolongs the survival of the host and transplanted graft in animal transplant models of liver, kidney, heart, bone marrow, small bowel and pancreas, lung and trachea, skin, cornea, and limb.

In animals, tacrolimus suppresses some humoral immunity and, to a greater extent, cell-mediated reactions such as allograft rejection, delayed-type hypersensitivity, collagen-induced arthritis, experimental allergic encephalomyelitis, and graft vs host disease.

Tacrolimus inhibits T-lymphocyte activation, although the exact mechanism of action is not known. Evidence suggests that the drug binds to an intracellular protein, FKBP-12. A complex of tacrolimus-FKBP-12, calcium, calmodulin, and calcineurin is then formed, and the phosphatase activity of calcineurin is inhibited. This effect may prevent the generation of nuclear factor of activated T-cells (NF-AT), a nuclear component thought to initiate gene transcription for the formation of lymphokines (interleukin-2, gamma interferon). The net result is the inhibition of T-lymphocyte activation (ie, immunosuppression).

➤*Pharmacokinetics:*

Absorption – Absorption of tacrolimus from the GI tract after oral administration is variable. The absolute bioavailability of tacrolimus was about 17% in adult kidney transplant patients, about 22% in adult liver transplant patients, and about 18% in healthy volunteers. Tacrolimus maximum blood concentrations (C_{max}) and area under the curve (AUC) appeared to increase in a dose-proportional fashion in 18 fasted healthy volunteers receiving a single oral dose of 3, 7, and 10 mg.

In kidney transplant patients, tacrolimus trough concentrations from 3 to 30 ng/mL measured at 10 to 12 hours postdose (C_{min}) and in liver transplant patients over a concentration range of 10 to 60 ng/mL correlated well with the AUC.

Food effects: The rate and extent of tacrolimus absorption were greatest under fasted conditions. The rate and extent of tacrolimus absorption were greatest under fasted conditions. The presence and composition of food decreased the rate and extent of tacrolimus absorption. The effect was most pronounced with a high-fat meal (848 kcal, 46% fat): Mean AUC and C_{max} were decreased 37% and 77%, respectively; T_{max} was lengthened 5-fold. A high-carbohydrate meal (668 kcal, 85% carbohydrate) decreased mean AUC and mean C_{max} by 28% and 65%, respectively.

Distribution – The plasma protein binding of tacrolimus is approximately 99%. Tacrolimus is bound mainly to albumin and alpha-1-acid glycoprotein and has a high level of association with erythrocytes. The distribution of tacrolimus between whole blood and plasma depends on several factors, such as hematocrit, temperature at the time of plasma separation, drug concentration, and plasma protein concentration. In a US study, the ratio of whole blood concentration to plasma concentration averaged 35 (range, 12 to 67).

Metabolism – Tacrolimus is extensively metabolized by the mixed-function oxidase system, primarily the cytochrome P450 system (CYP3A). A metabolic pathway leading to the formation of 8 possible metabolites has been proposed. Demethylation and hydroxylation were identified as the primary mechanisms of biotransformation in vitro. The major metabolite identified is 13-demethyl tacrolimus.

Excretion – The mean clearance following IV administration of tacrolimus is 0.04, 0.083, and 0.053 L/hr/kg in healthy volunteers, adult kidney transplant patients, and adult liver transplant patients, respectively. Less than 1% of the dose administered is excreted unchanged in urine.

After IV administration, fecal elimination accounted for about 92.4% and the elimination half-life was about 48.1 hours, whereas it was about

TACROLIMUS — INJECTION

43.5 hours based on tacrolimus concentrations. When administered orally, fecal elimination accounted for about 92.6%, urinary elimination accounted for about 2.3%, and the elimination half-life was about 31.9 hours, whereas it was about 48.4 hours based on tacrolimus concentrations. The pharmacokinetic parameters of tacrolimus have been determined following IV and oral administration in healthy volunteers, kidney transplant, and liver transplant patients.

Pharmacokinetic Parameters of Tacrolimus

Population	N	Route (dose)	C_{max} (ng/mL)	T_{max} (hr)	AUC (ng•hr/mL)	t½ (hr)	Clearance (L/hr/kg)	Vd (L/kg)
Healthy volunteers	8	IV (0.025 mg/kg/4 hr)	—	—	≈ 598[a]	≈ 34.2	≈ 0.04	≈ 1.91
	16	PO (5 mg)	≈ 29.7	≈ 1.6	≈ 243[b]	≈ 34.8	≈ 0.041[c]	≈ 1.94[c]
Kidney transplant patients	26	IV (0.02 mg/kg/12 hr)	—	—	≈ 294[d]	≈ 18.8	≈ 0.083	1.41
		PO (0.2 mg/kg/day)	≈ 19.2	3	≈ 203[d]	NA[e]	NA	NA
		PO (0.3 mg/kg/day)	≈ 24.2	1.5	≈ 288[d]	NA	NA	NA
Liver transplant patients	17	IV (0.05 mg/kg/12 hr)	—	—	≈ 3300[d]	≈ 11.7	≈ 0.053	≈ 0.85
		PO (0.3 mg/kg/day)	≈ 68.5	≈ 2.3	≈ 519[d]	NA	NA	NA

[a] AUC_{0-120}
[b] AUC_{0-72}
[c] Corrected for individual bioavailability.
[d] $AUC_{0-\infty}$
[e] NA = Not available
– = Not applicable

Special populations –

Children: Trough concentrations obtained from 31 children younger than 12 years of age showed that children need higher doses than adults to achieve similar trough concentrations (see Administration and Dosage).

Hepatic insufficiency: The mean clearance was substantially lower and half-life was prolonged in patients with severe hepatic dysfunction.

Contraindications

Hypersensitivity to tacrolimus; hypersensitivity to HCO-60 polyoxyl 60 hydrogenated castor oil (used in vehicle for injection).

Warnings

➤*Insulin-dependent post-transplant diabetes mellitus (PTDM):* Insulin-dependent PTDM was reported in 20% of tacrolimus-treated kidney patients without pretransplant history of diabetes mellitus in the Phase III study. The median time to onset of PTDM was 68 days. Insulin dependence was reversible in 15% of these PTDM patients at 1 year and in 50% at 2 years post-transplant. Black and Hispanic kidney transplant patients were at an increased risk of development of PTDM.

Insulin-dependent PTDM was reported in 18% and 11% of tacrolimus-treated liver transplant patients and was reversible in 45% and 31% of these patients at 1 year post-transplant, in the US and European randomized studies, respectively. Hyperglycemia was associated with the use of tacrolimus in 47% and 33% of liver transplant recipients in the US and European randomized studies, respectively, and may require treatment.

➤*Nephrotoxicity:* Tacrolimus can cause neurotoxicity and nephrotoxicity, particularly when used in high doses. Nephrotoxicity has been noted in approximately 52% of kidney transplantation patients and in 36% to 40% of liver transplantation patients receiving the drug. More overt nephrotoxicity is seen early after transplantation, characterized by increasing serum creatinine and a decrease in urine output. Closely monitor patients with impaired renal function; the dosage may need to be reduced. In patients with persistent elevations of serum creatinine who are unresponsive to dosage adjustments, consider changing to another immunosuppressive therapy. Take care in using tacrolimus with other nephrotoxic drugs; in particular, to avoid excess nephrotoxicity, do not use simultaneously with cyclosporine. Discontinue tacrolimus or cyclosporine at least 24 hours prior to initiating the other. In the presence of elevated tacrolimus or cyclosporine concentrations, usually delay dosing with the other drug (see Drug Interactions).

➤*Hyperkalemia:* Mild to severe hyperkalemia that may require treatment has been noted in 31% of kidney transplant recipients and in 13% to 45% of liver transplant recipients treated with tacrolimus. Monitor serum potassium levels and do not use potassium-sparing diuretics therapy.

➤*Neurotoxicity:* Neurotoxicity, including tremor, headache, and other changes in motor function, mental status, and sensory function occurred in approximately 55% of liver transplant recipients. Tremor occurred more often in tacrolimus-treated kidney transplant patients (54%) compared with cyclosporine-treated patients. Tremor and headache have been associated with high whole-blood concentrations of tacrolimus and may respond to dosage adjustment. Seizures have occurred in adult and pediatric patients. Coma and delirium also have been associated with high plasma concentrations of tacrolimus.

➤*Lymphomas:* As with other immunosuppressants, patients receiving tacrolimus are at increased risk of developing lymphomas and other malignancies, particularly of the skin. The risk appears to be related to the intensity and duration of immunosuppression rather than to the use of any specific agent. A lymphoproliferative disorder (LPD) related to Epstein-Barr virus (EBV) infection has been reported in immunosuppressed organ transplant recipients. The risk of LPD appears greatest in young children who are at risk for primary EBV infection while immunosuppressed or who are switched to tacrolimus following long-term immunosuppressive therapy. Because of the danger of oversuppression of the immune system, which can increase susceptibility to infection, use combination immunosuppressant therapy with caution.

➤*Myocardial hypertrophy:* Myocardial hypertrophy has been reported in association with the administration of tacrolimus and is generally manifested by echocardiographically demonstrated concentric increases in left ventricular posterior wall and interventricular septum thickness. Hypertrophy has been observed in infants, children, and adults. This condition appears reversible in most cases following dose reduction or discontinuance of therapy. In a group of 20 patients with pre- and post-treatment echocardiograms who showed evidence of myocardial hypertrophy, mean tacrolimus whole blood concentrations during the period prior to diagnosis of myocardial hypertrophy ranged from 11 to 53 ng/mL in infants, 4 to 46 ng/mL in children, and 11 to 24 ng/mL in adults.

➤*Hypersensitivity reactions:* A few patients receiving the injection have experienced anaphylactic reactions. Although the exact cause of these reactions is not known, other drugs with castor oil derivatives in the formulation have been associated with anaphylaxis in a small percentage of patients. Because of this potential risk of anaphylaxis, reserve the injection for patients who are unable to take capsules.

Continuously observe patients receiving the injection for at least the first 30 minutes following the start of the infusion and at frequent intervals thereafter. If signs or symptoms of anaphylaxis occur, stop the infusion. Have an aqueous solution of epinephrine available at the bedside as well as a source of oxygen. Refer to Management of Acute Hypersensitivity Reactions.

➤*Renal/Hepatic function impairment:* Use lower doses for patients with renal insufficiency (see Administration and Dosage).

The use of tacrolimus in liver transplant recipients experiencing posttransplant hepatic impairment may be associated with increased risk of developing renal insufficiency related to high whole-blood levels of tacrolimus. Monitor these patients closely and consider dosage adjustments. Use lower doses in these patients (see Administration and Dosage).

➤*Carcinogenesis:* An increased incidence of malignancy is a recognized complication of immunosuppression in recipients of organ transplants. The most common forms of neoplasms are non-Hodgkin's lymphomas and carcinomas of the skin. As with other immunosuppressive therapies, the risk of malignancies in tacrolimus recipients may be higher than in the healthy population. Lymphoproliferative disorders associated with Epstein-Barr virus infection have been seen. It has been reported that reduction or discontinuation of immunosuppression may cause the lesions to regress (see also Lymphomas).

➤*Fertility impairment:* Tacrolimus, given orally at 1 mg/kg (0.7 to 1.4 times the recommended clinical dose range of 0.1 to 0.2 mg/kg/day) to male and female rats prior to and during mating, as well as to dams during gestation and lactation, was associated with embryolethality and with adverse effects on female reproduction. Effects on female reproductive function (parturition) and embryolethal effects were indicated by a higher rate of pre-implantation loss and increased numbers of undelivered and nonviable pups. When given at 3.2 mg/kg, tacrolimus was associated with maternal and paternal toxicity, as well as reproductive toxicity including marked adverse effects on estrus cycles, parturition, pup viability, and pup malformations.

➤*Pregnancy: Category C.* In reproduction studies in rats and rabbits, adverse effects on the fetus were observed mainly at dose levels that were toxic to dams. Tacrolimus at oral doses of 0.32 and 1 mg/kg during organogenesis in rabbits was associated with maternal toxicity as well as an increase in incidence of abortions; these doses are equivalent to 0.5 to 1 times and 1.6 to 3.3 times the recommended clinical dose range (0.1 to 0.2 mg/kg). At the higher dose only, an increased incidence of malformations and developmental variations also was seen. Tacrolimus, at oral doses of 3.2 mg/kg during organogenesis in rats, was associated with maternal toxicity and caused an increase in late resorptions, decreased numbers of live births, and decreased pup weight and viability. Oral tacrolimus (1 and 3.2 mg/kg) to pregnant rats after organogenesis and during lactation was associated with reduced pup weights.

There are no adequate and well-controlled studies in pregnant women. Tacrolimus is transferred across the placenta. The use of tacrolimus during pregnancy has been associated with neonatal hyperkalemia and renal dysfunction. Use during pregnancy only if the potential benefit to the mother justifies potential risk to the fetus.

➤*Lactation:* Tacrolimus is excreted in breast milk; avoid nursing.

➤*Children:* Successful liver transplants have been performed in pediatric patients (up to 16 years of age) using tacrolimus. Pediatric patients generally require higher doses to maintain blood trough levels of tacrolimus similar to adult patients (see Administration and Dosage).

Precautions

➤*Monitoring:* Regularly assess serum creatinine, potassium, and fasting glucose. Perform routine monitoring of metabolic and hematologic systems as clinically warranted.

➤*Hypertension:* Hypertension is a common adverse effect of tacrolimus therapy. Mild or moderate hypertension is more frequently reported than

TACROLIMUS — INJECTION

severe hypertension. Antihypertensive therapy may be required; the control of blood pressure can be accomplished with any of the common antihypertensive agents. Because tacrolimus may cause hyperkalemia, avoid potassium-sparing diuretics. While calcium-channel blocking agents can be effective in treating tacrolimus-associated hypertension, take care because interference with tacrolimus metabolism may require a dosage reduction (see Drug Interactions).

Drug Interactions

➤*CYP450 system:* Because tacrolimus is metabolized mainly by the cytochrome P450 3A enzyme systems, substances known to inhibit these enzymes may affect the metabolism or increase bioavailability of tacrolimus with resultant increases or decreases in whole blood or plasma levels. Monitoring of blood levels and appropriate dosage adjustments are essential when such drugs are used concomitantly.

Tacrolimus Drug Interactions

Precipitant drug	Object drug*		Description
Nephrotoxic agents (eg, aminoglycosides, amphotericin B, cisplatin, cyclosporine)	Tacrolimus	↑	Because of the potential for additive or synergistic impairment of renal function, take care when administering tacrolimus with drugs that may be associated with renal dysfunction. Coadministration with cyclosporine resulted in additive/synergistic nephrotoxicity; tacrolimus blood levels also may be increased. Give the first tacrolimus dose no sooner than 24 hours after the last cyclosporine dose.
Bromocriptine, Cimetidine, Cisapride, Chloramphenicol, Danazol, Ethinyl estradiol, Methylprednisolone, Metoclopromide, Metronidazole, Nefazodone, Omeprazole, Protease inhibitors, Macrolide antibiotics (eg, clarithromycin, erythromycin, troleandomycin), Calcium channel blockers (eg,diltiazem, nicardepine, nifedipine, verapamil), Antifungal Agents (eg, clotrimazole, fluconazole, itraconazole, ketoconazole, miconazole)	Tacrolimus	↑	These agents may increase tacrolimus blood levels, increasing risk of toxicity.
Carbamazepine, Fosphenytoin, Phenobarbital, Phenytoin Antibiotics (eg, rifabutin, rifampin, rifapentine)	Tacrolimus	↓	These agents may decrease tacrolimus blood levels.
St. John's wort	Tacrolimus	↓	St. John's wort induces CYP3A4 and P-glycoprotein. Because tacrolimus is a substrate for CYP3A4, tacrolimus blood levels may decrease.
Tacrolimus	Mycophenolate mofetil	↑	Mycophenolate trough plasma concentrations may be elevated, increasing risk of side effects.
Tacrolimus	Vaccines	↓	Immunosuppressants may affect vaccination. Therefore, during treatment with tacrolimus, vaccination may be less effective. Avoid the use of live vaccines (eg, measles, mumps, rubella, oral polio, BCG, yellow fever, TY 21a typhoid).

* ↑ = Object drug increased. ↓ = Object drug decreased.

➤*Drug/Food interactions:* See Drug Interactions for more information.

Coadministered grapefuit juice has been reported to increase tacrolimus blood trough concentrations in liver transplant patients.

Adverse Reactions

Tacrolimus Adverse Reactions in Kidney and Liver Transplant Patients (%)[a]

	Liver transplant patients		Kidney transplant patients	
Adverse reaction	Tacrolimus (n = 514)	CBIR (n = 515)	Tacrolimus (n = 205)	CBIR (n = 207)
Cardiovascular				
Chest pain	—	—	19	13
Hypertension[b]	38-47	43-56	50	52
CNS				
Dizziness	—	—	19	16
Headache[b]	37-64	26-60	44	38
Insomnia	32-64	23-68	32	30
Paresthesia	17-40	17-30	23	16
Tremor[b]	48-56	32-46	54	34
GI				
Anorexia	7-34	5-24	—	—
Constipation	23-24	21-27	35	43
Diarrhea	37-72	27-47	44	41
Dyspepsia	—	—	28	20
LFT abnormal	6-36	5-30	—	—
Nausea	32-46	27-37	38	36
Vomiting	14-27	11-15	29	23
GU				
BUN increased[b]	12-30	9-22	—	—
Creatinine increased[b]	24-39	19-25	45	42
Kidney function abnormal[b]	36-40	23-27	—	—
Oliguria	18-19	12-15	—	—
Urinary tract infection	16-21	18-19	34	35
Hemic/Lymphatic				
Anemia	5-47	1-38	30	24
Leukocytosis	8-32	8-26	—	—
Leukopenia	—	—	15	17
Thrombocytopenia	14-24	19-20	—	—
Metabolic/ Nutritional				
Diabetes mellitus[b]	—	—	24	9
Hyperglycemia[b]	33-47	22-38	22	16
Hyperkalemia[b]	13-45	9-26	31	32
Hyperlipemia	—	—	31	38
Hypokalemia	13-29	16-34	22	25
Hypomagnesemia	16-48	9-45	34	17
Hypophosphatemia	—	—	49	53
Respiratory				
Atelectasis	5-28	4-30	—	—
Cough increased	—	—	18	15
Dyspnea	5-29	4-23	22	18
Pleural effusion	30-36	32-35	—	—
Skin/Appendages				
Pruritus	15-36	7-20	15	7
Rash	10-24	4-19	17	12
Miscellaneous				
Abdominal pain	29-59	22-54	33	31
Arthralgia	—	—	25	24
Ascites	7-27	8-22	—	—
Asthenia	11-52	7-48	34	30
Back pain	17-30	17-29	24	20
Edema	—	—	18	19
Fever	19-48	22-56	29	29
Infection	—	—	45	49
Pain	24-63	22-57	32	30
Peripheral edema	12-26	14-26	36	48

[a] Data are pooled from separate US and European studies and are not necessarily comparable.
[b] See Precautions or Warnings.

Liver transplant patients – The principal adverse reactions of tacrolimus are tremor, headache, diarrhea, hypertension, nausea, and renal dysfunction. These occur with oral and IV administration and may respond to a reduction in dosing. Diarrhea was sometimes associated with other GI complaints such as nausea and vomiting.

Hyperkalemia, hypomagnesemia, and hyperuricemia have occurred. Hyperglycemia has been noted in many patients; some may require insulin therapy (see Warnings and Precautions).

Kidney transplant patients – The most common adverse reactions reported in kidney transplant patients were infection, tremor, hypertension, decreased renal function, constipation, diarrhea, headache, abdominal pain, and insomnia. The following adverse events were reported in more than 3% and less than 15% incidence in liver or kidney transplant recipients receiving tacrolimus.

TACROLIMUS — INJECTION

➤*Cardiovascular:* Angina pectoris; chest pain; deep thrombophlebitis; abnormal ECG; hemorrhage; hypotension; postural hypotension; peripheral vascular disorder; phlebitis; tachycardia; thrombosis; vasodilation.

➤*CNS:* Abnormal dreams; agitation; amnesia; anxiety; confusion; convulsions; depression; dizziness; emotional lability; encephalopathy; hallucinations; hypertonia; incoordination; myoclonus; nervousness; neuropathy; psychosis; somnolence; thinking abnormal.

➤*Dermatologic:* Acne; alopecia; exfoliative dermatitis; fungal dermatitis; herpes simplex; hirsutism; skin discoloration; skin disorder; skin ulcer; sweating.

➤*Endocrine:* Cushing's syndrome; diabetes mellitus (see Warnings).

➤*GI:* Anorexia; cholangitis; cholestatic jaundice; dyspepsia; dysphasia; esophagitis; flatulence; gastritis; GI hemorrhage; GGT increase; GI perforation; hepatitis; ileus; increased appetite; jaundice; liver damage; liver function test abnormal; oral moniliasis; rectal disorder; stomatitis.

➤*GU:* Albuminuria; cystitis; dysuria; hematuria; hydronephrosis; kidney failure; kidney tubular necrosis; nocturia; pyuria; toxic nephropathy; oliguria; urinary frequency; urinary incontinence; vaginitis.

➤*Hematologic / Lymphatic:* Coagulation disorder; ecchymosis; hypochromic anemia; leukocytosis; leukopenia; polycythemia; prothrombin decreased; serum iron decreased; thrombocytopenia.

➤*Metabolic / Nutritional:* Acidosis; alkaline phosphatase increased; alkalosis; ALT increased; AST increased; bicarbonate decreased; bilirubinemia; BUN increased; dehydration; GGT increased; healing abnormal; hypercalcemia; hypercholesterolemia; hyperlipidemia; hyperphosphatemia; hyperuricemia; hypervolemia; hypocalcemia; hypoglycemia; hypophosphatemia; hyponatremia; hypoproteinemia; lactic dehydrogenase increase; weight gain.

➤*Musculoskeletal:* Arthralgia; cramps; generalized spasm; joint disorder; leg cramps; myalgia; myasthenia; osteoporosis.

➤*Respiratory:* Asthma; bronchitis; cough increased; lung disorder; pneumothorax; pulmonary edema; pharyngitis; pneumonia; respiratory disorder; rhinitis; sinusitis; voice alteration.

➤*Special senses:* Abnormal vision; amblyopia; ear pain; otitis media; tinnitus.

➤*Miscellaneous:* Abdomen enlarged; abscess; accidental injury; allergic reaction; cellulitis; chills; flu syndrome; generalized edema; hernia; peritonitis; photosensitivity reaction; sepsis.

There have been rare spontaneous reports of myocardial hypertrophy associated with clinically manifested ventricular dysfunction in patients receiving tacrolimus therapy.

Postmarketing – The following have been reported: Increased amylase including pancreatitis, hearing loss including deafness, leukoencephalopathy, thrombocytopenic purpura, hemolytic-uremic syndrome, acute renal failure, Stevens-Johnson syndrome, stomach ulcer, glycosuria, cardiac arrhythmia, gastroenteritis.

Overdosage

There is minimal experience with overdosage. Acute overdosages of up to 30 times the intended dose have been reported. Almost all cases have been asymptomatic and all patients recovered with no sequelae. In patients who have received inadvertent overdosage of tacrolimus, no adverse reactions different from those reported in patients receiving therapeutic doses have been described. Follow general supportive measures and systemic treatment in all cases of overdosage. Refer to General Management of Acute Overdosage. Based on the poor aqueous solubility and extensive erythrocyte and plasma protein binding, it is anticipated that tacrolimus is not dialyzable to any significant extent; there is no experience with charcoal hemoperfusion.

Patient Information

Inform patients of the need for repeated appropriate lab tests while they are receiving tacrolimus. Give patients complete dosage instructions, advise them of potential risks during pregnancy and inform them of the increased risk of neoplasia.

Inform patients that changes in dosage should not be undertaken without first consulting their physician.

Inform patients that tacrolimus can cause diabetes mellitus and advise them of the need to see their physician if they develop frequent urination or increased thirst or hunger.

SIROLIMUS

Rx	**Rapamune** (Wyeth Laboratories)	**Tablets:** 1 mg	Sucrose, lactose. (RAPAMUNE 1 mg). White, triangular. In 100s and *Redipak* UD 100s.
		2 mg	Sucrose, lactose. (RAPAMUNE 2 mg) Yellow to beige, triangular. In 100s and *Redipak* 100s.
		Solution, oral: 1 mg/mL	Ethanol. In 60 mL fill with oral syringe adaptor.

SIROLIMUS — ORAL

WARNING

Increased susceptibility to infection and the possible development of lymphoma may result from immunosuppression. Only physicians experienced in immunosuppressive therapy and management of renal transplant patients should use sirolimus. Patients receiving the drug should be managed in facilities equipped and staffed with adequate laboratory and supportive medical resources. The physician responsible for maintenance therapy should have complete information requisite for the follow-up of the patient.

Indications

➤*Renal transplant:* For the prophylaxis of organ rejection in patients receiving renal transplants. See Administration and Dosage for more information.

The safety and efficacy of cyclosporine withdrawal in high-risk patients have not been adequately studied and it is therefore not recommended. This includes patients with Banff grade 3 acute rejection or vascular rejection prior to cyclosporine withdrawal, those who are dialysis-dependent, or with serum creatinine greater than 4.5 mg/dL, black patients, retransplants, multi-organ transplants, and patients with high panel of reactive antibodies.

➤*Unlabeled uses:* Treatment of psoriasis.

Administration and Dosage

➤*Approved by the FDA:* September 15, 1999.

Sirolimus is to be administered orally once daily.

It is recommended that sirolimus be used in a regimen with cyclosporine and corticosteroids. Cyclosporine withdrawal is recommended 2 to 4 months after transplantation in patients at low to moderate immunological risk.

➤*Bioequivalence:* The 2 mg sirolimus oral solution has been demonstrated to be clinically equivalent to 2 mg sirolimus oral tablets; hence, are interchangeable on a mg to mg basis. However, it is not known whether higher doses of sirolimus oral solution are therapeutically equivalent to higher doses of tablets on a mg to mg basis (see Pharmacokinetics).

➤*Sirolimus and cyclosporine combination therapy:* The initial dose of sirolimus should be administered as soon as possible after transplantation. For de novo transplant recipients, a loading dose of sirolimus of 3 times the maintenance dose should be given. A daily maintenance dose of 2 mg is recommended for use in renal transplant patients, with a loading dose of 6 mg.

Although a daily maintenance dose of 5 mg, with a loading dose of 15 mg was used in clinical trials of the oral solution and was shown to be safe and effective, no efficacy advantage over the 2 mg dose could be established for renal transplant patients. Patients receiving 2 mg of sirolimus oral solution per day demonstrated an overall better safety profile than did patients receiving 5 mg of sirolimus oral solution per day.

➤*Sirolimus following cyclosporine withdrawal:* Initially, patients considered for cyclosporine withdrawal should be receiving sirolimus and cyclosporine combination therapy. At 2 to 4 months following transplantation, cyclosporine should be progressively discontinued over 4 to 8 weeks and the sirolimus dose should be adjusted to obtain whole blood trough concentrations within the range of 12 to 24 ng/mL (chromatographic method). Therapeutic drug monitoring should not be the sole basis for adjusting sirolimus therapy. Careful attention should be made to clinical signs/symptoms, tissue biopsy, and laboratory parameters. Cyclosporine inhibits the metabolism and transport of sirolimus, and consequently, sirolimus concentrations will decrease when cyclosporine is discontinued unless the sirolimus dose is increased. The sirolimus dose will need to be approximately 4–fold higher to account for both the absence of the pharmacokinetic interaction (approximately 2–fold increase) and the augmented immunosuppressive requirement in the absence of cyclosporine (approximately 2–fold increase).

Frequent sirolimus dose adjustments based on non-steady-state sirolimus concentrations can lead to overdosing or underdosing because sirolimus has a long half-life. Once the sirolimus maintenance dose is adjusted, patients should be retained on the new maintenance dose at least for 7 to 14 days before further dosage adjustment with concentration monitoring. In most patients, dose adjustments can be based on simple proportion: new sirolimus dose = current dose × (target concentration / current concentration). A loading dose should be considered in addition to a new maintenance dose when it is necessary to considerably increase sirolimus trough concentrations: Sirolimus loading dose = 3 x (new maintenance dose − current maintenance dose). The maximum sirolimus dose administered on any day should not exceed 40 mg. If an estimated daily dose exceeds 40 mg due to the addition of a loading dose, the loading dose should be administered over 2 days. Sirolimus trough concentrations should be monitored at least 3 to 4 days after a loading dose(s).

➤*Food effects:* To minimize the variability of exposure to sirolimus, this drug should be taken consistently with or without food. Grapefruit juice reduces CYP3A4-mediated metabolism of sirolimus and must not be administered with sirolimus or used for dilution.

➤*Timing of cyclosporine:* It is recommended that sirolimus be taken 4 hours after administration of cyclosporine oral solution (modified) or cyclosporine capsules (modified).

SIROLIMUS — ORAL

➤*Dosage adjustments:* The initial dosage in patients greater than or equal to 13 years who weigh less than 40 kg should be adjusted, based on body surface area, to 1 mg/m²/day. The loading dose should be 3 mg/m².

Hepatic/Renal function impairment – It is recommended that the maintenance dose of sirolimus be reduced by approximately one third in patients with hepatic impairment. It is not necessary to modify the sirolimus loading dose. Dosage need not be adjusted because of impaired renal function.

➤*Blood concentration monitoring:* See Precautions for more information.

➤*Instructions for dilution and administration of sirolimus oral solution:*

Bottles – The amber oral dose syringe should be used to withdraw the prescribed amount of sirolimus oral solution from the bottle. Empty the correct amount of sirolimus from the syringe into only a glass or plastic container holding at least 2 ounces (¼ cup, 60 mL) of water or orange juice. No other liquids, including grapefruit juice, should be used for dilution. Stir vigorously and drink at once. Refill the container with an additional volume (minimum of 4 ounces [½ cup, 120 mL]) of water or orange juice, stir vigorously, and drink at once.

Pouches – When using the pouch, squeeze the entire contents of the pouch into only a glass or plastic container holding at least 2 ounces (¼ cup, 60 mL) of water or orange juice. No other liquids, including grapefruit juice, should be used for dilution. Stir vigorously and drink at once. Refill the container with an additional volume (minimum of 4 ounces [½ cup, 120 mL]) of water or orange juice, stir vigorously, and drink at once.

➤*Storage/Stability:* Sirolimus oral solution bottles and pouches should be stored protected from light and refrigerated at 2° to 8°C (36° to 46°F). Once the bottle is opened, the contents should be used within 1 month. If necessary, the patient may store both the pouches and the bottles at room temperatures up to 25°C (77°F) for a short period of time (up to 24 hours for the pouches and not more than 15 days for the bottles).

An amber syringe and cap are provided for dosing and the product may be kept in the syringe for a maximum of 24 hours at room temperatures up to 25°C (77°F) or refrigerated at 2° to 8°C (36° to 46°F). The syringe should be discarded after 1 use. After dilution, the preparation should be used immediately.

Sirolimus oral solution provided in bottles may develop a slight haze when refrigerated. If such a haze occurs allow the product to stand at room temperature and shake gently until the haze disappears. The presence of this haze does not affect the quality of the product.

Sirolimus tablets should be stored at 20° to 25°C (68° to 77°F). Use cartons to protect blister cards and strips from light. Dispense in a tight, light-resistant container.

Actions

➤*Pharmacology:* Sirolimus inhibits T lymphocyte activation and proliferation that occurs in response to antigenic and cytokine (interleukin [IL]-2, IL-4, and IL-15) stimulation by a mechanism that is distinct from that of other immunosuppressants. Sirolimus also inhibits antibody production. In cells, sirolimus binds to the immunophilin, FK Binding Protein-12 (FKBP-12), to generate an immunosuppressive complex. The sirolimus:FKBP-12 complex has no effect on calcineurin activity. This complex binds to and inhibits the activation of the mammalian target of rapamycin (mTOR), a key regulatory kinase. This inhibition suppresses cytokine-driven T-cell proliferation, inhibiting the progression from the G_1 to the S phase of the cell cycle.

Studies in experimental models show that sirolimus prolongs allograft (kidney, heart, skin, islet, small bowel, pancreatico-duodenal, and bone marrow) survival in mice, rats, pigs, or primates. Sirolimus reverses acute rejection of heart and kidney allografts in rats and prolonged the graft survival in presensitized rats. In some studies, the immunosuppressive effect of sirolimus lasted up to 6 months after discontinuation of therapy. This tolerization effect is alloantigen specific.

In rodent models of autoimmune disease, sirolimus suppresses immune-mediated events associated with systemic lupus erythematosus, collagen induced arthritis, autoimmune type 1 diabetes, autoimmune myocarditis, experimental allergic encephalomyelitis, graft-versus-host disease, and autoimmune uveoretinitis.

➤*Pharmacokinetics:*

Absorption –

Following administration of sirolimus oral solution, sirolimus is rapidly absorbed, with a mean time-to-peak concentration (t_{max}) of approximately 1 hour after a single dose in healthy subjects and approximately 2 hours after multiple oral doses in renal transplant recipients. The systemic availability of sirolimus was estimated to be approximately 14% after the administration of sirolimus oral solution. The mean bioavailability of sirolimus after administration of the tablet is about 27% higher relative to the oral solution. Sirolimus oral tablets are not bioequivalent to the oral solution; however, clinical equivalence has been demonstrated at the 2-mg dose level (see Administration and Dosage). Sirolimus concentrations, following the administration of sirolimus oral solution to stable renal transplant patients, are dose proportional between 3 and 12 mg/m².

Food effects: In 22 healthy volunteers receiving sirolimus oral solution, a high-fat meal (861.8 kcal, 54.7% fat) altered the bioavailability characteristics of sirolimus. Compared to fasting, a 34% decrease in the peak blood sirolimus concentration (C_{max}), a 3.5-fold increase in the time-to-peak concentration (t_{max}), and a 35% increase in total exposure (AUC) was observed. After administration of sirolimus tablets and a high-fat meal in 24 healthy volunteers, C_{max}, t_{max}, and AUC showed increases of 65%, 32%, and 23%, respectively. To minimize variability, both sirolimus oral solution and tablets should be taken consistently with or without food (see Administration and Dosage).

Distribution – The mean (± SD) blood-to-plasma ratio of sirolimus was 36 (± 17.9) in stable renal allograft recipients, indicating that sirolimus is extensively partitioned into formed blood elements. The mean volume of distribution (V_{ss}/F) of sirolimus is 12 ± 7.52 L/kg. Sirolimus is extensively bound (approximately 92%) to human plasma proteins. In man, the binding of sirolimus was shown mainly to be associated with serum albumin (97%), α_1-acid glycoprotein, and lipoproteins.

Metabolism – Sirolimus is a substrate for both cytochrome P450 3A4 (CYP3A4) and P-glycoprotein. Sirolimus is extensively metabolized by O-demethylation or hydroxylation. Seven (7) major metabolites, including hydroxy, demethyl, and hydroxydemethyl, are identifiable in whole blood. Some of these metabolites are also detectable in plasma, fecal, and urine samples. Glucuronide and sulfate conjugates are not present in any of the biologic matrices. Sirolimus is the major component in human whole blood and contributes to more than 90% of the immunosuppressive activity.

Excretion – After a single dose of (^{14}C) sirolimus in healthy volunteers, the majority (91%) of radioactivity was recovered from the feces, and only a minor amount (2.2%) was excreted in urine.

Special populations –

Hepatic function impairment: Sirolimus (15 mg) was administered as a single oral dose to 18 subjects with normal hepatic function and to 18 patients with Child-Pugh class A or B hepatic impairment, in which hepatic impairment was primary and not related to an underlying systemic disease.

Sirolimus Pharmacokinetic Parameters (Mean ± SD) in 18 Healthy Subjects and 18 Patients with Hepatic Impairment (15 Mg Single Dose: Oral Solution)

Population	$C_{max,ss}$[a] (ng/mL)	t_{max} (hr)	$AUC_{0-\infty}$ (ng•hr/mL)	CL/F/WT (mL/hr/kg)
Healthy subjects	78.2 ± 18.3	0.82 ± 0.17	970 ± 272	215 ± 76
Hepatic impairment	77.9 ± 23.1	0.84 ± 0.17	1567 ± 616	144 ± 62

[a] As measured by LC/MS/MS.

Compared with the values in the normal hepatic group, the hepatic impairment group had higher mean values for sirolimus AUC (61%) and $t_{½}$ (43%) and had lower mean values for sirolimus CL/F/WT (33%). The mean $t_{½}$ increased from 79 ± 12 hours in subjects with normal hepatic function to 113 ± 41 hours in patients with impaired hepatic function. The rate of absorption of sirolimus was not altered by hepatic disease, as evidenced by C_{max} and t_{max} values. However, hepatic diseases with varying etiologies may show different effects and the pharmacokinetics of sirolimus in patients with severe hepatic dysfunction is unknown. Dosage adjustment is recommended for patients with mild to moderate hepatic impairment (see Administration and Dosage).

Children: Limited pharmacokinetic data are available in pediatric patients.

Sirolimus Pharmacokinetic Parameters (Mean ± SD) in Pediatric Patients with Stable Chronic Renal Failure Maintained on Hemodialysis or Peritoneal Dialysis (1, 3, 9, 15 mg/m² Single Dose)

Age group (years)	n	t_{max} (hr)	$t_{½}$ (hr)	CL/F/WT (mL/hr/kg)
5 to 11	9	1.1 ± 0.5	71 ± 40	580 ± 450
12 to 18	11	0.79 ± 0.17	55 ± 18	450 ± 232

Pharmacokinetics in renal transplant patients –

Sirolimus oral solution: Mean pharmacokinetic parameters for sirolimus oral solution given daily in combination with cyclosporine and corticosteroids in renal transplant patients are summarized below based on data collected at months 1, 3, and 6 after transplantation. There were no significant differences in any of these parameters as measured by the liquid chromatographic/tandem mass spectrometric method (LC/MS/MS) with respect to treatment group or month.

Sirolimus Pharmacokinetic Parameters (Mean ± SD) in Renal Transplant Patients (Multiple Dose Oral Solution)[a,b]

N	Dose	$C_{max,ss}$[c] (ng/mL)	$t_{max,ss}$ (hr)	$AUC_{\tau,ss}$[c] (ng•hr/mL)	CL/F/WT[d] (mL/hr/kg)
19	2 mg	12.2 ± 6.2	3.01 ± 2.4	158 ± 70	182 ± 72
23	5 mg	37.4 ± 21	1.84 ± 1.3	396 ± 193	221 ± 143

[a] Sirolimus administered 4 hours after cyclosporine oral solution (modified) (eg, *Neoral* oral solution) or cyclosporine capsules (modified) (*Neoral* soft gelatin capsules).
[b] As measured by the Liquid Chromatographic/Tandem Mass Spectrometric Method (LC/MS/MS).
[c] These parameters were dose normalized prior to the statistical comparison.
[d] CL/F/WT = oral dose clearance.

Whole blood sirolimus trough concentrations, as measured by immunoassay, (mean ± SD) for the 2 mg/day and 5 mg/day dose groups were 8.6 ± 4.0 ng/mL (n = 226) and 17.3 ± 7.4 ng/mL (n = 219), respectively. Whole blood trough sirolimus concentrations, as measured by LC/MS/MS, were significantly correlated (r^2 = 0.96) with $AUC_{\tau,ss}$. Upon repeated twice-daily administration without an initial loading dose in a multiple-dose study, the average trough concentration of sirolimus increases approximately 2- to 3-fold over the initial 6 days of therapy at which time steady state is

SIROLIMUS — ORAL

reached. A loading dose of 3 times the maintenance dose will provide near steady-state concentrations within 1 day in most patients. The mean ± SD terminal elimination half life ($t_{½}$) of sirolimus after multiple dosing in stable renal transplant patients was estimated to be about 62 ± 16 hours.

Sirolimus tablets: Pharmacokinetic parameters as measured by the liquid chromatographic/tandem mass spectrometric method (LC/MS/MS) for sirolimus tablets administered daily in combination with cyclosporine and corticosteroids in renal transplant patients are summarized below based on data collected at months 1 and 3 after transplantation.

Sirolimus Pharmacokinetic Parameters (Mean ± SD) in Renal Transplant Patients (Multiple Dose Tablets)[a,b]

N	Dose	$C_{max,ss}$[c] (ng/mL)	$t_{max,ss}$ (hr)	$AUC_{\tau,ss}$[c] (ng•hr/mL)	CL/F/WT[d] (mL/hr/kg)
17	Oral solution	14.4 ± 5.3	2.12 ± 0.84	194 ± 78	173 ± 50
13	Tablets	15 ± 4.9	3.46 ± 2.4	230 ± 67	139 ± 63

[a] Sirolimus administered 4 hours after cyclosporine oral solution (modified) (eg, *Neoral* oral solution) or cyclosporine capsules (modified) (*Neoral* soft gelatin capsules).
[b] As measured by the Liquid Chromatographic/Tandem Mass Spectrometric Method (LC/MS/MS).
[c] These parameters were dose normalized prior to the statistical comparison.
[d] CL/F/WT = oral dose clearance.

Whole blood sirolimus trough concentrations (mean ± SD), as measured by immunoassay, for the 2 mg oral solution and 2 mg tablets over 6 months, were 8.9 ± 4.4 ng/mL (n = 172) and 9.5 ± 3.9 ng/mL (n = 179), respectively. Whole blood trough sirolimus concentrations, as measured by LC/MS/MS, were significantly correlated (r^2 = 0.85) with $AUC_{\tau,ss}$. Mean whole blood sirolimus trough concentrations in patients receiving either sirolimus oral solution or sirolimus tablets with a loading dose of 3 times the maintenance dose achieved steady-state concentrations within 24 hours after the start of dose administration.

Average Sirolimus Doses and Sirolimus Trough Concentrations (Mean ± SD) in Renal Transplant Patients After Multiple Dose Tablet Administration

	Sirolimus with cyclosporine therapy[a]	Sirolimus following cyclosporine withdrawal[a]
Sirolimus dose (mg/day)		
Months 4 to 12	2.1 ± 0.7	8.2 ± 4.2
Months 12 to 24	2 ± 0.8	6.4 ± 3
Sirolimus C_{min}, (ng/mL)[b]		
Months 4 to 12	10.7 ± 3.8	23.3 ± 5
Months 12 to 24	11.2 ± 4.1	22.5 ± 4.8

[a] 215 patients were randomized to each group.
[b] Expressed by immunoassay and equivalence.

The withdrawal of cyclosporine and concurrent increases in sirolimus trough concentrations to steady-state required approximately 6 weeks. Larger sirolimus doses were required due to the absence of the inhibition of sirolimus metabolism and transport by cyclosporine and to achieve higher target concentrations during concentration-controlled administration following cyclosporine withdrawal.

Contraindications

Hypersensitivity to sirolimus or its derivatives or any component of the drug product.

Warnings

➤*Infection / Lymphoma / Malignancy:* Increased susceptibility to infection and the possible development of lymphoma and other malignancies, particularly of the skin, may result from immunosuppression (see Adverse Reactions). Oversuppression of the immune system can also increase susceptibility to infection including opportunistic infections, fatal infections, and sepsis. Only physicians experienced in immunosuppressive therapy and management of organ transplant patients should use sirolimus. Patients receiving the drug should be managed in facilities equipped and staffed with adequate laboratory and supportive medical resources. The physician responsible for maintenance therapy should have complete information requisite for the follow-up of the patient.

➤*Hyperlipidemia:* See Precautions for more information.

➤*Renal effects:* In studies 1 and 2, from month 6 through months 24 and 36, respectively, mean serum creatinine was increased and mean glomerular filtration rate was decreased in patients treated with sirolimus and cyclosporine compared with those treated with cyclosporine and placebo or azathioprine controls. The rate of decline in renal function was greater in patients receiving sirolimus and cyclosporine compared with control therapies.

➤*Lung transplantation - Bronchial anastomotic dehiscence:* Cases of bronchial anastomotic dehiscence, most fatal, have been reported in de novo lung transplant patients when sirolimus has been used as part of an immunosuppressive regimen.

➤*Hypersensitivity reactions:* Hypersensitivity reactions, including anaphylactic/anaphylactoid reactions, have been associated with the administration of sirolimus (see Adverse Reactions).

➤*Renal function impairment:* See Precautions for more information.

➤*Hepatic function impairment:*

Liver transplantation - Excess mortality, graft loss, and hepatic artery thrombosis (HAT) – The use of sirolimus in combination with tacrolimus was associated with excess mortality and graft loss in a study in de novo liver transplant recipients. Many of these patients had evidence of infection at or near the time of death.

In this and another study in de novo liver transplant recipients, the use of sirolimus in combination with cyclosporine or tacrolimus was associated with an increase in HAT; most cases of HAT occurred within 30 days post-transplantation and most led to graft loss or death. The safety and efficacy of sirolimus as immunosuppressive therapy have not been established in liver or lung transplant patients, and therefore, such use is not recommended.

➤*Carcinogenesis:* Carcinogenicity studies were conducted in mice and rats. In an 86-week female mouse study at dosages of 0, 12.5, 25 and 50/6 (dosage lowered from 50 to 6 mg/kg/day at week 31 due to infection secondary to immunosuppression) there was a statistically significant increase in malignant lymphoma at all dose levels (approximately 16 to 135 times the clinical doses adjusted for body surface area) compared to controls. In a second mouse study at dosages of 0, 1, 3 and 6 mg/kg (approximately 3 to 16 times the clinical dose adjusted for body surface area), hepatocellular adenoma and carcinoma (males), were considered sirolimus related. In the 104-week rat study at dosages of 0, 0.05, 0.1, and 0.2 mg/kg/day (approximately 0.4 to 1 times the clinical dose adjusted for body surface area), there was a statistically significant increased incidence of testicular adenoma in the 0.2 mg/kg/day group.

As usual for patients with increased risk for skin cancer, exposure to sunlight and UV light should be limited by wearing protective clothing and using a sunscreen with a high protective factor.

➤*Fertility impairment:* Reductions in testicular weights or histological lesions (eg, tubular atrophy and tubular giant cells) were observed in rats following dosages of 0.65 mg/kg (approximately 1 to 3 times the clinical doses adjusted for body surface area) and above and in a monkey study at 0.1 mg/kg (approximately 0.4 to 1 times the clinical doses adjusted for body surface area) and above. Sperm counts were reduced in male rats following the administration of sirolimus for 13 weeks at a dosage of 6 mg/kg (approximately 12 to 32 times the clinical doses adjusted for body surface area), but showed improvement by 3 months after dosing was stopped.

➤*Pregnancy: Category C.* Sirolimus was embryo/feto toxic in rats at dosages of 0.1 mg/kg and above (approximately 0.2 to 0.5 the clinical doses adjusted for body surface area). Embryo/feto toxicity was manifested as mortality and reduced fetal weights (with associated delays in skeletal ossification). However, no teratogenesis was evident. In combination with cyclosporine, rats had increased embryo/feto mortality compared to sirolimus alone. There were no effects on rabbit development at the maternally toxic dosage of 0.05 mg/kg (approximately 0.3 to 0.8 times the clinical doses adjusted for body surface area). There are no adequate and well controlled studies in pregnant women. Effective contraception must be initiated before sirolimus therapy, during sirolimus therapy, and for 12 weeks after sirolimus therapy has been stopped. Sirolimus should be used during pregnancy only if the potential benefit outweighs the potential risk to the embryo/fetus.

➤*Lactation:* Sirolimus is excreted in trace amounts in milk of lactating rats. It is not known whether sirolimus is excreted in human milk. The pharmacokinetic and safety profiles of sirolimus in infants are not known. Because many drugs are excreted in human milk and because of the potential for adverse reactions in nursing infants from sirolimus, a decision should be made whether to discontinue nursing or to discontinue the drug, taking into account the importance of the drug to the mother.

➤*Children:* The safety and efficacy of sirolimus in pediatric patients below the age of 13 years have not been established.

Precautions

➤*Monitoring:* It is prudent to monitor blood sirolimus levels in patients likely to have altered drug metabolism, in patients greater than or equal to 13 years old who weigh less than 40 kg, in patients with hepatic impairment, and during concurrent administration of potent CYP3A4 inducters and inhibitors (see Drug Interactions). Renal function, cholesterol, and triglyceride monitoring is also recommended.

Renal function should be closely monitored during the administration of sirolimus in combination with cyclosporine since long-term administration can be associated with deterioration of renal function. Appropriate adjustment of the immunosuppression regimen, including discontinuation of sirolimus or cyclosporine, should be considered in patients with elevated or increasing serum creatinine levels. Caution should be exercised when using other drugs which are known to impair renal function. In patients with low to moderate immunological risk continuation of combination therapy with cyclosporine beyond 4 months following transplantation should only be considered when the benefits outweigh the risks of this combination for the individual patients.

➤*Lipids:* The use of sirolimus in renal transplant patients was associated with increased serum cholesterol and triglycerides that may require treatment.

Any patient who is administered sirolimus should be monitored for hyperlipidemia using laboratory tests and if hyperlipidemia is detected, subsequent interventions such as diet, exercise, and lipid-lowering agents, as outlined by the National Cholesterol Education Program guidelines, should be initiated.

SIROLIMUS — ORAL

HMG-CoA reductase inhibitors/Fibrate – During sirolimus therapy with cyclosporine, patients administered an HMG-CoA reductase inhibitor or fibrate should be monitored for the possible development of rhabdomyolysis and other adverse effects as described in the respective monographs for these agents.

➤*Antimicrobial prophylaxis:* Cases of *Pneumocystis carinii* pneumonia have been reported in patients not receiving antimicrobial prophylaxis. Therefore, antimicrobial prophylaxis for *Pneumocystis carinii* pneumonia should be administered for 1 year following transplantation. Cytomegalovirus (CMV) prophylaxis is recommended for 3 months after transplantation, particularly for patients at increased risk for CMV disease.

➤*Interstitial lung disease:* Cases of interstitial lung disease (including pneumonitis, and infrequently bronchiolitis obliterans organizing pneumonia [BOOP] and pulmonary fibrosis), some fatal, with no identified infectious etiology have occurred in patients receiving immunosuppressive regimens including sirolimus. In some cases, the interstitial lung disease has resolved upon discontinuation or dose reduction of sirolimus. The risk may be increased as the trough sirolimus level increases (see Adverse Reactions).

Drug Interactions

Sirolimus Drug Interactions			
Precipitant drug	Object drug*		Description
Cyclosporine	Sirolimus	⬆	Sirolimus plasma concentrations may be increased, resulting in increased toxicity. Administer sirolimus 4 hours after cyclosporine to prevent variations in sirolimus concentrations.
CYP3A4 inhibitors such as: Bromocriptine, Cimetidine, Cisapride, Clarithromycin, Clotrimazole, Danazol, Erythromycin, Fluconazole, Itraconazole, Metoclopramide, Nicardipine, Troleandomycin, Verapamil, Protease inhibitors (eg, ritonavir, indinavir)	Sirolimus	⬆	Concomitant use may decrease the metabolism of sirolimus and increase sirolimus levels because of CYP3A4 inhibition.
CYP3A4 inducers such as: Carbamazepine, Phenobarbital, Phenytoin, Rifabutin, Rifapentine, St. John's Wort	Sirolimus	⬇	Concomitant use may increase metabolism of sirolimus decrease sirolimus levels because of CYP3A4 induction.
Diltiazem	Sirolimus	⬆	Sirolimus C_{max}, T_{max}, and AUC were increased 1.4-, 1.3-, and 1.6-fold, respectively, following coadministration of sirolimus and diltiazem. If diltiazem is administered, monitor sirolimus; a dose adjustment may be necessary.
Azole antifungal agents	Sirolimus	⬆	Plasma sirolimus concentrations may be elevated, increasing the risk of toxicity. Monitor sirolimus plasma concentrations and observe the patient for toxicity when starting or stopping an azole antifungal agent. Adjust the dose of sirolimus as needed.
Rifampin	Sirolimus	⬇	Rifampin greatly increased sirolimus oral-dose clearance by 5.5-fold, which represents mean decreases in AUC and C_{max} of about 82% and 71%, respectively. Consider alternative therapeutic agents with less enzyme induction potential where rifampin is indicated.

Sirolimus Drug Interactions			
Precipitant drug	Object drug*		Description
Sirolimus	Vaccines	⬇	Immunosuppressants may affect response to vaccination. Vaccination may be less effective in patients during treatment with sirolimus. Avoid live vaccines.

* ⬆ = Object drug increased. ⬇ = Object drug decreased.

➤*Drug/Food interactions:* Grapefruit juice reduces CYP3A4-mediated metabolism of sirolimus and must not be used for dilution (see Administration and Dosage).

Adverse Reactions

➤*Sirolimus oral solution:* Specific adverse reactions associated with the administration of sirolimus oral solution occurred at a significantly higher frequency than in the respective control group. For both sirolimus oral solution 2 mg/day and 5 mg/day these include hypercholesterolemia, hyperlipemia, hypertension, and rash; for sirolimus oral solution 2 mg/day acne; and for sirolimus oral solution 5 mg/day anemia, arthralgia, diarrhea, hypokalemia, and thrombocytopenia. The elevations of triglycerides and cholesterol and decreases in platelets and hemoglobin occurred in a dose-related manner in patients receiving sirolimus.

Patients maintained on sirolimus oral solution 5 mg/day, when compared to patients on sirolimus oral solution 2 mg/day, demonstrated an increased incidence of the following adverse reactions: Anemia, leukopenia, thrombocytopenia, hypokalemia, hyperlipemia, fever, and diarrhea.

Adverse Reactions Occurring at a Frequency of ≥ 20% in Any Treatment Group in Prevention of Acute Renal Rejection Trials (%) at ≥ 12 Months Posttransplantation for Studies 1 And 2[a]

Adverse reaction	Sirolimus oral solution 2 mg/day		Sirolimus oral solution 5 mg/day		Azathioprine 2 to 3 mg/kg/day	Placebo
	Study 1 (n = 281)	Study 2 (n = 218)	Study 1 (n = 269)	Study 2 (n = 208)	Study 1 (n = 160)	Study 2 (n = 124)
Miscellaneous						
Abdominal pain	28%	29%	30%	36%	29%	30%
Asthenia	38%	22%	40%	28%	37%	28%
Back pain	16%	23%	26%	22%	23%	20%
Chest pain	16%	18%	19%	24%	16%	19%
Fever	27%	23%	33%	34%	33%	35%
Headache	23%	34%	27%	34%	21%	31%
Pain	24%	33%	29%	29%	30%	25%
Cardiovascular						
Hypertension	43%	45%	39%	49%	29%	48%
GI						
Constipation	28%	36%	34%	38%	37%	31%
Diarrhea	32%	25%	42%	35%	28%	27%
Dyspepsia	17%	23%	23%	25%	24%	34%
Nausea	31%	25%	36%	31%	39%	29%
Vomiting	21%	19%	25%	25%	31%	21%
Hematologic/lymphatic						
Anemia	27%	23%	37%	33%	29%	21%
Leukopenia	9%	9%	15%	13%	20%	8%
Thrombocytopenia	13%	14%	20%	30%	9%	9%
Metabolic/nutritional						
Creatinine increased	35%	39%	37%	40%	28%	38%
Edema	24%	20%	16%	18%	23%	15%
Hypercholesteremia (see Warnings and Precautions)	38%	43%	42%	46%	33%	23%
Hyperkalemia	15%	17%	12%	14%	24%	27%
Hyperlipemia (see Warnings and Precautions)	38%	45%	44%	57%	28%	23%
Hypokalemia	17%	11%	21%	17%	11%	9%
Hypophosphatemia	20%	15%	23%	19%	20%	19%
Peripheral edema	60%	54%	64%	58%	58%	48%
Weight gain	21%	11%	15%	8%	19%	15%
Musculoskeletal						
Arthralgia	25%	25%	27%	31%	21%	18%
CNS						
Insomnia	14%	13%	22%	14%	18%	8%
Tremor	31%	21%	30%	22%	28%	19%

SIROLIMUS — ORAL

Adverse Reactions Occurring at a Frequency of ≥ 20% in Any Treatment Group in Prevention of Acute Renal Rejection Trials (%) at ≥ 12 Months Posttransplantation for Studies 1 And 2[a]						
	Sirolimus oral solution 2 mg/day		Sirolimus oral solution 5 mg/day		Azathioprine 2 to 3 mg/kg/day	Placebo
Adverse reaction	Study 1 (n = 281)	Study 2 (n = 218)	Study 1 (n = 269)	Study 2 (n = 208)	Study 1 (n = 160)	Study 2 (n = 124)
Respiratory						
Dyspnea	22%	24%	28%	30%	23%	30%
Pharyngitis	17%	16%	16%	21%	17%	22%
Upper respiratory tract infection	20%	26%	24%	23%	13%	23%
Dermatologic						
Acne	31%	22%	20%	22%	17%	19%
Rash	12%	10%	13%	20%	6%	6%
GU						
Urinary tract infection	20%	26%	23%	33%	31%	26%

[a] Patients received cyclosporine and corticosteroids.

With longer term follow-up, the adverse reaction profile remained similar. Some new reactions became significantly different among the treatment groups. For reactions which occurred at a frequency of greater than or equal to 20% by 24 months for study 1 and 36 months for study 2, only the incidence of edema became significantly higher in both sirolimus groups as compared with the control group. The incidence of headache became significantly more common in the sirolimus 5 mg/day group as compared with control therapy.

At 24 months for study 1, the following treatment-emergent infections were significantly different among the treatment groups: Bronchitis, Herpes simplex, pneumonia, pyelonephritis, and upper respiratory infections. In each instance, the incidence was highest in the sirolimus 5 mg/day group, lower in the sirolimus 2 mg/ day group and lowest in the azathioprine group. Except for upper respiratory infections in the sirolimus 5 mg/day cohort, the remainder of reactions occurred with a frequency of less than 20%.

At 36 months in study 2, only the incidence of treatment-emergent Herpes simplex was significantly different among the treatment groups, being higher in the sirolimus 5 mg/day group than either of the other groups.

➤*Incidence of malignancies:* The table below summarizes the incidence of malignancies in the 2 controlled trials for the prevention of acute rejection. At 24 (study 1) and 36 months (study 2) there were no significant differences among treatment groups.

Incidence (%) of Malignancies in Studies 1 (24 Months) and Study 2 (36 Months) Posttransplant[a,b]						
	Sirolimus oral solution 2 mg/day		Sirolimus oral solution 5 mg/day		Azathioprine 2 to 3 mg/day	Placebo
Malignancy	Study 1 (n = 284)	Study 2 (n = 227)	Study 1 (n = 274)	Study 2 (n = 219)	(n = 161)	(n = 130)
Lymphoma/ lymphoproliferative disease	0.7%	1.8%	1.1%	3.2%	0.6	0.8
Skin carcinoma						
Any squamous cell[c]	0.4%	2.7%	2.2%	0.9%	3.8%	3.0%
Any basal cell[c]	0.7%	2.2%	1.5%	1.8%	2.5%	5.3%
Melanoma	0.0%	0.4%	0.0%	1.4%	0.0%	0.0%
Miscellaneous/ not specified	0.0%	0.0%	0.0%	0.0%	0.0%	0.8%
Total	1.1%	4.4%	3.3%	4.1%	4.3%	7.7%
Other malignancy	1.1%	2.2%	1.5%	1.4%	0.6%	2.3%

[a] Patients received cyclosporine and corticosteroids.
[b] Includes patients who prematurely discontinued treatment.
[c] Patients may be counted in more than 1 category.

Among the adverse reactions that were reported at a rate of greater than or equal to 3% and less than 20% at 12 months, the following were more prominent in patients maintained on sirolimus 5 mg/day, when compared to patients on sirolimus 2 mg/day: Epistaxis, lymphocele, insomnia, thrombotic thrombocytopenic purpura (hemolytic-uremic syndrome), skin ulcer, increased LDH, hypotension, facial edema.

➤*Adverse reactions reported with greater than or equal to 3% and less than 20% incidence in patients in any sirolimus treatment group in the 2 controlled clinical trials for the prevention of acute rejection:*

Cardiovascular – Atrial fibrillation, congestive heart failure, hemorrhage, hypervolemia, hypotension, palpitation, peripheral vascular disorder, postural hypotension, syncope, tachycardia, thrombophlebitis, thrombosis, vasodilatation, venous thromboembolism.

CNS – Anxiety, confusion, depression, dizziness, emotional lability, hypertonia, hypesthesia, hypotonia, insomnia, neuropathy, paresthesia, somnolence.

Dermatologic – Fungal dermatitis, hirsutism, pruritus, skin hypertrophy, skin ulcer, sweating.

Endocrine – Cushing's syndrome, diabetes mellitus, glycosuria.

GI – Anorexia, dysphagia, eructation, esophagitis, flatulence, gastritis, gastroenteritis, gingivitis, gum hyperplasia, ileus, liver function tests abnormal, mouth ulceration, oral moniliasis, stomatitis.

GU – Albuminuria, bladder pain, dysuria, hematuria, hydronephrosis, impotence, kidney pain, kidney tubular necrosis, nocturia, oliguria, pyelonephritis, pyuria, scrotal edema, testis disorder, toxic nephropathy, urinary frequency, urinary incontinence, urinary retention.

Hematologic/Lymphatic – Ecchymosis, leukocytosis, lymphadenopathy, polycythemia, thrombotic thrombocytopenic purpura (hemolytic-uremic syndrome).

Metabolic/Nutritional – Acidosis, alkaline phosphatase increased, BUN increased, creatine phosphokinase increased, dehydration, healing abnormal, hypercalcemia, hyperglycemia, hyperphosphatemia, hypocalcemia, hypoglycemia, hypomagnesemia, hyponatremia, lactic dehydrogenase increased, AST/SGOT increased, ALT increased, weight loss.

Musculoskeletal – Arthrosis, bone necrosis, leg cramps, myalgia, osteoporosis, tetany.

Respiratory – Asthma, atelectasis, bronchitis, cough increased, epistaxis, hypoxia, lung edema, pleural effusion, pneumonia, rhinitis, sinusitis.

Special senses – Abnormal vision, cataract, conjunctivitis, deafness, ear pain, otitis media, tinnitus.

Miscellaneous – Abdomen enlarged, abscess, ascites, cellulitis, chills, face edema, flu syndrome, generalized edema, hernia, herpes zoster infection, lymphocele, malaise, pelvic pain, peritonitis, sepsis.

Less frequently occurring adverse reactions included: Mycobacterial infections, Epstein-Barr virus infections, and pancreatitis.

Among the reactions which were reported at an incidence of greater than or equal to 3% and less than 20% by 24 months for study 1 and 36 months for study 2, tachycardia and Cushing's syndrome were reported significantly more commonly in both sirolimus groups as compared with the control therapy. Reactions that were reported more commonly in the sirolimus 5 mg/ day group than either the sirolimus 2 mg/day group or control group were: Abnormal healing, bone necrosis, chills, congestive heart failure, dysuria, hernia, hirsutism, urinary frequency, and lymphadenopathy.

➤*Tablets:* The safety profile of the tablet did not differ from that of the oral solution formulation. The incidence of adverse reactions up to 12 months was determined in a randomized, multicenter controlled trial (study 3) in which 229 renal transplant patients received sirolimus oral solution 2 mg once daily and 228 patients received sirolimus tablets 2 mg once daily. All patients were treated with cyclosporine and corticosteroids. The adverse reactions that occurred in either treatment group with an incidence of greater than or equal to 20% in study 3 are similar to those reported for studies 1 and 2. There was no notable difference in the incidence of these adverse reactions between treatment groups (oral solution versus tablets) in study 3, with the exception of acne, which occurred more frequently in the oral solution group, and tremor which occurred more frequently in the tablet group, particularly in black patients.

The adverse reactions that occurred in patients with an incidence of greater than or equal to 3% and less than 20% in either treatment group in study 3 were similar to those reported in studies 1 and 2. There was no notable difference in the incidence of these adverse reactions between treatment groups (oral solution vs tablets) in study 3, with the exception of hypertonia, which occurred more frequently in the oral solution group and diabetes mellitus which occurred more frequently in the tablet group. Hispanic patients in the tablet group experienced hyperglycemia more frequently than Hispanic patients in the oral solution group. In study 3 alone, menorrhagia, metrorrhagia, and polyuria occurred with an incidence of greater than or equal to 3% and less than 20%.

The clinically important opportunistic or common transplant-related infections were identical in all 3 studies and the incidences of these infections were similar in study 3 compared with studies 1 and 2. The incidence rates of these infections were not significantly different between the oral solution and tablet treatment groups in study 3.

In study 3 (at 12 months), there were 2 cases of lymphoma/ lymphoproliferative disorder in the oral solution treatment group (0.8%) and 2 reported cases of lymphoma/lymphoproliferative disorder in the tablet treatment group (0.8%). These differences were not statistically significant and were similar to the incidences observed in studies 1 and 2.

➤*Sirolimus following cyclosporine withdrawal:* The incidence of adverse reactions was determined through 36 months in a randomized, multicenter controlled trial (Study 4) in which 215 renal transplant patients received sirolimus as a maintenance regimen following cyclosporine withdrawal and 215 patients received sirolimus with cyclosporine therapy. All patients were treated with corticosteroids. The safety profile prior to randomization (start of cyclosporine withdrawal) was similar to that of the 2 mg sirolimus groups in studies 1, 2, and 3. Following randomization (at 3 months) patients who had cyclosporine eliminated from their therapy experienced significantly higher incidences of abnormal liver function tests (including increased AST/SGOT and increased ALT/SGPT), hypokalemia, thrombocytopenia, abnormal healing, ileus, and rectal disorder. Conversely, the incidence of hypertension, cyclosporine toxicity, increased creatinine, abnormal kidney function, toxic nephropathy, edema, hyperkalemia, hyperuricemia, and gum hyperplasia was significantly higher in patients who remained on cyclosporine than those who had cyclosporine withdrawn from therapy. Mean systolic and diastolic blood pressure improved significantly following cyclosporine withdrawal.

SIROLIMUS — ORAL

In study 4, at 36 months, the incidence of Herpes zoster infection was significantly lower in patients receiving sirolimus following cyclosporine withdrawal compared with patients who continued to receive sirolimus and cyclosporine.

The incidence of malignancies in study 4 is presented in the table below. In study 4, the incidence of lymphoma/lymphoproliferative disease was similar in all treatment groups. The overall incidence of malignancy was higher in patients receiving sirolimus plus cyclosporine compared with patients who had cyclosporine withdrawn.

Incidence (%) of Malignancies in Study 4 at 36 Months Posttransplant[a,b]

Malignancy	Nonrandomized (n = 95)	Sirolimus with cyclosporine therapy (n = 215)	Sirolimus following cyclosporine withdrawal (n = 215)
Lymphoma/ lymphoproliferative disease	1.1%	1.4%	0.5%
Skin carcinoma			
Any squamous cell[c]	1.1%	1.9%	2.3%
Any basal cell[c]	3.2%	4.7%	2.3%
Melanoma	0.0%	0.5%	0.0%
Miscellaneous/ not specified	1.1%	0.9%	0.0%
Total	4.2%	6.5%	3.7%
Other malignancy	1.1%	3.3%	1.4%

[a] Patients received cyclosporine and corticosteroids.
[b] Includes patients who prematurely discontinued treatment.
[c] Patients may be counted in more than 1 category.

➤*Other clinical experience:* Cases of interstitial lung disease (including pneumonitis, and infrequently bronchiolitis obliterans organizing pneumonia [BOOP] and pulmonary fibrosis), some fatal, with no identified infectious etiology have occurred in patients receiving immunosuppressive regimens including sirolimus. In some cases, the interstitial lung disease has resolved upon discontinuation or dose reduction of sirolimus. The risk may be increased as the trough sirolimus level increases.

There have been reports of neutropenia and rare reports of pancytopenia. Hypersensitivity reactions, including anaphylactic/anaphylactoid reactions, have been associated with the administration of sirolimus.

Hepatotoxicity has been reported, including fatal hepatic necrosis with elevated sirolimus trough levels.

Abnormal healing following transplant surgery has been reported, including fascial dehiscence and anastomotic disruption (e.g., wound, vascular, airway, ureteral, biliary).

Overdosage

➤*Symptoms:* Reports of overdose with sirolimus have been received; however, experience has been limited. In general, the adverse effects of overdose are consistent with those listed in the Adverse Reactions section (see Adverse Reactions).

➤*Treatment:* General supportive measures should be followed in all cases of overdose. Based on the poor aqueous solubility and high erythrocyte binding of sirolimus, it is anticipated that sirolimus is not dialyzable to any significant extent. In mice and rats, the acute oral lethal dose was greater than 800 mg/kg.

Patient Information

Patients should be given complete dosage instructions (see Patient Instructions). Women of childbearing potential should be informed of the potential risks during pregnancy and that they should use effective contraception prior to initiation of sirolimus therapy, during sirolimus therapy and for 12 weeks after sirolimus therapy has been stopped (see Warnings, Pregnancy).

Patients should be told that exposure to sunlight and UV light should be limited by wearing protective clothing and using a sunscreen with a high protection factor because of the increased risk for skin cancer (see Warnings).

➤*Patient instructions for sirolimus oral solution administration:*

Bottles –

1.) Open the solution bottle. Remove the safety cap by squeezing the tabs on the cap and twisting counterclockwise.

Pouches –

1.) Before opening the pouch, squeeze the pouch from the neck area to push the contents into the lower part of the pouch.
2.) Unused pouches should be stored in the refrigerator.

INTERFERON ALFA-2a, RECOMBINANT (rIFN-A; IFLrA)

Rx	**Roferon-A** (Hoffman La-Roche)	**Prefilled syringes:** 3 million IU/syringe[1]	In 0.5 mL single-use, prefilled syringes. In 1s and 6s.
		6 million IU/syringe[1]	In 0.5 mL single-use, prefilled syringes. In 1s and 6s.
		9 million IU/syringe[1]	In 0.5 mL single-use, prefilled syringes. In 1s and 6s.

[1] With NaCl, polysorbate 80, benzyl alcohol, and ammonium acetate.

INTERFERON ALFA-2A, RECOMBINANT — INJECTION

WARNING

Alpha interferons, including interferon alfa-2a, recombinant, cause or aggravate fatal or life-threatening neuropsychiatric, autoimmune, ischemic, and infectious disorders. Closely monitor patients with periodic clinical and laboratory evaluations. Withdraw patients with persistently severe or worsening signs or symptoms of these conditions from therapy. In many, but not all, cases these disorders resolve after stopping interferon alfa-2a, recombinant therapy.

Indications

Interferon alfa-2a, recombinant is indicated for the treatment of chronic hepatitis C, hairy cell leukemia, and AIDS-related Kaposi sarcoma in patients 18 years of age or older. In addition, it is indicated for chronic phase, Philadelphia chromosome (Ph) positive chronic myelogenous leukemia (CML) patients who are minimally pretreated (within 1 year of diagnosis).

➤*Chronic hepatitis C:* Interferon alfa-2a, recombinant is indicated for use in patients with chronic hepatitis C, diagnosed by hepatitis C virus (HCV) antibody or a history of exposure to hepatitis C who have compensated liver disease and are 18 years of age or older. Perform a liver biopsy and a serum test for the presence of antibody to HCV to establish the diagnosis of chronic hepatitis C. Exclude other causes of hepatitis, including hepatitis B, prior to therapy with interferon alfa-2a, recombinant.

➤*AIDS-related Kaposi sarcoma:* Interferon alfa-2a, recombinant is indicated for the treatment of AIDS-related Kaposi sarcoma in a select group of patients. In determining whether a patient should be treated, assess the likelihood of response based on the clinical manifestations of HIV infection, including prior opportunistic infections, presence of B symptoms, CD_4 count, and the manifestations of Kaposi sarcoma requiring treatment.

➤*Unlabeled uses:* Treatment of metastatic melanoma. Designated as an orphan drug for renal cell carcinoma and chronic myelogenous leukemia (CML).

Administration and Dosage

➤*Administration:* Interferon alfa-2a, recombinant vials are administered either subcutaneously or intramuscularly (IM). The interferon alfa-2a, recombinant prefilled syringe is administered subcutaneously only, due to the length of the syringe needle (one-half inch) provided in the packaging.

➤*Chronic hepatitis C:* The recommended dosage of interferon alfa-2a, recombinant for the treatment of chronic hepatitis C is 3 million units 3 times a week administered subcutaneously or IM for 12 months (48 to 52 weeks). As an alternative, patients may be treated with an induction dose of 6 million units 3 times weekly for the first 3 months (12 weeks) followed by 3 million units 3 times weekly for 9 months (36 weeks). Normalization of serum ALT generally occurs within a few weeks after initiation of treatment in responders. Approximately 90% of patients who respond to interferon alfa-2a do so within the first 3 months of treatment; however, patients responding to interferon alfa-2a with a reduction in ALT should complete 12 months of treatment. Patients who have no response to interferon alfa-2a within the first 3 months of therapy are not likely to respond with continued treatment; consider treatment discontinuation in these patients.

Patients who tolerate and partially or completely respond to therapy with interferon alfa-2a, recombinant but relapse following its discontinuation may be retreated. Retreatment with either 3 million units 3 times weekly or with 6 million units 3 times weekly for 6 to 12 months may be considered.

Temporary dose reduction by 50% is recommended in patients who do not tolerate the prescribed dose. If adverse reactions resolve, treatment with the original prescribed dose can be reinitiated. In patients who cannot tolerate the reduced dose, cessation of therapy, at least temporarily, is recommended.

➤*Hairy cell leukemia:* Prior to initiation of therapy, perform tests to quantitate peripheral blood hemoglobin, platelets, granulocytes, and hairy cells and bone marrow hairy cells. Monitor these parameters periodically (eg, monthly) during treatment to determine whether response to treatment has occurred. If a patient does not respond within 6 months, discontinue treatment. If a response to treatment does occur, continue treatment until no further improvement is observed and these laboratory parameters have been stable for approximately 3 months. Patients with hairy cell leukemia have been treated for up to 24 consecutive months. The optimal duration of treatment for this disease has not been determined.

The induction dose of interferon alfa-2a, recombinant is 3 million units daily for 16 to 24 weeks, administered as an subcutaneous or IM injection. Subcutaneous administration is particularly suggested for, but not limited to, thrombocytopenic patients (platelet count less than 50,000) or patients at risk for bleeding. The recommended maintenance dose is 3 million units 3 times a week. Dose reduction by one half or withholding of individual doses may be needed when severe adverse reactions occur. The use of doses greater than 3 million units is not recommended in hairy cell leukemia.

INTERFERON ALFA-2A, RECOMBINANT — INJECTION

➤*AIDS-related Kaposi sarcoma:* Interferon alfa-2a is useful for the treatment of AIDS-related Kaposi sarcoma in a select group of patients. In determining whether a patient should be treated, assess the likelihood of response based on the clinical manifestations of HIV infection and the manifestations of Kaposi sarcoma requiring treatment.

Perform indicator lesion measurements and total lesion count before initiation of therapy. Periodically monitor (eg, monthly) these parameters during treatment to determine whether response to treatment or disease stabilization has occurred. When disease stabilization or a response to treatment occurs, continue treatment until there is no further evidence of tumor or until discontinuation is required because of a severe opportunistic infection or adverse reactions. The optimal duration of treatment for this disease has not been determined.

The recommended induction dose of interferon alfa-2a, recombinant is 36 million units daily for 10 to 12 weeks, administered as an IM or subcutaneous injection. Subcutaneous administration is particularly suggested for, but not limited to, patients who are thrombocytopenic (platelet count less than 50,000) or who are at risk for bleeding. The recommended maintenance dose is 36 million units 3 times a week. If severe reactions occur, modify the dose (50% reduction) or temporarily discontinue therapy until the adverse reactions abate. An escalating schedule of 3, 9, and 18 million units each daily for 3 days, followed by 36 million units daily for the remainder of the 10- to 12-week induction period has also produced equivalent therapeutic benefit with some amelioration of the acute toxicity in some patients.

➤*Ph-positive CML in chronic phase:* Prior to initiation of therapy, make a diagnosis of Philadelphia chromosome positive CML in chronic phase by the appropriate peripheral blood, bone marrow, and other diagnostic testing. Regularly monitor (eg, monthly) hematologic parameters. Since significant cytogenetic changes are not readily apparent until after hematologic response has occurred, and usually not until several months of therapy have elapsed, cytogenetic monitoring may be performed at less frequent intervals. Achievement of complete cytogenetic response has been observed up to 2 years following the start of interferon alfa-2a, recombinant treatment.

The recommended initial dose of interferon alfa-2a, recombinant is 9 million units daily administered as an subcutaneous or IM injection. Based on clinical experience, short-term tolerance may be improved by gradually increasing the dose of interferon alfa-2a, recombinant over the first week of administration from 3 million units daily for 3 days to 6 million units daily for 3 days to the target dose of 9 million units daily for the duration of the treatment period.

The optimal dose and duration of therapy have not yet been determined. Even though the median time to achieve a complete hematologic response was 5 months in study MI400, hematologic responses have been observed up to 18 months after treatment start. Continue treatment until disease progression. If severe adverse reactions occur, a treatment interruption or a reduction in either the dose or the frequency of injections may be necessary to achieve the individual maximally tolerated dose.

Limited data are available on the use of interferon alfa-2a, recombinant in children with CML. In 1 report of 15 children with Ph-positive, adult-type CML doses between 2.5 to 5 million units/m²/day given IM were tolerated. In another study, severe adverse reactions, including deaths, were noted in children with previously untreated Ph-negative, juvenile CML, who received interferon doses of 30 million units/m²/day.

➤*Storage/Stability:* Store the injectable solution and the prefilled syringe in the refrigerator at 2° to 8°C (36° to 46°F). Do not freeze or shake.

Actions

➤*Pharmacology:* The mechanism by which interferon alfa-2a, recombinant, or any other interferon, exerts antitumor or antiviral activity is not clearly understood. However, it is believed that direct antiproliferative action against tumor cells, inhibition of virus replication, and modulation of the host immune response play important roles in antitumor and antiviral activity.

The biological activities of interferon alfa-2a, recombinant are species-restricted (ie, they are expressed in a very limited number of species other than humans). As a consequence, preclinical evaluation of interferon alfa-2a, recombinant has involved in vitro experiments with human cells and some in vivo experiments. Using human cells in culture, interferon alfa-2a, recombinant has been shown to have antiproliferative and immunomodulatory activities that are very similar to those of the mixture of interferon alfa subtypes produced by human leukocytes. In vivo, interferon alfa-2a, recombinant has been shown to inhibit the growth of several human tumors growing in immunocompromised (nude) mice. Because of its species-restricted activity, it has not been possible to demonstrate antitumor activity in immunologically intact syngeneic tumor model systems, where effects on the host immune system would be observable. However, such antitumor activity has been repeatedly demonstrated with, for example, mouse interferon-alfa in transplantable mouse tumor systems. The clinical significance of these findings is unknown.

Serum-neutralizing activity, determined by a highly sensitive enzyme immunoassay, and a neutralization bioassay, was detected in approximately 25% of all patients who received interferon alfa-2a. Antibodies to human leukocyte interferon may occur spontaneously in certain clinical conditions (cancer, systemic lupus erythematosus, herpes zoster) in patients who have never received exogenous interferon. The significance of the appearance of serum neutralizing activity is not known.

➤*Pharmacokinetics:*

Absorption/Distribution – The serum concentrations of interferon alfa-2a, recombinant reflected a large intersubject variation in both healthy volunteers and patients with disseminated cancer.

The pharmacokinetics of interferon alfa-2a, recombinant after single IM doses to patients with disseminated cancer were similar to those found in healthy volunteers. Dose proportional increases in serum concentrations were observed after single doses up to 198 million units. There were no changes in the distribution or elimination of interferon alfa-2a, recombinant during twice-daily (0.5 to 36 million units), once-daily (1 to 54 million units), or 3 times weekly (1 to 136 million units) dosing regimens up to 28 days of dosing. Multiple IM doses of interferon alfa-2a, recombinant resulted in an accumulation of 2 to 4 times the single-dose serum concentrations. There is no pharmacokinetic information in patients with chronic hepatitis C, hairy cell leukemia, AIDS-related Kaposi sarcoma, and CML.

Metabolism/Excretion – The metabolism of interferon alfa-2a, recombinant is consistent with that of alfa interferons in general. Alfa interferons are totally filtered through the glomeruli and undergo rapid proteolytic degradation during tubular reabsorption, rendering a negligible reappearance of intact alfa interferon in the systemic circulation. Small amounts of radiolabeled interferon alfa-2a, recombinant appear in the urine of isolated rat kidneys, suggesting near complete reabsorption of interferon alfa-2a, recombinant catabolites. Liver metabolism and subsequent biliary excretion are considered minor pathways of elimination for alfa interferons.

In healthy people, interferon alfa-2a, recombinant exhibited an elimination half-life of 3.7 to 8.5 hours (mean, 5.1 hours), volume of distribution at steady-state of 0.223 to 0.748 L/kg (mean, 0.4 L/kg), and a total body clearance of 2.14 to 3.62 mL/min/kg (mean, 2.79 mL/min/kg) after a 36 million units (2.2×10^8 pg) intravenous (IV) infusion. After IM and subcutaneous administrations of 36 million units, peak serum concentrations ranged from 1,500 to 2,580 pg/mL (mean, 2,020 pg/mL) at a mean time to peak of 3.8 hours and from 1,250 to 2,320 pg/mL (mean, 1,730 pg/mL) at a mean time to peak of 7.3 hours, respectively. The apparent fraction of the dose absorbed after IM injection was greater than 80%.

Contraindications

Hypersensitivity to alfa interferon, benzyl alcohol, or any component of the product.

Warnings

➤*Psychological effects:* Depression and suicidal behavior, including suicidal ideation, suicidal attempts, and suicides, have been reported in association with treatment with alfa interferons, including interferon alfa-2a, recombinant. Inform patients to be treated with interferon alfa-2a, recombinant that depression and suicidal ideation may be adverse reactions of treatment and advise them to report these adverse reactions immediately to their health care providers. Closely monitor patients receiving interferon alfa-2a, recombinant therapy for the occurrence of depressive symptomatology. Consider cessation of treatment for patients experiencing depression. Although dose reduction or treatment cessation may lead to resolution of the depressive symptomatology, depression may persist and suicides have occurred after withdrawing therapy.

➤*CNS effects:* CNS adverse reactions have been reported in a number of patients. These reactions included decreased mental status, dizziness, impaired memory, agitation, manic behavior, and psychotic reactions. More severe obtundation and coma have been rarely observed. Most of these abnormalities were mild and reversible within a few days to 3 weeks upon dose reduction or discontinuation of interferon alfa-2a, recombinant therapy. Careful periodic neuropsychiatric monitoring of all patients is recommended.

➤*Special risk patients:* Use interferon alfa-2a, recombinant with caution in patients with severe preexisting cardiac disease, severe renal or hepatic disease, seizure disorders, or compromised CNS function.

Do not treat patients with a history of autoimmune hepatitis or a history of autoimmune disease and patients who are immunosuppressed transplant recipients with interferon alfa-2a, recombinant. Controlled studies of interferon alfa-2a, recombinant therapy in patients with advanced cirrhosis or decompensated liver disease have not been performed. In chronic hepatitis C, initiation of alfa-interferon therapy, including interferon alfa-2a, recombinant, has been reported to cause transient liver abnormalities, which can result in increased ascites, hepatic failure, or death in patients with poorly compensated liver disease.

➤*Cardiac effects:* Administer interferon alfa-2a, recombinant with caution to patients with cardiac disease or with any history of cardiac illness. Acute, self-limited toxicities (ie, fever, chills) frequently associated with interferon alfa-2a, recombinant administration may exacerbate preexisting cardiac conditions. Rarely, myocardial infarction (MI) has occurred in patients receiving interferon alfa-2a, recombinant. Cases of cardiomyopathy have been observed on rare occasions in patients treated with alfa interferons.

➤*GI effects:* Infrequently, severe or fatal GI hemorrhage has been reported in association with alfa-interferon therapy.

➤*Hematologic effects:* Alpha interferons suppress bone marrow function and may result in severe cytopenias including very rare events of aplastic anemia. It is advised that complete blood counts (CBC) be obtained pretreatment and monitored routinely during therapy. Discontinue alpha interferon therapy in patients who develop severe decreases in neutrophil (less than 0.5×10^9/L) or platelet counts (less than 25×10^9/L).

INTERFERON ALFA-2A, RECOMBINANT — INJECTION

Exercise caution when administering interferon alfa-2a, recombinant to patients with myelosuppression or when interferon alfa-2a, recombinant is used in combination with other agents that are known to cause myelosuppression. Synergistic toxicity has been observed when interferon alfa-2a, recombinant is administered in combination with zidovudine (AZT). The effects of interferon alfa-2a, recombinant when combined with other drugs used in the treatment of AIDS-related disease are not known.

➤*Hyperglycemia:* Hyperglycemia has been observed rarely in patients treated with interferon alfa-2a, recombinant. Measure symptomatic patients' blood glucose and follow-up accordingly. Patients with diabetes mellitus may require adjustment of their antidiabetic regimen.

➤*Visceral AIDS-related Kaposi sarcoma:* Do not use interferon alfa-2a, recombinant for the treatment of visceral AIDS-related Kaposi sarcoma associated with rapidly progressive or life-threatening disease.

➤*Benzyl alcohol:* The injectable solutions contain benzyl alcohol; do not use in patients with a known allergy to benzyl alcohol. This product is not indicated for use in neonates or infants; do not use in patients in that age group. There have been rare reports of death in neonates and infants associated with excessive exposure to benzyl alcohol. There have been reports of permanent neuropsychiatric deficits and multiple system organ failure associated with benzyl alcohol in neonates and infants. The amount of benzyl alcohol at which toxicity or adverse reactions may occur in neonates or infants is not known.

➤*Ophthalmologic disorders:* Decrease or loss of vision; retinopathy, including macular edema; retinal artery or vein thrombosis; retinal hemorrhages and cotton wool spots; optic neuritis; and papilledema are induced or aggravated by treatment with interferon alfa-2a or other alpha interferons. All patients should receive an eye examination at baseline. Patients with preexisting ophthalmologic disorders (eg, diabetic or hypertensive retinopathy) should receive periodic ophthalmologic exams during interferon alpha treatment. Give a prompt and complete eye exam to any patient who develops ocular symptoms. Discontinue interferon alfa-2a treatment in patients who develop new or worsening ophthalmologic disorders.

➤*Lab test abnormalities:* Leukopenia and elevation of hepatic enzymes occurred frequently but were rarely dose limiting. Thrombocytopenia occurred less frequently. Proteinuria and increased cells in urinary sediment were also seen infrequently. Dose-limiting hepatic or renal toxicities were unusual. Infrequently, severe renal toxicities, sometimes requiring renal dialysis, have been reported with alfa-interferon therapy alone or in combination with IL-2.

➤*Mutagenesis:* A chromosomal defect following the addition of human leukocyte interferon to lymphocyte cultures from a patient suffering from a lymphoproliferative disorder has been reported.

➤*Fertility impairment:* Interferon alfa-2a, recombinant has been studied for its effect on fertility in Macaca mulatta (rhesus monkeys). Nonpregnant rhesus females treated with interferon alfa-2a, recombinant at doses of 5 and 25 million units/kg/day have shown menstrual cycle irregularities, including prolonged or shortened menstrual periods and erratic bleeding; these cycles were considered to be anovulatory on the basis that reduced progesterone levels were noted and that expected increases in preovulatory estrogen and luteinizing hormones were not observed. These monkeys returned to a normal menstrual rhythm following discontinuation of treatment.

➤*Pregnancy:* *Category C.* Safe use in human pregnancy has not been established. Therefore, use interferon alfa-2a, recombinant during pregnancy only if the potential benefit justifies the potential risk to the fetus. Information from primate studies showed dose-related menstrual irregularities and an increased incidence of spontaneous abortions. Decreases in serum estradiol and progesterone concentrations have been reported in women treated with human leukocyte interferon. Therefore, fertile women should not receive interferon alfa-2a, recombinant unless they are using effective contraception during the therapy period.

The injectable solution contains benzyl alcohol. The excipient benzyl alcohol can be transmitted via the placenta. Take the possibility of toxicity into account in premature infants after the administration of interferon alfa-2a, recombinant solution for injection immediately prior to birth or cesarean delivery.

Interferon alfa-2a, recombinant has been shown to demonstrate a statistically significant increase in abortifacient activity in rhesus monkeys when given at approximately 20 to 500 times the human dose. A study in pregnant rhesus monkeys treated with 1, 5, or 25 million units/kg/day of interferon alfa-2a, recombinant in their early to midfetal period (days 22 to 70 of gestation) has failed to demonstrate teratogenic activity for interferon alfa-2a, recombinant.

There are no adequate and well-controlled studies in pregnant women.

➤*Lactation:* It is not known whether this drug is excreted in human milk. Because many drugs are excreted in human milk and because of the potential for serious adverse reactions in breast-feeding infants from interferon alfa-2a, recombinant, make a decision to discontinue breast-feeding or the drug, taking into account the importance of the drug to the mother.

➤*Children:* Use of interferon alfa-2a, recombinant in children with Ph-positive adult-type CML is supported by evidence from adequate and well-controlled studies of interferon alfa-2a, recombinant in adults with additional data from the literature on the use of alfa interferon in children with CML. A published report on 15 children with Ph-positive adult-type CML suggests a safety profile similar to that seen in adult CML; clinical responses were also observed.

For all other indications, safety and efficacy have not been established in patients younger than 18 years of age.

The injectable solutions are not indicated for use in neonates or infants; do not use in patients in that age group. There have been rare reports of death in neonates and infants associated with excessive exposure to benzyl alcohol.

Precautions

➤*Monitoring:* Perform complete blood with differential platelet counts and clinical chemistry tests before initiation of interferon alfa-2a, recombinant therapy and at appropriate periods during therapy. Since responses of hairy cell leukemia, AIDS-related Kaposi sarcoma, chronic hepatitis C, and CML are not generally observed for 1 to 3 months after initiation of treatment, very careful monitoring for severe depression of blood cell counts is warranted during the initial phase of treatment.

Take electrocardiograms before and during the course of treatment in those patients who have preexisting cardiac abnormalities or who are in advanced stages of cancer.

For patients being treated for chronic hepatitis C, evaluate serum ALT before therapy to establish baselines and repeat at week 2 and monthly thereafter following initiation of therapy for monitoring clinical response. Patients with neutrophil count less than 1,500/mm^3, platelet count less than 75,000/mm^3, hemoglobin less than 10 g/dL, and creatinine greater than 1.5 mg/dL were excluded from several major chronic hepatitis C studies; carefully monitor patients with these laboratory abnormalities if they are treated with interferon alfa-2a, recombinant.

In all instances where the use of interferon alfa-2a, recombinant is considered for chemotherapy, evaluate the need and usefulness of the drug against the risk of adverse reactions. Most adverse reactions are reversible if detected early. If severe reactions occur, reduce the dosage or discontinue the drug, and take appropriate corrective measures according to the clinical judgment of the health care provider. Carry out reinstitution of interferon alfa-2a, recombinant therapy with caution and adequate consideration of the further need for the drug, and be alert to possible recurrence of toxicity. The minimum effective doses of interferon alfa-2a, recombinant for treatment of hairy cell leukemia, AIDS-related Kaposi sarcoma, and CML have not been established.

➤*Interchangeability:* Variations in dosage and adverse reactions exist among different brands of interferon. Therefore, do not use different brands of interferon in a single treatment regimen.

➤*Autoimmune disease:* Rare cases of autoimmune diseases including thrombocytopenia, vasculitis, Raynaud phenomenon, rheumatoid arthritis, lupus erythematosus, and rhabdomyolysis have been observed in patients treated with alpha interferons. Closely monitor any patient developing an autoimmune disorder during treatment and, if appropriate, discontinue treatment.

➤*Lab test abnormalities:* Patients with preexisting thyroid abnormalities may be treated if normal thyroid-stimulating hormone (TSH) levels can be maintained by medication. Testing of TSH levels in these patients is recommended at baseline and every 3 months following initiation of therapy.

➤*Hazardous tasks:* Caution patients receiving high-dose alfa interferon against performing tasks that require complete mental alertness such as operating machinery or driving a motor vehicle. Inform patients to be treated with interferon alfa-2a, recombinant that depression and suicidal ideation may be side effects of treatment and advise them to report these side effects immediately to their doctors.

Drug Interactions

➤*CYP450 system:* Alfa interferons may affect the oxidative metabolic process by reducing the activity of hepatic microsomal cytochrome enzymes in the P-450 group. Although the clinical relevance is still unclear, take this into account when prescribing concomitant therapy with drugs metabolized by this route.

Interferon alfa-2a Drug Interactions

Precipitant drug	Object drug*		Description
Interferon alfa-2a	Theophylline	↑	Reduced clearance of theophylline following coadministration has been reported.
Interferon alfa-2a	Neurotoxic, hematotoxic or cardiotoxic drugs	↑	Effects of previously or coadministered drugs may be increased by interferons.
Interferon alfa-2a	Interleukin-2	↑	Potential risk of renal failure.
Interferon alfa-2a	CNS drugs	↔	Interactions could occur following coadministration of centrally acting drugs.

* ↑ = Object drug increased. ↔ = Undetermined clinical effect.

Adverse Reactions

➤*Psychological effects:* See Warnings for more information.

➤*Chronic hepatitis C:* Adverse reactions associated with the 3 million units dose include the following:

Cardiovascular – Arrhythmia (1%).

INTERFERON ALFA-2A, RECOMBINANT — INJECTION

CNS – Headache (52%), dizziness (13%), paresthesia (7%), confusion (7%), concentration impaired (4%), and change in taste or smell (3%).

Dermatologic – Injection site reaction (29%), partial alopecia (19%), rash (8%), dry skin or pruritus (7%), hematoma (1%), psoriasis (less than 1%), cutaneous eruptions (less than 1%), eczema (less than 1%), and seborrhea (less than 1%).

GI – Nausea/vomiting (33%), diarrhea (20%), anorexia (14%), abdominal pain (12%), flatulence (3%), liver pain (3%), digestion impaired (2%), and gingival bleeding (2%).

Psychiatric – Depression (16%), irritability (15%), insomnia (14%), anxiety (5%), and behavior disturbances (3%).

Pulmonary – Dryness or inflammation of oropharynx (6%), epistaxis (4%), rhinitis (3%), and sinusitis (less than 1%).

Miscellaneous – Conjunctivitis (4%), menstrual irregularity (2%), and visual acuity decreased (less than 1%).

Flu-like symptoms: Fatigue (58%), myalgia/arthralgia (51%), flu-like symptoms (33%), fever (28%), chills (23%), asthenia (6%), sweating (5%), leg cramps (3%), and malaise (1%). Patients receiving 6 million units 3 times weekly experienced a higher incidence of severe psychiatric reactions (9%) than those receiving 3 million units 3 times weekly (6%) in 2 large US studies. In addition, more patients withdrew from these studies when receiving 6 million units 3 times weekly (11%) than when receiving 3 million units 3 times weekly (7%). Up to half of patients receiving 3 million units or 6 million units 3 times weekly withdrawing from the study experienced depression or other psychiatric adverse reactions. At higher doses anxiety, sleep disorders, and irritability were observed more frequently. An increased incidence of fatigue, myalgia/arthralgia, headache, fever, chills, alopecia, sleep disturbances, and dry skin or pruritus was also generally observed during treatment with higher doses of interferon alfa-2a, recombinant.

Generally there were fewer adverse reactions reported in the second 6 months of treatment than in the first 6 months for patients treated with 3 million units 3 times weekly. Patients tolerant of initial therapy with interferon alfa-2a, recombinant generally tolerate retreatment at the same dose, but tend to experience more adverse reactions at higher doses.

Infrequent adverse reactions (greater than 1% but less than 3% incidence) included the following: cold feeling, cough, muscle cramps, diaphoresis, dyspnea, eye pain, reactivation of herpes simplex, lethargy, edema, sexual dysfunction, shaking, skin lesions, stomatitis, tooth disorder, urinary tract infection, and weakness in extremities.

➤*Hairy cell leukemia:*

Cardiovascular – All reactions (39%). Chest pain (11%), edema (11%), and hypertension (11%).

CNS – CNS (all reactions) (39%). Dizziness (21%), depression (16%), sleep disturbance (10%), decreased mental status (10%), anxiety (6%), lethargy (6%), visual disturbance (6%) and confusion (5%).

Peripheral nervous system (all reactions) (23%). Paresthesia (12%) and numbness (12%).

Dermatologic – All reactions (79%). Skin rash (44%), diaphoresis (22%), partial alopecia (17%), dry skin (17%), and pruritus (13%).

GI – All reactions (69%). Anorexia (43%), nausea/vomiting (39%), and diarrhea (34%).

Musculoskeletal – All reactions (73%). Myalgia (71%), joint or bone pain (25%), and arthritis or polyarthritis (5%).

Pulmonary – All reactions (40%). Coughing (16%), dyspnea (12%), and pneumonia (11%).

Respiratory – All reactions (45%). Throat irritation (21%), rhinorrhea (12%), and sinusitis (11%).

Miscellaneous –

Constitutional (100%): Fever (92%), fatigue (86%), headache (64%), chills (64%), weight loss (33%), dizziness (21%), and flu-like symptoms (16%).

Pain (34%): Pain (24%) and pain in back (16%).

Rare: Rarely (less than 5%), CNS effects, including gait disturbance, nervousness, syncope, and vertigo, as well as cardiac adverse reactions, including murmur, thrombophlebitis, and hypotension, were reported. Adverse reactions that occurred rarely, and may have been related to underlying disease, included ecchymosis, epistaxis, bleeding gums, and petechiae. Urticaria and inflammation at the site of injection were also rarely observed.

➤*AIDS-related Kaposi sarcoma:*

Cardiovascular – Chest pain (4%) and hypotension (4%).

CNS – Dizziness (40%), decreased mental status (17%), depression (16%), paresthesia (8%), confusion (8%), diaphoresis (7%), visual disturbances (5%), sleep disturbances (5%), and numbness (3%).

Dermatologic – Partial alopecia (22%), rash (11%), and dry skin or pruritus (5%).

GI – Anorexia (65%), nausea (51%), diarrhea (42%), emesis (17%), and abdominal pain (15%).

Pulmonary – Coughing (27%), dyspnea (11%), and edema (9%).

Miscellaneous – Weight loss (25%), change in taste (25%), dryness or inflammation of the oropharynx (14%), night sweats (8%), and rhinorrhea (4%).

Flu-like symptoms: Fatigue (95%), fever (74%), myalgia (69%), headache (66%), chills (41%), and arthralgia (24%).

Occasionally (less than 3%) nervous system reactions, including anxiety, nervousness, emotional lability, vertigo, and forgetfulness, as well as cardiac adverse reactions, including palpitations and arrhythmia, were reported. Other adverse reactions that occurred occasionally (less than 3%) and may have been related to underlying disease included sinusitis, constipation, chest congestion, pneumonia, urticaria, and flatulence. Adverse reactions that occurred rarely (less than 1%) included ataxia, seizures, cyanosis, gastric distress, bronchospasm, pain at injection site, earache, eye irritation, and rhinitis. Miscellaneous adverse reactions, such as poor coordination, lethargy, muscle contractions, neuropathy, tremor, involuntary movement, syncope, aphasia, aphonia, dysarthria, amnesia, weakness, and flushing of skin, were observed in less than 0.5% of patients. Cases of cardiomyopathy have been observed on rare occasions in patients treated with alfa interferons.

➤*CML:* For patients with CML, the percentage of adverse reactions, whether related to drug therapy or not, experienced by patients treated with rIFNalfa-2a is provided. Severe adverse reactions were observed in 66% and 31% of patients on study DM84-38 and MI400, respectively. Dose reduction and temporary cessation of therapy were required frequently. Permanent cessation of interferon alfa-2a, recombinant due to intolerable adverse reactions, was required in 15% and 23% of patients on studies DM84-38 and MI400, respectively.

Cardiovascular – Dysrhythmia (7%).

CNS – Headache (44%), depression (28%), decreased mental status (16%), dizziness (11%), sleep disturbances (11%), paresthesia (8%), involuntary movements (7%), and visual disturbance (6%).

Dermatologic – Hair changes (including alopecia) (18%), skin rash (18%), sweating (15%), dry skin (7%), and pruritus (7%).

GI – Anorexia (48%), nausea/vomiting (37%), and diarrhea (37%).

Pulmonary – Coughing (19%), dyspnea (8%).

Miscellaneous –

Flu-like symptoms: Fever (92%), asthenia or fatigue (88%), myalgia (68%), chills (63%), arthralgia/bone pain (47%) and headache (44%). Uncommon adverse reactions (less than 4%) reported in clinical studies included chest pain, syncope, hypotension, impotence, alterations in taste or hearing, confusion, seizures, memory loss, disturbances of libido, bruising, and coagulopathy. Miscellaneous adverse reactions that were rarely observed included Coombs' positive hemolytic anemia, aplastic anemia, hypothyroidism, cardiomyopathy, hypertriglyceridemia, and bronchospasm.

➤*Other investigational studies:* The following infrequent adverse reactions have been reported in greater than or equal to 1 of the approved clinical indications and with the investigational use of interferon alfa-2a, recombinant (less than 5%): pancreatitis, colitis, GI hemorrhage, stomatitis, thyroid dysfunction (including hypothyroidism and hyperthyroidism), diabetes (in some patients requiring insulin therapy), and pneumonitis (some cases responding to interferon cessation and corticosteroid therapy). In addition to the adverse reactions noted, other adverse reactions that occurred included: abdominal fullness, hypermotility, hepatitis, gait disturbance, hallucinations, encephalopathy, psychomotor retardation, coma, stroke, transient ischemic attacks, dysphasia, sedation, apathy, irritability, hyperactivity, claustrophobia, loss of libido, congestive heart failure, myocardial infarction, Raynaud phenomenon, hot flashes, tachypnea, ischemic retinopathy, excessive salivation, and anaphylactic reactions. These adverse reactions occurred rarely (less than 1%).

The following reactions have been rarely observed (less than 3%) in some patients receiving interferon alfa-2a, recombinant: autoimmune diseases (ie, vasculitis, arthritis, hemolytic anemia, and lupus erythematosus syndrome). The mechanism by which these reactions develop and their relationship to interferon alfa-2a, recombinant therapy are unclear. Similar reactions have been reported for other types of interferon.

Lab test abnormalities – The percentage of patients with chronic hepatitis C, hairy cell leukemia, AIDS-related Kaposi sarcoma, and CML who experienced a significant abnormal laboratory test value (National Cancer Institute [NCI] or World Health Organization [WHO] grades III or IV) at least once during their treatment with interferon alfa-2a, recombinant is shown in the following table:

Significant Abnormal Laboratory Test Values

	Chronic hepatitis C	Hairy cell leukemia	AIDS-related Kaposi sarcoma	CML[c]	
				US study	Non-US study
	(n = 203); 3 million units 3 times a week	(n = 218)	(n = 241)	(n = 91)	(n = 219)
Alkaline phosphatase	0%	3%	11%	3%	1%
Anemia (Hb)	0%	31% [a]	27%	15%	4%
AST	NAP [d]	9%	40%	5%	1%
Leukopenia	1.5%	45% [a]	49%	20%	3%
LDH[f]	NAP [d]	< 1%	10%	NA [e]	NA [e]
Neutropenia	10%	68% [a]	52%	22%	0%
Proteinuria	0%	10% [b]	< 1%	NA [e]	NA [e]
Thrombocytopenia	4.5%	62% [a]	35%	27%	5%

[a] In the majority of patients, initial hematologic laboratory test values were abnormal due to their underlying disease.
[b] Ten percent (10%) of the patients experienced a proteinuria greater than 1+ at least once.
[c] Patients enrolled in the 2 clinical studies receiving at least 1 dose of interferon alfa-2a, recombinant.
[d] NAP = Not applicable.
[e] NA = Not assessed.
[f] LDH = Lactate dehydrogenase.

INTERFERON ALFA-2A, RECOMBINANT — INJECTION

Chronic hepatitis C: The incidence of neutropenia (WHO grades III or IV) was over twice as high in those treated with 6 million units 3 times weekly (21%) as those treated with 3 million units 3 times weekly (10%).

Hairy cell leukemia: Increases in serum phosphorus (greater than or equal to 1.6 mmol/L) and serum uric acid (greater than or equal to 9.1 mg/dL) were observed in 9% and 10% of patients, respectively. The increase in serum uric acid is likely to be related to the underlying disease. Decreases in serum calcium (less than or equal to 1.9 mmol/L) and serum phosphorus (less than or equal to 0.9 mmol/L) were seen in 28% and 22% of patients, respectively.

CML: In the 2 clinical studies, a severe or life-threatening anemia was seen in up to 15% of patients. A severe or life-threatening leukopenia and thrombocytopenia were observed in up to 20% and 27% of patients, respectively. Changes were usually reversible when therapy was discontinued. One case of aplastic anemia and 1 case of Coombs' positive hemolytic anemia were seen in 310 patients treated with rIFN alfa-2a in clinical studies. Severe cytopenias led to discontinuation of therapy in 4% of all interferon alfa-2a, recombinant-treated patients.

Transient increases in liver transaminases or alkaline phosphatase of any intensity were seen in up to 50% of patients during treatment with interferon alfa-2a, recombinant. Only 5% of patients had a severe or life-threatening increase in AST. In the clinical studies, such abnormalities required termination of therapy in less than 1% of patients.

Overdosage

There are no reports of overdosage, but repeated large doses of interferon can be associated with profound lethargy, fatigue, prostration, and coma. Hospitalize such patients for observation and give appropriate supportive treatment.

Patient Information

Caution patients not to change brands of interferon without medical consultation, as a change in dosage may result. Inform patients regarding the potential benefits and risks attendant to the use of interferon alfa-2a, recombinant. If home use is determined to be desirable by the health care provider, give instructions on appropriate use, including review of the contents of the enclosed patient information sheet. Patients should be well hydrated, especially during the initial stages of treatment.

Thoroughly instruct patients in the importance of proper disposal procedures and caution them against reusing syringes and needles. If home use is prescribed, supply a puncture-resistant container for the disposal of used syringes and needles to the patient. Provide directions for disposal of the full container.

PEGINTERFERON ALFA-2a

Rx	**Pegasys** (Roche)	**Injection:** 180 mcg	In 1 mL single-use vials[a] and 0.5 mL prefilled syringes.[b] Available in vial[c] and prefilled syringe[d] monthly convenience packs.

[a] With sodium chloride 8 mg, polysorbate 80 0.05 mg, and benzyl alcohol 10 mg.
[b] With sodium chloride 4 mg, polysorbate 80 0.025 mg, and benzyl alcohol 5 mg.
[c] Contains 4 single-use vials, four 1 mL syringes with needles, and 8 alcohol swabs.
[d] Contains 4 single-use prefilled syringes, 4 needles, and 4 alcohol swabs.

PEGINTERFERON ALFA-2a – INJECTION

For complete and comparative prescribing information, refer to the ribavirin monograph.

WARNING

Alpha interferons, including peginterferon alfa-2a, may cause or aggravate fatal or life-threatening neuropsychiatric, autoimmune, ischemic, and infectious disorders. Monitor patients closely with periodic clinical and laboratory evaluations. Withdraw therapy in patients with persistently severe or worsening signs or symptoms of these conditions. In many, but not all, cases these disorders resolve after stopping peginterferon alfa-2a therapy.

Combination therapy with ribavirin – Ribavirin may cause birth defects and/or death of the fetus. Extreme care must be taken to avoid pregnancy in women taking peginterferon alfa-2a and in female partners of men taking peginterferon alfa-2a. Ribavirin causes hemolytic anemia. The anemia associated with ribavirin therapy may result in a worsening of cardiac disease. Because ribavirin is genotoxic and mutagenic, consider it a potential carcinogen.

Indications

➤*Chronic hepatitis B:* For the treatment of adult patients with HBeAg-positive and HBeAG-negative chronic hepatitis B virus (HBV) infection who have compensated liver disease and evidence of viral replication and liver inflammation.

➤*Chronic hepatitis C:* For the treatment of adults with chronic hepatitis C virus (HCV) infection who have compensated liver disease and have not been previously treated with interferon alpha. Patients in whom efficacy was demonstrated included patients with compensated liver disease and histological evidence of cirrhosis (Child-Pugh class A), and patients with HIV disease that is clinically stable (ie, antiretroviral therapy not required, receiving stable antiretroviral therapy).

➤*Unlabeled uses:* Renal cell carcinoma, chronic myelogenous leukemia.

Administration and Dosage

➤*Approved by the FDA:* October 16, 2002.

➤*Treatment duration:* There are no safety and efficacy data on treatment of chronic HCV or HBV for longer than 48 weeks. For patients with HCV, consider discontinuing therapy after 12 to 24 weeks of therapy if the patient has failed to demonstrate an early virologic response, defined as undetectable HCV ribonucleic acid (RNA) or at least a 2 $\log_{10}$ reduction from baseline in HCV RNA titer by 12 weeks of therapy.

➤*Self-injection:* A patient should only self-inject peginterferon alfa-2a if the health care provider determines that it is appropriate, the patient agrees to medical follow-up as necessary, and training in proper injection technique has been provided to the patient.

➤*Chronic HBV:*

Monotherapy – 180 mcg (1 mL vial or 0.5 mL prefilled syringe) once weekly for 48 weeks by subcutaneous administration in the abdomen or thigh.

➤*Chronic HCV:*

Monotherapy – 180 mcg (1 mL vial or 0.5 mL prefilled syringe) once weekly for 48 weeks by subcutaneous administration in the abdomen or thigh.

Combination therapy with ribavirin – 180 mcg (1 mL vial or 0.5 mL prefilled syringe) subcutaneously once weekly. The recommended dose of ribavirin and duration for peginterferon alfa-2a/ribavirin therapy is based on viral genotype (see the following table).

The daily dose of ribavirin is 800 to 1,200 mg administered orally in 2 divided doses. Individualize the dose to the patient depending on baseline disease characteristics (eg, genotype), response to therapy, and tolerability of the regimen.

Peginterferon Alfa-2a and Ribavirin Dosing Recommendations

Genotype	Peginterferon alfa-2a dose	Ribavirin dose	Duration
Genotypes 1, 4	180 mcg	< 75 kg = 1,000 mg	48 weeks
		≥ 75 kg = 1,200 mg	48 weeks
Genotypes 2, 3	180 mcg	800 mg	24 weeks

Genotypes 2 and 3 showed no increased response to treatment beyond 24 weeks. Data on genotypes 5 and 6 are insufficient for dosing recommendations.

➤*Chronic HCV with HIV coinfection:*

Monotherapy – 180 mcg (1 mL vial or 0.5 mL prefilled syringe) once weekly for 48 weeks by subcutaneous administration in the abdomen or thigh.

Combination therapy with ribavirin – 180 mcg subcutaneously once weekly and ribavirin 800 mg daily given orally in 2 divided doses for a total of 48 weeks, regardless of genotype. Because ribavirin absorption increases when administered with a meal, patients are advised to take ribavirin with food.

➤*Dose modifications:* If severe adverse reactions or laboratory abnormalities develop during combination ribavirin/peginterferon alfa-2a therapy, modify, or discontinue if appropriate, the dose until the adverse reactions abate. If intolerance persists after dose adjustment, discontinue ribavirin/peginterferon alfa-2a therapy.

When dose modification is required for moderate to severe adverse reactions (clinical and/or laboratory), initial dose reduction to 135 mcg (0.75 mL for the vials or adjustment to the corresponding graduation mark for the syringes) is generally adequate. However, in some cases, dose reduction to 90 mcg (0.5 mL for the vials or adjustment to the corresponding graduation mark for the syringes) may be needed. Following improvement of the adverse reaction, re-escalation of the dose may be considered.

Peginterferon Alfa-2a Hematological Dose Modification Guidelines

Laboratory values	Peginterferon alfa-2a dose	Discontinue peginterferon alfa-2a
ANC[a] ≥ 750/mm^3	Maintain 180 mcg	ANC < 500/mm^3, suspend treatment until ANC values return to more than 1,000/mm^3; reinstitute at 90 mcg and monitor ANC.
ANC < 750/mm^3	Reduce to 135 mcg	
Platelet ≥ 50,000/mm^3	Maintain 180 mcg	Platelet count < 25,000/mm^3
Platelet < 50,000/mm^3	Reduce to 90 mcg	

[a] ANC = absolute neutrophil count.

PEGINTERFERON ALFA-2a – INJECTION

Ribavirin Dosage Modification Guidelines		
Laboratory values	Reduce only ribavirin dosage to 600 mg/day[a]	Discontinue ribavirin
Hgb[b] in patients with no cardiac disease	< 10 g/dL	< 8.5 g/dL
Hgb in patients with history of stable cardiac disease	≥ 2 g/dL decrease in Hgb during any 4-week period treatment	< 12 g/dL despite 4 weeks at reduced dose

[a] One 200 mg tablet in the morning and two 200 mg tablets in the evening.
[b] Hgb = hemoglobin.

Once ribavirin has been withheld because of a laboratory abnormality or clinical manifestation, an attempt may be made to restart ribavirin at 600 mg daily and further increase the dosage to 800 mg daily depending upon the health care provider's judgment. However, it is not recommended that ribavirin be increased to the original dose (1,000 or 1,200 mg).

Guidelines for Modification or Discontinuation of Peginterferon Alfa-2a and for Scheduling Visits for Patients With Depression

	Initial management (4 to 8 weeks)		Depression		
Depression severity	Dose modification	Visit schedule	Remains stable	Improves	Worsens
Mild	No change.	Evaluate once weekly by visit and/or phone.	Continue weekly visit schedule.	Resume normal visit schedule.	(See moderate or severe depression)
Moderate	Decrease peginterferon alfa-2a dose to 135 mcg (in some cases, dose reduction to 90 mcg may be needed).	Evaluate once weekly (office visit at least every other week).	Consider psychiatric consultation. Continue reduced dosing.	If symptoms improve and are stable for 4 weeks, may resume normal visit schedule. Continue reduced dosing or return to normal dose.	(See severe depression)
Severe	Discontinue peginterferon alfa-2a permanently.	Obtain immediate psychiatric consultation.	Psychiatric therapy necessary.		

➤*Renal function impairment:* In patients with end-stage renal disease requiring hemodialysis, dose reduction to peginterferon alfa-2a 135 mcg is recommended. Monitor signs and symptoms of interferon toxicity closely. Do not use ribavirin in patients with creatinine clearance (Ccr) less than 50 mL/min.

➤*Hepatic function impairment:* If ALT increases are progressive despite dose reduction or accompanied by increased bilirubin or evidence of hepatic decompensation, discontinue therapy immediately.

Chronic HBV – In chronic HBV patients with elevations in ALT (greater than 5 times the upper limit of normal [ULN]), perform more frequent monitoring of liver function and consider either reducing the dose of peginterferon alfa-2a to 135 mcg or temporarily discontinuing treatment. After peginterferon alfa-2a dose reduction or withholding, therapy can be resumed after ALT flares subside.

Chronic HCV – In chronic HCV patients with progressive ALT increases above baseline values, reduce the dose of peginterferon alfa-2a to 135 mcg and perform more frequent monitoring of liver function. After peginterferon alfa-2a dose reduction or withholding, therapy can be resumed after ALT flares subside.

In patients with persistent, severe (ALT greater than 10 times above the ULN) hepatitis B flares, give consideration to discontinuation of treatment.

➤*Storage/Stability:* Refrigerate at 2° to 8°C (36° to 46°F). Do not freeze or shake. Protect from light. Vials and prefilled syringes are for single use only. Discard any unused portion.

Actions

➤*Pharmacology:* Interferons bind to specific receptors on the cell surface initiating intracellular signaling via a complex cascade of protein-protein interactions leading to rapid activation of gene transcription. Interferon-stimulated genes modulate many biological effects, including the inhibition of viral replication in infected cells, inhibition of cell proliferation, and immunomodulation. The clinical relevance of these in vitro activities is not known.

Peginterferon alfa-2a stimulates the production of effector proteins, such as serum neopterin and 2′,5′-oligoadenylate synthetase.

➤*Pharmacokinetics:*

Absorption/Distribution – Maximum serum concentrations (C_{max}) and area under the plasma concentration-time curve (AUC) increased in a non-linear dose-related manner following administration of 90 to 270 mcg of peginterferon alfa-2a. C_{max} occurs between 72 and 96 hours postdose. Week 48 mean trough concentrations (16 ng/mL; range, 4 to 28) at 168 hours post-dose are approximately 2-fold higher than week 1 mean trough concentrations (9 ng/mL; range, 0 to 15). Steady-state serum levels are reached within 5 to 8 weeks of once-weekly dosing. The peak-to-trough ratio at week 48 is approximately 2.

Effect of food on absorption of ribavirin: Bioavailability of a single oral dose of ribavirin was increased by coadministration with a high-fat meal. The absorption was slowed (time to maximum concentration was doubled), and the $AUC_{0-192\ h}$ and C_{max} increased by 42% and 66%, respectively, when ribavirin was taken with a high-fat meal compared with fasting conditions. Because ribavirin absorption increases when administered with a meal, advise patients to take ribavirin with food.

Metabolism/Excretion – The mean systemic clearance in healthy subjects given peginterferon alfa-2a was 94 mL/h, which is approximately 100-fold lower than that for interferon alfa-2a. The mean terminal half-life after subcutaneous dosing in patients with chronic HCV was 80 hours (range, 50 to 140 hours) compared with 5.1 hours (range, 3.7 to 8.5 hours) for interferon alfa-2a.

Special populations –

Renal function impairment: In patients with end-stage renal disease undergoing hemodialysis, there is a 25% to 45% reduction in peginterferon alfa-2a clearance.

The pharmacokinetics of ribavirin following administration of ribavirin have not been studied in patients with renal impairment and there are limited data from clinical trials on administration of ribavirin in patients with Ccr less than 50 mL/min. Therefore, do not treat patients with Ccr less than 50 mL/min with ribavirin.

Elderly: The AUC was increased from 1,295 to 1,663 ng•h/mL in subjects older than 62 years of age taking peginterferon alfa-2a 180 mcg, but peak concentrations were similar (9 vs 10 ng/mL) in those older and younger than 62 years of age.

Children: In a population pharmacokinetics study, 14 children 2 to 8 years of age with chronic HCV received peginterferon alfa-2a based on their body surface area (BSA) of the child × 180 mcg/1.73 m^2. The clearance of peginterferon alfa-2a in children was nearly 4-fold lower compared with the clearance reported in adults.

Steady-state trough levels in children with the BSA-adjusted dosing were similar to trough levels observed in adults with 180 mcg fixed dosing. Time to reach the steady state in children is approximately 12 weeks, whereas in adults, steady state is reached within 5 to 8 weeks. In these children receiving the BSA-adjusted dose, the mean exposure AUC during the dosing interval is predicted to be 25% to 70% higher than that observed in adults receiving 180 mcg fixed dosing. The safety and efficacy of peginterferon alfa-2a in patients younger than 18 years of age have not been established.

Contraindications

Hypersensitivity to peginterferon alfa-2a or any of its components; autoimmune hepatitis; hepatic decompensation (Child-Pugh score greater than 6 [class B and C]) in cirrhotic patients before or during treatment; hepatic decompensation with Child-Pugh score greater than or equal to 6 in cirrhotic chronic HCV patients coinfected with HIV before or during treatment; in neonates and infants because it contains benzyl alcohol. Benzyl alcohol is associated with an increased incidence of neurologic and other complications that are sometimes fatal in neonates and infants.

➤*Combination therapy with ribavirin:* Hypersensitivity to ribavirin or any component of the tablet; women who are pregnant; men whose female partners are pregnant; patients with hemoglobinopathies (eg, thalassemia major, sickle cell anemia).

Warnings

➤*Neuropsychiatric reactions:* Life-threatening or fatal neuropsychiatric reactions may manifest in patients receiving peginterferon alfa-2a therapy and include suicide, suicidal ideation, homicidal ideation, depression, relapse of drug addiction, and drug overdose. These reactions may occur in patients with and without previous psychiatric illness.

Use peginterferon alfa-2a with extreme caution in patients who report history of depression. Neuropsychiatric adverse reactions observed with alpha interferon treatment include aggressive behavior, psychoses, hallucinations, bipolar disorders, and mania. Monitor all patients for evidence of depression and other psychiatric symptoms. Advise patients to report any sign or symptom of depression or suicidal ideation to their health care provider. In severe cases, stop therapy immediately and institute psychiatric intervention.

➤*Infections:* Serious and severe bacterial infections, some fatal, have been observed in patients treated with alpha interferons, including peginterferon alfa-2a. Some of the infections have been associated with neutropenia. Discontinue peginterferon alfa-2a in patients who develop severe infections and institute appropriate antibiotic therapy.

➤*Bone marrow toxicity:* Peginterferon alfa-2a suppresses bone marrow function and may result in severe cytopenias. Ribavirin may potentiate the neutropenia and lymphopenia induced by alpha interferons including peginterferon alfa-2a. Very rarely, alpha interferons may be associated with aplastic anemia. Obtain complete blood cell counts (CBCs) pretreatment and monitor routinely during therapy.

Use peginterferon alfa-2a and ribavirin with caution in patients with baseline neutrophil counts less than 1,500 cells/mm^3, baseline platelet counts less than 90,000 cells/mm^3, or baseline hemoglobin (Hgb) less than 10 g/dL. Discontinue peginterferon alfa-2a therapy, at least temporarily, in patients who develop severe decreases in neutrophil and/or platelet counts.

Severe neutropenia and thrombocytopenia occur with a greater incidence in HIV-coinfected patients than monoinfected patients and may result in serious infections or bleeding.

PEGINTERFERON ALFA-2a – INJECTION

➤*Cardiovascular effects:* Hypertension, supraventricular arrhythmias, chest pain, and myocardial infarction have been observed in patients treated with peginterferon alfa-2a.

Administer peginterferon alfa-2a with caution to patients with preexisting cardiac disease. Because cardiac disease may be worsened by ribavirin-induced anemia, do not use ribavirin in patients with a history of significant or unstable cardiac disease.

Fatal and nonfatal myocardial infarctions have been reported in patients with anemia caused by ribavirin. Assess patients for underlying cardiac disease before initiation of ribavirin therapy. Before treatment, administer electrocardiograms to patients with preexisting cardiac disease and monitor these patients during therapy. If there is any deterioration of cardiovascular status, suspend or discontinue therapy. Because cardiac disease may be worsened by drug-induced anemia, do not use ribavirin in patients with a history of significant or unstable cardiac disease.

➤*Hepatitis exacerbations:* Exacerbations of hepatitis during hepatitis B therapy are not uncommon and are characterized by transient and potentially severe increases in serum ALT. Chronic HBV patients experienced transient acute exacerbations (flares) of hepatitis B (ALT elevation greater than 10-fold higher than the ULN) during peginterferon alfa-2a treatment (12% and 18%) and posttreatment (7% and 12%) in HBeAg-negative and HBeAg-positive patients, respectively. Marked transaminase flares while on peginterferon alfa-2a therapy have been accompanied by other liver test abnormalities. Monitor liver function more frequently in patients experiencing ALT flares. Consider peginterferon alfa-2a dose reduction in patients experiencing transaminase flares. If ALT increases are progressive despite reduction of peginterferon alfa-2a dose or are accompanied by increased bilirubin or evidence of hepatic decompensation, discontinue peginterferon alfa-2a immediately.

➤*Endocrine disorders:* Peginterferon alfa-2a causes or aggravates hypothyroidism and hyperthyroidism. Hyperglycemia, hypoglycemia, and diabetes mellitus have been observed to develop in patients treated with peginterferon alfa-2a. Do not begin peginterferon alfa-2a therapy in patients with these conditions at baseline who cannot be effectively treated by medication. Patients who develop these conditions during treatment and cannot be controlled with medication may require discontinuation of peginterferon alfa-2a therapy.

➤*Autoimmune disorders:* Development or exacerbation of autoimmune disorders, including hepatitis, idiopathic thrombocytopenia purpura, interstitial nephritis, myositis, psoriasis, rheumatoid arthritis, systemic lupus erythematosus, thrombotic thrombocytopenic purpura, and thyroiditis, have been reported in patients receiving alpha interferons. Use peginterferon alfa-2a therapy with caution in patients with autoimmune disorders.

➤*Pulmonary disorders:* Bronchiolitis obliterans, dyspnea, interstitial pneumonitis, pneumonia, pulmonary infiltrates, and sarcoidosis, some resulting in respiratory failure and/or death, may be induced or aggravated by peginterferon alfa-2a or alpha interferon therapy. Discontinue peginterferon alfa-2a treatment in patients who develop persistent or unexplained pulmonary infiltrates or pulmonary function impairment.

➤*Colitis:* Ulcerative and hemorrhagic/ischemic colitis, sometimes fatal, has been observed within 12 weeks of starting alpha interferon treatment. Abdominal pain, bloody diarrhea, and fever are the typical manifestations of colitis. Immediately discontinue peginterferon alfa-2a if these symptoms develop. The colitis usually resolves within 1 to 3 weeks of discontinuation of alpha interferon.

➤*Pancreatitis:* Pancreatitis, sometimes fatal, has occurred during alpha interferon and ribavirin treatment. Suspend peginterferon alfa-2a and ribavirin if symptoms or signs suggestive of pancreatitis are observed. Discontinue peginterferon alfa-2a and ribavirin in patients diagnosed with pancreatitis.

➤*Ophthalmologic disorders:* Decrease or loss of vision; retinopathy, including macular edema; retinal artery or vein thrombosis; retinal hemorrhages and cotton wool spots; optic neuritis; and papilledema are induced or aggravated by treatment with peginterferon alfa-2a or other alpha interferons. Give all patients an eye examination at baseline. Give patients with preexisting ophthalmologic disorders (eg, diabetic, hypertensive retinopathy) periodic ophthalmologic exams during interferon alfa treatment. Give any patient who develops ocular symptoms a prompt and complete eye examination. Discontinue peginterferon alfa-2a treatment in patients who develop new or worsening ophthalmologic disorders.

➤*Hemolytic anemia:* The primary toxicity of ribavirin is hemolytic anemia. Hgb less than 10 g/dL was observed in approximately 13% of ribavirin and peginterferon alfa-2a–treated patients in chronic HCV clinical trials. The anemia associated with ribavirin occurs within 1 to 2 weeks of initiation of therapy with maximum drop in Hgb observed during the first 8 weeks. Because the initial drop in Hgb may be significant, it is advised that Hgb or hematocrit be obtained pretreatment and at week 2 and week 4 of therapy or more frequently if clinically indicated. Follow patients as clinically appropriate.

➤*Hypersensitivity reactions:* Severe acute hypersensitivity reactions (eg, anaphylaxis, angioedema, bronchoconstriction, urticaria) have been rarely observed during alpha interferon and ribavirin therapy. If such reactions occur, discontinue therapy with peginterferon alfa-2a and ribavirin and immediately institute appropriate medical therapy.

➤*Renal function impairment:* A 25% to 45% higher exposure to peginterferon alfa-2a is seen in subjects undergoing hemodialysis. In patients with impaired renal function, closely monitor for signs and symptoms of interferon toxicity. Adjust doses of peginterferon alfa-2a accordingly. Use peginterferon alfa-2a with caution in patients with Ccr less than 50 mL/min.

It is recommended that renal function be evaluated in all patients started on ribavirin. Do not administer ribavirin to patients with Ccr less than 50 mL/min.

➤*Hepatic function impairment:* Chronic HCV patients with cirrhosis may be at risk of hepatic decompensation and death when treated with alpha interferons, including peginterferon alfa-2a. Cirrhotic chronic HCV patients coinfected with HIV receiving highly active antiretroviral therapy (HAART) and interferon alfa-2a with or without ribavirin appear to be at increased risk for the development of hepatic decompensation, compared with patients not receiving HAART. In study 6, among 129 chronic HCV/HIV cirrhotic patients receiving HAART, 14 (11%) of these patients across all treatment arms developed hepatic decompensation, resulting in 6 deaths. All 14 patients were on nucleoside reverse transcriptase inhibitors (NRTIs), including abacavir, didanosine, lamivudine, stavudine, and zidovudine. These small numbers of patients do not permit discrimination between specific NRTIs for the associated risk. During treatment, closely monitor patients' clinical status and hepatic function, and discontinue peginterferon alfa-2a treatment if decompensation (Child-Pugh score at least 6) is observed.

➤*Mutagenesis:*

Combination therapy with ribavirin: Ribavirin is genotoxic and mutagenic.

➤*Fertility impairment:* Peginterferon alfa-2a may impair fertility in women. Prolonged menstrual cycles and/or amenorrhea were observed in female cynomolgus monkeys given subcutaneous injections of 600 mcg/kg/dose (7,200 mcg/m^2/dose) of peginterferon alfa-2a every other day for 1 month, at approximately 180 times the recommended weekly human dose for a 60 kg person (based on BSA). Menstrual cycle irregularities were accompanied by a decrease and delay in the peak 17β-estradiol and progesterone levels following administration of peginterferon alfa-2a to female monkeys. A return to normal menstrual rhythm followed cessation of treatment. Every other day dosing with 100 mcg/kg (1,200 mcg/m^2) of peginterferon alfa-2a (equivalent to approximately 30 times the recommended human dose) had no effects on cycle duration or reproductive hormone status.

The effects of peginterferon alfa-2a on male fertility have not been studied. However, no adverse reactions on fertility were observed in male rhesus monkeys treated with nonpegylated interferon alfa-2a for 5 months at dosages up to 25 × 10^6 units/kg/day.

Combination therapy with ribavirin: Ribavirin has shown reversible toxicity in animal studies of male fertility.

➤*Elderly:* Younger patients have higher virologic response rates than older patients. Clinical studies of peginterferon alfa-2a alone or in combination with ribavirin did not include sufficient numbers of subjects 65 years of age and older to determine whether they respond differently from younger subjects. Adverse reactions related to alpha interferons, such as CNS, cardiac, and systemic (eg, flu-like) effects, may be more severe in the elderly; exercise caution when using peginterferon alfa-2a in this population. Peginterferon alfa-2a and ribavirin are known to be excreted by the kidney, and the risk of toxic reactions to this therapy may be greater in patients with impaired renal function. Because elderly patients are more likely to have decreased renal function, take care in dose selection; it may be useful to monitor renal function. Use peginterferon alfa-2a with caution in patients with Ccr less than 50 mL/min. Do not administer ribavirin to patients with Ccr less than 50 mL/min.

➤*Pregnancy: Category C.* Peginterferon alfa-2a has not been studied for its teratogenic effects. Nonpegylated interferon alfa-2a treatment of pregnant Rhesus monkeys at approximately 20 to 500 times the human weekly dose resulted in a statistically significant increase in abortions. No teratogenic effects were seen in the offspring delivered at term. Assume peginterferon alfa-2a to have abortifacient potential. There are no adequate and well-controlled studies of peginterferon alfa-2a in pregnant women. Use peginterferon alfa-2a during pregnancy only if the potential benefit justifies the potential risk to the fetus. Peginterferon alfa-2a is recommended for use in women of childbearing potential only when they are using effective contraception during therapy.

Combination therapy with ribavirin – Category X. Significant teratogenic and/or embryocidal effects have been demonstrated in all animal species exposed to ribavirin. Ribavirin therapy is contraindicated in women who are pregnant and in the male partners of women who are pregnant.

Ribavirin may cause birth defects and/or death in the exposed fetus. Take extreme care to avoid pregnancy in women and in female partners of men taking peginterferon alfa-2a and ribavirin combination therapy. Do not start ribavirin therapy unless a report of a negative pregnancy test has been obtained immediately prior to initiation of therapy. Women of childbearing potential and men must use 2 forms of effective contraception during treatment and for at least 6 months after conclusion of treatment. Routine monthly pregnancy tests must be performed during this time.

Ribavirin pregnancy registry – A ribavirin pregnancy registry has been established to monitor maternal and fetal outcomes of pregnancies of women and female partners of men exposed to ribavirin during treatment and for 6 months following cessation of treatment. Health care providers and patients are strongly encouraged to report such cases by calling 1-800-593-2214.

➤*Lactation:* It is not known whether peginterferon alfa-2a or ribavirin or its components are excreted in human milk. The effect of orally ingested peginterferon alfa-2a or ribavirin from breast milk on the breast-feeding infant has not been evaluated. Because of the potential for adverse reactions

PEGINTERFERON ALFA-2a – INJECTION

from the drug in breast-feeding infants, decide whether to discontinue breast-feeding or peginterferon alfa-2a and ribavirin treatment.

➤*Children:* The safety and efficacy of peginterferon alfa-2a alone or in combination with ribavirin in patients younger than 18 years of age have not been established.

Benzyl alcohol – Peginterferon alfa-2a contains benzyl alcohol. Benzyl alcohol has been reported to be associated with an increased incidence of neurological and other complications that can be fatal in neonates and infants.

Precautions

➤*Monitoring:* Before beginning peginterferon alfa-2a or peginterferon alfa-2a and ribavirin combination therapy, standard hematological and biochemical laboratory tests are recommended for all patients. Pregnancy screening for women of childbearing potential must be performed. Monitor all patients for evidence of depression and other psychiatric symptoms. In patients with impaired renal function, closely monitor for signs and symptoms of interferon toxicity. Patients with preexisting ophthalmologic disorders (eg, diabetic or hypertensive retinopathy) should receive periodic ophthalmologic exams during interferon-alfa treatment. Before treatment, administer electrocardiograms to patients with preexisting cardiac disease, and monitor during therapy.

After initiation of therapy, perform hematological tests at 2 and 4 weeks, and perform biochemical tests at 4 weeks. Perform additional testing periodically during therapy. In the clinical studies, the CBC (including Hgb level, white blood cell count [WBC], and platelet count) and chemistries (including liver function tests and uric acid) were measured at 1, 2, 4, 6, and 8, and then every 4 to 6 weeks, or more frequently if abnormalities were found. Thyrotropin (TSH) was measured every 12 weeks. Perform monthly pregnancy testing during combination therapy and for 6 months after discontinuing therapy.

➤*Fever:* While fever is commonly caused by peginterferon alfa-2a therapy, other causes of persistent fever must be ruled out, particularly in patients with neutropenia.

➤*Clinical study criteria:* The following entrance criteria used for the clinical studies of peginterferon alfa-2a may be considered as a guideline to acceptable baseline values for initiation of treatment:

- platelet count greater than or equal to 90,000 cells/mm^3 (as low as 75,000 cells/mm^3 in HCV patients with cirrhosis or 70,000 cells/mm^3 in patients with chronic HCV and HIV)
- ANC greater than or equal to 1,500 cells/mm^3
- serum creatinine concentration less than 1.5 times the ULN
- TSH and thyroxine (T_4) within normal limits or adequately controlled thyroid function
- CD4+ cell count at least 200 cells/mcL or CD4+ cell count at least 100 cells/mcL but less than 200 cells/mcL and HIV-1 RNA less than 5,000 copies/mL in patients coinfected with HIV
- Hgb at least 12 g/dL for women and at least 13 g/dL for men in chronic HCV monoinfected patients
- Hgb at least 11 g/dL for women and at least 12 g/dL for men in patients with chronic HCV and HIV

➤*Special risk:* The safety and efficacy of peginterferon alfa-2a alone or in combination with ribavirin have not been established for the treatment of chronic HCV in the following instances:

- those who have failed alpha interferon- or alpha interferon and ribavirin treatment
- liver or other organ transplant recipients
- hepatitis B patients coinfected with HCV or HIV
- hepatitis C patients coinfected with HBV or HIV with a CD4+ cell count less than 100 cells/mcL

Exercise caution when initiating treatment in any patient with baseline risk of severe anemia (eg, spherocytosis, history of GI bleeding).

➤*Lab test abnormalities:*

Hematologic abnormalities – Peginterferon alfa-2a treatment was associated with decreases in WBC, ANC, lymphocytes, and platelet counts often starting within the first 2 weeks of treatment. Dose reduction is recommended in patients with hematologic abnormalities.

Hepatic effects – In chronic HCV, transient elevations in ALT (2- to 5-fold above baseline) were observed in some patients receiving peginterferon alfa-2a, and were not associated with deterioration of other liver function tests. When the increase in ALT levels is progressive despite dose reduction or is accompanied by increased bilirubin, discontinue peginterferon alfa-2a therapy.

Unlike hepatitis C, during hepatitis B therapy follow-up, transient elevations in ALT of 5 to 10 times the ULN were observed in 25% and 27% and of greater than 10 times the ULN were observed in 12% and 18%, of HBeAg-negative and HBeAg-positive patients, respectively. These ALT elevations have been accompanied by other liver test abnormalities.

Immunogenicity –

Chronic HBV: Twenty-nine percent (42/143) of hepatitis B patients treated with peginterferon alfa-2a for 24 weeks developed binding antibodies to interferon alfa-, as assessed by an enzyme-linked immunosorbent assay (ELISA). Thirteen percent of patients (19/143) receiving peginterferon alfa-2a developed low-titer neutralizing antibodies (using an assay with a sensitivity of 100 interferon neutralizing units/mL).

Chronic HCV: Nine percent (71/834) of patients treated with peginterferon alfa-2a with or without ribavirin developed binding antibodies to interferon alfa-2a, as assessed by an ELISA. Three percent of patients (25/835) receiving peginterferon alfa-2a with or without ribavirin developed low-titer neutralizing antibodies (using an assay of a sensitivity of 100 interferon neutralizing units/mL).

➤*Hazardous tasks:* Caution patients who develop dizziness, confusion, somnolence, and fatigue to avoid driving or operating machinery.

Drug Interactions

Peginterferon Alfa-2a Drug Interactions			
Precipitant drug	Object drug		Description
Peginterferon alfa-2a	Methadone	↑	Concomitant treatment with peginterferon alfa-2a once weekly for 4 weeks was associated with methadone levels that were 10% to 15% higher than at baseline.
Peginterferon alfa-2a	NRTIs (eg, didanosine, zidovudine, stavudine)	↑	Coadministration may increase toxicities, such as hematologic toxicities. Cases of hepatic decomposition (some fatal) were observed.
Peginterferon alfa-2a	Theophylline	↑	Coadministration with peginterferon alfa-2a was associated with an inhibition of CYP1A2 and a 25% increase in theophylline AUC. Monitor theophylline levels and adjust dose as needed.

Adverse Reactions

Peginterferon alfa-2a alone or in combination with ribavirin causes a broad variety of serious adverse reactions. The most common life-threatening or fatal reactions induced or aggravated by peginterferon alfa-2a and ribavirin were depression, suicide, relapse of drug abuse/overdose, and bacterial infections, each occurring at a frequency of less than 1%. Hepatic decompensation occurred in 2% (10/574) of chronic HCV/HIV patients.

➤*Hepatitis C studies:* In all hepatitis C studies, 1 or more serious adverse reaction occurred in 10% of chronic HCV monoinfected patients and in 19% of chronic HCV/HIV patients receiving peginterferon alfa-2a alone or in combination with ribavirin. The most common serious adverse reaction (3% in chronic HCV and 5% in chronic HCV/HIV) was bacterial infection (eg, endocarditis, osteomyelitis, pneumonia, pyelonephritis, sepsis). Other serious adverse reactions occurred at a frequency of less than 1% and included aggression, angina, anxiety, aplastic anemia, arrhythmia, autoimmune phenomena (eg, hyperthyroidism, hypothyroidism, sarcoidosis, systemic lupus erythematosus, rheumatoid arthritis), cerebral hemorrhage, cholangitis, colitis, coma, corneal ulcer, diabetes mellitus, drug abuse and drug overdose, fatty liver, GI bleeding, hepatic dysfunction, myositis, pancreatitis, peptic ulcer, peripheral neuropathy, psychosis, pulmonary embolism, suicidal ideation, suicide, and thrombotic thrombocytopenic purpura.

Nearly all hepatitis C patients in clinical trials experienced 1 or more adverse reaction. The most commonly reported adverse reactions were psychiatric reactions, including anxiety, depression, insomnia, and irritability, and flu-like symptoms (eg, fatigue, headache, myalgia, pyrexia, rigors). Other common reactions were alopecia, anorexia, arthralgia, diarrhea, injection site reactions, nausea and vomiting, and pruritus.

Overall, 11% of chronic HCV monoinfected patients receiving 48 weeks of therapy with peginterferon alfa-2a either alone or in combination with ribavirin discontinued therapy; 16% of chronic HCV/HIV coinfected patients discontinued therapy. The most common reasons for discontinuation of therapy were psychiatric, flu-like syndrome (eg, lethargy, fatigue, headache), dermatologic, and GI disorders and laboratory abnormalities (thrombocytopenia, neutropenia, and anemia).

Overall, 39% of patients with chronic HCV or chronic HCV/HIV required modification of peginterferon alfa-2a and/or ribavirin therapy. The most common reason for dose modification of peginterferon alfa-2a in chronic HCV and chronic HCV/HIV patients was for laboratory abnormalities: neutropenia (20% and 27%, respectively) and thrombocytopenia (4% and 6%, respectively). The most common reason for dose modification of ribavirin in chronic HCV and chronic HCV/HIV patients was anemia (22% and 16%, respectively).

Peginterferon alfa-2a dose was reduced in 12% of patients receiving ribavirin 1,000 to 1,200 mg for 48 weeks and in 7% of patients receiving ribavirin 800 mg for 24 weeks. Ribavirin dose was reduced in 21% of patients receiving ribavirin 1,000 to 1,200 mg for 48 weeks and 12% in patients receiving ribavirin 800 mg for 24 weeks.

Chronic HCV monoinfected patients treated for 24 weeks with peginterferon alfa-2a and ribavirin 800 mg were observed to have lower incidence of serious adverse reactions (3% vs 10%), Hgb less than 10 g/dL (3% vs 15%), dose modification of peginterferon alfa-2a (30% vs 36%) and ribavirin (19% vs 38%), and of withdrawal from treatment (5% vs 15%), compared with patients treated for 48 weeks with peginterferon alfa-2a and ribavirin 1,000 or 1,200 mg. On the other hand, the overall incidence of adverse reactions appeared to be similar in the 2 treatment groups.

Because clinical trials are conducted under widely varying and controlled conditions, adverse reaction rates observed in clinical trials of a drug cannot be directly compared with rates in the clinical trials of another drug. Also, the adverse reaction rates listed here may not predict the rates observed in a broader patient population in clinical practice.

PEGINTERFERON ALFA-2a – INJECTION

Peginterferon Alfa-2a Adverse Reactions in Chronic HCV Patients (≥ 5%)

	Chronic hepatitis C monotherapy (pooled studies 1 to 3)		Chronic hepatitis C combination therapy (study 4)	
Adverse reaction	Peginterferon alfa-2a 180 mcg (48 weeks)[a] (n = 559)	Interferon alfa 2a recombinant[a,b] (n = 554)	Peginterferon alfa-2a 180 mcg + ribavirin 1,000 or 1,200 mg (48 weeks) (n = 451)	Interferon alfa-2b, recombinant + ribavirin 1,000 or 1,200 mg (48 weeks) (n = 443)
CNS				
Concentration impairment	8%	10%	10%	13%
Depression	18%	19%	20%	28%
Dizziness (excluding vertigo)	16%	12%	14%	14%
Fatigue/ Asthenia	56%	57%	65%	68%
Headache	54%	58%	43%	49%
Insomnia	19%	23%	30%	37%
Irritability/ Anxiety/ Nervousness	19%	22%	33%	38%
Memory impairment	5%	4%	6%	5%
Mood alteration	3%	2%	5%	6%
Dermatologic				
Alopecia	23%	30%	28%	33%
Dermatitis	8%	3%	16%	13%
Dry skin	4%	3%	10%	13%
Eczema	1%	1%	5%	4%
Increased sweating	6%	7%	6%	5%
Pruritus	12%	8%	19%	18%
Rash	5%	4%	8%	5%
Endocrine				
Hypothyroidism	3%	2%	4%	5%
GI				
Abdominal pain	15%	15%	8%	9%
Diarrhea	16%	16%	11%	10%
Dry mouth	6%	3%	4%	7%
Dyspepsia	< 1%	1%	6%	5%
Nausea/ Vomiting	24%	33%	25%	29%
Hematologic[c]				
Anemia	2%	1%	11%	11%
Lymphopenia	3%	5%	14%	12%
Neutropenia	21%	8%	27%	8%
Thrombocytopenia	5%	2%	5%	< 1%
Metabolic/Nutritional				
Anorexia	17%	17%	24%	26%
Weight decrease	4%	3%	10%	10%
Musculoskeletal				
Arthralgia	28%	29%	22%	23%
Back pain	9%	10%	5%	5%
Myalgia	37%	38%	40%	49%
Resistance mechanism disorders				
Overall	10%	6%	12%	10%
Respiratory				
Cough	4%	3%	10%	7%
Dyspnea	4%	2%	13%	14%
Dyspnea, exertional	< 1%	< 1%	4%	7%
Miscellaneous				
Blurred vision	4%	2%	5%	2%
Injection site reaction	22%	18%	23%	16%
Pain	11%	12%	10%	9%
Pyrexia	37%	41%	41%	55%
Rigors	35%	44%	25%	37%

[a] Pooled studies 1, 2, and 3.
[b] Either 3 million units or 6 million units 3 times a week for 12 weeks, followed by 3 million units 3 times a week for 36 weeks of interferon alfa-2a, recombinant.
[c] Severe hematologic abnormalities (lymphocytes $< 0.5 \times 10^9$/L; Hgb < 10 g/dL; neutrophils $< 0.75 \times 10^9$/L; platelets $< 50 \times 10^9$/L).

Chronic HCV with HIV coinfection – The adverse reaction profile of coinfected patients treated with peginterferon alfa-2a and ribavirin in study 6 was generally similar to that shown for monoinfected patients in study 4. Events occurring more frequently in coinfected patients were neutropenia (40%), anemia (14%), thrombocytopenia (8%), weight decrease (16%), and mood alteration (9%).

Chronic HBV – In clinical trials of 48-week treatment duration, the adverse reaction profile of peginterferon alfa-2a in chronic HBV was similar to that seen in chronic HCV peginterferon alfa-2a monotherapy use, except for exacerbations of hepatitis. Six percent of peginterferon alfa-2a-treated patients in the hepatitis B studies experienced 1 or more serious adverse reactions.

The most common or important serious adverse reactions in the hepatitis B studies were infections (appendicitis, influenza, sepsis, tuberculosis), hepatitis B flares, anaphylactic shock, thrombotic thrombocytopenic purpura.

The most commonly observed adverse reactions were pyrexia (54% vs 4%), headache (27% vs 9%), fatigue (24% vs 10%), myalgia (26% vs 4%), alopecia (18% vs 2%), and anorexia (16% vs 3%) in the peginterferon alfa-2a and lamivudine groups respectively.

Overall 5% of hepatitis B patients discontinued peginterferon alfa-2a therapy and 40% of patients required modification of peginterferon alfa-2a dose. The most common reason for dose modification in patients receiving peginterferon alfa-2a therapy was for laboratory abnormalities including neutropenia (20%), thrombocytopenia (13%), and ALT disorders (11%).

➤*Lab test abnormalities:* The laboratory test values observed in the hepatitis B trials (except where noted below) were similar to those seen in the peginterferon alfa-2a monotherapy hepatitis C trials.

ALT elevations –

Chronic HBV: Transient ALT elevations are common during hepatitis B therapy with peginterferon alfa-2a. Twenty-five percent and 27% of patients experienced elevations of 5 to 10 times the ULN and 12% and 18% had elevations of greater than 10 times the ULN during treatment of HBeAg-negative and HBeAg-positive disease, respectively. Flares have been accompanied by elevations of total bilirubin and alkaline phosphatase and less commonly with prolongation of prothrombin time and reduced albumin levels. Eleven percent of patients had dose modifications due to ALT flares and less than 1% of patients were withdrawn from treatment.

ALT flares of 5 to 10 times the ULN occurred in 13% and 16% of patients, while ALT flares of greater than 10 times the ULN occurred in 7% and 12% of patients in HBeAg-negative and HBeAg-positive disease, respectively, after discontinuation of peginterferon alfa-2a therapy.

Chronic HCV: One percent of patients in the hepatitis C trials experienced marked elevations (5- to 10-fold above the ULN) in ALT levels during treatment and follow-up. On occasion, these transaminase elevations were associated with hyperbilirubinemia and were managed by dose reduction or discontinuation of study treatment. Liver function test abnormalities were generally transient. One case was attributed to autoimmune hepatitis, which persisted beyond study medication discontinuation.

PEGINTERFERON ALFA-2a – INJECTION

Hemoglobin – In hepatitis C studies, the Hgb concentration decreased below 12 g/dL in 17% (median Hgb reduction of 2.2 g/dL) of monotherapy and 52% (median Hgb reduction of 3.7 g/dL) of combination therapy patients. Severe anemia (Hgb less than 10 g/dL) was encountered in 13% of all patients receiving combination therapy and in 2% of chronic HCV patients and 8% of chronic HCV/HIV patients receiving peginterferon alfa-2a monotherapy. Dose modification for anemia in ribavirin recipients treated for 48 weeks occurred in 22% of chronic HCV patients and 16% of chronic HCV/HIV patients.

Immunogenicity –
Chronic HBV: See Precautions for more information.
Chronic HCV: See Precautions for more information.

Lymphocytes – Decreases in lymphocyte count are induced by interferon alpha therapy. Peginterferon alfa-2a plus ribavirin combination therapy induced decreases in median total lymphocyte counts (56% in chronic HCV and 40% in chronic HCV/HIV, with median decrease of 1,170 cells/mm^3 in chronic HCV and 800 cells/mm^3 in chronic HCV/HIV). In hepatitis C studies, lymphopenia was observed during monotherapy (81%) and combination therapy with peginterferon alfa-2a and ribavirin (91%). Severe lymphopenia (less than 0.5×10^9/L) occurred in approximately 5% of all monotherapy patients and 14% of all combination peginterferon alfa-2a and ribavirin therapy recipients. Dose adjustments were not required by protocol. The clinical significance of the lymphopenia is not known.

In chronic HCV with HIV coinfection, CD4 counts decreased 29% from baseline (median decreases of 137 cells/mm^3), and CD8 counts decreased 44% from baseline (median decrease of 389 cells/mm^3) in the peginterferon alfa-2a plus ribavirin combination therapy arm. Median lymphocyte CD4 and CD8 counts returned to pretreatment levels after 4 to 12 weeks of the cessation of therapy. CD4 percent did not decrease during treatment.

Neutrophils – In the hepatitis C studies, decreases in neutrophil count below normal were observed in 95% of all patients treated with peginterferon alfa-2a either alone or in combination with ribavirin. Severe, potentially life-threatening neutropenia (ANC less than 0.5×10^9/L) occurred in 5% of chronic HCV patients and 12% of chronic HCV/HIV patients receiving peginterferon alfa-2a either alone or in combination with ribavirin. Modification of peginterferon alfa-2a dose for neutropenia occurred in 17% of patients receiving peginterferon alfa-2a monotherapy and 22% of patients receiving peginterferon alfa-2a/ribavirin combination therapy. In the chronic HCV/HIV patients, 27% required modification of interferon dosage for neutropenia. Two percent of patients with chronic HCV and 10% of patients with chronic HCV/HIV required permanent reductions of peginterferon alfa-2a dosage, and less than 1% required permanent discontinuation. Median neutrophil counts returned to pretreatment levels 4 weeks after cessation of therapy.

Platelets – In hepatitis C studies, platelet counts decreased in 52% of chronic HCV patients and 51% of chronic HCV/HIV patients treated with peginterferon alfa-2a alone (median decrease of 41% and 35% from baseline, respectively), and in 33% of chronic HCV patients and 47% of chronic HCV/HIV patients receiving combination therapy with ribavirin (median decrease of 30% from baseline). Moderate to severe thrombocytopenia (less than 50,000/mm^3) was observed in 4% of chronic HCV and 8% of chronic HCV/HIV patients. Median platelet counts returned to pretreatment levels 4 weeks after the cessation of therapy.

Postmarketing – The following adverse reactions have been identified and reported during postapproval use of peginterferon alfa-2a therapy: hearing impairment, hearing loss.

Triglycerides – Triglyceride levels are elevated in patients receiving alpha interferon therapy and were elevated in the majority of patients participating in clinical studies receiving either peginterferon alfa-2a alone or in combination with ribavirin. Random levels greater than or equal to 400 mg/dL were observed in about 20% of chronic HCV patients. Severe elevations of triglycerides (more than 1,000 mg/dL) occurred in 2% of monoinfected patients. In HCV/HIV coinfected patients, fasting levels at least 400 mg/dL were observed in up to 36% of patients receiving either peginterferon alfa-2a alone or in combination with ribavirin. Severe elevations of triglycerides (more than 1,000 mg/dL) occurred in 7% of coinfected patients.

Thyroid function – Peginterferon alfa-2a alone or in combination with ribavirin was associated with the development of abnormalities in thyroid laboratory values, some with associated clinical manifestations. In hepatitis C studies, hypothyroidism or hyperthyroidism requiring treatment, dose modification, or discontinuation occurred in 4% and 1% of peginterferon alfa-2a treated patients and 4% and 2% of peginterferon alfa-2a- and ribavirin-treated patients, respectively. Among the patients who developed thyroid abnormalities during peginterferon alfa-2a treatment, approximately half still had abnormalities during the follow-up period.

Overdosage

➤*Symptoms:* There is limited experience with overdosage. The maximum dosage received by any patient was 7 times the intended dosage of peginterferon alfa-2a (180 mcg/day for 7 days). There were no serious reactions attributed to overdosages. Weekly doses of up to 630 mcg have been administered to patients with cancer. Dose-limiting toxicities were fatigue, elevated liver enzymes, neutropenia, and thrombocytopenia.

➤*Treatment:* There is no specific antidote for peginterferon alfa-2a. Hemodialysis and peritoneal dialysis are not effective.

Patient Information

Direct patients receiving peginterferon alfa-2a alone or in combination with ribavirin in its appropriate use, inform them of the benefits and risks associated with treatment, and refer them to the peginterferon alfa-2a and, if applicable, ribavirin medication guides.

Peginterferon alfa-2a and ribavirin combination therapy must not be used by women who are pregnant or by men whose female partners are pregnant. Do not initiate ribavirin therapy until a report of a negative pregnancy test has been obtained immediately before starting therapy. Advise women of childbearing potential and men with female partners of childbearing potential of the teratogenic/embryocidal risks, and instruct them to practice effective contraception during ribavirin therapy and for 6 months posttherapy. Advise patients to notify their health care provider immediately in the event of a pregnancy.

Women of childbearing potential and men must use 2 forms of effective contraception during treatment and during the 6 months after treatment has been stopped; routine monthly pregnancy tests must be performed during this time.

To monitor maternal and fetal outcomes of pregnant women exposed to ribavirin, a ribavirin pregnancy registry has been established. Strongly encourage patients to register by calling 1-800-593-2214.

Advise patients that laboratory evaluations are required before starting therapy and periodically thereafter. Instruct patients to remain well hydrated, especially during the initial stages of treatment. Advise patients to take ribavirin with food.

Inform patients that it is not known if therapy with peginterferon alfa-2a alone or in combination with ribavirin will prevent transmission of HCV or HBV infection to others or prevent cirrhosis, liver failure, or liver cancer that might result from HCV or HBV infection.

Caution patients who develop dizziness, confusion, somnolence, and fatigue to avoid driving or operating machinery.

If home use is prescribed, supply a puncture-resistant container for the disposal of used needles and syringes to the patients. Thoroughly instruct patients in the importance of proper disposal; caution against any reuse of needles and syringes. Advise patients to dispose of the full container according to the directions provided by their health care provider.

Advise patients to report any signs or symptoms of depression or suicidal ideation to their health care provider.

INTERFERON ALFA-2b, RECOMBINANT (IFN-alpha 2; rIFN-α2; α-2-interferon)

Rx	**Intron A**[a] (Schering)	**Powder for injection:**[b] 5 million IU/vial	In vials with 1 mL diluent vial.[c]
		10 million IU/vial	In vials with 2 mL diluent vial.[c]
		18 million IU/vial	In vials with 1 mL diluent vial.[c]
		25 million IU/vial	In vials with 5 mL diluent vial.[c]
		50 million IU/vial	In vials with 1 mL diluent vial.[c]
		Injection:[d] 3 million IU/dose	In multidose pens (6 doses; 22.5 million IU/1.5 mL per pen) with needles.
		5 million IU/dose	In multidose pens (6 doses; 37.5 million IU/1.5 mL per pen) with needles.
		10 million IU/dose	In multidose pens (6 doses; 75 million IU/1.5 mL per pen) with needles.
		Solution for injection:[d] 3 million IU/vial	In vials, Pak-3 (6 vials, 6 syringes).
		5 million IU/vial	In vials, Pak-5 (6 vials, 6 syringes).
		10 million IU/vial	In vials, Pak-10 (6 vials, 6 syringes).
		18 million IU/vial	In multidose vials (22.8 million IU/3.8 mL per vial).
		25 million IU/vial	In multidose vials (32 million IU/3.2 mL per vial).

[a] Not all dosage forms and strengths are appropriate for some indications.
[b] Each milliliter includes 1 mg human albumin, 20 mg glycine, 2.3 mg sodium phosphate dibasic, 0.55 mg sodium phosphate monobasic.
[c] Diluent is bacteriostatic water for injection containing 0.9% benzyl alcohol as a preservative.
[d] Each milliliter contains 7.5 mg sodium chloride, 1.8 mg sodium phosphate dibasic, 1.3 mg sodium phosphate monobasic, 0.1 mg EDTA, 0.1 mg polysorbate 80, and 1.5 mg m-cresol as a preservative.

INTERFERON ALFA-2b RECOMBINANT — INJECTION

WARNING

Alpha interferons, including interferon alfa-2b, recombinant, cause or aggravate fatal or life-threatening neuropsychiatric, autoimmune, ischemic, and infectious disorders. Patients should be monitored closely with periodic clinical and laboratory evaluations. Patients with persistently severe or worsening signs or symptoms of these conditions should be withdrawn from therapy. In many but not all cases these disorders resolve after stopping interferon alfa-2b, recombinant therapy. See Warnings and Adverse Reactions.

Indications

➤*Hairy cell leukemia:* For injection is indicated for the treatment of patients 18 years of age or older with hairy cell leukemia.

➤*Malignant melanoma:* Adjuvant to surgical treatment in patients 18 years of age or older with malignant melanoma who are free of disease but at high risk for systemic recurrence, within 56 days of surgery.

➤*Follicular lymphoma:* For the initial treatment of clinically aggressive follicular non-Hodgkin's lymphoma in conjunction with anthracycline-containing combination chemotherapy in patients 18 years of age or older. Efficacy of interferon alfa-2b, recombinant in patients with low-grade, low-tumor burden follicular non-Hodgkin's lymphoma has not been demonstrated.

➤*Condylomata acuminata:* For intralesional treatment of selected patients 18 years of age or older with condylomata acuminata involving external surfaces of the genital and perianal areas (see Administration and Dosage).

➤*AIDS-related Kaposi's sarcoma:* For the treatment of selected patients 18 years of age or older with AIDS-related Kaposi's sarcoma. The likelihood of response to interferon alfa-2b, recombinant therapy is greater in patients who are without systemic symptoms, who have limited lymphadenopathy and who have a relatively intact immune system as indicated by total CD4 count.

➤*Chronic hepatitis C:* For the treatment of chronic hepatitis C in patients 18 years of age or older with compensated liver disease who have a history of blood or blood-product exposure and/or are hepatitis C virus (HCV) antibody-positive. Studies in these patients demonstrated that interferon alfa-2b, recombinant therapy can produce clinically meaningful effects on this disease, manifested by normalization of serum alanine aminotransferase (ALT) and reduction in liver necrosis and degeneration.

Serum creatinine should be normal or near normal.

Monitoring – Prior to initiation of interferon alfa-2b, recombinant therapy, CBC and platelet counts should be evaluated in order to establish baselines for monitoring potential toxicity. These tests should be repeated at weeks 1 and 2 following initiation of interferon alfa-2b, recombinant therapy, and monthly thereafter. Serum ALT should be evaluated at ≈ 3-month intervals to assess response to treatment (see Administration and Dosage).

Thyroid abnormalities – Patients with preexisting thyroid abnormalities may be treated if thyroid-stimulating hormone (TSH) levels can be maintained in the normal range by medication. TSH levels must be within normal limits upon initiation of interferon alfa-2b, recombinant treatment and TSH testing should be repeated at 3 and 6 months (see Precautions, Laboratory Tests).

➤*Chronic hepatitis B:* For the treatment of chronic hepatitis B in patients 1 year of age or older with compensated liver disease. Patients who have been serum HBsAg-positive for at least 6 months and have evidence of HBV replication (serum HBeAg-positive) with elevated serum ALT are candidates for treatment. Studies in these patients demonstrated that interferon alfa-2b, recombinant therapy can produce virologic remission of this disease (loss of serum HBeAg), and normalization of serum aminotransferases. interferon alfa-2b, recombinant therapy resulted in the loss of serum HBsAg in some responding patients.

Monitoring – Patients with causes of chronic hepatitis other than chronic hepatitis B or chronic hepatitis C should not be treated with interferon alfa-2b recombinant for injection. CBC and platelet counts should be evaluated prior to initiation of interferon alfa-2b, recombinant therapy in order to establish baselines for monitoring potential toxicity. These tests should be repeated at treatment weeks 1, 2, 4, 8, 12, and 16. Liver function tests, including serum ALT, albumin, and bilirubin, should be evaluated at treatment weeks 1, 2, 4, 8, 12, and 16. HBeAg, HBsAg, and ALT should be evaluated at the end of therapy, as well as 3- and 6-months posttherapy, since patients may become virologic responders during the 6-month period following the end of treatment. In clinical studies, 39% (15/38) of responding patients lost HBeAg 1 to 6 months following the end of interferon alfa-2b, recombinant therapy. Of responding patients who lost HBsAg, 58% (7/12) did so 1- to 6-months posttreatment.

A transient increase in ALT > 2 × baseline value (flare) can occur during interferon alfa-2b, recombinant therapy for chronic hepatitis B. In clinical trials in adults and pediatrics, this flare generally occurred 8 to 12 weeks after initiation of therapy and was more frequent in interferon alfa-2b, recombinant responders (adults 63%, 24/38; pediatrics 59%, 10/17) than in nonresponders (adults 27%, 13/48; pediatrics 35%, 19/55). However, in adults and pediatrics, elevations in bilirubin > 3 mg/dL (> 2 times ULN) occurred infrequently (adults 2%, 2/86; pediatrics 3%, 2/72) during therapy. When ALT flare occurs, in general, interferon alfa-2b, recombinant therapy should be continued unless signs and symptoms of liver failure are observed. During ALT flare, clinical symptomatology and liver function tests including ALT, prothrombin time, alkaline phosphatase, albumin, and bilirubin, should be monitored at ≈ 2-week intervals (see Warnings).

➤*Unlabeled uses:* Treatment of mycosis fungoides; essential thrombocythemia; ovarian and cervical carcinoma; renal cell carcinoma; basal and squamous cell skin cancer; bladder tumors (local use for superficial tumors); chronic myelogenous leukemia; cutaneous T-cell lymphoma; non-Hodgkin lymphoma; essential thrombocytosis; chronic granulocytic leukemia; melanoma; multiple myeloma; acute leukemias; carcinoid tumor; Hodgkin disease; cytomegalovirus; herpes simplex; papillomaviruses; rhinoviruses; varicella zoster; Behçet syndrome; hypereosinophilic syndrome; polycythemia vera.

Administration and Dosage

➤*Important:* Interferon alfa-2b, recombinant for injection dosing regimens are different for each of the following indications described in this section of the product information sheet. Interferon alfa-2b, recombinant solution for injection multidose pen contains a prefilled, multidose cartridge for subcutaneous administration.

It is designed to deliver doses as required using a simple dial mechanism. The needles provided in the packaging should be used for the interferon alfa-2b, recombinant solution for injection multidose pen only. A new needle is to be used each time a dose is delivered using the pen. Each interferon alfa-2b, recombinant solution for injection multidose pen is for individual patient use only.

➤*Hairy cell leukemia:* 2 million IU/m^2 administered intramuscularly or subcutaneously 3 times a week for up to 6 months. The 50 million IU strength of the interferon alfa-2b, recombinant powder for injection is not to be used for the treatment of hairy cell leukemia. Higher doses are not recommended. Responding patients may benefit from continued treatment.

If severe adverse reactions develop, the dosage should be modified (50% reduction) or therapy should be temporarily discontinued until the adverse reactions abate. If persistent or recurrent intolerance develops following adequate dosage adjustment, or disease progresses, interferon alfa-2b, recombinant treatment should be discontinued. The minimum effective interferon alfa-2b, recombinant dose has not been established.

➤*Malignant melanoma:* The recommended interferon alfa-2b, recombinant treatment regimen includes induction treatment 5 consecutive days per week for 4 weeks as an intravenous (IV) infusion at a dose of 20 million IU/m^2, followed by maintenance treatment 3 times per week for 48 weeks as a subcutaneous (SC) injection, at a dose of 10 million IU/m^2.

In the clinical trial, the median daily interferon alfa-2b, recombinant doses administered to patients were 19.1 million IU/m^2 during the induction phase and 9.1 million IU/m^2 during the maintenance phase.

Regular laboratory testing should be performed to monitor laboratory abnormalities for the purposes of dose modification (see Precautions, Laboratory Tests). If adverse reactions develop during interferon alfa-2b, recombinant treatment, particularly if granulocytes decrease to < 500/mm^3 or ALT/AST rises to > 5 × upper limit of normal, treatment should be temporarily discontinued until the adverse reactions abate. Interferon alfa-2b, recombinant treatment should be restarted at 50% of the previous dose. If intolerance persists after dose adjustments or if granulocytes decrease to < 250/mm^3 or ALT/AST rises to > 10 × upper limit of normal, interferon alfa-2b, recombinant therapy should be discontinued.

➤*Follicular lymphoma:* 5 million IU subcutaneously 3 times per week for up to 18 months in conjunction with an anthracycline-containing chemotherapy regimen.

In published reports, the doses of myelosuppressive drugs were reduced by 25% from those utilized in a full-dose CHOP regimen, and cycle length increased by 33% (eg, from 21 to 28 days) when an alfa interferon was added to the regimen. The dosing regimen should be modified for evidence of serious toxicity. The following dose modification guidelines for hematologic toxicity were used in the clinical trial: The chemotherapy regimen was delayed if either the neutrophil count was < 1500/mm^3 or the platelet count was < 75,000/mm^3. Administration of interferon alfa-2b, recombinant was temporarily interrupted for a neutrophil count < 1000/mm^3, or a platelet count < 50,000/mm^3, or reduced by 50% to 2.5 MIU 3 times a week for a neutrophil count > 1000/mm^3 but < 1500/mm^3.

Reinstitution of the initial interferon alfa-2b, recombinant dose (5 million IU 3 times a week) was tolerated after resolution of hematologic toxicity (≥ 1500/mm^3).

Interferon alfa-2b, recombinant therapy should be discontinued if AST exceeds > 5 × the upper limit of normal or serum creatinine > 2 mg/dL (see Warnings).

➤*Condylomata acuminata:* The 10 million IU vial of interferon alfa-2b, recombinant powder for injection must be reconstituted with 1 mL of diluent for interferon alfa-2b, recombinant for injection (bacteriostatic water for injection). Do not reconstitute the 10 million IU vial of interferon alfa-2b, recombinant powder for injection with more than 1 mL of diluent since the injection would be subpotent. Do not use the 3 million, 5 million, 18 million, 25 million, or 50 million IU vials of interferon alfa-2b, recombinant powder for injection for the treatment of condylomata acuminata since the resulting reconstituted solution would be either hypertonic or an inappropriate concentration. Do not use the 3 million IU vial or the 18 million IU multidose vial of interferon alfa-2b, recombinant solution for injection for the intralesional treatment of condylomata acuminata since the concentrations are inappropriate for such use.

Inject 1 million IU of interferon alfa-2b, recombinant for injection (either 0.1 mL of reconstituted 10 million IU interferon alfa-2b, recombinant pow-

INTERFERON ALFA-2b RECOMBINANT — INJECTION

der for injection or 0.1 mL of the 5 million IU, 10 million IU, or 25 million IU strengths of interferon alfa-2b, recombinant solution for injection, each having a final concentration of 10 million IU/mL) into each lesion 3 times per week on alternate days, for 3 weeks. The injection should be administered intralesionally using a tuberculin or similar syringe and a 25- to 30-gauge needle. The needle should be directed at the center of the base of the wart and at an angle almost parallel to the plane of the skin (approximating that in the commonly used PPD test). This will deliver the interferon to the dermal core of the lesion, infiltrating the lesion and causing a small wheal. Care should be taken not to go beneath the lesion too deeply; subcutaneous injection should be avoided, since this area is below the base of the lesion. Do not inject too superficially since this will result in possible leakage, infiltrating only the keratinized layer, and not the dermal core. As many as 5 lesions can be treated at one time. To reduce side effects, interferon alfa-2b, recombinant injections may be administered in the evening, when possible. Additionally, acetaminophen may be administered at the time of injection to alleviate some of the potential side effects.

The maximum response usually occurs 4 to 8 weeks after initiation of the first treatment course. If results at 12 to 16 weeks after the initial treatment course has concluded are not satisfactory, a second course of treatment using the above dosage schedule may be instituted providing that clinical symptoms and signs, or changes in laboratory parameters (liver function tests, WBC, and platelets) do not preclude such a course of action.

Patients with 6 to 10 condylomata may receive a second (sequential) course of treatment at the above dosage schedule, to treat up to 5 additional condylomata per course of treatment. Patients with > 10 condylomata may receive additional sequences depending on how large a number of condylomata are present.

➤*AIDS-related Kaposi's sarcoma:* 30 million IU/m^2 three times a week administered subcutaneously or intramuscularly. The 18 million and 25 million IU multidose strengths of the interferon alfa-2b, recombinant solution for injection should not be used for the treatment of AIDS-related Kaposi's sarcoma since the concentrations are inappropriate.

The selected dosage regimen should be maintained unless the disease progresses rapidly or severe intolerance is manifested. If severe adverse reactions develop, the dosage should be modified (50% reduction) or therapy should be temporarily discontinued until the adverse reactions abate. When patients initiate therapy at 30 million IU/m^2 3 times a week, the average dose tolerated at the end of 12 weeks of therapy is 110 million IU/week and 75 million IU/week at the end of 24 weeks of therapy.

When disease stabilization or a response to treatment occurs, treatment should continue until there is no further evidence of tumor or until discontinuation is required by evidence of a severe opportunistic infection or adverse effect.

➤*Chronic hepatitis C:* 3 million IU 3 times a week administered subcutaneously or intramuscularly. In patients tolerating therapy with normalization of ALT at 16 weeks of treatment, interferon alfa-2b, recombinant therapy should be extended to 18 to 24 months (72 to 96 weeks) at 3 million IU 3 times a week to improve the sustained response rate (see Pharmacology). Patients who do not normalize their ALTs after 16 weeks of therapy rarely achieve a sustained response with extension of treatment. Consideration should be given to discontinuing these patients from therapy.

If severe adverse reactions develop during interferon alfa-2b, recombinant treatment, the dose should be modified (50% reduction) or therapy should be temporarily discontinued until the adverse reactions abate. If intolerance persists after dose adjustment, interferon alfa-2b, recombinant therapy should be discontinued.

➤*Chronic hepatitis B:*

Adults – 30 to 35 million IU per week, administered subcutaneously or intramuscularly, either as 5 million IU daily or as 10 million IU 3 times a week for 16 weeks.

Children – 3 million IU/m^2 3 times a week for the first week of therapy followed by dose escalation to 6 million IU/m^2 3 times a week (maximum of 10 million IU 3 times a week) administered subcutaneously for a total therapy duration of 16 to 24 weeks.

If severe adverse reactions or laboratory abnormalities develop during interferon alfa-2b, recombinant therapy the dose should be modified (50% reduction), or discontinued if appropriate, until the adverse reactions abate. If intolerance persists after dose adjustment, interferon alfa-2b, recombinant therapy should be discontinued.

For patients with decreases in white blood cell, granulocyte, or platelet counts, the following guidelines for dose modification should be followed:

Interferon alfa-2b dose	White blood cell count	Granulocyte count	Platelet count
Reduce 50%	< 1.5 × 10^9/L	< 0.75 × 10^9/L	< 50 × 10^9/L
Permanently discontinue	< 1 × 10^9/L	< 0.5 × 10^9/L	< 25 × 10^9/L

Interferon alfa-2b, recombinant therapy was resumed at up to 100% of the initial dose when white blood cell, granulocyte, and/or platelet counts returned to normal or baseline values.

➤*Preparation and administration for intramuscular, subcutaneous, or intralesional reconstitution:* Inject the amount of diluent (bacteriostatic water for injection) stated below (diluent is supplied in either a vial or syringe), into the interferon alfa-2b, recombinant vial. Swirl gently to hasten complete dissolution of the powder. The appropriate interferon alfa-2b, recombinant dose should then be withdrawn and injected intramuscularly, subcutaneously, or intralesionally (see Patient Information for detailed instructions). After preparation and administration of the interferon alfa-2b, recombinant injection, it is essential to follow the procedure for proper disposal of syringes and needles (see Patient Information for detailed instructions).

Interferon alfa-2b, recombinant powder for injection is not indicated for use in infants and should not be used in pediatric patients in this age group because when reconstituted with the provided diluent it contains benzyl alcohol (see Warnings).

➤*Preparation and administration for intravenous infusion:* The infusion solution should be prepared immediately prior to use. Based on the desired dose, the appropriate vial strength(s) of interferon alfa-2b, recombinant powder for injection should be reconstituted with the diluent provided. The appropriate interferon alfa-2b, recombinant dose should then be withdrawn and injected into a 100 mL bag of 0.9% Sodium Chloride Injection, USP. The final concentration of interferon alfa-2b, recombinant for injection should be not less than 10 million IU/100 mL. The prepared solution should be infused over a 20-minute period.

Interferon alfa-2b, recombinant powder for injection					
	5 million IU	10 million IU	18 million IU	25 million IU	50 million IU[2]
Chronic hepatitis B	1 mL	1 mL			
Chronic hepatitis C					
Hairy cell leukemia	1 mL	2 mL		5 mL	
AIDS-related Kaposi sarcoma					1 mL
Condylomata acuminata		1 mL*			
Malignant melanoma					
Induction phase[1]	1 mL	1 mL	1 mL	5 mL	1 mL
Maintenance phase	1 mL	1 mL	1 mL		1 mL
Follicular lymphoma	1 mL	1 mL		5 mL	

* Important: For patients with condylomata acuminata, reconstitute the 10 million IU vial with only 1 mL of the diluent provided to reach a final concentration of 10 million IU/mL to be administered intralesionally.

[1] Based on the desired dose, the appropriate vial strengths should be reconstituted and administered intravenously.

[2] This vial strength should be used only for the treatment of patients with AIDS-related Kaposi's sarcoma or malignant melanoma since the concentration is inappropriate for all other indications.

Please refer to the Patient Information Sheet for detailed, step-by-step instructions on how to inject the interferon alfa-2b, recombinant solution for injection dose. After administration of interferon alfa-2b, recombinant solution for injection, it is essential to follow the procedure for proper disposal of syringes and needles.

➤*Preparation and administration of interferon alfa-2b, recombinant solution for injection:* The appropriate interferon alfa-2b, recombinant dose should be withdrawn from the vial and injected intramuscularly, subcutaneously, or intralesionally (5 million IU and 10 million IU vials, and 25 million IU multidose vials only). After administration of interferon alfa-2b, recombinant solution for injection, it is essential to follow the procedure for proper disposal of syringes and needles (see Patient Information for detailed instructions).

Interferon alfa-2b, recombinant solution for injection					
	3 million IU	5 million IU	10 million IU	18 million IU multidose*	25 million IU multidose[1]
Chronic hepatitis B		✓	✓		✓[3]
Chronic hepatitis C	✓			✓	
Hairy cell leukemia	✓	✓	✓	✓	✓
Condylomata acuminata		✓	✓		✓
Malignant melanoma	✓[2]	✓	✓	✓[2]	✓[4]
Follicular lymphoma		✓			✓

* This is a multidose vial which contains a total of 22.8 MIU of interferon alfa-2b, recombinant per 3.8 mL in order to provide the delivery of six 0.5 mL doses, each containing 3 MIU of interferon alfa-2b, recombinant for injection (for a label strength of 18 MIU).

[1] This is a multidose vial which contains a total of 32 MIU of interferon alfa-2b, recombinant per 3.2 mL in order to provide the delivery of five 0.5 mL doses, each containing 5 MIU of interferon alfa-2b, recombinant for injection (for a label strength of 25 MIU).

[2] Use only for dose reduction.

[3] Use only for the 5 MIU daily regimen.

[4] Use only for maintenance treatment.

INTERFERON ALFA-2b RECOMBINANT — INJECTION

Interferon alfa-2b, recombinant solution in multidose pens			
	3 million IU/ 0.2 mL*	5 million IU/ 0.2 mL**	10 million IU/ 0.2 mL***
Chronic hepatitis B		✓	✓
Chronic hepatitis C	✓		
Hairy cell leukemia	✓	✓	
Malignant melanoma			✓
Follicular lymphoma		✓	

* The 3 MIU multidose pen contains a total of 22.5 MIU of interferon alfa-2b, recombinant per 1.5 mL in order to provide the delivery of six 0.2 mL doses, each containing 3 MIU of interferon alfa-2b, recombinant solution for injection (for a label strength of 18 MIU).

** The 5 MIU multidose pen contains a total of 37.5 MIU of interferon alfa-2b, recombinant per 1.5 mL in order to provide the delivery of six 0.2 mL doses, each containing 5 MIU of interferon alfa-2b, recombinant solution for injection (for a label strength of 30 MIU).

*** The 10 MIU multidose pen contains a total of 75 MIU of interferon alfa-2b, recombinant per 1.5 mL in order to provide the delivery of six 0.2 mL doses, each containing 10 MIU of interferon alfa-2b, recombinant solution for injection (for a label strength of 60 MIU).

➤*Important:* The 3 million IU vial and the 18 million IU multidose vial of interferon alfa-2b, recombinant solution for injection are not to be used for chronic hepatitis B or condylomata acuminata. The multidose pen should not be used for condylomata acuminata. The 10 million IU vial of interferon alfa-2b, recombinant solution for injection should not be used for chronic hepatitis C. Interferon alfa-2b, recombinant solution for injection should not be used for AIDS-Related Kaposi's Sarcoma since the concentrations are inappropriate. Interferon alfa-2b, recombinant solution for injection is not recommended for intravenous administration and should not be used for the induction phase of malignant melanoma (see Administration and Dosage, Condylomata acuminata and AIDS-related Kaposi's sarcoma).

Parenteral drug products should be inspected visually for particulate matter and discoloration prior to administration, whenever solution and container permit. Interferon alfa-2b, recombinant for injection may be administered using either sterilized glass or plastic disposable syringes.

Interferon alfa-2b, recombinant solution for injection is not recommended for intravenous administration.

➤*Storage/Stability:* Store interferon alfa-2b, recombinant powder for injection both before and after reconstitution between 2° and 8°C (36° and 46°F).

Stability – Interferon alfa-2b, recombinant powder for injection provided in vials ranging from 3 to 50 million IU per vial, is stable at 45°C (113°F) for up to 7 days. After reconstitution with diluent (bacteriostatic water for injection), the solution is stable for 1 month at 2° to 8°C (36° to 46°F). The reconstituted solution is clear and colorless to light yellow.

Interferon alfa-2b, recombinant solution for injection multidose pens provided in strengths ranging from 18 to 60 million IU per pen is stable at 30°C (86°F) for up to 2 days. Interferon alfa-2b, recombinant solution for injection provided in vials ranging from 3 to 25 million IU per vial, is stable at 35°C (95°F) for up to 7 days and at 30°C (86°F) for up to 14 days. The solution is clear and colorless.

Actions

➤*Pharmacology:* The interferons are a family of naturally occurring small proteins and glycoproteins with molecular weights of ≈ 15,000 to 27,600 daltons produced and secreted by cells in response to viral infections and to synthetic or biological inducers.

Interferons exert their cellular activities by binding to specific membrane receptors on the cell surface. Once bound to the cell membrane, interferons initiate a complex sequence of intracellular events. In vitro studies demonstrated that these include the induction of certain enzymes, suppression of cell proliferation, immunomodulating activities such as enhancement of the phagocytic activity of macrophages and augmentation of the specific cytotoxicity of lymphocytes for target cells, and inhibition of virus replication in virus-infected cells.

In a study using human hepatoblastoma cell line, HB 611, the in vitro antiviral activity of alfa interferon was demonstrated by its inhibition of hepatitis B virus (HBV) replication.

➤*Pharmacokinetics:* The mean serum interferon alfa-2b, recombinant concentrations following intramuscular and subcutaneous injections were comparable. The maximum serum concentrations obtained via these routes were ≈ 18 to 116 IU/mL and occurred 3 to 12 hours after administration. The elimination half-life of interferon alfa-2b, recombinant for injection following both intramuscular and subcutaneous injections was ≈ 2 to 3 hours. Serum concentrations were undetectable by 16 hours after the injections.

After intravenous administration, serum interferon alfa-2b, recombinant concentrations peaked (135 to 273 IU/mL) by the end of the 30-minute infusion, then declined at a slightly more rapid rate than after intramuscular or subcutaneous drug administration, becoming undetectable 4 hours after the infusion. The elimination half-life was ≈ 2 hours.

Urine interferon alfa-2b, recombinant concentrations following a single dose (5 million IU/m^2) were not detectable after any of the parenteral routes of administration. This result was expected since preliminary studies with isolated and perfused rabbit kidneys have shown that the kidney may be the main site of interferon catabolism.

Contraindications

Hypersensitivity to interferon alfa or any component of the injection.

Warnings

➤*Special risk patients:* Moderate to severe adverse experiences may require modification of the patient's dosage regimen, or in some cases termination of interferon alfa-2b, recombinant therapy. Because of the fever and other "flu-like" symptoms associated with interferon alfa-2b, recombinant administration, it should be used cautiously in patients with debilitating medical conditions, such as those with a history of pulmonary disease (eg, chronic obstructive pulmonary disease), or diabetes mellitus prone to ketoacidosis. Caution should also be observed in patients with coagulation disorders (eg, thrombophlebitis, pulmonary embolism) or severe myelosuppression.

Patients with platelet counts of < 50,000/mm^3 should not be administered interferon alfa-2b, recombinant for injection intramuscularly, but instead by subcutaneous administration.

Interferon alfa-2b, recombinant therapy should be used cautiously in patients with a history of cardiovascular disease. Those patients with a history of myocardial infarction and/or previous or current arrhythmic disorder who require interferon alfa-2b, recombinant therapy should be closely monitored (see Laboratory tests). Cardiovascular adverse experiences, which include hypotension, arrhythmia, or tachycardia of 150 beats per minute or greater, and rarely, cardiomyopathy and myocardial infarction have been observed in some interferon alfa-2b, recombinant treated patients. Some patients with these adverse events had no history of cardiovascular disease. Transient cardiomyopathy was reported in ≈ 2% of the AIDS-related Kaposi's sarcoma patients treated with interferon alfa-2b recombinant for injection. Hypotension may occur during interferon alfa-2b, recombinant administration, or up to 2 days posttherapy, and may require supportive therapy including fluid replacement to maintain intravascular volume.

Supraventricular arrhythmias occurred rarely and appeared to be correlated with preexisting conditions and prior therapy with cardiotoxic agents. These adverse experiences were controlled by modifying the dose or discontinuing treatment, but may require specific additional therapy.

➤*CNS effects:* Depression and suicidal behavior including suicidal ideation, suicidal attempts, and completed suicides have been reported in association with treatment with alfa interferons, including interferon alfa-2b, recombinant therapy. Patients with a preexisting psychiatric condition, especially depression, or a history of severe psychiatric disorder should not be treated with interferon alfa-2b, recombinant for injection. Interferon alfa-2b, recombinant therapy should be discontinued for any patient developing severe depression or other psychiatric disorder during treatment. Obtundation and coma have also been observed in some patients, usually elderly, treated at higher doses. While these effects are usually rapidly reversible upon discontinuation of therapy, full resolution of symptoms has taken up to 3 weeks in a few severe episodes. Narcotics, hypnotics, or sedatives may be used concurrently with caution and patients should be closely monitored until the adverse effects have resolved.

➤*Thyroid abnormalities:* Infrequently, patients receiving interferon alfa-2b, recombinant therapy developed thyroid abnormalities, either hypothyroid or hyperthyroid. The mechanism by which interferon alfa-2b, recombinant for injection may alter thyroid status is unknown. Patients with preexisting thyroid abnormalities whose thyroid function cannot be maintained in the normal range by medication should not be treated with interferon alfa-2b, recombinant interferon alfa-2b, recombinant for injection. Prior to initiation of interferon alfa-2b, recombinant therapy, serum TSH should be evaluated. Patients developing symptoms consistent with possible thyroid dysfunction during the course of interferon alfa-2b, recombinant therapy should have their thyroid function evaluated and appropriate treatment instituted. Therapy should be discontinued for patients developing thyroid abnormalities during treatment whose thyroid function cannot be normalized by medication. Discontinuation of interferon alfa-2b, recombinant therapy has not always reversed thyroid dysfunction occurring during treatment.

➤*Hepatoxicity:* Hepatotoxicity, including fatality, has been observed in interferon alfa treated patients, including those treated with interferon alfa-2b, recombinant for injection. Any patient developing liver function abnormalities during treatment should be monitored closely and if appropriate, treatment should be discontinued.

➤*Pulmonary effects:* Pulmonary infiltrates, pneumonitis and pneumonia, including fatality, have been observed in interferon alfa treated patients, including those treated with interferon alfa-2b, recombinant for injection. The etiologic explanation for these pulmonary findings has yet to be established. Any patient developing fever, cough, dyspnea, or other respiratory symptoms should have a chest X-ray taken. If the chest X-ray shows pulmonary infiltrates or there is evidence of pulmonary function impairment, the patient should be closely monitored, and, if appropriate, interferon alfa treatment should be discontinued. While this has been reported more often in patients with chronic hepatitis C treated with interferon alfa, it has also been reported in patients with oncologic diseases treated with interferon alfa.

➤*Ophthalmic effects:* Retinal hemorrhages, cotton-wool spots, and retinal artery or vein obstruction have been observed rarely in patients treated with interferon alfa, including those treated with interferon alfa-2b, recombinant

INTERFERON ALFA-2b RECOMBINANT — INJECTION

for injection. The etiologic explanation for these findings has not yet been established. These events appear to occur after use of the drug for several months, but also have been reported after shorter treatment periods. Diabetes mellitus or hypertension have been present in some patients. Any patient complaining of changes in visual acuity or visual fields, or reporting other ophthalmologic symptoms during treatment with interferon alfa-2b, recombinant for injection, should have an eye examination. Because the retinal events may have to be differentiated from those seen with diabetic or hypertensive retinopathy, a baseline ocular examination is recommended prior to treatment with interferon in patients with diabetes mellitus or hypertension.

➤*Autoimmune disease:* Rare cases of autoimmune diseases including thrombocytopenia, vasculitis, Raynaud's phenomenon, rheumatoid arthritis, lupus erythematosus, and rhabdomyolysis have been observed in patients treated with alfa interferons, including patients treated with interferon alfa-2b, recombinant for injection. In very rare cases the event resulted in fatality. The mechanism by which these events develop and their relationship to interferon alfa therapy is not clear. Any patient developing an autoimmune disorder during treatment should be closely monitored and, if appropriate, treatment should be discontinued.

➤*Hyperglycemia:* Diabetes mellitus and hyperglycemia have been observed rarely in patients treated with interferon alfa-2b, recombinant for injection. Symptomatic patients should have their blood glucose measured and followed up accordingly. Patients with diabetes mellitus may require adjustment of their antidiabetic regimen.

➤*Product selection:* The 50 million IU strength of the interferon alfa-2b, recombinant powder for injection is not to be used for the treatment of hairy cell leukemia, condylomata acuminata, follicular lymphoma, chronic hepatitis C, or chronic hepatitis B. The 3 million, 5 million, 18 million, and 25 million IU strengths of the interferon alfa-2b, recombinant powder for injection are not to be used for the intralesional treatment of condylomata acuminata since the dilution required for the intralesional use would result in a hypertonic solution.

The interferon alfa-2b, recombinant multidose pens, the 3 million IU vial, and the 18 million IU multidose vial of interferon alfa-2b, recombinant solution for injection are not to be used for the treatment of condylomata acuminata.

The interferon alfa-2b, recombinant multidose pens and the 18 million and 25 million IU multidose vials of interferon alfa-2b, recombinant solution for injection are not to be used for the treatment of AIDS-related Kaposi's sarcoma. Interferon alfa-2b, recombinant solution for injection is not recommended for the intravenous treatment of malignant melanoma.

➤*AIDS-related Kaposi's sarcoma:* Interferon alfa-2b, recombinant therapy should not be used for patients with rapidly progressive visceral disease (see Pharmacology). Also of note, there may be synergistic adverse effects between interferon alfa-2b, recombinant for injection and zidovudine. Patients receiving concomitant zidovudine have had a higher incidence of neutropenia than that expected with zidovudine alone. Careful monitoring of the WBC count is indicated in all patients who are myelosuppressed and in all patients receiving other myelosuppressive medications. The effects of interferon alfa-2b, recombinant for injection when combined with other drugs used in the treatment of AIDS-related disease are unknown.

➤*Hypersensitivity reactions:* Acute serious hypersensitivity reactions (eg, urticaria, angioedema, bronchoconstriction, anaphylaxis) have been observed rarely in interferon alfa-2b, recombinant treated patients; if such an acute reaction develops, the drug should be discontinued immediately and appropriate medical therapy instituted. Transient rashes have occurred in some patients following injection, but have not necessitated treatment interruption.

➤*Hepatic function impairment:*

Chronic hepatitis C and chronic hepatitis B – Patients with decompensated liver disease, autoimmune hepatitis or a history of autoimmune disease, and patients who are immunosuppressed transplant recipients should not be treated with interferon alfa-2b, recombinant for injection. There are reports of worsening liver disease, including jaundice, hepatic encephalopathy, hepatic failure, and death following interferon alfa-2b, recombinant therapy in such patients. Therapy should be discontinued for any patient developing signs and symptoms of liver failure.

Chronic hepatitis B patients with evidence of decreasing hepatic synthetic functions, such as decreasing albumin levels or prolongation of prothrombin time, who nevertheless meet the entry criteria to start therapy, may be at increased risk of clinical decompensation if a flare of aminotransferases occurs during interferon alfa-2b, recombinant treatment. In such patients, if increases in ALT occur during interferon alfa-2b, recombinant therapy for chronic hepatitis B, they should be followed carefully including close monitoring of clinical symptomatology and liver function tests, including ALT, prothrombin time, alkaline phosphatase, albumin, and bilirubin. In considering these patients for interferon alfa-2b, recombinant therapy, the potential risks must be evaluated against the potential benefits of treatment.

Benzyl alcohol – Interferon alfa-2b, recombinant powder for injection when reconstituted with the provided diluent (bacteriostatic water for injection) contains benzyl alcohol. There have been rare reports of death in infants associated with excessive exposure to benzyl alcohol. The amount of benzyl alcohol at which toxicity or adverse effects may occur in infants is not known. Interferon alfa-2b, recombinant powder for injection is not indicated for use in infants and should not be used in pediatric patients in this age group.

➤*Fertility impairment:* Interferon may impair fertility. In studies of interferon administration in nonhuman primates, menstrual cycle abnormalities have been observed. Decreases in serum estradiol and progesterone concentrations have been reported in women treated with human leukocyte interferon. Therefore, fertile women should not receive interferon alfa-2b, recombinant therapy unless they are using effective contraception during the therapy period. Interferon alfa-2b, recombinant therapy should be used with caution in fertile men.

➤*Pregnancy: Category C.* Interferon alfa-2b, recombinant for injection has been shown to have abortifacient effects in Macaca mulatta (rhesus monkeys) at 7.5, 15, and 30 million IU/kg (90, 180, and 360 times the intramuscular or subcutaneous dose of 2 million IU/m^2). Although abortion was observed in all dose groups, it was only statistically significant at the mid- and high-dose groups. There are no adequate and well-controlled studies in pregnant women. Interferon alfa-2b, recombinant therapy should be used during pregnancy only if the potential benefit justifies the potential risk to the fetus.

➤*Lactation:* It is not known whether this drug is excreted in human milk. However, studies in mice have shown that mouse interferons are excreted into the milk. Because of the potential for serious adverse reactions from the drug in nursing infants, a decision should be made whether to discontinue nursing or to discontinue interferon alfa-2b, recombinant therapy, taking into account the importance of the drug to the mother.

➤*Children:* Safety and effectiveness in pediatric patients below the age of 18 years have not been established for indications other than chronic hepatitis B.

Chronic hepatitis B – Safety and effectiveness in pediatric patients ranging in age from 1 to 17 years have been established based upon one controlled clinical trial. Safety and effectiveness in pediatric patients below the age of 1 year have not been established.

Interferon alfa-2b, recombinant powder for injection when reconstituted with the provided diluent (bacteriostatic water for injection) contains benzyl alcohol and is not indicated for use in infants. There have been rare reports of death in infants associated with excessive exposure to benzyl alcohol. The amount of benzyl alcohol at which toxicity or adverse effects may occur in infants is not known (see Chronic hepatitis B).

Precautions

➤*Monitoring:* In addition to those tests normally required for monitoring patients, the following laboratory tests are recommended for all patients on interferon alfa-2b, recombinant therapy, prior to beginning treatment and then periodically thereafter.

- Standard hematologic tests — including hemoglobin, complete and differential white blood cell counts, and platelet count.
- Blood chemistries — electrolytes, liver function tests, and TSH.

Those patients who have preexisting cardiac abnormalities and/or are in advanced stages of cancer should have electrocardiograms taken prior to and during the course of treatment.

Baseline chest X-rays are suggested and should be repeated if clinically indicated.

For malignant melanoma patients, differential WBC count and liver function tests should be monitored weekly during the induction phase of therapy and monthly during the maintenance phase of therapy.

For specific recommendations in chronic hepatitis C and chronic hepatitis B, see Indications

While fever may be related to the flu-like syndrome reported commonly in patients treated with interferon, other causes of persistent fever should be ruled out.

➤*Psoriasis:* There have been reports of interferon, including interferon alfa-2b, recombinant for injection, exacerbating preexisting psoriasis; therefore, interferon alfa-2b, recombinant therapy should be used in these patients only if the potential benefit justifies the potential risk.

➤*Interchangeability:* Variations in dosage, routes of administration, and adverse reactions exist among different brands of interferon. Therefore, do not use different brands of interferon in any single treatment regimen.

➤*Lab test abnormalities:* Mild-to-moderate leukopenia and elevated serum liver enzyme levels have been reported with intralesional administration of interferon alfa-2b, recombinant for injection (see Adverse Reactions); therefore, the monitoring of these laboratory parameters should be considered.

Drug Interactions

Interferon Alfa-2b Drug Interactions

Precipitant drug	Object drug*		Description
Interferon alfa-2b	Theophyllines	↑	Concomitant use significantly reduces theophylline clearance (33% to 81%), resulting in a 100% increase in serum theophylline levels.
Interferon alfa-2b	Zidovudine	↑	There may be synergistic adverse effects between interferon alfa-2b and zidovudine. Patients have had a higher incidence of neutropenia than that expected with zidovudine alone. Carefully monitor WBC count in myelosuppressed patients or those receiving myelosuppressive agents.

* ↑ = Object drug increased.

INTERFERON ALFA-2b RECOMBINANT — INJECTION

Adverse Reactions

The most frequently reported adverse reactions were "flu-like" symptoms, particularly fever, headache, chills, myalgia, and fatigue. More severe toxicities are observed generally at higher doses and may be difficult for patients to tolerate.

In addition, the following spontaneous adverse experiences have been reported during the marketing surveillance of interferon alfa-2b, recombinant for injection: Nephrotic syndrome, pancreatitis, renal failure, and renal insufficiency. Very rarely, interferon alfa-2b, recombinant used alone or in combination with ribavirin capsules may be associated with aplastic anemia.

Treatment-related adverse reactions by indication

Percentage (%) of patients[1]

	Malignant melanoma	Follicular lymphoma	Hairy cell leukemia	Condylomata acuminata	AIDS-related Kaposi sarcoma		Chronic hepatitis C[5]	Chronic hepatitis B Adults		Chronic hepatitis B Pediatrics
Dosing regimens	20 MIU/m^2 induction (IV) 10 MIU/m^2 maintenance (SC)	5 MIU 3 times a week/SC	2 MIU/m^2 3 times a week/SC	1 MIU/lesion	30 MIU/m^2 3 times a week/SC	35 MIU once daily/SC	3 MIU 3 times a week	5 MIU once daily	10 MIU 3 times a week	6 MIU/m^2 3 times a week
Adverse reaction	n = 143	n = 135	n = 145	n = 352	n = 74	n = 29	n = 183	n = 101	n = 78	n = 116
Application site disorders			20%							
Injection site inflammation	-	1%	-	-	-	-	5%	3%	-	-
Other (≤ 5%)	Burning, injection site bleeding, injection site pain, injection site reaction (5% in chronic hepatitis B pediatrics), itching									
Hematologic (< 5%)	Anemia, anemia hypochromic, granulocytopenia, hemolytic anemia, leukopenia, lymphocytosis, neutropenia (9% in chronic hepatitis C, 14% in chronic hepatitis B pediatrics), thrombocytopenia (10% in chronic hepatitis C) (bleeding 8% in malignant melanoma), thrombocytopenic purpura									
Miscellaneous										
Facial edema	-	1%	-	< 1%	-	10%	< 1%	3%	1%	< 1%
Weight decrease	3%	13%	< 1%	< 1%	5%	3%	10%	2%	5%	3%
Other (5%)	Allergic reaction, cachexia, dehydration, earache, hernia, edema, hypercalcemia, hyperglycemia, hypothermia, inflammation nonspecific, lymphadenitis, lymphadenopathy, mastitis, periobital edema, poor peripheral circulation, peripheral edema (6% in follicular lymphoma), phlebitis superficial, scrotal/penile edema, thirst, weakness, weight increase									
Cardiovascular (< 5%)	Angina, arrhythmia, atrial fibrillation, bradycardia, cardiac failure, cardiomegaly, cardiomyopathy, coronary artery disorder, extrasystoles, heart valve disorder, hematoma, hypertension (9% in chronic hepatitis C), hypotension, palpitations, phlebitis, postural hypotension, pulmonary embolism, Raynaud's disease, tachycardia, thrombosis, varicose vein									
Endocrine (< 5%)	Aggravation of diabetes mellitus, goiter, gynecomastia, hyperglycemia, hyperthyroidism, hypertriglyceridemia, hypothyroidism, virilism									
Flu-like symptoms										
Fever	81%	56%	68%	56%	47%	55%	34%	66%	86%	94%
Headache	62%	21%	39%	47%	36%	21%	43%	61%	44%	57%
Chills	54%	-	46%	45%	-	-	-	-	-	-
Myalgia	75%	16%	39%	44%	34%	28%	43%	59%	40%	27%
Fatigue	96%	8%	61%	18%	84%	48%	23%	75%	69%	71%
Increased sweating	6%	13%	8%	2%	4%	21%	4%	1%	1%	3%
Asthenia	-	63%	7%	-	11%	-	40%	5%	15%	5%
Rigors	2%	7%	-	-	30%	14%	16%	38%	42%	30%
Arthralgia	6%	8%	8%	9%	-	3%	16%	19%	8%	15%
Dizziness	23%	-	12%	9%	7%	24%	9%	13%	10%	8%
Influenza-like symptoms	10%	18%	37%	-	45%	79%	26%	5%	-	< 1%
Back pain	-	15%	19%	6%	1%	3%	-	-	-	-
Dry mouth	1%	2%	19%	-	22%	28%	5%	6%	5%	-
Chest pain	2%	8%	< 1%	< 1%	1%	28%	4%	4%	-	-
Malaise	6%	-	-	14%	5%	-	13%	9%	6%	3%
Pain (unspecified)	15%	9%	18%	3%	3%	3%	-	-	-	-
Other (< 5%)	Chest pain substernal, rhinitis, rhinorrhea									
GI										
Diarrhea	35%	19%	18%	2%	18%	45%	13%	19%	8%	12%
Anorexia	69%	21%	19%	1%	38%	41%	14%	43%	53%	43%
Nausea	66%	24%	21%	17%	28%	21%	19%	50%	33%	18%
Taste alteration	24%	2%	13%	< 1%	5%	7%	2%	10%	-	-
Abdominal pain	2%	20%	< 5%	1%	5%	21%	16%	5%	4%	23%
Loose stools	-	1%	-	< 1%	-	10%	2%	2%	-	2%
Vomiting	[2]	32%	6%	2%	11%	14%	8%	7%	10%	27%
Constipation	1%	14%	< 1%	-	1%	10%	4%	5%	-	2%
Gingivitis	2%[3]	7%[3]	-	-	-	14%	-	1%	-	-
Dyspepsia	-	2%	-	2%	4%	-	7%	3%	8%	3%
Other (< 5%)	Abdominal ascites, abdominal distension, colitis, dysphagia, eructation, esophagitis, flatulence, gallstones, gastric ulcer, gastritis, gastroenteritis, gastrointestinal disorder (7% in follicular lymphoma), gastrointestinal hemorrhage, gastrointestinal mucosal discoloration, gingival bleeding, gum hyperplasia, halitosis, hemorrhoids, increased appetite, increased saliva, intestinal disorder, melena, mouth ulceration, mucositis, oral hemorrhage, oral leukoplakia, rectal bleeding after stool, rectal hemorrhage, stomatitis, stomatitis ulcerative, taste loss, tongue disorder, tooth disorder									

INTERFERON ALFA-2b RECOMBINANT — INJECTION

Treatment-related adverse reactions by indication										
	Percentage (%) of patients[1]									
	Malignant melanoma	Follicular lymphoma	Hairy cell leukemia	Condylomata acuminata	AIDS-related Kaposi sarcoma		Chronic hepatitis C[5]	Chronic hepatitis B		
								Adults		Pediatrics
Dosing regimens	20 MIU/m² induction (IV) 10 MIU/m² maintenance (SC)	5 MIU 3 times a week/SC	2 MIU/m² 3 times a week/SC	1 MIU/lesion	30 MIU/m² 3 times a week/SC	35 MIU once daily/SC	3 MIU 3 times a week	5 MIU once daily	10 MIU 3 times a week	6 MIU/m² 3 times a week
Adverse reaction	n = 143	n = 135	n = 145	n = 352	n = 74	n = 29	n = 183	n = 101	n = 78	n = 116
Hepatic/biliary (< 5%)	Abnormal hepatic function tests, biliary pain, bilirubinemia, hepatitis, increased lactate dehydrogenase, increased transaminases (AST/ALT) (elevated AST 63% in malignant melanoma and 24% in follicular lymphoma), jaundice, right upper quadrant pain (15% in chronic hepatitis C), and very rarely, hepatic encephalopathy, hepatic failure, and death									
Musculoskeletal										
Musculoskeletal pain	-	18%	-	-	-	-	21%	9%	1%	10%
Other (< 5%)	Arteritis, arthritis, arthritis aggravated, arthrosis, bone disorder, bone pain, carpal tunnel syndrome, hyporeflexia, leg cramps, muscle atrophy, muscle weakness, polyarteritis nodosa, tendinitis, rheumatoid arthritis, spondylitis									
CNS/Psychiatric										
Depression	40%	9%	6%	3%	9%	28%	19%	17%	6%	4%
Paresthesia	13%	13%	6%	1%	3%	21%	5%	6%	3%	< 1%
Impaired concentration	-	1%	-	< 1%	3%	14%	3%	8%	5%	3%
Amnesia	[4]	1%	< 5%	-	-	14%	-	-	-	-
Confusion	8%	2%	< 5%	4%	12%	10%	1%	-	-	2%
Hypoesthesia	-	1%	< 5%	1%	-	10%	-	-	-	-
Irritability	1%	1%	-	-	-	-	13%	16%	12%	22%
Somnolence	1%	2%	< 5%	3%	3%	-	33%[6]	14%	9%	5%
Anxiety	1%	9%	5%	< 1%	1%	3%	5%	2%	-	3%
Insomnia	5%	4%	-	< 1%	3%	3%	12%	11%	6%	8%
Nervousness	1%	1%	-	1%	-	3%	2%	3%	-	3%
Decreased libido	1%	1%	< 5%	-	-	-	1%	5%	1%	
Other (< 5%)	Abnormal coordination, abnormal dreaming, abnormal gait, abnormal thinking, aggravated depression, aggressive reaction, agitation (7% in chronic hepatitis B pediatrics), alcohol intolerance, apathy, aphasia, ataxia, Bell's palsy, CNS dysfunction, coma, convulsions, delirium, dysphonia, emotional lability, extrapyramidal disorder, feeling of ebriety, flushing, hearing disorder, hearing impairment, hot flashes, hyperesthesia, hyperkinesia, hypertonia, hypokinesia, impaired consciousness, labyrinthine disorder, loss of consciousness, manic depression, manic reaction, migraine, neuralgia, neuritis, neuropathy, neurosis, paresis, paroniria, parosmia, personality disorder, polyneuropathy, psychosis, speech disorder, stroke, suicidal ideation, suicide attempt, syncope, tinnitus, tremor, twitching, vertigo (8% in follicular lymphoma)									
Reproduction system disorders (< 5%)	Amenorrhea (12% in follicular lymphoma), dysmenorrhea, impotence, leukorrhea, menorrhagia, menstrual irregularity, pelvic pain, penis disorder, sexual dysfunction, uterine bleeding, vaginal dryness									
Resistance mechanism disorders										
Moniliasis	-	1%	-	< 1%	-	17%	-	-	-	-
Herpes simplex	1%	2%	-	1%	-	3%	1%	5%	-	-
Other (< 5%)	Abscess, conjunctivitis, fungal infection, hemophilus, herpes zoster, infection, infection bacterial, infection nonspecific (7% in follicular lymphoma), infection parasitic, otitis media, sepsis, stye, trichomonas, upper respiratory tract infection, viral infection (7% in chronic hepatitis C)									
Respiratory										
Dyspnea	15%	14%	< 1%	-	1%	34%	3%	5%	-	-
Coughing	6%	13%	< 1%	-	-	31%	1%	4%	-	5%
Pharyngitis	2%	8%	< 5%	1%	1%	31%	3%	7%	1%	7%
Sinusitis	1%	4%	-	-	-	21%	2%	-	-	-
Nonproductive coughing	2%	7%	-	-	-	14%	0%	1%	-	-
Nasal congestion	1%	7%	-	1%	-	10%	< 1%	4%	-	-
Other (≤ 5%)	Asthma, bronchitis (10% in follicular lymphoma), bronchospasm, cyanosis, epistaxis (7% in chronic hepatitis B pediatrics), hemoptysis, hypoventilation, laryngitis, lung fibrosis, pleural effusion, orthopnea, pleural pain, pneumonia, pneumonitis, pneumothorax, rales, respiratory disorder, respiratory insufficiency, sneezing, tonsillitis, tracheitis, wheezing									
Dermatologic										
Dermatitis	1%	-	8%	-	-	-	2%	1%	-	-
Alopecia	29%	23%	8%	-	12%	31%	28%	26%	38%	17%
Pruritus	-	10%	11%	1%	7%	-	9%	6%	4%	3%
Rash	19%	13%	25%	-	9%	10%	5%	8%	1%	5%
Dry skin	1%	3%	9%	-	9%	10%	4%	3%	-	< 1%
Other (< 5%)	Abnormal hair texture, acne, cellulitis, cyanosis of the hand, cold and clammy skin, dermatitis lichenoides, eczema, epidermal necrolysis, erythema, erythema nodosum, folliculitis, furunculosis, increased hair growth, lacrimal gland disorder, lacrimation, lipoma, maculopapular rash, melanosis, nail disorders, nonherpetic cold sores, pallor, peripheral ischemia, photosensitivity, pruritus genital, psoriasis, psoriasis aggravated, purpura (5% in chronic hepatitis C), rash erythematous, sebaceous cyst, skin depigmentation, skin discoloration, skin nodule, urticaria, vitiligo									

INTERFERON ALFA-2b RECOMBINANT — INJECTION

Treatment-related adverse reactions by indication										
Percentage (%) of patients[1]										
	Malignant melanoma	Follicular lymphoma	Hairy cell leukemia	Condylomata acuminata	AIDS-related Kaposi sarcoma		Chronic hepatitis C[5]	Chronic hepatitis B		
								Adults		Pediatrics
Dosing regimens	20 MIU/m² induction (IV) 10 MIU/m² maintenance (SC)	5 MIU 3 times a week/SC	2 MIU/m² 3 times a week/SC	1 MIU/lesion	30 MIU/m² 3 times a week/SC	35 MIU once daily/SC	3 MIU 3 times a week	5 MIU once daily	10 MIU 3 times a week	6 MIU/m² 3 times a week
Adverse reaction	n = 143	n = 135	n = 145	n = 352	n = 74	n = 29	n = 183	n = 101	n = 78	n = 116
Urinary system disorders (< 5%)	Albumin/protein in urine, cystitis, dysuria, hematuria, incontinence, increased BUN, micturition disorder, micturition frequency, nocturia, polyuria (10% in follicular lymphoma), renal insufficiency, urinary tract infection (5% in chronic hepatitis C)									
Ophthalmic (< 5%)	Abnormal vision, blurred vision, diplopia, dry eyes, eye pain, nystagmus, photophobia									

[1] Dash (-) indicates not reported.
[2] Vomiting was reported with nausea as a single term.
[3] Includes stomatitis/mucositis.
[4] Amnesia was reported with confusion as a single term.
[5] Percentages based upon a summary of all adverse events during 18 to 24 months of treatment.
[6] Predominantly lethargy.

➤*Hairy cell leukemia:* The adverse reactions most frequently reported during clinical trials in 145 patients with hairy cell leukemia were the "flu-like" symptoms of fever (68%), fatigue (61%), and chills (46%).

➤*Malignant melanoma:* The interferon alfa-2b, recombinant dose was modified because of adverse events in 65% (n = 93) of the patients. Interferon alfa-2b, recombinant therapy was discontinued because of adverse events in 8% of the patients during induction and 18% of the patients during maintenance. The most frequently reported adverse reaction was fatigue which was observed in 96% of patients. Other adverse reactions that were recorded in > 20% of interferon alfa-2b, recombinant treated patients included neutropenia (92%), fever (81%), myalgia (75%), anorexia (69%), vomiting/nausea (66%), increased SGOT (63%), headache (62%), chills (54%), depression (40%), diarrhea (35%), alopecia (29%), altered taste sensation (24%), dizziness/vertigo (23%), and anemia (22%).

Adverse reactions classified as severe or life threatening (ECOG Toxicity Criteria grade 3 or 4) were recorded in 66% and 14% of interferon alfa-2b, recombinant treated patients, respectively. Severe adverse reactions recorded in > 10% of interferon alfa-2b, recombinant treated patients included neutropenia/leukopenia (26%), fatigue (23%), fever (18%), myalgia (17%), headache (17%), chills (16%), and increased AST (14%). Grade 4 fatigue was recorded in 4% and grade 4 depression was recorded in 2% of interferon alfa-2b, recombinant treated patients. No other grade 4 AE was reported in more than 2 interferon alfa-2b, recombinant treated patients. Lethal hepatotoxicity occurred in 2 interferon alfa-2b, recombinant treated patients early in the clinical trial. No subsequent lethal hepatotoxicities were observed with adequate monitoring of liver function tests (see Precautions, Laboratory tests).

➤*Follicular lymphoma:* Ninety-six percent of patients treated with CHVP plus interferon alfa-2b, recombinant therapy and 91% of patients treated with CHVP alone reported an adverse event of any severity. Asthenia, fever, neutropenia, increased hepatic enzymes, alopecia, headache, anorexia, "flu-like" symptoms, myalgia, dyspnea, thrombocytopenia, paresthesia, and polyuria occurred more frequently in the CHVP plus interferon alfa-2b, recombinant treated patients than in patients treated with CHVP alone. Adverse reactions classified as severe or life threatening (World Health Organization grade 3 or 4) recorded in > 5% of CHVP plus interferon alfa-2b, recombinant treated patients included neutropenia (34%), asthenia (10%), and vomiting (10%). The incidence of neutropenic infection was 6% in CHVP plus interferon alfa-2b, recombinant vs 2% in CHVP alone. One patient in each treatment group required hospitalization.

Twenty-eight percent of CHVP plus interferon alfa-2b, recombinant treated patients had a temporary modification/interruption of their interferon alfa-2b, recombinant therapy, but only 13 patients (10%) permanently stopped interferon alfa-2b, recombinant therapy because of toxicity. There were 4 deaths on study; two patients committed suicide in the CHVP plus interferon alfa-2b, recombinant arm and two patients in the CHVP arm had unwitnessed sudden death. Three patients with hepatitis B (one of whom also had alcoholic cirrhosis) developed hepatotoxicity leading to discontinuation of interferon alfa-2b, recombinant. Other reasons for discontinuation included intolerable asthenia (5/135), severe flu symptoms (2/135), and one patient each with exacerbation of ankylosing spondylitis, psychosis, and decreased ejection fraction.

➤*Condylomata acuminata:* Eighty-eight percent (311/352) of patients treated with interferon alfa-2b, recombinant for injection for condylomata acuminata who were evaluable for safety, reported an adverse reaction during treatment. The incidence of the adverse reactions reported increased when the number of treated lesions increased from one to five. All 40 patients who had five warts treated, reported some type of adverse reaction during treatment.

Adverse reactions and abnormal laboratory test values reported by patients who were retreated were qualitatively and quantitatively similar to those reported during the initial interferon alfa-2b, recombinant treatment period.

➤*AIDS-related Kaposi's sarcoma:* In patients with AIDS-related Kaposi's sarcoma, some type of adverse reaction occurred in 100% of the 74 patients treated with 30 million IU/m² 3 times a week and in 97% of the 29 patients treated with 35 million IU per day.

Of these adverse reactions, those classified as severe (World Health Organization grade 3 or 4) were reported in 27% to 55% of patients. Severe adverse reactions in the 30 million IU/m² 3 times a week study included: Fatigue (20%), influenza-like symptoms (15%), anorexia (12%), dry mouth (4%), headache (4%), confusion (3%), fever (3%), myalgia (3%), and nausea and vomiting (1% each). Severe adverse reactions for patients who received the 35 million IU every day included: Fever (24%), fatigue (17%), influenza-like symptoms (14%), dyspnea (14%), headache (10%), pharyngitis (7%), and ataxia, confusion, dysphagia, GI hemorrhage, abnormal hepatic function, increased AST, myalgia, cardiomyopathy, face edema, depression, emotional lability, suicide attempt, chest pain, and coughing (1 patient each). Overall, the incidence of severe toxicity was higher among patients who received the 35 million IU per day dose.

➤*Chronic hepatitis C:* Two studies of extended treatment (18 to 24 months) with interferon alfa-2b, recombinant for injection show that ≈ 95% of all patients treated experience some type of adverse event and that patients treated for extended duration continue to experience adverse events throughout treatment. Most adverse events reported are mild to moderate in severity. However, 29/152 (19%) of patients treated for 18 to 24 months experienced a serious adverse event compared to 11/163 (7%) of those treated for 6 months. Adverse events which occur or persist during extended treatment are similar in type and severity to those occurring during short-course therapy.

Of the patients achieving a complete response after 6 months of therapy, 12/79 (15%) subsequently discontinued interferon alfa-2b, recombinant treatment during extended therapy because of adverse events, and 23/79 (29%) experienced severe adverse events (WHO grade 3 or 4) during extended therapy.

➤*Chronic hepatitis B:*

Adults – In patients with chronic hepatitis B, some type of adverse reaction occurred in 98% of the 101 patients treated at 5 million IU every day and 90% of the 78 patients treated at 10 million IU TIW. Most of these adverse reactions were mild to moderate in severity, were manageable, and were reversible following the end of therapy.

Adverse reactions classified as severe (causing a significant interference with normal daily activities or clinical state) were reported in 21% to 44% of patients. The severe adverse reactions reported most frequently were the "flu-like" symptoms of fever (28%), fatigue (15%), headache (5%), myalgia (4%), rigors (4%), and other severe "flu-like" symptoms which occurred in 1% to 3% of patients. Other severe adverse reactions occurring in more than one patient were alopecia (8%), anorexia (6%), depression (3%), nausea (3%), and vomiting (2%).

To manage side effects, the dose was reduced, or interferon alfa-2b, recombinant therapy was interrupted in 25% to 38% of patients. Five percent of patients discontinued treatment due to adverse experiences.

Children – In pediatric patients the most frequently reported adverse events were those commonly associated with interferon treatment; flu-like symptoms (100%), gastrointestinal system disorders (46%), and nausea and vomiting (40%). Neutropenia (13%) and thrombocytopenia (3%) were also reported. None of the adverse events were life threatening. The majority were moderate to severe and resolved upon dose reduction or drug discontinuation.

INTERFERON ALFA-2b RECOMBINANT — INJECTION

Lab test abnormalities –

Abnormal laboratory test values by indication										
Percentage (%) of patients[1]										
	Malignant melanoma	Follicular lymphoma	Hairy cell leukemia	Condylomata acuminata	AIDS-related Kaposi sarcoma		Chronic hepatitis C	Chronic hepatitis B		
								Adults		Pediatrics
Dosing regimens	20 MIU/m_2 induction (IV) 10 MIU/m_2 Maintenance (SC)	5 MIU 3 times a week/SC	2 MIU/m_2 3 times a week/SC	1MIU/lesion	30 MIU/m^2 3 times a week/SC	35 MIU once daily/SC	3 MIU 3 times a week	5 MIU once daily	10MIU 3 times a week	6 MIU/m^2 3 times a week
Laboratory tests	n = 143	n = 135	n = 145	n = 352	n = 69 to 73	n = 26 to 28	n = 140 to 171	n = 96 to 101	n = 75 to 103	n = 113 to 115
Hemoglobin	22%	8%	NA*	-	1%	15%	26%[7]	32%[1]	23%*	17%[2]
White blood cell count	[6]	-	NA	17%	10%	22%	26%[3]	68%[3]	34%[3]	9%[3]
Platelet count	15%	13%	NA	-	0%	8%	15%[4]	12%[4]	5%[4]	1%[4]
Serum creatinine	3%	2%	0%	-	-	-	6%	3%	0%	3%
Alkaline phosphatase	13%	-	4%	-	-	-	-	8%	4%	0%
Lactate dehydrogenase	1%	-	0%	-	-	-	-	-	-	-
Serum urea nitrogen	12%	4%	0%	-	-	-	-	2%	0%	2%
AST	63%	24%	4%	12%	11%	41%	-	-	-	-
ALT	2%	-	13%	-	10%	15%	-	-	-	-
Granulocyte count										
Total	92%	36%	NA	-	31%	39%	45%[6]	75%[6]	61%[6]	70%[6]
1000 to < 1500/mm^3	66%	-	-	-	-	-	32%	30%	32%	43%
750 to < 1000/mm^3	-	21%	-	-	-	-	10%	24%	18%	18%
500 to < 750/mm^3	25%	-	-	-	-	-	1%	17%	9%	7%
< 500/mm^3	1%	13%	-	-	-	-	2%	4%	2%	2%

* NA = not applicable. Patients' initial hematologic laboratory test values were abnormal due to their condition.
[1] Decrease of ≥ 2 g/dL.
[2] Decrease of ≥ 2 g/dL; 14% 2 to < 3 g/dL; 3% ≥ 3 g/dL.
[3] Decrease to < 3000/mm^3.
[4] Decrease to < 70,000/mm^3.
[5] Neutrophils plus bands.
[6] White blood cell count was reported as neutropenia.
[7] Decrease of ≥ 2 g/dL; 20% 2 to < 3 g/dL; 6% ≥ 3 g/dL.

Patient Information

Patients receiving interferon alfa-2b, recombinant treatment should be directed in its appropriate use, informed of benefits and risks associated with treatment, and referred to the Patient Information. This information is intended to aid in the safe and effective use of this medication. It is not a disclosure of all possible adverse or intended effects.

If home use is prescribed, a puncture-resistant container for the disposal of used syringes and needles should be supplied to the patient. Patients should be thoroughly instructed in the importance of proper disposal and cautioned against any reuse of needles and syringes. The full container should be disposed of according to the directions provided by the physician.

Patients should be cautioned not to change brands of interferon without medical consultation as a change in dosage may result.

Patients receiving high interferon alfa-2b, recombinant doses should be cautioned against performing tasks that would require complete mental alertness, such as operating machinery or driving a motor vehicle.

The most common adverse experiences occurring with interferon alfa-2b, recombinant therapy are "flu-like" symptoms, such as fever, headache, fatigue, anorexia, nausea, or vomiting (see Adverse Reactions) and appear to decrease in severity as treatment continues. Some of these "flu-like" symptoms may be minimized by bedtime administration. Antipyretics may be used to prevent or partially alleviate the fever and headache. Another common adverse experience is thinning of the hair.

It is advised that patients be well hydrated, especially during the initial stages of treatment.

PEGINTERFERON ALFA-2B

Rx	**PEG-Intron**[a] (Schering)	**Powder for injection, lyophilized:** 50 mcg/0.5 mL when reconstituted	In 2 mL vials[b] with 1 mL diluent vial, 2 syringes, and 2 alcohol swabs and *Redipen*[c] with 1 B-D needle and 2 alcohol swabs.
		80 mcg/0.5 mL when reconstituted	In 2 mL vials[b] with 1 mL diluent vial, 2 syringes, and 2 alcohol swabs and *Redipen*[c] with 1 B-D needle and 2 alcohol swabs.
		120 mcg/0.5 mL when reconstituted	In 2 mL vials[b] with 1 mL diluent vial, 2 syringes, and 2 alcohol swabs and *Redipen*[c] with 1 B-D needle and 2 alcohol swabs.
		150 mcg/0.5 mL when reconstituted	In 2 mL vials[b] with 1 mL diluent vial, 2 syringes, and 2 alcohol swabs and *Redipen*[c] with 1 B-D needle and 2 alcohol swabs.

[a] Effective October 22, 2001, *PEG-Intron* only will be made available through the *PEG-Intron* Access Assurance program. Pharmacists must obtain an order authorization number prior to placing an order with their wholesaler. To obtain this number, call (888) 437-2608 to provide the patient's Access Assurance ID# and the quantity to be dispensed (maximum 4 units). Patients without an Access Assurance ID# also may call this number to enroll. Next, contact the wholesaler and provide the authorization number and order information.

[b] Contains 1.11 mg dibasic and monobasic sodium phosphate, 0.074 mg polysorbate 80, and 59.2 mg sucrose.

[c] Contains 1.013 mg dibasic and monobasic sodium phosphate, 0.0675 mg polysorbate 80, and 54 mg sucrose.

PEGINTERFERON ALFA-2B — INJECTION

WARNING

Alpha interferons, including peginterferon alfa-2b, may cause or aggravate fatal or life-threatening neuropsychiatric, autoimmune, ischemic, and infectious disorders. Closely monitor patients with periodic clinical and laboratory evaluations. Withdraw patients with persistently severe or worsening signs or symptoms of these conditions from therapy. In many, but not all cases, these disorders resolve after stopping peginterferon alfa-2b therapy (see Precautions, Adverse Reactions).

Ribavirin use – Ribavirin may cause birth defects and/or death of the unborn child. Take extreme care to avoid pregnancy in female patients and in female partners of male patients. Ribavirin causes hemolytic anemia. The anemia associated with ribavirin therapy may result in a worsening of cardiac disease. Ribavirin is genotoxic and mutagenic; consider it a potential carcinogen (see Ribavirin monograph for additional information and warnings).

Indications

➤*Chronic hepatitis C:* For use alone or in combination with ribavirin capsules for the treatment of chronic hepatitis C in patients with compensated liver disease who have not been previously treated with interferon alpha and are at least 18 years of age.

When used in combination with ribavirin, refer to ribavirin monograph for additional prescribing information.

➤*Unlabeled uses:* Treatment of renal cell carcinoma, chronic myelogenous leukemia (CML), metastatic melanoma.

Administration and Dosage

➤*Approved by the FDA:* January 22, 2001.

There are no safety and efficacy data on treatment for longer than 1 year. Instruct patient to self-inject only if the physician determines that it is appropriate, the patient agrees to medical follow-up as necessary, and the patient receives training in proper injection technique.

➤*Monotherapy:* 1 mcg/kg/week subcutaneously for 1 year. Administer the dose on the same day of the week. Base initial dosing on the patient's weight as described in the following table.

Recommended Dosing of Peginterferon Alfa-2b

Redipen or vial strength to use (mcg/0.5 mL)	Body weight (kg)	Amount of peginterferon alfa-2b to administer (mcg)	Volume[a] of peginterferon alfa-2b to administer (mL)
50	≤ 45	40	0.4
	46 to 56	50	0.5
80	57 to 72	64	0.4
	73 to 88	80	0.5
120	89 to 106	96	0.4
	107 to 136	120	0.5
150	137 to 160	150	0.5

[a] When reconstituted as directed.

➤*Peginterferon alfa-2b/Ribavirin capsules combination therapy:* When administered in combination with ribavirin capsules, the recommended dose of peginterferon alfa-2b is 1.5 mcg/kg/week. The volume of peginterferon alfa-2b to be injected depends on the strength of peginterferon alfa-2b and the patient's body weight.

Recommended Peginterferon Alfa-2b Combination Therapy Dosing

Redipen or vial strength to use (mcg/0.5 mL)	Body weight (kg)	Amount of peginterferon alfa-2b to administer (mcg)	Volume[a] of peginterferon alfa-2b to administer (mL)
50	< 40	50	0.5
80	40 to 50	64	0.4
	51 to 60	80	0.5
120	61 to 75	96	0.4
	76 to 85	120	0.5
150	> 85	150	0.5

[a] When reconstituted as directed.

The recommended dose of ribavirin capsules is 800 mg/day in 2 divided doses; 2 capsules (400 mg) with breakfast and 2 capsules (400 mg) with dinner. Do not use ribavirin capsules in patients with Ccr less than 50 mL/min.

➤*Discontinuation:* It is recommended that patients receiving peginterferon alfa-2b alone or in combination with ribavirin be discontinued from therapy if hepatitis C virus (HCV) viral levels remain high after 6 months of therapy.

➤*Dose reduction:* If a serious adverse reaction develops during the course of treatment (see Warnings, Precautions), discontinue or modify the dosage of peginterferon alfa-2b and/or ribavirin capsules until the adverse reaction abates or decreases in severity. If persistent or recurrent serious adverse reactions develop despite adequate dosage adjustment, discontinue treatment. Decreases in hemoglobin, neutrophils, and platelets may require dose reduction or permanent discontinuation from therapy. For guidelines for dose modifications and discontinuation based on laboratory parameters, see the tables below. In the combination therapy trial, dose reductions occurred among 42% of patients receiving peginterferon alfa-2b 1.5 mcg/kg/ribavirin capsules 800 mg/day, including 57% of those patients 60 kg or less.

Guidelines for Modification or Discontinuation of Peginterferon Alfa-2b or Peginterferon Alfa-2b/Ribavirin Capsules and for Scheduling Visits for Patients with Depression

	Initial management (4 to 8 weeks)		Depression		
Depression severity[a]	Dose modification	Visit schedule	Remains stable	Improves	Worsens
Mild	No change.	Evaluate once/week by visit or phone.	Continue weekly visit schedule.	Resume normal visit schedule.	(See moderate or severe depression.)
Moderate	Decrease IFN dose 50%.	Evaluate once/week (office visit at least every other week).	Consider psychiatric consultation. Continue reduced dosing.	If symptoms improve and are stable for 4 weeks, may resume normal visit schedule. Continue reduced dosing or return to normal dose.	(See severe depression.)
Severe	Discontinue IFN/R permanently.	Obtain immediate psychiatric consultation.	Psychiatric therapy necessary.		

[a] See DSM-IV for definitions.

Guidelines for Dose Modification and Discontinuation of Peginterferon Alfa-2b or Peginterferon Alfa-2b/Ribavirin Capsules for Hematologic Toxicity

Laboratory values		Peginterferon alfa-2b	Ribavirin capsules
Hemoglobin[a]	< 10 g/dL	—	Decrease by 200 mg/day
	< 8.5 g/dL	Permanently discontinue	Permanently discontinue
WBC	$< 1.5 \times 10^9/L$	Reduce dose by 50%	—
	$< 1 \times 10^9/L$	Permanently discontinue	Permanently discontinue
Neutrophils	$< 0.75 \times 10^9/L$	Reduce dose by 50%	—
	$< 0.5 \times 10^9/L$	Permanently discontinue	Permanently discontinue
Platelets	$< 80 \times 10^9/L$	Reduce dose by 50%	—
	$< 50 \times 10^9/L$	Permanently discontinue	Permanently discontinue

[a] For patients with a history of stable cardiac disease receiving peginterferon alfa-2b in combination with ribavirin capsules, reduce the peginterferon alfa-2b dose by half and the ribavirin capsule dose by 200 mg/day if a more than 2 g/dL decrease in hemoglobin is observed during any 4-week period. Permanently discontinue peginterferon alfa-2b and ribavirin capsules if patient has hemoglobin levels less than 12 g/dL after this ribavirin dose reduction.

➤*Reconstitution:* Visually inspect the solution for particulate matter and discoloration prior to administration. The reconstituted solution should be clear and colorless. Do not use the solution if discolored or cloudy or if particulates are present. The prepared solution is to be injected subcutaneously.

Redipen – To reconstitute the lyophilized peginterferon alfa-2b in the *Redipen*, hold the *Redipen* upright (dose button down) and press the two halves of the pen together until there is an audible click. Gently invert the pen to mix the solution. Do not shake. Keeping the pen upright, attach the supplied needle and select the appropriate peginterferon alfa-2b dose by pulling back on the dosing button until the dark bands are visible and turning the button until the dark band is aligned with the correct dose. The *Redipen* is for single use only.

Vials – Reconstitute the peginterferon alfa-2b lyophilized product with only 0.7 mL of supplied diluent (sterile water for injection). The diluent vial is for single use only. Discard the remaining diluent. Do not add any other medication to solutions containing peginterferon alfa-2b, and do not reconstitute peginterferon alfa-2b with other diluents. Swirl gently to hasten complete dissolution of the powder.

PEGINTERFERON ALFA-2B — INJECTION

➤*Storage/Stability:*

Redipen – Store at 2° to 8°C (36° to 46°F). After reconstitution, use the solution immediately, or it may be stored up to 24 hours at 2° to 8°C (36° to 46°F). The reconstituted solution contains no preservative and is clear and colorless. Do not freeze.

Vials – Store at 25°C (77°F); excursions permitted to 15° to 30°C (59° to 86°F). After reconstitution with supplied diluent, use the solution immediately, or it may be stored up to 24 hours at 2° to 8°C (36° to 46°F). The reconstituted solution contains no preservative and is clear and colorless. Do not freeze.

Actions

➤*Pharmacology:* The biological activity of peginterferon alfa-2b is derived from its interferon alfa-2b moiety. Interferons exert their cellular activities by binding to specific membrane receptors on the cell surface and initiating a complex sequence of intracellular events. These include the induction of certain enzymes, suppression of cell proliferation, immunomodulating activities, such as enhancement of the phagocytic activity of macrophages and augmentation of the specific cytotoxicity of lymphocytes for target cells, and inhibition of virus replication in virus-infected cells.

➤*Pharmacokinetics:*

Absorption/Distribution – Following a single subcutaneous dose of peginterferon alfa-2b, the mean absorption half-life ($t_{½}$ k_a) was 4.6 hours. Maximal serum concentrations (C_{max}) occur between 15 and 44 hours postdose and are sustained for up to 48 to 72 hours. The C_{max} and AUC measurements of peginterferon alfa-2b increase in a dose-related manner. After multiple dosing, there is an increase in bioavailability of peginterferon alfa-2b. Week 48 mean trough concentrations (320 pg/mL; range, 0, 2960) are approximately 3-fold higher than week 4 mean trough concentrations (94 pg/mL; range, 0, 416).

Metabolism/Excretion – The mean peginterferon alfa-2b elimination half-life is approximately 40 hours (range, 22 to 60 hours) in patients with HCV infection. The apparent clearance of peginterferon alfa-2b is estimated to be approximately 22 mL/h•kg. Renal elimination accounts for 30% of the clearance. Single-dose peginterferon alfa-2b pharmacokinetics following a 1 mcg/kg subcutaneous dose suggest the clearance of peginterferon alfa-2b is reduced by approximately 50% in patients with impaired renal function (Ccr less than 50 mL/min).

Pegylation of interferon alfa-2b produces a product (peginterferon alfa-2b) whose clearance is lower than that of nonpegylated interferon alfa-2b. When compared with interferon alfa-2b, peginterferon alfa-2b (1 mcg/kg) has an approximately 7-fold lower mean apparent clearance and a 5-fold greater mean half-life, permitting a reduced dosing frequency. At effective therapeutic doses, peginterferon alfa-2b has approximately 10-fold greater C_{max} and 50-fold greater AUC than interferon alfa-2b.

Contraindications

➤*Peginterferon alfa-2b:* Hypersensitivity to peginterferon alfa-2b or any component of the product; autoimmune hepatitis; decompensated liver disease.

➤*Peginterferon alfa-2b/Ribavirin capsules combination:* Hypersensitivity to ribavirin capsules or any other component of the product; pregnant women; men whose female partners are pregnant; patients with hemoglobinopathies (eg, thalassemia major, sickle-cell anemia).

Warnings

➤*Neuropsychiatric events:* Life-threatening or fatal neuropsychiatric events, including suicide, suicidal and homicidal ideation, depression, relapse of drug addiction/overdose, and aggressive behavior have occurred in patients with and without a previous psychiatric disorder during peginterferon alfa-2b treatment and follow-up. Psychoses, hallucinations, bipolar disorders, and mania have been observed in patients treated with alpha interferons. Use peginterferon alfa-2b with extreme caution in patients with a history of psychiatric disorders. Advise patients to report immediately any symptoms of depression and/or suicidal ideation to their prescribing physicians. Physicians should monitor all patients for evidence of depression and other psychiatric symptoms. In severe cases, stop peginterferon alfa-2b immediately and institute psychiatric intervention.

➤*Bone marrow toxicity:* Peginterferon alfa-2b suppresses bone marrow function, sometimes resulting in severe cytopenias. Discontinue peginterferon alfa-2b in patients who develop severe decreases in neutrophil or platelet counts. Ribavirin may potentiate the neutropenia induced by interferon alpha. Very rarely, alpha interferons may be associated with aplastic anemia.

➤*Colitis:* Fatal and nonfatal ulcerative or hemorrhagic/ischemic colitis have been observed within 12 weeks of the start of alpha interferon treatment. Abdominal pain, bloody diarrhea, and fever are the typical manifestations. Immediately discontinue peginterferon alfa-2b in patients who develop these symptoms and signs. The colitis usually resolves within 1 to 3 weeks of discontinuation of alpha interferons.

➤*Pancreatitis:* Fatal and nonfatal pancreatitis have been observed in patients treated with alpha interferons. Suspend peginterferon alfa-2b therapy in patients with signs and symptoms suggestive of pancreatitis, and discontinue in patients diagnosed with pancreatitis.

➤*Pulmonary disorders:* Dyspnea, pulmonary infiltrates, pneumonia, bronchiolitis obliterans, interstitial pneumonitis, and sarcoidosis, some resulting in respiratory failure and/or patient deaths, may be induced or aggravated by peginterferon alfa-2b or alpha-interferon therapy. Recurrence of respiratory failure has been observed with interferon rechallenge. Suspend peginterferon alfa-2b combination treatment in patients who develop pulmonary infiltrates or pulmonary function impairment. Closely monitor patients who resume interferon treatment.

➤*Endocrine disorders:* Peginterferon alfa-2b causes or aggravates hypothyroidism and hyperthyroidism. Hyperglycemia has been observed in patients treated with peginterferon alfa-2b. Diabetes mellitus has been observed in patients treated with alpha interferons. Do not begin peginterferon alfa-2b therapy in patients with these conditions who cannot be effectively treated by medication. Do not continue peginterferon alfa-2b therapy in patients who develop these conditions during treatment and cannot be controlled with medication.

➤*Cardiovascular events:* Cardiovascular events, including hypotension, arrhythmia, tachycardia, cardiomyopathy, angina pectoris, and MI have been observed in patients treated with peginterferon alfa-2b. Use peginterferon alfa-2b cautiously in patients with cardiovascular disease. Closely monitor patients with a history of MI and arrhythmic disorder who require peginterferon alfa-2b therapy. Do not treat patients with a history of significant or unstable cardiac disease with peginterferon/ribavirin capsules combination therapy.

➤*Autoimmune disorders:* Development or exacerbation of autoimmune disorders (eg, thyroiditis, thrombocytopenia, rheumatoid arthritis, interstitial nephritis, systemic lupus erythematosus, psoriasis) has been observed in patients receiving peginterferon alfa-2b. Use peginterferon alfa-2b with caution in patients with autoimmune disorders.

➤*Ophthalmologic disorders:* Decrease or loss of vision, retinopathy (including macular edema), retinal artery or vein thrombosis, retinal hemorrhages and cotton wool spots, optic neuritis, and papilledema may be induced or aggravated by treatment with peginterferon alfa-2b or other alpha interferons. All patients should receive an eye examination at baseline. Patients with preexisting ophthalmologic disorders (eg, diabetic or hypertensive retinopathy) should receive periodic ophthalmologic exams during interferon alpha treatment. Any patient who develops ocular symptoms should receive a prompt and complete eye examination. Discontinue peginterferon alfa-2b treatment in patients who develop new or worsening ophthalmologic disorders.

➤*Anemia:* Ribavirin caused hemolytic anemia in 10% of peginterferon alfa-2b/ribavirin capsule-treated patients within 1 to 4 weeks of initiation of therapy. Obtain complete blood counts pretreatment and at weeks 2 and 4 of therapy or more frequently if clinically indicated. Anemia associated with ribavirin capsule therapy may result in a worsening of cardiac disease. Decrease in dosage or discontinuation of ribavirin capsules may be necessary.

➤*Hypersensitivity reactions:* Serious, acute hypersensitivity reactions (eg, urticaria, angioedema, bronchoconstriction, anaphylaxis) rarely have been observed during alpha interferon therapy. If such a reaction develops during treatment with peginterferon alfa-2b, discontinue treatment and immediately institute appropriate medical therapy. Transient rashes do not necessitate interruption of treatment.

➤*Renal function impairment:* Increases in serum creatinine levels have been observed in patients treated with interferons, including peginterferon alfa-2b therapy. Closely monitor patients with impairment of renal function for signs and symptoms of interferon toxicity, including increases in serum creatinine, and adjust doses of peginterferon alfa-2b accordingly. Use peginterferon alfa-2b with caution in patients with Ccr less than 50 mL/min. Do not use ribavirin in patients with Ccr less than 50 mL/min.

➤*Fertility impairment:* Irregular menstrual cycles were observed in female cynomolgus monkeys given subcutaneous injections of 4239 mcg/m^2 peginterferon alfa-2b every other day for 1 month (at approximately 345 times the recommended weekly human dose based on body surface area). These effects included transiently decreased serum levels of estradiol and progesterone, suggestive of anovulation. Normal menstrual cycles and serum hormone levels resumed in these animals 2 to 3 months following cessation of peginterferon alfa-2b treatment. Every other day dosing with 262 mcg/m^2 (approximately 21 times the recommended weekly human dose) had no effects on cycle duration or reproductive hormone status. The effects of peginterferon alfa-2b on male fertility have not been studied.

➤*Elderly:* In general, younger patients tend to respond better than older patients to interferon-based therapies. However, clinical studies of peginterferon alfa-2b alone or in combination with ribavirin capsules did not include sufficient numbers of subjects 65 years of age and older to determine whether they respond differently than younger subjects. Treatment with alpha interferons, including peginterferon alfa-2b, is associated with neuropsychiatric, cardiac, pulmonary, GI, and systemic (flu-like) adverse effects. Because these adverse reactions may be more severe in the elderly, exercise caution in the use of peginterferon alfa-2b in this population. This drug is known to be substantially excreted by the kidney. Because elderly patients are more likely to have decreased renal function, the risk of toxic reactions to this drug may be greater in patients with impaired renal function. Do not use ribavirin capsules in patients with Ccr less than 50 mL/min. When using peginterferon alfa-2b/ribavirin therapy, also refer to the ribavirin capsules medication guide.

➤*Pregnancy:* *Category C.* Assume that peginterferon alfa-2b has abortifacient potential. There are no adequate and well-controlled studies in pregnant women. Use during pregnancy only if the potential benefit justifies the potential risk to the fetus. Peginterferon alfa-2b is recommended for use in fertile women only when they are using effective contraception during the treatment period.

If pregnancy occurs in a patient or partner of a patient during treatment with peginterferon alfa-2b and ribavirin capsules during the 6 months after treatment cessation, physicians should report such cases by calling (800) 727-7064.

PEGINTERFERON ALFA-2B — INJECTION

*Use with ribavirin – Category X.*See the Warning box for more information.

➤*Lactation:* It is not known whether the components of peginterferon alfa-2b are excreted in human milk. Because of the potential for adverse reactions from the drug in nursing infants, decide whether to discontinue nursing or discontinue the treatment, taking into account the importance of the product to the mother.

➤*Children:* Safety and efficacy in patients younger than 18 years of age have not been established.

Precautions

➤*Monitoring:* Patients on peginterferon alfa-2b or peginterferon alfa-2b/ribavirin capsules combination therapy should have hematology and blood chemistry testing before the start of treatment and then periodically thereafter. Measure HCV RNA at 6 months of treatment. Discontinue peginterferon alfa-2b or peginterferon alfa-2b/ribavirin capsules combination therapy in patients with persistent high viral levels. Administer an ECG to patients who have preexisting cardiac abnormalities before treatment with peginterferon alfa-2b/ribavirin capsules.

➤*Immunogenicity:* Approximately 2% of patients receiving peginterferon alfa-2b or interferon alfa-2b with or without ribavirin capsules developed low-titer (160 or less) neutralizing antibodies to peginterferon alfa-2b or interferon alfa-2b. The clinical and pathological significance of the appearance of serum neutralizing antibodies is unknown.

➤*Organ transplants:* The safety and efficacy of peginterferon alfa-2b alone or in combination with ribavirin capsules for the treatment of hepatitis C in patients who have received liver or other organ transplants have not been studied. Preliminary data indicate that interferon alpha therapy may be associated with an increased rate of kidney graft rejection. Liver graft rejection also has been reported, but a causal association to interferon alpha therapy has not been established.

➤*Triglycerides:* Elevated triglyceride levels have been observed in patients treated with interferons, including peginterferon alfa-2b therapy. Manage elevated triglyceride levels as clinically appropriate. Hypertriglyceridemia may result in pancreatitis. Consider discontinuation of peginterferon alfa-2b therapy for patients with persistently elevated triglycerides (ie, triglycerides greater than 1000 mg/dL) associated with symptoms of potential pancreatitis, such as abdominal pain, nausea, or vomiting.

➤*Lab test abnormalities:* Peginterferon alfa-2b alone or in combination with ribavirin capsules may cause severe decreases in neutrophil and platelet counts and hematologic, endocrine (eg, thyroid-stimulating hormone [TSH]), and hepatic abnormalities. In 10% of patients treated with peginterferon alfa-2b, ALT levels rose 2- to 5-fold above baseline. The elevations were transient and were not associated with deterioration of other liver functions.

Adverse Reactions

➤*Monotherapy:* Nearly all study patients in clinical trials experienced 1 or more adverse events. In the peginterferon alfa-2b monotherapy trial, the incidence of serious adverse events was similar (approximately 12%) in all treatment groups. In the peginterferon alfa-2b/ribavirin capsules trial, the incidence of serious adverse events was 17% in the peginterferon alfa-2b/ribavirin capsules groups compared with 14% in the interferon alfa-2b/ribavirin capsules group.

In many, but not all cases, adverse events resolved after dose reduction or discontinuation of therapy. Some patients experienced ongoing or new serious adverse events during the 6-month, follow-up period. In the peginterferon alfa-2b/ribavirin capsules trial, 13 patients experienced life-threatening psychiatric events (suicidal ideation or attempt) and 1 patient committed suicide.

➤*Mortality:* There have been 5 patient deaths that occurred in clinical trials: 1 suicide in a patient receiving peginterferon alfa-2b monotherapy and 1 suicide in a patient receiving peginterferon alfa-2b/ribavirin capsules combination therapy; 2 deaths among patients receiving interferon alfa-2b monotherapy (1 murder/suicide and 1 sudden death); and 1 patient death in the interferon alfa-2b/ribavirin capsules group (motor vehicle accident).

➤*Discontinuation:* Overall, 10% to 14% of patients receiving peginterferon alfa-2b, alone or in combination with ribavirin capsules, discontinued therapy compared with 6% treated with interferon alfa-2b alone and 13% treated with interferon alfa-2b in combination with ribavirin capsules. The most common reasons for discontinuation of therapy were related to psychiatric, systemic (eg, fatigue, headache), or GI adverse events.

➤*Combination therapy:* In the combination therapy trial, dose reductions caused by adverse reactions occurred in 42% of patients receiving peginterferon alfa-2b (1.5 mcg/kg)/ribavirin capsules and in 34% of those receiving interferon alfa-2b/ribavirin capsules. The majority of patients (57%) weighing 60 kg or less receiving peginterferon alfa-2b (1.5 mcg/kg)/ribavirin capsules required dose reduction. Reduction of interferon was dose-related (peginterferon alfa-2b 1.5 mcg/kg greater than peginterferon alfa-2b 0.5 mcg/kg or interferon alfa-2b), 40%, 27%, 28%, respectively. Dose reduction for ribavirin capsules was similar across all 3 groups, 33% to 35%. The most common reasons for dose modifications were neutropenia (18%) or anemia (9%). Other common reasons included depression, fatigue, nausea, and thrombocytopenia.

In the peginterferon alfa-2b/ribavirin capsules combination trial, the most common adverse events were psychiatric, occurring among 77% of patients and included most commonly depression, irritability, and insomnia, each reported by approximately 30% to 40% of subjects in all treatment groups. Suicidal behavior (eg, ideation, attempts, suicides) occurred in 2% of all patients during treatment or during follow-up after treatment cessation.

Peginterferon alfa-2b induced fatigue or headache in approximately two thirds of patients and induced fever or rigors in approximately 50% of the patients. The severity of some of these systemic symptoms (eg, fever, headache) tended to decrease as treatment continued. The incidence tends to be higher with peginterferon alfa-2b than with interferon alfa-2b therapy alone or in combination with ribavirin capsules.

Application-site inflammation and reaction (eg, bruising, itchiness, irritation) occurred at approximately twice the incidence with peginterferon alfa-2b therapies (in up to 75% of patients) compared with interferon alfa-2b. However, injection-site pain was infrequent (2% to 3%) in all groups.

Other common adverse events in the peginterferon alfa-2b/ribavirin capsules group included alopecia (36%), anorexia (32%), arthralgia (34%), myalgia (56%), nausea (43%), pruritus (29%), and weight loss (29%).

➤*Severe adverse reactions:* In the peginterferon alfa-2b monotherapy trial, the incidence of severe adverse events was 13% in the interferon alfa-2b group and 17% in the peginterferon alfa-2b groups. In the peginterferon alfa-2b/ribavirin capsules combination therapy trial, the incidence of severe adverse events was 23% in the interferon alfa-2b/ribavirin capsules group and 31% to 34% in the peginterferon alfa-2b/ribavirin capsules groups. The incidence of life-threatening adverse events was 1% or less across all groups in the monotherapy and combination therapy trials.

Peginterferon Alfa-2b Adverse Events Occurring in > 5% of Patients[a]

	Study 1		Study 2	
Adverse reaction	Peginterferon alfa-2b 1 mcg/kg (n = 297)	Interferon alfa-2b 3 MIU (n = 303)	Peginterferon alfa-2b (1.5 mcg/kg)/ ribavirin capsules (n = 511)	Interferon alfa-2b/ ribavirin capsules (n = 505)
CNS				
Agitation	2	2	8	5
Anxiety/ Emotional lability/ Irritability	28	34	47	47
Concentration impaired	10	8	17	21
Depression	29	25	31	34
Dizziness	12	10	21	17
Fatigue/ Asthenia	52	54	66	63
Headache	56	52	62	58
Insomnia	23	23	40	41
Nervousness	4	3	6	6
Dermatologic				
Alopecia	22	22	36	32
Dry skin	11	9	24	23
Flushing	6	3	4	3
Pruritus	12	8	29	28
Rash	6	7	24	23
Sweating increased	6	7	11	7
GI				
Abdominal pain	15	11	13	13
Anorexia	20	17	32	27
Constipation	1	3	5	5
Diarrhea	18	16	22	17
Dry mouth	6	7	12	8
Dyspepsia	6	7	9	8
Nausea	26	20	43	33
Vomiting	7	6	14	12
Hematologic				
Anemia	0	0	12	17
Leukopenia	< 1	0	6	5
Neutropenia	6	2	26	14
Thrombocytopenia	7	< 1	5	2
Musculoskeletal				
Arthralgia	23	27	34	28
Musculoskeletal pain	28	22	21	19
Myalgia	54	53	56	50
Respiratory				
Coughing	8	5	23	16
Dyspnea	4	2	26	24
Pharyngitis	10	7	12	13
Rhinitis	2	2	8	6
Sinusitis	7	7	6	5
Miscellaneous				
Chest pain	6	4	8	7
Conjunctivitis	4	2	4	5

PEGINTERFERON ALFA-2B — INJECTION

Peginterferon Alfa-2b Adverse Events Occurring in > 5% of Patients[a]				
	Study 1		Study 2	
Adverse reaction	Peginterferon alfa-2b 1 mcg/kg (n = 297)	Interferon alfa-2b 3 MIU (n = 303)	Peginterferon alfa-2b (1.5 mcg/kg)/ ribavirin capsules (n = 511)	Interferon alfa-2b/ ribavirin capsules (n = 505)
Fever	22	12	46	33
Hepatomegaly	6	5	4	4
Hypothyroidism	5	3	5	4
Infection, fungal	< 1	3	6	1
Infection, viral	11	10	12	12
Injection-site inflammation/ reaction	47	20	75	49
Malaise	7	6	4	6
Menstrual disorder	4	3	7	6
Right upper quadrant pain	8	8	12	6
Rigors	23	19	48	41
Taste perversion	< 1	2	9	4
Vision blurred	2	3	5	6
Weight decrease	11	13	29	20

[a] Patients reporting 1 or more adverse event. A patient may have reported more than 1 adverse event within a body system/organ class category.

Many patients continued to experience adverse events several months after discontinuation of therapy. By the end of the 6-month follow-up period, the incidence of ongoing adverse events by body class in the peginterferon alfa-2b 1.5/ribavirin capsules group was 33% (psychiatric), 20% (musculoskeletal), and 10% (for endocrine and GI). In approximately 10% to 15% of patients, weight loss, fatigue, and headache had not resolved.

➤*Cardiovascular:* Angina, cardiomyopathy, MI, pericardial effusion, supraventricular arrhythmias, transient ischemic attack (1% or less).

➤*CNS:* Aggressive reaction, loss of consciousness, nerve palsy (facial, oculomotor), psychosis, relapse of drug addiction/overdose, severe depression, suicidal ideation, suicide attempt (1% or less).

➤*Dermatologic:* Aggravated psoriasis, injection-site necrosis, phototoxicity, urticaria, vasculitis (1% or less).

➤*Hematologic:* Autoimmune thrombocytopenia with or without purpura, neutropenia (1% or less).

➤*Metabolic:* Gout, hyperglycemia (1% or less).

➤*Respiratory:* Bronchiolitis obliterans, emphysema, pleural effusion (1% or less).

➤*Special senses:* Blindness, decreased visual acuity, optic neuritis, retinal artery or vein thrombosis, retinal ischemia (1% or less).

➤*Miscellaneous:* Gastroenteritis, hyperthyroidism, hypothyroidism, infection (eg, pneumonia, abscess, sepsis, cellulitis), interstitial nephritis, lupus-like syndrome, pancreatitis, rheumatoid arthritis, sarcoidosis (1% or less).

➤*Lab test abnormalities:*

Hemoglobin – Ribavirin capsules induced a decrease in hemoglobin levels in approximately two thirds of patients. Hemoglobin levels decreased to less than 11 g/dL in approximately 30% of patients. Severe anemia (less than 8 g/dL) occurred in less than 1% of patients. Dose modification was required in 9% and 13% of patients in the peginterferon alfa-2b/ribavirin capsule and interferon alfa-2b/ribavirin capsule groups, respectively. Hemoglobin levels become stable by treatment week 4 to 6 on average. Hemoglobin levels return to baseline between 4 and 12 weeks posttreatment. In the peginterferon alfa-2b monotherapy trial, hemoglobin decreases were generally mild and dose modifications were rarely necessary.

Neutrophils – Decreases in neutrophil counts were observed in a majority of patients treated with peginterferon alfa-2b alone (70%) or as combination therapy with ribavirin capsules (85%) and interferon alfa-2b/ribavarin capsules (60%). Severe and potentially life-threatening neutropenia (less than 0.5×10^9/L) occurred in 1% of patients treated with peginterferon alfa-2b monotherapy, 2% of patients treated with interferon alfa-2b/ribavirin capsules, and in 4% of patients treated with peginterferon alfa-2b/ribavirin capsules. Two percent of patients receiving peginterferon alfa-2b monotherapy and 18% of patients receiving peginterferon alfa-2b/ribavirin capsules required modification of interferon dosage. Few patients (1% or less) required permanent discontinuation of treatment. Neutrophil counts generally return to pretreatment levels within 4 weeks of cessation of therapy.

Platelets – Platelet counts decrease in approximately 20% of patients treated with peginterferon alfa-2b alone or with ribavirin capsules and in 6% of patients treated with interferon alfa-2b/ribavirin capsules. Severe decreases in platelet counts (less than 50,000/mm^3) occur in less than 1% of patients. Patients may require discontinuation or dose modification as a result of platelet decreases. In the peginterferon alfa-2b/ribavirin capsules combination therapy trial, 1% or 3% of patients required dose modification of interferon alfa-2b or peginterferon alfa-2b, respectively. Platelet counts generally returned to pretreatment levels within 4 weeks of the cessation of therapy.

Thyroid function – Development of TSH abnormalities, with and without clinical manifestations, are associated with interferon therapies. Clinically apparent thyroid disorders occur among patients treated with either interferon alfa-2b or peginterferon alfa-2b (with or without ribavirin capsules) at a similar incidence (5% for hypothyroidism and 3% for hyperthyroidism). Subjects developed new-onset TSH abnormalities while on treatment and during the follow-up period. At the end of the follow-up period, 7% of subjects still had abnormal TSH values.

Bilirubin and uric acid – In the peginterferon alfa-2b/ribavirin capsules trial, 10% to 14% of patients developed hyperbilirubinemia and 33% to 38% developed hyperuricemia in association with hemolysis. Six patients developed mild to moderate gout.

➤*Postmarketing:*

Cardiovascular – Cardiac ischemia.

CNS – Peripheral neuropathy, seizures, vertigo.

Dermatologic – Erythema multiforme, Stevens-Johnson syndrome, toxic epidermal necrolysis.

Metabolic – Renal failure, renal insufficiency.

Special senses – Hearing impairment, hearing loss.

Miscellaneous – Rhabdomyolysis, stomatitis.

Overdosage

There is limited experience with overdosage. In the clinical studies, a few patients accidentally received a dose greater than that prescribed. There were no instances in which a participant in the monotherapy or combination therapy trials received more than 10.5 times the intended dose of peginterferon alfa-2b. The maximum dose received by any patient was 3.45 mcg/kg weekly over a period of approximately 12 weeks. The maximum known overdosage of ribavirin capsules was an intentional ingestion of 10 g (fifty 200 mg capsules). There were no serious reactions attributed to these overdosages. In cases of overdosing, symptomatic treatment and close observation of the patient are recommended.

Patient Information

Direct patients receiving peginterferon alfa-2b alone or in combination with ribavirin capsules in its appropriate use, inform them of the benefits and risks associated with treatment, and refer them to the medication guide.

Advise patients to use a puncture-resistant container for the disposal of used syringes, needles, and the *Redipen*. Thoroughly instruct patients in the importance of proper disposal, and caution them against any reuse of needles, syringes, or the *Redipen*. Instruct patients to dispose of the full container in accordance with state and local laws.

Inform patients that there are no data evaluating whether peginterferon alfa-2b therapy will prevent transmission of HCV infection to others. Also, it is not known if treatment with peginterferon alfa-2b will cure hepatitis C or prevent cirrhosis, liver failure, or liver cancer that may be the result of infection with HCV.

Advise patients that laboratory evaluations are required before starting therapy and periodically thereafter. It is advised that patients be well-hydrated, especially during the initial stages of treatment. Flu-like symptoms associated with administration of peginterferon alfa-2b may be minimized by bedtime administration or by use of antipyretics.

Inform patients that ribavirin may cause birth defects and/or death of the unborn child. Extreme care must be taken to avoid pregnancy in female patients and in female partners of male patients during treatment with combination peginterferon alfa-2b/ribavirin capsules therapy and for 6 months posttherapy. Do not initiate combination peginterferon alfa-2b/ribavirin capsule therapy until a report of a negative pregnancy test has been obtained immediately prior to initiation of therapy. It is recommended that patients undergo monthly pregnancy tests during therapy and for 6 months posttherapy.

INTERFERON ALFA-2b, RECOMBINANT AND RIBAVIRIN COMBINATION

Rx	**Rebetron** (Schering)	**Injection/Capsules (combination packages):** 3 million IU interferon alfa-2b, recombinant/0.5 mL and 200 mg ribavirin	*Patients* ≤ *75 kg*: *Intron A* (injection): In single-dose vials (6s), one 18 million IU multidose vial, or one 18 million IU multidose pen. *Rebetol* (capsules): (REBETOL 200 MG). White. In 70s.
			Patients > 75 kg: *Intron A* (injection): In single-dose vials (6s), one 18 million IU multidose vial, or one 18 million IU multidose pen. *Rebetol* (capsules): (REBETOL 200 MG). White. In 84s.
			Dose reduction: *Intron A* (injection): In single-dose vials (6s), one 18 million IU multidose vial, or one 18 million IU multidose pen. *Rebetol* (capsules): (REBETOL 200 MG). White. In 42s.

INTERFERON ALFA-2b, RECOMBINANT AND RIBAVIRIN COMBINATION

For complete and comparative prescribing information, refer to the individual interferon alfa-2b and ribavirin monographs.

WARNING

Combination ribavirin/interferon alfa-2b therapy is contraindicated in women who are pregnant and in the male partners of women who are pregnant. Extreme care must be taken to avoid pregnancy during therapy and for 6 months after completion of treatment in female patients, and in female partners of male patients who are taking combination ribavirin/interferon alfa-2b therapy. Women of childbearing potential and men must use 2 reliable forms of effective contraception during treatment and during the 6-month posttreatment follow-up period. Significant teratogenic or embryocidal effects have been demonstrated for ribavirin in all animal species studied. Ribavirin monotherapy is not effective for the treatment of chronic hepatitis C and should not be used for this indication. Alpha interferons, including interferon alfa-2b, cause or aggravate fatal or life-threatening neuropsychiatric, autoimmune, ischemic, and infectious disorders. Closely monitor patients with periodic clinical and laboratory elevations. Withdraw patients from therapy who have persistently severe or worsening signs or symptoms of these conditions. In many, but not all cases, these disorders resolve after stopping interferon alfa-2b therapy.

Indications

➤*Hepatitis C:* Treatment of chronic hepatitis C in patients with compensated liver disease previously untreated with alpha interferon or who have relapsed following alpha interferon therapy.

See the Warning box for more information.

Administration and Dosage

Administer interferon alfa-2b SC and ribavirin orally without regard to food. Hydrate patients well, especially during initial treatment stages.

➤*Pregnancy:* See the Warning box for more information.

➤*Recommended dose:*

Recommended Interferon Alfa-2b/Ribavirin Combination Dosing

Body weight	Ribavirin	Interferon alfa-2b injection
≤ 75 kg	400 mg am PO 600 mg pm PO	3 million IU 3 times/week SC
> 75 kg	600 mg am PO 600 mg pm PO	

➤*Dose modifications:* If severe adverse reactions or laboratory abnormalities develop during combination therapy, modify the dose, or discontinue if appropriate, until the adverse reactions abate. If intolerance persists after dose adjustment, discontinue therapy.

It is recommended that patients who experience moderate depression (persistent low mood, loss of interest, poor self image, or hopelessness) have their interferon alfa-2b dose temporarily reduced or be considered for medical therapy. Discontinue treatment in patients experiencing severe depression or suicidal ideation/attempt from combination therapy and follow closely with appropriate medical management.

Interferon Alfa-2b/Ribavirin Combination Dose Modification Guidelines

Parameter	Dose reduction[1] ribavirin - 600 mg/day, interferon alfa-2b - 1.5 million IU 3 times/week	Permanent discontinuation of combination treatment
Hemoglobin	< 10 g/dL (reduce ribavirin) *Cardiac history patients only:* ≥ 2 g/dL decrease during any 4-week period during treatment (reduce ribavirin/ interferon alfa-2b)	< 8.5 g/dL *Cardiac history patients only:* < 12 g/dL after 4 weeks of dose reduction
White blood count	< 1.5 × 10^9/L (reduce interferon alfa-2b)	< 1 × 10^9/L

Interferon Alfa-2b/Ribavirin Combination Dose Modification Guidelines

Parameter	Dose reduction[1] ribavirin - 600 mg/day, interferon alfa-2b - 1.5 million IU 3 times/week	Permanent discontinuation of combination treatment
Neutrophil count	< 0.75 × 10^9/L (reduce interferon alfa-2b)	< 0.5 × 10^9/L
Platelet count	< 50 × 10^9/L (reduce interferon alfa-2b)	< 25 × 10^9/L

[1] Medication to be reduced in dose is shown in parentheses.

➤*Administration of interferon alfa-2b injection:* At the discretion of the physician, the patient may self-administer interferon alfa-2b.

Withdraw the appropriate dose from the vial or set on the multidose pen and inject SC. After administration, follow the procedure for proper disposal of syringes and needles.

Administration of Interferon Alfa-2b Injection

Vial/Pen label strength	Fill volume	Concentration
3 million IU vial	0.5 mL	3 million IU/0.5 mL
18 million IU multidose vial[1]	3.8 mL	3 million IU/0.5 mL
18 million IU multidose pen[2]	1.5 mL	3 million IU/0.2 mL

[1] This is a multidose vial that contains 22.8 million IU of interferon alfa-2b/3.8 mL in order to provide the delivery of six 0.5 mL doses, each containing 3 million IU of interferon alfa-2b (for a label strength of 18 million IU).

[2] This is a multidose pen that contains a 22.5 million IU of interferon alfa-2b/1.5 mL in order to provide the delivery of six 0.2 mL doses, each containing 3 million IU of interferon alfa-2b (for a label strength of 18 million IU).

➤*Treatment duration:* The recommended duration of treatment for patients previously untreated with interferon is 24 to 48 weeks. Individualize the duration of treatment to the patient depending on baseline disease characteristics, response to therapy, and tolerability of the regimen. After 24 weeks of treatment, assess virologic response. Consider treatment discontinuation in any patient who has not achieved an HCV RNA below the limit of detection of the assay by 24 weeks. There are no safety and efficacy data on treatment for > 48 weeks in the previously untreated patient population.

➤*Storage/Stability:* Interferon alfa-2b injection in vials is stable at 35°C (95°F) for ≤ 7 days and at 30°C (86°F) for ≤ 14 days; the multidose pen is stable at 30°C (86°F) for ≤ 2 days.

Refrigerate the combination package or the individual cartons between 2° and 8°C (36° and 46°F). The ribavirin carton may alternately be stored at 25°C (77°F).

Precautions

➤*Monitoring:* The following laboratory tests are recommended for all patients on combination therapy, prior to beginning treatment and then periodically thereafter: Standard hematologic tests including hemoglobin (pretreatment, week 2 and week 4 of therapy, and as clinically appropriate), complete and differential white blood cell counts, and platelet count; liver function tests and TSH; pregnancy including monthly monitoring for women of childbearing potential.

➤*Cardiac disease:* Administer therapy with caution to patients with preexisting cardiac disease. Assess patients before commencement of therapy and appropriately monitor them during therapy. If there is any deterioration of cardiovascular status, stop therapy.

➤*Renal function impairment:* Administer with caution in patients with Ccr < 50 mL/min.

Patient Information

Advise patients (male and female) to practice adequate contraception (2 reliable forms) during combination therapy and to notify the physician in the event of pregnancy.

Advise female patients of the need to perform a pregnancy test monthly during therapy and for 6 months post-therapy.

INTERFERON ALFACON-1

Rx	**Infergen** (InterMune)	**Injection:** 9 mcg	Preservative free. In 0.3 mL single-dose vials.
		15 mcg	Preservative free. In 0.5 mL single-dose vials.

INTERFERON ALFACON-1 — INJECTION

For complete and comparative prescribing information on interferon-alfa 2a and -alfa 2b, refer to the individual monographs.

WARNING

Alpha interferons, including interferon alfacon-1, cause or aggravate fatal or life-threatening neuropsychiatric, autoimmune, ischemic, and infectious disorders.

Patients should be monitored closely with periodic clinical and laboratory evaluations. Patients with persistently severe or worsening symptoms of these conditions should be withdrawn from therapy. In many but not all cases, these disorders resolve after stopping interferon alfacon-1 therapy.

Indications

➤*Chronic hepatis C:* Interferon alfacon-1 is indicated for the treatment of chronic hepatitis C virus (HCV) infection in patients 18 years of age or older with compensated liver disease who have anti-HCV serum antibodies or the presence of HCV RNA. Other causes of hepatitis, such as viral hepatitis B or autoimmune hepatitis should be ruled out prior to initiation of therapy with interferon alfacon-1. In some patients with chronic HCV infection, interferon alfacon-1 normalizes serum ALT, reduces serum HCV RNA concentrations to undetectable quantities (less than 100 copies/mL), and improves liver histology.

Administration and Dosage

➤*Approved by the FDA:* October 6, 1997.

➤*Recommended dose:* 9 mcg 3 times a week administered SC as a single injection for 24 weeks. At least 48 hours should elapse between doses of interferon alfacon-1.

Patients who tolerated previous interferon therapy and did not respond or relapsed following its discontinuation may be subsequently treated with 15 mcg of interferon alfacon-1 three times a week administered subcutaneously as a single injection for up to 48 weeks (see illustrated Medication Guide for instructions).

There are significant differences in specific activities among interferons. Health care providers should be aware that changes in interferon brand may require adjustments of dosage or change in route of administration. Patients should be warned not to change brands of interferon without medical consultation. Patients should also be instructed by their physician not to reduce the dosage of interferon alfacon-1 prior to medical consultation.

➤*Dose reduction:* For patients who experience a severe adverse reaction on interferon alfacon-1, dosage should be withheld temporarily. If the adverse reaction does not become tolerable, therapy should be discontinued. Dose reduction to 7.5 mcg may be necessary following an intolerable adverse event. In the pivotal study, 11% of patients (26 per 231) who initially received interferon alfacon-1 at a dose of 9 mcg (0.3 mL) were dose reduced to 7.5 mcg (0.25 mL).

If adverse reactions continue to occur at the reduced dosage, the physician may discontinue treatment or reduce dosage further. However, decreased efficacy may result from continued treatment at dosages less than 7.5 mcg.

During subsequent treatment with 15 mcg of interferon alfacon-1, up to 36% of patients required dose reductions in 3 mcg increments.

➤*Storage/Stability:* Interferon alfacon-1 should be stored in the refrigerator at 2° to 8°C (36° to 46°F). Do not freeze. Avoid vigorous shaking and exposure to direct sunlight. Just prior to injection, interferon alfacon-1 may be allowed to reach room temperature.

Actions

➤*Pharmacology:* Interferons are a family of naturally occurring small protein molecules with molecular weights of 15,000 to 21,000 daltons that are produced and secreted by cells in response to viral infections or to various synthetic and biological inducers. Two major classes of interferons have been identified (ie, type I and type II). Type I interferons include a family of greater than 25 alpha interferons as well as beta interferon and omega interferon. While all alpha interferons have similar biological effects, not all the activities are shared by each alpha interferon and, in many cases, the extent of activity varies substantially for each interferon subtype.

All type I interferons share common biological activities generated by binding of interferon to the cell-surface receptor, leading to the production of several interferon-stimulated gene products. Type I interferons induce pleiotropic biologic responses which include antiviral, antiproliferative and immunomodulatory effects, regulation of cell surface major histocompatibility antigen (HLA class I and class II) expression and regulation of cytokine expression. Examples of interferon-stimulated gene products include 2′5′ oligoadenylate synthetase (2′5′ OAS) and β-2 microglobulin.

The antiviral, antiproliferative, natural killer (NK) cell activation, and gene-induction activities of interferon alfacon-1 have been compared with other recombinant alpha interferons in in vitro assays and have demonstrated similar ranges of activity. Interferon alfacon-1 exhibited at least 5 times higher specific activity in vitro than interferon alfa-2a and interferon alfa-2b. Comparison of interferon alfacon-1 with a WHO international potency standard for recombinant interferon alfa (83/514) revealed that the specific activity of interferon alfacon-1 in both an in vitro antiviral cytopathic effect assay and an antiproliferative assay was 1×10^9 units/mg. However, correlation between in vitro activity and clinical activity of any interferon is unknown.

➤*Pharmacokinetics:* The pharmacokinetic properties of interferon alfacon-1 have not been evaluated in patients with chronic hepatitis C. Pharmacokinetic profiles were evaluated in healthy volunteer subjects after subcutaneous injection of 1, 3, or 9 mcg interferon alfacon-1. Plasma levels of interferon alfacon-1 after subcutaneous administration of any dose were too low to be detected by either ELISA or by inhibition of viral cytopathic effect. However, analysis of interferon alfacon-1-induced cellular products (induction of 2′5′ OAS and β-2 microglobulin) after treatment in these subjects revealed a statistically significant, dose-related increase in the area under the curve (AUC) for the levels of 2′5′ OAS or β-2 microglobulin induced over time ($P < 0.001$ for all comparisons). Concentrations of 2′5′ OAS were maximal at 24 hours after dosing, while serum levels of β-2 microglobulin appeared to reach a maximum 24 to 36 hours after dosing. The dose-response relationships observed for 2′5′ OAS and β-2 microglobulin were indicative of biological activity after subcutaneous administration of 1 to 9 mcg interferon alfacon-1.

Contraindications

Hypersensitivity to alpha interferons, to *E. coli*-derived products, or to any component of the product.

Warnings

➤*General:* Treatment with interferon alfacon-1 should be administered under the guidance of a qualified physician, and may lead to moderate-to-severe adverse experiences requiring dose reduction, temporary dose cessation, or discontinuation of further therapy.

➤*Discontinuation:* Withdrawal from study for adverse events occurred in 7% of patients initially treated with 9 mcg interferon alfacon-1 (including 4% due to psychiatric events). Withdrawal from study due to adverse events occurred in 5% of patients subsequently treated with 15 mcg interferon alfacon-1 for 24 weeks and 11% of patients subsequently treated with 15 mcg interferon alfacon-1 for 48 weeks.

➤*CNS effects:* Severe psychiatric adverse events may manifest in patients receiving therapy with alpha interferon, including interferon alfacon-1. Depression, suicidal ideation, and suicide attempt may occur. The incidence of psychiatric events of suicidal ideation was small (1%) for patients treated with 9 mcg interferon alfacon-1 compared to the overall incidence (55%) of psychiatric events. Interferon alfacon-1 should be used with caution in patients who report a history of depression and physicians should monitor all patients for evidence of depression. Physicians should inform patients of the possible development of depression prior to initiation of interferon alfacon-1 therapy, and patients should report any sign or symptom of depression immediately. Other prominent psychiatric adverse events may also occur, including nervousness, anxiety, emotional lability, abnormal thinking, agitation, or apathy.

Since the use of type I interferons has been associated with depression, interferon alfacon-1 therapy should not be used in patients with a history of severe psychiatric disorders and should be discontinued in patients developing severe depression, suicidal ideation, or other severe psychiatric disorders.

➤*Cardiac effects:* Interferon alfacon-1 should be administered with caution to patients with preexisting cardiac disease. Hypertension and supraventricular arrhythmias, chest pain and MI have been associated with interferon therapies.

Interferon alfacon-1 should be used with caution in patients with a history of cardiac disease. Hypertension (5%), tachycardia (4%), and palpitation (3%) were the most common cardiovascular adverse events reported for 9 mcg interferon alfacon-1 therapy, with 1% of patients reporting tachyarrhythmias which were dose limiting.

➤*Bone marrow toxicity:* Alpha interferons suppress bone marrow function and may result in severe cytopenias including very rare events of aplastic anemia. It is advised that complete blood counts be obtained pretreatment and monitored routinely during therapy. Alpha interferon therapy should be discontinued in patients who develop severe decreases in neutrophil (less than 0.5×10^9/L) or platelet counts (less than 50×10^9/L).

➤*Ophthalmologic disorders:* Decrease or loss of vision, retinopathy including macular edema, retinal artery or vein thrombosis, retinal hemorrhages and cotton wool spots, optic neuritis, and papilledema are induced or aggravated by treatment with interferon alfacon-1 or other alpha interferons. All patients should receive an eye examination at baseline. Patients with preexisting ophthalmologic disorders (eg, diabetic or hypertensive retinopathy) should receive periodic ophthalmologic exams during interferon alpha treatment. Any patient who develops ocular symptoms should receive a prompt and complete eye examination. Interferon alfacon-1 therapy should be discontinued in patients who develop new or worsening ophthalmologic disorders.

➤*Hypersensitivity reactions:* Serious acute hypersensitivity reactions have been reported in rare instances following treatment with alpha interferons. If hypersensitivity reactions occur (eg, urticaria, angioedema, bron-

INTERFERON ALFACON-1 — INJECTION

choconstriction, anaphylaxis), the drug should be discontinued immediately and appropriate medical treatment instituted.

➤*Hepatic function impairment:* No studies with interferon alfacon-1 have been conducted in patients with decompensated hepatic disease. Patients with decompensated hepatic disease should not be treated with interferon alfacon-1, and patients who develop symptoms of hepatic decompensation, such as jaundice, ascites, coagulopathy, or decreased serum albumin, should halt further interferon therapy.

➤*Elderly:* Clinical studies of interferon alfacon-1 did not include sufficient numbers of subjects aged 65 years and over to determine whether they respond differently than younger subjects. Other reported clinical experience has not identified differences in responses between the elderly and younger patients. However, treatment with interferons, including interferon alfacon-1, is associated with psychiatric, cardiac, and systemic (flu-like) adverse effects. Since decreased hepatic, renal or cardiac function, concomitant disease and the use of other drug therapies in elderly patients may produce adverse reactions of greater severity, caution should be exercised in the use of interferon alfacon-1 in this population.

➤*Pregnancy: Category C.* Interferon alfacon-1 has been shown to have embryolethal or abortifacient effects in golden Syrian hamsters when given at 135 times the human dose and in cynomolgus and rhesus monkeys when given at 9 to 81 times (based on body surface area) the human dose. There are no adequate and well-controlled studies in pregnant women. Interferon alfacon-1 should not be used during pregnancy. If a woman becomes pregnant or plans to become pregnant while taking interferon alfacon-1, she should be informed of the potential hazards to the fetus. Males and females treated with interferon alfacon-1 should be advised to use effective contraception.

➤*Lactation:* It is not known whether interferon alfacon-1 is excreted in human milk. Because many drugs are excreted in human milk, caution should be exercised if interferon alfacon-1 is administered to a nursing woman. The effect on the nursing neonate of oral interferon alfacon-1 in breast milk has not been evaluated.

➤*Children:* The safety and effectiveness of interferon alfacon-1 have not been established in patients younger than 18 years. Interferon alfacon-1 therapy is not recommended in pediatric patients.

Precautions

➤*Monitoring:* Laboratory tests are recommended for all patients on interferon alfacon-1 therapy, prior to beginning treatment (baseline), 2 weeks after initiation of therapy, and periodically thereafter during the 24 or 48 weeks of therapy at the discretion of the physician. Following completion of interferon alfacon-1 therapy, any abnormal test values should be monitored periodically. The entrance criteria that were used for the clinical study of interferon alfacon-1 may be considered as a guideline to acceptable baseline values for initiation of treatment:

- Platelet count greater than or equal to 75×10^9/L.
- Hemoglobin concentration greater than or equal to 100 g/L.
- ANC greater than or equal to $1,500 \times 10^6$/L.
- Serum creatinine concentration less than 180 mcmol/L (less than 2 mg/dL) or creatinine clearance greater than 0.83 mL/second (greater than 50 mL/min).
- Serum albumin concentration greater than or equal to 25 g/L.
- Bilirubin within normal limits.
- TSH and T_4 within normal limits.

Neutropenia, thrombocytopenia, hypertriglyceridemia, and thyroid disorders have been reported with administration of interferon alfacon-1. Therefore, these laboratory parameters should be monitored closely.

➤*Autoimmune disease:* Exacerbation of autoimmune disease has been reported in patients receiving type I interferon therapy. Interferon alfacon-1 should not be used in patients with autoimmune hepatitis and should be used with caution in patients with other autoimmune disorders.

➤*Fever:* While fever may be related to the flu-like symptoms reported in patients treated with interferon alfacon-1, when fever occurs, other possible causes of persistent fever should be ruled out.

➤*Endocrine disorders:* Interferon alfacon-1 should be administered with caution to patients with a history of endocrine disorders. Abnormal thyroid-stimulating hormone (TSH) and free thyroxine (T_4) level with hypothyroidism occurred in 4% of patients administered 9 mcg interferon alfacon-1, and thyroid supplements were required in approximately two-thirds of those patients.

➤*Special risk:* Interferon alfacon-1 should be used cautiously in patients with abnormally low peripheral blood cell counts or who are receiving agents that are known to cause myelosuppression. Transplantation patients, or other chronically immunosuppressed patients, should receive interferon alfacon-1 therapy with caution.

Drug Interactions

Interferon Alfacon-1 Drug Interactions

Precipitant Drug	Object Drug*		Description
Interferon alfacon-1	Myelosuppressive agents	↑	Use caution when administering with other agents known to cause myelosuppression.
Myelosuppressive agents	Interferon alfacon-1		

Interferon Alfacon-1 Drug Interactions

Precipitant Drug	Object Drug*		Description
Interferon alfacon-1	Drugs metabolized by cytochrome P450	↔	Use caution when administering to patients who are receiving agents metabolized via cytochrome P450, and monitor closely for changes in therapeutic and/or toxic levels of these concomitant drugs.

* ↑ = Object drug increased. ↔ = Undetermined clinical effect.

Adverse Reactions

➤*Most frequent:* Most adverse events were mild to moderate in severity and abated with cessation of therapy. Flu-like symptoms (ie, headache, fatigue, fever, rigors, myalgia, increased sweating, and arthralgia) were the most frequently reported treatment-related adverse reactions. Most were short lived and could be treated symptomatically.

➤*Depression:* Depression, usually mild to moderate in severity, was reported in 26% of patients who received 9 mcg interferon alfacon-1 and was the most common adverse event resulting in study drug discontinuation.

Patient Incidence of Adverse Events in Phase 3 Clinical Trials Regardless of Attribution[a]

Body system/ Preferred term	Initial treatment[b]		Subsequent treatment[b]	
	Interferon alfacon-1 9 mcg	IFN α-2b	Interferon alfacon-1 15 mcg, 24 weeks	Interferon alfacon-1 15 mcg, 48 weeks
	(n = 231)	(n = 236)	(n = 165)	(n = 168)
	% of patients		% of patients	
Application site				
Injection site erythema	23%	15%	17%	22%
Injection site pain	9%	3%	8%	11%
Injection site ecchymosis	6%	7%	5%	5%
Miscellaneous				
Fatigue	69%	67%	65%	71%
Fever	61%	45%	58%	55%
Rigors	57%	45%	62%	66%
Body pain	54%	45%	39%	51%
Influenza-like symptoms[c]	15%	11%	8%	8%
Pain chest	13%	14%	5%	9%
Hot flushes	13%	7%	7%	4%
Malaise	11%	10%	2%	5%
Asthenia	9%	11%	10%	7%
Edema peripheral	9%	8%	4%	3%
Access pain	8%	9%	1%	1%
Allergic reaction	7%	5%	3%	4%
Weight decrease	5%	7%	5%	2%
Cardiovascular				
Hypertension	5%	3%	2%	4%
Palpitation	3%	6%	5%	2%
CNS/PNS				
Headache	82%	83%	78%	80%
Insomnia	39%	30%	24%	28%
Dizziness	22%	25%	18%	25%
Paresthesia	13%	10%	9%	9%
Hypoesthesia	10%	8%	8%	10%
Amnesia	10%	6%	2%	5%
Hypertonia	7%	10%	6%	6%
Somnolence	4%	8%	6%	7%
Confusion	4%	6%	4%	5%
Hyperesthesia	1%	1%	1%	5%
Endocrine				
Abnormal thyroid test	9%	5%	4%	6%
GI				
Abdominal pain	41%	40%	24%	32%
Nausea	40%	36%	30%	36%
Diarrhea	29%	24%	24%	22%

INTERFERON ALFACON-1 — INJECTION

Patient Incidence of Adverse Events in Phase 3 Clinical Trials Regardless of Attribution[a]

Body system/ Preferred term	Initial treatment[b]		Subsequent treatment[b]	
	Interferon alfacon-1 9 mcg	IFN α-2b	Interferon alfacon-1 15 mcg, 24 weeks	Interferon alfacon-1 15 mcg, 48 weeks
	(n = 231)	(n = 236)	(n = 165)	(n = 168)
	% of patients		% of patients	
Anorexia	24%	17%	21%	14%
Dyspepsia	21%	18%	12%	10%
Vomiting	12%	11%	13%	11%
Constipation	9%	6%	5%	6%
Flatulence	8%	9%	6%	5%
Toothache	7%	7%	3%	7%
Saliva decreased	6%	7%	4%	1%
Hemorrhoids	6%	3%	1%	2%
Stomatitis ulcerative	3%	4%	2%	6%
Gingivitis	2%	3%	1%	5%
Special senses				
Tinnitus	6%	4	4	2
Earache	5%	7%	5%	5%
Otitis	2%	5%	1%	3%
Taste perversion	3%	6%	3%	5%
Hematologic				
Granulocytopenia	23%	25%	42%	39%
Thrombocytopenia	19%	16%	18%	18%
Leukopenia	15%	13%	19%	28%
Lymphadenopathy	6%	8%	4%	4%
Ecchymosis	6%	4%	4%	2%
Lymphocytosis	5%	7%	11%	5%
PT increased	3%	5%	1%	0%
Anemia	2%	3%	2%	6%
Hepatic				
Liver tenderness	5%	3%	6%	2%
Hepatomegaly	3%	5%	5%	2%
Metabolic/nutritional				
Hypertriglyceridemia	6%	7%	5%	5%
Musculoskeletal				
Myalgia	58%	56%	51%	55%
Arthralgia	51%	44%	43%	46%
Back pain	42%	37%	29%	23%
Limb pain	26%	25%	13%	23%
Skeletal pain	14%	14%	10%	12%
Neck pain	14%	13%	8%	5%
Musculoskeletal disorder	4%	4%	7%	4%
Psychiatric				
Nervousness	31%	29%	16%	22%
Depression	26%	25%	18%	19%
Anxiety	19%	18%	9%	14%
Emotional lability	12%	11%	6%	3%
Thinking abnormal	8%	12%	10%	20%
Agitation	6%	6%	4%	4%
Libido decreased	5%	5%	5%	4%
Apathy	2%	3%	4%	5%
GU (female)				
Dysmenorrhea	9%	9%	2%	7%
Vaginitis	8%	2%	5%	5%
Menstrual disorder	6%	5%	2%	5%
Menorrhagia	3%	0%	2%	5%
Moniliasis genital	2%	6%	2%	0%
Breast mass	0%	3%	0%	5%
Pain beast	0%	5%	2%	0%
Resistance mechanism				
Infection	3%	5%	2%	6%
Respiratory				
Pharyngitis	34%	31%	17%	21%
Upper respiratory tract infection	31%	34%	16%	18%
Cough	22%	17%	12%	11%
Sinusitis	17%	22%	12%	16%
Rhinitis	13%	16%	7%	9%
Respiratory tract congestion	12%	7%	4%	9%
Upper respiratory tract congestion	10%	14%	7%	9%
Epistaxis	8%	12%	6%	6%
Dyspnea	7%	12%	8%	7%
Bronchitis	6%	6%	2%	1%
Dermatologic				
Alopecia	14%	25%	10%	13%
Pruritus	14%	14%	11%	10%
Rash	13%	15%	13%	10%
Sweating increased	12%	11%	13%	11%
Erythema	6%	6%	7%	9%
Dry skin	6%	5%	2%	5%
Wound	4%	7%	3%	4%
Ophthalmic				
Conjunctivitis	8%	8%	4%	6%
Eye pain	5%	6%	4%	2%
Abnormal vision	3%	5%	5%	5%

[a] Only events that occurred at a frequency of greater than or equal to 5% in any treatment group are included. Patients can appear more than once in this table. Because the 2 studies were conducted at different times with nonidentical patient groups, the adverse events profile for the subsequent treatment study is not directly comparable to the initial treatment study.

[b] Adverse events reported in patients during treatment or posttreatment observation in the pivotal initial treatment and subsequent treatment studies are listed regardless of attribution to treatment.

[c] Influenza-like symptoms: Presumed viral etiology.

Overdosage

In interferon alfacon-1 trials, the maximum overdose reported was a dose of 150 mcg interferon alfacon-1 administered subcutaneous in a patient enrolled in a phase 1 advanced malignancy trial. The patient received 10 times the prescribed dosage for 3 days. The patient experienced a mild increase in anorexia, chills, fever, and myalgia. Increases in ALT (15 to 127 Units/L), aspartate transaminase (AST) (15 to 164 Units/L), and lactic dehydrogenase (LDH) (183 to 281 Units/L) were reported. These laboratory values returned to normal or to the patient's baseline values within 30 days.

Patient Information

If home use is determined to be desirable by the physician, instructions on appropriate use should be given by a health care professional. The patient must be instructed as to the proper dosage and administration. Information included in the Medication Guide should be fully reviewed with the patient; it is not a disclosure of all, or possible, adverse effects. The most common adverse reactions occurring with interferon alfacon-1 therapy are flu-like symptoms including fatigue, fever, rigors, headache, arthralgia, myalgia, and increased sweating. Nonnarcotic analgesics and bedtime administration of interferon alfacon-1 may be used to prevent or lessen some of these symptoms. Additionally, patients must be thoroughly instructed in the importance of proper disposal procedures and cautioned against the reuse of needles, syringes, or re-entry of the drug product. A puncture-resistant container for the disposal of used syringes and needles should be used by the patient and should be disposed of according to the directions provided by the health care provider.

INTERFERON ALFA-N3 (HUMAN LEUKOCYTE DERIVED)

Rx	**Alferon N** (Interferon Sciences, Inc.)	**Injection:** 5 million IU/ml	8 mg NaCl, 1.74 mg Na phosphate dibasic, 0.2 mg K phosphate monobasic, 0.2 mg KCl. In 1 ml vials.

INTERFERON ALFA-n3 — INJECTION

Indications

➤*Condylomata acuminata:* For the intralesional treatment of refractory or recurring external condylomata acuminata in patients 18 years of age or older (see Administration and Dosage).

The physician should select patients for treatment with interferon alfa-n3 (human leukocyte derived) after consideration of a number of factors: The locations and sizes of the lesions, past treatment and response thereto, and the patient's ability to comply with the treatment regimen. Interferon alfa-n3 (human leukocyte derived) is particularly useful for patients who have not responded satisfactorily to other treatment modalities (eg, podophyllin resin, surgery, laser or cryotherapy).

Administration and Dosage

➤*Approved by the FDA:* 1989.

➤*Recommended dose:* 0.05 mL (250,000 IU) per wart. Interferon alfa-n3 (human leukocyte derived) should be administered twice weekly for up to 8 weeks. The maximum recommended dose per treatment session is 0.5 mL (2.5 million IU). Interferon alfa-n3 (human leukocyte derived) should be injected into the base of each wart, preferably using a 30 gauge needle. For large warts, interferon alfa-n3 (human leukocyte derived) may be injected at several points around the periphery of the wart, using a total dose of 0.05 mL per wart.

➤*Duration of therapy:* Genital warts usually begin to disappear after several weeks of treatment with interferon alfa-n3 (human leukocyte derived). Treatment should continue for a maximum of 8 weeks. In clinical trials with interferon alfa-n3 (human leukocyte derived), many patients who had partial resolution of warts during treatment experienced further resolution of their warts after cessation of treatment. Of the patients who had complete resolution of warts due to treatment, half the patients had complete resolution of warts by the end of the treatment and half had complete resolution of warts during the 3 months after cessation of treatment. Thus, it is recommended that no further therapy (interferon alfa-n3 [human leukocyte derived] or conventional therapy) be administered for 3 months after the initial 8-week course of treatment unless the warts enlarge or new warts appear. Studies to determine the safety and efficacy of a second course of treatment with interferon alfa-n3 (human leukocyte derived) have not been conducted.

➤*Storage / Stability:* Interferon alfa-n3 (human leukocyte derived) should be stored at 2° to 8°C (36° to 46°F). Do not freeze. Do not shake.

Actions

➤*Pharmacology:* Interferons are naturally occurring proteins with antiviral, antiproliferative and immunoregulatory properties. They are produced and secreted in response to viral infections and to a variety of other synthetic and biological inducers. Four major families of interferons have been identified: Alpha, beta, gamma and omega. The interferon alpha family contains 13 different nonallelic molecular species. Their molecular weights range from 16,000 to 27,000 daltons.

Interferons bind to specific membrane receptors on cell surfaces. Interferon alfa-n3 has been shown to bind to the same receptors as Interferon alfa-2b. The receptors have a high degree of selectivity for the binding of human but not mouse interferon. This correlates with the high species specificity found in laboratory studies.

Binding of interferon to membrane receptors initiates a series of events including induction of protein synthesis. These actions are followed by a variety of cellular responses, including inhibition of virus replication and suppression of cell proliferation. Immunomodulation, including enhancement of phagocytosis by macrophages, augmentation of the cytotoxicity of lymphocytes and enhancement of human leukocyte antigen expression occurs in response to exposure to interferons. One or more of these activities may contribute to the therapeutic effect of interferon.

➤*Pharmacokinetics:* In a study of intralesional use of interferon alfa-n3 (human leukocyte derived) for the treatment of condylomata acuminata, plasma concentrations of interferon were below the detection limit of the assay, ie, less than 3 IU/mL. Minor systemic effects (eg, myalgias, fever, and headaches) were noted, indicating that some of the injected interferon entered the systemic circulation (see Adverse Reactions).

Contraindications

Hypersensitivity to human interferon alpha proteins or any component of the product. The product is also contraindicated in patients who have anaphylactic sensitivity to mouse immunoglobulin (IgG), egg protein or neomycin.

Warnings

➤*Special risk patients:* Because of the fever and other "flu-like" symptoms associated with interferon alfa-n3 (human leukocyte derived) (see Adverse Reactions), it should be used cautiously in patients with debilitating medical conditions such as cardiovascular disease (eg, unstable angina and uncontrolled congestive heart failure), severe pulmonary disease (eg, chronic obstructive pulmonary disease), or diabetes mellitus with ketoacidosis.

Interferon alfa-n3 (human leukocyte derived) should be used cautiously in patients with coagulation disorders (eg, thrombophlebitis, pulmonary embolism and hemophilia), severe myelosuppression, or seizure disorders. Acute, serious hypersensitivity reactions (eg, urticaria, angioedema, bronchoconstriction, and anaphylaxis) have not been observed in patients receiving interferon alfa-n3 (human leukocyte derived). However, if such reactions develop, drug administration should be discontinued immediately and appropriate medical therapy should be instituted.

Because this product is made from human blood, it may carry a risk of transmitting infectious agents (eg, viruses) and theoretically, the Creutzfeldt-Jakob disease (CJD) agent.

➤*Fertility impairment:* In studies with adult females, interferon alpha has been shown to affect the menstrual cycle and decrease serum estradiol and progesterone levels.

Interferon alfa-n3 (human leukocyte derived) should be used with caution in fertile men. Fertile women should be cautioned to use effective contraception while being treated with interferon alfa-n3 (human leukocyte derived).

➤*Pregnancy: Category C.* Animal reproduction studies have not been conducted with interferon alfa-n3 (human leukocyte derived). It is also not known whether interferon alfa-n3 (human leukocyte derived) can cause fetal harm when administered to a pregnant woman or can affect reproductive capacity. Interferon alfa-n3 (human leukocyte derived) should be given to a pregnant woman only if clearly needed.

Changes in the menstrual cycle and abortions have been reported to occur in non-human primates given extremely high doses of recombinant interferon alpha. In these studies, Macaca mulatta (rhesus monkeys) were given interferon daily by intramuscular injection. Abortifacient effects were noted when the recombinant interferon alpha was given daily during early to mid-gestation at intramuscular doses of 978 times the average intralesional dose of interferon alfa-n3 (human leukocyte derived) (360 times the maximum recommended dose).

➤*Lactation:* It is not known whether interferon alfa-n3 (human leukocyte derived) is excreted in human milk. Studies in mice have shown that mouse interferons are excreted in milk. Because many drugs are excreted in human milk and because of the potential for serious adverse reactions in nursing infants, a decision should be made whether to discontinue nursing or to not initiate drug treatment, taking into account the importance of the drug to the mother and the potential risks to the infant.

➤*Children:* Safety and effectiveness have not been established in patients less than 18 years of age.

Precautions

➤*Interchangeability:* Patients being treated with interferon alfa-n3 (human leukocyte derived) should be informed of the benefits and risks associated with the treatment. Because the manufacturing process, strength, and type of interferon (eg, natural, human leukocyte interferon versus single-species recombinant interferon) may vary for different interferon formulations, changing brands may require a change in dosage. Therefore, physicians are cautioned not to change from one interferon product to another without considering these factors.

Adverse Reactions

➤*Adverse reactions in patients with condylomata acuminata:* The "flu-like" adverse reactions, consisting of fever, myalgias, or headache, occurred primarily after the first treatment session and were reported by 30% of the patients. The frequency of "flu-like" adverse reactions abated with repeated dosing of interferon alfa-n3 (human leukocyte derived) so that the incidences due to interferon alfa-n3 (human leukocyte derived) and placebo were similar after 3 to f4 weeks of treatment (after 6 to 8 treatment sessions). "Flu-like" symptoms were relieved by administration of acetaminophen.

Adverse reactions were reported at least once during the course of treatment in the following percentages of patients in each treatment group:

Percent of patients with adverse reactions		
Adverse reactions	Interferon alfa-n3 (n = 104)	Placebo (n = 85)
Autonomic nervous system		
Sweating	2%	1%
Vasovagal reaction	2%	0%
Miscellaneous		
Fever	40%	19%
Chills	14%	2%
Fatigue	14%	6%
Malaise	9%	9%
Dermatologic		
Generalized pruritus	2%	0%
CNS/peripheral nervous system		
Dizziness	9%	4%
Insomnia	2%	1%

INTERFERON ALFA-n3 — INJECTION

Percent of patients with adverse reactions		
Adverse reactions	Interferon alfa-n3 (n = 104)	Placebo (n = 85)
GI		
Nausea	4%	7%
Vomiting	3%	0%
Dyspepsia/ heartburn	3%	1%
Diarrhea	2%	2%
Musculoskeletal		
Arthralgia	5%	1%
Back pain	4%	1%
Myalgias	45%	15%
Headache	31%	15%
Psychiatric		
Depression	2%	1%
Nasopharyngeal		
Drainage	2%	2%

Most of the systemic adverse reactions were mild or moderate. Severe systemic adverse reactions were reported by 18% of interferon alfa-n3 (human leukocyte derived)-treated patients and 13% of placebo-treated patients (not a statistically significant difference). Most of the severe systemic adverse reactions reported were "flu-like". Other severe systemic adverse reactions included back pain, insomnia, and sensitivity to allergens. Those adverse reactions which were reported by 1% of patients treated with interferon alfa-n3 (human leukocyte derived) in the double-blind trial include: Left groin lymph node swelling, tongue hyperaesthesia, thirst, tingling of legs/feet, hot sensation on bottom of feet, strange taste in mouth, increased salivation, heat intolerance, visual disturbances, pharyngitis, sensitivity to allergens, muscle cramps, nosebleed, throat tightness, and papular rash on neck. Additional adverse reactions which were reported by 1% of patients treated with placebo include: Pharyngitis, oral pain, penile discharge, cold, knuckle stiffness, herpes outbreak, cough, disorientation, and weight/appetite loss.

Additional adverse reactions which occurred only in open clinical trials of intralesional use of interferon alfa-n3 (human leukocyte derived) for treatment of condylomata acuminata were herpes labialis, hot flashes, nervousness, decrease in concentration, dysuria, photosensitivity, and swollen lymph nodes. These reactions occurred in 1% of the patients. One patient with a history of epilepsy, who was not taking anticonvulsant medication, had a grand mal seizure while being treated with interferon alfa-n3 (human leukocyte derived); this seizure was judged to be unrelated to interferon alfa-n3 (human leukocyte derived) administration.

➤*Local:* The frequency of application site disorders (such as itching and pain) for patients treated with interferon alfa-n3 (human leukocyte derived) was significantly less than that reported with placebo (12% versus 26%). No severe application site disorders were reported by patients treated with interferon alfa-n3 (human leukocyte derived), while 7% of placebo-treated patients reported severe disorders.

➤*Lab test abnormalities:* Abnormalities were seen with statistically equivalent frequencies in both the interferon alfa-n3 (human leukocyte derived) and placebo groups. None of the laboratory abnormalities were considered clinically significant. The abnormalities in the interferon alfa-n3 (human leukocyte derived)-treated patients consisted primarily of decreased WBC (11%). Decreases also occurred in 4% of the placebo patients (not a statistically significant difference). The abnormalities in interferon alfa-n3 (human leukocyte derived)-treated patients involved increases of only one WHO grade.

➤*Adverse reactions in patients with cancer:* The following adverse reactions were reported at least once (the percentage of patients experiencing the reaction is indicated in parenthesis): Chills (87%), fever (81%), anorexia (68%), malaise (65%), nausea (48%), vomiting (29%), myalgias (16%), arthralgia (10%), chest pains (10%), soreness at injection site (10%), sleepiness (10%), headache (10%), diarrhea (6%), fatigue (6%), low blood pressure (6%), sore mouth/stomatitis (6%), and blurred vision (6%). Those adverse reactions which were each reported by only one patient treated with interferon alfa-n3 (human leukocyte derived) include the following: Stiff shoulders, flushed face, edema, dry mouth, mucositis, coughing, numbness, numbness in hands, numbness in fingers, pain on ocular rotation, shakes/shivers, ringing in ears, cramps, constipation, muscle soreness, confusion, lightheadedness, depression, upset stomach, and sweating. The following adverse reactions were reported as severe by at least 1 patient (the percentage of patients experiencing the reaction is indicated in parentheses): Fever (55%), malaise (54%), anorexia (45%), chills (45%), nausea (16%), myalgias (13%), vomiting (10%), fatigue (6%), low blood pressure (6%), chest pains (6%), sore mouth/stomatitis (6%), headache (3%), diarrhea (3%), sleepiness (3%), arthralgia (3%), blurred vision (3%), stiff shoulders (3%), numbness (3%), pain on ocular rotation (3%), muscle soreness (3%), confusion (3%), lightheadedness (3%), depression (3%), and sweating (3%).

The number and percentage of patients with cancer who experienced a significant abnormal laboratory test value (values that changed from WHO Grades 0, 1, or 2 at baseline to WHO Grades 3 or 4 during or after treatment) at least once during the trials are shown in the following table:

Abnormal laboratory test values	
	Cancer (n = 31)
Hemoglobin level	2 (7%)
White blood cell count	1 (3%)
Platelet count	1 (3%)
GGT	1 (6%)
AST	1 (3%)
Alkaline phosphatase	2 (8%)
Total bilirubin	1 (4%)

Patient Information

Patients should be informed of the early signs of hypersensitivity reactions including hives, generalized urticaria, tightness of the chest, wheezing, hypotension and anaphylaxis, and should be advised to contact their physician if these symptoms occur.

Patients being treated with interferon alfa-n3 (human leukocyte derived) should be informed of benefits and risks associated with treatment. Patients should be cautioned not to change brands of interferon without medical consultation, as a change in dosage may occur.

INTERFERON GAMMA-1B

Rx	**Actimmune** (InterMune Pharm.)	**Injection:** 100 mcg (2 million IU)/0.5 ml	Preservative free. In single-dose vials.[a]

[a] With 20 mg mannitol, 0.36 mg sodium succinate, 0.05 mg polysorbate 20.

INTERFERON GAMMA-1B — INJECTION

Indications

➤*Chronic granulomatous disease:* For reducing the frequency and severity of serious infections associated with chronic granulomatous disease.

➤*Malignant osteopetrosis:* For delaying time to disease progression in patients with severe, malignant osteopetrosis.

Administration and Dosage

➤*Recommended dose:* 50 mcg/m^2 (1 million IU/m^2) for patients whose body surface area is > 0.5 m^2 and 1.5 mcg/kg/dose for patients whose body surface area is ≥ 0.5 m^2. Note that the above activity is expressed in International Units (1 million IU/50 mcg). This is equivalent to what was previously expressed as units (1.5 million U/50 mcg). Injections should be administered subcutaneously 3 times weekly (for example, Monday, Wednesday, Friday). The optimum sites of injection are the right and left deltoid and anterior thigh. Interferon gamma-1b can be administered by a physician, nurse, family member or patient when trained in the administration of subcutaneous injections.

➤*Preservative-Free:* The formulation does not contain a preservative. A vial of interferon gamma-1b is suitable for a single dose only. The unused portion of any vial should be discarded.

➤*Maximum dose:* Higher doses are not recommended. Safety and efficacy has not been established for interferon gamma-1b given in doses greater than or less than the recommended dose of 50 mcg/m^2. The minimum effective dose of interferon gamma-1b has not been established.

➤*Dose reduction:* If severe reactions occur, the dosage should be modified (50% reduction) or therapy should be discontinued until the adverse reaction abates.

➤*Administration:* Interferon gamma-1b may be administered using either sterilized glass or plastic disposable syringes.

➤*Storage/Stability:* Vials of interferon gamma-1b must be placed in a 2° to 8°C (36° to 46°F) refrigerator immediately upon receipt to ensure optimal retention of physical and biochemical integrity. Do not freeze. Avoid excessive or vigorous agitation. Do not shake. An unentered vial of interferon gamma-1b should not be left at room temperature for a total time exceeding 12 hours prior to use. Vials exceeding this time period should not be returned to the refrigerator; such vials should be discarded.

Actions

➤*Pharmacology:* Interferons are a family of functionally related, species-specific, proteins synthesized by eukaryotic cells in response to viruses and a variety of natural and synthetic stimuli. The most striking differences between interferon-gamma and other classes of interferon concern the immunomodulatory properties of this molecule. While gamma, alpha and beta interferons share certain properties, interferon-gamma has potent phagocyte-activating effects not seen with other interferon preparations. These effects include the generation of toxic oxygen metabolites within phagocytes in vitro, which are capable of mediating the intracellular killing of selected microorganisms such as *Staphylococcus aureus*, *Toxoplasma gondii*, *Leishmania donovani*, *Listeria monocytogenes*, and *Mycobacterium avium intracellulare*.

INTERFERON GAMMA-1B — INJECTION

Clinical studies in patients using interferon-gamma, have revealed a broad range of biological activities including the enhancement of the oxidative metabolism of tissue macrophages, enhancement of antibody-dependent cellular cytotoxicity (ADCC) and natural killer (NK) cell activity. Additionally, effects on Fc receptor expression on monocytes and major histocompatibility antigen expression have been noted.

To the extent that interferon-gamma is produced by antigen-stimulated T lymphocytes and regulates the activity of immune cells, it is appropriate to characterize interferon-gamma as a lymphokine of the interleukin type. There is growing evidence that interferon-gamma interacts functionally with other interleukin molecules such as interleukin-2 and that all of the interleukins form part of a complex, lymphokine regulatory network. For example, interferon-gamma and interleukin-4 appear to reciprocally interact to regulate murine IgE levels; interferon-gamma can suppress IgE levels in humans. Interferon-gamma also inhibits the production of collagen at the transcription level in human systems.

With respect to chronic granulomatous disease (an inherited disorder characterized by deficient phagocyte oxidative metabolism), pilot clinical trials of the systemic administration of interferon gamma-1b in patients with chronic granulomatous disease provided evidence for a treatment-related enhancement of phagocyte function including elevation of superoxide levels and improved killing of *Staphylococcus aureus*.

In severe, malignant osteopetrosis (another inherited disorder characterized by an osteoclast defect leading to bone overgrowth and deficient phagocyte oxidative metabolism), a treatment-related enhancement of superoxide production by phagocytes was observed in situ. Interferon gamma-1b was found to enhance osteoclast function in vitro.

➤*Pharmacokinetics:* The intravenous, intramuscular, and subcutaneous pharmacokinetics of interferon gamma-1b have been investigated in 24 healthy male subjects following single-dose administration of 100 mcg/m^2. Interferon gamma-1b is rapidly cleared after intravenous administration (1.4 L/min) and slowly absorbed after intramuscular or subcutaneous injection. After intramuscular or subcutaneous injection, the apparent fraction of dose absorbed was > 89%. The mean elimination half-life after intravenous administration of 100 mcg/m^2 in healthy male subjects was 38 minutes. The mean elimination half-lives for intramuscular and subcutaneous dosing with 100 mcg/m^2 were 2.9 and 5.9 hours, respectively. Peak plasma concentrations, determined by ELISA, occurred approximately 4 hours (1.5 ng/mL) after intramuscular dosing and 7 hours (0.6 ng/mL) after subcutaneous dosing. Multiple-dose subcutaneous pharmacokinetic studies were conducted in 38 healthy male subjects. There was no accumulation of interferon gamma-1b after 12 consecutive daily injections of 100 mcg/m^2. Pharmacokinetic studies in patients with chronic granulomatous disease have not been performed.

Trace amounts of interferon-gamma were detected in the urine of squirrel monkeys following intravenous administration of 500 mcg/kg. Interferon-gamma was not detected in the urine of healthy human volunteers following administration of 100 mcg/m^2 of interferon gamma-1b by the intravenous, intramuscular and subcutaneous routes. In vitro perfusion studies utilizing rabbit livers and kidneys demonstrate that these organs are capable of clearing interferon-gamma from perfusate. Studies of the administration of interferon-gamma to nephrectomized mice and squirrel monkeys demonstrate a reduction in clearance of interferon-gamma from blood; however, prior nephrectomy did not prevent elimination.

Contraindications

Hypersensitivity to interferon-gamma, *E. coli*-derived products, or any component of the product.

Warnings

➤*Cardiac effects:* Interferon gamma-1b should be used with caution in patients with preexisting cardiac disease, including symptoms of ischemia, congestive heart failure or arrhythmia. No direct cardiotoxic effect has been demonstrated but it is possible that acute and transient "flu-like" or constitutional symptoms such as fever and chills frequently associated with interferon gamma-1b administration at doses of 250 mcg/m^2/day or higher may exacerbate preexisting cardiac conditions.

➤*CNS effects:* Caution should be exercised when treating patients with known seizure disorders or compromised central nervous system function. CNS adverse reactions including decreased mental status, gait disturbance and dizziness have been observed, particularly in patients receiving doses > 250 mcg/m^2/day. Most of these abnormalities were mild and reversible within a few days upon dose reduction or discontinuation of therapy.

➤*Hematologic effects:* Caution should be exercised when administering interferon gamma-1b to patients with myelosuppression. Reversible neutropenia and elevation of hepatic enzymes can be dose limiting above 250 mcg/m^2/day. Thrombocytopenia and proteinuria have also been seen rarely.

➤*Hypersensitivity reactions:* Acute serious hypersensitivity reactions have not been observed in patients receiving interferon gamma-1b; however, if such an acute reaction develops, the drug should be discontinued immediately and appropriate medical therapy instituted. Transient cutaneous rashes have occurred in some patients following injection but have rarely necessitated treatment interruption.

➤*Fertility impairment:* Female cynomolgus monkeys treated with daily subcutaneous doses of 30 or 150 mcg/kg interferon gamma-1b (approximately 20 and 100 times the human dose) exhibited irregular menstrual cycles or absence of cyclicity during treatment. Similar findings were not observed in animals treated with 3 mcg/kg interferon gamma-1b. No studies have been performed assessing any potential effects of interferon gamma-1b on male fertility.

➤*Pregnancy: Category C.* Interferon gamma-1b has shown an increased incidence of abortions in primates when given in doses approximately 100 times the human dose. A study in pregnant primates treated with intravenous doses, 2 to 100 × the human dose failed to demonstrate teratogenic activity for interferon gamma-1b. There are no adequate and well-controlled studies in pregnant women. Interferon gamma-1b should be used during pregnancy only if the potential benefit justifies the potential risk to the fetus. In addition, studies evaluating recombinant murine interferon-gamma in pregnant mice, revealed increased incidences of uterine bleeding and abortifacient activity and decreased neonatal viability at maternally toxic doses. The clinical significance of this latter observation with recombinant murine interferon-gamma tested in a homologous system is uncertain.

➤*Lactation:* It is not known whether interferon gamma-1b is excreted in human milk. Because many drugs are excreted in human milk and because of the potential for serious adverse reactions in nursing infants from interferon gamma-1b, a decision should be made whether to discontinue nursing or to discontinue the drug, dependent upon the importance of the drug to the mother.

➤*Children:* Safety and effectiveness in children under the age of 1 year have not been established in patients with chronic granulomatous disease.

Precautions

➤*Monitoring:* In addition to those tests normally required for monitoring patients with chronic granulomatous disease and osteopetrosis, the following laboratory tests are recommended for all patients on interferon gamma-1b therapy prior to the beginning of and at 3-month intervals during treatment.

- Hematologic tests, including complete blood counts, differential and platelet counts
- Blood chemistries, including renal and liver function tests
- Urinalysis.

Drug Interactions

➤*CYP450 system:* Preclinical studies in rodents using species-specific interferon-gamma have demonstrated a decrease in hepatic microsomal cytochrome P450 concentrations. This could potentially lead to a depression of the hepatic metabolism of certain drugs that utilize this degradative pathway.

Adverse Reactions

The following data on adverse reactions are based on the subcutaneous administration of interferon gamma-1b at a dose of 50 mcg/m^2, three times weekly, in patients with chronic granulomatous disease (CGD) during an investigational trial in the United States and Europe.

The most common adverse events from this investigational trial of patients with chronic granulomatous disease are shown in the following table.

Interferon Gamma-1B Adverse Reactions

Clinical toxicity	Percent of patients: Interferon gamma-1B CGD (n = 63)	Placebo CGD (n = 65)
Fever	52%	28%
Headache	33%	9%
Rash	17%	6%
Chills	14%	0%
Injection site erythema or tenderness	14%	2%
Fatigue	14%	11%
Diarrhea	14%	12%
Vomiting	13%	5%
Nausea	10%	2%
Myalgia	6%	0%
Arthralgia	2%	0%
Injection site pain	0%	2%

Miscellaneous adverse reactions which occurred infrequently in patients with CGD and may have been related to underlying disease included back pain (2% vs 0%), abdominal pain (8% vs 3%) and depression (3% vs 0%) for interferon gamma-1b- and placebo-treated patients, respectively.

Similar safety data were observed in 34 patients with severe, malignant osteopetrosis.

➤*Interferon gamma-1b evaluated in additional disease state:* Interferon gamma-1b has also been evaluated in additional disease states in studies in which patients have generally received higher doses (> 100 mcg/m^2/day) administered by intramuscular injection or intravenous infusion. All of the previously described adverse reactions which occurred in patients with chronic granulomatous disease have also been observed in patients receiving higher doses. Adverse reactions not observed in patients with chronic granulomatous disease receiving doses < 100 mcg/m^2/day but seen rarely in patients receiving interferon gamma-1b in other studies include:

Cardiovascular – Hypotension, syncope, tachyarrhythmia, heart block, heart failure, and myocardial infarction.

CNS – Confusion, disorientation, gait disturbance, parkinsonian symptoms, seizure, hallucinations, and transient ischemic attacks.

INTERFERON GAMMA-1B — INJECTION

GI – Hepatic insufficiency, gastrointestinal bleeding, and pancreatitis.

Hematologic – Deep venous thrombosis and pulmonary embolism.

Lab test abnormalities – The incidence of abnormal hematologic, coagulation, hepatic and renal laboratory tests were similar between interferon gamma-1b and placebo treatment groups in the chronic granulomatous disease trial.

Metabolic – Hyponatremia and hyperglycemia.

Pulmonary – Tachypnea, bronchospasm, and interstitial pneumonitis.

Renal – Reversible renal insufficiency.

Miscellaneous – Exacerbation of dermatomyositis.

No neutralizing antibodies to interferon gamma-1b have been detected in any chronic granulomatous disease patients receiving interferon gamma-1b.

Patient Information

Patients being treated with interferon gamma-1b or their parents should be informed regarding the potential benefits and risks associated with treatment. If home use is determined to be desirable by the physician, instructions on appropriate use should be given, including review of the contents of the patient information insert. This information is intended to aid in the safe and effective use of the medication. It is not a disclosure of all possible adverse or intended effects.

If home use is prescribed, a puncture resistant container for the disposal of used syringes and needles should be supplied to the patient. Patients should be thoroughly instructed in the importance of proper disposal and cautioned against any reuse of needles and syringes. The full container should be disposed of according to the directions provided by the physician.

The most common adverse experiences occurring with interferon gamma-1b therapy are "flu-like" or constitutional symptoms such as fever, headache, chills, myalgia or fatigue (see Adverse Reactions) which may decrease in severity as treatment continues. Some of the "flu-like" symptoms may be minimized by bedtime administration. Acetaminophen may be used to prevent or partially alleviate the fever and headache.

The long-term effects of interferon gamma-1b therapy on growth, development or other parameters are not known.

INTERFERON BETA

Indications

➤*Multiple sclerosis (MS):* Treatment of MS. See individual monographs for specific indications.

Actions

➤*Pharmacology:* **Interferon beta-1a** is a 166 amino acid glycoprotein. It is produced by mammalian cells (Chinese hamster ovary cells) into which the human interferon beta gene has been introduced. The amino acid sequence of interferon beta-1a is identical to that of natural human interferon beta. **Interferon beta-1b** is manufactured by bacterial fermentation of a strain of *Escherichia coli* that bears a genetically engineered plasmid containing the gene for human interferon $beta_{ser17}$. Interferon beta-1b is a purified protein that has 165 amino acids. It does not include the carbohydrate side chains found in the natural material.

Interferons are a family of naturally occurring proteins and glycoproteins that are produced by eukaryotic cells in response to viral infection and other biological inducers. Interferon beta is produced by various cell types including fibroblasts and macrophages. Three major classes of interferons have been identified: Alpha, beta, and gamma; they each have overlapping yet distinct biologic activities.

Interferon beta has antiviral, antiproliferative, and immunoregulatory activities. The mechanisms by which it exerts its actions in MS are not clearly understood. However, it is known that the binding of interferon beta to its receptors initiates a complex cascade of intracellular events that leads to the expression of numerous interferon-induced gene products and markers, including 2′,5′-oligoadenylate synthetase, beta 2-microglobulin, and neopterin, which may mediate some of the biological activities.

➤*Pharmacokinetics:*

Interferon beta-1a – Biological response markers (eg, neopterin and β_2-microglobulin) are induced by interferon beta-1a following parenteral doses of 15 to 75 mcg in healthy subjects and treated patients. Biological response marker levels increase within 12 hours of dosing and remain elevated for at least 4 days. Peak biological response marker levels are typically observed 48 hours after dosing.

Interferon Beta-1a Pharmacokinetic Parameters[a]				
Route	Mean C_{max} (IU/mL)	T_{max} (h)	Mean AUC (IU•h/mL)	t½ (h)
IM	4.9	3 to 15	65	10
SC[b]	5.1	16 (median)	294	69

[a] Data are pooled from different studies and are not necessarily comparable.
[b] Based on a single dose of 60 mcg.

Interferon beta-1b – Because serum concentrations of interferon beta-1b are low or not detectable following SC administration of up to 0.25 mg, pharmacokinetic information in patients with MS receiving the recommended dose is not available. Following single and multiple daily SC administrations of 0.5 mg (16 mIU) to healthy volunteers (n = 12), serum concentrations were generally less than 100 IU/mL. Peak serum concentrations occurred between 1 to 8 hours, with a mean peak serum concentration of 40 IU/mL. Bioavailability, based on a total dose of 0.5 mg given as 2 SC injections at different sites, was approximately 50%.

After IV administration (0.006 to 2 mg), similar pharmacokinetic profiles were obtained from healthy volunteers (n = 12) and from patients with diseases other than MS (n = 142). In patients receiving single IV doses up to 2 mg, increases in serum concentrations were dose-proportional. Mean serum clearance values ranged from 9.4 to 28.9 mL/min/kg and were independent of dose. Mean terminal elimination half-life values ranged from 8 minutes to 4.3 hours and mean steady-state volume of distribution values ranged from 0.25 to 2.88 L/kg. IV dosing 3 times/week for 2 weeks resulted in no accumulation of interferon beta-1b in the serum of patients. Pharmacokinetic parameters after single and multiple IV doses were comparable.

Following SC administration every other day, biologic response marker levels increased significantly above baseline 6 to 12 hours after the first dose. Peak biologic response marker levels usually occur between 40 and 124 hours after dosing and remain elevated for at least 7 days.

Contraindications

Hypersensitivity to natural or recombinant interferon beta, human albumin, or any other component of the formulations.

Warnings

➤*Chronic progressive MS:* The safety and efficacy of interferon beta in chronic progressive MS have not been evaluated.

➤*Depression:* Use interferon beta with caution in patients with depression or other mood disorders, conditions that are common with MS. Depression and suicide have been reported in patients receiving interferon compounds. Depression, suicidal ideation, and suicidal attempts are known to occur at an increased frequency in patients receiving interferon compounds. Additionally, there have been postmarketing reports of depression, suicidal ideation, and/or development of new or worsening pre-existing psychiatric disorders, including psychosis. Some of these patients improved upon cessation of dosing.

Advise patients treated with interferon beta to immediately report any symptoms of depression or suicidal ideation. If a patient develops depression or other severe psychiatric symptoms, consider cessation of therapy.

➤*Injection-site necrosis (ISN):* ISN has been reported. Typically, ISN occurs within the first 4 months of therapy, although postmarketing reports have been received of ISN occurring over 1 year after initiation of therapy. Necrosis may occur at a single or multiple injection sites. The necrotic lesions are typically 3 cm or less in diameter, but larger areas have been reported. Generally, the necrosis has extended only to subcutaneous fat. However, there also are reports of necrosis extending to and including fascia overlaying muscle. In some lesions where biopsy results are available, vasculitis has been reported. For some lesions, debridement and, infrequently, skin grafting have been required.

As with any open lesion, it is important to avoid infection and, if it occurs, to treat the infection. Time to healing varied depending on the severity of the necrosis at the time of treatment. In most cases, healing was associated with scarring.

Some patients have experienced healing of necrotic skin lesions while **interferon beta-1b** therapy continued; others have not. Whether to discontinue therapy following a single site of necrosis is dependent on the extent of necrosis. For patients who continue therapy with interferon beta-1b after ISN has occurred, do not administer interferon beta -1b into the affected area until it is fully healed. If multiple lesions occur, discontinue therapy until healing occurs.

Periodically re-evaluate patient understanding and use of aseptic self-injection techniques, particularly if ISN has occurred.

➤*Anaphylaxis:* Anaphylaxis has been reported as a rare complication of interferon beta use. Other allergic reactions have included dyspnea, bronchospasm, tongue edema, orolingual edema, skin rash, and urticaria, and have ranged from mild to severe without a clear relationship to dose or duration of exposure. Several allergic reactions, some severe, have occurred after prolonged use.

➤*Decreased peripheral blood counts:* Decreased peripheral blood counts in all cell lines, including rare pancytopenia and thrombocytopenia, have been reported from postmarketing experience. Some cases of thrombocytopenia have had nadirs below 10,000/mcL. Some cases reoccur with rechallenge. Monitor patients for signs of these disorders.

➤*Albumin (human):* Some of these products contain albumin, a derivative of human blood. Based on effective donor screening and product manufacturing processes, it carries an extremely remote risk for transmission of viral diseases. A theoretical risk for transmission of Creutzfeldt-Jakob disease (CJD) also is considered extremely remote. No cases of transmission of viral diseases or CJD have been identified for albumin.

➤*Special risk patients:* Exercise caution when administering **interferon beta-1a** to patients with pre-existing seizure disorders. Seizures have been associated with the use of beta interferons. A relationship between occurrence of seizures and the use of interferon beta has not been established. Leukopenia and new or worsening thyroid abnormalities have developed in some patients treated with interferon beta. Regular monitoring for these conditions is recommended.

INTERFERON BETA

➤*Cardiac disease:* Closely monitor patients with cardiac disease, such as angina, CHF, or arrhythmia, for worsening of their clinical condition during initiation and continued treatment. While interferon beta does not have any known direct-acting cardiac toxicity, during the postmarketing period infrequent cases of CHF, cardiomyopathy, and cardiomyopathy with CHF have been reported in patients without known predisposition to these events and without other known etiologies being established. In rare cases, these events have been temporally related to the administration of interferon beta. In some of these instances, recurrence upon rechallenge was observed.

➤*Hepatic function impairment:* Severe liver dysfunction, leading to hepatic failure requiring liver transplantation, has been reported very rarely in patients taking interferon beta. Symptomatic hepatic dysfunction (including hepatitis), primarily presenting as jaundice, has been reported as a rare complication of use. Asymptomatic elevation of hepatic transaminases (particularly ALT) is common with interferon therapy. Initiate therapy with caution in patients with active liver disease, alcohol abuse, increased serum ALT (greater than 2.5 times the upper limit of normal [ULN]), or a history of significant liver disease. Consider dose reduction if ALT rises above 5 times the ULN. The dose may be re-escalated gradually once the enzyme levels have normalized. Stop treatment if jaundice or other clinical symptoms of liver dysfunction appear.

➤*Fertility impairment:* Menstrual irregularities were observed in monkeys administered **interferon beta-1a** at a dose 100 times the recommended weekly human dose. Anovulation and decreased serum progesterone levels also were noted transiently in some animals. These effects were reversible after discontinuation of the drug.

➤*Pregnancy: Category C.* There are no adequate and well-controlled studies in pregnant women. Abortifacient activity has been shown in animals and 6 spontaneous abortions were reported in patients on interferon beta therapy during the clinical trials. If the patient becomes pregnant or plans to become pregnant while taking interferon beta, apprise the patient of the potential hazards to the fetus and recommend that the patient discontinue therapy.

➤*Lactation:* It is not known whether interferon beta is excreted in breast milk. Decide whether to discontinue nursing or discontinue the drug, taking into account the importance of the drug to the mother.

➤*Children:* Safety and efficacy in children younger than 18 years of age have not been established.

Precautions

➤*Monitoring:* In addition to the laboratory tests normally required for monitoring patients with MS, blood cell counts and liver function tests are recommended at baseline and regular intervals (1, 3, and 6 months) following introduction of interferon beta therapy and then periodically thereafter in the absence of clinical symptoms. Thyroid function tests are recommended every 6 months in patients with a history of thyroid dysfunction or as clinically indicated. Patients with myelosuppression may require more intensive monitoring of complete blood cell counts, with differential and platelet counts.

➤*Self-administration:* Instruct patients in injection techniques to ensure the safe self-administration of interferon beta. A patient information sheet is provided with the product.

➤*Flu-like symptoms complex:* Flu-like symptoms, including headache, fever, fatigue, rigors, chest pain, back pain, and myalgia, have been commonly reported with interferon beta therapy. Symptoms usually occur 4 hours after injection and subside within 24 hours. Acetaminophen or NSAIDs prior to and/or following injection may help to prevent or treat these symptoms.

➤*Autoimmune disorders:* Autoimmune disorders of multiple target organs have been reported postmarketing, including idiopathic thrombocytopenia, hyper- and hypothyroidism, and rare cases of autoimmune hepatitis. Monitor patients for signs of these disorders and implement appropriate treatment when observed.

➤*Hepatic injury:* Hepatic injury, including elevated serum hepatic enzyme levels and hepatitis, some of which have been severe, has been reported postmarketing. In some patients, a recurrence of elevated serum levels of hepatic enzymes has occurred upon rechallenge. In some cases, these events have occurred in the presence of other drugs associated with hepatic injury. The potential of additive effects from multiple drugs or other hepatotoxic agents (eg, alcohol) has not been determined. Monitor patients for signs of hepatic injury and exercise caution when interferons are used concomitantly with other drugs associated with hepatic injury.

➤*Immunogenicity:* As with all therapeutic proteins, there is a potential for immunogenicity. Antibodies to interferon beta have developed during therapy. The relationship between antibody formation and clinical safety or efficacy is unknown.

➤*Latex sensitivity:* Administer with caution to patients with a possible history of latex sensitivity; packaging may contain dry natural rubber.

➤*Photosensitivity:* Photosensitization (photoallergy or phototoxicity) may occur; therefore, caution patients to take protective measures (ie, sunscreens, protective clothing) against exposure to sunlight or ultraviolet light (eg, tanning beds) until tolerance is determined.

Drug Interactions

➤*Myelosuppressive agents:* Because of the potential of **interferon beta-1a** to cause neutropenia and lymphopenia, proper monitoring is required if administered concomitantly with myelosuppressive agents.

Adverse Reactions

The most serious adverse reactions associated with interferon beta therapy were depression, suicidal ideation, and ISN (see Warnings). The most commonly reported adverse reactions were asthenia, flu-like symptoms complex (see Precautions), headache, injection site reaction, lymphopenia (lymphocytes less than 1500/mm^3), and pain. The most frequently reported adverse reactions resulting in clinical intervention (ie, discontinuation of therapy, adjustment in dosage, or the need for concomitant medication to treat an adverse reaction symptom) were asthenia, depression, flu-like symptoms complex, hypertonia, injection site reactions, increased liver enzymes, leukopenia, and myasthenia.

Interferon Beta Adverse Reactions (%)[a]

		Rebif		
Adverse reactions	*Avonex* (n = 351)	22 mcg 3 times/week (n = 189)	44 mcg 3 times/week (n = 184)	Interferon beta-1b (n = 1115)
Cardiovascular				
Hypertension	–	–	–	7
Migraine	5	–	–	–
Palpitations	–	–	–	4
Peripheral edema	–	–	–	15
Peripheral vascular disorder	–	–	–	6
Tachycardia	–	–	–	4
Vasodilation	2	–	–	8
CNS				
Anxiety	–	–	–	10
Asthenia	24	–	–	61
Convulsions	–	5	4	–
Depression	18	–	–	–
Dizziness	14	–	–	24
Fatigue	–	33	41	–
Headache	58	65	70	57
Incoordination	–	5	4	21
Nervousness	–	–	–	7
Hypertonia	–	7	6	50
Sleep difficulty	–	–	–	24
Somnolence		4	5	
Dermatologic				
Alopecia	4	–	–	4
Rash (erythematous, maculopapular)	–	5-7	4-5	24
Skin disorder	–	–	–	12
Sweating	–	–	–	8
GI				
Abdominal pain	8	22	20	19
Constipation	–	–	–	20
Diarrhea	–	–	–	19
Dry mouth	–	1	5	
Dyspepsia	–	–	–	14
Nausea	23	–	–	27
GU				
Dysmenorrhea[b]	–	–	–	7
Impotence[c]	–	–	–	9
Menorrhagia[b]	–	–	–	8
Metrorrhagia[b]	–	–	–	11
Prostatic disorder[c]	–	–	–	3
Urinary frequency	–	2	7	7
Urinary incontinence	–	4	2	–
Urinary urgency	–	–	–	13
Urine constituents, abnormal	3			–
UTI	17	–	–	–
Hemic/Lymphatic				
ANC < 1500/mm^3	–	–	–	14
Anemia	4	3	5	–
Leukopenia	–	28	36	–
Lymphadenopathy	–	11	12	8
Lymphocytes < 1500/mm^3	–	–	–	88
Thrombocytopenia	–	2	8	–
WBC < 3000/mm^3	–	–	–	14
Hepatic				
ALT > 5 × baseline	–	20	27	10
AST > 5 × baseline	–	10	17	3
Bilirubinemia	–	3	2	–
Hepatic function abnormal	–	4	9	–

INTERFERON BETA

Interferon Beta Adverse Reactions (%)[a]

Adverse reactions	*Avonex* (n = 351)	*Rebif* 22 mcg 3 times/week (n = 189)	*Rebif* 44 mcg 3 times/week (n = 184)	Interferon beta-1b (n = 1115)
Musculoskeletal				
Arthralgia	9	–	–	31
Back pain	–	23	25	–
Myalgia	29	25	25	27
Myasthenia	–	–	–	46
Skeletal pain	–	15	10	–
Respiratory				
Bronchitis	8	–	–	-
Dyspnea	–	–	–	7
Sinusitis	14	–	–	-
Upper respiratory tract infection	14	–	–	-
Special senses				
Eye disorder	4	–	–	–
Vision abnormal	–	7	13	–
Xerophthalmia	–	3	1	–
Miscellaneous				
Chest pain	5	6	8	11
Chills	19	–	–	25
Fever	20	25	28	36
Flu-like symptoms	49	56	59	60
Infection	7	–	–	–
ISN/inflammation/ ecchymosis	6	1	3	5
Injection site reaction/pain	3-8	89	92	85
Leg cramps	–	–	–	4
Malaise	–	4	5	8
Pain	23	–	–	51
Rigors	–	6	13	–
Thyroid disorder	–	4	6	–
Toothache	3	–	–	–
Weight gain		–	–	7

[a] Data are pooled from separate studies and are not necessarily comparable.
[b] Premenopausal patients.Male patients
– = Not reported.

➤*Postmarketing:*

Interferon beta-1a –

Cardiovascular: CHF, cardiomyopathy, cardiomyopathy with CHF.

CNS: New or worsening psychiatric disorders, seizures in patients without history.

GU: Menorrhagia, metrorrhagia.

Hematologic: Decreased peripheral blood counts, including pancytopenia (rare); thrombocytopenia (some cases with nadirs below 10,000/mcL and have reoccurred upon rechallenge); idiopathic thrombocytopenia.

Hepatic: Autoimmune hepatitis; hepatic injury, including elevated serum hepatic enzyme levels; hepatitis.

Miscellaneous: Anaphylaxis, hyper- and hypothyroidism.

Interferon beta-1b –

Cardiovascular: Cardiomyopathy, deep vein thrombosis, pulmonary embolism.

CNS: Ataxia, confusion, convulsion, depersonalization, emotional lability, paresthesia.

Dermatologic: Pruritus, skin discoloration, urticaria.

Endocrine: Hypothyroidism, hyperthyroidism, thyroid dysfunction.

GU: UTI, urosepsis.

Hemic/Lymphatic: Anemia, thrombocytopenia.

Metabolic/Nutritional: Gamma GT increase, hypocalcemia, hyperuricemia, triglyceride increase.

Respiratory: Bronchospasm, pneumonia.

Miscellaneous: Fatal capillary leak syndrome (may appear in patients with a pre-existing monoclonal gammopathy); hepatitis; pancreatitis; vomiting.

Patient Information

➤*Instruction on self-injection technique and procedures:* Instruct patients in the use of aseptic technique when administering interferon beta. Give appropriate instruction for reconstitution of the product and self-injection, including careful review of the patient information sheet that is provided. If possible, perform the first injection under the supervision of an appropriately qualified health care professional.

➤*Dosage schedule:* Caution patients not to change the dosage or the schedule of administration without medical consultation.

➤*Disposal:* Caution patients against the re-use of needles or syringes and instruct them in safe disposal procedures. Supply the patient with a puncture-resistant container for disposal of used needles/syringes along with instructions for safe disposal of containers.

➤*Injection site reactions:* Injection site reactions may occur at least one time during therapy. In general, these are transient and do not require discontinuation of therapy, but carefully assess the nature and severity of all reported reactions. Periodically re-evaluate patient understanding and use of aseptic self-injection technique and procedures.

Advise patients to promptly report any break in the skin, which may be associated with blue-black discoloration, swelling, or drainage of fluid from the injection site, prior to continuing interferon beta therapy.

➤*Flu-like symptoms:* Flu-like symptoms are common following initiation of therapy. Symptoms of flu syndrome are most prominent at the initiation of therapy and decrease in frequency with continued treatment. Concurrent use of analgesics and/or antipyretics may help ameliorate flu-like symptoms on treatment days.

➤*Depression/Suicide:* Caution patients to report depression or suicidal ideation.

➤*Abortifacient potential:* Advise patients about the abortifacient potential.

➤*Photosensitivity:* Advise patients to avoid prolonged exposure to sunlight or sunlamps; interferon beta may cause photosensitivity.

➤*Latex sensitivity:* Some of the packaging may contain latex; caution patients with a possible history of latex allergy.

INTERFERON BETA-1A

Rx	**Rebif** (Serono)	**Injection**: 8.8 mcg per 0.2 mL (2.4 million units)	Preservative-free. In prefilled single-use syringes. In *Titration Pack* 6s.[a]
		22 mcg per 0.5 mL (6 million units)	Preservative-free. In prefilled single-use syringes. In 12s.[b]
		44 mcg per 0.5 mL (12 million units)	Preservative-free. In prefilled single-use syringes. In 1s, 3s, and 12s.[c]
Rx	**Avonex** (Biogen Idec)	**Powder for injection, lyophilized**: 33 mcg (6.6 million units [30 mcg/vial when reconstituted])	Preservative-free. In administration dose packs (single-use vial with diluent [sterile water for injection], alcohol wipes, gauze pad, syringe, *Micro Pin* vial access pin, needle, and bandage).[d]
		Prefilled syringe: 30 mcg per 0.5 mL	Albumin-free. In administration dose packs (single-use syringe, needle, reclose-able accessory pouch, alcohol wipes, gauze pads, and bandages).[e]

[a] With 0.8 mg human albumin, 10.9 mg mannitol, 0.16 mg sodium acetate in water for injection.
[b] With 2 mg human albumin, 27.3 mg mannitol, 0.4 mg sodium acetate in water for injection.
[c] With 4 mg human albumin, 27.3 mg mannitol, 0.4 mg sodium acetate in water for injection.
[d] With 16.5 mg human albumin, 6.4 mg sodium chloride, 6.3 mg dibasic sodium phosphate, 1.3 mg monobasic sodium phosphate/vial.
[e] With 0.79 mg sodium acetate trihydrate, 0.25 mg glacial acetic acid, 15.8 mg arginine HCl, 0.025 mg polysorbate 20 in water for injection.

INTERFERON BETA-1A — INJECTION

Indications

➤*Multiple sclerosis (MS):* Interferon beta-1a is indicated for the treatment of patients with relapsing forms of multiple sclerosis to slow the accumulation of physical disability and decrease the frequency of clinical exacerbations . Patients with multiple sclerosis in whom efficacy has been demonstrated include patients who have experienced a first clinical episode and have magnetic resonance imaging (MRI) features consistent with multiple sclerosis. Safety and efficacy in patients with chronic progressive multiple sclerosis have not been established.

Administration and Dosage

➤*Approved by the FDA:* May 17, 1996.

➤*Avonex*: The recommended dosage of *Avonex* is 30 mcg injected intramuscularly (IM) once a week.

Avonex is intended for use under the guidance and supervision of a health care provider. Patients may self-inject only if their health care providers determine that it is appropriate and with medical follow-up, as necessary, after proper training in IM injection technique. Sites for injection include the thigh or upper arm.

INTERFERON BETA-1A — INJECTION

Reconstitution of Avonex vials – Use appropriate aseptic technique during the preparation of *Avonex*. To reconstitute lyophilized *Avonex*, use a sterile syringe and *Micro Pin* to inject 1.1 mL of the supplied diluent, sterile water for injection, into the *Avonex* vial. Gently swirl the vial of *Avonex* to dissolve the drug completely. Do not shake. The reconstituted solution should be clear to slightly yellow without particles. Visually inspect the reconstituted product prior to use. Discard the product if it contains particulate matter or is discolored. Each vial of reconstituted solution contains 30 mcg/mL interferon beta-1a. Withdraw 1 mL of reconstituted solution from the vial into a sterile syringe. Replace the cover on the *Micro Pin* and attach the sterile 23-gauge, 1.25 inch needle and inject the solution IM. The *Avonex* and diluent vials are for single-use only; discard unused portions.

Using Avonex prefilled syringes – Hold the *Avonex* prefilled syringe upright (rubber cap facing up). Remove the protective cover by turning and gently pulling the rubber cap in a clockwise motion. Attach the 23-gauge, 1.25 inch needle and inject the solution IM. The *Avonex* prefilled syringe is for single use only.

➤*Rebif*: Dosages of *Rebif* shown to be safe and effective are 22 and 44 mcg injected subcutaneously 3 times/week. Administer *Rebif*, if possible, at the same time (preferably in the late afternoon or evening) on the same 3 days (eg, Monday, Wednesday, Friday) at least 48 hours apart each week. Generally, start patients at 20% of the prescribed dose 3 times/week and increase over a 4-week period to the targeted dose, either 22 or 44 mcg 3 times/week (see the following table). Following the administration of each dose, discard any residual product remaining in the syringe in a safe and proper manner.

Schedule for Patient Titration

	Recommended titration (% of final)	Titration dose for *Rebif* 22 mcg	Titration dose for *Rebif* 44 mcg	Injection volume
Weeks 1 to 2	20%	4.4 mcg	8.8 mcg	0.1 mL
Weeks 3 to 4	50%	11 mcg	22 mcg	0.25 mL
Weeks 5+	100%	22 mcg	44 mcg	0.5 mL

Leukopenia or elevated liver function tests may necessitate dose reductions of 20% to 50% until toxicity is resolved.

Rebif is intended for use under the guidance and supervision of a health care provider. It is recommended that health care providers or qualified medical personnel train patients in the proper technique for self-administering subcutaneous injections using the prefilled syringe. Advise patients to rotate sites for subcutaneous injections. Concurrent use of analgesics and/or antipyretics may help ameliorate flu-like symptoms on treatment days. Visually inspect *Rebif* for particulate matter and discoloration prior to administration.

➤*Storage/Stability:*

Avonex –

30 mcg lyophilized powder vial: Store vials of *Avonex* in a 2° to 8°C (36° to 46°F) refrigerator. Should refrigeration be unavailable, store interferon beta-1a below 25°C (77°F) and away from heat and light for a period of up to 30 days. Do not freeze. Do not use beyond the expiration date stamped on the vial. Following reconstitution, it is recommended the product be used as soon as possible within 6 hours stored at 2° to 8°C (36° to 46°F). Do not freeze reconstituted interferon beta-1a.

30 mcg prefilled syringe: Avonex in prefilled syringes must be stored in a 2° to 8°C (36° to 46°F) refrigerator. Once removed from the refrigerator, allow *Avonex* in a prefilled syringe to warm to room temperature (approximately 30 minutes); use within 12 hours. Do not use external heat sources such as hot water to warm *Avonex* in a prefilled syringe. Do not expose to high temperatures. Do not freeze. Protect from light. Do not use beyond the expiration date stamped on the syringe.

Rebif – Store *Rebif* refrigerated between 2° to 8°C (36° to 46°F). Do not freeze. If a refrigerator is not available, store *Rebif* at or below 25°C (77°F) for up to 30 days and away from heat and light.

Do not use beyond the expiration date printed on packages.

INTERFERON BETA-1B

Rx	**Betaseron** (Berlex)	**Powder for injection, lyophilized**: 0.3 mg	Preservative-free. In single-use 3 mL capacity vials with 1.2 mL prefilled syringe of diluent (sodium chloride 0.54%)[a], alcohol prep pads, and vial adaptor with attached needle for each drug vial. In blister unit 15s.

[a] With 15 mg human albumin, 15 mg mannitol/vial.

INTERFERON BETA-1B — INJECTION

Indications

➤*Multiple sclerosis:* For the treatment of relapsing forms of multiple sclerosis to reduce the frequency of clinical exacerbations.

Administration and Dosage

➤*Approved by the FDA:* July 23, 1993.

➤*Recommended dose:* 0.25 mg injected subcutaneously every other day. Generally, patients should be started at 0.0625 mg (0.25 mL) subcutaneously every other day, and increased over a 6-week period to 0.25 mg (1 mL) every other day (see table below).

Schedule for dose titration

	Recommended titration	Interferon beta-1b dose	Volume
Weeks 1 to 2	25%	0.0625 mg	0.25 mL
Weeks 3 to 4	50%	0.125 mg	0.5 mL
Weeks 5 to 6	75%	0.1875 mg	0.75 mL
Week 7+	100%	0.25 mg	1 mL

➤*Preparation for administration:* To reconstitute lyophilized interferon beta-1b for injection, attach the prefilled syringe containing the diluent (Sodium Chloride, 0.54% solution) to the interferon beta-1b vial using the vial adapter. Slowly inject 1.2 mL of diluent into the interferon beta-1b vial. Gently swirl the vial to dissolve the drug completely; do not shake. Foaming may occur during reconstitution or if the vial is swirled or shaken too vigorously. If foaming occurs, allow the vial to sit undisturbed until the foam settles. Visually inspect the reconstituted product before use; discard the product if it contains particulate matter or is discolored. Keeping the syringe and vial adapter in place, turn the assembly over so the vial is on top. Withdraw the appropriate dose of interferon beta-1b solution. Remove the vial from the vial adapter before injecting interferon beta-1b. One mL of reconstituted interferon beta-1b solution contains 0.25 mg of interferon beta-1b/mL.

Interferon beta-1b is intended for use under the guidance and supervision of a physician. It is recommended that physicians or qualified medical personnel train patients in the proper technique for self-administering subcutaneous injections. Patients should be advised to rotate sites for subcutaneous injections. Concurrent use of analgesics and/or antipyretics may help ameliorate flu-like symptoms on treatment days. Interferon beta-1b should be visually inspected for particulate matter and discoloration prior to administration.

➤*Storage/Stability:* The reconstituted product contains no preservative. Before reconstitution with diluent, store interferon beta-1b at room temperature 25°C (77°F). Excursions of 15° to 30°C (59° to 86°F) are permitted. After reconstitution, if not used immediately, the product should be refrigerated and used within 3 hours. Avoid freezing.

ETANERCEPT

Rx	**Enbrel** (Amgen)	**Injection**: 50 mg/mL	Preservative free. Single-use prefilled syringe. In 0.98 mL prefilled single-use syringe with 27 gauge, ½ inch needle. Carton contains 4 prefilled syringes.[a]
		Powder for Injection, lyophilized: 25 mg	Preservative-free. With syringe, needle, alcohol swabs, plunger, and diluent (1 mL sterile bacteriostatic water for injection contains 0.9% benzyl alcohol). Carton contains 4 dose trays. In multiple-use vials.[b]

[a] With 10 mg/mL sucrose, 5.8 mg/mL sodium chloride, 5.3 mg/mL L-arginine hydrochloride, 2.6 mg/mL sodium phosphate, monobasic, monohydrate, and 0.9 mg/mL sodium phosphate, dibasic, anhydrous.

[b] With 40 mg mannitol, 10 mg sucrose, 1.2 mg tromethamine.

ETANERCEPT — INJECTION

Indications

➤*Ankylosing spondylitis:* For reducing signs and symptoms in patients with active ankylosing spondylitis.

➤*Plaque psoriasis:* For treatment of adult patients 18 years of age or older with chronic moderate to severe plaque psoriasis who are candidates for systemic therapy or phototherapy.

➤*Polyarticular-course juvenile rheumatoid arthritis (JRA):* For reducing signs and symptoms of moderately to severely active polyarticular-course JRA in patients who have had an inadequate response to 1 or more disease-modifying antirheumatic drugs (DMARDs).

➤*Psoriatic arthritis:* For reducing signs and symptoms, inhibiting the progression of structural damage of active arthritis, and improving physical

ETANERCEPT — INJECTION

function in patients with psoriatic arthritis. Etanercept can be used in combination with methotrexate in patients who do not respond adequately to methotrexate alone.

➤*Rheumatoid arthritis (RA):* For reducing signs and symptoms, inducing major clinical response, and inhibiting the progression of structural damage, and improving physical function in patients with moderately to severely active RA. Etanercept can be initiated in combination with methotrexate or used alone.

➤*Unlabeled uses:* Crohn disease.

Administration and Dosage

➤*Approved by the FDA:* November 2, 1998.

➤*JRA patients (children 4 to 17 years of age):* 0.8 mg/kg per week (up to a maximum of 50 mg per week). For pediatric patients weighing 63 kg (138 pounds) or more, administer the weekly dose of 50 mg using the prefilled syringe. For pediatric patients weighing more than 31 to 62 kg (68 to 136 pounds), administer the total weekly dose as 2 subcutaneous injections, either on the same day or 3 or 4 days apart using the multiple-use vial. Administer the dose for pediatric patients weighing less than 31 kg (68 pounds) as a single subcutaneous injection once weekly using the correct volume from the multiple-use vial. Glucocorticoids, nonsteroidal anti-inflammatory drugs (NSAIDs), or analgesics may be continued during treatment with etanercept. Concurrent use with methotrexate and higher doses of etanercept have not been studied in pediatric patients.

➤*Plaque psoriasis (adults):* A 50 mg dose given twice weekly (administered 3 or 4 days apart) for 3 months followed by a reduction to a maintenance dose of 50 mg per week. Administer the recommended dose subcutaneously, using 50 mg/mL single-use prefilled syringes.

Starting doses of etanercept 25 or 50 mg/week were also shown to be efficacious. The proportion of responders were related to etanercept dosage.

➤*RA, ankylosing spondylitis, and psoriatic arthritis (adults):* 50 mg per week given as 1 subcutaneous injection using a 50 mg/mL single-use prefilled syringe, or as two 25 mg injections given either on the same day or 3 or 4 days apart. Methotrexate, glucocorticoids, salicylates, NSAIDs, or analgesics may be continued during treatment with etanercept. Based on a study of etanercept 50 mg twice weekly in patients with RA that suggested higher incidence of adverse reactions but similar American College of Rheumatology (ACR) response rates, doses greater than 50 mg per week are not recommended.

➤*Storage / Stability:*

Single-use prefilled syringe – Do not use a prefilled syringe beyond the expiration date stamped on the carton or syringe barrel label. The prefilled syringes must be refrigerated at 2° to 8°C (36° to 46°F). Do not freeze. Keep the etanercept prefilled syringes in the original carton to protect from light until the time of use. Do not shake.

Multiple-use vial – Do not use a dose tray beyond the date stamped on the carton, dose tray label, vial label, or diluent syringe label. The dose tray containing etanercept (sterile powder) must be refrigerated at 2° to 8°C (36° to 46°F). Do not freeze. Reconstituted solutions of etanercept prepared with the supplied bacteriostatic water for injection (0.9% benzyl alcohol), using a 25-gauge needle, may be stored for up to 14 days if refrigerated at 2° to 8°C (36° to 46°F). Discard reconstituted solution after 14 days. Product stability and sterility cannot be ensured after 14 days.

Actions

➤*Pharmacology:* Etanercept binds specifically to tumor necrosis factor (TNF) and blocks its interaction with cell-surface TNF receptors (TNFRs). TNF is a naturally occurring cytokine that is involved in normal inflammatory and immune responses. It plays an important role in the inflammatory processes of RA, polyarticular course JRA, and ankylosing spondylitis and the resulting joint pathology. In addition, TNF plays a role in the inflammatory process of plaque psoriasis. Elevated levels of TNF are found in involved tissues and fluids of patients with RA, psoriatic arthritis, ankylosing spondylitis, and plaque psoriasis.

Two distinct TNFRs, a 55 kilodalton protein (p55) and a 75 kilodalton protein (p75), exist naturally as monomeric molecules on cell surfaces and in soluble forms. Biological activity of TNF is dependent upon binding to either cell surface TNFR.

Etanercept is a dimeric soluble form of the p75 TNFR that can bind to 2 TNF molecules. It inhibits the activity of TNF in vitro and has been shown to affect several animal models of inflammation, including murine, collagen-induced arthritis. Etanercept inhibits binding of both TNF α and TNF β (lymphotoxin alpha [LT α]) to cell surface TNFRs, rendering TNF biologically inactive. Cells expressing transmembrane TNF that bind etanercept are not lysed in vitro in the presence or absence of complement.

Etanercept can also modulate biological responses that are induced or regulated by TNF, including expression of adhesion molecules responsible for leukocyte migration (ie, E-selectin and, to a lesser extent, intercellular adhesion molecule-1 [ICAM-1]), serum levels of cytokines (eg, IL-6), and serum levels of matrix metalloproteinase-3 (MMP-3 or stromelysin).

➤*Pharmacokinetics:*

Absorption / Distribution – After administration of etanercept 25 mg by a single subcutaneous injection to 25 patients with RA, a maximum serum concentration (C_{max}) of 1.1 ± 0.6 mcg/mL and time to C_{max} of 69 ± 34 hours was observed in these patients following a single 25 mg dose. After 6 months of twice-weekly 25 mg doses in these same RA patients, the mean C_{max} was 2.4 ± 1 mcg/mL (n = 23). Patients exhibited a 2- to 7-fold increase in peak serum concentrations and approximate 4-fold increase in area under the curve ($AUC_{0-72\,h}$) (range, 1- to 17-fold) with repeated dosing. Serum concentrations in patients with RA have not been measured for periods of dosing that exceed 6 months.

In another study, serum concentration profiles at steady-state were comparable among patients with RA treated with etanercept 50 mg once weekly and those treated with etanercept 25 mg twice weekly. The mean (± standard deviation) C_{max}, minimum serum concentration (C_{min}), and partial AUC were 2.4 ± 1.5 mg/L, 1.2 ± 0.7 mg/L, and 297 ± 166 mg•h/L, respectively, for patients treated with etanercept 50 mg once weekly (n = 21); and 2.6 ± 1.2 mg/L, 1.4 ± 0.7 mg/L, and 316 ± 135 mg•h/L for patients treated with etanercept 25 mg twice weekly (n = 16). Serum concentrations in patients with RA have not been measured for periods of dosing that exceed 6 months. The pharmacokinetic parameters in patients with plaque psoriasis were similar to those seen in patients with RA.

Metabolism / Excretion – After administration of etanercept 25 mg by a single subcutaneous injection to 25 patients with RA, a mean ± standard deviation half-life of 102 ± 30 hours was observed with a clearance of 160 ± 80 mL/h.

Contraindications

Sepsis or known hypersensitivity to etanercept or any of its components.

Warnings

➤*Serious infections:* In postmarketing reports, serious infections and sepsis, including fatalities, have been reported with the use of etanercept. Many of the serious infections have occurred in patients on concomitant immunosuppressive therapy that, in addition to their underlying disease, could predispose them to infections. Rare cases of tuberculosis have been observed in patients treated with TNF antagonists, including etanercept. Closely monitor patients who develop a new infection while undergoing treatment with etanercept. Discontinue administration of etanercept if a patient develops a serious infection or sepsis. Do not initiate treatment with etanercept in patients with active infections including chronic or localized infections. Exercise caution when considering the use of etanercept in patients with a history of recurring infections or with underlying conditions that may predispose patients to infections such as advanced or poorly controlled diabetes.

➤*Neurologic effects:* Treatment with etanercept and other agents that inhibit TNF have been associated with rare cases of new onset or exacerbation of CNS-demyelinating disorders, some presenting with mental status changes and some associated with permanent disability. Cases of transverse myelitis, optic neuritis, multiple sclerosis, and new onset or exacerbation of seizure disorders have been observed in association with etanercept therapy. The causal relationship to etanercept therapy remains unclear. While no clinical trials have been performed evaluating etanercept therapy in patients with multiple sclerosis, other TNF antagonists administered to patients with multiple sclerosis have been associated with increases in disease activity. Exercise caution in considering the use of etanercept in patients with preexisting or recent-onset CNS-demyelinating disorders.

➤*Hematologic effects:* Rare reports of pancytopenia including aplastic anemia, some with a fatal outcome, have been reported in patients treated with etanercept. The causal relationship to etanercept therapy remains unclear. Although no high-risk group has been identified, exercise caution in patients being treated with etanercept who have a history of significant hematologic abnormalities. Advise all patients to seek immediate medical attention if they develop signs and symptoms suggestive of blood dyscrasias or infection (eg, persistent fever, bruising, bleeding, pallor) while on etanercept. Consider discontinuation of etanercept therapy in patients with confirmed significant hematologic abnormalities.

See Drug Interactions for more information.

➤*Malignancies:* In the controlled portions of clinical trials of all the TNF-blocking agents, more cases of lymphoma have been observed among patients receiving the TNF blocker compared with control patients. During the controlled portions of etanercept trials, 3 lymphomas were observed among 4,509 etanercept-treated patients versus 0 among 2,040 control patients (mean duration of controlled treatment ranged from 3 to 24 months). In the controlled and open-label portions of clinical trials of etanercept in RA patients, 9 lymphomas were observed in 5,723 patients over approximately 11,201 patient-years of therapy. This is 3-fold higher than that expected in the general population. While patients with RA or psoriasis, particularly those with highly active disease, may be at a higher risk (up to several fold) for the development of lymphoma, the potential role of TNF-blocking therapy in the development of malignancies is not known.

➤*Hypersensitivity reactions:* Allergic reactions associated with administration of etanercept during clinical trials have been reported in less than 2% of patients. If an anaphylactic reaction or other serious allergic reaction occurs, discontinue administration of etanercept immediately and initiate appropriate therapy.

Latex allergy – The needle cover of the prefilled syringe contains natural rubber (latex), which may cause allergic reactions in individuals sensitive to this substance.

➤*Elderly:* A total of 480 RA patients and 89 plaque psoriasis patients 65 years of age and older have been studied in clinical trials. No overall differences in safety or efficacy were observed between these patients and younger patients. Because there is a higher incidence of infections in the elderly population in general, use caution in treating the elderly.

➤*Pregnancy: Category B.* Developmental toxicity studies have been performed in rats and rabbits at doses ranging from 60- to 100-fold higher than the human dose and have revealed no evidence of harm to the fetus due to etanercept. There are, however, no studies in pregnant women. Because ani-

ETANERCEPT — INJECTION

mal reproduction studies are not always predictive of human response, use this drug during pregnancy only if clearly needed.

Pregnancy registry – To monitor outcomes of pregnant women exposed to etanercept, a pregnancy registry has been established. Health care providers are encouraged to register patients by calling 1-877-311-8972.

➤*Lactation:* It is not known whether etanercept is excreted in human milk or absorbed systemically after ingestion. Because many drugs and immunoglobulins are excreted in human milk, and because of the potential for serious adverse reactions in breast-feeding infants from etanercept, decide whether to discontinue breast-feeding or to discontinue the drug.

➤*Children:* Etanercept is indicated for treatment of polyarticular-course JRA in patients who have had an inadequate response to 1 or more DMARDs. Etanercept has not been studied in children younger than 4 years of age.

The safety and efficacy of etanercept in pediatric patients with plaque psoriasis have not been studied.

Precautions

➤*Heart failure:* Two large clinical trials evaluating the use of etanercept in the treatment of heart failure were terminated early because of lack of efficacy. Results of 1 study suggested higher mortality in patients treated with etanercept compared with placebo. Results of the second study did not corroborate these observations. Analyses did not identify specific factors associated with increased risk of adverse outcomes in heart failure patients treated with etanercept. There have been postmarketing reports of worsening of congestive heart failure (CHF), with and without identifiable precipitating factors, in patients taking etanercept. There have also been rare reports of new onset CHF, including CHF in patients without known preexisting cardiovascular disease. Some of these patients have been younger than 50 years of age. Exercise caution when using etanercept in patients who also have heart failure, and monitor patients carefully.

➤*Immunosuppression:* Anti-TNF therapies, including etanercept, affect host defenses against infections and malignancies because TNF mediates inflammation and modulates cellular immune responses. In a study of 49 patients with RA treated with etanercept, there was no evidence of depression of delayed-type hypersensitivity, depression of immunoglobulin levels, or change in enumeration of effector cell populations. The impact of treatment with etanercept on the development and course of malignancies and active or chronic infections is not fully understood. The safety and efficacy of etanercept in patients with immunosuppression or chronic infections have not been evaluated.

➤*Benzyl alcohol:* Benzyl alcohol, a preservative contained in the diluent supplied for multiple vials, has been associated with a fatal "gasping syndrome" in premature infants.

➤*Vaccinations:* Most psoriatic arthritis patients receiving etanercept were able to mount effective B-cell immune responses to pneumococcal polysaccharide vaccine, but titers in aggregate were moderately lower, and fewer patients had 2-fold rises in titers compared with patients not receiving etanercept. The clinical significance of this is unknown. Patients receiving etanercept may receive concurrent vaccinations, except for live vaccines. No data are available on the secondary transmission of infection by live vaccines in patients receiving etanercept.

It is recommended that JRA patients, if possible, be brought up to date with all immunizations in agreement with current immunization guidelines prior to initiating etanercept therapy. Patients with a significant exposure to varicella virus should temporarily discontinue etanercept therapy and be considered for prophylactic treatment with varicella-zoster immune globulin.

➤*Autoantibodies:* Treatment with etanercept may result in the formation of autoantibodies and, rarely, in the development of a lupus-like syndrome that may resolve following withdrawal of etanercept. If a patient develops symptoms and findings suggestive of a lupus-like syndrome following treatment with etanercept, discontinue treatment and carefully evaluate the patient.

Drug Interactions

➤*Sulfasalazine:* Patients in a clinical study who were on established therapy with sulfasalazine, to which etanercept was added, were noted to develop a mild decrease in mean neutrophil counts, in comparison with groups treated with either etanercept or sulfasalazine alone. The clinical significance of this observation is unknown.

➤*Anakinra:* In a study in which patients with active RA were treated for up to 24 weeks with concurrent etanercept and anakinra therapy, a 7% rate of serious infections was observed, which was higher than that observed with etanercept alone (0%). Two percent of patients treated concurrently with etanercept and anakinra developed neutropenia (ANC less than 1×10^9/L).

Adverse Reactions

➤*Injection site reactions:* In controlled trials in rheumatologic indications, approximately 37% of patients treated with etanercept developed injection site reactions. In controlled trials in patients with plaque psoriasis, 14% of patients treated with etanercept developed injection site reactions during the first 3 months of treatment. All injection site reactions were described as mild to moderate (eg, erythema or itching, pain, swelling) and generally did not necessitate drug discontinuation. Injection site reactions generally occurred in the first month and subsequently decreased in frequency. The mean duration of injection site reactions was 3 to 5 days. Seven percent of patients experienced redness at a previous injection site when subsequent injections were given. In postmarketing experience, injection site bleeding and bruising have also been observed in conjunction with etanercept therapy.

➤*Infections:* In controlled trials, there were no differences in rates of infection among RA, psoriatic arthritis, ankylosing spondylitis, and plaque psoriasis patients treated with etanercept and those treated with placebo (or methotrexate for RA and psoriatic arthritis patients). The most common type of infection was upper respiratory tract infection, which occurred at a rate of approximately 20% among both etanercept- and placebo-treated patients in RA, psoriatic arthritis, and ankylosing spondylitis trials, and at a rate of approximately 12% among both etanercept- and placebo-treated patients in plaque psoriasis trials in the first 3 months of treatment.

In placebo-controlled trials in RA, psoriatic arthritis, ankylosing spondylitis, and plaque psoriasis, no increase in the incidence of serious infections was observed (approximately 1% in both placebo- and etanercept-treated groups). In all clinical trials in RA, serious infections experienced by patients included pyelonephritis, bronchitis, septic arthritis, abdominal abscess, cellulitis, osteomyelitis, wound infection, pneumonia, foot abscess, leg ulcer, diarrhea, sinusitis, and sepsis. The rate of serious infections has not increased in open-label extension trials and is similar to that observed in etanercept- and placebo-treated patients from controlled trials. Serious infections, including sepsis and death, have also been reported during postmarketing use of etanercept. Some have occurred within a few weeks after initiating treatment with etanercept. Many of the patients had underlying conditions (eg, diabetes, congestive heart failure, history of active or chronic infections) in addition to their RA. Data from a sepsis clinical trial not specifically in patients with RA suggest that etanercept treatment may increase mortality in patients with established sepsis.

In patients who received both etanercept and anakinra for up to 24 weeks, the incidence of serious infections was 7%. The most common infections consisted of bacterial pneumonia (4 cases) and cellulitis (4 cases). One patient with pulmonary fibrosis and pneumonia died due to respiratory failure.

In postmarketing experience in rheumatologic indications, infections have been observed with various pathogens including viral, bacterial, fungal, and protozoal organisms. Infections have been noted in all organ systems and have been reported in patients receiving etanercept alone or in combination with immunosuppressive agents.

In clinical trials in plaque psoriasis, serious infections experienced by etanercept-treated patients have included cellulitis, gastroenteritis, pneumonia, abscess, and osteomyelitis.

➤*Malignancies:* Patients have been observed in clinical trials with etanercept for over 5 years. Among 4,462 RA patients treated with etanercept in clinical trials for a mean of 27 months (approximately 10,000 patient-years of therapy), 9 lymphomas were observed for a rate of 0.09 cases per 100 patient-years. This is 3-fold higher than the rate of lymphomas expected in the general population based on the Surveillance, Epidemiology, and End Results Database. An increased rate of lymphoma up to several fold has been reported in the RA patient population, and may be further increased in patients with more severe disease activity. Sixty-seven malignancies, other than lymphoma, were observed. Of these, the most common malignancies were colon, breast, lung, and prostate, which were similar in type and number to what would be expected in the general population. Analysis of the cancer rates at 6-month intervals suggest constant rates over 5 years of observation.

In the placebo-controlled portions of the psoriasis studies, 8 of 933 patients who received etanercept at any dose were diagnosed with a malignancy compared with 1 of 414 patients who received placebo. Among the 1,261 patients with psoriasis who received etanercept at any dose in the controlled and uncontrolled portions of the psoriasis studies (1,062 patient-years), a total of 22 patients were diagnosed with 23 malignancies: 9 patients with noncutaneous solid tumors, 12 patients with 13 nonmelanoma skin cancers (8 basal, 5 squamous), and 1 patient with non-Hodgkin lymphoma. Among the placebo-treated patients (90 patient-years of observation), 1 patient was diagnosed with 2 squamous cell cancers. The size of the placebo group and limited duration of the controlled portions of studies precludes the ability to draw firm conclusions.

➤*Immunogenicity:* Patients with RA, psoriatic arthritis, ankylosing spondylitis, or plaque psoriasis were tested at multiple time points for antibodies to etanercept. Antibodies to the TNF receptor portion or other protein components of the etanercept drug product, all non-neutralizing, were detected at least once in sera of approximately 6% of adult patients with RA, psoriatic arthritis, ankylosing spondylitis, or plaque psoriasis. These antibodies were all non-neutralizing. No apparent correlation of antibody development to clinical response or adverse reactions was observed. Results from JRA patients were similar to those seen in adult RA patients treated with etanercept. The long-term immunogenicity of etanercept is unknown.

➤*Autoantibodies:* Patients with RA had serum samples tested for autoantibodies at multiple time points. In RA studies 1 and 2, the percentage of patients evaluated for antinuclear antibodies (ANA) who developed new positive ANA (titer greater than or equal to 1:40) was higher in patients treated with etanercept (11%) than in placebo-treated patients (5%). The percentage of patients who developed new positive antidouble-stranded deoxyribonucleic acid (DNA) antibodies was also higher by radioimmunoassay (15% of patients treated with etanercept compared with 4% of placebo-treated patients) and by crithidia lucilae assay (3% of patients treated with etanercept compared with none of placebo-treated patients). The proportion of patients treated with etanercept who developed anticardiolipin antibodies was similarly increased compared with placebo-treated patients. In study 3, no pattern of increased autoantibody development was seen in etanercept patients compared with methotrexate patients.

ETANERCEPT — INJECTION

➤*Other adverse reactions:* The following table summarizes events reported in at least 3% of all patients with higher incidence in patients treated with etanercept compared with controls in placebo-controlled RA trials (including the combination methotrexate trial) and relevant events from study 3. In placebo-controlled plaque psoriasis trials, the percentages of patients reporting injection site reactions were lower in the placebo dose group (6.4%) than in the etanercept dose groups (15.5%) in studies 1 and 2. Otherwise, the percentages of patients reporting adverse reactions in the 50 mg twice a week dose group were similar to those observed in the 25 mg twice a week dose group or placebo group. In psoriasis study 1, there were no serious adverse reactions of worsening psoriasis following withdrawal of study drug. However, adverse reactions of worsening psoriasis, including 3 serious adverse reactions, were observed during the course of the clinical trials. Urticaria and noninfectious hepatitis were observed in a small number of patients, and angioedema was observed in 1 patient in clinical studies. Urticaria and angioedema have also been reported in spontaneous postmarketing reports. Adverse reactions in psoriatic arthritis, ankylosing spondylitis, and plaque psoriasis trials were similar to those reported in RA clinical trials.

Etanercept Adverse Reactions in RA Patients[a]

	Placebo-controlled		Active-controlled (Study 3)	
Adverse reaction	Placebo[b] (n = 152)	Etanercept (n = 349)	Methotrexate (n = 217)	Etanercept (n = 415)
CNS				
Dizziness	5%	7%	11%	8%
Headache	13%	17%	27%	24%
Dermatologic				
Alopecia	1%	1%	12%	6%
Rash	3%	5%	23%	14%
GI				
Abdominal pain	3%	5%	10%	10%
Dyspepsia	1%	4%	10%	11%
Mouth ulcer	1%	2%	14%	6%
Nausea	10%	9%	29%	15%
Vomiting	-	3%	8%	5%
Respiratory				
Cough	3%	6%	6%	5%
Pharyngitis	5%	7%	9%	6%
Pneumonitis (methotrexate lung)	-	-	2%	0%
Respiratory disorder	1%	5%	NA	NA
Sinusitis	2%	3%	3%	5%
Upper respiratory tract infection[c]	16%	29%	39%	31%
Miscellaneous				
Asthenia	3%	5%	12%	11%
Infection (total) [c]	32%	35%	72%	64%
Injection site reaction	10%	37%	7%	34%
Non-upper respiratory tract infection (non-URI) [c]	32%	38%	60%	51%
Peripheral edema	3%	2%	4%	8%

[a] Includes data from the 6-month study in which patients received concurrent methotrexate therapy.

[b] The duration of exposure for patients receiving placebo was less than the etanercept-treated patients.

[c] Infection (total) includes data from all 3 placebo-controlled trials. Non–upper respiratory tract infection and upper respiratory tract infection include data only from the 2 placebo-controlled trials where infections were collected separately from adverse reactions (placebo, n = 110; etanercept, n = 213).

In controlled trials of RA and psoriatic arthritis, rates of serious adverse reactions were seen at a frequency of approximately 5% among etanercept- and control-treated patients. In controlled trials of plaque psoriasis, rates of serious adverse reactions were seen at a frequency of less than 1.5% among etanercept- and placebo-treated patients in the first 3 months of treatment. Among patients with RA in placebo-controlled, active-controlled, and open-label trials of etanercept, malignancies and infections were the most common serious adverse reactions observed. Other infrequent serious adverse reactions observed in RA, psoriatic arthritis, ankylosing spondylitis, and plaque psoriasis clinical trials are listed by body system:

Cardiovascular – Deep vein thrombosis, heart failure, hypertension, hypotension, myocardial infarction, myocardial ischemia, thrombophlebitis.

CNS – Cerebral ischemia, depression, multiple sclerosis.

Dermatologic – Worsening psoriasis.

GI – Appendicitis, cholecystitis, GI hemorrhage, pancreatitis.

GU – Kidney calculus, membranous glomerulonephropathy.

Hematologic / Lymphatic – Lymphadenopathy.

Musculoskeletal – Bursitis, polymyositis.

Respiratory – Dyspnea, pulmonary embolism, sarcoidosis.

Miscellaneous – In a randomized, controlled trial in which 51 patients with RA received etanercept 50 mg twice weekly and 25 patients received etanercept 25 mg twice weekly, the following serious adverse reactions were observed in the 50 mg twice-weekly arm: GI bleeding, normal pressure hydrocephalous, seizure, and stroke. No serious adverse reactions were observed in the 25 mg arm.

➤*JRA:* Severe adverse reactions reported in 69 JRA patients 4 to 17 years of age included varicella, gastroenteritis, depression/personality disorder, cutaneous ulcer, and esophagitis/gastritis, group A streptococcal septic shock, type 1 diabetes mellitus, and soft tissue and postoperative wound infection.

Forty-three of 69 (62%) children with JRA experienced an infection while receiving etanercept during 3 months of the study (part 1, open-label), and the frequency and severity of infections were similar in 58 patients completing 12 months of open-label extension therapy. The types of infections reported in JRA patients were generally mild and consistent with those commonly seen in outpatient pediatric populations. Two JRA patients developed varicella infection and signs and symptoms of aseptic meningitis that resolved without sequelae.

The following adverse reactions were reported more commonly in 69 JRA patients receiving 3 months of etanercept compared with the 349 adult RA patients in placebo-controlled trials. These included headache (19% of patients, 1.7 events per patient year), nausea (9%, 1 event per patient year), abdominal pain (19%, 0.74 events per patient year), and vomiting (13%, 0.74 events per patient year).

In postmarketing experience, the following additional serious adverse reactions have been reported in pediatric patients: abscess with bacteremia, coagulopathy, cutaneous vasculitis, optic neuritis, pancytopenia, seizures, transaminase elevations, tuberculous arthritis, andurinary tract infection. The frequency of these events and their causal relationship to etanercept therapy are unknown.

➤*Heart failure:* See Precautions for more information.

➤*Postmarketing:*

Cardiovascular – Chest pain, new-onset congestive heart failure, stroke, vasodilation (flushing).

CNS – Fatigue, paresthesias, seizures and CNS events suggestive of multiple sclerosis or isolated demyelinating conditions such as transverse myelitis or optic neuritis.

Dermatologic – Cutaneous vasculitis, pruritus, subcutaneous nodules, urticaria.

GI – Altered sense of taste, anorexia, diarrhea, dry mouth, intestinal perforation.

Hematologic – Adenopathy, anemia, aplastic anemia, leukopenia, neutropenia, pancytopenia, thrombocytopenia.

Musculoskeletal – Joint pain, lupus-like syndrome with manifestations including rash consistent with subacute or discoid lupus.

Ophthalmic – Dry eyes, ocular inflammation.

Respiratory – Dyspnea, interstitial lung disease, pulmonary disease, worsening of prior lung disorder.

Miscellaneous – Angioedema, fever, flu syndrome, generalized pain, weight gain.

Patient Information

Etanercept is provided as a single-use prefilled syringe or multiple-use vial. The needle cover on the single-use prefilled syringe contains dry natural rubber (latex), which should not be handled by persons sensitive to this substance. If a patient or caregiver is to administer etanercept, instruct the patient or caregiver in injection techniques and how to measure and administer the correct dose. The first injection should be performed under the supervision of a qualified health care provider. Assess the patient's or caregiver's ability to inject subcutaneously. Instruct patients and caregivers in the technique as well as proper syringe and needle disposal, and caution them against reuse of needles and syringes. Use a puncture-resistant container for disposal of needles and syringes. If the product is intended for multiple use, additional syringes, needles, and alcohol swabs will be required.

ANAKINRA

Rx	**Kineret** (Amgen)	**Injection:** 100 mg/0.67 mL	Preservative-free. Sodium chloride, EDTA. In 1 mL single-use prefilled syringe with 27-gauge needle.

ANAKINRA — INJECTION

Indications

➤*Rheumatoid arthritis (RA):* For the reduction in signs and symptoms of moderately to severely active RA in patients 18 years of age and older who have failed 1 or more disease-modifying antirheumatic drugs (DMARDs). Anakinra can be used alone or in combination with DMARDs other than tumor necrosis factor (TNF)-blocking agents.

Administration and Dosage

➤*Approved by the FDA:* November 14, 2001.

The recommended dose of anakinra is 100 mg/day administered daily by SC injection. Higher doses did not result in a higher response. Administer the dose at approximately the same time every day.

➤*Storage/Stability:* Do not use anakinra beyond the expiration date shown on the carton. Store anakinra in the refrigerator at 2° to 8°C (36° to 46°F). Do not freeze or shake. Protect from light.

Do not use the prefilled syringe if particulates or discoloration are observed. Discard any unused portions; anakinra is preservative free.

Actions

➤*Pharmacology:* Anakinra is a recombinant, nonglycosylated form of the human interleukin-1 receptor antagonist (IL-1Ra). Anakinra differs from native human IL-1Ra in that it has the addition of a single methionine residue at its amino terminus. Anakinra consists of 153 amino acids and has a molecular weight of 17.3 kilodaltons. It is produced by recombinant DNA technology using an *Escherichia coli* bacterial expression system.

Anakinra blocks the biologic activity of IL-1 by competitively inhibiting IL-1 binding to the interleukin-1 type I receptor (IL-1RI), which is expressed in a wide variety of tissues and organs.

IL-1 production is induced in response to inflammatory stimuli and mediates various physiologic responses including inflammatory and immunological responses. IL-1 has a broad range of activities, including cartilage degradation by its induction of the rapid loss of proteoglycans and stimulation of bone resorption. The levels of the naturally occurring IL-1Ra in synovium and synovial fluid from RA patients are not sufficient to compete with the elevated amount of locally produced IL-1.

➤*Pharmacokinetics:* The absolute bioavailability of anakinra after a 70 mg SC bolus injection in healthy subjects (n = 11) is 95%. In subjects with RA, maximum plasma concentrations of anakinra occurred 3 to 7 hours after SC administration of anakinra at clinically relevant doses (1 to 2 mg/kg; n = 18); the terminal half-life ranged from 4 to 6 hours. In RA patients, no unexpected accumulation of anakinra was observed after daily SC doses for up to 24 weeks. The estimated anakinra clearance increased with increasing Ccr and body weight.

Special populations –

Renal function impairment: The mean plasma clearance of anakinra decreased 70% to 75% in normal subjects with severe or end-stage renal disease (defined as Ccr less than 30 mL/min, as estimated from serum creatinine levels). No formal studies have been conducted examining the pharmacokinetics of anakinra administered SC in RA patients with renal impairment.

Contraindications

Known hypersensitivity to *E. coli*-derived proteins, anakinra, or any component of the product.

Warnings

➤*Infections:* Anakinra has been associated with an increased incidence of serious infections (2%) vs placebo (less than 1%). Discontinue administration of anakinra if a patient develops a serious infection. Do not initiate treatment with anakinra in patients with active infections. The safety and efficacy of anakinra in immunocompromised patients or in patients with chronic infections have not been evaluated. In a 24-week study of concurrent etanercept and anakinra therapy, the rate of serious infections in the combination arm (7%) was higher than with etanercept alone (0%). The combination of anakinra and etanercept did not result in higher ACR response rates compared to etanercept alone. Coadministration of anakinra and etanercept has not demonstrated increased clinical benefit. Carefully monitor patients when considering initiation of anakinra therapy concurrently with etanercept therapy.

➤*Immunosuppression:* The impact of treatment with anakinra on active and/or chronic infections and the development of malignancies is unknown.

➤*Vaccinations:* No data are available on the effects of vaccination in patients receiving anakinra. Do not give live vaccines concurrently with anakinra. No data are available on the secondary transmission of infections by live vaccines in patients receiving anakinra. Because anakinra interferes with normal immune response mechanisms to new antigens such as vaccines, vaccination may not be effective in patients receiving anakinra.

➤*Hematologic events:* See Adverse Reactions for more information.

➤*Hypersensitivity reactions:* Hypersensitivity reactions associated with anakinra administration are rare. If a severe hypersensitivity reaction occurs, discontinue anakinra administration and initiate appropriate therapy.

➤*Renal function impairment:* This drug is known to be substantially excreted by the kidney; the risk of toxic reactions to this drug may be greater in patients with impaired renal function.

➤*Elderly:* Greater sensitivity of some older individuals cannot be ruled out. Because there is a higher incidence of infections in the elderly population in general, use caution in treating the elderly.

➤*Pregnancy: Category B.* Reproductive studies have been conducted with anakinra on rats and rabbits at doses up to 100 times the human dose and have revealed no evidence of impaired fertility or harm to the fetus. However, there are no adequate and well-controlled studies in pregnant women. Because animal reproduction studies are not always predictive of human response, use anakinra during pregnancy only if clearly needed.

➤*Lactation:* It is not known whether anakinra is secreted in human milk. Because many drugs are secreted in human milk, exercise caution if anakinra is administered to nursing women.

➤*Children:* The safety and efficacy of anakinra in patients with juvenile RA have not been established.

Precautions

➤*Monitoring:* Assess neutrophil counts prior to initiating anakinra treatment, while receiving anakinra monthly for 3 months, and quarterly for a period up to 1 year thereafter.

➤*Immunogenicity:* In 2 studies, 26% of patients tested positive for anti-anakinra antibodies at month 12 in a highly sensitive, anakinra-binding biosensor assay. Of the 1318 subjects with available data at week 12 or later, 1% were seropositive in a cell-based bioassay for antibodies capable of neutralizing the biologic effects of anakinra. Two of the 15 of these subjects were positive for neutralizing antibodies at more than 1 time point up to the week 52 visit and 4 were positive at week 52. No correlation between antibody development, clinical response, or adverse events was observed. The long-term immunogenicity of anakinra is unknown.

Adverse Reactions

Anakinra Adverse Reactions Occurring in ≥ 5% of RA Patients (%)		
Adverse reaction	Anakinra 100 mg/day (n = 1565)	Placebo (n = 733)
Injection-site reaction	71	29
Worsening of RA	19	29
Upper respiratory tract infection	14	17
Headache	12	9
Nausea	8	7
Diarrhea	7	5
Sinusitis	7	7
Arthralgia	6	6
Influenza-like symptoms	6	6
Pain, abdominal	5	5

The most serious adverse reactions were serious infection and neutropenia, particularly when used in combination with TNF-blocking agents. The most common adverse reaction with anakinra is injection-site reactions (ISRs). These reactions were the most common reason for withdrawing from studies.

➤*Infections:* In 2 combined studies, the incidence of infection was 39% in the anakinra-treated patients and 37% in placebo-treated patients. The incidence of serious infections was 2% in anakinra-treated patients and 1% in placebo-treated patients over 6 months. The incidence of serious infection over 1 year was 3% in anakinra-treated patients and 2% in patients receiving placebo. These infections consisted primarily of bacterial events such as cellulitis, pneumonia, and bone and joint infections, rather than unusual, opportunistic, fungal, or viral infections. Patients with asthma appeared to be at higher risk of developing serious infections; anakinra 4% vs placebo 0%. Most patients continued on study drug after the infection resolved. There were no on-study deaths caused by serious infectious episodes in either study.

In 2 studies in which patients were receiving etanercept and anakinra for up to 24 weeks, the incidence of serious infections was 7%. The common infections consisted of bacterial pneumonia (4 cases) and cellulitis (4 cases). One patient with pulmonary fibrosis and pneumonia died because of respiratory failure.

➤*Hematologic:* In placebo-controlled studies with anakinra, treatment was associated with small reductions in the mean values for total white blood count, platelets, and ANC, and a small increase in the mean eosinophil differential percentage.

In all placebo-controlled studies, 8% of patients receiving anakinra had decreases in ANC of at least 1 WHO toxicity grade, compared with 2% of placebo patients. Nine anakinra-treated patients (0.4%) developed neutropenia (ANC less than 1×10^9/L). Additional patients treated with anakinra plus etanercept (2%) developed ANC less than 1×10^9/L. One neutropenic patient developed cellulitis and recovered with antibiotic therapy.

➤*Malignancies:* Twenty-three malignancies of various types were observed in 2730 RA patients treated in clinical trials with anakinra for up to 60 months. The observed rates and incidences were similar to those expected for the population studied.

➤*Injection-site reaction:* The most common and consistently reported treatment-related adverse event associated with anakinra is an ISR. The majority of ISRs were reported as mild. These typically lasted for 14 to 28 days and were characterized by: Erythema, ecchymosis, inflammation, and/or pain. In 2 studies, 71% of patients developed an ISR, which was typically reported within the first 4 weeks of therapy. The development of ISRs

ANAKINRA — INJECTION

in patients who had not previously experienced ISRs was uncommon after the first month of therapy.

Patient Information

Instruct patients and their caregivers on the proper dosage and administration of anakinra. Provide all patients with the "Information for Patients and Caregivers" insert.

Inform patients of the signs and symptoms of allergic and other adverse drug reactions, and advise patients on appropriate actions. Thoroughly instruct patients and their caregivers on the importance of proper disposal and caution against the reuse of needles, syringes, and drug product. Have a puncture-resistance container available for the patient for the disposal of used syringes.

ADALIMUMAB

Rx	**Humira** (Abbott)	Injection: 40 mg per 0.8 mL	Preservative free. In prefilled syringes (the needle cover contains latex) and alcohol preps.

ADALIMUMAB — INJECTION

WARNING

Risk of infection – Tuberculosis (frequently disseminated or extrapulmonary at clinical presentation), invasive fungal infections, and other opportunistic infections have been observed in patients receiving adalimumab. Some of these infections have been fatal. Antituberculosis treatment of patients with latent tuberculosis infection reduces the risk of reactivation in patients receiving treatment with adalimumab. However, active tuberculosis has developed in patients receiving adalimumab whose screening for latent tuberculosis infection was negative. Patients should be evaluated for latent tuberculosis infection with a tuberculin skin test. Treatment of latent tuberculosis infection should be initiated prior to therapy with adalimumab. Patients receiving adalimumab for signs and symptoms of active tuberculosis, including patients who are tuberculin skin test negative, should be monitored.

Indications

➤*Rheumatoid arthritis (RA):* For reducing signs and symptoms, inducing major clinical response, inhibiting the progression of structural damage, and improving physical function in adult patients with moderately to severely active RA. Adalimumab may be used alone or in combination with methotrexate or other disease-modifying antirheumatic drugs (DMARDs).

➤*Psoriatic arthritis:* For reducing signs and symptoms of active arthritis in patients with psoriatic arthritis. Adalimumab may be used alone or in combination with DMARDs.

➤*Unlabeled uses:* Treatment of Crohn disease and plaque psoriasis.

Administration and Dosage

➤*Approved by the FDA:* December 31, 2002.

➤*Dosage:* The recommended dosage of adalimumab for adult patients with RA or psoriatic arthritis is 40 mg administered every other week as a subcutaneous injection. In RA, some patients not taking concomitant methotrexate may derive additional benefit from increasing the dosing frequency of adalimumab to 40 mg every week.

➤*Concomitant medications:* Methotrexate, glucocorticoids, salicylates, nonsteroidal anti-inflammatory drugs (NSAIDs), analgesics, or other DMARDs may be continued during treatment with adalimumab.

➤*Latex allergy:* The needle cover of the syringe contains dry rubber (latex), which should not be handled by persons sensitive to this substance.

➤*Self-administration:* Adalimumab is intended for use under the guidance and supervision of a health care provider. Patients may self-inject adalimumab if their health care provider determines that it is appropriate and with medical follow-up, as necessary, after proper training in injection technique.

Patients using the prefilled syringes should be instructed to inject the full amount in the syringe (0.8 mL), which provides adalimumab 40 mg.

Injection sites should be rotated, and injections should never be given into areas where the skin is tender, bruised, red, or hard.

The solution in the syringe should be carefully inspected visually for particulate matter and discoloration prior to subcutaneous administration. If particulates and discolorations are noted, the product should not be used. Adalimumab does not contain preservatives; therefore, unused portions of drug remaining from the syringe should be discarded.

Instructions for activating the needle stick device – Cartons for institutional use contain a syringe and needle with a needle protection device. To activate the needle stick protection device after injection, hold the syringe in one hand and, with the other hand, slide the outer protective shield over the exposed needle until it locks into place.

➤*Storage/Stability:* Do not use beyond the expiration date on the container. Adalimumab must be refrigerated at 2° to 8°C (36° to 46°F). Do not freeze. Protect the prefilled syringe from exposure to light. Store in the original carton until time of administration.

Actions

➤*Pharmacology:* Adalimumab binds specifically to tumor necrosis factor (TNF)-alpha and blocks its interaction with the p55 and p75 cell surface TNF receptors. Adalimumab also lyses surface TNF-expressing cells in vitro in the presence of complement. Adalimumab does not bind or inactivate lymphotoxin (TNF-beta). TNF is a naturally occurring cytokine that is involved in normal inflammatory and immune responses. Elevated levels of TNF are found in the synovial fluid of RA and psoriatic arthritis patients, and they play an important role in the pathologic inflammation and joint destruction that are hallmarks of these diseases.

Adalimumab also modulates biological responses that are induced or regulated by TNF, including changes in the levels of adhesion molecules responsible for leukocyte migration (ELAM-1, VCAM-1, and ICAM-1 with an IC_{50} of 1 to 2×10^{-10}M).

Pharmacodynamics – After treatment with adalimumab, a rapid decrease in levels of acute-phase reactants of inflammation (C-reactive protein [CRP] and erythrocyte sedimentation rate) and serum cytokines (IL-6) was observed, compared with baseline in patients with RA. Serum levels of matrix metalloproteinases (MMP-1 and MMP-3) that produce tissue remodeling responsible for cartilage destruction also were decreased after adalimumab administration.

➤*Pharmacokinetics:*

Absorption – The maximum serum concentration and the time to reach the maximum concentration were 4.7 ± 1.6 mcg/mL and 131 ± 56 hours, respectively, following a single subcutaneous administration of adalimumab 40 mg to healthy adult subjects. The average absolute bioavailability of adalimumab estimated from 3 studies following a single 40 mg subcutaneous dose was 64%. The pharmacokinetics of adalimumab were linear over the dose range of 0.5 to 10 mg/kg following a single intravenous dose.

Adalimumab mean steady-state trough concentrations of approximately 5 mcg/mL and 8 to 9 mcg/mL were observed without and with methotrexate, respectively. The serum adalimumab trough levels at steady state increased approximately proportionally with dose following 20, 40, and 80 mg every other week and every week subcutaneous dosing.

Distribution – The single-dose pharmacokinetics of adalimumab were determined in several studies with IV doses ranging from 0.25 to 10 mg/kg. The distribution volume ranged from 4.7 to 6 L. Adalimumab concentrations in the synovial fluid from 5 RA patients ranged from 31% to 96% of those in serum.

Metabolism – Population pharmacokinetic analyses revealed there was a trend toward higher apparent clearance of adalimumab in the presence of anti-adalimumab antibodies and lower clearance with increasing age in patients 40 to 75 years of age and older.

Minor increases in apparent clearance also were predicted in patients receiving doses lower than the recommended dose and in patients with high rheumatoid factor or CRP concentrations. These increases are not likely to be clinically important.

Excretion – The systemic clearance of adalimumab is approximately 12 mL/h. The mean terminal half-life was approximately 2 weeks, ranging from 10 to 20 days across studies.

In long-term studies with dosing longer than 2 years, there was no evidence of changes in clearance over time.

Contraindications

Known hypersensitivity to adalimumab or any of its components.

Warnings

➤*Risk of infection:* Serious infections, sepsis, tuberculosis, and rare cases of opportunistic infections, including fatalities, have been reported with the use of TNF-blocking agents, including adalimumab. Many of the serious infections have occurred in patients on concomitant immunosuppressive therapy that, in addition to their RA, could predispose them to infections.

Do not initiate treatment with adalimumab in patients with active infections, including chronic or localized infections. Closely monitor patients who develop a new infection while undergoing treatment with adalimumab. Discontinue administration of adalimumab if a patient develops a serious infection. Exercise caution when considering the use of adalimumab in patients with a history of recurrent infection or underlying conditions that may predispose them to infections or in patients who have resided in regions where tuberculosis and histoplasmosis are endemic. Carefully consider the benefits and risks of adalimumab treatment before initiation of adalimumab therapy.

➤*Use with anakinra:* Serious infections were seen in clinical studies with concurrent use of anakinra (an interleukin-1 antagonist) and another TNF-blocking agent, with no added benefit. Because of the nature of the adverse reactions seen with this combination therapy, similar toxicities may also result from the combination of anakinra and other TNF-blocking agents. Therefore, the combination of adalimumab and anakinra is not recommended.

➤*Neurologic events:* Use of TNF-blocking agents, including adalimumab, has been associated with rare cases of new onset or exacerbation of clinical symptoms and/or radiographic evidence of demyelinating disease. Exercise

ADALIMUMAB — INJECTION

caution in considering the use of adalimumab in patients with preexisting or recent-onset CNS demyelinating disorders.

➤*Malignancies:* In the controlled portions of clinical trials of some TNF-blocking agents, including adalimumab, more cases of malignancies have been observed among patients receiving those TNF blockers compared with control patients. During the controlled portions of adalimumab trials in patients with moderately to severely active RA, malignancies, other than lymphoma and nonmelanoma skin cancer, were observed at a rate (95% CI) of 0.7 (0.4, 1.3) per 100 patient-years among 1,922 adalimumab-treated patients versus a rate of 0.4 (0.1, 1.2) per 100 patient-years among 947 control patients (median duration of treatment of 5.6 months for adalimumab-treated patients and 5.2 months for control-treated patients). The size of the control group and limited duration of the controlled portions of studies precludes the ability to draw firm conclusions. In the controlled and uncontrolled open-label portions of the clinical trials of adalimumab, the more frequently observed malignancies, other than lymphoma and nonmelanoma skin cancer, were breast, colon, prostate, lung, and uterine. These malignancies in adalimumab- and control-treated patients were similar in type and number to what would be expected in the general population. During the controlled portions of adalimumab RA trials, the rate (95% CI) of nonmelanoma skin cancers was 0.9 (0.56, 1.55) per 100 patient-years among adalimumab-treated patients and 0.3 (0.07, 1.07) per 100 patient-years among control patients. The potential role of TNF-blocking therapy in the development of malignancies is not known.

In the controlled portions of clinical trials of all the TNF-blocking agents, more cases of lymphoma have been observed among patients receiving TNF-blockers compared with control patients. In controlled trials in patients with RA, 2 lymphomas were observed among 1,922 adalimumab-treated patients versus 1 among 947 control patients. In combining the controlled and uncontrolled open-label portions of these clinical trials with a median duration of approximately 3 years, including 3,042 patients and more than 8,500 patient-years of therapy, the observed rate of lymphomas is approximately 0.15 per 100 patient-years. This is approximately 4-fold higher than expected in the general population. Rates in clinical trials for adalimumab cannot be compared with rates of clinical trials of other TNF blockers and may not predict the rates observed in a broader patient population. Patients with RA, particularly those with highly active disease, are at a higher risk for the development of lymphoma.

➤*Hematologic events:* Rare reports of pancytopenia, including aplastic anemia, have been reported with TNF-blocking agents. Adverse reactions of the hematologic system, including medically significant cytopenia (eg, thrombocytopenia, leukopenia), have been reported infrequently with adalimumab. The causal relationship of these reports to adalimumab remains unclear. Advise patients to seek immediate medical attention if they develop signs and symptoms suggestive of blood dyscrasias or infection (eg, persistent fever, bruising, bleeding, pallor) while on adalimumab. Consider discontinuation of adalimumab therapy in patients with confirmed significant hematologic abnormalities.

➤*Hypersensitivity reactions:* In postmarketing experience, anaphylaxis has been reported rarely following adalimumab administration. If an anaphylactic or other serious allergic reaction occurs, discontinue administration of adalimumab immediately and institute appropriate therapy. In clinical trials of adalimumab, allergic reactions overall (eg, allergic rash, anaphylactoid reaction, fixed drug reaction, nonspecified drug reaction, urticaria) have been observed in approximately 1% of patients.

➤*Elderly:* A total of 519 patients 65 years of age and older, including 107 patients 75 years of age and older, received adalimumab in clinical studies. No overall difference in efficacy was observed between these subjects and younger subjects.

The frequency of serious infection and malignancy among adalimumab-treated subjects older than 65 years of age was higher than for those younger than 65 years of age. Because there is a higher incidence of infections and malignancies in the elderly population in general, use caution when treating the elderly.

➤*Pregnancy: Category B.* An embryofetal perinatal developmental toxicity study has been performed in cynomolgus monkeys at doses up to 100 mg/kg (266 times human area under the curve [AUC] when given adalimumab 40 mg subcutaneous with methotrexate every week or 373 times human AUC when given adalimumab 40 mg subcutaneous without methotrexate) and has revealed no evidence of harm to the fetuses caused by adalimumab.

There are no adequate and well-controlled studies in pregnant women. Because animal reproduction and developmental studies are not always predictive of human response, use adalimumab during pregnancy only if clearly needed.

Pregnancy registry – To monitor outcomes of pregnant women exposed to adalimumab, a pregnancy registry has been established. Health care providers are encouraged to register patients by calling 1-877-311-8972.

➤*Lactation:* It is not known whether adalimumab is excreted in human milk or absorbed systemically after ingestion. Because many drugs and immunoglobulins are excreted in human milk, and because of the potential for serious adverse reactions in breast-feeding infants from adalimumab, decide whether to discontinue breast-feeding or the drug, taking into account the importance of the drug to the mother.

➤*Children:* Safety and efficacy of adalimumab in children have not been established.

Precautions

➤*Monitoring:* Closely monitor patients who develop a new infection while undergoing treatment with adalimumab. Monitor patients for signs and symptoms of active tuberculosis, including patients who are tuberculin skin test negative. Monitor heart failure patients carefully.

➤*Tuberculosis:* As observed with other TNF-blocking agents, tuberculosis associated with the administration of adalimumab in clinical trials has been reported. While cases were observed at all doses, the incidence of tuberculosis reactivations was increased particularly at doses of adalimumab that were higher than the recommended dose.

Before initiation of therapy with adalimumab, evaluate patients for active or latent tuberculosis infection with a tuberculin skin test. If latent infection is diagnosed, institute appropriate prophylaxis in accordance with the Centers for Disease Control and Prevention guidelines. Instruct patients to seek medical advice if signs or symptoms (eg, persistent cough, wasting/weight loss, low grade fever) suggestive of a tuberculosis infection occur.

➤*Congestive heart failure (CHF):* Cases of worsening CHF and new-onset CHF have been reported with TNF blockers. Cases of worsening CHF have also been observed with adalimumab. Adalimumab has not been formally studied in patients with CHF; however, in clinical trials of another TNF blocker, a higher rate of serious CHF-related adverse reactions was observed. Exercise caution when using adalimumab in patients who have heart failure and monitor them carefully.

➤*Immunosuppression:* The possibility exists for TNF-blocking agents, including adalimumab, to affect host defenses against infections and malignancies because TNF mediates inflammation and modulates cellular immune responses. In a study of 64 patients with RA treated with adalimumab, there was no evidence of depression of delayed-type hypersensitivity, depression of immunoglobulin levels, or change in enumeration of effector T- and B-cells and NK-cells, monocyte/macrophages, and neutrophils. The impact of treatment with adalimumab on the development and course of malignancies, as well as active and/or chronic infections, is not fully understood. The safety and efficacy of adalimumab in patients with immunosuppression have not been evaluated.

➤*Autoimmunity:* Treatment with adalimumab may result in the formation of autoantibodies and, rarely, in the development of a lupus-like syndrome. If a patient develops symptoms suggestive of a lupus-like syndrome following treatment with adalimumab, discontinue treatment.

Drug Interactions

➤*Methotrexate:* Methotrexate reduced adalimumab apparent clearance after single and multiple dosing 29% and 44%, respectively.

Adalimumab has been studied in RA patients taking concomitant methotrexate. The data do not suggest the need for dose adjustment of either adalimumab or methotrexate.

➤*Immunizations:* No data are available on the effects of vaccination in patients receiving adalimumab. Do not give live vaccines concurrently with adalimumab. No data are available on the secondary transmission of infection by live vaccines in patients receiving adalimumab.

➤*Anakinra:* Coadministration of anakinra (an interleukin-l antagonist) and another TNF-blocking agent has been associated with an increased risk of serious infections, an increased risk of neutropenia, and no additional benefit compared with these medicinal products alone. Therefore, the combination of anakinra with other TNF-blocking agents, including adalimumab, also may result in similar toxicities.

Adverse Reactions

The most serious adverse reactions were serious infections, neurologic events, and malignancies.

The most common adverse reactions with adalimumab were injection site reactions. In placebo-controlled trials, 20% of patients treated with adalimumab developed injection site reactions (eg, erythema and/or itching, hemorrhage, pain or swelling), compared with 14% of patients receiving placebo. Most injection site reactions were described as mild and generally did not necessitate drug discontinuation.

The proportion of patients who discontinued treatment because of adverse reactions during the double-blind, placebo-controlled portion of studies I, II, III, and IV was 7% for patients taking adalimumab and 4% for placebo-treated patients. The most common adverse reactions leading to discontinuation of adalimumab were clinical flare reaction (0.7%), rash (0.3%), and pneumonia (0.3%).

➤*Infections:* In placebo-controlled RA trials, the rate of infection was 1 per patient year in the adalimumab-treated patients and 0.9 per patient year in the placebo-treated patients. The infections consisted primarily of upper respiratory tract infections, bronchitis, and urinary tract infections. Most patients continued on adalimumab after the infection resolved. The incidence of serious infections was 0.04 per patient year in adalimumab-treated patients and 0.02 per patient year in placebo-treated patients. Serious infections observed included pneumonia, septic arthritis, prosthetic and postsurgical infections, erysipelas, cellulitis, diverticulitis, and pyelonephritis.

In completed and ongoing global clinical studies that include more than 13,000 patients, the overall rate of tuberculosis is approximately 0.26 per 100 patient-years. In over 4,500 patients in the United States and Canada, the rate is approximately 0.07 per 100 patient-years. These studies include reports of miliary, lymphatic, peritoneal, and pulmonary tuberculosis. Most of the cases of tuberculosis occurred within the first 8 months after initiation of therapy and may reflect recrudescence of latent disease. Cases of opportunistic infections have also been reported in these clinical trials at an overall rate of approximately 0.075 per 100 patient-years. Some cases of opportunistic infections and tuberculosis have been fatal. In postmarketing experience, infections have been observed with various pathogens, including viral, bacterial, fungal, and protozoal organisms. Infections have been noted

ADALIMUMAB — INJECTION

in all organ systems and have been reported in patients receiving adalimumab alone or in combination with immunosuppressive agents.

➤*Malignancies:* More cases of malignancy have been observed in adalimumab-treated patients compared with control-treated patients in clinical trials.

➤*Autoantibodies:* In the RA controlled trials, 12% of patients treated with adalimumab and 7% of placebo-treated patients that had negative baseline antinuclear antibody titers developed positive titers at week 24. Two patients out of 3,046 treated with adalimumab developed clinical signs suggestive of new-onset lupus-like syndrome. The patients improved following discontinuation of therapy. No patients developed lupus nephritis or CNS symptoms. The impact of long-term treatment with adalimumab on the development of autoimmune diseases is unknown.

➤*Immunogenicity:* Patients in studies I, II, and III were tested at multiple time points for antibodies to adalimumab during the 6- to 12-month period. Approximately 5% (58 of 1,062) of adult RA patients receiving adalimumab developed low-titer antibodies to adalimumab at least once during treatment, which were neutralizing in vitro. Patients treated with concomitant methotrexate had a lower rate of antibody development than patients on adalimumab monotherapy (1% vs 12%). No apparent correlation of antibody development to adverse reactions was observed. With monotherapy, patients receiving every other week dosing may develop antibodies more frequently than those receiving weekly dosing. In patients receiving the recommended dosage of 40 mg every other week as monotherapy, the American College of Rheumatology 20 response was lower among antibody-positive patients than among antibody-negative patients. The long-term immunogenicity of adalimumab is unknown.

The data reflect the percentage of patients whose test results were considered positive for antibodies to adalimumab in an enzyme-linked immunosorbent assay and are highly dependent on the sensitivity and specificity of the assay. Additionally, the observed incidence of antibody positivity in an assay may be influenced by several factors, including sample handling, timing of sample collection, concomitant medications, and underlying disease. For these reasons, comparison of the incidence of antibodies to adalimumab with the incidence of antibodies to other products may be misleading.

➤*Other adverse reactions:* The following table summarizes reactions reported at a rate of at least 5% in patients treated with adalimumab 40 mg every other week, compared with placebo and with an incidence higher than placebo. Adverse reaction rates in patients treated with adalimumab 40 mg weekly were similar to rates in patients treated with adalimumab 40 mg every other week. In study III, the types and frequencies of adverse reactions in the second-year open-label extension were similar to those observed in the 1-year double-blind portion.

Adalimumab (≥ 5%) Adverse Reactions

Adverse reaction	Adalimumab 40 mg subcutaneous every other week (n = 705)	Placebo (n = 690)
Cardiovascular		
Hypertension	5%	3%
CNS		
Headache	12%	8%
GI		
Abdominal pain	7%	4%
Nausea	9%	8%
GU		
Hematuria	5%	4%
Urinary tract infection	8%	5%
Laboratory tests[a]		
Alkaline phosphatase increased	5%	3%
Hypercholesterolemia	6%	4%
Hyperlipidemia	7%	5%
Laboratory test abnormal	8%	7%
Respiratory		
Flu syndrome	7%	6%
Sinusitis	11%	9%
Upper respiratory tract infection	17%	13%
Miscellaneous		
Accidental injury	10%	8%
Back pain	6%	4%
Injection site pain	12%	12%
Injection site reaction[b]	8%	1%
Rash	12%	6%

[a] Laboratory test abnormalities were reported as adverse reactions in European trials.
[b] Does not include erythema or itching, hemorrhage, pain, or swelling.

➤*Other infrequent serious adverse reactions:* Other infrequent serious adverse reactions occurring at an incidence of less than 5% in RA patients treated with adalimumab were as follows.

Cardiovascular – Arrhythmia, atrial fibrillation, cardiovascular disorder, chest pain, CHF, coronary artery disorder, heart arrest, hypertensive encephalopathy, myocardial infarction, palpitation, pericardial effusion, pericarditis, syncope, tachycardia, vascular disorder.

CNS – Confusion, multiple sclerosis, paresthesia, subdural hematoma, tremor.

Dermatologic – Cellulitis, erysipelas, herpes zoster.

Endocrine – Parathyroid disorder.

GI – Cholecystitis, cholelithiasis, esophagitis, gastroenteritis, GI disorder, GI hemorrhage, hepatic necrosis, vomiting.

GU – Cystitis, kidney calculus, menstrual disorder, pyelonephritis.

Hematologic/Lymphatic – Agranulocytosis, granulocytopenia, leukopenia, lymphoma-like reaction, pancytopenia, polycythemia.

Metabolic/Nutritional – Dehydration, healing abnormal, ketosis, paraproteinemia, peripheral edema.

Musculoskeletal – Arthritis, bone disorder, bone fracture (not spontaneous), bone necrosis, joint disorder, muscle cramps, myasthenia, pyogenic arthritis, synovitis, tendon disorder.

Respiratory – Asthma, bronchospasm, dyspnea, lung disorder, lung function decreased, pleural effusion, pneumonia.

Special senses – Cataract.

Miscellaneous – Adenoma, carcinomas (eg, breast, GI, skin, urogenital), fever, infection, lupus erythematosus syndrome, lymphoma and melanoma, pain in extremity, pelvic pain, sepsis, surgery, thorax pain, thrombosis leg-, tuberculosis reactivated.

➤*Postmarketing:* Adverse reactions have been reported during postapproval use of adalimumab. Because these reactions are reported voluntarily from a population of uncertain size, it is not always possible to reliably estimate their frequency or establish a causal relationship to adalimumab exposure.

Dermatologic – Cutaneous vasculitis.

Hematologic – Thrombocytopenia.

Hypersensitivity – Anaphylaxis.

Respiratory – Interstitial lung disease, including pulmonary fibrosis.

Overdosage

➤*Treatment:* The maximum tolerated dose of adalimumab has not been established in humans. Multiple doses up to 10 mg/kg have been administered to patients in clinical trials without evidence of dose-limiting toxicities. In case of overdosage, it is recommended that the patient be monitored for any signs or symptoms of adverse reactions or effects and institute appropriate symptomatic treatment immediately.

Patient Information

Ensure that the first injection is performed under the supervision of a qualified health care provider. If a patient or caregiver is to administer adalimumab, instruct them in injection techniques and assess their ability to inject subcutaneously to ensure the proper administration of adalimumab. Use a puncture-resistant container for disposal of needles and syringes. Instruct patients or caregivers in the technique as well as proper syringe and needle disposal, and caution them against reuse of these items.

INFLIXIMAB

Rx	**Remicade** (Centocor)	**Powder for injection, lyophilized:** 100 mg	Sucrose 500 mg. Preservative-free. In 20 mL single-use vials.

INFLIXIMAB — INJECTION

WARNING

Risk of infections – Tuberculosis (frequently disseminated or extrapulmonary at clinical presentation), invasive fungal infections, and other opportunistic infections have been observed in patients receiving infliximab. Some of these infections have been fatal. Antituberculosis treatment of patients with a reactive tuberculin skin test reduces the risk of tuberculosis reactivation in patients receiving treatment with infliximab. However, active tuberculosis has developed in patients receiving infliximab who were tuberculin skin test negative prior to receiving infliximab.

Evaluate patients for latent tuberculosis infection with a tuberculosis skin test. Initiate treatment of latent tuberculosis infections prior to therapy with infliximab. Monitor patients receiving infliximab for signs and symptoms of active tuberculosis, including patients who are tuberculin skin test negative.

Hepatosplenic T-cell lymphomas – Rare postmarketing cases of hepatosplenic T-cell lymphoma have been reported in adolescent and young adult patients with Crohn disease treated with infliximab. This rare type of T-cell lymphoma has a very aggressive disease course and is usually fatal. All of these hepatosplenic T-cell lymphomas with infliximab have occurred in patients on concomitant treatment with azathioprine or 6-mercaptopurine.

Indications

➤*Ankylosing spondylitis:* For reducing signs and symptoms in patients with active ankylosing spondylitis.

➤*Crohn disease, moderate to severe:* For reducing the signs and symptoms and inducing and maintaining clinical remission in adult and pediatric patients with moderately to severely active Crohn disease who have had inadequate responses to conventional therapy.

Infliximab is indicated for the reduction in the number of draining enterocutaneous and rectovaginal fistulas and maintaining fistula closure in patients with fistulizing Crohn disease.

➤*Psoriatic arthritis:* For reducing signs and symptoms of active arthritis in patients with psoriatic arthritis.

➤*Rheumatoid arthritis, moderate to severe:* In combination with methotrexate, for reducing signs and symptoms, inhibiting the progression of structural damage, and improving physical function in patients with moderately to severely active rheumatoid arthritis.

➤*Ulcerative colitis:* For reducing signs and symptoms, achieving clinical remission and mucosal healing, and eliminating corticosteroid use in patients with moderately to severely active ulcerative colitis who have had an inadequate response to conventional therapy.

➤*Unlabeled uses:* For possible treatment of plaque psoriasis, psoriasis, juvenile arthritis, and severe pediatric Crohn disease.

Administration and Dosage

➤*Approved by the FDA:* August 24, 1998.

➤*Ankylosing spondylitis:* 5 mg/kg given as an intravenous (IV) infusion, followed by additional similar doses 2 and 6 weeks after the first infusion, and every 6 weeks thereafter.

➤*Crohn disease or fistulizing Crohn disease:*

Adults – 5 mg/kg given as an induction regimen at 0, 2, and 6 weeks, followed by a maintenance regimen of 5 mg/kg every 8 weeks thereafter for the treatment of adults with moderately to severely active Crohn disease or fistulizing Crohn disease. For adult patients who respond and then lose their response, consider treatment with 10 mg/kg. Patients who do not respond by week 14 are unlikely to respond with continued dosing; consider discontinuing infliximab in these patients.

Children – 5 mg/kg given as an IV induction regimen at 0, 2, and 6 weeks followed by a maintenance regimen of 5 mg/kg every 8 weeks for moderately to severely active Crohn disease.

➤*Psoriatic arthritis:* 5 mg/kg given as an IV infusion, followed by additional similar doses at 2 and 6 weeks after the first infusion, and every 8 weeks thereafter. Infliximab can be used with or without methotrexate.

➤*Rheumatoid arthritis:* 3 mg/kg given as an IV infusion, followed by additional similar doses at 2 and 6 weeks after the first infusion, and every 8 weeks thereafter. Give infliximab in combination with methotrexate. For patients who have incomplete responses, consider adjusting the dose up to 10 mg/kg or treating as often as every 4 weeks, bearing in mind that risk of serious infections is increased at higher doses.

➤*Ulcerative colitis:* 5 mg/kg given as an induction regimen at 0, 2, and 6 weeks, followed by a maintenance regimen of 5 mg/kg every 8 weeks thereafter for the treatment of moderately to severely active ulcerative colitis.

➤*Preparation and administration instructions:* Infliximab vials do not contain antibacterial preservatives. Therefore, use the vials after reconstitution immediately. Do not reenter or store them. The diluent to be used for reconstitution is 10 mL of sterile water for injection. The total dose of the reconstituted product must be further diluted to 250 mL with 0.9% sodium chloride injection. The infusion concentration should range between 0.4 and 4 mg/mL. Begin the infliximab infusion within 3 hours of preparation.

1.) Calculate the dose and the number of infliximab vials needed. Each infliximab vial contains infliximab 100 mg. Calculate the total volume of reconstituted infliximab solution required.
2.) Reconstitute each infliximab vial with 10 mL of sterile water for injection, using a syringe equipped with a 21-gauge or smaller needle. Remove the flip-top from the vial and wipe the top with an alcohol swab. Insert the syringe needle into the vial through the center of the rubber stopper and direct the stream of sterile water for injection to the glass wall of the vial. Do not use the vial if the vacuum is not present. Gently swirl the solution by rotating the vial to dissolve the lyophilized powder. Avoid prolonged or vigorous agitation. Do not shake. Foaming of the solution on reconstitution is not unusual. Allow the reconstituted solution to stand for 5 minutes. The solution should be colorless to light yellow and opalescent and may develop a few translucent particles because infliximab is a protein. Do not use if opaque particles, discoloration, or other foreign particles are present.
3.) Dilute the total volume of the reconstituted infliximab solution dose to 250 mL with 0.9% sodium chloride injection by withdrawing a volume of 0.9% sodium chloride injection equal to the volume of reconstituted infliximab from the 0.9% sodium chloride injection 250 mL bottle or bag. Slowly add the total volume of reconstituted infliximab solution to the 250 mL infusion bottle or bag. Gently mix.
4.) The infusion solution must be administered for a period of not less than 2 hours and must use an infusion set with an inline, sterile, nonpyrogenic, low-protein-binding filter (pore size of 1.2 mcm or less). Do not store any unused portion of the infusion solution for reuse.
5.) No physical biochemical compatibility studies have been conducted to evaluate the coadministration of infliximab with other agents. Do not infuse infliximab concomitantly in the same IV line with other agents.

➤*Storage / Stability:* Store the lyophilized product under refrigeration at 2° to 8°C (36° to 46°F). Do not freeze. Do not use beyond the expiration date. This product contains no preservative.

Actions

➤*Pharmacology:* Infliximab neutralizes the biological activity of TNF-α by binding with high affinity to the soluble and transmembrane forms of TNF-α and inhibits binding of TNF-α with its receptors. Infliximab does not neutralize TNFβ (lymphotoxin-α), a related cytokine that utilizes the same receptors as TNF-α. Biological activities attributed to TNF-α include the following: induction of proinflammatory cytokines such as interleukins 1 and 6; enhancement of leukocyte migration by increasing endothelial layer permeability and expression of adhesion molecules by endothelial cells and leukocytes; activation of neutrophil and eosinophil functional activity; induction of acute phase reactants and other liver proteins, as well as tissue-degrading enzymes produced by synoviocytes and/or chondrocytes. Cells expressing transmembrane TNF-α bound by infliximab can be lysed in vitro or in vivo. Infliximab inhibits the functional activity of TNF-α in a wide variety of in vitro bioassays utilizing human fibroblasts, endothelial cells, neutrophils, B and T lymphocytes, and epithelial cells. Anti–TNF-α antibodies reduce disease activity in the cotton-top tamarin colitis model, and decrease synovitis and joint erosions in a murine model of collagen-induced arthritis. Infliximab prevents disease in transgenic mice that develop polyarthritis as a result of constitutive expression of human TNF-α, and, when administered after disease onset, allows eroded joints to heal.

Pharmacodynamics – Elevated concentrations of TNF-α have been found in involved tissues and fluids of patients with rheumatoid arthritis, Crohn disease, ulcerative colitis, ankylosing spondylitis, and psoriatic arthritis. In rheumatoid arthritis, treatment with infliximab reduced infiltration of inflammatory cells in inflamed areas of the joint as well as expression of molecules mediating cellular adhesion (E-selectin, intercellular adhesion molecule-1, and vascular cell adhesion molecule-1, chemoattraction (interleukin-8 and monocyte chemotactic protein, and tissue degradation (matrix metalloproteinase 1 and 3). In Crohn disease, treatment with infliximab reduced infiltration of inflammatory cells and TNF-α production in inflamed areas of the intestine and reduced the proportion of mononuclear cells from the lamina propria able to express TNF-α and interferon.

After treatment with infliximab, patients with rheumatoid arthritis or Crohn disease exhibited decreased levels of serum interleukin-6 and C-reactive protein (CRP) compared with baseline. Peripheral blood lymphocytes from infliximab-treated patients showed no significant decrease in number or in proliferative responses to in vitro mitogenic stimulation when compared with cells from untreated patients. In psoriatic arthritis, treatment with infliximab resulted in a reduction of the number of T cells and blood vessels in the synovium and psoriatic skin, as well as a reduction of macrophages in the synovium. The relationship between these pharmacodynamic activities and the mechanism(s) by which infliximab exerts its clinical effects is unknown.

➤*Pharmacokinetics:*

Absorption / Distribution – Single IV infusions of 3 to 20 mg/kg showed a linear relationship between the dose administered and the maximum serum concentration. The volume of distribution at steady state was independent of dose and indicated that infliximab was distributed primarily within the vascular compartment.

Following an initial dose of infliximab, repeated infusions at 2 and 6 weeks resulted in predictable concentration-time profiles following each treatment.

INFLIXIMAB — INJECTION

No systemic accumulation of infliximab occurred upon continued repeated treatment with 3 or 10 mg/kg at 4- or 8-week intervals. At 8 weeks after a maintenance dose of 3 to 10 mg/kg of infliximab, median infliximab serum concentrations ranged from approximately 0.5 to 6 mcg/mL; however, infliximab concentrations were not detectable (less than 0.1 mcg/mL) in patients who became positive for antibodies to infliximab.

Excretion – Pharmacokinetic results for doses of 3 to 10 mg/kg in rheumatoid arthritis and 5 mg/kg in Crohn disease indicate that the terminal half-life of infliximab is 8 to 9.5 days. Development of antibodies to infliximab increased infliximab clearance.

Contraindications

Do not administer infliximab at doses greater than 5 mg/kg to patients with moderate to severe heart failure. In a randomized study evaluating infliximab in patients with moderate to severe heart failure (New York Heart Association [NYHA] functional Class III/IV), infliximab treatment at 10 mg/kg was associated with an increased incidence of death and hospitalization because of worsening heart failure.

Do not administer infliximab to patients with known hypersensitivity to any murine proteins or other component of the product.

Warnings

➤*Risk of infections:* Serious infections, including sepsis and pneumonia, have been reported in patients receiving TNF-blocking agents. Some of these infections have been fatal. Many of the serious infections in patients treated with infliximab have occurred in patients on concomitant immunosuppressive therapy that, in addition to their underlying disease, could predispose them to infections.

Do not give infliximab to patients with a clinically important, active infection. Exercise caution when considering the use of infliximab in patients with chronic infections or histories of recurrent infection. Monitor patients for signs and symptoms of infection while on or after treatment with infliximab. Closely monitor new infections. If a patient develops a serious infection, discontinue infliximab therapy.

Cases of tuberculosis, histoplasmosis, coccidioidomycosis, listeriosis, pneumocytosis, tuberculosis, and other bacterial, mycobacterial, and fungal infections have been observed in patients receiving infliximab. For patients who have resided in regions where histoplasmosis or coccidioidomycosis is endemic, carefully consider the benefits and risks of infliximab treatment before initiation of infliximab therapy.

See Drug Interactions for more information.

➤*Heart failure:* Infliximab has been associated with adverse outcomes in patients with heart failure; use in patients with heart failure only after consideration of other treatment options. The results of a randomized study evaluating the use of infliximab in patients with heart failure (NYHA functional Class III/IV) suggested higher mortality in patients who received infliximab 10 mg/kg and higher rates of cardiovascular adverse reactions at doses of 5 and 10 mg/kg. There have been postmarketing reports of worsening heart failure, with and without identifiable precipitating factors, in patients taking infliximab. There also have been rare postmarketing reports of new onset heart failure, including heart failure in patients without known preexisting cardiovascular disease. Some of these patients were younger than 50 years of age. If a decision is made to administer infliximab to patients with heart failure, closely monitor them during therapy, and discontinue infliximab if new or worsening symptoms of heart failure appear.

➤*Hematologic events:* Cases of leukopenia, neutropenia, thrombocytopenia, and pancytopenia, some with a fatal outcome, have been reported in patients receiving infliximab. The causal relationship to infliximab therapy remains unclear. Although no high-risk group(s) has been identified, exercise caution in patients being treated with infliximab who have ongoing or histories of significant hematologic abnormalities. Advise all patients to seek immediate medical attention if they develop signs and symptoms suggestive of blood dyscrasias or infection (eg, persistent fever) while on infliximab. Consider discontinuation of infliximab therapy in patients who develop significant hematologic abnormalities.

➤*Neurologic events:* Infliximab and other agents that inhibit TNF have been associated in rare cases with optic neuritis, seizure, and new onset or exacerbation of clinical symptoms and/or radiographic evidence of CNS-demyelinating disorders, including multiple sclerosis and CNS manifestations of systemic vasculitis. Exercise caution when considering the use of infliximab in patients with preexisting or recent onset of CNS-demyelinating or seizure disorders. Consider discontinuation of infliximab in patients who develop significant CNS adverse reactions.

➤*Malignancies:* In the controlled portions of clinical trials of some TNF-blocking agents including infliximab, more malignancies have been observed in patients receiving those TNF-blockers compared with control patients. During the controlled portions of infliximab trials in patients with moderately to severely active rheumatoid arthritis, Crohn disease, psoriatic arthritis, ankylosing spondylitis, and ulcerative colitis, 14 patients were diagnosed with malignancies among 2,897 infliximab-treated patients versus 1 among 1,262 control patients (at a rate of 0.65/100 patient-years among infliximab-treated patients versus a rate of 0.13/100 patient-years among control patients), with median duration of follow-up 0.5 years for infliximab-treated patients and 0.4 years for control patients. Of these, the most common malignancies were breast, colorectal, and melanoma. The rate of malignancies among infliximab-treated patients was similar to that expected in the general population whereas the rate in control patients was lower than expected. In the controlled portions of clinical trials of all the TNF-blocking agents, more cases of lymphoma have been observed among patients receiving a TNF-blocker compared with control patients.

In an exploratory clinical trial evaluating the use of infliximab in patients with moderate to severe chronic obstructive pulmonary disease (COPD), more malignancies were reported in infliximab-treated patients compared with control patients. All patients had a history of heavy smoking.

The potential role of TNF-blocking therapy in the development of malignancies is not known. Rates in clinical trials for infliximab cannot be compared with rates in clinical trials of other TNF-blockers and may not predict rates observed in a broader patient population. Exercise caution in considering infliximab treatment in patients with a history of malignancy or in continuing treatment in patients who develop malignancy while receiving infliximab.

➤*Hepatotoxicity:* Severe hepatic reactions, including acute liver failure, jaundice, hepatitis, and cholestasis, have been reported rarely in postmarketing data in patients receiving infliximab. Autoimmune hepatitis has been diagnosed in some of these cases. Severe hepatic reactions occurred between 2 weeks to more than a year after initiation of infliximab; elevations in hepatic aminotransferase levels were not noted prior to discovery of the liver injury in many of these cases. Some of these cases were fatal or necessitated liver transplantation. Evaluate patients with symptoms or signs of liver dysfunction for evidence of liver injury. If jaundice and/or marked liver enzyme elevations (eg, greater than or equal to 5 times the upper limit of normal [ULN]) develop, discontinue infliximab and undertake a thorough investigation of the abnormality. As with other immunosuppressive drugs, use of infliximab has been associated with reactivation of hepatitis B in patients who are chronic carriers of this virus (ie, surface-antigen positive). Appropriately evaluate chronic carriers of hepatitis B and monitor prior to the initiation of and during treatment with infliximab. In clinical trials, mild or moderate elevations of ALT and AST have been observed in patients receiving infliximab without progression to severe hepatic injury.

➤*Hypersensitivity reactions:* Infliximab has been associated with hypersensitivity reactions that varied in times of onset and required hospitalization in some cases. Most hypersensitivity reactions, which include urticaria, dyspnea, and/or hypotension, have occurred during or within 2 hours of infliximab infusion. However, in some cases, serum sickness-like reactions have been observed in patients with Crohn disease 3 to 12 days after infliximab therapy was reinstituted following an extended period without infliximab treatment. Symptoms associated with these reactions include fever, rash, headache, sore throat, myalgias, polyarthralgias, hand and facial edema, and/or dysphagia. These reactions were associated with marked increase in antibodies to infliximab, loss of detectable serum concentrations of infliximab, and possible loss of drug efficacy. For severe reactions, discontinue infliximab. Medications for the treatment of hypersensitivity reactions (eg, acetaminophen, antihistamines, corticosteroids, epinephrine) should be available for immediate use in the event of a reaction.

➤*Elderly:* In clinical trials of rheumatoid arthritis, no overall differences were observed in efficacy or safety in the 181 patients 65 years of age or older compared with younger patients, although the incidence of serious adverse reactions in patients 65 years of age or older was higher in both infliximab and control groups compared with younger patients. In Crohn disease, ulcerative colitis, ankylosing spondylitis, and psoriatic arthritis studies, there were insufficient numbers of patients 65 years of age or older to determine whether they respond differently from patients 18 to 65 years of age. Because there is a higher incidence of infections in the elderly population in general, use caution in treating the elderly.

➤*Pregnancy: Category B.* Because infliximab does not crossreact with TNF-α in species other than humans and chimpanzees, animal reproduction studies have not been conducted with infliximab.

It is not known if infliximab can cause fetal harm when administered to a pregnant woman or can affect reproduction capacity. Give infliximab to a pregnant woman only if clearly needed.

➤*Lactation:* It is not known if infliximab is excreted in human milk or absorbed systemically after ingestion. Because many drugs and immunoglobulins are excreted in human milk, and because of the potential for adverse reactions in breast-feeding infants from infliximab, decide whether to discontinue breast-feeding or the drug, taking into account the importance of the drug to the mother.

➤*Children:* Safety and efficacy of infliximab in patients with juvenile rheumatoid arthritis and in pediatric patients with Crohn disease have not been established.

Precautions

➤*Monitoring:* Monitor patients for signs and symptoms of infection during or after treatment with infliximab. Closely monitor new infections. If a patient develops a serious infection, discontinue infliximab therapy. Closely monitor patients who develop new or worsening symptoms of heart failure. Appropriately evaluate and monitor chronic carriers of hepatitis B prior to the initiation of and during treatment with infliximab. Closely monitor patients with heart failure during therapy, and discontinue infliximab if new or worsening symptoms of heart failure appear.

➤*Immunogenicity:* Treatment with infliximab can be associated with the development of antibodies to infliximab. The incidence of antibodies to infliximab in patients given a 3-dose induction regimen followed by maintenance dosing was approximately 10% as assessed through 1 to 2 years of infliximab treatment. A higher incidence of antibodies to infliximab was observed in patients with Crohn disease receiving infliximab after drug-free intervals greater than 16 weeks. The majority of antibody-positive patients had low titers. Patients who were antibody positive were more likely to have higher rates of clearance and reduced efficacy and to experience an infusion reaction than were patients who were antibody negative. Antibody development was lower among patients with rheumatoid arthritis and Crohn dis-

INFLIXIMAB — INJECTION

ease receiving immunosuppressant therapies such as 6-mercaptopurine/azathioprine or methotrexate.

➤*Autoimmunity:* Treatment with infliximab may result in the formation of autoantibodies and, rarely, in the development of a lupus-like syndrome. If a patient develops symptoms suggestive of a lupus-like syndrome after treatment with infliximab, discontinue treatment.

➤*Vaccinations:* See Drug Interactions for more information.

Drug Interactions

➤*Anakinra:* Coadministration of etanercept (another TNF-α–blocking agent) and anakinra (an interleukin-1 antagonist) has been associated with an increased risk of serious infections, and an increased risk of neutropenia and the combination has no additional benefit compared with these medicinal products alone. Other TNF-α–blocking agents (including infliximab) used in combination with anakinra also may result in similar toxicities. Therefore, the combination of infliximab and anakinra is not recommended.

➤*Vaccinations:* No data are available on the response to vaccination or on the secondary transmission of infection by live vaccines in patients receiving anti-TNF therapy. It is recommended that live vaccines not be given concurrently.

Adverse Reactions

The data described herein reflect exposure to infliximab in 3,263 patients (1,304 patients with rheumatoid arthritis, 1,106 patients with Crohn disease, 202 with ankylosing spondylitis, 150 with psoriatic arthritis, 484 with ulcerative colitis, and 17 patients with other conditions), including 1,484 patients exposed beyond 30 weeks and 296 exposed beyond 1 year. The most common reason for discontinuation of treatment was infusion-related reactions (eg, dyspnea, flushing, headache, rash). Adverse reactions have been reported in a higher proportion of patients with rheumatoid arthritis receiving the 10 mg/kg dose than the 3 mg/kg dose; however, no differences were observed in the frequency of adverse reactions between the 5 and 10 mg/kg doses in patients with Crohn disease.

➤*Infusion-related reactions:*

Acute infusion reactions – An infusion reaction was defined in clinical trials as any adverse reaction occurring during the infusion or within 1 to 2 hours after the infusion. Approximately 20% of infliximab-treated patients in all clinical trials experienced infusion reactions compared with approximately 10% of placebo-treated patients. Among all infliximab infusions, 3% were accompanied by nonspecific symptoms such as fever or chills, 1% were accompanied by cardiopulmonary reactions (primarily chest pain, hypotension, hypertension, or dyspnea), and less than 1% were accompanied by pruritus, urticaria, or the combined symptoms of pruritus/urticaria and cardiopulmonary reactions. Serious infusion reactions occurred in less than 1% of patients and included anaphylaxis, convulsions, erythematous rash, and hypotension. Approximately 3% of patients discontinued infliximab because of infusion reactions, and all patients recovered with treatment and/or discontinuation of infusion. Infliximab infusions beyond the initial infusion were not associated with a higher incidence of reactions.

Patients who became positive for antibodies to infliximab were more likely (approximately 2- to 3-fold) to have an infusion reaction than were those who were negative. Use of concomitant immunosuppressant agents appeared to reduce the frequency of antibodies to infliximab and infusion reactions.

Reactions following readministration – In a study where 37 of 41 patients with Crohn disease were retreated with infliximab following a 2- to 4-year period without infliximab treatment, 10 patients experienced adverse reactions, manifesting 3 to 12 days following infusion, of which 6 were considered serious. Signs and symptoms included the following: myalgia and arthralgia with fever and/or rash, with some patients also experiencing pruritus; facial, hand, or lip edema; dysphagia; urticaria; sore throat; headache. Patients experiencing these adverse reactions had not experienced infusion-related adverse reactions associated with initial infliximab therapy. These adverse reactions occurred in 39% (9 of 23) who had received liquid formulation, which no longer is in use, and 7% (1 of 14) of patients who received lyophilized formulation. The clinical data are not adequate to determine if occurrence of these reactions is due to differences in formulation. Patients' signs and symptoms improved substantially or resolved with treatment in all cases. There are insufficient data on the incidence of these events after drug-free intervals of 1 to 2 years. However, these reactions have been observed only infrequently in clinical trials and postmarketing surveillance with retreatment intervals up to 1 year.

➤*Infections:* In infliximab clinical studies, treated infections were reported in 36% of infliximab-treated patients (average of 51 weeks of follow-up) and in 25% of placebo-treated patients (average of 37 weeks of follow-up). The infections most frequently reported were respiratory tract infections (including sinusitis, pharyngitis, and bronchitis) and urinary tract infections. Among infliximab-treated patients, serious infections included pneumonia, cellulitis, abscess, skin ulceration, sepsis, and bacterial infection. In all clinical trials, 7 opportunistic infections were reported; 2 cases each of coccidioidomycosis (1 case was fatal) and histoplasmosis (1 case was fatal), and 1 case each of pneumocystosis, nocardiosis, and cytomegalovirus. Tuberculosis was reported in 14 patients, 4 of whom died because of miliary tuberculosis. Other cases of tuberculosis, including disseminated tuberculosis, also have been reported postmarketing. Most of these cases of tuberculosis occurred within the first 2 months after initiation of therapy with infliximab and may reflect recrudescence of latent disease. In the 1-year, placebo-controlled studies RA I and RA II, 5.3% of patients receiving infliximab every 8 weeks with methotrexate developed serious infections as compared with 3.4% of placebo patients receiving methotrexate. Of 924 patients receiving infliximab, 1.7% developed pneumonia and 0.4% developed tuberculosis, when compared with 0.3% and 0% in the placebo arm, respectively. In a shorter (22-week) placebo-controlled study of 1,082 RA patients randomized to receive placebo, 3 or 10 mg/kg of infliximab infusions at 0, 2, and 6 weeks, followed by every 8 weeks with methotrexate, serious infections were more frequent in the infliximab 10 mg/kg group (5.3%) than the 3 mg/kg or placebo groups (1.7% in both). During the 54-week Crohn's II Study, 15% of patients with fistulizing Crohn disease developed a new fistula-related abscess.

In infliximab clinical studies in patients with ulcerative colitis, infections treated with antimicrobials were reported in 19% of infliximab-treated patients (average of 27 weeks of follow-up) and in 14% of placebo-treated patients (average 22 weeks of follow-up). The types of infections, including serious infections, reported in patients with ulcerative colitis were similar to those reported in other clinical studies.

In postmarketing experience, infections have been observed with various pathogens including viral, bacterial, fungal, and protozoal organisms. Infections have been noted in all organ systems and have been reported in patients receiving infliximab alone or in combination with immunosuppressive agents.

➤*Autoantibodies/Lupus-like syndrome:* See Precautions for more information.

➤*Malignancies:* Malignancies, including non-Hodgkin lymphoma and Hodgkin disease, have also been reported in patients receiving infliximab during post-approval use.

See Warnings for more information.

➤*Patients with heart failure:* See Warnings for more information.

➤*Immunogenicity:* See Precautions for more information.

➤*Hepatotoxicity:* See Warnings for more information.

➤*Other adverse reactions:* Safety data are available from 3,263 infliximab-treated patients, including 1,304 with rheumatoid arthritis, 1,106 with Crohn disease, 484 with ulcerative colitis, 202 with ankylosing spondylitis, 150 with psoriatic arthritis, and 17 with other conditions. Adverse reactions reported in 5% or more of all patients with rheumatoid arthritis receiving 4 or more infusions are in the following table. The types and frequencies of adverse reactions observed were similar in infliximab-treated patients with rheumatoid arthritis, ankylosing spondylitis, psoriatic arthritis, and Crohn disease, except for abdominal pain, which occurred in 26% of infliximab-treated patients with Crohn disease. In the studies of Crohn disease, there were insufficient numbers and duration of follow-up for patients who never received infliximab to provide meaningful comparisons.

Infliximab Adverse Reactions Occurring in 5% or More of Patients Receiving 4 or More Infusions for Rheumatoid Arthritis

	Placebo (n = 350)	Infliximab (n = 1,129)
Average weeks of follow-up	59	66
Cardiovascular		
Hypertension	5%	7%
CNS		
Fatigue	7%	9%
Headache	14%	18%
Dermatologic		
Pruritus	2%	7%
Rash	5%	10%
GI		
Abdominal pain	8%	12%
Diarrhea	12%	12%
Dyspepsia	7%	10%
Nausea	20%	21%
GU		
Moniliasis	3%	5%
Urinary tract infection	6%	8%
Musculoskeletal		
Arthralgia	7%	8%
Back pain	5%	8%
Respiratory		
Bronchitis	9%	10%
Coughing	8%	12%
Pharyngitis	8%	12%
Rhinitis	5%	8%
Sinusitis	8%	14%
Upper respiratory tract infection	25%	32%
Miscellaneous		
Fever	4%	7%
Pain	7%	8%

INFLIXIMAB — INJECTION

The most common serious adverse reactions observed in clinical trials were infections. Other serious, medically relevant adverse reactions of 0.2% or more or clinically significant adverse reactions by body system were as follows:

Cardiovascular – Arrhythmia, bradycardia, brain infarction, cardiac arrest, circulatory failure, hypotension, myocardial infarction, pulmonary embolism, syncope, tachycardia, thrombophlebitis.

CNS – Confusion, dizziness, meningitis, neuritis, peripheral neuropathy, suicide attempt.

Dermatologic – Increased sweating, ulceration.

GI – Constipation, GI hemorrhage, ileus, intestinal obstruction, intestinal perforation, intestinal stenosis, pancreatitis, peritonitis, proctalgia.

GU – Menstrual irregularity, renal calculus, renal failure.

Hematologic/Lymphatic – Anemia, hemolytic anemia, leukopenia, pancytopenia, thrombocytopenia.

Hepatic – Biliary pain, cholecystitis, cholelithiasis, hepatitis.

Musculoskeletal – Intervertebral disk herniation, tendon disorder.

Respiratory – Adult respiratory distress syndrome, lower respiratory tract infection (including pneumonia), pleural effusion, pleurisy, pulmonary edema, respiratory insufficiency.

Miscellaneous – Allergic reaction; basal cell, breast, lymphoma neoplasms; cellulitis; dehydration; diaphragmatic hernia; edema; lymphadenopathy; sepsis; serum sickness; surgical/procedural sequela.

Postmarketing adverse reactions – The following adverse reactions have been reported during postmarketing use of infliximab: Guillain-Barré syndrome, idiopathic thrombocytopenic purpura, interstitial pneumonitis/fibrosis, neuropathies (additional neurologic events also have been observed), pericardial effusion, systemic and cutaneous vasculitis, thrombotic thrombocytopenic purpura, and transverse myelitis. Because these reactions are reported voluntarily from a population of uncertain size, it is not always possible to reliably estimate frequency or establish a causal relationship to infliximab exposure.

In postmarketing experience, cases of anaphylactic-like reactions, including laryngeal/pharyngeal edema and severe bronchospasm, and seizure have been associated with infliximab administration.

Malignancies, including non-Hodgkin lymphoma and Hodgkin disease, also have been reported in patients receiving infliximab during postapproval use.

In postmarketing experience, infections have been observed with various pathogens, including viral, bacterial, fungal, and protozoal organisms. Infections have been noted in all organ systems and have been reported in patients receiving infliximab alone or in combination with immunosuppressive agents.

Overdosage

➤*Treatment:* In case of overdosage, monitor the patient for any signs or symptoms of adverse reactions or effects, and institute appropriate symptomatic treatment immediately.

Patient Information

➤*What health concerns should I talk to my doctor about?:* Before receiving your first treatment with infliximab you should tell your doctor if you:

- Have or think you may have any kind of infection. The infection could be in only one place in your body (such as an open cut or sore), or an infection that affects your whole body (such as the flu). Having an infection could put you at risk for serious side effects from infliximab.
- Have an infection that will not go away or a history of infection that keeps coming back.
- Have had tuberculosis, or if you recently have been with anyone who might have tuberculosis. Your doctor will examine you for tuberculosis and perform a skin test. If your doctor thinks that you are at risk for tuberculosis, he or she may start treating you for tuberculosis before you begin infliximab therapy.
- Have lived in or visited an area of the country where an infection called histoplasmosis or coccidioidomycosis (an infection caused by a fungus that affects the lungs) is common. If you do not know if the area you live in is one where histoplasmosis or coccidioidomycosis is common, ask your doctor.
- Have or have previously had heart failure or other heart conditions.
- Have or have had a condition that affects your nervous system, like multiple sclerosis or Guillain-Barré syndrome, or experience any numbness or tingling, or have had a seizure.
- Are pregnant or breast-feeding.
- Have recently received or are scheduled to receive a vaccine.

➤*How often will I receive infliximab?:*

Rheumatoid arthritis – If you are receiving infliximab for rheumatoid arthritis you will receive your first dose followed by additional doses at 2 and 6 weeks after the first dose. You then will receive a dose every 8 weeks. Your doctor will monitor your response to infliximab and may change your dose or dose you more frequently (as often as every 4 weeks).

Crohn disease or fistulizing Crohn disease – If you are receiving infliximab for active Crohn disease or fistulizing Crohn disease, you will receive your first dose followed by additional doses at 2 and 6 weeks after the first dose. You then will receive a dose every 8 weeks. Your doctor will monitor your response to infliximab and may change your dose.

Ulcerative colitis – If you are receiving infliximab for psoriatic arthritis you will receive your first dose followed by additional doses at 2 and 6 weeks after the first dose. You will then receive a dose every 8 weeks.

Ankylosing spondylitis – If you are receiving infliximab for ankylosing spondylitis, you will receive your first dose followed by additional doses at 2 and 6 weeks after the first dose. You then will receive a dose every 6 weeks.

Psoriatic arthritis – If you are receiving infliximab for psoriatic arthritis, you will receive your first dose followed by additional doses at 2 and 6 weeks after the first dose. You will then receive a dose every 8 weeks.

ABATACEPT

Rx	**Orencia** (Bristol-Myers Squibb)	**Powder for injection, lyophilized**: 250 mg	500 mg maltose, 17.2 mg monobasic sodium phosphate, 14.6 mg sodium chloride. In single-use vials with syringe.

ABATACEPT — INJECTION

Indications

➤*Rheumatoid arthritis (RA):* For reducing signs and symptoms, inducing major clinical response, slowing the progression of structural damage, and improving physical function in adults with moderately to severely active RA who have had an inadequate response to one or more disease-modifying antirheumatic drugs (DMARDs), such as methotrexate or tumor necrosis factor (TNF) antagonists. Abatacept may be used as monotherapy or concomitantly with DMARDs other than TNF antagonists.

Do not administer abatacept concomitantly with TNF antagonists. Abatacept is not recommended for use concomitantly with anakinra.

Administration and Dosage

➤*Approved by the FDA:* December 23, 2005.

➤*Dosage:* Abatacept should be administered as a 30 minute intravenous (IV) infusion at the dose specified in the following table. Following the initial administration, abatacept should be given at 2 and 4 weeks after the first infusion, then every 4 weeks thereafter. Abatacept may be used as monotherapy or concomitantly with DMARDs other than TNF antagonists.

Abatacept Dosing		
Body weight	Dose	Number of 250 mg vials
< 60 kg	500 mg	2
60 to 100 kg	750 mg	3
> 100 kg	1 g	4

Use aseptic technique.

➤*Preparation for administration:* Each vial provides abatacept 250 mg for administration. The abatacept powder in each vial must be reconstituted with 10 mL sterile water for injection using only the silicone-free disposable syringe provided with each vial and an 18 to 21 gauge needle. If the abatacept powder is accidentally reconstituted using a siliconized syringe, the solution may develop a few translucent particles. Discard any solutions prepared using siliconized syringes.

If the silicone-free disposable syringe is dropped or becomes contaminated, use a new silicone-free disposable syringe from inventory. For information on obtaining additional silicone-free disposable syringes, contact Bristol-Myers Squibb at 1-800-ORENCIA.

During reconstitution, to minimize foam formation in solutions of abatacept, the vials should be rotated with gentle swirling until the contents are completely dissolved. Avoid prolonged or vigorous agitation. Do not shake. The solution should be clear and colorless to pale yellow. Do not use if opaque particles, discoloration, or other foreign particles are present.

1.) To reconstitute abatacept powder, remove the flip-top from the vial and wipe the top with an alcohol swab. Insert the syringe needle into the vial through the center of the rubber stopper and direct the stream of sterile water for injection to the glass wall of the vial. Do not use the vial if the vacuum is not present. Rotate the vial with gentle swirling until the contents are completely dissolved.
2.) Upon complete dissolution of the lyophilized powder, the vial should be vented with a needle to dissipate any form that may be present. After reconstitution, each milliliter will contain 25 mg (250 mg per 10 mL).
3.) The reconstituted abatacept solution must be further diluted to 100 mL as follows. From a 100 mL infusion bag or bottle, withdraw a volume of 0.9% sodium chloride injection equal to the volume of the reconstituted abatacept vials (for 2 vials remove 20 mL, for 3 vials remove 30 mL, for 4 vials, remove 40 mL). Slowly add the reconstituted abatacept solution from each vial into the infusion bag or bottle using the same silicone-free disposable syringe provided with each vial. Gently mix. The concentration of the fully diluted abatacept solution in the infusion bag or bottle will be approximately 5, 7.5, or 10 mg of abatacept per mL of solution, depending on whether 2, 3, or 4 vials of abatacept are used. Any unused portion in the vials must be immediately discarded.

ABATACEPT — INJECTION

Administration – Prior to administration, the abatacept solution should be inspected visually for particulate matter and discoloration. Discard the solution if any particulate matter or discoloration is observed.

The entire fully diluted abatacept solution should be administered over a period of 30 minutes and must be administered with an infusion set and a sterile nonpyrogenic, low–protein-binding filter (pore size of 0.2 to 1.2 mcm).

The infusion of the fully diluted abatacept solution must be completed within 24 hours of reconstitution of the abatacept vials. The fully diluted abatacept solution must be stored at room temperature or refrigerated at 2° to 8°C (36° to 46°F) before use.

Incompatibilities – Abatacept should not be infused concomitantly in the same IV line with other agents. No physical or biochemical compatibility studies have been conducted to evaluate the coadministration of abatacept with other agents.

➤*Storage/Stability:* Refrigerate at 2° to 8°C (36° to 46°F). Do not use beyond the expiration date. Protect the vials from light by storing in the original package until time of use.

Actions

➤*Pharmacology:* Abatacept, a selective costimulation modulator, inhibits T-cell (T lymphocyte) activation by binding to CD80 and CD86, thereby blocking interaction with CD28. This interaction provides a costimulatory signal necessary for full activation of T lymphocytes, implicated in the pathogenesis of rheumatoid arthritis (RA). Activated T lymphocytes are found in the synovium of patients with RA.

In vitro, abatacept decreases T-cell proliferation and inhibits the production of the cytokines tumor necrosis factor alpha (TNF-α), interferon-γ, and interleukin-2. In a rat collagen-induced arthritis model, abatacept suppresses inflammation, decreases anticollagen antibody production, and reduces antigen specific production of interferon-γ. The relationship of these biological response markers to the mechanisms by which abatacept exerts its effects in RA is unknown.

Pharmacodynamics – In clinical trials with abatacept at doses approximating 10 mg/kg, decreases were observed in serum levels of soluble interleukin-2 receptor, interleukin-6, rheumatoid factor, C-reactive protein, matrix metalloproteinase-3, and TNF-α. The relationship of these biological response markers to the mechanisms by which abatacept exerts its effects in RA is unknown.

➤*Pharmacokinetics:*

Special populations –

Body weight: Population pharmacokinetic analyses in RA patients revealed that there was a trend toward higher clearance of abatacept with increasing body weight. The pharmacokinetics of abatacept were studied in healthy adult subjects after a single 10 mg/kg IV infusion and in RA patients after multiple 10 mg/kg IV infusions (see the following table).

Abatacept Pharmacokinetic Parameters (Mean, Range) in Healthy Subjects and RA Patients after 10 mg/kg IV Infusion(s)

Pharmacokinetic parameter	Healthy subjects (after 10 mg/kg single dose) n = 13	RA patients (after 10 mg/kg multiple doses[a]) n = 14
Peak concentration (C_{max}) (mcg/mL)	292 (175 to 427)	295 (171 to 398)
Terminal half-life (days)	16.7 (12 to 23)	13.1 (8 to 25)
Systemic clearance (mL/h/kg)	0.23 (0.16 to 0.3)	0.22 (0.13 to 0.47)
Volume of distribution (L/kg)	0.09 (0.06 to 0.13)	0.07 (0.02 to 0.13)

[a] Multiple IV infusions were administered at days 1, 15, 30, and monthly thereafter.

The pharmacokinetics of abatacept in RA patients and healthy subjects appeared to be comparable. In RA patients, after multiple IV infusions, the pharmacokinetics of abatacept showed proportional increases of C_{max} and AUC over the dose range of 2 to 10 mg/kg. At 10 mg/kg, serum concentration appeared to reach a steady state by day 60 with a mean (range) trough concentration of 24 (1 to 66) mcg/mL. No systemic accumulation of abatacept occurred upon continued repeated treatment with 10 mg/kg at monthly intervals in RA patients.

Contraindications

Known hypersensitivity to abatacept or any of its components.

Warnings

➤*Concomitant use with TNF antagonists:* In controlled clinical trials, patients receiving concomitant abatacept and TNF antagonist therapy experienced more infections (63%) and serious infections (4.4%) compared with patients treated with only TNF antagonists (43% and 0.8%, respectively). These trials failed to demonstrate an important enhancement of efficacy with coadministration of abatacept with TNF antagonist; therefore, concurrent therapy with abatacept and a TNF antagonist is not recommended. While transitioning from TNF antagonist therapy to abatacept therapy, monitor patients for signs of infection.

➤*Hypersensitivity reactions:* See Adverse Reactions for more information.

➤*Carcinogenesis:* In a mouse carcinogenicity study, weekly subcutaneous injections of 20, 65, or 200 mg/kg of abatacept administered each week for up to 84 weeks in males and 88 weeks in females were associated with increases in the incidence of malignant lymphomas (all doses) and mammary gland tumors (intermediate- and high-dose in females). The mice from this study were infected with murine leukemia virus and mouse mammary tumor virus. These viruses are associated with an increased incidence of lymphomas and mammary gland tumors, respectively, in immunosuppressed mice. The doses used in these studies were 0.8-, 2- and 3-fold, the human exposure at 10 mg/kg, respectively, based on area under the curve (AUC). The relevance of these findings to the clinical use of abatacept is unknown. In a 1-year toxicity study in cynomolgus monkeys, abatacept was administered IV once weekly at doses up to 50 mg/kg (9-fold the human exposure at 10 mg/kg dose based on AUC). Abatacept was not associated with any significant drug-related toxicity. Reversible pharmacological effects consisted of minimal transient decreases in serum immunoglobulin and minimal to severe lymphoid depletion of germinal centers in the spleen and/or lymph nodes. No evidence of lymphomas or preneoplastic morphologic changes was observed, despite the presence of a virus (lymphocryptovirus) known to cause these lesions in immunosuppressed monkeys within the time frame of this study. The relevance of these findings to the clinical use of abatacept is unknown.

➤*Elderly:* The frequency of serious infection and malignancy among abatacept-treated patients older than 65 years of age was higher than for those younger than 65 years of age. Because there is a higher incidence of infections and malignancies in the elderly population in general, caution should be used when treating the elderly.

➤*Pregnancy: Category C.* At a dose of 200 mg/kg (11-fold a human 10 mg/kg dose based on AUC), alterations of immune function consisted of a 9-fold increase in the T-cell dependent antibody response in female pups and inflammation of the thyroid in 1 female pup out of 10 males and 10 females evaluated. Whether these findings indicate a risk for development of autoimmune diseases in humans exposed in utero to abatacept has not been determined. Abatacept was shown to cross the placenta. Because animal reproduction studies are not always predictive of human response, abatacept should be used during pregnancy only if clearly needed. There are no adequate and well-controlled studies in pregnant women.

➤*Lactation:* Abatacept has been shown to be present in rat milk. It is not known whether abatacept is excreted in human milk or absorbed systemically after ingestion. Because many drugs are excreted in human milk, and because of the potential for serious adverse reactions in breast-feeding infants from abatacept, possibly including effects on the developing immune system, decide whether to discontinue breast-feeding or the drug, taking into account the importance of the drug to the mother.

➤*Children:* Safety and efficacy of abatacept in children have not been established.

Precautions

➤*Infections:* Exercise caution when considering the use of abatacept in patients with a history of recurrent infections, underlying conditions that may predispose them to infections, or chronic, latent, or localized infections. Closely monitor patients who develop a new infection while undergoing treatment with abatacept. Discontinue administration of abatacept if a patient develops a serious infection. A higher rate of serious infections has been observed in patients treated with concurrent TNF antagonists and abatacept.

Prior to initiating immunomodulatory therapies, including abatacept, screen patients for latent tuberculosis infection with a tuberculin skin test. Abatacept has not been studied in patients with a positive tuberculosis screen, and the safety of abatacept in individuals with latent tuberculosis infection is unknown. Treat patients testing positive in tuberculosis screening by standard medical practice prior to therapy with abatacept.

➤*Immunizations:* Do not give live vaccines concurrently with abatacept or within 3 months of its discontinuation. No data are available on the secondary transmission of infection from persons receiving live vaccines to patients receiving abatacept. The efficacy of vaccination in patients receiving abatacept is not known. Based on its mechanism of action, abatacept may blunt the efficacy of some immunizations.

➤*Chronic obstructive pulmonary disease (COPD):* COPD patients treated with abatacept developed adverse reactions more frequently than those treated with placebo, including COPD exacerbations, cough, rhonchi, and dyspnea. Undertake use of abatacept with caution in patients with RA and COPD and monitor such patients for worsening of their respiratory status.

➤*Immunosuppression:* The possibility exists for drugs inhibiting T-cell activation, including abatacept, to affect host defenses against infections and malignancies because T cells mediate cellular immune responses. The impact of treatment with abatacept on the development and course of malignancies is not fully understood. In clinical trials, a higher rate of infections was seen in abatacept-treated patients compared with placebo.

Drug Interactions

Formal drug interaction studies have not been conducted with abatacept.

➤*TNF antagonists:* Coadministration of a TNF antagonist with abatacept has been associated with an increased risk of serious infections and no significant additional efficacy over use of the TNF antagonists alone. Concurrent therapy with abatacept and TNF antagonists is not recommended.

ABATACEPT — INJECTION

➤*Anakinra:* There is insufficient experience to assess the safety and efficacy of abatacept coadministered with anakinra, and therefore such use is not recommended.

Adverse Reactions

The most serious adverse reactions were serious infections and malignancies. The most commonly reported adverse reactions (occurring in at least 10% of patients treated with abatacept) were headache, upper respiratory tract infection, nasopharyngitis, and nausea.

The adverse reactions most frequently resulting in clinical intervention (interruption or discontinuation of abatacept) were caused by infection. The most frequently reported infections resulting in dose interruption were upper respiratory tract infection (1%), bronchitis (0.7%), and herpes zoster (0.7%). The most frequent infections resulting in discontinuation were pneumonia (0.2%), localized infection (0.2%), and bronchitis (0.1%).

Because clinical trials are conducted under widely varying and controlled conditions, adverse reaction rates observed in clinical trials of a drug cannot be directly compared with rates in the clinical trials of another drug and may not predict the rates observed in a broader patient population in clinical practice.

The data described herein reflect exposure to abatacept in patients with active RA in placebo-controlled studies (1,955 patients with abatacept, 989 with placebo). The studies had either a double-blind, placebo-controlled period of 6 months (258 patients with abatacept, 133 with placebo) or 1 year (1,697 patients with abatacept, 856 with placebo). A subset of these patients received concomitant biologic DMARD therapy, such as a TNF-blocking agent (204 patients with abatacept, 134 with placebo).

➤*Infections:* In the placebo-controlled trials, infections were reported in 54% of abatacept-treated patients and 48% of placebo-treated patients. The most commonly reported infections (reported in 5% to 13% of patients) were upper respiratory tract infection, nasopharyngitis, sinusitis, urinary tract infection, influenza, and bronchitis. Other infections reported in fewer than 5% of patients at a higher frequency (more than 0.5%) with abatacept compared with placebo were rhinitis, herpes simplex, and pneumonia.

Serious infections were reported in 3% of patients treated with abatacept and 1.9% of patients treated with placebo. The most common (0.2% to 0.5%) serious infections reported with abatacept were pneumonia, cellulitis, urinary tract infection, bronchitis, diverticulitis, and acute pyelonephritis.

➤*Malignancies:* In the placebo-controlled portions of the clinical trials (1,955 patients for a median of 12 months), the overall frequencies of malignancies were similar in the abatacept- and placebo-treated patients (1.3% and 1.1%, respectively). However, more cases of lung cancer were observed in abatacept-treated patients (4, 0.2%) than placebo-treated patients (0). In the cumulative abatacept clinical trials (placebo-controlled and uncontrolled, open-label) a total of 8 cases of lung cancer (0.21 cases per 100 patient years) and 4 lymphomas (0.10 cases per 100 patient-years) were observed in 2,688 patients (3,827 patient-years). The rate observed for lymphoma is approximately 3.5-fold higher than expected in an age- and gender-matched general population based on the Surveillance, Epidemiology, and End Results Database. Patients with RA, particularly those with highly active disease, are at a higher risk for the development of lymphoma. Other malignancies included skin, breast, bile duct, bladder, cervical, endometrial, lymphoma, melanoma, myelodysplastic syndrome, ovarian, prostate, renal, thyroid, and uterine cancers. The potential role of abatacept in the development of malignancies in humans is unknown.

➤*Acute infusion reactions:* Acute infusion-related reactions (adverse reactions occurring within 1 hour of the start of the infusion) in studies 3, 4, and 5 were more common in the abatacept-treated patients than the placebo patients (9% for abatacept, 6% for placebo). The most frequently reported reactions (1% to 2%) were dizziness, headache, and hypertension.

Acute infusion-related reactions that were reported in more than 0.1% and 1% or less of patients treated with abatacept included cardiopulmonary symptoms, such as hypotension, increased blood pressure, and dyspnea; other symptoms included nausea, flushing, urticaria, cough, hypersensitivity, pruritus, rash, and wheezing. Most of these reactions were mild to moderate. Fewer than 1% of abatacept-treated patients discontinued because of an acute infusion-related reaction. In controlled trials, 6 abatacept-treated patients compared with 2 placebo-treated patients discontinued study treatment because of acute infusion-related reactions.

Hypersensitivity reactions – Of 2,688 patients treated with abatacept in clinical trials, there were 2 cases of anaphylaxis or anaphylactoid reactions. Other reactions potentially associated with drug hypersensitivity, such as hypotension, urticaria, and dyspnea, each occurred in less than 0.9% of abatacept-treated patients and generally occurred within 24 hours of abatacept infusion. Appropriate medical support measures for the treatment of hypersensitivity reactions should be available for immediate use in the event of a reaction.

➤*COPD:* In study 5, there were 37 patients with COPD who were treated with abatacept and 17 COPD patients who were treated with placebo. The COPD patients treated with abatacept developed adverse reactions more frequently than those treated with placebo (97% versus 88%, respectively). Respiratory disorders occurred more frequently in abatacept-treated patients compared with placebo-treated patients (43% versus 24%, respectively) including COPD exacerbation, cough, rhonchi, and dyspnea. A higher percentage of abatacept-treated patients developed a serious adverse reaction compared with placebo-treated patients (27% versus 6%), including COPD exacerbation (3 of 37 patients [8%]) and pneumonia (1 of 37 patients [3%]).

➤*Other adverse reactions:* Adverse reactions occurring in 3% or more of patients and at least 1% more frequently in abatacept-treated patients during placebo-controlled RA studies are summarized in the following table.

Abatacept Adverse Reactions in RA Studies (≥ 3%)

Adverse Reaction	Abatacept (n = 1,955)[a]	Placebo (n = 989)[b]
Back pain	7%	6%
Cough	8%	7%
Dizziness	9%	7%
Dyspepsia	6%	4%
Headache	18%	13%
Hypertension	7%	4%
Nasopharyngitis	12%	9%
Pain in extremity	3%	2%
Rash	4%	3%
Urinary tract infection	6%	5%

[a] Includes 204 patients on concomitant biologic DMARDs (adalimumab, anakinra, etanercept, or infliximab).
[b] Includes 134 patients on concomitant biologic DMARDs (adalimumab, anakinra, etanercept, or infliximab).

➤*Immunogenicity:* Antibodies directed against the entire abatacept molecule or to the cytotoxic T-lymphocyte-associated antigen 4 (CTLA-4) portion of abatacept were assessed by enzyme-linked immunoabsorbent assays (ELISA) in RA patients for up to 2 years following repeated treatment with abatacept. Thirty-four of 1,993 (1.7%) patients developed binding antibodies to the entire abatacept molecule or to the CTLA-4 portion of abatacept. Because trough levels of abatacept can interfere with assay results, a subset analysis was performed. In this analysis it was observed that 9 of 154 (5.8%) patients that had discontinued treatment with abatacept for more than 56 days developed antibodies.

Samples with confirmed binding activity to CTLA-4 were assessed for the presence of neutralizing antibodies in a cell-based luciferase reporter assay. Six of 9 (67%) evaluable patients were shown to possess neutralizing antibodies. No correlation of antibody development to clinical response or adverse reactions was observed.

The data reflect the percentage of patients whose test results were positive for antibodies to abatacept in specific assays, and are highly dependent on the sensitivity and specificity of the assays. Additionally, the observed incidence of antibody positivity in an assay may be influenced by several factors, including sample handling, timing of sample collection, concomitant medication, and underlying disease. For these reasons, comparison of the incidence of antibodies to abatacept with the incidence of antibodies to other products may be misleading.

Overdosage

Abatacept is administered as an IV infusion under medically controlled conditions. Doses up to 50 mg/kg have been administered without apparent toxic effect.

➤*Treatment:* In case of overdosage, it is recommended that the patient be monitored for any signs or symptoms of adverse reactions and appropriate symptomatic treatment instituted.

Patient Information

Patients should be provided the abatacept *Patient Information* leaflet and provided an opportunity to read it prior to each treatment session. Because caution should be exercised in administering abatacept to patients with active infections, it is important that the patient's overall health be assessed at each visit and any questions resulting from the patient's reading of the *Patient Information* be discussed.

THALIDOMIDE

Rx	**Thalomid**[a] (Celgene)	**Capsules:** 50 mg	(Celgene/50 mg). White, opaque. In blister pack 28s and 280s.
		100 mg	(Celgene/100 mg). Tan. In blister pack 28s and 140s.
		200 mg	(Celgene/200 mg). Blue. In blister pack 28s and 84s.

[a] Available only to be prescribed and dispensed under the terms of the System for Thalidomide Education and Prescribing Safety (S.T.E.P.S.) restricted distribution program.

THALIDOMIDE — ORAL

WARNING

Severe, life-threatening human birth defects – If thalidomide is taken during pregnancy, it can cause severe birth defects or death to a fetus. Thalidomide should never be used by women who are pregnant or who could become pregnant while taking the drug. Even a single dose (1 capsule [50, 100, 200 mg]) taken by a pregnant woman can cause severe birth defects. Because of this toxicity and in an effort to make the chance of fetal exposure to thalidomide as negligible as possible, thalidomide is approved for marketing only under a special restricted distribution program approved by the Food and Drug Administration (FDA). This is called the S.T.E.P.S. program. Under this restricted distribution program, only prescribers and pharmacists registered with the program are allowed to prescribe and dispense the product. In addition, patients must be advised of, agree to, and comply with the requirements of the S.T.E.P.S. program in order to receive the product.

Prescribers – Thalidomide may be prescribed only by licensed prescribers who are registered in the S.T.E.P.S. program and understand the risk of teratogenicity if thalidomide is used during pregnancy. The following major human fetal abnormalities related to thalidomide administration during pregnancy have been documented: amelia (absence of limbs), phocomelia (short limbs), hypoplasticity of the bones, absence of bones, external ear abnormalities (including anotia, micro pinna, small or absent external auditory canals), facial palsy, eye abnormalities (anophthalmos, microphthalmos), and congenital heart defects. Alimentary tract, urinary tract, and genital malformations also have been documented. Mortality at or shortly after birth has been reported at about 40%. Effective contraception must be used for at least 4 weeks before beginning thalidomide therapy, during therapy, and for 4 weeks following discontinuation of therapy. Reliable contraception is indicated even where there has been a history of infertility, unless the patient has had a hysterectomy or has been postmenopausal for at least 24 months. Because thalidomide is present in the semen of patients receiving the drug, a male patient receiving thalidomide must always use a latex condom during any sexual contact with women of childbearing potential even if he has undergone a successful vasectomy. Two reliable forms of contraception must be used simultaneously unless continuous abstinence from reproductive heterosexual sexual intercourse is the chosen method. Refer women of childbearing potential to a qualified provider of contraceptive methods, if needed. Sexually mature women who have not undergone a hysterectomy or who have not been postmenopausal for at least 24 consecutive months (ie, who have had menses at some time in the preceding 24 consecutive months) are considered to be women of childbearing potential. Before starting treatment, administer a pregnancy test (sensitivity of at least 50 milliunits/mL) to women of childbearing potential. Perform the test within the 24 hours prior to beginning therapy. A prescription for thalidomide for a woman of childbearing potential must not be issued by the prescriber until a written report of a negative pregnancy test has been obtained by the prescriber. Once treatment has started, test for pregnancy weekly during the first month of use, then monthly thereafter in women with regular menstrual cycles. If menstrual cycles are irregular, test for pregnancy every 2 weeks. Perform pregnancy testing and counseling if a patient misses her period or if there is any abnormality in menstrual bleeding. If pregnancy occurs during thalidomide treatment, discontinue the drug immediately. Report any suspected fetal exposure to thalidomide to the FDA immediately via the MedWatch number at 1-800-FDA-1088 and also to the manufacturer. Refer the patient to an obstetrician/gynecologist experienced in reproductive toxicity for further evaluation and counseling.

Female patients – Thalidomide is contraindicated in women of childbearing potential unless alternative therapies are considered inappropriate and the patient meets ALL of the following conditions (ie, she is essentially unable to become pregnant while on thalidomide therapy):

- She understands and can reliably carry out instructions.
- She is capable of complying with the mandatory contraceptive measures, pregnancy testing, patient registration, and patient survey as described in the S.T.E.P.S. program.
- She has received both oral and written warnings of the hazards of taking thalidomide during pregnancy and of exposing a fetus to the drug.
- She has received both oral and written warnings of the risk of possible contraception failure and of the need to use 2 reliable forms of contraception simultaneously, unless continuous abstinence from reproductive heterosexual intercourse is the chosen method. Sexually mature women who have not undergone a hysterectomy or who have not been postmenopausal for at least 24 consecutive months (ie, who have had menses at some time in the preceding 24 consecutive months) are considered to be women of childbearing potential.

WARNING (cont.)

- She acknowledges, in writing, her understanding of these warnings and of the need for using 2 reliable methods of contraception for 4 weeks prior to starting thalidomide therapy, during thalidomide therapy, and for 4 weeks after stopping thalidomide therapy.
- She has had a negative pregnancy test, with a sensitivity of at least 50 milliunits/mL, within the 24 hours prior to beginning therapy.
- If the patient is between 12 and 18 years of age, her parent or legal guardian must have read this material and agreed to ensure compliance with the above.

Male patients – Thalidomide is contraindicated in sexually mature men unless the patient meets ALL of the following conditions:

- He understands and can reliably carry out instructions.
- He is capable of complying with the mandatory contraceptive measures that are appropriate for men, patient registration, and patient survey as described in the S.T.E.P.S. program.
- He has received both oral and written warnings of the hazards of taking thalidomide and exposing a fetus to the drug.
- He has received both oral and written warnings of the risk of possible contraception failure and of the need to use barrier contraception when having sexual intercourse with women of childbearing potential, even if he has undergone successful vasectomy.
- He acknowledges, in writing, his understanding of these warnings and of the need to use barrier contraception (latex condom), even if he has undergone successful vasectomy, when having sexual intercourse with women of childbearing potential. Sexually mature women who have not undergone a hysterectomy or who have not been postmenopausal for at least 24 consecutive months (ie, who have had menses at some time in the preceding 24 consecutive months) are considered to be women of childbearing potential.
- If the patient is between 12 and 18 years of age, his parent or legal guardian must have read this material and agreed to ensure compliance with the above.

Venous thromboembolic events – The use of thalidomide in multiple myeloma results in an increased risk of venous thromboembolic events, such as deep venous thrombosis and pulmonary embolus. This risk increases significantly when thalidomide is used in combination with standard chemotherapeutic agents, including dexamethasone. In one controlled trial, the rate of venous thromboembolic events was 22.5% in patients receiving thalidomide in combination with dexamethasone, compared with 4.9% in patients receiving dexamethasone alone ($P = 0.002$). Patients and health care providers are advised to be observant for the signs and symptoms of thromboembolism. Instruct patients to seek medical care if they develop symptoms such as shortness of breath, chest pain, or arm or leg swelling. Preliminary data suggest that patients who are appropriate candidates may benefit from concurrent prophylactic anticoagulation or aspirin treatment.

Indications

➤*Multiple myeloma:* In combination with dexamethasone, for the treatment of patients with newly diagnosed multiple myeloma.

Efficacy is based on response rates. There are no controlled trials demonstrating a clinical benefit, such as an improvement in survival.

➤*Erythema nodosum leprosum (ENL):*

Acute treatment – Acute treatment of the cutaneous manifestations of moderate to severe ENL. Not indicated as monotherapy for such ENL treatment in the presence of moderate to severe neuritis.

Maintenance therapy – Maintenance therapy for prevention and suppression of the cutaneous manifestations of ENL recurrence.

➤*Unlabeled uses:* Treatment of graft-versus-host disease (GVHD) after bone marrow transplantation; refractory multiple myeloma; primary brain tumors; appetite stimulant for cachexia in advanced cancer; aphthous ulcers; prostate cancer (in combination with docetaxel).

Orphan status – Clinical manifestations of mycobacterial infection caused by mycobacterium tuberculosis and nontuberculous mycobacteria; Crohn disease; HIV-associated wasting syndrome; Kaposi sarcoma; lupus erythematosus; multiple myeloma; myelofibrosis with myeloid metaplasia; primary brain malignancies; treatment and maintenance of reactional lepromatous leprosy; treatment and prevention of GVHD; treatment and prevention of recurrent aphthous stomatitis and treatment and prevention of recurrent aphthous ulcer in severely, terminally immunocompromised patients.

Administration and Dosage

➤*Approved by the FDA:* July 16, 1998.

THALIDOMIDE — ORAL

See the Warning box for more information.

➤*Multiple myeloma:* Administered in combination with dexamethasone in 28-day treatment cycles. Administer 200 mg orally once daily with water, preferably at bedtime and at least 1 hour after the evening meal. The dosage of dexamethasone is 40 mg daily administered orally on days 1 to 4, 9 to 12, and 17 to 20 every 28 days.

Patients who develop side effects such as constipation, oversedation, or peripheral neuropathy may benefit by either temporarily discontinuing the drug or continuing at a lower dose. With the abatement of these side effects, the drug may be started at a lower dose, or at the previous dose based on clinical judgement.

➤*ENL:* Initiate dosing at 100 to 300 mg/day, once daily with water, preferably at bedtime and at least 1 hour after the evening meal. Start patients weighing less than 50 kg (110 lb) at the low end of the dose range.

In patients with a severe cutaneous ENL reaction, or in those who have previously required higher doses to control the reaction, thalidomide dosing may be initiated at higher dosages, up to 400 mg/day once daily at bedtime or in divided doses with water at least 1 hour after meals.

In patients with moderate to severe neuritis associated with a severe ENL reaction, corticosteroids may be started concomitantly with thalidomide. Steroid usage can be tapered and discontinued when the neuritis has ameliorated.

Continue dosing with thalidomide until signs and symptoms of active reaction have subsided, usually at least 2 weeks. Patients may then be tapered off medication in 50 mg decrements every 2 to 4 weeks.

Maintain patients who have a documented history of requiring prolonged maintenance treatment to prevent the recurrence of cutaneous ENL or who flare during tapering on the minimum dose necessary to control the reaction. Attempt tapering of medication every 3 to 6 months, in decrements of 50 mg every 2 to 4 weeks.

➤*Dispensing instructions:* This product is only supplied to pharmacists registered with the S.T.E.P.S. program (see Warning Box). Pharmacists note: Before dispensing thalidomide, activate the authorization number on every prescription by calling the manufacturer's customer center at 1-888-423-5436 and obtain a confirmation number. Write the confirmation number on the prescription. Accept a thalidomide prescription only if it has been issued within the previous 7 days (telephone prescriptions are not permitted); dispense no more than a 4-week (28-day) supply. A new prescription is required for further dispensing. Dispense blister packs intact (capsules cannot be repackaged). Dispense subsequent prescriptions only if fewer than 7 days of therapy remain on the previous prescription, and educate all staff pharmacists about the dispensing procedure for thalidomide.

➤*Storage/Stability:* Store at 25°C (77°F); excursions permitted to 15° to 30°C (59° to 86°F). Protect from light.

Actions

➤*Pharmacology:* Thalidomide is an immunomodulatory agent with a spectrum of activity that is not fully characterized. In patients with ENL, the mechanism of action is not fully understood.

Data suggest that the immunologic effects of this compound can vary substantially under different conditions, but may be related to suppression of excessive tumor necrosis factor-alpha (TNF-α) production and down-modulation of selected cell surface adhesion molecules involved in leukocyte migration. For example, administration of thalidomide has been reported to decrease circulating levels of TNF-α in patients with ENL; however, it also has been shown to increase plasma TNF-α levels in HIV-seropositive patients.

➤*Pharmacokinetics:*

Absorption/Distribution – The absolute bioavailability of oral thalidomide has not yet been characterized in human subjects because of its poor aqueous solubility. In studies of healthy volunteers and subjects with Hansen disease, the mean time to peak plasma concentrations (T_{max}) of thalidomide ranged from 2.9 to 5.7 hours, indicating that thalidomide is slowly absorbed from the GI tract. While the extent of absorption as measured by AUC is proportional to the dose in healthy subjects, the C_{max} increased in a less than proportional manner (see table below). This lack of C_{max} dose proportionality, coupled with the observed increase in T_{max} values, suggests that the poor solubility of thalidomide in aqueous media may be hindering the rate of absorption.

Various Thalidomide Pharmacokinetic Parameters (mean)

Population/Single dose	$AUC_{0-\infty}$ (mcg•h/mL)	C_{max} (mcg/mL)	T_{max} (h)	Half-life (h)
Healthy subjects (n = 14)				
50 mg	4.9	0.62	2.9	5.52
200 mg	18.9	1.76	3.5	5.53
400 mg	36.4	2.82	4.3	7.29
Patients with Hansen disease (n = 6)				
400 mg	46.4	3.44	5.7	6.86

Coadministration of thalidomide with a high-fat meal causes minor (less than 10%) changes in the observed AUC and C_{max} values; however, it causes an increase in T_{max} to approximately 6 hours. The extent of plasma protein binding of thalidomide is unknown.

Metabolism – The exact metabolic route and fate of thalidomide is not known. Thalidomide does not appear to be hepatically metabolized to any large extent, but appears to undergo nonenzymatic hydrolysis in plasma to multiple metabolites. In a repeat dose study in which 200 mg was given to 10 healthy females for 18 days, thalidomide showed similar pharmacokinetic profiles on the first and last day of dosing. Thalidomide does not appear to induce or inhibit its own metabolism.

Excretion – As indicated in the table above, the mean elimination half-life ranges from approximately 5 to 7 hours after a single dose and is not altered by multiple dosing. Thalidomide has a renal clearance of 1.15 mL/min with less than 0.7% of the dose excreted in the urine as unchanged drug. Following a single dose, urinary levels of thalidomide were undetectable 48 hours after dosing. Although thalidomide is thought to be hydrolyzed to a number of metabolites, only a very small amount (0.02% of the administered dose) of 4-OH-thalidomide was identified in the urine of subjects 12 to 24 hours after dosing.

Contraindications

Pregnancy (*Category X*; see Warning Box and Warnings); hypersensitivity to the drug and its components.

Warnings

➤*Severe birth defects:* See Warning Box.

➤*Drowsiness and somnolence:* Thalidomide frequently causes drowsiness and somnolence. Instruct patients to avoid situations where drowsiness may be a problem and not to take other medications that may cause drowsiness without adequate medical advice. Advise patients about the possible impairment of mental or physical abilities required for the performance of hazardous tasks, such as driving a car or operating other complex or dangerous machinery.

➤*Peripheral neuropathy:* Thalidomide is known to cause nerve damage that may be permanent. Peripheral neuropathy is a common, potentially severe, and irreversible side effect of treatment with thalidomide. Peripheral neuropathy generally occurs following chronic use over a period of months; however, reports following relatively short-term use also exist. The correlation with cumulative dose is unclear. Symptoms may occur some time after thalidomide treatment has been stopped and may resolve slowly or not at all. Few reports of neuropathy have arisen in the treatment of ENL despite long-term thalidomide treatment. However, the inability clinically to differentiate thalidomide neuropathy from the neuropathy often seen in Hansen disease makes it difficult to determine accurately the incidence of thalidomide-related neuropathy in ENL patients.

Examine patients at monthly intervals for the first 3 months of therapy to enable the clinician to detect early signs of neuropathy, which include numbness, tingling, or pain in the hands and feet. Evaluate patients periodically thereafter during treatment. Regularly counsel, question, and evaluate patients for signs or symptoms of peripheral neuropathy. Give consideration to electrophysiological testing, consisting of measurement of sensory nerve action potential amplitudes at baseline and thereafter every 6 months in an effort to detect asymptomatic neuropathy. If symptoms of drug-induced neuropathy develop, discontinue thalidomide immediately to limit further damage, if clinically appropriate. Usually reinitiate thalidomide treatment only if the neuropathy returns to baseline status.

See Drug Interactions for more information.

➤*Dizziness/Orthostatic hypotension:* Thalidomide may cause dizziness and orthostatic hypotension. Advise patients to sit upright for a few minutes prior to standing up from a recumbent position.

➤*Neutropenia:* Decreased white blood cell counts, including neutropenia, have been reported. Do not initiate treatment with an absolute neutrophil count (ANC) of less than 750/mm^3. Monitor white blood cell count and differential on an ongoing basis, especially in patients who may be more prone to neutropenia, such as patients who are HIV-seropositive. If ANC decreases to less than 750/mm^3 while on treatment, reevaluate the patient's medication regimen and, if the neutropenia persists, consider withholding thalidomide if clinically appropriate.

➤*HIV patients:* In a randomized, placebo-controlled trial of thalidomide in HIV-seropositive patients, plasma HIV RNA levels were found to increase. A similar trend was observed in a second study conducted in patients who were HIV-seropositive. The clinical significance of this increase is unknown. Both studies were conducted prior to availability of highly active antiretroviral therapy. Until the clinical significance of this finding in HIV-seropositive patients is further understood, measure viral load after the first and third months of treatment and every 3 months thereafter.

➤*Hansen disease patients:* Data suggest that these patients, relative to healthy subjects, may have an increased bioavailability of thalidomide. The increase is reflected in an increased AUC and in increased peak plasma levels. Clinical significance is unknown.

➤*Thrombotic events:* Thrombotic events have been reported in patients treated with thalidomide. Patients with neoplastic and various inflammatory conditions being treated with thalidomide may have an increased incidence of pulmonary embolism, deep vein thrombophlebitis, thrombophlebitis, or thrombosis. It is not known if concomitant therapy with other medications, including anticancer agents, are a contributing factor.

➤*Hypersensitivity reactions:* Hypersensitivity to thalidomide has been reported. Signs and symptoms have included the occurrence of erythematous macular rash, possibly associated with fever, tachycardia, and hypotension. May necessitate interruption of therapy if severe. If the reaction recurs when dosing is resumed, discontinue thalidomide. Refer to Management of Acute Hypersensitivity Reactions.

➤*Pregnancy: Category X.*

See the Warning box for more information.

THALIDOMIDE — ORAL

➤*Lactation:* It is not known whether thalidomide is excreted in breast milk. Because of the potential for serious adverse reactions in nursing infants from thalidomide, decide whether to discontinue nursing or to discontinue the drug, taking into account the importance of the drug to the mother.

➤*Children:* No pharmacokinetic data are available in subjects younger than 18 years of age. Safety and efficacy in patients younger than 12 years of age have not been established.

Precautions

➤*Monitoring:* Have pregnancy testing (sensitivity of at least 50 mIU/mL) performed on women of childbearing potential. Perform the test within the 24 hours prior to beginning thalidomide therapy, weekly during the first month of use, then monthly thereafter in women with regular menstrual cycles or every 2 weeks in women with irregular menstrual cycles. Also perform pregnancy testing if a patient misses her period or if there is any abnormality in menstrual bleeding (see Warnings).

➤*Exposure:* The only type of thalidomide exposure known to result in drug-associated birth defects are as a result of direct oral ingestion of thalidomide. Currently, no specific data are available regarding the cutaneous absorption or inhalation of thalidomide in women of childbearing potential and whether these exposures may result in any birth defects. Instruct patients not to handle extensively or open thalidomide capsules and to maintain storage of capsules in blister packs until ingestion. If there is contact with non-intact thalidomide capsules or the powder contents, wash the exposed area with soap and water.

Thalidomide has been shown to be present in the serum and semen of patients receiving thalidomide. If health care providers or other care givers are exposed to body fluids from patients receiving thalidomide, utilize appropriate precautions, such as wearing gloves to prevent the potential cutaneous exposure to thalidomide or wash the exposed area with soap and water.

➤*Bradycardia:* Bradycardia in association with thalidomide use has been reported. There have been reports of cases of bradycardia requiring medical interventions. The clinical significance is unknown.

➤*Serious dermatological reactions:* Serious dermatologic reactions, including Stevens-Johnson syndrome and toxic epidermal necrolysis, which may be fatal, have been reported. Discontinue thalidomide if a skin rash occurs and only resume following appropriate clinical evaluation. If the rash is exfoliative, purpuric, or bullous, or if Stevens-Johnson syndrome or toxic epidermal necrolysis is suspected, do not resume use of thalidomide.

➤*Seizures:* Seizures, including grand mal convulsions, have been reported during postapproval use of thalidomide. During therapy with thalidomide, closely monitor patients with a history of seizures or with other risk factors for the development of seizures for clinical changes that could precipitate acute seizure activity.

➤*Drug abuse and dependence:* Physical and psychological dependence has not been reported in patients taking thalidomide. However, as with other tranquilizers/hypnotics, thalidomide has been reported to create habituation to its soporific effects.

➤*Photosensitivity:* Photosensitization (photoallergy or phototoxicity) may occur; therefore, caution patients to take protective measures (ie, sunscreens, protective clothing) against exposure to sunlight or ultraviolet light (eg, tanning beds) until tolerance is determined.

Drug Interactions

Thalidomide Drug Interactions

Precipitant drug	Object drug*		Description
Thalidomide	Alcohol Barbiturates Chlorpromazine Reserpine	↑	Thalidomide may enhance sedative activity of these agents.
Thalidomide	Medication associated with peripheral neuropathy (eg, metronidazole, vincristine, isoniazid)	↑	Symptoms of peripheral neuropathy may be enhanced when thalidomide is taken with other medications known to cause peripheral neuropathy. Use caution when administering concomitantly.
Medication associated with peripheral neuropathy (eg, metronidazole, vincristine, isoniazid)	Thalidomide		

* ↑ = Object drug increased.

➤*Drugs that interfere with hormonal contraceptives:* Concomitant use of carbamazepine, griseofulvin, HIV-protease inhibitors, modafinil, penicillins, rifabutin, rifampin, phenytoin, or certain herbal supplements such as St. John's wort with hormonal contraceptive agents may reduce the effectiveness of the contraception for up to 1 month after discontinuation of these concomitant therapies. Therefore, women requiring treatment with 1 or more of these drugs must use 2 other effective or highly effective methods of contraception or abstain from heterosexual sexual contact while taking thalidomide.

➤*Drug/Food interactions:* See Actions for more information.

Adverse Reactions

See the Warning box for more information.

Thalidomide is associated with bradycardia, dizziness/orthostatic hypotension, drowsiness/somnolence, HIV viral load increase, hypersensitivity, neutropenia, and peripheral neuropathy (see Warnings and Precautions). Dizziness, rash, and somnolence are the most commonly observed adverse events associated with the use of thalidomide.

All adverse events listed in the following table were mild to moderate in severity, and none resulted in discontinuation. Events that were more frequent in the placebo-treated group are not included.

Thalidomide Adverse Reactions (%)

Adverse reaction	All ARs reported in ENL patients 50 to 300 mg/day (n = 24)	ARs reported in ≥ 3 HIV-seropositive patients: Thalidomide 100 mg/day (n = 36)	Thalidomide 200 mg/day (n = 32)	Placebo (n = 35)
CNS				
Agitation	0	0	9.4	0
Dizziness	4.2	19.4	18.7	0
Headache	12.5	16.7	18.7	11.4
Insomnia	0	0	9.4	5.7
Nervousness	0	2.8	9.4	0
Neuropathy	0	8.3	0	0
Paresthesia	0	5.6	15.6	11.4
Somnolence	37.5	36.1	37.5	11.4
Tremor	4.2	0	0	0
Vertigo	8.3	0	0	0
Dermatologic				
Acne	0	11.1	3.1	0
Dermatitis, fungal	4.2	5.6	9.4	0
Nail disorder	4.2	0	3.1	0
Pruritus	8.3	2.8	6.3	5.7
Rash	20.8	25	25	31.4
Rash, maculopapular	4.2	16.7	18.7	5.7
Sweating	0	0	12.5	11.4
GI				
Abdominal pain	4.2	2.8	3.1	11.4
Anorexia	0	2.8	9.4	5.7
Constipation	4.2	2.8	9.4	0
Diarrhea	4.2	11.1	18.7	17.1
Dry mouth	0	8.3	9.4	5.7
Flatulence	0	8.3	0	5.7
Liver function tests (multiple abnormalities)	0	0	9.4	0
Nausea	4.2	0	12.5	2.9
Oral moniliasis	4.2	11.1	6.3	0
Tooth pain	4.2	0	0	0
GU				
Albuminuria	0	8.3	3.1	5.7
Hematuria	0	11.1	0	2.9
Impotence	8.3	2.8	0	0
Hematologic/Lymphatic				
Anemia	0	5.6	12.5	8.6
Leukopenia	0	16.7	25	8.6
Lymphadenopathy	0	5.6	12.5	8.6
Metabolic/Endocrine				
AST increased	0	2.8	12.5	5.7
Edema, peripheral	4.2	8.3	3.1	0
Hyperlipemia	0	5.6	9.4	2.9
Respiratory				
Pharyngitis	4.2	8.3	6.3	5.7
Rhinitis	4.2	0	0	11.4
Sinusitis	4.2	8.3	3.1	5.7
Miscellaneous				
Accidental injury	4.2	5.6	0	2.9
Asthenia	8.3	5.6	21.9	2.9
Back pain	4.2	5.6	0	0
Chills	4.2	0	9.4	11.4
Facial edema	4.2	0	0	0
Fever	0	19.4	21.9	17.1
Infection	0	8.3	6.3	2.9
Malaise	8.3	0	0	0
Neck pain	4.2	0	0	0
Neck rigidity	4.2	0	0	0
Pain	8.3	0	3.1	5.7

THALIDOMIDE — ORAL

Other adverse events observed in ENL patients – Thalidomide in doses no more than 400 mg/day has been administered investigationally in the US over a 19-year period in 1465 patients with ENL. The published literature describes the treatment of an additional 1678 patients. All reported events are included except those already listed in the previous table. Because of the fact that these data were collected from uncontrolled studies, the incidence rate cannot be determined.

➤*Cardiovascular:* Bradycardia; hypertension; hypotension; peripheral vascular disorder; tachycardia; vasodilation.

➤*CNS:* Abnormal thinking; agitation; amnesia; anxiety; causalgia; circumoral paresthesia; confusion; depression; euphoria; hyperesthesia; insomnia; nervousness; neuralgia; neuritis; neuropathy; paresthesia; peripheral neuritis; psychosis.

➤*Dermatologic:* Acne; alopecia; dry skin; eczematous rash; exfoliative dermatitis; ichthyosis; perifollicular thickening; photosensitivity; skin necrosis; seborrhea; sweating; urticaria; vesiculobullous rash.

➤*GI:* Anorexia; appetite increase/weight gain; dry mouth; dyspepsia; enlarged liver; eructation; flatulence; intestinal obstruction; vomiting.

➤*GU:* Hematuria; orchitis; proteinuria; pyuria; urinary frequency.

➤*Hematologic / Lymphatic:* Eosinophilia; ESR decrease; granulocytopenia; hypochromic anemia; leukemia; leukocytosis; leukopenia; MCV elevated; RBC abnormal; spleen palpable; thrombocytopenia.

➤*Lab test abnormalities:* ALT increased; BUN increased; creatinine increased; decreased creatinine clearance; electrolyte abnormalities; increased liver function tests; LDH increased; phosphorus decreased.

➤*Metabolic:* ADH inappropriate; alkaline phosphatase; amyloidosis; bilirubinemia; cyanosis; diabetes; edema; hyperglycemia; hyperkalemia; hyperuricemia; hypocalcemia; hypoproteinemia.

➤*Musculoskeletal:* Arthritis; bone tenderness; hypertonia; joint disorder; leg cramps; myalgia; myasthenia; periosteal disorder.

➤*Respiratory:* Cough; emphysema; epistaxis; pulmonary embolus; rales; upper respiratory tract infection; voice alteration.

➤*Special senses:* Amblyopia; deafness; dry eye; eye pain; tinnitus.

➤*Miscellaneous:* Abdomen enlarged; fever; upper extremity pain.

➤*Other adverse events observed in HIV-seropositive patients:*

Cardiovascular – Angina pectoris; arrhythmia; atrial fibrillation; bradycardia; cerebral ischemia; cerebrovascular accident; CHF; deep thrombophlebitis; heart arrest; heart failure; hypertension; hypotension; MI; murmur; palpitation; pericarditis; peripheral vascular disorder; postural hypotension; syncope; tachycardia; thrombophlebitis; thrombosis.

CNS – Abnormal gait; ataxia; decreased libido; decreased reflexes; dementia; dysesthesia; dyskinesia; emotional lability; hostility; hypalgesia; hyperkinesia; incoordination; meningitis; neurologic disorder; tremor; vertigo.

Dermatologic – Angioedema; benign skin neoplasm; eczema; herpes simplex; incomplete Stevens-Johnson syndrome; nail disorder; photosensitivity reaction; pruritus; psoriasis; skin discoloration; skin disorder.

GI – Cholangitis; cholestatic jaundice; colitis; dyspepsia; dysphagia; esophagitis; gastroenteritis; GI disorder; GI hemorrhage; gum disorder; hepatitis; pancreatitis; parotid gland enlargement; periodontitis; stomatitis; tongue discoloration; tooth disorder.

Hematologic / Lymphatic – Aplastic anemia; macrocytic anemia; megaloblastic anemia; microcytic anemia.

Metabolic – Avitaminosis; bilirubinemia; dehydration; hypercholesteremia; hypoglycemia; increased alkaline phosphatase; increased lipase; increased serum creatinine; peripheral edema.

Musculoskeletal – Myalgia; myasthenia.

Respiratory – Apnea; bronchitis; lung disorder; lung edema; pneumonia (including *Pneumocystis carinii* pneumonia); rhinitis.

Special senses – Conjunctivitis; eye disorder; lacrimation disorder; retinitis; taste perversion.

Miscellaneous – AIDS; allergic reaction; ascites; cellulitis; chest pain; chills and fever; cyst; decreased CD4 count; facial edema; flu syndrome; hernia; hormone level altered; moniliasis; sarcoma; sepsis; viral infection.

Other adverse events in the published literature or reported from other sources – The following additional events have been identified either in the published literature or from spontaneous reports from other sources: Acute renal failure; amenorrhea; aphthous stomatitis; bile duct obstruction; carpal tunnel; chronic myelogenous leukemia; diplopia; dysesthesia; dyspnea; enuresis; erythema nodosum; erythroleukemia; foot drop; galactorrhea; gynecomastia; hangover effect; hypomagnesemia; hypothyroidism; lymphedema; lymphopenia; metrorrhagia; migraine; myxedema; nodular sclerosing Hodgkin disease; nystagmus; oliguria; pancytopenia; petechiae; purpura; Raynaud syndrome; stomach ulcer; suicide attempt.

➤*Postmarketing:*

Cardiovascular – Cardiac arrhythmias including atrial fibrillation; bradycardia; EKG abnormalities; sick sinus syndrome; tachycardia.

CNS – Changes in mental status or mood including depression and suicide attempts; disturbances in consciousness including lethargy, loss of consciousness, or stupor; seizures including grand mal convulsions; status epilepticus; syncope.

Hematologic / Lymphatic – Decreased white blood cell counts including neutropenia and febrile neutropenia; changes in prothrombin time.

Metabolic / Endocrine – Electrolyte imbalance including hypercalcemia and hypocalcemia; hyperkalemia and hypokalemia; hyponatremia; hypothyroidism; increased alkaline phosphatase.

Miscellaneous – Erythema multiforme; pleural effusion.

Overdosage

There have been 3 cases of overdose reported, all attempted suicides. There have been no reported fatalities in doses of at least 14.4 g, and all patients recovered without reported sequelae.

Patient Information

See Warning Box.

Instruct patients about the potential teratogenicity of thalidomide and the precautions that must be taken to preclude fetal exposure as per the S.T.E.P.S. program and boxed Warnings. Take thalidomide only as prescribed in compliance with all of the provisions of the S.T.E.P.S. Restricted Distribution Program.

Instruct patients not to extensively handle or open thalidomide capsules and to maintain storage of capsules in blister packs until ingestion.

Instruct patients not to share medication with anyone else.

Thalidomide frequently causes drowsiness and somnolence. Instruct patients to avoid situations where drowsiness may be a problem and not to take other medications that may cause drowsiness without adequate medical advice. Advise patients as to the possible impairment of mental or physical abilities required for the performance of hazardous tasks, such as driving a car or operating other complex machinery. Thalidomide may potentiate the somnolence caused by alcohol.

Thalidomide may cause photosensitivity (sensitivity to sunlight). Instruct patients to avoid prolonged exposure to the sun and other ultraviolet light. Instruct patients to use sunscreens and wear protective clothing until tolerance is determined.

Thalidomide can cause peripheral neuropathies that may be initially signaled by numbness, tingling, pain, or a burning sensation in the feet or hands. Instruct patients to report such occurrences to their prescriber immediately.

Thalidomide may cause dizziness and orthostatic hypotension. Instruct patients to sit upright for a few minutes prior to standing from a recumbent position.

Patients are not permitted to donate blood while taking thalidomide. In addition, instruct male patients not to donate sperm while taking thalidomide.

LENALIDOMIDE

Rx	**Revlimid** (Celgene)	**Capsules:** 5 mg lenalidomide	(REV 5 mg). White. 30s and 100s.
		10 mg lenalidomide	(REV 10 mg). Blue/Green and pale yellow. In 30s and 100s.

LENALIDOMIDE — ORAL

WARNING

Warnings:

1.) Potential for human birth defects
2.) Hematologic toxicity (neutropenia and thrombocytopenia)
3.) Deep vein thrombosis and pulmonary embolism

Warning: Potential for human birth defects – Lenalidomide is an analog of thalidomide. Thalidomide is a known human teratogen that causes severe, life-threatening human birth defects. If lenalidomide is taken during pregnancy, it may cause birth defects or death to a fetus. Advise women to avoid pregnancy while taking lenalidomide.

Special prescribing requirements: Because of this potential toxicity and to avoid fetal exposure to lenalidomide, lenalidomide is only available under a special restricted distribution program, RevAssist. Under this program, only health care providers and pharmacists registered with the program are able to prescribe and dispense the product. In addition, lenalidomide is only dispensed to patients who are registered and meet all the conditions of the RevAssist program.

Please see the following information for health care providers and patients about this restricted distribution program.

Celgene's RevAssist program description:

Lenalidomide is prescribed only by licensed health care providers who are registered in the RevAssist program and understand the potential risk of teratogenicity if lenalidomide is used during pregnancy.

Effective contraception must be used by patients for at least 4 weeks before beginning lenalidomide therapy, during therapy, during dose interruptions, and for 4 weeks following discontinuation of therapy. Reliable contraception is indicated even if the patient has a history of infertility, unless infertility is due to hysterectomy or because the patient has been postmenopausal naturally for at least 24 consecutive months. Two reliable forms of contraception must be used simultaneously unless continuous abstinence from heterosexual sexual contact is the chosen method. Refer women of childbearing potential a qualified provider of contraceptive methods, if needed. Sexually mature women who have not undergone a hysterectomy or who have not been postmenopausal naturally for at least 24 consecutive months (ie, who have had menses at some time in the preceding 24 consecutive months) are considered to be women of childbearing potential.

Before prescribing lenalidomide, women of childbearing potential should have 2 negative pregnancy tests (sensitivity of at least 50 milliunits/mL). Perform the first test within 10 to 14 days, and the second test within 24 hours prior to prescribing lenalidomide. A prescription for lenalidomide for a woman of childbearing potential must not be issued by the health care provider until negative pregnancy tests have been verified by the health care provider.

It is not known whether lenalidomide is present in the semen of patients receiving the drug. Therefore, men receiving lenalidomide must always use a latex condom during any sexual contact with women of childbearing potential even if they have undergone a successful vasectomy.

Once treatment has started and during dose interruptions, pregnancy testing for women of childbearing potential should occur weekly during the first 4 weeks of use, then should be repeated every 4 weeks in women with regular menstrual cycles. If menstrual cycles are irregular, the pregnancy testing should occur every 2 weeks. Perform pregnancy testing and counseling if a patient misses her period or if there is any abnormality in her pregnancy test or in her menstrual bleeding. Lenalidomide treatment must be discontinued during this evaluation.

Pregnancy test results should be verified by the health care provider and the pharmacist prior to dispensing any prescription.

If pregnancy does occur during lenalidomide treatment, lenalidomide must be discontinued immediately.

Any suspected fetal exposure to lenalidomide should be reported to the FDA via the MedWatch number at 1-800-FDA-1088 and also to Celgene Corporation at 1-888-4CELGEN. Refer the patient to an obstetrician/gynecologist experienced in reproductive toxicity for further evaluation and counseling.

Lenalidomide should be used in women of childbearing potential only when the patient meets all of the following conditions (ie, she is unable to become pregnant while on lenalidomide therapy):

- She appears to understand the risks associated with the drug and is thought to be able to reliably carry out instructions.
- She is capable of complying with the contraceptive measures, pregnancy testing, patient registration, and patient survey as described in the RevAssist program.
- She has received both oral and written warnings of the potential risks of taking lenalidomide during pregnancy and of exposing a fetus to the drug.
- She has received both oral and written warnings of the risk of possible contraception failure and of the need to use 2 reliable forms of contraception simultaneously, unless continuous abstinence from heterosexual sexual contact is the chosen method. Sexually mature women who have not undergone a hysterectomy or who have not been postmenopausal for at least 24 consecutive months (ie, who have had menses at some time in the preceding 24 consecutive months) are considered to be women of childbearing potential.
- She acknowledges, in writing, her understanding of these warnings and of the need for using 2 reliable methods of contraception for 4 weeks prior to beginning lenalidomide therapy, during lenalidomide therapy, during dose interruptions and for 4 weeks after discontinuation of lenalidomide therapy.
- She has had 2 negative pregnancy tests with a sensitivity of at least 50 milliunits/mL, within 10 to 14 days and 24 hours prior to beginning therapy.
- If the patient is between 12 and 18 years of age, her parent or legal guardian is to read the educational materials and agree to try to ensure compliance with all conditions.

Lenalidomide should be used in sexually active men when the patient meets all of the following conditions:

- He appears to understand the risks associated with the drug and is thought to be able to reliably carry out instructions.
- He is capable of complying with the contraceptive measures that are appropriate for men, patient registration, and patient survey as described in the RevAssist program.
- He has received both oral and written warnings of the potential risks of taking lenalidomide and exposing a fetus to the drug.
- He has received both oral and written warnings of the risk of possible contraception failure and that it is unknown whether lenalidomide is present in semen. He has been instructed that he must always use a latex condom during any sexual contact with women of childbearing potential, even if he has undergone a successful vasectomy.
- He acknowledges, in writing, his understanding of these warnings and of the need to use a latex condom during any sexual contact with women of childbearing potential, even if he has undergone a successful vasectomy. Women of childbearing potential are considered to be sexually mature women who have not undergone a hysterectomy or who have not been postmenopausal for at least 24 consecutive months (ie, who have had menses at any time in the preceding 24 consecutive months).
- If the patient is between 12 and 18 years of age, his parent or legal guardian are to read the educational materials and agree to try to ensure compliance with all conditions.

Hematologic toxicity (neutropenia and thrombocytopenia) – This drug is associated with significant neutropenia and thrombocytopenia in patients with del(5q) myelodysplastic syndrome (MDS). Eighty percent of patients had to have a dose delay/reduction during the major study for the indication. Thirty-four percent of patients had to have a second dose delay/reduction. Grade 3 or 4 hematologic toxicity was seen in 80% of patients enrolled in the study. Patients on therapy should have their complete blood counts monitored weekly for the first 8 weeks of therapy and at least monthly thereafter. Patients may require dose interruption and/or reduction. Patients may require use of blood product support and/or growth factors.

Deep vein thrombosis (DVT) and pulmonary embolism (PE) – This drug has demonstrated a significantly increased risk of DVT and PE in patients with multiple myeloma who were treated with lenalidomide combination therapy. Patients and physicians are advised to be observant for the signs and symptoms of thromboembolism. Instruct patients to seek medical care if they develop symptoms such as shortness of breath, chest pain, or arm or leg swelling. It is not known whether prophylactic anticoagulation or antiplatelet therapy prescribed in conjunction with lenalidomide may lessen the potential for venous thromboembolic events. The decision to take prophylactic measures should be done carefully after an assessment of an individual patient's underlying risk factors.

Information about lenalidomide and the RevAssist program can be obtained at http://www.revlimid.com or by calling the manufacturer's toll free number 1-888-4CELGEN.

Indications

➤*Transfusion-dependent anemia:* For the treatment of patients with transfusion-dependent anemia due to low- or intermediate-1 risk MDS associated with a deletion 5q cytogenetic abnormality with or without additional cytogenetic abnormalities.

LENALIDOMIDE — ORAL

Administration and Dosage

➤*Approved by the FDA:* December 27, 2005.

➤*Recommended dose:* The recommended starting dose of lenalidomide is 10 mg with water daily. Patients should not break, chew, or open the capsules.

➤*Dose adjustments:*

Patients who are dosed initially at 10 mg and who experience thrombocytopenia should have their dosage adjusted as follows –

Lenalidomide 10 mg Dosage Adjustments Due to Thrombocytopenia	
Platelet counts	Recommended course
If thrombocytopenia develops within 4 weeks of starting treatment at 10 mg daily	
If baseline is 100,000/mcL or greater	
When platelets fall to fewer than 50,000/mcL	Interrupt lenalidomide treatment
When platelets return to 50,000/mcL or greater	Resume lenalidomide at 5 mg daily
If baseline is less than 100,000/mcL	
When platelets fall to 50% of baseline value	Interrupt lenalidomide treatment
If baseline is 60,000/mcL or greater and returns to 50,000/mcL or greater	Resume lenalidomide at 5 mg daily
If baseline is less than 60,000/mcL and returns to 30,000/mcL or more	Resume lenalidomide at 5 mg daily
If thrombocytopenia develops after 4 weeks of starting treatment at 10 mg daily	
When platelets are less than 30,000/mcL or less than 50,000/mcL and platelet transfusions	Interrupt lenalidomide treatment
When platelets return to 30,000/mcL or more (without hemostatic failure)	Resume lenalidomide at 5 mg daily

Patients who experience thrombocytopenia at 5 mg daily should have their dosage adjusted as follows –

Lenalidomide 5 mg Dosage Adjustments Due to Thrombocytopenia	
Platelet count	Recommended course
If thrombocytopenia develops during treatment at 5 mg daily	
When platelets are 30,000/mcL or less or 50,000/mcL or less and platelet transfusions	Interrupt lenalidomide treatment
When platelets return to 30,000/mcL or more (without hemostatic failure)	Resume lenalidomide at 5 mg every other day

Patients who are dosed initially at 10 mg and experience neutropenia should have their dosage adjusted as follows –

Lenalidomide 10 mg Dosage Adjustments Due to Neutropenia	
Neutrophil count	Recommended course
If neutropenia develops within 4 weeks of starting treatment at 10 mg daily	
If baseline ANC[a] is 1,000/mcL or greater	
When neutrophils fall to less than 750/mcL	Interrupt lenalidomide treatment
When neutrophils return to 1,000/mcL or greater	Resume lenalidomide at 5 mg daily
If baseline ANC is less than 1,000/mcL	
When neutrophils fall to less than 500/mcL	Interrupt lenalidomide treatment
When neutrophils return to 500/mcL or greater	Resume lenalidomide at 5 mg daily
If neutropenia develops after 4 weeks of starting treatment at 10 mg daily	
When neutrophils are less than 500/mcL for 7 days or more or neutrophils are less than 500/mcL associated with fever (38.5°C [101°F] or greater)	Interrupt lenalidomide treatment
When neutrophils return to 500/mcL or more	Resume lenalidomide at 5 mg daily

[a] ANC = absolute neutrophil count.

Patients who experience neutropenia at 5 mg daily should have their dosage adjusted as follows: –

Lenalidomide 5 mg Dosage Adjustments Due to Neutropenia	
Neutrophil count	Recommended course
If neutropenia develops during treatment at 5 mg daily	
When neutrophils are less than 500/mcL for 7 days or more or neutrophils are less than 500/mcL associated with fever (38.5°C [101°F] or greater)	Interrupt lenalidomide treatment
When neutrophils return to 500/mcL or more	Resume lenalidomide at 5 mg every other day

➤*Renal function impairment:* This drug is known to be substantially excreted by the kidney, and the risk of toxic reactions to this drug may be greater in patients with impaired renal function. Because elderly patients are more likely to have decreased renal function, take care in dose selection and monitor renal function.

➤*Storage/Stability:* Store at 25°C (77°F); excursions permitted to 15° to 30°C (59° to 86°F).

Actions

➤*Pharmacology:* The mechanism of action of lenalidomide remains to be fully characterized. Lenalidomide possesses immunomodulatory and antiangiogenic properties. Lenalidomide inhibited the secretion of proinflammatory cytokines and increased the secretion of anti-inflammatory cytokines from peripheral blood mononuclear cells. Lenalidomide inhibited cell proliferation with varying efficacy (IC50s) in some but not all cell lines. Of cell lines tested, lenalidomide was effective in inhibiting growth of Namalwa cells (a human B cell lymphoma cell line with a deletion of 1 chromosome 5) but was much less effective in inhibiting growth of KG-1 cells (human myeloblastic cell line, also with a deletion of 1 chromosome 5) and other cell lines without chromosome 5 deletions. Lenalidomide inhibited the expression of cyclooxygenase-2 (COX-2) but not COX-1 in vitro.

➤*Pharmacokinetics:*

Absorption – Lenalidomide, in healthy volunteers, is rapidly absorbed following oral administration with maximum plasma concentrations (C_{max}) occurring between 0.625 and 1.5 hours postdose. Coadministration with food does not alter the extent of absorption (area under the curve [AUC]) but does reduce the C_{max} 36%. The pharmacokinetic disposition of lenalidomide is linear. C_{max} and AUC increase proportionately with increases in dose. Multiple dosing at the recommended dose-regimen does not result in drug accumulation.

Pharmacokinetic sampling in MDS patients was not performed. In multiple myeloma patients, C_{max} occurred between 0.5 and 4 hours postdose both on days 1 and 28. AUC and C_{max} values increase proportionally with dose following single and multiple doses. Exposure (AUC) in multiple myeloma patients is 57% higher than in healthy men.

Distribution – In vitro (^{14}C)-lenalidomide binding to plasma proteins is approximately 30%.

Metabolism/Excretion – The metabolic profile of lenalidomide in humans has not been studied. In healthy volunteers, approximately two thirds of lenalidomide is eliminated unchanged through urinary excretion. The process exceeds the glomerular filtration rate and therefore is partially or entirely active. Half-life of elimination is approximately 3 hours.

Special populations –

Renal function impairment: The pharmacokinetics of lenalidomide in MDS patients with renal dysfunction have not been determined. In multiple myeloma patients, those with mild renal impairment had an AUC 56% greater than those with normal renal function.

Contraindications

Lenalidomide is contraindicated in any patients who have demonstrated hypersensitivity to the drug or its components.

➤*Pregnancy and women of childbearing potential:* Because of its structural similarities to thalidomide, a known human teratogen, lenalidomide is contraindicated in pregnant women and women capable of becoming pregnant. When there is no alternative, women of childbearing potential may be treated with lenalidomide provided adequate precautions are taken to avoid pregnancy. Women must commit either to abstain continuously from heterosexual sexual intercourse or to use 2 methods of reliable birth control, including at least 1 highly effective method (eg, intrauterine device [IUD], hormonal contraception, tubal ligation, partner's vasectomy) and 1 additional effective method (eg, latex condom, diaphragm, cervical cap), beginning 4 weeks prior to initiating treatment with lenalidomide, during therapy with lenalidomide, during therapy delay, and continuing for 4 weeks following discontinuation of lenalidomide therapy. If hormonal or IUD contraception is medically contraindicated, 2 other effective or highly effective methods may be used.

LENALIDOMIDE — ORAL

Women of childbearing potential being treated with lenalidomide should have pregnancy testing (sensitivity of at least 50 milliunits/mL). The first test should be performed within 10 to 14 days and the second test within 24 hours prior to beginning lenalidomide therapy and then weekly during the first month of lenalidomide, then monthly thereafter in women with regular menstrual cycles or every 2 weeks in women with irregular menstrual cycles. Perform pregnancy testing and counseling if a patient misses her period or if there is any abnormality in menstrual bleeding. If pregnancy occurs, lenalidomide must be immediately discontinued. Under these conditions, refer the patient to an obstetrician/gynecologist experienced in reproductive toxicity for further evaluation and counseling.

Warnings

➤*Hematologic toxicity (neutropenia and thrombocytopenia):* This drug is associated with significant neutropenia and thrombocytopenia in patients with del(5q) MDS. Eighty percent of patients had to have a dose delay or reduction during the major study for the indication. Thirty-four percent of patients had to have a second dose delay/reduction. Grade 3 or 4 hematologic toxicity was seen in 80% of patients enrolled in the study. In the 48% of patients who developed grade 3 or 4 neutropenia, the median time to onset was 42 days (range, 14 to 411 days), and the median time to documented recovery was 17 days (range, 2 to 170 days). In the 54% of patients who developed grade 3 or 4 thrombocytopenia, the median time to onset was 28 days (range, 8 to 290 days), and the median time to documented recovery was 22 days (range, 5 to 224 days). Patients on therapy should have their complete blood cell counts monitored weekly for the first 8 weeks of therapy and at least monthly thereafter. Patients may require dose interruption and/or reduction. Patients may require use of blood product support and/or growth factors.

➤*DVT and PE:* See the Warning box for more information.

➤*Renal function impairment:* No formal studies have been conducted in patients with renal impairment. This drug is known to be excreted by the kidney, and the risk of adverse reactions to this drug may be greater in patients with impaired renal function. Patients with renal insufficiency were excluded from the clinical trials, and those who developed renal insufficiency during the clinical trials had the drug held. Take care in dose selection and monitor renal function.

➤*Elderly:* Lenalidomide has been used in clinical trials in patients up to 95 years of age. Of the 148 patients with del(5q) MDS enrolled in the major study, 38% were 65 years of age and older, while 33% were 75 years of age and older. Although the overall frequency of adverse reactions (100%) was the same in patients over 65 years of age as in younger patients, the frequency of serious adverse reactions was higher in patients older than 65 years of age than in younger patients (54% vs 33%). A greater proportion of patients older than 65 years of age discontinued from the clinical studies because of adverse reactions than the proportion of younger patients (27% vs 16%). No differences in efficacy were observed between patients older than 65 years of age and younger patients.

This drug is known to be substantially excreted by the kidney, and the risk of toxic reactions to this drug may be greater in patients with impaired renal function. Because elderly patients are more likely to have decreased renal function, take care in dose selection and monitor renal function.

➤*Pregnancy: Category X.* (See Black Box Warning.) Lenalidomide is an analogue of thalidomide. Thalidomide is a known human teratogen that causes life-threatening human birth defects. Lenalidomide may cause fetal harm when administered to a pregnant woman. Advise women of childbearing potential to avoid pregnancy while on lenalidomide. Use 2 effective contraceptive methods during therapy, during therapy interruptions and for at least 4 weeks after completing therapy.

There are no adequate and well-controlled studies in pregnant women.

Because of this potential toxicity and to avoid fetal exposure to lenalidomide, lenalidomide is only available under a restricted distribution program. This program is called RevAssist.

Lenalidomide has been shown to have an embryocidal effect in rabbits at a dose of 50 mg/kg (approximately 120 times the human dose of 10 mg based on body surface area).

An embryo-fetal development study in rats revealed no teratogenic effects at the highest dose of 500 mg/kg (approximately 600 times the human dose of 10 mg based on body surface area). At 100, 300, or 500 mg/kg/day there was minimal maternal toxicity that included slight, transient reduction in mean body weight gain and food intake. However this animal model may not adequately address the full spectrum of the potential embryofetal developmental effects of lenalidomide.

A pre- and postnatal development study in rats revealed few adverse effects on the offspring of female rats treated with lenalidomide at doses up to 500 mg/kg (approximately 600 times the human dose of 10 mg based on body surface area). The male offspring exhibited slightly delayed sexual maturation and the female offspring had slightly lower body weight gains during gestation when bred to male offspring. Reproductive effects of lenalidomide have not been thoroughly assessed. The structural similarity of lenalidomide to thalidomide, a known human teratogen, suggests a potential risk to the developing fetus.

Because of the structural similarity to thalidomide, a known human teratogen, and the lack of sufficient information regarding lenalidomide's teratogenic potential, lenalidomide is contraindicated in women who are or may become pregnant, are not using the 2 required types of birth control, or are not continually abstaining from reproductive heterosexual sexual intercourse. Lenalidomide should not be used by women who are pregnant or who could become pregnant while taking the drug. If pregnancy does occur during treatment, the drug should be immediately discontinued. Under these conditions, refer the patient to an obstetrician/gynecologist experienced in reproductive toxicity for further evaluation and counseling. Any suspected fetal exposure to lenalidomide should be reported to the FDA via the MedWatch program at 1-800-FDA-1088 and also to Celgene Corporation at 1-888-4CELGEN (1-888-423-5436).

➤*Lactation:* It is not known whether this drug is excreted in human milk. Because many drugs are excreted in human milk and because of the potential for adverse reactions in breast-feeding infants from lenalidomide, decide whether to discontinue breast-feeding or to discontinue the drug, taking into account the importance of the drug to the mother.

➤*Children:* Safety and efficacy in pediatric patients younger than 18 years of age have not been established.

Precautions

➤*Monitoring:* Perform a complete blood cell count, including white blood cell count with differential, platelet count, hemoglobin, and hematocrit weekly for the first 8 weeks of lenalidomide treatment and monthly thereafter to monitor for cytopenias.

Drug Interactions

None well documented.

Adverse Reactions

A total of 148 patients received at least 1 dose of lenalidomide 10 mg in the del(5q) MDS clinical study. At least 1 adverse reaction was reported in all of the 148 patients who were treated with the 10 mg starting dose of lenalidomide. The most frequently reported adverse reactions were related to blood and lymphatic system disorders, skin and subcutaneous tissue disorders, GI disorders, and general disorders and administrative site conditions.

Thrombocytopenia (61.5%; 91/148) and neutropenia (58.8%; 87/148) were the most frequently reported adverse reactions observed. The next most common adverse reactions observed were diarrhea (48.6%; 72/148), pruritis (41.9%; 62/148), rash (35.8%; 53/148) and fatigue (31.1%; 46/148). The following table summarizes the adverse reactions that were reported in at least 5% of the lenalidomide treated patients in the del(5q) MDS clinical study. The second table summarizes the most frequently observed grade 3 and 4 adverse reactions regardless of relationship to treatment with lenalidomide. In the single-arm studies conducted, it is often not possible to distinguish adverse reactions that are drug-related and those that reflect the patient's underlying disease.

Lenalidomide Adverse Reactions	
Adverse reaction[a]	N = 148
Cardiovascular	
Hypertension[b]	9 (6.1%)
Palpitations	8 (5.4%)
CNS	
Depression	8 (5.4%)
Dizziness	29 (19.6%)
Fatigue	46 (31.1%)
Headache	29 (19.6%)
Hypoasthesia	10 (6.8%)
Insomnia	15 (10.1%)
Peripheral neuropathy[b]	8 (5.4%)
Rigors	9 (6.1%)
Dermatologic	
Dry skin	21 (14.2%)
Ecchymosis	8 (5.4%)
Erythema	8 (5.4%)
Night sweats	12 (8.1%)
Pruritus	62 (41.9%)
Rash[b]	53 (35.8%)
Sweating increased	10 (6.8%)
GI	
Abdominal pain[b]	18 (12.2%)
Abdominal pain upper	12 (8.1%)
Constipation	35 (23.6%)
Diarrhea[b]	72 (48.6%)
Dry mouth	10 (6.8%)
Dysgeusia	9 (6.1%)
Loose stools	9 (6.1%)
Nausea	35 (23.6%)
Vomiting[b]	15 (10.1%)
GU	
Dysuria	10 (6.8%)
Urinary tract infection[b]	16 (10.8%)

LENALIDOMIDE — ORAL

Lenalidomide Adverse Reactions	
Adverse reaction[a]	N = 148
Hematologic/Lymphatic	
Anemia[b]	17 (11.5%)
Febrile neutropenia	8 (5.4%)
Leukopenia[b]	12 (8.1%)
Neutropenia	87 (58.8%)
Thrombocytopenia	91 (61.5%)
Metabolic/Nutritional	
Anorexia	15 (10.1%)
Hypokalemia	16 (10.8%)
Hypomagnesemia	9 (6.1%)
Musculoskeletal	
Arthralgia	32 (21.6%)
Back pain	31 (20.9%)
Muscle cramp	27 (18.2%)
Myalgia	13 (8.8%)
Pain in limb	16 (10.8%)
Respiratory	
Bronchitis[b]	9 (6.1%)
Cough	29 (19.6%)
Dyspnea[b]	25 (16.9%)
Dyspnoea exertional	10 (6.8%)
Epistaxis	22 (14.9%)
Nasopharyngitis	34 (23%)
Pharyngitis	23 (15.5%)
Pneumonia[b]	17 (11.5%)
Rhinitis[b]	10 (6.8%)
Sinusitis[b]	12 (8.1%)
Upper respiratory tract infection[b]	22 (14.9%)
Miscellaneous	
Acquired hypothyroidism	10 (6.8%)
ALT increased	12 (8.1%)
Asthenia	22 (14.9%)
Cellulitis	8 (5.4%)
Chest pain	8 (5.4%)
Contusion	12 (8.1%)
Edema[b]	15 (10.1%)
Edema peripheral	30 (20.3%)
Pain[b]	10 (6.8%)
Peripheral swelling	12 (8.1%)
Pyrexia	31 (20.9%)

[a] System organ classes and preferred terms are coded using the Medical Dictionary for Regulatory Activities (MedDRA). A patient with multiple occurrences of an adverse reaction is counted only once in the adverse reaction category.
[b] Not otherwise specified.

Lenalidomide Grade 3 and 4 Adverse Reactions[a]	
Adverse Reaction[b]	N = 148
Patients with at least 1 grade 3/4 adverse reaction	131 (88.5%)
Cardiovascular	
Pulmonary embolism	3 (2%)
Pulmonary hypertension[c]	2 (1.4%)
CNS	
Dizziness	4 (2.7%)
Fatigue	7 (4.7%)
Headache	2 (1.4%)
Syncope	2 (1.4%)
Dermatologic	
Pruritus	3 (2%)
Rash[c]	10 (6.8%)

Lenalidomide Grade 3 and 4 Adverse Reactions[a]	
Adverse Reaction[b]	N = 148
GI	
Diarrhea[c]	5 (3.4%)
Nausea	6 (4.1%)
Vomiting[c]	2 (1.4%)
Hematologic/Lymphatic	
Anemia[c]	9 (6.1%)
Febrile neutropenia	6 (4.1%)
Granulocytopenia	3 (2%)
Leukopenia[c]	8 (5.4%)
Neutropenia	79 (53.4%)
Pancytopenia	3 (2%)
Thrombocytopenia	74 (50%)
Musculoskeletal	
Arthralgia	2 (1.4%)
Back pain	7 (4.7%)
Muscle cramp	3 (2%)
Pain in limb	2 (1.4%)
Respiratory	
Dyspnea	7 (4.7%)
Epistaxis	2 (1.4%)
Hypoxia	2 (1.4%
Pleural effusion	2 (1.4%)
Pneumonia[c]	11 (7.4%)
Pneumonitis[c]	2 (1.4%)
Respiratory distress	3 (2%)
Respiratory tract infection	2 (1.4%)
Upper respiratory tract infection	2 (1.4%)
Miscellaneous	
Asthenia	2 (1.4%)
Chest pain	3 (2%)
Multi-organ failure	2 (1.4%)
Pyrexia	5 (3.4%)
Sepsis	4 (2.7%)
Sweating increased	2 (1.4%)

[a] Adverse reactions with frequency of at least 1% in the 10 mg Overall group. Grade 3 and 4 are based on National Cancer Institute Common Toxicity Criteria version 2.
[b] Preferred Terms are coded using the MedDRA dictionary. A patient with multiple occurrences of an adverse reaction is counted only once in the adverse reaction category.
[c] Not otherwise specified.

In other clinical studies of lenalidomide in MDS patients, the following serious adverse reactions (regardless of relationship to study drug treatment) not described in the tables were reported:

➤*Cardiovascular:* Angina pectoris, aortic disorder, atrial fibrillation, atrial fibrillation aggravated, bradycardia, cardiac arrest, cardiac failure, cardiac failure congestive, cardio-respiratory arrest, cardiogenic shock, cardiomyopathy, deep vein thrombosis, hypotension, ischemia, myocardial infarction, myocardial ischemia, pulmonary edema, supraventricular arrhythmia, tachyarrhythmia, thrombophlebitis superficial, thrombosis, ventricular dysfunction.

➤*CNS:* Aphasia, cerebellar infarction, cerebral infarction, cerebrovascular accident, confusional state, depressed level of consciousness, dysarthria, fall, gait abnormal, migraine, spinal cord compression, subarachnoid hemorrhage, transient ischemic attack, vertigo.

➤*Dermatologic:* Acute febrile neutrophilic dermatosis.

➤*GI:* Colitis ischemic, colonic polyp, diverticulitis, dysphagia, gastritis, gastroenteritis, gastroesophageal reflux disease, GI hemorrhage, intestinal perforation, irritable bowel syndrome, melena, obstructive inguinal hernia, pancreatitis, pancreatitis due to biliary obstruction, perirectal abscess, rectal hemorrhage, small intestinal obstruction, upper GI hemorrhage.

➤*Hematologic/Lymphatic:* Acute leukemia, acute myeloid leukemia, anemia, bone marrow depression, coagulopathy, hemolysis, hemolytic anemia, lymphoma, refractory anemia, splenic infarction, warm type hemolytic anemia.

➤*Hepatic:* Cholecystitis, cholecystitis acute, hepatic failure, hyperbilirubinemia.

➤*Lab test abnormalities:* Blood creatinine increased, culture negative, hemoglobin decreased, liver function tests abnormal, troponin I increased.

➤*Metabolic/Nutritional:* Dehydration, gout, hypernatremia, hypoglycemia.

LENALIDOMIDE — ORAL

➤*Musculoskeletal:* Arthritis, arthritis aggravated, chondrocalcinosis pyrophosphate, gouty arthritis, neck pain, rigors.

➤*Renal:* Azotemia, calculus ureteric, hematuria, renal failure, renal failure acute, renal mass.

➤*Respiratory:* Bronchitis, chronic obstructive airways disease exacerbated, dyspnea exacerbated, interstitial lung disease, lobar pneumonia, lung infiltration, respiratory failure, sinusitis, sinusitis acute, wheezing.

➤*Miscellaneous:* Bacteremia, Basedow disease, bronchoalveolar carcinoma, central line infection, cervical vertebral fracture, clostridial infection, disease progression, ear infection, *Enterobacter* sepsis, femoral neck fracture, femur fracture, fractured pelvis, fungal infection, herpes viral infection, hip fracture, hypersensitivity, infection, influenza, intermittent pyrexia, kidney infection, *Klebsiella* sepsis, localized infection, lung cancer metastatic, nodule, oral infection, overdose, pelvic pain, postprocedural hemorrhage, prostate cancer metastatic, *Pseudomonas* infection, rib fracture, road traffic accident, septic shock, spinal compression fracture, *Staphylococcal* infection, sudden death, transfusion reaction, urosepsis.

Overdosage

No cases of overdose have been reported during the clinical studies.

Patient Information

Counsel patients on lenalidomide's potential risk of teratogenicity because of its structural similarity to thalidomide. Under the RevAssist program, patients may only acquire a prescription for lenalidomide therapy through a controlled distribution program through contracted pharmacies. Women of childbearing potential will be educated and counseled on the requirements of the RevAssist program and the precautions to be taken to preclude fetal exposure to lenalidomide. Patients should become familiar with the lenalidomide RevAssist educational materials, Patient Medication Guide, and direct any questions to their physician or pharmacist prior to starting lenalidomide therapy.

➤*Warning: potential for human birth defects:* Lenalidomide is an analogue of thalidomide. Thalidomide is a known human teratogen that causes life-threatening human birth defects. If lenalidomide is taken during pregnancy, it may cause birth defects or death to a fetus. Advise women to avoid pregnancy while on lenalidomide.

MITOXANTRONE HYDROCHLORIDE

For complete prescribing information, see the Mitoxantrone monograph in the Antineoplastics chapter.

HYDROXYCHLOROQUINE SULFATE

Rx	**Hydroxychloroquine Sulfate** (Various, eg, Geneva, Mylan, Teva, Watson)	**Tablets:** 200 mg (equivalent to 155 mg base)	In 100s, 500s, and 1000s.
Rx	**Plaquenil** (Sanofi Synthelabo)		(PLAQUENIL). White to off-white. Film-coated. In 100s.

HYDROXYCHLOROQUINE SULFATE — ORAL

WARNING

Physicians should completely familiarize themselves with the complete contents of the package insert before prescribing hydroxychloroquine.

Indications

➤*Lupus erythematosus:* For the treatment of chronic discoid and systemic lupus erythematosus (SLE) in patients who have not responded satisfactorily to drugs with less potential for serious side effects.

➤*Malaria:* For the suppressive treatment and treatment of acute attacks of malaria caused by *Plasmodium vivax*, *P. malariae*, *P. ovale*, and susceptible strains of *P. falciparum*.

➤*Rheumatoid arthritis (RA):* For the treatment of acute or chronic RA in patients who have not responded satisfactorily to drugs with less potential for serious side effects.

Administration and Dosage

➤*Approved by the FDA:* April 18, 1955.

➤*Lupus erythematosus:* Initially, 400 mg once or twice daily in adults, continued for several weeks or months depending on response. For prolonged maintenance therapy, a smaller dose (200 to 400 mg daily) frequently will suffice. The incidence of retinopathy reportedly has been higher when the maintenance dose is exceeded.

➤*RA:*

Initial dosage – 400 to 600 mg daily, taken with a meal or a glass of milk. Side effects may require temporary reduction. Later (usually from 5 to 10 days), dose may be increased gradually to optimum response level, often without return of side effects.

Maintenance dosage – When a good response is obtained (usually in 4 to 12 weeks), reduce dosage by 50% and continue at a level of 200 to 400 mg daily. Incidence of retinopathy is higher when this dose is exceeded.

Duration of therapy – The compound is cumulative and requires several weeks to exert therapeutic effects; minor side effects may occur early. Maximum effects may not be obtained for several months. If objective improvement (reduced joint swelling, increased mobility) does not occur within 6 months, discontinue the drug. Safe use of hydroxychloroquine to treat juvenile rheumatoid arthritis (JRA) has not been established.

Relapse – If relapse occurs after drug withdrawal, resume therapy or continue on an intermittent schedule if there are no ocular contraindications.

Corticosteroid dose reduction – Corticosteroids and salicylates may be used with this compound; generally they can be decreased gradually or eliminated after hydroxychloroquine has been used for several weeks. When gradual reduction of steroid dosage is indicated, reduce (every 4 to 5 days) dose of cortisone by no more than 5 to 15 mg; hydrocortisone by 5 to 10 mg; prednisolone and prednisone by 1 to 2.5 mg; methylprednisolone and triamcinolone by 1 to 2 mg; or dexamethasone by 0.25 to 0.5 mg.

➤*Malaria:* Hydroxychloroquine sulfate 200 mg is equivalent to 155 mg hydroxychloroquine base and 250 mg chloroquine phosphate.

Children's doses – Expressed in mg/kg, these should not exceed the recommended adult dose.

Suppression –

Adults: 310 mg base weekly on the same day each week. Begin 1 to 2 weeks prior to exposure; continue for 4 weeks after leaving endemic area. If suppressive therapy is not begun prior to exposure, double the initial loading dose (adults – 620 mg base; children – 10 mg base/kg) and give in 2 doses, 6 hours apart.

Children: Administer 5 mg base/kg weekly, up to a maximum adult dose.

Children's Hydroxychloroquine Dose Based on Age

Age (years)	Hydroxychloroquine base equivalent
< 1	37.5 mg
1 to 3	75 mg
4 to 6	100 mg
7 to 10	150 mg
11 to 16	225 mg

Acute attack –

Hydroxychloroquine Dose in Acute Malarial Attack

Dose	Time	Dosage (mg of base) Adults	Children
Initial dose	Day 1	620 mg	10 mg/kg
2nd dose	6 hours later	310 mg	5 mg/kg
3rd dose	Day 2	310 mg	5 mg/kg
4th dose	Day 3	310 mg	5 mg/kg

An alternative method, using a single dose of 620 mg base, has also been proven effective.

➤*Storage/Stability:* Store at room temperature, up to 30°C (86°F). Dispense in a tight, light-resistant container.

Actions

➤*Pharmacology:* Inhibition of heme polymerization appears crucial for antimalarial action. Hydroxychloroquine binds initially to heme and then prevents further heme polymerization by incorporating as heme-quinoline complexes into growing heme polymer chains. It is unknown whether the accumulation of heme, heme-quinoline complexes, or both suffices to kill the parasites or if other actions of the antimalarial quinolones are required.

➤*Pharmacokinetics:*

Absorption/Distribution – Pharmacokinetics of hydroxychloroquine are similar to chloroquine. Both drugs are absorbed very rapidly and almost completely after oral administration. Hydroxychloroquine is distributed widely into body tissues and concentrates in the spleen, liver, kidney, melanin-containing tissues, lungs, and, to a lesser extent, the spinal cord and brain. It has a large apparent volume of distribution (more than 100 L/kg). It is bound approximately 60% to plasma proteins.

Metabolism/Excretion – Chloroquine is extensively metabolized in the liver. The renal clearance is approximately half of its total systemic clearance. Renal excretion is increased by acidification of the urine. The terminal half-life ranges from 30 to 60 days, and traces of the drug can be found in the urine for years after a therapeutic regimen.

Contraindications

Retinal or visual field changes attributable to any 4-aminoquinoline compound; hypersensitivity to 4-aminoquinoline compounds; long-term therapy in children.

Warnings

➤*Psoriasis:* Use in patients with psoriasis may precipitate a severe attack. Porphyria may be exacerbated. Do not use unless the benefit to the patient outweighs possible risks.

➤*Ophthalmic effects:* Irreversible retinal damage has been observed in some patients who had received long-term or high-dosage 4-aminoquinoline therapy for discoid and SLE or RA. Retinopathy has been reported to be dose-related. When prolonged therapy is contemplated, perform initial (baseline) and periodic (every 3 months) ophthalmologic examinations (including visual acuity, expert slit-lamp, funduscopic, and visual field tests). If there is any indication of abnormality in the visual acuity, visual field, or retinal macular areas (eg, pigmentary changes, loss of foveal reflex) or any visual symptoms (eg, light flashes or streaks) not fully explainable by difficulties of accommodation or corneal opacities, discontinue drug immediately and observe patient for possible progression (see Adverse Reactions).

Retinal changes – See Adverse Reactions for more information.

Chloroquine retinopathy – Methods recommended for early diagnosis of "chloroquine retinopathy" consist of (1) funduscopic examination of macula for fine pigmentary disturbances or loss of the foveal reflex and (2) examination of central visual field with a small red test object for pericentral or paracentral scotoma or determination of retinal thresholds to red. Regard unexplained visual symptoms (eg, light flashes or streaks) as possible manifestations of retinopathy.

➤*Muscular weakness:* Examine patients on long-term therapy periodically, and test knee and ankle reflexes to detect evidence of muscular weakness. If weakness occurs, discontinue drug.

➤*Renal/Hepatic function impairment:* Use with caution.

➤*Pregnancy:* According to *Drugs in Pregnancy and Lactation* by Briggs, the pregnancy risk factor is a *C*. The Centers for Disease Control and Prevention recommends use for prophylaxis in pregnant women who are traveling to areas with chloroquine-sensitive *P. falciparum* malaria.

Avoid use during pregnancy, except in the suppression of malaria when the benefit outweighs the possible hazard. Chloroquine administered IV to pregnant mice rapidly crossed the placenta, accumulated selectively in the melanin structures of the fetal eyes, and was retained in the ocular tissues for 5 months after the drug was eliminated from the rest of the body.

➤*Lactation:* The drug has been detected in breast milk from 2 mothers receiving 400 mg daily doses for SLE or RA.

➤*Children:* Children are especially sensitive to 4-aminoquinolines. A number of fatalities have been reported following ingestion of chloroquine in small doses (0.75 g or 1 g in one 3-year-old).

Safe use of the drug in the treatment of JRA and SLE has not been established.

Precautions

➤*Monitoring:* Perform periodic blood cell counts during prolonged therapy. If a severe blood disorder appears, consider discontinuation. Use caution in glucose-6-phosphate dehydrogenase (G-6-PD) deficiency.

➤*Hepatic disease:* Use with caution in patients with hepatic disease or in conjunction with hepatotoxic drugs.

➤*Alcoholism:* Use with caution in patients with alcoholism.

➤*Dermatologic reactions:* Dermatologic reactions may occur; exercise care when given to any patient receiving a drug with significant tendency to produce dermatitis.

HYDROXYCHLOROQUINE SULFATE — ORAL

➤*Toxic symptoms:* If serious toxic symptoms occur, administer ammonium chloride (8 g daily in divided doses for adults) 3 or 4 days a week for several months after therapy has been stopped; acidification of the urine increases renal excretion by 20% to 90%. Exercise caution in renal function impairment and/or metabolic acidosis.

Drug Interactions

Hydroxychloroquine Drug Interactions			
Precipitant drug	Object drug*		Description
Cimetidine	Aminoquinolones (eg, hydroxychloroquine)	↑	The hydroxychloroquine dose may need to be lowered during coadministration because of increased pharmacologic effects of the hydroxychloroquine.
Aminoquinolones (eg, hydroxychloroquine)	Beta-blockers (eg, metoprolol)	↑	Plasma concentrations and cardiovascular effects of certain beta-blockers may be increased. Carefully monitor patients when hydroxychloroquine is started or stopped with concomitant use of certain beta-blockers (eg, metoprolol). Consider use of an alternative beta-blocker (eg, atenolol).
Aminoquinolones (eg, hydroxychloroquine)	Cyclosporine	↑	Elevated cyclosporine concentrations may occur, increasing the risk of nephrotoxicity. Consider monitoring cyclosporine and serum creatinine levels. Adjust cyclosporine dose accordingly.
Aminoquinolones (eg, hydroxychloroquine)	Digoxin	↑	Serum levels and actions of digoxin may be increased. Monitor for signs/symptoms of digoxin toxicity; reduce dosage if necessary.
Aminoquinolones (eg, hydroxychloroquine)	Magnesium salts	↓	Oral magnesium salts may decrease the absorption and effect of hydroxychloroquine. The antacid activity of magnesium salts also may be reduced. Separate doses of each drug by 2 to 4 hours. It may be necessary to increase the hydroxychloroquine dose.
Aminoquinolones (eg, hydroxychloroquine)	Mefloquine	↑	Coadministration may lead to an increased risk of seizures.

* ↑ = Object drug increased. ↓ = Object drug decreased.

Adverse Reactions

The following have occurred with 1 or more of the 4-aminoquinoline compounds.

➤*Cardiovascular:* Cardiomyopathy has been reported rarely with high daily doses of hydroxychloroquine.

➤*CNS:* Ataxia; convulsions; dizziness; emotional changes; headache; irritability; nerve deafness; nervousness; nightmares; nystagmus; psychosis; tinnitus; vertigo.

➤*Dermatologic:* Alopecia; bleaching of hair; photosensitivity; precipitation of nonlight-sensitive psoriasis; pruritus; skin and mucosal pigmentation; skin eruptions (urticarial, morbilliform, lichenoid, maculopapular, purpuric, erythema annulare centrifugum, Stevens-Johnson syndrome, acute generalized exanthematous pustulosis, and exfoliative dermatitis).

➤*GI:* Abdominal cramps; anorexia; diarrhea; nausea; vomiting. Isolated cases of abnormal liver function and fulminant hepatic failure.

➤*Hematologic:* Agranulocytosis; aplastic anemia; hemolysis in individuals with G-6-PD deficiency; leukopenia; thrombocytopenia.

➤*Musculoskeletal:* Skeletal muscle palsies, myopathy, or neuromyopathy leading to progressive weakness and atrophy of proximal muscle groups which may be associated with mild sensory changes, depression of tendon reflexes, and abnormal nerve conduction.

➤*Ophthalmic:*

Ciliary body – See Warnings. Disturbance of accommodation with blurred vision. This reaction is dose-related and reversible with cessation of therapy.

Cornea – Decreased corneal sensitivity; punctate to lineal opacities; transient edema. The corneal changes, with or without accompanying symptoms (eg, blurred vision, halos around lights, photophobia), are fairly common but reversible. Corneal deposits may appear as early as 3 weeks following initiation of therapy. The incidence of corneal changes and visual side effects appears to be considerably lower with hydroxychloroquine than with chloroquine.

Retina – Abnormal pigmentation (mild pigment stippling to a "bull's eye" appearance); atrophy; edema; elevated retinal threshold to red light in macular, paramacular, and peripheral retinal areas; increased macular recovery time following exposure to a bright light (photo-stress test); loss of foveal reflex.

Retinopathy – The most common visual symptoms attributed to retinopathy are: Reading and seeing difficulties (ie, words, letters, or parts of objects missing); photophobia; blurred distance vision; missing or blacked out areas in the central or peripheral visual field; light flashes and streaks. Retinopathy appears to be dose related and has occurred within several months (rarely) to several years of daily therapy; a few cases have been reported several years after the drug was discontinued.

Patients with retinal changes may have visual symptoms or may be asymptomatic (with or without visual field changes). Rarely, scotomatous vision or field defects may occur without obvious retinal change. Retinopathy may progress even after the drug is discontinued. In a number of patients, early retinopathy (macular pigmentation sometimes with central field defects) diminished or regressed completely after therapy was discontinued. Paracentral scotoma to red targets ("premaculopathy") is indicative of early retinal dysfunction, which is usually reversible with cessation of therapy.

A small number of cases of retinal changes have occurred in patients who received only hydroxychloroquine. These usually consisted of alteration in retinal pigmentation that was detected on periodic ophthalmologic examination; visual field defects also were present in some. A case of delayed retinopathy has been reported with vision loss starting 1 year after the drug was discontinued.

Other fundus changes – Attenuation of retinal arterioles; fine granular pigmentary disturbances in the peripheral retina; optic disc pallor and atrophy; prominent choroidal patterns in advanced stage.

Visual field defects – Central scotoma with decreased visual acuity; field constriction (rare); pericentral or paracentral scotoma.

➤*Miscellaneous:* Weight loss; lassitude; exacerbation or precipitation of porphyria.

Overdosage

➤*Symptoms:* Toxic symptoms may occur within 30 minutes and consist of headache, drowsiness, visual disturbances, cardiovascular collapse, and convulsions, followed by sudden and early respiratory and cardiac arrest. Electrocardiogram may reveal atrial standstill, nodal rhythm, prolonged intraventricular conduction time, and progressive bradycardia leading to ventricular fibrillation and/or arrest. Rarely, these symptoms occur with lower doses in hypersensitive patients.

➤*Treatment:* Treatment is symptomatic and must be prompt, with immediate evacuation of the stomach by emesis or gastric lavage. Treatment includes usual supportive measures. Refer to General Management of Acute Overdosage. Activated charcoal, in a dose at least 5 times the estimated dose ingested, may inhibit further intestinal absorption if introduced by stomach tube after lavage within 30 minutes after ingestion. Control convulsions before attempting gastric lavage. If caused by cerebral stimulation, attempt cautious administration of an ultrashort-acting barbiturate; if caused by anoxia, correct with oxygen, artificial respiration, or, in shock with hypotension, use vasopressor therapy. Perform tracheal intubation or tracheostomy followed by gastric lavage if necessary. Exchange transfusions have been used to reduce the level of the drug in the blood. Closely observe, for at least 6 hours, patients surviving the acute phase who are asymptomatic. Fluids may be forced. Sufficient ammonium chloride (8 g daily in divided doses for adults) administered for a few days will acidify the urine and help promote urinary excretion.

Patient Information

May cause GI upset; instruct patients to take with food or milk.

Instruct patients to notify physician if any of the following occur: Blurring or other vision changes; ringing in the ears or hearing loss; fever; sore throat; unusual bleeding or bruising; unusual pigmentation (blue-black) of the skin; muscle weakness; bleaching or loss of hair; mood or mental changes.

Advise the patient to stop taking this medicine for RA if there is no improvement (reduced joint swelling, increased mobility) within 6 months.

If RA recurs after the medicine has been stopped, this medicine may be resumed or taken on a periodic basis if there are no existing vision problems.

This medicine may cause dizziness. Instruct patients to use caution while driving or performing other tasks requiring alertness, coordination, or physical dexterity.

Lab tests, including eye exams, may be required to monitor therapy. Instruct patients to be sure to keep appointments.

WARNING

Signs of gold toxicity include the following: Fall in hemoglobin, leukopenia < 4000 WBC/mm^3, granulocytes < 1500/mm^3, platelets < 100,000 to 150,000/mm^3, proteinuria, hematuria, pruritus, rash, stomatitis or persistent diarrhea. Review recommended laboratory work results before instituting therapy and before each injection or written prescription for oral gold. See patient before each injection to determine presence or absence of adverse reactions; some of these can be severe or even fatal. Physicians planning to use gold compounds should be experienced with chrysotherapy and thoroughly familiar with both toxicity and benefits of gold.

Explain the possibility of adverse reactions to patients before starting therapy.

Advise patients to report promptly any toxicity symptoms (see Patient Information).

Indications

➤*Rheumatoid arthritis:*

Parenteral – Active early rheumatoid arthritis, both adult and juvenile types (cases not adequately controlled by other anti-inflammatory agents or conservative measures). Use only as one part of therapy program; alone, it is not a complete treatment.

Oral – Management of adults with active classical or definite rheumatoid arthritis (ARA criteria) with insufficient therapeutic response to or intolerant of an adequate trial of full doses of one or more NSAIDs. Add **auranofin** to baseline program; include non-drug therapies.

➤*Unlabeled uses:* Alternative or adjuvant to corticosteroids in treatment of pemphigus. For psoriatic arthritis in patients who do not tolerate or respond to NSAIDs.

Actions

➤*Pharmacology:* Gold suppresses or prevents, but does not cure, arthritis and synovitis. It is taken up by macrophages, resulting in inhibition of phagocytosis and possibly, lysosomal enzyme activity. Gold decreases concentrations of rheumatoid factor and immunoglobulins. The exact mode of action in rheumatoid arthritis is unknown; however, gold compounds may decrease synovial inflammation and retard cartilage and bone destruction. No substantial evidence exists that gold induces remission of rheumatoid arthritis.

Therapeutic effects from gold compounds occur slowly. Early improvement, often limited to reduction in morning stiffness, may begin after 6 to 8 weeks of treatment with **gold sodium thiomalate**, but beneficial effects may not be observed until after months of therapy. Therapeutic effects from **auranofin** may be seen after 3 to 4 months of treatment, but in some patients, not before 6 months.

➤*Pharmacokinetics:* Due to differences in administration routes (IM vs oral), dosage regimens (weekly vs daily), and actual quantity of gold administered to the patient, expect differences in the pharmacokinetic parameters of injectable and oral gold.

Parenteral gold compounds are water soluble. **Aurothioglucose** is an oily suspension; suspension results in delayed IM absorption. Both are similar in biologic and pharmacokinetic behavior.

After initial injection, serum levels of gold rise sharply and decline over the next week. Peak levels of aqueous preparations are higher and decline faster than oily preparations. After a standard weekly dose, considerable individual variation in levels of gold has been found. Small amounts are found in the serum for months after discontinuation.

Although parenteral gold is widely distributed in body tissues, highest concentrations occur in the reticuloendothelial system and in adrenal and renal cortices. Binding of gold to red blood cells from injectable gold compounds is lower compared with **auranofin**-derived gold. Blood to synovial fluid ratios are similar, ≈ 1.7:1, and synovial fluid levels are ≈ 50% of the blood concentrations. No correlation between blood-gold concentrations and safety or efficacy has been established.

Major pharmacokinetic differences are summarized in the table below:

Pharmacokinetics of Auranofin and Injectable Gold Compounds

<table>
<tr><th>Drug</th><th>Gold content (%)</th><th>Absorbed (%)</th><th>Time to peak (h)</th><th>Mean steady-state plasma levels (mcg/mL)</th><th>Protein binding (%)</th><th>Plasma half-life (days)</th><th>Excreted in urine (%)</th><th>Excreted in feces (%)</th></tr>
<tr><td>Auranofin</td><td>29</td><td>25 (15-33)</td><td>1-2</td><td>0.2-1</td><td>60</td><td>26 (21-31)</td><td>60[a]</td><td>85-95</td></tr>
<tr><td>Aurothioglucose</td><td rowspan="2">50</td><td rowspan="2">nd</td><td>4-6</td><td rowspan="2">1-5</td><td rowspan="2">95-99</td><td>3-27 (single dose)
14-40 (3rd dose)</td><td rowspan="2">70</td><td rowspan="2">30</td></tr>
<tr><td>Gold sodium thiomalate</td><td>2-6</td><td>up to 168 (11th dose)</td></tr>
</table>

[a] 60% of the absorbed gold (15% of administered dose). nd – No data.

Contraindications

➤*Parenteral:* Hypersensitivity to any component; uncontrolled diabetes mellitus; severe debilitation; renal disease; hepatic dysfunction or history of infectious hepatitis; marked hypertension; uncontrolled CHF; systemic lupus erythematosus; agranulocytosis or hemorrhagic diathesis; blood dyscrasias; patients recently radiated; those with severe toxicity from previous exposure to gold or other heavy metals; urticaria; eczema; colitis; pregnancy (see Warnings).

➤*Oral:* A history of any of the following gold-induced disorders: Anaphylactic reactions, necrotizing enterocolitis, pulmonary fibrosis, exfoliative dermatitis, bone marrow aplasia or other severe hematologic disorders; pregnancy (see Warnings).

Warnings

➤*Active disease:* When cartilage and bone damage has already occurred, gold cannot reverse structural damage to joints caused by previous disease. The greatest potential benefit occurs in patients with active synovitis, particularly in its early stage.

➤*Thrombocytopenia:* Thrombocytopenia has occurred in 1% to 3% of patients treated with **auranofin**, some of whom developed bleeding. It appears peripheral in origin and is usually reversible upon withdrawal. Onset is not related to duration of therapy; its course may be rapid. Monitor platelet counts at least monthly; however, if a precipitous decline in platelets or a platelet count < 100,000/mm^3 occurs or if signs and symptoms of thrombocytopenia (eg, purpura, ecchymoses or petechiae) occur, immediately withdraw auranofin and other therapies; obtain additional platelet counts. Do not reinstate auranofin unless thrombocytopenia resolves and studies show that it was not due to gold therapy.

➤*Immediate effects:* Immediate effects following injection, or at any time during therapy include the following: anaphylactic shock, syncope, bradycardia, thickening of the tongue, difficulty swallowing or breathing, and angioneurotic edema. These effects may occur immediately after injection or as late as 10 minutes after injection. If such effects occur, discontinue treatment.

➤*Renal/Hepatic function impairment:* Weigh the potential benefits of using **auranofin** in patients with progressive renal disease or significant hepatocellular disease against potential risks of gold toxicity on compromised organ systems and the difficulty in quickly detecting and correctly attributing the toxic effect.

➤*Carcinogenesis:* Renal adenomas developed in rats receiving injectable gold at doses higher and more frequent than recommended human doses. Sarcomas at the injection site occurred in some rats.

Studies demonstrated a significant increase in the frequency of renal tubular cell karyomegaly and cytomegaly, renal adenoma, and malignant renal epithelial tumors in animals treated with **auranofin** and **gold sodium thiomalate**.

➤*Elderly:* Tolerance to gold usually decreases with advancing age.

➤*Pregnancy: Category C.* Gold crosses the placenta. The placenta showed gold deposits; smaller amounts were detected in fetal liver and kidneys.

Gold therapy is usually contraindicated in pregnant patients. Warn the patient about the hazards of becoming pregnant while on gold therapy. Rheumatoid arthritis frequently improves when a patient becomes pregnant. Do not superimpose the potential nephrotoxicity of gold on the increased renal burden which normally occurs in pregnancy. Discontinue therapy upon recognition of pregnancy, if possible. Consider slow excretion of gold and its persistence in body tissues after discontinuing treatment when a woman receiving gold plans to become pregnant.

Animals – **Gold sodium thiomalate** was teratogenic during the organogenic period in small animals when given in doses 140 to 175 times the usual human dose. **Auranofin** showed impaired food intake, decreased maternal and fetal weights, and increased resorptions, abortions, and congenital abnormalities, mainly abdominal defects (eg, gastroschisis, umbilical hernia).

There are no adequate, well controlled studies in pregnant women.Use only when benefits outweigh potential hazards to the fetus.

➤*Lactation:* Injectable gold is excreted in breast milk. Following **auranofin** administration, gold is excreted in the milk of rodents; human data are not available. Trace amounts appear in the serum and red blood cells of nursing offspring. This may cause rashes, nephritis, hepatitis and hematologic aberrations in nursing infants. Decide whether to discontinue nursing or to discontinue parenteral gold, taking into account the importance of the drug to the mother. Nursing during auranofin therapy is not recommended. Consider the slow excretion and persistence of gold in the mother even after therapy is discontinued.

➤*Children:* Safety and efficacy for use of **aurothioglucose** in children < 6 years of age have not been established.**Auranofin** is not recommended for use in children; safety and efficacy have not been established (however, see Administration and Dosage).

Precautions

➤*Monitoring:* Before instituting treatment, rule out pregnancy; perform CBC with differential, platelet, hemoglobin, WBC and erythrocyte counts, urinalysis and renal and liver function tests. Perform urinalysis for protein and sediment changes prior to each injection. Perform CBC, including platelet estimation, before every second injection (every 2 weeks) throughout treatment. Purpura or ecchymoses always require a platelet count. Inquire regarding pruritus, rash, sore mouth, metallic taste and indigestion before each injection. Observe patient at least 15 minutes after each injection. For patients on auranofin, monitor CBC with differential, platelet count and urinalysis at least monthly.

Rapid reduction of hemoglobin, granulocytes < 1500/mm^3, leukopenia < 4000 WBC/mm^3, eosinophilia > 5%, platelets < 100,000 to 150,000/mm^3, albuminuria, hematuria, rash, dermatitis, pruritus, skin eruption, stomatitis, persistent diarrhea, jaundice or petechiae are signs of possible gold toxicity. Do not give additional therapy unless further studies show these abnormalities to be caused by conditions other than gold toxicity. Monitor patients with GI symptoms for GI bleeding (**auranofin**).

➤*Proteinuria:*

Auranofin – Proteinuria has developed in 3% to 9% of auranofin patients. If clinically significant proteinuria or microscopic hematuria is found, immediately stop auranofin and other therapies with the potential to cause proteinuria or microscopic hematuria.

Aurothioglucose – Patients with HLA-D locus histocompatibility antigens DRw2 and DRw3 may have a genetic predisposition to develop certain toxic reactions, such as proteinuria, during treatment with gold or D-penicillamine. Use aurothioglucose with caution in patients with compromised cardiovascular or cerebral circulation.

➤*Concomitant antirheumatic therapy:* Use of salicylates, NSAIDs and systemic corticosteroids may be continued when parenteral gold therapy is instituted. After improvement begins, slowly discontinue analgesics and NSAIDs as symptoms permit. Do not use penicillamine with gold salts.

➤*Nonvasomotor postinjection reaction:* Arthralgia may occur for a day or two after injection; it usually subsides after the first few injections. The mechanism of the transient increase in rheumatic symptoms after gold injection is unknown. These reactions are usually mild, but occasionally may be so severe that treatment is stopped prematurely.

➤*Special risk:* Control diabetes mellitus or CHF before gold therapy begins.

Extreme caution is indicated in patients with any of the following: History of blood dyscrasias such as agranulocytopenia or anemia caused by drug sensitivity; allergy or hypersensitivity to medications; skin rash; previous kidney or liver disease; marked hypertension; compromised cerebral or cardiovascular circulation.

Weigh the potential benefits of using auranofin in patients with inflammatory bowel disease, skin rash or history of bone marrow depression against potential risks of gold toxicity on compromised organ systems and the difficulty in quickly detecting and correctly attributing the toxic effect.

Drug Interactions

➤*Phenytoin:* One report suggests coadministration with auranofin may increase phenytoin blood levels.

Adverse Reactions

Adverse reactions to gold therapy may occur during treatment or many months after discontinuation. Incidence of toxic reactions is apparently unrelated to gold plasma levels, but may relate to cumulative body content of gold. Higher than conventional dosages may increase occurrence and severity of toxicity. Adverse reactions are most frequent when cumulative dose is 400 to 800 mg (**gold sodium thiomalate**) or 300 to 500 mg (**aurothioglucose**). **Auranofin** appears to cause fewer adverse reactions than injectable gold; however, therapeutic efficacy may also be less.

Adverse Reactions of Oral vs Parenteral Gold (%)

Adverse reaction	Auranofin (oral gold) (n = 445)	Injectable gold (n = 445)
Diarrhea	42.5	13
Rash	26	39
Stomatitis	13	18
Anemia	3.1	2.7
Elevated liver function tests	1.9	1.7
Leukopenia	1.3	2.2
Proteinuria	0.9	5.4
Thrombocytopenia	0.9	2.2
Pulmonary	0.2	0.2

➤*Dermatologic:* Dermatitis is the most common reaction to **injectable gold** and second most common to **auranofin**. Any eruption, especially pruritic, is considered to be a reaction until proven otherwise. Rash, urticaria (auranofin, 1 to 3%) and angioedema (auranofin, < 0.1%) may occur. Pruritus (auranofin, 17%) often exists before dermatitis, and is a warning of reaction. Erythema, and occasionally more severe reactions, such as papular, vesicular and exfoliative dermatitis leading to alopecia and nail shedding, may occur. Chrysiasis (gray-to-blue pigmentation caused by gold deposits in tissues) has occurred, especially on photoexposed areas. Gold dermatitis may be aggravated by exposure to sunlight or an actinic rash may develop.

➤*Renal:* Gold may produce a nephrotic syndrome or glomerulitis with proteinuria and hematuria; these are usually relatively mild and subside completely if recognized early and treatment is discontinued. They may become severe and chronic if treatment continues after onset. Acute renal failure secondary to acute tubular necrosis, acute nephritis or degeneration of proximal tubular epithelium may occur; perform regular urinalysis and discontinue treatment immediately if proteinuria or hematuria develop. Hematuria (1% to 3%) and proteinuria (3% to 9%) occur with **auranofin**.

➤*Hematologic:*

Auranofin – Thrombocytopenia (with or without purpura), leukopenia, eosinophilia, anemia (1% to 3%); neutropenia (0.1% to 1%); agranulocytosis, pancytopenia, hypoplastic anemia, aplastic anemia, pure red cell aplasia (< 0.1%). Granulocytopenia; panmyelopathy; hemorrhagic diathesis. Constantly monitor patients throughout treatment for blood dyscrasias of the formed elements of the blood (see Warnings and Precautions). Though rare, these reactions have potentially serious consequences. These reactions may occur separately or in combination at any time during treatment.

➤*Hepatic:* Elevated liver enzymes (**auranofin** 1% to 3%), jaundice (auranofin < 0.1%) with or without cholestasis, hepatitis with jaundice, toxic hepatitis, intrahepatic cholestasis.

➤*GI:*

Auranofin – Diarrhea/loose stools (50%), generally manageable by reducing the dose (eg, from 6 to 3 mg/day), and only 6% need permanent drug discontinuation; abdominal pain (14%); nausea (10%); anorexia, flatulence, dyspepsia (3% to 9%); constipation, dysgeusia (1% to 3%); GI bleeding, melena, positive stool for occult blood (0.1% to 1%); ulcerative enterocolitis (can be severe or fatal), dysphagia (< 0.1%).

Aurothioglucose – Nausea, vomiting, anorexia, abdominal cramps, ulcerative enterocolitis (can be severe or fatal), colitis (rare).

➤*CNS:* Confusion; hallucinations; seizures.

➤*Miscellaneous:* Iritis, corneal ulcers and gold deposits in ocular tissues (**gold sodium thiomalate**; rare). These include deposits in the lens or cornea unassociated clinically with eye disorders or visual impairment (**auranofin** incidence < 0.1%). Acute yellow atrophy; encephalitis; immunological destruction of the synovia; EEG abnormalities; peripheral neuropathy (auranofin < 0.1%) with and without fasciculations or neuritis; partial or complete hair loss (auranofin 1% to 3%); fever; headache (aurothioglucose rare); sensorimotor effects (including Guillain-Barre syndrome) and elevated spinal fluid protein have occurred (gold sodium thiomalate rare).

Mucous membranes – Stomatitis, the second most common adverse reaction with **injectable gold,** is also seen with **auranofin** (13%). It may be manifested by shallow ulcers on buccal membranes, on borders of tongue and on palate or in pharynx and may be the only adverse reaction or occur with dermatitis. Diffuse glossitis or gingivitis may develop. Metallic taste may precede these reactions. Careful oral hygiene is important. Inflammation of upper respiratory tract, pharyngitis, gastritis, colitis, tracheitis, vaginitis and rarely, conjunctivitis (auranofin 3% to 9%) have been reported. Glossitis (auranofin 1% to 3%), gingivitis (auranofin 0.1% to 1%) and thickening of the tongue have occurred.

Pulmonary – Pulmonary injury may be shown by gold bronchitis, interstitial pneumonitis (**auranofin** < 0.1%) or fibrosis, fever and partial or complete hair loss.

Nitritoid and allergic (parenteral) – Reactions of the "nitritoid type" may resemble anaphylactoid effects. Flushing, fainting, dizziness and sweating are most frequent. Other symptoms may include nausea, vomiting, malaise, headache and weakness.

Management of adverse reactions – Discontinue immediately if toxic reactions occur. Minor complications (ie, localized dermatitis, mild stomatitis, slight proteinuria) generally require no other therapy and resolve spontaneously with therapy suspension. For mild reactions, it may be sufficient to briefly stop use and then resume with smaller doses. Moderately severe skin and mucous membrane reactions often benefit from topical corticosteroids, oral antihistamines and anesthetic lotions.

If stomatitis or dermatitis become severe or more generalized, systemic corticosteroids (generally, 10 to 40 mg prednisone daily in divided doses) may provide symptomatic relief.

For serious renal, hematologic, pulmonary and enterocolitic complications, use high doses of systemic corticosteroids (40 to 100 mg prednisone daily in divided doses). The duration of corticosteroid treatment varies. Larger doses and a longer treatment period may be required than for dermatologic reactions. Often this treatment may be required for many months because of the slow elimination of gold from the body. Therapy may also be required for months when adverse effects are unusually severe or progressive.

In high-dose gold patients whose serious adverse reactions do not improve with high-dose corticosteroids, or who develop significant steroid-related adverse reactions, a chelating agent may be given to enhance gold excretion (eg, dimercaprol, penicillamine). Monitor patients given dimercaprol carefully; untoward reactions may occur. Corticosteroids and a chelating agent may be coadministered. Adjunctive use of an anabolic steroid with other drugs (eg, dimercaprol, penicillamine, corticosteroids) may contribute to recovery of bone marrow deficiency.

Do not reinstitute after severe or idiosyncratic reactions: After resolution of mild reactions, reduced doses may be given. If test dose of 5 mg is well tolerated, give progressively larger doses (5 to 10 mg increments) at weekly to monthly intervals until 25 to 50 mg is reached.

Overdosage

➤*Symptoms:* Overdosage from too rapid increases in dosing are manifested by rapid appearance of toxic reactions, particularly renal damage (eg, hematuria, proteinuria), and hematologic effects (eg, thrombocytopenia, granulocytopenia). Other toxic effects include fever, nausea, vomiting, diarrhea and skin disorders (eg, papulovesicular lesions, urticaria and exfoliative dermatitis, all with severe pruritus).

Auranofin overdosage – Auranofin overdosage experience is limited. A 50-year-old female took 27 mg daily for 10 days and developed encephalopathy and peripheral neuropathy. Auranofin was discontinued, and she eventually recovered.

➤*Treatment:* Promptly discontinue; give dimercaprol. Use specific supportive therapy for renal/hematologic complications. Refer to General Management of Acute Overdosage. Chelating agents are used with injectable gold; consider their use also for **auranofin** overdosage. In acute overdosage, immediately induce emesis or perform gastric lavage with supportive therapy.

Patient Information

Patient package insert is available with **auranofin**.

Notify physician of the following: Itching, rash, sore mouth, indigestion, metallic taste, easy bruising or nosebleed.

Increased joint pain may continue 1 or 2 days after an injection and usually subsides after the first few injections.

Chrysiasis (gray-to-blue pigmentation) may occur, especially on photoexposed areas. Minimize exposure to sunlight or artificial ultraviolet light.

Observe careful oral hygiene in conjunction with therapy.

Warn women of childbearing potential of the risks of using gold therapy during pregnancy.

AURANOFIN (29% Gold)

Rx	**Ridaura** (SK-Beecham)	**Capsules:** 3 mg	(Ridaura SKF). Tan and brown. In 60s.

AURANOFIN — ORAL

For complete and comparative prescribing information, refer to the Gold Compounds group monograph.

WARNING

Auranofin contains gold and, like other gold-containing drugs, can cause gold toxicity, signs of which include: Fall in hemoglobin, leukopenia < 4000 WBC/mm^3, granulocytes < 1500/mm^3, decrease in platelets < 150,000/mm^3, proteinuria, hematuria, pruritus, rash, stomatitis or persistent diarrhea. Therefore, the results of recommended laboratory work (see Precautions) should be reviewed before writing each auranofin prescription. Like other gold preparations, auranofin is only indicated for use in selected patients with active rheumatoid arthritis. Physicians planning to use auranofin should be experienced with chrysotherapy and should throughly familiarize themselves with the toxicity and benefits of auranofin. In addition, the following precautions should be routinely employed: The possibility of adverse reactions should be explained to patients before starting therapy. Patients should be advised to report promptly any symptoms suggesting toxicity (see Precautions).

Indications

➤*Rheumatoid arthritis:* Auranofin is indicated in the management of adults with active classical or definite rheumatoid arthritis (ARA criteria) who have had an insufficient therapeutic response to, or are intolerant of, an adequate trial of full doses of one or more nonsteroidal anti-inflammatory drugs. Auranofin should be added to a comprehensive baseline program, including nondrug therapies.

Unlike anti-inflammatory drugs, auranofin does not produce an immediate response. Therapeutic effects may be seen after 3 to 4 months of treatment, although improvement has not been seen in some patients before 6 months.

When cartilage and bone damage have already occurred, gold cannot reverse structural damage to joints caused by previous disease. The greatest potential benefit occurs in patients with active synovitis, particularly in its early stage.

In controlled clinical trials comparing auranofin with injectable gold, auranofin was associated with fewer dropouts due to adverse reactions, while injectable gold was associated with fewer dropouts for inadequate or poor therapeutic effect. Physicians should consider these findings when deciding on the use of auranofin in patients who are candidates for chrysotherapy.

➤*Unlabeled uses:* Alternative or adjuvant to corticosteroids in treatment of pemphigus. For psoriatic arthritis in patients who do not tolerate or respond to NSAIDs.

Administration and Dosage

➤*Approved by the FDA:* May 24, 1985.

➤*Usual adult dosage:* The usual adult dosage of auranofin is 6 mg daily, given either as 3 mg twice daily or 6 mg once daily. Initiation of therapy at dosages exceeding 6 mg daily is not recommended because it is associated with an increased incidence of diarrhea. If response is inadequate after 6 months, an increase to 9 mg (3 mg 3 times daily) may be tolerated. If response remains inadequate after a 3 month trial of 9 mg daily, auranofin therapy should be discontinued. Safety at dosages exceeding 9 mg daily has not been studied.

➤*Transferring from injectable gold:* In controlled clinical studies, patients on injectable gold have been transferred to auranofin by discontinuing the injectable agent and starting oral therapy with auranofin, 6 mg daily. When patients are transferred to auranofin, they should be informed of its adverse reaction profile, in particular the GI reactions (see Precautions). At 6 months, control of disease activity of patients transferred to auranofin and those maintained on the injectable agent was not different. Data beyond 6 months are not available.

➤*Storage/Stability:* Store between 15° and 30°C (59° and 86°F). Dispense in a tight, light-resistant container.

AUROTHIOGLUCOSE (Approximately 50% Gold)

Rx	**Aurothioglucose** (Parenta)	**Injection Suspension:** 50 mg/ mL	In 10 mL multidose vials.[a]
Rx	**Solganal** (Schering)		In 10 mL vials.

[a] In sesame oil with 2% aluminum monostearate and 1 mg propylparaben.

AUROTHIOGLUCOSE — INJECTION

For complete and comparative prescribing information, refer to the Gold Compounds group monograph.

WARNING

Physicians planning to use aurothioglucose suspension should throughly familiarize themselves with its toxicity and its benefits. The possibility of toxic reactions should always be explained to the patient before starting therapy. Patients should be warned to report promptly any symptom suggesting toxicity. Before each injection of aurothioglucose suspension, the physician should review the results of laboratory work and see the patient to determine the presence or absence of adverse reactions, since some of these can be severe or even fatal. Signs of gold toxicity include the following: Fall in hemoglobin, leukopenia < 4000 WBC/mm^3, proteinuria, hematuria, pruritus, rash, stomatitis or persistent diarrhea.

Indications

➤*Rheumatoid arthritis:* Aurothioglucose injectable suspension is indicated for the adjunctive treatment of early active rheumatoid arthritis (both of the adult and juvenile types) not adequately controlled by other anti-inflammatory agents and conservative measures. In chronic, advanced cases of rheumatoid arthritis, gold therapy is less valuable.

Antirheumatic measures such as salicylates and other anti-inflammatory drugs (both steroidal and nonsteroidal) may be continued after initiation of gold therapy. After improvement commences, these measures may be discontinued slowly as symptoms permit. (See Precautions and Administration and Dosage.)

➤*Unlabeled uses:* Alternative or adjuvant to corticosteroids in treatment of pemphigus. For psoriatic arthritis in patients who do not tolerate or respond to NSAIDs.

Administration and Dosage

➤*Adults:* The usual dosage schedule for the intramuscular administration of aurothioglucose injectable suspension is as follows: First dose, 10 mg; second and third doses, 25 mg; fourth and subsequent doses, 50 mg. The interval between doses is 1 week. The 50 mg dose is continued at weekly intervals until 0.8 to 1.0 g aurothioglucose injectable suspension has been given. If the patient has improved and has exhibited no sign of toxicity, the 50 mg dose may be continued many months longer, at 3- to 4-week intervals. A weekly dose above 50 mg is usually unnecessary and contraindicated; the tendency in gold therapy is toward lower dosage. With this in mind, it may eventually be established that a 25 mg dose is the one of choice. If no improvement has been demonstrated after a total administration of 1.0 g of aurothioglucose injectable suspension, the necessity for gold therapy should be reevaluated.

➤*Children 6 to 12 Years:* One fourth of the adult dose, governed chiefly by body weight, not to exceed 25 mg per dose.

AUROTHIOGLUCOSE — INJECTION

Safety and effectiveness in children below the age of 6 years have not been established.

➤*Preparation and administration:* Aurothioglucose injectable suspension should be injected intramuscularly (preferably intragluteally), never intravenously. The patient should be lying down and should remain recumbent for approximately 10 minutes after the injection. The vial should be thoroughly shaken in order to suspend all of the active material. Heating the vial to body temperature (by immersion in warm water) will facilitate drawing the suspension into the syringe. An 18-gauge, 1½-inch needle is recommended for depositing the preparation deep into the muscular tissue. For obese patients, an 18-gauge, 2-inch needle may be used. The site usually selected for injection is the upper outer quadrant of the gluteal region.

Shake the vial in horizontal position before the dose is withdrawn. Needle and syringe must be dry. The patient should be observed for at least 15 minutes following each injection.

➤*Storage/Stability:* Shake well before using. Store between 0° and 30°C (32° and 86°F). Protect from light. Store in carton until contents are used.

GOLD SODIUM THIOMALATE (≈ 50% Gold)

Rx	**Gold Sodium Thiomalate** (Parenta)	**Injection:** 50 mg/ml[a]	In 2 ml and 1 ml fill in 2 ml single-dose vials and 10 ml multiple-dose vials.
Rx	**Aurolate** (Pasadena)		In 2 and 10 ml vials.
Rx	**Myochrysine** (Taylor)		In 2 and 10 ml vials.

[a] With 0.5% benzyl alcohol.

GOLD SODIUM THIOMALATE — INJECTION

For complete and comparative prescribing information, refer to the Gold Compounds group monograph.

WARNING

Physicians planning to use gold sodium thiomalate should thoroughly familiarize themselves with its toxicity and its benefits. The possibility of toxic reactions should always be explained to the patient before starting therapy. Patients should be warned to report promptly any symptoms suggesting toxicity. Before each injection of gold sodium thiomalate, the physician should review the results of laboratory work, and see the patient to determine the presence or absence of adverse reactions since some of these can be severe or even fatal.

Indications

➤*Rheumatoid arthritis:* Gold sodium thiomalate is indicated in the treatment of selected cases of active rheumatoid arthritis is both adult and juvenile type. The greatest benefit occurs in the early active stage. In late stages of the illness when cartilage and bone damage have occurred, gold can only check the progression of rheumatoid arthritis and prevent further structural damage to joints. It cannot repair damage caused by previously active disease.

Gold sodium thiomalate should be used only as one part of a complete program of therapy; alone it is not a complete treatment.

Administration and Dosage

Gold sodium thiomalate should be administered only by intramuscular injection, preferably intragluteally. It should be given with the patient lying down. He should remain recumbent for ≈ 10 minutes after the injection.

Therapeutic effects from gold sodium thiomalate occur slowly. Early improvement, often limited to a reduction in morning stiffness, may begin after 6 to 8 weeks of treatment, but beneficial effects may not be observed until after months of therapy.

➤*Adults:* For the adult of average size the following dosage schedule is suggested:

Weekly Injections
1st injection: 10 mg.
2nd injection: 25 mg.
3rd and subsequent injections, 25 to 50 mg until there is toxicity or major clinical improvement, or, in the absence of either of these, the cumulative dose of gold sodium thiomalate reaches 1 g.

➤*Duration of therapy:* Gold sodium thiomalate is continued until the cumulative dose reaches 1 g unless toxicity or major clinical improvement occurs. If significant clinical improvement occurs before a cumulative dose of 1 g has been administered, the dose may be decreased or the interval between injections increased as with maintenance therapy. Maintenance doses of 25 to 50 mg every other week for 2 to 20 weeks are recommended. If the clinical course remains stable, injections of 25 to 50 mg may be given every third and subsequently every fourth week indefinitely. Some patients may require maintenance treatment at intervals of 1 to 3 weeks. Should the arthritis exacerbate during maintenance therapy, weekly injections may be resumed temporarily until disease activity is suppressed.

➤*Treatment failure:* Should a patient fail to improve during initial therapy (cumulative dose of 1 g), several options are available.

1.) The patient may be considered to be unresponsive and gold sodium thiomalate is discontinued.
2.) The same dose (25 to 50 mg) of gold sodium thiomalate may be continued for ≈ 10 additional weeks.
3.) The dose of gold sodium thiomalate may be increased by increments of 10 mg every 1 to 4 weeks, not to exceed 100 mg in single injection.

If significant clinical improvement occurs using option 2 or 3, the maintenance schedule described above should be initiated. If there is no significant improvement or if toxicity occurs, therapy with gold sodium thiomalate should be stopped. The higher the individual dose of gold sodium thiomalate, the greater the risk of gold toxicity. Selection of one of these options for chrysotherapy should be based upon a number of factors, including the physician's experience with gold salt therapy, the course of the patient's condition, the choice of alternative treatments, and the availability of the patient for the close supervision required.

➤*Juvenile rheumatoid arthritis:* The pediatric dose of gold sodium thiomalate is proportional to the adult dose on a weight basis. After the initial test dose of 10 mg, the recommended dose for children is 1 mg/kg body weight, not to exceed 50 mg for a single injection. Otherwise, the guidelines given above for administration to adults also apply to children.

➤*Concomitant drug therapy:* Gold salts should not be used concomitantly with penicillamine.

The safety of coadministration with cytotoxic drugs has not been established. Other measures, such as salicylates, other nonsteroidal anti-inflammatory drugs, or systemic corticosteroids, may be continued when gold sodium thiomalate is initiated. After improvement commences, analgesic and anti-inflammatory drugs may be discontinued slowly as symptoms permit.

➤*Storage/Stability:* Protect from light.
Store container in carton until contents have been used.

METHOTREXATE (Amethopterin; MTX)

See the Methotrexate monograph in the Antineoplastic Agents chapter.

SULFASALAZINE

See the Sulfasalazine monograph in the GI chapter.

LEFLUNOMIDE

Rx	**Leflunomide** (Various, eg, Apotex, Barr, Sandoz, Teva)	**Tablets:** 10 mg	May contain lactose. In 30s, 100s, and 1,000s.
Rx	**Arava** (Hoechst Marion Roussel)		Lactose. (ZBN). White. Film coated. In 30s and 100s.
Rx	**Leflunomide** (Various, eg, Apotex, Barr, Sandoz, Teva)	**Tablets:** 20 mg	May contain lactose. In 30s, 100s, and 1,000s.
Rx	**Arava** (Hoechst Marion Roussel)		Lactose, yellow ferric oxide. (ZBO). Light yellow, triangular. Film coated. In 30s and 100s.
Rx	**Arava** (Hoechst Marion Roussel)	**Tablets:** 100 mg	Lactose. (ZBP). White. Film coated. In 3-count blister packs.

LEFLUNOMIDE — ORAL

WARNING

Pregnancy must be excluded before the start of treatment with leflunomide. Leflunomide is contraindicated in pregnant women, or women of childbearing potential who are not using reliable contraception. Leflunomide can cause fetal harm when administered to a pregnant woman. Pregnancy must be avoided during leflunomide treatment or prior to the completion of the drug elimination procedure after leflunomide treatment.

Indications

➤*Rheumatoid arthritis:* Leflunomide is indicated in adults for the treatment of active rheumatoid arthritis (RA) to reduce signs and symptoms, to inhibit structural damage as evidenced by x-ray erosions and joint-space narrowing, and to improve physical function.

Administration and Dosage

➤*Approved by the FDA:* September 10, 1998.

➤*Loading dose:* Due to the long half-life in patients with RA and recommended dosing interval (24 hours), a loading dose is needed to provide steady-state concentrations more rapidly. It is recommended that leflunomide therapy be initiated with a loading dose of one 100 mg tablet per day for 3 days. Elimination of the loading dose regimen may decrease the risk of adverse reactions. This could be especially important for patients at increased risk of hematologic or hepatic toxicity, such as those receiving concomitant treatment with methotrexate or other immunosuppressive agents, or on such medications in the recent past.

➤*Maintenance therapy:* Daily dosing of 20 mg is recommended for treatment of patients with rheumatoid arthritis. A small cohort of patients (n = 104) treated with 25 mg/day experienced a greater incidence of side effects: Alopecia, weight loss, liver enzyme elevations. Doses higher than 20 mg/day are not recommended. If dosing at 20 mg/day is not well tolerated clinically, the dose may be decreased to 10 mg daily. Liver enzymes should be monitored and dose adjustments may be necessary. Due to the prolonged half-life of the active metabolite of leflunomide, patients should be carefully observed after dose reduction since it may take several weeks for metabolite levels to decline.

➤*Hepatic function impairment:* Guidelines for dose adjustment or discontinuation based on the severity and persistence of ALT elevation are recommended as follows: For confirmed ALT elevations between 2- and 3-fold ULN, dose reduction to 10 mg/day may allow continued administration of leflunomide under close monitoring. If elevations between 2- and 3-fold ULN persist despite dose reduction or if ALT elevations of greater than 3-fold ULN are present, leflunomide should be discontinued and cholestyramine or charcoal should be administered with close monitoring, including retreatment with cholestyramine or charcoal as indicated.

In clinical trials, leflunomide treatment as monotherapy or in combination with methotrexate was associated with elevations of liver enzymes, primarily ALT and AST, in a significant number of patients; these effects were generally reversible. Most transaminase elevations were mild (less than or equal to 2-fold ULN) and usually resolved while continuing treatment. Marked elevations (greater than 3-fold ULN) occurred infrequently and reversed with dose reduction or discontinuation of treatment. The following table shows liver enzyme elevations seen with monthly monitoring in clinical trials US301 and MN301. It was notable that the absence of folate use in MN302 was associated with a considerably greater incidence of liver enzyme elevation on methotrexate.

➤*Storage/Stability:* Store at 25°C (77°F); excursions permitted to 15° to 30°C (59° to 86°F). Protect from light.

Actions

➤*Pharmacology:* Leflunomide is an isoxazole immunomodulatory agent which inhibits dihydroorotate dehydrogenase (an enzyme involved in de novo pyrimidine synthesis) and has antiproliferative activity. Several in vivo and in vitro experimental models have demonstrated an anti-inflammatory effect.

➤*Pharmacokinetics:*

Absorption – Following oral administration, leflunomide is metabolized to an active metabolite M1, which is responsible for essentially all of its activity in vivo. Plasma levels of leflunomide are occasionally seen at very low levels. Studies of the pharmacokinetics of leflunomide have primarily examined the plasma concentrations of this active metabolite.

Following oral administration, peak levels of the active metabolite, M1, occurred between 6 to 12 hours after dosing. Due to the very long half-life of M1 (approximately 2 weeks), a loading dose of 100 mg for 3 days was used in clinical studies to facilitate the rapid attainment of steady-state levels of M1. Without a loading dose, it is estimated that attainment of steady-state plasma concentrations would require nearly 2 months of dosing. The resulting plasma concentrations following both loading doses and continued clinical dosing indicate that M1 plasma levels are dose proportional.

Pharmacokinetic parameters for M1 after administration of leflunomide at doses of 5, 10, and 25 mg/day for 24 weeks to patients (n = 54) with rheumatoid arthritis (mean ± SD) (Study YU204)

Parameter	Maintenance (loading) dose		
	5 mg (50 mg)	10 mg (100 mg)	25 mg (100 mg)
C_{24} (day 1) (mcg/mL)[1]	4 ± 0.6	8.4 ± 2.1	8.5 ± 2.2
C_{24} (ss) (mcg/mL)[2]	8.8 ± 2.9	18 ± 9.6	63 ± 36
$t_{1/2}$ (days)	15 ± 3	14 ± 5	18 ± 9

[1] Concentration at 24 hours after loading dose.
[2] Concentration at 24 hours after maintenance doses at steady-state.

Relative to an oral solution, leflunomide tablets are 80% bioavailable. Coadministration of leflunomide tablets with a high-fat meal did not have a significant impact on M1 plasma levels.

Distribution – M1 has a low volume of distribution (Vss = 0.13 L/kg) and is extensively bound (greater than 99.3%) to albumin in healthy subjects. Protein binding has been shown to be linear at therapeutic concentrations. The free fraction of M1 is slightly higher in patients with rheumatoid arthritis and approximately doubled in patients with chronic renal failure; the mechanism and significance of these increases are unknown.

Metabolism – Leflunomide is metabolized to one primary (M1) and many minor metabolites. Of these minor metabolites, only 4-trifluoromethylaniline (TFMA) is quantifiable, occurring at low levels in the plasma of some patients. The parent compound is rarely detectable in plasma. At the present time, the specific site of leflunomide metabolism in man is unknown. In vivo and in vitro studies suggest a role for both the GI wall and the liver in drug metabolism. No specific enzyme has been identified as the primary route of metabolism for leflunomide; however, hepatic cytosolic and microsomal cellular fractions have been identified as sites of drug metabolism.

Excretion – The active metabolite M1 is eliminated by further metabolism and subsequent renal excretion as well as by direct biliary excretion. In a 28-day study of drug elimination (n = 3) using a single dose of radiolabeled compound, approximately 43% of the total radioactivity was eliminated in the urine and 48% was eliminated in the feces. Subsequent analysis of the samples revealed the primary urinary metabolites to be leflunomide glucuronides and an oxanilic acid derivative of M1. The primary fecal metabolite was M1. Of these 2 routes of elimination, renal elimination is more significant over the first 96 hours, after which fecal elimination begins to predominate. In a study involving the intravenous administration of M1, the clearance was estimated to be 31 mL/hr.

In small studies using activated charcoal (n = 1) or cholestyramine (n = 3) to facilitate drug elimination, the in vivo plasma half-life of M1 was reduced from greater than 1 week to approximately 1 day. The active metabolite of leflunomide is eliminated slowly from the plasma. In instances of any serious toxicity from leflunomide, including hypersensitivity, use of a drug elimination procedure is highly recommended to reduce the drug concentration more rapidly after stopping leflunomide therapy. Similar reductions in plasma half-life were observed for a series of volunteers (n = 96) enrolled in pharmacokinetic trials who were given cholestyramine. This suggests that biliary recycling is a major contributor to the long elimination half-life of M1. Studies with both hemodialysis and CAPD (chronic ambulatory peritoneal dialysis) indicate that M1 is not dialyzable.

Special populations –

Renal function impairment: In single dose studies in patients (n = 6) with chronic renal insufficiency requiring either chronic ambulatory peritoneal dialysis (CAPD) or hemodialysis, neither had a significant impact on circulating levels of M1. The free fraction of M1 was almost doubled, but the mechanism of this increase is not known. In light of the fact that the kidney plays a role in drug elimination, and without adequate studies of lefluno-

LEFLUNOMIDE — ORAL

mide use in subjects with renal insufficiency, caution should be used when leflunomide is administered to these patients.

Hepatic function impairment: Studies of the effect of hepatic insufficiency on M1 pharmacokinetics have not been done. Given the need to metabolize leflunomide into the active species, the role of the liver in drug elimination/recycling, and the possible risk of increased hepatic toxicity, the use of leflunomide in patients with hepatic insufficiency is not recommended.

Contraindications

Hypersensitivity to leflunomide or any of the other components of the medication.

Leflunomide is contraindicated in women who are or may become pregnant. If this drug is used during pregnancy, or if the patient becomes pregnant while taking this drug, the patient should be apprised of the potential hazard to the fetus.

Warnings

➤*Immunosuppression potential / bone marrow suppression:* Leflunomide is not recommended for patients with severe immunodeficiency, bone marrow dysplasia, or severe, uncontrolled infections. In the event that a serious infection occurs, it may be necessary to interrupt therapy with leflunomide and administer cholestyramine or charcoal. Medications like leflunomide that have immunosuppression potential may cause patients to be more susceptible to infections, including opportunistic infections. Rarely, severe infections including sepsis, which may be fatal, have been reported in patients receiving leflunomide. Most of the reports were confounded by concomitant immunosuppressant therapy or comorbid illness which, in addition to rheumatoid disease, may predispose patients to infection.

There have been rare reports of pancytopenia, agranulocytosis, and thrombocytopenia in patients receiving leflunomide alone. These events have been reported most frequently in patients who received concomitant treatment with methotrexate or other immunosuppressive agents, or who had recently discontinued these therapies; in some cases, patients had a history of a significant hematologic abnormality.

See Precautions for more information.

If evidence of bone marrow suppression occurs in a patient taking leflunomide, treatment with leflunomide should be stopped, and cholestyramine or charcoal should be used to reduce the plasma concentration of leflunomide active metabolite.

In any situation in which the decision is made to switch from leflunomide to another antirheumatic agent with a known potential for hematologic suppression, it would be prudent to monitor for hematologic toxicity, because there will be overlap of systemic exposure to both compounds. Leflunomide washout with cholestyramine or charcoal may decrease this risk, but also may induce disease worsening if the patient had been responding to leflunomide treatment.

➤*Hepatotoxicity:* Rare cases of severe liver injury, including cases with fatal outcome, have been reported during treatment with leflunomide. Most cases of severe liver injury occur within 6 months of therapy in a setting of multiple risk factors for hepatotoxicity (liver disease, other hepatotoxins).

See Precautions for more information.

Liver enzyme elevations > 3-fold upper limits of normal (ULN)								
	US301			MN301			MN302*	
	LEF	PL	MTX	LEF	PL	SSZ	LEF	MTX
ALT								
> 3-fold ULN	8	3	5	2	1	2	13	83
(n %)	(4.4%)	(2.5%)	(2.7%)	(1.5%)	(1.1%)	(1.5%)	(2.6%)	(16.7%)
Reversed to ≤ 2-fold ULN	8	3	5	2	1	2	12	82
Timing of elevation								
0 to 3 months	6	1	1	2	1	2	7	27
4 to 6 months	1	1	3	–	–	–	1	34
7 to 9 months	1	1	1	–	–	–	–	16
10 to 12 months	–	–	–	–	–	–	5	6

* Only 10% of patients in MN302 received folate. All patients in US301 received folate.

In a 6-month study of 263 patients with persistent active rheumatoid arthritis despite methotrexate therapy, and with normal LFTs, leflunomide was added to a group of 133 patients starting at 10 mg per day and increased to 20 mg as needed. An increase in ALT greater than or equal to 3 times the ULN was observed in 3.8% of patients compared to 0.8% in 130 patients continued on methotrexate with placebo added.

➤*Malignancy:* The risk of malignancy, particularly lymphoproliferative disorders, is increased with the use of some immunosuppression medications. There is a potential for immunosuppression with leflunomide. No apparent increase in the incidence of malignancies and lymphoproliferative disorders was reported in the clinical trials of leflunomide, but larger and longer-term studies would be needed to determine whether there is an increased risk of malignancy or lymphoproliferative disorders with leflunomide.

➤*Drug elimination procedure:* The following drug elimination procedure is recommended to achieve nondetectable plasma levels less than 0.02 mg/L (0.02 mcg/mL) after stopping treatment with leflunomide:

1.) Administer cholestyramine 8 g 3 times daily for 11 days. (The 11 days do not need to be consecutive unless there is a need to lower the plasma level rapidly.)
2.) Verify plasma levels less than 0.02 mg/L (0.02 mcg/mL) by 2 separate tests at least 14 days apart. If plasma levels are higher than 0.02 mg/L, additional cholestyramine treatment should be considered.

Without the drug elimination procedure, it may take up to 2 years to reach plasma M1 metabolite levels less than 0.02 mg/L due to individual variation in drug clearance.

➤*Hypersensitivity reactions:* Rare cases of Stevens-Johnson syndrome and toxic epidermal necrolysis have been reported in patients receiving leflunomide. If a patient taking leflunomide develops any of these conditions, leflunomide therapy should be stopped, and a drug elimination procedure is recommended.

➤*Renal function impairment:* See Actions for more information.

➤*Hepatic function impairment:* See Actions for more information.

➤*Carcinogenesis:* Male mice in a 2-year bioassay exhibited an increased incidence in lymphoma at an oral dose of 15 mg/kg, the highest dose studied (1.7 times the human M1 exposure based on AUC). Female mice in the same study exhibited a dose-related increased incidence of bronchoalveolar adenomas and carcinomas combined beginning at 1.5 mg/kg (approximately 1/10 the human M1 exposure based on AUC). The significance of the findings in mice relative to the clinical use of leflunomide is not known.

➤*Mutagenesis:* 4-trifluoromethylaniline (TFMA), a minor metabolite of leflunomide, was mutagenic in the Ames assay and in the HGPRT gene mutation assay and was clastogenic in the in vitro assay for chromosome aberrations in the Chinese hamster cells. TFMA was not clastogenic in the in vivo mouse micronucleus assay nor in the in vivo cytogenetic test in Chinese hamster bone marrow cells.

➤*Pregnancy:* Category X.

See the Warning box for more information.

Use in women of childbearing potential – There are no adequate and well-controlled studies evaluating leflunomide in pregnant women. However, based on animal studies, leflunomide may increase the risk of fetal death or teratogenic effects when administered to a pregnant woman. Women of childbearing potential must not be started on leflunomide until pregnancy is excluded and it has been confirmed that they are using reliable contraception. Before starting treatment with leflunomide, patients must be fully counseled on the potential for serious risk to the fetus.

The patient must be advised that if there is any delay in onset of menses or any other reason to suspect pregnancy, they must notify the physician immediately for pregnancy testing, and if positive, the physician and patient must discuss the risk to the pregnancy. It is possible that rapidly lowering the blood level of the active metabolite, by instituting the drug elimination procedure described below, at the first delay of menses may decrease the risk to the fetus from leflunomide.

Upon discontinuing leflunomide, it is recommended that all women of childbearing potential undergo the drug elimination procedure described above. Women receiving leflunomide treatment who wish to become pregnant must discontinue leflunomide and undergo the drug elimination procedure described above, which includes verification of M1 metabolite plasma levels less than 0.02 mg/L (0.02 mcg/mL). Human plasma levels of the active metabolite (M1) less than 0.02 mg/L (0.02 mcg/mL) are expected to have minimal risk based on available animal data.

Use in males – Available information does not suggest that leflunomide would be associated with an increased risk of male-mediated fetal toxicity. However, animal studies to evaluate this specific risk have not been conducted. To minimize any possible risk, men wishing to father a child should consider discontinuing use of leflunomide and taking cholestyramine 8 g 3 times daily for 11 days.

Leflunomide, when administered orally to rats during organogenesis at a dose of 15 mg/kg, was teratogenic (most notably anophthalmia or microophthalmia and internal hydrocephalus). The systemic exposure of rats at this dose was approximately 1/10 the human exposure level based on AUC. Under these exposure conditions, leflunomide also caused a decrease in the maternal body weight and an increase in embryolethality with a decrease in fetal body weight for surviving fetuses. In rabbits, oral treatment with 10 mg/kg of leflunomide during organogenesis resulted in fused, dysplastic sternebrae. The exposure level at this dose was essentially equivalent to the maximum human exposure level based on AUC. At a 1 mg/kg dose, leflunomide was not teratogenic in rats and rabbits.

When female rats were treated with 1.25 mg/kg of leflunomide beginning 14 days before mating and continuing until the end of lactation, the offspring exhibited marked (greater than 90%) decreases in postnatal survival. The systemic exposure level at 1.25 mg/kg was approximately 1/100 the human exposure level based on AUC.

➤*Lactation:* Leflunomide should not be used by nursing mothers. It is not known whether leflunomide is excreted in human milk. Many drugs are excreted in human milk, and there is a potential for serious adverse reactions in nursing infants from leflunomide. Therefore, a decision should be made whether to proceed with nursing or to initiate treatment with leflunomide, taking into account the importance of the drug to the mother.

➤*Children:* The safety and efficacy of leflunomide in the pediatric population have not been studied. Use of leflunomide in patients less than 18 years of age is not recommended.

Precautions

➤*Monitoring:*

Hematologic monitoring – At minimum, patients taking leflunomide should have platelet, white blood cell count, and hemoglobin or hemacrit monitored at baseline and monthly for 6 months following initiation of therapy and every 6 to 8 weeks thereafter.

Bone marrow suppression monitoring – If used concomitantly with immunosuppressants such as methotrexate, chronic monitoring should be monthly.

Liver enzyme monitoring – ALT must be performed at baseline and monitored at monthly intervals during the first 6 months, then, if stable, every 6 to 8 weeks thereafter. In addition, if leflunomide and methotrexate are given concomitantly, ACR guidelines for monitoring methotrexate liver toxicity must be followed with ALT, AST, and serum albumin testing every month.

➤*Renal effects:* Due to a specific effect on the brush border of the renal proximal tubule, leflunomide has a uricosuric effect. A separate effect of hypophosphaturia is seen in some patients. These effects have not been seen together, nor have there been alterations in renal function.

➤*Need for drug elimination:* The active metabolite of leflunomide is eliminated slowly from the plasma. In instances of any serious toxicity from leflunomide, including hypersensitivity, use of a drug elimination procedure is highly recommended to reduce the drug concentration more rapidly after stopping leflunomide therapy. If hypersensitivity is the suspected clinical mechanism, more prolonged cholestyramine or charcoal administration may be necessary to achieve rapid and sufficient clearance. The duration may be modified based on the clinical status of the patient.

See Warnings for more information.

➤*Vaccinations:* No clinical data are available on the efficacy and safety of vaccinations during leflunomide treatment. Vaccination with live vaccines is, however, not recommended. The long half-life of leflunomide should be considered when contemplating administration of a live vaccine after stopping leflunomide.

Drug Interactions

➤*Warfarin:* Increased INR (International Normalized Ratio) when leflunomide and warfarin were coadministered has been rarely reported.

Leflunomide Drug Interactions

Precipitant drug	Object drug*		Description
Cholestyramine Charcoal	Leflunomide	⬇	Coadministration resulted in a rapid and significant decrease in the active metabolite of leflunomide.
Rifampin	Leflunomide	⬆	Following concomitant administration of a single dose of leflunomide to subjects receiving multiple doses of rifampin, M1 peak levels were increased (40%).
Leflunomide	Hepatotoxic drugs	⬆	Increased side effects may occur when leflunomide is given concomitantly with hepatotoxic substances. This is also to be considered when leflunomide treatment is followed by such drugs without a drug elimination procedure. Concomitant use of leflunomide with methotrexate resulted in a 2- to 3-fold elevation in liver enzymes in 5 of 30 patients. All elevations resolved, 2 with continuation of both drugs and 3 after discontinuation of leflunomide. A > 3-fold increase was seen in another 5 patients. All of these also resolved, 2 with continuation of both drugs and 3 after discontinuation of leflunomide. Three patients met "ACR criteria" for liver biopsy.
Leflunomide	NSAIDs	⬆	In vitro, M1 caused an increase (13% to 50%) in the free fraction of diclofenac and ibuprofen. In vitro studies indicate that M1 inhibits cytochrome P450 2C9, which is responsible for the metabolism of many NSAIDs. The clinical significance of this finding is unknown.
Leflunomide	Tolbutamide	⬌	In vitro, M1 caused increases (13% to 50%) in the free fraction of tolbutamide at concentrations in the clinical range. The clinical significance of this finding is unknown.

* ⬆ = Object drug increased. ⬇ = Object drug decreased.
⬌ = Undetermined clinical effect.

Adverse Reactions

Adverse reactions associated with the use of leflunomide in RA include diarrhea, elevated liver enzymes (ALT and AST), alopecia, and rash. In the controlled studies, the following adverse reactions were reported, regardless of causality.

Percentage of patients with adverse reactions greater than or equal to 3% in any leflunomide-treated group

	All RA studies	Placebo-controlled trials				Active-controlled trials	
		MN301 and US301				MN302*	
Adverse reaction	LEF (n = 1339)[1]	LEF (n = 315)	PBO (n = 210)	SSZ (n = 133)	MTX (n = 182)	LEF (n = 501)	MTX (n = 498)
Miscellaneous							
Allergic reaction	2%	5%	2%	0%	6%	1%	2%
Asthenia	3%	6%	4%	5%	6%	3%	3%
Flu syndrome	2%	4%	2%	0%	7%	0%	0%
Infection, upper respiratory	4%	0%	0%	0%	0%	0%	0%
Injury accident	5%	7%	5%	3%	11%	6%	7%
Pain	2%	4%	2%	2%	5%	1%	< 1%
Abdominal pain	6%	5%	4%	4%	8%	6%	4%
Back pain	5%	6%	3%	4%	9%	8%	7%
Cardiovascular							
Hypertension[2]	10%	9%	4%	4%	3%	10%	4%
New onset of hypertension		1%	< 1%	0%	2%	2%	< 1%
Chest pain	2%	4%	2%	2%	4%	1%	2%
GI							
Anorexia	3%	3%	2%	5%	2%	3%	3%
Diarrhea	17%	27%	12%	10%	20%	22%	10%
Dyspepsia	5%	10%	10%	9%	13%	6%	7%
Gastroenteritis	3%	1%	1%	0%	6%	3%	3%
Abnormal liver enzymes	5%	10%	2%	4%	10%	6%	17%
Nausea	9%	13%	11%	19%	18%	13%	18%
GI/abdominal pain	5%	6%	4%	7%	8%	8%	8%
Mouth ulcer	3%	5%	4%	3%	10%	3%	6%
Vomiting	3%	5%	4%	4%	3%	3%	3%
Metabolic/Nutritional							
Hypokalemia	1%	3%	1%	1%	1%	1%	< 1%
Weight loss[3]	4%	2%	1%	2%	0%	2%	2%
Musculoskeletal							
Arthralgia	1%	4%	3%	0%	9%	< 1%	1%
Leg cramps	1%	4%	2%	2%	6%	0%	0%
Joint disorder	4%	2%	2%	2%	2%	8%	6%
Synovitis	2%	< 1%	1%	0%	2%	4%	2%
Tenosynovitis	3%	2%	0%	1%	2%	5%	1%
CNS							
Dizziness	4%	5%	3%	6%	5%	7%	6%
Headache	7%	13%	11%	12%	21%	10%	8%
Paresthesia	2%	3%	1%	1%	2%	4%	3%
Respiratory							
Bronchitis	7%	5%	2%	4%	7%	8%	7%
Increased cough	3%	4%	5%	3%	6%	5%	7%
Respiratory infection	15%	21%	21%	20%	32%	27%	25%
Pharyngitis	3%	2%	1%	2%	1%	3%	3%
Pneumonia	2%	3%	0%	0%	1%	2%	2%
Rhinitis	2%	5%	2%	4%	3%	2%	2%
Sinusitis	2%	5%	5%	0%	10%	1%	1%
Dermatologic							
Alopecia	10%	9%	1%	6%	6%	17%	10%
Eczema	2%	1%	1%	1%	1%	3%	2%
Pruritus	4%	5%	2%	3%	2%	6%	2%
Rash	10%	12%	7%	11%	9%	11%	10%
Dry skin	2%	3%	2%	2%	0%	3%	1%
GU							
Urinary tract infection	5%	5%	7%	4%	2%	5%	6%

* Only 10% of patients in MN302 received folate. All patients in US301 received folate; none in MN301.

[1] Includes all controlled and uncontrolled trials with leflunomide.

[2] Hypertension as a preexisting condition was overrepresented in all leflunomide treatment groups in phase III trials. Analysis of new onset of hypertension revealed no difference among the treatment groups.

[3] In a meta-analysis of all phase II and III studies, during the first 6 months in patients receiving leflunomide, 10% lost 10 to 19 lbs (24 cases per 100 patient years) and 2% lost at least 20 lbs (4 cases/100 patient years). Of patients receiving leflunomide, 4% lost 10% of their baseline weight during the first 6 months of treatment.

LEFLUNOMIDE — ORAL

In addition, the following adverse reactions have been reported in 1% to less than 3% of the RA patients in the leflunomide treatment group in controlled clinical trials.

➤*Cardiovascular:* Angina pectoris, migraine, palpitation, tachycardia, vasculitis, vasodilation, varicose vein.

➤*CNS:* Anxiety, depression, dry mouth, insomnia, neuralgia, neuritis, sleep disorder, sweat, vertigo.

➤*Dermatologic:* Acne, contact dermatitis, fungal dermatitis, hair discoloration, hematoma, herpes simplex, herpes zoster, nail disorder, skin nodule, subcutaneous nodule, maculopapular rash, skin disorder, skin discoloration, ulcer skin.

➤*Endocrine:* Diabetes mellitus, hyperthyroidism.

➤*GI:* Cholelithiasis, colitis, constipation, esophagitis, flatulence, gastritis, gingivitis, melena, oral moniliasis, pharyngitis, salivary gland enlarged, stomatitis (or aphthous stomatitis), tooth disorder.

➤*GU:* Albuminuria, cystitis, dysuria, hematuria, menstrual disorder, vaginal moniliasis, prostate disorder, urinary frequency, vaginal moniliasis.

➤*Hematologic:* Anemia (including iron deficiency anemia), ecchymosis.

➤*Metabolic/Nutritional:* Creatine phosphokinase increased, peripheral edema, hyperglycemia, hyperlipidemia.

➤*Musculoskeletal:* Arthrosis, bursitis, muscle cramps, myalgia, bone necrosis, bone pain, tendon rupture.

➤*Respiratory:* Asthma, dyspnea, epistaxis, lung disorder.

➤*Special senses:* Blurred vision, cataract, conjunctivitis, eye disorder, taste perversion.

➤*Miscellaneous:* Abscess, cyst, fever, hernia, malaise, pain, neck pain, pelvic pain.

Other less common adverse events seen in clinical trials include: 1 case of anaphylactic reaction occurred in Phase 2 following rechallenge of drug after withdrawal due to rash (rare); urticaria; eosinophilia; transient thrombocytopenia (rare); and leukopenia less than 2000 WBC/mm^3 (rare).

➤*Adverse reactions during second year of treatment:* Adverse reactions during a second year of treatment with leflunomide in clinical trials were consistent with those observed during the first year of treatment and occurred at a similar or lower incidence.

CNS – Peripheral neuropathy.

Dermatologic – Erythema multiforme, Stevens-Johnson syndrome, toxic epidermal necrolysis.

GI – Pancreatitis.

Hematologic – Agranulocytosis, leukopenia, neutropenia, pancytopenia, thrombocytopenia.

Hepatic – Hepatitis, jaundice/cholestasis, severe liver injury such as hepatic failure and acute hepatic necrosis that may be fatal.

Hypersensitivity – Angioedema.

Respiratory – Interstitial lung disease.

Miscellaneous – Opportunistic infections, severe infections including sepsis that may be fatal.

Overdosage

➤*Symptoms:* There have been reports of chronic overdose in patients taking leflunomide at daily doses up to 5 times the recommended daily dose and reports of acute overdose in adults and children. There were no adverse reactions reported in the majority of case reports of overdose. Adverse reactions were consistent with the safety profile for leflunomide. The most frequent adverse reactions observed were diarrhea, abdominal pain, leukopenia, anemia, and elevated liver function tests.

➤*Treatment:* In the event of a significant overdose or toxicity, cholestyramine or charcoal administration is recommended to accelerate elimination. The active metabolite of leflunomide is eliminated slowly from the plasma. In instances of any serious toxicity from leflunomide, including hypersensitivity, use of a drug elimination procedure is highly recommended to reduce the drug concentration more rapidly after stopping leflunomide therapy. If hypersensitivity is the suspected clinical mechanism, more prolonged cholestyramine or charcoal administration may be necessary to achieve rapid and sufficient clearance. The duration may be modified based on the clinical status of the patient. Studies with both hemodialysis and CAPD (chronic ambulatory peritoneal dialysis) indicate that M1, the primary metabolite of leflunomide, is not dialyzable).

Patient Information

The potential for increased risk of birth defects should be discussed with female patients of childbearing potential. It is recommended that physicians advise women that they may be at increased risk of having a child with birth defects if they are pregnant when taking leflunomide, become pregnant while taking leflunomide, or do not wait to become pregnant until they have stopped taking leflunomide and followed the drug elimination procedure.

Patients should be advised of the possibility of rare, serious skin reactions. Patients should be instructed to inform their physicians promptly if they develop a skin rash or mucous membrane lesions.

Patients should be advised of the potential hepatotoxic effects of leflunomide and of the need for monitoring liver enzymes.

Patients should be instructed to notify their physicians if they develop symptoms such as unusual tiredness, abdominal pain, or jaundice.

Patients should be advised that they may develop a lowering of their blood counts and should have frequent hematologic monitoring. This is particularly important for patients who are receiving other immunosuppressive therapy concurrently with leflunomide, who have recently discontinued such therapy before starting treatment with leflunomide, or who have had a history of significant hematologic abnormality. Patients should be instructed to notify their physicians promptly if they notice symptoms of pancytopenia (eg, easy bruising or bleeding, recurrent infections, fever, paleness, unusual tiredness).

KERATINOCYTE GROWTH FACTORS

PALIFERMIN

Rx	**Kepivance** (Amgen)	**Powder for injection:** 6.25 mg	Sucrose. Preservative-free. Single-use vials.

PALIFERMIN — INJECTION

Indications

➤*Oral mucositis:* Palifermin is indicated to decrease the incidence and duration of severe oral mucositis in patients with hematologic malignancies who are receiving myelotoxic therapy requiring hematopoietic stem cell support.

Administration and Dosage

➤*Approved by the FDA:* December 15, 2004.

➤*Recommended dose:* The recommended dosage of palifermin is 60 mcg/kg/day, administered as an intravenous (IV) bolus injection for 3 consecutive days before and 3 consecutive days after myelotoxic therapy, for a total of 6 doses.

➤*Premyelotoxic therapy:* Administer the first 3 doses prior to myelotoxic therapy, with the third dose 24 to 48 hours before myelotoxic therapy.

➤*Postmyelotoxic therapy:* Administer the last 3 doses following myelotoxic therapy; administer the first of these doses after, but on the same day of, hematopoietic stem cell infusion and at least 4 days after the most recent administration of palifermin.

➤*Preparation for administration:* Do not use palifermin beyond the date stamped on the vial label.

Reconstitute palifermin lyophilized powder only with sterile water for injection (not supplied). Aseptically reconstitute palifermin by slowly injecting sterile water for injection 1.2 mL (not supplied) to yield a final concentration of 5 mg/mL. Gently swirl the contents during dissolution. Do not shake or vigorously agitate the vial.

Generally, dissolution of palifermin takes less than 3 minutes.

Do not filter the reconstituted solution during preparation or administration.

➤*Administration:* Administer palifermin by IV bolus injection. If heparin is used to maintain an IV line, use saline to rinse the line prior to and after palifermin administration because palifermin has been shown to bind to heparin in vitro.

➤*Storage/Stability:* Store the dispensing pack containing palifermin lyophilized powder in its carton and refrigerate at 2° to 8°C (36° to 46°F). Protect from light. Keep vials in pack until time of use.

The reconstituted solution contains no preservatives and is intended for single use only. Following reconstitution, it is recommended that the product be used immediately. If not used immediately, the reconstituted solution of palifermin may be stored refrigerated in its carton at 2° to 8°C (36° to 46°F) for up to 24 hours. Prior to injection, palifermin may be allowed to reach room temperature for a maximum of 1 hour, but it should be protected from light. Discard palifermin left at room temperature for more than 1 hour. Do not freeze the reconstituted solution.

Actions

➤*Pharmacology:* KGF is an endogenous protein in the fibroblast growth factor (FGF) family that binds to the KGF receptor. Binding of KGF to its receptor has been reported to result in proliferation, differentiation, and migration of epithelial cells. The KGF receptor, 1 of 4 receptors in the FGF family, has been reported to be present on epithelial cells in many tissues examined, including the tongue, buccal mucosa, esophagus, stomach, intestine, salivary gland, lung, liver, pancreas, kidney, bladder, mammary gland, skin (hair follicles and sebaceous gland), and the lens of the eye. The KGF receptor has been reported to not be present on cells of the hematopoietic lineage. Endogenous KGF is produced by mesenchymal cells and is upregulated in response to epithelial tissue injury.

Palifermin has been shown to enhance the growth of human epithelial tumor cell lines in vitro at concentrations at least 10 mcg/mL (more than 15-fold higher than average therapeutic concentrations in humans). In nude mouse xenograft models, 3 consecutive daily treatments of palifermin at doses of 1,500 and 4,000 mcg/kg (25- and 67-fold higher than the recommended human dose, respectively) repeated weekly for 4 to 6 weeks were associated with a dose-dependent increase in the growth rate of 1 of 7 KGF receptor-expressing human tumor cell lines.

PALIFERMIN — INJECTION

➤*Pharmacokinetics:*

Absorption/Distribution – The pharmacokinetics of palifermin were studied in healthy subjects and patients with hematologic malignancies. After single IV doses of 20 to 250 mcg/kg (healthy subjects) and 60 mcg/kg (cancer patients), palifermin concentrations declined rapidly (over 95% decrease) in the first 30 minutes postdose. A slight increase or plateau in concentration occurred at approximately 1 to 4 hours, followed by a terminal decline phase. Palifermin exhibited linear pharmacokinetics with extravascular distribution.

Metabolism/Excretion – On average, total body clearance appeared to be 2- to 4-fold higher and volume of distribution at steady state to be 2-fold higher in cancer patients compared with healthy subjects after a 60 mcg/kg single dose of palifermin. The elimination half-life was similar between healthy subjects and cancer patients (average, 4.5 hours; range, 3.3 to 5.7 hours). No accumulation of palifermin occurred after 3 consecutive daily doses of 20 and 40 mcg/kg in healthy volunteers or 60 mcg/kg in cancer patients.

Pharmacodynamics – Epithelial cell proliferation was assessed by Ki67 immunohistochemical staining in healthy subjects. A 3-fold or greater increase in Ki67 staining was observed in buccal biopsies from 3 of 6 healthy subjects given palifermin at 40 mcg/kg/day IV for 3 days, when measured 24 hours after the third dose. Dose-dependent epithelial cell proliferation was observed in healthy subjects given single IV doses of 120 to 250 mcg/kg 48 hours post-dosing.

Contraindications

Hypersensitivity to *E. coli*-derived proteins, palifermin, or any other component of the product.

Warnings

➤*Fertility impairment:* When palifermin was administered IV daily to male and female rats prior to and during mating, reproductive performance, fertility, and sperm assessment parameters were not affected at dosages up to 100 mcg/kg/day. Systemic toxicity (clinical signs of toxicity and/or body weight effects), decreased epididymal sperm counts, and increased postimplantation loss were observed at dosages 300 mcg/kg/day or higher (5-fold higher than the recommended human dosage). Increased preimplantation loss and a decreased fertility index were observed at a palifermin dosage of 1,000 mcg/kg/day.

➤*Pregnancy: Category C.* Palifermin has been shown to be embryotoxic in rabbits and rats when given in doses that are 2.5 and 8 times the human dose, respectively.

Increased postimplantation loss and decreased fetal body weights were observed when palifermin was administered to pregnant rabbits from days 6 to 18 of gestation at IV dosages 150 mcg/kg/day or higher (2.5-fold higher than the recommended human dosage). However, treatment with these doses also was associated with maternal toxicity (clinical signs and reductions in body weight gain/food consumption). No evidence of developmental toxicity was observed in rabbits at dosages up to 60 mcg/kg/day.

Increased postimplantation loss, decreased fetal body weight, and/or increased skeletal variations were observed when palifermin was administered to pregnant rats from days 6 to 17 or 19 of gestation at IV dosages 500 mcg/kg/day or higher (more than 8-fold higher than the recommended human dose). Treatment with these doses was also frequently associated with maternal toxicity (clinical signs and body weight effects). No evidence of developmental toxicity was observed in rats at dosages up to 300 mcg/kg/day.

There are no adequate and well-controlled studies in pregnant women. Use palifermin during pregnancy only if the potential benefit justifies the potential risk to the fetus.

➤*Lactation:* It is not known whether palifermin is excreted in human milk. Because many drugs are excreted in human milk, exercise caution when palifermin is administered to a breast-feeding woman.

➤*Children:* The safety and efficacy of palifermin in pediatric patients have not been established.

Precautions

➤*Potential for stimulation of tumor growth:* The safety and efficacy of palifermin have not been established in patients with nonhematologic malignancies. The effects of palifermin on stimulation of KGF receptor-expressing, nonhematopoietic tumors in patients are not known. Palifermin has been shown to enhance the growth of human epithelial tumor cell lines in vitro and to increase the rate of tumor cell line growth in a human carcinoma xenograft model.

Drug Interactions

➤*Heparin:* Palifermin has been shown to bind to heparin in vitro. Therefore, if heparin is used to maintain an IV line, use saline to rinse the line prior to and after palifermin administration.

➤*Chemotherapy:* Do not administer palifermin within 24 hours before, during infusion of, or within 24 hours after administration of myelotoxic chemotherapy. In a clinical trial, administration of palifermin within 24 hours of chemotherapy resulted in increased severity and duration of oral mucositis.

Adverse Reactions

Safety data are based upon 409 patients with hematologic malignancies (NHL, Hodgkin disease, AML, ALL, CML, CLL, or multiple myeloma) who received palifermin and 241 patients who received placebo in 3 randomized, placebo-controlled clinical studies and a pharmacokinetic study. Patients received palifermin either before, or before and after, regimens of myelotoxic chemotherapy, with or without TBI, followed by PBPC support. The patients were predominantly between 41 and 60 years of age (median age, 48 years), male (62%), and white (83%). NHL was the most common malignancy, followed by Hodgkin disease, multiple myeloma, and leukemia.

➤*Serious adverse reactions:* The most common serious adverse reaction attributed to palifermin was skin rash, which was reported in less than 1% (3/409) of patients treated with palifermin. Grade 3 skin rashes occurred in 14 patients, 9 of 409 (3%) receiving palifermin and 5 of 241 (2%) receiving placebo. In 7 patients (5 palifermin, 2 placebo), study drug was discontinued because of skin rash. Other serious adverse reactions occurred at a similar rate in patients who received palifermin (20%) or placebo (21%). The most frequently reported serious adverse reactions in palifermin and placebo-treated patients were fever, GI events, and respiratory events.

➤*Most common:* The most common adverse reactions attributed to palifermin were dysesthesia, oral toxicities (eg, alteration of taste, dysesthesia, tongue discoloration, tongue thickening), pain arthralgias, and skin toxicities (eg, edema, erythema, pruritus, rash). The median time-to-onset of cutaneous toxicity was 6 days following the first of 3 consecutive daily doses of palifermin, with a median duration of 5 days. In patients receiving palifermin, dysesthesia (including hyperesthesia, hypesthesia, and paresthesia) was usually localized to the perioral region, whereas in patients receiving placebo, dysesthesias were more likely to occur in extremities. Adverse reactions occurring more frequently in palifermin-treated patients as compared with placebo-treated patients (a higher incidence of at least 5%) are listed in the following table.

Adverse Reactions (≥ 5%) with Palifermin		
Adverse reaction	Palifermin (n = 409)	Placebo (n = 241)
CNS		
Dysesthesia (hyperesthesia/hypesthesia/paresthesia)	12%	7%
Dermatologic		
Erythema	32%	22%
Pruritus	35%	24%
Rash	62%	50%
GI		
Mouth/tongue thickness or discoloration	17%	8%
Taste altered	16%	8%
Metabolic		
Elevated serum amylase (grade 3/4)	62% (38%)	54% (31%)
Elevated serum lipase (grade 3/4)	28% (11%)	23% (5%)
Musculoskeletal		
Arthralgia	10%	5%
Miscellaneous		
Edema	28%	21%
Fever	39%	34%
Pain	16%	11%

➤*Cardiovascular:* In a phase 1, placebo-controlled study in patients undergoing hematopoietic transplantation and receiving palifermin (3 doses premyelotoxic therapy and 3 doses posttransplant), the proportion of palifermin-treated patients reporting an adverse reaction of hypertension in the palifermin 60 mcg/kg/day and 80 mcg/kg/day cohorts was greater than in the placebo group (2/15 [13%], 2/14 [14%], and 2/23 [9%] patients, respectively). These reactions were transient and did not require treatment discontinuation in any patient. In an integrated analysis of adverse reactions across palifermin studies in the hematology transplant setting, hypertensive events were reported in 30/409 palifermin (7%) patients and 13/241 placebo (5%) patients.

➤*Miscellaneous:*

Proteinuria – In a placebo-controlled study conducted in 145 patients with metastatic colorectal cancer receiving multicycle chemotherapy (5-fluorouracil/leucovorin), serial urine specimens were collected for 27 placebo-treated and 54 palifermin-treated patients. Among the 54 palifermin-treated patients, 9 patients with a baseline urinalysis negative for protein subsequently developed 2+ or greater proteinuria after treatment with palifermin. Among the 27 placebo-treated patients evaluated, none developed 2+ or greater proteinuria. Because of the study design, the number of cycles with urine analysis data collected was higher in the palifermin-treated patients. In addition, for the 9 patients with proteinuria, underlying medical conditions known to be associated with proteinuria were present at baseline. A causal relationship between palifermin and proteinuria has not been established.

➤*Lab test abnormalities:* Reversible elevations in serum lipase and amylase, which did not require treatment intervention, are shown in the preceding table. In general, peak increases were observed during the period of cytotoxic therapy and returned to baseline by the day of PBPC infusion. Fractionation of amylase revealed it to be predominantly salivary in origin.

Immunogenicity – As with all therapeutic proteins, there is a potential for immunogenicity. The clinical significance of antibodies to palifermin is unknown but may include lessened activity and/or cross-reactivity with other members of the FGF family of growth factors.

A sensitive electrochemiluminescence-based binding assay was performed on posttreatment sera from 645 patients treated with palifermin in clinical

PALIFERMIN — INJECTION

studies. Twelve (2%) of these 645 patients tested positive for antibodies to palifermin following treatment. None of the samples had evidence of neutralizing activity in a cell-based assay.

The incidence of antibody positivity is highly dependent on the specific assay and its sensitivity. Additionally, the observed incidence of antibody positivity in an assay may be influenced by several factors, including sample handling, timing of sample collection, concomitant medications, and underlying disease. For these reasons, comparison of the incidence of antibodies to palifermin with the incidence of antibodies to other products may be misleading.

Overdosage

The maximum amount of palifermin that can be safely administered in a single dose has not been determined. Single doses of 250 mcg/kg have been administered IV to 8 healthy volunteers without severe or serious adverse reactions. Five of 14 patients receiving 6 dosages of 80 mcg/kg/day administered IV over 2 weeks (3 doses preceding and 3 doses following myeloablative chemotherapy/TBI) experienced serious or severe adverse reactions. These reactions were consistent with those observed at the recommended dose but were generally more severe.

Patient Information

Inform patients of the possible side effects of palifermin, including mucocutaneous adverse effects. These include rash, erythema, edema, pruritus, oral/perioral dysesthesia, tongue discoloration, tongue thickening, and alteration of taste. Instruct patients to report these side effects, or any others, to their health care provider.

The safety and efficacy of palifermin have not been established in patients with nonhematologic malignancies. Inform patients of the evidence of tumor growth and stimulation in cell culture and in animal models of nonhematopoietic human tumors.

ANTIHISTAMINE-CONTAINING PREPARATIONS

otc	**Dermamycin** (Pfeiffer)	**Cream**: 2% diphenhydramine HCl, parabens, polyethylene glycol monostearate, propylene glycol	In 28.35 g.
		Spray: 2% diphenhydramine HCl, 1% menthol, alcohol, methylparaben	In 60 mL.
otc	**Maximum Strength Benadryl Itch Relief** (Pfeiffer)	**Cream**: 2% diphenhydramine HCl, 0.1% zinc acetate, parabens, aloe vera	In 14.2 g.
		Stick: 2% diphenhydramine HCl, 0.1% zinc acetate, 73.5% alcohol, aloe vera	In 14 mL.
otc	**Anti-Itch** (Taro)	**Cream**: 2% diphenhydramine HCl, 0.1% zinc acetate, parabens	In 28.4 g.
otc	**Ziradryl** (Parke-Davis)	**Lotion**: 1% diphenhydramine HCl, 2% zinc oxide, 2% alcohol, camphor, parabens	In 180 mL.
otc	**Benadryl** (Parke-Davis)	**Cream**: 1% diphenhydramine HCl, parabens in a greaseless base	In 15 g.
		Spray, non-aerosol: 1% diphenhydramine HCl, 85% alcohol	In 60 mL.
otc	**Caladryl** (Parke-Davis)	**Cream**: 1% diphenhydramine HCl, 8% calamine, parabens, camphor	In 45 g.
		Lotion: 1% diphenhydramine HCl, 8% calamine, camphor, 2% alcohol	In 75 and 180 mL.
otc	**Di-Delamine** (Commerce)	**Gel and Spray, non-aerosol**: 1% diphenhydramine HCl, 0.5% tripelennamine HCl, 0.12% benzalkonium Cl, menthol, EDTA	**Gel**: In 37.5 g. **Spray**: In 120 mL.
otc	**Sting-Eze** (Wisconsin Pharm.)	**Concentrate**: Diphenhydramine HCl, camphor, phenol, benzocaine, eucalyptol	In 15 mL.
otc	**Medacote** (Dal-Med)	**Lotion**: 1% pyrilamine maleate, dimethyl polysiloxane, zinc oxide, menthol and camphor in a greaseless base	In 120 mL.
otc	**Derma-Pax** (Recsei Labs)	**Lotion**: 0.44% pyrilamine maleate, 0.06% chlorpheniramine, 1% benzyl alcohol, 35% isopropanol, chlorobutanol	In 120 mL and pt.
otx	**Z-Xtra** (Magna)	**Lotion**: 2.07 mg pyrilamine maleate, 41.35 mg zinc oxide/mL. Benzocaine, apple blossom oil, silicone oil, lanolin oil, Wysteria oil, isopropanol, camphor, menthol, parabens	In 118 mL.
otc	**Calamycin** (Pfeiffer)	**Lotion**: Zinc oxide and 10% calamine, benzocaine, chloroxylenol, pyrilamine maleate, 2% isopropyl alcohol	In 120 mL.
otc	**Benadryl Itch Stopping Maximum Strength** (Warner Wellcome)	**Gel**: 2% diphenhydramine HCl, 1% zinc acetate, camphor, parabens	In 118 g.
otc	**Dermarest** (Del)	**Gel**: 2% diphenhydramine HCl, 2% resorcinol, aloe vera gel, benzalkonium chloride, EDTA, menthol, methylparaben, propylene glycol	In 29.25 and 56.25 g.
otc	**Dermarest Plus** (Del)	**Gel**: 2% diphenhydramine HCl, 1% menthol, aloe vera gel, benzalkonium chloride, isopropyl alcohol, methylparaben, propylene glycol	In 15 and 30 g.
		Spray: 2% diphenhydramine HCl, 1% menthol, aloe vera gel, benzalkonium chloride, methylparaben, propylene glycol, SD alcohol 40, EDTA	In 15 and 30 g.
otc	**Clearly Cala-gel** (Tec Labs)	**Gel**: Diphenhydramine HCl, zinc acetate, menthol, EDTA	Clear. In 180 g.
otc	**Benadryl Itch Relief** (GlaxoWellcome)	**Spray**: 2% diphenhydramine HCl, 0.1% zinc acetate, 73.6% alcohol, aloe vera	In 59 mL.
otc	**Benadryl Itch Relief Children's** (GlaxoWellcome	**Cream**: 1% diphenhydramine HCl, 0.1% zinc acetate, aloe vera, cetyl alcohol, parabens	In 14.2 g.
		Spray: 1% diphenhydramine HCl, 0.1% zinc acetate, 73.6% alcohol, aloe vera, povidone	In 59 mL.
otc	**Benadryl Itch Stopping Spray, Extra Strength** (Warner Lambert	**Spray**: 2% diphenhydramine HCl, 0.1% zinc acetate, 73.5% v/v alcohol, glycerin, tromethamine	In 59 mL.
otc	**Benadryl Itch Stopping Spray, Original Strength** (Warner Lambert)	**Spray**: 1% diphenhydramine HCl, 0.1% zinc acetate, 73.6% v/v alcohol, glycerin, tromethamine	In 59 mL.

ANTIHISTAMINE-CONTAINING PREPARATIONS — TOPICAL

Indications

Temporary relief of itching due to minor skin disorders, ivy, sumac and oak poisoning, sunburn, insect bites (nonpoisonous) and stings.

Actions

➤*Pharmacology:* Topical antihistamines have some local anesthetic activity and are used to relieve itching. Some transdermal absorption may occur, but not in sufficient quantities to produce systemic side effects. They may cause local irritation and sensitization, especially with prolonged use. Refer to Antihistamine monograph in Respiratory Drugs chapter for further information on systemic antihistamines.

Warnings

➤*Do not apply:* To blistered, raw or oozing areas of the skin, or around the eyes or other mucous membranes (eg, nose, mouth).

Precautions

➤*For external use only:* Avoid contact with the eyes.

➤*Discontinue use:* If the condition persists, recurs after a few days or irritation develops.

➤*Avoid prolonged use:* For more than 7 days or use on extensive skin areas.

DOXEPIN HCl

Rx	**Zonalon** (Bioglan)	**Cream**: 5%	Cetyl alcohol, petrolatum, benzyl alcohol, titanium dioxide. In 30 g.

DOXEPIN HYDROCHLORIDE — TOPICAL

For information on the systemic use of doxepin, refer to the individual monographs in the CNS Drugs chapter.

Indications

➤*Pruritus:* Short-term (up to 8 days) management of moderate pruritus in adult patients with atopic dermatitis or lichen simplex chronicus.

Administration and Dosage

➤*Approved by the FDA:* April 1, 1994.

For topical, dermatologic use only. Not for ophthalmic, oral, or intravaginal use.

Apply a thin film of doxepin cream 4 times each day with at least a 3- to 4-hour interval between applications. There are no data to establish the safety and effectiveness of doxepin cream when used for greater than 8 days. Chronic use beyond 8 days may result in higher systemic levels and should be avoided. Use of doxepin cream for longer than 8 days may result in an increased likelihood of contact sensitization.

The risk for sedation may increase with greater body surface area application of doxepin cream. Clinical experience has shown that drowsiness is significantly more common in patients applying doxepin cream to over 10% of body surface area; therefore, especially caution patients with greater than 10% of body surface area affected concerning possible drowsiness and other systemic adverse effects of doxepin. If excessive drowsiness occurs, it may be necessary to do 1 or more of the following: Reduce the body surface area treated, reduce the number of applications per day, reduce the amount of cream applied, or discontinue the drug.

➤*Occlusive dressing:* Occlusive dressings may increase the absorption of most topical drugs; therefore, do not use occlusive dressings with doxepin cream.

➤*Storage/Stability:* Store at or below 27°C (80°F).

DOXEPIN HYDROCHLORIDE — TOPICAL

Actions

➤*Pharmacology:* Although doxepin does have H1 and H2 histamine receptor blocking actions, the exact mechanism by which doxepin exerts its antipruritic effect is unknown. Doxepin cream can produce drowsiness in significant numbers of patients, and this sedation may reduce awareness, including awareness of pruritic symptoms.

➤*Pharmacokinetics:*

Absorption – In 19 pruritic eczema patients treated with doxepin cream, plasma doxepin concentrations ranged from nondetectable to 47 ng/mL from percutaneous absorption. Plasma levels from topical application of doxepin cream can result in CNS and other systemic side effects.

Metabolism/Excretion – Once absorbed into the systemic circulation, doxepin undergoes hepatic metabolism that results in conversion to pharmacologically active desmethyldoxepin. Further glucuronidation results in urinary excretion of the parent drug and its metabolites. Desmethyldoxepin has a half-life that ranges from 28 to 52 hours and is not affected by multiple dosing. Plasma levels of both doxepin and desmethyldoxepin are highly variable and are poorly correlated with dosage. Wide distribution occurs in body tissues including lungs, heart, brain, and liver. Renal disease, genetic factors, age, and other medications affect the metabolism and subsequent elimination of doxepin.

Contraindications

Untreated narrow angle glaucoma or a tendency to urinary retention; sensitivity to any of its components.

Warnings

➤*Drowsiness:* See Administration and Dosage for more information.

The sedating effects of alcoholic beverages, antihistamines, and other CNS depressants may be potentiated when doxepin cream is used.

If excessive drowsiness occurs, it may be necessary to reduce the frequency of applications, the amount of cream applied, and/or the percentage of body surface area treated, or discontinue the drug. However, the efficacy with reduced frequency of applications has not been established. Keep this product away from the eyes.

➤*Hypersensitivity reactions:* Use of doxepin cream can cause Type IV hypersensitivity reactions (contact sensitization) to doxepin.

➤*Elderly:* Clinical studies of doxepin cream did not include sufficient numbers of subjects aged 65 years and over to determine whether they respond differently from younger subjects. Other reported clinical experience has not identified differences in responses between the elderly and younger patients. In general, dose selection for an elderly patient should be cautious, usually starting at the low end of the dosing range, reflecting the greater frequency of decreased hepatic, renal or cardiac function, and of concomitant disease or other drug therapy.

The extent of renal excretion of doxepin has not been determined. Because elderly patients are more likely to have decreased renal function, take care in dose selections.

Sedating drugs may cause confusion and oversedation in the elderly; elderly patients generally should be observed closely for confusion and oversedation when started on doxepin cream. An 80-year-old male nursing home patient developed probable systemic anticholinergic toxicity which included urinary retention and delirium after doxepin cream had been applied to his arms, legs and back 3 times daily for 2 days.

➤*Pregnancy: Category B.*

There are no adequate and well-controlled studies in pregnant women. Use this drug during pregnancy only if clearly needed.

➤*Lactation:* Doxepin is excreted in human milk after oral administration. It is possible that doxepin may also be excreted in human milk following topical application of doxepin cream.

One case has been reported of apnea and drowsiness in a nursing infant whose mother was taking an oral dosage form of doxepin.

Because of the potential for serious adverse reactions in nursing infants from doxepin, a decision should be made whether to discontinue nursing or to discontinue the drug, taking into account the importance of the drug to the mother.

➤*Children:* The use of doxepin cream in pediatric patients is not recommended. Safe conditions for use of doxepin cream in children have not been established. One case has been reported of a 2.5-year-old child who developed somnolence, grand mal seizure, respiratory depression, ECG abnormalities, and coma after treatment with doxepin cream. A total of 27 g had been applied over 3 days for eczema. He was treated with supportive care, activated charcoal, and systemic alkalization, and he recovered.

Precautions

➤*Hazardous tasks:*

Drowsiness – See Warnings for more information.

Drug Interactions

➤*Drugs metabolized by P450 2D6:* Concomitant use of tricyclic antidepressants with drugs that can inhibit cytochrome P450 2D6 may require lower doses than usually prescribed for either the tricyclic antidepressant or the other drug. It is desirable to monitor TCA plasma levels whenever a TCA is going to be coadministered with another drug known to be an inhibitor of P450 2D6.

➤*MAO inhibitors:* Serious side effects and even death have been reported following the concomitant use of certain drugs with MAO inhibitors. Therefore, discontinue MAO inhibitors at least 2 weeks prior to the cautious initiation of therapy with doxepin cream. The exact length of time may vary and is dependent upon the particular MAO inhibitor being used, the length of time it has been administered, and the dosage involved.

➤*Cimetidine:* Serious anticholinergic symptoms (ie, severe dry mouth, urinary retention and blurred vision) have been associated with elevations in the serum levels of tricyclic antidepressant when cimetidine therapy is initiated. Additionally, higher than expected tricyclic antidepressant levels have been observed when they are begun in patients already taking cimetidine.

➤*CNS depressants:* See Warnings for more information.

➤*Tolazamide:* A case of severe hypoglycemia has been reported in a type 2 diabetes patient maintained on tolazamide (1 g/day) 11 days after the addition of oral doxepin (75 mg/day).

Adverse Reactions

➤*Controlled clinical trials:*

Systemic adverse effects – In controlled clinical trials of patients treated with doxepin cream, the most common systemic adverse event reported was drowsiness. Drowsiness occurred in 71 of 330 (22%) of patients treated with doxepin cream compared to 7 of 334 (2%) of patients treated with vehicle cream. Drowsiness resulted in the premature discontinuation of the drug in approximately 5% of patients treated with doxepin cream in controlled clinical trials.

Local site adverse effects – In controlled clinical trials of patients treated with doxepin cream, the most common local site adverse event reported was burning or stinging at the site of application. These occurred in 76 of 330 (23%) of patients treated with doxepin cream compared to 54 of 334 (16%) of patients treated with vehicle cream. Most of these reactions were categorized as "mild"; however, approximately 25% of patients who reported burning and/or stinging reported the reaction as "severe". Four patients treated with doxepin cream withdrew from the study because of the burning and/or stinging.

Doxepin Adverse Reactions (≥ 1%)		
Adverse reaction	Doxepin (n = 330)	Vehicle (n = 334)
Burning/stinging	76 (23%)	54 (16.2%)
Dizziness[a]	7 (2.1%)	3 (0.9%)
Drowsiness	71 (21.5%)	7 (2.1%)
Dry mouth[b]	32 (9.7%)	4 (1.2%)
Edema	4 (1.2%)	1 (0.3%)
Exacerbated eczema	10 (3%)	8 (2.4%)
Fatigue/ tiredness	10 (3%)	5 (1.5%)
Headache	3 (0.9%)	14 (4.2%)
Mental emotional changes	6 (1.8%)	1 (0.3%)
Other application site reaction[c]	10 (3%)	16 (4.8%)
Pruritus[d]	13 (3.9%)	20 (6%)
Taste perversion[e]	5 (1.5%)	1 (0.3%)

[a] Includes reports of "lightheadedness" and "dizziness/vertigo."
[b] Includes reports of "dry lips", "dry throat", and "thirst."
[c] Includes reports of "increased irritation at application site."
[d] Includes reports of "pruritus exacerbated."
[e] Includes reports of "bitter taste" and "metallic taste in mouth."

Adverse events occurring in 0.5% to less than 1% of doxepin-cream-treated patients in the controlled clinical trials included nervousness/anxiety, tongue numbness, fever, and nausea.

➤*Postmarketing experience:* Twenty-six cases of allergic contact dermatitis have been reported in patients using doxepin cream, 20 of which were documented by positive patch test to doxepin 5% cream.

Overdosage

➤*Symptoms:* Should overdosage with topical application of doxepin cream occur, the signs and symptoms may include cardiac dysrhythmias, severe hypotension, convulsions, and CNS depression, including coma. Changes in the electrocardiogram, particularly in QRS axis or width, are clinically significant indicators of tricyclic antidepressant toxicity.

Other signs of overdose may include confusion, disturbed concentration, transient visual hallucinations, dilated pupils, agitation, hyperactive reflexes, stupor, drowsiness, muscle rigidity, vomiting, hypothermia, hyperpyrexia, or any other doxepin topical adverse reactions.

➤*Treatment:*

General recommendations – Obtain an ECG, and immediately initiate cardiac monitoring. Protect the patient's airway, establish an IV line, and initiate gastric decontamination. A minimum of 6 hours of observation with cardiac monitoring and observation for signs of CNS or respiratory depression, hypotension, cardiac dysrhythmias and/or conduction blocks, and seizures is strongly advised. If signs of toxicity occur at any time during this period, extended monitoring is recommended. There are case reports of patients succumbing to fatal dysrhythmias late after overdose; these patients had clinical evidence of significant poisoning prior to death and

DOXEPIN HYDROCHLORIDE — TOPICAL

most received inadequate gastrointestinal decontamination. Monitoring of plasma drug levels should not guide management of the patient.

Cardiovascular – A maximal limb-lead QRS duration of greater than or equal to 0.1 seconds may be the best indication of the severity of the overdose. Use IV sodium bicarbonate to maintain the serum pH in the range of 7.45 to 7.55. If the pH response is inadequate, hyperventilation may also be used. Concomitant use of hyperventilation and sodium bicarbonate should be done with extreme caution, with frequent pH monitoring. A pH greater than 7.6 or a pCO_2 less than 20 mm Hg is undesirable. Dysrhythmias unresponsive to sodium bicarbonate therapy/hyperventilation may respond to lidocaine, bretylium or phenytoin.

Type 1A and 1C antiarrhythmics are generally contraindicated (eg, quinidine, disopyramide, and procainamide).

In rare instances, hemoperfusion may be beneficial in acute refractory cardiovascular instability in patients with acute toxicity. However, hemodialysis, peritoneal dialysis, exchange transfusions, and forced diuresis generally have been reported as ineffective in tricyclic antidepressant poisoning.

CNS – In patients with CNS depression, early intubation is advised because of the potential for abrupt deterioration. Control seizures with benzodiazepines, or if these are ineffective, other anticonvulsants (eg, phenobarbital, phenytoin). Physostigmine is not recommended except to treat life-threatening symptoms that have been unresponsive to other therapies, and then only in consultation with a poison control center.

Pediatric management – The principles of management of child and adult overdosages are similar. It is strongly recommended that the physician contact the local poison control center for specific pediatric treatment.

Patient Information

Since drowsiness may occur with the use of doxepin cream, warn patients of the possibility and caution them against driving a car or operating dangerous machinery while using this drug. Also caution patients that their responses to alcohol may be potentiated.

ANTI-INFECTIVES, TOPICAL

Antibiotic Agents

GENTAMICIN SULFATE

Rx	**Gentamicin** (Various, eg, Fougera)	**Ointment**: 0.1% (as base)	May contain white petrolatum, parabens. In 15 g.
		Cream: 0.1% (as base)	May contain propylene glycol, parabens. In 15 g.

GENTAMICIN SULFATE — TOPICAL

Indications

➤*Primary skin infections:* Impetigo contagiosa, superficial folliculitis, ecthyma, furunculosis, sycosis barbae, and pyoderma gangrenosum.

➤*Secondary skin infections:* Infectious eczematoid dermatitis, pustular acne, pustular psoriasis, infected seborrheic dermatitis, infected contact dermatitis (including poison ivy), infected excoriations, and bacterial superinfections of fungal or viral infections.

➤*Other infections:* Treatment of infected skin cysts and certain other skin abscesses when preceded by incision and drainage to permit adequate contact between the antibiotic and the infecting bacteria. Good results have been obtained in the treatment of infected stasis and other skin ulcers, infected superficial burns, paronychia, infected insect bites and stings, infected lacerations and abrasions, and wounds from minor surgery. Patients sensitive to neomycin can be treated with gentamicin, although regular observation of patients sensitive to topical antibiotics is advisable when such patients are treated with any topical antibiotic.

➤*Ointment:* Gentamicin sulfate ointment helps retain moisture and has been useful in infection on dry eczematous or psoriatic skin.

➤*Cream:* For wet, oozing primary infections and greasy, secondary infections, such as pustular acne or infected seborrheic dermatitis. If a water-washable preparation is desired, gentamicin sulfate cream is preferable.

Administration and Dosage

➤*Approved by the FDA:* February 18, 1982.

➤*Adults and children over 1 year of age:* A small amount of gentamicin sulfate cream or ointment should be applied gently to the lesions three or four times daily. The area treated may be covered with a gauze dressing if desired. In impetigo contagiosa, the crusts should be removed before application of gentamicin sulfate to permit maximum contact between the antibiotic and the infection. Care should be exercised to avoid further contamination of the infected skin. Infected stasis ulcers have responded well to gentamicin sulfate under gelatin packing.

➤*Storage/Stability:* Store between 2° and 30°C (36° and 86°F).

Actions

➤*Pharmacology:* Gentamicin sulfate, a wide-spectrum antibiotic, provides highly effective topical treatment in primary and secondary bacterial infections of the skin. Gentamicin sulfate may clear infections that have not responded to other topical antibiotic agents. In impetigo contagiosa and other primary skin infections, treatment three or four times daily with gentamicin sulfate usually clears the lesions promptly. In secondary skin infections, gentamicin sulfate facilitates the treatment of the underlying dermatosis by controlling the infection. Bacteria susceptible to the action of gentamicin sulfate include sensitive strains of streptococci (group A beta-hemolytic, alpha-hemolytic), *Staphylococcus aureus* (coagulase-positive, coagulase-negative, and some penicillinase-producing strains), and the gram-negative bacteria, *Pseudomonas aeruginosa*, *Aerobacter aerogenes*, *Escherichia coli*, *Proteus vulgaris*, and *Klebsiella pneumoniae*.

Contraindications

History of sensitivity reactions to any of its components.

Precautions

➤*Superinfection:* Use of topical antibiotics occasionally allows overgrowth of nonsusceptible organisms, including fungi. If this occurs, or if irritation, sensitization, or superinfection develops, treatment with gentamicin should be discontinued and appropriate therapy instituted.

Adverse Reactions

In patients with dermatoses treated with gentamicin, irritation (erythema and pruritus) that did not usually require discontinuance of treatment has been reported in a small percentage of cases. There was no evidence of irritation or sensitization, however, in any of these patients patch-tested subsequently with gentamicin on normal skin. Possible photosensitization has been reported in several patients but could not be elicited in these patients by reapplication of gentamicin followed by exposure to ultraviolet radiation.

BACITRACIN

otc	**Bacitracin** (Various, eg, Fougera, Ivax, Rugby)	**Ointment**: 500 units/g	May contain mineral oil or white petrolatum. In 14, 28, 120, and 454 g and UD 144s.

BACITRACIN ZINC — TOPICAL

Indications

➤*Topical infection:* A first aid antibiotic to help prevent infection in minor cuts, scrapes, and burns.

Administration and Dosage

➤*Directions:*

1.) Clean the affected area.
2.) Apply a small amount of product (an amount equal to the surface area of the tip of a finger) on the area 1 to 3 times daily. Do not use longer than 1 week unless directed by a physician.
3.) The affected area may be covered with a sterile bandage.

➤*Storage/Stability:* Store at 15° to 25°C (59° to 77°F). See the box or crimp of tube for the expiration date.

Actions

➤*Pharmacology:* Bacitracin is believed to be bactericidal or bacteriostatic in action depending on the concentration of the drip and the susceptibility of the organism. Bacitracin inhibits cell-wall synthesis by preventing amino acids and nucleotides into the cell. Absorption is reported to be negligible following topical administration.

Contraindications

Known hypersensitivity to any of the ingredients; use in the eyes.

Warnings

➤*Systemic therapy:* Deeper cutaneous infections may require systemic antibiotic therapy in addition to local treatment. Use caution when applying over large areas of the body for deep puncture wounds, animal bites, or serious burns.

➤*External use:* Bacitracin zinc is for external use only. Do not use in or near the eyes, nose, mouth, mucous membranes, or apply over large areas of the body.

➤*Hypersensitivity reactions:* Stop use if a rash or other allergic reaction occurs.

➤*Pregnancy: Category C.* There are no adequate and well controlled studies in pregnant women. Use during pregnancy only when clearly needed.

➤*Lactation:* It is not known whether bacitracin is excreted in breast milk. Use caution when applying on a breastfeeding woman.

BACITRACIN ZINC — TOPICAL

Adverse Reactions

Rash; hypersensitivity reaction (rare).

Patient Information

For external use only.

Do not use:
- In the eyes
- If you are allergic to any of the ingredients
- Over large areas of the body
- Longer than 1 week unless directed by a doctor

Ask a doctor before use in case of deep or puncture wounds, animal bites, or serious burns

Stop use and ask a doctor if:
- The condition persists or gets worse.
- A rash or other allergic reaction develops.

Keep out of reach of children. If swallowed, get medical help or contact a poison control center right away.

AZELAIC ACID

Rx	**Azelex** (Allergan)	**Cream:** 20%	Glycerin, cetearyl alcohol, benzoic acid. In 30 and 50 g.
Rx	**Finacea** (Berlex Labs)	**Gel:** 15%	Benzoic acid, EDTA. In 30 g.

AZELAIC ACID — TOPICAL

Indications

➤*Cream:* For the topical treatment of mild-to-moderate inflammatory acne vulgaris.

➤*Gel:* For topical treatment of inflammatory papules and pustules of mild to moderate rosacea. Patients should be instructed to avoid spicy foods, thermally hot foods and drinks, alcoholic beverages, and to use only very mild soaps or soapless cleansing lotion for facial cleansing.

Administration and Dosage

➤*Approved by the FDA:* September 13, 1995.

➤*Cream:* After the skin is thoroughly washed and patted dry, a thin film of azelaic acid should be gently but thoroughly massaged into the affected areas twice daily, in the morning and evening. The hands should be washed following application. The duration of use of azelaic acid can vary from person to person and depends on the severity of the acne. Improvement of the condition occurs in the majority of patients with inflammatory lesions within 4 weeks.

➤*Gel:* Massage a thin layer gently into the affected areas on the face twice daily, in the morning and evening. Azelaic acid gel, 15%, has only been studied up to 12 weeks in patients with mild to moderate rosacea.

➤*Storage/Stability:*

Gel – Store at 25°C (77°F); excursions permitted between 15° to 30°C (59° to 86°F).

Cream – Store between 15° to 30°C (59° to 86°F). Protect from freezing.

Actions

➤*Pharmacology:* The exact mechanism of action of azelaic acid is not known. The following in vitro data are available, but their clinical significance is unknown. Azelaic acid has been shown to possess antimicrobial activity against *Propionibacterium acnes* and *Staphylococcus epidermidis.* The antimicrobial action may be attributable to inhibition of microbial cellular protein synthesis. A normalization of keratinization leading to an anticomedonal effect of azelaic acid may also contribute to its clinical activity. Electron microscopic and immunohistochemical evaluation of skin biopsies from human subjects treated with azelaic acid demonstrated a reduction in the thickness of the stratum corneum, a reduction in number and size of keratohyalin granules, and a reduction in the amount and distribution of filaggrin (a protein component of keratohyalin) in epidermal layers. This is suggestive of the ability to decrease microcomedo formation.

➤*Pharmacokinetics:*

Cream – Following a single application of azelaic acid to human skin in vitro, azelaic acid penetrates into the stratum corneum (approximately 3% to 5% of the applied dose) and other viable skin layers (up to 10% of the dose is found in the epidermis and dermis). Negligible cutaneous metabolism occurs after topical application. Approximately 4% of the topically applied azelaic acid is systemically absorbed. Azelaic acid is mainly excreted unchanged in the urine but undergoes some oxidation to shorter chain dicarboxylic acids. The observed half-lives in healthy subjects are approximately 45 minutes after oral dosing and 12 hours after topical dosing, indicating percutaneous absorption rate-limited kinetics. Azelaic acid is a dietary constituent (whole grain cereals and animal products), and can be formed endogenously from longer-chain dicarboxylic acids, metabolism of oleic acid, and oxidation of monocarboxylic acids. Endogenous plasma concentration (20 to 80 ng/mL) and daily urinary excretion (4 to 28 mg) of azelaic acid are highly dependent on dietary intake, After topical treatment with azelaic acid in humans, plasma concentration and urinary excretion of azelaic acid are not significantly different from baseline levels.

Gel – The percutaneous absorption of azelaic acid after topical application of azelaic acid gel, 15%, could not be reliably determined. Mean plasma azelaic acid concentrations in rosacea patients treated with azelaic acid gel, 15%, twice daily for at least 8 weeks are in the range of 42 to 63.1 ng/mL. These values are within the maximum concentration range of 24 to 90.5 ng/mL observed in rosacea patients treated with vehicle only. This indicates that azelaic acid gel, 15%, does not increase plasma azelaic acid concentration beyond the range derived from nutrition and endogenous metabolism.

In vitro and human data suggest negligible cutaneous metabolism of ^{3}H-azelaic acid 20% cream after topical application. Azelaic acid is mainly excreted unchanged in the urine, but undergoes some β-oxidation to shorter chain dicarboxylic acids.

Contraindications

Hypersensitivity to any of its components.

Warnings

➤*Hypopigmentation:* There have been isolated reports of hypopigmentation after use of azelaic acid. Since azelaic acid has not been well studied in patients with dark complexions, these patients should be monitored for early signs of hypopigmentation.

➤*Pregnancy: Category B.*

Embryotoxic effects were observed in Segment 1 and Segment 11 oral studies with rats receiving 2500 mg/kg/day of azelaic acid. Similar effects were observed in Segment 11 studies in rabbits given 150 to 500 mg/kg/day and in monkeys given 500 mg/kg/day. The doses at which these effects were noted were all within toxic dose ranges for the dams. No teratogenic effects were observed. There are, however, no adequate and well controlled studies in pregnant women. Because animal reproduction studies are not always predictive of human response, this drug should be used during pregnancy only if clearly needed.

➤*Lactation:* Equilibrium dialysis was used to assess human milk partitioning in vitro. At an azelaic acid concentration of 25 mcg/mL, the milk/plasma distribution coefficient was 0.7 and the milk/buffer distribution was 1), indicating that passage of drug into maternal milk may occur. Since less than 4% of a topically applied dose of azelaic acid is systemically absorbed, the uptake of azelaic acid into maternal milk is not expected to cause a significant change from baseline azelaic acid levels in the milk. However, caution should be exercised when azelaic acid is administered to a nursing mother.

➤*Children:*

Cream – Safety and efficacy in pediatric patients under 12 years of age have not been established.

Gel – Safety and efficacy of azelaic acid, 15%, in pediatric patients have not been established.

Precautions

➤*Hypersensitivity:* If sensitivity or severe irritation develop with the use of azelaic acid treatment should be discontinued and appropriate therapy instituted.

Drug Interactions

None known.

Adverse Reactions

➤*Cream:* During US clinical trials with azelaic acid, adverse reactions were generally mild and transient in nature. The most common adverse reactions occurring in approximately 1% to 5% of patients were pruritus, burning, stinging and tingling. Other adverse reactions such as erythema, dryness, rash, peeling, irritation, dermatitis, and contact dermatitis were reported in less than 1% of subjects. There is the potential for experiencing allergic reactions with use of azelaic acid. In patients using azelaic acid formulations, the following additional adverse experiences have been reported rarely: Worsening of asthma, vitiligo depigmentation, small depigmented spots, hypertrichosis, reddening (signs of keratosis pilaris), and exacerbation of recurrent herpes labialis.

➤*Gel:*

Cutaneous Adverse Reactions Occurring In ≥ 1% of Subjects In the Rosacea Trials by Treatment Group and Maximum Intensity*

	Azelaic acid gel, 15% n = 333 (100%)			Vehicle n = 331 (100%)		
Adverse reaction	Mild (n = 86) (26%)	Moderate (n = 44) (13%)	Severe (n = 20) (6%)	Mild (n = 49) (15%)	Moderate (n = 27) (8%)	Severe (n = 5) (2%)
Burning/ stinging/ tingling	66 (20%)	30 (9%)	12 (4%)	8 (2%)	6 (2%)	2 (1%)
Pruritus	24 (7%)	14 (4%)	3 (1%)	9 (3%)	6 (2%)	0 (0%)

AZELAIC ACID — TOPICAL

Cutaneous Adverse Reactions Occurring In ≥ 1% of Subjects In the Rosacea Trials by Treatment Group and Maximum Intensity*						
	Azelaic acid gel, 15% n = 333 (100%)			Vehicle n = 331 (100%)		
Adverse reaction	Mild (n = 86) (26%)	Moderate (n = 44) (13%)	Severe (n = 20) (6%)	Mild (n = 49) (15%)	Moderate (n = 27) (8%)	Severe (n = 5) (2%)
Scaling/ dry skin/ xerosis	21 (6%)	8 (2%)	4 (1%)	33 (10%)	12 (4%)	1 (0%)
Erythema/ irritation	6 (2%)	6 (2%)	1 (0%)	8 (2%)	4 (1%)	2 (1%)
Edema	3 (1%)	2 (1%)	0 (0%)	3 (1%)	0 (0%)	0 (0%)
Contact dermatitis	2 (1%)	2 (1%)	0 (0%)	1 (0%)	0 (0%)	0 (0%)
Acne	2 (1%)	1 (0%)	0 (0%)	1 (0%)	0 (0%)	0 (0%)
Seborrhea	2 (1%)	0 (0%)	0 (0%)	0 (0%)	0 (0%)	0 (0%)
Photosensitivity	1 (0%)	0 (0%)	0 (0%)	3 (1%)	1 (0%)	1 (0%)
Skin disease	1 (0%)	0 (0%)	0 (0%)	1 (0%)	2 (1%)	0 (0%)

* Subjects may have greater than 1 cutaneous adverse reaction; thus, the sum of the frequencies of preferred terms may exceed the number of subjects with at least 1 cutaneous adverse reaction.

Azelaic acid gel, 15%, and its vehicle caused irritant reactions at the application site in human dermal safety studies. Azelaic acid gel, 15%, caused significantly more irritation than its vehicle in a cumulative irritation study. Some improvement in irritation was demonstrated over the course of the clinical studies, but this improvement might be attributed to subject dropouts. No phototoxicity or photoallergenicity were reported in human dermal safety studies.

In patients using azelaic acid formulations, the following additional adverse reactions have been reported rarely: Worsening of asthma, vitiligo depigmentation, small depigmented spots, hypertichosis, reddening (signs of keratosis pilaris), and exacerbation of recurrent herpes labialis.

Overdosage

➤*Gel:* Azelaic acid gel, 15%, is intended for cutaneous use only. If pronounced local irritation occurs, patients should be directed to discontinue use and appropriate therapy should be instituted.

Patient Information

➤*Cream:* Patients should be told:

1.) To use azelaic acid for the full prescribed treatment period.
2.) To avoid the use of occlusive dressings or wrappings.
3.) To keep azelaic acid away from the mouth, eyes and other mucous membranes. If it does come in contact with the eyes, they should wash their eyes with large amounts of water and consult a physician if eye irritation persists.
4.) If they have dark complexions, to report abnormal changes in skin color to their physician.
5.) Due in part to the low pH of azelaic acid, temporary skin irritation (pruritus, burning, or stinging) may occur when azelaic acid is applied to broken or inflamed skin, usually at the start of treatment. However, this irritation commonly subsides if treatment is continued. If it continues, azelaic acid should be applied only once a day, or the treatment should be stopped until these effects have subsided. If troublesome irritation persists, use should be discontinued, and patients should consult their physician.

➤*Gel:* Azelaic acid gel, 15%, is to be used only as directed by the physician.

Azelaic acid gel, 15%, is for external use only. It is not to be used orally, intravaginally, or for the eyes.

Cleanse affected area(s) with a very mild soap or a soapless cleansing lotion and pat dry with a soft towel before applying azelaic acid gel, 15%. Avoid alcoholic cleansers, tinctures and astringents, abrasives and peeling agents.

Avoid contact of azelaic acid gel, 15%, with the mouth, eyes, and other mucous membranes. If it does come in contact with the eyes, wash the eyes with large amounts of water and consult a physician if eye irritation persists.

The hands should be washed following application of azelaic acid gel, 15%.

Cosmetics may be applied after azelaic acid gel, 15%, has dried.

Skin irritation (eg, pruritus, burning, stinging) may occur during use of azelaic acid gel, 15%, usually during the first few weeks of treatment. If irritation is excessive or persists, use of azelaic acid gel, 15%, should be discontinued, and patients should consult their physician.

Avoid any foods and beverages that might provoke erythema, flushing, and blushing (including spicy food, alcoholic beverages, and thermally hot drinks, including hot coffee and tea).

Patients should report abnormal changes in skin color to their physician.

Avoid the use of occlusive dressings or wrappings.

BENZOYL PEROXIDE

Rx	**Benzoyl Peroxide 2½ Wash** (Various, eg, Glades)	**Liquid**: 2.5%	In 237 mL.
Rx	**Benzac AC Wash 2½** (Galderma)		Glycerin, water based. In 240 mL.
Rx	**Triaz** (Medicis)	**Liquid**: 3%	Glycerin, petrolatum, lavender extract, menthol. In 170.3 and 340.2 g.
Rx	**Brevoxyl Creamy Wash** (Stiefel)	**Liquid**: 4%	Glycerin, castor oil, parabens, mineral oil. In 170 g.
Rx	**Benzac AC Wash 5** (Galderma)	**Liquid**: 5%	Glycerin, water based. In 240 mL.
Rx	**Benzac W Wash 5** (Galderma)		Water based. In 120 and 240 mL.
Rx	**Benzoyl Peroxide 5% Wash** (Various, eg, Glades)		In 118, 148, and 237 mL.
Rx	**Triaz** (Medicis)	**Liquid**: 6%	Glycerin, petrolatum, lavender extract, menthol. In 170.3 and 340.2 g.
Rx	**Brevoxyl Creamy Wash** (Stiefel)	**Liquid**: 8%	Glycerin, castor oil, parabens, mineral oil. In 170 g.
Rx	**Triaz** (Medicis)	**Liquid**: 9%	Glycerin, white petrolatum, zinc lactate, lavender extract, menthol. In 340.2 g.
Rx	**Benzac AC Wash 10** (Galderma)	**Liquid**: 10%	Glycerin, water based. In 240 mL.
Rx	**Benzac W Wash 10** (Galderma)		Water based. In 240 mL.
Rx	**Benzoyl Peroxide 10% Wash** (Various, eg, Glades)		In 148 and 237 mL.
otc	**Oxy Oil-Free Maximum Strength Acne Wash** (GlaxoSmithKline)		Parabens, diazolidinyl urea. In 237 mL.
otc	**PanOxyl** (Stiefel)	**Bar**: 5%	Soap free. Cetostearyl alcohol, glycerin, castor oil, mineral oil. In 113 g.
otc	**PanOxyl** (Stiefel)	**Bar**: 10%	Soap free. Cetostearyl alcohol, glycerin, castor oil, mineral oil. In 113 g.
Rx	**Desquam-X 10** (Westwood Squibb)		Lactic acid, EDTA, sorbitol. In 106 g.
Rx	**Zoderm** (Doak)	**Cleanser**: 4.5%	Urea, glycerin, cetyl alcohol, glyceryl stearate, EDTA. In 400 mL.
		6.5%	Urea, glycerin, cetyl alcohol, glyceryl stearate, EDTA. In 400 mL.
		8.5%	Urea, glycerin, cetyl alcohol, glyceryl stearate, EDTA. In 400 mL.
otc	**Neutrogena Clear Pore** (Neutrogena)	**Cleanser/Mask**: 3.5%	Glycerin, titanium dioxide, EDTA, menthol. In 125 mL.
Rx	**Triaz Cleanser** (Medicis)	**Lotion**: 3%	Glycerin, glycolic acid, petrolatum, zinc lactate, menthol. In 170 and 340 g.
Rx	**Brevoxyl 4 Cleansing** (Stiefel)	**Lotion**: 4%	Cetyl alcohol. In 297 g.
Rx[a]	**Benzoyl Peroxide** (Various, eg, Thames)	**Lotion**: 5%	In 30 mL.
Rx	**Triaz Cleanser** (Medicis)	**Lotion**: 6%	Glycerin, glycolic acid, petrolatum, zinc lactate, menthol. In 170 and 340 g.

BENZOYL PEROXIDE

Rx	**Brevoxyl 8 Cleansing** (Stiefel)	**Lotion:** 8%	Cetyl alcohol. In 297 g.
Rx[a]	**Benzoyl Peroxide** (Various, eg, Thames)	**Lotion:** 10%	In 30 mL.
Rx	**Triaz Cleanser** (Medicis)		Glycerin, glycolic acid, petrolatum, zinc lactate, menthol. In 85, 170, and 340 g.
Rx	**Zoderm** (Doak)	**Cream:** 4.5%	Urea, glyceryl stearate, cetearyl alcohol, cetyl alcohol, EDTA. In 125 mL.
		6.5%	Urea, glyceryl stearate, cetearyl alcohol, cetyl alcohol, EDTA. In 125 mL.
		8.5%	Urea, glyceryl stearate, cetearyl alcohol, cetyl alcohol, EDTA. In 125 mL.
otc	**Clearasil Maximum Strength Acne Treatment** (Boots Healthcare)	**Cream:** 10%	Parabens. Vanishing. In 18 g.
Rx[a]	**Benzoyl Peroxide** (Various, eg, Glades)	**Gel:** 2.5%	In 60 g.
Rx	**Benzac W 2½** (Galderma)		EDTA, water based. In 60 and 90g.
Rx	**Benzac AC 2½** (Galderma)		Glycerin, EDTA, water based. In 60 and 90 g.
Rx	**PanOxyl AQ 2½** (Stiefel)		EDTA, methylparaben, glycerin. In 57 and 113 g.
Rx	**Triaz** (Medicis)	**Gel:** 3%	Glycerin, zinc lactate, EDTA. In 42.5 g.
Rx	**Brevoxyl-4** (Stiefel)	**Gel:** 4%	Cetyl alcohol, stearyl alcohol. In 42.5 and 90 g.
Rx	**Zoderm** (Doak)	**Gel:** 4.5%	Urea, EDTA, glycerin. In 125 mL.
Rx[a]	**Benzoyl Peroxide** (Various, eg, Glades)	**Gel:** 5%	In 60 and 90 g.
Rx	**Benzac AC 5** (Galderma)		Glycerin, EDTA, water based. In 60 and 90 g.
Rx	**Benzac 5** (Galderma)		12% alcohol. In 60 g.
Rx	**Benzac W 5** (Galderma)		EDTA, water based. In 60 and 90 g.
Rx	**Desquam-E 5** (Westwood Squibb)		EDTA, water based. In 42.5 g.
Rx	**Desquam-X 5** (Westwood Squibb)		EDTA, water based. In 42.5 and 85 g.
Rx	**PanOxyl 5** (Stiefel)		12% alcohol. In 56.7 and 113.4 g.
Rx	**PanOxyl AQ 5** (Stiefel)		Methylparaben, glycerin, EDTA. In 56.7 and 113.4 g.
Rx	**Triaz** (Medicis)	**Gel:** 6%	Glycerin, cetyl stearyl alcohol, zinc lactate, EDTA. In 42.5 g.
Rx	**Zoderm** (Doak)	**Gel:** 6.5%	Urea, EDTA, glycerin. In 125 mL.
Rx	**Clinac BPO** (Ferndale)	**Gel:** 7%	EDTA. In 45 and 90 g.
Rx	**Brevoxyl-8** (Stiefel)	**Gel:** 8%	Cetyl alcohol, stearyl alcohol. In 42.5 and 90 g.
Rx	**Zoderm** (Doak)	**Gel:** 8.5%	Urea, EDTA, glycerin. In 125 mL.
Rx	**Triaz** (Medicis)	**Gel:** 9%	Cetyl stearyl alcohol, glycolic acid, zinc lactate, EDTA. In 42.5 g.
otc	**Acne Clear** (Altaire)	**Gel:** 10%	EDTA. In 45 g.
Rx[a]	**Benzoyl Peroxide** (Various, eg, Glades)		In 60 and 90 g.
Rx	**Benzac AC 10** (Galderma)		Glycerin, EDTA, water based. In 60 and 90 g.
Rx	**Benzac 10** (Galderma)		12% alcohol. In 60 g.
Rx	**Benzac W 10** (Galderma)		Water based. In 60 and 90 g.
Rx	**Benzagel Wash** (Dermik)		14% alcohol. In 60 g.
Rx	**Desquam-E 10** (Westwood Squibb)		EDTA, water based. In 42.5 g.
Rx	**Desquam-X 10** (Westwood Squibb)		EDTA, water based. In 42.5 and 85 g.
Rx	**PanOxyl 10** (Stiefel)		20% alcohol. In 56.7 and 113.4 g.
Rx	**PanOxyl AQ 10** (Stiefel)		Methylparaben, EDTA, glycerin. In 56.7 and 113.4 g.
Rx	**Triaz** (Medicis)		Glycerin, glycolic acid, cetyl stearyl alcohol, zinc lactate, EDTA. In 42.5 g.

[a] Product available *otc* or *Rx*, depending on product labeling.

BENZOYL PEROXIDE — TOPICAL

Indications

➤*Acne:* Treatment of mild to moderate acne vulgaris.

Administration and Dosage

➤*Cleansers:* Wash once or twice daily. Wet skin areas to be treated prior to administration. Rinse thoroughly and pat dry. Control amount of drying or peeling by modifying dose frequency or concentration. Adjust frequency of use to obtain the desired clinical response. Clinically visible improvement will normally occur by the third week of therapy. Maximum lesion reduction may be expected after approximately 8 to 12 weeks of drug use. Continuing use of the drug is normally required to maintain a satisfactory clinical response.

➤*Other doseforms:* Apply once or twice daily. After cleansing skin, smooth small amount over affected area. If bothersome dryness or peeling occurs, reduce dose frequency or drug concentration. If excessive stinging or burning occurs after any single application, remove with mild soap and water; resume use the next day.

➤*Storage/Stability:* Store at room temperature 15° to 30°C (59° to 86°F).

Actions

➤*Pharmacology:* The effectiveness of benzoyl peroxide in the treatment of acne vulgaris is primarily attributable to its antibacterial activity, especially with respect to *Propionibacterium acnes*, the predominant organism in sebaceous follicles and comedones. The antibacterial activity of this compound is presumably because of the release of active or free-radical oxygen capable of oxidizing bacterial proteins. In acne patients treated topically with benzoyl peroxide, resolution of the acne usually coincides with reduction in the levels of *P. acnes* and free fatty acids (FFA). Mild desquamation is another observed action of topically applied benzoyl peroxide and may also play a role in the drug's effectiveness in acne. Studies also indicate that topical benzoyl peroxide may exert a sebostatic effect with a resultant reduction of skin surface lipids.

➤*Pharmacokinetics:* Benzoyl peroxide is absorbed by the skin, where it is metabolized to benzoic acid and then excreted as benzoate in the urine.

Contraindications

Hypersensitivity to benzoyl peroxide or any components of the products. Cross-sensitivity may occur with benzoic acid derivatives (see Precautions).

Warnings

➤*Sun exposure:* When using this product, avoid unnecessary sun exposure and use a sunscreen.

➤*Carcinogenesis:* Based upon considerable evidence, benzoyl peroxide is not considered to be a carcinogen. However, in one study, using mice known to be highly susceptible to cancer, there was evidence for benzoyl peroxide as a tumor promoter. The clinical significance of this is unknown.

BENZOYL PEROXIDE — TOPICAL

➤*Pregnancy: Category C.* It is not known whether benzoyl peroxide can cause fetal harm when administered to a pregnant woman or can affect reproductive capacity. However, there are no available data on the effect of benzoyl peroxide on the later growth, development, and functional maturation of the unborn child. Use in pregnant women only if clearly needed.

➤*Lactation:* It is not known whether this drug is excreted in breast milk. Administer with caution to nursing mothers.

➤*Children:* Safety and efficacy in children younger than 12 years of age have not been established.

Precautions

➤*External use only:* Avoid contact with eyes, eyelids, lips, mucous membranes, and highly inflamed or damaged skin. If accidental contact occurs, rinse with water.

➤*Irritation:* If severe irritation develops, consult a doctor, discontinue use, and institute appropriate therapy. After the reaction clears, treatment may often be resumed with less frequent application.

➤*Bleaching effect:* Benzoyl peroxide is an oxidizing agent; it may bleach hair and colored fabric.

➤*Cross-sensitization:* With benzoic acid derivatives (eg, cinnamon, certain topical anesthetics), cross-sensitization may occur.

Drug Interactions

➤*Tretinoin:* Concomitant use may cause significant skin irritation.

Adverse Reactions

Excessive drying, manifested by marked peeling, erythema, possible edema, and allergic contact sensitization/dermatitis.

Overdosage

➤*Symptoms:* Excessive scaling, erythema, or edema.

➤*Treatment:* Discontinue use. If reaction is caused by excessive use and not allergy, cautiously reinstate at reduced dosage after signs and symptoms subside. To hasten resolution of adverse effects, use emollients, cool compresses, and/or topical corticosteroids.

Patient Information

Keep away from eyes, mouth, inside of nose and mucous membranes. If contact occurs, rinse with water.

May cause transitory feeling of warmth or slight stinging. Expect dryness and peeling; if excessive redness or discomfort occurs, decrease or discontinue use temporarily. If excessive irritation develops, discontinue use and contact a physician.

Avoid other sources of skin irritation (eg, sunlight, sun lamps, other topical acne medications) unless directed by a physician.

Avoid contact with hair or colored fabric; bleaching may occur.

Normal use of water-based cosmetics is permissible.

BENZOYL PEROXIDE COMBINATIONS

Rx	**Sulfoxyl Regular** (Stiefel)	**Lotion**: 5% benzoyl peroxide, 2% sulfur	Stearic acid, zinc laurate. In 59 mL.
Rx	**Sulfoxyl Strong** (Stiefel)	**Lotion**: 10% benzoyl peroxide, 5% sulfur	Stearic acid, zinc laurate. In 59 mL.
Rx	**Duac** (Stiefel)	**Gel**: 5% benzoyl peroxide, 1% clindamycin	EDTA, glycerin, methylparaben. In 45 g.
Rx	**BenzaClin** (Dermik)		In 25 g.
Rx	**Erythromycin-Benzoyl Peroxide** (Various, eg, Clay-Park)	**Gel**: 5% benzoyl peroxide, 3% erythromycin	In 23 and 46 g.
Rx	**Benzamycin** (Dermik)		20% alcohol. In 0.8, 23, and 46 g.
Rx	**Benzamycin Pak** (Dermik)		SD alcohol 40B. In 0.8 g pouches. In 60s.

BENZOYL PEROXIDE COMBINATIONS — TOPICAL

Indications

➤*Acne vulgaris:* Topical treatment of acne vulgaris.

➤*Acne vulgaris, inflamed (Duac* only): Topical treatment of inflammatory acne vulgaris.

Administration and Dosage

➤*Sulfoxyl Lotion,* regular and strong: Apply the medication to the affected areas once a day during the first week, and then twice daily thereafter as tolerated. Adjust frequency of use to desired clinical response. Cleanse the affected areas with a nonmedicated soap prior to application. Improvement is typically seen by the third week of therapy. Maximum lesion reduction can be seen in approximately 8 to 12 weeks. Continue use of drug to maintain satisfactory response.

➤*Duac*: Apply once daily in the evening to the affected areas after the skin is thoroughly washed and patted dry.

➤*Benzamycin/Benzamycin Pak* and *BenzaClin*: Apply twice daily, morning and evening to affected areas after the skin is thoroughly washed and patted dry.

➤*Preparation of gel:*

Benzamycin Pak – Instruct patient to mix 2 separate components in foil pouch before applying this medication.

BenzaClin – Prior to dispensing, add purified water to the vial of powder (up to the mark) and shake until contents dissolve. Add this solution to the gel and stir until homogenous.

Benzamycin – Prior to dispensing, add ethyl alcohol (70%) to the vial of powder (up to the mark) and shake until contents dissolve. Add this solution to the gel and stir until homogenous.

➤*Storage/Stability:*

Sulfoxyl Lotion regular and strong – Store at room temperature 15° to 30°C (59° to 86°F). Shake well.

Duac – Before dispensing, store in a cold place preferably a refrigerator, between 2° to 8°C (36° to 46°F). Do not freeze. Once dispensed, store in room temperature up to 25°C (77°F) with a 2 month expiration date, discard any unused medication.

Benzamycin Pak – Store at room temperature 20° to 25°C (68° to 77°F). Keep away from heat and any open flame.

Benzamycin, BenzaClin – Prior to reconstitution store at room temperature 20° to 25°C (68° to 77°F). After reconstitution, store refrigerated at 2° to 8°C (36° to 46°F). Do not freeze. Following mixing, *BenzaClin* gel is good for 2 months. *Benzamycin* is good for 3 months; discard any unused medication after expiration date.

Actions

➤*Pharmacology:*

Benzoyl peroxide – Benzoyl peroxide is an antibacterial agent and has been shown to be effective against *Propionibacterium acnes*, an anaerobe found in sebaceous follicles and comedones. The antibacterial action of benzoyl peroxide is believed to be due to the release of active oxygen, it also has a keratolytic and desquamative effect, which may also contribute to its efficacy. When benzoyl peroxide is applied to the skin, it is absorbed and converted to benzoic acid.

Erythromycin/Clindamycin – Erythromycin and clindamycin are antibiotics that reduce lesions of acne vulgaris in part due to the antibacterial activity; however, the exact mechanism is not fully known. Erythromycin and clindamycin act by inhibition of protein synthesis in susceptible organisms by reversibly binding to 50 S ribosomal subunits, thereby inhibiting translocation of aminoacyl transfer-RNA and inhibiting polypeptide synthesis. Antagonism has been demonstrated in vitro between erythromycin, lincomycin, chloramphenicol, and clindamycin.

➤*Pharmacokinetics:* Benzoyl peroxide has been shown to be absorbed by the skin where it is converted to benzoic acid. Less than 2% of the dose enters systemic circulation as benzoic acid. Mean systemic bioavailability of topical clindamycin is suggested to be less than 1%.

Drug resistance – There are reports of an increase of *Propionibacterium acnes* resistance to clindamycin in the treatment of acne. In patients with *P. acnes* resistant to clindamycin, the clindamycin component may provide no additional benefit beyond benzoyl peroxide alone.

Contraindications

History of hypersensitivity to erythromycin, clindamycin, benzoyl peroxide, sulfur, or to any of its components.

➤*Duac/BenzaClin*: Hypersensitivity to any of its components or to lincomycin; history of regional enteritis, ulcerative colitis, or antibiotic-associated colitis.

Warnings

➤*Colitis:* Orally and parenterally administered antibacterial agents, including erythromycin and clindamycin have been associated with severe colitis, which may result in patient death. Use of the topical formulation results in absorption of the antibiotic from the skin surface. Diarrhea, bloody diarrhea, and colitis (including pseudomembranous colitis) have been reported with topical and systemic use of antibiotics. The colitis is characterized by severe persistent diarrhea and severe abdominal cramps and may be associated with the passage of blood and mucus. Endoscopic examination may reveal pseudomembranous colitis, stool culture for *Clostridium difficile* and stool assay for *C. difficile* toxin may be helpful diagnostically. When severe diarrhea occurs, discontinue the drug and institute therapeutic mea-

BENZOYL PEROXIDE COMBINATIONS — TOPICAL

sures. Diarrhea, colitis, and pseudomembranous colitis have been known to occur up to several weeks after cessation of oral and parenteral antibiotic therapy.

Mild cases of pseudomembranous colitis usually respond to drug discontinuation. In moderate to severe cases, consider management with fluids and electrolytes, protein supplementation and treatment with an antibacterial drug clinically effective against *C. difficile* colitis.

➤*Concomitant therapy:* Use concomitant topical acne therapy with caution because a possible cumulative irritancy effect may occur, especially with the use of peeling, desquamating, or abrasive agents. Clindamycin and erythromycin containing products should not be used in combination. In vitro studies have shown antagonism between these 2 antimicrobials. The clinical significance of this is not known.

➤*Carcinogenesis:* Benzoyl peroxide has been shown to be a tumor promoter and progression agent in a number of animal studies. The clinical significance of this is unknown. Benzoyl peroxide in acetone at doses of 5 to 10 mg administered twice per week induced skin tumors in transgenic mice in a study using 20 weeks of topical treatment.

➤*Mutagenesis:* Benzoyl peroxide has been found to cause DNA strand breaks in a variety of mammalian cell types, to be mutagenic in *Salmonella typhimurium* tests by some but not all investigators, and to cause sister chromatid exchanges in Chinese hamster ovary cells.

➤*Pregnancy: Category C.* There are no adequate and well-controlled trials in pregnant women. Use during pregnancy only if clearly needed.

➤*Lactation:* It is not known whether erythromycin, clindamycin, sulfur, or benzoyl peroxide is excreted in human milk after topical application. However, erythromycin and clindamycin is excreted in human milk following oral and parenteral administration. Because of the potential for serious adverse reactions in nursing infants, a decision should be made whether to discontinue nursing or to discontinue the drug, taking into account the importance of the drug to the mother.

➤*Children:* Safety and efficacy in children younger than 12 years of age have not been established.

Precautions

➤*For external use:* Use externally only. Avoid contact with the eyes, nose, mouth, and mucous membranes. Benzoyl peroxide may cause bleaching when in contact with hair, fabrics, or carpeting.

➤*Superinfection:* The use of antibiotic agents (especially prolonged or repeated therapy) may be associated with the overgrowth of nonsusceptible organisms including fungi. Such overgrowth may lead to a secondary infection. If this occurs, discontinue use and take appropriate measures.

Adverse Reactions

Topical Antibiotic and Benzoyl Peroxide Combination Adverse Reactions (%)[a]

Adverse reaction	*BenzaClin* gel (N = 420)	*Benzamycin* gel	*Benzamycin Pak* gel (N = 236)	*Duac* gel (N = 397) (mild to moderate)	Erythromycin-benzoyl peroxide gel	*Sulfoxyl* lotion, *Regular* and *Strong*
Application site reaction	3	—	—	—	—	—
Blepharitis	—	—	1.7	—	—	—
Burning sensation	—	✓	2.5	5/< 1	✓	—
Dry skin	12	3	7.6	19/1	3	—
Erythema	1	✓	2.5	26/5	✓	5
Eye inflammation	—	✓	—	—	✓	—
Eye irritation	—	✓	—	—	✓	—
Face inflammation	—	✓	—	—	✓	—
Irritation	—	✓	—	—	✓	—
Itching	—	✓	—	—	✓	—
Nose inflammation	—	✓	—	—	✓	—
Oiliness	—	✓	—	—	✓	—
Peeling	2	✓	0.5	17/2	✓	5
Photosensitivity reaction (eg, sunburn, stinging with sun exposure	1	—	1.3	—	—	—
Pruritus	2	—	1.7	—	—	—
Skin discoloration	—	✓	—	—	✓	—
Stinging			2.5	—	—	—
Tenderness	—	✓	—	—	✓	—
Urticarial reaction	—	3	—	—	3	—

[a] All events; data are pooled from separate studies and are not necessarily comparable.
— = not applicable
✓ = Incidence not provided.

Patient Information

Benzoyl peroxide may bleach hair, fabrics, or carpets.

Patients should not use any other topical acne preparation unless otherwise directed by a physician.

This medication is to be used externally. Avoid eyes, nose, mouth, and mucous membranes.

Inform patients to mix the *Benzamycin Pak* prior to use. The medication is dispensed in a foil pouch containing medication in 2 separate compartments. Mix contents thoroughly in palm of hand prior to application.

Excessive or prolonged exposure to sunlight should be limited.

After application of medicine, be sure to wash hands.

BenzaClin should be stored in a refrigerator; discard any unused portion after 2 months. *Duac* should be stored at room temperature with a 2 month expiration. *Benzamycin* should be refrigerated and discarded after 3 months.

CLINDAMYCIN, TOPICAL

Rx	**Clindamycin Phosphate** (Various, eg, Fougera)	Gel: 1%	In 30 and 60 g.
Rx	**Cleocin T** (Pharmacia & Upjohn)		Methylparaben. In 30 and 60 g.
Rx	**Clindagel** (Galderma)		Methylparaben. In 7.5, 42, and 77 g.
Rx	**ClindaMax** (PharmaDerm)		Methylparaben. In 30 and 60 g.
Rx	**Clindamycin Phosphate** (Various, eg, Fougera)	Lotion: 1%	In 60 mL.
Rx	**Cleocin T** (Pharmacia & Upjohn)		2.5% cetostearyl alcohol, glycerin, 2.5% isostearyl alcohol, 0.3% methylparaben. In 60 mL.
Rx	**ClindaMax** (PharmaDerm)		2.5% cetostearyl alcohol, glycerin, 2.5% isostearyl alcohol, 0.3% methylparaben. In 60 mL.

CLINDAMYCIN, TOPICAL

Rx	**Clindamycin Phosphate** (Various, eg, Fougera, Morton Groves)	**Solution, topical:** 1%	In 30 and 60 mL.
Rx	**Cleocin T** (Pharmacia & Upjohn)		50% isopropyl alcohol. In 30 and 60 mL and single-use pledget applicators.
Rx	**Clindets** (Stiefel Labs)		52% isopropyl alcohol. In 1 mL pledgets.
Rx	**Evoclin** (Connetics)	**Foam:** 1%	Cetyl alcohol, dehydrated alcohol (ethanol 58%), stearyl alcohol. In 50 g.[a]

[a] Pressurized with a hydrocarbon (propane/butane) propellant.

CLINDAMYCIN PHOSPHATE — TOPICAL

Indications

➤*Acne:* Treatment of acne vulgaris. In view of the potential for diarrhea, bloody diarrhea, and pseudomembranous colitis, consider whether other agents are more appropriate.

Administration and Dosage

➤*Approved by the FDA:* July 9, 1980.

Apply a thin film of clindamycin topical solution, topical lotion, or topical gel (except *Clindagel*) twice daily to the affected area.

Apply a thin film of *Clindagel* gel or clindamycin topical foam once daily to the affected areas. Use enough to cover the affected area lightly.

➤*Pledget:* More than 1 pledget may be used. Each pledget should be used only once and then discarded. Remove pledget from foil just before use. Do not use if the seal is broken.

➤*Foam:* Apply once daily to affected area after the skin is washed with mild soap and allowed to dry fully. Use enough to cover the entire affected area.

➤*Storage/Stability:*

Gel –

Cleocin T: Store at controlled room temperature, 20° to 25°C (68° to 77°F). Protect from freezing.

Clindagel: Store at controlled room temperature, 20° to 25°C (68° to 77°F); excursions permitted between 15° and 30°C (59° and 86°F). Do not store in direct sunlight.

Clindamax : Store at controlled room temperature, 15° to 30°C (59° to 86°F). Protect from freezing.

Lotion –

Clindamax lotion: Store at controlled room temperature, 15° to 30°C (59° to 86°F). Protect from freezing.

Cleocin T lotion: Store at controlled room temperature, 20° to 25°C (68° to 77°F). Protect from freezing.

Foam –

Evoclin: Flammable. Avoid fire, flame, or smoking during and immediately following application.

Contents under pressure. Do not puncture or incinerate. Do not expose to heat or store at temperature above 49°C (120°F).

Keep out of the reach of children.

Solution –

Cleocin T: Store at controlled room temperature, 20° to 25°C (68° to 77°F). Protect from freezing.

Clindets: Store at controlled room temperature, 15° to 30°C (59° to 86°F).

Actions

➤*Pharmacology:* Although clindamycin phosphate is inactive in vitro, rapid in vivo hydrolysis converts this compound to the antibacterially active clindamycin.

Cross resistance has been demonstrated between clindamycin and lincomycin.

Antagonism has been demonstrated between clindamycin and erythromycin.

Clindamycin activity has been demonstrated in comedones from acne patients. Clindamycin in vitro inhibits all *Propionibacterium acnes* cultures tested (minimum inhibitory concentrations [MICs], 0.4 mcg/mL). Free fatty acids on the skin surface have been decreased from approximately 14% to 2% following application of clindamycin.

➤*Pharmacokinetics:*

Absorption/Distribution – Following multiple topical applications of clindamycin phosphate at a concentration equivalent to clindamycin 10 mg/mL in an isopropyl alcohol and water solution, very low levels of clindamycin are present in the serum (0 to 3 ng/mL), and less than 0.2% of the dose is recovered in urine as clindamycin.

The mean concentration of antibiotic activity in extracted comedones after application of clindamycin topical solution for 4 weeks was 597 mcg/g of comedonal material (range, 0 to 1,490).

Clindagel: In an open-label, parallel-group study of 24 patients with acne vulgaris, once-daily topical administration of approximately 3 to 12 g/day of clindamycin gel for 5 days resulted in peak plasma clindamycin concentrations that were less than 5.5 ng/mL.

Foam: In an open-label, parallel-group study in 24 patients with acne vulgaris, 12 patients (3 men and 9 women) applied 4 g of clindamycin foam once daily for 5 days, and 12 patients (7 men and 5 women) applied 4 g of *Clindagel* (1%) once daily for 5 days. On day 5, the mean peak drug concentration (C_{max}) and area under the curve ($AUC_{0\ to\ 12}$) were 23% and 9% lower, respectively, for clindamycin foam than for clindamycin 1% topical gel.

Excretion –

Gel: Following multiple applications of clindamycin gel, less than 0.04% of the total dose was excreted in the urine.

Foam: Following multiple applications of clindamycin foam, less than 0.024% of the total dose was excreted unchanged in the urine over 12 hours on day 5.

➤*Microbiology:* Although clindamycin phosphate is inactive in vitro, rapid in vivo hydrolysis converts this compound to clindamycin, which has antibacterial activity. Clindamycin inhibits bacteria protein synthesis at the ribosomal level by binding to the 50S ribosomal subunit and affecting the process of peptide chain initiation. In vitro studies indicated that clindamycin inhibited all tested *Propionibacterium acnes* cultures at an MIC of 0.4 mcg/mL. Cross-resistance has been demonstrated between clindamycin and erythromycin.

Contraindications

Hypersensitivity to preparations containing clindamycin or lincomycin, history of regional enteritis or ulcerative colitis, or history of antibiotic-associated colitis.

Warnings

➤*Colitis:* Orally and parenterally administered clindamycin has been associated with severe colitis, which may result in patient death. Use of the topical formulation of clindamycin results in absorption of the antibiotic from the skin surface. Diarrhea, bloody diarrhea, and colitis (including pseudomembranous colitis) have been reported with the use of topical and systemic clindamycin.

Studies indicate a toxin(s) produced by *Clostridia* is a primary cause of antibiotic-associated colitis. The colitis is usually characterized by severe persistent diarrhea and severe abdominal cramps and may be associated with the passage of blood and mucus. Endoscopic examination may reveal pseudomembranous colitis. Stool culture for *Clostridium difficile* and stool assay for *C. difficile* toxin may be helpful diagnostically.

When significant diarrhea occurs, discontinue the drug. Consider large bowel endoscopy to establish a definitive diagnosis in cases of severe diarrhea.

Antiperistaltic agents (eg, opiates, diphenoxylate with atropine) may prolong and worsen the condition. Vancomycin has been found to be effective in the treatment of antibiotic-associated pseudomembranous colitis produced by *C. difficile*. The usual adult dosage is 500 mg to 2 g of vancomycin orally per day in 3 to 4 divided doses administered for 7 to 10 days. Cholestyramine or colestipol resins bind vancomycin in vitro. If a resin and vancomycin are to be administered concurrently, it may be advisable to separate the time of administration of each drug.

Diarrhea, colitis, and pseudomembranous colitis have been observed to begin up to several weeks following cessation of oral and parenteral therapy with clindamycin.

Foam – Mild cases of pseudomembranous colitis usually respond to drug discontinuation alone. In moderate to severe cases, consider management with fluids and electrolytes, protein supplementation, and treatment with an antibacterial drug clinically effective against *C. difficile* colitis.

➤*Pregnancy:* *Category B.*

There are no adequate and well-controlled studies in pregnant women. Because animal reproduction studies are not always predictive of human response, use this drug during pregnancy only if clearly needed.

➤*Lactation:* It is not known whether clindamycin is excreted in human milk. However, orally and parenterally administered clindamycin has been reported to appear in breast milk. Because of the potential for serious adverse reactions in breast-feeding infants, decide whether to discontinue breast-feeding or the drug, taking into account the importance of the drug to the mother.

➤*Children:* Safety and efficacy in children younger than 12 years of age have not been established.

Precautions

➤*For external use only:* Clindamycin topical solution (including pledgets) contains an alcohol base that will cause burning and irritation of the eye. In the event of accidental contact with sensitive surfaces (eg, abraded skin, eye, mucous membranes), bathe with copious amounts of cool tap water. The solution has an unpleasant taste; exercise caution when applying medication around the mouth.

Avoid contact of clindamycin foam with eyes. If contact occurs, rinse eyes thoroughly with water.

➤*Special risk:* Prescribe clindamycin with caution in atopic individuals.

CLINDAMYCIN PHOSPHATE — TOPICAL

Drug Interactions

➤*Neuromuscular-blocking agents:* Clindamycin has been shown to have neuromuscular-blocking properties that may enhance the action of other neuromuscular-blocking agents; use clindamcyin with caution in patients receiving such agents.

Adverse Reactions

See Warnings for more information.

Abdominal pain and GI disturbances, as well as gram-negative folliculitis, have been reported in association with the use of topical formulations of clindamycin.

➤*Dermatologic:*

Topical Clindamycin Adverse Reactions

Treatment-emergent adverse reaction	Number of patients reporting reactions		
	Solution (n = 553) (%)	Gel (n = 148) (%)	Lotion (n = 160) (%)
Burning	62 (11%)	15 (10%)	17 (11%)
Burning/itching	60 (11%)	NR[a]	NR
Dryness	105 (19%)	34 (23%)	29 (18%)
Erythema	86 (16%)	10 (7%)	22 (14%)
Itching	36 (7%)	15 (10%)	17 (11%)
Oiliness/Oily skin	8 (1%)	26 (18%)	12[b] (10%)
Peeling	61 (11%)	NR	11 (7%)

[a] NR = not recorded.
[b] Of 126 subjects.

➤*Clindagel:*

***Clindagel* Adverse Reactions in ≥ 1% of Patients**

Adverse reaction	Number (%) of patients	
	Clindagel (once daily) (n = 168)	Vehicle gel (once daily) (n = 84)
Contact dermatitis	0 (0%)	1 (1.2%)
Dermatitis	0 (0%)	1 (1.2%)
Dry skin	0 (0%)	0 (0%)
Erythematous rash	0 (0%)	0 (0%)
Folliculitis	0 (0%)	1 (1.2%)
Fungal dermatitis	0 (0%)	1 (1.2%)
Peeling	1 (0.6%)	0 (0%)
Photosensitivity reaction	0 (0%)	1 (1.2%)
Pruritus	1 (0.6%)	1 (1.2%)
Skin and appendage disorders	0 (0%)	1 (1.2%)

➤*Foam:*

Clindamycin Foam Adverse Reactions Occurring in ≥ 1% of Patients

Adverse reaction	Number (%) of patients	
	Clindamycin foam (n = 439)	Vehicle foam (n = 154)
Application site burning	27 (6%)	14 (9%)
Application site dryness	4 (1%)	5 (3%)
Application site pruritus	5 (1%)	5 (3%)
Application site reaction, not otherwise specified	3 (1%)	4 (3%)
Headache	12 (3%)	1 (1%)

Overdosage

➤*Symptoms:* Topically applied clindamycin may be absorbed in sufficient amounts to produce systemic effects.

Patient Information

This medicine is for external use only. Advise patients to avoid contact with the eyes because burning or irritation can occur. Advise patients to wash the area with cool tap water if contact with the eyes or sensitive surfaces (eg, mucous membranes, scraped skin) occurs.

Advise patients that this medicine is not for ophthalmic, oral, or intravaginal use.

Advise patients that this medicine has an unpleasant taste and to use caution when applying this medicine around the mouth.

Advise patients to keep clindamycin out of the reach of children.

Advise patients to contact their doctors at once if severe diarrhea, stomach cramps/pain, or bloody stools occur. This could be a symptom of a serious side effect requiring immediate medical attention. Advise patients not to treat diarrhea without consulting their doctors.

➤*Foam:* Contents under pressure. Advise patients not to puncture or incinerate container, expose to heat, or store at temperatures above 49°C (120°F).

Advise patients not to dispense clindamycin foam directly onto hands or face, because the foam will begin to melt on contact with warm skin.

ERYTHROMYCIN, TOPICAL

Rx	**Erythromycin** (Various, eg, Morton Grove)	**Solution:** 2%	Contains alcohol. In 60 mL.
Rx	**A/T/S** (Medicis)		66% alcohol. In 60 mL.
Rx	**Eryderm 2%** (Abbott)		77% alcohol. In 60 mL with applicator.
Rx	**A/T/S** (Medicis)	**Gel:** 2%	92% alcohol. In 30 g.
Rx	**Emgel** (GlaxoSmithKline)		77% alcohol. In 27 and 50 g.
Rx	**Erythromycin** (Various, eg, Glades)		Contains alcohol. In 30 and 60 g.
Rx	**Akne-Mycin** (Healthpoint)	**Ointment:** 2%	Cetostearyl alcohol, petrolatum, mineral oil. In 25 g.
Rx	**Ery Pads** (Glades)	**Pledgets:** 2%	60.5% alcohol. In 60s.

ERYTHROMYCIN — TOPICAL

Indications

➤*Acne:* For the treatment of acne vulgaris.

Administration and Dosage

➤*Gel:* Erythromycin topical gel should be applied sparingly as a thin film to affected area(s) once or twice a day after the skin is thoroughly cleansed and patted dry. If there has been no improvement after 6 to 8 weeks, or if the condition becomes worse, treatment should be discontinued and the physician should be reconsulted. Spread the medication lightly rather than rubbing it in. There are no data directly comparing the safety and efficacy of twice-daily versus daily dosing.

➤*Topical solution:* Apply to the affected area(s) each morning and evening after the skin is thoroughly washed with warm water and soap and patted dry. Use enough solution to thoroughly wet the affected area(s). The hands should be washed after application. Acne lesions on the face, neck, shoulder, chest and back may be treated in this manner.

When using the *Dab-O-Matic* applicator to apply erythromycin topical solution, it should be moistened first by holding the bottle upside down and pressing once on the applicator surface with a clean finger. Then erythromycin topical solution can be applied with the applicator to the affected area(s) using a dabbing motion. The bottle should be closed tightly after each use.

➤*Pledgets:* Rub over the affected area twice a day after skin is thoroughly washed with warm water and soap and patted dry. Acne lesions on the face, neck, shoulder, chest, and back may be treated in this manner. Additional pledgets may be used, if needed. Each pledget should be used once and discarded. Close jar tightly after each use.

➤*Ointment:* Apply to the affected area twice daily, morning and evening.

➤*Storage/Stability:*

Gel – This medication is flammable; keep away from heat and flame. Store and dispense in original container. Keep tube tightly closed. Store between 15° and 25°C (59° and 77°F).

ERYTHROMYCIN — TOPICAL

Topical solution – This medication is flammable; keep away from heat and flame. Store in tight, light-resistant container at controlled room temperature, 15° to 30°C (59° to 86°F).

Pledgets – Keep jar tightly closed. Store at controlled room temperature, between 15° and 30°C (59° and 86°F).

Ointment – Store below 27°C (80°F).

Actions

➤*Pharmacology:* The exact mechanism by which topical erythromycin reduces lesions of acne vulgaris is not fully known; however, the effect appears to be caused by part to the antibacterial activity of the drug.

➤*Microbiology:* Erythromycin acts by inhibition of protein synthesis in susceptible organisms by reversibly binding to 50 S ribosomal subunits, thereby inhibiting translocation of aminoacyl transfer-RNA and inhibiting polypeptide synthesis. Antagonism has been demonstrated in vitro between erythromycin, and lincomycin, chloramphenicol, and clindamycin.

Contraindications

Hypersensitivity to erythromycin or to any of the other listed ingredients in the various preparations.

Warnings

➤*Pseudomembranous colitis:* Pseudomembranous colitis has been reported with nearly all antibacterial agents, including erythromycin, and may range in severity from mild to life-threatening. Therefore, it is important to consider this diagnosis in patients who present with diarrhea subsequent to the administration of antibacterial agents.

Treatment with antibacterial agents alters the normal flora of the colon and may permit overgrowth of clostridia. Studies indicate that a toxin produced by *Clostridium difficile* is 1 primary cause of "antibiotic-associated" colitis.

After the diagnosis of pseudomembranous colitis has been established, therapeutic measures should be initiated. Mild cases of pseudomembranous colitis usually respond to drug discontinuation alone. In moderate to severe cases, consider management with fluids and electrolytes, protein supplementation, and treatment with an antibacterial drug clinically effective against *C. difficile* colitis.

➤*Pregnancy: Category C* (topical solution) and *Category B* (other topical preparations).

There are no adequate and well-controlled studies in pregnant women. Because animal reproduction studies are not always predictive of human response, only use this drug in pregnancy if clearly needed. Erythromycin has been reported to cross the placental barrier in humans, but fetal plasma levels are generally low.

The safe use of topical erythromycin during pregnancy has not been established.

➤*Lactation:* It is not known whether erythromycin is excreted in human milk after topical application of gel, pledgets, or ointment. Erythromycin topical solution is excreted in breast milk, and erythromycin is excreted in human milk following oral and parenteral erythromyin administration. Therefore, caution should be exercised when erythromycin is administered to a breast-feeding woman.

The safe use of topical erythromycin during lactation has not been established.

➤*Children:* Safety and efficacy in children have not been established.

Precautions

➤*For external use only:* These formulations of erythromycin are for topical use only; they are not for ophthalmic use. Keep them out of the eyes, nose, and mouth and all mucous membranes. Use concomitant topical therapy with caution because a possible cumulative irritancy effect may occur, especially with the use of peeling, desquamating or abrasive agents.

Avoid contact with eyes and all mucous membranes.

➤*Superinfection:* The use of antibiotic agents may be associated with the overgrowth of antibiotic-resistant organisms. If this occurs, discontinue administration of the drug and take appropriate measures.

Adverse Reactions

The following local adverse reactions have been reported occasionally: peeling, dryness, burning, itching, desquamation, erythema, and oiliness. Irritation of the eyes and tenderness of the skin have also been reported with the topical use of erythromycin. A generalized urticarial reaction, possibly related to the use of erythromycin, which required systemic steroid therapy has been reported.

➤*Dermatologic:*

Gel – In controlled clinical trials, the incidence of burning associated with erythromycin topical gel was approximately 25%.

Ointment – In clinical trials, there was 1 report of a possible contact sensitization, which could not be confirmed. There were isolated reports of skin irritation, such as erythema and peeling.

Patient Information

- Patients should wash, rinse, and dry affected areas before application.
- Advise patients to wash their hands after application of medicine.
- This medication is to be used as directed by the physician. It is for external use only. Patients should avoid contact with the eyes, nose, mouth, and all mucous membranes.
- This medication should not be used for any disorder other than that for which it was prescribed.
- Patients should not use any other topical acne medication unless otherwise directed by their physicians.
- Patients should report to their physicians any signs of local adverse reactions.

METRONIDAZOLE

Rx	**MetroLotion** (Galderma)	**Lotion:** 0.75%	Benzyl alcohol, stearyl alcohol, glycerin, mineral oil. In 59 mL.
Rx	**Metronidazole** (Fougera)	**Cream:** 0.75%	Glycerin, benzyl alcohol, lactic acid. In 45 g.
Rx	**MetroCream** (Galderma)		Glycerin, benzyl alcohol. In 45 g.
Rx	**Noritate** (Dermik Labs)	**Cream:** 1%	Parabens, glycerin. In 30 g.
Rx	**MetroGel** (Galderma)	**Gel:** 0.75%	Parabens, EDTA. In 28.4 and 45 g.

METRONIDAZOLE — TOPICAL

Indications

➤*Rosacea:* Treatment of inflammatory papules, pustules, and erythema of rosacea.

➤*Unlabeled uses:* Topical metronidazole has been used as a gel or 1% solution or suspension to treat infected decubitus ulcers; perioral dermatitis has been treated with topical metronidazole gel or cream.

Administration and Dosage

Apply and rub in a thin film once (1% cream) or twice daily, morning and evening, to entire affected areas after washing.

Cleanse areas to be treated before application of topical metronidazole. Patients may use cosmetics after application of topical metronidazole 5 minutes after allowing medication to dry.

➤*Storage/Stability:* Store at controlled room temperature, 15° to 30°C (59° to 86°F) for 0.75% cream and gel; and 20° to 25°C (68° to 77°F) for 0.75% lotion and 1% cream.

Actions

➤*Pharmacology:* Metronidazole is classified therapeutically as an antiprotozoal and antibacterial agent. The mechanisms by which topical metronidazole acts in reducing inflammatory lesions of acne rosacea are unknown, but may include an antibacterial or an anti-inflammatory effect.

➤*Pharmacokinetics:* Bioavailability studies on administration of 1 g topical metronidazole (7.5 mg metronidazole) to the faces of 10 rosacea patients showed a maximum serum concentration of 66 ng/mL. This is about 100 times less than concentrations afforded by a single 250 mg oral tablet. Three patients had no detectable serum concentrations of metronidazole. The mean dose of gel applied during clinical studies was 600 mg (4.5 mg metronidazole) per application. Therefore, under normal usage levels, the formulation affords minimal serum concentrations. The time to peak plasma concentration (T_{max}) with detectable metronidazole was 8 to 12 hours after topical application.

Contraindications

History of hypersensitivity to metronidazole, parabens, or other ingredients.

Warnings

➤*Carcinogenesis:* In several long-term studies in mice, oral doses of approximately 225 mg/m²/day or greater (approximately 37 times the human topical dose on a mg/m² basis) were associated with an increase in pulmonary tumors and lymphomas. Several long-term oral studies in the rat have shown statistically significant increases in mammary and hepatic tumors at doses more than 885 mg/m²/day (144 times the topical human dose).

In 1 study, using albino hairless mice, intraperitoneal administration of metronidazole at a dose of 45 mg/m²/day (approximately 7 times the human topical dose on a mg/m² basis) was associated with an increase in ultraviolet radiation-induced skin carcinogenesis. Neither dermal carcinogenicity nor photocarcinogenicity studies have been performed with any topical metronidazole.

➤*Mutagenesis:* A dose-related increase in the frequency of micronuclei was observed in mice after intraperitoneal injections. An increase in chromosomal aberrations in peripheral blood lymphocytes was reported in patients with Crohn disease who were treated with 200 to 1,200 mg/day of metronidazole for 1 to 24 months.

METRONIDAZOLE — TOPICAL

➤*Pregnancy: Category B.* There has been no experience to date with the use of topical metronidazole in pregnant women. Metronidazole crosses the placental barrier and enters the fetal circulation rapidly. Since oral metronidazole is a carcinogen in some rodents, use during pregnancy only if clearly needed.

➤*Lactation:* After oral administration, metronidazole is excreted in breast milk in concentrations similar to those in plasma. Even though metronidazole blood levels are significantly lower than those achieved after oral metronidazole, discontinue nursing or the drug, taking into account the importance of the drug to the mother.

➤*Children:* Safety and efficacy in children have not been established.

Precautions

➤*Conjunctivitis:* Conjunctivitis associated with topical use of metronidazole on the face has been reported.

➤*For external use only:* Tearing of the eyes has occurred; avoid eye contact. If a reaction suggesting local irritation occurs, direct patients to use the medication less frequently, discontinue use temporarily, or discontinue use until further instructions.

➤*Blood dyscrasia:* Metronidazole is a nitroimidazole; use with care in patients with evidence of, or history of, blood dyscrasia.

Drug Interactions

➤*Anticoagulants:* Drug interactions are less likely with topical administration but should be kept in mind when topical metronidazole is prescribed for patients who are receiving anticoagulant treatment. Oral metronidazole may potentiate the anticoagulant effect of warfarin and coumarin resulting in a prolongation of prothrombin time.

Adverse Reactions

Topical Metronidazole Adverse Events (%)[a]

Adverse reaction	0.75% cream	1% cream (N = 200)	0.75% lotion (N = 71)	0.75% gel
Acne	–	✓	–	–
Burning/stinging	–	–	1	✓
Conjunctivitis	–	✓	–	–
Constipation	–	✓	–	–
Contact dermatitis	–	–	3	–
Dryness	✓	✓	0	✓
Erythema	< 3		6	
Eye irritation (eg, watering/ tearing)	✓	✓	✓	✓
Headache	–	✓	–	–
Local allergic reaction	–	✓	3	–
Metallic taste	✓	–	✓	✓
Nausea	✓	✓	✓	✓
Paresthesia	–	✓		–
Pruritus	< 3	–	1	–
Rash	–	✓	–	–
Severe flare of comedonal acne	–	✓	–	–
Skin irritation	< 3	✓	✓	✓
Tingling/ numbness of extremities	✓	✓	✓	✓
Transient redness	✓	–	✓	✓
Worsening of rosacea	< 3	✓	1	–

[a] All events; data are pooled from separate studies and are not necessarily comparable.
✓ = Incidence not provided.
– = not applicable.

Patient Information

For external use only. Avoid contact with the eyes.

Cleanse affected area(s) before applying the medication. Report any adverse reaction or irritation to your physician.

May apply cosmetics to face after medication is dry.

MUPIROCIN (Pseudomonic Acid A)

Rx	**Mupirocin** (Various, eg, Clay-Park, Teva)	**Ointment:** 2%	In a polyethylene glycol base. In 15, 22, and 30 g.
Rx	**Bactroban** (GlaxoSmithKline)	**Ointment:** 2% (20 mg/g)	Polyethylene glycol base. In 22 g.
Rx	**Centany** (OrthoNeutrogena)	**Ointment:** 2%	In a base containing castor oil and hard fat. In 15 and 30 g.
Rx	**Bactroban** (GlaxoSmithKline)	**Cream:** 2% mupirocin (2.15% as calcium)	Oil/water base. Benzyl alcohol, cetyl alcohol, stearyl alcohol. In 15 and 30 g.
Rx	**Bactroban Nasal** (GlaxoSmithKline)	**Ointment:** 2% mupirocin (2.15% as calcium)	Glycerin esters. In 1 g.

MUPIROCIN (Pseudomonic Acid A) — TOPICAL

Indications

➤*Topical Infection:*

Topical ointment – Impetigo caused by *Staphylococcus aureus*, beta-hemolytic streptococcus, and *Streptococcus pyogenes*.

Topical cream – Treatment of secondarily infected traumatic skin lesions (up to 10 cm in length or 100 cm^2 in area) caused by susceptible strains of *S. aureus* and *S. pyogenes*.

Nasal – Eradication of nasal colonization with methicillin-resistant *S. aureus* in adult patients and health care workers as part of a comprehensive infection control program to reduce infection risk among patients at high risk of methicillin-resistant *S. aureus* infection during institutional outbreaks of infections with this pathogen.

➤*Unlabeled uses:* Topical mupirocin may be effective in treating diaper dermatitis caused by *Candida*.

Administration and Dosage

➤*Topical ointment:* Apply a small amount to the affected area 3 times daily. The area may be covered with gauze dressing. Reevaluate those not showing a response in 3 to 5 days.

➤*Topical cream:* Apply a small amount to the affected area 3 times daily for 10 days. The area may be covered with gauze dressing. Reevaluate those not showing a response in 3 to 5 days.

➤*Nasal (12 years of age and older):* Divide approximately one half of the ointment from the single-use tube between the nostrils and apply twice daily (morning and evening) for 5 days.

After application, close nostrils by pressing together and releasing sides of the nose repeatedly for about 1 minute. The single-use tube will deliver a total of approximately 0.5 g of the ointment (approximately 0.25 g/nostril).

➤*Storage/Stability:* Store the topical ointment between 20° and 25°C (68° to 77°F), and store the nasal ointment and topical cream at or below 25°C (77°F). Do not freeze the cream.

Actions

➤*Pharmacology:* Mupirocin is an antibacterial agent produced by fermentation using the organism *Pseudomonas fluorescens*. Mupirocin is considered a topical antibacterial structurally unrelated to other agents, inhibits bacterial protein synthesis by reversibly and specifically binding to bacterial isoleucyl transfer-RNA synthetase. Mupirocin demonstrates no in vitro cross-resistance with other antimicrobials. However, when resistance does occur, it appears to result from the production of a modified isoleucyl-tRNA synthetase. High level plasmid-mediated resistance (MIC greater than 1024 mcg/mL) has been reported in some strains of *S. aureus* and coagulase negative staphylococci.

➤*Pharmacokinetics:*

Absorption/Distribution –

Cream: Systemic absorption of mupirocin through human intact skin is minimal. Systemic absorption was studied following application of mupirocin cream 3 times/day for 5 days to various skin lesions (greater than 10 cm in length or 100 cm^2 in area) in 16 adults (29 to 60 years of age) and 10 children (3 to 12 years of age). Some systemic absorption was observed by detection of the metabolite, monic acid in urine. More frequent occurrence of percutaneous absorption in children (90%) was found compared with adults (44%). However, urinary concentrations in children and adults were within range. Mupirocin is highly protein bound (more than 97%), and the effect of wound secretions on the MICs of mupirocin has not been determined.

Ointment: Mupirocin ointment applied to the lower arm of healthy male subjects followed by occlusion for 24 hours showed no measurable systemic absorption (less than 1.1 ng mupirocin/mL of whole blood).

Nasal: Following single or repeated intranasal applications of 0.2 g of mupirocin nasal 3 times/day for 3 days to adults showed no evidence of systemic absorption. A study in neonates and premature infants indicated that, unlike adults, significant systemic absorption occurred following intranasal administration. Mupirocin nasal has not been adequately studied in children less than 12 years of age.

MUPIROCIN (Pseudomonic Acid A) — TOPICAL

Metabolism / Excretion – Any mupirocin reaching the systemic circulation is rapidly metabolized, predominantly to inactive monic acid which is eliminated by renal excretion and demonstrates no antibacterial activity. The elimination half-life after IV administration was 20 to 40 minutes for mupirocin and 30 to 80 minutes for monic acid.

➤*Microbiology:* The aerobic isolates of *Staphylococcus aureus* (including methicillin-resistant and β-lactamase producing strains), *S. epidermidis, S. saprophyticus*, and *Streptococcus pyogenes* are susceptible to mupirocin in vitro. Mupirocin also has been found to be active against certain gram-negative bacteria.

Contraindications

Hypersensitivity reactions to any components of the products.

Warnings

➤*For external use only:* Avoid mucosal surfaces and contact with the eyes.

➤*Pregnancy: Category B.* There are no adequate and well-controlled studies in pregnant women. Use during pregnancy only if clearly needed.

➤*Lactation:* It is not known whether mupirocin is excreted in breast milk. Exercise caution when administering to a nursing woman.

➤*Children:* Safety and efficacy of mupirocin ointment and cream have been established in children 2 months to 16 years of age.

Safety in children younger than 12 years of age has not been established for mupirocin nasal.

Precautions

➤*Open wounds:* Polyethylene glycol can be absorbed from open wounds and damaged skin and is excreted by the kidney. Do not use if absorption of large quantities of polyethylene glycol is possible, especially if there is evidence of moderate or severe renal impairment.

➤*Prophylaxis:* There are insufficient data at this time to recommend use of mupirocin nasal for general prophylaxis of any infection in any patient population or to establish that this product is safe and effective as part of an intervention program to prevent autoinfection of high-risk patients from their own nasal colonization.

➤*Sensitivity reaction:* If a reaction suggesting sensitivity or chemical irritation occurs, discontinue treatment and institute appropriate alternative therapy.

➤*Superinfection:* Prolonged use of antibiotics may result in overgrowth of nonsusceptible organisms, including fungi.

Drug Interactions

Do not use mupirocin nasal concurrently with any other nasal products.

Adverse Reactions

Topical ointment – Burning, stinging, or pain (1.5%); itching (1%); rash, nausea, erythema, dry skin, tenderness, swelling, contact dermatitis, and increased exudate (less than 1%); systemic reactions (rare).

Topical cream – Headache (1.7%); rash, nausea (1.1%); abdominal pain, burning at application site, cellulitis, dermatitis, dizziness, pruritus, secondary wound infection, and ulcerative stomatitis (less than 1%).

Secondarily infected eczema: Adverse events thought to be possibly or probably drug-related are as follows: Nausea (4.9%); headache and burning at application site (3.6%); pruritus (2.4%); 1 report each of abdominal pain, bleeding secondary to eczema, pain secondary to eczema, hives, dry skin, and rash.

Nasal – Headache (9%); rhinitis (6%); respiratory disorder including upper respiratory tract congestion (5%); pharyngitis (4%); taste perversion (3%); burning/stinging, cough (2%); pruritus (1%); blepharitis, diarrhea, dry mouth, ear pain, epistaxis, nausea, rash (less than 1%).

Patient Information

This medication is for external use only. Avoid eyes and mucosal membranes.

Stop the medication and contact your doctor if irritation, severe itching or rash occurs.

If no improvement is seen within 3 to 5 days, contact your doctor.

The treated area may be covered by a gauze dressing.

➤*Nasal:* Press the sides of the nose together and gently massage after application to spread the ointment throughout the inside of the nostrils.

ANTIBIOTIC COMBINATIONS

	Product and Distributor	Polymyxin B Sulfate (units/g)	Neomycin (mg/g)[1]	Bacitracin Zinc (units/g)	Other	How Supplied
otc	**Lanabiotic Ointment** (Combe)	10,000	3.5	500	40 mg lidocaine	Aloe, lanolin, mineral oil, petrolatum. In 28 g.
otc	**Tri-Biozene Ointment** (Reese)				10 mg pramoxine HCl/g	White petrolatum. In 15 g.
otc	**Neosporin Plus Pain Relief Ointment** (Pfizer)					White petrolatum. In 15 and 30 g.
otc	**Betadine First Aid Antibiotics Plus Moisturizer Ointment** (Purdue Frederick)			500		Cholesterolized ointment base. In 14 g.
otc	**Double Antibiotic Ointment** (Fougera)					In ≈ 15 and ≈ 30 g, UD 0.9 g (144s).
otc	**Polysporin Ointment** (Pfizer)					White petrolatum base. In ≈ 15 and ≈ 30 g.
otc	**Betadine Plus First Aid Antibiotics and Pain Reliever Ointment** (Purdue Frederick)				10 mg pramoxine HCl/g	Cholesterolized ointment base. In 14 g.
otc	**Neosporin Plus Pain Relief Cream** (Pfizer)		3.5		10 mg pramoxine HCl/g	Methylparaben, mineral oil, white petrolatum. In 15 g.
otc	**Neosporin Original Ointment** (Pfizer)	5000		400		Cocoa butter, cottonseed oil, olive oil, white petrolatum. In 14 and 28 g, UD 0.9 g (10s).
otc	**Triple Antibiotic Ointment** (Various, eg, Alpharma)					In 15, 30, and 454 g.

[1] As base; equivalent to 5 mg neomycin sulfate.

ANTIBIOTIC COMBINATIONS — TOPICAL

Indications

➤*Topical infection / Pain:* Used as a first aid to help prevent skin infection and for the temporary relief of pain in minor cuts, wounds, scrapes, and burns.

Administration and Dosage

Clean the affected area. Apply a small amount of the antibiotic on the area 1 to 3 times/day. Do not use for longer than 1 week unless consulted by a physician. The affected area may be covered with a sterile bandage.

Actions

➤*Pharmacology:* The topical anti-infectives may be either bactericidal or bacteriostatic. Most inhibit protein synthesis. **Bacitracin** inhibits cell-wall synthesis.

Contraindications

Known sensitivity to any of the ingredients; use in the eyes.

Warnings

➤*Systemic therapy:* Deeper cutaneous infections may require systemic antibiotic therapy in addition to local treatment. Use caution when applying over large areas of the body for deep puncture wounds, animal bites, or serious burns.

➤*Neomycin toxicity:* Because of the potential nephrotoxicity and ototoxicity of neomycin, use with care in treating extensive burns, trophic ulceration, or other extensive conditions where absorption is possible. Do not apply more than once daily in burn cases where more than 20% of the body is affected. Especially if the patient has impaired renal function.

➤*External use:* For external use only. Do not use in or near the eyes, nose, mouth, mucous membranes, or apply over large areas of the body.

➤*Pregnancy: Category C* (bacitracin zinc/neomycin). There are no adequate and well-controlled studies in pregnant women. Use only when clearly needed and when the potential benefits outweigh the unknown potential hazards to the fetus. Ototoxicity is known to occur after oral, parenteral, and topical neomycin; however, it has not been reported to affect in utero exposure. Cranial nerve toxicity has been reported in the fetus follow-

Antibiotic Agents

ANTIBIOTIC COMBINATIONS — TOPICAL

ing exposure to other aminoglycosides (eg, kanamycin, streptomycin) and may potentially occur with neomycin.

Category B (polymyxin B). There are no adequate and well-controlled studies in pregnant women. Use during pregnancy only if clearly needed.

➤*Lactation:* It is not known whether **bacitracin zinc**, **polymyxin B**, or **neomycin** are excreted in breast milk. Exercise caution when applying on a breastfeeding woman. Neomycin has been reported to be excreted into the milk of lactating cows and ewes after a single 10 mg/kg IM dose; also small amounts of other aminoglycosides (eg, gentamicin) are excreted into breast milk and absorbed by the nursing infant.

➤*Children:* Safety and efficacy in children younger than 2 years of age have not been established.

Precautions

➤*Neomycin hypersensitivity:* Chronic application of neomycin sulfate to inflamed skin of individuals with allergic contact dermatitis and chronic dermatoses (eg, chronic otitis externa, stasis dermatitis) increases the possibility of sensitization. Low grade reddening with swelling, dry scaling, itching, or a failure to heal are usually manifestations of this hypersensitivity. Discontinue use if these symptoms appear and avoid neomycin-containing products thereafter.

➤*Superinfection:* Prolonged use of antibiotics may result in overgrowth of nonsusceptible organisms, particularly fungi. Such overgrowth may lead to a secondary infection. Discontinue the drug and take appropriate measures if superinfection occurs.

Adverse Reactions

Bacitracin ointment – Allergic contact dermatitis has occurred.

Neomycin – Hypersensitivity (see Precautions); ototoxicity and nephrotoxicity have occurred (see Warnings).

Patient Information

Discontinue use of medication if rash or other allergic reaction develops or if condition persists or worsens.

For external use only. Cleanse affected area prior to application of medicine.

Notify physician if condition worsens or if rash or irritation develops.

Not for prolonged use. Do not use for longer than 1 week unless directed by a physician.

Antifungal Agents

BUTENAFINE HCl

otc	**Lotrimin Ultra** (Schering Plough)	**Cream:** 1% butenafine hydrochloride	Benzyl alcohol, cetyl alcohol, glycerin, white petrolatum. In 12 and 24 g.
Rx	**Mentax** (Bertek)		Benzyl and cetyl alcohol, glycerin, white petrolatum. In 15 and 30 g.

BUTENAFINE HYDROCHLORIDE — TOPICAL

Indications

➤*Topical infections:* For the treatment of the following dermatologic infections: Tinea (pityriasis) versicolor due to *M. furfur* (formerly *P. orbiculare*), interdigital tinea pedis (athlete's foot), tinea corporis (ringworm) and tinea cruris (jock itch) due to *E. floccosum*, *T. mentagrophytes*, *T. rubrum*, and *T. tonsurans*.

Administration and Dosage

➤*Approved by the FDA:* October 18, 1996.

➤*Tinea (pityriasis) versicolor:* Apply once daily for 2 weeks.

➤*Interdigital tinea pedis:* Apply twice daily for 7 days or once daily for 4 weeks.

➤*Tinea corporis or tinea cruris:* Apply once daily for 2 weeks.

Sufficient butenafine hydrochloride cream should be applied to cover affected areas and immediately surrounding skin of patients with tinea versicolor, interdigital tinea pedis, tinea corporis, and tinea cruris.

If a patient shows no clinical improvement after the treatment period, the diagnosis and therapy should be reviewed.

➤*Storage/Stability:* Store between 5° and 30°C (41° and 86°F).

Actions

➤*Pharmacokinetics:*

Absorption/Distribution – In 1 study conducted in healthy subjects for 14 days, 6 g of butenafine hydrochloride cream 1% was applied once daily to the dorsal skin (3000 cm^2) of 7 subjects, and 20 g of the cream was applied once daily to the arms, trunk and groin areas (10,000 cm^2) of another 12 subjects. After 14 days of topical applications, the 6 g dose group yielded a mean peak plasma butenafine hydrochloride concentration, C_{max}, of 1.4 ± 0.8 ng/mL, occurring at a mean time to the peak plasma concentration, t_{max}, of 15 ± 8 hours, and a mean area under the plasma concentration-time curve, $AUC_{0\text{-}24\,hrs}$ of 23.9 ± 11.3 ng•hr/mL. For the 20 g dose group, the mean C_{max} was 5 ± 2 ng/mL, occurring at a mean t_{max} of 6 ± 6 hours, and the mean $AUC_{0\text{-}24\,hrs}$ was 87.8 ± 45.3 ng•hr/mL. A biphasic decline of plasma butenafine hydrochloride concentrations was observed with the half-lives estimated to be 35 hours and greater than 150 hours, respectively.

At 72 hours after the last dose application, the mean plasma concentrations decreased to 0.3 ± 0.2 ng/mL for the 6 g dose group and 1.1 ± 0.9 ng/mL for the 20 g dose group. Low levels of butenafine hydrochloride remained in the plasma 7 days after the last dose application (mean: 0.1 ± 0.2 ng/mL for the 6 g dose group, and 0.7 ± 0.5 ng/mL for the 20 g dose group). The total amount (or % dose) of butenafine hydrochloride absorbed through the skin into the systemic circulation has not been quantitated.

In 11 patients with tinea pedis, butenafine hydrochloride cream 1% was applied by the patients to cover the affected and immediately surrounding skin area once daily for 4 weeks, and a single blood sample was collected between 10 and 20 hours following dosing at 1, 2, and 4 weeks after treatment. The plasma butenafine hydrochloride concentration ranged from undetectable to 0.3 ng/mL.

In 24 patients with tinea cruris, butenafine hydrochloride cream 1% was applied by the patients to cover the affected and immediately surrounding skin area once daily for 2 weeks (mean average daily dose: 1.3 ± 0.2 g). A single blood sample was collected between 0.5 and 65 hours after the last dose, and the plasma butenafine hydrochloride concentration ranged from undetectable to 2.52 ng/mL (mean ± SD: 0.91 ± 0.15 ng/mL). Four weeks after cessation of treatment, the plasma butenafine hydrochloride concentration ranged from undetectable to 0.28 ng/mL.

Metabolism/Excretion – It was determined that the primary metabolite in urine was formed through hydroxylation at the terminal t-butyl side-chain.

➤*Microbiology:* Butenafine hydrochloride is a benzylamine derivative with a mode of action similar to that of the allylamine class of antifungal drugs. Butenafine hydrochloride is hypothesized to act by inhibiting the epoxidation of squalene, thus blocking the biosynthesis of ergosterol, an essential component of fungal cell membranes. The benzylamine derivatives, like the allylamines, act at an earlier step in the ergosterol biosynthesis pathway than the azole class of anti-fungal drugs. Depending on the concentration of the drug and the fungal species tested, butenafine hydrochloride may be fungicidal in vitro. However, the clinical significance of these in vitro data is unknown.

Butenafine hydrochloride has been shown to be active against most strains of the following microorganisms, both in vitro and in clinical infections: *Epidermophyton floccosum*, *Malassezia furfur*, *Trichophyton mentagrophytes*, *Trichophyton rubrum*, and *trichophyton tonsurans*.

Contraindications

Known or suspected sensitivity to butenafine hydrochloride cream 1% or any of its components.

Warnings

➤*For dermatologic use only:* Butenafine hydrochloride cream 1% is not for ophthalmic, oral, or intravaginal use.

➤*Pregnancy:* *Category B*.

➤*Lactation:* It is not known if butenafine hydrochloride is excreted in human milk. Because many drugs are excreted in human milk, caution should be exercised in prescribing butenafine hydrochloride cream 1% to a nursing woman. Nursing mothers should avoid application of butenafine hydrochloride cream 1% to the breast.

➤*Children:* Safety and efficacy in pediatric patients below the age of 12 years have not been studied. Use of butenafine hydrochloride cream 1% in pediatric patients 12 to 16 years of age is supported by evidence from adequate and well-controlled studies of butenafine hydrochloride cream 1% in adults.

Precautions

➤*Irritation/diagnosis:* Butenafine hydrochloride cream 1% is for external use only. If irritation or sensitivity develops with the use of butenafine hydrochloride cream 1%, treatment should be discontinued and appropriate therapy instituted. Diagnosis of the disease should be confirmed either by culture or an appropriate medium, (except *M. furfur* [formerly *P. orbiculare*]) or by direct microscopic examination of infected superficial epidermal tissue in a solution of potassium hydroxide.

➤*Mucous membranes:* Use butenafine hydrochloride cream 1% as directed by the physician, and avoid contact with the eyes, nose, and mouth, and other mucous membranes.

➤*Special risk:* Patients who are known to be sensitive to allylamine antifungals should use butenafine hydrochloride cream 1% with caution, since cross-reactivity may occur.

Drug Interactions

None known.

Adverse Reactions

In controlled clinical trials, 9 (approximately 1%) of 815 patients treated with butenafine hydrochloride cream 1%, reported adverse reactions related to the skin. These included burning/stinging, itching, and worsening of the condition. No patient treated with butenafine hydrochloride cream 1% discontinued treatment due to an adverse reaction. In the vehicle-treated patients, 2 of 718 patients discontinued because of treatment site adverse reactions, 1 of which was severe burning/stinging and itching at the site of application.

BUTENAFINE HYDROCHLORIDE — TOPICAL

In uncontrolled clinical trials, the most frequently reported adverse reactions in patients treated with butenafine hydrochloride cream 1% were contact dermatitis, erythema, irritation, and itching, each occurring in less than 2% of patients.

➤*Hypersensitivity:* In provocative testing in over 200 subjects, there was no evidence of allergic contact sensitization for either cream or vehicle base for butenafine hydrochloride cream 1%.

Patient Information

Use butenafine hydrochloride cream 1% as directed by the physician. The hands should be washed after applying the medication to the affected area(s). Avoid contact with the eyes, nose, mouth, and other mucous membranes. Butenafine hydrochloride cream 1% is for external use only.

Dry the affected area(s) thoroughly before application if you wish to apply butenafine hydrochloride cream 1% after bathing.

Use the medication for the full treatment time recommended by the physician, even though symptoms may have improved. Notify the physician if there is no improvement after the end of the prescribed treatment period, or sooner, if the condition worsens (see below).

Inform the physician if the area of application shows signs of increased irritation, redness, itching, burning, blistering, swelling, or oozing.

Avoid the use of occlusive dressings unless otherwise directed by the physician.

Do not use this medication for any disorder other than that for which it was prescribed.

CICLOPIROX

Rx	**Ciclopirox** (Fougera)	**Cream:** 0.77%	Water miscible base. 1% benzyl alcohol, cetyl alcohol, mineral oil, stearyl alcohol, myristyl alcohol. In 15, 30, and 90 g.
Rx	**Loprox** (Medicis)		Water miscible base. 1% benzyl alcohol, cetyl alcohol, stearyl alcohol, myristyl alcohol, mineral oil. In 15, 30, and 90 g.
Rx	**Loprox** (Medicis)	**Gel:** 0.77%	Isopropyl alcohol. In 30, 45, and 100 g.
		Shampoo: 1%	In 120 mL.
Rx	**Ciclopirox** (Various, eg, Fougera)	**Suspension, topical:** 0.77%	In 30 and 60 mL bottles.
Rx	**Loprox** (Medicis)		Stearyl alcohol, cetyl alcohol, mineral oil, myristyl alcohol, benzyl alcohol, lactic acid. In 30 and 60 mL.
Rx	**Penlac Nail Lacquer** (Dermik Labs.)	**Solution, topical:** 8%	Isopropyl alcohol. In 3.3 and 6.6 mL with brushes.

CICLOPIROX — TOPICAL

Indications

➤*Nail lacquer topical solution:* As a component of a comprehensive management program for topical treatment of immunocompetent patients with mild to moderate onychomycosis of fingernails and toenails, without lunula involvement, due to *Trichophyton rubrum*. The comprehensive management program includes removal of the unattached, infected nails as frequently as monthly, by a health care provider who has special competence in the diagnosis and treatment of nail disorders, including minor nail procedures.

➤*Lotion and cream:* For the topical treatment of the following dermal infections: tinea pedis, tinea cruris, and tinea corporis due to *Trichophyton rubrum*, *T. mentagrophytes*, *Epidermophyton floccosum*, and *Microsporum canis*; cutaneous candidiasis (moniliasis) due to *Candida albicans*; and tinea (pityriasis) versicolor due to *Malassezia furfur*.

➤*Gel:* For the topical treatment of interdigital tinea pedis and tinea corporis due to *T. rubrum*, *T. mentagrophytes*, or *E. floccosum*; and seborrheic dermatitis of the scalp.

➤*Shampoo:* For the treatment of seborrheic dermatitis of the scalp in adults.

Administration and Dosage

➤*Approved by the FDA:* December 30, 1982.

➤*Nail lacquer topical solution:* Use as a component of a comprehensive management program for onychomycosis. Removal of the unattached, infected nail, as frequently as monthly, by a health care provider, weekly trimming by the patient, and daily application of the medication are all integral parts of this therapy. Give careful consideration of the appropriate nail management program to patients with diabetes.

➤*Lotion and cream:* Gently massage into the affected and surrounding skin areas twice daily, in the morning and evening. Clinical improvement with relief of pruritus and other symptoms usually occurs within the first week of treatment. If a patient shows no clinical improvement after 4 weeks of treatment with ciclopirox the diagnosis should be redetermined. Patients with tinea versicolor usually exhibit clinical and mycological clearing after 2 weeks of treatment.

➤*Gel:*

Superficial dermatophyte infections – Gently massage into the affected areas and surrounding skin twice daily, in the morning and evening, immediately after cleaning or washing the areas to be treated. Interdigital tinea pedis and tinea corporis should be treated for 4 weeks. If a patient shows no clinical improvement after 4 weeks of treatment, the diagnosis should be reviewed.

Seborrheic dermatitis of the scalp – Apply to affected scalp areas twice daily, in the morning and evening, for 4 weeks. Clinical improvement usually occurs within the first week with continuing resolution of signs and symptoms through the fourth week of treatment. If a patient shows no clinical improvement after 4 weeks of treatment, the diagnosis should be reviewed.

➤*Shampoo:* Wet hair and apply approximately 5 mL of ciclopirox shampoo to the scalp. Up to 10 mL may be used for long hair. Lather and leave on hair and scalp for 3 minutes. Avoid contact with eyes. Rinse off. Repeat treatment twice per week for 4 weeks, with an minimum of 3 days between applications. If a patient shows no clinical improvement after 4 weeks of treatment, the diagnosis should be reviewed.

➤*Storage/Stability:*

Nail lacquer topical solution – Protect from light (eg, store the bottle in the carton after every use).

Store ciclopirox 8% topical solution nail lacquer at room temperature between 15° and 30°C (59° and 86°F).

Caution: Flammable. Keep away from heat and flame.

Lotion – Store between 5° and 25°C (41° and 77°F).

Cream, gel, and shampoo – Store at controlled room temperature, 15° to 30°C (59° to 86°F).

Actions

➤*Pharmacology:* Ciclopirox olamine is a broad-spectrum antifungal agent that inhibits the growth of pathogenic dermatophytes, yeasts, and *M. furfur*. Ciclopirox exhibits fungicidal activity in vitro against isolates of *T. rubrum*, *T. mentagrophytes*, *E. floccosum*, *M. canis*, and *C. albicans*.

Ciclopirox acts by chelation of polyvalent cations (Fe^{3+} or Al^{3+}) resulting in the inhibition of the metal-dependent enzymes that are responsible for the degradation of peroxides within the fungal cell.

In vitro studies showed that ciclopirox inhibited the formation of 5-lipoxygenase-inflammatory mediators (5-HETE and LTB_4) and also inhibited PGE_2 release in a cell culture model. In vivo ciclopirox inhibited inflammation in an arachidonic acid-induced murine ear edema model. The clinical significance of these findings is unknown.

➤*Pharmacokinetics:*

Lotion and cream – Penetration studies in human cadaverous skin from the back, with ciclopirox 0.77% cream with tagged ciclopirox showed the presence of 0.8% to 1.6% of the dose in the stratum corneum 1.5 to 6 hours after application. The levels in the dermis were still 10 to 15 times above the minimum inhibitory concentrations.

Pharmacokinetic studies in men with radiolabeled ciclopirox solution in polythylene glycol 400 showed an average of 1.3% absorption of the dose when it was applied topically to 750 cm^2 on the back followed by occlusion for 6 hours. The biological half-life was 1.7 hours and excretion occurred via the kidney. Two days after application, only 0.01% of the dose applied could be found in the urine. Fecal excretion was negligible. Autoradiographic studies with human cadaver skin showed that ciclopirox penetrates into the hair and through the epidermis and hair follicles into the sebaceous glands and dermis, while a portion of the drug remains in the stratum corneum.

Gel – A comparative study of the pharmacokinetics of ciclopirox 0.77% gel and 0.77% cream in 18 healthy males indicated that systemic absorption of ciclopirox from ciclopirox gel was higher than that of ciclopirox cream. A 5 g dose of ciclopirox gel produced a mean (± SD) peak serum concentration of 25.02 (± 20.6) ng/mL total ciclopirox and 5 g of ciclopirox cream produced 18.62 (± 13.56) ng/mL total ciclopirox. Approximately 3% of the applied ciclopirox was excreted in the urine within 48 hours after application, with a renal elimination half-life of about 5.5 hours. In a study of ciclopirox gel, 16 men with moderate to severe tinea cruris applied approximately 15 g/day of the gel for 14.5 days. The mean (± SD) dose-normalized values of C_{max} for total ciclopirox in serum were 100 (± 42) ng/mL on day 1 and 238 (± 144) ng/mL on day 15. During the 10 hours after dosing on day 1, approximately 10% of the administered dose was excreted in the urine.

Nail lacquer topical solution – As demonstrated in pharmacokinetic studies in animals and man, ciclopirox olamine is rapidly absorbed after oral administration and completely eliminated in all species via feces and urine. Most of the compound is excreted either unchanged or as glucuronide. After

CICLOPIROX — TOPICAL

oral administration of 10 mg of radiolabeled drug (14C-ciclopirox) to healthy volunteers, approximately 96% of the radioactivity was excreted renally within 12 hours of administration. Ninety-four percent (94%) of the renally excreted radioactivity was in the form of glucuronides. Thus, glucuronidation is the main metabolic pathway of this compound.

Systemic absorption of ciclopirox was determined in 5 patients with dermatophytic onychomycoses, after application of ciclopirox 8% topical solution nail lacquer to all 20 digits and adjacent 5 mm of skin once daily for 6 months. Random serum concentrations and 24 hour urinary excretion of ciclopirox olamine were determined at 2 weeks and at 1, 2, 4, and 6 months after initiation of treatment and 4 weeks posttreatment. In this study, ciclopirox serum levels ranged from 12 to 80 ng/mL. Based on urinary data, mean absorption of ciclopirox from the dosage form was less than 5% of the applied dose. One month after cessation of treatment, serum and urine levels of ciclopirox olamine were below the limit of detection.

In 2 vehicle-controlled trials, patients applied ciclopirox 8% topical solution nail lacquer to all toenails and affected fingernails. Out of a total of 66 randomly selected patients on active treatment, 24 had detectable serum ciclopirox concentrations at some point during the dosing interval (range, 10 to 24.6 ng/mL). It should be noted that 11 of these 24 patients used concomitant medication containing ciclopirox as ciclopirox 0.77% cream.

The penetration of the ciclopirox 8% topical solution nail lacquer was evaluated in an in vitro investigation. Radiolabeled ciclopirox applied once to onychomycotic toenails that were avulsed demonstrated penetration up to a depth of approximately 0.4 mm. As expected, nail plate concentrations decreased as a function of nail depth. The clinical significance of these findings in nail plates is unknown. Nail bed concentrations were not determined.

Contraindications

Hypersensitivity to any of its components.

Warnings

➤*For external use only:* Ciclopirox is not for ophthalmic, oral, or intravaginal use.

➤*Nail lacquer topical solution:* For use on nails and immediately adjacent skin only.

➤*Mutagenesis:*

Nail lacquer topical solution: The following in vitro genotoxicity tests have been conducted with ciclopirox: evaluation of gene mutation in Ames *Salmonella* and *Escherichia coli* assays (negative); chromosome aberration assays in V79 Chinese hamster lung fibroblasts, with and without metabolic activation (positive); gene mutation assay in the HGPRT-test with V79 Chinese hamster lung fibroblasts (negative); unscheduled DNA synthesis in human A549 cells (negative); and BALB/c3T3 cell transformation assay (negative). In an in vivo Chinese hamster bone marrow cytogenetic assay, ciclopirox was negative for chromosome aberrations at 5,000 mg/kg.

The following in vitro genotoxicity tests were conducted with ciclopirox 8% topical solution nail lacquer: Ames *Salmonella* test (negative); unscheduled DNA synthesis in the rat hepatocytes (negative); cell transformation assay in BALB/c3T3 cell assay (positive). The positive response of the lacquer formulation in the BALB/c3T3 test was attributed to its butyl monoester of poly] resin component (*Gantrez* ES-435), which also tested positive in this test. The cell transformation assay may have been confounded because of the film-forming nature of the resin. *Gantrez* ES-435 tested nonmutagenic in both the in vitro mouse lymphoma forward mutation assay with or without activation and unscheduled DNA synthesis assay in rat hepatocytes.

Lotion, cream, and gel: The following in vitro and in vivo genotoxicity tests have been conducted with ciclopirox olamine: studies to evaluate gene mutation in the Ames *Salmonella*/Mammalian Microsome Assay (negative) and Yeast *S. cerevisiae* Assay (negative) and studies to evaluate chromosome aberrations in vivo in the Mouse Dominant Lethal Assay and in the Mouse Micronucleus Assay at 500 mg/kg (negative). The following battery of in vitro genotoxicity tests were conducted with ciclopirox: a chromosome aberration assay in V79 Chinese Hamster Cells, with and without metabolic activation (positive); and a primary DNA damage assay (ie, unscheduled DNA Synthesis Assay in A548 Human Cells [negative]) and a gene mutation assay in the HGPRT-test with V79 Chinese Hamster Cells (negative). An in vitro Cell Transformation Assay in BALB/C3T3 Cells was negative for cell transformation. In an in vivo Chinese Hamster Bone Marrow Cytogenetic Assay, ciclopirox was negative for chromosome aberrations at 5,000 mg/kg.

➤*Pregnancy: Category B.* There are no adequate or well-controlled studies of topically applied ciclopirox in pregnant women. Use during pregnancy only if the potential benefit justifies the potential risk to the fetus.

➤*Lactation:* It is not known whether this drug is excreted in human milk. Since many drugs are excreted in human milk, exercise caution when is administering to a nursing woman.

➤*Children:*

Nail lacquer topical solution – Safety and efficacy in pediatric patients have not been established.

Gel and shampoo – Safety and efficacy in pediatric patients younger than 16 years of age have not been established.

Cream and lotion – Safety and efficacy in pediatric patients younger than 10 years of age have not been established.

Precautions

➤*Hypersensitivity:* If a reaction suggesting sensitivity or chemical irritation should occur with the use of ciclopirox, discontinue treatment and institute appropriate therapy.

➤*Diabetes:* So far there is no relevant clinical experience with patients with type 1 diabetes or who have diabetic neuropathy. Carefully consider the risk of removal of the unattached, infected nail by the health care provider and trimming by the patient, before prescribing to patients with a history of type 1 diabetes mellitus or diabetic neuropathy.

➤*Gel:* A transient burning sensation may occur, especially after application to sensitive areas. Avoid contact with eyes. Efficacy of ciclopirox gel in immunosuppressed individuals has not been studied. Seborrheic dermatitis in association with acne, atopic dermatitis, parkinsonism, psoriasis, and rosacea has not been studied with ciclopirox gel. Efficacy in the treatment of plantar and vesicular types of tinea pedis has not been established.

Drug Interactions

➤*Systemic antifungals:* No studies have been conducted to determine whether ciclopirox might reduce the efficacy of systemic antifungal agents for onychomycosis. Therefore, the concomitant use of ciclopirox 8% topical solution and systemic antifungal agents for onychomycosis is not recommended.

Adverse Reactions

➤*Nail lacquer topical solution:*

Dermatologic – In the vehicle-controlled clinical trials conducted in the US, 9% (30/327) of patients treated with ciclopirox topical solution nail lacquer and 7% (23/328) of patients treated with vehicle reported treatment-emergent adverse reactions considered by the investigator to be causally related to the test material.

The incidence of these adverse reactions within each body system was similar between the treatment groups except for dermatologic; 8% (27/327) and 4% (14/328) of subjects in the ciclopirox and vehicle groups reported at least 1 adverse reaction, respectively. The most common were rash-related adverse events: periungual erythema and erythema of the proximal nail fold were reported more frequently in patients treated with ciclopirox 8% topical solution nail lacquer (5% [16/327]) than in patients treated with vehicle (1% [3/328]). Other treatment-emergent adverse reactions thought to be causally related included nail disorders such as shape change, irritation, ingrown toenail, and discoloration.

The incidence of nail disorders was similar between the treatment groups (2% [6/327] in the ciclopirox 8% topical solution nail lacquer group and 2% [7/328] in the vehicle group). Moreover, application site reactions and/or burning of the skin occurred in 1% of patients treated with ciclopirox 8% topical solution nail lacquer (3/327) and vehicle (4/328).

A 21-Day Cumulative Irritancy study was conducted under conditions of semi-occlusion. Mild reactions were seen in 46% of patients with the ciclopirox 8% topical solution nail lacquer, 32% with the vehicle and 2% with the negative control, but all were reactions of mild transient erythema. There was no evidence of allergic contact sensitization for either the ciclopirox 8% topical solution nail lacquer or the vehicle base. In the vehicle-controlled studies, 1 patient treated with ciclopirox 8% topical solution nail lacquer discontinued treatment due to a rash localized to the palm (causal relation to test material undetermined).

Use of ciclopirox 8% topical solution nail lacquer for 48 additional weeks was evaluated in an open-label extension study conducted in patients previously treated in the vehicle-controlled studies. Three percent (9/281) of subjects treated with ciclopirox 8% topical solution nail lacquer experienced at least 1 treatment-emergent adverse reaction that the investigator thought was causally related to the test material. Mild rash in the form of periungual erythema (1% [2/281]) and nail disorders (1% [4/281]) were the most frequently reported. Four patients discontinued because of treatment-emergent adverse reactions. Two of the 4 had events considered to be related to test material: 1 patient's great toenail "broke away" and another had an elevated creatine phosphokinase level on day 1 (after 48 weeks of treatment with vehicle in the previous vehicle-controlled study).

➤*Lotion:*

Dermatologic – In the controlled clinical trial with 89 patients using ciclopirox lotion and 89 patients using the vehicle, the incidence of adverse reactions was low. Those considered possibly related to treatment or occurring in more than 1 patient were pruritus, which occurred in 2 patients using ciclopirox lotion and 1 patient using the lotion vehicle, and burning, which occurred in 1 patient using ciclopirox lotion.

➤*Cream:*

Dermatologic – In all controlled clinical studies with 514 patients using ciclopirox cream and in 296 patients using the vehicle cream, the incidence of adverse reactions was low. This included pruritus at the site of application in 1 patient and worsening of the clinical signs and symptoms in another patient using ciclopirox cream, and burning in 1 patient and worsening of the clinical signs and symptoms in another patient using the vehicle cream.

➤*Gel:*

Dermatologic – In clinical trials, 140 (39%) of 359 subjects treated with ciclopirox gel reported adverse reactions, irrespective of relationship to test materials, that resulted in 8 subjects discontinuing treatment. The most frequent reaction reported was skin burning sensation upon application, which occurred in approximately 34% of seborrheic dermatitis patients and 7% of tinea pedis patients. Adverse reactions occurring between 1% to 5% were contact dermatitis and pruritus. Other reactions that occurred in less than 1% included dry skin, acne, rash, alopecia, pain upon application, eye pain, and facial edema.

Patient Information

➤*Nail lacquer topical solution:* Patients should have detailed instructions regarding the use of ciclopirox 8% topical solution nail lacquer as a

CICLOPIROX — TOPICAL

component of a comprehensive management program for onychomycosis in order to achieve maximum benefit with the use of this product.

Tell the patient to:
1.) Use ciclopirox 8% topical solution nail lacquer as directed by a health care provider.
2.) Avoid contact with eyes and mucous membranes.
3.) Avoid contact with skin other than skin immediately surrounding the treated nail(s).

Apply ciclopirox 8% topical solution nail lacquer evenly over the entire nail plate and 5 mm of surrounding skin. If possible, apply ciclopirox 8% topical solution nail lacquer to the nail bed, hyponychium, and the under surface of the nail plate when it is free of the nail bed (eg, onycholysis). Contact with the surrounding skin may produce mild, transient irritation (redness).

Do not use this medication for any disorder other than that for which it is prescribed.

Discuss your treatment plan with your doctor for regular removal of the unattached, infected nail.

Before using this medication, tell your doctor if you are pregnant or nursing, are a type 1 diabetic or have diabetic neuropathy, have a history of immunosuppression, are immunocompromised (eg, received an organ transplant), require medication to control epilepsy, use or require topical corticosteroids on a repeated monthly basis, or use steroid inhalers on a regular basis.
1.) Avoid contact with the eyes and mucous membranes.
2.) Removal of the unattached, infected nail, as frequently as monthly, by a doctor is needed with use of this medication. Inform a doctor if you have diabetes or problems with numbness in your toes or fingers for consideration of the appropriate nail management program (before trimming your nails or removing nail material).
3.) Inform your doctor if the area of application shows signs of increased irritation (ie, redness, itching, burning, blistering, swelling, oozing).
4.) Up to 48 weeks of daily applications with ciclopirox 8% topical solution nail lacquer and professional removal, as frequently as monthly, of the unattached, infected nail are considered the full treatment time to achieve a clear or almost clear nail (defined as 10% or less residual nail involvement). Six months of therapy with professional removal of the unattached, infected nail may be required before initial improvement of symptoms is noticed.
5.) A completely clear nail may not be achieved with use of this medication. In clinical studies, less than 12% of patients were able to achieve either a clear or almost clear toenail.
6.) Do not use nail polish or other nail cosmetic products on the treated nails.
7.) Avoid use near heat or open flame because product is flammable.

Patient Instructions – Before starting treatment, remove any loose nail or nail material using nail clippers or nail files. If you have diabetes or problems with numbness in your toes or fingers, talk to your doctor before trimming your nails or removing any nail material.

Apply once daily (preferably at bedtime) to all affected nails with the applicator brush provided. Apply the lacquer evenly over the entire nail. Where possible, apply nail lacquer to the underside of the nail and to the skin beneath it. Allow lacquer to dry (approximately 30 seconds) before putting on socks or stockings. After applying medication, wait 8 hours before taking a bath or shower.

Apply ciclopirox 8% topical solution nail lacquer daily over the previous coat.

Once a week, remove the ciclopirox 8% topical solution nail lacquer with alcohol. Remove as much as possible of the damaged nail using nail clippers or nail files.

Repeat process (steps 2 through 4).

To prevent screw cap from sticking to the bottle, do not allow solution to get into the bottle threads.

To prevent the solution from drying out, bottle should be closed tightly after every use.

To protect from light, replace bottle into carton after each use.

➤*Lotion:*
1.) Use the medication for the full treatment time even though signs/symptoms may have improved; notify your doctor if there is no improvement after 4 weeks.
2.) Inform your doctor if the area of application shows signs of increased irritation (ie, redness, itching, burning, blistering, swelling, oozing) indicative of possible sensitization.
3.) Avoid the use of occlusive wrappings or dressings.

CLOTRIMAZOLE

otc/ Rx[1]	**Clotrimazole** (Various, eg Taro)	**Cream:** 1%	1% benzyl alcohol, cetostearyl alcohol. Vanishing base. In 15, 30, 45, and 2 x 45 g tubes.
otc	**Cruex** (Novartis Consumer Health)		1% benzyl alcohol, cetostearyl alcohol. In 15 g.
otc	**Lotrimin AF** (Schering-Plough)		Benzyl alcohol, cetearyl alcohol. In 12 and 24 g.
otc	**Desenex** (Novartis Consumer Health)		1% benzyl alcohol, cetostearyl alcohol. In 15 and 30 g.
otc	**Lotrimin AF** (Schering-Plough)	**Lotion:** 1%	Benzyl alcohol, cetearyl alcohol. In 20 mL.
otc/ Rx[1]	**Clotrimazole** (Various, eg Taro)	**Solution, topical:** 1%	PEG 400. In 30 mL.
otc	**Lotrimin AF** (Schering-Plough)		PEG. In 10 mL.

[1] Products are available *OTC* or *Rx*, depending on product labeling.

CLOTRIMAZOLE — TOPICAL

Indications

➤*Fungal infections:*

OTC products – Clotrimazole is an antifungal that cures most jock itch (tinea cruris), athlete's foot (tinea pedis), and ringworm (tinea corporis) due to *Trichophyton rubrum*, *Trichophyton mentagrophytes*, *Epidermophyton floccosum*, and *Microsporum canis*. Relieves itching, burning, cracking, and discomfort which can accompany these conditions.

Rx products – Topical treatments of candidiasis due to *Candida albicans* and tinea versicolor due to *Malassezia furfur*.

Administration and Dosage

➤*OTC products:*

Directions – Not effective on scalp or nails.

Adults and children 2 years of age and older: Use tip of cap to break the seal and open the tube. Wash the affected skin with soap and water and dry completely before applying.

• *Jock itch* – Apply a thin layer over affected area morning and evening for 2 weeks or as directed by a doctor

• *Athlete's foot and ringworm* – Apply a thin layer over affected area morning and evening for 4 weeks or as directed by a doctor. For athlete's foot, pay special attention to the spaces between the toes. Wear well-fitting, ventilated shoes and change shoes and socks at least once a day.

➤*Rx products:* Gently massage sufficient clotrimazole into the affected and surrounding skin areas twice a day, in the morning and evening.

Clinical improvement, with relief of pruritus, usually occurs within the first week of treatment with clotrimazole. If the patient shows no clinical improvement after 4 weeks of treatment with clotrimazole, the diagnosis should be reviewed.

➤*Storage/Stability:* Store between 20° and 25°C (68°and 77°F). Do not use if seal is broken or is not visible. See tube crimp for lot number and expiration date.

Actions

➤*Pharmacology:* Clotrimazole is a broad-spectrum antifungal agent that is used for the treatment of dermal infections caused by various species of pathogenic dermatophytes, yeasts, and *Malassezia furfur*. The primary action of clotrimazole is against dividing and growing organisms.

In vitro, clotrimazole exhibits fungistatic and fungicidal activity against isolates of *Trichophyton rubrum*, *Trichophyton mentagrophytes*, *Epidermophyton floccosum*, *Microsporum canis*, and *Candida* species, including *Candida albicans*. In general, the in vitro activity of clotrimazole corresponds to that of tolnaftate and griseofulvin against the mycelia of dermatophytes (*Trichophyton*, *Microsporum*, and *Epidermophyton*), and to that of the polyenes (amphotericin B and nystatin) against budding fungi (*Candida*). Using an in vivo (mouse) and an in vitro (mouse kidney homogenate) testing system, clotrimazole and miconazole were equally effective in preventing the growth of the pseudomycelia and mycelia of *Candida albicans*.

➤*Pharmacokinetics:* Clotrimazole appears to be well absorbed in humans following oral administration and is eliminated mainly as inactive metabolites. Following topical and vaginal administration, however, clotrimazole appears to be minimally absorbed.

Six hours after the application of radioactive clotrimazole 1% cream and 1% solution onto intact and acutely inflamed skin, the concentration of clotrimazole varied from 100 mcg/cm^3, in the stratum corneum to 0.5 to 1 mcg/cm^3 in the stratum reticulare, and 0.1 mcg/cm^3 in the subcutis. No measurable amount of radioactivity (less than 0.001 mcg/mL) was found in the serum within 48 hours after application under occlusive dressing of 0.5 mL of the solution or 0.8 g of the cream. Only 0.5% or less of the applied radioactivity was excreted in the urine.

Contraindications

Hypersensitivity to any of their components.

CLOTRIMAZOLE — TOPICAL

Warnings

➤*Pregnancy: Category B.* The disposition of ^{14}C-clotrimazole has been studied in humans and animals. Clotrimazole is very poorly absorbed following dermal application or intravaginal administration to humans.

In clinical trials, use of vaginally applied clotrimazole in pregnant women in their second and third trimesters has not been associated with ill effects. There are, however, no adequate and well-controlled studies in pregnant women during the first trimester of pregnancy.

High oral doses of clotrimazole in rats and mice ranging from 50 to 120 mg/kg resulted in embryotoxicity (possibly secondary to maternal toxicity), impairment of mating, decreased litter size and number of viable young and decreased pup survival to weaning. However, clotrimazole was not teratogenic in mice, rabbits and rats at oral doses up to 200, 180, and 100 mg/kg, respectively. Oral absorption in the rat amounts to approximately 90% of the administered dose.

Because animal reproduction studies are not always predictive of human response, this drug should be used only if clearly indicated during the first trimester of pregnancy.

➤*Lactation:* It is not known whether this drug is excreted in human milk. Because many drugs are excreted in human milk, caution should be exercised when clotrimazole is used by a nursing woman.

➤*Children:* Do not use in children younger than 2 years of age unless directed by a physician.

Precautions

➤*Monitoring:* If there is lack of response to clotrimazole, appropriate microbiological studies should be repeated to confirm the diagnosis and rule out other pathogens before instituting another course of antimycotic therapy.

➤*Sensitivity:* If irritation or sensitivity develops with the use of clotrimazole, treatment should be discontinued and appropriate therapy instituted.

➤*For external use only:* For external use only. Avoid contact with the eyes.

Drug Interactions

None known.

Adverse Reactions

➤*Dermatologic:* Erythema, stinging, blistering, peeling, edema, pruritus, urticaria, burning, and general skin irritation.

Overdosage

Acute overdosage with topical application of clotrimazole is unlikely and would not be expected to lead to a life-threatening situation.

Patient Information

This information is intended to aid in the safe and effective use of this medication. It is not a disclosure of all possible adverse or intended effects.

For external use only.

Keep out of reach of children. If swallowed, get medical help or contact a poison control center right away.

Use the medication for the full treatment time even though the symptoms may have improved. Notify the physician if there is no improvement after 4 weeks of treatment.

Inform the physician if the area of application shows signs of increased irritation (eg, redness, itching, burning, blistering, swelling, oozing) indicative of possible sensitization.

Avoid use of occlusive wrappings/dressings.

Avoid sources of infection or reinfection.

➤*Do not use:*
- In or near the mouth or the eyes.
- For vaginal yeast infections.
- On nails or scalp.

ECONAZOLE NITRATE

Rx	**Econazole Nitrate** (Various, eg, Fougera, Taro)	**Cream:** 1%	In 15, 30, and 85 g.
Rx	**Spectazole** (Ortho Pharm. Corp.)		Water miscible base. Mineral oil. In 15, 30, and 85 g.

ECONAZOLE NITRATE — TOPICAL

Indications

➤*Fungal infection:* For treatment of tinea pedis, tinea cruris, and tinea corporis caused by *Trichophyton rubrum*, *Trichophyton mentagrophytes*, *Trichophyton tonsurans*, *Microsporum canis*, *Microsporum audouini*, *Microsporum gypseum*, and *Epidermophyton floccosum* in the treatment of cutaneous candidiasis, and in the treatment of tinea versicolor.

Administration and Dosage

➤*Approved by the FDA:* December 23, 1982.

Sufficient econazole nitrate cream should be applied to cover affected areas once daily in patients with tinea pedis, tinea cruris, tinea corporis, and tinea versicolor, and twice daily (morning and evening) in patients with cutaneous candidiasis.

Early relief of symptoms is experienced by the majority of patients and clinical improvement may be seen fairly soon after treatment is begun; however, candidal infections and tinea cruris and corporis should be treated for 2 weeks and tinea pedis for 1 month in order to reduce the possibility of recurrence. If a patient shows no clinical improvement after the treatment period, the diagnosis should be redetermined. Patients with tinea versicolor usually exhibit clinical and mycological clearing after 2 weeks of treatment.

➤*Storage / Stability:* Store econazole nitrate cream below 30°C (86°F).

Actions

➤*Pharmacokinetics:*

Absorption – After topical application to the skin of healthy subjects, systemic absorption of econazole nitrate is extremely low.

Distribution – Although most of the applied drug remains on the skin surface, drug concentrations were found in the stratum corneum which, by far, exceeded the minimum inhibitory concentration for dermatophytes. Inhibitory concentrations were achieved in the epidermis and as deep as the middle region of the dermis.

Excretion – Less than 1% of the applied dose was recovered in the urine and feces.

➤*Microbiology:* Econazole nitrate has been shown to be active against most strains of the following microorganisms, both in vitro and in clinical infections.

Dermatophytes
- *Epidermophyton floccosum*
- *Microsporum audouini*
- *Microsporum canis*
- *Microsporum gypseum*
- *Trichophyton mentagrophytes*
- *Trichophyton rubrum*
- *Trichophyton tonsurans*
- *Trichophyton verrucosum*

Yeasts
- *Candida albicans*
- *Candida guillermondii*
- *Candida parapsilosis*
- *Candida tropicalis*
- *Malassezia furfur*

Contraindications

Hypersensitivity to econazole or any of its ingredients.

Warnings

➤*For external use only:* Econazole nitrate is not for ophthalmic use.

➤*Pregnancy: Category C.* Econazole nitrate should be used in the first trimester of pregnancy only when the physician considers it essential to the welfare of the patient. The drug should be used during the second and third trimesters of pregnancy only if clearly needed.

➤*Lactation:* It is not known whether econazole nitrate is excreted in human milk. Following oral administration of econazole nitrate to lactating rats, econazole and/or metabolites were excreted in milk and were found in nursing pups. Also, in lactating rats receiving large oral doses (40 or 80 times the human dermal dose), there was a reduction in postpartum viability of pups and survival to weaning; however, at these high doses, maternal toxicity was present and may have been a contributing factor. Caution should be exercised when econazole nitrate is administered to a nursing woman.

Precautions

➤*Sensitivity:* If a reaction suggesting sensitivity or chemical irritation should occur, use of the medication should be discontinued.

Adverse Reactions

During clinical trials, approximately 3% of patients treated with econazole nitrate 1% cream reported side effects thought possibly to be due to the drug, consisting mainly of burning, itching, stinging, and erythema. One case of pruritic rash has also been reported.

Overdosage

Overdosage of econazole nitrate in humans has not been reported to date. In mice, rats, guinea pigs and dogs, the oral LD_{50} values were found to be 462, 668, 272, and greater than 160 mg/kg, respectively.

Patient Information

For external use only. Avoid introduction of econazole nitrate cream into the eyes.

GENTIAN VIOLET TOPICAL

otc	**Gentian Violet** (Various, eg, Humco)	**Solution, topical:** 1%	In 30 mL.
		2%	In 30 mL.

GENTIAN VIOLET — TOPICAL

Indications

➤*Topical infection:* An antiseptic for the external treatment of abrasions, minor cuts, surface injuries, and superficial fungus infections of the skin.

Administration and Dosage

Clean and apply directly to the wound or use a cotton-tipped applicator once or twice daily. Do not bandage.

Actions

➤*Pharmacology:* Gentian violet is an antibacterial and antifungal dye. It is active against some gram-positive bacteria, especially *Staphylococcus* species. It inhibits the growth of *Candida*, *Cryptococcus*, *Epidermophyton*, and *Trichophyton*. Because of its staining properties and the availability of effective alternatives, gentian violet has generally been replaced in practice by other agents.

Warnings

➤*General:* This medication is for external use only. Medication will stain skin and clothing. Do not apply to an ulcerative lesion as this may result in "tattooing" of the skin. Do not use in the eyes. In case of deep or puncture wounds or serious burns, consult a physician. If redness, irritation, swelling or pain persists or increases, or if infection occurs, discontinue use and consult a physician.

Overdosage

In case of accidental ingestion, seek professional assistance or contact a poison control center immediately.

Patient Information

Gentian violet topical solution is an antiseptic for the external treatment of abrasions, minor cuts, surface injuries, and superficial fungus infections of the skin.

This medication contains gentian violet 1% or 2%, ethyl alcohol 10% (preservative), and purified water.

This medication is for external use only. Medication will stain skin and clothing. Do not apply to an ulcerative lesion as this may result in "tattooing" of the skin. Do not use in the eyes. In case of deep or puncture wounds or serious burns, consult a physician. If redness, irritation, swelling or pain persists or increases, or if infection occurs, discontinue use and consult a physician.

SERTACONAZOLE NITRATE

Rx	**Ertaczo** (OrthoNeutrogena)	**Cream:** 2%	Lt. mineral oil, methylparaben. In 15 and 30 g tubes.

SERTACONAZOLE NITRATE — TOPICAL

Indications

➤*Tinea pedis:* For the topical treatment of interdigital tinea pedis in immunocompetent patients 12 years of age and older, caused by *Trichophyton rubrum*, *Trichophyton mentagrophytes*, and *Epidermophyton floccosum*.

Administration and Dosage

➤*Approved by the FDA:* December 10, 2003.

Apply twice daily for 4 weeks. Sufficient sertaconazole nitrate 2% cream should be applied to cover both the affected areas between the toes and the immediately surrounding healthy skin of patients with interdigital tinea pedis. If a patient shows no clinical improvement 2 weeks after the treatment period, the diagnosis should be reviewed.

➤*Storage/Stability:* Store at 25°C (77°F); excursions permitted to 15° to 30°C (59° to 86°F).

Actions

➤*Pharmacokinetics:* In a multiple-dose pharmacokinetic study that included 5 male patients with interdigital tinea pedis (range of diseased area, 42 to 140 cm^2; mean, 93 cm^2), sertaconazole nitrate 2% cream was applied topically every 12 hours for a total of 13 doses to the diseased skin (0.5 g sertaconazole nitrate per 100 cm^2). Sertaconazole concentrations in plasma measured by serial blood sampling for 72 hours after the 13th dose were below the limit of quantitation (2.5 ng/mL) of the analytical method used.

➤*Microbiology:* Sertaconazole is an antifungal that belongs to the imidazole class of antifungals. While the exact mechanism of action of this class of antifungals is not known, it is believed that they act primarily by inhibiting the cytochrome P-450-dependent synthesis of ergosterol. Ergosterol is a key component of the cell membrane of fungi, and lack of this component leads to fungal cell injury primarily by leakage of key constituents in the cytoplasm from the cell.

Activity in vivo – Sertaconazole nitrate has been shown to be active against isolates of the following microorganisms in clinical infections: *Trichophyton rubrum*, *Trichophyton mentagrophytes*, and *Epidermophyton floccosum*.

Contraindications

Sensitivity to sertaconazole nitrate or any of its components or to other imidazoles.

Warnings

➤*For external use only:* Sertaconazole nitrate 2% cream is not indicated for ophthalmic, oral, or intravaginal use.

➤*Hypersensitivity reactions:* Physicians should exercise caution when prescribing sertaconazole nitrate 2% cream to patients known to be sensitive to imidazole antifungals, since cross-reactivity may occur.

➤*Pregnancy: Category C.* In an oral peripostnatal study in rats, a reduction in live birth indices and an increase in the number of still-born pups was seen at 80 and 160 mg/kg/day.

There are no adequate and well-controlled studies that have been conducted on topically applied sertaconazole nitrate 2% cream in pregnant women. Because animal reproduction studies are not always predictive of human response, sertaconazole nitrate 2% cream should be used during pregnancy only if clearly needed.

➤*Lactation:* It is not known if sertaconazole is excreted in human milk. Because many drugs are excreted in human milk, caution should be exercised when prescribing sertaconazole nitrate 2% cream to a nursing woman.

➤*Children:* The efficacy and safety have not been established in pediatric patients below the age of 12 years.

Precautions

➤*Sensitivity:* Sertaconazole nitrate 2% cream is for use on the skin only. If irritation or sensitivity develops, treatment should be discontinued and appropriate therapy instituted.

➤*Diagnosis:* Diagnosis of the disease should be confirmed either by direct microscopic examination of infected superficial epidermal tissue in a solution of potassium hydroxide or by culture on an appropriate medium.

➤*Special risk:* Physicians should exercise caution when prescribing sertaconazole nitrate 2% cream to patients known to be sensitive to imidazole antifungals, since cross-reactivity may occur.

Drug Interactions

None known.

Adverse Reactions

➤*Dermatologic:* In clinical trials, cutaneous adverse events occurred in 7 of 297 (2%) patients (2 of them severe) receiving sertaconazole nitrate 2% cream and in 7 of 291 (2%) patients (2 of them severe) receiving vehicle. These reported cutaneous adverse events included contact dermatitis, dry skin, burning skin, application site reaction and skin tenderness.

In a dermal sensitization study, 8 of 202 evaluable patients tested with sertaconazole nitrate 2% cream and 4 of 202 evaluable patients tested with vehicle, exhibited a slight erythematous reaction in the challenge phase. There was no evidence of cumulative irritation or contact sensitization in a repeated insult patch test involving 202 healthy volunteers. In non-US postmarketing surveillance for sertaconazole nitrate 2% cream, the following cutaneous adverse events were reported: Contact dermatitis, erythema, pruritus, vesiculation, desquamation, and hyperpigmentation.

Overdosage

Overdosage with sertaconazole nitrate 2% cream has not been reported to date. Sertaconazole nitrate 2% cream is intended for topical dermatologic use only. It is not for oral, ophthalmic, or intravaginal use.

Patient Information

Use sertaconazole nitrate 2% cream as directed by the physician. The hands should be washed after applying the medication to the affected area(s). Avoid contact with the eyes, nose, mouth and other mucous membranes. Sertaconazole nitrate 2% cream is for external use only.

Dry the affected area(s) thoroughly before application, if you wish to use sertaconazole nitrate 2% cream after bathing.

Use the medication for the full treatment time recommended by the physician, even though symptoms may have improved. Notify the physician if there is no improvement after the end of the prescribed treatment period, or sooner, if the condition worsens.

Inform the physician if the area of application shows signs of increased irritation, redness, itching, burning, blistering, swelling or oozing.

SERTACONAZOLE NITRATE — TOPICAL

Avoid the use of occlusive dressings unless otherwise directed by the physician.

Do not use this medication for any disorder other than that for which it was prescribed.

KETOCONAZOLE

Rx	**Ketoconazole** (Teva)	**Cream:** 2% in an aqueous vehicle[1]	Cetyl alcohol, stearyl alcohol, sodium sulfite. In 15, 30, and 60 g.
Rx	**Nizoral** (McNeil)		In 15, 30, and 60 g.
otc	**Nizoral A-D** (McNeil Consumer)	**Shampoo:** 1%	In 207 mL.
Rx	**Ketoconazole** (Clay-Park)	**Shampoo:** 2%	In 118 mL.
Rx	**Nizoral** (McNeil)	**Shampoo:** 2% in an aqueous suspension	In 120 mL.

[1] With sodium sulfite.

KETOCONAZOLE — TOPICAL

Indications

➤*Fungal infections:*

Cream – Tinea corporis (ringworm), tinea cruris (jock itch) and tinea pedis (athlete's foot) caused by *Trichophyton rubrum, T. mentagrophytes* and *E. floccosum*; tinea (pityriasis) versicolor caused by *P. orbiculare* (*M. furfur*); cutaneous candidiasis caused by *Candida* sp.; seborrheic dermatitis.

Shampoo – Reduction of scaling due to dandruff.

Administration and Dosage

➤*Cream:*

Cutaneous candidiasis, tinea corporis, tinea cruris and tinea (pityriasis) versicolor – Apply once daily to cover the affected and immediate surrounding area. Clinical improvement may be seen fairly soon after treatment is begun; however, treat candidal infections and tinea cruris and corporis for 2 weeks in order to reduce the possibility of recurrence. Patients with tinea versicolor usually require 2 weeks of treatment. Patients with tinea pedis require 6 weeks of treatment.

Seborrheic dermatitis – Apply to the affected area twice daily for 4 weeks or until clinical clearing. If a patient shows no clinical improvement after the treatment period, redetermine the diagnosis.

➤*Shampoo:*

Dandruff – Moisten hair and scalp thoroughly with water. Apply sufficient shampoo to produce enough lather to wash scalp and hair and gently massage it over the entire scalp area for ≈ 1 minute. Rinse hair thoroughly with warm water. Repeat, leaving shampoo on scalp for an additional 3 minutes. After the second thorough rinse, dry hair with towel or warm air flow. Shampoo twice a week for 4 weeks with at least 3 days between each shampooing, and then intermittently as needed to maintain control.

➤*Storage/Stability:* Do not store above room temperature (25°C; 77°F); protect from light.

Actions

➤*Pharmacology:* Ketoconazole is a broad spectrum antifungal agent. In vitro studies suggest it impairs ergosterol synthesis, which is a vital component of fungal cell membranes. The therapeutic effect in seborrheic dermatitis and dandruff may be due to reduction of *Pityrosporum ovale* (*Malassezia ovale*).

➤*Microbiology:* Ketoconazole inhibits the growth of the following common dermatophytes and yeasts by altering the permeability of the cell membrane. Dermatophytes: *Trichophyton rubrum, T. mentagrophytes, T. tonsurans, Microsporum canis, M. audouini, M. gypseum* and *Epidermophyton floccosum*. Yeasts: *Candida albicans, C. tropicalis, P. ovale* (*M. ovale*); and *P. orbiculare* (*M. furfur*, the organism responsible for tinea versicolor). Development of resistance to the drug has not been reported.

Contraindications

Hypersensitivity to any component of the product.

Warnings

➤*Pregnancy: Category C.* There are no adequate and well controlled studies in pregnant women. Use during pregnancy only if the potential benefits outweigh the potential hazards to the fetus.

➤*Lactation:* Safety for use in the nursing mother has not been established; however, exercise caution when applying on a nursing woman.

➤*Children:* Safety and efficacy in children have not been established.

Precautions

➤*For external use only:* Avoid contact with the eyes.

➤*Sensitivity:* Discontinue if sensitivity or chemical irritation occurs.

➤*Sulfite sensitivity:* The cream contains sulfites that may cause allergic-type reactions including anaphylactic symptoms and life-threatening or less severe asthmatic episodes in certain susceptible persons. The overall prevalence of sulfite sensitivity in the general population is unknown and probably low. It is seen more frequently in asthmatic or atopic nonasthmatic persons.

Adverse Reactions

Cream – Severe irritation, pruritus, stinging (approximately 5%); painful allergic reaction (one patient).

Shampoo – Increase in normal hair loss, irritation (less than 1%); abnormal hair texture; scalp pustules; mild dryness of skin; itching; oiliness/dryness of hair and scalp.

Overdosage

➤*Shampoo:* In the event of ingestion, employ supportive measures, including gastric lavage with sodium bicarbonate. Refer to General Management of Acute Overdosage.

Patient Information

For external use only. Avoid contact with the eyes.

➤*Shampoo:* Removal of the curl from permanently waved hair may occur.

MICONAZOLE NITRATE

otc	**Tetterine** (S.S.S. Company)	**Ointment:** 2%	Petrolatum. In 28.4 g.
otc	**Miconazole Nitrate** (Taro)	**Cream:** 2%	Benzoic acid, mineral oil, apricot kernal oil. In 15 and 30 g.
otc	**Micatin** (Ortho)		Mineral oil. In 15 and 30 g.
Rx	**Monistat-Derm** (Ortho)		Water miscible, mineral oil base. In 15, 30 and 90 g.
otc	**Neosporin AF** (Pfizer Consumer Healthcare)		Mineral oil. In 14 g.
otc	**Micatin** (Ortho)	**Powder:** 2%	In 90 g.
otc	**Lotrimin AF** (Schering-Plough)		Talc. In 90 g.
otc	**Zeasorb-AF** (Stiefel)		In 70 g.
otc	**Lotrimin AF** (Schering-Plough)	**Spray Powder:** 2%	10% SD alcohol 40. In 100 g
otc	**Micatin** (Ortho)		Alcohol. Available with and without deodorant. In 90 g.
otc	**Prescription Strength Desenex** (Ciba)		10% SD alcohol 40-B, aloe vera gel. In 90 mL.
otc	**Ting** (Heritage)		10% SD alcohol 40, aloe vera gel. In 85 g.
otc	**Micatin** (Ortho)	**Spray Liquid:** 2%	Alcohol. In 105 mL.
otc	**Lotrimin AF** (Schering-Plough)		17% SD alcohol 40. In 113 mL.
otc	**Neosporin AF** (Schering-Plough)		Alcohol. In 105 g.
otc	**Prescription Strength Desenex** (Ciba)		15% SD alcohol 40-B. In 105 mL.
otc	**Fungoid Tincture** (Pedinol)	**Solution:** 2%	Alcohol. In 7.39 and 29.57 mL with brush applicator.
otc	**Zeasorb-AF** (Stiefel)	**Gel:** 2%	Alcohol. In 24 g.

MICONAZOLE NITRATE — TOPICAL

Indications

Treatment of athlete's foot (tinea pedis), jock itch (tinea cruris) and ringworm (tinea corporis). For effective relief of the itching, burning, cracking and scaling which can accompany these conditions.

Administration and Dosage

➤*Approved by the FDA:* June 30, 1999.

Clean the affected area and dry thoroughly. Shake spray can well, hold 4 to 6 inches from skin. Apply or spray a thin layer of the product over affected area twice daily (morning and night) or as directed by a doctor. Supervise children in the use of this product.

For athlete's foot, pay special attention to the spaces between the toes. Wear well-fitting, ventilated shoes and change shoes and socks at least once daily. For athlete's foot or ringworm, use daily for 4 weeks. For jock itch, use daily for 2 weeks. If condition persists longer, consult a doctor. Supervise children in the use of this product. This product is not effective on the scalp or nails.

➤*Storage/Stability:* Store at room temperature, 15° to 30°C (59°to 86°F).

Sprays – Contents under pressure. Do not puncture or incinerate. Flammable mixture, do not use near fire or flame. Do not expose to heat or temperatures above 49°C (120°F). Use only as directed. Intentional misuse by deliberately concentrating and inhaling the contents can be harmful or fatal.

Warnings

➤*For external use only:* Avoid contact with the eyes or other mucous membranes.

➤*Irritation:* If irritation occurs, discontinue use and consult a doctor. Use only as directed.

➤*Pregnancy:* If pregnant ask a health professional before use.

➤*Lactation:* If breastfeeding, ask a health professional before use.

➤*Children:* Do not use on children under 2 years of age unless directed by a doctor. Keep this and all drugs out of the reach of children. In case of accidental ingestion, seek professional assistance or contact a poison control center immediately.

NAFTIFINE HCl

Rx	**Naftin** (Allergan Herbert)	**Cream:** 1%	In 15, 30 and 60 g.
		Gel: 1%	In 20, 40 and 60 g.

NAFTIFINE HYDROCHLORIDE — TOPICAL

Indications

➤*Fungal infection:* For the topical of tinea pedis, tinea cruris, and tinea corporis caused by the organisms *Trichophyton rubrum, Trichophyton mentagrophytes, Trichophyton tonsurans*†, and *Epidermophyton floccosum*.

Administration and Dosage

➤*Approved by the FDA:* February 29, 1988.

A sufficient quantity of naftifine should be gently massaged into the affected and surrounding skin areas once a day in the morning and evening. The hands should be washed after application.

If no clinical improvement is seen after 4 weeks of treatment with naftifine hydrochloride gel or cream 1%, the patient should be re-evaluated.

➤*Storage/Stability:*

Gel – Store at room temperature.

Cream – Store below 30°C (86°F).

Actions

➤*Pharmacology:* Naftifine hydrochloride is a synthetic, allylamine derivative. The following in vitro data are available, but their clinical significance is unknown. Naftifine hydrochloride has been shown to exhibit fungicidal activity in vitro against a broad spectrum of organisms including *Trichophyton rubrum, Trichophyton mentagrophytes, Trichophyton tonsurans, Epidermophyton floccosum*, and *Microsporum canis, Microsporum audouini*, and *Microsporum gypseum*; and fungistatic activity against *Candida* species including *Candida albicans*. Naftifine hydrochloride gel and cream 1% have only been shown to be clinically effective against the disease entities listed in the Indications.

Although the exact mechanism of action against fungi is not known, naftifine hydrochloride appears to interfere with sterol biosynthesis by inhibiting the enzyme squalene 2,3-epoxidase. This inhibition of enzyme activity results in decreased amounts of sterols, especially ergosterol, and a corresponding accumulation of squalene in the cells.

➤*Pharmacokinetics:* In vitro and in vivo bioavailability studies have demonstrated that naftifine penetrates the stratum corneum in sufficient concentration to inhibit the growth of dermatophytes.

Following a single topical application of 1% naftifine cream to the skin of healthy subjects, systemic absorption was approximately 6% of the applied dose.

Following single topical applications of ^{3}H-labeled naftifine gel 1% to the skin of healthy subjects, up to 4.2% of the applied dose was absorbed. Naftifine and/or its metabolites are excreted via the urine and feces with a half-life of approximately two to three days.

Contraindications

Hypersensitivity to any of its components.

Warnings

➤*For external use only:* Naftifine hydrochloride gel and cream 1% are for topical use only and not for ophthalmic use.

➤*Pregnancy: Category B.* There are no adequate and well-controlled studies in pregnant women. This drug should be used during pregnancy only if clearly needed.

➤*Lactation:* It is not known whether this drug is excreted in human milk. Because many drugs are excreted in human milk, caution should be exercised when naftifine hydrochloride gel or cream 1% is administered to a nursing woman.

➤*Children:* Safety and effectiveness in pediatric patients have not been established.

Precautions

➤*Irritation/diagnosis:* Naftifine hydrochloride gel and cream 1% are for external use only. If irritation or sensitivity develop with the use of naftifine hydrochloride gel or cream 1%, treatment should be discontinued and appropriate therapy instituted. Diagnosis of the disease should be confirmed either by direct microscopic examination of a mounting of infected tissue in a solution of potassium hydroxide or by culture on an appropriate medium.

Adverse Reactions

➤*Gel:*

Dermatologic – During clinical trials, the incidence of adverse reactions was as follows: Burning/stinging (5%), itching (1%), erythema (0.5%), rash (0.5%), skin tenderness (0.5%).

➤*Cream:*

Dermatologic – During clinical trials, the incidence of adverse reactions was as follows: Burning/stinging (6%), dryness (3%), erythema (2%), itching (2%), local irritation (2%).

Patient Information

Avoid the use of occlusive dressings or wrappings unless otherwise directed by the physician.

Keep naftifine hydrochloride gel or cream 1% away from the eyes, nose, mouth and other mucous membranes.

NYSTATIN

Rx	**Nystatin** (Various, eg, Major, NMC)	**Cream:** 100,000 units per g	In 15 and 30 g.
Rx	**Mycostatin** (Westwood Squibb)		Aqueous vanishing cream base. In 15 and 30 g.
Rx	**Nilstat** (Lederle)		Aqueous vanishing cream base. In 15 and 240 g.
Rx	**Nystatin** (Various, eg, Goldline, Major, Moore, NMC)	**Ointment:** 100,000 units per g	In 15 and 30 g.
Rx	**Mycostatin** (Westwood Squibb)		Polyethylene and mineral oil gel base. In 15 and 30 g.
Rx	**Nilstat** (Lederle)		Light mineral oil and plastibase 50W. In 15 g.
Rx	**Nystatin** (Various, eg, Par)	**Powder:** 100,000 units per g	Dispersed in talc. In 15 and 60 g.
Rx	**Mycostatin** (Westwood Squibb)		Dispersed in talc. In 15 g.
Rx	**Nystop** (Paddock)		Dispersed in talc. In 15 and 30 g.
Rx	**Pedi-Dri** (Pedinol)		Dispersed in talc. In 56.7 g.

† Efficacy for these organisms in this organ system was studied in fewer than 10 infections.

NYSTATIN — TOPICAL

Indications

➤*Mycotic infections:* Treatment of cutaneous or mucocutaneous mycotic infections, caused by *Candida (Monilia) albicans* and other *Candida* species. Conditions such as athlete's foot (dermatophytosis), perleche, paronychia, intertrigo, diaper rash, and other cutaneous lesions can be expected to respond. The cream is usually preferred to the ointment in moniliasis involving intertriginous areas.

Administration and Dosage

➤*Nystatin cream and ointment:* Apply liberally to the affected areas twice daily or as indicated until healing is complete. Nystatin cream is usually preferred to nystatin ointment in candidiasis involving intertriginous areas; very moist lesions, however, are best treated with nystatin topical powder.

➤*Nystatin topical powder:* Apply to candidal lesions 2 or 3 times daily until lesions have healed. For fungal infection of the feet caused by *Candida* species, the powder should be dusted freely on the feet as well as in shoes and socks.

➤*Storage/Stability:*

Cream and topical powder – Store at controlled room temperature 15° to 30°C (59° to 86°F). Avoid exposure to excessive heat, 40°C (104°F). Keep out of reach of children.

Ointment – Store at room temperature not exceeding 25°C (77°F). Avoid excessive heat.

Actions

➤*Pharmacology:* Nystatin is an antibiotic with antifungal activity against a wide variety of yeasts and yeast-like fungi. It probably acts by binding to sterols in the cell membrane of the fungus with a resultant change in membrane permeability, allowing leakage of intracellular components. Nystatin is a polyene antibiotic of undetermined structural formula that is obtained from *Streptomyces noursei* and is the first well tolerated antifungal antibiotic of dependable efficacy for the treatment of cutaneous, oral and intestinal infections caused by *Candida (Monilia) albicans* and other *Candida* species. Nystatin exhibits no appreciable activity against bacteria.

Nystatin provides specific therapy for all localized forms of candidiasis. Symptomatic relief is rapid, often occurring within 24 to 72 hours after the initiation of treatment. Cure is effected both clinically and mycologically in most cases of localized candidiasis.

Contraindications

History of hypersensitivity to any component.

Warnings

➤*Adverse reactions:* Nystatin is virtually nontoxic and nonsensitising and is well-tolerated by all age groups including debilitated infants, even on prolonged administration. Large oral doses have occasionally produced diarrhea and gastrointestinal disturbance. If local sensitization develops, treatment should be discontinued.

Precautions

➤*Hypersensitivity:* Should a reaction of hypersensitivity occur, the drug should be immediately withdrawn and appropriate measures taken.

➤*For external use only:* This preparation is not for ophthalmic use.

Overdosage

Treatment of overdosage should be symptomatic and supportive.

OXICONAZOLE NITRATE

Rx	**Oxistat** (GlaxoWellcome)	**Cream:** 1%	White petrolatum, propylene glycol, stearyl alcohol NF, cetyl alcohol NF, 0.2% benzoic acid. In 15, 30 and 60 g tubes.
		Lotion: 1%	White petrolatum, propylene glycol, stearyl alcohol NF, cetyl alcohol NF, 0.2% benzoic acid. In 30 mL.

OXICONAZOLE NITRATE — TOPICAL

Indications

➤*Fungal infections:* For the treatment of the following dermal infections: Tinea pedis, tinea cruris, and tinea corporis due to *Trichophyton rubrum*, *Trichophyton mentagrophytes*, or *Epidermophyton floccosum*.

Cream – For the treatment of tinea (pityriasis) versicolor due to *Malassezia furfur*.

Oxiconazole cream may be used in children for tinea corporis, tinea cruris, tinea pedis, and tinea (pityriasis) versicolor; however, these indications for which oxiconazole cream has been shown to be effective rarely occur in children younger than 12 years of age.

Administration and Dosage

➤*Approved by the FDA:* August 18, 1997.

Oxiconazole cream or lotion should be applied to affected and immediately surrounding areas once to twice daily in patients with tinea pedia, tinea corporis, or tinea cruris.

➤*Cream:* Oxiconazole cream should be applied once daily in the treatment of tinea (pityriasis) versicolor. Tinea corporis, tinea cruris, and tinea (pityriasis) versicolor should be treated for 2 weeks and tinea pedis for 1 month to reduce the possibility of recurrence. If a patient shows no clinical improvement after the treatment period, the diagnosis should be reviewed.

Note – Tinea (pityriasis) versicolor may give rise to hyperpigmented or hypopigmented patches on the trunk that may extend to the neck, arms, and upper thighs. Treatment of the infection may not immediately result in restoration of pigment to the affected sites. Normalization of pigment following successful therapy is variable and may take months, depending on individual skin type and incidental sun exposure. Although tinea (pityriasis) versicolor is not contagious, it may recur because the organism that causes the disease is part of the normal skin flora.

➤*Storage/Stability:* Store between 15° and 30°C (59° and 86°F).

Actions

➤*Pharmacokinetics:* The penetration of oxiconazole nitrate into different layers of the skin was assessed using an in vitro permeation technique with human skin. Five hours after application of 2.5 mg/cm^2 of oxiconazole nitrate cream onto human skin, the concentration of oxiconazole nitrate was demonstrated to be 16.2 mcmol in the epidermis, 3.64 mcmol in the upper corium, and 1.29 mcmol in the deeper corium. Systemic absorption of oxiconazole nitrate is low. Using radiolabeled drug, less than 0.3% of the applied dose of oxiconazole nitrate was recovered in the urine of volunteer subjects up to 5 days after application of the cream formulation.

➤*Microbiology:* Oxiconazole nitrate is an imidazole derivative whose antifungal activity is derived primarily from the inhibition of ergosterol biosynthesis, which is critical for cellular membrane integrity. It has in vitro activity against a wide range of pathogenic fungi.

Oxiconazole has been shown to be active against most strains of the following organisms both in vitro and in clinical infections at indicated body sites (see Indications): *Epidermophyton floccosum, Trichophyton mentagrophytes, Trichophyton rubrum*, and *Malassezia furfur*.

Contraindications

Hypersensitivity to any of their components.

Warnings

➤*For external use only:* Oxiconazole cream and lotion are not for ophthalmic or intravaginal use.

➤*Fertility impairment:* Reproductive studies revealed no impairment of fertility in rats at oral doses of 3 mg/kg per day in females (1 time the human dose based on mg/m^2) and 15 mg/kg per day in males (4 times the human dose based on mg/m^2). However, at doses above this level, the following effects were observed: A reduction in the fertility parameters of males and females, a reduction in the number of sperm in vaginal smears, extended estrous cycle, and a decrease in mating frequency.

➤*Pregnancy: Category B.* There are no adequate and well-controlled studies in pregnant women. This drug should be used during pregnancy only if clearly needed.

➤*Lactation:* Because oxiconazole is excreted in human milk, caution should be exercised when the drug is administered to a nursing woman.

➤*Children:* Oxiconazole cream may be used in pediatric patients for tinea corporis, tinea cruris, tinea pedis, and tinea (pityriasis) versicolor; however, these indications for which oxiconazole cream has been shown to be effective rarely occur in children < 12 years of age.

Precautions

➤*Irritation:* Oxiconazole cream and lotion are for external dermal use only. Avoid introduction of oxiconazole cream or lotion into the eyes or vagina. If a reaction suggesting sensitivity or chemical irritation should occur with the use of oxiconazole cream or lotion, treatment should be discontinued and appropriate therapy instituted. If signs of epidermal irritation should occur, the drug should be discontinued.

Drug Interactions

None known.

Adverse Reactions

➤*Cream:* During clinical trials, of 955 patients treated with oxiconazole nitrate cream, 1%, 41 (4.3%) reported adverse reactions thought to be related to drug therapy. These reactions included pruritus (1.6%); burning (1.4%); irritation and allergic contact dermatitis (0.4% each); folliculitis (0.3%); erythema (0.2%); and papules, fissure, maceration, rash, stinging, and nodules (0.1% each).

OXICONAZOLE NITRATE — TOPICAL

➤*Lotion:* In a controlled, multicenter clinical trial of 269 patients treated with oxiconazole nitrate lotion, 1%, 7 (2.6%) reported adverse reactions thought to be related to drug therapy. These reactions included burning and stinging (0.7% each) and pruritus, scaling, tingling, pain, and dyshidrotic eczema (0.4% each).

Overdosage

When 5% oxiconazole cream (5 times the concentration of the marketed product) was applied at a rate of 1 g/kg to ≈ 10% of body surface area of a group of 40 male and female rats for 35 days, 3 deaths and severe dermal inflammation were reported. No overdoses in humans have been reported with use of oxiconazole nitrate cream or lotion.

Patient Information

Use oxiconazole as directed by the physician. The hands should be washed after applying the medication to the affected area(s). Avoid contact with the eyes, nose, mouth, and other mucous membranes. Oxiconazole is for external use only.

Use the medication for the full treatment time recommended by the physician, even though symptoms may have improved. Notify the physician if there is no improvement after 2 to 4 weeks, or sooner if the condition worsens (see below).

Inform the physician if the area of application shows signs of increased irritation, itching, burning, blistering, swelling, or oozing.

Avoid the use of occlusive dressings unless otherwise directed by the physician.

Do not use this medication for any disorder other than that for which it was prescribed.

SULCONAZOLE NITRATE

Rx	**Exelderm** (Westwood Squibb)	**Cream:** 1%	In 15, 30 and 60 g tubes.
		Solution: 1%	In 30 mL.

SULCONAZOLE NITRATE — TOPICAL

Indications

➤*Fungal infections:*

Cream – For the treatment of tinea pedis (athlete's foot), tinea cruris, and tinea corporis caused by *Trichophyton rubrum*, *Trichophyton mentagrophytes*, *Epidermophyton floccosum*, and *Microsporum canis* (Efficacy for this organism in the organ system was studied in less than 10 infections), and for the treatment of tinea versicolor.

Solution – For the treatment of tinea cruris and tinea corporis caused by *Trichophyton rubrum*, *Trichophyton mentagrophytes*, *Epidermophyton floccosum*, and *Microsporum canis*; and for the treatment of tinea versicolor. Effectiveness has not been proven in tinea pedis (athlete's foot).

Administration and Dosage

➤*Approved by the FDA:* February 28, 1989.

If significant clinical improvement is not seen after 4 weeks of treatment, an alternate diagnosis should be considered.

➤*Cream:* A small amount of cream should be gently massaged into the affected and surrounding skin areas once or twice daily, except in tinea pedis, where administration should be twice daily.

Early relief of symptoms is experienced by the majority of patients and clinical improvement may be seen fairly soon after treatment is begun; however, tinea corporis/cruris and tinea versicolor should be treated for 3 weeks and tinea pedis for 4 weeks to reduce the possibility of recurrence.

➤*Solution:* A small amount of the solution should be gently massaged into the affected and surrounding skin areas once or twice daily.

Symptomatic relief usually occurs within a few days after starting sulconazole nitrate solution, 1%, and clinical improvement usually occurs within 1 week. To reduce the possibility of recurrence, tinea cruris, tinea corporis, and tinea versicolor should be treated for 3 weeks.

➤*Storage/Stability:* Avoid excessive heat, above 40°C (104°F), and protect from light.

Actions

➤*Pharmacology:* Sulconazole nitrate is an imidazole derivative that inhibits the growth of the common pathogenic dermatophytes including *Trichophyton rubrum*, *Trichophyton mentagrophytes*, *Epidermophyton floccosum*, and *Microsporum canis*. It also inhibits the organism responsible for tinea versicolor, *Malassezia furfur*, and certain gram positive bacteria.

Contraindications

Hypersensitivity to any of the ingredients.

Warnings

➤*Pregnancy: Category C.* Sulconazole nitrate has been shown to be embryotoxic in rats when given in doses 125 times the human dose (in mg/kg). The drug at this dose given orally to rats also resulted in prolonged gestation and dystocia. Several females died during the perinatal period, most likely due to labor complications. Sulconazole nitrate was not teratogenic in rats or rabbits at oral doses of 50 mg/kg/day.

There are no adequate and well-controlled studies in pregnant women. Sulconazole nitrate should be used during pregnancy only if the potential benefit justifies the potential risk to the fetus.

➤*Lactation:* It is not known whether this drug is excreted in human milk. Because many drugs are excreted in human milk, caution should be exercised when sulconazole nitrate is administered to a nursing woman.

➤*Children:* Safety and effectiveness have not been established.

Precautions

➤*For external use only:* Avoid contact with the eyes. If irritation develops, the solution or cream should be discontinued and appropriate therapy instituted.

Adverse Reactions

➤*Cream:* There were no systemic effects and only infrequent cutaneous adverse reactions in 1185 patients treated with sulconazole nitrate cream in controlled clinical trials. Approximately 3% of these patients reported itching, 3% burning or stinging, and 1% redness. These complaints did not usually interfere with treatment.

➤*Solution:* There were no systemic effects and only infrequent cutaneous adverse reactions in 370 patients treated with sulconazole nitrate solution in controlled clinical trials. Approximately 1% of these patients reported itching and 1% burning or stinging. These complaints did not usually interfere with treatment.

Patient Information

Use sulconazole nitrate as directed by the physician, only use it externally, and avoid contact with the eyes.

TERBINAFINE HCl

otc	**DesenexMyax** (Novartis)	**Cream:** 1%	Benzyl alcohol, stearyl alcohol, cetyl alcohol. In 24 g.
otc	**Lamisil AT** (Novartis)		With benzyl alcohol, cetyl alcohol and stearyl alcohol. In 15 and 30 g.
otc	**Lamisil AT** (Novartis)	**Spray:** 1%	Ethanol, propylene glycol. In 30 mL.

TERBINAFINE HYDROCHLORIDE — TOPICAL

Indications

➤*Dermatologic infections:* For the topical treatment of the following dermatologic infections: Tinea (pityriasis) versicolor due to *Malassezia furfur* (formerly *Pityrosporum ovale*), and tinea pedis (athlete's foot), tinea cruris (jock itch), or tinea corporis (ringworm), due to *Trichophyton rubrum*, *Trichophyton mentagrophytes*, or *Epidermophyton floccosum* (see Administration and Dosage). Diagnosis of disease should be confirmed either by culture (except *Malassezia furfur* [formerly *Pityrosporum ovale*]) or direct microscopic examination of scrapings from infected tissue mounted in a solution of potassium hydroxide.

Administration and Dosage

➤*Terbinafine hydrochloride cream or spray:*

For adults and children 12 years and over – Use the tip of the cap to break the seal and open the tube of the cream. For the cream or spray use the following directions. Wash the affected skin with soap and water and dry completely before applying. For athlete's foot, wear well-fitting, ventilated shoes. Change shoes and socks at least once daily. For athlete's foot between the toes only, apply twice a day (morning and night) for 1 week or as directed by a doctor. For athlete's foot on the bottom or sides of the foot, apply twice a day (morning and night) for 2 weeks or as directed by a doctor. For jock

TERBINAFINE HYDROCHLORIDE — TOPICAL

itch and ringworm, apply once a day (morning or night) for 1 week or as directed by a doctor. Wash hands after each use.

Children under 12 years of age – Ask a doctor.

➤*Storage/Stability:*

Terbinafine hydrochloride cream – Store between 5° and 30°C (41° to 86°F). See box or tube crimp for lot number and expiration date. Do not use if seal on tube is broken or is not visible.

Terbinafine hydrochloride spray – Store at 8° to 25°C (46° to 77°F).

Actions

➤*Pharmacokinetics:*

Absorption – In a study of 10 patients with tinea cruris, once-daily application of terbinafine hydrochloride solution for 7 days (total amount of terbinafine hydrochloride applied averaged 0.8 g) resulted in plasma concentrations of terbinafine of up to 21 ng/mL on day 7, representing ≈ 2% of plasma concentrations achieved with a 250 mg terbinafine hydrochloride tablet. Plasma concentrations of the N-demethylated metabolite of terbinafine ranged up to 14 ng/mL in these patients. In subjects with healthy skin, neither the parent nor the N-demethylated metabolite were detected in the plasma following once-daily dosing for seven days with 0.3 g of 1% terbinafine hydrochloride solution.

Distribution – The skin pharmacokinetics of terbinafine hydrochloride solution, delivered by spray was compared to the 1% cream in 36 healthy subjects following both single and multiple applications (≈ 5 mg of terbinafine hydrochloride was applied to roughly a 190 cm^2 area on the back). Maximum mean total stratum corneum drug concentrations (C_{max}) averaged 720 and 810 ng/cm^2 on days 1 and 7, respectively. No significant differences in total stratum corneum AUC (area under the curve), C_{max} and half-life were seen between the 1% spray and the 1% cream after 1 or 7 days of treatment. Similar skin levels of terbinafine are achieved by delivery of terbinafine hydrochloride solution from the spray bottle or from application of terbinafine hydrochloride cream.

Metabolism – It is unknown whether or not there is any significant skin metabolism of topically applied terbinafine. Radiolabeled studies with oral dosage forms indicate that terbinafine is highly metabolized into a number of metabolites which undergo conjugation and excretion into the urine. The primary metabolite seen in the urine (10% of the oral dose) is N-demethyl terbinafine.

Excretion – The half-life of terbinafine when absorbed through the skin, regardless of the method of topical administration, is ≈ 21 hours. Approximately 75% of cutaneously absorbed terbinafine is eliminated in the urine, predominately as metabolites.

➤*Microbiology:* Terbinafine hydrochloride is a synthetic allylamine derivative. Terbinafine hydrochloride is hypothesized to act by inhibiting the epoxidation of squalene, thus blocking the biosynthesis of ergosterol, an essential component of fungal cell membranes. The allylamine derivatives, like the benzylamines, act at an earlier step in the ergosterol biosynthesis pathway than the azole class of antifungal drugs. Depending on the concentration of the drug and the fungal species tested in vitro, terbinafine hydrochloride may be fungicidal. However, the clinical significance of in vitro data is unknown.

Terbinafine has been shown to be active against most strains of the following organisms both in vitro and in clinical infections as described in Indications: *Epidermophyton floccosum*, *Malassezia furfur* (formerly *Pityrosporum ovale*), *Trichophyton mentagrophytes*, and *Trichophyton rubrum*.

Contraindications

Known or suspected hypersensitivity to terbinafine or any other of its components.

Warnings

➤*For external use only:* Terbinafine is not for ophthalmic, oral, or intravaginal use.

➤*Pregnancy: Category B.*

There are no adequate and well-controlled studies in pregnant women. Only use terbinafine hydrochloride if clearly indicated during pregnancy.

➤*Lactation:* After a single oral dose of 500 mg of terbinafine hydrochloride to 2 volunteers, the total dose of terbinafine secreted in human milk during the 72-hour post-dosing period was 0.65 mg in 1 person and 0.15 mg in the other. The total excretion of terbinafine in human milk was 0.13% and 0.03% of the administered dose, respectively. This 500 mg dose represents about 50 times the percutaneous exposure as described in the previous paragraph. The concentrations of the N-demethylated metabolite measured in the human milk of these 2 volunteers were below the detection limit of the assay used (150 ng/mL of milk).

Because of the small amount of data on human neonatal exposure, a decision should be made whether to discontinue nursing or to discontinue the drug, taking into account the importance of the drug to the mother.

Nursing mothers should avoid application of terbinafine hydrochloride solution to the breast.

➤*Children:* Safety and efficacy have not been established in children.

Drug Interactions

None known.

Adverse Reactions

➤*Local:* Burning or irritation (1.3%); itching (1.1%); skin exfoliation (1%); rash (0.9%).

Patient Information

Use terbinafine hydrochloride as directed by the physician and avoid contact with the eyes, nose, mouth, or other mucous membranes. The spray form should not be used on the face. In case of accidental contact with the eyes, rinse eyes thoroughly with running water and consult a physician if any symptoms persist.

Use the medication for the full treatment time even though symptoms may have improved.

Inform the physician if the area of application shows signs of increased irritation or possible sensitization (redness, itching, burning, blistering, swelling, or oozing).

Avoid the use of occlusive dressings unless otherwise directed by the physician.

TOLNAFTATE

otc	**Tolnaftate** (Various, eg, Fougera, Goldline, IDE, Moore, Parmed, NMC, Rugby, UDL)	**Cream:** 1%	In 15 g.
otc	**Absorbine Athlete's Foot Cream** (W.F. Young)		Parabens. In 21.3 g.
otc	**Genaspor** (Goldline)		In 15 g.
otc	**Tinactin** (Schering-Plough)		In 15 and 30 g.
otc	**Tinactin for Jock Itch** (Schering-Plough)		Petrolatum, mineral oil. In 15 g.
otc	**Ting** (Fisons)		In 15 g.
otc	**Tolnaftate** (Various, eg, Copley, Fougera, Goldline, Major, Moore, Parmed, Rugby)	**Solution:** 1%	In 10 mL.
otc	**Tinactin** (Schering-Plough)		In 10 mL.
otc	**Aftate for Athlete's Foot** (Schering-Plough)	**Gel:** 1%	In 15 g.
otc	**Aftate for Jock Itch** (Schering-Plough)		In 15 g.
otc	**Tolnaftate** (Various)	**Powder:** 1%	In 45 g.
otc	**Quinsana Plus** (Stephan)		Cornstarch, talc. In 90 g.
otc	**Tinactin** (Schering-Plough)		Cornstarch, talc. In 45 and 90 g.
otc	**Aftate for Athlete's Foot** (Schering-Plough)	**Spray Powder:** 1%	14% alcohol, talc. In 105 g.
otc	**Aftate for Jock Itch** (Schering-Plough)		14% alcohol. In 105 g.
otc	**Tinactin** (Schering-Plough)		14% alcohol, talc. **Deodorant:** In 100 g. **Regular:** In 100, 150 g.
otc	**Tinactin for Jock Itch** (Schering-Plough)		14% alcohol, talc. In 100 g.
otc	**Absorbine Footcare** (W.F. Young)	**Spray Liquid:** 1%	Acetone, chloroxylenol, menthol, wormwood oil. In 59.2 and 118.3 mL.
otc	**Aftate for Athlete's Foot** (Schering-Plough)		36% alcohol. In 120 mL.
otc	**Tinactin** (Schering-Plough)		36% alcohol. In 120 mL.

TOLNAFTATE — TOPICAL

Indications

➤*Fungal infection:* Treatment of tinea pedis (athlete's foot), cruris (jock itch) or corporis (ringworm) due to infection with *Trichophyton rubrum, T. mentagrophytes, T. tonsurans, Microsporum canis, M. audouini,* and *Epidermophyton floccosum* and for tinea versicolor due to *Malassezia furfur.*

In onychomycosis, in chronic scalp infections in which fungi are numerous and widely distributed in skin and hair follicles, where kerion has formed and in fungus infections of palms and soles, use tolnaftate concurrently for adjunctive local benefit in these lesions.

Powder and powder aerosol – Also effective prophylactically against athlete's foot.

Administration and Dosage

Only small quantities are required. Treatment twice a day for 2 or 3 weeks is usually adequate, although 4 to 6 weeks may be required if the skin has thickened. Continue treatment to maintain remission.

The choice of vehicle is important for these products. Ointments, creams, and liquids are used as primary therapy. In general, powders are used as adjunctive therapy, but they may be acceptable as primary therapy in very mild conditions.

Before applying tolnaftate, wash the affected area with soap and water and dry thoroughly. Then apply enough medicine to cover the affected area.

➤*For athlete's foot and ringworm:* Use daily for 4 weeks.

➤*For jock itch:* Use daily for 2 weeks.

➤*Dosing:*

Aerosol powder, aerosol solution, liquid spray, cream, gel, powder, or topical solution –

For fungus infections:

• *Adults and children 2 years of age and older* – Apply to the affected area(s) of the skin 2 times per day (morning and night).

• *Children younger than 2 years of age* – Use is not recommended except under the advice and supervision of a doctor.

Athlete's foot: Pay special attention to the spaces between the toes when applying tolnaftate.

To prevent athlete's foot, apply the powder or liquid or powder spray forms of this medicine once or twice daily (morning and/or night).

For athlete's foot, wear well-fitting, ventilated shoes; change shoes and socks at least once a day.

Powder: If powder is used on the feet, sprinkle it between the toes, on feet, and in socks and shoes.

Aerosol powder: Shake well before using.

From a distance of 6 to 10 inches, spray the powder on the affected areas. If it is used on the feet, spray it between toes, on feet, and in socks and shoes.

Do not inhale the powder.

Do not use near heat, open flame, or while smoking.

Solution: If the solution becomes a solid, it may be dissolved by warming the closed container of medicine in warm water.

Aerosol solution or liquid spray: Shake well before using.

From a distance of 6 to 10 inches, spray the solution on the affected area. If it is used on the feet, spray it between toes and on feet.

Do not inhale the vapors from the spray.

Do not use near heat, open flame, or while smoking.

Premeasured unit-dose swabs: Hold the swab vertically with the color band tip upwards. Bend the tip at the color band to one side until it snaps.

Discard swab after use.

➤*Storage/Stability:* Store at controlled room temperature 15° to 30°C (59° to 86°F). Store away from excessive heat, direct light, and cold.

Do not puncture, break, or burn the aerosol powder or aerosol solution container. Do not store at temperatures above 48.9°C (120°F).

Solution – Store at controlled room temperature 15° to 30°C (59° to 86°F). Store away from excessive heat, direct light, and cold.

The solution solidifies at low temperatures and liquifies readily when warmed, retaining its potency. Protect from freezing.

Actions

➤*Pharmacology:* Effective in the treatment of superficial fungal infections of the skin.

Warnings

➤*Discontinuation:* If symptoms do not improve after 10 days of use as recommended by the labeling, discontinue use unless otherwise directed.

➤*Sensitization or irritation:* Persons younger than 18 years of age or those with sensitive or allergic skin should only use as directed by a doctor. Discontinue treatment if sensitization or irritation develops.

➤*Nail/Scalp infections:* Not recommended for these infections except as adjunctive therapy to systemic treatment.

➤*Children:* Do not use in children younger than 2 years of age.

Precautions

➤*For external use only:* Keep out of the eyes.

➤*Prophylaxis:* To help prevent reinfection after the period of treatment with this medicine, the powder or spray powder forms of tolnaftate may be used each day after bathing and carefully drying the affected area.

➤*Reevaluate patient:* If no improvement or worsening occurs after 4 weeks, reevaluate patient.

Adverse Reactions

➤*Sensitivity:* A few cases of sensitization have been confirmed; mild irritation has occurred.

➤*Local:* A mild temporary stinging may be expected when applying the aerosol solution form of tolnaftate.

Patient Information

For external use only. Avoid contact with the eyes.

Before applying tolnaftate, wash the affected area with soap and water and dry thoroughly. Then apply enough medicine to cover the affected area.

Do not miss any doses.

Stop use and ask a doctor:

- If irritation occurs.
- If there is no improvement within 4 weeks (for athlete's foot and ringworm) or within 2 weeks (for jock itch).

➤*Dosing:* Some products are not affected on the scalp or nails. See individual product labeling.

Persons younger than 18 years of age or those with highly sensitive or allergic skin should only use as directed by a doctor. Tell your doctor if you have ever had an allergic reaction to tolnaftate or if you are allergic to any other substances, such as preservatives or dyes.

Supervise children in the use of this product.

If you are pregnant, planning to become pregnant, or breastfeeding, ask a doctor before using this medicine.

Tell your doctor if you are using any other topical prescription or nonprescription (OTC) medicine that will be applied to the same area of skin.

Keep out of reach of children. If swallowed, get medical help or contact a poison control center right away.

To prevent athlete's foot, apply the powder or liquid or powder spray forms of this medicine once or twice daily (morning and/or night).

For athlete's foot, wear well-fitting, ventilated shoes; change shoes and socks at least once a day.

UNDECYLENIC ACID AND DERIVATIVES

otc	**Caldesene** (Fisons)	**Powder:** 10% calcium undecylenate	In 60 and 120 g.
otc	**Cruex** (Ciba Consumer)		Talc. In 45 g.
otc	**Cruex Aerosol** (Ciba Consumer)	**Powder:** 19% total undecylenate as undecylenic acid and zinc undecylenate	Menthol, talc. In 54, 105 and 165 g.
otc	**Desenex** (Ciba Consumer)	**Powder:** 25% total undecylenate as undecylenic acid and zinc undecylenate	Talc. In 45 g.
otc	**Phicon F** (T.E. Williams)	**Cream:** 8% undecylenic acid, 0.05% pramoxine HCl	In 60 g.
otc	**Blis-To-Sol** (Oakhurst)	**Powder:** 12% zinc undecylenate	Bentonite, talc, zinc oxide. In 60 g.
otc	**Cruex** (Ciba Consumer)	**Cream:** 20% total undecylenate as undecylenic acid and zinc undecylenate	Lanolin, parabens, white petrolatum. In 15 g.
otc	**Elon Dual Defense Anti-Fungal Formula** (Dartmouth)	**Solution:** 25% undecylenic acid	Alcohol. In 30 mL.
otc	**Fungoid AF** (Pedinol)	**Solution:** 25% undecylenic acid	In 30 mL.
otc	**Gordochom** (Gordon)	**Solution:** 25% undecylenic acid and chloroxylenol in an oily base.	In 30 mL.
otc	**Desenex** (Ciba Consumer)	**Soap:** Undecylenic acid	In 97.5 g.

UNDECYLENIC ACID — TOPICAL

Indications

➤*Fungal infections:* Undecylenic acid eliminates fungal infections of the skin by inhibiting the growth and reproduction of fungal cells.

Undecylenic acid is formulated to cure most ringworm (tinea corporis) and athlete's foot (tinea pedis) affecting the finger and toe areas, including the skin around the nails. Undecylenic acid also helps to relieve the itching, scaling, cracking, burning, redness, soreness, irritations, and other related discomforts which may accompany these conditions.

This product is not effective on scalp or nails.

Administration and Dosage

➤*Directions:* Clean affected area with soap and warm water and dry thoroughly. Apply a thin layer of undecylenic acid solution over affected area twice daily (morning and night) or as directed by a doctor.

The choice of vehicle is important for these products. Ointments, creams, and liquids are used as primary therapy. In general, powders are used as adjunctive therapy, but they may be acceptable as primary therapy in very mild conditions.

Athlete's foot – For athlete's foot pay special attention to spaces between the toes. Wear well-fitting, ventilated shoes, and change shoes and socks at least once daily.

Athlete's foot and ringworm – For athlete's foot and ringworm, use daily for 4 weeks. If condition persists longer, consult a doctor.

➤*Storage/Stability:* Protect from freezing. If freezing occurs, warm to room temperature 21° to 27°C (70° to 80°F).

Actions

➤*Pharmacology:* Eliminates fungal infections of the skin by inhibiting the growth and reproduction of fungal cells.

Warnings

➤*For external use only:* Avoid contact with eyes.

➤*Accidental ingestion:* Stop use and contact a physician, emergency care facility or poison control center immediately for advice in case of accidental ingestion.

➤*Children:* Keep this and all medication out of the reach of children.

Do not use on children under 2 years of age unless directed by a doctor. If irritation occurs or if there is no improvement within 4 weeks, discontinue use and consult a doctor.

Patient Information

➤*General information about undecylenic acid:* For many years, physicians and pharmacists have recommended undecylenic acid for treating infections of the nails and surrounding tissue. However, in 1994 the FDA ruled that no over-the-counter antifungal product is effective on the nails. It was the FDA's opinion that products available without a prescription could not penetrate the nails, and were therefore ineffective in treating them. A statement reading "this product not effective on scalp or nails" was subsequently required on the labels of all over the counter antifungal products.

➤*Important tips on using undecylenic acid:* Use undecylenic acid as soon as an infection is detected. This will kill fungus before it gets out of control and prevents it from spreading to other areas.

ANTIFUNGAL COMBINATIONS

otc	**SteriNail** (Dr. Nordyke's Labs)	**Solution**: Undecylenic acid tolnaftate, propylene glycol, acetone, acetic acid, pripionic acid, benzyl alcohol, eucalyptol and benzyl acetate	In 30 mL. 3-step kit includes SteriScrub (28.35 g) and SteriBrush.
otc	**Blis-To-Sol** (Chattem)	**Liquid**: 1% tolnaftate	In 30 mL.
Rx	**Bensal HP** (7 Oaks Pharmaceutical Co.)	**Ointment**: 6% benzoic acid and 3% salicylic acid	Extract of oak bark. In 15 and 30 g tubes and 30 and 60 g jars.
otc	**Whitfield's** (Various, eg, Dixon-Shane, Fougera, Goldline, Lannett, Lilly, Moore, NMC, Rugby, URL)		In 30 g and 1 lb.
otc	**Blis-To-Sol** (Chattem)	**Powder**: 12% zinc undecylenate	Talc, zinc oxide. In 60 g.
Rx	**Versiclear** (Hope Pharmaceuticals)	**Lotion**: 25% sodium thiosulfate, 1% salicylic acid, 10% isopropyl alcohol, menthol, propylene glycol, EDTA and colloidal alumina	In 120 mL.
Rx	**Castellani Paint Modified** (Pedinol)	**Liquid**: Basic fuchsin, phenol, resorcinol and acetone	In 30 and 480 mL.
		Also available as a colorless solution with alcohol and without basic fuchsin.	In 30 and 480 mL.
otc	**Fungi-Nail** (Kramer)	**Liquid**: 1% resorcinol, 2% salicylic acid, 2% chloroxylenol, 0.5% benzocaine, 50% isopropyl alcohol	In 30 mL.

ANTIFUNGAL COMBINATIONS — TOPICAL

Active Ingredients

The principal active components of these formulations include:

➤*Antifungal agents: UNDECYLENIC ACID* (see individual monograph), *SODIUM PROPIONATE, BENZOIC ACID, SODIUM THIOSULFATE.*

➤*Other components include:*

SALICYLIC ACID – For its topical keratolytic action (see individual monograph).

BORIC ACID – As an astringent and antiseptic.

CHLOROXYLENOL – As an antiseptic.

BENZOCAINE – As an anesthetic (see individual monograph).

MENTHOL and PHENOL – For their antipruritic, anesthetic and antiseptic effects.

RESORCINOL – As an antipruritic and antiseptic.

CHLOROPHYLL DERIVATIVES – To promote healing, although there is no evidence to support this effect. These agents do have a deodorant action.

BASIC FUCHSIN – For its antifungal and antibacterial activity.

➤*Note:* The choice of vehicle is important for these products. Ointments, creams and liquids are used as primary therapy. In general, powders are used as adjunctive therapy, but they may be acceptable as primary therapy in very mild conditions.

Antiseptics and Germicides

BENZALKONIUM CHLORIDE (BAC)

otc	**Pedi-Pro** (Pedinol)	**Powder**: 1%	Menthol. In 56.7 g.
otc	**Benzalkonium Chloride** (Various, eg, A-A Spectrum)	**Concentrate**: 17%	In 500 mL and 4 L.
otc	**Benza** (Century)	**Solution**: 1:750	In 60 and 120 mL.
otc	**Ony-Clear** (Pedinol Pharmacal)	**Solution, topical**: 1%	Urea. In 30 mL with brush-on applicator.
otc	**Zephiran** (Sanofi Winthrop)	**Solution, aqueous**: 1:750	In 240 mL and gal.
		Disinfectant concentrate: 17%	In 120 mL and gal.
		Tincture: 1:750	In gal.
		Tissue: 1:750. With chlorothymol, isopropyl alcohol and alcohol (20%)	In individual single use packets.
otc	**Mycocide NS** (Woodward)	**Solution**: Benzalkonium chloride, propylene glycol, diazolidinyl urea, methylparaben	In 30 mL.

BENZALKONIUM CHLORIDE (BAC)

otc	**no more germies towelettes** (Johnson & Johnson)	**Towelettes:** Benzalkonium chloride, aloe vera gel, EDTA, methylparaben, 15% SD alcohol 40.	In 24 individually wrapped towelettes.

BENZALKONIUM CHLORIDE — TOPICAL

Indications

➤*Aqueous solutions:* For the antisepsis of skin, mucous membranes, and wounds. They are used for preoperative preparation of the skin, surgeons' hand and arm soaks, treatment of wounds, preservation of ophthalmic solutions, irrigations of the eye, body cavities, bladder, urethra, and vaginal douching.

➤*1% topical solution:* To soften and rejuvenate nails. The topical 1% solution also softens and rejuvenates feet and helps guard against bacterial contamination that potentially can cause skin infection.

➤*0.13% topical solution:* External first aid antiseptic.

➤*1% topical foot powder:* To help guard against bacterial contamination that potentially can cause skin infection. This medication is a drying, absorbing, and deodorizing topical powder.

Administration and Dosage

➤*Aqueous solutions:*

Directions for use – Liberal use of the solution is recommended to compensate for any adsorption of benzalkonium chloride by cotton or other materials.

Preoperative preparation of skin: Benzalkonium chloride solutions 1:750 is recommended as an antiseptic for use on unbroken skin in the preoperative preparation of the surgical field. Detergents and soaps should be thoroughly rinsed from the skin before applying benzalkonium chloride solutions. The detergent action of benzalkonium chloride solutions, particularly when used alternately with alcohol, leaves the skin smooth and clean. When benzalkonium chloride solutions are applied by friction (using several changes of sponges), dirt, skin fats, desquamating epithelium, and superficial bacteria are effectively removed, thus exposing the underlying skin to the antiseptic activity of the solutions.

Recommended dilutions – For specific directions, see below.

Surgery:
- *Preoperative preparation of skin* – Aqueous solution 1:750.
- *Surgeons' hand and arm soaks* – Aqueous solution 1:750.
- *Irrigation of deep infected wounds* – Aqueous solution 1:3000 to 1:20,000.
- *Denuded skin and mucous membranes* – Aqueous solution 1:5000 to 1:10,000.

Obstetrics and gynecology:
- *Preoperative preparation of skin* – Aqueous solution 1:750.
- *Vaginal douche and irrigation* – Aqueous solution 1:2000 to 1:5000.
- *Postepisiotomy care* – Aqueous solution 1:5000 to 1:10,000.
- *Breast and nipple hygiene* – Aqueous solution 1:1000 to 1:2000.

Urology:
- *Bladder and urethral irrigation* – Aqueous solution 1:5000 to 1:20,000.
- *Bladder retention lavage* – Aqueous solution 1:20,000 to 1:40,000.

Dermatology:
- *Oozing and open infections* – Aqueous solution 1:2000 to 1:5000.
- *Wet dressings by irrigation or open dressing* – Use in occlusive dressings is inadvisable. Aqueous solution 1:5000 or less.

Ophthalmology:
- *Eye irrigation* – Aqueous solution 1:5000 to 1:10,000.
- *Preservation of ophthalmic solutions* – Aqueous solution 1:5000 to 1:7500.

Correct use of benzalkonium chloride – Benzalkonium chloride solutions must be prepared, stored and used correctly to achieve and maintain their antiseptic action. Serious inactivation and contamination of benzalkonium chloride solutions may occur with misuse.

Correct diluent: Sterile Water for Injection is recommended for irrigation of body cavities.

Sterile distilled water is recommended for irrigating traumatized tissue and in the eye.

Resin deionized water should not be used because the deionizing resins can carry pathogens (especially gram-negative bacteria): They also inactivate quaternary ammonium compounds.

Stored water is not recommended since it may contain many organisms.

Saline should not be used since it may decrease the antibacterial potency of benzalkonium chloride solutions.

Incompatibilities: Anionic detergents and soaps should be thoroughly rinsed from the skin or other areas prior to use of benzalkonium chloride solutions because they reduce its antibacterial activity.

Serum and protein material also decrease the activity of benzalkonium chloride.

Corks should not be used to stopper bottles containing benzalkonium chloride solutions.

Fibers or fabrics absorb benzalkonium chloride. Examples are: Cotton; wool; rubber materials; gauze sponges; rayon.

Applicators or sponges, intended for a skin prep, should be stored separately and dipped in benzalkonium chloride solutions immediately before use.

Under certain circumstances the following commonly encountered substances are incompatible with benzalkonium chloride solutions: Iodine; silver nitrate; fluorescein; nitrates; peroxide; lanolin; potassium permanganate; aluminum; caramel; kaolin; pine oil; zinc sulfate; zinc oxide; yellow oxide of mercury.

Dilutions of Benzalkonium Chloride Aqueous Solution 1:750		
Final dilution	Benzalkonium chloride aqueous solution 1:750 (parts)	Sterile water for injection or sterile distilled water (parts)
1:1000	3	1
1:2000	3	5
1:2500	3	7
1:3000	3	9
1:4000	3	13
1:5000	3	17
1:10,000	3	37
1:20,000	3	77
1:40,000	3	157

➤*1% topical solution:* Clean and dry affected areas. Apply a small amount to the affected area twice a day, morning and evening, or as recommended by a podiatrist or physician.

➤*0.13% topical solution:* 0.13% topical solution is for adults and children 2 years of age or older. Clean the affected area. Apply a small amount of 0.13% topical solution on the area 1 to 3 times daily. The area may be covered with a sterile bandage. If bandaged, the patient should let it dry first. For children under 2 years of age, the patient should consult a physician.

Soaps and anionic detergents may deactivate the effects of this product.

➤*1% topical foot powder:* For best results, use twice a day, morning and evening. Gently squeeze the bottle or shake powder onto feet, between toes, in socks, shoes and sneakers to help guard against bacterial contamination and to aid in the drying, absorbing moisture, deodorizing, and cooling of the feet.

➤*Storage / Stability:*

Aqueous solutions – Store at 25°C (77°F); excursions permitted to 15° to 30°C (59° to 86°F).

1% topical solution and foot powder – Store at controlled room temperature 15° to 30°C (59° to 86°F).

Actions

➤*Pharmacology:* Benzalkonium chloride solutions are rapidly acting anti-infective agents with a moderately long duration of action. They are active against bacteria and some viruses, fungi, and protozoa. Bacterial spores are considered to be resistant. Solutions are bacteriostatic or bactericidal according to their concentration. The exact mechanism of bactericidal action is unknown but is thought to be due to enzyme inactivation. Activity generally increases with increasing temperature and pH. Gram-positive bacteria are more susceptible than gram-negative bacteria.

Highest Dilution of Benzalkonium Chloride Aqueous Solutions Destroying The Organism in 10 Minutes but Not in 5 Minutes	
Organisms	20°C (68°F)
Streptococcus pyogenes	1:75,000
Staphylococcus aureus	1:52,500
Salmonella typhosa	1:37,500
Escherichia coli	1:10,500

Pseudomonas is the most resistant gram-negative genus. Using the AOAC Use-Dilution Confirmation Method, no growth was obtained when *Staphylococcus aureus*, *Salmonella choleraesuis*, and *Pseudomonas aeruginosa* (strain PRD-10) were exposed for 10 minutes at 20°C (68°F) to benzalkonium chloride aqueous solution 1:750.

Benzalkonium chloride aqueous solution 1:750 has been shown to retain its bactericidal activity following autoclaving for 30 minutes at 15 lb pressure, freezing, and then thawing.

The tubercle bacillus may be resistant to aqueous benzalkonium chloride solutions.

Benzalkonium chloride solutions also demonstrate deodorant, wetting, detergent, keratolytic, and emulsifying activity.

Contraindications

Use in occlusive dressings, casts, and anal or vaginal packs; sensitivity to any of the ingredients in the product.

BENZALKONIUM CHLORIDE — TOPICAL

Warnings

➤*Soaps/anionic detergents:* Since benzalkonium chloride is inactivated by soaps and anionic detergents, thorough rinsing is necessary if these agents are employed prior to their use.

➤*Aqueous solutions:* Sterile water for injection should be used as diluent in preparing diluted aqueous solutions intended for use on deep wounds or for irrigation of body cavities. Otherwise, freshly distilled water should be used. Tap water, containing metallic ions and organic matter, may reduce antibacterial potency. Resin deionized water should not be used since it may contain pathogenic bacteria.

Organic, inorganic, and synthetic materials and surfaces may adsorb sufficient quantities of benzalkonium chloride to significantly reduce its antibacterial potency in solutions. This has resulted in serious contamination of benzalkonium chloride solutions with viable pathogenic bacteria. Solutions should not be stored in bottles stoppered with cork closures, but rather in those equipped with appropriate screw-caps. Cotton, wool, rayon, and other materials should not be stored in benzalkonium chloride solutions. Gauze sponges and fiber pledgets used to apply solutions of benzalkonium chloride to the skin should be sterilized and stored in separate containers. Only immediately prior to application should they be immersed in benzalkonium chloride solutions.

Antiseptics such as benzalkonium chloride solutions must not be relied upon to achieve complete sterilization, because they do not destroy bacterial spores and certain viruses, including the etiologic agent of infectious hepatitis, and may not destroy *Mycobacterium tuberculosis* and other rare bacterial strains.

If solutions stronger than 1:3000 enter the eyes, irrigate immediately and repeatedly with water. Prompt medical attention should then be obtained. Concentrations greater than 1:5000 should not be used on mucous membranes, with the exception of the vaginal mucosa.

➤*Accidental ingestion:* In case of accidental ingestion, the patient should seek professional assistance or contact a poison control center immediately.

Precautions

➤*Preoperative antisepsis:* In preoperative antisepsis of the skin, benzalkonium chloride solutions should not be permitted to remain in prolonged contact with the patient's skin. Avoid pooling of the solution on the operating table.

➤*Inflamed/irritated tissues:* Benzalkonium chloride solutions that are used on inflamed or irritated tissues must be more dilute than those used on normal tissues.

➤*Preoperative preparation:* Benzalkonium chloride solutions used in skin preparation have a tendency to "run off" the skin. It may be preferable to use alternately with alcohol in preoperative preparation of the skin.

Preoperative periorbital skin or head prep should be performed only before the patient, or eye, is anesthetized.

Overdosage

➤*Symptoms:* If benzalkonium chloride solution, particularly a concentrated solution, is ingested, marked local irritation of the GI tract, manifested by nausea and vomiting, may occur. Signs of systemic toxicity include restlessness, apprehension, weakness, confusion, dyspnea, cyanosis, collapse, convulsions, and coma. Death occurs as a result of paralysis of the respiratory muscles.

➤*Treatment:* Immediate administration of several glasses of a mild soap solution, milk, or egg whites beaten in water is recommended. This may be followed by gastric lavage with a mild soap solution. Alcohol should be avoided as it promotes absorption.

To support respiration, the airway should be clear and oxygen should be administered, employing artificial respiration if necessary. If convulsions occur, a short-acting barbiturate may be given parenterally with caution.

Patient Information

➤*1% topical solution, 0.13% topical solution, 1% topical foot powder:* This medication is for external use only. Keep out of the reach of children. Do not use in the eyes or apply over large areas of the body. In cases of deep or puncture wounds, animal bites, or serious burns, consult a podiatrist, physician, or pharmacist. Stop use and consult a podiatrist, physician, or pharmacist if redness, swelling or pain persists or increases or if the condition persists, gets worse or if irritation occurs. Do not use in large quantities, particularly over raw surfaces or blistered areas. The 1% topical foot powder is not for use for longer than 1 week unless directed by a podiatrist, physician, or pharmacist. Do not bandage. Do not use if known to be sensitive to any of the ingredients in this product.

In case of accidental ingestion, seek professional assistance or contact your poison control center immediately.

CHLORHEXIDINE GLUCONATE

otc	**BactoShield 2** (Amsco)	**Solution:** 2% with 4% isopropyl alcohol	In 960 mL.
otc	**Dyna-Hex 2 Skin Cleanser** (Western Medical)	**Liquid:** 2% with 4% isopropyl alcohol	In 120, 240, 480 and 960 mL and gal.
otc	**Betasept** (Purdue Frederick)	**Liquid:** 4% with 4% isopropyl alcohol	In 946 mL.
otc	**Dyna-Hex Skin Cleanser** (Western Medical)		In 120, 240 and 480 mL and gal.
otc	**Exidine Skin Cleanser** (Baxter Health Care)		In 120 and 240 mL, qt and gal.
otc	**Hibiclens Antiseptic/ Antimicrobial Skin Cleanser** (Stuart)		In 120, 240, 480, and 960 mL.
otc	**Hibistat Germicidal Hand Rinse** (Stuart)	**Rinse:** 0.5% with 70% isopropanol and emollients	In 120 and 240 mL.
otc	**Hibistat Towelettes** (Stuart)	**Wipes:** 0.5% with 70% isopropanol	In 50s.
otc	**Hibiclens** (Stuart)	**Sponge/Brush:** 4% with 4% isopropyl alcohol	In unit-of-use 22 mL.
otc	**Bactoshield** (Amsco)	**Foam:** 4% with 4% isopropyl alcohol	In 180 mL aerosol.

CHLORHEXIDINE GLUCONATE — TOPICAL

Indications

➤*Cleanser:* As a surgical hand scrub, skin wound and general skin cleanser, health care personnel hand wash, and for preoperative skin preparation. Chlorhexidine gluconate significantly reduces the number of microorganisms on the hands and forearms prior to surgery or patient care.

Administration and Dosage

➤*Approved by the FDA:* August 13, 1986.

➤*Surgical hand scrub (brush-sponge and nail cleaner):*
1.) Open package and clean under nails with the nail pick provided. Nails should be maintained with a 1 millimeter free edge.
2.) Wet hands and forearms to the elbows with warm water.
3.) Wet sponge and squeeze to work up lather with about 5 mL of chlorhexidine gluconate.
4.) Discard brush-sponge.
5.) Rinse hands and forearms thoroughly and dry with a sterile towel.

➤*Skin wound and general skin cleansing:* Wounds that involve more than the superficial layers of the skin should not be routinely treated with chlorhexidine gluconate. Chlorhexidine gluconate should not be used for repeated general skin cleansing of large body areas except in those patients whose underlying condition makes it necessary to reduce the bacterial population of the skin. To use, thoroughly rinse the area to be cleansed with water. Apply the minimum amount of chlorhexidine gluconate necessary to cover the skin or wound area and wash gently. Rinse thoroughly again.

➤*Healthcare personnel hand wash:* Wet hands with water. Dispense approximately 5 mL of chlorhexidine gluconate into cupped hands and wash in a vigorous manner for 15 seconds. Rinse and thoroughly dry.

➤*Preoperative skin preparation:* Apply chlorhexidine gluconate liberally to surgical site and swab for at least 2 minutes. Dry with a sterile towel. Repeat procedure for an additional 2 minutes and dry with a sterile towel.

➤*Storage/Stability:* Store between 20° to 25°C (68° to 77°F). Avoid freezing and excessive heat above 40°C (104°F). Keep out of the reach of children.

Warnings

➤*For external use only:* For external use only. Keep out of eyes, ears, and mouth. Chlorhexidine gluconate should not be used as a preoperative skin preparation of the face or head. Misuse of products containing chlorhexide gluconate has been reported to cause serious and permanent eye injury when it has been permitted to enter and remain in the eye during surgical procedures. If chlorhexidine gluconate should contact these areas, rinse out promptly and thoroughly with cold water. Avoid contact with meninges. Do not use in the genital area.

➤*Deep wounds:* Do not use chlorhexidine gloconate routinely if you have wounds that involve more than the superficial layers of the skin.

➤*Sensitivity:* Chlorhexidine gluconate should not be used by persons who have a sensitivity to it or its components.

CHLORHEXIDINE GLUCONATE — TOPICAL

➤*Deafness:* Chlorhexidine gluconate has been reported to cause deafness when instilled in the middle ear through perforated ear drums.

➤*Hypersensitivity reactions:* Irritation, sensitization, and generalized allergic reactions have been reported with chlorhexidine-containing products, especially in the genital areas. If adverse reactions occur and last more than 72 hours, discontinue use immediately and, if severe, contact a physician.

➤*Children:* Keep out of reach of children. If swallowed, get medical help or contact a poison control center right away.

Adverse Reactions

Irritation, sensitization, and generalized allergic reactions have been reported with chlorhexidine-containing products, especially in the genital areas. If adverse reactions occur and last more than 72 hours, discontinue use immediately and, if severe, contact a physician.

Overdosage

In case of accidental ingestion, seek professional assistance or contact a poison control center immediately. If swallowed, get medical help or contact a poison control center right away.

Patient Information

When using this product, keep out of eyes, ears and mouth. May cause serious and permanent eye injury if permitted to enter or allowed to remain.

If contact occurs, rinse with cold water right away.

Do not use routinely if you have wounds which involve more than the superficial layers of the skin.

Stop use and ask a doctor if irritation, sensitization or allergic reaction occurs and lasts more than 72 hours.

Keep out of reach of children. If swallowed, get medical help or contact a poison control center right away.

GLUTARALDEHYDE

otc	**Cidex**[1] (J & J Medical)	**Solution:** 2%	In qt, gal and 2.5 gal.[3]
otc	**Cidex Plus 28**[2] (J & J Medical)	**Solution:** 3.2%	In qt, gal and 2.5 gal.[4]

[1] Activated dialdehyde is stable for 14 days after activation.
[2] Long-life activated dialdehyde is stable for 28 days after activation.
[3] Vial of activator contains solid sodium salts as buffer to adjust pH to 8.2 to 8.9.
[4] Vial of activator contains aqueous potassium salts as buffer to adjust pH to 7.2 to 7.8.

GLUTARALDEHYDE — TOPICAL

Indications

➤*Sterilant:* For use as a sterilant, disinfectant, and precleaning agent. When used or reused, according to Directions for use, at full strength for a maximum of 14 days at 25°C (77°F) with an immersion time of at least 10 hours.

➤*Precleaning agent compatibility: Cidex Solution* and *Cidex Plus 28 Day Solution* are compatible with enzymatic detergents (eg, *Enzol Enzymatic Detergent*), which are mild in pH, low foaming, and easily rinsed from equipment. Detergents that are either highly acidic or alkaline are contraindicated as precleaning agents since improper rinsing could affect the efficacy of the *Cidex Solution* by altering its pH.

Administration and Dosage

➤*Direction for use:*

Activation – Activate the *Cidex Solution* or *Cidex Plus 28 Day Solution* by adding the entire contents of the *Activator Vial* that is attached to the *Cidex Solution* or *Cidex Plus 28 Day Solution* container. Shake well. Activated solution immediately changes color to green, thereby indicating solution is ready to use. *Cidex Solution* or *Cidex Plus 28 Day Solution* is intended for use in manual (bucket and tray) systems made from polypropylene, ABS, polyethylene, glass-filled polypropylene or specially molded polycarbonate plastics. Record the date of activation (mixing date) and expiration date on the *Cidex Solution* or *Cidex Plus 28 Day Solution* container label in the space provided, in a log book or a label affixed to any secondary container used for the activated solution.

Cleaning/decontamination – Blood and other body fluids must be thoroughly cleaned from surfaces, lumens, and objects before application of the disinfectant or sterilant. Blood and other body fluids should be autoclaved and disposed of according to all applicable federal, state and local regulations for infectious waste disposal.

For complete disinfection or sterilization of medical instruments and equipment, thoroughly clean, rinse and rough dry objects before immersing in *Cidex Solution* or *Cidex Plus 28 Day Solution*. Cleanse and rinse the lumens of hollow instruments before filling with *Cidex Solution* or *Cidex Plus 28 Day Solution*. Refer to the reusable device manufacturer's labeling for additional instructions on disassembly, decontamination, cleaning and leak testing of their equipment.

Usage –

Sterilization (bucket/tray manual system): Immerse medical equipment/device completely in *Cidex Solution* or *Cidex Plus 28 Day Solution* for a minimum of 10 hours at 25°C (77°F) to eliminate all microorganisms including *Clostridium sporogenes* and *Bacillus subtilis* spores. Remove equipment from the solution using sterile technique and rinse thoroughly with sterile water following the rinsing instructions below.

High level disinfection (bucket/tray manual system): Immerse medical equipment/device completely in *Cidex Solution* for a minimum of 45 minutes or *Cidex Plus 28 Day Solution* for a minimum of 20 minutes at 25°C (77°F) at to destroy all pathogenic microorganisms, except for large numbers of bacterial endospores, but including *Mycobacterium tuberculosis* (quantitative TB method). Remove devices and equipment from the solution and rinse thoroughly following the rinsing instructions below.

Intermediate level disinfection (bucket/tray manual system): Immerse medical equipment/device completely in *Cidex Solution* or *Cidex Plus 28 Day Solution* for a minimum of 10 minutes at 20° to 25°C (68° to 77°F) to destroy all vegetative bacteria, except for large numbers of *Mycobacterium tuberculosis*, but including *Pseudomonas aeruginosa*, pathogenic fungi, and viruses (poliovirus type 1; adenovirus type 2; herpes simplex type 1,2; HIV-1 (AIDS virus); influenza type A [WS/33]; vaccinia; coronavirus; cytomegalovirus; rhinovirus type 14; coxsachlevirus B-1 (for 28-day solution) on inanimate surfaces.

A 10-minute immersion at 20°C (68°F) will kill 87.9% of *Mycobacterium tuberculosis* (quantitative TB method) for *Cidex Solution* and 99.6% of *Mycobacterium tuberculosis* for *Cidex Plus 28 Day Solution*.

A 10-minute immersion at 25°C (77°F) will kill 99.8% of *Mycobacterium tuberculosis* (quantitative TB method) for *Cidex Solution* and 99.98% of *Mycobacterium tuberculosis* for *Cidex Plus 28 Day Solution*.

Remove devices and equipment from the solution and rinse thoroughly following the rinsing instructions below.

Rinsing instructions: Following immersion in *Cidex Solution* or *Cidex Plus 28 Day Solution*, thoroughly rinse the equipment or medical device by immersing it completely in 3 separate copious volumes of water. Each rinse should be a minimum of 1 minute in duration unless otherwise noted by the device or equipment manufacturer. Use fresh portions of water for each rinse. Discard the water following each rinse. Do not reuse the water for rinsing or any other purpose as it will be contaminated with glutaraldehyde.

Reusage:

• *Cidex Solution* – *Cidex Solution* has also demonstrated efficacy in the presence of 2% organic soil contamination and a simulated amount of microbiological burden during reuse. This solution may be used and reused within the limitations indicated above for up to 14 days after activation. Do not use activated solution beyond 14 days. Efficacy of this product during its use-life must be verified by the *Cidex Solution Test Strip* to determine that the minimum effective concentration (MEC) of 1.5% is present.

• *Cidex Plus 28 Day Solution* – *Cidex Plus 28 Day Solution* has also demonstrated efficacy in the presence of 2% organic soil contamination and a simulated amount of microbiological burden during reuse. This solution may be used and reused within the limitations indicated above for up to 28 days after activation. Do not use activated solution beyond 28 days. Efficacy of this product during its use-life must be verified by the *Cidex Plus Solution Test Strip* to determine that the minimum effective concentration (MEC) of 2.1% is present.

Monitoring of germicide to ensure specifications are met – During the usage of *Cidex Solution* or *Cidex Plus 28 Day Solution*, as a high or intermediate level disinfectant or sterilant, it is recommended that a thermometer and timer be utilized to ensure that the optimum usage conditions are met. In addition, it is recommended that the *Cidex Solution* or *Cidex Plus 28 Day Solution* be tested with the *Cidex Solution Test Strip* or *Cidex Plus Solution Test Strip* prior to each usage. This is to ensure that the appropriate concentration of glutaraldehyde is present and to guard against a dilution which may lower the effectiveness of the solution below its MEC. The pH of the activated solution may also be periodically checked to verify that the pH of the solution is between 7.5 and 8.1.

➤*Storage/Stability:* Prior to activation, *Cidex Solution* or *Cidex Plus 28 Day Solution* should be stored in its original sealed container at controlled room temperature 15° to 30°C (59° to 86°F).

Once the *Cidex Solution* or *Cidex Plus 28 Day Solution* has been activated, it should be stored in the original container until transferred to the closed containers in which the immersion for disinfection or sterilization is to take place. Containers should be stored in a well ventilated, low traffic area at controlled room temperature.

The use period for activated *Cidex Solution* or *Cidex Plus 28 Day Solution* is for no longer than 14 days or 28 days respectively, following activation or as indicated by the *Cidex Solution Test Strip* or *Cidex Plus Solution Test Strip*. Once activated, the solution requires no further dilution prior to its usage.

Material compatibility – *Cidex Solution* and *Cidex Plus 28 Day Solution* are recommended for usage, respectively, with medical devices made from the materials shown below. Care must be taken with medical and dental equipment such as anesthesia and respiratory therapy tubing, dental mirrors and burs. These devices may be damaged when cleaned with a highly alkaline detergent, poorly rinsed after disinfection, stored wet or dried at temperatures exceeding 41°C (105°F).

GLUTARALDEHYDE — TOPICAL

Cidex Solution Compatible Materials

Metals	Plastics	Elastomers
Chrome plate[1]	Polysulfone[1]	Polychloroprene (neoprene)[1]
Copper[1]	Teflon[1]	Polyurethane[1]
Monel[1]	Polyethylene lerephthalate (polyester)[3]	Black natural rubber[7]
Nickel plate[1]	Polymethylmethacrylate (acrylic)[3]	Red natural rubber[7]
Nickel silver alloy[1]	Polystyrene[3]	Silicone rubber (Silastic)[7]
Platinum[1]	Polyvinylchloride (PVC)[3]	
Silver solder[1]	Polycarbonate[4]	
Tungsten[1]	Acrylonitrile-butadiene-styrene (ABS)[7]	
70–30 solder[1]	Nylon[7]	
Aluminum[2]	Polyethylene[7]	
Gold plate[2]	Polypropylene[7]	
Silver plate[2]		
Anodized aluminum[5]		
Brass[5]		
Carbon steel[7]		
Stainless steel[7]		

[1] Represents 8 hours of continuous contact with *Cidex Solution.*
[2] Represents 10 hours of total contact with *Cidex Solution* over 20 disinfection cycles.
[3] Represents 20 hours of total contact with *Cidex Solution* over 20 disinfection cycles.
[4] Represents 40 hours of total contact with *Cidex Solution* over 40 disinfection cycles.
[5] Represents 144 hours of continuous contact with *Cidex Solution* .
[6] Represents 283 hours of total contact with *Cidex Solution* over 20 disinfection cycles.
[7] Represents 336 hours of total contact with *Cidex Solution* over 20 disinfection cycles.

Cidex Plus 28 Day Solution Compatible Materials

Metals	Plastics	Elastomers
Carbon steel[2]	Acrylonitrile-butadiene-styrene (ABS)[2]	Black rubber[2]
Stainless steel[2]	Polyvinylchloride (PVC)[2]	Red rubber[2]
Brass[2]	Polystyrene[1]	Polyurethane[1]
Nickel plate[2]	Polyethylene[2]	Silicone rubber[1]
Chrome plate[2]	Polypropylene[2]	
Aluminum[2]	Polysulfone[1]	
Anodized aluminum[1]	Polymethylmethacrylate (acrylic)[1]	
Copper[2]	Polyethylene lerephthalate (polyester)[1]	
Nickel silver alloy[2]		
Gold plate[1]		
Silver plate[1]		

[1] Represents 10 hours of continuous contact with *Cidex Plus 28 Day Solution* over 20 disinfection cycles.
[2] Represents 672 hours of continuous exposure with *Cidex Plus 28 Day Solution* over the 28–day use cycle of the disinfectant.

Cidex Plus 28 Day Solution is not recommended for disinfection of 1 piece molded, solvent bonded or sonic welded polycarbonate equipment. Stress cracking has been observed after repeated treatments.

Disposal information –

Germicide disposal: Discard residual solution in drain. Flush thoroughly with water.

Container disposal: Do not reuse empty container. Wrap container and put in trash.

Actions

➤*Microbiology:*

Spectrum of activity[1]

Bacteria		Fungi	Viruses	
Spores	Vegetative Organisms		Non-enveloped	Enveloped
Bacillus subtilus	*Staphylococcus aureus*	*Trichophyton mentagrophytes*	Poliovirus Type 1	Coronavirus
Clostridium sporogenes	*Salmonella choleraesuis*		Rhinovirus Type 14	Cytomegalovirus
	Pseudomonas aeruginosa		Adenovirus Type 2	Influenza virus (Type A/WS/33)
	Mycobacterium tuberculosis		Vaccinia	HIV-1 (AIDS Virus)
			Coxsackievirus B-1[2]	Herpes simplex types 1 and 2

[1] Testing for *Cidex Solution* was done after 14 days of simulated reuse using prescribed testing methods, while *Cidex Plus 28 Day Solution* was done after 28 days of simulated reuse.
[2] Tested with 28-day solution only.

Contraindications

For sterilizing reusable medical devices that are compatible with other available methods of sterilization that can be biologically monitored (eg, heat, ethylene oxide, or peroxide gas plasma), or critical devices intended for single use (eg, catheters); as a high level disinfection of a semi-critical device when sterilization is practical.

➤*Endoscope usage:* *Cidex Activated Dialdehyde Solution* or *Cidex Plus 28 Day Solution* is not the method of choice for sterilization of rigid endoscopes which the device manufacturer indicates are compatible with steam sterilization. In general, glutaraldehyde solutions that do not contain surfactants (eg, *Cidex Solution* or *Cidex Activated Dialdehyde Solution*) are more appropriate for flexible endoscopes, since glutaraldehyde solutions containing sufactants (eg, *Cidex Formula 7 Solution* or *Cidex Plus 28 Day Solution*) are more difficult to rinse from the devices. However, these surfactant containing disinfectants may be used for reprocessing of flexible endoscopes, if a validated protocol for rinsing and leak testing is employed.

➤*Polycarbonate equipment usage:* *Cidex Plus 28 Day Solution* is not recommended for disinfection of 1 piece molded, solvent bonded or sonic welded polycarbonate equipment. Stress cracking has been observed after repeated procedures.

Warnings

Cidex Activated Dialdehyde Solution or *Cidex Plus 28 Day Solution* is hazardous to humans and domestic animals.

➤*Danger:* Keep out of the reach of children.

➤*Contains glutaraldehyde:* Direct contact is corrosive to exposed tissue, causing eye damage and skin irritation/damage. Do not get into eyes, on skin or on clothing.

Avoid contamination of food.

Use in well ventilated area in closed containers.

In case of contact, immediately flush eyes or skin with plenty of water for at least 15 minutes. For eyes, get medical attention.

Harmful if swallowed. Drink large quantities of water and call a physician immediately.

Probable mucosal damage from oral exposure may contraindicate the use of gastric lavage.

Precautions

➤*Safety instructions:* Disposable latex gloves, eye protection, face masks, and liquid-proof gowns should be worn when cleaning and sterilizing/disinfecting soiled devices and equipment.

Contaminated, reusable devices must be thoroughly cleaned prior to disinfection or sterilization, since residual contamination will decrease effectiveness of the germicide.

The reusable device manufacturer should provide the user with a validated reprocessing procedure for that device using *Cidex Solution* or *Cidex Plus 28 Day Solution*.

The use of *Cidex Solution* or *Cidex Plus 28 Day Solution* in automated endoscope washers must be part of a validated reprocessing procedure provided by the washer manufacturer. Contact the manufacturer of the endoscope washer for instructions on the maximum number of reprocessing cycles which may be used before refilling with fresh *Cidex Solution* or *Cidex Plus 28 Day Solution*. Use *Cidex Solution Test Strips* or *Cidex Solution Plus Test Strips* to monitor glutaraldehyde concentration before each cycle to detect unexpected dilution.

HEXACHLOROPHENE

Rx	**pHisoHex** (Winthrop Pharm.)	**Liquid:** 3%	Petrolatum, lanolin, PEG. In 150 mL, pt and gal and UD 8 mL (50s).

HEXACHLOROPHENE — TOPICAL

Indications

➤*Bacteriostatic skin cleanser:* For use as a surgical scrub and a bacteriostatic skin cleanser. It may also be used to control an outbreak of gram-positive infection where other infection control procedures have been unsuccessful. Use only as long as necessary for infection control.

Administration and Dosage

➤*Surgical Hand Scrub:*

1.) Wet hands and forearms with water. Apply approximately 5 mL of hexachlorophene over the hands and rub into a copious lather by adding small amounts of water. Spread suds over hands and forearms and scrub well with a wet brush for 3 minutes. Pay particular attention to the nails and interdigital spaces. A separate nail cleaner may be used. Rinse thoroughly under running water.
2.) Apply 5 mL of hexachlorophene to hands again and scrub as above for another 3 minutes. Rinse thoroughly with running water and dry.
3.) For repeat surgical scrubs during the day, scrub thoroughly with the same amount of hexachlorophene for 3 minutes only. Rinse thoroughly with water and dry.

➤*Bacteriostatic Cleansing:* Wet hands with water. Dispense approximately 5 mL of hexachlorophene into the palm, work up a lather with water and apply to area to be cleansed.

Rinse thoroughly after each washing.

Infant Care – Hexachlorophene should not be used routinely for bathing infants. See Warnings.

Use of baby skin products containing alcohol may decrease the antibacterial action of hexachlorophene.

➤*Storage/Stability:* Store at room temperature up to 25° C (77°F).

Prolonged direct exposure of hexachlorophene to strong light may cause brownish surface discoloration but does not affect its antibacterial or detergent properties. Shaking will disperse the color. If hexachlorophene is spilled or splashed on porous surfaces, rinse off to avoid discoloration.

Hexachlorophene should not be dispensed from, or stored in, containers with ordinary metal parts. A special type of stainless steel must be used or undesirable discoloration of the product or oxidation of metal may occur.

Directions For Cleaning Dispensers – Before initial installation and use, run an antiseptic, such as an aqueous solution of benzalkonium chloride, NF, 1:500 to 1:750, or alcohol, through the working parts; rinse with sterile water. At weekly intervals thereafter, remove dispenser and pour off remainder of hexachlorophene emulsion. Rinse empty dispenser with water. Run water through the working parts by operating the dispenser. Sanitize as described above. Rinse thoroughly with sterile water.

Actions

➤*Pharmacology:* Hexachlorophene is a bacteriostatic cleansing agent. It cleanses the skin thoroughly and has bacteriostatic action against staphylococci and other gram-positive bacteria. Cumulative antibacterial action develops with repeated use. Cleansing with alcohol or soaps containing alcohol removes the antibacterial residue.

Detectable blood levels of hexachlorophene following absorption through intact skin have been found in subjects who regularly scrubbed with hexachlorophene emulsion 3%. (See Warnings.)

Hexachlorophene has the same slight acidity as normal skin (pH value 5.0 to 6.0).

Contraindications

On burned or denuded skin; as an occlusive dressing, wet pack, or lotion; routinely for prophylactic total body bathing; as a vaginal pack or tampon; or on any mucous membranes; sensitivity to any of its components; primary light sensitivity to halogenated phenol derivatives because of the possibility of cross-sensitivity to hexachlorophene.

Warnings

➤*Monitoring:* Patients should be closely monitored and use should be immediately discontinued at the first sign of any of the symptoms described below.

➤*Rapid absorption:* Rapid absorption of hexachlorophene may occur with resultant toxic blood levels when preparations containing hexachlorophene are applied to skin lesions such as ichthyosis congenita, the dermatitis of Letterer-Siwe's syndrome, or other generalized dermatological conditions. Application to burns has also produced neurotoxicity and death.

➤*Cerebral irritability:* Hexachlorophene should be discontinued promptly if signs or symptoms of cerebral irritability occur. Infants, especially those who weigh less than 1,200 g and those with a gestational age of less than 35 weeks or those with dermatoses, are particularly susceptible to hexachlorophene absorption. Systemic toxicity may be manifested by signs of stimulation (irritation) of the central nervous system, sometimes with convulsions.

➤*Infant adverse reactions:* Infants have developed dermatitis, irritability, generalized clonic muscular contractions and decerebrate rigidity following application of a 6% hexachlorophene powder. Examination of brainstems of those infants revealed vacuolization like that which can be produced in newborn experimental animals following repeated topical application of 3% hexachlorophene. Moreover, a study of histologic sections of premature infants who died of unrelated causes has shown a positive correlation between hexachlorophene baths and lesions in white matter of brains.

➤*Fertility impairment:* Topical exposure of neonatal rats to 3% hexachlorophene solution caused reduced fertility in 7-month-old males, due to inability to ejaculate.

➤*Pregnancy: Category C.* There are no adequate and well-controlled studies in pregnant women. Hexachlorophene should be used during pregnancy only if the potential benefit justifies potential risk to the fetus. Hexachlorophene is not recommended as an antiseptic lubricant for vaginal exams during labor because appreciable amounts have been detected in maternal and cord serum.

Hexachlorophene has been shown to be teratogenic and embryotoxic in rats when given by mouth or instilled into the vagina in large doses.

Administration of 500 mg/kg diet or 20 to 30 mg/kg bw/day by gavage to rats caused some malformations (angulated ribs, cleft palate, micro and anophthalmia) and reduction in litter size.

Teratogenic – Placental transfer and excretion in milk of hexachlorophene has been demonstrated in rats.

Hexachlorophene is embryotoxic and produces some teratogenic effects.

➤*Lactation:* It is not known whether this drug is excreted in human milk. Because many drugs are excreted in human milk and because of the potential for serious adverse reactions in nursing infants from hexachlorophene, a decision should be made whether to discontinue nursing or to discontinue the drug taking into account the importance of the drug to the mother.

➤*Children:* Hexachlorophene should not be used routinely for bathing premature or term infants.

Precautions

➤*Eye contact:* Avoid accidental contact of hexachlorophene with the eyes.

If contact occurs, promptly rinse thoroughly with water. To assist in the detection of ocular irritation, applications to the head and periorbital skin areas should be performed only in responsive patients with unanesthetized eyes.

➤*After use:* Rinse thoroughly after use, especially from sensitive areas such as the scrotum and perineum.

➤*For external use only:* Hexachlorophene is intended for external use only. If swallowed, hexachlorophene is harmful, especially to infants and children. Hexachlorophene should not be poured into measuring cups, medicine bottles, or similar containers since it may be mistaken for baby formula or other medications.

Adverse Reactions

Dermatitis and photosensitivity. Sensitivity to hexachlorophene is rare; however, persons who have developed photoallergy to similar compounds also may become sensitive to hexachlorophene.

In persons with highly sensitive skin, the use of hexachlorophene may at times produce a reaction characterized by redness or mild scaling or dryness, especially when it is combined with such mechanical factors as excessive rubbing or exposure to heat or cold.

Overdosage

➤*Symptoms:* The accidental ingestion of hexachlorophene in amounts from 1 oz to 4 oz has caused anorexia, vomiting, abdominal cramps, diarrhea, dehydration, convulsions, hypotension, and shock, and in several reported instances, fatalities.

➤*Treatment:* If patients are seen early, the stomach should be evacuated by emesis or gastric lavage. Olive oil or vegetable oil (60 mL or 2 fl oz) may then be given to delay absorption of hexachlorophene, followed by a saline cathartic to hasten removal. Treatment is symptomatic and supportive; intravenous fluids (5 percent dextrose in physiologic saline solution) may be given for dehydration. Any other electrolyte derangement should be corrected. If marked hypotension occurs, vasopressor therapy is indicated. Use of opiates may be considered if gastrointestinal symptoms (cramping, diarrhea) are severe. Scheduled medical or surgical procedures should be postponed until the patient's condition has been evaluated and stabilized.

IODINE COMPOUNDS

IODINE

otc	**Iodine Topical** (Various, eg, AA–Spectrum)	**Solution**: 2% iodine and 2.4% sodium iodide in purified water	In 500 and 4000 mL.
otc[1]	**Strong Iodine (Lugol's Solution)** (Various, eg, Lannett)	**Solution**: 5% iodine and 10% potassium iodide in water	In pt and gal.
otc	**Iodine Tincture** (Various, eg, Century, Lannett)	**Solution**: 2% iodine and 2.4% sodium iodide in 47% alcohol, purified water	In pt and gal.
otc	**Strong Iodine Tincture** (Various, eg, A-A Spectrum)	**Solution**: 7% iodine and 5% potassium iodide in 83% alcohol	In 500 and 4000 mL.

[1] Some of these products may be available *Rx*, depending on distributor discretion.

IODINE — TOPICAL

Indications

➤*Antiseptic:* Iodine preparations are used externally for their broad microbicidal spectrum against bacteria, fungi, viruses, spores, protozoa and yeasts. Iodine may be used to disinfect intact skin preoperatively. Potassium iodide is added to increase the solubility of the iodine. Sodium iodide is present to stabilize the tincture and make it miscible with water in all proportions.

Contraindications

Hypersensitivity to iodine.

Warnings

➤*For external use only:* Avoid contact with the eyes and mucous membranes.

➤*Highly toxic if ingested:* Sodium thiosulfate is the most effective chemical antidote.

➤*Staining:* Iodine preparations stain skin and clothing.

➤*Occlusive dressings:* Do not use.

POVIDONE IODINE

otc	**Povidone-Iodine** (Various, eg, Humco, IDE, Major)	**Ointment**: 10%	In 30 g and lb.
		Solution: 10%	In pt and gal.
		Liquid: 10%	In pt.
		Spray: 10%	In 2 oz.
otc	**Betadine** (Purdue Frederick)	**Aerosol**: 5%. Glycerin, dibasic sodium phosphate	In 88.7 mL.
		Gel (vaginal): 10%. Polyethylene glycols.	In 18 and 90 g w/vaginal applicator.
		Ointment: 10%. Polyethylene glycols.	In 28 g tube, lb jar and 0.94 and 3.8 g packets.
		Skin cleanser, foam: 7.5%. Ammonium nonoxynol-4-sulfate, lauramide DEA	In 170 g.
		Solution: 10%. Citric acid, dibasic sodium phosphate, glycerin	In 15, 120 and 237 mL, pt, qt, gal and 30 mL packets.
		Solution, swab aid: 10%. Citric acid, dibasic sodium phosphate, glycerin	In 100s.
		Solution, swabsticks: 10%. Citric acid, dibasic sodium phosphate, glycerin	In packets of 1 (200s) or 3 (50s).
		Surgical scrub: 7.5%. Ammonium nonoxynol-4-sulfate, lauramide DEA	In pt with or without pump, qt, gal and 15 mL packets.
otc	**Betagen** (Goldline)	**Ointment**: 1/5 available iodine. PEG-8 and PEG-75	In 28.35 g and lb.
		Solution: 10%	In pt and gal.
		Surgical scrub: 7.5%	In pt.
otc	**Biodine Topical 1%** (Major)	**Solution**: 1% iodine	In pt and gal.
otc	**Etodine** (Fougera)	**Ointment**: 1% available iodine	In 30 g, lb and 0.94 g (144s).
otc	**Mallisol** (Hauck)	**Ointment**	In 1 g packets.
otc	**Minidyne** (Pedinol)	**Solution**: 10%. Citric acid and sodium phosphate dibasic	In 15 mL.
otc	**Polydine** (Century)	**Ointment**	In 30 and 120 g & lb.
		Scrub	In 30, 120 and 240 mL, pt and gal.
		Solution	In 30, 120 and 240 mL, pt and gal.
otc	**Povidine** (Various, eg, Barre-National, Moore, Rugby)	**Ointment**: 10%	In 28.4 g and lb.
		Solution: 10%	In pt and gal.
		Surgical scrub: 5.5	In pt and gal.

POVIDONE-IODINE — TOPICAL

Indications

➤*Professional and hospital use:*

Ointment, swabs, aerosol spray – Povidone-iodine kills pathogens in primary or secondary topical infection, first-, second-, and third-degree burns, surgical incisions, decubitus or stasis ulcers, and traumatic lesions.

Use prophylactically to help prevent microbial infection in incisions, burns, and topical lesions.

Surgical scrub – Povidone-iodine surgical scrub is used for preparation of the skin prior to surgery, to help reduce bacteria that potentially can cause skin infection, for handwashing to reduce bacteria on the skin, and to reduce the number of microorganisms on the hands and forearms prior to surgery or patient care.

Swabsticks – This medication is for professional and hospital use as an bactericidal/virucidal antiseptic.

➤*Over-the-counter (OTC) products:* First aid to help prevent infection in minor cuts, scrapes, and burns.

Administration and Dosage

➤*Professional and hospital use:*

Ointment – Apply directly to affected area as needed. The affected area may be bandaged.

Swabs – Tear notch; pull top of packette up and away, exposing pad. Use the pad to swab area thoroughly. Repeat on the other side if necessary. Use 1 time only.

Aerosol spray – Hold container about 10 inches from skin. Press valve firmly with index finger, spraying to cover desired area. Allow to dry. Replace cap after use. If actuator clogs, remove and soak in warm water.

POVIDONE-IODINE — TOPICAL

Surgical scrub –
Surgical hand scrub:
1.) Wet hands with water.
2.) Pour about 5 mL (1 teaspoonful) of scrub on the palm of the hand and spread over both hands.
3.) Without adding more water, scrub thoroughly for about 5 minutes.
4.) Use a brush if desired. Clean thoroughly under fingernails.
5.) Add a little water and develop copious suds. Rinse thoroughly under running water.
6.) Repeat the entire procedure using another 5 mL of scrub.
Patient preoperative skin preparation:
1.) After the skin area is shaved, wet it with water.
2.) Apply scrub (1 mL is sufficient to cover an area of 20 to 30 square inches), develop lather, and scrub thoroughly for about 5 minutes.
3.) Rinse off using sterile gauze saturated with water.
4.) Paint the area with povidone-iodine solution or spray with povidone-iodine aerosol spray and allow to dry.

Swabsticks – Tear at notch; pull top of packette across, exposing end of swabstick. Remove povidone-iodine solution swabstick and apply as needed. Use 1 time only.

➤*OTC products:*

Solution, ointment – Clean the affected area. Apply a small amount of this product to the area 1 to 3 times daily. The area may be covered with a sterile bandage. If bandaged, let dry first.

Skin cleanser solution – Wet skin and apply a sufficient amount to work up a rich, golden lather. Allow lather to remain for about 3 minutes and rinse off. Repeat 2 to 3 times a day or as directed by a physician.

➤*Storage/Stability:* Patients should avoid storing at excessive heat. Store in original container.

This medication does not stain skin and natural fabrics. Contents of aerosol spray are under pressure.

Aerosol spray – This product contains dry natural rubber. The contents are under pressure. The hole in the bottom is part of the aerosol system. The product contains no chlorofluorocarbons.

Warnings

➤*External use only:* Povidone-iodine topical products are for external use only. Do not use these products in the eyes or over large areas of the body. Avoid spraying the aerosol in the eyes.

➤*Preoperative prepping:* In preoperative prepping, avoid "pooling" beneath the patient.

➤*Long term use:* Do not use these products for longer than 1 week unless directed by a doctor.

Prolonged exposure may cause irritation, or, rarely, severe skin reactions.

➤*Heating:* Do not heat prior to application.

Ask a doctor before use if the patient has deep or puncture wounds or serious burns.

Patient Information

Povidone-iodine topical products are for external use only.

Do not use these products in the eyes or over large areas of the body.

Avoid spraying the aerosol in the eyes.

In preoperative prepping, avoid "pooling" beneath the patient.

Do not use these products for longer than 1 week unless directed by a doctor.

Prolonged exposure may cause irritation, or, rarely, severe skin reactions.

Do not heat prior to application.

MERCURY COMPOUNDS

THIMEROSAL (49% mercury)

otc	**Thimerosal** (Lannett)	**Solution:** 1:1000	Stainless. In pt and gal.
otc	**Mersol** (Century Pharm.)	**Tincture:** 1:1000 with 50% alcohol	In 120 mL, pt and gal.

THIMEROSAL (49% mercury) — TOPICAL

Indications

➤*Antiseptic:* For antisepsis of the skin prior to surgery and for first aid treatment.

Administration and Dosage

Apply locally 1 to 3 times a day.

Actions

➤*Pharmacology:* An organomercurial antiseptic with sustained bacteriostatic and fungistatic activity against common pathogens.

Contraindications

Hypersensitivity to thimerosal.

Precautions

➤*For external use only:* Avoid contact with the eyes.

➤*Prolonged repeated applications:* Frequent or prolonged use or application to large areas may cause serious mercury poisoning.

➤*Incompatibilities:* Thimerosal is incompatible with strong acids, salts of heavy metals, potassium permanganate and iodine; do not use in combination with or immediately following their application.

➤*Discontinue:* If redness, swelling, pain, infection, rash, or irritation persists or increases, discontinue and consult physician.

Adverse Reactions

➤*Hypersensitivity:* Some individuals are hypersensitive to the thio or mercuri radicals. Symptoms include erythematous, papular and vesicular eruptions over the application area.

Overdosage

For ingestion of the tincture, consider alcohol and acetone content.

➤*Treatment:* Supportive therapy. Refer to General Management of Acute Overdosage.

OXYCHLOROSENE SODIUM

otc	**Clorpactin WCS-90** (Guardian)	**Powder for Solution:** 2 g sodium oxychlorosene	In 2 g bottles (5s).

OXYCHLOROSENE SODIUM — TOPICAL

Indications

➤*Localized infection:* Used for treating localized infections, particularly when resistant organisms are present; to remove necrotic debris in massive infections or from radiation necrosis; to counteract odorous discharges; as a preoperative and postoperative irrigant and for the cleansing and disinfection of fistulae, sinus tract, empyemas, and wounds.

Administration and Dosage

Apply by irrigations, instillation, spray, soaks or wet compresses, preferably thoroughly cleansing with gravity flow irrigation or syringe to provide copious quantities of fresh solution to remove organic wastes and debris. Also for preoperative skin preparation and postoperative protection. Apply topically as the 0.4% solution in water or isotonic saline. Use dilutions of 0.1% to 0.2% in urology and ophthalmology.

Add the powder to the required amount of cool or lukewarm water (not hot). Saline solution may be used where indicated. Stir or shake for a minute or two. Allow solution to stand for several minutes, then stir (or shake) for an additional 2 or 3 minutes. The solution may be used as such (disregarding any residue still left) or it may be allowed to settle for several minutes and the clear solution decanted for use.

This entire procedure should require no more than 10 to 15 minutes, and the resultant solution has been shown to contain more than 95% of the hypochlorous acid (based on the theoretical evaluation).

To endeavor to dissolve the product completely would require an hour or even more and offer no advantage.

➤*Storage/Stability:* Oxychlorosene sodium solutions should be used as soon as possible after preparation. If, however, the solution must be stored, it should be kept refrigerated at 4° to 8°C (39.2° to 46.5°F) in a capped or sealed plastic or glass container with a non-metallic cap, and used within 14 days of preparation. If stored at room temperature of 23°C (73.4°F), solutions should be used within 7 days after preparation.

Actions

➤*Pharmacology:* Oxychlorosene is a complex of the sodium salt of dodecylbenzenesulfonic acid and hypochlorous acid. Its action is markedly cidal, rapid and complete against both gram-negative and gram-positive bacteria, fungi, yeast, mold, viruses and spores.

Contraindications

Infection sites not exposed to direct contact with the solution; systemic use.

Precautions

➤*Bladder/eye installation:* Instillation of 0.2% solution, particularly into the bladder or into the eye, may cause severe discomfort. Pretreat the eye with a topical anesthetic. In the bladder, use a 0.1% concentration for the first treatment, instilling the solution to the capacity of the bladder without over-distention.

SILVER NITRATE

Rx	**Silver Nitrate** (Gordon Labs)	**Ointment:** 10%	Petrolatum base. In 30 g.
		Solution: 10%	In 30 mL.
		25%	In 30 mL.
		50%	In 30 mL.

SILVER NITRATE — TOPICAL

Indications

To treat indolent wounds, destroy exuberant granulations, freshen the edges of ulcers and fissures, touch the bases of vesicular, bullous or aphthous lesions and provide styptic action.

➤*10% Ointment:*

Podiatry – To treat neurovascular helomas; to cauterize and destroy small nerve endings and blood vessels. It forms a protective covering after the removal of corns and calluses.

➤*10% Solution:* Impetigo vulgaris.

Podiatry – Helomas.

➤*25% Solution:* Pruritus.

Podiatry – Plantar warts.

➤*50% Solution:*

Podiatry – Plantar warts; granulation tissue; papillomatous growths; granuloma pyogenicum.

➤*Unlabeled uses:* Concentrations of 0.1% to 0.5% are used as wet dressings in burns and on lesions.

Administration and Dosage

➤*Ointment:* Apply in apertured pad on affected area for ≈ 5 days, as needed.

➤*Solution:* Apply a cotton applicator dipped in solution on the affected area or lesion 2 or 3 times a week for 2 or 3 weeks, as needed.

Actions

➤*Pharmacology:* Silver nitrate is a strong caustic and escharotic providing antisepetic, astringent, germicidal, local (epithelial) stimulant or caustic action externally.

The attachment of silver to a reactive group of a protein sharply decreases the protein's solubility; the protein's conformation may also be altered and denaturation may occur. Precipitation of the protein generally results. At low concentrations of silver, precipitation is confined to proteins in the interstices and an astringent action occurs. At high concentrations, membrane and intracellular structures are damaged and there is a casutic or corrosive effect.

Because silver ions attach so readily to the various groups of proteins, the ions are captured before they diffuse far into tissues. Precipitation of silver as silver chloride also limits extent of ion movement. Thus, local effects of silver are self-limiting and spread of damage occurs only when the dose overwhelms the capacity of tissues to fix the ion at the application site. Antiseptic effects of silver may derive in part from the reaction with bacterial and viral proteins.

Contraindications

Application on wounds, cuts or broken skin.

Warnings

➤*Skin discoloration:* Prolonged or frequent use may permanently discolor skin due to deposition of reduced silver. However, topical silver nitrate for local application to suppress granulation tissue apparently does not produce argyria.

➤*Staining of clothes:* Will stain clothing and linens.

➤*Electrolyte abnormalities:* If wet dressings are used over extensive areas or prolonged periods, electrolyte abnormalities can result. Sodium and chloride leach into the dressing and hyponatremia or hypochloremia can occur. Absorbed nitrate can cause methemoglobinemia.

Precautions

➤*Irritation:* Discontinue use if redness or irritation occurs.

➤*For external use only:* Avoid contact with the eyes.

Overdosage

➤*Symptoms:* The fatal dose of silver nitrate may be as low as 2 g. Oral intake of silver nitrate causes a local corrosive effect including pain and burning of mouth, salivation, vomiting, diarrhea progressing to anuria, shock, coma, convulsions and death. Blackening of skin and mucous membranes occurs (sometimes permanent).

➤*Treatment:* Give NaCl in water, 10 g/L, to precipitate silver Cl. Follow with catharsis, including NaCl solution. Also attend to shock and methemoglobinemia if present.

If splashed in eyes, wash with copious amounts of water and see a physician.

SODIUM HYPOCHLORITE

otc	**Dakin's** (Century Pharm.)	**Solution:** 0.25%	In pt.
		0.5%	In pt and gal.

SODIUM HYPOCHLORITE — TOPICAL

Indications

➤*Antiseptic:* Applied topically to the skin as an antiseptic.

Actions

➤*Pharmacology:* Sodium hypochlorite has germicidal, deodorizing and bleaching properties. It is effective against vegetative bacteria and viruses, and also, to some degree, against spores and fungi.

Precautions

➤*Chemical burns:* May be produced; avoid skin or eye contact with this solution.

TRICLOSAN (Irgasan)

otc	**Oxy ResiDon't** (SK Beecham)	**Liquid:** 0.6%, diazolidinyl urea	In 240 mL
otc	**no more germies** (J & J)	**Soap:** 0.25%, PEG, EDTA	In 237 mL
otc	**Septi-Soft** (Calgon Vestal)	**Solution:** 0.25%. With glycerin, emollients	In 240 mL, qt, gal.
otc	**Septisol** (Calgon Vestal)		In 240 mL, qt, gal.
otc	**Stridex Face Wash** (Sterling Health)	**Solution:** 1% triclosan	Glycerin, EDTA. Alcohol free. In 237 mL.
otc	**Clearasil Daily Face Wash** (Procter & Gamble)	**Liquid:** 0.3% triclosan	Aloe vera gel, glycerin, EDTA. In 135 mL.
otc	**ASC Lotionized** (Geritrex)		Aloe vera gel, sweet almond oil, parabens, tartrazine. In 8 oz.

TRICLOSAN (Irgasan) — TOPICAL

Indications

➤*Skin cleanser:*

Septi-Soft – Skin cleanser. May use as hand/body wash, shampoo, bed or towel bath.

Septisol – Healthcare personnel handwash and skin degermer.

Administration and Dosage

Dispense a small amount (5 mL) on hands, rub thoroughly for 30 seconds, rinse thoroughly, dry.

➤*Septi-Soft:* May also be used as hand or body wash, shampoo, bed or towel bath.

Actions

➤*Pharmacology:* Triclosan, a bis-phenol disinfectant, is a bacteriostatic agent with activity against a wide range of gram-positive and gram-negative bacteria.

Contraindications

Use on burned or denuded skin or mucous membranes; routine prophylactic total body bathing.

➤*Septi-Soft:* Not a surgical scrub; do not use in preparation for surgery.

Precautions

For external use only. Avoid contact with the eyes.

MISCELLANEOUS ANTISEPTICS

otc	**Stat•One Isopropyl Rubbing Alcohol** (Continental)	**Gel**: 70% isopropyl rubbing alcohol	In 28.4 g.
otc	**Stat•One Hydrogen Peroxide** (Continental)	**Gel**: 3% hydrogen peroxide	In 28.4 g.
otc	**Kleen-Handz** (American Medical)	**Solution**: 62% SD alcohol	Aloe vera, purified water. In 60 mL.
otc	**S.T. 37** (Numark Labs)	**Solution**: 0.1% hexylresorcinol	Glycerin, EDTA. In 236.5 and 473 mL.
otc	**Mercurochrome** (Humco)	**Solution**: 2% merbromin	In 30 mL.
otc	**Tincture of Green Soap** (Paddock)	**Liquid**: With 28% to 32% alcohol	In gal.
otc	**Antiseptic Wound & Skin Cleanser** (MPM Medical)	**Liquid**: 0.1% benzethonium chloride	EDTA, glycerin, methylparaben. In 120 mL.
otc	**Stat•One Hydrogen Peroxide** (Continental)	**Gel**: 3% hydrogen peroxide	In 28.4 g.
otc	**Stat•One Isopropyl Rubbing Alcohol** (Continental)	**Gel**: 70% isopropyl rubbing alcohol	In 28.4 g.
otc	**B.F.I. Antiseptic** (Numark Labs)	**Powder**: 16% bismuth-formic-iodide, zinc phenol sulfonate, potassium alum, bismuth subgallate, boric acid, menthol, eucalyptol, thymol	In 35.4 g.
otc	**Alco-Gel** (Tweezerman)	**Gel**: 60% ethyl alcohol	In 60 and 480 g.
Rx	**Arzol Silver Nitrate Applicators** (Arzol)	**Applicator**: 75% silver nitrate and 25% potassium nitrate	In 100s.

Antiviral Agents

ACYCLOVIR (Acycloguanosine)

Rx	**Zovirax** (Biovail)	**Ointment**: 5% (50 mg/g)	In a polyethylene glycol base. In 15 g tubes.
		Cream: 5% (50 mg/g)	Cetostearyl alcohol, mineral oil, in an aqueous cream base. In 2 g tubes.

ACYCLOVIR — TOPICAL

Indications

➤*Herpes virus:*

Ointment – Management of initial genital herpes and in limited non-life-threatening mucocutaneous herpes simplex virus infections in immunocompromised patients.

Cream – Treatment of recurrent herpes labialis (cold sores) in adults and adolescents (12 years of age and older).

Administration and Dosage

➤*Approved by the FDA:* 1984.

➤*Ointment:* Apply sufficient quantity to adequately cover all lesions every 3 hours 6 times per day for 7 days. The dose size per application will vary depending upon the total lesion area but should approximate a one-half inch ribbon of ointment per 4 square inches of surface area. A finger cot or rubber glove should be used when applying acyclovir to prevent autoinoculation of other body sites and transmission of infection to other persons. Therapy should be initiated as early as possible following onset of signs and symptoms.

➤*Cream:* Apply 5 times per day for 4 days (ie, during the prodrome or when lesions appear). For adolescents 12 years of age and older, the dosage is the same as in adults.

➤*Storage/Stability:*

Ointment – Store at 15° to 25°C (59° to 77°F) in a dry place.

Cream – Store at or below 25°C (77°F); excursions permitted to 15° to 30°C (59° to 86°F).

Actions

➤*Pharmacology:*

Virology –

Mechanism of antiviral action: Acyclovir is a synthetic purine nucleoside analogue with in vitro and in vivo inhibitory activity against herpes simplex virus types 1 (HSV-1), 2 (HSV-2), and varicella-zoster virus (VZV). The inhibitory activity of acyclovir is highly selective due to its affinity for the enzyme thymidine kinase (TK) encoded by HSV and VZV. This viral enzyme converts acyclovir into acyclovir monophosphate, a nucleotide analogue. The monophosphate is further converted into diphosphate by cellular guanylate kinase and into triphosphate by a number of cellular enzymes. In vitro, acyclovir triphosphate stops replication of herpes viral DNA. This is accomplished in 3 ways:

1.) Competitive inhibition of viral DNA polymerase,
2.) Incorporation into and termination of the growing viral DNA chain, and
3.) Inactivation of the viral DNA polymerase. The greater antiviral activity of acyclovir against HSV compared to VZV is due to its more efficient phosphorylation by the viral TK.

Drug resistance: Resistance of HSV and VZV to acyclovir can result from qualitative and quantitative changes in the viral TK and/or DNA polymerase. Clinical isolates of HSV and VZV with reduced susceptibility to acyclovir have been recovered from immunocompromised patients, especially with advanced HIV infection. While most of the acyclovir-resistant mutants isolated thus far from immunocompromised patients have been found to be TK-deficient mutants, other mutants involving the viral TK gene (TK partial and TK altered) and DNA polymerase have been isolated. TK-negative mutants may cause severe disease in infants and immunocompromised adults. The possibility of viral resistance to acyclovir should be considered in patients who show poor clinical response during therapy.

➤*Pharmacokinetics:*

Ointment – A study included 11 patients with localized varicella-zoster. In this uncontrolled study, acyclovir was detected in the blood of 9 patients and in the urine of all patients tested. Acyclovir levels in plasma ranged from less than 0.01 to 0.28 mcg/mL in 8 patients with normal renal function, and from less than 0.01 to 0.78 mcg/mL in 1 patient with impaired renal function. Acyclovir excreted in the urine ranged from less than 0.02% to 9.4% of the daily dose. Therefore, systemic absorption of acyclovir after topical application is minimal.

Cream –

Adults: A clinical pharmacology study was performed with acyclovir cream in adult volunteers to evaluate the percutaneous absorption of acyclovir. In

ACYCLOVIR — TOPICAL

this study, which included 6 male volunteers, the cream was applied to an area of 710 cm^2 on the backs of the volunteers 5 times daily at intervals of 2 hours for a total of 4 days. The weight of cream applied and urinary excretion of acyclovir were measured daily. Plasma concentration of acyclovir was assayed 1 hour after the final application. The average daily urinary excretion of acyclovir was approximately 0.04% of the daily applied dose. Plasma acyclovir concentrations were below the limit of detection (0.01 mcM) in 5 subjects and barely detectable (0.014 mcM) in 1 subject. Systemic absorption of acyclovir from acyclovir cream is minimal in adults.

Contraindications

Hypersensitivity or chemical intolerance to the components of the formulation.

Warnings

➤*Cutaneous use only:* Acyclovir ointment or cream is intended for cutaneous use only and should not be used in the eye.

➤*Pregnancy: Category B.* Acyclovir should be used during pregnancy only if the potential benefit justifies the potential risk to the fetus.

➤*Lactation:* It is not known whether topically applied acyclovir is excreted in breast milk. Systemic exposure following topical administration is minimal. After oral administration of acyclovir, acyclovir concentrations have been documented in breast milk in 2 women and ranged from 0.6 to 4.1 times the corresponding plasma levels. These concentrations would potentially expose the nursing infant to a dose of acyclovir up to 0.3 mg/kg per day. Nursing mothers who have active herpetic lesions near or on the breast should avoid nursing.

➤*Children:*

Ointment – Safety and effectiveness in pediatric patients have not been established.

Cream – Safety and effectiveness in pediatric patients less than 12 years of age have not been established.

Precautions

➤*Ointment:* The recommended dosage, frequency of applications, and length of treatment should not be exceeded. There exist no data which demonstrate that the use of acyclovir ointment 5% will either prevent transmission of infection to other persons or prevent recurrent infections when applied in the absence of signs and symptoms. Acyclovir ointment 5% should not be used for the prevention of recurrent HSV infections. Although clinically significant viral resistance associated with the use of acyclovir ointment 5% has not been observed, this possibility exists.

➤*Cream:* Acyclovir cream is intended for cutaneous use only and should not be used in the eye or inside the mouth or nose. Acyclovir cream should only be used on herpes labialis on the affected external aspects of the lips and face. Because no data are available, application to human mucous membranes is not recommended. Acyclovir cream has a potential for irritation and contact sensitization. The effect of acyclovir cream has not been established in immunocompromised patients.

Drug Interactions

None known.

Adverse Reactions

➤*Ointment:* In the controlled clinical trials, mild pain (including transient burning and stinging) was reported by about 30% of patients in both the active and placebo arms; treatment was discontinued in 2 of these patients. Local pruritus occurred in 4% of these patients. In all studies, there was no significant difference between the drug and placebo group in the rate or type of reported adverse reactions nor were there any differences in abnormal clinical laboratory findings.

➤*Observed during clinical practice:*

Dermatologic – Pruritus, rash.

Miscellaneous – Edema or pain at the application site.

➤*Cream:* In 5 double-blind, placebo-controlled trials, 1124 patients were treated with acyclovir cream and 1161 with placebo (vehicle) cream. Acyclovir cream was well tolerated; 5% of patients on acyclovir cream and 4% of patients on placebo reported local application site reactions.

The most common adverse reactions at the site of topical application were dry lips, desquamation, dryness of skin, cracked lips, burning skin, pruritus, flakiness of skin, and stinging on skin; each event occurred in less than 1% of patients receiving acyclovir cream and vehicle. Three patients on acyclovir cream and 1 patient on placebo discontinued treatment due to an adverse event.

An additional study, enrolling 22 healthy adults, was conducted to evaluate the dermal tolerance of acyclovir cream compared with vehicle using single occluded and semi-occluded patch testing methodology. Both acyclovir cream and vehicle showed a high and cumulative irritation potential. Another study, enrolling 251 healthy adults, was conducted to evaluate the contact sensitization potential of acyclovir cream using repeat insult patch testing methodology. Of 202 evaluable subjects, possible cutaneous sensitization reactions were observed in the same 4 (2%) subjects with both acyclovir cream and vehicle, and these reactions to both acyclovir cream and vehicle were confirmed in 3 subjects upon rechallenge. The sensitizing ingredient(s) has not been identified.

The safety profile in patients 12 to 17 years of age was similar to that observed in adults.

➤*Observed during clinical practice:*

Dermatologic – Contact dermatitis, eczema, application site reactions including signs and symptoms of inflammation.

Miscellaneous – Angioedema, anaphylaxis.

Overdosage

Overdosage by topical application is unlikely.

Patient Information

Use only for cold sores. For external use only.

PENCICLOVIR

Rx	**Denavir** (Novartis)	**Cream:** 1% (10 mg/g)	Cetostearyl alcohol, mineral oil, white petrolatum. In 1.5 g tubes.

PENCICLOVIR — TOPICAL

Indications

➤*Herpes labialis:* Treatment of recurrent herpes labialis (cold sores) in adults.

Administration and Dosage

➤*Approved by the FDA:* September 24, 1996.

Apply every 2 hours during waking hours for a period of 4 days. Treatment should be started as early as possible (ie, during the prodrome or when lesions appear).

➤*Storage/Stability:* Store at controlled room temperature, 20° to 25°C (68° to 77°).

Actions

➤*Pharmacokinetics:* Measurable penciclovir concentrations were not detected in plasma or urine of healthy male volunteers (n = 12) following single or repeat application of the 1% cream at a dose of 180 mg penciclovir daily (approximately 67 times the estimated usual clinical dose).

➤*Microbiology:* The antiviral compound penciclovir has in vitro inhibitory activity against herpes simplex virus types 1 (HSV-1) and 2 (HSV-2). In cells infected with HSV-1 or HSV-2, viral thymidine kinase phosphorylates penciclovir to a monophosphate form which, in turn, is converted to penciclovir triphosphate by cellular kinases. In vitro studies demonstrate that penciclovir triphosphate inhibits HSV polymerase competitively with deoxyguanosine triphosphate. Consequently, herpes viral DNA synthesis and, therefore, replication are selectively inhibited.

Drug resistance – Penciclovir-resistant mutants of HSV can result from qualitative changes in viral thymidine kinase or DNA polymerase. The most commonly encountered acyclovir-resistant mutants that are deficient in viral thymidine kinase are also resistant to penciclovir.

Contraindications

Hypersensitivity to the product or any of its components.

Warnings

➤*Carcinogenesis:* Two-year carcinogenicity studies were conducted with famciclovir (the oral prodrug of penciclovir) in rats and mice. An increase in the incidence of mammary adenocarcinoma (a common tumor in female rats of the strain used) was seen in female rats receiving 600 mg/kg/day (approximately 395 × the maximum theoretical human exposure to penciclovir following application of the topical product, based on area under the plasma concentration curve comparisons [24 hr• AUC]).

➤*Mutagenesis:* An increase in clastogenic responses was seen with penciclovir in the L5178Y mouse lymphoma cell assay (at doses ≥ 1,000 mcg/mL) and, in human lymphocytes incubated in vitro at doses ≥ 250 mcg/mL. When tested in vivo, penciclovir caused an increase in micronuclei in mouse bone marrow following the intravenous administration of doses ≥ 500 mg/kg (≥ 810 x the maximum human dose, based on body surface area conversion).

➤*Fertility impairment:* Testicular toxicity was observed in multiple animal species (rats and dogs) following repeated intravenous administration of penciclovir (160 mg/kg/day and 100 mg/kg/day, respectively, approximately 1,155 and 3,255 x the maximum theoretical human AUC). Testicular changes seen in both species included atrophy of the seminiferous tubules and reductions in epididymal sperm counts and/or an increased incidence of sperm with abnormal morphology or reduced motility. Adverse testicular effects were related to an increasing dose or duration of exposure to penciclovir.

➤*Pregnancy: Category B.* There are no adequate and well-controlled studies in pregnant women. Use during pregnancy only if clearly needed.

➤*Lactation:* There is no information on whether penciclovir is excreted in human milk after topical administration. However, following oral administration of famciclovir (the oral prodrug of penciclovir) to lactating rats, penciclovir was excreted in breast milk at concentrations higher than those seen

PENCICLOVIR — TOPICAL

in the plasma. Therefore, a decision should be made whether to discontinue the drug, taking into account the importance of the drug to the mother. There are no data on the safety of penciclovir in newborns.

➤*Children:* Safety and effectiveness in pediatric patients have not been established.

Precautions

➤*General:* Penciclovir should only be used on herpes labialis on the lips and face. Because no data are available, application to human mucous membranes is not recommended. Particular care should be taken to avoid application in or near the eyes since it may cause irritation. The effect of penciclovir has not been established in immunocompromised patients.

Adverse Reactions

In two double-blind, placebo-controlled trials, 1516 patients were treated with penciclovir cream and 1541 with placebo. The most frequently reported adverse event was headache, which occurred in 5.3% of the patients treated with penciclovir and 5.8% of the placebo-treated patients. The rates of reported local adverse reactions are shown in the data below. One or more local adverse reactions were reported by 2.7% of the patients treated with penciclovir and 3.9% of placebo-treated patients.

Local Adverse Reactions Reported in Phase III Trials

	Penciclovir (n = 1516) %	Placebo (n = 1541) %
Application site reaction	1.3%	1.8%
Hypesthesia/local anesthesia	0.9%	1.4%
Taste perversion	0.2%	0.3%
Pruritus	0%	0.3%
Pain	0%	0.1%
Rash (erythematous)	0.1%	0.1%
Allergic reaction	0%	0.1%

Two studies, enrolling 108 healthy subjects, were conducted to evaluate the dermal tolerance of 5% penciclovir cream (a 5-fold higher concentration than the commercial formulation) compared to vehicle using repeated occluded patch testing methodology. The 5% penciclovir cream induced mild erythema in approximately one-half of the subjects exposed, an irritancy profile similar to the vehicle control in terms of severity and proportion of subjects with a response. No evidence of sensitization was observed.

BORIC ACID

otc	**Boric Acid** (Various, eg, Clay-Park, IDE, Major, Moore, Rugby, URL)	**Ointment**: 10%	In 30 and 60 g and lb.

BORIC ACID — TOPICAL

Indications

➤*Skin irritation:* A soothing application for chafed skin, abrasions, burns and other skin irritations.

Administration and Dosage

➤*For external use only:* For external use only. Avoid contact with the eyes.

➤*Dosage:* Apply directly to affected area once or twice daily.

Burn Preparations

MAFENIDE

Rx	**Sulfamylon** (Bertek)	**Solution, topical**: 5% mafenide (as acetate)	In 50 g packets for reconstitution.
Rx	**Sulfamylon** (Dow B. Hickam)	**Cream**: 85 mg (as acetate) per g	EDTA, cetyl alcohol, stearyl alcohol, parabens. sodium metabisulfite. In 37, 114 and 411 g.

MAFENIDE ACETATE — TOPICAL

Indications

➤*Burn treatment:* For adjunctive therapy of patients with second- and third-degree burns; for use as an adjunctive topical antimicrobial agent to control bacterial infection when used under moist dressings over meshed autografts on excised burn wounds.

Administration and Dosage

➤*Cream:* Prompt institution of appropriate measures for controlling shock and pain is of prime importance. The burn wounds are then cleansed and debrided, and mafenide acetate cream is applied with a sterile gloved hand. Satisfactory results can be achieved with application of the cream once or twice daily, to a thickness of ≈ 1⁄16 inch; thicker application is not recommended. The burned areas should be covered with mafenide acetate cream at all times. Therefore, whenever necessary, the cream should be reapplied to any areas from which it has been removed (eg, by patient activity). The routine of administration can be accomplished in minimal time, since dressings usually are not required. If individual patient demands make them necessary, however, only a thin layer of dressing should be used.

When feasible, the patient should be bathed daily, to aid in debridement. A whirlpool bath is particularly helpful, but the patient may be bathed in bed or in a shower.

The duration of therapy with mafenide acetate cream depends on each patient's requirements. Treatment is usually continued until healing is progressing well or until the burn site is ready for grafting. Mafenide acetate cream should not be withdrawn from the therapeutic regimen while there is the possibility of infection. However, if allergic manifestations occur during treatment with mafenide acetate cream, discontinuation of treatment should be considered.

If acidosis occurs and becomes difficult to control, particularly in patients with pulmonary dysfunction, discontinuing therapy with mafenide acetate cream for 24 to 48 hours while continuing fluid therapy may aid in restoring acid-base balance.

➤*Solution:*

Preparation of solution – Mafenide acetate topical solution is supplied as a powder and is to be reconstituted with Sterile Water for Irrigation, USP or 0.9% Sodium Chloride Irrigation, USP. Aseptic techniques should be observed during preparation of the solution. Premeasured quantities of 50 g of mafenide acetate powder are provided in packets. The entire quantity of mafenide acetate should be emptied into a suitable container that contains 1000 mL of Sterile Water for Irrigation, USP or 0.9% Sodium Chloride Irrigation, USP and mixed until completely dissolved. The resulting mafenide acetate, USP 5% solution should be filtered through a 0.22 micron sterilizing grade filter prior to use. The reconstituted/filtered solution should be used within 48 hours after preparation. Not for injection. For topical use only.

Use of the solution – The grafted area should be covered with 1 layer of fine mesh gauze. An 8-ply burn dressing should be cut to the size of the graft and wetted with mafenide acetate solution using an irrigation syringe or irrigation tubing until leaking is noticeable. If irrigation tubing is used, the tubing should be placed over the burn dressing in contact with the wound and covered with a second piece of 8-ply dressing. The irrigation dressing should be secured with a bolster dressing and wrapped as appropriate. The gauze dressing should be kept wet. In clinical studies, this has been accomplished by irrigating with a syringe or injecting the solution into the irrigation tubing every 4 hours or as necessary. If irrigation tubing is not used, the gauze dressing may be moistened every 6 to 8 hours or as necessary to keep wet.

Wound dressings may be left undisturbed, except for the irrigations, for up to 5 days. Additional soaks may be initiated until graft take is complete. Maceration of skin may result from wet dressings applied for intervals as short as 24 hours. Treatment is usually continued until autograft vascularization occurs and healing is progressing (typically occurring in about 5 days). Safety and efficacy have not been established for more than 5 days for an individual grafting procedure.

If allergic manifestations occur during treatment with mafenide acetate solution, discontinuation of treatment should be considered. If acidosis occurs and becomes difficult to control, particularly in patients with pulmonary dysfunction, discontinuing the soaks with the mafenide acetate solution for 24 to 48 hours may aid in restoring acid-base balance (see Precautions). Dressing changes and monitoring the site for bacterial growth during this interruption should be adjusted accordingly.

➤*Storage/Stability:*

Cream – Avoid exposure to excessive heat (temperatures above 40°C or 104°F).

Solution –

Packets: Store packets in a dry place at room temperature 15° to 30°C (59° to 86°F).

Prepared solution: Store at room temperature 15° to 30°C (59° to 86°F). Use within 48 hours of preparation.

Actions

➤*Pharmacology:* The mechanism of action of mafenide is not known, but is different from that of the sulfonamides. Mafenide is not antagonized by pABA, serum, pus or tissue exudates, and there is no correlation between bacterial sensitivities to mafenide and to the sulfonamides. Its activity is not altered by changes in the acidity of the environment.

Cream – Mafenide acetate cream, applied topically, produces a marked reduction in the bacterial population present in the avascular tissues of second- and third-degree burns. Reduction in bacterial growth after application of mafenide acetate cream has also been reported to permit spontaneous healing of deep partial-thickness burns, and thus prevent conversion of burn wounds from partial thickness to full thickness. It should be noted, however, that delayed eschar separation has occurred in some cases.

Solution – The osmolality of the 5% topical solution is ≈ 340 mOsm/kg.

➤*Pharmacokinetics:*

Absorption/Distribution –

Cream: Applied topically, mafenide acetate cream diffuses through devascularized areas and is absorbed.

Clinical studies have shown that when applied topically to burns as an 11.2% mafenide acetate cream, blood levels of the parent drug peaked at 2 hours following application, ranging from 26 to 197 mcg/mL for single doses of 14 to 77 g of mafenide acetate.

Solution: Applied topically, mafenide acetate solution diffuses through devascularized areas. Approximately 80% of a mafenide acetate dose is delivered to burned tissue over 4 hours following topical application of the 5% solution.

Cream and solution: Following application of mafenide acetate cream and solution, peak mafenide concentrations in human burned skin tissue occur at 2 and 4 hours, respectively. Peak tissue concentrations are similar following administration of the solution or cream.

Metabolism/Excretion –

Cream: Mafenide acetate cream is rapidly converted to a metabolite (p-carboxybenzenesulfonamide) which is cleared through the kidneys. Mafenide acetate is active in the presence of pus and serum, and its activity is not altered by changes in the acidity of the environment.

Solution: Once absorbed, mafenide is rapidly converted to an inactive metabolite (p-carboxybenzenesulfonamide) which is cleared through the kidneys. Metabolite levels peaked at 3 hours, ranging from 10 to 340 mcg/mL. Twenty-four hours after application, combined parent and metabolite blood levels had fallen to pretreatment levels.

➤*Microbiology:*

Antibacterial activity – Mafenide acetate exerts bacteriostatic action against many gram-negative and gram-positive organisms, including *Pseudomonas aeruginosa* and certain strains of anaerobes.

Contraindications

Hypersensitivity to mafenide.

Warnings

➤*Fatal hemolytic anemia:* Fatal hemolytic anemia with disseminated intravascular coagulation, presumably related to a glucose-6-phosphate dehydrogenase deficiency, has been reported following therapy with mafenide acetate.

➤*Fungal colinization:* Fungal colonization in and below the eschar may occur concomitantly with reduction of bacterial growth in the burn wound. However, fungal dissemination through the infected burn wound is rare.

MAFENIDE ACETATE — TOPICAL

➤*Hypersensitivity reactions:* Mafenide acetate cream should be administered with caution to patients with history of hypersensitivity to mafenide. It is not known whether there is cross-sensitivity to other sulfonamides.

➤*Renal function impairment:* Mafenide acetate cream should be used with caution in burn patients with acute renal failure.

➤*Pregnancy: Category C.* Animal reproduction studies have not been conducted with mafenide acetate. It is also not known whether mafenide acetate can cause fetal harm when administered to a pregnant woman or can affect reproduction capacity. Therefore, the preparation is not recommended for the treatment of women of childbearing potential, unless the burned area covers greater than 20% of the total body surface, or the need for the therapeutic benefit of mafenide acetate is, in the physician's judgment, greater than the possible risk to the fetus.

➤*Lactation:* It is not known whether mafenide acetate is excreted in human milk. Because many drugs are excreted in human milk and because of the potential for serious adverse reaction in nursing infants from mafenide acetate, a decision should be made whether to discontinue nursing or to discontinue the drug, taking into account the importance of the drug to the mother.

➤*Children:*

Solution – The safety and efficacy of mafenide acetate for solution have been established in the age groups 3 months to 16 years.

Precautions

➤*Monitoring:* Mafenide acetate and its metabolite, p-carboxybenzenesulfonamide, inhibit carbonic anhydrase, which may result in metabolic acidosis, usually compensated by hyperventilation. In the presence of impaired renal function, high blood levels of mafenide acetate and its metabolite may exaggerate the carbonic anhydrase inhibition. Therefore, close monitoring of acid-base balance is necessary, particularly in patients with extensive second-degree or partial-thickness burns and in those with pulmonary or renal dysfunction. Some burn patients treated with mafenide acetate have also been reported to manifest an unexplained syndrome of masked hyperventilation with resulting respiratory alkalosis (slightly alkaline blood pH, low arterial pCO_2, and decreased total CO_2); change in arterial pO_2 is variable. The etiology and significance of these findings are unknown.

➤*For external use only:* For external use only. Avoid contact with eyes.

➤*Superinfection:* Use may result in bacterial or fungal overgrowth of nonsusceptible organisms. Such overgrowth may lead to a secondary infection. Appropriate measures should be taken if superinfection occurs.

➤*Sulfite sensitivity:* Mafenide acetate cream contains sodium metabisulfite, a sulfite that may cause allergic-type reactions including anaphylactic symptoms and life-threatening or less severe asthmatic episodes in certain susceptible people. The overall prevalence of sulfite sensitivity in the general population is unknown and probably low. Sulfite sensitivity is seen more frequently in asthmatic than in nonasthmatic people.

Adverse Reactions

In the clinical setting of severe burns, it is often difficult to distinguish between an adverse reaction to mafenide acetate and burn sequelae. In a clinical study of pediatric patients with acute burns requiring autografts who received mafenide acetate solution in addition to double antibiotic solution (DAB) wound therapy (neomycin sulfate 40 mg and polymyxin B 200,000 U/L), the incidence of rash (4.6%) and itching (2.8%) in the group that received mafenide acetate solution was not different from that experienced with DAB dressings alone (5.7% and 1.3%, respectively).

From other clinical settings, a single case of bone marrow depression and a single case of an acute attack of porphyria have been reported following therapy with mafenide acetate. Fatal hemolytic anemia with disseminated intravascular coagulation, presumably related to a glucose-6-phosphate dehydrogenase deficiency, has been reported following therapy with mafenide acetate. The following adverse reactions have been reported with topical mafenide acetate therapy:

➤*Allergic:* Rash, itching, facial edema, swelling, hives, blisters, erythema, and eosinophilia.

➤*Dermatologic:*

Cream – The most frequently reported reaction was pain on application or a burning sensation. Rare occurrences are excoriation of new skin, and bleeding of skin.

Solution – Pain or burning sensation, rash and pruritus (often localized to the area covered by the wound dressing), erythema, skin maceration from prolonged wet dressings, facial edema, swelling, hives, blisters, eosinophilia.

➤*Metabolic:* Acidosis, increase in serum chloride.

➤*Respiratory:* Tachypnea or hyperventilation, decrease in arterial pCO_2.

➤*Miscellaneous:* Accidental ingestion of mafenide acetate cream has been reported to cause diarrhea.

Patient Information

Notify physician if condition worsens, if irritation occurs, or if hyperventilation occurs.

NITROFURAZONE

Rx	**Nitrofurazone** (Various, eg, Clay-Park)	**Topical Solution:** 0.2%	In pt and gal.
Rx	**Furacin** (Roberts)		In 480 mL.
Rx	**Nitrofurazone** (Various, eg, Clay-Park)	**Ointment (soluble):** 0.2%	In 480 g.
Rx	**Furacin Soluble Dressing** (Roberts)		In a polyethylene glycol base. In 28, 56 and 454 g.
Rx	**Furacin** (Roberts)	**Cream:** 0.2%	Cetyl alcohol, mineral oil, parabens. Water-miscible base. In 28 g.

NITROFURAZONE — TOPICAL

Indications

➤*Burn treatment:* For adjunctive therapy of patients with second- and third-degree burns when bacterial resistance to other agents is a real or potential problem.

➤*Skin grafting:* In skin grafting where bacterial contamination may cause graft rejection or donor site infection particularly in hospitals with historical resistant bacteria epidemics.

Administration and Dosage

➤*Topical cream:* Apply directly to the lesion, or first place on gauze. Reapply once daily or every few days, depending on the usual dressing technique.

➤*Soluble dressing:*

Burns – Apply directly to the lesion with a spatula, or first place on gauze. Impregnated gauze may be used. Reapply depending on the preferred dressing technique. Flushing the dressing with sterile saline facilitates its removal.

Preparation of impregnated gauze –

Sterile gauze strips: Sterile gauze strips are placed in a tray and covered with nitrofurazone soluble dressing. Repeat the procedure, adding several layers of gauze for each layer of nitrofurazone soluble dressing. Sprinkling a little sterile water on each layer of dressing will minimize any color change from autoclaving. Cover the tray very loosely and autoclave at 121°C (249.8°F) for 30 minutes at 15 to 20 pounds pressure.

Bandage rolls: To impregnate bandage rolls, place some nitrofurazone soluble dressing in the bottom of a glass jar. Stand rolls on end. Place more nitrofurazone soluble dressing on top. Cover top of jar with aluminum foil. Autoclave at 121°C (249.8°F) for 45 minutes at 15 to 20 pounds pressure. Do not store impregnated bandage rolls for more than 24 hours.

Autoclaving more than once is not recommended.

➤*Storage/Stability:* Avoid exposure to direct sunlight, strong fluorescent lighting, alkaline materials, and excessive heat (greater than 40°C; 104°F).

Actions

➤*Pharmacology:* Nitrofurazone is a nitrofuran that is bactericidal for most pathogens commonly causing surface infections, including *Staphylococcus aureus*, *Streptococcus*, *Escherichia coli*, *Clostridium perfringens*, *Aerobacter aerogenes*, and *Proteus*.

Nitrofurazone inhibits a number of bacterial enzymes, especially those involved in the aerobic and anaerobic degradation of glucose and pyruvate. The activity appears to involve the pyruvate dehydrogenase system as well as citrate synthetase, malate dehydrogenase, glutathione reductase, and pyruvate decarboxylase. Glutathione reductase inhibition may be caused by control of pentose phosphate metabolism. Although nitrofurazone inhibits a variety of enzymes, it is not considered to be a general enzyme inactivator since many enzymes are not inhibited by this compound.

Contraindications

Known sensitization to any of the components of this preparation is a contraindication for use.

Warnings

➤*Renal function impairment:*

Soluble dressing – Nitrofurazone soluble dressing should be used with caution in patients with known or suspected renal impairment. The polyethylene glycols in the base can be absorbed through denuded skin and may not be excreted normally by the compromised kidney. This may lead to symptoms of progressive renal impairment such as increased BUN, anion gap, and metabolic acidosis.

➤*Carcinogenesis:* Nitrofurazone has been shown to produce mammary tumors when fed at high doses to female Sprague-Dawley rats. The relevance of this to topical use in humans is unknown. Dietary dosage levels of 60 and 30 mg/kg/day shortened the onset time of the typical mammary gland tumors associated with older female rats. These tumors exhibited the same histological characteristics seen in the spontaneously occurring tumors, and were seen only in the female animals. No mammary tumors were seen in rats treated with nitrofurazone orally in the diet for 1 year at

NITROFURAZONE — TOPICAL

levels of ≈ 11 mg/kg/day. Spermatogenic arrest was noted in the male rats in dietary dosage levels of ≥ 30 mg/kg/day, after 1 year on test.

➤*Pregnancy: Category C.* Nitrofurazone has been shown to have an embryocidal effect in rabbits when given in oral doses 30 times the human dose. There are no adequate and well-controlled studies in pregnant women. Nitrofurazone should be used during pregnancy only if the potential benefit justifies the potential risk to the fetus.

➤*Lactation:* It is not known whether this drug is excreted in human milk. Because many drugs are excreted in human milk and because of the potential for tumorigenicity shown for nitrofurazone in animal studies, a decision should be made whether to discontinue nursing or to discontinue the drug, taking into account the importance of the drug to the mother.

➤*Children:* Safety and effectiveness in pediatric patients have not been established.

Precautions

➤*Superinfection:* Use of topical antimicrobials like nitrofurazone occasionally allows overgrowth of nonsusceptible organisms including fungi. If this occurs, or if irritation, sensitization or superinfection develops, treatment with nitrofurazone should be discontinued and appropriate therapy instituted.

Adverse Reactions

➤*Allergic:* Allergic reactions to nitrofurazone should be treated symptomatically.

➤*Dermatologic:* Instances of clinical skin reactions have been reported for patients treated with nitrofurazone formulations. Symptoms appear as varying degrees of contact dermatitis such as rash, pruritus, and local edema. Although the exact incidence of such reactions is difficult to determine, historically, a survey of world literature and clinical data indicates an overall incidence of ≈ 1%.

Overdosage

➤*Symptoms:* The oral administration of nitrofurazone for 7 days to rats at extremely high dosage levels of 240 mg/kg/day produced severe hepatorenal lesions whereas only renal changes were seen when the dosage level was reduced to 60 mg/kg/day for 60 days.

Dogs treated orally with nitrofurazone for 400 days at levels of 11 mg/kg/day showed no toxic effects related to drug treatment.

The single IV administration in dogs of 20, 35, or 75 mg/kg nitrofurazone produced clinical signs of lacrimation, salivation, emesis, diarrhea, excitation, weakness, ataxia, and weight loss, whereas 100 mg/kg produced convulsions and death.

Patient Information

➤*Topical cream:* Patients should be told to use nitrofurazone topical cream only as directed by a physician. Patients should be advised to discontinue the drug and contact a physician should rash or irritation occur.

SILVER SULFADIAZINE

Rx	**SSD Cream** (Boots)	**Cream:** 10 mg per g in a water-miscible base[1]	Cetyl alcohol. In 25, 50, 85, 400 and 1000 g.
Rx	**Silvadene** (Hoescht Marion Roussel)		In 20, 50, 85, 400 and 1000 g.
Rx	**Thermazene** (Sherwood)		In 50, 400 and 1000 g.
Rx	**SSD AF Cream** (Boots)		In 50, 400 and 1000 g.

[1] Contains white petrolatum, stearyl alcohol, 0.3% methylparaben.

SILVER SULFADIAZINE — TOPICAL

Indications

➤*Burn treatment:* As an adjunct for the prevention and treatment of wound sepsis in patients with second- and third-degree burns.

Administration and Dosage

For topical use only. Not for ophthalmic use.

➤*Administration:* Prompt institution of appropriate regimens for care of the burned patient is of prime importance and includes the control of shock and pain. The burn wounds are then cleansed and debrided, and silver sulfadiazine cream is applied under sterile conditions. The burn areas should be covered with silver sulfadiazine cream at all times. The cream should be applied once to twice daily to a thickness of approximately 1⁄16 inch. Whenever necessary, the cream should be reapplied to any areas from which it has been removed by patient activity. Administration may be accomplished in minimal time because dressings are not required. However, if individual patient requirements make dressings necessary, they may be used.

➤*Hydrotherapy:* Reapply immediately after hydrotherapy.

➤*Duration of therapy:* Treatment with silver sulfadiazine cream should be continued until satisfactory healing has occurred, or until the burn site is ready for grafting. The drug should not be withdrawn from the therapeutic regimen while there remains the possibility of infection except if a significant adverse reaction occurs.

➤*Storage/Stability:* Store at controlled room temperature 15° to 30°C (59° to 86°F).

Actions

➤*Pharmacology:* Silver sulfadiazine has broad antimicrobial activity. It is bactericidal for many gram-negative and gram-positive bacteria as well as being effective against yeast. Results from in vitro testing are listed below.

Sufficient data have been obtained to demonstrate that silver sulfadiazine will inhibit bacteria that are resistant to other antimicrobial agents and that the compound is superior to sulfadiazine.

Studies using radioactive micronized silver sulfadiazine, electron microscopy, and biochemical techniques have revealed that the mechanism of action of silver sulfadiazine on bacteria differs from silver nitrate and sodium sulfadiazine. Silver sulfadiazine acts only on the cell membrane and cell wall to produce its bactericidal effect.

Results of In Vitro Testing with Silver Sulfadiazine Cream 1% Concentration of Silver Sulfadiazine Number of Sensitive Strains/Total Number of Strains Tested

Genus and species	50 mcg/mL	100 mcg/mL
Pseudomonas aeruginosa	130/130	130/130
Xanthomonas (Pseudomonas) maltophilia	7/7	7/7
Enterobacter species	48/50	50/50
Enterobacter cloacae	24/24	24/24
Klebsiella species	53/54	54/54
Escherichia coli	63/63	63/63
Serratia species	27/28	28/28
Proteus mirabilis	53/53	53/53
Morganella morganii	10/10	10/10
Providencia rettgeri	2/2	2/2
Providencia species	1/1	1/1
Proteus vulgaris	2/2	2/2
Citrobacter species	10/10	10/10
Acinetobacter calcoaceticus	10/11	11/11
Staphylococcus aureus	100/101	100/101
Staphylococcus epidermidis	51/51	51/51
β-hemolytic *Streptococcus*	4/4	4/4
Enterococcus species	52/53	53/53
Corynebacterium diphtheriae	2/2	2/2
Clostridium perfringens	0/2	2/2
Candida albicans	43/50	50/50

Silver sulfadiazine is not a carbonic anhydrase inhibitor and may be useful in situations where such agents are contraindicated.

Contraindications

Hypersensitivity to silver sulfadiazine or any of the other ingredients in the preparation; pregnant women approaching or at term; on premature infants; on newborn infants during the first 2 months of life.

Warnings

➤*Cross-sensitivity:* There is potential cross-sensitivity between silver sulfadiazine and other sulfonamides. If allergic reactions attributable to treatment with silver sulfadiazine occur, continuation of therapy must be weighed against the potential hazards of the particular allergic reaction.

➤*Hemolysis:* The use of silver sulfadiazine cream in some cases of glucose-6-phosphate dehydrogenase-deficient individuals may be hazardous, as hemolysis may occur.

➤*Renal/Hepatic function impairment:* If hepatic and renal functions become impaired and elimination of drug decreases, accumulation may occur and discontinuation of silver sulfadiazine cream should be weighed against the therapeutic benefit being achieved.

➤*Pregnancy: Category B.* There are no adequate and well-controlled studies in pregnant women. Use during pregnancy only if clearly justified. Use of silver sulfadiazine is contraindicated in pregnant women approaching or at term.

SILVER SULFADIAZINE — TOPICAL

➤*Lactation:* It is not known whether silver sulfadiazine is excreted in human milk. However, sulfonamides are known to be excreted in human milk, and all sulfonamide derivatives are known to increase the possibility of kernicterus. Because of the possibility for serious adverse reactions in nursing infants from sulfonamides, a decision should be made whether to discontinue nursing or to discontinue the drug, taking into account the importance of the drug to the mother.

➤*Children:* Safety and effectiveness in pediatric patients have not been established. Use of silver sulfadiazine is contraindicated in premature infants or in newborn infants during the first 2 months of life.

Precautions

➤*Topical proteolytic enzymes:* In considering the use of topical proteolytic enzymes in conjunction with silver sulfadiazine cream, the possibility should be noted that silver may inactive such enzymes.

➤*Lab test abnormalities:* In the treatment of burn wounds involving extensive areas of the body, the serum sulfa concentrations may approach adult therapeutic levels (8% to 12%). Therefore, in these patients it would be advisable to monitor serum sulfa concentrations. Renal function should be carefully monitored and the urine should be checked for sulfa crystals. Absorption of the propylene glycol vehicle has been reported to affect serum osmolality, which may affect the interpretation of laboratory tests.

➤*Superinfection:* Fungal proliferation in and below the eschar may occur. However, the incidence of clinically reported fungal superinfection is low.

Adverse Reactions

Reduction in bacterial growth after application of topical antibacterial agents has been reported to permit spontaneous healing of deep partial-thickness burns by preventing conversion of the partial thickness to full thickness by sepsis. However, reduction in bacterial colonization has caused delayed separation, in some cases necessitating escharotomy in order to prevent contracture.

Absorption of silver sulfadiazine varies depending upon the percent of body surface area and the extent of the tissue damage. Although few have been reported, it is possible that any adverse reaction associated with sulfonamides may occur.

➤*Dermatologic:* Infrequently occurring events include skin necrosis, erythema multiforme, skin discoloration, burning sensation, rashes, and interstitial nephritis.

➤*Hematologic:* Several cases of transient leukopenia have been reported in patients receiving silver sulfadiazine therapy. Leukopenia associated with silver sulfadiazine administration is primarily characterized by decreased neutrophil count. Maximal white blood cell depression occurs within 2 to 4 days of initiation of therapy. Rebound to normal leukocyte levels follows onset within 2 to 3 days. Recovery is not influenced by continuation of silver sulfadiazine therapy. The incidence of leukopenia in various reports averages about 20%. A higher incidence of leukopenia has been seen in patients treated concurrently with cimetidine.

➤*Miscellaneous:* Some of the reactions that have been associated with sulfonamides are as follows: Blood dyscrasias including agranulocytosis, aplastic anemia, thrombocytopenia, leukopenia, and hemolytic anemia; dermatologic and allergic reactions, including Stevens-Johnson syndrome and exfoliative dermatitis; GI reactions; hepatitis and hepatocellular necrosis; CNS reactions; toxic nephrosis.

CHLOROXINE

Rx	**Capitrol** (Westwood Squibb)	**Shampoo:** 2%	In 120 mL.

CHLOROXINE — TOPICAL

Indications

➤*Dandruff/seborheic dermatitis:* Treatment of dandruff and mild to moderately severe seborrheic dermatitis of the scalp.

Administration and Dosage

Massage thoroughly into wet scalp. Allow lather to remain on scalp for 3 minutes; rinse. Repeat application and rinse. Two treatments per week are usually sufficient.

Actions

➤*Pharmacology:* A synthetic antibacterial compound; also has antifungal activity. Chloroxine reduces excess scaling in patients with scaling or seborrheic dermatitis.

Contraindications

Hypersensitivity to any of the ingredients. Do not use on acutely inflamed lesions.

Warnings

➤*Pregnancy: Category C.* Safety for use during pregnancy has not been established. Use only when clearly needed and when the potential benefits outweigh the potential hazards to the fetus.

➤*Lactation:* It is not known whether the drug is excreted in breast milk. Exercise caution when administering to a nursing woman.

➤*Children:* Safety and efficacy for use in children have not been established.

Precautions

➤*For external use only:* Avoid contact with eyes; if contact occurs, flush with cool water.

Adverse Reactions

➤*Dermatologic:* Irritation and burning of the scalp and adjacent areas have occurred. Discoloration of light colored hair has occurred.

Patient Information

For external use only. Avoid contact with eyes.

If irritation, burning or rash occurs, discontinue use.

May discolor blond, gray or bleached hair.

ANTI-INFLAMMATORY AGENTS

Corticosteroids, Topical

Indications

➤*Relief of inflammatory and pruritic manifestations of corticosteroid-responsive dermatoses:* Some of the conditions in which topical corticosteroids have been proven effective include: Contact dermatitis, atopic dermatitis, nummular eczema, stasis eczema, asteatotic eczema, lichen planus, lichen simplex chronicus, insect and arthropod bite reactions, first- and second-degree localized burns and sunburns.

➤*Alternative/Adjunctive treatment:* Psoriasis, seborrheic dermatitis, severe diaper rash, disidrosis, nodular prurigo, chronic discoid lupus erythematosus, alopecia areata, lymphocytic infiltration of the skin, mycosis fungoides and familial benign pemphigus of Hailey-Hailey.

➤*Possibly effective in the following conditions:* Bullous pemphigoid, cutaneous mastocytosis, lichen sclerosus et atrophicus and vitiligo.

Topical corticosteroids relieve inflammatory symptoms associated with dermatophyte and yeast infections of the skin and may be used concomitantly with antifungal agents for initial treatment.

The use of topical corticosteroids in combination with antibiotics in secondary infected dermatoses remains controversial.

➤*Nonprescription hydrocortisone preparations:* Temporary relief of itching associated with minor skin irritations, inflammation and rashes due to eczema, insect bites, poison ivy, poison oak, poison sumac, soaps, detergents, cosmetics, jewelry, seborrheic dermatitis, psoriasis and external genital and anal itching.

Administration and Dosage

➤*Usual dose:* Apply sparingly to affected areas 2 to 4 times daily.

➤*General considerations:* Topical corticosteroids have a repository effect; with continuous use, one or two applications per day may be as effective as three or more. Many clinicians advise applying twice daily until clinical response is achieved, and then only as frequently as needed to control the condition.

Short term or intermittent therapy using high potency agents (eg, every other day, 3 to 4 consecutive days per week, or once per week) may be more effective and cause fewer adverse effects than continuous regimens using lower potency products.

Do not discontinue treatment abruptly. After long-term use or after using a potent agent, in order to prevent a rebound effect, switch to a less potent agent or alternate use of topical corticosteroids and emollient products.

Use low potency agents in children, on large areas, and on body sites especially prone to steroid damage such as the face, scrotum, axilla, flexures and skin folds. Reserve higher potency agents for areas and conditions resistant to treatment with milder agents; they may be alternated with milder agents.

Perform appropriate clinical and laboratory tests if a topical corticosteroid is used for long periods or over large areas of the body.

Treatment with very high potency topical corticosteroids should not exceed 2 consecutive weeks and the total dosage should not exceed 50 g per week because of the potential for these drugs to suppress the HPA axis.

➤*Occlusive dressing technique:*

1.) Soak the area in water or wash it well.
2.) While the skin is still moist, gently rub medication into the affected areas.
3.) Cover the area with a plastic wrap (eg, *Saran Wrap*, *Handi Wrap*). Alternatively, plastic gloves may be used for hands, plastic bags for feet, or a bathing cap for scalp.
4.) Seal edges with tape or bandage, ensuring that the wrap adheres closely to the skin.
5.) Leave in place overnight or at least 6 hours. Do not use for more than 12 hours in a 24 hour period. Do not use this technique with very high potency topical corticosteroids.

Actions

➤*Pharmacology:* Topical corticosteroids are adrenocorticosteroid derivatives incorporated into a vehicle suitable for application to skin or external mucous membranes. Modifications of the essential 4-ring steroid structure such as hydroxylation, methylation, fluorination or esterification are often made to increase lipid solubility and potency and decrease mineralocorticoid effects.

The primary therapeutic effects of the topical corticosteroids are due to their anti-inflammatory activity which is non-specific (ie, they act against most causes of inflammation including mechanical, chemical, microbiological and immunological).

Topically applied corticosteroids diffuse across cell membranes to interact with cytoplasmic receptors located in both the dermal and intradermal cells. The intracellular effects are similar to those that occur with systemically administered corticosteroids.

At the cellular level, corticosteroids appear to induce phospholipase A_2 inhibitory proteins (lipocortins), thus depressing formation, release and activity of the endogenous mediators of inflammation such as prostaglandins, kinins, histamine, liposomal enzymes and the complement system.

When corticosteroids are applied to inflamed skin, they inhibit the migration of macrophages and leukocytes into the area by reversing vascular dilation and permeability. The clinical result is a decrease in edema, erythema and pruritus.

By suppressing DNA synthesis, topically applied corticosteroids have an antimitotic effect on epidermal cells. This property is useful in proliferative disorders such as psoriasis, but also can be demonstrated in normal skin.

➤*Pharmacokinetics:* The amount of corticosteroid absorbed from the skin depends on the intrinsic properties of the drug itself, the vehicle used, the duration of exposure and the surface area and condition of the skin to which it is applied. In general, absorption will be enhanced by increased skin temperature, hydration, application to inflamed or denuded skin, intertriginous areas (eg, eyelids, groin, axilla) or skin surfaces with a thin stratum corneum layer (eg, face, scrotum). Palms, soles and crusted surfaces are less permeable. Occlusive dressings greatly enhance skin penetration and, therefore, increase drug absorption.

Infants and children have a higher total body surface to body weight ratio that decreases with age. Therefore, proportionately more topically applied medications will be absorbed systemically in this population, putting them at a greater risk for systemic effects.

Following topical absorption, corticosteroids enter the systemic circulation and are metabolized and excreted via pathways described for systemically administered corticosteroids.

Vehicles – Ointments are more occlusive and are preferred for dry scaly lesions. Use creams on oozing lesions or in intertriginous areas where the occlusive effects of ointments may cause maceration and folliculitis. Creams are often preferred by patients for aesthetic reasons even though their water content makes them more drying than ointments. Gels, aerosols, lotions and solutions are useful on hairy areas. Urea enhances the penetration of hydrocortisone and selected steroids by hydrating the skin. As a general rule, ointments and gels are more potent than creams or lotions. However, optimized vehicles that have been formulated for some products have demonstrated equal potency in cream, gel and ointment forms. Steroid impregnated tapes are useful for occlusive therapy in small areas.

Occlusive dressings – Occlusive dressings such as a plastic wrap increase skin penetration approximately tenfold by increasing the moisture content of the stratum corneum. Occlusion can be beneficial in resistant cases but it may also lead to sweat retention and increased bacterial and fungal infections. Additionally, increased absorption of the corticosteroid may produce systemic side effects. Therefore, do not use occlusive dressings for more than 12 hours per day and when using very potent topical corticosteroids.

Relative potency – The relative potency of a product depends on several factors including the characteristics and concentration of the drug and the vehicle used. Vasoconstrictor assays are used to measure the relative potency of the commercially available products. The estimated relative potency of selected topical corticosteroid preparations is given in the following table. Ranking is based on vasoconstrictor assays of brand name products. In some cases, generic "equivalents" have less vasoconstrictive activity.

Relative Potency of Selected Topical Corticosteroid Products

Drug		Dosage Form	Strength
I.	*Very high potency*		
	Augmented betamethasone dipropionate	Ointment	0.05%
	Clobetasol propionate	Cream, Ointment	0.05%
	Diflorasone diacetate	Ointment	0.05%
	Halobetasol propionate	Cream, Ointment	0.05%
II.	*High potency*		
	Amcinonide	Cream, Lotion, Ointment	0.1%
	Augmented betamethasone dipropionate	Cream	0.05%
	Betamethasone dipropionate	Cream, Ointment	0.05%
	Betamethasone valerate	Ointment	0.1%
	Desoximetasone	Cream, Ointment	0.25%
		Gel	0.05%
	Diflorasone diacetate	Cream, Ointment (emollient base)	0.05%
	Fluocinolone acetonide	Cream	0.2%
	Fluocinonide	Cream, Ointment, Gel	0.05%
	Halcinonide	Cream, Ointment	0.1%
	Triamcinolone acetonide	Cream, Ointment	0.5%
III.	*Medium potency*		
	Betamethasone benzoate	Cream, Gel, Lotion	0.025%
	Betamethasone dipropionate	Lotion	0.05%
	Betamethasone valerate	Cream	0.1%
	Clocortolone pivalate	Cream	0.1%
	Desoximetasone	Cream	0.05%
	Fluocinolone acetonide	Cream, Ointment	0.025%
	Flurandrenolide	Cream, Ointment	0.025%
		Cream, Ointment, Lotion	0.05%
		Tape	4 mcg/cm^2
	Fluticasone propionate	Cream	0.05%
		Ointment	0.005%
	Hydrocortisone butyrate	Ointment, Solution	0.1%
	Hydrocortisone valerate	Cream, Ointment	0.2%
	Mometasone furoate	Cream, Ointment, Lotion	0.1%
	Triamcinolone acetonide	Cream, Ointment, Lotion	0.025%
		Cream, Ointment, Lotion	0.1%
IV.	*Low potency*		
	Aclometasone dipropionate	Cream, Ointment	0.05%
	Desonide	Cream	0.05%
	Dexamethasone	Aerosol	0.01%
		Aerosol	0.04%
	Dexamethasone sodium phosphate	Cream	0.1%
	Fluocinolone acetonide	Cream, Solution	0.01%
	Hydrocortisone	Lotion	0.25%
		Cream, Ointment, Lotion, Aerosol	0.5%
		Cream, Ointment, Lotion, Solution	1%
		Cream, Ointment, Lotion	2.5%
	Hydrocortisone acetate	Cream, Ointment	0.5%
		Cream, Ointment	1%

Contraindications

Hypersensitivity to any component; monotherapy in primary bacterial infections such as impetigo, paryonchia, erysipelas, cellulitis, angular cheilitis, erythrasma (clobetasol), treatment of rosacea, perioral dermatitis or acne; use on the face, groin or axilla (very high or high potency agents); ophthalmic use (prolonged ocular exposure may cause steroid-induced glaucoma and cataracts). When applied to the eyelids or skin near the eyes, the drug may enter the eyes.

Warnings

➤*Pregnancy: Category C.* Corticosteroids are teratogenic in animals when administered systemically at relatively low dosages. The more potent corticosteroids are teratogenic after dermal application in animals. There are no adequate and well controlled studies in pregnant women. Therefore, use during pregnancy only if the potential benefits outweigh the potential hazards to the fetus. In pregnant patients, do not use extensively; do not use in large amounts or for prolonged periods of time.

➤*Lactation:* It is not known whether topical corticosteroids could result in sufficient systemic absorption to produce detectable quantities in breast milk. Systemic corticosteroids are secreted into breast milk in quantities not likely to have a deleterious effect on the infant. Nevertheless, exercise caution when administering topical corticosteroids to a nursing mother.

➤*Children:* Children may be more susceptible to topical corticosteroid-induced hypothalamic-pituitary-adrenal (HPA) axis suppression and Cushing's syndrome than adults because of a larger skin surface area to body weight ratio.

HPA axis suppression, Cushing's syndrome and intracranial hypertension have occurred in children receiving topical corticosteroids. Manifestations of adrenal suppression include linear growth retardation, delayed weight gain, low plasma cortisol levels and absence of response to ACTH stimulation. Manifestations of intracranial hypertension include bulging fontanelles, headaches and bilateral papilledema.

Limit administration to the least amount compatible with effective therapy. Chronic corticosteroid therapy may interfere with the growth and development of children.

Do not use potent topical corticosteroids to treat diaper dermatoses in infants.

Safety and efficacy of augmented betamethasone dipropionate, clobetasol, fluticasone propionate, desoximetasone and halobetasol propionate are not established.

Precautions

➤*Systemic effects:* Systemic absorption of topical corticosteroids has produced reversible HPA axis suppression, Cushing's syndrome, hyperglycemia and glycosuria. Conditions that augment systemic absorption include the application of the more potent steroids, use over large surface areas, prolonged use and the addition of occlusive dressings.

Periodically evaluate patients for evidence of HPA axis suppression by using morning plasma cortisol, urinary free cortisol and ACTH stimulation tests. If HPA axis suppression is noted, attempt to withdraw the drug, reduce the frequency of application, substitute a less potent steroid or use a sequential approach with the occlusive technique. Also test for impairment of thermal homeostasis.

Recovery of HPA axis function and thermal homeostasis are generally prompt and complete upon discontinuation of the drug. Infrequently, signs and symptoms of steroid withdrawal may occur, requiring supplemental systemic corticosteroids.

Clobetasol suppresses the HPA axis at doses as low as 2 g per day.

Children – They may absorb proportionally larger amounts of topical corticosteroids and may be more susceptible to systemic toxicity (see Warnings).

As a general rule, little effect on the HPA axis will occur with use of a potent topical corticosteroid in amounts of less than 50 g weekly for an adult and 15 g weekly for a small child, without occlusion. To cover the adult body one time requires 12 to 26 g.

For information regarding systemic corticosteroids, refer to the Adrenal Cortical Steroids, Glucocorticoids group monograph in the Endocrine and Metabolic Agents chapter.

➤*Local irritation:* If local irritation develops, discontinue use and institute appropriate therapy. Medications containing alcohol may produce dry skin or burning sensations/irritation in open lesions. Allergic contact dermatitis is usually diagnosed by observing failure to heal rather than noting clinical exacerbation as with most topical products not containing corticosteroids. Corroborate such an observation with diagnostic patch testing.

Skin atrophy – This is common and may be clinically significant in 3 to 4 weeks with potent preparations. Atrophy occurs most readily at sites where percutaneous absorption is high.

Take care when using periorbitally or in the genital area. Avoid use of high potency topical corticosteroids on the face and in intertriginous areas because of resulting striae.

➤*Psoriasis:* Do not use topical corticosteroids as sole therapy in widespread plaque psoriasis.

In rare instances, treatment (or withdrawal of treatment) of psoriasis with corticosteroids is thought to have provoked the pustular form of the disease.

➤*Atrophic changes:* Certain areas of the body, such as the face, groin and axillae, are more prone to atrophic changes than other areas of the body following treatment with corticosteroids. Frequent observation of the patient is important if these areas are to be treated.

➤*Infections:* In the presence of an infection, institute therapy with an antifungal or antibacterial agent. If a favorable response does not occur promptly, discontinue the corticosteroid until the infection has been controlled. Treating skin infections with topical corticosteroids can extensively worsen the infection.

➤*For external use only:* Avoid inhalation of aerosols, ingestion or contact with eyes.

➤*Vehicles:* Many topical corticosteroids are in specially formulated bases designed to maximize their release and potency. Mixing with other bases or vehicles may affect potency far beyond that normally expected from the dilution. Exercise caution before mixing; if necessary, contact the manufacturer to determine if there may be an incompatibility.

➤*Occlusive therapy:* Discontinue the use of occlusive dressings if infection develops, and institute appropriate antimicrobial therapy.

Occasionally, a patient may develop a sensitivity reaction to a particular occlusive dressing material or adhesive; a substitute material may be necessary.

Do not use occlusive dressings in **augmented betamethasone dipropionate, betamethasone dipropionate, clobetasol, halobetasol propionate** and **mometasone** treatment regimens.

Adverse Reactions

➤*Local:* Burning; itching; irritation; erythema; dryness; folliculitis; hypertrichosis; pruritus; acneiform eruptions; hypopigmentation; perioral dermatitis; allergic contact dermatitis; numbness of fingers; stinging and cracking/tightening of skin; maceration of the skin; secondary infection; skin atrophy; striae; miliaria; telangiectasia. These may occur more frequently with occlusive dressings.

Also, there have been reports of development of pustular psoriasis from chronic plaque psoriasis following reduction or discontinuation of potent topical corticosteroids.

Sensitivity to a particular dressing material or adhesive may occur occasionally.

➤*Systemic:* Systemic absorption of topical corticosteroids has produced reversible HPA axis suppression, manifestations of Cushing's syndrome, hyperglycemia and glycosuria (see Precautions). This is more likely to occur with occlusive dressings and with the more potent steroids. Patients with liver failure or children (see Warnings) may be at at higher risk. Lightheadedness and hives have been reported rarely.

Following prolonged application around the eyes, cataracts and glaucoma may develop. In diffusely atrophied skin, blood vessels may become visible on the skin surface; telangiectasia and purpura may occur at the site of trauma.

The risk of adverse reactions may be minimized by changing to a less potent agent, reducing the dosage or using intermittent therapy.

Overdosage

Topical corticosteroids can be absorbed in sufficient amounts to produce systemic effects (see Precautions).

Patient Information

Apply ointments, creams or gels sparingly in a light film; rub in gently. Washing or soaking the area before application may increase drug penetration.

To use a lotion, solution or gel on your scalp, part your hair, apply a small amount of the medicine on the affected area and rub it in gently. Protect the area from washing, clothing, rubbing, etc until the lotion dries. You may wash your hair as usual but not right after applying the medicine.

To apply aerosols, shake well and spray on affected area holding container about 3 to 6 inches away. Spray for about 2 seconds to cover an area the size of your hand. Take care not to inhale the vapors. If you are spraying your face or near your face, cover your eyes.

Use only as directed. Do not put bandages, dressing, cosmetics or other skin products over the treated area unless directed by your physician.

Notify your physician if the condition being treated gets worse, or if burning, swelling or redness develop.

Avoid prolonged use around the eyes, in the genital and rectal areas, on the face, armpits and in skin creases unless directed by your physician. Avoid contact with the eyes.

If you forget a dose, apply it as soon as you remember and continue on your regular schedule. If it is almost time for the next application, wait and continue on your regular schedule. Do not apply double doses.

For parents of pediatric patients: Do not use tight-fitting diapers or plastic pants on a child treated in the diaper area; these garments may work like occlusive dressings and cause more of the drug to be absorbed into your child's body.

ALCLOMETASONE DIPROPIONATE

Rx	**Alclometasone Dipropionate** (Various, eg, Taro)	**Ointment:** 0.05%	In 15, 45, and 60 g.
Rx	**Aclovate** (GlaxoWellcome)		Hexylene glycol, white wax, propylene glycol stearate, white petrolatum. In 15 and 45 g.
Rx	**Alclometasone Dipropionate** (E. Fougera)	**Cream:** 0.05%	Hydrophilic, emollient base. White petrolatum, cetostearyl alcohol. In 15, 45, and 60 g.
Rx	**Aclovate** (GlaxoWellcome)		Hydrophilic, emollient base. Propylene glycol, white petrolatum, glyceryl stearate, PEG-100 stearate, chlorocresol. In 15 and 45 g.

ALCLOMETASONE DIPROPIONATE — TOPICAL

Complete prescribing information begins in the Topical Corticosteroids group monograph.

AMCINONIDE

Rx	**Amcinonide** (Taro)	**Ointment:** 0.1%	White petrolatum, benzyl alcohol 2.2%. In 15, 30, and 60 g.
Rx	**Cyclocort** (Astellas)		White petrolatum, benzyl alcohol 2%. In 15, 30, and 60 g.
Rx	**Amcinonide** (Taro)	**Cream:** 0.1%	Benzyl alcohol, glycerin. In 4, 15, 30, and 60 g.
Rx	**Cyclocort** (Astellas)		Hydrophilic base. Benzyl alcohol 2%, glycerin. In 15, 30, and 60 g.
Rx	**Cyclocort** (Astellas)	**Lotion:** 0.1%	Hydrophilic base. Benzyl alcohol 1%, glycerin. In 20 and 60 mL.

AMCINONIDE — TOPICAL

Complete prescribing information begins in the Topical Corticosteroids group monograph.

AUGMENTED BETAMETHASONE DIPROPIONATE

Rx	**Betamethasone Dipropionate, Augmented** (Various, eg, Alpharma, Fougera, Warrick)	**Ointment:** 0.05%	In an optimized vehicle. Propylene glycol, propylene glycol stearate, white wax, white petrolatum. In 15, 45, and 50 g.
Rx	**Diprolene** (Schering)		In an optimized vehicle. Propylene glycol, propylene glycol stearate, white wax, white petrolatum. In 15 and 45 g.
Rx	**Betamethasone Dipropionate, Augmented** (Various, eg, Fougera, Sandoz)	**Cream:** 0.05%	Propylene glycol, sorbitol solution, white petrolatum. In 15 and 50 g.
Rx	**Diprolene AF** (Schering)		Emollient base. Chlorocresol, propylene glycol, white petrolatum, white wax. In 15 and 45 g.
Rx	**Betamethasone Dipropionate, Augmented** (Various, eg, Fougera, Sandoz)	**Gel:** 0.05%	Propylene glycol. In 15 and 50 g.
Rx	**Diprolene** (Schering)		Propylene glycol. In 15 and 45 g.
Rx	**Diprolene** (Schering)	**Lotion:** 0.05%	30% isopropyl alcohol, hydroxypropylcellulose, propylene glycol. In 30 and 60 mL.

AUGMENTED BETAMETHASONE DIPROPIONATE — TOPICAL

Complete prescribing information begins in the Topical Corticosteroids group monograph.

Corticosteroids, Topical

BETAMETHASONE DIPROPIONATE

Rx	**Betamethasone Dipropionate** (Various, eg, NMC)	**Ointment**: 0.05%	In 15 and 45 g.
Rx	**Diprosone** (Schering)		Mineral oil, white petrolatum. In 15 and 45 g.
Rx	**Maxivate** (Westwood Squibb)		Mineral oil, white petrolatum.
Rx	**Betamethasone Dipropionate** (Various, eg, NMC, Schein)	**Cream**: 0.05%	In 15 and 45 g.
Rx	**Diprosone** (Schering)		Hydrophilic, emollient. Mineral oil, white petrolatum, chlorocresol, propylene glycol. In 15 and 45 g.
Rx	**Maxivate** (Westwood Squibb)		Hydrophilic base. Mineral oil, white petrolatum, polyethylene glycol, chlorocresol. In 15 and 45 g.
Rx	**Teladar** (Dermol)		Mineral oil, white petrolatum, polyethylene glycol, 4 chloro-m-cresol, propylene glycol. In 15 and 45 g.
Rx	**Betamethasone Dipropionate** (Various, eg, Goldline, Major, Moore, Rugby)	**Lotion**: 0.05%	In 20 and 60 mL.
Rx	**Diprosone** (Schering)		46.8% alcohol. In 30 mL.
Rx	**Maxivate** (Westwood Squibb)		Isopropyl alcohol. In 60 mL.
Rx	**Diprosone** (Schering)	**Aerosol**: 0.1%	10% isopropyl alcohol, mineral oil. In 85 g.

BETAMETHASONE DIPROPIONATE — TOPICAL

Complete prescribing information begins in the Topical Corticosteroids group monograph.

BETAMETHASONE VALERATE

Rx	**Betamethasone Valerate** (Various, eg, Genetco, Goldline, Major, Taro)	**Ointment**: 0.1%	In 15 and 45 g.
Rx	**Psorion Cream** (ICN)	**Cream**: 0.05%	Mineral oil, white petrolatum, propylene glycol. In 15 and 45 g.
Rx	**Betamethasone Valerate** (Various, eg, Genetco, Major, Moore, Taro)	**Cream**: 0.1%	In 15 and 45 g.
Rx	**Beta-Val** (Lemmon)		Aqueous, vanishing base. Mineral oil, white petrolatum, 4-chloro-m-cresol. In 15 and 45 g.
Rx	**Betamethasone Valerate** (Various, eg, Moore)	**Lotion**: 0.1%	In 60 mL.
Rx	**Beta-Val** (Lemmon)		47.5% isopropyl alcohol. In 60 mL.
Rx	**Luxiq** (Connetics)	**Foam**: 1.2 mg/g	60.4% ethanol, cetyl alcohol, stearyl alcohol. In 100 g.
Rx	**Betamethasone Valerate** (Paddock)	**Powder for compounding**	In micronized 5 and 10 g.

BETAMETHASONE VALERATE — TOPICAL

Complete prescribing information begins in the Topical Corticosteroids group monograph.

CLOBETASOL PROPIONATE

Rx	**Clobetasol Propionate** (Various, eg, Copley, NMC Labs)	**Ointment**: 0.05%	In 15, 30, and 45 g.
Rx	**Temovate** (GlaxoWellcome)		White petrolatum, sorbitan sesquioleate. In 15, 30, and 45 g.
Rx	**Cormax** (Watson)		White petrolatum, sorbitan sesquioleate. In 15 and 45 g.
Rx	**Embeline** (Healthpoint)		White petrolatum. In 15, 30, 45, and 60 g.
Rx	**Clobetasol Propionate** (Various, eg, Copley, NMC Labs)	**Cream**: 0.05%	In 15, 30, and 45 g.
Rx	**Cormax** (Watson)		White petrolatum, cetyl alcohol, stearyl alcohol, lanolin oil, parabens. In 30 and 45 g.
Rx	**Embeline** (Healthpoint)		White petrolatum, cetyl alcohol, stearyl alcohol, lanolin oil, parabens. In 15, 30, 45, and 60 g.
Rx	**Temovate** (GlaxoWellcome)		Chlorocresol. In 15, 30, and 45 g.
Rx	**Temovate Emollient** (Glaxo-Wellcome)		Emollient base. In 15, 30, and 60 g.
Rx	**Embeline E, 0.05%** (Healthpoint)		Cetostearyl alcohol. In 15, 30, and 60 g tubes.
Rx	**Clobex** (Galderma)	**Lotion**: 0.05%	Mineral oil. In 15, 30, 59, and 118 mL.
Rx	**Embeline** (Healthpoint)	**Scalp application**: 0.05%	40% isopropyl alcohol. In 25 and 50 mL.
Rx	**Temovate** (GlaxoWellcome)		39.3% isopropyl alcohol. In 25 and 50 mL.
Rx	**Clobetasol Propionate** (Various, eg, Fougera, Glades)	**Gel**: 0.05%	In 15, 30, and 60 g.
Rx	**Embeline** (Healthpoint)		In 15, 30, and 60 g.
Rx	**Temovate** (GlaxoWellcome)		In 15, 30, and 60 g.
Rx	**Olux** (Connetics)	**Foam**: 0.05%	60% ethanol, cetyl alcohol, stearyl alcohol. In 100g.
Rx	**Clobex** (Galderma)	**Shampoo**: 0.05%	Alcohol. In 118 mL.
Rx	**Clobex** (Galderma)	**Spray**: 0.05%	Alcohol. In 60 mL.
Rx	**Clobetasol Propionate** (Taro)	**Solution**: 0.05%	39.3% isopropyl alcohol. In 25 and 50 mL.

CLOBETASOL PROPIONATE — TOPICAL

Complete prescribing information begins in the Topical Corticosteroids group monograph.

CLOCORTOLONE PIVALATE

Rx	**Cloderm** (Hermal)	**Cream**: 0.1%	Water-washable, emollient base. White petrolatum, mineral oil, EDTA, parabens. In 15 and 45 g.

CLOCORTOLONE PIVALATE — TOPICAL

Complete prescribing information begins in the Topical Corticosteroids group monograph.

DESONIDE

Rx	**Desonide** (Various, eg, Copley, Goldline, Major, Moore, Rugby, Taro)	**Ointment**: 0.05%	In 15 and 60 g.
Rx	**DesOwen** (Owen/Galderma)		Mineral oil. In 15 and 60 g.
Rx	**Tridesilon** (Clay-Park Lab)		White petrolatum. In 15 and 60 g.
Rx	**Desonide** (Taro)	**Cream**: 0.05%	Methylparaben, mineral oil, white petrolatum. In 15 and 60 g.
Rx	**DesOwen** (Owen/Galderma)		In 15 and 60 g.
Rx	**Tridesilon** (Clay-Park Lab)		White petrolatum, alcohol, glycerin, mineral oil, methylparaben. In 15 and 60 g.
Rx	**Desonide** (Various, eg, Fougera, Glades)	**Lotion**: 0.05%	May contain light mineral oil, cetyl alcohol, stearyl alcohol, parabens, EDTA. In 59 and 118 mL.
Rx	**DesOwen** (Owen/Galderma)		Light mineral oil, parabens, EDTA. In 60 and 120 mL.
Rx	**LoKara** (PharmaDerm)		Light mineral oil, cetyl alcohol, stearyl alcohol, parabens, EDTA. In 59 and 118 mL.

DESONIDE — TOPICAL

Complete prescribing information begins in the Topical Corticosteroids group monograph.

DESOXIMETASONE

Rx	**Topicort** (Taro)	**Ointment**: 0.25%	White petrolatum, sorbitan sesquioleate. In 15 and 60 g.
Rx	**Desoximetasone** (Various, eg, Taro)	**Cream**: 0.05%	Emollient base. White petrolatum, lanolin alcohols, mineral oil, EDTA. In 15 and 60 g.
Rx	**Topicort LP** (Taro)		Emollient. White petrolatum, mineral oil, lanolin alcohols, EDTA. In 15 and 60 g.
Rx	**Desoximetasone** (Various, eg, Taro)	**Cream**: 0.25%	Emollient base. White petrolatum, lanolin alcohols, mineral oil. In 15 and 60 g.
Rx	**Topicort** (Taro)		Emollient. White petrolatum, mineral oil, lanolin alcohols. In 15, 60, 120 g.
Rx	**Topicort** (Taro)	**Gel**: 0.05%	20% SD alcohol 40, EDTA, docusate sodium, trolamine. In 15 and 60 g.

DESOXIMETASONE — TOPICAL

Complete prescribing information begins in the Topical Corticosteroids group monograph.

DEXAMETHASONE

Rx	**Decaspray** (Merck)	**Aerosol**: 0.04%	In 25 g.

Complete prescribing information begins in the Topical Corticosteroids group monograph.

DEXAMETHASONE SODIUM PHOSPHATE

Rx	**Decadron Phosphate** (Merck)	**Cream**: 0.1%	Greaseless base. Mineral oil, EDTA, 0.15% methylparaben, 0.1% sorbic acid. In 15 and 30 g.

Complete prescribing information begins in the Topical Corticosteroids group monograph.

DIFLORASONE DIACETATE

Rx	**ApexiCon** (PharmaDerm)	**Ointment**: 0.05%	White petrolatum. In 30 and 60 g.
Rx	**Diflorasone Diacetate** (Taro)		In 15, 30, and 60 g tubes.
Rx	**Maxiflor** (Allergan)		Emollient, occlusive base. Lanolin alcohol, white petrolatum. In 15, 30 and 60 g.
Rx	**Psorcon E** (Dermik)		Emollient, occlusive base. Lanolin alcohol, white petrolatum. In 15, 30 and 60 g.
Rx	**ApexiCon E** (PharmaDerm)	**Cream**: 0.05%	Stearyl alcohol, mineral oil, cetyl alcohol. In 30 and 60 g.
Rx	**Diflorasone Diacetate** (Taro)		In 15, 30, and 60 g tubes.
Rx	**Florone** (Dermik)		Emulsified, hydrophilic base. Propylene glycol. In 30 and 60 g.
Rx	**Florone E** (Dermik)		Emollient, hydrophilic vanishing base. Mineral oil. In 15, 30 and 60 g.
Rx	**Maxiflor** (Allergan)		Emulsified, hydrophilic base. 15% propylene glycol. In 15, 30 and 60 g.
Rx	**Psorcon E** (Dermik)		Hydrophilic base. Stearyl alcohol, cetyl alcohol, mineral oil. In 15 and 30 g.

DIFLORASONE DIACETATE — TOPICAL

Complete prescribing information begins in the Topical Corticosteroids group monograph.

FLUOCINOLONE ACETONIDE

Rx	**Fluocinolone** (Various, eg, Fougera, Goldline, Moore)	**Ointment**: 0.025%	In 15 and 60 g.
Rx	**Synalar** (Syntex)		White petrolatum. In 15, 30 and 425 g.
Rx	**Fluocinolone** (Various, eg, Fougera, Geneva, Goldline, Major, Moore, NMC)	**Cream**: 0.01%	In 15 and 60 g.
Rx	**Flurosyn** (Rugby)		Washable. Parabens. In 15, 60, 425 g.
Rx	**Synalar** (Syntex)		Water-washable, aqueous base. Mineral oil, EDTA, parabens. In 30 and 425 g.
Rx	**Fluocinolone** (Various, eg, Fougera, Geneva, Goldline, Major, Moore)	**Cream**: 0.025%	In 15 and 60 g.
Rx	**Flurosyn** (Rugby)		Washable. Parabens. In 15, 60, 425 g.
Rx	**Synalar** (Syntex)		Water-washable, aqueous base. Mineral oil, EDTA, parabens. In 30, 60 and 425 g.
Rx	**Fluocinolone** (Various, eg, Fougera, Goldline, Major, Moore, Rugby)	**Solution**: 0.01%	In 20 and 60 mL.
Rx	**Synalar** (Syntex)		Water-washable base. In 20, 60 mL.
Rx	**Capex** (Galderma)	**Shampoo**: 0.01%	In 12 mg capsule with shampoo base to be mixed by pharmacist before dispensing. 5.48 mg dibasic calcium phosphate dihydrate. In 180 mL.
Rx	**Derma-Smoothe/FS** (Hill)	**Oil**: 0.01%	A blend of oils, including mineral oil and peanut oil. In 120 mL.

FLUOCINOLONE ACETONIDE — TOPICAL

Complete prescribing information begins in the Topical Corticosteroids group monograph.

FLUOCINONIDE

Rx	**Fluocinonide** (Various, eg, Goldline, Lemmon, Taro)	**Cream**: 0.05%	In 15, 30, 60 and 120 g.
Rx	**Fluocinonide "E" Cream** (Various, eg, Goldline, Taro, URL)		In 15, 30, 60 and 120 g.
Rx	**Fluonex** (ICN)		Greaseless, anhydrous, water-washable. In 15 and 30 g.
Rx	**Lidex** (Syntex)		Water-miscible, emollient, hydrophilic, anhydrous, greaseless. In 15, 30, 60 and 120 g.
Rx	**Lidex-E** (Syntex)		Water-washable, aqueous emollient base. Mineral oil. In 15, 30 and 60 g.
Rx	**Vanos** (Medicis)	**Cream**: 0.1%	In 30 and 60 g.
Rx	**Fluocinonide** (Various, eg, Lemmon, Rugby, Taro)	**Ointment**: 0.05%	In 15, 30 and 60 g.
Rx	**Lidex** (Syntex)		Occlusive, emollient. White petrolatum. In 15, 30, 60 and 120 g.
Rx	**Fluocinonide** (Various, eg, Fougera, Goldline, Lemmon, Major, Moore)	**Solution**: 0.05%	In 60 mL.
Rx	**Lidex** (Syntex)		35% alcohol. In 20 and 60 mL.
Rx	**Fluocinonide** (Various, eg, Fougera, Lemmon, Moore)	**Gel**: 0.05%	In 60 g.
Rx	**Lidex** (Syntex)		Water-miscible, greaseless. EDTA. In 15, 30, 60, and 120 g.

FLUOCINONIDE — TOPICAL

Complete prescribing information begins in the Topical Corticosteroids group monograph.

FLURANDRENOLIDE

Rx	**Cordran** (Oclassen)	**Ointment**: 0.05%	White petrolatum. In 15, 30 and 60 g.
Rx	**Cordran SP** (Oclassen)	**Cream**: 0.05%	Emulsified base. Mineral oil. In 15, 30 and 60 g.
Rx	**Flurandrenolide** (Various, eg, Barre-National)	**Lotion**: 0.05%	In 60 mL.
Rx	**Cordran** (Oclassen)		Oil-in-water base. Mineral oil, glycerin, menthol, benzyl alcohol. In 15 and 60 mL.
Rx	**Cordran** (Oclassen)	**Tape**: 4 mcg per square cm	In 24" x 3" and 80" x 3" rolls.

FLURANDRENOLIDE — TOPICAL

Complete prescribing information begins in the Topical Corticosteroids group monograph.

FLUTICASONE PROPIONATE

Rx	**Fluticasone Propionate** (Sandoz)	**Cream**: 0.05%	Cetostearyl alcohol, mineral oil. In 15, 30, and 60 g tubes.
	Cutivate (GlaxoSmithKline)		Mineral oil base. Imidurea. In 15, 30 and 60 g.
Rx	**Fluticasone Propionate** (Fougera)	**Ointment**: 0.005%	In 15, 30, and 60 g tubes.
	Cutivate (GlaxoSmithKline)		In 15 and 60 g.
Rx	**Cutivate** (GlaxoSmithKline)	**Lotion**: 0.05%	Cetostearyl alcohol, parabens. In 60 mL.

FLUTICASONE PROPIONATE — TOPICAL

Complete prescribing information begins in the Topical Corticosteroids group monograph.

HALCINONIDE

Rx	**Halog** (Westwood-Squibb)	**Ointment:** 0.1%	Polyethylene and mineral oil gel base. In 15, 30, 60 and 240 g.
Rx	**Halog** (Westwood-Squibb)	**Cream:** 0.1%	Titanium dioxide, cetyl alcohol. In 15, 30, 60 and 240 g.
Rx	**Halog-E** (Westwood-Squibb)		Water-washable, greaseless, hydrophilic, vanishing, emollient. White petrolatum. In 30 and 60 g.
Rx	**Halog** (Westwood-Squibb)	**Solution:** 0.1%	EDTA. In 20 and 60 mL.

HALCINONIDE — TOPICAL

Complete prescribing information begins in the Topical Corticosteroids group monograph.

HALOBETASOL PROPIONATE

Rx	**Halobetasol Propionate** (Various, eg, Clay Park, Fougera, Taro)	**Ointment:** 0.05%	In 15 and 50 g.
Rx	**Ultravate** (Westwood Squibb)		Petrolatum. In 15 and 45 g.
Rx	**Halobetasol Propionate** (Various, eg, Clay Park, Fougera, Glades)	**Cream:** 0.05%	In 15 and 50 g.
Rx	**Ultravate** (Westwood Squibb)		Glycerin, diazolidinyl urea. In 15 and 45 g.

HALOBETASOL PROPIONATE — TOPICAL

Complete prescribing information begins in the Topical Corticosteroids group monograph.

HYDROCORTISONE

Rx[a]	**Hydrocortisone** (Various, eg, Carolina Medical, Fougera, Parmed, Rugby[b], URL)	**Ointment:** 0.5%	In 30 g.
otc	**Cortizone•5** (Pfizer Consumer)		White petrolatum. In 28 g.
Rx[a]	**Hydrocortisone** (Various, eg, Carolina Medical[c], Fougera, Major, Parmed, Rugby, URL)	**Ointment:** 1%	In 20, 30, and 120 g and lb.
otc	**Hydrocortisone with Aloe** (G & W Labs)		Mineral oil, white petrolatum, parabens. In 28.4 g.
otc	**HydroSkin** (Rugby)		Mineral oil, white petrolatum base. In 28.4 g.
otc	**Cortizone•10** (Pfizer Consumer)		White petrolatum. In 30 g.
Rx	**Hycort** (Everett)		White petrolatum and mineral oil base. In 30 g.
otc	**Tegrin-HC** (Block)		Mineral oil, white petrolatum. In 28 g.
Rx	**1% HC** (C & M)		Washable. Petrolatum base. In 15, 20, 30, 60, 120, and 240 g and lb.
Rx	**Hydrocortisone** (Various, eg, Major, Parmed, Rugby, URL)	**Ointment:** 2.5%	In 20 g.
Rx	**Hytone** (Dermik)		Emollient base. Mineral oil, white petrolatum. In 30 g.
Rx[a]	**Hydrocortisone** (Various, eg, Fougera, Geneva, Major, Roberts Hauck, Rugby[b], URL)	**Cream:** 0.5%	In 15, 30, and 120 g and lb.
otc	**Cortizone for Kids** (Pfizer)		Parabens, cetearyl alcohol, glycerin, white petrolatum. In 14 g.
otc	**Delcort** (Roberts Med)		In 1 g packets.
otc	**Dermolate** (Schering-Plough)		Greaseless, vanishing. Petrolatum, mineral oil, chlorocresol. In 15 and 30 g.
otc	**HydroTex** (Syosset)		In 30 and 60 g.
Rx[a]	**Hydrocortisone** (Various, eg, Fougera, Geneva, Goldline, Major, Moore, Parmed, Roberts Hauck, Rugby, URL[b])	**Cream:** 1%	In 20, 30, and 120 g and lb.
otc	**HydroSkin** (Rugby)		Mineral oil, lanolin alcohol, cetyl alcohol, parabens. In 113.4 g.
Rx	**Ala-Cort** (Del-Ray)		Glycerin. In 30 and 90 g.
otc	**Maximum Strength Bactine** (Miles Inc.)		Glycerin, lt. mineral oil, methylparaben, white petrolatum. In 30 g.
Rx	**Cort-Dome** (Miles Inc.)		Glycerin, white petrolatum, lt. mineral oil, methylparaben. In 30 g.
Rx	**Delcort** (Roberts Med)		In 1 g packets.
Rx	**Hi-Cor 1.0** (C & M)		Washable. Petrolatum, glycerin. In 15, 20, 30, 60, 120, and 240 g and lb.
Rx	**Hytone** (Dermik)		Water-washable. Cholesterol. In 30 and 120 g.
otc	**Procort** (Roberts)		In 30 g.
Rx	**Synacort** (Syntex)		Mineral oil. In 15, 30, and 60 g.
otc	**Maximum Strength KeriCort-10** (Bristol-Myers Squibb)		Parabens, cetyl alcohol, stearyl alcohol. In 56.7 g.
otc	**Cortaid Intensive Therapy** (Pharmacia & Upjohn)		Alcohol, parabens. In 56 g tubes.
otc	**Cortizone-10** (Pfizer Consumer)		Aloe, cetearyl alcohol, glycerin, mineral oil, parabens, petrolatum. In 14, 28, and 57 g.
otc	**Cortizone-10 Plus** (Pfizer Consumer)		Alcohol, aloe, glycerin, mineral oil, parabens, petrolatum. In 28 and 57 g.
otc	**Cortizone-10 External Anal Itch** (Pfizer Consumer)		Cetearyl alcohol, glycerin mineral oil, parabens, petrolatum. In 28 g.

HYDROCORTISONE

Rx	**Hydrocortisone** (Various, eg, Geneva, Goldline, King, Major, Moore, NMC, Rugby, URL)	**Cream:** 2.5%	In 20 and 30 g and lb.
Rx	**Anusol-HC** (Salix)		Water-washable. Benzyl and stearyl alcohols, petrolatum, EDTA. In 30 g.
Rx	**Eldecort** (ICN)		Lt. mineral oil, propylene glycol, allantoin. In 15 and 30 g.
Rx	**Hi-Cor 2.5** (C & M)		Washable. Petrolatum, glycerin. In 15, 20, 30, 60, 120, and 240 g and lb.
Rx	**Hydrocort** (Parmed)		In 20 and 30 g and lb.
Rx	**Hytone** (Dermik)		Water-washable base. Cholesterol. In 30 and 60 g.
Rx	**Synacort** (Syntex)		Mineral oil. In 30 g.
Rx	**proctoCream•HC 2.5%** (Schwarz Pharma)		Glyceryl monostearate, glycerin, stearyl alcohol, benzyl alcohol. In 30 g tubes.
Rx	**Cetacort** (Owen/Galderma)	**Lotion:** 0.25%	Parabens. In 120 mL.
Rx[a]	**Hydrocortisone** (Various, eg, Goldline, Mericon, Parmed, Rugby, URL)	**Lotion:** 0.5%	In 30, 60, and 120 mL.
Rx	**Cetacort** (Owen/Galderma)		Parabens. In 60 mL.
otc[a]	**Hydrocortisone** (Various, eg, Geneva, Glades, Mericon)	**Lotion:** 1%	In 120 mL.
otc	**HydroSkin** (Rugby)		Cetyl alcohol, parabens. In 118 mL.
Rx	**Acticort 100** (Baker Cummins)		In 60 mL.
Rx	**Ala-Cort** (Del-Ray)		Lt. mineral oil, glycerin. In 118 mL.
Rx	**LactiCare-HC** (Stiefel)		Lt. mineral oil, lactic acid. In 120 mL.
Rx	**Ala-Scalp** (Del-Ray)	**Lotion:** 2%	Isopropyl alcohol, benzalkonium chloride. In 30 mL.
Rx	**Hydrocortisone** (Glades)	**Lotion:** 2.5%	Stearyl alcohol, cetyl alcohol, lt. mineral oil. In 59 and 120 mL.
Rx	**Hytone** (Dermik)		Cholesterol, triethanolamine. In 60 mL.
Rx	**LactiCare-HC** (Stiefel)		Lt. mineral oil, lactic acid. In 60 mL.
otc	**Scalpicin** (Combe)	**Liquid:** 1%	Menthol, SD alcohol 40. In 45, 75, and 120 mL.
otc	**T/Scalp** (Neutrogena)		Greaseless. In 60 and 600 mL.
otc	**Extra Strength CortaGel** (Norstar)	**Gel:** 1%	Greaseless. EDTA. In 15 and 30 g.
Rx	**Alcortin** (Primus)	**Gel:** 2%	Alcohols, glycerin. In 2 g tubes.
Rx	**Penecort** (Allergan)	**Solution:** 1%	Alcohol, petrolatum, propylene glycol. In 30 and 60 mL.
Rx	**Texacort** (GenDerm)		Lipid free. 33% SD alcohol 40-2. In 30 mL.
Rx	**Texacort** (JSJ Pharm[d])	**Solution:** 2.5%	Alcohol. In 30 mL.
otc	**Maximum Strength Cortaid** (Pharmacia & Upjohn)	**Pump spray:** 1%	55% alcohol, glycerin, methylparaben. In 45 mL.
otc	**Procort** (Roberts)	**Spray:** 1%	In 45 mL.
otc	**Cortizone-10 Quickshot** (Pfizer Consumer)		Alcohols. In 44 mL.
otc	**Maximum Strength Cortaid Faststick** (Pharmacia & Upjohn)	**Stick, roll-on:** 1%	55% alcohol, glycerin, methylparaben. In 14 g.

[a] Products are available *otc* or *Rx* depending on product labeling.
[b] Also available with aloe.
[c] In *Absorbase* (a water-in-oil emulsion of cholesterolized petrolatum and purified water).
[d] JSJ Pharmaceuticals, 3655 Route 202, Suite 116, Doylestown PA 18901; 1-(267) 880-2360; FAX 1-(215) 348-9186.

HYDROCORTISONE — TOPICAL

Complete prescribing information begins in the Topical Corticosteroids group monograph.

HYDROCORTISONE ACETATE

otc	**Lanacort-5** (Combe)	**Ointment:** 0.5%	Acetylated lanolin alcohols, aloe, petrolatum. In 15 g.
otc	**Corticaine** (UCB)	**Cream:** 0.5%	Greaseless. Glycerin, EDTA, menthol, parabens. In 30 g.
otc	**Cortaid with Aloe** (Pharmacia & Upjohn)		Aloe vera, parabens. In 15 and 30 g.
otc	**Cortef Feminine Itch** (Pharmacia & Upjohn)		Vanishing. Aloe vera, parabens. In 15 g.
otc	**Lanacort-5 Creme** (Combe)		Aloe, parabens. In 15 and 22.5 g.
otc	**Tucks** (Pfizer Consumer Health)	**Ointment:** 1%	Parabens, mineral oil, white petrolatum. In 19.8 g.
otc	**Maximum Strength Cortaid** (Pharmacia & Upjohn)		Mineral oil, parabens, cholesterol, white petrolatum. In 30 g.
otc	**Maximum Strength Hydrocortisone Acetate** (Clay-Park Labs)		Aloe extract, white petrolatum. In 28 g.
Rx[a]	**Hydrocortisone Acetate** (Various, eg, Thames)	**Cream:** 1%	Mineral oil, parabens. In 20, 30 and 120 g.
otc	**Gynecort Female Creme** (Combe)		Parabens, sorbitol, zinc pyrithione. In 15 g.
otc	**Lanacort 10 Creme** (Combe)		Parabens. In 15 and 30 g.
otc	**Maximum Strength Cortaid** (Pharmacia & Upjohn)		Parabens, glycerin, white petrolatum. In 15 g.
otc	**Maximum Strength Caldecort** (Ciba Self-Medication)		Cetostearyl alcohol, white petrolatum. In 14 g.
Rx	**U-cort** (Taro)		10% Urea, alcohol, EDTA. In 28.35 and 7 g.

[a] Products are available *otc* or *Rx* depending on product labeling.

HYDROCORTISONE ACETATE — TOPICAL

Complete prescribing information begins in the Topical Corticosteroids group monograph.

HYDROCORTISONE PROBUTATE

Rx	**Pandel** (Collagenex)	**Cream:** 0.1%	In 15, 45, and 80 g.

HYDROCORTISONE BUTYRATE

Rx	**Hydrocortisone Butyrate** (Taro)	**Ointment:** 0.1%	Mineral oil. In 5, 10, 15, 30, and 45 g.
Rx	**Locoid** (Ferndale)		Mineral oil. In 15 and 45 g.
Rx	**Hydrocortisone Butyrate** (Taro)	**Cream:** 0.1%	In a hydrophilic base. Alcohol, lt. mineral oil, parabens, white petrolatum. In 5, 10, 15, 30, and 45 g.
Rx	**Locoid** (Ferndale)		Alcohol, mineral oil, parabens, white petrolatum. In 15 and 45 g.
Rx	**Locoid Lipocream** (Ferndale)		Alcohol, mineral oil, parabens, white petrolatum. In 15 and 45 g.
Rx	**Hydrocortisone Butyrate** (Taro)	**Solution:** 0.1%	50% isopropyl alcohol, glycerin. In 20 and 60 mL.
Rx	**Locoid** (Ferndale)		50% alcohol, glycerin. In 20 and 60 mL.

HYDROCORTISONE BUTYRATE — TOPICAL

Complete prescribing information begins in the Topical Corticosteroids group monograph.

HYDROCORTISONE VALERATE

Rx	**Hydrocortisone Valerate** (Taro)	**Ointment:** 0.2%	Hydrophilic base. White petrolatum, alcohol, mineral oil. In 15, 45, and 60 g.
	Westcort (Westwood Squibb)		Hydrophilic base. White petrolatum, mineral oil. In 15, 45, and 60 g.
Rx	**Hydrocortisone Valerate** (Copley)	**Cream:** 0.2%	Hydrophlic base. White petrolatum, alcohol. In 15, 45, and 60 g.
	Westcort (Westwood Squibb)		Hydrophilic base. White petrolatum. In 15, 45, 60, and 120 g.

HYDROCORTISONE VALERATE — TOPICAL

Complete prescribing information begin in the Topical Corticosteroids group monograph.

MOMETASONE FUROATE

Rx	**Mometasone Furoate** (Various, eg, Sandoz, Taro)	**Ointment:** 0.1%	In 15 and 45 g.
Rx	**Elocon** (Schering)		White petrolatum. In 15 and 45 g.
Rx	**Mometasone Furoate** (Clay Park)	**Cream:** 0.1%	White petrolatum, stearyl alcohol. In 15 and 45 g.
Rx	**Elocon** (Schering)		White petrolatum. In 15 and 45 g.
Rx	**Elocon** (Schering)	**Lotion:** 0.1%	40% isopropyl alcohol. In 27.5 and 55 mL.
Rx	**Mometasone Furoate** (Clay Park)	**Topical solution:** 0.1%	40% isopropyl alcohol, glycerin. In 30 and 60 mL.

MOMETASONE FUROATE — TOPICAL

Complete prescribing information begins in the Topical Corticosteroids group monograph.

PREDNICARBATE

Rx	**Dermatop E** (Dermik)	**Cream:** 0.1% prednicarbate	White petrolatum, mineral oil, EDTA, lanolin alcohols, cetostearyl alcohol, lactic acid. In 15 and 60 g.
		Ointment: 0.1% prednicarbate	White petrolatum, glycerin. In 15 and 60 g.

PREDNICARBATE — TOPICAL

Complete prescribing information begins in the Topical Corticosteroids group monograph.

TRIAMCINOLONE ACETONIDE

Rx	**Triamcinolone Acetonide** (Various, eg, Fougera, Goldline, Moore, URL)	**Ointment:** 0.025%	In 15, 80 and 454 g.
Rx	**Flutex** (Syosset)		White petrolatum, mineral oil. In 28, 57 and 113 g.
Rx	**Kenalog** (Westwood Squibb)		In *Plastibase* (polyethylene, mineral oil gel base). In 15, 80 and 240 g.
Rx	**Triamcinolone Acetonide** (Various, eg, Fougera, Goldline, Moore, NMC, URL)	**Ointment:** 0.1%	In 15 and 80 g and lb.
Rx	**Aristocort** (Fujisawa)		White petrolatum. In 15, 60 and 240 g.
Rx	**Aristocort A** (Fujisawa)		White petrolatum. In 15 and 60 g.
Rx	**Flutex** (Syosset)		White petrolatum, mineral oil. In 28, 57 and 113 g.
Rx	**Kenalog** (Westwood Squibb)		In *Plastibase* (polyethylene, mineral oil gel base). In 15, 60, 80 and 240 g.
Rx	**Triamcinolone Acetonide** (Various, eg, URL)	**Ointment:** 0.5%	In 15 g.
Rx	**Aristocort** (Fujisawa)		White petrolatum base. In 15 and 240 g.
Rx	**Flutex** (Syosset)		White petrolatum, mineral oil. In 28, 57 and 113 g.
Rx	**Kenalog** (Westwood Squibb)		In *Plastibase* (polyethylene, mineral oil gel base). In 20 g.
Rx	**Triamcinolone Acetonide** (Various, eg, Goldline, Major, Moore, Schein, URL)	**Cream:** 0.025%	In 15, 80 and 454 g.
Rx	**Aristocort** (Fujisawa)		In 15 & 60 g & lb.
Rx	**Aristocort A** (Fujisawa)		Water-washable. 2% benzyl alcohol. In 15 & 60 g.
Rx	**Flutex** (Syosset)		Mineral oil, lanolin alcohol, sodium bisulfite. In 15, 30, 60, 120 and 240 g.
Rx	**Kenalog** (Westwood Squibb)		Vanishing base. White petrolatum. In 15, 80, 240 g.

TRIAMCINOLONE ACETONIDE

Rx	**Triamcinolone Acetonide** (Various, eg, Fougera, Goldline)	**Cream**: 0.1%	In 15, 80 and 454 g.
Rx	**Aristocort** (Fujisawa)		In 15, 60 and 240 g and lb.
Rx	**Aristocort A** (Fujisawa)		Water-washable base. Glycerin, 2% benzyl alcohol. In 15, 60 and 240 g.
Rx	**Delta-Tritex** (Dermol)		In 30 and 80 g.
Rx	**Flutex** (Syosset)		Mineral oil, lanolin alcohol, sodium bisulfite. In 15, 30, 60, 120 and 240 g.
Rx	**Kenalog** (Westwood Squibb)		Vanishing base. White petrolatum. In 15, 60, 80 & 240 g.
Rx	**Kenonel** (Marnel)		In 20 g.
Rx	**Triderm** (Del-Rey)		Mineral oil. In 30 and 90 g.
Rx	**Triamcinolone Acetonide** (Various, eg, Fougera, Goldline, Moore, URL)	**Cream**: 0.5%	In 15 g.
Rx	**Aristocort** (Fujisawa)		In 15 and 240 g.
Rx	**Aristocort A** (Fujisawa)		Water-washable base. 2% benzyl alcohol. In 15 g.
Rx	**Flutex** (Syosset)		Mineral oil, lanolin alcohol, sodium bisulfite. In 15, 30, 60, 120 and 240 g.
Rx	**Kenalog** (Westwood Squibb)		Vanishing base. White petrolatum. In 20 g.
Rx	**Triamcinolone Acetonide** (Various, eg, Major, Morton Grove, Rugby)	**Lotion**: 0.025%	In 60 mL.
Rx	**Kenalog** (Westwood Squibb)		In 60 mL.
Rx	**Triamcinolone Acetonide** (Various, eg, Goldline, Morton Grove, Moore, PBI)	**Lotion**: 0.1%	In 60 mL.
Rx	**Kenalog** (Westwood Squibb)		In 15 and 60 mL.
Rx	**Delta-Tritex** (Dermol)	**Ointment**: 0.1%	In 30 g.
Rx	**Kenalog** (Westwood Squibb)	**Aerosol**: (2 sec. spray)	10.3% alcohol. In 23 and 63 g.

TRIAMCINOLONE ACETONIDE — TOPICAL

Complete prescribing information begins in the Topical Corticosteroids group monograph.

CORTICOSTEROID COMBINATIONS

	Product & Distributor	Hydrocortisone (%)	Clioquinol (%)	Pramoxine (%)	Other Content and How Supplied
Rx	**Hydrocortisone with Clioquinol Cream** (Various, eg, Moore, Rugby)	0.5	3		In 30 g.
Rx	**Ala-Quin Cream** (Del-Ray)				Glycerin. In 30 g.
Rx	**Hydrocortisone with Clioquinol Cream** (Various, eg, Goldline, Moore, Rugby, Schein, URL)	1	3		In 20, 30 and 300 g.
Rx	**Corque Cream** (Geneva)	1	3		In 20 g.
Rx	**Hysone Cream** (Roberts Med)	1	3		In 20 g tube.
Rx	**Hydrocortisone with Clioquinol Ointment** (Various, eg, Moore, Rugby)	1	3		In 20 and 30 g.
Rx	**1 + 1-F Creme** (Dunhall)	1	3	1	Mineral oil, lanolin alcohol, parabens. In 30 g.
Rx	**Analpram-HC Cream** (Ferndale)	1[1]		1	0.1% potassium sorbate, 0.1% sorbic acid. In 30 g.
Rx	**Enzone Cream** (UAD)				Hydrophilic. 0.1% K sorbate, 0.1% sorbic acid. In 30 g.
Rx	**Pramosone Cream** (Ferndale)				Hydrophilic base. 0.1% potassium sorbate, 0.1% sorbic acid. In 30, 60 and 120 g.
Rx	**ProctoCream-HC Cream** (Reed & Carnrick)				Hydrophilic base. Propylene glycol. In 30 g
Rx	**Pramosone Ointment** (Ferndale)				Emollient base. White petrolatum. In 30 and 120 g.
Rx	**Pramosone Lotion** (Ferndale)				Hydrophilic. Glycerin, 0.1% potassium sorbate, 0.1% sorbic acid. In 60, 120, 240 mL.
Rx	**Epifoam Aerosol Foam** (Schwarz Pharma)				Parabens, propylene glycol. In 10 g.
Rx	**ProctoFoam-HC Aerosol Foam** (Reed & Carnrick)				Hydrophilic base. Parabens. In 10 g.
Rx	**Cortane-B Lotion** (Blansett)	1		1	0.1% chloroxylenol. Benzalkonium Cl. In 60 mL.
Rx	**Carmol HC Cream** (Doak)	1[1]			Water-washable, vanishing. 10% urea, sodium metabisulfite. In 30 and 120 g.
Rx	**Hydrocortison Iodoquinol 1% Cream** (Various, eg, Cypress, Glades)	1			1% iodoquinol. In 30 g.
Rx	**Vytone Cream** (Aventis)	1			Greaseless. 1% iodoquinol, propylene glycol, cetyl alcohol. In 30 g.
Rx	**Novacort Gel** (Primus)	2		1	Alcohols, aloe, glycerin. In 29 g tubes.
Rx	**Alcortin** (Primus)	2			1% iodoquinol. Alcohols, aloe, glycerin. In 2 g.

CORTICOSTEROID COMBINATIONS

	Product & Distributor	Hydrocortisone (%)	Clioquinol (%)	Pramoxine (%)	Other Content and How Supplied
Rx	**Analpram-HC Cream** (Ferndale)	2.5[1]		1	In 30 g.
Rx	**Pramosone Cream** (Ferndale)				Hydrophilic. 0.1% K sorbate, 0.1% sorbic acid. In 30, 120 g.
Rx	**Pramosone Ointment** (Ferndale)				Emollient base. White petrolatum. In 30 and 120 g.
Rx	**Pramosone Lotion** (Ferndale)				Hydrophilic. Glycerin, 0.1% potassium sorbate, 0.1% sorbic acid. In 60 and 120 mL.
Rx	**Zone-A Forte Lotion** (UAD)				Hydrophilic. Glycerin, triethanolamine, 0.1% K sorbate, 0.1% sorbic acid. In 60 mL.
Rx	**Lidocaine/Hydrocortisone Cream** (River's Edge)	0.5[1]			3% lidocaine hydrochloride, aluminum sulfate, alcohols, glycerin, lt. mineral oil, parabens, petrolatum. In 28.5 and 85 g.
Rx	**AnaMantle HC Cream** (Bradley)				3% lidocaine HCl, cetyl alcohol, light mineral oil, parabens, glycerin, stearyl alcohol, petrolatum. In kits of 7 g tubes with single-use applicators (14s).
Rx	**Lida-Mantle-HC Cream** (Doak)				3% lidocaine HCl, glycerin, parabens. In 30 g.
Rx	**LidaMantle HC Lotion** (Doak)				3% lidocaine HCl, cetyl alcohol, mineral oil, methylparaben, petrolatum. In 177 mL.
otc	**HC Derma-Pax Liquid** (Recsei)	0.5[1]			0.44% pyrilamine maleate, 0.06% chlorpheniramine maleate, 1% benzyl alcohol, 35% isopropanol, 25% chlorobutanol. In 60 and 120 mL.
otc	**Massengill Medicated Towelettes** (SK-Beecham)				Diazolidinyl urea, parabens, propylene glycol. In 10 and 16 softcloth towelettes.

[1] Hydrocortisone acetate.

CORTICOSTEROID COMBINATIONS — TOPICAL

These products contain corticosteroids in combination with various other components. They are indicated for a variety of specific and nonspecific dermatoses. For further information see individual monographs. Components of these formulations include:

Active Ingredients

➤*CORTICOSTEROID:* Used for their anti-inflammatory, antipruritic and vasoconstrictive effects.

➤*CLIOQUINOL, IODOQUINOL, TRIACETIN, CLOTRIMAZOLE, NYSTATIN, POLYMYXIN B SULFATE, BACITRACIN ZINC, CETYLPYRIDINIUM Cl and CHLOROXYLENOL:* Used for their antifungal, antibacterial and anti-eczematous effects.

➤*LIDOCAINE:* Used as a local anesthetic.

➤*UREA:* This is a mild keratolytic and hydrates dry skin.

➤*CHLORPHENIRAMINE:* This is an antihistamine.

➤*BENZOYL PEROXIDE:* Used for its peeling and drying effects.

CORTICOSTEROID AND ANTIBIOTIC COMBINATIONS

		Dosage form	Corticosteroid	Neomycin sulfate	Other	Base/How Supplied
Rx	**Cortisporin** (Monarch)	Cream	0.5% hydrocortisone acetate	0.5%	10,000 units polymyxin B sulfate and neomycin sulfate equiv. to 3.5 mg neomycin base per g; white, liquid petrolatum; 0.25% methylparaben	In 7.5 g.
Rx	**Myco-Biotic** II (Moore)		0.1% triamcinolone acetonide		Aqueous vanishing. 100,000 units nystatin per g, white petrolatum	In 15, 30 and 60 g and lb.
Rx	**Hydrocortisone-Neomycin** (Various)	Ointment	1% hydrocortisone	0.5%	White petrolatum, mineral oil	In 20 g.
Rx	**Cortisporin** (Monarch)		1% hydrocortisone		400 units bacitracin zinc, white petrolatum, and 5000 units polymyxin B sulfate and neomycin sulfate equiv. to 3.5 mg neomycin base per g	In 15 g.

Consider the information for Topical Corticosteroids, Antibiotics and Antifungals when using these products (see individual monographs).

CORTICOSTEROID AND ANTIFUNGAL COMBINATIONS

		Dosage form	Corticosteroid	Antifungal	Base/How Supplied
Rx	**Clotrimazole and Betamethasone Dipropionate** (Fougera)	Cream	0.05% betamethasone (as dipropionate)	1% clotrimazole	Mineral oil, white petrolatum, cetearyl alcohol, benzyl alcohol. In 15 and 45 g.
Rx	**Lotrisone** (Schering)				Hydrophilic. Mineral oil, white petrolatum, benzyl alcohol. In 15 and 45 g.
Rx	**Nystatin-Triamcinolone Acetonide** (Various, eg, Fougera, Taro)		0.1% triamcinolone acetonide	100,000 units nystatin per g	In 15, 30 and 60 g and UD 1.5 g.
Rx	**Mycogen** II (Goldline)				In 15, 30, 60 and 120 g.
Rx	**Mycolog**-II (B-M Squibb)				Vanishing base. White petrolatum. In 15, 30, 60 and 120 g.
Rx	**Myconel** (Marnel)				In 20 g.
Rx	**Myco-Triacet** II (Lemmon)				Aqueous, vanishing base. White petrolatum, parabens. In 15, 30 and 60 g.
Rx	**Tri-Statin** II (Rugby)				Vanishing base. White petrolatum. In 15, 30 and 60 g.
Rx	**Clotrimazole and Betamethasone Dipropionate** (Fougera)	Lotion	0.05% betamethasone (as dipropionate)	1% clotrimazole	Hydrophilic. Mineral oil, white petrolatum, alcohols. In 30 mL.
Rx	**Lotrisone** (Schering)				Hydrophilic. Mineral oil, white petrolatum, alcohols. In 30 mL.
Rx	**Nystatin-Triamcinolone Acetonide** (Various, eg, Fougera)	Ointment	0.1% triamcinolone acetonide	100,000 units nystatin per g	In 15, 30 and 60 g.
Rx	**Mycogen** II (Goldline)				In 15, 30 and 60 g.
Rx	**Mycolog**-II (B-M Squibb)				Mineral oil, gel base. In 15, 30, 60 and 120 g.
Rx	**Myco-Triacet** II (Lemmon)				Vanishing base. White petrolatum and mineral oil. In 15 and 30 g.

Consider the information given for Topical Corticosteroids and for Topical Antifungals when using these products.

ANTI-PSORIATIC AGENTS

In addition to the products described here, other products for treatment of psoriasis include: Coal tar; corticosteroids; salicylic acid. Refer to individual monographs.

ANTHRALIN (Dithranol)

Rx	**Dritho-Scalp** (Summers Labs)	**Cream:** 0.5%	White petrolatum, cetostearyl alcohol. In 50 g.
Rx	**Anthralin** (Rising Pharmaceuticals)	**Cream:** 1%	In 50 g.
Rx	**Psoriatec** (Sirius)		In 50 g.

ANTHRALIN — TOPICAL

Indications

➤*Psoriasis:* Treatment of quiescent or chronic psoriasis of the scalp. Continue treatment until the skin is entirely clear (ie, when there is nothing to feel with the fingers and the texture is normal).

Administration and Dosage

Generally, it is recommended that anthralin be applied once a day or as directed by a health care provider. Anthralin is known to be a potential skin irritant. The irritant potential of anthralin is directly related to the strength being used, the time of contact, and each patient's individual tolerance. Therefore, where the response to anthralin treatment has not previously been established, always commence treatment using a short contact time of 5 to 10 minutes for at least 1 week. When a short contact time is used initially, it can be increased stepwise to 20 to 30 minutes before removing the cream by thoroughly washing or showering.

➤*1% cream:*

For the skin – Apply sparingly only to the psoriatic lesions and rub gently and carefully into the skin. Avoid applying an excessive quantity, which may cause unnecessary soiling and staining of the clothing or bed linen. At the end of each period of treatment, rinse the skin thoroughly with cool to lukewarm water before washing with soap. The margins of the lesions may gradually become stained purple/brown as treatment progresses, but this will disappear after cessation of treatment.

For the scalp – Wash the hair with shampoo, rinse with water, and apply anthralin 1% cream while the hair is still damp. Rub the cream well into the psoriatic lesions. Keep anthralin 1% cream away from the eyes. Take care to avoid application of the cream to uninvolved scalp margins. Rinse hair and scalp thoroughly with cool to lukewarm water and then shampoo the hair and scalp to remove any surplus cream (which may have changed in color). This treatment may be repeated on alternate days if necessary.

➤*0.5% scalp cream:* Apply as directed and remove by washing or showering. The optimal period of contact will vary according to the strength used and the patient's response to treatment.

Comb the hair to remove scalar debris and, after suitably parting, apply anthralin only to the lesions and rub in well, taking care to prevent the cream spreading onto the forehead.

Keep anthralin well away from the eyes.

Avoid application of the cream to uninvolved scalp margins. Remove any unintended residue that may be deposited behind the ears. At the end of each period of contact, wash the hair and scalp to remove any surplus cream (which may have become red/brown in color).

Always wash hands thoroughly after use.

➤*Storage / Stability:* Store at controlled room temperature, 15° to 30°C (59° to 86°F). Keep out of reach of children.

Actions

➤*Pharmacology:* Although the precise mechanism of anthralin's antipsoriatic action is not fully understood, in vitro evidence suggests that its antimitotic effect results from inhibition of DNA synthesis. Additionally, the chemically reducing properties of anthralin may upset oxidative metabolic processes, providing a further slowing down of epidermal mitosis.

Absorption has not been finally determined, but in a limited clinical study of anthralin cream, no traces of anthraquinone metabolites were detected in the urine of subjects treated; however, caution is advised in patients with renal disease.

Contraindications

Acute or actively inflamed psoriatic eruptions; hypersensitivity to any of the ingredients.

Warnings

➤*For external use only:* Avoid contact with the eyes or mucous membranes. Exercise caution when applying anthralin cream to the face or intertriginous skin areas. Anthralin should not normally be applied to intertriginous skin areas and high strengths should not be used on these sites. Remove any unintended residue that may be deposited behind the ears. Avoid applying to the folds and creases of the skin.

ANTHRALIN — TOPICAL

➤*Sensitivity reaction:* Discontinue use if a sensitivity reaction occurs or if excessive irritation develops on uninvolved skin areas.

➤*Pregnancy: Category C.* Animal reproduction studies have not been conducted with anthralin. It is also not known whether anthralin can cause fetal harm when administered to a pregnant woman or can affect reproduction capacity. Anthralin should be given to a pregnant woman only if clearly needed.

➤*Lactation:* It is not known whether this drug is excreted in human milk. Because many drugs are excreted in milk and because of the potential for tumorigenicity shown for anthralin in animal studies, decide whether to discontinue breastfeeding or the drug, taking into account the importance of the drug to the mother.

➤*Children:* Safety and efficacy in pediatric patients have not been established.

Precautions

➤*Staining:* Anthralin may stain the hair; apply sparingly and carefully to psoriatic lesions only. Contact with fabrics, plastics, and other materials may cause staining and should be avoided. To prevent the possibility of discoloration, always rinse the bath/shower with hot water immediately after washing/showering and then use a suitable cleanser to remove any deposit on the surface of the bath or shower. To prevent the possibility of staining clothing or bed linen while gaining experience in using anthralin, it may be advisable to use protective dressings. Always wash hands thoroughly after use.

➤*Long-term use of topical corticosteroids:* Because long-term use of topical corticosteroids may destabilize psoriasis, and withdrawal may also give rise to a "rebound" phenomenon, allow an interval of at least 1 week between the discontinuance of such steroids and the commencement of anthralin therapy. Application of petrolatum or a suitably bland emollient may be useful during the intervening period.

Drug Interactions

➤*Topical corticosteroids:* Because long-term use of topical corticosteroids may destabilize psoriasis, and withdrawal may also give rise to a "rebound" phenomenon, allow an interval of at least 1 week between the discontinuance of such steroids and the commencement of anthralin therapy.

Adverse Reactions

Very few instances of contact allergic reactions to anthralin have been reported. However, transient primary irritation of the healthy or uninvolved skin surrounding the treated lesions is more frequently seen and may occasionally be severe. Application of anthralin must be restricted to the psoriatic lesions. If the initial treatment produces excessive soreness or if the lesions spread, reduce frequency of application and, in extreme cases, discontinue use and consult health care provider. Some temporary discoloration of hair and fingernails may arise during the period of treatment but should be minimized by careful application. Anthralin may stain skin, hair, or fabrics. Staining of fabrics may be permanent, so contact should be avoided.

Patient Information

Anthralin cream is for external use only. It is not for ophthalmic use. Avoid contact with the eyes or mucous membranes. Use care when applying anthralin cream to any facial area, uninvolved scalp margins, behind the ears, or in other sensitive areas such as skin folds. As with any other prescription drug, discontinue use if you experience any unexpected reaction or discomfort and immediately consult your doctor.

➤*Staining:* Anthralin cream may stain skin, hair, or fabrics. Some temporary discoloration of hair and nails may arise during the period of treatment but should be minimized by careful application. Staining of fabrics may be permanent, so contact should be avoided.

➤*Avoiding staining to clothes, bath or shower:* As anthralin cream may stain, follow directions carefully to avoid exposure to clothes, bath, or shower.

Clothing – Thoroughly rinse exposed clothing with cool or lukewarm water only. Wash with detergent and water as usual. The suggested water temperature should be warm (not above 86°F) or cold.

Bath and shower – To reduce the possibility of discoloration to the bath or shower, always rinse well with cool or lukewarm water only. Use a suitable cleaner to remove any deposit left on the surface.

➤*Application to skin:*

1.) While avoiding normal skin, apply small amount to the psoriatic lesions. Thoroughly and carefully rub the cream into the skin until it no longer smears.
2.) Immediately following application, wash your hands with cool or lukewarm water only.
3.) Leave anthralin cream on for the prescribed amount of time. Your doctor may recommend a short contact period at first, and then gradually increase the contact time
4.) After prescribed amount of time, rinse anthralin cream off the skin thoroughly using cool or lukewarm water only. Avoid hot water and soaps as they could cause product to stain or irritate.
5.) After anthralin cream has been thoroughly washed off, shower using soap and water.

➤*Application to scalp:*

1.) Wash the hair with shampoo and rinse with water.
2.) Part the hair away from the psoriatic scalp lesion. Apply anthralin cream and rub thoroughly into the psoriatic scalp lesions while the hair is still damp. Remove any unintended residue that may be deposited behind the ears.
3.) Immediately following application, wash your hands with cool or lukewarm water only.
4.) Leave anthralin cream on the prescribed amount of time. Your doctor may recommend a short contact period at first, and then gradually increase the contact time.
5.) After prescribed amount of time, rinse hair and scalp with cool or lukewarm water only. Avoid hot water and shampoo as they could cause product to stain or irritate.
6.) Following thorough removal of anthralin cream, shampoo and water may be used on the hair and scalp.

CALCIPOTRIENE

Rx	**Dovonex** (Westwood Squibb)	**Ointment:** 0.005%	In 30, 60 and 100 g.
		Cream: 0.005%	In 30, 60 and 100 g.
		Solution: 0.005%	Menthol. In 60 mL.

CALCIPOTRIENE — TOPICAL

Indications

➤*Plaque Psoriasis:* Calcipotriene cream and ointment are indicated for the treatment of plaque psoriasis in adults. The safety and effectiveness of topical calcipotriene in dermatoses other than psoriasis have not been established.

➤*Psoriasis of the scalp:* Calcipotriene scalp solution is indicated for the topical treatment of chronic, moderately severe psoriasis of the scalp. The safety and effectiveness of topical calcipotriene in dermatoses other than psoriasis have not been established.

Administration and Dosage

➤*Approved by the FDA:* December 29, 1993.

For topical dermatologic use only.

➤*Cream and ointment:* Apply a thin layer of calcipotriene cream or ointment to the affected skin once or twice daily and rub in gently and completely. The safety and efficacy of calcipotriene cream have been demonstrated in patients treated for 8 weeks.

➤*Scalp solution:* Comb the hair to remove scaly debris and after suitably parting, apply calcipotriene scalp solution twice daily, only to the lesions, and rub in gently and completely, taking care to prevent the solution spreading onto the forehead. The safety and efficacy of calcipotriene scalp solution have been demonstrated in patients treated for 8 weeks.

Keep calcipotriene scalp solution well away from the eyes. Avoid application of the solution to uninvolved scalp margins. Always wash hands thoroughly after use.

➤*Storage/Stability:* Store at controlled room temperature 15° to 25°C (59° to 77°F). Do not freeze. Avoid exposing the scalp solution to sunlight. Keep out of reach of children.

Scalp solution – Drug product is flammable. Keep away from open flame.

Actions

➤*Pharmacology:* In humans, the natural supply of vitamin D depends mainly on exposure to the ultraviolet rays of the sun for conversion of 7-dehydrocholesterol to vitamin D_3 (cholecalciferol) in the skin. Calcipotriene is a synthetic analog of vitamin D_3.

Vitamin D3 receptors, proteins that bind chemically to calcitriol, occur in many parts of the body, including the skin cells known as keratinocytes. The scaly red patches of psoriasis are caused by the abnormal growth and production of the keratinocytes. Calcipotriene regulates skin cell production and development.

Although the precise mechanism of calcipotriene's antipsoriatic action is not fully understood, in vitro evidence suggests that calcipotriene is roughly equipotent to the natural vitamin in its effects on proliferation and differentiation of a variety of cell types. Calcipotriene has also been shown, in animal studies, to be 100-200 times less potent in its effects on calcium utilization than the natural hormone.

➤*Pharmacokinetics:*

Absorption/Distribution – There is evidence that maternal 1,25-dihydroxy vitamin D_3 (calcitriol) may enter the fetal circulation, but it is not known whether it is excreted in human milk. The systemic disposition of calcipotriene is expected to be similar to that of the naturally occurring vitamin.

Cream and Ointment: Clinical studies with radiolabelled ointment indicate that approximately 6% (±3%, SD) of the applied dose of calcipotriene is absorbed systemically when the ointment is applied topically to psoriasis

CALCIPOTRIENE — TOPICAL

plaques or 5% (±2.6%, SD) when applied to normal skin, and much of the absorbed active is converted to inactive metabolites within 24 hours of application.

Scalp Solution: Clinical studies with radiolabelled calcipotriene solution indicate that less than 1% of the applied dose of calcipotriene is absorbed through the scalp when the solution (2.0 mL) is applied topically to normal skin or psoriasis plaques (160 cm^2) for 12 hours, and that much of the absorbed calcipotriene is converted to inactive metabolites within 24 hours of application.

Metabolism / Excretion – Vitamin D and its metabolites are transported in the blood, bound to specific plasma proteins. After entering the bloodstream, it is metabolized in the liver and kidneys to its active form, the hormone calcitriol. The active form of the vitamin, 1,25-dihydroxy vitamin D_3 (calcitriol), is known to be recycled via the liver and excreted in the bile. Calcipotriene metabolism following systemic uptake is rapid, and occurs via a similar pathway to the natural hormone.

The primary metabolites are much less potent than the parent compound.

Contraindications

➤*Cream and ointment:* Hypersensitivity to any of the components of the preparation; hypercalcemia or evidence of vitamin D toxicity. Do not use calcipotriene cream and ointment on the face.

➤*Scalp solution:* Acute psoriatic eruptions; hypersensitivity to any of the components of the preparations; hypercalcemia or evidence of vitamin D toxicity.

Warnings

➤*Scalp Solution:* Avoid contact with the eyes or mucous membranes. Discontinue use if a sensitivity reaction occurs or if excessive irritation develops on uninvolved skin areas.

Drug product is flammable. Keep away from open flame.

➤*Elderly:*

Ointment only – Of the total number of patients in clinical studies of calcipotriene ointment, approximately 12% were 65 or older, while approximately 4% were 75 or older. The results of an analysis of severity of skin-related adverse events showed a statistically significant difference for subjects over 65 years (more severe) compared to those under 65 years (less severe).

➤*Pregnancy: Category C.* Studies of teratogenicity were done by the oral route where bioavailability is expected to be approximately 40–60% of the administered dose. In rabbits, increased maternal and fetal toxicity were noted at a dosage of 12 mcg/kg/day (132 mcg/m^2/day); a dosage of 36 mcg/kg/day (396 mcg/m^2/day) resulted in a significant increase in the incidence of incomplete ossification of the pubic bones and forelimb phalanges of fetuses. In a rat study, a dosage of 54 mcg/kg/day (318 mcg/m^2/day) resulted in a significantly increased incidence of skeletal abnormalities (enlarged fontanelles and extra ribs). The enlarged fontanelles are most likely due to calcipotriene's effect upon calcium metabolism. The estimated maternal and fetal no-effect exposure levels in the rat (43.2 mcg/m^2/day) and rabbit (17.6 mcg/m^2/day) studies are approximately equal to the expected human systemic exposure level (18.5 mcg/m^2/day) from dermal application. There are no adequate and well-controlled studies in pregnant women. Therefore, calcipotriene should be used during pregnancy only if the potential benefit justifies the potential risk to the fetus.

➤*Lactation:* There is evidence that maternal 1,25–dihydroxy vitamin D3 (calcitriol) may enter the fetal circulation, but it is not known whether it is excreted in human milk. The systemic disposition of calcipotriene is expected to be similar to that of the naturally occurring vitamin. Because many drugs are excreted in human milk, caution should be exercised when calcipotriene cream, ointment, or scalp solution is administered to a nursing woman.

➤*Children:* Safety and effectiveness of calcipotriene in pediatric patients have not been established. Because of a higher ratio of skin surface area to body mass, pediatric patients are at greater risk than adults of systemic adverse effects when they are treated with topical medication.

Precautions

➤*Irritation:* Use of calcipotriene may cause irritation of lesions and surrounding uninvolved skin. If irritation develops, calcipotriene should be discontinued.

➤*Hypercalcemia:* Reversible elevation of serum calcium has occurred with use of topical calcipotriene. If elevation in serum calcium outside the normal range should occur, discontinue treatment until normal calcium levels are restored.

Adverse Reactions

➤*Cream and ointment:* In controlled clinical trials, the most frequent adverse reactions reported for calcipotriene cream and ointment were burning, itching, and skin irritation, which occurred in approximately 10%-15% of patients. Erythema, dry skin, peeling, rash, dermatitis, worsening of psoriasis including development of facial/scalp psoriasis were reported in 1% to 10% of patients. Other experiences reported in less than 1% of patients included skin atrophy, hyperpigmentation, hypercalcemia, and folliculitis. Once daily dosing has not been shown to be superior in safety to twice daily dosing.

➤*Scalp solution:* In controlled clinical trials, the most frequent adverse reactions reported to be related to calcipotriene scalp solution use were transient burning, stinging and tingling, which occurred in approximately 23% of patients. Rash was reported in about 11% of patients. Dry skin, irritation and worsening of psoriasis was reported in 1%-5% of patients. Skin atrophy, hyperpigmentation, hypercalcemia, and folliculitis were not observed in these studies, but cannot be excluded.

Overdosage

Topically applied calcipotriene can be absorbed in sufficient amounts to produce systemic effects. Elevated serum calcium has been observed with excessive use of topical calcipotriene. If elevation in serum calcium should occur, discontinue treatment until normal calcium levels are restored.

Patient Information

This medication is to be used as directed by the physician and should not be used for any disorder other than that for which it was prescribed. It is for external use only. Avoid contact with the face or eyes. As with any topical medication, patients should wash hands after application. Patients should report to their physician any signs of local adverse reactions.

CALCIPOTRIENE AND BETAMETHASONE DIPROPIONATE

Rx	**Taclonex** (Warner Chilcott)	**Ointment:** 0.005% calcipotriene, 0.064% betamethasone dipropionate	Mineral oil, white petrolatum. In 15, 30, and 60 g.

CALCIPOTRIENE AND BETAMETHASONE DIPROPIONATE — TOPICAL

Indications

➤*Psoriasis vulgaris:* For the topical treatment of psoriasis vulgaris in adults 18 years of age and older for up to 4 weeks.

Administration and Dosage

➤*Approved by the FDA:* January 9, 2006.

Apply an adequate layer of ointment to the affected area(s) once daily for up to 4 weeks. The ointment should be rubbed in gently and completely. The maximum weekly dose should not exceed 100 g. Treatment of more than 30% body surface area is not recommended. Ointment should not be applied to the face, axillae, or groin.

➤*Storage / Stability:* Store ointment between 20° and 25°C (68° to 77°F); excursions permitted between 15° and 30°C (59° to 86°F). Keep out of reach of children.

METHOTREXATE (Amethopterin; MTX)

See the Methotrexate monograph in the Antineoplastic Agents chapter.

SELENIUM SULFIDE

otc	**Selenium Sulfide** (Various, eg, Rugby)	**Lotion/Shampoo:** 1%	In 210 mL.
otc	**Head & Shoulders Intensive Treatment** (Procter & Gamble)		In 400 mL.
otc	**Selsun Blue Medicated Treatment** (Chattem)		Menthol. In 325 mL.
Rx	**Selenium Sulfide** (Various, eg, Clay-Park)	**Lotion:** 2.5%	In 120 mL.
Rx	**Selsun** (Abbott)		In 120 mL.

SELENIUM SULFIDE — TOPICAL

Indications

➤*Dandruff, seborrheic dermatitis of the scalp, tinea versicolor:* For the treatment of dandruff, seborrheic dermatitis of the scalp, and tinea versicolor.

➤*Unlabeled uses:* Adjunctive therapy for tinea capitis.

Administration and Dosage

➤*Dandruff and seborrheic dermatitis:* For the usual case, 2 applications each week for 2 weeks will afford control. After this, the lotion or shampoo may be used at less frequent intervals: Weekly, every 2 weeks, or even every 3 or 4 weeks in some cases. The preparation should not be applied more frequently than required to maintain control.

SELENIUM SULFIDE — TOPICAL

➤*Tinea versicolor:* Apply to affected areas and lather with a small amount of water. Allow product to remain on skin for 10 minutes, then rinse the body thoroughly. Repeat this procedure once a day for 7 days.

➤*Application instructions:* Keep tightly capped. Shake well before using. Product may damage jewelry; remove jewelry before use.

Dandruff and seborrheic dermatitis of the scalp –

1.) Massage about 5 or 10 mL (1 or 2 teaspoonfuls) of shampoo into wet scalp.
2.) Allow to remain on scalp for 2 to 3 minutes.
3.) Rinse scalp thoroughly.
4.) Repeat application and rinse thoroughly.
5.) After treatment, wash hands well.
6.) Repeat treatments as directed by physician.

Tinea versicolor –

1.) Apply to affected areas and lather with a small amount of water.
2.) Allow to remain on skin for 10 minutes.
3.) Rinse body thoroughly.
4.) Repeat this procedure once a day for 7 days.

➤*Selenium sulfide lotion/shampoo 1%:* Use at least twice per week or as directed by a doctor. For maximum dandruff control, use every time hair is shampooed.

If used on bleached, tinted, grey, or permed hair, rinse for 5 minutes in cool running water.

➤*Storage/Stability:* Store at controlled room temperature 15° to 30°C (59° to 86°F).

Protect from heat. Keep tightly closed.

Keep this and all medications out of the reach of children.

Actions

➤*Pharmacology:* Selenium sulfide appears to have a cytostatic effect on cells of the epidermis and follicular epithelium, thus reducing corneocyte production.

Contraindications

Allergies to any of its components.

Warnings

➤*Hypersensitivity reactions:* If sensitivity reactions occur, discontinue use.

➤*Pregnancy: Category C* (tinea versicolor). When used on body surfaces for the treatment of tinea versicolor, selenium sulfide is classified as pregnancy *Category C*. Under ordinary circumstances, selenium sulfide lotion should not be used for the treatment of tinea versicolor in pregnant women.

Animal reproduction studies have not been conducted with selenium sulfide. It is also not known whether selenium sulfide can cause fetal harm when applied to body surfaces of a pregnant woman or can affect reproduction capacity.

➤*Children:* Safety and effectiveness in infants have not been established.

Precautions

➤*Acute inflammation/exudation:* Do not use when acute inflammation or exudation is present as increased absorption may occur.

➤*For external use only:* Avoid contact with the eyes.

➤*Irritation:* Selenium sulfide may irritate the skin, especially in the genital area and in skin folds. Rinse these areas thoroughly after application.

Adverse Reactions

➤*In decreasing order of severity:* Skin irritation; occasional reports of increase in amount of normal hair loss; discoloration of hair (can be avoided or minimized by thorough rinsing of hair after treatment).

As with other shampoos, oiliness or dryness of hair and scalp may occur.

Overdosage

➤*Symptoms:* Selenium sulfide shampoos have generally low toxicity if ingested. Nausea, vomiting, and diarrhea usually occur after oral ingestion. There may also be a burning sensation in the mouth and a garlic-like taste/smell to the breath. The detergents found in selenium sulfide shampoos may act as emetics, thereby preventing significant GI absorption of selenium.

➤*Treatment:* There have been no documented reports of serious toxicity in humans resulting from acute ingestion of selenium sulfide; however, acute toxicity studies in animals suggest that ingestion of large amounts could result in potential human toxicity. For this reason, evacuation of the stomach contents should be considered in cases of acute oral ingestion.

Patient Information

Application to skin or scalp may produce skin irritation or sensitization. If sensitivity reactions occur, use should be discontinued. May be irritating to mucous membranes of the eyes and contact with this area should be avoided. Thoroughly rinse after application.

For external use only. Do not use on broken skin or inflamed areas. If allergic reactions occur, discontinue use. Avoid getting shampoo or lotion in eyes or in contact with genital area as it may cause irritation and burning.

May damage jewelry; remove before using.

If using before or after bleaching, tinting, or permanent waving, rinse hair for at least 5 minutes in cool running water.

When applied to the body for treatment of tinea versicolor, selenium sulfide may produce skin irritation, especially in the genital area and where skin folds occur. These areas should be thoroughly rinsed after application.

Keep out of the reach of children. If swallowed, get medical help or contact a poison control center right away.

➤*Shampoo:* Ask a doctor before use if you have seborrheic dermatitis in areas other than the scalp.

For color-treated or permed hair, rinse thoroughly.

Stop use and ask a doctor if condition worsens or does not improve after regular use of this product as directed.

ANTISEBORRHEIC PRODUCTS

Antiseborrheic Combinations

Active Ingredients

➤*SALICYLIC ACID and SULFUR (see individual monographs):* These are used for antiseborrheic and keratolytic/keratoplastic actions.

➤*TAR PREPARATIONS, PYRITHIONE ZINC (see individual monographs) and MYRISTYLTRIMETHYLAMMONIUM BROMIDE:* These are used for their antipruritic, antibacterial or antiseborrheic actions.

➤*MENTHOL:* This is used as an antipruritic.

➤*BENZALKONIUM CHLORIDE, ISOPROPYL ALCOHOL, PHENOL and MENTHOL:* These are used as antiseptics.

➤*IODOQUINOL and BENZYL ALCOHOL:* These are antimicrobial agents.

Precautions

➤*For external use only:* Avoid contact with eyes; in case of contact, flush with water.

➤*Irritation/Staining/Discoloration:* If undue skin irritation develops or increases, discontinue use and consult physician. Preparations containing tar may temporarily discolor blond, bleached or tinted hair. Slight staining of clothing may also occur.

ANTISEBORRHEIC SHAMPOOS

otc	**Maximum Strength Meted** (GenDerm)	**Shampoo:** 5% sulfur and 3% salicylic acid	In 118 mL.
otc	**MG217 Medicated Tar-Free Shampoo** (Triton)		In 4 and 8 oz.
otc	**MG400** (Triton)	**Shampoo:** 3% salicylic acid, 5% colloidal sulfur in Guy-Base II.	In 240 mL and pt.
otc	**Scalpicin** (Combe)	**Shampoo:** 3% salicylic acid, menthol	SD alcohol 40. In 45 and 75 mL.
otc	**Sebex** (Rugby)	**Shampoo:** 2% sulfur and 2% salicylic acid	In 118 mL.
otc	**Sulfoam** (Doak)	**Shampoo:** 2% sulfur	In 237 mL.
otc	**P & S** (Baker Cummins)	**Shampoo:** 2% salicylic acid	In 120 mL.
otc	**Neutrogena T/Sal** (Triton)	**Shampoo:** 2% salicylic acid, 2% solubilized coal tar extract	In 135 mL.
otc	**Ionil** (Owen/Galderma)	**Shampoo:** Salicylic acid, benzalkonium chloride, EDTA	In 120 and 240 mL, pt and qt.
otc	**X•Seb** (Baker Cummins)	**Shampoo:** 4% salicylic acid	In 120 mL.
otc	**Tarsum** (Summers)	**Shampoo/Gel:** 10% crude coal tar and 5% salicylic acid	In 120 and 240 mL.
otc	**X•Seb T** (Baker Cummins)	**Shampoo:** 10% coal tar solution, 4% salicylic acid	In 120 mL.

ANTISEBORRHEIC SHAMPOOS

otc	**X•Seb T Plus** (Ivax)	**Shampoo**: 10% coal tar solution, 0.4% salicylic acid, EDTA	In 118 and 236 mL.
otc	**Ionil T** (Owen/Galderma)	**Shampoo**: Coal tar solution, salicylic acid, benzalkonium chloride	In 120 and 240 mL, pt and qt.
otc	**Sebaquin** (Summers)	**Shampoo**: 3% iodoquinol, lanolin	In 120 mL.
otc	**X•Seb Plus** (Baker Cummins)	**Shampoo**: 1% pyrithione zinc and 2% salicylic acid	In 120 mL.

Complete prescribing information begins in the Antiseborrheic Combinations introduction.

MEDICATED HAIR DRESSINGS

Rx	**Sal-Oil-T** (Syosset)	**Solution**: 10% crude coal tar, 6% salicylic acid, vegetable oil	In 59.14 mL.
otc	**P & S** (Baker Cummins)	**Liquid**: Phenol, mineral oil and glycerin	In 120 and 240 mL.

Complete prescribing information begins in the Antiseborrheic Combinations introduction.

ARNICA

ARNICA

otc	**Arnica** (Various, eg, Humco)	**Tincture**: 20%	In 30, 60, 120 mL, pt, gal.

ARNICA — TOPICAL

Indications

➤*Pain:* Relief of pain from sprains and bruises; of doubtful value.

Administration and Dosage

Apply locally with massage 2 or 3 times daily.

Precautions

➤*For external use only:* Avoid getting into eyes or mucous membranes.

➤*Irritation:* Do not apply to irritated skin or if excessive irritation develops.

Adverse Reactions

Arnica is an irritant to mucous membranes; when ingested, it has produced severe gastroenteritis, nervous disturbances, tachycardia, bradycardia and collapse.

Arnica may cause dermatitis in sensitive persons.

ASTRINGENTS

ALUMINUM ACETATE SOLUTION (Burow's or Modified Burow's Solution)

otc	**Buro-Sol** (Doak)	**Powder**: 0.23% aluminum acetate	In 12 packets.
otc	**Burow's Solution** (Various, eg, Paddock)	Aluminum acetate solution	In 480 mL.
otc	**Bluboro Powder** (Allergan Herbert)	Aluminum sulfate and calcium acetate. One packet or tablet in a pint of water produces a modified 1:40 Burow's solution. Apply every 15 to 30 minutes for 4 to 8 hours.	**Powder packets**: 1.8 g. In 12s and 100s.
otc	**Domeboro Powder and Tablets** (Miles)		**Effervescent tablets**: In 12s and 100s.
			Powder packets: In 12s and 100s.
otc	**Pedi-Boro Soak Paks** (Pedinol)		**Powder packets**: 2.7 g. In 12s and 100s.
otc	**Bite Rx** (International Lab. Tech. Corp.)[a]	**Solution**: 0.5% w/w aluminum acetate	Benzalkonium chloride. In 120 mL.

[a] (954) 893-1118

ALUMINUM ACETATE SOLUTION (Burow's or Modified Burow's Solution) — TOPICAL

Indications

➤*Inflammatory conditions of the skin:* An astringent wet dressing for relief of inflammatory conditions of the skin, such as insect bites, poison ivy, swelling, allergy, bruises and athlete's foot.

Precautions

➤*Discontinue use:* If intolerance, irritation or extension of inflammatory condition being treated occurs. If symptoms persist more than 7 days, discontinue use and consult physician.

➤*Do not use plastic:* Do not use plastic nor any other impervious material to prevent evaporation.

➤*For external use only:* Avoid contact with the eyes.

Drug Interactions

➤*Collagenase:* The enzyme activity of topical collagenase may be inhibited by aluminum acetate solution because of the metal ion and low pH. Cleanse the site of the solution with repeated washings of normal saline before applying the enzyme ointment.

HAMAMELIS WATER (Witch Hazel)

otc	**Witch Hazel** (Various, eg, Humco, Lannett)	**Liquid**	In 120 and 240 mL, pt and gal.
otc	**A•E•R** (Birchwood)	**Pads**: 50%. 12.5% glycerin, methylparaben, benzalkonium chloride	In 40s.

HAMAMELIS WATER — TOPICAL

Indications

➤*Anal/Vaginal irritation:* Temporary relief of anal or vaginal irritation and itching, hemorrhoids, postepisiotomy discomfort, and hemorrhoidectomy discomfort.

Administration and Dosage

➤*Directions:* When practical, cleanse the affected area with mild soap and warm water and rinse thoroughly. Gently dry by patting or blotting with toilet tissue or soft cloth before each application of this product.

Gently apply to the affected area by patting and then discard.

Apply to the affected area up to 6 times daily or after each bowel movement.

Children under 12 years of age – Consult a doctor.

➤*Storage/Stability:* Store at 15° to 30°C (59° to 86°F).

Actions

➤*Pharmacology:* Hamamelis water is a mild astringent prepared from twigs of *Hamamelis virginiana*; the distillate is then adjusted with an appropriate amount of alcohol.

Warnings

➤*Worsened conditions:* If condition worsens or does not improve within 7 days, consult a physician.

➤*Bleeding:* In case of bleeding, consult a physician promptly.

Precautions

➤*For external use only:* For external use only. Avoid contact with eyes.

Antiseborrheic Combinations

HAMAMELIS WATER — TOPICAL

Patient Information

Consult a doctor if condition worsens or does not improve within 7 days, in case of bleeding, or before exceeding the recommended dosage.

Do not put this product into the rectum using fingers or any mechanical device or applicator.

Keep out of the reach of children. If swallowed, get medical help or contact a poison control center right away.

CLEANSERS

Anti-Acne

MEDICATED BAR CLEANSERS

otc	**Clearasil Antibacterial Soap** (Procter & Gamble)	**Bar:** Triclosan	In 92 g.
otc	**Oxy Medicated Soap** (SmithKline Beecham)	**Bar:** 1% triclosan, EDTA	In 97.5 g.
otc	**Stri-Dex Cleansing Bar** (Sterling Health)	**Bar:** 1% triclosan, lanolin alcohol, EDTA	In 105 g.
otc	**Salicylic Acid Cleansing** (Stiefel)	**Bar:** 2% salicylic acid, EDTA	In 113 g.
otc	**Sulfur Soap** (Stiefel)	**Bar:** 10% precipitated sulfur, EDTA	In 116 g.
otc	**Fostex Acne Medication Cleansing** (Westwood Squibb)	**Bar:** 2% salicylic acid, EDTA	In 106 g.
otc	**Salicylic Acid and Sulfur Soap** (Stiefel)	**Bar:** 10% precipitated sulfur, 3% salicylic acid, EDTA	In 116 g.
otc	**SAStid Soap** (Stiefel)	**Bar:** 10% precipitated sulfur, EDTA	In 116 g.
otc	**Aveeno Cleansing for Acne-Prone Skin** (Rydelle)	**Bar:** Salicylic acid, colloidal oatmeal, glycerin and titanium dioxide	Soap free. In 90 g.

ABRASIVE CLEANSERS

otc	**Pernox Lathering Abradant Scrub** (Westwood Squibb)	**Lotion:** Sulfur, salicylic acid	In 141 g.
otc	**Pernox Scrub for Oily Skin** (Westwood Squibb)	**Cleanser:** Sulfur, salicylic acid, EDTA	Regular or lemon scent. In 56 and 113 g.
otc	**Brasivol** (Stiefel)	**Cleanser:** Aluminum oxide particles in a surfactant cleansing base	In fine (153 g), medium (180 g) and rough (195 g) textures.
otc	**Ionax** (Galderma)	**Scrub:** Benzalkonium chloride, SD alcohol 40	Lemon scented. In 60 and 120 g.
otc	**Seba-Nil Cleansing Mask** (Galderma)	**Scrub:** SD alcohol-40, castor oil, methylparaben	In 105 g.
otc	**PROPApH Peel-off Acne Mask** (Del Pharm.)	**Mask:** 2% salicylic acid, polyvinyl alcohol, parabens, SD alcohol 40, vitamin E acetate	In 60 mL.

LIQUID CLEANSERS

otc	**Stridex Anti-Bacterial Foaming Wash** (Blistex)	1% triclosan, parabens, glycerin, meadow foam oil, peppermint oil, spearmint oil, aloe, menthol	In 177 mL.
otc	**Clearasil Medicated Deep Cleanser** (Procter & Gamble)	0.5% salicylic acid and 42% alcohol, menthol, EDTA, aloe vera gel, hydrogenated castor oil	In 229 mL.
otc	**Clearasil Acne-Fighting Pads** (Procter & Gamble)	2% salicylic acid, alcohol, EDTA, aloe	In 65s.
otc	**PROPApH Astringent Cleanser Maximum Strength** (Del)	**Liquid:** 2% salicylic acid, aloe vera gel, 55.1% SD alcohol 40-2	In 355 mL.
otc	**Clearasil Double Textured Pads** (Procter & Gamble)	**Regular Strength:** 2% salicylic acid, 40% alcohol, glycerin, aloe vera gel, disodium EDTA	In 32s and 40s.
		Maximum Strength: 2% salicylic acid, 40% alcohol, aloe vera gel, menthol, disodium EDTA	In 32s and 40s.
otc	**Stri-Dex Pads** (Sterling Health)	**Regular Strength:** 0.5% salicylic acid, 28% SD alcohol, citric acid, menthol	In 55s.
		Maximum Strength: 2% salicylic acid, 44% SD alcohol, citric acid, menthol	In 55s and 90s. Dual textured in 32s.
		Oil Fighting Formula: 2% salicylic acid, citric acid, menthol, 54% SD alcohol	In 55 Super Scrub pads.
		Sensitive Skin: 0.5% salicylic acid, citric acid, aloe vera gel, menthol, 28% SD alcohol	In 55s.
otc	**Oxy Medicated Cleanser and Pads** (SK-Beecham)	**Regular Strength Pads:** 0.5% salicylic acid, 40% alcohol, citric acid, menthol, propylene glycol	**Pads:** In 50s and 90s.
		Maximum Strength Pads: 2% salicylic acid, 50% alcohol, citric acid, menthol, propylene glycol	In 50s and 90s.
		Sensitive Skin Pads: 0.5% salicylic acid, 22% alcohol, disodium lauryl sulfosuccinate, menthol, trisodium EDTA	In 50s and 90s.
otc	**Ionax Astringent Cleanser** (Galderma)	Salicylic acid, EDTA, isopropyl alcohol	In 240 mL.
otc	**Drytex Lotion** (C & M)	Salicylic acid, 10% acetone, 40% isopropyl alcohol, tartrazine	In 240 mL.
otc	**Seba-Nil Oily Skin Cleanser** (Galderma)	SD alcohol 40, acetone	In 240 and 473 mL.
otc	**Tyrosum Cleanser** (Summers)	50% isopropanol, 10% acetone, 2% polysorbate 80	**Liquid:** In 120 mL and pt.
			Packets: In 24s and 50s.
otc	**Acno Cleanser** (Baker Cummins)	60% isopropyl alcohol, EDTA	In 240 mL.
Rx	**Xerac AC** (Person & Covey)	6.25% aluminum chloride-hexahydrate in 96% anhydrous ethyl alcohol	In 35 and 60 mL.
otc	**Exact** (Premier)	2% salicylic acid, propylene glycol, aloe vera gel, disodium EDTA, menthol, parabens, glycerin, diazolidinyl urea	In 118 mL.
otc	**Neutrogena Oil-free Acne Wash** (Neutrogena)	2% salicylic acid, EDTA, propylene glycol, tartrazine, aloe extract	In 180 mL.

LIQUID CLEANSERS

otc	**Neutrogena Antiseptic Cleanser for Acne-Prone Skin** (Neutrogena)	Benzethonium chloride, butylene glycol, methylparaben, menthol, peppermint oil, eucalyptus oil, corn-mint oil, rosemary oil, witch hazel extract, camphor	In 135 mL.
otc	**PROPApH Cleansing for Sensitive Skin** (Del Pharm.)	**Pads**: 0.5% salicylic acid, SD alcohol 40, EDTA, menthol, aloe vera gel	In 45s.
otc	**PROPApH Cleansing Maximum Strength** (Del Pharm)	**Pads**: 2% salicylic acid, SD alcohol 40, propylene glycol, EDTA, menthol, aloe vera gel	In 45s.
otc	**PROPApH Foaming Face Wash** (Del Pharm.)	2% salicylic acid, EDTA, menthol, aloe vera gel	Alcohol-, oil-, and soap-free. In 180 mL.
otc	**Oil of Olay Foaming Face Wash Liquid** (Procter & Gamble)	Potassium cocoyl hydrolyzed collagen, glycerin, EDTA	Regular and sensitive skin formulas: In 90 mL tubes and 210 mL pump.

SOAP FREE CLEANSERS

These products are recommended for patients with sensitive, dry or irritated skin, who may react adversely to common soap products. Some products may be useful for patients with atopic dermatitis, diaper dermatitis and other eczematous skin conditions. Therapeutic cleansers include "soap free" cleansers, which may be adjusted to a neutral pH and are less irritating to sensitive skin, and "modified" soap products, which may contain emollient components or may be adjusted to a neutral or slightly acidic pH.

otc	**Aquanil Cleanser** (Person & Covey)	**Lotion**: Lipid free. Glycerin, cetyl, stearyl and benzyl alcohol, sodium laureth sulfate, xanthan gum	In 240 and 480 mL.
otc	**Bacti-Cleanse** (Pedinol)	**Lotion**: Benzalkonium chloride, mineral oil, isopropyl palmitate, cetyl alcohol, glycerine, glyceryl stearate, PEG 100 stearate, dimethicone, diazolidinyl urea, parabens, DMDM hydantoin, EDTA	In 453.6 mL.
otc	**Derm-Cleanse** (Yers Pharm)	**Liquid**: Soap free. Sodium lauryl sulfate, mineral oil, propylene glycol, hydroxyethylcellulose, EDTA	In 240 mL.
otc	**Drytergent** (C & M)	**Liquid**: TEA-dodecylbenzenesulfonate, boric acid, lauramide DEA, propylene glycol, tartrazine	In 240 and 480 mL.
otc	**Free & Clear** (Pharmaceutical Specialties)	**Shampoo**: Ammonium laureth sulfate, disodium cocamido MEA sulfsosuccinate, cocamidopropyl hydroxysultaine, cocamide DEA, PEG-120 methyl glucose dioleate, EDTA, potassium sorbate, citric acid	Dye free. In 240 mL
otc	**Green Soap** (Paddock)	**Liquid**: Soybean oil, potassium salt, ethanol	For skin and hair. In 3780 mL.
otc	**Lowila Cake** (Westwood Squibb)	**Bar**: Soap free. Dextrin, sodium lauryl sulfoacetate, boric acid, urea, sorbitol, mineral oil, PEG-14 M, lactic acid, cellulose gum, DSS	In 112.5 g.
otc	**Cetaphil** (Galderma)	**Bar**: Soap-free. Petrolatum	In 127 g.
		Bar, antibacterial: Soap-free. Triclosan, petrolatum	In 127 g.
		Cleanser: Cetyl alcohol, stearyl alcohol, parabens	In 236 mL.
		Cream: Lipid free. Cetyl alcohol, stearyl alcohol, sodium lauryl sulfate, propylene glycol, parabens	In 480 g.
		Lotion: Cetyl alcohol, propylene glycol, sodium lauryl sulfate, stearyl alcohol, parabens	In 120, 240, 480 mL.
otc	**Ancet** (C & M)	**Liquid**: Sodium lauryl sulfate, lauramide DEA, propylene glycol, hydroxyethyl ethylcellulose, PCMX	In 240 mL.
otc	**Ceta** (C & M)	**Liquid**: Soap free. Propylene glycol, hydroxyethylcellulose, cetyl and cetearyl alcohols, sodium lauryl sulfate, parabens	In 240 mL.
otc	**pHisoDerm** (Chattem)	**Liquid**: Soap free. Sodium octoxynol-2 ethane sulfonate solution, petrolatum, octoxynol-3, mineral oil (with lanolin alcohol and oleyl alcohol), cocamide MEA, imidazolidinyl urea, sodium benzoate, tetrasodium EDTA and methylcellulose	Regular formula: Scented and unscented. In 150, 270, 480 mL and gal.
			Oily skin formula: In 150 and 480 mL.
otc	**pHisoDerm For Baby** (Chattem)	**Liquid**: Sodium octoxynol-2 ethane sulfonate solution, petrolatum, octoxynol-3, mineral oil (with lanolin alcohol and oleyl alcohol), cocamide MEA, imidazolidinyl urea, sodium benzoate, tetrasodium EDTA and methylcellulose. pH adjusted with hydrochloric acid.	In 150 and 270 mL.
otc	**Spectro-Jel** (Recsei)	**Gel**: Soap free. Iodo-methyl-cellulose, carboxypolymethylene, cetyl alcohol, sorbitan monooleate, fumed silica, triethanolamine stearate, glycol polysiloxane, propylene glycol, glycerine and 5% isopropyl alcohol	In 127.5 mL, pt and gal.
otc	**Lobana Body Shampoo** (Ulmer)	**Liquid**: Chloroxylenol in a mild sudsing base with conditioners and emollients	In 240 mL and gal.
otc	**Tersaseptic** (Doak)	**Shampoo/Liquid**: DEA-lauryl sulfate, lauramide DEA, propylene glycol, ethoxydiglycol, PEG-12 distearate, EDTA, triclosan, citric acid	In 475 mL.
otc	**Lobana Liquid Lather** (Ulmer)	**Body wash**: Sodium laureth sulfate, sodium lauroyl sarcosinate, sodium myristyl sarcosinate, lauramide DEA, linoleamide DEA, octyl hydroxystearate, polyquarternium 7, tetrasodium EDTA, quaternium 15, sodium chloride, citric acid	In 240 mL and gal.
otc	**Neutrogena Non-Drying Cleansing** (Neutrogena)	**Lotion**: Glycerin, caprylic/capric triglyceride, PEG-20 almond glycerides, cetyl recinoleate, isohexadecane, TEA-cocoyl glutamate, PEG-20 methyl glucose sesquistearate, methyl glucose sesquistearate, stearyl alcohol, cetyl alcohol, EDTA, dipotassium glycyrrhizate, stearyl glycyrrhetinate, bisabolol, parabens, acrylates/C 10-30 alkyl acrylate crosspolymer, triethanolamine, diazolidinyl urea	In 165 mL.
otc	**SFC** (Stiefel)	**Lotion**: Soap free. PEG-75, stearyl alcohol, sodium cocoyl isethionate, parabens	In 237 and 480 mL.
otc	**Cetaklenz** (Geritrex)	**Cleanser**: Cetyl alcohol, propylene glycol, sodium lauryl sulfate, stearyl alcohol, DMDM hydantoin, parabens	Fragrance free. In 120 mL.

MODIFIED BAR SOAPS

otc	**pHisoDerm Cleansing Bar** (Chattem)	**Bar**: Sodium tallowate, sodium cocoate, petrolatum, glycerin, lanolin, sodium chloride, BHT, EDTA, titanium dioxide	Scented or unscented. In 99 g.
otc	**Oilatum Soap** (Stiefel)	**Bar**: Sodium tallowate, sodium cocoate, peanut oil, octyl hydroxystearate, lecithin, NaCl, PEG-14M, titanium dioxide, o-tolyl biguanide, EDTA, sodium borohydride, glyceryl oleate, corn oil, t-butyl hydroquinone, propylene glycol	Scented or unscented. In 120 and 240 g.
otc	**Neutrogena Dry Skin Soap** (Neutrogena Corp.)	**Bar**: TEA-stearate, triethanolamine, sodium tallowate, glycerin, sodium cocoate, sodium ricinoleate, TEA-oleate, laneth-10 acetate, cocamide DEA, nonoxynol 12, PEG-5 octanoate, tocopherol	Transparent. Scented or unscented. In 105 and 165 (scented only) g.
otc	**Neutrogena Oily Skin Soap** (Neutrogena Corp.)	**Bar**: TEA-stearate, triethanolamine, sodium tallowate, glycerin, sodium lauroyl sarcosinate, sodium cocoate, sodium ricinoleate, witch hazel, tocopherol	Transparent. Scented. In 105 g.
otc	**Neutrogena Soap** (Neutrogena Corp.)	**Bar**: TEA-stearate, triethanolamine, glycerin, sodium tallowate, sodium cocoate, sodium ricinoleate, TEA-oleate, cocamide DEA, tocopherol	Transparent. Scented or unscented. In 105 and 165 g.
otc	**Neutrogena Cleansing for Acne-Prone Skin** (Neutrogena Corp.)	**Bar**: TEA-stearate, triethanolamine, glycerin, sodium tallowate, sodium cocoate, TEA-oleate, sodium ricinoleate, acetylated lanolin alcohol, cocamide DEA, TEA lauryl sulfate, tocopherol	Transparent, nonmedicated. In 105 g.
otc	**Ambi 10** (Kiwi Brands)	**Bar**: Triclosan, sodium tallowate, PEG-20, titanium dioxide	In 99 g.
otc	**Alpha Keri Moisturizing Soap** (Bristol-Myers)	**Bar**: Sodium tallowate, sodium cocoate, mineral oil, lanolin oil, PEG-75, glycerin, titanium dioxide, sodium chloride, BHT, EDTA	Nondetergent, emollient. In 120 g.
otc	**Purpose Soap** (Johnson & Johnson)	**Bar**: Sodium tallowate, sodium cocoate, glycerin, NaCl, BHT, EDTA	In 108 and 180 g.

MODIFIED BAR SOAPS

otc	**Nivea Moisturizing Creme Soap** (Beiersdorf)	**Bar:** Sodium tallowate, sodium cocoate, glycerin, petrolatum, titanium dioxide, NaCl, octyldodecanol, macadamia nut oil, aloe, sodium thiosulfate, lanolin alcohol, pentasodium pentetate, EDTA, BHT, beeswax	In 90 and 150 g.
otc	**Cuticura Medicated Soap** (DEP Corp.)	**Bar:** 1% triclocarban, sodium tallowate, sodium cocoate, glycerin, mineral oil, petrolatum, sodium chloride, tetrasodium EDTA, sodium bicarbonate, magnesium silicate and iron oxides	Phosphorus free. Emollient. Mildly antibacterial. In 97.5 and 142 g.
otc	**Formula 405** (Doak)	**Bar:** Sodium tallowate, sodium cocoate, Doak Additive A, PPG-20 methyl glucose ether, titanium dioxide, trochlorocarbanilide, pentasodium pentetate, EDTA	Fragrance free. In 100 g.

COUNTERIRRITANTS

CAPSAICIN

otc	**Capsin** (Fleming)	**Lotion:** 0.025%	Benzyl alcohol, propylene glycol, denatured alcohol. In 59 mL.
otc	**Capsin** (Fleming)	**Lotion:** 0.075%	Benzyl alcohol, propylene glycol, denatured alcohol. In 59 mL.
otc	**Capsaicin** (Various, eg, Alpharma, Ferndale, Ivax)	**Cream:** 0.025%	In 45 and 60 g.
otc	**Pain Doctor** (Fougera)		25% methyl salicylate, 10% menthol, propylene glycol, parabens. In 60 g.
otc	**Zostrix** (Rodlen Labs)	**Cream:** 0.025% in an emollient base	In 45 and 90 g.
otc	**Capzasin•P** (Chattem)	**Cream:** 0.035%	Alcohols, petrolatum. In 42.5 g.
otc	**Capsaicin** (Various, eg, Alpharma, Ferndale, Ivax)	**Cream:** 0.075%	In 60 g.
otc	**Rid•a•Pain•HP** (Pfeiffer)		Alcohols, parabens. In 45 g.
otc	**Zostrix-HP** (Rodlen Labs)	**Cream:** 0.075% in an emollient base	In 30 and 60 g.
otc	**Capzasin•HP** (Chattem)	**Cream:** 0.1%	Alcohols, petrolatum. In 42.5 g.
otc	**Axsain** (Rodlen Labs)	**Cream:** 0.25% in an emollient base	Lidocaine, benzyl alcohol, cetyl alcohol, white petrolatum. In 60 g tubes.
otc	**Dolorac** (GenDerm)		Benzyl alcohol, cetyl alcohol. In 28 g tubes.
otc	**R-Gel** (Healthline Labs)	**Gel:** 0.025%	EDTA. In 15 and 30 g.
otc	**Pain-X** (B.F. Ascher)	**Gel:** 0.05%	5% menthol, 4% camphor, alcohol, parabens. In 42.5 g.
otc	**No Pain-HP** (Young Again Products)	**Roll-on:** 0.075%	In 60 mL.

CAPSAICIN — TOPICAL

Indications

➤*Muscle/Joint pain:* For the temporary relief of minor aches and pains of muscles and joints associated with backache, strains, sprains, arthritis, rheumatoid arthritis and osteoarthritis. For use in treating neuralgias, consult a physician.

➤*Unlabeled uses:* Capsaicin is being investigated for use in other disorders including psoriasis, vitiligo, and intractable pruritus, as well as postmastectomy and postamputation neuroma (phantom limb syndrome), vulvar vestibulitis, apocrine chromhidrosis, and reflex sympathetic dystrophy.

Administration and Dosage

➤*Directions:* For persons under 18 years of age, consult a physician before using.

Adults – Apply a thin film of capsaicin to affected area 3 to 4 times daily. A burning sensation may occur upon application, but generally disappears with regular use. Application schedules of less than 3 to 4 times a day or for less than 2 weeks may not provide optimum pain relief. Unless treating hands, wash hands thoroughly after each application.

➤*Storage/Stability:* Store at room temperature 15° to 30°C (59° to 86°F).

Actions

➤*Pharmacology:* Capsaicin is a natural chemical derived from plants of the solanaceae family. Although the precise mechanism of action is not fully understood, evidence suggests that the drug renders skin and joints insensitive to pain by depleting and preventing reaccumulation of Substance P in peripheral sensory neurons. Substance P is thought to be the principal chemomediator of pain impulses from the periphery to the central nervous system.

Warnings

For external use only. Do not apply to wounds or to damaged or irritated skin. Do not wrap tightly. Do not get on mucous membranes, into eyes or on contact lenses. If this occurs, rinse the affected area thoroughly with water. Discontinue use of this product and consult your doctor if condition worsens or does not improve after regular use, if blistering occurs, or if severe burning persists. Do not apply heat to the treated area immediately before or after applications as this may increase the burning sensation. If you have difficulty breathing or swallowing as a result of using this product, consult your doctor immediately. Keep this and all drugs out of the reach of children. In case of accidental ingestion, seek professional assistance or contact a poison control center immediately.

Adverse Reactions

No systemic side effects have been attributed to capsaicin. A localized burning sensation may be experienced upon application. This sensation, typically mild, generally subsides with regular use. Continue to use capsaicin consistently as directed, unless the burning sensation becomes too painful to tolerate. Heat and excessive perspiration may intensify the burning sensation; therefore, do not apply immediately before or after activities such as bathing, swimming, sunbathing, or strenuous exercise. Generally, the more you use capsaicin as directed, the more likely you are to obtain maximum relief and minimize the burning sensation. Other adverse reactions include stinging; erythema; cough; respiratory tract irritation.

Patient Information

Doctors prescribe capsaicin for the relief of pain from arthritis and painful neuralgias. For use in painful neuralgias, consult a physician.

Regular and frequent application is essential. Proper use of capsaicin is essential for maximum pain relief. Capsaicin must be applied regularly and frequently, as directed, to deplete the supply of Substance P in nerve cells and prevent it from building up again. Because it takes time for Substance P to be depleted, relief occurs gradually. To achieve optimum pain relief, be sure to apply capsaicin daily as directed. Relief may be delayed, or may not occur, if cream is applied less often.

Apply to the painful area regularly (3 to 4 times a day).

Do not apply to wounds or to damaged or irritated skin. Do not tightly wrap or bandage the treated area. Do not apply heat to the treated area.

Apply just enough cream to cover the affected area with a thin layer, and gently massage into the skin until fully absorbed.

Wash hands thoroughly after use to avoid spreading cream to the eyes, mucous membranes, or other sensitive areas of the body. Since trace amounts of capsaicin may remain on hands even after washing, avoid touching mucous membranes, eyes, or contact lenses after use. If capsaicin gets into the eyes, it will cause a burning sensation, but has not been reported to cause any harm. Flush eyes with water. Avoid exposure of cream to contact lenses.

If you are treating your hands with capsaicin, wait 30 minutes after applying before washing hands.

Avoid thick application. Be sure to massage the cream into the skin until no residue remains. Avoid inhaling airborne material from dried residue, which can cause coughing, sneezing, tearing, and/or throat or respiratory irritation. If difficulty breathing or swallowing occurs, contact a physician.

If condition worsens or does not improve after 14 to 28 days, discontinue use of this product and consult your physician.

Indications

➤*Dichloroacetic acid:* Verrucae (warts); calluses; hard and soft corns; xanthoma palpebrarum; seborrheic keratoses; ingrown nails; cysts and benign erosion of the cervix; endocervicitis; epistaxis.

➤*Monochloroacetic and trichloroacetic acid:* Removal of verrucae.

The CDC recommends trichloroacetic acid as an alternative regimen to cryotherapy for treatment of external genital/perianal warts and vaginal and anal warts.

Actions

➤*Pharmacology:* Rapidly penetrates and cauterizes skin, keratin and other tissues. Monochloroacetic acid is more deeply destructive than trichloroacetic acid.

Contraindications

Treatment of malignant or premalignant lesions; hypersensitivity to any component.

Warnings

➤*Cauterant properties:* These acids are powerful keratolytics and cauterants. Restrict use to areas where these effects are desired. May cause severe burning, inflammation or tenderness of skin.

➤*Cervical lesions:* A careful diagnosis and possibly a biopsy is required to rule out malignancy; treatment is contraindicated in the event of positive findings.

➤*Normal tissue:* Apply only to the lesion being treated. To prevent acid from spreading onto normal skin, apply petrolatum around the area to be treated. If any acid is spilled on normal tissue or if too much acid is applied, remove immediately and wash with water. Sodium bicarbonate may be applied as a local antidote.

MONOCHLOROACETIC ACID

Rx	**Mono-Chlor** (Gordon)	**Liquid**: 80%	In 15 mL.

MONOCHLOROACETIC ACID — TOPICAL

For Monochloroacetic Acid prescribing information, see the Chloroacetic Acids group monograph.

Administration and Dosage

Remove callus tissue. Apply to verruca. Apply bandage and allow to remain in place for 5 to 6 days. Remove verruca tissue and reapply as needed. If crystallization of liquid occurs, place capped bottle in hot water to redissolve.

TRICHLOROACETIC ACID

Rx	**Tri-Chlor** (Gordon)	**Liquid**: 80%	In 15 mL.

TRICHLOROACETIC ACID — TOPICAL

Complete prescribing information begins in the Chloroacetic Acids group monograph.

Indications

➤*Condylomata:* To aid in the elimination of condylomata.

The Centers for Disease Control (CDC) recommends trichloroacetic acid as an alternative regimen to cryotherapy for treatment of external genital/perianal warts and vaginal and anal warts.

Administration and Dosage

For external use only. Debride callous tissue. Apply to condyloma. Cover with suitable dressing for 5 to 6 days. Reapply as needed. If crystallization of liquid occurs, place capped bottle in hot water to redissolve.

PODOFILOX

Rx	**Condylox** (Oclassen)	**Topical Gel:** 0.5% podofilox	Alcohol. In 3.5 mL aluminum tubes.
Rx	**Podofilox** (Various, eg, Paddock, Watson)	**Topical Solution:** 0.5% podofilox	95% alcohol. In 3.5 mL.
Rx	**Condylox** (Oclassen)		Alcohol. In 3.5 mL bottles.

PODOFILOX — TOPICAL

Indications

➤*Warts:* Podofilox gel is indicated for the topical treatment of anogenital warts (external genital warts [condyloma acuminatum]) and perianal warts. It is not indicated for the treatment of mucous membrane warts (see Precautions).

Podofilox topical solution is indicated for for the topical treatment of anogenital warts (external genital warts [condyloma acuminatum]). It is not indicated for the treatment of perianal warts or for the treatment of mucous membrane warts (see Precautions).

Administration and Dosage

➤*Approved by the FDA:* March 13, 1997.

Apply twice daily every 12 hours (eg, morning and evening) for 3 consecutive days, then withhold use for 4 consecutive days. This 1-week cycle of treatment may be repeated until there is no visible wart tissue for a maximum of 4 cycles. If there is incomplete response after 4 treatment cycles, discontinue treatment and consider alternative treatment. Safety and efficacy of more than 4 treatment cycles have not been established. There is no evidence to suggest that more frequent application will increase efficacy, but additional applications would be expected to increase the rate of local adverse reactions and systemic absorption.

➤*Gel:* Podofilox gel should be applied to the warts with the applicator tip or finger. Application on the surrounding normal tissue should be minimized. Treatment should be limited to ≤ 10 cm^2 of wart tissue and to no more than 0.5 g of the gel/day.

Care should be taken to allow the gel to dry before allowing the return of opposing skin surfaces to their normal positions. Patients should be instructed to wash their hands thoroughly before and after each application.

➤*Topical solution:* Podofilox solution is applied to the warts with a cotton-tipped applicator supplied with the drug. The drug-dampened applicator should be touched to the wart to be treated, applying the minimum amount of solution necessary to cover the lesion. Treatment should be limited to less than 10 cm^2 of wart tissue, and to no more than 0.5 mL of the solution/day.

Care should be taken to allow the solution to dry before allowing the return of opposing skin surfaces to their normal positions. After each treatment, the used applicator should be carefully disposed of and the patient should wash his or her hands.

➤*Storage / Stability:* Store at controlled room temperature between 15° to 30°C (59° to 86°F). Avoid excessive heat. Do not freeze.

Actions

➤*Pharmacology:* Treatment of genital warts with podofilox results in necrosis of visible wart tissue. The exact mechanism of action is unknown.

➤*Pharmacokinetics:*

Absorption / Distribution – In systemic absorption studies in 52 patients, topical application of 0.05 mL of an ethanolic solution containing 0.5% podofilox to external genitalia did not result in detectable serum levels. Applications of 0.1 to 1.5 mL resulted in peak serum levels of 1 to 17 ng/mL 1 to 2 hours after application.

Excretion – The elimination half-life ranged from 1 to 4.5 hours. The drug was not found to accumulate after multiple treatments.

Contraindications

Hypersensitivity or intolerance to any components of the formulation.

Warnings

➤*Cutaneous use only:* Avoid contact with the eyes. If contact with the eyes occurs, patients should immediately flush the eyes with copious quantities of water and seek medical advice.

➤*Flammable:* Drug product is flammable. Keep away from open flame.

➤*Mutagenesis:* Results from the mouse micronucleus in vivo assay using podofilox 0.5% solution at doses up to 25 mg/kg (75 mg/m^2), indicate that podofilox should be considered a potential clastogen (a chemical that induces disruption and breakage of chromosomes).

➤*Pregnancy: Category C.* Podofilox was not teratogenic in the rabbit following topical application of up to 0.21/mg/kg (5 times the maximum human dose) once daily for 13 days. The scientific literature contains references that podofilox solution is embryotoxic in rats when administered systemically in a dose ≈ 250 times the recommended maximum human dose.

Teratogenicity and embryotoxicity have not been studied with intravaginal application. Many antimitotic drug products are known to be embryotoxic. There are no adequate and well-controlled studies in pregnant women. Podofilox should be used during pregnancy only if the potential benefit justifies the potential risk to the fetus.

➤*Lactation:* It is not known whether this drug is excreted in human milk. Because of the potential for serious adverse reactions in nursing infants from podofilox, a decision should be made whether to discontinue nursing or to discontinue the drug, taking into account the importance of the drug to the mother.

➤*Children:* Safety and efficacy in pediatric patients have not been established.

Precautions

➤*Mucous membrane warts:* Data is not available on the safe and effective use of this product for treatment of warts occurring on mucous membranes of the genital area (including the urethra, rectum and vagina). The recommended method of application, frequency of application, and duration of usage should not be exceeded (see Administration and Dosage).

Adverse Reactions

➤*Gel:* In clinical trials with podofilox 0.5%, the local adverse reactions listed below were reported during the treatment of anogenital warts. The severity of local adverse reactions were predominantly mild or moderate and did not increase during the treatment period. Severe reactions were most frequent within the first 2 weeks of treatment.

Adverse reaction	Mild	Moderate	Severe
Bleeding	19.2%	3%	0.7%
Burning	37.1%	25.9%	11.5%
Erosion	27%	20.8%	8.9%
Inflammation	32.2%	30.4%	9.3%
Itching	32.2%	16%	7.8%
Pain	23.7%	20.4%	11.5%

Local – Other local adverse reactions reported included stinging (7%), and erythema (5%); less commonly reported local adverse events included desquamation, scabbing, discoloration, tenderness, dryness, crusting, fissures, soreness, ulceration, swelling/edema, tingling, rash, and blisters.

Miscellaneous – The most common systemic adverse event reported during the clinical studies was headache (7%).

➤*Topical solution:* In clinical trials, the following local adverse reactions were reported at some point during treatment. Reports of burning and pain were more frequent and of greater severity in women and than in men.

Adverse reaction	Males	Females
Burning	64%	78%
Erosion	67%	67%
Inflammation	71%	63%
Itching	50%	65%
Pain	50%	72%

Adverse effects reported in less than 5% of the patients included pain with intercourse, insomnia, tingling, bleeding, tenderness, chafing, malodor, dizziness, scarring, vesicle formation, crusting edema, dryness/peeling, foreskin irretraction, hematuria, vomiting and ulceration.

Overdosage

➤*Symptoms:* Topically applied podofilox may be absorbed systemically (see Pharmacokinetics). Toxicity reported following systemic administration of podofilox in investigational use for cancer treatment included nausea, vomiting, fever, diarrhea, bone marrow depression, and oral ulcers. Following 5 to 10 daily IV doses of 0.5 to 1 mg/kg/day, significant hematological toxicity occurred but was reversible. Other toxicities occurred at lower doses. Toxicity reported following systemic administration of podophyllum resin included nausea, vomiting, fever, diarrhea, peripheral neuropathy, altered mental status, lethargy, coma, tachypnea, respiratory failure, leukocytosis, pancytosis, hematuria, renal failure and seizures.

➤*Treatment:* Treatment of topical overdosage should include washing the skin free of any remaining drug and symptomatic and supportive therapy.

Patient Information

Only use this medication as directed by the health care provider. Instruct patients to wash their hands thoroughly before and after each application. It is for external use only. Avoid contact with the eyes. Advise patients not to use this medication for any disorder other than that for which it was prescribed. Patients should report any signs of adverse reactions to the health care provider. If no improvement is observed after 4 weeks of treatment, discontinue the medication and consult the health care provider.

PODOPHYLLUM RESIN (Podophyllin)

Rx	**Podocon-25** (Paddock)	**Liquid:** 25% podophyllum resin in tincture of benzoin	In 15 mL.
Rx	**Podofin** (Syosset)		In 15 mL.

PODOPHYLLIN — TOPICAL

Indications

➤*Warts:* For the removal of soft genital (venereal) warts (condylomata acuminata).

Administration and Dosage

Podophyllin is to be applied only by a physician. It is not to be dispensed to the patient. Thoroughly cleanse affected area. Use supplied applicator to apply podophyllin sparingly to lesion. Avoid contact with healthy tissue. Allow to dry thoroughly. Only intact (no bleeding) lesions should be treated. As podophyllin is a powerful caustic and severe irritant, it is recommended the first application of podophyllin be left in contact for only a short time (30 to 40 minutes) to determine patient's sensitivity. To avoid systemic absorption, time of contact should be minimum time necessary to produce the desired result (1 to 4 hours, depending on condition of lesion and of patient), the physician developing his own experience and technique. Large areas or numerous warts should not be treated at once.

After treatment time has elapsed, remove dried podophyllin thoroughly with alcohol or soap and water.

➤*Storage / Stability:* Store at room temperature 15° to 30°C (59° to 86°F) in tight, light-resistant containers.

Actions

➤*Pharmacology:* Podophyllin resin is a cytotoxic agent that has been used topically in the treatment of genital warts. It arrests mitosis in metaphase, an effect it shares with other cytotoxic agents such as the vinca alkaloids. The active agent is podophyllotoxin, whose concentration varies with the type of podophyllin used; the American source normally containing one-fourth the amount of podophyllotoxin as the Indian source.

Contraindications

In diabetics, patients using steroids, or with poor blood circulation. Do not use podophyllin on bleeding warts, moles, birthmarks or unusual warts with hair growing from them. It is recommended that podophyllin not be used during pregnancy (see Warnings).

Warnings

Podophyllin is a powerful caustic and severe irritant. Keep away from the eyes; if eye contact occurs, flush with copious amounts of warm water and consult physician or poison control center immediately for advice.

➤*Pregnancy:* There have been reports of complications associated with the topical use of podophyllin on condylomata of pregnant patients including birth defects, fetal death and stillbirth. In the absence of controlled safety studies, podophyllin remains contraindicated for use on pregnant patients.

➤*Lactation:* It is not known whether podophyllin is excreted in human milk following topical application. In the absence of controlled safety studies, podophyllin remains contraindicated for use on nursing patients.

Precautions

➤*Irritation / Inflammation:* Do not use podophyllin if wart or surrounding tissue is inflamed or irritated.

Adverse Reactions

The use of topical podophyllin has been known to result in paresthesia, polyneuritis, paralytic ileus, pyrexia, leukopenia, thrombocytopenia, coma, and death.

DIAPER RASH PRODUCTS

METHIONINE

Rx[a]	**Methionine** (Various, eg, Mason, Tyson & Assoc.)	**Tablets:** 500 mg	In 30s and 60s.
Rx	**M-Caps** (Pal-Pak)	**Capsules:** 200 mg	In 1000s.
Rx	**Uracid** (Wesley)		In 1000s.

[a] Products available *otc* or *Rx*, depending on product labeling.

METHIONINE — ORAL

For dietary supplement prescribing information, see the Nutritional Agents chapter.

Indications

➤*Dermatological conditions:* Treatment of diaper rash in infants and for control of odor; dermatitis and ulceration caused by ammoniacal urine in incontinent adults.

Administration and Dosage

➤*Diaper rash caused by ammoniacal urine:* 75 mg in warm formula or other liquid, 3 or 4 times daily or 3 to 5 days. In severe cases or when the infant is older than 1 year old it may be necessary to double the dosage the first two days of treatment.

➤*Control of odor in incontinent adults:* 200 to 500 mg, 3 or 4 times daily after meal.

Actions

➤*Pharmacology:* The acid-producing effect of methionine on urine pH creates an ammonia free urine.

Contraindications

A history of liver disease; large doses of methionine may exaggerate the toxemia of the disease.

Precautions

➤*Protein intake:* Excessive methionine added alone to the diet over extended periods may result in a less than normal weight gain in infants when protein intake is insufficient. Maintain adequate protein intake during therapy and do not exceed the recommended dosage.

Patient Information

Take with food, milk or other liquid.

DIAPER RASH PRODUCTS, TOPICAL

otc	**Paladin** (Pal Midwest Ltd[a])	**Ointment:** Petrolatum, starch, lanolin, zinc oxide, mineral oil, boric acid, bees wax, vitamin A and D concentrate	In 2 oz.
otc	**Diaper Rash** (Various, eg, Goldline, Rugby)	**Ointment:** Zinc oxide, cod liver oil, lanolin, methylparaben, petrolatum, talc	In 113 g.
otc	**A and D Medicated** (Schering-Plough)	**Ointment:** White petrolatum, zinc oxide, benzyl alcohol, cod liver oil, light mineral oil, propylparabens, vitamins A and D	In 113 g.
otc	**A+D Ointment with Zinc Oxide** (Schering-Plough)	**Ointment:** 1% dimethicone, 10% zinc oxide, aloe, benzyl alcohol, vitamins A and D, cod liver oil, light mineral oil, synthetic beeswax	In 81 g.
otc	**Bottom Better** (InnoVisions)	**Ointment:** 49% petrolatum, 15.5% lanolin, lanolin alcohols, EDTA, parabens	In 3.75 g packets (18).
otc	**Vitamin A & Vitamin D** (Geritrex)	**Ointment:** Vitamin A and vitamin D in a base of lanolin, white petrolatum, paraffin	In 410 g.
otc	**Desitin** (Leeming)	**Ointment:** 40% zinc oxide, cod liver oil, talc, petrolatum, lanolin, methylparaben	In 30, 60, 120, 240, and 270 g.
otc	**Diaper Guard** (Del)	**Ointment:** 1% dimethicone, 66% white petrolatum, cocoa butter, parabens, vitamins A, D_3 and E, zinc oxide	In 49.6 and 99.2 g.
otc	**Diaparene Diaper Rash** (Lehn & Fink)	**Ointment:** Zinc oxide, petrolatum, parabens, imidazolidinyl urea	In 60 g.
otc	**Flanders Buttocks** (Flanders Inc.)	**Ointment:** Zinc oxide, castor oil, balsam peru	In 60 g.
otc	**Desitin Creamy** (Pfizer)	**Ointment:** 10% zinc oxide, mineral oil, white petrolatum, parabens	In 57 g.

DIAPER RASH PRODUCTS, TOPICAL

otc	**Soothe & Cool** (Medline[b])	**Cream**: 5% dimethicone, 5% zinc oxide, lanolin, cetyl alcohol, vitamins A, D, and E	In 118 mL.
otc	**Diaparene Baby** (Lehn & Fink)	**Cream**: Mineral oil, petrolatum, aloe, EDTA, diazolidinyl urea, parabens	In 60 g.
otc	**Amerigel** (Amerx Health Care Corp.)	**Lotion**: Glycerin, lemon oil, parabens, oak extract (oakin).	In 228 g.
otc	**Dyprotex** (Blistex)	**Pads**: 40% micronized zinc oxide, 37.6% petrolatum, 2.5% dimethicone, cod liver oil, aloe	In 3 pads (9 applications) and 8 pads (24 applications).
otc	**Diaparene Cornstarch Baby** (Lehn & Fink)	**Powder**: Corn starch, aloe	In 120, 270, and 420 g.
otc	**Mexsana Medicated** (Schering-Plough)	**Powder**: Kaolin, eucalyptus oil, camphor, corn starch, lemon oil, zinc oxide	In 90, 187.5 and 330 g.
otc	**Desitin with Zinc Oxide** (Pfizer)	**Powder**: 88.2% cornstarch, 10% zinc oxide	In 28 and 397 g.
otc	**Gold Bond Medicated Baby Powder** (Chattem)	**Powder**: Talc, zinc oxide	In 113 and 283 g.
otc	**Gold Bond Cornstarch Plus Medicated Baby Powder** (Chattem)	**Powder**: Cornstarch, zinc oxide, kaolin	In 113 and 283 g.
otc	**Gold Bond Triple Action Medicated Baby Powder** (Chattem)	**Powder**: 89% talc, 10% zinc oxide	In 113 and 283 g.

[a] Pal Midwest Ltd, P.O. Box 624, Rockford, IL 61101; (815) 965-2981; fax (815) 332-3366.
[b] Medline Industries, Inc., One Medline Place, Mundelein, IL, 60060-4486; 1-(800)-MEDLINE; fax 1-(800) 351-1512.

DIAPER RASH PRODUCTS — TOPICAL

Indications

➤*Diaper rash / Ammonia dermatitis:* For use in diaper rash or ammonia dermatitis.

Active Ingredients

The principal active components of these formulations include:

➤*EUCALYPTOL:* Antimicrobial agent. Minimizes bacterial proliferation.

➤*ZINC OXIDE:* For drying.

➤*CAMPHOR:* A local anesthetic. Relieves pain, itching and irritation.

➤*BALSAM PERU:* It is claimed to promote wound healing or tissue repair, but effectiveness has not been conclusively demonstrated.

➤*CALCIUM CARBONATE and KAOLIN:* Used for their moisture absorbing abilities.

➤*PROTECTANTS and LUBRICANTS:* To minimize chafing and irritation.

DIAPER RASH COMBINATIONS

Rx	**Vusion** (Barrier Therapeutics[a])	**Ointment**: 0.25% miconazole nitrate, 15% zinc oxide, and 81.35% white petrolatum	In 30 g tubes.

[a] Barrier Therapeutics, 600 College Rd., Ste 3200, Princeton, NJ 08540; (609) 945-1200; http://www.barriertherapeutics.com.

MICONAZOLE/ZINC OXIDE — TOPICAL

Indications

➤*Diaper dermatitis:* For the adjunctive treatment of diaper dermatitis only when complicated by documented candidiasis (microscopic evidence of pseudohyphae and/or budding yeast) in immunocompetent children 4 weeks of age and older. A positive fungal culture for *Candida albicans* is not adequate evidence of candidial infection since colonization with *C. albicans* can result in a positive culture. Establish the presence of candidial infection by microscopic evaluation prior to initiating treatment.

See Administration and Dosage for more information.

Administration and Dosage

➤*Approved by the FDA:* February 16, 2006.

➤*Before use:* Before applying the ointment, gently cleanse the skin with lukewarm water and pat dry with a soft towel. Avoid using any scented soaps, shampoos, or lotions on the diaper area.

➤*Recommended use:* Apply to the affected area at each diaper change for 7 days. Gently apply a thin layer of ointment to the diaper area with the fingertips. Do not rub into skin as this may cause additional irritation. Thoroughly wash hands after applying the ointment.

➤*Duration:* Continue treatment for the full 7 days, even if there is improvement. The safety when used for longer than 7 days is not known.

➤*Additional treatment measures:* Use ointment as part of a treatment regimen that includes measures directed at the underlying diaper dermatitis, including gentle cleansing of the diaper area and frequent diaper changes.

Do not use ointment as a substitute for frequent diaper changes or to prevent the occurrence of diaper dermatitis, because preventative use may result in the development of drug resistance.

➤*Storage / Stability:* Store at controlled room temperature, between 20° and 25°C (68° and 77°F); excursions are permitted between 15° and 30°C (59° and 86°F). Keep out of the reach of children.

DRYING AGENTS

ALUMINUM CHLORIDE (HEXAHYDRATE)

Rx	**Aluminum Chloride (Hexahydrate)** (Glades)	**Solution**: 20% in 88.5% SD alcohol 40-2	In 37.5 mL bottle and 35 and 60 mL *Dab-O-Matic* applicator bottle.
Rx	**Drysol** (Person & Covey)	**Solution**: 20% in 93% SD alcohol 40	In 37.5 mL or 35 and 60 mL with *Dab-O-Matic* applicator.

ALUMINUM CHLORIDE (HEXAHYDRATE) — TOPICAL

Indications

➤*Hyperhidrosis:* An astringent used as an aid in the management of hyperhidrosis.

Administration and Dosage

➤*Directions:* Apply to the affected area once daily, only at bedtime. To help prevent irritation, the area should be completely dry prior to application. Do not apply aluminum chloride (hexahydrate) to broken, irritated, or recently shaved skin.

➤*Dab-O-Matic* Bottle: Apply from the applicator to the affected area.

➤*Plastic bottle:* Apply with fingers or a moistened cotton ball to the affected area.

➤*For maximum effect:* May cover the treated area with a saran wrap held in place by a snug fitting "T" or body shirt, mitten, or sock. Never hold saran in place with tape.

Wash the treated area the following morning.

Excessive sweating may be stopped after 2 or more treatments. Thereafter, apply aluminum chloride (hexahydrate) once or twice a week or as needed.

➤*Storage/Stability:* Store between 15° to 30°C (59° to 86°F).

Keep cap tightly closed when not in use to prevent evaporation.

Warnings

➤*Sensitivity:* If irritation or sensitization occurs, discontinue use or consult with a physician.

➤*For external use only:* Avoid contact with eyes.

Adverse Reactions

May produce a burning or prickling sensation.

Patient Information

If irritation or sensitization occurs, discontinue use or consult with a physician.

For external use only. Avoid contact with eyes

Aluminum chloride (hexahydrate) may be harmful to certain metals and fabrics.

Do not use near open flame.

FORMALDEHYDE

Rx	**Formalyde-10** (Pedinol)	**Spray:** 10%	SD-40 alcohol. In 60 mL.
Rx	**Lazer Formalyde** (Pedinol)	**Solution:** 10%	In 90 mL.

FORMALDEHYDE — TOPICAL

Indications

➤*Odor/Perspiration of the feet:* Safeguards against offensive odor and dries excessive moisture of feet. Drying agent for pre- and post-surgical removal of warts or for non-surgical laser treatment of warts where dryness is required.

Administration and Dosage

➤*Directions:*

Spray – Spray once a day to affected areas or as directed by a podiatrist, dermatologist or physician. Keep cap closed tightly. Do not shake the bottle.

Solution – Apply with the roll-on applicator once a day to affected areas, or as directed by your podiatrist, dermatologist, or physician. Do not shake the bottle with the cap removed. Keep cap closed tightly.

➤*Storage/Stability:* Store at controlled room temperature 15° to 30°C (59° to 86°F).

Contraindications

Sensitivity to any ingredients in formaldehyde spray or solution.

Warnings

➤*Children:* Safety and effectiveness in pediatric patients have not been established.

Precautions

For external use only. Harmful if swallowed. Contact a local poison control center immediately. Keep out of the reach of children. Avoid contact and keep away from face, eyes, nose and mucous membranes. Check skin for sensitivity to formaldehyde prior to application since it may be irritating and sensitizing to the skin of some patients. If redness or irritation persists, consult your podiatrist, dermatologist or physician.

ENZYME PREPARATIONS

COLLAGENASE

Rx	**Collagenase Santyl** (Ross)	**Ointment:** 250 units collagenase enzyme/g.	White petrolatum. In 15 and 30 g.

COLLAGENASE — TOPICAL

Indications

➤*Dermal ulcers:* For debriding chronic dermal ulcers and severely burned areas.

Administration and Dosage

Collagenase ointment should be applied once daily (or more frequently if the dressing becomes soiled, as from incontinence). When clinically indicated, crosshatching thick eschar with a No. 10 blade allows collagenase ointment more surface contact with necrotic debris. It is also more desirable to remove, with forceps and scissors, as much loosened detritus as can be done readily. Use collagenase ointment in the following manner:

➤*Instructions for use:*

1.) Prior to application the wound should be cleansed of debris and digested material by gently rubbing with a gauze pad saturated with normal saline solution, or with the desired cleansing agent compatible with collagenase ointment, followed by a normal saline solution rinse.
2.) Whenever infection is present, it is desirable to use an appropriate topical antibiotic powder. The antibiotic should be applied to the wound prior to the application of collagenase ointment. Should the infection not respond, therapy with collagenase ointment should be discontinued until remission of the infection.
3.) Collagenase ointment may be applied directly to the wound or to a sterile gauze pad, which is then applied to the wound and properly secured.
4.) Use of the collagenase ointment should be terminated when debridement of necrotic tissue is completed and granulation tissue is well established.

➤*Storage/Stability:* Do not store above 25°C (77°F). Sterility is guaranteed until the tube is opened.

Actions

➤*Pharmacology:* Since collagen accounts for 75% of the dry weight of skin tissue, the ability of collagenase to digest collagen in the physiological pH and temperature range makes it particularly effective in the removal of detritus. Collagenase thus contributes towards the formation of granulation tissue and subsequent epithelization of dermal ulcers and severely burned areas. Collagen in healthy tissue or in newly formed granulation tissue is not attacked.

Contraindications

Local or systemic hypersensitivity to collagenase.

Precautions

➤*Monitoring:* Monitor debilitated patients closely for systematic bacterial infections because of the theoretical possibility that debriding enzymes may increase the risk of bacteremia.

➤*External use only:* Avoid contact with the eyes.

➤*Compatible/Incompatible solutions:* The optimal pH range of collagenase is 6 to 8. Higher or lower pH conditions will decrease the enzyme's activity and appropriate precautions should be taken. The enzymatic activity is also adversely affected by certain detergents, and heavy metal ions such as mercury and silver which are used in some antiseptics. When it is suspected such materials have been used, the site should be carefully cleansed by repeated washings with normal saline before collagenase ointment is applied. Soaks containing metal ions or acidic solutions should be avoided because of the metal ion and low pH. Cleansing materials such as hydrogen peroxide, Dakin's solution, and normal saline are compatible with the collagenase ointment.

➤*Erythema:* A slight transient erythema has been noted occasionally in the surrounding tissue, particularly when collagenase ointment was not confined to the wound. Therefore, apply the ointment carefully within the area of the wound.

➤*Children:* Safety and efficacy in pediatric patients have not been established.

Adverse Reactions

➤*Hypersensitivity:* No allergic sensitivity or toxic reactions have been noted in clinical use when used as directed. However, 1 case of systemic manifestations of hypersensitivity to collagenase in a patient treated for more than 1 year with a combination of collagenase and cortisone has been reported.

COLLAGENASE — TOPICAL

Overdosage

➤*Treatment:* If deemed necessary, the enzymes may be inactivated by washing the area with povidone iodine.

ENZYME COMBINATIONS, TOPICAL

Rx	**Granul-Derm** (Qualitest)	**Aerosol**: 0.1 mg trypsin, 72.5 mg balsam peru, and 650 mg castor oil per 0.82 mL	In 113.4 g.
Rx	**Granulex** (Bertek)	**Aerosol**: 0.12 mg trypsin, 87 mg balsam peru, and 788 mg castor oil per g	In 113.4 g.
Rx	**Ethezyme** (Ethex)	**Ointment**: 1.1 × 10^6 units papain and 100 mg urea per g	Hydrophilic base. EDTA, glycerin, parabens. In 30 g.
Rx	**Accuzyme** (Healthpoint)	**Ointment**: 8.3 × 10^5 units papain and 100 mg urea per g	Hydrophilic base. Glycerin, parabens. In 30 g.
Rx	**Ethezyme 830** (Ethex)		Hydrophilic base. EDTA, glycerin, parabens. In 30 g.
Rx	**Gladase** (Smith & Nephew)		Glycerin, parabens. In 30 g.
Rx	**Papain-Urea-Chlorophyllin** (Cypress)	**Ointment**: ≥ 521,700 units papain, 10% urea, 0.5% chlorophyllin copper complex sodium per g	Glycerin, parabens. In 30 g.
Rx	**Gladase-C** (Smith & Nephew)		Boric acid, glyceryl stearate, glycerin, stearyl alcohol, parabens. In 6 and 30 g.
Rx	**Panafil** (Healthpoint)		Hydrophilic base. Boric acid, chlorobutanol (anhydrous), propylene glycol, stearyl alcohol, white petrolatum. In 30 g.
Rx	**Panafil** (Healthpoint)	**Spray**: ≥ 521,700 units papain, 10% urea, 0.5% chlorophyllin copper complex sodium per g	Ceteary alcohol, glycerin, lactose (anhydrous), mineral oil, parabens. In 33 mL.
Rx	**Accuzyme** (Healthpoint)	**Spray**: 8.3 × 10^5 units papain and 10% urea per g	Anhydrous lactose, cetearyl alcohol, glycerin, mineral oil, parabens. In 33 mL.

ENZYME COMBINATIONS — TOPICAL

Indications

➤*Topical lesions:* For debridement of necrotic tissue and liquefication of slough in acute and chronic lesions such as pressure ulcers, varicose, diabetic, and decubitus ulcers, burns, postoperative wounds, pilonidal cyst wounds, carbuncles, and miscellaneous traumatic or infected wounds. Also stimulates vascular bed activity to improve epithelization.

Administration and Dosage

➤*Cleansing:* Cleanse the wound prior to application with wound cleanser or saline. For papain-containing products, avoid cleansing with hydrogen peroxide solution because it may inactivate papain.

➤*Aerosol:* Shake well. Hold upright and approximately 12 inches from the area to be treated. Press valve and coat wound rapidly. Wound may be left unbandaged or a wet dressing may be applied. Apply 2 to 3 times daily, or as often as necessary. To remove, wash gently with water.

➤*Ointment:* Apply ointment directly to the wound, cover with appropriate dressing, and secure into place. Daily or twice daily applications are preferred. Irrigate the wound at each redressing to remove any accumulation of liquefied necrotic material.

Longer intervals between redressings (2 or 3 days) have proved satisfactory, and ointment may be applied under pressure dressings.

➤*Spray:* In accordance with good wound care practices, protect the periwound with a skin protectant of choice to prevent and/or reduce maceration and irritation caused by drainage from the wound. When practicable, daily or twice daily changes of dressings are preferred. Longer intervals between redressings (2 or 3 days) have proved satisfactory, and spray may be applied under pressure dressings.

Instructions for use – Shake well. Upon initial use only, the spray pump will need to be primed. Begin first time use by holding spray upright directly over the wound, and prime the pump 6 to 8 times.

Once the pump has been primed, hold the spray bottle approximately 2 to 3 inches from the wound and use even, firm, and consistent pressure to dispense product. When sprayed from the appropriate distance, the spray should appear in a nickel-sized diameter.

Completely cover the wound site with spray. The wound should not be visible under the product. Cover wound with appropriate dressing of choice (eg, saline-moistened gauze, semi-occlusive dressings), and secure into place.

Spray is designed to be used at an angle; however, as the product is dispensed, it may be necessary to hold the spray bottle in an upright position to achieve a full pump.

➤*Storage/Stability:*

Aerosol – Do not store above 120°F.

Ointment – Store at 15° to 30°C (59° to 86°F).

Spray – Store upright at 20° to 25°C (68° to 77°F) for *Panafil* and 8° to 15°C (46° to 59°F) for *Accuzyme*. Do not refrigerate.

Contraindications

Sensitivity to papain or any other components of these preparations.

Warnings

➤*Arterial clots:* Do not spray aerosol products on fresh arterial clots.

➤*For external use only:* Avoid contact with the eyes.

➤*Transient burning:* Transient burning may occur upon application.

➤*Papain:* Papain may be inactivated by the salts of heavy metals such as lead, silver, and mercury. Avoid contact with medications containing these metals.

Adverse Reactions

Generally well-tolerated and nonirritating. A transient burning sensation may be experienced by a small percentage of patients upon application. Occasionally, the profuse exudate from enzymatic digestion may irritate the skin. In such cases, more frequent dressing changes will alleviate discomfort until exudate decreases.

Patient Information

Changing the dressing more often may help if irritation occurs.

In sensitive areas, temporary stinging or burning sensation may occur.

IMMUNOMODULATORS, TOPICAL

IMIQUIMOD

Rx	**Aldara** (3M Pharm)	**Cream**: 5%	Cetyl alcohol, stearyl alcohol, white petrolatum, benzyl alcohol, parabens. In single-use packets. In boxes of 12.

IMIQUIMOD — TOPICAL

Indications

➤*Actinic keratosis:* For the topical treatment of clinically typical, nonhyperkeratotic, nonhypertrophic actinic keratoses on the face or scalp in immunocompetent adults.

➤*Superficial basal cell carcinoma:* For the topical treatment of biopsy-confirmed, primary superficial basal cell carcinoma (sBCC) in immunocompetent adults, with a maximum tumor diameter of 2 cm, located on the trunk (excluding anogenital skin), neck, or extremities (excluding hands and feet), only when surgical methods are medically less appropriate and patient follow-up can be reasonably assured. Establish the histological diagnosis of sBCC prior to treatment because safety and efficacy of imiquimod 5% cream have not been established for other types of basal cell carcinomas, including nodular, morpheaform (fibrosing or sclerosing) types.

➤*Genital and perianal warts:* For the treatment of external genital and perianal warts/condyloma acuminata in patients 12 years of age or older.

Administration and Dosage

➤*Approved by the FDA:* February 27, 1997.

➤*For external use only:* Imiquimod cream is not for ophthalmic use.

➤*Actinic keratosis:* Apply 2 times per week for 16 weeks to a defined treatment area on the face or scalp (but not both concurrently). The treatment area should be one contiguous area of approximately 25 cm^2 (eg, 5 cm × 5 cm). Apply imiquimod cream to the entire treatment area (eg, forehead, scalp, one cheek).

Administration – Before applying the cream, wash the treatment area with mild soap and water and allow the area to dry thoroughly (at least

IMIQUIMOD — TOPICAL

10 minutes). Apply no more than 1 packet of imiquimod cream to the contiguous treatment area at each application. Imiquimod cream is applied prior to normal sleeping hours, and left on the skin for approximately 8 hours, after which time the cream is removed by washing the area with mild soap and water. Rub the cream into the treatment area until the cream is no longer visible. Avoid contact with the eyes, lips and nostrils. Examples of 2 times per week application schedules are Monday and Thursday, or Tuesday and Friday prior to sleeping hours. Imiquimod cream treatment should continue for the full 16 weeks. However, do not extend the treatment period beyond 16 weeks due to missed doses or rest periods. Local skin reactions in the treatment area are common. Patients should contact their health care providers if they experience any sign or symptom in the treatment area that restricts or prohibits their daily activity or makes continued application of the cream difficult. A rest period of several days may be taken if required by the patient's discomfort or severity of the local skin reaction. Demonstrate the technique for proper dose administration to maximize the benefit of imiquimod cream therapy. Handwashing before and after cream application is recommended.

Carefully reevaluate lesions that do not respond to therapy and reconsider management.

➤*sBCC:* Apply 5 times per week for 6 weeks to a biopsy-confirmed sBCC. The target tumor should have a maximum diameter of no more than 2 cm and be located on the trunk (excluding anogenital skin), neck, or extremities (excluding hands and feet). The treatment area should include a 1 cm margin of skin around the tumor.

Administration – Imiquimod cream is to be applied 5 times per week, prior to normal sleeping hours, and left on the skin for approximately 8 hours. Before applying the cream, wash the treatment area with mild soap and water and allow the area to dry thoroughly. Apply sufficient cream to cover the treatment area, including one centimeter of skin surrounding the tumor. Rub the cream into the treatment area until the cream is no longer visible. Avoid contact with the eyes. Following the treatment period, remove the cream by washing the area with mild soap and water. An example of a 5 times per week application schedule is to apply imiquimod cream, once per day, Monday through Friday, prior to sleeping hours. Imiquimod cream treatment should continue for 6 weeks. Local skin reactions in the treatment area are common. Patients should contact their health care providers if they experience any sign or symptom in the treatment area that restricts or prohibits their daily activity or makes continued application of the cream difficult. A rest period of several days may be taken if required by the patient's discomfort or severity of the local skin reaction. Demonstrate the technique for proper dose administration to maximize the benefit of imiquimod cream therapy. Handwashing before and after cream application is recommended.

Early clinical clearance: Early clinical clearance cannot be adequately assessed until resolution of local skin reactions. It is appropriate to have the first follow-up visit at approximately 12 weeks posttreatment to assess the treatment site for clinical clearance. Local skin reactions or other findings (eg, infection) may require that a patient be seen sooner than the 12-week posttreatment visit. If there is clinical evidence of persistent tumor at the 12-week posttreatment assessment, consider a biopsy or other alternative intervention; the safety and efficacy of a repeat course of imiquimod cream treatment have not been established. If any suspicious lesion arises in the treatment area at any time after 12 weeks, the patient should seek a medical evaluation.

Target Tumor Diameter	Size of Cream Droplet to Be Used (diameter)	Approximate Amount of Cream to Be Used
0.5 to < 1 cm	4 mm	10 mg
≥ 1 to < 1.5 cm	5 mm	25 mg
≥ 1.5 to 2 cm	7 mm	40 mg

➤*Genital and perianal warts:*

Administration – Imiquimod cream is to be applied 3 times per week, prior to normal sleeping hours, and left on the skin for 6 to 10 hours. Instruct patients to apply imiquimod cream to external genital/perianal warts. A thin layer is applied to the wart area and rubbed in until the cream is no longer visible. The application site is not to be occluded. Following the treatment period, remove the cream by washing the treated area with mild soap and water. Examples of 3 times per week application schedules are: Monday, Wednesday, Friday; or Tuesday, Thursday, Saturday application prior to sleeping hours. Continue imiquimod cream treatment until there is total clearance of the genital/perianal warts or for a maximum of 16 weeks.

Demonstrate the technique for proper dose administration to maximize the benefit of imiquimod cream therapy. Handwashing before and after cream application is recommended. Local skin reactions (erythema) at the treatment site are common. A rest period of several days may be taken if required by the patient's discomfort or severity of the local skin reaction. Treatment may resume once the reaction subsides.

Nonocclusive dressings such as cotton gauze or cotton underwear may be used in the management of skin reactions.

➤*Storage/Stability:* Store below 25°C (77°F). Avoid freezing.

Actions

➤*Pharmacology:*

Actinic keratosis – The mechanism of action of imiquimod cream in treating actinic keratosis lesions is unknown. In a study of 18 patients with actinic keratosis comparing imiquimod cream with vehicle, increases from baseline in week 2 biomarker levels were reported for CD3, CD4, CD8, CD11c, and CD68 for imiquimod cream treated patients; however, the clinical relevance of these findings is unknown.

sBCC – The mechanism of action of imiquimod cream in treating sBCC lesions is unknown. An open label study in 6 subjects with sBCC suggests that treatment with imiquimod cream may increase the infiltration of lymphocytes, dendritic cells, and macrophages into the tumor lesion; however, the clinical significance of these findings is unknown.

Genital and perianal warts – Imiquimod is an immune response modifier. Imiquimod has no direct antiviral activity in cell culture. A study in 22 patients with genital/perianal warts comparing imiquimod and vehicle shows that imiquimod induces mRNA encoding cytokines including interferon-α at the treatment site. In addition HPVL1 mRNA and HPV DNA are significantly decreased following treatment. However, the clinical relevance of these findings is unknown.

➤*Pharmacokinetics:*

Absorption – Systemic absorption of imiquimod was observed across the affected skin of 12 patients with genital/perianal warts, with an average dose of 4.6 mg. Mean peak drug concentration of approximately 0.4 ng/mL was seen during the study. Mean urinary recoveries of imiquimod and metabolites combined over the whole course of treatment, expressed as percent of the estimated applied dose, were 0.11 and 2.41% in the men and women, respectively.

Systemic absorption of imiquimod across the affected skin of 58 patients with actinic keratosis was observed with a dosing frequency of 3 applications per week for 16 weeks.

Mean Serum Imiquimod Concentration Following Administration of the Last Topical Dose During Week 16	
Amount of imiquimod cream applied	Mean peak serum imiquimod concentration (C_{max})
12.5 mg (1 packet)	0.1 ng/mL
25 mg (2 packets)	0.2 ng/mL
75 mg (6 packets)	3.5 ng/mL

Metabolism/Excretion – The application surface area was not controlled when more than 1 packet was used. Dose proportionality was not observed. However, it appears that systemic exposure may be more dependent on surface area of application than amount of applied dose. The apparent half-life was approximately 10 times greater with topical dosing than the 2 hour apparent half-life seen following subcutaneous dosing, suggesting prolonged retention of drug in the skin. Mean urinary recoveries of imiquimod and metabolites combined were 0.08% and 0.15% of the applied dose in the group using 75 mg (6 packets) for men and women, respectively, following 3 applications per week for 16 weeks.

Contraindications

Sensitivity reactions to any of its components. Discontinue if hypersensitivity to any of its ingredients is noted.

Warnings

➤*Other types of basal cell carcinomas:* The diagnosis of sBCC should be confirmed prior to treatment, since safety and efficacy of imiquimod cream have not been established for other types of basal cell carcinomas, including nodular, morpheaform (fibrosing or sclerosing) types and is not recommended for treatment of BCC subtypes other than the superficial variant (ie, sBCC). Patients with sBCC treated with imiquimod cream are recommended to have regular follow-up of the treatment site.

Estimated Clinical Clearance Rates for sBCC				
Follow-up visit after 12-week posttreatment assessment	No. of subjects who remained clinically clear	No. of subjects with sBCC recurrence	No. of subjects who discontinued at this visit with no sBCC[a]	Estimated rate of patients who clinically cleared and remained clear[b]
Month 3	153	4	5	87%
Month 6	149	4	0	85%
Month 12	143	2	4	84%
Month 24	139	4	0	79%

[a] Reasons for discontinuation included death, noncompliance, entry criteria violations, personal reasons, and treatment of nearby sBCC tumor.
[b] Estimated rate of patients who clinically cleared and remained clear are estimated based on the time to event analysis employing the life table method beginning with the rate of clinical clearance at 12 weeks posttreatment.

➤*Human papilloma viral disease:* Imiquimod cream has not been evaluated for the treatment of urethral, intravaginal, cervical, rectal, or intra-anal human papilloma viral disease and is not recommended for these conditions.

➤*Carcinogenesis:* In a dermal mouse carcinogenicity study, imiquimod cream (up to 5 mg/kg/application imiquimod or 0.3% imiquimod cream) was applied to the backs of mice 3 times per week for 24 months. A statistically significant increase in the incidence of liver adenomas and carcinomas was noted in high dose male mice compared with control male mice (251 × maximum recommended human dose [MRHD] based on weekly AUC comparisons). An increased number of skin papillomas was observed in vehicle cream control group animals at the treated site only. The quantitative com-

IMIQUIMOD — TOPICAL

position of the vehicle cream used in the dermal mouse carcinogenicity study is the same as the vehicle cream used for imiquimod cream, minus the active moiety (imiquimod).

➤*Elderly:* No overall differences in safety or efficacy were observed between these patients and younger patients. No other clinical experience has identified differences in responses between the elderly and younger patients, but greater sensitivity of some older individuals cannot be ruled out.

➤*Pregnancy: Category C.* Systemic embryofetal development studies were conducted in rats and rabbits. Oral dosages of 1, 5, and 20 mg/kg/day imiquimod were administered during the period of organogenesis (gestational days 6 to 15) to pregnant female rats. In the presence of maternal toxicity, fetal effects noted at 20 mg/kg/day [8 × MRHD based on body surface area (BSA) comparisons] included increased resorptions, decreased fetal body weights, delays in skeletal ossification, bent limb bones, and 2 fetuses in 1 litter (2 of 1,567 fetuses) demonstrated exencephaly, protruding tongues, and low-set ears. No treatment related effects on embryofetal toxicity or teratogenicity were noted at 5 mg/kg/day (55 × MRHD based on AUC comparisons).

A combined fertility and peri- and postnatal development study was conducted in rats. Oral doses of 1, 1.5, 3, and 6 mg/kg/day imiquimod were administered to male rats from 70 days prior to mating through the mating period and to female rats from 14 days prior to mating through parturition and lactation. No effects on growth, fertility, reproduction, or postnatal development were noted at dosages up to 6 mg/kg/day (87 × MRHD based on AUC comparisons), the highest dose evaluated in this study. In the absence of maternal toxicity, bent limb bones were noted in the F1 fetuses at a dose of 6 mg/kg/day (87 × MRHD based on AUC comparisons). This fetal effect was also noted in the oral rat embryofetal development study conducted with imiquimod. No treatment related effects on teratogenicity were noted at 3 mg/kg/day (41 × MRHD based on AUC comparisons).

There are no adequate and well-controlled studies in pregnant women. Use imiquimod cream during pregnancy only if the potential benefit justifies the potential risk to the fetus.

➤*Lactation:* It is not known whether topically applied imiquimod is excreted in breast milk.

➤*Children:* Safety and efficacy in patients with external genital/perianal warts younger than 12 years of age have not been established.

Actinic keratosis and sBCC are not conditions generally seen within the pediatric population. The safety and efficacy of imiquimod cream for actinic keratosis or sBCC in patients younger than 18 years of age have not been established.

Precautions

➤*Immunosuppressed patients:* The safety and efficacy of imiquimod cream in immunosuppressed patients have not been established.

➤*Previous drug or surgical treatment:* Imiquimod cream administration is not recommended until the skin is completely healed from any previous drug or surgical treatment.

➤*Inflammatory conditions:* Imiquimod has the potential to exacerbate inflammatory conditions of the skin.

➤*Actinic keratosis:* Safety and efficacy have not been established for imiquimod cream in the treatment of actinic keratosis with repeated use (ie, more than one treatment course) in the same 25 cm^2 area.

The safety of imiquimod cream applied to areas of skin greater than 25 cm^2 (eg, 5 cm × 5 cm) for the treatment of actinic keratosis has not been established.

➤*sBCC:* The safety and efficacy of treating sBCC lesions on the face, head and anogenital area have not been established.

Basal cell nevus syndrome or xeroderma pigmentosum – The efficacy and safety of imiquimod cream have not been established for patients with basal cell nevus syndrome or xeroderma pigmentosum.

➤*Genital and perianal warts:* Local skin reactions (erythema) at the treatment site are common. A rest period of several days may be taken if required by the patient's discomfort or severity of the local skin reaction. Treatment may resume once the reaction subsides.

➤*Nonocclusive dressings:* Nonocclusive dressings such as cotton gauze or cotton underwear may be used in the management of skin reactions.

➤*Photosensitivity:* Avoid exposure to sunlight (including sunlamps) or minimize it during use of imiquimod cream because of concern for heightened sunburn susceptibility. Warn patients to use protective clothing (hat) when using imiquimod cream. Advise patients with sunburn not to use imiquimod cream until fully recovered. Patients who may have considerable sun exposure (eg, due to their occupations) and those patients with inherent sensitivity to sunlight should exercise caution when using imiquimod cream. Phototoxicity has not been adequately assessed for imiquimod cream. The enhancement of ultraviolet carcinogenicity is not necessarily dependent on phototoxic mechanisms. Despite the absence of observed phototoxicity in humans, imiquimod cream shortened the time to skin tumor formation in an animal photoco-carcinogenicity study. Therefore, it is prudent for patients to minimize or avoid natural or artificial sunlight exposure.

Adverse Reactions

Dermal safety studies involving induction and challenge phases produced no evidence that imiquimod cream causes photoallergenicity or contact sensitization in healthy skin; however, cumulative irritancy testing revealed the potential for imiquimod cream to cause irritation, and in the clinical studies application site reactions were reported in a significant percentage of study patients. Phototoxicity testing was incomplete as wavelengths in the UVB range were not included and imiquimod cream has peak absorption in the UVB range (320 nm) of the light spectrum.

➤*Actinic keratosis:* The data described below reflect exposure to imiquimod cream or vehicle in 436 patients enrolled in 2 double-blind, vehicle-controlled, 2 times per week studies. Patients applied imiquimod cream or vehicle to a 25 cm^2 contiguous treatment area on the face or scalp 2 times per week for 16 weeks.

Summary of All Adverse Reactions Reported by > 1% of Patients in the Combined 2 Times Per Week Studies

Body system/Preferred term	Imiquimod 2 times per week (n = 215)	Vehicle 2 times per week (n = 221)
Application site reaction	71 (33%)	32 (14.5%)
Cardiovascular		
Atrial fibrillation	3 (1.4%)	2 (0.9%)
Chest pain	1 (0.5%)	4 (1.8%)
Hypertension	3 (1.4%)	5 (2.3%)
CNS		
Dizziness	3 (1.4%)	1 (0.5%)
Dermatologic	47 (21.9%)	42 (19%)
Alopecia	3 (1.4%)	0
Dermatitis	3 (1.4%)	7 (3.2%)
Eczema	4 (1.9%)	3 (1.4%)
Hyperkeratosis	19 (8.8%)	12 (5.4%)
Photosensitivity reaction	2 (0.9%)	4 (1.8%)
Pruritus	2 (0.9%)	3 (1.4%)
Rash	5 (2.3%)	5 (2.3%)
Skin disorder	6 (2.8%)	7 (3.2%)
Verruca	1 (0.5%)	3 (1.4%)
GI		
Diarrhea	6 (2.8%)	2 (0.9%)
Dyspepsia	6 (2.8%)	4 (1.8%)
Gastroesophageal reflux	3 (1.4%)	3 (1.4%)
Nausea	3 (1.4%)	3 (1.4%)
Vomiting	3 (1.4%)	1 (0.5%)
GU	8 (3.7%)	10 (4.5%)
Urinary tract infection	3 (1.4%)	1 (0.5%)
Metabolic and nutritional		
Hypercholesterolemia	4 (1.9%)	0
Musculoskeletal		
Arthralgia	2 (0.9%)	4 (1.8%)
Arthritis	2 (0.9%)	3 (1.4%)
Myalgia	3 (1.4%)	3 (1.4%)
Skeletal pain	1 (0.5%)	3 (1.4%)
Ophthalmic		
Conjunctivitis	1 (0.5%)	3 (1.4%)
Eye abnormality	4 (1.9%)	1 (0.5%)
Eye infection	0	3 (1.4%)
Respiratory		
Bronchitis	2 (0.9%)	3 (1.4%)
Coughing	6 (2.8%)	10 (4.5%)
Pharyngitis	4 (1.9%)	4 (1.8%)
Pulmonary congestion	1 (0.5%)	3 (1.4%)
Rhinitis	7 (3.3%)	8 (3.6%)
Sinusitis	16 (7.4%)	14 (6.3%)
Upper respiratory tract infection	33 (15.3%)	27 (12.2%)
Miscellaneous		
Abrasion NOS[a]	7 (3.3%)	5 (2.3%)
Back pain	3 (1.4%)	2 (0.9%)
Basal cell carcinoma	5 (2.3%)	5 (2.3%)
Carcinoma squamous	8 (3.7%)	5 (2.3%)
Cyst NOS	0	4 (1.8%)
Fatigue	3 (1.4%)	2 (0.9%)
Fever	3 (1.4%)	0
Headache	11 (5.1%)	7 (3.2%)
Hernia NOS	4 (1.9%)	1 (0.5%)
Herpes simplex	4 (1.9%)	4 (1.8%)

IMIQUIMOD — TOPICAL

Summary of All Adverse Reactions Reported by > 1% of Patients in the Combined 2 Times Per Week Studies

Body system/Preferred term	Imiquimod 2 times per week (n = 215)	Vehicle 2 times per week (n = 221)
Inflicted injury	19 (8.8%)	21 (9.5%)
Influenza-like symptoms	4 (1.9%)	4 (1.8%)
Pain	3 (1.4%)	3 (1.4%)
Postoperative pain	3 (1.4%)	4 (1.8%)
Resistance mechanism disorders	9 (4.2%)	11 (5%)
Rigors	3 (1.4%)	0
Viral infection	3 (1.4%)	2 (0.9%)

[a] NOS = not otherwise specified.

Summary of All Application Site Reactions Reported by > 1% of Patients in the Combined 2 Times Per Week Studies

Included term	Imiquimod 2 times per week (n = 215)	Vehicle 2 times per week (n = 221)
Bleeding at target site	7 (3.3%)	1 (0.5%)
Burning at remote site	4 (1.9%)	0 (0%)
Burning at target site	12 (5.6%)	4 (1.8%)
Induration at remote site	3 (1.4%)	0 (0%)
Induration at target site	5 (2.3%)	3 (1.4%)
Irritation at remote site	3 (1.4%)	0 (0%)
Itching at remote site	7 (3.3%)	3 (1.4%)
Itching at target site	44 (20.5%)	15 (6.8%)
Pain at target site	5 (2.3%)	2 (0.9%)
Stinging at target site	6 (2.8%)	2 (0.9%)
Tenderness at target site	4 (1.9%)	3 (1.4%)

Local skin reactions were collected independently of the adverse reaction "application site reaction" in an effort to provide a better picture of the specific types of local reactions that might be seen. The most frequently reported local skin reactions were erythema, flaking/scaling/dryness, and scabbing/crusting. The prevalence and severity of local skin reactions that occurred during controlled studies are shown in the following table.

Local Skin Reactions in the Treatment Area as Assessed by the Investigator (Percentage of Patients) 2 Times Per Week Application

	Mild/Moderate/Severe		Severe	
	Imiquimod cream (n = 215)	Vehicle (n = 220)	Imiquimod cream (n = 215)	Vehicle (n = 220)
Edema	106 (49%)	22 (10%)	0	0
Erosion/Ulceration	103 (48%)	20 (9%)	5 (2%)	0
Erythema	209 (97%)	206 (93%)	38 (18%)	5 (2%)
Flaking/Scaling/Dryness	199 (93%)	199 (91%)	16 (7%)	7 (3%)
Scabbing/Crusting	169 (79%)	92 (42%)	18 (8%)	4 (2%)
Vesicles	19 (9%)	2 (1%)	0	0
Weeping/Exudate	45 (22%)	3 (1%)	0	0

The adverse reactions that most frequently resulted in clinical intervention (eg, rest periods, withdrawal from study) were local skin and application site reactions. Overall, in the clinical studies, 2% (5/215) of patients discontinued for local skin/application site reactions. Of the 215 patients treated, 35 patients (16%) on imiquimod cream and 3 of 220 patients (1%) on vehicle cream had at least 1 rest period. Of these imiquimod cream patients, 32 (91%) resumed therapy after a rest period.

In the actinic keratosis studies, 22 of 678 imiquimod treated patients developed treatment site infections that required a rest period off imiquimod cream and were treated with antibiotics (19 with oral and 3 with topical).

➤*sBCC:* The data described below reflect exposure to imiquimod cream or vehicle in 364 patients enrolled in 2 double-blind, vehicle-controlled, 5 times per week studies. Patients applied imiquimod cream or vehicle 5 times per week for 6 weeks. The incidence of adverse reactions reported by greater than 1% of subjects during the 6 week treatment period is summarized in the following table.

Summary of All Adverse Reactions Reported by > 1% of Patients in the Combined 5 Times Per Week Studies

Body system/ Preferred term	Imiquimod 5 times per week (n = 185)	Vehicle 5 times per week (n = 179)
Application site disorders		
Application site reaction	52 (28.1%)	5 (2.8%)
Cardiovascular		
Hypertension	5 (2.7%)	1 (0.6%)
CNS		
Anxiety	2 (1.1%)	1 (0.6%)
Dizziness	2 (1.1%)	1 (0.6%)
Headache	14 (7.6%)	4 (2.2%)
Dermatologic		
Hyperkeratosis	3 (1.6%)	2 (1.1%)
Rash	3 (1.6%)	1 (0.6%)
Skin disorder	1 (0.5%)	3 (1.7%)
GI		
Abdominal pain	1 (0.5%)	2 (1.1%)
Diarrhea	1 (0.5%)	2 (1.1%)
Dyspepsia	3 (1.6%)	2 (1.1%)
GI disorder NOS[a]	1 (0.5%)	2 (1.1%)
Nausea	2 (1.1%)	0
Tooth disorder	0	2 (1.1%)
Metabolic/Nutritional		
Gout	2 (1.1%)	0
Musculoskeletal		
Skeletal pain	3 (1.6%)	2 (1.1%)
Respiratory		
Coughing	3 (1.6%)	1 (0.6%)
Pharyngitis	2 (1.1%)	1 (0.6%)
Rhinitis	5 (2.7%)	1 (0.6%)
Sinusitis	4 (2.2%)	1 (0.6%)
Upper respiratory tract infection	6 (3.2%)	2 (1.1%)
Miscellaneous		
Aggravated allergy	2 (1.1%)	1 (0.6%)
Back pain	7 (3.8%)	1 (0.6%)
Chest pain	2 (1.1%)	0
Fatigue	4 (2.2%)	2 (1.1%)
Fever	3 (1.6%)	0
Infection	1 (0.5%)	3 (1.7%)
Infection fungal	2 (1.1%)	2 (1.1%)
Inflicted injury	3 (1.6%)	3 (1.7%)
Lymphadenopathy	5 (2.7%)	1 (0.6%)
Pain	3 (1.6%)	2 (1.1%)
Procedural site reaction	2 (1.1%)	3 (1.7%)

[a] NOS = not otherwise specified.

In controlled clinical studies, the most frequently reported adverse reactions were local skin and application site reactions including erythema, edema, induration, erosion, flaking/scaling, scabbing/crusting, itching and burning at the application site. The incidence of the application site reactions reported by greater than 1% of the subjects during the 6 week treatment period is summarized in the following table.

IMIQUIMOD — TOPICAL

Summary of All Application Site Reactions Reported by > 1% of Patients in the Combined 5 Times Per Week Studies		
Included term	Imiquimod 5 times per week (n = 185)	Vehicle 5 times per week (n = 179)
Bleeding at target site	4 (2.2%)	0
Burning at target site	11 (5.9%)	2 (1.1%)
Erythema at remote site	3 (1.6%)	0
Infection at target site	2 (1.1%)	0
Itching at target site	30 (16.2%)	1 (0.6%)
Pain at target site	6 (3.2%)	0
Papule(s) at target site	3 (1.6%)	0
Tenderness at target site	2 (1.1%)	0
Tingling at target site	1 (0.5%)	2 (1.1%)

Local skin reactions were collected independently of the adverse reaction "application site reaction" in an effort to provide a better picture of the specific types of local reactions that might be seen. The prevalence and severity of local skin reactions that occurred during controlled studies are shown in the following table.

Most Intense Local Skin Reactions in the Treatment Area as Assessed by the Investigator (Percentage of Patients) 5 Times Per Week Application				
	Mild/Moderate		Severe	
	Imiquimod cream (n = 184)	Vehicle (n = 178)	Imiquimod cream (n = 184)	Vehicle (n = 178)
Edema	71%	36%	7%	0%
Erosion	54%	14%	13%	0%
Erythema	69%	95%	31%	2%
Flaking/Scaling	87%	76%	4%	0%
Induration	78%	53%	6%	0%
Scabbing/Crusting	64%	34%	19%	0%
Ulceration	34%	3%	6%	0%
Vesicles	29%	2%	2%	0%

The adverse reactions that most frequently resulted in clinical intervention (eg, rest periods, withdrawal from study) were local skin and application site reactions; 10% (19/185) of patients received rest periods. The average number of doses not received per patient due to rest periods was 7 doses with a range of 2 to 22 doses; 79% of patients (15/19) resumed therapy after a rest period. Overall, in the clinical studies, 2% (4/185) of patients discontinued for local skin/application site reactions.

In the sBCC studies, 17 of 1,266 (1.3%) imiquimod-treated patients developed treatment site infections that required a rest period off imiquimod cream and were treated with antibiotics.

➤*External genital warts:* In controlled clinical trials for genital warts, the most frequently reported adverse reactions were those of local skin and application site reactions; some patients also reported systemic reactions. These reactions were usually mild to moderate in intensity; however, severe reactions were reported with 3 times a week application. These reactions were more frequent and more intense with daily application than with 3 times a week application. Overall, in the 3 times a week application clinical studies, 1.2% (4 out of 327) of the patients discontinued due to local skin/application site reactions. The incidence and severity of local skin reactions during controlled clinical trials are shown in the following table:

Wart Site Reaction as Assessed by Investigator (Percentage of Patients) 3 Times Per Week Application								
	Mild/ Moderate/ Severe				Severe			
	Women		Men		Women		Men	
	Imiquimod cream (n = 114)	Vehicle (n = 99)	Imiquimod cream (n = 156)	Vehicle (n = 157)	Imiquimod cream (n = 114)	Vehicle (n = 99)	Imiquimod cream (n = 156)	Vehicle (n = 157)
Edema	20 (18%)	5 (5%)	19 (12%)	1 (1%)	1 (1%)	0 (0%)	0 (0%)	0 (0%)
Erosion	35 (31%)	8 (8%)	47 (30%)	10 (6%)	1 (1%)	0 (0%)	2 (1%)	0 (0%)

Wart Site Reaction as Assessed by Investigator (Percentage of Patients) 3 Times Per Week Application								
	Mild/ Moderate/ Severe				Severe			
	Women		Men		Women		Men	
	Imiquimod cream (n = 114)	Vehicle (n = 99)	Imiquimod cream (n = 156)	Vehicle (n = 157)	Imiquimod cream (n = 114)	Vehicle (n = 99)	Imiquimod cream (n = 156)	Vehicle (n = 157)
Erythema	74 (65%)	21 (21%)	90 (58%)	34 (22%)	4 (4%)	0 (0%)	6 (4%)	0 (0%)
Excoriation/ Flaking	21 (18%)	8 (8%)	40 (26%)	12 (8%)	0 (0%)	0 (0%)	1 (1%)	0 (0%)
Induration	6 (5%)	2 (2%)	11 (7%)	3 (2%)	0 (0%)	0 (0%)	0 (0%)	0 (0%)
Scabbing	4 (4%)	0 (0%)	20 (13%)	4 (3%)	0 (0%)	0 (0%)	0 (0%)	0 (0%)
Ulceration	9 (8%)	1 (1%)	7 (4%)	1 (1%)	3 (3%)	0 (0%)	0 (0%)	0 (0%)
Vesicles	3 (3%)	0 (0%)	3 (2%)	0 (0%)	0 (0%)	0 (0%)	0 (0%)	0 (0%)

Remote site skin reactions were also reported in men and women treated 3 times a week with imiquimod 5% cream. The severe remote site skin reactions reported for women were erythema (3%), ulceration (2%), and edema (1%); and for men, erosion (2%), and erythema, edema, induration, and excoriation/flaking (each 1%).

Adverse reactions judged to be probably or possibly related to imiquimod cream reported by greater than 5% of patients are listed in the following table; also included are soreness, influenza-like symptoms, and myalgia.

Three Times Per Week Application				
	Women		Men	
	Imiquimod 5% cream (n = 117)	Vehicle (n = 103)	Imiquimod 5% cream (n = 156)	Vehicle (n = 158)
Fungal infection[a]	11%	3%	2%	1%
Application site disorders:				
Application site reactions				
Wart site:				
Burning	26%	12%	9%	5%
Itching	32%	20%	22%	10%
Pain	8%	2%	2%	1%
Soreness	3%	0%	0%	1%
Systemic reactions:				
Headache	4%	3%	5%	2%
Influenza-like symptoms	3%	2%	1%	0%
Myalgia	1%	0%	1%	1%

[a] Incidences reported without regard to causality with imiquimod cream.

Adverse reactions judged to be possibly or probably related to imiquimod cream and reported by greater than 1% of patients included:

CNS – Headache.

GI – Diarrhea.

Local –

Wart site reactions: Burning, hypopigmentation, irritation, itching, pain, rash, sensitivity, soreness, stinging, tenderness.

Remote site reactions: Bleeding, burning, itching, pain, tenderness, tinea cruris.

Musculoskeletal – Myalgia.

Miscellaneous – Fatigue, fever, influenza-like symptoms.

Overdosage

➤*Symptoms:* Persistent topical overdosing of imiquimod 5% cream could result in severe local skin reactions. The most clinically serious adverse reaction reported following multiple oral imiquimod doses of greater than 200 mg (equivalent to imiquimod content of greater than 16 packets) was hypotension which resolved following oral or IV fluid administration.

Patient Information

This medication is to be used as directed by a doctor. It is for external use only. Avoid eye contact.

Do not bandage the treatment area or otherwise cover or wrap as to be occlusive.

Some reports have been received of localized hypopigmentation and hyperpigmentation following imiquimod use. Follow-up information suggests that these skin color changes may be permanent in some patients.

IMIQUIMOD — TOPICAL

➤*Actinic keratosis:* It is recommended that the treatment area be washed with mild soap and water 8 hours following imiquimod cream application.

It is common for patients to experience local skin reactions (can range from mild to severe in intensity) during treatment with imiquimod cream, and these reactions may extend beyond the application site onto the surrounding skin. Skin reactions generally decrease in intensity or resolve after cessation of imiquimod cream therapy. Potential local skin reactions include erythema, edema, vesicles, erosion/ulceration, weeping/exudate, flaking/scaling/dryness, and scabbing/crusting. Most patients using imiquimod cream for the treatment of actinic keratosis experience erythema, flaking/scaling/dryness and scabbing/crusting at the application site with normal dosing. Patients may also experience application site reactions such as itching and/or burning. Local skin reactions may be of such an intensity that patients may require rest periods from treatment. Treatment with imiquimod cream can be resumed after the skin reaction has subsided, as determined by the doctor. Patients should contact their doctors promptly if they experience any sign or symptom at the application site that restricts or prohibits their daily activity or makes continued application of the cream difficult.

Because of local skin reactions, during treatment and until healed, the treatment area is likely to appear noticeably different from normal skin. The skin surrounding the treatment area may also be affected, but less intensely so.

Avoid contact with the eyes, lips, and nostrils.

Use of sunscreen is encouraged; minimize or avoid exposure to natural or artificial sunlight (tanning beds or UVA/B treatment) while using imiquimod cream.

During treatment, subclinical actinic keratosis lesions may become apparent in the treatment area and may subsequently resolve.

Discard partially used packets and do not reuse.

Dosing is twice weekly for the full 16 weeks, unless otherwise directed by the doctor. However, the treatment period should not be extended beyond 16 weeks due to missed doses or rest periods.

➤*sBCC:* It is recommended that the treatment area be washed with mild soap and water 8 hours following imiquimod cream application.

Most patients using imiquimod cream for the treatment of sBCC experience erythema, edema, induration, erosion, scabbing/crusting, and flaking/scaling at the application site with normal dosing. These local skin reactions generally decrease in intensity or resolve after cessation of imiquimod cream therapy. Patients may also experience application site reactions such as itching and/or burning. Local skin reactions may be of such an intensity that patients may require rest periods from treatment. Treatment with imiquimod cream can be resumed after the skin reaction has subsided, as determined by the doctor.

During treatment and until healed, affected skin is likely to appear noticeably different from normal skin.

It is prudent for patients to minimize or avoid exposure to natural or artificial sunlight.

The clinical outcome of therapy can be determined after regeneration of the treated skin, approximately 12 weeks after the end of treatment.

Patients should contact their doctors if they experience any sign or symptom at the application site that restricts or prohibits their daily activity or makes continued application of the cream difficult.

Patients with sBCC treated with imiquimod cream are recommended to have regular follow-up to reevaluate the treatment site.

➤*External genital warts:* It is recommended that the treatment area be washed with mild soap and water 6 to 10 hours following imiquimod 5% cream application.

It is common for patients to experience local skin reactions such as erythema, erosion, excoriation/flaking, and edema at the site of application or surrounding areas. Most skin reactions are mild to moderate. Severe skin reactions can occur and should be reported promptly to the doctor. Should severe local skin reaction occur, remove the cream by washing the treatment area with mild soap and water. Treatment with imiquimod cream can be resumed after the skin reaction has subsided.

Avoid sexual (genital, anal, oral) contact while the cream is on the skin.

Application of imiquimod 5% cream in the vagina is considered internal and should be avoided. Women should take special care if applying the cream at the opening of the vagina because local skin reactions on the delicate moist surfaces can result in pain or swelling, and may cause difficulty in passing urine.

Uncircumcised men treating warts under the foreskin should retract the foreskin and clean the area daily.

Be aware that new warts may develop during therapy; imiquimod is not a cure.

The effect of imiquimod cream on the transmission of genital/perianal warts is unknown.

Imiquimod cream may weaken condoms and vaginal diaphragms; therefore, concurrent use is not recommended.

TACROLIMUS

Rx	**Protopic** (Astellas Pharma[a])	**Ointment:** 0.03%	Mineral oil, white petrolatum. In 30, 60, and 100 g.
		0.1%	Mineral oil, white petrolatum. In 30, 60, and 100 g.

[a] Astellas Pharma, 3 Parkway North Center, Deerfield, IL 60016; 800-888-7704; http://www.astellas.com.

TACROLIMUS — TOPICAL

Tacrolimus is also available as a capsule for organ rejection prophylaxis; see the Biologic and Immunologic Agents chapter.

WARNING

Long-term safety of topical calcineurin inhibitors has not been established.

Although a causal relationship has not been established, rare cases of malignancy (ie, skin cancer and lymphoma) have been reported in patients treated with topical calcineurin inhibitors, including tacrolimus ointment.

Therefore:
- Avoid continuous long-term use of topical calcineurin inhibitors, including tacrolimus ointment, in any age group, and limit application to areas of involvement with atopic dermatitis.
- Tacrolimus ointment is not indicated for use in children younger than 2 years of age. Only tacrolimus 0.03% ointment is indicated for use in children 2 to 15 years of age.

Indications

➤*Atopic dermatitis (moderate to severe):* Tacrolimus ointment, both 0.03% and 0.1% for adults, and only 0.03% for children 2 to 15 years of age, is indicated as second-line therapy for the short-term and noncontinuous chronic treatment of moderate to severe atopic dermatitis in nonimmunocompromised adults and children who have failed to respond adequately to other topical prescription treatments for atopic dermatitis, or when those treatments are not advisable.

➤*Unlabeled uses:* Treatment of vitiligo in children; facial, flexural, and intertriginous psoriasis.

Administration and Dosage

➤*Approved by the FDA:* December 8, 2000.

➤*Adults:*

0.03% and 0.1% ointment – Apply a thin layer to the affected skin twice daily. The minimum amount should be rubbed in gently and completely to control signs and symptoms of atopic dermatitis. Stop using when signs and symptoms of atopic dermatitis resolve.

If signs and symptoms (eg, itch, rash, redness) do not improve within 6 weeks, patients should be reexamined to confirm the diagnosis of atopic dermatitis.

➤*Children (2 to 15 years of age):*

0.03% ointment – Apply a thin layer to the affected skin twice daily. The minimum amount should be rubbed in gently and completely to control signs and symptoms of atopic dermatitis. Stop using when signs and symptoms of atopic dermatitis resolve.

If signs and symptoms (eg, itch, rash, redness) do not improve within 6 weeks, patients should be reexamined by their health care provider to confirm the diagnosis of atopic dermatitis.

➤*Long-term use:* See the Warning box for more information.

➤*Occlusive dressing:* The safety of tacrolimus ointment under occlusion, which may promote systemic exposure, has not been evaluated. Tacrolimus 0.03% and 0.1% ointment should not be used with occlusive dressings.

➤*Storage/Stability:* Store at room temperature 25°C (77°F); excursions are permitted to 15° to 30°C (59° to 86°F).

Actions

➤*Pharmacology:* The mechanism of action of tacrolimus in atopic dermatitis is not known. While the following have been observed, the clinical significance of these observations in atopic dermatitis is not known. It has been demonstrated that tacrolimus inhibits T-lymphocyte activation by first binding to an intracellular protein, FKBP-12. A complex of tacrolimus-FKBP-12, calcium, calmodulin, and calcineurin is then formed and the phosphatase activity of calcineurin is inhibited. This effect has been shown to prevent the dephosphorylation and translocation of nuclear factor of activated T-cells (NF-AT), a nuclear component thought to initiate gene transcription for the formation of lymphokines (eg, interleukin-2, gamma interferon). Tacrolimus also inhibits the transcription for genes that encode IL-3, IL-4, IL-5, GM-CSF, and TNF-α, all of which are involved in the early stages of T-cell activation. Additionally, tacrolimus has been shown to inhibit the release of pre-formed mediators from skin mast cells and basophils, and to down regulate the expression of FcERI on Langerhans cells.

➤*Pharmacokinetics:*

Absorption –

Adults: The pooled results from 3 pharmacokinetic studies in 88 adult atopic dermatitis patients indicate that tacrolimus is minimally absorbed after the topical application of tacrolimus ointment. Peak tacrolimus blood concentrations ranged from undetectable to 20 ng/mL after single or multiple doses of tacrolimus 0.03% and 0.1% ointment, with 85% (75 of 88) of the patients having peak blood concentrations less than 2 ng/mL. In general, as treatment continued, systemic exposure declined as the skin returned to

TACROLIMUS — TOPICAL

normal. In clinical studies with periodic blood sampling, a similar distribution of tacrolimus blood levels was also observed in adult patients, with 90% (1,253 of 1,391) of patients having a blood concentration less than 2 ng/mL.

The absolute bioavailability of tacrolimus in atopic dermatitis patients is approximately 0.5%. In adults with an average of 53% body surface area (BSA) treated, exposure area under the curve (AUC) of tacrolimus ointment is approximately 30-fold less than that seen with oral immunosuppressive doses in kidney and liver transplant patients.

Mean peak tacrolimus blood concentrations following oral administration (0.3 mg/kg/day) in adult kidney transplant (n = 26) and liver transplant (n = 17) patients are 24.2 ± 15.8 ng/mL and 68.5 ± 30 ng/mL, respectively. The lowest tacrolimus blood level at which systemic effects (eg, immunosuppression) can be observed is not known.

Children: In a pharmacokinetic study of 14 pediatric atopic dermatitis patients between the ages of 2 and 5 years, peak blood concentrations of tacrolimus ranged from undetectable to 14.8 ng/mL after single or multiple doses of tacrolimus 0.03% ointment, with 86% (12 of 14) of patients having peak blood concentrations below 2 ng/mL throughout the study.

The highest peak concentration was observed in 1 patient with 82% BSA involvement on day 1 following application of tacrolimus 0.03% ointment. The peak concentrations for this subject were 14.8 ng/mL on day 1 and 4.1 ng/mL on day 14. Mean peak tacrolimus blood concentrations following oral administration in children with a history of liver transplant (n = 9) were 43.4 ± 27.9 ng/mL.

In a similar pharmacokinetic study with 61 enrolled children (6 to 12 years of age) with atopic dermatitis, peak tacrolimus blood concentrations ranged from undetectable to 5.3 ng/mL after single or multiple doses of tacrolimus 0.1% ointment, with 91% (52 of 57) of evaluable patients having peak blood concentrations below 2 ng/mL throughout the study period. When detected, systemic exposure generally declined as treatment continued.

In clinical studies with periodic blood sampling, a similar distribution of tacrolimus blood levels was also observed, with 98% (509 of 522) of children having a blood concentration below 2 ng/mL.

Distribution – The plasma protein binding of tacrolimus is approximately 99% and is independent of concentration over a range of 5 to 50 ng/mL. Tacrolimus is bound mainly to albumin and alpha-1-acid glycoprotein, and has a high level of association with erythrocytes. The distribution of tacrolimus between whole blood and plasma depends on several factors, such as hematocrit, temperature at the time of plasma separation, drug concentration, and plasma protein concentration. In a US study, the ratio of whole blood concentration to plasma concentration averaged 35 (range, 12 to 67).

There was no evidence based on blood concentrations that tacrolimus accumulates systemically upon intermittent topical application for periods of up to 1 year. As with other topical calcineurin inhibitors, it is not known whether tacrolimus is distributed into the lymphatic system.

Metabolism – Tacrolimus is extensively metabolized by the mixed-function oxidase system, primarily the cytochrome P-450 system (CYP3A). A metabolic pathway leading to the formation of 8 possible metabolites has been proposed. Demethylation and hydroxylation were identified as the primary mechanisms of biotransformation in vitro. The major metabolite identified in incubations with human liver microsomes is 13-demethyl tacrolimus. In in vitro studies, a 31-demethyl metabolite has been reported to have the same activity as tacrolimus.

Excretion – The mean clearance following intravenous (IV) administration of tacrolimus is 0.04, 0.083, and 0.053 L/h/kg in healthy volunteers, adult kidney transplant patients, and adult liver transplant patients, respectively. Less than 1% of the dose administered is excreted unchanged in urine.

In a mass balance study of IV administered radiolabeled tacrolimus to 6 healthy volunteers, the mean recovery of radiolabel was 77.8% ± 12.7%. Fecal elimination accounted for 92.4 ± 1%, and the elimination half-life based on radioactivity was 48.1 ± 15.9 hours, whereas it was 43.5 ± 11.6 hours based on tacrolimus concentrations. The mean clearance of radiolabel was 0.029 ± 0.015 L/h/kg, and the clearance of tacrolimus was 0.029 ± 0.009 L/h/kg.

When administered orally, the mean recovery of the radiolabel was 94.9% ± 30.7%. Fecal elimination accounted for 92.6 ± 30.7%, urinary elimination accounted for 2.3 ± 1.1%, and the elimination half-life based on radioactivity was 31.9 ± 10.5 hours, whereas it was 48.4 ± 12.3 hours based on tacrolimus concentrations. The mean clearance of radiolabel was 0.226 ± 0.116 L/h/kg and clearance of tacrolimus 0.172 ± 0.088 L/h/kg.

Contraindications

History of hypersensitivity to tacrolimus or any other component of the ointment.

Warnings

➤*Infections/Lymphomas/Skin Malignancies:* Prolonged systemic use of calcineurin inhibitors for sustained immunosuppression in animal studies and transplant patients following systemic administration has been associated with an increased risk of infections, lymphomas, and skin malignancies. These risks are associated with the intensity and duration of immunosuppression.

Based on the preceding information and the mechanism of action, there is a concern about potential risk with the use of topical calcineurin inhibitors, including tacrolimus ointment. While a causal relationship has not been established, rare cases of skin malignancy and lymphoma have been reported in patients treated with topical calcineurin inhibitors, including tacrolimus ointment.

➤*Immunocompromised patients:* Do not use tacrolimus ointment in immunocompromised adults and children.

➤*Long-term use:* If signs and symptoms of atopic dermatitis do not improve within 6 weeks, reexamine the patient and confirm the diagnosis.

The safety of tacrolimus ointment has not been established beyond 1 year of noncontinuous use.

➤*Renal effects:* Rare postmarketing cases of acute renal failure have been reported in patients treated with tacrolimus ointment. Systemic absorption is more likely to occur in patients with epidermal barrier defects, especially when tacrolimus is applied to large BSAs. Exercise caution in patients predisposed to renal function impairment.

➤*Carcinogenesis:* A 104-week dermal carcinogenicity study was performed in mice with tacrolimus ointment (0.03% to 3%), equivalent to tacrolimus doses of 1.1 to 118 mg/kg/day or 3.3 to 354 mg/m^2/day. In the study, the incidence of skin tumors was minimal and the topical application of tacrolimus was not associated with skin tumor formation under ambient room lighting. However, a statistically significant elevation in the incidence of pleomorphic lymphoma in high-dose male (25 of 50) and female animals (27 of 50) and in the incidence of undifferentiated lymphoma in high-dose female animals (13 of 50) was noted in the mouse dermal carcinogenicity study. Lymphomas were noted in the mouse dermal carcinogenicity study at a daily dose of 3.5 mg/kg (tacrolimus 0.1% ointment) (26 times MRHD based on AUC comparisons). No drug-related tumors were noted in the mouse dermal carcinogenicity study at a daily dose of 1.1 mg/kg (tacrolimus 0.03% ointment) (10 times MRHD based on AUC comparisons).

In a 52-week photocarcinogenicity study, the median time to onset of skin tumor formation was decreased in hairless mice following chronic topical dosing with concurrent exposure to ultraviolet (UV) radiation (40 weeks of treatment followed by 12 weeks of observation) with tacrolimus ointment at greater than or equal to 0.1% of tacrolimus.

➤*Fertility impairment:* Reproductive toxicology studies were not performed with topical tacrolimus. In studies of oral tacrolimus, no impairment of fertility was seen in male and female rats. Tacrolimus, given orally at 1 mg/kg (0.12 times MRHD based on BSA) to male and female rats, prior to and during mating, as well as to dams during gestation and lactation, was associated with embryolethality and with adverse effects on female reproduction. Effects on female reproductive function (parturition) and embryolethal effects were indicated by a higher rate of preimplantation loss and increased numbers of undelivered and nonviable pups. When given at 3.2 mg/kg (0.43 times MRHD based on BSA), tacrolimus was associated with maternal and paternal toxicity as well as reproductive toxicity, including marked adverse effects on estrus cycles, parturition, pup viability, and pup malformations.

➤*Pregnancy:* Category C.

Teratogenic – Reproduction studies were carried out with systemically administered tacrolimus in rats and rabbits. Adverse reactions on the fetus were observed mainly at oral dose levels that were toxic to dams. Tacrolimus at oral doses of 0.32 and 1 mg/kg (0.04 to 0.12 times MRHD based on BSA) during organogenesis in rabbits was associated with maternal toxicity as well as an increase in incidence of abortions. At the higher dose only, an increased incidence of malformations and developmental variations was also seen. Tacrolimus, at oral doses of 3.2 mg/kg during organogenesis in rats, was associated with maternal toxicity and caused an increase in late resorptions, decreased numbers of live births, and decreased pup weight and viability. Tacrolimus, given orally at 1 and 3.2 mg/kg (0.04 to 0.12 times MRHD based on BSA) to pregnant rats after organogenesis and during lactation, was associated with reduced pup weights.

There are no adequate and well-controlled studies of systemically administered tacrolimus in pregnant women. Tacrolimus is transferred across the placenta. The use of systemically administered tacrolimus during pregnancy has been associated with neonatal hyperkalemia and renal dysfunction. Only use tacrolimus ointment during pregnancy if the potential benefit to the mother justifies a potential risk to the fetus.

➤*Lactation:* Although systemic absorption of tacrolimus following topical applications of tacrolimus ointment is minimal relative to systemic administration, it is known that tacrolimus is excreted in human milk. Because of the potential for serious adverse reactions in breast-feeding infants from tacrolimus, decide whether to discontinue breast-feeding or the drug, taking into account the importance of the drug to the mother.

➤*Children:* Tacrolimus ointment is not indicated for children younger than 2 years of age.

Only the lower concentration, 0.03%, of tacrolimus ointment is recommended for use as a second-line therapy for short-term and noncontinuous chronic treatment of moderate to severe atopic dermatitis in nonimmunocompromised children 2 to 15 years of age who have failed to respond adequately to other topical prescription treatments for atopic dermatitis, or when those treatments are not advisable.

The long-term safety and effects of tacrolimus ointment on the developing immune system are unknown.

Four studies were conducted involving a total of about 4,400 patients 2 to 15 years of age: one 12-week, randomized, vehicle-controlled study and 3 open-label safety studies of 1 to 3 years' duration. About 2,500 of these patients were 2 to 6 years of age.

In these studies, the most common adverse reactions associated with tacrolimus ointment application in children were skin burning and pruritus. In addition to skin burning and pruritus, the less common events (less than 5%) of varicella zoster (mostly chickenpox) and vesiculobullous rash were more frequent in patients treated with tacrolimus 0.03% ointment compared with vehicle. In the open-label safety studies, the incidence of adverse reactions, including infections, did not increase with increased duration of study drug exposure or amount of ointment used. In about 4,400 children treated with tacrolimus ointment, 24 (0.5%) were reported with eczema herpeticum.

TACROLIMUS — TOPICAL

Because the safety and efficacy of tacrolimus ointment have not been established in children younger than 2 years of age, its use in this age group is not recommended.

In an open-label study, immune response to a 23-valent pneumococcal polysaccharide vaccine was assessed in 23 children 2 to 12 years of age with moderate to severe atopic dermatitis treated with tacrolimus 0.03% ointment. Protective antibody titers developed in all patients. Similarly, in a 7-month, double-blind trial, the vaccination response to meningococcal serogroup C was equivalent in children 2 to 11 years of age with moderate to severe atopic dermatitis treated with tacrolimus 0.03% ointment (n = 121) or a hydrocortisone ointment regimen (n = 111) and in healthy children (n = 44).

Precautions

➤*Monitoring:* Monitor patients who develop lymphadenopathy to ensure that the lymphadenopathy resolves.

➤*Premalignant/Malignant skin conditions:* Avoid the use of tacrolimus ointment on premalignant and malignant skin conditions. Some malignant skin conditions, such as cutaneous T-cell lymphoma, may mimic atopic dermatitis.

➤*Netherton syndrome:* The use of tacrolimus ointment in patients with Netherton syndrome or other skin diseases in which there is the potential for increased systemic absorption of tacrolimus is not recommended. The safety of tacrolimus ointment has not been established in patients with generalized erythroderma.

➤*Local symptoms:* The use of tacrolimus ointment may cause local symptoms such as skin burning (burning sensation, stinging, soreness) or pruritus. Localized symptoms are most common during the first few days of tacrolimus ointment application and typically improve as the lesions of atopic dermatitis resolve. With tacrolimus 0.1% ointment, 90% of the skin burning events had a duration between 2 minutes and 3 hours (median, 15 minutes). Ninety percent of the pruritus events had a duration between 3 minutes and 10 hours (median, 20 minutes).

➤*Bacterial and viral skin infections:* Before commencing treatment with tacrolimus ointment, cutaneous bacterial or viral infections at treatment sites should be resolved. Studies have not evaluated the safety and efficacy of tacrolimus ointment in the treatment of clinically infected atopic dermatitis.

While patients with atopic dermatitis are predisposed to superficial skin infections, including eczema herpeticum (Kaposi varicelliform eruption), treatment with tacrolimus ointment may be independently associated with an increased risk of varicella zoster virus infection (chickenpox or shingles), herpes simplex virus infection, or eczema herpeticum.

➤*Lymphadenopathy:* In clinical studies, 112 of 13,494 (0.8%) cases of lymphadenopathy were reported and were usually related to infections (particularly of the skin) and noted to resolve upon appropriate antibiotic therapy. Of these 112 cases, the majority had either a clear etiology or were known to resolve. Transplant patients receiving immunosuppressive regimens (eg, systemic tacrolimus) are at increased risk for developing lymphoma; therefore, patients who receive tacrolimus ointment and develop lymphadenopathy should have the etiology of their lymphadenopathy investigated. In the absence of a clear etiology for the lymphadenopathy, or in the presence of acute infectious mononucleosis, discontinue tacrolimus ointment. Monitor patients who develop lymphadenopathy to ensure that the lymphadenopathy resolves.

➤*Photosensitivity:* During the course of treatment, patients should minimize or avoid natural or artificial sunlight exposure, even while tacrolimus is not on the skin. It is not known whether tacrolimus ointment interferes with skin response to UV damage.

Drug Interactions

Tacrolimus (Topical) Drug Interactions

Precipitant drug	Object drug[a]		Description
CYP3A4 inhibitors (eg, calcium channel blockers, cimetidine, erythromycin, itraconazole, ketoconazole, fluconazole)	Tacrolimus	↑	Use with caution.
Tacrolimus	Alcohol	↑	Risk of transient facial flushing may be increased. Avoid alcohol during topical tacrolimus.

[a] ↑ = Object drug increased.

Adverse Reactions

No phototoxicity or photoallergenicity was detected in clinical studies with 12 and 216 healthy volunteers, respectively. One out of 198 healthy volunteers showed evidence of sensitization in a contact sensitization study.

In three 12-week, randomized, vehicle-controlled studies and 4 safety studies, 655 and 9,163 patients, respectively, were treated with tacrolimus ointment. The duration of follow-up for adults and children in the safety studies is tabulated in the following table:

Tacrolimus Duration of Follow-up in 4 Open-Label Safety Studies

Time on study	Adults	Children	Total
< 1 year	4,682	4,481	9,163
≥ 1 year	1,185	1,349	2,534
≥ 2 years	200	275	475
≥ 3 years	118	182	300

The following table depicts the adjusted incidence of adverse reactions pooled across the 3 identically designed 12-week controlled studies for patients in vehicle, tacrolimus 0.03% ointment, and tacrolimus 0.1% ointment treatment groups. The following table also depicts the unadjusted incidence of adverse reactions in 4 safety studies, regardless of relationship to study drug.

Tacrolimus Adverse Reactions

	12-week, randomized, double-blind, phase 3 studies 12-week adjusted incidence rate (%)					Open-label studies (up to 3 years) Tacrolimus 0.1% and 0.03% ointment incidence rate (%)		
	Adults			Children		Adults	Children	Total
	Vehicle (n = 212)	Tacrolimus 0.03% ointment (n = 210)	Tacrolimus 0.1% ointment (n = 209)	Vehicle (n = 116)	Tacrolimus 0.03% ointment (n = 118)	(n = 4,682)	(n = 4,481)	(n = 9,163)
Cardiovascular								
Hypertension	0%	0%	1%	0%	0%	2%	0%	1%
CNS								
Asthenia	1%	2%	3%	0%	0 %	1%	0%	1%
Depression	1%	2%	1%	0%	0%	1%	0%	1%
Headache[a]	11%	20%	19%	8%	5%	13%	9%	11%
Hyperesthesia[a]	1%	3%	7%	0%	0%	2%	0 %	1%
Insomnia	3%	4%	3%	1%	1 %	2%	0%	1%
Paresthesia	1%	3%	3%	0%	0%	2%	1%	2%
Dermatologic								
Acne[a]	2%	4%	7%	1%	0%	3%	2%	3%
Alopecia	0%	1%	1%	0%	0%	1%	1%	1%
Cellulitis	1%	1%	1%	0%	0%	1%	1%	1%
Contact dermatitis	1%	3%	3%	3%	4%	2%	2%	2%
Dry skin	7%	3%	3%	0%	1%	1%	1%	1%
Eczema	2%	2%	2%	0%	0%	1%	0%	1%
Eczema herpeticum	0%	1%	1%	0%	2%	0%	0%	0%
Exfoliative dermatitis	3%	3%	1%	0%	0%	0%	1%	0%
Folliculitis[a]	1%	6%	4%	0%	2%	4%	2%	3%
Fungal dermatitis	0%	2%	1%	3%	0%	2%	4%	3%
Maculopapular rash	2%	2%	2%	3%	0%	4%	1%	1%
Pruritus[a]	37%	46%	46%	27%	41%	25%	19%	22%
Pustular rash	2%	3%	4%	3%	2%	2%	7%	5%
Rash[a]	1%	5%	2%	4%	2%	2%	3%	3%
Skin burning[a]	26%	46%	58%	29%	43%	28%	20%	24%

TACROLIMUS — TOPICAL

Tacrolimus Adverse Reactions								
	12-week, randomized, double-blind, phase 3 studies 12-week adjusted incidence rate (%)					Open-label studies (up to 3 years) Tacrolimus 0.1% and 0.03% ointment incidence rate (%)		
	Adults			Children		Adults	Children	Total
	Vehicle (n = 212)	Tacrolimus 0.03% ointment (n = 210)	Tacrolimus 0.1% ointment (n = 209)	Vehicle (n = 116)	Tacrolimus 0.03% ointment (n = 118)	(n = 4,682)	(n = 4,481)	(n = 9,163)
Skin disorder	2%	2%	1%	1%	4%	2%	2%	2%
Skin erythema	20%	25%	28%	13%	12%	12%	7%	9%
Skin infection	11%	12%	5%	14%	10%	9%	10%	12%
Skin neoplasm benign[b]	1%	1%	1%	0%	0%	1%	2%	2%
Skin tingling[a]	2%	3%	8%	1%	2%	2%	1%	1%
Sunburn	1%	2%	1%	0%	0%	2%	1%	1%
Urticaria	3%	3%	6%	1%	1%	3%	4%	4%
Varicella zoster/ herpes zoster[c]	0%	1%	0%	0%	5%	1%	2%	2%
Vesiculobullous rash[a]	3%	3%	2%	0%	4%	2%	1%	1%
GI								
Abdominal pain	3%	1%	1%	2%	3%	1%	3%	2%
Diarrhea	3%	3%	4%	2%	5%	2%	4%	3%
Dyspepsia[a]	1%	1%	4%	0%	0%	2%	2%	2%
Gastroenteritis	1%	2%	2%	3%	0%	2%	4%	3%
Nausea	4%	3%	2%	0%	1%	2%	1%	2%
Periodontal abscess	1%	0%	1%	0%	0%	1%	1%	1%
Tooth disorder	0%	1%	1%	1%	0%	2%	1%	1%
Vomiting	0%	1%	1%	7%	6%	1%	4%	3%
GU								
Dysmenorrhea	2%	4%	4%	0%	0%	2%	1%	1%
Urinary tract infection	0%	0%	1%	0%	0%	2%	1%	2%
Musculoskeletal								
Arthralgia	1%	1%	3%	2%	0%	2%	1%	2%
Back pain[a]	0%	2%	2%	1%	1%	3%	0%	2%
Myalgia[a]	0%	3%	2%	0%	0%	2%	1%	1%
Metabolic								
Face edema	2%	2%	1%	2%	1%	1%	1%	1%
Peripheral edema	2%	4%	3%	0%	0%	2%	0%	1%
Respiratory								
Asthma	4%	6%	4%	6%	6%	4%	13%	8%
Bronchitis	0%	2%	2%	3%	3%	4%	4%	4%
Cough increased	2%	1%	1%	14%	18%	3%	10%	6%
Pharyngitis	3%	3%	4%	11%	6%	4%	12%	8%
Pneumonia	0%	1%	1%	2%	0%	1%	3%	2%
Rhinitis	4%	3%	2%	2%	6%	2%	4%	3%
Sinusitis[a]	1%	4%	2%	8%	3%	6%	7%	6%
Special senses								
Conjunctivitis	0%	2%	2%	2%	1%	3%	3%	3%
Ear pain	1%	0%	1%	0%	1%	0%	1%	1%
Otitis media	4%	0%	1%	6%	12%	2%	11%	6%
Miscellaneous								
Accidental injury	4%	3%	6%	3%	6%	6%	8%	7%
Alcohol intolerance[a]	0%	3%	7%	0%	0%	4%	0%	2%
Allergic reaction	8%	12%	6%	8%	4%	9%	13%	11%
Cyst[a]	0%	1%	3%	0%	0%	1%	0%	1%
Exacerbation of untreated area	1%	0%	1%	1%	0%	1%	1%	1%
Fever	4%	4%	1%	13%	21%	2%	14%	8%
Flu-like symptoms[a]	19%	23%	31%	25%	28%	22%	34%	28%
Herpes simplex	4%	4%	4%	2%	0%	4%	3%	3%
Infection	1%	1%	2%	9%	7%	6%	10%	8%
Lack of drug effect	1%	1%	0%	1%	1%	6%	6%	6%
Lymphadenopathy	2%	2%	1%	0%	3%	1%	2%	1%
Pain	1%	2%	1%	0%	1%	2%	1%	2%
Procedural complication	1%	0%	0%	1%	0%	1%	1%	1%

[a] May be reasonably associated with the use of this drug product.
[b] Generally "warts."
[c] All the herpes zoster cases in the pediatric 12-week study and the majority of cases in the open-label studies in children were reported as chickenpox.

TACROLIMUS — TOPICAL

➤*Other adverse reactions (0.2% to less than 1%):*

Cardiovascular – Chest pain, syncope, tachycardia, valvular heart disease, vasodilatation.

CNS – Abnormal thinking, anxiety, chills, dizziness, hypertonia, malaise, migraine, vertigo.

Dermatologic – Cutaneous moniliasis, furunculosis, leukoderma, nail disorder, photosensitivity reaction, seborrhea, skin carcinoma, skin discoloration, skin hypertrophy, skin ulcer, sweating.

GI – Anorexia, colitis, constipation, cramps, gastritis, GI disorder, hernia, mouth ulceration, oral moniliasis, rectal disorder, stomatitis, taste perversion, tooth caries.

GU – Cystitis, moniliasis, vaginal moniliasis, vaginitis.

Hematologic – Anemia, bilirubinemia, ecchymosis, hypercholerestemia.

Metabolic – Dehydration, edema, hypothyroidism.

Musculoskeletal – Arthritis, arthrosis, bone disorder, bursitis, joint disorder, neck pain, tendon disorder.

Respiratory – Dry mouth/nose, dyspnea, epistaxis, laryngitis, lung disorder.

Special senses – Abnormal vision, blepharitis, cataract, conjunctival edema, dry eyes, ear disorder, eye pain, otitis externa.

Miscellaneous – Abscess, anaphylactoid reaction, breast neoplasm benign, neoplasm benign, unintended pregnancy.

➤*Postmarketing:* The following adverse reactions have been identified during postapproval use of tacrolimus ointment. Because these reactions are reported voluntarily from a population of uncertain size, it is not always possible to reliably estimate their frequency or establish a causal relationship to drug exposure.

CNS – Seizures.

Dermatologic – Rosacea.

Renal – Acute renal failure in patients with or without Netherton syndrome, renal function impairment.

Miscellaneous – Basal cell carcinoma, bullous impetigo, lymphomas, malignant melanoma, osteomyelitis, septicemia, squamous cell carcinoma.

Overdosage

Ointment is not for oral use. Oral ingestion of tacrolimus ointment may lead to adverse reactions associated with systemic administration of tacrolimus. If oral ingestion occurs, patients should seek medical advice.

Patient Information

Tacrolimus ointment should only be used as directed and only for the disorder for which it was prescribed.

Tacrolimus ointment is for external use only.

As with any topical medication, patients or caregivers should wash hands after application if hands are not an area for treatment.

While using tacrolimus ointment, the patient should minimize or avoid exposure to natural or artificial sunlight (tanning beds or UVA/B treatment).

Patients should report any signs of adverse reactions to their physician.

Before applying tacrolimus after a bath or shower, patients should be sure the skin is completely dry.

PIMECROLIMUS

Rx	**Elidel** (Novartis)	**Cream:** 1%	In 30, 60, and 100 g tubes.

PIMECROLIMUS — TOPICAL

WARNING

Long-term safety of topical calcineurin inhibitors has not been established.

Although a causal relationship has not been established, rare cases of malignancy (eg, skin and lymphoma) have been reported in patients treated with topical calcineurin inhibitors including pimecrolimus cream.

Therefore,

- Continuous long-term use of topical calcineurin inhibitors, including pimecrolimus cream, in any age group should be avoided, and application limited to areas of involvement with atopic dermatitis.
- Pimecrolimus cream is not indicated for use in children less than 2 years of age.

Indications

➤*Atopic dermatitis:* Pimecrolimus cream 1% is indicated as second-line therapy for short-term and noncontinuous chronic treatment of mild-to-moderate atopic dermatitis in nonimmunocompromised patients 2 years of age and older who have failed to respond adequately to other topical prescription treatments or when those treatments are not advisable.

Administration and Dosage

➤*Approved by the FDA:* December 14, 2001.

➤*Dose:* Apply a thin layer of pimecrolimus cream to the affected skin twice daily. The patient or caregiver should stop using pimecrolimus when signs and symptoms (eg, itch, rash, and redness) resolve and should be instructed on what actions to take if symptoms recur.

If signs and symptoms persist beyond 6 weeks, the patient should be re-examined by their healthcare provider to confirm the diagnosis of atopic dermatitis.

➤*Long-term use:* See the Warning box for more information.

➤*Occlusive dressing:* The safety of pimecrolimus cream under occlusion, which may promote systemic exposure, has not been evaluated. Pimecrolimus cream should not be used with occlusive dressings.

➤*Storage/Stability:* Store at 25°C (77°F); excursions permitted to 15° to 30°C (59° to 86°F). Do not freeze.

Actions

➤*Pharmacology:*

Mechanism of action/pharmacodynamics – The mechanism of action of pimecrolimus in atopic dermatitis is not known. While the following have been observed, the clinical significance of these observations in atopic dermatitis is not known. It has been demonstrated that pimecrolimus binds with high affinity to macrophilin-12 (FKBP-12) and inhibits the calcium-dependent phosphatase, calcineurin. As a consequence, it inhibits T cell activation by blocking the transcription of early cytokines. In particular, pimecrolimus inhibits at nanomolar concentrations interleukin-2 and interferon gamma (Th1-type) and interleukin-4 and interleukin-10 (Th2-type) cytokine synthesis in human T cells. In addition, pimecrolimus prevents the release of inflammatory cytokines and mediators from mast cells in vitro after stimulation by antigen/IgE.

➤*Pharmacokinetics:*

Absorption – In adult patients being treated for atopic dermatitis (13% to 62% body surface area [BSA] involvement) for periods up to a year, blood concentrations of pimecrolimus are routinely either at or below the limit of quantification of the assay (less than 0.5 ng/mL). In those subjects with detectable blood levels they are routinely less than 2 ng/mL and show no sign of drug accumulation with time. Because of the low systemic absorption of pimecrolimus following topical application the calculation of standard pharmacokinetic measures (eg, AUC, C_{max}, $t_{½}$) cannot be reliably done.

Distribution – In vitro studies of the protein binding of pimecrolimus indicate that it is 74% to 87% bound to plasma proteins.

Metabolism – Following the administration of a single oral radiolabeled dose of pimecrolimus numerous circulating O-demethylation metabolites were seen. Studies with human liver microsomes indicate that pimecrolimus is metabolized in vitro by the CYP3A sub-family of metabolizing enzymes. No evidence of skin mediated drug metabolism was identified in vivo using the minipig or in vitro using stripped human skin.

Excretion – Based on the results of the aforementioned radiolabeled study, following a single oral dose of pimecrolimus approximately 81% of the administered radioactivity was recovered, primarily in the feces (78.4%) as metabolites. Less than 1% of the radioactivity found in the feces was due to unchanged pimecrolimus.

Contraindications

Hypersensitivity to pimecrolimus or any of the components of the cream.

Warnings

➤*Local reactions:* The use of pimecrolimus cream may cause local symptoms such as skin burning. Localized symptoms are most common during the first few days of pimecrolimus cream application and typically improve as the lesions of atopic dermatitis resolve. Most application site reactions lasted no more than 5 days, were mild to moderate in severity, and started within 1 to 5 days of treatment (see Adverse Reactions).

➤*Carcinogenesis:* In a 2-year rat dermal carcinogenicity study using pimecrolimus cream, a statistically significant increase in the incidence of follicular cell adenoma of the thyroid was noted in low-, mid-, and high-dose male animals compared to vehicle and saline control male animals. Follicular cell adenoma of the thyroid was noted in the dermal rat carcinogenicity study at the lowest dose of 2 mg/kg/day (0.2% pimecrolimus cream; 1.5 times the maximum recommended human dose [MRHD] based on AUC comparisons). No increase in the incidence of follicular cell adenoma of the thyroid was noted in the oral carcinogenicity study in male rats up to 10 mg/kg/day (66 times MRHD based on AUC comparisons). However, oral studies may not reflect continuous exposure or the same metabolic profile as by the dermal route. In a mouse dermal carcinogenicity study using pimecrolimus in an ethanolic solution, no increase in incidence of neoplasms was observed in the skin or other organs up to the highest dose of 4 mg/kg/day (0.32% pimecrolimus in ethanol) 27 times MRHD based on AUC comparisons. However, lymphoproliferative changes (including lymphoma) were noted in a 13-week repeat dose dermal toxicity study conducted in mice using pimecrolimus in an ethanolic solution at a dose of 25 mg/kg/day (47 times MRHD based on AUC comparisons). No lymphoproliferative changes were noted in this study at a dose of 10 mg/kg/day (17 times MRHD based on AUC comparisons). However, the latency time to lymphoma formation was shortened to 8 weeks after dermal administration of pimecrolimus dissolved in ethanol at a dose of 100 mg/kg/day (179 to 217 times MRHD based on AUC comparisons).

PIMECROLIMUS — TOPICAL

In a mouse oral (gavage) carcinogenicity study, a statistically significant increase in the incidence of lymphoma was noted in high-dose male and female animals compared to vehicle control male and female animals. Lymphomas were noted in the oral mouse carcinogenicity study at a dose of 45 mg/kg/day (258 to 340 times MRHD based on AUC comparisons). No drug-related tumors were noted in the mouse oral carcinogenicity study at a dose of 15 mg/kg/day (60 to 133 times MRHD based on AUC comparisons). In an oral (gavage) rat carcinogenicity study, a statistically significant increase in the incidence of benign thymoma was noted in 10 mg/kg/day pimecrolimus-treated male and female animals compared to vehicle-control treated male and female animals. In addition, a significant increase in the incidence of benign thymoma was noted in another oral (gavage) rat carcinogenicity study in 5 mg/kg/day pimecrolimus-treated male animals compared to vehicle control-treated male animals. No drug-related tumors were noted in the rat oral carcinogenicity study at a dose of 1 mg/kg/day male animals (1.1 times MRHD based on AUC comparisons) and at a dose of 5 mg/kg/day for female animals (21 times MRHD based on AUC comparisons).

In a 52-week dermal photo-carcinogenicity study, the median time to onset of skin tumor formation was decreased in hairless mice following chronic topical dosing with concurrent exposure to UV radiation (40 weeks of treatment followed by 12 weeks of observation) with the pimecrolimus cream vehicle alone. No additional effect on tumor development beyond the vehicle effect was noted with the addition of the active ingredient, pimecrolimus, to the vehicle cream.

➤*Pregnancy: Category C.* There are no adequate and well-controlled studies of topically administered pimecrolimus in pregnant women. The experience with pimecrolimus cream when used by pregnant women is too limited to permit assessment of the safety of its use during pregnancy.

A combined oral fertility and embryofetal developmental study was conducted in rats and an oral embryofetal developmental study was conducted in rabbits. Pimecrolimus was administered during the period of organogenesis (2 weeks prior to mating until gestational day 16 in rats, gestational days 6 to 18 in rabbits) up to dose levels of 45 mg/kg/day in rats and 20 mg/kg/day in rabbits. In the absence of maternal toxicity, indicators of embryofetal toxicity (postimplantation loss and reduction in litter size) were noted at 45 mg/kg/day (38 times MRHD based on AUC comparisons) in the oral fertility and embryofetal developmental study conducted in rats. No malformations in the fetuses were noted at 45 mg/kg/day (38 times MRHD based on AUC comparisons) in this study. No maternal toxicity, embryotoxicity or teratogenicity were noted in the oral rabbit embryofetal developmental toxicity study at 20 mg/kg/day (3.9 times MRHD based on AUC comparisons), which was the highest dose tested in this study.

An oral peri- and postnatal developmental study was conducted in rats. Pimecrolimus was administered from gestational day 6 through lactational day 21 up to a dose level of 40 mg/kg/day. Only 2 of 22 females delivered live pups at the highest dose of 40 mg/kg/day. Postnatal survival, development of the F1 generation, their subsequent maturation and fertility were not affected at 10 mg/kg/day (12 times MRHD based on AUC comparisons), the highest dose evaluated in this study.

Pimecrolimus was transferred across the placenta in oral rat and rabbit embryofetal developmental studies.

There are, however, no adequate and well-controlled studies in pregnant women. Because animal reproduction studies are not always predictive of human response, this drug should be used only if clearly needed during pregnancy.

➤*Lactation:* It is not known whether this drug is excreted in human milk. Because of the potential for serious adverse reactions in nursing infants from pimecrolimus, a decision should be made whether to discontinue nursing or to discontinue the drug, taking into account the importance of the drug to the mother.

➤*Children:* Pimecrolimus cream may be used in pediatric patients 2 years of age and older. Three phase 3 pediatric studies were conducted involving 1114 patients 2 to 17 years of age. Two studies were 6-week randomized vehicle-controlled studies with a 20-week open-label phase, and 1 was a vehicle-controlled long-term (up to 1 year) safety study with the option for sequential topical corticosteroid use. Of these patients 542 (49%) were 2 to 6 years of age. In the short-term studies, 11% of pimecrolimus patients did not complete these studies and 1.5% of pimecrolimus patients discontinued due to adverse events. In the 1-year study, 32% of pimecrolimus patients did not complete this study and 3% of pimecrolimus patients discontinued due to adverse events. Most discontinuations were due to unsatisfactory therapeutic effect.

The most common local adverse event in the short-term studies of pimecrolimus cream in pediatric patients ages 2 to 17 was application site burning (10% vs 13% vehicle); the incidence in the long-term study was 9% pimecrolimus vs 7% vehicle (see Adverse Reactions). Adverse events that were more frequent (greater than 5%) in patients treated with pimecrolimus cream compared to vehicle were headache (14% vs 9%) in the short-term trial. Nasopharyngitis (26% vs 21%), influenza (13% vs 4%), pharyngitis (8% vs 3%), viral infection (7% vs 1%), pyrexia (13% vs 5%), cough (16% vs 11%), and headache (25% vs 16%) were increased over vehicle in the 1-year safety study (see Adverse Reactions). In 843 patients ages 2 to 17 years treated with pimecrolimus cream, 9 (0.8%) developed eczema herpeticum (5 on pimecrolimus cream alone and 4 on pimecrolimus cream used in sequence with corticosteroids). In 211 patients on vehicle alone, there were no cases of eczema herpeticum. The majority of adverse events were mild to moderate in severity.

Pimecrolimus cream is not recommended for use in pediatric patients below the age of 2 years. Two phase 3 studies were conducted involving 436 infants age 3 months to 23 months. One 6-week randomized vehicle-controlled study with a 20-week open-label phase and 1 long-term safety study were conducted. In the 6-week study, 11% of pimecrolimus and 48% of vehicle patients did not complete this study; no patient in either group discontinued due to adverse events. Infants on pimecrolimus cream had an increased incidence of some adverse events compared to vehicle. In the 6-week vehicle-controlled study these adverse events included pyrexia (32% vs 13% vehicle), URI (24% vs 14%), nasopharyngitis (15% vs 8%), gastroenteritis (7% vs 3%), otitis media (4% vs 0%), and diarrhea (8% vs 0%). In the open-label phase of the study, for infants who switched to pimecrolimus cream from vehicle, the incidence of the above-cited adverse events approached or equaled the incidence of those patients who remained on pimecrolimus cream. In the 6-month safety data, 16% of pimecrolimus and 35% of vehicle patients discontinued early and 1.5% of pimecrolimus and 0% of vehicle patients discontinued due to adverse events. Infants on pimecrolimus cream had a greater incidence of some adverse events as compared to vehicle. These included pyrexia (30% vs 20%), upper respiratory tract infection (21% vs 17%), cough (15% vs 9%), hypersensitivity (8% vs 2%), teething (27% vs 22%), vomiting (9% vs 4%), rhinitis (13% vs 9%), viral rash (4% vs 0%), rhinorrhea (4% vs 0%), and wheezing (4% vs 0%).

The effects of pimecrolimus cream on the developing immune system in infants are unknown.

Precautions

➤*Lymphadenopathy:* In clinical studies, 14 cases of lymphadenopathy (0.9%) were reported while using pimecrolimus cream. These cases of lymphadenopathy were usually related to infections and noted to resolve upon appropriate antibiotic therapy. Of these 14 cases, the majority had either a clear etiology or were known to resolve. Patients who receive pimecrolimus cream and who develop lymphadenopathy should have the etiology of their lymphadenopathy investigated. In the absence of a clear etiology for the lymphadenopathy, or in the presence of acute infectious mononucleosis, discontinuation of pimecrolimus cream should be considered. Patients who develop lymphadenopathy should be monitored to ensure that the lymphadenopathy resolves.

➤*Active cutaneous viral infections:* Pimecrolimus cream 1% should not be applied to areas of active cutaneous viral infections.

➤*Topical infection:* Studies have not evaluated the safety and efficacy of pimecrolimus cream in the treatment of clinically infected atopic dermatitis. Before commencing treatment with pimecrolimus cream, clinical infections at treatment sites should be cleared.

While patients with atopic dermatitis are predisposed to superficial skin infections including eczema herpeticum (Kaposi's varicelliform eruption), treatment with pimecrolimus cream may be associated with an increased risk of varicella-zoster virus infection (chickenpox or shingles), herpes simplex virus infection, or eczema herpeticum. In the presence of these skin infections, the balance of risks and benefits associated with pimecrolimus cream use should be evaluated.

➤*Skin papilloma or warts:* In clinical studies, 15 cases of skin papilloma or warts (1%) were observed in patients using pimecrolimus cream. The youngest patient was age 2 and the oldest was age 12. In cases where there is worsening of skin papillomas or they do not respond to conventional therapy, discontinuation of pimecrolimus cream should be considered until complete resolution of the warts is achieved.

➤*Netherton's syndrome:* The use of pimecrolimus cream in patients with Netherton's syndrome is not recommended due to the potential for increased systemic absorption of pimecrolimus.

➤*Immunocompromised patients:* There are no data to support use of pimecrolimus in immunocompromised patients.

➤*Photosensitivity:* The enhancement of ultraviolet carcinogenicity is not necessarily dependent on phototoxic mechanisms. Despite the absence of observed phototoxicity in humans (see Adverse Reactions), pimecrolimus cream shortened the time to skin tumor formation in an animal photocarcinogenicity study (see Warnings, Carcinogenesis). Therefore, it is prudent for patients to minimize or avoid natural or artificial sunlight exposure.

Drug Interactions

Potential interactions between pimecrolimus and other drugs, including immunizations, have not been systematically evaluated. Due to the very low blood levels of pimecrolimus detected in some patients after topical application, systemic drug interactions are not expected, but cannot be ruled out. The concomitant administration of known CYP3A family of inhibitors in patients with widespread or erythrodermic disease should be done with caution. Some examples of such drugs are erythromycin, itraconazole, ketoconazole, fluconazole, calcium channel blockers, and cimetidine.

Adverse Reactions

In a 1-year safety study in pediatric patients age 2 to 17 years old involving sequential use of pimecrolimus cream and a topical corticosteroid, 43% of pimecrolimus patients and 68% of vehicle patients used corticosteroids during the study. Corticosteroids were used for more than 7 days by 34% of pimecrolimus patients and 54% of vehicle patients. An increased incidence of impetigo, skin infection, superinfection (infected atopic dermatitis), rhinitis, and urticaria were found in the patients that had used pimecrolimus cream and topical corticosteroid sequentially as compared to pimecrolimus cream alone.

In 3 randomized, double-blind vehicle-controlled pediatric studies and 1 active-controlled adult study, 843 and 328 patients respectively, were treated with pimecrolimus cream. In these clinical trials, 48 (4%) of the 1171 pimecrolimus patients and 13 (3%) of 408 vehicle-treated patients discontinued therapy due to adverse events. Discontinuations for AEs were primarily due to application site reactions, and cutaneous infections. The most common application site reaction was application site burning, which occurred in 8% to 26% of patients treated with pimecrolimus cream.

PIMECROLIMUS — TOPICAL

The following table depicts the incidence of adverse reactions pooled across the 2 identically designed 6-week studies with their open label extensions and the 1-year safety study for pediatric patients ages 2 to 17. Data from the adult active-controlled study is also included in this table. Adverse reactions are listed regardless of relationship to study drug.

Treatment Emergent Adverse Events in Pimecrolimus Treatment Groups (≥ 1%)

Adverse event	Pediatric patients[a] vehicle-controlled (6 weeks)		Pediatric patients[a] open-label (20 weeks)	Pediatric patients[a] vehicle-controlled (1 year)		Adult active comparator (1 year)
	Pimecrolimus (n = 267)	Vehicle (n = 136)	Pimecrolimus (n = 335)	Pimecrolimus (n = 272)	Vehicle (n = 75)	Pimecrolimus (n = 328)
≥ 1 adverse event	68.2	71.3	72	84.6	74.7	78
Dermatological						
Skin infection NOS[b]	3	5.1	5.4	2.2	4	6.4
Impetigo	1.9	2.2	3.6	4	5.3	2.4
Folliculitis	1.1	0.7	0.9	2.2	4	6.1
Molluscum contagiosum	0.7	0	1.2	1.8	0	0
Skin papilloma	0.4	0	0.6	3.3	< 1	0
Herpes simplex dermatitis	0	0	0.3	1.5	0	0.6
Urticaria	1.1	0	0.3	0.4	< 1	0.9
Acne NOS	0	0.7	0.3	1.5	< 1	1.8
GI						
Gastroenteritis NOS	0	2.2	0.6	7.4	2.7	1.8
Abdominal pain, upper	4.1	4.4	3	5.5	6.7	0.3
Sore throat	3.4	3.7	5.4	8.1	5.3	3.7
Vomiting NOS	3	4.4	4.2	6.6	8	0.6
Diarrhea NOS	1.1	0.7	0.6	7.7	5.3	2.1
Nausea	0.4	2.2	1.2	4	6.7	1.8
Abdominal pain NOS	0.4	0.7	1.5	4.4	4	0.3
Toothache	0.4	0.7	0.6	2.6	1.3	0.6
Constipation	0.4	0	0.6	3.7	< 1	0
Loose stools	0	0.7	1.2	< 1	< 1	0
Musculoskeletal						
Back pain	0.4	1.5	0.3	< 1	0	1.8
Arthralgias	0	0	0.3	1.1	1.3	1.5
Respiratory						
Upper respiratory tract infection NOS	14.2	13.2	19.4	4.8	8	4.3
Nasopharyngitis	10.1	7.4	19.6	26.5	21.3	7.6
Sinusitis	1.1	0.7	3.3	2.2	1.3	0.6
Pneumonia NOS	1.1	0.7	1.5	0	1.3	0.3
Pharyngitis NOS	0.7	1.5	0.9	8.1	2.7	0.9
Pharyngitis streptococcal	0.7	1.5	3	0	< 1	0
Bronchitis NOS	0.4	2.2	1.2	10.7	8	2.4
Upper respiratory tract infection viral NOS	0.4	0	0.9	1.5	0	0.3
Bronchitis acute NOS	0	0	0	1.5	0	0
Cough	11.6	8.1	9.3	15.8	10.7	2.4
Nasal congestion	2.6	1.5	1.8	1.5	1.3	0.6
Rhinorrhea	1.9	0.7	0.9	0.4	1.3	0
Asthma aggravated	1.5	2.2	3.9	1.1	1.3	0
Sinus congestion	1.1	0.7	0.6	< 1	< 1	0.9
Rhinitis	0.4	0	1.5	4.4	6.7	2.1
Wheezing	0.4	0.7	1.2	0.7	< 1	0
Asthma NOS	0.7	0.7	3.3	3.7	2.7	2.4
Epistaxis	0	0.7	0	3.3	1.3	0.3
Dyspnea NOS	0	0	0	1.8	1.3	0.6
Special senses						
Ear infection NOS	2.2	1.5	5.7	3.3	1.3	0.6
Otitis media	2.2	0.7	3	2.9	5.3	0.6
Eye infection NOS	0	0	0	1.1	< 1	0.3
Conjunctivitis NEC	0.7	0.7	2.1	2.2	4	3
Earache	0.7	0.7	0	2.9	2.7	0
Miscellaneous						
Influenza	3	0.7	6.6	13.2	4	9.8
Bacterial infection	1.5	2.2	1.2	1.1	0	1.8
Staphylococcal infection	0.4	3.7	2.1	0	< 1	0.9
Herpes simplex	0.4	0	1.2	3.3	2.7	4
Tonsillitis NOS	0.4	0	0.9	6.3	0	0.6
Viral infection NOS	0.7	0.7	0.3	6.6	1.3	0
Chickenpox	0.7	0	0.9	2.9	4	0.3
Tonsillitis acute NOS	0	0	0	2.6	0	0
Application site burning	10.4	12.5	1.5	8.5	6.7	25.9
Pyrexia	7.5	8.8	12.2	12.5	5.3	1.2
Application site reaction NOS	3	5.1	2.1	3.3	2.7	14.6
Application site irritation	3	5.9	0.9	0.4	4	6.4
Influenza-like illness	0.4	0	0.6	1.8	2.7	1.8
Application site erythema	0.4	0	0	2.2	0	2.1
Application site pruritus	1.1	1.5	0.6	1.8	0	5.5
Dysmenorrhea	1.1	0	1.5	1.1	1.3	1.2
Hypersensitivity NOS	4.1	4.4	4.8	5.1	1.3	3.4
Accident NOS	1.1	0.7	0.3	< 1	1.3	0
Laceration	0.7	0.7	1.5	< 1	< 1	0
Headache	13.9	8.8	11.3	25.4	16	7

[a] Ages 2 to 17 years.

Overdosage

➤*Treatment:* If oral ingestion occurs, medical advice should be sought.

Patient Information

Patients should use pimecrolimus cream as directed by the physician. Pimecrolimus cream is for external use on the skin only. As with any topical medication, patients or caregivers should wash hands after application if hands are not an area for treatment.

Patients should minimize or avoid exposure to natural or artificial sunlight (tanning beds or UVA/B treatment) while using pimecrolimus cream.

Patients should not use this medication for any disorder other than that for which it was prescribed.

Patients should report any signs or symptoms of adverse reactions to their physician.

Therapy should be discontinued after signs and symptoms of atopic dermatitis have resolved. Treatment with pimecrolimus should be resumed at the first signs or symptoms of recurrence.

Use of pimecrolimus may cause reactions at the site of application such as a mild to moderate feeling of warmth or sensation of burning. Patients should see a physician if an application site reaction is severe or persists for more than 1 week.

The patient should contact the physician if no improvement in the atopic dermatitis is seen following 6 weeks of treatment, or if at any time the condition worsens.

DICLOFENAC SODIUM

Rx	**Solaraze** (SkyePharma)	**Gel:** 3%[a]	Benzyl alcohol. In 25 and 50 g.

[a] 1 g contains 30 mg diclofenac sodium

DICLOFENAC SODIUM — TOPICAL

For information on CNS and ophthalmic/otic uses of diclofenac sodium, refer to individual monographs.

Indications

➤*Actinic keratoses (AK):* For the topical treatment of AK. Sun avoidance is indicated during therapy.

Administration and Dosage

Apply gel to lesion areas twice daily. It is to be smoothed onto the affected skin gently. The amount needed depends upon the size of the lesion site. Assure that enough gel is applied to adequately cover each lesion. Normally, 0.5 g of gel is used on each 5 cm × 5 cm lesion site. The recommended duration of therapy is from 60 to 90 days. Complete healing of the lesion(s) or optimal therapeutic effect may not be evident for up to 30 days following cessation of therapy. Lesions that do not respond to therapy must be carefully reevaluated and management reconsidered.

➤*Storage/Stability:* Store at controlled room temperatures (15° to 30°C; 59° to 86°F). Protect from heat. Avoid freezing.

Actions

➤*Pharmacology:* The mechanism of action of diclofenac in the treatment of AK is unknown. The contribution to efficacy of individual components of the vehicle has not been established.

➤*Pharmacokinetics:*

Absorption – When diclofenac is applied topically, it is absorbed into the epidermis. In a study in patients with compromised skin (mainly atopic dermatitis and other dermatitic conditions) of the hands, arms, or face, ≈ 10% of the applied dose (2 g of 3% gel over 100 cm^2) of diclofenac was absorbed systemically in normal and compromised epidermis after 7 days, with 4 times daily applications.

After topical application of 2 g diclofenac 3 times daily for 6 days to the calf of the leg in healthy subjects, diclofenac could be detected in plasma. The systemic bioavailability after topical application of diclofenac is lower than after oral dosing.

Blood drawn at the end of treatment from 60 patients with AK lesions treated with topical diclofenac in 3 adequate and well-controlled clinical trials were assayed for diclofenac levels. Each patient was administered 0.5 g diclofenac gel twice a day for ≤ 105 days. There were ≤ three 5 cm × 5 cm treatment sites per patient on the face, forehead, hands, forearm, and scalp. Serum concentrations of diclofenac were on the average ≤ 20 ng/mL. These data indicate that systemic absorption of diclofenac in patients treated topically with diclofenac is much lower than that occurring after oral daily dosing of diclofenac sodium.

Distribution – Diclofenac binds tightly to serum albumin. Diclofenac's volume of distribution following oral administration is ≈ 550 mL/kg.

Metabolism – Biotransformation of diclofenac following oral administration involves conjugation at the carboxyl group of the side chain or single or multiple hydroxylations resulting in several phenolic metabolites, most of which are converted to glucuronide conjugates. Two of these phenolic metabolites are biologically active; however, to a much smaller extent than diclofenac. Metabolism following topical administration is thought to be similar to that after oral administration. The small amounts of diclofenac and its metabolites appearing in the plasma following topical administration makes the quantification of specific metabolites imprecise.

Excretion – Diclofenac and its metabolites are excreted mainly in the urine after oral dosing. Systemic clearance of diclofenac from plasma is ≈ 263 mL/min. The terminal plasma half-life is 1 to 2 hours. Four of the metabolites also have short terminal half-lives of 1 to 3 hours.

Contraindications

Patients with a known hypersensitivity to diclofenac, benzyl alcohol, polyethylene glycol monomethyl ether 350, or hyaluronate sodium.

Warnings

➤*Hypersensitivity reactions:* As with other NSAIDs, anaphylactoid reactions may occur in patients without prior exposure to diclofenac. Administer diclofenac with caution to patients with the aspirin triad. The triad typically occurs in asthmatic patients who experience rhinitis with or without nasal polyps, or who exhibit severe, potentially fatal bronchospasm after taking aspirin or other NSAIDs.

➤*Carcinogenesis:* A photocarcinogenicity study with ≤ 0.035% diclofenac in the vehicle gel was conducted in hairless mice at topical doses ≤ 2.8 mg/kg/day. Median tumor onset was earlier in the 0.035% group.

➤*Elderly:* Of the 211 subjects treated with diclofenac in controlled clinical studies, 143 subjects were ≥ 65 years of age. Of those 143 subjects, 55 subjects were ≥ 75 years of age. No overall differences in safety or effectiveness were observed between these subjects and younger subjects, and other reported clinical experience has not identified differences in responses between the elderly and younger patients, but greater sensitivity of some older individuals cannot be ruled out.

➤*Pregnancy: Category B.* The safety of diclofenac gel has not been established during pregnancy. However, there are no adequate and well-controlled studies performed with diclofenac alone at oral doses ≤ 20 mg/kg/day (15 times the estimated systemic human exposure) in mice, 10 mg/kg/day (15 times the estimated systemic human exposure) in rats, and 10 mg/kg/day (30 times the estimated systemic human exposure) in rabbits have revealed no evidence of teratogenicity despite the induction of maternal toxicity. In rats, maternally toxic doses were associated with dystocia, prolonged gestation, reduced fetal weights and growth, and reduced fetal survival.

Diclofenac has been shown to cross the placental barrier in mice and rats. However, there are no adequate and well-controlled studies in pregnant women. Because animal reproduction studies are not always predictive of human response, do not use during pregnancy unless the benefits to the mother justify the potential risk to the fetus. Because of the risk to the fetus resulting in premature closure of the ductus arteriosus, avoid diclofenac in late pregnancy.

The effects of diclofenac on labor and delivery in pregnant women are unknown. Because of the known effects of prostaglandin-inhibiting drugs on the fetal cardiovascular system (closure of ductus arteriosus), avoid use of diclofenac during late pregnancy. As with other NSAIDs, it is possible that diclofenac may inhibit uterine contractions and delay parturition.

➤*Lactation:* Because of the potential for serious adverse reactions in nursing infants from diclofenac, a decision should be made whether to discontinue nursing or to discontinue the drug, taking into account the importance of the drug to the mother.

➤*Children:* AK is not a condition seen within the pediatric population; do not use diclofenac gel in children.

Precautions

Do not allow gel to come in contact with the eyes. The safety of the concomitant use of sunscreens, cosmetics, or other topical medications and diclofenac is unknown.

➤*Special risk:* Use diclofenac gel with caution in patients with active GI ulceration or bleeding and severe renal or hepatic impairments. Do not apply to open skin wounds, infections, or exfoliative dermatitis.

Drug Interactions

➤*NSAIDs:* Although the systemic absorption of diclofenac is low, minimize concomitant oral administration of other NSAIDs such as aspirin at anti-inflammatory/analgesic doses.

Adverse Reactions

Of the 423 patients evaluable for safety in adequate and well-controlled trials, 211 were treated with diclofenac and 212 were treated with vehicle gel. Eighty-seven percent of the diclofenac-treated patients and 84% of the vehicle-treated patients experienced ≥ 1 adverse reactions during the studies. The majority of these reactions were mild-to-moderate in severity and resolved upon discontinuation of therapy.

Of the 211 patients treated with diclofenac, 82% experienced adverse reactions involving skin and the application site compared to 75% of the vehicle-treated patients. Application site reactions were the most frequent adverse reactions in both groups. Contact dermatitis, rash, dry skin, and exfoliation (scaling) were significantly more prevalent in the diclofenac group than in the vehicle-treated patients.

Eighteen percent of diclofenac-treated patients and 4% of vehicle-treated patients discontinued from the clinical trials because of adverse reactions (whether considered related to treatment or not). These discontinuations were mainly caused by skin irritation or related cutaneous adverse reactions.

Adverse Reactions Reported During Diclofenac Phase 3 Clinical Trials for 60- and 90-day Treatments (%)

	60-day treatment		90-day treatment	
Adverse reaction	Diclofenac (n = 48)	Gel vehicle (n = 49)	Diclofenac (n = 114)	Gel vehicle (n = 114)
Cardiovascular				
Chest pain	2	0	1	0
Hypertension	2	0	1	0
Phlebitis	0	2	0	0
CNS				
Anxiety	0	2	0	1
Dizziness	0	0	0	4
Hypokinesia	2	0	0	0
Headache	0	6	7	6
Migraine	0	2	1	0

DICLOFENAC SODIUM — TOPICAL

Adverse Reactions Reported During Diclofenac Phase 3 Clinical Trials for 60- and 90-day Treatments (%)				
	60-day treatment		90-day treatment	
Adverse reaction	Diclofenac (n = 48)	Gel vehicle (n = 49)	Diclofenac (n = 114)	Gel vehicle (n = 114)
Dermatologic				
Acne	0	2	0	1
Application site reaction	75	71	84	70
Acne	0	4	1	0
Alopecia	2	0	1	1
Contact dermatitis	19	4	33	4
Dry skin	27	12	25	17
Edema	4	0	3	0
Exfoliation	6	4	24	13
Hyperesthesia	0	0	3	1
Pain	15	22	26	30
Paresthesia	8	4	20	20
Photosensitivity reaction	0	2	3	0
Pruritus	31	59	52	45
Rash	35	20	46	17
Vesiculobullous rash	0	0	4	1
Contact dermatitis	2	0	0	0
Dry skin	0	4	3	0
Herpes simplex	0	2	0	0
Maculopapular rash	0	2	0	0
Pain	2	2	1	0
Pruritus	4	6	4	1
Rash	2	10	4	0
Skin carcinoma	0	6	2	2
Skin nodule	0	2	0	0
Skin ulcer	2	0	1	0
GI				
Abdominal pain	2	0	1	0
Constipation	0	0	0	2
Diarrhea	2	0	2	3
Dyspepsia	2	0	3	4
Lab test abnormalities				
Increased creatine phosphokinase	0	0	4	1
Increased creatinine	2	2	0	1
Hypercholesteremia	0	2	1	0
Hyperglycemia	0	2	1	0
AST increased	0	0	3	0
ALT increased	0	0	2	0
Musculoskeletal				
Back pain	4	0	2	2
Arthralgia	2	0	0	2
Arthrosis	2	0	0	0
Myalgia	2	0	3	1
Respiratory				
Asthma	2	0	0	0
Dyspnea	2	0	2	0
Pharyngitis	2	8	2	4
Pneumonia	2	0	0	1
Rhinitis	2	2	2	2
Sinusitis	0	0	2	0
Miscellaneous				
Accidental injury	0	0	4	2
Allergic reaction	0	0	1	3
Asthenia	0	0	2	0
Chills	0	2	0	0
Edema	0	2	0	0
Flu syndrome	10	6	1	4
Infection	4	6	4	5
Neck pain	0	0	2	0
Pain	2	0	2	2
Conjunctivitis	2	0	4	1
Eye pain	0	2	2	0
Hematuria	0	0	2	1
Procedure	0	0	0	3

DICLOFENAC SODIUM — TOPICAL

➤*Dermatologic:* Skin hypertrophy, paresthesia, seborrhea, urticaria, application site reactions (skin carcinoma, hypertonia, skin hypertrophy lacrimation disorder, maculopapular rash, purpuric rash, vasodilation) (less than 1%).

Overdosage

➤*Treatment:* In the event of oral ingestion of diclofenac gel, resulting in significant systemic side effects, it is recommended that the stomach be emptied by vomiting or lavage. Forced diuresis may theoretically be beneficial because the drug is excreted in the urine. The effect of dialysis or hemoperfusion in the elimination of diclofenac (99% protein-bound) remains unproven. In addition to supportive measures, the use of oral activated charcoal may help to reduce the absorption of diclofenac. Give supportive and symptomatic treatment for complications such as renal failure, convulsions, GI irritation, and respiratory depression.

Patient Information

In clinical studies, localized dermal side effects such as contact dermatitis, exfoliation, dry skin, and rash were found in patients treated with diclofenac at a higher incidence than in those with placebo.

Patients should understand the importance of monitoring and follow-up evaluation, the signs and symptoms of dermal adverse reactions, and the possibility of irritant or allergic contact dermatitis. If severe dermal reactions occur, treatment with diclofenac may be interrupted until the condition subsides.

Avoid exposure to sunlight and the use of sunlamps.

Safety and efficacy of the use of diclofenac together with other dermal products, including cosmetics, sunscreens, and other topical medications on the area being treated have not been studied.

SALICYLIC ACID

otc	**Panscol** (Baker Cummins)	**Ointment**: 3%	In 90 g.
otc	**MG217 Sal-Acid Ointment** (Triton)	**Ointment**: 3% with vitamin E	In 2 oz.
otc	**Fostex** (Bristol Products)	**Cream**: 2% with etetic acid, stearyl alcohol	In 118 g.
Rx	**Salex** (Healthpoint)	**Cream**: 6%	Alcohols, glycerin, parabens. In 400 g bottles.
otc	**Panscol** (Baker Cummins)	**Lotion**: 3%	In 120 mL.
Rx	**Salex** (Healthpoint)	**Lotion**: 6%	In 414 mL.
otc	**Fung-O** (S.S.S. Company)	**Liquid**: 17% salicylic acid, 2% alcohol and 68% ether	In 15 mL w/drop applicator.
otc	**Mosco** (Medtech)	**Liquid**: 17.6% in a flexible collodion base with 33% alcohol and 65.5% ether	In 10 mL.
otc	**Dr Scholl's Wart Remover Kit** (Schering-Plough)	**Liquid**: 17% in a flexible collodion with 17% alcohol, 52% ether, acetone	In 10 mL with brush and cushions.
otc	**Occlusal-HP** (GenDerm)	**Liquid**: 17% in a polyacrylic vehicle with isopropyl alcohol	In 10 mL with brush applicator.
otc	**Compound W** (Whitehall)	**Liquid**: 17% with collodion, 21.2% alcohol, 63.6% ether, camphor, castor oil, menthol	In 9 mL.
otc	**DuoFilm** (Schering-Plough)	**Liquid**: 17% in flexible collodion with 15.8% alcohol, castor oil, 42.6% ether	In 15 mL with brush applicator.
otc	**Maximum Strength Wart Remover** (Glades)	**Liquid**: 17% with 29% alcohol, castor oil in a flexible collodion	In 13.3 mL with applicator.
otc	**Off-Ezy Wart Remover Kit** (Del Pharm)	**Liquid**: 17% in collodion-like vehicle with 21% alcohol and 65% ether, acetone	In 13.5 mL with skin buffer and applicator.
otc	**Off-Ezy Corn & Callus Remover Kit** (Del Pharm)	**Liquid**: 17% in collodion-like vehicle with 21% alcohol and 65% ether, acetone	In 13.5 mL with callus smoother and corn cushions.
otc	**Wart-Off** (Pfizer)	**Liquid**: 17% in flexible collodion with 26.35% alcohol, propylene glycol dipelargonate	In 15 mL with applicator.
otc	**Salactic Film** (Pedinol)	**Liquid**: 17% in collodion-like vehicle	In 15 mL with brush applicator.
otc	**Gordofilm** (Gordon)	**Liquid**: 16.7% in flexible collodion	In 15 mL with brush applicator.
otc	**Freezone** (Whitehall)	**Liquid**: 13.6% in a collodion-like vehicle, 20.5% alcohol, 64.8% ether, castor oil	In 9 mL.
otc	**Dr Scholl's Corn/Callus Remover** (Schering-Plough)	**Liquid**: 12.6% in flexible collodion with 18% alcohol, 55% ether, acetone, hydrogenated vegetable oil	In 10 mL with 3 cushions.
otc	**Hydrisalic** (Pedinol)	**Gel**: 6%	Alcohol. In 28.35 g.
otc	**Sal-Plant** (Pedinol)	**Gel**: 17% in collodion-like vehicle	In 14 g.
otc	**Compound W** (Whitehall)	**Gel**: 17% with 67.5% alcohol, camphor, castor oil, collodion, colloidal silicon dioxide, hydroxypropyl cellulose, hypophosphorous acid, polysorbate 80	In 7 g.
otc	**DuoPlant** (Schering-Plough)	**Gel**: 17% in flexible collodion with 57.6% alcohol, 16.42% ether, ethyl lactate, hydroxypropyl cellulose, polybutene	In 14.2 g.
otc	**Keralyt** (Summers)	**Gel**: 6%, 21% SD-40 alcohol	In 28.4 g.
otc	**Psor-a-set** (Hogil)	**Soap**: 2%	In 97.5 g.
otc	**DuoFilm** (Schering-Plough)	**Transdermal patch**: 40% in a rubber-based vehicle	In 18s (containing 3 sizes).
otc	**Trans-Ver-Sal PlantarPatch** (Doak)	**Transdermal patch**: 15% with karaya, PEG-300, propylene glycol, quaternium-15	20 mm patches in 25s with 25 securing tapes and one emery file.
otc	**Trans-Ver-Sal PediaPatch** (Doak)	**Transdermal patch**: 15% in karaya gum base	In 6 mm (20s) with bandage tapes.
otc	**Trans-Ver-Sal AdultPatch** (Doak)	**Transdermal patch**: 15% with karaya, PEG-300, propylene glycol, quaternium-15	6 or 12 mm patches in 40s with 42 securing tapes and one emery file.
otc	**Mediplast** (Beiersdorf)	**Plaster**: 40%	2″ × 3″ patches in 2s and 25s.
otc	**Sal-Acid** (Pedinol)	**Plaster**: 40% in a plaster vehicle	In 14s.

SALICYLIC ACID

otc	**Dr Scholl's Advanced Pain Relief Corn Removers** (Schering-Plough)	**Disk:** 40% in a rubber-based vehicle	In 6s with cushions.
otc	**Dr Scholl's Callus Removers** (Schering-Plough)		In 4s with 6 pads and 4s with 4 pads (extra-thick).
otc	**Dr Scholl's Clear Away Plantar** (Schering-Plough)		In 24s with cushions.
otc	**Dr Scholl's Clear Away** (Schering-Plough)		In 18s with cover-up disks.
otc	**Dr Scholl's Corn Removers** (Schering-Plough)		In 9s (pads and disks) as regular, extra-thick, soft, small, waterproof and ultra-thin and 6s (pads and disks) as wrap-around.
otc	**Dr Scholl's Moisturizing Corn Remover Kit** (Schering-Plough)		In 6s with moisturizing cream and cushions.
otc	**Dr Scholl's Clear Away OneStep** (Schering-Plough)	**Strips:** 40% in a rubber-based vehicle	In 14s.
otc	**Dr Scholl's OneStep Corn Removers** (Schering-Plough)		In 6s.
otc	**Compound W for Kids** (Medtech)	**Pad:** 40% in a plaster vehicle	Lanolin, rubber. In 12s.

SALICYLIC ACID — TOPICAL

Indications

➤*Hyperkeratotic skin disorders:* A topical aid in the removal of excessive keratin in hyperkeratotic skin disorders, including common and plantar warts, psoriasis, calluses and corns.

➤*Unlabeled uses:* The use of a 40% salicylic acid disk covered with an adhesive strip has been used to aid in the removal of inaccessible splinters in children.

Administration and Dosage

Apply to affected area. May soak in warm water for 5 minutes prior to use to hydrate skin and enhance the effect. Remove any loose tissue with brush, wash cloth or emery board and dry thoroughly.

In general, for treatment of warts, improvement should occur in 1 to 2 weeks; maximum resolution may be expected after 4 to 6 weeks, although application for up to 12 weeks may be necessary. If skin irritation develops or there is no improvement after several weeks, contact a physician.

➤*Storage/Stability:* Some products are flammable; keep away from fire or flame. Keep bottle tightly capped and store at room temperature away from heat.

Actions

➤*Pharmacology:* Salicylic acid is the only *otc* product considered safe and effective by the FDA for use as a keratolytic for corns, calluses and warts. Salicylic acid produces desquamation of the horny layer of skin, while not affecting the structure of the viable epidermis, by dissolving intercellular cement substance. The keratolytic action causes the cornified epithelium to swell, soften, macerate and then desquamate.

Salicylic acid is keratolytic at concentrations of approximately 2% to 6%. These concentrations are generally used for treatment of dandruff, seborrhea and psoriasis. Concentrations of 5% to 17% in collodion are safe and effective for the removal of common and plantar warts; up to 40% in plasters is used to remove warts, corns and calluses.

Salicylic acid preparations, alone or in combination, have also been used to treat dandruff, seborrheic dermatitis, acne, tinea infections and psoriasis.

➤*Pharmacokinetics:*

Absorption/Distribution – In a study of the percutaneous absorption of salicylic acid in four patients with extensive active psoriasis, peak serum salicylate levels never exceeded 5 mg/dl even though more than 60% of the applied salicylic acid was absorbed. Systemic toxic reactions are usually associated with much higher serum levels (30 to 40 mg/dl). Peak serum levels occurred within 5 hours of the topical application under occlusion.

Metabolism/Excretion – The major urinary metabolites identified after topical administration differ from those after oral salicylate administration; those derived from percutaneous absorption contain more salicylate glucuronides (42%) and less salicyluric (52%) and salicylic acid (6%).

Contraindications

Sensitivity to salicylic acid; prolonged use, especially in infants, diabetics, and patients with impaired circulation; use on moles, birthmarks or warts with hair growing from them, genital or facial warts or warts on mucous membranes, irritated skin or any area that is infected or reddened.

Warnings

➤*Salicylate toxicity:* Prolonged use over large areas, especially in young children and those patients with significant renal or hepatic impairment, could result in salicylism. Limit the area to be treated and be aware of signs of salicylate toxicity (eg, nausea, vomiting, dizziness, loss of hearing, tinnitus, lethargy, hyperpnea, diarrhea, psychic disturbances). In the event of salicylic acid toxicity, discontinue use.

➤*Special risk patients:* Do not use if diabetic or poor blood circulation exists.

➤*Pregnancy: Category C.* There are no adequate and well controlled studies in pregnant women. Use during pregnancy only if the potential benefit justifies the potential risk to the fetus.

Precautions

➤*For external use only:* Avoid contact with eyes, mucous membranes and normal skin surrounding warts. If contact with eyes or mucous membranes occurs, immediately flush with water for 15 minutes. Avoid inhaling vapors.

Drug Interactions

Interactions have been reported with both topical and oral salicylates. Refer to the Salicylates monograph for a complete listing.

Adverse Reactions

Local irritation may occur from contact with normal skin surrounding the affected area. If irritation occurs, temporarily discontinue use and take care to apply only to wart site when treatment is resumed.

Patient Information

For external use only. Avoid contact with eyes, face, genitals, mucous membranes and normal skin surrounding warts.

Medication may cause reddening or scaling of skin when used on open skin lesions.

Contact with clothing, fabrics, plastics, wood, metal or other materials may cause damage; avoid contact.

SULFUR PREPARATIONS

otc	**Sulpho-Lac Acne Medication** (Doak)	**Cream:** 5% sulfur	27% zinc sulfate, 53% Vleminckx's solution base. Greaseless. In 28.35 and 50 g.
otc	**Acne Lotion 10** (C & M)	**Lotion:** 10% colloidal sulfur	22.5% isopropyl alcohol. Tinted. Aqueous. In 60 mL.
otc	**Liquimat** (Galderma)	**Lotion:** 4% sulfur	22% SD alcohol 40, cetyl alcohol. Assorted tints. In 45 mL.
otc	**Sulpho-Lac** (Doak)	**Soap:** 5% sulfur	In a coconut and tallow oil soap base. In 85 g.
otc	**Sulmasque** (C & M)	**Mask:** 6.4% sulfur	With 15% isopropyl alcohol, methylparaben. In 150 g.

SULFUR — TOPICAL

Indications

➤*Dandruff:*

Shampoo – Relieves the itching and scalp flaking associated with dandruff.

For men, women, and children over 2 years of age. Daily shampooing may be helpful if scalp is oily.

➤*Acne:*

Soap – Aids in the treatment of mild acne and oily skin.

Softens the hard shell of acne blemishes, helps dissolve and remove blackheads, washes away excess oils which may cause blackheads, and refreshes skin.

Administration and Dosage

➤*Shampoo:* Shake well. Wet hair and vigorously massage a small amount of sulfur topical medicated antidandruff shampoo into hair and scalp working up a lather. Rinse thoroughly with warm water. Repeat procedure.

➤*Soap:* Use twice daily. Work up lather with hands or washcloth and apply to affected areas without scrubbing. Let dry about 1 minute, rinse thoroughly, and pat dry.

Actions

➤*Pharmacology:* Sulfur, a keratolytic, provides peeling and drying actions. Although it may help to resolve comedones, it may also promote the development of new ones by increasing horny cell adhesion.

Warnings

➤*Shampoo:* For external use only. Avoid contact with the eyes; if this happens, rinse thoroughly with water. If condition worsens or does not improve after regular use of this product as directed, consult a physician. Do not use on children under 2 years of age except as directed by a physician.

➤*Soap:* Use with other topical acne medications at the same time or immediately following use of this product may increase dryness or irritation of the skin. If this occurs, use only 1 medication unless directed by a doctor. Do not get into eyes.

Patient Information

Stop use and ask doctor if excessive skin irritation develops or increases.

Keep out of reach of children. If swallowed, get medical help or contact a poison control center immediately.

KERATOLYTIC AGENT COMBINATION

otc	**Gets-It** (Oakhurst)	**Liquid:** Salicylic acid, zinc chloride and collodion in ≈ 35% ether and ≈ 28% alcohol	In 12 mL.

ACNE PRODUCTS, COMBINATIONS

		Sulfur	Salicylic Acid	Resorcinol	Other Content	How Supplied
otc	**Finac Lotion** (C & M)		2%		22.5% isopropyl alcohol, propylene glycol, acetone	In 60 mL.
otc	**PROPApH Cleansing Lotion for Normal/Combination Skin** (Del)		0.5%		SD alcohol 40, menthol, EDTA	In 180 mL (lotion) and 45s (pads).
otc	**PROPApH Cleansing Pads** (Del)		0.5%		SD alcohol 40, EDTA, menthol	In 45s.
otc	**PROPApH Cleansing for Oily Skin Lotion** (Del)		0.6%		SD alcohol 40, EDTA, menthol	In 180 mL.
Rx	**Clenia Cream** (Upsher-Smith)	5%			10% sodium sulfacetamide, parabens, EDTA	In 28 g tubes.
Rx	**Clenia Foam** (Upsher-Smith)	5%			10% sodium sulfacetamide, parabens, EDTA	In 170 and 340 mg bottles.
Rx	**Rosac Cream** (Stiefel)	5%			10% sodium sulfacetamide, benzyl alcohol, cetostearyl alcohol, EDTA	In 45 g.
Rx	**Sodium Sulfacetamide 10% and Sulfur 5%** (Glades)	5%			10% sodium sulfacetamide, cetyl alcohol, benzyl alcohol, EDTA	In 30 mL tube and 25 mL.
Rx	**Zetacet Topical Suspension** (Stiefel)	5%			10% sodium sulfacetamide, cetyl alcohol, benzyl alcohol, EDTA	In 30 g.
Rx	**Zetacet Wash** (Stiefel)	5%			10% sodium sulfacetamide, alcohols, EDTA, parabens, white petrolatum	In 170.1 and 340.2 g.
Rx	**Avar Cleanser** (Sirius)	5%			10% sodium sulfacetamide, cetyl alcohol, stearyl alcohol	In 226.8 g.
Rx	**Avar-e Emollient Cream** (Sirius)	5%			10% sodium sulfacetamide, glycerin, EDTA, benzyl alcohol, cetyl alcohol	In 45 g.
Rx	**Avar-e Green Cream** (Sirius)	5%			10% sodium sulfacetamide, glycerin, EDTA, benzyl alcohol, cetyl alcohol	For color correction. In 45 g.
Rx	**Avar Gel** (Sirius)	5%			10% sodium sulfacetamide, EDTA, benzyl alcohol	In 45 g.
Rx	**Avar Green Gel** (Sirius)	5%			10% sodium sulfacetamide, EDTA, benzyl alcohol	For color correction. In 45 g.
Rx	**Plexion Cleansing Cloths** (Medicis)	5%			10% sodium sulfacetamide, glycerine, glyceryl stearate, stearyl alcohol, propylene glycol, propylene glycol oleate, cetyl alcohol, EDTA, parabens, decolorized aloe vera gel	In 30s.
Rx	**Plexion Cleanser** (Medicis)	5%			10% sodium sulfacetamide, cetyl alcohol, stearyl alcohol, EDTA, parabens	In 170 and 340 g.
Rx	**Plexion TS Topical Suspension** (Medicis)	5%			10% sodium sulfacetamide, mineral oil, glyceryl stearate, propylene glycol, benzyl alcohol, cetyl alcohol, stearyl alcohol, EDTA, sodium thiosulfate, coco-glycerides	In 30s.
Rx	**Plexion SCT Cream** (Medicis)	5%			10% sodium sulfacetamide, witch hazel, benzyl alcohol	In 120 g.
Rx	**Rosanil Cleanser** (Galderma)	5%			10% sodium sulfacetamide, EDTA, light mineral oil, parabens	In 170 g.
Rx	**Rosula Gel** (Doak)	5%			10% sodium sulfacetamide in a 10% urea vehicle	In 45 mL.
Rx	**Vanocin** (Stratus)	5%			10% sodium sulfacetamide, benzyl alcohol, cetyl alcohol, EDTA, parabens, stearyl alcohol	In 30 and 60 g.
Rx	**Sulfacet-R Lotion** (Dermik)	5%			10% sodium sulfacet amide, parabens	Tinted. In 25 mL.
Rx	**Novacet Lotion** (Genderm)	5%			10% sodium sulfacetamide, cetyl alcohol, benzyl alcohol, EDTA, sodium thiosulfate	In 30 mL.
otc	**Acno Lotion** (Baker Cummins)	3%				Greaseless. In 120 mL.
otc	**Acnotex Lotion** (C & M)	8%		2%	20% isopropyl alcohol	In 60 mL.
otc	**Acnomel Cream** (Numark)	8%		2%	11% alcohol	In 28 g.
otc	**Adult Acnomel Cream** (Numark)	8%		2%	15% alcohol, propylene glycol	Tinted. In 28 g.
otc	**Medicated Acne Cleanser** (C & M)	4%		2%		In 129 g.
otc	**Sulforcin Lotion** (Galderma)	5%		2%	11.65% SD alcohol 40, methylparaben	In 120 mL.

ACNE PRODUCTS, COMBINATIONS

		Sulfur	Salicylic Acid	Resorcinol	Other Content	How Supplied
otc	**Rezamid Lotion** (Summers)	5%		2%	28% alcohol	In 56.7 mL.
otc	**R/S Lotion** (Summers)					In 56.7 mL.
otc	**Clearasil Clearstick Maximum Strength** (Procter & Gamble)		2%		39% alcohol, menthol, EDTA	For regular and sensitive skin. In 35 mL.
otc	**Clearasil Double Clear Maximum Strength Pads** (Procter & Gamble)		2%		40% alcohol, witch hazel distillate, menthol	In 32s.
otc	**Fostex Acne Cleansing Cream** (Westwood Squibb)		2%		Stearyl alcohol, EDTA	In 118 g.
otc	**Oxy Night Watch Maximum Strength Lotion** (SK-Beecham)		2%		Cetyl alcohol, EDTA, parabens, stearyl alcohol	In 60 mL.
otc	**PROPApH Acne Maximum Strength Cream** (Del)		2%		Lanolin alcohol, cetearyl alcohol, EDTA, menthol, stearyl alcohol	In 19.5 g.
otc	**Sal-Clens Acne Cleanser Gel** (C & M)		2%			In 240 g.
otc	**Sebasorb Lotion** (Summers)		2%		10% attapulgite	In 45 mL.
otc	**Stridex Clear Gel** (Sterling Health)		2%		9.3% SD alcohol	In 30 g.
otc	**Clearasil Clearstick Regular Strength** (Procter & Gamble)		1.25%		39% alcohol, aloe vera gel, menthol, disodium EDTA	In 35 mL.
otc	**Clearasil Double Clear Pads Regular Strength** (Procter & Gamble)		1.25%		40% alcohol, witch hazel distillate, menthol	In 32s.
otc	**Oxy Night Watch Sensitive Skin Lotion** (SK-Beecham)		1%		Cetyl alcohol. EDTA, stearyl alcohol, parabens	In 60 mL.
otc	**RA Lotion** (Medco Lab)			3%	43% alcohol	In 120, 240, and 480 mL.
otc	**Clearasil Adult Care Cream** (Procter & Gamble)				Sulfur, resorcinol, 10% alcohol, parabens	In 17 g.
Rx	**Klaron** (Dermik)				10% sodium sulfacetamide, propylene glycol, polyethylene glycol 400, methylparaben, EDTA	In 59 mL.
Rx	**Seb-Prev** (Glades)				10% sodium sulfacetamide, propylene glycol, methylparaben, EDTA	In 118 mL.
Rx	**Rosula NS Medicated Pads** (Doak)				10% sodium sulfacetamide, 10% urea, sodium EDTA, sodium thiosulfate	In 30s.

[a] Sirius Laboratories, Inc., 100 Fairway Drive, Suite 130, Vernon Hills, IL 60061; (847) 968–2424.

ACNE PRODUCTS, COMBINATIONS — TOPICAL

Active Ingredients

These products contain keratolytics and astringents to aid in removing keratin and to dry the skin. Many products also have hydroalcoholic or organic solvent bases to aid in removal of sebum. Individual components include:

➤*ANTIMICROBIAL:* Sodium thiosulfate and sodium sulfacetamide.

➤*ANTISEPTIC:* Ethanol, isopropyl alcohol, phenol, sulfur and acetone.

➤*KERATOLYTICS:* Salicylic acid, resorcinol and sulfur.

➤*PROTECTIVES and ADSORBANTS:* Zinc oxide.

Hydrocortisone-containing acne products are listed under Topical Corticosteroid Combinations.

LOCAL ANESTHETICS, TOPICAL

In addition to the single entity products listed in this section, other products containing topical local anesthetics are listed in other sections, based on their specific uses. These include: Anorectal Preparations and Ophthalmic Local Anesthetics (see individual monographs).

Indications

Because of the diversity of uses of these products, the following is a general discussion. For information on specific applications of individual products, consult the manufacturer's package literature.

➤*Skin disorders:* For topical anesthesia in local skin disorders, including: Pruritus and pain due to minor burns, skin manifestations of systemic disease (eg, chickenpox), prickly heat, abrasions, sunburn, plant poisoning, insect bites, eczema; local analgesia on normal, intact skin (EMLA).

➤*Mucous membranes:* For local anesthesia of accessible mucous membranes, including: Oral, nasal and laryngeal mucous membranes; respiratory or urinary tracts. Also for the treatment of pruritus ani, pruritus vulvae and hemorrhoids.

Administration and Dosage

➤*Topical:* Apply to the affected area as needed. Ointments and creams can be applied to gauze or to a bandage prior to applying to the skin.

➤*Mucous membranes:* Dosage varies and depends upon the area to be anesthetized, vascularity of tissues, individual tolerance and technique of anesthesia. Administer the lowest dose possible that still provides adequate anesthesia. Apply to affected areas using the proper technique (see individual manufacturer inserts).

In debilitated, elderly patients or children, administer lower concentrations.

A combination of tetracaine 0.5%, epinephrine 1:2000 and cocaine 11.8% (also known as TAC) in a liquid topical formulation has been used for minor skin lacerations, especially of the face and scalp. Other preparations include cocaine 11.8% and epinephrine 1:1000, and lidocaine 4%, epinephrine 1:1000 and tetracaine 0.5%, both utilizing methylcellulose for a more viscous gel formulation. Use results in decreased pain on application, allowing for better compliance and tolerance of repair procedure. This may be beneficial in patients who cannot tolerate injection anesthesia or those who are difficult to control (eg, children). A commercial preparation of lidocaine and prilocaine (EMLA) was developed for a similar purpose (increased absorption in children) on intact skin. However, toxic effects are also more likely to occur in infants and children with all of these preparations.

The use of the lidocaine/prilocaine combination appears to be beneficial as a pretreatment in decreasing the pain of DPT vaccinations (and presumably other vaccinations) in infants. The cream is applied at the injection site with occlusive dressing for at least 60 minutes prior to the vaccination.

Actions

➤*Pharmacology:* Local anesthetics inhibit conduction of nerve impulses from sensory nerves. This action results from an alteration of the cell membrane permeability to ions. Although poorly absorbed through the intact epidermis (except for the lidocaine/prilocaine mixture; penetration and subsequent systemic absorption is enhanced over use of each agent alone), these agents are readily absorbed from mucous membranes. When skin permeability has been increased by abrasions or ulcers, the absorption and, subsequently, the efficacy of local anesthetics improves; however, the incidence of side effects also increases. Onset, depth and duration of dermal analgesia provided by the lidocaine/prilocaine mixture depends primarily on duration of application.

Topical Local Anesthetics: Indications, Dose, Strength, Peak Effect and Duration						
Local anesthetics, topical	Indications		Maximum adult dose (mg)	Available or recommended strengths (%)	Peak[a] effect (minutes)	Duration[a] of effect (minutes)
	Skin	Mucous membrane				
Amides	✓		25	0.5-1	< 5	15-45
Dibucaine						
Lidocaine	✓	✓	†[b]	2-5	2-5	15-45
Esters	✓	✓		0.5-20	< 5	15-45
Benzocaine						
Butamben picrate	✓			1		
Cocaine		✓	50-200	4-10	1-5	30-60
Tetracaine	✓	✓	50	0.5-2	3-8	30-60
Miscellaneous		✓	100	0.5-1	< 10	< 60
Dyclonine						
Pramoxine	✓		200	1	3-5	
Lidocaine/Prilocaine	✓			2.5/2.5	60-120	60-120

[a] Based primarily on application to mucous membranes.
[b] Variable depending on doseform.

Contraindications

Hypersensitivity to any component of these products; ophthalmic use.

Warnings

➤*Systemic effects:* Use the lowest dose effective for anesthesia to avoid high plasma levels and serious adverse effects. Repeated doses of **lidocaine** and **dyclonine** may cause significant increases in blood levels with each repeated dose because of slow accumulation of the drug or its metabolites. Have resuscitative equipment available for immediate use. Lidocaine/prilocaine is not recommended for use on mucous membranes because of its much greater absorption through this area than through intact skin, potentially resulting in serious adverse effects.

➤*Methomoglobinemia:* **Benzocaine**, **lidocaine** and **prilocaine** should not be used in those rare patients with congenital or idiopathic methemoglobinemia and in infants younger than 12 months of age who are receiving treatment with methemoglobin-inducing agents. Very young patients or patients with glucose-6–phosphate deficiencies are more susceptible to methemoglobinemia.

➤*Ototoxic effects:* **Lidocaine/prilocaine** has an ototoxic effect when instilled into the middle ear of animals, but not when used in the external auditory canal. Do not use this combination in any situation where penetration or migration beyond the tympanic membrane into the middle ear is possible.

➤*Hepatic function impairment:* Patients with severe hepatic disease, because of their inability to metabolize local anesthetics normally, are at greater risk of developing toxic plasma concentrations of lidocaine and prilocaine.

➤*Pregnancy:* *Category B* (lidocaine); *Category C* (benzocaine, cocaine, dyclonine, tetracaine). Safety for use during pregnancy has not been established. Use in women of childbearing potential, and particularly in early pregnancy, only when the potential benefits outweigh the potential hazards to the fetus.

➤*Lactation:* Lidocaine, and probably prilocaine, are excreted in breast milk. Exercise caution when administering any of these drugs to a nursing woman.

➤*Children:* Safety and efficacy of dyclonine and tetracaine have not been established in children younger than 12 years of age. Do not use benzocaine in infants less than 1 year of age. Dosages in children should be reduced commensurate with age, body weight and physical condition.

Precautions

➤*For external or mucous membrane use only:* Do not use in the eyes.

➤*Minimal effective dose:* Reactions and complications are best averted by using the minimal effective dose. Not for prolonged use. Give debilitated or elderly patients, acutely ill patients and children dosages commensurate with their age, size and physical condition.

➤*Severe shock / heartblock:* Use **lidocaine** and **dyclonine** with caution.

➤*Traumatized mucosa:* Use cautiously in persons with known drug sensitivities or in patients with severely traumatized mucosa and sepsis in the region of the application. If irritation or rash occurs, discontinue treatment and institute appropriate therapy.

➤*Oral use:* Topical anesthetics may impair swallowing and enhance danger of aspiration. Do not ingest food for 1 hour after anesthetic use in mouth or throat. This is particularly important in children because of their frequency of eating.

➤*Tartrazine sensitivity:* Some of these products contain tartrazine, which may cause allergic-type reactions (including bronchial asthma) in susceptible individuals. Although the incidence of tartrazine sensitivity in the general population is low, it is frequently seen in patients who also have aspirin hypersensitivity. Specific products containing tartrazine are identified in the product listings.

➤*Sulfite sensitivity:* Some of these products contain sulfites which may cause allergic-type reactions including anaphylactic symptoms and life-threatening or less severe asthmatic episodes in certain susceptible persons. The overall prevalence of sulfite sensitivity in the general population is unknown and probably low. Sulfite sensitivity is seen more frequently in asthmatic or atopic non-asthmatic persons. Specific products containing sulfites are identified in the product listings.

Drug Interactions

➤*Class I antiarrhythmic agents:* Use with caution in patients receiving Class I antiarrhythmic drugs (such as tocainide and mexiletine) because the toxic effects are additive and potentially synergistic.

➤*Drug / Lab test interactions:* Dyclonine topical solutions should not be used in cystoscopic procedures following intravenous pyelography because an iodine precipitate occurs which interferes with visualization.

Adverse Reactions

Adverse reactions are, in general, dose-related and may result from high plasma levels due to excessive dosage or rapid absorption, hypersensitivity, idiosyncrasy or diminished tolerance. (See Overdosage.)

➤*Hypersensitivity:* Cutaneous lesions; urticaria; edema; contact dermatitis; bronchospasm; shock; anaphylactoid reactions. The detection of sensitivity by skin testing is of doubtful value.

➤*Local:* Burning; stinging; tenderness; sloughing.

➤*Miscellaneous:* Urethritis with and without bleeding. In a few case reports, methemoglobinemia characterized by cyanosis has followed topical application of **benzocaine** or **lidocaine/prilocaine** and may be more common with prilocaine (see Warnings). Seizures in children have occurred from overuse of **oral lidocaine**.

Overdosage

➤*Symptoms:* Reactions due to overdosage (high plasma levels) are systemic and involve the CNS (convulsions) or the cardiovascular system (hypotension).

CNS – Reactions are excitatory or depressant, and may be characterized by: Nervousness; apprehension; euphoria; confusion; dizziness; lightheadedness; tinnitus; blurred vision; vomiting; sensations of heat, cold or numbness; twitching; tremors; drowsiness; convulsions; unconsciousness; respiratory depression or arrest. Excitatory reactions may be very brief or not occur at all; in this case, first sign of toxicity may be drowsiness, merging into unconsciousness and respiratory arrest.

Cardiovascular – Reactions are depressant, and may be characterized by: Hypotension; myocardial depression; bradycardia; cardiac arrest; cardiovascular collapse.

➤*Treatment:* Maintain airway and support ventilation. Cardiovascular support consists of vasopressors, preferably those that stimulate the myocardium, IV fluids and perhaps blood transfusions. Control convulsions by slow IV of 0.1 mg/kg diazepam or 10 to 50 mg succinylcholine, with continued use of oxygen. Refer to General Management of Acute Overdosage.

Methemoglobinemia – This may be treated with methylene blue 1%, 1 to 2 mg/kg IV over 10 minutes (refer to individual monograph).

Patient Information

Do not ingest food for 1 hour following use of oral topical anesthetic preparations in the mouth or throat. Topical anesthesia may impair swallowing, thus enhancing the danger of aspiration.

Numbness of the tongue or buccal mucosa may increase the danger of biting trauma. Do not eat or chew gum while the mouth or throat area is anesthetized.

When lidocaine/prilocaine is used, the patient should be aware that the production of dermal analgesia may be accompanied by the block of all sensations in the treated skin. For this reason, the patient should avoid inadvertent trauma to the treated area by scratching, rubbing, or exposure to extreme hot or cold temperatures until complete sensation has returned.

Amide Local Anesthetics

DIBUCAINE

otc	**Dibucaine** (Various, eg, IDE, Moore)	**Ointment**: 1%	In 30 g.
otc	**Nupercainal** (Ciba Consumer)		Acetone, sodium bisulfite, lanolin, mineral oil, white petrolatum. In 30 and 60 g.

DIBUCAINE HEMORRHOIDAL — TOPICAL

Complete prescribing information begins in the Local Anesthetics, Topical group monograph.

Indications

➤*Topical pain:* For prompt, temporary relief of pain, itching and burning due to hemorrhoids or other anorectal disorders. May also be used topically for temporary relief of pain and itching associated with sunburn, minor burns, cuts, scrapes, insect bites or minor skin irritation.

Administration and Dosage

➤*Adults:* When practical, cleanse the affected area with mild soap and warm water and rinse thoroughly. Gently dry by patting or blotting with toilet tissue or a soft cloth before application of this product. Puncture tube seal with cap or sharp object. Apply externally to the affected area up to 3 or 4 times daily.

➤*Children 2 to 12 years:* Do not use except under the advice and supervision of a physician.

➤*Infants younger than 2 years of age or less than 35 lbs body weight:* Do not use on infants younger than 2 years of age or less than 35 lbs body weight.

➤*Storage/Stability:* Store between 15° to 30°C (59° to 86°F). Keep this and all medication out of the reach of children.

LIDOCAINE HYDROCHLORIDE

otc	**Zilactin-L** (Zila)	**Liquid**: 2.5%	79.3% alcohol. In 10 mL.
Rx	**Numby Stuff** (Iomed)	**Solution, topical**: 2% For iontophoretic dermal delivery.	1:100,000 epinephrine/30 mL multiple-unit fliptop vial.
Rx	**LidoSite Topical System** (Vyteris)	**Patch**: 10% for iontophoretic delivery.	0.1% epinephrine, EDTA, sodium metabisulfite. Topical system includes 1 **Lidosite** controller and 25 **Lidosite** patches.
Rx	**Lidocaine HCl** (Moore)	**Ointment**: 5%	In 50 g.
otc	**Solarcaine Aloe Extra Burn Relief** (Schering-Plough)	**Cream**: 0.5%	Aloe, lanolin oil, lanolin, camphor, propylparaben, eucalyptus oil, EDTA, menthol, tartrazine. In 120 g.
Rx	**Lidocaine Hydrochloride** (River's Edge)	**Cream**: 3%	Alcohols, aluminum sulfate, glycerin, lt. mineral oil, parabens, petrolatum. In 28.35 and 85 g.
Rx	**LidaMantle** (Doak Dermatologics)		Cetyl alcohol, stearyl alcohol, glycerin, petrolatum, parabens, light mineral oil. In 28 and 85 g.
otc	**L-M-X4** (Ferndale)	**Cream**: 4%	Benzyl alcohol. In 5 and 30 g.
otc	**Lidosense 4** (River's Edge)		Benzyl alcohol. In 5, 15, and 30 g.
Rx	**Lidocaine Hydrochloride** (River's Edge)	**Lotion**: 3%	Aluminum sulfate, alcohols, glycerin, lt. mineral oil, parabens, petrolatum. In 177 mL.
otc	**Solarcaine Aloe Extra Burn Relief** (Schering-Plough)	**Gel**: 0.5%	Aloe vera gel, glycerin, EDTA, isopropyl alcohol, menthol, diazolidinyl urea, tartrazine. In 120 and 240 g.
otc	**Burn-O-Jel** (S.S.S. Company)		Aloe vera gel, EDTA, glycerin, ethyl alcohol. In 85 g.
otc	**Xylocaine** (AstraZeneca)	**Gel**: 2%	Parabens. In 5 and 30 mL.
otc	**DermaFlex** (Zila)	**Gel**: 2.5%	79% alcohol. In 15 g.
otc	**Solarcaine Aloe Extra Burn Relief** (Schering-Plough)	**Spray**: 0.5%	Aloe vera gel, glycerin, EDTA, diaolidinyl urea, vitamin E, parabens. In 135 mg.
Rx	**Lidocaine HCl Topical**[a] (Various, eg, Moore, Roxane)	**Solution**: 4% For topical anesthesia of accessible mucous membranes of the oral and nasal cavities and proximal portions of the digestive tract.	In 50 mL.[a]
Rx	**Xylocaine** (Astra)		Parabens. In 50 mL.
Rx	**Lidocaine 2% Viscous**[b] (Various, eg, Moore, Roxane)	**Solution**: 2% For topical anesthesia of irritated or inflamed mucous membranes of the mouth and pharynx. Also used to reduce gagging during the taking of x-rays or dental impressions.	In 50 and 100 mL and UD 20 mL.[abc]
Rx	**Xylocaine Viscous** (Astra)		Sodium carboxymethylcellulose, parabens, saccharin. In 100 and 450 mL.
Rx	**Anestacon** (PolyMedica)	**Jelly**: 2% For prevention and control of pain in procedures involving the male and female urethra, for topical treatment of painful urethritis and as an anesthetic lubricant for endotracheal intubation.	1% hydroxypropylmethylcellulose, 0.01% benzalkonium chloride. In 15 and 240 mL disposable units.
Rx	**Lidocaine HCl** (IMS)	**Jelly**: 2%	Preservative-free. In UD 5, 10, and 20 mL single-use vials. In 25s.
Rx	**Dentipatch** (Noven)	**Patch**: 23 mg/2 cm^2 patch For production of mild topical anesthesia of accessible mucous membranes of the mouth prior to superficial dental procedures.	Aspartame. In 50s or 100s.
		46.1 mg/2 cm^2 patch For production of mild topical anesthesia of accessible mucous membranes of the mouth prior to superficial dental procedures.	Aspartame. In 50s and 100s.
Rx	**Lidoderm** (Endo)	**Patch**: 10 × 14 cm. 5% lidocaine. For relief of pain associated with postherpetic neuralgia	EDTA, glycerin, parabens, polyvinyl alcohol. In 5s.

[a] May contain parabens.
[b] May contain sodium carboxymethylcellulose.
[c] May contain saccharin.

LIDOCAINE HYDROCHLORIDE — TOPICAL

Complete prescribing information begins in the Local Anesthetics, Topical group monograph.

[illegible]ications

[illegible]xicity: Lidocaine HCl 4% and 5% creams are not recommended in [illegible]l situation in which penetration or migration beyond the tym[illegible]nbrane into the middle ear is possible because of ototoxic effects [illegible]in animal studies.

➤*Anorectal discomfort:*

Cream 5% – For the temporary relief of local discomfort, including pain and itching, soreness or burning associated with anorectal disorders.

➤*Anesthetic lubricant for intubation:*

Jelly and ointment – Lidocaine HCl 2% jelly is useful as an anesthetic lubricant for endotracheal intubation (oral and nasal).

Amide Local Anesthetics

LIDOCAINE HYDROCHLORIDE — TOPICAL

Lidocaine HCl 5% ointment is also useful as an anesthetic lubricant for intubation.

➤*Oropharynx anesthetic:*

Ointment – For production of anesthesia of accessible mucous membrane of the oropharynx.

➤*Skin discomfort/irritation:*

Cream 4% and ointment 2.5% and 5% – For the temporary relief of pain associated with minor cuts and abrasions of the skin, minor burns, including sunburn, minor skin irritation or abrasions of the skin, and insect bites.

Cream 3% – Pruritus, pruritic eczemas, abrasions, minor burns, insect bites, pain, soreness and discomfort due to pruritus ani, pruritus vulvae, hemorrhoids, anal fissures, and similar conditions of the skin and mucous membranes.

➤*Urethral pain:*

Jelly – For prevention and control of pain in procedures involving the male and female urethra and for topical treatment of painful urethritis.

➤*Unlabeled uses:* Used intranasally in treatment of migraines.

Administration and Dosage

➤*Approved by the FDA:* November 1948.

➤*Adults:*

Cream 4% and 5% – A thick layer of lidocaine cream is applied to intact skin.

When lidocaine cream is used concomitantly with other products containing local anesthetic agents, the amount absorbed from all formulations must be considered. The amount absorbed in the case of lidocaine cream is determined by the area over which it is applied and the duration of application. Although the incidence of systemic adverse reactions with lidocaine cream is very low, caution should be exercised, particularly when applying it over large areas and leaving it on for longer than 2 hours. The incidence of systemic adverse reactions can be expected to be directly proportional to the area and time of exposure.

Cream 3% – Apply a thin film to the affected area 2 or 3 times daily.

Ointment 5% – A single application should not exceed 5 g of lidocaine 5% ointment, containing 250 mg of lidocaine base (equivalent chemically to approximately 300 mg of lidocaine hydrochloride). This is roughly equivalent to squeezing a 6 inch length of ointment from the tube. In a 70 kg adult this dose equals 3.6 mg/kg (1.6 mg/lb) lidocaine base. No more than one-half tube, approximately 17 to 20 g of ointment or 850 to 1000 mg lidocaine base, should be administered in any 1 day.

Although the incidence of adverse effects with lidocaine 5% ointment is quite low, caution should be exercised, particularly when employing large amounts, since the incidence of adverse effects is directly proportional to the total dose of local anesthetic agent administered.

For medical use, apply topically for adequate control of symptoms. The use of a sterile gauze pad is suggested for application to broken skin tissue.

In dentistry, apply to previously dried oral mucosa. Subsequent removal of excess saliva with cotton rolls or saliva ejector minimizes dilution of the ointment, permits maximum penetration, and minimizes the possibility of swallowing the topical ointment.

For use in connection with the insertion of new dentures, apply to all denture surfaces contacting mucosa.

Jelly – The dosage varies and depends upon the area to be anesthetized, vascularity of the tissues, individual tolerance, and the technique of anesthesia. The lowest dosage needed to provide effective anesthesia should be administered. Dosages should be reduced for children and for elderly and debilitated patients. Although the incidence of adverse effects with lidocaine 2% jelly is quite low, caution should be exercised, particularly when employing large amounts, since the incidence of adverse effects is directly proportional to the total dose of local anesthetic agent administered.

For surface anesthesia of the adult urethra: When using lidocaine 2% jelly 30 mL tubes, sterilize the plastic cone for 5 minutes in boiling water, cool, and attach to the tube. The cone may be gas sterilized or cold sterilized, as preferred. The lidocaine 2% jelly syringes do not require sterilization. The syringes are prefilled sterile disposable units packaged in presterilized trays.

• *Male patients* – Slowly instill approximately 15 mL (300 mg of lidocaine HCl) into the urethra or until the patient has a feeling of tension. A penile clamp is then applied for several minutes at the corona. An additional dose of not more than 15 mL (300 mg) can be instilled for adequate anesthesia.

Prior to sounding or cystoscopy, a penile clamp should be applied for 5 to 10 minutes to obtain adequate anesthesia. A total dose of 30 mL (600 mg) is usually required to fill and dilate the male urethra. Prior to catheterization, smaller volumes of 5 to 10 mL (100 to 200 mg) are usually adequate for lubrication.

Female patients: Slowly instill 3 to 5 mL (60 to 100 mg of lidocaine HCl) of the jelly into the urethra. If desired, some jelly may be deposited on a cotton swab and introduced into the urethra. In order to obtain adequate anesthesia, several minutes should be allowed prior to performing urological procedures.

Lubrication for endotracheal intubation: Apply a moderate amount of jelly to the external surface of the endotracheal tube shortly before use. Care should be taken to avoid introducing the product into the lumen of the tube. Do not use the jelly to lubricate endotracheal stylettes. There have been rare reports concerning the inner lumen occlusion (see Warnings and Adverse Reactions). It is also recommended that use of endotracheal tubes with dried jelly on the external surface be avoided for lack of lubricating effect.

Maximum dosage: No more than 600 mg or 30 mL of lidocaine 2% jelly should be given in any 12-hour period.

➤*Children:*

Cream – A thick layer is applied to intact skin. A single application of lidocaine cream in a child weighing less than 10 kg should not be applied over an area greater than 100 cm^2. A singles application cream in children weighing between 10 kg and 20 kg should not be applied over an area greater than 600 cm^2. When applying lidocaine cream to young children, care must be taken to maintain careful observation of the child to prevent accidental ingestion of lidocaine cream.

Ointment and jelly – It is difficult to recommend a maximum dose of any drug for children since this varies as a function of age and weight. For children less than 10 years old who have a normal lean body mass and a normal lean body development, the maximum dose may be determined by the application of one of the standard pediatric drug formulas (eg, Clark's rule). For example, in a child of 5 years weighing 50 lbs, the dose of lidocaine hydrochloride should not exceed 75 to 100 mg when calculated according to Clark's rule. In any case, the maximum amount of lidocaine administered should not exceed 4.5 mg/kg (2 mg/lb) of body weight.

➤*Storage/Stability:*

Cream and ointment – Store at controlled room temperature 15° and 30°C (59° to 86°F). Protect from freezing. Keep container closed tightly at all times when not in use.

Jelly – Store at controlled room temperature 20° to 25°C (68° to 77°F) (see USP).

LIDOCAINE — TRANSDERMAL

Indications

➤*Postherpetic neuralgia:* For relief of pain associated with postherpetic neuralgia. It should be applied only to intact skin.

Administration and Dosage

➤*Recommended dose:* Apply the patch to intact skin to cover the most painful area. Apply up to 3 patches, only once for up to 12 hours within a 24 hour period. Patches may be cut into smaller sizes with scissors prior to removal of the release liner. Clothing may be worn over the area of application.

➤*Special risk patients:* Smaller areas of treatment are recommended in a debilitated patient, or a patient with impaired elimination.

➤*Irritation/Burning sensation:* If irritation or a burning sensation occurs during application, remove the patch(es) and do not reapply until the irritation subsides.

➤*Concomitant topical anesthetics:* When a lidocaine patch is used concomitantly with other products containing local anesthetic agents, the amount absorbed from all formulations must be considered.

➤*Storage/Stability:* Store at 25°C (77°F); excursions permitted to 15° to 30°C (59° to 86°F).

Ester Local Anesthetics

BENZOCAINE

otc	**Americaine Anesthetic** (Fisons)	**Spray:** 20%	In 60 mL.
otc	**Benz-O-Sthetic** (Geritrex)		In 56 g.
otc	**Boil-Ease** (Del)	**Ointment:** 20% with camphor, lanolin, eucalyptus oil, menthol, petrolatum, phenol	In 30 g.
otc	**Dermoplast** (Medtech)	**Spray:** 20% with 0.5% menthol, methylparaben, aloe, lanolin	In 59 mL.
otc	**Dermoplast Antibacterial** (Medtech)	**Spray:** 20% with 0.2% benzethonium Cl, menthol, methylparaben, aloe, lanolin	In 59 mL.
otc	**Lanacane** (Combe)	**Spray:** 20% with 0.1% benzethonium Cl, 36% ethanol, aloe extract	In 113 mL.

Ester Local Anesthetics

BENZOCAINE

otc	**Solarcaine Medicated First Aid Spray** (Schering-Plough)	**Spray:** 20% with 0.13% triclosan, alcohol	In 90 mL.
otc	**Dermoplast** (Whitehall-Robins)	**Lotion:** 8% with 0.5% menthol, aloe, glycerin, parabens, lanolin	In 90 mL.
otc	**Solarcaine** (Schering-Plough)	**Aerosol:** 20% with 0.13% triclosan, 35% SD alcohol 40, tocopheryl acetate	In 90 and 120 mL.
otc	**Bicozene** (Sandoz)	**Cream:** 6% with 1.67% resorcinol, castor oil, glycerin	In 30 g.
otc	**Foille Plus** (Blistex)	**Aerosol:** 20% with 12% alcohol	In 105 mL.
otc	**Foille** (Blistex)	**Spray:** 5% with 0.63% chloroxylenol	In 97.5 mL.
otc	**Benzocaine** (Various, eg, IDE)	**Cream:** 5%	In 480 g.
otc	**Foille Medicated First Aid** (Blistex)	**Ointment:** 5% with 0.1% chloroxylenol, benzyl alcohol, EDTA in corn oil base	In 3.5 and 28 g.
		Aerosol: 5% with 0.6% chloroxylenol, benzyl alcohol in corn oil base	In 92 mL.
otc	**Chigger-Tox** (Scherer)	**Liquid:** Benzocaine with benzyl benzoate and green soap in an isopropanol base	In 30 mL.
otc	**Solarcaine** (Schering-Plough)	**Lotion:** Benzocaine with triclosan, mineral oil, alcohol, aloe extract, tocopheryl acetate, menthol, camphor, parabens, EDTA	In 120 mL.
otc	**Lanacane** (Combe)	**Cream:** 6% with 0.1% benzethonium Cl, aloe, parabens, castor oil, glycerin, isopropyl alcohol	In 28 and 56 g.
otc	**Maximum Strength Anbesol** (Whitehall)	**Liquid:** 20%	50% alcohol, saccharin. In 9 mL.
otc	**Anbesol Cold Sore Therapy** (Wyeth Consumer Health)	**Ointment:** 20% with 1% allantoin, 3% camphor, 64.9% petrolatum, aloe, benzyl alcohol, parabens, menthol, vitamin E	In 7.1 g.
otc	**Hurricaine** (Beutlich)	**Gel:** 20%	60% alcohol, saccharin. In 7 g.
		Spray: 20% For oral and mucosal anesthesia to control pain and suppress the gag reflex.	Cherry flavor. In 60 mL.
Rx	**Americaine Anesthetic Lubricant** (Fisons)	**Gel:** 20% For use as a lubricant and anesthetic on intratracheal catheters and pharyngeal and nasal airways; on nasogastric and endoscopic tubes; urinary catheters; laryngoscopes; proctoscopes; sigmoidoscopes; vaginal specula.	0.1% benzethonium chloride. In 30 g and UD 2.5 g.
otc	**Orajel Mouth-Aid** (Del)	**Liquid:** 20%	0.1% cetylpyridinium Cl, 70% ethyl alcohol, tartrazine, saccharin. In 13.5 mL.
		Gel: 20%	0.02 benzalkonium Cl, 0.1% zinc Cl, EDTA, saccharin. In 5.6 and 10 g.

BENZOCAINE — TOPICAL

Complete prescribing information begins in the Local Anesthetics, Topical group monograph.

Indications

➤*Topical pain:*

Anesthetic lubricant – For general use as a lubricant and topical anesthetic on intratracheal catheters and pharyngeal and nasal airways to obtund the pharyngeal and tracheal reflexes; on nasogastric and endoscopic tubes; urinary catheters; laryngoscopes; proctoscopes; sigmoidoscopes; and vaginal specula.

Cream – For temporary relief of minor skin irritations.

Cream and paste 20% – For temporary pain relief of mouth and gum sores, mouth pain, canker sores, cold sores, fever blisters, minor irritation of the mouth caused by dentures or orthodontic appliances.

Gel – For temporary relief of pain associated with minor dental procedures, canker sores, fever blisters, braces, cold sores, dentures, teething, toothaches, gum pain, minor irritation, sore mouth, and sore throat.

Lubricant 5% or 4% – Helps in temporarily prolonging the time until ejaculation. Safe for use with prophylactics.

➤*Liquid:* For temporary relief of pain associated with:

Medical indications – Minor cuts and burns, nasal packing, nasal biopsies, passing nasogastric tubes, mucositis, stomatitis, thrush, head and neck examinations, condylomata, culdocentesis, proctoscopic exams.

Dental indications – Injections, rubber dams, suture removal, instrumentation, arch bar removal, minor mouth irritation, banding a molar, removal of mobile deciduous teeth, deep scalings, localized gingival curettage, denture discomfort, and post-operation discomfort.

➤*Ointment:* For the temporary relief of local pain, itching, and soreness associated with hemorrhoids and anorectal inflammation.

Anbesol ointment – For temporary relief of pain associated with fever blisters and cold sores.

➤*Spray:* For oral and mucosal anesthesia to control pain and to suppress the gag reflex. For oral or mucosal application.

Administration and Dosage

➤*Anesthetic lubricant:* Apply evenly to exterior of tube or instrument prior to use.

➤*Cream, gel, paste (for oral pain):* To open tube, cut the tip of the tube on the score mark with scissors.

Adults and children 2 years of age and older – Apply to the affected area, allow to remain in place at least 1 minute, and then spit out. Use up to 4 times daily or as directed by a doctor or dentist.

Cream (for toothache pain): Squeeze a 1 inch strip of cream onto finger or cotton swab. Apply it to affected cavity and around gum surrounding the teeth before bedtime. The cream will stay in place for extended duration of relief.

Children under 2 years of age – Consult a doctor or dentist. For infants under the age of 4 months, there is no recommended dosage or treatment except under the advice and supervision of a doctor or dentist.

20% strengths – Do not use more than 4 times in a 24-hour period unless directed by a doctor or dentist.

Do not use for more than 7 days unless directed by a doctor or dentist.

Genital desensitizer – Apply a small amount to head and shaft of penis before intercourse, or use as directed by a doctor. Wash product off after intercourse.

➤*Liquid:* Apply to area to be anesthetized. Anesthesia is accomplished within 15 to 30 seconds.

➤*Ointment (for hemorrhoids):* Do not put this product into the rectum by using fingers or any mechanical device or applicator. Do not exceed the recommended dosage unless directed to do so by a doctor.

➤*Ointment (for fever blister and cold sores):*

Adults and children 2 years of age and older – Apply to the affected area not more than 3 or 4 times daily.

➤*Spray (for oral and mucosal pain):* Firmly insert disposable extension tube into hole on side of spray can valve. The extension tube is designed to fit securely.

Hold spray extension tube tip 1 to 2 inches away from area to be anesthetized. Spray ½ second. Repeat if necessary. Anesthesia is accomplished in 15 to 30 seconds.

Adults and children 2 years of age and older – Apply to the affected area. Gargle, swish around mouth, or allow to remain in place no longer than 30 seconds and then spit out. Use up to 4 times daily or as directed by a doctor or dentist. Supervise children under the age of 12 years in the use of this product.

Ester Local Anesthetics

BENZOCAINE — TOPICAL

Children under 2 years of age – Consult a doctor or dentist. For infants under the age of 4 months, there is no recommended dosage or treatment except under the advice and supervision of a doctor or dentist.

➤*Storage/Stability:* Store at room temperature 20° to 25°C (68° to 77°F).

Lubricant – Store at 15° to 25°C (59° to 77°F).

Spray – Do not store at temperatures above 49°C (120°F).

COCAINE

c-ii	**Cocaine HCl** (Roxane)	**Topical Solution**: 4%	In 10 mL multidose and UD 4 mL.
		10%	In 10 mL multidose and UD 4 mL.
c-ii	**Cocaine Viscous** (Roxane)	**Topical Solution**: 4%	In 10 mL multidose and UD 4 mL.
		10%	In 10 mL multidose bottles and UD 4 mL.
c-ii	**Cocaine HCl** (Mallinckrodt)	**Powder**	In 5 and 25 g.

COCAINE HYDROCHLORIDE — TOPICAL

Indications

➤*Topical anesthesia:* For the introduction of local (topical) anesthesia of accessible mucous membranes of the oral, laryngeal and nasal cavities.

Administration and Dosage

The dosage varies and depends upon the area to be anesthetized, vascularity of the tissues, individual tolerance, and the technique of anesthesia. The lowest dosage needed to provide effective anesthesia should be administered. Dosages should be reduced for children and for elderly and debilitated patients. Cocaine hydrochloride topical solution can be administered by means of cotton applicators or packs, instilled into a cavity, or as a spray.

➤*Storage/Stability:* Store at controlled room temperature 15° to 30°C (59° to 86°F).

Actions

➤*Pharmacology:* Cocaine blocks the initiation or conduction of the nerve impulse following local application, thereby effecting local anesthetic action.

➤*Pharmacokinetics:* Cocaine is absorbed from all sites of application, including mucous membranes and the gastrointestinal mucosa. Cocaine is degraded by plasma esterases, with the half-life in the plasma being ≈ 1 hour.

Contraindications

Known history of hypersensitivity to the drug or to the components of the topical solution.

Warnings

➤*Resuscitative equipment:* Resuscitative equipment and drugs should be immediately available when any local anesthetic is used.

➤*Pregnancy:* *Category C.* Animal reproduction studies have not been conducted with cocaine. It is also not known whether cocaine can cause fetal harm when administered to a pregnant woman or can affect reproduction capacity. Cocaine should be given to a pregnant woman only if needed.

Precautions

➤*Special risk:* The lowest dosage that results in effective anesthesia should be used to avoid high plasma levels and serious adverse effects. Debilitated, elderly patients, acutely ill patients, and children should be given reduced doses commensurate with their age and physical status.

Cocaine hydrochloride topical solution should be used with caution in patients with severely traumatized mucosa and sepsis in the region of the proposed application. Use with caution in persons with known drug sensitivities.

Adverse Reactions

Adverse reactions may be due to high plasma levels as a result of excessive and rapid absorption of the drug. Reactions are systemic in nature and involve the central nervous system or the cardiovascular system. A small number of reactions may result from hypersensitivity, idiosyncrasy or diminished tolerance on the part of the patient.

➤*Cardiovascular:* Small doses of cocaine slow the heart rate, but after moderate doses, the rate is increased due to central sympathetic stimulation.

➤*CNS:* CNS reactions are excitatory or depressant and may be characterized by nervousness, restlessness and excitement. Tremors and eventually clonicotonic convulsions may result. Emesis may occur. Central stimulation is followed by depression, with death resulting from respiratory failure.

Cocaine is pyrogenic, augmenting heat production in stimulating muscular activity and causing vasoconstriction which decreases heat loss. Cocaine is known to interfere with the uptake of norepinephrine by adrenergic nerve terminals, producing sensitization to catecholamines, causing vasoconstriction and mydriasis.

➤*Ophthalmic:* Cocaine causes sloughing of the corneal epithelium, causing clouding, pitting, and occasionally ulceration of the cornea. The drug is not meant for ophthalmic use.

Overdosage

The fatal dose of cocaine has been approximated at 1.2 g, although severe toxic effects have been reported from doses as low as 20 mg.

➤*Symptoms:* The symptoms of cocaine poisoning are referable to the CNS, namely the patient becomes excited, restless, garrulous, anxious and confused. Enhanced reflexes, headache, rapid pulse, irregular respiration, chills, rise in body temperature, mydriasis, exophthalmos, nausea, vomiting and abdominal pain are noticed. In severe overdoses, delirium, Cheyne-Stokes respiration, convulsions, unconsciousness, and death from respiratory arrest result. Acute poisoning by cocaine is rapid in developing.

➤*Treatment:* The specific treatment of acute cocaine poisoning is the intravenous administration of a short-acting barbiturate or diazepam. Artificial respiration may be necessary. It is important to limit absorption of the drug. If entrance of the drug into circulation can be checked, and respiratory exchange maintained, the prognosis is favorable since cocaine is eliminated fairly rapidly.

PRAMOXINE HYDROCHLORIDE

otc	**AmLactin AP** (Upsher-Smith)	**Cream**: 1%	12% lactic acid, light mineral oil, cetyl alcohol, glycerin, parabens. In 140 g.
otc	**Prax** (Ferndale)		Hydrophilic base with glycerin, cetyl alcohol, white petrolatum. In 30 and 113.4 g and 1 lb.
otc	**Tronothane HCl** (Abbott)		Water miscible base with cetyl alcohol, glycerin, parabens. In 28.4 g.
otc	**Sarna Ultra** (Stiefel)		0.5% menthol, 30% petrolatum, benzyl alcohol. In 56.6 g.
otc	**Prax** (Ferndale)	**Lotion**: 1%	Hydrophilic base with mineral oil, cetyl alcohol, glycerin, lanolin, 0.1% potassium sorbate, 0.1% sorbic acid. In 15, 120 and 240 mL.
otc	**Sarna Sensitive Anti-Itch** (Stiefel)		Benzyl alcohol, cetyl alcohol, petrolatum. Fragrance free. In 222 mL.
otc	**PrameGel** (Bioglan)	**Gel**: 1%	Emollient base with 0.5% menthol, benzyl alcohol, SD alcohol 40. In 118 g.
otc	**Itch-X** (Ascher & Co.)		10% benzyl alcohol, aloe vera gel, diazolidinyl urea, SD alcohol 40, parabens. In 35.4 g.
otc	**Itch-X** (Ascher & Co.)	**Spray**: 1%	10% benzyl alcohol, aloe vera gel, SD alcohol 40. In 60 mL.
otc	**Bactine Pain Relieving Cleansing** (Bayer)	**Wipes**: 1%	0.13% benzalkonium chloride, EDTA. In 16s.
otc	**ProctoFoam NS** (Schwarz Pharma)	**Aerosol Foam**: 1%	In 15 g with applicator.

PRAMOXINE HYDROCHLORIDE — TOPICAL

Complete prescribing information begins in the Local Anesthetics, Topical group monograph.

Indications

➤*Topical pain:*

Foam – For temporary relief of pain and itching associated with hemorrhoids.

Gel and spray – For the temporary relief of pain and itching associated with rashes, minor skin irritations, allergic itches, sunburn, hives, minor burns, insect bites, poison ivy, poison oak and poison sumac.

Lotion – Pramoxine lotion is specially formulated to give prompt, temporary relief from dry itching skin and pain due to minor burns, abrasions and other irritated skin conditions, and to use as an anogenital cleansing lotion.

Non-caine and paraben-free, pramoxine lotion is less irritating and can be used on sensitive skin.

Pramoxine lotion is also applied as a rectal wipe for relief from discomfort and pain in hemorrhoids, fissures, anogenital pruritus, bowel movements, and various dermatologic skin disorders. In addition to use for the pain and discomfort associated with hemorrhoids and fissures, pramoxine lotion is also used following rectal surgery.

Administration and Dosage

➤*Foam:*

Directions – Shake well before use. Dispense pramoxine foam onto a clean tissue or pad and apply externally to the affected area up to 5 times daily.

Adults: When practical, cleanse the affected area with mild soap and warm water and rinse thoroughly. Gently dry by patting or blotting with toilet tissue or a soft cloth before application of pramoxine foam.

Children younger than 12 years of age: Consult a physician.

➤*Gel, spray:*

Adults and children 2 years of age and older – Apply to affected area not more than 3 to 4 times daily.

Children younger than 2 years of age – Consult a physician.

➤*Lotion:*

Adults and children 2 years of age and older – Apply to affected area not more than 3 to 4 times daily.

Children – Consult a physician.

Anogenital cleansing – For cleansing of anogenital area, spread pramoxine lotion on cotton or tissue and wipe affected area.

➤*Storage/Stability:* Store pramoxine products at controlled room temperature 15° to 30°C (59° to 86°F).

Keep these and all medicines out of the reach of children.

Foam – Store upright. Do not refrigerate. Do not store at temperatures above 48.8°C (120°F).

Spray – Flammable. Keep away from fire or flame.

LOCAL ANESTHETICS, TOPICAL COMBINATIONS

otc	**Detane** (Del)	**Gel**: 7.5% benzocaine, carbomer 940, PEG 400	In 15 g.
otc	**Sting-Kill** (Kiwi)	**Swabs**: 18.9% benzocaine, 0.9% menthol	In 0.5 & 14 mL.
Rx	**Cetacaine** (Cetylite)	14% benzocaine, 2% tetracaine HCl, 2% butamben and 0.5% benzalkonium chloride with 0.005% cetyl dimethyl ethyl ammonium bromide in a bland water soluble base	**Gel**: In 29 g.
			Liquid: In 56 mL.
			Ointment: In 37 g.
			Aerosol: In 56 g.
otc	**Aerocaine** (Aeroceuticals)	**Aerosol**: 13.6% benzocaine with 0.5% benzethonium Cl	In 15 and 75 mL.
otc	**Aerotherm** (Aeroceuticals)		In 150 mL.
otc	**Anbesol** (Whitehall)	**Liquid**: 6.3% benzocaine with 0.5% phenol, povidone-iodine, 70% alcohol, camphor, menthol	In 9.3 & 22.2 mL.
		Gel: 6.3% benzocaine, 0.5% phenol, 70% alcohol	In 7.5 g.
Rx	**Lidocaine/Prilocaine** (Various, eg, Hi-Tech, Sandoz)	**Cream**: 2.5% lidocaine, 2.5% prilocaine	In 5, 15, and 30 g.
Rx	**EMLA** (Astra)	**Cream**: 2.5% lidocaine, 2.5% prilocaine	In 5 g with *Tegaderm* dressings and 30 g.
otc	**Vagisil** (Combe)	**Cream**: Benzocaine and resorcin with lanolin alcohol, parabens, trisodium HEDTA, mineral oil and sodium sulfite	In 30 and 60 g.
otc	**Unguentine Maximum Strength** (Lee)	**Cream**: 5% benzocaine, 2% resorcinol.	Alcohols, methylparaben, mineral oil. In 28.3 g.
otc	**Chiggerex** (Scherer)	**Ointment**: Benzocaine with camphor, menthol	In 50 g.
otc	**Skeeter Stik** (Triton)	**Liquid**: 4% lidocaine with 2% phenol in an isopropyl alcohol base	In 14 mL.
otc	**Bactine Pain Relieving Cleansing** (Bayer)	**Spray**: 2.5% lidocaine, 0.13% benzalkonium chloride, EDTA	In 150 mL.
otc	**Bactine Antiseptic Anesthetic** (Bayer)	2.5% lidocaine HCl, 0.13% benzalkonium chloride, EDTA, 3.17% alcohol	**Aerosol**: In 90 g.
			Spray: In 60, 120 and 480 mL.
otc	**Unguentine Plus** (Mentholatum)	**Cream**: 2% lidocaine HCl with 2% chloroxylenol and 0.5% phenol, parabens, mineral oil	In 30 g.
otc	**Medi-Quik** (Mentholatum)	**Aerosol**: Lidocaine HCl and benzalkonium chloride	In 90 mL.
		Spray: 2% lidocaine, 0.13% benzalkonium chloride, 0.2% camphor, benzyl alcohol	In 85 mL.
otc	**Dr. Scholl's Cracked Heel Relief** (Schering-Plough)	**Cream**: 2% lidocaine, 0.13% benzethonium Cl	Aloe. In 89 mL.
otc	**ProTech First-Aid Stik** (Triton)	**Liquid**: 2.5% lidocaine HCl, 10% povidone iodine	In 14 mL dab-on applicator.
Rx	**Synera** (Ferndale Labs)	**Patch**: 70 mg lidocaine, 70 mg tetracaine, polyvinyl alcohol, sorbitan monopalmitate, parabens	In 2s and 10s.
otc	**TheraPatch Cold Sore** (LecTec)	**Patch**: 4% lidocaine HCl, 0.5% camphor, aloe vera, eucalyptus oil, glycerin	In 21s.
Rx	**EMLA Anesthetic** (AstraZeneca)	**Disc**: 1 g EMLA emulsion (2.5% lidocaine, 2.5% prilocaine). Contact surface ≈ 10 cm^2	In 2s and 10s.
otc	**Campho-Phenique Cold Sore Treatment and Scab Relief** (Bayer)	**Cream**: 1% pramoxine hydrochloride	30% petrolatum, alcohols, EDTA, glycerin, parabens, ureas. Mint flavor. In 6.5 g.

Refer to the general discussion of these products beginning in the Local Anesthetics, Topical group monograph.

MISCELLANEOUS TOPICAL ANESTHETICS

Rx	**Ethyl Chloride** (Gebauer)	**Spray:** Chloroethane **Indications:** Topical vapo-coolant to control pain associated with minor surgical procedures (eg, lancing boils, incision and drainage of small abscesses), athletic injuries, injections and for treatment of myofascial pain, restricted motion and muscle spasm	In 100 g metal tubes, 105 mL *Spra-Pak* and 120 mL bottles (fine, medium, and coarse spray).
Rx	**Fluro-Ethyl** (Gebauer)	**Aerosol spray:** 25% ethyl chloride and 75% dichlorotetrafluoroethane **Indications:** Topical refrigerant anesthetic to control pain associated with minor surgical procedures, dermabrasion, injections, contusions and minor strains	In 270 mL.
Rx	**Gebauer's Spray and Stretch** (Gebauer)	**Spray:** Tetrafluoroethane and pentafluoropropane **Indications:** Vapo-coolant for topical application in management of myofascial pain, restricted motion, muscle spasm, and minor sports injuries	In 103.5 mL.
otc	**Aerofreeze** (Graham-Field)	**Spray:** Trichloromonofluoromethane and dichlorodifluoromethane **Indications:** Topical anesthesia for preinjection, skin planing, dermabrasion and minor surgical procedures; for treatment of strains, sprains and muscle spasms	In 240 mL.

Complete prescribing information begins in the Local Anesthetics, Topical group monograph.

MINOXIDIL

MINOXIDIL

otc	**Rogaine** (Pharmacia & Upjohn)	**Solution:** 2%	In 60 mL bottle with multiple applicators.
otc	**Minoxidil Extra Strength for Men** (Apotex)	**Solution:** 5%	30% alcohol. In 60 mL bottles (1s and 2s).
otc	**Rogaine Extra Strength for Men** (Pharmacia & Upjohn)		Alcohol. In two 60 mL bottles w/ dropper and sprayer applicators.

MINOXIDIL — TOPICAL

Indications

➤*Alopecia:* Treatment of androgenetic alopecia, expressed in males as baldness of the vertex of the scalp and in females as diffuse hair loss or thinning of the frontoparietal areas. At least 4 months of twice-daily applications are generally required before evidence of hair growth can be expected.

➤*Unlabeled uses:* Although further study is needed, topical minoxidil may be useful in the treatment of alopecia areata (a systemic disease in which patches of hair fall out over a period of a few days; any part of the body may be involved).

Actions

➤*Pharmacology:* To study the potential for systemic effects of topical minoxidil, 3 concentrations (1%, 2% and 5%) applied twice daily were compared to low oral doses (2.5 and 5 mg given once daily) and placebo in hypertensive patients in a double-blind, controlled trial. The 5 mg oral dose had readily detectable effects, including a fall in diastolic pressure of about 5 mmHg and an increase in heart rate of 7 bpm. No other group had a clear effect, although there was some evidence of a weak and inconsistent effect in the 2.5 mg oral, and possibly the 5% topical, treatments.

➤*Pharmacokinetics:*

Absorption – Topical minoxidil has poor absorption, averaging ≈ 1.4% (range 0.3% to 4.5%) from normal intact scalp, and about 2% in the hypertensive patients, whose scalps were shaved.

In a comparison of topical and oral absorption, peak serum levels of unchanged drug after 1 mL twice a day of 2% solution (the maximum recommended dose) averaged 5.8% (range, 1.4% to 12.7%) of the level observed after 2.5 mg orally twice a day. Similarly, in the hypertension study where patients had shaved scalps, mean concentrations after 1 mL twice a day of 2% topical solution (1.7 ng/mL) were 1⁄20 the concentrations seen after daily oral doses of 2.5 mg (32.8 ng/mL) or 5 mg (59.2 ng/mL). Blood levels obtained in the large controlled hair growth trials averaged less than 2 ng/mL for the 2% solution (range, up to 30 ng/mL). If more than the recommended dose is applied to inflamed skin in an individual with relatively high absorption, blood levels with systemic effects might rarely be obtained.

Serum levels resulting from topical administration are governed by the drug's percutaneous absorption rate. Following cessation of topical dosing, ≈ 95% of systemically absorbed minoxidil is eliminated within 4 days.

Contraindications

Hypersensitivity to any component of the preparation.

Warnings

➤*Pregnancy: Category C.* Adequate and well-controlled studies have not been conducted in pregnant women. Do not administer to a pregnant woman.

➤*Lactation:* Because of the potential for adverse effects in nursing infants from minoxidil absorption, do not apply on a nursing woman.

➤*Children:* Safety and efficacy in patients younger than 18 years of age have not been established.

Precautions

➤*Monitoring:* Give a history and physical examination to patients being considered for topical minoxidil. Advise of the potential risk; the patient and physician should decide that the benefits outweigh the risks.

Monitor patients ≥ 1 month after starting topical minoxidil and ≥ 6 months thereafter. If systemic effects occur, discontinue use.

➤*Sensitive surfaces:* This product contains an alcohol base that will cause burning and irritation of the eyes. In the event of accidental contact with sensitive surfaces (eg, eyes, abraded skin, mucous membranes), bathe the area with large amounts of cool tap water.

➤*Inhalation:* Avoid inhaling the spray mist.

➤*For topical use only:* Accidental ingestion could lead to adverse systemic effects.

Adverse Reactions

➤*Cardiovascular:* Edema; chest pain; blood pressure increases/decreases; palpitations; pulse rate increases/decreases (1.5%; placebo, 1.6%).

➤*CNS:* Headache; dizziness; faintness; lightheadedness (3.4%; placebo, 3.5%).

➤*Dermatologic:* Irritant dermatitis; allergic contact dermatitis (7.4%; placebo 5.4%); eczema; hypertrichosis; local erythema; pruritus; dry skin/scalp flaking; exacerbation of hair loss; alopecia.

➤*Endocrine:* Menstrual changes, breast symptoms (0.5%; placebo, 0.5%).

➤*GI:* Diarrhea, nausea, vomiting (4.3%; placebo, 6.6%).

➤*GU:* Urinary tract infections, renal calculi, urethritis, prostatitis, epididymitis, vaginitis, vulvitis, vaginal discharge, itching (0.9%; placebo, 0.8% to 1.1%); sexual dysfunction.

➤*Hematologic:* Lymphadenopathy, thrombocytopenia, anemia (0.3; placebo, 0.6%).

➤*Hypersensitivity:* Nonspecific allergic reactions, hives, allergic rhinitis, facial swelling, sensitivity (1.3%; placebo, 1%).

➤*Metabolic:* Edema, weight gain (1.2%; placebo, 1.3%).

➤*Musculoskeletal:* Fractures, back pain, tendinitis, aches and pains (2.6%; placebo, 2.2%).

➤*Psychiatric:* Anxiety, depression, fatigue (0.4%; placebo, 1%).

➤*Respiratory:* Bronchitis, upper respiratory tract infection, sinusitis (7.2%; placebo, 8.6%).

➤*Special senses:* Conjunctivitis, ear infection, vertigo (1.2%; placebo, 1.2%); visual disturbances, including decreased visual acuity.

Overdosage

Increased systemic absorption of minoxidil topical solution may potentially occur if frequent or larger doses than directed are used or if the drug is applied to large surface areas of the body or areas other than the scalp. There are no known cases of minoxidil overdosage resulting from topical administration.

Patient Information

➤*Important information about the use of regular strength topical solution for men:* Minoxidil topical solution is indicated to regrow hair on top of the scalp.

If your amount of hair loss is more than that shown on the side of the carton, regular strength topical solution for men may not work for you.

Avoid contact with eyes. In case of accidental contact, rinse with large amounts of cool tap water.

Keep out of the reach of children. Do not use on babies or children. In case of accidental ingestion, seek professional assistance or contact a poison control center immediately.

MINOXIDIL — TOPICAL

Keep the carton and educational booklet. They contain important information.

➤*Important information about extra strength topical solution for men:*
- Provides more hair regrowth than regular strength topical solution for men.
- Results may occur at 2 months with twice-daily usage. For some men, it may take at least 4 months for results to be seen.

➤*Important information about minoxidil topical solution for women:*
- Two percent minoxidil.
- Hair regrowth treatment.

Minoxidil topical solution for women is medically proven to regrow hair. Minoxidil topical solution is the only hair regrowth product ever prescribed by doctors for men and women.

➤*Who should not use minoxidil topical solution?:*

Topical solution for men – Do not use:
- If you are a woman (may grow facial hair and may be harmful if used during pregnancy or breastfeeding).
- If you are not sure of the reason for your hair loss.
- If you are younger than 18 years of age. Not for babies or children.
- If you are using other medicines on the scalp.
- If you have no family history of hair loss.
- If you have sudden or patchy hair loss.
- If you have a red, inflamed, infected, irritated or painful scalp.

Extra strength topical solution for men – Women should not use minoxidil extra strength topical solution because studies have shown it works no better in women than minoxidil for women. Some women may also grow facial hair. In addition, minoxidil extra strength topical solution may be harmful if used during pregnancy or breastfeeding.

Topical solution for women: Minoxidil topical solution will not prevent or improve hair loss related to pregnancy or to the recently discontinued use of birth control pills.

Do not use minoxidil for women if hair loss is patchy as shown below. You should ask your doctor if you are unsure of the cause of your hair loss.

Minoxidil: Minoxidil topical solution should not be used on babies or on children younger than 18 years old.

Minoxidil will not prevent or improve hair loss which may occur with the use of some prescription and nonprescription medications, certain severe nutritional problems (very low body iron; too much vitamin A intake), low thyroid states (hypothyroidism), chemotherapy, or diseases which cause scarring of the scalp. Also, minoxidil topical solution will not improve hair loss due to damage from the use of hair care products which cause scarring or deep burns of the scalp, or hair grooming methods such as cornrowing or ponytails which require pulling the hair tightly back from the scalp.

Do not use if you are not sure of the reason for your hair loss.

EFLORNITHINE HYDROCHLORIDE

Rx	**Vaniqa** (SkinMedica)	**Cream:** 13.9%	Parabens, mineral oil, alcohols. In 30 g.

EFLORNITHINE HYDROCHLORIDE — TOPICAL

For information on IV use of eflornithine as an antiprotozoal, refer to the specific monograph in the Systemic Anti-Infectives chapter.

Indications

➤*Reduction of facial hair:* For the reduction of unwanted facial hair in women.

Administration and Dosage

➤*Approved by the FDA:* July 27, 2000.

Apply a thin layer of eflornithine HCl to affected areas of the face and adjacent involved areas under the chin and rub in thoroughly. Do not wash treated area for at least 4 hours. Use twice daily at least 8 hours apart or as directed by a physician. The patient should continue to use hair removal techniques as needed in conjunction with eflornithine HCl. (Eflornithine HCl should be applied at least 5 minutes after hair removal.) Cosmetics or sunscreens may be applied over treated areas after cream has dried.

➤*Storage / Stability:* Store at 25°C (77°F); excursions permitted to 15° to 30°C (59° to 86°F) Do not freeze. See tube crimp and carton end for expiration date and lot number.

Actions

➤*Pharmacology:* There are no studies examining the inhibition of the enzyme ornithine decarboxylase (ODC) in human skin following the application of topical eflornithine. However, there are studies in the literature that report the inhibition of ODC activity in skin following oral eflornithine. It is postulated that topical eflornithine HCl irreversibly inhibits skin ODC activity. This enzyme is necessary in the synthesis of polyamines. Animal data indicate that inhibition of ornithine decarboxylase inhibits cell division and synthetic functions, which affect the rate of hair growth. Eflornithine HCl cream has been shown to retard the rate of hair growth in nonclinical and clinical studies.

➤*Pharmacokinetics:*

Absorption / Distribution – The mean percutaneous absorption of eflornithine in women with unwanted facial hair, from a 13.9% w/w cream formulation, is less than 1% of the radioactive dose, following either single or multiple doses under conditions of clinical use, that included shaving within 2 hours before radiolabeled dose application in addition to other forms of cutting or plucking and tweezing to remove facial hair. Steady state was reached within 4 days of twice daily application. The apparent steady-state plasma $t_{½}$ of eflornithine was ≈ 8 hours. Following twice-daily application of 0.5 g of the cream (total dose 1 g/day; 139 mg as anhydrous eflornithine HCl), under conditions of clinical use in women with unwanted facial hair (n = 10), the steady-state C_{max}, C_{trough} and area under the plasma concentration curve (AUC_{12hr}) were ≈ 10 ng/mL, 5 ng/mL, and 92 ng•hr/mL, respectively, expressed in terms of the anhydrous free base of eflornithine HCl. At steady state, the dose-normalized peak concentrations (C_{max}) and the extent of daily systemic exposure (AUC) of eflornithine following twice-daily application of 0.5 g of the cream (total dose 1 g/day) is estimated to be ≈ 100- and 60-fold lower, respectively, when compared to 370 mg/day once daily oral doses.

Metabolism / Excretion – This compound is not known to be metabolized and is primarily excreted unchanged in the urine.

Contraindications

Sensitivity to any components of the preparation.

Warnings

➤*Hypersensitivity reactions:* Discontinue use if hypersensitivity occurs.

➤*Carcinogenesis:* In a 12-month photocarcinogenicity study in hairless albino mice, animals treated with the vehicle alone showed an increased incidence of skin tumors induced by exposure to ultraviolet (UVA/UVB) light, whereas mice treated topically with eflornithine HCl cream at doses up to 600 mg/kg (19 × the maximum recommended human dose [MRHD] based on body surface area [BSA]) showed an incidence of skin tumors equivalent to untreated-control animals.

➤*Fertility impairment:* In a peri/postnatal study in rats, eflornithine HCl administered in the drinking water was associated with maternal toxicity and reduced pup weights at doses of at least 625 mg/kg (40 × the MRHD based on BSA) and a slightly reduced fertility index, which was considered to be of questionable biological significance, at 1698 mg/kg (110 × the MRHD based on BSA). No effects were seen with an oral dose of 223 mg/kg (14 × the MRHD based on BSA). In the latter study, the multiples of the human exposure are likely much higher, since eflornithine is well absorbed orally in rats, whereas minimal absorption occurs in humans treated topically.

➤*Pregnancy: Category C.* In the first dermal embryo-fetal development study in rats treated with eflornithine HCl cream, 13.9% (in which no precautions were taken to prevent ingestion of drug from application sites), maternal toxicity and fetal effects including reduced numbers of live fetuses, decreased fetal weights, and delayed ossification and development of the viscera were observed at doses of 225 and 450 mg/kg (15 × and 29 × the MRHD based on BSA, respectively). When the study was repeated under conditions that avoided ingestion from application sites, no maternal, fetal or teratogenic effects were observed at doses up to 450 mg/kg (29 × the MRHD based on BSA). In the first study in which no precautions were taken to prevent ingestion, circulating plasma levels were 11- to 14- fold higher than in the second study in which ingestion was prevented. In a dermal embryo-fetal development study in rabbits treated with eflornithine HCl cream no adverse maternal or fetal effects occurred at doses up to 90 mg/kg (11 × the MRHD based on BSA). Significant dermal irritation, as well as possible ingestion of eflornithine HCl cream occurred at 300 mg/kg/day (36 × the MRHD based on BSA) and was associated with maternal deaths, abortions, increased fetal resorptions, and reduced fetal weights. Fetotoxicity in the absence of maternal toxicity has been reported in oral studies with eflornithine with fetal no-effect doses of 80 mg/kg in rats and 45 mg/kg in rabbits. In these studies, no evidence of teratogenicity was observed in rats given up to 200 mg/kg or in rabbits given up to 135 mg/kg.

Although eflornithine HCl cream was not formally studied in pregnant patients, 22 pregnancies occurred during the trials. Nineteen of these pregnancies occurred while patients were using eflornithine HCl. Of the 19 pregnancies, there were 9 healthy infants, 4 spontaneous abortions, 5 induced/elective abortions, and 1 birth defect (Down's syndrome to a 35 year-old). Because there are no adequate and well-controlled studies in pregnant women, the risk/benefit ratio of using eflornithine HCl in women with unwanted facial hair who are pregnant should be weighed carefully with serious consideration for either not implementing or discontinuing use of eflornithine HCl cream.

➤*Lactation:* It is not known whether or not eflornithine HCl is excreted in human milk. Caution should be exercised when eflornithine HCl is administered to a nursing woman.

➤*Children:* The safety and effectiveness of this product have not been established in pediatric patients younger than 12 years of age.

EFLORNITHINE HYDROCHLORIDE — TOPICAL

Precautions

For external use only. Transient stinging or burning may occur when applied to abraded or broken skin.

Adverse Reactions

Adverse Reactions That Occured at > 1%			
	Vehicle-controlled studies		Vehicle-controlled and open-label studies
Adverse Reaction	Eflornithine HCl cream (n = 393)	Vehicle (n = 201)%	Eflornithine HCl cream (n = 1373)
Acne	21.3%	21.4%	10.8%
Alopecia	1.5%	2.5%	1.3%
Anorexia	1%	2%	0.7%
Asthenia	0%	1%	0.3%
Burning skin	4.3%	2%	3.5%
Dizziness	1.5%	1.5%	1.3%
Dry skin	1.8%	3%	3.3%
Dyspepsia	2.5%	2%	1.9%
Erythema (redness)	1.3%	0%	2.5%
Facial edema	0.3%	3%	0.7%
Folliculitis	0.5%	0%	1%
Hair ingrown	0.3%	2%	0.9%
Headache	3.0%	5%	4%
Nausea	0.5%	1%	0.7%
Pruritus (itching)	3.8%	4%	3.1%
Pseudofolliculitis barbae	16.3%	15.4%	4.9%
Rash	2.8%	0%	1.5%
Skin irritation	1%	1%	1.8%
Stinging skin	7.9%	2.5%	4.1%
Tingling skin	3.6%	1.5%	2.2%
Vertigo	0.3%	1%	0.1%

➤*Dermatologic:* Treatment-related skin adverse events that occurred in less than 1% of the subjects treated with eflornithine HCl are the following: Bleeding skin, cheilitis, contact dermatitis, swelling of lips, herpes simplex, numbness and rosacea.

➤*Lab test abnormalities:* No laboratory test abnormalities have been consistently found to be associated with eflornithine HCl cream. In an open-labeled study, some patients showed an increase in their transaminases; however, the clinical significance of these findings is not known.

Overdosage

Overdosage information with eflornithine HCl cream is unavailable. Given the low percutaneous penetration of this drug, overdosage via the topical route is not expected (see Pharmacokinetics).

➤*Treatment:* However, should very high topical doses (eg, multiple tubes per day) or oral ingestion be encountered (a 30 g tube contains 4.2 g of eflornithine HCl), the patient should be monitored, and appropriate supportive measures administered as necessary.

Patient Information

➤*Who should not use eflornithine HCl cream?:* You should not use eflornithine HCl cream if you are allergic to any of the ingredients in the cream. All ingredients are listed on the tube and at the beginning of this leaflet.

You should not use eflornithine HCl cream if you are younger than 12 years of age.

➤*What should you tell your doctor before using eflornithine HCl cream?:* If you are allergic to any of the ingredients, tell your doctor.

If you are pregnant or plan to become pregnant, discuss with your doctor whether you should use eflornithine HCl cream during pregnancy. No clinical studies have been performed in pregnant women.

If you are breastfeeding, consult your doctor before using eflornithine HCl cream. It is not known if eflornithine HCl cream is passed to infants through breast milk.

If you are taking any prescription medicines, nonprescription medicines or using any facial or skin creams, check with your physician before use of eflornithine HCl cream.

➤*What are the possible side effects of eflornithine HCl cream?:* Eflornithine HCl cream may cause temporary redness, stinging, burning, tingling or rash on areas of the skin where it is applied. Folliculitis (hair bumps) may also occur. If these persist, consult your doctor.

PHOTOCHEMOTHERAPY

AMINOLEVULINIC ACID HYDROCHLORIDE

Rx	**Levulan Kerastick** (DUSA)	**Solution, topical:** 20% (354 mg aminolevulinic acid HCl)	48% v/v ethanol, isopropyl alcohol. In 4s, 6s, and 12s. Applicator contains 2 glass ampules and an applicator tip. One ampule contains 1.5 mL solution vehicle, the other ampule contains 354 mg aminolevulinic acid HCl.

AMINOLEVULINIC ACID HYDROCHLORIDE — TOPICAL

Indications

➤*Non-hyperkeratotic actinic keradoses:* For the treatment of non-hyperkeratotic actinic keratoses of the face or scalp.

➤*Unlabeled uses:* (In conjunction with a photodynamic therapy.) Barrett's esophagus; Bowen's disease; epidermodysplasia verruciformis; intraepithelial neoplasma of the lower genital tract; nevus sebaceus; mycosis fungoides; actinic cheilitis; premalignant epithelial lesions of the oral cavity; intraepithelial neoplasia and associated human papillomavirus of the uterine cervix; oral leukoplakia; multifocal superficial transitional cell carcinoma of the upper urinary tract; vulvar lichen sclerosus; advanced-stage esophageal cancer; non-melanoma skin malignancies of the eyelid; squamous cell carcinoma; Kaposi's sarcoma; xeroderma pigmentosum; aids in diagnosis of basal cell carcinomas.

Administration and Dosage

➤*Approved by the FDA:* December 3, 1999.

Aminolevulinic acid HCl for topical solution is intended for direct application to individual lesions diagnosed as actinic keratoses and not to perilesional skin. This product is not intended for application by patients or unqualified medical personnel. Application should involve either scalp or face lesions, but not both simultaneously. The recommended treatment frequency is 1 application of the aminolevulinic acid HCl topical solution and 1 dose of illumination per treatment site per 8-week treatment session. Each individual aminolevulinic acid HCl should be used for only 1 patient. Photodynamic therapy for actinic keratoses with aminolevulinic acid HCl for topical solution is a 2 stage process involving application of the product to the target lesions with aminolevulinic acid HCl, followed 14 to 18 hours later by illumination with blue light using the *BLU-U* Blue Light Photodynamic Therapy Illuminator. The second visit, for illumination, must take place in the 14 to 18 hour window following application. Patients in clinical trials usually received application in the late afternoon, with illumination the following morning.

Schedule for Aminolevulinic Acid and Blue Light Administration	
Aminolevulinic acid topical solution application	Time window for blue light illumination
6 am	8 pm to midnight
7 am	9 pm to 1 am
8 am	10 pm to 2 am
9 am	11 pm to 3 am
10 am	Midnight to 4 am
11 am	1 am to 5 am
12 pm	2 am to 6 am
1 pm	3 am to 7 am
2 pm	4 am to 8 am
3 pm	5 am to 9 am
4 pm	6 am to 10 am
5 pm	7 am to 11 am
6 pm	8 am to noon
7 pm	9 am to 1 pm
8 pm	10 am to 2 pm
9 pm	11 am to 3 pm
10 pm	Noon to 4 pm

Treated lesions that have not completely resolved after 8 weeks may be treated a second time with aminolevulinic acid HCl for topical solution photodynamic therapy. Patients did not receive follow-up past 12 weeks after the initial treatment, so the incidence of recurrence of treated lesions past 12 weeks and the role of further treatment is not known.

AMINOLEVULINIC ACID HYDROCHLORIDE — TOPICAL

➤*Step A:*

Aminolevulinic acid HCl for topical solution application – Actinic keratoses targeted for treatment should be clean and dry prior to application of aminolevulinic acid HCl topical solution.

Preparation: The aminolevulinic acid HCl topical solution should be prepared as follows:

1.) Hold the aminolevulinic acid HCl so that the applicator cap is pointing up.

• *Aminolevulinic acid HCl preparation* – Following solution admixture, remove the cap from the aminolevulinic acid HCl. The dry applicator tip should be dabbed on a gauze pad until uniformly wet with solution.

Application: Apply the solution directly to the target lesions by dabbing gently with the wet applicator tip. Enough solution should be applied to uniformly wet the lesion surface, including the edges without excess running or dripping. The effect of aminolevulinic acid HCl topical solution on ocular tissues is unknown. Aminolevulinic acid HCl topical solution should not be applied to the periorbital area or allowed to contact ocular or mucosal surfaces. Once the initial application has dried, apply again in the same manner. The aminolevulinic acid HCl topical solution must be used immediately following preparation (dissolution) due to the instability of the activated product. If the solution application is not completed within 2 hours of activation, the applicator should be discarded and new aminolevulinic acid HCl for topical solution used.

Photosensitization of the treated lesions will take place over the next 14 to 18 hours. The actinic keratoses should not be washed during this time. The patient should be advised to wear a wide-brimmed hat or other protective apparel to shade the treated actinic keratosis lesions from sunlight or other bright light sources until *BLU-U* treatment. The patient should be advised to reduce light exposure if the sensations of stinging or burning are experienced.

If for any reason the patient cannot be given *BLU-U* treatment during the prescribed time after aminolevulinic acid HCl topical solution application, he or she may nonetheless experience sensations of stinging or burning if the photosensitized actinic keratoses are exposed to sunlight or prolonged or intense light at that time. The patient should be advised to wear a wide-brimmed hat or other protective apparel to shade the treated actinic keratosis lesions from sunlight or other bright light sources until at least 40 hours after the application of aminolevulinic acid HCl topical solution. The patient should be advised to reduce light exposure if the sensations of stinging or burning are experienced.

➤*Step B:*

Administration of BLU-U treatment 14 to 18 hours after application of aminolevulinic acid HCl topical solution – At the visit for light illumination, the actinic keratoses to be treated should be gently rinsed with water and patted dry. Photoactivation of actinic keratoses treated with aminolevulinic acid HCl topical solution is accomplished with *BLU-U* illumination from the *BLU-U* Blue Light Photodynamic Therapy Illuminator. A 1000 second (16 minutes 40 seconds) exposure is required to provide a 10 J/cm^2 light dose. During light treatment, both patients and medical personnel should be provided with blue blocking protective eyewear, as specified in the *BLU-U* Operating Instructions, to minimize ocular exposure. Please refer to the *BLU-U* Operating Instructions for further information on conducting the light treatment. Patients should be advised that transient stinging or burning at the target lesion sites occurs during the period of light exposure.

If blue light treatment with the *BLU-U* Blue Light Photodynamic Therapy Illuminator is interrupted or stopped for any reason, it should not be restarted and the patient should be advised to protect the treated lesions from exposure to sunlight or prolonged or intense light for at least 40 hours after application of the aminolevulinic acid HCl topical solution from the first visit.

➤*For patients with facial lesions:*

1.) The *BLU-U* Blue Light Photodynamic Therapy Illuminator is positioned so that the base is slightly above the patient's shoulder, parallel to the patient's face.
2.) The *BLU-U* is positioned around the patient's head so the entire surface area to be treated lies between 2 inches and 4 inches from the *BLU-U* surface.
   a.) The patient's nose should be no closer than 2 inches from the surface;
   b.) The patient's forehead and cheeks should be no further than 4 inches from the surface;
   c.) The sides of the patient's face and the patient's ears should be no closer than 2 inches from the *BLU-U* surface.

A chin rest may be used to provide support for the patient's head during treatment.

➤*For patients with scalp lesions:*

1.) The knobs on either side of the *BLU-U* are loosened and the *BLU-U* is rotated to a horizontal position.
2.) The *BLU-U* is positioned around the patient's head so the entire surface area to be treated lies between 2 inches and 4 inches from the *BLU-U* surface.
   a.) The patient's scalp should be no closer than 2 inches from the surface;
   b.) The patient's scalp should be no further than 4 inches from the surface;
   c.) The sides of the patient's face and the patient's ears should be no closer than 2 inches from the *BLU-U* surface.

A chin rest may be used to provide support for the patient's head during treatment.

Aminolevulinic acid HCl for topical solution is not intended for use with any device other than the *BLU-U* blue light photodynamic illuminator. Use of aminolevulinic acid HCl for topical solution without subsequent *BLU-U* illumination is not recommended.

➤*Storage / Stability:* Store at 25°C (77°F); excursions permitted to 15° to 30°C (59° to 86°F). Aminolevulinic acid HCl for topical solution should be used immediately following preparation (dissolution). Solution application must be completed within 2 hours of preparation. An applicator that has been prepared must be discarded 2 hours after mixing (dissolving) and new aminolevulinic acid HCl for topical solution used, if needed.

Actions

➤*Pharmacology:* The metabolism of aminolevulinic acid HCl (ALA) is the first step in the biochemical pathway resulting in heme synthesis. Aminolevulinic acid HCl is not a photosensitizer, but rather a metabolic precursor of protoporphyrin IX (PpIX), which is a photosensitizer. The synthesis of ALA is normally tightly controlled by feedback inhibition of the enzyme, ALA synthetase, presumably by intracellular heme levels. ALA, when provided to the cell, bypasses this control point and results in the accumulation of PpIX, which is converted into heme by ferrochelatase through the addition of iron to the PpIX nucleus.

According to the presumed mechanism of action, photosensitization following application of aminolevulinic acid HCl occurs through the metabolic conversion of ALA to PpIX, which accumulates in the skin to which aminolevulinic acid HCl has been applied. When exposed to light of appropriate wavelength and energy, the accumulated PpIX produces a photodynamic reaction, a cytotoxic process dependent upon the simultaneous presence of light and oxygen. The absorption of light results in an excited state of the porphyrin molecule, and subsequent spin transfer from PpIX to molecular oxygen generates singlet oxygen, which can further react to form superoxide and hydroxyl radicals. Photosensitization of actinic (solar) keratosis lesions using the aminolevulinic acid HCl, plus illumination with the *BLU-U* Blue Light Photodynamic Therapy Illuminator (*BLU-U*), is the basis for aminolevulinic acid HCl photodynamic therapy (PDT).

➤*Pharmacokinetics:* ALA is not indicated for internal use, but has been administered orally for some unlabeled uses.

In a human pharmacokinetic study (n = 6) using a 128 mg dose of sterile intravenous ALA HCl and oral ALA HCl (equivalent to 100 mg ALA) in which plasma ALA and PpIX were measured, the mean half-life of ALA was 0.7 ± 0.18 hours after the oral dose and 0.83 ± 0.05 hours after the intravenous dose. The oral bioavailability of ALA was 50% to 60% with a mean C_{max} of 4.65 ± 0.94 mcg/mL. PpIX concentrations were low and were detectable only in 42% of the plasma samples. PpIX concentrations in plasma were quite low relative to ALA plasma concentrations, and were below the level of detection (10 ng/mL) after 10 to 12 hours.

ALA does not exhibit fluorescence, while PpIX has a high fluorescence yield. Time-dependent changes in surface fluorescence have been used to determine PpIX accumulation and clearance in actinic keratosis lesions and perilesional skin after application of aminolevulinic acid HCl topical solution in 12 patients. Peak fluorescence intensity was reached in 11 ± 1 hour in actinic keratoses and 12 ± 1 hour in perilesional skin. The mean clearance half-life of fluorescence for lesions was 30 ± 10 hours and 28 ± 6 hours for perilesional skin. The fluorescence in perilesional skin was similar to that in actinic keratoses. Therefore, aminolevulinic acid HCl topical solution should only be applied to the affected skin.

Contraindications

Cutaneous photosensitivity at wavelengths of 400 to 450 nm; porphyria or known allergies to porphyrins; sensitivity to any of the components of the aminolevulinic acid HCl for topical solution.

Warnings

➤*For topical use only:* The aminolevulinic acid HCl for topical solution contains alcohol and is intended for topical use only. Do not apply to the eyes or to mucous membranes. Excessive irritation may be experienced if this product is applied under occlusion.

➤*Mutagenesis:* At least 1 report in the literature has noted genotoxic effects in cultured rat hepatocytes after ALA exposure with PpIX formation. Other studies have documented oxidative DNA damage in vivo and in vitro as a result of ALA exposure.

➤*Pregnancy: Category C.* Animal reproduction studies have not been conducted with ALA HCl. It is also not known whether aminolevulinic acid HCl topical solution can cause fetal harm when administered to a pregnant woman or can affect reproductive capacity. Aminolevulinic acid HCl topical solution should be given to a pregnant woman only if clearly needed.

➤*Lactation:* The levels of ALA or its metabolites in the milk of subjects treated with aminolevulinic acid HCl topical solution have not been measured. Because many drugs are excreted in human milk, caution should be exercised when aminolevulinic acid HCl topical solution is administered to a nursing woman.

Precautions

➤*Coagulation disorders:* Aminolevulinic acid HCl for topical solution has not been tested on patients with inherited or acquired coagulation defects.

➤*Photodamaged skin:* Application of aminolevulinic acid HCl topical solution to perilesional areas of photodamaged skin of the face or scalp may result in photosensitization. Upon exposure to activating light from the *BLU-U* Blue Light Photodynamic Therapy Illuminator, such photosensitized skin may produce a stinging or burning sensation and may become erythematous or edematous in a manner similar to that of actinic keratoses

AMINOLEVULINIC ACID HYDROCHLORIDE — TOPICAL

treated with aminolevulinic acid HCl. Because of the potential for skin to become photosensitized, aminolevulinic acid HCl for topical solution should be used by a qualified health professional to apply drug only to actinic keratoses and not perilesional skin.

➤*Photosensitivity:* During the time period between the application of aminolevulinic acid HCl topical solution and exposure to activating light from the *BLU-U* Blue Light Photodynamic Therapy Illuminator, the treatment site will become photosensitive. After aminolevulinic acid HCl topical solution application, patients should avoid exposure of the photosensitive treatment sites to sunlight or bright indoor light (eg, examination lamps, operating room lamps, tanning beds, or lights at close proximity) during the period prior to blue light treatment. Exposure may result in a stinging or burning sensation and may cause erythema or edema of the lesions. Before exposure to sunlight, patients should, therefore, protect treated lesions from the sun by wearing a wide-brimmed hat or similar head covering of light-opaque material. Sunscreens will not protect against photosensitivity reactions caused by visible light. It has not been determined if perspiration can spread aminolevulinic acid HCl topical solution outside the treatment site to eye or surrounding skin.

Drug Interactions

There have been no formal studies of the interaction of aminolevulinic acid HCl for topical solution with any other drugs, and no drug-specific interactions were noted during any of the controlled clinical trials. It is, however, possible that concomitant use of other known photosensitizing agents such as griseofulvin, thiazide diuretics, sulfonylureas, phenothiazines, sulfonamides, and tetracyclines might increase the photosensitivity reaction of actinic keratoses treated with the aminolevulinic acid HCl for topical solution.

Adverse Reactions

In Phase 3 studies, no non-cutaneous adverse events were found to be consistently associated with aminolevulinic acid HCl topical solution application followed by blue light exposure.

Photodynamic therapy response – The constellation of transient local symptoms of stinging or burning, itching, erythema and edema as a result of aminolevulinic acid HCl topical solution plus *BLU-U* treatment was observed in all clinical studies of aminolevulinic acid HCl for topical solution photodynamic therapy for actinic keratoses treatment. Stinging or burning subsided between 1 minute and 24 hours after the *BLU-U* Blue Light Photodynamic Therapy Illuminator was turned off, and appeared qualitatively similar to that perceived by patients with erythropoietic protoporphyria upon exposure to sunlight. There was no clear drug dose or light dose dependent change in the incidence or severity of stinging or burning.

In 2 Phase 3 trials, the sensation of stinging or burning appeared to reach a plateau at 6 minutes into the treatment. Severe stinging or burning at 1 or more lesions being treated was reported by at least 50% of patients at some time during treatment. The majority of patients reported that all lesions treated exhibited at least slight stinging or burning. Less than 3% of patients discontinued light treatment due to stinging or burning.

The most common changes in lesion appearance after aminolevulinic acid HCl for topical solution photodynamic therapy were erythema and edema. In 99% of active treatment patients, some or all lesions were erythematous shortly after treatment, while in 79% of vehicle treatment patients, some or all lesions were erythematous. In 35% of active treatment patients, some or all lesions were edematous, while no vehicle-treated patients had edematous lesions. Both erythema and edema resolved to baseline or improved by 4 weeks after therapy. Aminolevulinic acid HCl topical solution application to photodamaged perilesional skin resulted in photosensitization of photodamaged skin and in a photodynamic response.

➤*Other localized cutaneous adverse experiences:*

Post-Pdt Cutaneous Adverse Reactions ALA-018/ALA-019

	Face				Scalp			
	Aminolevulinic acid (n = 139)		Vehicle (n = 41)		Aminolevulinic acid (n = 42)		Vehicle (n = 21)	
Adverse reaction	Mild/moderate	Severe	Mild/moderate	Severe	Mild/moderate	Severe	Mild/moderate	Severe
Scaling/crusting	71%	1%	12%	0%	64%	2%	19%	0%
Pain	1%	0%	0%	0%	0%	0%	0%	0%
Tenderness	1%	0%	0%	0%	2%	0%	0%	0%
Itching	25%	1%	7%	0%	14%	7%	19%	0%
Edema	1%	0%	0%	0%	0%	0%	0%	0%
Ulceration	4%	0%	0%	0%	2%	0%	0%	0%
Bleeding/hemorrhage	4%	0%	0%	0%	2%	0%	0%	0%
Hypo-/hyper-pigmentation	22%		20%		36%		33%	

Post-Pdt Cutaneous Adverse Reactions ALA-018/ALA-019

	Face				Scalp			
	Aminolevulinic acid (n = 139)		Vehicle (n = 41)		Aminolevulinic acid (n = 42)		Vehicle (n = 21)	
Adverse reaction	Mild/moderate	Severe	Mild/moderate	Severe	Mild/moderate	Severe	Mild/moderate	Severe
Vesiculation	4%	0%	0%	0%	5%	0%	0%	0%
Pustules	4%	0%	0%	0%	0%	0%	0%	0%
Oozing	1%	0%	0%	0%	0%	0%	0%	0%
Dysesthesia	2%	0%	0%	0%	0%	0%	0%	0%
Scabbing	2%	1%	0%	0%	0%	0%	0%	0%
Erosion	14%	1%	0%	0%	2%	0%	0%	0%
Excoriation	1%	0%	0%	0%	0%	0%	0%	0%
Wheal/flare	7%	1%	0%	0%	2%	0%	0%	0%
Skin disorder NOS	5%	0%	0%	0%	12%	0%	5%	0%

➤*Adverse reactions reported by body system:* In the Phase 3 studies, 7 patients experienced a serious adverse event. All were deemed remotely or not related to treatment. No clinically significant patterns of clinical laboratory changes were observed for standard serum chemical or hematologic parameters in any of the controlled clinical trials.

Overdosage

➤*Aminolevulinic acid HCl for topical solution overdose:* Aminolevulinic acid HCl for topical solution overdose have not been reported. In the unlikely event that the drug is ingested, monitoring and supportive care are recommended. The patient should be advised to avoid incidental exposure to intense light sources for at least 40 hours. The consequences of exceeding the recommended topical dosage are unknown.

➤*BLU-U* light overdose: There is no information on overdose of blue light from the *BLU-U* Blue Light Photodynamic Therapy Illuminator following aminolevulinic acid HCl for topical solution application.

Patient Information

➤*Aminolevulinic acid HCl photodynamic therapy for actinic keratoses:* The first step in aminolevulinic acid HCl photodynamic therapy (PDT) for actinic keratoses is application of the aminolevulinic acid HCl for topical solution to actinic keratoses located on the patient's face or scalp. After aminolevulinic acid HCl for topical solution is applied to the actinic keratoses in the doctor's office, the patient will be told to return the next day. During this time the actinic keratoses will become sensitive to light (photosensitive). Care should be taken to keep the treated actinic keratoses dry and out of bright light. After aminolevulinic acid HCl topical solution is applied, it is important for the patient to wear light-protective clothing, such as a wide-brimmed hat, when exposed to sunlight or sources of light. Fourteen to 18 hours after application of aminolevulinic acid HCl topical solution the patient will return to the doctor's office to receive blue light treatment, which is the second and final step in the treatment. Prior to blue light treatment, the actinic keratoses will be rinsed with tap water. The patient will be given goggles to wear as eye protection during the blue light treatment. The blue light is of low intensity and will not heat the skin. However, during the light treatment, which lasts for approximately 17 minutes, the patient will experience sensations of tingling, stinging, prickling or burning of the treated lesions. These feelings of discomfort should improve at the end of the light treatment. Following treatment, the actinic keratoses and, to some degree, the surrounding skin, will redden, and swelling and scaling may also occur. However, these lesion changes are temporary and should completely resolve by 4 weeks after treatment.

➤*Photosensitivity:* After aminolevulinic acid HCl topical solution is applied to the actinic keratoses in the doctor's office, the patient should avoid exposure of the photosensitive actinic keratoses to sunlight or bright indoor light (eg, from examination lamps, operating room lamps, tanning beds, or lights at close proximity) during the period prior to blue light treatment. If the patient feels stinging or burning on the actinic keratoses, exposure to light should be reduced. Before going into sunlight, the patient should protect treated lesions from the sun by wearing a wide-brimmed hat or similar head covering of light-opaque material. Sunscreens will not protect the patient against photosensitivity reactions.

If for any reason the patient cannot return for blue light treatment during the prescribed period after application of aminolevulinic acid HCl topical solution (14 to 18 hours), the patient should call the doctor. The patient should also continue to avoid exposure of the photosensitized lesions to sunlight or prolonged or intense light for at least 40 hours. If stinging or burning is noted, exposure to light should be reduced.

WARNING

Methoxsalen with ultraviolet (UV) radiation is to be used only by physicians with competence in diagnosis and treatment of psoriasis and vitiligo, and with special training and experience in photochemotherapy. Constantly supervise such therapy. For psoriasis, restrict photochemotherapy to patients with severe, recalcitrant, disabling psoriasis not adequately responsive to other therapies, and only when diagnosis is supported by biopsy. Because of possible ocular damage, skin aging, and skin cancer (including melanoma), inform patient of risks.

For specific warnings, precautions, indications, and instructions related to photopheresis, consult the *UVAR Photopheresis System* operator's manual before using *Uvadex*.

These are potent drugs, capable of producing severe burns if improperly used. Read entire monograph before prescribing or dispensing these medications.

Never dispense methoxsalen lotion to a patient. The lotion should be applied only by a physician under controlled conditions for light exposure and subsequent light shielding.

Caution – Do not use *Oxsoralen-Ultra* interchangeably with *8-MOP* without retitration of the patient. This new dosage form of methoxsalen exhibits significantly greater bioavailability and earlier photosensitization onset time than previous dosage forms. Treat patients in accordance with dosimetry specifically recommended for this product. Determine minimum phototoxic dose (MPD) and phototoxic peak time after drug administration prior to onset of photochemotherapy with this dosage form.

Indications

➤*Oxsoralen-Ultra, 8-MOP*: Symptomatic control of severe recalcitrant disabling psoriasis not responsive to other therapy when the diagnosis has been supported by biopsy. Administer only in conjunction with a schedule of controlled doses of long wave UV radiation.

➤*Oxsoralen (lotion), 8-MOP*, trioxsalen: With long wave UV radiation for repigmentation of idiopathic vitiligo.

➤*8-MOP, Uvadex*: For extracorporeal administration with long wave UV radiation of white blood cells (photopheresis) and the *UVAR Photopheresis System* in the palliative treatment of the skin manifestations of cutaneous T-cell lymphoma (CTCL) that is unresponsive to other forms of treatment. Refer to the *UVAR Photopheresis System* operator's manual for specific warnings, precautions, indications, and instructions related to photopheresis.

➤*Trioxsalen:* For increasing tolerance to sunlight and for enhancing pigmentation.

Actions

➤*Pharmacology:* Normal skin pigmentation is due to melanin formed by the oxidation of tyrosine to DOPA (dihydroxyphenylalanine). Melanin must be activated by radiant energy in the form of UV light, preferably between 290 and 380 nm. The combination treatment regimen of psoralen (P) and UV radiation of 320 to 400 nm wavelength (UVA) is known by the acronym PUVA. Skin reactivity to UVA radiation is markedly enhanced by the ingestion of methoxsalen.

Oral **methoxsalen** reaches the skin via the blood, and UVA penetrates well into the skin. If sufficient cell injury occurs in the skin, an inflammatory reaction occurs. The most obvious manifestation of this reaction is delayed erythema, which may not begin for several hours and peaks at 48 to 72 hours. The inflammation is followed over several days to weeks by repair, which is manifested by increased melanization of the epidermis and thickening of the stratum corneum.

The exact mechanism of action of psoralens in the process of melanogenesis is not known. The action of these drugs depends upon the presence of functional melanocytes and their proliferation (mitotic activation) by the photoactivated psoralen. One belief is that exposure of methoxsalen-treated patients to UV light thickens the stratum corneum, induces an inflammatory reaction, and increases the amount of melanin in exposed areas. The exact mechanism of action of methoxsalen with the epidermal melanocytes and keratinocytes is not known.

Methoxsalen acts as a photosensitizer; subsequent exposure to UVA can lead to cell injury. In the treatment of psoriasis, the mechanism is assumed to be DNA photodamage and resulting decrease in cell proliferation, but other vascular, leukocyte, or cell regulatory mechanisms may also be involved. The best known biochemical reaction of methoxsalen is with DNA. Methoxsalen, upon photoactivation, conjugates and forms covalent bonds with DNA, which leads to the formation of both monofunctional (addition to a single strand of DNA) and bifunctional (cross-linking of psoralen to both strands of DNA) adducts. Reactions with proteins have also been described.

➤*Pharmacokinetics:* Oral psoralen is > 95% absorbed from the GI tract. Concomitant administration with food increases peak serum concentrations.

Oxsoralen-Ultra Capsules – *Oxsoralen-Ultra Capsules* reach peak drug levels in 0.5 to 4 hours (mean, 1.8 hours) when given with 8 ounces of milk. Maximum bioavailability of *8-MOP* is reached in 1.5 to 3 hours (mean, 2 hours) and may last up to 8 hours. Detectable methoxsalen levels were observed up to 12 hours post-dose. Half-life is ≈ 2 hours. Photosensitivity studies demonstrate a short peak photosensitivity time of 1.5 to 2.1 hours for *Oxsoralen-Ultra Capsules*.

Methoxsalen is reversibly bound to serum albumin and is preferentially taken up by epidermal cells. It is rapidly metabolized. Accumulation does not occur during continuous use; metabolism occurs in hepatic microsomal enzymes. Approximately 95% is excreted in urine within 24 hours; 4% to 10% is excreted in feces.

Trioxsalen possesses greater activity than methoxsalen, yet its median lethal dose is 6 times that of methoxsalen.

Contraindications

Idiosyncratic reactions to psoralen compounds; melanoma or a history of melanoma; invasive squamous cell carcinomas; aphakia (increased risk of retinal damage because of the absence of lenses); patients possessing a specific history of a light-sensitive disease state; diseases associated with photosensitivity including porphyria, acute lupus erythematosus, porphyria cutanea tarda, erythropoietic protoporphyria, variegate porphyria, xeroderma pigmentosum, leukoderma of infectious origin, and in albinism; concomitant use with any preparation having internal or external photosensitizing capacity.

➤*Oral trioxsalen and methoxsalen lotion:* Children ≤ 12 years of age.

Warnings

➤*Skin burning:* Serious burns from either UVA or sunlight (even through window glass) can result if recommended drug dosage or exposure schedules are exceeded or protective covering or sunscreens are not used. The blistering of the skin sometimes encountered after UV exposure generally heals without complication or scarring. Suitable covering of the area of application or a topical sunblock should follow the therapeutic UVA exposure.

➤*Cataracts:* Exposure to large doses of UVA light causes cataracts in animals. Oral methoxsalen exacerbates this toxicity. Serum methoxsalen concentrations are substantially lower after extracorporeal methoxsalen treatment than after oral methoxsalen treatment. The concentration of methoxsalen in the lens is proportional to the serum level. If the lens is exposed to UVA during the presence of methoxsalen in the lens, photochemical action may lead to irreversible binding of methoxsalen to proteins and the DNA components of the lens. However, if the lens is shielded from UVA, the methoxsalen will diffuse out of the lens in a 24-hour period. Emphatically instruct patients to wear UVA-absorbing, wraparound sunglasses for the 24 hours following ingestion of methoxsalen, whether exposed to direct or indirect sunlight in the open, or through window glass.

Among patients using proper eye protection, there is no evidence for a significantly increased risk of cataracts in association with PUVA therapy. Of 1380 patients, 35 have developed cataracts in the 5 years since their first PUVA treatment, an incidence comparable to that expected in a population of this size and age distribution. No relationship between PUVA dose and cataract risk has been noted.

➤*Actinic degeneration:* Exposure to sunlight or UV radiation may prematurely age skin.

➤*Cardiac disease:* Do not treat patients with cardiac disease or who may be unable to tolerate prolonged standing or exposure to heat stress in a vertical UVA chamber.

➤*UVA dosage:* Total cumulative safe UVA dosage over long periods of time is not established.

Do not increase the dosage of **trioxsalen** and exposure time. To prevent harmful effects, instruct patient to adhere to prescribed dosage schedule and procedure.

➤*Hepatic function impairment:* Because hepatic biotransformation is necessary for drug urinary excretion, treat patients with hepatic insufficiency with caution.

➤*Carcinogenesis:* In a prospective study of 1380 patients given PUVA therapy for psoriasis, 237 patients developed 1422 cutaneous squamous cell cancers. This appears greatest among patients who are fair-skinned or who had pre-PUVA exposure to prolonged tar and UVB treatment, ionizing radiation, or arsenic.

A study in 690 patients for up to 4 years showed no increase in risk of nonmelanoma skin cancer. However, patients had significantly less PUVA exposure. There is no evidence of an increased risk of melanoma in PUVA patients, but there is a need for continued evaluation of melanoma risk in these patients.

In a study in Indian patients treated for 4 years for vitiligo, 12% developed keratoses, but not cancer, in the depigmented, vitiliginous areas.

➤*Pregnancy:* *Category C.* It is not known whether psoralens can cause fetal harm when administered to a pregnant woman or can affect reproduction capacity. Use only if clearly needed.

Category D (*Uvadex* only). Methoxsalen may cause fetal harm when given to a pregnant woman. Doses of 80 to 160 mg/kg/day given during organogenesis caused significant fetal toxicity in rats. The lowest of these doses, 80 mg/kg/day, is over 4000 times greater than a single dose of methoxsalen on a mg/m^2 basis. Fetal toxicity was associated with significant maternal weight loss, anorexia, and increased relative liver weight. Signs of fetal toxicity included increased fetal mortality, increased resorptions, late fetal death, fewer fetuses per litter, and decreased fetal weight. Methoxsalen caused an increase in skeletal malformation and variations at doses of ≥ 80 mg/kg/day. There are no adequate and well-controlled studies of methoxsalen in pregnant women. If methoxsalen is used during pregnancy, or if the patient becomes pregnant while receiving methoxsalen, apprise the patient of the potential hazard to the fetus. Advise women of childbearing potential to avoid becoming pregnant.

➤*Lactation:* It is not known whether these agents are excreted in breast milk. Exercise caution when administering to a nursing woman.

➤*Children:* Safety of **methoxsalen** use has not been established. Potential hazards include possible carcinogenicity and cataractogenicity, and probable actinic degeneration. Oral **trioxsalen** and **methoxsalen** lotion are contraindicated in children ≤ 12 years of age.

Precautions

➤*Monitoring:* Perform the following before therapy: CBC (hemoglobin or hematocrit; WBC, and if abnormal, a differential count), antinuclear antibodies, liver and renal function tests (creatinine or blood urea nitrogen), and ophthalmologic examination; retest in 6 to 12 months and conduct additional tests at more extended time periods as indicated. Conduct ophthalmologic examinations yearly after the start of therapy.

➤*Basal cell carcinoma:* Diligently observe and treat patients exhibiting multiple basal cell carcinomas or having a history of basal cell carcinomas.

➤*Vitiligo therapy:* Do not increase the dosage of methoxsalen above 0.6 mg/kg; overdosage may result in serious burning of the skin. Protect eyes and skin from sun.

➤*Furocoumarin-containing foods:* No clinical reports or tests verify that more severe reactions may result from concomitant ingestion of furocoumarin-containing foods, but warn the patient that eating limes, figs, parsley, parsnips, mustard, carrots, and celery might be dangerous.

➤*PUVA erythema/sunburn differences:* PUVA-induced inflammation differs from sunburn or UVB phototherapy in several ways. The percent transmission of UVB varies between 0% to 34% through skin, whereas UVA varies between 1% to 80% transmission; thus, UVA is transmitted to a larger percent through the skin. The in situ depth of photochemistry is deeper within the tissue because UVA is transmitted further into the skin. The DNA lesions induced by PUVA are very different from UV-induced thymine dimers and may lead to a DNA cross-link. The DNA lesion may be more problematic to the cell because cross-links are more lethal and psoralen-DNA photoproducts may be "new" or unfamiliar substrates for DNA repair enzymes. DNA synthesis is also suppressed longer after PUVA. The time course of delayed erythema is different with PUVA and may not involve the usual mediators seen in sunburn. PUVA-induced redness may be just beginning at 24 hours, when UVB erythema has already passed its peak. The erythema dose-response curve is also steeper for PUVA. Compared to equally erythemogenic doses of UVB, the histologic alterations induced by PUVA show more dermal vessel damage and longer duration of epidermal and dermal abnormalities.

Exercise special care in treating patients who are receiving concomitant therapy (either topically or systemically) with known photosensitizing agents such as **anthralin**, **coal tar** or **coal tar derivatives**, **griseofulvin**, **phenothiazines**, **nalidixic acid**, **halogenated salicylanilides** (bacteriostatic soaps), **sulfonamides**, **tetracyclines**, **thiazides**, and certain organic staining dyes such as **methylene blue**, **toluidine blue**, **rose bengal**, and **methyl orange**.

Adverse Reactions

Severe burns and blisters can result from excessive sunlight or sunlamp UV exposure.

Basal cell epitheliomas have been removed from exposed and unexposed areas.

Nausea is common (10%).

Other effects of **methoxsalen** include the following: Nervousness; insomnia; psychological depression; edema; dizziness; headache; malaise; hypopigmentation; vesiculation and bullae formation; nonspecific rash; herpes simplex; miliaria; urticaria; folliculitis; GI disturbances; cutaneous tenderness; leg cramps; hypotension; extension of psoriasis and depression; gastric discomfort.

➤*Combined methoxsalen/UVA therapy:*

Pruritus (≈ 10%): Alleviate with frequent application of bland emollients or other topical agents; severe pruritus may require systemic treatment. If pruritus is unresponsive, shield pruritic areas from further UVA exposure until the condition resolves. If intractable pruritus is generalized, discontinue UVA treatment until pruritus disappears.

Erythema: Mild, transient erythema 24 to 48 hours after PUVA therapy is expected; it indicates a therapeutic interaction between methoxsalen and UVA. Shield any area showing moderate erythema during subsequent UVA exposures until the erythema has resolved. Erythema greater than Grade 2, which appears within 24 hours after UVA treatment may signal a potentially severe burn. Erythema may worsen progressively over the next 24 hours since peak erythemal reaction characteristically occurs 48 hours or later after methoxsalen ingestion. Protect the patient from further UVA exposures and sunlight; monitor closely.

Uvadex: Side effects of photopheresis (*Uvadex* used with the *UVAR Photopheresis System*) were primarily related to hypotension secondary to changes in extracorporeal volume (> 1%). In one study, 6 serious cardiovascular adverse experiences were reported in 5 patients (10%). Five of these 6 events were not related to photopheresis and did not interfere with the scheduled photopheresis treatments. One patient (2%) with ischemic heart disease had an arrhythmia after the first day of photopheresis, but this resolved by the next day. Six infections were also reported in 5 patients. Two of the 6 events were Hickman catheter infections in 1 patient, which did not interrupt the scheduled photopheresis. The other 4 infections were not related to photopheresis and did not interfere with scheduled treatments.

Overdosage

Induce emesis within the first 2 to 3 hours after ingestion of methoxsalen, since maximum blood levels are reached by this time. Follow accepted procedures for treatment of severe burns. Keep the individual in a darkened room for ≥ 24 hours or until cutaneous reactions subside. There are no known reports of overdosage with extracorporeal administration of methoxsalen.

This does not apply to topical use. In the unlikely event that the lotion is ingested, follow standard procedures for poisoning, including gastric lavage. Protection from UVA or daylight for hours or days would also be necessary.

Patient Information

Use **topical methoxsalen** only on small, well-defined lesions that can be protected by clothing or sunscreen (≥ SPF 15) from subsequent exposure to radiant energy. If used to treat vitiligo of face or hands, keep the treated area protected from light by use of protective clothing or sunscreens. The area of application may be highly photosensitive for several days and may result in severe burns if exposed to additional UV or sunlight.

➤*Before methoxsalen ingestion:* Do not sunbathe during the 24 hours prior to methoxsalen ingestion and UV exposure. Sunburn may prevent an accurate evaluation of the patient's response to photochemotherapy.

➤*After methoxsalen ingestion:* Wear UVA-absorbing wraparound sunglasses during daylight for 24 hours to prevent cataracts (see Warnings). The protective eyewear must prevent entry of stray radiation to the eyes, including that which may enter from the sides of the eyewear. Visual discrimination should be permitted by the eyewear for patient well-being and comfort.

Avoid sun exposure, even through window glass or cloud cover, for ≥ 8 hours after methoxsalen ingestion. If sun exposure cannot be avoided, wear protective devices such as a hat and gloves, or apply sunscreens that filter out UVA radiation (eg, sunscreens with SPF ≥ 15). Apply sunscreens to all areas that might be exposed to the sun (including lips). Do not apply sunscreens to areas affected by psoriasis until after treatment in the UVA chamber.

➤*Before PUVA therapy:* Certain other medicines can make the patient more sensitive to the combination drug and light treatment. In addition, certain other medical conditions can be aggravated by this treatment. Before starting treatment, the patient should be sure to tell his/her physician if experiencing any of the following: Severe reaction to *Oxsoralen-Ultra*; recent or planned x-ray treatment; history of skin cancer, eye problems such as cataracts or loss of the lens of the eyes, liver problems, heart or blood pressure problems, any medical condition that requires the patient to stay out of the sun such as lupus erythematosus; or are taking any drugs (either prescription or nonprescription).

Some drugs can increase the patient's sensitivity to UV light either from the sun or man-made sources. Examples of such drugs include major tranquilizers, sulfa drugs for the treatment of infection or diabetes, tetracycline, antibiotics, griseofulvin products, thiazide-containing diuretics (blood pressure or water elimination drugs), and certain antibacterial or deodorant soaps.

➤*During PUVA therapy:* Wear total UVA-absorbing/blocking goggles mechanically designed to give maximal ocular protection. Failure to do so may increase the risk of cataract formation. A radiometer can verify elimination of UVA transmission through the goggles.

Protect abdominal skin, breasts, genitalia, and other sensitive areas for approximately one-third of the initial exposure time until tanning occurs. Unless affected by disease, shield male genitalia.

➤*After combined methoxsalen/UVA therapy:* Wear UVA-absorbing wraparound sunglasses during the daylight for 24 hrs after therapy. Do not sunbathe for 48 hrs after therapy. Erythema or burning because of photochemotherapy and sunburn are additive.

➤*PUVA therapy risks:* Premature skin aging may result from prolonged PUVA therapy, especially in those individuals who tan poorly. This problem is similar to excessive exposure to sunlight. There is an increased risk of developing non-fatal skin cancer. This risk is greater for individuals who fall into the following categories: Fair skin that burns rather than tans; prior treatment with x-rays, grenz rays, or arsenic; prior coal tar and UVB treatment.

Even though the physician will be examining the patient, the patient should routinely and completely examine himself/herself for small growths on his/her skin or skin sores that will not heal. Immediately report such observations to the physician.

Minimize or avoid nausea by taking the drug with milk or food, or by dividing into 2 doses, taken 30 minutes apart.

Do not exceed prescribed dosage or exposure time.

Avoid furocoumarin-containing foods (eg, limes, figs, parsley, parsnips, mustard, carrots, celery).

Psoralens

METHOXSALEN (8–Methoxypsoralen)

Rx	**8-MOP** (ICN Pharmaceuticals)	**Capsules**: 10 mg	In 50s.
Rx	**Oxsoralen-Ultra** (ICN Pharmaceuticals)	**Capsules, soft gelatin**: 10 mg	(ICN 650). Green. In 50s.
Rx	**Uvadex** (Therakos)	**Solution**: 20 mcg/mL	Alcohol (0.05 mL). In 10 mL vials.
Rx	**Oxsoralen** (ICN Pharmaceuticals, Inc.)	**Lotion**: 1% (10 mg/mL)	Acetone. Alcohol (71%). In 30 mL.

METHOXSALEN — ORAL

For complete prescribing information, refer to the Psoralens group monograph.

WARNING

Methoxsalen with UV radiation should be used only by physicians who have special competence in the diagnosis and treatment of psoriasis and who have special training and experience in photochemotherapy. The use of psoralen and ultraviolet (UV) radiation therapy should be under constant supervision of such a physician. For the treatment of patients with psoriasis, photochemotherapy should be restricted to patients with severe, recalcitrant, disabling psoriasis which is not adequately responsive to other forms of therapy, and only when the diagnosis has been supported by biopsy. Because of the possibilities of ocular damage, aging of the skin, and skin cancer (including melanoma), the patient should be fully informed by the physician of the risks inherent in this therapy.

8-MOP capsules – When methoxsalen is used in combination with photopheresis, refer to the UVAR System Operator's Manual for specific warnings, cautions, indications, and instructions related to photopheresis.

Caution – Oxsoralen-Ultra (methoxsalen soft gelatin capsules) should not be used interchangeably with *8-MOP* (methoxsalen hard gelatin capsules). This new dosage form of methoxsalen (*Oxsoralen-Ultra*) exhibits significantly greater bioavailability and earlier photosensitization onset time than previous methoxsalen dosage forms. Patients should be treated in accordance with the dosimetry specifically recommended for this product. The minimum phototoxic dose (MPD) and phototoxic peak time after drug administration prior to the onset of photochemotherapy with this dosage form should be determined.

8-MOP capsules may not be interchanged with *Oxsoralen-Ultra* capsules without retitration of the patient.

Indications

➤*Psoriasis:* For the symptomatic control of severe, recalcitrant, disabling psoriasis not adequately responsive to other forms of therapy and when the diagnosis has been supported by biopsy. Methoxsalen is intended to be administered only in conjunction with a schedule of controlled doses of long-wave UV radiation.

➤*8-MOP* capsules: For the repigmentation of idiopathic vitiligo.

Photopheresis (methoxsalen with long-wave UV radiation of white blood cells) is indicated for use with UVAR system in the palliative treatment of the skin manifestations of cutaneous T-cell lymphoma (CTCL) in persons who have not been responsive to other forms of treatment.

While this dosage form of methoxsalen has been approved for use in combination with photopheresis, *Oxsoralen Ultra* capsules have not been approved for that use.

Administration and Dosage

➤*Approved by the FDA:* October 30, 1986.

➤*8-MOP* capsules:

Vitiligo therapy –

Drug dosage: 2 capsules (10 mg each) in 1 dose taken with milk or in food 2 to 4 hours before UV light exposure.

Light exposure: The exposure time to sunlight should be comply with the following guide:

	Basic Skin Color		
Exposure	Light	Medium	Dark
Initial exposure	15 min	20 min	25 min
Second exposure	20 min	25 min	30 min
Third exposure	25 min	30 min	35 min
Fourth exposure	30 min	35 min	40 min

• *Subsequent exposure* – Gradually increase exposure based on erythema and tenderness of the amelanotic skin.

Therapy should be on alternate days and never on 2 consecutive days.

➤*Caution:* Methoxsalen soft gelatin capsules (*Oxsoralen-Ultra*) represent a new dose form. This new dosage form exhibits significantly greater bioavailability and earlier photosensitization onset time than previous methoxsalen dosage forms. Each patient should be evaluated by determining the minimum phototoxic dose (MPD) and phototoxic peak time after drug administration prior to onset of photochemotherapy with this dosage form. Human bioavailability studies have indicated that the following drug-dosage and administration directions are to be used as a guideline only.

➤*Psoriasis therapy:*

Drug dosage –

Initial therapy: The methoxsalen soft gelatin capsules (*Oxsoralen-Ultra*) should be taken 1½ to 2 hours before UVA exposure; methoxsalen hard gelatin capsules (*8-MOP*) should be taken 2 hours before exposure. Methoxsalen should be taken with some low-fat food or milk according to the following tables:

• *Oxsoralen-Ultra –*

Patient's Weight		Dose
(kg)	(lbs)	(mg)
< 30	< 66	10
30 to 50	66 to 110	20
51 to 65	112 to 143	30
66 to 80	146 to 176	40
81 to 90	179 to 198	50
91 to 115	201 to 254	60
> 115	> 254	70

• *8-MOP* capsules –

Patient's Weight		Dose
(kg)	(lbs)	(mg)
< 30	< 66	10
30 to 50	66 to 110	20
51 to 65	111 to 145	30
66 to 80	146 to 175	40
81 to 90	176 to 200	50
91 to 115	201 to 250	60
> 115	> 250	70

Initial exposure – The initial UVA exposure energy level and corresponding time of exposure is determined by the patient's skin characteristics for sunburning and tanning as follows:

Skin type	History	Recommended joules/cm^2
I	Always burn, never tan (patients with erythrodermic psoriasis are to be classed as type I for determination of UVA dosage)	0.5 J/cm^2
II	Always burn, but sometimes tan	1 J/cm^2
III	Sometimes burn, but always tan	1.5 J/cm^2
IV	Never burn, always tan	2 J/cm^2
Skin type	Physician examination	J/cm^2
V*	Moderately pigmented	2.5 J/cm^2
VI*	Blacks	3 J/cm^2

* Patients with natural pigmentation of these types should be classified into a lower skin type category if the sunburning history so indicates.

Oxsoralen-Ultra: If the MPD is done, start at half the MPD.

Dosage directions: Additional drug dosage directions are as follows:

• *Weight change* – In the event that the weight of a patient changes during treatment such that he falls into an adjacent weight range/dose category, no change in the dose of methoxsalen is usually required. If, in the physician's opinion, however, a weight change is sufficiently great to modify the drug dose, then an adjustment in the time of exposure to UVA should be made.

• *Dose/week* – The number of doses/week of methoxsalen capsules will be determined by the patient's schedule of UVA exposures. In no case should treatments be given more often than once every other day because the full extent of phototoxic reactions may not be evident until 48 hours after each exposure.

• *Dosage increase* – Dosage may be increased by 10 mg after the 15th treatment under the proper conditions.

➤*UVA radiation source specifications and information:*

Irradiance uniformity – The following specifications should be met with the window of the detector held in a vertical plane:

Vertical variation: For readings taken at any point along the vertical center axis of the chamber (to within 15 cm from the top and bottom), the lowest reading should not be less than 70% of the highest reading.

Horizontal variation: Throughout any specific horizontal plane, the lowest reading must be at least 80% of the highest reading, excluding the peripheral 3 cm of the patient treatment space.

UVA exposure dosimetry measurements – The maximum radiant exposure or irradiance (within ± 15 %) of UVA (320 to 400 nanometers) delivered to the patient should be determined by using an appropriate radiometer calibrated to be read in J/cm^2 or mW/cm^2. In the absence of a standard measuring technique approved by the National Bureau of Standards, the system

METHOXSALEN — ORAL

should use a detector corrected to a cosine spatial response. The use and recalibration frequency of such a radiometer for a specific UVA irradiator chamber should be specified by the manufacturer because the UVA dose (exposure) is determined by the design of the irradiator, the number of lamps, and the age of the lamp. If irradiance is measured, the radiometer reading in mW/cm^2 is used to calculate the exposure time in minutes to deliver the required UVA in J/cm^2 to a patient in the UVA irradiator cabinet.

Exposure time: The equation to calculate exposure time is the following: Exposure time (minutes) = desired UVA dose (J/cm^2)/0.06 × irradiance (mW/cm^2).

Overexposure due to human error should be minimized by using an accurate automatic timing device, which is set by the operator and controlled by energizing and deenergizing the UVA irradiator lamp. The timing device calibration interval should be specified by the manufacturer. Safety systems should be included to minimize the possibility of delivering a UVA exposure which exceeds the prescribed dose, in the event the timer or radiometer should malfunction.

UVA spectral output distribution – The spectral distributions of the lamps should meet the following specifications:

Wavelength Band (nanometers)	Output[1]
< 310	< 1
310 to 320	1 to 3
320 to 330	4 to 8
330 to 340	11 to 17
340 to 350	18 to 25
350 to 360	19 to 28
360 to 370	15 to 23
370 to 380	8 to 12
380 to 390	3 to 7
390 to 400	1 to 3

[1] As a percentage of total irradiance between 320 and 400 nanometers.

➤*PUVA treatment protocol:*

Oxsoralen-Ultra capsules – These methoxsalen capsules reach their maximum bioavailability in 1½ to 2 hours after ingestion.

Oxsoralen-Ultra vs *8-MOP* capsules – On average, the serum level achieved with *Oxsoralen-Ultra* is twice that obtained with *8-MOP* (formerly *Oxsoralen*) and reach their peak concentration in less than half the time of the *8-MOP* capsules.

As a result, the mean MED J/cm^2 for the *Oxsoralen-Ultra* capsules is substantially less than that required for *8-MOP*).

Photosensitivity studies demonstrate a peak photosensitivity of 1.5 to 2.1 hours for *Oxsoralen-Ultra* capsules.

Initial exposure – The initial UVA exposures should be conducted according to the guidelines presented above.

Clearing phase – Specific recommendations for patient treatment are as follows:

Skin types I, II, and III: Patients with skin types I, II, and III may be treated 2 or 3 times/week. UVA exposure may be held constant or increased by up to 1 J/cm^2 at each treatment, according to the patient's response. If erythema occurs, however, do not increase exposure time until erythema resolves. The severity and extent of the patient's erythema may be used to determine whether the next exposure should be shortened, omitted, or maintained at the previous dosage (see Adverse Reactions).

Skin types IV, V, and VI: Patients with skin types IV, V, and VI may be treated 2 or 3 times/week. UVA exposure may be held constant or increased by up to 1.5 J/cm^2 at each treatment unless erythema occurs. If erythema occurs, follow instructions outlined above in procedures for patients with skin types I, II, and III.

Erythrodermic psoriasis: Patients with erythrodermic psoriasis should be treated with special attention because preexisting erythema may obscure observations of possible treatment-related phototoxic erythema. These patients may be treated 2 or 3 times/week, as a type I patient.

Miscellaneous situations: If there is no response after a total of 10 treatments, the exposure of UVA energy may be increased by an additional 0.5 to 1 J/cm^2 above the prior incremental increases for each treatment (eg, a patient whose exposure dose is being increased by 1 J/cm^2 may now have all subsequent doses increased by 1.5 to 2 J/cm^2).

If there is no response, or only minimal response, after 15 treatments, the dosage of methoxsalen may be increased by 10 mg (a one-time increase in dosage). This increased dosage may be continued for the remainder of the course of treatment but should not be exceeded.

If a patient misses a treatment, the UVA exposure time of the next treatment should not be increased. If more than 1 treatment is missed, reduce the exposure by 0.5 J/cm^2 for each treatment missed.

If the lower extremities are not responding as well as the rest of the body and do not show erythema, cover all other body areas and give 25% of the present exposure dose as an additional exposure to the lower extremities. This additional exposure to the lower extremities should be terminated if erythema develops on these areas.

• *Nonresponsive psoriasis* – If a patient's generalized psoriasis is not responding, or if the condition appears to be worsening during treatment, the possibility of a generalized phototoxic reaction should be considered. This may be confirmed by the improvement of the condition following temporary discontinuance of this therapy for 2 weeks. If no improvement occurs during the interruption of treatment, this patient may be considered a treatment failure.

Alternative exposure schedule – As an alternative to increasing the UVA exposure at each treatment, the following schedule may be followed. This schedule may reduce the total number of J/cm^2 received by the patient over the entire course of therapy. Incremental increases in UVA exposure for all patients may range from 0.5 to 1.5 J/cm^2, according to the patient's response to therapy. Once Grade 2 clearing has been reached and the patient is progressing adequately, UVA dosage is held constant. This dosage is maintained until Grade 4 clearing is reached. If the rate of clearing significantly decreases, exposure dosage may be increased at each treatment (0.1 to 1.5 J/cm^2) until Grade 3 clearing and a satisfactory progress rate is attained. The UVA exposure will be held constant again until Grade 4 clearing is attained. These increases may be used also if the rate of clearing significantly decreases between Grade 3 and Grade 4 response. However, the possibility of a phototoxic reaction should be considered; see previous information. In summary, this schedule raises slightly the increments (J/cm^2) of UVA dosage, but limits these increases to those periods when the patient is not responding adequately. Otherwise, the UVA exposure is held at the lowest effective dose.

Maintenance phase – The goal of maintenance treatment is to keep the patient as symptom-free as possible with the least amount of UVA exposure.

Schedule of exposures: When patients have achieved 95% clearing, or Grade 4 response, they may be placed on the maintenance schedules described below (M_1 to M_4), in sequence. It is recommended that each maintenance schedule be adhered to for at least 2 treatments (unless erythema or psoriatic flare occurs, in which case see below).

Maintenance schedules:

Maintenance Schedules	
M_1	Once/week
M_2	Once/2 weeks
M_3	Once/3 weeks
M_4	As needed (ie, for flares)

Length of exposure – The UVA exposure for the first maintenance treatment of any schedule (except M_4 as noted above) is the same as that of the patient's last treatment under the previous schedule. For skin types I to IV, however, it is recommended that the maximum UVA dosage during maintenance treatments not exceed the following:

Skin Types	Joules/cm^2/treatment
I	12
II	14
III	18
IV	22

If the patient develops erythema or new lesions of psoriasis, proceed as follows:

Erythema: During maintenance therapy, the patient's tan and threshold dose for erythema may gradually decrease. If maintenance treatments produce significant erythema, the exposure to UVA should be decreased by 25% until further treatments no longer produce erythema.

Psoriasis: If the patient develops new areas of psoriasis during maintenance therapy (but still is classified as having a Grade 4 response), the exposure to UVA may be increased by 0.5 to 1.5 J/cm^2 at each treatment; this is appropriate for all types of patients. These increases are continued until the psoriasis is brought under control and the patient is again clear. The exposure being administered when this clearing is reached should be used for further maintenance treatment.

Flares during maintenance – If the patient flares during maintenance treatment (develops psoriasis on greater than 5% of the originally involved areas of the body), his maintenance treatment schedule may be changed to the preceding maintenance or clearing schedule. The patient may be kept on his schedule until again 95% clear. If the original maintenance treatment schedule is unable to control the psoriasis, the schedule may be changed to a more frequent regimen. If a flare occurs within less than 6 weeks after the last treatment, 25% of the maximum exposure received during the clearing phase, with the clearing schedule received during the clearing phase, may be used and then proceed with the clearing schedule previously followed for this patient. (At 95% clearing, follow regular maintenance until the optimum maintenance schedule is determined for the patient.) If more than 6 weeks have elapsed since the last treatment was given, treat patients as if they were beginning therapy insofar as exposure dosages are concerned, since their threshold for erythema may have decreased.

Grades of Erythema	
Grade	Erythema level
0	No erythema
1	Minimally perceptible erythema (faint pink)
2	Marked erythema but with no edema
3	Fiery erythema with edema
4	Fiery erythema with edema and blistering

Psoralens

METHOXSALEN — ORAL

Response to therapy		
Grade	Criteria	% improvement (compared to original extent of disease)
−1	Psoriasis worse	0%
0	No change	0%
1	Minimal improvement, slightly less scale, or erythema	5% to 20%
2	Definite improvement, partial flattening of all plaques, less scaling, and less erythema	20% to 50%
3	Considerable improvement, nearly complete flattening of all plaques, but borders of plaques still palpable	50% to 95%
4	Clearing, complete flattening of plaques including borders (plaques may be outlined by pigmentation)	95%

➤*Storage/Stability:* Store at 25°C (77°F); excursion permitted to 15° to 30°C (59° to 86°F).

METHOXSALEN — INJECTION

For complete prescribing information, refer to the Psoralens group monograph.

WARNING

Methoxsalen should be used only by physicians who have special competence in the diagnosis and treatment of cutaneous T-cell lymphoma and have special training and experience in the *UVAR* or *UVAR XTS Photopheresis System*. Consult the *UVAR Photopheresis System* operator's manual before using this product.

Indications

➤*Cutaneous T-cell lymphoma:* For extracorporeal administration with the *UVAR Photopheresis System* in the palliative treatment of skin manifestations of cutaneous T-cell lymphoma (CTCL) that is unresponsive to other forms of treatment.

Administration and Dosage

➤*Normal treatment schedule:* Give methoxsalen on 2 consecutive days every 4 weeks for a minimum of 7 treatment cycles (6 months). The total dose of methoxsalen used with the *UVAR Photopheresis System* in conjunction with *Uvadex* is substantially lower (approximately 200 times) than that used with oral administration.

➤*Accelerated treatment schedule:* If the assessment of the patient during the fourth treatment cycle (approximately 3 months) reveals an increased skin score from the baseline score, the frequency of treatment may be increased to 2 consecutive treatments every 2 weeks. If a 25% improvement in the skin score is attained after 4 consecutive weeks, the regular treatment schedule may resume. Patients who are maintained in the accelerated treatment schedule may receive a maximum of 20 cycles. There is no clinical evidence to show that treatment with methoxsalen for more than 6 months or using a different schedule provides additional benefit. In a study, 15 of the 17 responses were seen within 6 months of treatment, and only 2 patients responded to treatment after 6 months.

➤*Instruction for administration:* Each methoxsalen treatment involves collection of leukocytes, photoactivation, and reinfusion of photoactivated cells. During each photopheresis treatment performed with the *UVAR system*, 10 mL (200 mcg) of methoxsalen is injected directly into the photoactivation bag during the first buffy coat collection cycle. At the end of 6 cycles, a total of 740 mL (240 mL of buffy coat, 300 mL of plasma, and 200 mL of normal saline priming fluid) is collected and mixed with the 200 mcg of methoxsalen present in the photoactivation bag. After photoactivation, the cells are reinfused. Consult the *UVAR Photopheresis System* operator's manual before using this product.

During treatments with the *UVAR XTS System*, the dosage of methoxsalen for each treatment will be calculated according to the treatment volume (displayed on the XTS display panel). The prescribed amount of methoxsalen will be injected into the recirculation bag prior to the Photoactivation Phase using the following formula:

Treatment Volume × 0.017 = mL of methoxsalen for each treatment.

➤*Storage/Stability:* Store between 15° and 30°C (59° and 86°F).

METHOXSALEN — TOPICAL

For complete prescribing information, refer to the Psoralens group monograph.

WARNING

Methoxsalen lotion is a potent drug capable of producing severe burns if improperly used. It should be applied only by a physician under controlled conditions for light exposure and subsequent light shielding. This preparation should never be dispensed to a patient.

Indications

➤*Vitiligo:* Repigmenting agent in vitiligo, used in conjunction with controlled doses of UVA (320 to 400 nm) or sunlight.

Administration and Dosage

Apply lotion to a small, well-defined, vitiliginous lesion, then expose this area to UVA light. Initial exposure time must not exceed one half the minimal erythema dose.

Regulate treatment intervals by erythema response (once a week or less, depending on the results).

Pigmentation may begin after a few weeks; significant repigmentation may take up to 6 to 9 months. Periodic treatment may be needed to retain the new pigment.

Essentially, idiopathic vitiligo is reversible, but not equally in every patient. Individualize treatment. Repigmentation varies in completeness, time of onset, and duration; it occurs more rapidly on fleshy regions such as the face, abdomen, and buttocks, and less rapidly over bony areas such as the dorsum of the hands and feet.

Protect the hands and fingers of the person applying the medication with gloves or finger cots to avoid photosensitization and possible burns.

➤*Protect form light:* Instruct patient to keep the treated areas protected from light by use of protective clothing or sunscreening agents. The area of application may be highly photosensitive for several days and may result in severe burn injury if exposed to additional UV or sunlight.

➤*Storage/Stability:* Store at 25°C (77°F); excursions permitted to 15° to 30°C (59° to 88°F).

Tar-Containing Preparations

TAR DERIVATIVES, SHAMPOOS

otc	**DHS Tar** (Person & Covey)	**Shampoo:** 0.5% coal tar	**Liquid:** In 120, 240 & 480 mL.
			Gel: In 240 g.
otc	**Tera-Gel** (Geritrex)	**Shampoo:** 0.5% coal tar	EDTA, parabens. In 114 mL.
otc	**PC-Tar** (Geritrex)	**Shampoo:** 1% coal tar	EDTA. In 180 mL.
otc	**Zetar** (Dermik)	**Shampoo:** 1% coal tar	In 177 mL.
otc	**Doak Tar** (Doak)	**Shampoo:** 1.2% coal tar	Isopropyl alcohol. In 237 mL.
otc	**Ionil T Plus** (Healthpoint)	**Shampoo:** 2% coal tar	In 120 and 240 mL.
otc	**Neutrogena T/Gel Original** (Neutrogena Corp.)	**Shampoo:** 2% coal tar extract	In 132, 255, 480 mL.

TAR DERIVATIVES, SHAMPOOS

otc	**Pentrax** (Medicis)	**Shampoo:** 5% coal tar	In 236 mL.
otc	**Creamy Tar** (Genesis)	**Shampoo:** 6.65% coal tar solution, 0.67% crude coal tar (2% coal tar)	In 240 mL.
otc	**MG 217 Medicated Tar** (Triton)	**Shampoo:** 15% coal tar solution (3% coal tar)	In 120 and 240 mL.
otc	**Polytar** (Stiefel)	**Shampoo:** 4.5% polytar (coal tar solution, solubilized crude coal tar equivalent to 0.5% coal tar).	Lanolin. In 177 and 355 mL.

TAR DERIVATIVES SHAMPOOS — TOPICAL

Indications

➤*Itchy conditions of the body and scalp:* For treatment of scalp psoriasis, seborrheic dermatitis, dandruff, cradle-cap, and other oily, itchy conditions of the body and scalp.

Administration and Dosage

Refer to specific product labeling. Rub shampoo liberally into wet hair and scalp. Leave on for several minutes. Rinse thoroughly. Repeat and rinse. Depending on product, use from once daily to at least twice a week or as directed by a physician. For severe scalp problems, use daily.

Actions

➤*Pharmacology:* Tar derivatives have antiseptic, antibacterial, and antiseborrheic properties and loosen and soften scales and crusts.

Contraindications

Acute inflammation; open or infected lesions.

Warnings

➤*Carcinogenesis:* High concentrations of some chemicals in coal tar may cause cancer. However, concentrations of 0.5% to 5% appear to be safe.

➤*Children:* Use on children less than 2 years of age only as directed by a physician.

Precautions

➤*For external use only:* Avoid contact with eyes. If contact occurs, rinse eyes thoroughly with water. Do not use in or around the rectum or in the genital or groin area.

➤*Irritation:* Discontinue if irritation develops and contact a physician. In rare instances, temporary discoloration of blond, bleached, or tinted hair may occur.

➤*If condition worsens or does not improve:* After regular use as directed, if excessive dryness or any undesirable effect occurs, discontinue use and contact physician.

➤*Other treatment:* Do not use this product with other forms of psoriasis therapy, such as ultraviolet radiation or prescription drugs, unless directed to do so by a physician.

➤*Photosensitivity:* Use caution in exposing skin to sunlight after application. It may increase sunburn for up to 24 hours after application.

Adverse Reactions

Minor dermatologic side effects include rash or burning sensation. Photosensitivity may occur. May discolor skin.

Patient Information

For external use only. Avoid contact with the eyes.

Use caution in the sunlight after applying; it may increase the tendency to sunburn up to 24 hours after application.

Do not use for prolonged periods without consulting physician.

If condition covers a large part of the body, consult a physician before using.

TAR-CONTAINING PRODUCTS, BATH PREPARATIONS

otc	**Balnetar** (Westwood Squibb)	**Liquid:** 2.5% coal tar in mineral oil, lanolin oil	In 221 mL.
otc	**Cutar Emulsion** (Summers)	**Liquid:** 7.5% LCD (1.5% coal tar) in mineral oil, lanolin alcohols extract, parabens	In 177 mL and 1 gal.
otc	**Doak Tar Oil** (Doak)	**Oil:** 2% doak tar distillate (equivalent to 0.8% coal tar), mineral oil	In 237 mL.

TAR-CONTAINING PRODUCTS, BATH PREPARATIONS — TOPICAL

Indications

➤*Pruritic dermatoses:* These products contain tar derivatives, which have keratoplastic, antieczematous, and antipruritic effects. They are used as adjuncts in a wide range of pruritic dermatoses including psoriasis and seborrheic dermatitis.

Administration and Dosage

➤*Directions:* Add to bath water. Soak 10 to 20 minutes and then pat dry.

Contraindications

Hypersensitivity to any ingredient of the product.

Warnings

➤*Carcinogenesis:* High concentrations of some chemicals in coal tar may cause cancer. However, concentrations of 0.5% to 5% appear to be safe.

Precautions

➤*For external use only:* Avoid contact with the eyes. If contact occurs, rinse with water and contact physician.

➤*Use caution:* To avoid slipping in the bathtub.

➤*Staining:* May occur on plastic or fiberglass tubs.

➤*Irritation:* If irritation persists, discontinue use. Coal tar may cause allergic irritation.

➤*Application considerations:* Do not apply to acutely inflamed or broken skin or to the genital or rectal areas.

➤*Photosensitivity:* Coal tar is photosensitizing; for 24 hours after use, avoid exposure to direct sunlight or sunlamps.

Adverse Reactions

Dermatitis; allergic sensitization; folliculitis; photosensitization (see Precautions).

Patient Information

Discontinue use and consult with physician if condition worsens or does not improve after regular use, covers a large area of the body, or causes irritation or allergic reaction.

Discontinue use and consult with physician if used for a prolonged period of time.

TAR-CONTAINING PRODUCTS, MISCELLANEOUS

otc	**Medotar** (Medco)	**Ointment:** 1% coal tar	Octoxynol-5, zinc oxide, white petrolatum. In 454 g.
otc	**Taraphilic** (Medco)	**Ointment:** 1% coal tar distillate	Stearyl alcohol, petrolatum, parabens. In 454 g.
otc	**MG217 Medicated Tar** (Triton)	**Ointment:** 10% coal tar solution USP (equivalent to 2% coal tar)	Petrolatum, cetyl alcohol. In 107 g.
otc	**Fototar** (ICN Pharm)	**Cream:** coal tar extract (equivalent to 2% coal tar)	Emollient moisturizing base. In 85 and 454 g.
otc	**MG217 Medicated Tar Lotion** (Triton)	**Lotion:** 5% coal tar solution (equivalent to 1% coal tar)	Moisturizing base. Cetyl alcohol, mineral oil. In 120 mL.
otc	**Oxipor VHC** (Medtech)	**Lotion:** 25% coal tar solution (equivalent to 5% coal tar)	79% alcohol. In 56 mL.

TAR-CONTAINING PRODUCTS, MISCELLANEOUS

otc	**Packer's Pine Tar** (GenDerm)	**Soap:** Pine tar, pine oil	Soap base. In 99 g.
otc	**Polytar** (Stiefel)	**Soap:** 2.5% coal tar solution (equivalent to 0.5% coal tar)	Glycerin, ethyl alcohol, peanut oil. In 113 g.

TAR-CONTAINING PRODUCTS, MISCELLANEOUS — TOPICAL

Indications

➤*Psoriasis/Seborrheic dermatitis:* For the relief and control of itching, irritation, and skin flaking associated with psoriasis and seborrheic dermatitis.

Administration and Dosage

Refer to specific product labeling. Depending on product, use from 1 to 4 times/day.

Contraindications

Hypersensitivity to any ingredient in the product.

Warnings

➤*Carcinogenesis:* High concentrations of some chemicals in coal tar may cause cancer. However, concentrations of 0.5% to 5% appear to be safe.

Precautions

➤*For external use only:* Avoid contact with the eyes. If contact occurs, rinse eyes thoroughly with water and contact physician.

➤*Application considerations:* Do not apply preparations to acutely inflamed or broken skin or to the genital or rectal areas except on the advice of a physician.

➤*Discoloration/Staining:* Staining of clothing may occur which is normally removed by standard laundry methods. Use on the scalp may cause temporary staining of light colored hair.

➤*Other treatment:* Do not use with other forms of psoriasis therapy (eg, ultraviolet radiation, drug therapy) unless directed to do so by a physician.

➤*Flammable:* Some coal tar products are extremely flammable. Keep away from fire and flame.

➤*Photosensitivity:* Avoid exposure to sunlight for up to 24 hours as it may increase tendency to sunburn. Do not use on patients who have a disease characterized by photosensitivity (eg, lupus erythematosus, sunlight allergy).

Patient Information

Do not use for prolonged periods without consulting physician.

If condition worsens or does not improve after regular use, consult physician.

If condition covers a large part of the body, consult physician before using.

PIGMENT AGENTS

DIHYDROXYACETONE

otc	**Chromelin Complexion Blender** (Summers)	**Suspension:** 5%	Isopropyl alcohol, propylene glycol. In 30 mL.

DIHYDROXYACETONE — TOPICAL

Indications

➤*Idiopathic vitiligo:* Used to darken light or unpigmented areas of skin affected by vitiligo, scars, and other causes.

Administration and Dosage

Use applicator top to apply evenly to areas of skin to be darkened. Allow to remain on the skin at least 3 hours before washing. The first effects appear in about 6 hours after initial application. To achieve a darker color, repeat application instructions once or twice in 24 hours, more often if darker color is desired. The coloration will last 3 to 10 days with gradual and even fading. To prevent darkening of skin surrounding treated areas, take a damp tissue and gently wipe off any dihydroxyacetone (DHA) that has overlapped onto normally pigmented skin. Maintenance applications of once a day or every other day should be sufficient.

Actions

➤*Pharmacology:* The mechanism of action is not fully understood; however, DHA may involve a reaction (similar to that caused by sun exposure) with amino acids in the stratum corneum of the skin to produce a brownish color. As the concentration of the drug increases, so does the pigmentation.

Precautions

➤*For external use only:* Avoid contact with hair, eyes, eyelids, abraded skin, and clothes.

➤*Sun exposure:* Use sunscreen before exposing treated areas to the sun.

Adverse Reactions

➤*Dermatologic:* Rashes with erythema and allergic dermatitis; skin irritation or sensitivity (rare).

Patient Information

Use sunscreen before exposing treated skin to the sun.

Use applicator to evenly apply to affected areas to be treated; to prevent darkening of skin in surrounding areas, take a damp cloth to wipe off excess.

Do not wash the treated area for 3 hours after application.

First application takes about 6 hours to develop color.

Cosmetics may be applied on treated areas.

May stain clothing; let treated areas dry.

HYDROQUINONE

otc	**Eldopaque** (ICN)	**Cream:** 2%	With sunblock. In 14.2 and 28.4 g.
otc	**Esoterica Facial** (Medicis)		Octyl dimethyl PABA, benzophenone, stearyl alcohol, sodium bisulfite, parabens, EDTA. In 90 g.
otc	**Esoterica Regular** (Medicis)		Light mineral oil, stearyl alcohol, parabens, sodium bisulfite, EDTA. In 90 g.
otc	**Esoterica Sunscreen** (Medicis)		3.3% padimate O, 2.5% oxybenzone, mineral oil, parabens, sodium bisulfite, EDTA. In 85 g.
otc	**Solaquin** (ICN)		With sunscreens. In 28.4 g.

HYDROQUINONE

Rx	**Hydroquinone** (Various, eg, Ethex, Glades)	**Cream:** 4%	May contain EDTA, parabens, mineral oil, sodium metabisulfite. In 28.35 g.
Rx	**Hydroquinone with Sunscreen** (Various, eg, Ethex, Glades)		May contain padimate O, dioxybenzone, oxybenzone, octyl methoxycinnamate, octyl dimethyl-p-aminobenzoate, cetearyl alcohol, vitamin E, parabens, mineral oil, cetearyl alcohol, stearyl alcohol, lactic acid, EDTA, sodium metabisulfite. In 28.35 g.
Rx	**Claripel** (Stiefel)		Cetostearyl alcohol, EDTA, parabens, octyl methoxycinnamate, avobenzone, oxybenzone, sodium metabisulfite, stearyl alcohol, glycerin. In 45 g.
Rx	**Eldopaque Forte** (ICN)		In a sunblock base. Talc, light mineral oil, EDTA, sodium metabisulfite. In 28.4 g.
Rx	**Eldoquin-Forte** (ICN)		In a vanishing base. Light mineral oil, propylparaben, sodium metabisulfite. In 28.4 g.
Rx	**EpiQuin Micro** (SkinMedica)		Vitamins A, E, and C, cetyl alcohol, benzyl alcohol, EDTA, glycerin, methylparaben, sodium metabisulfite. In 30 g.
Rx	**Glyquin** (ICN)		In a vanishing base. Padimate O, oxybenzone, octyl methoxycinnamate, methylparaben. SPF 15. In 28 g.
Rx	**Glyquin-XM** (ICN)		In a vanishing base. Octocrylene, oxybenzone, avobenzone, vitamin E, methylparaben, EDTA. SPF 15. In 28 g.
Rx	**Solaquin Forte** (ICN)		In a vanishing base. Dioxybenzone, padimate O, oxybenzone, EDTA, sodium metabisulfite, cetearyl alcohol, stearyl alcohol, lactic acid. In 28.4 g.
Rx	**Lustra** (Medicis)		Glycerin, alcohol, cetyl alcohol, cetearyl alcohol, benzyl alcohol, sodium metabisulfite, EDTA. In 28.4 g.
Rx	**Lustra-AF** (Medicis)		Glycerin, alcohol, cetyl alcohol, cetearyl alcohol, benzyl alcohol, sodium metabisulfite, EDTA, octyl methoxycinnamate, avobenzone. In 28.4 g.
Rx	**Nuquin HP** (Stratus)		Octyl methoxycinnamate, glycerin, cetyl alcohol, cetostearyl alcohol, stearyl alcohol, sodium metabisulfite. In 14.2, 28.4, and 56.7 g.
Rx	**Melquin HP** (Stratus)		In a vanishing base. Mineral oil, petrolatum, cetostearyl alcohol, glycerin, sodium metabisulfite. In 14.2 and 28.4 g.
Rx	**Melpaque HP** (Stratus)		In a sunblocking base. Mineral oil, parabens, EDTA, sodium metabisulfite, talc. Tinted. In 14.2 and 28.4 g.
Rx	**Hydroquinone** (Glades)	**Solution:** 3%	SD alcohol 40-B, isopropyl alcohol. In 29 mL with applicator.
otc	**NeoStrata Skin Lightening** (NeoStrata)	**Gel:** 2%	Denatured alcohol. sodium bisulfite, EDTA. In 4.8 g.
Rx	**Hydroquinone** (Glades)	**Gel:** 3%	Hydroalcoholic base. Padimate O, dioxybenzone, EDTA, sodium metabisulfite. In 30 g.
Rx	**Hydroquinone** (Glades)	**Gel:** 4%	Hydroalcoholic base. Padimate O, dioxybenzone, alcohol, EDTA, sodium metabisulfite. In 28.35 g.
Rx	**Solaquin Forte** (ICN)		Hydroalcoholic base. Padimate O, dioxybenzone, EDTA, alcohol, sodium metabisulfite. In 28.4 g.
Rx	**Aclaro** (Harmony)	**Emulsion:** 4%	Alcohols, EDTA. In 50 mL spray bottles.

HYDROQUINONE — TOPICAL

Indications

➤*Hyperpigmented skin:* For the gradual temporary bleaching of hyperpigmented skin conditions such as chloasma, melasma, freckles, senile lentigines and other unwanted areas of melanin hyperpigmentation.

Administration and Dosage

Hydroquinone cream, gel, and topical solution should be applied to the affected area(s) and rubbed in well twice daily or as directed by a physician to achieve maximum therapeutic potential. However, *Melpaque HP 4%* should not be rubbed in. Hydroquinone bleaching is faster, more dependable, and easier if the treated area is protected from ultraviolet light. During the day, an effective broad-spectrum sunscreen should be used and unnecessary solar exposure avoided, or protective clothing should be worn to cover bleached skin in order to prevent repigmentation from occurring. There is no recommended dosage for children younger than 12 years of age except under the advice and supervision of a physician. Keep container tightly closed. Note that slight darkening of hydroquinone products is normal and does not affect the potency of the products.

➤*Neostrata HQ* gel and *HQ Plus* gel: Apply sparingly to affected areas once or twice daily. Use only as directed by a physician. Depigmentation is a gradual process, and results should be expected within 12 weeks of daily use. If no improvement is seen within 8 weeks, discontinue use. To maintain results, use several times a week or as directed by a physician.

For best results, use with sunscreen or avoid exposure to sunlight. Keep tube tightly closed to ensure airtight seal.

Actions

➤*Pharmacology:* Topical application of hydroquinone produces a reversible depigmentation of the skin by inhibition of the enzymatic oxidation of tyrosine to 3,4-dihydroxyphenylalanine (dopa) and suppression of other melanocyte metabolic processes. Exposure to sunlight or ultraviolet light will cause repigmentation of bleached areas.

In addition to hydroquinone, some products contain sunscreens (eg, octyl dimethyl PABA, ethyl dihydroxypropyl PABA, dioxybenzone, oxybenzone).

Contraindications

Hypersensitivity to hydroquinone or any other ingredients of the products. The safety of topical hydroquinone use during pregnancy or in children (less than or equal to 12 years old) has not been established.

Warnings

➤*Bleaching:* Hydroquinone is a skin-bleaching agent which may produce unwanted cosmetic effects if not used as directed. The physician should be familiar with the contents of this monograph before prescribing or dispensing this medication.

➤*Irritation:* To evaluate possible susceptibility to irritation, or sensitivity, each patient should begin by applying the medication to a small portion of unbroken skin at or near the pigmented area (approximately 1 cm^2) over a period of several days. If no irritation occurs within 24 hours, begin treatment. Minor redness is not necessarily a contraindication, but treatment should be discontinued if itching, excessive inflammation, or vesicle formation occurs. Use of hydroquinone products in paranasal and infraorbital areas increases the chance of irritation. If no improvement is seen after 2 months of treatment, use of this product should be discontinued.

➤*Sun exposure:* Sunscreen use is an essential aspect of hydroquinone therapy since even minimal sunlight exposure stimulates melanocyte activity. The sunscreens in some hydroquinone products provide the necessary sun protection during skin bleaching activity. During the depigmentation maintenance treatment subsequent to the intensive depigmentation therapy, sun exposure of the bleached skin should be avoided to prevent repigmentation.

➤*For external use only:* Avoid contact with eyes. In case of accidental contact, patient should rinse eyes thoroughly with water and contact physician. A bitter taste and antiseptic effect may occur if applied to the lips.

➤*Pregnancy: Category C.* Animal reproduction studies have not been conducted with topical hydroquinone. It is also not known whether hydroquinone can cause fetal harm when used topically on a pregnant woman or affect reproductive capacity. It is not known to what degree, if any, topical hydroquinone is absorbed systemically. Topical hydroquinone should be used in pregnant women only when clearly indicated. Consult with a physician if you are pregnant or intend to become pregnant within 3 months.

➤*Lactation:* It is not known whether topical hydroquinone is absorbed or excreted in human milk. Caution is advised when topical hydroquinone is used by a nursing mother.

➤*Children:* See Administration and Dosage for more information.

HYDROQUINONE — TOPICAL

Precautions

➤*Sensitivity:* This medication is for external use only. A mild, transient stinging may occur in people with sensitive skin. Do not use on broken or irritated skin. Discontinue use if irritation or rash occurs. Avoid contact with eyes and mucous membranes. In case of contact, rinse thoroughly with water.

Do not use near eyes. Use in paranasal and infraorbital areas increases the chance of irritation.

➤*Peroxide:* Concurrent use of peroxide may result in transient dark staining of skin areas due to oxidation of hydroquinone. Staining can be removed by discontinuing concurrent use and by normal soap cleansing.

➤*Sulfite sensitivity:* Some of these products may contain sodium metabisulfite, a sulfite that may cause serious allergic-type reactions (eg, hives, itching, wheezing, anaphylaxis, serious asthma attacks) in certain susceptible persons. Although the overall prevalence of sulfite sensitivity in the general population is probably low, it is seen more frequently in asthmatics or atopic nonasthmatics.

Adverse Reactions

No systemic adverse reactions have been reported. Occasional hypersensitivity (localized contact dermatitis) may occur, in which case the medication should be discontinued and the physician notified immediately.

Overdosage

There have been no systemic reactions from the use of topical hydroquinone. However, treatment should be limited to relatively small areas of the body at one time since some patients experience a transient skin reddening and a mild burning sensation which does not preclude treatment.

Patient Information

For external use only. Avoid contact with eyes.

Do not use on irritated, denuded or damaged skin.

Discontinue use and consult physician if rash or irritation develops.

MONOBENZONE

Rx	**Benoquin** (ICN)	**Cream:** 20%[a]	Cetyl alcohol, propylene glycol. In 35.4 g.

[a] In a water washable base.

MONOBENZONE — TOPICAL

Indications

➤*Idiopathic vitiligo:* For treatment of final depigmentation in extensive vitiligo.

Monobenzone is a potent depigmenting agent, not a mild cosmetic bleach. Do not use except for indication.

Administration and Dosage

Apply and rub into the pigmented areas to be treated 2 or 3 times/day. Depigmentation is usually observed after 1 to 4 months of therapy. If satisfactory results have not been obtained within 4 months, discontinue treatment. When the desired degree of depigmentation is obtained, apply only as often as needed to maintain (usually only 2 times/week).

➤*Storage / Stability:* Store at 25°C (77°F).

Actions

➤*Pharmacology:* Monobenzone is the monobenzyl ether of hydroquinone whose mechanism of action is not fully understood. The topical application of monobenzone increases the excretion of melanin from the melanocytes. Monobenzone may cause destruction of melanocytes and permanent depigmentation. This effect is erratic and may take 1 to 4 months to occur while existing melanin is lost with normal sloughing of the stratum corneum. Hyperpigmented skin appears to fade more rapidly than does normal skin and exposure to sunlight reduces the depigmenting effect of the drug. The histology of the skin after depigmentation with topical monobenzone is the same as that seen in vitiligo; the epidermis is normal except for the absence of identifiable melanocytes.

Contraindications

Freckling; hyperpigmentation because of photosensitization following use of certain perfumes or following inflammation of the skin; melasma (chloasma) of pregnancy; cafe-au-lait spots; pigmented nevi; malignant melanoma; pigment resulting from pigments other than melanin, including bile, silver, and artificial pigments; hypersensitivity to monobenzone or any ingredients of the product.

Warnings

➤*Skin sensitivity:* Following therapy with monobenzone, the skin will be sensitive for the rest of the patient's life. Use sunscreens during exposure.

➤*Discontinue use:* Discontinue use when irritation, a burning sensation, or dermatitis occur.

➤*For external use only:* Avoid contact with eyes, hair, and abraded skin.

➤*Pregnancy: Category C.* It is not known whether the drug can cause fetal harm when used topically on a pregnant woman. Use only when clearly needed.

➤*Lactation:* It is not known whether monobenzone is absorbed or excreted in breast milk. Use with caution in nursing mothers.

➤*Children:* Safety and efficacy in children younger than 12 years of age have not been established.

Adverse Reactions

➤*Dermatologic:* Mild, transient skin irritation and sensitization, including erythematous and eczematous reactions. Discontinue use if irritation, a burning sensation, or dermatitis occur. Areas of normal skin distant to the site of monobenzone application have frequently become depigmented. In addition, irregular, excessive, unsightly, and permanent depigmentation has frequently occurred.

Patient Information

Inform patient that depigmentation in areas of normal skin distant to the site of application may become irregular, excessive, unsightly, and frequently permanent.

Use sunscreens during sun exposure.

For external use only, avoid contact with the eyes and abraded skin.

Discontinue use and contact physician if irritation, a burning sensation, or dermatitis occurs.

PIGMENT AGENT COMBINATIONS

Rx	**Tri-Luma** (Galderma)	**Cream:** 0.01% fluocinolone acetonide, 4% hydroquinone, 0.05% tretinoin	Cetyl alcohol, glycerin, parabens, sodium metabisulfite, stearyl alcohol. In 30 g.
Rx	**Solage** (Galderma)	**Topical solution:** 2% mequinol, 0.01% tretinoin	Ethyl alcohol, EDTA. In 30 mL.

PIGMENT AGENT COMBINATIONS — TOPICAL

Indications

➤*Tri-Luma:* Short-term treatment of moderate to severe melasma of the face, in the presence of measures for sun avoidance, including the use of sunscreens.

➤*Solage:* Treatment of solar lentigines as an adjunct to a comprehensive skin care and sun avoidance program. Efficacy of daily use longer than 24 weeks has not been established.

Administration and Dosage

➤*Tri-Luma:* Apply once daily at night. Apply at least 30 minutes before bedtime. Gently wash the face and neck with a mild cleanser. Rinse and pat the skin dry. Apply a thin film of the cream to the hyperpigmented areas of melasma including about ½ inch of healthy-appearing skin surrounding each lesion. Rub lightly and uniformly into the skin. Do not use occlusive dressing. During the day, use a sunscreen of SPF 30 and wear protective clothing. Avoid sunlight exposure. Patients may use moisturizers and/or cosmetics during the day.

➤*Solage:* Apply to the solar lentigines using the applicator tip while avoiding application to the surrounding skin. Use twice daily, morning and evening, at least 8 hours apart. Patients should not shower or bathe the treatment area for at least 6 hours after application.

➤*Storage / Stability:* Store at controlled room temperature (20° to 25°C; 68° to 77°F).

Tri-Luma – Keep tightly closed. Protect from freezing.

Solage – Protect from light by continuing to store in the carton after opening.

Actions

➤*Pharmacology:*

Tri-Luma – One of the components is hydroquinone, a depigmenting agent, which may interrupt 1 or more steps in the tyrosine-tyrosinase pathway of melanin synthesis. However, the mechanism of action of the active ingredients in the treatment of melasma is unknown.

Solage – The mechanism of action of mequinol is unknown. Although mequinol is a substrate for the enzyme tyrosinase and acts as a competitive inhibitor of the formation of melanin precursors, the clinical significance of these findings is unknown. The mechanism of action of tretinoin as a depigmenting agent also is unknown.

➤*Pharmacokinetics:*

Tri-Luma – Percutaneous absorption of unchanged tretinoin, hydroquinone, and fluocinolone acetonide into the systemic circulation of 2 groups of healthy volunteers (n = 59) was found to be minimal following 8 weeks of daily application of 1 or 6 g.

PIGMENT AGENT COMBINATIONS — TOPICAL

Solage – The percutaneous absorption of tretinoin and the systemic exposure to tretinoin and mequinol were assessed in healthy subjects (n = 8) following 2 weeks of twice daily topical treatment with *Solage*. Approximately 0.8 mL was applied to a 400 cm^2 area of the back, corresponding to a dose of 37.3 mcg/cm^2 for mequinol and 0.23 mcg/cm^2 for tretinoin. The percutaneous absorption of tretinoin was approximately 4.4%, and systemic concentrations did not increase over endogenous levels. The mean C_{max} for mequinol was 9.92 ng/mL and the T_{max} was 2 hours.

Contraindications

Hypersensitivity, allergy or intolerance to the product or any of its components; pregnancy or use in women of childbearing potential (*Solage* only).

Warnings

➤*Ochronosis:* Hydroquinone (contained in *Tri Luma*) may produce exogenous ochronosis, a gradual blue-black darkening of the skin, whose occurrence should prompt discontinuation of therapy. The majority of patients developing this condition are black, but it may also occur in Caucasians and Hispanics.

➤*Eczema:* Tretinoin has been reported to cause severe irritation on eczematous skin and should be used only with utmost caution in patients with this condition.

➤*Irritation:*

Solage – *Solage* may cause skin irritation, erythema, burning, stinging or tingling, peeling, and pruritus. If the degree of such local irritation warrants, patients should be directed to use less medication, decrease the frequency of application, discontinue use temporarily, or discontinue use altogether.

Tri-Luma – *Tri-Luma* contains hydroquinone and tretinoin that may cause mild to moderate irritation. Local irritation such as skin reddening, peeling, mild burning sensation, dryness, and pruritus may be expected at the site of application. Transient skin reddening or mild burning sensation does not preclude treatment. If a reaction suggests hypersensitivity or chemical irritation, discontinue the medication.

➤*Vitiligo:* *Solage* should be used with caution by patients with a history or family history of vitiligo.

➤*Adrenal suppression:* *Tri-Luma* contains the corticosteroid fluocinolone acetonide. Systemic absorption of topical corticosteroids can produce reversible hypothalamic-pituitary-adrenal (HPA) axis suppression with the potential for glucocorticosteroid insufficiency after withdrawal of treatment. Manifestations of Cushing syndrome, hyperglycemia, and glucosuria can also be produced by systemic absorption of topical corticosteroid while on treatment. If HPA axis suppression is noted, the use of *Tri-Luma* should be discontinued. Recovery of HPA axis function generally occurs upon discontinuation of topical corticosteroids.

➤*Hypersensitivity reactions:* Cutaneous hypersensitivity to the active ingredients of *Tri-Luma* has been reported in the literature. In a patch test study to determine sensitization potential in 221 healthy volunteers, 3 volunteers developed sensitivity reactions to *Tri-Luma* or its components.

➤*Carcinogenesis:*

Tri-Luma: Studies of hydroquinone in animals have demonstrated some evidence of carcinogenicity. The carcinogenic potential of hydroquinone in humans is unknown. Studies in hairless albino mice suggest that concurrent exposure to tretinoin may enhance the tumorigenic potential of carcinogenic doses of UVB and UVA light from a solar simulator. Published studies have demonstrated that hydroquinone is a mutagen and a clastogen.

Solage: In a photocarcinogenicity study in mice administered *Solage*, median time to onset of tumors decreased.

➤*Pregnancy:* *Category C* (*Tri-Luma*), *Category X* (*Solage*).

Tri-Luma – *Tri-Luma* contains the teratogen tretinoin, which may cause embryofetal death, altered fetal growth, congenital malformations, and potential neurologic deficits. There are no adequate and well-controlled studies in pregnant women. *Tri-Luma* should be used during pregnancy only if the potential benefit justifies the potential risk to the fetus.

Solage – The combination of mequinol and tretinoin may cause fetal harm when administered to a pregnant woman. Due to the known effects of these active ingredients, *Solage* should not be used in women of childbearing potential. No adequate or well-controlled trials have been conducted with *Solage* in pregnant women.

➤*Lactation:* Corticosteroids (contained in *Tri-Luma*), when systemically administered, appear in human milk. It is not known if the other ingredients in *Tri-Luma* or *Solage* are excreted in human milk. Exercise caution when administering to a nursing woman.

➤*Children:* Safety and efficacy in pediatric patients have not been established. *Solage* should not be used on children.

Precautions

➤*Weather extremes:* Weather extremes such as wind or cold may be more irritating to patients using *Solage*.

➤*Photosensitivity:* *Solage* should not be administered if the patient is also taking drugs known to be photosensitizers (eg, thiazides, tetracyclines, fluoroquinolones, phenothiazines, sulfonamides) because of the possibility of augmented phototoxicity. Because of heightened burning susceptibility, exposure to sunlight (including sunlamps) to treated areas should be avoided or minimized. Patients must be advised to use protective clothing and comply with a comprehensive sun avoidance program. Patients with sunburn should be advised not to use *Solage* until fully recovered. Patients who may have considerable sun exposure because of their occupation and those patients with inherent sensitivity to sunlight should exercise particular caution.

➤*Sulfite sensitivity:* *Tri-Luma* contains sodium metabisulfite, which may cause allergic-type reactions, including anaphylactic symptoms and life-threatening/less severe asthmatic episodes in susceptible people. The overall prevalence in the general population is unknown and probably low. It is seen more frequently in asthmatic or atopic nonasthmatic people.

Drug Interactions

➤*Topical preparations:* Concomitant topical products with a strong skin drying effect, products with high concentrations of alcohol, astringents, spices or lime, medicated soaps or shampoos, permanent wave solutions, electrolysis, hair depilatories or waxes, or other preparations that might dry or irritate the skin should be used with caution in patients being treated with *Solage* because they may increase irritation.

➤*Photosensitizers:* Avoid drugs known to be photosensitizers (eg, thiazides, tetracyclines, fluoroquinolones, phenothiazines, sulfonamides) because of the possibility of augmented phototoxicity.

Adverse Reactions

➤*Tri-Luma:* The most frequently reported events were erythema, desquamation, burning, dryness, and pruritus at the site of application. The majority of these events were mild to moderate in severity.

Tri-Luma **Adverse Reactions (≥ 1% of Patients; n = 161)**	
Adverse reaction	Incidence
Erythema	41
Desquamation	38
Burning	18
Dryness	14
Pruritus	11
Acne	5
Paresthesia	3
Telangiectasia	3
Hyperesthesia	2
Pigmentary changes	2
Irritation	2
Papules	1
Acne-like rash	1
Rosacea	1
Dry mouth	1
Rash	1
Vesicles	1

The following local adverse reactions have been reported infrequently with topical corticosteroids. They may occur more frequently with the use of occlusive dressings, especially with higher potency corticosteroids. These reactions are listed in an approximate decreasing order of occurrence: Burning, itching, irritation, dryness, folliculitis, acneiform eruptions, hypopigmentation, perioral dermatitis, allergic contact dermatitis, secondary infection, skin atrophy, striae, miliaria.

Tri-Luma contains hydroquinone, which may produce exogenous ochronosis, a gradual blue-black darkening of the skin, whose occurrence should prompt discontinuation of therapy.

Cutaneous hypersensitivity to the active ingredients of *Tri-Luma* has been reported in the literature. In a patch test study to determine sensitization potential in 221 healthy volunteers, 3 volunteers developed sensitivity reactions to *Tri-Luma* or its components.

➤*Solage:* The most frequent adverse reactions were erythema (49%); burning, stinging, or tingling (26%); desquamation (14%); pruritus (12%); skin irritation (5%).

Some patients experienced temporary hypopigmentation of treated lesions (5%) or of the skin surrounding treated lesions (7%); 89% had resolution of hypopigmentation upon discontinuation of treatment to the lesion, and/or re-instruction on proper application to the lesion only. Another 8% of patients with hypopigmentation events had resolution within 120 days after the end of treatment, and 2.8% had persistence of hypopigmentation beyond 120 days. Approximately 6% of patients discontinued study participation with *Solage* because of adverse reactions. These discontinuations were due primarily to skin redness (erythema) or related cutaneous adverse reactions.

Solage **Adverse Events (> 1%)**	
Adverse event	Incidence
Erythema	44.6
Burning/Stinging/Tingling	21.9
Desquamation	12.6
Pruritus	11
Skin irritation	7.3
Halo hypopigmentation	6.2
Hypopigmentation	4.1
Dry skin	3.1
Rash	2.5
Crusting	2.4
Rash vesicular bullae	2.1
Dermatitis	2

PIGMENT AGENT COMBINATIONS — TOPICAL

Overdosage

If applied excessively, no more rapid or better results will be obtained and marked redness, peeling, discomfort, or hypopigmentation may occur. Oral ingestion of *Solage* may lead to the same adverse effects as those associated with excessive oral intake of vitamin A (hypervitaminosis A). If oral ingestion occurs, the patient should be monitored, and appropriate supportive measures administered as necessary. The maximal no-effect level for oral administration of *Solage* in rats was 5 mL/kg (30 mg/m^2). Clinical signs observed were attributed to the high alcohol content (77%) of the drug formulation.

Patient Information

Solage should not be used in women of childbearing potential or in pregnant women.

Exposure to sunlight, sunlamp, or UV light should be avoided. Patients who are consistently exposed to sunlight or skin irritants either through their work environment or habits should exercise particular caution. Sunscreen and protective covering (such as the use of a hat) over the treated areas should be used.

Sunscreen use is an essential aspect of melasma therapy, as even minimal sunlight sustains melanocytic activity.

Weather extremes such as heat or cold may be irritating to patients. Because of the drying effect of *Tri-Luma*, a moisturizer may be applied to the face in the morning after washing.

Application should be kept away from the eyes, nose, or angles of the mouth because the mucosa is much more sensitive than the skin to the irritant effect. If local irritation persists or becomes severe, application of the medication should be discontinued and the health care provider consulted. Allergic contact dermatitis, blistering, crusting, and severe burning or swelling of the skin, and irritation of the mucous membranes of the eyes, nose, and mouth require medical attention. If the medication is applied excessively, marked redness, peeling, or discomfort may occur.

POISON IVY PRODUCTS

POISON IVY TREATMENT PRODUCTS

otc	**Maximum Strength Ivarest** (Blistex)	**Cream:** 14% calamine and 2% diphenhydramine HCl[a]	Lanolin oil, petrolatum, propylene glycol. In 56 g.
otc	**Zanfel** (Zanfel Labs)	**Cream:** Polyethylene granules, nonoxynol-9, disodium EDTA, triethanolamine	In 30 g.
otc	**Calamine** (Various, eg, Goldline, Major, Moore)	**Lotion:** 6.97% calamine, 6.97% zinc oxide	Glycerin. In 118, 240, and 480 mL.
otc	**Phenolated Calamine** (Humco)	**Lotion:** Calamine, zinc oxide	Glycerin, 1% liquefied phenol. In 177 mL.
otc	**Caladryl** (Pfizer)	**Lotion:** 8% calamine, 1% pramoxine HCl	Alcohol, camphor, diazolidinyl urea, parabens. In 177 mL.
otc	**Ivy Super Dry** (Ivy Corp)	**Liquid:** 2% zinc acetate, 10% benzyl alcohol, 35% isopropanol, menthol, camphor	Glycerin, parabens. In 177 mL.
otc	**Ivy-Dry** (Ivy Corp)	**Lotion:** 2% zinc acetate, 12.5% isopropanol	Glycerin, methylparaben. In 118 mL.
otc	**Caladryl Clear** (Pfizer)	**Lotion:** 1% pramoxine HCl, 0.1% zinc acetate	Alcohol, camphor, diazolidinyl urea, parabens. In 177 mL.
otc	**Anti-Itch Gel** (Band-Aid)	**Gel:** 0.45% camphor	37% SD alcohol 23 A. In 60 g.
otc	**Itch Relief Gel Spritz** (Band-Aid)	**Spray:** 0.5% camphor	Benzyl alcohol, glycerin, SD alcohol 40 B (43%). In 56 g.
otc	**Ivy Soothe** (Enviroderm)	**Cream:** 1% hydrocortisone	Parabens, cetyl alcohol, glycerin, white petrolatum. In 28 g.
otc	**Zanfel** (Zanfel Labs)	**Wash:** Polyethylene granules, sodium lauroyl sarcosinate, nonoxynol-9, EDTA, triethanolamine	In 30 mL.

[a] Do not use with other products that contain diphenhydramine.

POISON IVY TREATMENT PRODUCTS — TOPICAL

For other products used for relief of symptoms associated with contact dermatoses, see also: Antihistamine-Containing Preparations, Topical; Local Anesthetics, Topical; Corticosteroids, Topical.

Indications

➤*Ivy, oak, sumac poisoning:* For the relief of itching, pain, and discomfort of ivy, oak, and sumac poisoning. Some products are also recommended for insect bites and other minor skin irritations.

Administration and Dosage

Please refer to individual product labeling for specific information. Apply to affected area 3 to 4 times daily as needed.

Shake calamine lotions well before using.

Active Ingredients

The principal active components of these products include:

➤*Antimicrobial:* Benzyl alcohol.

➤*Antiseptic:* Phenol, isopropyl alcohol, benzalkonium chloride, camphor, menthol, zinc oxide.

➤*Protectants/Astringents:* Calamine, zinc oxide.

➤*Local anesthetics/Analgesics:* Benzocaine, camphor, pramoxine, menthol, phenylcarbinol (benzyl alcohol), methyl salicylate.

➤*Antipruritics:* Benzyl alcohol, camphor.

➤*Antihistamines:* Diphenhydramine.

Precautions

➤*For external use only:* Do not use in the eyes. If the condition for which these preparations are used persists or recurs, or if rash, irritation or sensitivity develops, discontinue use and consult physician.

➤*Irritation:* Do not use on blistered or broken skin.

➤*Application considerations:* Do not use on large areas of the body.

➤*Children:* Most of these products are not recommended for use on children younger than 2 years of age.

Ivy Super Dry is not recommended for use in children younger than 6 years of age.

➤*Sulfite sensitivity:* Some of these products contain sulfites that may cause allergic-type reactions, including anaphylactic symptoms and life-threatening/less severe asthmatic episodes in susceptible persons. The overall prevalence in the general population is unknown and probably low. It is seen more frequently in asthmatic or atopic nonasthmatic persons.

POISON IVY PREVENTATIVES

otc	**Tecnu Outdoor Skin Cleanser** (Tec Labs)	**Lotion:** Deodorized mineral spirits, propylene glycol, octylphenoxypolyethoxyethanol, mixed fatty acid soap	In 118 and 355 mL.
otc	**Ivy Stat** (Tec Labs)	**Gel:** 1% hydrocortisone	Propylene glycol, menthol, SD alcohol 40-B. In 89 mL.
otc	**Ivy Block** (EnviroDerm)	**Lotion:** 5% bentoquatam	Benzyl alcohol, methylparaben, SDA 40 denatured alcohol. In 118 mL.
otc	**Ivy Cleanse** (EnviroDerm)	**Wipes:** Isopropyl and cetyl alcohol	In packet of 12 individually wrapped towelettes.

POISON IVY PREVENTATIVES — TOPICAL

Indications

➤*Poison ivy, oak, and sumac:* For the removal of the toxic oils that cause rash and itching of poison ivy, oak, and sumac from affected skin; and to stop the irritant from spreading.

Administration and Dosage

Please refer to individual product labeling for more specific information.

➤*Tecnu:* Use within the first few hours after exposure or as soon as the rash appears. Use before smoking, going to the bathroom, and at day's end to minimize spreading oils.

Before rash has started – Apply to exposed, dry skin within 2 to 8 hours after exposure to poison plant. Rub vigorously for 2 minutes to remove oils. If hypersensitive, wash entire body. Rinse skin clean with cool running water or wipe off with a cloth; repeat.

As soon as rash appears – Rub on affected skin and surrounding areas or to entire body for best results for 2 minutes. Avoid breaking skin. Rinse off with cool running water to remove cleanser and oils. If itching persists, reapply and rinse in a very warm shower (not a bath). Towel dry gently. Repeat as needed and before bedtime.

To clean clothing and equipment – Saturate contaminated, dry clothing. Let soak for several minutes. Launder clothing by itself as usual with detergent and hot water. Wipe off equipment and tools with a clean cloth saturated with the cleanser. Then wipe off or rinse with running water. Clean hands with cleanser after handling contaminated items.

➤*Ivy Block (6 years of age and older):* Shake well before use. Apply 15 minutes before risk of exposure. Avoid intentional contact with poison ivy, oak, and sumac. Remove with soap and water after risk of exposure. Apply every 4 hours for continued protection or sooner if needed.

➤*IvyStat (2 years of age and older):*

Step 1 – Cleanse affected skin with exfoliate. Rub gently for 15 to 30 seconds. Rinse off with running water and towel dry gently. Repeat as needed and before bedtime.

Step 2 – Apply 1% hydrocortisone gel and rub thoroughly into skin 3 to 4 times/day as needed. If itching recurs, repeat steps 1 and 2.

➤*Ivy Cleanse:* Immediately wipe exposed skin areas with towelette; discard. Avoid contaminating cleansed areas. Clean hands with fresh towelette.

Precautions

➤*Irritation:* Do not apply to deep puncture wounds, burns, or oozing areas of skin. May irritate sensitive skin.

➤*For external use only:* Do not use in eyes or near other mucous membranes.

➤*Hydrocortisone:* Do not use within 3 days of using hydrocortisone ointments on affected areas.

➤*Colorfastness:* May cause colorfastness when used on clothing. Check for colorfastness of fabric first by testing a corner of the fabric.

Adverse Reactions

➤*Dermatologic:* Rash; may irritate sensitive skin.

Patient Information

Advise patient to discontinue use and consult doctor if symptoms persist for more than 7 days or if redness, irritation, increased itching, or infection occurs.

Advise patient that this product is for external use only.

Advise patient to launder clothing and decontaminate exposed pets, tools, etc.

PYRIMIDINE ANTAGONIST, TOPICAL

FLUOROURACIL

Rx	**Carac** (Dermik)	**Cream:** 0.5%	Glycerin, parabens. In 30 g.
Rx	**Fluoroplex** (Allergan)	**Cream:** 1%	Benzyl alcohol, emulsifying wax, and mineral oil. In 30 g.
Rx	**Efudex** (ICN Pharmaceuticals)	**Cream:** 5%	Parabens in a white petrolatum base. In 25 and 40 g.
Rx	**Fluoroplex** (Allergan)	**Solution:** 1%	In 30 mL dropper bottle.
Rx	**Fluorouracil** (Taro)	**Solution:** 2%	In 10 mL.
Rx	**Efudex** (ICN Pharmaceuticals)		EDTA, and parabens. In 10 mL dropper bottle.
Rx	**Fluorouracil** (Taro)	**Solution:** 5%	In 10 mL.
Rx	**Efudex** (ICN Pharmaceuticals)		EDTA, and parabens. In 10 mL dropper bottle.

FLUOROURACIL — TOPICAL

For complete and comparative prescribing information, refer to the Fluorouracil and Floxuridine group monograph.

Indications

➤*Actinic/Solar keratoses:* For the topical treatment of multiple actinic or solar keratoses of the face and anterior scalp.

➤*Unlabeled uses:* A 1% solution of fluorouracil in 70% ethanol and the 5% cream have been used in the treatment of condylomata acuminata.

Administration and Dosage

➤*0.5% cream:* Fluorouracil cream should be applied once a day to the skin where actinic keratosis lesions appear, using enough to cover the entire area with a thin film. Fluorouracil cream should not be applied near the eyes, nostrils or mouth. Fluorouracil cream should be applied 10 minutes after thoroughly washing, rinsing, and drying the entire area. Fluorouracil cream may be applied using the fingertips. Immediately after application, the hands should be thoroughly washed. Fluorouracil should be applied up to 4 weeks as tolerated. Continued treatment up to 4 weeks results in greater lesion reduction. Local irritation is not markedly increased by extending treatment from 2 to 4 weeks, and is generally resolved within 2 weeks of cessation of treatment.

➤*1% cream or topical solution:* The patient should be instructed to apply sufficient medication to cover the entire face or other affected areas.

Apply medication twice daily with nonmetallic applicator or fingertips and wash hands afterwards. A treatment period of 2 to 6 weeks is usually required.

Increasing the frequency of application and a longer period of administration with fluorouracil cream or topical solution may be required on areas other than the head and neck.

When fluorouracil cream or topical solution is applied to keratotic skin, a response occurs with the following sequence: Erythema, usually followed by scaling, tenderness, erosion, ulceration, necrosis and re-epithelization. When the inflammatory reaction reaches the erosion, ulceration and necrosis stages, the use of the drug should be terminated. Responses may sometimes occur in areas which appear clinically normal. These may be sites of subclinical actinic (solar) keratosis which the medication is affecting.

The reaction to topical fluorouracil 1% cream or lotion may be unsightly in treated areas during therapy, and, in some cases, for several weeks following cessation of therapy.

➤*Storage/Stability:* Store ointment or 0.5% cream at controlled room temperature 20° to 25°C (68° to 77°F).

Store 1% cream and solution at 15° to 30°C (59° to 86°F).

Actions

➤*Pharmacology:* There is evidence that the metabolism of fluorouracil in the anabolic pathway blocks the methylation reaction of deoxyuridylic acid to thymidylic acid. In this manner, fluorouracil interferes with the synthesis of deoxyribonucleic acid (DNA) and to a lesser extent inhibits the formation of ribonucleic acid (RNA). Since DNA and RNA are essential for cell division and growth, the effect of fluorouracil may be to create a thymine deficiency that provokes unbalanced growth and death of the cell. The effects of DNA and RNA deprivation are most marked on those cells that grow more rapidly and take up fluorouracil at a more rapid rate. The contribution to efficacy or safety of individual components of the vehicle has not been established.

➤*Pharmacokinetics:* A multiple-dose, randomized, open-label, parallel study was performed in 21 patients with actinic keratoses. Twenty patients had pharmacokinetic samples collected: 10 patients treated with *Carac* and 10 treated with *Efudex* 5% cream. Patients were treated for a maximum of 28 days with *Carac*, 1 g once daily in the morning; or *Efudex* 5% cream, 1 g twice daily, in the morning and evening. Steady-state plasma concentrations and the amounts of fluorouracil in urine resulting from the topical application of either product were measured. Three patients who received *Carac* and 9 patients who received *Efudex* 5% cream had measurable plasma fluorouracil levels; however, only 1 patient receiving *Carac* and 6 patients receiving *Efudex* 5% cream had a sufficient number of data points to calculate mean pharmacokinetic parameters.

Plasma Pharmacokinetic Summary

PK parameter	*Carac* cream (n = 1)	*Efudex* (mean ± SD) (n = 6)
C_{max}	0.77 ng/mL	11.49 ± 8.24 ng/mL
t_{max}	1 hour	1.03 ± 0.028 hours
AUC (0-24)	2.8 ng•hr/mL	22.39 ± 7.89 ng•hr/mL

Five of 10 patients receiving *Carac* and 9 of 10 patients receiving *Efudex* 5% cream had measurable urine fluorouracil levels.

FLUOROURACIL — TOPICAL

Urine Pharmacokinetic Summary		
PK parameter	*Carac* (mean ± SD) (range) (n = 10)	*Efudex* (mean ± SD) (range) (n = 10)
Cum Ae*	2.74 ± 5.22 mcg (range: 0 to 15.02)	119.83 ± 94.8 mcg (range: 0 to 329.87)
Max excretion rate (min-max)	0.19 ± 0.52 mcg/hr (range: 0 to 1.67)	40.27 ± 47.14 mcg/hr (range: 0 to 164.5)

Both *Carac* and *Efudex* 5% cream demonstrated low measurable plasma concentrations for fluorouracil when administered under steady-state conditions. Cumulative urinary excretion of fluorouracil was low for *Carac* and for *Efudex*, corresponding to 0.055% and 0.24% of the applied doses, respectively.

Contraindications

Fluorouracil may cause fetal harm when administered to a pregnant woman. Fluorouracil is contraindicated in women who are or may become pregnant. If this drug is used during pregnancy, or if the patient becomes pregnant while taking this drug, the patient should be apprised of the potential hazard to the fetus.

No adequate and well-controlled studies have been conducted in pregnant women with either topical or parenteral forms of fluorouracil. One birth defect (ventricular septal defect) and cases of miscarriage have been reported when fluorouracil was applied to mucous membrane areas. Multiple birth defects have been reported in the fetus of a patient treated with intravenous fluorouracil.

Animal reproduction studies have not been conducted with fluorouracil. Fluorouracil, the active ingredient, has been shown to be teratogenic in mice, rats, and hamsters when administered parenterally at doses ≥ 10, 15 and 33 mg/kg/day, respectively, (4, 11 and 20 times, respectively, the maximum recommended human dose [MRHD] based on body surface area [BSA]). Fluorouracil was administered during the period of organogenesis for each species. Embryolethal effects occurred in monkeys at parenteral doses greater than 40 mg/kg/day (65 times the MRHD based on BSA) administered during the period of organogenesis.

Fluorouracil should not be used in patients with dihydropyrimidine dehydrogenase (DPD) enzyme deficiency. A large percentage of fluorouracil is catabolized by the enzyme dihydropyrimidine dehydrogenase (DPD). DPD enzyme deficiency can result in shunting of fluorouracil to the anabolic pathway, leading to cytotoxic activity and potential toxicities. Rarely, life-threatening toxicities such as stomatitis, diarrhea, neutropenia, and neurotoxicity have been reported with intravenous administration of fluorouracil in patients with DPD enzyme deficiency.

A case of life-threatening systemic toxicity has been reported with the topical use of fluorouracil 5% in a patient with DPD enzyme deficiency. Symptoms included severe abdominal pain, bloody diarrhea, vomiting, fever, and chills. Physical examination revealed stomatitis, erythematous skin rash, neutropenia, thrombocytopenia, inflammation of the esophagus, stomach, and small bowel. Although this case was observed with 5% fluorouracil cream, it is unknown whether patients with profound DPD enzyme deficiency would develop systemic toxicity with lower concentrations of topically applied fluorouracil.

Fluorouracil is contraindicated in patients with known hypersensitivity to any of its components.

Warnings

➤*DPD enzyme deficiency:* See Contraindications for more information.

➤*Mucous membranes:* Avoid applications to mucous membranes due to the possibility of local inflammation and ulceration.

➤*Occlusive dressing:* If an occlusive dressing is used, there may be an increase in the incidence of inflammatory reactions in the adjacent normal skin.

➤*Hypersensitivity reactions:* The potential for a delayed hypersensitivity reaction to fluorouracil exists. Patch testing to prove hypersensitivity may be inconclusive.

➤*Mutagenesis:* Studies with fluorouracil have shown positive effects in in vitro and in vivo tests for mutagenicity.

Fluorouracil produced morphological transformation of cells in in vitro cell transformation assays. Morphological transformation was also produced in an in vitro assay by a metabolite of fluorouracil, and the transformed cells produced malignant tumors when injected into immunosuppressed syngeneic mice. Fluorouracil has been shown to exert mutagenic activity in yeast cells, *Bacillus subtilis*, and Drosophila assays. In addition, fluorouracil has produced chromosome damage at concentrations of 1 and 2 mcg/mL in an in vitro hamster fibroblast assay, was positive in a microwell mouse lymphoma assay, and was positive in in vivo micronucleus assays in rats and mice following intraperitoneal administration. Some patients receiving cumulative doses of 0.24 to 1 g of fluorouracil parenterally have shown an increase in numerical and structural chromosome aberrations in peripheral blood lymphocytes.

➤*Fertility impairment:* Studies with fluorouracil have shown positive effects on impairment of fertility in in vivo animal studies.

Fluorouracil has been shown to impair fertility after parenteral administration in rats. Fluorouracil administered at intraperitoneal doses of 125 and 250 mg/kg has been shown to induce chromosomal aberrations and changes in chromosome organization of spermatogonia in rats. In mice, single-dose intravenous and intraperitoneal injections of fluorouracil have been reported to kill differentiated spermatogonia and spermatocytes at a dose of 500 mg/kg and produce abnormalities in spermatids at 50 mg/kg.

➤*Elderly:* No significant differences in safety and efficacy measures were demonstrated in patients older than 65 years of age compared to all other patients.

➤*Pregnancy: Category X.*

Teratogenic – See Contraindications.

➤*Lactation:* It is not known whether fluorouracil is excreted in human milk. Because many drugs are excreted in human milk and because of the potential for serious adverse reactions in nursing infants from fluorouracil, a decision should be made whether to discontinue nursing or to discontinue the drug, taking into account the importance of the drug to the mother.

➤*Children:* Actinic keratosis is not a condition seen within the pediatric population, except in association with rare genetic diseases. Fluorouracil should not be used in children. The safety and effectiveness of fluorouracil have not been established in patients younger than 18 years of age.

Precautions

➤*Ulcerated/Inflamed skin:* There is a possibility of increased absorption through ulcerated or inflamed skin.

➤*Lab test abnormalities:* To rule out the presence of a frank neoplasm, a biopsy may be considered for those areas failing to respond to treatment or recurring after treatment.

➤*Photosensitivity:* The patient should avoid prolonged exposure to sunlight or other forms of ultraviolet irradiation during treatment with fluorouracil, as the intensity of the reaction may be increased.

Adverse Reactions

The following were adverse reactions considered to be drug-related and occurring with a frequency of ≥ 1% with fluorouracil: Application site reaction (94.6%), and eye irritation (5.4%).

Summary of Facial Irritation Signs and Symptoms - Pooled Phase 3 Studies					
Adverse reaction	Active 1 week n = 85 (n %)	Active 2 week n = 87 (n %)	Active 4 week n = 85 (n %)	All active treatments n = 257 (n %)	Vehicle treatments n = 127 (n %)
Burning	51 (60%)	70 (80.5%)	71 (83.5%)	192 (74.7%)	28 (22%)
Dryness	59 (69.4%)	76 (87.4%)	79 (92.9%)	214 (83.3%)	60 (47.2%)
Edema	12 (14.1%)	28 (32.2%)	51 (60%)	91 (35.4%)	6 (4.7%)
Erosion	21 (24.7%)	38 (43.7%)	54 (63.5%)	113 (44%)	17 (13.4%)
Erythema	76 (89.4%)	82 (94.3%)	82 (96.5%)	240 (93.4%)	76 (59.8%)
Pain	26 (30.6%)	34 (39.1%)	52 (61.2%)	112 (43.6%)	7 (5.5%)

During clinical trials, irritation generally began on day 4 and persisted for the remainder of treatment. Severity of facial irritation at the last treatment visit was slightly below baseline for the vehicle group, mild to moderate for the 1 week active treatment group, and moderate for the 2- and 4-week active treatment groups. Mean severity declined rapidly for each active group after completion of treatment and was below baseline for each group at the week 2 posttreatment follow-up visit.

Thirty-one patients (12% of those treated with fluorouracil in the phase 3 clinical studies) discontinued study treatment early due to facial irritation. Except for 3 patients, discontinuation of treatment occurred on or after day 11 of treatment.

Eye irritation adverse events, described as mild to moderate in intensity, were characterized as burning, watering, sensitivity, stinging and itching. These adverse events occurred across all treatment arms in 1 of the 2 phase 3 studies.

Summary of All Adverse Reactions Reported in ≥ 1% of Patients in The Combined Active Treatment and Vehicle Groups - Pooled Phase 3 Studies 9721 and 9722 combined					
Adverse reaction	Active 1 week n = 85 (n %)	Active 2 week n = 87 (n %)	Active 4 week n = 85 (n %)	All active treatments n = 257 (n %)	Vehicle treatments n = 127 (n %)
Dermatologic	78 (91.8%)	83 (95.4%)	82 (96.5%)	243 (94.6%)	85 (66.9%)
Application site reaction	78 (91.8%)	83 (95.4%)	82 (96.5%)	243 (94.6%)	83 (65.4%)
Skin irritation	1 (1.2%)	0	2 (2.4%)	3 (1.2%)	0
Musculoskeletal	1 (1.2%)	1 (1.1%)	1 (1.2%)	3 (1.2%)	5 (3.9%)
Muscle soreness	0	0	0	0	2 (1.6%)

FLUOROURACIL — TOPICAL

Summary of All Adverse Reactions Reported in ≥ 1% of Patients in The Combined Active Treatment and Vehicle Groups - Pooled Phase 3 Studies 9721 and 9722 combined

Adverse reaction	Active 1 week n = 85 (n %)	Active 2 week n = 87 (n %)	Active 4 week n = 85 (n %)	All active treatments n = 257 (n %)	Vehicle treatments n = 127 (n %)
Ophthalmic	6 (7.1%)	4 (4.6%)	6 (7.1%)	16 (6.2%)	6 (4.7%)
Eye irritation	5 (5.9%)	3 (3.4%)	6 (7.1%)	14 (5.4%)	3 (2.4%)
Respiratory	5 (5.9%)	0	1 (1.2%)	6 (2.3%)	0 (4.7%)
Sinusitis	4 (4.7%)	0	0	4 (1.6%)	2 (1.6%)
Miscellaneous	7 (8.2%)	6 (6.9%)	12 (14.1%)	25 (9.7%)	15 (11.8%)
Headache	3 (3.5%)	2 (2.3%)	3 (3.5%)	8 (3.1%)	3 (2.4%)
Common cold	4 (4.7%)	0	2 (2.4%)	6 (2.3%)	3 (2.4%)
Allergy	0	2 (2.3%)	1 (1.2%)	3 (1.2%)	2 (1.6%)
Upper respiratory infection	0	0	0	0	2 (1.6%)

➤*Adverse experiences reported by body system:* In the phase 3 studies, no serious adverse event was considered related to study drug. A total of 5 patients, 3 in the active treatment groups and 2 in the vehicle group, experienced at least one serious adverse event. Three patients died as a result of adverse event(s) considered unrelated to study drug (stomach cancer, myocardial infarction and cardiac failure).

Posttreatment clinical laboratory tests other than pregnancy tests were not performed during the phase 3 clinical studies. Clinical laboratory tests were performed during conduct of a phase 2 study of 104 patients and 21 patients in a phase 1 study. No abnormal serum chemistry, hematology, or urinalysis results in these studies were considered clinically significant.

➤*1% cream and topical solution:* Pain, pruritus, burning, irritation, inflammation, allergic contact dermatitis and telangiectasia have been reported. Occasionally, hyperpigmentation and scarring have also been reported.

Overdosage

Ordinarily, topical overdosage will not cause acute problems. If fluorouracil is accidentally ingested, induce emesis and gastric lavage. Administer symptomatic and supportive care as needed. If contact is made with the eye, flush with copious amounts of water.

Patient Information

This medication is to be used as directed.

This medication should not be used for any disorder other than that for which it was prescribed.

It is for external use only.

Avoid contact with the eyes, eyelids, nostrils, and mouth.

Cleanse affected area and wait 10 minutes before applying fluorouracil.

Wash hands immediately after applying fluorouracil.

Avoid prolonged exposure to sunlight or other forms of ultraviolet irradiation during treatment, as the intensity of the reaction may be increased.

Most patients using fluorouracil get skin reactions where the medicine is used. These reactions include redness, dryness, burning, pain, erosion (loss of the upper layer of skin), and swelling. Irritation at the application site may persist for 2 or more weeks after therapy is discontinued. Treated areas may be unsightly during and after therapy.

If you develop abdominal pain, bloody diarrhea, vomiting, fever, or chills while on fluorouracil therapy, stop the medication and contact your physician and/or pharmacist.

Report any side effects to the physician and/or pharmacist.

PYRITHIONE ZINC

PYRITHIONE ZINC

otc	**Dermazinc** (Dermalogix)	**Shampoo:** 0.25%	Parabens. In 240 mL.
otc	**Zincon** (Medtech)	**Shampoo:** 1%	Propylene glycol. In 118 and 240 mL.
otc	**Head & Shoulders** (Procter & Gamble)		Cetyl and benzyl alcohol. In "normal to oily" and "normal to dry" formulas. In 200, 400, and 750 mL.
otc	**Head & Shoulders Dry Scalp** (Procter & Gamble)		Cetyl and benzyl alcohol. In regular and conditioning formulas. In 200, 400, 750, and 1000 mL.
otc	**DHS Zinc** (Person & Covey)	**Shampoo:** 2%	In 240 and 360 mL.
otc	**Denorex Everyday Dandruff** (Medtech)		Propylene glycol, menthol. In 118 and 240 mL.
otc	**ZNP Bar** (Stiefel)	**Soap:**[a] 2%	Cetostearyl alcohol. In 119 g.

[a] Also contains corn starch, glycerin, hydrogenated castor oil, and mineral oil.

PYRITHIONE ZINC — TOPICAL

Indications

➤*Hyperkeratotic skin conditions:* Pyrithione zinc products relieve the symptoms of itching, flaking, and inflammation caused by psoriasis, eczema, dandruff, lichen planus, seborrheic dermatitis, and other hyperkeratotic skin conditions of the face, body, and scalp. It also may help prevent recurrence of symptoms.

Administration and Dosage

➤*Shampoo:* Shake well. Apply shampoo; lather, rinse, and repeat. Use at least twice weekly for best results.

➤*Soap:* Use on affected areas in place of regular soap. Work up a rich lather using warm water and massage into affected areas; rinse well, then repeat. Use twice weekly for best results. May be used as a shampoo.

➤*Storage/Stability:* Store at room temperature, 20° to 25°C (68° to 77°F).

Actions

➤*Pharmacology:* Pyrithione zinc, a cytostatic agent, reduces cell turnover rate. Its action is thought to be due to a nonspecific toxicity for epidermal cells. The compound strongly binds to hair and external skin layers.

Warnings

➤*For external use only:* Keep out of eyes; if contact occurs, rinse thoroughly with water.

➤*Children:* Do not use on children younger than 2 years of age unless directed by a doctor.

Adverse Reactions

Irritation of the skin (rare).

Patient Information

For external use only.

Ask a doctor before use if you have a condition that covers a large area of the body.

When using this product, avoid contact with the eyes. If contact occurs, rinse eyes thoroughly with water.

Stop use and ask a doctor if:
- Condition worsens.
- Condition does not improve after regular use of this product as directed.

Keep out of the reach of children. If swallowed, get medical help or contact a poison control center right away.

RETINOIDS

ADAPALENE

Rx	**Differin** (Galderma)	**Cream:** 0.1%	EDTA, parabens, glycerin. In 45 g.
		Gel: 0.1%	EDTA, methyl paraben. In 45 g.

ADAPALENE — TOPICAL

Indications

➤*Acne vulgaris:* For the topical treatment of acne vulgaris.

Administration and Dosage

➤*Approved by the FDA:* May 31, 1996.

Apply once a day to affected areas after washing in the evening before retiring. A mild, transitory sensation of warmth or slight stinging may occur shortly after application.

A thin film should be applied, avoiding eyes, lips, and mucous membranes.

During the early weeks of therapy, an apparent exacerbation of acne may occur. This is due to the action of the medication on previously unseen lesions and should not be considered a reason to discontinue therapy. Therapeutic results should be noticed after 8 to 12 weeks of treatment.

➤*Storage/Stability:* Store at controlled room temperature 20° to 25°C (68° to 77°F). Protect from freezing.

Actions

➤*Pharmacology:* Adapalene is a chemically stable, retinoid-like compound.

Biochemical and pharmacological profile studies have demonstrated that adapalene is a modulator of cellular differentiation, keratinization, and inflammatory processes all of which represent important features in the pathology of acne vulgaris.

Mechanistically, adapalene binds to specific retinoic acid nuclear receptors but does not bind to the cytosolic receptor protein. Although the exact mode of action of adapalene is unknown, it is suggested that topical adapalene may normalize the differentiation of follicular epithelial cells resulting in decreased microcomedone formation.

➤*Pharmacokinetics:*

Absorption/Distribution – Absorption of adapalene through human skin is low.

Only trace amounts (less than 0.25 ng/mL) of parent substance have been found in the plasma of acne patients following chronic topical application of adapalene in controlled clinical trials.

Cream: In a pharmacokinetic study with 6 acne patients treated once daily for 5 days with 2 g of adapalene cream applied to 1000 cm^2 of acne-involved skin, there were no quantifiable amounts (limit of quantification = 1.35 ng/mL) of adapalene in the plasma samples from any patient.

Excretion – Excretion appears to be primarily by the biliary route.

Contraindications

Hypersensitivity to adapalene or any of the components in the vehicle.

Warnings

➤*Hypersensitivity reactions:* Use of adapalene should be discontinued if hypersensitivity to any of the ingredients is noted.

➤*Carcinogenesis:* Carcinogenicity studies with adapalene have been conducted in mice at topical doses of 0.3, 0.9, and 2.6 mg/kg/day and in rats at oral doses of 0.15, 0.5, and 1.5 mg/kg/day (≈ 4 to 75 times the maximal daily human topical dose). In the oral study, positive linear trends were observed in the incidence of follicular cell adenomas and carcinomas in the thyroid glands of female rats, and in the incidence of benign and malignant pheochromocytomas in the adrenal medullas of male rats.

No photocarcinogenicity studies were conducted. Animal studies have shown an increased risk of skin neoplasms with adapalene cream, tumorigenic risk with the use of pharmacologically similar drugs (eg, retinoids) when exposed to UV irradiation in the laboratory or to sunlight. Although the significance of these studies to human use is not clear, patients should be advised to avoid or minimize exposure to either sunlight or artificial UV irradiation sources.

Cream: Carcinogenicity studies with adapalene have been conducted in mice at topical doses of 0.4, 1.3, and 4 mg/kg/day, and in rats at oral doses of 0.15, 0.5, and 1.5 mg/kg/day. These doses are up to 8 times (mice) and 6 times (rats) (in terms of $mg/m^2/day$) the maximum potential exposure at the recommended topical human dose (MRHD), assumed to be 2.5 g adapalene cream, which is ≈ 1.5 mg/m^2 adapalene. In the oral study, increased incidence of benign and malignant pheochromocytomas in the adrenal medullas of male rats was observed.

➤*Pregnancy:* Category C.

Teratogenic – No teratogenic effects were seen in rats at oral doses of adapalene 0.15 to 5 mg/kg/day, up to 120 times the maximal daily human topical dose (for adapalene cream up to 20 times the MRHD based on mg/m^2 comparisons). However, adapalene administered orally at doses of ≥ 25 mg/kg, (100 times the MRHD for rats or 200 times MRHD for rabbits) has been shown to be teratogenic. Cutaneous route teratology studies conducted in rats and rabbits at doses of 0.6, 2, and 6 mg/kg/day, up to 150 times the maximal daily human topical dose; for adapalene cream, 24 times the MRHD for rats, or 48 times the MRHD for rabbits, exhibited no fetotoxicity and only minimal increases in supernumerary ribs in rats. There are no adequate and well-controlled studies in pregnant women. Adapalene should be used during pregnancy only if the potential benefit justifies the potential risk to the fetus.

➤*Lactation:* It is not known whether this drug is excreted in human milk. Because many drugs are excreted in human milk, caution should be exercised when adapalene is administered to a nursing woman.

➤*Children:* Safety and efficacy in pediatric patients below the age of 12 have not been established.

Precautions

➤*For external use only:* Avoid contact with the eyes, lips, angles of the nose, and mucous membranes. The product should not be applied to cuts, abrasions, eczematous skin, or sunburned skin.

As with other retinoids, use of "waxing" as a depilatory method should be avoided on skin treated with adapalene.

➤*Local adverse reactions:* Certain cutaneous signs and symptoms such as erythema, dryness, scaling, burning or pruritus may be experienced during treatment. These are most likely to occur during the first 2 to 4 weeks; with the cream they are mostly mild to moderate in intensity and will usually lessen with continued use of the medication. Depending upon the severity of adverse events, patients should be instructed to reduce the frequency of application or discontinue use.

➤*Photosensitivity:* Patients with sunburn should be advised not to use the product until fully recovered. If a reaction suggesting sensitivity or chemical irritation occurs, use of the medication should be discontinued. Exposure to sunlight, including sunlamps, should be minimized during the use of adapalene. Patients who normally experience high levels of sun exposure, and those with inherent sensitivity to sun, should be warned to exercise caution. Use of sunscreen products and protective clothing over treated areas is recommended when exposure cannot be avoided. Weather extremes, such as wind or cold, also may be irritating to patients under treatment with adapalene.

Drug Interactions

As adapalene has the potential to produce local irritation in some patients, concomitant use of other potentially irritating topical products (medicated or abrasive soaps and cleansers, soaps and cosmetics that have a strong drying effect, and products with high concentrations of alcohol, astringents, spices, or lime) should be approached with caution.

Particular caution should be exercised in using preparations containing sulfur, resorcinol, or salicylic acid in combination with adapalene. If these preparations have been used, it is advisable not to start therapy with adapalene until the effects of such preparations in the skin have subsided.

Adverse Reactions

➤*Gel:* Some adverse effects such as erythema, scaling, dryness, pruritus, and burning will occur in 10% to 40% of patients with adapalene gel. Pruritus or burning immediately after application also occurs in ≈ 20% of patients with adapalene gel. The following additional adverse experiences were reported in ≈ 1% or less of patients: Skin irritation, burning/stinging, erythema, sunburn, and acne flares. These are most commonly seen during the first month of therapy and decrease in frequency and severity thereafter. All adverse effects with use of adapalene during clinical trials were reversible upon discontinuation of therapy.

➤*Cream:* In controlled clinical trials, local cutaneous irritation was monitored in 285 acne patients who used adapalene cream once daily for 12 weeks. The frequency and severity of erythema, scaling, dryness, pruritis, and burning were assessed during these studies. The incidence of local cutaneous irritation with adapalene cream from the controlled clinical studies is provided in the following table.

Incidence of Local Cutaneous Irritation With Adapalene Cream From Controlled Clinical Studies (N = 285)				
	None	Mild	Moderate	Severe
Erythema	52% (148)	38% (108)	10% (28)	< 1% (1)
Scaling	58% (166)	35% (100)	6% (18)	< 1% (1)
Dryness	48% (136)	42% (121)	9% (26)	< 1 (2)
Pruritus (persistent)	74% (211)	21% (61)	4% (12)	< 1% (1)
Burning/ stinging	71% (202)	24% (69)	4% (12)	< 1% (2)

Other reported local cutaneous adverse events in patients who used adapalene cream once daily included: Sunburn (2%), skin discomfort-burning and stinging (1%), and skin irritation (1%). Events occurring in less than 1% of patients treated with adapalene cream included: Acne flare, dermatitis and contact dermatitis, eyelid edema, conjunctivitis, erythema, pruritus, skin discoloration, rash, and eczema.

Overdosage

Adapalene is intended for cutaneous use only. If the medication is applied excessively, no more rapid or better results will be obtained and marked redness, peeling, or discomfort may occur. The acute oral toxicity of adapalene in mice and rats is greater than 10 mL/kg. Chronic ingestion of the drug may lead to the same side effects as those associated with excessive oral intake of vitamin A.

Patient Information

This medication is to be used only as directed by the physician.

It is for external use only.

Avoid contact with the eyes, lips, angles of the nose, and mucous membranes.

Cleanse area with a mild or soapless cleanser before applying this medication.

Moisturizers may be used if necessary; however, products containing alpha hydroxy or glycolic acids should be avoided.

Exposure of the eye to this medication may result in reactions such as swelling, conjunctivitis, and eye irritation.

ADAPALENE — TOPICAL

This medication should not be applied to cuts, abrasions, eczematous or sunburned skin.

Wax epilation should not be performed on treated skin due to the potential for skin erosions.

During the early weeks of therapy, an apparent exacerbation of acne may occur. This is due to the action of this medication on previously unseen lesions and should not be considered a reason to discontinue therapy. Overall clinical benefit may be noticed after 2 weeks of therapy, but at least 8 weeks are required to obtain consistent beneficial effects.

First Generation Retinoids

TRETINOIN (trans-Retinoic Acid; Vitamin A Acid)

Rx	**Renova** (Ortho Dermatological)	**Cream:** 0.02%	Parabens, benzyl alcohol, cetyl alcohol, stearyl alcohol, EDTA. In 40 g.
Rx	**Tretinoin** (Alpharma, Spear Dermatology)	**Cream:** 0.025%	May contain stearyl alcohol. In 20 and 45 g.
Rx	**Altinac** (Upsher-Smith)		Stearyl alcohol. In 20 and 45 g.
Rx	**Avita** (Bertek)		Stearyl alcohol. In 20 and 45 g.
Rx	**Retin-A** (Ortho)		Hydrophilic vehicle. In 20 and 45 g.
Rx	**Tretinoin** (Spear Dermatology)	**Cream:** 0.05%	Stearyl alcohol. In 20 and 45 g.
Rx	**Altinac** (Upsher-Smith)		Stearyl alcohol. In 20 and 45 g.
Rx	**Renova** (Ortho Dermatological)		Methylparaben, stearyl alcohol, EDTA. In 20, 40, and 60 g.
Rx	**Retin-A** (Ortho)		Hydrophilic vehicle. In 20 and 45 g.
Rx	**Tretinoin** (Spear Dermatology)	**Cream:** 0.1%	Stearyl alcohol. In 20 and 45 g.
Rx	**Altinac** (Upsher-Smith)		Stearyl alcohol. In 20 and 45 g.
Rx	**Retin-A** (Ortho)		Stearyl alcohol. In 20 and 45 g.
Rx	**Tretinoin** (Spear Dermatology)	**Gel:** 0.01%	Alcohol. In 15 and 45 g.
Rx	**Retin-A** (Ortho)		90% alcohol. In 15 and 45 g.
Rx	**Tretinoin** (Spear Dermatology)	**Gel:** 0.025%	Alcohol. In 15 and 45 g.
Rx	**Avita** (Bertek)		83% ethanol. In 20 and 45 g.
Rx	**Retin-A** (Ortho)		90% alcohol. In 15 and 45 g.
Rx	**Retin-A Micro** (Ortho)	**Gel:** 0.04%	Glycerin, EDTA, propylene glycol, benzyl alcohol. In 20 and 45 g.
Rx	**Retin-A Micro** (Ortho)	**Gel:** 0.1%	Glycerin, EDTA, propylene glycol, benzyl alcohol. In 20 and 45 g.
Rx	**Retin-A** (Ortho)	**Liquid:** 0.05%	55% alcohol. In 28 mL.

TRETINOIN — TOPICAL

Indications

➤*Acne (except Renova):* Topical treatment of acne vulgaris.

➤*Renova:*

Dermatologic conditions –

0.02% cream: Adjunctive agent for use in the mitigation (palliation) of fine wrinkles in patients who use comprehensive skin care and sun avoidance programs.

0.05% cream: Adjunctive agent for use in the mitigation (palliation) of fine wrinkles, mottled hyperpigmentation, and tactile roughness of facial skin in patients who do not achieve such palliation using comprehensive skin care and sun avoidance programs alone.

➤*Unlabeled uses:* Treatment of hyperpigmentation of photoaged skin, postinflammatory, hyperpigmentation, melasma, and facial actinic keratoses.

Administration and Dosage

➤*Acne treatment:* Apply once a day before bedtime or in the evening . Cover the entire affected area lightly.

Closely monitor alterations of vehicle, drug concentration, or dose frequency. During the early weeks of therapy, an apparent exacerbation of inflammatory lesions may occur due to the action of the medication on deep, previously undetected lesions; this is not a reason to discontinue therapy.

Therapeutic results should be seen after 2 to 3 weeks, but may not be optimal until after 6 weeks. Once lesions have responded satisfactorily, maintain therapy with less frequent applications or other dosage forms.

Patients may use cosmetics, but thoroughly cleanse area to be treated before applying medication.

➤*Liquid:* Apply with fingertip, gauze pad, or cotton swab. Do not oversaturate gauze or cotton to the extent that liquid will run into unaffected areas.

➤*Gel:* Excessive application results in "pilling" of the gel, which minimizes the likelihood of overapplication by the patient.

➤*Renova:* Gently wash face with a mild soap, pat the skin dry, and wait 20 to 30 minutes before applying. Apply tretinoin to the face once a day in the evening, using only enough to cover the entire affected area lightly. Apply a pea-sized amount of cream to cover the entire face. Take caution to avoid contact with eyes, ears, nostrils, and mouth.

For best results, do not apply another skin care product or cosmetic for at least 1 hour after applying tretinoin.

Do not wash face for at least 1 hour after applying tretinoin.

Application of tretinoin may cause a transitory feeling of warmth or slight stinging.

Mitigation (palliation) of fine facial wrinkling, mottled hyperpigmentation, and tactile roughness may occur gradually over the course of therapy. Up to 6 months of therapy may be required before the effects are seen. Most of the improvement noted with tretinoin is seen during the first 24 weeks of therapy. Thereafter, therapy primarily maintains the improvement noticed during the first 24 weeks.

Patients treated with tretinoin may use cosmetics, but the areas to be treated should be cleansed thoroughly before the medication is applied.

➤*Storage/Stability:* Store between 15° to 25°C (59° to 77°F).

Actions

➤*Pharmacology:* Tretinoin is a retinoid metabolite of vitamin A. Although the exact mode of action of tretinoin is unknown, current evidence suggests that topical tretinoin decreases cohesiveness of follicular epithelial cells with decreased microcomedo formation. Additionally, tretinoin stimulates mitotic activity and increases turnover of follicular epithelial cells, causing extrusion of the comedones.

➤*Pharmacokinetics:*

Absorption – The transdermal absorption of tretinoin from various topical formulations ranged from 1% to 31% of applied dose, depending on whether it was applied to healthy or dermatitic skin. In vitro and in vivo pharmacokinetic studies with tretinoin cream and gel indicated that less than 0.3% of the topically applied dose is bioavailable. Circulating plasma levels of tretinoin are only slightly elevated above those found in healthy normal controls. Estimates of in vivo bioavailability of *Retin-A Micro* following single and multiple daily applications, for a period of 28 days with the 0.1% gel, were approximately 0.82% and 1.41%, respectively. When percutaneous absorption of *Renova* was assessed in healthy male subjects (n = 14) after a single application, as well as after repeated daily applications for 28 days, the absorption of tretinoin was less than 2% and endogenous concentrations of tretinoin and its major metabolites were unaltered.

Contraindications

Hypersensitivity to any component of the product; discontinue if hypersensitivity to any ingredient is noted.

Warnings

➤*For external use only:* Keep tretinoin away from the eyes, mouth, angles of the nose, and mucous membranes.

➤*Renova:*

Mitigating effects – Tretinoin has shown no mitigating effects on significant signs of chronic sun exposure (eg, coarse or deep wrinkling, skin yellowing, lentigines, telangiectasia, skin laxity, keratinocytic atypia, melanocytic atypia, dermal elastosis).

Tretinoin 0.02% cream has shown no mitigating effects on tactile roughness or mottled hyperpigmentation.

Tretinoin does not eliminate wrinkles, repair sun damaged skin, reverse photoaging, or restore a more youthful or younger dermal histologic pattern.

Many patients achieve desired palliative effect on fine wrinkling, mottled hyperpigmentation, and tactile roughness of facial skin with the use of comprehensive skin care and sun avoidance programs including sunscreens, protective clothing, and nonprescription emollient creams.

Long-term use – Tretinoin is a dermal irritant, and the results of continued irritation of the skin for greater than 48 weeks are not known. There is

TRETINOIN — TOPICAL

evidence of atypical changes in melanocytes and keratinocytes and of increased dermal elastosis in some patients treated with tretinoin 0.05% for longer than 52 weeks.

➤*Pregnancy:* *Category C.* Oral tretinoin is teratogenic. There are no adequate and well-controlled studies in pregnant women. Use during pregnancy only if the potential benefit justifies the potential risk. Do not use *Renova* and *Avita* during pregnancy.

Topical tretinoin in animal teratogenicity tests has generated equivocal results. There is evidence of teratogenicity (shortened or kinked tail) of topical tretinoin in Wistar rats at doses greater than 1 mg/kg/day (200 times the recommended human topical clinical dose) Anomalies (humerus: short 13%, bent 6%; os parietal incompletely ossified 14%) also have been reported in rats when 10 mg/kg/day was dermally applied.

There are other reports in New Zealand White rabbits with doses of approximately 80 times the recommended human topical clinical dose of an increased incidence of domed head and hydrocephaly, typical of retinoid-induced fetal malformations in this species

In contrast, several well-controlled animal studies have shown that dermally applied tretinoin was not teratogenic at doses of 100 and 200 times the recommended human topical clinical dose in rats and rabbits, respectively.

Dermal tretinoin has been shown to be fetotoxic in rabbits when administered in doses 100 times the recommended topical human clinical dose.

Thirty cases of temporally associated congenital malformations have been reported during 2 decades of clinical use of another formulation of topical tretinoin (acne preparation). Although no definite pattern of teratogenicity and no causal association has been established from these cases, 5 of the reports describe the rare birth defect category holoprosencephaly (defects associated with incomplete midline development of the forebrain). The significance of these spontaneous reports in terms of risk to the fetus is unknown.

➤*Lactation:* It is not known whether this drug is excreted in breast milk. Exercise caution when tretinoin is administered to a nursing mother.

➤*Children:*

Renova – Safety and efficacy in patients less than 18 years of age have not been established.

Precautions

➤*Irritation:* Tretinoin may induce severe local erythema, pruritus, burning, stinging, and peeling at the application site. If the degree of local irritation warrants, use medication less frequently or discontinue use temporarily or completely. Tretinoin may cause severe irritation to eczematous skin; use with caution in patients with this condition.

➤*Photosensitivity:* It is advisable to "rest" a patient's skin until effects of keratolytic agents subside before beginning tretinoin. Minimize exposure to sunlight and sunlamps, and advise patients with sunburn not to use tretinoin until fully recovered because of heightened susceptibility to sunlight as a result of tretinoin use. Patients who undergo considerable sun exposure due to occupation and those with inherent sun sensitivity should exercise particular caution. Use sunscreen products and wear protective clothing over treated areas. Weather extremes, such as wind and cold, also may irritate treated areas.

Drug Interactions

➤*Sulfur, resorcinol, benzoyl peroxide, or salicylic acid:* Cautiously use concomitant topical medications because of possible interactions with tretinoin. Significant skin irritation may result. It also is advisable to "rest" a patient's skin until the effects of such preparations subside before use of tretinoin is begun.

➤*Topical preparations:* Cautiously use medicated or abrasive soaps and cleansers, soaps and cosmetics that have a strong drying effect, and products with high concentrations of alcohol, astringents, spices, or lime, permanent wave solutions, electrolysis, hair depilatories or waxes, and products that may irritate the skin in patients being treated with tretinoin because they may increase irritation.

➤*Photosensitizers:* Do not use tretinoin if the patient also is taking drugs known to be photosensitizers (eg, thiazides, tetracyclines, fluoroquinolones, phenothiazines, sulfonamides) because of the possibility of augmented phototoxicity.

Adverse Reactions

Almost all patients reported 1 or more local reactions such as peeling, dry skin, burning, stinging, erythema, and pruritus during therapy with tretinoin.

Sensitive skin may become excessively red, edematous, blistered, or crusted. If these effects occur, discontinue medication until skin integrity is restored or adjust to a tolerable level. True contact allergy is rare.

Temporary hyperpigmentation or hypopigmentation has been reported with repeated application. Some individuals have a heightened susceptibility to sunlight while under treatment.

All adverse effects have been reversible upon discontinuation.

Overdosage

➤*Symptoms:* Application of larger amounts of medication than recommended has not been shown to lead to more rapid or better results, and marked redness, peeling, or discomfort may occur. Oral ingestion of the drug may lead to the same side effects as those associated with excessive oral intake of vitamin A.

Patient Information

➤*Renova*: Apply only as an adjunct to a comprehensive skin care and sun avoidance program. Apply a moisturizing sunscreen with a minimum SPF of 15 every morning when being treated with tretinoin. Avoid direct sun exposure as much as possible and totally avoid sunlamps while using tretinoin. Do not use if sunburned or if eczema or other chronic skin conditions exist. Do not use if inherently sensitive to sunlight or if also taking other drugs that increase sensitivity to sunlight.

Do not use if pregnant, attempting to become pregnant, or at high risk of pregnancy.

A majority of patients will lose most mitigating effects on fine wrinkles, mottled hyperpigmentation, and tactile roughness of facial skin with discontinuation of a comprehensive skin care and sun avoidance program including tretinoin; however, the safety and efficacy of tretinoin daily use for greater than 48 weeks have not been established.

ISOTRETINOIN (13-cis-Retinoic Acid)

Rx	**Accutane** (Roche)	**Capsules:**[a] 10 mg	(ACCUTANE 10 ROCHE). Light pink. In UD 10s.
		20 mg	(ACCUTANE 20 ROCHE). Maroon. In UD 10s.
		40 mg	(ACCUTANE 40 ROCHE). Yellow. In UD 10s.
Rx	**Amnesteem** (Bertek)	**Capsules:** 10 mg	(I10). Reddish brown. In 30s and 100s.
Rx	**Claravis** (Barr Laboratories)		(BARR 934). Lt. gray. In blister pack 30s and 100s.
Rx	**Amnesteem** (Bertek)	**Capsules:** 20 mg	(I20). Reddish brown and cream. In 30s and 100s.
Rx	**Claravis** (Barr Laboratories)		(BARR 935). Brown-orange. In blister pack 30s and 100s.
Rx	**Amnesteem** (Bertek)	**Capsules:** 40 mg	(I40). Orange brown. In 30s and 100s.
Rx	**Claravis** (Barr Laboratories)		(BARR 936). Lt. orange. In blister pack 30s and 100s.
Rx	**Sotret** (Ranbaxy)	**Capsules, soft gel:** 10 mg	(5R). Parabens. Lt. Pink. In 30s and 100s.
		20 mg	(6R). Parabens. Maroon. In 30s and 100s.
		30 mg	(8R). Parabens. Golden yellow. In 30s and 100s.
		40 mg	(7R). Parabens. Yellow. In 30s and 100s.

[a] Capsule contains suspension of drug in soybean oil; also contains parabens and EDTA.

ISOTRETINOIN — ORAL

WARNING

Isotretinoin must not be used by females who are pregnant or who may become pregnant while undergoing treatment. Although not every fetus exposed to isotretinoin has resulted in a deformed child, there is an extremely high risk that a deformed infant can result if pregnancy occurs while taking isotretinoin in any amount even for short periods of time. Potentially, any fetus exposed during pregnancy can be affected. Presently, there is no accurate means of determining, after isotretinoin exposure, which fetus has been affected and which fetus has not been affected.

Major human fetal abnormalities related to isotretinoin administration have been documented. There is an increased risk of spontaneous abortion. In addition, premature births have been reported.

Documented external abnormalities – Skull abnormality; ear abnormalities (including anotia, micropinna, small or absent external auditory canals); eye abnormalities (including microphthalmia); facial dymorphia; cleft palate.

Documented internal abnormalities – CNS abnormalities (including cerebral abnormalities, cerebellar malformation, hydrocephalus, microcephaly, cranial nerve deficit); cardiovascular abnormalities; thymus gland abnormality; parathyroid hormone deficiency. In some cases, death has occurred with certain of the abnormalities previously noted.

Cases of IQ scores less than 85 with or without obvious CNS abnormalities have also been reported.

Isotretinoin is contraindicated in females of childbearing potential unless the patient meets all of the following conditions:

- Must not be pregnant or breastfeeding.
- Must be capable of complying with the mandatory contraceptive measures required for isotretinoin therapy and understand behaviors associated with an increased risk of pregnancy.
- Must be reliable in understanding and carrying out instructions.

Accutane from Roche Pharmaceuticals must be prescribed under the System to Manage *Accutane* Related Teratogenicity (SMART). Similar programs from different manufacturers include: Isotretinoin Medication Program: Alerting you to the Risks of Teratogenicity (IMPART) for *Sotret* from Ranbaxy Pharmaceuticals; the System to Prevent Isotretinoin-Related Issues of Teratogenicity (SPIRIT) for *Amnesteem* from Bertek Pharmaceuticals; and the Adverse Event Learning & Education Regarding Teratogenicity (ALERT) for *Claravis* from Barr Laboratories.

To prescribe isotretinoin, the prescriber must obtain a supply of yellow self-adhesive isotretinoin qualification stickers. To obtain these stickers:

1.) Read the booklet entitled System to Manage *Accutane*-Related Teratogenicity (SMART) Guide to Best Practices. Similar booklets from different manufacturers include: Isotretinoin Medication Program: Alerting you to the Risks of Teratogenicity (IMPART) for *Sotret* from Ranbaxy Pharmaceuticals; the System to Prevent Isotretinoin-Related Issues of Teratogenicity (SPIRIT) for *Amnesteem* from Bertek Pharmaceuticals; and The Adverse Event Learning & Education Regarding Teratogenicity (ALERT) for *Claravis* from Barr Laboratories.
2.) Sign and return the completed SMART for *Accutane* letter of understanding. Similar letters from different manufacturers include: IMPART for *Sotret* from Ranbaxy Pharmaceuticals; SPIRIT for *Amnesteem* from Bertek Pharmaceuticals; and ALERT for *Claravis* from Barr Laboratories containing the following prescriber checklist:

- I know the risk and severity of fetal injury/birth defects from isotretinoin.
- I know how to diagnose and treat the various presentations of acne.
- I know the risk factors for unplanned pregnancy and the effective measures for avoidance of unplanned pregnancy.
- It is the informed patient's responsibility to avoid pregnancy during isotretinoin therapy and for 1 month after stopping isotretinoin. To help patients have the knowledge and tools to do so: Before beginning treatment of female patients with isotretinoin I will refer for expert, detailed pregnancy prevention counseling and prescribing, reimbursed by the manufacturer, or I have the expertise to perform this function and elect to do so.
- I understand, and will properly use throughout the isotretinoin treatment course, the SMART for *Accutane* procedures for isotretinoin, including monthly pregnancy avoidance counseling, pregnancy testing and use of the yellow self-adhesive isotretinoin qualification stickers. Similar programs from different manufacturers include IMPART for *Sotret* from Ranbaxy Pharmaceuticals, SPIRIT for *Amnesteem* from Bertek Pharmaceuticals, and ALERT for *Claravis* from Barr Laboratories.

3.) To use the yellow self-adhesive isotretinoin qualification sticker: Isotretinoin should not be prescribed or dispensed to any patient (male or female) without a yellow self-adhesive isotretinoin qualification sticker.

WARNING (cont.)

For female patients, the yellow self-adhesive isotretinoin qualification sticker signifies that she:

- Must have had 2 negative urine or serum pregnancy tests with a sensitivity of at least 25 milliunit/mL before receiving the initial isotretinoin prescription. The first test (a screening test) is obtained by the prescriber when the decision is made to pursue qualification of the patient for isotretinoin. The second pregnancy test (a confirmation test) should be done during the first 5 days of the menstrual period immediately preceding the beginning of isotretinoin therapy. For patients with amenorrhea, the second test should be done at least 11 days after the last act of unprotected sexual intercourse (without using 2 effective forms of contraception). Each month of therapy, the patient must have a negative result from a urine or serum pregnancy test. A pregnancy test must be repeated every month prior to the female patient receiving each prescription.
- Must have selected and have committed to use 2 forms of effective contraception simultaneously, at least 1 of which must be a primary form, unless absolute abstinence is the chosen method, or the patient has undergone a hysterectomy. Patients must use 2 forms of effective contraception for at least 1 month prior to initiation of isotretinoin therapy, during isotretinoin therapy, and for 1 month after discontinuing isotretinoin therapy. Counseling about contraception and behaviors associated with an increased risk of pregnancy must be repeated on a monthly basis.

Effective forms of contraception include both primary and secondary forms of contraception. Primary forms of contraception include the following: Tubal ligation, partner's vasectomy, intrauterine devices, birth control pills, and topical/injectable/implantable/insertable hormonal birth control products. Secondary forms of contraception include diaphragms, latex condoms, and cervical caps; each must be used with a spermicide.

Any birth control method can fail. Therefore, it is critically important that women of childbearing potential use 2 effective forms of contraception simultaneously. A drug interaction that decreases effectiveness of hormonal contraceptives has not been entirely ruled out for isotretinoin. Although hormonal contraceptives are highly effective, there have been reports of pregnancy from women who have used oral contraceptives, as well as topical/injectable/implantable/insertable hormonal birth control products. These reports occurred while these patients were taking isotretinoin. These reports are more frequent for women who use only a single method of contraception. Patients must receive written warnings about the rates of possible contraception failure (included in patient education kits).

Prescribers are advised to consult the monograph of any medication administered concomitantly with hormonal contraceptives, since some medications may decrease the effectiveness of these birth control products. Patients should be prospectively cautioned not to self-medicate with the herbal supplement St. John's wort because a possible interaction has been suggested with hormonal contraceptives based on reports of breakthrough bleeding on oral contraceptives shortly after starting St. John's wort. Pregnancies have been reported by users of combined hormonal contraceptives who also used some form of St. John's wort.

- Must have signed a patient information/consent form that contains warnings about the risk of potential birth defects if the fetus is exposed to isotretinoin.
- Must have been informed of the purpose and importance of participating in the isotretinoin survey and have been given the opportunity to enroll.

The yellow self-adhesive isotretinoin qualification sticker documents that the female patient is qualified, and includes the date of qualification, patient gender, cut-off date for filling the prescription, and up to a 30-day supply limit with no refills.

These yellow self-adhesive isotretinoin qualification stickers should also be used for male patients.

If a pregnancy does occur during treatment of a woman with isotretinoin, the prescriber and patient should discuss the desirability of continuing the pregnancy. Prescribers are strongly encouraged to report all cases of pregnancy to the manufacturer's program specialist who will be available to discuss pregnancy information, or prescribers may contact the Food and Drug Administration MedWatch Program at 1-800-FDA-1088.

Isotretinoin should be prescribed only by prescribers who have demonstrated special competence in the diagnosis and treatment of severe recalcitrant nodular acne, are experienced in the use of systemic retinoids, have read the SMART for *Accutane* Guide to Best Practices. Similar guides from different manufacturers include: IMPART for *Sotret* from Ranbaxy Pharmaceuticals, SPIRIT for *Amnesteem* from Bertek Pharmaceuticals, and ALERT for *Claravis* from Barr Laboratories. A signed letter of understanding should be returned and completed for SMART for *Accutane*. Similar letters from different manufacturers include: IMPART for *Sotret* from Ranbaxy Pharmaceuticals, SPIRIT for *Amnesteem* from Bertek Pharmaceuticals, and ALERT for *Claravis* from Barr Laboratories, yellow self-adhesive isotretinoin qualification stickers obtained. Isotretinoin should not be prescribed or dispensed without a yellow self-adhesive isotretinoin qualification sticker.

ISOTRETINOIN — ORAL

WARNING (cont.)

Information for pharmacists – Isotretinoin must only be dispensed:
- In no more than a 30-day supply.
- Only on presentation of an isotretinoin prescription with a yellow self-adhesive isotretinoin qualification sticker.
- Within 7 days of the qualification date.
- Refills require a new prescription with a yellow self-adhesive isotretinoin qualification sticker.
- No telephone or computerized prescriptions are permitted.

An isotretinoin medication guide must be given to the patient each time isotretinoin is dispensed, as required by law. This isotretinoin medication guide is an important part of the risk-management program for the patient.

Indications

➤*Severe recalcitrant nodular acne:* For the treatment of severe recalcitrant nodular acne. Nodules are inflammatory lesions with a diameter of greater than or equal to 5 mm. The nodules may become suppurative or hemorrhagic. "Severe," by definition, means "many" as opposed to "few or several" nodules. Because of significant adverse effects associated with its use, isotretinoin should be reserved for patients with severe nodular acne who are unresponsive to conventional therapy, including systemic antibiotics. In addition, isotretinoin is indicated only for those females who are not pregnant, because isotretinoin can cause severe birth defects (see the Warning box for more information).

A single course of therapy for 15 to 20 weeks has been shown to result in complete and prolonged remission of disease in many patients. If a second course of therapy is needed, it should not be initiated until at least 8 weeks after completion of the first course, because experience has shown that patients may continue to improve while off isotretinoin. The optimal interval before retreatment has not been defined for patients who have not completed skeletal growth. Decreased bone mineral density and premature epiphyseal closure have been reported in pediatric patients taking isotretinoin.

➤*Unlabeled uses:* Derivatives of vitamin A, the retinoids, have reported activity in treating specific premalignant lesions and reducing incidence of second primary tumors in patients with prior head and neck, lung, or liver cancers.

Administration and Dosage

➤*Approved by the FDA:* May 7, 1982.

Isotretinoin should be administered with a meal.

The recommended dosage range for isotretinoin is 0.5 to 1 mg/kg given in 2 divided doses with food daily for 15 to 20 weeks. In studies comparing 0.1, 0.5, and 1 mg/kg/day, it was found that all dosages provided initial clearing of disease, but there was a greater need for retreatment with the lower dosages. During treatment, the dose may be adjusted according to response of the disease or the appearance of clinical side effects—some of which may be dose related. Adult patients whose disease is very severe with scarring or is primarily manifested on the trunk may require dose adjustments up to 2 mg/kg/day, as tolerated. Failure to take isotretinoin with food will significantly decrease absorption. Before upward dose adjustments are made, the patients should be questioned about their compliance with food instructions.

The safety of once-daily dosing with isotretinoin has not been established. Once-daily dosing is not recommended.

If the total nodule count has been reduced by more than 70% prior to completing 15 to 20 weeks of treatment, the drug may be discontinued. After a period of 2 months or more off therapy, and if warranted by persistent or recurring severe nodular acne, a second course of therapy may be initiated. The optimal interval before retreatment has not been defined for patients who have not completed skeletal growth. Long-term use of isotretinoin, even in low doses, has not been studied, and is not recommended. It is important that isotretinoin be given at the recommended doses for no longer than the recommended duration. The effect of long-term use of isotretinoin on bone loss is unknown. Isotretinoin has been shown to decrease bone mineral density, cause hyperostosis and premature epiphyseal closure.

Contraceptive measures must be followed for any subsequent course of therapy.

Isotretinoin Dosing by Body Weight (Based On Administration With Food)

Body weight		Total mg/day		
Kilograms	Pounds	0.5 mg/kg	1 mg/kg	2 mg/kg[a]
40	88	20	40	80
50	110	25	50	100
60	132	30	60	120
70	154	35	70	140
80	176	40	80	160
90	198	45	90	180
100	220	50	100	200

[a] Adult patients whose disease is very severe with scarring or is primarily manifested on the trunk may require dose adjustments up to 2 mg/kg/day, as tolerated. The recommended dosage range is 0.5 to 1 mg/kg/day.

➤*Information for pharmacists:* See the Warning box for more information.

➤*Storage/Stability:* Store at 15° to 30°C (59° to 86°F). Protect from light.

Actions

➤*Pharmacology:* Isotretinoin is a retinoid, which, when administered in pharmacologic dosages of 0.5 to 1 mg/kg/day, inhibits sebaceous gland function and keratinization. The exact mechanism of action of isotretinoin is unknown.

Nodular acne – Clinical improvement in nodular acne patients occurs in association with a reduction in sebum secretion. The decrease in sebum secretion is temporary and is related to the dose and duration of treatment with isotretinoin, and reflects a reduction in sebaceous gland size and an inhibition of sebaceous gland differentiation.

➤*Pharmacokinetics:*

Absorption – Due to its high lipophilicity, oral absorption of isotretinoin is enhanced when given with a high-fat meal. In a crossover study, 74 healthy adult subjects received a single 80 mg oral dose (2 times 40 mg capsules) of isotretinoin under fasted and fed conditions. Both peak plasma concentration (C_{max}) and the total exposure (AUC) of isotretinoin were more than doubled following a standardized high-fat meal when compared with isotretinoin given under fasted conditions. The observed elimination half-life was unchanged. This lack of change in half-life suggests that food increases the bioavailability of isotretinoin without altering its disposition. The time to peak concentration (t_{max}) was also increased with food and may be related to a longer absorption phase. Therefore, isotretinoin capsules should always be taken with food. Clinical studies have shown that there is no difference in the pharmacokinetics of isotretinoin between patients with nodular acne and healthy subjects with normal skin.

Pharmacokinetic Parameters of Isotretinoin Mean (%Cv), N = 74

Isotretinoin 2 × 40 mg capsules	$AUC_{0-\infty}$ (ng•hr/mL)	C_{max} (ng/mL)	t_{max} (hr)	$t_{½}$ (hr)
Fed*	10,004 (22%)	862 (22%)	5.3 (77%)	21 (39%)
Fasted	3,703 (46%)	301 (63%)	3.2 (56%)	21 (30%)

* Eating a standardized high-fat meal.

Distribution – Isotretinoin is more than 99.9% bound to plasma proteins, primarily albumin.

Metabolism – Following oral administration of isotretinoin, at least 3 metabolites have been identified in human plasma: 4-oxo-isotretinoin, retinoic acid (tretinoin), and 4-oxo-retinoic acid (4-oxo-tretinoin). Retinoic acid and 13-cis-retinoic acid are geometric isomers and show reversible interconversion. The administration of one isomer will give rise to the other. Isotretinoin is also irreversibly oxidized to 4-oxo-isotretinoin, which forms its geometric isomer 4-oxo-tretinoin.

After a single 80 mg oral dose of isotretinoin to 74 healthy adult subjects, concurrent administration of food increased the extent of formation of all metabolites in plasma when compared to the extent of formation under fasted conditions.

All of these metabolites possess retinoid activity that is in some in vitro models more than that of the parent isotretinoin. However, the clinical significance of these models is unknown. After multiple oral dose administration of isotretinoin to adult cystic acne patients (greater than or equal to 18 years), the exposure of patients to 4-oxo-isotretinoin at steady-state under fasted and fed conditions was approximately 3.4 times higher than that of isotretinoin.

In vitro studies indicate that the primary P450 isoforms involved in isotretinoin metabolism are 2C8, 2C9, 3A4, and 2B6. Isotretinoin and its metabolites are further metabolized into conjugates, which are then excreted in urine and feces.

Excretion – Following oral administration of an 80 mg dose of ^{14}C-isotretinoin as a liquid suspension, ^{14}C activity in blood declined, with a half-life of 90 hours. The metabolites of isotretinoin and any conjugates are ultimately excreted in the feces and urine in relatively equal amounts (total of 65% to 83%). After a single 80 mg oral dose of isotretinoin to 74 healthy adult subjects under fed conditions, the mean ± SD elimination half-lives ($t_{½}$) of isotretinoin and 4-oxo-isotretinoin were 21 ± 8.2 hours and 24 ± 5.3 hours, respectively. After both single and multiple doses, the observed accumulation ratios of isotretinoin ranged from 0.9 to 5.43 in patients with cystic acne.

Contraindications

➤*Pregnancy:* *Category X.* Isotretinoin must not be used by females who are pregnant or who may become pregnant while undergoing treatment the (See the Warning box for more information).

➤*Allergic reactions:* Hypersensitivity to this medication or to any of its components. *Accutane* and *Sotret* isotretinoin capsules should not be given to patients who are sensitive to parabens, which are used as preservatives in the gelatin capsule.

Warnings

➤*Psychiatric disorders:* Isotretinoin may cause depression, psychosis and, rarely, suicidal ideation, suicide attempts, suicide, and aggressive or violent behaviors. Discontinuation of isotretinoin therapy may be insufficient; further evaluation may be necessary. No mechanism of action has been established for these events.

➤*Pseudotumor cerebri:* Isotretinoin use has been associated with a number of cases of pseudotumor cerebri (benign intracranial hypertension), some of which involved concomitant use of tetracyclines. Concomitant treatment with tetracyclines should therefore be avoided. Early signs and symptoms of

ISOTRETINOIN — ORAL

pseudotumor cerebri include papilledema, headache, nausea and vomiting, and visual disturbances. Patients with these symptoms should be screened for papilledema and, if present, they should be told to discontinue isotretinoin immediately and be referred to a neurologist for further diagnosis and care.

➤*Pancreatitis:* Acute pancreatitis has been reported in patients with either elevated or normal serum triglyceride levels. In rare instances, fatal hemorrhagic pancreatitis has been reported. Isotretinoin should be stopped if hypertriglyceridemia cannot be controlled at an acceptable level or if symptoms of pancreatitis occur.

➤*Lipids:* Elevations of serum triglycerides in excess of 800 mg/dL have been reported in patients treated with isotretinoin. Marked elevations of serum triglycerides were reported in approximately 25% of patients receiving isotretinoin in clinical trials. In addition, approximately 15% developed a decrease in high-density lipoproteins and about 7% showed an increase in cholesterol levels. In clinical trials, these effects on triglycerides, HDL, and cholesterol were reversible upon cessation of isotretinoin therapy. Some patients have been able to reverse triglyceride elevation by reduction in weight, restriction of dietary fat and alcohol, and reduction in dose while continuing isotretinoin.

Blood lipid determinations should be performed before isotretinoin is given and then at intervals until the lipid response to isotretinoin is established, which usually occurs with 4 weeks. Especially careful consideration must be given to risk/benefit for patients who may be at high risk during isotretinoin therapy (patients with diabetes, obesity, increased alcohol intake, lipid metabolism disorder or familial history of lipid metabolism disorder). If isotretinoin therapy is instituted, more frequent checks of serum values for lipids or blood sugar are recommended.

See Precautions for more information.

The cardiovascular consequences of hypertriglyceridemia associated with isotretinoin are unknown.

➤*Hearing impairment:* Impaired hearing has been reported in patients taking isotretinoin; in some cases, the hearing impairment has been reported to persist after therapy has been discontinued. Mechanism(s) and causality for this event have not been established. Patients who experience tinnitus or hearing impairment should discontinue isotretinoin treatment and be referred to specialized care for further evaluation.

➤*Inflammatory bowel disease:* Isotretinoin has been associated with inflammatory bowel disease (including regional ileitis) in patients without a history of intestinal disorders. In some instances, symptoms have been reported to persist after isotretinoin treatment has been stopped. Patients experiencing abdominal pain, rectal bleeding or severe diarrhea should discontinue isotretinoin immediately.

➤*Skeletal:*

Bone mineral density – Effects of multiple courses of isotretinoin on the developing musculoskeletal system are unknown. There is some evidence that long-term, high-dose, or multiple courses of therapy with isotretinoin have more of an effect than a single course of therapy on the musculoskeletal system. In an open-label clinical trial (n = 217) of a single course of therapy with isotretinoin for severe recalcitrant nodular acne, bone density measurements at several skeletal sites were not significantly decreased (lumbar spine change greater than −4% and total hip change greater than −5%) or were increased in the majority of patients. One patient had a decrease in lumbar spine bone mineral density greater than 4% based on unadjusted data. Sixteen (7.9%) patients had decreases in lumbar spine bone mineral density greater than 4%, and all the other patients (92%) did not have significant decreases or had increases (adjusted for body mass index). Nine patients (4.5%) had a decrease in total hip bone mineral density greater than 5% based on unadjusted data. Twenty-one (10.6%) patients had decreases in total hip bone mineral density greater than 5%, and all the other patients (89%) did not have significant decreases or had increases (adjusted for body mass index). Follow-up studies performed in 8 of the patients with decreased bone mineral density for up to 11 months thereafter demonstrated increasing bone density in 5 patients at the lumbar spine, while the other 3 patients had lumbar spine bone density measurements below baseline values. Total hip bone mineral densities remained below baseline (range −1.6% to −7.6%) in 5 of 8 patients (62.5%).

In a separate open-label extension study of 10 patients, ages 13 to 18 years, who started a second course of isotretinoin 4 months after the first course, 2 patients showed a decrease in mean lumbar spine bone mineral density up to 3.25%.

Spontaneous reports of osteoporosis, osteopenia, bone fractures, and delayed healing of bone fractures have been seen in the isotretinoin population. While causality to isotretinoin has not been established, an effect cannot be ruled out. Longer-term effects have not been studied. It is important that isotretinoin be given at the recommended doses for no longer than the recommended duration.

Hyperostosis – A high prevalence of skeletal hyperostosis was noted in clinical trials for disorders of keratinization with a mean dose of 2.24 mg/kg/day. Additionally, skeletal hyperostosis was noted in 6 of 8 patients in a prospective study of disorders of keratinization. Minimal skeletal hyperostosis and calcification of ligaments and tendons have also been observed by x-rays in prospective studies of nodular acne patients treated with a single course of therapy at recommended doses. The skeletal effects of multiple isotretinoin treatment courses for acne are unknown.

In a clinical study of 217 pediatric patients (12 to 17 years) with severe recalcitrant nodular acne, hyperostosis was not observed after 16 to 20 weeks of treatment with approximately 1 mg/kg/day of isotretinoin given in 2 divided doses. Hyperostosis may require a longer time frame to appear. The clinical course and significance remain unknown.

Premature epiphyseal closure – There are spontaneous reports of premature epiphyseal closure in acne patients receiving recommended doses of isotretinoin. The effect of multiple course of isotretinoin on epiphyseal closure is unknown.

➤*Vision impairment:* Visual problems should be carefully monitored. All isotretinoin patients experiencing visual difficulties should discontinue isotretinoin treatment and have an ophthalmological examination.

Corneal opacities – Corneal opacities have occurred in patients receiving isotretinoin for acne and more frequently when higher drug dosages were used in patients with disorders of keratinization. All isotretinoin patients experiencing visual difficulties should discontinue the drug and have an ophthalmologic examination. The corneal opacities that have been observed in clinical trial patients treated with isotretinoin have either completely resolved or were resolving at follow-up 6 to 7 weeks after discontinuation of the drug.

Decreased night vision – A number of cases of decreased night vision have occurred during isotretinoin therapy and in some instances the event has persisted after therapy was discontinued. Because the onset in some patients was sudden, patients should be advised of this potential problem and warned to be cautious when driving or operating any vehicle at night. Visual problems should be carefully monitored.

➤*Hepatotoxicity:* Clinical hepatitis considered to be possibly or probably related to isotretinoin therapy has been reported. Additionally, mild-to-moderate elevations of liver enzymes have been observed in approximately 15% of individuals treated during clinical trials, some of which normalized with dosage reduction or continued administration of the drug. If normalization does not readily occur or if hepatitis is suspected during treatment with isotretinoin, the drug should be discontinued and the etiology further investigated.

➤*Hypersensitivity reactions:* Anaphylactic reactions and other allergic reactions have been reported. Cutaneous allergic reactions and serious cases of allergic vasculitis, often with purpura (bruises and red patches) of the extremities and extracutaneous involvement (including renal) have been reported. Severe allergic reaction necessitates discontinuation of therapy and appropriate medical management.

➤*Carcinogenesis:* In male and female Fischer 344 rats given oral isotretinoin at dosages of 8 or 32 mg/kg/day (1.3 to 5.3 times the recommended clinical dose of 1 mg/kg/day, respectively, after normalization for total body surface area) for greater than 18 months, there was a dose-related increased incidence of pheochromocytoma relative to controls. The incidence of adrenal medullary hyperplasia was also increased at the higher dosage in both sexes. The relatively high level of spontaneous pheochromocytomas occurring in the male Fischer 344 rat makes it an equivocal model for study of this tumor; therefore, the relevance of this tumor to the human population is uncertain.

➤*Mutagenesis:* The Ames test was conducted with isotretinoin in 2 laboratories. The results of the tests in 1 laboratory were negative while in the second laboratory a weakly positive response (less than 1.6 background) was noted in *S. typhimurium* TA100 when the assay was conducted with metabolic activation.

➤*Fertility impairment:* In dogs, testicular atrophy was noted after treatment with oral isotretinoin for approximately 30 weeks at dosages of 20 or 60 mg/kg/day (10 or 30 times the recommended clinical dose of 1 mg/kg/day, respectively, after normalization for total body surface area). In general, there was microscopic evidence for appreciable depression of spermatogenesis but some sperm were observed in all testes examined and in no instance were completely atrophic tubules seen.

➤*Elderly:* Clinical studies of isotretinoin did not include sufficient numbers of subjects aged 65 years and over to determine whether they respond differently from younger subjects. Although reported clinical experience has not identified differences in responses between elderly and younger patients, effects of aging might be expected to increase some risks associated with isotretinoin therapy (eg, decreased bone mineral density, hepatotoxicity, elevated triglycerides).

➤*Pregnancy:* Category X.

See the Warning box for more information.

➤*Lactation:* It is not known whether this drug is excreted in human milk. Because of the potential for adverse reactions, nursing mothers should not receive isotretinoin.

➤*Children:* The use of isotretinoin in pediatric patients younger than 12 years of age has not been studied. The use of isotretinoin for the treatment of severe recalcitrant nodular acne in pediatric patients ages 12 to 17 years should be given careful consideration, especially for those patients where a known metabolic or structural bone disease exists.

Precautions

➤*Monitoring:*

CPK – Some patients undergoing vigorous physical activity while on isotretinoin therapy have experienced elevated CPK levels; however, the clinical significance is unknown. There have been rare postmarketing reports of rhabdomyolysis, some associated with strenuous physical activity. In a clinical trial of 217 pediatric patients (12 to 17 years) with severe recalcitrant nodular acne, transient elevations in CPK were observed in 12% of patients, including those undergoing strenuous physical activity in association with reported musculoskeletal adverse events such as back pain, arthralgia, limb injury, or muscle sprain. In these patients, approximately half of the CPK elevations returned to normal within 2 weeks and half returned to normal within 4 weeks. No cases of rhabdomyolysis were reported in this trial.

ISOTRETINOIN — ORAL

Glucose – Certain patients receiving isotretinoin have experienced problems in the control of their blood sugar. In addition, new cases of diabetes have been diagnosed during isotretinoin therapy, although no causal relationship has been established.

Lipids – Pretreatment and follow-up blood lipids should be obtained under fasting conditions. After consumption of alcohol, at least 36 hours should elapse before these determinations are made. It is recommended that these tests be performed at weekly or biweekly intervals until the lipid response to isotretinoin is established. The incidence of hypertriglyceridemia is 1 patient in 4 on isotretinoin therapy.

Liver function tests – Since elevations of liver enzymes have been observed during clinical trials, and hepatitis has been reported, pretreatment and follow-up liver function tests should be performed at weekly or biweekly intervals until the response to isotretinoin has been established. Mild-to-moderate elevations of liver enzymes have been observed in approximately 15% of individuals treated during clinical trials, some of which normalized with dosage reduction or continued administration of the drug. If normalization does not readily occur, or if hepatitis is suspected during treatment with isotretinoin, the drug should be discontinued and the etiology further investigated.

Pregnancy test – Female patients of childbearing potential must have negative results from 2 urine or serum pregnancy tests with a sensitivity of at least 25 milliunit/mL before receiving the initial isotretinoin prescription. The first test is obtained by the prescriber when the decision is made to pursue qualification of the patient for isotretinoin (a screening test). The second pregnancy test (a confirmation test) should be done during the first 5 days of the menstrual period immediately preceding the beginning of isotretinoin therapy. For patients with amenorrhea, the second test should be done at least 11 days after the last act of unprotected sexual intercourse (without using 2 effective forms of contraception).

Each month of therapy, the patient must have a negative result from a urine or serum pregnancy test. A pregnancy test must be repeated each month prior to the female patient receiving each prescription.

➤*The isotretinoin pregnancy prevention and risk-management programs:* The *Accutane* Pregnancy Prevention and Risk Management Programs consist of the System to Manage *Accutane* Related Teratogenicity (SMART) and the *Accutane* Pregnancy Prevention Program (PPP). SMART for *Accutane* should be followed for prescribing isotretinoin with the goal of preventing fetal exposure to isotretinoin. Similar programs from different manufacturers include: Isotretinoin Medication Program: Alerting you to the Risks of Teratogenicity (IMPART) and the *Sotret* Program to Prevent Pregnancy (PPP) from Ranbaxy Pharmaceuticals; the System to Prevent Isotretinoin-Related Issues of Teratogenicity (SPIRIT) and the *Amnesteem* Pregnancy Prevention Initiative from Bertek Pharmaceuticals; and the Adverse Event Learning & Education Regarding Teratogenicity (ALERT) for *Claravis* from Barr Laboratories.

See the Warning box for more information.

➤*Special risk:* Although an effect of isotretinoin on bone loss is not established, physicians should use caution when prescribing isotretinoin to patients with a genetic predisposition for age-related osteoporosis, a history of childhood osteoporosis conditions, osteomalacia, or other disorders of bone metabolism. This would include patients diagnosed with anorexia nervosa and those who are on chronic drug therapy that causes drug-induced osteoporosis/osteomalacia or affects vitamin D metabolism, such as systemic corticosteroids and any anticonvulsant.

Patients may be at increased risk when participating in sports with repetitive impact where the risks of spondylolisthesis with and without pars fractures and hip growth plate injuries in early and late adolescence are known. There are spontaneous reports of fractures or delayed healing in patients while on treatment with isotretinoin or following cessation of treatment with isotretinoin while involved in these activities. While causality to isotretinoin has not been established, an effect cannot be ruled out.

Drug Interactions

➤*Microdosed progesterone preparations:* Microdosed progesterone preparations ("minipills" that do not contain an estrogen) may be an inadequate method of contraception during isotretinoin therapy. Although other hormonal contraceptives are highly effective, there have been reports of pregnancy from women who have used combined oral contraceptives, as well as topical/injectable/implantable/insertable hormonal birth control products. These reports are more frequent for women who use only a single method of contraception. It is not known if hormonal contraceptives differ in their effectiveness when used with isotretinoin. Therefore, it is critically important for women of childbearing potential to select and commit to use 2 forms of effective contraception simultaneously, at least 1 of which must be a primary form, unless absolute abstinence is the chosen method, or the patient has undergone a hysterectomy. Patients must use 2 forms of effective contraception for at least 1 month prior to initiation of isotretinoin therapy, during isotretinoin therapy, and for 1 month after discontinuing isotretinoin therapy. Counseling about contraception and behaviors associated with an increased risk of pregnancy must be repeated on a monthly basis. Effective forms of contraception include both primary and secondary forms of contraception. Primary forms of contraception include the following: Tubal ligation, partner's vasectomy, intrauterine devices, birth control pills, and injectable/implantable/insertable hormonal birth control products. Secondary forms of contraception include diaphragms, latex condoms, and cervical caps; each must be used with a spermicide.

➤*Tetracyclines:* Concomitant treatment with isotretinoin and tetracyclines should be avoided because isotretinoin use has been associated with a number of cases of pseudotumor cerebri (benign intracranial hypertension), some of which involved concomitant use of tetracyclines.

➤*Vitamin A:* Because of the relationship of isotretinoin to vitamin A, patients should be advised against taking vitamin supplements containing vitamin A to avoid additive toxic effects.

➤*Phenytoin:* Isotretinoin has not been shown to alter the pharmacokinetics of phenytoin in a study in 7 healthy volunteers. These results are consistent with the in vitro finding that neither isotretinoin nor its metabolites induce or inhibit the activity of the CYP2C9 human hepatic P450 enzyme. Phenytoin is known to cause osteomalacia. No formal clinical studies have been conducted to assess if there is an interactive effect on bone loss between phenytoin and isotretinoin. Therefore, caution should be exercised when using these drugs together.

➤*Systemic corticosteroids:* Systemic corticosteroids are known to cause osteoporosis. No formal clinical studies have been conducted to assess if there is an interactive effect on bone loss between systemic corticosteroids and isotretinoin. Therefore, caution should be exercised when using these drugs together.

Adverse Reactions

➤*Dose relationship:* Cheilitis and hypertriglyceridemia are usually dose related. Most adverse reactions reported in clinical trials were reversible when therapy was discontinued; however, some persisted after cessation of therapy (eg, depression, psychosis, suicidal ideation, suicide attempts, suicide, aggressive or violent behavior, hearing impairment, inflammatory bowel disease, decreased night vision).

Cardiovascular – Palpitation, tachycardia, vascular thrombotic disease, stroke.

CNS – Pseudotumor cerebri, dizziness, drowsiness, headache, insomnia, lethargy, malaise, nervousness, paresthesias, seizures, stroke, syncope, weakness.

Dermatologic – Acne fulminans, alopecia (which in some cases persists), bruising, cheilitis (dry lips), dry mouth, dry nose, dry skin, epistaxis, eruptive xanthomas, flushing, fragility of skin, hair abnormalities, hirsutism, hyperpigmentation and hypopigmentation, infections (including disseminated herpes simplex), nail dystrophy, paronychia, peeling of palms and soles, photoallergic/photosensitizing reactions, pruritus, pyogenic granuloma, rash (including facial erythema, seborrhea, and eczema), sunburn susceptibility increased, sweating, urticaria, vasculitis (including Wegener's granulomatosis), abnormal wound healing (delayed healing or exuberant granulation tissue with crusting).

Endocrine – Hypertriglyceridemia, alterations in blood sugar levels.

GI – Inflammatory bowel disease, hepatitis, pancreatitis, bleeding and inflammation of the gums, colitis, esophagitis, esophageal ulceration, ileitis, nausea, other nonspecific gastrointestinal symptoms.

GU – Glomerulonephritis, nonspecific urogenital findings, abnormal menses.

Hematologic – Allergic reactions (cutaneous, allergic vasculitis, often with purpura of the extremities and extra cutaneous involvement [including renal]), anemia, thrombocytopenia, neutropenia, rare reports of agranulocytosis.

Lab test abnormalities – Elevation of plasma triglycerides, decrease in serum high-density lipoprotein (HDL) levels, elevations of serum cholesterol during treatment.

Increased alkaline phosphatase, AST, ALT, GGTP or LDH.

Elevation of fasting blood sugar, elevations of CPK, hyperuricemia.

Decreases in red blood cell parameters, decreases in white blood cell counts (including severe neutropenia and rare reports of agranulocytosis), elevated sedimentation rates, elevated platelet counts, thrombocytopenia.

White cells in the urine, proteinuria, microscopic or gross hematuria.

Musculoskeletal – Skeletal hyperostosis, calcification of tendons and ligaments, premature epiphyseal closure, decreases in bone mineral density, musculoskeletal symptoms (sometimes severe) including back pain and arthralgia, transient pain in the chest, arthritis, tendonitis, other types of bone abnormalities, elevations of CPK/rare reports of rhabdomyolysis.

Ophthalmic – Corneal opacities, decreased night vision which may persist, cataracts, color vision disorder, conjunctivitis, dry eyes, eyelid inflammation, keratitis, optic neuritis, photophobia, visual disturbances.

Psychiatric – Suicidal ideation, suicide attempts, suicide, depression, psychosis, aggression, violent behaviors, emotional instability.

Of the patients reporting depression, some reported that the depression subsided with discontinuation of therapy and recurred with reinstitution of therapy.

Respiratory – Bronchospasms (with or without a history of asthma), respiratory tract infection, voice alteration.

Special senses – Hearing impairment, tinnitus.

Miscellaneous – Allergic reactions, including vasculitis, systemic hypersensitivity, edema, fatigue, lymphadenopathy, weight loss.

Overdosage

Because an overdose would be expected to result in higher levels of isotretinoin in semen than found during a normal treatment course, male patients should use a condom, or avoid reproductive sexual activity with a female who is or might become pregnant, for 30 days after the overdose. All patients with isotretinoin overdose should not donate blood for at least 30 days.

First Generation Retinoids

ISOTRETINOIN — ORAL

➤*Symptoms:* In humans, overdose has been associated with vomiting, facial flushing, cheilosis, abdominal pain, headache, dizziness, and ataxia. All symptoms quickly resolved without apparent residual effects.

Patient Information

Females of childbearing potential should be instructed that they must not be pregnant when isotretinoin therapy is initiated, and that they should use 2 forms of effective contraception 1 month before starting isotretinoin, while taking isotretinoin, and for 1 month after isotretinoin has been stopped. They should also sign a consent form prior to beginning isotretinoin therapy. They should be given an opportunity to enroll in the isotretinoin survey and to review the patient videotapes provided by the manufacturer to the prescriber. The videos include information about contraception, the most common reasons that contraception fails, and the importance of using 2 forms of effective contraception when taking teratogenic drugs and comprehensive information about types of potential birth defects which could occur if a woman who is pregnant takes isotretinoin at any time during pregnancy. Female patients should be seen by their prescribers monthly and have a urine or serum pregnancy test performed each month during treatment to confirm negative pregnancy status before another isotretinoin prescription is written.

Isotretinoin is found in the semen of male patients taking isotretinoin, but the amount delivered to a female partner would be about 1 million times lower than an oral dose of 40 mg. While the no-effect limit for isotretinoin-induced embryopathy is unknown, 20 years of postmarketing reports include 4 with isolated defects compatible with features of retinoid exposed fetuses. None of these cases had the combination of malformations characteristic of retinoid exposure, and all had other possible explanations for the defects observed.

Patients may report mental health problems or family history of psychiatric disorders. These reports should be discussed with the patient or the patient's family. A referral to a mental health professional may be necessary. The physician should consider whether or not isotretinoin therapy is appropriate in this setting. Isotretinoin may cause depression, psychosis and, rarely, suicidal ideation, suicide attempts, suicide, and aggressive or violent behaviors.

Patients should be informed that they must not share isotretinoin with anyone else because of the risk of birth defects and other serious adverse events.

Patients should not donate blood during therapy and for 1 month following discontinuance of the drug because the blood might be given to a pregnant woman whose fetus must not be exposed to isotretinoin.

Patients should be reminded to take isotretinoin with a meal. To decrease the risk of esophageal irritation, patients should swallow the capsules with a full glass of liquid.

Patients should be informed that transient exacerbation (flare) of acne has been seen, generally during the initial period of therapy.

Wax epilation and skin resurfacing procedures (such as dermabrasion, laser) should be avoided during isotretinoin therapy and for at least 6 months thereafter due to the possibility of scarring. Isotretinoin may cause abnormal wound healing.

Patients should be advised to avoid prolonged exposure to UV rays or sunlight.

Patients should be informed that they may experience decreased tolerance to contact lenses during and after therapy.

Patients should be informed that approximately 16% of patients treated with isotretinoin in a clinical trial developed musculoskeletal symptoms (including arthralgia) during treatment. In general, these symptoms were mild to moderate, but occasionally required discontinuation of the drug. Transient pain in the chest has been reported less frequently. In the clinical trial, these symptoms generally cleared rapidly after discontinuation of isotretinoin, but in some cases persisted. There have been rare postmarketing reports of elevated CPK levels/rhabdomyolysis, some associated with strenuous physical activity.

Pediatric patients and their caregivers should be informed that approximately 29% (104/358) of pediatric patients treated with isotretinoin developed back pain. Back pain was severe in 13.5% (14/104) of the cases and occurred at a higher frequency in female than male patients. Arthralgias were experienced in 22% (79/358) of pediatric patients. Arthralgias were severe in 7.6% (6/79) of patients. Appropriate evaluation of the musculoskeletal system should be done in patients who present with these symptoms during or after a course of isotretinoin. Consideration should be given to discontinuation of isotretinoin if any significant abnormality is found.

Neutropenia and rare cases of agranulocytosis have been reported. Isotretinoin should be discontinued if clinically significant decreases in white cell counts occur.

Second Generation Retinoids

ACITRETIN

Rx	**Soriatane** (Connetics)	**Capsules**[a]: 10 mg	(SORIATANE 10). Brown/white. In 30s.
		25 mg	(SORIATANE 25). Brown/yellow. In 30s.

[a] Capsule shells contain gelatin, iron oxide, titanium dioxide, and may also contain benzyl alcohol.

ACITRETIN — ORAL

WARNING

Acitretin causes birth defects. Female patients must not get pregnant.

Acitretin must not be used by females who are pregnant, or who intend to become pregnant during therapy or at any time for at least 3 years following discontinuation of therapy. Acitretin also must not be used by females who may not use reliable contraception while undergoing treatment or for at least 3 years following discontinuation of treatment. Acitretin is a metabolite of etretinate, and major human fetal abnormalities have been reported with the administration of etretinate and acitretin. Potentially, any fetus exposed can be affected.

Clinical evidence has shown that concurrent ingestion of acitretin and ethanol has been associated with the formation of etretinate, which has a longer elimination half-life than acitretin. Because the longer elimination half-life of etretinate would increase the duration of teratogenic potential for female patients, ethanol must not be ingested by female patients either during treatment with acitretin or for 2 months after cessation of therapy. This allows for elimination of acitretin, thus removing the substrate for transesterification to etretinate. The mechanism of the metabolic process for conversion of acitretin to etretinate has not been fully defined. It is not known whether substances other than ethanol are associated with transesterification.

Acitretin has been shown to be embryotoxic or teratogenic in rabbits, mice, and rats at doses of 0.6, 3, and 15 mg/kg, respectively. These doses are approximately 0.2, 0.3, and 3 times the maximum recommended therapeutic dose, respectively, based on a mg/m^2 comparison.

Major human fetal abnormalities associated with acitretin or etretinate administration have been reported including meningomyelocele, meningoencephalocele, multiple synostoses, facial dysmorphia, syndactylies, absence of terminal phalanges, malformations of hip, ankle and forearm, low set ears, high palate, decreased cranial volume, cardiovascular malformation, and alterations of the skull and cervical vertebrae.

Acitretin should be prescribed only by those who have special competence in the diagnosis and treatment of severe psoriasis, are experienced in the use of systemic retinoids, and understand the risk of teratogenicity.

Important information for women of childbearing potential – Acitretin should be considered only for women with severe psoriasis unresponsive to other therapies or whose clinical condition contraindicates the use of other treatments.

WARNING (cont.)

Females of reproductive potential must not be given a prescription for acitretin until pregnancy is excluded. Acitretin is contraindicated in females of reproductive potential unless the patient meets all of the following conditions:

- Must have had 2 negative urine or serum pregnancy tests with a sensitivity of at least 25 mIU/mL before receiving the initial acitretin prescription. The first test (a screening test) is obtained by the prescriber when the decision is made to pursue acitretin therapy. The second pregnancy test (a confirmation test) should be done during the first 5 days of the menstrual period immediately preceding the beginning of acitretin therapy. For patients with amenorrhea, the second test should be done at least 11 days after the last act of unprotected sexual intercourse (without using 2 effective forms of contraception [birth control] simultaneously). Timing of pregnancy testing throughout the treatment course should be monthly or individualized based on the prescriber's clinical judgment.
- Must have selected and have committed to use 2 effective forms of contraception (birth control) simultaneously, at least 1 of which must be a primary form, unless absolute abstinence is the chosen method, or the patient has undergone a hysterectomy or is clearly postmenopausal.
- Patients must use 2 effective forms of contraception (birth control) simultaneously for at least 1 month prior to initiation of acitretin therapy, during acitretin therapy, and for at least 3 years after discontinuing acitretin therapy. An acitretin patient referral form is available so that patients can receive an initial free contraceptive counseling session and pregnancy testing. Counseling about contraception and behaviors associated with an increased risk of pregnancy must be repeated on a regular basis by the prescriber. To encourage compliance with this recommendation, a limited supply of the drug should be prescribed. Effective forms of contraception include both primary and secondary forms of contraception. Primary forms of contraception include the following: Tubal ligation, partner's vasectomy, intrauterine devices, birth control pills, and injectable/implantable/insertable/topical hormonal birth

ACITRETIN — ORAL

WARNING (cont.)

control products. Secondary forms of contraception include diaphragms, latex condoms, and cervical caps; each secondary form must be used with a spermicide. Any birth control method can fail. Therefore, it is critically important that women of childbearing potential use 2 effective forms of contraception (birth control) simultaneously. It has not been established if there is a pharmacokinetic interaction between acitretin and combined oral contraceptives. However, it has been established that acitretin interferes with the contraceptive effect of microdosed progestin preparations. Microdosed "minipill" progestin preparations are not recommended for use with acitretin. It is not known whether other progestational contraceptives, such as implants and injectables, are adequate methods of contraception during acitretin therapy. Prescribers are advised to consult the package insert of any medication administered concomitantly with hormonal contraceptives, since some medications may decrease the effectiveness of these birth control products. Patients should be prospectively cautioned not to self-medicate with the herbal supplement St. John's wort because a possible interaction has been suggested with hormonal contraceptives based on reports of breakthrough bleeding on oral contraceptives shortly after starting St. John's wort. Pregnancies have been reported by users of combined hormonal contraceptives who also used some form of St. John's wort.

- Must have signed a Patient Agreement/Informed Consent for Female Patients that contains warnings about the risk of potential birth defects if the fetus is exposed to acitretin, about contraceptive failure, and about the fact that they must not ingest beverages or products containing ethanol while taking acitretin and for 2 months after acitretin treatment has been discontinued.

If pregnancy does occur during acitretin therapy or at any time for at least 3 years following discontinuation of acitretin therapy, the prescriber and patient should discuss the possible effects on the pregnancy. The available information is as follows:

Acitretin, the active metabolite of etretinate, is teratogenic and is contraindicated during pregnancy. The risk of severe fetal malformations is well established when systemic retinoids are taken during pregnancy. Pregnancy must also be prevented after stopping acitretin therapy, while the drug is being eliminated to below a threshold blood concentration that would be associated with an increased incidence of birth defects. Because this threshold has not been established for acitretin in humans and because elimination rates vary among patients, the duration of post-therapy contraception to achieve adequate elimination cannot be calculated precisely. It is strongly recommended that contraception be continued for at least 3 years after stopping treatment with acitretin, based on the following considerations:

- In the absence of transesterification to form etretinate, greater than 98% of the acitretin would be eliminated within 2 months, assuming a mean elimination half-life of 49 hours.
- In cases where etretinate is formed, as has been demonstrated with concomitant administration of acitretin and ethanol, greater than 98% of the etretinate formed would be eliminated in 2 years, assuming a mean elimination half-life of 120 days, and greater than 98% of the etretinate formed would be eliminated in 3 years, based on the longest demonstrated elimination half-life of 168 days. However, etretinate was found in plasma and subcutaneous fat in 1 patient reported to have had sporadic alcohol intake, 52 months after she stopped acitretin therapy.
- Severe birth defects have been reported where conception occurred during the time interval when the patient was being treated with acitretin and/or etretinate. In addition, severe birth defects have also been reported when conception occurred after the mother completed therapy. These cases have been reported both prospectively (before the outcome was known) and retrospectively (after the outcome was known). The events below are listed without distinction as to whether the reported birth defects are consistent with retinoid-induced embryopathy or not.
- There have been 318 prospectively reported cases involving pregnancies and the use of etretinate, acitretin or both. In 238 of these cases, the conception occurred after the last dose of etretinate (103 cases), acitretin (126) or both (9). Fetal outcome remained unknown in approximately one-half of these cases, of which 62 were terminated and 14 were spontaneous abortions. Fetal outcome is known for the other 118 cases and 15 of the outcomes were abnormal (including cases of absent hand/wrist, clubfoot, GI malformation, hypocalcemia, hypotonia, limb malformation, neonatal apnea/anemia, neonatal ichthyosis, placental disorder/death, undescended testicle and 5 cases of premature birth). In the 126 prospectively reported cases where conception occurred after the last dose of acitretin only, 43 cases involved conception at least 1 year but less than 2 years after the last dose. There were 3 reports of abnormal outcomes out of these 43 cases (involving limb malformation, GI tract malformations and premature birth). There were only 4 cases where conception occurred at least 2 years after the last dose but there were no reports of birth defects in these cases.

WARNING (cont.)

- There is also a total of 35 retrospectively reported cases where conception occurred at least 1 year after the last dose of etretinate, acitretin or both. From these cases there are 3 reports of birth defects when the conception occurred at least 1 year but less than 2 years after the last dose of acitretin (including heart malformations, Turner's Syndrome, and unspecified congenital malformations) and 4 reports of birth defects when conception occurred 2 or more years after the last dose of acitretin (including foot malformation, cardiac malformations [2 cases] and unspecified neonatal and infancy disorder). There were 3 additional abnormal outcomes in cases where conception occurred 2 or more years after the last dose of etretinate (including chromosome disorder, forearm aplasia, and stillbirth).
- Females who have taken etretinate must continue to follow the contraceptive recommendations for etretinate. Etretinate is no longer marketed in the US; for information, call the manufacturer at 1-800-526-6367.
- Patients should not donate blood during and for at least 3 years following the completion of acitretin therapy because women of childbearing potential must not receive blood from patients being treated with acitretin.

Important information for males taking acitretin – Patients should not donate blood during and for at least 3 years following acitretin therapy because women of childbearing potential must not receive blood from patients being treated with acitretin.

Samples of seminal fluid from 3 male patients treated with acitretin and 6 male patients treated with etretinate have been assayed for the presence of acitretin. The maximum concentration of acitretin observed in the seminal fluid of these men was 12.5 ng/mL. Assuming an ejaculate volume of 10 mL, the amount of drug transferred in semen would be 125 ng, which is 1/200,000 of a single 25 mg capsule. Thus, although it appears that residual acitretin in seminal fluid poses little, if any, risk to a fetus while a male patient is taking the drug or after it is discontinued, the no-effect limit for teratogenicity is unknown and there is no registry for birth defects associated with acitretin. The available data are as follows:

There have been 25 cases of reported conception when the male partner was taking acitretin. The pregnancy outcome is known in 13 of these 25 cases. Of these, 9 reports were retrospective and 4 were prospective (meaning the pregnancy was reported prior to knowledge of the outcome).

- When acitretin treatment was given at time of conception, there were 5 deliveries of healthy neonates (4 of 5 cases were prospective), 5 spontaneous abortions, and 1 induced abortion.
- When acitretin was discontinued approximately 4 weeks prior to conception, there was 1 induced abortion (with malformation pattern not typical of retinoid embryopathy [bilateral cystic hygromas of neck, hypoplasia of lungs bilateral, pulmonary atresia, VSD with overriding truncus arteriosus]).
- When acitretin was discontinued approximately 6 to 8 months prior to conception, there was 1 spontaneous abortion.

For all patients – An acitretin medication guide must be given to the patient each time acitretin is dispensed, as required by law.

Hepatotoxicity – Of the 525 patients treated in US clinical trials, 2 had clinical jaundice with elevated serum bilirubin and transaminases considered related to acitretin treatment. Liver function test results in these patients returned to normal after acitretin was discontinued. Two of the 1289 patients treated in European clinical trials developed biopsy-confirmed toxic hepatitis. A second biopsy in one of these patients revealed nodule formation suggestive of cirrhosis. One patient in a Canadian clinical trial of 63 patients developed a 3-fold increase of transaminases. A liver biopsy of this patient showed mild lobular disarray, multifocal hepatocyte loss and mild triaditis of the portal tracts compatible with acute reversible hepatic injury. The patient's transaminase levels returned to normal 2 months after acitretin was discontinued.

The potential of acitretin therapy to induce hepatotoxicity was prospectively evaluated using liver biopsies in an open-label study of 128 patients. Pretreatment and posttreatment biopsies were available for 87 patients. A comparison of liver biopsy findings before and after therapy revealed 49 (58%) patients showed no change, 21 (25%) improved and 14 (17%) patients had a worsening of their liver biopsy status. For 6 patients, the classification changed from class 0 (no pathology) to class I (normal fatty infiltration; nuclear variability and portal inflammation; both mild); for 7 patients, the change was from class I to class II (fatty infiltration, nuclear variability, portal inflammation and focal necrosis; all moderate to severe); and for 1 patient, the change was from class II to class IIIb (fibrosis, moderate to severe). No correlation could be found between liver function test result abnormalities and the change in liver biopsy status, and no cumulative dose relationship was found.

Elevations of AST, ALT, GGT (GGTP) or LDH have occurred in approximately 1 in 3 patients treated with acitretin. Of the 525 patients treated in clinical trials in the US, treatment was discontinued in 20 (3.8%) due to elevated liver function test results. If hepatotoxicity is suspected during treatment with acitretin, the drug should be discontinued and the etiology further investigated.

ACITRETIN — ORAL

WARNING (cont.)

Ten of 652 patients treated in US clinical trials of etretinate, of which acitretin is the active metabolite, had clinical or histologic hepatitis considered to be possibly or probably related to etretinate treatment. There have been reports of hepatitis-related deaths worldwide; a few of these patients had received etretinate for 1 month or less before presenting with hepatic symptoms or signs.

Indications

➤*Psoriasis:* For the treatment of severe psoriasis in adults. Because of significant adverse effects associated with its use, acitretin should be prescribed only by physicians knowledgeable in the systemic use of retinoids. In females of reproductive potential, acitretin should be reserved for nonpregnant patients who are unresponsive to other therapies or whose clinical condition contraindicates the use of other treatments.

Most patients experience relapse of psoriasis after discontinuing therapy. Subsequent courses, when clinically indicated, have produced results similar to the initial course of therapy.

➤*Unlabeled uses:* Darier's disease, palmoplantar pustulosis, lichen planus (30 mg/day for 4 weeks, titrated to 10 to 50 mg/day for 12 weeks total); children with lamellar ichthyosis, non-bullous, and bullous ichthyosiform erythroderma, Sjogren-Larsson syndrome (0.47 mg/kg/day); additional studies indicate mild to marked improvement in lichen sclerosus et atrophicus of the vulva and palmoplantar lichen nitidus.

Administration and Dosage

➤*Approved by the FDA:* October 28, 1996.

Individualization of dosage is required to achieve maximum therapeutic response while minimizing side effects. Acitretin therapy should be initiated at 25 or 50 mg/day, given as a single dose with the main meal. Maintenance doses of 25 to 50 mg/day may be given dependent upon an individual patient's response to initial treatment. Relapses may be treated as outlined for initial therapy.

When acitretin is used with phototherapy, the prescriber should decrease the phototherapy dose, dependent on the patient's individual response.

Females who have taken etretinate (*Tegison*) must continue to follow the contraceptive recommendations for etretinate.

➤*Information for pharmacists:* An acitretin medication guide must be given to the patient each time acitretin is dispensed, as required by law.

➤*Storage/Stability:* Store between 15° and 25°C (59° and 77°F). Protect from light. Avoid exposure to high temperatures and humidity after the bottle is opened.

Actions

➤*Pharmacology:* The mechanism of action of acitretin is unknown.

➤*Pharmacokinetics:*

Absorption – Oral absorption of acitretin is optimal when given with food. For this reason, acitretin was given with food in all of the following studies. After administration of a single 50 mg oral dose of acitretin to 18 healthy subjects, maximum plasma concentrations ranged from 196 to 728 ng/mL (mean: 416 ng/mL) and were achieved in 2 to 5 hours (mean: 2.7 hours). The oral absorption of acitretin is linear and proportional with increasing doses from 25 to 100 mg. Approximately 72% (range: 47% to 109%) of the administered dose was absorbed after a single 50 mg dose of acitretin was given to 12 healthy subjects.

Distribution – Acitretin is more than 99.9% bound to plasma proteins, primarily albumin.

Metabolism – Following oral absorption, acitretin undergoes extensive metabolism and interconversion by simple isomerization to its 13-cis form (cis-acitretin). The formation of cis-acitretin relative to parent compound is not altered by dose or fed/fast conditions of oral administration of acitretin. Both parent compound and isomer are further metabolized into chain-shortened breakdown products and conjugates which are excreted. Following multiple-dose administration of acitretin, steady-state concentrations of acitretin and cis-acitretin in plasma are achieved within approximately 3 weeks.

Excretion – The chain-shortened metabolites and conjugates of acitretin and cis-acitretin are ultimately excreted in the feces (34% to 54%) and urine (16% to 53%). The terminal elimination half-life of acitretin following multiple-dose administration is 49 hours (range 33 to 96 hours), and that of cis-acitretin under the same conditions is 63 hours (range 28 to 157 hours). The accumulation ratio of the parent compound is 1.2; that of cis-acitretin is 6.6.

Special populations –

Renal function impairment: Plasma concentrations of acitretin were significantly lower (59.3%) in end-stage renal failure subjects (n = 6) when compared to age-matched controls, following single 50 mg oral doses. Acitretin was not removed by hemodialysis in these subjects.

Elderly: In a multiple-dose study in healthy young (n = 6) and elderly (n = 8) subjects, a 2-fold increase in acitretin plasma concentrations were seen in elderly subjects, although the elimination half-life did not change.

Psoriasis: In an 8-week study of acitretin pharmacokinetics in patients with psoriasis, mean steady-state trough concentrations of acitretin increased in a dose proportional manner with dosages ranging from 10 to 50 mg daily. Acitretin plasma concentrations were nonmeasurable (less than 4 ng/mL) in all patients 3 weeks after cessation of therapy.

Contraindications

Pregnancy *Category X.*

Severely impaired liver or kidney function; chronic abnormally elevated blood lipid values.

An increased risk of hepatitis has been reported to result from combined use of methotrexate and etretinate. Consequently, the combination of methotrexate with acitretin is also contraindicated.

Since both acitretin and tetracyclines can cause increased intracranial pressure, their combined use is contraindicated.

Acitretin is contraindicated in cases of hypersensitivity to the preparation (acitretin or excipients) or to other retinoids.

Warnings

➤*Pancreatitis:* Lipid elevations occur in 25% to 50% of patients treated with acitretin. Triglyceride increases sufficient to be associated with pancreatitis are much less common, although fatal fulminant pancreatitis has been reported. There have been rare reports of pancreatitis during acitretin therapy in the absence of hypertriglyceridemia.

➤*Pseudotumor cerebri:* Acitretin and other retinoids administered orally have been associated with cases of pseudotumor cerebri (benign intracranial hypertension). Some of these events involved concomitant use of isotretinoin and tetracyclines. However, the event seen in a single acitretin patient was not associated with tetracycline use. Early signs and symptoms include papilledema, headache, nausea and vomiting and visual disturbances. Patients with these signs and symptoms should be examined for papilledema and, if present, should discontinue acitretin immediately and be referred for neurological evaluation and care. Since both acitretin and tetracyclines can cause increased intracranial pressure, their combined use is contraindicated.

➤*Ophthalmologic effects:* The eyes and vision of 329 patients treated with acitretin were examined by ophthalmologists. The findings included dry eyes (23%), irritation of eyes (9%) and brow and lash loss (5%). The following were reported in less than 5% of patients: Bell's palsy, blepharitis and/or crusting of lids, blurred vision, conjunctivitis, corneal epithelial abnormality, cortical cataract, decreased night vision, diplopia, itchy eyes or eyelids, nuclear cataract, pannus, papilledema, photophobia, posterior subcapsular cataract, recurrent sties and subepithelial corneal lesions.

Any patient treated with acitretin who is experiencing visual difficulties should discontinue the drug and undergo ophthalmologic evaluation.

➤*Hyperostosis:* In adults receiving long-term treatment with acitretin, appropriate examinations should be periodically performed in view of possible ossification abnormalities. Because the frequency and severity of iatrogenic bony abnormality in adults is low, periodic radiography is only warranted in the presence of symptoms or long-term use of acitretin. If such disorders arise, the continuation of therapy should be discussed with the patient on the basis of a careful risk/benefit analysis. In clinical trials with acitretin, patients were prospectively evaluated for evidence of development or change in bony abnormalities of the vertebral column, knees, and ankles.

➤*Vertebral results:* Of 380 patients treated with acitretin, 15% had preexisting abnormalities of the spine which showed new changes or progression of preexisting findings. Changes included degenerative spurs, anterior bridging of spinal vertebrae, diffuse idiopathic skeletal hyperostosis, ligament calcification and narrowing and destruction of a cervical disc space.

De novo changes (formation of small spurs) were seen in 3 patients after 1½ to 2½ years.

➤*Skeletal appendicular results:* Six of 128 patients treated with acitretin showed abnormalities in the knees and ankles before treatment that progressed during treatment. In 5 patients, these changes involved the formation of additional spurs or enlargement of existing spurs. The sixth patient had degenerative joint disease which worsened. No patients developed spurs de novo. Clinical complaints did not predict radiographic changes.

➤*Lipids and possible cardiovascular effects:* Blood lipid determinations should be performed before acitretin is administered and again at intervals of 1 to 2 weeks until the lipid response to the drug is established, usually within 4 to 8 weeks. In patients receiving acitretin during clinical trials, 66% and 33% experienced elevation in triglycerides and cholesterol, respectively. Decreased high density lipoproteins (HDL) occurred in 40% of patients. These effects of acitretin were generally reversible upon cessation of therapy.

Patients with an increased tendency to develop hypertriglyceridemia included those with disturbances of lipid metabolism, diabetes mellitus, obesity, increased alcohol intake, or a familial history of these conditions. Because of the risk of hypertriglyceridemia, serum lipids must be more closely monitored in high-risk patients and during long-term treatment.

Hypertriglyceridemia and lowered HDL may increase a patient's cardiovascular risk status. Although no causal relationship has been established, there have been postmarketing reports of acute MI or thromboembolic events in patients on acitretin therapy. In addition, elevation of serum triglycerides to greater than 800 mg/dL has been associated with fatal fulminant pancreatitis. Therefore, dietary modifications, reduction in acitretin dose, or drug therapy should be employed to control significant elevations of triglycerides. If, despite these measures, hypertriglyceridemia and low HDL levels persist, the discontinuation of acitretin should be considered.

➤*Hepatotoxicity:* See the Warning box for more information.

➤*Carcinogenesis:* An 80-week carcinogenesis study in mice has been completed with etretinate, the ethyl ester of acitretin. Blood level data obtained during this study demonstrated that etretinate was metabolized to acitretin

ACITRETIN — ORAL

and that blood levels of acitretin exceeded those of etretinate at all times studied. In the etretinate study, an increased incidence of blood vessel tumors (hemangiomas and hemangiosarcomas at several different sites) was noted in male, but not female, mice at doses approximately one-half the maximum recommended human therapeutic dose based on a mg/m^2 comparison.

➤*Fertility impairment:* Chronic toxicity studies in dogs revealed testicular changes (reversible mild to moderate spermatogenic arrest and appearance of multinucleated giant cells) in the highest dosage group (50 then 30 mg/kg/day).

➤*Elderly:* Clinical studies of acitretin did not include sufficient numbers of subjects aged 65 and older to determine whether they respond differently than younger subjects. Other reported clinical experience has not identified differences in responses between the elderly and younger patients. In general, dose selection for an elderly patient should be cautious, usually starting at the low end of the dosing range, reflecting the greater frequency of decreased hepatic, renal, or cardiac function, and of concomitant disease or other drug therapy. A 2-fold increase in acitretin plasma concentrations was seen in healthy elderly subjects compared with young subjects, although the elimination half-life did not change.

➤*Pregnancy:* *Category X.*

Teratogenic – See the Warning box for more information.

Nonteratogenic – In rats dosed at 3 mg/kg/day (approximately one-half the maximum recommended therapeutic dose based on a mg/m^2 comparison), slightly decreased pup survival and delayed incisor eruption were noted. At the next lowest dose tested, 1 mg/kg/day, no treatment-related adverse effects were observed.

➤*Lactation:* Studies on lactating rats have shown that etretinate is excreted in the milk. There is 1 prospective case report where acitretin is reported to be excreted in human milk. Therefore, nursing mothers should not receive acitretin prior to or during nursing because of the potential for serious adverse reactions in nursing infants.

➤*Children:* Safety and efficacy in pediatric patients have not been established. No clinical studies have been conducted in pediatric patients. Ossification of interosseous ligaments and tendons of the extremities, skeletal hyperostoses, decreases in bone mineral density, and premature epiphyseal closure have been reported in children taking other systemic retinoids, including etretinate, a metabolite of acitretin. A causal relationship between these effects and acitretin has not been established. While it is not known that these occurrences are more severe or more frequent in children, there is concern in pediatric patients because of the implications for growth potential.

Precautions

➤*Monitoring:* If significant abnormal laboratory results are obtained, either dosage reduction with careful monitoring or treatment discontinuation is recommended, depending on clinical judgment.

Blood sugar – Some patients receiving retinoids have experienced problems in the control of their blood sugar. In addition, new cases of diabetes have been diagnosed during retinoid therapy, including diabetic ketoacidosis. In diabetics, blood sugar levels should be monitored very carefully.

Lipids – In clinical studies, the incidence of hypertriglyceridemia was 66%, hypercholesterolemia was 33% and that of decreased HDL was 40%. Pretreatment and follow-up measurements should be obtained under fasting conditions. It is recommended that these tests be performed weekly or every other week until the lipid response to acitretin has stabilized.

Liver function tests – Elevations of AST, ALT, or LDH were experienced by approximately 1 in 3 patients treated with acitretin. It is recommended that these tests be performed prior to initiation of acitretin therapy, at 1- to 2-week intervals until stable and thereafter at intervals as clinically indicated. Acitretin is contraindicated in patients with severely impaired liver or kidney function and in patients with chronic abnormally elevated blood lipid values.

➤*Females of reproductive potential:* See the Warning box for more information.

➤*Psychiatric symptoms:* Depression or other psychiatric symptoms such as aggressive feelings or thoughts of self-harm have been reported. These events, including self-injurious behavior, have been reported in patients taking other systemically administered retinoids, as well as in patients taking acitretin. Since other factors may have contributed to these events, it is not known if they are related to acitretin. Patients should be counseled to stop taking acitretin and notify their prescriber immediately if they experience psychiatric symptoms.

➤*Worsening symptoms:* Patients should be advised that a transient worsening of psoriasis is sometimes seen during the initial treatment period. Patients should be advised that they may have to wait 2 to 3 months before they get the full benefit of acitretin, although some patients may achieve significant improvements within the first 8 weeks of treatment as demonstrated in clinical trials.

➤*Contact lenses:* Patients should be advised that they may experience decreased tolerance to contact lenses during the treatment period and sometimes after treatment has stopped.

➤*Blood donation:* Patients should not donate blood during and for at least 3 years following therapy because acitretin can cause birth defects and women of childbearing potential must not receive blood from patients being treated with acitretin.

➤*Photosensitivity:* Patients should avoid the use of sun lamps and excessive exposure to sunlight (nonmedical UV exposure) because the effects of UV light are enhanced by retinoids.

➤*Phototherapy:* Significantly lower doses of phototherapy are required when acitretin is used because acitretin-induced effects on the stratum corneum can increase the risk of erythema (burning).

➤*Special risk:* Caution is advised in patients with severely impaired liver or kidney function.

➤*Hazardous tasks:* Decreased night vision has been reported with acitretin therapy. Patients should be advised of this potential problem and warned to be cautious when driving or operating any vehicle at night. Visual problems should be carefully monitored.

Drug Interactions

Acitretin Drug Interactions

Precipitant drug	Object drug*		Description
Acitretin	Glyburide	↔	Possible potentiation of blood glucose lowering effect of glyburide in 3 of 7 subjects. Careful supervision is recommended.
Acitretin	Methotrexate	↑	Increased risk of hepatitis with combined use. Concomitant use is contraindicated.
Acitretin	Oral contraceptives (progestin only)	↓	It has been established that acitretin interferes with the contraceptive effect of microdosed progestin "minipill" preparations. It is not known if there is an interaction with combined oral contraceptives.
Acitretin	Phenytoin	↑	The protein binding of phenytoin may be decreased.
Ethanol	Acitretin	↑	Etretinate formation has occurred with concomitant ingestion of alcohol and acitretin. Etretinate has a much longer half-life than acitretin (≈ 120 days) which appears to be a result of storage in adipose tissue (see Pharmacokinetics).
Acitretin	Tetracyclines	↑	Concomitant use is contraindicated due to the increased risk for increased intracranial pressure.
Tetracyclines	Acitretin		
Acitretin	Vitamin A and oral retinoids	↑	Avoid coadministration because of the increased risk of hypervitaminosis A.
Vitamin A and oral retinoids	Acitretin		

* ↑ = Object drug increased. ↓ = Object drug decreased.
↔ = Undetermined clinical effect.

Adverse Reactions

Hypervitaminosis A produces a wide spectrum of signs and symptoms primarily of the mucocutaneous, musculoskeletal, hepatic, neuropsychiatric, and central nervous systems. Many of the clinical adverse reactions reported to date with acitretin administration resemble those of the hypervitaminosis A syndrome.

➤*Adverse events/postmarketing reports:* In addition to the events listed in the tables for the clinical trials, the following adverse events have been identified during postapproval use of acitretin. Because these events are reported voluntarily from a population of uncertain size, it is not always possible to reliably estimate their frequency or establish a causal relationship to drug exposure.

Cardiovascular – Acute myocardial infarction, thromboembolism, stroke

CNS – Myopathy with peripheral neuropathy has been reported during acitretin therapy. Both conditions improved with discontinuation of the drug.

Dermatologic – Thinning of the skin, skin fragility and scaling may occur all over the body, particularly on the palms and soles; nail fragility is frequently observed.

GU – Vulvo-vaginitis due to *Candida albicans.*

Psychiatric – Aggressive feelings or suicidal thoughts have been reported. These events, including self-injurious behavior, have been reported in patients taking other systemically administered retinoids, as well as in patients taking acitretin. Since other factors may have contributed to these events, it is not known if they are related to acitretin.

➤*Clinical trials:* During clinical trials with acitretin, 513/525 (98%) of patients reported a total of 3545 adverse events. One-hundred sixteen (22%) patients left studies prematurely, primarily because of adverse experiences involving the mucous membranes and skin. Three (3) patients died. Two of the deaths were not drug related (pancreatic adenocarcinoma and lung cancer); the other patient died of an acute MI, considered remotely related to drug therapy.

In clinical trials, acitretin has been associated with elevations in liver function test results or triglyceride levels and hepatitis.

ACITRETIN — ORAL

Adverse Events Frequently Reported During Clinical Trials; Percent of Patients Reporting (N = 525)

Body system	> 75%	50% to 75%	25% to 50%	10% to 25%
CNS				
Rigors				✓
Dermatologic				
Alopecia		✓		
Dry skin			✓	
Erythematous rash				✓
Hyperesthesia				✓
Nail disorder			✓	
Paresthesia				✓
Paronychia				✓
Pruritus			✓	
Skin atrophy				✓
Skin peeling		✓		
Sticky skin				✓
Mucous membranes				
Cheilitis	✓			
Dry mouth				✓
Epistaxis				✓
Rhinitis			✓	
Musculoskeletal				
Arthralgia				✓
Spinal hyperostosis (progression of existing lesions)				✓
Ophthalmic				
Xerophthalmia				✓

Adverse Events Less Frequently Reported During Clinical Trials (Some of Which May Bear No Relationship to Therapy); Percent of Patients Reporting (N = 525)

Body system	1% to 10%	< 1%
Cardiovascular		
Chest pain		✓
Cyanosis		✓
Flushing	✓	
Increased bleeding time		✓
Intermittent claudication		✓
Peripheral ischemia		✓
CNS (also see psychiatric)		
Abnormal gait		✓
Headache	✓	
Migraine		✓
Neuritis		✓
Pseudotumor cerebri (intracranial hypertension)		✓
Pain	✓	
Dermatologic		
Abnormal skin odor	✓	
Acne		✓
Abnormal hair texture	✓	
Breast pain		✓
Bullous eruption	✓	
Cyst		✓
Cold/clammy skin	✓	
Dermatitis	✓	
Eczema		✓
Fungal infection		✓
Furunculosis		✓
Hair discoloration		✓
Herpes simplex		✓
Hyperkeratosis		✓
Hypertrichosis		✓
Hypoesthesia		✓
Impaired healing		✓
Increased sweating	✓	
Infection	✓	
Otitis externa		✓
Otitis media		✓
Photosensitivity reaction		✓
Psoriasis aggravated		✓
Psoriasiform rash	✓	
Purpura	✓	
Pyogenic granuloma	✓	
Rash	✓	
Seborrhea	✓	
Skin fissures	✓	
Skin ulceration	✓	
Sunburn	✓	
Scleroderma		✓
Skin nodule		✓
Skin hypertrophy		✓
Skin disorder		✓
Skin irritation		✓
Sweat gland disorder		✓
Urticaria		✓
Verrucae		✓
GI		
Abdominal pain	✓	
Constipation		✓
Diarrhea	✓	
Dyspepsia		✓
Esophagitis		✓
Gastritis		✓
Gastroenteritis		✓
Glossitis		✓
Hemorrhoids		✓
Melena		✓
Nausea		✓
Tenesmus		✓
Tongue disorder		✓
Tongue ulceration		✓
GU		
Abnormal urine		✓
Dysuria		✓
Penis disorder		✓
Hepatic		
Hepatic function abnormal		✓
Hepatitis		✓
Jaundice		✓
Mucous membranes		
Altered saliva		✓
Anal disorder		✓
Gingival bleeding	✓	
Gingivitis	✓	
Gum hyperplasia		✓
Hemorrhage		✓
Increased saliva		✓
Pharyngitis		✓
Stomatitis	✓	
Thirst	✓	
Ulcerative stomatitis	✓	

ACITRETIN — ORAL

Adverse Events Less Frequently Reported During Clinical Trials (Some of Which May Bear No Relationship to Therapy); Percent of Patients Reporting (N = 525)		
Body system	1% to 10%	< 1%
Musculoskeletal		
Arthritis	✓	
Arthrosis	✓	
Back pain	✓	
Bone disorder		✓
Hypertonia	✓	
Myalgia	✓	
Olecranon bursitis		✓
Osteodynia	✓	
Peripheral joint hyperostosis (progression of existing lesions)	✓	
Spinal hyperostosis (new lesions)		✓
Tendonitis		✓
Ophthalmic		
Abnormal/blurred vision	✓	
Abnormal lacrimation		✓
Blepharitis	✓	
Chalazion		✓
Conjunctival hemorrhage		✓
Conjunctivitis/irritation	✓	
Corneal epithelial abnormality	✓	
Corneal ulceration		✓
Decreased night vision/night blindness	✓	
Diplopia		✓
Ectropion		✓
Eye abnormality	✓	
Eye pain	✓	
Itchy eyes and lids		✓
Papilledema		✓
Photophobia	✓	
Recurrent sties		✓
Subepithelial corneal lesions		✓
Psychiatric		
Anxiety		✓
Depression	✓	
Dysphonia		✓
Insomnia	✓	
Libido decreased		✓
Nervousness		✓
Somnolence		✓
Reproductive		
Atrophic vaginitis		✓
Leukorrhea		✓
Respiratory		
Coughing		✓
Increased sputum	✓	✓
Laryngitis		✓
Sinusitis	✓	
Special senses		
Ceruminosis		✓
Deafness		✓
Earache	✓	
Taste loss	✓	
Taste perversion	✓	
Tinnitus	✓	
Miscellaneous		
Alcohol tolerance		✓
Anorexia	✓	
Dizziness		✓
Edema	✓	
Fatigue	✓	
Fever		✓
Hot flashes	✓	
Increased appetite	✓	
Influenza-like symptoms		✓
Malaise		✓
Moniliasis		✓
Muscle weakness		✓
Weight increase		✓

Lab test abnormalities – Acitretin therapy induces changes in liver function tests in a significant number of patients. Elevations of AST, ALT or LDH were experienced by approximately 1 in 3 patients treated with acitretin. In most patients, elevations were slight to moderate and returned to normal either during continuation of therapy or after cessation of treatment. In patients receiving acitretin during clinical trials, 66% and 33% experienced elevation in triglycerides and cholesterol, respectively. Decreased high density lipoproteins (HDL) occurred in 40%. Transient, usually reversible elevations of alkaline phosphatase have been observed.

Abnormal Laboratory Test Results Reported During Clinical Trials Percent of Patients Reporting				
Body system	50% to 75%	25% to 50%	10% to 25%	1% to 10%
Electrolytes				
Increased phosphorus			✓	
Decreased phosphorus				✓
Increased potassium			✓	
Decreased potassium				✓
Increased sodium			✓	
Decreased sodium				✓
Increased and decreased magnesium			✓	
Increased and decreased calcium				✓
Increased and decreased chloride				✓
GU				
Acetonuria			✓	
Glycosuria				✓
Hematuria			✓	
Proteinuria				✓
RBC in urine			✓	
WBC in urine		✓		
Hematologic				
Increased reticulocytes		✓		
Decreased hematocrit			✓	
Increased bands				✓
Increased basophils				✓
Decreased hemoglobin			✓	
Increased eosinophils				✓

ACITRETIN — ORAL

Abnormal Laboratory Test Results Reported During Clinical Trials Percent of Patients Reporting				
Body system	50% to 75%	25% to 50%	10% to 25%	1% to 10%
Decreased WBC			✓	
Increased haptoglobin			✓	
Increased hematocrit				✓
Increased hemoglobin				✓
Increased neutrophils			✓	
Increased WBC			✓	
Increased lymphocytes				✓
Increased monocytes				✓
Decreased haptoglobin				✓
Decreased lymphocytes				✓
Decreased neutrophils				✓
Decreased reticulocytes				✓
Increased or decreased platelets				✓
Increased or decreased RBC				✓
Hepatic				
Increased alkaline phosphatase			✓	
Increased cholesterol		✓		
Increased globulin				✓
Increased direct bilirubin			✓	
Increased total bilirubin				✓
Increased LDH		✓		
Increased AST		✓		
Increased GGTP			✓	
Increased total protein				✓
Increased ALT		✓		
Increased and decreased serum albumin				✓
Decreased HDL cholesterol		✓		
Renal				
Increased BUN				✓
Increased creatinine				✓
Increased uric acid			✓	
Miscellaneous				
Increased CPK		✓		
Decreased fasting blood sugar			✓	
Increased and decreased iron				✓
Increased triglycerides	✓			
Increased fasting blood sugar		✓		
Increased high occult blood			✓	

Overdosage

➤*Symptoms:* Symptoms of overdose are identical to acute hypervitaminosis A (ie, headache and vertigo). The acute oral toxicity (LD_{50}) of acitretin in both mice and rats was greater than 4000 mg/kg.

In one reported case of overdose, a 32-year-old male with Darier's disease took 21 × 25 mg capsules (525 mg single dose). He vomited several hours later but experienced no other ill effects.

➤*Treatment:* In the event of acute overdosage, acitretin must be withdrawn at once.

All female patients of childbearing potential who have taken an overdose of acitretin must have a pregnancy test at the time of overdose and be counseled regarding birth defects and contraceptive use for at least 3 years' duration after the overdose.

Patient Information

➤*Females of reproductive potential:* Acitretin can cause severe birth defects. Female patients must not be pregnant when acitretin therapy is initiated, they must not become pregnant while taking acitretin, and for at least 3 years after stopping acitretin, so that the drug can be eliminated to below a blood concentration that would be associated with an increased incidence of birth defects. Because this threshold has not been established for acitretin in humans and because elimination rates vary among patients, the duration of posttherapy contraception to achieve adequate elimination cannot be calculated precisely.

Females of reproductive potential should also be advised that they must not ingest beverages or products containing ethanol while taking acitretin and for 2 months after acitretin treatment has been discontinued. This allows for elimination of the acitretin which can be converted to etretinate in the presence of alcohol.

Female patients should be advised that any method of birth control can fail, including tubal ligation, and that microdosed progestin "minipill" preparations are not recommended for use with acitretin. Data from 1 patient who received a very low-dosed progestin contraceptive (levonorgestrel 0.03 mg) had a significant increase of the progesterone level after 3 menstrual cycles during acitretin treatment.

Female patients should sign a consent form prior to beginning acitretin therapy.

➤*All patients:* Depression or other psychiatric symptoms such as aggressive feelings or thoughts of self-harm have been reported. These events, including self-injurious behavior, have been reported in patients taking other systemically administered retinoids, as well as in patients taking acitretin. Since other factors may have contributed to these events, it is not known if they are related to acitretin. Patients should be counseled to stop taking acitretin and notify their prescriber immediately if they experience psychiatric symptoms.

Patients should be advised that a transient worsening of psoriasis is sometimes seen during the initial treatment period. Patients should be advised that they may have to wait 2 to 3 months before they get the full benefit of acitretin, although some patients may achieve significant improvements within the first 8 weeks of treatment as demonstrated in clinical trials.

Patients should be advised that they may experience decreased tolerance to contact lenses during the treatment period and sometimes after treatment has stopped.

Patients should not donate blood during and for at least 3 years following therapy because acitretin can cause birth defects and women of childbearing potential must not receive blood from patients being treated with acitretin.

Because of the relationship of acitretin to vitamin A, patients should be advised against taking vitamin A supplements in excess of minimum recommended daily allowances to avoid possible additive toxic effects.

ACITRETIN — ORAL

Patients should avoid the use of sun lamps and excessive exposure to sunlight (nonmedical UV exposure) because the effects of UV light are enhanced by retinoids.

Patients should be advised that they must not give their acitretin capsules to any other person.

ALITRETINOIN

Rx	**Panretin** (Ligand)	**Gel:** 0.1%	Dehydrated alcohol. In 60 g tubes.

ALITRETINOIN — TOPICAL

Indications

➤*Kaposi's sarcoma (KS) cutaneous lesions:* Topical treatment of cutaneous lesions in patients with AIDS-related KS.

➤*Unlabeled uses:* Treatment of refractory cutaneous T-cell lymphoma.

Administration and Dosage

➤*Approved by the FDA:* February 2, 1999.

Do not use occlusive dressings with alitretinoin gel.

Initially apply 2 times/day to cutaneous KS lesions. The application frequency can be gradually increased to 3 or 4 times/day, according to individual lesion tolerance. If application site toxicity occurs, the application frequency can be reduced. If severe irritation occurs, application of drug can be discontinued for a few days until the symptoms subside.

Apply sufficient gel to cover the lesion with a generous coating. Allow the gel to dry for 3 to 5 minutes before covering with clothing. Because unaffected skin may become irritated, avoid application of the gel to healthy skin surrounding the lesions. In addition, do not apply the gel on or near mucosal surfaces of the body.

A response of KS lesions may be seen as soon as 2 weeks after initiation of therapy, but most patients require longer application. With continued application, further benefit may be attained. Some patients have required over 14 weeks to respond. In clinical trials, alitretinoin gel was applied for up to 96 weeks. Continue alitretinoin gel as long as the patient is deriving benefit.

Actions

➤*Pharmacology:* Alitretinoin (9-cis-retinoic acid) is a naturally occurring endogenous retinoid that binds to and activates all known intracellular retinoid receptor subtypes (RARα, RARβ, RARγ, RXRα, RXRβ, and RXRγ). Once activated, these receptors function as transcription factors that regulate the expression of genes that control the process of cellular differentiation and proliferation in healthy and neoplastic cells. Alitretinoin inhibits the growth of KS cells in vitro.

➤*Pharmacokinetics:* There is indirect evidence that absorption of 9-cis-retinoic acid is not extensive. Plasma concentrations were evaluated during clinical studies in patients with cutaneous lesions of AIDS-related KS after repeated multiple daily dose application of alitretinoin gel for up to 60 weeks. The range of 9-cis-retinoic acid plasma concentrations in these patients was similar to the range of circulating, naturally occurring 9-cis-retinoic acid plasma concentrations in untreated healthy volunteers.

Although there are no detectable plasma concentrations of 9-cis-retinoic acid metabolites after topical application of alitretinoin gel, in vitro studies indicate that the drug is metabolized to 4-hydroxy-9-cis-retinoic acid and 4-oxo-9-cis-retinoic acid by CYP 2C9, 3A4, 1A1, and 1A2 enzymes. In vivo, 4-oxo-9-cis-retinoic acid is the major circulating metabolite following oral administration of 9-cis-retinoic acid.

Contraindications

Hypersensitivity to retinoids or to any of the ingredients of the product; when systemic anti-KS therapy is required (eg, more than 10 new KS lesions in the prior month, symptomatic lymphedema, symptomatic pulmonary KS, symptomatic visceral involvement).

Warnings

➤*Systemic therapy:* Alitretinoin gel is not a systemic therapy; therefore, it cannot treat visceral KS, nor prevent the development of new KS lesions where it has not been applied. Alitretinoin is not indicated when systemic anti-KS therapy is required (see Contraindications). There is no experience to date using alitretinoin gel with systemic anti-KS treatment.

➤*Pregnancy: Category D.* Alitretinoin gel could cause fetal harm if significant absorption were to occur in a pregnant woman. 9-cis-retinoic-acid is teratogenic in rabbits and mice. An increased incidence of fused sternebrae, and limb and craniofacial defects occurred in rabbits given oral doses of 0.5 mg/kg/day (about 5 times the estimated daily human topical dose on a mg/m^2 basis) during the period of organogenesis. Oral 9-cis-retinoic acid also was embryocidal, as indicated by early resorptions and postimplantation loss when it was given to rabbits during the period of organogenesis at doses of 1.5 mg/kg/day and to rats at doses of 5 mg/kg/day. It is not known whether topical alitretinoin gel can modulate endogenous 9-cis-retinoic acid levels in a pregnant woman nor whether systemic exposure is increased by application to ulcerated lesions or by duration of treatment. There are no adequate and well-controlled studies in pregnant women. If alitretinoin gel is used during pregnancy, or if the patient becomes pregnant while taking the drug, apprise the patient of the potential hazard to the fetus. Advise women of childbearing potential to avoid becoming pregnant.

➤*Lactation:* It is not known whether alitretinoin or its metabolites are excreted in breast milk. Because of the potential for adverse reactions from alitretinoin gel in nursing infants, mothers should discontinue nursing prior to using the drug.

➤*Children:* Safety and efficacy in children have not been established.

Precautions

➤*Response:* In the clinical trials, responses were seen as early as 2 weeks; however, most patients required 4 to 8 weeks of treatment, and some patients did not experience significant improvement until 14 weeks or more of treatment. The cumulative percentage of patients who achieved a response was less than 1% at 2 weeks, 10% at 4 weeks, and 28% at 8 weeks.

➤*Cutaneous T-cell lymphoma:* Alitretinoin gel is indicated for topical treatment of KS. Patients with cutaneous T-cell lymphoma were less tolerant of topical alitretinoin gel; 5 of 7 patients had 6 episodes of treatment-limiting toxicities (grade 3 dermal irritation) with alitretinoin gel (0.01% or 0.05%).

➤*Photosensitivity:* Retinoids as a class have been associated with photosensitivity. There were no reports of photosensitivity associated with the use of alitretinoin gel in clinical studies. Nonetheless, because in vitro data indicate that 9-cis-retinoic acid may have a weak photosensitizing effect, advise patients to minimize exposure of treated areas to sunlight and sunlamps during the use of alitretinoin gel.

Drug Interactions

➤*DEET:* Do not use products that contain DEET (N,N-diethyl-m-toluamide), a common component of insect repellent products, while using alitretinoin gel. Animal toxicology studies showed increased DEET toxicity when DEET was included as part of the formulation.

Adverse Reactions

Adverse events associated with the use of alitretinoin gel in patients with AIDS-related KS occurred almost exclusively at the site of application. The dermal toxicity begins as erythema; with continued application, erythema may increase and edema may develop. Dermal toxicity may become treatment-limiting, with intense erythema, edema, and vesiculation. Adverse events are usually mild to moderate in severity; they led to withdrawal from the study in only 7% of the patients. Severe local (application site) skin adverse events occurred in about 10% of patients in the US study (vs 0% in the control group).

Alitretinoin Application Site Reactions (≥ 5%)

	Study 1		Study 2	
Adverse reaction	Alitretinoin gel (n = 134)	Vehicle gel (n = 134)	Alitretinoin gel (n = 36)	Vehicle gel (n = 46)
Rash (eg, erythema, scaling, irritation, redness, rash, dermatitis)	77	11	25	4
Pain (eg, burning, pain)	34	7	0	4
Pruritus (eg, itching)	11	4	8	4
Exfoliative dermatitis (eg, flaking, peeling, desquamation, exfoliation)	9	2	3	0
Skin disorder (eg, excoriation, cracking, scabbing, crusting, drainage, eschar, fissure, oozing)	8	1	0	0
Paresthesia (eg, stinging, tingling)	3	0	22	7
Edema (eg, swelling, inflammation)	8	3	3	0

Overdosage

Systemic toxicity following acute overdosage with topical application of alitretinoin gel is unlikely because of limited systemic plasma levels observed with normal therapeutic doses. There is no specific antidote for overdosage.

Patient Information

Advise patients against applying gel on or near mucosal surfaces of the body such as eyes, nostrils, mouth, lips, vagina, tip of the penis, rectum, or anus.

Advise patients against using insect repellents containing DEET or other products containing DEET while using alitretinoin.

Instruct patients to keep out of reach of children.

Product contains alcohol; keep away from open flame.

Do not administer to patients who are pregnant or breastfeeding. Instruct patients to take precautions to avoid becoming pregnant while using altretinoin. If the patient is pregant, thinking of becoming pregnant, or breastfeeding, advise them to speak with their health care provider for more information.

ALITRETINOIN — TOPICAL

Inform patients that KS lesions can appear and affect other parts of their body, including internal organs (eg, lungs and intestines). Advise patients to regularly consult their health care provider about the status of their KS disease, especially if they note changes.

Alitretinoin does not treat lung or intestinal KS.

Alitretinoin does not prevent the appearance of new KS lesions or the increased growth of KS lesions not treated with alitretinoin.

Alitretinoin does not treat extremity swelling associated with KS.

Instruct patients to avoid applying the gel to areas of healthy skin around a KS lesion. Exposure of healthy skin to alitretinoin may cause unnecessary irritation or redness.

Instruct patients to avoid showering, bathing, or swimming for at least 3 hours after any application, if possible.

Instruct patients to avoid covering the KS lesions treated with gel with any bandage or material other than loose clothing.

Instruct patients to avoid prolonged exposure of the treated area to sunlight or other ultraviolet light (eg, tanning lamps).

Instruct patients to avoid the use of other topical products on treated KS lesions. Mineral oil may be used between alitretinoin applications in order to help prevent excessive dryness or itching. Mineral oil should not be applied for at least 2 hours before or after the application of alitretinoin.

Instruct patients to avoid scratching the treated areas.

Instruct patients to always use the cap to close the tube tightly after each use.

TAZAROTENE

Rx	**Tazorac** (Allergan)	**Cream:** 0.05%	1% benzyl alcohol, EDTA, medium chain triglycerides, mineral oil. In 15, 30, and 60 g.
Rx	**Avage** (Allergan)	**Cream:** 0.1%	1% benzyl alcohol, EDTA, medium chain triglycerides, mineral oil. In 15 and 30 g.
Rx	**Tazorac** (Allergan)		1% benzyl alcohol, EDTA, medium chain triglycerides, mineral oil. In 15, 30, and 60 g.
Rx	**Tazorac** (Allergan)	**Gel:** 0.05%	1% benzyl alcohol, EDTA. In 30 and 100 g.
		0.1%	1% benzyl alcohol, EDTA. In 30 and 100 g.

TAZAROTENE — TOPICAL

Indications

➤*Tazorac cream:*

Acne – Topical treatment of patients with acne vulgaris (0.1% only).

Psoriasis – For the topical treatment of patients with plaque psoriasis.

➤*Tazorac gel:*

Acne – Topical treatment of patients with facial acne vulgaris of mild to moderate severity (0.1% only).

Psoriasis – Topical treatment of patients with stable plaque psoriasis of up to 20% body surface area involvement.

The efficacy of tazarotene in the treatment of acne previously treated with other retinoids or resistant to oral antibiotics has not been established.

➤*Avage:*

Wrinkling, hyper- and hypopigmentation, lentigines – As an adjunctive agent for use in the mitigation (palliation) of facial fine wrinkling, facial mottled hyper- and hypopigmentation, and benign facial lentigines in patients who use comprehensive skin care and sunlight avoidance programs. This product does not eliminate or prevent wrinkles, repair sun-damaged skin, reverse photoaging, or restore more youthful or younger skin.

- *Avage* has not demonstrated a mitigating effect on significant signs of chronic sunlight exposure such as coarse or deep wrinkling, tactile roughness, telangiectasia, skin laxity, keratinocytic atypia, melanocytic atypia, or dermal elastosis.
- *Avage* should be used under medical supervision as an adjunct to a comprehensive skin care and sunlight avoidance program that includes the use of effective sunscreens (minimum SPF 15) and protective clothing.
- Neither the safety nor the effectiveness of *Avage* for the prevention or treatment of actinic keratoses, skin neoplasms, or lentigo maligna has been established.
- Neither the safety nor the efficacy of using *Avage* daily for greater than 52 weeks has been established, and daily use beyond 52 weeks has not been systematically and histologically investigated in adequate and well-controlled trials.

Administration and Dosage

➤*Approved by the FDA:* June 13, 1997.

For topical use only. Not for ophthalmic, oral, or intravaginal use.

Application may cause excessive irritation in the skin of certain sensitive individuals. In cases where it has been necessary to temporarily discontinue therapy or where the dosing has been reduced to a lower concentration (in patients with psoriasis) or to an interval the patient can tolerate, therapy can be resumed, or the drug concentration or frequency of application can be increased as the patient becomes able to tolerate the treatment. Closely monitor frequency of application by careful observation of the clinical therapeutic response and skin tolerance. Efficacy has not been established for less than once daily dosing frequencies

➤*Acne:* Cleanse the face gently. After the skin is dry, apply a thin film of tazarotene (2 mg/cm^2) once a day in the evening to the skin where acne lesions appear. Use enough to cover the entire affected area. Tazarotene was investigated for up to 12 weeks during clinical trials for acne.

➤*Psoriasis:* Apply tazarotene once a day in the evening to psoriatic lesions, using enough (2 mg/cm^2) to cover only the lesion with a thin film. The gel should cover no more than 20% of body surface area. If a bath or shower is taken prior to application, dry the skin before applying. If emollients are used, apply them at least 1 hour before *Tazorac* cream. Because unaffected skin may be more susceptible to irritation, carefully avoid application of tazarotene to these areas. It is recommended that treatment start with the 0.05% cream with strength increase to 0.1% if tolerated and medically indicated. Tazarotene gel was investigated for up to 12 months during clinical trials for psoriasis.

➤*Wrinkling, hyper- and hypopigmentation, lentigines:* Apply a pea-sized amount once a day at bedtime to lightly cover the entire face including the eyelids if desired. Facial moisturizers may be used as frequently as desired. Remove any makeup before applying the cream to the face. If the face is washed or a bath or shower is taken prior to application, the skin should be dry before applying the cream. If emollients or moisturizers are used, they can be applied before or after application of tazarotene cream, ensuring that the first cream or lotion has absorbed into the skin and has dried completely. Closely monitor frequency of application by careful observation of the clinical therapeutic response and skin tolerance. If the frequency of dosing is reduced, it should be noted that efficacy at a reduced frequency of application has not been established. The duration of the mitigating effects on facial fine wrinkling, mottled hypo- and hyperpigmentation, and benign facial lentigines following discontinuation has not been studied.

➤*Storage / Stability:*

Tazorac and Avage cream – Store at 25°C (77°F). Excursions permitted from -5° to 30°C (23° to 86°F).

Gel – Tazarotene gel should be stored at 25°C (77°F). Excursion permitted to 15° to 30°C (59° to 86°F).

Actions

➤*Pharmacology:* Tazarotene is a retinoid prodrug that is converted to its active form, tazarotenic acid, by rapid de-esterification in most biological systems. Tazarotenic acid binds to all 3 members of the retinoic acid receptor (RAR) family (RARα, RARβ and RARγ), but shows relative selectivity for RARβ and RARγ and may modify gene expression. The clinical significance of these findings is unknown.

The mechanism of tazarotene action is not defined. Tazarotene inhibited corneocyte accumulation in rhino mouse skin and cross-linked envelope formation in cultured human keratinocytes. Topical tazarotene blocks induction of mouse epidermal ornithine decarboxylase (ODC) activity, which is associated with cell proliferation and hyperplasia. In cell culture and in vitro models of skin, tazarotene suppresses expression of MRP8, a marker of inflammation present in the epidermis of psoriasis subjects at high levels. In human keratinocyte cultures, it inhibits cornified envelope formation, whose build-up is an element of psoriatic scale. Tazarotene also induces the expression of a gene that may be a growth suppressor in human keratinocytes and that may inhibit epidermal hyperproliferation in treated plaques. The clinical significance of these findings is unknown.

➤*Pharmacokinetics:*

Absorption / Distribution – Following topical application, tazarotene undergoes esterase hydrolysis to form its active metabolite, tazarotinic acid. Little parent compound can be detected in the plasma. Tazarotenic acid is highly bound to plasma proteins (more than 99%).

Cream: In a multiple dose study with a once-daily dose for 14 consecutive days in 9 psoriatic patients, measured doses of tazarotene 0.1% cream were applied to involved skin without occlusion. The C_{max} of tazarotenic acid was 2.31 ng/mL occurring 8 hours after the final dose, and the $AUC_{0\text{-}24h}$ was 31.2 ng•h/mL on day 15 in the 5 patients who were administered clinical doses of 2 mg cream/cm^2.

Tazarotene cream 0.1% was applied once daily to the face (N = 8) or to 15% of body surface area (N = 10) of female patients with moderate to severe acne vulgaris. The mean C_{max} and AUC values of tazarotenic acid peaked at day 15 for both dosing groups during a 29-day treatment period. Mean C_{max} and $AUC_{0\text{-}24h}$ values of tazarotenic acid from patients in the 15% body surface area dosing group were more than 10 times higher than those from patients in the face-only dosing group. In the face-only group, the C_{max} and $AUC_{0\text{-}24h}$ of tazarotenic acid on day 15 were 0.1 ng/mL and 1.54 ng•h/mL, respectively, whereas in the 15% body surface area dosing group, the C_{max} and $AUC_{0\text{-}24h}$ of tazarotenic acid on day 15 were 1.2 ng/mL and 17.01 ng•h/mL, respectively. The steady state pharmacokinetics of tazarotenic acid had been reached by day 8 in the face-only and by day 15 in the 15% body surface area dosing groups.

Tazarotene cream 0.1% was topically applied once daily to the face or to 15% of body surface area over 4 weeks in patients with fine wrinkling and mottled hyperpigmentation. In the "face-only" dosing group, the maximum average C_{max} and $AUC_{0\text{-}24h}$ values of tazarotenic acid occurred on day 15 with C_{max} and $AUC_{0\text{-}24h}$ of tazarotenic acid being 0.236 ng/mL and 2.44 ng•h/mL, respectively. The mean C_{max} and $AUC_{0\text{-}24h}$ values of tazarotenic acid from patients in the 15% body surface area dosing group were approximately 10 times higher than those from patients in the face-only dosing group. The single highest C_{max} throughout the study period was 3.43 ng/mL on day 29 from patients in the 15% body surface area dosing group.

Gel: Studies following a single, topical dose of tazarotene determined that systemic absorption of the total dose was less than 1% without occlusion in psoriatic patients and approximately 5% under occlusion in healthy patients. Another study found the C_{max} and AUC for the 0.1% gel to be 40% higher than the 0.05% gel. Systemic absorption of 2 mg/cm^2 doses of 0.1% gel applied topically without occlusion was less than 1% after 7 days of therapy when applied to 20% of the total body surface area (BSA) of healthy patients and was about 15% after 14 days when applied to approximately 13% of total BSA in psoriatic patients. The results of these in vivo studies refer to the active metabolite only.

An in vitro percutaneous absorption study indicated that about 4% to 5% of the applied dose was in the stratum corneum (tazarotene:metabolite, 5:1) and 2% to 4% was in the viable epidermis-dermis layer (tazarotene:metabolite, 2:1) 24 hours after topical application of the gel.

Metabolism / Excretion – The half-life of the metabolite following topical application of tazarotene is approximately 18 hours and is similar among

TAZAROTENE — TOPICAL

healthy and psoriatic patients. The parent drug and metabolite are further metabolized and eliminated through urinary and fecal pathways.

Contraindications

Pregnancy; hypersensitivity to any components of the product.

Warnings

➤*Carcinogenesis:* In evaluation of photocarcinogenicity, median time to onset of tumors was decreased and the number of tumors increased in hairless mice following chronic topical dosing with intercurrent exposure to ultraviolet radiation at tazarotene concentrations of 0.001%, 0.005%, and 0.01% for up to 40 weeks.

➤*Fertility impairment:* There was a significant decrease in the number of estrous stages and an increase in developmental effects at oral doses up to 2 mg/kg/day. That dose produced an $AUC_{0\text{-}24h}$ that was 6.7 times the maximum $AUC_{0\text{-}24h}$ in patients treated with 2 mg/cm^2 of tazarotene cream 0.1% over 15% body surface area for signs of fine wrinkling and mottled hyperpigmentation.

➤*Pregnancy:* *Category X.* In rabbits, topical tazarotene caused retinoid malformations, including spina bifida, hydrocephaly, and heart anomalies.

As with other retinoids, when tazarotene was given orally to experimental animals, developmental delays were seen in rats, and teratogenic effects and postimplantation loss were observed in rats and rabbits at doses producing 2.1 and 52 times, respectively, the maximum $AUC_{0\text{-}24h}$ in patients treated with 2 mg/cm^2 of tazarotene cream 0.1% over 15% body surface area for fine wrinkling and mottled hyperpigmentation.

In a study of the effect of oral tazarotene on fertility and early embryonic development in rats, decreased number of implantation sites, decreased litter size, decreased number of live fetuses, and decreased fetal body weights, all classic developmental effects of retinoids, were observed when female rats were administered 2 mg/kg/day from 15 days before mating through gestation day 7. A low incidence of retinoid-related malformations at that dose were reported to be related to treatment. That dose produced an $AUC_{0\text{-}24h}$ that was 6.7 times the maximum $AUC_{0\text{-}24h}$ in patients treated with 2 mg/cm^2 of tazarotene cream 0.1% over 15% body surface area for signs of fine wrinkling and mottled hyperpigmentation.

Tazarotene is contraindicated in women who are or may become pregnant. If this drug is used during pregnancy or if the patient becomes pregnant while taking this drug, discontinue treatment and apprise the patient of the potential hazard to the fetus. Warn women of childbearing potential of the potential risk and to use adequate birth-control measures when using tazarotene. Consider the possibility that a woman of childbearing potential is pregnant at the time of institution of therapy. Obtain a negative result for a pregnancy test having a sensitivity down to at least 50 mIU/mL for human chorionic gonadotropin (hCG) within 2 weeks prior to tazarotene therapy, which should begin during a normal menstrual period.

➤*Lactation:* Tazarotene is excreted in breast milk of rats. It is not known whether this drug is excreted in human milk. Exercise caution when tazarotene is administered to a breast-feeding woman.

➤*Children:*

Tazorac – The safety and efficacy of tazarotene cream have not been established in patients with psoriasis under the age of 18 years or in patients with acne under the age of 12 years.

Avage – The safety and efficacy of tazarotene cream have not been established in patients under the age of 17 years with facial fine wrinkling, facial mottled hypo- and hyperpigmentation, and benign facial lentigines.

Gel – The safety and efficacy of tazarotene have not been established in pediatric patients under the age of 12 years.

Precautions

➤*For external use only:* Apply only to the affected areas. Avoid contact with eyes, eyelids (*Tazorac* only), and mouth. If contact with the eyes occurs, rinse thoroughly with water. The safety of use of tazarotene gel over more than 20% of body surface area has not been established in psoriasis or acne.

➤*Eczematous skin:* Do not use retinoids on eczematous skin, as they may cause severe irritation.

➤*Dermatologic medications and cosmetics:* Avoid those medications and cosmetics that have a strong drying effect. It also is advisable to "rest" a patient's skin until the effects of such preparations subside before use of tazarotene is begun

➤*Photosensitizers (eg, thiazides, tetracyclines, fluoroquinolones, phenothiazines, sulfonamides):* Administer with caution if the patient is also taking drugs known to be photosensitizers because of the increased possibility of augmented photosensitivity.

➤*Discontinue:* If pruritus, burning, skin redness, or peeling is excessive, discontinue until the integrity of the skin is restored, or reduce the dosing to an interval the patient can tolerate. However, efficacy at reduced frequency of application has not been established. Alternatively, patients with psoriasis who are being treated with *Tazorac* 1% cream can be switched to the lower concentration (0.05%).

➤*Weather extremes:* Wind or cold may be more irritating to patients using tazarotene.

➤*Lentigo maligna:* Some facial pigmented lesions are not lentigines, but rather lentigo maligna, a type of melanoma. Facial pigmented lesions of concern should be carefully assessed by a qualified physician (eg, dermatologist) before application of *Avage*. Do not treat lentigo maligna with *Avage*.

➤*Photosensitivity:* Photosensitization (photoallergy or phototoxicity) may occur; therefore, caution patients to take protective measures (ie, sunscreens, protective clothing) against exposure to sunlight or ultraviolet light (eg, tanning beds) until tolerance is determined.

Because of heightened burning susceptibility, avoid exposure to sunlight (including sunlamps) unless deemed medically necessary; in such cases, minimize exposure during the use of tazarotene. Warn patients to use sunscreens (minimum SPF 15) and protective clothing when using tazarotene. Advise patients with sunburn not to use tazarotene until fully recovered. Patients who may have considerable sun exposure because of their occupation and those patients with inherent sensitivity to sunlight should exercise particular caution when using tazarotene.

In human dermal safety studies, tazarotene did not induce allergic contact sensitization, phototoxicity, or photoallergy.

Drug Interactions

Concomitant dermatologic medications and cosmetics that have a strong drying effect should be avoided. It is also advisable to "rest" a patient's skin until the effects of such preparations subside before use of tazarotene is begun.

Adverse Reactions

The most frequent adverse events with tazarotene are limited to the skin and include the following:

➤*Gel:*

Acne: Desquamation, burning/stinging, dry skin, erythema, pruritus (10% to 30%); irritation, skin pain, fissuring, localized edema, skin discoloration (1% to 10%).

Psoriasis: Pruritus, burning/stinging, erythema, worsening of psoriasis, irritation, skin pain (10% to 30%); rash, desquamation, irritant contact dermatitis, skin inflammation, fissuring, bleeding, dry skin (1% to 10%). In general, the incidence of adverse events with 0.05% gel was 2% to 5% lower than that seen with 0.1% gel.

Increases in psoriasis worsening and sun-induced erythema were noted in some patients over months 4 to 12, as compared with the first 3 months of a 1-year study.

➤*Tazorac cream:*

Acne: Desquamation, dry skin, erythema, burning sensation (10% to 30%); pruritus, irritation, face pain, stinging (1% to 5%).

Psoriasis: Pruritus, erythema, burning (10% to 23%); irritation, desquamation, stinging, contact dermatitis, dermatitis, eczema, worsening of psoriasis, skin pain, rash, hypertriglyceridemia, dry skin, skin inflammation, peripheral edema (more than 1% to less than 10%).

Tazorac 0.1% cream was associated with a somewhat greater degree of local irritation than the 0.05% cream. In general, the rates of irritation adverse events reported during psoriasis studies with 0.1% cream were 1% to 4% higher than those reported for the 0.05% cream.

➤*Avage cream:* Desquamation (40%); erythema (34%); burning sensation (26%); dry skin (16%); skin irritation, pruritus (10%); irritant contact dermatitis (8%); stinging, acne, rash (3%); cheilitis (1%). A few patients reported adverse events at week 0; however, for patients who were treated with *Avage*, the highest number of new reports for each adverse event was at week 2. When combining data from the 2 pivotal studies, 5.3% of patients in the tazarotene group and 0.9% of patients in the vehicle group discontinued because of adverse events. Overall, 3.5% of patients in the tazarotene group and 2.8% of patients in the vehicle group reported adverse events (including edema, irritation, and inflammation) directly related to the eye or eyelid. The majority of these conditions were mild.

Overdosage

➤*Symptoms:* Excessive topical use of tazarotene may lead to marked redness, peeling, or discomfort.

Oral ingestion of the drug may lead to the same adverse effects as those associated with excessive oral intake of vitamin A (hypervitaminosis A) or other retinoids.

➤*Treatment:* If oral ingestion occurs, monitor the patient and administer appropriate supportive measures as necessary. Refer to General Management of Acute Overdosage.

Patient Information

Do not use tazarotene if you are pregnant, plan to become pregnant, or may become pregnant because of the potential harm to the unborn child. Talk with your doctor about effective birth control if you are a woman who is able to become pregnant. If you become pregnant while using tazarotene, contact your physician immediately.

Do not use tazarotene if you have a sunburn, eczema, or other continuing skin conditions.

Do not use tazarotene if you are sensitive to sunlight.

For best results, if emollients or moisturizers are used, they can be applied before or after tazarotene cream, ensuring that the first cream or lotion has absorbed into the skin and dried completely.

Avoid sunlight and other medicines that may increase your sensitivity to sunlight. Avoidance of excessive sun exposure and the use of sunscreens with protective measures (hat, visor) are recommended. In the morning, apply a moisturizing sunscreen SPF 15 or greater.

Refer to patient package insert for additional patient information.

➤*Avage:* Apply only a small, pea-sized amount (about ¼ inch or 5 mm diameter) of *Avage* to your face at one time.

Avage does not remove or prevent wrinkles or repair sun-damaged skin.

TAZAROTENE — TOPICAL

➤*Tazorac:* Apply a thin film to your psoriasis areas once a day in the evening.

Usually your acne will begin to improve in about 4 weeks. Continue to use *Tazorac* for up to 12 weeks as directed by your doctor.

REXINOIDS

BEXAROTENE

Rx	**Targretin** (Ligand Pharmaceuticals)	**Gel:** 1%	Dehydrated alcohol. In 60 g.

BEXAROTENE — TOPICAL

Bexarotene is also available as a soft gelatin capsule for the treatment of cutaneous T-cell lymphoma (CTCL). Refer to the Antineoplastic Agents chapter.

Indications

➤*Cutaneous T cell lymphoma:* For the topical treatment of cutaneous lesions in patients with cutaneous T-cell lymphoma (CTCL) (Stage IA and IB) who have refractory or persistent disease after other therapies or who have not tolerated other therapies.

Administration and Dosage

➤*Approved by the FDA:* December 29, 1999.

➤*Dose:* Bexarotene should be initially applied once every other day for the first week. Increase the application frequency at weekly intervals to once daily, then twice daily, then 3 times daily and finally 4 times daily according to individual lesion tolerance. Generally, patients were able to maintain a dosing frequency of 2 to 4 times/day. Most responses were seen at dosing frequencies of 2 times/day and higher. If application site toxicity occurs, the application frequency can be reduced. Should severe irritation occur, application of drug can be temporarily discontinued for a few days until the symptoms subside (see Warnings).

Apply sufficient gel to cover the lesion with a generous coating. Allow the gel to dry before covering with clothing. Because unaffected skin may become irritated, avoid application of the gel to normal skin surrounding the lesions. In addition, do not apply the gel near mucosal surfaces of the body.

A response may be seen as soon as 4 weeks after initiation of therapy but most patients require longer application. With continued application, further benefit may be attained. The longest onset time for the first response among the responders was 392 days based on the Composite Assessment of Index Lesion Severity in the multicenter study. In clinical trials, bexarotene was applied for up to 172 weeks.

➤*Duration of therapy:* Continue bexarotene as long as the patient is deriving benefit.

➤*Occlusive dressings:* Do not use occlusive dressings with bexarotene.

➤*Storage/Stability:* Store at 25°C (77°F); with excursions permitted to 15° to 30°C (59° to 86°F) (see USP). Avoid exposing to high temperatures and humidity after the tube is opened. Protect from light.

Actions

➤*Pharmacology:* Bexarotene selectively binds and activates retinoid X receptor subtypes (RXRα, RXRβ, RXRγ). RXRs can form heterodimers with various receptor partners such as retinoic acid receptors (RARs), vitamin D receptor, thyroid receptor, and peroxisome proliferator activator receptors (PPARs). Once activated, these receptors function as transcription factors that regulate the expression of genes that control cellular differentiation and proliferation. Bexarotene inhibits the growth in vitro of some tumor cell lines of hematopoietic and squamous cell origin. It also induces tumor regression in vivo in some animal models. The exact mechanism of action of bexarotene in the treatment of CTCL is unknown.

➤*Pharmacokinetics:*

Absorption/Distribution – Plasma concentrations of bexarotene were determined during clinical studies in patients with CTCL or following repeated single or multiple-daily dose applications of bexarotene 1% for up to 132 weeks. Plasma bexarotene concentrations were generally less than 5 ng/mL and did not exceed 55 ng/mL. However, only 2 patients with very intense dosing regimens (greater than 40% BSA lesions and 4 times daily dosing) were sampled. Plasma bexarotene concentrations and the frequency of detecting quantifiable plasma bexarotene concentrations increased with increasing percent body surface area treated and increasing quantity of bexarotene applied. The sporadically observed and generally low plasma bexarotene concentrations indicated that, in patients receiving doses of low-to-moderate intensity, there is a low potential for significant plasma concentrations following repeated application of bexarotene. Bexarotene is highly bound (greater than 99%) to plasma proteins. The plasma proteins to which bexarotene binds have not been elucidated, and the ability of bexarotene to displace drugs bound to plasma proteins and the ability of drugs to displace bexarotene binding have not been studied (see Precautions). The uptake of bexarotene by organs or tissues has not been evaluated.

Metabolism – Four bexarotene metabolites have been identified in plasma following oral administration of bexarotene: 6- and 7-hydroxy-bexarotene and 6- and 7-oxo-bexarotene. In vitro studies suggest that cytochrome P450 3A4 is the major cytochrome P450 responsible for formation of the oxidative metabolites and that the oxidative metabolites may be glucuronidated. The oxidative metabolites are active in in vitro assays of retinoid receptor activation, but the relative contribution of the parent and any metabolites to the efficacy and safety of bexarotene gel is unknown.

Excretion – The renal elimination of bexarotene and its metabolites was examined in patients with type 2 diabetes mellitus following oral administration of bexarotene. Neither bexarotene nor its metabolites were excreted in urine in appreciable amounts.

Contraindications

Hypersensitivity to bexarotene or other components of the product.

Warnings

➤*Renal function impairment:* No formal studies have been conducted with bexarotene in patients with renal insufficiency. Urinary elimination of bexarotene and its known metabolites is a minor excretory pathway for bexarotene (less than 1% of an orally administered dose), but because renal insufficiency can result in significant protein binding changes, and bexarotene is more than 99% protein bound, pharmacokinetics may be altered in patients with renal insufficiency.

➤*Hepatic function impairment:* No specific studies have been conducted with bexarotene in patients with hepatic insufficiency. Because less than 1% of the dose of oral bexarotene is excreted in the urine unchanged and there is in vitro evidence of extensive hepatic contribution to bexarotene elimination, hepatic impairment would be expected to lead to greatly decreased clearance.

➤*Elderly:* Of the total patients with CTCL in clinical studies of bexarotene, 62% were younger than 65 years of age, and 38% were ≥ 65 years of age. No overall differences in safety were observed between patients ≥ 65 years and younger patients, but greater sensitivity of some older individuals to bexarotene cannot be ruled out. Responses to bexarotene were observed across all age group decades, without preference for any individual age group decade.

➤*Pregnancy: Category X.* Bexarotene 1% may cause fetal harm when administered to a pregnant woman.

Bexarotene must not be given to a pregnant woman or a woman who intends to become pregnant. If a woman becomes pregnant while taking bexarotene, bexarotene must be stopped immediately and the woman given appropriate counseling.

Bexarotene caused malformations when administered orally to pregnant rats during days 7 to 17 of gestation. Developmental abnormalities included incomplete ossification at 4 mg/kg/day and cleft palate, depressed eye bulge/microphthalmia, and small ears at 16 mg/kg/day. At doses greater than 10 mg/kg/day, bexarotene caused developmental mortality. The no-effect oral dose in rats was 1 mg/kg/day. Plasma bexarotene concentrations in patients with CTCL applying bexarotene 1% were generally less than one hundredth the C_{max} associated with dysmorphogenesis in rats, although some patients had C_{max} levels that were approximately one-eighth the concentration associated with dysmorphogenesis in rats.

Women of childbearing potential should be advised to avoid becoming pregnant when bexarotene is used. The possibility that a woman of childbearing potential is pregnant at the time therapy is instituted should be considered. A negative pregnancy test (eg, serum beta-human chorionic gonadotropin, beta-HCG) with a sensitivity of at least 50 mIU/L should be obtained within 1 week prior to bexarotene therapy, and the pregnancy test must be repeated at monthly intervals while the patient remains on bexarotene. Effective contraception must be used for 1 month prior to the initiation of therapy, during therapy and for at least 1 month following discontinuation of therapy; it is recommended that 2 reliable forms of contraception be used simultaneously unless abstinence is the chosen method. Male patients with sexual partners who are pregnant, possibly pregnant, or who could become pregnant must use condoms during sexual intercourse while applying bexarotene and for at least 1 month after the last dose of drug. Bexarotene therapy should be initiated on the second or third day of a normal menstrual period. No more than a 1 month supply of bexarotene should be given to the patient so that the results of pregnancy testing can be assessed and counseling regarding avoidance of pregnancy and birth defects can be reinforced.

➤*Lactation:* It is not known whether bexarotene is excreted in human milk. Because many drugs are excreted in human milk and because of the potential for serious adverse reactions in nursing infants from bexarotene, a decision should be made whether to discontinue nursing or to discontinue the drug, taking into account the importance of the drug to the mother.

➤*Children:* Safety and effectiveness in pediatric patients have not been established.

Precautions

➤*Protein binding:* Bexarotene is highly bound (greater than 99%) to plasma proteins. The plasma proteins to which bexarotene binds have not been elucidated, and the ability of bexarotene to displace drugs bound to plasma proteins and the ability of drugs to displace bexarotene binding have not been studied.

➤*Special risk:* Bexarotene should be used with caution in patients with a known hypersensitivity to other retinoids. No clinical instances of cross-reactivity have been noted.

➤*Photosensitivity:* Retinoids as a class have been associated with photosensitivity. In vitro assays indicate that bexarotene is a potential photosensitizing agent. There were no reports of photosensitivity in patients in the clinical studies. Patients should be advised to minimize exposure to sunlight and artificial ultraviolet light during the use of bexarotene.

BEXAROTENE — TOPICAL

Drug Interactions

➤*Vitamin A:* In clinical studies, patients were advised to limit vitamin A intake to ≤ 15,000 IU/day. Because of the relationship of bexarotene to vitamin A, patients should be advised to limit vitamin A supplements to avoid potential additive toxic effects.

➤*DEET:* Patients who are applying bexarotene should not concurrently use products that contain DEET (N,N-diethyl-m-toluamide), a common component of insect repellent products. An animal toxicology study showed increased DEET toxicity when DEET was included as part of the formulation.

➤*CYP-450 system:* On the basis of the metabolism of bexarotene by cytochrome P450 3A4, concomitant ketoconazole, itraconazole, erythromycin and grapefruit juice could increase bexarotene plasma concentrations. Similarly, based on data that gemfibrozil increases bexarotene concentrations following oral bexarotene administration, concomitant gemfibrozil could increase bexarotene plasma concentrations. However, due to the low systemic exposure to bexarotene after low to moderately intense gel regimens (see Pharmacokinetics), increases that occur are unlikely to be of sufficient magnitude to result in adverse effects.

Adverse Reactions

The safety of bexarotene has been assessed in clinical studies of 117 patients with CTCL who received bexarotene for up to 172 weeks. In the multicenter open-label study, 50 patients with CTCL received bexarotene for up to 98 weeks. The mean duration of therapy for these 50 patients was 199 days. The most common adverse events reported with an incidence at the application site of at least 10% in patients with CTCL were rash, pruritus, skin disorder, and pain.

Adverse events leading to dose reduction or study drug discontinuation in at least 2 patients were rash, contact dermatitis, and pruritus.

Of the 49 patients (98%) who experienced any adverse event, most experienced events categorized as mild (9 patients, 18%) or moderate (27 patients, 54%). There were 12 patients (24%) who experienced at least 1 moderately severe adverse event. The most common moderately severe events were rash (7 patients, 14%) and pruritus (3 patients, 6%). Only 1 patient (2%) experienced a severe adverse event (rash).

In the patients with CTCL receiving bexarotene, adverse events reported regardless of relationship to study drug at an incidence of ≥ 5% are presented below.

A similar safety profile for bexarotene was demonstrated in the Phase I to II program. For the 67 patients enrolled in the Phase I to II program, the mean duration of treatment was 436 days (range 12 to 1203 days). As in the multicenter study, the most common adverse events regardless of relationship to study drug in the Phase I to II program were rash (78%), pain (40%), and pruritus (40%).

Incidence of All Adverse Reactions*and Application Site Adverse Reactions With Incidence ≥ 5% for All Application Frequencies of Bexarotene Topical Gel in The Multicenter Ctcl Study

Adverse reaction	All adverse reactions n = 50 (n %)	Application site adverse reactions n = 50 (n %)
Cardiovascular		
Edema	5 (10%)	0
Peripheral edema	3 (6%)	0
CNS		
Paresthesia	3 (6%)	3 (6%)
Dermatologic		
Contact dermatitis[1]	7 (14%)	4 (8%)
Exfoliative dermatitis	3 (6%)	0
Pruritus[2]	18 (36%)	9 (18%)
Rash[3]	36 (72%)	28 (56%)
Maculopapular rash	3 (6%)	0
Skin disorder (NOS)[4]	13 (26%)	9 (18%)
Sweating	3 (6%)	0
Hema/lymphatic		
Leukopenia	3 (6%)	0
Lymphadenopathy	3 (6%)	0
WBC abnormal	3 (6%)	0
Metabolic-nutritional		
Hyperlipemia	5 (10%)	0
Respiratory		
Cough increased	3 (6%)	0
Pharyngitis	3 (6%)	0
Miscellaneous		
Asthenia	3 (6%)	0
Headache	7 (14%)	0
Infection	9 (18%)	0
Pain	15 (30%)	9 (18%)

* Regardless of association with treatment.
[1] Includes investigator terms such as contact dermatitis, irritant contact dermatitis, irritant dermatitis.
[2] Includes investigator terms such as pruritus, itching, itching of lesion.
[3] Includes investigator terms such as erythema, scaling, irritation, redness, rash, dermatitis.
[4] Includes investigator terms such as skin inflammation, excoriation, sticky or tacky sensation of skin; NOS = Not Otherwise Specified.

Overdosage

➤*Symptoms:* Systemic toxicity following acute overdosage with topical application of bexarotene is unlikely because of low systemic plasma levels observed with normal therapeutic doses.

➤*Treatment:* There is no specific antidote for overdosage.

There has been no experience with acute overdose of bexarotene in humans. Any overdose with bexarotene should be treated with supportive care for the signs and symptoms exhibited by the patient.

SCABICIDES/PEDICULICIDES

CROTAMITON

Rx	**Eurax** (Bristol-Myers Squibb)	**Cream:** 10%	Vanishing base. Cetyl alcohol. In 60 g.
		Lotion: 10%	Emollient base. Cetyl alcohol. In 60 and 454 g.

CROTAMITON — TOPICAL

Indications

➤*Scabies/Pruritus:* For eradication of scabies (*Sarcoptes scabiei*) and for symptomatic treatment of pruritic skin.

Administration and Dosage

➤*Approved by the FDA:* June, 26 2003.

➤*Lotion:* Shake well before using.

➤*Scabies:* Thoroughly massage into the skin of the whole body from the chin down, paying particular attention to all folds and creases. A second application is advisable 24 hours later. Clothing and bed linen should be changed the next morning. A cleansing bath should be taken 48 hours after the last application.

➤*Pruritus:* Massage gently into affected areas until medication is completely absorbed. Repeat as needed.

➤*Storage/Stability:* Store at room temperature.

Actions

➤*Pharmacology:* Crotamiton has scabicidal and antipruritic actions. The mechanisms of these actions are not known.

Contraindications

Crotamiton should not be applied topically to patients who develop a sensitivity or are allergic to it or who manifest a primary irritation response to topical medications.

Warnings

➤*Irritation:* If severe irritation or sensitization develops, treatment with this product should be discontinued and appropriate therapy instituted.

➤*Pregnancy: Category C.* Animal reproduction studies have not been conducted with crotamiton. It is also not known whether crotamiton can cause fetal harm when applied topically to a pregnant woman or can affect reproduction capacity. Crotamiton should be given to a pregnant woman only if clearly needed.

➤*Children:* Safety and effectiveness in children have not been established.

Precautions

➤*General:* Crotamiton should not be applied in the eyes or mouth because it may cause irritation. It should not be applied to acutely inflamed skin or raw or weeping surfaces until the acute inflammation has subsided.

CROTAMITON — TOPICAL

Adverse Reactions

Allergic sensitivity or primary irritation reactions may occur in some patients.

Overdosage

➤*Acute toxicity (after accidental oral administration in children):*

Highest known doses ingested –

Cream: Children — 2 g (age 1½ years).

Lotion: 1 ounce (age 2 years.) A death was reported but cause was not confirmed.

Oral LD_{50} in animals (mg/kg); rats, 2212; mice, 2011.

➤*Symptoms:*

Oral ingestion – Burning sensation in the mouth, irritation of the buccal, esophageal and gastric mucosa, nausea, vomiting, abdominal pain.

➤*Treatment:* There is no specific antidote if taken orally. General measures to eliminate the drug and reduce its absorption, combined with symptomatic treatment, are recommended.

Patient Information

Take a routine bath or shower. Thoroughly massage crotamiton cream or lotion into the skin from the chin to the toes including folds and creases.

A second application is advisable 24 hours later.

This 60 gram tube or bottle is sufficient for two applications.

Clothing and bed linen should be changed the next day. Contaminated clothing and bed linen may be dry-cleaned, or washed in the hot cycle of the washing machine.

A cleansing bath should be taken 48 hours after the last application.

LINDANE (Gamma Benzene Hexachloride)

Rx	**Lindane** (Various, eg, Alpharma, Major)	**Lotion:** 1%	In 30 and 59 mL, and pharmacy-size only pint.
		Shampoo: 1%	In 30 and 59 mL, and pharmacy-size only pint.

LINDANE (Gamma Benzene Hexachloride) — TOPICAL

WARNING

Only use lindane in patients who cannot tolerate or have failed first-line treatment with safer medications for the treatment of scabies.

Neurologic toxicity – Seizures and deaths have been reported following lindane use with repeat or prolonged application, but also in rare cases following a single application used according to directions. Exercise caution when using lindane in infants, children, the elderly, and individuals with other skin conditions (eg, atopic dermatitis, psoriasis) and in those who weigh less than 110 lbs (50 kg) as they may be at risk of serious neurotoxicity.

Contraindications – See Contraindications for more information.

Proper use – Instruct patients on the proper use of lindane, the amount to apply, how long to leave it on, and avoiding retreatment. Inform patients that itching occurs after the successful killing of scabies and is not necessarily an indication for retreatment with lindane.

Indications

➤*Lotion:* For the treatment of scabies (*Sarcoptes scabiei*) only in patients who cannot tolerate or who have failed other treatments.

➤*Shampoo:* For the treatment of head lice (*Pediculosis humanis capitis*), crab lice (*Pthirus pubis*), and their ova only in patients who cannot tolerate or who have failed other treatments.

Administration and Dosage

All patients must be provided a medication guide each time lindane is dispensed.

Washing of all recently worn clothing, underwear, pajamas, sheets, pillows, and towels is very important. Do not administer orally. Instruct caregivers to wear gloves or wash hands immediately after applying the lotion or shampoo. Inform patient that itching occurs after the successful killing of scabies or lice and it is not necessarily an indication for retreatment with lindane. Lindane does not prevent infestation or reinfestation and should not be used to ward off a possible infestation.

➤*Scabies (lotion):* Apply a thin layer of lotion over all skin (ie, entire trunk, extremities, soles of feet, underneath finger nails) from the neck down. Wash hands immediately or use gloves when applying lindane. One ounce (30 mL) is sufficient for an average adult. Do not prescribe more than 2 ounces (60 mL) for larger adults. Apply once and wash off in 8 to 12 hours. Do not retreat unless instructed to do so by a physician; 1 application of lindane is generally successful. Do not cover areas where medication is applied. Treat sexual contacts concurrently.

Patient may bathe prior to application; however, wait at least 1 hour after bathing before applying lindane to skin. Wet and warm skin may increase absorption, leading to toxicity (eg, seizures).

➤*Head lice/crab lice (shampoo):* Apply shampoo directly to dry hair without adding water. Work thoroughly into the hair and allow to remain in place for 4 minutes only. Give special attention to the fine hairs along the neck. After 4 minutes, add small quantities of water to hair until a good lather forms. Immediately rinse all lather away. Towel briskly and then remove nits with nit comb or tweezers. Do not cover the hair with shower cap or towel. Avoid unnecessary contact of lather with other body surfaces. Do not prescribe more than 2 ounces (60 mL) for larger adults. Do not retreat or use as a routine shampoo. Treat sexual contacts concurrently.

Actions

➤*Pharmacology:* An ectoparasiticide and ovicide effective against *Sarcoptes scabiei* (scabies). Parasiticidal action is exerted direct absorbtion into the parasites and their ova.

➤*Pharmacokinetics:* Approximately 10% systemic absorption of a lindane acetone solution was reported when applied to the forearm of human subjects and left in place for 24 hours. A blood level of 290 ng/mL was associated with convulsions following the accidental ingestion of a lindane-containing product. It was found that the greatest peak blood level of 64 ng/mL occurred 6 hours after total body application of lindane in 1 of 8 nonscabietic pediatric patients. The half-life in blood was determined to be approximately 18 hours. Data available suggest that lindane has a rapid distribution phase followed by a longer β-elimination phase.

Contraindications

Premature neonates, because their skin may be more permeable than that of full-term infants and their liver enzymes may not be sufficiently developed; patients with known seizure disorders; hypersensitivity to lindane or any component of the products; crusted (Norwegian) scabies and other skin conditions (eg, atopic dermatitis, psoriasis) that may increase systemic absorption.

Warnings

➤*Absorption:* Simultaneous application of creams, ointments, or oils may enhance absorption.

➤*Neurotoxicity:* Seizures and deaths have been reported following lindane use with repeat or prolonged application, but also in rare cases following a single application. Infants, children, the elderly, individuals with other skin conditions, and those who weigh less than 110 lbs (50 kg) may be at greater risk of serious neurotoxicity. Give careful consideration before prescribing lindane to patients with conditions that may increase the risk of seizure, such as HIV infection, history of head trauma or a prior seizure, CNS tumor, the presence of severe hepatic cirrhosis, excessive use of alcohol, abrupt withdrawal from alcohol or sedatives, as well as concomitant use of medications known to lower seizure threshold.

➤*Deaths:* Serious outcomes such as hospitalization and disability or death has occurred. In approximately 20% of the total reported cases, lindane was reported to have been used according to the labeled directions. Of these cases, 13 deaths were reported, many cases of which were remote from the time of actual lindane use. Lindane toxicity, verified by autopsy, was the cause of 1 infant's death and was the cause of death reported for an adult who ingested it orally in a successful suicide. The direct causes of death for the other cases were attributed to reasons other than lindane. Most of these adverse events occurred with lindane lotion.

➤*Fertility impairment:* The number of spermatids in the testes of rats 2 weeks after oral administration of a single dose of 30 mg/kg body weight (12 times the estimated human exposure) was significantly reduced compared with the control rats.

➤*Elderly:* There have been no studies of lindane in the elderly. There are 4 postmarketing reports of deaths in elderly patents who were treated for scabies with lindane. Two patients died within 24 hours of lindane application, and the third patient died 41 days after application of lindane, having suffered a seizure on the day of death. A fourth patient died of an unreported cause of death on the same day that lindane treatment for scabies was administered.

➤*Pregnancy: Category C.* Give lindane to pregnant women only if clearly needed. There are no adequate and well-controlled studies in pregnant women. There are no known maternal or fetal health risks if the scabies is not treated. Lindane is lipophilic and may accumulate in the placenta. There has been a single case report of a stillborn infant following multiple maternal exposures to lindane during pregnancy. The relationship of the maternal exposures to the fetal outcome is unknown.

Animal data suggest that lindane exposure of the fetus may increase the likelihood of neurologic developmental abnormalities. The immature central nervous system (as in the fetus) may have increased susceptibility to the effects of the drug.

When rats received lindane in the diet from day 6 of gestation through day 10 of lactation, reduced pup survival, decreased pup weight and decreased weight gains during lactation, increased motor activity, and decreased motor activity habituation were seen in pups at 5.6 mg/kg. An increased number of stillborn pups was seen at 8 mg/kg, and increased pup mortality was seen at 5.6 mg/kg.

➤*Lactation:* Lindane is lipophilic and is present in human breast milk, but exact quantities are not known. There may be a risk of toxicity if lindane is ingested from breast milk, or from skin absorption from mother to baby in the course of breastfeeding when lindane is applied topically to the chest area. Advise nursing mothers who require treatment with lindane of the potential risks. Counsel them to avoid large areas of skin-to-skin contact with the infant

LINDANE (Gamma Benzene Hexachloride) — TOPICAL

while lindane is applied, as well as to interrupt breastfeeding, with expression and discarding of milk, for at least 24 hours following use.

➤*Children:* Animal data demonstrated increased risk of adverse events in the young across species. Pediatric patients have a higher surface to volume ratio and may be at risk of greater systemic exposure when lindane is applied to the body. Infants and children may be at an even higher risk due to immaturity of organ systems such as skin and liver. Use lindane with extreme caution in patients who weigh less than approximately 110 lbs (50 kg) and especially in infants.

Precautions

➤*For external use only:* Avoid contact with eyes; if this occurs, immediately flush eyes with water.

➤*Oils:* Oils may enhance absorption of lindane. Avoid using oil treatment, oil-based hair dressings, or conditioners before and after applying lindane.

Drug Interactions

Use lindane with caution with drugs that lower seizure threshold. These drugs may include the following: Antipsychotics, antidepressants, theophylline, cyclosporine, mycophenolate mofetil, tacrolimus capsules, penicillins, imipenem, quinolone antibiotics, chloroquine sulfate, pyrimethamine, isoniazid, meperidine, radiographic contrast agents, centrally active anticholinesterases, methocarbamol.

Adverse Reactions

Lindane has been reported to cause CNS stimulation ranging from dizziness to seizures. Although seizures were almost always associated with ingestion or misuse of the product (to include repeat treatment), seizures and deaths have been reported when lindane was used according to directions. Irritant dermatitis from contact with this product has also been reported.

➤*Postmarketing experience:* Alopecia, dermatitis, headache, pain, paresthesia, pruritus, and urticaria. The relationship of some of these events to lindane therapy is unknown.

Overdosage

➤*Symptoms:* Overdosage or oral ingestion can cause CNS excitation and, if taken in sufficient quantities, seizures may occur. A blood level of 290 ng/mL was associated with convulsions following the accidental ingestion of a lindane-containing product.

➤*Treatment:* If accidental ingestion occurs, institute prompt gastric emptying. However, because oils favor absorption, give saline cathartics for intestinal evacuation rather than oil laxatives. If CNS manifestations occur, administer pentobarbital, phenobarbital, or diazepam. Refer to General Management of Acute Overdosage.

Patient Information

The skin should be clean and without any other lotion, cream, or oil on it. Oils can make lindane go through the skin faster and possibly increase the risk of neurotoxicity (eg, seizures).

Wait at least 1 hour after bathing or showering before putting lindane on the skin.

Wet or warm skin can make lindane go through skin faster; make sure skin is dry and cool before application.

Put lotion under fingernails after trimming the fingernails short, because scabies are very likely to remain there. A toothbrush can be used to apply the lotion under the fingernails. Immediately after use, wrap the toothbrush in paper and throw away.

Use only a single application, applied as a very thin layer over all skin from the neck down.

Do not use any covering over the applied lindane that does not breathe (eg, diapers with plastic lining, plastic clothes, tight clothes, or blankets).

Wash the lindane completely off after 8 to 12 hours. Never leave lindane on the skin for more than 12 hours. Warm, but not hot water can be used.

Wash all recently worn clothing, underwear, pajamas, used sheets, pillow cases, and towels in very hot water or dry-clean.

The patient may still itch after using lindane, even after all the scabies (insects) are dead.

For external use only (oral ingestion can lead to serious CNS toxicity). Do not apply to face. Avoid eyes; if there is contact, flush well with water for several minutes. Avoid unnecessary skin contact or contact with mucous membranes (eg, nose, mouth). Wear rubber gloves, particularly when applying to more than 1 person.

Notify physician if condition worsens or if itching, redness, swelling, burning, or skin rash occurs.

Avoid use on open cuts and extensive excoriations.

Treat sexual contacts simultaneously.

Lindane does not prevent infestation or reinfestation and should not be used to ward off a possible infestation.

A lindane medication guide must be given to the patient each time lindane is dispensed.

MALATHION

Rx	**Ovide** (Taro)	**Lotion:** 0.5%[a]	In 59 mL.

[a] In a vehicle of 78% isopropyl alcohol, terpineol, dipentene, and pine needle oil.

MALATHION — TOPICAL

Indications

➤*Head lice:* For patients infected with *Pediculus humanus capitis* (head lice and their ova) of the scalp hair.

Administration and Dosage

➤*Approved by the FDA:* August 2, 1982.

Close eyes tightly during product application. If accidentally placed in the eye, flush immediately with water. Use only on scalp hair.

1.) Apply malathion lotion on dry hair in an amount just sufficient to thoroughly wet the hair and scalp. Pay particular attention to the back of the head and neck while applying malathion. Wash hands after applying to scalp.
2.) Allow hair to dry naturally; use no electric heat source, and allow hair to remain uncovered.
3.) After 8 to 12 hours, the hair should be shampooed.
4.) Rinse and use a fine-toothed (nit) comb to remove dead lice and eggs.
5.) If lice are still present after 7 to 9 days, repeat with a second application of malathion.
6.) Further treatment is generally not necessary. Other family members should be evaluated by a physician to determine if infested, and if so, receive treatment.

➤*Storage/Stability:* Store at controlled room temperature 20° to 25°C (68° to 77°F).

Flammable. Keep away from heat and open flame. Keep out of the reach of children.

Actions

➤*Pharmacology:* Malathion is an organophosphate agent which acts as a pediculicide by inhibiting cholinesterase activity in vivo. Inadvertent transdermal absorption of malathion has occurred from its agricultural use. In such cases, acute toxicity was manifested by excessive cholinergic activity (ie, increased sweating, salivary and gastric secretion, GI and uterine motility, and bradycardia). Because the potential for transdermal absorption of malathion from malathion lotion is not known at this time, strict adherence to the dosing instructions regarding its use in children, method of application, duration of exposure, and frequency of application is required.

Contraindications

In neonates and infants because their scalps are more permeable and may have increased absorption of malathion; do not use on individuals known to be sensitive to malathion or to any of the ingredients in the vehicle.

Warnings

➤*Flammable:* Malathion lotion is flammable. The lotion and wet hair should not be exposed to open flames or electric heat sources, including hair dryers and electric curlers. Do not smoke while applying lotion or while hair is wet. Allow hair to dry naturally and to remain uncovered after application of malathion lotion.

➤*Irritation:* If malathion comes into contact with the eyes, flush immediately with water. Consult a physician if eye irritation persists.

If skin irritation occurs, discontinue use of product until irritation clears. Reapply the malathion, and if irritation reoccurs, consult a physician.

Slight stinging sensations may occur with the use of malathion.

Close eyes tightly during product application. If accidentally placed in the eye, flush immediately with water. Use only on scalp hair.

➤*Mutagenesis:* Although mutagenesis has not been studied in malathion lotion, malathion has been shown to be genotoxic in a number of in vitro and in vivo mutation and clastogenicity assays.

➤*Pregnancy: Category B.* There was no evidence of teratogenicity in studies in rats and rabbits at doses up to 900 mg/kg/day and 100 mg/kg/day malathion, respectively. A study in rats failed to show any gross fetal abnormalities attributable to feeding malathion up to 2500 ppm (approximately 200 mg/kg/day) in the diet during a 3-generation evaluation period. These doses were approximately 2 to 10 times higher than the anticipated human dose (based on body surface area and assuming 100% bioavailability). Because animal reproduction studies are not always predictive of human responses, this drug should be used (or handled) during pregnancy only if clearly needed.

➤*Lactation:* Malathion in an acetone vehicle has been reported to be absorbed through human skin to the extent of 8% of the applied dose. However, percutaneous absorption from the malathion, 0.5% formulation has not been studied, and it is not known whether malathion is excreted in human milk. Because many drugs are excreted in human milk, caution should be exercised when malathion is administered to (or handled by) a nursing mother.

➤*Children:* The safety and efficacy of malathion in children younger than 6 years of age have not been established via well controlled trials. Malathion lotion should only be used on children under the direct supervision of an adult.

MALATHION — TOPICAL

Adverse Reactions

➤*Dermatologic:* Malathion has been shown to be irritating to the skin and scalp. Accidental contact with the eyes can result in mild conjunctivitis. It is not known if malathion has the potential to cause contact allergic sensitization.

Overdosage

➤*Symptoms:* Malathion, although a weaker cholinesterase inhibitor than some other organophosphates, may be expected to exhibit the same symptoms of cholinesterase depletion after accidental ingestion orally.

Severe respiratory distress is the major and most serious symptom of organophosphate poisoning.

➤*Treatment:* Severe respiratory distress may require artificial respiration, and atropine may be needed to counteract the symptoms of cholinesterase depletion.

Consideration should be given, as part of the treatment program, to the high concentration of isopropyl alcohol in the vehicle.

If accidentally swallowed, vomiting should be induced promptly or the stomach lavaged with 5% sodium bicarbonate solution.

Repeat analyses of serum and RBC cholinesterase may assist in establishing the diagnosis and formulating a long-range prognosis.

Patient Information

Malathion is flammable. The lotion and hair wet with lotion should not be exposed to open flames or electric heat sources, including hair dryers and electric curlers. Do not smoke while applying lotion or while hair is wet. The person applying malathion lotion should wash hands after application. Allow hair to dry naturally and to remain uncovered after application of malathion lotion.

Malathion should only be used on children under the direct supervision of an adult. Children should be warned to stay away from lighted cigarettes, open flames, and electric heat sources while the hair is wet.

In case of accidental ingestion of malathion lotion by mouth, seek medical attention immediately.

If you are pregnant or nursing, contact your physician before using malathion.

If malathion comes into contact with the eyes, flush immediately with water. Consult a physician if eye irritation persists or if visual changes occur.

If skin irritation occurs, wash scalp and hair immediately. If the irritation clears, malathion lotion may be reapplied. If irritation reoccurs, consult a physician.

Slight stinging sensations may be produced when using malathion lotion.

Apply malathion on the scalp hair in an amount just sufficient to thoroughly wet hair and scalp. Pay particular attention to the back of the head and neck when applying malathion. Anyone applying malathion should wash hands immediately after the application process is complete.

Allow hair to dry naturally and to remain uncovered. Shampoo hair after 8 to 12 hours, again paying attention to the back of the head and neck while shampooing.

Rinse hair and use a fine-toothed (nit) comb to remove dead lice and eggs.

If lice are still present after 7 to 9 days, repeat with a second application of malathion.

Further treatment is generally not necessary. Other family members should be evaluated by a physician to determine if infested, and if so, receive treatment.

PERMETHRIN

Rx	**Permethrin** (Various, eg, Clay-Park)	**Cream:** 5%	In 60 g tubes.
Rx	**Elimite** (Allergen)		Lanolin alcohols, coconut oil, mineral oil. In 60 g tubes.
Rx	**Acticin** (Bertek)		Coconut oil, lanolin alcohols, light mineral oil. In 60 g tubes.
otc	**Permethrin** (Various, eg, Alpharma)	**Lotion:** 1%	In 60 mL with comb.

PERMETHRIN — TOPICAL

Indications

➤*Cream:* For the treatment of scabies (*Sarcoptes scabiei*) infestation.

➤*Lotion/Cream rinse:* For the treatment of head lice (*Pediculus humanus capitis*) and its nits (eggs).

➤*Liquid:* For the treatment of infestation with *Pediculus humanus* var. *capitis* (the head louse) and its nits (eggs). Treatment for recurrences is required in less than 1% of patients since the ovicidal activity may be supplemented by residual persistence in the hair. If live lice are observed 7 or more days following the initial application, give a second application.

➤*Unlabeled uses:* Permethrin appears to be effective for the topical treatment of papulopustular rosacea.

Administration and Dosage

➤*Scabies (cream):* Thoroughly massage cream into the skin from the head to the soles of the feet. Scabies rarely infest the scalp of adults, although the hairline, neck, temple, and forehead may be infested in infants and geriatric patients. Remove the cream by washing (shower or bath) after 8 to 14 hours. Treat infants on the scalp, temple, and forehead. One application is generally curative. Usually 30 g is sufficient for an average adult.

Patients often experience pruritus after treatment. This is rarely a sign of treatment failure and is not an indication for retreatment. Demonstrable living mites after 14 days indicate that retreatment is necessary.

➤*Head lice (lotion/cream rinse):* Apply to hair after washing with shampoo; rinse with water and towel dry. Apply a sufficient amount to saturate hair and scalp (especially behind the ears and nape of neck). Leave on hair for no longer than 10 minutes, then rinse with water. A single application is generally sufficient; however, if lice are observed within 7 days after application, apply a second treatment. Remove any remaining nits with the nit comb provided.

➤*Storage/Stability:* Store at 15° to 25°C (59° to 77°F).

Actions

➤*Pharmacology:* Permethrin is a pyrethroid active against lice, ticks, mites, and fleas. It acts on the parasites' nerve cell membranes to disrupt the sodium channel current, resulting in delayed repolarization and paralysis of the pests.

➤*Pharmacokinetics:* Permethrin is rapidly metabolized by ester hydrolysis to inactive metabolites that are excreted primarily in the urine. Although the amount of permethrin absorbed after a single application of the 5% cream has not been determined precisely, preliminary data suggest it is 2% or less of the amount applied. Residual persistence is detectable on the hair for at least 10 days following a single application.

Contraindications

Hypersensitivity to any synthetic pyrethroid or pyrethrin, or to any component of the product. If hypersensitivity develops, discontinue use.

Warnings

➤*Carcinogenesis:* Species-specific increases in pulmonary adenomas, a common benign tumor of mice, were seen in the mouse studies. In 1 study, incidence of pulmonary alveolar-cell carcinomas and benign liver adenomas increased only in female mice when permethrin was given in their food at a concentration of 5000 ppm.

➤*Pregnancy: Category B.* There are no adequate and well-controlled studies in pregnant women. Use during pregnancy only if clearly needed.

➤*Lactation:* It is not known whether this drug is excreted in breast milk. Because of the evidence for tumorigenic potential of permethrin in animal studies, consider discontinuing nursing temporarily or withholding the drug while the mother is nursing.

➤*Children:* Safety and efficacy for use in children younger than 2 months of age have not been established.

Precautions

➤*For external use only:* Do not use near eyes, mucous membranes (ie, nose, mouth, vagina), or ingest orally. If infestation of eyelashes or eyebrows occurs, consult physician.

➤*Asthmatics:* Permethrin may cause breathing difficulties or exacerbate asthmatic episodes.

➤*Pruritus, erythema, and edema:* These often accompany scabies and head lice infestation. Treatment with permethrin may temporarily exacerbate these conditions.

Adverse Reactions

The most frequent adverse reaction is pruritus. Usually a consequence of scabies or head lice infestation itself, it may be temporarily aggravated following treatment.

➤*Cream:* Mild transient burning/stinging (10%); itching (7%); tingling, numbness, erythema, or rash (2% or less).

Postmarketing reactions – Headache, fever, dizziness, abdominal pain, diarrhea, nausea, vomiting (5%); seizure (rare).

➤*Lotion/Cream rinse:* Itching, redness, swelling of scalp.

Overdosage

If ingested, perform gastric lavage and employ general supportive measures. Excessive topical use may result in increased irritation and erythema.

Patient Information

For external use only. Avoid contact with the mucous membranes (eg, nose, mouth, vagina). May be irritating to the eyes. Avoid contact with the eyes; flush with water immediately if eye contact with the drug occurs.

Itching, redness, or swelling of the scalp may occur; notify physician if irritation persists.

PERMETHRIN — TOPICAL

Patient instructions and information are available with the product. Do not exceed the prescribed dosage.

Inform patients that they may still experience pruritus after treatment. This is rarely a sign of treatment failure or an indication for retreatment.

Inform patients on the importance of washing in hot water all personal articles susceptible to infestation (eg, sheets, pillows, clothing, combs, brushes). It is recommended to thoroughly vacuum rooms.

MISCELLANEOUS PEDICULICIDES

otc	**Tisit**[a] (Pfeiffer)	**Lotion**: 0.3% pyrethrins, 2% piperonyl butoxide	In 59 and 118 mL.
otc	**Tisit** (Pfeiffer)	**Gel**: 0.3% pyrethrins, 3% piperonyl butoxide	In 30 mL.
otc	**Klout** (PediaMed)	**Shampoo**: Acetic acid, isopropanol, sodium laureth sulfate	Parabens. In 118.3 mL with comb.
otc	**A-200** (Hogil)	**Shampoo**: 0.33% pyrethrins, 4% piperonyl butoxide	In 59 and 118 mL with comb, and in 118 mL kits containing comb and lice control spray.
otc	**Pronto** (Del)		Benzyl alcohol, decyl alcohol, isopropyl alcohol. In 60 and 120 mL with comb.
otc	**Pyrinyl Plus** (Rugby)		Benzyl alcohol. In 59 mL.
otc	**RID** (Bayer)		SD alcohol. In 60, 120, and 240 mL, and 120 mL kits containing gel, comb, and lice control spray.
otc	**Tisit** (Pfeiffer)		In 59 and 118 mL with comb.
otc	**Lice Treatment** (Goldline)		Benzyl alcohol. In 59 and 118 mL with comb.
otc	**RID** (Bayer)	**Mousse**: 0.33% pyrethrins, 4% piperonyl butoxide	Cetearyl alcohol, SD alcohol, isobutane. In 165 mL with comb.

[a] Contains petroleum distillate and piperonyl butoxide equivalent to 1.6% ether.

MISCELLANEOUS PEDICULICIDES — TOPICAL

Indications

➤*Lice:* Treatment of infestations of head lice, body lice, and pubic (crab) lice and their eggs.

Administration and Dosage

Administration and dosage varies. Refer to individual package inserts for information.

Contraindications

Hypersensitivity to ingredients; ragweed sensitized persons (pyrethrins and permethrins).

Precautions

➤*For external use only:* Harmful if swallowed or inhaled. May be irritating to the eyes and mucous membranes (eg, nose, mouth, vagina). In case of contact with eyes, flush with water. Discontinue use and notify physician if irritation or infection occurs.

➤*Infestation of eyelashes or eyebrows:* Do not use in these areas; consult physician.

➤*Reinfestation:* To prevent reinfestation, sterilize or treat all brushes/combs, towels, clothing, and bedding concurrently. It is recommended that all rooms inhabited by infected patients be thoroughly vacuumed. A second treatment may need to be repeated in 7 to 10 days to kill any newly hatched lice.

➤*Pubic lice:* May be transmitted by sexual contact. Treat sexual partners simultaneously.

WOUND HEALING AGENTS

BECAPLERMIN

Rx	**Regranex** (Johnson & Johnson Wound Management)	**Gel**: 100 mcg	Parabens. In 2, 7.5 and 15 g multi-use tubes.

BECAPLERMIN — TOPICAL

Indications

➤*Diabetic neuropathic ulcers:* For the treatment of lower extremity diabetic neuropathic ulcers that extend into the subcutaneous tissue or beyond and have an adequate blood supply. When used as an adjunct to, and not a substitute for, good ulcer care practices, including initial sharp debridement, pressure relief, and infection control, becaplermin increases the incidence of complete healing of diabetic ulcers.

Administration and Dosage

➤*Approved by the FDA:* December 16, 1997.

The amount of becaplermin to be applied will vary depending upon the size of the ulcer area. To calculate the length of gel to apply to the ulcer, measure the greatest length of the ulcer by the greatest width of the ulcer in either inches or centimeters. Use the formulas below to calculate the length of gel in inches and centimeters.

➤*Calculating amount in inches:* To calculate the length of gel in inches to be applied daily, multiply the length times the width times 0.6 for a 15 or 7.5 g tube. For a 2 g tube, multiply the length times the width times 1.3.

Using the calculation, each square inch of ulcer surface will require ≈⅔ inch length of gel squeezed from a 15 g or 7.5 g tube, or ≈ 1⅓ inch length of the gel from a 2 g tube. For example, if the ulcer measures 1 inch by 2 inches, then a 1 inch length of gel should be used for 15 g or 7.5 g tubes (1×2× 0.6 = 1½) and 2¾ inch gel length should be used for the 2 g tube (1×2×1.3 = 2¾).

➤*Calculating amount in centimeters:* To calculate the length of gel in centimeters to be applied daily, multiply the length times the width ÷ 4 for a 15 or 7.5 g tube. For a 2 g tube, multiply the length times the width ÷ 2.

Using the calculations for ulcer size in centimeters, each square centimeter of ulcer surface will require ≈ a 0.25 cm length of gel squeezed from a 15 g or 7.5 g tube, or ≈ 0.5 cm length of gel from a 2 g tube. For example, if the ulcer measures 4 cm by 2 cm, then a 2 cm length of gel should be used for 15 g or 7.5 g tube ([4×2]÷4=2) and a 4 cm length of gel should be used for 2 g tube ([4×2]÷2=4).

The amount of becaplermin to be applied should be recalculated by the physician or wound care giver at weekly or biweekly intervals depending on the rate of change in ulcer area. The weight of becaplermin from 7.5 g and 15 g tubes is 0.65 g per inch length and 0.25 g per cm length.

To apply becaplermin, the calculated length of gel should be squeezed on to a clean measuring surface (eg, wax paper). The measured becaplermin is transferred from the clean measuring surface using an application aid and then spread over the entire ulcer area to yield a thin continuous layer of ≈ 1⁄16 of an inch thickness. The site(s) of application should then be covered by a saline-moistened dressing and left in place for ≈ 12 hours. The dressing should then be removed and the ulcer rinsed with saline or water to remove residual gel and covered again with a second moist dressing (without becaplermin) for the remainder of the day. Becaplermin should be applied once daily to the ulcer until complete healing has occurred. If the ulcer does not decrease in size by ≈ 30% after 10 weeks of treatment or complete healing has not occurred in 20 weeks, continued treatment with becaplermin should be reassessed. The step-by-step instructions for applying becaplermin for home administration are described in Patient Information.

➤*Storage/Stability:* Store refrigerated, 2° to 8°C (36° to 46°F). Do not freeze. Do not use the gel after the expiration date at the bottom of the tube.

Actions

➤*Pharmacology:* Becaplermin has biological activity similar to that of endogenous platelet-derived growth factor, which includes promoting the chemotactic recruitment and proliferation of cells involved in wound repair and enhancing the formation of granulation tissue.

➤*Pharmacokinetics:* Ten patients with Stage III or IV (as defined in the International Association of Enterostomal Therapy [IAET] guide to chronic wound staging), lower extremity diabetic ulcers received topical applications of becaplermin 0.01% at a dose range of 0.32 to 2.95 mcg/kg (7 mcg/cm^2) daily for 14 days. Six patients had nonquantifiable PDGF levels at baseline and throughout the study, 2 patients had PDGF levels at baseline which did not increase substantially, and 2 patients had PDGF levels that increased sporadically above their baseline values during the 14-day study period.

Systemic bioavailability of becaplermin was less than 3% in rats with full thickness wounds receiving single or multiple (5 days) topical applications of 127 mcg/kg (20.1 mcg/cm^2 of wound area) of becaplermin.

Contraindications

Known hypersensitivity to any component of this product (eg, parabens); known neoplasm(s) at the site(s) of application.

BECAPLERMIN — TOPICAL

Warnings

➤*Nonsterile:* Becaplermin is a nonsterile, low bioburden preserved product. Therefore, it should not be used in wounds that close by primary intention.

➤*Pregnancy: Category C.* Animal reproduction studies have not been conducted with becaplermin. It is also not known whether becaplermin can cause fetal harm when administered to a pregnant woman or can affect reproductive capacity. Becaplermin should be given to pregnant women only if clearly needed.

➤*Lactation:* It is not known whether becaplermin is excreted in human milk. Because many drugs are secreted in human milk, caution should be exercised when becaplermin is administered to nursing women.

➤*Children:* Safety and efficacy of becaplermin in children younger than 16 years of age have not been established.

Precautions

For external use only.

➤*Sensitivity:* If application site reactions occur, the possibility of sensitization or irritation caused by parabens or m-cresol should be considered.

➤*Exposed joints, tendons, ligaments, and bone:* The effects of becaplermin on exposed joints, tendons, ligaments, and bone have not been established in humans. In preclinical studies, rats injected at the metatarsals with 3 or 10 mcg/site (≈ 60 or 200 mcg/kg) of becaplermin every other day for 13 days displayed histological changes indicative of accelerated bone remodeling consisting of periosteal hyperplasia and subperiosteal bone resorption and exostosis. The soft tissue adjacent to the injection site had fibroplasia with accompanying mononuclear cell infiltration reflective of the ability of PDGF to stimulate connective tissue growth.

Drug Interactions

None known.

Adverse Reactions

Patients receiving becaplermin, placebo, and good ulcer care alone had a similar incidence of ulcer-related adverse events such as infection, cellulitis, or osteomyelitis. However, erythematous rashes occurred in 2% of patients treated with becaplermin and placebo, and none in patients receiving good ulcer care alone. The incidence of cardiovascular, respiratory, musculoskeletal, and central and peripheral nervous system disorders was not different across all treatment groups. Mortality rates were also similar across all treatment groups. Patients treated with becaplermin did not develop neutralizing antibodies against becaplermin.

Patient Information

Patients should be advised that hands should be washed thoroughly before applying becaplermin.

The tip of the tube should not come into contact with the ulcer or any other surface; the tube should be recapped tightly after each use.

A cotton swab, tongue depressor, or other application aid should be used to apply becaplermin.

Becaplermin should only be applied once a day in a carefully measured quantity (see Administration and Dosage). The measured quantity of gel should be spread evenly over the ulcerated area to yield a thin continuous layer of ≈1⁄16 of an inch thickness. The measured length of the gel to be squeezed from the tube should be adjusted according to the size of the ulcer. The amount of becaplermin to be applied daily should be recalculated at weekly or biweekly intervals by the physician or wound caregiver.

➤*Step-by-step instructions for application of becaplermin are as follows:*

- Squeeze the calculated length of gel on to a clean, firm, nonabsorbable surface (eg, wax paper).
- With a clean cotton swab, tongue depressor, or similar application aid, spread the measured becaplermin over the ulcer surface to obtain an even layer.
- Cover with a saline-moistened gauze dressing.

After ≈ 12 hours, the ulcer should be gently rinsed with saline or water to remove residual gel and covered with a saline-moistened gauze dressing (without becaplermin).

It is important to use becaplermin together with a good ulcer care program, including a strict non-weightbearing program.

Excess application of becaplermin has not been shown to be beneficial.

Becaplermin should be stored in the refrigerator. Do not freeze becaplermin.

Becaplermin should not be used after the expiration date on the bottom, crimped end of the tube.

CHLOROPHYLL DERIVATIVES

otc	**Chloresium** (Rystan)	**Ointment:** 0.5% chlorophyllin copper complex in a hydrophilic base	In 30 and 120 g and lb.
		Solution: 0.2% chlorophyllin copper complex in isotonic saline	In 240 and 960 mL.

CHLOROPHYLL DERIVATIVES — TOPICAL

Refer to the Gastrointestinal Agents chapter for additional information.

Indications

➤*Dermatoses:* Arteriosclerotic, diabetic and varicose ulcers; trophic decubitus ulcers and chronic ulcers of nonspecific origin; malignant lesions (where deodorization is desired); traumatic injuries; skin grafting and skin defects; thermal, chemical and irradiation injuries; a wide variety of dermatoses.

Administration and Dosage

➤*Ointment:* Apply generously and cover with gauze, linen or other appropriate dressing. For best results, do not change dressings more often than every 48 to 72 hours.

➤*Solution:* Apply full strength as continuous wet dressing, or instill directly into sinus tracts, fistulae, deep ulcers or cavities.

Actions

➤*Pharmacology:* Aids wound healing by helping to produce a clean, granulating wound base for epithelialization or skin grafting. It also soothes inflamed, painful tissues and controls wound odor, even in malignant lesions. This is a true deodorizing, not a masking, action.

Adverse Reactions

Sensitivity reactions (rare); itching; irritation.

DEXTRANOMER

otc	**Debrisan** (Johnson & Johnson)	**Beads**	In 25, 60 and 120 g containers and 4 g packets (in 7s and 14s).
		Paste	Premixed, sterile. In 10 g packets (6s).

DEXTRANOMER — TOPICAL

Indications

➤*Topical ulcers:* For use in cleaning wet ulcers and wounds such as venous stasis ulcers, decubitus ulcers, infected traumatic and surgical wounds and infected burns.

Administration and Dosage

➤*Application:* Debride and clean the wound (dextranomer is not an enzyme and will not debride). Leave cleansed area moist. Apply to at least a thickness of ¼ inch to achieve desired suction effects. Cover area with a dry dressing and close on all sides.

➤*Removal:* When saturated, dextranomer changes colors and should be removed. Removal should be as complete as possible and is best achieved by irrigation. Vigorous irrigation (ie, soaking or whirlpool) may be necessary to remove patches that adhere to the wound surface.

➤*Paste:* May be needed for hard to reach areas or irregular body surfaces.

Mix beads with glycerin either on the dry dressing or in a receptacle or use premixed paste. Do not mix with any substance but glycerin. (See package insert for complete procedure.) Dress wound in the usual manner. Mix a fresh paste for each application. Do not reuse.

➤*Reapply:* Dextranomer beads or paste should be reapplied every 12 hours or more frequently if necessary. Reduce number of applications as exudate diminishes. Discontinue applications when the area is free of exudate and edema, or when a healthy granulation base is present. Consult physician if condition worsens or persists beyond 14 to 21 days.

Actions

➤*Pharmacology:* Dextranomer's ability to remove exudates rapidly and continuously from the surface of the wound results in a reduction of inflammation and edema. In vitro evidence suggests that the suction forces created by the drug may remove bacteria and inflammatory exudates from the surface of the wound.

Dextranomer is a hydrophilic dextran polymer in the form of tiny beads or paste. The hydrophilic beads absorb approximately 4 mL of fluid per 1 g of beads. The beads swell to approximately 4 times their original size. This swelling causes significant suction forces and capillary action in the spaces between the beads. This action continues as long as unsaturated beads or paste are in proximity to the wound.

When applied to the surface of wet ulcers or wounds, dextranomer removes various exudates and particles that impede tissue repair. Low molecular weight components of wound exudates are drawn up within the beads or paste, while higher molecular weight components (plasma proteins and fibrinogen) are found between the swollen beads. Removal of these latter components (particularly fibrin and fibrinogen) retards eschar formation.

Precautions

➤*For external use only:* Avoid contact with the eyes.

DEXTRANOMER — TOPICAL

➤*Wound packing:* When treating cratered decubitus ulcers, do not pack wound tightly. Allow for expansion of beads. Maceration of surrounding skin may result if occlusive dressings are used.

➤*Removal of dextranomer:* Do not use dextranomer in deep fistulas, sinus tracts or any body cavity where complete removal is not assured.

Remove the beads or paste once they are saturated. This avoids encrustation which makes removal more difficult. All dextranomer must be removed before any surgical procedures to close the wound (ie, graft or flap).

➤*Edema reduction:* Wounds may appear larger during the first few days of treatment due to reduction of edema.

➤*Dry wounds:* Not effective in cleansing dry wounds.

➤*Complete healing:* Not all wounds require treatment with dextranomer to complete healing. When the wound is no longer wet and a healthy granulation base is established, discontinue dextranomer.

➤*Treatment of the underlying condition:* This (eg, venous or arterial flow, pressure) should proceed concurrently with the use of dextranomer.

Adverse Reactions

Upon application or removal of beads, transitory pain, bleeding, blistering and erythema have occurred. Severe infections have been associated with administration in both diabetic and immunosuppressed patients.

Patient Information

For external use only. Avoid contact with the eyes.

EMOLLIENTS

DEXPANTHENOL

otc	**Panthoderm** (Jones Medical)	**Cream:** 2% in a water miscible base	In 30 and 60 g.

DEXPANTHENOL — TOPICAL

Indications

➤*Dermatological conditions:* Relieves itching and aids healing of skin in mild eczemas and dermatoses; itching skin, minor wounds, stings, bites, poison ivy, poison oak (dry stage) and minor skin irritations. Also used in infants and children for diaper rash, chafing and mild skin irritations.

Administration and Dosage

For external use only. Avoid contact with the eyes.

Apply to affected areas once or twice daily.

UREA (Carbamide)

Rx	**Keralac** (Doak)	**Ointment:** 50%	Vitamin E, lactic acid, zinc pyrithione, glycerin, EDTA, cetyl alcohol. In 45 g.
otc	**Aquacare** (Menley & James)	**Cream:** 10%	Petrolatum, glycerin, lanolin oil, mineral oil, lanolin alcohol, benzyl alcohol. In 75 g.
otc	**Carmol 20** (Doak)	**Cream:** 20%	Nonlipid vanishing cream base. In 90 g and lb.
otc	**Gormel Creme** (Gordon)		Mineral oil, parabens. In 75, 120 g, lb.
otc	**Lanaphilic** (Medco)		Petrolatum, lanolin oil, PPG, lactic acid, parabens. In lb.
otc	**Ureacin-20** (Pedinol)		Lactic acid, glycerin, mineral oil, parabens, EDTA. In 75 g.
Rx	**Urea** (Various, eg, Clay Park, Hi-Tech)	**Cream:** 40%	Mineral oil, petrolatum, cetyl alcohol. In 28.35 and 198.6 g.
Rx	**Carmol 40** (Doak)		Mineral oil, petrolatum, cetyl alcohol. In 28.35 and 85 g.
Rx	**Gordon's Urea 40%** (Gordon)		Petrolatum base. In 30 g.
Rx	**Vanamide** (Dermik)		Light mineral oil, cetyl alcohol, petrolatum. In 85 and 199 g.
Rx	**Keralac** (Doak)	**Cream:** 50%	Cetyl alcohol, EDTA, lactic acid. In 142 and 255 g.
otc	**Aquacare** (Menley & James)	**Lotion:** 10%	Mineral oil, petrolatum, parabens. In 240 mL.
otc	**Carmol 10** (Doak)		In 180 mL.
otc	**Ureacin-10** (Pedinol)		EDTA, parabens, lactic acid. In 240 mL.
otc	**Ultra Mide 25** (Baker Cummins)	**Lotion:** 25%	Mineral oil, glycerin, lanolin, EDTA. In 240 mL.
Rx	**Urea** (River's Edge)	**Lotion:** 35%	Cetyl alcohol, EDTA, lactic acid. In 207 and 325 mL.
Rx	**Keralac** (Doak)		Cetyl alcohol, EDTA, lactic acid. In 207 and 325 mL.
Rx	**Urea** (Various, eg, Clay Park, Hi-Tech)	**Lotion:** 40%	Mineral oil, petrolatum, cetyl alcohol. In 236.6 mL.
Rx	**Urea** (Clay Park)	**Gel:** 40%	Glycerin, EDTA. In 15 mL.
Rx	**Carmol 40** (Doak)		Glycerin, EDTA. In 15 mL.
Rx	**Keralac** (Doak)	**Gel:** 50%	EDTA, lactic acid. In 18 mL
Rx	**Umecta** (JSJ[a])	**Suspension, topical:** 40%	*Helianthus annuus* oil, EDTA. In 283.4 g.
Rx	**Umecta** (JSJ[a])	**Emulsion:** 40%	*Helianthus annuus* oil, EDTA. In 113.5 g.
Rx	**Keralac Nailstik** (Doak)	**Solution, topical:** 50%	EDTA. In carton of 6 nailsticks, each containing 2.4 mL.

[a] JSJ Pharmaceuticals, 3655 Route 202, Suite 116, Doylestown, PA 18901; 800-499-4468.

UREA — TOPICAL

Indications

➤*Urea 40% and 50%:* For debridement and promotion of normal healing of hyperkeratotic surface lesions, particularly where healing is retarded by local infection, necrotic tissue, fibrinous or purulent debris, or eschar. Urea is useful for the treatment of hyperkeratotic conditions such as dry, rough skin; dermatitis; psoriasis; xerosis; ichthyosis; eczema; keratosis; keratoderma; and corns and calluses; as well as damaged, ingrown, and devitalized nails.

➤*Urea 10% and 20%:* For moisturizing and softening dry, cracked, calloused rough and hardened skin of feet, hands, or elbows.

Administration and Dosage

➤*Urea 40% and 50%:* Apply urea cream, lotion, ointment, or gel to affected areas twice per day, or as directed by a health care provider. Rub in until completely absorbed. Protect surrounding tissue.

Apply to diseased or damaged nail tissue twice per day, or as directed by a health care provider. If desired, cover with adhesive bandage or gauze and secure with adhesive tape.

When applying to diseased or damaged nail surfaces, use an ample amount. Cover as previously described. You can also remove a "finger" from a plastic or vinyl glove and slip over the bandage-covered site. Secure glove finger with additional adhesive tape. Keep dry and occlusive for 3 to 7 days.

➤*Urea 10% and 20%:* Massage into dry skin areas once daily or as prescribed by a health care provider.

➤*Storage/Stability:* Store at controlled room temperature 15° to 30°C (59° to 86°F).

Protect from freezing. Keep this and all medications out of the reach of children.

VITAMIN E, TOPICAL

otc	**Vitamin E** (Various, eg, Nature's Bounty)	**Cream**	In 60 g.
otc	**Vitec** (Pharmaceutical Specialities)	**Cream:** dl-alpha tocopheryl acetate in a vanishing cream base, cetearyl alcohol, sorbitol, propylene glycol, simethicone, glyceryl monostearate, PEG monostearate	In 120 g.
otc	**Vite E Creme** (Gordon)	**Cream:** 50 mg dl-alpha tocopheryl acetate per g	In lb.
otc	**Vitamin E** (Various, eg, Nature's Bounty)	**Lotion**	In 120 mL.
otc	**Palomar "E"** (Pal Midwest)	**Ointment:** Vitamin E, boric acid, beeswax, lanolin, mineral oil, petroleum, starch, zinc oxide	In 2 oz.
otc	**Coppertone Aloe Aftersun Lotion** (Schering-Plough)	**Lotion:** Vitamin E, aloe, glyceryl, lanolin, paraben, EDTA, jojoba oil, cocoa butter, mineral oil	In 473 mL.
otc	**Vitamin E** (Various, eg, Mission, Nature's Bounty)	**Oil**	In 30 and 60 mL.[a]

[a] May or may not contain aloe.

VITAMIN E — TOPICAL

Indications

➤*Dermatological conditions:* Temporary relief of minor skin disorders such as diaper rash, burns, sunburn and chapped or dry skin.

Administration and Dosage

For external use only. Avoid contact with the eyes.

Apply a thin layer over affected area.

VITAMINS A, D and E, TOPICAL

otc	**Vitamin A & D** (Various, eg, Goldline, Rugby)	**Ointment**	In 60 g and lb.
otc	**A and D** (Schering-Plough)	**Ointment:** Fish liver oil, cholecalciferol, lanolin, petrolatum, mineral oil	In 45, 120, 480 g, 75 g pump dispenser.
otc	**Caldesene** (Fisons)	**Ointment:** Cod liver oil (vitamins A and D), 15% zinc oxide, lanolin oil, 54% petrolatum, parabens, talc	In 37.5 g.
otc	**Comfortine** (Dermik)	**Ointment:** Vitamins A and D, lanolin, zinc oxide, chloroxylenol, iron oxides, lanolin alcohol, mineral oil, triethanolamine, vegetable oil	In 45 and 120 g.
otc	**Desitin** (Pfizer)	**Ointment:** Cod liver oil (vit A & D), 40% zinc oxide, talc, petrolatum-lanolin base	In 30, 60, 120, 240, 270 g.
otc	**Lobana Peri-Garde** (Ulmer)	**Ointment:** Vitamins A, D and E and chloroxylenol in an emollient base	In 240 g.
otc	**Clocream** (Roberts)	**Cream:** Cod liver oil (vitamins A and D), cholecalciferol, vitamin A palmitate, cottonseed oil, glycerin, parabens, mineral oil	Vanishing base. In 30 g.
otc	**Lazer Creme** (Pedinol)	**Cream:** Vitamins A (3333.3 units/g) and E (116.67 units/g)	In 60 g.
otc	**Lobana Derm-Ade** (Ulmer)	**Cream:** Vitamins A, D and E, moisturizers, emollients, silicone	Vanishing base. In 270 g.
otc	**Retinol** (Nature's Bounty)	**Cream:** 100,000 IU vitamin A, glycol stearate, mineral oil, propylene glycol, lanolin oil, propylene glycol stearate SE, lanolin alcohol, retinol, parabens, EDTA	In 60 g.
otc	**Retinol-A** (Young Again Products)	**Cream:** 300,000 IU vitamin A palmitate per 30 g.	In 60 g.
otc	**Aloe Grande** (Gordon)	**Lotion:** Vitamins A (3333.3 units/g) and E (50 units/g), petrolatum, mineral oil, sodium lauryl sulfate, oleic acid, parabens, triethanolamine, aloe	In 240 mL.
otc	**Coppertone Cool Beads** (Schering-Plough)	**Lotion:** Vitamins A and E, aloe vera, glycol, EDTA, lactose	In 340 g.

VITAMINS A, D and E — TOPICAL

Indications

➤*Dermatological conditions:* For temporary relief of discomfort due to minor burns, sunburn, windburn, abrasions, chapped or chafed skin and other minor non-infected skin irritations including diaper rash and irritations associated with ileostomy and colostomy skin drainage.

Administration and Dosage

Apply locally to affected skin with gentle massage.

Warnings

➤*For external use only:* Avoid contact with the eyes.

➤*Worsened condition:* If the condition for which these preparations is used worsens or does not improve within 7 days, consult a physician.

EMOLLIENTS, MISCELLANEOUS

otc	**Balmex** (Block)	**Ointment:** 11.3% zinc oxide, aloe vera gel, parabens, mineral oil	In 30, 60, 120, and 454 g.
otc	**Allercreme Ultra Emollient** (Carme)	**Cream:** Mineral oil, petrolatum, lanolin, lanolin alcohol, lanolin oil, glycerin, glyceryl stearate, PEG-100 stearate, squalane, parabens	Unscented. In 60 g.
otc	**AmLactin** (Upsher-Smith)	**Cream:** 12% ammonium lactate	In 140, 225, and 400 g.
otc	**Geri-Hydrolac** (Geritrex)		Mineral oil, petrolatum, parabens. In 140 g.
Rx	**Lac Hydrin** (Wootwood Squibb)		Cetyl alcohol, glycerin, glyceryl stearate, lt. mineral oil, parabens. In 280 and 385 g.
Rx	**LAC-Lotion** (Paddock)	**Cream:** 12% ammonium lactate (12% lactic acid neutralized with ammonium hydroxide), light mineral oil, cetyl alcohol, parabens, glycerin	In 225 and 400 g.
otc	**AquaBalm** (Quintessa)	**Cream:** Petrolatum, methyl glucate dioleate, propylene glycol, DMDM hydantoin, iodopropynyl butylcarbamate	Fragrance free. In 114 g.
otc	**Aqua Glycolic Face** (Merz)	**Cream:** Cetyl ricinoleate, C12-15 alkyl benzoate, glycolic acid, hyaluronic acid, ceresin, ammonium glycolate, glyceryl stearate, PEG-100 stearate, sorbitan stearate, sorbitol, propylene glycol, diazolidinyl urea, parabens, magnesium aluminum silicate, dimethicone, xanthan gum, trisodium EDTA	In 50 mL.

EMOLLIENTS, MISCELLANEOUS

otc	**Aveeno Moisturizing** (Rydelle)	**Cream:** 1% colloidal oatmeal, glycerin, petrolatum, dimethicone, phenylcarbinol	In 120 g.
otc	**Catrix Correction** (Donell DerMedex)	**Cream:** Dipentaerythrityl, hexacaprylate/hexacaprate, sesame oil, *Catrix* (bovine-derived complex mucopolysaccharide), ceteareth-20, glycerin, caprylic/capric triglyceride, glycereth-7, dimethicone, xanthan gum, tocopheryl linoleate, alanine, glycine, urea, EDTA, imidazolidinyl urea, parabens, phenoxyethanol, orange oil, cardamon oil, titanium dioxide	In 36.9 g.
otc	**Complex 15 Face** (Schering-Plough)	**Cream:** Caprylic/capric triglyceride, squalane, glycerin, glyceryl stearate, lecithin, PEG-50 stearate, propylene glycol, dimethicone, diazolidinyl urea, carbomer-934P, EDTA	In 75 g.
otc	**Complex 15 Hand & Body** (Schering-Plough)	**Cream:** Mineral oil, glycerin, squalane, caprylic/capric triglyceride, glycol stearate, PEG-50, carboxylic acid sterol ester, glyceryl stearate, lecithin, dimethicone, diazolidinyl urea, carbomer-934, EDTA	In 120 g.
otc	**Curel Moisturizing** (Bausch & Lomb)	**Cream:** Glycerin, petrolatum, dimethicone, parabens	In 90 g.
otc	**Cutemol** (Summers)	**Cream:** Allantoin, mineral oil, acetylated lanolin, lanolin alcohols extract, mineral wax, beeswax, sorbitan sesquioleate, parabens	In 60 and 240 g.
otc	**DML Forte** (Person & Covey)	**Cream:** Petrolatum, PPG-2 myristyl ether propionate, glyceryl stearate, glycerin, simethicone, benzyl alcohol, silica, EDTA, sodium carbomer 1342	In 113 g.
otc	**Geri-Hydrolac** (Geritrex)	**Cream:** Ammonium lactate (equivalent to 12% lactic acid), light mineral oil, petrolatum, propylene glycol, glycerin, cetyl alcohol, parabens	In 140 g.
otc	**Hydrisinol** (Pedinol)	**Cream:** Sulfonated hydrogenated castor oil, hydrogenated vegetable oil	In 120 g and lb.
otc	**Hydrocerin** (Geritrex)	**Cream:** Petrolatum, mineral oil, mineral wax, ceresin lanolin alcohol, parabens	In 480 g.
otc	**Kerasal AL** (Taro Consumer)	**Cream:** Ammonium lactate, lt. mineral oil, glycerin, propylene glycol, cetyl alcohol, glyceryl monostearate, polyoxyethylene 100 stearate, magnesium aluminum silicate, methylcellulose, polyoxyl 40 stearate, laureth-4, parabens	May contain ammonium hydroxide and lactic acid. In 42 g.
otc	**Keri Creme** (Westwood Squibb)	**Cream:** Mineral oil, lanolin alcohol, talc, sorbitol, ceresin, propylene glycol, magnesium stearate, glyceryl oleate, parabens	In 75 g.
otc	**Kinerase** (Valeant)	**Cream:** 0.1% N^6-furfuryladenine, stearic acid, cetyl alcohol, safflower oil, stearyl alcohol, aloe vera, parabens, imidazolidinyl urea, ascorbic acid	In 40 and 80 g.
otc	**Kinerase Intensive Eye Cream** (ICN Pharm)	**Cream:** 0.125% kinetin, safflower seed oil, cetyl alcohol, urea, parabens	In 20 g.
otc	**Lanolor** (Westwood Squibb)	**Cream:** Lanolin oil, glyceryl stearates, propylene glycol, sodium lauryl sulfate, simethicone, polyoxyl 40 stearate, cetyl esters wax, methylparaben	In 60 and 240 g.
otc	**Lubriderm** (Warner-Lambert)	**Cream:** Mineral oil, petrolatum, lanolin, lanolin alcohol, lanolin oil, glycerin, glyceryl stearate, PEG-100 stearate, sorbitan laurate, parabens	Scented and unscented. In 81 g.
otc	**Neutrogena Norwegian Formula Hand** (Neutrogena)	**Cream:** Glycerin, sodium cetearyl sulfate, sodium sulfate, parabens	Scented and unscented. In 56.7 g.
Rx	**Lactinol-E Creme** (Pedinol)	**Cream:** 10% lactic acid, 3,500 units/30 g vitamin E	In 56.7 g.
otc	**Lactrex 12%** (SDR Pharmaceuticals)	**Cream:** 12% lactic acid, petrolatum, EDTA	In 184 g.
otc	**Lady Esther** (Menley & James)	**Cream:** Mineral oil	In 120 g
otc	**Nouriva Repair** (Ferndale)	**Cream:** Petrolatum, paraffin, mineral oil, sorbitan oleate, carnauba wax, ceramide 3, cholesterol, glycerin, oleic acid, palmitic acid, acrylates/C 10-30 albyl acrylate crosspolymer, tromethamine	In 30 g.
otc	**Nutraderm** (Owen/Galderma)	**Cream:** Mineral oil, sorbitan stearate, stearyl alcohol, sorbitol, citric acid, cetyl esters wax, sodium lauryl sulfate, dimethicone, parabens, diazolidinyl urea	In 90, 240, and 480 g.
otc	**Pacquin Medicated** (Pfizer)	**Cream:** Dimethicone, glycerin, cetyl alcohol, parabens	In 227 g.
otc	**Pacquin Dry Skin** (Pfizer)	**Cream:** Glycerin, cetyl alcohol, parabens	In 227 g.
otc	**Pacquin Plus** (Pfizer)	**Cream:** Glycerin, lanolin, cetyl alcohol, parabens	In 227 g.
otc	**Pacquin Plus with Aloe** (Pfizer)	**Cream:** Aloe vera gel, mineral oil, petrolatum, synthetic beeswax, cetyl alcohol, lanolin, dimethicone, stearic acid, methylparaben	In 227 g.
otc	**Pacquin Skin Cream with Aloe** (Pfizer)	**Cream:** Aloe vera gel, mineral oil, petrolatum, synthetic beeswax, cetyl alcohol, methylparaben	In 227 g.
otc	**Penecare** (Reed & Carnrick)	**Cream:** Lactic acid, mineral oil, imidurea	In 120 g.
otc	**Pedi-Vit-A Creme** (Pedinol)	**Cream:** 100,000 units vitamin A per 30 g	In 60 g.
otc	**Pen•Kera** (B.F. Ascher)	**Cream:** Glycerin, mineral oil, sorbitan stearate, urea, wheat germ glycerides, carbomer 940, triethanolamine, DMDM hydantoin, diazolidinyl urea	Dye and fragrance free. In 237 mL.
otc	**Phicon** (T.E. Williams)	**Cream:** 250 units vitamin A and 66.7 units E per g, aloe vera, 5% pramoxine hydrochloride	In 60 g.
otc	**Polysorb Hydrate** (Fougera)	**Cream:** Sorbitan sesquioleate in a wax and petrolatum base	In 56.7 g and lb.
otc	**Pretty Feet and Hands** (B.F. Ascher)	**Cream:** Mineral oil, glyceryl stearate, stearyl alcohol, cetyl alcohol, aloe vera gel, parabens	In 88.7 mL.
otc	**Penecare** (Reed & Carnrick)	**Lotion:** Lactic acid, imidurea	In 240 mL.
otc	**Allercreme Skin** (Carme)	**Lotion:** Mineral oil, sorbitol, triethanolamine, parabens	In 240 mL.
otc	**Aloe Vesta** (ConvaTec)	**Lotion:** 3% dimethicone	Alcohols, aloe, glycerin, petrolatum. In 60 mL.
otc	**AmLactin** (Upsher-Smith)	**Lotion:** 12% ammonium lactate, parabens, light mineral oil	In 225 and 400 g.
Rx	**Ammonium Lactate** (Glades)	**Lotion:** Ammonium lactate (equiv. to 12% lactic acid), light mineral oil, glyceryl stearate, glycerin, cetyl alcohol, parabens	In 225 and 400 g.

EMOLLIENTS, MISCELLANEOUS

otc	**Aqua Glycolic Hand & Body** (Merz)	**Lotion**: Glycolic acid, ammonium glycolate, cetyl alcohol, glyceryl stearate, PEG-100 stearate, C12-15 alkyl benzoate, mineral oil, stearyl alcohol, magnesium aluminum silicate, xanthan gum, parabens, disodium EDTA	In 177 mL.
otc	**Aquanil** (Person & Covey)	**Lotion**: Glycerin, benzyl alcohol, sodium laureth sulfate, stearyl alcohol, xanthan gum	In 240 and 480 mL.
otc	**Aveeno** (Rydelle)	**Lotion**: 1% colloidal oatmeal, glycerin, phenylcarbinol, petrolatum, dimethicone, benzyl alcohol	In 240 mL.
otc	**Balmex Emollient** (Macsil)	**Lotion**: Lanolin oil, silicone, Balsam Peru, glycerol monostearate	In 180 mL.
otc	**Choice DM Daily Moisturizing** (Bristol-Myers Squibb)	**Lotion**: Petrolatum, glycerin, dimethicone, steareth-2, cetyl alcohol, benzyl alcohol, laureth-23, magnesium aluminum silicate, carbomer, potassium sorbate, sodium hydroxide, aloe	Fragrance free. In 226.8 g.
otc	**Complex 15 Hand & Body** (Schering-Plough)	**Lotion**: Caprylic/capric triglyceride, PEG-50 stearate, squalane, carboxylic acid sterol ester, diazolidinyl urea, glycerin, glyceryl stearate, lecithin, dimethicone, glycol stearate, carbomer-934P, EDTA	Unscented. In 30 mL.
otc	**Corn Huskers** (Warner-Lambert)	**Lotion**: 6.7% glycerin, 5.7% SD alcohol 40, algin, guar gum, methylparaben	In 120 and 210 mL.
otc	**Dermasil** (Unilever)	**Lotion**: Dimethicone, mineral oil, glycerin, sunflower seed oil, borage seed oil, cetyl alcohol, lanolin alcohol, sweet almond oil, rose extract, sandalwood oil, EDTA, parabens	In 472 mL.
otc	**Derma Viva** (Rugby)	**Lotion**: Mineral oil, glyceryl stearate, laureth-4, lanolin oil, PEG-100 stearate, PEG-40 stearate, PEG-4 dilaurate, trolamine, DSS, parabens	In 237 mL.
otc	**DML** (Person & Covey)	**Lotion**: Petrolatum, glycerin, dimethicone, benzyl alcohol, volatile silicone, glyceryl stearate, palmitic acid, carbomer 941, xanthan gum	Unscented. In 240 and 480 mL.
otc	**Emollia** (Gordon Labs)	**Lotion**: Mineral oil, propylene glycol, white wax, sodium lauryl sulfate, oleic acid, parabens	In 120 and 240 mL and gal.
otc	**Epilyt** (Stiefel)	**Lotion concentrate**: Propylene glycol, glycerin, oleic acid, lactic acid	In 118 mL.
otc	**Esotérica Dry Skin Treatment** (SK-Beecham)	**Lotion**: Propylene glycol, dicaprylate/dicaprate, mineral oil, glyceryl stearate, cetyl esters wax, hydrolyzed animal protein, dimethicone, TEA-carbomer-941, parabens	In 37.5 mL.
otc	**Eucerin Moisturizing** (Beiersdorf)	**Lotion**: Mineral oil, PEG-40 sorbitan peroleate, lanolin acid glycerin ester, sorbitol, propylene glycol, cetyl palmitate, lanolin alcohol	Unscented. In 52.5, 120, and 240 mL, pt and gal.
otc	**Geri-Hydrolac 5%** (Geritrex)	**Lotion**: 5% lactic acid buffered with ammonium hydroxide, cetyl alcohol, dimethicone, EDTA, glycerin, parabens, petrolatum	In 237 mL.
otc	**Geri SS** (Geritrex)	**Lotion**: Mineral oil, propylene glycol, cetearyl alcohol, petrolatum, glycerin, dimethicone, colloidal oatmeal, hydrogenated castor oil, parabens, stearyl alcohol, EDTA, lemon oil, tocopheryl acetate	In 240 g.
otc	**Geri-Soft** (Geritrex)	**Lotion**: Mineral oil, propylene glycol, cetearyl alcohol, sorbitol, petrolatum, dimethicone, lanolin, castor oil, stearic acid, parabens, stearyl alcohol, EDTA, lemon oil	In 240 g.
otc	**Gold Bond Medicated Triple Action Relief** (Chattem)	**Lotion**: 5% dimethicone, 0.15% menthol	Aloe, cetyl alcohol, EDTA, glycerin, parabens, petrolatum, stearyl alcohol. In 236 mL.
otc	**Hydrisea** (Pedinol)	**Lotion**: 8% Dead Sea salts concentrate, NaCl, MgCl, KCl, CaCl, mineral oil, propylene glycol, sorbitan stearate, glyceryl stearate, PEG-75 lanolin, EDTA, imidazolidinyl urea, tartrazine, parabens	In 120 mL.
otc	**Hydrisinol** (Pedinol)	**Lotion**: Sulfonated castor oil, hydrogenated vegetable oil, propylene glycol stearate SE, mineral oil, lanolin, lanolin alcohol, sesame oil, sunflower oil, aloe, triethanolamine, sorbitan stearate, parabens, hydroxyethyl cellulose	In 240 mL.
otc	**Hydrocerin** (Geritrex)	**Lotion**: EDTA, lanolin, parabens, mineral oil, PEG-40 sorbitan, peroleate, propylene glycol, sorbitol, water	In 240 g.
otc	**Keri Original** (Bristol-Myers Squibb)	**Lotion**: Mineral oil, glycerin, PEG-40 stearate, glyceryl stearate, PEG-100 stearate, PEG-4 dilaurate, laureth-4, aloe, sunflower seed oil, tocopheryl acetate, parabens, fragrance, DMDM hydantoin, EDTA	Scented and unscented. In 241 g.
otc	**Keri Advanced** (Bristol-Myers Squibb)	**Lotion**: Glycerin, stearic acid, hydrogenated polyisobutene, petrolatum, cetyl alcohol, aloe, tocopheryl acetate, dimethicone, PEG-100 stearate, parabens, PEG-5 soya sterol, magnesium aluminum silicate, phenoxyethanol, EDTA, diazolidinyl urea, fragrance	Oil free. In 241 g.
otc	**Keri Age Defy & Protect** (Bristol-Myers Squibb)	**Lotion**: 7.5% octinoxate, 2% oxybenzone, cetearyl alcohol, glycerin, ammonium lactate, dimethicone, tocopheryl, EDTA	With alpha hydroxy and SPF +15. In 425 g.
otc	**Keri Light** (Bristol Myers Squibb)	**Lotion**: Glycerin, stearyl alcohol, ceteareth–20, cetearyl octanoate, stearyl heptanoate, squalane, parabens, carbomer-934	In 195 and 390 mL.
otc	**Keri Nourishing Shea Butter** (Bristol Myers Squibb)	**Lotion**: Mineral oil, glycerin, shea butter, vitamin E acetate, parabens, sunflower seed oil, EDTA, aloe	In 425 g.
otc	**Keri Sensitive Skin** (Bristol Myers Squibb)	**Lotion**: Glycerin, hydrogenated polyisobutane, petrolatum, cetyl alcohol, aloe barbadensis gel, vitamin E acetate, EDTA, parabens	In 241 g.
otc	**Keri Shave Minimizing** (Bristol-Myers Squibb)	**Lotion**: Glycerin, cetearyl alcohol, mineral oil, petrolatum, SD alcohol 40-B, DMDM hydantoin, glyceryl dilaurate, dimethicone, aluminum starch octenyl-succinate, fragrance, parabens, cyclomethicone, sangulsorba officinalis root extract, hydrolyzed soy protein	In 425 g.
otc	**Kinerase** (Valeant)	**Lotion**: 0.1% N^6-furfuryladenine, glycerin, stearyl alcohol, safflower oil, cetyl alcohol, aloe, parabens, corn oil, vitamin E acetate, ascorbic acid, retinyl palmitate	In 40 and 80 mL.
Rx	**Lac-Hydrin** (Westwood Squibb)	**Lotion**: 12% ammonium lactate (12% lactic acid neutralized with ammonium hydroxide), light mineral oil, cetyl alcohol, parabens	In 150 and 360 mL.
otc	**Lac-Hydrin Five** (Westwood Squibb)	**Lotion**: Lactic acid, glycerin, petrolatum, squalane, steareth-2, PCE-21-stearyl ether, propylene glycol dioctanoate, dimethicone, cetyl palmitate, diazolidinyl urea	Unscented. In 120 and 240 mL.
otc	**LactiCare** (Stiefel)	**Lotion**: Lactic acid, mineral oil, sodium hydroxide, glyceryl stearate, PEG-100 stearate, carbomer-940, DMDM hydantoin	In 222 and 345 mL.
otc	**Lobana Body** (Ulmer)	**Lotion**: Mineral oil, triethanolamine stearate, lanolin, propylene glycol, and parabens	In 120 and 240 mL and gal.
otc	**Lubriderm** (Warner-Lambert)	**Lotion**: Mineral oil, petrolatum, sorbitol, lanolin, lanolin alcohol, triethanolamine, and parabens	Scented and unscented. In 75, 120, 240, 360, 480 mL.
otc	**Lubriderm Daily Moisture with SPF 15** (Pfizer Consumer Health)	**Lotion**: 7.5% octinoxate, 4% octisalate, 3% oxybenzone	In 100, 177, 296, and 473 mL.

EMOLLIENTS, MISCELLANEOUS

otc	**Lubriderm Skin Nourishing with Sea Kelp Extract** (Pfizer Consumer)	**Lotion:** Glycerin, glyceryl stearate SE, cetyl alcohol, emulsifying wax, petrolatum, caprylic/capric triglyceride, castor oil, octyldodecanol, dimethicone, diazolidinyl urea, propylene glycol, xanthan gum, disodium EDTA, fragrance, giant kelp leaf extract, iodopropynyl butylcarbamate	In 100, 177, and 473 mL.
otc	**Lubriskin** (Geritrex)	**Lotion:** Mineral oil, petrolatum, lanolin, lanolin alcohol, cetearyl alcohol, castor oil, triethanolamine, stearyl alcohol, propylene glycol, parabens, EDTA	In 240 g.
otc	**Neutrogena Body** (Neutrogena)	**Lotion:** Glyceryl stearate, PEG-100 stearate, imidazolidinyl urea, carbomer-954, parabens, sodium lauryl sulfate, triethanolamine	Scented and unscented. In 240 mL.
otc	**Nivea After Tan** (Beiersdorf)	**Lotion:** SD alcohol 40B, mineral oil, PEG-40 castor oil, glyceryl stearate, parabens, aloe extract, lanolin alcohol, imidazolidinyl urea, phenoxyethanol, triethanolamine, chamomile extract, carbomer, simethicone	In 120 mL.
otc	**Nivea Moisturizing Extra Enriched** (Beiersdorf)	**Lotion:** Mineral oil, PEG-40 sorbitan peroleate, glycerin, polyglyceryl-3 diisostearate, petrolatum, glyceryl lanolate, lanolin alcohol, phenoxyethanol	In 120, 240, and 360 mL.
otc	**Nutraderm** (Owen/Galderma)	**Lotion:** Mineral oil, sorbitan stearate, stearyl alcohol, sodium lauryl sulfate, carbomer 940, diazolidinyl urea, parabens, triethanolamine	In 240 and 480 mL.
otc	**Shepard's Cream** (Dermik)	**Lotion:** Glycerin, sesame oil, vegetable oil, SD alcohol 40-B, propylene glycol, ethoxydiglycol, triethanolamine, glyceryl stearate, simethicone, monoglyceride citrate, parabens	Unscented. In 240 and 480 mL.
otc	**Therapeutic Bath** (Goldline)	**Lotion:** Mineral oil, glyceryl stearate, PEG-100 stearate, propylene glycol, PEG-40 stearate, laureth-4, PEG-4 dilaurate, lanolin oil, parabens, carbomer 934, trolamine, DSS	In 236 mL.
otc	**Ultra Derm** (Baker Cummins)	**Lotion:** Mineral oil, petrolatum, lanolin oil, glycerin, propylene glycol, glyceryl stearate, PEG-50 stearate, propylene glycol stearate SE, sorbitan laurate, potassium sorbate, phosphoric acid, EDTA	In 240 mL.
otc	**Vaseline Intensive Care** (Unilever)	**Lotion:** Ethylhexyl p-methoxycinnamate, (SPF5). Glycerin, sunflower seed oil, cetyl alcohol, corn oil, methylparaben, EDTA	In 325 mL.
otc	**Wibi** (Owen/Galderma)	**Lotion:** Glycerin, SD alcohol 40, PEG-4, PEG-6-32 stearate, PEG-6-32, carbomer-940, PEG-75, parabens, triethanolamine, menthol	In 240 and 480 mL.
otc	**Wondra** (Richardson-Vicks)	**Lotion:** Petrolatum, lanolin acid, glycerin, EDTA, hydrogenated vegetable glycerides phosphate, carbomer, dimethicone, imidazolidinyl urea, EDTA, titanium dioxide, parabens	Scented and unscented. In 300 mL.
otc	**Xeroderm** (Dermol)	**Lotion:** Mineral oil, acetylate lanolin alcohol, cetyl alcohol, glycerin, triethanolamine, parabens, imidazolidinyl urea	In 267 mL.
otc	**Collastin Oil Free Moisturizer** (Dermol)	**Lotion:** Soluble collagen, hydrolyzed elastin	In 60 mL.
otc	**Eucerin Plus** (Beiersdorf)	**Lotion:** Mineral oil, hydrogenated castor oil, 5% sodium lactate, 5% urea, glycerin, lanolin alcohol	In 177 mL.
Rx	**Lactinol** (Pedinol)	**Lotion:** 10% lactic acid	In 237 mL.
otc	**Hawaiian Tropic Cool Aloe With I.C.E.** (Tanning Research)	**Gel:** Lidocaine, menthol, aloe, SD alcohol 40, diazolidinyl urea, EDTA, vitamins A and E, tartrazine	In 360 g.
otc	**Coppertone Aloe Vera Gel** (Schering-Plough)	**Gel:** Aloe vera, glycerin, parabens, EDTA	Alcohol free. In 454 g.
otc	**Neutrogena Body** (Neutrogena)	**Oil:** Sesame oil, PEG-40 sorbitan peroleate	In 240 mL.
otc	**Nivea Skin** (Beiersdorf)	**Oil:** Mineral oil, lanolin, petrolatum, glyceryl lanolate, lanolin alcohol	In 240 mL.
otc	**Eucerin Itch-Relief Moisturizing Spray** (Beiersdorf)	**Spray:** 0.15% menthol, glycerin, mineral oil, cetyl alcohol, *Oenothera biennis* (evening primrose oil)	In 200 mL.
otc	**Aloe Vesta** (ConvaTec)	**Spray:** 36% petrolatum, hexamethyldisiloxane, *Softisan* 649, mineral oil, aloe extract	In 60 g.
otc	**Sardoettes** (Schering-Plough)	**Towelettes:** Mineral oil, tocopherol, beta-carotene	In 25s.

EMOLLIENTS, MISCELLANEOUS — TOPICAL

Indications

➤*Dry, itchy skin:* These preparations lubricate and moisturize the skin, counteracting dryness and itching.

EMOLLIENT BATH PREPARATIONS

otc	**ActiBath Effervescent Tablets** (Jergens)	20% colloidal oatmeal	In 4s.
otc	**Aveeno Shave Gel** (Rydelle)	Oatmeal flour	In 210 g.
otc	**Nutra•Soothe** (Pertussin)	Colloidal oatmeal, light mineral oil	In individual oil (9) and oatmeal powder packets (9).
otc	**Nutraderm Bath Oil** (Owen/Galderma)	Mineral oil, lanolin oil, PEG-4 dilaurate, benzophenone-3, butylparaben	In 240 mL.
otc	**Sardo Bath & Shower Oil** (Schering-Plough)	Mineral oil, tocopherol	In 112.5 mL.
otc	**Ultra Derm Bath Oil** (Baker Cummins)	Mineral oil, lanolin oil, octoxynol-3	In 240 mL.
otc	**Alpha Keri Therapeutic Bath Oil** (Westwood)	Mineral oil, lanolin oil, PEG-4 dilaurate, benzophenone-3	In 120 and 240 mL and pt.
otc	**Therapeutic Bath Oil** (Goldline)		In 473 mL.
otc	**Geri-Silk Bath Oil** (Geritrex)	Mineral oil, PEG-4 dilaurate, lanolin oil, D&C Green #6, fragrance	In 237 mL.

EMOLLIENT BATH PREPARATIONS

otc	**LubraSol Bath Oil** (Pharmaceutical Specialties)	Mineral oil, lanolin oil, PEG-200 dilaurate, oxybenzone	In 240 mL.
otc	**Domol Bath & Shower Oil** (Miles)	Di-isopropyl sebacate, mineral oil	In 240 mL.
otc	**Lubriderm Bath Oil** (Warner-Lambert)	Mineral oil, PPG-15, stearyl ether oleth-2, nonoxynol-5	In 480 mL.
otc	**Cameo Oil** (Medco)	Mineral oil, PEG-8 dioleate, lanolin oil	Unscented. In 240, 480, and 960 mL.
otc	**RoBathol Bath Oil** (Pharmaceutical Specialties)	Cottonseed oil, alkyl aryl polyether alcohol	Lanolin free. Dye free. In 240 mL, pt, and gal.
otc	**Esoterica Soap** (Medicis)	Sodium tallowate, sodium cocoate, mineral oil, acacia, sodium cocoyl isethionate, lauramide DEA, potassium oleate, titanium dioxide, pentasodium pentetate, tetra sodium etidronate	In 85 g.
otc	**Dermasil Lotion** (Chesebrough-Ponds)	Glycerin, dimethicone, sunflower seed oil, petrolatum, borage seed oil, vitamin E acetate, vitamin A palmitate, vitamin D_3, corn oil, EDTA, methylparaben	In 120 and 240 mL.
otc	**Aveeno Shower & Bath Oil** (Rydelle)	5% colloidal oatmeal, mineral oil, glyceryl stearate, PEG 100 stearate, laureth-4, benzyl alcohol, silica benzaldehyde	In 240 mL.

EMOLLIENT BATH PREPARATIONS — TOPICAL

Indications

➤*Dermatoses:* These products contain colloidal solids and various oils which act as emollients. They are recommended for relief of minor skin irritations and pruritus associated with common dermatoses and dry skin conditions.

Precautions

➤*For external use only:* Avoid contact with the eyes; if this occurs, flush with clear water.

Use caution – To avoid slipping in tub when using bath oils.

Do not use – On acutely inflamed areas.

PROTECTANTS

ZINC OXIDE

otc	**Dr. Smith's Adult Care** (Beta Dermaceuticals)	**Ointment**: 10%	Petrolatum, lanolin, mineral oil, olive oil. In 85 g.
otc	**Dr. Smith's Diaper Ointment** (Beta Dermaceuticals)		Petrolatum, lanolin, mineral oil, olive oil. In 85 g.
otc	**Zinc Oxide** (Various, eg, Moore, Paddock, Rugby)	**Ointment**: 20%	In 30 and 60 g and lb.

ZINC OXIDE — TOPICAL

Indications

Zinc oxide diaper rash ointment promotes healing, protects skin and relieves chafing.

In addition to healing diaper rash, zinc oxide ointment is indicated for treating many everyday skin problems. It promotes healing, protects, and helps seal out wetness. Use for minor burns, cuts, and scrapes.

Administration and Dosage

If diaper rash is present or at the first sign of redness, chafing, or minor skin irritation, apply zinc oxide ointment 3 or more times daily as needed.

To help prevent diaper rash apply zinc oxide ointment to the diaper area before you have to, especially at bedtime when exposure to wet diapers may be prolonged.

For superficial non-infected wounds and burns, apply a thin layer of zinc oxide, using a gauze dressing if necessary.

➤*Storage/Stability:* Store between 15° and 30°C (59° and 86°F).

PROTECTANTS, MISCELLANEOUS

otc	**Hydropel** (C & M)	**Ointment**: 30% silicone, 10% hydrophobic starch derivative, petrolatum	In 60 g and lb.
otc	**Silicone No. 2** (C & M)	**Ointment**: 10% silicone in petrolatum, hydrophobic starch derivative, methylparaben	In 30 and 480 g.
otc	**White Cloverine Salve** (Medtech)	**Ointment**: 97% white petrolatum, rectified turpentine oil, white wax	In 30 g.
otc	**Kerodex** (Whitehall)	**Cream**: #51-Bentonite, calcium carbonate, cellulose gum, chloroxylenol, glycerin, iron oxides, isopropyl alcohol, kaolin, parabens, petrolatum, sodium lauryl sulfate, spermaceti. Nongreasy invisible barrier for dry or oily work	In 113 g.
		Cream: #71-Calcium carbonate, cetrimonium bromide, iron oxide, isopropyl alcohol, kaolin, parabens, mineral oil, paraffin, petrolatum, sodium hexametaphosphate, sodium lauryl sulfate, zinc oxide. Nongreasy invisible water repellent barrier for wet work	In 113 g.
otc	**Elon Barrier Protectant** (Dartmouth)	**Liquid**: Paraffinum, liquidum, isopropyl palmitate, cetearyl alcohol, polyglyceryl-2 dipolyhydroxystearate, propylene glycol, cetearyl glucoside, C12-15 alkyl benzoate, stearic acid, bisabolol, petrolatum, phenoxyethanol, PEG-30 dipolyhydroxystearate, PEG-40 stearate, parabens, hamamelis virginiana, denatured alcohol.	In 28 g.
otc	**BlisterGard** (Medtech)	**Liquid**: 6.7% alcohol, pyroxylin solution, oil of cloves, 8-hydroxyquinoline	In 30 mL.
otc	**New-Skin** (Medtech)		In 10 and 30 mL bottle and 3.5 mL tube.
otc	**Skin Shield** (Del)	**Liquid**: 0.75% dyclonine HCl, 0.2% benzethonium chloride, acetone, castor oil, 10% SD alcohol 40. Waterproof.	In 13.3 mL.
otc	**New-Skin Antiseptic** (Medtech)	**Spray Liquid**: Pyroxylin solution, acetone ACS, oil of cloves, 8-hydroxyquinoline, 4.2% alcohol	In 28.5 g.
otc	**Sprayzoin** (Geritrex)	**Spray**: Benzoin compound, ethyl alcohol	In 118 mL.
otc	**Aerozoin** (Graham Field)	**Spray**: 30% tincture of benzoin compound, 44.8% isopropyl alcohol	In 105 mL.
otc	**Benzoin** (Various, eg, Humco, Lannett)	**Tincture**	In 60 and 120 mL, pt and gal.

PROTECTANTS, MISCELLANEOUS

otc	**Benzoin Compound** (Various, eg, Century, Geritrex. Humco, Lannett, Paddock, Purepac)	**Tincture:** Benzoin, aloe, storax, tolu balsam, 74% to 80% alcohol	In 30, 60 and 120 mL, pt and gal.
otc	**TinBen** (Ferndale)	**Tincture:** Benzoin, 75% to 83% alcohol	In 120 mL.
otc	**TinCoBen** (Ferndale)	**Tincture:** Benzoin, aloe, tolu balsam, storax, 77% alcohol	In 120 mL.
otc	**Pro-Q** (CollaGenex)	**Foam:** Dimethicone, glycerin, parabens	In 75 and 161 mL.

PROTECTANTS, MISCELLANEOUS — TOPICAL

Indications

➤*Dermatological conditions:* To protect skin against contact irritants.

Contraindications

Do not use silicone on wet, exudative lesions or inflamed or abraded skin.

SUNSCREENS

SUNSCREENS

		SPF		
otc	**Hawaiian Tropic Baby Faces Sunblock** (Tanning Research)	30+	**Lotion:** Titanium dioxide, octyl methoxycinnamate, octocrylene, benzophenone-3, octyl salicylate	PABA free. Waterproof. In 120 mL.
otc	**SolBar PF** (Person & Covey)	30+	**Cream:** Oxybenzone, octyl methoxycinnamate, octocrylene	PABA free. Waterproof. In 120 g.
otc	**Coppertone Sport** (Schering-Plough)	30+	**Lotion:** Ethylhexyl, p-methoxycinnamate, oxybenzone, 2-ethylhexyl salicylate, homosalate. Parabens, aloe	PABA free. Waterproof. In 118 mL.
otc	**Hawaiian Tropic Sunblock** (Tanning Research)	30+	**Lotion:** Titanium dioxide, octyl methoxycinnamate, benzophenone-3, octyl salicylate, octocrylene	PABA free. Waterproof. In 120 and 300 mL.
otc	**Coppertone Moisturizing Sunblock** (Schering-Plough)	30+	**Lotion:** Ethylhexyl p-methoxycinnamate, 2-ethylhexyl salicylate, octocrylene, oxybenzone	PABA free. Waterproof. In 120 and 300 mL.
otc	**Coppertone Shade Sunblock** (Schering-Plough)	30+	**Lotion:** Ethylhexyl p-methoxycinnamate, 2-ethylhexyl salicylate, oxybenzone, homosalate. Sorbitol, benzyl alcohol, aloe, vitamin E, parabens, jojoba oil, EDTA, phenethyl alcohol	PABA free. Waterproof. In 118 mL.
otc	**Coppertone Water Babies** (Schering-Plough)	30+	**Lotion:** Ethylhexyl p-methoxycinnamate, 2-ethylhexyl salicylate, oxybenzone, homosalate. Alcohol, aloe, parabens	PABA free. Waterproof. In 118 mL.
otc	**Water Babies UVA/UVB Sunblock** (Schering-Plough)	30+	**Lotion:** Ethylhexyl p-methoxycinnamate, 2-ethylhexyl salicylate, octocrylene, oxybenzone	PABA free. Waterproof. In 120 mL.
otc	**Hawaiian Tropic Just For Kids Sunblock** (Tanning Research)	30+	**Lotion:** Octyl methoxycinnamate, benzophenone-3, octyl salicylate, octocrylene, titanium dioxide	PABA free. Waterproof, all day protection. In 88.7 mL.
otc	**Coppertone Kids** (Schering-Plough)	30+	**Lotion:** Ethylhexyl p-methoxycinnamate, 2-ethylhexyl salicylate, oxybenzone, homosalate. Sorbitol, benzyl alcohol, aloe, jojoba oil, parabens	PABA free. Waterproof. In 237 mL.
otc	**Vaseline Intensive Care Blockout** (Chesebrough Ponds)	30+	**Lotion:** Padimate, ethylhexyl p-methoxycinnamate, oxybenzone, 2-ethylhexyl salicylate, titanium dioxide	Waterproof. In 120 mL.
otc	**Bullfrog Sunblock** (Chattem)	30+	**Gel:** Benzophenone-3, octocrylene, octyl methoxycinnamate. Aloe, vitamin E, isostearyl alcohol	PABA free. Waterproof, all day protection. In 120 g.
otc	**Hawaiian Tropic Baby Faces Sunblock** (Tanning Research)	30+	**Lotion:** Octyl methoxycinnamate, benzophenone-3, octyl salicylate, titanium dioxide, octocrylene	PABA free. Waterproof, all day protection. In 60, 120 and 300 mL.
otc	**Hawaiian Tropic Sunblock** (Tanning Research)	30+	**Lotion:** Homosalate, octyl methoxycinnamate, benzophenone-3, menthyl anthranilate, octyl salicylate	PABA free. Waterproof, all day protection. In 120 mL.
otc	**Coppertone Oil Free** (Schering-Plough)	30	**Lotion:** Ethylhexyl p-methoxycinnamate, oxybenzone, 2-ethylhexyl salicylate, homosalate. Parabens, EDTA, glyceryl	PABA free. Waterproof. In 118 mL.
otc	**Coppertone Water Babies** (Schering-Plough)	30	**Lotion:** Ethylhexyl p-methoxycinnamate, oxybenzone, 2-ethylhexyl salicylate, homosalate. Glyceryl, alcohol, parabens	PABA free. Waterproof. In 118 mL.
otc	**Neutrogena No-Stick Sunscreen** (Neutrogena)	30	**Cream:** 7.5% octyl methoxycinnamate, 15% homosalate, 6% benzophenone-3, 5% octyl salicylate	EDTA, parabens, diazolidinyl urea. In 118 g.
otc	**Tl•Screen** (Pedinol)	30	**Lotion:** 7.5% octyl methoxycinnamate, 6% oxybenzone, 5% octyl salicylate, 7.5% octocrylene	PABA free. Waterproof. In 120 mL.
otc	**PreSun Active** (Bristol-Myers)	30	**Gel:** Octyl methoxycinnamate, oxybenzone, octyl salicylate. 69% SD alcohol 40	PABA free. Waterproof, non-greasy. In 120 mL.
otc	**PreSun Ultra** (Westwood Squibb)	30	**Lotion:** 7.5% octyl methoxycinnamate, 5% octyl salicylate, 3% oxybenzone, 3% avobenzone	In 120 mL.
otc	**PreSun Ultra** (Westwood Squibb)	30	**Gel:** 7.5% octyl methoxycinnamate, 5% octyl salicylate, 6% oxybenzone, 3% avobenzone	65.5% SD alcohol 40. In 120 mL.
otc	**Sundown Sunblock** (Johnson & Johnson)	30	**Lotion:** Octyl methoxycinnamate, octyl salicylate, oxybenzone, titanium dioxide	PABA free. Waterproof, non-greasy. In 120 mL.
otc	**Bain de Soleil All Day for Kids** (Procter & Gamble)	30	**Lotion:** Ethylhexyl p-methoxycinnamate, 2-ethylhexyl 2-cyano-3, 3-diphenylacrylate, oxybenzone, titanium dioxide. Stearyl alcohol, vitamin E, EDTA	PABA free. Waterproof. In 120 mL.
otc	**Bain de Soleil All Day Waterproof Sunblock** (Procter & Gamble)	30	**Lotion:** Ethylhexyl p-methoxycinnamate, 2-ethylhexyl 2-cyano-3, 3-diphenylacrylate, oxybenzone, titanium dioxide. Stearyl alcohol, vitamin E, EDTA	PABA free. Waterproof, non-greasy, all day protection. In 120 mL.
otc	**Coppertone Moisturizing Sunblock** (Schering-Plough)	30	**Lotion:** Ethylhexyl p-methoxycinnamate, oxybenzone, 2-ethylhexyl salicylate, homosalate	PABA free. Waterproof. In 120 and 240 mL.
otc	**Coppertone Sport** (Schering-Plough)	30	**Lotion:** Ethylhexyl p-methoxycinnamate, oxybenzone, 2-ethylhexyl salicylate	PABA free. Waterproof. In 120 mL.
otc	**Shade Sunblock** (Schering-Plough)	30	**Stick:** Ethylhexyl p-methoxycinnamate, oxybenzone, 2-ethylhexyl salicylate, homosalate	Waterproof. In 18 g.

SUNSCREENS

		SPF		
otc	**Shade Sunblock** (Schering-Plough)	30	**Lotion**: Ethylhexyl p-methoxycinnamate, 2-ethylhexyl salicylate, homosalate, oxybenzone	Waterproof. In 120 mL.
otc	**Shade Sunblock** (Schering-Plough)	30	**Gel**: Ethylhexyl p-methoxycinnamate, homosalate, oxybenzone. 73% SD alcohol 40	Waterproof. Oil free. In 120 g.
otc	**Water Babies UVA/UVB Sunblock** (Schering-Plough)	30	**Lotion**: Ethylhexyl p-methoxycinnamate, 2-ethylhexyl salicylate, homosalate, oxybenzone	PABA free. Waterproof. In 120 and 240 mL.
otc	**Hawaiian Tropic Just For Kids Sunblock** (Tanning Research)	30	**Lotion**: Homosalate, octyl methoxycinnamate, benzophenone-3, menthyl anthranilate, octyl salicylate	PABA free. Waterproof, all day protection. In 88.7 mL.
otc	**Hawaiian Tropic Sport Sunblock** (Tanning Research)	30	**Lotion**: Octyl methoxycinnamate, octocrylene, benzophenone-3, octyl salicylate, titanium dioxide	PABA free. Waterproof, all day protection. In 88.7 mL.
otc	**SolBar PF** (Person & Covey)	30	**Liquid**: 10% octocrylene, 7.5% octyl methoxycinnamate, 6% oxybenzone. 77% SD alcohol 40	PABA free. In 114 mL.
otc	**Bain de Soleil SPF 30 + Color** (Procter & Gamble)	30	**Lotion**: Octocrylene, octyl methoxycinnamate, oxybenzone. Mineral oil, cetyl alcohol, EDTA	Waterproof. In 118 mL.
otc	**Coppertone Kids Sunblock** (Schering-Plough)	30	**Lotion**: Octocrylene, ethylhexyl p-methoxycinnamate, oxybenzone, 2-ethylhexyl salicylate	PABA free. Waterproof. In 120 and 240 mL.
otc	**Tréo** (Biopharm Lab)	30	**Lotion**: Octocrylene, octyl methoxycinnamate, benzophenone-3, octyl salicylate. Isostearyl alcohol, diazolidinyl urea, propylparabens. Also contains 0.05% citronella oil as an insect repellent	PABA free. Waterproof. In 118 mL.
otc	**Coppertone Kids Spray 'n Splash**(Schering-Plough)	30	**Spray**: Ethylhexyl p-methoxycinnamate, oxybenzone, 2-ethylhexyl salicylate, homosalate. Parabens, EDTA	PABA free. Waterproof. In 236 mL.
otc	**Coppertone To Go Sunblock** (Schering-Plough)	30	**Spray**: Ethylhexyl p-methoxycinnamate, oxybenzone, 2-ethylhexyl salicylate, homosalate. Alcohol	PABA free. Waterproof. In 112 mL.
otc	**Coppertone Sport Sunblock Spray** (Schering-Plough)	30	**Spray**: Ethylhexyl p-methoxycinnamate, oxybenzone, 2-ethylhexyl salicylate, homosalate. Alcohol	PABA free. Waterproof. In 112 mL.
otc	**Coppertone Moisturizing Sunblock** (Schering-Plough)	25	**Lotion**: Ethylhexyl p-methoxycinnamate, oxybenzone, 2-ethylhexyl salicylate, homosalate	PABA free, Waterproof. In 120 mL.
otc	**Vaseline Intensive Care Moisturizing Sunblock** (Chesebrough Ponds)	25	**Lotion**: Ethylhexyl p-methoxycinnamate, oxybenzone, 2-ethylhexyl salicylate. Glycerin, aloe vera gel, C12-15 alkyl benzoate, cetyl alcohol, petrolatum, vitamin E, parabens, EDTA	PABA free. Waterproof. In 118 mL.
otc	**Neutrogena Sunblock Stick** (Neutrogena)	25	**Stick**: Octyl methoxycinnamate, benzophenone-3, octyl salicylate. Castor oil, cetearyl alcohol, propylparaben, shea butter	PABA free. Waterproof. In 12.6 g.
otc	**PreSun Moisturizing Sunscreen with Keri** (Bristol-Myers)	25	**Lotion**: Octyl methoxycinnamate, oxybenzone, octyl salicylate. Petrolatum, cetyl alcohol, diazolidinyl urea	Waterproof. In 120 mL.
otc	**PreSun for Kids Spray Mist** (Bristol-Myers)	23	Waterproof. In 105 mL.	
otc	**Eucerin Dry Skin Care Daily Facial** (Beiersdorf)	20	**Lotion**: Ethylhexyl p-methoxycinnamate, titanium dioxide, 2-phenylbenzimidazole-5-sulfonic acid, 2-ethylhexyl salicylate. Mineral oil, cetearyl alcohol, castor oil, lanolin alcohol, EDTA	In 120 mL.
otc	**Hawaiian Tropic Baby Faces** (Tanning Research)	20	**Gel**: Octyl methoxycinnamate, octocrylene, benzophenone-3, menthyl anthranilate	PABA free. Waterproof. In 120 g.
otc	**TI•Screen Sports** (Pedinol)	20	**Gel**: 7.5% octinoxate, 6% oxybenzone, 5% octisalate, 2% avobenzone	70% alcohol. In 120 mL.
otc	**Bullfrog Sunblock** (Chattem)	18	**Gel**: Octocrylene, benzophenone-3, octyl methoxycinnamate. Isostearyl alcohol, vitamin E, aloe	PABA free. Waterproof, all day protection. In 120 g.
otc	**Bullfrog** (Chattem)	18	**Stick**: Benzophenone-3, octyl methoxycinnamate. Isostearyl alcohol, aloe, hydrogenated vegetable oil, vitamin E	Waterproof. In 16.5 g.
otc	**Bullfrog Extra Moisturizing Gel** (Chattem)	18	**Gel**: Benzophenone-3, octocrylene, octyl methoxycinnamate. Vitamin E, aloe	PABA free. Waterproof, all day protection. In 90 g.
otc	**Bullfrog Sport Lotion** (Chattem)	18	**Lotion**: Benzophenone-3, octocrylene, octyl methoxycinnamate, octyl salicylate, titanium dioxide. Diazolidinyl urea, EDTA, parabens, vitamin E, aloe	Waterproof, all day protection. In 120 mL.
otc	**Bullfrog for Kids** (Chattem)	18	**Gel**: Octocrylene, octyl methoxycinnamate, octyl salicylate. Vitamin E, aloe, C12-15 alcohols benzoate	Waterproof, non-greasy, all day protection. In 60 g.
otc	**Neutrogena Chemical-Free Sunblocker** (Neutrogena)	17	**Lotion**: Titanium dioxide. Parabens, diazolidinyl urea, shea butter	PABA free. In 120 mL.
otc	**SUNPRuF 17** (C & M)	17	**Gel**: 7.8% octyl methoxycinnamate, 5.2% octyl salicylate	Oil free, water-resistant. In 120 g.
otc	**TI•Screen Sunless** (Pedinol)	17	**Creme**: 7.5% octyl methoxycinnamate, 3% benzophenone-3. Mineral oil, alcohols, PEG-100, parabens	In 118 mL.
otc	**TI•Baby Natural** (Pedinol)	16	**Lotion**: 5% titanium dioxide	PABA free. Waterproof. In 120 mL.
otc	**TI•Screen Natural** (Pedinol)	16	**Lotion**: 5% titanium dioxide	PABA free. Waterproof. In 120 mL.
otc	**Hawaiian Tropic 15 Plus Sunblock** (Tanning Research)	15+	**Lotion**: Menthyl anthranilate, octyl methoxycinnamate, benzophenone-3	PABA free. Waterproof, all day protection. In 7.5, 15, 60, 120, 240 and 300 mL.
otc	**Hawaiian Tropic 15 Plus** (Tanning Research)	15+	**Gel**: Octyl methoxycinnamate, octocrylene, benzophenone-3, menthyl anthranilate	PABA free. Waterproof, all day protection. In 120 g.
otc	**TI•Screen** (Pedinol)	15+	**Lotion**: 7.5% ethylhexyl p-methoxycinnamate, 5% oxybenzone	PABA free. Water resistant. In 120 mL.
otc	**TI•Lite** (Pedinol)	15	**Cream**: 7.5% ethylhexyl p-methoxycinnamate, 2% titanium dioxide. Cetyl alcohol, phenethyl alcohol, parabens, EDTA	In 60 g.
otc	**Aquaderm** (Baker Cummins)	15	**Cream**: 7.5% octyl methoxycinnamate, 6% oxybenzone	In 105 g.
otc	**SolBar PF Sunscreen** (Person & Covey)	15	**Liquid**: 7.5% octyl methoxycinnamate, 5% oxybenzone. 76% SD alcohol 40	PABA free. In 120 mL.
otc	**SUNPRuF 15** (C & M)	15	**Lotion**: 7.5% octyl methoxycinnamate, 5% benzophenone-3	PABA free. Water-resistant. In 240 mL.

SUNSCREENS

		SPF		
otc	**Bain de Soleil SPF 15 + Color** (Procter & Gamble)	15	**Lotion**: Octyl methoxycinnamate, octocrylene, oxybenzone. Mineral oil, cetyl alcohol, EDTA	Waterproof. In 118 mL.
otc	**Catrix Correction** (Donell DerMedex)	15	**Cream**: Octyl methoxycinnamate, menthyl anthranilate, benzophenone 3, titanium dioxide. Sesame oil, cetearyl alcohol, urea, EDTA, imidazolidinyl urea, parabens	PABA free. In 39 g.
otc	**Oil of Olay Daily UV Protectant** (Procter & Gamble)	15	**Cream**: Octyl methoxycinnamate, titanium dioxide. Phenylbenzimidazole sulfonic acid, glycerin, cetyl alcohol, imidazolidinyl urea, parabens, EDTA, castor oil	Scented or unscented. In 51 g.
otc	**Bain de Soleil All Day Waterproof Sunblock** (Procter & Gamble)	15	**Lotion**: Ethylhexyl p-methoxycinnamate, 2-ethylhexyl 2-cyano-3, 3-diphenylacrylate, oxybenzone, titanium dioxide. Stearyl alcohol, vitamin E, EDTA	PABA free. Waterproof, non-greasy, all day protection. In 120 mL.
otc	**Coppertone Sport** (Schering-Plough)	15	**Lotion**: Ethylhexyl p-methoxycinnamate, oxybenzone	PABA free. Waterproof. In 120 mL.
otc	**Shade Sunblock** (Schering-Plough)	15	**Gel**: Ethylhexyl p-methoxycinnamate, oxybenzone. 75% SD alcohol 40	Waterproof. Oil free. In 120 g.
otc	**Vaseline Intensive Care Sport Sunblock** (Chesebrough Ponds)	15	**Lotion**: Ethylhexyl p-methoxycinnamate, oxybenzone, C12-15 alkyl benzoate. Aloe vera gel, vitamin E, EDTA	PABA free. Waterproof, non-greasy. In 118 mL.
otc	**Coppertone Kids Sunblock** (Schering-Plough)	15	**Lotion**: Ethylhexyl p-methoxycinnamate, oxybenzone, 2-ethylhexyl salicylate, homosalate	PABA free. Waterproof. In 120 and 240 mL.
otc	**Coppertone Moisturizing Sunblock** (Schering-Plough)	15	**Lotion**: Ethylhexyl p-methoxycinnamate, oxybenzone	PABA free. Waterproof. In 120, 240 and 300 mL.
otc	**Faces Only Moisturizing Sunblock by Coppertone** (Schering-Plough)	15	**Lotion**: Ethylhexyl p-methoxycinnamate, oxybenzone	PABA free. In 55.5 mL.
otc	**Oil of Olay Daily UV Protectant** (Procter & Gamble)	15	**Lotion**: Ethylhexyl p-methoxycinnamate, 2-phenylbenzimidazole-5-sulfonic acid, titanium dioxide. Cetyl alcohol, imidazolidinyl urea, parabens, EDTA, castor oil, tartrazine	PABA free. Greaseless. Scented or unscented. In 105 and 157.7 mL.
otc	**Vaseline Intensive Care Ultra Violet Daily Defense** (Chesebrough Ponds)	15	**Lotion**: Ethylhexyl p-methoxycinnamate, oxybenzone. Vitamin E, cetyl alcohol, acetylated lanolin alcohol, parabens, EDTA	PABA free. Non-greasy. In 120 and 300 mL.
otc	**Hawaiian Tropic Sport Sunblock** (Tanning Research)	15	**Lotion**: Octyl methoxycinnamate, benzophenone-3, octocrylene	PABA free. Waterproof, all day protection. In 88.7 mL.
otc	**Neutrogena Intensified Day Moisture** (Neutrogena)	15	**Cream**: Octyl methoxycinnamate, 2-phenylbenzimidazole sulfonic acid, titanium dioxide. Cetyl alcohol, diazolidinyl urea, parabens, EDTA	PABA free. In 67.5 g.
otc	**Ray Block** (Del Ray)	15	**Lotion**: 5% octyl dimethyl PABA, 3% benzophenone-3. SD alcohol	In 118.3 mL.
otc	**Solex A15 Clear Lotion** (Dermol)	15	**Lotion**: 5% octyl dimethyl PABA, 33% benzophenone. SD alcohol	Non-oily. In 120 mL.
otc	**Johnson's Baby Sunblock** (Johnson & Johnson)	15	**Lotion**: Titanium dioxide. Hydrogenated castor oil, EDTA, hydroxylated lanolin, zinc oxide, mineral oil	PABA free. Waterproof. In 120 mL.
otc	**Total Eclipse Oily and Acne Prone Skin Sunscreen** (Triangle Labs)	15	**Lotion**: Padimate O, oxybenzone, glyceryl PABA. 77% alcohol	In 120 mL.
otc	**Total Eclipse Moisturizing** (Triangle Labs)	15	**Lotion**: Padimate O, oxybenzone, octyl salicylate	In 120 mL.
otc	**Shade UVAGuard** (Schering-Plough)	15	**Lotion**: 7.5% octyl methoxycinnamate, 3% avobenzone, 3% oxybenzone	Waterproof. In 120 mL.
otc	**SolBar Plus 15** (Person & Covey)	15	**Cream**: 4% oxybenzone, 2% dioxybenzone, 6% octyl dimethyl PABA	In 113 g.
otc	**PreSun Moisturizing Sunscreen with Keri** (Bristol-Myers)	15	**Lotion**: Octyl dimethyl PABA, oxybenzone. Cetyl alcohol, diazolidinyl urea	Waterproof. In 120 mL.
otc	**SolBar PF** (Person & Covey)	15	**Cream**: 7.5% octyl methoxycinnamate, 5% oxybenzone	PABA free. In 222 g.
otc	**Sundown Sunblock** (Johnson & Johnson)	15	**Lotion**: Octyl methoxycinnamate, oxybenzone, octyl salicylate, titanium dioxide	PABA free. Waterproof, non-greasy. In 120 mL.
otc	**Water Babies UVA/UVB Sunblock** (Schering-Plough)	15	**Lotion**: Ethylhexyl p-methoxycinnamate, oxybenzone	PABA free. Waterproof. In 120 mL.
otc	**DML Facial Moisturizer** (Person & Covey)	15	**Cream**: 8% octyl methoxycinnamate, 4% oxybenzone. Benzyl alcohol, petrolatum, EDTA	In 45 g.
otc	**Hawaiian Tropic Self Tanning Sunblock** (Tanning Research)	15	**Cream**: Octyl methoxycinnamate, benzophenone-3. Aloe, cetyl alcohol, stearyl alcohol, cocoa butter, parabens, vitamin E	PABA free. In 93.75 mL.
otc	**Nivea Sun** (Beiersdorf)	15	**Lotion**: Octyl methoxycinnamate, octyl salicylate, benzophenone-3, 2-phenylbenzimidazole-5-sulfonic acid	PABA free. Waterproof. In 120 mL.
otc	**Neutrogena Moisture** (Neutrogena)	15	**Lotion**: Octyl methoxycinnamate, benzophenone-3. Parabens, diazolidinyl urea	PABA free. In sheer tint and untinted. In 120 mL.
otc	**Neutrogena Sunblock** (Neutrogena)	15	**Cream**: Octyl methoxycinnamate, octyl salicylate, menthyl anthranilate, titanium dioxide. Mineral oil, propylparaben	PABA free. Waterproof. In 67.5 g.
otc	**Tréo** (Biopharm Lab)	15	**Lotion**: Octocrylene, octyl methoxycinnamate, benzophenone-3, octyl salicylate. Isostearyl alcohol, diazolidinyl urea, propylparabens. Also contains 0.05% citronella oil as an insect repellent	PABA free. Waterproof. In 118 mL.
otc	**Coppertone Oil Free** (Schering-Plough)	15	**Lotion**: Ethylhexyl p-methoxycinnamate, oxybenzone. Aloe, parabens, EDTA	PABA free. Waterproof. In 118 and 237 mL.
otc	**Coppertone Sport Sunblock Spray** (Schering-Plough)	15	**Spray**: Ethylhexyl p-methoxycinnamate, 2-ethylhexyl salicylate, homosalate, oxybenzone. Alcohol	PABA free. Waterproof. In 112 mL.
otc	**Hawaiian Tropic 10 Plus** (Tanning Research)	10+	**Lotion**: Octyl methoxycinnamate, benzophenone-3, menthyl anthranilate	PABA free. Waterproof, all day protection. In 120 mL.
otc	**Original Eclipse Sunscreen** (Triangle Labs)	10	**Lotion**: Padimate O, glyceryl PABA	In 120 mL.
otc	**Scar Cream Maximum Strength** (Clay-Park Labs)	10	**Cream**: 7.5% octyl methoxycinnamate, 5% octyl salicylate.	Alcohols, mineral oil, parabens, urea. In 28 g.
otc	**Hawaiian Tropic 8 Plus** (Tanning Research)	8+	**Gel**: Octyl methoxycinnamate, benzophenone-3, menthyl anthranilate	PABA free. Waterproof, all day protection. In 120 g.

SUNSCREENS

		SPF		
otc	**Vaseline Intensive Care No Burn No Bite** (Chesebrough Ponds)	8	**Lotion**: Ethylhexyl p-methoxycinnamate, oxybenzone	PABA free. Waterproof. In 180 mL.
otc	**TI•Screen** (Pedinol)	8	**Lotion**: 6% ethylhexyl p-methoxycinnamate, 2% oxybenzone	PABA free. Water resistant. In 120 mL.
otc	**Bain de Soleil All Day Waterproof Sunfilter** (Procter & Gamble)	8	**Lotion**: 2-ethylhexyl 2-cyano-3, 3-diphenylacrylate, ethylhexyl p-methoxycinnamate, titanium dioxide. Stearyl alcohol, vitamin E, EDTA	PABA free. Waterproof, non-greasy, all day protection. In 120 mL.
otc	**Coppertone Moisturizing Sunscreen** (Schering-Plough)	8	**Lotion**: Ethylhexyl p-methoxycinnamate, oxybenzone	PABA free. Waterproof. In 120 and 240 mL.
otc	**Coppertone Oil Free** (Schering-Plough)	8	**Lotion**: Ethylhexyl p-methoxycinnamate, oxybenzone. Aloe, parabens, vitamin E, EDTA	PABA free. Waterproof. In 118 mL.
otc	**Coppertone Sport** (Schering-Plough)	8	**Lotion**: Ethylhexyl p-methoxycinnamate, oxybenzone	PABA free. Waterproof. In 120 mL.
otc	**Bain de Soleil SPF 8 + Color** (Procter & Gamble)	8	**Lotion**: Octyl methoxycinnamate, octocrylene. Mineral oil, cetyl alcohol, EDTA	Waterproof. In 118 mL.
otc	**Neutrogena Glow Sunless Tanning** (Neutrogena)	8	**Lotion**: Octyl methoxycinnamate. Cetyl alcohol, diazolidinyl urea, parabens, EDTA	PABA free. In 120 mL.
otc	**Neutrogena Sunblock** (Neutrogena)	8	**Cream**: Octyl methoxycinnamate, menthyl anthranilate, titanium dioxide. Mineral oil	PABA free. Waterproof. In 67.5 g.
otc	**Sundown Sunscreen** (Johnson & Johnson)	8	**Lotion**: Octyl methoxycinnamate, octyl salicylate, oxybenzone, titanium dioxide	PABA free. Waterproof. In 120 mL.
otc	**Tréo** (Biopharm Lab)	8	**Lotion**: Octocrylene, octyl methoxycinnamate, benzophenone-3, octyl salicylate. Isostearyl alcohol, diazolidinyl urea, propylparabens. Also contains 0.05% citronella oil as an insect repellent	PABA free. Waterproof. In 118 mL.
otc	**Hawaiian Tropic Protective Tanning** (Tanning Research)	6	**Lotion**: Titanium dioxide	PABA free. Waterproof. In 240 mL.
otc	**Coppertone Moisturizing Sunscreen** (Schering-Plough)	6	**Lotion**: Ethylhexyl p-methoxycinnamate, oxybenzone	PABA free. Waterproof. In 120 mL.
otc	**Faces Only Clear Sunscreen by Coppertone** (Schering-Plough)	6	**Gel**: Ethylhexyl p-methoxycinnamate, oxybenzone	PABA free. In 55.5 g.
otc	**Hawaiian Tropic Protective Tanning Dry** (Tanning Research)	6	**Oil**: 2-ethylhexyl p-methoxycinnamate, homosalate, menthyl anthranilate	Waterproof. In 180 mL.
			Gel: Phenylbenzimidazole, sulfonic acid, benzophenone-4	In 180 g.
otc	**Neutrogena Moisture** (Neutrogena)	5	**Lotion**: Octyl methoxycinnamate. Petrolatum, cetyl alcohol, parabens, diazolidinyl urea, EDTA, cetyl alcohol	PABA free. In 60 and 120 mL.
otc	**Bain de Soleil Mega Tan** (Procter & Gamble)	4	**Lotion**: Ethylhexyl p-methoxycinnamate, 2-ethylhexyl salicylate. Lanolin, cocoa butter, palm oil, aloe, DMDM hydantoin, xanthan gum, shea butter, EDTA	Waterproof. In 120 mL.
otc	**Bain de Soleil Orange Gelée** (Procter & Gamble)	4	**Gel**: Ethylhexyl p-methoxycinnamate, 2-ethylhexyl salicylate	PABA free. In 93.75 g.
otc	**Bain de Soleil Tropical Deluxe** (Procter & Gamble)	4	**Lotion**: Ethylhexyl p-methoxycinnamate, 2-ethylhexyl salicylate. Cetyl alcohol, EDTA	PABA free. Waterproof. In 240 mL.
otc	**Coppertone Moisturizing Suntan** (Schering-Plough)	4	**Lotion**: Ethylhexyl p-methoxycinnamate, oxybenzone	PABA free. Waterproof. In 120 and 240 mL.
otc	**Hawaiian Tropic Dark Tanning with Sunscreen** (Tanning Research)	4	**Oil**: Ethylhexyl p-methoxycinnamate, octyl dimethyl PABA	Waterproof. In 240 mL.
			Gel: Phenylbenzimidazole, sulfonic acid	PABA free. In 240 g.
otc	**Tropical Blend Dark Tanning** (Schering-Plough)	4	**Lotion**: Ethylhexyl p-methoxycinnamate, oxybenzone	Waterproof. In 240 mL.
			Oil: Padimate O, oxybenzone	Waterproof. In 240 mL.
otc	**Coppertone Sport** (Schering-Plough)	4	**Lotion**: Ethylhexyl p-methoxycinnamate, oxybenzone	PABA free. Waterproof. In 120 mL.
otc	**Coppertone Tan Magnifier Suntan** (Schering-Plough)	4	**Lotion**: Ethylhexyl p-methoxycinnamate	PABA free. In 120 mL.
			Gel: 2-phenylbenzimidazole-5-sulfonic acid	PABA free. In 120 g.
otc	**Bain de Soleil All Day** (Procter & Gamble)	4	**Lotion**: 2-ethylhexyl 2-cyano-3, 3-diphenylacrylate, ethylhexyl p-methoxycinnamate, titanium dioxide. Stearyl alcohol, vitamin E, EDTA	PABA free. Waterproof. In 120 mL.
otc	**Tropical Blend Dry Oil** (Schering-Plough)	4	**Oil**: Homosalate, oxybenzone	Non-greasy. In 180 mL.
otc	**Tropical Blend Tan Magnifier** (Schering-Plough)	4	**Oil**: Triethanolmine salicylate	Waterproof. In 240 mL.
otc	**Coppertone Gold Dark Tanning Oil** (Schering Plough)	4	**Spray**: Homosalate, oxybenzone. Aloe, vitamin E, mineral oil, paraben	In 236 mL.
otc	**Coppertone Gold Dark Tanning Exotic Oil** (Schering-Plough)	*	**Spray**: Homosalate. Mineral oil, coconut oil, olive oil, macadamia nut oil, cocoa butter, vitamin E, lanolin oil, sweet almond oil, jojoba oil, aloe	In 236 mL.
otc	**Q.T. Quick Tanning Suntan by Coppertone** (Schering-Plough)	2	**Lotion**: Ethylhexyl p-methoxycinnamate, dihydroxyacetone	PABA free. In 120 mL.
otc	**Coppertone Moisturizing Suntan** (Schering-Plough)	2	**Oil**: Homosalate	PABA free. Waterproof. In 120 mL.
otc	**Tropical Blend Dark Tanning** (Schering-Plough)	2	**Lotion/Oil**: Homosalate	Waterproof. In 240 mL.
otc	**Tropical Blend Dry Oil** (Schering-Plough)	2	**Oil**: Homosalate	Non-greasy. In 180 mL.
otc	**Hawaiian Tropic Dark Tanning** (Tanning Research)	2	**Gel**: Phenylbenzimidazole sulfonic acid	In 240 mL.
			Oil: 2-ethylhexyl methoxycinnamate, octyl dimethyl PABA	Waterproof. In 240 mL.
otc	**Coppertone Tan Magnifier Suntan** (Schering-Plough)	2	**Oil**: Triethanolamine salicylate	PABA free. In 120 mL.
otc	**Tropical Blend Tan Magnifier** (Schering-Plough)	2	**Oil**: Triethanolamine salicylate	Waterproof. In 240 mL.

SUNSCREENS

		SPF		
otc	**Coppertone Gold Tan Magnifier Oil** (Schering-Plough)	2	**Oil**: Triethanolamine salicylate. Glycerin, aloe, lanolin oil, cocoa butter, macadamia nut oil, olive oil, sweet almond oil, vitamin E, jojoba oil, coconut oil, parabens	In 236 mL.
otc	**Coppertone Gold Dark Tanning Sandproof Dry Oil** (Schering-Plough)	2	**Spray**: Homosalate. Aloe, vitamin E, mineral oil, paraben	In 236 mL.
otc	**A-Fil** (GenDerm)	*	**Cream**: 5% menthyl anthranilate, 5% titanium dioxide	In 45 g.
otc	**RVPaque** (ICN)	*	**Cream**: Red petrolatum, zinc oxide, cinoxate	Water resistant. Greaseless. Tinted. In 15 and 37.5 g.
otc	**Coppertone Sunless Tanner Spray** (Schering-Plough)	*	**Spray, non-aerosol**: Aloe vera, vitamin E, glycerin	In 118 mL.
otc	**Hawaiian Tropic 45 Plus Sunblock Lip Balm** (Tanning Research)	30+	**Lip balm**: Octyl methoxycinnamate, benzophenone-3, octyl salicylate, titanium dioxide, menthyl anthranilate	PABA free. Waterproof. Tropical, mint and cherry flavors. In 4.2 g.
otc	**Herpecin-L** (Chattem)	30+ 30	**Lip balm**: 7.5% octyl methoxycycinnamate, 6% oxybenzone, 5% octyl salicylate, 1% dimethicone. Beeswax, petrolatum, zinc oxide	In 2.8 g.
otc	**Blistex Ultra Protection** (Blistex)	30	**Lip balm**: Octyl methoxycinnamate, oxybenzone, octyl salicylate, menthyl anthranilate, homosalate, dimethicone	PABA free. Water resistant. In 4.2 g.
otc	**Coppertone Little Licks** (Schering-Plough)	30	**Lip balm**: Ethylhexyl p-methoxycinnamate, oxybenzone, 2-ethylhexyl salicylate. Paraben, aloe, saccharin	Waterproof. Cherry flavor. In 4.2 g.
otc	**Water Babies Little Licks by Coppertone** (Schering-Plough)	30	**Lip Balm**: Ethylhexyl p-methoxycinnamate, oxybenzone, 2-ethylhexyl salicylate	PABA free. Waterproof. In 4.5 g.
otc	**Stay Moist Lip Conditioner** (Stanback)	15+	**Lip balm**: Padimate O, oxybenzone. Aloe vera, vitamin E	Tropical fruit flavor. In 4.8 g.
otc	**TI•Screen** (Pedinol)	15+	**Lip balm**: 7.5% ethylhexyl p-methoxycinnamate, 5% oxybenzone. Petrolatum	PABA free. In 4.5 g.
otc	**Catrix Lip Saver** (Donell DerMedex)	15	**Lip Balm**: Allantoin, ethylhexyl p-methoxycinnamate, oxybenzone. Mineral oil, castor oil, petrolatum, vitamin E, propylparabon	PABA free. In 4.5 g.
otc	**ChapStick Sunblock 15 Petroleum Jelly Plus** (Robins)	15	**Ointment**: 89% white petrolatum, 7% padimate O, 3% oxybenzone. Aloe, lanolin	In 10 g.
otc	**Chapstick Sunblock 15** (Robins)	15	**Lip balm**: 7% padimate O, 3% oxybenzone. 0.5% cetyl alcohol, 44% petrolatums, 0.5% lanolin, 0.5% isopropyl myristate, parabens, mineral oil, titanium dioxide	In 4.25 g.
otc	**Eclipse Lip and Face Protectant** (Triangle Labs)	15	**Stick**: Padimate O, oxybenzone	In 4.5 g.
otc	**Neutrogena Lip Moisturizer** (Neutrogena)	15	**Lip balm**: Octyl methoxycinnamate, benzophenone-3. Corn oil, castor oil, mineral oil, lanolin oil, petrolatum, lanolin, stearyl alcohol	PABA free. In 4.5 g.
otc	**Daily Conditioning Treatment** (Blistex)	15	**Lip balm**: 7.5% padimate O, 3.5% oxybenzone, cetyl alcohol, aloe, cocoa butter, lanolin, vitamins A and E, petrolatum	In 7 g.
otc	**Blistex** (Blistex)	10	**Lip balm**: 6.6% padimate O, 2.5% oxybenzone. 2% dimethicone, cocoa butter, lanolin, parabens, mineral oil, petrolatum	Regular, mint, berry flavors. In 4.5 g.

SUNSCREENS — TOPICAL

Indications

➤*Sunburn prevention:* Overexposure to the sun may cause premature skin aging and skin cancer. The liberal and regular use of these products may help reduce the occurrence of these harmful effects.

For persons with conditions such as systemic lupus erythematosus, solar urticaria, erythropoietic protoporphyria or those taking photosensitizing drugs. Following is a partial list of drugs that may cause photosensitivity:

- Antihistamines (eg, cyproheptadine, diphenhydramine)
- Anti-infectives (eg, tetracyclines, nalidixic acid, sulfonamides)
- Antineoplastic agents (eg, fluorouracil, methotrexate, procarbazine)
- Antipsychotic agents (eg, phenothiazines, haloperidol)
- Diuretics (eg, thiazides, acetazolamide, amiloride)
- Hypoglycemic agents (eg, sulfonylureas)
- Nonsteroidal anti-inflammatory drugs (eg, phenylbutazone, ketoprofen, naproxen)
- Miscellaneous (eg, bergamot oils, etc, used in cosmetics; coal tar; psoralens; amiodarone; oral contraceptives; quinidine; disopyramide; gold salts; isotretinoin; captopril; carbamazepine)

Administration and Dosage

Apply liberally to all exposed areas (2 mg/cm^2 is recommended) at least 30 minutes prior to sun exposure (up to 2 hours for aminobenzoic acid and its esters) to allow for penetration and binding to the skin. Reapply after swimming or excessive sweating.

➤*Children:* Do not use sunscreens on infants younger than 6 months of age. Do not use SPFs as low as 2 or 3 on children younger than 2 years of age.

➤*Sun protection factor (SPF):* Sunscreen products include SPF ratings. This factor indicates the amount of increased resistance to sunburning the product provides, relative to unprotected skin. The SPF value is based on a numerical index designed to tell how much protection from the sun a product will provide. The SPF value is defined as the ratio of the amount of energy required to produce a minimal erythema dose (MED) or minimal sunburn through a film of a sunscreen drug product to the amount of energy required to produce the same MED without any treatment. (Example: Using a product with an SPF value of 6 would permit 6 times as much sun exposure.) Base product selection on the patient's history of response to sun exposure.

Recommended Sunscreen Product Guide[a]

Skin type	Patient characteristics[b]	Suggested product SPF
I	Always burns easily; rarely tans	20 to 30
II	Always burns easily; tans minimally	12 to < 20
III	Burns moderately; tans gradually	8 to < 12
IV	Burns minimally; always tans well	4 to < 8
V	Rarely burns; tans profusely	2 to < 4
VI[c]	Never burns; deeply pigmented (insensitive)	None indicated

[a] Based on the FDA's tentative final monograph (TFM) for sunscreen products.
[b] Based on first 45 to 60 minutes sun exposure after winter season or no sun exposure.
[c] This skin type not included in TFM.

➤*Waterproof formulas:* Maintain sunburn protection after being in the water up to 80 minutes.

➤*Water resistant formulas:* Maintain sunburn protection after being in the water up to 40 minutes.

Sweat resistant formulas – Maintain protection after 30 minutes or less of continuous heavy perspiration.

SPFs greater than 15 were not recommended by the 1978 FDA advisory panel on sunscreens. However, the agency issued a tentative final monograph on this product class in May 1993, and is proposing an upper limit for SPF values of 30. Scientific evidence shows a point of diminishing returns at levels above SPF 30; any benefits that might be derived from using sunscreens with SPFs greater than 30 are negligible. An SPF of at least 15 for most individuals is recommended by the Skin Cancer Foundation.

In addition to the products listed on the following pages, there are other sunscreens available from various cosmetic manufacturers.

Actions

➤*Pharmacology:* Sunscreens provide either a chemical or a physical barrier to sunlight. These agents help to prevent sunburn, actinic keratosis, premature aging, photosensitivity reactions, and to reduce incidences of skin cancer. Chemical sunscreens act by absorbing ultraviolet (UV) radiation in the medium wavelength range of 290 to 320 nm (UVB range). This is the spectrum of UV radiation primarily responsible for sunburning and

SUNSCREENS — TOPICAL

inducing skin cancer. UVA may augment the carcinogenic effects of UVB. Long wavelength UV radiation in the 320 to 400 nm (UVA range) can cause tanning and is responsible for most photosensitivity reactions that occur with many drugs, plants, soaps and cosmetics; it is also a major risk factor for serious skin damage. UVA irradiation can exceed that of UVB by 10- to 1,000-fold. UVA deeply penetrates into the dermis; UVB is primarily absorbed in the epidermis. There has been discussion of dividing UVA into UVA I (340 to 400 nm) and UVA II (320 to 340 nm); besides UVB, UVA II may cause the most skin damage. Physical sunscreens reflect or scatter light in both the visible and UV spectrum (290 to 700 nm), preventing penetration of the skin.

UV radiation in the 200 to 290 nm band is known as UVC; although little reaches the earth from the sun, some artificial sources emit UVC. UVC is thought to cause some erythema of the skin.

Sunscreen effectiveness is dependent on UV absorption spectrum, concentration, vehicle and ability to withstand swimming or sweating.

Sunscreen Ingredients

	Sunscreens	UV spectrum (nm)	Concentrations (%)
Chemical	*Benzophenones*	UVA and UVB	
	Oxybenzone	270 to 350	2 to 6
	Dioxybenzone	260 to 380[a]	3
	PABA and PABA esters	UVB	
	p-aminobenzoic acid	260 to 313	5 to 15
	Ethyl dihydroxy propyl PABA	280 to 330	1 to 5
	Padimate O (octyl dimethyl PABA)	290 to 315	1.4 to 8
	Glyceryl PABA	264 to 315	2 to 3
	Cinnamates	UVB[b]	
	Cinoxate	270 to 328	1 to 3
	Ethylhexyl p-methoxycinnamate	290 to 320	2 to 7.5
	Octocrylene	250 to 360	7 to 10
	Octyl methoxycinnamate	290-320	—
	Salicylates	UVB[c]	
	Ethylhexyl salicylate	280 to 320	3 to 5
	Homosalate	295 to 315	4 to 15
	Octyl salicylate	280 to 320	3 to 5
	Miscellaneous	UVB	
	Menthyl anthranilate	260 to 380[d]	3.5 to 5
	Digalloyl trioleate	270 to 320	2 to 5
	Avobenzone (butyl-methoxy-dibenzoylmethane; Parsol 1789)	UVA 320 to 400	3

Sunscreen Ingredients

	Sunscreens	UV spectrum (nm)	Concentrations (%)
Physical	Titanium dioxide	290 to 700	2 to 25
	Red petrolatum	290 to 365[e]	30 to 100
	Zinc oxide	290 to 700	—

[a] Values available when used in combination with other screens.
[b] Some UVA spectrum.
[c] Primarily UVB, but has about ⅓ the absorbency of PABA.
[d] Values are for concentrations higher than normally found in nonprescription drugs.
[e] At 334 nm, 16% UV radiation is transmitted; at 365 nm, 58% is transmitted.

Precautions

➤*Sensitivity:* Avoid prolonged exposure to sun and to tanning lamps. Sunsensitive persons particularly should exercise caution. If irritation or sensitization occurs, discontinue use.

Do not use sunscreens containing PABA or its derivatives if sensitive to benzocaine, procaine, sulfonamides, thiazides, PABA or PABA esters.

➤*For external use only:* Avoid contact with eyes.

➤*Vehicle:* Do not use sunscreens in highly alcoholic vehicles on eczematous or inflamed skin.

➤*PABA:* May cause a permanent yellow stain on clothing.

➤*Vitamin D deficiency:* May occur in elderly patients; sunscreens that block UV-B may block cutaneous vitamin D synthesis.

➤*UV exposure:* The amount of UV exposure is influenced by many factors (eg, time of day, season, latitude, altitude, atmospheric conditions). UVB radiation is strongest between 10 am and 2 pm; UVA is relatively constant. Each 1,000 foot increase in altitude adds 4% to UV light intensity. Reflectance from water depends on the angle of exposure, with almost 100% when the sun is directly overhead. Fresh snow reflects approximately 85% to 100% of UV light, and sand reflects 20% to 25%.

Adverse Reactions

Contact dermatitis may develop with PABA or its esters (especially glyceryl PABA), benzophenones and cinnamates. Physical sunscreens are occlusive; miliaria or folliculitis may occur.

Patient Information

Follow directions on product container concerning frequency of application; reapply after swimming or sweating. Reapplication does not extend the protection period.

➤*For external use only:* Do not swallow. Avoid contact with the eyes.

Discontinue use if signs of irritation or rash appear.

PABA may permanently stain clothing yellow.

Wear protective eye coverings or sunglasses; UV light can cause corneal damage.

OINTMENT AND LOTION BASES

otc	**Lanaphilic** (Medco)	**Ointment**: Stearyl alcohol, white petrolatum, isopropyl palmitate, lanolin oil, propylene glycol, sorbitol, sodium lauryl sulfate, parabens	In lb.
otc	**Lanaphilic w/Urea 10%** (Medco)	**Ointment**: Urea, stearyl alcohol, white petrolatum, isopropyl palmitate, lanolin oil, sorbitol, propylene glycol, sodium lauryl sulfate, lactic acid, parabens	In lb.
otc	**Petrolatum** (Carolina Medical)	**Ointment**: Petrolatum, mineral oil, ceresin wax, woolwax alcohol	In 430 g.
otc	**Absorbase** (Carolina Medical)	**Ointment**: Petrolatum, mineral oil, ceresin wax, woolwax alcohol, potassium sorbate	Unscented. In 114 and 454 g.
otc	**Hydrophilic** (Rugby)	**Ointment**: White petrolatum, stearyl alcohol, propylene glycol, sodium lauryl sulfate, parabens	In 454 g.
otc	**Aquabase** (Paddock)	**Ointment**: Petrolatum, mineral oil, mineral wax, woolwax alcohol, sorbitan sesquioleate	Unscented. Dye free. In 454 g.
otc	**Aquaphilic** (Medco)	**Ointment**: Stearyl alcohol, white petrolatum, isopropyl palmitate, sorbitol, propylene glycol, sodium lauryl sulfate, parabens	In lb.
otc	**Aquaphilic w/Carbamide 10% and 20%** (Medco)	**Ointment**: Urea, stearyl alcohol, white petrolatum, isopropyl palmitate, propylene glycol, sorbitol, sodium lauryl sulfate, lactic acid, parabens	In lb.
otc	**Aquaphor Healing Ointment** (Beiersdorf)	**Ointment**: Petrolatum, mineral oil, lanolin, alcohol, panthenol, glycerin.	In 10 and 50 g tubes and 99 and 396 g jars.
otc	**Polyethylene Glycol** (Medco)	**Ointment**: Water soluble greaseless base with PEG-8 and PEG-75	In lb.
otc	**Solumol** (C & M)	**Ointment**: Petrolatum, mineral oil, cetearyl alcohol, sodium lauryl sulfate, glycerin, propylene glycol	In lb.
otc	**Unibase** (Warner Chilcott)	**Ointment**: Nongreasy, water removable base with white petrolatum, glycerin, sodium lauryl sulfate, propylparaben. Will absorb 30% of its weight in water	In lb.
otc	**Acid Mantle** (Doak)	**Cream**: Water, cetearyl alcohol, sodium lauryl sulfate, sodium cetearyl sulfate, glycerin, petrolatum, synthetic beeswax, mineral oil, methylparaben, aluminum sulfate, calcium acetate, white potato dextrin	In 120 g.
otc	**Velvachol** (Owen/Galderma)	**Cream**: Water miscible vehicle containing petrolatum, mineral oil, stearyl alcohol, sodium lauryl sulfate, cholesterol, parabens	In lb.
otc	**Dermabase** (Paddock)	**Cream**: Mineral oil, petrolatum, cetostearyl alcohol, propylene glycol, sodium lauryl sulfate, isopropyl palmitate, imidazolidinyl urea, parabens	In 454 g.
otc	**Dermovan** (Owen/Galderma)	**Cream**: Nonionic, water miscible vanishing cream vehicle containing glyceryl stearate, stearamidoethyl diethylamine, glycerin, mineral oil, cetyl esters, parabens	In lb.

OINTMENT AND LOTION BASES

otc	**Hydrocream Base** (Paddock)	**Cream:** Petrolatum, mineral oil, mineral wax, woolwax alcohol, cholesterol, imidazolidinyl urea, parabens	In 454 g.
otc	**Eucerin** (Beiersdorf)	**Cream:** Petrolatum, mineral oil, mineral wax, woolwax alcohol	In 60, 120, 240 and 480 g.
otc	**Hydrocerin** (Geritrex)	**Cream:** Petrolatum, mineral oil, lanolin alcohol, parabens	In 120 g.
otc	**Vanicream** (Pharmaceutical Specialties)	**Cream:** White petrolatum, cetearyl alcohol, ceteareth-20, sorbitol solution, propylene glycol, simethicone, glyceryl monostearate, polyethylene glycol monostearate	In 120 g and lb.
otc	**Nutraderm** (Owen/Galderma)	**Lotion:** Mineral oil, sorbitan stearate, stearyl alcohol, sodium lauryl sulfate, cetyl alcohol, carbomer-940, parabens, triethanolamine	In 240 and 480 mL.
otc	**Hydrocerin** (Geritrex)	**Lotion:** Mineral oil, lanolin alcohol, parabens	In 473 mL.
otc	**Vehicle/N** (Neutrogena)	**Solution:** 45% SD alcohol 40, laureth-4, propylene glycol, 4% isopropyl alcohol	In 50 mL with applicator.
otc	**Vehicle/N Mild** (Neutrogena)	**Solution:** 37.5% SD alcohol 40, laureth-4, 5% isopropyl alcohol	In 50 mL with applicator.
otc	**Solvent-G** (Syosset)	**Liquid:** 55% SD alcohol 40B, laureth-4, isopropyl alcohol, propylene glycol	In 50 mL.

OINTMENT AND LOTION BASES — TOPICAL

Indications

➤*Bases:* These products are used as bases for incorporation of various active ingredients in extemporaneously compounded dermatological prescriptions.

RUBS AND LINIMENTS

Indications

➤*Topical pain:* These products are used for relief of pain of muscular aches, neuralgia, rheumatism, arthritis, sprains and like conditions, when skin is intact.

Contraindications

Allergy to components of any formulation or to salicylates.

Warnings

➤*For external use only:* Avoid contact with eyes and mucous membranes.

Precautions

➤*Apply to affected parts only:* Do not apply to irritated skin; if excessive irritation develops, discontinue use. If pain persists for more than 7 to 10 days, or if redness is present, or in conditions affecting children younger than 10 years of age, consult a physician.

➤*Heat therapy:* Do not use an external source of heat (eg, heating pad) with these agents since irritation or burning of the skin may occur.

➤*Protective covering:* Applying a tight bandage or wrap over these agents is not recommended since increased absorption may occur.

Drug Interactions

➤*Anticoagulants:* An enhanced anticoagulant effect (eg, increased prothrombin time) occurred in several patients receiving an anticoagulant and using topical methylsalicylate concurrently.

Adverse Reactions

If applied to large skin areas, salicylate side effects may occur, such as tinnitus, nausea or vomiting. Toxic if ingested.

Counterirritants may cause local irritation, especially in patients with sensitive skin.

GELS, CREAMS AND OINTMENTS

otc	**Aspercreme Cream** (Chattem)	10% trolamine salicylate	In 37.5, 90, and 150 g.
otc	**Flex-Power Performance Sports** (Flex-Power)		Cetyl alcohol, EDTA, parabens, glycerols, stearyl alcohol, sodium metabisulfite. Citrus light and clean scents. In 120 g.
otc	**Mobisyl Creme** (Ascher)		In 35.4, 100, and 227 g.
otc	**Myoflex Creme** (Fisons)		In 60, 120, and 240 g and lb.
otc	**Sportscreme** (Chattem)		In 37.5 and 90 g.
otc	**Panalgesic Cream** (E.C. Robins/Poythress)	35% methyl salicylate, 4% menthol	In 120 g.
otc	**Icy Hot Cream** (Chattem)	30% methyl salicylate, 10% menthol, carbomer, cetyl esters wax, emulsifying wax, trolamine	In 37.5 and 90 g.
otc	**ArthriCare Triple-Medicated Gel** (Commerce)	30% methyl salicylate, 1.25% menthol, 0.7% methyl nicotinate, isopropyl alcohol, propylene glycol, hydroxypropylmethylcellulose, DSS	In 90 g.
otc	**Musterole Deep Strength Rub** (Schering-Plough)	30% methyl salicylate, 0.5% methyl nicotinate and 3% menthol	In 37 and 90 g.
otc	**Ben-Gay Ultra Strength Cream** (Pfizer)	30% methyl salicylate, 10% menthol, 4% camphor, EDTA, glyceryl stearate SE, anhydrous lanolin, polysorbate 80, potassium carbomer and stearate, triethanolamine carbomer and stearate	In 35 g.
otc	**Arthritis Formula Ben-Gay** (Pfizer)	30% methyl salicylate, 8% menthol, glyceryl stearate SE, anhydrous lanolin, polysorbate 85, potassium stearate, sorbitan tristearate, xanthan gum	In 35 g.
otc	**Exocaine Plus Rub** (Commerce Drug)	30% methyl salicylate	In 39 and 120 g.
otc	**Icy Hot Chill Stick** (Chattem)	30% methyl salicylate, 10% menthol	Hydrogenated castor oil, stearyl alcohol. In 49 g.
otc	**Icy Hot Balm** (Chattem)	29% methyl salicylate, 7.6% menthol, paraffin, white petrolatum	In 105 g.
otc	**Exocaine Medicated Rub** (Commerce)	25% methyl salicylate, clove oil, eucalyptus oil, lanolin, cetyl alcohol, glycerin, glyceryl, menthol, parabens	In 120 g.
otc	**Improved Analgesic Ointment** (Rugby)	18.3% methyl salicylate, 16% menthol	In 36, 85 and 454 g.
otc	**Ben-Gay Original Ointment** (Pfizer)	18.3% methyl salicylate, 16% menthol, anhydrous lanolin, microcrystalline wax, synthetic bees wax	In 35 and 90 g.
otc	**Pain Bust•RII** (Continental)	17% methyl salicylate, 12% menthol	In 90 g.

GELS, CREAMS AND OINTMENTS

otc	**Arthritis Hot Creme** (Chattem)	15% methyl salicylate, 10% menthol, glyceryl stearate, carbomer 934, lanolin, PEG-100 stearate, propylene glycol, trolamine, parabens	In 90 g.
otc	**Icy Hot Arthritis Therapy Gel** (Chattem)	0.025% capsaicin, parabens, aloe vera, alcohol, wax, soybean oil	In 70.8 g.
otc	**Deep-Down Rub** (SK-Beecham)	15% methyl salicylate, 5% menthol, 0.5% camphor, 40.5% SD alcohol	In 37.5 and 90 g.
otc	**Minit-Rub** (Bristol-Myers)	15% methyl salicylate, 3.5% menthol, 2.3% camphor, anhydrous lanolin	In 45 and 90 g.
otc	**Thera-gesic Cream** (Mission)	15% methyl salicylate, menthol, dimethylpolysiloxane, glycerin, carbopol, triethanolamine, parabens	In 90 and 150 g.
otc	**Ziks Cream** (Nodum)	12% methyl salicylate, 1% menthol, 0.025% capsaicin, cetyl alcohol	In 60 g.
otc	**Gordogesic Creme** (Gordon)	10% methyl salicylate, propylene glycol, mineral oil, white wax, triethanolamine, parabens	In 75 g and lb.
otc	**Methagual** (Gordon)	8% methyl salicylate, 2% guaiacol, petrolatum, white wax, parabens	In 60 g and lb.
otc	**Blue Gel Muscular Pain Reliever** (Rugby)	Menthol	In 240 g.
otc	**Eucalyptamint Maximum Strength Ointment** (Ciba)	16% menthol, lanolin, eucalyptus oil	In 60 mL.
otc	**Flexall Ultra Plus** (Chattem)	16% menthol, 10% methyl salicylate, 3.1% camphor in aloe vera gel base, eucalyptus oil, glycerin, peppermint oil, alcohol	In 70.8 g.
otc	**Maximum Strength Flex-all 454** (Chattem)	16% menthol, aloe vera gel, eucalyptus oil, methyl salicylate, peppermint oil, SD alcohol 38-B, thyme oil	In 90 g.
otc	**Bayer Muscle and Joint Cream** (Bayer)	10% menthol, 4% camphor, 30% methyl salicylate, EDTA, glyceryl, lanolin, stearyl alcohol	In 56 and 114 g.
otc	**Eucalyptamint Gel** (Ciba Consumer)	8% menthol, eucalyptus oil, SD 3A alcohol	In 60 g.
otc	**Wonder Ice Gel** (Pedinol)	5.25% menthol	In 113 and 473 g.
otc	**Double Ice ArthriCare Gel** (Commerce)	4% menthol, 3.1% camphor, aloe vera gel, carbomer 940, dioctylsodium sulfosuccinate, isopropyl alcohol, propylene glycol, triethanolamine	In 90 g.
otc	**Absorbine Power Gel** (W.F. Young)	4% menthol	In 88 g.
otc	**Mineral Freez Gel** (Geritrex)	2% menthol	Alcohol. In 226.8 g.
otc	**Pain Gel Plus** (Mentholatum Co.)	4% menthol, aloe, vitamin E	In 57 g.
otc	**Vanishing Scent Ben-Gay** (Pfizer)	2.5% menthol, alcohol, camphor	In 120 g.
otc	**Odor Free ArthriCare Rub** (Commerce)	1.25% menthol, 0.25% methyl nicotinate, 0.025% capsaicin, aloe vera gel, carbomer 940, DMDM hydantoin, emulsifying wax, glyceryl stearate SE, isopropyl alcohol, myristyl propionate, propylparaben, triethanolamine	In 90 g.
otc	**Sōltice Quick-Rub** (Oakhurst)	5.1% menthol, 5.1% camphor	Eucalyptus oil, glycerin, methyl salicylate. In 37 and 85 g.
otc	**Dermal-Rub Balm** (Hauck)	Methyl salicylate, camphor, racemic menthol, cajuput oil	In 30 g and lb.
otc	**Analgesic Balm** (Various, eg, URL)	Methyl salicylate, menthol	In 30 and 454 g.
otc	**Analgesic Balm-GRX** (Geritrex)	14% methyl salicylate, 6% menthol	In 28 g.
otc	**TheraFlu Vapor Stick Cough & Muscle Aches** (Novartis)	4.8% camphor, 2.6% menthol, cetyl alcohol, eucalyptus oil, parabens	In 51 g.
otc	**Vicks VapoRub Cream** (Richardson-Vicks)	4.7% camphor, 2.6% menthol, 1.2% eucalyptus oil, cedarleaf oil, EDTA, glycerin, imidazolidinyl urea, cetyl and stearyl alcohols, parabens, nutmeg oil, titanium dioxide, spirits of turpentine	In 45, 60, 90 and 180 g.
otc	**Methalgen Cream** (Alra)	Camphor, menthol, methyl salicylate, oil of mustard	In 60 and 480 g.
otc	**Therapeutic Mineral Ice Exercise Formula Gel** (Bristol-Myers)	4% menthol, ammonium hydroxide, carbomer 934P or 934, cupric sulfate, isopropyl alcohol, thymol	In 90 g.
otc	**Ben-Gay Vanishing Scent Gel** (Pfizer)	3% menthol, benzophenone-4, camphor, diazolidinyl urea, EDTA, isopropyl alcohol, potassium carbomer 940	In 35 g.
otc	**Blue Ice Gel** (Geritrex)	2% menthol	Isopropyl alcohol. In 227 g.
otc	**Therapy Ice** (Major)	**Gel**: 2% menthol	Isopropyl alcohol. In 226.8 g.
otc	**Sportscreme Ice Gel** (Thompson)	2% menthol, carbomer 934, styrene/acrylate copolymer, triethanolamine, 38% SD alcohol 40	In 227 g.
otc	**Therapeutic Mineral Ice Gel** (Bristol-Myers)	2% menthol, ammonium hydroxide, carbomer 934, cupric sulfate, isopropyl alcohol, thymol	In 105, 240, and 480 g.
otc	**Flex-all 454 Gel** (Chattem)	Menthol in an aloe vera gel, methyl salicylate, alcohol, allantoin, boric acid, carbomer 940, diazolidinyl urea, iodine, polysorbate 60, propylene glycol, potassium iodide, triethanolamine, eucalyptus oil, glycerin, parabens	In 60, 120, and 240 g.
otc	**Eucalyptamint** (Ciba Consumer)	**Gel**: 8% menthol	

LIQUIDS

otc	**Extra Strength Absorbine Jr. Liquid** (W.F. Young)	4% menthol	In 59 and 118 mL.

LOTIONS AND LINIMENTS

otc	**Aspercreme Rub Lotion** (Thompson)	10% trolamine salicylate, cetyl alcohol, glyceryl stearate, lanolin, parabens, potassium phosphate, propylene glycol, sodium lauryl sulfate, stearic acid	In 180 mL.
otc	**Panalgesic Gold Liniment** (ECR Pharm)	55% methyl salicylate, 3.1% camphor, 1.25% menthol, 18.6% emollient oils, 22% alcohol	In 120 mL.
otc	**Gordobalm** (Gordon)	Menthol, camphor, methyl salicylate, 16% isopropyl alcohol, tragacanth, thymol, acetone, eucalyptus oil, tartrazine	In 120 mL and gal.
otc	**Heet Liniment** (Whitehall)	15% methyl salicylate, 3.6% camphor, capsicum oleoresin (as 0.025% capsaicin), acetone, 70% alcohol	In 68.5 and 150 mL.
otc	**Banalg Hospital Strength Lotion** (Forest)	14% methyl salicylate, 3% menthol	In 60 mL.
otc	**Banalg Lotion** (Forest)	4.9% methyl salicylate, 2% camphor, 1% menthol	In 60 and 480 mL.
otc	**Extra Strength Absorbine Jr.** (W.F. Young)	4% natural menthol	In 60 mL.
otc	**Absorbine Jr. Liniment** (W.F. Young)	1.27% menthol, plant extracts of calendula, echinacea and wormwood, iodine, potassium iodide, thymol, acetone, chloroxylenol	In 60 and 120 mL.
otc	**Arth-Rx Topical Analgesic Lotion** (Phillips Gulf)	0.5% methyl nicotinate, 0.025% capsaicin, aloe vera gel, extracts of arnica, rue, chamomile, boswellia	In 90 mL roll-on applicator.
otc	**Yager's Liniment** (Oakhurst Company)	3.1% camphor, 8.3% turpentine, clove oil	In 120 and 240 mL.

SPRAYS

otc	**Sports Spray** (Mentholatum)	35% methyl salicylate, 10% menthol, 5% camphor, 58% alcohol	In 85 g.

PATCHES

otc	**BENGAY** (Pfizer)	**Patch**: 1.4% menthol	Glycerin. In regular and large sizes. In 1s.
otc	**Icy Hot Back Pain Relief** (Chattem)	**Patch**: 5% menthol	Glycerin. In 5s.
otc	**Icy Hot Pop & Peel** (Chattem)		Glycerin. In 5s.

TOPICAL COMBINATIONS, MISCELLANEOUS

TOPICAL COMBINATIONS, MISCELLANEOUS

otc	**Boyol Salve** (Pfeiffer)	**Salve**: 10% ichthammol, benzocaine, lanolin, petrolatum	In 30 g.
otc	**Dermadrox** (Geritrex)	**Ointment**: Aluminum hydroxide gel, zinc chloride, lanolin, calcium carbonate, vitamin A in a hydrophilic ointment base *For relief of minor skin irritations such as chafing, interico and galling.*	In 113 g.
otc	**Wonderful Dream** (Wonderful Dream Salve Corp.)	**Salve**: Phenyl mercury nitrate 1:5000, oil of tar, turpentine, olive oil, linseed oil, posin, burgundy pitch, camphor, beeswax, mutton tallow	In 34 g.
otc	**Dr. Dermi-Heal** (Quality)	**Ointment**: 1% allantoin, zinc oxide, Balsam Peru, castor oil, petrolatum *For relief of diaper rash, chafing, minor burns, bed sores, external vaginal itching and irritation, ostomy irritation and heat rash.*	In 75 g.
otc	**Saratoga** (Blair)	**Ointment**: Zinc oxide, boric acid, eucalyptol, acetylated lanolin alcohols, white petrolatum, white beeswax *For temporary relief of itching and minor skin irritations, chapped and chafed skin, diaper rash, bed sores, mild burns.*	In 28 and 60 g.
otc	**Unguentine** (Mentholatum)	**Ointment**: 1% phenol, petrolatum, oleostearine, zinc oxide, eucalyptus oil, thyme oil *For pain relief in minor burns.*	In 30 g.
otc	**Amerigel** (Amerx Health Care Corp.)	**Ointment**: Meadowsweet extract, oakbark extract, polyethylene glycol 400, polyethylene glycol 3350, zinc acetate. *For stage I-IV pressure ulcers, stasis ulcers, diabetic skin ulcers, post-surgical incisions, 1st and 2nd degree burns, cuts, and abrasions.*	In 28.3 g.
Rx	**Mimyx** (Stiefel)	**Cream**: Betaine, olive oil, glycerin, pentylene glycol, palm glycerides, vegetable oil, squalane, hydroxyethyl cellulose, carbomer, xanthan gum. *To manage and relieve the burning and itching experienced with various types of dermatoses, including atopic dermatitis, allergic contact dermatitis, and radiation dermatitis.*	Preservative-free. In 70 g.
otc	**Ostiderm** (Pedinol)	**Lotion**: Aluminum sulfate, zinc oxide *For foot odor/excessive moisture.*	In 42.5 mL.
		Roll-On: Aluminum chlorohydrate, camphor, alcohol, EDTA, diazolidinyl urea, *Safeguards against offensive odor and dries excessive moisture of the feet.*	In 88.7 mL.
otc	**Men-Phor** (Geritrex Corp.)	**Lotion**: 0.5% camphor, 0.5% menthol, carbopol, cetearyl alcohol, cetyl alcohol, hydantoin, castor oil, petrolatum. *To provide temporary relief for dry itching skin, sunburn, insect bites, and pruritus.*	In 222 mL.
otc	**Sarna Anti-Itch** (Stiefel)	**Lotion**: 0.5% camphor, 0.5% menthol, carbomer 940, DMDM hydantoin, glyceryl stearate, PEG-8 stearate, PEG-100 stearate, petrolatum *For relief of dry, itching skin, sunburn, poison ivy and poison oak.*	In 222 mL.
otc	**Schamberg's** (C & M)	**Lotion**: Zinc oxide, 0.15% menthol, 1% phenol, peanut oil and lime water *For the temporary relief of itching.*	In 480 mL.

TOPICAL COMBINATIONS, MISCELLANEOUS

otc	**Soothaderm** (Pharmakon)	**Lotion**: 2.07 mg pyrilamine maleate, 2.08 mg benzocaine and 41.35 mg zinc oxide per mL, simethicone, parabens, propylene glycol, camphor, menthol *For relief of itching due to chickenpox, diaper rash, insect bites, poison ivy/oak, prickly heat and sunburn.*	In 118 mL.
otc	**Florida Sunburn Relief** (Pharmacel)	**Lotion**: 3% benzyl alcohol, 0.4% phenol, 0.2% camphor, 0.15% menthol *For relief of pain due to sunburn.*	In 60 mL.
otc	**Outgro** (Whitehall)	**Solution**: 25% tannic acid, 5% chlorobutanol, 83% isopropyl alcohol *For temporary pain relief of ingrown toenails.*	In 9.3 mL.
otc	**Stypto-Caine** (Pedinol)	**Solution**: 250 mg aluminum chloride, 2.5 mg tetracaine HCl, 1 mg oxyquinoline sulfate per g with glycerin *To stop bleeding in minor cuts.*	In 59 mL.
otc	**Campho-Phenique** (Sterling Health)	**Liquid**: 10.8% camphor, 4.7% phenol, eucalyptus oil, light mineral oil *To relieve pain and combat infections.*	In 22.5, 45 and 120 mL.
otc	**Oxyzal Wet Dressing** (Gordon)	**Liquid**: Oxyquinoline sulfate, benzalkonium Cl 1:2000 *For minor infections.*	In 30, 120 and 480 mL.
otc	**Campho-Phenique** (Sterling Health)	**Gel**: 4.7% phenol, 10.8% camphor, colloidal silicon dioxide, eucalyptus oil, glycerin, light mineral oil *Pain relief in cold sores, fever blisters, cuts, scrapes, burns and insect bites.*	In 6.9 and 15 g.
otc	**Topic** (Syntex)	**Gel**: 5% benzyl alcohol, camphor, menthol, 30% isopropyl alcohol *For temporary relief of itching from poison oak/ivy, insect bites, eczema, minor skin allergies and heat rash.*	In 60 g.
otc	**Mederma** (Merz)	**Gel**: Water (purified), PEG-4, onion (allium cepa) extract, xanthan gum, allantoin, fragrance, methylparaben, sorbic acid. *Helps scars appear softer and smoother.*	In 50g.
otc	**Aluminum Paste** (Paddock)	**Ointment**: 10% metallic aluminum *An occlusive skin protectant.*	White petrolatum base. In lb.
otc	**Sarna Anti-Itch** (Stiefel)	**Foam**: 0.5% camphor, 0.5% menthol, carbomer 940, DMDM hydantoin, glyceryl stearate, PEG-8 and PEG-100 stearate, petrolatum *For relief of dry, itching skin.*	In 99 g.
otc	**ProTech First-Aid Stik** (Triton)	**Liquid**: 10% povidone-iodine, 2.5% lidocaine HCl *For cleaning and pain relief of cuts, scrapes and burns.*	In 14 mL.
otc	**Proderm Topical** (Dow B. Hickam)	**Dressing**: 650 mg castor oil and 72.5 mg Balsam Peru per 0.82 mL *For prevention and management of decubitus ulcers.*	In 113.4 g.
otc	**Dome-Paste** (Miles)	**Wound dressing**: Zinc oxide, calamine, gelatin *For conditions of extremities (eg, varicose ulcers) requiring protection.*	3″ by 10 yd or 4″ by 10 yd bandages.
otc	**Breezee Mist Foot Powder** (Pedinol)	**Powder**: Isobutane, talc, aluminum chlorohydrate, cyclomethicone, isopropyl myristate. propylene carbonate, stearalkonium hectorite, undecylenic acid, fragrance, menthol *Cooling formula soothes and helps keep feet dry and odor free.*	In 113 g aerosol can.
otc	**Columbia Antiseptic Powder** (F.C. Sturtevant[a])	**Powder**: Zinc oxide, talc, carbolic acid, boric acid.	In 30 and 420 g.
Rx	**Scarlet Red Ointment Dressings** (Sherwood Medical)	**Wound dressings**: 5% scarlet red, lanolin, olive oil and petrolatum in fine mesh absorbent gauze *For epithelialization of donor sites, burns and wounds.*	In 5″ x 9″ strips.

[a] The F.C. Sturtevant Company, P.O. Box 607, Bronxville, NY 10708; 914-337-5131, 888–871-5661; fax 914-337-5309; http://www.columbiapowder.com

TOPICAL COMBINATIONS, MISCELLANEOUS

Active Ingredients

Principal active ingredients of these formulations include:

➤*BORIC ACID, OXYQUINOLINE and BENZALKONIUM Cl:* Used as antiseptics.

➤*ZINC OXIDE and ALUMINUM:* Provide astringent and topical protectant actions.

➤*CAMPHOR, EUCALYPTOL, MENTHOL and PHENOL:* Used as antipruritics, mild local anesthetics and counterirritants.

➤*BENZOCAINE and LIDOCAINE:* Local anesthetics.

➤*PYRILAMINE MALEATE:* An antihistamine.

➤*CASTOR OIL (RICINUS OIL), GLYCERIN and MINERAL OIL:* Used as emollients.

➤*BENZYL ALCOHOL:* Used as an antipruritic.

➤*BISMUTH SUBNITRATE:* Used as a skin protectant.

➤*BALSAM PERU:* Used to stimulate tissue growth.

➤*BIEBRICH SCARLET RED:* Used to promote wound healing.

➤*ICHTHAMMOL:* Used as an anti-infective.

DRESSINGS AND GRANULES

FLEXIBLE HYDROACTIVE DRESSINGS AND GRANULES

otc	**IntraSite** (Smith & Nephew)	**Gel**: 2% graft T starch copolymer, 78% water, 20% propylene glycol. Sterile amorphous hydrogel dressing	In UD 25 g (10s).
otc	**Shur-Clens** (Calgon Vestal)	**Solution**: 20% poloxamer 188	In UD 100 and 200 mL.
otc	**FlexiGel Strands** (Smith-Nephew)	**Absorbent wound dressing**	Single-use absorbent matrix. 6 g unit. In 10s.
otc	**DuoDerm** (ConvaTec)	**Dressings, sterile**: 4″ x 4″, 6″ x 8″, 8″ x 8″ and 8″ x 12″	In 3s (8″ x 12″ only), 5s and 20s
		Dressing, adhesive border: 4″ x 4″ 8″ x 8″	In 5s. In 3s.
		Granules, sterile: 5 g per tube	In 5s.
		Paste, sterile	In 30 g tube.
otc	**DuoDerm CGF** (ConvaTec)	**Control gel formula dressing, sterile**: 4″ x 4″, 6″ x 6″, 8″ x 8″	In 5s.
		Control gel formula border dressing, sterile: 2.5″ x 2.5″, 4″ x 4″, 6″ x 6″, 4″ x 5″, 6″ x 7″ with adhesive borders	In 5s.
otc	**DuoDerm Extra Thin** (ConvaTec)	**Control gel formula dressing, extra thin, sterile**: 4″ x 4″, 6″ x 6″	In 10s.

FLEXIBLE HYDROACTIVE DRESSINGS AND GRANULES

otc	**Sorbsan** (Dow B. Hickam)	**Pads, sterile:** Calcium alginate fiber 2" x 2", 3" x 3", 4" x 4" and 4" x 8"	In 1s.
		Wound packing fibers, sterile: Calcium alginate fiber. 12" (2 g)	In 1s.

FLEXIBLE HYDROACTIVE DRESSINGS AND GRANULES — TOPICAL

Indications

➤*Dressings:* For the local management of: Dermal ulcers; pressure ulcers; leg ulcers; superficial wounds (eg, minor abrasions, donor sites, second-degree burns); protective dressings; postoperative wounds.

➤*Granules:* For use in the local management of exudating dermal ulcers in association with the dressings.

➤*Paste:* For use in association with *DuoDerm* dressings for local management of exudating dermal ulcers.

Administration and Dosage

Clean and prepare the wound site before application. See package labeling for wound management and application/removal instructions for the dressing and granules. Dressings are designed to remain in place from 1 to 7 days.

Actions

➤*Pharmacology:* The dressings interact with wound exudate producing a soft moist gel at the wound surface enabling removal of the dressing with little or no damage to newly formed tissues. They are designed to remain in place from 1 to 7 days.

Contraindications

Dermal ulcers involving muscle, tendon or bone; ulcers resulting from infection, such as tuberculosis, syphilis and deep fungal infections; lesions in patients with active vasculitis, such as periarteritis nodosa, systemic lupus erythematosus and cryoglobulinemia; third-degree burns; clinically infected wounds.

Precautions

➤*Excess exudate:* In the presence of excess exudate, the ability of the dressings to remain in place with less frequent leakage may be improved by applying the granules directly into the wound site. Used in this way, with the dressings, the granules may reduce the frequency of dressing change.

➤*Odor:* Wounds often have a characteristic disagreeable odor. The odor usually disappears following wound cleansing.

➤*Wound deterioration:* When using any occlusive dressing, the wound will increase in size and depth during the initial phase as the necrotic debris is cleaned away.

➤*Infection:* If clinical infection develops, discontinue DuoDerm and institute appropriate treatment. Restart *DuoDerm* when the infection has been eradicated.

IRRIGATING SOLUTIONS

PHYSIOLOGICAL IRRIGATING SOLUTIONS

Rx	**0.45% Sodium Chloride Irrigation** (Abbott)	**Solution:** 450 mg sodium chloride per 100 mL	In 250 and 500 mL and 1, 1.5, 2 and 3 L.
Rx	**0.9% Sodium Chloride Irrigation** (Abbott)	**Solution:** 900 mg sodium chloride per 100 mL	In 100, 250 and 500 mL and 1, 1.5, 2 and 3 L.
Rx	**Ringer's Irrigation** (Various, eg, McGaw)	**Solution:** 860 mg sodium chloride, 30 mg potassium chloride, 33 mg calcium chloride per 100 mL	In 1 L.
Rx	**Tis-U-Sol** (Baxter)	**Solution:** 800 mg NaCl, 40 mg KCl, 20 mg magnesium sulfate, 8.75 mg dibasic sodium phosphate heptahydrate and 6.25 mg monobasic potassium phosphate per 100 mL	In 1 L.
Rx	**Lactated Ringer's Irrigation** (Abbott)	**Solution:** 600 mg sodium chloride, 310 mg sodium lactate, anhydrous, 30 mg potassium chloride, 20 mg calcium chloride, dihydrate per 100 mL	In 300 mL.
Rx	**Physiolyte** (American McGaw)	**Solution:** 530 mg NaCl, 370 mg sodium acetate, 500 mg sodium gluconate, 37 mg KCl and 30 mg magnesium Cl per 100 mL	In 1 L.
Rx	**PhysioSol** (Hospira)	**Solution:** 526 mg NaCl, 222 mg sodium acetate, 502 mg sodium gluconate, 37 mg KCl and 30 mg magnesium chloride hexahydrate per 100 mL	In 250 and 500 mL and 1 L.
Rx	**Cytosol** (Cytosol Ophthalmics)	**Solution:** 48 mg calcium chloride, 30 mg magnesium chloride, 75 mg potassium chloride, 390 mg sodium acetate, 640 mg sodium chloride, 170 mg sodium citrate per 100 mL	In 200 and 500 mL.
Rx	**Saf-Clens** (Calgon Vestal)	**Spray:** Meroxapol 105, NaCl, potassium sorbate NF, DMDM hydantoin	In 177 mL.

PHYSIOLOGICAL IRRIGATING SOLUTIONS — TOPICAL

Indications

➤*Irrigation:* For general irrigation, washing and rinsing purposes which permit use of a sterile, nonpyrogenic electrolyte solution.

Administration and Dosage

The dose depends on the capacity or surface area of the structure to be irrigated and the nature of the procedure. When used as a vehicle for other drugs, follow manufacturer's recommendations.

➤*Storage/Stability:* Avoid excessive heat. Do not freeze. Store at 25°C (77°F); however, brief exposure to 40°C (104°F) does not cause adverse effects.

Contraindications

Irrigation during electrosurgical procedures.

Warnings

➤*For irrigation only:* Not for injection.

➤*Absorption:* Irrigating fluids enter the systemic circulation in relatively large volumes and must be regarded as a systemic drug. Absorption of large amounts can cause fluid or solute overloading resulting in dilution of serum electrolyte concentrations, overhydration, congested states or pulmonary edema.

➤*Dilutional states:* The risk of dilutional states is inversely proportional to the electrolyte concentrations of administered parenteral solutions. The risk of solute overload causing congested states with peripheral and pulmonary edema is directly proportional to the electrolyte concentrations of such solutions.

➤*Do not heat:* Do not heat to higher than 66°C (higher than 150°F).

➤*Pregnancy: Category C.* It is not known whether these solutions can cause fetal harm when administered to a pregnant woman or can affect reproduction capacity. Give to a pregnant woman only if clearly needed.

Precautions

➤*Continuous irrigation:* Observe caution when solution is used for continuous irrigation or allowed to "dwell" inside body cavities because of possible absorption into the blood stream and circulatory overload.

➤*Aseptic technique:* This is essential for irrigation of body cavities, wounds and urethral catheters or for wetting dressings that come in contact with body tissues.

➤*Accidental contamination:* Careless technique may transmit infection.

➤*Containers:* When used as a "pour" irrigation, do not allow any part of the contents to contact the surface below the outer protected thread area of the semi-rigid wide mouth container. When used via irrigation equipment, attach the administration set promptly. Discard unused portions and use a fresh container for the start-up of each cycle or repeat procedure. For repeated irrigations of urethral catheters, use a separate container for each patient.

➤*Displaced catheters/drainage tubes:* This can lead to irrigation or infiltration of unintended structures or cavities.

➤*Additives:* May be incompatible. When introducing additives, use aseptic technique, mix thoroughly and do not store.

➤*Tissue distention/disruption:* Excessive volume or pressure during irrigation of closed cavities may cause undue distention or disruption of tissues.

Adverse Reactions

Should any adverse reaction occur, discontinue the irrigant, evaluate the patient, institute appropriate countermeasures and save the remainder of the fluid for examination.

Overdosage

In overhydration or solute overload, reevaluate and institute corrective measures.

➤*General Considerations in Topical Ophthalmic Drug Therapy:* Proper administration is essential to optimal therapeutic response. In many instances, health professionals may be too casual when instructing patients on proper use of ophthalmics. The administration technique used often determines drug safety and efficacy.

- The normal eye retains ≈ 10 mcL of fluid (adjusted for blinking). The average dropper delivers 25 to 50 mcL/drop. The value of more than one drop is questionable.
- Minimize systemic absorption of ophthalmic drops by compressing lacrimal sac for 3 to 5 minutes after instillation. This retards passage of drops via nasolacrimal duct into areas of potential absorption such as nasal and pharyngeal mucosa.
- Because of rapid lacrimal drainage and limited eye capacity, if multiple drop therapy is indicated, the best interval between drops is 5 minutes. This ensures that the first drop is not flushed away by the second or that the second is not diluted by the first.
- Topical anesthesia will increase the bioavailability of ophthalmic agents by decreasing the blink reflex and the production and turnover of tears.
- Factors that may increase absorption from ophthalmics include lax eyelids of some patients, usually the elderly, which creates a greater reservoir for retention of drops, and hyperemic or diseased eyes.
- Eyecup use is discouraged due to risk of contamination.
- Ophthalmic suspensions mix with tears less rapidly and remain in the cul-de-sac longer than solutions.
- Ophthalmic ointments maintain contact between the drug and ocular tissues by slowing the clearance rate to as little as 0.5% per minute. Ophthalmic ointments provide maximum contact between drug and external ocular tissues.
- Ophthalmic ointments may impede delivery of other ophthalmic drugs to the affected side by serving as a barrier to contact.
- Ointments may blur vision during the waking hours. Use with caution in conditions where visual clarity is critical (eg, operating motor equipment, reading) or use at bedtime.
- Monitor expiration dates closely. Do not use outdated medication.
- Solutions and ointments are frequently misused. Do not assume that patients know how to maximize safe and effective use of these agents. Combine appropriate patient education and counseling with prescribing and dispensing of ophthalmics.

Topical application is the most common route of administration for ophthalmic drugs. Advantages include convenience, simplicity, noninvasive nature and the ability of the patient to self-administer. Because of blood and aqueous losses of drug, topical medications do not typically penetrate in useful concentrations to posterior ocular structures and therefore are of no therapeutic benefit for diseases of retina, optic nerve and other posterior segment structures.

➤*Ingredients:* The following inactive agents may be present in ophthalmic products:

PRESERVATIVES – Preservatives destroy or inhibit multiplication of microorganisms introduced into the product by accident and are as follows:

Benzalkonium Cl, benzethonium Cl, cetylpyridinium Cl, chlorobutanol, EDTA, mercurial preservatives (phenylmercuric nitrate, phenyl mercuric acetate, thimerosal), methyl/propylparabens, phenylethyl alcohol, sodium benzoate, sodium propionate, sorbic acid.

VISCOSITY-INCREASING AGENTS – Viscosity-increasing agents slow drainage of the product from the eye, thus increasing retention time of the active drug. Increased bioavailability may result. Viscosity-increasing agents are as follows:

Carboxymethylcellulose sodium, dextran 70, gelatin, glycerin, hydroxyethylcellulose, hydroxypropyl methylcellulose, methylcellulose, PEG, poloxamer 407, polysorbate 80, propylene glycol, polyvinyl alcohol, polyvinylpyrrolidone (povidone).

ANTIOXIDANTS – Antioxidants prevent or delay deterioration of products by oxygen in the air and are as follows:

EDTA, sodium bisulfite, sodium metabisulfite, sodium thiosulfate, thiourea.

WETTING AGENTS – Wetting agents reduce surface tension, allowing drug solution to spread over eye and are as follows.

Polysorbate 20 and 80, poloxamer 282, tyloxapol.

BUFFERS – Buffers help maintain ophthalmic products in the range of pH 6 to 8, which is the comfortable range for ophthalmic instillation and are as follows:

Acetic acid, boric acid, phosphoric acid, potassium bicarbonate, potassium borate and tetraborate, potassium carbonate, potassium citrate, potassium phosphates, sodium acetate, sodium bicarbonate, sodium biphosphate, sodium borate, sodium carbonate, sodium citrate, sodium hydroxide, sodium phosphate, hydrochloric acid.

TONICITY AGENTS – Tonicity agents help the ophthalmic product solutions to be isotonic with natural tears. Products in the sodium chloride equivalence range of 0.9% ± 0.2% are considered isotonic and will help prevent ocular pain and tissue damage. A range of 0.6% to 1.8% is usually comfortable for ophthalmic use. Tonicity agents are as follows:

Buffers, dextran 40 and 70, dextrose, glycerin, potassium Cl, propylene glycol, sodium Cl.

➤*Packaging Standards:* To help reduce confusion in labeling and identification of various topical ocular medications, drug packaging standards have been proposed. When fully implemented by the ophthalmic drug industry, the standard colors for drug labels and bottle caps will include the following:

Ophthalmic Drug Packaging Standards

Therapeutic class	Proposed color
Beta blockers	Yellow, blue or both
Mydriatics and cycloplegics	Red
Miotics	Green
Nonsteroidal anti-inflammatory agents	Grey
Anti-infectives	Brown, tan

➤*Medications:*

Solutions and suspensions – Most topical ocular preparations are commercially available as solutions or suspensions that are applied directly to the eye from the bottle, which serves as the eye dropper. Avoid touching the dropper tip to the eye because this can lead to contamination of the medication and may also cause ocular injury. Resuspend suspensions (notably, many ocular steroids) by shaking to provide an accurate dosage of drug.

Recommended procedures for administration of solutions or suspensions –

- Wash hands thoroughly before administration.
- Tilt head backward or lie down and gaze upward.
- Gently grasp lower eyelid below eyelashes and pull the eyelid away from the eye to form a pouch.
- Place dropper directly over eye. Avoid contact of the dropper with the eye, finger or any surface.
- Look upward just before applying a drop.
- After instilling the drop, look downward for several seconds.
- Release the lid slowly and close eyes gently.
- With eyes closed, apply gentle pressure with fingers to the inside corner of eye for 3 to 5 min. This retards drainage of solution from intended solution.
- Do not rub the eye or squeeze the eyelid. Minimize blinking.
- Do not rinse the dropper.
- Do not use eye drops that have changed color or contain a precipitate.
- If more than one type of ophthalmic drop is used, wait ≥ 5 minutes before administering the second agent.
- When the instillation of eye drops is difficult (eg, pediatric patients, adults with particularly strong blink reflex), the close-eye method may be used. This involves lying down, placing the prescribed number of drops on the eyelid in the inner corner of the eye, then opening eye so that drops will fall into the eye by gravity.

Ointments – The primary purpose for an ophthalmic ointment vehicle is to prolong drug contact time with the external ocular surface. This is particularly useful for treating children, who may "cry out" topically applied solutions, and for medicating ocular injuries, such as corneal abrasions, when the eye is to be patched. Administer solutions before ointments. Ointments preclude entry of subsequent drops.

Recommended procedures for administration of ointments –

- Wash hands thoroughly before administration.
- Holding the ointment tube in the hand for a few minutes will warm the ointment and facilitate flow.
- When opening the ointment tube for the first time, squeeze out and discard the first 0.25 inch of ointment as it may be too dry.
- Tilt head backward or lie down and gaze upward.
- Gently pull down the lower eyelid to form a pouch.
- Place 0.25 to 0.5 inch of ointment with a sweeping motion inside the lower eyelid by squeezing the tube gently and slowly release the eyelid.
- Close the eye for 1 to 2 minutes and roll the eyeball in all directions.
- Temporary blurring of vision may occur. Avoid activities requiring visual acuity until blurring clears.
- Remove excessive ointment around the eye or ointment tube tip with a tissue.
- If using more than one kind of ointment, wait about 10 minutes before applying the second drug.

Gels – Ophthalmic gels are similar in viscosity and clinical usage to ophthalmic ointments. Pilocarpine (*Pilopine HS*) is currently the only ophthalmic preparation available in gel form, and it is intended to serve as a "sustained-release" pilocarpine, requiring only once-daily administration (at bedtime).

Sprays – Although not commercially available, some practitioners use mydriatics or cycloplegics, alone or in combination, administered as a spray to the eye to dilate the pupil or for cycloplegic examination. This is most often used for pediatric patients, and the solution is administered using a sterile perfume atomizer.

Lid scrubs – Commercially available eyelid cleansers or antibiotic solutions or ointments can be applied directly to the lid margin for the treatment of noninfectious blepharitis. This is best accomplished by applying the medication to the end of a cotton-tipped applicator and then scrubbing the eyelid margin several times daily. The gauze pads supplied with commercially available eyelid cleansers are also convenient.

➤*Devices:*

Contact lenses – Soft contact lenses can absorb water-soluble drugs and release them over prolonged periods of time. This has the clinical advantage of promoting sustained-release solutions or suspensions that would otherwise be removed quickly from the external ocular tissues. Soft contact lenses as delivery devices are most often used in the management of dry eye disorders, but the technique is occasionally used for the treatment of ocular infections, including corneal ulcers.

Corneal shields – A non-cross-linked, homogenized, porcine scleral collagen shield is available (*Bio-Cor Fyodoror Collagen Corneal Shield*). This is placed as a bandage on the cornea following surgery or injury, protecting and lubricating the cornea. Topical antibiotics have been used with the shield to promote healing of corneal ulcers.

Cotton pledgets – Small pieces of cotton can be saturated with ophthalmic solutions and placed in the conjunctival sac. These devices allow a prolonged ocular contact time with solutions that are normally administered topically into the eye. The clinical use of pledgets is usually reserved for mydriatic solutions such as cocaine or phenylephrine. This drug delivery method promotes maximum mydriasis in an attempt to break posterior synechiae or to dilate sluggish pupils.

Filter paper strips – Sodium fluorescein and rose bengal dyes are commercially available as drug-impregnated filter paper strips. The strips help ensure sterility of sodium fluorescein which, when prepared in solution, can become easily contaminated with Pseudomonas aeruginosa. These dyes are used diagnostically to disclose corneal injuries, infections such as herpes simplex, and dry eye disorders.

Artificial tear inserts – A rod-shaped pellet of hydroxypropyl cellulose without preservative (*Lacrisert*), is inserted into the inferior conjunctival sac with a specially designed applicator. Following placement, the device absorbs fluid, swells and then releases the nonmedicated polymer to the eye for up to 24 hours. The device is designed as a sustained-release artificial tear for the treatment of dry eye disorders.

Membrane-bound inserts – A membrane-controlled drug delivery system (*Ocusert*) delivers a constant quantity of pilocarpine to the eye for up to 1 week. Placed onto the bulbar conjunctiva under the upper or lower eyelid, it is a useful substitute for pilocarpine drops or gel in glaucoma patients who cannot comply with more frequent instillation or in those with ocular or visual side effects from pilocarpine solutions.

AGENTS FOR GLAUCOMA

Glaucoma is a condition of the eye in which an elevation of the intraocular pressure (IOP) leads to progressive cupping and atrophy of the optic nerve head, deterioration of the visual fields, and, ultimately, blindness. Primary open-angle glaucoma is the most common type of glaucoma. Angle-closure glaucoma and congenital glaucoma are treated primarily by surgical methods, although short-term drug therapy is used to decrease IOP prior to surgery.

Drugs used in the therapy of primary open-angle glaucoma include a variety of agents with different mechanisms of action. The therapeutic goal in treating glaucoma is reducing the elevated IOP, a major risk factor in the pathogenesis of glaucomatous visual field loss. The higher the level of IOP, the greater the likelihood of glaucomatous visual field loss and optic nerve damage. Reduction of IOP may be accomplished by: 1) Decreasing the rate of production of aqueous humor, or 2) increasing the rate of outflow (drainage) of aqueous humor from the anterior chamber of the eye.

The 6 groups of agents used in therapy of primary open-angle glaucoma are listed in the table, which summarizes their mechanism of decreasing IOP, effects on pupil size and ciliary muscle, and duration of action.

Agents for Glaucoma

Drug	Strength	Duration (h)	Decrease aqueous production	Increase aqueous outflow	Effect on pupil	Effect on ciliary muscle
Sympathomimetics						
Apraclonidine[1]	0.5%-1%	7-12	+++	NR	NR	NR
Epinephrine	0.1%-2%	12	+	++	mydriasis	NR
Dipivefrin	0.1%	12	+	++	mydriasis	NR
Brimonidine	0.2%	12	++	++	NR	NR
Beta blockers						
Betaxolol	0.25%-0.5%	12	+++	NR	NR	NR
Carteolol	1%	12	+++	nd	NR	NR
Levobunolol	0.25%-0.5%	12- 24	+++	NR	NR	NR
Metipranolol	0.3%	12-24	+++	+	NR	NR
Timolol	0.25%-0.5%	12- 24	+++	+	NR	NR
Miotics, direct-acting						
Acetylcholine[2]	1%	10-20 min	NR	+++	miosis	accommodation
Carbachol [2]	0.75%-3%	6-8	NR	+++	miosis	accommodation
Pilocarpine[3]	0.25%-10%	4-8	NR	+++	miosis	accommodation
Miotics, cholinesterase inhibitors						
Physostigmine	0.25%-0.5%	12-36	NR	+++	miosis	accommodation
Demecarium	0.125%-0.25%	days/wk	NR	+++	miosis	accommodation
Echothiophate	0.03%-0.25%	days/wk	NR	+++	miosis	accommodation
Carbonic anhydrase inhibitors						
Dichlorphenamide[4]	50 mg	6-12	+++	NR	NR	NR
Acetazolamide[4]	125-500 mg	8-12	+++	NR	NR	NR
Methazolamide[4]	25-50 mg	10-18	+++	NR	NR	NR
Dorzolamide[5]	2%	≈ 8	+++	NR	NR	NR
Prostaglandin analog						
Latanoprost	.005%	24	NR	+++	NR	NR

* +++ = significant activity ++ = moderate activity + = some activity NR = no activity reported nd = No data available

[1] 1% used only to decrease IOP in surgery.

[2] Intraocular administration only for miosis during surgery; carbachol also available as a topical agent.

[3] Also available as a gel and an insert; the duration of these doseforms is longer (18 to 24 hours and 1 week, respectively) than the solution.

[4] Systemic agents; for detailed information, see group monograph in Cardiovascular section.

[5] Topical ophthalmic agent.

➤*Sympathomimetic agents:* Sympathomimetic agents (adrenergic agonists) have both α and β activity (apraclonidine is a relatively selective alpha adrenergic agonist). They lower IOP mainly by increasing outflow and reducing production of aqueous humor. Epinephrine is used as an adjunct to miotic or beta-blocker therapy; however, it is also used as primary therapy, especially in young patients or patients with cataracts. The combination of a miotic and a sympathomimetic will have additive effects in lowering IOP.

Dipivefrin HCl is a prodrug that is metabolized to epinephrine in vivo. The IOP-lowering and intraocular effects are qualitatively and quantitatively similar to epinephrine; however, extraocularly, dipivefrin may be better tolerated and have a lower incidence of adverse effects.

➤*Beta-adrenergic blocking agents:* Beta-adrenergic blocking agents may be used alone or in conjunction with other agents. They may be more effective than either pilocarpine or epinephrine alone and have the advantage of not affecting either pupil size or accommodation. They lower IOP by decreasing the rate of aqueous production.

➤*Miotics (direct-acting):* Direct-acting miotics were considered the first step in glaucoma therapy. They have now yielded to the beta-blockers. Pilocarpine is a useful adjunctive agent that is additive to the beta-blockers, carbonic anhydrase inhibitors, or sympathomimetics. Dosage and frequency of administration must be individualized. Patients with darkly pigmented irides may require higher strengths of pilocarpine.

➤*Miotics (cholinesterase inhibitors):* Cholinesterase inhibitor miotics include both reversible/short-acting (eg, physostigmine) and irreversible/long-acting (eg, echothiophate) agents that enhance the effects of endogenous acetylcholine by inactivation of the enzyme acetylcholinesterase. These agents are more potent and longer-acting than the direct-acting cholinergic agents. Side effects and systemic toxicity are more common and of greater significance. Using a direct-acting cholinergic and a cholinesterase inhibitor provides no improvement in response.

➤*Carbonic anhydrase inhibitors:* Carbonic anhydrase inhibitors are administered systemically, except for the topical agent dorzolamide. IOP is lowered by suppressing the secretion of aqueous humor (inflow). Systemic carbonic anhydrase inhibitors are used as adjunctive therapy and do not replace topical therapy.

➤*Hyperosmotic agents:* Hyperosmotic agents (mannitol, urea, glycerin, and isosorbide) are administered systemically and are useful in lowering IOP in acute situations. These agents lower IOP by creating an osmotic gradient between the ocular fluids and plasma. They are not for chronic use.

➤*Prostaglandin analogs:* Prostaglandin analogs increase uveoscleral outflow through a new mechanism of action, selective prostenoid receptor agonism. Latanoprost, currently the only agent available in this class, can be used concomitantly with other topical ophthalmic drug products to reduce IOP.

Alpha Adrenergic Agonist

BRIMONIDINE TARTRATE

Rx	**Brimonidine Tartrate** (Various, eg, Bausch & Lomb, Falcon)	**Solution:** 0.2%	In 5, 10, 15 mL.
Rx	**Alphagan P** (Allergan)	**Solution:** 0.1%	In 5, 10, and 15 mL bottles.[a]
		0.15%	In 5, 10, and 15 mL bottles.[a]

[a] With 0.005% *Purite;* boric acid; potassium chloride; sodium borate; sodium chloride; hydrochloric acid and/or sodium hydroxide to adjust pH.

BRIMONIDINE TARTRATE — OPHTHALMIC

Refer to Topical Ophthalmic Drugs introduction for complete and comparative prescribing information.

Indications

➤*Intraocular pressure (IOP):* For lowering intraocular pressure in patients with open-angle glaucoma or ocular hypertension. The IOP-lowering efficacy of brimonidine tartrate ophthalmic solution diminishes over time in some patients. This loss of effect appears with a variable time of onset in each patient and should be closely monitored.

Administration and Dosage

➤*Approved by the FDA:* March 16, 2001.

➤*Dose:* Instill 1 drop in the affected eye(s) 3 times daily, approximately 8 hours apart.

➤*Concomitant therapy:* May be used concomitantly with other topical ophthalmic drug products to lower intraocular pressure. If more than 1 topical ophthalmic product is being used, the products should be administered at least 5 minutes apart.

➤*Storage/Stability:* Store between 15° and 25°C (59° to 77°F). Keep out of the reach of children.

Actions

➤*Pharmacology:* Brimonidine tartrate is an alpha adrenergic receptor agonist. It has a peak ocular hypotensive effect occurring at 2 hours post-dosing. Fluorophotometric studies in animals and humans suggest that brimonidine tartrate has a dual mechanism of action by reducing aqueous humor production and increasing uveoscleral outflow.

➤*Pharmacokinetics:*

Absorption/Distribution – After ocular administration of either a 0.1% or 0.2% solution, plasma concentrations peaked within 0.5 to 2.5 hours and declined with a systemic half-life of approximately 2 hours.

Metabolism/Excretion – In humans, systemic metabolism of brimonidine is extensive. It is metabolized primarily by the liver. Urinary excretion is the major route of elimination of the drug and its metabolites. Approximately 87% of an orally administered radioactive dose was eliminated within 120 hours, with 74% found in the urine.

Contraindications

Hypersensitivity to brimonidine tartrate or any component of this medication; patients receiving monoamine oxidase (MAO) inhibitor therapy.

Warnings

➤*Renal/Hepatic function impairment:* Brimonidine tartrate has not been studied in patients with hepatic or renal impairment; caution should be used in treating such patients.

➤*Pregnancy: Category B.*

Teratogenic – There are no adequate and well-controlled studies of brimonidine tartrate in pregnant women; however in animal studies, brimonidine crossed the placenta and entered into the fetal circulation to a limited extent. Brimonidine tartrate should be used during pregnancy only if the potential benefit to the mother justifies the potential risk to the fetus.

➤*Lactation:* It is not known whether brimonidine tartrate is excreted in human milk, although in animal studies, brimonidine tartrate has been shown to be excreted in breast milk. A decision should be made whether to discontinue nursing or to discontinue the drug, taking into account the importance of the drug to the mother.

➤*Children:* In a well-controlled clinical study in pediatric glaucoma patients (ages 2 to 7 years), the most commonly observed adverse reactions with brimonidine tartrate ophthalmic 0.2% dosed 3 times daily were somnolence (50% to 83% in patients ages 2 to 6 years) and decreased alertness. In pediatric patients 7 years of age or older (greater than 20 kg), somnolence appears to occur less frequently (25%). Approximately 16% of patients on brimonidine tartrate ophthalmic solution discontinued from the study due to somnolence.

The safety and efficacy of brimonidine tartrate ophthalmic solution have not been studied in pediatric patients below the age of 2 years. Brimonidine tartrate ophthalmic solution is not recommended for use in pediatric patients under the age of 2 years.

Precautions

➤*Monitoring:* Patients prescribed IOP-lowering medication should be routinely monitored for IOP.

➤*Special risk:* Although brimonidine tartrate had minimal effect on blood pressure of patients in clinical studies, caution should be exercised in treating patients with severe cardiovascular disease.

Brimonidine tartrate should be used with caution in patients with depression, cerebral or coronary insufficiency, Raynaud's phenomenon, orthostatic hypotension or thromboangiitis obliterans. During the studies there was a loss of effect in some patients. The IOP-lowering efficacy observed with brimonidine tartrate ophthalmic solution during the first month of therapy may not always reflect the long-term level of IOP reduction.

➤*Hazardous tasks:* As with other drugs in this class, brimonidine tartrate may cause fatigue or drowsiness in some patients. Patients who engage in hazardous activities should be cautioned of the potential for a decrease in mental alertness.

Drug Interactions

Brimonidine Drug Interactions

Precipitant Drug	Object Drug*		Description
Brimonidine	Beta blockers, antihypertensives, cardiac glycosides	↑	Because alpha-agonists, as a class, may reduce pulse and blood pressure, use caution with concomitant drugs such as beta-blockers (ophthalmic and systemic), antihypertensives, and/or cardiac glycosides.
Brimonidine	CNS depressants (eg, alcohol, barbiturates, opiates, sedatives or anesthetics)	↑	Consider the possibility of an additive or potentiating effect with CNS depressants.
Brimonidine	MAOIs	↑	Coadministration is contraindicated.
Tricyclic antidepressants	Brimonidine	↓	Tricyclic antidepressants can affect the metabolism and uptake of circulating amines.

* ↑ = Object drug increased. ↓ = Object drug decreased.

Adverse Reactions

➤*0.1% and 0.15% ophthalmic solution:*

Adverse reactions occurring in approximately 10% to 20% of subjects – Allergic conjunctivitis, conjunctival hyperemia, and eye pruritus.

Adverse reactions occurring in approximately 5% to 9% of subjects – Burning sensation, conjunctival folliculosis, hypertension, oral dryness, and visual disturbance.

Reactions occurring in approximately 1% to 4% of subjects – Allergic reaction, asthenia, blepharitis, bronchitis, conjunctival edema, conjunctival hemorrhage, conjunctivitis, cough, dizziness, dyspepsia, dyspnea, epiphora, eye discharge, eye dryness, eye irritation, eye pain, eyelid edema, eyelid erythema, flu syndrome, follicular conjunctivitis, foreign body sensation, headache, pharyngitis, photophobia, rash, rhinitis, sinus infection, sinusitis, superficial punctate keratopathy, visual field defect, vitreous floaters, and worsened visual acuity.

The following reactions were reported in less than 1% of subjects – Corneal erosion, insomnia, nasal dryness, somnolence, and taste perversion.

➤*0.2% ophthalmic solution:*

Adverse events occurring in approximately 10% to 30% – In descending order of incidence, adverse events included oral dryness, ocular hyperemia, burning and stinging, headache, blurring, foreign body sensation, fatigue/drowsiness, conjunctival follicles, ocular allergic reactions, and ocular pruritus.

Reactions occurring in approximately 3% to 9% – In descending order, adverse events included corneal staining/erosion, photophobia, eyelid erythema, ocular ache/pain, ocular dryness, tearing, upper respiratory tract symptoms, eyelid edema, conjunctival edema, dizziness, blepharitis, ocular

BRIMONIDINE TARTRATE — OPHTHALMIC

irritation, gastrointestinal symptoms, asthenia, conjunctival blanching, abnormal vision and muscular pain.

Adverse reactions reported in less than 3% – Lid crusting, conjunctival hemorrhage, abnormal taste, insomnia, conjunctival discharge, depression, hypertension, anxiety, palpitations, nasal dryness, and syncope.

Postmarketing – The following reactions have been identified during postmarketing use of brimonidine tartrate 0.2% in clinical practice. Because they are reported voluntarily from a population of unknown size, estimates of the frequency cannot be made. The reactions, which have been chosen for inclusion due to either their seriousness, frequency of reporting, possible causal connection to brimonidine tartrate, or a combination of these factors, include: Bradycardia; hypotension; iritis; miosis; skin reactions (including erythema, eyelid pruritus, rash, and vasodilation); and tachycardia. Apnea, bradycardia, hypotension, hypothermia, hypotonia, and somnolence have been reported in infants receiving brimonidine tartrate.

Overdosage

No information is available on overdosage in humans. Treatment of an oral overdose includes supportive and symptomatic therapy; a patent airway should be maintained.

Patient Information

The preservative in brimonidine tartrate 0.2%, benzalkonium chloride, may be absorbed by soft contact lenses. Patients wearing soft contact lenses should be instructed to wait at least 15 minutes after instilling brimonidine tartrate to insert soft contact lenses.

As with other drugs in this class, brimonidine tartrate may cause fatigue or drowsiness in some patients. Patients who engage in hazardous activities should be cautioned of the potential for a decrease in mental alertness.

APRACLONIDINE HCl

Rx	**Iopidine** (Alcon)	**Solution**: 1%	0.01% benzalkonium chloride. In 0.1 mL (2s).
		Solution: 0.5%	0.01% benzalkonium chloride. In 5 mL and 10 mL *Drop-Tainers.*

APRACLONIDINE HYDROCHLORIDE — OPHTHALMIC

Refer to Topical Ophthalmic Drugs introduction for complete and comparative prescribing information.

Indications

➤*0.5% solution:* For short-term adjunctive therapy in patients on maximally tolerated medical therapy who require additional IOP reduction. Patients on maximally tolerated medical therapy who are treated with apraclonidine ophthalmic solution to delay surgery should have frequent follow-up examinations and treatment should be discontinued if the IOP rises significantly.

The addition of apraclonidine ophthalmic solution to patients already using 2 aqueous suppressing drugs (ie, beta blocker plus carbonic anhydrase inhibitor) as part of their maximally tolerated medical therapy may not provide additional benefit. This is because apraclonidine ophthalmic solution is an aqueous suppressing drug and the addition of a third aqueous suppressant may not significantly reduce IOP.

The IOP-lowering efficacy of apraclonidine ophthalmic solution diminishes over time in some patients. This loss of effect, or tachyphylaxis, appears to be an individual occurrence with a variable time of onset and should be closely monitored. The benefit for most patients is less than 1 month.

➤*1% solution:* To control or prevent post-surgical elevations in intraocular pressure (IOP) that occur in patients after argon laser trabeculoplasty, argon laser iridotomy, or Nd:YAG posterior capsulotomy.

Administration and Dosage

➤*Approved by the FDA:* December 31, 1987.

Not for injection into the eye. Not for oral ingestion.

➤*0.5% solution:* Instill 1 to 2 drops of apraclonidine ophthalmic solution in the affected eye(s) 3 times daily. Because apraclonidine ophthalmic solution will be used with other ocular glaucoma therapies, practice an approximate 5-minute interval between instillation of each medication to prevent washout of the previous dose.

➤*1% solution:* Instill 1 drop of apraclonidine in the scheduled operative eye 1 hour before initiating anterior segment laser surgery and instill a second drop to the same eye immediately upon completion of the laser surgical procedure. Use a separate container for each single-drop dose, and discard each container after use.

➤*Storage/Stability:* Store between 2° to 25°C (36° to 77°F). Protect from freezing and light.

Actions

➤*Pharmacology:* Apraclonidine is a relatively selective alpha-2-adrenergic agonist and does not have significant membrane stabilizing (local anesthetic) activity. When instilled in the eye, apraclonidine ophthalmic solution, has the action of reducing elevated, as well as normal IOP, whether or not accompanied by glaucoma. Ophthalmic apraclonidine has minimal effect on cardiovascular parameters.

➤*Pharmacokinetics:*

Absorption –

0.5%: The onset of action of apraclonidine can usually be noted within 1 hour, and maximum IOP reduction occurs about 3 hours after instillation.

Topical use of apraclonidine ophthalmic solution leads to systemic absorption. Studies of apraclonidine 0.5% ophthalmic solution dosed 1 drop 3 times a day in both eyes for 10 days in healthy volunteers yielded mean peak and trough concentrations of 0.9 ng/mL and 0.5 ng/mL, respectively.

1%: The onset of action with apraclonidine 1% can usually be noted within 1 hour and the maximum IOP reduction usually occurs 3 to 5 hours after application of a single dose.

Metabolism – The half-life of apraclonidine 0.5% ophthalmic solution was calculated to be 8 hours.

Contraindications

Hypersensitivity to apraclonidine or any other component of this medication, as well as systemic clonidine; patients receiving monoamine oxidase (MAO) inhibitors.

Warnings

➤*Hypersensitivity reactions:* Use of apraclonidine ophthalmic solution can lead to an allergic-like reaction characterized wholly or in part by the symptoms of hyperemia, pruritus, discomfort, tearing, foreign body sensation, and edema of the lids and conjunctiva. Discontinue apraclonidine ophthalmic solution therapy if ocular allergic-like symptoms occur.

➤*Renal function impairment:* Although the topical use of apraclonidine ophthalmic solution has not been studied in renal failure patients, structurally related clonidine undergoes a significant increase in half-life in patients with severe renal impairment. Close monitoring of cardiovascular parameters in patients with impaired renal function is advised if they are candidates for topical apraclonidine therapy. Close monitoring of cardiovascular parameters in patients with impaired liver function is also advised as the systemic dosage form of clonidine is partly metabolized in the liver.

➤*Elderly:* No overall differences in safety and effectiveness have been observed between elderly and younger patients.

➤*Pregnancy: Category C.* Apraclonidine has been shown to have an embryocidal effect in rabbits when given in an oral dose of 3 mg/kg (60 and 150 times the maximum recommended human dose for 0.5% and 1% solutions, respectively). Dose related maternal toxicity was observed in pregnant rats at 0.3 mg/kg (6 and 15 times the maximum recommended human dose for 0.5% and 1% solutions, respectively). There are no adequate and well controlled studies in pregnant women. Use apraclonidine ophthalmic solution during pregnancy only if the potential benefit justifies the potential risk to the fetus.

➤*Lactation:* It is not known whether this drug is excreted in human milk. Because many drugs are excreted in human milk, exercise caution when apraclonidine ophthalmic solution is administered to a nursing woman.

➤*Children:* Safety and effectiveness in pediatric patients have not been established.

Precautions

➤*Monitoring:* Periodically monitor the visual fields of glaucoma patients on maximally tolerated medical therapy who are treated with apraclonidine ophthalmic solution to delay surgery.

Since apraclonidine is a potent depressor of IOP, closely monitor patients who develop exaggerated reduction in IOP.

Topical ocular administration of 2 drops of 0.5%, 1% and 1.5% apraclonidine ophthalmic solution to New Zealand albino rabbits 3 times daily for 1 month resulted in sporadic and transient instances of minimal corneal edema in the 1.5% group only; no histopathological changes were noted in those eyes. No adverse ocular effects were observed in cynomolgus monkeys treated with 2 drops of 1.5% solution applied 3 times daily for 3 months. No corneal changes were observed in 320 humans given at least 1 dose of 1% apraclonidine ophthalmic solution.

➤*Special risk:* Use apraclonidine ophthalmic solution with caution in patients with coronary insufficiency, recent myocardial infarction, cerebrovascular disease, chronic renal failure, Raynaud's disease, or thromboangiitis obliterans. Caution and monitoring of depressed patients are advised since apraclonidine has been infrequently associated with depression.

While the topical administration of apraclonidine ophthalmic solution had minimal effect on heart rate or blood pressure in clinical studies evaluating glaucoma patients and patients undergoing anterior segment laser surgery, the preclinical pharmacology profile of this drug suggests that caution should be observed in treating patients with severe cardiovascular disease, including hypertension.

1% – Consider the possibility of a vasovagal attack occurring during laser surgery and use caution in patients with a history of such episodes.

➤*Hazardous tasks:* Apraclonidine can cause dizziness and somnolence. Warn patients who engage in hazardous activities requiring mental alertness of the potential for a decrease in mental alertness while using apraclonidine.

Alpha Adrenergic Agonist

APRACLONIDINE HYDROCHLORIDE — OPHTHALMIC

Drug Interactions

Apraclonidine Drug Interactions			
Precipitant drug	Object drug*		Description
Apraclonidine	Cardiovascular agents	⬇	Since apraclonidine may reduce pulse and blood pressure, caution in using cardiovascular drugs is advised. Patients using cardiovascular drugs concurrently with apraclonidine 0.5% should have pulse and blood pressures frequently monitored.
Apraclonidine	MAO inhibitors	⬆	Apraclonidine should not be used in patients receiving MAO inhibitors (see Contraindications).

* ⬆ = Object drug increased. ⬇ = Object drug decreased.

Do not use apraclonidine in patients receiving MAO inhibitors. Although no specific drug interactions with topical glaucoma drugs or systemic medications were identified in clinical studies of apraclonidine 0.5% ophthalmic solution, consider the possibility of an additive or potentiating effect with CNS depressants (alcohol, barbiturates, opiates, sedatives, anesthetics). Tricyclic antidepressants have been reported to blunt the hypotensive effect of systemic clonidine. It is not known whether the concurrent use of these agents with apraclonidine can lead to a reduction in IOP-lowering effect. No data on the level of circulating catecholamines after apraclonidine withdrawal are available. Caution, however, is advised in patients taking tricyclic antidepressants which can affect the metabolism and uptake of circulating amines. Exercise caution with simultaneous use of clonidine and other similar pharmacologic agents.

An additive hypotensive effect has been reported with the combination of systemic clonidine and neuroleptic therapy. Systemic clonidine may inhibit the production of catecholamines in response to insulin-induced hypoglycemia and mask the signs and symptoms of hypoglycemia.

Adverse Reactions

➤*0.5% solution:* In clinical studies the overall discontinuation rate related to apraclonidine 0.5% ophthalmic solution was 15%. The most commonly reported events leading to discontinuation included (in decreasing order of frequency) hyperemia, pruritus, tearing, discomfort, lid edema, dry mouth, and foreign body sensation.

The following adverse reactions (incidences) were reported in clinical studies of apraclonidine 0.5% ophthalmic solution as being possibly, probably, or definitely related to therapy:

Ocular – The following adverse reactions were reported in 5% to 15% of patients: Discomfort, hyperemia, and pruritus.

The following adverse reactions were reported in 1% to 5% of patients: Blanching, blurred vision, conjunctivitis, discharge, dry eye, foreign body sensation, lid edema, and tearing.

The following adverse reactions were reported in less than 1% of patients: Abnormal vision, blepharitis, blepharoconjunctivitis, conjunctival edema, conjunctival follicles, corneal erosion, corneal infiltrate, corneal staining, edema, irritation, keratitis, keratopathy, lid disorder, lid erythema, lid margin crusting, lid retraction, lid scales, pain, photophobia.

Nonocular – Dry mouth occurred in approximately 10% of the patients.

The following adverse reactions were reported in less than 3% of patients: Abnormal coordination, asthenia, arrhythmia, asthma, chest pain, constipation, contact dermatitis, depression, dermatitis, dizziness, dry nose, dyspnea, facial edema, headache, insomnia, malaise, myalgia, nausea, nervousness, paresthesia, parosmia, peripheral edema, pharyngitis, rhinitis, somnolence, and taste perversion.

Postmarketing – The following events have been identified during postmarketing use of apraclonidine 0.5% ophthalmic solution in clinical practice. Because they are reported voluntarily from a population of unknown size, estimates of frequency cannot be made. The events, which have been chose for inclusion due to either their seriousness, frequency of reporting, possible causal connection to apraclonidine 0.5% ophthalmic solution, or a combination of these factors, include bradycardia.

➤*1% solution:* The following adverse events, occurring in less than 2% of patients, were reported in association with the use of apraclonidine ophthalmic solution in laser surgery: conjunctival blanching, irregular heart rate, mydriasis, nasal decongestion, ocular inflammation, ocular injection, and upper lid elevation.

The following adverse events were observed in investigational studies dosing apraclonidine ophthalmic solution once or twice daily for up to 28 days in nonlaser studies:

CNS – Decreased libido, dream disturbances, insomnia, irritability.

GI – Abdominal pain, diarrhea, emesis, stomach discomfort.

Ophthalmic – Allergic response, blurred or dimmed vision, burning, conjunctival blanching, conjunctival microhemorrhage, discomfort, dryness, foreign body sensation, hypotony, itching, mydriasis, upper lid elevation.

Miscellaneous – Body heat sensation, chest heaviness or burning, clammy or sweaty palms, dry mouth, extremity pain or numbness, fatigue, head cold sensation, headache, increased pharyngeal secretion, nasal burning or dryness, paresthesia, pruritus not associated with rash, shortness of breath, taste abnormalities.

Overdosage

➤*Symptoms:* Ingestion of apraclonidine 0.5% ophthalmic solution has been reported to cause bradycardia, drowsiness, and hypothermia.

Accidental or intentional ingestion of oral clonidine has been reported to cause apnea, arrhythmias, asthenia, bradycardia, conduction defects, diminished or absent reflexes, dryness of the mouth, hypotension, hypothermia, hypoventilation, irritability, lethargy, miosis, pallor, respiratory depression, sedation or coma, seizure, somnolence, transient hypertension, and vomiting.

➤*Treatment:* Treatment of an oral overdose includes supportive and symptomatic therapy; maintain a patent airway. Hemodialysis is of limited value, since a maximum of 5% of circulating drug is removed.

Patient Information

Do not touch dropper tip to any surface as this may contaminate the contents.

Apraclonidine can cause dizziness and somnolence. Warn patients who engage in hazardous activities requiring mental alertness of the potential for a decrease in mental alertness, physical dexterity, or coordination while using apraclonidine.

Sympathomimetics

DIPIVEFRIN HYDROCHLORIDE (Dipivalyl epinephrine)

Rx	**Dipivefrin HCl** (Various, eg, Falcon)	**Solution:** 0.1%	In 5, 10 and 15 mL.
Rx	**Propine** (Allergan)		In 5, 10 & 15 mL C Cap Compliance Cap B.I.D.[1]

[1] With 0.005% benzalkonium chloride, sodium chloride, EDTA and hydrochloric acid.

DIPIVEFRIN HYDROCHLORIDE — OPHTHALMIC

Refer to Topical Ophthalmic Drugs introduction for more complete and comparative information.

Indications

➤*Glaucoma:* Initial therapy for the control of intraocular pressure in chronic open-angle glaucoma. Patients responding inadequately to other antiglaucoma therapy may respond to addition of dipivefrin.

Administration and Dosage

➤*Initial glaucoma therapy:* One drop in the eye(s) every 12 hours.

➤*Replacement with dipivefrin:* When patients are being transferred to dipivefrin from antiglaucoma agents other than epinephrine, on the first day continue the previous medication and add 1 drop of dipivefrin in each eye every 12 hours. On the following day, discontinue the previously used antiglaucoma agent and continue with dipivefrin.

In transferring patients from conventional epinephrine therapy to dipivefrin, simply discontinue the epinephrine medication and institute the dipivefrin regimen.

➤*Addition of dipivefrin:* When patients on other antiglaucoma agents require additional therapy, add 1 drop of dipivefrin every 12 hours.

➤*Concomitant therapy:* For difficult to control patients, the addition of dipivefrin to other agents such as pilocarpine, carbachol, echothiophate iodide, or acetazolamide has been shown to be effective.

➤*Storage/Stability:* Store in tight, light-resistant container at 15° to 25°C (59° to 77°F).

Actions

➤*Pharmacology:* Dipivefrin ophthalmic solution is a prodrug of epinephrine formed by the diesterification of epinephrine and pivalic acid. The addition of pivaloyl groups to the epinephrine molecule enhances its lipophilic character and as a consequence, its penetration into the anterior chamber.

Dipivefrin is converted to epinephrine inside the human eye by enzyme hydrolysis. The liberated epinephrine, an adrenergic agonist, appears to exert its action by decreasing aqueous production and by enhancing outflow facility. The dipivefrin prodrug delivery system is a more efficient way of delivering the therapeutic effects of epinephrine, with fewer side effects than are associated with conventional epinephrine therapy.

The onset of action with 1 drop of dipivefrin occurs about 30 minutes after treatment, with maximum effect seen at about 1 hour.

Sympathomimetics

DIPIVEFRIN HYDROCHLORIDE — OPHTHALMIC

Contraindications

Narrow angles since any dilation of the pupil may predispose the patient to an attack of angle-closure glaucoma. This product is contraindicated in patients who are hypersensitive to any of its components.

Warnings

➤*Pregnancy:* Category B. There are no adequate and well-controlled studies in pregnant women. Because animal reproduction studies are not always predictive of human response, use this drug during pregnancy only if clearly needed.

➤*Lactation:* It is not known whether this drug is excreted in human milk. Because many drugs are excreted in human milk, exercise caution when dipivefrin ophthalmic solution is administered to a breast-feeding woman.

➤*Children:* Safety and effectiveness in pediatric patients have not been established.

Precautions

➤*Aphakic patients:* Macular edema has been shown to occur in up to 30% of aphakic patients treated with epinephrine. Discontinuation of epinephrine generally results in reversal of the maculopathy.

➤*Animal studies:* Rabbit studies indicated a dose-related incidence of meibomian gland retention cysts following topical administration of both dipivefrin and epinephrine.

Adverse Reactions

➤*Cardiovascular:* Tachycardia, arrhythmias, and hypertension have been reported with ocular administration of epinephrine.

➤*Local:* The most frequent side effects reported with dipivefrin alone were infection in 6.5% of patients and burning and stinging in 6%. Follicular conjunctivitis, eye pain, mydriasis, blurry vision, eye pruritus, headache, and allergic reaction to dipivefrin have been reported. Epinephrine therapy can lead to adrenochrome deposits in the conjunctiva and cornea.

Alpha-Adrenergic Antagonist

DAPIPRAZOLE HYDROCHLORIDE

Rx	**Rēv-Eyes** (Storz/Lederle)	**Powder, lyophilized:** 25 mg (0.5% solution when reconstituted)	In vial with 5 mL diluent and dropper.[1]

[1] With 2% mannitol, 0.4% hydroxypropyl methylcellulose, 0.01% EDTA, 0.01% benzalkonium chloride and sodium chloride.

DAPIPRAZOLE HYDROCHLORIDE — OPHTHALMIC

Refer to Topical Ophthalmic Drugs introduction for more complete and comparative information.

Indications

➤*Mydriasis:* Treatment of iatrogenically induced mydriasis produced by adrenergic (phenylephrine) or parasympatholytic (tropicamide) agents.

Administration and Dosage

Instill 2 drops into the conjunctiva of each eye followed 5 minutes later by an additional 2 drops. Administer after the ophthalmic examination to reverse the diagnostic mydriasis.

Shake container for several minutes to ensure mixing.

➤*Storage / Stability:* Store at room temperature 15° to 30°C (59° to 86°F) for 21 days after reconstitution.

Actions

➤*Pharmacology:* Dapiprazole acts through blocking the alpha-adrenergic receptors in smooth muscle and produces miosis through an effect on the dilator muscle of the iris.

The drug does not have any significant activity on ciliary muscle contraction and, therefore, does not induce a significant change in the anterior chamber depth or the thickness of the lens.

Contraindications

When constriction is undesirable, such as acute iritis; hypersensitivity to any component of this preparation.

Warnings

➤*For topical ophthalmic use only.:* Not for injection.

➤*Frequency of use:* Do not use in the same patient more frequently than once a week.

➤*IOP reduction:* Not indicated for the reduction of IOP or in the treatment of open-angle glaucoma.

➤*Vision reduction:* May cause difficulty in dark adaptation and may reduce field of vision. Patients should exercise caution in night driving or when performing other activities in poor illumination.

➤*Pregnancy:* Category B. There are no adequate and well controlled studies in pregnant women. Use during pregnancy only when clearly needed and when potential benefits outweigh the potential hazards to the fetus.

➤*Lactation:* It is not known whether this drug is excreted in breast milk. Exercise caution when dapiprazole is administered to a nursing woman.

➤*Children:* Safety and efficacy for use in children have not been established.

Adverse Reactions

Conjunctival injection lasting 20 minutes (greater than 80%); burning on instillation (≈ 50%); ptosis, lid erythema, lid edema, chemosis, itching, punctate keratitis, corneal edema, browache, photophobia, headaches (10% to 40%); dryness of the eye, tearing, blurring of vision (less frequent).

Patient Information

May cause difficulty in dark adaptation and may reduce field of vision. Exercise caution when driving at night or performing other activities in poor illumination.

To avoid contamination, do not touch tip of container to any surface.

Do not use in the same patient more frequently than once a week.

Discard any solution that is not clear and colorless.

Beta-Adrenergic Blocking Agents

Refer to the general discussion of these products in the Topical Ophthalmic Introduction for more complete and comparative information.

Indications

➤*Glaucoma:* Lowering intraocular pressure (IOP) in patients with chronic open-angle glaucoma.

For specific approved indications, refer to individual drug monographs.

Administration and Dosage

➤*Concomitant therapy:* If IOP is not controlled with these agents, institute concomitant pilocarpine, other miotics, dipivefrin or systemic carbonic anhydrase inhibitors.

Use of epinephrine with topical β-blockers is controversial. Some reports indicate initial effectiveness of the combination decreases over time (see Drug Interactions).

➤*Monitoring:* The IOP-lowering response to betaxolol and timolol may require a few weeks to stabilize.

Because of diurnal IOP variations in individual patients, satisfactory response to once-a-day therapy is best determined by measuring IOP at different times during the day.

Actions

➤*Pharmacology:* Timolol, levobunolol, carteolol and metipranolol are noncardioselective (β_1 and β_2) β-blockers; betaxolol and levobetaxolol are cardioselective (β_1) β-blockers. Topical β-blockers do not have significant membrane-stabilizing (local anesthetic) actions or intrinsic sympathomimetic activity. They reduce elevated and normal IOP, with or without glaucoma.

The exact mechanism of ocular antihypertensive action is not established, but it appears to be a reduction of aqueous production. However, some studies show a slight increase in outflow facility with timolol and metipranolol.

These agents reduce IOP with little or no effect on pupil size or accommodation. Blurred vision and night blindness often associated with miotics are not associated with these agents. The inability to see around lenticular opacities when the pupil is constricted is avoided. These agents may be absorbed systemically (see Warnings).

➤*Pharmacokinetics:*

Pharmacokinetics of Ophthalmic β-Adrenergic Blocking Agents

Drug	β-receptor selectivity	Onset (min)	Maximum effect (hr)	Duration (hr)
Carteolol	β_1 and β_2	nd[a]	2	12
Betaxolol	β_1	≤ 30	2	12
Levobunolol	β_1 and β_2	less than 60	2 to 6	≤ 24
Metipranolol	β_1 and β_2	≤ 30	≈ 2	24
Timolol	β_1 and β_2	≤ 30	1 to 2	≤ 24
Levobetaxolol	β_1	≤ 30	2	≈ 12

[a] nd = No data

Contraindications

Bronchial asthma, a history of bronchial asthma or severe chronic obstructive pulmonary disease; sinus bradycardia; second-degree and third-degree

AV block; overt cardiac failure; cardiogenic shock; hypersensitivity to any component of the products.

Warnings

➤*Systemic absorption:* These agents may be absorbed systemically. The same adverse reactions found with systemic β-blockers (see group monograph in Cardiovascular section) may occur with topical use. For example, severe respiratory reactions and cardiac reactions, including death due to bronchospasm in asthmatics, and rarely, death associated with cardiac failure, have been reported with topical β-blockers.

➤*Cardiovascular:* Timolol may decrease resting and maximal exercise heart rate even in healthy subjects.

Cardiac failure – Sympathetic stimulation may be essential for circulation support in diminished myocardial contractility; its inhibition by β-receptor blockade may precipitate more severe failure.

In patients without history of cardiac failure, continued depression of myocardium with β-blockers may lead to cardiac failure. Discontinue at the first sign or symptom of cardiac failure.

➤*Non-allergic bronchospasm:* Patients with a history of chronic bronchitis, emphysema, etc, should receive β-blockers with caution; they may block bronchodilation produced by catecholamine stimulation of β_2-receptors.

➤*Major surgery:* Withdrawing β-blockers before major surgery is controversial. Beta-receptor blockade impairs the heart's ability to respond to β-adrenergically mediated reflex stimuli. This may augment the risk of general anesthesia. Some patients on β-blockers have had protracted severe hypotension during anesthesia. Difficulty restarting and maintaining heartbeat has been reported. In elective surgery, gradual withdrawal of β-blockers may be appropriate.

The effects of β-blocking agents may be reversed by β-agonists such as isoproterenol, dopamine, dobutamine, or levarterenol.

➤*Diabetes mellitus:* Administer with caution to patients subject to spontaneous hypoglycemia or to diabetic patients (especially labile diabetics). Beta-blocking agents may mask signs and symptoms of acute hypoglycemia.

➤*Thyroid:* Beta-adrenergic blocking agents may mask clinical signs of hyperthyroidism (eg, tachycardia). Manage patients suspected of developing thyrotoxicosis carefully to avoid abrupt withdrawal of β-blockers, which might precipitate thyroid storm.

➤*Cerebrovascular insufficiency:* Because of potential effects of β-blockers on blood pressure and pulse, use with caution in patients with cerebrovascular insufficiency. If signs or symptoms suggesting reduced cerebral blood flow develop, consider alternative therapy.

➤*Carcinogenesis:* In female mice receiving oral metipranolol doses of 5, 50 and 100 mg/kg/day, the low dose had an increased number of pulmonary adenomas.

➤*Pregnancy: Category C.* There have been no adequate and well controlled studies in pregnant women. Use during pregnancy only if the potential benefits outweigh potential hazards to the fetus.

Carteolol – Increased resorptions and decreased fetal weights occurred in rabbits and rats at maternal doses ≈ 1052 and 5264 times the maximum human dose, respectively. A dose-related increase in wavy ribs was noted in the developing rat fetus when pregnant rats received doses ≈ 212 times the maximum human dose.

Betaxolol – In oral studies with rats and rabbits, evidence of post-implantation loss was seen at dose levels above 12 mg/kg and 128 mg/kg, respectively. Betaxolol was not teratogenic, however, and there were no other adverse effects on reproduction at subtoxic dose levels.

Levobunolol – Fetotoxicity was observed in rabbits at doses 200 and 700 times the glaucoma dose.

Metipranolol – Increased fetal resorption, fetal death and delayed development occurred in rabbits receiving 50 mg/kg orally during organogenesis.

Timolol – Doses of 1000 mg/kg/day (142,000 times the maximum recommended human ophthalmic dose) were maternotoxic in mice and resulted in increased fetal resorptions. Increased fetal resorptions were also seen in rabbits at 14,000 times the systemic exposure following the maximum recommended human ophthalmic dose, in this case without apparent maternotoxicity.

Levobetaxolol – There was evidence of drug-related postimplantation loss in rabbits with levobetaxolol at 12 mg/kg/day and sternebrae malformations at 4 mg/kg/day. No other adverse effects on reproduction were noted at subtoxic dose levels.

➤*Lactation:* It is not known whether betaxolol, levobunolol or metipranolol are excreted in breast milk. Systemic β-blockers and topical and ophthalmic timolol maleate are excreted in milk. Carteolol is excreted in breast milk of animals. Exercise caution when administering to a nursing mother.

Because of the potential for serious adverse reactions from timolol in nursing infants, decide whether to discontinue nursing or discontinue the drug taking into account the importance of the drug to the mother.

➤*Children:* Safety and efficacy for use in children have not been established.

Precautions

➤*Angle-closure glaucoma:* The immediate objective is to reopen the angle, requiring constriction of the pupil with a miotic. These agents have little or no effect on the pupil. When they are used to reduce elevated IOP in angle-closure glaucoma, use with a miotic.

➤*Muscle weakness:* Beta-blockade may potentiate muscle weakness consistent with certain myasthenic symptoms (eg, diplopia, ptosis, generalized weakness). Timolol has increased muscle weakness in some patients with myasthenic symptoms or myasthenia gravis.

➤*Long-term therapy:* In long-term studies (2 and 3 years), no significant differences in mean IOP were observed after initial stabilization.

➤*Sulfite sensitivity:* Some of these products contain sulfites which may cause allergic-type reactions (eg, hives, itching, wheezing, anaphylaxis) in certain susceptible persons. Although the overall prevalence of sulfite sensitivity in the general population is probably low, it is seen more frequently in asthmatics or atopic nonasthmatics.

Drug Interactions

Ophthalmic Beta Blocker Drug Interactions

Precipitant drug	Object drug*		Description
Beta blockers, ophthalmic	Beta blockers, oral	↑	Use topical beta blockers with caution because of the potential for additive effects on systemic and ophthalmic beta-blockade.
Beta blockers, ophthalmic	Calcium antagonists	↑	Possible cases of hypotension, left ventricular failure, and atrioventricular conduction disturbances may occur from coadministration of timolol maleate and calcium antagonists. Avoid use in patients with impaired cardiac function.
Beta blockers, ophthalmic	Catecholamine-depleting drugs (eg, reserpine)	↑	Use of reserpine with ophthalmic beta blockers can cause additive effects and the production of hypotension or marked bradycardia, which may result in syncope, vertigo, or postural hypotension. Close observation is recommended.
Catecholamine-depleting drugs (eg, reserpine)	Beta blockers, ophthalmic		
Beta blockers, ophthalmic	Digitalis	↑	Coadministration of ophthalmic beta blockers with digitalis and calcium antagonists may have additive effects in prolonging atrioventricular conduction time.
Digitalis	Beta blockers, ophthalmic		
Quinidine	Beta blockers, ophthalmic	↑	Decreased heart rate has been reported during combined treatment with timolol maleate and quinidine, possibly because quinidine inhibits the metabolism of timolol maleate via the P450 enzyme, CYP2D6.
Beta blockers	Phenothiazine compounds	↑	Potential additive hypotensive effects due to mutual inhibition of metabolism.

* ↑ = Object drug increased.

Other drugs that may interact with systemic β-adrenergic blocking agents may also interact with ophthalmic agents. For further information, refer to the β-blocker group monograph in the Cardiovasculars chapter.

Adverse Reactions

➤*The following have occurred with ophthalmic β_1 and β_2 (nonselective) blockers:*

Cardiovascular – Arrhythmia; syncope; heart block; cerebral vascular accident; cerebral ischemia; congestive heart failure; palpitation.

CNS – Headache; depression.

Dermatologic – Hypersensitivity, including localized and generalized rash.

Endocrine – Masked symptoms of hypoglycemia in insulin-dependent diabetics (see Warnings).

GI – Nausea.

Ophthalmic – Keratitis; blepharoptosis; visual disturbances including refractive changes (due to withdrawal of miotic therapy in some cases); diplopia; ptosis.

Respiratory – Bronchospasm (predominantly in patients with preexisting bronchospastic disease); respiratory failure.

➤*Carteolol:*

Ophthalmic – Transient irritation, burning, tearing, conjunctival hyperemia, edema (≈ 25%); blurred/cloudy vision; photophobia; decreased night vision; ptosis; blepharoconjunctivitis; abnormal corneal staining; corneal sensitivity.

Systemic – Bradycardia; decreased blood pressure; arrhythmia; heart palpitation; dyspnea; asthenia; headache; dizziness; insomnia; sinusitis; taste perversion.

➤*Betaxolol:*

Cardiovascular – Bradycardia; heart block; CHF.

CNS – Dizziness; vertigo; headaches; depression; lethargy; increase in signs and symptoms of myasthenia gravis.

Ophthalmic – Brief discomfort (25%); occasional tearing (5%). Rare: Decreased corneal sensitivity; erythema; itching; corneal punctate staining; keratitis, anisocoria; photophobia; edema.

Pulmonary – Pulmonary distress characterized by dyspnea, bronchospasm, thickened bronchial secretions, asthma, and respiratory failure.

Miscellaneous – Taste and smell perversions; hives; toxic epidermal necrolysis; hair loss; glossitis; insomnia.

➤*Metipranolol:*

Ophthalmic – Transient local discomfort; conjunctivitis; eyelid dermatitis; blepharitis; blurred vision; tearing; browache; abnormal vision; photophobia; edema; uveitis.

Systemic – Allergic reaction; headache; asthenia; hypertension; MI; atrial fibrillation; angina; palpitation; bradycardia; nausea; rhinitis; dyspnea; epistaxis; bronchitis; coughing; dizziness; anxiety; depression; somnolence; nervousness; arthritis; myalgia; rash.

➤*Levobetaxolol:*

Cardiovascular – Bradycardia, heart block, hypertension, hypotension, tachycardia, vascular anomaly (less than 2%).

CNS – Anxiety, dizziness, hypertonia, vertigo (less than 2%).

Dermatologic – Alopecia, dermatitis, psoriasis (less than 2%).

Endocrine – Diabetes, hypothyroidism (less than 2%).

GI – Constipation, dyspepsia (less than 2%).

GU – Breast abscess, cystitis (less than 2%).

Metabolic/Nutritional – Gout, hypercholesteremia, hyperlipidemia (less than 2%).

Musculoskeletal – Arthritis, tendonitis (less than 2%).

Ophthalmic – Transient ocular discomfort upon instillation (11%); transient blurred vision (≈ 2%); cataracts, vitreous disorders (less than 2%).

Pulmonary – Pulmonary distress characterized by bronchitis, dyspnea, pharyngitis, pneumonia, rhinitis, and sinusitis (less than 2%).

Special senses – Ear pain, otitis media, taste perversion, tinnitus (less than 2%).

Miscellaneous – Accidental injury, headache, infection (less than 2%).

➤*Levobunolol:*

Cardiovascular – Effects may resemble timolol.

CNS – Ataxia, dizziness, headache, lethargy (rare).

Dermatologic – Urticaria, pruritus (rare).

Ophthalmic – Transient burning/stinging (≤ 33%); blepharoconjunctivitis (≤ 5%); iridocyclitis (rare); decreased corneal sensitivity.

➤*Timolol:*

Cardiovascular – Bradycardia; arrhythmia; hypotension; syncope; heart block; cerebral vascular accident; cerebral ischemia; heart failure; palpitation; cardiac arrest.

CNS – Dizziness; depression; fatigue; lethargy; hallucinations; confusion.

Ophthalmic – Ocular irritation including conjunctivitis; blepharitis; keratitis; blepharoptosis; decreased corneal sensitivity; visual disturbances including refractive changes; diplopia; ptosis.

Respiratory – Bronchospasm (mainly in patients with preexisting bronchospastic disease); respiratory failure; dyspnea.

Miscellaneous – Aggravation of myasthenia gravis; alopecia; nausea; localized and generalized rash; urticaria; impotence; decreased libido; masked symptoms of hypoglycemia in diabetics; diarrhea.

➤*Systemic β-adrenergic blocker-associated reactions:* Consider potential effects with ophthalmic use (see Warnings).

Overdosage

If ocular overdosage occurs, flush eye(s) with water or normal saline. If accidentally ingested, efforts to decrease further absorption may be appropriate (gastric lavage).

The most common signs and symptoms of overdosage from systemic β-blockers are bradycardia, hypotension, bronchospasm and acute cardiac failure. If these occur, discontinue therapy and initiate appropriate supportive therapy.

Patient Information

Transient stinging/discomfort is relatively common; notify physician if severe.

Do not touch dropper tip to any surface; do not use with contact lenses in eyes.

LEVOBUNOLOL HYDROCHLORIDE

Rx	**Levobunolol** (Various, eg, Bausch & Lomb)	**Solution:** 0.25%	In 5 and 10 mL.
Rx	**Betagan Liquifilm** (Allergan)		In 5 and 10 mL dropper bottles with B.I.D. *C Cap.*[1]
Rx	**Levobunolol** (Various, eg, Bausch & Lomb, Falcon)	**Solution:** 0.5%	In 5, 10, and 15 mL.
Rx	**Betagan Liquifilm** (Allergan)		In 2 mL bottles with standard cap and 5, 10, and 15 mL with B.I.D. and Q.D. *C Cap.*[1]

[1] With 1.4% polyvinyl alcohol; 0.004% benzalkonium chloride; sodium metabisulfite; EDTA; sodium phosphate, dibasic; potassium phosphate, monobasic; NaCl; hydrochloric acid; sodium hydroxide.

LEVOBUNOLOL HYDROCHLORIDE — OPHTHALMIC

For complete and comparative prescribing information, refer to the Beta-Adrenergic Blocking Agents group monograph.

Indications

➤*Elevated IOP:* Lowering IOP in chronic open-angle glaucoma or ocular hypertension.

Administration and Dosage

➤*Usual dose:*

0.5% solution – 1 to 2 drops in the affected eye(s) once a day.

0.25% solution – 1 to 2 drops in the affected eye(s) twice daily. In patients with more severe or uncontrolled glaucoma, the 0.5% solution can be administered twice a day. As with any new medication, carefully monitor patients.

Dosages greater than 1 drop of 0.5% levobunolol twice daily are not generally more effective. If IOP is not at a satisfactory level on this regimen, concomitant therapy can be instituted. Do not administer ≥ 2 topical ophthalmic beta-adrenergic blocking agents simultaneously.

➤*Storage/Stability:* Store at controlled room temperature 15° to 30°C (59° to 86°F). Keep container tightly closed. Protect from light.

BETAXOLOL HYDROCHLORIDE

Rx	**Betaxolol HCl** (Various, Akorn, Falcon)	**Solution:** 5.6 mg (equiv. to 5 mg base) per mL (0.5%)	In 2.5, 5, 10, and 15 mL.
Rx	**Betoptic** (Alcon)		In 2.5, 5, 10, and 15 mL *Drop-Tainer* dispensers.[1]
Rx	**Betoptic S** (Alcon)	**Suspension:** 2.8 mg (equiv. to 2.5 mg base) per mL (0.25%)	In 2.5, 5, 10, and 15 mL *Drop-Tainer* dispensers.[2]

[1] With 0.01% benzalkonium chloride, NaCl, hydrochloric acid and/or sodium hydroxide, EDTA.

[2] With 0.01% benzalkonium chloride, mannitol, poly sulfonic acid, hydrochloric acid or sodium hydroxide, EDTA.

BETAXOLOL HYDROCHLORIDE — OPHTHALMIC

For complete and comparative prescribing information, refer to the Beta-Adrenergic Blocking Agents group monograph.

Indications

➤*Elevated intraocular pressure:* Treatment of ocular hypertension and chronic open-angle glaucoma. May be used alone or in combination with other antiglaucoma drugs.

Administration and Dosage

The recommended dose is 1 to 2 drops in the affected eye(s) twice daily. In some patients, the intraocular-pressure-lowering responses to betaxolol hydrochloride ophthalmic solution or suspension may require a few weeks to stabilize. As with any new medication, careful monitoring of patients is advised.

If the intraocular pressure of the patient is not adequately controlled on this regimen, concomitant therapy with pilocarpine and other miotics, or epinephrine or carbonic anhydrase inhibitors can be instituted.

Do not touch dropper tip to any surface as this may contaminate the solution.

➤*Storage/Stability:* Store at room temperature.

Suspension – Shake well before using.

METIPRANOLOL HYDROCHLORIDE

Rx	**Metipranolol** (Falcon)	**Solution**: 0.3%	In 5 and 10 mL.[1]
Rx	**OptiPranolol** (Bausch & Lomb)		In 5 and 10 mL dropper bottles.[2]

[1] With 0.004% benzalkonium chloride, povidone, hydrochloric acid, NaCl,EDTA.

[2] With 0.004% benzalkonium chloride, glycerin , povidone, hydrochloric acid, NaCl, sodium hydroxide and/or hydrochloric acid, EDTA.

METIPRANOLOL — OPHTHALMIC

For complete and comparative prescribing information, refer to the Beta-Adrenergic Blocking Agents group monograph.

Indications

➤*Elevated intraocular pressure:* Treatment of elevated intraocular pressure (IOP) in patients with ocular hypertension or open-angle glaucoma.

Administration and Dosage

➤*Approved by the FDA:* December 29, 1989.

The recommended dose is 1 drop of metipranolol ophthalmic solution in the affected eye(s) twice daily.

If the patient's IOP is not at a satisfactory level on this regimen, use of more frequent administration or a larger dose of metipranolol ophthalmic solution is not known to be of benefit. Concomitant therapy to lower IOP can be instituted.

➤*Storage / Stability:* Store between 15° to 30°C (59° to 86°F). Replace cap immediately after use.

CARTEOLOL HYDROCHLORIDE

Rx	**Carteolol HCl** (Various, eg, Akorn, Falcon)	**Solution**: 1%	In 5, 10, and 15 mL.
Rx	**Ocupress** (Novartis Pharmaceuticals)		In 5, 10, and 15 mL dispenser bottles.[a]

[a] With 0.005% benzalkonium chloride; NaCl; sodium phosphate, dibasic and monobasic.

CARTEOLOL HYDROCHLORIDE — OPHTHALMIC

For complete and comparative prescribing information, refer to the Beta-Adrenergic Blocking Agents group monograph.

Indications

➤*Elevated IOP:* Lowering of IOP in chronic open-angle glaucoma and intraocular hypertension.

Administration and Dosage

➤*Approved by the FDA:* May 23, 1990.

➤*Usual dose:* Instill 1 drop in affected eye(s) twice daily. If the patient's IOP is not at a satisfactory level on this regimen, concomitant therapy can be instituted.

➤*Storage / Stability:* Store at 15° to 25°C (59° to 77°F) (room temperature) and protect from light.

TIMOLOL MALEATE, OPHTHALMIC

Rx	**Timolol Maleate** (Various, eg, Akorn, Bausch & Lomb, Falcon, Fougera)	**Solution**: 0.25%	In 2.5, 5, 10, and 15 mL.
Rx	**Betimol**[a] (Vistakon[b])		In 5, 10, and 15 mL.[c]
Rx	**Timoptic**[d] (Merck)		Preservative free. In UD 60s *Ocudose*.[e]
Rx	**Timoptic**[d] (Merck)		In 5 and 10 mL *Ocumeters*.[f]
Rx	**Timolol Maleate** (Various, eg, Akorn, Bausch & Lomb, Falcon, Fougera)	**Solution**: 0.5%	In 2.5, 5, 10, and 15 mL.
Rx	**Betimol**[a] (Vistakon[b])		In 5, 10, and 15 mL.[c]
Rx	**Istalol**[d] (Ista Pharm)		In 5 mL.[g]
Rx	**Timoptic**[d] (Merck)		Preservative free. In UD 60s *Ocudose*.[e]
Rx	**Timoptic**[d] (Merck)		In 5 and 10 mL *Ocumeters*.[g]
Rx	**Timolol GFS**[d] (Falcon)	**Solution, gel-forming**: 0.25%	In 2.5 and 5 mL.[h]
Rx	**Timoptic-XE**[d] (Merck)		In 5 mL *Ocumeters*.[h]
Rx	**Timolol GFS**[d] (Falcon)	**Solution, gel-forming**: 0.5%	In 2.5 and 5 mL.[h]
Rx	**Timoptic-XE**[d] (Merck)		In 5 mL *Ocumeters*.[h]

[a] As hemihydrate.
[b] Vistakon Pharmaceuticals, Jacksonville, FL 32256
[c] With 0.01% benzalkonium chloride and monosodium and disodium phosphate dihydrate.
[d] As maleate.
[e] Preservative free; use immediately after opening; discard remaining contents. With monobasic and dibasic sodium phosphate and sodium hydroxide.
[f] With 0.01% benzalkonium chloride, sodium hydroxide, and monobasic and dibasic sodium phosphate.
[g] With 0.005% benzalkonium chloride, monobasic sodium phosphate monohydrate, 0.47% potassium sorbate, and sodium hydroxide.
[h] With 0.012% benzododecinium bromide.

TIMOLOL MALEATE — OPHTHALMIC

For complete and comparative prescribing information, refer to the Beta-Adrenergic Blocking Agents group monograph.

Indications

➤*Elevated intraocular pressure (IOP):* Treatment of elevated IOP in patients with ocular hypertension or open-angle glaucoma.

Administration and Dosage

➤*Approved by the FDA:* November 5, 1986.

Since in some patients the pressure-lowering response to timolol may require a few weeks to stabilize, evaluation should include a determination of IOP after approximately 4 weeks of treatment with timolol.

➤*Timolol ophthalmic gel-forming solution (Timoptic-XE):*

Administration – Instruct patients to invert the closed container and shake once before each use. It is not necessary to shake the container more than once. Administer other topically applied ophthalmic medications at least 10 minutes before timolol ophthalmic gel-forming solution.

Dosage – Instill 1 drop in the affected eye(s) once daily.

Concomitant therapy – Dosages higher than 1 drop of timolol 0.5% ophthalmic gel-forming solution once daily have not been studied. If the patient's IOP is still not at a satisfactory level on this regimen, concomitant therapy may be considered. The concomitant use of 2 topical beta-adrenergic blocking agents is not recommended.

➤*Timolol ophthalmic solution (Timoptic):*

Dosage – The usual starting dosage is 1 drop of timolol 0.25% in the affected eye(s) twice daily. If the clinical response is not adequate, the dosage may be changed to 1 drop of 0.5% solution in the affected eye(s) twice daily. If the IOP is maintained at satisfactory levels, the dosage schedule may be changed to 1 drop once daily in the affected eye(s). Because of diurnal variations in IOP, satisfactory response to the once-a-day dosage is best determined by measuring the IOP at different times during the day.

Concomitant therapy – Dosages above 1 drop of timolol 0.5% twice daily generally have not been shown to produce further reduction in IOP. If the patient's IOP is still not at a satisfactory level on this regimen, concomitant therapy with other agent(s) for lowering IOP can be instituted. The concomitant use of 2 topical beta-adrenergic blocking agents is not recommended.

➤*Timolol ophthalmic solution (Istalol):*

Dosage – The starting dosage is 1 drop of 0.5% in the affected eye(s) once daily in the morning.

Concomitant therapy – If the patient's IOP is not at a satisfactory level on this regimen, concomitant therapy with other agent(s) for lowering IOP can be instituted. The concomitant use of 2 topical beta-adrenergic blocking agents is not recommended.

➤*Timolol preservative-free ophthalmic solution in dispenser (Timoptic in Ocudose):*

TIMOLOL MALEATE — OPHTHALMIC

Administration – Preservative-free timolol in dispenser is a sterile solution that does not contain a preservative. The solution from 1 individual unit is to be used immediately after opening for administration to 1 or both eyes. Because sterility cannot be guaranteed after the individual unit is opened, discard the remaining contents immediately after administration.

Dosage – The usual starting dosage is 1 drop of preservative-free timolol 0.25% in a dispenser in the affected eye(s) administered twice daily. Apply enough gentle pressure on the individual container to obtain a single drop of solution. If the clinical response is not adequate, the dosage may be changed to 1 drop of 0.5% solution in the affected eye(s) administered twice daily. If the IOP is maintained at satisfactory levels, the dosage schedule may be changed to 1 drop once daily in the affected eye(s). Because of diurnal variations in IOP, satisfactory response to the once-a-day dosage is best determined by measuring the IOP at different times during the day.

Concomitant therapy – Dosages above 1 drop of timolol 0.5% ophthalmic solution twice daily generally have not been shown to produce further reduction in IOP. If the patient's IOP is still not at a satisfactory level on this regimen, concomitant therapy with other agent(s) for lowering IOP can be instituted taking into consideration that the preparation(s) used concomitantly may contain 1 or more preservatives. The concomitant use of 2 topical beta-adrenergic blocking agents is not recommended.

➤*Storage / Stability:*

Timolol ophthalmic gel-forming solution and timolol ophthalmic solution – Store between 15° and 30°C (59° and 86°F). Protect from freezing. Protect from light.

Timolol ophthalmic solution (Istalol) – Store between 15° and 25°C (59° and 77°F).

Timolol preservative-free ophthalmic solution in dispenser – Store at room temperature, 15° to 30°C (59° to 86°F). Protect from freezing. Protect from light.

Because evaporation can occur through the unprotected polyethylene unit dose container and prolonged exposure to direct light can modify the product, keep the unit dose container in the protective foil overwrap and use within 1 month after the foil package has been opened.

LEVOBETAXOLOL HYDROCHLORIDE OPHTHALMIC

Rx	**Betaxon** (Alcon)	**Suspension, ophthalmic:** 0.5% as base (5.6 mg/mL)	0.01% benzalkonium chloride, EDTA, hydrochloric acid, boric acid. In 5, 10, and 15 mL *Drop-tainers.*

LEVOBETAXOLOL HYDROCHLORIDE — OPHTHALMIC

For complete and comparative prescribing information, refer to the Beta-Adrenergic Blocking Agents group monograph.

Indications

➤*Elevated intraocular presure:* For lowering intraocular pressure in patients with chronic open-angle glaucoma or ocular hypertension.

Administration and Dosage

➤*Approved by the FDA:* February 24, 2000.

The recommended dose is 1 drop in the affected eye(s) twice daily. In some patients, the intraocular pressure lowering responses to levobetaxolol hydrochloride ophthalmic suspension may require a few weeks to stabilize. As with any new medication, careful monitoring of patients is advised. The concomitant use of 2 topical beta-adrenergic agents is not recommended.

➤*Storage / Stability:* Store upright 4° to 25°C (39° to 77°F). Protect from light. Shake well before using.

Refer to the Topical Ophthalmic Drugs introduction and Agents for Glaucoma introduction for a general discussion of these products. For information on the oral use of pilocarpine, refer to the monograph in the Mouth and Throat Products section.

Indications

➤*Carbachol, topical; pilocarpine:*

Glaucoma – To decrease elevated IOP in glaucoma.

➤*Acetylcholine; carbachol, intraocular:*

Miosis – To induce miosis during surgery.

See individual monographs for specific indications.

Actions

➤*Pharmacology:* The direct-acting miotics are parasympathomimetic (cholinergic) drugs which duplicate the muscarinic effects of acetylcholine. When applied topically, these drugs produce pupillary constriction, stimulate the ciliary muscles and increase aqueous humor outflow facility. Miosis, produced through contraction of the iris sphincter, causes increased tension on the scleral spur (reducing outflow resistance) and opening of the trabecular meshwork spaces facilitating outflow. With the increase in outflow facility, there is a decrease in intraocular pressure (IOP). Topical ophthalmic instillation of acetylcholine causes no discernible response as cholinesterase destroys the molecule more rapidly than it can penetrate the cornea; therefore, acetylcholine is only used intraocularly.

Miosis Induction of Direct-Acting Miotics

Miotic	Onset	Peak	Duration
Acetylcholine, intraocular	seconds	—	10 min
Carbachol			
Intraocular	seconds	2 to 5 min	1 to 2 days
Topical	10 to 20 min	—	4 to 8 hours
Pilocarpine, topical	10 to 30 min	—	4 to 8 hours

Contraindications

Hypersensitivity to any component of the formulation; where constriction is undesirable (eg, acute iritis, acute or anterior uveitis, some forms of secondary glaucoma, pupillary block glaucoma, acute inflammatory disease of the anterior chamber).

Warnings

➤*Corneal abrasion:* Use carbachol with caution in the presence of corneal abrasion to avoid excessive penetration.

➤*Pregnancy:* *Category C* (carbachol, pilocarpine). Safety for use during pregnancy has not been established. Use only when clearly needed.

➤*Lactation:* It is not known whether these drugs are excreted in breast milk; exercise caution when administering to a nursing woman.

➤*Children:* Safety and efficacy for use in children have not been established.

Precautions

➤*Systemic reactions:* Caution is advised in patients with acute cardiac failure, bronchial asthma, peptic ulcer, hyperthyroidism, GI spasm, urinary tract obstruction, Parkinson's disease, recent MI, hypertension or hypotension.

➤*Retinal detachment:* Retinal detachment has been caused by miotics in susceptible individuals, in individuals with preexisting retinal disease or in those who are predisposed to retinal tears. Fundus examination is advised for all patients prior to initiation of therapy.

➤*Miosis:* Miosis usually causes difficulty in dark adaptation. Advise patients to use caution while night driving or performing hazardous tasks in poor light.

➤*Angle-closure:* Although withdrawal of the peripheral iris from the anterior chamber angle by miosis may reduce the tendency for narrow-angle closure, miotics can occasionally precipitate angle closure by increasing resistance to aqueous flow from posterior to anterior chamber.

➤*Pilocarpine ocular system (Ocusert):* Carefully consider and evaluate patients with acute infectious conjunctivitis or keratitis prior to use.

Drug Interactions

➤*Nonsteroidal anti-inflammatory agents (NSAIDs), topical:* Although studies with acetylcholine chloride or carbachol revealed no interference, and there is no known pharmacological basis for an interaction, there have been reports that these drugs have been ineffective when used in patients treated with topical NSAIDs.

Adverse Reactions

➤*Acetylcholine:*

Ophthalmic – Corneal edema; clouding; decompensation.

Systemic – Bradycardia; hypotension; flushing; breathing difficulties; sweating.

➤*Carbachol:*

Ophthalmic – Transient stinging and burning; corneal clouding; persistent bullous keratopathy; postoperative iritis following cataract extraction with intraocular use; retinal detachment; transient ciliary and conjunctival injection; ciliary spasm with resultant temporary decrease of visual acuity.

Systemic – Headache; salivation; GI cramps; vomiting; diarrhea; asthma; syncope; cardiac arrhythmia; flushing; sweating; epigastric distress; tightness in bladder; hypotension; frequent urge to urinate.

➤*Pilocarpine:*

Ophthalmic – Transient stinging and burning; tearing; ciliary spasm; conjunctival vascular congestion; temporal, peri- or supra-orbital headache; superficial keratitis; induced myopia (especially in younger individuals who have recently started administration); blurred vision; poor dark adaptation; reduced visual acuity in poor illumination in older individuals and in individuals with lens opacity. A subtle corneal granularity has occurred with pilocarpine gel. Lens opacity (prolonged use), retinal detachment (rare; see Precautions).

Systemic – Hypertension, tachycardia, bronchiolar spasm, pulmonary edema, salivation, sweating, nausea, vomiting, diarrhea (rare).

Pilocarpine ocular system (Ocusert): Conjunctival irritation, including mild erythema with or without a slight increase in mucus secretion with first use. These symptoms tend to lessen or disappear after the first week of therapy. Ciliary spasm may occur with pilocarpine usage but is not a contraindication to continued therapy unless the induced myopia is debilitating to the patient. Rarely, a sudden increase in pilocarpine effects has been reported during use.

Irritation from pilocarpine has been infrequently encountered and may require cessation of therapy. True allergic reactions are uncommon, but require discontinuation of therapy. Corneal abrasion and visual impairment have been reported.

Overdosage

Should accidental overdosage in the eye(s) occur, flush with water.

➤*Treatment:* Treatment includes usual supportive measures. Refer to General Management of Acute Overdosage. Observe patients for signs of toxicity (eg, salivation, lacrimation, sweating, nausea, vomiting, diarrhea). If these occur, anticholinergics (atropine) may be necessary. Bronchial constriction may be a problem in asthmatic patients.

Patient Information

May sting upon instillation, especially first few doses.

May cause headache, browache and decreased night vision. Use caution while night driving or performing hazardous tasks in poor light.

To avoid contamination, do not touch tip of container to any surface. Replace cap after using. Keep bottle tightly closed when not in use. Discard solution after expiration date.

ACETYLCHOLINE CHLORIDE, INTRAOCULAR

Rx	**Miochol-E** (Novartis Pharmaceuticals)	**Solution:** 1:100 acetylcholine chloride when reconstituted	In 2 mL dual chamber univial (lower chamber 20 mg lyophilized acetylcholine chloride and 56 mg mannitol; upper chamber 2 mL electrolyte diluent[1] and sterile water for injection).

[1] Sodium chloride, potassium chloride, magnesium chloride hexahydrate, calcium chloride dihydrate.

ACETYLCHOLINE CHLORIDE — OPHTHALMIC

For complete and comparative prescribing information, refer to the Miotics, Direct-Acting group monograph.

Indications

➤*Miosis:* To obtain miosis of the iris in seconds after delivery of the lens in cataract surgery, in penetrating keratoplasty, iridectomy and other anterior segment surgery where rapid miosis may be required.

Administration and Dosage

With a new needle of sturdy gauge, 18 to 20, draw all the solution into a dry, sterile syringe. Replace needle with a suitable atraumatic cannulae for intraocular irrigation.

The acetylcholine chloride solution is instilled into the anterior chamber before or after securing one or more sutures. Instillation should be gentle and parallel to the iris face and tangential to pupil border.

If there are no mechanical hindrances, the pupil starts to constrict in seconds and the peripheral iris is drawn away from the angle of the anterior chamber. Any anatomical hindrance to miosis must be released to permit the desired effect of the drug. In most cases, 0.5 to 2 mL produces satisfactory miosis.

In cataract surgery, use acetylcholine chloride only after delivery of the lens.

➤*Preparation for administration:* Aqueous solutions of acetylcholine chloride are unstable. Prepare solution immediately before use. Do not use solution which is not clear and colorless. Discard any solution that has not been used.

➤*Storage / Stability:* Keep from freezing. Store at controlled room temperature 15° to 30°C (59° to 86°F).

CARBACHOL, INTRAOCULAR

Rx	**Carbastat** (Novartis Ophthalmics)	**Solution:** 0.01%	In 1.5 mL vials.[1]
Rx	**Miostat** (Alcon)		In 1.5 mL vials.[1]

[1] With 0.64% sodium chloride, 0.075% potassium chloride, 0.048% calcium chloride dihydrate, 0.03% magnesium chloride hexahydrate, 0.39% sodium acetate trihydrate, 0.17% sodium citrate dihydrate, sodium hydroxide, hydrochloric acid.

CARBACHOL — INTRAOCULAR

For complete and comparative prescribing information, refer to the Miotics, Direct-Acting group monograph.

Indications

➤*Miosis:* Intraocular use for miosis during surgery.

Administration and Dosage

For single-dose intraocular use only. Discard unused portion.

Open under aseptic conditions only.

Gently instill no more than 0.5 mL into the anterior chamber before or after securing sutures. Miosis is usually maximal 2 to 5 minutes after application.

➤*Storage / Stability:* Store at room temperature 15° to 30°C (59° to 86°F).

CARBACHOL, TOPICAL

Rx	**Isopto Carbachol** (Alcon)	**Solution:** 0.75%	In 15 and 30 mL *Drop-Tainers.*[1]
		1.5%	In 15 and 30 mL *Drop-Tainers.*[1]
		2.25%	In 15 mL *Drop-Tainers.*[1]
Rx	**Isopto Carbachol** (Alcon)	3%	In 15 and 30 mL *Drop-Tainers.*[1]
Rx	**Carboptic** (Optopics)		In 15 mL.[2]

[1] With 0.005% benzalkonium chloride, 1% hydroxypropyl methylcellulose, sodium chloride, boric acid and sodium borate.

[2] With benzalkonium chloride, polyvinyl alcohol and sodium phosphate dibasic and monobasic.

CARBACHOL — TOPICAL

For complete prescribing information, refer to the Miotics, Direct-Acting group monograph.

Indications

➤*Glaucoma:* For lowering intraocular pressure in the treatment of glaucoma.

Administration and Dosage

Instill 2 drops into eye(s) up to 3 times daily.

➤*Storage / Stability:* Store at 8° to 27°C (46° to 80°F).

PILOCARPINE HYDROCHLORIDE

Rx	**Isopto Carpine** (Alcon)	**Solution:** 0.25%	In 15 mL.[1]
Rx	**Pilocarpine hydrochloride** (Various, eg, Rugby)	**Solution:** 0.5%	In 15 and 30 mL.
Rx	**Isopto Carpine** (Alcon)		In 15 and 30 mL.[1]
Rx	**Pilocar** (Novartis Ophthalmics)		In 15 mL.[2]
Rx	**Pilocarpine hydrochloride** (Various, eg, Alcon, Goldline, Rugby)	**Solution:** 1%	In 2, 15 and 30 mL and UD 1 mL.
Rx	**Akarpine** (Akorn)		In 15 mL.
Rx	**Isopto Carpine** (Alcon)		In 15 and 30 mL.[1]
Rx	**Pilocar** (Novartis Ophthalmics)		In 15 mL and 1 mL dropperettes.[2]

Miotics, Direct-Acting

PILOCARPINE HYDROCHLORIDE

Rx	**Pilocarpine hydrochloride** (Various eg, Alcon, Goldline, Rugby)	**Solution:** 2%	In 2, 15, and 30 mL.
Rx	**Akarpine** (Akorn)		In 15 mL dropper bottles.
Rx	**Isopto Carpine** (Alcon)		In 15 and 30 mL.[1]
Rx	**Pilocar** (Novartis Ophthalmics)		In 15 mL, twin-pack (2 × 15 mL) and 12 × 1 mL dropperettes.[2]
Rx	**Isopto Carpine** (Alcon)	**Solution:** 3%	In 15 mL and 30 mL.[1]
Rx	**Pilocarpine hydrochloride** (Various, eg, Alcon, Goldline, Rugby)	**Solution:** 4%	In 2, 15 and 30 mL.
Rx	**Akarpine** (Akorn)		In 15 mL dropper bottles.
Rx	**Isopto carpine** (Alcon)		In 15 and 30 mL.[1]
Rx	**Pilocar** (Novartis Ophthalmics)		In 15 mL, twin-pack (2 × 15 mL) and 12 × 1 mL dropperettes.[2]
Rx	**Isopto Carpine** (Alcon)	**Solution:** 5%	In 15 mL.[1]
Rx	**Pilocarpine hydrochloride** (Various, eg, Rugby)	**Solution:** 6%	In 15 mL.
Rx	**Isopto Carpine** (Alcon)		In 15 and 30 mL.[1]
Rx	**Pilocar** (Novartis Ophthalmics)		In 15 mL.[3]
Rx	**Pilocarpine hydrochloride** (Alcon)	**Solution:** 8%	In 2 mL.
Rx	**Isopto Carpine** (Alcon)		In 15 mL.
Rx	**Isopto Carpine** (Alcon)	**Solution:** 10%	In 15 mL.[1]
Rx	**Pilopine HS** (Alcon)	**Gel:** 4%	In 3.5 g.[6]

[1] With 0.5% hydroxypropyl methylcellulose and 0.01% benzalkonium chloride.
[2] With dydroxypropyl methylcellulose, benzalkonium chloride and EDTA.
[3] With polyvinyl alcohol, benzalkonium chloride and EDTA.
[4] With 0.004% benzalkonium chloride, EDTA, povidone, PEG and hydroxyethyl cellulose.
[5] With dydroxypropyl methylcellulose, 0.01% benzalkonium chloride and EDTA.
[6] With 0.008% benzalkonium chloride, carbopol 940 and EDTA.

PILOCARPINE — OCULAR

For complete and comparative prescribing information, refer to the Miotics, Direct-Acting group monograph.

Indications

➤*Chronic simple glaucoma:* Chronic simple glaucoma, especially open-angle glaucoma. Patients may be maintained on pilocarpine as long as intraocular pressure (IOP) is controlled and there is no deterioration in the visual fields.

Chronic angle-closure glaucoma.

➤*Acute (angle-dose) glaucoma:* Alone, or in combination with other miotics, β-adrendergic blocking agents, epinephrine, carbonic anhydrase inhibitors or hyperosmotic agents to decrease IOP prior to surgery.

Pre- and postoperative intraocular tension.

➤*Mydriasis:* Mydriasis caused by mydriatic or cycloplegic agents.

Administration and Dosage

➤*Solution:*

Initial – 1 or 2 drops 3 to 4 times a daily. The frequency of instillation and the concentration are determined by patient response. Individuals with heavily pigmented irides may require higher strengths.

➤*Gel:* Apply a 0.5 inch ribbon in the lower conjunctival sac of affected eye(s) once daily at bedtime. If other glaucoma medication is also used at bedtime, use drops at least 5 minutes before the gel.

➤*Storage / Stability:* Do not freeze. Store at room temperature.

Miotics, Cholinesterase Inhibitors

ECHOTHIOPHATE IODIDE, OPHTHALMIC

Rx	**Phospholine Iodide** (Wyeth-Ayerst)	**Powder for Reconstitution:** 6.25 mg to make 0.125%	With 5 mL diluent.[a]

[a] With potassium acetate, 0.55% chlorobutanol and 1.2% mannitol.

ECHOTHIOPHATE IODIDE — OPHTHALMIC

Indications

➤*Glaucoma:* Chronic open-angle glaucoma; subacute or chronic angle-closure glaucoma after iridectomy or where surgery is refused or contraindicated; certain nonuveitic secondary types of glaucoma, especially glaucoma following cataract surgery.

➤*Accommodative esotropia:* For concomitant esotropias with a significant accommodative component.

Administration and Dosage

➤*Glaucoma:*

Dosage regimen – The dosage regimen prescribed should call for the lowest concentration that will control the intraocular pressure around-the-clock. Where tonometry around-the-clock is not feasible, it is suggested that appointments for tension-taking be made at different times of the day so that inadequate control may be more readily detected. Two doses a day are preferred to one in order to maintain as smooth a diurnal tension curve as possible, although a single dose per day or every other day has been used with satisfactory results. Because of the long duration of action of the drug, it is never necessary or desirable to exceed a schedule of twice a day. The daily dose or 1 of the 2 daily doses should always be instilled just before retiring to avoid inconvenience due to the miosis.

Early chronic simple glaucoma – Echothiophate iodide solution 0.03% instilled twice a day, just before retiring and in the morning, may be prescribed advantageously for cases of early chronic simple glaucoma that are not controlled around-the-clock with other less-potent agents. Because of prolonged action, control during the night and early morning hours may then sometimes be obtained. A change in therapy is indicated if, at any time, the tension fails to remain at an acceptable level on this regimen.

Advanced chronic simple glaucoma and glaucoma secondary to cataract surgery – These cases may respond satisfactorily to echothiophate iodide 0.03% twice a day as above. When the patient is being transferred to echothiophate iodide solution because of unsatisfactory control with pilocarpine, carbachol, epinephrine, etc, one of the higher strengths, 0.06%, 0.125%, or 0.25% will usually be needed. In this case, a brief trial with the 0.03% eyedrops will be advantageous in that the higher strengths will then be more easily tolerated.

Concomitant therapy – Echothiophate iodide solution may be used concomitantly with epinephrine, a carbonic anhydrase inhibitor, or both.

➤*Accommodative esotropia (pediatric use):*

Diagnosis – One drop of 0.125% may be instilled once a day in both eyes on retiring, for a period of 2 or 3 weeks. If the esotropia is accommodative, a favorable response will usually be noted which may begin within a few hours.

Treatment – Echothiophate iodide is prescribed at the lowest concentration and frequency which gives satisfactory results. After the initial period of treatment for diagnostic purposes, the schedule may be reduced to 0.125% every other day or 0.06% every day. These dosages can often be gradually lowered as treatment progresses. The 0.03% strength has proven to be effective in some cases. The maximum usually recommended dosage is 0.125% once a day, although more intensive therapy has been used for short periods.

Duration of treatment –

Diagnosis: In diagnosis, only a short period is required and little time will be lost in instituting other procedures if the esotropia proves to be unresponsive.

Treatment: In therapy, there is no definite limit so long as the drug is well tolerated. However, if the eyedrops, with or without eyeglasses, are gradually withdrawn after about a year or two and deviation recurs, surgery should be considered. As with other miotics, tolerance may occasionally develop after prolonged use. In such cases, a rest period will restore the original activity of the drug.

➤*Storage / Stability:* Store under refrigeration (2° to 8°C).

Reconstituted product may be stored at room temperature (≈ 25°C) for up to 4 weeks.

ECHOTHIOPHATE IODIDE — OPHTHALMIC

Actions

➤*Pharmacology:* Echothiophate iodide is a long-acting cholinesterase inhibitor for topical use which enhances the effect of endogenously liberated acetylcholine in iris, ciliary muscle, and other parasympathetically innervated structures of the eye. It thereby causes miosis, increase in facility of outflow of aqueous humor, fall in intraocular pressure, and potentiation of accommodation.

Echothiophate iodide will depress both plasma and erythrocyte cholinesterase levels in most patients after a few weeks of eyedrop therapy.

Contraindications

Active uveal inflammation; most cases of angle-closure glaucoma, due to the possibility of increasing angle block; hypersensitivity to the active or inactive ingredients.

Warnings

➤*Pregnancy: Category C.* Animal reproduction studies have not been conducted with echothiophate iodide. It is also not known whether echothiophate iodide can cause fetal harm when administered to a pregnant woman or can affect reproduction capacity. Echothiophate iodide should be given to a pregnant woman only if clearly needed.

➤*Lactation:* Because of the potential for serious adverse reactions in nursing infants from echothiophate iodide, a decision should be made whether to discontinue nursing or to discontinue the drug, taking into account the importance of the drug to the mother.

Precautions

➤*Monitoring:* Gonioscopy is recommended prior to initiation of therapy. Routine examinations to detect lens opacity should accompany clinical use of echothiophate iodide solution.

➤*Systemic effects:* While systemic effects are infrequent, proper use of the drug requires digital compression of the nasolacrimal ducts for a minute or two following instillation to minimize drainage into the nasal chamber with its extensive absorption area. To prevent possible skin absorption, hands should be washed following instillation.

Temporary discontinuance of medication is necessary if cardiac irregularities occur.

Temporary discontinuance of medication is necessary if salivation, urinary incontinence, diarrhea, profuse sweating, muscle weakness, or respiratory difficulties occur.

➤*Insecticides/Pesticides:* Patients receiving echothiophate iodide who are exposed to carbamateor organophosphate-type insecticides and pesticides (eg, professional gardeners, farmers, workers in plants manufacturing or formulating such products) should be warned of the additive systemic effects possible from absorption of the pesticide through the respiratory tract or skin. During periods of exposure to such pesticides, the wearing of respiratory masks, and frequent washing and clothing changes may be advisable.

➤*Special risk:* Where there is a quiescent uveitis or a history of this condition, anticholinesterase therapy should be avoided or used cautiously because of the intense and persistent miosis and ciliary muscle contraction that may occur.

Anticholinesterase drugs should be used with extreme caution, if at all, in patients with marked vagotonia, bronchial asthma, spastic GI disturbances, peptic ulcer, pronounced bradycardia and hypotension, recent MI, epilepsy, parkinsonism, and other disorders that may respond adversely to vagotonic effects.

Anticholinesterase drugs should be employed prior to ophthalmic surgery only as a considered risk because of the possible occurrence of hyphemia.

Echothiophate iodide should be used with great caution, if at all, where there is a prior history of retinal detachment.

Drug Interactions

Echothiophate iodide solution potentiates other cholinesterase inhibitors such as succinylcholine or organophosphate and carbamate insecticides. Patients undergoing systemic anticholinesterase treatment should be warned of the possible additive effects of echothiophate iodide.

Succinylcholine should be administered only with great caution, if at all, prior to or during general anesthesia to patients receiving anticholinesterase medication because of possible respiratory or cardiovascular collapse.

Caution should be observed in treating glaucoma with echothiophate iodide in patients who are at the same time undergoing treatment with systemic anticholinesterase medications for myasthenia gravis, because of possible adverse additive effects.

Adverse Reactions

➤*Cardiovascular:* Cardiac irregularities.

➤*Ophthalmic:* Although the relationship, if any, of retinal detachment to the administration of echothiophate iodide has not been established, retinal detachment has been reported in a few cases during the use of echothiophate iodide in adult patients without a history of this disorder.

Stinging, burning, lacrimation, lid muscle twitching, conjunctival and ciliary redness, browache, induced myopia with visual blurring may occur.

Activation of latent iritis or uveitis may occur.

Iris cysts may form, and if treatment is continued, may enlarge and obscure vision. This occurrence is more frequent in children. The cysts usually shrink upon discontinuance of the medication, reduction in strength of the drops or frequency of instillation. Rarely, they may rupture or break free into the aqueous. Regular examinations are advisable when the drug is being prescribed for the treatment of accommodative esotropia.

Prolonged use may cause conjunctival thickening, obstruction of nasolacrimal canals.

Lens opacities occurring in patients under treatment for glaucoma with echothiophate iodide solution have been reported and similar changes have been produced experimentally in healthy monkeys. Routine examinations should accompany clinical use of the drug.

Paradoxical increase in intraocular pressure may follow anticholinesterase instillation. This may be alleviated by prescribing a sympathomimetic mydriatic such as phenylephrine.

Carbonic Anhydrase Inhibitors

Refer to the Topical Ophthalmic Drugs introduction for more complete information.

Indications

➤*Elevated intraocular pressure (IOP):* Treatment of elevated IOP in patients with ocular hypertension or open-angle glaucoma.

Actions

➤*Pharmacology:* Dorzolamide and brinzolamide are carbonic anhydrase inhibitors for ophthalmic use. Carbonic anhydrase (CA) is an enzyme found in many tissues of the body, including the eye. It catalyzes the reversible reaction involving the hydration of carbon dioxide and the dehydration of carbonic acid. In humans, CA exists as a number of isoenzymes, the most active being CA-II, found primarily in red blood cells (RBCs), but also in other tissues. Inhibition of CA in the ciliary processes of the eye decreases aqueous humor secretion, presumably by slowing the formation of bicarbonate ions with subsequent reduction in sodium and fluid transport. The result is a reduction in intraocular pressure (IOP). Dorzolamide and brinzolamide reduce elevated IOP by inhibiting CA-II. Elevated IOP is a major risk factor in the pathogenesis of optic nerve damage and glaucomatous visual field loss.

➤*Pharmacokinetics:* When topically applied, dorzolamide and brinzolamide reach the systemic circulation and accumulate in RBCs during chronic dosing as a result of binding to CA-II. Extensive distribution into RBCs yields a long half-life, ≈ 3.5 to 4 months. The parent drugs form a single N-desethyl metabolite that inhibits CA-II less potently than the parent drug, but also inhibits CA-I. The metabolite also accumulates in RBCs, where it binds primarily to CA-I. Plasma concentrations of parent and metabolite are generally below the assay limit of quantitation. Plasma protein binding is moderate (≈ 33%) for dorzolamide and ≈ 60% for brinzolamide. These agents are primarily excreted unchanged in the urine, and the metabolite also is excreted in urine.

Contraindications

Hypersensitivity to any component of these products.

Warnings

➤*Systemic effects:* Dorzolamide and brinzolamide are sulfonamides and, although administered topically, are absorbed systemically. Therefore, the same types of adverse reactions attributable to systemic sulfonamides may occur with topical administration of these agents (refer to the systemic Sulfonamides monograph in the Anti-Infectives chapter). Fatalities have occurred, although rarely, because of severe reactions to sulfonamides including Stevens-Johnson syndrome, toxic epidermal necrolysis, fulminant hepatic necrosis, agranulocytosis, aplastic anemia, and other blood dyscrasias. Sensitization may recur when a sulfonamide is readministered regardless of the route of administration. If signs of serious reactions or hypersensitivity occur, discontinue the use of this preparation.

➤*Renal/Hepatic function impairment:* These agents have not been studied in patients with severe renal impairment (Ccr less than 30 mL/min). However, because dorzolamide, brinzolamide, and their metabolites are excreted predominantly by the kidney, these agents are not recommended in such patients.

Dorzolamide and brinzolamide have not been studied in patients with hepatic impairment and should be used with caution in such patients.

➤*Carcinogenesis:* In a 2-year study of dorzolamide administered orally to male and female Sprague-Dawley rats, urinary bladder papillomas were seen in male rats in the highest dosage group of 20 mg/kg/day (250 times the recommended human ophthalmic dose); papillomas were not seen in rats given oral doses equivalent to ≈ 12 times the recommended dose. The increased incidence of urinary bladder papillomas is a class effect of CA inhibitors in rats.

➤*Elderly:* Of all the patients in dorzolamide clinical studies, 44% were ≥ 65 years of age, and 10% were ≥ 75 years of age. No overall differences in efficacy or safety were observed between these patients and younger patients, but greater sensitivity of some older individuals to the product cannot be ruled out.

➤*Pregnancy: Category C.* Maternal toxicity and a significant increase in the number of fetal variations (eg, malformations of the vertebral bodies) was seen in animals at doses greater than 20 times the recommended human ophthalmic dose. These malformations occurred at doses that caused metabolic acidosis with decreased body weight gain in dams and decreased fetal weights. There are no adequate and well controlled studies in pregnant women. Use during pregnancy only if the potential benefit justifies the risk to the fetus.

➤*Lactation:* In lactating rats, decreases in body weight gain were seen in offspring with these agents at oral doses greater than 94 times the recommended human ophthalmic dose. A slight delay in postnatal development (incisor eruption, vaginal canalization, and eye openings), secondary to lower fetal body weight, also was noted with dorzolamide.

It is not known whether this drug is excreted in breast milk. Because of the potential for serious adverse reactions in nursing infants, decide whether to discontinue nursing or to discontinue the drug, taking into account the importance of the drug to the mother.

➤*Children:* Safety and efficacy in children have not been established.

Precautions

➤*Corneal endothelium effects:* Carbonic anhydrase activity has been observed in both the cytoplasm and around the plasma membranes of the corneal endothelium. The effect of continued administration of dorzolamide or brinzolamide on the corneal endothelium has not been fully evaluated.

➤*Acute angle-closure glaucoma:* The management of patients with acute angle-closure glaucoma requires therapeutic interventions in addition to ocular hypotensive agents. Dorzolamide and brinzolamide have not been studied in patients with acute angle-closure glaucoma.

➤*Ocular effects:* Local ocular adverse effects, primarily conjunctivitis and lid reactions, were reported with chronic administration of dorzolamide. Many of these reactions had the clinical appearance and course of an allergic-type reaction that resolved upon discontinuation of drug therapy. If such reactions are observed, discontinue the drug and evaluate the patient before considering restarting the drug.

➤*Concomitant oral CA inhibitors:* There is a potential for an additive effect on the known systemic effects of CA inhibition in patients receiving an oral CA inhibitor and dorzolamide or brinzolamide. Concomitant administration of ophthalmic and oral CA inhibitors is not recommended.

➤*Bacterial keratitis:* There have been reports of bacterial keratitis associated with the use of topical ophthalmic products in multiple-dose containers. These containers had been inadvertently contaminated by patients who, in most cases, had a concurrent corneal disease or a disruption of the ocular epithelial surface. Serious damage to the eye and subsequent loss of vision may result from using contaminated solutions.

➤*Contact lenses:* The preservative used in these products, benzalkonium chloride, may be absorbed by soft contact lenses. Do not administer these agents while wearing soft contact lenses; reinsert lenses ≥ 15 minutes after drug administration.

Drug Interactions

Although acid-base and electrolyte disturbances were not reported in the clinical trials with dorzolamide and brinzolamide, these disturbances have been reported with oral CA inhibitors and have, in some instances, resulted in drug interactions (eg, toxicity associated with high-dose salicylate therapy). Therefore, consider the potential for such drug interactions in patients receiving either of these agents.

Adverse Reactions

➤*Dorzolamide:*

Miscellaneous – Ocular burning, stinging or discomfort immediately following administration (≈ 33%); bitter taste following administration (≈ 25%); superficial punctate keratitis (10% to 15%); signs and symptoms of ocular allergic reaction (≈ 10%); blurred vision, tearing, dryness, photophobia (≈ 1% to 5%); headache, nausea, asthenia/fatigue (infrequent); skin rashes, urolithiasis, iridocyclitis (rare).

➤*Brinzolamide:*

Miscellaneous – Blurred vision, bitter, sour, or unusual taste (≈ 5% to 10%); blepharitis, dermatitis, dry eye, foreign body sensation, headache, hyperemia, ocular discharge, ocular discomfort, ocular keratitis, ocular pain, ocular pruritus, rhinitis (1% to 5%); allergic reactions, alopecia, chest pain, conjunctivitis, diarrhea, diplopia, dizziness, dry mouth, dyspnea, dyspepsia, eye fatigue, hypertonia, keratoconjunctivitis, keratopathy, kidney pain, lid margin crusting or sticky sensation, nausea, pharyngitis, tearing, urticaria (less than 1%).

Overdosage

Electrolyte imbalance, development of an acidotic state and possible CNS effects may occur. Monitor serum electrolyte levels (particularly potassium) and blood pH levels. Significant lethality was observed in female rats and mice after single oral doses of 1927 and 1320 mg/kg of dorzolamide, respectively.

Patient Information

Dorzolamide and brinzolamide are sulfonamides and, although administered topically, are absorbed systemically. Therefore, the same types of adverse reactions that are attributable to systemic sulfonamides may occur with topical administration. Advise patients that if serious or unusual reactions or signs of hypersensitivity occur, they should discontinue use of the product and consult their physician.

Vision may be temporarily blurred. Instruct patients to exercise care in operating machinery or driving a motor vehicle.

Advise patients that if they develop any ocular reactions, particularly conjunctivitis and lid reactions, they should discontinue medication use and seek their physician's advice.

Instruct patients to avoid allowing the tip of the dispensing container to contact the eye or surrounding structures. Ocular solutions, if handled improperly or if the tip of the dispensing container contacts the eye or surrounding structures, can become contaminated by common bacteria known to cause ocular infections. Serious damage to the eye and subsequent loss of vision may result from using contaminated solutions.

Advise patients that if they develop an intercurrent ocular condition (eg, trauma, ocular surgery, infection), they should immediately seek their physician's advice concerning the continued use of the present multidose container.

If more than one topical ophthalmic drug is being used, administer the drugs at least 10 minutes apart.

DORZOLAMIDE HYDROCHLORIDE

Rx	**Trusopt** (Merck)	**Solution:** 2% (as base)	In 5 and 10 mL *Ocumeters.*[1]

[1] With 0.0075% benzalkonium chloride, hydroxyethylcellulose, sodium hydroxide, and mannitol.

DORZOLAMIDE HYDROCHLORIDE — OPHTHALMIC

For complete and comparative prescribing information, refer to the Carbonic Anhydrase Inhibitors group monograph.

Indications

➤*Elevated intraocular pressure (IOP):* Treatment of elevated IOP in patients with ocular hypertension or open-angle glaucoma.

Administration and Dosage

➤*Approved by the FDA:* December 9, 1994.

➤*Dosage:* One drop in the affected eye(s) 3 times daily.

➤*Concomitant therapy:* Dorzolamide may be used concomitantly with other topical ophthalmic drug products to lower intraocular pressure. If more than one ophthalmic drug is being used, administer the drugs at least 10 minutes apart.

➤*Storage/Stability:* Store at 15° to 30°C (59° to 86°F). Protect from light.

BRINZOLAMIDE

Rx	**Azopt** (Alcon)	**Suspension:** 1%	In 2.5, 5, 10, and 15 mL *Drop-Tainers.*[1]

[1] With 0.01% benzalkonium chloride, mannitol, carbomer 974P, tyloxapol, sodium chloride, hydrochloric acid and/or sodium hydroxide, and EDTA.

BRINZOLAMIDE — OPHTHALMIC

For complete and comparative prescribing information, refer to the Carbonic Anhydrase Inhibitors group monograph.

Indications

➤*Elevated intraocular pressure (IOP):* Treatment of elevated IOP in patients with ocular hypertension or open-angle glaucoma.

Administration and Dosage

➤*Approved by the FDA:* April 3, 1998.

➤*Dosage:* One drop in the affected eye(s) 3 times daily.

➤*Concomitant therapy:* Brinzolamide may be used concomitantly with other topical ophthalmic drug products to lower intraocular pressure. If more than one topical ophthalmic drug is being used, administer the drugs at least 10 minutes apart.

➤*Storage/Stability:* Store at 4° to 30°C (39° to 86°F). Shake well.

LATANOPROST

Rx	**Xalatan** (Pfizer)	**Solution:** 0.005%	Benzalkonium chloride 0.02%, sodium chloride. In 2.5 mL fill dropper bottles.

LATANOPROST — OPHTHALMIC

Refer to the Topical Ophthalmic Drugs introduction for more complete and comparative information.

Indications

➤*Elevated intraocular pressure:* For the reduction of elevated intraocular pressure in patients with open-angle glaucoma and ocular hypertension who are intolerant of other intraocular pressure lowering medications or insufficiently responsive (failed to achieve target IOP determined after multiple measurements over time) to another intraocular pressure lowering medication.

Administration and Dosage

➤*Approved by the FDA:* June 5, 1996.

The recommended dosage is 1 drop (1.5 mcg) in the affected eye(s) once daily in the evening.

The dosage of latanoprost sterile ophthalmic solution should not exceed once daily since it has been shown that more frequent administration may decrease the intraocular pressure lowering effect.

Reduction of the intraocular pressure starts approximately 3 to 4 hours after administration and the maximum effect is reached after 8 to 12 hours. Latanoprost may be used concomitantly with other topical ophthalmic drug products to lower intraocular pressure.

If more than 1 topical ophthalmic drug is being used, the drugs should be administered at least 5 minutes apart.

➤*Storage/Stability:* Protect from light. Store unopened bottle under refrigeration at 2° to 8°C (36° to 46°F). During shipment to the patient, the bottle may be maintained at temperatures up to 40°C (104°F) for a period not exceeding 8 days. Once a bottle is opened for use, it may be stored at room temperature up to 25°C (77°F) for 6 weeks.

Actions

➤*Pharmacology:* Latanoprost is a prostanoid selective FP receptor agonist which is believed to reduce the intraocular pressure by increasing the outflow of aqueous humor. Studies in animals and man suggest that the main mechanism of action is increased uveoscleral outflow. Elevated IOP represents a major risk factor for glaucomatous field loss. The higher the level of IOP, the greater the likelihood of optic nerve damage and visual field loss.

➤*Pharmacokinetics:*

Absorption – Latanoprost is absorbed through the cornea where the isopropyl ester prodrug is hydrolyzed to the acid form to become biologically active. Studies in man indicate that the peak concentration in the aqueous humor is reached about 2 hours after topical administration.

Distribution – The distribution volume in humans is 0.16 ± 0.02 L/kg. The acid of latanoprost could be measured in aqueous humor during the first 4 hours, and in plasma only during the first hour after local administration.

Metabolism – Latanoprost, an isopropyl ester prodrug, is hydrolyzed by esterases in the cornea to the biologically active acid. The active acid of latanoprost reaching the systemic circulation is primarily metabolized by the liver to the 1,2-dinor and 1,2,3,4-tetranor metabolites via fatty acid β-oxidation.

Excretion – The elimination of the acid of latanoprost from human plasma was rapid ($t_{1/2}$ = 17 minutes) after both intravenous and topical administration. Systemic clearance is approximately 7 mL/min/kg. Following hepatic β-oxidation, the metabolites are mainly eliminated via the kidneys. Approximately 88% and 98% of the administered dose is recovered in the urine after topical and intravenous dosing, respectively.

Contraindications

Known hypersensitivity to latanoprost, benzalkonium chloride or any other ingredients in this product.

Warnings

➤*Ocular pigment changes:* Latanoprost has been reported to cause changes to pigmented tissues. The most frequently reported changes have been increased pigmentation of the iris and periorbital tissue (eyelid) and increased pigmentation and growth of eyelashes. These changes may be permanent. Pigmentation is expected to increase as long as latanoprost is administered. After discontinuation of latanoprost, pigmentation of the iris is likely to be permanent while pigmentation of the periorbital tissue and eyelash changes have been reported to be reversible in some patients. Patients who receive treatment should be informed of the possibility of increased pigmentation. The effects of increased pigmentation beyond 5 years are not known.

Latanoprost sterile ophthalmic solution may gradually change eye color, increasing the amount of brown pigment in the iris by increasing the number of melanosomes (pigment granules) in melanocytes. The long-term effects on the melanocytes and the consequences of potential injury to the melanocytes or deposition of pigment granules to other areas of the eye are currently unknown. The change in iris color occurs slowly and may not be noticeable for several months to years. Patients should be informed of the possibility of iris color change.

Eyelid skin darkening has also been reported in association with the use of latanoprost.

Latanoprost may gradually change eyelashes and vellus hair; these changes include increased length, thickness, pigmentation, and number of lashes or hairs, and misdirected growth of eyelashes. Eyelash changes are usually reversible upon discontinuation of treatment.

Patients who are expected to receive treatment in only 1 eye should be informed about the potential for increased brown pigmentation of the iris, periorbital tissue, and eyelashes in the treated eye and thus, heterochromia between the eyes. They should also be advised of the potential for a disparity between the eyes in length, thickness, or number of eyelashes. These changes in pigmentation and lash growth may be permanent.

➤*Renal/Hepatic function impairment:* Latanoprost has not been studied in patients with renal or hepatic impairment and should therefore be used with caution in such patients.

➤*Mutagenesis:* Latanoprost was not mutagenic in bacteria, in mouse lymphoma or in mouse micronucleus tests. Chromosome aberrations were observed in vitro with human lymphocytes.

➤*Pregnancy: Category C.* Reproduction studies have been performed in rats and rabbits. In rabbits an incidence of 4 of 16 dams had no viable fetuses at a dose that was approximately 80 times the maximum human dose, and the highest nonembryocidal dose in rabbits was approximately 15 times the maximum human dose.

There are no adequate and well-controlled studies in pregnant women. Latanoprost should be used during pregnancy only if the potential benefit justifies the potential risk to the fetus.

➤*Lactation:* It is not known whether this drug or its metabolites are excreted in human milk. Because many drugs are excreted in human milk, caution should be exercised when latanoprost is administered to a nursing woman.

➤*Children:* Safety and effectiveness in pediatric patients have not been established.

Precautions

➤*Monitoring:* Latanoprost is hydrolyzed in the cornea. The effect of continued administration of latanoprost sterile ophthalmic solution on the corneal endothelium has not been fully evaluated. Latanoprost sterile ophthalmic solution may gradually increase the pigmentation of the iris. The eye color change is due to increased melanin content in the stromal melanocytes of the iris rather than to an increase in the number of melanocytes. This change may not be noticeable for several months to years. Typically the brown pigmentation around the pupil spreads concentrically towards the periphery of the iris and the entire iris or parts of the iris become more brownish. Neither nevi nor freckles of the iris appear to be affected by treatment. While treatment with latanoprost can be continued in patients who develop noticeably increased iris pigmentation, these patients should be examined regularly and, depending on the clinical situation, treatment may be stopped if increased pigmentation ensues.

During clinical trials, the increase in brown iris pigment has not been shown to progress further upon discontinuation of treatment, but the resultant color change may be permanent.

➤*Other forms of glaucoma:* There is limited experience with latanoprost in the treatment of angle closure, inflammatory or neovascular glaucoma.

➤*Infections:* There have been reports of bacterial keratitis associated with the use of multiple-dose containers of topical ophthalmic products. These containers had been inadvertently contaminated by patients who, in most cases, had a concurrent corneal disease or a disruption of the ocular epithelial surface.

➤*Contact lenses:* Contact lenses should be removed prior to the administration of latanoprost, and may be reinserted 15 minutes after administration.

➤*Special risk:*

Active intraocular inflammation (iritis/uveitis) – Latanoprost should be used with caution in patients with a history of intraocular inflammation (iritis/uveitis) and should generally not be used in patients with active intraocular inflammation.

Macular edema, including cystoid macular edema – Macular edema, including cystoid macular edema, has been reported during treatment with latanoprost. These reports have mainly occurred in aphakic patients, in pseudophakic patients with a torn posterior lens capsule, or in patients with known risk factors for macular edema. Latanoprost should be used with caution in patients who do not have an intact posterior capsule or who have known risk factors for macular edema.

Drug Interactions

In vitro studies have shown that precipitation occurs when eye drops containing thimerosal are mixed with latanoprost. If such drugs are used they should be administered with an interval of at least 5 minutes between applications.

Adverse Reactions

➤*Adverse reactions referred to in other sections:* Eyelash changes (increased length, thickness, pigmentation, and number of lashes); eyelid skin darkening; intraocular inflammation (iritis/uveitis); iris pigmentation changes; and macular edema, including cystoid macular edema.

LATANOPROST — OPHTHALMIC

➤*Adverse reactions in controlled clinical trials:* Local conjunctival hyperemia was observed; however, less than 1% of the patients treated with latanoprost required discontinuation of therapy because of intolerance to conjunctival hyperemia.

Ophthalmic – The ocular adverse reactions and ocular signs and symptoms reported in 5% to 15% of the patients on latanoprost sterile ophthalmic solution in the 6-month, multicenter, double-masked, active-controlled trials were blurred vision, burning and stinging, conjunctival hyperemia, foreign body sensation, itching, increased pigmentation of the iris, and punctate epithelial keratopathy.

In addition to the above listed ocular reactions/signs and symptoms, the following were reported in 1% to 4% of the patients: Dry eye, excessive tearing, eye pain, lid crusting, lid discomfort/pain, lid edema, lid erythema, and photophobia.

The following events were reported in less than 1% of the patients: Conjunctivitis, diplopia and discharge from the eye. During clinical studies, there were extremely rare reports of the following: Retinal artery embolus, retinal detachment, and vitreous hemorrhage from diabetic retinopathy.

Systemic – The most common systemic adverse reactions seen with latanoprost were upper respiratory tract infection/cold/flu which occurred at a rate of approximately 4%. Chest pain/angina pectoris, muscle/joint/back pain, and rash/allergic skin reaction each occurred at a rate of 1% to 2%.

➤*Postmarketing:* The following reactions have been identified during postmarketing use of latanoprost in clinical practice. Because they are reported voluntarily from a population of unknown size, estimates of frequency cannot be made. The reactions, which have been chosen for inclusion due to either their seriousness, frequency of reporting, possible causal connection to latanoprost, or a combination of these factors, include the following: Asthma and exacerbation of asthma; corneal edema and erosions; dyspnea; eyelash and vellus hair changes (increased length, thickness, pigmentation, and number); eyelid skin darkening; herpes keratitis; intraocular inflammation (iritis/uveitis); keratitis; macular edema, including cystoid macular edema; misdirected eyelashes sometimes resulting in eye irritation; and toxic epidermal necrolysis.

Overdosage

➤*Symptoms:* Apart from ocular irritation and conjunctival or episcleral hyperemia, the ocular effects of latanoprost administered at high doses are not known. Intravenous administration of large doses of latanoprost in monkeys has been associated with transient bronchoconstriction; however, in 11 patients with bronchial asthma treated with latanoprost, bronchoconstriction was not induced. Intravenous infusion of up to 3 mcg/kg in healthy volunteers produced mean plasma concentrations 200 times higher than during clinical treatment and no adverse reactions were observed. Intravenous dosages of 5.5 to 10 mcg/kg caused abdominal pain, dizziness, fatigue, hot flushes, nausea and sweating.

➤*Treatment:* If overdosage with latanoprost sterile ophthalmic solution occurs, treatment should be symptomatic.

Patient Information

Patients should be advised about the potential for increased brown pigmentation of the iris, which may be permanent. Patients should also be informed about the possibility of eyelid skin darkening, which may be reversible after discontinuation of latanoprost.

Patients should also be informed of the possibility of eyelash and vellus hair changes in the treated eye during treatment with latanoprost. These changes may result in a disparity between eyes in length, thickness, pigmentation, number of eyelashes or vellus hairs, or direction of eyelash growth. Eyelash changes are usually reversible upon discontinuation of treatment.

The increased pigmentation to the iris and eyelid, as well as the changes to the eyelashes, may be permanent.

Patients should be instructed to avoid allowing the tip of the dispensing container to contact the eye or surrounding structures because this could cause the tip to become contaminated by common bacteria known to cause ocular infections. Serious damage to the eye and subsequent loss of vision may result from using contaminated solutions.

Patients also should be advised that if they develop an intercurrent ocular condition (eg, trauma, or infection) or have ocular surgery, they should immediately seek their physician's advice concerning the continued use of the multidose container.

Patients should be advised that if they develop any ocular reactions, particularly conjunctivitis and lid reactions, they should immediately seek their physician's advice.

Patients should also be advised that latanoprost contains benzalkonium chloride which may be absorbed by contact lenses. Contact lenses should be removed prior to administration of the solution. Lenses may be reinserted 15 minutes following administration of latanoprost. If more than 1 topical ophthalmic drug is being used, the drugs should be administered at least 5 minutes apart.

TRAVOPROST

Rx	Travatan (Alcon)	Solution: 0.004%	0.015% benzalkonium chloride/mL, EDTA. In 2.5 mL *Drop-Tainers*.

TRAVOPROST — OPHTHALMIC

Indications

➤*Elevated intraocular pressure:* For the reduction of elevated intraocular pressure in patients with open-angle glaucoma or ocular hypertension who are intolerant of other intraocular pressure-lowering medications or insufficiently responsive (failed to achieve target IOP determined after multiple measurements over time) to another intraocular pressure-lowering medication.

Administration and Dosage

➤*Approved by the FDA:* March 16, 2001.

The recommended dosage is 1 drop in the affected eye(s) once daily in the evening. The dosage of travoprost should not exceed once daily since it has been shown that more frequent administration may decrease the intraocular pressure lowering effect.

Reduction of intraocular pressure starts approximately 2 hours after administration, and the maximum effect is reached after 12 hours.

Travoprost may be used concomitantly with other topical ophthalmic drug products to lower intraocular pressure. If more than 1 topical ophthalmic drug is being used, the drugs should be administered at least 5 minutes apart.

➤*Storage/Stability:* Store between 2° to 25°C (36° to 77°F). Discard the container within 6 weeks of removing it from the sealed pouch.

Actions

➤*Pharmacology:* Travoprost free acid is a selective FP prostanoid receptor agonist which is believed to reduce intraocular pressure by increasing uveoscleral outflow. The exact mechanism of action is unknown at this time.

➤*Pharmacokinetics:*

Absorption – Travoprost is absorbed through the cornea and is hydrolyzed to the active free acid. Data from 4 multiple-dose pharmacokinetic studies (totaling 107 subjects) have shown that plasma concentrations of the free acid are below 0.01 ng/mL (the quantitation limit of the assay) in two-thirds of the subjects. In those individuals with quantifiable plasma concentrations (n = 38), the mean plasma C_{max} was 0.018 ± 007 ng/mL (ranged 0.01 to 0.052 ng/mL) and was reached within 30 minutes. From these studies, travoprost is estimated to have a plasma half-life of 45 minutes. There was no difference in plasma concentrations between days 1 and 7, indicating steady-state was reached early and that there was no significant accumulation.

Metabolism – Travoprost, an isopropyl ester prodrug, is hydrolyzed by esterases in the cornea to its biologically active free acid. Systemically, travoprost free acid is metabolized to inactive metabolites via beta-oxidation of the α(carboxylic acid) chain to give the 1,2-dinor and 1,2,3,4-tetranor analogs, via oxidation of the 15-hydroxyl moiety, as well as via reduction of the 13, 14 double bond.

Excretion – Elimination of travoprost free acid from human plasma was rapid and levels were generally below the limit of quantification within 1 hour after dosing. The terminal elimination half-life of travoprost free acid was estimated from 14 subjects and ranged from 17 minutes to 86 minutes with the mean half-life of 45 minutes. Less than 2% of the topical ocular dose of travoprost was excreted in the urine within 4 hours as the travoprost free acid.

Contraindications

Known hypersensitivity to travoprost, benzalkonium chloride, or any other ingredients in this product. Travoprost may interfere with the maintenance of pregnancy and should not be used by women during pregnancy or by women attempting to become pregnant.

Warnings

➤*Ocular pigment changes:* Travoprost has been reported to cause changes to pigmented tissues. The most frequently reported changes have been increased pigmentation of the iris and periorbital tissue (eyelid) and increased pigmentation and growth of eyelashes. These changes may be permanent.

Travoprost may gradually change eye color, increasing the amount of brown pigmentation in the iris by increasing the number of melanosomes (pigment granules) in melanocytes. The long-term effects on the melanocytes and the consequences of potential injury to the melanocytes or deposition of pigment granules to other areas of the eye are currently unknown. The change in iris color occurs slowly and may not be noticeable for months to years. Patients should be informed of the possibility of iris color change.

Eyelid skin darkening has been reported in association with the use of travoprost.

Travoprost may gradually change eyelashes in the treated eye; these changes include increased length, thickness, pigmentation, or number of lashes. Patients who are expected to receive treatment in only 1 eye should be informed about the potential for increased brown pigmentation of the iris, periorbital or eyelid tissue, and eyelashes in the treated eye and thus heterochromia between the eyes. They should also be advised of the potential for a disparity between the eyes in length, thickness, or number of eyelashes.

➤*Mutagenesis:* Travoprost was not mutagenic in the Ames test, mouse micronucleus test and rat chromosome aberration assay. A slight increase in

TRAVOPROST — OPHTHALMIC

the mutant frequency was observed in 1 of 2 mouse lymphoma assays in the presence of rat S-9 activation enzymes.

➤*Fertility impairment:* Travoprost did not affect mating or fertility indices in male or female rats at subcutaneous doses up to 10 mcg/kg/day (250 times the maximum recommended human ocular dose [MRHOD] of 0.04 mcg/kg/day on a mcg/kg basis). At 10 mcg/kg/day, the mean number of corpora lutea was reduced, and the post-implantation losses were increased. These effects were not observed at 3 mcg/kg/day (75 times the MRHOD).

➤*Pregnancy:* *Category C.*

Teratogenic – Travoprost was teratogenic in rats, at an IV dose up to 10 mcg/kg/day (250 times the MRHOD), evidenced by an increase in the incidence of skeletal malformations as well as external and visceral malformations, such as fused sternebrae, domed head and hydrocephaly. Travoprost was not teratogenic in rats at IV doses up to 3 mcg/kg/day (75 times the MRHOD), and in mice at subcutaneous doses up to 1 mcg/kg/day (25 times the MRHOD). Travoprost produced an increase in post-implantation losses and a decrease in fetal viability in rats at IV doses greater than 3 mcg/kg/day (75 times the MRHOD) and in mice at subcutaneous doses greater than 0.3 mcg/kg/day (7.5 times the MRHOD).

In the offspring of female rats that received travoprost subcutaneously from day 7 of pregnancy to lactation day 21 at the doses of greater than or equal to 0.12 mcg/kg/day (3 times the MRHOD), the incidence of postnatal mortality was increased, and neonatal body weight gain was decreased. Neonatal development was also affected, evidenced by delayed eye opening, pinna detachment and preputial separation, and by decreased motor activity.

No adequate and well-controlled studies have been performed in pregnant women. Travoprost may interfere with the maintenance of pregnancy and should not be used by women during pregnancy or by women attempting to become pregnant.

Since prostaglandins are biologically active and may be absorbed through the skin, women who are pregnant or attempting to become pregnant should exercise appropriate precautions to avoid direct exposure to the contents of the bottle. In case of accidental contact with the contents of the bottle, thoroughly cleanse the exposed area with soap and water immediately.

➤*Lactation:* A study in lactating rats demonstrated that radiolabeled travoprost or its metabolites were excreted in milk. It is not known whether this drug or its metabolites are excreted in human milk. Because many drugs are excreted in human milk, caution should be exercised when travoprost is administered to a nursing woman.

➤*Children:* Safety and efficacy in pediatric patients have not been established.

Precautions

➤*Monitoring:* Patients may slowly develop increased brown pigmentation of the iris. This change may not be noticeable for months to years. Iris pigmentation changes may be more noticeable in patients with mixed colored irides (ie, blue-brown, grey-brown, yellow-brown, and green-brown); however, it has also been observed in patients with brown eyes. The color change is believed to be due to increased melanin content in the stromal melanocytes of the iris. The exact mechanism of action is unknown at this time. Typically, the brown pigmentation around the pupil spreads concentrically towards the periphery in affected eyes, but the entire iris or parts of it may become more brownish. Until more information about increased brown pigmentation is available, patients should be examined regularly and, depending on the situation, treatment may be stopped if increased pigmentation ensues.

➤*Infections:* There have been reports of bacterial keratitis associated with the use of multiple-dose containers of topical ophthalmic products. These containers had been inadvertently contaminated by patients who, in most cases, had a concurrent corneal disease or a disruption of the epithelial surface.

➤*Other forms of glaucoma:* Travoprost has not been evaluated for the treatment of angle closure, inflammatory or neovascular glaucoma.

➤*Contact lenses:* Travoprost should not be administered while wearing contact lenses.

Patients should be advised that travoprost contains benzalkonium chloride which may be absorbed by contact lenses. Contact lenses should be removed prior to the administration of the solution. Lenses may be reinserted 15 minutes following administration of travoprost.

➤*Special risk:* Travoprost should be used with caution in patients with a history of intraocular inflammation (iritis/uveitis) and should generally not be used in patients with active intraocular inflammation.

Macular edema, including cystoid macular edema, has been reported during treatment with prostaglandin $F_{2\alpha}$ analogues. These reports have mainly occurred in aphakic patients, pseudophakic patients with a torn posterior lens capsule, or in patients with known risk factors for macular edema. Travoprost should be used with caution in these patients.

Adverse Reactions

The most common ocular adverse event observed in controlled clinical studies with travoprost 0.004% was ocular hyperemia which was reported in 35% to 50% of patients. Approximately 3% of patients discontinued therapy due to conjunctival hyperemia.

Ocular adverse events reported at an incidence of 5% to 10% included decreased visual acuity, eye discomfort, foreign body sensation, pain, and pruritus.

Ocular adverse events reported at an incidence of 1% to 4% included, abnormal vision, blepharitis, blurred vision, cataract, cells, conjunctivitis, dry eye, eye disorder, flare, iris discoloration, keratitis, lid margin crusting, photophobia, subconjunctival hemorrhage, and tearing.

Nonocular adverse events reported at a rate of 1% to 5% were accidental injury, angina pectoris, anxiety, arthritis, back pain, bradycardia, bronchitis, chest pain, cold syndrome, depression, dyspepsia, gastrointestinal disorder, headache, hypercholesterolemia, hypertension, hypotension, infection, pain, prostate disorder, sinusitis, urinary incontinence, and urinary tract infection.

Patient Information

Patients should also be instructed to avoid allowing the tip of the dispensing container to contact the eye or surrounding structures because this could cause the tip to become contaminated by common bacteria known to cause ocular infections. Serious damage to the eye and subsequent loss of vision may result from using contaminated solutions.

Patients also should be advised that if they develop an intercurrent ocular condition (eg, trauma, infection) or have ocular surgery, they should immediately seek their physician's advice concerning the continued use of the multi-dose container.

Patients should be advised that if they develop any ocular reactions, particularly conjunctivitis and lid reactions, they should immediately seek their physician's advice.

If more than 1 topical ophthalmic drug is being used, the drugs should be administered at least 5 minutes apart.

Travoprost has been reported to cause changes to pigmented tissues. The most frequently reported changes have been increased pigmentation of the iris and periorbital tissue (eyelid) and increased pigmentation and growth of eyelashes. These changes may be permanent.

Travoprost should not be administered while wearing contact lenses.

Travoprost should be used with caution in patients with a history of intraocular inflammation (iritis/uveitis) and should generally not be used in patients with active intraocular inflammation.

BIMATOPROST

Rx	**Lumigan** (Allergan)	**Solution:** 0.03%	0.05 mg benzalkonium chloride/mL. In 2.5 and 5 mL.

BIMATOPROST — OPHTHALMIC

Indications

➤*Elevated intraocular pressure:* For the reduction of elevated intraocular pressure in patients with open angle glaucoma or ocular hypertension who are intolerant of other intraocular pressure (IOP) lowering medications or insufficiently responsive (failed to achieve target IOP determined after multiple measurements over time) to another intraocular pressure lowering medication.

Administration and Dosage

➤*Approved by the FDA:* March 16, 2001.

The recommended dosage is 1 drop in the affected eye(s) once daily in the evening. The dosage of bimatoprost ophthalmic solution should not exceed once daily since it has been shown that more frequent administration may decrease the intraocular pressure lowering effect.

Reduction of the intraocular pressure starts approximately 4 hours after the first administration with maximum effect reached within approximately 8 to 12 hours.

Bimatoprost may be used concomitantly with other topical ophthalmic drug products to lower intraocular pressure. If more than 1 topical ophthalmic drug is being used, the drugs should be administered at least 5 minutes apart.

➤*Storage/Stability:* Bimatoprost should be stored in the original container at 15° to 25°C (59° to 77°F).

Actions

➤*Pharmacology:* Bimatoprost is a prostamide, a synthetic structural analog of prostaglandin with ocular hypotensive activity. It selectively mimics the effects of naturally occurring substances, prostamides. Bimatoprost is believed to lower intraocular pressure (IOP) in humans by increasing outflow of aqueous humor through both the trabecular meshwork and uveoscleral routes. Elevated IOP presents a major risk factor for glaucomatous field loss. The higher the level of IOP, the greater the likelihood of optic nerve damage and visual field loss.

➤*Pharmacokinetics:*

Absorption – After 1 drop of bimatoprost ophthalmic solution 0.03% was administered once daily to both eyes of 15 healthy subjects for 2 weeks, blood concentrations peaked within 10 minutes after dosing and were below the lower limit of detection (0.025 ng/mL) in most subjects within 1.5 hours after dosing. Mean C_{max} and $AUC_{0\text{-}24hr}$ values were similar on days 7 and 14 at approximately 0.08 ng/mL and 0.09 ng•hr/mL, respectively, indicating that steady state was reached during the first week of ocular dosing. There was no significant systemic drug accumulation over time.

BIMATOPROST — OPHTHALMIC

Distribution – Bimatoprost is moderately distributed into body tissues with a steady-state volume of distribution of 0.67 L/kg. In human blood, bimatoprost resides mainly in the plasma. Approximately 12% of bimatoprost remains unbound in human plasma.

Metabolism – Bimatoprost is the major circulating species in the blood once it reaches the systemic circulation following ocular dosing. Bimatoprost then undergoes oxidation, N-deethylation and glucuronidation to form a diverse variety of metabolites.

Excretion – Following an intravenous dose of radiolabeled bimatoprost (3.12 mcg/kg) to 6 healthy subjects, the maximum blood concentration of unchanged drug was 12.2 ng/mL and decreased rapidly with an elimination half-life of approximately 45 minutes. The total blood clearance of bimatoprost was 1.5 L/hr/kg. Up to 67% of the administered dose was excreted in the urine while 25% of the dose was recovered in the feces.

Contraindications

Hypersensitivity to bimatoprost or any other ingredient in this product.

Warnings

➤*Ocular pigment changes:* Bimatoprost ophthalmic solution has been reported to cause changes to pigmented tissues. These reports include increased pigmentation and growth of eyelashes and increased pigmentation of the iris and periorbital tissue (eyelid). These changes may be permanent.

Bimatoprost may gradually change eye color, increasing the amount of brown pigment in the iris by increasing the number of melanosomes (pigment granules) in melanocytes. The long-term effects on the melanocytes and the consequences of potential injury to the melanocytes or deposition of pigment granules to other areas of the eye are currently unknown. The change in iris color occurs slowly and may not be noticeable for several months to years. Patients should be informed of the possibility of iris color change.

Eyelid skin darkening has also been reported in association with the use of bimatoprost.

Bimatoprost may gradually change eyelashes; these changes include increased length, thickness, pigmentation, and number of lashes.

Patients who are expected to receive treatment in only 1 eye should be informed about the potential for increased brown pigmentation of the iris, periorbital tissue, and eyelashes in the treated eye and thus, heterochromia between the eyes. They should also be advised of the potential for a disparity between the eyes in length, thickness, or number of eyelashes.

➤*Pregnancy: Category C.*

Teratogenic – In embryo/fetal developmental studies in pregnant mice and rats, abortion was observed at oral doses of bimatoprost which achieved at least 33 or 97 times, respectively, the intended human exposure based on blood AUC levels.

At doses 41 times the intended human exposure based on blood AUC levels, the gestation length was reduced in the dams, the incidence of dead fetuses, late resorptions, peri- and postnatal pup mortality was increased, and pup body weights were reduced.

There are no adequate and well-controlled studies of bimatoprost administration in pregnant women. Because animal reproductive studies are not always predictive of human response, bimatoprost should be administered during pregnancy only if the potential benefit justifies the potential risk to the fetus.

➤*Lactation:* It is not known whether bimatoprost is excreted in human milk, although in animal studies, bimatoprost has been shown to be excreted in breast milk. Because many drugs are excreted in human milk, caution should be exercised when bimatoprost is administered to a nursing woman.

➤*Children:* Safety and efficacy in children have not been established.

Precautions

➤*Monitoring:* Patients may slowly develop increased brown pigmentation of the iris. This change may not be noticeable for several months to years. Typically the brown pigmentation around the pupil is expected to spread concentrically towards the periphery in affected eyes, but the entire iris or parts of it may also become more brownish. Until more information about increased brown pigmentation is available, patients should be examined regularly and, depending on the clinical situation, treatment may be stopped if increased pigmentation ensues. The increase in brown iris pigment is not expected to progress further upon discontinuation of treatment, but the resultant color change may be permanent. Neither nevi nor freckles of the iris are expected to be affected by treatment.

➤*Infections:* There have been reports of bacterial keratitis associated with the use of multiple-dose containers of topical ophthalmic products. These containers had been inadvertently contaminated by patients who, in most cases, had a concurrent corneal disease or a disruption of the ocular epithelial surface.

➤*Other forms of glaucoma:* Bimatoprost has not been evaluated for the treatment of angle closure, inflammatory or neovascular glaucoma.

➤*Contact lenses:* Bimatoprost should not be administered while wearing contact lenses.

➤*Special risk:* Bimatoprost ophthalmic solution should be used with caution in patients with active intraocular inflammation (eg, uveitis).

Macular edema, including cystoid macular edema, has been reported during treatment with bimatoprost ophthalmic solution. Bimatoprost should be used with caution in aphakic patients, in pseudophakic patients with a torn posterior lens capsule, or in patients with known risk factors for macular edema.

Adverse Reactions

In clinical trials, the most frequent events associated with the use of bimatoprost ophthalmic solution occurring in approximately 15% to 45% of patients, in descending order of incidence, included conjunctival hyperemia, growth of eyelashes, and ocular pruritus. Approximately 3% of patients discontinued therapy due to conjunctival hyperemia.

Ocular adverse events occurring in approximately 3% to 10% of patients, in descending order of incidence, included ocular dryness, visual disturbance, ocular burning, foreign body sensation, eye pain, pigmentation of the periocular skin, blepharitis, cataract, superficial punctate keratitis, eyelid erythema, ocular irritation, and eyelash darkening. The following ocular adverse events reported in approximately 1% to 3% of patients, in descending order of incidence, included: Eye discharge, tearing, photophobia, allergic conjunctivitis, asthenopia, increases in iris pigmentation, and conjunctival edema. In less than 1% of patients, intraocular inflammation was reported as iritis.

Systemic adverse events reported in approximately 10% of patients were infections (primarily colds and upper respiratory tract infections). The following systemic adverse events reported in approximately 1% to 5% of patients, in descending order of incidence, included headaches, abnormal liver function tests, asthenia and hirsutism.

Overdosage

No information is available on overdosage in humans. If overdose with bimatoprost ophthalmic solution occurs, treatment should be symptomatic.

In oral (by gavage) mouse and rat studies, doses up to 100 mg/kg/day did not produce any toxicity. This dose expressed as mg/m^2 is at least 70 times higher than the accidental dose of 1 bottle of bimatoprost for a 10 kg child.

Patient Information

Patients should be informed that bimatoprost has been reported to cause increased growth and darkening of eyelashes and darkening of the skin around the eye in some patients. These changes may be permanent.

Some patients may slowly develop darkening of the iris, which may be permanent.

When only 1 eye is treated, patients should be informed of the potential for a cosmetic difference between the eyes in eyelash length, darkness or thickness, or color changes of the eyelid skin or iris.

Patients should be instructed to avoid allowing the tip of the dispensing container to contact the eye, surrounding structures, fingers, or any other surface in order to avoid contamination of the solution by common bacteria known to cause ocular infections. Serious damage to the eye and subsequent loss of vision may result from using contaminated solutions.

Patients should also be advised that if they develop an intercurrent ocular condition (eg, trauma, infection) or have ocular surgery, they should immediately seek their physician's advice concerning the continued use of the multi-dose container.

Patients should be advised that if they develop any ocular reactions, particularly conjunctivitis and eyelid reactions, they should immediately seek their physician's advice.

Contact lenses should be removed prior to instillation of bimatoprost and may be reinserted 15 minutes following its administration. Patients should be advised that bimatoprost contains benzalkonium chloride, which may be absorbed by soft contact lenses.

If more than 1 topical ophthalmic drug is being used, the drugs should be administered at least 5 minutes between applications.

Combinations

PILOCARPINE AND EPINEPHRINE

Rx	P_1E_1 (Alcon)	**Solution:** 1% pilocarpine HCl, 1% epinephrine bitartrate	In 15 mL *Drop-Tainers.*[1]
Rx	P_2E_1 (Alcon)	**Solution:** 2% pilocarpine HCl, 1% epinephrine bitartrate	In 15 mL *Drop-Tainers.*[1]
Rx	P_4E_1 (Alcon)	**Solution:** 4% pilocarpine HCl, 1% epinephrine bitartrate	In 15 mL *Drop-Tainers.*[1]
Rx	P_6E_1 (Alcon)	**Solution:** 6% pilocarpine HCl, 1% epinephrine bitartrate	In 15 mL *Drop-Tainers.*[1]

[1] With 0.01% benzalkonium chloride, methylcellulose, EDTA, chlorobutanol, polyethylene glycol and sodium bisulfite.

Combinations

PILOCARPINE AND EPINEPHRINE — OPHTHALMIC

Also refer to the general discussion of Miotics, Cholinesterase Inhibitors.

Indications

➤*Glaucoma:* Therapy of open-angle glaucoma.

For other specific indications, refer to the individual monographs.

Administration and Dosage

Instill 1 or 2 drops into the eye(s) 1 to 4 times daily. Determine concentration and frequency of instillation by severity of the glaucoma and by patient response.

Individuals with heavily pigmented irides may require larger doses.

➤*Storage/Stability:* Store at 8° to 30°C (46° to 86°F). Keep tightly closed. Do not use solution if it is brown or contains a precipitate. Protect from light and heat.

DORZOLAMIDE HYDROCHLORIDE AND TIMOLOL MALEATE

Rx	**Cosopt** (Merck)	**Solution:** 2% dorzolamide, 0.5% timolol	In 5 and 10 mL *Ocumeters.*[1]

[1] With 0.0075% benzalkonium chloride and mannitol.

DORZOLAMIDE HYDROCHLORIDE AND TIMOLOL MALEATE — OPHTHALMIC

Refer to the general discussion of Carbonic Anhydrase Inhibitors and Beta-adrenergic Blocking Agents.

Indications

➤*Elevated intraocular pressure (IOP):* Treatment of elevated IOP in patients with ocular hypertension or open-angle glaucoma.

Administration and Dosage

Instill one drop into the affected eye(s) two times daily. If more than one topical ophthalmic drug is being used, the drugs should be administered at least 10 minutes apart.

➤*Storage/Stability:* Store between 15° and 25°C (59° to 77°F). Protect from light.

NONSTEROIDAL ANTI-INFLAMMATORY AGENTS (NSAIDs)

Refer to the Topical Ophthalmic Drugs introduction for more complete and comparative information.

Indications

➤*Flurbiprofen, suprofen:* Inhibition of intraoperative miosis.

➤*Diclofenac:* Treatment of postoperative inflammation following cataract extraction.

➤*Ketorolac:* Relief of ocular itching caused by seasonal allergic conjunctivitis. Treatment of postoperative inflammation following cataract extraction.

➤*Unlabeled uses:*

Flurbiprofen – Topical treatment of cystoid macular edema, inflammation after cataract or glaucoma laser surgery and uveitis syndromes.

Actions

➤*Pharmacology:* Flurbiprofen, suprofen, diclofenac and ketorolac are NSAIDs available as ophthalmic solutions. Flurbiprofen and suprofen are phenylalkanoic acids, diclofenac is a phenylacetic acid and ketorolac tromethamine is a member of the pyrrolo-pyrrolle group; they have analgesic, antipyretic and anti-inflammatory activity. Their mechanism of action is believed to be through inhibition of the cyclo-oxygenase enzyme that is essential in the biosynthesis of prostaglandins.

In animals, prostaglandins are mediators of certain kinds of intraocular inflammation. Prostaglandins produce disruption of the blood-aqueous humor barrier, vasodilation, increased vascular permeability, leukocytosis and increased intraocular pressure (IOP). These agents have no significant effect on IOP.

Prostaglandins also appear to play a role in the miotic response produced during ocular surgery by constricting the iris sphincter independently of cholinergic mechanisms. These agents inhibit the miosis induced during the course of cataract surgery.

Contraindications

Hypersensitivity to the drugs or any component of the products.

➤*Flurbiprofen, suprofen:* Epithelial herpes simplex keratitis (dendritic keratitis).

➤*Diclofenac, ketorolac:* Patients wearing soft contact lenses (see Precautions).

Warnings

➤*Cross-sensitivity:* The potential for cross-sensitivity to acetylsalicylic acid and other NSAIDs exists. Use caution when treating individuals who have previously exhibited sensitivities to these drugs.

➤*Bleeding tendencies:* Systemic absorption occurs with drugs applied ocularly. With some NSAIDs, there exists the potential for increased bleeding time caused by interference with thrombocyte aggregation. There have been reports that ocularly applied NSAIDs may cause increased bleeding of ocular tissues (including hyphemas) in conjunction with ocular surgery. Use with caution in surgical patients with known bleeding tendencies or in patients taking drugs known to cause bleeding (eg, anticoagulants).

➤*Flank pain/Renal function impairment:* Use of oral suprofen has been associated with a syndrome of acute flank pain and generally reversible renal insufficiency, which may present as acute uric acid nephropathy. This syndrome occurs in ≈ 1 in 3500 patients and has been reported with as few as one to two doses of a 200 mg capsule.

➤*Pregnancy: Category C* (flurbiprofen, ketorolac, suprofen); *Category B* (diclofenac). **Flurbiprofen** is embryocidal, delays parturition, prolongs gestation, reduces weight and slightly retards fetal growth in rats at daily oral doses of ≥ 0.4 mg/kg (≈ 185 times the human daily topical dose).

Oral doses of **ketorolac** at 1.5 mg/kg (8.8 mg/m^2), which was half of the human oral exposure, administered after gestation day 17 caused dystocia and higher pup mortality in rats.

Oral doses of **suprofen** of up to 200 mg/kg/day in animals resulted in an increased incidence of fetal resorption associated with maternal toxicity. There was an increase in still-births and a decrease in postnatal survival in pregnant rats treated with ≥ 2.5 mg/kg/day.

Oral **diclofenac** in mice and rats crosses the placental barrier. In rats, maternally toxic doses were associated with dystocia, prolonged gestation and reduced fetal weights, growth and survival.

There are no adequate and well controlled studies in pregnant women. Use during pregnancy only if the potential benefits outweigh the potential hazards to the fetus.

➤*Lactation:* It is not known whether **flurbiprofen** is excreted in breast milk. Because of the potential for serious adverse reactions in nursing infants, decide whether to discontinue nursing or to discontinue the drug, taking into account the importance of the drug to the mother.

Suprofen is excreted in breast milk after a single oral dose. Based on measurements of plasma and milk levels in women taking oral suprofen, the milk concentration is ≈ 1% of the plasma level. Because systemic absorption may occur from topical ocular administration, consider discontinuing nursing while on suprofen; its safety in human neonates has not been established.

Exercise caution while **ketorolac** is administered to a nursing woman.

➤*Children:* Safety and efficacy for use in children have not been established.

Precautions

➤*Wound healing:* may be delayed with the use of flurbiprofen.

➤*Contact lenses:* Patients wearing hydrogel soft contact lenses who have used diclofenac concurrently have experienced ocular irritation manifested by redness and burning.

Drug Interactions

➤*Acetylcholine chloride and carbachol:* Although clinical and animal studies revealed no interference, and there is no known pharmacological basis for an interaction, both of these drugs have reportedly been ineffective when used in patients treated with flurbiprofen or suprofen.

Adverse Reactions

Most frequent – Transient burning and stinging upon instillation (diclofenac 15%, ketorolac ≈ 40%); other minor symptoms of ocular irritation.

Suprofen: Discomfort; itching; redness; allergy, iritis, pain, chemosis, photophobia, irritation, punctate epithelial staining (< 0.5%).

Diclofenac: Keratitis (28%, although most cases occurred in cataract studies prior to drug therapy); elevated IOP (15%, although most cases occurred post-surgery and prior to drug therapy); anterior chamber reaction; ocular allergy; nausea, vomiting (1%); viral infections (≤ 1%).

Ketorolac: Ocular irritation; allergic reactions; superficial keratitis; superficial ocular infections; eye dryness; corneal infiltrates; corneal ulcer; blurry vision.

Flurbiprofen – Increased bleeding tendency of ocular tissues in conjunction with ocular surgery.

Overdosage

Overdosage will not ordinarily cause acute problems. If accidentally ingested, drink fluids to dilute.

FLURBIPROFEN SODIUM

Rx	**Ocufen** (Allergan)	**Solution**: 0.03%	In 2.5 mL dropper bottles.[1]
Rx	**Flurbiprofen Sodium Ophthalmic** (Various, eg, Bausch & Lomb)		In 2.5 mL.[1]

[1] With 1.4% polyvinyl alcohol, 0.005% thimerosal and EDTA.

FLURBIPROFEN SODIUM — OPHTHALMIC

Complete and comparative prescribing information begins in the Ophthalmic NSAIDs group monograph.

Indications

For the inhibition of intraoperative miosis.

Administration and Dosage

➤*Approved by the FDA:* December 31, 1986.

A total of 4 drops of flurbiprofen sodium ophthalmic solution should be administered by instilling 1 drop approximately every 30 minutes beginning 2 hours before surgery.

➤*Storage/Stability:* Store between 15° to 25°C (59° to 79°F).

SUPROFEN

Rx	**Profenal** (Alcon)	**Solution**: 1%	In 2.5 mL *Drop-Tainers*.[1]

[1] With 0.005% thimerosal, 2% caffeine and EDTA.

SUPROFEN — OPHTHALMIC

Complete and comparative prescribing information begins in the Ophthalmic NSAIDs group monograph.

Indications

For inhibition of intraoperative miosis.

Administration and Dosage

On the day of surgery, instill 2 drops into the conjunctival sac at 3 hours, 2 hours and 1 hour prior to surgery. Two drops may be instilled into the conjunctival sac every 4 hours while awake the day preceding surgery.

➤*Storage/Stability:* Store at room temperature.

DICLOFENAC SODIUM

Rx	**Voltaren** (Novartis Pharmaceuticals)	**Solution**: 0.1%	In 2.5 and 5 mL dropper bottles.[1]

[1] With 1 mg/mL EDTA, boric acid, polyoxyl 35 castor oil, 2 mg/mL sorbic acid and tromethamine.

DICLOFENAC SODIUM — OPHTHALMIC

Complete and comparative prescribing information begins in the Ophthalmic NSAIDs group monograph.

Indications

For the treatment of postoperative inflammation in patients who have undergone cataract extraction and for the temporary relief of pain and photophobia in patients undergoing corneal refractive surgery.

Administration and Dosage

➤*Approved by the FDA:* March 28, 1991.

➤*Cataract surgery:* Apply 1 drop of solution to the affected eye, 4 times daily beginning 24 hours after cataract surgery and continuine throughout the first 2 weeks of the postoperative period.

➤*Corneal refractive surgery:* Apply 1 or 2 drops of solution to the operative eye within the hour prior to corneal refractive surgery. Within 15 minutes after surgery, apply 1 or 2 drops to the operative eye and continue 4 times daily for up to 3 days.

➤*Storage/Stability:* Store between 15° to 30°C (59° to 86°F). Protect from light. Dispense in original, unopened container only.

KETOROLAC TROMETHAMINE

Rx	**Acular LS** (Allergan)	**Solution**: 0.4%	In 5 mL dropper bottles.[a]
Rx	**Acular** (Allergan)	**Solution**: 0.5%	In 3, 5, and 10 mL dropper bottles.[b]
Rx	**Acular PF** (Allergan)		Preservative-free. In 0.4 mL single-use vials.[c]

[a] With 0.015% EDTA, 0.006% benzalkonium chloride, sodium chloride, hydrochloric acid, and/or sodium hydroxide.
[b] With 0.01% benzalkonium chloride, 0.1% EDTA, octoxynol 40, sodium chloride, hydrochloric acid, and/or sodium hydroxide.
[c] With sodium chloride, hydrochloric acid, and/or sodium hydroxide.

KETOROLAC TROMETHAMINE — OPHTHALMIC

Complete and comparative prescribing information begins in the Ophthalmic NSAIDs group monograph.

Indications

➤*0.5% solution:* For the temporary relief of ocular itching due to seasonal allergic conjunctivitis; for the treatment of postoperative inflammation in patients who have undergone cataract extraction.

➤*0.4% solution:* For the reduction of ocular pain and burning/stinging following corneal refractive surgery.

➤*Preservative-free solution:* For the treatment of ocular pain and photophobia following incisional refractive surgery. Results from clinical studies indicate that ketorolac tromethamine has no significant effect upon intraocular pressure.

Administration and Dosage

➤*Approved by the FDA:* November 9, 1992.

➤*Acular:*

Ocular itching – 1 drop (0.25 mg) 4 times/day.

Following cataract extraction – 1 drop to the affected eye(s) 4 times/day beginning 24 hours after cataract surgery and continuing through the first 2 weeks of the postoperative period.

➤*Acular LS:* 1 drop 4 times/day in the operated eye, as needed, for pain and burning/stinging for up to 4 days following corneal refractive surgery.

➤*Acular PF:* 1 drop 4 times/day in the operated eye, as needed, for pain and photophobia for up to 3 days after incisional refractive surgery.

➤*Storage/Stability:*

Acular and Acular PF – Store between 15° and 30°C (59° to 86°F). Protect from light.

Acular LS – Store between 15° and 25°C (59° to 77°F).

BROMFENAC OPHTHALMIC SOLUTION

Rx	**Xibrom** (Bausch & Lomb)	**Solution**: 0.09%	In 5 mL dropper bottles.[a]

[a] With benzalkonium chloride 0.05 mg/mL, EDTA 0.2 mg/mL, povidone 20 mg/mL, and sodium hydroxide.

BROMFENAC — OPHTHALMIC

Complete and comparative prescribing information begins in the Ophthalmic NSAIDs group monograph.

Indications

For the treatment of postoperative inflammation and the reduction of ocular pain in patients who have undergone cataract extraction.

Administration and Dosage

➤*Approved by the FDA:* March 24, 2005.

Instill 1 drop to the affected eye(s) 2 times daily beginning 24 hours after cataract surgery and continuing through the first 2 weeks of the postoperative period.

➤*Storage/Stability:* Store at 15° to 25°C (59° to 77°F).

NEPAFENAC

Rx	**Nevanac** (Alcon)	**Suspension:** 0.1%	In 3 mL.

NEPAFENAC — OPHTHALMIC

Indications

For the treatment of pain and inflammation associated with cataract surgery.

Administration and Dosage

➤*Approved by the FDA:* August 19, 2005.

Shake well before use. Apply 1 drop to the affected eye(s) 3 times daily beginning 1 day prior to cataract surgery; continue on the day of surgery, and through the first 2 weeks of the postoperative period.

Nepafenac may be administered in conjunction with other topical ophthalmic medications such as beta-blockers, carbonic anhydrase inhibitors, alpha-agonists, cycloplegics, and mydriatics.

➤*Storage/Stability:* Store at 2° to 25°C (36° to 77°F).

CORTICOSTEROIDS

Refer to the Topical Ophthalmics introduction for complete and comparative information on administration and use.

Indications

➤*Inflammatory conditions:* For the treatment of steroid-responsive inflammatory conditions of the palpebral and bulbar conjunctiva, cornea, lid, sclera and anterior segment of the globe, such as: Allergic conjunctivitis; acne rosacea; superficial punctate keratitis; herpes zoster keratitis; iritis; cyclitis; selected infective conjunctivitis; vernal conjunctivitis; episcleritis; epinephrine sensitivity; and anterior uveitis.

Ocular surgery – For treatment of postoperative inflammation following ocular surgery.

➤*Corneal injury:* For corneal injury from chemical, radiation or thermal burns or penetration of foreign bodies.

See individual monographs for specific indications and administration and dosage.

Administration and Dosage

Treatment duration varies with type of lesion and may extend from a few days to several weeks, depending on therapeutic response. If signs and symptoms fail to improve after 2 days, the patients should be re-evaluated. Relapse may occur if therapy is reduced too rapidly; taper over several days. Relapses, more common in chronic active lesions than in self-limited conditions, usually respond to retreatment.

Actions

➤*Pharmacology:* Topical corticosteroids exert an anti-inflammatory action. Aspects of the inflammatory process such as edema, fibrin deposition, capillary dilation, leukocyte migration, capillary proliferation, deposition of collagen, scar formation and fibroblastic proliferation are suppressed. Steroids inhibit inflammatory response to inciting agents of mechanical, chemical or immunological nature. Topical corticosteroids are effective in acute inflammatory conditions of the conjunctiva, sclera, cornea, lids, iris and anterior segment of the globe; and in ocular allergic conditions. In ocular disease, route of administration depends on site and extent of disorder.

The mechanism of the anti-inflammatory action is thought to be potentiation of epinephrine vasoconstriction, stabilization of lysosomal membranes, retardation of macrophage movement, prevention of kinin release, inhibition of lymphocyte and neutrophil function, inhibition of prostaglandin synthesis and, in prolonged use, decrease of antibody production.

Inhibiting fibroblastic proliferation may prevent symblepharon formation in chemical and thermal burns. Decreased scarring with clearer corneas after topical corticosteroids is a result of inhibiting fibroblastic proliferation and vascularization.

Contraindications

Acute epithelial herpes simplex keratitis (dendritic keratitis); fungal diseases of ocular structures; vaccinia, varicella and most other viral diseases of the cornea and conjunctiva; ocular tuberculosis; hypersensitivity; after uncomplicated removal of a superficial corneal foreign body; mycobacterial eye infection; acute, purulent, untreated eye infections that may be masked or enhanced by the presence of steroids (see Warnings).

➤*Medrysone:* Medrysone is not for use in iritis and uveitis; its efficacy has not been demonstrated.

Warnings

➤*Moderate-to-severe inflammation:* Use higher strengths for moderate-to-severe inflammations. In difficult cases of anterior segment eye disease, systemic therapy may be required. When deeper ocular structures are involved, use systemic therapy.

➤*Ocular damage:* Prolonged use may result in glaucoma, elevated IOP, optic nerve damage, defects in visual acuity and fields of vision, posterior subcapsular cataract formation or secondary ocular infections from pathogens liberated from ocular tissues. Check IOP and lens frequently if used for ≥ 10 days. In diseases that cause thinning of cornea or sclera, perforation has occurred with topical steroids.

➤*Cataract surgery:* The use of steroids after cataract surgery may delay healing and increase the incidence of bleb formation.

➤*Mustard gas keratitis or Sjögren's keratoconjunctivitis:* Topical steroids are not effective.

➤*Infections:* Prolonged use may result in secondary ocular infections caused by suppression of host response. Acute, purulent, untreated eye infections may be masked or the activity enhanced by steroids. Fungal infections of the cornea have been reported with long-term local steroid applications. Therefore, suspect fungal invasion in any persistent corneal ulceration where a steroid has been used or is being used. Take fungal cultures when appropriate.

Stromal herpes simplex keratitis treatment with steroid medication requires great caution; frequent slit-lamp microscopy is mandatory.

➤*Pregnancy: Category C.* There are no adequate and well controlled studies in pregnant women. Use only when clearly needed and when potential benefits outweigh potential hazards.

➤*Lactation:* Topically applied steroids are absorbed systemically. It is not known if sufficient systemic absorption occurs to produce detectable quantities in breast milk. Therefore, because of the potential for serious adverse reactions in nursing infants, decide whether to discontinue nursing or discontinue the drug, taking into account the importance of the drug to the mother.

➤*Children:* Safety and efficacy have not been established.

Fluorometholone – Safety and efficacy in children < 2 years of age have not been established.

Precautions

➤*Bacterial keratitis:* Bacterial keratitis associated with the use of multiple-dose containers of topical ophthalmic products has been reported. Containers had been inadvertently contaminated by patients who, in most cases, had a concurrent corneal disease or a disruption of the ocular epithelial surface. Serious damage to the eye and subsequent loss of vision may result from using contaminated preparations.

➤*Benzalkonium chloride:* Benzalkonium chloride is a preservative used in some of these products that may be absorbed by soft contact lenses. Patients wearing soft contact lenses should wait ≥ 15 minutes after instilling products containing this preservative before inserting their lenses.

➤*Sulfite sensitivity:* Some of these products contain sulfites that may cause allergic-type reactions (eg, hives, itching, wheezing, anaphylaxis) in certain susceptible people. Although the overall prevalence of sulfite sensitivity in the general population is probably low, it is seen more frequently in asthmatics or in atopic nonasthmatic people. Specific products containing sulfites are identified in the product listings.

Adverse Reactions

Glaucoma (elevated IOP) with optic nerve damage, loss of visual acuity and field defects; posterior subcapsular cataract formation; delayed wound healing; secondary ocular infection from pathogens, including herpes simplex and fungi liberated from ocular tissues; acute uveitis; perforation of globe where there is corneal or scleral thinning; exacerbation of viral, bacterial and fungal corneal infections; transient stinging or burning; chemosis; dry eyes; epiphora; photophobia; keratitis; conjunctivitis; corneal ulcers; mydriasis; ptosis; blurred vision, discharge, discomfort, ocular pain, foreign body sensation, hyperemia, pruritus (rimexolone). Rarely, filtering blebs have been reported with steroid use after cataract surgery.

➤*Systemic:* Systemic side effects may occur with extensive use (eg, hypercorticoidism) (see Adrenocortical Steroids group monograph in the Endocrine and Metabolic Agents chapter).

Patient Information

Medical supervision during therapy is recommended.

Instruct patients that use of contaminated ocular solutions can cause ocular infections and serious damage to the eye with subsequent loss of vision. To avoid contamination, do not touch applicator tip to any surface. Replace cap after using.

If improvement in the condition being treated does not occur within 2 days, or if pain, redness, itching or swelling of the eye occurs, discontinue medication and notify the physician. Take care not to discontinue prematurely.

Advise patients to immediately seek physician's advice concerning continued use of the present multidose container if they develop an intercurrent ocular condition (eg, trauma, ocular surgery, infection).

Benzalkonium chloride is absorbed by contact lenses. Do not administer medications containing benzalkonium chloride while wearing soft contact lenses. Instruct patients to wait ≥ 15 minutes after instilling medication before inserting their lenses.

FLUOROMETHOLONE

Rx	**Fluorometholone Ophthalmic Suspension** (Various, eg, Falcon)	**Suspension:** 0.1%	In 5, 10 and 15 mL.[1]
Rx	**FML** (Allergan)		In 5 and 10 mL.[2]
Rx	**Flarex** (Alcon)	**Suspension:** 0.1% fluorometholone acetate	In 2.5, 5 and 10 mL Drop-Tainers.[3]
Rx	**FML Forte** (Allergan)	**Suspension:** 0.25%	In 2, 5, 10 and 15 mL.[4]
Rx	**FML S.O.P.** (Allergan)	**Ointment:** 0.1%	In 3.5 g.[5]

[1] With 0.004% benzalkonium chloride, EDTA, polysorbate 80 and 1.4% polyvinyl alcohol.
[2] With 0.004% benzlkonium chloride, EDTA, polysorbate 80 and polyvinyl alcohol.
[3] With 0.01% benzalkonium chloride, EDTA, hydroxyethylcellulose and tyloxapol.
[4] With 0.005% benzalkonium chloride, EDTA, polysorbate 80 and 1.4% polyvinyl alcohol.
[5] With 0.0008% phenylmercuric acetate, white petrolatum, mineral oil and lanolin alcohol.

FLUOROMETHOLONE — OPHTHALMIC

Complete and comparative prescribing information begins in the Ophthalmic Corticosteroids group monograph.

Indications

➤*Ointment and suspension:* For the treatment of steroid-responsive inflammation of the palpebral and bulbar conjunctiva, cornea, and anterior segment of the globe.

Administration and Dosage

If signs and symptoms fail to improve after 2 days, the patient should be reevaluated.

➤*Ointment:* The dosing of fluorometholone ophthalmic ointment may be reduced, but care should be taken not to discontinue therapy prematurely. In chronic conditions, withdrawal of treatment should be carried out by gradually decreasing the frequency of applications.

A small amount (≈ ½ inch ribbon) of ointment should be applied to the conjunctival sac 1 to 3 times daily. During the initial 24 to 48 hours, the frequency of dosing may be increased to one application every 4 hours. Care should be taken not to discontinue therapy prematurely.

➤*Suspension:* Instill 1 drop into the conjunctival sac 2 to 4 times daily. During the initial 24 to 48 hours, the dosage may be increased to 1 application every 4 hours. Care should be taken not to discontinue therapy prematurely.

➤*Storage/Stability:*

Ointment – Store at or below 25°C (77°F). Avoid exposure to temperatures above 40°C (104°F).

Suspension – Store at controlled room temperature 15° to 30°C (59° to 86°F). Protect from freezing. Shake well before using. Keep bottle tightly closed when not in use.

FLUOROMETHOLONE ACETATE — OPHTHALMIC

Complete and comparative prescribing information begins in the Ophthalmic Corticosteroids group monograph.

Indications

For use in the treatment of steroid-responsive inflammatory conditions of the palpebral and bulbar conjunctiva, cornea, and anterior segment of the eye.

Administration and Dosage

➤*Approved by the FDA:* February 11, 1986.

Shake well before using. One to 2 drops instilled into the conjunctival sac(s) 4 times daily. During the initial 24 to 48 hours the dosage may be safely increased to 2 drops every 2 hours. If no improvement after 2 weeks, consult physician. Care should be taken not to discontinue therapy prematurely.

MEDRYSONE

Rx	**HMS** (Allergan)	**Suspension:** 1%	In 5 and 10 mL.[1]

[1] With 0.004% benzalkonium chloride, EDTA, 1.4% polyvinyl alcohol and hydroxypropyl methyl-cellulose.

MEDRYSONE — OPHTHALMIC

Complete and comparative prescribing information begins in the Ophthalmic Corticosteroids group monograph.

Indications

For the treatment of allergic conjunctivitis, vernal conjunctivitis, episcleritis, and epinephrine sensitivity.

Administration and Dosage

Shake well before using. Instill 1 drop in the conjunctival sac up to every 4 hours.

➤*Storage/Stability:* Store at temperatures up to 25°C (77°F). Protect from freezing.

PREDNISOLONE

Rx	**Pred Mild** (Allergan)	**Suspension:** 0.12% prednisolone acetate	In 5 and 10 mL.[1]
Rx	**Econopred** (Alcon)	**Suspension:** 0.125% prednisolone acetate	In 5 and 10 mL *Drop-Tainers.*[2]
Rx	**Econopred Plus** (Alcon)	**Suspension:** 1% prednisolone acetate	In 5 and 10 mL *Drop-Tainers.*[2]
Rx	**Pred Forte** (Allergan)		In 1, 5, 10 and 15 mL.[1]
Rx	**Prednisolone Acetate Ophthalmic** (Falcon)		In 10 and 15 mL.[2]
Rx	**Prednisolone Sodium Phosphate** (Various, eg, Schein)	**Solution:** 0.125% prednisolone sodium phosphate	In 5, 10 and 15 mL.
Rx	**AK-Pred** (Akorn)		In 5 and 10 mL.[3]
Rx	**Inflamase Mild** (Novartis Ophthalmics)		In 5 and 10 mL.[3]
Rx	**Prednisolone Sodium Phosphate** (Various, eg, Bausch & Lomb, Schein)	**Solution:** 1% prednisolone sodium phosphate	In 5, 10 and 15 mL.
Rx	**AK-Pred** (Akorn)		In 5, 10 and 15 mL.[3]
Rx	**Inflamase Forte** (Novartis Pharmaceuticals)		In 5, 10 and 15 mL.[3]

[1] With benzalkonium chloride, EDTA, polysorbate 80, hydroxypropyl methylcellulose and sodium bisulfite.
[2] With 0.01% benzalkonium chloride, EDTA, polysorbate 80, hydroxypropyl methylcellulose and glycerin.
[3] With 0.01% benzalkonium chloride and EDTA.

PREDNISOLONE ACETATE — OPHTHALMIC

Complete and comparative prescribing information begins in the Ophthalmic Corticosteroids group monograph.

Indications

Steroid responsive inflammatory conditions of the palpebral and bulbar conjunctiva, cornea, and anterior segment of the globe such as allergic conjunctivitis, acne rosacea, superficial punctate keratitis, herpes zoster keratitis, iritis, cyclitis, selected infective conjunctivitides, when the inherent hazard of steroid use is accepted to obtain an advisable diminution in edema and inflammation; corneal injury from chemical, radiation, or thermal burns, or penetration of foreign bodies.

Administration and Dosage

Shake well before using. Two drops topically in the eye(s) 4 times daily. In cases of bacterial infections, concomitant use of anti-infective agents is mandatory. Care should be taken not to discontinue therapy prematurely.

If signs and symptoms fail to improve after 2 days, the patient should be reevaluated.

The dosing of the suspension may be reduced, but take care not to discontinue therapy prematurely. In chronic conditions, carry out withdrawal of treatment by gradually decreasing the frequency of applications.

➤*Storage/Stability:* Store at 8° to 24°C (46° to 75°F) in an upright position.

PREDNISOLONE SODIUM PHOSPHATE — OPHTHALMIC

Complete and comparative prescribing information begins in the Ophthalmic Corticosteroids group monograph.

Indications

For the treatment of the following conditions: Steroid responsive inflammatory conditions of the palpebral and bulbar conjunctiva, cornea, and anterior segment of the globe, such as allergic conjunctivitis, acne rosacea, superficial punctate keratitis, herpes zoster keratitis, iritis, cyclitis, selected infective conjunctivitis when the inherent hazard of steroid use is accepted to obtain an advisable diminution in edema and inflammation; corneal injury from chemical, radiation, or thermal burns, or penetration of foreign bodies.

Prednisolone sodium phosphate 1% ophthalmic solution is recommended for moderate to severe inflammations, particularly when unusually rapid control is desired. In stubborn cases of anterior segment eye disease, systemic adrenocortical hormone therapy may be required. When the deeper ocular structures are involved, systemic therapy is necessary.

Administration and Dosage

Depending on the severity of inflammation, instill 1 or 2 drops of solution into the conjunctival sac up to every hour during the day and every 2 hours during the night as necessary as initial therapy. When a favorable response is observed, reduce dosage to 1 drop every 4 hours. Later, further reduction in dosage to 1 drop 3 to 4 times daily may suffice to control symptoms. The duration of treatment will vary with the type of lesion and may extend from a few days to several weeks, according to therapeutic response. Relapses, more common in chronic active lesions than in self-limiting conditions, usually respond to retreatment.

➤*Storage / Stability:* To be dispensed only in original, unopened container.

Store at controlled room temperature 15° to 25°C (59° to 77°F). Protect from light. Keep out of the reach of children.

DEXAMETHASONE SODIUM PHOSPHATE

Rx	**Dexamethasone Sodium Phosphate** (Various, eg, Bausch & Lomb, Schein, Zenith Goldline)	**Solution:** 0.1% dexamethasone phosphate (as sodium phosphate)	In 5 mL.
Rx	**Decadron Phosphate** (Merck)		In 5 mL *Ocumeters.*[1]
Rx	**Maxidex** (Alcon)	**Suspension:** 0.1% dexamethasone	In 5 and 15 mL *Drop-Tainers.*[2]
Rx	**Dexamethasone Sodium Phosphate** (Various, eg, Zenith Goldline)	**Ointment:** 0.05% dexamethasone phosphate (as sodium phosphate)	In 3.5 g.

[1] With polysorbate 80, EDTA, 0.1% sodium bisulfite, 0.25% phenylethanol, 0.02% benzalkonium chloride.
[2] With 0.01% benzalkonium chloride, EDTA, 0.5% hydroxypropylmethylcellulose, polysorbate 80.
[3] With lanolin anhydrous, parabens, PEG-400, white petrolatum and mineral oil.
[4] With white petrolatum and mineral oil.

DEXAMETHASONE SODIUM PHOSPHATE — OPHTHALMIC

Complete and comparative prescribing information begins in the Ophthalmic Corticosteroids group monograph.

Indications

➤*Inflammatory conditions:* Treatment of steroid-responsive inflammatory conditions of the palpebral and bulbar conjunctiva, cornea and anterior segment of the globe, such as allergic conjunctivitis, acne rosacea, superficial punctate keratitis, herpes zoster keratitis, iritis, selected infective conjunctivitis when the inherent hazard of steroid use is accepted to obtain advisable edema and inflammation diminution.

➤*Corneal injury:* Corneal injury from chemical, radiation or thermal burns or penetration of foreign bodies.

Administration and Dosage

➤*Solutions:* Instill 1 to 2 drops into the conjunctival sac every hour during the day and every 2 hours during the night as initial therapy. When a favorable response is observed, reduce dosage to 1 drop every 4 hours. Further reduction in dosage to 1 drop 3 or 4 times daily may suffice to control symptoms.

➤*Suspension:* Shake well before using. Instill 1 or 2 drops in the conjunctival sac(s). In severe disease, drops may be used hourly, being tapered to discontinuation as inflammation subsides. In mild disease, drops may be used ≤ 4 to 6 times daily.

➤*Ointment:* Apply a thin coating of ointment 3 to 4 times a day. When a favorable response is observed, reduce the number of daily applications to twice daily and later to once daily as a maintenance dose if this is sufficient to control symptoms.

The ointment is particularly convenient when an eye pad is used. It may also be the preparation of choice for patients in whom therapeutic benefit depends on prolonged contact of the active ingredients with ocular tissues.

RIMEXOLONE OPHTHALMIC

Rx	**Vexol** (Alcon)	**Suspension:** 1%	In 2.5, 5 and 10 mL *Drop-Tainers.*[1]

[1] With 0.01% benzalkonium chloride, polysorbate 80 and EDTA.

RIMEXOLONE — OPHTHALMIC

Complete and comparative prescribing information begins in the Ophthalmic Corticosteroids group monograph.

Indications

For the treatment of postoperative inflammation following ocular surgery and in the treatment of anterior uveitis.

Administration and Dosage

➤*Postoperative inflammation:* Apply 1 to 2 drops of rimexolone ophthalmic suspension into the conjunctival sac of the affected eye 4 times daily beginning 24 hours after surgery and continuing throughout the first 2 weeks of the postoperative period.

➤*Anterior uveitis:* Apply 1 to 2 drops of rimexolone ophthalmic suspension into the conjunctival sac of the affected eye every hour during waking hours for the first week, 1 drop every 2 hours during waking hours of the second week, and then taper until uveitis is resolved.

➤*Storage / Stability:* Store upright between 4° and 30°C (40° and 86°F). Shake well before using.

LOTEPREDNOL ETABONATE

Rx	**Lotemax** (Bausch & Lomb)	**Suspension:** 0.5%	In 2.5, 5, 10 and 15 mL.[1]
Rx	**Alrex** (Bausch & Lomb)	**Suspension:** 0.2%	In 5 and 10 mL.[1]

[1] With 0.01% benzalkonium chloride and EDTA.

LOTEPREDNOL ETABONATE — OPHTHALMIC

Complete and comparative prescribing information begins in the Ophthalmic Corticosteroids group monograph.

Indications

For the treatment of steroid responsive inflammatory conditions of the palpebral and bulbar conjunctiva, cornea and anterior segment of the globe such as allergic conjunctivitis, acne rosacea, superficial punctate keratitis, herpes zoster keratitis, iritis, cyclitis, selected infective conjunctivitides, when the inherent hazard of steroid use is accepted to obtain an advisable diminution in edema and inflammation.

Loteprednol etabonate 0.5% is also indicated for the treatment of postoperative inflammation following ocular surgery.

Loteprednol etabonate ophthalmic suspension 0.2% is indicated for the temporary relief of the signs and symptoms of seasonal allergic conjunctivitis.

Administration and Dosage

➤*Approved by the FDA:* March 9, 1998.

Shake vigorously before using.

➤*Allergic Conjunctivitis:* Instill one drop into the affected eye(s) 4 times daily.

➤*Steroid Responsive Disease Treatment:* Apply one to two drops of loteprednol etabonate 0.5% into the conjunctival sac of the affected eye(s) four times daily. During the initial treatment within the first week, the dosing may be increased, up to 1 drop every hour, if necessary. Care should be taken not to discontinue therapy prematurely. If signs and symptoms fail to improve after two days, the patient should be re-evaluated (see Precautions).

LOTEPREDNOL ETABONATE — OPHTHALMIC

➤*Post-Operative Inflammation:* Apply 1 to 2 drops of loteprednol etabonate into the conjunctival sac of the operated eye(s) 4 times daily beginning 24 hours after surgery and continuing throughout the first 2 weeks of the postoperative period.

➤*Storage/Stability:* Store upright between 15° to 25°C (59° to 77°F). Do not freeze. Keep out of reach of children.

FLUOCINOLONE ACETONIDE

Rx	**Retisert** (Bausch & Lomb)	**Implant:** 0.59 mg	In individual cartons.

FLUOCINOLONE ACETONIDE — OPHTHALMIC

Indications

➤*Uveitis:* For the treatment of chronic, noninfectious uveitis affecting the posterior segment of the eye.

Administration and Dosage

➤*Approved by the FDA:* April 8, 2005.

➤*Dosage of implant:* Fluocinolone is implanted surgically into the posterior segment of the affected eye through a pars plana incision. The implant contains 1 tablet of fluocinolone 0.59 mg. The implant is designed to release fluocinolone at a nominal initial rate of 0.6 mcg/day, decreasing over the first month to a steady state between 0.3 to 0.4 mcg/day within approximately 30 months. Following depletion of fluocinolone from the implant as evidenced by recurrence of uveitis, the fluocinolone implant may be replaced.

➤*Handling and disposal:* Caution should be exercised in handling fluocinolone ophthalmic in order to avoid damage to the implant, which may result in an increased rate of drug release from the implant. Thus, fluocinolone ophthalmic should be handled only by the suture tab. Care should be taken during implantation and explantation to avoid sheer forces on the implant that could disengage the silicone cup reservoir (which contains a fluocinolone tablet) from the suture tab. Aseptic technique should be maintained at all times prior to and during the surgical implantation procedure. Fluocinolone ophthalmic should not be resterilized by any method.

➤*Storage/Stability:* Store in the original container at 15° to 25°C (59° to 77°F). Protect from freezing.

Actions

➤*Pharmacology:* Corticosteroids inhibit the inflammatory response to a variety of inciting agents and may delay or slow healing. They inhibit the edema, fibrin deposition, capillary dilation, leukocyte migration, capillary proliferation, fibroblast proliferation, deposition of collagen, and scar formation associated with inflammation. There is no generally accepted explanation for the mechanism of action of ocular corticosteroids. However, corticosteroids are thought to act by the induction of phospholipase A_2 inhibitory proteins, collectively called lipocortins. It is postulated that these proteins control the biosynthesis of potent mediators of inflammation such as prostaglandins and leukotrienes by inhibiting the release of their common precursor arachidonic acid. Arachidonic acid is released from membrane phospholipids by phospholipase A_2. Corticosteroids are capable of producing a rise in intraocular pressure (IOP).

➤*Pharmacokinetics:*

Absorption/Distribution – In a subset of patients who received the intravitreal implant, and had blood samples taken at various times (weeks 1, 4, and 34) after implantation, plasma levels of fluocinolone were below the limit of detection (0.2 ng/mL) at all times. Aqueous and vitreous humor samples were assayed for fluocinolone in a further subset of patients. While detectable concentrations of fluocinolone were seen throughout the observation interval (up to 34 months), the concentrations were highly variable, ranging from below the limit of detection (0.2 ng/mL) to 589 ng/mL.

Contraindications

Contraindicated in most viral diseases of the cornea and conjunctiva, including epithelial herpes simplex keratitis (dendritic keratitis), vaccinia, and varicella, as well as in mycobacterial infections of the eye and fungal diseases of ocular structures; in individuals with known or suspected hypersensitivity to any of the ingredients in this preparation and to other corticosteroids.

Warnings

➤*Surgery complications:* As with any surgical procedure, there is risk involved. Potential complications accompanying intraocular surgery to place fluocinolone into the vitreous cavity may include, but are not limited to, the following: cataract formation, choroidal detachment, temporary decreased visual acuity, endophthalmitis, hypotony, increased IOP, exacerbation of intraocular inflammation, retinal detachment, vitreous hemorrhage, vitreous loss, and wound dehiscence.

➤*Visual acuity:* Following implantation of fluocinolone, nearly all patients will experience an immediate and temporary decrease in visual acuity in the implanted eye, which lasts for approximately 1 to 4 weeks postoperatively. This decrease in visual acuity is likely a result of the surgical procedure.

➤*Ocular damage:* Prolonged use of corticosteroids may result in glaucoma with damage to the optic nerve, in defects in visual acuity and fields of vision, and in posterior subcapsular cataract formation. Use steroids with caution in the presence of glaucoma. Patients must be monitored for elevated IOP.

➤*Intraocular pressure:* Based on clinical trials with fluocinolone, within 34 weeks postimplantation, approximately 60% of patients will require IOP-lowering medications to control IOP. Within an average postimplantation period of approximately 2 years, approximately 32% of patients are expected to require filtering procedures to control IOP.

➤*Cataract surgery:* Within an average postimplantation period of approximately 2 years, nearly all phakic eyes are expected to develop cataracts and require cataract surgery.

The use of steroids after cataract surgery may delay healing and increase the incidence of bleb formation.

➤*Infections:* Use of ocular steroids may prolong the course and may exacerbate the severity of many viral infections of the eye (including herpes simplex). Employment of a corticosteroid medication in the treatment of patients with a history of herpes simplex requires great caution.

Prolonged use of corticosteroids may suppress the host response and increase the hazard of secondary ocular infections. In acute purulent conditions of the eye, steroids may mask infection or enhance existing infection.

➤*Elderly:* No overall differences in safety and efficacy have been observed between elderly and younger patients.

➤*Pregnancy: Category C.*

Teratogenic – Corticosteroids generally are teratogenic in laboratory animals when administered systemically at relatively low dosage levels. Fluocinolone, when administered subcutaneously at a dose of 0.13 mg/kg/day (approximately 10,000 times the daily clinical dose of fluocinolone) during days 6 to 18 of pregnancy in the rabbit, induced abortion at the end of the third and at the beginning of the fourth gestational week. When administered subcutaneously to rats and rabbits during gestation at a maternal toxic dose of 50 mcg/kg/day (approximately 4,000 times the clinical dose of fluocinolone), fluocinolone caused abortions and malformations in a few surviving fetuses. There are no adequate and well-controlled studies in pregnant women. Use fluocinolone during pregnancy only if the potential benefit justifies the potential risk to the fetus.

➤*Lactation:* It is not known whether ocular administration of corticosteroids may result in sufficient systemic absorption to produce detectable quantities in human milk. Systemic steroids appear in human milk and may suppress growth, interfere with endogenous corticosteroid production, or cause other untoward effects. Exercise caution when fluocinolone is implanted in a breast-feeding woman.

➤*Children:* Safety and efficacy in pediatric patients younger than 12 years of age have not been established.

Precautions

➤*Handling and disposal:* As with all intraocular surgery, rigorously maintain sterility of the surgical field and fluocinolone. Caution should be exercised in handling fluocinolone ophthalmic in order to avoid damage to the implant, which may result in an increased rate of drug release from the implant. Fluocinolone ophthalmic should be handled only by the suture tab. Take care during implantation and explantation to avoid sheer forces on the implant that could disengage the silicone cup reservoir (which contains a fluocinolone tablet) from the suture tab. Fluocinolone ophthalmic should not be resterilized by any method.

➤*Bilateral implantation:* Because resistance to infections is known to be reduced by corticosteroids, do not carry out simultaneous bilateral implantation in order to limit the potential for bilateral postoperative infection.

➤*Special risk:* Use fluocinolone with caution in most viral diseases of the cornea and conjunctiva, including epithelial herpes simplex keratitis (dendritic keratitis), vaccinia, and varicella.

Adverse Reactions

➤*Ophthalmic:*

Ocular adverse reactions – Adverse reactions associated with ocular administration of corticosteroids include elevated IOP with possible development of glaucoma, optic nerve damage, visual acuity and field defects, posterior subcapsular cataract formation, delayed wound healing, and perforation of the globe where there is thinning of the sclera.

The development of secondary ocular infection (bacterial, fungal, and viral) has occurred after use of ophthalmic steroids. Fungal and viral infections of the cornea are particularly prone to develop coincidentally with long-term applications of steroids. Consider the possibility of fungal invasion in any persistent corneal ulceration where steroid treatment has been used.

The most frequently reported ocular adverse reactions in the overall study population were cataract, increased IOP, procedural complication, and eye pain. These reactions occurred in approximately 50% to 90% of patients. Procedural complication includes cataract fragments in the eye postoperatively, implant expulsion, injury, mechanical complication of implant, migration of implant, postoperative complications, postoperative wound complications, and wound dehiscence.

Based on clinical trials with fluocinolone, within an average postimplantation period of approximately 2 years, nearly all phakic eyes are expected to develop cataracts and require cataract surgery.

Within 34 weeks postimplantation, approximately 60% of patients will require IOP-lowering medications to control IOP. Within an average postim-

FLUOCINOLONE ACETONIDE — OPHTHALMIC

plantation period of approximately 2 years, approximately 32% of patients are expected to require filtering procedures to control IOP.

Ocular adverse reactions occurring in approximately 10% to 35% of patients included abnormal sensation in the eye, blurred vision, conjunctival hemorrhage, conjunctival hyperemia, dry eye, eye inflammation, eye irritation, eyelid edema, glaucoma, hypotony, increased tearing, maculopathy, pruritus, ptosis, reduced visual acuity, vitreous floaters, and vitreous hemorrhage.

Ocular adverse reactions occurring in approximately 5% to 9% of patients included blepharitis, choroidal detachment, conjunctival edema/chemosis, corneal edema, eye discharge, eye swelling, macular edema, photophobia, photopsia, retinal hemorrhage, visual disturbance, and vitreous opacities.

➤*Systemic:* The most frequently reported nonocular adverse reaction was headache (31%).

Other nonocular adverse reactions occurring in approximately 5% to 15% of patients were arthralgia, back pain, cough, dizziness, influenza, limb pain, nasopharyngitis, nausea, pain, pyrexia, rash, sinusitis, upper respiratory tract infection, and vomiting.

Patient Information

Fluocinolone is designed to locally treat inflammation in the eye, but it is not known to treat the underlying disease. Medication to treat the underlying disease may be prescribed concurrently as deemed appropriate by a physician. Advise patients to have ophthalmologic follow-up examinations of both eyes at appropriate intervals following implantation of fluocinolone.

As with any surgical procedure, there is risk involved. Potential complications accompanying intraocular surgery to place fluocinolone into the vitreous cavity may include, but are not limited to, the following: cataract formation, choroidal detachment, endophthalmitis, exacerbation of intraocular inflammation, hypotony, increased IOP, retinal detachment, temporary decreased visual acuity, vitreous hemorrhage, vitreous loss, and wound dehiscence.

Following implantation of fluocinolone, nearly all patients will experience an immediate and temporary decrease in visual acuity in the implanted eye that lasts for approximately 1 to 4 weeks postoperatively. This decrease in visual acuity likely is a result of the surgical implant procedure.

Based on clinical trials with fluocinolone, within 34 weeks postimplantation, approximately 60% of patients will require IOP-lowering medications to control IOP. Within an average postimplantation period of approximately 2 years, approximately 32% of patients are expected to require filtering procedures to control IOP.

Within an average postimplantation period of approximately 2 years, nearly all phakic eyes are expected to develop cataracts and require cataract surgery.

MAST CELL STABILIZERS

PEMIROLAST POTASSIUM

Rx	**Alamast** (Vistakon)	**Solution, ophthalmic:** 0.1% (1 mg/mL)	0.005% lauralkonium chloride, glycerin, dibasic and monobasic sodium phosphate, phosphoric acid, and/or sodium hydroxide. In 10 mL.

PEMIROLAST POTASSIUM — OPHTHALMIC

Indications

➤*Allergic conjunctivitis:* For the prevention of itching of the eye due to allergic conjunctivitis.

Administration and Dosage

➤*Approved by the FDA:* September 24, 1999.

The recommended dose is 1 to 2 drops in each affected eye 4 times daily.

Symptomatic response to therapy (decreased itching) may be evident within a few days, but frequently requires longer treatment (up to 4 weeks).

➤*Storage/Stability:* Store at 15° to 25°C (59° to 77°F).

Actions

➤*Pharmacology:* Pemirolast potassium is a mast cell stabilizer that inhibits the in vivo type I immediate hypersensitivity reaction.

In vitro and in vivo studies have demonstrated that pemirolast potassium inhibits the antigen-induced release of inflammatory mediators (eg, histamine, leukotriene C_4, D_4, E_4) from human mast cells.

In addition, pemirolast potassium inhibits the chemotaxis of eosinophils into ocular tissue and blocks the release of mediators from human eosinophils.

Although the precise mechanism of action is unknown, the drug has been reported to prevent calcium influx into mast cells upon antigen stimulation.

➤*Pharmacokinetics:*

Absorption/Distribution – Topical ocular administration of 1 to 2 drops of pemirolast potassium ophthalmic solution in each eye 4 times daily in 16 healthy volunteers for 2 weeks resulted in detectable concentrations in the plasma. The mean (± SE) peak plasma level of 4.7 ± 0.8 ng/mL occurred at 0.42 ± 0.05 hours and the mean $t_{1/2}$ was 4.5 ± 0.2 hours. When a single 10 mg pemirolast potassium dose was taken orally, a peak plasma concentration of 0.723 mcg/mL was reached.

Excretion – Following topical administration, about 10% to 15% of the dose was excreted unchanged in the urine.

Contraindications

Hypersensitivity to any of the ingredients of this product.

Warnings

➤*Administration:* For topical ophthalmic use only. Not for injection or oral use.

➤*Fertility impairment:* Pemirolast potassium had no effect on mating and fertility in rats at oral doses up to 250 mg/kg (≈ 20,000 fold the human dose at 2 drops/eye, 40 mcL/drop, 4 times a day for a 50 kg adult). A reduced fertility and pregnancy index occurred in the F_1 generation when F_0 dams were treated with 400 mg/kg pemirolast potassium during late pregnancy and lactation period (≈ 30,000 fold the human dose).

➤*Pregnancy: Category C.*

Teratogenic – Pemirolast potassium caused an increased incidence of thymic remnant in the neck, interventricular septal defect, fetuses with wavy rib, splitting of thoracic vertebral body, and reduced numbers of ossified sternebrae, sacral and caudal vertebrae, and metatarsi when rats were given oral doses ≥ 250 mg/kg (≈ 20,000-fold the human dose at 2 drops/eye, 40 mcL/drop, 4 times a day for a 50 kg adult) during organogenesis. Increased incidence of dilation of renal pelvis/ureter in the fetuses and neonates was also noted when rats were given an oral dose of 400 mg/kg pemirolast potassium (≈ 30,000-fold the human dose). Pemirolast potassium was not teratogenic in rabbits given oral doses up to 150 mg/kg (≈ 12,000-fold the human dose) during the same time period. There are no adequate and well-controlled studies in pregnant women. Because animal reproductive studies are not always predictive of human response, pemirolast potassium ophthalmic solution should be used during pregnancy only if the benefit outweighs the risk.

Nonteratogenic – Pemirolast potassium produced increased pre- and postimplantation losses, reduced embryo/fetal and neonatal survival, decreased neonatal body weight, and delayed neonatal development in rats receiving an oral dose at 400 mg/kg (≈ 30,000-fold the human dose). Pemirolast potassium also caused a reduction in the number of corpus lutea, the number of implantations, and number of live fetuses in the F_1 generation in rats when F_0 dams were given oral dosages ≥ 250 mg/kg (≈ 20,000-fold the human dose) during late gestation and the lactation period.

➤*Lactation:* Pemirolast potassium is excreted in the milk of lactating rats at concentrations higher than those in plasma. It is not known whether pemirolast potassium is excreted in human milk. Because many drugs are excreted in human milk, caution should be exercised when pemirolast potassium ophthalmic solution is administered to a nursing woman.

➤*Children:* Safety and effectiveness in pediatric patients below the age of 3 years have not been established.

Adverse Reactions

➤*Less than 5%:* The following ocular and non-ocular adverse reactions were reported at an incidence of less than 5%:

Ophthalmic – Burning, dry eye, foreign body sensation, and ocular discomfort.

Miscellaneous – Allergy, back pain, bronchitis, cough, dysmenorrhea, fever, sinusitis, and sneezing/nasal congestion.

➤*Miscellaneous:* In clinical studies lasting up to 17 weeks with pemirolast potassium ophthalmic solution, headache, rhinitis, and cold/flu symptoms were reported at an incidence of 10% to 25%. The occurrence of these side effects was generally mild. Some of these events were similar to the underlying ocular disease being studied.

Overdosage

No accounts of pemirolast potassium ophthalmic solution overdose were reported following topical ocular application.

Oral ingestion of the contents of a 10 mL bottle would be equivalent to 10 mg of pemirolast potassium.

Patient Information

For topical ophthalmic use only. Not for injection or oral use.

To prevent contaminating the dropper tip and solution, do not touch the eyelids or surrounding areas with the dropper tip. Keep the bottle tightly closed when not in use.

Patients should be advised not to wear contact lenses if their eyes are red. Pemirolast potassium ophthalmic solution should not be used to treat contact lens related irritation. The preservative in pemirolast potassium ophthalmic solution, lauralkonium chloride, may be absorbed by soft contact lenses. Patients who wear soft contact lenses and whose eyes are not red should be instructed to wait at least 10 minutes after instilling pemirolast potassium before they insert their contact lenses.

NEDOCROMIL SODIUM

Rx	**Alocril** (Allergan)	**Solution, ophthalmic:** 2% (20 mg/mL)	0.01% benzalkonium Cl, 0.5% NaCl, 0.05% EDTA. In 5 mL w/ dropper tip.

NEDOCROMIL SODIUM — OPHTHALMIC

Indications

➤*Allergic conjunctivitis:* For the treatment of itching associated with allergic conjunctivitis.

Administration and Dosage

➤*Approved by the FDA:* December 15, 1999.

1 or 2 drops in each eye twice a day. Use at regular intervals.

Continue treatment throughout the period of exposure (ie, until the pollen season is over or until exposure to the offending allergen is terminated), even when symptoms are absent.

➤*Storage/Stability:* Store between 2° to 25°C (36° to 77°F). Keep tightly closed and out of the reach of children.

Actions

➤*Pharmacology:* Nedocromil sodium is a mast cell stabilizer. It inhibits the release of mediators from cells involved in hypersensitivity reactions. Decreased chemotaxis and decreased activation of eosinophils have also been demonstrated.

In vitro studies with adult human bronchoalveolar cells showed that nedocromil sodium inhibits histamine release from a population of mast cells as belonging to the mucosal subtype and beta-glucuronidase release from macrophages.

➤*Pharmacokinetics:* Nedocromil sodium exhibits low systemic absorption, with less than 4% of the total dose systemically absorbed following multiple dosing. Absorption is mainly through the nasolacrimal duct rather than through the conjunctiva. It is not metabolized and is eliminated primarily unchanged in urine (70%) and feces (30%).

Contraindications

Hypersensitivity to nedocromil sodium or to any of the other ingredients.

Warnings

➤*Pregnancy: Category B.* Reproduction studies performed in mice, rats, and rabbits using a subcutaneous dose of 100 mg/kg/day (greater than 1,600 times the maximum recommended human daily ocular dose on a mg/kg basis) revealed no evidence of teratogenicity or harm to the fetus caused by nedocromil sodium. However there are no adequate and well-controlled studies in pregnant women. Because animal reproduction studies are not always predictive of human response, use nedocromil sodium during pregnancy only if clearly needed.

➤*Lactation:* After IV administration to lactating rats, nedocromil was excreted in milk. It is not known whether this drug is excreted in human milk. Exercise caution when nedocromil sodium is administered to nursing women.

➤*Children:* Safety and efficacy in children younger than 3 years of age have not been established.

Adverse Reactions

The most frequently reported adverse experience was headache (≈ 40%). Ocular burning, irritation and stinging, unpleasant taste, nasal congestion (10% to 30%); asthma, conjunctivitis, eye redness, photophobia, rhinitis (1% to 10%).

Patient Information

Instruct patients to refrain from wearing contact lenses while exhibiting the signs and symptoms of allergic conjunctivitis.

LODOXAMIDE TROMETHAMINE

Rx	**Alomide** (Alcon)	**Solution:** 0.1%	In 10 mL *Drop-Tainers.*

LODOXAMIDE TROMETHAMINE — OPHTHALMIC

Indications

Treatment of the ocular disorders referred to by the terms vernal keratoconjunctivitis, vernal conjunctivitis, and vernal keratitis.

Administration and Dosage

➤*Approved by the FDA:* September 23, 1993.

The dose for adults and children greater than 2 years of age is one to two drops in each affected eye 4 times daily for up to 3 months.

➤*Storage/Stability:* Store at 15° to 27°C (59° to 80°F).

Actions

➤*Pharmacology:* Lodoxamide tromethamine is a mast cell stabilizer that inhibits the in vivo Type I immediate hypersensitivity reaction. Lodoxamide therapy inhibits the increases in cutaneous vascular permeability that are associated with reagin or IgE and antigen-mediated reactions.

In vitro studies have demonstrated the ability of lodoxamide to stabilize rodent mast cells and prevent antigen-stimulated release of histamine. In addition, lodoxamide prevents the release of other mast cell inflammatory mediators (ie, SRS-A, slow-reacting substances of anaphylaxis, also known as the peptido-leukotrienes) and inhibits eosinophil chemotaxis. Although lodoxamide's precise mechanism of action is unknown, the drug has been reported to prevent calcium influx into mast cells upon antigen stimulation.

➤*Pharmacokinetics:* The disposition of 14C-lodoxamide was studied in six healthy adult volunteers receiving a 3 mg (50 mCi) oral dose of lodoxamide. Urinary excretion was the major route of elimination. The elimination half-life of 14C-lodoxamide was 8.5 hours in urine. In a study conducted in twelve healthy adult volunteers, topical administration of lodoxamide tromethamine ophthalmic solution 0.1%, one drop in each eye four times per day for ten days, did not result in any measurable lodoxamide plasma levels at a detection limit of 2.5 ng/mL.

Contraindications

Hypersensitivity to any component of this product.

Warnings

➤*Contact lenses:* As with all ophthalmic preparations containing benzalkonium chloride, patients should be instructed not to wear soft contact lenses during treatment with lodoxamide tromethamine ophthalmic solution.

➤*Mutagenesis:* No evidence of mutagenicity or genetic damage was seen in the Ames *Salmonella* Assay, Chromosomal Aberration in CHO Cells Assay, or Mouse Forward Lymphoma Assay. In the BALB/c-3T3 Cells Transformation Assay, some increase in the number of transformed foci was seen at high concentrations (greater than 4000 mcg/mL).

➤*Pregnancy: Category B.* Reproduction studies with lodoxamide tromethamine administered orally to rats and rabbits in doses of 100 mg/kg/day (more than 5000 times the proposed human clinical dose) produced no evidence of developmental toxicity. There are, however, no adequate and well-controlled studies in pregnant women. Because animal reproduction studies are not always predictive of human response, lodoxamide tromethamine ophthalmic solution 0.1% should be used during pregnancy only if clearly needed.

➤*Lactation:* It is not known whether lodoxamide tromethamine is excreted in human milk. Because many drugs are excreted in human milk, caution should be exercised when lodoxamide tromethamine ophthalmic solution 0.1% is administered to nursing women.

➤*Children:* Safety and effectiveness in pediatric patients below the age of 2 have not been established.

Precautions

➤*Ocular effects:* Patients may experience a transient burning or stinging upon instillation of lodoxamide tromethamine ophthalmic solution. Should these symptoms persist, the patient should be advised to contact the prescribing physician.

Adverse Reactions

During clinical studies of lodoxamide tromethamine ophthalmic solution 0.1%, the most frequently reported ocular adverse experiences were transient burning, stinging, or discomfort upon instillation, which occurred in approximately 15% of the subjects. Other ocular events occurring in 1% to 5% of the subjects included ocular itching/pruritus, blurred vision, dry eye, tearing/discharge, hyperemia, crystalline deposits, and foreign body sensation. Events that occurred in less than 1% of the subjects included corneal erosion/ulcer, scales on lid/lash, eye pain, ocular edema/swelling, ocular warming sensation, ocular fatigue, chemosis, corneal abrasion, anterior chamber cells, keratopathy/keratitis, blepharitis, allergy, sticky sensation, and epitheliopathy.

Nonocular events reported were headache (1.5%) and (at less than 1%) heat sensation, dizziness, somnolence, nausea, stomach discomfort, sneezing, dry nose, and rash.

Overdosage

➤*Symptoms:* There have been no reports of lodoxamide tromethamine opthalmic solution 0.1% overdose following topical ocular application. Accidental overdose of an oral preparation of 120 to 180 mg of lodoxamide resulted in a temporary sensation of warmth, profuse sweating, diarrhea, lightheadedness, and a feeling of stomach distension; no permanent adverse effects were observed. Side effects reported following systemic oral administration of 0.1 mg to 10 mg of lodoxamide include a feeling of warmth or flushing, headache, dizziness, fatigue, sweating, nausea, loose stools, and urinary frequency/urgency.

➤*Treatment:* The physician may consider emesis in the event of accidental ingestion.

Patient Information

As with all opthalmic preparations containing benzalkonium chloride, patients should be instructed not to wear soft contact lenses during treatment with lodoxamide.

CROMOLYN SODIUM

Rx	**Crolom** (Dura)	**Solution:** 4%	In 2.5 and 10 mL bottles with controlled drop tip.
Rx	**Cromolyn Sodium Ophthalmic Solution** (Akorn)		In 10 mL with controlled dropper tip.
Rx	**Cromolyn Sodium Ophthalmic Solution** (Falcon)		In 10 and 15 mL.
Rx	**Cromolyn Sodium Ophthalmic** (Teva)		In 10 mL.

CROMOLYN SODIUM — OPHTHALMIC

Indications

Treatment of vernal keratoconjunctivitis, vernal conjunctivitis, and vernal keratitis.

Administration and Dosage

The dose is 1 to 2 drops in each eye 4 to 6 times a day at regular intervals.

Symptomatic response to therapy (decreased itching, tearing, redness, and discharge) is usually evident within a few days, but longer treatment for up to 6 weeks is sometimes required. Once symptomatic improvement has been established, therapy should be continued for as long as needed to sustain improvement.

If required, corticosteroids may be used concomitantly with cromolyn sodium ophthalmic solution.

➤*Storage/Stability:* Store between 15° to 30°C (59° to 86°F). Protect from light. Store in original carton. Keep tightly closed.

Keep out of reach of children.

Actions

➤*Pharmacology:* In vitro and in vivo animal studies have shown that cromolyn sodium inhibits the degranulation of sensitized mast cells which occurs after exposure to specific antigens. Cromolyn sodium acts by inhibiting the release of histamine and SRS-A (slow-reacting substance of anaphylaxis) from the mast cell.

Another activity demonstrated in vitro is the capacity of cromolyn sodium to inhibit the degranulation of non-sensitized rat mast cells by phospholipase A and the subsequent release of chemical mediators. Another study showed that cromolyn sodium did not inhibit the enzymatic activity of released phospholipase A on its specific substrate.

➤*Pharmacokinetics:*

Absorption/Distribution – Cromolyn sodium is poorly absorbed. When multiple doses of cromolyn sodium ophthalmic solution are instilled into healthy rabbit eyes, less than 0.07% of the administered dose of cromolyn sodium is absorbed into the systemic circulation (presumably by way of the eye, nasal passages, buccal cavity and gastrointestinal tract). Trace amounts (less than 0.01%) of the cromolyn sodium dose penetrate into the aqueous humor and clearance from this chamber is virtually complete within 24 hours after treatment is stopped.

Excretion – In healthy volunteers, analysis of drug excretion indicates that approximately 0.03% of cromolyn sodium is absorbed following administration to the eye.

Contraindications

Hypersensitivity to cromolyn sodium or to any of the other ingredients.

Warnings

➤*Pregnancy:* Category B.

Teratogenic – Reproduction studies with cromolyn sodium administered subcutaneously to pregnant mice and rats at maximum daily doses of 540 mg/kg (1620 mg/m^2) and 164 mg/kg (984 mg/m^2), respectively, and intravenously to rabbits at a maximum daily dose of 485 mg/kg (5820 mg/m^2) produced no evidence of fetal malformation. These doses represent approximately 57, 35, and 205 times the maximum daily human dose, respectively, on a mg/m^2 basis. Adverse fetal effects (increased resorption and decreased fetal weight) were noted only at the very high parenteral doses that produced maternal toxicity. There are, however, no adequate and well-controlled studies in pregnant women. Because animal reproduction studies are not always predictive of human response, this drug should be used during pregnancy only if clearly needed.

➤*Lactation:* It is not known whether this drug is excreted in human milk. Because many drugs are excreted in human milk, caution should be exercised when cromolyn sodium ophthalmic solution is administered to a nursing woman.

➤*Children:* Safety and effectiveness in pediatric patients below the age of 4 years have not been established.

Precautions

➤*Ocular effects:* Patients may experience a transient stinging or burning sensation following application of cromolyn sodium ophthalmic solution.

➤*Usage:* Do not exceed the recommended frequency of administration. Advise patients that the effect of cromolyn sodium ophthalmic solution therapy is dependent upon its administration at regular intervals, as directed.

Adverse Reactions

➤*Hypersensitivity:* Immediate hypersensitivity reactions have been reported rarely and include dyspnea, edema, and rash.

➤*Ophthalmic:* The most frequently reported adverse reaction attributed to the use of cromolyn sodium ophthalmic solution, on the basis of reoccurrence following readministration, is transient ocular stinging or burning upon instillation.

The following adverse reactions have been reported as infrequent events. It is unclear whether they are attributed to the drug: Conjunctival injection; watery eyes; itchy eyes; dryness around the eye; puffy eyes; eye irritation; styes.

Patient Information

Users of contact lenses should refrain from wearing lenses while exhibiting the signs and symptoms of vernal keratoconjunctivitis, vernal conjunctivitis, or vernal keratitis. Do not wear contact lenses during treatment with cromolyn sodium ophthalmic solution.

➤*Special tips:*

1.) Avoid placing cromolyn sodium ophthalmic solution directly on the cornea (the area just over the pupil), because it is especially sensitive. You will find the administration of the eye drops more comfortable if you place the drops just inside the lower eyelid as shown in the figure above.
2.) To avoid contamination of the solution, do not touch the dropper tip to the eye, fingers, or any other surface. Replace cap after use. It is recommended that any remaining contents be discarded after the treatment period described by your physician.
3.) Store between 15° to 30°C (59° to 86°F). Protect from light; store in original carton.
4.) Keep tightly closed and out of the reach of children.
5.) Do not use with any other ocular medication unless directed by your physician. Do not wear contact lenses during treatment with cromolyn sodium ophthalmic solution.

OPHTHALMIC DECONGESTANTS

Refer to the Topical Ophthalmic Drugs introduction for more complete information.

Indications

Refer to individual product listings for specific indications.

Actions

➤*Pharmacology:* The effects of sympathomimetic agents on the eye include: Pupil dilation, increase in outflow of aqueous humor and vasoconstriction (α-adrenergic effects); relaxation of the ciliary muscle and a decrease in the formation of aqueous humor (β-adrenergic effects). Hydroxyamphetamine dilates the pupil, probably by stimulating the dilator muscles of the iris.

Strong (α) vasoconstriction preparations (phenylephrine 2.5% and 10%; hydroxyamphetamine) cause vasoconstriction and pupillary dilation for diagnostic eye exams, during surgery and to prevent synechiae formation in uveitis. Weak sympathomimetic solutions (phenylephrine 0.12%; naphazoline; tetrahydrozoline) are used as ophthalmic decongestants (vasoconstriction of conjunctival blood vessels) for symptomatic relief of minor eye irritations. Epinephrine is used for open-angle glaucoma and is not included in this monograph (see Epinephrine monograph in the Agents for Glaucoma section).

Ophthalmic Vasoconstrictors/Mydriatics

Vasoconstrictor/ Mydriatic	Duration of action (hr)	Available concentration	Prescription status
Hydroxyamphetamine	few hours	1%	Rx
Naphazoline	3 to 4	0.012%	otc
		0.02%	otc
		0.03%	otc
		0.1%	Rx
Oxymetazoline	4 to 6	0.025%	otc
Phenylephrine	0.5 to 1.5	0.12%	otc
	—	2.5%	Rx
	—	10%	Rx
Tetrahydrozoline	1 to 4	0.05%	otc

Contraindications

Hypersensitivity to any of these agents; narrow-angle glaucoma or anatomically narrow (occludable) angle and no glaucoma; prior to peripheral iridectomy in eyes capable of angle closure because mydriatic action may precipitate angle block.

➤*Phenylephrine 10%:* Patients with insulin-dependent diabetes; hypertensive patients; generalized arteriosclerosis; aneurysms; preexisting cardiovascular diseases; infants, small children with low body weight; elderly patients.

Warnings

➤*Anesthetics:* Discontinue prior to use of anesthetics which sensitize the myocardium to sympathomimetics (eg, cyclopropane, halothane).

Local anesthetics can increase absorption of topically applied drugs; exercise caution when applying prior to use of phenylephrine. However, use of a local anesthetic prior to phenylephrine 2.5% or 10% may help prevent pain.

➤*Overuse:* Overuse may produce increased redness of the eye.

➤*Pregnancy: Category C.* Safety for use during pregnancy is not established. Use only if clearly needed and if the potential benefits outweigh potential hazards to the fetus.

➤*Lactation:* Safety for use during breastfeeding has not been established. Use caution when administering to a nursing woman.

➤*Children:* Safety and efficacy have not been established. Phenylephrine 10% is contraindicated in infants.

Precautions

➤*Narrow-angle glaucoma:* Ordinarily, any mydriatic is contraindicated in patients with glaucoma. However, when temporary pupil dilation may free adhesions, or when vasoconstriction of intrinsic vessels may lower intraocular tension, these advantages may temporarily outweigh danger from coincident pupil dilation.

➤*Rebound congestion:* Rebound congestion may occur with frequent or extended use of ophthalmic vasoconstrictors. This may be of importance when there is retinal detachment or prior to cataract surgery. Rebound miosis has occurred in older persons 1 day after receiving phenylephrine; reinstillation produced a reduction in mydriasis.

➤*Systemic absorption:* Exceeding recommended dosages of these agents or applying **phenylephrine** 2.5% to 10% solutions to the instrumented, traumatized, diseased or postsurgical eye or adnexa, or to patients with suppressed lacrimation, as during anesthesia, may result in the absorption of sufficient quantities to produce a systemic vasopressor response.

➤*Pigment floaters:* Older individuals may develop transient pigment floaters in the aqueous humor 30 to 45 minutes after instillation of phenylephrine. The appearance may be similar to anterior uveitis or to a microscopic hyphema.

➤*Potentially hazardous tasks:* **Phenylephrine** may cause temporary blurred or unstable vision; observe caution while driving or performing other hazardous tasks.

➤*Special risk:* Use with caution in the presence of hypertension, diabetes, hyperthyroidism, cardiovascular abnormalities, arteriosclerosis.

➤*Sulfite sensitivity:* Some of these products contain sulfites that may cause allergic-type reactions (eg, hives, itching, wheezing, anaphylaxis) in certain susceptible persons. Although the overall prevalence of sulfite sensitivity in the general population is probably low, it is seen more frequently in asthmatics or in atopic nonasthmatic persons.

Drug Interactions

Ophthalmic Sympathomimetic Drug Interactions

Precipitant drug	Object drug*		Description
Anesthetics	Ophthalmic sympathomimetics	↑	Cautiously use anesthetics that sensitize the myocardium to sympathomimetics (eg, cyclopropane, halothane). Local anesthetics can increase absorption of topical drugs; exercise caution when applying prior to use of phenylephrine.
Beta blockers	Ophthalmic sympathomimetics	↑	Systemic side effects may occur more readily in patients taking these drugs.
MAOIs	Ophthalmic sympathomimetics	↑	When given with, or up to 21 days after MAOIs, exaggerated adrenergic effects may result. Supervise and adjust dosage carefully.

* ↑ = Object drug increased.

Also consider drug interactions that may occur with systemic use of the sympathomimetics (see Vasopressors Used for Shock).

Adverse Reactions

➤*Ophthalmic:* Transitory stinging on initial instillation; blurring of vision; mydriasis; increased redness; irritation; discomfort; blurring; punctate keratitis; lacrimation; increased IOP.

Phenylephrine – Phenylephrine may cause rebound miosis and decreased mydriatic response to therapy in older persons.

➤*Cardiovascular:* Palpitation; tachycardia; cardiac arrhythmia; hypertension; ventricular arrhythmias (ie, premature ventricular contractions); reflex bradycardia; coronary occlusion; pulmonary embolism; subarachnoid hemorrhage; myocardial infarction; stroke; death associated with cardiac reactions. Headache or browache may occur.

Phenylephrine 10% – Significant elevation of blood pressure is rare but can occur after conjunctival instillation. Exercise caution with elderly patients and children of low body weight. Carefully monitor the blood pressure of these patients. (See Warnings and Contraindications.) There have been rare reports of the development of serious cardiovascular reactions, including ventricular arrhythmias and myocardial infarctions. These episodes, some fatal, have usually occurred in elderly patients with preexisting cardiovascular diseases.

➤*Miscellaneous:* Headache; blanching; tremor; trembling; sweating; dizziness; nausea; nervousness; drowsiness; weakness; hyperglycemia.

Overdosage

➤*Hydroxyamphetamine:* If ocular overdosage occurs, dilute pilocarpine (1%) may be administered. If accidentally ingested, sedation is indicated. Further treatment is symptomatic.

Patient Information

Do not use beyond 48 to 72 hours without consulting a physician.

If irritation, blurring or redness persists, or if severe eye pain, headache, vision changes, floating spots, dizziness, decrease in body temperature, drowsiness, acute eye redness or pain with light exposure occur, discontinue use and consult a physician.

Do not use if you have glaucoma except under the advice of a physician.

Refer to the Topical Ophthalmic Introduction for more complete information.

➤*Potentially hazardous tasks:* Phenylephrine may cause temporary blurred or unstable vision; observe caution while driving or performing other hazardous tasks.

TETRAHYDROZOLINE HYDROCHLORIDE

otc	**Tetrahydrozoline HCl** (Various, eg, Moore, Rugby, Steris)	**Solution:** 0.05%	In 15 and 30 mL.
otc	**Collyrium Fresh** (Wyeth-Ayerst)		In 15 mL.[1]
otc	**Geneye** (Goldline)		In 15 mL.[3]
otc	**Geneye Extra** (Goldline)		In 15 mL.[4]
otc	**Murine Plus** (Ross)		In 15 and 30 mL.[5]
otc	**Optigene 3** (Pfeiffer)		In 15 mL.[3]
otc	**Tetrasine** (Optopics)		In 15 and 22.5 mL.
otc	**Tetrasine Extra** (Optopics)		In 15 mL.[4]

[1] With 0.01% benzalkonium chloride and EDTA.
[2] With 0.01% benzalkonium chloride and 0.1% EDTA.
[3] With benzalkonium chloride and EDTA.
[4] With 1% polyethylene glycol 400, benzalkonium chloride and EDTA.
[5] With 0.013% benzalkonium chloride, 0.1% EDTA and 1% PEG-400.

TETRAHYDROZOLINE HYDROCHLORIDE — OPHTHALMIC

For complete and comparative prescribing information, refer to the Ophthalmic Decongestants group monograph.

Indications

➤*Ocular redness:* Relieves redness of the eye due to minor eye irritations.

Administration and Dosage

➤*Directions:* Instill 1 to 2 drops in the affected eye(s) up to 4 times daily.

➤*Storage / Stability:* Store at room temperature 15° to 30°C (59° to 86°F). If solution changes color or becomes cloudy, do not use.

PHENYLEPHRINE HYDROCHLORIDE

otc	**Relief** (Allergan)	**Solution**: 0.12%	Preservative free. In UD 0.3 mL.[1]
Rx	**Phenylephrine HCl** (Various)	**Solution**: 2.5%	In 15 mL.
Rx	**AK-Dilate** (Akorn)		In 2 and 15 mL.[2]
Rx	**Mydfrin 2.5%** (Alcon)		In 3 and 5 mL *Drop-Tainers*.[3]
Rx	**Neo-Synephrine** (Sanofi Winthrop)		In 15 mL.[4]
Rx	**Phenylephrine HCl** (Various, eg, Iolab, Steris)	**Solution**: 10%	In 2 and 5 mL.
Rx	**AK-Dilate** (Akorn)		In 2 and 5 mL.[2]
Rx	**Neo-Synephrine** (Sanofi Winthrop)		In 5 mL.[5]
Rx	**Neo-Synephrine Viscous** (Sanofi Winthrop)		In 5 mL.[6]

[1] With 1.4% polyvinyl alcohol and EDTA.
[2] With benzalkonium chloride.
[3] With 0.01% benzalkonium chloride, EDTA and sodium bisulfite.
[4] With 1:7500 benzalkonium chloride.
[5] With 1:10,000 benzalkonium chloride.
[6] With 1:10,000 benzalkonium chloride and methylcellulose.

PHENYLEPHRINE HYDROCHLORIDE — OPHTHALMIC

For complete and comparative prescribing information, refer to the Ophthalmic Decongestants group monograph.

Indications

➤*2.5% and 10% solutions:* For use as a decongestant and vasoconstrictor and for pupil dilatation in uveitis (posterior synechiae), wide angle glaucoma, prior to surgery, refraction, ophthalmoscopic examination, and diagnostic procedures.

➤*0.12% solution:* Used to relieve redness of the eye due to minor eye irritations and as a lubricant to prevent further irritation or to relieve dryness of the eye.

Administration and Dosage

Do not touch dropper tip to any surface, since this may contaminate the solution.

➤*Vasoconstriction and pupil dilatation:* Phenylephrine hydrochloride 2.5% and 10% ophthalmic solutions are especially useful when rapid and powerful dilatation of the pupil without cycloplegia and reduction of congestion in the capillary bed are desired. A drop of a suitable topical anesthetic may be applied, followed in a few minutes by 1 drop of phenylephrine hydrochloride ophthalmic solution on the upper limbus. The anesthetic prevents stinging and consequent dilution of the solution by lacrimation. It may occasionally be necessary to repeat the instillation after 1 hour, again preceded by the use of the topical anesthetic.

➤*Uveitis:*

Posterior synechiae – Phenylephrine hydrochloride 2.5% and 10% ophthalmic solutions may be used in patients with uveitis when synechiae are present or may develop. The formation of synechiae may be prevented by the use of these solutions and atropine or other cycloplegics to produce wide dilatation of the pupil. It should be emphasized, however, that the vasoconstrictor effect of phenylephrine hydrochloride may be antagonistic to the increase of local blood flow in uveal infection.

To free recently formed posterior synechiae, 1 drop of phenylephrine hydrochloride ophthalmic solution may be applied to the upper surface of the cornea and be repeated as necessary, not to exceed 3 times. Treatment may be continued the following day, if necessary. In the interim, hot compresses should be applied for 5 or 10 minutes 3 times a day, with 1 drop of a 1% or 2% solution of atropine sulfate before and after each series of compresses.

➤*Glaucoma:*

10% solution and 10% viscous solution – In certain patients with glaucoma, temporary reduction of intraocular tension may be attained by producing vasoconstriction of the intraocular vessels; this may be accomplished by placing 1 drop of the 10% ophthalmic solutions on the upper surface of the cornea. This treatment may be repeated as often as necessary. Phenylephrine hydrochloride 2.5% and 10% ophthalmic solutions may be used with miotics in patients with wide angle glaucoma. It reduces the difficulties experienced by the patient because of the small field produced by miosis, and still it permits and often supports the effect of the miotic in lowering the intraocular pressure. Hence, there may be marked improvement in visual acuity after using phenylephrine hydrochloride ophthalmic solutions in conjunction with miotic drugs.

➤*Surgery:* When a short-acting mydriatic is needed for wide dilatation of the pupil before intraocular surgery, phenylephrine hydrochloride 2.5% and 10% ophthalmic solutions may be applied topically from 30 to 60 minutes before the operation.

➤*Refraction:* Prior to determination of refractive errors, phenylephrine hydrochloride 2.5% ophthalmic solution may be used effectively with homatropine hydrobromide, atropine sulfate, or a combination of homatropine and cocaine hydrochloride.

Adults – One drop of the preferred cycloplegic is placed in each eye, followed in 5 minutes by 1 drop of phenylephrine hydrochloride 2.5% ophthalmic solution and in 10 minutes by another drop of the cycloplegic. In 50 to 60 minutes, the eyes are ready for refraction.

Children – For older pediatric patients, a drop of atropine sulfate 1% is placed in each eye, followed in 10 to 15 minutes by 1 drop of phenylephrine hydrochloride 2.5% ophthalmic solution and in 5 to 10 minutes by a second drop of atropine sulfate 1%. In 1 to 2 hours, the eyes are ready for refraction.

For a "one application method", phenylephrine hydrochloride 2.5% ophthalmic solution may be combined with a cycloplegic to elicit synergistic action. The additive effect varies depending on the patient. Therefore, when using a "one application method", it may desirable to increase the concentration of the cycloplegic.

➤*Ophthalmoscopic examination:* One drop of phenylephrine hydrochloride 2.5% ophthalmic solution is placed in each eye. Sufficient mydriasis to permit examination is produced in 15 to 30 minutes. Dilatation lasts from 1 to 3 hours.

➤*Diagnostic procedures:*

Provocative test for angle block in patients with glaucoma – The 2.5% ophthalmic solution may be used as a provocative test when latent increased intraocular pressure is suspected. Tension is measured before application of phenylephrine hydrochloride and again after dilatation. A 3 to 5 mm of mercury rise in pressure suggests the presence of angle block in patients with glaucoma; however, failure to obtain such a rise does not preclude the presence of glaucoma from other causes.

Shadow test (retinoscopy) – When dilatation of the pupil without cycloplegic action is desired for the shadow test, phenylephrine hydrochloride 2.5% ophthalmic solution may be used alone.

Blanching test – One or 2 drops of phenylephrine hydrochloride 2.5% ophthalmic solution should be applied to the injected eye. After 5 minutes, examine for perilimbal blanching. If blanching occurs, the congestion is superficial and probably does not indicate iritis.

➤*0.12% solution:* Instill 1 or 2 drops in the affected eye up to 4 times daily.

➤*Storage/Stability:* Prolonged exposure to air or strong light may cause oxidation and discoloration. Do not use if the solution changes color, becomes cloudy, or contains a precipitate.

OXYMETAZOLINE HYDROCHLORIDE

otc	**OcuClear** (Schering-Plough)	**Solution**: 0.025%	In 30 mL.[1]
otc	**Visine L.R.** (Pfizer)		In 15 and 30 mL.[1]

[1] With 0.01% benzalkonium chloride and 0.1% EDTA.

OXYMETAZOLINE HYDROCHLORIDE — OPHTHALMIC

For complete and comparative prescribing information, refer to the Ophthalmic Decongestants group monograph.

Indications

➤*Redness:* For relief of redness of the eye due to minor eye irritations.

Administration and Dosage

➤*Adults and children 6 years of age and older:* Instill 1 or 2 drops in the affected eye(s) every 6 hours.

➤*Storage/Stability:* Do not use if solution changes color or becomes cloudy.

NAPHAZOLINE HYDROCHLORIDE

otc	**20/20 Eye Drops** (S.S.S. Company)	**Drops**: 0.012%	In 15 mL.[a]
otc	**All Clear** (Bausch & Lomb)	**Solution**: 0.012%	In 15 mL.[b]
otc	**Allerest Eye Drops** (Novartis Ophthalmic)		In 15 mL.[c]
otc	**Clear Eyes** (Ross)		In 15 and 30 mL.[a]
otc	**Clear Eyes Seasonal Relief** (Medtech)		In 15 and 30 mL.[d]
otc	**Clear Eyes for Dry Eyes Plus Redness Relief** (Medtech)		In 15 mL.[e]
otc	**Naphcon** (Alcon)		In 15 mL.[f]
otc	**VasoClear** (Novartis Ophthalmics)	**Solution**: 0.02%	In 15 mL.[g]
otc	**All Clear AR** (Bausch & Lomb)	**Solution**: 0.03%	In 15 mL.[h]
otc	**Comfort Eye Drops** (Pilkington/Barnes Hind)		In 15 mL.[i]
otc	**Maximum Strength Allergy Drops** (Bausch & Lomb)		In 15 mL.[h]
Rx	**Naphazoline HCl** (Various, eg, Goldline)	**Solution**: 0.1%	In 15 mL.
Rx	**AK-Con** (Akorn)		In 15 mL.[f]
Rx	**Albalon** (Allergan)		In 15 mL.[j]
Rx	**Nafazair** (Bausch & Lomb)		In 15 mL.[f]
Rx	**Naphcon Forte** (Alcon)		In 15 mL *Drop-Tainers*.[f]

[a] With benzalkonium chloride, EDTA, 0.2% glycerin.
[b] With 0.2% PEG 300, 0.01% benzalkonium chloride, EDTA.
[c] With benzalkonium chloride, EDTA.
[d] With benzalkonium chloride, EDTA, 0.25% zinc sulfate, 0.2% glycerin.
[e] With 0.8% hypromellose, 0.25% glycerin, benzalkonium chloride, EDTA.
[f] With 0.01% benzalkonium chloride, EDTA.
[g] With 0.01% benzalkonium chloride, 0.25% polyvinyl alcohol, 1% PEG-400, EDTA.
[h] With 0.01% benzalkonium chloride, 0.5% hydroxypropyl methylcellulose and EDTA.
[i] With 0.005% benzalkonium chloride and 0.02% EDTA.
[j] With 0.004% benzalkonium chloride, EDTA, 1.4% polyvinyl alcohol.

NAPHAZOLINE HYDROCHLORIDE — OPHTHALMIC

For complete and comparative prescribing information, refer to the Ophthalmic Decongestants group monograph.

Indications

➤*Redness:* To soothe, refresh and remove redness due to minor eye irritations such as smoke, smog, sunglare, wearing contact lenses, allergies or swimming.

Administration and Dosage

Instill 1 or 2 drops into the conjunctival sac of affected eye(s) every 3 to 4 hours, up to 4 times daily.

➤*Storage/Stability:* Do not use if solution changes color or becomes cloudy.

OPHTHALMIC ANTIHISTAMINES

OLOPATADINE HYDROCHLORIDE

Rx	**Patanol** (Alcon)	**Solution**: 0.1%	In 5 mL *Drop-Tainer* dispenser.[a]
Rx	**Olopatadine Hydrochloride** (Alcon)	**Solution**: 0.2%	In 2.5 mL fill in 4 mL bottle.[b]

[a] With benzalkonium chloride.
[b] With benzalkonium chloride 0.01%, EDTA, povidone, dibasic sodium phosphate, sodium chloride, hydrochloric acid/sodium hydroxide.

OLOPATADINE HYDROCHLORIDE — OPHTHALMIC

Indications

➤*Allergic conjunctivitis:* For temporary prevention of itching of the eye due to allergic conjunctivitis.

Administration and Dosage

The recommended dose is 1 to 2 drops in each affected eye 2 times per day at an interval of 6 to 8 hours (0.1% solution); 1 drop in each affected eye once a day (0.2% solution).

➤*Storage/Stability:* Store at 36° to 77°F (2° to 25°C).

Actions

➤*Pharmacology:* Olopatadine is an inhibitor of histamine release from the mast cell and a relatively selective histamine H_1-antagonist that inhibits the in vivo and in vitro type 1 immediate hypersensitivity reaction. Olopatadine is devoid of effects on alpha-adrenergic, dopamine, muscarinic type 1 and 2, and serotonin receptors.

➤*Pharmacokinetics:* Olopatadine has low systemic exposure. Plasma concentrations are generally below the quantitation limit of the assay (less than 0.5 ng/mL). Samples in which olopatadine is quantifiable are typically found within 2 hours of dosing and range from 0.5 to 1.3 ng/mL. The half-life in plasma is approximately 3 hours, and elimination is predominantly through renal excretion. Approximately 60% to 70% of the dose is recovered in the urine as parent drug. Two metabolites, the mono-desmethyl and the N-oxide, were detected at low concentrations in the urine.

Contraindications

Hypersensitivity to any component of this product.

Warnings

➤*Pregnancy: Category C.* Olopatadine was not found to be teratogenic in rats and rabbits. There are no adequate and well controlled studies in pregnant women. Use this drug in pregnant women only if the potential benefit to the mother justifies the potential risk to the embryo or fetus.

➤*Lactation:* Olopatadine has been identified in the milk of nursing rats following oral administration. It is not known whether topical ocular administration could result in sufficient systemic absorption to produce detectable quantities in breast milk. Exercise caution when olopatadine is administered to a nursing mother.

➤*Children:* Safety and effectiveness in pediatric patients younger than 3 years of age have not been established.

Precautions

➤*Administration:* Not for injection. Do not instill olopatadine while wearing contact lenses.

Adverse Reactions

➤*Ophthalmic:* Burning or stinging, dry eye, foreign body sensation, hyperemia, keratitis, lid edema, pruritus (less than 5%).

➤*Miscellaneous:* Headache (7%); asthenia, cold syndrome, pharyngitis, rhinitis, sinusitis, taste perversion (less than 5%).

Patient Information

To prevent contaminating the dropper tip and solution, do not touch the eyelids and surrounding areas with the dropper tip of the bottle.

Keep bottle tightly closed when not in use.

EMEDASTINE DIFUMARATE

Rx	**Emadine** (Alcon)	**Solution**: 0.05%	Benzalkonium chloride. In 5 mL.

EMEDASTINE DIFUMARATE — OPHTHALMIC

Indications

➤*Allergic conjunctivitis:* For the temporary relief of the signs and symptoms of allergic conjunctivitis.

Administration and Dosage

➤*Approved by the FDA:* December 29, 1997.

The recommended dose is 1 drop in the affected eye up to 4 times daily.

➤*Storage/Stability:* Store at 4° to 30°C (39° to 86°F).

EMEDASTINE DIFUMARATE — OPHTHALMIC

Actions

➤*Pharmacology:* Emedastine is a relatively selective, histamine H_1 antagonist. In vitro examinations of emedastine's affinity for histamine receptors (H_1: Ki = 1.3 nM, H_2: Ki = 49,067 nM, and H_3: Ki = 12,430 nM) demonstrate relative selectivity for the H_1 histamine receptor. In vivo studies have shown concentration-dependent inhibition of histamine-stimulated vascular permeability in the conjunctiva following topical ocular administration. Emedastine appears to be devoid of effects on adrenergic, dopaminergic and serotonin receptors.

➤*Pharmacokinetics:*

Absorption – Following topical administration in man, emedastine was shown to have low systemic exposure. In a study involving 10 healthy volunteers dosed bilaterally twice daily for 15 days with emedastine difumarate, plasma concentrations of the parent compound were generally below the quantitation limit of the assay (less than 0.3 ng/mL). Samples in which emedastine was quantifiable ranged from 0.3 to 0.49 ng/mL.

Metabolism/Excretion – The elimination half-life of oral emedastine in plasma is 3 to 4 hours. Approximately 44% of the oral dose is recovered in the urine over 24 hours with only 3.6% of the dose excreted as parent drug. Two primary metabolites, 5- and 6-hydroxyemedastine, are excreted in the urine as both free and conjugated forms. The 5'-oxoanalogs of 5- and 6-hydroxyemedastine and the N-oxide are also formed as minor metabolites.

Contraindications

Hypersensitivity to the solution or any of its components.

Warnings

➤*Administration:* Emedastine difumarate is for topical use only and not for injection or oral use.

➤*Pregnancy: Category B.* Teratology and perinatal and postnatal studies have been conducted with emedastine difumarate in rats and rabbits. At 15,000 times the maximum recommended ocular human use level, emedastine difumarate was shown not to be teratogenic in rats and rabbits and no effects on peri/postnatal development were observed in rats. However, at 70,000 times the maximum recommended ocular human use level, emedastine difumarate was shown to increase the incidence of external, visceral and skeletal anomalies in rats. There are, however, no adequate and well-controlled studies in pregnant women. Because animal studies are not always predictive of human response, this drug should be used during pregnancy only if clearly needed.

➤*Lactation:* Emedastine has been identified in breast milk in rats following oral administration. It is not known whether topical ocular administration could result in sufficient systemic absorption to produce detectable quantities in breast milk. Nevertheless, caution should be exercised when emedastine difumarate is administered to a nursing mother.

➤*Children:* Safety and effectiveness in pediatric patients less than 3 years of age have not been established.

Adverse Reactions

In controlled clinical studies of emedastine difumarate ophthalmic solution 0.05% lasting for 42 days, the most frequent adverse reaction was headache (11%).

➤*Adverse reactions reported in less than 5% of patients:* The following adverse reactions were reported in less than 5% of patients: Abnormal dreams, asthenia, bad taste in the mouth, blurred vision, burning or stinging, corneal infiltrates, corneal staining, dermatitis, discomfort, dry eye, foreign body sensation, hyperemia, keratitis, pruritus, rhinitis, sinusitis and tearing. Some of these events were similar to the underlying disease being studied.

Overdosage

➤*Symptoms:* Somnolence and malaise have been reported following daily oral administration. Oral ingestion of the contents of a 15 mL dispenser would be equivalent to 7.5 mg.

➤*Treatment:* In case of overdosage, treatment is symptomatic and supportive.

Patient Information

To prevent contaminating the dropper tip and solution, care should be taken not to touch the eyelids or surrounding areas with the dropper tip of the bottle. Keep the bottle tightly closed when not in use. Do not use if the solution has become discolored.

Patients should be advised not to wear a contact lens if their eye is red. Emedastine difumarate should not be used to treat contact lens-related irritation. The preservative in emedastine difumarate, benzalkonium chloride, may be absorbed by soft contact lenses. Patients who wear soft contact lenses, and whose eyes are not red, should be instructed to wait at least 10 minutes after instilling emedastine difumarate before they insert their contact lenses.

AZELASTINE HYDROCHLORIDE

Rx	**Optivar** (MedPointe Healthcare[1])	**Solution:** 0.5 mg/mL (equiv. to 0.457 mg azelastine base)	0.125 mg benzalkonium chloride, EDTA dihydrate, hydroxypropylmethylcellulose, sodium hydroxide. In 10 mL containers with 6 mL solution with dropper.

[1] MedPointe Healthcare Inc., 265 Davidson Avenue, Suite 300, Somerset, NJ 08873–4120; (732) 564–2200; http://www.medpointeinc.com.

AZELASTINE HYDROCHLORIDE — OPHTHALMIC

For more comparative information, see Azelastine HCl in the Antihistamines group monograph.

Indications

➤*Allergic conjunctivitis:* For the treatment of itching of the eye associated with allergic conjunctivitis.

Administration and Dosage

➤*Approved by the FDA:* October 1996.

The recommended dose is 1 drop instilled into each affected eye twice a day.

➤*Storage/Stability:* Store upright between 2° and 25°C (36° and 77°F).

Actions

➤*Pharmacology:* Azelastine hydrochloride is a relatively selective histamine H_1 antagonist and an inhibitor of the release of histamine and other mediators from cells (eg, mast cells) involved in the allergic response. Based on in vitro studies using human cell lines, inhibition of other mediators involved in allergic reactions (eg, leukotrienes, PAF) has been demonstrated with azelastine hydrochloride. Decreased chemotaxis and activation of eosinophils has also been demonstrated.

➤*Pharmacokinetics:*

Absorption – Absorption of azelastine following ocular administration was relatively low. A study in symptomatic patients receiving 1 drop of azelastine hydrochloride in each eye 2 to 4 times a day (0.06 to 0.12 mg azelastine hydrochloride) demonstrated plasma concentrations of azelastine hydrochloride to generally be between 0.02 and 0.25 ng/mL after 56 days of treatment. Three of 19 patients had quantifiable amounts of N-desmethylazelastine that ranged from 0.25 to 0.87 ng/mL at day 56.

Metabolism/Excretion – Based on IV and oral administration, the elimination half-life, steady-state volume of distribution and plasma clearance were 22 hours, 14.5 L/kg and 0.5 L/hr/kg, respectively. Approximately 75% of an oral dose of radiolabeled azelastine hydrochloride was excreted in the feces with less than 10% as unchanged azelastine. Azelastine hydrochloride is oxidatively metabolized to the principal metabolite, N-desmethylazelastine, by the cytochrome P450 enzyme system. In vitro studies in human plasma indicate that the plasma protein binding of azelastine and N-desmethylazelastine are approximately 88% and 97%, respectively.

Contraindications

Hypersensitivity to any of its components.

Warnings

➤*Administration:* Azelastine hydrochloride is for ocular use only and not for injection or oral use.

➤*Fertility impairment:* Reproduction and fertility studies in rats showed no effects on male or female fertility at oral doses of up to 25,000 times the maximum recommended ocular human use level. At 68.6 mg/kg/day (57,000 times the maximum recommended ocular human use level), the duration of the estrous cycle was prolonged and copulatory activity and the number of pregnancies were decreased. The numbers of corpora lutea and implantations were decreased; however, the implantation ratio was not affected.

➤*Elderly:* No overall differences in safety or efficacy have been observed between elderly and younger adult patients.

➤*Pregnancy: Category C.*

Teratogenic – Azelastine hydrochloride has been shown to be embryotoxic, fetotoxic, and teratogenic (external and skeletal abnormalities) in mice at an oral dose of 68.6 mg/kg/day (57,000 times the recommended ocular human use level). At an oral dose of 30 mg/kg/day (25,000 times the recommended ocular human use level), delayed ossification (undeveloped metacarpus) and the incidence of 14th rib were increased in rats. At 68.6 mg/kg/day (57,000 times the maximum recommended ocular human use level) azelastine hydrochloride caused resorption and fetotoxic effects in rats. The relevance to humans of these skeletal findings noted at only high drug exposure levels is unknown.

There are no adequate and well-controlled studies in pregnant women. Only use azelastine hydrochloride during pregnancy if the potential benefit justifies the potential risk to the fetus.

➤*Lactation:* It is not known whether azelastine hydrochloride is excreted in human milk. Because many drugs are excreted in human milk, exercise caution when administering azelastine hydrochloride to a nursing woman.

➤*Children:* Safety and efficacy in pediatric patients below the age of 3 years have not been established.

Adverse Reactions

In controlled multiple-dose studies where patients were treated for up to 56 days, the most frequently reported adverse reactions were transient eye burning/stinging (approximately 30%), headaches (approximately 15%) and bitter taste (approximately 10%). The occurrence of these events was generally mild.

AZELASTINE HYDROCHLORIDE — OPHTHALMIC

The following events were reported in 1% to 10% of patients: Asthma, conjunctivitis, dyspnea, eye pain, fatigue, influenza-like symptoms, pharyngitis, pruritus, rhinitis and temporary blurring. Some of these events were similar to the underlying disease being studied.

Patient Information

To prevent contaminating the dropper tip and solution, take care not to touch any surface, the eyelids or surrounding areas with the dropper tip of the bottle. Keep bottle tightly closed when not in use. This product is sterile when packaged.

Advise patients not to wear a contact lens if their eyes are red. Azelastine hydrochloride should not be used to treat contact lens-related irritation. The preservative in azelastine hydrochloride, benzalkonium chloride, may be absorbed by soft contact lenses. Instruct patients who wear soft contact lenses, and whose eyes are not red, to wait at least 10 minutes after instilling azelastine hydrochloride before they insert their contact lenses.

KETOTIFEN FUMARATE

Rx	**Zaditor** (Novartis Pharmaceuticals)	**Solution:** 0.025%	In 5 mL and 7.5 mL.[1]

[1] With glycerol, sodium hydroxide/hydrochloric acid, purified water, and benzalkonium chloride 0.01% as a preservative.

KETOTIFEN FUMARATE — OPHTHALMIC

Indications

➤*Allergic conjunctivitis:* For the temporary prevention of itching of the eye due to allergic conjunctivitis.

Administration and Dosage

➤*Approved by the FDA:* July 2, 1999.

The recommended dose is 1 drop in the affected eye(s) every 8 to 12 hours.

➤*Storage/Stability:* Store at 4° to 25°C (39° to 77°F)

Actions

➤*Pharmacology:* Ketotifen is a relatively selective, noncompetitive histamine antagonist (H_1-receptor) and mast cell stabilizer. Ketotifen inhibits the release of mediators from cells involved in hypersensitivity reactions. Decreased chemotaxis and activation of eosinophils have also been demonstrated.

In human conjunctival allergen-challenge studies, ketotifen fumarate was significantly more effective than placebo in preventing ocular itching associated with allergic conjunctivitis. The action of ketotifen occurs rapidly with an effect seen within minutes after administration.

Contraindications

Hypersensitivity to any component of this product.

Warnings

➤*Administration:* For topical ophthalmic use only. Not for injection or oral use.

➤*Fertility impairment:* Treatment of male rats with oral doses of ketotifen ≥ 10 mg/kg/day orally [6667 times the maximum recommended human ocular dose (MRHOD) of 0.0015 mg/kg/day on a mg/kg basis] for 70 days prior to mating resulted in mortality and a decrease in fertility. Treatment with ketotifen did not impair fertility in female rats receiving up to 50 mg/kg/day of ketotifen orally (33,333 times the MRHOD) for 15 days prior to mating.

➤*Pregnancy: Category C.* Oral treatment of pregnant rabbits during organogenesis with 45 mg/kg/day of ketotifen (30,000 times the MRHOD) resulted in an increased incidence of retarded ossification of the sternebrae. However, no effects were observed in rabbits treated with up to 15 mg/kg/day (10,000 times the MRHOD). Similar treatment of rats during organogenesis with 100 mg/kg/day of ketotifen (66,667 times the MRHOD) did not reveal any biologically relevant effects.

Oral treatment of pregnant rats (up to 100 mg/kg/day or 66,667 times the MRHOD) and rabbits (up to 45 mg/kg/day or 30,000 times the MRHOD) during organogenesis did not result in any biologically relevant embryofetal toxicity. In the offspring of the rats that received ketotifen orally from day 15 of pregnancy to day 21 postpartum at 50 mg/kg/day (33,333 times the MRHOD), a maternally toxic treatment protocol, the incidence of postnatal mortality was slightly increased, and body weight gain during the first 4 days postpartum was slightly decreased.

There are no adequate and well-controlled studies in pregnant women. Use during pregnancy only if the potential benefits outweigh the potential hazards to the fetus.

➤*Lactation:* Ketotifen fumarate has been identified in breast milk in rats following oral administration. It is not known whether topical ocular administration could result in sufficient systemic absorption to produce detectable quantities in breast milk. Nevertheless, caution should be exercised when ketotifen fumarate is administered to a nursing mother.

➤*Children:* Safety and efficacy in pediatric patients under the age of 3 years have not been established.

Adverse Reactions

In controlled clinical studies, conjunctival injection, headaches, and rhinitis were reported at an incidence of 10% to 25%. The occurrence of these side effects was generally mild. Some of these events were similar to the underlying ocular disease being studied.

The following ocular and nonocular adverse reactions were reported at an incidence of less than 5%:

➤*Ophthalmic:* Allergic reactions, burning or stinging, conjunctivitis, discharge, dry eyes, eye pain, eyelid disorder, itching, keratitis, lacrimation disorder, mydriasis, photophobia, and rash.

➤*Miscellaneous:* Flu syndrome, pharyngitis.

Overdosage

➤*Symptoms:* Oral ingestion of the contents of a 5 mL bottle would be equivalent to 1.725 mg of ketotifen fumarate. Clinical results have shown no serious signs or symptoms after the ingestion of up to 20 mg of ketotifen fumarate.

Patient Information

To prevent contaminating the dropper tip and solution, care should be taken not to touch the eyelids or surrounding areas with the dropper tip of the bottle. Keep the bottle tightly closed when not in use. Patients should be advised not to wear a contact lens if their eye is red. Ketotifen fumarate ophthalmic solution should not be used to treat contact lens-related irritation. The preservative in ketotifen fumarate ophthalmic solution, benzalkonium chloride, may be absorbed by soft contact lenses. Patients who wear soft contact lenses and whose eyes are not red, should be instructed to wait at least 10 minutes after instilling ketotifen fumarate ophthalmic solution before they insert their contact lenses.

EPINASTINE HYDROCHLORIDE

Rx	**Elestat** (Allergan)	**Solution, ophthalmic:** 0.05%	0.01% benzalkonium chloride, EDTA. In 8 and 15 mL.

EPINASTINE HYDROCHLORIDE — OPHTHALMIC

Indications

➤*Allergic conjunctavitis:* For the prevention of itching associated with allergic conjunctivitis.

Administration and Dosage

➤*Approved by the FDA:* October 16, 2003.

The recommended dosage is 1 drop in each eye twice a day.

Continue treatment throughout the period of exposure (ie, until the pollen season is over or until exposure to the offending allergen is terminated), even when symptoms are absent.

➤*Storage/Stability:* Store at 15° to 25°C (59° to 77°F). Keep bottle tightly closed and out of the reach of children.

Actions

➤*Pharmacology:* Epinastine is a topically active, direct H_1-receptor antagonist and an inhibitor of the release of histamine from the mast cell. Epinastine is selective for the histamine H_1-receptor and has affinity for the histamine H_2 receptor. Epinastine also possesses affinity for the α_1-, α_2-, and 5-HT_2-receptors. Epinastine does not penetrate the blood/brain barrier and, therefore, is not expected to induce side effects of the central nervous system.

➤*Pharmacokinetics:*

Absorption/Distribution – Fourteen subjects, with allergic conjunctivitis, received 1 drop of epinastine in each eye twice daily for 7 days. On day 7, average maximum epinastine plasma concentrations of 0.04 ± 0.014 ng/mL were reached after about 2 hours, indicating low systemic exposure. While these concentrations represented an increase over those seen following a single dose, the day 1 and day 7 area under the curve (AUC) values were unchanged, indicating that there is no increase in systemic absorption with multiple dosing. Epinastine is 64% bound to plasma proteins.

Metabolism/Excretion – The total systemic clearance is approximately 56 L/hr and the terminal plasma elimination half-life is about 12 hours. Epinastine is mainly excreted unchanged. About 55% of an intravenous dose is recovered unchanged in the urine with about 30% in feces. Less than 10% is metabolized. The renal elimination is mainly via active tubular secretion.

Contraindications

Hypersensitivity to epinastine or to any of the other ingredients.

EPINASTINE HYDROCHLORIDE — OPHTHALMIC

Warnings

➤*Administration:* Epinastine hydrochloride is for topical ophthalmic use only and not for injection or oral use.

➤*Mutagenesis:* Epinastine in newly synthesized batches was negative for mutagenicity in the Ames/*Salmonella* assay and in vitro chromosome aberration assay using human lymphocytes. Positive results were seen with early batches of epinastine in 2 in vitro chromosomal aberration studies conducted in 1980s with human peripheral lymphocytes and with V79 cells, respectively. Epinastine was negative in the in vivo clastogenicity studies, including the mouse micronucleus assay and chromosome aberration assay in Chinese hamsters. Epinastine was also negative in the cell transformation assay using Syrian hamster embryo cells, V79/HGPRT mammalian cell point mutation assay, and in vivo/in vitro unscheduled DNA synthesis assay using rat primary hepatocytes.

➤*Fertility impairment:* Epinastine had no effect on fertility of male rats. Decreased fertility in female rats was observed at an oral dose up to approximately 90,000 times the MROHD.

➤*Elderly:* No overall differences in safety or effectiveness have been observed between elderly and younger patients.

➤*Pregnancy: Category C.* There are, however, no adequate and well-controlled studies in pregnant women. Because animal reproduction studies are not always predictive of human response, epinastine ophthalmic solution should be used during pregnancy only if the potential benefit justifies the potential risk to the fetus.

Teratogenic – In an embryofetal developmental study in pregnant rats, maternal toxicity with no embryofetal effects was observed at an oral dose that was approximately 150,000 times the MROHD. Total resorptions and abortion were observed in an embryofetal study in pregnant rabbits at an oral dose that was approximately 55,000 times the MROHD. In both studies, no drug-induced teratogenic effects were noted.

Epinastine reduced pup body weight gain following an oral dose to pregnant rats that was approximately 90,000 times the MROHD.

➤*Lactation:* A study in lactating rats revealed excretion of epinastine in the breast milk. It is not known whether this drug is excreted in human milk. Because many drugs are excreted in human milk, caution should be exercised when epinastine ophthalmic solution is administered to a nursing woman.

➤*Children:* Safety and effectiveness in pediatric patients younger than the age of 3 years have not been established.

Precautions

➤*Contact lenses:* Advise patients not to wear a contact lenses if their eyes are red. Do not use epinastine to treat contact-lens-related irritation. The preservative in epinastine, benzalkonium chloride, may be absorbed by soft contact lenses. Contact lenses should be removed prior to instillation of epinastine and may be reinserted after 10 minutes following its administration.

➤*Administration:* Instruct patients to avoid allowing the tip of the dispensing container to contact the eye, surrounding structures, fingers, or any other surface in order to avoid contamination of the solution by common bacteria known to cause ocular infections. Serious damage to the eye and subsequent loss of vision may result from using contaminated solutions. Keep bottle tightly closed when not in use.

Adverse Reactions

The most frequently reported ocular adverse events occurring in approximately 1% to 10% of patients were burning sensation in the eye, folliculosis, hyperemia, and pruritus.

The most frequently reported non-ocular adverse events were infection (cold symptoms and upper respiratory tract infections) seen in approximately 10% of patients, and headache, rhinitis, sinusitis, increased cough, and pharyngitis seen in approximately 1% to 3% of patients.

Some of these events were similar to the underlying disease being studied.

Patient Information

Advise patients not to wear a contact lenses if their eyes are red. Do not use epinastine hydrochloride ophthalmic solution to treat contact-lens-related irritation. The preservative in epinastine, benzalkonium chloride, may be absorbed by soft contact lenses. Contact lenses should be removed prior to instillation of epinastine and may be reinserted after 10 minutes following its administration.

Instruct patients to avoid allowing the tip of the dispensing container to contact the eye, surrounding structures, fingers, or any other surface in order to avoid contamination of the solution by common bacteria known to cause ocular infections. Serious damage to the eye and subsequent loss of vision may result from using contaminated solutions.

Keep bottle closed tightly when not in use.

OPHTHALMIC DECONGESTANT/ANTIHISTAMINE COMBINATIONS

OPHTHALMIC DECONGESTANT/ANTIHISTAMINE COMBINATIONS

	Product & Distributor	Decongestant	Antihistamine	How Supplied
otc	**Zincfrin Solution** (Alcon)	phenylephrine HCl 0.12%		In 15 and 30 mL *Drop-Tainers.*[a]
otc	**Naphazoline HCl & Pheniramine Maleate Solution** (Various, eg, Moore)	naphazoline HCl 0.025%	pheniramine maleate 0.3%	In 15 mL.
otc	**Naphazoline Plus Solution** (Parmed)			In 15 mL.[b]
otc	**Naphcon-A Solution** (Alcon)			In 15 mL *Drop-Tainers.*[b]
otc	**Visine-A** (Pfizer Consumer Health)			EDTA. In 15 mL.
otc	**Opcon-A Solution** (Bausch & Lomb)	naphazoline HCl 0.027%	pheniramine maleate 0.315%	In 15 mL.[c]
otc	**Naphazoline HCl & Antazoline Phosphate Sodium** (Various, eg, Moore, Steris)	naphazoline HCl 0.05%	antazoline phosphate 0.5%	In 5 and 15 mL.
otc	**Visine Allergy Relief** (Pfizer)	tetrahydrozoline HCl 0.05%		In 15 and 30 mL.[d]
otc	**Geneye AC Allergy Formula** (Goldline)			In 15 mL.[e]

[a] With 0.01% benzalkonium Cl, polysorbate 80, 0.25% zinc sulfate.
[b] With 0.01% benzalkonium Cl, EDTA.
[c] With 0.5% hydroxypropyl methylcellulose, 0.01% benzalkonium CL, 0.1% EDTA, boric acid.
[d] With 0.01% benzalkonium Cl, 0.1% EDTA, 0.25% zinc sulfate.
[e] With 0.01% benzalkonium Cl, EDTA, 0.25% zinc sulfate.

OPHTHALMIC DECONGESTANT/ANTIHISTAMINE COMBINATIONS — OPHTHALMIC

Indications

➤*Itching/Redness:* Temporary relief of the minor eye symptoms of itching and redness caused by pollen, animal hair, etc.

Administration and Dosage

Recommendations vary. Refer to manufacturer package insert for instructions.

Warnings

➤*Antihistamines:* Topical antihistamines are potential sensitizers and may produce a local sensitivity reaction. Because they may produce angle closure, use with caution in persons with a narrow angle or a history of glaucoma.

CYCLOPLEGIC MYDRIATICS

Refer to the Topical Ophthalmic Drugs introduction for more complete and comparative information.

Indications

➤*Mydriasis/Cycloplegia:* For cycloplegic refraction and for dilating the pupil in inflammatory conditions of the iris and uveal tract. See individual monographs for specific indications.

Actions

➤*Pharmacology:* Anticholinergic agents block the responses of the sphincter muscle of the iris and the muscle of the ciliary body to cholinergic stimulation, producing pupillary dilation (mydriasis) and paralysis of accommodation (cycloplegia).

Cycloplegic Mydriatics

	Mydriasis		Cycloplegia		
Drug	Peak (min)	Recovery (days)	Peak (min)	Recovery (days)	Solution available
Atropine	30 - 40	7 - 10	60 - 180	6 - 12	0.5% - 2%
Homatropine	40 - 60	1 - 3	30 - 60	1 - 3	2% - 5%
Scopolamine	20 - 30	3 - 7	30 - 60	3 - 7	0.25%
Cyclopentolate	30 - 60	1	25 - 75	.25 - 1	0.5% - 2%
Tropicamide	20 - 40	0.25	20 - 35	< 0.25	0.5% - 1%

Contraindications

Primary glaucoma or a tendency toward glaucoma (eg, narrow anterior chamber angle); hypersensitivity to belladonna alkaloids or any component of the products; adhesions (synechiae) between the iris and the lens; children who have previously had a severe systemic reaction to atropine.

Warnings

For topical ophthalmic use only. Not for injection.

➤*Glaucoma:* Determine the intraocular tension and the depth of the angle of the anterior chamber before and during use to avoid glaucoma attacks.

➤*Elderly:* Use these products with caution in the elderly and others where increased IOP may be encountered.

➤*Pregnancy: Category C* (atropine, homatropine). Safety for use during pregnancy has not been established. Give to a pregnant woman only if clearly needed.

➤*Lactation:* Atropine and homatropine may be detectable, in very small amounts, in breast milk. Although this is controversial, according to the American Academy of Pediatrics, these agents are compatible with breastfeeding. It is not known if cyclopentolate is excreted in breast milk. Exercise caution when administering to a nursing woman.

➤*Children:* Excessive use in children and in certain susceptible individuals may product systemic toxic symptoms. Use with extreme caution in infants and small children.

Tropicamide and cyclopentolate may cause CNS disturbances, which may be dangerous in infants and children. Keep in mind the possibility of occurrence of psychotic reaction and behavioral disturbance due to hypersensitivity to anticholinergic drugs. Use with extreme caution. Increased susceptibility to cyclopentolate has been reported in infants, young children and in children with spastic paralysis or brain damage. Feeding intolerance may follow ophthalmic use of this product in neonates. It is recommended that feeding be withheld for 4 hours after examination. Do not use in concentrations > 0.5% in small infants.

Precautions

➤*Systemic effects:* Avoid excessive systemic absorption by compressing the lacrimal sac by digital pressure for 1 to 3 minutes after instillation.

➤*Down's syndrome/children with brain damage:* Use cycloplegics with caution. These patients may demonstrate a hyperreactive response to topical atropine.

➤*Hazardous tasks:* May produce drowsiness, blurred vision or sensitivity to light (due to dilated pupils); observe caution while driving or performing other tasks requiring alertness, coordination or physical dexterity.

➤*Sulfite sensitivity:* Some of these products contain sulfites which may cause allergic-type reactions (eg, hives, itching, wheezing, anaphylaxis) in certain susceptible persons. Although the overall prevalence of sulfite sensitivity in the general population is probably low, it is seen more frequently in asthmatics or in atopic nonasthmatic persons. Specific products containing sulfites are identified in the product listings.

Adverse Reactions

➤*Local:* Increased intraocular pressure; transient stinging/burning; irritation with prolonged use (eg, allergic lid reactions, hyperemia, follicular conjunctivitis, blepharoconjunctivitis, vascular congestion, edema, exudate, eczematoid dermatitis).

➤*Systemic:* Dryness of the mouth and skin; blurred vision; photophobia with or without corneal staining; tachycardia; headache; parasympathetic stimulation; somnolence; visual hallucinations.

Other toxic manifestations of anticholinergic drugs include: Skin rash; abdominal distention in infants; unusual drowsiness; hyperpyrexia; vasodilation; urinary retention; diminished GI motility; decreased secretion in salivary and sweat glands, pharynx, bronchii and nasal passages. Severe manifestations of toxicity include: Coma; medullary paralysis; death. Severe reactions are manifested by hypotension with progressive respiratory depression.

Cyclopentolate and tropicamide have been associated with psychotic reactions and behavioral disturbances in children. CNS disturbances have occurred in children on tropicamide. Ataxia, incoherent speech, restlessness, hallucinations, hyperactivity, seizures, disorientation as to time and place, and failure to recognize people have occurred with cyclopentolate.

Overdosage

➤*Ocular:* If ocular overdosage occurs, flush eye(s) with water or normal saline. Use of a topical miotic may be required. If accidentally ingested, induce emesis or gastric lavage.

➤*Systemic:* If symptoms develop (see Adverse Reactions), patients usually recover spontaneously when the drug is discontinued. In cases of severe toxicity, give physostigmine salicylate (see individual monograph). Have atropine (1 mg) available for immediate injection if physostigmine causes bradycardia, convulsions or bronchoconstriction.

➤*Cyclopentolate toxicity:* Cyclopentolate toxicity may cause exaggerated symptoms (see Adverse Reactions). When administration of the drug product is discontinued, the patient usually recovers spontaneously. In case of severe manifestation of toxicity, the antidote of choice is physostigmine salicylate.

Children – Slowly inject 0.5 mg physostigmine salicylate IV. If toxic symptoms persist and no cholinergic symptoms are produced, repeat at 5 minute intervals to a maximum cumulative dose of 2 mg.

Adults and adolescents – Slowly inject 2 mg physostigmine salicylate IV. A second dose of 1 to 2 mg may be given after 20 minutes if no reversal of toxic manifestations has occurred.

Patient Information

To avoid contamination, do not touch dropper tip to any surface. Replace cap after using.

May cause blurred vision. Do not drive or engage in any hazardous activities while the pupils are dilated.

May cause sensitivity to light. Protect eyes in bright illumination during dilation.

Keep out of the reach of children. These drugs should not be taken orally. Wash your own hands and the child's following administration.

If eye pain occurs, discontinue use and consult physician immediately.

Refer to the Topical Ophthalmics Introduction for more complete information on administration and use.

ATROPINE SULFATE

Rx	**Atropine Sulfate Ophthalmic** (Various, eg, Bausch & Lomb, Goldline)	**Ointment:** 1%	In 3.5 and UD 1 g.
Rx	**Isopto Atropine** (Alcon)	**Solution:** 0.5%	In 5 mL *Drop-Tainers.*[1]
Rx	**Atropine Sulfate** (Various, eg, Alcon)	**Solution:** 1%	In 2, 5 and 15 mL and UD 1 mL.
Rx	**Atropine-1** (Optopics)		In 2, 5 and 15 mL.
Rx	**Isopto Atropine** (Alcon)		In 5 and 15 mL *Drop-Tainers.*[1]
Rx	**Atropine Sulfate** (Alcon)	**Solution:** 2%	In 2 mL.

[1] With 0.01% benzalkonium chloride, 0.5% hydroxypropyl methylcellulose and boric acid.
[2] With 0.01% benzalkonium chloride, hydroxypropyl methylcellulose and boric acid.
[3] With benzalkonium chloride, EDTA and boric acid.

ATROPINE SULFATE — OPHTHALMIC

For complete and comparative prescribing information, refer to the Cycloplegic Mydriatics group monograph.

Indications

➤*Mydriasis/Cycloplegia:* For mydriasis or cycloplegia. For cycloplegic refraction, for pupillary dilation desired in inflammatory conditions of the iris and uveal tract.

Administration and Dosage

➤*Solution:* 1 or 2 drops in the eye(s) 3 times a day or as directed by a physician.

➤*Ointment:* A small amount in the conjunctival sac once or twice a day or as directed by a physician.

➤*Storage/Stability:* Store between 15° to 30°C (59° to 86°F). Use solution only if imprinted neckband is intact. Use ointment only if bottom ridge of tube cap is not exposed.

Keep out of reach of children.

SCOPOLAMINE HBr (Hyoscine HBr)

Rx	**Isopto Hyoscine** (Alcon)	**Solution:** 0.25%	In 5 and 15 mL *Drop-Tainers.*[1]

[1] With 0.01% benzalkonium chloride and 0.5% hydroxypropyl methylcellulose.

SCOPOLAMINE HBr (Hyoscine HBr) — OPHTHALMIC

For complete and comparative prescribing information, refer to the Cycloplegic Mydriatics group monograph.

Indications

➤*Mydriasis/Cycloplegia:* For cycloplegia and mydriasis in diagnostic procedures.

➤*Iridocyclitis:* For preoperative and postoperative states in the treatment of iridocyclitis.

Administration and Dosage

➤*Uveitis:* Instill 1 or 2 drops into the eye(s) up to 4 times daily.

➤*Refraction:* Instill 1 or 2 drops into the eye(s) 1 hour before refracting.

Compress the lacrimal sac by digital pressure for several minutes after instillation.

➤*Storage/Stability:* Protect from light. Store at 8° to 27°C (46° to 80°F).

HOMATROPINE HYDROBROMIDE

Rx	**Isopto Homatropine** (Alcon)	**Solution:** 2%	In 5 and 15 mL *Drop-Tainers.*[1]
Rx	**Homatropine HBr** (Various, eg, Alcon, Novartis Ophthalmics)	**Solution:** 5%	In 1, 2 and 5 mL.
Rx	**Isopto Homatropine** (Alcon)		In 5 and 15 mL *Drop-Tainers.*[1]

[1] With 0.01% benzalkonium chloride, 0.5% hydroxypropylmethylcellulose and polysorbate 80.

HOMATROPINE HYDROBROMIDE — OPHTHALMIC

For complete and comparative prescribing information, refer to the Cycloplegic Mydriatics group monograph.

Indications

For treatment of iritis and iridocyclitis, for relief of ciliary spasm, and also as an aid in refraction. It is frequently employed as a cycloplegic and mydriatic in preoperative and postoperative conditions.

Administration and Dosage

Usual dosage is 1 or 2 drops of the 2% or 5% solution in the eye(s) 2 or 3 times a day, modified at discretion of the physician.

Individuals with heavily pigmented irides may require larger doses.

➤*For refraction:* One or 2 drops of the 2% solution every 10 to 15 minutes for 5 doses or 1 or 2 drops of the 5% solution repeated in 15 minutes, modified at discretion of the physician.

➤*Children:* Use only the 2% strength.

➤*Storage/Stability:* Store at 15° to 30°C (5946° to 86°F).

TROPICAMIDE

Rx	**Tropicamide** (Various, eg, Bausch & Lomb)	**Solution:** 0.5%	In 2 and 15 mL.
Rx	**Mydriacyl** (Alcon)		In 15 mL *Drop-Tainers.*[1]
Rx	**Tropicacyl** (Akorn)		In 15 mL.[2]
Rx	**Tropicamide** (Various, eg, Bausch & Lomb)	**Solution:** 1%	In 15 mL.
Rx	**Mydriacyl** (Alcon)		In 3 and 15 mL *Drop-Tainers.*[1]
Rx	**Tropicacyl** (Akorn)		In 2 and 15 mL.[2]

[1] With 0.01% benzalkonium chloride and EDTA.
[2] With 0.1% benzalkonium chloride and EDTA.

TROPICAMIDE — OPHTHALMIC

For complete and comparative prescribing information, refer to the Cycloplegic Mydriatics group monograph.

Indications

➤*Mydriasis/Cycloplegia:* For mydriasis and cycloplegia for diagnostic procedures.

Administration and Dosage

➤*Approved by the FDA:* August 9, 1982.

For refraction, instill 1 or 2 drops of 1% solution in the eye(s); repeat in 5 minutes. If patient is not seen within 20 to 30 minutes, an additional drop may be instilled to prolong mydriatic effect. For examination of fundus, instill 1 or 2 drops of 0.5% solution 15 or 20 minutes prior to examination. Individuals with heavily pigmented irides may require higher strength or more doses. Mydriasis will reverse spontaneously with time, typically in 4 to 8 hours. However, in some cases, complete recovery may take up to 24 hours.

➤*Storage/Stability:* Store between 15° to 30°C (59° to 86°F). Do not refrigerate or store at high temperatures. Keep container closed tightly .

Do not use if imprinted neckband is not intact.

CYCLOPENTOLATE HYDROCHLORIDE

Rx	**Cyclogyl** (Alcon)	**Solution:** 0.5%	In 2, 5 and 15 mL *Drop-Tainers.*[1]
Rx	**Cyclopentolate HCl** (Various, eg, Steris)	**Solution:** 1%	In 2, 5 and 15 mL.
Rx	**AK-Pentolate** (Akorn)		In 1 and 15 mL.[1]
Rx	**Cyclogyl** (Alcon)		In 2, 5 and 15 mL.[1]
Rx	**Pentolair** (Bausch & Lomb)		In 2 and 15 mL squeeze bottles.[2]
Rx	**Cyclogyl** (Alcon)	**Solution:** 2%	In 2, 5 and 15 mL *Drop-Tainers.*[1]

[1] With 0.01% benzalkonium chloride, EDTA and boric acid.
[2] With 0.01% benzalkonium chloride and EDTA.

CYCLOPENTOLATE HYDROCHLORIDE — OPHTHALMIC

For complete and comparative prescribing information, refer to the Cycloplegic Mydriatics group monograph.

Indications

➤*Mydriasis/Cycloplegia:* Used to produce mydriasis and cycloplegia in diagnostic procedures.

Administration and Dosage

➤*Adults:* 1 or 2 drops of 0.5%, 1% or 2% solution in the eye, which may be repeated in 5 to 10 minutes if necessary. Complete recovery usually occurs in 24 hours. Complete recovery from mydriasis in some individuals may require several days.

➤*Children:* 1 or 2 drops of 0.5%, 1% or 2% solution in the eye which may be repeated 5 to 10 minutes later by a second application of 0.5% or 1% solution if necessary.

➤*Small infants:* A single instillation of 1 drop of 0.5% cyclopentolate in the eye. To minimize absorption, apply pressure over the nasolacrimal sac for 2 to 3 minutes. Observe infant closely for at least 30 minutes following instillation. Individuals with heavily pigmented irides may require higher strengths.

Individuals with heavily pigmented irides may require higher strengths.

➤*Storage/Stability:* Store at 8° to 27°C (46° to 80°F).

MYDRIATIC COMBINATIONS

Rx	**Cyclomydril** (Alcon)	**Solution:** 0.2% cyclopentolate HCl/1% phenylephrine HCl.	In 2 and 5 mL *Drop-Tainers.*[1]
Rx	**Murocoll-2** (Bausch & Lomb)	**Drops:** 0.3% scopolamine HBr/10% phenylephrine HCl.	In 5 mL.[2]

[1] With 0.01% benzalkonium chloride, EDTA and boric acid.
[2] With 0.01% benzalkonium chloride, sodium metabisulfite and EDTA.

MYDRIATIC COMBINATIONS — OPHTHALMIC

These combinations induce mydriasis that is considerably greater than that of either drug alone. See individual monographs for complete prescribing information.

Indications

➤*Cyclomydril:* Producation of mydriasis.

➤*Murocoll-2:* For mydriasis, cycloplegia and to break posterior synechiae in iritis.

Administration and Dosage

➤*Cyclomydril:* Instill 1 drop into each eye every 5 to 10 minutes, not to exceed 3 times.

➤*Murocoll-2:*

Mydriasis – 1 or 2 drops into eye(s); repeat in 5 minutes, if necessary.

Postoperatively – 1 or 2 drops into the eye(s) 3 or 4 times daily.

ANTIBIOTICS

Refer to the Topical Ophthalmic Drugs introduction for more complete information.

Indications

➤*Ocular infections:* Treatment of superficial ocular infections involving the conjunctiva or cornea (eg, conjunctivitis, keratitis, keratoconjunctivitis, corneal ulcers, blepharitis, blepharoconjunctivitis, acute meibomianitis and dacryocystitis) caused by strains of microorganisms susceptible to antibiotics.

➤*Erythromycin:* Prophylaxis of ophthalmia neonatorum due to Neisseria gonorrhoeae or Chlamydia trachomatis.

➤*Chloramphenicol:* Use only in those serious infections for which less potentially dangerous drugs are ineffective or contraindicated (see Warnings).

For a list of microorganisms usually susceptible to these agents, refer to systemic monographs in the Anti-infectives chapter.

Topical Ophthalmic Antibiotic Preparations

		Miscellaneous							Quinolones		Aminoglycosides			Sulfonamides	
	Organism/Infection	Bacitracin	Gramicidin	Polymyxin B	Erythromycin	Chloramphenicol	Trimethoprim	Oxytetracycline	Ciprofloxacin	Ofloxacin	Neomycin	Gentamicin	Tobramycin	Sodium Sulfacetamide	Sulfisoxazole
Gram-positive	*Staphylococcus sp.*	✓	✓						✓	✓		✓	✓		
	S. aureus	✓	✓		✓	✓	✓		✓	✓	✓	✓[a]	✓	✓	✓
	Streptococcus sp.	✓	✓			✓			✓	✓			✓	✓	✓
	S. pneumoniae	✓	✓		✓	✓	✓		✓	✓		✓[a]	✓	✓	✓
	α-*hemolytic streptococci* (viridans group)				✓									✓	✓
	β-*hemolytic streptococci*	✓										✓[a]	✓		
	S. pyogenes	✓			✓		✓		✓	✓		✓		✓	✓
	Corynebacterium sp.	✓	✓		✓						✓	✓	✓		
Gram-negative	*Escherichia coli*			✓		✓	✓	✓	✓	✓	✓	✓	✓	✓	✓
	Haemophilus aegyptius					✓	✓		✓	✓		✓	✓	✓	✓
	H. ducreyi					✓		✓	✓			✓	✓		
	H. influenzae or parainfluenzae			✓	✓	✓	✓	✓	✓	✓	✓	✓	✓	✓	✓
	Klebsiella sp					✓		✓	✓	✓	✓	✓	✓	✓	✓
	K. pneumoniae			✓			✓		✓	✓		✓	✓		
	Neisseria sp	✓				✓			✓		✓	✓	✓		
	N. gonorrhoeae	✓			✓[b]				✓	✓		✓	✓	✓	
	Proteus sp.						✓		✓	✓	✓	✓	✓	✓	✓
	Acinetobacter calcoaceticus								✓	✓		✓	✓		
	Enterobacter aerogenes			✓			✓	✓	✓	✓	✓	✓	✓		
	Enterobacter sp.					✓			✓	✓	✓	✓	✓	✓	✓
	Serratia marcescens						✓		✓	✓		✓	✓		
	Moraxella sp.					✓				✓		✓	✓		
	Chlamydia trachomatis				✓[b]				✓	✓				✓	✓
	Pasteurella tularensis							✓							
	Pseudomonas aeruginosa			✓					✓	✓		✓[a]	✓		
	Bartonella bacilliformis							✓							
	Bacteroides sp.							✓							
	Vibrio sp					✓		✓	✓	✓	✓	✓	✓	✓	
	Providencia sp.								✓						

[a] Increasing resistance has been seen.

[b] For prophylaxis.

Administration and Dosage

Administration and dosage varies for the individual products. Refer to the individual manufacturer inserts.

Contraindications

Hypersensitivity to any component of these products; epithelial herpes simplex keratitis (dendritic keratitis); vaccinia; varicella; mycobacterial infections of the eye; fungal diseases of the ocular structure; use of steroid combinations after uncomplicated removal of a corneal foreign body.

Warnings

➤*Sensitization:* Sensitization from the topical use of an antibiotic may contraindicate the drug's later systemic use in serious infections. For this reason, topical preparations containing antibiotics not ordinarily administered systemically are preferable.

Products with neomycin sulfate may cause cutaneous/conjunctival sensitization.

➤*Cross-sensitivity:* Allergic cross-reactions may occur that could prevent future use of any or all of the following antibiotics: kanamycin, neomycin, paromomycin, streptomycin, and possibly, gentamicin.

➤*Hematopoietic toxicity:* Hematopoietic toxicity has occurred occasionally with the systemic use of **chloramphenicol** and rarely with topical administration. It generally is a dose-related toxic effect on bone marrow, and usually is reversible on cessation of therapy. Rare cases of aplastic anemia, bone marrow hypoplasia, and death have been reported with prolonged (months to years) or frequent intermittent (over months and years) use of ocular chloramphenicol.

➤*Corneal healing:* Ophthalmic ointments may retard corneal epithelial healing.

➤*Pregnancy: Category B* (erythromycin, tobramycin), *Category C* (gentamicin, ciprofloxacin, ofloxacin, polymyxin B). Safety for use during pregnancy has not been established. Use only when clearly needed and when the potential benefits outweigh the potential hazards to the fetus.

➤*Lactation:* It is not known whether **ciprofloxacin** or **ofloxacin** appears in breast milk following ophthalmic use. Exercise caution when administering **ciprofloxacin** to a breast-feeding mother. Because of the potential for adverse reactions in breast-feeding infants from **ofloxacin, chloramphenicol**, and **tobramycin,** decide whether to discontinue breast-feeding or discontinue the drug, taking into account the importance of the drug to the mother.

➤*Children:* **Tobramycin** is safe and effective in children. Safety and efficacy of **fluoroquinolones** in infants younger than 1 year of age, and **polymyxin B/trimethoprim** in infants younger than 2 months have not been established.

Precautions

➤*Monitoring:* Perform culture and susceptibility testing during treatment.

➤*Systemic antibiotics:* In all except very superficial infections, supplement the topical use of antibiotics with appropriate systemic medication. Systemic aminoglycoside antibiotics require monitoring the total serum concentration (peak and trough).

➤*Crystalline precipitate:* A white crystalline precipitate located in the superficial portion of the corneal defect was observed in approximately 17% of patients on **ciprofloxacin**. Onset was within 1 to 7 days after starting therapy. The precipitate resolved in most patients within 2 weeks, and did not preclude continued use or adversely affect the clinical course or outcome.

➤*Superinfection:* Do not use topical antibiotics in deep-seated ocular infections or in those that are likely to become systemic. Use of antibiotics (especially prolonged or repeated therapy) may result in bacterial or fungal overgrowth of nonsusceptible organisms. Such overgrowth may lead to a secondary infection. Take appropriate measures if superinfection occurs.

➤*Sulfite sensitivity:* Some of these products contain sulfites that may cause allergic-type reactions (eg, hives, itching, wheezing, anaphylaxis) in certain susceptible people. Although the overall prevalence of sulfite sensitivity in the general population is probably low, it is seen more frequently in asthmatics or in atopic nonasthmatic people. Specific products containing sulfites are identified in the product listings.

Adverse Reactions

Sensitivity reactions such as transient irritation, burning, stinging, itching, inflammation, angioneurotic edema, urticaria, and vesicular and maculopapular dermatitis have occurred in some patients.

➤*Chloramphenicol:* Hematological reactions (including aplastic anemia) have been reported (see Warnings).

➤*Fluoroquinolones:* White crystalline precipitates; lid margin crusting; crystals/scales; foreign body sensation; conjunctival hyperemia; bad/bitter taste in mouth; corneal staining; keratopathy/keratitis; allergic reactions; lid edema; tearing; photophobia; corneal infiltrates; nausea; decreased vision; chemosis.

➤*Aminoglycosides:* Localized ocular toxicity and hypersensitivity, lid itching, lid swelling, and conjunctival erythema (less than 3% with tobramycin); bacterial/fungal corneal ulcers; nonspecific conjunctivitis; conjunctival epithelial defects; conjunctival hyperemia (gentamicin). Similar reactions may occur with the topical use of other aminoglycoside antibiotics.

Overdosage

➤*Symptoms:* Symptoms of tobramycin overdose include punctate keratitis, erythema, increased lacrimation, edema, and lid itching. These may be similar to adverse reactions.

➤*Treatment:* A topical overdose of **ciprofloxacin** may be flushed from the eyes with warm tap water.

Patient Information

Instruct patient to tilt head back, place medication in conjunctival sac, and close eyes. Patients should apply light finger pressure on lacrimal sac for 1 minute following instillation.

May cause temporary blurring of vision or stinging following administration. Advise patient to notify health care provider if stinging, burning, or itching becomes pronounced or if redness, irritation, swelling, decreasing vision, or pain persists or worsens.

To avoid contamination, instruct patient to not touch tip of container to any surface and replace cap after using.

In general, patients being treated for bacterial conjunctivitis should not wear contact lenses; however, if the health care provider considers contact lens use appropriate, wait at least 15 minutes after using any solutions containing benzalkonium chloride before inserting the lens, as it may be absorbed by the lens.

➤*Quinolones:* Advise patient to discontinue and to notify health care provider at the first sign of a skin rash or other allergic reaction.

CHLORAMPHENICOL

Rx	**Chloramphenicol** (Various, eg, Goldline,Schein)	**Solution**[a]: 5 mg/mL	In 7.5 and 15 mL.
Rx	**Chloramphenicol** (Various, eg, Schein)	**Ointment**: 10 mg/g	In 3.5 g.
Rx	**Chloromycetin** (Parke-Davis)	**Powder for solution**: 25 mg/vial.	Preservative free. In 15 mL with diluent.

[a] Refrigerate until dispensed.

CHLORAMPHENICOL — OPHTHALMIC

Complete and comparative prescribing information begins in the Ophthalmic Antibiotics group monograph.

WARNING

Bone marrow hypoplasia including aplastic anemia and death has been reported following local application of chloramphenicol. Chloramphenicol should not be used when less potentially dangerous agents would be expected to provide effective treatment.

Indications

➤*Ocular infections:* Only use chloramphenicol in those serious infections for which less potentially dangerous drugs are ineffective or contraindicated. Bacteriological studies should be performed to determine the causative organisms and their sensitivity to chloramphenicol (see Warning Box).

For the treatment of surface ocular infections involving the conjunctiva or cornea caused by chloramphenicol-susceptible organisms.

Chloramphenicol is active against the following common bacterial eye pathogens:
• *Staphylococcus aureus.*
• Streptococci, including *Streptococcus pneumoniae.*
• *Escherichia coli.*
• *Haemophilus influenzae.*
• *Klebsiella / Enterobacter* species.
• Moraxella lacunata (Morax-Axenfeld bacillus).
• *Neisseria* species.

The product does not provide adequate coverage against:
• *Pseudomonas aeruginosa.*
• *Serratia marcescens.*

Administration and Dosage

➤*Approved by the FDA:* September 25, 1985.

Two drops applied to the affected eye every 3 hours or more frequently if deemed advisable by the prescribing physician. Administration should be continued day and night for the first 48 hours, after which the interval between applications may be increased. Treatment should be continued for at least 48 hours after the eye appears normal.

➤*Directions for dispensing:* Prepare solution by adding sterile distilled water to the vial as follows:
• To prepare a 0.5% solution, add 5 mL of sterile water to the vial.
• To prepare a 0.25% solution, add 10 mL of sterile water to the vial.
• To prepare a 0.16% solution, add 15 mL of sterile water to the vial.

Solutions remain stable at room temperature for 10 days.

➤*Storage / Stability:* Store below 30°C (86°F).

ERYTHROMYCIN

Rx	**Erythromycin** (Various, eg, Akorn, Bausch & Lomb, Fougera, Goldline, Rugby)	**Ointment**: 0.5%	In 3.5 g.
Rx	**Ilotycin** (Dista)		In 3.5 g.[a]

[a] With white petrolatum and mineral oil.

ERYTHROMYCIN — OPHTHALMIC

Complete and comparative prescribing information begins in the Ophthalmic Antibiotics group monograph.

Indications

➤*Ocular infections:* For the treatment of superficial ocular infections involving the conjunctiva or cornea caused by organisms susceptible to erythromycin ophthalmic ointment.

For prophylaxis of ophthalmia neonatorum due to *N. gonorrhoeae* or *C. trachomatis.*

The effectiveness of erythromycin in the prevention of ophthalmia caused by penicillinase-producing *N. gonorrhoeae* is not established.

For infants born to mothers with clinically apparent gonorrhea, intravenous or intramuscular injections of aqueous crystalline penicillin G should be given; a single dose of 50,000 units for term infants or 20,000 units for infants of low birth weight. Topical prophylaxis alone is inadequate for these infants.

Administration and Dosage

➤*Approved by the FDA:* March 29, 1982.

ERYTHROMYCIN — OPHTHALMIC

In the treatment of superficial ocular infections, erythromycin ophthalmic ointment approximately 1 cm in length should be applied directly to the infected eye(s) up to 6 times daily, depending on the severity of the infection.

For prophylaxis of neonatal gonococcal or chlamydial ophthalmia, a ribbon of ointment approximately 1 cm in length should be instilled into each lower conjunctival sac. The ointment should not be flushed from the eye following instillation. A new tube should be used for each infant.

➤*Storage/Stability:* Store between 15° to 30°C (59° to 86°F).

GENTAMICIN SULFATE

Rx	**Gentamicin Ophthalmic** (Various, eg, Bausch & Lomb, Goldline, Rugby, Schein)	**Solution**: 3 mg/mL	In 5 and 15 mL.
Rx	**Garamycin** (Schering)		In 5 mL dropper bottles.[a]
Rx	**Genoptic** (Allergan)		In 1 and 5 mL dropper bottles.[b]
Rx	**Gentacidin** (Novartis Ophthalmics)		In 5 mL dropper bottles.[a]
Rx	**Gentamicin Sulfate Ophthalmic** (E. Fougera)	**Ointment**: 3 mg/g	In 3.5 g.[c]
Rx	**Garamycin** (Schering)		In 3.5 g.[d]
Rx	**Genoptic S.O.P.** (Allergan)		In 3.5 g.[d]
Rx	**Gentak** (Akorn)		In 3.5 g.[d]

[a] With 0.1 mg/mL benzalkonium chloride, sodium phosphate and NaCl.
[b] With benzalkonium chloride, 1.4% polyvinyl alcohol, EDTA, sodium phosphate dibasic, NaCl and hydrochloric acid or sodium hydroxide.
[c] In a base of white petrolatum and mineral oil.
[d] With white petrolatum and parabens.

GENTAMICIN SULFATE — OPHTHALMIC

Complete and comparative prescribing information begins in the Ophthalmic Antibiotics group monograph.

Indications

➤*Ocular infections:* For the topical treatment of ocular bacterial infections, including conjunctivitis, keratitis, keratoconjunctivitis, corneal ulcers, blepharitis, blepharoconjunctivitis, acute meibomianitis, and dacryocystitis caused by susceptible strains of the following microorganisms: *Staphylococcus aureus*, *Staphylococcus epidermidis*, *Streptococcus pyogenes*, *Streptococcus pneumoniae*, *Enterobacter aerogenes*, *Escherichia coli*, *Haemophilus influenzae*, *Klebsiella pneumoniae*, *Neisseria gonorrhoeae*, *Pseudomonas aeruginosa*, and *Serratia marcescens*.

Administration and Dosage

➤*Approved by the FDA:* July 26, 1984.

➤*Ophthalmic solution:* Instill 1 or 2 drops into the affected eye every 4 hours. In severe infections, dosage may be increased to as much as 2 drops once every hour.

➤*Ophthalmic ointment:* Apply a small amount (about ½ inch) to the affected eye 2 to 3 times a day.

➤*Storage/Stability:* Store gentamicin sulfate ophthalmic ointment and solution between 2° and 30°C (36° and 86°F).

TOBRAMYCIN

Rx	**Tobramycin** (Various, eg, Bausch & Lomb)	**Solution**: 0.3% tobramycin	In 5 mL bottle.[a]
Rx	**AKTob** (Akorn)		In 5 mL.[b]
Rx	**Defy** (Akorn)		In 5 mL.
Rx	**Tobrex** (Alcon)		In 5 mL *Drop-Tainers*.[c]
Rx	**Tobrex** (Alcon)	**Ointment**: 3 mg tobramycin per g	In 3.5 g.[d]

[a] With 0.01% benzalkonium Cl and boric acid.
[b] With 0.01% benzalkonium chloride, boric acid and sodium sulfate.
[c] With 0.01% benzalkonium chloride, tyloxapol and boric acid.
[d] With white petrolatum, mineral oil and 0.5% chlorobutanol.

TOBRAMYCIN — OPHTHALMIC

Complete and comparative prescribing information begins in the Ophthalmic Antibiotics group monograph.

Indications

➤*Ocular infections:* For the treatment of external infections of the eye and its adnexa caused by susceptible bacteria.

Administration and Dosage

➤*Approved by the FDA:* December 13, 1984.

➤*Solution:* In mild to moderate disease, instill 1 or 2 drops into the affected eye(s) every 4 hours. In severe infections, instill 2 drops into the eye(s) hourly until improvement, following which treatment should be reduced prior to discontinuation.

➤*Ointment:* In mild to moderate disease, apply a half-inch ribbon into the affected eye(s) 2 or 3 times per day. In severe infections, instill a half-inch ribbon into the affected eye(s) every 3 to 4 hours until improvement, following which treatment should be reduced prior to discontinuation.

➤*Storage/Stability:* Store at 8° to 27°C (46° to 80°F).

POLYMYXIN B

Rx	**Polymyxin B Sulfate Sterile** (Roerig)	**Powder for solution**: 500,000 units	In 20 mL vials.

POLYMYXIN B — OPHTHALMIC

Complete and comparative prescribing information begins in the Ophthalmic Antibiotics group monograph.

Indications

➤*Ocular infections:* For the topical and subconjunctival treatment of infections of the eye caused by susceptible strains of *Pseudomonas aeruginosa*.

Administration and Dosage

➤*Approved by the FDA:* September 30, 1994.

Dissolve 500,000 polymyxin B units in 20 to 50 mL sterile water for injection or sodium chloride injection for a 10,000 to 25,000 units/mL concentration.

For the treatment of *Pseudomonas aeruginosa* infections of the eye, a concentration of 0.1% to 0.25% (10,000 units to 25,000 units/mL) is administered 1 to 3 drops every hour, increasing the intervals as response indicates.

Subconjunctival injection of up to 10,000 units/day may be used for the treatment of *Pseudomonas aeruginosa* infections of the cornea and conjunctiva.

➤*Note:* Avoid total ophthalmic instillation over 25,000 units/kg/day.

➤*Storage/Stability:*

Before reconstitution – Store at controlled room temperature 15° to 30°C (59° to 86°F).

Protect from light. Retain in carton until time of use.

After reconstitution – Product must be stored under refrigeration, between 2° to 8°C (36° to 46°F) and any unused portion should be discarded after 72 hours.

BACITRACIN

Rx	**Bacitracin** (Various, eg, Goldline, Major, Schein, URL)	**Ointment**: 500 units/g	In 3.5 and 3.75 g.
Rx	**AK-Tracin** (Akorn)		Preservative free. In 3.5 g.[a]

[a] With white petrolatum and mineral oil.

BACITRACIN — OPHTHALMIC

Complete and comparative prescribing information begins in the Ophthalmic Antibiotics group monograph.

Indications

➤*Ocular infections:* Treatment of superficial ocular infections involving the conjunctiva or cornea (eg, conjunctivitis, keratitis, keratoconjunctivitis, corneal ulcers, blepharitis, blepharoconjunctivitis, acute meibomianitis and dacryocystitis) due to strains of microorganisms susceptible to antibiotics.

For a list of microorganisms usually susceptible to these agents, refer to systemic monographs in the Anti-infectives chapter.

Administration and Dosage

Administration and dosage varies for the individual products. Refer to the individual manufacturer inserts.

CIPROFLOXACIN HYDROCHLORIDE

Rx	**Ciprofloxacin** (Various, eg, Bausch & Lomb, Novax)	**Solution**: 3.5 mg/mL (equivalent to 3 mg base)	In 2.5, 5, and 10 mL dropper bottles.[a]
Rx	**Ciloxan** (Alcon)		In 2.5 and 5 mL *Drop-Tainers*[b].
Rx	**Ciloxan** (Alcon)	**Ointment**: 3.33 mg/g (equivalent to 3 mg base)	Mineral oil, white petrolatum. In 3.5 g.

[a] With 0.006% benzalkonium chloride, mannitol, and EDTA.

[b] With 0.006% benzalkonium chloride, 4.6% mannitol, and 0.05% EDTA.

CIPROFLOXACIN HYDROCHLORIDE — OPHTHALMIC

Complete and comparative prescribing information begins in the Ophthalmic Antibiotics group monograph.

Indications

➤*Ocular infections:* For the treatment of superficial ocular infections involving the conjunctiva or cornea (eg, conjunctivitis, keratitis, keratoconjunctivitis, corneal ulcers, blepharitis, blepharoconjunctivitis, acute meibomianitis, dacryocystitis) due to strains of microorganisms susceptible to antibiotics.

➤*Ophthalmic ointment:* For the treatment of bacterial conjunctivitis caused by susceptible strains of the microorganisms listed below:

Gram-positive – Staphylococcus aureus; Staphylococcus epidermidis; Streptococcus pneumoniae; Streptococcus (viridans group).

Gram-negative – Haemophilus influenzae.

➤*Ophthalmic solution:* For the treatment of infections caused by susceptible strains of the designated microorganisms in the conditions listed below:

Corneal ulcers –
- *Pseudomonas aeruginosa.*
- *Serratia marcescens* (efficacy for this organism was studied in fewer than 10 infections).
- *Staphylococcus aureus.*
- *Staphylococcus epidermidis.*
- *Streptococcus pneumoniae.*
- *Streptococcus* (viridans group) (efficacy for this organism was studied in fewer than 10 infections).

Conjunctivitis –
- *Haemophilus influenzae.*
- *Staphylococcus aureus*
- *Staphylococcus epidermidis.*
- *Streptococcus pneumoniae.*

Administration and Dosage

➤*Approved by the FDA:* May 30, 1998 (ointment); December 31, 1990 (solution).

➤*Ophthalmic ointment:* Apply a ½ inch ribbon into the conjunctival sac 3 times a day on the first 2 days, then apply a ½ inch ribbon 2 times a day for the next 5 days.

➤*Ophthalmic solution:*

Corneal ulcers – Instill 2 drops into the affected eye every 15 minutes for the first 6 hours and then 2 drops into the affected eye every 30 minutes for the remainder of the first day. On the second day, instill 2 drops in the affected eye hourly. On the third through the fourteenth day, place 2 drops in the affected eye every 4 hours. Treatment may be continued after 14 days if corneal re-epithelialization has not occurred.

Conjunctivitis – Instill 1 or 2 drops into the conjunctival sac(s) every 2 hours while awake for 2 days and 1 or 2 drops every 4 hours while awake for the next 5 days.

➤*Storage/Stability:*

Ophthalmic ointment – Store at 2° to 25°C (36° to 77°F).

Ophthalmic solution – Store at 2° to 30°C (36° to 86°F). Protect from light.

GATIFLOXACIN

Rx	**Zymar** (Allergan)	**Solution**: 0.3% (3 mg/mL)	In 2.5 and 5 mL dropper bottles.[a]

[a] With 0.005% benzalkonium chloride and EDTA.

GATIFLOXACIN — OPHTHALMIC

Complete and comparative prescribing information begins in the Ophthalmic Antibiotics group monograph.

Indications

Treatment of bacterial conjunctivitis caused by susceptible strains of the following organisms listed below:

➤*Gram positive bacteria: Cornyebacterium propinquum*†; *Staphylococcus aureus; S. epidermidis; Streptococcus mitis*†; *S. pneumoniae.*

➤*Gram negative bacteria: Haemophilus influenzae.*

Administration and Dosage

➤*Approved by the FDA:* March 28, 2003.

➤*Days 1 and 2:* Instill 1 drop in affected eye(s) every 2 hours while awake, up to 8 times/day.

➤*Days 3 through 7:* Instill 1 drop up to 4 times/day while awake.

➤*Storage/Stability:* Store between 15° to 25°C (59° to 77°F). Protect from freezing.

MOXIFLOXACIN HYDROCHLORIDE

Rx	**Vigamox** (Alcon)	**Solution**: 0.5% (5 mg/mL)	In 3 mL *Drop-Tainer*.[a]

[a] With boric acid, sodium chloride, and purified water.

MOXIFLOXACIN HYDROCHLORIDE — OPHTHALMIC

Complete and comparative prescribing information begins in the Ophthalmic Antibiotics group monograph.

Indications

For the treatment of bacterial conjunctivitis caused by susceptible strains of the following organisms:

➤*Aerobic gram-positive microorganisms: Corynebacterium* species†; *Micrococcus luteus*†; *Staphylococcus aureus; Staphylococcus epidermidis; Staphylococcus haemolyticus; Staphylococcus hominis; Staphylococcus warneri*†; *Streptococcus pneumoniae; Streptococcus* viridans group.

➤*Aerobic gram-negative microorganisms: Acinetobacter lwoffii*†; *Haemophilus influenzae; Haemophilus parainfluenzae*†.

➤*Other microorganisms: Chlamydia trachomatis.*

Administration and Dosage

➤*Approved by the FDA:* April 15, 2003.

Instill 1 drop in the affected eye 3 times a day for 7 days.

➤*Storage/Stability:* Store at 2° to 25°C (36° to 77°F).

† Efficacy for this organism was studied in fewer than 10 infections.

OFLOXACIN

Rx	**Ofloxacin** (Pacific Pharma)	**Solution:** 0.3% (3 mg/mL)	In 5 and 10 mL.[a]
Rx	**Ocuflox** (Allergan)		In 1, 5, and 10 mL.[a]

[a] With 0.005% benzalkonium chloride.

OFLOXACIN — OPHTHALMIC

Complete and comparative prescribing information begins in the Ophthalmic Antibiotics group monograph.

Indications

For the treatment of infections caused by susceptible strains of the following bacteria in the conditions listed below:

➤*Conjunctivitis:*

Gram-positive bacteria – Staphylococcus aureus; Staphylococcus epidermidis; Streptococcus pneumoniae.

Gram-negative bacteria – Enterobacter cloacae; Haemophilus influenzae; Proteus mirabilis; Pseudomonas aeruginosa.

➤*Corneal ulcers:*

Gram-positive bacteria – Staphylococcus aureus; Staphylococcus epidermidis; Streptococcus pneumoniae.

Gram-negative bacteria – Pseudomonas aeruginosa; Serratia marcescens (efficacy for this organism was studied in fewer than 10 infections).

Anaerobic species – Propionibacterium acnes.

Administration and Dosage

➤*Approved by the FDA:* July 30, 1993.

➤*Bacterial conjunctivitis:*

Recommended dosage regimen for the treatment of bacterial conjunctivitis	
Days 1 and 2	Instill 1 to 2 drops every 2 to 4 hours in the affected eye(s).
Days 3 through 7	Instill 1 to 2 drops 4 times daily.

➤*Bacterial corneal ulcer:*

Recommended Dosage Regimen for the Treatment of Bacterial Corneal Ulcer	
Days 1 and 2	Instill 1 to 2 drops into the affected eye every 30 minutes while awake. Awaken at approximately 4 and 6 hours after retiring and instill 1 to 2 drops.
Days 3 through 7 to 9	Instill 1 to 2 drops hourly while awake.
Days 7 to 9 through treatment completion	Instill 1 to 2 drops 4 times daily.

➤*Storage/Stability:* Store at 15° to 25°C (59° to 77°F).

LEVOFLOXACIN

Rx	**Quixin** (Santen)	**Solution:** 0.5% (5 mg/mL)	In 2.5 and 5 mL.[a]
Rx	**Iquix** (Santen)	**Solution:** 1.5% (15 mg/mL)	In 5 mL.

[a] With 0.005% benzalkonium chloride.

LEVOFLOXACIN — OPHTHALMIC

Complete and comparative prescribing information begins in the Ophthalmic Antibiotics group monograph.

Indications

For the treatment of bacterial conjunctivitis caused by susceptible strains of the following organisms:

➤*Aerobic gram-positive microorganisms: Corynebacterium* species (Efficacy for this organism was studied in fewer than 10 infections.); *Staphylococcus aureus* (methicillin-susceptible strains only); *Staphylococcus epidermidis* (methicillin-susceptible strains only); *Streptococcus pneumoniae*; *Streptococcus* (groups C/F); *Streptococcus* (group G); Viridans group streptococci.

➤*Aerobic gram-negative microorganisms: Acinetobacter lwoffii; Haemophilus influenzae; Serratia marcescens.*

Administration and Dosage

➤*Days 1 and 2:* Instill 1 to 2 drops in the affected eye(s) every 2 hours while awake up to 8 times per day.

➤*Days 3 through 7:* Instill 1 to 2 drops in the affected eye(s) every 4 hours while awake up to 4 times per day.

➤*Storage/Stability:* Store at 15° to 25°C (59° to 77°F).

Sulfonamides

Refer to Topical Ophthalmic Drugs introduction for more complete information.

Indications

➤*Ocular infections:* For conjunctivitis, corneal ulcer and other superficial ocular infections due to susceptible microorganisms.

➤*Trachoma:* As an adjunct to systemic sulfonamide therapy in the treatment of trachoma.

Administration and Dosage

Usual duration of treatment is 7 to 10 days.

➤*Solutions:*

Conjunctivitis or other superficial ocular infections – Instill 1 to 2 drops into the lower conjunctival sac(s) every 1 to 4 hours initially according to severity of infection. Dosages may be tapered by increasing the time interval between doses as the condition responds.

Trachoma – 2 drops every 2 hours. Concomitant systemic sulfonamide therapy is indicated.

Storage/Stability – Protect from light. On long standing, solutions will darken in color and should be discarded.

➤*Ointments:* Apply a small amount (0.5 inch) into the lower conjunctival sac(s) 3 to 4 times daily and at bedtime. Dosages may be tapered by increasing the time interval between doses as the condition responds. Or apply 0.5 to 1 inch into the conjunctival sac(s) at night in conjunction with the use of drops during the day, or before an eye is patched.

Storage/Stability – Store away from heat.

Actions

➤*Pharmacology:* Sulfonamides are bacteriostatic against a wide range of susceptible gram-positive and gram-negative microorganisms. Through competition with para-aminobenzoic acid (PABA), they restrict synthesis of folic acid which bacteria require for growth. For complete information, refer to the systemic sulfonamides monograph in the Anti-infectives chapter.

➤*Pharmacokinetics:* Sulfonamides do not appear to be appreciably absorbed from mucous membranes.

➤*Microbiology:* Topically applied sulfonamides are considered active against susceptible strains of the following common bacterial eye pathogens: *Escherichia coli, Staphylococcus aureus, Streptococcus pneumoniae, Streptococcus* (viridans group), *Haemophilus influenzae, Klebsiella* sp and *Enterobacter* sp.

Topically applied sulfonamides do not provide adequate coverage against *Neisseria* sp, *Serratia marcescens* and *Pseudomonas aeruginosa*. A significant percentage of staphylococcal isolates are completely resistant to sulfa drugs.

Contraindications

Hypersensitivity to sulfonamides or any component of the product; infants younger than 2 months of age; in epithelial herpes simplex keratitis (dendritic keratitis), vaccinia, varicella and many other viral diseases of the cornea and conjunctiva; mycobacterial infection or fungal diseases of the ocular structures; after uncomplicated removal of a corneal foreign body (steroid combinations).

Warnings

➤*Staphylococcus species:* A significant percentage of isolates are resistant to sulfa drugs.

➤*Hypersensitivity reactions:* Severe sensitivity reactions have been identified in individuals with no prior history of sulfonamide hypersensitivity (see Adverse Reactions).

➤*Pregnancy: Category C.* Safety for use during pregnancy has not been established. Use only when clearly needed and when potential benefits outweigh potential hazards to the fetus.

➤*Lactation:* Systemic sulfonamides are excreted in breast milk.

➤*Children:* Safety and efficacy not established. Contraindicated in infants younger than 2 months old.

Precautions

For topical ophthalmic use only. Not for injection.

➤*Epithelial healing:* Ophthalmic ointments may retard corneal wound healing.

➤*Sensitization:* Sensitization may occur when a sulfonamide is readministered, regardless of route. Cross-sensitivity between different sulfonamides may occur. If signs of sensitivity or other untoward reactions occur, discontinue use of the preparation.

➤*PABA:* PABA present in purulent exudates inactivates sulfonamides.

➤*Dry eye:* Use with caution in patients with severe dry eye.

➤*Superinfection:* Use of antibiotics (especially prolonged or repeated therapy) may result in bacterial or fungal overgrowth of nonsusceptible organisms. Such overgrowth may lead to a secondary infection. Take appropriate measures if this occurs.

➤*Sulfite sensitivity:* May cause allergic-type reactions (eg, hives, itching, wheezing, anaphylaxis) in certain susceptible people. Although overall prevalence in the general population is probably low, it is more common in asthmatics or in atopic nonasthmatics. Specific products containing sulfites are identified in product listings.

Drug Interactions

Silver preparations are incompatible with these solutions.

Adverse Reactions

Headache; local irritation; itching; periorbital edema, burning and transient stinging; bacterial and fungal corneal ulcers. As with all sulfonamide preparations, severe sensitivity reactions include rare occurrences of Stevens-Johnson syndrome, exfoliative dermatitis, toxic epidermal necrolysis, photosensitivity, fever, skin rash, GI disturbance and bone marrow depression; fatalities have occurred.

Patient Information

For topical use only.

To avoid contamination, do not touch tip of container to any surface.

Keep bottle tightly closed when not in use. Do not use if solution has darkened.

Notify physician if improvement is not seen after several days, if condition worsens, or if pain, increased redness, itching or swelling of the eye occurs or persists for longer than 48 hours. Do not discontinue use without consulting physician.

SULFISOXAZOLE DIOLAMINE

Rx	**Gantrisin** (Roche)	**Solution**: 4%	With 1:100,000 phenylmercuric nitrate. In 15 mL with dropper.

SULFISOXAZOLE DIOLAMINE — OPHTHALMIC

Complete and comparative prescribing information is found in the Sulfonamides group monograph.

Indications

➤*Ocular infections:* For conjunctivitis, corneal ulcer and other superficial ocular infections due to susceptible microorganisms.

➤*Trachoma:* As an adjunct to systemic sulfonamide therapy in the treatment of trachoma.

Administration and Dosage

Usual duration of treatment is 7 to 10 days.

➤*Solutions:*

Conjunctivitis or other superficial ocular infections – Instill 1 to 2 drops into the lower conjunctival sac(s) every 1 to 4 hours initially according to severity of infection. Dosages may be tapered by increasing the time interval between doses as the condition responds.

Trachoma – 2 drops every 2 hours. Concomitant systemic sulfonamide therapy is indicated.

➤*Storage/Stability:* Protect from light. On long standing, solutions will darken in color and should be discarded.

SULFACETAMIDE SODIUM

Rx	**Sulster** (Akorn)	**Solution**: 1%	In 5 and 10 mL.
Rx	**Sulfacetamide Sodium** (Various, eg, Bausch & Lomb, Fougera, Goldline, Moore, Optopics, Rugby, Steris, URL)	**Solution**: 10%	In 15 mL.
Rx	**AK-Sulf** (Akorn)		In 2, 5 and 15 mL.[a]
Rx	**Bleph-10** (Allergan)		In 2.5, 5 and 15 mL.[b]
Rx	**Ocusulf-10** (Optopics)		In 2, 5 and 15 mL.[c]
Rx	**Storz Sulf** (Lederle)		In 15 mL.
Rx	**Sulfacetamide Sodium** (Various, eg, Schein, Steris)	**Solution**: 30%	In 15 mL.
Rx	**Sodium Sulfacetamide** (Various, eg, Moore, URL)	**Ointment**: 10%	In 3.5 g
Rx	**AK-Sulf** (Akorn)		In 3.5 g.[d]
Rx	**Cetamide** (Alcon)		In 3.5 g.[e]

[a] 3.1 mg sodium thiosulfate pentahydrate, 5 mg methylcellulose, 0.5 mg methylparaben and 0.1 mg propylparaben per mL.
[b] With 1.4% polyvinyl alcohol, 0.005% benzalkonium chloride, polysorbate 80, sodium thiosulfate and EDTA.
[c] With parabens, 1.4% polyvinyl alcohol and sodium thiosulfate.
[d] With 0.5 mg methylparaben, 0.1 mg propylparaben, 0.25 mg benzalkonium chloride and petrolatum base per g.
[e] With 0.0008% phenylmercuric acetate, white petrolatum, mineral oil, petrolatum and lanolin alcohol.

SULFACETAMIDE SODIUM — OPHTHALMIC

Complete and comparative prescribing information begins in the Sulfonamides group monograph.

Indications

➤*Ocular infections:* For the treatment of conjunctivitis and other superficial ocular infections due to susceptible microorganisms, and as an adjunctive in systemic sulfonamide therapy of trachoma: *Escherichia coli*, *Staphylococcus aureus*, *Streptococcus pneumoniae*, *Streptococcus* (viridans group), *Haemophilus influenzae*, *Klebsiella* species, and *Enterobacter* species.

Topically applied sulfonamides do not provide adequate coverage against *Neisseria* species, *Serratia marcescens* and *Pseudomonas aeruginosa*. A significant percentage of staphylococcal isolates are completely resistant to sulfa drugs.

Administration and Dosage

➤*Conjunctivitis and other superficial ocular infections:* Instill 1 or 2 drops into the conjunctival sac(s) of the affected eye(s) every 2 to 3 hours initially. Dosages may be tapered by increasing the time interval between doses as the condition responds. The usual duration of treatment is 7 to 10 days.

➤*Trachoma:* Instill 2 drops into the conjunctival sac(s) of the affected eye(s) every 2 hours. Topical administration must be accompanied by systemic administration.

➤*Storage/Stability:* Store between 8° to 25°C (46° to 77°F).

Sulfonamide solutions, on long standing, will darken in color and should be discarded. Protect from light.

Keep out of reach of children.

COMBINATION ANTIBIOTIC PRODUCTS

	Product and Distributor	Polymyxin B Sulfate (units/g or mL)	Neomycin (mg/g or mL)	Bacitracin Zinc (units/g)	Other Antibiotics	How Supplied
Rx	**Neomycin and Polymyxin B Sulfates and Bacitracin Zinc Ophthalmic Ointment** (Various, eg, Bausch & Lomb, Fougera)	10,000	3.5[a]	400		White petrolatum, mineral oil. In 3.5 g.
Rx	**Neosporin Ophthalmic Ointment** (Monarch)					White petrolatum. In 3.5 g.
Rx	**Neomycin and Polymyxin B Sulfates and Gramicidin Ophthalmic Solution** (Various, eg, Bausch & Lomb, URL, Zenith Goldline)	10,000	1.75		0.025 mg/mL gramicidin	Sodium chloride, 0.5% alcohol, propylene glycol, hydrochloric acid, 0.001% thimerosal, poloxamer 188, ammonium hydroxide. In 10 mL.
Rx	**Neosporin Ophthalmic Solution** (Monarch)					Alcohol 0.5%, 0.001% thimerosal, propylene glycol, sodium chloride. In 10 mL *Drop Dose.*
Rx	**Bacitracin Zinc and Polymyxin B Sulfate Ophthalmic Ointment** (Bausch & Lomb)	10,000		500		White petrolatum, mineral oil. In 3.5 g.
Rx	**AK-Poly-Bac Ophthalmic Ointment** (Akorn)					White petrolatum, mineral oil. In 3.5 g.
Rx	**Polysporin Ophthalmic Ointment** (Monarch)					White petrolatum. In 3.5 g.
Rx	**Terramycin w/Polymyxin B Sulfate Ophthalmic Ointment** (Roerig)	10,000			5 mg/g oxytetracycline hydrochloride	White and liquid petrolatum. In 3.5 g.
Rx	**Terak with Polymyxin B Sulfate Ophthalmic Ointment** (Akorn)					White and liquid petrolatum. In 3.5 g.
Rx	**Trimethoprim Sulfate and Polymyxin B Sulfate Ophthalmic Solution** (Various, eg, Bausch and Lomb, Falcon)	10,000			1 mg/mL trimethoprim sulfate	In 10 mL.
Rx	**Polytrim Ophthalmic Solution** (Allergan)					0.04 mg/mL benzalkonium chloride, sodium chloride, sodium hydroxide. In 5 and 10 mL.

[a] Equivalent to 5 g neomycin sulfate.

COMBINATION ANTIBIOTIC PRODUCTS — OPHTHALMIC

Complete and comparative prescribing information begins in the Ophthalmic Antibiotics group monograph.

STEROID AND ANTIBIOTIC SOLUTIONS AND SUSPENSIONS

	Product & Distributor	Steroid	Antibiotic	Other Content	How Supplied
Rx	**Cortisporin Ophthalmic Suspension** (Monarch)	1% hydrocortisone	Neomycin sulfate equivalent to 0.35% neomycin base and 10,000 units/mL polymyxin B sulfate	0.001% thimerosal, cetyl alcohol, glyceryl monostearate, mineral oil, propylene glycol	In 7.5 mL *Drop Dose.*
Rx	**Poly-Pred Liquifilm Ophthalmic Suspension** (Allergan)	0.5% prednisolone acetate	Neomycin sulfate equivalent to 0.35% neomycin base and 10,000 units/mL polymyxin B sulfate	1.4% polyvinyl alcohol, 0.001% thimerosal, polysorbate 80, propylene glycol, sodium acetate	In 5 and 10 mL.
Rx	**Pred-G Ophthalmic Suspension** (Allergan)	1% prednisolone acetate	Gentamicin sulfate equivalent to 0.3% gentamicin base	0.005% benzalkonium chloride, 1.4% polyvinyl alcohol, EDTA, hydrochloric acid, hydroxypropyl methylcellulose, NaCl, polysorbate 80, sodium citrate dihydrate, sodium hydroxide	In 2, 5 and 10 mL.
Rx	**NeoDecadron Ophthalmic Solution** (Merck)	0.1% dexamethasone phosphate (as dexamethasone sodium phosphate)	Neomycin sulfate equivalent to 0.35% neomycin base	0.02% benzalkonium chloride, EDTA, hydrochloric acid, 0.1% sodium bisulfite, polysorbate 80, sodium borate, sodium citrate	In 5 mL *Ocumeters.*
Rx	**Neo-Dexameth Ophthalmic Solution** (Major)			0.01% benzalkonium chloride, EDTA, hydrochloric acid, polysorbate 80, sodium bisulfite, sodium borate, sodium citrate	In 5 mL.
Rx	**TobraDex Ophthalmic Suspension** (Alcon)	0.1% dexamethasone	0.3% tobramycin	0.01% benzalkonium chloride, EDTA, hydroxyethyl cellulose, NaCl, sodium hydroxide, tyloxapol	In 2.5, 5 and 10 mL *Drop-Tainers.*
Rx	**Neomycin and Polymyxin B Sulfates and Dexamethasone Ophthalmic Suspension** (Various, eg, Falcon)	0.1% dexamethasone	Neomycin sulfate equivalent to 0.35% neomycin base and 10,000 units/mL polymyxin B sulfate	0.004% benzalkonium chloride, 0.5% hydroxypropyl methylcellulose, hydrochloric acid, NaCl, polysorbate 20, sodium hydroxide	In 5 mL.
Rx	**Maxitrol Ophthalmic Suspension** (Alcon)				In 5 mL *Drop-Tainers.*
Rx	**Zylet Suspension** (Bausch & Lomb)	0.5% loteprednol etabonate	0.3% tobramycin	0.01% benzalkonium chloride, EDTA, glycerin, povidone, tyloxapol, sulfuric acid and/or sodium hydroxide	In 2.5, 5, and 10 mL.

STEROID AND ANTIBIOTIC SOLUTIONS AND SUSPENSIONS — OPHTHALMIC

Indications

➤*Inflammatory conditions:* For steroid-responsive inflammatory ocular conditions in which a corticosteroid is indicated and in which superficial bacterial infection or risk of infection exists.

For inflammatory conditions of the palpebral and bulbar conjunctiva, cornea and anterior segment of the globe in which the inherent risk of corticosteroid use in certain infective conjunctivitides is accepted to obtain a diminution in edema and inflammation. For chronic anterior uveitis and corneal injury from chemical, radiation or thermal burns, or penetration of foreign bodies.

The use of a combination drug with an anti-infective component is indicated when the risk of infection is high or when there is an expectation that potentially dangerous numbers of bacteria will be present in the eye.

Administration and Dosage

➤*Dexacidin:* Taper to discontinuation as inflammation subsides.

➤*Poly-Pred:* Reduce dose frequency as inflammation is brought under control.

➤*Pred-G:* Do not discontinue prematurely.

➤*Zylet:* Decrease gradually as warranted by improvement in clinical signs. Take care not to discontinue therapy prematurely.

Do not prescribe more than 20 mL initially; do not refill without further evaluation.

➤*Storage / Stability:* Store suspensions upright and shake well before using.

For complete dosage instructions, see individual manufacturer inserts.

STEROID AND ANTIBIOTIC OINTMENTS

	Product & Distributor	Steroid (per g)	Antibiotic (per g)	Other Content	How Supplied
Rx	**Ophthocort** (Parke-Davis)	0.5% hydrocortisone acetate	1% chloramphenicol, 10,000 units polymyxin B (as sulfate)	Liquid petrolatum, polyethylene	Preservative free. In 3.5 g.
Rx	**Bacitracin Zinc/Neomycin Sulfate/Polymyxin B Sulfate/Hydrocortisone** (Various, eg, Fougera)	1% hydrocortisone	Neomycin sulfate equivalent to 0.35% neomycin base, 400 units bacitracin zinc, 10,000 units polymyxin B sulfate		In 3.5 g.
Rx	**Cortisporin** (Glaxo Wellcome)			White petrolatum	In 3.5 g.
Rx	**Pred-G** (Allergan)	0.6% prednisolone acetate	Gentamicin sulfate equivalent to 0.3% gentamicin base	0.5% chlorobutanol, white petrolatum, mineral oil, petrolatum, lanolin alcohol	In 3.5 g.
Rx	**Neomycin/Polymyxin B Sulfate/Dexamethasone** (Various, eg, Fougera, Rugby)	0.1% dexamethasone	Neomycin sulfate equivalent to 0.35% neomycin base, 10,000 units polymyxin B sulfate		In 3.5 g.
Rx	**Maxitrol** (Alcon)			Parabens, white petrolatum, lanolin	In 3.5 g.

STEROID AND ANTIBIOTIC OINTMENTS — OPHTHALMIC

Indications

➤*Inflammatory conditions:* For steroid-responsive inflammatory ocular conditions in which a corticosteroid is indicated and in which bacterial infection or risk of infection exists.

For inflammatory conditions of the palpebral and bulbar conjunctiva, cornea and anterior segment of the globe in which the inherent risk of steroid use in certain infective conjunctivitis is accepted to obtain a diminution in edema and inflammation. For chronic anterior uveitis and corneal injury from chemical, radiation or thermal burns, or penetration of foreign bodies.

Administration and Dosage

Apply ointment to the affected eye(s) every 3 or 4 hours, depending on the severity of the condition.

Do not prescribe more than 8 g initially, and the prescription should not be refilled until further evaluation. For complete dosage instructions, see individual manufacturer inserts.

STEROID AND SULFONAMIDE COMBINATIONS

STEROID AND SULFONAMIDE COMBINATIONS, SUSPENSIONS AND SOLUTIONS

	Product & Distributor	Steroid	Sulfonamide	Other Content	How Supplied
Rx	**FML-S Suspension** (Allergan)	0.1% fluorometholone	10% sodium sulfacetamide	EDTA, 1.4% polyvinyl alcohol, 0.006% benzalkonium chloride, polysorbate 80, povidone, sodium thiosulfate and sodium chloride	In 5 and 10 mL.
Rx	**Blephamide Suspension** (Allergan)	0.2% prednisolone acetate	10% sodium sulfacetamide	EDTA, 1.4% polyvinyl alcohol, polysorbate 80, sodium thiosulfate, benzalkonium chloride	In 2.5, 5 and 10 mL.
Rx	**Metimyd Suspension** (Schering)	0.5% prednisolone acetate	10% sodium sulfacetamide	0.5% phenylethyl alcohol, 0.025% benzalkonium chloride, sodium thiosulfate, EDTA, tyloxapol	In 5 mL.
Rx	**Sulfacetamide Sodium and Prednisolone Sodium Phosphate** (Schein)	0.25% prednisolone sodium phosphate	10% sodium sulfacetamide	0.01% mg thimerosal, EDTA, boric acid	In 5 and 10 mL
Rx	**Sulster Solution** (Akorn)			0.01% thimerosal, EDTA	In 5 and 10 mL.
Rx	**Vasocidin Solution** (Novartis)			EDTA, 0.01% thimerosal, poloxamer 407	In 5 and 10 mL.

STEROID AND SULFONAMIDE COMBINATIONS, SUSPENSIONS AND SOLUTIONS — OPHTHALMIC

The information for steroid preparations and sulfonamide preparations must be considered when using these products. See individual monographs.

Indications

➤*Inflammation/Infection:* For corticosteroid-responsive inflammatory ocular conditions for which a corticosteroid is indicated and where superficial bacterial ocular infection or a risk of infection exists.

Administration and Dosage

➤*Solutions/Suspensions:* Instill 1 to 3 drops into the conjunctival sac(s) every 1 to 4 hours during the day and at bedtime until a favorable response is obtained.

Do not prescribe more than 20 mL initially or refill prescription without further evaluation.

For complete dosage instructions, see individual manufacturer inserts.

Storage/Stability – Protect from light. Do not freeze. Shake well before using. Do not use if solution or suspension has darkened. Clumping may occur on long standing at high temperatures.

➤*Ointments:* Apply a small amount (≈ ½ inch ribbon) into the conjunctival sac(s) 3 or 4 times daily and once at bedtime (or once or twice at night) until a favorable response is obtained.

Do not prescribe more than 8 g initially, and the prescription should not be refilled without further evaluation.

For complete dosage instructions, see individual manufacturer inserts.

Storage/Stability – Keep tightly closed. Store away from heat.

STEROID AND SULFONAMIDE COMBINATIONS, OINTMENTS

	Product & Distributor	Steroid	Sulfonamide	Other Content	How Supplied
Rx	**Blephamide** (Allergan)	0.2% prednisolone acetate	10% sodium sulfacetamide	0.0008% phenylmercuric acetate, mineral oil, white petrolatum, lanolin alcohol	In 3.5 g.

POVIDONE IODINE

Rx	**Betadine 5% Sterile Ophthalmic Prep Solution** (Alcon)	**Solution:** 5% povidone iodine	In 50 mL.[1]

[1] Glycerin, sodium chloride, sodium hydroxide and sodium phosphate.

POVIDONE IODINE — OPHTHALMIC

Indications

➤*Ophthalmic preoperative prep:* Used prior to eye surgery to prep the periocular region (lids, brow and cheek) and irrigate the ocular surface (cornea, conjunctiva and palpebral fornices).

Administration and Dosage

Transfer solution to a sterile prep cup. Apply to lashes and lid margins with sterile applicator, repeat once. Apply to lids, brow and cheek with sterile applicator, repeat 3 times. Irrigate cornea, conjunctiva and palpebral fornices with solution and leave in for 2 minutes; flush with sterile saline solution.

Actions

➤*Pharmacology:* Povidone iodine has broad-spectrum antimicrobial action.

Contraindications

Hypersensitivity to iodine.

Warnings

➤*For external use only:* Not for intraocular injection or irrigation.

➤*Pregnancy:* Category C. Safety for use during pregnancy has not been established. Use only when clearly needed.

➤*Lactation:* Because of the potential for adverse reactions in nursing infants, decide whether to discontinue nursing or discontinue the drug, taking into account the importance of the drug to the mother.

➤*Children:* Safety and efficacy have not been established.

Precautions

➤*Thyroid disorders:* Use caution in patients with thyroid disorders due to the possibility of iodine absorption.

Adverse Reactions

Local sensitivity has been exhibited by some individuals.

SILVER NITRATE

Rx	**Silver Nitrate** (Lilly)	**Solution:** 1%	With acetic acid and sodium acetate. In 100s (wax ampules).

SILVER NITRATE — OPHTHALMIC

Indications

➤*Ophthlamic neonatorum:* Prevention of gonorrheal ophthalmia neonatorum.

Administration and Dosage

Immediately after birth, clean the eyelids with steril absorbent cotton or gauze and sterile water. Use a separate pledget for each eye; wash unopened lids from the nose outward until free of blood, mucus or meconium. Next, separate the lids and instill 2 drops of 1% solutions. Elevate lids away from the eyeball so that a lake of silver nitrate may lie for ≥ 30 seconds between them, contacting the entire conjunctival sac.

The American Academy of Pediatrics has endorsed a statement from the Committee on Ophthalmia Neonatorum of the National Society for the prevention of Blindness, which does not recommend irrigation of the eyes following instillation of the silver nitrate.

➤*Storage/Stability:* Do not freeze. Do not use when cold. Protect from light.

Actions

➤*Pharmacology:* Silver nitrate ophthalmic solution is an anti-infective. In weak solutions, it is used as a germicide and astringent to mucous membranes. The germicidal action is due to precipitation of bacterial proteins by liberated silver ions.

Contraindications

Hypersensitivity to any component of the formulation.

Warnings

➤*Neonatal chlamydial conjunctivitis:* Silver nitrate has not been effective for the prevention of neonatal chlamydial conjunctivitis.

➤*Cauterization of cornea:* A 1% solution is considered optimal. Use with caution, since cauterization of the cornea and blindness may result, especially with repeated applications.

➤*Caustic/Irritant:* Silver nitrate is caustic and irritating to the skin and mucous membranes.

Precautions

➤*Staining:* Handle solutions carefully because they tend to stain skin and utensils. Stains may be removed from linen by applications of iodine tincture followed by sodium thiosulfate solution.

Drug Interactions

➤*Sulfonamide:* Sulfonamide preparations are incompatible with silver preparations.

Adverse Reactions

A mild chemical conjunctivitis should result from a properly performed Credé prophylaxis using silver nitrate. A more severe chemical conjunctivitis occurs in ≤ 20% of cases.

Overdosage

When ingested, silver nitrate is highly toxic to the GI tract and CNS. Swallowing can cause severe gastroenteritis that may be fatal. Sodium chloride may be used by gastric lavage to remove the chemical.

When a solution of ≥ 2% silver nitrate concentration is used in the eye, conjunctivits may be produced. Irrigate the eye with an isotonic solution of sodium chloride after solutions of silver nitrate stronger than 1% are instilled.

OPHTHALMIC ANTIFUNGALS

NATAMYCIN — OPHTHALMIC

Rx	**Natacyn** (Alcon)	**Suspension:** 5%	With 0.02% benzalkonium chloride. In 15 mL.

NATAMYCIN — OPHTHALMIC

Indications

➤*Ocular fungal infections:* For the treatment of fungal blepharitis, conjunctivitis, and keratitis caused by susceptible organisms including *Fusarium solani* keratitis. As in other forms of suppurative keratitis, initial and sustained therapy of fungal keratitis should be determined by the clinical diagnosis, laboratory diagnosis by smear and culture of corneal scrapings and drug response. Whenever possible the in vitro activity of natamycin against the responsible fungus should be determined. The effectiveness of natamycin as a single agent in fungal endophthalmitis has not been established.

Administration and Dosage

Shake well before using.

The preferred initial dosage in fungal keratitis is one drop of natamycin ophthalmic suspension, USP 5% instilled in the conjunctival sac at hourly or 2-hour intervals. The frequency of application can usually be reduced to 1 drop 6 to 8 times daily after the first 3 to 4 days. Therapy should generally be continued for 14 to 21 days or until there is resolution of active fungal keratitis. In many cases, it may be helpful to reduce the dosage gradually at 4 to 7 day intervals to assure that the replicating organism has been eliminated. Less frequent initial dosage (4 to 6 daily applications) may be sufficient in fungal blepharitis and conjunctivitis.

➤*Storage/Stability:* Store in refrigerator at 2° to 8°C (36° to 46°F) or at room temperature 8° to 24°C (46° to 75°F). Do not freeze. Avoid exposure to light and excessive heat.

Actions

➤*Pharmacology:* Natamycin is a tetraene polyene antibiotic derived from *Streptomyces natalensis*. It possesses in vitro activity against a variety of yeast and filamentous fungi, including *Candida*, *Aspergillus*, *Cephalosporium*, *Fusarium* and *Penicillium*. The mechanism of action appears to be through binding of the molecule to the sterol moiety of the fungal cell membrane. The polyenesterol complex alters the permeability of the membrane to produce depletion of essential cellular constituents. Although the activity against fungi is dose-related, natamycin is predominantly fungicidal. Natamycin is not effective in vitro against gram-positive or gram-negative bacteria. Topical administration appears to produce effective concentrations of natamycin within the corneal stroma but not in intraocular fluid. Systemic absorption should not be expected following topical administration of natamycin ophthalmic suspension, USP 5%. As with other polyene antibiotics, absorption from the gastrointestinal tract is very poor. Studies in rabbits receiving topical natamycin revealed no measurable compound in the aqueous humor or sera, but the sensitivity of the measurement was no greater than 2 mg/mL.

Contraindications

Hypersensitivity to any of its components.

NATAMYCIN — OPHTHALMIC

Warnings

➤*Pregnancy: Category C.* Animal reproduction studies have not been conducted with natamycin. It is also not known whether natamycin can cause fetal harm when administered to a pregnant woman or can affect reproduction capacity. Natamycin ophthalmic suspension, USP 5% should be given to a pregnant woman only if clearly needed.

➤*Lactation:* It is not known whether these drugs are excreted in human milk. Because many drugs are excreted in human milk, caution should be exercised when natamycin is administered to a nursing woman.

➤*Children:* Safety and effectiveness in pediatric patients have not been established.

Precautions

➤*Usage:* Failure of improvement of keratitis following 7 to 10 days of administration of the drug suggests that the infection may be caused by a microorganism not susceptible to natamycin. For topical eye use only; not for injection.

Continuation of therapy should be based on clinical re-evaluation and additional laboratory studies.

➤*Toxicity:* Adherence of the suspension to areas of epithelial ulceration or retention of the suspension in the fornices occurs regularly. There have only been a limited number of cases in which natamycin has been used; therefore, it is possible that adverse reactions of which we have no knowledge at present may occur. For this reason, patients on this drug should be monitored at least twice weekly. Should suspicion of drug toxicity occur, the drug should be discontinued.

Adverse Reactions

One case of conjunctival chemosis and hyperemia, thought to be allergic in nature, has been reported.

Patient Information

Do not touch dropper tip to any surface, as this may contaminate the suspension.

OPHTHALMIC ANTIVIRAL AGENTS

TRIFLURIDINE OPHTHALMIC

Rx	**Trifluridine** (Falcon)	**Solution:** 1%	In aqueous solution with NaCl, 0.001% thimerosal. In 7.5 mL.
Rx	**Viroptic** (Monarch)		In aqueous solution with NaCl and 0.001% thimerosal. In 7.5 mL Drop-Dose.

TRIFLURIDINE — OPHTHALMIC

Refer to the Topical Ophthalmics introduction for more complete and comparative information.

Indications

➤*Ocular viral infections:* For the treatment of primary keratoconjunctivitis and recurrent epithelial keratitis due to herpes simplex virus, types 1 and 2.

Administration and Dosage

➤*Approved by the FDA:* October 6, 1995.

Instill 1 drop of trifluridine ophthalmic solution onto the cornea of the affected eye every 2 hours while awake for a maximum daily dosage of 9 drops until the corneal ulcer has completely re-epithelialized. Following re-epithelialization, treatment for an additional 7 days of 1 drop every 4 hours while awake for a minimum daily dosage of 5 drops is recommended. If there are no signs of improvement after 7 days of therapy or complete re-epithelialization has not occurred after 14 days of therapy, other forms of therapy should be considered. Continuous administration of trifluridine for periods exceeding 21 days should be avoided because of potential ocular toxicity.

The recommended dosage and frequency of administration should not be exceeded.

➤*Storage/Stability:* Store under refrigeration 2° to 8°C (36° to 46°F).

Actions

➤*Pharmacology:* Trifluridine is a fluorinated pyrimidine nucleoside with in vitro and in vivo activity against herpes simplex virus, types 1 and 2 and vacciniavirus. Some strains of adenovirus are also inhibited in vitro.

Trifluridine is also effective in the treatment of epithelial keratitis that has not responded clinically to the topical adminstration of idoxuridine or when ocular toxicity or hypersensitivity to idoxuridine has occurred. In a smaller number of patients found to be resistant to topical vidarabine, trifluridine was also effective.

Trifluridine interferes with DNA synthesis in cultured mammalian cells. However, its antiviral mechanism of action is not completely known.

➤*Pharmacokinetics:*

Absorption – Systemic absorption of trifluridine following therapeutic dosing with trifluridine appears to be negligible. No detectable concentrations of trifluridine or 5-carboxy-2′-deoxyuridine were found in the sera of adult healthy subjects who had trifluridine instilled into their eyes 7 times daily for 14 consecutive days.

Contraindications

Hypersensitivity reactions or chemical intolerance to trifluridine.

Warnings

➤*Animal pharmacology and animal toxicology:* Corneal wound-healing studies in rabbits showed that trifluridine did not significantly retard closure of epithelial wounds. However, mild toxic changes such as intracellular edema of the basal cell layer, mild thinning of the overlying epithelium and reduced strength of stromal wounds were observed.

Whereas instillation of trifluridine into rabbit eyes during a subchronic toxicity study produced some degree of corneal epithelial thinning, a 12-month chronic toxicity study in rabbits in which trifluridine was instilled into eyes in intermittent, multiple, full-therapy courses showed no drug-related changes in the cornea.

➤*Carcinogenesis:* Lifetime carcinogenicity bioassays in rats and mice given daily SC doses of trifluridine have been performed. Rats tested at 1.5, 7.5, and 15 mg/kg/day had increased incidences of adenocarcinomas of the intestinal tract and mammary glands, hemangiosarcomas of the spleen and liver, carcinosarcomas of the prostate gland, and granulosa-thecal cell tumors of the ovary. Mice were tested at 1, 5, and 10 mg/kg/day; those given 10 mg/kg/day trifluridine had significantly increased incidences of adenocarcinomas of the intestinal tract and uterus. Those given 10 mg/kg/day also had a significantly increased incidence of testicular atrophy as compared to vehicle-control mice.

➤*Mutagenesis:* Trifluridine has been shown to exert mutagenic, DNA-damaging and cell-transforming activities in various standard in vitro test systems, and clastogenic activity in Vicia faba cells. It did not induce chromosome aberrations in bone marrow cells of male or female rats following a single SC dose of 100 mg/kg, but was weakly positive in female, but not in male, rats following daily SC administration at 700 mg/kg/day for 5 days.

Although the significance of these test results is not clear or fully understood, there exists the possibility that mutagenic agents may cause genetic damage in humans.

➤*Pregnancy: Category C.*

Teratogenic – Trifluridine was not teratogenic at doses up to 5 mg/kg/day (23 times the estimated human exposure) when given SC to rats and rabbits. However, fetal toxicity consisting of delayed ossification of portions of the skeleton occurred at dose levels of 2.5 and 5 mg/kg/day in rats and at 2.5 mg/kg/day in rabbits. In addition, both 2.5 and 5 mg/kg/day produced fetal death and resorption in rabbits. In both rats and rabbits, 1 mg/kg/day (5 times the estimated human exposure) was a no-effect level. There were no teratogenic or fetotoxic effects after topical application of trifluridine ophthalmic solution ($\approx$ 5 times the estimated human exposure) to the eyes of rabbits on the sixth through the 18th days of pregnancy. In a nonstandard test, trifluridine solution has been shown to be teratogenic when injected directly into the yolk sac of chicken eggs. There are no adequate and well-controlled studies in pregnant women. Trifluridine ophthalmic solution should be used during pregnancy only if the potential benefit justifies the potential risk to the fetus.

➤*Lactation:* It is unlikely that trifluridine is excreted in human milk after ophthalmic instillation of trifluridine because of the relatively small dosage ($\leq$ 5 mg/day), its dilution in body fluids and its extremely short half-life ($\approx$ 12 minutes). The drug should not be prescribed for nursing mothers unless the potential benefits outweigh the potential risks.

➤*Children:* Safety and efficacy in pediatric patients below 6 years of age have not been established.

Precautions

➤*Diagnosis:* Only prescribe trifluridine ophthalmic solution for patients who have a clinical diagnosis of herpetic keratitis.

➤*Irritation:* Trifluridine may cause mild local irritation of the conjunctiva and cornea when instilled, but these effects are usually transient.

➤*Resistance:* Although documented in vitro viral resistance to trifluridine has not been reported following multiple exposures to trifluridine, the possibility of the development of viral resistance exists.

Adverse Reactions

The most frequent adverse reactions reported during controlled clinical trials were mild, transient burning or stinging upon instillation (4.6%) and palpebral edema (2.8%). Other adverse reactions in decreasing order of reported frequency were superficial punctate keratopathy, epithelial keratopathy, hypersensitivity reaction, stromal edema, irritation, keratitis sicca, hyperemia, and increased intraocular pressure.

Overdosage

➤*Symptoms:* Overdosage by ocular instillation is unlikely because any excess solution should be quickly expelled from the conjunctival sac.

Acute overdosage by accidental oral ingestion of trifluridine has not occurred. However, should such ingestion occur, the 75 mg dosage of trifluridine in a 7.5 mL bottle of trifluridine is not likely to produce adverse effects.

TRIFLURIDINE — OPHTHALMIC

Single IV doses of 1.5 to 30 mg/kg/day in children and adults with neoplastic disease produce reversible bone marrow depression as the only potentially serious toxic effect and only after 3 to 5 courses of therapy. The acute oral LD_{50} in the mouse and rat was ≥ 4379 mg/kg.

GANCICLOVIR

Rx	**Vitrasert** (Bausch & Lomb Incorporated)	**Implant:** 4.5 mg	In individual unit boxes.

GANCICLOVIR — IMPLANT

Indications

➤*Cytomegalovirus (CMV) retinitis:* For the treatment of CMV retinitis in patients with acquired immune deficiency syndrome (AIDS).

Administration and Dosage

➤*Approved by the FDA:* March 4, 1996.

The ganciclovir implant is for intravitreal implantation only.

Each ganciclovir implant contains a minimum of 4.5 mg ganciclovir and is designed to release the drug over a 5– to 8–month period of time. Following depletion of ganciclovir from the ganciclovir implant, as evidenced by progression of retinitis, the ganciclovir implant may be removed or replaced.

➤*Handling and disposal:* Caution should be exercised in handling of the ganciclovir implant in order to avoid damage to the polymer coating on the implant, which may result in an increased rate of drug release. Thus, the ganciclovir implant should be handled only by the suture tab. Aseptic technique should be maintained at all times prior to and during the surgical implantation procedure.

Because the ganciclovir implant contains ganciclovir, which shares some of the properties of antitumor agents (ie, carcinogenicity, mutagenicity), consideration should be given to handling and disposal of the ganciclovir implant according to guidelines issued for antineoplastic drugs.

➤*Storage/Stability:* Store at controlled room temperature, 15° to 30°C (59° to 86°F). Protect from freezing, excessive heat, and light.

Actions

➤*Pharmacology:* Ganciclovir is a synthetic nucleoside analog of 2′-deoxyguanosine that inhibits replication of herpes viruses both in vitro and in vivo. Sensitive human viruses include CMV, herpes simplex virus (types 1 and 2), Epstein-Barr virus, and varicella zoster virus. Clinical studies have been limited to assessment of efficacy in patients with CMV infection.

Median effective inhibitory doses (ED_{50}) of ganciclovir for human CMV isolates tested in vitro in several cell lines ranged from 0.2 to 3 mcg/mL. The relationship between in vitro sensitivity of CMV to ganciclovir and clinical response has not been established. Ganciclovir inhibits mammalian cell proliferation in vitro at higher concentrations (10 to 60 mcg/mL) with bone marrow colony forming cells being the most sensitive (ID_{50} greater than 10 mcg/mL) of those cell types tested.

Emergence of viral resistance has been reported based on in vitro sensitivity testing of CMV isolates from patients receiving intravenous (IV) ganciclovir treatment. The prevalence of resistant isolates is unknown, and there is a possibility that some patients may be infected with strains of CMV resistant to ganciclovir. Therefore, consider the possibility of viral resistance in patients who show poor clinical response.

➤*Pharmacokinetics:*

Absorption/Distribution – In a clinical trial of ganciclovir implants, 26 patients (30 eyes) received a total of 39 primary implants and 12 exchange implants (performed 32 weeks after the implant was inserted or earlier if progression of CMV retinitis occurred). Because most of the exchanged implants were empty, the time the implant actually ran out of drug was unknown, and a precise in vivo release rate could not be calculated. However, approximate in vivo release rates could be determined for the exchanged implants, which ranged from 1 mcg/h to more than 1.62 mcg/h.

In 14 implants (3 exchanged, 11 autopsy) in which the in vivo release rate could accurately be calculated, the mean release rate was 1.4 mcg/h, with a range from 0.5 to 2.88 mcg/h. The mean vitreous drug levels in 8 eyes (4 collected at the time of retinal detachment surgery; 2 collected from autopsy eyes within 6 hours of death and prior to fixation; 2 collected from implant exchanges) was 4.1 mcg/mL.

Contraindications

Hypersensitivity to ganciclovir or acyclovir, and in patients with any contraindications for intraocular surgery, (eg, external infection, severe thrombocytopenia).

Warnings

➤*Extraocular CMV disease:* CMV retinitis may be associated with CMV elsewhere in the body. The ganciclovir implant provides localized therapy limited to the implanted eye. The ganciclovir implant does not provide treatment for systemic CMV disease. Monitor patients for extraocular CMV disease.

➤*Surgical risk:* As with any surgical procedure, there is risk involved. Potential complications accompanying intraocular surgery to place the ganciclovir implant into the vitreous cavity may include, but are not limited to, the following: vitreous loss, vitreous hemorrhage, cataract formation, retinal detachment, uveitis, endophthalmitis, and disease in visual acuity.

➤*Visual acuity:* Following implantation of the ganciclovir implant, nearly all patients will experience an immediate and temporary decrease in visual acuity in the implanted eye which lasts for approximately 2 to 4 weeks postoperatively. The decrease in visual acuity is likely a result of the surgical implant procedure.

➤*Carcinogenesis:* Ganciclovir was carcinogenic in the mouse at oral dosages of 20 and 1,000 mg/kg/day. At the dosage of 1,000 mg/kg/day, there was a significant increase in the incidence of tumors of the preputial gland in males, forestomach (nonglandular mucosa) in males and females, and reproductive tissues (ovaries, uterus, mammary gland, clitoral gland, vagina) and liver in females. At the dosage of 20 mg/kg/day, a slightly increased incidence of tumors was noted in the preputial and harderian glands in males, forestomach in males and females, and liver in females. Except for histiocytic sarcoma of the liver, ganciclovir-induced tumors were generally of epithelial or vascular origin. Although the preputial and clitoral glands, forestomach, and harderian glands of mice do not have human counterparts, ganciclovir should be considered a potential carcinogen in humans.

➤*Mutagenesis:* Ganciclovir increased mutations in mouse lymphoma cells and deoxyribonucleic acid (DNA) damage in human lymphocytes in vitro at concentrations between 50 to 500 and 250 to 2,000 mcg/mL, respectively. In mouse micronucleus assay, ganciclovir was clastogenic at doses of 150 and 500 mg/kg (IV) (2.8 to 10×human exposure based on area under the curve [AUC]) but not 50 mg/kg (exposure approximately comparable with the human based on AUC). Ganciclovir was not mutagenic in the Ames Salmonella assay at concentrations of 500 to 5,000 mcg/mL.

➤*Fertility impairment:* Ganciclovir caused decreased mating behavior, decreased fertility, and an increased incidence of embryolethality in female mice following IV dosages of 90 mg/kg/day. Ganciclovir caused decreased fertility in male mice and hypospermatogenisis in mice and dogs following daily oral or IV administration of doses ranging from 0.2 to 10 mg/kg.

➤*Pregnancy: Category C.* Ganciclovir has been shown to be teratogenic in rabbits and embryotoxic in rabbits and mice following IV administration. Fetal reabsorption was present in at least 85% of rabbits and mice administered 60 and 108 mg/kg/day, respectively. Effects observed in rabbits included: fetal growth retardation, embryolethality, teratogenicity, and/or maternal toxicity. Teratogenic changes included cleft palate, anophthalmia/microphthalmia, aplastic organs (kidney and pancreas), hydrocephaly, and brachygnathia. In mice, effects observed were maternal/fetal toxicity and embryolethality.

Daily IV doses of 90 mg/kg administered to female mice prior to mating, during gestation, and during lactation caused hypoplasia of the testes and seminal vesicles in the month-old male offspring, as well as pathologic changes in the nonglandular region of the stomach.

Although each ganciclovir implant contains 4.5 to 6.4 mg of ganciclovir, which is released locally in the vitreous, there are no adequate and well-controlled studies in pregnant women on the effects of the ganciclovir implant. Therefore, only use ganciclovir implant used during pregnancy if the potential benefit justifies the potential risk to the fetus.

➤*Lactation:* It is not known whether ganciclovir from the ganciclovir implant is excreted in human milk. Daily IV doses of 90 mg/kg administered to female mice prior to mating, during gestation, and during lactation caused hypoplasia of the testes and seminal vesicles in the month-old male offspring, as well as pathologic changes in the nonglandular region of the stomach. Because many drugs are excreted in human milk, and because carcinogenicity and teratogenicity effects occurred in animals treated with ganciclovir, instruct mothers to discontinue breast-feeding if they have the ganciclovir implant.

➤*Children:* Safety and efficacy in patients younger than below 9 years of age have not been established.

Precautions

➤*Monitoring:* Monitor patients for extraocular CMV disease.

➤*Handling:* As with all intraocular surgery, rigorously maintain sterility of the surgical field and the ganciclovir implant. maintained. Handle the ganciclovir implant only by the suture tab in order to avoid damaging the polymer coatings because this could affect release rate of ganciclovir inside the eye. Do not resterilize the ganciclovir implant by any method.

➤*Experienced surgeons:* A high level of surgical skill is required for implantation of the ganciclovir implant. A surgeon should have observed or assisted in surgical implantation of the ganciclovir implant prior to attempting the procedure.

➤*Retinal tamponade:* There is limited experience with retinal tamponade in conjunction with the ganciclovir implant.

Drug Interactions

No drug interactions have been observed with the ganciclovir implant.

Adverse Reactions

➤*Ophthalmic:* During clinical trials, the most frequent adverse reactions seen in patients treated with the ganciclovir implant involved the eye.

During the first 2 months following implantation, visual acuity loss of 3 lines or more, vitreous hemorrhage, and retinal detachments occurred in approximately 10% to 20% of patients. Cataract formation/lens opacities,

GANCICLOVIR — IMPLANT

macular abnormalities, intraocular pressure spikes, optic disk/nerve changes, hyphemas, and uveitis occurred in approximately 1% to 5%.

Adverse reactions with an incidence of less than 1% were: [angle closure glaucoma with anterior chamber swallowing, anterior chamber cell and flare, astigmatism, chemosis, choroidal folds, choroiditis, corneal dellen, cotton wool spots, endophthalmitis, gliosis, hemorrhage (other than vitreous), hypotony, keratopathy, microangiopathy, pellet extrusion from scleral wound, phthisis bulbi, retinal hole, retinal tear, retinopathy, sclerosis, severe postoperative inflammation, synechia, vitreous detachment, and vitreous traction].

Patient Information

Advise the patient that the ganciclovir implant is not a cure for CMV retinitis, and some immunocompromised patients may continue to experience progression of retinitis with the ganciclovir implant. Adise patients to have ophthalmologic follow-up examinations of both eyes at appropriate intervals following implantation of the ganciclovir implant.

As with any surgical procedure, there is risk involved. Potential complications accompanying intraocular surgery to place the ganciclovir implant into the vitreous cavity may include, but are not limited to, the following: intraocular infection or inflammation, detachment of the retina, and formation of cataract in the natural crystalline lens.

Following implantation of the ganciclovir implant, nearly all patients will experience an immediate and temporary decrease in visual acuity in the implanted eye which lasts for approximately 2 to 4 weeks. This decrease in visual acuity is likely a result of the surgical implant procedure.

The ganciclovir implant only treats eyes in which it has been implanted. Additionally, because CMV is a systemic disease, monitor patients for extraocular CMV infections (eg, pneumonitis, colitis) in the body.

Advise patients that ganciclovir has caused decreased sperm production in animals and may cause infertility in humans. Advise women of childbearing potential that ganciclovir causes birth defects in animals and should not be used during pregnancy. Also advise patients that ganciclovir has caused tumors in animals. Although there is no information from human studies, consider ganciclovir a potential carcinogen.

OPHTHALMIC IMMUNOLOGIC AGENTS

CYCLOSPORINE — OPHTHALMIC

Rx	**Restasis** (Allergan)	**Emulsion, ophthalmic:** 0.05%[1]	Preservative-free. In 0.4 mL single-use vials.

[1] With glycerin, castor oil, and polysorbate 80.

CYCLOSPORINE — OPHTHALMIC

Indications

➤*Increased tear production:* To increase tear production in patients whose tear production is presumed to be suppressed due to ocular inflammation associated with keratoconjunctivitis sicca. Increased tear production was not seen in patients currently taking topical anti-inflammatory drugs or using punctal plugs.

Administration and Dosage

➤*Approved by the FDA:* December 23, 2002.

Invert the unit dose vial a few times to obtain a uniform, white, opaque emulsion before using. Instill 1 drop of cyclosporine ophthalmic emulsion twice a day in each eye, approximately 12 hours apart. Cyclosporine can be used concomitantly with artificial tears, allowing a 15-minute interval between products. Discard vial immediately after use.

➤*Storage/Stability:* Store cyclosporine ophthalmic emulsion at 15° to 25°C (59° to 77°F). Keep out of the reach of children.

Actions

➤*Pharmacology:* Cyclosporine is an immunosuppressive agent when administered systemically.

In patients whose tear production is presumed to be suppressed due to ocular inflammation associated with keratoconjunctivitis sicca, cyclosporine emulsion is thought to act as a partial immunomodulator. The exact mechanism of action is not known.

➤*Pharmacokinetics:*

Absorption – Blood cyclosporin A concentrations were measured using a specific high-pressure liquid chromatography-mass spectrometry assay. Blood concentrations of cyclosporine, in all the samples collected, after topical administration of cyclosporine ophthalmic suspension 0.05%, twice daily, in humans for up to 12 months, were below the quantitation limit of 0.1 ng/mL. There was no detectable accumulation in blood during 12 months of treatment with cyclosporine ophthalmic emulsion.

Contraindications

In patients with active ocular infections; in patients with known or suspected hypersensitivity to any of the ingredients in the formulation.

Warnings

➤*Herpes keratitis:* Cyclosporine ophthalmic emulsion has not been studied in patients with a history of herpes keratitis.

➤*Carcinogenesis:* Systemic carcinogenicity studies were carried out in male and female mice and rats. In the 78-week oral (diet) mouse study, at doses of 1, 4, and 16 mg/kg/day, evidence of a statistically significant trend was found for lymphocytic lymphomas in females, and the incidence of hepatocellular carcinomas in mid-dose males significantly exceeded the control value.

In the 24-month oral (diet) rat study, conducted at 0.5, 2, and 8 mg/kg/day, pancreatic islet cell adenomas significantly exceeded the control rate in the low-dose level. The hepatocellular carcinomas and pancreatic islet cell adenomas were not dose related. The low doses in mice and rats are approximately 1000 and 500 times greater, respectively, than the daily human dose of 1 drop (28 mcL) of 0.05% cyclosporine ophthalmic emulsion twice daily into each eye of a 60 kg person (0.001 mg/kg/day), assuming that the entire dose is absorbed.

➤*Mutagenesis:* Cyclosporine has not been found to be mutagenic/genotoxic in the Ames test, V79-HGPRT Test, the micronucleus test in mice and Chinese hamsters, the chromosome-aberration tests in Chinese hamster bone marrow, the mouse dominant lethal assay, and the DNA-repair test in sperm from treated from treated mice. A study analyzing sister chromatid exchange (SCE) induction by cyclosporine using human lymphocytes in vitro gave indication of a positive effect (ie, induction of SCE).

➤*Pregnancy: Category C.*

There are no adequate and well-controlled studies of cyclosporine ophthalmic emulsion in pregnant women. Only administer cyclosporine ophthalmic emulsion to a pregnant woman if clearly needed.

Nonteratogenic – Adverse reactions were seen in reproduction in rats and rabbits only at dose levels toxic to dams. At toxic doses (rats at 30 mg/kg/day and rabbits at 100 mg/kg/day), cyclosporine oral solution was embryo- and fetotoxic as indicated by increased pre- and postnatal mortality and reduced fetal weight together with related skeletal retardations. These doses are 30,000 and 100,000 times greater, respectively, than the daily human dose of 1 drop (28 mcL) of 0.05% cyclosporine ophthalmic emulsion twice daily into each eye of a 60 kg person (0.001 mg/kg/day), assuming that the entire dose is absorbed.

No evidence of embryofetal toxicity was observed in rats or rabbits receiving cyclosporine at oral doses up to 17/mg/kg/day or 30 mg/kg/day, respectively, during organogenesis. These doses in rats and rabbits are approximately 17,000 and 30,000 times greater, respectively, than the daily human dose.

Offspring of rats receiving a 45 mg/kg/day oral dose of cyclosporine from day 15 of pregnancy until day 21 postpartum, a maternally toxic level, exhibited an increase in postnatal mortality; this dose is 45,000 times greater than the daily human topical dose, 0.001 mg/kg/day, assuming that the entire dose is absorbed. No adverse events were observed at oral doses up to 15 mg/kg/day (15,000 times greater than the daily human dose).

➤*Lactation:* Cyclosporine is known to be excreted in human milk following systemic administration, but excretion in human milk after topical treatment has not been investigated. Although blood concentrations are undetectable after topical administration of cyclosporine ophthalmic emulsion, caution should be exercised when cyclosporine ophthalmic emulsion is administered to a nursing woman.

➤*Children:* The safety and efficacy of cyclosporine ophthalmic emulsion have not been established in pediatric patients below 16 years of age.

Precautions

➤*Administration:* Cyclosporine ophthalmic emulsion is for ophthalmic use only.

Adverse Reactions

The most common adverse reaction following the use of cyclosporine ophthalmic emulsion was ocular burning (17%).

Other events reported in 1% to 5% of patients included conjunctival hyperemia, discharge, epiphora, eye pain, foreign body sensation, pruritus, stinging, and visual disturbance (most often blurring).

Patient Information

The emulsion from 1 individual single-use vial is to be used immediately after opening for administration to 1 or both eyes, and the remaining contents should be discarded immediately after administration.

Do not allow the tip of the vial to touch the eye or any surface, as this may contaminate the emulsion.

Cyclosporine ophthalmic emulsion should not be administered while wearing contact lenses. Patients with decreased tear production typically should not wear contact lenses. If contact lenses are worn, they should be removed prior to the administration of the emulsion. Lenses may be reinserted 15 minutes following administration of cyclosporine ophthalmic emulsion.

PEGAPTANIB SODIUM

Rx	**Macugen** (Eyetech)	**Injection:** 0.3 mg[a]	In 1 mL glass syringe. With 27-gauge needle and shield.

[a] Equivalent to 1.6 mg pegaptanib sodium (pegylated oligonucleotide) or 3.2 mg when expressed as the sodium salt form of the oligonucleotide moiety.

PEGAPTANIB SODIUM — OPHTHALMIC INJECTION

Indications

➤*Neovascular age-related macular degeneration (AMD):* For the treatment of neovascular (wet) age-related macular degeneration.

Administration and Dosage

➤*Approved by the FDA:* December 17, 2004.

Administer pegaptanib 0.3 mg once every 6 weeks by intravitreous injection into the eye to be treated.

The safety and efficacy of pegaptanib therapy administered to both eyes concurrently have not been studied.

➤*Administration:* Inspect pegaptanib visually for particulate matter and discoloration prior to administration. Administration of the syringe contents involves attaching the threaded plastic plunger rod to the rubber stopper inside the barrel of the syringe. Do not pull back on the plunger. The syringe needle cap is then removed to allow administration of the product.

Carry out the injection procedure under controlled aseptic conditions, which includes the use of sterile gloves, a sterile drape, and a sterile eyelid speculum (or equivalent). Give adequate anesthesia and a broad-spectrum microbicide prior to the injection.

➤*Storage/Stability:* Store in the refrigerator at 2° to 8°C (36° to 46°F). Do not freeze or shake vigorously.

Actions

➤*Pharmacology:* Pegaptanib is a selective vascular endothelial growth factor (VEGF) antagonist. VEGF is a secreted protein that selectively binds and activates its receptors located primarily on the surface of vascular endothelial cells. VEGF induces angiogenesis and increases vascular permeability and inflammation, all of which are thought to contribute to the progression of the neovascular (wet) form of AMD, a leading cause of blindness. VEGF has been implicated in blood retinal barrier breakdown and pathological ocular neovascularization.

Pegaptanib is an aptamer, a pegylated modified oligonucleotide, which adopts a 3-dimensional conformation that enables it to bind to extracellular VEGF. Under in vitro testing conditions, pegaptanib binds to the major pathological VEGF isoform, extracellular $VEGF_{165}$, thereby inhibiting $VEGF_{165}$ binding to its VEGF receptors. The inhibition of $VEGF_{164}$, the rodent counterpart of human $VEGF_{165}$, was effective at suppressing pathological neovascularization.

➤*Pharmacokinetics:*

Absorption – In animals, pegaptanib is slowly absorbed into the systemic circulation from the eye after intravitreous administration. The rate of absorption from the eye is the rate limiting step in the disposition of pegaptanib in animals and is likely to be the rate limiting step in humans.

In humans, a mean maximum plasma concentration of about 80 ng/mL occurs within 1 to 4 days after a 3 mg monocular dose (10 times the recommended dose). The mean area under the plasma concentration-time curve (AUC) is about 25 mcg•h/mL at this dose.

Distribution – Twenty-four hours after intravitreous administration of a radiolabeled dose of pegaptanib to both eyes of rabbits, radioactivity was mainly distributed in vitreous fluid, retina, and aqueous fluid. After intravitreous and intravenous administrations of radiolabeled pegaptanib to rabbits, the highest concentrations of radioactivity (excluding the eye for the intravitreous dose) were obtained in the kidney.

Metabolism/Excretion – In rabbits, the component nucleotide, 2-fluorouridine, is found in plasma and urine after single radiolabeled pegaptanib intravenous and intravitreous doses. In rabbits, pegaptanib is eliminated as parent drug and metabolites primarily in the urine.

Based on preclinical data, pegaptanib is metabolized by endo- and exonucleases.

In humans, after a 3 mg monocular dose (10 times the recommended dose), the average (± standard deviation) apparent plasma half life of pegaptanib is 10 (±4) days.

Special populations –

Renal function impairment: Dose adjustment for patients with renal impairment is not needed when administering the 0.3 mg dose.

Following a single 3 mg dose (10 times the recommended dose) in patients with severe (n = 7), moderate (n = 18), and mild (n = 10) renal impairment, the mean (CV%) pegaptanib AUC values were 37.8 (17%), 26.7 (31%), and 23.6 (21%) mcg•h/mL, respectively. The corresponding C_{max} values were 96.8 (23%), 81.6 (29.2%), and 66.5 (47%) ng/mL, respectively.

In patients with renal impairment, following administration of pegaptanib 3 mg doses every 6 weeks, the last detectable pegaptanib concentrations in plasma after the fourth dose were highly variable (ranging from 8 ng/mL to 66 ng/mL) and the variability was more pronounced in patients with severe renal impairment.

Contraindications

Ocular or periocular infections.

Warnings

➤*Endophthalmitis:* Intravitreous injections including those with pegaptanib have been associated with endophthalmitis. Utilize proper aseptic injection technique when administering pegaptanib. In addition, monitor patients during the week following the injection to permit early treatment, should an infection occur.

➤*Increased intraocular pressure:* Increases in intraocular pressure have been seen within 30 minutes of injection with pegaptanib. Therefore, monitor and manage intraocular pressure, as well as the perfusion of the optic nerve head.

➤*Mutagenesis:* Pegaptanib and its monomer component nucleotides (2'-MA, 2'-MG, 2'-FU, 2'-FC) were evaluated for genotoxicity in a battery of in vitro and in vivo assay systems. Pegaptanib, 2'-O-methyladenosine (2'-MA), and 2'-O-methylguanosine (2'-MG) were negative in all assay systems evaluated. 2'-fluorouridine (2'-FU) and 2'-fluorocytidine (2'-FC) were nonclastogenic and were negative in all *Salmonella typhimurium* tester strains, but produced a non-dose-related increase in revertant frequency in a single *Escherichia coli* tester strain. Pegaptanib, 2-FU, and 2-FC tested negative in cell transformation assays.

➤*Pregnancy: Category B.* There are no studies in pregnant women. The potential risk to humans is unknown. Use pegaptanib during pregnancy only if the potential benefit to the mother justifies the potential risk to the fetus.

➤*Lactation:* It is not known whether pegaptanib is excreted in human milk. Because many drugs are excreted in human milk, exercise caution when pegaptanib is administered to a nursing woman.

➤*Children:* Safety and effectiveness of pegaptanib in pediatric patients have not been studied.

Precautions

➤*Monitoring:* Following the injection, monitor patient's elevation in intraocular pressure and for endophthalmitis. Monitoring may consist of a check for perfusion of the optic nerve head immediately after the injection, tonometry within 30 minutes following the injection, and biomicroscopy between 2 and 7 days following the injection. Instruct patients to report any symptoms suggestive of endophthalmitis without delay.

➤*Administration:* For ophthalmic intravitreal injection only.

Drug Interactions

None known.

Adverse Reactions

Serious adverse events related to the injection procedure occurring in less than 1% of intravitreous injections included endophthalmitis, retinal detachment, and iatrogenic traumatic cataract.

The most frequently reported adverse events in patients treated with pegaptanib 0.3 mg for up to 2 years were anterior chamber inflammation, blurred vision, cataract, conjunctival hemorrhage, corneal edema, eye discharge, eye irritation, eye pain, hypertension, increased intraocular pressure, ocular discomfort, punctate keratitis, reduced visual acuity, visual disturbance, vitreous floaters, and vitreous opacities. These events occurred in approximately 10% to 40% of patients.

➤*The following events were reported in 6% to 10% of patients receiving pegaptanib 0.3 mg therapy:*

CNS – Dizziness, headache.

GI – Diarrhea, nausea.

Special senses – Blepharitis, conjunctivitis, photopsia, vitreous disorder.

Miscellaneous – Bronchitis, urinary tract infection.

➤*The following events were reported in 1% to 5% of patients receiving pegaptanib 0.3 mg therapy:*

Cardiovascular – Carotid artery occlusion, cerebrovascular accident, transient ischemic attack.

GI – Dyspepsia, vomiting.

Musculoskeletal – Arthritis, bone spur.

Special senses – Allergic conjunctivitis, conjunctival edema, corneal abrasion, corneal deposits, corneal epithelium disorder, endophthalmitis, eye inflammation, eyelid irritation, eye swelling, hearing loss, meibomianitis, mydriasis, periorbital hematoma, retinal edema, vitreous hemorrhage.

Miscellaneous – Chest pain, contact dermatitis, contusion, diabetes mellitus, pleural effusion, urinary retention, vertigo.

Overdosage

Doses of pegaptanib up to 10 times the recommended dosage of 0.3 mg have been studied. No additional adverse events have been noted, but there is decreased efficacy with doses above 1 mg.

Patient Information

In the days following pegaptanib administration, patients are at risk for the development of endophthalmitis. If the eye becomes red, sensitive to light, painful, or develops a change in vision, the patient should seek immediate care with their ophthalmologist.

VERTEPORFIN

Rx	**Visudyne** (QLT PhotoTherapeutics/Novartis Ophthalmics)	**Lyophilized cake for injection**: 15 mg (reconstituted to 2 mg/mL)	Egg phosphatidylglycerol. In single-use vials.

VERTEPORFIN — INJECTION

Indications

For the treatment of patients with predominantly classic subfoveal choroidal neovascularization due to age-related macular degeneration, pathologic myopia or presumed ocular histoplasmosis.

There is insufficient evidence to indicate verteporfin for the treatment of predominately occult subfoveal choroidal neovascularization.

➤*Unlabeled uses:* Treatment of psoriasis; psoriatic arthritis; rheumatoid arthritis; nonmelanoma skin cancers; circumscribed choroidal hemangioma.

Administration and Dosage

➤*Approved by the FDA:* April 12, 2000.

A course of verteporfin therapy is a 2-step process requiring administration of both drug and light.

The first step is the intravenous infusion of verteporfin. The second step is the activation of verteporfin with light from a nonthermal diode laser.

The physician should re-evaluate the patient every 3 months and if choroidal neovascular leakage is detected on fluorescein angiography, therapy should be repeated.

➤*Lesion size determination:* The greatest linear dimension (GLD) of the lesion is estimated by fluorescein angiography and color fundus photography. All classic and occult choroidal neovascularization (CNV), blood and/or blocked fluorescence, and any serous detachments of the retinal pigment epithelium should be included for this measurement. Fundus cameras with magnification within the range of 2.4 to 2.6X are recommended. The GLD of the lesion on the fluorescein angiogram must be corrected for the magnification of the fundus camera to obtain the GLD of the lesion on the retina.

➤*Spot size determination:* The treatment spot size should be 1,000 microns larger than the GLD of the lesion on the retina to allow a 500 micron border, ensuring full coverage of the lesion. The maximum spot size used in the clinical trials was 6400 microns.

The nasal edge of the treatment spot must be positioned at least 200 microns from the temporal edge of the optic disc, even if this will result in lack of photoactivation of CNV within 200 microns of the optic nerve.

➤*Verteporfin administration:* Reconstitute each vial of verteporfin with 7 mL of Sterile Water for Injection to provide 7.5 mL containing 2 mg/mL. Reconstituted verteporfin must be protected from light and used within 4 hours. It is recommended that reconstituted verteporfin be inspected visually for particulate matter and discoloration prior to administration. Reconstituted verteporfin is an opaque dark green solution.

The volume of reconstituted verteporfin required to achieve the desired dose of 6 mg/m^2 body surface area is withdrawn from the vial and diluted with 5% Dextrose for Injection to a total infusion volume of 30 mL. The full infusion volume is administered intravenously over 10 minutes at a rate of 3 mL/min, using an appropriate syringe pump and in-line filter. The clinical studies were conducted using a standard infusion line filter of 1.2 microns.

Precautions should be taken to prevent extravasation at the injection site. In the event of extravasation during infusion, the extravasation area must be thoroughly protected from direct light until the swelling and discoloration have faded in order to prevent the occurrence of a local burn which could be severe. If emergency surgery is necessary within 48 hours after treatment, as much of the internal tissue as possible should be protected from intense light.

➤*Light administration:* Initiate 689 nm wavelength laser light delivery to the patient 15 minutes after the start of the 10-minute infusion with verteporfin.

Photoactivation of verteporfin is controlled by the total light dose delivered. In the treatment of choroidal neovascularization, the recommended light dose is 50 J/cm^2 of neovascular lesion administered at an intensity of 600 mW/cm^2. This dose is administered over 83 seconds.

Light dose, light intensity, ophthalmic lens magnification factor and zoom lens setting are important parameters for the appropriate delivery of light to the predetermined treatment spot. Follow the laser system manuals for procedure set up and operation.

The laser system must deliver a stable power output at a wavelength of 689 ± 3 nm. Light is delivered to the retina as a single circular spot via a fiber optic and a slit lamp, using a suitable ophthalmic magnification lens.

The following laser systems have been tested for compatibility with verteporfin and are approved for delivery of a stable power output at a wavelength of 689 ± 3 nm: *Coherent Opal Photoactivator Laser Console* and *Modified Coherent LaserLink Adapter*, Manufactured by Lumenis, Inc, Santa Clara, CA; *Zeiss VISULAS 690s* laser and *VISULINK PDT/U* adapter, Manufactured by Carl Zeiss Inc, Thornwood, NY.

➤*Concurrent bilateral treatment:* The controlled trials only allowed treatment of one eye per patient. In patients who present with eligible lesions in both eyes, physicians should evaluate the potential benefits and risks of treating both eyes concurrently. If the patient has already received previous verteporfin therapy in one eye with an acceptable safety profile, both eyes can be treated concurrently after a single administration of verteporfin. The more aggressive lesion should be treated first, at 15 minutes after the start of infusion. Immediately at the end of light application to the first eye, the laser settings should be adjusted to introduce the treatment parameters for the second eye, with the same light dose and intensity as for the first eye, starting no later than 20 minutes from the start of infusion.

In patients who present for the first time with eligible lesions in both eyes without prior verteporfin therapy, it is prudent to treat only one eye (the most aggressive lesion) at the first course. One week after the first course, if no significant safety issues are identified, the second eye can be treated using the same treatment regimen after a second verteporfin infusion. Approximately 3 months later, both eyes can be evaluated and concurrent treatment following a new verteporfin infusion can be started if both lesions still show evidence of leakage.

➤*Spills and disposal:* Spills of verteporfin should be wiped up with a damp cloth. Skin and eye contact should be avoided due to the potential for photosensitivity reactions upon exposure to light. Use of rubber gloves and eye protection is recommended. All materials should be disposed of properly.

➤*Accidental exposure:* Because of the potential to induce photosensitivity reactions, it is important to avoid contact with the eyes and skin during preparation and administration of verteporfin. Any exposed person must be protected from bright light. Following injection with verteporfin, care should be taken to avoid exposure of skin or eyes to direct sunlight or bright indoor light for 5 days. In the event of extravasation during infusion, the extravasation area must be thoroughly protected from direct light until the swelling and discoloration have faded in order to prevent the occurrence of a local burn which could be severe. If emergency surgery is necessary within 48 hours after treatment, as much of the internal tissue as possible should be protected from intense light.

➤*Storage/Stability:* Store verteporfin between 20° and 25°C (68° to 77°F).

Actions

➤*Pharmacology:* Verteporfin therapy is a 2-stage process requiring administration of both verteporfin for injection and nonthermal red light.

Verteporfin is transported in the plasma primarily by lipoproteins. Once verteporfin is activated by light in the presence of oxygen, highly reactive, short-lived singlet oxygen and reactive oxygen radicals are generated. Light activation of verteporfin results in local damage to neovascular endothelium, resulting in vessel occlusion. Damaged endothelium is known to release procoagulant and vasoactive factors through the lipo-oxygenase (leukotriene) and cyclo-oxygenase (eicosanoids such as thromboxane) pathways, resulting in platelet aggregation, fibrin clot formation and vasoconstriction. Verteporfin appears to somewhat preferentially accumulate in neovasculature, including choroidal neovasculature. However, animal models indicate that the drug is also present in the retina. Therefore, there may be collateral damage to retinal structures following photoactivation including the retinal pigmented epithelium and outer nuclear layer of the retina. The temporary occlusion of CNV following verteporfin therapy has been confirmed in humans by fluorescein angiography.

➤*Pharmacokinetics:*

Metabolism/Excretion – Following intravenous infusion, verteporfin exhibits a bi-exponential elimination with a terminal elimination half-life of approximately 5 to 6 hours. The extent of exposure and the maximal plasma concentration are proportional to the dose between 6 and 20 mg/m^2. At the intended dose, pharmacokinetic parameters are not significantly affected by gender.

Verteporfin is metabolized to a small extent to its diacid metabolite by liver and plasma esterases. NADPH-dependent liver enzyme systems (including the cytochrome P450 isozymes) do not appear to play a role in the metabolism of verteporfin. Elimination is by the fecal route, with less than 0.01% of the dose recovered in urine.

Special populations –

Hepatic function impairment: In a study of patients with mild hepatic insufficiency (defined as having two abnormal hepatic function tests at enrollment), AUC and C_{max} were not significantly different from the control group, half-life however was significantly increased by approximately 20%.

Contraindications

Porphyria or a known hypersensitivity to any component of this preparation.

Warnings

➤*Light exposure:* Following injection with verteporfin, care should be taken to avoid exposure of skin or eyes to direct sunlight or bright indoor light for 5 days. In the event of extravasation during infusion, the extravasation area must be thoroughly protected from direct light until the swelling and discoloration have faded in order to prevent the occurrence of a local burn which could be severe. If emergency surgery is necessary within 48 hours after treatment, as much of the internal tissue as possible should be protected from intense light.

➤*Decrease in vision:* Patients who experience severe decrease of vision of 4 lines or more within 1 week after treatment should not be retreated, at least until their vision completely recovers to pretreatment levels and the potential benefits and risks of subsequent treatment are carefully considered by the treating physician.

➤*Lasers:* Use of incompatible lasers that do not provide the required characteristics of light for the photoactivation of verteporfin could result in

VERTEPORFIN — INJECTION

incomplete treatment due to partial photoactivation of verteporfin, overtreatment due to overactivation of verteporfin, or damage to surrounding normal tissue.

➤*Hepatic function impairment:* Verteporfin therapy should be considered carefully in patients with moderate to severe hepatic impairment or biliary obstruction since there is no clinical experience with verteporfin in such patients.

➤*Mutagenesis:* Photodynamic therapy (PDT) as a class has been reported to result in DNA damage including DNA strand breaks, alkali-labile sites, DNA degradation, and DNA-protein cross links which may result in chromosomal aberrations, sister chromatid exchanges (SCE), and mutations. In addition, other photodynamic therapeutic agents have been shown to increase the incidence of SCE in Chinese hamster ovary (CHO) cells irradiated with visible light and in Chinese hamster lung fibroblasts irradiated with near UV light, increase mutations and DNA-protein cross-linking in mouse L5178 cells, and increase DNA-strand breaks in malignant human cervical carcinoma cells, but not in normal cells. Verteporfin was not evaluated in these latter systems. It is not known how the potential for DNA damage with PDT agents translates into human risk.

➤*Elderly:* Approximately 90% of the patients treated with verteporfin in the clinical efficacy trials were greater than 65 years of age. A reduced treatment effect was seen with increasing age.

➤*Pregnancy:* *Category C.* There are no adequate and well-controlled studies in pregnant women. Only use verteporfin during pregnancy if the benefit justifies the potential risk to the fetus.

Teratogenic – Rat fetuses of dams administered verteporfin for injection intravenously at greater than or equal to 10 mg/kg/day during organogenesis (approximately 40-fold human exposure at 6 mg/m^2 based on AUC_{inf} in female rats) exhibited an increase in the incidence of anophthalmia/microphthalmia. Rat fetuses of dams administered 25 mg/kg/day (approximately 125-fold the human exposure at 6 mg/m^2 based on AUC_{inf} in female rats) had an increased incidence of wavy ribs and anophthalmia/microphthalmia.

In pregnant rabbits, a decrease in body weight gain and food consumption was observed in animals that received verteporfin for injection intravenously at greater than or equal to 10 mg/kg/day during organogenesis. The no observed adverse effect level (NOAEL) for maternal toxicity was 3 mg/kg/day (approximately 7-fold human exposure at 6 mg/m^2 based on body surface area). There were no teratogenic effects observed in rabbits at doses up to 10 mg/kg/day.

➤*Lactation:* It is not known whether verteporfin for injection is excreted in human milk. Because many drugs are excreted in human milk, caution should be exercised when verteporfin is administered to a woman who is nursing.

➤*Children:* Safety and effectiveness in pediatric patients have not been established.

Precautions

➤*Extravasation:* Standard precautions should be taken during infusion of verteporfin to avoid extravasation. Examples of standard precautions include, but are not limited to:

- A free-flowing intravenous (IV) line should be established before starting verteporfin infusion and the line should be carefully monitored.
- Due to the possible fragility of vein walls of some elderly patients, it is strongly recommended that the largest arm vein possible, preferably antecubital, be used for injection.
- Small veins in the back of the hand should be avoided.

If extravasation does occur, the infusion should be stopped immediately and cold compresses applied. Following injection with verteporfin, care should be taken to avoid exposure of skin or eyes to direct sunlight or bright indoor light for 5 days. In the event of extravasation during infusion, the extravasation area must be thoroughly protected from direct light until the swelling and discoloration have faded in order to prevent the occurrence of a local burn which could be severe. If emergency surgery is necessary within 48 hours after treatment, as much of the internal tissue as possible should be protected from intense light.

➤*Anesthesia:* There is no clinical data related to the use of verteporfin in anesthetized patients. At a greater than 10-fold higher dose given by bolus injection to anesthetized pigs, verteporfin caused severe hemodynamic effects, including death, probably as a result of complement activation. These effects were diminished or abolished by pretreatment with antihistamine, and they were not seen in conscious nonsedated pigs. Verteporfin resulted in a concentration-dependent increase in complement activation in human blood in vitro. At 10 mcg/mL (approximately 5 times the expected plasma concentration in human patients), there was mild to moderate complement activation. At greater than or equal to 100 mcg/mL, there was significant complement activation. Signs (chest pain, syncope, dyspnea, and flushing) consistent with complement activation have been observed in less than 1% of patients administered verteporfin. Patients should be supervised during verteporfin infusion.

Drug Interactions

Based on the mechanism of action of verteporfin, many drugs used concomitantly could influence the effect of verteporfin therapy. Possible examples include the following:

Calcium channel blockers, polymyxin B or radiation therapy could enhance the rate of verteporfin uptake by the vascular endothelium. Other photosensitizing agents (eg, tetracyclines, sulfonamides, phenothiazines, sulfonylurea hypoglycemic agents, thiazide diuretics and griseofulvin) could increase the potential for skin photosensitivity reactions. Compounds that quench active oxygen species or scavenge radicals, such as dimethyl sulfoxide, β-carotene, ethanol, formate and mannitol, would be expected to decrease verteporfin activity. Drugs that decrease clotting, vasoconstriction or platelet aggregation (eg, thromboxane A_2 inhibitors) could also decrease the efficacy of verteporfin therapy.

Adverse Reactions

The most frequently reported adverse events to verteporfin are injection site reactions (including extravasation and rashes) and visual disturbances (including blurred vision, decreased visual acuity and visual field defects). These events occurred in approximately 10% to 30% of patients. The following events, listed by body system, were reported more frequently with verteporfin therapy than with placebo therapy and occurred in 1% to 10% of patients.

➤*Cardiovascular:* Atrial fibrillation, hypertension, peripheral vascular disorder, varicose veins.

➤*CNS:* Hypesthesia, sleep disorder, vertigo.

➤*Dermatologic:* Eczema.

➤*GI:* Constipation, gastrointestinal cancers, nausea.

➤*GU:* Prostatic disorder.

➤*Hematologic/Lymphatic:* Anemia, white blood cell count decreased, white blood cell count increased.

➤*Hepatic:* Elevated liver function tests.

➤*Metabolic/Nutritional:* Albuminuria, creatinine increased.

➤*Musculoskeletal:* Arthralgia, arthrosis, myasthenia.

➤*Ophthalmic:* Blepharitis, cataracts, conjunctivitis/conjunctival injection, dry eyes, ocular itching, severe vision loss with or without subretinal or vitreous hemorrhage.

Severe vision decrease, equivalent of 4 lines or more, within 7 days after treatment has been reported in 1% to 5% of patients. Partial recovery of vision was observed in some patients.

➤*Respiratory:* Cough, pharyngitis, pneumonia.

➤*Special senses:* Decreased hearing, diplopia, lacrimation disorder.

➤*Miscellaneous:* Asthenia, back pain, fever, flu syndrome, photosensitivity reactions.

Photosensitivity reactions usually occurred in the form of skin sunburn following exposure to sunlight.

The higher incidence of back pain in the verteporfin group occurred primarily during infusion.

➤*Other adverse events:* The following adverse events have occurred either at low incidence (less than 1%) during clinical trials or have been reported during the use of verteporfin in clinical practice where these events were reported voluntarily from a population of unknown size and frequency of occurrence cannot be determined precisely. They have been chosen for inclusion based on factors such as seriousness, frequency of reporting, possible causal connection to verteporfin, or a combination of these factors:

Ophthalmic – Retinal detachment (nonrhegmatogenous), retinal or choroidal vessel nonperfusion.

Miscellaneous – Chest pain and other musculoskeletal pain during infusion, hypersensitivity reactions (which can be severe), syncope, severe allergic reactions with dyspnea and flushing, and vaso-vagal reactions.

Overdosage

Overdose of drug and/or light in the treated eye may result in nonperfusion of normal retinal vessels with the possibility of severe decrease in vision that could be permanent. An overdose of drug will also result in the prolongation of the period during which the patient remains photosensitive to bright light. In such cases, it is recommended to extend the photosensitivity precautions for a time proportional to the overdose.

Patient Information

Patients who receive verteporfin will become temporarily photosensitive after the infusion. Patients should wear a wrist band to remind them to avoid direct sunlight for 5 days. During that period, patients should avoid exposure of unprotected skin, eyes or other body organs to direct sunlight or bright indoor light. Sources of bright light include, but are not limited to, tanning salons, bright halogen lighting and high power lighting used in surgical operating rooms or dental offices. Prolonged exposure to light from light-emitting medical devices such as pulse oximeters should also be avoided for 5 days following verteporfin administration.

If treated patients must go outdoors in daylight during the first 5 days after treatment, they should protect all parts of their skin and their eyes by wearing protective clothing and dark sunglasses. UV sunscreens are not effective in protecting against photosensitivity reactions because photoactivation of the residual drug in the skin can be caused by visible light.

Patients should not stay in the dark and should be encouraged to expose their skin to ambient indoor light, as it will help inactivate the drug in the skin through a process called photobleaching.

OCULAR LUBRICANTS

otc	**Akwa Tears** (Akorn)	**Ointment**: White petrolatum, mineral oil, lanolin	Preservative free. In 3.5 g.
otc	**Dry Eyes** (Bausch & Lomb)		Preservative free. In 3.5 g.
otc	**Artificial Tears** (Rugby)	**Ointment**: White petrolatum, anhydrous liquid lanolin, mineral oil	In 3.5 g.
otc	**Duratears Naturale** (Alcon)		Preservative free. In 3.5 g.
otc	**HypoTears** (Novartis Ophthalmics)	**Ointment**: White petrolatum, light mineral oil	Preservative and lanolin free. In 3.5 g.
otc	**Puralube** (Fougera)		In 3.5 g.
otc	**Tears Renewed** (Akorn)		Preservative and lanolin free. In 3.5 g.
otc	**Stye** (Del Pharm)	**Ointment**: 55% white petrolatum, 32% mineral oil, boric acid, stearic acid, wheat germ oil	In 3.5 g.
otc	**Lacri-Lube NP** (Allergan)	**Ointment**: 55.5% white petrolatum, 42.5% mineral oil, 2% petrolatum/lanolin alcohol	Preservative free. In 0.7 g (UD 24s).
otc	**Refresh PM** (Allergan)	**Ointment**: 56.8% white petrolatum, 41.5% mineral oil, lanolin alcohols, sodium chloride	Preservative free. In 3.5 g.
otc	**Lacri-Lube S.O.P.** (Allergan)	**Ointment**: 56.8% white petrolatum, 42.5% mineral oil, chlorobutanol, lanolin alcohols	In 3.5 and 7 g.
otc	**Preservative Free Moisture Eyes PM** (Bausch & Lomb)	**Ointment**: 80% white petrolatum, 20% mineral oil	Preservative free. In 3.5 g.
otc	**LubriFresh P.M.** (Major)	**Ointment**: 83% white petrolatum, 15% mineral oil	Preservative free. Lanolin oil. In 3.5 g.

OCULAR LUBRICANTS — OPHTHALMIC

Refer to the Topical Ophthalmics introduction for more complete and comparative information.

Indications

➤*Ophthalmic lubrication:* Protection and lubrication of the eye.

Administration and Dosage

Pull down the lower lid of affected eye(s) and apply a small amount (0.25 inch) of ointment to the inside of the eyelid.

➤*Storage/Stability:* Store at room temperature 15° to 30°C (59° to 86°F). Store away from heat.

Actions

➤*Pharmacology:* These products serve as lubricants and emollients.

Contraindications

Hypersensitivity to any component of the products.

Patient Information

Do not touch tube tip to any surface since this may contaminate the product.

Do not use with contact lenses.

If eye pain, vision changes or continued redness or irritation occurs, or if the condition worsens or persists for > 72 hours, discontinue use and contact a physician.

TYLOXAPOL

otc	**Enuclene** (Alcon)	**Solution**: 0.25%	0.02% benzalkonium Cl. In 15 mL *Drop-Tainers.*

TYLOXAPOL — OPHTHALMIC

Indications

Tyloxapol solution is recommended for wearers of artificial eyes.

Tyloxapol solution lubricates, cleans, and wets the artificial eye, thereby increasing the wearing comfort to the patient.

Administration and Dosage

The drops should be used just as ordinary eye drops are used. With the artificial eye in place, drop 1 or 2 drops onto it, 3 or 4 times daily. The artificial eye may be removed periodically if advised by the physician and 2 or 3 drops applied to remove oily or mucous materials. The artificial eye is then rubbed between the fingers and rinsed with tap water. Then 1 or 2 drops may be applied to the artificial eye, either prior to or after reinsertion.

➤*Storage/Stability:* Store at 8° to 27°C (46° to 80°F).

Contraindications

Contraindicated in those persons who have shown hypersensitivity to any component of this preparation.

Patient Information

Do not touch dropper tip to any surface as this may contaminate the solution.

If irritation persists or increases, discontinue use and consult physician. Keep container tightly closed.

Keep out of reach of children.

ARTIFICIAL TEARS

ARTIFICIAL TEAR SOLUTIONS

otc	**20/20 Tears** (S.S.S. Co.)	**Drops**: 1.4% PVA, NaCl, KCl, 0.05% EDTA, 0.01% benzalkonium Cl.	In 0.5 fl oz.
otc	**Tears Again** (OcuSOFT Inc.[a])	**Drops**: 0.3% hydroxypropyl methylcellulose, boric acid, phosphoric acid, potassium chloride, sodium chloride *Dissipate* as a preservative	In 15 mL.
otc	**OptiZen** (InnoZen)	**Drops**: 0.5% polysorbate 80.	EDTA, NaCl, sodium phosphate, sorbic acid. In 10 mL.
otc	**Soothe** (Alimera Sciences[b])	**Drops**: 0.4% polysorbate 80, *Restoryl* (consists of 1% Drakeol-15 and 4.5% Drakeol-35)	EDTA. In 15 mL.
otc	**Visine Tears** (Pfizer Consumer)	**Drops**: 0.2% glycerin, 0.2% hypromellose, 1% polyethylene glycol 400	In 15 and 30 mL.
otc	**Visine Tears Preservative Free** (Pfizer Consumer)		Preservative-free. In 0.4 mL single-use containers.
otc	**Visine Pure Tears** (Pfizer Consumer)		In 9.5 mL single-drop dispenser.
otc	**Clear Eyes Contact Lens Relief** (Medtech)	**Drops**: 0.25% sorbic acid, 0.1% EDTA, sodium chloride, hypromellose, glycerin.	In 15 mL.
otc	**TheraTears** (Advanced Vision Research)	**Gel**: 1% carboxymethylcellulose sodium, KCl, sodium bicarbonate, NaCl, sodium phosphate.	In UD 28s.
otc	**Akwa Tears** (Akorn)	**Solution**: 0.01% benzalkonium Cl, 1.4% polyvinyl alcohol, sodium phosphate, EDTA, NaCl	In 15 mL.
otc	**Artificial Tears** (Various, eg, Rugby, Steris, URL)	**Solution**: 0.01% benzalkonium chloride. May also contain EDTA, NaCl, polyvinyl alcohol, hydroxypropyl methylcellulose	In 15 and 30 mL.

ARTIFICIAL TEAR SOLUTIONS

otc	**Computer Eye Drops** (Bausch & Lomb)	**Solution:** 0.01% benzalkonium chloride, 1% glycerin, NaCl, boric acid, EDTA	In 15 mL.
otc	**AquaSite** (Novartis Ophthalmics)	**Solution:** 0.2% PEG-400, 0.1% dextran 70, polycarbophil, NaCl, EDTA, sodium hydroxide	Preservative free. In 24 × 1 single dose and 15 mL multidose.
otc	**Artificial Tears Plus** (Various)	**Solution:** 1.4% polyvinyl alcohol, 0.6% povidone, 0.5% chlorobutanol, NaCl	In 15 mL.
otc	**Bion Tears** (Alcon)	**Solution:** 0.1% dextran 70, 0.3% hydroxypropyl methylcellulose 2910, NaCl, KCl, sodium bicarbonate	Preservative free. In single-use 0.45 mL containers (28s).
otc	**Celluvisc** (Allergan)	**Solution:** 1% carboxymethylcellulose, NaCl, KCl, sodium lactate	Preservative free. In 0.3 mL (UD 30s).
otc	**Comfort Tears** (Allergan)	**Solution:** Hydroxyethylcellulose, 0.005% benzalkonium chloride, 0.02% EDTA	In 15 mL.
otc	**Dry Eyes** (Bausch & Lomb)	**Solution:** 1.4% polyvinyl alcohol, 0.01% benzalkonium chloride, sodium phosphate, EDTA, NaCl	In 15 mL.
otc	**GenTeal** (Novartis Ophthalmics)	**Drops:** 0.3% hydroxypropyl methylcellulose, boric acid, phosphone acid, sodium chloride, sodium perborate	In 15 and 25 mL.
otc	**HypoTears** (Novartis Ophthalmics)	**Solution:** 1% polyvinyl alcohol, PEG-400, 1% dextrose, 0.01% benzalkonium Cl, EDTA	In 15 and 30 mL.
otc	**HypoTears PF** (Novartis Ophthalmics)	**Solution:** 1% polyvinyl alcohol, PEG-400, 1% dextrose, EDTA	Preservative free. In 0.6 mL (30s).
otc	**Isopto Plain** (Alcon)	**Solution:** 0.5% hydroxypropyl methylcellulose 2910, 0.01% benzalkonium chloride, NaCl, sodium phosphate, sodium citrate	In 15 mL *Drop-Tainers*.
otc	**Isopto Tears** (Alcon)		In 15 and 30 mL.
otc	**Just Tears** (Blairex)	**Solution:** Benzalkonium chloride, EDTA, 1.4% polyvinyl alcohol, NaCl, KCl	In 15 mL.
otc	**Liquifilm Tears** (Allergan)	**Solution:** 1.4% polyvinyl alcohol, 0.5% chlorobutanol, NaCl	In 15 and 30 mL.
otc	**Murine** (Ross)	**Solution:** 0.5% polyvinyl alcohol, 0.6% povidone, benzalkonium chloride, dextrose, EDTA, NaCl, sodium bicarbonate, sodium phosphate	In 15 and 30 mL.
otc	**Murocel** (Bausch & Lomb)	**Solution:** 1% methylcellulose, propylene glycol, NaCl, 0.046% methylparaben, 0.02% propylparaben, boric acid, sodium borate	In 15 mL.
otc	**Nu-Tears** (Optopics)	**Solution:** 1.4% polyvinyl alcohol, EDTA, sodium chloride, benzalkonium chloride, KCl	In 15 mL.
otc	**Nu-Tears II** (Optopics)	**Solution:** 1% polyvinyl alcohol, 1% PEG-400, EDTA, benzalkonium chloride	In 15 mL.
otc	**Preservative Free Moisture Eyes** (Bausch & Lomb)	**Solution:** 0.95% propylene glycol, boric acid, NaCl, KCl, sodium borate, edetate disodium	Preservative free. In 0.6 mL (UD 32s).
otc	**Puralube Tears** (Fougera)	**Solution:** 1% polyvinyl alcohol, 1% PEG 400, EDTA, benzalkonium Cl	In 15 mL.
otc	**Refresh** (Allergan)	**Solution:** 1.4% polyvinyl alcohol, 0.6% povidone, NaCl	Preservative free. In 0.3 mL (UD 30s, 50s).
otc	**Refresh Plus** (Allergan)	**Solution:** 0.5% carboxymethylcellulose sodium, KCl, NaCl	Preservative free. In 0.3 mL single-use containers (30s and 50s).
otc	**Refresh Tears** (Allergan)	**Solution:** 0.5% carboxymethylcellulose sodium	In 15 mL dropper bottles.
otc	**Clear Eyes for Dry Eyes** (Medtech)	**Solution:** 1% carboxymethylcellulose sodium, 0.25% glycerin	Boric acid, EDTA. In 15 mL.
otc	**OcuCoat** (Storz Ophthalmics)	**Solution:** 0.1% dextran 70, 0.8% hydroxypropyl methylcellulose, sodium phosphate, KCl, NaCl, 0.01% benzalkonium chloride, dextrose	In 15 mL.
otc	**OcuCoat PF** (Storz Ophthalmics)	**Solution:** 0.1% dextran 70, 0.8% hydroxypropyl methylcellulose, sodium phosphate, KCl, NaCl, dextrose	Preservative free. In 0.5 mL single-dose containers (28s).
otc	**TearGard** (Lee)	**Solution:** 0.25% sorbic acid, 0.1% EDTA, hydroxyethylcellulose	Thimerosal free. In 15 mL.
otc	**Teargen** (Zenith Goldline)	**Solution:** 0.01% benzalkonium Cl, EDTA, NaCl, polyvinyl alcohol	In 15 mL.
otc	**Teargen II** (Zenith Goldline)	**Solution:** 4 mg hydroxypropyl methylcellulose, 0.01% benzalkonium chloride, EDTA, KCl, NaCl, hydrochloric acid, sodium hydroxide.	In 15 mL.
otc	**Tearisol** (Novartis Ophthalmics)	**Solution:** 0.5% hydroxypropyl methylcellulose, 0.01% benzalkonium chloride, EDTA, boric acid, KCl	In 15 mL.
otc	**Tears Naturale** (Alcon)	**Solution:** 0.1% dextran 70, 0.01% benzalkonium chloride, 0.3% hydroxypropyl methylcellulose, NaCl, EDTA, hydrochloric acid, sodium hydroxide, KCl	In 15 and 30 mL.
otc	**Tears Naturale Free** (Alcon)	**Solution:** 0.3% hydroxypropyl methylcellulose 2910, 0.1% dextran 70, NaCl, KCl, sodium borate	Preservative free. In 0.6 mL single-use containers.
otc	**Tears Naturale II** (Alcon)	**Solution:** 0.1% dextran 70, 0.3% hydroxypropyl methylcellulose 2910, 0.001% polyquaternium-1, NaCl, KCl, sodium borate	In 15 and 30 mL *Drop-Tainers*.
otc	**Tears Naturale Forte** (Alcon)	**Solution:** 0.1% dextran 70, 0.3% hydroxypropyl methylcellulose, 0.2% glycerin, 0.001% polyquaternium-1, NaCl, KCl, sodium borate	In 15 and 30 mL.
otc	**Tears Plus** (Allergan)	**Solution:** 1.4% polyvinyl alcohol, NaCl, 0.6% povidone, 0.5% chlorobutanol	In 15 and 30 mL.
otc	**Tears Renewed** (Akorn)	**Solution:** 0.01% benzalkonium chloride, EDTA, 0.1% dextran 70, NaCl, 0.3% hydroxypropyl methylcellulose 2906	In 2, 15 and 30 mL.
otc	**Ultra Tears** (Alcon)	**Solution:** 1% hydroxypropyl methylcellulose 2910, 0.01% benzalkonium chloride, NaCl	In 15 mL.
otc	**Viva-Drops** (Vision Pharm)	**Solution:** Polysorbate 80, sodium chloride, EDTA, retinyl palmitate, mannitol, sodium citrate, pyruvate	Preservative free. In 10 and 15 mL.
otc	**Visine for Contacts** (Pfizer Consumer)	**Solution:** sterile isotonic solution with borate buffer system, hypromellose, glycerin	EDTA. In 15 and 30 mL.

[a] OcuSOFT Inc., P.O. Box 429, Richmond, TX 77406; (281) 342-3350.

[b] Alimera Sciences, 6120 Windward Parkway, Alpharetta, GA 30005; (678) 990-5740.

ARTIFICIAL TEAR — SOLUTIONS

Indications

➤*Ophthalmic lubricants:* These products offer tear-like lubrication for the relief of dry eyes and eye irritation associated with deficient tear production. Also used as ocular lubricants for artificial eyes.

Administration and Dosage

Instill 1 to 2 drops into eye(s) 3 or 4 times daily, as needed.

Actions

➤*Pharmacology:* These products contain balanced amounts of salts to maintain ocular tonicity (0.9% NaCl equivalent), buffers to adjust pH, viscosity agents to prolong eye contact time, and preservatives for sterility. See the Topical Ophthalmics introduction for a description and listing of these ingredients.

Patient Information

Do not touch the tip of the container or dropper to any surface. Close container immediately after use.

If headache, eye pain, vision changes, continued redness or irritation occurs, or if condition worsens or persists for longer than 3 days, discontinue use and consult a physician.

May cause mild stinging or temporary blurred vision.

Some of these products should not be used with soft contact lenses.

ARTIFICIAL TEAR INSERT

Rx	**Lacrisert** (Merck)	**Insert:** 5 mg hydroxypropyl cellulose	Preservative free. In 60s with applicator.

ARTIFICIAL TEAR — INSERT

Indications

➤*Dry eye syndromes, moderate to severe:* Keratoconjunctivityis sicca (especially in patients who remain symptomatic after an adequate trial of artivicial tear solutions); exposure keratitis; decreased corneal sensitivity; recurrent corneal erosions.

Administration and Dosage

Once daily, inserted into inferior cul-de-sac beneath the base of the tarsus, not in apposition to the cornea nor beneath the eyelid at the level of the tarsal plate. Individual patients may require twice-daily use for optimal results.

If not properly positioned, the insert will be expelled into the interpalpebral fissure, and may cause symptoms of a foreign body.

Occasionally, the insert is inadvertently expelled from the eye, espeically in patients with shallow conjunctival fornices. Caution the patient against rubbing the eyelid(s), especially upon awakening, so as not to dislodge or expel the insert. If required, another insert may be used. If transient blurred vision develops, the patient may want to remove the insert a few hours after insertion to avoid this.

Actions

➤*Pharmacology:* The hydroxypropyl cellulose insert acts to stabilize and thicken the precorneal tear film and prolong tear film breakup time, which is usually accelerated in patients with dry eye states. The insert also acts to lubricate and protect the eye.

Signs and symptoms resulting from moderate to severe dry eye syndromes, such as conjunctival hyperemia, corneal and conjunctival staining with rose bengal, exudation, itching, burning, foreign body sensation, smarting, photophobia, dryness and blurred or cloudy vision are reduced. Progressive visual deterioration may be retarded, halted or sometimes reversed.

➤*Pharmacokinetics:* Hydroxypropyl cellulose is a physiologically inert substance. Dissolution studies in rabbits showed that the inserts became softer within 1 hour after they were placed in the conjunctival sac. Most dissolved completely in 14 to 18 hours; with a single exception, all had disappeared by 24 hours after insertion. Similar dissolution of inserts was observed during prolonged use (up to 54 weeks).

Contraindications

Hypersensitivity to hydroxypropyl cellulose.

Adverse Reactions

The following have occurred, but in most instances were mild and transient: Transient blurring of vision; ocular discomfort or irritation; matting or stickiness of eyelashes; ohotophobia; hypersensitivity; edema of the eyelids; hyperemia.

Patient Information

May produce transient blurring of vision; exercise caution while operating hazardous machinery or driving a motor vehicle.

If improperly placed in the inferior cul-de-sac, corneal abrasion may result. Patient should practice insertion and removal in physician's office until proficiency is achieved.

Illustrated instructions are included in each package.

If symptoms worsen, remove insert and notify physician.

OPHTHALMIC PUNCTAL PLUGS

PUNCTAL PLUGS

Rx	**Herrick Lacrimal Plug** (Lacrimedics)	**Plug:** Silicone plug	In 0.3 and 0.5 mm sizes (packs of 2 plugs).
Rx	**Punctum Plug** (Eagle Vision)		In 0.5, 0.6, 0.7 and 0.8 mm sizes (packs of 2 plugs). Contains one inserter tool.

PUNCTAL PLUGS — OPHTHALMIC

Indications

➤*Keratitis sicca (dry eye):* Treatment of symptoms of dry eye (eg, redness, burning, reflex tearing, itching, foreign body sensation); after eye surgery to prevent complications due to dry eye; to enhance the efficacy of ocular medications; for patients experiencing dry eye-related contact lens problems.

Administration and Dosage

Plugs must be inserted by a physician or doctor of optometry.

Actions

➤*Pharmacology:* These flexible silicone plugs partially block the puncta and horizontal canaliculus and eliminate tear loss by this route.

Contraindications

Hypersensitivity to silicone; eye infection.

Precautions

➤*Injection path:* If injecting an anesthetic agent in the region of the canaliculus, maintain approximately a 5 mm distance between the injection path and the angular vessels.

➤*Dilation:* Do not dilate punctal opening greater than 1.2 mm.

➤*Irritation:* If irritation caused by plug insertion persists longer than several days, reexamine the patient and consider plug removal.

Patient Information

Do not press fingers on or near the eyelid. Use a cotton-tipped swab to remove "sleep" from the corner of eyes.

Do not attempt to replace a plug that has fallen out.

Relief may not occur immediately after insertion; some discomfort and tearing may occur for a few days.

OPHTHALMIC COLLAGEN IMPLANTS

COLLAGEN IMPLANTS

Rx	**Collagen Implant** (Lacrimedics)	**Implant:** Collagen implant	In 0.2, 0.3, 0.4, 0.5 and 0.6 mm sizes (72s).
Rx	**Temporary Punctal/Canalicular Collagen Implant** (Eagle Vision)		In 0.2, 0.3, 0.4, 0.5 and 0.6 mm sizes (72s).

COLLAGEN — IMPLANTS

Indications

➤*Dry eyes:* For the relief of dry eyes and secondary abnormalities such as conjunctivitis, corneal ulcer, pterygium, blepharitis, keratitis, red lid margins, recurrent chalazion, recurrent corneal erosion, filamentary keratitis and other noninfectious external eye diseases; to enhance the effect of ocular medications; treatment of symptoms of dry eye (eg, redness, burning, reflex tearing, itching, foreign body sensation); after eye surgery to prevent complications; for patients experiencing dry eye-related contact lens problems.

COLLAGEN — IMPLANTS

Administration and Dosage

Implants must be inserted by a physician or doctor of optometry. Placement of implants in all four canaliculi is recommended to prevent a false negative response.

Actions

➤*Pharmacology:* These absorbable implants partially block the puncta and horizontal canaliculus, eliminating tear loss by this route.

Contraindications

Tearing secondary to chronic dacryocystitis with mucopurulent discharge; allergy to bovine collagen; inflammation of eyelid; epiphoria.

Patient Information

Relief may not occur immediately after insertion.

No removal is necessary; implants dissolve within 7 to 10 days.

Reexamination is usually required within 14 days.

Successful treatment may indicate a need for permanent treatment (eg, non-dissolvable silicone plugs).

OPHTHALMIC HYPEROSMOLAR PREPARATIONS

SODIUM CHLORIDE, HYPERTONIC

otc	**Adsorbonac** (Alcon)	**Solution:** 2%	In 15 mL.[1]
otc	**Muro 128** (Bausch & Lomb)		In 15 mL.[2]
otc	**Adsorbonac** (Alcon)	**Solution:** 5%	In 15 mL.[1]
otc	**AK-NaCl** (Akorn)		In 15 mL.[3]
otc	**Muro 128** (Bausch & Lomb)		In 15 and 30 mL.[4]
otc	**AK-NaCl** (Akorn)	**Ointment:** 5%	Preservative free. In 3.5 g.[5]
otc	**Muro 128** (Bausch & Lomb)		In 3.5 g single and twin packs.[6]

[1] With povidone, hydroxyethylcellulose 2910, PEG-90M, poloxamer 188, 0.004% thimerosal, EDTA.
[2] With hydroxypropyl methylcellulose 2906, 0.046% methylparaben, 0.02% propylparaben, propylene glycol, boric acid.
[3] With hydroxypropyl methylcellulose, propylene glycol, 0.023% methylparaben, 0.01% propylparaben, boric acid.
[4] Boric acid, hydroxypropyl methylcellulose 2910, propylene glycol, 0.023% methylparaben, 0.01% propylparaben.
[5] With mineral oil, white petrolatum, lanolin oil.
[6] With mineral oil, white petrolatum, lanolin.

SODIUM CHLORIDE, HYPERTONIC — OPHTHALMIC

Indications

For the temporary relief of corneal edema.

Administration and Dosage

➤*Approved by the FDA:* May 17, 1985.

For ophthalmic use only.

➤*Sodium chloride ophthalmic ointment:* Pull down lower lid of the affected eye(s) and apply a small amount (≈ ¼ inch) of the ointment to the inside of the eyelid every 3 or 4 hours, or as directed by a doctor.

Note: Tubes are filled by weight (⅛ oz/3.5 g), not volume.

See crimp of tube for lot number and expiration date.

➤*Sodium chloride ophthalmic solution:* Instill 1 or 2 drops in the affected eye(s) every 3 or 4 hours, or as directed by a doctor.

➤*Storage/Stability:* Store between 15° to 30°C (59° to 86°F).

Do not freeze.

Keep tightly closed. Protect from light.

Sodium chloride ophthalmic ointment – Do not use if bottom ridge of tube cap is exposed and imprinted seal on box is broken or missing.

Sodium chloride ophthalmic solution – Store upright and immediately replace cap after use.

Do not use if imprinted neckband is not intact.

Actions

➤*Pharmacology:* A hypertonic (hyperosmolar) solution exerts an osmotic gradient greater than that present in the body tissues and fluids, so that water is drawn from the body tissues and fluids across semipermeable membranes. Applied topically to the eye, a hypertonicity agent creates an osmotic gradient which draws water out of the cornea.

Contraindications

Hypersensitivity to any component of the product.

Warnings

Do not use this product except under the advice and supervision of a doctor.

If you experience eye pain, changes in vision, continued redness or irritation of the eye, or if the condition worsens or persists, consult a doctor.

➤*Sodium chloride ophthalmic solution:* If the solution changes color or becomes cloudy, do not use.

Adverse Reactions

May cause temporary burning and irritation upon instillation.

Patient Information

To avoid contamination, do not touch tip of container to any surface. Replace cap after using.

Do not use this product except under the advice and supervision of a physician. If you experience eye pain, changes in vision, continued redness or irritation of the eye or if the condition worsens or persists, discontinue use and consult a physician.

Product may cause temporary burning and irritation when instilled into the eye.

If solution changes color or becomes cloudy, do not use.

CONTACT LENS PRODUCTS

➤*Contact lens guidelines:* Inadequate cleaning can lead to lens discoloration and lens surface buildup of protein, lipids, minerals and other environmental contaminants, which can contribute to giant papillary conjunctivitis (GPC), superficial punctate keratitis (SPK) and corneal abrasion. Irregular contact lens disinfection can cause severe ocular infection.

Contact Lens Guidelines

- Proper contact lens care will increase success and decrease complications.
- Cleaning does not disinfect lenses.
- Disinfecting does not clean lenses.
- Enzyme solutions are not a substitute for disinfection.
- Wash and rinse hands thoroughly before handling contact lenses.
- Do not insert contact lenses if eyes are red or irritated. If eyes become painful or vision worsens while wearing lenses, remove lenses and consult an eye-care practitioner immediately.
- Do not wear contact lenses while sleeping unless they have been prescribed for extended wear.
- For soft lens care, use only products designed for soft lenses.
- For rigid lens care, use only products designed for rigid lenses.
- Do not change or substitute products from a different manufacturer without consulting a doctor.
- Do not use non-sterile, home-prepared saline solutions unless recommended by your eye-care practitioner.
- Always follow label directions or doctor's recommendations.
- Do not store lenses in tap water.
- After removal, lenses must be cleaned, rinsed and disinfected before wearing again.
- Lenses that are stored> 12 hours may again require cleaning, rinsing and disinfection; consult package insert or eye care practitioner.
- Never use saliva to wet contact lenses.
- Keep lens care products out of the reach of children.
- Do not instill topical medications while contact lenses are being worn unless directed by a doctor.
- Do not get cosmetic lotions, creams or sprays in your eyes or on lenses. It is best to put on lenses before putting on makeup and remove them before removing makeup. Water-based cosmetics are less likely to damage lenses than oil-based products.
- Schedule and keep follow-up appointments with your eye-care practitioner (approximately every 6 to 12 months or as recommended).
- Contact lenses wear out with time and should be replaced regularly. Throw away disposable lenses after the recommended wearing period.
- Check with your eye-care practitioner regarding wearing lenses during sports activities.

➤*Contact lens materials:* Three types of contact lenses are manufactured: Hard, rigid gas permeable and soft.

➤*Hard contact lenses:* Hard contact lenses are made from polymethylmethacrylate (PMMA). PMMA does not transmit the oxygen needed for normal corneal integrity. Hard contact lenses have caused chronic corneal edema, corneal distortion, edematous corneal formations, spectacle blur, polymegathism and corneal abrasions. Because of these ocular complications, hard lenses are seldom the lens of choice for a new contact lens patient. Less than 1% of the contact lens population wear hard contact lenses.

➤*Rigid gas permeable lenses:* Approximately 20% of contact lens patients wear rigid gas permeable (RGP) lenses. These lenses are oxygen permeable; therefore, the RGP patient does not have the severe physiological complications of the hard lens patient. Several lens polymers with a high degree of oxygen permeability have been approved by the FDA for extended wear. RGP lenses provide the patient with good vision, durability and easy care.

➤*Soft contact lenses:* Soft contact lenses are made of hydroxyethylmethacrylate (HEMA), a plastic compound. The first soft lens was marketed in the US in 1971. Today, most soft lenses manufactured from HEMA contain 30% to 50% water.

Daily wear soft contact lenses are designed to be worn all day (12 to 14 hours), but must be removed nightly to be cleaned and disinfected. Extended wear soft lenses can be worn for ≥ 24 hours. The FDA and most eye care practitioners recommend a maximum wearing period of 7 days. The lenses must then be removed overnight for cleaning and disinfection. The major advantage of extended wear lenses is convenience. Daily wear soft lenses provide the same level of comfort and vision as extended wear soft lenses. The popularity of extended wear soft lenses has decreased due to the increased risk of infection.

➤*Disposable soft lenses:* Disposable soft lenses are designed to eliminate the complications of lens deposits by planned lens replacement. Lens deposits can interfere with vision, cause corneal irritation and contribute to ocular infection. In addition, disposable lenses offer the patient the convenience of reduced lens care.

Disposable lenses are approved for daily wear and extended wear. It is recommended that the lenses be discarded after a specified length of time; the physician will prescribe the replacement schedule for each patient. If a disposable lens is not discarded immediately after lens removal, it should be cleaned with a surfactant cleaner and stored in a disinfection solution.

➤*Contact Lens Care Products:* Products for use with contact lenses possess the same general characteristics of all ophthalmic products (eg, sterile, isotonic, free of particulate matter). Additionally, product formulations contain various components to achieve specific goals of contact lens care.

Although all contact lenses serve similar functions in correcting visual defects, each distinct type of lens material requires a unique lens care program. In selecting appropriate lens care solutions, it is essential to correctly identify the type of lens the patient is using.

➤*Hard and rigid gas permeable lenses:* Similar lens care is used for the hard and RGP lenses. Products include *wetting/soaking/disinfecting solutions*, cleaning agents and rewetting solutions.

When a rigid contact lens is removed from the eye, it may be covered with lipids, proteins, eye makeup and other debris. After removal, immediately clean the lens with a *surfactant cleaner*. Improper cleaning can contribute to a lens surface buildup that can interfere with vision and potentially cause corneal irritation.

Soak rigid lenses overnight in a *wetting/soaking/disinfecting solution*. This solution has four major functions:

1.) To enhance the lens surface wettability
2.) To maintain the lens hydration similar to that achieved during daily contact lens wear
3.) To disinfect the lens
4.) To act as a mechanical buffer between the lens and the cornea

It is not uncommon for a rigid lens patient to experience dryness after several hours of wear. This is especially true with RGP lens patients because of the hydrophobic nature of the lens material. *Rewetting drops* can provide temporary relief by rinsing some debris off the lens surface and rewetting the eye and the lens.

Many clinicians recommend the weekly use of an enzyme (papain) cleaner with RGP lenses. This weekly cleaning process is very effective in removing protein deposits from the lens surface. A protein film on an RGP lens can decrease vision and cause giant papillary conjunctivitis.

➤*Soft contact lenses:* Soft contact lens care systems are designed to clean, disinfect and rewet the lenses. The first step is cleaning. Cleaning the lens gently in the palm of the hand with a *daily surfactant cleaner* will remove fresh lipids, oils and other debris. Clean soft lenses thoroughly with a surfactant cleaner each time a lens is removed. After cleaning the lens, thoroughly rinse with a soft lens *rinsing/storage solution*. All *rinsing/storage solutions* contain 0.9% saline. Some are available with no preservatives in unit-dose vials or aerosol containers. Other saline solutions contain preservatives to decrease microorganism growth. Discourage use of saline made with salt tablets because of risk of contamination and infection (see Precautions).

Enzymatic cleaners – Enzymatic cleaners are generally used on a weekly basis. They more effectively remove protein deposits than surfactant cleaners because they contain proteolytic enzymes (papain, pancreatin or subtilisin). Most enzymes are dissolved directly in saline, but the subtilisin enzyme tablet can be dissolved in a hydrogen peroxide disinfection solution.

Disinfection – Disinfection is the most important step in soft lens care. Disinfection is achieved by using a thermal (heat) or chemical (cold) system.

Thermal disinfection: Thermal disinfection was the first system approved for soft contact lenses. A heat unit designed for soft lenses is used for 10 min at 80°C (176°F). This procedure will kill most microorganisms that are dangerous to the eye. Recently, Acanthamoeba keratitis has become a concern to many clinicians. Heat disinfection is the most effective procedure to successfully kill Acanthamoeba; however, heat disinfection cannot be used with all soft lens material. Also, continued use of heat can shorten soft lens life.

Chemical disinfection: The original chemical soft lens disinfection systems used thimerosal with either chlorhexidine or a quaternary ammonium compound. These systems had a high incidence of sensitivity reactions. Various hydrogen peroxide care systems are currently available in the US. Most systems require two steps to achieve disinfection and hydrogen peroxide neutralization; one other system combines disinfection and neutralization in a single step. Hydrogen peroxide (3%) is very effective and can be used with all soft lens polymers. However, hydrogen peroxide care systems can be complex and expensive. Do not substitute generic peroxide solutions for solutions formulated for contact lenses. They may be contaminated with heavy metals, have different concentrations of hydrogen peroxide or use stabilizers that may discolor soft lenses.

The two newest chemical soft lens care systems introduced into the US marketplace include *Opti-Free* by Alcon and *ReNu* by Bausch & Lomb. Polyquad (polyquaternium-1) and Dymed (polyammopropylbiguamide) are the disinfection agents utilized in these care systems. Both are simple to use and may therefore increase patient compliance. These two chemical systems have become the care system of choice for the majority of soft lens patients.

Recommended Disinfection Times For Soft Lenses by Product

System	Manufacturer	Disinfection time (minimum)	Neutralization time (minimum)
AOSEPT	Novartis Ophthalmics	6 hrs[1]	6 hrs[1]
Disinfecting Solution	Bausch & Lomb	4 hrs	none
Flex-Care	Alcon	4 hrs	none
MiraSept System	Alcon	10 min	10 min
Opti-Free	Alcon	4 hrs	none
Opti-Soft	Alcon	4 hrs	none
ReNu Multi-Purpose	Bausch & Lomb	4 hrs	none
Soft Mate Consept	Pilkington Barnes Hind	10 min	10 min

[1] One-step method: Disinfection and neutralization occur together for a total of 6 hours.

Soft lens rewetting solutions – Soft lens rewetting solutions permit the lubrication of the soft lens while it is on the eye. Most patients find these rewetting drops minimally effective in reducing the symptoms of dryness. Maximum relief can be achieved by removing the lens, cleaning it with a daily surfactant cleaner and thoroughly rinsing it with a rinsing/storage saline solution.

➤*Precautions:*

Acanthamoeba keratitis – Soft contact lens wearers who use homemade saline solution are at risk of developing Acanthamoebakeratitis, a serious and painful corneal infection that may cause blindness or impaired vision. Homemade saline solutions (nonsterile) may be used during thermal disinfection but NOT after.

Drug interference with contact lens use – Systemic medications may affect the physiology of the cornea, lids and tear system. In addition, many drugs may discolor soft contact lenses. Pharmacists and eye-care practitioners should be aware of the interaction of systemic medications and contact lenses.

Drug Interference With Contact Lens Use

Drug	RGP/Hard/Soft Lens	Action
Anticholinergics	RGP, hard, soft	Tear volume decreased
Antihistamines, sympathomimetics	RGP, hard, soft	Tear volume decreased, blink rate decreased
Chlorthalidone	RGP, hard, soft	Causes lid or corneal edema
Clomiphene	RGP, hard, soft	Causes lid or corneal edema
Diuretics, thiazide	RGP, hard, soft	Tear volume decreased
Dopamine	soft	Discoloration of contact lenses
Epinephrine, topical	soft	Discoloration of contact lenses
Fluorescein, topical	soft	Lens absorbs the yellow dye
Hypnotics, sedatives, muscle relaxants	RGP, hard, soft	Blink rate decreased
Iodine groups	soft	Discoloration of contact lenses
Nitrofurantoin	soft	Discoloration of contact lenses
Oral contraceptives	RGP, hard, soft	Increased stickiness of mucus; corneal lid edema due to fluid retention properties of estrogens
Phenazopyridine	soft	Discoloration of contact lenses
Phenolphthalein	soft	Discoloration of contact lenses

Drug Interference With Contact Lens Use

Drug	RGP/Hard/Soft Lens	Action
Phenylephrine	soft	Discoloration of contact lenses
Primidone	RGP, hard, soft	Causes lid or corneal edema
Rifampin	soft	Lens absorbs drug, causing orange discoloration
Sulfasalazine	soft	Yellow staining
Tetracycline	soft	Discoloration of contact lenses
Tricyclic antidepressants	RGP, hard, soft	Tear volume decreased

Products are listed on the following pages and are grouped as follows:

Contact Lens Solutions

Type of lens	Type of solution
Hard	Wetting Cleaning Cleaning/Soaking Wetting/Soaking Cleaning/Soaking/Wetting Rewetting
RGP	Disinfecting/Wetting/Soaking Cleaning Enzymatic Cleaners Cleaning/Disinfecting/Soaking Rewetting
Soft	Rinsing/Storage Chemical Disinfection Surfactant Cleaning Enzymatic Cleaners Rewetting

Hard (PMMA) Contact Lens Products

Refer to the general discussion of these products in the Contact Lens Products monograph.

Actions

➤*Pharmacology:* Conventional hard lenses are made of a rigid hydrophobic polymer, polymethylmethacrylate (PMMA). For optimum comfort, these lenses require care with separate wetting, cleaning and soaking solutions. Refer to the general discussion of these products in the Contact Lens Products monograph.

WETTING SOLUTIONS, HARD LENSES

otc	**Liquifilm Wetting** (Allergan)	**Solution:** 0.004% benzalkonium chloride, EDTA, hydroxypropyl methylcellulose, NaCl, KCl, polyvinyl alcohol	In 60 mL.
otc	**Sereine** (Optikem)	**Solution:** Buffered. 0.1% EDTA, 0.01% benzalkonium chloride	In 60 and 120 mL.
otc	**Wetting Solution** (Pilkington Barnes Hind)	**Solution:** Polyvinyl alcohol, 0.004% benzalkonium chloride, 0.02% EDTA	In 60 mL.

WETTING SOLUTIONS, HARD LENSES — OPHTHALMIC

Actions

➤*Pharmacology:* Wetting solutions contain surfactants to facilitate hydration of the hydrophobic hard lens surface. These solutions include methylcellulose and derivatives, polyvinyl alcohol, povidone, some newer polymers, preservatives and buffers. These agents increase solution viscosity and act as a physical cushioning agent between lens and cornea.

WETTING/SOAKING SOLUTIONS, HARD LENSES

otc	**Sereine** (Optikem)	**Solution:** Buffered, isotonic. 0.1% EDTA, 0.01% benzalkonium chloride	In 120 mL.
otc	**Soac-Lens** (Alcon)	**Solution:** Buffered. 0.004% thimerosal, 0.1% EDTA, wetting agents	In 118 mL.
otc	**Wet-N-Soak Plus** (Allergan)	**Solution:** Buffered, isotonic. 0.003% benzalkonium chloride, polyvinyl alcohol, EDTA	In 120 and 180 mL.

REWETTING SOLUTIONS, HARD LENSES

otc	**20/20 Lubricating and Rewetting Solution** (S.S.S. Co.)	**Drops:** 1.4% PVA, NaCl, KCl, 0.05% EDTA, 0.01% benzalkonium Cl.	In 0.5 fl oz.
otc	**Adapettes** (Alcon)	**Solution:** Buffered, isotonic. Povidone and other water-soluble polymers, sorbic acid, EDTA	Thimerosal free. In 15 mL.
otc	**Clerz 2** (Alcon)	**Solution:** Isotonic. Hydroxyethylcellulose, poloxamer 407, NaCl, KCl, sodium borate, boric acid, sorbic acid, EDTA	Thimerosal free. In 5, 15 and 30 mL.
otc	**Lens Lubricant** (Bausch & Lomb)	**Solution:** Buffered, isotonic. 0.004% thimerosal, 0.1% EDTA, povidone, polyoxyethylene	In 15 mL.
otc	**Opti-Tears** (Alcon)	**Solution:** Isotonic. 0.1% EDTA, 0.001% polyquaternium-1, dextran, NaCl, KCl, hydroxymethylcellulose	Thimerosal and sorbic acid free. In 15 mL.
otc	**Lens Drops** (Novartis Ophthalmics)	**Solution:** Buffered, isotonic. NaCl, carbamide, poloxamer 407, 0.2% EDTA, 0.15% sorbic acid.	Thimerosal free. In 15 mL.

REWETTING SOLUTIONS, HARD LENSES — OPHTHALMIC

Actions

➤*Pharmacology:* Rewetting solutions are intended for use directly in the eye in conjunction with a contact lens. These products improve wearing time by rehydrating the lens, which may become dry and contaminated during wear, although more benefit is obtained by actually removing and rewetting the lens. The principle components of these solutions are wetting agents.

CLEANING SOLUTIONS, HARD LENSES

otc	**LC-65** (Allergan)	**Solution:** Buffered. 0.001% thimerosal, EDTA	In 15 and 60 mL.
otc	**Opti-Clean** (Alcon)	**Solution:** Buffered, isotonic. Tween 21, hydroxyethylcellulose, polymeric cleaners, 0.004% thimerosal, 0.1% EDTA	In 12 and 20 mL.
otc	**Opti-Clean II** (Alcon)	**Solution:** Buffered, isotonic. Tween 21, polymeric cleaners, 0.1% EDTA, 0.001% polyquaternium-1	Thimerosal free. In 12 and 20 mL.
otc	**Resolve/GP** (Allergan)	**Solution:** Buffered. Cocoamphocarboxyglycinate, sodium lauryl sulfate, hexylene glycol, alkyl ether sulfate, fatty acid amide surfactants	Preservative free. In 30 mL.
otc	**Sereine** (Optikem)	**Solution:** Cocoamphodiacetate and glycols, 0.1% EDTA, 0.01% benzalkonium chloride	In 60 mL.
otc	**Titan** (Pilkington Barnes Hind)	**Solution:** Buffered. Nonionic cleaning agents, 2% EDTA, 0.13% potassium sorbate	In 30 mL.

Hard (PMMA) Contact Lens Products

CLEANING SOLUTIONS, HARD LENSES — OPHTHALMIC

Actions

➤*Pharmacology:* Cleaning solutions contain surfactant cleaners to facilitate removal of oleaginous, proteinaceous and other types of debris from the lens surface. To adequately clean, physically rub lens in the palm of the hand or between thumb and finger with solution for about 20 seconds and rinse with water or sterile saline solution.

CLEANING AND SOAKING SOLUTIONS, HARD LENSES

otc	**Clean-N-Soak** (Allergan)	**Solution:** Buffered. Surfactant cleaning agent with 0.004% phenylmercuric nitrate	In 120 mL.

CLEANING/SOAKING/WETTING SOLUTIONS, HARD LENSES

otc	**Total** (Allergan)	**Solution:** Buffered, isotonic. Polyvinyl alcohol, benzalkonium chloride, EDTA	In 60 and 120 mL.

Rigid Gas Permeable Contact Lens Products

Refer to the general discussion of these products in Contact Lens Products monograph.

Actions

➤*Pharmacology:*

Gas permeable hard lenses – Silicone/acrylate and fluoropolymers are used in rigid gas permeable (RGP) contact lenses. Lens care regimens include the use of a surfactant cleaner, enzyme cleaner and storage in a chemical disinfecting solution. Advise patients to follow the lens care protocol provided by the lens manufacturer or the instructions of their doctor.

DISINFECTING/WETTING/SOAKING SOLUTIONS, RGP LENSES

otc	**Boston Advance Comfort Formula** (Polymer Tech)	**Solution:** Buffered, slightly hypertonic. 0.00015% polyaminopropyl biguanide, 0.05% EDTA, cationic cellulose derivative polymer (wetting agent)	In 120 mL.
otc	**Boston Conditioning Solution** (Polymer Tech)	**Solution:** Buffered, slightly hypertonic, low viscosity. 0.05% EDTA, 0.006% chlorhexidine gluconate, cationic cellulose derivative polymer as wetting agent	In 120 mL.
otc	**Flex-Care Especially for Sensitive Eyes** (Alcon)	**Solution:** Buffered, isotonic. 0.1% EDTA, 0.005% chlorhexidine gluconate, NaCl, sodium borate, boric acid	Thimerosal free. In 118, 237 and 355 mL.
otc	**Stay-Wet 3** (Sherman)	**Solution:** 0.02% sodium bisulfite, 0.1% benzyl alcohol, 0.05% sorbic acid, 0.1% EDTA, sodium and potassium chloride salts containing polyvinyl pyrrolidone, polyvinyl alcohol, hydroxyethylcellulose	Thimerosal free. In 30 mL.
otc	**Stay-Wet 4** (Sherman)	**Solution:** 0.15% benzyl alcohol, 0.1% EDTA, NaCl, KCl, polyvinyl alcohol, hydroxyethyl cellulose	Thimerosal free. In 30 mL.
otc	**Wetting and Soaking Solution** (Bausch & Lomb)	**Solution:** Buffered, hypertonic. 0.006% chlorhexidine gluconate, 0.05% EDTA, cationic cellulose derivative polymer	Thimerosal free. In 118 mL.
otc	**Wet-N-Soak Plus** (Allergan)	**Solution:** Buffered, isotonic. 0.003% benzalkonium chloride, polyvinyl alcohol, EDTA	In 120 and 180 mL.

CLEANING SOLUTIONS, RGP LENSES

otc	**Boston Advance Cleaner** (Polymer Tech)	**Solution:** Concentrated homogenous surfactant. Alkyl ether sulfate, ethoxylated alkyl phenol, triquaternary cocoa-based phospholipid, silica gel	In 30 mL.
otc	**Boston Cleaner** (Polymer Tech)	**Solution:** Concentrated homogenous surfactant. Alkyl ether sulfate, silica gel, titanium dioxide	In 30 mL.
otc	**Concentrated Cleaner** (Bausch & Lomb)	**Solution:** Surfactant solution with alkyl ether sulfate and silica gel	Preservative free. In 30 mL.
otc	**Gas Permeable Daily Cleaner** (Pilkington Barnes Hind)	**Solution:** 0.13% potassium sorbate, 2% EDTA, ethoxylated polyoxypropylene glycol, tris (hydroxymethyl) amino methane, hydroxyethylcellulose	Thimerosal free. In 30 mL.
otc	**LC-65** (Allergan)	**Solution:** Buffered cleaning agent. 0.001% thimerosal and EDTA	In 15 and 60 mL.
otc	**Opti-Clean** (Alcon)	**Solution:** Buffered, isotonic. 0.004% thimerosal, 0.1% EDTA, Tween 21, hydroxyethylcellulose, *Microclens* polymeric cleaners	In 12 and 20 mL.
otc	**Opti-Clean II Especially for Sensitive Eyes** (Alcon)	**Solution:** Buffered, isotonic. 0.1% EDTA, 0.001% polyquaternium-1, *Microclens* polymeric cleaners, Tween 21	Thimerosal free. In 12 and 20 mL.
otc	**Resolve/GP** (Allergan)	**Solution:** Buffered. Cocoamphocarboxyglycinate, sodium lauryl sulfate, hexylene glycol, alkyl ether sulfate, fatty acid amide surfactants	Preservative free. In 30 mL.

ENZYMATIC CLEANERS, RGP LENSES

otc	**Boston One Step Liquid Enzymatic Cleaner** (Polymer Tech)	**Solution:** Proteolytic enzyme (subtilisin).	Preservative free. Contains glycerol. In 2.4 mL.
otc	**Opti-Zyme Enzymatic Cleaner Especially for Sensitive Eyes** (Alcon)	**Tablets:** Highly purified pork pancreatin. *To make solution for soaking, dilute in preserved saline or sterile unpreserved saline solution*	Preservative free. In 8s, 24s, 36s and 56s.
otc	**ProFree/GP Weekly Enzymatic Cleaner** (Allergan)	**Tablets:** Papain, NaCl, sodium carbonate, sodium borate, EDTA	In 16s and 24s with vials.

CLEANING/DISINFECTING/SOAKING SOLUTIONS, RGP LENSES

otc	**de • STAT 3** (Sherman)	**Solution:** 0.1% benzyl alcohol, 0.5% EDTA, lauryl sulfate salt of imidazoline, octylphenoxypolyethoxyethanol	Thimerosal free. In 118 mL.
otc	**de • STAT 4** (Sherman)	**Solution:** 0.3% benzyl alcohol, 0.5% EDTA, lauryl sulfate salt of imidazoline, octylphenoxypolyethoxyethanol	Thimerosal free. In 118 mL.
otc	**Boston Simplicity Multi-Action** (Polymer Technology)	**Solution:** PEO sorbitan monolaurate, silicone glycol copolymer, cellulosic viscosifier, derivatized PEG, 0.003% chlorhexidine gluconate, 0.0005% polyaminopropyl biguanide, 0.05% EDTA	In 60, 90, and 120 mL.

Rigid Gas Permeable Contact Lens Products

REWETTING SOLUTIONS, RGP LENSES

otc	**Boston Rewetting Drops** (Polymer Tech)	**Solution**: Buffered, slightly hypertonic. 0.006% chlorhexidine gluconate, 0.05% EDTA, cationic cellulose derivative polymer as wetting agent	In 10 mL.
otc	**Boston Simplicity** (Polymer Tech)	**Solution**: Buffered, slightly hypertonic. 0.003% chlorhexidine gluconate, 0.0005% polyaminopropyl guanide, 0.05% EDTA, PEO sorbitan monolaurate, betaine surfactant, silicone glycol copolymer, derivatized polyethylene glycol, cellulosic viscosifier.	In 120 mL.
otc	**Wet-N-Soak** (Allergan)	**Solution**: Borate buffered, isotonic. 0.006% WSCP, hydroxyethylcellulose	In 15 mL.

Soft (Hydrogel) Contact Lens Products

Refer to the general discussion of these products in the Contact Lens Products monograph.

WARNING

Do NOT use conventional (hard) lens solutions on soft contact lenses. Use caution in product selection. Not all products are intended for use on all types of soft lenses.

Actions

➤*Pharmacology:* Soft (hydrogel) contact lenses are made of hydrophilic polymers. Hydrogel lenses must be maintained in a hydrated state in physiological saline to prevent them from becoming brittle. Hydrogel lenses will absorb many substances; therefore, use only solutions specifically formulated for hydrogel lenses. In addition, these lenses must be disinfected either by heating in saline solution or by soaking in a chemical solution. Heating a lens in solutions used for chemical disinfection only may cause the lens to become opaque.

Soft lens solutions are especially formulated to be compatible with, and to meet the particular needs of, soft contact lenses. Of particular importance to soft lens care is the need for thorough cleaning to remove deposits which coat and may discolor the lens, especially when subjected to asepticizing by heating.

RINSING/STORAGE SOLUTIONS, SOFT CONTACT LENSES

Actions

➤*Pharmacology:* Use these solutions for rinsing and storage of hydrogel lenses in conjunction with heat disinfection. Prepared saline solutions may contain chelating agents (EDTA) which prevent calcium deposits from forming. Thimerosal-free preserved saline solutions may be used by patients sensitive to thimerosal or mercury containing compounds. Preservative free solutions are for patients intolerant to preservatives. Salt tablets are available to make saline solution; however, these solutions are nonsterile and contain no preservatives; use only with heat disinfection methods. Because cases of *Acanthamoebakeratitis* (a serious eye infection) have occurred in patients using homemade saline solutions, the use of salt tablets for soft contact lens storage/rinsing solution is not recommended.

PRESERVED SALINE SOLUTIONS, SOFT CONTACT LENSES

otc	**Alcon Saline Especially for Sensitive Eyes** (Alcon)	**Solution**: Buffered, isotonic. NaCl, borate buffer system, sorbic acid, EDTA	Thimerosal free. In 360 mL.
otc	**BarnesHind Saline for Sensitive Eyes** (Pilkington Barnes Hind)	**Solution**: Isotonic. 0.13% potassium sorbate, 0.025% EDTA	In 360 mL (2s).
otc	**MiraSept Step 2** (Alcon)	**Solution**: Boric acid, sodium borate, NaCl, EDTA, sodium pyruvate.	In 120 mL.
otc	**Opti-Soft** (Alcon)	**Solution**: Buffered, isotonic. 0.1% EDTA, 0.001% polyquaternium-1, NaCl, borate buffer system. For lenses with ≤ 45% water content	Thimerosal free. In 355 mL.
otc	**ReNu** (Bausch & Lomb)	**Solution**: Buffered, isotonic. 0.00003% polyaminopropyl biguanide, NaCl, boric acid, EDTA	In 355 mL.
otc	**Saline** (Bausch & Lomb)	**Solution**: Buffered, isotonic. 0.001% thimerosal, boric acid, NaCl, EDTA	In 355 mL.
otc	**Sensitive Eyes** (Bausch & Lomb)	**Solution**: Buffered, isotonic. 0.1% sorbic acid, 0.025% EDTA, NaCl, boric acid, sodium borate	Thimerosal free. In 118, 237 and 355 mL.
otc	**Sensitive Eyes Plus** (Bausch & Lomb)	**Solution**: Boric acid, sodium borate, KCl, NaCl, 0.00003% polyaminopropyl biguanide, 0.025% EDTA	In 118 and 355 mL.
otc	**SoftWear** (Novartis Ophthalmics)	**Solution**: Isotonic, NaCl, boric acid, sodium borate, sodium perborate (generating up to 0.006% hydrogen peroxide stabilized with phosphonic acid)	Thimerosal free. In 120, 240 and 360 mL.
otc	**Your Choice Sterile Preserved Saline Solution** (Amcon)	**Solution**: Isotonic. 0.1% sorbic acid, boric buffer, EDTA, NaCl	In 60 and 360 mL.

PRESERVATIVE FREE SALINE SOLUTIONS, SOFT CONTACT LENSES

otc	**Blairex Sterile Saline** (Blairex)	**Solution**: Buffered, isotonic. NaCl, boric acid, sodium borate	In 90, 240 and 360 mL aerosol.
otc	**Unisol Plus** (Alcon)		In 240 and 360 mL aerosol.
otc	**Your Choice Non-Preserved Saline Solution** (Amcon)		In 360 mL.
otc	**Novartis Ophthalmic Vision Saline** (Novartis Ophthalmics)	**Solution**: Buffered, isotonic. NaCl, boric acid, sodium borate	In 240 and 360 mL aerosol.
otc	**Lens Plus Sterile Saline** (Allergan)	**Solution**: Buffered, isotonic. NaCl, boric acid, nitrogen	In 90, 240 and 360 mL aerosol.
otc	**Oxysept 2** (Allergan)	**Solution**: Buffered, isotonic. NaCl, catalytic neutralizing agent, EDTA, mono-and dibasic sodium phosphates	In 15 mL single-use containers (25s).

SALT TABLETS FOR NORMAL SALINE, SOFT CONTACT LENSES

otc	**Marlin Salt System** (Marlin)	**Tablets**: 250 mg NaCl	In 200s with 27.7 mL bottle.

SALT TABLETS FOR NORMAL SALINE, SOFT CONTACT LENSES — OPHTHALMIC

Actions

➤*Pharmacology:* Reconstitute tablets in container provided with distilled, deionized or purified water; do not use mineral or tap water. These solutions are not sterile and are intended only for use in conjunction with heat disinfection regimens. Use only as a rinse priorto heat disinfection and as storage during heat disinfection. Not for use as a rinse after disinfection (eg, before lens placement in the eye). Not for use in the eye. See Precautions in the Contact Lens Products monograph.

Soft (Hydrogel) Contact Lens Products

SURFACTANT CLEANING SOLUTIONS, SOFT CONTACT LENSES

otc	**DURAcare** II (Blairex)	**Solution**: Buffered, hypertonic. 0.1% sodium bisulfite, 0.1% sorbic acid, 0.25% EDTA, salt buffers, ethylene/propylene oxide, octylphenoxypolyethoxyethanol, lauryl sulfate salt of imidazoline	Thimerosal free. In 30 mL.
otc	**LC-65** (Allergan)	**Solution**: Buffered. 0.001% thimerosal, EDTA	In 15 and 60 mL.
otc	**Novartis Ophthalmic Vision Cleaner for Sensitive Eyes** (Novartis Ophthalmics)	**Solution**: Cocoamphorcarboxyglycinate, sodium lauryl sulfate, hexylene glycol, 0.1% sorbic acid, 0.2% EDTA	In 15 mL.
otc	**Lens Plus Daily Cleaner** (Allergan)	**Solution**: Buffered. Cocoamphocarboxyglycinate, sodium lauryl sulfate, hexylene glycol, NaCl, sodium phosphate	Preservative free. In 15 and 30 mL.
otc	**MiraFlow Extra Strength** (Novartis Ophthalmics)	**Solution**: 15.7% isopropyl alcohol, poloxamer 407, amphoteric 10	Thimerosal free. In 12 and 20 mL.
otc	**Opti-Clean** (Alcon)	**Solution**: Buffered, isotonic. 0.004% thimerosal, 0.1% EDTA, Tween 21, hydroxyethyl cellulose, *Microclens* polymeric cleaners	In 12 and 20 mL.
otc	**Opti-Clean** II (Alcon)	**Solution**: Buffered, isotonic. 0.1% EDTA, 0.001% polyquaternium-1, *Microclens* polymeric cleaners, *Tween 21*	Thimerosal free. In 12 and 20 mL.
otc	**Opti-Free** (Alcon)	**Solution**: Buffered, isotonic. 0.01% EDTA, 0.001% polyquaternium-1, *Microclens* polymeric cleaners, *Tween 21*	Thimerosal free. In 12 and 20 mL.
otc	**Pliagel** (Alcon)	**Solution**: 0.25% sorbic acid, 0.5% EDTA, NaCl, KCl, poloxamer 407	In 25 mL.
otc	**Sensitive Eyes Daily Cleaner** (Bausch & Lomb)	**Solution**: Buffered, isotonic. 0.25% sorbic acid, 0.5% EDTA, NaCl, hydroxypropyl methylcellulose, poloxamine, sodium borate	In 20 mL.
otc	**Sensitive Eyes Saline/Cleaning** (Bausch & Lomb)	**Solution**: Buffered, isotonic. 0.15% sorbic acid, 0.1% EDTA, boric acid, poloxamine, sodium borate, NaCl	In 237 mL.

SURFACTANT CLEANING SOLUTIONS, SOFT CONTACT LENSES — OPHTHALMIC

Indications

Cleaning solutions are used for daily prophylactic cleaning to prevent the accumulation of proteinaceous (mucus) deposits and to remove other debris.

ENZYMATIC CLEANERS, SOFT CONTACT LENSES

otc	**Allergan Enzymatic** (Allergan)	**Tablets**: Papain, NaCl, sodium carbonate, sodium borate, EDTA. *To make solution for soaking, dilute in sterile saline.*	In 12s, 24s, 36s and 48s.
otc	**Enzymatic Cleaner for Extended Wear** (Alcon)	**Tablets**: Highly purified pork pancreatin. *To make solution for soaking, dilute in preserved saline or sterile unpreserved saline.*	In 12s.
otc	**Opti-zyme Enzymatic Cleaner Especially for Sensitive Eyes** (Alcon)		Preservative free. In 8s, 24s, 36s and 56s.
otc	**Vision Care Enzymatic Cleaner** (Alcon)		In 24s.
otc	**Opti-Free** (Alcon)	**Tablets**: Highly purified pork pancreatin. *To make solution for soaking, dilute in* Opti-Free *disinfecting solution.*	In 6s, 12s and 18s.
otc	**ReNu Effervescent Enzymatic Cleaner** (Bausch & Lomb)	**Tablets**: Subtilisin, polyethylene glycol, sodium carbonate, NaCl, tartaric acid. *To make solution for soaking, dilute in preserved saline or sterile unpreserved saline solution.*	In 10s, 20s and 30s.
otc	**ReNu Thermal Enzymatic Cleaner** (Bausch & Lomb)	**Tablets**: Subtilisin, sodium carbonate, NaCl, boric acid. *To make solution for heat disinfection directly in lens carrying case.*	In 16s.
otc	**Ultrazyme Enzymatic Cleaner** (Allergan)	**Tablets**: Effervescing, buffering and tableting agents. Subtilisin A. *To make solution for soaking, dilute in 3% hydrogen peroxide disinfecting solution.*	In 5s, 10s, 15s and 20s.
otc	**Complete Weekly Enzymatic Cleaner** (Allergan)	**Tablets**: Effervescing, buffering and tableting agents. Subtilisin A. *To make solution for soaking, dilute in sterile saline.*	In 8s.

ENZYMATIC CLEANERS, SOFT CONTACT LENSES — OPHTHALMIC

Actions

➤*Pharmacology:* Enzymatic cleaning, by soaking in a solution prepared from enzyme tablets, is recommended once weekly to remove protein and other lens deposits.

REWETTING SOLUTIONS, SOFT CONTACT LENSES

otc	**20/20 Lubricating and Rewetting Solution** (S.S.S. Co.)	**Drops**: 1.4% PVA, NaCl, KCl, 0.05% EDTA, 0.01% benzalkonium Cl.	In 0.5 fl oz.
otc	**Clerz Plus** (Alcon)	**Drops**: Buffered, isotonic, citrate buffer, NaCl, 0.05% EDTA, 0.001% polyquaternium-1, PEG-11	In 5, 8, and 10 mL.
otc	**Blairex Lens Lubricant** (Blairex)	**Solution**: Isotonic. 0.25% sorbic acid, 0.1% EDTA, borate buffer, NaCl, hydroxypropyl methylcellulose, glycerin	Thimerosal free. In 15 mL.

Soft (Hydrogel) Contact Lens Products

REWETTING SOLUTIONS, SOFT CONTACT LENSES

otc	**Clerz 2** (Alcon)	**Solution**: Isotonic. NaCl, KCl, hydroxyethylcellulose, poloxamer 407, sodium borate, boric acid, sorbic acid, EDTA	Thimerosal free. In 5 (2s), 15 and 30 mL.
otc	**Lens Lubricant** (Bausch & Lomb)	**Solution**: Buffered, isotonic. 0.004% thimerosal, 0.1% EDTA, povidone, polyoxyethylene	In 15 mL.
otc	**Lens Plus Rewetting Drops** (Allergan)	**Solution**: Buffered, isotonic. NaCl, boric acid	Preservative free. In 0.35 mL (30s).
otc	**Opti-Tears** (Alcon)	**Solution**: Isotonic. 0.1% EDTA, 0.001% polyquaternium-1, dextran, NaCl, KCl, hydroxypropyl methylcellulose	Thimerosal free. In 15 mL.
otc	**Opti-Free** (Alcon)	**Solution**: Isotonic. Citrate buffer, NaCl, 0.05% EDTA, 0.001% polyquaternium-1	In 10 and 20 mL.
otc	**Opti-One** (Alcon)		In 10 mL.
otc	**Sensitive Eyes Drops** (Bausch & Lomb)	**Solution**: Buffered. 0.1% sorbic acid, 0.025% EDTA, NaCl, boric acid, sodium borate	In 30 mL.
otc	**Lens Drops** (Novartis Ophthalmics)	**Solution**: Buffered, isotonic. NaCl, borate buffer, poloxamer 407, 0.2% EDTA, 0.15% sorbic acid, carbamide	In 15 mL.
otc	**Complete** (Allergan)	**Solution**: Buffered, isotonic. NaCl, 0.0001% polyhexamethylene biguanide, tromethamine, tyloxapol, EDTA	In 15 mL.

REWETTING SOLUTIONS, SOFT CONTACT LENSES — OPHTHALMIC

Actions

➤*Pharmacology:* May be used directly in the eye to rehydrate and improve comfort of hydrogel lenses.

CHEMICAL DISINFECTION SYSTEMS

Actions

➤*Pharmacology:* Chemical disinfection is an alternative to heat. Two-solution systems use separate disinfecting and rinsing solutions. One-solution systems use the same solution for rinsing and storage.

Warnings

➤*Heat disinfection:* Lenses must NOT be disinfected by heating when using these solutions.

HYDROGEN PEROXIDE-CONTAINING SYSTEMS, SOFT LENSES

otc	**MiraSept** (Alcon)	**Disinfecting Solution**: 3% hydrogen peroxide, sodium stannate, sodium nitrate	In 120 mL.
		Rinse and Neutralizer: Isotonic. Boric acid, sodium borate, NaCl, sodium pyruvate, EDTA	In 120 mL (2s).
otc	**Oxysept** (Allergan)	**Disinfecting Solution**: 3% hydrogen peroxide, sodium stannate, sodium nitrate, phosphate buffer	In 240 and 360 mL.
		Neutralizer Tablets: Catalase, buffering agents	In 12s (with *Oxy-Tab* cup) and 36s.
otc	**Ultra-Care** (Allergan)	**Disinfecting Solution**: 3% hydrogen peroxide, sodium stannate, sodium nitrate, phosphate buffer	In 120 and 360 mL.
		Neutralizer Tablets: Catalase, hydroxypropyl methylcellulose, buffering agents	In 12s and 36s with cup.
otc	**Quick CARE** (Novartis Ophthalmics)	**Disinfecting Solution**: Isopropanol, NaCl, polyoxypropylenepolyoxy ethylene block copolymer, disodium lauroamphodiacetate	In 15 mL.
		Rinse and Neutralizer: Isotonic. Sodium borate, boric acid, sodium perborate (generating up to 0.006% hydrogen peroxide), phosphonic acid	In 360 mL.
otc	**AOSEPT** (Novartis Ophthalmics)	**Disinfecting Solution**: 3% hydrogen peroxide, 0.85% NaCl, phosphonic acid, phosphate buffers	In 120, 240 and 360 mL.
		AODISC Neutralizer: Platinum-coated tablet	Tablet good for 100 uses or 3 months of daily use.[1]

[1] For use only with the AOSEPT system.

NON-HYDROGEN PEROXIDE-CONTAINING SYSTEMS, SOFT LENSES

otc	**Disinfecting Solution** (Bausch & Lomb)	**Solution**: Buffered, isotonic. 0.005% chlorhexidine, 0.1% EDTA, 0.001% thimerosal, NaCl, sodium borate, boric acid	In 355 mL.
otc	**Flex-Care Especially for Sensitive Eyes** (Alcon)	**Solution**: Buffered, isotonic. 0.1% EDTA, 0.005% chlorhexidine gluconate, NaCl, sodium borate, boric acid	In 360 mL.
otc	**Opti-Free** (Alcon)	**Solution**: Isotonic. 0.05% EDTA, 0.001% polyquaternium-1, citrate buffer, NaCl	Thimerosal free. In 118, 237 and 355 mL.
otc	**Opti-Free Express Multi-Purpose** (Alcon)	**Solution**: Isotonic. 0.0005% myristamidopropyl dimethylamine, 0.001% polyquaternium-1, citrate, NaCl, boric acid, sorbitol, EDTA	In 118 mL.
otc	**Opti-One Multi-Purpose** (Alcon)	**Solution**: Buffered, isotonic. 0.05% EDTA, 0.001% polyquaternium-1, sodium chloride, NaCl	In 118, 237, 355 and 473mL.
otc	**Complete All-In-One Solution** (Allergan)	**Solution**: Buffered, isotonic. NaCl, 0.0001% polyhexamethylene biguanide, EDTA	In 60, 120 and 360 mL.
otc	**ReNu Multi-Purpose** (Bausch & Lomb)	**Solution**: Isotonic. 0.00005% polyaminopropyl biguanide, 0.01% EDTA, NaCl, sodium borate, boric acid, poloxamine	In 118, 237 and 355 mL.

Refer to the Topical Ophthalmic Drugs introduction for more complete information.

Indications

Corneal anesthesia of short duration (eg, tonometry, gonioscopy, removal of corneal foreign bodies and sutures); short corneal and conjunctival procedures; cataract surgery; conjunctival and corneal scraping for diagnostic purposes; paracentesis of the anterior chamber.

Ophthalmic Uses of Local Anesthetics	
Route	Use
Injectable	Facial nerve block
	Retrobulbar anesthesia
	Eyelid infiltration
Topical	Gonioscopy
	Tonometry
	Fundus contact lens biomicroscopy
	Evaluation of corneal abrasions
	Forced duction testing
	Schirmer tear testing
	Electroretinography
	Lacrimal dilation and irrigation
	Contact lens fitting
	Superficial foreign body removal
	Minor surgery of conjunctiva
	Suture removal
	Corneal epithelial debridement

Actions

➤*Pharmacology:* Local anesthetics stabilize the neuronal membrane so the neuron is less permeable to ions. This prevents the initiation and transmission of nerve impulses, thereby producing the local anesthetic action.

Studies indicate that local anesthetics influence permeability of the nerve cell membrane by limiting sodium ion permeability by closing the pores through which the ions migrate in the lipid layer of the nerve cell membrane. This limitation prevents the fundamental change necessary for the generation of the action potential.

➤*Pharmacokinetics:* Tetracaine and proparacaine are approximately equally potent. They have a rapid onset of anesthesia beginning within 13 to 30 seconds following instillation; the duration of action is 15 to 20 minutes.

Contraindications

Hypersensitivity to similar drugs (ester-type local anesthetics), para-aminobenzoic acid or its derivatives or to any other ingredient in these preparations; prolonged use, especially for self-medication (not recommended).

Warnings

➤*For topical ophthalmic use only.:* Prolonged use may diminish duration of anesthesia, retard wound healing and cause corneal epithelial erosions(see Adverse Reactions).

➤*Systemic toxicity:* Systemic toxicity is rare with topical ophthalmic application of local anesthetics. It usually occurs as CNS stimulation followed by CNS and cardiovascular depression.

➤*Protection of the eye:* Protection of the eye from irritating chemicals, foreign bodies and rubbing during the period of anesthesia is very important. Thoroughly rinse tonometers soaked in sterilizing or detergent solutions with sterile distilled water before use. Advise the patient to avoid touching the eye until anesthesia has worn off. Because the "blink" reflex is temporarily eliminated, it is advised that the eye be covered with a patch following instillation.

➤*Pregnancy: Category C.* Safety for use during pregnancy has not been established. Use only when clearly needed and when potential benefits outweigh potential hazards to the fetus.

➤*Lactation:* Safety for use during lactation has not been established. Use only when clearly needed and when potential benefits outweigh potential hazards to the infant.

➤*Children:* Safety and efficacy for use in children have not been established.

Precautions

➤*Tolerance:* varies with the status of the patient; give debilitated, elderly or acutely ill patients doses commensurate with their weight, age and physical status.

➤*Reduced plasma esterase:* Use caution in patients with abnormal or reduced levels of plasma esterases.

➤*Special risk:* Use cautiously and sparingly in patients with known allergies, cardiac disease or hyperthyroidism.

Adverse Reactions

Prolonged ophthalmic use of topical anesthetics has been associated with corneal epithelial erosions, retardation or prevention of healing of corneal erosions and reports of severe keratitis and permanent corneal opacification with accompanying visual loss and scarring or corneal perforation. Inadvertent damage may be done to the anesthetized cornea and conjunctiva by rubbing an eye to which topical anesthetics have been applied.

➤*Tetracaine:* Transient stinging, burning and conjunctival redness may occur. A rare, severe, immediate type allergic corneal reaction has been reported characterized by acute diffuse epithelial keratitis with filament formation and sloughing of large areas of necrotic epithelium, diffuse stromal edema, descemetitis and iritis.

Rarely, local reactions including lacrimation, photophobia and chemosis have occurred.

➤*Proparacaine:* Local or systemic sensitivity occurs occasionally. At recommended concentration and dosage, proparacaine usually produces little or no initial irritation, stinging, burning, conjunctival redness, lacrimation or increased winking. However, some local irritation and stinging may occur several hours after instillation.

Rarely, a severe, immediate-type, hyperallergic corneal reaction may occur, which includes acute, intense and diffuse epithelial keratitis, a gray, ground-glass appearance, sloughing of large areas of necrotic epithelium, corneal filaments and, sometimes, iritis with descemetitis. Pupillary dilation or cycloplegic effects have been observed rarely.

Allergic contact dermatitis with drying and fissuring of the fingertips and softening and erosion of the corneal epithelium and conjunctival congestion and hemorrhage have been reported.

Patient Information

Avoid touching or rubbing the eye until the anesthesia has worn off because inadvertent damage may be done to the anesthetized cornea and conjunctiva.

To avoid contamination, do not touch dropper tip to any surface. Replace cap after using.

Do not use if discolored, cloudy or if it contains a precipitate. Protect from light.

Refer to the Topical Ophthalmics introduction for more complete information.

TETRACAINE

Rx	**Tetracaine HCl** (Various, eg, Alcon, Iolab, Optopics, Schein)	**Solution:** 0.5%	In 1, 2 and 15 mL.

[1] With 0.4% chlorobutanol and 0.75% sodium chloride.

TETRACAINE — OPHTHALMIC

Complete and comparative prescribing information begins in the Local Anesthetics, Topical group monograph.

Administration and Dosage

➤*Solution:* Instill 1 or 2 drops. Not for prolonged use.

➤*Storage/Stability:* Store at 8° to 27°C (46° to 80°F). Protect from light.

PROPARACAINE HYDROCHLORIDE

Rx	**Proparacaine HCl** (Various, eg, Moore, Raway, Rugby)	**Solution:** 0.5%	In 2, 15 mL and UD 1 mL.
Rx	**Alcaine** (Alcon)		In 15 mL *Drop-Tainers*.[1, 2]
Rx	**Ophthaine** (Apothecon)		In 15 mL.[3, 4]
Rx	**Ophthetic** (Allergan)		In 15 mL.[4, 5]

[1] With glycerin and 0.01% benzalkonium Cl.
[2] Refrigerate after opening.
[3] With glycerin, 0.2% chlorobutanol and benzalkonium Cl.
[4] Refrigerate.
[5] With 0.01% benzalkonium Cl, glycerin and sodium Cl.

PROPARACAINE HYDROCHLORIDE — OPHTHALMIC

Complete and comparative prescribing information begins in the Local Anesthetics, Topical group monograph.

Indications

➤*Anesthesia:* For topical anesthesia in ophthalmic practice. Representative ophthalmic procedures in which the preparation provides good local anesthesia include measurement of intraocular pressure (tonometry), removal of foreign bodies and sutures from the cornea, conjunctival scraping in diagnosis and gonioscopic examination; it is also indicated for use as a topical anesthetic prior to surgical operations such as cataract extraction.

Administration and Dosage

➤*Deep anesthesia as in cataract extraction:* Instill 1 drop every 5 to 10 minutes for 5 to 7 doses.

➤*Removal of sutures:* Instill 1 or 2 drops 2 or 3 minutes before removal of stitches.

➤*Removal of foreign bodies:* Instill 1 or 2 drops prior to operating.

➤*Tonometry:* Instill 1 or 2 drops immediately before measurement.

➤*Storage/Stability:* Store between 2° to 8°C (35° to 46°F). If solution shows more than a faint yellow color, it should not be used.

MISCELLANEOUS LOCAL ANESTHETIC COMBINATIONS

Rx	**Fluoracaine** (Akorn)	**Solution**: 0.5% proparacaine HCl and 0.25% fluorescein sodium	In 5 mL.[1,2]
Rx	**Fluorescein Sodium with Proparacaine HCl** (Pasadena)		In 5 mL with dropper.[3]
Rx	**Fluress** (Pilkington Barnes Hind)	**Solution**: 0.4% benoxinate HCl and 0.25% fluorescein sodium	In 5 mL with dropper.[4]
Rx	**Flurate** (Bausch & Lomb)		In 5 mL with dropper.[5]

[1] Refrigerate.
[2] With glycerin, povidone, polysorbate 80 and 0.01% thimerosal.
[3] With povidone, glycerin, EDTA and 0.01% thimerosal.
[4] With povidone, boric acid and 1% chlorobutanol.
[5] 1% chlorobutnol, povidone.

MISCELLANEOUS LOCAL ANESTHETIC COMBINATIONS — OPHTHALMIC

Complete and comparative prescribing information begins in the Local Anesthetics, Topical group monograph.

Indications

For procedures in which a topical ophthalmic anesthetic agent in conjunction with a disclosing agent is indicated: Corneal anesthesia of short duration (eg, tonometry, gonioscopy, removal of corneal foreign bodies); short corneal and conjunctival procedures.

Administration and Dosage

➤*Removal of foreign bodies or sutures; tonometry:* 1 to 2 drops (in single instillations) in each eye before operating.

➤*Deep ophthalmic anesthesia:*

Proparacaine/fluorescein – Instill 1 drop in each eye every 5 to 10 minutes for 5 to 7 doses. Use of an eye patch is recommended.

Benoxinate/fluorescein – Instill 2 drops into each eye at 90 second intervals for 3 instillations.

➤*Storage/Stability:* Protect from light.

OPHTHALMIC DIAGNOSTIC PRODUCTS

In addition to the following products, the ophthalmic vasoconstrictors, cycloplegic mydriatics and topical local anesthetics are used in diagnostic procedures (see individual monographs).

➤*Vasoconstrictors/Mydriatics:* With α-sympathomimetic activity cause dilation of the pupil and are used to facilitate ophthalmoscopic examination and other diagnostic procedures.

➤*Cycloplegic Mydriatics:* Cycloplegic Mydriatics (anticholinergics) cause both dilation of the pupil and paralysis of accommodation. These agents are used to facilitate refraction.

➤*Local Anesthetics:* Used to facilitate gonioscopy, tonometry and other procedures.

FLUORESCEIN SODIUM

Rx	**AK-Fluor** (Akorn)	**Injection**: 10%	In 5 mL amps and vials.
Rx	**Fluorescite** (Alcon)		In 5 mL amps with syringes.
Rx	**AK-Fluor** (Akorn)	**Injection**: 25%	In 2 mL amps and vials.
Rx	**Fluorescite** (Alcon)		In 2 mL amps.
Rx	**Fluorescein Sodium** (Various, eg, Alcon)	**Solution**: 2%	In 1, 2 and 15 mL.
otc	**Ful-Glo** (Sola/Barnes-Hind)	**Strips**: 0.6 mg	In 300s.
otc	**Fluorets** (Akorn)	**Strips**: 1 mg	In 100s.

FLUORESCEIN SODIUM — INJECTION

Indications

➤*Angiography/Angioscopy:* Indicated in diagnostic fluorescein angiography or angioscopy of the fundus and of the iris vasculature.

Administration and Dosage

Inject the contents of the ampul or vial rapidly into the antecubital vein, after taking precautions to avoid extravasation. A syringe filled with fluorescein is attached to transparent tubing and a 25-gauge scalp vein needle for injection. Insert the needle and draw the patient's blood to the hub of the syringe so that a small air bubble separates the patient's blood in the tubing from the fluorescein. With the room lights on, slowly inject the blood back into the vein while watching the skin over the needle tip. If the needle has extravasated, the patient's blood will be seen to bulge the skin; stop the injection before any fluorescein is injected. When assured that extravasation has not occurred, the room light may be turned off and the fluorescein injection completed. Luminescence appears in the retina and choroidal vessels in 9 to 14 seconds and can be observed by standard viewing equipment. If potential allergy is suspected, an intradermal skin test may be performed prior to IV administration (ie, 0.05 mL injected intradermally to be evaluated 30 to 60 minutes following injection). For children, the dose is calculated on the basis of 35 mg per 10 pounds of body weight.

➤*Storage/Stability:* Store at 15° to 25°C (59° to 77°F); protect from freezing.

Actions

➤*Pharmacology:* The yellowish green fluorescence of the product demarcates the vascular area under observation, distinguishing it from adjacent areas.

Contraindications

Hypersensitivity to any component of this preparation.

Warnings

➤*Extravasation:* Care must be taken to avoid extravasation during injection because the high pH of fluorescein solution can result in severe local tissue damage. The following complications resulting from extravasation of fluorescein have been noted to occur: sloughing of the skin, superficial phlebitis, subcutaneous granuloma, and toxic neuritis along the median curve in the antecubital area. Complications resulting from extravasation can cause severe pain in the arm for up to several hours. When significant extravasation occurs, discontinue the injection and implement conservative measures to treat damaged tissues and relieve pain.

➤*Pregnancy: Category C.* Avoid angiography on patients who are pregnant, especially those in first trimester. There have been no reports of fetal complications from fluorescein injection during pregnancy.

➤*Lactation:* Exercise caution when fluorescein injection is administered to a nursing woman.

➤*Children:* Safety and efficacy in children have not been established.

Precautions

➤*Special risk:* Exercise caution in patients with a history of allergy or bronchial asthma. An emergency tray including such items as 0.1% epinephrine for IV or IM use; an antihistamine, soluble steroid, and aminophylline for IV use; and oxygen should always be available in the event of possible reaction to fluorescein injection.

FLUORESCEIN SODIUM — INJECTION

Adverse Reactions

Nausea and headache, GI distress, syncope, vomiting, hypotension, and other symptoms and signs of hypersensitivity have occurred. Cardiac arrest, basilar artery ischemia, severe shock, convulsions, thrombophlebitis at the injection site and rare cases of death have been reported. Extravasation of the solution at the injection site causes intense pain at the site and a dull aching pain in the injected arm. Generalized hives and itching, bronchospasm, and anaphylaxis have been reported. A strong taste may develop after injection.

The most common reaction is nausea.

Patient Information

Skin will attain a temporary yellowish discoloration. Urine attains a bright yellow color. Discoloration of the skin fades in 6 to 12 hours; urine fluorescence in 24 to 36 hours.

FLUORESCEIN SODIUM — OPHTHALMIC

Indications

➤*Ophthalmic solution:* Fluorescein ophthalmic solution is indicated for the detection of corneal stippling, abrasions and ulcerations. Fluorescein ophthalmic solution is also indicated for detecting pressure points from contact lenses. Fluorescein ophthalmic solution is indicated for use in conjunction with certain applanation tonometers for measurement of intraocular pressure. This medication is also indicated for use in testing wound leakage (Seidel test).

➤*Ophthalmic strips:* Fluorescein ophthalmic strips are indicated for staining the anterior segment of the eye when fitting contact lenses, in disclosing corneal injury.

Fluorescein sodium ophthalmic strips are indicated for staining the anterior segment of the eye when:

- Delineating a corneal injury, herpetic lesion or foreign body.
- Determining the site of an intraocular injury.
- Fitting contact lenses.
- Making the fluorescein test to ascertain postoperative closure of the sclerocorneal (also referred to as cornecoscleral) wound in delayed anterior chamber reformation.
- Making the lacrimal drainage test.
- In applanation tonometry.

Administration and Dosage

➤*Ophthalmic solution:* One drop topically in the eye(s) followed by irrigation of excess as needed. Additional drops may be instilled if needed.

➤*Ophthalmic strips:* To open envelope, grasp pull tabs firmly and separate slowly. Separate the 2 strips by tearing off white tab end. To ensure full fluorescence and patient comfort, the fluorescein sodium ophthalmic strip impregnated tip should be moistened before application. One (1) or 2 drops of sterile, isotonic irrigation solution, sterile water, or other ophthalmic solution should be used for this purpose. While the patient looks down, stroke the tip across the bulbar conjunctiva or fornix. The patient should then blink several times after application to obtain the best results. For best results, patient should close lid tightly over strip until desired amount of staining is obtained. Another method is to retract upper lid and touch tip of strip to the bulbar conjunctiva on the temporal side until an adequate amount of stain is available for a clearly defined endpoint reading.

Note – Contents may not be sterile if individual strip package has been damaged or previously opened.

➤*Storage/Stability:*

Ophthalmic solution – Store at 8° to 30°C (46° to 80°F).

Keep out of the reach of children.

9 mg strips – Store at room temperature (approximately 25°C [77°F]).

Actions

➤*Pharmacology:* Fluorescein sodium is a dye which stains areas of denuded corneal and conjunctival epithelium.

Contraindications

Hypersensitivity to any component of this preparation; hypersensitivity to mercury-containing compounds.

Warnings

➤*Administration:* Fluorescein sodium is for topical ophthalmic external use only; it is not for injection.

➤*9 mg strips:* Never use fluorescein while the patient is wearing soft contact lenses because the lenses may become stained. Whenever fluorescein is used, flush the eyes with sterile, normal saline solution, and wait at least 1 hour before replacing the lenses.

➤*Hypersensitivity reactions:* Discontinue if sensitivity develops.

➤*Lactation:* Fluorescein has been demonstrated to be excreted in human milk. Caution should be exercised when fluorescein is administered to a nursing woman.

Precautions

➤*Usage:* This medication may stain soft contact lenses. Do not touch dropper tip to any surface, as this may contaminate the solution.

Patient Information

This medication may cause strong taste with use.

This medication may cause temporary yellowish discoloration of the skin. Urine will turn bright yellow. Discoloration of skin fades in 6 to 12 hours; urine, in 24 to 36 hours.

Soft contact lenses may become stained. Do not wear lenses while fluorescein is being used. Whenever fluorescein is used, flush the eyes with sterile normal solution and wait at least 1 hour before replacing the lenses.

FLUOREXON

otc	**Fluoresoft-0.35%** (Various, eg, Amcon, Con-cise Lens, Eye Care and Cure, Holles, Ocusoft)	**Solution:** 0.35%	Preservative-free. In 0.35 mL ampules. In 20s.

FLUOREXON — OPHTHALMIC

Indications

➤*Applanation tonometry:* For conducting the applanation tonometry procedure without removing the lens.

➤*Contact lens fitting aid:* For the assessment of proper fitting characteristics of hydrogel lenses. For quickly and accurately locating the optic zone in aphakic or low-plus lenses.

For the evaluation of corneal integrity of patients wearing hydrogel contact lenses. In many instances, arcuate staining will show definite correlation with the edge of the optic zone, indicating improper bearing surfaces.

➤*Tear break-up time test:* For use in place of sodium fluorescein when conducting the tear breakup time test.

➤*Toric lenses:* For locating the lathe-cut index markings (toric lenses). Use as directed for fitting contact lenses.

Administration and Dosage

Place 1 drop on the concave surface of the lens and place the lens immediately on the eye. Alternately, place 1 or 2 drops in the lower cul-de-sac and have the patient blink several times.

As the dye passes under the lens, observe a central dark zone of 6 to 9 mm in diameter (ie, a limbal fluorescent ring about 2 mm wide) that forms after each blink. If such staining pattern cannot be observed immediately, slide the lens upward by gently pushing it with a finger, causing the dye to penetrate under the lens as it slides back into normal position. Additional drops may be used if the fluorescence starts to dissipate after prolonged examination. When the examination is completed, rinse the eye and lens with saline. The lens may be reinserted immediately, as opposed to the long waiting period required after the use of fluorescein.

Begin the examination immediately after instillation of fluorexon drops. The material tends to dissipate readily with the tear flow, leading to a progressive reduction in fluorescence. Prolonged examination may require sequential application of drops.

➤*Applanation tonometry:* After seating the patient at the slit lamp and either removing the contact lens or displacing it to the side, instill a drop of proparacaine or similar topical anesthetic, followed 1 to 2 minutes later by a drop of fluorexon. Take the reading immediately after, followed by rinsing out the eye and replacing the contact lens.

➤*Storage/Stability:* Store below 24°C (75°F). Avoid direct sunlight. For one-time use only; discard ampule after use.

Actions

➤*Pharmacology:* Fluorexon is a large molecular weight fluorescent solution for use as a diagnostic and fitting aid for patients with hydrogel contact lenses. Fluorexon is used, with or without lens in place (when fluorescein is contraindicated), most commonly to avoid staining lenses. It may be used for soft and hard lenses.

Contraindications

Hypersensitivity to sodium fluorescein.

Warnings

➤*Contact lenses:* When used with lenses of greater than 55% hydration, some color may remain on lens. Remove by washing repeatedly with washing solution approved for the lens. Rinse with saline or water. Any residual coloring will wash out with the tear flow when the lens is reinserted in the eye. With highly hydrated lenses, the amount of coloring picked up will vary with exposure. Avoid unnecessary delays in examination procedure.

FLUOREXON — OPHTHALMIC

Precautions

➤*Hydrogen peroxide:* Do not use hydrogen peroxide solutions to clean or sterilize lenses until all traces of fluorexon are removed because this oxidizing agent can bind fluorexon molecules to the lens.

ROSE BENGAL

otc	**Rose Bengal** (Barnes-Hind)	**Strips:** 1.3 mg per strip	In 100s.
otc	**Rosets** (Akorn)		In 100s.

ROSE BENGAL — OPHTHALMIC

Indications

➤*Suspected corneal/conjunctival damage:* A diagnostic agent in routine ocular examinations or when superficial corneal or conjunctival tissue damage is suspected. Effective aid for diagnosis of keratitis, keratoconjunctivitis sicca, corrosions or abrasions, and for the detection of foreign bodies.

Administration and Dosage

Thoroughly saturate tip of strip with 2 or 3 drops of sterile ophthalmic solution. Touch bulbar conjunctiva or lower fornix with moistened strip. The patient should blink several times after application.

Actions

➤*Pharmacology:* Rose bengal is an iodine derivative of fluorescein and stains dead or degenerated epithelial cells (corneal and conjunctival) and the mucus of the precorneal tear film.

Contraindications

Hypersensitivity to rose bengal or any component of the formulation.

Precautions

➤*Irritation:* The solution may be irritating.

➤*Staining:* Rose bengal can stain eyelids, cheeks, fingers, and clothing in a concentration-dependent manner. Keeping the amount of dye at a minimum and irrigating the eye can help circumvent this problem.

Adverse Reactions

➤*Ophthalmic:* Irritation and discomfort.

INDOCYANINE GREEN

See the Indocyanine green monograph in the Diagnostic Aids chapter.

TEAR TEST STRIPS

Rx	**Schirmer Tear Test** (Various, eg, Alcon)	**Strips:** Sterile tear flow test strips	In 250s.

TEAR TEST STRIPS — OPHTHALMIC

Indications

➤*Schirmer Tear Test:*

Test I – To diagnose dry eye syndrome, to evaluate lacrimal gland function in contact lens wearers, to check tear production prior to eyelid surgery and prior to corneal transplantation and cataract surgery.

Test II – To assess the adequacy of reflex lacrimation.

➤*Sno-Strips:* To assess tear secretion.

Administration and Dosage

Perform test on eye before any topical medication (especially anesthetic) is administered or other procedures are carried out (eg, manipulation of eyelids).

➤*Schirmer Tear Tests:* Strips are placed at the junction of the middle and temporal one third of the eyelid margin. To avoid increased reflex lacrimation and pain, do not touch the cornea. After 5 minutes, remove the strips and measure the length of the moistened area. A value of less than 5 mm is very suggestive of a true dry eye state.

For the Schirmer II Tear Test, insert the strips in the usual manner. Gently irritate the nasal mucosa with a cotton-tip applicator to provoke relfex lacrimation. Remove the strips after 5 minutes. A value of less than 10 mm suggests that the patient is unable to produce reflex lacrimation and has demonstrated reflex secretion failure.

➤*Sno-Strips:* Apply to lower temporal lid margin of eye. The distance between the notch and shoulder of strip is 10 mm, which should be wetted in approximately 3 minutes. Repeat if greater than 5 minutes; greater than 10 minutes indicates reduced tear secretion.

OPHTHALMIC SURGICAL ADJUNCTS

TRYPAN BLUE OPHTHALMIC SOLUTION

Rx	**VisionBlue** (Dutch Ophthalmic)	**Solution:** 0.06%	0.5 mL in 2.25 mL single-use *Luer Lok* syringe.

TRYPAN BLUE — OPHTHALMIC SOLUTION

Indications

➤*Surgical Aid:* Aids in ophthalmic surgery by staining the anterior capsule of the lens.

Administration and Dosage

➤*Approved by the FDA:* December 16, 2004.

➤*Administration:* Trypan blue is packaged in a 2.25 mL syringe to which a blunt cannula must be attached.

After opening the eye, inject an air bubble into the anterior chamber of the eye to minimize dilution of trypan blue by the aqueous humor. Carefully apply trypan blue onto the anterior lens capsule using a blunt cannula. Sufficient staining is achieved as soon as the dye has contacted the capsule. Then irrigate the anterior chamber with balanced salt solution to remove all excess dye. An anterior capsulotomy can then be performed.

➤*Storage/Stability:* Store at 15° to 25°C (59° to 77°F). Protect from direct sunlight.

Actions

➤*Pharmacology:* Trypan blue selectively stains connective tissue structures in the human eye, such as the anterior lens capsule of the human crystalline lens.

Trypan blue is intended to be applied directly onto the anterior lens capsule, staining any portion of the capsule that comes in contact with the dye. Excess dye is washed out of the anterior chamber. The dye does not penetrate the capsule, permitting visualization of the anterior capsule in contrast to the nonstained lens cortex and inner lens material.

Contraindications

Trypan blue is contraindicated when a nonhydrated (dry state), hydrophilic acrylic intraocular lens (IOL) is planned to be inserted into the eye because the dye may be absorbed by and stain the IOL.

Warnings

➤*Carcinogenesis:* Trypan blue is carcinogenic in rats. Wister/Lewis rats developed lymphomas after receiving subcutaneous injections of trypan blue 1% dosed at 50 mg/kg every other week for 52 weeks (total dose approximately 1,250,000-fold the maximum recommended human dose of 0.06 mg per injection in a 60 kg person, assuming total absorption).

➤*Mutagenesis:* Trypan blue was mutagenic in the Ames test and caused DNA strand breaks in vitro.

➤*Elderly:* No overall differences in safety and efficacy have been observed between elderly and younger patients.

➤*Pregnancy: Category C.* Trypan blue is teratogenic in rats, mice, rabbits, hamsters, dogs, guinea pigs, pigs, and chickens. The majority of teratogenicity studies performed involve intravenous, intraperitoneal, or subcutaneous administration in the rat. The teratogenic dose is 50 mg/kg as a single dose or 25 mg/kg/day during embryogenesis in the rat. These doses are approximately 50,000- and 25,000-fold the maximum recommended human dose of 0.06 mg per injection in a 60 kg person, assuming total absorption. Characteristic anomalies included neural tube, cardiovascular, vertebral, tail, and eye defects. Trypan blue also caused an increase in postimplantation mortality and decreased fetal weight. In the monkey, trypan blue caused abortions with 1 or 2 daily doses of 50 mg/kg between the 20th through 25th days of pregnancy, but no apparent increase in birth defects (approximately 50,000-fold maximum recommended human dose of 0.06 mg per injection, assuming total absorption). There are no adequate and well-controlled

TRYPAN BLUE — OPHTHALMIC SOLUTION

studies in pregnant women. Give trypan blue to a pregnant woman only if the potential benefit justifies the potential risk to the fetus.

➤*Lactation:* It is not known whether this drug is excreted in human milk. Because many drugs are excreted in human milk, exercise caution when trypan blue is administered to a breast-feeding woman.

➤*Children:* The safety and efficacy of trypan blue have been established in pediatric patients. Use of trypan blue is supported by evidence from an adequate and well-controlled study in pediatric patients.

Precautions

➤*Irrigation:* After injection, immediately remove all excess trypan blue from the eye by thorough irrigation of the anterior chamber.

Drug Interactions

None known.

Adverse Reactions

Adverse reactions reported following use of trypan blue include discoloration of high water content hydrogen IOLs and inadvertent staining of the posterior lens capsule and vitreous face. Staining of the posterior lens capsule or the vitreous face is generally self limited, lasting up to 1 week.

SODIUM HYALURONATE

Rx	**Healon** (Kabi Pharmacia)	**Injection:** 10 mg/mL[1]	In 0.4, 0.55, 0.85 and 2 mL disp. syringes.
Rx	**Amvisc** (Chiron)	**Injection:** 12 mg/mL[2]	In 0.5 or 0.8 mL disp. syringe.
Rx	**Coease** (Advance Medical)		In 0.5 or 0.8 mL disposable syringes.
Rx	**Shellgel** (Cytosol Ophthalmics)		In 0.8 mL disposable syringes.
Rx	**Healon GV** (Kabi Pharmacia)	**Injection:** 14 mg/mL[1]	In 0.55 and 0.85 mL disp. syringes.
Rx	**Amvisc Plus** (Bausch & Lomb)	**Injection:** 16 mg/mL[2]	In 0.5 or 8 mL disp. syringe.
Rx	**AMO Vitrax** (Allergan)	**Injection:** 30 mg/mL[3]	In 0.65 mL disp. syringe.

[1] With 8.5 mg NaCl per mL.
[2] With 9 mg NaCl per mL.
[3] With 3.2 mg NaCl, 0.75 mg KCl, 0.48 mg calcium chloride, 0.3 mg magnesium chloride, 3.9 mg sodium acetate and 1.7 mg sodium citrate per mL.

SODIUM HYALURONATE — OPHTHALMIC

Indications

For use as a surgical aid to protect corneal endothelium during cataract extraction (extracapsular) procedures, intraocular lens (IOL) implantation and anterior segment surgery. When introduced in the anterior segment of the eye during these surgical procedures, sodium hyaluronate viscoelastic preparation serves to maintain a deep anterior chamber.

In addition, sodium hyaluronate viscoelastic preparation helps to push back the vitreous face and prevent formation of a post-operative flat chamber.

Administration and Dosage

Refrigerated sodium hyaluronate viscoelastic preparation should be allowed to attain room temperature (≈ 20 to 30 minutes) prior to use. Sodium hyaluronate viscoelastic preparation should be slowly and carefully introduced into the anterior segment of the eye using a cannula or needle.

Injection of sodium hyaluronate viscoelastic preparation can be performed either before or after delivery of the lens. Sodium hyaluronate viscoelastic preparation may also be used to coat surgical instruments and the intraocular lenses prior to insertion.

Additional sodium hyaluronate viscoelastic preparation can be injected during surgery to replace any sodium hyaluronate viscoelastic preparation lost during surgical manipulation (see Precautions).

➤*Storage/Stability:* Store in refrigerator (2° to 8°C; 36° to 46°F). Protect from freezing. Protect from light. Bring to room temperature prior to use (≈ 20 to 40 minutes).

Actions

➤*Pharmacology:* Sodium hyaluronate is a high molecular weight polysaccharide, composed of sodium glucuronate and N-acetyl-glucosamine which forms a repeating disaccharide unit by linking alternately beta 1-3 and beta 1-4 glycosidic bonds. The 1% viscous and transparent material, sodium hyaluronate, is a specific fraction of sodium hyaluronate, developed as an aid in ophthalmic surgery. It acts as a space occupying fluid that is replaced by the body's natural fluids.

Sodium hyaluronate is a physiological material that is widely distributed in the connective tissues of both animals and man. Chemically identical in all species, hyaluronate can be found in the vitreous and aqueous humor of the eye, the synovial fluid, the skin and the umbilical cord.

Sodium hyaluronate viscoelastic preparation has the following properties:
- High molecular weight (mass average molecular weight ≈ 3 million daltons)
- High viscosity

Contraindications

At present there are no known contraindications to the use of sodium hyaluronate viscoelastic material when used as recommended; care should be used in patients with hypersensitivity to any components in this material (see Precautions).

Warnings

➤*Compatibility:* Mixing of quaternary ammonium salts such as benzalkonium chloride with sodium hyaluronate results in the formation of a precipitate. The eye should not be irrigated with any solution containing benzalkonium chloride if sodium hyaluronate viscoelastic preparation is to be used during surgery.

Precautions

1.) Precautions normally associated with anterior segment surgical procedures should be observed.
2.) Preexisting glaucoma or compromised outflow and operative procedures and sequelae thereto, including enzymatic zonulysis, absence of an iridectomy, trauma to filtration structures, and by blood and lenticular remnants in the anterior chamber may increase post-operative intraocular pressure. Therefore,
   Do not overfill the eye chamber with sodium hyaluronate viscoelastic preparation.
   Remove all remaining sodium hyaluronate viscoelastic preparation by irrigation and/or aspiration at the close of surgery.
   Carefully monitor the intraocular pressure, especially during the immediate postoperative period. If a significant rise is observed, treat appropriately.
3.) Cannulas are intended for single patient use only. If reuse becomes necessary on the same patient during the surgical procedures, rinse the cannula thoroughly with sterile distilled water to remove all traces of residual material.
4.) Instilling excessive amounts of sodium hyaluronate viscoelastic preparation into the anterior segment of the eye may cause increased intraocular pressure.
5.) Use only if solution is clear.
6.) Avoid trapping air bubble.
7.) Sodium hyaluronate material is obtained from microbial fermentation by a purified proprietary process. Although precautions have been taken to make this device protein-free and it has been tested in animals for allergenic response, this device, used in susceptible persons, may produce allergenic responses.
8.) On rare occasions, viscoelastic products containing sodium hyaluronate have been observed to become slightly opaque or to form a slight precipitate upon instillation into the eye. The clinical significance, if any, of this phenomenon is not known. The physician should, however, be aware of this possibility, and, should it be observed, the cloudy or precipitated material should be removed by irrigation and/or aspiration.
9.) Sodium hyaluronate viscoelastic preparation is a highly purified substance extracted from bacterial cells. However, physicians should be aware of immunological, allergic and other potential risks of the type that can occur from the injection of any biological substance since the presence of minute quantities of impurities (eg, proteins) cannot be totally excluded.

Adverse Reactions

Sodium hyaluronate viscoelastic preparation is tolerated after injection into human eyes during ophthalmic surgical procedures. As with most viscoelastic ophthalmic materials, a transient rise in intraocular pressure has been reported in some cases.

Postoperative inflammatory reactions such as hypopyon and iritis have been reported with the use of ophthalmic viscoelastic materials, as well as incidents of corneal edema and corneal decompensation. Their relationship to the use of sodium hyaluronate has not been established.

In clinical trials, 298 patients were treated with sodium hyaluronate viscoelastic preparation and 224 patients were treated with sodium hyaluronate, an approved comparative device on the US market for more than 5 years. The incidences of adverse experiences that were reported in greater than 1% of the patients are shown in the table below.

SODIUM HYALURONATE — OPHTHALMIC

Sodium Hyaluronate Adverse Reactions Reported in > 1% of Patients

Adverse Reaction	Sodium hyaluronate viscoelastic preparation[1] n = 298 (%)	Control[1] n = 224 (%)
Increased intraocular pressure requiring treatment[2]	22 (7.4%)	17 (7.6%)
Superficial and conjunctival punctate keratitis	12 (4%)	5 (2.2%)
Cystoid macular edema	8 (2.7%)	2 (0.9%)
Posterior capsule opacity	8 (2.7%)	10 (4.5%)
Seidel phenomenon	4 (1.3%)	4 (1.8%)
Conjunctivitis	3 (1%)	3 (1.3%)
Corneal edema	3(1%)	0
Corneal erosion	3 (1%)	0
Sphincter damage	3 (1%)	1(0.4%)
Uveitis	3 (1%)	3 (1.3%)

[1] There is no statistically significant difference in the number of adverse events between the 2 treatment groups.
[2] Mean IOP sodium hyaluronate viscoelastic preparation = 36.7 mmHg (30 mmHg to 52 mmHg).Mean IOP control = 33.6 mmHg (28 mmHg to 48 mmHg).

Adverse reactions that occurred in less than 1% and in at least 2 patients include: Ocular hemorrhage, corneoscleral leak, suture related adverse reactions, vitreous in anterior chamber, hyphema and hematic Tyndall, synechlae, capsule rupture, and cyclytic membrane.

SODIUM HYALURONATE AND CHONDROITIN SULFATE

Rx	**Viscoat** (Alcon)	**Solution:** ≤ 40 mg sodium chondroitin sulfate, 30 mg sodium hyaluronate per mL	0.45 mg sodium dihydrogen phosphate hydrate, 2 mg disodium hydrogen phosphate, 4.3 mg sodium chloride per mL. In 0.5 mL disposable syringes.

SODIUM HYALURONATE AND CHONDROITIN SULFATE SOLUTION — OPHTHALMIC

Refer to the Sodium Hyaluronate monograph for more and comparative complete information.

Indications

➤*Surgical aid:* A surgical aid in anterior segment procedures including cataract extraction and intraocular lens implantation.

Administration and Dosage

Carefully introduce (using a 27-gauge cannula) into the anterior chamber. May inject prior to or following delivery of the crystalline lens. Instillation prior to lens delivery provides additional protection to corneal endothelium, protecting it from possible damage arising from surgical instrumentation. May also be used to coat intraocular lens and tips of surgical instruments prior to implantation surgery. May inject additional solution during anterior segment surgery to fully maintain the chamber or to replace solution lost during surgery. At the end of surgery, remove solution by thoroughly irrigating the eye with a balanced salt solution. Alternatively, the solution may be left in the eye when used as directed.

➤*Storage/Stability:* Store at 2° to 8°C (36° to 46°F). Do not freeze.

SODIUM HYALURONATE AND FLUORESCEIN SODIUM

Rx	**Healon Yellow** (Pharmacia)	**Solution:** 10 mg sodium hyaluronate, 0.005 mg fluorescein sodium per mL	8.5 mg NaCl, 0.28 mg disodium hydrogen phosphate dihydrate, 0.04 mg sodium dihydrogen phosphate hydrate per mL. In 0.55 or 0.85 mL disposable syringes with cannula.

SODIUM HYALURONATE AND FLUORESCEIN SODIUM SOLUTION — OPHTHALMIC

Refer to the Sodium Hyaluronate and Fluorescein Sodium monographs for more complete and comparative information.

Indications

➤*Surgical aid:* A surgical aid in anterior segment procedures including cataract extraction, intraocular lens (IOL) implantation and corneal transplant surgery. The fluorescein sodium facilitates visualization of the product during the surgical procedure.

Administration and Dosage

➤*Cataract surgery/IOL implantation:* Carefully introduce (using a 27–gauge cannula) into the anterior chamber. May inject prior to or following delivery of the lens. Instillation prior to lens delivery provides additional protection to corneal endothelium, protecting it from possible damage arising from removal of the cataractous lens. May also be used to coat the intraocular lens and surgical instruments prior to insertion. May inject additional solution during surgery to replace solution lost during surgical manipulation. Remove solution by irrigation or aspiration at the close of surgery.

➤*Corneal transplant surgery:* After removal of the corneal button, fill the anterior chamber with the solution. Then, suture the donor graft in place. May inject additional solution to replace solution lost during surgical manipulation. Remove solution by irrigation or aspiration at the close of surgery.

➤*Storage/Stability:* Store at 2° to 8°C (36° to 46°F). Allow to attain room temperature (approximately 30 min) prior to use. Do not freeze. Protect from light.

Precautions

➤*IOP:* Do not overfill the anterior segment as it may result in increased intraocular pressure, glaucoma or other ocular damage.

HYDROXYPROPYL METHYLCELLULOSE

Rx	**OcuCoat** (Storz)	**Solution:** 2%	In a balanced salt solution. In 1 mL syringe with cannula.
otc	**Gonak** (Akorn)	**Solution:** 2.5%	In 15 mL.[1]
otc	**Goniosol** (Novartis Ophthalmics)		In 15 mL.[1]

[1] With 0.01% benzalkonium chloride and EDTA.

HYDROXYPROPYL METHYLCELLULOSE SOLUTION — OPHTHALMIC

Indications

For professional use during gonioscopic examination.

Administration and Dosage

For use in the eyes only.

Fill gonioscopic prism with solution, as necessary.

➤*Storage/Stability:* Store between 15° to 30°C (59° to 86°F).

Keep this and all drugs out of the reach of children.

Warnings

To avoid contamination, do not touch tip of container to any surface. Replace cap after using. Not for use in conjunction with hot laser treatment. If solution changes color or becomes cloudy, do not use.

➤*Note:* If this solution dries on optical surfaces, let them stand in cool water before cleansing.

HYDROXYETHYLCELLULOSE

Rx	**Gonioscopic** (Alcon)	**Solution:** Hydroxyethylcellulose	0.004% thimerosal, 0.1% EDTA. In 15 mL *Drop-Tainers.*

HYDROXYETHYLCELLULOSE — OPHTHALMIC

Indications

➤*Gonioscopic bonding:* For use in bonding gonioscopic prisms to the eye.

Administration and Dosage

➤*Storage/Stability:* Store at room temperature 15° to 30°C (59° to 86°F).

BOTULINUM TOXIN TYPE A

For prescribing information, refer to the Botulinum Toxin monographs in the CNS chapter.

POLYDIMETHYLSILOXANE (Silicone Oil)

Rx	**AdatoSil 5000** (Escalon Ophthalmics)	**Injection:** Polydimethylsiloxane oil	In single-use 10 and 15 mL vials.

POLYDIMETHYLSILOXANE — OPHTHALMIC

Indications

➤*Retinal detachments:* Prolonged retinal tamponade in selected cases of complicated retinal detachments where other interventions are not appropriate for patient management. Complicated retinal detachments or recurrent retinal detachments occur most commonly in eyes with proliferative vitreoretinopathy (PVR), proliferative diabetic retinopathy (PDR), cytomegalovirus (CMV) retinitis, giant tears and following perforating injuries.

For primary use in detachments due to AIDS-related CMV retinitis and other viral infections.

Administration and Dosage

➤*Approved by the FDA:* November 7, 1994.

Polydimethylsiloxane can be used in conjunction with or following standard retinal surgical procedures including scleral buckle surgery, vitrectomy, membrane peeling and retinotomy or relaxing retinectomy.

Avoid introduction of air bubbles into the oil by careful withdrawal or decanting of the oil into the syringe. The oil can be injected into the vitreous from the syringe via a single use cannulated infusion line or syringe needle. Subretinal fluid can be drained with a flute needle concurrent with polydimethylsiloxane infusion. The vitreous space can be filled with the oil to between 80% and 100% while exchanging for fluid or air, taking necessary precautions to avoid high intraocular pressure from developing during the exchange. Because the polydimethylsiloxane is less dense than the eye aqueous fluid, a basal iridectomy at the 6 o'clock meridian (Ando iridectomy) is recommended to minimize oil induced pupillary block and early angle-closure glaucoma. Upon choice of the physician, it may be desirable to have the patient assume a face-down posture during the first 24 hours following surgery.

Monitor the patient closely for development of glaucoma, cataract and keratopathy complications and schedule for follow-up reexamination at regular intervals.

It is recommended that polydimethylsiloxane be removed at an appropriate interval within 1 year following instillation if the retina is stable, attached and without significant remnants of proliferation. Although there is insufficient clinical evidence to support justification for longer term tamponade, whether or not the oil should be removed in patients at high risk for redetachment or the development of phthisis and shrinkage due to hypotony must be determined individually by the physician. In order to minimize the number of invasive traumatic experiences for patients with AIDS and CMV retinitis at high risk for redetachment and who have a shortened expected lifespan, avoid silicone oil removal procedures if the patient concurs.

Polydimethylsiloxane can be removed from the posterior chamber by withdrawal with a normal 10 mL syringe and a wide bore 1 mm cannula. By repeated oil-fluid exchange most of the remaining small silicone oil droplets can subsequently be mobilized and removed from the eye. Alternatively, oil may be passively removed by infusion of an appropriate aqueous solution under the oil bubble, while allowing the oil to effuse out of a sclerotomy incision, or limbal incision in aphakic patients.

As there is a possible correlation between the migration of polydimethylsiloxane into the anterior chamber and the appearance of corneal changes such as edema, hazing or opacification, Descemet folds or decompensation, perform regular monitoring of the patient's corneal status and take early corrective action if necessary, including extraction of the oil from the anterior chamber. Large bubbles or droplets of oil in the anterior chamber can be removed manually by syringe. Further standard practice for medical treatment of the keratopathy is recommended.

Temporary pressure increases > 3 weeks after surgery that can normalize either spontaneously or that can be corrected by surgical treatment are those in which the polydimethylsiloxane causes a mechanical blockage of the pupil or inferior iridectomy or causes chamber angle closure by forcing its way anteriorly. In these situations some of the oil may be withdrawn to relieve the mechanical force of the oil interface. Presence of polydimethylsiloxane droplets in the anterior chamber may also cause a chronic outflow obstruction of the trabecular meshwork. In such situations elevated intraocular pressure can be managed with anti-glaucoma medication in the majority of outflow obstruction patients.

➤*Admixture incompatibility:* Do not admix with any other substances prior to injection.

➤*Storage / Stability:* Store at room or cool temperature (8° to 24°C; 46° to 75°F). Polydimethylsiloxane is supplied in a sterile vial intended for single use only and contains no preservative. Do not resterilize. Discard unused portions. Product should be discarded following expiration date.

Actions

➤*Pharmacology:* Polydimethylsiloxane, an oil that is injected into the vitreous space of the eye, is used as a prolonged retinal tamponade in select cases of retinal detachment.

Contraindications

Pseudophakic patients with silicone intraocular lens (silicone oil can chemically interact and opacify silicone elastomers).

Warnings

➤*Cataract:* Approximately 50% to 70% of phakic patients developed a cataract within 12 months of oil instillation. Approximately 33% of phakic AIDS CMV retinitis patients developed some degree of cataract within an average 4 to 5 month time frame from oil instillation.

➤*Anterior chamber oil migration:* In 17% to 20% of patients, oil emulsification or migration into the anterior chamber was observed. Migration into the anterior chamber occurred in both phakic and aphakic patients.

➤*Keratopathy:* From 8% to 20% of patients developed keratopathy (0.6%, AIDS patients). This complication occurred most frequently in aphakic patients (18% to 21%) and in the patients in whom oil had migrated into the anterior chamber (30%); the keratopathy in these cases was attributed to prolonged physical contact between the corneal endothelium and the silicone oil.

➤*Glaucoma:* Approximately 19% to 20% (0.06%, AIDS patients) of patients developed a persistent elevation in intraocular pressure (> 23 to 25 mm Hg). The neovascular glaucoma rate was about 8%. Moderate temporary postoperative increases occurred within the first 3 weeks of treatment. Thereafter, secondary ocular hypertension occurred by several mechanisms. Glaucoma complications occurred in approximately 30% of patients in which anterior chamber oil is noted. Patients with proliferative diabetic retinopathy were at highest risk for development of glaucoma following silicone oil instillation into the vitreous space.

Precautions

➤*Long-term use:* The safety and efficacy of long-term use have not been established.

Adverse Reactions

Most common – The most common adverse reactions include: Cataract (50% to 70%); anterior chamber oil migration (17% to 20%); keratopathy (8% to 20%); glaucoma (19% to 20%). See Warnings.

➤*Miscellaneous:* Other adverse reactions ranked by frequency of occurrence: Redetachment, optic nerve atrophy, rubeosis iritis, temporary IOP increase, macular pucker, vitreous hemorrhage, phthisis, traction detachment, angle block (> 2%); subretinal strands, retinal rupture, endophthalmitis, subretinal silicone oil, choroidal detachment, aniridia, PVR reproliferation, cystoid macular edema, enucleation (< 2%).

INTRAOCULAR IRRIGATING SOLUTIONS

Rx	**Balanced Salt Solution** (Various, eg, Akorn)	**Solution:** 0.64% NaCl, 0.075% KCl, 0.03% magnesium chloride, 0.048% calcium chloride, 0.39% sodium acetate, 0.17% sodium citrate and sodium hydroxide or hydrochloric acid	In 18 and 500 mL.
Rx	**BSS** (Alcon)		Preservative free. In 15, 30, 250 and 500 mL.

INTRAOCULAR IRRIGATING SOLUTIONS

Indications

➤*Irrigation:* For irrigation during various surgical procedures of the eyes. Some products may also be used for the ears, nose and throat (consult specific product labeling).

Administration and Dosage

Use balanced salt solution according to the established practices for each surgical procedure. Follow the manufacturer directions for the particular administration set to be used. For products with separate solutions for reconstitution, never use either Part I or Part II alone; this could result in damage to the eye.

➤*Storage / Stability:* Store at 8° to 30°C (46° to 86°F). Avoid excessive heat. Do not freeze. Discard prepared solution after 6 hours. Do not use if cloudy or if seal or packaging is damaged. Do not use reconstituted solution if it is discolored or contains a precipitate.

Actions

➤*Pharmacology:* Sterile irrigating solution is a sterile physiological balanced salt solution, each mL containing sodium chloride 0.64%, potassium chloride 0.075%, calcium chloride dihydrate 0.048%, magnesium chloride hexahydrate 0.03%, sodium acetate trihydrate 0.39%, sodium citrate dihydrate 0.17%, sodium hydroxide or hydrochloric acid (to adjust pH) and water. This solution is isotonic to ocular tissue and contains electrolytes required for normal cellular metabolic functions.

Warnings

➤*Route of administration:* Not for injection or IV infusion. Use aseptic technique only.

Precautions

➤*Preservative-free solutions:* Do not use for more than one patient.

INTRAOCULAR IRRIGATING SOLUTIONS

➤*Corneal clouding and edema:* Corneal clouding and edema have been reported following ocular surgery in which balanced salt solution was used as an irrigating solution. Take appropriate measures to minimize trauma to the cornea and other ocular tissues.

➤*Concomitant medication:* Addition of any medication to balanced salt solution may result in damage to intraocular tissue.

➤*Diabetics:* Studies suggest that intraocular irrigating solutions which are iso-osmotic with normal aqueous fluids should be used with caution in diabetic patients undergoing vitrectomy as intraoperative lens changes have been observed.

Adverse Reactions

When corneal endothelium is abnormal, irrigation or any other trauma may result in bullous keratopathy. Postoperative inflammatory reactions and corneal edema and decompensation have occurred. Relationship to balanced salt solution is not established.

OPHTHALMIC NON-SURGICAL ADJUNCTS

LID SCRUBS

otc	**Eye Scrub** (Novartis Ophthalmics)	**Solution:** PEG-200 glyceryl monotallowate, disodium laureth sulfosuccinate, cocoamidopropylamine oxide, PEG-78 glyceryl monococoate, benzyl alcohol, EDTA	In 240 mL.
otc	**OCuSOFT** (OCuSOFT)	**Solution:** PEG-80 sorbitan laurate, sodium trideceth sulfate, PEG-150 distearate, cocoamidopropyl hydroxysultaine, lauroamphocarboxyglycinate, sodium laureth-13 carboxylate, PEG-15 tallow polyamine, quaternium-15	Alcohol and dye free. In UD 30s (pads), 30, 120 and 240 mL and compliance kit (120 mL and 100 pads).

LID SCRUBS — OPHTHALMIC

Indications

➤*Eyelid cleansing:* To aid in the removal of oils, debris or desquamated skin.

Administration and Dosage

Close eye(s) and gently scrub on eyelid(s) and lashes using lateral side-to-side strokes; rinse thoroughly.

Precautions

For external use only. Do not instill directly into eye.

HAMAMELIS WATER

Rx	**Succus Cineraria Maritima** (Various)	**Solution:** Aqueous and glycerin solution of senecio compositae, hamamelis water, boric acid	In 7 mL.

HAMAMELIS WATER — OPHTHALMIC

Indications

➤*Optic opacity:* The manufacturer claims usefulness for the treatment of optic opacity caused by cataract. Not intended for use in glaucoma.

Administration and Dosage

Instill 2 drops morning and night into affected eye(s).

EXTRAOCULAR IRRIGATING SOLUTIONS

otc	**AK-Rinse** (Akorn)	**Solution:** Sodium carbonbate, KCl, boric acid, EDTA, 0.01% benzalkonium Cl	In 30 and 118 mL.
otc	**Blinx** (Akorn)	**Solution:** NaCl, KCl, sodium phosphate, 0.005% benzalkonium Cl, 0.02% EDTA	In 120 mL.
otc	**Collyrium for Fresh Eyes Wash** (Wyeth-Ayerst)	**Solution:** Boric acid, sodium borate, benzalkonium Cl	In 120 mL.
otc	**Dacriose** (Novartis Ophthalmics)	**Solution:** NaCl, KCl, sodium phosphate, sodium hydroxide, 0.01% benzalkonium Cl, EDTA	In 15 and 120 mL.
otc	**Eye Stream** (Alcon)	**Solution:** 0.64% NaCl, 0.075% KCl, 0.03% magnesium Cl hexahydrate, 0.048% calcium Cl dihydrate, 0.39% sodium acetate trihydrate, 0.17% sodium citrate dihydrate, 0.013% benzalkonium Cl	In 30 and 118 mL.
otc	**Eye Wash** (Goldline)	**Solution:** Boric acid, KCl, EDTA, anhydrous sodium carbonate, 0.01% benzalkonium Cl	In 118 mL.
otc	**Eye Irrigating Solution** (Rugby)	**Solution:** NaCl, mono- and dibasic sodium phosphate, benzalkonium Cl, EDTA	In 118 mL.
otc	**Irrigate Eye Wash** (Optopics)	**Solution:** NaCl, mono- and dibasic sodium phosphate, benzalkonium Cl, EDTA	In 118 mL.
otc	**Optigene** (Pfeiffer)	**Solution:** NaCl, mono- and dibasic sodium phosphate, EDTA, benzalkonium Cl	In 118 mL.
otc	**Visual-Eyes** (Optopics)	**Solution:** NaCl, mono- and dibasic sodium phosphate, benzalkonium Cl, EDTA	In 120 mL.

EXTRAOCULAR IRRIGATING SOLUTIONS — OPHTHALMIC

Indications

➤*Irrigation:* For irrigating the eye to help relieve irritation by removing loose foreign material, air pollutants (smog or pollen) or chlorinated water.

Administration and Dosage

➤*Solution:* Flush the affected eye(s) as needed, controlling the rate of flow of solution by pressure on the bottle.

➤*Eyecup:* Fill the sterile eyecup halfway with eye wash. Apply the cup tightly to the affected eye and tilt the head backward. Open eyes wide, rotate eye and blink several times to ensure that the solution completely floods the eye. Discard the wash. Rinse the cup with clean water and repeat the procedure with the other eye, if necessary.

Rinse the eyecup before and after every use. Avoid contamination of the rim or inside surfaces of the cup.

➤*Storage / Stability:* If solution changes color or becomes cloudy, do not use.

Actions

➤*Pharmacology:* These sterile isotonic solutions are for general ophthalmic use. Office uses include irrigating procedures following tonometry, gonioscopy, foreign body removal or use of fluorescein; they are also used to soothe and cleanse the eye. Because these solutions have a short contact time with the eye, they do not need to provide nutrients to cells. Unlike intraocular irrigants, irrigants for extraocular use contain preservatives which prevent bacteriostatic contamination. However, the preservatives are exceedingly toxic to the corneal endothelium and intraocular use of extraocular irrigating fluids is contraindicated.

Contraindications

Hypersensitivity to any component of the formulation; as a saline solution for rinsing and soaking contact lenses; injection or intraocular surgery.

Patient Information

If you experience pain, changes in vision, continued redness or irritation of the eye, or if the condition worsens or persists, consult a doctor.

Obtain immediate medical treatment for all open wounds in or near the eyes.

If solution changes color or becomes cloudy, do not use. Do not use these products with contact lenses.

To avoid contamination, do not touch tip of the container to any surface. Replace cap after using.

The otic preparations on the following pages are divided into groups as follows:
- Steroid and Antibiotic Combinations
- Miscellaneous Preparations
- Antibiotics

➤*Patient Information:* For use in the ear only. Avoid contact with the eyes.

Notify physician if burning or itching occurs or if condition persists.

Perforated tympanic membrane is considered a contraindication to the use of any medication in the external ear canal.

Proper use of ear drops –
- Wash hands thoroughly.
- Avoid touching the dropper to the ear or any other surface. For accuracy and to avoid contamination, have another person insert the ear drops when possible.
- Hold container in the hand for a few minutes to warm to near body temperature if it has been refrigerated.
- If the drops are in a suspension form, shake well for 10 seconds before using.
- Lie on your side or tilt the affected ear up for ease of administration.To allow the drops to run in:
  Adults-Hold the earlobe up and back.
  Children-Hold the earlobe down and back.
- Instill the prescribed number of drops in the ear.
- Do not insert the dropper into the ear.
- Keep the ear tilted for about 2 minutes, or insert a soft cotton plug, whichever is recommended.

Products used to soften, loosen and remove earwax –
- Do not use if ear drainage, discharge, pain, irritation or rash occurs.
- If you become dizzy, consult a physician.
- Do not use if injury or perforation of the ear drum exists or after ear surgery unless directed otherwise.
- Do not use for > 4 days; if excessive earwax remains after use of this product, consult a physician.
- Any wax remaining after treatment may be removed by gently flushing with warm water using a soft rubber bulb ear syringe.

Steroid and Antibiotic Combinations

Refer also to Patient Information in the Otic Product Preparations introduction for instructions on the use of these products.

Indications

Treatment of superficial bacterial infections of the external auditory canal.

➤*Suspension:* Also used to treat infections of mastoidectomy and fenestration cavities.

Administration and Dosage

The usual adult dose is 4 drops instilled 3 or 4 times daily.

Actions

➤*Pharmacology:*

In these combinations –

HYDROCORTISONE: Hydrocortisone is used for its antiallergic, antipruritic and anti-inflammatory effects.

ANTIBIOTICS: Antibiotics are used for their antibacterial actions.

Contraindications

Hypersensitivity to any component.

Precautions

➤*Superinfection:* Prolonged treatment may result in overgrowth of nonsusceptible organisms and fungi (eg, herpes simplex, vaccinia, varicella).

STEROID AND ANTIBIOTIC COMBINATIONS, SOLUTIONS

Rx	**Antibiotic Ear Solution** (Various, eg, Geneva)	**Solution**: 1% hydrocortisone, 5 mg neomycin sulfate[1], 10,000 units polymyxin B	In 10 mL.
Rx	**AntibiOtic** (Parnell)		In 10 mL.[2]
Rx	**Cortisporin Otic** (Monarch)		In 10 mL with dropper.[3]
Rx	**Ear-Eze** (Hyrex)		In 10 mL with dropper.[2]
Rx	**LazerSporin-C** (Pedinol)		In 10 mL with dropper.
Rx	**Otosporin** (Calmic)		In 10 mL with dropper.

[1] 5 mg neomycin sulfate is equivalent to 3.5 mg neomycin base.
[2] With propylene glycol, glycerin and potassium metabisulfite.
[3] With cupric sulfate, propylene glycol, glycerin and potassium metabisulfite.

STEROID AND ANTIBIOTIC COMBINATIONS, SOLUTIONS — OTIC

Complete and comparative prescribing information begins in the Steroid and Antibiotic Combinations monograph.

STEROID AND ANTIBIOTIC COMBINATIONS, SUSPENSIONS

Rx	**Antibiotic Ear Suspension** (Various, eg, Geneva)	**Suspension**: 1% hydrocortisone, 5 mg neomycin sulfate[1], 10,000 units polymyxin B	In 10 mL with dropper.
Rx	**Cortisporin Otic** (Glaxo Wellcome)		In 10 mL with dropper.[2]
Rx	**Octicair** (Bausch & Lomb)		In 10 mL with dropper.[3]
Rx	**Pediotic** (Glaxo Wellcome)		In 7.5 mL with dropper.[4]
Rx	**Neomycin/Polymyxin B Sulfates/Hydrocortisone Otic** (Steris)		In 10 mL with dropper.[2]
Rx	**Coly-Mycin S Otic** (Parke-Davis)	**Suspension**: 1% hydrocortisone, 4.71 neomycin sulfate[5]	With 3 mg colistin (as sulfate) and 0.05% thonzonium Br/mL. In 5 and 10 mL with dropper.[6]
Rx	**Cortisporin-TC Otic** (Monarch)	**Suspension**: 1% hydrocortisone, 3.3 mg neomycin sulfate	With 3 mg colistin (as sulfate) and 0.5 mg thonzonium bromide. In 10 mL with dropper
Rx	**Cipro HC Otic** (Alcon)	**Suspension**: 0.2% ciprofloxacin, 1% hydrocortisone per mL	Benzyl alcohol. In 10 mL.
Rx	**Ciprodex** (Alcon)	**Suspension**: 0.3% ciprofloxacin, 0.1% dexamethasone	Benzalkonium chloride, boric acid, EDTA. In 5 and 7.5 mL *Drop-Tainer*.

[1] 5 mg neomycin sulfate is equivalent to 3.5 mg neomycin base.
[2] With cetyl alcohol, propylene glycol, polysorbate 80 and thimerosal.
[3] With cetyl alcohol, polyoxyl 40 stearate, polysorbate 80, propylene glycol, sulfuric acid and benzalkonium Cl.
[4] With thimerosal, cetyl alcohol, glyceryl monostearate, mineral oil, polyoxyl 40 stearate and propylene glycol.
[5] 4.71 mg neomycin sulfate is equivalent to 3.3 mg neomycin base.
[6] With polysorbate 80, acetic acid, sodium acetate and thimerosal.

STEROID AND ANTIBIOTIC COMBINATIONS, SUSPENSIONS — OTIC

Complete and comparative prescribing information begins in the Steroid and Antibiotic Combinations group monograph.

MISCELLANEOUS OTIC PREPARATIONS

Rx	**Acetasol HC** (Barre-National)	**Solution:** 1% hydrocortisone, 2% acetic acid, 3% propylene glycol diacetate, 0.015% sodium acetate and 0.02% benzethonium chloride *Dose:* Insert saturated wick into ear; leave in for 24 hours, keeping moist with 3 to 5 drops every 4 to 6 hours. Keep moist for 24 hours. Remove wick and instill 5 drops 3 or 4 times daily	With 0.05% citric acid. In 10 mL with dropper.
Rx	**Hydrocortisone and Acetic Acid** (Taro)	**Solution:** 1% hydrocortisone, 2% acetic acid, 3% propylene glycol diacetate, 0.015% sodium acetate and 0.02% benzethonium chloride *Dose:* Adults – Insert saturated wick into ear; leave in for at least 24 hours, keeping moist with 3 to 5 drops every 4 to 6 hours. Wick may be removed after 24 hours, but continue to instill 5 drops 3 or 4 times daily as indicated. Children – 3 to 4 drops may be sufficient because of smaller ear canal capacity.	With 0.2% citric acid. In 10 mL dropper tip bottle.
otc	**EarSol-HC** (Parnell)	**Solution:** 1% hydrocortisone, 44% alcohol, propylene glycol, *Dermprotective Factor* yerba santa, benzyl benzoate *Dose:* Insert 4 to 6 drops into ear ≤ 3 to 4 times/day	In 30 mL.
Rx	**Cortic** (Everett)	**Drops:** 1% hydrocortisone, 1% pramoxine HCl, 0.1% chloroxylenol, 3% propylene glycol diacetate and benzalkonium chloride *Dose:* Insert saturated wick into ear; leave in for 24 hours, keeping moist with 3 to 5 drops every 4 to 6 hours. Remove wick and instill 5 drops 3 or 4 times daily	In 10 mL.
Rx	**Cortic-ND** (Everett)	**Drops:** 1% hydrocortisone, 1% pramoxine HCl, 0.1% chloroxylenol, and benzalkonium chloride *Dose:* Adults - 4 to 5 drops into affected ear tid or qid; infants and small children - 3 drops.	In 15 mL.
Rx	**Cortane-B Aqueous** (Blansett)	**Drops:** 1% hydrocortisone, 1% pramoxine HCl, 0.1% chloroxylenol *Dose:* 4 to 5 drops into affected ear tid or qid; infants and small children - 3 drops.	In 10 mL.
Rx	**Cortane-B Otic** (Blansett)	**Drops:** 1% hydrocortisone, 1% pramoxine HCl, 0.1% chloroxylenol *Dose:* 4 to 5 drops into affected ear tid or qid; infants and small children - 3 drops.	In 10 mL.
Rx	**Oti-Med** (Hyrex)	**Drops:** 0.1% chloroxylenol, 1% pramoxine HCl, 1% hydrocortisone, propylene glycol, benzalkonium Cl *Dose:* Adults - Instill 4 to 5 drops into affected ear 3 or 4 times daily. Children and infants - Instill 3 drops into affected ear 3 or 4 times daily.	In 10 mL vials.
Rx	**Tri-Otic** (Pharmics)	**Drops:** 0.1% chloroxylenol, 1% pramoxine HCl; 1% hydrocortisone	In 10 mL vials.
Rx	**Allergen Ear Drops** (Goldline)	**Solution:** 1.4% benzocaine, 5.4% antipyrine, glycerin *Dose:* Fill ear canal with 2 to 4 drops; insert saturated cotton pledget. Repeat 3 or 4 times daily, or up to once every 1 to 2 hours	In 15 mL with dropper.[1]
Rx	**Antipyrine and Benzocaine Otic** (URL)		In 15 mL with dropper.
Rx	**Auroguard Otic** (SDA)	**Solution:** 1.4% benzocaine, 5.4% antipyrine, glycerin, oxyquinoline sulfate *Dose:* Instill 2 to 4 drops into affected ear. Moisten cotton pledget with solution and gently insert into ear canal. Repeat 3 or 4 times daily.	In 15 mL.
Rx	**Americaine Otic** (Fisons)	**Solution:** 20% benzocaine, 0.1% benzethonium chloride, 1% glycerin, PEG 300 *Dose:* Instill 4 or 5 drops. Insert cotton pledget. Repeat every 1 to 2 hours	In 15 mL with dropper.
Rx	**Otocain** (Abana)		In 15 mL.
Rx	**Cresylate** (Recsei)	**Solution:** 25% m-cresyl acetate, 25% isopropanol, 1% chlorobutanol, 1% benzyl alcohol, 5% castor oil, propylene glycol *Dose:* 2 to 4 drops as required	In 15 mL with dropper and pt.
Rx	**Acetic Acid Otic** (Various, eg, Rugby)	**Solution:** 2% acetic acid with 3% propylene glycol diacetate, 0.02% benzethonium chloride, 0.015% sodium acetate *Dose:* Insert saturated wick; keep moist 24 hours. Remove wick and instill 5 drops 3 or 4 times daily	In 15 mL.
Rx	**Acetasol** (Barre)		In 15 mL.
Rx	**Acetic Acid 2% and Aluminum Acetate Otic Solution** (Bausch & Lomb)	**Solution:** 2% acetic acid in aluminum acetate solution *Dose:* Insert saturated wick; keep moist for 24 hours. Instill 4 to 6 drops every 2 to 3 hours	In 60 mL.
Rx	**Burow's Otic** (Rugby)		In 60 mL.
Rx	**Otic Domeboro** (Bayer)		In 60 mL with dropper.
Rx	**Borofair Otic** (Major)	**Solution:** 2% acetic acid, aluminum acetate	In 60 mL.
Rx	**Zoto-HC** (Horizon)	**Drops:** 1 mg chloroxylenol, 10 mg pramoxine HCl, 10 mg hydrocortisone, 3% propylene glycol diacetate, benzalkonium chloride. *Dose:* Instill 4 to 5 drops into affected ear 3 or 4 times daily	In 10 mL plastic dropper vials.
Rx	**Mediotic-HC** (Dayton)	**Drops:** 0.1 % chloroxylenol, 1% pramoxine HCl, 1% hydrocortisone, 0.01% benzalkonium chloride. *Dose:* Adults and children over 12 yr of age: Instill 4 to 5 drops into affected ear 3 or 4 times daily. Infants and children under 12 yr of age - Instill 3 drops in affected ear 3 or 4 times daily.	In 15 mL with dropper.
Rx	**Otomar-HC** (Marnel)	**Solution:** 1 mg chloroxylenol, 10 mg hydrocortisone, 10 mg pramoxine HCl per mL. *Dose:* Instill 5 drops into affected ear 3 or 4 times daily.	In 10 mL plastic dropper vials.
otc	**Auro-Dri** (Commerce)	**Solution:** 2.75% boric acid, isopropyl alcohol *Dose:* Instill 3 to 8 drops in each ear	In 30 mL with dropper.
otc	**Dri/Ear** (Pfeiffer)		In 30 mL.
otc	**Ear-Dry** (Scherer)		In 30 mL w/ dropper.
otc	**Star-Otic** (Stellar)	**Solution:** Nonaqueous acetic acid, Burow's solution, boric acid, propylene glycol *Dose:* Instill 2 to 3 drops before and after swimming or showering	In 15 mL with dropper.
otc	**Debrox** (Marion Merrell Dow)	**Drops:** 6.5% carbamide peroxide, glycerin, propylene glycol, sodium stannate *Dose:* Instill 5 to 10 drops twice daily for up to 4 days	In 30 mL with dropper.
otc	**Murine Ear** (Ross)	**Drops:** 6.5% carbamide peroxide, 6.3% alcohol, glycerin, polysorbate 20 *Dose:* Instill 5 to 10 drops twice daily for up to 4 days	In 15 mL.
otc	**Auro Ear Drops** (Commerce)	**Solution:** 6.5% carbamide peroxide in an anhydrous glycerine base *Dose:* Instill 5 to 10 drops twice daily for up to 4 days	In 15 mL.

MISCELLANEOUS OTIC PREPARATIONS

otc	**E•R•O Ear** (Scherer)	**Drops** 6.5% carbamide peroxide, anhydrous glycerin *Dose:* Instill 5 to 10 drops twice daily for up to 4 days	In 15 mL.
otc	**Mollifene Ear Wax Removing Formula** (Pfeiffer)		With propylene glycol and sodium stannate. In 15 mL with dropper.
otc	**Swim-Ear** (Fougera)	**Liquid:** 95% isopropyl alcohol, 5% anhydrous glycerin *Dose:* Instill 4 or 5 drops in affected ear after swimming, showering or bathing	In 30 mL.

[1] With oxyquinoline sulfate.

MISCELLANEOUS OTIC PREPARATIONS — OTIC

Indications

➤*In these combinations:*

HYDROCORTISONE and DESONIDE – Hydrocortisone and desonide are steroids used for their anti-inflammatory and antipruritic effects.

PHENYLEPHRINE – Phenylephrine is a vasoconstrictor which may be a decongestant.

ACETIC ACID, M-CRESYL ACETATE, BORIC ACID, BENZALKONIUM CHLORIDE, BENZETHONIUM CHLORIDE and ALUMINUM ACETATE (BUROW'S SOLUTION) – Acetic acid, M-cresyl acetate, boric acid, benzalkonium chloride, benzethonium chloride and aluminum acetate (Burow's Solution) provide antibacterial or antifungal action.

CARBAMIDE PEROXIDE and TRIETHANOLAMINE – Carbamide peroxide and triethanolamine emulsify and disperse ear wax.

GLYCERIN – Glycerin is a solvent and vehicle; it has emollient, hygroscopic and humectant properties.

BENZOCAINE – Benzocaine is a local anesthetic.

ANTIPYRINE – Antipyrine is an analgesic.

Otic Antibiotics

OFLOXACIN — OTIC

Rx	**Ofloxacin** (Various, eg, Allergan, Apotex, Bausch & Lomb, Falcon)	**Solution:** 0.3% (3 mg/mL)	In 5 and 10 mL dropper bottles.[a]
Rx	**Floxin Otic** (Daiichi)		In 5 and 10 mL dropper bottles.[b]

[a] With 0.005% benzalkonium chloride.

[b] With 0.0025% benzalkonium chloride, 0.9% sodium chloride.

OFLOXACIN — OTIC

Indications

For the treatment of infections caused by susceptible strains of the designated microorganisms in the specific conditions listed below:

➤*Otitis externa:* In adults and children ≥ 1 year of age, due to *Staphylococcus aureus* and *Pseudomonas aeruginosa*.

➤*Chronic suppurative otitis media:* In patients ≥ 12 years of age with perforated tympanic membranes due to *Staphylococcus aureus*, *Proteus mirabilis*, and *Pseudomonas aeruginosa*.

➤*Acute otitis media:* In children ≥ 1 year of age with tympanostomy tubes due to *Staphylococcus aureus*, *Streptococcus pneumoniae*, *Haemophilus influenzae*, *Moraxella catarrhalis*, and *Pseudomonas aeruginosa*.

Administration and Dosage

➤*Otitis externa:* The recommended dosage regimen for the treatment of otitis externa is:

Children 1 to 12 years of age – 5 drops (0.25 mL, 0.75 mg ofloxacin) instilled into the affected ear twice daily for 10 days.

Patients ≥ 12 years of age – 10 drops (0.5 mL, 1.5 mg ofloxacin) instilled into the affected ear twice daily for 10 days.

The solution should be warmed by holding the bottle in the hand for 1 or 2 minutes to avoid dizziness, which may result from the instillation of a cold solution. The patient should lie with the affected ear upward, and then the drops should be instilled. This position should be maintained for 5 minutes to facilitate penetration of the drops into the ear canal. Repeat, if necessary, for the opposite ear.

➤*Acute otitis media in children with tympanostomy tubes:* The recommended dosage regimen for the treatment of acute otitis media in children 1 to 12 years of age with tympanostomy tubes is:

5 drops (0.25 mL, 0.75 mg ofloxacin) instilled into the affected ear twice daily for 10 days. The solution should be warmed by holding the bottle in the hand for 1 or 2 minutes to avoid dizziness, which may result from the instillation of a cold solution. The patient should lie with the affected ear upward, and then the drops should be instilled. The tragus should then be pumped 4 times by pushing inward to facilitate penetration of the drops into the middle ear. This position should be maintained for 5 minutes. Repeat, if necessary, for the opposite ear.

➤*Chronic suppurative otitis media with perforated tympanic membranes:* The recommended dosage regimen for the treatment of chronic suppurative otitis media with perforated tympanic membranes in patients 12 years and older is 10 drops (0.5 mL, 1.5 mg ofloxacin) instilled into the affected ear twice daily for 14 days. The solution should be warmed by holding the bottle in the hand for 1 or 2 minutes to avoid dizziness, which may result from the instillation of a cold solution. The patient should lie with the affected ear upward, before instilling the drops. The tragus should then be pumped 4 times by pushing inward to facilitate penetration into the middle ear. This position should be maintained for 5 minutes. Repeat, if necessary, for the opposite ear.

➤*Storage/Stability:* Store at 15° to 25°C (59° to 77°F).

Actions

➤*Pharmacology:* Ofloxacin has in vitro activity against a wide range of gram-negative and gram-positive microorganisms. Ofloxacin exerts its antibacterial activity by inhibiting DNA gyrase, a bacterial topoisomerase. DNA gyrase is an essential enzyme, which controls DNA topology and assists in DNA replication, repair, deactivation, and transcription. Cross-resistance has been observed between ofloxacin and other fluoroquinolones. There is generally no cross-resistance between ofloxacin and other classes of antibacterial agents such as beta-lactams or aminoglycosides.

➤*Pharmacokinetics:* Drug concentrations in serum (in subjects with tympanostomy tubes and perforated tympanic membranes), in otorrhea, and in mucosa of the middle ear (in subjects with perforated tympanic membranes) were determined following otic administration of ofloxacin solution. In 2 single-dose studies, mean ofloxacin serum concentrations were low in adult patients with tympanostomy tubes, with and without otorrhea, after otic administration of a 0.3% solution (4.1 ng/mL (n = 3) and 5.4 ng/mL (n = 5), respectively). In adults with perforated tympanic membranes, the maximum serum drug level of ofloxacin detected was 10 ng/mL after administration of a 0.3% solution.

Ofloxacin was detectable in the middle ear mucosa of some adult subjects with perforated tympanic membranes (11 of 16 subjects). The variability of ofloxacin concentration in middle ear mucosa was high. The concentrations ranged from 1.2 to 602 mcg/g after otic administration of a 0.3% solution. Ofloxacin was present in high concentrations in otorrhea (389 to 2850 mcg/g, n = 13) 30 minutes after otic administration of a 0.3% solution in subjects with chronic suppurative otitis media and perforated tympanic membranes. However, the measurement of ofloxacin in the otorrhea does not necessarily reflect the exposure of the middle ear to ofloxacin.

➤*Microbiology:* Ofloxacin has been shown to be active against most strains of the following microorganisms, both in vitro and clinically in otic infections.

Aerobes, gram-positive – *Staphylococcus aureus* and *Streptococcus pneumoniae*.

Aerobes, gram-negative – *Haemophilus influenzae*, *Moraxella catarrhalis*, *Proteus mirabilis*, and *Pseudomonas aeruginosa*.

Contraindications

Hypersensitivity to ofloxacin, to other quinolones, or to any of the components in this medication.

Warnings

➤*Administration:* Ofloxacin otic solution is not for ophthalmic use or for injection.

➤*Hypersensitivity reactions:* Serious and occasionally fatal hypersensitivity (anaphylactic) reactions, some following the first dose, have been reported in patients receiving systemic quinolones, including ofloxacin. Some reactions were accompanied by cardiovascular collapse, loss of consciousness, angioedema (including laryngeal, pharyngeal or facial edema), airway obstruction, dyspnea, urticaria, and itching. If an allergic reaction to ofloxacin is suspected, stop the drug. Serious acute hypersensitivity reactions may require immediate emergency treatment. Oxygen and airway management, including intubation, should be administered as clinically indicated.

OFLOXACIN — OTIC

➤*Mutagenesis:* Ofloxacin was not mutagenic in the Ames test, the sister chromatid exchange assay (Chinese hamster and human cell lines), the unscheduled DNA synthesis (UDS) assay using human fibroblasts, the dominant lethal assay, or the mouse micronucleus assay. Ofloxacin was positive in the rat hepatocyte UDS assay, and in the mouse lymphoma assay.

➤*Pregnancy: Category C.*

Teratogenic – Ofloxacin has been shown to have an embryocidal effect in rats at a dose of 810 mg/kg/day and in rabbits at 160 mg/kg/day.

These dosages resulted in decreased fetal body weights and increased fetal mortality in rats and rabbits, respectively. Minor fetal skeletal variations were reported in rats receiving doses of 810 mg/kg/day. Ofloxacin has not been shown to be teratogenic at doses as high as 810 mg/kg/day and 160 mg/kg/day when administered to pregnant rats and rabbits, respectively.

Ofloxacin has not been shown to have any adverse effects on the developing embryo or fetus at doses relevant to the amount of ofloxacin that will be delivered ototopically at the recommended clinical doses.

Nonteratogenic – Additional studies in the rat demonstrated that doses up to 360 mg/kg/day during late gestation had no adverse effects on late fetal development, labor, delivery, lactation, neonatal viability, or growth of the newborn. There are, however, no adequate and well-controlled studies in pregnant women. Ofloxacin otic should be used during pregnancy only if the potential benefit justifies the potential risk to the fetus.

➤*Lactation:* In nursing women, a single 200 mg oral dose resulted in concentrations of ofloxacin in milk, which were similar to those found in plasma. It is not known whether ofloxacin is excreted in human milk following topical otic administration. Because of the potential for serious adverse reactions from ofloxacin in nursing infants, a decision should be made whether to discontinue nursing or to discontinue the drug, taking into account the importance of the drug to the mother.

➤*Children:* No changes in hearing function occurred in 30 children treated with ofloxacin otic and tested for audiometric parameters. Although safety and efficacy have been demonstrated in children ≥ 1 year of age, safety and efficacy in infants younger than 1 year of age have not been established. Although quinolones, including ofloxacin, have been shown to cause arthropathy in immature animals after systemic administration, young growing guinea pigs dosed in the middle ear with 0.3% ofloxacin otic solution for 1 month showed no systemic effects, quinolone-induced lesions, erosions of the cartilage in weight-bearing joints, or other signs of arthropathy.

Precautions

➤*Arthropathy:* The systemic administration of quinolones, including ofloxacin at doses much higher than given or absorbed by the otic route, has led to lesions or erosions of the cartilage in weight-bearing joints and other signs of arthropathy in immature animals of various species.

Young growing guinea pigs dosed in the middle ear with 0.3% ofloxacin otic solution showed no systemic effects, lesions, or erosions of the cartilage in weight-bearing joints, or other signs of arthropathy. No drug-related structural or functional changes of the cochlea and no lesions in the ossicles were noted in the guinea pig following otic administration of 0.3% ofloxacin for 1 month.

➤*Superinfection:* As with other anti-infective preparations, prolonged use may result in overgrowth of nonsusceptible organisms, including fungi. If the infection is not improved after 1 week, cultures should be obtained to guide further treatment. If otorrhea persists after a full course of therapy, or if 2 or more episodes of otorrhea occur within 6 months, further evaluation is recommended to exclude an underlying condition such as cholesteatoma, foreign body, or a tumor.

Drug Interactions

Specific drug interaction studies have not been conducted with ofloxacin otic.

Adverse Reactions

➤*Subjects with otitis externa:* The following treatment-related adverse reactions occurred in ≥ 1% of the subjects with intact tympanic membranes

Adverse reaction	Frequency (n = 229)
Application site reaction	3%
Dizziness	1%
Earache	1%
Pruritus	4%
Vertigo	1%

The following treatment-related adverse reactions were each reported in a single subject: Dermatitis; eczema; erythematous rash; follicular rash; rash; hypoaesthesia; tinnitus; dyspepsia; hot flushes; flushing; otorrhagia.

➤*Subjects with acute otitis media with tympanostomy tubes and subjects with chronic suppurative otitis media with perforated tympanic membranes:* The following treatment-related adverse reactions occurred in ≥ 1% of the subjects with nonintact tympanic membranes.

Adverse reaction	Frequency (n = 656)
Dizziness	1%
Earache	1%
Paraesthesia	1%
Pruritus	1%
Rash	1%
Taste perversion	7%

Other treatment-related adverse reactions reported in subjects with nonintact tympanic membranes included the following: Diarrhea (0.6%); nausea (0.3%); vomiting (0.3%); dry mouth (0.5%); headache (0.3%); vertigo (0.5%); otorrhagia (0.6%); tinnitus (0.3%); fever (0.3%). The following treatment-related adverse reactions were each reported in a single subject: Application site reaction; otitis externa; urticaria; abdominal pain; dysaesthesia; hyperkinesia; halitosis; inflammation; pain; insomnia; coughing; pharyngitis; rhinitis; sinusitis; tachycardia.

Patient Information

Avoid contaminating the applicator tip with material from the fingers or other sources. This precaution is necessary if the sterility of the drops is to be preserved. Systemic quinolones, including ofloxacin, have been associated with hypersensitivity reactions, even following a single dose. Discontinue use immediately and contact your physician at the first sign of a rash or allergic reaction.

➤*Otitis externa:* Prior to administration of ofloxacin otic in patients with otitis externa, the solution should be warmed by holding the bottle in the hand for 1 or 2 minutes to avoid dizziness which may result from the instillation of a cold solution. The patient should lie with the affected ear upward, and then the drops should be instilled. This position should be maintained for 5 minutes to facilitate penetration of the drops into the ear canal. Repeat, if necessary, for the opposite ear (see Administration and Dosage).

➤*Acute otitis media and chronic suppurative otitis media:* In children 1 to 12 years of age with acute otitis media with tympanostomy tubes and in patients with chronic suppurative otitis media with perforated tympanic membranes, prior to administration, the solution should be warmed by holding the bottle in the hand for 1 or 2 minutes to avoid dizziness which may result from the instillation of a cold solution. The patient should lie with the affected ear upward, and then the drops should be instilled. The tragus should then be pumped 4 times by pushing inward to facilitate penetration of the drops into the middle ear. This position should be maintained for 5 minutes. Repeat, if necessary, for the opposite ear (see Administration and Dosage).

The chemotherapeutic agents include a wide range of compounds that work by various mechanisms. Although development has been directed toward agents capable of selective actions on neoplastic tissues, those presently available manifest significant toxicity on normal tissues as a major complication of therapy. Thoroughly consider the risks vs benefits of therapy when using these agents.

Because of the complexities and dangers in cancer chemotherapy, use should be restricted to, or under the direct supervision of, physicians experienced in its use. In addition to drug therapy, surgical excision and radiation therapy also are employed when appropriate.

➤*Handling of cytotoxic agents:* Most antineoplastics are toxic compounds known to be carcinogenic, mutagenic, or teratogenic. Direct contact may cause irritation of the skin, eyes, and mucous membranes. Safe and aseptic handling of parenteral chemotherapeutic drugs by medical personnel involved in preparation and administration of these agents is mandatory. Potential risks from repeated contact with parenteral antineoplastics can be controlled by a combination of specific containment equipment and proper work techniques. The NIH Division of Safety brochure outlines recommendations for safe handling of these agents.

➤*Mechanisms of action:* The mechanism of action by which these agents suppress proliferation of neoplasms is not fully understood. Generally, they affect at least 1 stage of cell growth or replication. Those more active at 1 specific phase of cellular growth are referred to as *cell cycle specific* agents; those that are active on both proliferating and resting cells are *cell cycle nonspecific* agents. The selectivity of cytotoxic agents inversely follows cell cycle specificity. Rapidly dividing normal tissues including bone marrow, blood components, hair follicles, and mucous membranes of the GI tract may also experience major adverse effects.

➤*Alkylating agents:* These agents form highly reactive carbonium ions that react with essential cellular components, thereby altering normal biological function. Alkylating agents replace hydrogen atoms with an alkyl radical causing cross-linking and abnormal base pairing in deoxyribonucleic acid (DNA) molecules. They also react with sulfhydryl, phosphate, and amino groups resulting in multiple lesions in both dividing and nondividing cells. The resultant defective DNA molecules are unable to carry out normal cellular reproductive functions. Examples of alkylating agents include the following:

busulfan
carboplatin
carmustine
chlorambucil
cisplatin
cyclophosphamide
dacarbazine
estramustine
ifosfamide
lomustine
mechlorethamine
melphalan
pipobroman
streptozocin
thiotepa
uracil mustard

➤*Antimetabolites:* Antimetabolites include a diverse group of compounds that interfere with various metabolic processes, thereby disrupting normal cellular functions. These agents may act by 2 general mechanisms: By incorporating the drug, rather than a normal cellular constituent, into an essential chemical compound; or by inhibiting a key enzyme from functioning normally. Their primary benefit is the ability to disrupt nucleic acid synthesis. These agents work only on dividing cells during the S phase of nucleic acid synthesis and are most effective on rapidly proliferating neoplasms. Examples of antimetabolites include the following:

cytarabine
floxuridine
5-fluorouracil
fludarabine
gemcitabine
hydroxyurea
mercaptopurine
methotrexate
thioguanine

➤*Hormones:* These have been used to treat several types of neoplasms. Hormonal therapy interferes at the cellular membrane level with growth stimulatory receptor proteins. The mechanism of action, however, is still unclear. Adrenocortical steroids are used primarily for their suppressant effect on lymphocytes in leukemias and lymphomas and as a component in many combination regimens. The counterbalancing effect of androgens, estrogens, and progestins has been used to advantage in the therapy of malignancies of tissues dependent upon these sex-related hormones (eg, tumors of the breast, endometrium, prostate). These agents have the advantage of greater specificity for tissues responsive to their effects, thus inhibiting proliferation without a direct cytotoxic action.

Examples of hormone agents include the following:

aminoglutethimide
anastrozole
bicalutamide
diethylstilbestrol
estramustine
flutamide
goserelin
leuprolide
medroxyprogesterone
megestrol
mitotane
polyestradiol
tamoxifen
testolactone

➤*Antibiotic:* Antibiotic-type agents, unlike their anti-infective relatives, are capable of disrupting cellular functions of host (mammalian) tissues. Their primary mechanisms of action are to inhibit DNA-dependent RNA synthesis and to delay or inhibit mitosis. The antibiotics are cell cycle nonspecific. Examples of antineoplastic antibiotics include the following:

bleomycin
dactinomycin
daunorubicin
doxorubicin
idarubicin
mitomycin
mitoxantrone
pentostatin
plicamycin.

➤*Mitotic inhibitors:* Mitotic inhibitor mechanisms that are not fully understood. Podophyllotoxin derivatives inhibit DNA synthesis at specific phases of the cell cycle. Vinca alkaloids bind to tubulin, the subunits of the microtubules that form the mitotic spindle. This complex inhibits microtubule assembly, causing metaphase arrest. In contrast, paclitaxel enhances the polymerization of tubulin and induces the production of stable, nonfunctional microtubules, thus inhibiting cell replication. Podophyllotoxin derivatives include etoposide and teniposide. Vinca alkaloids include vinblastine, vincristine, and vinorelbine. A new class of agents called taxanes includes paclitaxel and docetaxel.

➤*Radiopharmaceuticals:* Radiopharmaceuticals exert direct toxic effects on exposed tissue via radiation emission. Primary activity is against metastatic disease. Examples include strontium-89, sodium iodide I 131, and chromic phosphate P 32.

➤*Biological response modifiers:* Biological response modifiers have complex antineoplastic, antiviral, and immunomodulating activities. It is believed that the antitumor activity of interferons is a result of a direct antiproliferative action against tumor cells and modulation of the host immune response. Examples of biological agents include the following:

aldesleukin (human interleukin-2)
interferon alfa-2a (recombinant DNA)
interferon alfa-2b (recombinant DNA)
interferon alfa-n3 (human leukocyte)
interferon gamma-1B (recombinant DNA)

➤*Miscellaneous:* Metabolism of altretamine is required for cytotoxicity, although the mechanisms are not clear. Asparaginase is an enzyme that inhibits protein synthesis of malignant cells by inhibiting asparagine, which is required for protein synthesis. Intravesical BCG is a suspension of *Mycobacterium bovis* that promotes a local inflammatory reaction in the urinary bladder and reduces cancerous lesions. Cladribine inhibits DNA synthesis and repair through a complex mechanism. Levamisole is an immunomodulator with complex effects. Procarbazine produces toxic metabolites, which induce chromosomal breakage. Tretinoin is a retinoid related to retinol (vitamin A), which induces cytodifferentiation. Porfimer is a photosensitivity agent. Topotecan and irinotecan are topoisomerase I inhibitors.

➤*Extravasation:* This occurs when IV fluid and medication leak into interstitial tissue. Damage resulting from extravasation of certain antineoplastic agents can range from painful erythematous swelling to full-thickness injury with deep necrotic lesions requiring surgical debridement and skin grafting.

Prevention of extravasation injury – This is based on careful, accurate IV drug administration. Avoid areas of previous irradiation and extremities with poor venous circulation for IV cannula placement. Dilute drugs properly and give at an appropriate rate.

Treatment – Treatment of extravasation includes immediate discontinuation of infusion and appropriate antidote administration. Goals of treatment are palliation and prevention of severe tissue damage. For further information regarding the instillation of a specific antidote, refer to individual product monographs. Consider surgical evaluation if an open wound occurs. Some practitioners recommend leaving the IV cannula in place to aspirate some of the chemotherapeutic agent and administering an antidote to the injured site. Others recommend immediate removal of the cannula and administration of the antidote by intradermal or SC injections. Immediate removal of the cannula followed by application of ice has also been recommended for all agents except etoposide, vinblastine, and vincristine (warm compresses are recommended for these agents). Apply the ice for 15 to 20 minutes every 4 to 6 hours for the first 72 hours. Elevate the affected area.

Hydrocortisone sodium succinate or dexamethasone sodium phosphate have been used on the extravasated site for their anti-inflammatory activity. However, these agents as well as other drugs (sodium bicarbonate, DMSO) are unproven for antidote use. Specific antidotes that are recommended include sodium thiosulfate for mechlorethamine and hyaluronidase for vincristine and vinblastine.

Drugs associated with severe local necrosis (vesicants) include the following –

dacarbazine
dactinomycin
daunorubicin
doxorubicin
epirubicin
idarubicin
mechlorethamine
mitomycin
streptozocin
vinblastine
vincristine
vinorelbine

➤*Nausea and vomiting:* These may be the most prominent adverse reactions of cancer chemotherapy from the patient's perspective. In clinical trials, 17% to 98% of patients reported emesis. At least 30% of patients experience acute emesis despite antiemetic therapy. Uncontrolled emesis may cause serious complications, including dehydration, malnutrition, metabolic disorders, esophageal injury, and aspiration. In addition, the patient's quality of life may be reduced significantly. Prevention and management of nausea and vomiting is an important aspect of cancer treatment.

Antineoplastics can be categorized according to their emetogenic potential based on the frequency of emesis. Level 1 is the least emetogenic, while Level 5 is the most emetogenic. Combining antineoplastic agents may increase the overall risk for emesis. For example, a combination of drugs with the risks factors of 2 + 2 + 2 may give a combined emetogenic risk of Level 3 (or 2 + 2 + 3 = 4 and 3 + 3 + 3 = 5).

Emetogenic Potential of Antineoplastics			
Level	Frequency of emesis	Chemotherapeutic agent	
1	< 10%	Bleomycin Busulfan (oral, < 4 mg/kg/day) Chlorambucil (oral) Cladribine Doxorubicin, liposomal Estramustine Floxuridine Fludarabine Hydroxyurea	Interferon alfa Melphalan (oral) Mercaptopurine Methotrexate ≤ 50 mg/m² Pentostatin Thioguanine (oral) Tretinoin Vinblastine Vincristine Vinorelbine
2	10% to 30%	Asparaginase Cytarabine (< 1000 mg/m²) Daunorubicin, liposomal Docetaxel Doxorubicin HCl (< 20 mg/m²) Etoposide Fluorouracil (< 1000 mg/m²) Denileukin diftitox	Gemcitabine Methotrexate (50 to 250 mg/m²) Mitomycin Paclitaxel Pegaspargase Teniposide Thiotepa Topotecan
3	30% to 60%	Aldesleukin Altretamine (oral) Capecitabine (oral) Cyclophosphamide (≤ 750 mg/m²) Cyclophosphamide (oral) Dactinomycin (≤ 1.5 mg/m²) Daunorubicin (≤ 50 mg/m²)	Doxorubicin HCl (20 to 60 mg/m²) Epirubicin Idarubicin Ifosfamide (≤ 1500 mg/m²) Methotrexate (250 to 1000 mg/m²) Mitoxantrone (< 15 mg/m²) Temozolomide
4	60% to 90%	Carboplatin Carmustine (≤ 250 mg/m²) Cisplatin (< 50 mg/m²) Cyclophosphamide (750 to 1500 mg/m²) Cytarabine (≥ 1000 mg/m²) Dactinomycin (> 1.5 mg/m²) Daunorubicin (> 50 mg/m²)	Doxorubicin HCl (> 60 mg/m²) Irinotecan Lomustine (≤ 60 mg/m²) Melphalan (IV) Methotrexate (≥ 1000 mg/m²) Mitoxantrone (≥ 15 mg/m²) Procarbazine
5	> 90%	Carmustine (> 250 mg/m²) Cisplatin (≥ 50 mg/m²) Cyclophosphamide (> 1500 mg/m²) Dacarbazine	Ifosfamide (> 1500 mg/m²) Lomustine (> 60 mg/m²) Mechlorethamine Streptozocin

The incidence of emesis with these and other agents varies greatly among individuals. Dose, schedule, concomitant therapy, other medical complications, and psychologic parameters may affect the incidence, as well.

Prevention and treatment – Prevention and treatment of nausea and vomiting should include measures such as dietary adjustment, restriction of activity, and positive support. However, if pharmacologic management is necessary, several agents or groups of agents may prove useful. Some drugs that have been used with varying degrees of success, either alone or in combination, include 5-HT_3 receptor antagonists (such as ondansetron, dolasetron, and granisetron), phenothiazines, butyrophenones, cannabinoids, corticosteroids, antihistamines, benzodiazepines, metoclopramide, and scopolamine.

CHEMOTHERAPY REGIMENS

Combinations of antineoplastic agents are frequently superior to single drug therapy in the management of many diseases, leading to higher response rates and increased duration of remissions. Using agents that work by differing mechanisms may improve antineoplastic efficacy. Neoplastic cells that acquire rapid resistance to a single agent by random mutation develop resistance less rapidly when treated with a combination of agents.

Selection of agents for combination chemotherapeutic regimens is based on mechanism of drug action, cell-cycle specificity of action, responsiveness to dosage schedules, and drug toxicity.

Many lists of chemotherapy regimens have been published; most sort the regimens by the malignancy treated. Acronyms and abbreviations used to describe chemotherapy regimens can be a source of confusion and inaccuracy. Practitioners should be cautious for several reasons, including the following: 1) a given acronym may refer to several different regimens, 2) different acronyms may be used for the same regimen, 3) abbreviations are frequently cited inconsistently in the literature, and 4) inaccuracies have been propagated in the literature when regimens were cited incorrectly. Referring to a regimen by an acronym or abbreviation may cause misunderstandings and misinterpretations, with potentially serious consequences. Whenever possible, acronyms and abbreviations should not be used to order drug regimens for patients. Use of abbreviations sacrifices clarity.

As a guide, a number of commonly used combination chemotherapeutic regimens are listed below. **Note:** CI = continuous IV infusion.

5 + 2

Use: Acute myelocytic leukemia (AML; reinduction). *Cycle*: 7 days. Regimen given once after an induction regimen has been used.

Regimen: Cytarabine 100-200 mg/m²/day CI, days 1 through 5 *with*
Daunorubicin 45 mg/m² IV, days 1 and 2
or
Mitoxantrone 12 mg/m² IV, days 1 and 2

7 + 3

Use: Acute myelocytic leukemia (AML; induction). *Cycle*: 7 days. Give 1 cycle only.

Regimen: Cytarabine 100-200 mg/m²/day CI, days 1 through 7
with
Daunorubicin 30 or 45 mg/m² IV, days 1 through 3
or
Idarubicin 12 mg/m² IV, days 1 through 3
or
Mitoxantrone 12 mg/m² IV, days 1 through 3

7 + 3 + 7

Use: Acute myelogenous leukemia (AML induction - adults). *Cycle*: 21 days. Give 1 cycle. If patient has persistent leukemia at day 21, give 1 to 2 additional cycles.

Regimen: Cytarabine 100 mg/m²/day CI, days 1 through 7
Daunorubicin 50 mg/m²/day IV, days 1 through 3
Etoposide 75 mg/m²/day IV, days 1 through 7

"8 in 1"

Use: Brain tumors (pediatrics). *Cycle*: 14 days

Regimen: Methylprednisolone 300 mg/m²/dose PO every 6 hours for 3 doses, day 1, starting at hour 0
Vincristine 1.5 mg/m² (2 mg maximum dose) IV, day 1, hour 0
Lomustine 100 mg/m²/day PO, day 1, hour 0
Procarbazine 75 mg/m²/day PO, day 1, hour 1
Hydroxyurea 3000 mg/m²/day PO, day 1, hour 2
Cisplatin 90 mg/m² IV, day 1, begin hour 3 (6-hour infusion)
Cytarabine 300 mg/m² IV, day 1, hour 9
Dacarbazine 150 mg/m² IV, day 1, hour 12

ABV

Use: Kaposi's sarcoma. *Cycle*: 28 days

Regimen: Doxorubicin 40 mg/m² IV, day 1
Bleomycin 15 units IV, days 1 and 15
Vinblastine 6 mg/m² IV, day 1

Use: Kaposi's sarcoma. *Cycle*: 28 days

Regimen: Doxorubicin 10 mg/m² IV, days 1 and 15
Bleomycin 15 units IV, days 1 and 15
Vincristine 1 mg IV, days 1 and 15

ABVD

Use: Lymphoma (Hodgkin's). *Cycle*: 28 days

Regimen: Doxorubicin 25 mg/m² IV, days 1 and 15
Bleomycin 10 units/m² IV, days 1 and 15
Vinblastine 6 mg/m² IV, days 1 and 15
with
Dacarbazine 375 mg/m² IV, days 1 and 15
or
Dacarbazine 150 mg/m² IV, days 1 through 5

AC

Use: Breast cancer. *Cycle*: 21 days

Regimen: Doxorubicin 60 mg/m² IV, day 1
Cyclophosphamide 600 mg/m² IV, day 1

Use: Sarcoma (bony). *Cycle*: 21 to 28 days

Regimen: Doxorubicin 30 mg/m²/day CI, days 1 through 3
Cisplatin 100 mg/m² IV, day 4

Use: Neuroblastoma (pediatrics). *Cycle*: 21 to 28 days

Regimen: Cyclophosphamide 150 mg/m²/day PO, days 1 through 7
Doxorubicin 35 mg/m² IV, day 8

AC/Paclitaxel, Sequential

Use: Breast cancer. *Cycle*: 21 days

Regimen: Give 4 cycles of AC regimen for breast cancer
followed by
Paclitaxel 175 mg/m² IV, day 1 for 4 cycles

ACE (CAE)

Use: Lung cancer (small cell). *Cycle*: 21 to 28 days

Regimen: Cyclophosphamide 1000 mg/m² IV, day 1
Doxorubicin 45 mg/m² IV, day 1
Etoposide 50 mg/m² IV, days 1 through 5

ACe

Use: Breast cancer. *Cycle*: 21 to 28 days

Regimen: Cyclophosphamide 200 mg/m²/day PO, days 3 through 6
Doxorubicin 40 mg/m² IV, day 1

AD

Use: Sarcoma (soft tissue). *Cycle*: 21 days

Regimen: Doxorubicin 45-60 mg/m² IV, day 1
Dacarbazine 200-250 mg/m² IV, days 1 through 5

AP

Use: Ovarian, endometrial cancer. *Cycle*: 21 to 28 days

Regimen: Doxorubicin 50-60 mg/m² IV, day 1
Cisplatin 50-60 mg/m² IV, day 1

ARAC-DNR

Use: Acute myelocytic leukemia (AML).

Regimen: Cytarabine 100 mg/m²/day CI, days 1 through 7
Daunorubicin 30 or 45 mg/m² IV, days 1 through 3
If leukemia is persistent, additional doses are given: Cytarabine on days 1 through 5, daunorubicin on days 1 and 2

B-CAVe

Use: Lymphoma (Hodgkin's). *Cycle*: 28 days

Regimen: Bleomycin 5 units/m² IV on days 1, 28, and 35
Lomustine 100 mg/m²/day PO on day 1
Doxorubicin 60 mg/m² IV on day 1
Vinblastine 5 mg/m² IV on day 1

BCVPP

Use: Lymphoma (Hodgkin's). *Cycle*: 28 days

Regimen: Carmustine 100 mg/m² IV, day 1
Cyclophosphamide 600 mg/m² IV, day 1
Vinblastine 5 mg/m² IV, day 1
Procarbazine 50 mg/m²/day PO, day 1
Procarbazine 100 mg/m²/day PO, days 2 through 10
Prednisone 60 mg/m²/day PO, days 1 through 10

BEACOPP

Use: Lymphoma (Hodgkin's). *Cycle*: 21 days

Regimen: Bleomycin 10 units/m² IV, day 8
Etoposide 100 mg/m² IV, days 1 through 3
Doxorubicin 25 mg/m² IV, day 1
Cyclophosphamide 650 mg/m² IV, day 1
Vincristine 1.4 mg/m² (2 mg maximum dose) IV, day 1
Procarbazine 100 mg/m²/day PO, days 1 through 7
Prednisone 40 mg/m²/day PO, days 1 through 14
Filgrastim 300-480 mcg/day SC, starting on day 8, give for at least 3 days or until leukocytes exceed 2000 cells/mm³ for 3 days

BEP

Use: Testicular cancer, germ cell tumors. *Cycle*: 21 days

Regimen: Bleomycin 30 units IV, days 2, 9, and 16
Etoposide 100 mg/m² IV, days 1 through 5
Cisplatin 20 mg/m² IV, days 1 through 5

Bicalutamide + LHRH-A

Use: Prostate cancer. *Cycle*: Ongoing

Regimen: Bicalutamide 50 mg PO daily
with
Goserelin acetate 3.6 mg/dose implant SC every 28 days
or
Leuprolide depot 7.5 mg/dose IM every 28 days

BIP

Use: Cervical cancer. *Cycle*: 21 days

Regimen: Bleomycin 30 units/day CI, day 1
Cisplatin 50 mg/m² IV, day 2
Ifosfamide 5000 mg/m²/day CI, day 2
Mesna 6000 mg/m²/cycle CI over 36 hours, day 2 (start with ifosfamide)

BOMP

Use: Cervical cancer. *Cycle*: 6 weeks

Regimen: Bleomycin 10 units IM, days 1, 8, 15, 22, 29, and 36
Vincristine 1 mg/m² (2 mg maximum dose) IV, days 1, 8, 22, and 29
Cisplatin 50 mg/m² IV, days 1 and 22
Mitomycin 10 mg/m² IV, day 1

CA

Use: Acute myelocytic leukemia (AML; induction - pediatrics). *Cycle*: 7 days. Give 2 cycles. If patient has persistent blasts at day 15, give a third cycle.

Regimen: Cytarabine 3000 mg/m²/dose IV every 12 hours for 4 doses, days 1 and 2
Asparaginase 6000 units/m² IM, at hour 42

CABO

Use: Head and neck cancer. *Cycle*: 21 days

Regimen: Cisplatin 50 mg/m² IV, day 4
Methotrexate 40 mg/m² IV, days 1 and 15
Bleomycin 10 units/dose IV, days 1, 8, and 15
Vincristine 2 mg/dose IV, days 1, 8, and 15

CAE - see ACE

CAF

Use: Breast cancer. *Cycle*: 28 days

Regimen: Cyclophosphamide 100 mg/m²/day PO, days 1 through 14
Doxorubicin 30 mg/m² IV, days 1 and 8
Fluorouracil 500 mg/m² IV, days 1 and 8

Use: Breast cancer. *Cycle*: 21 days

Regimen: Cyclophosphamide 500 mg/m² IV, day 1
Doxorubicin 50 mg/m² IV, day 1
Fluorouracil 500 mg/m² IV, day 1

CAL-G

Use: Acute lymphocytic leukemia (ALL induction - adult). *Cycle*: 4 weeks. Give 1 cycle only.

Regimen: Cyclophosphamide 1200 mg/m² IV, day 1
Daunorubicin 45 mg/m² IV, days 1 through 3
Vincristine 2 mg IV, days 1, 8, 15, and 22
Prednisone 60 mg/m²/day PO or IV, days 1 through 21
with
Asparaginase 6000 units/m²/day SC, days 5, 8, 11, 15, 18, and 22

CAMP

Use: Lung cancer (non-small cell). *Cycle*: 28 days

Regimen: Cyclophosphamide 300 mg/m^2/day IV, days 1 and 8
Doxorubicin 20 mg/m^2 IV, days 1 and 8
Methotrexate 15 mg/m^2 IV, days 1 and 8
Procarbazine 100 mg/m^2/day PO, days 1 through 10

CAP

Use: Lung cancer (non-small cell). *Cycle*: 28 days

Regimen: Cyclophosphamide 400 mg/m^2 IV, day 1
Doxorubicin 40 mg/m^2 IV, day 1
Cisplatin 60 mg/m^2 IV, day 1

Carbo-Tax

Use: Ovarian cancer. *Cycle*: 21 days

Regimen: Paclitaxel 175 mg/m^2 IV over 3 hours, day 1
Carboplatin IV dose by Calvert equation to AUC 7.5, day 1 (after paclitaxel)
or
Paclitaxel 185 mg/m^2 IV over 3 hours, day 1
Carboplatin IV dose by Calvert equation to AUC 6, day 1 (after paclitaxel)

CaT

Use: Adenocarcinoma (unknown primary), lung cancer (non-small cell), ovarian cancer. *Cycle*: 21 days

Regimen: Carboplatin IV dose by Calvert equation to AUC 7.5, day 1 or 2 (give after paclitaxel infusion)
with
Paclitaxel 175 mg/m^2 IV, day 1
or
Paclitaxel 135 mg/m^2/day CI over 24 hours, on day 1

CAV/EP

Use: Lung cancer (small cell). *Cycle*: 42 days for 3 cycles

Regimen: Cyclophosphamide 1000 mg/m^2 IV, day 1
Doxorubicin 50 mg/m^2 IV, day 1
Vincristine 1.2 mg/m^2 IV, day 1
Etoposide 100 mg/m^2/day IV, days 22 and 23 and 24
Cisplatin 25 mg/m^2/day IV, days 22 and 23 and 24

CAV (VAC)

Use: Lung cancer (small cell). *Cycle*: 21 days

Regimen: Cyclophosphamide 1000 mg/m^2 IV, day 1
Doxorubicin 40-50 mg/m^2 IV, day 1
Vincristine 1-1.4 mg/m^2 (2 mg maximum dose) IV, day 1

CAVE

Use: Lung cancer (small cell). *Cycle*: 21 days

Regimen: **Add to CAV:** Etoposide 100 mg/m^2 IV, days 2 through 4

CA-VP16

Use: Lung cancer (small cell). *Cycle*: 21 days

Regimen: Cyclophosphamide 1000 mg/m^2 IV, day 1
Doxorubicin 45 mg/m^2 IV, day 1
Etoposide 80 mg/m^2/day, days 1 through 3

CC

Uses: Ovarian cancer. *Cycle*: 28 days

Regimen: Cyclophosphamide 600 mg/m^2 IV, day 1
Carboplatin 300-350 mg/m^2 IV, day 1

CDB

Use: Melanoma. *Cycle*: 21 days

Regmen: Cisplatin 25 mg/m^2/day IV, days 1 through 3
Dacarbazine 220 mg/m^2 IV, days 1 through 3
Carmustine 150 mg/m^2 IV, day 1 of odd-numbered cycles only (eg, cycle 1, 3, 5)

CDDP/VP-16

Use: Brain tumors (pediatrics). *Cycle*: 21 days

Regimen: Cisplatin 90 mg/m^2 IV, day 1
Etoposide 150 mg/m^2 IV, days 3 and 4

CDE

Use: Lymphoma (HIV-related, non-Hodgkins - adult). *Cycle*: 28 days

Regimen: Cyclophosphamide 200 mg/m^2/day CI, days 1 through 4
Doxorubicin 12.5 mg/m^2/day CI, days 1 through 4
Etoposide 60 mg/m^2/day CI, days 1 through 4
Filgrastim 5 mcg/kg/day SC starting on day 6, at least 24 hours after the end of the CIs, and ending when the absolute neutrophil count (ANC) is at least 10,000 $cells/mm^3$

CEF

Use: Breast cancer. *Cycle*: 28 days

Regimen: Cyclophosphamide 75 mg/m^2/day PO, days 1 through 14
Epirubicin 60 mg/m^2 IV, days 1 and 8
Fluorouracil 500 mg/m^2 IV, days 1 and 8
Cotrimoxazole 2 tablets PO twice daily, days 1 through 28

CEPP(B)

Use: Lymphoma (non-Hodgkin's). *Cycle*: 28 days

Regimen: Cyclophosphamide 600-650 mg/m^2 IV, days 1 and 8
Etoposide 70-85 mg/m^2 IV, days 1 through 3
Prednisone 60 mg/m^2/day PO, days 1 through 10
may or may not give with
Bleomycin 15 units/m^2 IV, days 1 and 15

CEV

Use: Lung cancer (small cell). *Cycle*: 21 days

Regimen: Cyclophosphamide 1000 mg/m^2 IV, day 1
Etoposide 50 mg/m^2 IV, day 1
Etoposide 100 mg/m^2/day PO, days 2 through 5
Vincristine 1.4 mg/m^2 (2 mg maximum dose) IV, day 1

CF

Use: Adenocarcinoma, head and neck cancer. *Cycle*: 21 to 28 days

Regimen: Cisplatin 100 mg/m^2 IV, day 1
Fluorouracil 1000 mg/m^2/day CI, days 1 through 4 or days 1 through 5

Use: Head and neck cancer. *Cycle*: 21 to 28 days

Regimen: Carboplatin 400 mg/m^2 IV, day 1
Fluorouracil 1000 mg/m^2/day CI, days 1 through 4 or days 1 through 5

CFM - see CNF

CHAMOCA (Modified Bagshawe)

Use: Gestational trophoblastic neoplasm. *Cycle*: At least 18 days, as toxicity permits

Regimen: Hydroxyurea 500 mg/dose PO every 6 hours for 4 doses, day 1 (start at 6 am)
Dactinomycin 0.2 mg IV, days 1 through 3 (give at 7 pm)
Dactinomycin 0.5 mg IV, days 4 and 5 (give at 7 pm)
Cyclophosphamide 500 mg/m^2 IV, days 3 and 8 (give at 7 pm)
Vincristine 1 mg/m^2 IV (2 mg maximum dose), day 2 (give at 7 am)
Methotrexate 100 mg/m^2 IV push, day 2 (give at 7 pm)
Methotrexate 200 mg/m^2 IV over 12 hours, day 2 (give after IV push dose)
Leucovorin 14 mg/dose IM every 6 hours for 6 doses, days 3 through 5 (begin at 7 pm on day 3)
Doxorubicin 30 mg/m^2 IV, day 8 (give at 7 pm)

CHAP

Use: Ovarian cancer. *Cycle*: 28 days

Regimen: Cyclophosphamide 150 mg/m^2/day PO, days 2 through 8
or
Cyclophosphamide 400 mg/m^2/day IV, day 1
with
Altretamine 150 mg/m^2/day PO, days 2 through 8
Doxorubicin 30 mg/m^2 IV, day 1
Cisplatin 50-60 mg/m^2 IV, day 1

ChlVPP

Use: Lymphoma (Hodgkin's). *Cycle*: 28 days

Regimen: Chlorambucil 6 mg/m^2/day (10 mg/day maximum dose) PO, days 1 through 14
Vinblastine 6 mg/m^2 (10 mg/day maximum dose) IV, days 1 and 8
Procarbazine 100 mg/m^2/day (150 mg/day maximum dose) PO, days 1 through 14
Prednisone 40-50 mg/day PO, days 1 through 14*
*Note: Prednisolone is recommended in the British literature. In the US, prednisone is the preferred corticosteroid. The doses of these 2 corticosteroids are equivalent (ie, prednisone 40 mg PO = prednisolone 40 mg PO).

ChIVPP/EVA

Use: Lymphoma (Hodgkin's). *Cycle*: 28 days

Regimen: **See ChIVPP, except:**
Chlorambucil, Procarbazine, and Prednisone* days 1 through 7 and
Vinblastine day 1 only
with
Etoposide 200 mg/m^2 IV, day 8
Vincristine 2 mg IV, day 8
Doxorubicin 50 mg/m^2 IV, day 8
*Note: Prednisolone is recommended in the British literature. In the US, prednisone is the preferred corticosteroid. The doses of these 2 corticosteroids are equivalent (ie, prednisone 40 mg PO = prednisolone 40 mg PO).

CHOP

Use: Lymphoma (non-Hodgkin's), HIV-related lymphoma. *Cycle*: 21 to 28 days

Regimen: Cyclophosphamide 750 mg/m^2 IV, day 1
Doxorubicin 50 mg/m^2 IV, day 1
Vincristine 1.4 mg/m^2 (2 mg maximum dose) IV, day 1
Prednisone 100 mg/day PO, days 1 through 5

CHOP-BLEO

Use: Lymphoma (non-Hodgkin's). *Cycle*: 21 to 28 days

Regimen: **Add to CHOP:** Bleomycin 15 units/day IV, days 1 through 5

CISCA

Use: Bladder cancer. *Cycle*: 21 to 28 days

Regimen: Cyclophosphamide 650 mg/m^2 IV, day 1
Doxorubicin 50 mg/m^2 IV, day 1
Cisplatin 100 mg/m^2 IV, day 2

CISCA II /VB IV

Use: Germ cell tumors. *Cycle*: Individualized based on duration of myelosuppression

Regimen: Cyclophosphamide 500 mg/m^2 IV, days 1 and 2
Doxorubicin 40-45 mg/m^2 IV, days 1 and 2
Cisplatin 100-120 mg/m^2 IV, day 3
alternating with
Vinblastine 3 mg/m^2/day CI, days 1 through 5
Bleomycin 30 units/day CI, days 1 through 5

Cisplatin-Docetaxel

Use: Bladder cancer. *Cycle*: Every 7 days for 8 weeks

Regimen: Cisplatin 30 mg/m^2 IV, day 1
Docetaxel 40 mg/m^2 IV, day 4

Cisplatin-Fluorouracil

Use: Cervical cancer. *Cycle*: 21 days

Regimen: Cisplatin 75 mg/m^2 IV, day 1
followed by
Fluorouracil 1000 mg/m^2/day CI, for 96 hours total
Used in conjunction with
Radiation therapy

Use: Cervical cancer. *Cycle*: 28 days

Regimen: Cisplatin 50 mg/m^2 IV, day 1 starting 4 hours *before* external beam radiotherapy.
Fluorouracil 1000 mg/m^2/day CI, days 2 through 5

Cisplatin-Vinorelbine

Use: Cervical cancer. *Cycle*: 21 days

Regimen: Cisplatin 80 mg/m^2 IV, day 1
Vinorelbine 25 mg/m^2 IV, days 1 and 8

CLD-BOMP

Use: Cervical cancer. *Cycle*: 21 days

Regimen: Bleomycin 5 units/day CI, days 1 through 7
Cisplatin 10 mg/m^2 IV, days 1 through 7
Vincristine 0.7 mg/m^2 IV, day 7
Mitomycin 7 mg/m^2 IV, day 7

CMF

Use: Breast cancer. *Cycle*: 28 days

Regimen: Methotrexate 40-60 mg/m^2 IV, days 1 and 8
Fluorouracil 600 mg/m^2 IV, days 1 and 8
with
Cyclophosphamide 100 mg/m^2/day PO, days 1 through 14
or
Cyclophosphamide 750 mg/m^2 IV, day 1

CMF-IV

Use: Breast cancer. *Cycle*: 21 days

Regimen: Cyclophosphamide 600 mg/m^2 IV, day 1
Methotrexate 40 mg/m^2 IV, day 1
Fluorouracil 600 mg/m^2 IV, day 1

CMFP

Use: Breast cancer. *Cycle*: 28 days

Regimen: Cyclophosphamide 100 mg/m^2/day PO, days 1 through 14
Methotrexate 30-40 mg/m^2/day IV, days 1 and 8
Fluorouracil 400-600 mg/m^2/day IV, days 1 and 8
Prednisone 40 mg/m^2/day PO, days 1 through 14

CMFVP

Use: Breast cancer. *Cycle*: 28 days

Regimen: Cyclophosphamide 400 mg/m^2 IV, day 1
Methotrexate 30 mg/m^2 IV, days 1 and 8
Fluorouracil 400 mg/m^2 IV, days 1 and 8
Vincristine 1 mg IV, days 1 and 8
Prednisone 80 mg/day PO, days 1 through 7

C-MOPP - see COPP

CMV

Use: Bladder cancer. *Cycle*: 21 days

Regimen: Cisplatin 100 mg/m^2 IV, day 2 (at least 12 hours after methotrexate)
Methotrexate 30 mg/m^2 IV, days 1 and 8
Vinblastine 4 mg/m^2 IV, days 1 and 8

CNF

Use: Breast cancer. *Cycle*: 21 days

Regimen: Cyclophosphamide 500 mg/m^2 IV, day 1
Mitoxantrone 10 mg/m^2 IV, day 1
Fluorouracil 500 mg/m^2 IV, day 1

CNOP

Use: Lymphoma (non-Hodgkin's). *Cycle*: 21 to 28 days

Regimen: Cyclophosphamide 750 mg/m^2 IV, day 1
Mitoxantrone 12 mg/m^2 IV, day 1
Vincristine 1.4 mg/m^2 (2 mg maximum dose) IV, day 1
Prednisone 50 mg/m^2/day PO, days 1 through 5

COB

Use: Head and neck cancer. *Cycle*: 21 days

Regimen: Cisplatin 100 mg/m^2 IV, day 1
Vincristine 1 mg IV, days 2 and 5
Bleomycin 30 units/day CI, days 2 through 5

CODE

Use: Lung cancer (small cell). *Cycle*: 9 week regimen

Regimen: Cisplatin 25 mg/m^2 IV, every week for 9 weeks
Vincristine 1 mg/m^2 (2 mg maximum dose) IV weekly, weeks 1, 2, 4, 6, and 8
Doxorubicin 40 mg/m^2 IV weekly, weeks 1, 3, 5, 7, and 9
Etoposide 80 mg/m^2 IV day 1 of weeks 1, 3, 5, 7, and 9
Etoposide 80 mg/m^2/day PO, days 2 and 3 of weeks 1, 3, 5, 7, and 9
used in conjunction with
Prednisone 50 mg PO daily for 5 weeks, alternate days until chemotherapy completion, then taper over 2 weeks

COMLA

Use: Lymphoma (non-Hodgkin's). *Cycle*: 78-85 days

Regimen: Cyclophosphamide 1500 mg/m^2 IV, day 1
Vincristine 1.4 mg/m^2 (2 mg maximum dose) IV, days 1, 8, and 15
Methotrexate 120 mg/m^2 IV, days 22, 29, 36, 43, 50, 57, 64, and 71
Leucovorin 25 mg/m^2/dose PO every 6 hours for 4 doses, beginning 24 hours after each methotrexate dose
Cytarabine 300 mg/m^2 IV, days 22, 29, 36, 43, 50, 57, 64, and 71

COMP

Use: Lymphoma (Hodgkin's - pediatrics). *Cycle*: 28 days

Regimen: Cyclophosphamide 1200 mg/m^2 IV, day 1
Vincristine 2 mg/m^2 (2 mg maximum dose) IV, days 3, 10, 17, and 24
Methotrexate 300 mg/m^2 IV, day 12
Prednisone 60 mg/m^2/day (60 mg/day maximum) PO in 4 divided doses, days 3 through 30, then taper for 7 days

Cooper Regimen

Use: Breast cancer. *Cycle*: 36 weeks

Regimen: Cyclophosphamide 2 mg/kg/day PO, weeks 1 through 36
Methotrexate 0.7 mg/kg IV weekly, weeks 1 through 8
Methotrexate 0.7 mg/kg IV every other week, weeks 10, 12, 14, 16, 18, 20, 22, 24, 26, 28, 30, 32, 34, and 36
Fluorouracil 12 mg/kg IV weekly, weeks 1 through 8
Fluorouracil 12 mg/kg IV every other week, weeks 10, 12, 14, 16, 18, 20, 22, 24, 26, 28, 30, 32, 34, and 36
Vincristine 0.035 mg/kg IV (2 mg maximum dose) weekly, weeks 1 through 5
Vincristine 0.035 mg/kg IV monthly, weeks 8, 12, 16, 20, 24, 28, 32, and 36
Prednisone 0.75 mg/kg/day PO, days 1 through 10, then taper off over next 40 days

COP

Use: Lymphoma (non-Hodgkin's). *Cycle*: 14 to 28 days

Regimen: Cyclophosphamide 800-1000 mg/m^2 IV, day 1
Vincristine 2 mg IV, day 1
Prednisone 60 mg/m^2/day (or 100 mg/day) PO, days 1 through 5, then taper off over next 3 days

COPE

Use: Lung cancer (small cell). *Cycle*: 21 days

Regimen: Cyclophosphamide 750 mg/m^2 IV, day 1
Vincristine 2 mg/cycle IV, day 14
Cisplatin 50 mg/m^2 IV, day 2
Etoposide 100 mg/m^2 IV, days 1 through 3

COPE (Baby Brain I)

Use: Brain tumors (pediatrics). *Cycle*: 28 days, alternate cycles AABAAB

Regimen: **Cycle A:**
Vincristine 0.065 mg/kg (1.5 mg maximum dose) IV, days 1 and 8
Cyclophosphamide 65 mg/kg IV, day 1
Cycle B: Cisplatin 4 mg/kg IV, day 1
Etoposide 6.5 mg/kg IV, days 3 and 4

COPP (C-MOPP)

Use: Lymphoma (non-Hodgkin's or Hodgkin's). *Cycle*: 28 days

Regimen: Cyclophosphamide 450-650 mg/m^2 IV, days 1 and 8
Vincristine 1.4-2 mg/m^2 (2 mg maximum dose) IV, days 1 and 8
Procarbazine 100 mg/m^2/day PO, days 1 through 14
Prednisone 40 mg/m^2/day PO, cycles 1 and 4,* days 1 through 14
*Note: Some clinicians give prednisone with every cycle of COPP. The original clinical trials gave prednisone only with the first and fourth cycles.

CP

Use: Chronic lymphocytic leukemia (CLL). *Cycle*: 14 days

Regimen: Chlorambucil 30 mg/m^2/day PO, day 1
Prednisone 80 mg/day PO, days 1 through 5

Use: Ovarian cancer. *Cycle*: 21 to 28 days

Regimen: Cyclophosphamide 600-1000 mg/m^2 IV, day 1
Cisplatin 60-80 mg/m^2 IV, day 1

CT

Use: Ovarian cancer. *Cycle*: 21 days

Regimen: Cisplatin 75 mg/m^2 IV, day 2 (given after paclitaxel)
Paclitaxel 135 mg/m^2/day CI, day 1

CVD

Use: Malignant melanoma. *Cycle*: 21 days

Regimen: Cisplatin 20 mg/m^2 IV, days 2 through 5
Vinblastine 1.6 mg/m^2 IV, days 1 through 5
Dacarbazine 800 mg/m^2 IV, day 1

CVD + IL-2I

Use: Malignant melanoma. *Cycle*: 21 days

Regimen: Cisplatin 20 mg/m^2 IV, days 1 through 4
Vinblastine 1.6 mg/m^2 IV, days 1 through 4
Dacarbazine 800 mg/m^2 IV, day 1
Aldesleukin 9 million units/m^2/day CI, days 1 through 4
Interferon alfa 5 million units/m^2/day SC, days 1 through 5, 7, 9, 11, and 13

CVI (VIC)

Use: Lung cancer (non-small cell). *Cycle*: 28 days

Regimen: Carboplatin 300-350 mg/m^2 IV, day 1
Etoposide 60-100 mg/m^2 IV, days 1, 3, and 5
Ifosfamide 1500 mg/m^2 IV, days 1, 3, and 5
Mesna 400 mg/m^2 IV before ifosfamide given, days 1, 3, and 5
Mesna 1600 mg/m^2/day CI, days 1, 3, and 5 (give after mesna bolus)

CVP

Use: Lymphoma (non-Hodgkin's), chronic lymphocytic leukemia (CLL). *Cycle*: 21 days

Regimen: Cyclophosphamide 300-400 mg/m^2/day PO, days 1 through 5
Vincristine 1.4 mg/m^2 (2 mg maximum dose) IV, day 1
Prednisone 100 mg/m^2/day PO, days 1 through 5

CVPP

Use: Lymphoma (Hodgkin's). *Cycle*: 28 days

Regimen: Lomustine 75 mg/m^2/day PO, day 1
Vinblastine 4 mg/m^2 IV, days 1 and 8
Procarbazine 100 mg/m^2/day PO, days 1 through 14
Prednisone 40 mg/m^2/day PO, cycles 1 and 4, days 1 through 14

CYVADIC

Use: Sarcoma (bony or soft tissue). *Cycle*: 21 days

Regimen: Cyclophosphamide 500 mg/m^2 IV, day 1
Vincristine 1 mg/m^2 (2 mg maximum dose) IV, days 1 and 5
Doxorubicin 50 mg/m^2 IV, day 1
Dacarbazine 250 mg/m^2 IV, days 1 through 5

DA

Use: Acute myelocytic leukemia (AML; induction - pediatrics).

Regimen: Daunorubicin 45-60 mg/m^2 IV, days 1 through 3
Cytarabine 100 mg/m^2/day CI, days 1 through 7

DAT

Use: Acute myelocytic leukemia (AML; induction - pediatrics). *Cycle*: 14 to 21 days

Regimen: Daunorubicin 60 mg/m^2/day CI, days 5 through 7
Cytarabine 100 mg/m^2 IV every 12 hours, days 1 through 7
Thioguanine 100 mg/m^2/day PO, every 12 hours, day 1 through 7

DAV

Use: Acute myelocytic leukemia (AML; induction - pediatrics). *Cycle*: Give a single cycle.

Regimen: Daunorubicin 60 mg/m^2/day IV, days 3 through 5
Cytarabine 100 mg/m^2/day CI, days 1 through 2
Cytarabine 100 mg/m^2/dose IV every 12 hours for 12 doses, days 3 through 8
Etoposide 150 mg/m^2/day IV, days 6 through 8

DCT

Use: Acute myelocytic leukemia (AML; adult induction). *Cycle*: 7 days. Give once. May be given a second time based on individual response. Time between cycles not specified.

Regimen: Daunorubicin 40 mg/m^2 IV, days 1 through 3
Cytarabine 100 mg/m^2/dose IV every 12 hours, days 1 through 7
Thioguanine 100 mg/m^2/dose PO every 12 hours, days 1 through 7

DHAP

Use: Lymphoma (non-Hodgkin's). *Cycle*: 21 to 28 days

Regimen: Cisplatin 100 mg/m^2/day CI, day 1
Cytarabine 2000 mg/m^2 IV every 12 hours for 2 doses (total dose, 4000 mg/m^2), day 2
Dexamethasone 40 mg/day PO or IV, days 1 through 4

DI

Use: Sarcoma (soft-tissue). *Cycle*: 21 days

Regimen: Doxorubicin 50 mg/m^2/day IV, day 1
Ifosfamide 5000 mg/m^2/day CI, day 1 (after doxorubicin given)
Mesna 600 mg/m^2 IV bolus before ifosfamide infusion
Mesna 2500 mg/m^2/day CI over 36 hours

Docetaxel-Cisplatin

Use: Lung cancer (non-small cell). *Cycle*: 21 days

Regimen: Docetaxel 75 mg/m^2 IV, day 1
Cisplatin 75 mg/m^2 IV, day 1 (after docetaxel)

Dox → CMF, Sequential

Use: Breast cancer. *Cycle*: 21 days

Regimen: Doxorubicin 75 mg/m^2 IV, day 1 for 4 cycles
followed by
CMF-IV for 8 cycles

DTIC/Tamoxifen

Use: Malignant melanoma. *Cycle*: 21 days

Regimen: Dacarbazine 250 mg/m^2 IV, days 1 through 5
Tamoxifen 20 mg/m^2/day PO, days 1 through 5

DVP

Use: Acute lymphocytic leukemia (ALL; induction - pediatric). *Cycle*: 35 days. Give a single cycle.

Regimen: Daunorubicin 25 mg/m^2 IV, days 1, 8, and 15
Vincristine 1.5 mg/m^2 (2 mg maximum dose) IV, days 1, 8, 15, and 22
Prednisone 60 mg/m^2/day PO, days 1 through 28 then taper over next 14 days
used in conjunction with
intrathecal chemotherapy

EAP

Use: Gastric, small bowel cancer. *Cycle*: 21 to 28 days

Regimen: Etoposide 100-120 mg/m^2 IV, days 4 through 6
Doxorubicin 20 mg/m^2 IV, days 1 and 7
Cisplatin 40 mg/m^2 IV, days 2 and 8

EC

Use: Lung cancer. *Cycle*: 21 to 28 days

Regimen: Etoposide 100-120 mg/m^2 IV, days 1 through 3
Carboplatin 300-350 mg/m^2 IV, day 1
or
Carboplatin IV dose by Calvert equation to AUC 6, day 1

EFP

Use: Gastric, small bowel cancer. *Cycle*: 21 to 28 days

Regimen: Etoposide 80-100 mg/m^2 IV, days 1, 3, and 5
Fluorouracil 800-900 mg/m^2/day CI, days 1 through 5
Cisplatin 20 mg/m^2 IV, days 1 through 5

ELF

Use: Gastric cancer. *Cycle*: 21 to 28 days

Regimen: Etoposide 120 mg/m^2 IV, days 1 through 3
Leucovorin 300 mg/m^2 IV, days 1 through 3
Fluorouracil 500 mg/m^2 IV, days 1 through 3 (after leucovorin)

EMA 86

Use: Acute myelocytic leukemia (AML; adult induction). *Cycle*: Give a single cycle.

Regimen: Mitoxantrone 12 mg/m^2 IV, days 1 through 3
Etoposide 200 mg/m^2/day CI, days 8 through 10
Cytarabine 500 mg/m^2/day CI, days 1 through 3 and days 8 through 10

EP

Use: Testicular cancer. *Cycle*: 21 days

Regimen: Etoposide 100 mg/m^2 IV, days 1 through 5
Cisplatin 20 mg/m^2 IV, days 1 through 5

Use: Lung cancer, adenocarcinoma. *Cycle*: 21 to 28 days

Regimen: Etoposide 80-120 mg/m^2 IV, days 1 through 3
Cisplatin 80-100 mg/m^2 IV, day 1

ESHAP

Use: Lymphoma (non-Hodgkin's). *Cycle*: 21 to 28 days

Regimen: Methylprednisolone 250-500 mg/day IV, days 1 through 4 or 1 through 5
Etoposide 40-60 mg/m^2 IV, days 1 through 4
Cytarabine 2000 mg/m^2 IV, day 5 (after etoposide and cisplatin finished)
Cisplatin 25 mg/m^2/day CI, days 1 through 4

Estramustine/Vinblastine

Use: Prostate cancer. *Cycle*: 8 weeks

Regimen: Estramustine 10 mg/kg/day PO given in 3 divided doses, days 1 through 42
Vinblastine 4 mg/m^2 IV weekly, weeks 1 through 6

EVA

Use: Lymphoma (Hodgkin's). *Cycle*: 28 days

Regimen: Etoposide 100 mg/m^2 IV, days 1 through 3
Vinblastine 6 mg/m^2 IV, day 1
Doxorubicin 50 mg/m^2 IV, day 1

FAC

Use: Breast cancer. *Cycle*: 21 to 28 days

Regimen: Fluorouracil 500 mg/m^2 IV, days 1 and 8
Doxorubicin 50 mg/m^2 IV, day 1
Cyclophosphamide 500 mg/m^2 IV, day 1

FAM

Use: Adenocarcinoma, gastric cancer. *Cycle*: 8 weeks

Regimen: Fluorouracil 600 mg/m^2/day IV, days 1, 8, 29, and 36
Doxorubicin 30 mg/m^2/day IV, days 1 and 29
Mitomycin 10 mg/m^2 IV, day 1

FAMTX

Use: Gastric cancer. *Cycle*: 28 days

Regimen: Methotrexate 1500 mg/m^2 IV, day 1
Fluorouracil 1500 mg/m^2 IV, day 1 (give after methotrexate given)
Leucovorin 15 mg/m^2/dose PO every 6 hours for 8 doses (start 24 hours after methotrexate); increase dose to 30 mg/m^2/dose PO every 6 hours for 16 doses if 24-hour methotrexate level at least 2.5 mol/L
Doxorubicin 30 mg/m^2 IV, day 15

FAP

Use: Gastric cancer. *Cycle*: 5 weeks

Regimen: Fluorouracil 300 mg/m^2 IV, days 1 through 5
Doxorubicin 40 mg/m^2 IV, day 1
Cisplatin 60 mg/m^2 IV, day 1

F-CL (FU/LV)

Use: Colorectal cancer. *Cycle*: 4 to 8 weeks

Regimen: Fluorouracil 600 mg/m^2 IV, weekly for 6 weeks (after starting leucovorin), then 2-week rest period
Leucovorin 500 mg/m^2 IV, weekly for 6 weeks, then 2-week rest period
or
Fluorouracil 370-425 mg/m^2 IV, days 1 through 5 (after starting leucovorin)
Leucovorin 20 mg/m^2 IV, days 1 through 5

FEC

Use: Breast cancer. *Cycle*: 21 days

Regimen: Fluorouracil 500 mg/m^2 IV, day 1
Cyclophosphamide 500 mg/m^2 IV, day 1
Epirubicin 100 mg/m^2 IV, day 1

FED

Use: Lung cancer (non-small cell). *Cycle*: 21 days

Regimen: Fluorouracil 960 mg/m^2/day CI, days 2 through 4
Etoposide 80 mg/m^2 IV, days 2 through 4
Cisplatin 100 mg/m^2 IV, day 1

FL

Use: Prostate cancer. *Cycle*: Ongoing

Regimen: Flutamide 250 mg/dose PO every 8 hours
with
Leuprolide acetate 1 mg SC daily
or
Leuprolide depot 7.5 mg IM/dose, every 28 days
or
Leuprolide depot 22.5 mg IM/dose, every 3 months

Fle

Use: Colorectal cancer. *Cycle*: 1 year

Regimen: Fluorouracil 450 mg/m^2 IV, days 1 through 5
Fluorouracil 450 mg/m^2 IV weekly, weeks 5 through 52
Levamisole 50 mg/dose PO every 8 hours, days 1 through 3 of every other week for 1 year

FNC - see CNF

FU/LV - see F-CL

FU/LV/CPT-11

Use: Metastatic colorectal cancer.* *Cycle*: 42 days

Regimen: Fluorouracil 500 mg/m^2 IV, days 1, 8, 15, and 22
Leucovorin 20 mg/m^2 IV, days 1, 8, 15, and 22
Irinotecan 125 mg/m^2 IV, days 1, 8, 15, and 22
*Note: A recent study analysis found an increased risk of early deaths (within 60 days of initiating treatment) with use of this regimen. Specific risk factors that may have contributed to death were not identified. Intensive patient monitoring and dosage modification is recommended to reduce the risk of severe adverse effects.

FUP

Use: Gastric cancer. *Cycle*: 28 days

Regimen: Fluorouracil 1000 mg/m^2/day CI, days 1 through 5
Cisplatin 100 mg/m^2 IV, day 2

FZ

Use: Prostate cancer. *Cycle*: Ongoing

Regimen: Flutamide 250 mg/dose PO every 8 hours
with
Goserelin acetate 3.6 mg/dose implant SC every 28 days
or
Goserelin acetate 10.8 mg/dose implant SC every 12 weeks

Gemcitabine-Carboplatin

Use: Lung cancer (non-small cell). *Cycle*: 28 days

Regimen: Gemcitabine 1000 mg/m^2 or 1100 mg/m^2 IV, days 1 and 8
Carboplatin IV dose by Calvert equation to AUC 5, day 8

Gemcitabine-Cis

Use: Lung cancer (non-small cell). *Cycle*: 28 days

Regimen: Gemcitabine 1000-1200 mg/m^2 IV, days 1, 8, and 15
Cisplatin 100 mg/m^2/cycle IV, day 1, 2, or 15

Gemcitabine-Cisplatin

Use: Metastatic bladder cancer. *Cycle*: 28 days up to 6 cycles

Regimen: Gemcitabine 1000 mg/m^2 IV, days 1, 8, and 15
Cisplatin 70 mg/m^2 IV, day 2

Gemcitabine-Vinorelbine

Use: Lung cancer (non-small cell). *Cycle*: 21 days up to 6 cycles

Regimen: Gemcitabine 1200 mg/m^2 IV, days 1 and 8
Vinorelbine 30 mg/m^2 IV, days 1 and 8

Use: Lung cancer (non-small cell). *Cycle*: 28 days up to 6 cycles

Regimen: Gemcitabine 800 mg/m^2 or 1000 mg/m^2 IV, days 1, 8, and 15
Vinorelbine 20 mg/m^2 IV, days 1, 8, and 15

HDMTX

Use: Sarcoma (bony). *Cycle*: 1 to 4 weeks

Regimen: Methotrexate 8000-12,000 mg/m^2 (20,000 mg maximum dose) IV, day 1
Leucovorin 15 mg/m^2/dose PO or IV every 6 hours for 10 doses, beginning 20 to 30 hours after beginning of methotrexate infusion

Hexa-CAF

Use: Ovarian cancer. *Cycle*: 28 days

Regimen: Altretamine 150 mg/m^2/day PO, days 1 through 14
Cyclophosphamide 100-150 mg/m^2/day PO, days 1 through 14
Methotrexate 40 mg/m^2 IV, days 1 and 8
Fluorouracil 600 mg/m^2 IV, days 1 and 8

Hi-C DAZE

Use: Acute myelogenous leukemia (AML induction - pediatrics). *Cycle*: Give a single cycle.

Regimen: Daunorubicin 30 mg/m^2 IV, days 1 through 3
Cytarabine 3000 mg/m^2/dose IV every 12 hours, days 1 through 4 (total of 8 doses)
Etoposide 200 mg/m^2 IV, days 1 through 3 and days 6 through 8
5-azacytidine* 150 mg/m^2 IV, days 3 through 5 and days 8 through 10
*Note: 5-azacytidine is an investigational Group C drug. Although it is not currently marketed in the US, the product may be obtained from the NCI.

ICE - see MICE

ICE Protocol - see Idarubicin, Cytarabine, Etoposide

ICE-T

Use: Breast cancer, sarcoma, lung cancer (non-small cell). *Cycle*: 28 days

Regimen: Ifosfamide 1250 mg/m^2 IV, days 1 through 3
Carboplatin 300 mg/m^2 IV, day 1
Etoposide 80 mg/m^2 IV, days 1 through 3
Paclitaxel 175 mg/m^2 IV, day 4
with
Mesna 20% of ifosfamide dose IV before, then mesna 40% of ifosfamide dose PO given 4 and 8 hours after ifosfamide
or
Mesna 1250 mg/m^2 IV, days 1 through 3

IDA-based BF 12 - see Idarubicin, Cytarabine, Etoposide

Idarubicin, Cytarabine, Etoposide (ICE Protocol)

Use: Acute myelogenous leukemia (AML induction - adults). *Cycle*: Give a single cycle

Regimen: Idarubicin 6 mg/m^2 IV, days 1 through 5
Cytarabine 600 mg/m^2 IV, days 1 through 5
Etoposide 150 mg/m^2 IV, days 1 through 3

Idarubicin, Cytarabine, Etoposide (IDA-based BF 12)

Use: Acute myelogenous leukemia (AML induction - adults). *Cycle*: Usually 1 cycle used. A second cycle may be considered for patients with partial response. Time between cycles not specified.

Regimen: Idarubicin 5 mg/m^2 IV, days 1 through 5
Cytarabine 2000 mg/m^2/dose IV every 12 hours, days 1 through 5 (total of 10 doses)
Etoposide 100 mg/m^2 IV, days 1 through 5

IDMTX/6-MP

Use: Acute lymphocytic leukemia (ALL; consolidation - pediatrics). *Cycle*: 2 weeks, up to 12 cycles

Regimen: **Week 1:** Methotrexate 200 mg/m^2 IV bolus, day 1
Mercaptopurine 200 mg/m^2 IV bolus, day 1
then
Methotrexate 800 mg/m^2/day CI, day 1
Mercaptopurine 800 mg/m^2 IV over 8 hours, day 1
Leucovorin 5 mg/m^2/dose PO or IV every 6 hours for 5-13 doses, beginning 24 hours after methotrexate infusion finished.
Week 2: Methotrexate 20 mg/m^2 IM day 8
Mercaptopurine 50 mg/m^2 PO, days 8 through 14

IE

Use: Sarcoma (soft-tissue). *Cycle*: 21 days

Regimen: Ifosfamide 1800 mg/m^2 IV, days 1 through 5
Etoposide 100 mg/m^2 IV, days 1 through 5
with
Mesna 1800 mg/m^2 IV, days 1 through 5
or
Mesna 20% of ifosfamide dose prior to, then 4 and 8 hours after ifosfamide

IfoVP

Use: Sarcoma (osteosarcoma - pediatrics). *Cycle*: 21 days

Regimen: Ifosfamide 1800 mg/m^2 IV, days 1 through 5
Etoposide 100 mg/m^2 IV, days 1 through 5
Mesna 1800 mg/m^2 IV, days 1 through 5

Interleukin 2-Interferon alfa 2

Use: Renal cell carcinoma. *Cycle*: 56 days

Regimen: Aldesleukin 20 million units/m^2/dose SC 3 times weekly, weeks 1 and 4
Aldesleukin 5 million units/m^2/dose SC 3 times weekly, weeks 2, 3, 5, and 6
Interferon alfa 6 million units/m^2/dose SC once weekly, weeks 1 and 4
Interferon alfa 6 million units/m^2/dose SC 3 times weekly, weeks 2, 3, 5, and 6

IPA

Use: Hepatoblastoma (pediatrics). *Cycle*: 21 days

Regimen: Ifosfamide 500 mg/m^2 IV bolus, day 1
Ifosfamide 1000 mg/m^2/day CI, days 1 through 3
Cisplatin 20 mg/m^2 IV, days 4 through 8
Doxorubicin 30 mg/m^2/day CI, days 9 and 10

Linker Protocol

Use: Acute lymphocytic leukemia (ALL; induction and consolidation).

Regimen: **Remission induction**. Give 1 cycle only.
Daunorubicin 50 mg/m² IV, days 1 through 3
Vincristine 2 mg IV, days 1, 8, 15, and 22
Prednisone 60 mg/m²/day PO, days 1 through 28
Asparaginase 6000 units/m² IM, days 17 through 28
If residual leukemia in marrow on day 14:
Daunorubicin 50 mg/m² IV, day 15
If residual leukemia in marrow on day 28:
Daunorubicin 50 mg/m² IV, days 29 and 30
Vincristine 2 mg IV, days 29 and 36
Prednisone 60 mg/m²/day PO, days 29 through 42
Asparaginase 6000 units/m² IM, days 29 through 35
Consolidation therapy. *Cycle*: 28 days
Treatment A (cycles 1, 3, 5, and 7)
Daunorubicin 50 mg/m² IV, days 1 and 2
Vincristine 2 mg IV, days 1 and 8
Prednisone 60 mg/m²/day PO, days 1 through 14
Asparaginase 12,000 units/m² IM, days 2, 4, 7, 9, 11, and 14
Treatment B (cycles 2, 4, 6, and 8)
Teniposide 165 mg/m² IV, days 1, 4, 8, and 11
Cytarabine 300 mg/m² IV, days 1, 4, 8, and 11
Treatment C (cycle 9)
Methotrexate 690 mg/m² IV over 42 hours
Leucovorin 15 mg/m² IV every 6 hours for 12 doses (start at end of methotrexate infusion)

M-2

Use: Multiple myeloma. *Cycle*: 5 weeks

Regimen: Vincristine 0.03 mg/kg (2 mg maximum dose) IV, day 1
Carmustine 0.5 mg/kg IV, day 1
Cyclophosphamide 10 mg/kg IV, day 1
Prednisone 1 mg/kg/day PO, days 1 through 7, tapered over next 14 days
with
Melphalan 0.25 mg/kg/day PO, days 1 through 4
or
Melphalan 0.1 mg/kg/day PO, days 1 through 7 or days 1 through 10

MAC III

Use: Gestational trophoblastic neoplasm (high-risk). *Cycle*: 21 days

Regimen: Methotrexate 1 mg/kg IM, days 1, 3, 5, and 7
Leucovorin 0.1 mg/kg IM, days 2, 4, 6, and 8 (give 24 hours after each methotrexate dose)
Dactinomycin 0.012 mg/kg IV, days 1 through 5
Cyclophosphamide 3 mg/kg IV, days 1 through 5

MACC

Use: Lung cancer (non-small cell). *Cycle*: 21 days

Regimen: Methotrexate 30-40 mg/m² IV, day 1
Doxorubicin 30-40 mg/m² IV, day 1 (total cumulative dose 550 mg/m²)
Cyclophosphamide 400 mg/m² IV, day 1
Lomustine 30 mg/m²/day PO, day 1

MACOP-B

Use: Lymphoma (non-Hodgkin's). *Cycle*: Give only a single cycle

Regimen: Methotrexate 400 mg/m² IV weekly, weeks 2, 6, and 10
Leucovorin 15 mg/dose PO every 6 hours for 6 doses, begin 24 hours after each methotrexate dose
Doxorubicin 50 mg/m² IV weekly, weeks 1, 3, 5, 7, 9, and 11
Cyclophosphamide 350 mg/m² IV weekly, weeks 1, 3, 5, 7, 9, and 11
Vincristine 1.4 mg/m² (2 mg maximum dose) IV weekly, weeks 2, 4, 6, 8, 10, and 12
Bleomycin 10 units/m² IV weekly, weeks 4, 8, and 12
Prednisone 75 mg/day PO for 12 weeks, tapered over last 2 weeks

MAID

Use: Sarcoma (soft-tissue, bony). *Cycle*: 21 days

Regimen: Mesna 2500 mg/m²/day CI, days 1 through 4
Doxorubicin 15 mg/m²/day CI, days 1 through 4
Ifosfamide 2000 mg/m²/day CI, days 1 through 3
Dacarbazine 250 mg/m²/day CI, days 1 through 4

m-BACOD

Use: Lymphoma (non-Hodgkin's). *Cycle*: 21 days

Regimen: Bleomycin 4 units/m² IV, day 1
Doxorubicin 45 mg/m² IV, day 1
Cyclophosphamide 600 mg/m² IV, day 1
Vincristine 1 mg/m² (2 mg maximum dose) IV, day 1
Dexamethasone 6 mg/m²/day PO, days 1 through 5
Methotrexate 200 mg/m² IV, days 8 and 15
Leucovorin 10 mg/m²/dose PO every 6 hours for 8 doses, begin 24 hours after each methotrexate dose

m-BACOD (Reduced Dose)

Use: Lymphoma (non-Hodgkins) associated with HIV infection. *Cycle*: 21 days

Regimen: Methotrexate 200 mg/m² IV, day 15
Bleomycin 4 units/m² IV, day 1
Doxorubicin 25 mg/m² IV, day 1
Cyclophosphamide 300 mg/m² IV, day 1
Vincristine 1.4 mg/m² (2 mg maximum dose) IV, day 1
Dexamethasone 3 mg/m²/day PO, days 1 through 5

M-BACOD

Use: Lymphoma (non-Hodgkin's). *Cycle*: 21 days

Regimen: Bleomycin 4 units/m² IV, day 1
Doxorubicin 45 mg/m² IV, day 1
Cyclophosphamide 600 mg/m² IV, day 1
Vincristine 1 mg/m² (2 mg maximum dose) IV, day 1
Dexamethasone 6 mg/m²/day PO, days 1 through 5
Methotrexate 3000 mg/m² IV, day 15
Leucovorin 10 mg/m²/dose PO every 6 hours for 8 doses, begin 24 hours after each methotrexate dose

MBC

Use: Head and neck cancer. *Cycle*: 21 days

Regimen: Methotrexate 40 mg/m² IV, days 1 and 14
Bleomycin 10 units/m² IM or IV, days 1, 7, and 14
Cisplatin 50 mg/m² IV, day 4

MC

Use: Acute myelocytic leukemia (AML; adult induction). *Cycle*: Give a single cycle

Regimen: Mitoxantrone 12 mg/m² IV, days 1 through 3
Cytarabine 100-200 mg/m²/day CI or IV, days 1 through 7

MF

Use: Breast cancer. *Cycle*: 28 days

Regimen: Methotrexate 100 mg/m² IV, days 1 and 8
Fluorouracil 600 mg/m² IV, days 1 and 8, given 1 hour after methotrexate
Leucovorin 10 mg/m²/dose IV or PO every 6 hours for 6 doses, starting 24 hours after methotrexate

MICE (ICE)

Use: Sarcoma (adults, osteosarcoma - pediatrics), lung cancer. *Cycle*: 21 to 28 days

Regimen: Ifosfamide 1250-1500 mg/m² IV, days 1 through 3
Carboplatin 300-635 mg/m² IV, day 1 or 3
Etoposide 80-100 mg/m² IV, days 1 through 3
with
Mesna 1250 mg/m² IV, days 1 through 3
or
Mesna 20% of ifosfamide dose IV before, 4 hours after, and 8 hours after each ifosfamide infusion.

MINE

Use: Lymphoma (non-Hodgkin's). *Cycle*: 21 days

Regimen: Mesna 1330 mg/m² IV, days 1 through 3, given with Ifosfamide
Mesna 500 mg/dose PO, 4 hours after ifosfamide, days 1 through 3
Ifosfamide 1330 mg/m² IV, days 1 through 3
Mitoxantrone 8 mg/m² IV, day 1
Etoposide 65 mg/m² IV, days 1 through 3

MINE-ESHAP

Use: Lymphoma (non-Hodgkin's). *Cycle*: 21 days

Regimen: Give MINE for 6 cycles, then give ESHAP for 3 to 6 cycles

mini-BEAM

Use: Lymphoma (Hodgkin's). *Cycle*: 4 to 6 weeks

Regimen: Carmustine 60 mg/m² IV, day 1
Etoposide 75 mg/m² IV, days 2 through 5
Cytarabine 100 mg/m²/dose IV every 12 hours for 8 doses, days 2 through 5
Melphalan 30 mg/m² IV, day 6

MOBP

Use: Cervical cancer. *Cycle*: 6 weeks

Regimen:
Bleomycin 30 units/day CI, days 1 through 4
Vincristine 0.5 mg/m^2 IV, days 1 and 4
Cisplatin 50 mg/m^2 IV, days 1 and 22
Mitomycin 10 mg/m^2 IV, day 2

MOP

Use: Brain tumors (pediatrics). *Cycle*: 28 days.

Regimen:
Mechlorethamine 6 mg/m^2 IV, days 1 and 8
Vincristine 1.5 mg/m^2 (2 mg maximum dose) IV, days 1 and 8
Procarbazine 100 mg/m^2/day PO, days 1 through 14

MOPP

Use: Lymphoma (Hodgkin's). *Cycle*: 28 days

Regimen:
Mechlorethamine 6 mg/m^2 IV, days 1 and 8
Vincristine 1.4 mg/m^2 (2 mg maximum dose) IV, days 1 and 8
Procarbazine 100 mg/m^2/day PO, days 1 through 14
Prednisone 40 mg/m^2/day PO, cycles 1 and 4,* days 1 through 14
*Note: Some clinicians give prednisone with every cycle of MOPP. The original clinical trials gave prednisone only with the first and fourth cycles.

Use: Brain cancer (medulloblastoma). *Cycle*: 28 days

Regimen:
Mechlorethamine 3 mg/m^2 IV, days 1 and 8
Vincristine 1.4 mg/m^2 (2 mg maximum dose) IV, days 1 and 8
Prednisone 40 mg/m^2/day PO, days 1 through 10
Procarbazine 50 mg PO, day 1
Procarbazine 100 mg PO, day 2
Procarbazine 100 mg/m^2/day PO, days 3 through 10

MOPP/ABV

Use: Lymphoma (Hodgkin's). *Cycle*: 28 days

Regimen:
Mechlorethamine 6 mg/m^2 IV, day 1
Vincristine 1.4 mg/m^2 (2 mg maximum dose) IV, day 1
Procarbazine 100 mg/m^2/day PO, days 1 through 7
Prednisone 40 mg/m^2/day PO, days 1 through 14
Doxorubicin 35 mg/m^2 IV, day 8
Bleomycin 10 units/m^2 IV, day 8
Vinblastine 6 mg/m^2 IV, day 8

MOPP/ABVD

Use: Lymphoma (Hodgkin's). *Cycle*: 28 days

Regimen: Alternate MOPP and ABVD regimens every month

MP

Use: Multiple myeloma. *Cycle*: 21 to 28 days

Regimen:
Melphalan 8 mg/m^2/day PO, days 1 through 4
Prednisone 60 mg/m^2/day PO, days 1 through 4

Use: Prostate cancer. *Cycle*: 21 days

Regimen:
Mitoxantrone 12 mg/m^2 IV, day 1
Prednisone 5 mg/dose PO twice daily

MTX/6-MP

Use: Acute lymphocytic leukemia (ALL; continuation - pediatrics). *Cycle*: Ongoing, weeks 25 through 130

Regimen:
Methotrexate 20 mg/m^2 IM weekly
Mercaptopurine 50 mg/m^2/day PO
used in conjunction with
intrathecal therapy once every 12 weeks

MTX/6-MP/VP

Use: Acute lymphocytic leukemia (ALL; continuation - pediatrics). *Cycle*: Ongoing, 2 to 3 years

Regimen:
Methotrexate 20 mg/m^2/dose PO weekly
Mercaptopurine 75 mg/m^2/day PO
Vincristine 1.5 mg/m^2 IV once monthly
Prednisone 40 mg/m^2/day PO for 5 days each month

MTX-CDDPAdr

Use: Osteosarcoma (pediatrics). *Cycle*: 28 days

Regimen:
Methotrexate 12,000 mg/m^2 IV, days 1 and 8
Leucovorin 20 mg/m^2/dose IV every 3 hours for 8 doses then give PO every 6 hours for 8 doses (begin 16 hours after end of methotrexate infusion)
Cisplatin 75 mg/m^2 IV, day 15 of cycles 1 through 7
Cisplatin 120 mg/m^2 IV, day 15 of cycles 8 through 10
Doxorubicin 25 mg/m^2 IV, days 15 through 17 of cycles 1 through 7

MV

Use: Breast cancer. *Cycle*: 6 to 8 weeks

Regimen:
Mitomycin 20 mg/m^2 IV, day 1
Vinblastine 0.15 mg/kg IV, days 1 and 21

Use: Acute myelocytic leukemia (AML; induction). *Cycle*: Give 1 cycle. Second cycle may be considered if complete response not achieved.

Regimen:
Mitoxantrone 10 mg/m^2 IV, days 1 through 5
Etoposide 100 mg/m^2 IV, days 1 through 5

M-VAC

Use: Bladder cancer. *Cycle*: 28 days

Regimen:
Methotrexate 30 mg/m^2 IV, days 1, 15, and 22
Vinblastine 3 mg/m^2 IV, days 2, 15, and 22
Doxorubicin 30 mg/m^2 IV, day 2
Cisplatin 70 mg/m^2 IV, day 2

MVP

Use: Lung cancer (non-small cell). *Cycle*: 6 weeks

Regimen:
Mitomycin 8 mg/m^2 IV, day 1
Vinblastine 6 mg/m^2 IV, days 1 and 22
Cisplatin 50 mg/m^2 IV, days 1 and 22

MVPP

Use: Lymphoma (Hodgkin's). *Cycle*: 4 to 6 weeks

Regimen:
Mechlorethamine 6 mg/m^2 IV, days 1 and 8
Vinblastine 4 mg/m^2 IV, days 1 and 8
Procarbazine 100 mg/m^2/day PO, days 1 through 14
Prednisone 40 mg/m^2/day PO, cycles 1 and 4,* days 1 through 14
*Note: Some clinicians give prednisone with every cycle of MVPP. The original clinical trials gave prednisone only with the first and fourth cycles.

NFL

Use: Breast cancer. *Cycle*: 21 days

Regimen:
Mitoxantrone 12 mg/m^2 IV, day 1
Fluorouracil 350 mg/m^2 IV, days 1 through 3 after leucovorin
Leucovorin 300 mg IV, days 1 through 3
or
Mitoxantrone 10 mg/m^2 IV, day 1
Fluorouracil 1000 mg/m^2 CI, days 1 through 3 after leucovorin
Leucovorin 100 mg/m^2 IV, days 1 through 3

NOVP

Use: Lymphoma (Hodgkin's). *Cycle*: 21 days

Regimen:
Mitoxantrone 10 mg/m^2 IV, day 1
Vinblastine 6 mg/m^2 IV, day 1
Prednisone 100 mg/day PO, days 1 through 5
Vincristine 1.4 mg/m^2 (2 mg maximum dose) IV, day 8

OPA

Use: Lymphoma (Hodgkin's - pediatrics). *Cycle*: 15 days. Up to 2 cycles used. Time between cycles not specified.

Regimen:
Vincristine 1.5 mg/m^2 (2 mg maximum dose) IV, days 1, 8, and 15
Prednisone 60 mg/m^2/day PO in 3 divided doses, days 1 through 15
Doxorubicin 40 mg/m^2 IV, days 1 and 15

OPPA

Use: Lymphoma (Hodgkin's - pediatrics). *Cycle*: 15 days. Up to 2 cycles used. Time between cycles not specified.

Regimen: **Add to OPA:** Procarbazine 100 mg/m^2/day PO in 2-3 divided doses, days 1 through 15

PAC

Use: Ovarian, endometrial cancer. *Cycle*: 28 days

Regimen:
Cisplatin 50 mg/m^2 IV, day 1
Doxorubicin 50 mg/m^2 IV, day 1
Cyclophosphamide 500 mg/m^2 IV, day 1

PAC-I (Indiana Protocol)

Use: Ovarian cancer. *Cycle*: 21 days

Regimen:
Cisplatin 50 mg/m^2 IV, day 1 (total cumulative dose 300 mg/m^2)
Doxorubicin 50 mg/m^2 IV, day 1
Cyclophosphamide 750 mg/m^2 IV, day 1

PA-CI

Use: Hepatoblastoma (pediatrics). *Cycle*: 21 days

Regimen:
Cisplatin 90 mg/m^2 IV, day 1
Doxorubicin 20 mg/m^2 CI, days 2 through 5

Paclitaxel-Carboplatin-Etoposide

Use: Adenocarcinoma (unknown primary), lung cancer (small cell). *Cycle*: 21 days

Regimen: Paclitaxel 200 mg/m^2/day IV, day 1
Carboplatin IV dose by Calvert equation to AUC 6, day 1 (give after paclitaxel)
Etoposide 50 mg/day PO alternated with 100 mg/day PO, days 1 through 10

Paclitaxel-Vinorelbine

Use: Breast cancer. *Cycle*: 28 days

Regimen: Paclitaxel 135 mg/m^2 IV, day 1 (after vinorelbine infusion)
Vinorelbine 30 mg/m^2 IV, days 1 and 8

PC

Use: Lung cancer (non-small cell). *Cycle*: 21 days

Regimen: Paclitaxel 135 mg/m^2/day CI, day 1
Carboplatin IV dose by Calvert equation to AUC 7.5, day 2 (after paclitaxel)

Use: Lung cancer (non-small cell). *Cycle*: 21 days

Regimen: Paclitaxel 175 mg/m^2 IV, day 1
Cisplatin 80 mg/m^2 IV, day 1 after paclitaxel

Use: Bladder cancer. *Cycle*: 21 days

Regimen: Paclitaxel 200 or 225 mg/m^2/day IV, day 1
Carboplatin IV dose by Calvert equation to AUC 5-6, day 1 (after paclitaxel)

PCV

Use: Brain tumor. *Cycle*: 6 to 8 weeks

Regimen: Lomustine 110 mg/m^2/day PO, day 1
Procarbazine 60 mg/m^2/day PO, days 8 through 21
Vincristine 1.4 mg/m^2 (2 mg maximum dose) IV, days 8 and 29

PE

Use: Prostate cancer. *Cycle*: 21 days

Regimen: Paclitaxel 30 mg/m^2/day CI, days 1 through 4
Estramustine 600 mg/m^2/day PO given in 2-3 divided doses (start 24 hours before first paclitaxel infusion)

PFL

Use: Head and neck, gastric cancer. *Cycle*: 28 days

Regimen: Cisplatin 25 mg/m^2/day CI, days 1 through 5
Fluorouracil 800 mg/m^2/day CI, days 2 through 6
Leucovorin 500 mg/m^2/day CI, days 1 through 6

Use: Head and neck, gastric cancer. *Cycle*: 21 days

Regimen: Cisplatin 100 mg/m^2 IV, day 1
Fluorouracil 600-1000 mg/m^2/day CI, days 1 through 5
Leucovorin 50 mg/m^2/dose PO every 4-6 hours, days 1 through 6

POC

Use: Brain tumors (pediatrics). *Cycle*: 6 weeks

Regimen: Prednisone 40 mg/m^2/day PO, days 1 through 14
Vincristine 1.5 mg/m^2 (2 mg maximum dose), days 1, 8, and 15
Lomustine 100 mg/m^2/day PO, day 1

ProMACE

Use: Lymphoma (non-Hodgkin's). *Cycle*: 28 days

Regimen: Prednisone 60 mg/m^2/day PO, days 1 through 14
Methotrexate 750 mg/m^2 IV, day 14
Leucovorin 50 mg/m^2/dose IV every 6 hours for 5 doses, day 15 (start 24 hours after methotrexate)
Doxorubicin 25 mg/m^2 IV, days 1 and 8
Cyclophosphamide 650 mg/m^2 IV, days 1 and 8
Etoposide 120 mg/m^2 IV, days 1 and 8

ProMACE/cytaBOM

Use: Lymphoma (non-Hodgkin's). *Cycle*: 21 days

Regimen: Prednisone 60 mg/m^2/day PO, days 1 through 14
Doxorubicin 25 mg/m^2 IV, day 1
Cyclophosphamide 650 mg/m^2 IV, day 1
Etoposide 120 mg/m^2 IV, day 1
Cytarabine 300 mg/m^2 IV, day 8
Bleomycin 5 units/m^2 IV, day 8
Vincristine 1.4 mg/m^2 (2 mg maximum dose) IV, day 8
Methotrexate 120 mg/m^2 IV, day 8
Leucovorin 25 mg/m^2/dose PO every 6 hours for 4 doses (start 24 hours after methotrexate dose)
Cotrimoxazole DS 2 tablets PO twice daily, days 1 through 28

ProMACE/MOPP

Use: Lymphoma (non-Hodgkin's). *Cycle*: 28 days

Regimen: Prednisone 60 mg/m^2/day PO, days 1 through 14
Doxorubicin 25 mg/m^2 IV, day 1
Cyclophosphamide 650 mg/m^2 IV, day 1
Etoposide 120 mg/m^2 IV, day 1
Mechlorethamine 6 mg/m^2 IV, day 8
Vincristine 1.4 mg/m^2 (2 mg maximum dose) IV, day 8
Procarbazine 100 mg/m^2/day PO, days 8 through 14
Methotrexate 500 mg/m^2 IV, day 15
Leucovorin 50 mg/m^2/dose PO every 6 hours for 4 doses (start 24 hours after methotrexate dose)

Pt/VM

Use: Neuroblastoma (pediatrics). *Cycle*: 21 to 28 days

Regimen: Cisplatin 90 mg/m^2 IV, day 1
Teniposide 100 mg/m^2 IV, day 3

PVA

Use: Acute lymphocytic leukemia (ALL; induction - pediatrics). *Cycle*: 28 days. Give a single cycle.

Regimen: Prednisone 40 mg/m^2/day (60 mg maximum dose) PO, given in 3 divided doses, days 1 through 28
Vincristine 1.5 mg/m^2 (2 mg maximum dose) IV, days 1, 8, 15, and 22
with
Asparaginase 6000 units/m^2/dose IM, 3 times weekly for 2 weeks (ie, days 2, 5, 7, 9, 12, and 14)
or
Asparaginase 6000 units/m^2/dose IM, days 2, 5, 8, 12, 15, and 19
used in conjunction with
intrathecal therapy, day 1

PVB

Use: Testicular cancer, adenocarcinoma. *Cycle*: 21 days

Regimen: Cisplatin 20 mg/m^2 IV, days 1 through 5
Vinblastine 0.15 mg/kg IV, days 1 and 2
Bleomycin 30 units IV, days 2, 9, and 16

PVDA

Use: Acute lymphocytic leukemia (ALL; induction - pediatrics). *Cycle*: 28 days. Give a single cycle.

Regimen: Prednisone 40 mg/m^2/day PO, days 1 through 28
Vincristine 1.5 mg/m^2 (2 mg maximum dose) IV, days 1, 8, 15, and 22
Daunorubicin 25 mg/m^2 IV, days 1, 8, 15, and 22
Asparaginase 10,000 units/m^2 IM, days 2, 4, 6, 9, 11, 13, 16, 18, and 20 (ie, 3 times weekly for 12 doses)
used in conjunction with
intrathecal therapy

Sequential AC/Paclitaxel - see AC/Paclitaxel, Sequential

Sequential Dox ➡ CMF - see Dox ➡ CMF, Sequential

SMF

Use: Pancreatic cancer. *Cycle*: 8 weeks

Regimen: Streptozocin 1000 mg/m^2 IV, days 1, 8, 29, and 36
Mitomycin 10 mg/m^2 IV, day 1
Fluorouracil 600 mg/m^2 IV, days 1, 8, 29, and 36

Stanford V

Use: Lymphoma (Hodgkin's). *Cycle*: 28 days

Regimen: Mechlorethamine 6 mg/m^2 IV, day 1
Doxorubicin 25 mg/m^2 IV, days 1 and 15
Vinblastine 6 mg/m^2 IV, days 1 and 15
Vincristine 1.4 mg/m^2 (2 mg maximum dose) IV, days 8 and 22
Bleomycin 5 units/m^2 IV, days 8 and 22
Etoposide 60 mg/m^2 IV, days 15 and 16
Prednisone 40 mg/m^2/day PO, every other day continually for 10 weeks, then taper off by 10 mg every other day for next 14 days

TAD

Use: Acute myelocytic leukemia (AML; adult induction). *Cycle*: 21 days. Give 1 cycle only.

Regimen: Daunorubicin 60 mg/m^2 IV, days 3 through 5
Cytarabine 100 mg/m^2/day CI, days 1 and 2
Cytarabine 100 mg/m^2 IV every 12 hours, days 3 through 8
Thioguanine 100 mg/m^2/dose PO every 12 hours, days 3 through 9

Tamoxifen-Epirubicin

Use: Breast cancer. *Cycle*: 28 days for epirubicin for 6 cycles. Tamoxifen therapy continuous for 4 years.

Regimen: Tamoxifen 20 mg PO daily, continuously
Epirubicin 50 mg/m^2 IV, on days 1 and 8

TCF

Use: Esophageal cancer. *Cycle*: 28 days

Regimen: Paclitaxel 175 mg/m^2 IV, day 1
Cisplatin 20 mg/m^2 IV, days 1 through 5 (give after paclitaxel)
Fluorouracil 750 mg/m^2/day, CI days 1 through 5

TIP

Use: Head and neck, esophageal cancer. *Cycle*: 21 to 28 days

Regimen: Paclitaxel 175 mg/m^2 IV, day 1
Ifosfamide 1000 mg/m^2 IV, days 1 through 3
Mesna 400 mg/m^2 IV pre-ifosfamide, days 1 through 3
Mesna 200 mg/m^2 IV given 4 hours after ifosfamide, days 1 through 3
Cisplatin 60 mg/m^2 IV, day 1 (give after paclitaxel infusion)

TIT

Use: Acute lymphocytic leukemia (CNS prophylaxis - pediatrics).

Regimen: Doses are based on patient's age. Give during weeks 1, 2, 3, 7, 13, 19, and 25 of intensification and every 12 weeks during maintenance.
Age 1-2 years:
- Methotrexate 8 mg intrathecal
- Cytarabine 16 mg intrathecal
- Hydrocortisone 8 mg intrathecal

Age 2-3 years:
- Methotrexate 10 mg intrathecal
- Cytarabine 20 mg intrathecal
- Hydrocortisone 10 mg intrathecal

Age 3-9 years:
- Methotrexate 12 mg intrathecal
- Cytarabine 24 mg intrathecal
- Hydrocortisone 12 mg intrathecal

Age 9 years and older:
- Methotrexate 15 mg intrathecal
- Cytarabine 30 mg intrathecal
- Hydrocortisone 15 mg intrathecal

Topo/CTX

Use: Sarcomas (bony and soft-tissue - pediatrics). *Cycle*: 21 days

Regimen: Cyclophosphamide 250 mg/m^2 IV, days 1 through 5
Topotecan 0.75 mg/m^2 IV, days 1 through 5 after cyclophosphamide
Mesna 150 mg/m^2/dose IV before and 3 hours after each cyclophosphamide dose, days 1 through 5

Trastuzumab-Paclitaxel

Use: Breast cancer. *Cycle*: 21 days for at least 6 cycles

Regimen: Paclitaxel 175 mg/m^2/dose IV, day 1
Trastuzumab 4 mg/kg IV, day 1 first cycle only (loading dose)
Trastuzumab 2 mg/kg IV weekly, days 1, 8, and 15, except for day 1 of first cycle.

VAB-6

Use: Testicular cancer. *Cycle*: 21 to 28 days

Regimen: Cyclophosphamide 600 mg/m^2 IV, day 1
Dactinomycin 1 mg/m^2 IV, day 1
Vinblastine 4 mg/m^2 IV, day 1
Cisplatin 120 mg/m^2 IV, day 4
Bleomycin 30 units IV push, day 1 (omit from cycle 3)
then
Bleomycin 20 units/m^2/day CI, days 1 through 3 (omit from cycle 3)

VAC Pediatric

Use: Sarcoma (pediatrics). *Cycle*: 21 days

Regimen: Vincristine 2 mg/m^2 IV (2 mg maximum dose), day 1
Dactinomycin 1 mg/m^2 IV, day 1
Cyclophosphamide 600 mg/m^2 IV, day 1

VAC Pulse

Use: Sarcomas.

Regimen: Vincristine 2 mg/m^2 (2 mg maximum dose) IV weekly, for 12 weeks
Dactinomycin 0.015 mg/kg/day (0.5 mg/day maximum dose) CI, days 1 through 5, every 3 months for 5 courses
Cyclophosphamide 10 mg/kg/day IV or PO, days 1 through 7, every 6 weeks

VAC Standard

Use: Sarcomas.

Regimen: Vincristine 2 mg/m^2 (2 mg maximum dose) IV weekly, for 12 weeks
Dactinomycin 0.015 mg/kg/day (0.5 mg/day maximum dose) CI, days 1 through 5, every 3 months for 5 courses
Cyclophosphamide 2.5 mg/kg/day PO, daily for 2 years

VACAdr

Use: Sarcoma (bony and soft-tissue - pediatrics).

Regimen: Vincristine 1.5 mg/m^2 (2 mg maximum dose) IV, days 1, 8, 15, 22, 29, and 36
Cyclophosphamide 500 mg/m^2 IV, days 1, 8, 15, 22, 29, and 36
Doxorubicin 60 mg/m^2 IV, day 36
followed by 6 week rest period, then
Dactinomycin 0.015 mg/kg/day IV, days 1 through 5
Vincristine 1.5 mg/m^2 (2 mg maximum dose) IV, days 14, 21, 28, 35, and 42
Cyclophosphamide 500 mg/m^2 IV, days 14, 21, 28, 35, and 42
Doxorubicin 60 mg/m^2 IV, day 42 (give on day of final vincristine and cyclophosphamide doses)

VAD

Use: Multiple myeloma. *Cycle*: 3 to 4 weeks

Regimen: Vincristine 0.4 mg/day (dose is not in mg/m^2) CI, days 1 through 4
Doxorubicin 9 mg/m^2/day CI, days 1 through 4
Dexamethasone 40 mg/day PO, days 1 through 4, days 9 through 12, and days 17 through 20
*Note: After completing the first 2 cycles of VAD, some clinicians give dexamethasone only on days 1 through 4 of each cycle to reduce the risk of infection. Antibiotic prophylaxis with cotrimoxazole also has been used for this purpose.

Use: Acute lymphocytic leukemia. *Cycle*: 24 to 28 days

Regimen: Vincristine 0.4 mg/day (dose is not in mg/m^2) CI, days 1 through 4
Doxorubicin 9-12 mg/m^2/day CI, days 1 through 4
Dexamethasone 40 mg/day PO, days 1 through 4, days 9 through 12, and days 17 through 20

Use: Wilm's tumor (pediatrics). *Cycle*: 1 year. Give 1 cycle only.

Regimen 1: Vincristine 1.5 mg/m^2 (2 mg maximum dose) IV, weekly for first 10-11 weeks then every 3 weeks for 15 more weeks
with
Dactinomycin 1.5 mg/m^2 IV every 6 weeks, starting week 1 for 9 doses
Doxorubicin 40 mg/m^2 IV every 6 weeks for 26 weeks, starting week 4, for 9 doses

Regimen 2: Vincristine 1.5 mg/m^2 (2 mg maximum dose) IV, given every 6 weeks for 6 to 15 months
Dactinomycin 0.015 mg/kg/day IV for 5 doses, given every 6 weeks for 6 to 15 months
or
Dactinomycin 0.06 mg/kg IV, given every 6 weeks for 6 to 15 months
may or may not give with
Doxorubicin 60 mg/m^2 IV, given every 6 weeks for 6 to 15 months

VATH

Use: Breast cancer. *Cycle*: 21 days

Regimen: Vinblastine 4.5 mg/m^2 IV, day 1
Doxorubicin 45 mg/m^2 IV, day 1
Thiotepa 12 mg/m^2 IV, day 1
Fluoxymesterone 30 mg/day PO in 3 divided doses, throughout entire course

VBAP

Use: Multiple myeloma. *Cycle*: 21 days

Regimen:
Vincristine 1 mg/m² (2 mg maximum dose) IV, day 1
Carmustine 30 mg/m² IV, day 1
Doxorubicin 30 mg/m² IV, day 1
Prednisone 60 mg/m²/day PO, days 1 through 4

VBCMP

Use: Multiple myeloma. *Cycle*: 35 days

Regimen:
Vincristine 1.2 mg/m² (2 mg maximum dose) IV, day 1
Carmustine 20 mg/m² IV, day 1
Melphalan 8 mg/m²/day PO, days 1 through 4
Cyclophosphamide 400 mg/m² IV, day 1
Prednisone 40 mg/m²/day PO, days 1 through 7 of all cycles
with
Prednisone 20 mg/m²/day PO, days 8 through 14 of first 3 cycles only

VC

Use: Lung cancer (non-small cell).

Regimen:
Vinorelbine 30 mg/m² IV, weekly
Cisplatin 120 mg/m² IV, days 1 and 29, then give 1 dose every 6 weeks

VCAP

Use: Multiple myeloma. *Cycle*: 21 days

Regimen:
Vincristine 1 mg/m² (2 mg maximum dose) IV, day 1
Cyclophosphamide 125 mg/m²/day PO, days 1 through 4
Doxorubicin 30 mg/m² IV, day 1
Prednisone 60 mg/m²/day PO, days 1 through 4

VCMP - see VMCP

VD

Use: Breast cancer. *Cycle*: 21 days

Regimen:
Vinorelbine 25 mg/m² IV, days 1 and 8
Doxorubicin 50 mg/m² IV, day 1

VeIP

Use: Genitourinary cancer, testicular cancer. *Cycle*: 21 days

Regimen:
Vinblastine 0.11 mg/kg IV, days 1 and 2
Cisplatin 20 mg/m² IV, days 1 through 5
Ifosfamide 1200 mg/m² IV, days 1 through 5
Mesna 1200 mg/m²/day CI, days 1 through 5

VIC - see CVI

Vinorelbine-Cisplatin

Use: Lung cancer (non-small cell). *Cycle*: 42 days

Regimen:
Vinorelbine 30 mg/m² IV, weekly
Cisplatin 120 mg/m² IV, days 1 and 29 for first cycle; then day 1 of subsequent cycles

Vinorelbine-Doxorubicin

Use: Breast cancer. *Cycle*: 21 days

Regimen:
Vinorelbine 25 mg/m² IV, days 1 and 8
Doxorubicin 50 mg/m² IV, day 1

Vinorelbine-Gemcitabine

Use: Lung cancer (non-small cell). *Cycle*: 28 days

Regimen:
Vinorelbine 20 mg/m² IV, days 1, 8, and 15
Gemcitabine 800 mg/m² IV, days 1, 8, and 15

VIP

Use: Genitourinary cancer, testicular cancer. *Cycle*: 21 days

Regimen:
Etoposide 75 mg/m² IV, days 1 through 5
Cisplatin 20 mg/m² IV, days 1 through 5
Ifosfamide 1200 mg/m² IV, days 1 through 5
Mesna 1200 mg/m²/day CI, days 1 through 5

Use: Lung cancer (small cell). *Cycle*: 21 to 28 days

Regimen:
Ifosfamide 1200 mg/m² IV, days 1 through 4
Cisplatin 20 mg/m² IV, days 1 through 4
Mesna 120-300 mg/m² IV, day 1 (give before ifosfamide started)
Mesna 1200 mg/m²/day CI, days 1 through 4 (after mesna bolus given)
with
Etoposide 37.5 mg/m²/day PO, days 1 through 14
or
Etoposide 75 mg/m²/day IV, days 1 through 4

Use: Lung cancer (non-small cell). *Cycle*: 28 days

Regimen:
Ifosfamide 1000-1200 mg/m² IV, days 1 through 3
Cisplatin 100 mg/m² IV, days 1 and 8
Etoposide 60-75 mg/m² IV, days 1 through 3
with
Mesna 300 mg/m²/dose IV every 4 hours, days 1 through 4
or
Mesna 20% of ifosfamide dose IV before, 4 and 8 hours after ifosfamide

VM

Use: Breast cancer. *Cycle*: 6 to 8 weeks

Regimen:
Mitomycin 10 mg/m² IV, days 1 and 28 for 2 cycles, then day 1 only
Vinblastine 5 mg/m² IV, days 1, 14, 28, and 42 for 2 cycles, then days 1 and 21 only

VMCP

Use: Multiple myeloma. *Cycle*: 21 days

Regimen:
Vincristine 1 mg/m² (2 mg maximum dose) IV, day 1
Melphalan 6 mg/m²/day PO, days 1 through 4
Cyclophosphamide 125 mg/m²/day PO, days 1 through 4
Prednisone 60 mg/m²/day PO, days 1 through 4

VP

Use: Lung cancer (small cell). *Cycle*: 21 days

Regimen:
Etoposide 100 mg/m²/day IV, days 1 through 4
Cisplatin 20 mg/m² IV, days 1 through 4

V-TAD

Use: Acute myelocytic leukemia (AML; induction). *Cycle*: 7 days. Give 1 cycle. Up to 3 cycles have been given, but time between cycles is not specified.

Regimen:
Etoposide 50 mg/m² IV, days 1 through 3
Thioguanine 75 mg/m²/dose PO every 12 hours, days 1 through 5
Daunorubicin 20 mg/m² IV, days 1 and 2
Cytarabine 75 mg/m²/day CI, days 1 through 5

➤*NCI INVESTIGATIONAL AGENTS:* For further information, contact Pharmaceutical Management Branch, National Cancer Institute, Executive Plaza North, Room 804, 6130 Executive Blvd., Rockville, MD 20892, (301) 496-5725.

ALKYLATING AGENTS

Nitrogen Mustards

CHLORAMBUCIL

Rx	**Leukeran** (GlaxoSmithKline)	**Tablets:** 2 mg	(GX EG3 L). Brown. Film coated. In 50s.

CHLORAMBUCIL — ORAL

WARNING

Chlorambucil can severely suppress bone marrow function. Chlorambucil is a carcinogen in humans. Chlorambucil is probably mutagenic and teratogenic in humans. Chlorambucil produces human infertility.

Indications

➤*Leukemia/Lymphomas:* For the treatment of chronic lymphatic (lymphocytic) leukemia, malignant lymphomas including lymphosarcoma, giant follicular lymphoma, and Hodgkin disease. It is not curative in any of these disorders but may produce clinically useful palliation.

➤*Unlabeled uses:* Chlorambucil has shown activity in other malignancies such as ovarian and testicular carcinoma, non-Hodgkin lymphoma, and Waldenström macroglobulinemia. Treatment of polycythemia vera.

Administration and Dosage

➤*Approved by the FDA:* March 18, 1957.

➤*Initial and short courses of therapy:* The usual oral dosage is 0.1 to 0.2 mg/kg body weight daily for 3 to 6 weeks as required. This usually amounts to 4 to 10 mg/day for the average patient. The entire daily dose may be given at one time. These dosages are for initiation of therapy or for short courses of treatment. The dosage must be carefully adjusted according to the response of the patient and must be reduced as soon as there is an abrupt fall in the white blood cell count. Patients with Hodgkin disease usually require 0.2 mg/kg/day, whereas patients with other lymphomas or chronic lymphocytic leukemia usually require only 0.1 mg/kg/day. When lymphocytic infiltration of the bone marrow is present, or when the bone marrow is hypoplastic, the daily dose should not exceed 0.1 mg/kg (about 6 mg for the average patient).

Alternate schedules for the treatment of chronic lymphocytic leukemia employing intermittent, biweekly, or once-monthly pulse doses of chlorambucil

CHLORAMBUCIL — ORAL

have been reported. Intermittent schedules of chlorambucil begin with an initial single dose of 0.4 mg/kg. Doses are generally increased by 0.1 mg/kg until control of lymphocytosis or toxicity is observed. Subsequent doses are modified to produce mild hematologic toxicity. It is felt that the response rate of chronic lymphocytic leukemia to the biweekly or once-monthly schedule of chlorambucil administration is similar or better to that previously reported with daily administration and that hematologic toxicity was less than or equal to that encountered in studies using daily chlorambucil.

Radiation and cytotoxic drugs render the bone marrow more vulnerable to damage, and chlorambucil should be used with particular caution within 4 weeks of a full course of radiation therapy or chemotherapy. However, small doses of palliative radiation over isolated foci remote from the bone marrow will not usually depress the neutrophil and platelet count. In these cases chlorambucil may be given in the customary dosage.

➤*Maintenance:* It is presently felt that short courses of treatment are safer than continuous maintenance therapy, although both methods have been effective. It must be recognized that continuous therapy may give the appearance of "maintenance" in patients who are actually in remission and have no immediate need for further drug. If maintenance dosage is used, it should not exceed 0.1 mg/kg/day and may well be as low as 0.03 mg/kg/day. A typical maintenance dose is 2 to 4 mg/day, or less, depending on the status of the blood counts. It may, therefore, be desirable to withdraw the drug after maximal control has been achieved, since intermittent therapy reinstituted at time of relapse may be as effective as continuous treatment.

➤*Storage / Stability:* Store in a refrigerator at 2° to 8°C (36° to 46°F).

Actions

➤*Pharmacokinetics:*

Absorption – Chlorambucil is rapidly and completely absorbed from the GI tract. After single oral doses of 0.6 to 1.2 mg/kg, peak plasma chlorambucil levels C_{max} are reached within 1 hour and the terminal half-life $t_{1/2}$ of the parent drug is estimated at 1.5 hours.

Distribution – Chlorambucil and its metabolites are extensively bound to plasma and tissue proteins. In vitro, chlorambucil is 99% bound to plasma proteins, specifically albumin. Cerebrospinal fluid levels of chlorambucil have not been determined. Evidence of human teratogenicity suggests that the drug crosses the placenta.

Metabolism – Chlorambucil is extensively metabolized in the liver primarily to phenylacetic acid mustard which has antineoplastic activity. Chlorambucil and its major metabolite spontaneously degrade in vivo forming monohydroxy and dihydroxy derivatives.

Excretion – After a single dose of radiolabeled chlorambucil (^{14}C), approximately 15% to 60% of the radioactivity appears in the urine after 24 hours. Again, less than 1% of the urinary radioactivity is in the form of chlorambucil or phenylacetic acid mustard. In summary, the pharmacokinetic data suggest that oral chlorambucil undergoes rapid GI absorption and plasma clearance and that it is almost completely metabolized, having extremely low urinary excretion.

Contraindications

Resistance to the agent; hypersensitivity to chlorambucil. There may be cross-hypersensitivity (skin rash) between chlorambucil and other alkylating agents.

Warnings

➤*Hypersensitivity reactions:* See Adverse Reactions for more information.

➤*Carcinogenesis:* Because of its carcinogenic properties, do not give chlorambucil to patients with conditions other than chronic lymphatic leukemia or malignant lymphomas. Convulsions, infertility, leukemia, and secondary malignancies have been observed when chlorambucil was employed in the therapy of malignant and nonmalignant diseases.

There are many reports of acute leukemia arising in patients with both malignant and nonmalignant diseases following chlorambucil treatment. In many instances, these patients also received other chemotherapeutic agents or some form of radiation therapy. The quantitation of the risk of chlorambucil-induction of leukemia or carcinoma in humans is not possible. Evaluation of published reports of leukemia developing in patients who have received chlorambucil (and other alkylating agents) suggests that the risk of leukemogenesis increases with both chronicity of treatment and large cumulative doses. However, it has proved impossible to define a cumulative dose below which there is no risk of the induction of secondary malignancy. The potential benefits from chlorambucil therapy must be weighed on an individual basis against the possible risk of the induction of a secondary malignancy.

➤*Mutagenesis:* Chlorambucil has been shown to cause chromatid or chromosome damage in humans. Both reversible and permanent sterility have been observed in both sexes receiving chlorambucil.

➤*Fertility impairment:* A high incidence of sterility has been documented when chlorambucil is administered to prepubertal and pubertal males. Prolonged or permanent azoospermia has also been observed in adult males. While most reports of gonadal dysfunction secondary to chlorambucil have related to males, the induction of amenorrhea in females with alkylating agents is well documented and chlorambucil is capable of producing amenorrhea. Autopsy studies of the ovaries from women with malignant lymphoma treated with combination chemotherapy including chlorambucil have shown varying degrees of fibrosis, vasculitis, and depletion of primordial follicles.

➤*Pregnancy: Category D.* Chlorambucil can cause fetal harm when administered to a pregnant woman. Unilateral renal agenesis has been observed in 2 offspring whose mothers received chlorambucil during the first trimester. Urogenital malformations, including absence of a kidney, were found in fetuses of rats given chlorambucil. There are no adequate and well-controlled studies in pregnant women. If this drug is used during pregnancy, or if the patient becomes pregnant while taking this drug, apprise the patient of the potential hazard to the fetus. Advise women of childbearing potential to avoid becoming pregnant.

➤*Lactation:* It is not known whether this drug is excreted in human milk. Because many drugs are excreted in human milk and because of the potential for serious adverse reactions in nursing infants from chlorambucil, decide whether to discontinue nursing or discontinue the drug, taking into account the importance of the drug to the mother.

➤*Children:* The safety and efficacy in pediatric patients have not been established.

Precautions

➤*Monitoring:* Patients must be followed carefully to avoid life-endangering damage to the bone marrow during treatment. Perform weekly blood examinations to determine hemoglobin levels, total and differential leukocyte counts, and quantitative platelet counts. Also, during the first 3 to 6 weeks of therapy, it is recommended that white blood cell counts be made 3 or 4 days after each of the weekly complete blood counts. It has been suggested that in following patients it is helpful to plot the blood counts on a chart at the same time that body weight, temperature, spleen size, etc, are recorded. It is considered dangerous to allow a patient to go greater than 2 weeks without hematological and clinical examination during treatment.

➤*Bone marrow damage:* Many patients develop a slowly progressive lymphopenia during treatment. The lymphocyte count usually rapidly returns to normal levels upon completion of drug therapy. Most patients have some neutropenia after the third week of treatment and this may continue for up to 10 days after the last dose. Subsequently, the neutrophil count usually rapidly returns to normal. Severe neutropenia appears to be related to dosage and usually occurs only in patients who have received a total dosage of 6.5 mg/kg or more in one course of therapy with continuous dosing. About one-fourth of all patients receiving the continuous-dose schedule, and one-third of those receiving this dosage in 8 weeks or less may be expected to develop severe neutropenia.

While it is not necessary to discontinue chlorambucil at the first evidence of a fall in neutrophil count, it must be remembered that the fall may continue for 10 days after the last dose, and that as the total dose approaches 6.5 mg/kg, there is a risk of causing irreversible bone marrow damage. Decrease the dose of chlorambucil if leukocyte or platelet counts fall below normal values, and discontinue the dose for more severe depression.

Persistently low neutrophil and platelet counts or peripheral lymphocytosis suggest bone marrow infiltration. If confirmed by bone marrow examination, the daily dosage of chlorambucil should not exceed 0.1 mg/kg. Chlorambucil appears to be relatively free from GI side effects or other evidence of toxicity apart from the bone marrow-depressant action. In humans, single oral doses of 20 mg or more may produce nausea and vomiting.

➤*Radiation and chemotherapy:* Do not give chlorambucil at full dosages before 4 weeks after a full course of radiation therapy or chemotherapy because of the vulnerability of the bone marrow to damage under these conditions. If the pretherapy leukocyte or platelet counts are depressed from bone marrow disease process prior to institution of therapy, institute the treatment at a reduced dosage.

➤*Seizures:* Children with nephrotic syndrome and patients receiving high pulse doses of chlorambucil may have an increased risk of seizures. As with any potentially epileptogenic drug, exercise caution when administering chlorambucil to patients with a history of seizure disorder or head trauma, or to patients who are receiving other potentially epileptogenic drugs.

Drug Interactions

There are no known drug/drug interactions with chlorambucil.

Adverse Reactions

➤*CNS:* Tremors, muscular twitching, myoclonia, confusion, agitation, ataxia, flaccid paresis, and hallucinations have been reported as rare adverse reactions to chlorambucil that resolve upon discontinuation of drug. Rare, focal, or generalized seizures have been reported to occur in both children and adults at both therapeutic daily doses and pulse-dosing regimens, and in acute overdose.

➤*GI:* GI disturbances such as nausea and vomiting, diarrhea, and oral ulceration occur infrequently.

➤*Hematologic:* See Precautions for more information.

➤*Hypersensitivity:* Allergic reactions such as urticaria and angioneurotic edema have been reported following initial or subsequent dosing. Skin hypersensitivity (including rare reports of skin rash progressing to erythema multiforme, toxic epidermal necrolysis, and Stevens-Johnson syndrome) has been reported.

➤*Miscellaneous:* Other reported adverse reactions include pulmonary fibrosis, hepatotoxicity and jaundice, drug fever, peripheral neuropathy, interstitial pneumonia, sterile cystitis, infertility, leukemia, and secondary malignancies.

Overdosage

➤*Symptoms:* Reversible pancytopenia was the main finding of inadvertent overdoses of chlorambucil. Neurological toxicity ranging from agitated behavior and ataxia to multiple grand mal seizures has also occurred.

CHLORAMBUCIL — ORAL

➤*Treatment:* As there is no known antidote, closely monitor the blood picture and institute general supportive measures, together with appropriate blood transfusions, if necessary. Chlorambucil is not dialyzable.

Patient Information

Inform patients that the major toxicities of chlorambucil are related to hypersensitivity, drug fever, myelosuppression, hepatotoxicity, infertility, seizures, GI toxicity, and secondary malignancies. Patients should never be allowed to take the drug without medical supervision and should consult their doctor if they experience skin rash, bleeding, fever, jaundice, persistent cough, seizures, nausea, vomiting, amenorrhea, or unusual lumps/masses. Advise women of childbearing potential to avoid becoming pregnant.

CYCLOPHOSPHAMIDE

Rx	**Cyclophosphamide** (Gensia Sicor)	**Tablets:** 25 mg	Lactose. (54 639). Lt. blue. In 100s and UD 100s.
Rx	**Cytoxan** (Mead Johnson Oncology)		Lactose. White with blue flecks. In 100s.
Rx	**Cyclophosphamide** (Gensia Sicor)	**Tablets:** 50 mg	Lactose. (54 980). Lt. blue. In 100s and UD 100s.
Rx	**Cytoxan** (Mead Johnson Oncology)		Lactose. White with blue flecks. In 100s and 1000s.
Rx	**Cytoxan Lyophilized** (Mead Johnson Oncology)	**Powder for Injection:** 75 mg mannitol/100 mg cyclophosphamide	In 100, 200, 500 mg and 1 and 2 g vials.
Rx	**Neosar** (Gensia Sicor)	**Powder for Injection:** 82 mg sodium bicarbonate/100 mg cyclophosphamide	In 100, 200 and 500 mg and 1 and 2 g vials.

CYCLOPHOSPHAMIDE

Indications

➤*Malignant diseases:* Malignant lymphomas (stages III and IV of the Ann Arbor staging system), Hodgkin's disease, lymphocytic lymphoma (nodular or diffuse), mixed-cell type lymphoma, histiocytic lymphoma, Burkitt's lymphoma, neuroblastoma (disseminated disease), adenocarcinoma of the ovary, retinoblastoma, carcinoma of the breast.

➤*Multiple myeloma:* Treatment of multiple myeloma.

➤*Leukemias:* Chronic lymphocytic leukemia, chronic granulocytic leukemia (it is usually ineffective in acute blastic crisis), acute myelogenous and monocytic leukemia, acute lymphoblastic (stem-cell) leukemia in children (cyclophosphamide given during remission is effective in prolonging its duration).

➤*Mycosis fungoides:* Advanced disease.

➤*Nonmalignant disease-biopsy proven "minimal change" nephrotic syndrome in children:* Cyclophosphamide is useful in carefully selected cases of biopsy proven "minimal change" nephrotic syndrome in children but should not be used as primary therapy. In children whose disease fails to respond adequately to appropriate adrenocorticosteroid therapy or in whom the adrenocorticosteroid therapy produces or threatens to produce intolerable side effects, cyclophosphamide may induce a remission. Cyclophosphamide is not indicated for the nephrotic syndrome in adults or for any other renal disease.

➤*Unlabeled uses:* Variety of severe rheumatologic conditions: Wegener's granulomatosis, other steroid-resistant vasculidites and in some cases of severe progressive rheumatoid arthritis and systemic lupus erythematosus. Toxicity is limiting.

Cyclophosphamide (total dose 1 to 12 g) has been used to halt the progression of multiple sclerosis or decrease the frequency and duration of episodes. It has also been used in the treatment of polyarteritis nodosa using an initial dose of 2 mg/kg/day orally or 4 mg/kg/day IV. Cyclophosphamide (500 mg over 1 hour every 1 to 3 weeks), alone or in combination with corticosteroids, may be useful in the treatment of polymyositis.

Treatment of bronchogenic, small cell lung, endometrial, prostrate, and testicular carcinomas; sarcomas; bone marrow transplantation.

Administration and Dosage

➤*Malignant diseases (adults and children):*

IV – When used as the only oncolytic drug therapy, the initial course of cyclophosphamide for patients with no hematologic deficiency usually consists of 40 to 50 mg/kg given IV in divided doses over a period of 2 to 5 days. Other intravenous regimens include 10 to 15 mg/kg given every 7 to 10 days or 3 to 5 mg/kg twice weekly.

Oral – Oral cyclophosphamide dosing is usually in the range of 1 to 5 mg/kg/day for both initial and maintenance dosing. Many other regimens of intravenous and oral cyclophosphamide have been reported. Dosages must be adjusted in accord with evidence of antitumor activity or leukopenia. The total leukocyte count is a good, objective guide for regulating dosage. Transient decreases in the total white blood cell count to 2000 cells/mm^3 (following short courses) or more persistent reduction to 3000 cells/mm^3 (with continuing therapy) are tolerated without serious risk of infection if there is no marked granulocytopenia.

When cyclophosphamide is included in combined cytotoxic regimens, it may be necessary to reduce the dose of cyclophosphamide as well as that of the other drugs.

➤*Nonmalignant diseases (biopsy proven "minimal change" nephrotic syndrome in children):* An oral dose of 2.5 to 3 mg/kg daily for a period of 60 to 90 days is recommended. In males, the incidence of oligospermia and azoospermia increases if the duration of cyclophosphamide treatment exceeds 60 days. Treatment beyond 90 days increases the probability of sterility. Adrenocorticosteroid therapy may be tapered and discontinued during the course of cyclophosphamide therapy. See Precautions section concerning hematologic monitoring.

➤*Preparation of parenteral solution:* Lyophilized cyclophosphamide should be prepared for parenteral use by adding Bacteriostatic Water for Injection, USP (paraben preserved only) or Sterile Water for Injection, USP to the vial and shaking to dissolve. Use the quantity of diluent shown below to reconstitute the product.

Reconstitution of Cyclophosphamide

Dose strength	Quantity of diluent
100 mg	5 mL
200 mg	10 mL
500 mg	25 mL
1 g	50 mL
2 g	100 mL

Solutions of lyophilized cyclophosphamide may be injected intravenously, intramuscularly, intraperitoneally, or intrapleurally or they may be infused intravenously in the following: dextrose injection (5% dextrose), dextrose and sodium chloride injection (5% dextrose and 0.9% sodium chloride), 5% dextrose and Ringer's injection, lactated Ringer's injection, sodium chloride injection (0.45% sodium chloride), sodium lactate injection (⅙ molar sodium lactate).

Reconstituted lyophilized cyclophosphamide is chemically and physically stable for 24 hours at room temperature or for 6 days in the refrigerator; it does not contain any antimicrobial preservative and thus care must be taken to ensure the sterility of prepared solutions.

Lyophilized cyclophosphamide and cyclophosphamide prepared by adding Bacteriostatic Water for Injection, USP (paraben preserved only) should be used within 24 hours if stored at room temperature or within 6 days if stored under refrigeration.

If lyophilized cyclophosphamide and cyclophosphamide are not prepared by adding Bacteriostatic Water for Injection, USP (paraben preserved only), it is recommended that the solution be used promptly (preferably within 6 hours). The osmolarities of solutions of lyophilized cyclophosphamide, and normal saline are found in the following table:

Osmolarities of Lyophilized Cyclophosphamide Solutions and Normal Saline

	mOsm/L
Lyophilized cyclophosphamide	431
Cyclophosphamide	352
Normal saline	287

Lyophilized cyclophosphamide is slightly hypotonic.

Preparation of oral solution – Extemporaneous liquid preparations of cyclophosphamide for oral administration may be prepared by dissolving lyophilized cyclophosphamide in aromatic elixir, N.F. Such preparations should be stored under refrigeration in glass containers and used within 14 days.

➤*Storage/Stability:* Storage at or below 25°C (77°F) is recommended; this product will withstand brief exposure to temperatures up to 30°C (86°F) but should be protected from temperatures above 30°C (86°F).

Actions

➤*Pharmacology:* Cyclophosphamide is biotransformed principally in the liver to active alkylating metabolites by a mixed function microsomal oxidase system. These metabolites interfere with the growth of susceptible rapidly proliferating malignant cells. The mechanism of action is thought to involve cross-linking of tumor cell DNA.

CYCLOPHOSPHAMIDE

➤*Pharmacokinetics:*

Absorption – Cyclophosphamide is well absorbed after oral administration with a bioavailability greater than 75%.

Metabolism/Excretion – The unchanged drug has an elimination half-life of 3 to 12 hours. It is eliminated primarily in the form of metabolites, but from 5% to 25% of the dose is excreted in urine as unchanged drug. Several cytotoxic and noncytotoxic metabolites have been identified in urine and in plasma. Concentrations of metabolites reach a maximum in plasma 2 to 3 hours after an IV dose. Plasma protein binding of unchanged drug is low but some metabolites are bound to an extent greater than 60%. It has not been demonstrated that any single metabolite is responsible for either the therapeutic or toxic effects of cyclophosphamide. Although elevated levels of metabolites of cyclophosphamide have been observed in patients with renal failure, increased clinical toxicity in such patients has not been demonstrated.

Contraindications

Severely depressed bone marrow function; hypersensitivity to cyclophosphamide.

Warnings

➤*Urinary system:* Hemorrhagic cystitis may develop in patients treated with cyclophosphamide. Rarely, this condition can be severe and even fatal. Fibrosis of the urinary bladder, sometimes extensive, also may develop with or without accompanying cystitis. Atypical urinary bladder epithelial cells may appear in the urine. These adverse effects appear to depend on the dose of cyclophosphamide and the duration of therapy. Such bladder injury is thought to be due to cyclophosphamide metabolites excreted in the urine. Forced fluid intake helps to assure an ample output of urine, necessitates frequent voiding, and reduces the time the drug remains in the bladder. This helps to prevent cystitis. Hematuria usually resolves in a few days after cyclophosphamide treatment is stopped, but it may persist. Medical or surgical supportive treatment may be required, rarely, to treat protracted cases of severe hemorrhagic cystitis. It is usually necessary to discontinue cyclophosphamide therapy in instances of severe hemorrhagic cystitis.

➤*Cardiac toxicity:* Although a few instances of cardiac dysfunction have been reported following use of recommended doses of cyclophosphamide, no causal relationship has been established. Cardiotoxicity has been observed in some patients receiving high doses of cyclophosphamide ranging from 120 to 270 mg/kg administered over a period of a few days, usually as a portion of an intensive antineoplastic multidrug regimen or in conjunction with transplantation procedures. In a few instances with high doses of cyclophosphamide, severe, and sometimes fatal, congestive heart failure has occurred after the first cyclophosphamide dose. Histopathologic examination has primarily shown hemorrhagic myocarditis. Hemopericardium has occurred secondary to hemorrhagic myocarditis and myocardial necrosis. Pericarditis has been reported independent of any hemopericardiums.

No residual cardiac abnormalities, as evidenced by electrocardiogram or echocardiogram appear to be present in patients surviving episodes of apparent cardiac toxicity associated with high doses of cyclophosphamide.

Cyclophosphamide has been reported to potentiate doxorubicin-induced cardiotoxicity.

➤*Wound healing:* Cyclophosphamide may interfere with normal wound healing.

➤*Hypersensitivity reactions:* See Adverse Reactions for more information.

➤*Carcinogenesis:* Second malignancies have developed in some patients treated with cyclophosphamide used alone or in association with other antineoplastic drugs or modalities. Most frequently, they have been urinary bladder, myeloproliferative, or lymphoproliferative malignancies. Second malignancies most frequently were detected in patients treated for primary myeloproliferative or lymphoproliferative malignancies or nonmalignant disease in which immune processes are believed to be involved pathologically.

In some cases, the second malignancy developed several years after cyclophosphamide treatment had been discontinued. In a single breast cancer trial utilizing 2 to 4 times the standard dose of cyclophosphamide in conjunction with doxorubicin a small number of cases of secondary acute myeloid leukemia occurred within 2 years of treatment initiation. Urinary bladder malignancies generally have occurred in patients who previously had hemorrhagic cystitis. In patients treated with cyclophosphamide-containing regimens for a variety of solid tumors, isolated case reports of secondary malignancies have been published. One case of carcinoma of the renal pelvis was reported in a patient receiving long-term cyclophosphamide therapy for cerebral vasculitis. The possibility of cyclophosphamide-induced malignancy should be considered in any benefit-to-risk assessment for use of the drug.

➤*Fertility impairment:* Cyclophosphamide interferes with oogenesis and spermatogenesis. It may cause sterility in both sexes. Development of sterility appears to depend on the dose of cyclophosphamide, duration of therapy, and the state of gonadal function at the time of treatment. Cyclophosphamide-induced sterility may be irreversible in some patients.

Amenorrhea associated with decreased estrogen and increased gonadotropin secretion develops in a significant proportion of women treated with cyclophosphamide. Affected patients generally resume regular menses within a few months after cessation of therapy. Girls treated with cyclophosphamide during prepubescence generally develop secondary sexual characteristics normally and have regular menses. Ovarian fibrosis with apparently complete loss of germ cells after prolonged cyclophosphamide treatment in late prepubescence has been reported. Girls treated with cyclophosphamide during prepubescence subsequently have conceived.

Men treated with cyclophosphamide may develop oligospermia or azoospermia associated with increased gonadotropin but normal testosterone secretion. Sexual potency and libido are unimpaired in these patients. Boys treated with cyclophosphamide during prepubescence develop secondary sexual characteristics normally, but may have oligospermia or azoospermia and increased gonadotropin secretion. Some degree of testicular atrophy may occur. Cyclophosphamide-induced azoospermia is reversible in some patients, though the reversibility may not occur for several years after cessation of therapy. Men temporarily rendered sterile by cyclophosphamide have subsequently fathered healthy children.

➤*Pregnancy: Category D.* Cyclophosphamide can cause fetal harm when administered to a pregnant woman and such abnormalities have been reported following cyclophosphamide therapy in pregnant women. Abnormalities were found in 2 infants and a 6-month-old fetus born to women treated with cyclophosphamide. Ectrodactylia was found in 2 of the 3 cases. Healthy infants have also been born to women treated with cyclophosphamide during pregnancy, including the first trimester. If this drug is used during pregnancy, or if the patient becomes pregnant while taking (receiving) this drug, the patient should be apprised of the potential hazard to the fetus. Women of childbearing potential should be advised to avoid becoming pregnant.

➤*Lactation:* Cyclophosphamide is excreted in breast milk. Because of the potential for serious adverse reactions and the potential for tumorigenicity shown for cyclophosphamide in humans, a decision should be made whether to discontinue nursing or to discontinue the drug, taking into account the importance of the drug to the mother.

➤*Children:* The safety profile of cyclophosphamide in pediatric patients is similar to that of the adult population (see Adverse Reactions).

Precautions

➤*Monitoring:* During treatment, the patient's hematologic profile (particularly neutrophils and platelets) should be monitored regularly to determine the degree of hematopoietic suppression. Urine should also be examined regularly for red cells which may precede hemorrhagic cystitis.

➤*Immunosuppression:* Treatment with cyclophosphamide may cause significant suppression of immune responses. Serious, sometimes fatal, infections may develop in severely immunosuppressed patients. Cyclophosphamide treatment may not be indicated or should be interrupted or the dose reduced in patients who have or who develop viral, bacterial, fungal, protozoan, or helminthic infections.

➤*Special risk:* Special attention to the possible development of toxicity should be exercised in patients being treated with cyclophosphamide if any of the following conditions are present: leukopenia, thrombocytopenia, tumor cell infiltration of bone marrow, previous x-ray therapy, previous therapy with other cytotoxic agents, impaired hepatic function, impaired renal function.

Drug Interactions

If a patient has been treated with cyclophosphamide within 10 days of general anesthesia, the anesthesiologist should be alerted.

➤*Adrenalectomy:* Since cyclophosphamide has been reported to be more toxic in adrenalectomized dogs, adjustment of the doses of both replacement steroids and cyclophosphamide may be necessary for the adrenalectomized patient.

Cyclophosphamide Drug Interactions

Precipitant drug	Object drug*		Description
Allopurinol	Cyclophosphamide	↑	The myelosuppressive effects of cyclophosphamide may be enhanced, possibly increasing the risk of bleeding or infection.
Chloramphenicol	Cyclophosphamide	↓	Cyclophosphamide half-life may increase and metabolite concentrations may be decreased.
Phenobarbital	Cyclophosphamide	↓	The rate of metabolism and the leukopenic activity of cyclophosphamide reportedly are increased by chronic administration of high doses of phenobarbital.
Thiazide diuretics	Cyclophosphamide[a]	↑	Antineoplastic-induced leukopenia may be prolonged.
Cyclophosphamide	Anticoagulants	↑	Anticoagulant effect is increased.
Cyclophosphamide[a]	Digoxin	↓	Digoxin serum levels may be reduced.
Cyclophosphamide	Doxorubicin	↑	Doxorubicin-induced cardiotoxicity is potentiated.
Cyclophosphamide	Quinolone	↓	The antimicrobial effects of quinolones may be decreased.
Cyclophosphamide	Succinylcholine	↑	Neuromuscular blockade may be prolonged, because of inhibition of cholinesterase activity.

* ↑ = Object drug increased. ↓ = Object drug decreased.
[a] Cyclophosphamide used in combination with other antineoplastics.

Adverse Reactions

➤*Carcinogenesis:* See Warnings for more information.

CYCLOPHOSPHAMIDE

➤*Infections:* See Precautions for more information.

➤*Reproductive system:* See Warnings for more information.

➤*Dermatologic:* Alopecia occurs commonly in patients treated with cyclophosphamide. The hair can be expected to grow back after treatment with the drug or even during continued drug treatment, though it may be different in texture or color. Skin rash occurs occasionally in patients receiving the drug. Pigmentation of the skin and changes in nails can occur. Very rare reports of Stevens-Johnson syndrome and toxic epidermal necrolysis have been received during postmarketing surveillance; due to the nature of spontaneous adverse event reporting, a definitive causal relationship to cyclophosphamide has not been established.

➤*GI:* Nausea and vomiting commonly occur with cyclophosphamide therapy. Anorexia and, less frequently, abdominal discomfort or pain and diarrhea may occur. There are isolated reports of hemorrhagic colitis, oral mucosal ulceration and jaundice occurring during therapy. These adverse drug effects generally remit when cyclophosphamide treatment is stopped.

➤*GU:* See Warnings for more information.

Hemorrhagic ureteritis and renal tubular necrosis have been reported to occur in patients treated with cyclophosphamide. Such lesions usually resolve following cessation of therapy.

➤*Hematologic:* Leukopenia occurs in patients treated with cyclophosphamide, is related to the dose of drug, and can be used as a dosage guide. Leukopenia of less than 2000 cells/mm^3 develops commonly in patients treated with an initial loading dose of the drug, and less frequently in patients maintained on smaller doses. The degree of neutropenia is particularly important because it correlates with a reduction in resistance to infections. Fever without documented infection has been reported in neutropenic patients.

Thrombocytopenia or anemia develop occasionally in patients treated with cyclophosphamide. These hematologic effects usually can be reversed by reducing the drug dose or by interrupting treatment. Recovery from leukopenia usually begins in 7 to 10 days after cessation of therapy.

➤*Respiratory:* Interstitial pneumonitis has been reported as part of the postmarketing experience. Interstitial pulmonary fibrosis has been reported in patients receiving high doses of cyclophosphamide over a prolonged period.

➤*Miscellaneous:* Anaphylactic reactions have been reported; death has also been reported in association with this event. Possible cross-sensitivity with other alkylating agents has been reported. SIADH (syndrome of inappropriate ADH secretion) has been reported with the use of cyclophosphamide. Malaise and asthenia have been reported as part of the postmarketing experience.

Overdosage

No specific antidote for cyclophosphamide is known. Overdosage should be managed with supportive measures, including appropriate treatment for any concurrent infection, myelosuppression, or cardiac toxicity should it occur.

IFOSFAMIDE

Rx	**Ifosfamide** (American Pharmaceutical Partners)	**Powder for Injection:** 1 g	In single-dose vials.
Rx	**Ifex** (Mead Johnson Oncology)		In single-dose vials.[1]
Rx	**Ifosfamide** (American Pharmaceutical Partners)	**Powder for Injection:** 3 g	In single-dose vials.
Rx	**Ifex** (Mead Johnson Oncology)		In single-dose vials.[2]

[1] Includes 200 mg amps *Mesnex* (mesna).

[2] Includes 400 mg amps *Mesnex* (mesna).

IFOSFAMIDE — INJECTION

WARNING

Ifosfamide for injection should be administered under the supervision of a qualified physician experienced in the use of cancer chemotherapeutic agents. Urotoxic side effects, especially hemorrhagic cystitis, as well as CNS toxicities such as confusion and coma have been associated with the use of ifosfamide. When they occur, they may require cessation of ifosfamide therapy. Severe myelosuppression has been reported.

Indications

➤*Germ cell testicular cancer:* In combination with certain other approved antineoplastic agents for third-line chemotherapy of germ cell testicular cancer. It should ordinarily be used in combination with a prophylactic agent for hemorrhagic cystitis, such as mesna.

➤*Unlabeled uses:* Ifosfamide has shown activity in lung, breast, ovarian, pancreatic and gastric cancer, sarcomas, acute leukemias (except AML) and malignant lymphomas. Further studies are needed with ifosfamide alone and with other agents.

Treatment of soft-tissue, Ewing's and osteogenic sarcomas; non-Hodgkin's lymphomas; bladder and cervical carcinoma.

Administration and Dosage

➤*Approved by the FDA:* December 12, 1988.

Ifosfamide should be administered IV at a dose of 1.2 g/m^2/day for 5 consecutive days. Treatment is repeated every 3 weeks or after recovery from hematologic toxicity (platelets greater than or equal to 100,000/mcL, WBC greater than or equal to 4000/mcL). In order to prevent bladder toxicity, ifosfamide should be given with extensive hydration consisting of at least 2 L of oral or IV fluid per day. A protector, such as mesna, should also be used to prevent hemorrhagic cystitis. Ifosfamide should be administered as a slow IV infusion lasting a minimum of 30 minutes. Although ifosfamide has been administered to a small number of patients with compromised hepatic or renal function, studies to establish optimal dose schedules of ifosfamide in such patients have not been conducted.

➤*Preparation:* Injections are prepared for parenteral use by adding Sterile Water for Injection or Sterile Bacteriostatic Water for Injection (benzyl alcohol or parabens preserved), to the vial and shaking to dissolve. Use the quantity of diluent shown in the information following to constitute the product:

Reconstitution of Ifosfamide

Dosage strength	Quantity of diluent	Final concentration
1 g	20 mL	50 mg/mL
3 g	60 mL	50 mg/mL

Solutions of ifosfamide may be diluted further to achieve concentrations of 0.6 to 20 mg/mL in the following fluids: 5% Dextrose Injection, 0.9% Sodium Chloride Injection, Lactated Ringer's Injection, Sterile Water for Injection.

Because essentially identical stability results were obtained for Sterile Water admixtures as for the other admixtures (5% Dextrose Injection, 0.9% Sodium Chloride Injection, and Lactated Ringer's Injection), the use of large volume parenteral glass bottles, *Viaflex* bags or *PAB* bags that contain intermediate concentrations or mixtures of excipients (eg, 2.5% Dextrose Injection, 0.45% Sodium Chloride Injection, or 5% Dextrose and 0.9% Sodium Chloride Injection) is also acceptable.

➤*Storage/Stability:* Store at controlled room temperature 20° to 25°C (68° to 77°F). Protect from temperatures above 30°C (86°F).

Constituted or constituted and further diluted solutions of ifosfamide should be refrigerated and used within 24 hours.

Actions

➤*Pharmacology:* Ifosfamide has been shown to require metabolic activation by microsomal liver enzymes to produce biologically active metabolites. Activation occurs by hydroxylation at the ring carbon atom 4 to form the unstable intermediate 4-hydroxyifosfamide. This metabolite rapidly degrades to the stable urinary metabolite 4-ketoifosfamide. Opening of the ring results in formation of the stable urinary metabolite, 4-carboxyifosfamide. These urinary metabolites have not been found to be cytotoxic. N, N-bis (2-chloroethyl)-phosphoric acid diamide (ifosphoramide) and acrolein are also found. Enzymatic oxidation of the chloroethyl side chains and subsequent dealkylation produces the major urinary metabolites, dechloroethyl ifosfamide and dechloroethyl cyclophosphamide. The alkylated metabolites of ifosfamide have been shown to interact with DNA.

➤*Pharmacokinetics:*

Absorption/Distribution – Ifosfamide exhibits dose-dependent pharmacokinetics in humans.

Metabolism/Excretion – At single doses of 3.8 to 5 g/m^2, the plasma concentrations decay biphasically and the mean terminal elimination half-life is about 15 hours. At doses of 1.6 to 2.4 g/m^2/day, the plasma decay is monoexponential and the terminal elimination half-life is about 7 hours. Ifosfamide is extensively metabolized in humans, and the metabolic pathways appear to be saturated at high doses.

After administration of doses of 5 g/m^2 of ^{14}C labeled ifosfamide, from 70% to 86% of the dosed radioactivity was recovered in the urine, with about 61% of the dose excreted as parent compound. At doses of 1.6 to 2.4 g/m^2 only 12% to 18% of the dose was excreted in the urine as unchanged drug within 72 hours.

Contraindications

Severely depressed bone marrow function; hypersensitivity to ifosfamide.

Warnings

➤*Urotoxic side effects:* See Adverse Reactions for more information.

➤*Myelosuppression:* See Adverse Reactions for more information.

➤*CNS:* See Adverse Reactions for more information.

➤*Wound healing:* Ifosfamide may interfere with normal wound healing.

➤*Carcinogenesis:* Ifosfamide has been shown to be carcinogenic in rats, with female rats showing a significant incidence of leiomyosarcomas and mammary fibroadenomas.

➤*Mutagenesis:* The mutagenic potential of ifosfamide has been documented in bacterial systems in vitro and mammalian cells in vivo. In vivo, ifosfamide has induced mutagenic effects in mice and *Drosophila melano-*

IFOSFAMIDE — INJECTION

gaster germ cells, and has induced a significant increase in dominant lethal mutations in male mice as well as recessive sex-linked lethal mutations in *Drosophila*.

➤*Fertility impairment:* In pregnant mice, resorptions increased and anomalies were present at day 19 after a 30 mg/m^2 dose of ifosfamide was administered on day 11 of gestation. Embryolethal effects were observed in rats following the administration of 54 mg/m^2 doses of ifosfamide from the sixth through the fifteenth day of gestation and embryotoxic effects were apparent after dams received 18 mg/m^2 doses over the same dosing period. Ifosfamide is embryotoxic to rabbits receiving 88 mg/m^2/day doses from the sixth through the eighteenth day after mating. The number of anomalies was also significantly increased over the control group.

➤*Pregnancy: Category D.* Animal studies indicate that the drug is capable of causing gene mutations and chromosomal damage in vivo. Embryotoxic and teratogenic effects have been observed in mice, rats and rabbits at doses 0.05 to 0.075 times the human dose. Ifosfamide can cause fetal damage when administered to a pregnant woman. If ifosfamide is used during pregnancy, or if the patient becomes pregnant while taking this drug, the patient should be apprised of the potential hazard to the fetus.

➤*Lactation:* Ifosfamide is excreted in breast milk. Because of the potential for serious adverse events and the tumorigenicity shown for ifosfamide in animal studies, a decision should be made whether to discontinue nursing or to discontinue the drug, taking into account the importance of the drug to the mother.

➤*Children:* Safety and effectiveness in pediatric patients have not been established.

Precautions

➤*Monitoring:* During treatment, the patient's hematologic profile (particularly neutrophils and platelets) should be monitored regularly to determine the degree of hematopoietic suppression. Urine should also be examined regularly for red cells which may precede hemorrhagic cystitis.

➤*Special risk:* Ifosfamide should be given cautiously to patients with impaired renal function as well as to those with compromised bone marrow reserve, as indicated by the following: Leukopenia, granulocytopenia, extensive bone marrow metastases, prior radiation therapy, or prior therapy with other cytotoxic agents.

Drug Interactions

The physician should be alert for possible combined drug actions, desirable or undesirable, involving ifosfamide even though ifosfamide has been used successfully concurrently with other drugs, including other cytotoxic drugs.

Adverse Reactions

Ifosfamide Adverse Reactions

Adverse reaction	Incidence [a] (%)
Alopecia	83%
Nausea/vomiting	58%
Hematuria	46%
Gross hematuria	12%
CNS toxicity	12%
Infection	8%
Renal impairment	6%
Liver dysfunction	3%
Phlebitis	2%
Fever	1%
Allergic reaction	< 1%
Anorexia	< 1%
Cardiotoxicity	< 1%
Coagulopathy	< 1%
Constipation	< 1%
Dermatitis	< 1%
Diarrhea	< 1%
Fatigue	< 1%
Hypertension	< 1%
Hypotension	< 1%
Malaise	< 1%
Polyneuropathy	< 1%
Pulmonary symptoms	< 1%
Salivation	< 1%
Stomatitis	< 1%

[a] Based upon 2070 patients from the published literature in 30 single-agent studies.

➤*CNS:* CNS side effects were observed in 12% of patients treated with ifosfamide. Those most commonly seen were somnolence, confusion, depressive psychosis, and hallucinations. Other less frequent symptoms include dizziness, disorientation, and cranial nerve dysfunction. Seizures and coma with death were occasionally reported. The incidence of CNS toxicity may be higher in patients with altered renal function.

➤*GI:* Nausea and vomiting occurred in 58% of the patients who received ifosfamide. They were usually controlled by standard antiemetic therapy. Other GI side effects include anorexia, diarrhea, and in some cases, constipation.

➤*GU:* Urotoxicity consisted of hemorrhagic cystitis, dysuria, urinary frequency and other symptoms of bladder irritation. Hematuria occurred in 6% to 92% of patients treated with ifosfamide. The incidence and severity of hematuria can be significantly reduced by using vigorous hydration, a fractionated dose schedule and a protector such as mesna. At daily doses of 1.2 g/m^2 for 5 consecutive days without a protector, microscopic hematuria is expected in about one-half of the patients and gross hematuria in about 8% of patients.

➤*Hematologic:* Myelosuppression was dose related and dose limiting. It consisted mainly of leukopenia and, to a lesser extent, thrombocytopenia. A WBC count less than 3000/mcL is expected in 50% of the patients treated with ifosfamide single agent at doses of 1.2 g/m^2/day for 5 consecutive days. At this dose level, thrombocytopenia (platelets less than 100,000/ mcL) occurred in about 20% of the patients. At higher dosages, leukopenia was almost universal, and at total dosages of 10 to 12 g/m^2/cycle, one-half of the patients had a WBC count less than 1000/mcL and 8% of patients had platelet counts less than 50,000/mcL. Myelosuppression was usually reversible and treatment can be given every 3 to 4 weeks. When ifosfamide is used in combination with other myelosuppressive agents, adjustments in dosing may be necessary. Patients who experience severe myelosuppression are potentially at increased risk for infection. Anemia has been reported as part of postmarketing surveillance.

➤*Renal:* Renal toxicity occurred in 6% of the patients treated with ifosfamide as a single agent. Clinical signs, such as elevation in BUN or serum creatinine or decrease in creatinine clearance, were usually transient. They were most likely to be related to tubular damage. One episode of renal tubular acidosis which progressed into chronic renal failure was reported. Proteinuria and acidosis also occurred in rare instances. Metabolic acidosis was reported in 31% of patients in 1 study when ifosfamide was administered at doses of 2 to 2.5 g/m^2/day for 4 days. Renal tubular acidosis, Fanconi syndrome, renal rickets and acute renal failure have been reported. Close clinical monitoring of serum and urine chemistries including phosphorus, potassium, alkaline phosphatase and other appropriate laboratory studies is recommended. Appropriate replacement therapy should be administered as indicated.

➤*Miscellaneous:* Alopecia occurred in approximately 83% of the patients treated with ifosfamide as a single agent. In combination, this incidence may be as high as 100%, depending on the other agents included in the chemotherapy regimen. Increases in liver enzymes or bilirubin were noted in 3% of the patients. Other less frequent side effects included phlebitis, pulmonary symptoms, fever of unknown origin, allergic reactions, stomatitis, cardiotoxicity, and polyneuropathy.

Overdosage

➤*Treatment:* No specific antidote for ifosfamide is known. Management of overdosage would include general supportive measures to sustain the patient through any period of toxicity that might occur.

MECHLORETHAMINE HYDROCHLORIDE (Nitrogen Mustard; HN_2)

Rx	**Mustargen** (Merck)	**Powder for Injection:** 10 mg	In sets of 4 vials.

MECHLORETHAMINE HYDROCHLORIDE — INJECTION

WARNING

Administer mechlorethamine injection only under the supervision of a physician who is experienced in the use of cancer chemotherapeutic agents.

This drug is highly toxic, and both powder and solution must be handled and administered with care. Inhalation of dust or vapors and contact with skin or mucous membranes, especially those of the eyes, must be avoided. Avoid exposure during pregnancy. Due to the toxic properties of mechlorethamine (eg, corrosivity, carcinogenicity, mutagenicity, teratogenicity), review special handling procedures prior to handling and follow them diligently.

Extravasation of the drug into subcutaneous tissues results in a painful inflammation. The area usually becomes indurated and sloughing may occur. If leakage of drug is obvious, prompt infiltration of the area with sterile isotonic sodium thiosulfate (1/6 molar) and application of an ice compress for 6 to 12 hours may minimize the local reaction. For a 1/6 molar solution of sodium thiosulfate, use 4.14 g of sodium thiosulfate per 100 mL of Sterile Water for Injection or 2.64 g of anhydrous sodium thiosulfate per 100 mL or dilute 4 mL of Sodium Thiosulfate Injection (10%) with 6 mL of Sterile Water for Injection.

Indications

➤*Leukemia / Lymphomas / Polycythemia vera / Mycosis fungoides / Bronchogenic carcinoma (IV only):* For the palliative treatment of Hodgkin's disease (stages III and IV), lymphosarcoma, chronic myelocytic or chronic lymphocytic leukemia, polycythemia vera, mycosis fungoides, and bronchogenic carcinoma.

➤*Metastatic carcinoma:* Intrapleurally, intraperitoneally, or intrapericardially for the palliative treatment of metastatic carcinoma resulting in effusion.

➤*Unlabeled uses:* A topical mechlorethamine solution has been used to treat patients with mycosis fungoides.

Administration and Dosage

March 15, 1949.

Not for oral administration.

➤*IV administration:* The dosage of mechlorethamine varies with the clinical situation, the therapeutic response, and the magnitude of hematologic depression. A total dose of 0.4 mg/kg of body weight for each course usually is given either as a single dose or in divided doses of 0.1 to 0.2 mg/kg/day. Base dosage on ideal dry body weight. The presence of edema or ascites must be considered so that dosage will be based on actual weight unaugmented by these conditions.

The margin of safety in therapy with mechlorethamine is narrow, and considerable care must be exercised in the matter of dosage. Repeated examinations of blood are mandatory as a guide to subsequent therapy.

Within a few minutes after IV injection, mechlorethamine undergoes chemical transformation, combines with reactive compounds, and is no longer present in its active form in the bloodstream. Do not give subsequent courses until the patient has recovered hematologically from the previous course; this is best determined by repeated studies of the peripheral blood elements awaiting their return to normal levels. It is often possible to give repeated courses of mechlorethamine as early as 3 weeks after treatment.

➤*Preparation of solution:* Each vial of mechlorethamine contains 10 mg of mechlorethamine titurated with sodium chloride q.s. 100 mg. In neutral or alkaline aqueous solution, it undergoes rapid chemical transformation and is highly unstable. Although solutions prepared according to instructions are acidic and do not decompose as rapidly, they should be prepared immediately before each injection, since they will decompose on standing. When reconstituted, mechlorethamine is a clear, colorless solution. Do not use if the solution is discolored or if droplets of water are visible within the vial prior to reconstitution.

Using a sterile 10 mL syringe, inject 10 mL of Sterile Water for Injection or 10 mL Sodium Chloride Injection into a vial of mechlorethamine. With the needle (syringe attached) still in the rubber stopper, shake the vial several times to dissolve the drug completely. The resultant solution contains 1 mg of mechlorethamine/mL.

➤*Special handling:* This drug is highly toxic, and both powder and solution must be handled and administered with care. Because mechlorethamine is a powerful vesicant, it is intended primarily for IV use, and in most instances is given by this route. Inhalation of dust or vapors and contact with skin or mucous membranes, especially those of the eyes, must be avoided. Wear appropriate protective equipment when handling mechlorethamine. Should accidental eye contact occur, institute copious irrigation with water, normal saline or a balanced salt, ophthalmic, irrigating solution immediately, followed by prompt ophthalmologic consultation. Should accidental skin contact occur, the affected part must be irrigated immediately with copious amounts of water, for at least 15 minutes, followed by 2% sodium thiosulfate solution. Seek medical attention immediately. Destroy contaminated clothing.

➤*Technique for IV administration:* Withdraw into the syringe the calculated volume of solution required for a single injection. Dispose of any remaining solution after neutralization (see below). Although the drug may be injected directly into any suitable vein, it is injected preferably into the rubber or plastic tubing of a flowing IV infusion set. This reduces the possibility of severe local reactions due to extravasation or high concentration of the drug. Injecting the drug into the tubing rather than adding it to the entire volume of the infusion fluid minimizes a chemical reaction between the drug and the solution. The rate of injection apparently is not critical, provided it is completed within a few minutes.

➤*Intracavitary administration:* Nitrogen mustard has been used by intracavitary administration with varying success in certain malignant conditions for the control of pleural, peritoneal, and pericardial effusions caused by malignant cells.

The technique and the dose used by any of these routes varies. Therefore, if mechlorethamine is given by the intracavitary route, consult the published articles concerning such use. Because of the inherent risks involved, the physician should be experienced in the appropriate injection techniques, and be thoroughly aware of the indications, dosages, hazards, and precautions as set forth in the published literature. When using mechlorethamine by the intracavitary route, keep in mind the general precautions concerning this agent.

The usual dose of nitrogen mustard for intracavitary injection is 0.4 mg/kg of body weight, though 0.2 mg/kg (or 10 to 20 mg) has been used by the intrapericardial route. The solution is prepared, as previously described for IV injection, by adding 10 mL of Sterile Water for Injection or 10 mL of Sodium Chloride Injection to the vial containing 10 mg of mechlorethamine (amounts of diluent of 50 to 100 mL of normal saline have also been used). Change the position of the patient every 5 to 10 minutes for an hour after injection to obtain more uniform distribution of the drug throughout the serous cavity. The remaining fluid may be removed from the pleural or peritoneal cavity by paracentesis 24 to 36 hours later. Carefully follow the patient by clinical and x-ray examination to detect reaccumulation of fluid.

➤*Decontamination:* To clean rubber gloves, tubing, and glassware after giving mechlorethamine, soak them in an aqueous solution containing equal volumes of sodium thiosulfate (5%) and sodium bicarbonate (5%) for 45 minutes. Excess reagents and reaction products are washed away easily with water. Neutralize any unused injection solution by mixing with an equal volume of sodium thiosulfate/sodium bicarbonate solution. Allow the mixture to stand for 45 minutes. Treat vials that have contained mechlorethamine the same way with thiosulfate/bicarbonate solution before disposal.

➤*Storage / Stability:* Store at controlled room temperature 15° to 30°C (59° to 86°F). Protect from light and humidity. Solutions of mechlorethamine decompose on standing; therefore, prepare solutions of the drug immediately before use.

Actions

➤*Pharmacology:* Mechlorethamine, a biologic alkylating agent, has a cytotoxic action which inhibits rapidly proliferating cells.

➤*Pharmacokinetics:* In water or body fluids, mechlorethamine undergoes rapid chemical transformation and combines with water or reactive compounds of cells, so that the drug is no longer present in active form a few minutes after administration.

Contraindications

Infectious diseases; previous anaphylactic reactions to mechlorethamine.

Warnings

➤*Amyloidosis:* As nitrogen mustard therapy may contribute to extensive and rapid development of amyloidosis, only use it if foci of acute and chronic suppurative inflammation are absent.

➤*Carcinogenesis:* Therapy with alkylating agents such as mechlorethamine may be associated with an increased incidence of a second malignant tumor, especially when such therapy is combined with other antineoplastic agents or radiation therapy.

➤*Mutagenesis:* Mechlorethamine induced mutations in the Ames test, in *E. coli*, and *Neurospora crassa*. Mechlorethamine caused chromosome aberrations in a variety of plant and mammalian cells. Dominant lethal mutations were produced in ICR/Ha Swiss mice.

➤*Fertility impairment:* Mechlorethamine impaired fertility in the rat at a daily dose of 500 mg/kg IV for 2 weeks.

➤*Pregnancy: Category D.* Mechlorethamine can cause fetal harm when administered to a pregnant woman. Mechlorethamine has been shown to produce fetal malformations in the rat and ferret when given as single subcutaneous injections of 1 mg/kg (2 to 3 times the maximum recommended human dose). There are no adequate and well-controlled studies in pregnant women. If this drug is used during pregnancy, or if the patient becomes pregnant while taking this drug, apprise the patient of the potential hazard to the fetus. Advise women of childbearing potential to avoid becoming pregnant.

➤*Lactation:* It is not known whether this drug is excreted in human milk. Because many drugs are excreted in human milk and because of the potential for serious adverse reactions in nursing infants from mechlorethamine, make a decision whether to discontinue nursing or to discontinue the drug, taking into account the importance of the drug to the mother.

➤*Children:* Safety and efficacy in pediatric patients have not been established by well-controlled studies. Use of mechlorethamine in pediatric patients has been quite limited. Mechlorethamine has been used in Hodgkin's disease, stages III and IV, in combination with other oncolytic agents (MOPP schedule). The MOPP chemotherapy combination includes mechlorethamine, vincristine, procarbazine, and prednisone or prednisolone.

MECHLORETHAMINE HYDROCHLORIDE — INJECTION

Precautions

➤*Monitoring:* Many abnormalities of renal, hepatic, and bone marrow function have been reported in patients with neoplastic disease and receiving mechlorethamine. It is advisable to check renal, hepatic, and bone marrow functions frequently.

See Administration and Dosage for more information.

➤*Inoperable neoplasms/terminal stage:* Because of the toxicity of mechlorethamine, and the unpleasant side effects following its use, the potential risk and discomfort from the use of this drug in patients with inoperable neoplasms or in the terminal stage of the disease must be balanced against the limited gain obtainable. These gains will vary with the nature and the status of the disease under treatment. The routine use of mechlorethamine in all cases of widely disseminated neoplasms is to be discouraged.

➤*Tumors:* Tumors of bone and nervous tissue have responded poorly to therapy. Results are unpredictable in disseminated and malignant tumors of different types.

➤*Concomitant therapy:* Precautions must be observed with the use of mechlorethamine and x-ray therapy or other chemotherapy in alternating courses. Hematopoietic function is characteristically depressed by either form of therapy, and neither mechlorethamine following x-ray therapy nor x-ray therapy subsequent to the drug should be given until bone marrow function has recovered. In particular, irradiation of such areas as sternum, ribs, and vertebrae shortly after a course of nitrogen mustard may lead to hematologic complications.

➤*Immunosuppression:* Mechlorethamine has been reported to have immunosuppressive activity. Therefore, keep in mind that use of the drug may predispose the patient to bacterial, viral, or fungal infection.

➤*Hyperuricemia:* Hyperuricemia may develop during therapy with mechlorethamine. The problem of urate precipitation should be anticipated, particularly in the treatment of the lymphomas; institute adequate methods for control of hyperuricemia and direct careful attention toward adequate fluid intake before treatment.

➤*Hematologic:* The use of mechlorethamine in patients with leukopenia, thrombocytopenia, and anemia, due to invasion of the bone marrow by tumor carries a greater risk. In such patients, a good response to treatment, with disappearance of the tumor from the bone marrow, may be associated with improvement of bone marrow function. However, in the absence of a good response, or in patients who have been previously treated with chemotherapeutic agents, hematopoiesis may be further compromised, and leukopenia, thrombocytopenia, and anemia may become more severe and lead to the demise of the patient.

➤*Chronic lymphatic leukemia:* Because drug toxicity, especially sensitivity to bone marrow failure, seems to be more common in chronic lymphatic leukemia than in other conditions, give the drug with great caution in this condition, if at all.

Adverse Reactions

➤*Dermatologic:* Occasionally, a maculopapular skin eruption occurs, but this may be idiosyncratic and does not necessarily recur with subsequent courses of the drug. Erythema multiforme has been observed. Herpes zoster, a common complicating infection in patients with lymphomas, may first appear after therapy is instituted, and on occasion may be precipitated by treatment. Discontinue further treatment during the acute phase of this illness to avoid progression to generalized herpes zoster.

➤*GI:* Mechlorethamine is given preferably at night in case sedation for side effects is required. Nausea and vomiting usually occur 1 to 3 hours after use of the drug. Emesis may disappear in the first 8 hours, but nausea may persist for 24 hours. Nausea and vomiting may be so severe as to precipitate vascular accidents in patients with a hemorrhagic tendency. Premedication with antiemetics, in addition to sedatives, may help control severe nausea and vomiting. Anorexia, weakness, and diarrhea may also occur.

➤*GU:* Since the gonads are susceptible to mechlorethamine, treatment may be followed by delayed catamenia, oligomenorrhea, or temporary or permanent amenorrhea. Impaired spermatogenesis, azoospermia, and total germinal aplasia have been reported in male patients treated with alkylating agents, especially in combination with other drugs. In some instances, spermatogenesis may return in patients in remission, but this may occur only several years after intensive chemotherapy has been discontinued. Warn patients of the potential risk to their reproductive capacity.

➤*Hematologic:* The usual course of mechlorethamine (total dose of 0.4 mg/kg either given as a single IV dose or divided into 2 or 4 daily doses of 0.2 or 0.1 mg/kg, respectively) generally produces a lymphocytopenia within 24 hours after the first injection; significant granulocytopenia occurs within 6 to 8 days and lasts for 10 days to 3 weeks. Agranulocytosis appears to be relatively infrequent and recovery from leukopenia in most cases is complete within 2 weeks of the maximum reduction. Thrombocytopenia is variable, but the time course of the appearance and recovery from reduced platelet counts generally parallels the sequence of granulocyte levels. In some cases, severe thrombocytopenia may lead to bleeding from the gums and GI tract, petechiae, and small subcutaneous hemorrhages; these symptoms appear to be transient, and, in most cases, disappear with return to a normal platelet count. However, a severe and even uncontrollable depression of the hematopoietic system occasionally may follow the usual dose of mechlorethamine, particularly in patients with widespread disease and debility and in patients previously treated with other antineoplastic agents or x-ray. Persistent pancytopenia has been reported. In rare instances, hemorrhagic complications may be due to hyperheparinemia. Erythrocyte and hemoglobin levels may decline during the first 2 weeks after therapy but rarely significantly. Depression of the hematopoietic system may be found up to 50 days or more after starting therapy.

➤*Local:* Thrombosis and thrombophlebitis may result from direct contact of the drug with the intima of the injected vein. Avoid high concentration and prolonged contact with the drug, especially in cases of elevated pressure in the antebrachial vein (eg, in mediastinal tumor compression from severe vena cava syndrome).

➤*Miscellaneous:* Hypersensitivity reactions, including anaphylaxis, have been reported. Nausea, vomiting, and depression of formed elements in the circulating blood are dose-limiting side effects and usually occur with the use of full doses of mechlorethamine. Jaundice, alopecia, vertigo, tinnitus, and diminished hearing may occur infrequently. Rarely, hemolytic anemia associated with such diseases as the lymphomas and chronic lymphocytic leukemia may be precipitated by treatment with alkylating agents including mechlorethamine. Also, various chromosomal abnormalities have been reported in association with nitrogen mustard therapy.

Overdosage

➤*Symptoms:* With total doses exceeding 0.4 mg/kg of body weight for a single course, severe leukopenia, anemia, thrombocytopenia, and a hemorrhagic diathesis with subsequent delayed bleeding may develop. Death may follow.

➤*Treatment:* The only treatment in instances of excessive dosage appears to be repeated blood-product transfusions, antibiotic treatment of complicating infections, and general supportive measures.

MELPHALAN (L-PAM; L-Phenylalanine Mustard; L-Sarcolysin)

Rx	**Alkeran** (Celgene)	**Tablets:** 2 mg	(GX EH3 A). Lactose. White. Film-coated. In amber glass bottles. In 50s.
		Powder for Injection, lyophilized: 50 mg	In single-use vials[1] with 10 mL vial of sterile diluent.[2]

[1] With 20 mg povidone.

[2] Water for injection with 0.2 g sodium citrate, 6 mL propylene glycol and 0.52 mL ethanol.

MELPHALAN — ORAL

WARNING

Melphalan should be administered under the supervision of a qualified physician experienced in the use of cancer chemotherapeutic agents. Severe bone marrow suppression with resulting infection or bleeding may occur. Melphalan is leukemogenic in humans.

Melphalan produces chromosomal aberrations in vitro and in vivo and, therefore, should be considered potentially mutagenic in humans.

Indications

➤*Multiple myeloma/epithelial ovarian cancer:* For the palliative treatment of multiple myeloma and for the palliation of nonresectable epithelial carcinoma of the ovary.

➤*Unlabeled uses:* Treatment of breast cancer, testicular cancer, and bone marrow transplantation.

Administration and Dosage

➤*Multiple myeloma:* The usual oral dose is 6 mg daily. The entire daily dose may be given at 1 time. The dose is adjusted, as required, on the basis of blood counts done at approximately weekly intervals. After 2 to 3 weeks of treatment, the drug should be discontinued for up to 4 weeks during which time the blood count should be followed carefully. When the white blood cell and platelet counts are rising, a maintenance dose of 2 mg daily may be instituted. Because of the patient-to-patient variation in melphalan plasma levels following oral administration of the drug, several investigators have recommended that the dosage of melphalan be cautiously escalated until some myelosuppression is observed in order to ensure that potentially therapeutic levels of the drug have been reached.

Alternate regimens – Other dosage regimens have been used by various investigators. Investigators in 1 study have used an initial course of 10 mg/day for 7 to 10 days. They report that maximal suppression of the leukocyte and platelet counts occurs within 3 to 5 weeks and recovery within 4 to 8 weeks. Continuous maintenance therapy with 2 mg/day is instituted when the white blood cell count is greater than 4000 cells/mcL and the platelet count is greater than 100,000 cells/mcL. Dosage is adjusted to between 1 and 3 mg/day depending upon the hematological response. It is desirable to try to maintain a significant degree of bone marrow depression so as to keep the leukocyte count in the range of 3000 to 3500 cells/mcL.

One study reports starting treatment with 0.15 mg/kg/day for 7 days. This is followed by a rest period of at least 14 days, but it may be as long as 5 to 6 weeks. Maintenance therapy is started when the white blood cell and

MELPHALAN — ORAL

platelet counts are rising. The maintenance dose is 0.05 mg/kg/day or less and is adjusted according to the blood count.

Another study has shown that the use of melphalan in combination with prednisone significantly improves the percentage of patients with multiple myeloma who achieve palliation. One regimen has been to administer courses of melphalan at 0.25 mg/kg/day for 4 consecutive days (or, 0.2 mg/kg/day for 5 consecutive days) for a total dose of 1 mg/kg per course. These 4- to 5-day courses are then repeated every 4 to 6 weeks if the granulocyte count and the platelet count have returned to normal levels.

It is to be emphasized that response may be very gradual over many months; it is important that repeated courses or continuous therapy be given since improvement may continue slowly over many months, and the maximum benefit may be missed if treatment is abandoned too soon.

➤*Renal function impairment:* In patients with moderate-to-severe renal impairment, currently available pharmacokinetic data do not justify an absolute recommendation on dosage reduction to those patients, but it may be prudent to use a reduced dose initially.

➤*Epithelial ovarian cancer:* One commonly employed regimen for the treatment of ovarian carcinoma has been to administer melphalan at a dose of 0.2 mg/kg/day for 5 days as a single course. Courses are repeated every 4 to 5 weeks depending upon hematologic tolerance.

➤*Storage/Stability:* Store in a refrigerator, 2° to 8°C (36° to 46°F). Protect from light.

Actions

➤*Pharmacology:* Melphalan is an alkylating agent of the bischloroethylamine type. As a result, its cytotoxicity appears to be related to the extent of its interstrand cross-linking with DNA, probably by binding at the N^7 position of guanine. Like other bifunctional alkylating agents, it is active against both resting and rapidly dividing tumor cells.

➤*Pharmacokinetics:*

Absorption/Distribution – The pharmacokinetics of melphalan after oral administration has been extensively studied in adult patients. Plasma melphalan levels are highly variable after oral dosing, both with respect to the time of the first appearance of melphalan in plasma (range 0 to 6 hours) and to the peak plasma concentration (C_{max}) (range 70 to 4000 ng/mL, depending on the dose) achieved. These results may be due to incomplete intestinal absorption, a variable "first pass" hepatic metabolism, or to rapid hydrolysis. Five patients were studied after both oral and IV dosing with 0.6 mg/kg as a single bolus dose by each route. The areas under the plasma concentration-time curves (AUC) after oral administration averaged 61% ± 26% (± standard deviation; range 25% to 89%) of those following IV administration.

The steady-state volume of distribution of melphalan is 0.5 L/kg. Penetration into cerebrospinal fluid (CSF) is low. The extent of melphalan binding to plasma proteins ranges from 60% to 90%. Serum albumin is the major binding protein, while α_1-acid glycoprotein appears to account for about 20% of the plasma protein binding. Approximately 30% of melphalan is (covalently) irreversibly bound to plasma proteins. Interactions with immunoglobulins have been found to be negligible.

Metabolism/Excretion – In 18 patients given a single oral dose of 0.6 mg/kg of melphalan, the terminal plasma half-life ($t_{1/2}$) of parent drug was 1.5 ± 0.83 hours. The 24-hour urinary excretion of parent drug in these patients was 10% ± 4.5%, suggesting that renal clearance is not a major route of elimination of parent drug.

In a separate study in 18 patients given single oral doses of 0.2 to 0.25 mg/kg of melphalan, C_{max} and AUC, when dose adjusted to a dose of 14 mg, were (mean ± SD) 212 ± 74 ng/mL and 498 ± 137 ng•hr/mL, respectively. Elimination phase $t_{1/2}$ in these patients was approximately 1 hour and the median t_{max} was 1 hour.

Melphalan is eliminated from plasma primarily by chemical hydrolysis to monohydroxymelphalan and dihydroxymelphalan. Aside from these hydrolysis products, no other melphalan metabolites have been observed in humans. Although the contribution of renal elimination to melphalan clearance appears to be low, 1 pharmacokinetic study showed a significant positive correlation between the elimination rate constant for melphalan and renal function and a significant negative correlation between renal function and the area under the plasma melphalan concentration/time curve.

Contraindications

Prior resistance to this agent; hypersensitivity to melphalan.

Warnings

➤*Bone marrow suppression:* As with other nitrogen mustard drugs, excessive dosage will produce marked bone marrow suppression. Bone marrow suppression is the most significant toxicity associated with melphalan in most patients. Therefore, the following tests should be performed at the start of therapy and prior to each subsequent course of melphalan: Platelet count, hemoglobin, white blood cell count, and differential. Thrombocytopenia or leukopenia are indications to withhold further therapy until the blood counts have sufficiently recovered. Frequent blood counts are essential to determine optimal dosage and to avoid toxicity. Dose adjustment on the basis of blood counts at the nadir and day of treatment should be considered.

➤*Hypersensitivity reactions:* Hypersensitivity reactions, including anaphylaxis, have occurred rarely. These reactions have occurred after multiple courses of treatment and have recurred in patients who experienced a hypersensitivity reaction to IV melphalan. If a hypersensitivity reaction occurs, oral or IV melphalan should not be readministered.

➤*Renal function impairment:* See Administration and Dosage for more information.

Patients with azotemia should be closely observed, however, in order to make dosage reductions, if required, at the earliest possible time.

➤*Carcinogenesis:* Secondary malignancies, including acute nonlymphocytic leukemia, myeloproliferative syndrome, and carcinoma have been reported in patients with cancer treated with alkylating agents (including melphalan). Some patients also received other chemotherapeutic agents or radiation therapy. Precise quantitation of the risk of acute leukemia, myeloproliferative syndrome, or carcinoma is not possible. Published reports of leukemia in patients who have received melphalan (and other alkylating agents) suggest that the risk of leukemogenesis increases with chronicity of treatment and with cumulative dose. In 1 study, the 10-year cumulative risk of developing acute leukemia or myeloproliferative syndrome after melphalan therapy was 19.5% for cumulative doses ranging from 730 mg to 9652 mg. In this same study, as well as in an additional study, the 10-year cumulative risk of developing acute leukemia or myeloproliferative syndrome after melphalan therapy was less than 2% for cumulative doses less than 600 mg. This does not mean that there is a cumulative dose below which there is no risk of the induction of secondary malignancy. The potential benefits from melphalan therapy must be weighed on an individual basis against the possible risk of the induction of a second malignancy.

Adequate and well-controlled carcinogenicity studies have not been conducted in animals. However, intraperitoneal administration of melphalan in rats (5.4 to 10.8 mg/m²) and in mice (2.25 to 4.5 mg/m²) 3 times per week for 6 months followed by 12 months post dose observation produced peritoneal sarcoma and lung tumors, respectively.

➤*Mutagenesis:* Melphalan has been shown to cause chromatid or chromosome damage in humans. IM administration of melphalan at 6 and 60 mg/m² produced structural aberrations of the chromatid and chromosomes in bone marrow cells of Wistar rats.

➤*Fertility impairment:* Melphalan causes suppression of ovarian function in premenopausal women, resulting in amenorrhea in a significant number of patients. Reversible and irreversible testicular suppression have also been reported.

➤*Pregnancy: Category D.* Melphalan may cause fetal harm when administered to a pregnant woman. Melphalan was embryolethal and teratogenic in rats following oral (6 to 18 mg/m² per day for 10 days) and intraperitoneal (18 mg/m²) administration. Malformations resulting from melphalan included alterations of the brain (underdevelopment, deformation, meningocele, and encephalocele) and eye (anophthalmia and microphthalmos), reduction of the mandible and tail, as well as hepatocele (exomphaly).

There are no adequate and well-controlled studies in pregnant women. If this drug is used during pregnancy, or if the patient becomes pregnant while taking this drug, the patient should be apprised of the potential hazard to the fetus. Women of childbearing potential should be advised to avoid becoming pregnant.

➤*Lactation:* It is not known whether this drug is excreted in human milk. Melphalan should not be given to nursing mothers.

➤*Children:* The safety and efficacy of melphalan in pediatric patients have not been established.

Precautions

➤*Monitoring:* Periodic complete blood counts with differentials should be performed during the course of treatment with melphalan. At least 1 determination should be obtained prior to each treatment course.

See Warnings for more information.

➤*Prior radiation/chemotherapy:* Melphalan should be used with extreme caution in patients whose bone marrow reserve may have been compromised by prior irradiation or chemotherapy, or whose marrow function is recovering from previous cytotoxic therapy. If the leukocyte count falls below 3000 cells/mcL, or the platelet count below 100,000 cells/mcL, melphalan should be discontinued until the peripheral blood cell counts have recovered.

Drug Interactions

Melphalan Drug Interactions

Precipitant drug	Object drug*		Description
Cisplatin	Melphalan	↑	Cisplatin may affect melphalan kinetics by inducing renal dysfunction and subsequently altering melphalan clearance.
Nalidixic acid	Melphalan	↑	Incidence of severe hemorrhagic necrotic enterocolitis has been reported to increase in pediatric patients.
Melphalan	Carmustine	↑	Carmustine lung toxicity threshold may be reduced.
Melphalan	Cyclosporine	↑	An increase in the toxicity of cyclosporine, particularly nephrotoxicity, has been observed following coadministration.

* ↑ = Object drug increased.

MELPHALAN — ORAL

Adverse Reactions

➤*GI:* GI disturbances such as nausea and vomiting, diarrhea, and oral ulceration occur infrequently.

➤*Hematologic:* The most common side effect is bone marrow suppression. Although bone marrow suppression frequently occurs, it is usually reversible if melphalan is withdrawn early enough. However, irreversible bone marrow failure has been reported.

➤*Hepatic:* Hepatic disorders ranging from abnormal liver function tests to clinical manifestations such as hepatitis and jaundice have been reported.

➤*Hypersensitivity:* See Warnings for more information.

➤*Miscellaneous:* Pulmonary fibrosis and interstitial pneumonitis, skin hypersensitivity, vasculitis, alopecia, and hemolytic anemia.

Overdosage

➤*Symptoms:* Overdoses, including doses up to 50 mg/day for 16 days, have been reported. Immediate effects are likely to be vomiting, ulceration of the mouth, diarrhea, and hemorrhage of the GI tract. The principal toxic effect is bone marrow suppression. Hematologic parameters should be closely followed for 3 to 6 weeks.

➤*Treatment:* An uncontrolled study suggests that administration of autologous bone marrow or hematopoietic growth factors (ie, sargramostim, filgrastim) may shorten the period of pancytopenia. General supportive measures, together with appropriate blood transfusions and antibiotics, should be instituted as deemed necessary by the physician. This drug is not removed from plasma to any significant degree by hemodialysis.

Patient Information

Patients should be informed that the major toxicities of melphalan are related to bone marrow suppression, hypersensitivity reactions, GI toxicity, and pulmonary toxicity. The major long-term toxicities are related to infertility and secondary malignancies. Patients should never be allowed to take the drug without close medical supervision and should be advised to consult their physician if they experience skin rash, vasculitis, bleeding, fever, persistent cough, nausea, vomiting, amenorrhea, weight loss, or unusual lumps/masses. Women of childbearing potential should be advised to avoid becoming pregnant.

MELPHALAN — INJECTION

WARNING

Melphalan should be administered under the supervision of a qualified physician experienced in the use of cancer chemotherapeutic agents. Severe bone marrow suppression with resulting infection or bleeding may occur. Controlled trials comparing IV to oral melphalan have shown more myelosuppression with the IV formulation. Hypersensitivity reactions, including anaphylaxis, have occurred in approximately 2% of patients who received the IV formulation. Melphalan is leukemogenic in humans. Melphalan produces chromosomal aberrations in vitro and in vivo and, therefore, should be considered potentially mutagenic in humans.

Indications

➤*Multiple myeloma:* For the palliative treatment of patients with multiple myeloma for whom oral therapy is not appropriate.

➤*Unlabeled uses:* Treatment of breast cancer, testicular cancer, and bone marrow transplantation.

Administration and Dosage

➤*Approved by the FDA:* November 18, 1992.

The usual IV dose is 16 mg/m^2. Dosage reduction of up to 50% should be considered in patients with renal insufficiency (BUN greater than or equal to 30 mg/dL). The drug is administered as a single infusion over 15 to 20 minutes. Melphalan is administered at 2-week intervals for 4 doses, then, after adequate recovery from toxicity, at 4-week intervals. Available evidence suggests about one-third to one-half of the patients with multiple myeloma show a favorable response to the drug. Experience with oral melphalan suggests that repeated courses should be given since improvement may continue slowly over many months, and the maximum benefit may be missed if treatment is abandoned prematurely. Dose adjustment on the basis of blood cell counts at the nadir and day of treatment should be considered.

➤*Preparation for administration/stability:*

1.) Melphalan for injection must be reconstituted by rapidly injecting 10 mL of the supplied diluent directly into the vial of lyophilized powder using a sterile needle (20-gauge or larger needle diameter) and syringe. Immediately shake vial vigorously until a clear solution is obtained. This provides a 5 mg/mL solution of melphalan. Rapid addition of the diluent followed by immediate vigorous shaking is important for proper dissolution.
2.) Immediately dilute the dose to be administered in 0.9% Sodium Chloride Injection to a concentration not more than 0.45 mg/mL.
3.) Administer the diluted product over a minimum of 15 minutes.
4.) Complete administration within 60 minutes of reconstitution.

The time between reconstitution/dilution and administration of melphalan should be kept to a minimum because reconstituted and diluted solutions of melphalan are unstable. Over as short a time as 30 minutes, a citrate derivative of melphalan has been detected in reconstituted material from the reaction of melphalan with sterile diluent for melphalan. Upon further dilution with saline, nearly 1% label strength of melphalan hydrolyzes every 10 minutes.

➤*Storage/Stability:* Store at controlled room temperature 15° to 30°C (59° to 86°F) and protect from light.

A precipitate forms if the reconstituted solution is stored at 5°C (41°F). Do not refrigerate the reconstituted product.

Actions

➤*Pharmacology:* Melphalan is an alkylating agent of the bischloroethylamine type. As a result, its cytotoxicity appears to be related to the extent of its interstrand cross-linking with DNA, probably by binding at the N^7 position of guanine. Like other bifunctional alkylating agents, it is active against both resting and rapidly dividing tumor cells.

➤*Pharmacokinetics:*

Absorption/Distribution – The pharmacokinetics of melphalan after IV administration has been extensively studied in adult patients. Following injection, drug plasma concentrations declined rapidly in a biexponential manner with distribution phase and terminal elimination phase half-lives of approximately 10 and 75 minutes, respectively. Mean (±SD) peak melphalan plasma concentrations in myeloma patients given IV melphalan at doses of 10 or 20 mg/m^2 were 1.2 ± 0.4 and 2.8 ± 1.9 mcg/mL, respectively.

The steady-state volume of distribution of melphalan is 0.5 L/kg. Penetration into cerebrospinal fluid (CSF) is low. The extent of melphalan binding to plasma proteins ranges from 60% to 90%. Serum albumin is the major binding protein, while α_1-acid glycoprotein appears to account for approximately 20% of the plasma protein binding. Approximately 30% of the drug is (covalently) irreversibly bound to plasma proteins. Interactions with immunoglobulins have been found to be negligible.

Metabolism/Excretion – Melphalan is eliminated from plasma primarily by chemical hydrolysis to monohydroxymelphalan and dihydroxymelphalan. Aside from these hydrolysis products, no other melphalan metabolites have been observed in humans. Although the contribution of renal elimination to melphalan clearance appears to be low, one study noted an increase in the occurrence of severe leukopenia in patients with elevated BUN after 10 weeks of therapy.

Estimates of average total body clearance varied among studies, but typical values of approximately 7 to 9 mL/min/kg (250 to 325 mL/min/m^2) were observed. One study has reported that on repeat dosing of 0.5 mg/kg every 6 weeks, the clearance of melphalan decreased from 8.1 mL/min/kg after the first course, to 5.5 mL/min/kg after the third course, but did not decrease appreciably after the third course.

Contraindications

Prior resistance to this agent; hypersensitivity to melphalan.

Warnings

➤*Bone marrow suppression:* As with other nitrogen mustard drugs, excessive dosage will produce marked bone marrow suppression. Bone marrow suppression is the most significant toxicity associated with melphalan for injection in most patients. Therefore, the following tests should be performed at the start of therapy and prior to each subsequent dose of melphalan: Platelet count, hemoglobin, white blood cell count, and differential. Thrombocytopenia or leukopenia are indications to withhold further therapy until the blood counts have sufficiently recovered. Frequent blood counts are essential to determine optimal dosage and to avoid toxicity. Dose adjustment on the basis of blood counts at the nadir and day of treatment should be considered.

➤*Hypersensitivity reactions:* Hypersensitivity reactions including anaphylaxis have occurred in approximately 2% of patients who received the IV formulation. These reactions usually occur after multiple courses of treatment. Treatment is symptomatic. The infusion should be terminated immediately, followed by the administration of volume expanders, pressor agents, corticosteroids, or antihistamines at the discretion of the physician. If a hypersensitivity reaction occurs, IV should not be readministered since hypersensitivity reactions have also been reported with oral melphalan.

➤*Renal function impairment:* See Administration and Dosage for more information.

➤*Carcinogenesis:* Secondary malignancies, including acute nonlymphocytic leukemia, myeloproliferative syndrome, and carcinoma, have been reported in patients with cancer treated with alkylating agents (including melphalan). Some patients also received other chemotherapeutic agents or radiation therapy. Precise quantitation of the risk of acute leukemia, myeloproliferative syndrome, or carcinoma is not possible. Published reports of leukemia in patients who have received melphalan (and other alkylating agents) suggest that the risk of leukemogenesis increases with chronicity of treatment and with cumulative dose. In 1 study, the 10-year cumulative risk of developing acute leukemia or myeloproliferative syndrome after oral melphalan therapy was 19.5% for cumulative doses ranging from 730 to 9652 mg. In this same study, as well as in an additional study, the 10-year cumulative risk of developing acute leukemia or myeloproliferative syndrome after oral melphalan therapy was less than 2% for cumulative doses less than 600 mg. This does not mean that there is a cumulative dose below which there is no risk of the induction of secondary malignancy. The potential benefits from melphalan therapy must be weighed on an individual basis against the possible risk of the induction of a second malignancy.

Adequate and well-controlled carcinogenicity studies have not been conducted in animals. However, intraperitoneal (IP) administration of mel-

MELPHALAN — INJECTION

phalan in rats (5.4 to 10.8 mg/m^2) and in mice (2.25 to 4.5 mg/m^2) 3 times per week for 6 months followed by 12 months post-dose observation produced peritoneal sarcoma and lung tumors, respectively.

➤*Mutagenesis:* Melphalan has been shown to cause chromatid or chromosome damage in humans. IM administration of melphalan at 6 and 60 mg/m^2 produced structural aberrations of the chromatid and chromosomes in bone marrow cells of Wistar rats.

➤*Fertility impairment:* Melphalan causes suppression of ovarian function in premenopausal women, resulting in amenorrhea in a significant number of patients. Reversible and irreversible testicular suppression have also been reported.

➤*Pregnancy: Category D.* Melphalan may cause fetal harm when administered to a pregnant woman. While adequate animal studies have not been conducted with IV melphalan, oral (6 to 18 mg/m^2 per day for 10 days) and IP (18 mg/m^2) administration in rats was embryolethal and teratogenic. Malformations resulting from melphalan included alterations of the brain (underdevelopment, deformation, meningocele, and encephalocele) and eye (anophthalmia and microphthalmos), reduction of the mandible and tail, as well as hepatocele (exomphaly). There are no adequate and well-controlled studies in pregnant women. If this drug is used during pregnancy, or if the patient becomes pregnant while taking this drug, the patient should be apprised of the potential hazard to the fetus. Women of childbearing potential should be advised to avoid becoming pregnant.

➤*Lactation:* It is not known whether this drug is excreted in human milk. IV melphalan should not be given to nursing mothers.

➤*Children:* Safety and efficacy in pediatric patients have not been established.

Precautions

➤*Monitoring:* Periodic complete blood counts with differentials should be performed during the course of treatment with melphalan. At least 1 determination should be obtained prior to each dose.

See Warnings for more information.

➤*Prior radiation and chemotherapy:* Melphalan should be used with extreme caution in patients whose bone marrow reserve may have been compromised by prior irradiation or chemotherapy or whose marrow function is recovering from previous cytotoxic therapy.

Drug Interactions

Melphalan Drug Interactions

Precipitant drug	Object drug*		Description
Cisplatin	Melphalan	↑	Cisplatin may affect melphalan kinetics by inducing renal dysfunction and subsequently altering melphalan clearance.
Nalidixic acid	Melphalan	↑	Incidence of severe hemorrhagic necrotic enterocolitis has been reported to increase in pediatric patients.
Melphalan	Carmustine	↑	Carmustine lung toxicity threshold may be reduced.
Melphalan	Cyclosporine	↑	An increase in the toxicity of cyclosporine, particularly nephrotoxicity, has been observed following coadministration.

* ↑ = Object drug increased.

Adverse Reactions

➤*GI:* GI disturbances such as nausea and vomiting, diarrhea, and oral ulceration occur infrequently.

➤*Hematologic:* The most common side effect is bone marrow suppression. White blood cell count and platelet count nadirs usually occur 2 to 3 weeks after treatment, with recovery in 4 to 5 weeks after treatment. Irreversible bone marrow failure has been reported.

➤*Hepatic:* Hepatic toxicity, including veno-occlusive disease, has been reported. Hepatic disorders ranging from abnormal liver function tests to clinical manifestations such as jaundice and hepatitis have been reported.

➤*Hypersensitivity:* Acute hypersensitivity reactions including anaphylaxis were reported in 2.4% of 425 patients receiving melphalan for injection for myeloma. These reactions were characterized by urticaria, pruritus, edema, and in some patients, tachycardia, bronchospasm, dyspnea, and hypotension. These patients appeared to respond to antihistamine and corticosteroid therapy. If a hypersensitivity reaction occurs, IV or oral melphalan should not be readministered since hypersensitivity reactions have also been reported with oral melphalan.

➤*Miscellaneous:* Other reported adverse reactions include skin hypersensitivity, skin ulceration at injection site, skin necrosis rarely requiring skin grafting, vasculitis, alopecia, hemolytic anemia, allergic reaction, pulmonary fibrosis, and interstitial pneumonitis.

Overdosage

➤*Symptoms:* Overdoses resulting in death have been reported. Overdoses, including doses up to 290 mg/m^2 have produced the following symptoms: Severe nausea and vomiting, decreased consciousness, convulsions, muscular paralysis, and cholinomimetic effects. Severe mucositis, stomatitis, colitis, diarrhea, and hemorrhage of the GI tract occur at high doses (greater than 100 mg/m^2).

Elevations in liver enzymes and veno-occlusive disease occur infrequently. Significant hyponatremia caused by an associated inappropriate secretion of ADH syndrome has been observed. Nephrotoxicity and adult respiratory distress syndrome have been reported rarely. The principal toxic effect is bone marrow suppression.

➤*Treatment:* Hematologic parameters should be closely followed for 3 to 6 weeks. An uncontrolled study suggests that administration of autologous bone marrow or hematopoietic growth factors (ie, sargramostim, filgrastim) may shorten the period of pancytopenia. General supportive measures together with appropriate blood transfusions and antibiotics should be instituted as deemed necessary by the physician. This drug is not removed from plasma to any significant degree by hemodialysis or hemoperfusion. A pediatric patient survived a 254 mg/m^2 overdose treated with standard supportive care.

Patient Information

Patients should be informed that the major acute toxicities of melphalan are related to bone marrow suppression, hypersensitivity reactions, GI toxicity, and pulmonary toxicity. The major long-term toxicities are related to infertility and secondary malignancies. Patients should never be allowed to take the drug without close medical supervision and should be advised to consult their physicians if they experience skin rash, signs or symptoms of vasculitis, bleeding, fever, persistent cough, nausea, vomiting, amenorrhea, weight loss, or unusual lumps/masses. Women of childbearing potential should be advised to avoid becoming pregnant.

ESTRAMUSTINE PHOSPHATE SODIUM

Rx	**Emcyt** (Pharmacia)	**Capsules:** 140 mg (as estramustine phosphate)	White. In 100s.

ESTRAMUSTINE PHOSPHATE SODIUM — ORAL

Indications

➤*Metastatic/Progressive prostate cancer:* Palliative treatment of metastatic and/or progressive carcinoma of the prostate.

➤*Unlabeled uses:* Treatment of metastatic renal cell carcinoma.

Administration and Dosage

➤*Recommended daily dosage:* 14 mg/kg/day (ie, one 140 mg capsule for each 10 kg or 22 lb) given in 3 or 4 divided doses (dosage range, 10 to 16 mg/kg/day).

Take with water at least 1 hour before or 2 hours after meals.

Milk, milk products, and calcium-rich foods or drugs (such as calcium-containing antacids) must not be taken simultaneously with estramustine phosphate sodium.

➤*Duration of therapy:* Treat for 30 to 90 days before assessing the possible benefits of continued therapy. Continue therapy as long as response is favorable. Some patients have been maintained on therapy for more than 3 years at doses ranging from 10 to 16 mg/kg/day.

➤*Storage/Stability:* Refrigerate at 2° to 8°C (36° to 46°F). Capsules may be left out of the refrigerator for 24 to 48 hours without affecting potency.

Actions

➤*Pharmacology:* Estramustine phosphate combines estradiol and nornitrogen mustard by a carbamate link. The molecule is phosphorylated to make it water soluble. The intent of the molecule design was for the estradiol portion to facilitate the uptake of the alkylating agent into the hormone-sensitive prostate cancer cells. However, it was determined that estramustine does not function in vivo as an alkylating agent and not all of its effects can be attributed to the estrogenic hormones. Estramustine has been shown to have weaker estrogenic effects than estradiol. It has been called an antimicrotubule agent because it covalently binds to microtubule-associated proteins, thereby inhibiting microtubule assembly and eventually causing their disassembly.

➤*Pharmacokinetics:*

Absorption/Distribution – After oral administration, estramustine is well absorbed with a bioavailability of at least 75%. Estramustine phosphate is readily dephosphorylated during absorption, and the major metabolites in plasma are estramustine, the estrone analog, estradiol, and estrone.

ESTRAMUSTINE PHOSPHATE SODIUM — ORAL

Prolonged treatment produces elevated total plasma concentrations of estradiol that are within ranges similar to the elevated estradiol levels found in prostatic cancer patients given conventional estradiol therapy. Estrogenic effects, as demonstrated by changes in circulating levels of steroids and pituitary hormones, are similar in patients treated with either estramustine phosphate or conventional estradiol.

Metabolism / Excretion – Estramustine is found in the body mainly as estromustine (17-keto analog).

The metabolic urinary patterns of estradiol and the estradiol moiety of estramustine phosphate are very similar, although the metabolites derived from estramustine phosphate are excreted at a slower rate. The nornitrogen mustard and estradiol metabolites are excreted independently into the bile, feces, and urine.

Contraindications

Hypersensitivity to estradiol or nitrogen mustard.

Active thrombophlebitis or thromboembolic disorders, except where the actual tumor mass is the cause of the thromboembolic phenomenon and the benefits of therapy outweigh the risks.

Warnings

➤*Thrombosis:* The risk of thrombosis, including fatal and nonfatal myocardial infarction, increases in men receiving estrogens for prostatic cancer. Use with caution in patients with a history of thrombophlebitis, thrombosis or thromboembolic disorders, especially if they were associated with estrogen therapy. Use with caution in patients with cerebral vascular or coronary artery disease.

➤*Glucose tolerance:* Tolerance to glucose may be decreased; observe diabetic patients receiving this drug.

➤*Elevated blood pressure:* Blood pressure elevation may occur; monitor blood pressure periodically during therapy.

➤*Hypersensitivity reactions:* Allergic reactions and angioedema at times involving the airway have been reported.

➤*Hepatic function impairment:* Estramustine may be poorly metabolized in patients with impaired liver function. Administer with caution.

➤*Carcinogenesis:* Long-term continuous administration of estrogens in certain animal species increases frequency of carcinomas of the breast and liver. Compounds structurally similar are carcinogenic in mice.

➤*Mutagenesis:* Although testing by the Ames method failed to demonstrate mutagenicity for estramustine, both estradiol and nitrogen mustard are mutagenic. For this reason, and because some patients who had been impotent while on estrogen therapy have regained potency while taking the drug, advise use of contraceptive measures.

Precautions

➤*Fluid retention:* Exacerbation of pre-existing or incipient peripheral edema or congestive heart disease may occur in some patients. Other conditions potentially influenced by fluid retention, such as epilepsy, migraine, or renal dysfunction, require careful observation.

➤*Calcium / Phosphorus metabolism:* Calcium/Phosphorus metabolism may be influenced by estramustine; use with caution in patients with metabolic bone diseases associated with hypercalcemia or in patients with renal insufficiency.

➤*Gynecomastia / Impotence:* Gynecomastia and impotence are known estrogenic effects.

➤*Lab test abnormalities:* Certain endocrine and liver function tests may be affected by estrogen-containing drugs. Estramustine phosphate sodium may depress testosterone levels. Abnormalities of hepatic enzymes and of bilirubin have occurred. Perform such tests at appropriate intervals during therapy and repeat after the drug has been withdrawn for 2 months.

Drug Interactions

➤*Drug / Food interactions:* Milk, milk products, and calcium-rich foods or drugs may impair the absorption of estramustine phosphate sodium.

Adverse Reactions

Estramustine Phosphate Sodium Adverse Reactions

Adverse reactions	Estramustine phosphate sodium (11.5 to 15.9 mg/kg/day) (n = 93)	Diethylstilbestrol (3 mg/day) (n = 93)
Cardiovascular		
Cardiac arrest	0	2
Cerebrovascular accident	2	0
MI	3	1
Thrombophlebitis	3	7
Pulmonary emboli	2	5
CHF	3	2
CNS		
Lethargy alone	4	3
Depression	0	2
Emotional lability	2	0
Insomnia	3	0
Headache	1	1
Anxiety	1	0
Dermatologic		
Rash	1	4
Pruritus	2	2
Dry skin	2	0
Pigment changes	0	3
Easy bruising	3	0
Flushing	1	0
Night sweats	0	1
Fingertip (peeling skin)	1	0
Thinning hair	1	1
GI		
Nausea	15	8
Diarrhea	12	11
Minor GI upset	11	6
Anorexia	4	3
Flatulence	2	0
Vomiting	1	1
GI bleeding	1	0
Burning throat	1	0
Thirst	1	0
GU		
Breast tenderness	66	64
Breast enlargement		
Mild	60	54
Moderate	10	16
Marked	0	5
Respiratory		
Dyspnea	11	3
Upper respiratory discharge	1	1
Hoarseness	1	0
Special senses		
Pain in eyes	0	1
Tearing of eyes	1	1
Tinnitus	0	1
Laboratory test abnormalities		
Hematologic		
Leukopenia	4	2
Thrombopenia	1	2
Hepatic		
Bilirubin alone	1	5
Bilirubin and LDH	0	1
Bilirubin and AST	2	1
Bilirubin, LDH, AST	2	0
LDH and/or AST	31	28
Miscellaneous		
Hypercalcemia (transient)	0	1
Leg cramps	8	11
Edema	19	17
Chest pain	1	1
Hot flashes	0	1

Overdosage

Although there has been no experience with overdosage, it may produce pronounced manifestations of the adverse reactions. In the event of overdosage, evacuate gastric contents by gastric lavage and initiate symptomatic therapy. Monitor hematologic and hepatic parameters for at least 6 weeks after overdosage.

Patient Information

Because of the possibility of mutagenic effects, use contraceptive measures.

Take with water at least 1 hour before or 2 hours after meals.

Milk, milk products, and calcium-rich foods or drugs (such as calcium-containing antacids) must not be taken simultaneously with estramustine phosphate sodium.

CARMUSTINE (BCNU)

Rx	**BiCNU** (Bristol Labs Oncology)	**Powder for Injection, lyophilized**: 100 mg	Preservative-free. In single-dose vials with 3 mL sterile diluent.
Rx	**Gliadel** (Guilford Pharm.)	**Wafer**: 7.7 mg	Preservative-free. In single-dose treatment box with 8 individually pouched wafers.

CARMUSTINE — INJECTION

WARNING

Carmustine for injection should be administered under the supervision of a qualified physician experienced in the use of cancer chemotherapeutic agents.

Bone marrow suppression, notably thrombocytopenia and leukopenia, which may contribute to bleeding and overwhelming infections in an already compromised patient, is the most common and severe of the toxic effects of carmustine for injection (see Warnings and Adverse Reactions).

Since the major toxicity is delayed bone marrow suppression, blood counts should be monitored weekly for at least 6 weeks after a dose (see Adverse Reactions). At the recommended dosage, courses of carmustine for injection should not be given more frequently than every 6 weeks.

The bone marrow toxicity of carmustine for injection is cumulative and therefore dosage adjustment must be considered on the basis of nadir blood counts from prior dose (see Administration and Dosage).

Pulmonary toxicity from carmustine for injection appears to be dose related. Patients receiving greater than 1400 mg/m^2 cumulative dose are at significantly higher risk than those receiving less.

Delayed pulmonary toxicity can occur years after treatment, and can result in death, particularly in patients treated in childhood (see Adverse Reactions, and Warnings; Children).

Indications

As palliative therapy as a single agent or in established combination therapy with other approved chemotherapeutic agents in the following:

1.) Brain tumors (glioblastoma, brainstem glioma, medulloblastoma, astrocytoma, ependymoma, and metastatic brain tumors).
2.) Multiple myeloma in combination with prednisone.
3.) Hodgkin's disease as secondary therapy in combination with other approved drugs in patients who relapse while being treated with primary therapy, or who fail to respond to primary therapy.
4.) Non-Hodgkin's lymphomas as secondary therapy in combination with other approved drugs for patients who relapse while being treated with primary therapy, or who fail to respond to primary therapy.

➤*Unlabeled uses:* Treatment of hematopoietic stem cell transplantation (HSCT), mycosis fungoides, colorectal carcinoma, malignant melanoma.

Administration and Dosage

The recommended dose of carmustine for injection as a single agent in previously untreated patients is 150 to 200 mg/m^2 intravenously every 6 weeks. This may be given as a single dose or divided into daily injections such as 75 to 100 mg/m^2 on 2 successive days. When carmustine for injection is used in combination with other myelosuppressive drugs or in patients in whom bone marrow reserve is depleted, the doses should be adjusted accordingly.

Doses subsequent to the initial dose should be adjusted according to the hematologic response of the patient to the preceding dose. The following schedule is suggested as a guide to dosage adjustment:

Carmustine Injection Dosage Adjustment

Nadir after prior dose		
Leukocytes/mm^3	Platelets/mm^3	Percentage of prior dose to be given
> 4000	> 100,000	100%
3000 to 3999	75,000 to 99,999	100%
2000 to 2999	25,000 to 74,999	70%
< 2000	< 25,000	50%

A repeat course of carmustine for injection should not be given until circulating blood elements have returned to acceptable levels (platelets above 100,000/mm^3, leukocytes above 4000/mm^3), and this is usually in 6 weeks. Adequate number of neutrophils should be present on a peripheral blood smear. Blood counts should be monitored weekly and repeat courses should not be given before 6 weeks because the hematologic toxicity is delayed and cumulative.

➤*Administration precautions:* As with other potentially toxic compounds, caution should be exercised in handling carmustine for injection and preparing the solution of carmustine for injection. Accidental contact of reconstituted carmustine for injection with the skin has caused transient hyperpigmentation of the affected areas. The use of gloves is recommended. If carmustine for injection lyophilized material or solution contacts the skin or mucosa, immediately wash the skin or mucosa thoroughly with soap and water.

The reconstituted solution should be used intravenously only and should be administered by IV drip. Injection of carmustine for injection over shorter periods of time than 1 to 2 hours may produce intense pain and burning at the site of injection.

➤*Preparation of intravenous solutions:* First, dissolve carmustine for injection with 3 mL of the supplied sterile diluent (Dehydrated Alcohol Injection, USP). Second, aseptically add 27 mL Sterile Water for Injection, USP. Each mL of resulting solution contains 3.3 mg of carmustine for injection in 10% ethanol. Such solutions should be protected from light.

Reconstitution as recommended results in a clear, colorless to yellowish solution which may be further diluted with 5% Dextrose Injection, USP. Parenteral drug products should be inspected visually for particulate matter and discoloration prior to administration, whenever solution and container permit.

➤*Important note:* The lyophilized dosage formulation contains no preservatives and is not intended for use as a multiple dose vial.

➤*Storage/Stability:* Unopened vials of the dry drug must be stored in a refrigerator (2° to 8°C; 36° to 46°F). The recommended storage of unopened vials provides a stable product for 2 years. After reconstitution as recommended, carmustine for injection is stable for 8 hours at room temperature (25°C; 77°F), protected from light.

Vials reconstituted as directed and further diluted to a concentration of 0.2 mg/mL in 5% Dextrose Injection, USP, should be stored at room temperature, protected from light and utilized within 8 hours.

Glass containers were used for the stability data provided in this section. Only use glass containers for carmustine for injection administration.

Important note – Carmustine for injection has a low melting point (30.5° to 32°C; 86.9° to 89.6°F). Exposure of the drug to this temperature or above will cause the drug to liquefy and appear as an oil film on the vials. This is a sign of decomposition and vials should be discarded. If there is a question of adequate refrigeration upon receipt of this product, immediately inspect the larger vial in each individual carton. Hold the vial to the bright light for inspection. The carmustine for injection will appear as a very small amount of dry flakes or dry congealed mass. If this is evident, the carmustine for injection is suitable for use and should be refrigerated immediately.

Store dry powder in refrigerator (2° to 8°C; 36° to 46°F).

Actions

➤*Pharmacology:* Although it is generally agreed that carmustine alkylates DNA and RNA, it is not cross-resistant with other alkylators. As with other nitrosoureas, it may also inhibit several key enzymatic processes by carbamoylation of amino acids in proteins.

➤*Pharmacokinetics:* Intravenously administered carmustine is rapidly degraded, with no intact drug detectable after 15 minutes. However, in studies with C^{14}-labeled drug, prolonged levels of the isotope were detected in the plasma and tissue, probably representing radioactive fragments of the parent compound.

It is thought that the antineoplastic and toxic activities of carmustine may be due to metabolites. Approximately 60% to 70% of a total dose is excreted in the urine in 96 hours and about 10% as respiratory CO_2. The fate of the remainder is undetermined.

Because of the high lipid solubility and the relative lack of ionization at physiological pH, carmustine crosses the blood-brain barrier quite effectively. Levels of radioactivity in the CSF are ≥ 50% of those measured concurrently in plasma.

Contraindications

Hypersensitivity to carmustine.

Warnings

➤*Bone marrow suppression:* See the Warning box for more information.

➤*Pulmonary toxicity:* See the Warning box for more information.

➤*Long-term use:* Long-term use of nitrosoureas has been reported to be associated with the development of secondary malignancies.

➤*Ocular:* Carmustine for injection has been administered through an intraarterial intracarotid route; this procedure is investigational and has been associated with ocular toxicity.

➤*Renal/Hepatic function impairment:* Liver and renal function tests should be monitored periodically (see Adverse Reactions).

➤*Carcinogenesis:* Carmustine for injection is carcinogenic in rats and mice, producing a marked increase in tumor incidence in doses approximating those employed clinically. Nitrosourea therapy does have carcinogenic potential in humans (see Adverse Reactions).

➤*Fertility impairment:* Carmustine for injection also affects fertility in male rats at doses somewhat higher than the human dose.

➤*Pregnancy: Category D.* Carmustine for injection may cause fetal harm when administered to a pregnant woman. Carmustine for injection has been shown to be embryotoxic in rats and rabbits and teratogenic in rats when given in doses equivalent to the human dose. There are no adequate and well-controlled studies in pregnant women. If this drug is used during pregnancy, or if the patient becomes pregnant while taking (receiving) this drug, the patient should be apprised of the potential hazard to the fetus. Women of childbearing potential should be advised to avoid becoming pregnant.

CARMUSTINE — INJECTION

➤*Lactation:* It is not known whether this drug is excreted in human milk. Because of the potential for serious adverse events in nursing infants, nursing should be discontinued while taking carmustine for injection.

➤*Children:* Safety and effectiveness in children have not been established. Delayed onset pulmonary fibrosis occurring up to 17 years after treatment, has been reported in a long-term study of patients who received carmustine for injection in childhood and early adolescence (1 to 16 years of age). Eight out of the 17 patients (47%) who survived childhood brain tumors, including all the 5 patients initially treated at younger than 5 years of age, died of pulmonary fibrosis. Therefore, the risks and benefits of carmustine for injection therapy must be carefully considered, due to the extremely high risk of pulmonary toxicity (see Adverse Reactions, Pulmonary toxicity).

Precautions

➤*Monitoring:* In all instances where the use of carmustine for injection is considered for chemotherapy, the physician must evaluate the need and usefulness of the drug against the risks of toxic effects or adverse reactions. Most such adverse reactions are reversible if detected early. When such effects or reactions do occur, the drug should be reduced in dosage or discontinued and appropriate corrective measures should be taken according to the clinical judgment of the physician. Reinstitution of carmustine for injection therapy should be carried out with caution, and with adequate consideration of the further need for the drug and alertness as to possible recurrence of toxicity.

Due to delayed bone marrow suppression, blood counts should be monitored weekly for at least 6 weeks after a dose.

Baseline pulmonary function studies should be conducted along with frequent pulmonary function tests during treatment. Patients with a baseline below 70% of the predicted Forced Vital Capacity (FVC) or Carbon Monoxide Diffusing Capacity (DL_{CO}) are particularly at risk.

See Warnings for more information.

Drug Interactions

Carmustine Drug Interactions

Precipitant drug	Object drug*		Description
Cimetidine	Carmustine	⬆	Cimetidine may enhance the myelosuppressive effects of carmustine, possibly to the point of toxicity. Avoid if possible.
Carmustine	Digoxin	⬇	Digoxin serum levels may be reduced, and its actions may be decreased by a combination chemotherapy regimen including carmustine.
Carmustine	Phenytoin	⬇	Phenytoin serum concentrations may be decreased by a combination chemotherapy regimen including carmustine.

* ⬆ = Object drug increased. ⬇ = Object drug decreased.

Adverse Reactions

➤*GI:* Nausea and vomiting after IV administration of carmustine for injection are noted frequently. This toxicity appears within 2 hours of dosing, usually lasting 4 to 6 hours, and is dose related. Prior administration of antiemetics is effective in diminishing and sometimes preventing this side effect.

➤*Hematologic:* A frequent and serious toxicity of carmustine for injection is delayed myelosuppression. It usually occurs 4 to 6 weeks after drug administration and is dose related. Thrombocytopenia occurs at about 4 weeks postadministration and persists for 1 to 2 weeks. Leukopenia occurs at 5 to 6 weeks after a dose of carmustine for injection and persists for 1 to 2 weeks. Thrombocytopenia is generally more severe than leukopenia. However, both may be dose-limiting toxicities.

Carmustine for injection may produce cumulative myelosuppression, manifested by more depressed indices or longer duration of suppression after repeated doses.

The occurrence of acute leukemia and bone marrow dysplasias have been reported in patients following long-term nitrosourea therapy.

Anemia also occurs, but is less frequent and less severe than thrombocytopenia or leukopenia.

➤*Hepatic:* A reversible type of hepatic toxicity, manifested by increased transaminase, alkaline phosphatase, and bilirubin levels, has been reported in a small percentage of patients receiving carmustine for injection.

➤*Pulmonary:* Pulmonary toxicity characterized by pulmonary infiltrates and/or fibrosis has been reported to occur from 9 days to 43 months after treatment with carmustine for injection and related nitrosoureas. Most of these patients were receiving prolonged therapy with total doses of carmustine for injection greater than 1400 mg/m^2. However, there have been reports of pulmonary fibrosis in patients receiving lower total doses. Other risk factors include past history of lung disease and duration of treatment. Cases of fatal pulmonary toxicity with carmustine for injection have been reported.

Additionally, delayed onset pulmonary fibrosis occurring up to 17 years after treatment has been reported in a long-term study with 17 patients who received carmustine for injection in childhood and early adolescence (1 to 16 years) in cumulative doses ranging from 770 to 1800 mg/m^2 combined with cranial radiotherapy for intracranial tumors. Chest x-rays demonstrated pulmonary hypoplasia with upper zone contraction. Gallium scans were normal in all cases. Thoracic CT scans have demonstrated an unusual pattern of upper zone fibrosis. There was some late reduction of pulmonary function in all long-term survivors. This form of lung fibrosis may be slowly progressive and has resulted in death in some cases. In this long-term study, 8 of 17 died of delayed pulmonary lung fibrosis, including all those initially treated (5 of 17) at younger than 5 years of age.

➤*Renal:* Renal abnormalities consisting of progressive azotemia, decrease in kidney size and renal failure have been reported in patients who received large cumulative doses after prolonged therapy with carmustine for injection and related nitrosoureas. Kidney damage has also been reported occasionally in patients receiving lower total doses.

➤*Miscellaneous:* Accidental contact of reconstituted carmustine for injection with skin has caused burning and hyperpigmentation of the affected areas.

Rapid IV infusion of carmustine for injection may produce intensive flushing of the skin and suffusion of the conjunctiva within 2 hours, lasting about 4 hours. It is also associated with burning at the site of injection although true thrombosis is rare.

Neuroretinitis, chest pain, headache, allergic reaction, hypotension and tachycardia have been reported as part of ongoing surveillance.

Overdosage

No proven antidotes have been established for carmustine for injection overdosage.

Patient Information

Contraceptive measures are recommended during therapy.

CARMUSTINE — IMPLANT

WARNING

Delayed pulmonary toxicity can occur years after treatment and can result in death, particularly in patients treated in childhood.

Indications

As an adjunct to surgery and radiation in newly diagnosed high-grade malignant glioma patients; in recurrent glioblastoma multiforme patients as an adjunct to surgery.

➤*Unlabeled uses:* Topical carmustine has been shown to be effective in the treatment of primary cutaneous T-cell lymphoma (ie, mycosis fungoides and Sezary syndrome). Carmustine, alone or in combination therapy, has also shown some benefit in the management of malignant melanoma.

Administration and Dosage

It is recommended that 8 wafers be placed in the resection cavity if the size and shape of cavity allows. Should the size and shape not accommodate 8 wafers, the maximum number of wafers as allowed should be used to cover as much of the resection cavity as possible. Slight overlapping of the wafer is acceptable. Wafers broken in half may be used, but discard wafers broken in more than 2 pieces. Oxidized regenerated cellulose may be placed over the wafers to secure them against the cavity surface. After placement of the wafers, the resection cavity should be irrigated and the dura closed in a water-tight fashion.

➤*Preparation/Handling:* Use of double gloves is recommended because exposure to carmustine can cause severe burning and hyperpigmentation of the skin. Use surgical instruments dedicated to the handling of the wafers for implantation. Deliver the aluminum foil laminate pouches containing the wafer to the operating room and leave unopened until ready to implant the wafers.

➤*Storage/Stability:* Unopened foil pouches may be kept at ambient room temperature for a maximum of 6 hours at a time. Store at or below -20°C (-4°F).

Actions

➤*Pharmacology:* Carmustine alkylates deoxyribonucleic acid (DNA) and ribonucleic acid (RNA) and also inhibits several enzymes by carbamoylation of amino acids in proteins. Carmustine is not cross resistant with other alkylators. Antineoplastic and toxic activities may be caused by metabolites.

➤*Pharmacokinetics:* Wafers are biodegradable in the human brain when implanted into the cavity after tumor resection. The carmustine released from the wafer diffuses into the surrounding brain tissue. The rate of biodegradation is variable from patient to patient. A wafer remnant may be observed on brain imaging scans or at re-operation even though extensive degradation of all components has occurred. The absorption, distribution, metabolism, and excretion of the copolymer in humans is unknown.

Contraindications

Hypersensitivity to carmustine or to any components of the wafer formulation.

Warnings

➤*Hematologic:* The most frequent and serious toxic effect of injectable carmustine is delayed myelosuppression, which usually occurs 4 to 6 weeks after administration and is dose related (see Warning Box). Thrombocytopenia occurs at about 4 weeks postadministration and persists for 1 to

CARMUSTINE — IMPLANT

2 weeks. Leukopenia occurs at 5 to 6 weeks after a dose and persists for 1 to 2 weeks Thrombocytopenia is generally more severe than leukopenia; however, both may have dose-limiting toxicities.

➤*Ocular:* Carmustine administration through an intra-arterial intracarotid route is investigational and has been associated with ocular toxicity.

➤*Brain herniation:* Cases of intracerebral mass effect unresponsive to corticosteroids have been described in patients treated with the wafer, including one case leading to brain herniation.

➤*Seizures:* In the initial surgery trial, the incidence of seizures was 33.3% in patients receiving carmustine wafer and 37.5% in patients receiving placebo. Grand mal seizures occurred in 5% of wafer-treated patients and 4.2% of placebo-treated patients. The incidence of seizures within the first 5 days after wafer implantation was 2.5% in the wafer group and 4.2% in the placebo group. The time from surgery to the onset of the first postoperative seizure did not differ between the wafer and placebo-treated patients.

In the surgery for recurrent disease trial, the incidence of postoperative seizures was the same for the wafer treatment group and placebo (19%). Of the 22 patients, 54% of wafer-treated patients and 9% of placebo patients experienced the first new or worsened seizure within the first 5 postoperative days; the median time to onset was 3.5 days and 61 days, respectively.

➤*Brain edema:* Brain edema was noted in 22.5% of patients treated with the wafer and in 19.2% of placebo patients. Development of brain edema with mass effect (caused by tumor recurrence, intracranial infection, or necrosis) may necessitate re-operation and, in some cases, removal of the wafer or its remnants.

➤*Intracranial infection:* In the initial surgery trial, the incidence of brain abscess or meningitis was 5% in patients treated with carmustine wafer and 6% in patients receiving placebo. In the recurrent setting, the incidence of brain abscess or meningitis was 4% in patients treated with the wafer and 1% in patients receiving placebo.

➤*Obstructive hydrocephalus:* Avoid communication between the surgical resection cavity and the ventricular system to prevent the wafers from migrating into the ventricular system and causing obstructive hydrocephalus. If a communication exists larger than the diameter of a wafer, close it prior to wafer implantation.

➤*Carcinogenesis:* Carmustine injection is carcinogenic in rats and mice, producing a marked increase in tumor incidence in doses approximating those employed clinically. Nitrosourea therapy does have carcinogenic potential in humans. There were increases in tumor incidence in all treated animals, predominantly SC and lung neoplasms. Long-term use of nitrosoureas has been reported to be associated with the development of secondary malignancies.

➤*Mutagenesis:* Carmustine was mutagenic in vitro (Ames assay, human lymphoblast HGPRT assay) and clastogenic both in vitro (V79 hamster cell micronucleus assay) and in vivo (SCE assay in rodent brain tumors, mouse bone marrow micronucleus assay).

➤*Fertility impairment:* Carmustine injection affects fertility in male rats at doses somewhat higher than the human dose. Carmustine caused testicular degeneration at intraperitoneal doses of 8 mg/kg/week for 8 weeks (about 1.3 times the recommended human dose on a mg/m^2 basis) in male rats.

➤*Pregnancy: Category D.* Carmustine is embryotoxic and teratogenic in rats and embryotoxic in rabbits at dose levels equivalent to the human dose. Carmustine may cause fetal harm when administered to a pregnant woman. There are no adequate and well-controlled studies in pregnant women. If this drug is used during pregnancy, or if the patient becomes pregnant while taking this drug, advise her of the potential hazard to the fetus. Advise women of childbearing potential to avoid becoming pregnant.

➤*Lactation:* It is not known whether this drug is excreted in breast milk. Because of the potential for serious adverse reactions in breastfeeding infants from carmustine, discontinue nursing.

➤*Children:* Safety and efficacy for use in children have not been established. Delayed-onset pulmonary fibrosis occurring up to 17 years after treatment, has been reported in a long-term study of patients who received carmustine injection in childhood and early adolescence (1 to 16 years of age). Eight out of the 17 patients (47%) who survived childhood brain tumors, including all of the 5 patients initially treated at less than 5 years of age, died of pulmonary fibrosis. Therefore, the risks and benefits of carmustine injection therapy must be carefully considered, because of the extremely high risk of pulmonary toxicity (see Adverse Reactions).

Precautions

➤*Monitoring:* Monitor patients undergoing craniotomy for malignant glioma and implantation of the wafer closely for known complications of craniotomy, including seizures, intracranial infections, abnormal wound healing, and brain edema.

Computed tomography and magnetic resonance imaging of the head may demonstrate enhancement in the brain tissue surrounding the resection cavity after implantation of carmustine wafers. This enhancement may represent edema and inflammation caused by the wafer or tumor progression.

➤*Healing abnormalities:* The following healing abnormalities have been reported in clinical trials of carmustine wafer: Wound dehiscence, delayed wound healing, subdural, subgaleal, or wound effusions, and cerebrospinal fluid lead. In the initial surgery trial, healing abnormalities occurred in 15.8% of carmustine wafer-treated patients and in 11.7% of placebo recipients. Cerebrospinal fluid leaks occurred in 5% of carmustine wafer recipients and 0.8% of those given placebo. During surgery, obtain a water-tight dural closure to minimize the risk of cerebrospinal fluid leak.

In the surgery for recurrent disease trial, the incidence of healing abnormalities was 14% in carmustine-wafer treated patients and 5% in patients receiving placebo wafers.

Drug Interactions

Carmustine Drug Interactions

Precipitant drug	Object drug*		Description
Cimetidine	Carmustine	↑	Cimetidine may enhance the myelosuppressive effects of carmustine, possibly to the point of toxicity. Avoid if possible.
Carmustine	Digoxin	↓	Digoxin serum levels may be reduced, and its actions may be decreased by a combination chemotherapy regimen including carmustine.
Carmustine	Phenytoin	↓	Phenytoin serum concentrations may be decreased by a combination chemotherapy regimen including carmustine.

* ↑ = Object drug increased. ↓ = Object drug decreased.

Adverse Reactions

Adverse Events Observed in Patients Receiving Carmustine Wafer at Initial Surgery (≥ 5%)

Adverse reaction	Carmustine wafer (N = 120)	Placebo (N = 120)
Cardiovascular		
Deep thrombophlebitis	10	9
Pulmonary embolus	8	8
Hemorrhage	7	6
CNS		
Headache	28	37
Hemiplegia	41	44
Convulsion	33	38
Confusion	23	21
Brain edema	23	19
Aphasia	18	18
Depression	16	10
Somnolence	11	15
Speech disorder	11	8
Amnesia	9	10
Intracranial hypertension	9	2
Personality disorder	8	8
Anxiety	7	4
Facial paralysis	7	4
Neuropathy	7	10
Ataxia	6	4
Hypesthesia	6	5
Paresthesia	6	8
Thinking abnormal	6	8
Abnormal gait	5	5
Dizziness	5	9
Grand mal convulsion	5	4
Hallucinations	5	3
Insomnia	5	6
Tremor	5	7
Coma	4	5
Incoordination	3	7
Hypokinesia	2	7
Endocrine system		
Diabetes mellitus	5	4
Cushing syndrome	3	5
Alopecia	10	12
GI		
Nausea	22	17
Vomiting	21	16
Constipation	19	12
Abdominal pain	8	2
Diarrhea	5	4
Liver function tests abnormal	1	5

CARMUSTINE — IMPLANT

Adverse Events Observed in Patients Receiving Carmustine Wafer at Initial Surgery (≥ 5%)		
Adverse reaction	Carmustine wafer (N = 120)	Placebo (N = 120)
GU		
Urinary tract infection	8	11
Urinary incontinence	8	8
Metabolic/Nutritional disorders		
Healing abnormal	16	12
Peripheral edema	9	9
Respiratory		
Pneumonia	8	8
Dyspnea	3	7
Special senses		
Conjunctival edema	7	7
Abnormal vision	6	6
Visual field defect	5	7
Eye disorder	3	5
Diplopia	1	5
Miscellaneous		
Aggravation reaction[1]	82	79
Asthenia	22	15
Infection	18	20
Fever	18	18
Pain	13	15
Rash	12	11
Back pain	7	3
Face edema	6	5
Abscess	5	3
Accidental injury	5	7
Chest pain	5	0
Allergic reaction	2	5
Myasthenia	4	5

[1] Adverse events coded to "aggravation reaction" were usually events involving tumor/disease progression or general deterioration of condition (eg, condition/health/Karnofsky/neurological/physical deterioration).

Adverse Reactions: Carmustine Wafer vs Placebo for Recurrent Disease (≥ 4%)		
Adverse reaction	Wafer with carmustine (n=110; %)	Wafer without carmustine (n=112; %)
CNS		
Convulsion	19	19
Hemiplegia	19	20
Headache	15	13
Somnolence	14	11
Confusion	10	8
Aphasia	9	11
Stupor	6	6
Brain edema	4	1
Intracranial hypertension	4	6
Meningitis or abscess	4	1
Miscellaneous		
Urinary tract infection	21	17
Healing abnormal	14	5
Fever	12	8
Nausea and vomiting	8	6
Pain	7	1
Rash	5	4

➤*Cardiovascular:* Hypertension (3%); hypotension (1%).

➤*CNS:* Seizures, brain edema (see Warnings); hydrocephalus, depression (3%); abnormal thinking, ataxia, dizziness, insomnia, monoplegia (2%); coma, amnesia, diplopia, paranoid reaction (1%); cerebral hemorrhage and cerebral infarct (less than 1%).

➤*GI:* Diarrhea, constipation (2%); dysphagia, GI hemorrhage, fecal incontinence (1%).

➤*Hematologic / Lymphatic:* Thrombocytopenia, leukocytosis (1%).

➤*Metabolic / Nutritional:* Hyponatremia, hyperglycemia (3%); hypokalemia (1%).

➤*Respiratory:* Infection (2%); aspiration pneumonia (1%).

➤*Special senses:* Visual field defect (2%); eye pain (1%).

➤*Miscellaneous:* Healing abnormalities, intracranial infection (see Warnings and Precautions); peripheral edema, neck pain, rash, urinary incontinence (2%); accidental injury, back pain, allergic reaction, asthenia, chest pain, sepsis (1%).

Overdosage

No proven antidotes have been established for carmustine overdosage.

Patient Information

Contraceptive measures are recommended during therapy.

LOMUSTINE (CCNU)

Rx	**CeeNU** (Bristol Labs Oncology)	**Capsules:** 10 mg	Mannitol. Two-tone white. In 20s.
		40 mg	Mannitol. White/green. In 20s.
		100 mg	Mannitol. Two-tone green. In 20s.
		Dose Pack: Two 100 mg capsules, two 40 mg capsules and two 10 mg capsules.	

LOMUSTINE — ORAL

WARNING

Bone marrow suppression, notably thrombocytopenia and leukopenia, which may contribute to bleeding and overwhelming infections in an already compromised patient, is the most common and severe of the toxic effects of lomustine.

Because the major toxicity is delayed bone marrow suppression, monitor blood counts weekly for ≥ 6 weeks after a dose. At the recommended dosage, do not give courses of lomustine more frequently than every 6 weeks.

Bone marrow toxicity is cumulative. Consider dosage adjustments on the basis of nadir blood counts from prior dosage (see Administration and Dosage and Warnings).

Indications

➤*Brain Tumors:* Both primary and metastatic, in patients who have already received appropriate surgical and/or radiotherapeutic procedures.

➤*Hodgkin's Disease:* Secondary therapy in combination with other approved drugs in patients who relapse while being treated with primary therapy, or who fail to respond to primary therapy.

Administration and Dosage

➤*Adults and children:* The recommended dose in adults and children as a single agent in previously untreated patients is 130 mg/m^2 as a single oral dose every 6 weeks. In individuals with compromised bone marrow function, the dose should be reduced to 100 mg/m^2 every 6 weeks. When lomustine is used in combination with other myelosuppressive drugs, the doses should be adjusted accordingly.

Doses subsequent to the initial dose should be adjusted according to the hematologic response of the patient to the preceding dose.

Lomustine Dosage Adjustment		
Nadir after prior dose		
Leukocytes	Platelets	Percentage of prior dose to be given
> 4000	> 100,000	100%
3000 to 3999	75,000 to 99,999	100%
2000 to 2999	25,000 to 74,999	70%
< 2000	< 25,000	50%

A repeat course of lomustine should not be given until circulating blood elements have returned to acceptable levels (platelets above 100,000/mm^2, leukocytes above 4000/mm^2) and this is usually in 6 weeks. Adequate number of neutrophils should be present on a peripheral blood smear. Blood counts should be monitored weekly and repeat courses should not be given before 6 weeks because the hematologic toxicity is delayed and cumulative.

➤*Storage / Stability:* Store at room temperature in well closed containers. Avoid excessive heat (over 40°C; 104°F).

LOMUSTINE — ORAL

Actions

➤*Pharmacology:* Although it is generally agreed that lomustine alkylates DNA and RNA, it is not cross resistant with other alkylators. As with other nitrosoureas, it may also inhibit several key enzymatic processes by carbamoylation of amino acids in proteins.

➤*Pharmacokinetics:*

Absorption / Distribution – Because of the high lipid solubility and the relative lack of ionization at physiological pH, lomustine crosses the blood-brain barrier quite effectively. Levels of radioactivity in the CSF are 50% or greater than those measured concurrently in plasma.

Metabolism / Excretion – Following oral administration of radioactive lomustine at doses ranging from 30 mg/m^2 to 100 mg/m^2, about half of the radioactivity given was excreted in the form of degradation products within 24 hours.

The serum half-life of the metabolites ranges from 16 hours to 2 days. Tissue levels are comparable to plasma levels at 15 minutes after intravenous administration.

Contraindications

Hypersensitivity to lomustine.

Warnings

➤*Hematologic:* Since the major toxicity is delayed bone marrow suppression, blood counts should be monitored weekly for at least 6 weeks after a dose (see Adverse Reactions). At the recommended dosage, courses of lomustine should not be given more frequently than every 6 weeks.

See Administration and Dosage for more information.

➤*Pulmonary toxicity:* See Adverse Reactions for more information.

➤*Long-term use:* Long-term use of nitrosoureas has been reported to be possibly associated with the development of secondary malignancies.

➤*Carcinogenesis:* Lomustine is carcinogenic in rats and mice, producing a marked increase in tumor incidence in doses approximating those employed clinically. Nitrosourea therapy dose have carcinogenic potential in humans (see Adverse Reactions).

➤*Fertility impairment:* Lomustine also affects fertility in male rats at doses somewhat higher than the human dose.

➤*Pregnancy: Category D.* Lomustine can cause fetal harm when administered to a pregnant woman. Lomustine is embryotoxic and teratogenic in rats and embryotoxic in rabbits at dose levels equivalent to the human dose. There are no adequate and well controlled studies in pregnant women. If this drug is used during pregnancy, or if the patient becomes pregnant while taking (receiving) this drug, the patient should be apprised of the potential hazard to the fetus. Women of childbearing potential should be advised to avoid becoming pregnant.

➤*Lactation:* It is not known whether this drug is excreted in human milk. Because many drugs are excreted in human milk and because of the potential for serious adverse reactions in nursing infants from lomustine, a decision should be made whether to discontinue nursing or to discontinue the drug, taking into account the importance of the drug to the mother.

Precautions

➤*Monitoring:* Since lomustine may cause liver dysfunction, it is recommended that liver function tests be monitored periodically.

Renal function tests should also be monitored periodically.

➤*Lab test abnormalities:* See Administration and Dosage for more information.

Baseline pulmonary function studies should be conducted along with frequent pulmonary function tests during treatment. Patients with a baseline below 70% of the predicted Forced Vital Capacity (FVC) or Carbon Monoxide Diffusing Capacity (DL_{co}) are particularly at risk.

Adverse Reactions

➤*CNS:* Neurological reactions such as disorientation, lethargy, ataxia, and dysarthria have been noted in some patients receiving lomustine. However, the relationship to medication in these patients is unclear.

➤*GI:* Nausea and vomiting may occur 3 to 6 hours after an oral dose and usually lasts less than 24 hours. Prior administration of antiemetics is effective in diminishing and sometimes preventing this side effect. Nausea and vomiting can also be reduced if lomustine capsules is administered to fasting patients.

➤*Hematologic:* The most frequent and most serious toxicity of lomustine is delayed myelosuppression. It usually occurs 4 to 6 weeks after drug administration and is dose related. Thrombocytopenia occurs at about 4 weeks postadministration and persists for 1 to 2 weeks. Leukopenia occurs at 5 to 6 weeks after a dose of lomustine and persists for 1 to 2 weeks. Approximately 65% of patients receiving 130 mg/m^2 develop white blood counts below 5000 wbc/mm^3. 36% develop white blood counts below 3000 wbc/mm^3. Thrombocytopenia is generally more severe than leukopenia. However, both may be dose-limiting toxicities.

Lomustine may produce cumulative myelosuppression, manifested by more depressed indices or longer duration of suppression after repeated doses.

The occurrence of acute leukemia and bone marrow dysplasias have been reported in patients following long term nitrosourea therapy.

Anemia also occurs, but is less frequent and less severe than thrombocytopenia or leukopenia.

➤*Hepatic:* A reversible type of hepatic toxicity, manifested by increased transaminase, alkaline phosphatase and bilirubin levels, has been reported in a small percentage of patients receiving lomustine.

➤*Pulmonary:* Pulmonary toxicity characterized by pulmonary infiltrates and/or fibrosis has been reported rarely with lomustine. Onset of toxicity has occurred after an interval of 6 months or longer from the start of therapy with cumulative doses of lomustine usually greater than 1100 mg/m^2. There is one report of pulmonary toxicity at a cumulative dose of only 600 mg.

Delayed onset pulmonary fibrosis occurring up to 17 years after treatment has been reported in patients who received related nitrosoureas in childhood and early adolescence (1 to 16 years) combined with cranial radiotherapy for intracranial tumors. There appeared to be some late reduction of pulmonary function of all long-term survivors. This form of lung fibrosis may be slowly progressive and has resulted in death in some cases. In this long-term study of carmustine, all those initially treated at less than five years of age died of delayed pulmonary fibrosis.

➤*Renal:* Renal abnormalities consisting of progressive azotemia, decrease in kidney size and renal failure have been reported in patients who received large cumulative doses after prolonged therapy with lomustine. Kidney damage has also been reported occasionally in patients receiving lower total doses.

➤*Miscellaneous:* Stomatitis, alopecia, optic atrophy, and visual disturbances such as blindness have been reported infrequently.

Overdosage

No proven antidotes have been established for lomustine overdosage.

Patient Information

In order to provide the proper dose of lomustine, patients should be aware that there may be two or more different types and colors of capsules in the container dispensed by the pharmacist.

Patients should be told that lomustine is given as a single oral dose and will not be repeated for at least 6 weeks.

Patients should be told that nausea and vomiting usually last less than 24 hours, although loss of appetite may last for several days.

If any of the following reactions occur, notify the physician: fever, chills, sore throat, unusual bleeding or bruising, shortness of breath, dry cough, swelling of feet or lower legs, mental confusion, or yellowing of eyes and skin.

STREPTOZOCIN

Rx	**Zanosar** (Gensia Sicor)	**Powder for Injection:** 1 g (100 mg/ml)	In vials.

STREPTOZOCIN — INJECTION

WARNING

Streptozocin sterile powder should be administered under the supervision of a physician experienced in the use of cancer chemotherapeutic agents.

A patient need not be hospitalized but should have access to a facility with a laboratory and supportive resources sufficient to monitor drug tolerance and to protect and maintain a patient compromised by drug toxicity. Renal toxicity is dose-related and cumulative and may be severe or fatal. Other major toxicities are nausea and vomiting, which may be severe and at times treatment-limiting. In addition, liver dysfunction, diarrhea and hematological changes have been observed in some patients. Streptozocin is mutagenic. When administered parenterally, it has been found to be tumorigenic or carcinogenic in some rodents.

WARNING (cont.)

The physician must judge the possible benefit to the patient against the known toxic effects of this drug in considering the advisability of therapy with streptozocin. The physician should be familiar with the following text before making a judgment and beginning treatment.

Indications

➤*Metastatic islet cell carcinoma of the pancrease:* For the treatment of metastatic islet cell carcinoma of the pancreas. Responses have been obtained with both functional and nonfunctional carcinomas. Because of its inherent renal toxicity, therapy with this drug should be limited to patients with symptomatic or progressive metastatic disease.

➤*Unlabeled uses:* Treatment of Hodgkin disease, palliative treatment of metastatic carcinoid tumor, palliative treatment of colorectal cancer, pancreatic adenocarcinoma, metastatic pheochromocytoma.

STREPTOZOCIN — INJECTION

Administration and Dosage

Streptozocin sterile powder should be administered intravenously by rapid injection or short/prolonged infusion. It is not active orally. Although it has been administered intra-arterially, this is not recommended pending further evaluation of the possibility that adverse renal effects may be evoked more rapidly by this route of administration.

➤*Dosage schedules:* Two different dosage schedules have been employed successfully with streptozocin.

Daily schedule – The recommended dose for daily intravenous administration is 500 mg/m^2 of body surface area for 5 consecutive days every 6 weeks until maximum benefit or until treatment-limiting toxicity is observed. Dose escalation on this schedule is not recommended.

Weekly schedule – The recommended initial dose for weekly intravenous administration is 1000 mg/m^{2}of body surface area at weekly intervals for the first 2 courses (weeks). In subsequent courses, drug doses may be escalated in patients who have not achieved a therapeutic response and who have not experienced significant toxicity with the previous course of treatment. However, *a single dose of 1500 mg/m^{2}body surface area should not be exceeded*as a greater dose may cause azotemia. When administered on this schedule, the median time to onset of response is about 17 days and the median time to maximum response is about 35 days. The median total dose to onset of response is about 2000 mg/m^2 body surface area and the median total dose to maximum response is about 4000 mg/m^2 body surface area.

➤*Maintenance:* The ideal duration of maintenance therapy with streptozocin has not yet been clearly established for either of the above schedules.

➤*Response to therapy:* For patients with functional tumors, serial monitoring of fasting insulin levels allows a determination of biochemical response to therapy. For patients with either functional or nonfunctional tumors, response to therapy can be determined by measurable reductions of tumor size (reduction of organomegaly, masses, or lymph nodes).

➤*Reconstitution:* Reconstitute streptozocin with 9.5 mL of Dextrose Injection USP, or 0.9% Sodium Chloride Injection USP. The resulting pale-gold solution will contain 100 mg of streptozocin and 22 mg of citric acid per mL. Where more dilute infusion solutions are desirable, further dilution in the above vehicles is recommended. The total storage time for streptozocin after it has been placed in solution should not exceed 12 hours. This product contains no preservatives and is not intended as a multiple-dose vial.

➤*Storage/Stability:* Unopened vials of streptozocin should be stored at refrigeration temperatures (2° to 8°C; 35.6° to 46.4°F) and protected from light (preferably stored in carton).

Actions

➤*Pharmacology:* Streptozocin inhibits DNA synthesis in bacterial and mammalian cells. In bacterial cells, a specific interaction with cytosine moieties leads to degradation of DNA. The biochemical mechanism leading to mammalian cell death has not been definitely established; streptozocin inhibits cell proliferation at a considerably lower level than that needed to inhibit precursor incorporation into DNA or to inhibit several of the enzymes involved in DNA synthesis. Although streptozocin inhibits the progression of cells into mitosis, no specific phase of the cell cycle is particularly sensitive to its lethal effects.

Streptozocin is active in the L1210 leukemic mouse over a fairly wide range of parenteral dosage schedules. In experiments in many animal species, streptozocin induced a diabetes that resembles human hyperglycemic nonketotic diabetes mellitus. This phenomenon, which has been extensively studied, appears to be mediated through a lowering of beta cell nicotinamide adenine dinucleotide (NAD) and consequent histopathologic alteration of pancreatic islet beta cells.

➤*Pharmacokinetics:* The metabolism and the chemical dissociation of streptozocin that occurs under physiologic conditions has not been extensively studied. When administered intravenously to a variety of experimental animals, streptozocin disappears from the blood very rapidly. In all species tested, it was found to concentrate in the liver and kidney. As much as 20% of the drug (or metabolites containing an N-nitrosourea group) is metabolized or excreted by the kidney. Metabolic products have not yet been identified.

Warnings

➤*Topical exposure:* When exposed dermally, some rats developed benign tumors at the site of application of streptozocin. Consequently, streptozocin may pose a carcinogenic hazard following topical exposure if not properly handled (see Administration and Dosage).

➤*Renal toxicity:* Many patients treated with streptozocin sterile powder have experienced renal toxicity, as evidenced by azotemia, anuria, hypophosphatemia, glycosuria and renal tubular acidosis. Such toxicity is dose-related and cumulative and may be severe or fatal. Renal function must be monitored before and after each course of therapy. Serial urinalysis, blood urea nitrogen, plasma creatinine, serum electrolytes and creatinine clearance should be obtained prior to, at least weekly during, and for 4 weeks after drug administration. Serial urinalysis is particularly important for the early detection of proteinuria and should be quantitated with a 24 hour collection when proteinuria is detected. Mild proteinuria is one of the first signs of renal toxicity and may herald further deterioration of renal function. Reduction of the dose of streptozocin or discontinuation of treatment is suggested in the presence of significant renal toxicity. Adequate hydration may help reduce the risk of nephrotoxicity to renal tubular epithelium by decreasing renal and urinary concentration of the drug and its metabolites.

Use of streptozocin in patients with preexisting renal disease requires a judgment by the physician of potential benefit as opposed to the known risk of serious renal damage.

This drug should not be used in combination with or concomitantly with other potential nephrotoxins.

➤*Carcinogenesis:* When administered parenterally, it has been shown to induce renal tumors in rats and to induce liver tumors and other tumors in hamsters. Stomach and pancreatic tumors were observed in rats treated orally with streptozocin. Streptozocin has also been shown to be carcinogenic in mice.

➤*Mutagenesis:* Streptozocin is mutagenic in bacteria, plants, and mammalian cells.

➤*Fertility impairment:* Streptozocin adversely affected fertility when administered to male and female rats.

➤*Pregnancy: Category D.* Reproduction studies revealed that streptozocin is teratogenic in the rat and has abortifacient effects in rabbits. When administered intravenously to pregnant monkeys, it appears rapidly in the fetal circulation. There are no studies in pregnant women. Streptozocin should be used during pregnancy only if the potential benefit justifies the potential risk to the fetus.

➤*Lactation:* It is not known whether streptozocin is excreted in human milk. Because many drugs are excreted in human milk and because of the potential for serious adverse reactions in nursing infants, nursing should be discontinued in patients receiving streptozocin.

Precautions

➤*Monitoring:* Patients who are treated with streptozocin must be monitored closely, particularly for evidence of renal, hepatic, and hematopoietic toxicity. Renal function tests are described in the Warnings section. Patients should also be monitored closely for evidence of hematopoietic and hepatic toxicities. Complete blood counts and liver function tests should be done at least weekly. Dosage adjustments or discontinuance of the drug may be indicated, depending upon the degree of toxicity noted.

➤*Injection site reactions:* Streptozocin sterile powder is irritating to tissues. Extravasation may cause severe tissue lesions and necrosis.

Drug Interactions

Streptozocin may demonstrate additive toxicity when used in combination with other cytotoxic drugs. Streptozocin has been reported to prolong the elimination half-life of doxorubicin and may lead to severe bone marrow suppression; a reduction of the doxorubicin dosage should be considered in patients receiving streptozocin concurrently. The concurrent use of streptozocin and phenytoin has been reported in one case to result in reduced streptozocin cytotoxicity.

Adverse Reactions

➤*GI:* Most patients treated with streptozocin sterile powder have experienced severe nausea and vomiting, occasionally requiring discontinuation of drug therapy. Some patients experienced diarrhea.

➤*Hepatic:* A number of patients have experienced hepatic toxicity, as characterized by elevated liver enzyme (AST and LDH) levels and hypoalbuminemia.

➤*Hematologic:* Hematological toxicity has been rare, most often involving mild decreases in hematocrit values. However, fatal hematological toxicity with substantial reductions in leukocyte and platelet count has been observed.

➤*Metabolic:* Mild to moderate abnormalities of glucose tolerance have been noted in some patients treated with streptozocin. These have generally been reversible, but insulin shock with hypoglycemia has been observed.

➤*Renal:* See Warnings. Two cases of nephrogenic diabetes insipidus following therapy with streptozocin have been reported. One had spontaneous recovery and the second responded to indomethacin.

➤*Postmarketing experience:* Spontaneous reports have been received of local inflammation (ie, edema, erythema, burning, tenderness) following extravasation of the product. In most cases, these events resolved the same day or within a few days.

Overdosage

No specific antidote for streptozocin is known.

Patient Information

Confusion, lethargy, and depression have been reported in a limited number of patients receiving continuous intravenous infusion of streptozocin for 5 days. Patients should be informed that there may be a potential risk in driving or using complex machinery.

DACARBAZINE (DTIC; Imidazole Carboxamide)

Rx	**Dacarbazine** (Various, eg, American Pharmaceutical Partners, Bedford, Mayne, Gensia Sicor)	**Powder for injection:** 100 mg	May contain mannitol. In vials.
Rx	**DTIC-Dome** (Bayer)		May contain mannitol. In vials.
Rx	**Dacarbazine** (Various, eg, American Pharmaceutical Partners, Bedford, Mayne, Gensia Sicor)	**Powder for injection:** 200 mg	May contain mannitol. In vials.
Rx	**DTIC-Dome** (Bayer)		May contain mannitol. In vials.

DACARBAZINE — INJECTION

WARNING

It is recommended that dacarbazine for injection be administered under the supervision of a qualified physician experienced in the use of cancer chemotherapeutic agents.

Hemopoietic depression is the most common toxicity with dacarbazine for injection.

Hepatic necrosis has been reported.

Studies have demonstrated this agent to have a carcinogenic and teratogenic effect when used in animals.

In treatment of each patient, the physician must weigh carefully the possibility of achieving therapeutic benefit against the risk of toxicity.

Indications

➤*Metastatic malignant melanoma / Hodgkin's disease:* For the treatment of metastatic malignant melanoma. In addition, dacarbazine is also indicated for Hodgkin's disease as a secondary-line therapy when used in combination with other effective agents.

➤*Unlabeled uses:* In combination with cyclophosphamide and vincristine for malignant pheochromocytoma; in combination with other agents for the treatment of advanced metastatic soft tissue sarcoma; alone or in combination with other agents for the management of Kaposi sarcoma; treatment of soft-tissue sarcomas, neuroblastomas, fibrosarcomas, rhabdomyosarcoma, islet cell carcinomas, medullary carcinoma of the thyroid.

Administration and Dosage

➤*Approved by the FDA:* August 27, 1998.

➤*Malignant melanoma:* 2 to 4.5 mg/kg/day for 10 days. Treatment may be repeated at 4-week intervals.

An alternate recommended dosage is 250 mg/m^2 body surface/day IV for 5 days. Treatment may be repeated every 3 weeks.

➤*Hodgkin's disease:* 150 mg/m^2 body surface/day for 5 days, in combination with other effective drugs. Treatment may be repeated every 4 weeks. An alternative recommended dosage is 375 mg/m^2 body surface on day 1, in combination with other effective drugs, to be repeated every 15 days.

➤*Preparation of solution:* Dacarbazine for injection 100 mg/vial and 200 mg/vial are reconstituted with 9.9 mL and 19.7 mL, respectively, of Sterile Water for Injection. The resulting solution contains 10 mg/mL of dacarbazine, having a pH of 3 to 4. The calculated dose of the resulting solution is drawn into a syringe and administered only IV.

The reconstituted solution may be further diluted with 5% dextrose injection or sodium chloride injection and administered as an IV infusion.

➤*Storage / Stability:* Store in a refrigerator 2° to 8°C (36° to 46°F). Protect from light. Use within 8 hours of reconstitution.

After reconstitution and prior to use, the solution in the vial may be stored at 4°C (39.2°F) for up to 72 hours or at normal room conditions (temperature and light) for up to 8 hours. If the reconstituted solution is further diluted in 5% dextrose injection or sodium chloride injection the resulting solution may be stored at 4°C (39.2°F) for up to 24 hours or at normal room conditions for up to 8 hours.

Actions

➤*Pharmacology:* Although the exact mechanism of action of dacarbazine for injection is not known, the following 3 hypotheses have been offered:

- Inhibition of DNA synthesis by acting as a purine analog.
- Action as an alkylating agent.
- Interaction with sulfhydryl (SH) groups.

➤*Pharmacokinetics:*

Absorption / Distribution – After IV administration of dacarbazine for injection, the volume of distribution exceeds total body water content, suggesting localization in some body tissue, probably the liver. At therapeutic concentrations, dacarbazine is not appreciably bound to human plasma protein.

Metabolism / Excretion – Its disappearance from the plasma is biphasic with initial half-life of 19 minutes and a terminal half-life of 5 hours. In a patient with renal and hepatic dysfunctions, the half-lives were lengthened to 55 minutes and 7.2 hours.

The average cumulative excretion of unchanged dacarbazine in the urine is 40% of the injected dose in 6 hours. Dacarbazine is subject to renal tubular secretion rather than glomerular filtration.

In man, dacarbazine is extensively degraded. Besides unchanged dacarbazine, 5-aminoimidazole -4 carboxamide (AIC) is a major metabolite of dacarbazine excreted in the urine. AIC is not derived endogenously but from the injected dacarbazine, because the administration of radioactive dacarbazine labeled with ^{14}C in the imidazole portion of the molecule (dacarbazine-2-^{14}C) gives rise to AIC-2-^{14}C.

Contraindications

Hypersensitivity to dacarbazine.

Warnings

➤*Hemopoietic depression:* Hemopoietic depression is the most common toxicity with dacarbazine for injection, and involves primarily the leukocytes and platelets, although anemia may sometimes occur. Leukopenia and thrombocytopenia may be severe enough to cause death. The possible bone marrow depression requires careful monitoring of white blood cells, red blood cells, and platelet levels. Hemopoietic toxicity may warrant temporary suspension or cessation of therapy with dacarbazine for injection.

➤*Hepatotoxicity:* Hepatic toxicity accompanied by hepatic vein thrombosis and hepatocellular necrosis resulting in death, has been reported. The incidence of such reactions has been low; approximately 0.01% of patients treated. This toxicity has been observed mostly when dacarbazine for injection has been administered concomitantly with other antineoplastic drugs; however, it has also been reported in some patients treated with dacarbazine for injection alone.

➤*Hypersensitivity reactions:* Anaphylaxis can occur following the administration of dacarbazine for injection.

➤*Carcinogenesis:* Carcinogenicity of dacarbazine was studied in rats and mice. Proliferative endocardial lesions, including fibrosarcomas and sarcomas were induced by dacarbazine in rats. In mice, administration of dacarbazine resulted in the induction of angiosarcomas of the spleen.

➤*Pregnancy: Category C.*

Teratogenic – Dacarbazine for injection has been shown to be teratogenic in rats when given in doses 20 times the human daily dose on day 12 of gestation. Dacarbazine, when administered in 10 times the human daily dose to male rats (twice weekly for 9 weeks), did not affect the male libido; although, female rats mated to male rats had higher incidence of resorptions than controls. In rabbits, dacarbazine daily dose 7 times the human daily dose given on days 6 to 15 of gestation resulted in fetal skeletal anomalies. There are no adequate and well-controlled studies in pregnant women. Dacarbazine for injection should be used during pregnancy only if the potential benefit justifies the potential risk to the fetus.

➤*Lactation:* It is not known whether this drug is excreted in human milk. Because many drugs are excreted in human milk and because of the potential for tumorigenicity shown for dacarbazine for injection in animal studies, a decision should be made whether to discontinue nursing or to discontinue the drug, taking into account the importance of the drug to the mother.

Precautions

Hospitalization is not always necessary, but adequate laboratory study capability must be available. Extravasation of the drug SC during IV administration may result in tissue damage and severe pain. Local pain, burning sensation, and irritation at the site of injection may be relieved by locally applied hot packs.

Adverse Reactions

➤*Dermatologic:* Alopecia has been noted, as has facial flushing and facial paresthesia.

Erythematous and urticarial rashes have been observed infrequently after administration of dacarbazine for injection. Rarely, photosensitivity reactions may occur.

➤*GI:* Symptoms of anorexia, nausea, and vomiting are the most frequently noted of all toxic reactions. Over 90% of patients are affected with the initial few doses. The vomiting lasts 1 to 12 hours, and is incompletely and unpredictably palliated with phenobarbital or prochlorperazine. Rarely, intractable nausea and vomiting have necessitated discontinuance of therapy with dacarbazine for injection. Rarely, dacarbazine for injection has caused diarrhea. Some helpful suggestions include restricting the patient's oral intake of food for 4 to 6 hours prior to treatment. The rapid toleration of these symptoms suggests that a CNS mechanism may be involved, and usually these symptoms subside after the first 1 or 2 days.

➤*Lab test abnormalities:* There have been few reports of significant liver or renal function test abnormalities in man. However, these abnormalities have been observed more frequently in animal studies.

➤*Miscellaneous:* There are a number of minor toxicities that are infrequently noted. Patients have experienced an influenza-like syndrome of fever up to 39°C (102.2°F), myalgias and malaise. These symptoms occur usually after large single doses, may last for several days, and they may occur with successive treatments.

Overdosage

➤*Treatment:* Give supportive treatment and monitor blood cell counts.

DACARBAZINE — INJECTION

Patient Information

Advise patients of common side effects, which include the following: increased risk of infection or bleeding for 21 to 25 days after therapy; nausea, vomiting, or loss of appetite for 1 to 2 days after each dose (restricting food intake for 4 to 6 hours before treatment may help); reversible hair loss.

ALKYL SULFONATES

BUSULFAN

Rx	**Myleran** (GlaxoSmithKline)	**Tablets:** 2 mg	Lactose. (GX EF3 M). White. Film coated. In 25s.
Rx	**Busulfex** (Orphan Medical)	**Injection:** 6 mg/mL	In 10 mL single-use ampules with syringe filters.

BUSULFAN — ORAL

WARNING

Busulfan is a potent drug. Do not use it unless a diagnosis of chronic myelogenous leukemia (CML) has been adequately established and the responsible health care provider is knowledgeable in assessing response to chemotherapy.

Busulfan can induce severe bone marrow hypoplasia. Reduce or discontinue the dosage immediately at the first sign of any unusual depression of bone marrow function as reflected by an abnormal decrease in any of the formed elements of the blood. Perform a bone marrow examination if the bone marrow status is uncertain.

Malignant tumors and acute leukemias have been reported in patients who have received busulfan therapy, and this drug may be a human carcinogen. The World Health Organization (WHO) has concluded that there is a causal relationship between busulfan exposure and the development of secondary malignancies. Four cases of acute leukemia occurred among 243 patients treated with busulfan as adjuvant chemotherapy following surgical resection of bronchogenic carcinoma. All 4 cases were from a subgroup of 19 of these 243 patients who developed pancytopenia while taking busulfan 5 to 8 years before leukemia became clinically apparent. These findings suggest that busulfan is leukemogenic, although its mode of action is uncertain.

Indications

➤*CML:* Busulfan is indicated for the palliative treatment of chronic myelogenous (myeloid, myelocytic, granulocytic) leukemia.

➤*Unlabeled uses:* Other myeloproliferative disorders, including severe thrombocytosis and polycythemia vera, myelofibrosis; bone marrow transplantation (BMT).

Administration and Dosage

➤*Approved by the FDA:* June 26, 1954.

Busulfan is administered orally. The usual adult dose range for remission induction is 4 to 8 mg, total dose, daily. Dosing on a weight basis is the same for children and adults, approximately 60 mcg/kg of body weight or 1.8 mg/m^2 of body surface, daily. Because the rate of fall of the leukocyte count is dose related, reserve daily doses exceeding 4 mg daily for patients with the most compelling symptoms; the greater the total daily dose, the greater the possibility of inducing bone marrow aplasia.

A decrease in the leukocyte count is not usually seen during the first 10 to 15 days of treatment. The leukocyte count may actually increase during this period; do not interpret it as resistance to the drug, and do not increase the dose. Because the leukocyte count may continue to fall for more than 1 month after discontinuing the drug, it is important that busulfan be discontinued prior to the total leukocyte count falling into the normal range. When the total leukocyte count has declined to approximately 15,000/mcL, withhold the drug.

With a constant dose of busulfan, the total leukocyte count declines exponentially; a weekly plot of the leukocyte count on semilogarithmic graph paper aids in predicting the time when therapy should be discontinued. With the recommended dose of busulfan, a normal leukocyte count is usually achieved in 12 to 20 weeks.

During remission, the patient is examined at monthly intervals and treatment resumed with the induction dosage when the total leukocyte count reaches approximately 50,000/mcL. When remission is less than 3 months, maintenance therapy of 1 to 3 mg daily may be advisable in order to keep the hematological status under control and prevent rapid relapse.

➤*Handling/Disposal:* Consider procedures for proper handling and disposal of anticancer drugs. Several guidelines on this subject have been published.

There is no general agreement that all of the procedures recommended in the guidelines are necessary or appropriate.

➤*Storage/Stability:* Store at 25°C (77°F); excursions are permitted to 15° to 30°C (59° to 77°F).

Actions

➤*Pharmacology:* In aqueous media, busulfan undergoes a wide range of nucleophilic substitution reactions. While this chemical reactivity is relatively nonspecific, alkylation of the deoxyribonucleic acid (DNA) is thought to be an important biological mechanism for its cytotoxic effect. Coliphage T7 exposed to busulfan had the DNA crosslinked by intrastrand crosslinkages, but no interstrand linkages were found.

The metabolic fate of busulfan has been studied in rats and humans using ^{14}C- and ^{35}S-labeled materials. In humans, as in the rat, almost all of the radioactivity in ^{35}S-labeled busulfan is excreted in the urine in the form of ^{35}S-methanesulfonic acid. No unchanged drug was found in human urine, although a small amount has been reported in rat urine. It was demonstrated that the formation of methanesulfonic acid in vivo in the rat was not caused by a simple hydrolysis of busulfan to 1, 4-butanediol because only about 4% of 2, 3-^{14}C-busulfan was excreted as carbon dioxide, whereas 2, 3-^{14}C-1, 4-butanediol was converted almost exclusively to carbon dioxide. The predominant reaction of busulfan in the rat is the alkylation of sulfhydryl groups (particularly cysteine and cysteine-containing compounds) to produce a cyclic sulfonium compound, which is the precursor of the major urinary metabolite of the 4-carbon portion of the molecule, 3-hydroxytetrahydrothiophene-1, 1-dioxide. This has been termed a "sulfur-stripping" action of busulfan, and it may modify the function of certain sulfur-containing amino acids, polypeptides, and proteins; whether this action makes an important contribution to the cytotoxicity of busulfan is unknown.

The biochemical basis for acquired resistance to busulfan is largely a matter of speculation. Although altered transport of busulfan into the cell is one possibility, increased intracellular inactivation of the drug before it reaches the DNA is also possible. Experiments with other alkylating agents have shown that resistance to this class of compounds may reflect an acquired ability of the resistant cell to repair alkylation damage more effectively.

➤*Pharmacokinetics:*

Absorption/Distribution – Busulfan is a small, highly lipophilic molecule that easily crosses the blood brain barrier. Following absorption, 32% and 47% of busulfan are bound to plasma proteins and red blood cells, respectively. Busulfan is reported to have a volume of distribution of 0.64 ± 0.12 L/kg in adults.

Busulfan absorption from the GI tract is essentially complete. This has been demonstrated in radioactive studies after both intravenous (IV) and oral administration of ^{35}S-busulfan, ^{14}C-busulfan and ^{3}H-busulfan. Following the IV administration of a single therapeutic dose of ^{35}S-busulfan, there was rapid disappearance of radioactivity from the blood, and 90% to 95% of the ^{35}S-label disappeared within 3 to 5 minutes after injection.

A study compared a single 2 mg IV bolus injection with a single oral dose of a 2 mg tablet of nonradioactive busulfan in 8 adult patients 13 to 60 years of age. The study demonstrated mean bioavailability of 80% in adults with large interpatient variability ranging from 47% to 103%. However, mean bioavailability for 8 children 18 months to 6 years of age was 68%, ranging from 22% to 120%.

In another study, busulfan 2, 4, and 6 mg given as a single oral dose on consecutive days (starting with the lowest dose) in 5 adult patients, the mean dose-normalized (to 2 mg dose) area under the plasma concentration time curve (AUC) was about 130 ng•h/mL, while the mean intrapatient and interpatient variability was approximately 16% and 21%, respectively. Busulfan was eliminated with a plasma terminal elimination half-life of approximately 2.6 hours, and demonstrated linear kinetics within the range of 2 to 6 mg for both the maximum plasma concentration (C_{max}) and AUC. The mean C_{max} for the 2, 4, and 6 mg doses (after dose normalization to 2 mg) was approximately 30 ng/mL. A recent study of 4 to 8 mg as single oral doses in 12 patients showed that the mean ± standard deviation (SD) C_{max} (after dose normalization to 4 mg) was 68.2 ± 24.4 ng/mL, occurring at approximately 0.9 hours, and the mean ± SD AUC (after dose normalization to 4 mg) was 269 ± 62 ng•h/mL. These results are consistent with previous results. In addition, the mean ± SD elimination half-life was 2.69 ± 0.49 hours.

Currently, there are no available data on the effect of food on busulfan bioavailability.

Metabolism/Excretion – After oral or IV administration of ^{35}S-busulfan to humans, 45% to 60% of the radioactivity was recovered in the urine in the 48 hours after administration; the majority of the total urinary excretion occurred in the first 24 hours. In humans, more than 95% of the urinary ^{35}S-label occurs as ^{35}S-methanesulfonic acid. Oral and IV administration of 1, 4-^{14}C-busulfan showed the same rapid initial disappearance of plasma radioactivity with a subsequent low-level plateau as observed following the administration of ^{35}S-labeled drug. Cumulative radioactivity in the urine after 48 hours was 25% to 30% of the administered dose (contrasting with 45% to 60% for ^{35}S-busulfan) and suggests a slower excretion of the alkylating portion of the molecule and its metabolites than for the sulfonoxymethyl moieties. Regardless of the route of administration, 1, 4-^{14}C-busulfan yielded a complex mixture of at least 12 radiolabeled metabolites in urine; the main metabolite being 3-hydroxytetrahydrothiophene-1, 1-dioxide. Pharmacokinetic studies employing ^{3}H-busulfan labeled on the tetramethylene chain confirmed a rapid initial clearance of the radioactivity from plasma, irrespective of whether the drug was given orally or IV.

Busulfan clearance in adult patients is 2.4 to 2.6 mL/min/kg. The elimination of busulfan appears to be independent of renal function. This probably

BUSULFAN — ORAL

reflects the extensive metabolism of the drug in the liver because less that 2% of the administered dose is excreted in the urine unchanged within 24 hours. Busulfan metabolism occurs in the liver and is mediated by gluthathione-S-transferase. The drug is metabolized by enzymatic activity to at least 12 metabolites, among which tetrahydrothiophene, tetrahydrothiophene 12-oxide, sulfolane, and 3-hydroxysulfolane were identified. These metabolites do not have cytotoxic activity.

There is no experience with the use of dialysis in an attempt to modify the clinical toxicity of busulfan. One technical difficulty would derive from the extremely poor water solubility of busulfan. Additionally, all studies of the metabolism of busulfan employing radiolabeled materials indicate rapid chemical reactivity of the parent compound with prolonged retention of some of the metabolites (particularly the metabolites arising from the "alkylating" portion of the molecule). The efficacy of dialysis at removing significant quantities of unreacted drug would be expected to be minimal in such a situation.

Special populations –

Renal function impairment: The impact of hemodialysis on the clearance of busulfan was determined in a patient with chronic renal failure undergoing autologous stem cell transplantation. The apparent oral clearance of busulfan during a 4-hour hemodialysis session was increased 65%, but the 24-hour oral clearance of busulfan was increased only 11%.

The incidence of venoocclusive disease was higher (33.3% vs 3%) in patients with busulfan $AUC_{0\text{-}6h}$ greater than 1,500 mcM•min (C_{ss} greater than 900 mcg/mL) compared with patients with busulfan $AUC_{0\text{-}6h}$ less than 1,500 mcM•min (C_{ss} less than 900 mcg/L).

Children: The bioavailability of oral busulfan shows large intrapatient variability ranging from 22% to 120% (mean 68%) in children. Plasma clearance is reported to be 2 to 4 times higher in children than adults when receiving 1 mg/kg every 6 hours for 4 days. Oral dosing children according to body surface yields AUC and C_{max} values and the colony stimulating factor-:plasma ratio similar to those seen in adults. Busulfan is reported to have a volume of distribution of 1.15 + 0.52 L/kg in children.

Obese patients: Obesity has been reported to increase busulfan clearance. Consider dosing based on body surface area or adjusted ideal body weight (defined as an ideal body weight plus 25% of the difference between actual and ideal body weight) in obese patients.

Drug interactions: Itraconazole reduced busulfan clearance by up to 25% in patients receiving itraconazole compared with patients who did not receive itraconazole. Higher busulfan exposure caused by concomitant itraconazole or metronidazole could lead to toxic plasma levels in some patients. Fluconazole had no effect on the clearance of busulfan. Patients treated with concomitant cyclophosphamide and busulfan with phenytoin pretreatment have increased cyclophosphamide and busulfan clearance, which may lead to decreased concentrations of cyclophosphamide and busulfan. However, busulfan clearance may be reduced in the presence of cyclophosphamide alone, presumably because of competition for glutathione.

Diazepam had no effect on the clearance of busulfan.

No information is available regarding the penetration of busulfan into brain or cerebrospinal fluid.

Contraindications

Busulfan is contraindicated in patients in whom a definitive diagnosis of CML has not been firmly established.

Busulfan is contraindicated in patients who have previously suffered a hypersensitivity reaction to busulfan or any other component of the preparation.

Warnings

➤*Hematologic effects:* The most frequent, serious side effect of treatment with busulfan is the induction of bone marrow failure (which may or may not be anatomically hypoplastic), resulting in severe pancytopenia. The pancytopenia caused by busulfan may be more prolonged than that induced with other alkylating agents. It is generally thought that the usual cause of busulfan-induced pancytopenia is the failure to stop administration of the drug soon enough; individual idiosyncrasy to the drug does not seem to be an important factor. Use busulfan with extreme caution and exceptional vigilance in patients whose bone marrow reserve may have been compromised by prior irradiation or chemotherapy, or whose marrow function is recovering from previous cytotoxic therapy. Although recovery from busulfan-induced pancytopenia may take from 1 month to 2 years, this complication is potentially reversible; vigorously support the patient through any period of severe pancytopenia.

The most consistent, dose-related toxicity is bone marrow suppression. This may be manifested by anemia, leukopenia, thrombocytopenia, or any combination of these. It is imperative that patients be instructed to promptly report the development of fever, sore throat, signs of local infection, bleeding from any site, or symptoms suggestive of anemia. Any one of these findings may indicate busulfan toxicity; however, they also may indicate transformation of the disease to acute blastic form. Because busulfan may have a delayed effect, it is important to withdraw the medication temporarily at the first sign of an abnormally large or exceptionally rapid fall in any of the formed elements of the blood. Never allow patients to take the drug without close medical supervision.

➤*Pulmonary effects:* A rare, important complication of busulfan therapy is the development of bronchopulmonary dysplasia with pulmonary fibrosis. Symptoms have been reported to occur within 8 months to 10 years after initiation of therapy, the average duration of therapy being 4 years. The histologic findings associated with busulfan lung mimic those seen following pulmonary irradiation. Clinically, patients have reported the insidious onset of cough, dyspnea, and low-grade fever. In some cases, however, onset of symptoms may be acute. Pulmonary function studies have revealed diminished diffusion capacity and decreased pulmonary compliance. It is important to exclude more common conditions (such as opportunistic infections or leukemic infiltration of the lungs) with appropriate diagnostic techniques. If measures such as exfoliative cytology, sputum cultures, and virologic studies fail to establish an etiology for pulmonary infiltrates, lung biopsy may be necessary to establish the diagnosis. Treatment of established, busulfan-induced pulmonary fibrosis is unsatisfactory; in most cases, the patients have died within 6 months after the diagnosis was established. There is no specific therapy for this complication. Discontinue busulfan if this lung toxicity develops. The administration of corticosteroids has been suggested, but the results have not been impressive or uniformly successful.

Pulmonary toxicity consistent with idiopathic pneumonia syndrome commonly occurs following high-dose of busulfan, often in combination with cyclophosphamide, as part of a preparatory regimen for BMT. The syndrome usually manifests within 3 months of transplantation.

➤*Cardiac effects:* Cardiac tamponade has been reported in a small number of patients with thalassemia (2% in 1 series) who received busulfan and cyclophosphamide as the preparatory regimen for BMT. In this series, the cardiac tamponade often was fatal. Abdominal pain and vomiting preceded the tamponade in most patients.

➤*Hepatic effects:* Hepatic venoocclusive disease (HVOD), which may be life-threatening, has been reported in patients receiving busulfan, usually in combination with cyclophosphamide or other chemotherapeutic agents prior to BMT. Possible risk factors for the development of HVOD include the following: total busulfan dose exceeding 16 mg/kg based on ideal body weight; concurrent use of multiple, alkylating agents.

A clear cause-and-effect relationship with busulfan has not been demonstrated. Periodic measurement of serum transaminases, alkaline phosphatase, and bilirubin is indicated for early detection of hepatotoxicity. A reduced incidence of HVOD and other regimen-related toxicities have been observed in patients treated with high dose busulfan and cyclophosphamide when the first dose of cyclophosphamide has been delayed for more than 24 hours after the last dose of busulfan.

➤*Cellular dysplasia:* Busulfan may cause cellular dysplasia in many organs in addition to the lung. Cytologic abnormalities characterized by giant, hyperchromatic nuclei have been reported in adrenal glands, bone marrow, lymph nodes, pancreas, and thyroid, liver. This cytologic dysplasia may be severe enough to cause difficulty in interpretation of exfoliative cytologic examinations from the bladder, breast, lung, and the uterine cervix.

➤*Carcinogenesis:* Malignant tumors and acute leukemias have been reported in patients who have received busulfan therapy; this drug may be a human carcinogen. The WHO has concluded that there is a causal relationship between busulfan exposure and the development of secondary malignancies. Four cases of acute leukemia occurred among 243 patients treated with busulfan as adjuvant chemotherapy following surgical resection of bronchogenic carcinoma. All 4 cases were from a subgroup of 19 of these 243 patients who developed pancytopenia while taking busulfan 5 to 8 years before leukemia became clinically apparent. These findings suggest that busulfan is leukemogenic, although its mode of action is uncertain.

➤*Mutagenesis:* In addition to the widespread epithelial dysplasia that has been observed during busulfan therapy, chromosome aberrations have been reported in cells from patients receiving busulfan. Busulfan is mutagenic in mice, and, possibly, in humans.

➤*Fertility impairment:* Ovarian suppression and amenorrhea with menopausal symptoms commonly occur during busulfan therapy in premenopausal patients. Busulfan has been associated with ovarian failure, including failure to achieve puberty in women. Busulfan interferes with spermatogenesis in experimental animals, and there have been clinical reports of azoospermia, sterility, and testicular atrophy in men.

➤*Elderly:* Clinical studies of busulfan did not include sufficient numbers of subjects 65 years of age and older to determine whether they respond differently from younger subjects. Other reported clinical experience has not identified differences in responses between the elderly and younger patients. In general, use caution in dose selection for an elderly patient, usually starting at the low end of the dosing range, reflecting the greater frequency of decreased cardiac, hepatic, or renal function and of concomitant disease or other drug therapy.

➤*Pregnancy: Category D.* Busulfan may cause fetal harm when administered to a pregnant woman. Although there have been a number of cases reported where apparently healthy children have been born after busulfan treatment during pregnancy, 1 case has been cited in which a malformed baby was delivered by a mother treated with busulfan. During the pregnancy that resulted in the malformed infant, the mother received x-ray therapy early in the first trimester, mercaptopurine until the third month, then busulfan until delivery. In pregnant rats, busulfan produces sterility in male and female offspring because of the absence of germinal cells in testes and ovaries. Germinal cell aplasia or sterility in offspring of mothers receiving busulfan during pregnancy has not been reported in humans. There are no adequate and well-controlled studies in pregnant women. If this drug is used during pregnancy, or if the patient becomes pregnant while taking this drug, apprise the patient of the potential hazard to the fetus. Advise women of childbearing potential to avoid becoming pregnant.

Nonteratogenic – There have been reports in the literature of small infants being born after the mothers received busulfan during pregnancy, in particular, during the third trimester. One case was reported in which an infant had mild anemia and neutropenia at birth after busulfan was administered to the mother from the eighth week of pregnancy to term.

BUSULFAN — ORAL

➤*Lactation:* It is not known whether this drug is excreted in breast milk. Because of the potential for tumorigenicity shown for busulfan in animal and human studies, decide whether to discontinue breast-feeding or the drug, taking into account the importance of the drug to the mother.

➤*Children:* Dosing on a weight basis is the same for children and adults, approximately 60 mcg/kg of body weight or 1.8 mg/m^2 of body surface, daily. Because the rate of fall of the leukocyte count is dose related, reserve daily doses exceeding 4 mg for patients with the most compelling symptoms; the greater the total daily dose, the greater the possibility of inducing bone marrow aplasia.

Precautions

➤*Monitoring:* It is recommended that evaluation of the hemoglobin or hematocrit, total white blood cell count and differential count, and quantitative platelet count be obtained weekly while the patient is on busulfan therapy. In cases in which the cause of fluctuation in the formed elements of the peripheral blood is obscure, bone marrow examination may be useful for evaluation of marrow status. A decision to increase, decrease, continue, or discontinue a given dose of busulfan must be based not only on the absolute hematologic values, but also on the rapidity with which changes are occurring. The dosage of busulfan may need to be reduced if this agent is combined with other drugs whose primary toxicity is myelosuppression. Occasional patients may be unusually sensitive to busulfan administered at standard dosage and suffer neutropenia or thrombocytopenia after a relatively short exposure to the drug. Do not use busulfan where facilities for complete blood counts, including quantitative platelet counts, are not available at weekly (or more frequent) intervals.

➤*Bone marrow suspension:* The most consistent, dose-related toxicity is bone marrow suppression. This may be manifested by anemia, leukopenia, thrombocytopenia, or any combination of these. It is imperative to instruct patients to promptly report the development of fever, sore throat, signs of local infection, bleeding from any site, or symptoms suggestive of anemia. Any one of these findings may indicate busulfan toxicity; however, they also may indicate transformation of the disease to acute blastic form. Because busulfan may have a delayed effect, it is important to withdraw the medication temporarily at the first sign of an abnormally large or exceptionally rapid fall in any of the formed elements of the blood. Never allow patient to take the drug without close medical supervision.

➤*Seizures:* Seizures have been observed in patients receiving higher than recommended doses of busulfan. As with any potentially epileptogenic drug, exercise caution when administering busulfan to patients with a history of seizure disorder or head trauma, or to patients receiving other potentially epileptogenic drugs. Some investigators have used prophylactic anticonvulsant therapy in this setting.

➤*Vaccinations:* Avoid administration of live vaccines to immunocompromised patients.

Drug Interactions

Busulfan may cause additive myelosuppression when used with other myelosuppressive drugs.

Busulfan-induced pulmonary toxicity may be additive to the effects produced by other cytotoxic agents.

The concomitant systemic administration of itraconazole to patients receiving high-dose busulfan may result in reduced busulfan clearance. Monitor patients for signs of busulfan toxicity when itraconazole is used concomitantly with busulfan. The coadministration of metronidazole and high-dose busulfan may result in increased trough levels of busulfan, and, therefore, it is not recommended.

Busulfan Drug Interactions

Precipitant drug	Object drug[a]		Description
Cyclophosphamide	Busulfan	↑	Coadministration may cause a decrease in busulfan clearance.
Itraconazole	Busulfan	↑	Itraconazole reduced busulfan clearance up to 25%. This may result in toxic busulfan levels. Monitor closely.
Metronidazole	Busulfan	↑	Metronidazole may increase busulfan trough concentrations, increasing the risk of serious toxicities. Coadministration is not recommended.
Phenytoin	Busulfan	↓	Patients treated with concomitant cyclophosphamide and busulfan with phenytoin pretreatment have increased cyclophosphamide and busulfan clearance.

[a] ↑ = Object drug increased. ↓ = Object drug decreased.

Adverse Reactions

➤*Cardiovascular:* Cardiac tamponade has been reported in a small number of patients with thalassemia who received busulfan and cyclophosphamide as the preparatory regimen for BMT. In this series, the cardiac tamponade often was fatal. Abdominal pain and vomiting preceded the tamponade in most patients.

One case of endocardial fibrosis has been reported in a 79-year-old woman who received a total dose of busulfan 7,200 mg over a period of 9 years for the management of CML. At autopsy, she had endocardial fibrosis of the left ventricle in addition to interstitial pulmonary fibrosis.

➤*CNS:* Seizures have been observed in patients receiving higher than recommended doses of busulfan. As with any potentially epileptogenic drug, exercise caution when administering busulfan to patients with a history of seizure disorder or head trauma, or to patients receiving other potentially epileptogenic drugs. Some investigators have used prophylactic anticonvulsant therapy in this setting.

➤*Dermatologic:* Hyperpigmentation is the most common adverse skin reaction and occurs in 5% to 10% of patients, particularly those with a dark complexion.

➤*Hematologic:* The most frequent, serious, toxic effect of busulfan is dose-related myelosuppression, resulting in leukopenia, thrombocytopenia, and anemia. Myelosuppression is most frequently the result of a failure to discontinue dosage in the face of an undetected decrease in leukocyte or platelet counts.

Aplastic anemia (sometimes irreversible) has been reported rarely, often following long-term conventional doses and high doses of busulfan.

➤*Hepatic:* HVOD, which may be life-threatening, has been reported in patients receiving busulfan, usually in combination with cyclophosphamide or other chemotherapeutic agents prior to BMT.

➤*Metabolic:* In a few cases, a clinical syndrome closely resembling adrenal insufficiency and characterized by anorexia, melanoderma, nausea, severe fatigue, vomiting, weakness, and weight loss has developed after prolonged busulfan therapy. The symptoms have sometimes been reversible when busulfan was withdrawn. Adrenal responsiveness to exogenously administered adrenocorticotropic hormone usually has been normal. However, pituitary function testing with metyrapone revealed a blunted urinary 17-hydroxycorticosteroid excretion in 2 patients. Following the discontinuation of busulfan (which was associated with clinical improvement), rechallenge with metyrapone revealed normal pituitary-adrenal function.

Hyperuricemia and/or hyperuricosuria are not uncommon in patients with CML. Additional rapid destruction of granulocytes may accompany the initiation of chemotherapy and increase the urate pool. Adverse reactions can be minimized by increased hydration, urine alkalinization, and the prophylactic administration of a xanthine oxidase inhibitor such as allopurinol.

➤*Ophthalmic:* Busulfan is capable of inducing cataracts in rats; there have been several reports indicating that this is a rare complication in humans.

➤*Pulmonary:* Interstitial pulmonary fibrosis has been reported rarely, but it is a clinically significant adverse reaction when observed and calls for immediate discontinuation of further administration of the drug. The role of corticosteroids in arresting or reversing the fibrosis has been reported to be beneficial in some cases and without effect in others.

➤*Miscellaneous:* Other reported adverse reactions include the following: alopecia, cheilosis, cholestatic jaundice, dryness of the oral mucous membranes, erythema multiforme, erythema nodosum, excessive dryness and fragility of the skin with anhidrosis, gynecomastia, myasthenia gravis, porphyria cutanea tarda, urticaria. Most of these are single case reports, and in many, a clear cause-and-effect relationship with busulfan has not been demonstrated.

➤*Adverse reactions observed during clinical practice:* The following reactions have been identified during postapproval use of busulfan. Because they are reported voluntarily from a population of unknown size, estimates of frequency cannot be made. These reactions have been chosen for inclusion because of a combination of their seriousness, frequency of reporting, or potential causal connection to busulfan.

Dermatologic – Rash; an increased local cutaneous reaction has been observed in patients receiving radiotherapy soon after busulfan.

Hematologic / Lymphatic – Aplastic anemia.

Hepatic – Centrilobular sinusoidal fibrosis, hepatocellular atrophy, hepatocellular necrosis, HVOD, hyperbilirubinemia.

Ophthalmic – Cataracts, corneal thinning, lens changes.

Respiratory – Pneumonia.

Miscellaneous – Infection, mucositis, sepsis.

Overdosage

➤*Symptoms:* GI toxicity with diarrhea, mucositis, nausea, and vomiting and has been observed when busulfan was used in association with BMT.

Oral median lethal doses (LD_{50}) in mice are singles doses of busulfan 120 mg/kg. Two distinct types of toxic response are seen at median lethal doses given intraperitoneally. Within a matter of hours, there are signs of stimulation of the CNS with convulsions and death on the first day. Mice are more sensitive to this effect than rats. With doses at the LD_{50} there is also delayed death because of damage to the bone marrow. At 3 times the LD_{50}, atrophy of the mucosa of the large intestine is found after a week, whereas that of the small intestine is little affected. After doses in the order of 10 times those used therapeutically were added to the diet of rats, irreversible cataracts were produced after several weeks. Small doses had no such effect.

➤*Treatment:* There is no known antidote to busulfan. The principal toxic effects are bone marrow depression and pancytopenia. Closely monitor the hematologic status and institute vigorous supportive measures if necessary. Gastric lavage followed by administration of charcoal would be indicated if ingestion were recent. Dialysis may be considered in the management of overdose as there is 1 report of successful dialysis of busulfan. The 1 report

BUSULFAN — ORAL

of the impact of hemodialysis on the oral clearance was in a patient with chronic renal failure undergoing autologous peripheral stem cell transplantation for non-Hodgkin lymphoma. A 4-hour hemodialysis session increased the apparent oral clearance of busulfan by about 65%. The factors that favor hemodialysis of busulfan include the following: low molecular weight, low plasma protein binding, and a blood-to-plasma partition ratio of close to 1. However, with a 4-hour hemodialysis, the mean daily (24 hours) oral clearance of busulfan was only increased about 10%.

Patient Information

Inform patients beginning therapy with busulfan of the importance of having periodic blood counts and of immediate reporting of any unusual fever or bleeding. Aside from the major toxicity of myelosuppression, instruct patients to report any difficulty in breathing, congestion, or persistent cough. Tell patients that diffuse pulmonary fibrosis is an infrequent, but serious and potentially life-threatening, complication of long-term busulfan therapy. Alert patients to report any signs of abrupt weakness, anorexia, melanoderma, nausea and vomiting, unusual fatigue, and weight loss that could be associated with a syndrome resembling adrenal insufficiency. Never allow patients to take the drug without medical supervision, and inform them that other encountered toxicities to busulfan include amenorrhea, drug hypersensitivity, dryness of the mucous membranes, infertility, skin hyperpigmentation, and, rarely, cataract formation. Advise women of childbearing potential to avoid becoming pregnant. Explain the increased risk of a second malignancy to the patient.

BUSULFAN — INJECTION

WARNING

Busulfan injection is a potent cytotoxic drug that causes profound myelosuppression at the recommended dosage. It should be administered under the supervision of a qualified health care provider who is experienced in allogeneic hematopoietic stem-cell transplantation, the use of cancer chemotherapeutic drugs, and the management of patients with severe pancytopenia. Appropriate management of therapy and complications is only possible when adequate diagnostic and treatment facilities are readily available.

Indications

➤*Chronic myelogenous leukemia (CML):* For use in combination with cyclophosphamide as a conditioning regimen prior to allogeneic hematopoietic progenitor cell transplantation for CML.

Administration and Dosage

➤*Approved by the FDA:* February 4, 1999.

When busulfan injection is administered as a component of the busulfan/cyclophosphamide conditioning regimen prior to bone marrow or peripheral blood progenitor cell replacement, the recommended doses are as follows:

➤*Adults:* The usual adult dosage is 0.8 mg/kg of ideal body weight (IBW) or actual body weight (ABW), whichever is lower, administered every 6 hours for 4 days (a total of 16 doses). For obese or severely obese patients, busulfan should be administered based on adjusted ideal body weight (AIBW). IBW should be calculated as follows (height in cm, and weight in kg):

$$\text{IBW (kg; men)} = 50 + 0.91 \times (\text{height in cm} - 152)$$

$$\text{IBW (kg; women)} = 45 + 0.91 \times (\text{height in cm} - 152)$$

AIBW should be calculated as follows:

$$\text{AIBW} = \text{IBW} + 0.25 \times (\text{actual weight} - \text{IBW})$$

Cyclophosphamide is given on each of 2 days as a 1-hour infusion at a dose of 60 mg/kg beginning on bone marrow transplantation (BMT) day −3, no sooner than 6 hours following the 16th dose of busulfan.

Busulfan clearance is best predicted when the busulfan dose is administered based on AIBW. Dosing busulfan based on ABW, IBW, or other factors can produce significant differences in busulfan clearance among lean, healthy, and obese patients.

Busulfan should be administered intravenously (IV) via a central venous catheter as a 2-hour infusion every 6 hours × 4 consecutive days for a total of 16 doses. All patients should be premedicated with phenytoin because busulfan is known to cross the blood-brain barrier and induce seizures. Phenytoin reduces busulfan plasma area under the curve (AUC) 15%. Use of other anticonvulsants may result in higher busulfan plasma AUCs and an increased risk of venoocclusive disease or seizures. In cases where other anticonvulsants must be used, plasma busulfan exposure should be monitored. Antiemetics should be administered prior to the first dose of busulfan and continued on a fixed schedule through administration of busulfan. Where available, pharmacokinetic monitoring may be considered to further optimize therapeutic targeting.

➤*Children:* See Warnings for more information.

➤*Dose adjustment based on therapeutic drug monitoring:* Instructions for measuring the AUC of busulfan at dose 1 (see Blood Sample Collection for AUC Determination) and the formula for adjustment of subsequent doses to achieve the desired target AUC (1,125 mcM•min) follow:

$$\text{Adjusted dose (mg)} = \frac{\text{actual dose (mg)} \times \text{target AUC (mcM•min)}}{\text{actual AUC (mcM•min)}}$$

➤*Blood sample collection for AUC determination:* Calculate the AUC (mcM•min) based on blood samples collected at the following time points:

For dose 1 – Two hours (end of infusion), 4 and 6 hours (immediately prior to the next scheduled busulfan administration). Actual sampling times should be recorded.

For doses other than dose 1 – Pre-infusion (baseline), 2 hours (end of infusion), 4 and 6 hours (immediately prior to the next scheduled busulfan administration).

AUC calculations based on fewer than the 3 specified samples may result in inaccurate AUC determinations.

For each scheduled blood sample, collect 1 to 3 mL of blood into heparinized (Na or Li heparin) *Vacutainer* tubes. The blood samples should be placed on wet ice immediately after collection and should be centrifuged (at 4°C [39.2°F]) within 1 hour. The plasma, harvested into appropriate cryovial storage tubes, should be frozen immediately at −20°C (−4°F). All plasma samples should be sent in a frozen state (on dry ice) to the assay laboratory for the determination of plasma busulfan concentrations.

Calculation of AUC – Busulfan AUC calculations may be made using the following instructions and appropriate standard pharmacokinetic formula:

Dose 1 AUC_∞ calculation:

$AUC_\infty = AUC_{0\text{-}6h} + AUC_{extrapolated}$, where $AUC_{0\text{-}6h}$ should be estimated using the linear trapezoidal rule, and AUC extrapolated can be computed by taking the ratio of the busulfan concentration at hour 6 and the terminal elimination rate constant, λ_z. The λ_z must be calculated from the terminal elimination phase of the busulfan concentration versus time curve. An "O" predose busulfan concentration should be assumed and used in the calculation of AUC.

If the AUC is assessed subsequent to dose 1, steady-state AUC_{ss} ($AUC_{0\text{-}6h}$) should be estimated from the trough, 2-, 4-, and 6-hour concentrations using the linear trapezoidal rule.

➤*Instructions for drug administration and blood sample collection for therapeutic drug monitoring:* An administration set with minimal residual hold-up (priming) volume (1 to 3 mL) should be used for drug infusion to ensure accurate delivery of the entire prescribed dose and to ensure accurate collection of blood samples for therapeutic drug monitoring and dose adjustment.

Prime the administration set tubing with drug solution to allow accurate documentation of the start time of busulfan infusion. Collect the blood sample from a peripheral IV line to avoid contamination with infusing drug. If the blood sample is taken directly from the existing central venous catheter (CVC), do not collect the blood sample while the drug is infusing to ensure that the end of infusion sample is not contaminated with any residual drug. At the end of infusion (2 hours), disconnect the administration tubing and flush the CVC line with 5 mL of normal saline prior to the collection of the end of infusion sample from the CVC port. Collect the blood samples from a different port than that used for the busulfan infusion. When recording the busulfan infusion stop time, do not include the time required to flush the indwelling catheter line. Discard the administration tubing at the end of the 2-hour infusion.

➤*Preparation and administration precautions:* An administration set with minimal residual hold-up volume (2 to 5 mL) should be used for product administration.

As with other cytotoxic compounds, caution should be exercised in handling and preparing the solution of busulfan. Skin reactions may occur with accidental exposure. The use of gloves is recommended. If busulfan or diluted busulfan solution contacts the skin or mucosa, wash the skin or mucosa thoroughly with water.

Busulfan is a clear, colorless solution. Parenteral drug products should be visually inspected for particulate matter and discoloration prior to administration whenever the solution and container permit. If particulate matter is seen in the busulfan ampule, the drug should not be used.

➤*Preparation for IV administration:* Busulfan must be diluted prior to use with either 0.9% sodium chloride injection (normal saline) or 5% dextrose injection (D5W). The diluent quantity should be 10 times the volume of busulfan, ensuring that the final concentration of busulfan is approximately greater than or equal to 0.5 mg/mL. Calculation of the dose for a 70 kg patient, would be performed as follows.

$$\frac{\text{(70 kg patient)} \times \text{(0.8 mg/kg)}}{\text{(6 mg/mL)}} = \text{busulfan 9.3 mL (56 mg total dose)}$$

To prepare the final solution for infusion, add busulfan 9.3 mL to 93 mL of diluent (normal saline or D5W) as calculated: (busulfan 9.3 mL) × (10) = 93 mL of either diluent plus busulfan 9.3 mL to yield a final concentration of busulfan 0.54 mg/mL (9.3 mL × 6 mg/mL ÷ 102.3 mL = 0.54 mg/mL).

All transfer procedures require strict adherence to aseptic techniques, preferably employing a vertical laminar flow safety hood while wearing gloves and protective clothing. In accordance with pharmacy practices, filter busulfan using the 5 micron syringe filter provided with each package, using 1 filter per ampule. If using the enclosed syringe filter in the forward flow direction, the calculated volume of busulfan should allow for approximately 0.16 mL of residual busulfan that will remain in the filter.

Do not put the busulfan into an IV bag or large-volume syringe that does not contain normal saline of D5W. Always add the busulfan to the diluent, not

BUSULFAN — INJECTION

the diluent to the busulfan. Mix thoroughly by inverting several times. Use of syringe filters other than the specific type included in this package with each ampule is not recommended. Do not use polycarbonate syringes or polycarbonate filter needles with busulfan.

Infusion pumps should be used to administer the diluted busulfan solution. Set the flow rate of the pump to deliver the entire prescribed busulfan dose over 2 hours. Prior to and following each infusion, flush the catheter line with approximately 5 mL of 0.9% sodium chloride injection or 5% dextrose injection. Do not infuse concomitantly with another IV solution of unknown compatibility.

Warning – Rapid infusion of busulfan has not been tested and is not recommended.

➤*Storage/Stability:* Unopened ampules of busulfan are stable until the date indicated on the package when stored under refrigeration at 2° to 8°C (36° to 46°F).

Busulfan diluted in 0.9% sodium chloride injection or 5% dextrose injection is stable at room temperature (25°C [73°F]) for up to 8 hours, but the infusion must be completed within that time. Busulfan diluted in 0.9% sodium chloride injection is stable at refrigerated conditions (2° to 8°C [6° to 46°F]) for up to 12 hours, but the infusion must be completed within that time.

Actions

➤*Pharmacology:*

Mechanism of action – Busulfan is a bifunctional alkylating agent in which 2 labile methanesulfonate groups are attached to opposite ends of a 4-carbon alkyl chain. In aqueous media, busulfan hydrolyzes to release the methanesulfonate groups. This produces reactive carbonium ions that can alkylate deoxyribonucleic acid (DNA). DNA damage is thought to be responsible for much of the cytotoxicity of busulfan.

➤*Pharmacokinetics:*

Distribution – Studies of distribution, metabolism, and elimination of busulfan have not been done; however, the literature on oral busulfan is relevant.

Busulfan achieves concentrations in the cerebrospinal fluid approximately equal to those in plasma. Irreversible binding to plasma elements, primarily albumin, has been estimated to be 32.4 ± 2.2%, which is consistent with the reactive electrophilic properties of busulfan.

Metabolism – Busulfan is predominantly metabolized by conjugation with glutathione, both spontaneously and by glutathione S-transferase catalysis. This conjugate undergoes further extensive oxidative metabolism in the liver.

Excretion – Following administration of ^{14}C-labeled busulfan to humans, approximately 30% of the radioactivity was excreted into the urine over 48 hours; negligible amounts were recovered in feces. The incomplete recovery of radioactivity may be caused by to the formation of long-lived metabolites or nonspecific alkylation of macromolecules.

The pharmacokinetics of busulfan were studied in 59 patients participating in a prospective trial of a busulfan-cyclophosphamide preparatory regimen prior to allogeneic hematopoietic progenitor stem-cell transplantation. Patients received busulfan 0.8 mg/kg every 6 hours for a total of 16 doses over 4 days. Fifty-five of 59 patients (93%) administered busulfan maintained AUC values below the target value (less than 1,500 mcM•min).

Steady-State Pharmacokinetic Parameters Following Busulfan Infusion (0.8 mg/kg; n = 59)

	Mean	CV (%)[a]	Range
C_{max} (ng/mL)[b]	1,222	18%	496 to 1,684
AUC (mcM•min)	1,167	20%	556 to 1,673
CL (mL/min/kg)[c]	2.52	25%	1.49 to 4.31

[a] CV = coefficient of variation.
[b] C_{max} = maximum plasma concentration.
[c] CL = clearance normalized to actual body weight for all patients.

Contraindications

History of hypersensitivity to any of its components.

Warnings

➤*Hematologic:* The most frequent serious consequence of treatment with busulfan at the recommended dose and schedule is profound myelosuppression, occurring in all patients. Severe granulocytopenia, thrombocytopenia, anemia, or any combination thereof may develop. Monitor frequent complete blood counts, including white blood cell differentials and quantitative platelet counts, during treatment and until recovery is achieved. Absolute neutrophil counts (ANCs) dropped below 0.5 × 10^9/L at a median of 4 days posttransplant in 100% of patients treated in the busulfan clinical trial. The ANC recovered at a median of 13 days following allogeneic transplantation when prophylactic granulocyte colony-stimulating factor (G-CSF) was used in the majority of patients.

Thrombocytopenia (less than 25,000/mm^3 or requiring platelet transfusion) occurred at a median of 5 to 6 days in 98% of patients. Anemia (hemoglobin less than 8 g/dL) occurred in 69% of patients. Use antibiotic therapy and platelet and red blood cell support when medically indicated.

➤*Neurological:* Seizures have been reported in patients receiving high-dose oral busulfan at doses producing plasma drug levels similar to those achieved following the recommended dosage of busulfan. Despite prophylactic therapy with phenytoin, 1 seizure (1/42 patients) was reported during an autologous transplantation clinical trial of busulfan. This episode occurred during the cyclophosphamide portion of the conditioning regimen, 36 hours after the last busulfan dose. Initiate anticonvulsant prophylactic therapy prior to busulfan treatment. Exercise caution when administering the recommended dose of busulfan to patients with a history of a seizure disorder or head trauma, or who are receiving other potentially epileptogenic drugs.

➤*Hepatic:* Current literature suggests that high busulfan AUC values (greater than 1,500 mcM•min) may be associated with an increased risk of developing hepatic venoocclusive disease (HVOD). Patients who have received prior radiation therapy, at least 3 cycles of chemotherapy, or a prior progenitor cell transplant may be at increased risk of developing HVOD with the recommended busulfan dose and regimen. Based on clinical examination and laboratory findings, HVOD was diagnosed in 8% (5/61) of patients treated with busulfan in the setting of allogeneic transplantation, was fatal in 2/5 cases (40%), and yielded an overall mortality from HVOD in the entire study population of 2/61 (3%). Three of the 5 patients diagnosed with HVOD were retrospectively found to meet the Jones criteria. The incidence of HVOD reported in the literature from the randomized, controlled trials was 7.7% to 12%.

➤*Cardiac:* Cardiac tamponade has been reported in children with thalassemia (8/400 or 2% in 1 series) who received high doses of oral busulfan and cyclophosphamide as the preparatory regimen for hematopoietic progenitor cell transplantation. Six of the 8 children died, and 2 were saved by rapid pericardiocentesis. Abdominal pain and vomiting preceded the tamponade in most patients. No patients treated in the busulfan clinical trials experienced cardiac tamponade.

➤*Pulmonary:* Bronchopulmonary dysplasia with pulmonary fibrosis is a rare but serious complication following chronic busulfan therapy. The average onset of symptoms is 4 years after therapy (range, 4 months to 10 years).

➤*Carcinogenesis:* The IV administration of busulfan (48 mg/kg given as biweekly doses of 12 mg/kg, or 30% of the total busulfan dose on a mg/m^2 basis) increased the incidence of thymic and ovarian tumors in mice. Four cases of acute leukemia occurred among 19 patients who became pancytopenic in a 243-patient study incorporating busulfan as adjuvant therapy following surgical resection of bronchogenic carcinoma. Clinical appearance of leukemia was observed 5 to 8 years after oral busulfan treatment. Busulfan is a presumed human carcinogen.

➤*Mutagenesis:* Busulfan is a mutagen and a clastogen. In in vitro tests it caused mutations in *Salmonella typhimurium* and *Drosophila melanogaster*. Chromosomal aberrations induced by busulfan have been reported in vivo (rats, mice, hamsters, and humans) and in vitro (rodent and human cells).

➤*Fertility impairment:* Ovarian suppression and amenorrhea commonly occur in premenopausal women undergoing chronic, low-dose busulfan therapy for CML. Busulfan depleted oocytes of female rats. Busulfan induced sterility in male rats and hamsters. Sterility, azoospermia, and testicular atrophy have been reported in men.

The solvent dimethylacetamide (DMA) also may impair fertility. A DMA daily dose of 0.45 g/kg given to rats for 9 days (equivalent to 44% of the daily dose of DMA contained in the recommended dose of busulfan on a mg/m^2 basis) significantly decreased spermatogenesis in rats. A single subcutaneous dose of 2.2 g/kg (27% of the total DMA dose contained in busulfan on a mg/m^2 basis) 4 days after insemination terminated pregnancy in 100% of tested hamsters.

➤*Pregnancy: Category D.* Busulfan may cause fetal harm when administered to a pregnant woman. Busulfan produced teratogenic changes in the offspring of mice, rats, and rabbits when given during gestation. Malformations and anomalies included significant alterations in the musculoskeletal system, body weight gain, and size. In pregnant rats, busulfan produced sterility in male and female offspring because of the absence of germinal cells in the testes and ovaries. The solvent DMA also may cause fetal harm when administered to a pregnant woman. In rats, DMA doses of 400 mg/kg/day (approximately 40% of the daily dose of DMA in the busulfan dose on a mg/m^2 basis) given during organogenesis caused significant developmental anomalies. The most striking abnormalities included anasarca, cleft palate, vertebral anomalies, rib anomalies, and serious anomalies of the vessels of the heart. There are no adequate and well-controlled studies of busulfan or DMA in pregnant women. If busulfan is used during pregnancy, or if the patient becomes pregnant while receiving busulfan, inform the patient of the potential hazard to the fetus. Advise women of childbearing potential to avoid becoming pregnant.

➤*Lactation:* It is not known whether this drug is excreted in breast milk. Because many drugs are excreted in breast milk, and because of the potential for tumorigenicity shown for busulfan in human and animal studies, decide whether to discontinue breast-feeding or the drug, taking into account the importance of the drug to the mother.

➤*Children:* The efficacy of busulfan in the treatment of CML has not been specifically studied in children. An open-label, uncontrolled study evaluated the pharmacokinetics of busulfan in 24 children receiving busulfan as part of a conditioning regimen administered prior to hematopoietic progenitor cell transplantation for a variety of malignant hematologic (n = 15) or non-malignant diseases (n = 9). Patients ranged in age from 5 months to 16 years of age (median, 3 years of age). Busulfan dosing was targeted to achieve an AUC of 900 to 1,350 mcM•min, with an initial dose of 0.8 or 1 mg/kg (based on ABW) if the patient was older than 4 years of age or 4 years of age and younger, respectively. The dose was adjusted based on plasma concentration after completion of dose 1.

Patients received busulfan doses every 6 hours as a 2-hour infusion over 4 days for a total of 16 doses, followed by cyclophosphamide 50 mg/kg once

BUSULFAN — INJECTION

daily for 4 days. After 1 rest day, hematopoietic progenitor cells were infused. All patients received phenytoin as seizure prophylaxis. The target AUC (900 to 1,350 ± 5% mcM•min) for busulfan was achieved at dose 1 in 71% (17/24) of patients. Steady-state pharmacokinetic testing was performed at doses 9 and 13. Busulfan levels were within the target range for 21 of 23 evaluable patients.

All 24 patients experienced neutropenia (ANC less than 0.5×10^9/L) and thrombocytopenia (platelet transfusions or platelet count less than 20,000/mm^3). Seventy-nine percent (19/24) of patients experienced lymphopenia (absolute lymphocyte count less than 0.1×10^9). In 23 patients, the ANC recovered to more than 0.5×10^9/L (median time to recovery = BMT day +13; range = BMT day +9 to +22). One patient who died on day +20 had not recovered to an ANC greater than 0.5×10^9/L.

Four (17%) patients died during the study. Two patients died within 28 days of transplant; 1 with pneumonia and capillary leak syndrome, and the other with pneumonia and venoocclusive disease. Two patients died prior to day 100; 1 because of progressive disease and 1 because of multiorgan failure.

Adverse reactions were reported in all 24 patients during the study period (BMT day −10 through BMT day +28) or poststudy surveillance period (day +29 through +100). These included vomiting (100%), nausea (83%), stomatitis (79%), HVOD (21%), graft-versus-host disease (GVHD) (25%), and pneumonia (21%).

Based on the results of this 24-patient clinical trial, a suggested dosing regimen of busulfan in children is shown in the following dosing nomogram:

Busulfan Dosing Nomogram

Patient's ABW	Busulfan dosage
≤ 12 kg	1.1 (mg/kg)
> 12 kg	0.8 (mg/kg)

Simulations based on a pediatric population pharmacokinetic model indicate that approximately 60% of children will achieve a target busulfan exposure (AUC) between 900 to 1,350 mcM•min with the first dose of busulfan using this dosing nomogram. Therapeutic drug monitoring and dose adjustment following the first dose of busulfan is recommended.

Precautions

➤*Monitoring:* Monitor patients receiving busulfan daily with a complete blood count, including differential count and quantitative platelet count, until engraftment has been demonstrated.

To detect hepatotoxicity, which may herald the onset of HVOD, evaluate serum transaminases, alkaline phosphatase, and bilirubin daily through BMT day +28.

➤*Hematologic:* See Warnings for more information.

➤*Cytologic dysplasia:* Busulfan may cause cellular dysplasia in many organs. Cytologic abnormalities characterized by giant, hyperchromatic nuclei have been reported in lymph nodes, pancreas, thyroid, adrenal glands, liver, lungs, and bone marrow. This cytologic dysplasia may be severe enough to cause difficulty in interpretation of exfoliative cytologic examinations of the lungs, bladder, breast, and the uterine cervix.

Drug Interactions

Busulfan Drug Interactions

Precipitant drug	Object drug[a]		Description
Acetaminophen	Busulfan	⬆	Because busulfan is eliminated from the body via conjugation with glutathione, use of acetaminophen prior to (< 72 hours) or concurrently with busulfan may result in reduced busulfan clearance based on the known property of acetaminophen to decrease glutathione levels in the blood and tissues.
Cyclophosphamide	Busulfan	⬆	Cardiac tamponade, which was often fatal, has been reported in a small number of patients with thalassemia (2% in 1 series) who received high doses of busulfan and cyclophosphamide (see Precautions).
Itraconazole	Busulfan	⬇	Itraconazole decreases busulfan clearance up to 25% and may produce AUCs > 1,500 mcM•min in some patients.
Phenytoin	Busulfan	⬆	Phenytoin increases the clearance of busulfan ≥ 15%, possibly caused by the induction of glutathione-S-transferase.
Thioguanine	Busulfan	⬆	In 1 study, ≈ 3.6% of patients receiving continuous (6 to 45 months) concomitant therapy for treatment of CML had esophageal varices associated with abnormal liver function tests. Liver biopsies performed in 33% of these patients all showed evidence of nodular regenerative hyperplasia. Use with caution in long-term continuous therapy.

[a] ⬆ = Object drug increased. ⬇ = Object drug decreased.

Adverse Reactions

DMA, the solvent used in the busulfan formulation, was studied in 1962 as a potential cancer chemotherapy drug. In a phase 1 trial, the maximum tolerated dose (MTD) was 14.8 g/m^2/day for 4 days. The daily recommended dose of busulfan contains DMA equivalent to 42% of the MTD on a mg/m^2 basis. The dose-limiting toxicities in the phase 1 study were hepatotoxicity as evidenced by increased AST levels and neurological symptoms as evidenced by hallucinations. The hallucinations had a pattern of onset at 1 day postcompletion of DMA administration and were associated with electroencephalogram changes. The lowest dose at which hallucinations were recognized was equivalent to 1.9 times that delivered in a conditioning regimen utilizing busulfan 0.8 mg/kg every 6 hours × 16 doses. Other neurological toxicities included confusion, lethargy, and somnolence. The relative contribution of DMA and/or other concomitant medications to neurologic and hepatic toxicities observed with busulfan is difficult to ascertain.

Treatment with busulfan at the recommended dose and schedule will result in profound myelosuppression in 100% of patients, including anemia, granulocytopenia, thrombocytopenia, or a combined loss of formed elements of the blood.

Summary of the Incidence (20%) of Nonhematologic Adverse Reactions Through BMT Day +28 in Patients Who Received Busulfan Prior to Allogeneic Hematopoietic Progenitor Cell Transplantation

Nonhematological adverse reactions[a]	Incidence (%)
Cardiovascular	
Hypertension	36%
Tachycardia	44%
Thrombosis	33%
Vasodilation	25%
CNS	
Anxiety	72%
Depression	23%
Dizziness	30%
Insomnia	84%
Dermatologic	
Pruritus	28%
Rash	57%
GI	
Abdominal enlargement	23%
Abdominal pain	72%
Anorexia	85%
Constipation	38%
Diarrhea	84%
Dry mouth	26%
Dyspepsia	44%
Nausea	98%
Rectal disorder	25%
Stomatitis (mucositis)	97%
Vomiting	95%
Metabolic/Nutritional	
AST elevation	31%
Creatinine increased	21%
Edema	36%
Hyperbilirubinemia	49%
Hyperglycemia	66%
Hypocalcemia	49%
Hypokalemia	64%
Hypomagnesemia	77%

BUSULFAN — INJECTION

Summary of the Incidence (20%) of Nonhematologic Adverse Reactions Through BMT Day +28 in Patients Who Received Busulfan Prior to Allogeneic Hematopoietic Progenitor Cell Transplantation

Nonhematological adverse reactions[a]	Incidence (%)
Respiratory	
Cough	28%
Dyspnea	25%
Epistaxis	25%
Lung disorder	34%
Rhinitis	44%
Miscellaneous	
Allergic reaction	26%
Asthenia	51%
Back pain	23%
Chest pain	26%
Chills	46%
Edema, general	28%
Fever	80%
Headache	69%
Inflammation at injection site	25%
Pain	44%

[a] Includes all reported adverse reactions regardless of severity (toxicity grades 1 to 4).

The following sections describe clinically significant reactions occurring in the busulfan clinical trials, regardless of drug attribution.

➤*Cardiovascular:* Mild or moderate tachycardia was reported in 44% of patients. In 7 patients (11%), it was first reported during busulfan administration. Other rhythm abnormalities, which were all mild or moderate, included arrhythmia (5%), atrial fibrillation (2%), ventricular extrasystoles (2%), and third-degree heart block (2%). Mild or moderate thrombosis occurred in 33% of patients, and all episodes were associated with the central venous catheter. Hypertension was reported in 36% of patients and was grade 3/4 in 7%. Hypotension occurred in 11% of patients and was grade 3/4 in 3%. Mild vasodilation (flushing and hot flashes) was reported in 25% of patients. Other cardiovascular events included cardiomegaly (5%), mild electrocardiogram abnormality (2%), grade 3/4 left-sided heart failure in 1 patient (2%), and moderate pericardial effusion (2%). These reactions were reported primarily in the postcyclophosphamide phase.

➤*CNS:* The most commonly reported adverse reactions of the CNS were insomnia (84%), anxiety (75%), dizziness (30%), and depression (23%). Severity was mild or moderate except for 1 patient (1%) who experienced severe insomnia. One patient (1%) developed a life-threatening cerebral hemorrhage and a coma as a terminal event following multiorgan failure after HVOD. Other reactions considered severe included delirium (2%), agitation (2%), and encephalopathy (2%). The overall incidence of confusion was 11% and 5% of patients were reported to have experienced hallucinations. The patient who developed delirium and hallucination on the allogeneic study had onset of confusion at the completion of busulfan. The overall incidence of lethargy in the allogeneic busulfan clinical trial was 7%, and somnolence was reported in 2%. One patient (2%) treated in an autologous transplantation study experienced a seizure while receiving cyclophosphamide, despite prophylactic treatment with phenytoin.

➤*Dermatologic:* Rash (57%) and pruritus (28%) were reported; both conditions were predominantly mild. Alopecia was mild in 15% of patients; mild vesicular rash and vesiculobullous rash were reported in 10% of patients. Moderate maculopapular rash and skin discoloration was reported in 8% of patients. Acne was reported in 7% of patients. Exfoliative dermatitis was reported in 5% of patients. Erythema nodosum and moderate alopecia were reported in 2% of patients.

➤*GI:* GI toxicities were frequent and generally considered to be related to the drug. Few were categorized as serious. Mild or moderate nausea occurred in 92% of patients in the allogeneic clinical trial, and mild or moderate vomiting occurred in 95% through BMT day 28; nausea was severe in 7% of patients. The incidence of vomiting during busulfan administration (BMT day −7 to −4) was 43% in the allogeneic clinical trial. Grade 3 to 4 stomatitis developed in 26% of the participants, and grade 3 esophagitis developed in 2%. Grade 3 to 4 diarrhea was reported in 5% of the allogeneic study participants, while mild or moderate diarrhea occurred in 75%. Mild or moderate constipation occurred in 38% of patients; ileus developed in 8% of patients and was severe in 2% of patients. Forty-four percent of patients reported mild or moderate dyspepsia. Two percent of patients experienced mild hematemesis. Pancreatitis developed in 2% of patients. Mild or moderate rectal discomfort occurred in 24% of patients. Severe anorexia occurred in 21% of patients and was mild/moderate in 64% of patients.

➤*Hematologic:* At the indicated dose and schedule, busulfan produced profound myelosuppression in 100% of patients. Following hematopoietic progenitor cell infusion, recovery of neutrophil counts to greater than or equal to 500 cells/mm^3 occurred at median day 13 when prophylactic G-CSF was administered to the majority of participants on the study. The median number of platelet transfusions per patient on study was 6, and the median number of red blood cell transfusions on study was 4. Prolonged prothrombin time was reported in 1 patient (2%).

➤*Hepatic:* Hyperbilirubinemia occurred in 49% of patients in the allogeneic BMT trial. Grade 3/4 hyperbilirubinemia occurred in 30% of patients within 28 days of transplantation and was considered life-threatening in 5% of these patients. Hyperbilirubinemia was associated with GVHD in 6 patients and with HVOD in 5 patients. Grade 3/4 AST elevations occurred in 7% of patients. Alkaline phosphatase increases were mild or moderate in 15% of patients. Mild or moderate jaundice developed in 12% of patients, and mild or moderate hepatomegaly developed in 6% of patients.

HVOD – See Warnings for more information.

➤*Metabolic/Nutritional:* Hyperglycemia was observed in 67% of patients and grade 3/4 hyperglycemia was reported in 15%. Hypomagnesemia was mild or moderate in 77% of patients; hypokalemia was mild or moderate in 62% and severe in 2% of patients; hypocalcemia was mild or moderate in 46% and severe in 3% of patients; hypophosphatemia was mild or moderate in 17% of patients; and hyponatremia was reported in 2% of patients.

➤*Renal:* Creatinine was mildly or moderately elevated in 21% of patients. BUN was increased in 3% of patients and to a grade 3/4 level in 2% of patients. Seven percent of patients experienced dysuria, 15% experienced oliguria, and 8% experienced hematuria. There were 4 (7%) grade 3/4 cases of hemorrhagic cystitis in the allogeneic clinical trial.

➤*Respiratory:* Mild or moderate dyspnea occurred in 25% of patients and was severe in 2% of patients. One patient (2%) experienced severe hyperventilation; and in 2 (3%) additional patients it was mild or moderate. Mild rhinitis and mild or moderate cough were reported in 44% and 28% of patients, respectively. Mild epistaxis events were reported in 25% of patients. Three patients (5%) on the allogeneic study developed documented alveolar hemorrhage. All required mechanical ventilatory support and all died. Nonspecific interstitial fibrosis was found on wedge biopsies performed with video-assisted thoracoscopy in 1 patient on the allogeneic study who subsequently died from respiratory failure on BMT day +98. Other pulmonary events, reported as mild or moderate, included pharyngitis (18%), hiccup (18%), asthma (8%), hemoptysis (3%), pleural effusion (3%), sinusitis (3%), atelectasis (2%), and hypoxia (2%).

➤*Miscellaneous:* Other reported reactions included headache (mild or moderate 64%, severe 5%), abdominal pain (mild or moderate 69%, severe 3%), asthenia (mild or moderate 49%, severe 2%), unspecified pain (mild or moderate 43%, severe 2%), allergic reaction (mild or moderate 24%, severe 2%), injection site inflammation (mild or moderate 25%), injection site pain (mild or moderate 15%), chest pain (mild or moderate 26%), back pain (mild or moderate 23%), myalgia (mild or moderate 16%), arthralgia (mild or moderate 13%), and ear disorder in 3%.

GVHD – GVHD developed in 18% of patients (11/61) receiving allogeneic transplants; it was severe in 3% and mild or moderate in 15% of patients. There were 3 deaths (5%) attributed to GVHD.

Edema – Patients receiving allogeneic transplant exhibited some form of edema (79%), hypervolemia, or documented weight increase (8%); all events were reported as mild or moderate.

Infection/Fever – Fifty-one percent of patients experienced at least 1 episode of infection. Pneumonia was fatal in 1 patient (2%) and life-threatening in 3% of patients. Fever was reported in 80% of patients; it was mild or moderate in 78% and severe in 3% of patients. Forty-six percent of patients experienced chills.

Deaths – There were 2 deaths through BMT day +28 in the allogeneic transplant setting. There were an additional 6 deaths BMT day +29 through BMT day +100 in the allogeneic transplant setting.

Overdosage

There is no known antidote to busulfan other than hematopoietic progenitor cell transplantation. In the absence of hematopoietic progenitor cell transplantation, the recommended dosage for busulfan would constitute an overdose of busulfan. The principal toxic effect is profound bone marrow hypoplasia/aplasia and pancytopenia but the CNS, liver, lungs, and GI tract may be affected. Closely monitor the hematologic status and institute vigorous supportive measures as medically indicated. Survival after a single dose of busulfan 140 mg tablets in an 18 kg, 4-year-old child has been reported. Inadvertent administration of a greater-than-normal dose of oral busulfan (2.1 mg/kg; total dose of 23.3 mg/kg) occurred in a 2-year-old child prior to a scheduled BMT without sequelae. An acute dose of 2.4 g was fatal in a 10-year-old boy. There is 1 report that busulfan is dialyzable, thus consider dialysis in the case of overdose. Busulfan is metabolized by conjugation with glutathione, thus administration of glutathione may be considered.

Patient Information

Explain the increased risk of a second malignancy to the patient.

ALTRETAMINE (Hexamethylmelamine)

Rx	**Hexalen** (MGI Pharma)	**Capsules**: 50 mg	Lactose. (USB001 Hexalen 50 mg). Clear. In 100s.

ALTRETAMINE (Hexamethylmelamine) — ORAL

WARNING

Administer only under the supervision of a physician experienced in the use of antineoplastic agents.

Monitor peripheral blood counts at least monthly, prior to the initiation of each course of altretamine therapy and as clinically indicated (see Adverse Reactions).

Because of the possibility of altretamine-related neurotoxicity, perform neurologic examination regularly during administration (see Adverse Reactions).

Indications

➤*Ovarian cancer:* For use as a single agent in the palliative treatment of patients with persistent or recurrent ovarian cancer following first-line therapy with a cisplatin- or alkylating agent-based combination.

Administration and Dosage

Altretamine may be administered either for 14 or 21 consecutive days in a 28 day cycle at a dose of 260 mg/m^2/day. Give the total daily dose as 4 divided oral doses after meals and at bedtime.

Temporarily discontinue altretamine (for ≥ 14 days) and subsequently restart at 200 mg/m^2/day for any of the following situations: GI intolerance unresponsive to symptomatic measures; WBC < 2000/mm^3 or granulocyte count < 1000/mm^3; platelet count < 75,000/mm^3; progressive neurotoxicity.

If neurologic symptoms fail to stabilize on the reduced dose schedule, discontinue altretamine indefinitely.

Actions

➤*Pharmacology:* Altretamine, formerly known as hexamethylmelamine, is a synthetic cytotoxic antineoplastic s-triazine derivative. The precise mechanism by which altretamine exerts its cytotoxic effect is unknown, although a number of theoretical possibilities have been studied. Structurally, altretamine resembles the alkylating agent triethylenemelamine, yet in vitro tests for alkylating activity of altretamine and its metabolites have been negative. Altretamine is efficacious for certain ovarian tumors resistant to classical alkylating agents. Metabolism of altretamine is a requirement for cytotoxicity. Synthetic monohydroxymethylmelamines and products of altretamine metabolism in vitro and in vivo can form covalent adducts with tissue macromolecules including DNA, but the relevance of these reactions to antitumor activity is unknown.

➤*Pharmacokinetics:* Altretamine is well absorbed following oral administration, but undergoes rapid and extensive demethylation in the liver, producing variations in altretamine plasma levels. The principal metabolites are pentamethylmelamine and tetramethylmelamine. After oral administration to 11 patients with advanced ovarian cancer in doses of 120 to 300 mg/m^2, peak plasma levels were reached between 0.5 and 3 hours, varying from 0.2 to 20.8 mg/L. Half-life of the β-phase of elimination ranged from 4.7 to 10.2 hours. Altretamine and metabolites show binding to plasma proteins. The free fractions of altretamine, pentamethylmelamine and tetramethylmelamine are 6%, 25% and 50%, respectively.

Following oral administration of 4 mg/kg, urinary recovery was 61% at 24 hours and 90% at 72 hours. Human urinary metabolites were N-demethylated homologues of altretamine with < 1% unmetabolized altretamine excreted at 24 hours. After intraperitoneal administration to mice, tissue distribution was rapid in all organs, reaching a maximum at 30 minutes. The excretory organs (liver and kidney) and the small intestine showed high concentrations, whereas relatively low concentrations were found in other organs, including the brain.

Contraindications

Hypersensitivity to altretamine.

Pre-existing severe bone marrow depression or severe neurologic toxicity; however, altretamine has been administered safely to patients heavily pretreated with cisplatin or alkylating agents including patients with preexisting cisplatin neuropathies. Careful monitoring of neurologic function in these patients is essential.

Warnings

➤*Neurotoxicity:* Altretamine causes mild to moderate neurotoxicity. Peripheral neuropathy and CNS symptoms (eg, mood disorders, disorders of consciousness, ataxia, dizziness, vertigo) have occurred. They are more likely to occur in patients receiving continuous high-dose daily altretamine than moderate-dose altretamine administered on an intermittent schedule. Neurologic toxicity appears to be reversible when therapy is discontinued. It has been suggested that the incidence and severity of neurotoxicity may be decreased by concomitant administration of pyridoxine, but this remains unproven. Perform a neurologic examination prior to the initiation of each course of therapy.

➤*Hematologic:* Altretamine causes mild to moderate dose-related myelosuppression. Leukopenia < 3000 WBC/mm^3 occurred in < 15% of patients on a variety of intermittent or continuous dose regimens; < 1% had leukopenia < 1000 WBC/mm^3. Thrombocytopenia < 50,000 platelets/mm^3 was seen in < 10% of patients. When given in doses of 8 to 12 mg/kg/day over a 21 day course, nadirs of leukocyte and platelet counts were reached by 3 to 4 weeks, and normal counts were regained by 6 weeks. With continuous administration at doses of 6 to 8 mg/kg/day, nadirs are reached in 6 to 8 weeks (median). Monitor peripheral blood counts prior to the initiation of each course of therapy, monthly, and as clinically indicated. Adjust the dose as necessary (see Administration and Dosage).

➤*Mutagenesis:* Altretamine was weakly mutagenic when tested in strain TA100 of *Salmonella typhimurium*.

➤*Fertility impairment:* Altretamine administered to female rats 14 days prior to breeding through the gestation period had no adverse effect on fertility, but it decreased postnatal survival at 120 mg/m^2/day and was embryocidal at 240 mg/m^2/day. Administration of 120 mg/m^2/day to male rats for 60 days prior to mating resulted in testicular atrophy, reduced fertility and a possible dominant lethal mutagenic effect. Male rats treated with 450 mg/m^2/day for 10 days had decreased spermatogenesis and atrophy of testes, seminal vesicles and ventral prostate.

➤*Pregnancy: Category D.* Altretamine is embryotoxic and teratogenic in rats and rabbits when given at doses 2 and 10 times the human dose, and it may cause fetal damage when administered to a pregnant woman. If altretamine is used during pregnancy, or if the patient becomes pregnant while taking the drug, apprise the patient of the potential hazard to the fetus. Advise women to avoid becoming pregnant.

➤*Lactation:* It is not known whether altretamine is excreted in breast milk. Because there is a possibility of toxicity in nursing infants secondary to altretamine treatment of the mother, it is recommended that breastfeeding be discontinued if the mother is treated with altretamine.

➤*Children:* Safety and efficacy in children have not been established.

Precautions

➤*Nausea and vomiting:* With continuous high-dose daily altretamine, nausea and vomiting of gradual onset occur frequently. In most instances, these symptoms are controllable with antiemetics; at times, however, the severity requires dose reduction or, rarely, discontinuation of therapy. In some instances, a tolerance of these symptoms develops after several weeks of therapy. The incidence and severity of nausea and vomiting are reduced with moderate-dose administration of altretamine. In two clinical studies of single-agent altretamine using a moderate, intermittent dose and schedule, only 1 patient (1%) discontinued altretamine due to severe nausea and vomiting.

Drug Interactions

Altretamine Drug Interactions

Precipitant drug	Object drug*		Description
Cimetidine	Altretamine	↑	Cimetidine, an inhibitor of microsomal drug metabolism, increased altretamine's half-life and toxicity in a rat model.
Altretamine	Monoamine oxidase inhibitors	↑	Monoamine oxidase inhibitors and concurrent altretamine may cause severe orthostatic hypotension. Four patients, all > 60 years of age, experienced symptomatic hypotension after 4 to 7 days of concomitant therapy.

* ↑ = Object drug increased.

Adverse Reactions

The most common adverse reactions are: Nausea and vomiting (see Precautions); peripheral neuropathy, CNS symptoms and myelosuppression (see Warnings).

Altretamine Adverse Reactions in Previously Treated Ovarian Cancer Patients (n = 70)

Adverse reaction	Incidence (%)
GI	
Nausea and vomiting	
Mild to moderate	32
Severe	1
Increased alkaline phosphatase	9
Hematologic	
Leukopenia	
WBC 2000 to 2999/mm^3	4
WBC < 2000/mm^3	1
Thrombocytopenia	
Platelets 75,000 to 99,000/mm^3	6
Platelets < 75,000/mm^3	3
Anemia	
Mild	20
Moderate to severe	13

ALTRETAMINE (Hexamethylmelamine) — ORAL

Altretamine Adverse Reactions in Previously Treated Ovarian Cancer Patients (n = 76)	
Adverse reaction	Incidence (%)
Neurologic	
Peripheral sensory neuropathy	
Mild	22
Moderate to severe	9
Anorexia and fatigue	1
Seizures	1
Renal	
Serum creatinine 1.6 to 3.75 mg/dl	7
BUN	
25-40 mg/dl	5
41-60 mg/dl	3
Greater than 60 mg/dl	1

THIOTEPA (Triethylenethiophosphoramide; TSPA; TESPA)

Rx	**Thioplex** (Amgen)	**Powder for injection, lyophilized:** 15 mg	In vials.
Rx	**Thiotepa** (Sicor)		In single-dose vials.
Rx	**Thiotepa** (Sicor)	**Powder for injection, lyophilized:** 30 mg	In single-dose vials.

THIOTEPA — INJECTION

Indications

Thiotepa has been tried with varying results in the palliation of a wide variety of neoplastic diseases. However, the most consistent results have been seen in the following tumors: adenocarcinoma of the breast; adenocarcinoma of the ovary; for controlling intracavitary effusions secondary to diffuse or localized neoplastic diseases of various serosal cavities; for the treatment of superficial papillary carcinoma of the urinary bladder.

While now largely superseded by other treatments, thiotepa has been effective against other lymphomas, such as lymphosarcoma and Hodgkin's disease.

➤*Unlabeled uses:* Prevention of ptergium recurrence after postoperative β-irradiation, autologous bone marrow transplantation.

Administration and Dosage

➤*Approved by the FDA:* December 22, 1994.

Dosage must be carefully individualized. A slow response to thiotepa does not necessarily indicate a lack of effect. Therefore, increasing the frequency of dosing may only increase toxicity. After maximum benefit is obtained by initial therapy, it is necessary to continue the patient on maintenance therapy (1- to 4-week intervals). In order to continue optimal effect, maintenance doses should not be administered more frequently than weekly in order to preserve correlation between dose and blood counts.

➤*Preparation and administration precautions:* Thiotepa is a cytotoxic anticancer drug, and, as with other potentially toxic compounds, caution should be exercised in handling and preparation of thiotepa. Skin reactions associated with accidental exposure to thiotepa may occur. The use of gloves is recommended. If thiotepa solution contacts the skin, immediately wash the skin thoroughly with soap and water. If thiotepa contacts mucous membranes, the membranes should be flushed thoroughly with water.

➤*Preparation of solution:* Thiotepa should be reconstituted with 1.5 or 3 mL of sterile water for injection resulting in a drug concentration of approximately 10 mg/mL.

Thiotepa Quantities and Concentration					
Label claim (mg/vial)	Actual content (mg/vial)	Amount of diluent to be added (mL)	Approximate withdrawable volume (mL)	Approximate withdrawable amount (mg/vial)	Approximate reconstituted concentration (mg/mL)
15	15.6	1.5	1.4	14.7	10.4
30	31.2	3	2.8	29.4	10.4

The reconstituted solution is hypotonic and should be further diluted with sodium chloride injection (0.9% sodium chloride) before use.

When reconstituted with sterile water for injection, solutions of thiotepa for injection should be stored in a refrigerator and used within 8 hours. Reconstituted solutions further diluted with sodium chloride injection should be used immediately.

In order to eliminate haze, filter solutions through a 0.22 micron filter† prior to administration. Filtering does not alter solution potency. Reconstituted solutions should be clear. Solutions that remain opaque or precipitate after filtration should not be used.

➤*Initial and maintenance doses:* Initially the higher dose in the given range is commonly administered. The maintenance dose should be adjusted weekly on the basis of pretreatment control blood counts and subsequent blood counts.

➤*IV administration:* Thiotepa may be given by rapid IV administration in doses of 0.3 to 0.4 mg/kg. Doses should be given at 1- to 4-week intervals.

➤*Intracavitary administration:* The dosage recommended is 0.6 to 0.8 mg/kg. Administration is usually effected through the same tubing which is used to remove the fluid from the cavity involved.

➤*Intravesical administration:* Patients with papillary carcinoma of the bladder are dehydrated for 8 to 12 hours prior to treatment. Then 60 mg of thiotepa in 30 to 60 mL of sodium chloride injection is instilled into the bladder by catheter. For maximum effect, the solution should be retained for 2 hours. If the patient finds it impossible to retain 60 mL for 2 hours, the dose may be given in a volume of 30 mL. If desired, the patient may be positioned every 15 minutes for maximum area contact. The usual course of treatment is once a week for 4 weeks. The course may be repeated if necessary, but second and third courses must be given with caution since bone marrow depression may be increased. Deaths have occurred after intravesical administration, caused by bone marrow depression from systemically absorbed drug.

➤*Storage/Stability:* Store in refrigerator between 2° to 8°C (36° to 46°F). Protect from light at all times.

Actions

➤*Pharmacology:* Thiotepa is a cytotoxic agent of the polyfunctional type, related chemically and pharmacologically to nitrogen mustard. The radiomimetic action of thiotepa is believed to occur through the release of ethylenimine radicals which, like irradiation, disrupt the bonds of DNA. One of the principal bond disruptions is initiated by alkylation of guanine at the N-7 position, which severs the linkage between the purine base and the sugar and liberates alkylated guanines.

➤*Pharmacokinetics:* TEPA, which possesses cytotoxic activity, appears to be the major metabolite of thiotepa found in human serum and urine. Urinary excretion of ^{14}C-labeled thiotepa and metabolites in a 34-year-old patient with metastatic carcinoma of the cecum who received a dose of 0.3 mg/kg IV was 63%. Thiotepa and TEPA in urine each accounts for less than 2% of the administered dose.

The pharmacokinetics of thiotepa and TEPA in 13 female patients (45 to 84 years) with advanced stage ovarian cancer receiving 60 mg and 80 mg thiotepa by IV infusion on subsequent courses given at 4-week intervals are presented in the following table:

Pharmacokinetics of Thiotepa and TEPA				
Pharmacokinetic parameters (units)	Thiotepa		TEPA	
	60 mg	80 mg	60 mg	80 mg
Peak serum concentration (ng/mL)	1331 ± 119	1828 ± 135	273 ± 46	353 ± 46
Elimination half-life (hr)	2.4 ± 0.3	2.3 ± 0.3	17.6 ± 3.6	15.7 ± 2.7
Area under the curve (ng/hr/mL)	2832 ± 412	4127 ± 668	4789 ± 1022	7452 ± 1667
Total body clearance (mL/min)	446 ± 63	419 ± 56	—	—

Contraindications

Hypersensitivity (allergy) to this preparation.

Therapy is probably contraindicated in cases of existing hepatic, renal, or bone marrow damage. However, if the need outweighs the risk in such patients, thiotepa may be used in low dosage, and accompanied by hepatic, renal and hemopoietic function tests.

Warnings

➤*Hematologic:* Death from septicemia and hemorrhage has occurred as a direct result of hematopoietic depression by thiotepa.

Thiotepa is highly toxic to the hematopoietic system. A rapidly falling white blood cell or platelet count indicates the necessity for discontinuing or reduc-

† Polysulfone membrane (*Gelman's Sterile Acrodisc*, Single Use) or triton-free mixed ester of cellulose/PVC (*Millipore's MILLEX*-GS Filter Unit).

THIOTEPA — INJECTION

ing the dosage of thiotepa. Weekly blood and platelet counts are recommended during therapy and for at least 3 weeks after therapy has been discontinued.

➤*Carcinogenesis:* Like many alkylating agents, thiotepa has been reported to be carcinogenic when administered to laboratory animals. Carcinogenicity is shown most clearly in studies using mice, but there is some evidence of carcinogenicity in man. In patients treated with thiotepa, cases of myelodysplastic syndromes and acute nonlymphocytic leukemia have been reported.

In mice, repeated IP administration of thiotepa (1.15 or 2.3 mg/kg 3 times per week for 52 or 43 weeks, respectively) produced a significant increase in the combined incidence of squamous cell carcinomas of the skin, preputial gland, and ear canal, and combined incidence of lymphoma and lymphocytic leukemia. In other studies in mice, repeated IP administration of thiotepa (4 or 8 mg/kg 3 times per week for 4 weeks followed by a 20-week observation period or 1.8 mg/kg 3 times per week for 4 weeks followed by a 35-week observation period) resulted in an increased incidence of lung tumors. In rats, repeated IP administration of thiotepa (0.7 or 1.4 mg/kg 3 times per week for 52 or 34 weeks, respectively) produced significant increases in the incidence of squamous cell carcinomas of the skin or ear canal, combined hematopoietic neoplasms, and uterine adenocarcinomas. Thiotepa given IV to rats (1 mg/kg once per week for 52 weeks) produced an increased incidence of malignant tumors (abdominal cavity sarcoma, lymphosarcoma, myelosis, seminoma, fibrosarcoma, salivary gland hemangioendothelioma, mammary sarcoma, pheochromocytoma) and benign tumors.

The lowest reported carcinogenic dose in mice (1.15 mg/kg, 3.68 mg/m^2) is approximately 7-fold less than the maximum recommended human therapeutic dose based on body-surface area. The lowest reported carcinogenic dose in rats (0.7 mg/kg, 4.9 mg/m^2) is approximately 6-fold less than the maximum recommended human therapeutic dose based on body surface area.

➤*Mutagenesis:* Thiotepa was mutagenic in in vitro assays in *Salmonella typhimurium*, *E. coli*, Chinese hamster lung and human lymphocytes. Chromosomal aberrations and sister chromatid exchanges were observed in vitro with thiotepa in bean root tips, human lymphocytes, Chinese hamster lung, and monkey lymphocytes. Mutations were observed with oral thiotepa in mouse at doses greater than 2.5 mg/kg (8 mg/m^2). The mouse micronucleus test was positive with IP administration of greater than 1 mg/kg (3.2 mg/m^2). Other positive in vivo chromosomal aberration or mutation assays included *Drosophila melanogaster*, Chinese hamster marrow, murine marrow, monkey lymphocyte, and murine germ cell.

➤*Fertility impairment:* Thiotepa impaired fertility in male mice at oral or IP doses greater than or equal to 0.7 mg/kg (2.24 mg/m^2), approximately 12-fold less than the maximum recommended human therapeutic dose based on body surface area. Thiotepa (0.5 mg) inhibited implantation in female rats when instilled into the uterine cavity. Thiotepa interfered with spermatogenesis in mice at IP doses greater than or equal to 0.5 mg/kg (1.6 mg/m^2), approximately 17-fold less than the maximum recommended human therapeutic dose based on body surface area. Thiotepa interfered with spermatogenesis in hamsters at an IP dose of 1 mg/kg (4.1 mg/m^2), approximately 7-fold less than the maximum recommended human therapeutic dose based on body surface area.

➤*Pregnancy: Category D.* Thiotepa can cause fetal harm when administered to a pregnant woman. Thiotepa given by the IP route was teratogenic in mice at doses greater than or equal to 1 mg/kg (3.2 mg/m^2), approximately 8-fold less than the maximum recommended human therapeutic dose based on body-surface area. Thiotepa given by the IP route was teratogenic in rats at doses ≥ 3 mg/kg (21 mg/m^2), approximately equal to the maximum recommended human therapeutic dose based on body surface area. Thiotepa was lethal to rabbit fetuses at a dose of 3 mg/kg (41 mg/m^2), approximately 2 times the maximum recommended human therapeutic dose based on body surface area. Patients of childbearing potential should be advised to avoid pregnancy. There are no adequate and well-controlled studies in pregnant women. If thiotepa is used during pregnancy, or if pregnancy occurs during thiotepa therapy, the patient and partner should be apprised of the potential hazard to the fetus.

➤*Lactation:* It is not known whether thiotepa is excreted in human milk. Because many drugs are excreted in human milk and because of the potential for tumorigenicity shown for thiotepa in animal studies, a decision should be made whether to discontinue nursing or to discontinue the drug, taking into account the importance of the drug to the mother.

➤*Children:* Safety and efficacy in pediatric patients have not been established.

Precautions

➤*Monitoring:* The most reliable guide to thiotepa toxicity is the white blood cell count. If this falls to 3000 or less, the dose should be discontinued. Another good index of thiotepa toxicity is the platelet count; if this falls to 150,000, therapy should be discontinued. Red blood cell count is a less accurate indicator of thiotepa toxicity. If the drug is used in patients with hepatic or renal damage (see Contraindications), regular assessment of hepatic and renal function tests are indicated.

➤*Bone marrow depression:* The serious complication of excessive thiotepa therapy, or sensitivity to the effects of thiotepa, is bone marrow depression. If proper precautions are not observed, thiotepa may cause leukopenia, thrombocytopenia, and anemia.

Drug Interactions

It is not advisable to combine, simultaneously or sequentially, cancer chemotherapeutic agents or a cancer chemotherapeutic agent and a therapeutic modality having the same mechanism of action. Therefore, thiotepa combined with other alkylating agents such as nitrogen mustard or cyclophosphamide or thiotepa combined with irradiation would serve to intensify toxicity rather than to enhance therapeutic response. If these agents must follow each other, it is important that recovery from the first agent, as indicated by white blood cell count, be complete before therapy with the second agent is instituted.

Other drugs which are known to produce bone marrow depression should be avoided.

Adverse Reactions

In addition to its effect on the blood-forming elements (see Warnings and Precautions), thiotepa may cause other adverse reactions.

➤*Allergic:* Rash, urticaria, laryngeal edema, asthma, anaphylactic shock, wheezing.

➤*CNS:* Dizziness, headache, blurred vision.

➤*Dermatologic:* Dermatitis, alopecia. Skin depigmentation has been reported following topical use.

➤*GI:* Nausea, vomiting, abdominal pain, anorexia.

➤*GU:* Amenorrhea, interference with spermatogenesis.

➤*Local:* Contact dermatitis, pain at the injection site.

➤*Renal:* Dysuria, urinary retention. There have been rare reports of chemical cystitis or hemorrhagic cystitis following intravesical, but not parenteral administration of thiotepa.

➤*Respiratory:* Prolonged apnea has been reported when succinylcholine was administered prior to surgery, following combined use of thiotepa and other anticancer agents. It was theorized that this was caused by decrease of pseudocholinesterase activity caused by the anticancer drugs.

➤*Special senses:* Conjunctivitis.

➤*Miscellaneous:* Fatigue, weakness. Febrile reaction and discharge from a subcutaneous lesion may occur as the result of breakdown of tumor tissue.

Overdosage

➤*Symptoms:* Hematopoietic toxicity can occur following overdose, manifested by a decrease in the white cell count or platelets. Red blood cell count is a less accurate indicator of thiotepa toxicity. Bleeding manifestations may develop. The patient may become more vulnerable to infection, and less able to combat such infection.

Dosages within and minimally above the recommended therapeutic doses have been associated with potentially life-threatening hematopoietic toxicity. Thiotepa has a toxic effect on the hematopoietic system that is dose related.

➤*Treatment:* Thiotepa is dialyzable.

There is no known antidote for overdosage with thiotepa. Transfusions of whole blood or platelets have proven beneficial to the patient in combating hematopoietic toxicity.

Patient Information

The patient should notify the physician in the case of any sign of bleeding (eg, epistaxis, easy bruising, change in color of urine, black stool) or infection (eg, fever, chills) or for possible pregnancy to patient or partner.

Effective contraception should be used during thiotepa therapy if either the patient or the partner is of childbearing potential.

METHOTREXATE (Amethopterin; MTX)

Rx	**Methotrexate** (Various, eg, Major, Roxane, UDL)	**Tablets:** 2.5 mg	In 36s, 100s, and UD 20s.
Rx	**Rheumatrex Dose Pack** (STADA)		(LLM1). Yellow, scored. In 5, 7.5, 10, 12.5, and 15 mg/week dose packs.
Rx	**Trexall** (Barr)	**Tablets:** 5 mg	Lactose. (b 927/5). Green, oval, scored. Film-coated. In 30s, 60s, and 100s.
		7.5	Lactose (b 928/7½). Blue, oval, scored. Film-coated. In 30s, 60s, and 100s.
		10 mg	Lactose. (b 929/10). Pink, oval, scored. Film-coated. In 30s, 60s, and 100s.
		15 mg	Lactose. (b 945/15). Purple, oval, scored. Film-coated. In 30s, 60s, and 100s.
Rx	**Methotrexate Sodium** (Various, eg, American Pharmaceutical Partners[a], Bedford Labs)	**Injection:** 25 mg/mL (as base)	Preservative free. In 2, 4, 8, 10, 20, and 40 mL single-use vials.
Rx	**Methotrexate Sodium** (Various, eg, American Pharmaceutical Partners, Xanodyne)		In 2 and 10 mL vials.[b]
Rx	**Methotrexate LPF Sodium** (Xanodyne)		Preservative free. In 2, 4, and 10 mL single-use vials.[c]
Rx	**Methotrexate Sodium** (Various, eg, American Pharmaceutical Partners, Xanodyne)	**Powder for Injection, lyophilized:** 1 g (as base)	Preservative free. In single-use vials.[d]

[a] The 2, 4, 8, 10, 20, and 40 mL solutions contain approximately 0.43, 0.86, 1.72, 2.15, 4.3, and 8.6 mEq sodium per vial, respectively.
[b] Contains 0.9% benzyl alcohol as a preservative; must not be used for intrathecal or high dose therapy.
[c] The 2, 4, and 10 mL vials contain approximately 0.43, 0.86, and 2.15 mEq sodium per vial, respectively.
[d] Approximately 0.14 mEq sodium in the 20 mg vial; 7 mEq sodium in the 1 g vial.

METHOTREXATE — ORAL

WARNING

The high dose regimens recommended for osteosarcoma require meticulous care.

Deaths – Use methotrexate only in life-threatening neoplastic diseases, or in patients with psoriasis or rheumatoid arthritis (RA) with severe, recalcitrant, disabling disease that is not adequately responsive to other forms of therapy. Deaths have occurred with the use of methotrexate in malignancy, psoriasis, and RA. Closely monitor patients for bone marrow, liver, lung, and kidney toxicities.

Bone marrow depression: Marked bone marrow depression may occur with resultant anemia, leukopenia, or thrombocytopenia.

Unexpectedly severe (sometimes fatal) bone marrow suppression, aplastic anemia, and GI toxicity have occurred with coadministration of methotrexate (usually in high dosage) along with some NSAIDs (see Precautions, Drug Interactions).

Monitoring – Periodic monitoring for toxicity, including CBC with differential and platelet counts, and liver and renal function testing is mandatory. Periodic liver biopsies may be indicated in some situations. Monitor patients at increased risk for impaired methotrexate elimination (eg, renal dysfunction, pleural effusions, ascites) more frequently (see Precautions).

Liver – Methotrexate causes hepatotoxicity, fibrosis, and cirrhosis, but generally only after prolonged use. Acutely, liver enzyme elevations are frequent, usually transient and asymptomatic, and also do not appear predictive of subsequent hepatic disease. Liver biopsy after sustained use often shows histologic changes, and fibrosis and cirrhosis have occurred; these latter lesions often are not preceded by symptoms or abnormal liver function tests (see Precautions). For this reason, periodic liver biopsies are usually recommended for psoriatic patients who are under long-term treatment. Persistent abnormalities in liver function tests may precede appearance of fibrosis or cirrhosis in the RA population.

Methotrexate-induced lung disease – Methotrexate-induced lung disease is a potentially dangerous lesion that may occur acutely at any time during therapy and has occurred at doses as low as 7.5 mg/week. It is not always fully reversible. Pulmonary symptoms (especially a dry, nonproductive cough) may require interruption of treatment and careful investigation.

Pregnancy – Fetal death and/or congenital anomalies have occurred; do not use in women of childbearing potential unless benefits outweigh possible risks. Pregnant women with psoriasis or RA should not receive methotrexate (see Contraindications).

Renal use – Use methotrexate in patients with impaired renal function with extreme caution, and at reduced dosages, because renal dysfunction will prolong elimination.

GI – Diarrhea and ulcerative stomatitis require interruption of therapy; hemorrhagic enteritis and death from intestinal perforation may occur.

Diluents – Do not use methotrexate formulations and diluents containing preservatives for intrathecal or experimental high dose MTX therapy.

WARNING (cont.)

Malignant lymphomas – Malignant lymphomas, which may regress following withdrawal of methotrexate, may occur in patients receiving low-dose methotrexate and, thus, may not require cytotoxic treatment. Discontinue methotrexate first and, if the lymphoma does not regress, appropriate treatment should be instituted.

Tumor lysis syndrome – Like other cytotoxic drugs, methotrexate may induce tumor lysis syndrome in patients with rapidly growing tumors.

Skin reactions – Severe, occasionally fatal skin reactions have been reported following single or multiple doses of methotrexate. Reactions have occurred within days of methotrexate administration. Recovery has been reported with discontinuation of therapy.

Potentially fatal opportunistic infections – Potentially fatal opportunistic infections, especially *Pneumocystis carinii* pneumonia, may occur with methotrexate therapy.

Radiotherapy – Methotrexate given concomitantly with radiotherapy may increase the risk of soft tissue necrosis and osteonecrosis.

Severe reactions – Because of the possibility of severe toxic reactions (which can be fatal), fully inform patients of the risks involved and assure constant supervision.

Indications

➤*Antineoplastic chemotherapy:* Treatment of gestational choriocarcinoma, chorioadenoma destruens, and hydatidiform mole.

Methotrexate alone or in combination with other anticancer agents for treatment of breast cancer, epidermoid cancers of the head and neck, advanced mycosis fungoides (cutaneous T-cell lymphoma) and lung cancer, particularly squamous cell and small cell types; in combination therapy in the treatment of advanced-stage non-Hodgkin lymphomas.

Methotrexate in high doses followed by leucovorin rescue in combination with other chemotherapeutic agents is effective in prolonging relapse-free survival in patients with nonmetastatic osteosarcoma who have undergone surgical resection or amputation for the primary tumor.

➤*Psoriasis:* Symptomatic control of severe, recalcitrant, disabling psoriasis that is not adequately responsive to other forms of therapy but only when the diagnosis has been established, as by biopsy and/or after dermatologic consultation. It is important to ensure that a psoriasis "flare" is not due to an undiagnosed concomitant disease affecting immune responses.

➤*RA:* Management of selected adults with severe, active RA (ACR criteria), or children with active polyarticular-course juvenile rheumatoid arthritis (JRA) who have had an insufficient therapeutic response to, or are intolerant of, an adequate trial of first-line therapy including full dose NSAIDs.

➤*Unlabeled uses:* Used as maintenance regimen for Wegener granulomatosis; dermatomyositis; relapsing-remitting multiple sclerosis; myositis; ulcerative colitis; refractory Crohn disease; uveitis; systemic lupus erythematosus; psoriatic arthritis.

Administration and Dosage

Oral administration is often preferred when low doses are being administered.

➤*Choriocarcinoma and similar trophoblastic diseases:* Administer 15 to 30 mg orally daily for a 5 day course. Repeat courses 3 to 5 times, as required, with rest periods of 1 or more weeks between courses, until any toxic

METHOTREXATE — ORAL

symptoms subside. Evaluate the effectiveness of therapy by 24 hour quantitative analysis of urinary chorionic gonadotropin hormone (hCG), which should return to normal or less than 50 IU/24 hr usually after the third or fourth course and is usually followed by a complete resolution of measurable lesions in 4 to 6 weeks. One to 2 courses of methotrexate after normalization of hCG is usually recommended. Careful clinical assessment is essential before each course. Cyclic combination therapy with other antitumor drugs may be useful.

Since hydatidiform mole may precede choriocarcinoma, prophylaxis chemotherapy with methotrexate has been recommended. Chorioadenoma destruens is an invasive form of hydatidiform mole. Administer methotrexate in doses similar to those for choriocarcinoma.

➤*Leukemia:* Acute lymphatic (lymphoblastic) leukemia in children and young adolescents is most responsive. In young adults and older patients, clinical remission is more difficult to obtain and early relapse is more common.

When used for induction, methotrexate in doses of 3.3 mg/m^2, in combination with prednisone 60 mg/m^2 given daily, produced remission in 50% of patients, usually within 4 to 6 weeks. Corticosteroid therapy, in combination with other antileukemic drugs or in cyclic combinations with methotrexate included, has appeared to produce rapid and effective remissions. Methotrexate in combination with other agents is the drug of choice for maintenance of remissions. When remission is achieved and supportive care has produced general clinical improvement, initiate maintenance therapy as follows: Give methotrexate orally 2 times weekly in total weekly doses of 30 mg/m^2. If relapse occurs, repeat initial induction regimen.

➤*Lymphomas (Burkitt Tumor, Stages I and II):* 10 to 25 mg/day orally for 4 to 8 days. In Stage III, give methotrexate concomitantly with other antitumor agents. Treatment in all stages generally consists of several courses with 7 to 10 day rest periods. Lymphosarcomas in Stage III may respond to combined drug therapy with methotrexate given in doses of 0.625 to 2.5 mg/kg/day.

➤*Mycosis fungoides (cutaneous T-cell lymphoma):* Methotrexate therapy produces clinical responses in 50% of cases. Dosage in early stages is usually 5 to 50 mg once weekly. Dose reduction or cessation is guided by patient response and hematologic monitoring. Methotrexate has also been administered twice weekly in doses ranging from 15 to 37.5 mg in patients who have responded poorly to weekly therapy. Combination chemotherapy regimens that include IV methotrexate administered at higher doses with leucovorin rescue have been utilized in advanced stages of the disease.

➤*Psoriasis, RA, and JRA:*

Adult RA – Recommended starting dosage schedules (methotrexate sodium tablets for oral administration are available):

1.) Single oral doses of 7.5 mg once weekly.
2.) Divided oral doses of 2.5 mg at 12-hour intervals for 3 doses given as a course once weekly.

Polyarticular-course JRA – The recommended starting dose is 10 mg/m^2 given once weekly. For either adult RA or polyarticular-course JRA, dosages may be adjusted gradually to achieve an optimal response. Limited experience shows a significant increase in the incidence and severity of serious toxic reactions, especially bone marrow suppression, at doses greater than 20 mg/week in adults. Although there is experience with doses up to 30 mg/m^2/week in children, there are too few published data to assess how doses over 20 mg/m^2/week might affect the risk of serious toxicity in children. Experience does suggest, however, that children receiving 20 to 30 mg/m^2/week (0.65 to 1 mg/kg/week) may have better absorption and fewer GI side effects if methotrexate is administered either IM or subcutaneously.

Therapeutic response usually begins within 3 to 6 weeks and the patient may continue to improve for another 12 weeks or more.

The optimal duration of therapy is unknown. Limited data available from long-term studies in adults indicate that the initial clinical improvement is maintained for at least 2 years with continued therapy. When methotrexate is discontinued, the arthritis usually worsens within 3 to 6 weeks.

Weekly therapy may be instituted to provide doses over a range of 5 to 15 mg administered as a single weekly dose. All schedules should be continually tailored to the individual patient. An initial test dose may be given prior to the regular dosing schedule to detect any extreme sensitivity to adverse effects. Maximal myelosuppression usually occurs in 7 to 10 days.

Psoriasis – Recommended starting dose schedules:

1.) Weekly single oral dose schedule: 10 to 25 mg/week until adequate response is achieved.
2.) Divided oral dose schedule: 2.5 mg at 12-hour intervals for 3 doses.

Dosages in each schedule may be gradually adjusted to achieve optimal clinical response; 30 mg/week should not ordinarily be exceeded.

Once optimal clinical response has been achieved, each dosage schedule should be reduced to the lowest possible amount of drug and to the longest possible rest period. The use of methotrexate may permit the return to conventional topical therapy, which should be encouraged.

➤*Storage / Stability:* Store at controlled room temperature (20° to 25°C; 68° to 77°F); excursions permitted to 15° to 30°C (59° to 86°F). Protect from light.

Actions

➤*Pharmacology:* Methotrexate competitively inhibits dihydrofolic acid reductase. Dihydrofolates must be reduced to tetrahydrofolates by this enzyme before they can be utilized as carriers of one-carbon groups in the synthesis of purine nucleotides and thymidylate. Therefore, methotrexate interferes with DNA synthesis, repair, and cellular replication.

Actively proliferating tissues such as malignant cells, bone marrow, fetal cells, buccal and intestinal mucosa, and cells of the urinary bladder are generally more sensitive to this effect of methotrexate. Cellular proliferation in malignant tissue is greater than in most normal tissue; thus, methotrexate may impair malignant growth without irreversibly damaging normal tissues.

The original rationale for high-dose methotrexate therapy was based on the concept of selective rescue of normal tissues by leucovorin. More recent evidence suggests that high-dose methotrexate may also overcome methotrexate resistance caused by impaired active transport, decreased affinity of dihydrofolic acid reductase for methotrexate, increased levels of dihydrofolic acid reductase resulting from gene amplification, or decreased polyglutamation of methotrexate. The actual mechanism of action is unknown.

➤*Pharmacokinetics:*

Absorption / Distribution – In adults, oral absorption appears to be dose-dependent. After oral doses of 30 mg/m^2 or less, methotrexate is generally well absorbed with a mean bioavailability of about 60%. The absorption of doses greater than 80 mg/m^2 is significantly less, possibly due to a saturation effect. Peak serum levels are usually reached in 1 to 2 hours. In leukemic children, oral absorption reportedly varies widely (23% to 95%). A 20-fold difference between highest and lowest peak levels was reported. Significant interindividual variability was also noted in time to peak concentration and fraction of dose absorbed. Food delayed absorption and reduced peak concentration.

Following oral administration of methotrexate in doses of 6.4 to 11.2 mg/m^2/week in pediatric patients with JRA, mean serum concentrations were approximately 0.59 micromolar at 1 hour, 0.44 micromolar at 2 hours, and 0.29 micromolar at 3 hours. Methotrexate competes with reduced folates for active transport across cell membranes by means of a single carrier-mediated active transport process. At serum concentrations greater than 100 micromolar, passive diffusion becomes a major pathway by which effective intracellular concentrations can be achieved. Approximately 50% of the absorbed drug is bound to serum protein. Methotrexate does not penetrate the blood-cerebrospinal fluid barrier in therapeutic amounts. High CSF drug concentrations may be attained by direct intrathecal administration.

Metabolism / Excretion – After absorption, methotrexate undergoes hepatic and intracellular metabolism to polyglutamated forms which can be converted back to methotrexate by hydrolase enzymes. These polyglutamates act as inhibitors of dihydrofolate reductase and thymidylate synthetase. Small amounts of methotrexate polyglutamates may remain in tissues for extended periods. The retention and prolonged drug action of these active metabolite(s) vary among different cells, tissues, and tumors. A small amount of metabolism to 7-hydroxymethotrexate may occur at doses commonly prescribed. Accumulation of this metabolite may become significant at the high doses used in osteogenic sarcoma. The aqueous solubility of 7-hydroxymethotrexate is threefold to fivefold lower than the parent compound. Methotrexate is partially metabolized by intestinal flora after oral administration.

The terminal half-life is approximately 3 to 10 hours for patients receiving treatment for psoriasis, RA, or low-dose antineoplastic therapy (less than 30 mg/m^2). For patients on high doses, the terminal half-life is 8 to 15 hours. In pediatric patients receiving methotrexate for acute lymphocytic leukemia (6.3 to 30 mg/m^2), or for JRA (3.75 to 26.2 mg/m^2), the terminal half-life has been reported to range from 0.7 to 5.8 hours or 0.9 to 2.3 hours, respectively.

Renal excretion is the primary route of elimination and is dependent upon dosage and route of administration. With IV administration, 80% to 90% of the administered dose is excreted unchanged in the urine within 24 hours. There is limited biliary excretion of 10% or less. Enterohepatic recirculation of methotrexate has been proposed. Renal excretion occurs by glomerular filtration and active tubular secretion. Impaired renal function, as well as concurrent use of drugs such as weak organic acids that also undergo tubular secretion, can markedly increase serum levels. Excellent correlation has been reported between methotrexate clearance and endogenous creatinine clearance.

Clearance rates vary widely and are generally decreased at higher doses. Delayed drug clearance is one of the major factors responsible for toxicity because the toxicity for normal tissues appears more dependent upon the duration of exposure to the drug rather than the peak level achieved. When a patient has delayed drug elimination due to compromised renal function or other causes, methotrexate serum concentrations may remain elevated for prolonged periods.

The potential for toxicity from high-dose regimens or delayed excretion is reduced by leucovorin calcium during the final phase of methotrexate plasma elimination. Guidelines for monitoring serum methotrexate levels, and for adjustment of leucovorin dosing to reduce the risk of toxicity, are provided in Administration and Dosage.

Contraindications

Hypersensitivity to the drug.

Patients with psoriasis or RA with alcoholism, alcoholic liver disease, or other chronic liver disease should not receive methotrexate. Patients with psoriasis or RA who have overt or laboratory evidence of immunodeficiency syndromes should not receive methotrexate.

Patients with psoriasis or RA who have pre-existing blood dyscrasias (eg, bone marrow hypoplasia, leukopenia, thrombocytopenia, significant anemia) should not receive methotrexate.

➤*Pregnancy:* Methotrexate can cause fetal death or teratogenic effects when administered to a pregnant woman. Methotrexate is contraindicated in pregnant women with psoriasis or RA and should be used in the treatment of neoplastic diseases only when the potential benefit outweighs the risk to the fetus. Women of childbearing potential should not be started on methotrexate until pregnancy is excluded and should be fully counseled on the serious risk to the fetus should they become pregnant while undergoing treatment. Pregnancy should be avoided if either partner is receiving methotrexate; during and for a minimum of 3 months after therapy for male patients, and during and for at least 1 ovulatory cycle after therapy for female patients.

METHOTREXATE — ORAL

Lactation – Because of the potential for serious adverse reactions from methotrexate in breastfed infants, it is contraindicated in nursing mothers.

Warnings

➤*Toxic effects:* Toxic effects, potentially serious, may be related in frequency and severity to dose or frequency of administration, but have been seen at all doses. These effects can occur at any time during therapy; follow patients closely. Most adverse reactions are reversible if detected early. When reactions occur, reduce dosage or discontinue drug and take appropriate corrective measures; this could include use of leucovorin calcium. Use caution if therapy is reinstituted. Consider further need for the drug and possibility of recurrence of toxicity.

➤*Renal function impairment:* Methotrexate is excreted principally by the kidneys. Its use in impaired renal function may result in accumulation of toxic amounts or additional renal damage. Determine the patient's renal status prior to and during therapy. Exercise caution should significant renal impairment occur. Reduce or discontinue drug dosage until renal function improves or is restored. The potential for toxicity from high dose regimens or delayed excretion is reduced by the administration of leucovorin calcium during the final phase of methotrexate plasma elimination.

➤*Carcinogenesis:* Non-Hodgkin lymphoma and other tumors have been reported in patients receiving low-dose oral methotrexate. However, there have been instances of malignant lymphoma arising during treatment with low-dose oral methotrexate that have regressed completely following withdrawal of methotrexate without requiring active antilymphoma treatment.

➤*Mutagenesis:* Although there is evidence that the drug causes chromosomal damage to animal somatic cells and human bone marrow cells, the clinical significance remains uncertain. Weigh the benefits against this potential risk before using methotrexate alone or in combination with other drugs, especially in children or young adults.

➤*Fertility impairment:* Impairment of fertility, oligospermia, and menstrual dysfunction in humans has been reported during and for a short period after cessation of therapy.

➤*Elderly:* Clinical pharmacology has not been well studied in these patients. Due to diminished hepatic and renal function and decreased folate stores in this population, consider relatively low doses. Closely monitor for early signs of toxicity.

Since decline in renal function may be associated with increases in adverse events and serum creatinine measurements may overestimate renal function in the elderly, more accurate methods (ie, creatinine clearance) should be considered. Elderly patients should be closely monitored for early signs of hepatic, bone marrow, and renal toxicity. Postmarketing experience suggests that the occurrence of bone marrow suppression, thrombocytopenia, and pneumonitis may increase with age.

➤*Pregnancy: Category X.* See Contraindications for more information.

➤*Lactation:* See Contraindications for more information.

➤*Children:* Safety and efficacy in children have not been established, other than in cancer chemotherapy and in polyarticular-course JRA.

Precautions

➤*Monitoring:* Baseline assessment should include complete blood count with differential and platelet counts; hepatic enzymes; renal function tests; and chest x-ray. During therapy of RA and psoriasis, monitoring of these parameters is recommended: Hematology at least monthly, renal function and liver function every 1 to 2 months. More frequent monitoring is usually indicated during antineoplastic therapy. During initial or changing doses, or during periods of increased risk of elevated methotrexate blood levels (eg, dehydration), more frequent monitoring may be indicated. Pulmonary function tests may be useful if methotrexate-induced lung disease is suspected, especially if baseline measurements are available. Appropriate steps should be taken to avoid conception during methotrexate therapy.

Hepatic – A relationship between abnormal liver function tests and fibrosis or cirrhosis of the liver has not been established. Transient liver function test abnormalities are observed frequently after methotrexate administration and are usually not cause for modification of methotrexate therapy. Persistent liver function test abnormalities or depression of serum albumin may indicate serious liver toxicity; they require evaluation.

RA: Liver function tests should be performed at baseline and at 4 to 8 week intervals in patients receiving methotrexate for RA. Pretreatment liver biopsy should be performed for patients with a history of excessive alcohol consumption, persistently abnormal baseline liver function test values, or chronic hepatitis B or C infection. During therapy, liver biopsy should be performed if there are persistent liver function test abnormalities or there is a decrease in serum albumin below the normal range (in the setting of well-controlled RA).

➤*Organ system toxicity:*

GI – If vomiting, diarrhea, or stomatitis occur, which may result in dehydration, discontinue methotrexate until recovery occurs. Use with extreme caution in the presence of peptic ulcer disease or ulcerative colitis.

Hematologic – Methotrexate can suppress hematopoiesis and cause anemia, aplastic anemia, pancytopenia, leukopenia, neutropenia and/or thrombocytopenia. Use with caution, if at all, in patients with malignancy and preexisting hematopoietic impairment. In controlled clinical trials in RA (n = 128), leukopenia (WBC less than 3000/mm^3) was seen in 2 patients, thrombocytopenia (platelets less than 100,000/mm^3) in 6 patients, and pancytopenia in 2 patients.

In psoriasis and RA, methotrexate should be stopped immediately if there is a significant drop in blood counts. In the treatment of neoplastic diseases, continue methotrexate only if potential benefit warrants risk of severe myelosuppression. Evaluate those with profound granulocytopenia and fever immediately; they usually require parenteral broad-spectrum antibiotics.

Hepatic – See the Warning box for more information.
Psoriasis: See the Warning box for more information.
RA: See the Warning box for more information.

Infection or immunologic states – Use with extreme caution in the presence of active infection; usually contraindicated in patients with overt or laboratory evidence of immunodeficiency syndromes. Hypogammaglobulinemia occurs rarely.

See the Warning box for more information.

Neurologic – There have been reports of leukoencephalopathy following IV administration of methotrexate to patients who have had craniospinal irradiation. Serious neurotoxicity, frequently manifested as generalized or focal seizures, has been reported with unexpectedly increased frequency among pediatric patients with acute lymphoblastic leukemia who were treated with intermediate-dose IV methotrexate (1 g/m^2). Symptomatic patients were commonly noted to have leukoencephalopathy and/or microangiopathic calcifications on diagnostic imaging studies. Chronic leukoencephalopathy has also occurred in patients who received repeated doses of high-dose methotrexate with leucovorin rescue even without cranial irradiation. Discontinuation of methotrexate does not always result in complete recovery.

A transient acute neurologic syndrome has been observed in patients treated with high dosage regimens. Manifestations of this stroke-like encephalopathy may include confusion, hemiparesis, transient blindness, seizures, and coma. The exact cause is unknown.

Pulmonary – Pulmonary symptoms (especially a dry, nonproductive cough) or a nonspecific pneumonitis occurring during therapy indicate a potentially dangerous lesion and require interruption of treatment and careful investigation. The typical patient presents with fever, cough, dyspnea, hypoxemia, and an infiltrate on chest x-ray; infection (including pneumonia) needs to be excluded. This lesion can occur at all dosages.

Renal – Methotrexate may cause renal damage that may lead to acute renal failure. High doses used in the treatment of osteosarcoma may cause renal damage leading to acute renal failure. Nephrotoxicity is due primarily to the precipitation of methotrexate and 7-hydroxymethotrexate in the renal tubules. Close attention to renal function including adequate hydration, urine alkalinization and measurement of serum methotrexate and creatinine levels are essential for safe administration.

Skin – See the Warning box for more information.

➤*Vaccines:* Immunization may be ineffective when given during methotrexate therapy. Immunization with live virus vaccines is generally not recommended. Disseminated vaccinia infections after smallpox immunization have occurred in patients receiving methotrexate.

➤*Debility:* Use with extreme caution in the presence of debility.

➤*Pleural effusions or ascites:* Methotrexate exits slowly from third space compartments (eg, pleural effusions or ascites). This results in a prolonged terminal plasma half-life and unexpected toxicity. In patients with significant third space accumulations, evacuate the fluid before treatment and monitor plasma methotrexate levels.

➤*Psoriasis lesions:* Lesions of psoriasis may be aggravated by concomitant exposure to ultraviolet radiation. Radiation dermatitis and sunburn may be "recalled" by the use of methotrexate.

➤*Folate deficiency:* Folate deficiency states may increase methotrexate toxicity.

Drug Interactions

➤*NSAIDS/Salicylates:* Nonsteroidal anti-inflammatory drugs (NSAIDs) should not be administered prior to or concomitantly with the high doses of methotrexate used in the treatment of osteosarcoma. Concomitant administration of some NSAIDs with high-dose methotrexate therapy has been reported to elevate and prolong serum methotrexate levels, resulting in deaths from severe hematologic and GI toxicity.

Caution should be used when NSAIDs and salicylates are administered concomitantly with lower doses of methotrexate. These drugs have been reported to reduce the tubular secretion of methotrexate in an animal model and may enhance its toxicity.

➤*Salicylates, phenylbutazone, phenytoin, sulfonamides, probenecid:* Methotrexate is partially bound to serum albumin, and toxicity may be increased because of displacement by certain drugs, such as salicylates, phenylbutazone, phenytoin, and sulfonamides. Renal tubular transport is also diminished by probenecid; use of methotrexate with this drug should be carefully monitored.

➤*Cisplatin:* In the treatment of patients with osteosarcoma, caution must be exercised if high-dose methotrexate is administered in combination with a potentially nephrotoxic chemotherapeutic agent (eg, cisplatin).

➤*Mercaptopurine:* Methotrexate increases the plasma levels of mercaptopurine. The combination of methotrexate and mercaptopurine may therefore require dose adjustment.

➤*Oral antibiotics:* Oral antibiotics such as tetracycline, chloramphenicol, and nonabsorbable broad-spectrum antibiotics, may decrease intestinal absorption of methotrexate or interfere with the enterohepatic circulation by inhibiting bowel flora and suppressing metabolism of the drug by bacteria.

➤*Hepatotoxic agents:* The potential for increased hepatotoxicity when methotrexate is administered with other hepatotoxic agents has not been evaluated. However, hepatotoxicity has been reported in such cases. Therefore, patients receiving concomitant therapy with methotrexate and other

METHOTREXATE — ORAL

potential hepatotoxins (eg, azathioprine, retinoids, sulfasalazine) should be monitored closely for possible increased risk of hepatotoxicity.

Methotrexate Drug Interactions

Precipitant drug	Object drug[a]		Description
Aminoglycosides, oral	Methotrexate	⬇	The antitumorigenic actions of methotrexate may be decreased, but not predictably. Consider parenteral methotrexate if oral aminoglycosides are being coadministered.
Charcoal	Methotrexate	⬇	Charcoal can reduce absorption of methotrexate and remove it from systemic circulation. Depending on the clinical situation, this will reduce the effectiveness or toxicity of methotrexate.
Chloramphenicol	Methotrexate	⬇	Oral chloramphenicol may decrease intestinal absorption of methotrexate or interfere with the enterohepatic circulation by inhibiting bowel flora and suppressing metabolism of the drug by bacteria.
Folic acid	Methotrexate	⬇	Vitamin preparations containing folic acid or its derivatives may decrease responses to systemically administered methotrexate.
NSAIDs	Methotrexate	⬆	Concomitant administration of some NSAIDs with high dose methotrexate has been reported to elevate and prolong serum methotrexate levels, resulting in deaths from severe hematologic and GI toxicity. NSAIDs may reduce tubular secretion of methotrexate and enhance toxicity. Monitor renal impairment that could predispose to methotrexate toxicity, for signs of methotrexate toxicity, and methotrexate levels if indicated.
Penicillins	Methotrexate	⬆	Serum methotrexate concentrations may be elevated, increasing the risk of toxicity. Monitor for methotrexate toxicity and measure methotrexate concentrations twice a week for at least the first 2 weeks. If a broad-spectrum antibiotic is needed, ceftazidime may be less likely to interact.
Probenecid	Methotrexate	⬆	Methotrexate plasma levels, therapeutic effects, and toxicity may be enhanced. Monitor methotrexate concentrations and adjust dose accordingly.
Salicylates	Methotrexate	⬆	Increased toxic effects of methotrexate may occur. Salicylates may reduce tubular secretion of methotrexate and enhance toxicity. Consider monitoring methotrexate levels.
Sulfonamides	Methotrexate	⬆	Sulfonamides may increase the risk of methotrexate-induced bone marrow suppression. Methotrexate may predispose patients to trimethoprim-sulfamethoxazole (TMP-SMZ)-induced megaloblastic anemia. Closely monitor patients for signs of hematologic toxicity.
Methotrexate	Sulfonamides		
Tetracyclines	Methotrexate	⬆	Methotrexate concentrations may be elevated, increasing the risk of toxicity (eg, bone marrow suppression). If tetracyclines cannot be avoided in patients receiving high-dose methotrexate, closely monitor methotrexate plasma concentrations and patients for signs and symptoms of toxicity.
Trimethoprim	Methotrexate	⬆	Trimethoprim may increase the risk of methotrexate-induced bone marrow suppression and megaloblastic anemia. If this drug combination cannot be avoided, closely monitor for signs of hematologic toxicity.
Methotrexate	Digoxin	⬇	Serum levels of digoxin may be reduced and actions may be decreased. Monitor patient for signs of reduction in pharmacologic effect of digoxin and increase digoxin dose if necessary. Serum level monitoring may facilitate tailoring dosage.
Methotrexate	Phenytoin	⬇	Serum concentrations of phenytoin may be decreased, resulting in a loss of therapeutic effect. Monitor phenytoin serum levels and adjust the phenytoin dosage appropriately. IV phenytoin may be useful.
Methotrexate	Theophylline	⬆	Methotrexate may decrease the clearance of theophylline. Theophylline levels should be monitored when used concomitantly with methotrexate.
Methotrexate	Thiopurines (eg, azathioprine)	⬆	The actions of thiopurines may be enhanced. Reduced thiopurine dosage may be used during coadministration with methotrexate.

[a] ⬆ = Object drug increased. ⬇ = Object drug decreased.

➤*Drug/Food interactions:* Food may delay the absorption and reduce the peak concentration of methotrexate.

Adverse Reactions

The incidence and severity of acute side effects are generally related to dose and dosing frequency. See also Precautions section under "Organ System Toxicity."

The most common adverse reactions are: Ulcerative stomatitis; leukopenia; nausea; abdominal distress; malaise; fatigue; chills; fever; dizziness; decreased resistance to infection.

➤*Cardiovascular:* Pericarditis, pericardial effusion, hypotension, and thromboembolic events (including arterial thrombosis, cerebral thrombosis, deep vein thrombosis, retinal vein thrombosis, thrombophlebitis, and pulmonary embolus).

➤*CNS:* Headaches; drowsiness; blurred vision; aphasia; hemiparesis; paresis; convulsions; transient blindness; speech impairment, including dysarthria. Following low doses, there have been occasional reports of transient subtle cognitive dysfunction, mood alteration, unusual cranial sensations, leukoencephalopathy, or encephalopathy.

After intrathecal use, the CNS toxicity that may occur can be classified as follows:

1.) Acute chemical arachnoiditis (headache, back pain, nuchal rigidity, fever);
2.) subacute myelopathy (paraparesis/paraplegia with involvement of spinal nerve roots);
3.) chronic leukoencephalopathy (confusion, irritability, somnolence, ataxia, dementia, seizures, and coma).

➤*Dermatologic:* Erythematous rashes; pruritus; urticaria; photosensitivity; pigmentary changes; alopecia; ecchymosis; telangiectasia; acne; furunculosis; erythema multiforme; toxic epidermal necrolysis; Stevens-Johnson syndrome; skin necrosis; skin ulceration; exfoliative dermatitis; photosensitivity; "burning of skin lesions"; rash; plaque erosions (rare).

➤*GI:* Gingivitis; stomatitis; pharyngitis; anorexia; nausea; vomiting; diarrhea; hematemesis; melena; GI ulceration and bleeding; enteritis; pancreatitis.

➤*GU:* Renal failure; azotemia; cystitis; hematuria; severe nephropathy; defective oogenesis or spermatogenesis; transient oligospermia; menstrual dysfunction and vaginal discharge; infertility; abortion; fetal defects; gynecomastia; dysuria; vaginal discharge.

➤*Hematologic:* Bone marrow depression; leukopenia; thrombocytopenia; suppressed hematopoiesis causing anemia; aplastic anemia; pancytopenia; neutropenia; decreased hematocrit; lymphadenopathy and lymphoproliferative disorders (including reversible); hypogammaglobulinemia (rare).

➤*Hepatic:* Hepatotoxicity; acute hepatitis; chronic fibrosis; cirrhosis; decrease in serum albumin; liver enzyme elevations.

➤*Musculoskeletal:* Stress fracture, arthralgias, chest pain.

➤*Pulmonary:* Chronic interstitial obstructive pulmonary disease has occasionally occurred; deaths from respiratory fibrosis, respiratory failure, and

METHOTREXATE — ORAL

interstitial pneumonitis have been reported. Upper respiratory infections, coughing, and epistaxis have occurred.

➤*Special senses:* Conjunctivitis; serious visual changes of unknown etiology; eye discomfort; tinnitus.

➤*Miscellaneous:* Rare reactions related to the use of methotrexate include arthralgia/myalgia, diabetes, osteoporosis and sudden death. Cases of anaphylactoid reactions have occurred; nodulosis; vasculitis, loss of libido/impotence; reversible lymphomas; tumor lysis syndrome; soft tissue necrosis; osteonecrosis; sweating.

Infection – The following also occurred. Infections, pneumonia, sepsis, nocardiosis, histoplasmosis, cryptococcosis, herpes zoster, herpes simplex hepatitis, and disseminated herpes simplex. There have been case reports of sometimes fatal opportunistic infections. *Pneumocystis carinii* pneumonia was the most common infection.

Overdosage

➤*Symptoms:* Reports of oral overdose often indicate accidental daily administration instead of weekly (single or divided doses). Symptoms commonly reported following oral overdose include those symptoms and signs reported at pharmacologic doses, particularly hematologic and GI reaction. For example, leukopenia, thrombocytopenia, anemia, pancytopenia, bone marrow suppression, mucositis, stomatitis, oral ulceration, nausea, vomiting, GI ulceration, and GI bleeding. In some cases, no symptoms were reported. There have been reports of death following overdose. In these cases, events such as sepsis or septic shock, renal failure, and aplastic anemia were also reported.

➤*Treatment:* Leucovorin (citrovorum factor) is used to diminish the toxicity and counteract the effect of inadvertent overdosages of methotrexate. Administer leucovorin as promptly as possible. As the time interval between administration and leucovorin rescue increases, leucovorin's effectiveness in counteracting toxicity diminishes. Monitoring of the serum methotrexate concentration is essential in determining the optimal dose and duration of leucovorin treatment.

In cases of massive overdosage, hydration and urinary alkalinization may be necessary to prevent the precipitation of methotrexate and its metabolites in the renal tubules. Neither hemodialysis nor peritoneal dialysis improves methotrexate elimination. Effective clearance of methotrexate has been reported with acute intermittent hemodialysis using a high-flux dialyzer.

Patient Information

Avoid alcohol, salicylates, and prolonged exposure to sunlight or sunlamps (particularly patients with psoriasis).

Use contraceptive measures during and for at least 3 months (males) or 1 ovulatory cycle (females) after cessation of therapy. The risk of effects on reproduction should be discussed with both males and females on methotrexate.

Notify physician if any of the following occurs: Diarrhea; abdominal pain; black stools; fever and chills; sore throat; sores in or around the mouth; cough; yellow discoloration of the skin or eyes; swelling of the feet or legs; joint pain. May cause nausea, vomiting, loss of appetite, hair loss, skin rash, fever, or dizziness. Notify the physician if these effects persist.

Inform patients of the early signs of toxicity, of the need to see their physician promptly if they occur, and the need for close follow-up, including laboratory tests to monitor toxicity.

METHOTREXATE SODIUM — INJECTION

WARNING

Methotrexate should be used only by physicians whose knowledge and experience include the use of antimetabolite therapy.

Because of the possibility of serious toxic reactions (which can be fatal):
Methotrexate should be used only in life-threatening neoplastic diseases, or in patients with psoriasis or rheumatoid arthritis (RA) with severe, recalcitrant, disabling disease which is not adequately responsive to other forms of therapy.
Deaths have been reported with the use of methotrexate in the treatment of malignancy, psoriasis, and RA.
Patients should be closely monitored for bone marrow, liver, lung and kidney toxicities.
Patients should be informed by their physicians of the risks involved and be under a physician's care throughout therapy.

The use of methotrexate high-dose regimens recommended for osteosarcoma requires meticulous care. High-dose regimens for other neoplastic diseases are investigational, and a therapeutic advantage has not been established.

Methotrexate formulations and diluents containing preservatives must not be used for intrathecal or high-dose methotrexate therapy.

1.) Methotrexate has been reported to cause fetal death or congenital anomalies. Therefore, it is not recommended for women of childbearing potential unless there is clear medical evidence that the benefits can be expected to outweigh the considered risks. Pregnant women with psoriasis or RA should not receive methotrexate.
2.) Methotrexate elimination is reduced in patients with impaired renal function, ascites, or pleural effusions. Such patients require especially careful monitoring for toxicity, and require dose reduction or, in some cases, discontinuation of methotrexate administration.
3.) Unexpectedly severe (sometimes fatal) bone marrow suppression and GI toxicity have been reported with concomitant administration of methotrexate (usually in high dosage) along with some nonsteroidal anti-inflammatory drugs (NSAIDs).
4.) Methotrexate causes hepatotoxicity, fibrosis and cirrhosis, but generally only after prolonged use. Acutely, liver enzyme elevations are frequently seen. These are usually transient and asymptomatic, and also do not appear predictive of subsequent hepatic disease. Liver biopsy after sustained use often shows histologic changes, and fibrosis and cirrhosis have been reported; these latter lesions may not be preceded by symptoms or abnormal liver function tests in the psoriasis population. For this reason, periodic liver biopsies are usually recommended for psoriatic patients who are under long-term treatment. Persistent abnormalities in liver function tests may precede appearance of fibrosis or cirrhosis in the RA population.
5.) Methotrexate-induced lung disease is a potentially dangerous lesion, which may occur acutely at any time during therapy and which has been reported at doses as low as 7.5 mg/week. It is not always fully reversible. Pulmonary symptoms (especially a dry, nonproductive cough) may require interruption of treatment and careful investigation.
6.) Diarrhea and ulcerative stomatitis require interruption of therapy; otherwise, hemorrhagic enteritis and death from intestinal perforation may occur.
7.) Malignant lymphomas, which may regress following withdrawal of methotrexate, may occur in patients receiving low-dose methotrexate and, thus, may not require cytotoxic treatment. Discontinue methotrexate first and, if the lymphoma does not regress, institute appropriate treatment.

WARNING (cont.)

1.) Like other cytotoxic drugs, methotrexate may induce "tumor lysis syndrome" in patients with rapidly growing tumors. Appropriate supportive and pharmacologic measures may prevent or alleviate this complication.
2.) Severe, occasionally fatal, skin reactions have been reported following single or multiple doses of methotrexate. Reactions have occurred within days of methotrexate administration. Recovery has been reported with discontinuation of therapy.
3.) Potentially fatal opportunistic infections, especially *Pneumocystis carinii* pneumonia, may occur with methotrexate therapy.
4.) Methotrexate given concomitantly with radiotherapy may increase the risk of soft tissue necrosis and osteonecrosis.

Indications

➤*Antineoplastic chemotherapy:* Treatment of gestational choriocarcinoma, chorioadenoma destruens and hydatidiform mole.

In acute lymphocytic leukemia, methotrexate is indicated in the prophylaxis of meningeal leukemia and is used in maintenance therapy in combination with other chemotherapeutic agents. Methotrexate is also indicated in the treatment of meningeal leukemia.

Methotrexate is used alone or in combination with other anticancer agents in the treatment of breast cancer, epidermoid cancers of the head and neck, advanced mycosis fungoides (cutaneous T cell lymphoma), and lung cancer, particularly squamous cell and small cell types. Methotrexate is also used in combination with other chemotherapeutic agents in the treatment of advanced stage non-Hodgkin's lymphomas.

Methotrexate in high doses followed by leucovorin rescue in combination with other chemotherapeutic agents is effective in prolonging relapse-free survival in patients with nonmetastatic osteosarcoma who have undergone surgical resection or amputation for the primary tumor.

➤*Psoriasis:* Methotrexate is indicated in the symptomatic control of severe, recalcitrant, disabling psoriasis that is not adequately responsive to other forms of therapy, but only when the diagnosis has been established, as by biopsy and/or after dermatologic consultation. It is important to ensure that a psoriasis "flare" is not due to an undiagnosed concomitant disease affecting immune responses.

➤*RA:* Methotrexate is indicated in the management of selected adults with severe, active, classical or definite RA (American Rheumatism Association [ARA] criteria), or children with active polyarticular-course juvenile RA, who have had an insufficient therapeutic response to, or are intolerant of, an adequate trial of first-line therapy, including full-dose NSAIDs.

➤*Unlabeled uses:* Treatment of testicular carcinoma, bladder carcinoma, prevention of acute graft-versus-host disease (GVHD).

Administration and Dosage

➤*Approved by the FDA:* March 3, 1982.

Oral administration is often preferred when low doses are being administered, since absorption is rapid, and effective serum levels are obtained. Methotrexate sodium injection and methotrexate for injection may be given by the IM, IV, intra-arterial or intrathecal route. However, the preserved formulation contains benzyl alcohol and must not be used for intrathecal or high-dose therapy.

➤*Choriocarcinoma and similar trophoblastic diseases:* Methotrexate is administered IM in doses of 15 to 30 mg daily for a 5-day course. Such courses are usually repeated for 3 to 5 times as required, with rest periods of

METHOTREXATE SODIUM — INJECTION

1 or more weeks interposed between courses, until any manifesting toxic symptoms subside. The effectiveness of therapy is ordinarily evaluated by 24-hour quantitative analysis of urinary chorionic gonadotropin (hCG), which should return to normal or less than 50 Units per 24 hr usually after the third or fourth course and usually be followed by a complete resolution of measurable lesions in 4 to 6 weeks. One to 2 courses of methotrexate after normalization of hCG is usually recommended. Before each course of the drug, careful clinical assessment is essential. Cyclic combination therapy of methotrexate with other antitumor drugs has been reported as being useful.

Since hydatidiform mole may precede choriocarcinoma, prophylactic chemotherapy with methotrexate has been recommended.

Chorioadenoma destruens is considered to be an invasive form of hydatidiform mole. Methotrexate is administered in these disease states in doses similar to those recommended for choriocarcinoma.

➤*Leukemia:* Methotrexate, alone or in combination with steroids, was used initially for induction of remission in acute lymphoblastic leukemias. More recently, corticosteroid therapy, in combination with other antileukemic drugs or in cyclic combinations with methotrexate included, has appeared to produce rapid and effective remissions. When used for induction, methotrexate in doses of 3.3 mg/m^2 in combination with 60 mg/m^2 of prednisone, given daily, produced remissions in 50% of patients treated, usually within a period of 4 to 6 weeks. Methotrexate in combination with other agents appears to be the drug of choice for securing maintenance of drug-induced remissions. When remission is achieved and supportive care has produced general clinical improvement, maintenance therapy is initiated, as follows: Methotrexate is administered 2 times weekly IM in total weekly doses of 30 mg/m^2. It has also been given in doses of 2.5 mg/kg IV every 14 days. If and when relapse does occur, reinduction of remission can again usually be obtained by repeating the initial induction regimen.

➤*Meningeal leukemia:* In the treatment or prophylaxis of meningeal leukemia, methotrexate must be administered intrathecally. Preservative-free methotrexate is diluted to a concentration of 1 mg/mL in an appropriate sterile, preservative-free medium such as 0.9% Sodium Chloride Injection.

Intrathecal methotrexate administration at a dose of 12 mg/m^2 (maximum 15 mg) has been reported to result in low CSF methotrexate concentrations and reduced efficacy in children and high concentrations and neurotoxicity in adults. The following dosage regimen is based on age instead of body surface area:

Methotrexate Dosing According to Age for the Treatment of Meningeal Leukemia

Age (years)	Dose (mg)
< 1	6
1	8
2	10
3 or older	12

Because the CSF volume and turnover may decrease with age, a dose reduction may be indicated in elderly patients.

For the treatment of meningeal leukemia, intrathecal methotrexate may be given at intervals of 2 to 5 days. However, administration at intervals of less than 1 week may result in increased subacute toxicity. Methotrexate is administered until the cell count of the cerebrospinal fluid returns to normal. At this point one additional dose is advisable. For prophylaxis against meningeal leukemia, the dosage is the same as for treatment except for the intervals of administration. On this subject, it is advisable for the physician to consult the medical literature.

➤*Mycosis fungoides (cutaneous T cell lymphoma):* Therapy with methotrexate as a single agent appears to produce clinical response in up to 50% of patients treated. Dosage in early stages is usually 5 to 50 mg once weekly. Dose reduction or cessation is guided by patient response and hematologic monitoring. Methotrexate has also been administered twice weekly in doses ranging from 15 to 37.5 mg in patients who have responded poorly to weekly therapy. Combination chemotherapy regimens that include IV methotrexate administered at higher doses with leucovorin rescue have been utilized in advanced stages of the disease.

➤*Osteosarcoma:* An effective adjuvant chemotherapy regimen requires the administration of several cytotoxic chemotherapeutic agents. In addition to high-dose methotrexate with leucovorin rescue, these agents may include doxorubicin, cisplatin, and the combination of bleomycin, cyclophosphamide and dactinomycin (BCD) in the doses and schedule shown below. The starting dose for high-dose methotrexate treatment is 12 g/m^2. If this dose is not sufficient to produce a peak serum methotrexate concentration of 1,000 mcM (10^{-3} mol/L) at the end of the methotrexate infusion, the dose may be escalated to 15 g/m^2 in subsequent treatments. If the patient is vomiting or is unable to tolerate oral medication, leucovorin is given IV or IM at the same dose and schedule.

Osteosarcoma Chemotherapy Regimens: Dose and Schedules

Drug*	Dose*	Treatment week after surgery
Methotrexate	12 g/m^2 IV as 4-hour infusion (starting dose)	4, 5, 6, 7, 11, 12, 15, 16, 29, 30, 44, 45
Leucovorin	15 mg orally every 6 hours for 10 doses starting at 24 hours after start of methotrexate infusion	
Doxorubicin[1] as a single drug	30 mg/m^2/day IV × 3 days	8, 17
Doxorubicin[1]	50 mg/m^2 IV	20, 23, 33, 36
Cisplatin[1]	100 mg/m^2	20, 23, 33, 36
Bleomycin[1]	15 Units/m^2 IV × 2 days	2, 13, 26, 39, 42
Cyclophosphamide[1]	600 mg/m^2 IV × 2 days	2, 13, 26, 39, 42
Dactinomycin[1]	0.6 mg/m^2 IV × 2 days	2, 13, 26, 39, 42

* Link MP, Goorin AM, Miser AW, et al: The effect of adjuvant chemotherapy on relapse-free survival in patients with osteosarcoma of the extremity. *N Engl J Med* 1986; 314(25):1600-06.
[1] For the information following, please see respective monographs for each drug for full prescribing information. Dosage modifications may be necessary because of drug-induced toxicity.

When these higher doses of methotrexate are to be administered, the following safety guidelines should be closely observed.

➤*Guidelines for methotrexate therapy with leucovorin rescue:* Administration of methotrexate should be delayed until recovery if any of the following occurs:

- The WBC count is less than 1,500/mcL.
- The neutrophil count is less than 200/mcL.
- The platelet count is less than 75,000/mcL.
- The serum bilirubin level is greater than 1.2 mg/dL.
- The ALT level is greater than 450 units.
- Mucositis is present, until there is evidence of healing.
- Persistent pleural effusion is present; this should be drained dry prior to infusion.

Adequate renal function must be documented.

1.) Serum creatinine must be normal, and creatinine clearance must be greater than 60 mL/min, before initiation of therapy.
2.) Serum creatinine must be measured prior to each subsequent course of therapy. If serum creatinine has increased by 50% or more compared to a prior value, the creatinine clearance must be measured and documented to be greater than 60 mL/min (even if the serum creatinine is still within the normal range).

Patients must be well hydrated, and must be treated with sodium bicarbonate for urinary alkalinization.

1.) Administer 1,000 mL/m^2 of IV fluid over 6 hours prior to initiation of the methotrexate infusion. Continue hydration at 125 mL/m^2/hr (3 L/m^2/day) during the methotrexate infusion, and for 2 days after the infusion has been completed.
2.) Alkalinize urine to maintain pH above 7 during methotrexate infusion and leucovorin calcium therapy. This can be accomplished by the administration of sodium bicarbonate orally or by incorporation into a separate IV solution.

Repeat serum creatinine and serum methotrexate 24 hours after starting methotrexate and at least once daily until the methotrexate level is below 5×10^{-8} mol/L (0.05 mcM).

The table below provides guidelines for leucovorin calcium dosage based upon serum methotrexate levels (see guidelines below).

Leucovorin Rescue Schedules Following Treatment with Higher Doses of Methotrexate

Clinical situation	Laboratory findings	Leucovorin dosage and duration
Normal methotrexate elimination	Serum methotrexate level approximately 10 mcM at 24 hours after administration, 1 mcM at 48 hours, and < 0.2 mcM at 72 hours.	15 mg orally, IM, or IV every 6 hours for 60 hours (10 doses starting at 24 hours after start of methotrexate infusion).
Delayed late methotrexate elimination	Serum methotrexate level remaining above 0.2 mcM at 72 hours, and > 0.05 mcM at 96 hours after administration.	Continue 15 mg orally, IM, or IV every 6 hours, until methotrexate level is < 0.05 mcM.

METHOTREXATE SODIUM — INJECTION

Leucovorin Rescue Schedules Following Treatment with Higher Doses of Methotrexate		
Clinical situation	Laboratory findings	Leucovorin dosage and duration
Delayed early methotrexate elimination or evidence of acute renal injury	Serum methotrexate level of 50 mcM or more at 24 hours, or 5 mcM or more at 48 hours after administration, or a 100% or greater increase in serum creatinine level at 24 hours after methotrexate administration (eg, an increase from 0.5 mg/dL to a level of 1 mg/dL or more).	150 mg IV every 3 hours, until methotrexate level is < 1 mcM; then 15 mg IV every 3 hours until methotrexate level is < 0.05 mcM

Patients who experience delayed early methotrexate elimination are likely to develop nonreversible oliguric renal failure. In addition to appropriate leucovorin therapy, these patients require continuing hydration and urinary alkalinization, and close monitoring of fluid and electrolyte status, until the serum methotrexate level has fallen to below 0.05 mcM and the renal failure has resolved. If necessary, acute, intermittent hemodialysis with a high-flux dialyzer may also be beneficial in these patients.

Some patients will have abnormalities in methotrexate elimination, or abnormalities in renal function following methotrexate administration, which are significant but less severe than the abnormalities described above. These abnormalities may or may not be associated with significant clinical toxicity. If significant clinical toxicity is observed, leucovorin rescue should be extended for an additional 24 hours (total 14 doses over 84 hours) in subsequent courses of therapy. The possibility that the patient is taking other medications which interact with methotrexate (eg, medications which may interfere with methotrexate binding to serum albumin, or elimination) should always be reconsidered when laboratory abnormalities or clinical toxicities are observed.

Caution – Do not administer leucovorin intrathecally.

➤*Psoriasis, RA, and juvenile rheumatoid arthritis (JRA):*

Adult RA – See Methotrexate-Oral.

Polyarticular-course JRA – The recommended starting dose is 10 mg/m^2 given once weekly. For either adult RA or polyarticular-course JRA, dosages may be adjusted gradually to achieve an optimal response. Limited experience shows a significant increase in the incidence and severity of serious toxic reactions, especially bone marrow suppression, at doses greater than 20 mg/week in adults. Although there is experience with doses up to 30 mg/m^2/week in children, there are too few published data to assess how doses over 20 mg/m^2/week might affect the risk of serious toxicity in children. Experience does suggest, however, that children receiving 20 to 30 mg/m^2/week (0.65 to 1 mg/kg/week) may have better absorption and fewer GI side effects if methotrexate is administered either IM or subcutaneously.

Therapeutic response usually begins within 3 to 6 weeks and the patient may continue to improve for another 12 weeks or more.

The optimal duration of therapy is unknown. Limited data available from long-term studies in adults indicate that the initial clinical improvement is maintained for at least 2 years with continued therapy. When methotrexate is discontinued, the arthritis usually worsens within 3 to 6 weeks.

All schedules should be continually tailored to the individual patient. An initial test dose may be given prior to the regular dosing schedule to detect any extreme sensitivity to adverse effects. Maximal myelosuppression usually occurs in 7 to 10 days.

Psoriasis – Recommended starting dose schedules (see also Methotrexate-Oral): Weekly single IM or IV dose schedule: 10 to 25 mg/week until adequate response is achieved.

Dosages in each schedule may be gradually adjusted to achieve optimal clinical response; 30 mg/week should not ordinarily be exceeded.

Once optimal clinical response has been achieved, each dosage schedule should be reduced to the lowest possible amount of drug and to the longest possible rest period. The use of methotrexate may permit the return to conventional topical therapy, which should be encouraged.

➤*Reconstitution of lyophilized powders:* Reconstitute immediately prior to use.

Methotrexate sodium for injection should be reconstituted with an appropriate sterile, preservative-free medium such as 5% Dextrose Solution or Sodium Chloride Injection. Reconstitute the 20 mg vial to a concentration no greater than 25 mg/mL. The 1 g vial should be reconstituted with 19.4 mL to a concentration of 50 mg/mL. When high doses of methotrexate are administered by IV infusion, the total dose is diluted in 5% Dextrose Solution.

For intrathecal injection, reconstitute to a concentration of 1 mg/mL with an appropriate sterile, preservative-free medium such as Sodium Chloride Injection.

➤*Dilution instructions for liquid methotrexate sodium injection products:*

Methotrexate sodium injection, isotonic liquid (contains preservative) – If desired, the solution may be further diluted with a compatible medium such as Sodium Chloride Injection. Storage for 24 hours at a temperature of 21° to 25°C (69° to 77°F) results in a product which is within 90% of label potency.

Methotrexate sodium injection, isotonic liquid (preservative-free, for single use only) – If desired, the solution may be further diluted immediately prior to use with an appropriate sterile, preservative-free medium such as 5% Dextrose Solution or Sodium Chloride Injection.

➤*Storage/Stability:* Store at controlled room temperature 20° to 25°C (68° to 77°F); excursions permitted to 15° to 30°C (59° to 86°F). Protect from light.

Actions

➤*Pharmacology:* Methotrexate inhibits dihydrofolic acid reductase. Dihydrofolates must be reduced to tetrahydrofolates by this enzyme before they can be utilized as carriers of 1-carbon groups in the synthesis of purine nucleotides and thymidylate. Therefore, methotrexate interferes with DNA synthesis, repair, and cellular replication. Actively proliferating tissues such as malignant cells, bone marrow, fetal cells, buccal and intestinal mucosa, and cells of the urinary bladder are in general more sensitive to this effect of methotrexate. When cellular proliferation in malignant tissues is greater than in most normal tissues, methotrexate may impair malignant growth without irreversible damage to healthy tissues.

Methotrexate in high doses, followed by leucovorin rescue, is used as a part of the treatment of patients with nonmetastatic osteosarcoma. The original rationale for high-dose methotrexate therapy was based on the concept of selective rescue of normal tissues by leucovorin. More recent evidence suggests that high-dose methotrexate may also overcome methotrexate resistance caused by impaired active transport, decreased affinity of dihydrofolic acid reductase for methotrexate, increased levels of dihydrofolic acid reductase resulting from gene amplification, or decreased polyglutamation of methotrexate. The actual mechanism of action is unknown.

➤*Pharmacokinetics:*

Absorption – Methotrexate is generally completely absorbed from parenteral routes of injection. After IM injection, peak serum concentrations occur in 30 to 60 minutes. As in leukemic pediatric patients, a wide interindividual variability in the plasma concentrations of methotrexate has been reported in pediatric patients with JRA.

Distribution – After IV administration, the initial volume of distribution is approximately 0.18 L/kg (18% of body weight) and steady-state volume of distribution is approximately 0.4 to 0.8 L/kg (40% to 80% of body weight). Methotrexate competes with reduced folates for active transport across cell membranes by means of a single carrier-mediated active transport process. At serum concentrations greater than 100 mcM, passive diffusion becomes a major pathway by which effective intracellular concentrations can be achieved. Methotrexate in serum is approximately 50% protein bound. Laboratory studies demonstrate that it may be displaced from plasma albumin by various compounds including sulfonamides, salicylates, tetracyclines, chloramphenicol, and phenytoin.

Methotrexate does not penetrate the blood-cerebrospinal fluid barrier in therapeutic amounts when given orally or parenterally. High CSF concentrations of the drug may be attained by intrathecal administration.

Metabolism – After absorption, methotrexate undergoes hepatic and intracellular metabolism to polyglutamated forms which can be converted back to methotrexate by hydrolase enzymes. These polyglutamates act as inhibitors of dihydrofolate reductase and thymidylate synthetase. Small amounts of methotrexate polyglutamates may remain in tissues for extended periods. The retention and prolonged drug action of these active metabolites vary among different cells, tissues and tumors. A small amount of metabolism to 7-hydroxymethotrexate may occur at doses commonly prescribed. Accumulation of this metabolite may become significant at the high doses used in osteogenic sarcoma. The aqueous solubility of 7-hydroxymethotrexate is 3- to 5-fold lower than the parent compound.

Excretion – Renal excretion is the primary route of elimination and is dependent upon dosage and route of administration. With IV administration, 80% to 90% of the administered dose is excreted unchanged in the urine within 24 hours. There is limited biliary excretion amounting to 10% or less of the administered dose. Enterohepatic recirculation of methotrexate has been proposed.

Renal excretion occurs by glomerular filtration and active tubular secretion. Nonlinear elimination due to saturation of renal tubular reabsorption has been observed in psoriatic patients at doses between 7.5 and 30 mg. Impaired renal function, as well as concurrent use of drugs such as weak organic acids that also undergo tubular secretion, can markedly increase methotrexate serum levels. Excellent correlation has been reported between methotrexate clearance and endogenous creatinine clearance.

Methotrexate clearance rates vary widely and are generally decreased at higher doses. Delayed drug clearance has been identified as 1 of the major factors responsible for methotrexate toxicity. It has been postulated that the toxicity of methotrexate for normal tissues is more dependent upon the duration of exposure to the drug rather than the peak level achieved. When a patient has delayed drug elimination due to compromised renal function, a third-space effusion, or other causes, methotrexate serum concentrations may remain elevated for prolonged periods. In pediatric patients receiving methotrexate for acute lymphocytic leukemia (6.3 to 30 mg/m^2), or for JRA (3.75 to 26.2 mg/m^2), the terminal half-life has been reported to range from 0.7 to 5.8 hours or 0.9 to 2.3 hours, respectively.

METHOTREXATE SODIUM — INJECTION

The terminal half-life reported for methotrexate is approximately 3 to 10 hours for patients receiving treatment for psoriasis, or RA or low-dose antineoplastic therapy (less than 30 mg/m^2). For patients receiving high doses of methotrexate, the terminal half-life is 8 to 15 hours.

The potential for toxicity from high-dose regimens or delayed excretion is reduced by the administration of leucovorin calcium during the final phase of methotrexate plasma elimination. Pharmacokinetic monitoring of methotrexate serum concentrations may help identify those patients at high risk for methotrexate toxicity and aid in proper adjustment of leucovorin dosing. Guidelines for monitoring serum methotrexate levels, and for adjustment of leucovorin dosing to reduce the risk of methotrexate toxicity, are available.

Contraindications

Methotrexate can cause fetal death or teratogenic effects when administered to a pregnant woman. Methotrexate is contraindicated in pregnant women with psoriasis or RA and should be used in the treatment of neoplastic diseases only when the potential benefit outweighs the risk to the fetus. Women of childbearing potential should not be started on methotrexate until pregnancy is excluded and should be fully counseled on the serious risk to the fetus should they become pregnant while undergoing treatment. Pregnancy should be avoided if either partner is receiving methotrexate; during and for a minimum of 3 months after therapy for male patients, and during and for at least 1 ovulatory cycle after therapy for female patients.

Because of the potential for serious adverse reactions from methotrexate in breastfed infants, it is contraindicated in nursing mothers.

Patients with psoriasis or RA with alcoholism, alcoholic liver disease or other chronic liver disease should not receive methotrexate.

Patients with psoriasis or RA who have overt or laboratory evidence of immunodeficiency syndromes should not receive methotrexate.

Patients with psoriasis or RA who have preexisting blood dyscrasias, such as bone marrow hypoplasia, leukopenia, thrombocytopenia or significant anemia, should not receive methotrexate.

Patients with a known hypersensitivity to methotrexate should not receive the drug.

Warnings

➤*Intrathecal use/high dose:* Methotrexate formulations and diluents containing preservatives must not be used for intrathecal or high-dose methotrexate therapy.

➤*Renal effects:* High doses of methotrexate used in the treatment of osteosarcoma may cause renal damage leading to acute renal failure. Nephrotoxicity is due primarily to the precipitation of methotrexate and 7-hydroxymethotrexate in the renal tubules. Close attention to renal function including adequate hydration, urine alkalinization and measurement of serum methotrexate and creatinine levels are essential for safe administration.

➤*Hepatic effects:* Methotrexate has the potential for acute (elevated transaminases) and chronic (fibrosis and cirrhosis) hepatotoxicity. Chronic toxicity is potentially fatal; it generally has occurred after prolonged use (generally 2 years or more) and after a total dose of at least 1.5 g. In studies in psoriatic patients, hepatotoxicity appeared to be a function of total cumulative dose and appeared to be enhanced by alcoholism, obesity, diabetes and advanced age. An accurate incidence rate has not been determined; the rate of progression and reversibility of lesions is not known. Special caution is indicated in the presence of preexisting liver damage or impaired hepatic function.

In psoriasis, liver function tests, including serum albumin, should be performed periodically prior to dosing, but are often normal in the face of developing fibrosis or cirrhosis. These lesions may be detectable only by biopsy. The usual recommendation is to obtain a liver biopsy at pretherapy or shortly after initiation of therapy (2 to 4 months), at a total cumulative dose of 1.5 g, and after each additional 1 to 1.5 g. Moderate fibrosis or any cirrhosis normally leads to discontinuation of the drug; mild fibrosis normally suggests a repeat biopsy in 6 months. Milder histologic findings such as fatty change and low-grade portal inflammation are relatively common pretherapy. Although these mild changes are usually not a reason to avoid or discontinue methotrexate therapy, the drug should be used with caution.

In RA, age at first use of methotrexate and duration of therapy have been reported as risk factors for hepatotoxicity; other risk factors, similar to those observed in psoriasis, may be present in RA but have not been confirmed to date. Persistent abnormalities in liver function tests may precede appearance of fibrosis or cirrhosis in this population. There is a combined reported experience in 217 RA patients with liver biopsies both before and during treatment (after a cumulative dose of at least 1.5 g) and in 714 patients with a biopsy only during treatment. There are 64 (7%) cases of fibrosis and 1 (0.1%) case of cirrhosis. Of the 64 cases of fibrosis, 60 were deemed mild. The reticulin stain is more sensitive for early fibrosis, and its use may increase these figures. It is unknown whether even longer use will increase these risks.

Liver function tests should be performed at baseline and at 4- to 8-week intervals in patients receiving methotrexate for RA. Pretreatment liver biopsy should be performed for patients with a history of excessive alcohol consumption, persistently abnormal baseline liver function test values or chronic hepatitis B or C infection. During therapy, liver biopsy should be performed if there are persistent liver function test abnormalities or there is a decrease in serum albumin below the normal range (in the setting of well-controlled RA). If the results of a liver biopsy show mild changes (Roenigk grades I, II, IIIa), methotrexate may be continued and the patient monitored as per recommendations listed above. Methotrexate should be discontinued in any patient who displays persistently abnormal liver function tests and refuses liver biopsy or in any patient whose liver biopsy shows moderate-to-severe changes (Roenigk grade IIIb or IV).

➤*Carcinogenesis:* Non-Hodgkin's lymphoma and other tumors have been reported in patients receiving low-dose oral methotrexate. However, there have been instances of malignant lymphoma arising during treatment with low-dose oral methotrexate, which have regressed completely following withdrawal of methotrexate, without requiring active antilymphoma treatment. Benefits should be weighed against the potential risks before using methotrexate alone or in combination with other drugs, especially in children or young adults.

➤*Fertility impairment:* It has been reported to cause impairment of fertility, oligospermia and menstrual dysfunction in humans, during and for a short period after cessation of therapy.

➤*Elderly:* Clinical studies of methotrexate did not include sufficient numbers of subjects aged 65 years and older to determine whether they respond differently from younger subjects. In general, dose selection for an elderly patient should be cautious, reflecting the greater frequency of decreased hepatic and renal function, decreased folate stores, concomitant disease or other drug therapy (ie, that interfere with renal function, methotrexate or folate metabolism) in this population. Since decline in renal function may be associated with increases in adverse events and serum creatinine measurements may overestimate renal function in the elderly, more accurate methods (ie, creatinine clearance) should be considered. Serum methotrexate levels may also be helpful. Elderly patients should be closely monitored for early signs of hepatic, bone marrow, and renal toxicity. In chronic use situations, certain toxicities may be reduced by folate supplementation. Postmarketing experience suggests that the occurrence of bone marrow suppression, thrombocytopenia, and pneumonitis may increase with age.

➤*Pregnancy: Category X.* Methotrexate causes embryotoxicity, abortion, and fetal defects in humans.

Methotrexate can cause fetal death or teratogenic effects when administered to a pregnant woman. Methotrexate is contraindicated in pregnant women with psoriasis or RA and should be used in the treatment of neoplastic diseases only when the potential benefit outweighs the risk to the fetus. Women of childbearing potential should not be started on methotrexate until pregnancy is excluded and should be fully counseled on the serious risk to the fetus should they become pregnant while undergoing treatment. Pregnancy should be avoided if either partner is receiving methotrexate; during and for a minimum of 3 months after therapy for male patients, and during and for at least 1 ovulatory cycle after therapy for female patients.

➤*Lactation:* Because of the potential for serious adverse reactions from methotrexate in breastfed infants, it is contraindicated in nursing mothers.

➤*Children:* Safety and efficacy in children have been established only in cancer chemotherapy and in polyarticular-course JRA.

Published clinical studies evaluating the use of methotrexate in children and adolescents (ie, patients 2 to 16 years of age) with JRA demonstrated safety comparable to that observed in adults with RA.

Methotrexate injectable formulations containing the preservative benzyl alcohol are not recommended for use in neonates. There have been reports of fatal "gasping syndrome" in neonates (children less than 1 month of age) following the administrations of IV solutions containing the preservative benzyl alcohol. Symptoms including a striking onset of gasping respiration, hypotension, bradycardia, and cardiovascular collapse.

Precautions

➤*Monitoring:* Patients undergoing methotrexate therapy should be closely monitored so that toxic effects are detected promptly. Baseline assessment should include a complete blood count with differential and platelet counts, hepatic enzymes, renal function tests, and a chest x-ray. During therapy of RA and psoriasis, monitoring of these parameters is recommended: Hematology at least monthly, renal function and liver function every 1 to 2 months. More frequent monitoring is usually indicated during antineoplastic therapy. During initial or changing doses, or during periods of increased risk of elevated methotrexate blood levels (eg, dehydration), more frequent monitoring may also be indicated.

Toxic effects: Methotrexate has the potential for serious toxicity. Toxic effects may be related in frequency and severity to dose or frequency of administration but have been seen at all doses. Because they can occur at any time during therapy, it is necessary to follow patients on methotrexate closely. Most adverse reactions are reversible if detected early. When such reactions do occur, the drug should be reduced in dosage or discontinued, and appropriate corrective measures should be taken. If necessary, this could include the use of leucovorin calcium or acute, intermittent hemodialysis with a high-flux dialyzer. If methotrexate therapy is reinstituted, it should be carried out with caution, with adequate consideration of further need for the drug and with increased alertness as to possible recurrence of toxicity.

➤*Neurologic:* There have been reports of leukoencephalopathy following IV administration of methotrexate to patients who have had craniospinal irradiation. Serious neurotoxicity, frequently manifested as generalized or focal seizures, has been reported with unexpectedly increased frequency among pediatric patients with acute lymphoblastic leukemia who were treated with intermediate-dose IV methotrexate (1 g/m^2). Symptomatic patients were commonly noted to have leukoencephalopathy or microangiopathic calcifications on diagnostic imaging studies. Chronic leukoencephalopathy has also been reported in patients who received repeated doses of high-dose methotrexate with leucovorin rescue even without cranial irradiation. Discontinuation of methotrexate does not always result in complete recovery.

METHOTREXATE SODIUM — INJECTION

A transient acute neurologic syndrome has been observed in patients treated with high-dosage regimens. Manifestations of this stroke-like encephalopathy may include confusion, hemiparesis, seizures and coma. The exact cause is unknown.

After the intrathecal use of methotrexate, the CNS toxicity which may occur can be classified as follows: Acute chemical arachnoiditis manifested by such symptoms as headache, back pain, nuchal rigidity, and fever; subacute myelopathy characterized by paraparesis/paraplegia associated with involvement with 1 or more spinal nerve roots; chronic leukoencephalopathy manifested by confusion, irritability, somnolence, ataxia, dementia, seizures and coma. This condition can be progressive and even fatal.

➤*Pulmonary:* Pulmonary symptoms (especially a dry, nonproductive cough) or a nonspecific pneumonitis occurring during methotrexate therapy may be indicative of a potentially dangerous lesion and require interruption of treatment and careful investigation. Although clinically variable, the typical patient with methotrexate-induced lung disease presents with fever, cough, dyspnea, hypoxemia, and an infiltrate on chest x-ray; infection needs to be excluded. This lesion can occur at all dosages.

➤*Skin:* Severe, occasionally fatal, dermatologic reactions, including toxic epidermal necrolysis, Stevens-Johnson syndrome, exfoliative dermatitis, skin necrosis, and erythema multiforme, have been reported in children and adults, within days of oral, IM, IV, or intrathecal methotrexate administration. Reactions were noted after single or multiple, low, intermediate or high doses of methotrexate in patients with neoplastic and nonneoplastic diseases.

➤*Pleural effusions or ascites:* Methotrexate exits slowly from third space compartments (eg, pleural effusions or ascites). This results in a prolonged terminal plasma half-life and unexpected toxicity. In patients with significant third-space accumulations, it is advisable to evacuate the fluid before treatment and to monitor plasma methotrexate levels.

➤*Psoriasis lesions:* Lesions of psoriasis may be aggravated by concomitant exposure to ultraviolet radiation. Radiation dermatitis and sunburn may be "recalled" by the use of methotrexate.

➤*Debility:* Methotrexate should be used with extreme caution in the presence of debility.

➤*Gastrointestinal:* If vomiting, diarrhea, or stomatitis occur, which may result in dehydration, methotrexate should be discontinued until recovery occurs. Methotrexate should be used with extreme caution in the presence of peptic ulcer disease or ulcerative colitis.

➤*Hematologic:* Methotrexate can suppress hematopoiesis and cause anemia, aplastic anemia, pancytopenia, leukopenia, neutropenia, or thrombocytopenia. In patients with malignancy and preexisting hematopoietic impairment, the drug should be used with caution, if at all. In controlled clinical trials in RA (n = 128), leukopenia (WBC less than 3,000/mm^3) was seen in 2 patients, thrombocytopenia (platelets less than 100,000/mm^3) in 6 patients, and pancytopenia in 2 patients.

In psoriasis and RA, methotrexate should be stopped immediately if there is a significant drop in blood counts. In the treatment of neoplastic diseases, methotrexate should be continued only if the potential benefit warrants the risk of severe myelosuppression. Patients with profound granulocytopenia and fever should be evaluated immediately and usually require parenteral broad-spectrum antibiotic therapy.

➤*Infection or immunologic states:* Methotrexate should be used with extreme caution in the presence of active infection, and is usually contraindicated in patients with overt or laboratory evidence of immunodeficiency syndromes. Immunization may be ineffective when given during methotrexate therapy. Immunization with live virus vaccines is generally not recommended. There have been reports of disseminated vaccinia infections after smallpox immunization in patients receiving methotrexate therapy. Hypogammaglobulinemia has been reported rarely.

See Adverse Reactions for more information.

➤*Lab test abnormalities:* Transient liver function test abnormalities are observed frequently after methotrexate administration and are usually not cause for modification of methotrexate therapy. Persistent liver function test abnormalities, or depression of serum albumin may be indicators of serious liver toxicity and require evaluation.

A relationship between abnormal liver function tests and fibrosis or cirrhosis of the liver has not been established for patients with psoriasis. Persistent abnormalities in liver function tests may precede appearance of fibrosis or cirrhosis in the RA population.

Pulmonary function tests may be useful if methotrexate-induced lung disease is suspected, especially if baseline measurements are available.

Drug Interactions

➤*NSAIDS / Salicylates:* Nonsteroidal anti-inflammatory drugs (NSAIDs) should not be administered prior to or concomitantly with the high doses of methotrexate used in the treatment of osteosarcoma. Concomitant administration of some NSAIDs with high-dose methotrexate therapy has been reported to elevate and prolong serum methotrexate levels, resulting in deaths from severe hematologic and GI toxicity.

Caution should be used when NSAIDs and salicylates are administered concomitantly with lower doses of methotrexate. These drugs have been reported to reduce the tubular secretion of methotrexate in an animal model and may enhance its toxicity.

➤*Salicylates, phenylbutazone, phenytoin, sulfonamides, probenecid:* Methotrexate is partially bound to serum albumin, and toxicity may be increased because of displacement by certain drugs, such as salicylates, phenylbutazone, phenytoin, and sulfonamides. Renal tubular transport is also diminished by probenecid; use of methotrexate with this drug should be carefully monitored.

➤*Cisplatin:* In the treatment of patients with osteosarcoma, caution must be exercised if high-dose methotrexate is administered in combination with a potentially nephrotoxic chemotherapeutic agent (eg, cisplatin).

➤*Mercaptopurine:* Methotrexate increases the plasma levels of mercaptopurine. The combination of methotrexate and mercaptopurine may therefore require dose adjustment.

➤*Oral antibiotics:* Oral antibiotics such as tetracycline, chloramphenicol, and nonabsorbable broad-spectrum antibiotics, may decrease intestinal absorption of methotrexate or interfere with the enterohepatic circulation by inhibiting bowel flora and suppressing metabolism of the drug by bacteria.

➤*Hepatotoxic agents:* The potential for increased hepatotoxicity when methotrexate is administered with other hepatotoxic agents has not been evaluated. However, hepatotoxicity has been reported in such cases. Therefore, patients receiving concomitant therapy with methotrexate and other potential hepatotoxins (eg, azathioprine, retinoids, sulfasalazine) should be monitored closely for possible increased risk of hepatotoxicity.

Methotrexate Drug Interactions

Precipitant drug	Object drug[a]		Description
Aminoglycosides, oral	Methotrexate	⬇	The antitumorigenic actions of methotrexate may be decreased, but not predictably. Consider parenteral methotrexate if oral aminoglycosides are being coadministered.
Chloramphenicol	Methotrexate	⬇	Oral chloramphenicol may decrease intestinal absorption of methotrexate or interfere with the enterohepatic circulation by inhibiting bowel flora and suppressing metabolism of the drug by bacteria.
Folic acid	Methotrexate	⬇	Vitamin preparations containing folic acid or its derivatives may decrease responses to systemically administered methotrexate.
NSAIDs	Methotrexate	⬆	Concomitant administration of some NSAIDs with high dose methotrexate has been reported to elevate and prolong serum methotrexate levels, resulting in deaths from severe hematologic and GI toxicity. NSAIDs may reduce tubular secretion of methotrexate and enhance toxicity. Monitor renal impairment that could predispose to methotrexate toxicity, for signs of methotrexate toxicity, and methotrexate levels if indicated.
Penicillins	Methotrexate	⬆	Serum methotrexate concentrations may be elevated, increasing the risk of toxicity. Monitor for methotrexate toxicity and measure methotrexate concentrations twice a week for at least the first 2 weeks. If a broad-spectrum antibiotic is needed, ceftazidime may be less likely to interact.
Probenecid	Methotrexate	⬆	Methotrexate plasma levels, therapeutic effects, and toxicity may be enhanced. Monitor methotrexate concentrations and adjust dose accordingly.
Salicylates	Methotrexate	⬆	Increased toxic effects of methotrexate may occur. Salicylates may reduce tubular secretion of methotrexate and enhance toxicity. Consider monitoring methotrexate levels.

METHOTREXATE SODIUM — INJECTION

Methotrexate Drug Interactions			
Precipitant drug	Object drug[a]		Description
Sulfonamides	Methotrexate	↑	Sulfonamides may increase the risk of methotrexate-induced bone marrow suppression. Methotrexate may predispose patients to trimethoprim-sulfamethoxazole (TMP-SMZ)-induced megaloblastic anemia. Closely monitor patients for signs of hematologic toxicity.
Methotrexate	Sulfonamides		
Tetracyclines	Methotrexate	↑	Methotrexate concentrations may be elevated, increasing the risk of toxicity (eg, bone marrow suppression). If tetracyclines cannot be avoided in patients receiving high-dose methotrexate, closely monitor methotrexate plasma concentrations and patients for signs and symptoms of toxicity.
Trimethoprim	Methotrexate	↑	Trimethoprim may increase the risk of methotrexate-induced bone marrow suppression and megaloblastic anemia. If this drug combination cannot be avoided, closely monitor for signs of hematologic toxicity.
Methotrexate	Digoxin	↓	Serum levels of digoxin may be reduced and actions may be decreased. Monitor patient for signs of reduction in pharmacologic effect of digoxin and increase digoxin dose if necessary. Serum level monitoring may facilitate tailoring dosage.
Methotrexate	Phenytoin	↓	Serum concentrations of phenytoin may be decreased, resulting in a loss of therapeutic effect. Monitor phenytoin serum levels and adjust the phenytoin dosage appropriately. IV phenytoin may be useful.
Methotrexate	Theophylline	↑	Methotrexate may decrease the clearance of theophylline. Theophylline levels should be monitored when used concomitantly with methotrexate.
Methotrexate	Thiopurines (eg, azathioprine)	↑	The actions of thiopurines may be enhanced. Reduced thiopurine dosage may be used during coadministration with methotrexate.

[a] ↑ = Object drug increased. ↓ = Object drug decreased.

Adverse Reactions

The most frequently reported adverse reactions include ulcerative stomatitis, leukopenia, nausea, and abdominal distress. Other frequently reported adverse effects are malaise, undue fatigue, chills and fever, dizziness and decreased resistance to infection.

➤*Adverse reactions in oncology setting:*

Cardiovascular – Pericarditis, pericardial effusion, hypotension, and thromboembolic events (including arterial thrombosis, cerebral thrombosis, deep vein thrombosis, retinal vein thrombosis, thrombophlebitis, and pulmonary embolus).

CNS – Headaches, drowsiness, blurred vision, transient blindness, speech impairment including dysarthria and aphasia, hemiparesis, paresis and convulsions have also occurred following administration of methotrexate. Following low doses, there have been occasional reports of transient subtle cognitive dysfunction, mood alteration, unusual cranial sensations, leukoencephalopathy, or encephalopathy.

Dermatologic – Erythematous rashes, pruritus, urticaria, photosensitivity, pigmentary changes, alopecia, ecchymosis, telangiectasia, acne, furunculosis, erythema multiforme, toxic epidermal necrolysis, Stevens-Johnson syndrome, skin necrosis, and exfoliative dermatitis.

GI – Gingivitis, pharyngitis, stomatitis, anorexia, nausea, vomiting, diarrhea, hematemesis, melena, GI ulceration and bleeding, enteritis, pancreatitis.

GU – Severe nephropathy or renal failure, azotemia, cystitis, hematuria, proteinuria; defective oogenesis or spermatogenesis, transient oligospermia, menstrual dysfunction, vaginal discharge and gynecomastia; infertility, abortion, fetal death, fetal defects.

Hepatic – Hepatotoxicity, acute hepatitis, chronic fibrosis and cirrhosis, hepatic failure, decrease in serum albumin, liver enzyme elevations.

Hematologic/Lymphatic – Suppressed hematopoiesis, anemia, aplastic anemia, pancytopenia, leukopenia, neutropenia, thrombocytopenia, agranulocytosis, eosinophilia, lymphadenopathy, and lymphoproliferative disorders (including reversible).

Hypogammaglobulinemia has been reported rarely.

Musculoskeletal – Stress fracture.

Ophthalmic – Conjunctivitis, serious visual changes of unknown etiology.

Pulmonary – Respiratory fibrosis, respiratory failure, alveolitis, interstitial pneumonitis deaths have been reported, and chronic interstitial obstructive pulmonary disease has occasionally occurred.

Miscellaneous –

Infection: There have been case reports of sometimes fatal opportunistic infections in patients receiving methotrexate therapy for neoplastic and non-neoplastic diseases. *Pneumocystis carinii* pneumonia was the most common opportunistic infection. There have also been reports of infections, pneumonia, cytomegalovirus infection, including cytomegaloviral pneumonia, sepsis, fatal sepsis, nocardiosis; histoplasmosis, cryptococcosis, *Herpes zoster*, *H. simplex* hepatitis, and disseminated *H. simplex*. Other rarer reactions related to or attributed to the use of methotrexate such as nodulosis; vasculitis; arthralgia/myalgia; loss of libido/impotence; diabetes; osteoporosis; sudden death; lymphoma, including reversible lymphomas; tumor lysis syndrome; soft tissue necrosis; and osteonecrosis. Anaphylactoid reactions have been reported.

➤*Adverse reactions in double-blind RA studies:*

Incidence greater than 10% – Elevated liver function tests 15%, nausea/vomiting 10%.

Incidence 3% to 10% – Stomatitis, thrombocytopenia (platelet count less than 100,000/mm^3).

Incidence 1% to 3% – Rash/pruritus/dermatitis, diarrhea, alopecia, leukopenia (WBC less than 3,000/mm^3), pancytopenia, dizziness.

Two other controlled trials of patients (n = 680) with RA on 7.5 mg to 15 mg/week oral doses showed an incidence of interstitial pneumonitis of 1%.

Other less common reactions included decreased hematocrit, headache, upper respiratory tract infection, anorexia, arthralgias, chest pain, coughing, dysuria, eye discomfort, epistaxis, fever, infection, sweating, tinnitus, and vaginal discharge.

➤*Adverse reactions in JRA studies:* The approximate incidences of adverse reactions reported in pediatric patients with JRA treated with oral, weekly doses of methotrexate (5 to 20 mg/m^2/week or 0.1 to 0.65 mg/kg/week) were as follows (virtually all patients were receiving concomitant nonsteroidal anti-inflammatory drugs, and some also were taking low-dose corticosteroids): Elevated liver function tests, 14%; GI reactions (eg, nausea, vomiting, diarrhea), 11%; stomatitis, 2%; leukopenia, 2%; headache, 1.2%; alopecia, 0.5%; dizziness, 0.2%; and rash, 0.2%. Although there is experience with dosing up to 30 mg/m^2/week in JRA, the published data for doses above 20 mg/m^2/week are too limited to provide reliable estimates of adverse reaction rates.

Overdosage

➤*Symptoms:* Symptoms of intrathecal overdosage are generally CNS symptoms, including headache, nausea and vomiting, seizure and convulsion, and acute toxic encephalopathy. In some cases, no symptoms were reported. There have been reports of death following intrathecal overdose. In these cases, cerebellar herniation associated with increased intracranial pressure, and acute toxic encephalopathy have also been reported.

➤*Treatment:* Leucovorin is indicated to diminish the toxicity and counteract the effect of inadvertently administered overdosages of methotrexate. Leucovorin administration should begin as promptly as possible. As the time interval between methotrexate administration and leucovorin initiation increases, the effectiveness of leucovorin in counteracting toxicity decreases. Monitoring of the serum methotrexate concentration is essential in determining the optimal dose and duration of treatment with leucovorin.

In cases of massive overdosage, hydration and urinary alkalinization may be necessary to prevent the precipitation of methotrexate or its metabolites in the renal tubules. Generally speaking, neither hemodialysis nor peritoneal dialysis have been shown to improve methotrexate elimination. However, effective clearance of methotrexate has been reported with acute intermittent hemodialysis using a high-flux dialyzer (Wall, SM et al. *Am J Kidney Dis* 28(6): 846-854, 1996).

Accidental intrathecal overdosage may require intensive systemic support, high-dose systemic leucovorin, alkaline diuresis and rapid CSF drainage and ventriculolumbar perfusion.

There are published case reports of IV and intrathecal carboxypeptidase G2 treatment to hasten clearance of methotrexate in cases of overdose.

Patient Information

Patients should be informed of the early signs and symptoms of toxicity, of the need to see their physicians promptly if they occur, and the need for close follow-up, including periodic laboratory tests to monitor toxicity.

Both the physician and pharmacist should emphasize to the patient that the recommended dose is taken weekly in RA and psoriasis, and that mistaken daily use of the recommended dose has led to fatal toxicity. Patients should be encouraged to read the Patient Instructions sheet within the dose pack. Prescriptions should not be written or refilled on an as-needed basis.

Patients should be informed of the potential benefit and risk in the use of methotrexate. The risk of effects on reproduction should be discussed with both male and female patients taking methotrexate.

PEMETREXED

Rx	**Alimta** (Eli Lilly)	**Powder for injection, lyophilized:** 500 mg	500 mg mannitol. In single-use vials.

PEMETREXED — INJECTION

Indications

➤*Malignant pleural mesothelioma (MPM):* In combination with cisplatin for the treatment of patients with MPM whose disease is unresectable or who are otherwise not candidates for curative surgery.

➤*Non-small cell lung cancer (NSCLC):* As a single-agent for the treatment of patients with locally advanced or metastatic NSCLC after prior chemotherapy.

Administration and Dosage

➤*Approved by the FDA:* February 5, 2004.

For intravenous (IV) infusion only.

➤*Malignant pleural mesothelioma:* The recommended dose of pemetrexed is 500 mg/m² administered as an IV infusion over 10 minutes on day 1 of each 21-day cycle. The recommended dose of cisplatin is 75 mg/m² infused over 2 hours beginning approximately 30 minutes after the end of pemetrexed administration. Give patients hydration consistent with local practice prior to and/or after receiving cisplatin. Refer to cisplatin monograph for more information.

➤*Non-small cell lung cancer (NSCLC):* The recommended dose of pemetrexed is 500 mg/m² administered as an IV infusion over 10 minutes on day 1 of each 21-day cycle.

➤*Premedication regimen:*

Corticosteroid – Skin rash has been reported more frequently in patients not pretreated with a corticosteroid. Pretreatment with dexamethasone (or equivalent) reduces the incidence and severity of cutaneous reaction. In clinical trials, dexamethasone 4 mg was given by mouth twice daily the day before, the day of, and the day after pemetrexed administration.

Vitamin supplementation – To reduce toxicity, instruct patients treated with pemetrexed to take a low-dose oral folic acid preparation or multivitamin with folic acid on a daily basis. At least 5 daily doses of folic acid must be taken during the 7-day period preceding the first dose of pemetrexed; dosing should continue during the full course of therapy and for 21 days after the last dose of pemetrexed. Patients must also receive 1 intramuscular (IM) injection of vitamin B_{12} during the week preceding the first dose of pemetrexed and every 3 cycles thereafter. Subsequent vitamin B_{12} injections may be given the same day as pemetrexed. In clinical trials, the dose of folic acid studied ranged from 350 to 1,000 mcg, and the dose of vitamin B_{12} was 1,000 mcg. The most commonly used dose of oral folic acid in clinical trials was 400 mcg.

➤*Dose adjustment:* Discontinue pemetrexed therapy if a patient experiences any hematologic or nonhematologic grade 3 or 4 toxicity after 2 dose reductions (except grade 3 transaminase elevations), or immediately if grade 3 or 4 neurotoxicity is observed.

Hematologic toxicities – Dose adjustments at the start of a subsequent cycle should be based on nadir hematologic counts or maximum nonhematologic toxicity from the preceding cycle of therapy. Treatment may be delayed to allow sufficient time for recovery. Do not have patients begin a new cycle of treatment unless the absolute neutrophil count (ANC) is 1,500 cells/mm³ or more, the platelet count is 100,000 cells/mm³ or more, and creatine clearance (Ccr) is 45 mL/min or more. Upon recovery, retreat patients using the guidelines in the following table, which are suitable for using pemetrexed as a single agent or in combination with cisplatin:

Dose Reduction for Pemetrexed (Single-Agent or in Combination) and Cisplatin - Hematologic Toxicities	
Nadir ANC < 500/mm³ and nadir platelets ≥ 50,000/mm³	75% of previous dose (both drugs)
Nadir platelets < 50,000/mm³ regardless of nadir ANC	50% of previous dose (both drugs)

Nonhematologic toxicities – If patients develop nonhematologic toxicities (excluding neurotoxicity) grade 3 or higher (except grade 3 transaminase elevations), withhold pemetrexed until toxicities resolve to less than or equal to the patient's pretherapy value. Resume treatment according to guidelines in the following table:

Dose Reduction for Pemetrexed (Single-Agent or in Combination) and Cisplatin - Nonhematologic Toxicities[a,b]		
	Dose of pemetrexed (mg/m²)	Dose of cisplatin (mg/m²)
Any grade 3[c] or 4 toxicities except mucositis	75% of previous dose	75% of previous dose
Any diarrhea requiring hospitalization (irrespective of grade) or grade 3 or 4 diarrhea	75% of previous dose	75% of previous dose
Grade 3 or 4 mucositis	50% of previous dose	100% of previous dose

[a] NCI Common Toxicity Criteria (CTC).
[b] Excluding neurotoxicity.
[c] Except grade 3 transaminase elevation.

Neurotoxicity – In the event of neurotoxicity, the recommended dose adjustments for pemetrexed and cisplatin are shown in the following table. Discontinue therapy if grade 3 or 4 neurotoxicity is experienced.

Dose Reduction for Pemetrexed (Single-Agent or in Combination) and Cisplatin - Neurotoxicity		
CTC grade	Dose of pemetrexed (mg/m²)	Dose of cisplatin (mg/m²)
0 to 1	100% of previous dose	100% of previous dose
2	100% of previous dose	50% of previous dose

➤*Renal function impairment:* In clinical studies, patients with Ccr 45 mL/min or higher required no dose adjustments other than those recommended for all patients. Insufficient numbers of patients with Ccr less than 45 mL/min have been treated to make dosage recommendations for this group of patients. Therefore, do not administer pemetrexed to patients whose Ccr is less than 45 mL/min using the standard Cockcroft and Gault formula (see following paragraph) or GFR measured by Tc99m-DPTA serum clearance method:

Males: [140 − age in years] × actual body weight (kg)/72 × serum creatinine (mg/dL) = mL/min.

Females: Estimated Ccr for males × 0.85.

Concomitant use with nonsteroid anti-inflammatory drugs (NSAIDS) – Exercise caution when administering pemetrexed concurrently with NSAIDs to patients whose Ccr is less than 80 mL/min. Patients with mild to moderate renal insufficiency should avoid taking NSAIDs with short elimination half-lives for a period of 2 days before, the day of, and 2 days following administration of pemetrexed. In the absence of data regarding potential interaction between pemetrexed and NSAIDs with longer half-lives, all patients taking these NSAIDs should interrupt dosing for at least 5 days before, the day of, and 2 days following pemetrexed administration. If coadministration of an NSAID is necessary, closely monitor patients for toxicity, especially myelosuppression and renal and GI toxicity.

➤*Preparation for IV infusion administration:*

1.) Use aseptic technique during the reconstitution and further dilution of pemetrexed for IV infusion administration.
2.) Calculate the dose and the number of pemetrexed vials needed. Each vial contains pemetrexed 500 mg. The vial contains an excess of pemetrexed to facilitate delivery of label amount.
3.) Reconstitute 500 mg vials with 20 mL of 0.9% sodium chloride injection (preservative-free) to create a solution containing pemetrexed 25 mg/mL. Gently swirl each vial until the powder is completely dissolved. The resulting solution is clear and ranges in color from colorless to yellow or green-yellow without adversely affecting product quality. The pH of the reconstituted pemetrexed solution is between 6.6 and 7.8. Further dilution is required.
4.) Visually inspect parenteral drug products for particulate matter and discoloration prior to administration. Do not administer if particulate matter is observed.
5.) Further dilute the appropriate volume of reconstituted pemetrexed solution to 100 mL with 0.9% sodium chloride injection (preservative-free) and administered as an IV infusion over 10 minutes.
6.) Chemical and physical stability of reconstituted and infusion solutions of pemetrexed were demonstrated for up to 24 hours following initial reconstitution, when stored at refrigerated or ambient room temperature and lighting. When prepared as directed, reconstitution and infusion solutions of pemetrexed contain no antimicrobial preservatives. Discard any unused portion.

Admixture incompatibilities – Reconstitution and further dilution prior to IV infusion is only recommended with 0.9% sodium chloride injection (preservative-free). Pemetrexed is physically incompatible with diluents containing calcium, including lactated Ringer injection and Ringer injection, and therefore these should not be used. Coadministration of pemetrexed with other drugs and diluents has not been studied, and therefore is not recommended.

➤*Storage / Stability:* Store at 25°C (77°F); excursions permitted to 15° to 30°C (59° to 86°F).

Chemical and physical stability of reconstituted and infusion solutions of pemetrexed were demonstrated for up to 24 hours following initial reconstitution when stored refrigerated at 2° to 8°C (36° to 46°F) or at 25°C (77°F); excursions permitted to 15° to 30°C (59° to 86°F). When prepared as directed, reconstituted and infusion solutions of pemetrexed contain no antimicrobial preservatives. Discard unused portion.

Actions

➤*Pharmacology:* Pemetrexed is an antifolate containing the pyrrolopyrimidine-based nucleus that exerts its antineoplastic activity by disrupting folate-dependent metabolic processes essential for cell replication. In vitro studies have shown that pemetrexed inhibits thymidylate synthase (TS), dihydrofolate reductase (DHFR), and glycinamide ribonucleotide formyltransferase (GARFT), all folate-dependent enzymes involved in the de novo biosynthesis of thymidine and purine nucleotides. Pemetrexed is transported into cells by both the reduced folate carrier and membrane folate binding protein transport systems. Once in the cell, pemetrexed is converted

PEMETREXED — INJECTION

to polyglutamate forms by the enzyme folylpolyglutamate synthetase. The polyglutamate forms are retained in cells and are inhibitors of TS and GARFT. Polyglutamation is a time- and concentration-dependent process that occurs in tumor cells and, to a lesser extent, in normal tissues. Polyglutamated metabolites have an increased intracellular half-life resulting in prolonged drug action in malignant cells.

Preclinical studies have shown that pemetrexed inhibits the in vitro growth of mesothelioma cell lines (MSTO-211H, NCI-H2052). Studies with the MSTO-211H mesothelioma cell line showed synergistic effects when pemetrexed was combined concurrently with cisplatin.

ANCs following single-agent administration of pemetrexed to patients not receiving folic acid and vitamin B_{12} supplementation were characterized using population pharmacodynamic analyses. Severity of hematologic toxicity, as measured by the depth of the ANC nadir, is inversely proportional to the systemic exposure of pemetrexed. It was also observed that lower ANC nadirs occurred in patients with elevated baseline cystathionine or homocysteine concentrations. The levels of these substances can be reduced by folic acid and vitamin B_{12} supplementation. There is no cumulative effect of pemetrexed exposure on ANC nadir over multiple treatment cycles.

Time to ANC nadir with pemetrexed systemic exposure (AUC), varied between 8 to 9.6 days over a range of exposures from 38.3 to 316.8 mcg•hr/mL. Return to baseline ANC occurred 4.2 to 7.5 days after the nadir over the same range of exposures.

➤*Pharmacokinetics:*

Absorption / Distribution –

Pemetrexed total AUC and maximum plasma concentration (C_{max}) increase proportionally with dose. Pemetrexed has a steady-state volume of distribution of 16.1 L. In vitro studies indicate that pemetrexed is approximately 81% bound to plasma proteins. Binding is not affected by degree of renal impairment.

Metabolism / Excretion – Pemetrexed is not metabolized to an appreciable extent.

Pemetrexed is primarily eliminated in the urine, with 70% to 90% of the dose recovered unchanged within the first 24 hours following administration. The total systemic clearance of pemetrexed is 91.8 mL/min and the elimination half-life of pemetrexed is 3.5 hours in patients with normal renal function (Ccr of 90 mL/min). The clearance decreases, and exposure (AUC) increases, as renal function decreases.

The pharmacokinetics of pemetrexed do not change over multiple treatment cycles.

The pharmacokinetics of pemetrexed in special populations were examined in about 400 patients in controlled and single arm studies.

Contraindications

History of severe hypersensitivity reaction to pemetrexed or any other ingredient used in the formulation.

Warnings

➤*Bone marrow suppression:* Pemetrexed can suppress bone marrow function, manifested by neutropenia, thrombocytopenia, and anemia; myelosuppression is usually the dose-limiting toxicity. Dose reductions for subsequent cycles are based on nadir ANC, platelet count, and maximum nonhematologic toxicity seen in the previous cycle.

➤*Folate and vitamin B_{12} supplementation:* See Administration and Dosage for more information.

➤*Renal function impairment:* See Administration and Dosage for more information.

One patient with severe renal impairment (Ccr 19 mL/min) who did not receive folic acid and vitamin B_{12} died of drug-related toxicity following administration of pemetrexed alone.

➤*Hepatic function impairment:* Dose adjustments based on hepatic impairment experienced during treatment with pemetrexed may be required.

➤*Mutagenesis:* Pemetrexed was clastogenic in the in vivo micronucleus assay in mouse bone marrow, but was not mutagenic in multiple in vitro tests (Ames assay, CHO cell assay).

➤*Fertility impairment:* Pemetrexed administered at IV dosages of 0.1 mg/kg/day or greater to male mice (about 1/1,666 the recommended human dosage on a mg/m^2 basis) resulted in reduced fertility, hypospermia, and testicular atrophy.

➤*Pregnancy: Category D.* Pemetrexed may cause fetal harm when administered to a pregnant woman. Pemetrexed was fetotoxic and teratogenic in mice at intraperitoneal doses of 0.2 mg/kg (0.6 mg/m^2) or 5 mg/kg (15 mg/m^2) when given on gestation days 6 through 15. Pemetrexed caused fetal malformations (incomplete ossification of talus and skull bone) at 0.2 mg/kg (about 1/833 the recommended IV human dose on a mg/m^2 basis), and cleft palate at 5 mg/kg (about 1/33 the recommended IV human dose on a mg/m^2 basis). Embryotoxicity was characterized by increased embryo-fetal deaths and reduced litter sizes. There are no studies of pemetrexed in pregnant women. Advise patients to avoid becoming pregnant. If pemetrexed is used during pregnancy, or if the patient becomes pregnant while taking pemetrexed, apprise the patient of the potential hazard to the fetus.

➤*Lactation:* It is not known whether pemetrexed or its metabolites are excreted in human milk. Because many drugs are excreted in human milk, and because of the potential for serious adverse reactions in nursing infants from pemetrexed, it is recommended that nursing be discontinued if the mother is treated with pemetrexed.

➤*Children:* The safety and efficacy of pemetrexed in pediatric patients have not been established.

Precautions

➤*Monitoring:* Perform complete blood cell counts, including platelet counts, on all patients receiving pemetrexed. Monitor patients for nadir and recovery (which were tested in the clinical study before each dose and on days 8 and 15 of each cycle). Patients should not begin a new cycle of treatment unless the ANC is 1,500 cells/mm^3 or greater, the platelet count is 100,000 cells/mm^3 or greater, and Ccr is 45 mL/min or higher. Perform periodic chemistry tests to evaluate renal and hepatic function.

➤*Cutaneous reaction:* Skin rash has been reported more frequently in patients not pretreated with a corticosteroid in clinical trials. Pretreatment with dexamethasone (or equivalent) reduces the incidence and severity of cutaneous reaction.

➤*Pleural effusion or ascites:* The effect of third space fluid, such as pleural effusion and ascites, on pemetrexed is unknown. In patients with clinically significant third space fluid, consider draining the effusion prior to pemetrexed administration.

Extravasation risk – Pemetrexed is not a vesicant. There is no specific antidote for extravasation of pemetrexed. To date, there have been few reported cases of pemetrexed extravasation, and they were not assessed as serious by the investigator. Manage pemetrexed extravasation with local standard practice for extravasation as with other nonvesicants.

➤*Special risk:* Pemetrexed is known to be primarily excreted by the kidney. Decreased renal function will result in reduced clearance and greater exposure (AUC) to pemetrexed compared with patients with normal renal function. Cisplatin coadministration with pemetrexed has not been studied in patients with moderate renal impairment.

Drug Interactions

Pemetrexed Drug Interactions			
Precipitant drug	Object drug[a]		Description
Nephrotoxic agents	Pemetrexed	↑	Coadministration of nephrotoxic drugs could result in delayed clearance of pemetrexed. Coadministration of substances that also are tubularly secreted (eg, probenecid) could potentially result in delayed clearance of pemetrexed.
NSAIDs (eg, ibuprofen)	Pemetrexed	↑	Daily ibuprofen doses of 400 mg 4 times/day reduce pemetrexed's clearance about 20% (and increase AUC 20%) in patients with normal renal function. Use caution when administering ibuprofen concurrently with pemetrexed to patients with mild to moderate renal insufficiency (Ccr 45 to 79 mL/min), and avoid giving NSAIDs with short elimination half-lives 2 days before, the day of, and 2 days following pemetrexed administration. Interrupt dosing in all patients taking NSAIDs with long elimination half-lives for at least 5 days before, the day of, and 2 days following pemetrexed administration. If coadministration of an NSAID is necessary, closely monitor patients for toxicity, especially myelosuppression and renal and GI toxicity.

[a] ↑ = Object drug increased.

Pemetrexed is primarily eliminated unchanged renally as a result of glomerular filtration and tubular secretion. Co-administration of nephrotoxic drugs could result in delayed clearance of pemetrexed. Co-administration of substances that are also tubularly secreted (eg, probenecid) could potentially result in delayed clearance of pemetrexed.

Adverse Reactions

➤*MPM:* In the following table, adverse reactions occurring in at least 5% patients are shown along with important reactions (renal failure, infection) occurring at lower rates. Adverse reactions equally or more common in the cisplatin group are not included. The adverse reactions more common in the pemetrexed group were primarily hematologic effects, fever and infection, stomatitis/pharyngitis, and rash/desquamation.

PEMETREXED — INJECTION

Adverse Reactions[a] in Fully Supplemented Patients Receiving Pemetrexed Plus Cisplatin for MPM (% Incidence)						
	Pemetrexed/Cisplatin (n = 168)			Cisplatin (n = 163)		
Adverse reaction	All grades	Grade 3	Grade 4	All grades	Grade 3	Grade 4
Cardiovascular						
Thrombosis/embolism	7%	4%	2%	4%	3%	1%
CNS						
Mood alteration/ depression	14%	1%	0%	9%	1%	0%
Neuropathy/sensory	17%	0%	0%	15%	1%	0%
GI						
Anorexia	35%	2%	0%	25%	1%	0%
Constipation	44%	2%	1%	39%	1%	0%
Dehydration	7%	3%	1%	1%	1%	0%
Diarrhea without colostomy	26%	4%	0%	16%	1%	0%
Dysphagia/ esophagitis/ odynophagia	6%	1%	0%	6%	0%	0%
Nausea	84%	11%	1%	79%	6%	0%
Stomatitis/pharyngitis	28%	2%	1%	9%	0%	0%
Vomiting	58%	10%	1%	52%	4%	1%
Hematologic						
Anemia	33%	5%	1%	14%	0%	0%
Febrile neutropenia	1%	1%	0%	1%	0%	0%
Leukopenia	55%	14%	2%	20%	1%	0%
Neutropenia	58%	19%	5%	16%	3%	1%
Thrombocytopenia	27%	4%	1%	10%	0%	0%
Renal						
Creatinine elevation	16%	1%	0%	12%	1%	0%
Renal failure	2%	0%	1%	1%	0%	0%
Miscellaneous						
Allergic reaction/ Hypersensitivity	2%	0%	0%	1%	0%	0%
Chest pain	40%	8%	1%	30%	5%	1%
Dyspnea	66%	10%	1%	62%	5%	2%
Fatigue	80%	17%	0%	74%	12%	1%
Fever	17%	0%	0%	9%	0%	0%
Infection without neutropenia	11%	1%	1%	4%	0%	0%
Infection with grade 3 or 4 neutropenia	6%	1%	0%	4%	0%	0%
Infection/febrile neutropenia, other	3%	1%	0%	2%	0%	0%
Other constitutional symptoms	11%	2%	1%	8%	1%	1%
Rash/Desquamation	22%	1%	0%	9%	0%	0%

[a] Refer to NCI CTC Version 2.0.

The following table compares the incidence (percentage of patients) of CTC grade 3 or 4 toxicities in patients who received vitamin supplementation with daily folic acid and vitamin B_{12} from the time of enrollment in the study (fully supplemented) with the incidence in patients who never received vitamin supplementation (never supplemented) during the study in the pemetrexed plus cisplatin arm.

Selected Grade 3 or 4 Adverse Reactions Comparing Fully Supplemented vs Never Supplemented Patients in the Pemetrexed Plus Cisplatin Arm (% Incidence)		
Adverse reaction regardless of causality[a] (%)	Fully supplemented patients (n = 168)	Never supplemented patients (n = 32)
Cardiovascular		
Hypertension	11%	3%
Thrombosis/embolism	6%	3%
GI		
Anorexia	2%	9%
Diarrhea without colostomy	4%	9%
Nausea	12%	31%
Vomiting	11%	34%
Hematologic		
Febrile neutropenia	1%	9%
Infection with grade 3 or 4 neutropenia	1%	6%
Neutropenia	24%	38%
Thrombocytopenia	5%	9%
Miscellaneous		
Chest pain	8%	6%
Dehydration	4%	9%
Fatigue	17%	25%
Fever	0%	6%

[a] Refer to NCI CTC criteria for laboratory and nonlaboratory values for each grade of toxicity (Version 2.0). For fully supplemented patients treated with pemetrexed plus cisplatin, the incidence of CTC grade 3/4 fatigue, leukopenia, neutropenia, and thrombocytopenia were greater in patients 65 years of age or older as compared to patients younger than 65 years of age. No relevant effect of pemetrexed safety because of gender or race was identified, except an increased incidence of rash in men (24%) compared with women (16%).

➤*NSCLC:* The following table provides the clinically relevant undesirable effects that have been reported in 265 patients randomly assigned to receive single-agent pemetrexed with folic acid and vitamin B_{12} supplementation and 276 patients randomly assigned to receive single-agent docetaxel. All patients were diagnosed with locally advanced or metastatic NSCLC and had received prior chemotherapy.

Adverse Reactions in Patients Receiving Pemetrexed vs Docetaxel in NSCLC CTC Grades (% Incidence)						
	Pemetrexed (n = 265)			Docetaxel (n = 276)		
Adverse reaction	All grades	Grade 3	Grade 4	All grades	Grade 3	Grade 4
Cardiovascular						
Cardiac ischemia	3%	2%	1%	2%	< 1%	0%
Thrombosis/embolism	4%	2%	1%	3%	2%	1%
CNS						
Mood alteration/ depression	11%	0%	< 1%	10%	1%	0%
Neuropathy/sensory	29%	2%	0%	32%	1%	0%
Dermatologic						
Alopecia	11%	NA	NA	42%	NA	NA
Rash/desquamation	17%	0%	0%	9%	0%	0%
GI						
Anorexia	62%	4%	1%	58%	7%	< 1%
Constipation	30%	0%	0%	23%	1%	0%
Diarrhea without colostomy	21%	< 1%	0%	34%	4%	0%
Dysphagia/ esophagitis/ odynophagia	5%	1%	< 1%	7%	1%	0%
Nausea	39%	4%	0%	25%	3%	0%
Stomatitis/pharyngitis	20%	1%	0%	23%	1%	0%
Vomiting	25%	2%	0%	19%	1%	0%
Hematologic						
Anemia	33%	6%	2%	33%	6%	< 1%
Febrile neutropenia	2%	1%	1%	14%	10%	3%
Leukopenia	13%	4%	< 1%	34%	17%	11%
Neutropenia	11%	3%	2%	45%	8%	32%
Thrombocytopenia	9%	2%	0%	1%	1%	0%
Hepatic						
ALT elevation	10%	2%	1%	2%	< 1%	0%
AST elevation	8%	< 1%	1%	1%	< 1%	0%
Musculoskeletal						
Arthralgia	8%	< 1%	0%	13%	3%	0%
Myalgia	13%	2%	0%	20%	3%	0%
Renal						
Creatinine elevation	3%	0%	0%	1%	0%	0%
Decreased Ccr	5%	1%	0%	1%	0%	0%
Renal failure	< 1%	0%	0%	< 1%	0%	0%
Respiratory						
Dyspnea	72%	14%	4%	74%	17%	9%
Miscellaneous						
Allergic reaction/ hypersensitivity	8%	0%	0%	8%	1%	< 1%
Chest pain	38%	6%	< 1%	32%	7%	< 1%
Dehydration	3%	1%	0%	4%	1%	0%

PEMETREXED — INJECTION

Adverse Reactions in Patients Receiving Pemetrexed vs Docetaxel in NSCLC CTC Grades (% Incidence)						
	Pemetrexed (n = 265)			Docetaxel (n = 276)		
Adverse reaction	All grades	Grade 3	Grade 4	All grades	Grade 3	Grade 4
Edema	19%	< 1%	0%	24%	< 1%	0%
Fatigue	87%	14%	2%	81%	16%	1%
Fever	26%	1%	< 1%	19%	< 1%	0%
Infection/febrile neutropenia (other)	6%	2%	0%	2%	< 1%	0%
Infection with grade 3 or grade 4 neutropenia	< 1%	0%	0%	6%	4%	1%
Infection without neutropenia	23%	5%	< 1%	17%	3%	1%
Other constitutional symptoms	8%	1%	1%	6%	1%	< 1%

Clinically relevant grade 3 and grade 4 laboratory toxicities were similar between integrated phase 2 results from 3 single-agent pemetrexed studies (n = 164) and the phase 3 single-agent pemetrexed study described above, with the exception of neutropenia (12.8% vs 5.3%, respectively) and ALT elevation (15.2% vs 1.9%, respectively). These differences were likely because of differences in the patient population, since the phase 2 studies included chemo-naive and heavily pretreated breast cancer patients with preexisting liver metastases and/or abnormal baseline liver tests.

The incidence of CTC grade 3/4 hypertension was the only finding demonstrating an age difference in patients treated with pemetrexed and was greater in patients 65 years of age or older compared with younger patients. There are insufficient numbers of nonwhite patients to assess ethnic differences. The incidence of CTC grade 3/4 dyspnea was higher in men for both treatment arms.

Overdosage

➤*Symptoms:* There have been few cases of pemetrexed overdose. Reported toxicities included neutropenia, anemia, thrombocytopenia, mucositis, and rash. Anticipated complications of overdose include bone marrow suppression as manifested by neutropenia, thrombocytopenia, and anemia. In addition, infection with or without fever, diarrhea, and mucositis may be seen.

➤*Treatment:* If an overdose occurs, institute general supportive measures as deemed necessary by the treating health care provider.

In clinical trials, leucovorin was permitted for CTC grade 4 leukopenia lasting 3 days or longer, CTC grade 4 neutropenia lasting 3 days or longer, and immediately for CTC grade 4 thrombocytopenia, bleeding associated with grade 3 thrombocytopenia, or grade 3 or 4 mucositis. The following IV doses and schedules of leucovorin were recommended for IV use: 100 mg/m^2 IV once, followed by 50 mg/m^2 IV every 6 hours for 8 days.

The ability of pemetrexed to be dialyzed is unknown.

Patient Information

Read the patient information leaflet that comes with pemetrexed before you start treatment and each time you are treated with pemetrexed. There may be new information. This information does not take the place of talking to your doctor about your medical condition or treatment. Talk to your doctor if you have any questions about pemetrexed.

You must take folic acid and vitamin B_{12} while receiving this medication. Talk with your doctor.

Lab tests will be required to monitor therapy. Be sure to keep appointments.

Do not take any over-the-counter or prescription medications without talking with your doctor. This includes any herbal preparations or dietary supplements.

CAPECITABINE

Rx	**Xeloda** (Roche)	**Tablets:** 150 mg	Lactose. (Xeloda 150). Light peach, oblong. Film-coated. In 60s.
		500 mg	Lactose. (Xeloda 500). Peach, oblong. Film-coated. In 120s.

CAPECITABINE — ORAL

WARNING

Warfarin interaction – Frequently monitor the anticoagulant response (international normalized ratio [INR] or prothrombin time [PT]) of patients receiving concomitant capecitabine and oral coumarin-derivative anticoagulant therapy in order to adjust the anticoagulant dose accordingly. A clinically important capecitabine-warfarin drug interaction was demonstrated in a clinical pharmacology trial. Altered coagulation parameters and/or bleeding, including death, have been reported in patients taking capecitabine concomitantly with coumarin-derivative anticoagulants such as warfarin and phenprocoumon. Postmarketing reports have shown clinically significant increases in PT and INR in patients who were stabilized on anticoagulants at the time capecitabine was introduced. These events occurred within several days and up to several months after initiating capecitabine therapy and, in a few cases, within 1 month after stopping capecitabine. These events occurred in patients with and without liver metastases. Age older than 60 years and a diagnosis of cancer independently predispose patients to an increased risk of coagulopathy.

Indications

➤*Colorectal cancer:* Capecitabine is indicated as a single agent for adjuvant treatment in patients with Duke stage C colon cancer who have undergone complete resection of the primary tumor when treatment with fluoropyrimidine therapy alone is preferred. Capecitabine was noninferior to 5-fluorouracil and leucovorin for disease-free survival. Although neither capecitabine nor combination chemotherapy prolongs overall survival, combination chemotherapy has been demonstrated to improve disease-free survival compared with 5-fluorouracil/leucovorin. Consider these results when prescribing single-agent capecitabine in the adjuvant treatment of Duke stage C colon cancer.

Capecitabine is indicated as first-line treatment of patients with metastatic colorectal carcinoma when treatment with fluoropyrimidine therapy alone is preferred. Combination chemotherapy has shown a survival benefit compared with 5-fluorouracil/leucovorin alone. A survival benefit over 5-fluorouracil/leucovorin has not been demonstrated with capecitabine monotherapy. Use of capecitabine instead of 5-fluorouracil/leucovorin in combinations has not been adequately studied to ensure safety or preservation of the survival advantage.

➤*Breast cancer:* Capecitabine in combination with docetaxel is indicated for the treatment of patients with metastatic breast cancer after failure of prior anthracycline-containing chemotherapy.

Capecitabine monotherapy is indicated for the treatment of patients with metastatic breast cancer resistant to both paclitaxel and an anthracycline–containing chemotherapy regimen or resistant to paclitaxel and for whom further anthracycline therapy is not indicated (eg, patients who have received cumulative doses of 400 mg/m^2 of doxorubicin or doxorubicin equivalents). Resistance is defined as progressive disease while on treatment, with or without an initial response, or relapse within 6 months of completing treatment with an anthracycline-containing adjuvant regimen.

➤*Unlabeled uses:* As adjuvant treatment for pancreatic cancer.

Administration and Dosage

➤*Approved by the FDA:* April 30, 1998.

The recommended dosage of capecitabine is 1,250 mg/m^2 administered orally twice daily (morning and evening; equivalent to 2,500 mg/m^2 total daily dose) for 2 weeks followed by a 1-week rest period given as 3-week cycles. Capecitabine tablets should be swallowed with water within 30 minutes after a meal. In combination with docetaxel, the recommended dose of capecitabine is 1,250 mg/m^2 twice daily for 2 weeks followed by a 1-week rest period, combined with docetaxel at 75 mg/m^2 as a 1-hour intravenous (IV) infusion every 3 weeks. Premedication, according to the docetaxel labeling, should be started prior to docetaxel administration for patients receiving the capecitabine plus docetaxel combination. The following table provides the total daily dose by body surface area and the number of tablets to be taken at each dose.

Adjuvant treatment in patients with Duke stage C colon cancer is recommended for a total of 6 months (ie, capecitabine 1,250 mg/m^2 orally twice daily for 2 weeks followed by a 1-week rest period), given as 3-week cycles for a total of 8 cycles (24 weeks).

Capecitabine Dose Calculation According to Body Surface Area			
Dosage level 1,250 mg/m^2 twice a day		Number of tablets per dose (morning and evening)	
Surface area (m^2)	Total daily[a] dose (mg)	150 mg	500 mg
≤ 1.25	3,000	0	3
1.26 to 1.37	3,300	1	3
1.38 to 1.51	3,600	2	3
1.52 to 1.65	4,000	0	4
1.66 to 1.77	4,300	1	4
1.78 to 1.91	4,600	2	4
1.92 to 2.05	5,000	0	5
2.06 to 2.17	5,300	1	5
≥ 2.18	5,600	2	5

[a] Total daily dose divided by 2 to allow equal morning and evening doses.

➤*Dose modification guidelines:* Capecitabine dosage may need to be individualized to optimize patient management. Patients should be carefully monitored for toxicity and doses of capecitabine should be modified as

CAPECITABINE — ORAL

necessary to accommodate individual patient tolerance to treatment. Toxicity due to capecitabine administration may be managed by symptomatic treatment, dose interruptions, and adjustment of capecitabine dose. Once the dose has been reduced it should not be increased at a later time.

Capecitabine combination therapy with docetaxel –

Capecitabine in Combination with Docetaxel Dose Reduction Schedule

Toxicity NCIC grades[a]	Grade 2	Grade 3	Grade 4
1st appearance	Grade 2 occurring during the 14 days of capecitabine treatment: Interrupt capecitabine treatment until resolved to grade 0 to 1. Treatment may be resumed during the cycle at the same dose of capecitabine. Doses of capecitabine missed during a treatment cycle are not to be replaced. Prophylaxis for toxicities should be implemented where possible. Grade 2 persisting at the time the next capecitabine/docetaxel treatment is due: Delay treatment until resolved to grade 0 to 1, then continue at 100% of the original capecitabine and docetaxel dose. Prophylaxis for toxicities should be implemented where possible.	Grade 3 occurring during the 14 days of capecitabine treatment: Interrupt the capecitabine treatment until resolved to grade 0 to 1. Treatment may be resumed during the cycle at 75% of the capecitabine dose. Doses of capecitabine missed during a treatment cycle are not to be replaced. Prophylaxis for toxicities should be implemented where possible. Grade 3 persisting at the time the next capecitabine/docetaxel treatment is due: Delay treatment until resolved to grade 0 to 1. For patients developing grade 3 toxicity at any time during the treatment cycle, upon resolution to grade 0 to 1, subsequent treatment cycles should be continued at 75% of the original capecitabine dose and at 55 mg/m^2 of docetaxel. Implement prophylaxis for toxicities where possible.	Discontinue treatment unless the treating health care provider considers it to be in the best interest of the patient to continue with capecitabine at 50% of original dose.
2nd appearance of same toxicity	Grade 2 occurring during the 14 days of capecitabine treatment: Interrupt capecitabine treatment until resolved to grade 0 to 1. Treatment may be resumed during the cycle at 75% of original capecitabine dose. Doses of capecitabine missed during a treatment cycle are not to be replaced. Implement prophylaxis for toxicities where possible. Grade 2 persisting at the time the next capecitabine/docetaxel treatment is due: Delay treatment until resolved to grade 0 to 1. For patients developing 2nd occurrence of grade 2 toxicity at any time during the treatment cycle, upon resolution to grade 0 to 1, subsequent treatment cycles should be continued at 75% of the original capecitabine dose and at 55 mg/m^2 of docetaxel. Implement prophylaxis for toxicities where possible.	Grade 3 occurring during the 14 days of capecitabine treatment: Interrupt the capecitabine treatment until resolved to grade 0 to 1. Treatment may be resumed during the cycle at 50% of the capecitabine dose. Doses of capecitabine missed during a treatment cycle are not to be replaced. Implement prophylaxis for toxicities where possible. Grade 3 persisting at the time the next capecitabine/docetaxel treatment is due: Delay treatment until resolved to grade 0 to 1. For patients developing grade 3 toxicity at any time during the treatment cycle, upon resolution to grade 0 to 1, subsequent treatment cycles should be continued at 50% of the original capecitabine dose and the docetaxel discontinued. Implement prophylaxis for toxicities where possible.	Discontinue treatment.
3rd appearance of same toxicity	Grade 2 occurring during the 14 days of capecitabine treatment: Interrupt capecitabine treatment until resolved to grade 0 to 1. Treatment may be resumed during the cycle at 50% of the original capecitabine dose. Doses of capecitabine missed during a treatment cycle are not to be replaced. Prophylaxis for toxicities should be implemented where possible. Grade 2 persisting at the time the next capecitabine/docetaxel treatment is due: Delay treatment until resolved to grade 0 to 1. For patients developing 3rd occurrence of grade 2 toxicity at any time during the treatment cycle, upon resolution to grade 0 to 1, subsequent treatment cycles should be continued at 50% of the original capecitabine dose and the docetaxel discontinued. Implement prophylaxis for toxicities where possible.	Discontinue treatment.	
4th appearance of same toxicity	Discontinue treatment.		

[a] National Cancer Institute of Canada (NCIC) Common Toxicity Criteria were used except for hand-and-foot syndrome.

Capecitabine monotherapy –

Recommended Dose Modifications with Capecitabine Monotherapy

Toxicity NCIC grades[a]	During a course of therapy	Dose adjustment for next treatment (% of starting dose)
Grade 1	Maintain dose level	Maintain dose level
	Grade 2	
1st appearance	Interrupt until resolved to grade 0 to 1	100%
2nd appearance	Interrupt until resolved to grade 0 to 1	75%
3rd appearance	Interrupt until resolved to grade 0 to 1	50%
4th appearance	Discontinue treatment permanently	
	Grade 3	
1st appearance	Interrupt until resolved to grade 0 to 1	75%
2nd appearance	Interrupt until resolved to grade 0 to 1	50%
3rd appearance	Discontinue treatment permanently	

Recommended Dose Modifications with Capecitabine Monotherapy

Toxicity NCIC grades[a]	During a course of therapy	Dose adjustment for next treatment (% of starting dose)
	Grade 4	
1st appearance	Discontinue permanently or if the health care provider deems it to be in the patient's best interest to continue, interrupt until resolved to grade 0 to 1	50%

[a] NCIC Common Toxicity Criteria were used except for the hand-and-foot syndrome.

Dosage modifications are not recommended for grade 1 events. Therapy with capecitabine should be interrupted upon the occurrence of a grade 2 or 3 adverse experience. Once the adverse event has resolved or decreased in intensity to grade 1, then capecitabine therapy may be restarted at full dose or as adjusted according to the previous tables. If a grade 4 experience occurs, therapy should be discontinued or interrupted until resolved or decreased to grade 1, and therapy should be restarted at 50% of the original dose. Doses of capecitabine omitted for toxicity are not replaced or restored; instead the patient should resume the planned treatment cycles.

CAPECITABINE — ORAL

➤*Special populations:*

Renal function impairment – No adjustment to the starting dose of capecitabine is recommended in patients with mild renal impairment (creatinine clearance = 51 to 80 mL/min [Cockroft and Gault]). In patients with moderate renal impairment (baseline creatinine clearance = 30 to 50 mL/min), a dose reduction to 75% of the capecitabine starting dose when used as monotherapy or in combination with docetaxel (from 1,250 mg/m^2 to 950 mg/m^2 twice daily) is recommended. Subsequent dose adjustment is recommended as outlined in the preceding tables if a patient develops a grade 2 to 4 adverse event. The starting dose adjustment recommendations for patients with moderate renal impairment apply both to capecitabine monotherapy and capecitabine in combination use with docetaxel.

➤*Storage/Stability:* Store at 25°C (77°F); excursions permitted to 15° to 30°C (59° to 86°F). Keep tightly closed.

Actions

➤*Pharmacology:* Capecitabine is relatively noncytotoxic in vitro. This drug is enzymatically converted to 5-fluorouracil in vivo.

Both normal and tumor cells metabolize 5-fluorouracil to 5-fluoro-2'-deoxyuridine monophosphate and 5-fluorouridine triphosphate. These metabolites cause cell injury by 2 different mechanisms. First, 5-fluoro-2'-deoxyuridine monophosphate and the folate cofactor, N^{5-10}-methylenetetrahydrofolate, bind to thymidylate synthase to form a covalently bound ternary complex. This binding inhibits the formation of thymidylate from 2'-deoxy-uridylate. Thymidylate is the necessary precursor of thymidine triphosphate, which is essential for the synthesis of deoxyribonucleic acid (DNA), so that a deficiency of this compound can inhibit cell division. Second, nuclear transcriptional enzymes can mistakenly incorporate 5-fluorouridine triphosphate in place of uridine triphosphate during the synthesis of ribonucleic acid (RNA). This metabolic error can interfere with RNA processing and protein synthesis.

➤*Pharmacokinetics:*

Absorption – Capecitabine is readily absorbed from the GI tract. Capecitabine reached peak blood levels in about 1.5 hours (T_{max}) with peak 5-fluorouracil levels occurring slightly later, at 2 hours. Food reduced both the rate and extent of absorption of capecitabine with mean maximum plasma concentration (C_{max}) and area under the curve ($AUC_{0-\infty}$) decreased by 60% and 35%, respectively. The C_{max} and $AUC_{0-\infty}$ of 5-fluorouracil were also reduced by food by 43% and 21%, respectively. Food delayed T_{max} of both parent and 5-fluorouracil by 1.5 hours.

The pharmacokinetics of capecitabine and its metabolites have been evaluated in about 200 cancer patients over a dosage range of 500 to 3,500 mg/m^2/day. Over this range, the pharmacokinetics of capecitabine and its metabolite, 5'-deoxy-5-fluorocytidine were dose proportional and did not change over time. The increases in the AUCs of 5'-deoxy-5-fluorouridine and 5-fluorouracil, however, were greater than proportional to the increase in dose, and the AUC of 5-fluorouracil was 34% higher on day 14 than on day 1.

The interpatient variability in the C_{max} and AUC of 5-fluorouracil was greater than 85%.

Distribution – Plasma protein binding of capecitabine and its metabolites is less than 60% and is not concentration-dependent. Capecitabine was primarily bound to human albumin (approximately 35%).

Metabolism – Capecitabine is extensively metabolized enzymatically to 5-fluorouracil. The enzyme dihydropyrimidine dehydrogenase hydrogenates 5-fluorouracil, the product of capecitabine metabolism, to the much less toxic 5-fluoro-5,6-dihydro-fluorouracil. Dihydropyrimidinase cleaves the pyrimidine ring to yield 5-fluoro-ureido-propionic acid. Finally, beta-ureido-propionase cleaves 5-fluoro-ureido-propionic acid to alpha-fluoro-beta-alanine, which is cleared in the urine.

Excretion – Capecitabine and its metabolites are predominantly excreted in urine; 95.5% of administered capecitabine dose is recovered in urine. Fecal excretion is minimal (2.6%). The major metabolite excreted in urine is alpha-fluoro-beta-alanine, which represents 57% of the administered dose. About 3% of the administered dose is excreted in urine as unchanged drug.

The elimination half-life of both parent capecitabine and 5-fluorouracil was about three fourths of an hour.

Special populations –

Renal function impairment: Following oral administration of 1,250 mg/m^2 capecitabine twice a day to cancer patients with varying degrees of renal impairment, patients with moderate (creatinine clearance = 30 to 50 mL/min) and severe (creatinine clearance less than 30 mL/min) renal impairment showed 85% and 258% higher systemic exposure to alpha-fluoro-beta-alanine on day 1 compared with healthy renal function patients (creatinine clearance greater than 80 mL/min). Systemic exposure to 5'-deoxy-5-fluorouridine was 42% and 71% greater in moderately and severely renal impaired patients, respectively, than in healthy patients. Systemic exposure to capecitabine was about 25% greater in both moderately and severely renal impaired patients. Capecitabine is contraindicated in patients with severe renal impairment (creatinine clearance less than 30 mL/min [Cockroft and Gault]).

Hepatic function impairment: Capecitabine has been evaluated in 13 patients with mild to moderate hepatic dysfunction due to liver metastases defined by a composite score, including bilirubin, AST/ALT, and alkaline phosphatase following a single 1,255 mg/m^2 dose of capecitabine. Both $AUC_{0-\infty}$ and C_{max} of capecitabine increased by 60% in patients with hepatic dysfunction compared with patients with healthy hepatic function (n = 14). The $AUC_{0-\infty}$ and C_{max} of 5-fluorouracil were not affected. In patients with mild to moderate hepatic dysfunction due to liver metastases, exercise caution when capecitabine is administered. The effect of severe hepatic dysfunction on capecitabine is not known.

Contraindications

Capecitabine is contraindicated in patients who have a known hypersensitivity to capecitabine or to any of its components. Capecitabine is contraindicated in patients who have a known hypersensitivity to 5-fluorouracil. Capecitabine is contraindicated in patients with known dihydropyrimidine dehydrogenase (DPD) deficiency. Capecitabine is contraindicated in patients with severe renal impairment (creatinine clearance less than 30 mL/min [Cockroft and Gault]).

Warnings

➤*Coagulopathy:* See Black Box Warning for more information.

➤*Diarrhea:* Capecitabine can induce diarrhea, sometimes severe. Carefully monitor patients with severe diarrhea and give fluid and electrolyte replacement if they become dehydrated. In 875 patients with either metastatic breast or colorectal cancer who received capecitabine monotherapy, the median time to first occurrence of grade 2 to 4 diarrhea was 34 days (range, 1 to 369 days). The median duration of grade 3 to 4 diarrhea was 5 days. NCIC grade 2 diarrhea is defined as an increase of 4 to 6 stools/day or nocturnal stools, grade 3 diarrhea as an increase of 7 to 9 stools/day or incontinence and malabsorption, and grade 4 diarrhea as an increase of greater than or equal to 10 stools/day or grossly bloody diarrhea or the need for parenteral support. If grade 2, 3, or 4 diarrhea occurs, immediately interrupt administration of capecitabine until the diarrhea resolves or decreases in intensity to grade 1. Following a reoccurrence of grade 2 diarrhea or occurrence of any grade 3 or 4 diarrhea, decrease subsequent doses of capecitabine. Standard antidiarrheal treatments (eg, loperamide) are recommended.

Necrotizing enterocolitis (typhlitis) has been reported.

➤*Renal function impairment:* Patients with moderate renal impairment at baseline require dose reduction. Carefully monitor patients with mild and moderate renal impairment at baseline for adverse reactions. Prompt interruption of therapy with subsequent dose adjustments is recommended if a patient develops a grade 2 to 4 adverse reaction. Once the adverse reaction has resolved or decreased in intensity to grade 1, then capecitabine therapy may be restarted at full dose or reduced by 25% for each subsequent appearance of grade 2 toxicity. With the fourth appearance of grade 2 toxicity, discontinue treatment permanently. Interrupt therapy with capecitabine upon the occurrence of a grade 3 adverse experience. Once the adverse reaction has resolved or decreased in intensity to grade 1, then capecitabine therapy may be restarted at 75% of starting dose or reduced by 25% for the second appearance of a grade 3 adverse experience. Discontinue treatment permanently at the third appearance. If a grade 4 experience occurs, discontinue therapy permanently or interrupt until resolved or decreased to grade 1, and then restart at 50% of the original dose if it is in the patient's best interest to continue. Doses of capecitabine omitted for toxicity are not replaced or restored; instead the patient should resume the planned treatment cycles.

➤*Hepatic function impairment:* Carefully monitor patients with mild to moderate hepatic dysfunction due to liver metastases when capecitabine is administered. The effect of severe hepatic dysfunction on the disposition of capecitabine is not known.

➤*Mutagenesis:* Capecitabine was not mutagenic in vitro to bacteria (Ames test) or mammalian cells (Chinese hamster V79/HPRT gene mutation assay). Capecitabine was clastogenic in vitro to human peripheral blood lymphocytes but not clastogenic in vivo to mouse bone marrow (micronucleus test). Fluorouracil causes mutations in bacteria and yeast. Fluorouracil also causes chromosomal abnormalities in the mouse micronucleus test in vivo.

➤*Fertility impairment:* In studies of fertility and general reproductive performance in mice, oral capecitabine dosages of 760 mg/kg/day disturbed estrus and consequently caused a decrease in fertility. In mice who became pregnant, no fetuses survived this dose. The disturbance in estrus was reversible. In males, this dose caused degenerative changes in the testes, including decreases in the number of spermatocytes and spermatids. In separate pharmacokinetic studies, this dose in mice produced 5'-deoxy-5-fluorouridine AUC values about 0.7 times the corresponding values in patients administered the recommended daily dose.

➤*Elderly:* Patients 80 years of age or older may experience a greater incidence of grade 3 or 4 adverse reactions. In 875 patients with either metastatic breast of colorectal cancer who received capecitabine monotherapy, 62% of the 21 patients greater than or equal to 80 years of age treated with capecitabine experienced a treatment-related grade 3 or 4 adverse reaction: Diarrhea in 6 (28.6%), nausea in 3 (14.3%), hand-and-foot syndrome in 3 (14.3%), and vomiting in 2 (9.5%) patients. Among the 10 patients 70 years of age and older (no patients were older than 80 years of age) treated with capecitabine in combination with docetaxel, 30% (3 out of 10) of patients experienced grade 3 or 4 diarrhea and stomatitis, and 40% (4 out of 10) experienced grade 3 hand-and-foot syndrome.

Among the 67 patients 60 years of age and older receiving capecitabine in combination with docetaxel, the incidence of grade 3 or 4 treatment-related adverse reactions, treatment-related serious adverse reactions, withdrawals due to adverse reactions, treatment discontinuations due to adverse reactions, and treatment discontinuations within the first 2 treatment cycles was higher than in the less than 60 years of age patient group.

In 995 patients receiving capecitabine as adjuvant therapy for Duke stage C colon cancer after resection of the primary tumor, 41% of the 398 patients 65 years of age and older treated with capecitabine experienced a treatment-related grade 3 or 4 adverse reaction: hand-and-foot syndrome in 75 (18.8%), diarrhea in 52 (13.1%), stomatitis in 12 (3%), neutropenia/granulocytopenia

CAPECITABINE — ORAL

in 11 (2.8%), vomiting in 6 (1.5%), and nausea in 5 (1.3%) patients. In patients 65 years of age and older (all randomized population; capecitabine 188 patients, 5-fluorouracil/leucovorin 208 patients) treated for Duke stage C colon cancer after resection of the primary tumor, the hazard ratios for disease-free survival and overall survival for capecitabine compared with 5-fluorouracil/leucovorin were 1.01 (95% CI, 0.8 to 1.27) and 1.04 (95% CI, 0.79 to 1.37), respectively.

Pay particular attention to monitoring the adverse effects of capecitabine in the elderly.

➤*Pregnancy: Category D.* Advise women of childbearing potential to avoid becoming pregnant while receiving treatment with capecitabine.

Capecitabine may cause fetal harm when given to a pregnant woman. Capecitabine at dosages of 198 mg/kg/day during organogenesis caused teratogenic malformations and embryo death in mice. In separate pharmacokinetic studies, this dose in mice produced 5′-deoxy-5-fluorouridine AUC values about 0.2 times the corresponding values in patients administered the recommended daily dose. Teratogenic malformations in mice included cleft palate, anophthalmia, microphthalmia, oligodactyly, polydactyly, syndactyly, kinky tail, and dilation of cerebral ventricles. At dosages of 90 mg/kg/day, capecitabine given to pregnant monkeys during organogenesis caused fetal death. This dose produced 5′-deoxy-5-fluorouridine AUC values about 0.6 times the corresponding values in patients administered the recommended daily dose. There are no adequate and well-controlled studies in pregnant women using capecitabine. If the drug is used during pregnancy, or if the patient becomes pregnant while receiving this drug, apprise the patient of the potential hazard to the fetus. Advise women of childbearing potential to avoid becoming pregnant while receiving treatment with capecitabine.

➤*Lactation:* Lactating mice given a single oral dose of capecitabine excreted significant amounts of capecitabine metabolites into the milk. Because of the potential for serious adverse reactions in breast-feeding infants from capecitabine, it is recommended that breast-feeding be discontinued when receiving capecitabine therapy.

➤*Children:* The safety and efficacy of capecitabine in patients younger than 18 years of age have not been established.

Precautions

➤*Monitoring:* A health care provider experienced in the use of cancer chemotherapeutic agents should monitor patients receiving therapy with capecitabine. Most adverse reactions are reversible and do not need to result in discontinuation, although doses may need to be withheld or reduced.

➤*Hand-and-foot syndrome:* Hand-and-foot syndrome (palmar-plantar erythrodysesthesia or chemotherapy-induced acral erythema) is a cutaneous toxicity. Median time to onset was 79 days (range, 11 to 360 days) with a severity range of grades 1 to 3 for patients receiving capecitabine monotherapy in the metastatic setting. Grade 1 is characterized by any of the following: numbness, dysesthesia/paresthesia, tingling, painless swelling or erythema of the hands and/or feet, and/or discomfort that does not disrupt normal activities. Grade 2 hand-and-foot syndrome is defined as painful erythema and swelling of the hands and/or feet, and/or discomfort affecting the patient's activities of daily living. Grade 3 hand-and-foot syndrome is defined as moist desquamation, ulceration, blistering or severe pain of the hands and/or feet, and/or severe discomfort that causes the patient to be unable to work or perform activities of daily living. If grade 2 or 3 hand-and-foot syndrome occurs, interrupt administration of capecitabine until the event resolves or decreases in intensity to grade 1. Following grade 3 hand-and-foot syndrome, decrease subsequent doses of capecitabine.

➤*Cardiotoxicity:* The cardiotoxicity observed with capecitabine includes myocardial infarction/ischemia, angina, dysrhythmias, cardiac arrest, cardiac failure, sudden death, electrocardiographic changes, and cardiomyopathy. These adverse reactions may be more common in patients with a history of coronary artery disease.

➤*DPD:* Rarely, unexpected, severe toxicity (eg, stomatitis, diarrhea, neutropenia and neurotoxicity) associated with 5-fluorouracil has been attributed to a deficiency of DPD activity. A link between decreased levels of DPD and increased, potentially fatal, toxic effects of 5-fluorouracil therefore cannot be excluded.

➤*Hyperbilirubinemia:* In 875 patients with either metastatic breast or colorectal cancer who received at least 1 dose of capecitabine 1,250 mg/m^2 twice daily as monotherapy for 2 weeks followed by a 1-week rest period, grade 3 (1.5 to 3 × ULN) hyperbilirubinemia occurred in 15.2% (n = 133) of patients and grade 4 (greater than 3 × ULN) hyperbilirubinemia occurred in 3.9% (n = 34) of patients. Of 566 patients who had hepatic metastases at baseline and 309 patients without hepatic metastases at baseline, grade 3 or 4 hyperbilirubinemia occurred in 22.8% and 12.3%, respectively. Of the 167 patients with grade 3 or 4 hyperbilirubinemia, 18.6% (n = 31) also had postbaseline elevations (grades 1 to 4, without elevations at baseline) in alkaline phosphatase and 27.5% (n = 46) had postbaseline elevations in transaminases at any time (not necessarily concurrent). The majority of these patients, 64.5% (n = 20) and 71.7% (n = 33), had liver metastases at baseline. In addition, 57.5% (n = 96) and 35.3% (n = 59) of the 167 patients had elevations (grades 1 to 4) at both prebaseline and postbaseline in alkaline phosphatase or transaminases, respectively. Only 7.8% (n = 13) and 3% (n = 5) had grade 3 or 4 elevations in alkaline phosphatase or transaminases.

In the 596 patients treated with capecitabine as first-line therapy for metastatic colorectal cancer, the incidence of grade 3 or 4 hyperbilirubinemia was similar to the overall clinical trial safety database of capecitabine monotherapy. The median time to onset for grade 3 or 4 hyperbilirubinemia in the colorectal cancer population was 64 days and median total bilirubin increased from 8 mcm/L at baseline to 13 mcm/L during treatment with capecitabine. Of the 136 colorectal cancer patients with grade 3 or 4 hyperbilirubinemia, 49 patients had grade 3 or 4 hyperbilirubinemia as their last measured value, of which 46 had liver metastases at baseline.

In 251 patients with metastatic breast cancer who received a combination of capecitabine and docetaxel, grade 3 (1.5 to 3 × ULN) hyperbilirubinemia occurred in 7% (n = 17) and grade 4 (greater than 3 × ULN) hyperbilirubinemia occurred in 2% (n = 5).

If drug-related grade 2 to 4 elevations in bilirubin occur, immediately interrupt administration of capecitabine until the hyperbilirubinemia resolves or decreases in intensity to grade 1. NCIC grade 2 hyperbilirubinemia is defined as 1.5 × normal, grade 3 hyperbilirubinemia as 1.5 to 3 × normal and grade 4 hyperbilirubinemia as greater than 3 × normal.

➤*Hematologic:* In 875 patients with either metastatic breast or colorectal cancer who received a dose of 1,250 mg/m^2 administered twice daily as monotherapy for 2 weeks followed by a 1-week rest period, 3.2%, 1.7%, and 2.4% of patients had grade 3 or 4 neutropenia, thrombocytopenia, or decreases in hemoglobin, respectively. In 251 patients with metastatic breast cancer who received a dose of capecitabine in combination with docetaxel, 68% had grade 3 or 4 neutropenia, 2.8% had grade 3 or 4 thrombocytopenia, and 9.6% had grade 3 or 4 anemia.

Drug Interactions

Capecitabine Drug Interactions

Precipitant drug	Object drug[a]		Description
Antacids	Capecitabine	↑	When 20 mL of an aluminum hydroxide- and magnesium hydroxide–containing antacid was administered immediately after capecitabine, AUC and C_{max} increased by 16% and 35%, respectively, for capecitabine and by 18% and 22%, respectively, for 5′-deoxy-5-fluorocytidine.
Leucovorin	Capecitabine	↑	The concentration of 5-fluorouracil is increased and its toxicity may be enhanced by leucovorin. Deaths from severe enterocolitis, diarrhea, and dehydration have been reported in elderly patients receiving weekly leucovorin and fluorouracil.
Capecitabine	Phenytoin	↑	Carefully monitor phenytoin levels in patients taking capecitabine. The phenytoin dose may need to be reduced. The mechanism of interaction is presumed to be inhibition of the CYP2C9 isoenzyme by capecitabine or its metabolites.
Capecitabine	Warfarin	↑	Altered coagulation parameters and/or bleeding have been reported in patients taking capecitabine concomitantly with warfarin. Monitor patients regularly for PT or INR alterations and adjust anticoagulant dose as necessary.

[a] ↑ = Object drug increased.

➤*Drug/Food interactions:* In all clinical trials, patients were instructed to administer capecitabine within 30 minutes after a meal. Since current safety and efficacy data are based upon administration with food, it is recommended that capecitabine be administered with food. Capecitabine tablets should be swallowed with water within 30 minutes after a meal.

Adverse Reactions

➤*Adjuvant colon cancer:* The following table shows the adverse reactions occurring in at least 5% of patients from one phase 3 trial in patients with Duke stage C colon cancer who received at least 1 dose of study medication and had at least 1 safety assessment. A total of 995 patients were treated with 1,250 mg/m^2 twice a day of capecitabine administered for 2 weeks followed by a 1-week rest period, and 974 patients were administered 5-fluorouracil and leucovorin (20 mg/m^2 leucovorin IV followed by 425 mg/m^2 IV bolus 5-fluorouracil, on days 1 to 5, every 28 days). The median duration of treatment was 164 days for capecitabine-treated patients and 145 days for 5-fluorouracil/leucovorin–treated patients. A total of 112 (11%) and 73 (7%) capecitabine and 5-fluorouracil/leucovorin–treated patients, respectively, discontinued treatment because of adverse reactions. A total of 18 deaths due to all causes occurred either on study or within 28 days of receiving study drug: 8 (0.8%) patients randomized to capecitabine and 10 (1%) randomized to 5-fluorouracil/leucovorin.

The second table that follows shows grade 3/4 laboratory abnormalities occurring in at least 1% of patients from 1 phase 3 trial in patients with Duke stage C colon cancer who received at least 1 dose of study medication and had at least 1 safety assessment.

CAPECITABINE — ORAL

Adverse Reactions in Patients Treated with Capecitabine or 5-Fluorouracil/Leucovorin for Colon Cancer in the Adjuvant Setting (≥ 5%)

	Adjuvant treatment for colon cancer (N = 1,969)			
	Capecitabine (n = 995)		5-Fluorouracil/Leucovorin (n = 974)	
Adverse reaction	All grades	Grade 3/4	All grades	Grade 3/4
CNS				
Asthenia	10%	< 1%	10%	1%
Dizziness	6%	< 1%	6%	—
Fatigue	16%	< 1%	16%	1%
Headache	5%	< 1%	6%	< 1%
Lethargy	10%	< 1%	9%	< 1%
Dermatologic				
Alopecia	6%	—	22%	< 1%
Erythema	6%	1%	5%	< 1%
Hand-and-foot syndrome	60%	17%	9%	< 1%
Rash	7%	—	8%	—
GI				
Abdominal pain	14%	3%	16%	2%
Anorexia	9%	< 1%	11%	< 1%
Constipation	9%	—	11%	< 1%
Diarrhea	47%	12%	65%	14%
Dysgeusia	6%	—	9%	—
Dyspepsia	6%	< 1%	5%	—
Nausea	34%	2%	47%	2%
Stomatitis	22%	2%	60%	14%
Upper abdominal pain	7%	< 1%	7%	< 1%
Vomiting	15%	2%	21%	2%
Hematologic				
Neutropenia	2%	< 1%	8%	5%
Respiratory				
Epistaxis	2%	—	5%	—
Special senses				
Conjunctivitis	5%	< 1%	6%	< 1%
Miscellaneous				
Pyrexia	7%	< 1%	9%	< 1%

Grade 3/4 Laboratory Abnormalities in Patients Receiving Capecitabine Monotherapy for Adjuvant Treatment of Colon Cancer (≥ 1%)

Adverse reaction	Capecitabine (n = 995) Grade 3/4	IV 5-Fluorouracil/ Leucovorin (n = 974) Grade 3/4
Decreased calcium	2.3%	2.2%
Decreased hemoglobin	1%	1.2%
Decreased lymphocytes	13%	13%
Decreased neutrophils[a]	2.2%	26.2%
Decreased neutrophils/granulocytes	2.4%	26.4%
Decreased platelets	1%	0.7%
Increased ALT	1.6%	0.6%
Increased bilirubin[b]	20%	6.3%
Increased calcium	1.1%	0.7%

[a] The incidence of grade 3/4 white blood cells abnormalities was 1.3% in the capecitabine arm and 4.9% in the IV 5-fluorouracil/leucovorin.

[b] It should be noted that grading was according to NCIC CTC Version 1 (May, 1994). In the NCIC-CTC Version 1, hyperbilirubinemia grade 3 indicates a bilirubin value of 1.5 to 3 × ULN range, and grade 4 value of greater than 3 × ULN. The NCI CTC Version 2 and above define a grade 3 bilirubin value of greater than 3 to 10 × ULN, and grade 4 values greater than 10 × ULN.

➤*Metastatic colorectal cancer:* The following table shows the adverse reactions occurring in greater than or equal to 5% of patients from pooling the 2 phase 3 trials in first line metastatic colorectal cancer. A total of 596 patients with metastatic colorectal cancer were treated with 1,250 mg/m^2 twice a day of capecitabine administered for 2 weeks followed by a 1-week rest period, and 593 patients were administered 5-fluorouracil and leucovorin in the Mayo regimen (20 mg/m^2 leucovorin IV followed by 425 mg/m^2 IV bolus 5-fluorouracil, on days 1 to 5, every 28 days). In the pooled colorectal database the median duration of treatment was 139 days for capecitabine-treated patients and 140 days for 5-fluorouracil/leucovorin-treated patients. A total of 78 (13%) and 63 (11%) capecitabine and 5-fluorouracil/leucovorin-treated patients, respectively, discontinued treatment because of adverse reactions/intercurrent illness. A total of 82 deaths due to all causes occurred either on study or within 28 days of receiving study drug: 50 (8.4%) patients randomized to capecitabine and 32 (5.4%) randomized to 5-fluorouracil/leucovorin.

Phase 3 Colorectal Trials with Capecitabine vs 5-Fluorouracil/ Leucovorindence Related or Unrelated to Treatment (≥ 5%)

	Capecitabine (n = 596)			5-Fluorouracil/Leucovorin (n = 593)		
Number of patients with greater than 1 adverse reaction	Total %	Grade 3 %	Grade 4 %	Total %	Grade 3 %	Grade 4 %
	96	52	9	94	45	9
CNS						
Depression	5%	—[a]	—[a]	4%	< 1%	—[a]
Dizziness[c]	8%	< 1%	—[a]	8%	< 1%	—[a]
Fatigue/Weakness	42%	4%	—[a]	46%	4%	—[a]
Headache	10%	1%	—[a]	7%	—[a]	—[a]
Insomnia	7%	—[a]	—[a]	7%	—[a]	—[a]
Mood alteration	5%	—[a]	—[a]	6%	< 1%	—[a]
Peripheral sensory neuropathy	10%	—[a]	—[a]	4%	—[a]	—[a]
Dermatologic						
Alopecia	6%	—[a]	—[a]	21%	< 1%	—[a]
Dermatitis	27%	1%	—[a]	26%	1%	—[a]
Hand-and-foot syndrome	54%	17%	NA[b]	6%	1%	NA
Skin discoloration	7%	< 1%	—[a]	5%	—[a]	—[a]
GI						
Abdominal pain	35%	9%	< 1%	31%	5%	—[a]
Constipation	14%	1%	< 1%	17%	1%	—[a]
Diarrhea	55%	13%	2%	61%	10%	2%
GI hemorrhage	6%	1%	< 1%	3%	1%	—[a]
GI motility disorder	10%	< 1%	—[a]	7%	< 1%	—[a]
Ileus	6%	4%	1%	5%	2%	1%
Nausea	43%	4%	—[a]	51%	3%	< 1%
Oral discomfort	10%	—[a]	—[a]	10%	—[a]	—[a]
Stomatitis	25%	2%	< 1%	62%	14%	1%
Taste disturbance	6%	1%	—[a]	11%	< 1%	1%
Upper GI inflammatory disorders	8%	< 1%	—[a]	10%	1%	—[a]
Vomiting	27%	4%	< 1%	30%	4%	< 1%
Hematologic/Lymphatic						
Anemia	80%	2%	< 1%	79%	1%	< 1%
Neutropenia	13%	1%	2%	46%	8%	13%
Metabolic						
Appetite decreased	26%	3%	< 1%	31%	2%	< 1%
Dehydration	7%	2%	< 1%	8%	3%	1%
Edema	15%	1%	—[a]	9%	1%	—[a]
Musculoskeletal						
Arthralgia	8%	1%	—[a]	6%	1%	—[a]
Back pain	10%	2%	—[a]	9%	< 1%	—[a]
Respiratory						
Cough	7%	< 1%	1%	8%	—[a]	—[a]
Dyspnea	14%	1%	—[a]	10%	< 1%	1%
Epistaxis	3%	< 1%	—[a]	6%	—[a]	—[a]
Pharyngeal disorder	5%	—[a]	—[a]	5%	—[a]	—[a]
Sore throat	2%	—[a]	—[a]	6%	—[a]	—[a]
Special senses						
Eye irritation	13%	—[a]	—[a]	10%	< 1%	—[a]
Vision abnormal	5%	—[a]	—[a]	2%	—[a]	—[a]
Miscellaneous						
Chest pain	6%	1%	—[a]	6%	1%	< 1%
Hyperbilirubinemia	48%	18%	5%	17%	3%	3%
Pain	12%	1%	—[a]	10%	1%	—[a]
Pyrexia	18%	1%	—[a]	21%	2%	—[a]
Venous thrombosis	8%	3%	< 1%	6%	2%	—[a]
Viral infection	5%	< 1%	—[a]	5%	< 1%	—[a]

[a] Not observed.

[b] NA = Not applicable.

[c] Excluding vertigo.

➤*Breast cancer combination:* The following data are shown for the combination study with capecitabine and docetaxel in patients with metastatic breast cancer. In the capecitabine and docetaxel combination arm the treatment was capecitabine administered orally 1,250 mg/m^2 twice daily as intermittent therapy (2 weeks of treatment followed by 1 week without treatment) for at least 6 weeks and docetaxel administered as a 1-hour IV infusion at a dose of 75 mg/m^2 on the first day of each 3-week cycle for at least 6 weeks. In the monotherapy arm, docetaxel was administered as a 1-hour IV infusion at a dose of 100 mg/m^2 on the first day of each 3-week cycle for at least 6 weeks. The mean duration of treatment was 129 days in the combination arm and 98 days in the monotherapy arm. A total of 66 patients (26%) in the combination arm and 49 (19%) in the monotherapy arm withdrew from the study because of adverse reactions. The percentage of patients requiring dose reductions due to adverse reactions were 65% in the combination arm and 36% in the monotherapy arm. The percentage of

CAPECITABINE — ORAL

patients requiring treatment interruptions due to adverse reactions in the combination arm was 79%. Treatment interruptions were part of the dose modification scheme for the combination therapy arm but not for the docetaxel monotherapy-treated patients.

Adverse Reactions Considered Related or Unrelated to Treatment in Capecitabine and Docetaxel Combination vs Docetaxel Monotherapy Study (≥ 5%)

	Capecitabine 1,250 mg/m² twice daily with docetaxel 75 mg/m²/3 weeks (n = 251)			Docetaxel 100 mg/m²/3 weeks (n = 255)		
Adverse reaction	Total %	Grade 3 %	Grade 4 %	Total %	Grade 3 %	Grade 4 %
Number of patients with at least 1 adverse reaction	99	76.5	29.1	97	57.6	31.8
CNS						
Asthenia	26%	4%	< 1%	25%	6%	—[a]
Depression	5%	—[a]	—[a]	5%	1%	—[a]
Dizziness	12%	—[a]	—[a]	8%	< 1%	—[a]
Fatigue	22%	4%	—[a]	27%	6%	—[a]
Headache	15%	3%	—[a]	15%	2%	—[a]
Hypoaesthesia	4%	< 1%	—[a]	8%	< 1%	—[a]
Insomnia	8%	—[a]	—[a]	10%	< 1%	—[a]
Lethargy	7%	—[a]	—[a]	6%	2%	—[a]
Paresthesia	12%	< 1%	—[a]	16%	1%	—[a]
Peripheral neuropathy	6%	—[a]	—[a]	10%	1%	—[a]
Weakness	16%	2%	—[a]	11%	2%	—[a]
Dermatologic						
Alopecia	41%	6%	—[a]	42%	7%	—[a]
Dermatitis	8%	—[a]	—[a]	11%	1%	—[a]
Hand-and-foot syndrome	63%	24%	NA[b]	8%	1%	NA
Nail discoloration	6%	—[a]	—[a]	4%	< 1%	—[a]
Nail disorder	14%	2%	—[a]	15%	—[a]	—[a]
Onycholysis	5%	1%	—[a]	5%	1%	—[a]
Pruritus	4%	—[a]	—[a]	5%	—[a]	—[a]
Rash erythematous	9%	< 1%	—[a]	5%	—[a]	—[a]
GI						
Abdominal pain	30%	< 3%	< 1%	24%	2%	—[a]
Anorexia	13%	1%	—[a]	11%	< 1%	—[a]
Constipation	20%	2%	—[a]	18%	—[a]	—[a]
Diarrhea	67%	14%	< 1%	48%	5%	< 1%
Dry mouth	6%	< 1%	—[a]	5%	—[a]	—[a]
Dyspepsia	14%	—[a]	—[a]	8%	1%	—[a]
Nausea	45%	7%	—[a]	36%	2%	—[a]
Stomatitis	67%	17%	< 1%	43%	5%	—[a]
Taste disturbance	16%	< 1%	—[a]	14%	< 1%	—[a]
Vomiting	35%	4%	1%	24%	2%	—[a]
Infection						
Oral candidiasis	7%	< 1%	—[a]	8%	< 1%	—[a]
Upper respiratory tract	4%	—[a]	—[a]	5%	1%	—[a]
Urinary tract	6%	< 1%	—[a]	4%	—[a]	—[a]
Laboratory test abnormalities						
Anemia	80%	7%	3%	83%	5%	< 1%
Hyperbilirubinemia	20%	7%	2%	6%	2%	2%
Leukopenia	91%	37%	24%	88%	42%	33%
Lymphocytopenia	99%	48%	41%	98%	44%	40%
Neutropenia/ Granulocytopenia	86%	20%	49%	87%	10%	66%
Thrombocytopenia	41%	2%	1%	23%	1%	2%
Metabolic/Nutritional						
Appetite decreased	10%	—[a]	—[a]	5%	—[a]	—[a]
Dehydration	10%	2%	—[a]	7%	< 1%	< 1%
Edema	33%	< 2%	—[a]	34%	< 3%	1%
Weight decreased	7%	—[a]	—[a]	5%	—[a]	—[a]
Musculoskeletal						
Arthralgia	15%	2%	—[a]	24%	3%	—[a]
Back pain	12%	< 1%	—[a]	11%	3%	—[a]
Bone pain	8%	< 1%	—[a]	10%	2%	—[a]
Myalgia	15%	2%	—[a]	25%	2%	—[a]
Respiratory						
Cough	13%	1%	—[a]	22%	< 1%	—[a]
Dyspnea	14%	2%	< 1%	16%	2%	—[a]
Epistaxis	7%	< 1%	—[a]	6%	—[a]	—[a]
Pleural effusion	2%	1%	—[a]	7%	4%	—[a]

Adverse Reactions Considered Related or Unrelated to Treatment in Capecitabine and Docetaxel Combination vs Docetaxel Monotherapy Study (≥ 5%)

	Capecitabine 1,250 mg/m² twice daily with docetaxel 75 mg/m²/3 weeks (n = 251)			Docetaxel 100 mg/m²/3 weeks (n = 255)		
Adverse reaction	Total %	Grade 3 %	Grade 4 %	Total %	Grade 3 %	Grade 4 %
Number of patients with at least 1 adverse reaction	99	76.5	29.1	97	57.6	31.8
Rhinorrhea	5%	—[a]	—[a]	3%	—[a]	—[a]
Sore throat	12%	2%	—[a]	11%	< 1%	—[a]
Special senses						
Conjunctivitis	5%	—[a]	—[a]	4%	—[a]	—[a]
Eye irritation	5%	—[a]	—[a]	1%	—[a]	—[a]
Lacrimation increased	12%	—[a]	—[a]	7%	< 1%	—[a]
Miscellaneous						
Chest pain (noncardiac)	4%	< 1%	—[a]	6%	2%	—[a]
Flushing	5%	—[a]	—[a]	5%	—[a]	—[a]
Influenza-like illness	5%	—[a]	—[a]	5%	—[a]	—[a]
Lymphoedema	3%	< 1%	—[a]	5%	1%	—[a]
Neutropenic fever	16%	3%	13%	21%	5%	16%
Pain	7%	< 1%	—[a]	5%	1%	—[a]
Pain in limb	13%	< 1%	—[a]	13%	2%	—[a]
Pyrexia	28%	2%	—[a]	34%	2%	—[a]

[a] Not observed.
[b] NA = Not applicable.

➤*Breast cancer capecitabine monotherapy:* The following data are shown for the study in stage IV breast cancer patients who received a dose of 1,250 mg/m² administered twice daily for 2 weeks followed by a 1-week rest period. The mean duration of treatment was 114 days. A total of 13 out of 162 patients (8%) discontinued treatment because of adverse reactions/intercurrent illness.

Adverse Reactions Considered Remotely, Possibly, or Probably Related to Capecitabine Treatment in the Single Arm Trial in Stage IV Breast Cancer

	Phase 2 trial in stage IV breast cancer (n = 162)		
Adverse reaction	Total	Grade 3	Grade 4
CNS			
Dizziness	8%	—[a]	—[a]
Fatigue	41%	8%	—[a]
Headache	9%	1%	—[a]
Insomnia	8%	—[a]	—[a]
Paresthesia	21%	1%	—[a]
Dermatologic			
Dermatitis	37%	1%	—[a]
Hand-and-foot syndrome	57%	11%	NA[b]
Nail disorder	7%	—[a]	—[a]
GI			
Abdominal pain	20%	4%	—[a]
Anorexia	23%	3%	—[a]
Constipation	15%	1%	—[a]
Diarrhea	57%	12%	3%
Dyspepsia	8%	—[1]	—[a]
Nausea	53%	4%	—[a]
Stomatitis	24%	7%	—[a]
Vomiting	37%	4%	—[a]
Hematologic			
Anemia	72%	3%	1%
Lymphopenia	94%	44%	15%
Neutropenia	26%	2%	2%
Thrombocytopenia	24%	3%	1%
Metabolic			
Dehydration	7%	4%	1%
Edema	9%	1%	—[a]
Musculoskeletal			
Myalgia	9%	—[a]	—[a]
Miscellaneous			
Eye irritation	15%	—[a]	—[a]
Hyperbilirubinemia	22%	9%	2%
Pain in limb	6%	1%	—[a]

CAPECITABINE — ORAL

Adverse Reactions Considered Remotely, Possibly, or Probably Related to Capecitabine Treatment in the Single Arm Trial in Stage IV Breast Cancer			
	Phase 2 trial in stage IV breast cancer (n = 162)		
Adverse reaction	Total	Grade 3	Grade 4
Pyrexia	12%	1%	—[a]

[a] Not observed.
[b] NA = Not applicable.

➤*Capecitabine and docetaxel in combination:* Shown by body system are the clinically relevant adverse reactions in less than 5% of patients in the overall clinical trial safety database of 251 patients (study details) reported as related to the administration of capecitabine in combination with docetaxel and that were clinically at least remotely relevant. In parentheses is the incidence of grade 3 and 4 occurrences of each adverse reaction.

It is anticipated that the same types of adverse reactions observed in the capecitabine monotherapy studies may be observed in patients treated with the combination of capecitabine plus docetaxel.

Cardiovascular – Hypotension (1.2%), postural hypotension (0.8%), supraventricular tachycardia (0.39%), syncope (1.2%), venous phlebitis and thrombophlebitis (0.39%).

CNS – Ataxia (0.39%), polyneuropathy (0.39%), migraine (0.39%).

GI – Ileus (0.39%), necrotizing enterocolitis (0.39%), esophageal ulcer (0.39%), hemorrhagic diarrhea (0.8%), taste loss (0.8%).

Hematologic/Lymphatic – Agranulocytosis (0.39%), prothrombin decreased (0.39%).

Hepatic – Abnormal liver function tests, hepatic coma, hepatic failure, hepatotoxicity, jaundice (0.39%).

Miscellaneous – Bronchopneumonia (0.39%), hypersensitivity (1.2%), neutropenic sepsis (2.39%), renal failure (0.39%), sepsis (0.39%).

➤*Capecitabine monotherapy metastatic breast and colorectal cancer:* Shown by body system are the clinically relevant adverse reactions in less than 5% of patients in the overall clinical trial safety database of 875 patients (phase 3 colorectal studies [596 patients], phase 2 colorectal study [34 patients], phase 2 breast cancer studies [245 patients]) reported as related to the administration of capecitabine and that were clinically at least remotely relevant. In parentheses is the incidence of grade 3 or 4 occurrences of each adverse reaction.

Cardiovascular – Atrial fibrillation, bradycardia, cerebrovascular accident, extrasystoles, hypertension, myocarditis, tachycardia, ventricular extrasystoles (0.1%), hypotension, pulmonary embolism (0.2%), pericardial effusion.

CNS – Ataxia, insomnia (0.5%), confusion, depression, difficulty walking, dysphasia, encephalopathy, irritability, tremor (0.1%), abnormal coordination, dysarthria, loss of consciousness (0.2%), impaired balance, sedation, vertigo.

Dermatologic – Nail disorder, photosensitivity reaction, sweating increased (0.1%), pruritus, radiation recall syndrome, skin ulceration (0.2%).

GI – Abdominal distension, ascites, dysphagia, gastric ulcer, gastroenteritis, proctalgia, toxic dilation of intestine (0.1%), ileus (0.3%).

Hematologic/Lymphatic – Leukopenia (0.2%), bone marrow depression, coagulation disorder, lymphoedema, pancytopenia (0.1%), idiopathic thrombocytopenia purpura (1%).

Hepatic – Cholestatic hepatitis, hepatic fibrosis, hepatitis (0.1%), abnormal liver function tests.

Metabolic/Nutritional – Cachexia, increased weight (0.4%), hypertriglyceridemia (0.1%), edema, hypokalemia, hypomagnesemia.

Musculoskeletal – Arthritis, bone pain, myalgia (0.1%), muscle weakness.

Respiratory – Cough, epistaxis, hemoptysis, respiratory distress (0.1%), asthma, bronchitis, bronchopneumonia, pneumonia (0.2%), dyspnea.

Miscellaneous – Laryngitis (1%), chest pain, fungal infections (including candidiasis) (0.2%), chest mass, collapse, drug hypersensitivity, fibrosis, hoarseness, hot flushes, influenza-like illness, pain, thirst (0.1%), renal impairment (0.6%), keratoconjunctivitis, sepsis (0.3%), conjunctivitis, hemorrhage.

Postmarketing: Hepatic failure, lacrimal duct stenosis.

Overdosage

➤*Symptoms:* The manifestations of acute overdose would include nausea, vomiting, diarrhea, GI irritation and bleeding, and bone marrow depression.

➤*Treatment:* Medical management of overdose should include customary supportive medical interventions aimed at correcting the presenting clinical manifestations. Although no clinical experience using dialysis as a treatment for capecitabine overdose has been reported, dialysis may be of benefit in reducing circulating concentrations of 5′-deoxy-5-fluorouridine, a low-molecular weight metabolite of the parent compound.

Patient Information

Inform patients and patients' caregivers of the expected adverse effects of capecitabine, particularly nausea, vomiting, diarrhea, and hand-and-foot syndrome, and make them aware that patient specific dose adaptations during therapy are expected and necessary. Encourage patients to recognize the common grade 2 toxicities associated with capecitabine treatment.

➤*Diarrhea:* Instruct patients experiencing grade 2 or greater diarrhea (an increase of 4 to 6 stools/day or nocturnal stools) to stop taking capecitabine immediately. Standard antidiarrheal treatments (eg, loperamide) are recommended.

➤*Nausea:* Instruct patients experiencing grade 2 or greater nausea (food intake significantly decreased but able to eat intermittently) to stop taking capecitabine immediately. Initiation of symptomatic treatment is recommended.

➤*Vomiting:* Instruct patients experiencing grade 2 or greater vomiting (2 to 5 episodes in a 24-hour period) to stop taking capecitabine immediately. Initiation of symptomatic treatment is recommended.

➤*Hand-and-foot syndrome:* Instruct patients experiencing grade 2 or greater hand-and-foot syndrome (painful erythema and swelling of the hands and/or feet and/or discomfort affecting the patients' activities of daily living) to stop taking capecitabine immediately.

➤*Stomatitis:* Instruct patients experiencing grade 2 or greater stomatitis (painful erythema, edema or ulcers of the mouth or tongue, but able to eat) to stop taking capecitabine immediately. Initiation of symptomatic treatment is recommended.

➤*Fever and neutropenia:* Instruct patients who develop a fever of 38°C (100.5°F) or greater or other evidence of potential infection to call their health care provider.

CYTARABINE

Rx	**Cytarabine** (Mayne)	**Injection:** 20 mg/mL	In 5 mL single- and multi-[a] dose vials and preservative free 50 mL flip-top vial (pharmacy bulk package).
Rx	**Tarabine PFS** (Adria)		Preservative free. In 5 mL single vials and 50 mL bulk package vials.
Rx	**Cytarabine** (Various, eg, Bedford, Gensia)	**Powder for Injection:** 100 mg	In vials.
		500 mg	In vials.
		1 g	In vials.
		2 g	In vials.
Rx	**DepoCyt** (Enzon)	**Injection:** 10 mg/ml (liposomal)[b]	Preservative free. In 5 ml vials.

[a] With 0.9% benzyl alcohol.
[b] In Sodium Chloride 0.9% w/v in Water for Injection.

CYTARABINE — INJECTION

WARNING

Conventional cytarabine – Only physicians experienced in cancer chemotherapy should use cytarabine for injection and cytarabine sterile powder for injection.

For induction therapy, patients should be treated in a facility with laboratory and supportive resources sufficient to monitor drug tolerance and protect and maintain a patient compromised by drug toxicity. The main toxic effect of cytarabine for injection is bone marrow suppression with leukopenia, thrombocytopenia, and anemia. Less serious toxicity includes nausea, vomiting, diarrhea and abdominal pain, oral ulceration, and hepatic dysfunction.

The physician must judge possible benefit to the patient against known toxic effects of this drug in considering the advisability of therapy with cytarabine for injection. Before making this judgment or beginning treatment, the physician should be familiar with the following text.

Liposome injection – Intrathecal cytarabine liposome injection should be administered only under the supervision of a qualified physician experienced in the use of intrathecal cancer chemotherapeutic agents. Appropriate management of complications is possible only when adequate diagnostic and treatment facilities are readily available. In all clinical studies, chemical arachnoiditis, a syndrome manifested primarily by nausea, vomiting, headache, and fever was a common adverse event. If left untreated, chemical arachnoiditis may be fatal. The incidence and severity of chemical arachnoiditis can be reduced by coadministration of dexamethasone. Patients receiving intrathecal cytarabine should be treated concurrently with dexamethasone to mitigate the symptoms of chemical arachnoiditis.

Indications

➤*Conventional cytarabine:* Cytarabine solution for injection and cytarabine powder for injection, in combination with other approved anticancer drugs, is indicated for remission induction in acute nonlymphocytic leukemia of adults and pediatric patients. It has also been found useful in the treatment of acute lymphocytic leukemia and the blast phase of chronic myelocytic leukemia. Intrathecal administration of cytarabine injection (preservative-free preparations only) is indicated in the prophylaxis and treatment of meningeal leukemia.

➤*Liposome injection:* For the intrathecal treatment of lymphomatous meningitis. This indication is based on demonstration of increased complete response rate compared to unencapsulated cytarabine. There are no controlled trials that demonstrate a clinical benefit resulting from this treatment, such as improvement in disease-related symptoms, or increased time to disease progression, or increased survival.

➤*Unlabeled uses:* Treatment of Hodgkin disease; bone marrow transplantation.

Administration and Dosage

Cytarabine solution for injection and sterile powder for injection are not active orally. The schedule and method of administration varies with the program of therapy to be used. Cytarabine may be given by IV infusion or injection, SC, or intrathecally (preservative-free preparation only).

Patients can tolerate higher total doses when they receive the drug by rapid IV injection as compared with slow infusion. This phenomenon is related to the drug's rapid inactivation and brief exposure of susceptible normal and neoplastic cells to significant levels after rapid injection. Normal and neoplastic cells seem to respond in somewhat parallel fashion to these different modes of administration and no clear-cut clinical advantage has been demonstrated for either.

➤*Acute nonlymphocytic leukemia:* In the induction therapy of acute nonlymphocytic leukemia, the usual cytarabine dose in combination with other anticancer drugs is 100 mg/m^2/day by continuous IV infusion (days 1 to 7) or 100 mg/m^2 IV every 12 hours (days 1 to 7).

➤*Meningeal leukemia:* Cytarabine injections have been used intrathecally in acute leukemia in doses ranging from 5 mg/m^2 to 75 mg/m^2 of body surface area. The frequency of administration varied from once a day for 4 days to once every 4 days. The most frequently used dose was 30 mg/m^2 every 4 days until cerebrospinal fluid findings were normal, followed by 1 additional treatment. The dosage schedule is usually governed by the type and severity of central nervous system manifestations and the response to previous therapy.

If used intrathecally, do not use a diluent containing benzyl alcohol. Many clinicians reconstitute with autologous spinal fluid or preservative-free 0.9% sodium chloride injection, and use immediately.

Intrathecal use – Cytarabine solution for injection and sterile powder for injection given intrathecally may cause systemic toxicity, and careful monitoring of the hemopoietic system is indicated. Modification of other antileukemic therapy may be necessary. Major toxicity is rare. The most frequently reported reactions after intrathecal administration were nausea, vomiting and fever; these reactions are mild and self-limiting. Paraplegia has been reported. Necrotizing leukoencephalopathy occurred in 5 children; these patients had also been treated with intrathecal methotrexate and hydrocortisone, as well as by central nervous system radiation. Isolated neurotoxicity has been reported. Blindness occurred in 2 patients in remission whose treatment had consisted of combination systemic chemotherapy, prophylactic central nervous system radiation and intrathecal cytarabine.

When cytarabine is administered both intrathecally and IV within a few days, there is an increased risk of spinal cord toxicity; however, in serious life-threatening disease, concurrent use of IV and intrathecal cytarabine is left to the discretion of the treating physician.

Focal leukemic involvement of the CNS may not respond to intrathecal cytarabine and may better be treated with radiotherapy.

➤*Sterile powder for injection:*

Reconstitution – The 100 mg vial may be reconstituted with 5 mL of Bacteriostatic Water for Injection with benzyl alcohol 0.945% w/v added as preservative. The resulting solution contains 20 mg of cytarabine per mL. (Do not use Bacteriostatic Water for Injection with benzyl alcohol 0.945% w/v as a diluent for intrathecal use).

The 500 mg vial may be reconstituted with 10 mL Bacteriostatic Water for Injection with benzyl alcohol 0.945% w/v added as preservative. The resulting solution contains 50 mg of cytarabine per mL. (Do not use Bacteriostatic Water for Injection with benzyl alcohol 0.945% w/v as a diluent for intrathecal use).

The 1 g vial may be reconstituted with 10 mL of Bacteriostatic Water for Injection with benzyl alcohol 0.945% w/v added as preservative. The resulting solution contains 100 mg of cytarabine per mL. (Do not use Bacteriostatic Water for Injection with benzyl alcohol 0.945% w/v as a diluent for intrathecal use).

The 2 g vial may be reconstituted with 20 mL of Bacteriostatic Water for Injection with benzyl alcohol 0.945% w/v added as preservative. The resulting solution contains 100 mg of cytarabine per mL. (Do not use Bacteriostatic Water for Injection with benzyl alcohol 0.945% w/v as a diluent for intrathecal use).

If used intrathecally many clinicians reconstitute with preservative-free 0.9% sodium chloride injection and use immediately.

➤*Liposome injection:*

Preparation of intrathecal cytarabine – Intrathecal cytarabine liposome injection is a cytotoxic anticancer drug and, as with other potentially toxic compounds, caution should be used in handling intrathecal cytarabine. The use of gloves is recommended. If intrathecal cytarabine suspension contacts the skin, wash immediately with soap and water. If it contacts mucous membranes, flush thoroughly with water. Intrathecal cytarabine particles are more dense than the diluent and have a tendency to settle with time. Vials of intrathecal cytarabine should be allowed to warm to room temperature and gently agitated or inverted to re-suspend the particles immediately prior to withdrawal from the vial. Avoid aggressive agitation. No further reconstitution or dilution is required.

Intrathecal cytarabine administration – Intrathecal cytarabine liposome injection should be withdrawn from the vial immediately before administration. Intrathecal cytarabine liposome injection is a single-use vial and does not contain any preservative; intrathecal cytarabine liposome injection should be used within 4 hours of withdrawal from the vial. Unused portions of each vial should be discarded properly. Do not save any unused portions for later administration. Do not mix intrathecal cytarabine with any other medications.

In-line filters must not be used when administering intrathecal cytarabine liposome injection. Intrathecal cytarabine is administered directly into the cerebral spinal fluid (CSF) via an intraventricular reservoir or by direct injection into the lumbar sac. Intrathecal cytarabine should be injected slowly over a period of 1 to 5 minutes. Following drug administration by lumbar puncture, the patient should be instructed to lie flat for 1 hour. Patients should be observed by the physician for immediate toxic reactions.

Patients should be started on dexamethasone 4 mg twice daily either by mouth or IV for 5 days beginning on the day of intrathecal cytarabine injection.

Intrathecal cytarabine liposome injection must only be administered by the intrathecal route.

Further dilution of intrathecal cytarabine liposome injection is not recommended.

Lymphomatous meningitis – For the treatment of lymphomatous meningitis, intrathecal cytarabine liposome formulation 50 mg (1 vial of intrathecal cytarabine) is recommended to be given according to the following schedule:

Induction therapy: Liposomal cytarabine, 50 mg, administered intrathecally (intraventricular or lumbar puncture) every 14 days for 2 doses (weeks 1 and 3).

Consolidation therapy: Liposomal cytarabine, 50 mg, administered intrathecally (intraventricular or lumbar puncture) every 14 days for 3 doses (weeks 5, 7, and 9) followed by 1 additional dose at week 13.

Maintenance: Liposomal cytarabine, 50 mg, administered intrathecally (intraventricular or lumbar puncture) every 28 days for 4 doses (weeks 17, 21, 25, and 29).

If drug-related neurotoxicity develops, the dose should be reduced to 25 mg. If it persists, treatment with intrathecal cytarabine should be discontinued.

➤*Chemical stability of infusion solutions:* Chemical stability studies were performed by ultraviolet assay on cytarabine injection in infusion solutions. These studies showed that when reconstituted cytarabine or cytarabine solution for injection was added to Sterile Water for Injection, 5% Dextrose Injection or Sodium Chloride Injection, 94% to 96% of the cytarabine was present after 192 hours storage at room temperature.

➤*Storage/Stability:*

Solution for injection – Store cytarabine solution for injection at controlled room temperature 15° to 30°C (59° to 86°F). Protect from light. Retain in carton until time of use.

CYTARABINE — INJECTION

Sterile powder for injection – Store at 25°C (77°F); excursions permitted to 15° to 30°C (59° to 86°F).

The pH of the reconstituted cytarabine for injection solutions is about 5. Solutions reconstituted with Bacteriostatic Water for Injection with benzyl alcohol 0.945% w/v may be stored at controlled room temperature, 20° to 25°C (68° to 77°F) for 48 hours. Discard any solutions in which a slight haze develops. Solutions reconstituted without a preservative should be used immediately.

Liposome injection – Refrigerate at 2° to 8°C (36° to 46°F). Protect from freezing and avoid aggressive agitation.

Actions

➤*Pharmacology:* Cytarabine is cytotoxic to a wide variety of proliferating mammalian cells in culture. It exhibits cell phase specificity, primarily killing cells undergoing DNA synthesis (S-phase) and under certain conditions blocking the progression of cells from the G_1 phase to the S-phase. Although the mechanism of action is not completely understood, it appears that cytarabine acts through the inhibition of DNA polymerase. A limited, but significant, incorporation of cytarabine into both DNA and RNA has also been reported. Extensive chromosomal damage, including chromatoid breaks, have been produced by cytarabine and malignant transformation of rodent cells in culture has been reported. Deoxycytidine prevents or delays (but does not reverse) the cytotoxic activity.

Cytarabine is metabolized by deoxycytidine kinase and other nucleotide kinases to the nucleotide triphosphate, an effective inhibitor of DNA polymerase; it is inactivated by a pyrimidine nucleoside deaminase, which converts it to the nontoxic uracil derivative. It appears that the balance of kinase and deaminase levels may be an important factor in determining sensitivity or resistance of the cell to cytarabine.

Cytarabine is capable of obliterating immune responses in man during administration with little or no accompanying toxicity. Suppression of antibody responses to *E. coli*-VI antigen and tetanus toxoid have been demonstrated. This suppression was obtained during both primary and secondary antibody responses.

Cytarabine also suppressed the development of cell-mediated immune responses such as delayed hypersensitivity skin reaction to dinitrochlorobenzene. However, it had no effect on already established delayed hypersensitivity reactions.

Following 5-day courses of intensive therapy with cytarabine solution for injection or sterile powder for injection, the immune response was suppressed, as indicated by the following parameters: Macrophage ingress into skin windows; circulating antibody response following primary antigenic stimulation; lymphocyte blastogenesis with phytohemagglutinin. A few days after termination of therapy there was a rapid return to normal.

Liposome injection –

Mechanism of action: Intrathecal cytarabine liposome injection is a sustained-release formulation of the active ingredient cytarabine designed for direct administration into the CSF. Cytarabine is a cell cycle phase-specific antineoplastic agent, affecting cells only during the S-phase of cell division. Intracellularly, cytarabine is converted into cytarabine-5'-triphosphate (ara-CTP), which is the active metabolite. The mechanism of action is not completely understood, but it appears that ara-CTP acts primarily through inhibition of DNA polymerase. Incorporation into DNA and RNA may also contribute to cytarabine cytotoxicity. Cytarabine is cytotoxic to a wide variety of proliferating mammalian cells in culture.

➤*Pharmacokinetics:*

Absorption/Distribution –

Solution for injection and sterile powder for injection: Cytarabine is rapidly metabolized and is not effective orally; less than 20% of the orally administered dose is absorbed from the GI tract.

Relatively constant plasma levels can be achieved by continuous IV infusion.

After SC or IM administration of cytarabine labeled with tritium, peak plasma levels of radioactivity are achieved about 20 to 60 minutes after injection and are considerably lower than those after IV administration.

Cerebrospinal fluid levels of cytarabine are low in comparison to plasma levels after single IV injection. However, in 1 patient in whom cerebrospinal levels were examined after 2 hours of constant IV infusion, levels approached 40% of the steady state plasma level. With intrathecal administration, levels of cytarabine in the cerebrospinal fluid declined with a first order half-life of about 2 hours. Because cerebrospinal fluid levels of deaminase are low, little conversion to 1-β-D-arabinofuranosyluracil (ara-U) was observed.

Liposome injection: The pharmacokinetics of liposomal cytarabine administered intrathecally to patients at a 50 mg dose every 2 weeks is currently under investigation. However, preliminary analysis of the pharmacokinetic data show that following intrathecal cytarabine administration in patients, in either the lumbar sac or by intraventricular reservoir, peak levels of free cytarabine were observed within 5 hours in both the ventricle and lumbar sac. These peak levels were followed by a biphasic elimination profile with a terminal phase half-life of 100 to 263 hours over a dose range of 12.5 mg to 75 mg. In contrast, intrathecal administration of 30 mg of free cytarabine showed a biphasic CSF concentration profile with a terminal phase half-life of 3.4 hours. Since the transfer rate of cytarabine from the CSF to plasma is slow and the conversion of cytarabine to ara-U in the plasma is fast, systemic exposure to cytarabine was negligible following intrathecal administration of intrathecal cytarabine, 50 mg or 75 mg.

Metabolism/Excretion –

Solution for injection and powder for injection: Following rapid IV injection of cytarabine labeled with tritium, the disappearance from plasma is biphasic. There is an initial distributive phase with a half-life of about 10 minutes, followed by a second elimination phase with a half-life of about 1 to 3 hours. After the distributive phase, more than 80% of plasma radioactivity can be accounted for by the inactive metabolite ara-U. Within 24 hours about 80% of the administered radioactivity can be recovered in the urine, approximately 90% of which is excreted as ara-U.

Liposome injection: The primary route of elimination of intrathecal cytarabine liposome injection is metabolism to the inactive compound ara-U (1-β-D-arabinofuranosyluracil or uracilarabinoside), followed by urinary excretion of ara-U. In contrast to systemically administered cytarabine, which is rapidly metabolized to ara-U, conversion to ara-U in the CSF is negligible after intrathecal administration because of the significantly lower cytidine deaminase activity in the CNS tissues and CSF. The CSF clearance rate of cytarabine is similar to the CSF bulk flow rate of 0.24 mL/min.

Contraindications

Hypersensitivity to cytarabine or any component of the formulation; active meningeal infection (liposomal cytarabine only).

Warnings

➤*Hematologic:* Cytarabine is a potent bone-marrow suppressant. Therapy should be started cautiously in patients with preexisting drug-induced bone marrow suppression. Patients receiving this drug must be under close medical supervision and, during induction therapy, should have leukocyte and platelet counts performed daily. Bone marrow examinations should be performed frequently after blasts have disappeared from the peripheral blood. Facilities should be available for management of complications, possibly fatal, of bone marrow suppression (infection resulting from granulocytopenia and other impaired body defenses, and hemorrhage secondary to thrombocytopenia). One case of anaphylaxis that resulted in acute cardiopulmonary arrest and required resuscitation has been reported. This occurred immediately after the IV administration of cytarabine solution for injection or powder for injection.

➤*Experimental doses:* Severe and at times fatal CNS, GI, and pulmonary toxicity (different from that seen with conventional therapy regimens of cytarabine) has been reported following some experimental dose schedules for cytarabine solution for injection and sterile powder for injection. These reactions include reversible corneal toxicity, and hemorrhagic conjunctivitis, which may be prevented or diminished by prophylaxis with a local corticosteroid eye drop; cerebral and cerebellar dysfunction, including personality changes, somnolence and coma, usually reversible; severe gastrointestinal ulceration, including pneumatosis cystoides intestinalis leading to peritonitis; sepsis and liver abscess; pulmonary edema, liver damage with increased hyperbilirubinemia; bowel necrosis; and necrotizing colitis. Rarely, severe skin rash, leading to desquamation has been reported. Complete alopecia is more commonly seen with experimental high dose therapy than with standard treatment programs using cytarabine solution for injection or powder for injection. If experimental high-dose therapy is used, do not use a preparation or diluent containing benzyl alcohol.

Cases of cardiomyopathy with subsequent death have been reported following experimental high dose therapy with cytarabine in combination with cyclophosphamide when used for bone marrow transplant preparation.

A syndrome of sudden respiratory distress, rapidly progressing to pulmonary edema and radiographically pronounced cardiomegaly has been reported following experimental high dose therapy with cytarabine used for the treatment of relapsed leukemia from 1 institution in 16 of 72 patients. The outcome of this syndrome can be fatal.

➤*Benzyl alcohol:* Benzyl alcohol is contained in the diluent for this product. Benzyl alcohol has been reported to be associated with a fatal "gasping syndrome" in premature infants.

➤*Delayed progressive ascending paralysis:* Two patients with childhood acute myelogenous leukemia who received intrathecal and IV cytarabine solution for injection or sterile powder for injection at conventional doses (in addition to a number of other concomitantly administered drugs) developed delayed progressive ascending paralysis resulting in death in 1 of the 2 patients.

➤*Liposome injection:* See the Warning box for more information.

Death – During the clinical studies, 2 deaths related to intrathecal liposomal cytarabine were reported. One patient died after developing encephalopathy 36 hours after an intraventricular dose of intrathecal cytarabine, 125 mg. This patient was receiving concurrent whole-brain irradiation and had previously received systemic chemotherapy with cyclophosphamide, doxorubicin, and fluorouracil, as well as intraventricular methotrexate. The other patient received intrathecal cytarabine 50 mg by the intraventricular route and developed focal seizures progressing to status epilepticus. This patient died approximately 8 weeks after the last dose of study medication. The death of 1 additional patient was considered "possibly" related to intrathecal cytarabine. He was a 63-year-old with extensive lymphoma involving the nasopharynx, brain, and meninges with multiple neurologic deficits who died of apparent disease progression 4 days after his second dose of intrathecal cytarabine.

Intrathecal use – After intrathecal administration of free cytarabine, the most frequently reported reactions are nausea, vomiting and fever. Intrathecal administration of free cytarabine may cause myelopathy and other neurologic toxicity and can rarely lead to a permanent neurologic deficit. Administration of intrathecal cytarabine in combination with other chemotherapeutic agents or with cranial/spinal irradiation may increase this risk of neurotoxicity.

Blockage to CSF flow may result in increased free cytarabine concentrations in the CSF and an increased risk of neurotoxicity.

CYTARABINE — INJECTION

➤*Hypersensitivity reactions:* One case of anaphylaxis that resulted in acute cardiopulmonary arrest and required resuscitation has been reported. This occurred immediately after the IV administration of cytarabine for injection.

Liposome injection – Anaphylactic reactions following IV administration of free cytarabine have been reported.

➤*Renal/Hepatic function impairment:* The human liver apparently detoxifies a substantial fraction of an administered dose. In particular, patients with renal or hepatic function impairment may have a higher likelihood of CNS toxicity after high-dose cytarabine solution for injection or sterile powder for injection treatment. Use the drug with caution and possibly at reduced dose in patients whose liver or kidney function is poor.

➤*Mutagenesis:*

Solution for injection and sterile powder for injection: Extensive chromosomal damage, including chromatoid breaks, has been produced by cytarabine, and malignant transformation of rodent cells in culture has been reported.

Liposome injection: The active ingredient of intrathecal cytarabine liposome injection, cytarabine, was mutagenic in in vitro tests and was clastogenic in vitro (chromosome aberrations and SCE in human leukocytes) and in vivo (chromosome aberrations and SCE assay in rodent bone marrow, mouse micronucleus assay). Cytarabine caused the transformation of hamster embryo cells and rat H43 cells in vitro. Cytarabine was clastogenic to meiotic cells; a dose-dependent increase in sperm-head abnormalities and chromosomal aberrations occurred in mice given intraperitoneal cytarabine.

➤*Pregnancy:*

Cytarabine solution for injection and sterile powder for injection – Category D. Cytarabine can cause fetal harm when administered to a pregnant woman. Cytarabine causes abnormal cerebellar development in the neonatal hamster and is teratogenic to the rat fetus. There are no adequate and well-controlled studies in pregnant women. Women of childbearing potential should be advised to avoid becoming pregnant.

A review of the literature has shown 32 reported cases where cytarabine solution for injection or sterile powder for injection was given during pregnancy, either alone or in combination with other cytotoxic agents:

Eighteen healthy infants were delivered. Four of these had first trimester exposure. Five infants were premature or of low birth weight. Twelve of the 18 healthy infants were followed up at ages ranging from 6 weeks to 7 years, and showed no abnormalities. One apparently healthy infant died at 90 days of gastroenteritis.

Two cases of congenital abnormalities have been reported, one with upper and lower distal limb defects, and the other with extremity and ear deformities. Both of these cases had first trimester exposure.

There were 7 infants with various problems in the neonatal period, including pancytopenia; transient depression of WBC, hematocrit or platelets; electrolyte abnormalities; transient eosinophilia; and 1 case of increased IgM levels and hyperpyrexia possibly due to sepsis. Six of the 7 infants were also premature. The child with pancytopenia died at 21 days of sepsis.

Therapeutic abortions were done in 5 cases. Four fetuses were grossly healthy, but one had an enlarged spleen and another showed Trisomy C chromosome abnormality in the chorionic tissue.

Because of the potential for abnormalities with cytotoxic therapy, particularly during the first trimester, a patient who is or who may become pregnant while on cytarabine solution for injection or sterile powder for injection should be apprised of the potential risk to the fetus and the advisability of pregnancy continuation. There is a definite, but considerably reduced risk if therapy is initiated during the second or third trimester. Although healthy infants have been delivered to patients treated in all 3 trimesters of pregnancy, follow-up of such infants would be advisable.

➤*Lactation:*

Solution for injection and sterile powder for injection – It is not known whether this drug is excreted in human milk. Because many drugs are excreted in human milk, and because of the potential for serious adverse reactions in nursing infants from cytarabine, a decision should be made whether to discontinue nursing or to discontinue the drug, taking into account the importance of the drug to the mother.

Liposome injection – It is not known whether cytarabine is excreted in human milk following intrathecal cytarabine liposome injection administration. The systemic exposure to free cytarabine following intrathecal treatment with intrathecal cytarabine was negligible. Despite the low apparent risk, because many drugs are excreted in human milk and because of the potential for serious adverse reactions in nursing infants, the use of intrathecal cytarabine is not recommended in nursing women.

➤*Children:*

Solution for injection and sterile powder for injection – Cytarabine solution for injection and sterile powder for injection, in combination with other approved anticancer drugs, is indicated for remission induction in acute nonlymphocytic leukemia of pediatric patients.

Liposome injection – The safety and efficacy of intrathecal cytarabine liposome injection in pediatric patients has not been established.

Precautions

➤*Monitoring:*

Solution for injection and sterile powder for injection – Patients receiving cytarabine must be monitored closely. Frequent platelet and leukocyte counts and bone marrow examinations are mandatory. Consider suspending or modifying therapy when drug-induced marrow depression has resulted in a platelet count under 50,000 or a polymorphonuclear granulocyte count under 1000/mm^3. Counts of formed elements in the peripheral blood may continue to fall after the drug is stopped and reach lowest values after drug-free intervals of 12 to 24 days. When indicated, restart therapy when definite signs of marrow recovery appear (on successive bone marrow studies). Patients whose drug is withheld until "normal" peripheral blood values are attained may escape from control.

Periodic checks of bone marrow, liver and kidney functions should be performed in patients receiving cytarabine.

Like other cytotoxic drugs, cytarabine may induce hyperuricemia secondary to rapid lysis of neoplastic cells. The clinician should monitor the patient's blood uric acid level and be prepared to use such supportive and pharmacologic measures as might be necessary to control this problem.

Liposome injection – Intrathecal cytarabine liposome injection has the potential of producing serious toxicity. All patients receiving intrathecal cytarabine should be treated concurrently with dexamethasone to mitigate the symptoms of chemical arachnoiditis. Toxic effects may be related to a single dose or to cumulative administration. Because toxic effects can occur at any time during therapy (although they are most likely within 5 days of drug administration), patients receiving intrathecal therapy with intrathecal cytarabine liposome injection should be monitored continuously for the development of neurotoxicity. If patients develop neurotoxicity, subsequent doses of intrathecal cytarabine should be reduced, and intrathecal cytarabine should be discontinued if toxicity persists.

Although significant systemic exposure to free cytarabine following intrathecal treatment is not expected, some effect on bone marrow function cannot be excluded. Systemic toxicity due to IV administration of cytarabine consists primarily of bone marrow suppression with leukopenia, thrombocytopenia, and anemia. Accordingly, careful monitoring of the hematopoietic system is advised.

➤*Rapid administration:* When large IV doses are given quickly, patients are frequently nauseated and may vomit for several hours postinjection. This problem tends to be less severe when the drug is infused.

➤*Acute pancreatitis:* Acute pancreatitis has been reported to occur in a patient receiving cytarabine for injection by continuous infusion and in patients being treated with cytarabine for injection who have had prior treatment with L-asparaginase.

➤*Neoplastic meningitis:* Some patients with neoplastic meningitis receiving treatment with intrathecal cytarabine may require concurrent radiation or systemic therapy with other chemotherapeutic agents; this may increase the rate of adverse events.

➤*CSF elevations:* Transient elevations in CSF protein and white blood cells have been observed in patients following intrathecal cytarabine administration and have also been noted after intrathecal treatment with methotrexate or cytarabine.

Drug Interactions

Cytarabine Drug Interactions

Precipitant drug	Object drug[a]		Description
Cytarabine	Digoxin	⬇	Combination chemotherapy (including cytarabine) may decrease digoxin absorption even several days after stopping chemotherapy. Digoxin capsules and digitoxin do not appear to be affected.
Cytarabine	Gentamicin	⬇	An in vitro interaction between gentamicin and cytarabine showed a cytarabine-related antagonism for the susceptibility of K. pneumoniae strains. This study suggests that in patients on cytarabine being treated with gentamicin for a K. pneumoniae infection, the lack of a prompt therapeutic response may indicate the need for reevaluation of antibacterial therapy.

[a] ⬇ = Object drug decreased.

➤*Digoxin:* Reversible decreases in steady-state plasma digoxin concentrations and renal glycoside excretion were observed in patients receiving beta-acetyldigoxin and chemotherapy regimens containing cyclophosphamide, vincristine and prednisone with or without cytarabine solution for injection or sterile powder for injection or procarbazine. Steady-state plasma digitoxin concentrations did not appear to change. Therefore, monitoring of plasma digoxin levels may be indicated in patients receiving similar combination chemotherapy regimens. The utilization of digitoxin for such patients may be considered as an alternative.

➤*Gentamicin:* An in vitro interaction study between gentamicin and cytarabine showed a cytarabine-related antagonism for the susceptibility of *K. pneumoniae* strains. This study suggests that in patients on cytarabine being treated with gentamicin for a *K. pneumoniae* infection, the lack of a prompt therapeutic response may indicate the need for reevaluation of antibacterial therapy.

CYTARABINE — INJECTION

➤*Fluorocytosine:* Clinical evidence in 1 patient showed possible inhibition of fluorocytosine efficacy during therapy with cytarabine solution for injection or sterile powder for injection. This may be due to potential competitive inhibition of its uptake.

➤*Drug/Lab test interactions:*

Liposome injection – See Precautions for more information.

Adverse Reactions

➤*Conventional cytarabine:*

Hematologic – Because cytarabine is a bone-marrow suppressant, anemia, leukopenia, thrombocytopenia, megaloblastosis and reduced reticulocytes can be expected as a result of administration with cytarabine. The severity of these reactions are dose and schedule dependent. Cellular changes in the morphology of bone marrow and peripheral smears can be expected. Following 5-day constant infusions or acute injections of 50 mg/m^2 to 600 mg/m^2, white cell depression follows a biphasic course. Regardless of initial count, dosage level, or schedule, there is an initial fall starting the first 24 hours with a nadir at days 7 to 9. This is followed by a brief rise which peaks around the twelfth day. A second and deeper fall reaches nadir at days 15 to 24. Then there is rapid rise to above baseline in the next 10 days. Platelet depression is noticeable at 5 days with a peak depression occurring between days 12 to 15. Thereupon, a rapid rise to above baseline occurs in the next 10 days.

Infection (solution for injection and sterile powder for injection) – Viral, bacterial, fungal, parasitic, or saprophytic infections, in any location in the body may be associated with the use of cytarabine for injection or sterile powder for injection alone or in combination with other immunosuppressive agents following immunosuppressant doses that affect cellular or humoral immunity. These infections may be mild, but can be severe and at times fatal.

Cytarabine (Ara-C) syndrome – A cytarabine syndrome has been described. It is characterized by fever, myalgia, bone pain, occasionally chest pain, maculopapular rash, conjunctivitis and malaise. It usually occurs 6 to 12 hours following drug administration. Corticosteroids have been shown to be beneficial in treating or preventing this syndrome. If the symptoms of the syndrome are deemed treatable, corticosteroids should be contemplated as well as continuation of therapy with cytarabine solution for injection or sterile powder for injection.

Most frequent adverse reactions – Anorexia; oral and anal inflammation or ulceration; rash; nausea; thrombophlebitis; vomiting; hepatic dysfunction; bleeding (all sites); diarrhea; fever. Nausea and vomiting are most frequent following rapid IV injection.

Less frequent adverse reactions – Sepsis; esophageal ulceration; conjunctivitis (may occur with rash); esophagitis; pneumonia; dizziness; cellulitis at injection site; chest pain; alopecia; skin ulceration; pericarditis; anaphylaxis (see Warnings); urinary retention; bowel necrosis; allergic edema; renal dysfunction; abdominal pain; pruritus; neuritis; pancreatitis; shortness of breath; neural toxicity; freckling; urticaria; sore throat; jaundice; headache.

➤*Experimental doses:*

Miscellaneous – See Warnings for more information.

Two patients with adult acute nonlymphocytic leukemia developed peripheral motor and sensory neuropathies after consolidation with high-dose cytarabine solution for injection or sterile powder for injection, daunorubicin, and asparaginase. Patients treated with high-dose cytarabine solution for injection or sterile powder for injection should be observed for neuropathy since dose schedule alterations may be needed to avoid irreversible neurologic disorders.

Ten patients treated with experimental intermediate doses of cytarabine solution for injection or sterile powder for injection (1 g/m^2) with and without other chemotherapeutic agents (meta-AMSA, daunorubicin, etoposide) at various dose regimens developed a diffuse interstitial pneumonitis without clear cause that may have been related to the cytarabine.

Two cases of pancreatitis have been reported following experimental doses of cytarabine and numerous other drugs. Cytarabine could have been the causative agent.

➤*Liposome injection:* Arachnoiditis is an expected and well-documented side effect of both neoplastic meningitis and of intrathecal chemotherapy. For clinical studies of intrathecal cytarabine, chemical arachnoiditis was defined as the occurrence of any one of the symptoms of neck rigidity, neck pain, meningism, or any 2 of the symptoms of nausea, vomiting, headache, fever, back pain, or CSF pleocytosis; the grade assigned to an episode of chemical arachnoiditis was the highest severity grade of its component symptoms. Since most of the adverse events reported in the trials were transient episodes associated with drug exposure, the incidence of these events is best expressed by drug cycle. A cycle of treatment for all treatment groups was defined as the 14-day period between intrathecal cytarabine doses. The duration of reported symptoms was from 1 to 5 days. Although it was sometimes difficult to distinguish between drug-related chemical arachnoiditis, infectious meningitis, or disease progression, greater than 90% of the chemical arachnoiditis cases reported occurred within 48 hours of the administration of intrathecal drug, indicating a drug etiology.

In the early study, chemical arachnoiditis was observed in 100% of cycles without dexamethasone prophylaxis; with concurrent administration of dexamethasone, chemical arachnoiditis was observed in 33% of cycles. Patients receiving intrathecal liposome injection should be treated concurrently with dexamethasone to mitigate the symptoms of chemical arachnoiditis.

Comparison of adverse events occurring in greater than or equal to 10% of patients, by cycle –

Patients with Lymphomatous Meningitis Receiving Intrathecal Cytarabine Liposome Injection or Cytarabine (Ara-C) in the Randomized Study

	All adverse reactions %		Grade 3 or 4 adverse reactions %	
Body system/ adverse reaction	Intrathecal cytarabine liposome injection (n = 74)	Cytarabine (n = 45)	Intrathecal cytarabine liposome injection (n = 74)	Cytarabine (n = 45)
CNS	45%	53%	18%	18%
Confusion	14%	7%	4%	2%
Somnolence	12%	11%	4%	2%
Abnormal gait	4%	11%	1%	2%
GI	27%	44%	7%	9%
Nausea*	11%	16%	0%	4%
Vomiting*	12%	18%	3%	2%
Constipation	7%	11%	0%	0%
Hematologic	19%	22%	11%	13%
Neutropenia	9%	11%	8%	11%
Thrombocytopenia	8%	16%	5%	11%
Anemia	1%	13%	1%	4%
Metabolic/nutritional	16%	24%	0%	0%
Peripheral edema	7%	11%	0%	0%
GU	11%	20%	3%	2%
Urinary incontinence	3%	11%	0%	0%
Special senses	16%	18%	1%	2%
Miscellaneous	53%	60%	18%	22%
Headache	28%	9%	5%	2%
Asthenia	19%	33%	5%	9%
Fever*	11%	24%	4%	0%
Back pain*	7%	11%	0%	2%
Pain	11%	20%	3%	0%

* Components of chemical arachnoiditis.

Overdosage

➤*Conventional cytarabine:* There is no antidote for overdosage of cytarabine solution for injection or sterile powder for injection. Doses of 4.5 g/m^2 by IV infusion over 1 hour every 12 hours for 12 doses has caused an unacceptable increase in irreversible CNS toxicity and death. Single doses as high as 3 g/m^2 have been administered by rapid IV infusion without apparent toxicity.

➤*Liposome injection:* No overdosages with intrathecal cytarabine have been reported. An overdose with intrathecal cytarabine may be associated with severe chemical arachnoiditis including encephalopathy.

In an early uncontrolled study without dexamethasone prophylaxis, single doses up to 125 mg were administered. One patient at the 125 mg dose level died of encephalopathy 36 hours after receiving an intraventricular dose of intrathecal cytarabine. This patient, however, was also receiving concomitant whole brain irradiation and had previously received intraventricular methotrexate.

There is no antidote for overdose of intrathecal cytarabine or unencapsulated cytarabine released from intrathecal cytarabine. Exchange of CSF with isotonic saline has been carried out in a case of intrathecal overdose of free cytarabine, and such a procedure may be considered in the case of intrathecal cytarabine overdose. Management of overdose should be directed at maintaining vital functions.

Patient Information

Patients should be informed about the expected adverse events of headache, nausea, vomiting, and fever, and about the early signs and symptoms of neurotoxicity. The importance of concurrent dexamethasone administration should be emphasized at the initiation of each cycle of intrathecal cytarabine treatment. Patients should be instructed to seek medical attention if signs or symptoms of neurotoxicity develop, or if oral dexamethasone is not well tolerated.

FLUOROURACIL (5-Fluorouracil; 5-FU)

Rx	**Fluorouracil** (Various, eg, American Pharmaceutical Partners)	**Injection:** 50 mg/ml	In 10, 20, and 100 ml vials and 10 ml amps.
Rx	**Adrucil** (Gensia Sicor)		In 10, 50, and 100 ml vials.

FLUOROURACIL — INJECTION

WARNING

It is recommended that fluorouracil injection be given only by or under the supervision of a qualified physician who is experienced in cancer chemotherapy and who is well versed in the use of potent antimetabolites. Because of the possibility of severe toxic reactions, it is recommended that patients be hospitalized at least during the initial course of therapy.

These instructions should be thoroughly reviewed before administration of fluorouracil.

Indications

➤*Cancer:* For the palliative management of carcinoma of the colon, rectum, breast, stomach, and pancreas.

➤*Unlabeled uses:* Treatment of ovarian, cervical, bladder, hepatic, prostate, endometrial, esophageal, and head and neck carcinoma.

Administration and Dosage

➤*General instructions:* Fluorouracil injection should be administered only intravenously, using care to avoid extravasation. No dilution is required.

All dosages are based on the patient's actual weight. However, the estimated lean body mass (dry weight) is used if the patient is obese or if there has been a spurious weight gain due to edema, ascites, or other forms of abnormal fluid retention.

It is recommended that prior to treatment each patient be carefully evaluated in order to estimate as accurately as possible the optimum initial dosage of fluorouracil.

➤*Initial dosage:* 12 mg/kg is given intravenously once daily for 4 successive days. The daily dose should not exceed 800 mg. If no toxicity is observed, 6 mg/kg are given on the sixth, eight, tenth, and twelfth days unless toxicity occurs. No therapy is given on the fifth, seventh, ninth, and eleventh days. Therapy is to be discontinued at the end of the twelfth day, even if no toxicity has become apparent.

Rarely, unexpected, severe toxicity (eg, stomatitis, diarrhea, neutropenia, neurotoxicity) associated with 5-fluorouracil has been attributed to deficiency of dipyrimidine dehydrogenase activity. A few patients have been rechallenged with 5-fluorouracil and despite 5-fluorouracil dose lowering, toxicity recurred and progressed with worse morbidity. Absence of this catabolic enzyme appears to result in prolonged clearance of 5-fluorouracil. Poor risk patients or those who are not in an adequate nutritional state should receive 6 mg/kg/day for 3 days. If no toxicity is observed, 3 mg/kg may be given on the fifth, seventh, and ninth days unless toxicity occurs. No therapy is given on the fourth, sixth, or eighth days. The daily dose should not exceed 400 mg.

A sequence of injections on either schedule constitutes a "course of therapy".

➤*Maintenance therapy:* In instances where toxicity has not been a problem, it is recommended that therapy be continued using either of the following schedules:

1.) Repeat dosage of first course every 30 days after the last day of the previous course of treatment.
2.) When toxic signs resulting from the initial course of therapy have subsided, administer a maintenance dosage of 10 to 15 mg/kg/week as a single dose. Do not exceed 1 g/week.

The patient's reaction to the previous course of therapy should be taken into account in determining the amount of the drug to be used, and the dosage should be adjusted accordingly. Some patients have received from 9 to 45 courses of treatment during periods which ranged from 12 to 60 months.

➤*Pharmacy bulk package:* Not for direct infusion.

Although the fluorouracil solution may discolor slightly during storage, the potency and safety are not adversely affected.

The 100 mL pharmacy bulk package is for use in the pharmacy admixture service only. It should be inserted into a ring sling (plastic hanging device) and suspended as a unit in the vertical laminar flow hood. Use only if clear and seal is intact and undamaged.

Only a single entry through the vial closure should be made. Swab vial stopper with an antiseptic solution. Insert a sterile dispensing set or transfer device into the vial which allows measured distribution of the contents. After piercing the stopper, promptly dispense contents of the pharmacy bulk package through the sterile transfer device or dispensing set. If dispensing cannot be performed promptly, discard contents no later than 4 hours after initial entry.

The above process should be carried out under a laminar flow hood using aseptic technique. Care should be exercised to protect personnel from aerosolized drug.

➤*Storage / Stability:* Store at 15° to 30°C (59° to 86°F). Do not freeze. Protect from light. Retain in carton until time of use. Discard any unused portion.

Actions

➤*Pharmacology:* There is evidence that the metabolism of fluorouracil in the anabolic pathway blocks the methylation reaction of deoxyuridylic acid to thymidylic acid. In this manner fluorouracil interferes with the synthesis of deoxyribonucleic acid (DNA) and to a lesser extent inhibits the formation of ribonucleic acid (RNA). Since DNA and RNA are essential for cell division and growth, the effect of fluorouracil may be to create a thymine deficiency which provokes unbalanced growth and death of the cell. The effects of DNA and RNA deprivation are most marked in those cells which grow more rapidly and which take up fluorouracil at a more rapid rate.

➤*Pharmacokinetics:*

Absorption / Distribution – Following IV injection, fluorouracil distributes into tumors, intestinal mucosa, bone marrow, liver and other tissues throughout the body. In spite of its limited lipid solubility, fluorouracil diffuses readily across the blood-brain barrier and distributes into cerebrospinal fluid and brain tissue.

Metabolism – The catabolic metabolism of fluorouracil results in degradation products (eg, CO_2 urea and α-fluoro-β-alanine) which are inactive.

Excretion – 7% to 20% of the parent drug is excreted unchanged in the urine in 6 hours; of this over 90% is excreted in the first hour. The remaining percentage of the administered dose is metabolized, primarily in the liver. The inactive metabolites are excreted in the urine over the next 3 to 4 hours. When fluorouracil is labeled in the 6 carbon position, thus preventing the ^{14}C metabolism to CO_2, approximately 90% of the total radioactivity is excreted in the urine. When fluorouracil is labeled in the 2 carbon position approximately 90% of the total radioactivity is excreted in expired CO_2. Ninety percent (90%) of the dose is accounted for during the first 24 hours following IV administration.

Following IV administration of fluorouracil, the mean half-life of elimination from plasma is approximately 16 minutes, with a range of 8 to 20 minutes, and is dose dependent. No intact drug can be detected in the plasma 3 hours after an IV injection.

Contraindications

Poor nutritional state; depressed bone marrow function; potentially serious infections; hypersensitivity to fluorouracil.

Warnings

➤*Special risk patients:* Use with extreme caution in poor risk patients with a history of high-dose pelvic irradiation or previous use of alkylating agents, those who have a widespread involvement of bone marrow by metastatic tumors or those with impaired hepatic or renal function.

➤*Toxic reactions:* Rarely, unexpected, severe toxicity (eg, stomatitis, diarrhea, neutropenia, neurotoxicity) associated with 5-fluorouracil has been attributed to deficiency of dipyrimidine dehydrogenase activity. A few patients have been rechallenged with 5-fluorouracil and despite 5-fluorouracil dose lowering, toxicity recurred and progressed with worse morbidity. Absence of this catabolic enzyme appears to result in prolonged clearance of 5-fluorouracil.

➤*Combination therapy:* Any form of therapy which adds to the stress of the patient, interferes with nutrition or depresses bone marrow function will increase the toxicity of fluorouracil.

➤*Mutagenesis:* Oncogenic transformation of fibroblasts from mouse embryo has been induced in vitro by fluorouracil, but the relationship between oncogenicity and mutagenicity is not clear. Fluorouracil has been shown to be mutagenic to several strains of *Salmonella typhimurium*, including TA 1535, TA 1537, and TA 1538, and to *Saccharomyces cerevisiae*, although no evidence of mutagenicity was found with *Salmonella typhimurium* strains TA 92, TA 98, and TA 100. In addition, a positive effect was observed in the micronucleus test on bone marrow cells of the mouse, and fluorouracil at very high concentrations produced chromosomal breaks in hamster fibroblasts in vitro.

➤*Fertility impairment:* Fluorouracil has not been adequately studied in animals to permit an evaluation of its effects on fertility and general reproductive performance. However, doses of 125 or 250 mg/kg administered intraperitoneally have been shown to induce chromosomal aberrations and changes in chromosomal organization of spermatogonia in rats. Spermatogonial differentiation was also inhibited by fluorouracil, resulting in transient infertility. However, in studies with a strain of mouse which is sensitive to the induction of sperm head abnormalities after exposure to a range of chemical mutagens and carcinogens, fluorouracil did not produce any abnormalities at oral doses of up to 80 mg/kg/day. In female rats, fluorouracil, administered intraperitoneally at weekly doses of 25 or 50 mg/kg for 3 weeks during the pre-ovulatory phase of oogenesis, significantly reduced the incidence of fertile matings, delayed the development of pre- and postimplantation embryos, increased the incidence of pre-implantation lethality and induced chromosomal anomalies in these embryos. In a limited study in rabbits, a single 25 mg/kg dose of fluorouracil or 5 daily doses of 5 mg/kg had no effect on ovulation, appeared not to affect implantation and had only a limited effect in producing zygote destruction. Compounds such as fluorouracil, which interfere with DNA, RNA and protein synthesis, might be expected to have adverse effects on gametogenesis.

FLUOROURACIL — INJECTION

➤*Pregnancy:* Category D.

Teratogenic – Fluorouracil may cause fetal harm when administered to a pregnant woman. Fluorouracil has been shown to be teratogenic in laboratory animals. Fluorouracil exhibited maximum teratogenicity when given to mice as single intraperitoneal injections of 10 to 40 mg/kg on day 10 or 12 of gestation. Similarly, intraperitoneal doses of 12 to 37 mg/kg given to rats between days 9 and 12 of gestation and IM doses of 3 to 9 mg given to hamsters between days 8 and 11 of gestation were teratogenic. Malformations included cleft palates, skeletal defects, and deformed appendages, paws, and tails. The dosages which were teratogenic in animals are 1 to 3 times the maximum recommended human therapeutic dose. In monkeys, divided doses of 40 mg/kg given between days 20 and 24 of gestation were not teratogenic.

There are no adequate and well-controlled studies with fluorouracil in pregnant women. While there is no evidence of teratogenicity in humans due to fluorouracil, it should be kept in mind that other drugs which inhibit DNA synthesis (eg, methotrexate, aminopterin) have been reported to be teratogenic in humans. Women of childbearing potential should be advised to avoid becoming pregnant. If the drug is used during pregnancy, or if the patient becomes pregnant while taking the drug, the patient should be told of the potential hazard to the fetus. Fluorouracil should be used during pregnancy only if the potential benefit justifies the potential risk to the fetus.

Nonteratogenic – Fluorouracil has not been studied in animals for its effects on peri- and postnatal development. However, fluorouracil has been shown to cross the placenta and enter into fetal circulation in the rat. Administration of fluorouracil has resulted in increased resorption and embryolethality in rats. In monkeys, maternal doses higher than 40 mg/kg resulted in abortion of all embryos exposed to fluorouracil. Compounds which inhibit DNA, RNA and protein synthesis might be expected to have adverse effects on peri- and postnatal development.

➤*Lactation:* It is not known whether fluorouracil is excreted in human milk. Because fluorouracil inhibits DNA, RNA and protein synthesis, mothers should not nurse while receiving this drug.

➤*Children:* Safety and efficacy in pediatric patients have not been established.

Precautions

➤*Monitoring:* White blood counts with differential are recommended before each dose.

➤*Severe toxicity:* Fluorouracil is a highly toxic drug with a narrow margin of safety. Therefore, patients should be carefully supervised, since therapeutic response is unlikely to occur without some evidence of toxicity. Severe hematological toxicity, gastrointestinal hemorrhage and even death may result from the use of fluorouracil despite meticulous selection of patients and careful adjustment of dosage. Although severe toxicity is more likely in poor risk patients, fatalities may be encountered occasionally even in patients in relatively good condition.

➤*Discontinuation:* Therapy is to be discontinued promptly whenever 1 of the following signs of toxicity appears:

- Stomatitis or esophagopharyngitis, at the first visible sign.
- Leukopenia (WBC less than 3500), or a rapidly falling white blood count.
- Vomiting, intractable.
- Diarrhea, frequent bowel movements or watery stools.
- Gastrointestinal ulceration and bleeding.
- Thrombocytopenia, (platelets less than 100,000).
- Hemorrhage from any site.

➤*Hand/Foot syndrome:* The administration of 5-fluorouracil has been associated with the occurrence of palmar-plantar erythrodysesthesia syndrome, also known as hand-foot syndrome. This syndrome has been characterized as a tingling sensation of hands and feet which may progress over the next few days to pain when holding objects or walking. The palms and soles become symmetrically swollen and erythematous with tenderness of the distal phalanges, possibly accompanied by desquamation. Interruption of therapy is followed by gradual resolution over 5 to 7 days. Although pyridoxine has been reported to ameliorate the palmar-plantar erythrodysesthesia syndrome, its safety and effectiveness have not been established.

Drug Interactions

➤*Leucovorin calcium:* Leucovorin calcium may enhance the toxicity of fluorouracil.

Adverse Reactions

➤*GI:* Stomatitis and esophagopharyngitis (which may lead to sloughing and ulceration), diarrhea, anorexia, nausea, and emesis are commonly seen during therapy.

➤*Hematologic:* Leukopenia usually follows every course of adequate therapy with fluorouracil. The lowest white blood cell counts are commonly observed between the ninth and fourteenth days after the first course of treatment, although uncommonly the maximal depression may be delayed for as long as 20 days. By the thirtieth day the count has usually returned to the normal range.

➤*Dermatologic:* Alopecia and dermatitis may be seen in a substantial number of cases. The dermatitis most often seen is a pruritic maculopapular rash usually appearing on the extremities and less frequently on the trunk. It is generally reversible and usually responsive to symptomatic treatment.

➤*Other adverse reactions:*

Allergic – Anaphylaxis and generalized allergic reactions.

Cardiovascular – Myocardial ischemia, angina.

CNS – Acute cerebellar syndrome (which may persist following discontinuance of treatment), nystagmus, headache.

Dermatologic – Dry skin, fissuring, photosensitivity, as manifested by erythema or increased pigmentation of the skin; vein pigmentation; palmar-plantar erythrodysesthesia syndrome, as manifested by tingling of the hands and feet following by pain, erythema, and swelling.

GI – Gastrointestinal ulceration and bleeding.

Hematologic – Pancytopenia, thrombocytopenia, agranulocytosis, anemia.

Ophthalmic – Lacrimal duct stenosis, visual changes, lacrimation, photophobia.

Psychiatric – Disorientation, confusion, euphoria.

Miscellaneous – Thrombophlebitis, epistaxis, nail changes (including loss of nails).

Overdosage

The possibility of overdosage with fluorouracil is unlikely in view of the mode of administration. Nevertheless, the anticipated manifestations would be nausea, vomiting, diarrhea, gastrointestinal ulceration and bleeding, bone marrow depression (including thrombocytopenia, leukopenia and agranulocytosis). No specific antidotal therapy exists. Patients who have been exposed to an overdose of fluorouracil should be monitored hematologically for at least 4 weeks. Should abnormalities appear, appropriate therapy should be utilized.

Patient Information

Patients should be informed of expected toxic effects, particularly oral manifestations. Patients should be alerted to the possibility of alopecia as a result of therapy and should be informed that it is usually a transient effect.

FLOXURIDINE

Rx	**Floxuridine** (Bedford)	**Powder for Injection, lyophilized:** 500 mg	In 5 ml vials.
Rx	**FUDR** (Roche)		In 5 ml vials.

FLOXURIDINE — INJECTION

WARNING

It is recommended that floxuridine be given only by or under the supervision of a qualified physician who is experienced in cancer chemotherapy and intraarterial drug therapy and is well versed in the use of potent antimetabolites.

Because of the possibility of severe toxic reactions, all patients should be hospitalized for initiation of the first course of therapy.

Indications

➤*GI adenocarcinoma metastatic to the liver:* For the palliative management of gastrointestinal adenocarcinoma metastatic to the liver, when given by continuous regional intra-arterial infusion in carefully selected patients who are considered incurable by surgery or other means. Patients with known disease extending beyond an area capable of infusion via a single artery should, except in unusual circumstances, be considered for systemic therapy with other chemotherapeutic agents.

➤*Unlabeled uses:* Treatment of tumors of the liver, ovaries, or kidneys.

Administration and Dosage

➤*Reconstitution:* Each vial must be reconstituted with 5 mL of sterile water for injection to yield a solution containing ≈ 100 mg of floxuridine/mL. The calculated daily dose(s) of the drug is then diluted with 5% dextrose or 0.9% sodium chloride injection to a volume appropriate for the infusion apparatus to be used. The administration of floxuridine is best achieved with the use of an appropriate pump to overcome pressure in large arteries and to ensure a uniform rate of infusion.

➤*Dosage:* The recommended therapeutic dosage schedule of floxuridine by continuous arterial infusion is 0.1 to 0.6 mg/kg/day. The higher dosage ranges (0.4 mg to 0.6 mg) are usually employed for hepatic artery infusion because the liver metabolizes the drug, thus reducing the potential for systemic toxicity. Therapy can be given until adverse reactions appear (see Precautions). When these side effects have subsided, therapy may be resumed. The patient should be maintained on therapy as long as response to floxuridine continues.

➤*Storage/Stability:* The sterile powder should be stored at 15° to 30°C (59° to 86°F). Reconstituted vials should be stored under refrigeration (2° to 8°C, 36° to 46°F) for not more than 2 weeks.

FLOXURIDINE — INJECTION

Actions

➤*Pharmacology:* When floxuridine is given by rapid intra-arterial injection it is apparently rapidly catabolized to 5-fluorouracil. Thus, rapid injection of floxuridine produces the same toxic and antimetabolic effects as does 5-fluorouracil. The primary effect is to interfere with the synthesis of deoxyribonucleic acid (DNA) and to a lesser extent inhibit the formation of ribonucleic acid (RNA). However, when floxuridine is given by continuous intra-arterial infusion its direct anabolism to floxuridine-monophosphate is enhanced, thus increasing the inhibition of DNA.

Floxuridine is metabolized in the liver. The drug is excreted intact and as urea, fluorouracil, alpha-fluoro-beta-ureidopropionic acid, dihydrofluorouracil, alpha-fluoro-beta-guanidopropionic acid, and alpha-fluoro-beta-alanine in the urine; it is also expired as respiratory carbon dioxide.

Contraindications

Poor nutritional state; depressed bone marrow function; potentially serious infections.

Warnings

➤*Combination therapy:* Any form of therapy which adds to the stress of the patient, interferes with nutrition or depresses bone marrow function will increase the toxicity of floxuridine.

➤*Renal/Hepatic function impairment:* Floxuridine should be used with extreme caution in poor risk patients with impaired hepatic or renal function or a history of high-dose pelvic irradiation or previous use of alkylating agents. The drug is not intended as an adjuvant to surgery.

➤*Mutagenesis:* Oncogenic transformation of fibroblasts from mouse embryo has been induced in vitro by floxuridine, but the relationship between oncogenicity and mutagenicity is not clear. Floxuridine has also been shown to be mutagenic in human leukocytes in vitro and in the Drosophila test system. In addition, 5-fluorouracil, to which floxuridine is catabolized when given by intra-arterial injection, has been shown to be mutagenic in in vitro tests.

➤*Fertility impairment:* The effects of floxuridine on fertility and general reproductive performance have not been studied in animals. However, because floxuridine is catabolized to 5-fluorouracil, it should be noted that 5-fluorouracil has been shown to induce chromosomal aberrations and changes in chromosome organization of spermatogonia in rats at doses of 125 or 250 mg/kg, administered intraperitoneally. Spermatogonial differentiation was also inhibited by fluorouracil, resulting in transient infertility. In female rats, fluorouracil, administered intraperitoneally at doses of 25 or 50 mg/kg during the preovulatory phase of oogenesis, significantly reduced the incidence of fertile matings, delayed the development of pre- and postimplantation embryos, increased the incidence of preimplantation lethality and induced chromosomal anomalies in these embryos. Compounds such as floxuridine, which interfere with DNA, RNA and protein synthesis, might be expected to have adverse effects on gametogenesis.

➤*Pregnancy: Category D.* There are no adequate and well-controlled studies with floxuridine in pregnant women. If this drug is used during pregnancy or if the patient becomes pregnant while taking (receiving) this drug, the patient should be apprised of the potential hazard to the fetus. Women of childbearing potential should be advised to avoid becoming pregnant.

Teratogenic – Floxuridine has been shown to be teratogenic in the chick embryo, mouse (at doses of 2.5 to 100 mg/kg) and rat (at doses of 75 to 150 mg/kg). Malformations included cleft palates, skeletal defects and deformed appendages, paws and tails. The dosages which were teratogenic in animals are 3.2- to 125-times the recommended human therapeutic dose. There are no adequate and well-controlled studies with floxuridine in pregnant women. While there is no evidence of teratogenicity in humans due to floxuridine, it should be kept in mind that other drugs which inhibit DNA synthesis (eg, methotrexate and aminopterin) have been reported to be teratogenic in humans. Floxuridine should be used during pregnancy only if the potential benefit justifies the potential risk to the fetus.

Nonteratogenic – Floxuridine has not been studied in animals for its effects on peri- and postnatal development. However, compounds which inhibit DNA, RNA, and protein synthesis might be expected to have adverse effects on peri- and postnatal development.

➤*Lactation:* It is not known whether floxuridine is excreted in human milk. Because floxuridine inhibits DNA and RNA synthesis, mothers should not nurse while receiving this drug.

➤*Children:* Safety and effectiveness in pediatric patients have not been established.

Precautions

➤*Monitoring:* Careful monitoring of the white blood count and platelet count is recommended.

➤*Special risk:* Sterile floxuridine is a highly toxic drug with a narrow margin of safety. Therefore, patients should be carefully supervised since therapeutic response is unlikely to occur without some evidence of toxicity. Severe hematological toxicity, gastrointestinal hemorrhage, and even death may result from the use of floxuridine despite meticulous selection of patients and careful adjustment of dosage. Although severe toxicity is more likely in poor risk patients, fatalities may be encountered occasionally even in patients in relatively good condition.

Discontinuation – Therapy is to be discontinued promptly whenever 1 of the following signs of toxicity appears:

- Myocardial ischemia.
- Stomatitis or esophagopharyngitis, at the first visible sign.
- Leukopenia (WBC under 3500) or a rapidly falling white blood count.
- Vomiting, intractable.
- Diarrhea, frequent bowel movements or watery stools.
- Gastrointestinal ulceration and bleeding.
- Thrombocytopenia (platelets under 100,000).
- Hemorrhage from any site.

Adverse Reactions

Adverse reactions to the arterial infusion of floxuridine are generally related to the procedural complications of regional arterial infusion, which include arterial aneurysm, arterial ischemia, arterial thrombosis, embolism, fibromyositis, thrombophlebitis, hepatic necrosis, abscesses, infection at catheter site, bleeding at catheter site, and catheter blocked, displaced or leaking.

➤*Cardiovascular:* Myocardial ischemia.

➤*Dermatologic:* Alopecia, dermatitis, nonspecific skin toxicity, rash, and the more common adverse reaction of localized erythema.

➤*GI:* Some of the most common adverse reactions to the drug in general include nausea, vomiting, diarrhea, enteritis, and stomatitis. Other gastrointestinal reactions include duodenal ulcer, duodenitis, gastritis, bleeding, gastroenteritis, glossitis, pharyngitis, anorexia, cramps, abdominal pain; possible intra- and extrahepatic biliary sclerosis, as well as acalculous cholecystitis.

➤*Lab test abnormalities:* The more common laboratory abnormalities are anemia, leukopenia, thrombocytopenia and elevations of alkaline phosphatase, serum transaminase, serum bilirubin and lactic dehydrogenase. Other abnormalities include BSP, prothrombin, total proteins, sedimentation rate and thrombopenia.

➤*Miscellaneous:* Fever, lethargy, malaise, weakness.

Overdosage

The possibility of overdosage with floxuridine is unlikely in view of the mode of administration. Nevertheless, the anticipated manifestations would be nausea, vomiting, diarrhea, gastrointestinal ulceration and bleeding, bone marrow depression (including thrombocytopenia, leukopenia and agranulocytosis). No specific antidotal therapy exists. Patients who have been exposed to an overdosage of floxuridine should be monitored hematologically for at least 4 weeks. Should abnormalities appear, appropriate therapy should be utilized. In mice, the acute intravenous floxuridine LD_{50} was 880 ± 51 mg/kg. Similarly, in rats, rabbits, and dogs, the acute intravenous floxuridine LD_{50} was 670 ± 73 mg/kg, 94 ± 19.6 mg/kg, and 157 ± 46 mg/kg, respectively.

Patient Information

Patients should be informed of expected toxic effects, particularly oral manifestations. Patients should be alerted to the possibility of alopecia as a result of therapy and should be informed that it is usually a transient effect.

GEMCITABINE HYDROCHLORIDE

Rx	**Gemzar** (Eli Lilly)	**Powder for Injection, lyophilized:** 200 mg	Mannitol. In 10 mL single-use vials.
		1 g	Mannitol. In 50 mL single-use vials.

GEMCITABINE HYDROCHLORIDE — INJECTION

Indications

➤*Breast cancer:* In combination with paclitaxel as first-line treatment of patients with metastatic breast cancer after failure of prior anthracycline-containing adjuvant chemotherapy, unless anthracyclines were clinically contraindicated.

➤*Non-small cell lung cancer:* In combination with cisplatin as first-line treatment of patients with inoperable, locally advanced (Stage IIIA or IIIB), or metastatic (Stage IV) non-small cell lung cancer.

➤*Pancreatic cancer:* As first-line treatment for patients with locally advanced (nonresectable Stage II or Stage III) or metastatic (Stage IV) adenocarcinoma of the pancreas. Gemcitabine is indicated for patients previously treated with 5-fluorouracil.

➤*Unlabeled uses:* Treatment of bladder cancer, biliary cancer, relapsed or refractory testicular cancer, squamous cell carcinoma of the head and neck, ovarian cancer.

Administration and Dosage

➤*Approved by the FDA:* May 15, 1996.

Gemcitabine is for IV use only. Gemcitabine may be administered on an outpatient basis.

➤*Single-agent use:*

Pancreatic cancer – Administer gemcitabine by IV infusion at a dose of 1,000 mg/m^2 over 30 minutes once weekly for up to 7 weeks (or until toxicity necessitates reducing or holding a dose), followed by a week of rest from

GEMCITABINE HYDROCHLORIDE — INJECTION

treatment. Subsequent cycles should consist of infusions once weekly for 3 consecutive weeks out of every 4 weeks.

Dose modifications – Dosage adjustment is based upon the degree of hematologic toxicity experienced by the patient. Clearance in women and the elderly is reduced, and women were somewhat less able to progress to subsequent cycles.

Monitor patients receiving gemcitabine prior to each dose with a complete blood count (CBC), including differential and platelet count. If marrow suppression is detected, modify or suspend therapy according to the guidelines in the table below.

Dosage reduction guidelines			
Absolute granulocyte count (× 10^6/L)		Platelet count (× 10^6/L)	% of full dose
≥ 1,000	and	≥ 100,000	100
500 to 999	or	50,000 to 99,000	75
< 500	or	< 50,000	Hold

Perform laboratory evaluation of renal and hepatic function, including transaminases and serum creatinine, prior to initiation of therapy and periodically thereafter. Administer gemcitabine with caution in patients with evidence of significant renal or hepatic impairment.

Patients treated with gemcitabine who complete an entire cycle of therapy may have the dose for subsequent cycles increased 25%, provided that the absolute granulocyte count (AGC) and platelet nadirs exceed 1,500 × 10^6/L and 100,000 × 10^6/L, respectively, and if nonhematologic toxicity has not been greater than World Health Organization (WHO) grade 1. If patients tolerate the subsequent course of gemcitabine at the increased dose, the dose for the next cycle can be further increased 20%, provided again that the AGC and platelet nadirs exceed 1,500 × 10^6/L and 100,000 × 10^6/L, respectively, and that nonhematologic toxicity has not been greater than WHO grade 1.

➤*Combination use:*

Non-small cell lung cancer – Two schedules have been investigated, and the optimum schedule has not been determined. With the 4-week schedule, administer gemcitabine intravenously at 1,000 mg/m^2 over 30 minutes on days 1, 8, and 15 of each 28-day cycle. Cisplatin should be administered intravenously at 100 mg/m^2 on day 1 after the infusion of gemcitabine. With the 3-week schedule, administer gemcitabine intravenously at 1,250 mg/m^2 over 30 minutes on days 1 and 8 of each 21-day cycle. Administer cisplatin at a dose of 100 mg/m^2 intravenously after the infusion of gemcitabine on day 1. See cisplatin monograph for cisplatin administration and hydration guidelines.

Dose modifications: Dosage adjustments for hematologic toxicity may be required for gemcitabine and for cisplatin. Gemcitabine dosage adjustment for hematological toxicity is based on the granulocyte and platelet counts taken on the day of therapy. Monitor patients receiving gemcitabine prior to each dose with a CBC, including differential and platelet counts. If marrow suppression is detected, modify or suspend therapy according to the guidelines given under Single-agent use. For cisplatin dosage adjustment, see cisplatin monograph.

In general, for severe (grade 3 or 4) nonhematological toxicity, except alopecia and nausea/vomiting, hold or decrease therapy with gemcitabine plus cisplatin 50% depending on the judgment of the treating physician. During combination therapy with cisplatin, carefully monitor serum creatinine, serum potassium, serum calcium, and serum magnesium (grade 3/4 serum creatinine toxicity for gemcitabine plus cisplatin was 5% vs 2% for cisplatin alone).

Breast cancer – Administer gemcitabine intravenously at a dose of 1,250 mg/m^2 over 30 minutes on days 1 and 8 of each 21-day cycle. Administer paclitaxel at 175 mg/m^2 on day 1 as a 3-hour IV infusion before gemcitabine administration. Monitor patients prior to each dose with a CBC, including differential counts. Patients should have an absolute granulocyte count at least 1,500 x 10^6/L and a platelet count at least 100,000 x 10^6/L prior to each cycle.

Dose modifications: Gemcitabine dosage adjustments for hematological toxicity is based on the granulocyte and platelet counts taken on day 8 of therapy. If marrow suppression is detected, modify gemcitabine dosage according to the guidelines below.

Day 8 Dosage Reduction Guidelines for Gemcitabine Hydrochloride in Combination with Paclitaxel			
Absolute granulocyte count (x 10^6 /L)		Platelet count (x 10^6/L)	% of full dose
≥ 1200	and	> 75,000	100
1,000 to 1,199	or	50,000 to 75,000	75
700 to 999	and	≥ 50,000	50
< 700	or	< 50,000	Hold

In general, for severe (Grade 3 or 4) nonhematological toxicity, except alopecia and nausea/vomiting, decrease therapy with gemcitabine 50% depending on the judgment of the treating physician. For paclitaxel dosage adjustment, see paclitaxel monograph.

Dilution – The recommended diluent for reconstitution of gemcitabine is 0.9% sodium chloride injection without preservatives. Because of solubility considerations, the maximum concentration for gemcitabine upon reconstitution is 40 mg/mL. Reconstitution at concentrations greater than 40 mg/mL may result in incomplete dissolution and should be avoided.

Reconstitution: To reconstitute, add 5 mL 0.9% sodium chloride injection to the 200 mg vial or 25 mL 0.9% sodium chloride injection to the 1 g vial. Shake to dissolve. These dilutions each yield a gemcitabine concentration of 38 mg/mL, which includes accounting for the displacement volume of the lyophilized powder (0.26 mL for the 200 mg vial or 1.3 mL for the 1 g vial). The total volume upon reconstitution will be 5.26 or 26.3 mL, respectively. Complete withdrawal of the vial contents will provide 200 mg or 1 g of gemcitabine, respectively. The appropriate amount of drug may be administered as prepared or further diluted with 0.9% sodium chloride injection to concentrations as low as 0.1 mg/mL.

➤*Storage/Stability:* Store at controlled room temperature (20° to 25°C [68° to 77°F]).

When prepared as directed, gemcitabine solutions are stable for 24 hours at controlled room temperature (20° to 25°C [68° to 77°F]). Discard unused portion. Do not refrigerate solutions of reconstituted gemcitabine, as crystallization may occur.

Actions

➤*Pharmacology:* Gemcitabine exhibits cell phase specificity, primarily killing cells undergoing DNA synthesis (S-phase) and also blocking the progression of cells through the G1/S-phase boundary. Gemcitabine is metabolized intracellularly by nucleoside kinases to the active diphosphate (dFdCDP) and triphosphate (dFdCTP) nucleosides. The cytotoxic effect of gemcitabine is attributed to a combination of 2 actions of the diphosphate and the triphosphate nucleosides, which leads to inhibition of DNA synthesis. First, gemcitabine diphosphate inhibits ribonucleotide reductase, which is responsible for catalyzing the reactions that generate the deoxynucleoside triphosphates for DNA synthesis. Inhibition of this enzyme by the diphosphate nucleoside causes a reduction in the concentrations of deoxynucleotides, including dCTP. Second, gemcitabine triphosphate competes with dCTP for incorporation into DNA. The reduction in the intracellular concentration of dCTP (by the action of the diphosphate) enhances the incorporation of gemcitabine triphosphate into DNA (self-potentiation). After the gemcitabine nucleoside is incorporated into DNA, only 1 additional nucleoside is added to the growing DNA strands. After this addition, there is inhibition of further DNA synthesis. DNA polymerase epsilon is unable to remove the gemcitabine nucleotide and repair the growing DNA strands (masked chain termination). In CEM T lymphoblastoid cells, gemcitabine induces internucleosomal DNA fragmentation, one of the characteristics of programmed cell death.

Gemcitabine demonstrated dose-dependent synergistic activity with cisplatin in vitro. No effect of cisplatin on gemcitabine triphosphate accumulation or DNA double-strand breaks was observed. In vivo, gemcitabine showed activity in combination with cisplatin against the LX-1 and CALU-6 human lung xenografts, but minimal activity was seen with the NCI-H460 or NCI-H520 xenografts. Gemcitabine was synergistic with cisplatin in the Lewis lung murine xenograft. Sequential exposure to gemcitabine 4 hours before cisplatin produced the greatest interaction.

➤*Pharmacokinetics:*

Absorption/Distribution – Volume of distribution of gemcitabine was 50 L/m^2 following infusions lasting less than 70 minutes, indicating that gemcitabine, after short infusions, is not extensively distributed into tissues. For long infusions, the volume of distribution rose to 370 L/m^2, reflecting slow equilibration of gemcitabine within the tissue compartment.

Gemcitabine plasma protein binding is negligible.

Metabolism/Excretion – Gemcitabine disposition was studied in 5 patients who received a single 1,000 mg/m^2/30 minute infusion of radiolabeled drug. Within 1 week, 92% to 98% of the dose was recovered, almost entirely in the urine. Gemcitabine (less than 10%) and the inactive uracil metabolite, 2′-deoxy-2′,2′-difluorouridine (dFdU), accounted for 99% of the excreted dose. The metabolite dFdU is also found in plasma.

Clearance was affected by age and gender. Differences in either clearance or volume of distribution based on patient characteristics or the duration of infusion result in changes in half-life and plasma concentrations.

Gemcitabine Clearance and Half-life for the "Typical" Patient				
Age	Clearance men (L/hr/m^2)	Clearance women (L/hr/m^2)	Half-life[a] men (min)	Half-life[a] women (min)
29	92.2	69.4	42	49
45	75.7	57	48	57
65	55.1	41.5	61	73
79	40.7	30.7	79	94

[a] Half-life for patients receiving a short infusion (less than 70 minutes).

Gemcitabine half-life for short infusions ranged from 32 to 94 minutes, and the value for long infusions varied from 245 to 638 minutes, depending on age and gender, reflecting a greatly increased volume of distribution with longer infusions. The lower clearance in women and the elderly results in higher concentrations of gemcitabine for any given dose.

The maximum plasma concentrations of dFdU (inactive metabolite) were achieved up to 30 minutes after discontinuation of the infusions, and the metabolite is excreted in urine without undergoing further biotransformation. The metabolite did not accumulate with weekly dosing but could with decreased renal function.

The active metabolite, gemcitabine triphosphate, can be extracted from peripheral blood mononuclear cells. The half-life of the terminal phase for gemcitabine triphosphate from mononuclear cells ranges from 1.7 to 19.4 hours.

Contraindications

Hypersensitivity to the drug.

GEMCITABINE HYDROCHLORIDE — INJECTION

Warnings

➤*Infusion time:* Prolongation of the infusion time beyond 60 minutes and more frequently than weekly dosing has been shown to increase toxicity.

➤*Hematologic effects:* Gemcitabine can suppress bone marrow function as manifested by leukopenia, thrombocytopenia, and anemia, and myelosuppression is usually the dose-limiting toxicity. Monitor patients for myelosuppression during therapy. Dosage adjustment is based upon the degree of hematologic toxicity experienced by the patient.

➤*Pulmonary effects:* Pulmonary toxicity has been reported with the use of gemcitabine. In cases of severe lung toxicity, discontinue gemcitabine therapy immediately and institute appropriate supportive care measures.

➤*Renal/Hepatic function impairment:* Use gemcitabine with caution in patients with preexisting renal impairment or hepatic insufficiency.

Renal effects – Hemolytic uremic syndrome (HUS) and/or renal failure have been reported following 1 or more doses of gemcitabine. Renal failure leading to death or requiring dialysis, despite discontinuation of therapy, has been rarely reported. The majority of the cases of renal failure leading to death were caused by HUS.

Hepatic effects – Serious hepatotoxicity, including liver failure and death, has been reported very rarely in patients receiving gemcitabine alone or in combination with other potentially hepatotoxic drugs.

➤*Mutagenesis:* Gemcitabine induced forward mutations in vitro in a mouse lymphoma (L5178Y) assay and was clastogenic in an in vivo mouse micronucleus assay.

➤*Fertility impairment:* Gemcitabine intraperitoneal doses of 0.5 mg/kg/day (about 0.14% the human dose on a mg/m^2 basis) in male mice had an effect on fertility with moderate to severe hypospermatogenesis, decreased fertility, and decreased implantations. In female mice, fertility was not affected but maternal toxicities were observed at 1.5 mg/kg/day IV (about 0.5% the human dose on a mg/m^2 basis) and fetotoxicity or embryolethality was observed at 0.25 mg/kg/day IV (about 0.077% the human dose on a mg/m^2 basis).

➤*Elderly:* See Actions for more information.

➤*Pregnancy: Category D.* Gemcitabine can cause fetal harm when administered to a pregnant woman. Gemcitabine is embryotoxic causing fetal malformations (eg, cleft palate, incomplete ossification) at doses of 1.5 mg/kg/day in mice (about 1/200 the recommended human dose on a mg/m^2 basis). Gemcitabine is fetotoxic, causing fetal malformations (eg, fused pulmonary artery, absence of gall bladder) at doses of 0.1 mg/kg/day in rabbits (about 1/600 the recommended human dose on a mg/m^2 basis). Embryotoxicity was characterized by decreased fetal viability, reduced live litter sizes, and developmental delays. There are no studies of gemcitabine in pregnant women. If gemcitabine is used during pregnancy or if the patient becomes pregnant while taking gemcitabine, apprise the patient of the potential hazard to the fetus.

➤*Lactation:* It is not known whether gemcitabine or its metabolites are excreted in human milk. Because many drugs are excreted in human milk and because of the potential for serious adverse reactions from gemcitabine in nursing infants, warn the mother and decide whether to discontinue nursing or to discontinue the drug, taking into account the importance of the drug to the mother and the potential risk to the infant.

➤*Children:* Gemcitabine has not been studied in pediatric patients. Safety and effectiveness in pediatric patients have not been established.

Precautions

➤*Monitoring:* Patients receiving therapy with gemcitabine should be monitored closely by a physician experienced in the use of cancer chemotherapeutic agents. Most adverse events are reversible and do not need to result in discontinuation, although doses may need to be withheld or reduced. There was a greater tendency in women, especially older women, not to proceed to the next cycle.

Perform laboratory evaluation of renal and hepatic function prior to initiation of therapy and periodically thereafter.

See Administration and Dosage for more information.

➤*Gender:* Gemcitabine clearance is affected by gender. In the single agent safety database (n = 979 patients), however, there is no evidence that unusual dose adjustments (other than those recommended) are necessary in women. In general, in single agent studies of gemcitabine adverse reaction rates were similar in men and women, but women, especially older women, were more likely not to proceed to a subsequent cycle and to experience grade 3 or 4 neutropenia and thrombocytopenia.

Adverse Reactions

➤*Single-agent use:* Myelosuppression is the principal dose-limiting toxicity with gemcitabine therapy. Dosage adjustments for hematologic toxicity are frequently needed.

Selected WHO-graded Adverse Events in Patients Receiving Single Agent Gemcitabine (WHO grades [% incidence])*

	All patients[a]			Pancreatic cancer patients[b]			Discontinuations (%)[c]
Adverse reaction	All grades	Grade 3	Grade 4	All grades	Grade 3	Grade 4	All patients
Laboratory, hematologic[d]							
Anemia	68%	7%	1%	73%	8%	2%	< 1%
Leukopenia	62%	9%	< 1%	64%	8%	1%	< 1%
Neutropenia	63%	19%	6%	61%	17%	7%	—
Thrombocytopenia	24%	4%	1%	36%	7%	< 1%	< 1%
Hepatic							< 1%
Alkaline phosphatase	55%	7%	2%	77%	16%	4%	
ALT	68%	8%	2%	72%	10%	1%	
AST	67%	6%	2%	78%	12%	5%	
Bilirubin	13%	2%	< 1%	26%	6%	2%	
Renal							< 1%
BUN	16%	0%	0%	15%	0%	0%	
Creatinine	8%	< 1%	0%	6%	0%	0%	
Hematuria	35%	< 1%	0%	23%	0%	0%	
Proteinuria	45%	< 1%	0%	32%	< 1%	0%	
Non-laboratory[e]							
Alopecia	15%	< 1%	0%	16%	0%	0%	0%
Constipation	23%	1%	< 1%	31%	3%	< 1%	0%
Diarrhea	19%	1%	0%	30%	3%	0%	0%
Dyspnea	23%	3%	< 1%	10%	0%	< 1%	< 1%
Fever	41%	2%	0%	38%	2%	0%	< 1%
Hemorrhage	17%	< 1%	< 1%	4%	2%	< 1%	< 1%
Infection	16%	1%	< 1%	10%	2%	< 1%	< 1%
Nausea and vomiting	69%	13%	1%	71%	10%	2%	< 1%
Pain	48%	9%	< 1%	42%	6%	< 1%	< 1%
Paresthesias	10%	< 1%	0%	10%	< 1%	0%	0%
Rash	30%	< 1%	0%	28%	< 1%	0%	< 1%
Somnolence	11%	< 1%	< 1%	11%	2%	< 1%	< 1%
Stomatitis	11%	< 1%	0%	10%	< 1%	0%	< 1%

* Grade based on criteria from the WHO.
[a] N = 699 to 974; all patients with laboratory or nonlaboratory data.
[b] N = 161 to 241; all pancreatic cancer patients with laboratory or nonlaboratory data.
[c] N = 979.
[d] Regardless of causality.
[e] Table includes nonlaboratory data with incidence for all patients at least 10%. For approximately 60% of the patients, non-laboratory events were graded only if assessed to be possibly drug-related.

GEMCITABINE HYDROCHLORIDE — INJECTION

Selected WHO-graded Adverse Events From Comparative Trial of Gemcitabine and 5-FU in Pancreatic Cancer (WHO grades [% incidence])*

Adverse reaction	Gemcitabine[a] All grades	Gemcitabine[a] Grade 3	Gemcitabine[a] Grade 4	5-FU[b] All grades	5-FU[b] Grade 3	5-FU[b] Grade 4
Laboratory[c], hematologic						
Anemia	65%	7%	3%	45%	0%	0%
Leukopenia	71%	10%	0%	15%	2%	0%
Neutropenia	62%	19%	7%	18%	2%	3%
Thrombocytopenia	47%	10%	0%	15%	2%	0%
Hepatic						
Alkaline phosphatase	71%	16%	0%	64%	10%	3%
ALT	72%	8%	2%	38%	0%	0%
AST	72%	10%	2%	52%	2%	0%
Bilirubin	16%	2%	2%	25%	6%	3%
Renal						
BUN	8%	0%	0%	10%	0%	0%
Creatinine	2%	0%	0%	0%	0%	0%
Hematuria	13%	0%	0%	0%	0%	0%
Proteinuria	10%	0%	0%	2%	0%	0%
Non-laboratory[d]						
Alopecia	18%	0%	0%	16%	0%	0%
Constipation	10%	3%	0%	11%	2%	0%
Diarrhea	24%	2%	0%	31%	5%	0%
Dyspnea	6%	0%	0%	3%	0%	0%
Fever	30%	0%	0%	16%	0%	0%
Hemorrhage	0%	0%	0%	2%	0%	0%
Infection	8%	0%	0%	3%	2%	0%
Nausea and vomiting	64%	10%	3%	58%	5%	0%
Pain	10%	2%	0%	7%	0%	0%
Paresthesias	2%	0%	0%	2%	0%	0%
Rash	24%	0%	0%	13%	0%	0%
Somnolence	5%	2%	0%	7%	2%	0%
Stomatitis	14%	0%	0%	15%	0%	0%

* Grade based on criteria from the WHO.
[a] N = 58 to 63; all gemcitabine patients with laboratory or nonlaboratory data.
[b] N = 61 to 63; all 5-FU patients with laboratory or nonlaboratory data.
[c] Regardless of causality.
[d] Nonlaboratory events were graded only if assessed to be possibly drug-related.

Allergic – Bronchospasm was reported for less than 2% of patients. Anaphylactoid reaction has been reported rarely. Do not administer gemcitabine to patients with a known hypersensitivity to this drug.

Cardiovascular – During clinical trials, 2% of patients discontinued therapy with gemcitabine due to cardiovascular events such as myocardial infarction, cerebrovascular accident, arrhythmia, and hypertension. Many of these patients had a history of cardiovascular disease (see Postmarketing).

CNS – There was a 10% incidence of mild paresthesias and a less than 1% rate of severe paresthesias.

Dermatologic – Rash was reported in 30% of patients. The rash was typically a macular or finely granular maculopapular pruritic eruption of mild to moderate severity involving the trunk and extremities. Pruritus was reported in 13% of patients. Alopecia, usually minimal, was reported 15% of patients.

GI – Nausea and vomiting were commonly reported (69%) but were usually of mild to moderate severity. Severe nausea and vomiting (WHO grade 3 or 4) occurred in less than 15% of patients. Diarrhea was reported by 19% of patients, and stomatitis by 11% of patients.

Hematologic – In studies in pancreatic cancer, myelosuppression is the dose-limiting toxicity with gemcitabine, but less than 1% of patients discontinued therapy for either anemia, leukopenia, or thrombocytopenia. Red blood cell transfusions were required by 19% of patients. The incidence of sepsis was less than 1%. Petechiae or mild blood loss (hemorrhage), from any cause, was reported in 16% of patients; less than 1% of patients required platelet transfusions. Monitor patients for myelosuppression during gemcitabine therapy and modify or suspend dosage according to the degree of hematologic toxicity.

Hepatic – In clinical trials, gemcitabine was associated with transient elevations of one or both serum transaminases in approximately 70% of patients, but there was no evidence of increasing hepatic toxicity with either longer duration of exposure to gemcitabine or with greater total cumulative dose. Serious hepatotoxicity, including liver failure and death, has been reported very rarely in patients receiving gemcitabine alone or in combination with other potentially hepatotoxic drugs (see Postmarketing).

Renal – In clinical trials, mild proteinuria and hematuria were commonly reported. Clinical findings consistent with the hemolytic uremic syndrome (HUS) were reported in 6 of 2,429 patients (0.25%) receiving gemcitabine in clinical trials. Four patients developed HUS on gemcitabine therapy, 2 immediately posttherapy. Consider the diagnosis of HUS if the patient develops anemia with evidence of microangiopathic hemolysis as indicated by elevation of bilirubin or LDH, reticulocytosis, severe thrombocytopenia, and/or evidence of renal failure (elevation of serum creatinine or BUN). Discontinue gemcitabine therapy immediately. Renal failure may not be reversible even with discontinuation of therapy and dialysis may be required.

Respiratory – In clinical trials, dyspnea, unrelated to underlying disease, has been reported in association with gemcitabine therapy. Dyspnea was occasionally accompanied by bronchospasm. Pulmonary toxicity has been reported with the use of gemcitabine (see Pulmonary under Postmarketing experience). The etiology of these effects is unknown. If such effects develop, discontinue gemcitabine. Early use of supportive care measures may help ameliorate these conditions.

Miscellaneous – Edema (13%), peripheral edema (20%), and generalized edema (less than 1%) were reported. Less than 1% of patients discontinued because of edema.

Injection-site related events were reported for 4% of patients. There were not reports of injection-site necrosis. Gemcitabine is not a vesicant.

The overall incidence of fever was 41%. This is in contrast to the incidence of infection (16%) and indicates that gemcitabine may cause fever in the absence of clinical infection. Fever was frequently associated with other flu-like symptoms and was usually mild and clinically manageable.

"Flu syndrome" was reported for 19% of patients. Individual symptoms of fever, asthenia, anorexia, headache, cough, chills, and myalgia were commonly reported. Fever and asthenia were also reported frequently as isolated symptoms. Insomnia, rhinitis, sweating, and malaise were reported infrequently. Less than 1% of patients discontinued due to flu-like symptoms.

Infections were reported for 16% of patients. Sepsis was rarely reported (less than 1%).

➤*Combination Use in non-small cell lung cancer:*

Selected CTC-graded Adverse Events From Comparative Trial of Gemcitabine Plus Cisplatin vs Single-agent Cisplatin in NSCLC (CTC grades [% incidence])*

Adverse reaction	Gemcitabine plus cisplatin[a] All grades	Gemcitabine plus cisplatin[a] Grade 3	Gemcitabine plus cisplatin[a] Grade 4	Cisplatin[b] All grades	Cisplatin[b] Grade 3	Cisplatin[b] Grade 4
Laboratory[c], hematologic						
Anemia	89%	22%	3%	67%	6%	1%
Leukopenia	82%	35%	11%	25%	2%	1%
Lymphocytes	75%	25%	18%	51%	12%	5%
Neutropenia	79%	22%	35%	20%	3%	1%
Thrombocytopenia	85%	25%	25%	13%	3%	1%
Platelet transfusions[d]	21%			< 1%		
RBC transfusion[d]	39%			13%		
Hepatic						
Transaminase	22%	2%	1%	10%	1%	0%
Alkaline phosphatase	19%	1%	0%	13%	0%	0%
Renal						
Creatinine	38%	4%	< 1%	31%	2%	< 1%
Hematuria	15%	0%	0%	13%	0%	0%
Proteinuria	23%	0%	0%	18%	0%	0%
Other laboratory						
Hyperglycemia	30%	4%	0%	23%	3%	0%
Hypocalcemia	18%	2%	0%	7%	0%	< 1%
Hypomagnesemia	30%	4%	3%	17%	2%	0%
Nonlaboratory[e]						
Alopecia	53%	1%	0%	33%	0%	0%
Constipation	28%	3%	0%	21%	0%	0%
Diarrhea	24%	2%	2%	13%	0%	0%
Dyspnea	12%	4%	3%	11%	3%	2%
Fever	16%	0%	0%	5%	0%	0%
Hemorrhage	14%	1%	0%	4%	0%	0%
Hypotension	12%	1%	0%	7%	1%	0%
Infection	18%	3%	2%	12%	1%	0%
Local	15%	0%	0%	6%	0%	0%
Nausea	93%	25%	2%	87%	20%	< 1%
Neuro cortical	16%	3%	1%	9%	1%	0%
Neuro headache	14%	0%	0%	7%	0%	0%
Neuro hearing	25%	6%	0%	21%	6%	0%
Neuro mood	16%	1%	0%	10%	1%	0%

GEMCITABINE HYDROCHLORIDE — INJECTION

Selected CTC-graded Adverse Events From Comparative Trial of Gemcitabine Plus Cisplatin vs Single-agent Cisplatin in NSCLC (CTC grades [% incidence])*

	Gemcitabine plus cisplatin[a]			Cisplatin[b]		
Adverse reaction	All grades	Grade 3	Grade 4	All grades	Grade 3	Grade 4
Neuro motor	35%	12%	0%	15%	3%	0%
Neuro sensory	23%	1%	0%	18%	1%	0%
Rash	11%	0%	0%	3%	0%	0%
Stomatitis	14%	1%	0%	5%	0%	0%
Vomiting	78%	11%	12%	71%	10%	9%

* Grade based on Common Toxicity Criteria (CTC). Table includes data for adverse events with incidence at least 10% in either arm.
[a] N = 217 to 253; all gemcitabine plus cisplatin patients with laboratory or nonlaboratory data. Gemcitabine at 1,000 mg/m^2 on days 1, 8, and 15 and cisplatin at 100 mg/m^2 on day 1 every 28 days.
[b] N = 213 to 248; all cisplatin patients with laboratory or nonlaboratory data. Cisplatin at 100 mg/m^2 on day 1 every 28 days.
[c] Regardless of causality.
[d] Percent of patients receiving transfusions. Percent transfusions are not CTC-graded events.
[e] Nonlaboratory events were graded only if assessed to be possibly drug-related.

Selected WHO-graded Adverse Events From Comparative Trial of Gemcitabine Plus Cisplatin vs Etoposide Plus Cisplatin in NSCLC (WHO grades [% incidence])*

	Gemcitabine plus cisplatin[a]			Etoposide plus cisplatin[b]		
Adverse reaction	All grades	Grade 3	Grade 4	All grades	Grade 3	Grade 4
Laboratory[c], hematologic						
Anemia	88%	22%	0%	77%	13%	2%
Leukopenia	86%	26%	3%	87%	36%	7%
Neutropenia	88%	36%	28%	87%	20%	56%
Platelet transfusions[d]	3%			8%		
RBC transfusions[d]	29%			21%		
Thrombocytopenia	81%	39%	16%	45%	8%	5%
Hepatic						
Alkaline phosphatase	16%	0%	0%	11%	0%	0%
ALT	6%	0%	0%	12%	0%	0%
AST	3%	0%	0%	11%	0%	0%
Bilirubin	0%	0%	0%	0%	0%	0%
Renal						
BUN	6%	0%	0%	4%	0%	0%
Creatinine	2%	0%	0%	2%	0%	0%
Hematuria	22%	0%	0%	10%	0%	0%
Proteinuria	12%	0%	0%	5%	0%	0%
Nonlaboratory[e,f]						
Alopecia	77%	13%	0%	92%	51%	0%
Constipation	17%	0%	0%	15%	0%	0%
Diarrhea	14%	1%	1%	13%	0%	2%
Dyspnea	1%	0%	1%	3%	0%	0%
Fever	6%	0%	0%	3%	0%	0%
Hemorrhage	9%	0%	3%	3%	0%	3%
Infection	28%	3%	1%	21%	8%	0%
Nausea and vomiting	96%	35%	4%	86%	19%	7%
Paresthesias	38%	0%	0%	16%	2%	0%
Rash	10%	0%	0%	3%	0%	0%
Somnolence	3%	0%	0%	3%	2%	0%
Stomatitis	20%	4%	0%	18%	2%	0%

* Grade based on criteria from the WHO.
[a] N = 67 to 69; all gemcitabine plus cisplatin patients with laboratory or nonlaboratory data. Gemcitabine at 1,250 mg/m^2 on days 1 and 8 and cisplatin at 100 mg/m^2 on day 1 every 21 days.
[b] N = 57 to 63; all cisplatin plus etoposide patients with laboratory or nonlaboratory data. Cisplatin at 100 mg/m^2 on day 1 and IV etoposide at 100 mg/m^2 on days 1, 2, and 3 every 21 days.
[c] Regardless of causality.
[d] Percent of patients receiving transfusions. Percent transfusions are not WHO-graded events.
[e] Nonlaboratory events were graded only if assessed to be possibly drug-related.
[f] Pain data were not collected.

➤*Combination use in breast cancer:* The safety data occurrences of at least 10% (all grades) from the gemcitabine plus paclitaxel vs paclitaxel study in breast cancer are presented below.

Adverse Events From Comparative Trial of Gemcitabine Hydrochloride Plus Paclitaxel vs Single-agent Paclitaxel in Breast Cancer[a] (CTC Grades [% incidence])

	Gemcitabine plus paclitaxel (n = 262)			Paclitaxel (n = 259)		
Adverse reaction	All grades	Grade 3	Grade 4	All grades	Grade 3	Grade 4
Laboratory[b], hematologic						
Anemia	69%	6%	1%	51%	3%	< 1%
Leukopenia	21%	10%	1%	12%	2%	0%
Neutropenia	69%	31%	17%	31%	4%	7%
Thrombocytopenia	26%	5%	< 1%	7%	< 1%	< 1%
Hepatobiliary						
ALT	18%	5%	< 1%	6%	< 1%	0%
AST	16%	2%	0%	5%	< 1%	0%
Nonlaboratory[c]						
Alopecia	90%	14%	4%	92%	19%	3%
Anorexia	17%	0%	0%	12%	< 1%	0%
Arthralgia	24%	3%	0%	22%	2%	< 1%
Bone pain	11%	2%	0%	10%	< 1%	0%
Constipation	11%	< 1%	0%	12%	0%	0%
Diarrhea	20%	3%	0%	13%	2%	0%
Fatigue	40%	6%	< 1%	28%	1%	< 1%
Fever	13%	< 1%	0%	3%	0%	0%
Myalgia	33%	4%	0%	33%	3%	< 1%
Neuropathy, motor	15%	2%	< 1%	10%	< 1%	0%
Neuropathy, sensory	64%	5%	< 1%	58%	3%	0%
Nausea	50%	1%	0%	31%	2%	0%
Pain, other	11%	< 1%	0%	8%	< 1%	0%
Rash/ Desquamation	11%	< 1%	< 1%	5%	0%	0%
Stomatitis/ Pharyngitis	13%	1%	< 1%	8%	< 1%	0%
Vomiting	29%	2%	0%	15%	2%	0%

[a] Grade based on CTC Version 2.0 (all grades at least 10%).
[b] Regardless of causality.
[c] Nonlaboratory events were graded only if assessed to be possibly drug-related.

The following are the clinically relevant adverse events that occurred in more than 1% and less than 10% (all grades) of patients on either arm. In parentheses are the incidences of Grade 3 and 4 adverse events (gemcitabine plus paclitaxel vs paclitaxel): Febrile neutropenia (5% vs 1.2%), infection (0.8% vs 0.8%), dyspnea (1.9% vs 0%), and allergic reaction/hypersensitivity (0% vs 0.8%).

➤*Postmarketing experience:*

Cardiovascular – CHF and MI have been reported very rarely with the use of gemcitabine. Arrhythmias, predominantly supraventricular in nature, have been reported very rarely.

Dermatologic – Cellulitis and nonserious injection site reactions in the absence of extravasation have been rarely reported.

Hepatic – Serious hepatotoxicity including liver failure and death has been reported very rarely in patients receiving gemcitabine alone or in combination with other potentially hepatotoxic drugs.

Respiratory – Parenchymal toxicity, including interstitial pneumonitis, pulmonary fibrosis, pulmonary edema, and adult respiratory distress syndrome (ARDS), has been reported rarely following 1 or more doses of gemcitabine administered to patients with various malignancies. Some patients experienced the onset of pulmonary symptoms up to 2 weeks after the last gemcitabine dose. Respiratory failure and death occurred very rarely in some patients despite discontinuation of therapy.

Renal – Hemolytic uremic syndrome (HUS) and/or renal failure have been reported following 1 or more doses of gemcitabine. Renal failure leading to death or requiring dialysis, despite discontinuation of therapy, has been rarely reported. The majority of the cases of renal failure leading to death were caused by HUS.

Vascular disorders – Vascular toxicity reported with gemcitabine includes clinical signs of vasculitis, which has been reported very rarely. Gangrene has also been reported very rarely.

Overdosage

There is no known antidote for overdoses of gemcitabine. Myelosuppression, paresthesias, and severe rash were the principal toxicities seen when a single dose as high as 5,700 mg/m^2 was administered by IV infusion over

Pyrimidine Analogs

GEMCITABINE HYDROCHLORIDE — INJECTION

30 minutes every 2 weeks to several patients in a Phase 1 study. In the event of suspected overdose, monitor the patient with appropriate blood counts and give supportive therapy as necessary.

Purine Analogs and Related Agents

CLADRIBINE (2-chlorodeoxyadenosine; CdA)

Rx	**Cladribine** (Bedford)	**Solution for Injection**: 1 mg/ml	9 mg NaCl/ml. In 10 ml fill in a 20 ml single-use vial.
Rx	**Leustatin** (Ortho Biotech)		Preservative free. In 10 ml or 10 ml fill in 20 ml single-use vials.

CLADRIBINE — INJECTION

WARNING

Cladribine should be administered under the supervision of a qualified physician experienced in the use of antineoplastic therapy. Suppression of bone marrow function should be anticipated. This is usually reversible and appears to be dose dependent. Serious neurological toxicity (including irreversible paraparesis and quadraparesis) has been reported in patients who received cladribine by continuous infusion at high doses (4 to 9 times the recommended dose for hairy cell leukemia). Neurologic toxicity appears to demonstrate a dose relationship; however, severe neurological toxicity has been reported rarely following treatment with standard cladribine dosing regimens.

Acute nephrotoxicity has been observed with high doses of cladribine (4 to 9 times the recommended dose for hairy cell leukemia), especially when given concomitantly with other nephrotoxic agents/therapies.

Indications

➤*Hairy cell leukemia:* For the treatment of active hairy cell leukemia as defined by clinically significant anemia, neutropenia, thrombocytopenia or disease-related symptoms.

➤*Unlabeled uses:* Treatment of chronic lymphocytic leukemia; non-Hodgkin's lymphoma; acute myeloid leukemia.

Administration and Dosage

➤*Approved by the FDA:* February 26, 1993.

➤*Usual dose:* The recommended dose and schedule of cladribine for active hairy cell leukemia is as a single course given by continuous infusion for 7 consecutive days at a dose of 0.09 mg/kg/day. Deviations from this dosage regimen are not advised. If the patient does not respond to the initial course of cladribine for hairy cell leukemia, it is unlikely that they will benefit from additional courses. Physicians should consider delaying or discontinuing the drug if neurotoxicity or renal toxicity occurs.

➤*Special risk:* Specific risk factors predisposing to increased toxicity from cladribine have not been defined. In view of the known toxicities of agents of this class, it would be prudent to proceed carefully in patients with known or suspected renal insufficiency or severe bone marrow impairment of any etiology. Patients should be monitored closely for hematologic and non-hematologic toxicity.

➤*Preparation and administration of IV solutions:* Cladribine must be diluted with the designated diluent prior to administration. Since the drug product does not contain any antimicrobial preservative or bacteriostatic agent, aseptic technique and proper environmental precautions must be observed in preparation of cladribine solutions.

To prepare a single daily dose – Add the calculated dose (0.09 mg/kg or 0.09 mL/kg) of cladribine to an infusion bag containing 500 mL of 0.9% Sodium Chloride Injection, USP. Infuse continuously over 24 hours. Repeat daily for a total of 7 consecutive days. The use of 5% dextrose as a diluent is not recommended because of increased degradation of cladribine. Admixtures of cladribine are chemically and physically stable for at least 24 hours at room temperature under normal room fluorescent light in PVC infusion containers. Since limited compatibility data are available, adherence to the recommended diluents and infusion systems is advised.

Method	Dose of cladribine injection	Recommended diluent	Quantity of diluent
24 hour infusion method	1 (day) × 0.09 mg/kg	0.9% sodium chloride injection, USP	500 mL

To prepare a 7-day infusion – The 7-day infusion solution should only be prepared with bacteriostatic 0.9% sodium chloride injection (0.9% benzyl alcohol preserved). In order to minimize the risk of microbial contamination, both cladribine and the diluent should be passed through a sterile 0.22µ disposable hydrophilic syringe filter as each solution is being introduced into the infusion reservoir. First add the calculated dose of cladribine (7 days times 0.09 mg/kg or mL/kg) to the infusion reservoir through the sterile filter. Then add a calculated amount of bacteriostatic 0.9% sodium chloride injection (0.9% benzyl alcohol preserved) also through the filter to bring the total volume of the solution to 100 mL. After completing solution preparation, clamp off the line, disconnect and discard the filter. Aseptically aspirate air bubbles from the reservoir as necessary using the syringe and a dry second sterile filter or a sterile vent filter assembly. Reclamp the line and discard the syringe and filter assembly. Infuse continuously over 7 days. Solutions prepared with bacteriostatic sodium chloride injection for individuals weighing more than 85 kg may have reduced preservative effectiveness due to greater dilution of the benzyl alcohol preservative. Admixtures for the 7-day infusion have demonstrated acceptable chemical and physical stability for at least 7 days in the *SIMS Deltec Medication Cassette Reservoir*.

Method	Dose of cladribine injection	Recommended diluent	Quantity of diluent
7-day infusion method (use sterile 0.22µ filter when preparing infusion solution)	7 (days) × 0.09 mg/kg	Bacteriostatic 0.9% sodium chloride injection, USP (0.9% benzyl alcohol)	quantity required up to 100 mL

IV admixture incompatibility – Because limited compatibility data are available, adherence to the recommended diluents and infusion systems is advised. Solutions containing cladribine should not be mixed with other intravenous drugs or additives or infused simultaneously via a common intravenous line, since compatibility testing has not been performed. Preparations containing benzyl alcohol should not be used in neonates. Benzyl alcohol is a constituent of the recommended diluent for the 7-day infusion solution. Benzyl alcohol has been reported to be associated with a fatal "gasping syndrome" in premature infants.

➤*Storage/Stability:* Care must be taken to ensure the sterility of prepared solutions. Once diluted, solutions of cladribine should be administered promptly or stored in the refrigerator 2° to 8°C (36° to 46° F) for no more than 8 hours prior to start of administration. Vials of cladribine are for single-use only. Any unused portion should be discarded in an appropriate manner (see Handling and disposal).

Parenteral drug products should be inspected visually for particulate matter and discoloration prior to administration, whenever solution and container permit. A precipitate may occur during the exposure of cladribine to low temperatures; it may be resolubilized by allowing the solution to warm naturally to room temperature and by shaking vigorously. Do not heat or microwave.

When stored in refrigerated conditions between 2° to 8°C (36° to 46°F) protected from light, unopened vials of cladribine are stable until the expiration date indicated on the package. Freezing does not adversely affect the solution. If freezing occurs, thaw naturally to room temperature. Do not heat or microwave. Once thawed, the vial of cladribine is stable until expiry if refrigerated. Do not refreeze. Once diluted, solutions containing cladribine should be administered promptly or stored in the refrigerator (2° to 8°C) for no more than 8 hours prior to administration.

Actions

➤*Pharmacology:* The selective toxicity of 2-chloro-2′-deoxy-β-D-adenosine towards certain normal and malignant lymphocyte and monocyte populations is based on the relative activities of deoxycytidine kinase and deoxynucleotidase. Cladribine passively crosses the cell membrane. In cells with a high ratio of deoxycytidine kinase to deoxynucleotidase, it is phosphorylated by deoxycytidine kinase to 2-chloro-2′-deoxy-β-D-adenosine monophosphate (2-CdAMP). Since 2-chloro-2′-deoxy-β-D-adenosine is resistant to deamination by adenosine deaminase and there is little deoxynucleotide deaminase in lymphocytes and monocytes, 2-CdAMP accumulates intracellularly and is subsequently converted into the active triphosphate deoxynucleotide, 2-chloro-2′-deoxy-β-D-adenosine triphosphate (2-CdATP). It is postulated that cells with high deoxycytidine kinase and low deoxynucleotidase activities will be selectively killed by 2-chloro-2′-deoxy-β-D-adenosine as toxic deoxynucleotides accumulate intracellularly.

Cells containing high concentrations of deoxynucleotides are unable to properly repair single-strand DNA breaks. The broken ends of DNA activate the enzyme poly (ADP-ribose) polymerase resulting in NAD and ATP depletion and disruption of cellular metabolism. There is evidence, also, that 2-CdATP is incorporated into the DNA of dividing cells, resulting in impairment of DNA synthesis. Thus, 2-chloro-2′-deoxy-β-D-adenosine can be distinguished from other chemotherapeutic agents affecting purine metabolism in that it is cytotoxic to both actively dividing and quiescent lymphocytes and monocytes, inhibiting both DNA synthesis and repair.

➤*Pharmacokinetics:* In a clinical investigation, 17 patients with hairy cell leukemia and normal renal function were treated for 7 days with the recommended treatment regimen of cladribine injection (0.09 mg/kg/day) by continuous intravenous infusion. The mean steady-state serum concentration was estimated to be 5.7 ng/mL with an estimated systemic clearance of 663.5 mL/hr/kg when cladribine was given by continuous infusion over 7 days. In hairy cell leukemia patients, there does not appear to be a relationship between serum concentrations and ultimate clinical outcome.

In another study, 8 patients with hematologic malignancies received a 2-hour infusion of cladribine injection (0.12 mg/kg). The mean end-of-infusion plasma cladribine concentration was 48 ± 19 ng/mL. For 5 of these patients, the disappearance of cladribine could be described by either a biphasic or triphasic decline. For these patients with normal renal function, the mean terminal half-life was 5.4 hours. Mean values for clearance and steady-state volume of distribution were 978 ± 422 mL/hr/kg and 4.5 ± 2.8 L/kg, respectively.

CLADRIBINE — INJECTION

Plasma concentrations are reported to decline multiexponentially after intravenous infusions with terminal half-lives ranging from approximately 3 to 22 hours. In general, the apparent volume of distribution of cladribine is very large (mean approximately 9 L/kg), indicating an extensive distribution of cladribine in body tissues. The mean half-life of cladribine in leukemic cells has been reported to be 23 hours.

Cladribine penetrates into cerebrospinal fluid. One report indicates that concentrations are approximately 25% of those in plasma.

Cladribine is bound approximately 20% to plasma proteins.

Except for some understanding of the mechanism of cellular toxicity, no other information is available on the metabolism of cladribine in humans. An average of 18% of the administered dose has been reported to be excreted in urine of patients with solid tumors during a 5-day continuous intravenous infusion of 3.5 to 8.1 mg/m²/day of cladribine. The effect of renal and hepatic impairment on the elimination of cladribine has not been investigated in humans.

Contraindications

Hypersensitivity to this drug or any of its components.

Warnings

➤*Bone marrow suppression:* Severe bone marrow suppression, including neutropenia, anemia and thrombocytopenia, has been commonly observed in patients treated with cladribine, especially at high doses. At initiation of treatment, most patients in the clinical studies had hematologic impairment as a manifestation of active hairy cell leukemia. Following treatment with cladribine, further hematologic impairment occurred before recovery of peripheral blood counts began. During the first 2 weeks after treatment initiation, mean platelet count, ANC, and hemoglobin concentration declined and subsequently increased with normalization of mean counts by day 12, week 5 and week 8, respectively. The myelosuppressive effects of cladribine were most notable during the first month following treatment. Forty-four percent (44%) of patients received transfusions with RBCs and 14% received transfusions with platelets during month 1. Careful hematologic monitoring, especially during the first 4 to 8 weeks after treatment with cladribine, is recommended (see Precautions).

➤*Fever:* Fever (greater than or equal to 100°F) was associated with the use of cladribine in approximately two-thirds of patients (131/196) in the first month of therapy. Virtually all of these patients were treated empirically with parenteral antibiotics. Overall, 47% (93/196) of all patients had fever in the setting of neutropenia (ANC less than or equal to 1000), including 62 patients (32%) with severe neutropenia (ie, ANC less than or equal to 500).

Fever was a frequently observed side effect during the first month of study. Since the majority of fevers occurred in neutropenic patients, patients should be closely monitored during the first month of treatment and empiric antibiotics should be initiated as clinically indicated. Although 69% of patients developed fevers, less than ⅓ of febrile events were associated with documented infection. Given the known myelosuppressive effects of cladribine, practitioners should carefully evaluate the risks and benefits of administering this drug to patients with active infections.

➤*Nephrotoxicity/Neurotoxicity:* In a Phase I investigational study using cladribine in high doses (4 to 9 times the recommended dose for hairy cell leukemia) as part of a bone marrow transplant conditioning regimen, which also included high dose cyclophosphamide and total body irradiation, acute nephrotoxicity and delayed onset neurotoxicity were observed. Thirty-one (31) poor-risk patients with drug-resistant acute leukemia in relapse (29 cases) or non-Hodgkins lymphoma (2 cases) received cladribine for 7 to 14 days prior to bone marrow transplantation. During infusion, 8 patients experienced GI symptoms. While the bone marrow was initially cleared of all hematopoietic elements, including tumor cells, leukemia eventually recurred in all treated patients. Within 7 to 13 days after starting treatment with cladribine, 6 patients (19%) developed manifestations of renal dysfunction (eg, acidosis, anuria, elevated serum creatinine) and 5 required dialysis. Several of these patients were also being treated with other medications having known nephrotoxic potential. Renal dysfunction was reversible in 2 of these patients. In the 4 patients whose renal function had not recovered at the time of death, autopsies were performed; in 2 of these, evidence of tubular damage was noted. Eleven (11) patients (35%) experienced delayed onset neurologic toxicity. In the majority, this was characterized by progressive irreversible motor weakness (paraparesis/quadriparesis), of the upper or lower extremities, first noted 35 to 84 days after starting high-dose therapy with cladribine. Noninvasive testing (electromyography and nerve conduction studies) was consistent with demyelinating disease. Severe neurologic toxicity has also been noted with high doses of another drug in this class.

Axonal peripheral polyneuropathy was observed in a dose escalation study at the highest dose levels (approximately 4 times the recommended dose for hairy cell leukemia) in patients not receiving cyclophosphamide or total body irradiation. Severe neurological toxicity has been reported rarely following treatment with standard cladribine dosing regimens.

In patients with hairy cell leukemia treated with the recommended treatment regimen (0.09 mg/kg/day for 7 consecutive days), there have been no reports of nephrologic toxicities.

➤*Death:* Of the 196 hairy cell leukemia patients entered in the 2 trials, there were 8 deaths following treatment. Of these, 6 were of infectious etiology, including 3 pneumonias, and 2 occurred in the first month following cladribine therapy. Of the 8 deaths, 6 occurred in previously treated patients who were refractory to α-interferon.

➤*Mutagenesis:* As expected for compounds in this class, the actions of cladribine yield DNA damage. In mammalian cells in culture, cladribine caused the accumulation of DNA strand breaks. Cladribine was also incorporated into DNA of human lymphoblastic leukemia cells. Cladribine was not mutagenic in vitro (Ames and Chinese hamster ovary cell gene mutation tests) and did not induce unscheduled DNA synthesis in primary rat hepatocyte cultures. However, cladribine was clastogenic both in vitro (chromosome aberrations in Chinese hamster ovary cells) and in vivo (mouse bone marrow micronucleus test).

➤*Fertility impairment:* When administered intravenously to cynomolgus monkeys, cladribine has been shown to cause suppression of rapidly generating cells, including testicular cells. The effect on human fertility is unknown.

➤*Pregnancy: Category D.* Cladribine should not be given during pregnancy. Cladribine is teratogenic in mice and rabbits and consequently has the potential to cause fetal harm when administered to a pregnant woman. A significant increase in fetal variations was observed in mice receiving 1.5 mg/kg/day (4.5 mg/m²) and increased resorptions, reduced litter size and increased fetal malformations were observed when mice received 3 mg/kg/day (9 mg/m²). Fetal death and malformations were observed in rabbits that received 3 mg/kg/day (33 mg/m²). No fetal effects were seen in mice at 0.5 mg/kg/day (1.5 mg/m²) or in rabbits at 1 mg/kg/day (11 mg/m²).

Although there is no evidence of teratogenicity in humans due to cladribine, other drugs which inhibit DNA synthesis (eg, methotrexate and aminopterin) have been reported to be teratogenic in humans. Cladribine has been shown to be embryotoxic in mice when given at doses equivalent to the recommended dose.

There are no adequate and well-controlled studies in pregnant women. If cladribine is used during pregnancy, or if the patient becomes pregnant while taking this drug, the patient should be apprised of the potential hazard to the fetus. Women of child-bearing age should be advised to avoid becoming pregnant.

➤*Lactation:* It is not known whether this drug is excreted in human milk. Because many drugs are excreted in human milk and because of the potential for serious adverse reactions in nursing infants from cladribine, a decision should be made whether to discontinue nursing or discontinue the drug, taking into account the importance of the drug for the mother.

➤*Children:* Safety and effectiveness in pediatric patients have not been established. In a Phase I study involving patients 1 to 21 years old with relapsed acute leukemia, cladribine was given by continuous intravenous infusion in doses ranging from 3 to 10.7 mg/m²/day for 5 days (one-half to twice the dose recommended in hairy cell leukemia). In this study, the dose-limiting toxicity was severe myelosuppression with profound neutropenia and thrombocytopenia. At the highest dose (10.7 mg/m²/day), 3 of 7 patients developed irreversible myelosuppression and fatal systemic bacterial or fungal infections. No unique toxicities were noted in this study.

See Administration and Dosage for more information.

Precautions

➤*Monitoring:* Cladribine is a potent antineoplastic agent with potentially significant toxic side effects. It should be administered only under the supervision of a physician experienced with the use of cancer chemotherapeutic agents. Patients undergoing therapy should be closely observed for signs of hematologic and non-hematologic toxicity. Periodic assessment of peripheral blood counts, particularly during the first 4 to 8 weeks post-treatment, is recommended to detect the development of anemia, neutropenia and thrombocytopenia and for early detection of any potential sequelae (eg, infection or bleeding). As with other potent chemotherapeutic agents, monitoring of renal and hepatic function is also recommended, especially in patients with underlying kidney or liver dysfunction.

➤*Tymor lysis syndrome:* Rare cases of tumor lysis syndrome have been reported in patients treated with cladribine with other hematologic malignancies having a high tumor burden.

➤*Special risk:* See Administration and Dosage for more information.

Drug Interactions

There are no known drug interactions with cladribine. Caution should be exercised if cladribine is administered before, after, or in conjunction with other drugs known to cause immunosuppression or myelosuppression.

Adverse Reactions

Most frequent – Safety data are based on 196 patients with hairy cell leukemia: The original cohort of 124 patients plus an additional 72 patients enrolled at the same 2 centers after the original enrollment cutoff. In month 1 of the hairy cell leukemia clinical trials, severe neutropenia was noted in 70% of patients, fever in 69%, and infection was documented in 28%. Other adverse experiences reported frequently during the first 14 days after initiating treatment included fatigue (45%), nausea (28%), rash (27%), headache (22%) and injection site reactions (19%). Most nonhematologic adverse experiences were mild to moderate in severity.

Myelosuppression – Myelosuppression was frequently observed during the first month after starting treatment. Neutropenia (ANC less than 500 times 10^6/L) was noted in 70% of patients, compared with 26% in whom it was present initially. Severe anemia (hemoglobin less than 8.5 g/dL) developed in 37% of patients, compared with 10% initially and thrombocytopenia (platelets less than 20 times 10^9/L) developed in 12% of patients, compared to 4% in whom it was noted initially.

Infection/Fever – During the first month, 54 of 196 patients (28%) exhibited documented evidence of infection. Serious infections (eg, septicemia, pneumonia) were reported in 6% of all patients; the remainder were mild or moderate. Several deaths were attributable to infection and/or complications

CLADRIBINE — INJECTION

related to the underlying disease. During the second month, the overall rate of documented infection was 6%; these infections were mild to moderate and no severe systemic infections were seen. After the third month, the monthly incidence of infection was either less than or equal to that of the months immediately preceding cladribine therapy.

During the first month, 11% of patients experienced severe fever (ie, greater than or equal to 104°F). Documented infections were noted in fewer than one-third of febrile episodes. Of the 196 patients studied, 19 were noted to have a documented infection in the month prior to treatment. In the month following treatment, there were 54 episodes of documented infection: 23 (42%) were bacterial, 11 (20%) were viral and 11 (20%) were fungal. Seven (7) of 8 documented episodes of herpes zoster occurred during the month following treatment. Fourteen (14) of 16 episodes of documented fungal infections occurred in the first 2 months following treatment. Virtually all of these patients were treated empirically with antibiotics.

Prolonged depressed CD4 counts – Analysis of lymphocyte subsets indicates that treatment with cladribine is associated with prolonged depression of the CD4 counts. Prior to treatment, the mean CD4 count was 766/mcL. The mean CD4 count nadir, which occurred 4 to 6 months following treatment, was 272/mcL. Fifteen (15) months after treatment, mean CD4 counts remained below 500/mcL. CD8 counts behaved similarly, though increasing counts were observed after 9 months. The clinical significance of the prolonged CD4 lymphopenia is unclear.

Prolonged bone marrow hypocellularity – Another event of unknown clinical significance includes the observation of prolonged bone marrow hypocellularity. Bone marrow cellularity of less than 35% was noted after 4 months in 42 of 124 patients (34%) treated in the 2 pivotal trials. This hypocellularity was noted as late as day 1010. It is not known whether the hypocellularity is the result of disease related marrow fibrosis or if it is the result of cladribine toxicity. There was no apparent clinical effect on the peripheral blood counts.

➤*Dermatologic:* The vast majority of rashes were mild and occurred in patients who were receiving or had recently been treated with other medications (eg, allopurinol or antibiotics) known to cause rash.

➤*GI:* Most episodes of nausea were mild, not accompanied by vomiting, and did not require treatment with antiemetics. In patients requiring antiemetics, nausea was easily controlled, most frequently with chlorpromazine.

➤*Adverse reactions in greater than 5% of patients:* Adverse reactions reported during the first 2 weeks following treatment initiation (regardless of relationship to drug) by greater than 5% of patients included:

Cardiovascular – Edema (6%), tachycardia (6%)

CNS – Headache (22%), dizziness (9%), insomnia (7%).

Dermatologic – Rash (27%), injection site reactions (19%), pruritus (6%), pain (6%), erythema (6%).

GI – Nausea (28%), decreased appetite (17%), vomiting (13%), diarrhea (10%), constipation (9%), abdominal pain (6%).

Hematologic / Lymphatic – Purpura (10%), petechiae (8%), epistaxis (5%).

Musculoskeletal – Myalgia (7%), arthralgia (5%).

Respiratory – Abnormal breath sounds (11%), cough (10%), abnormal chest sounds (9%), shortness of breath (7%).

Miscellaneous – Fever (69%), fatigue (45%), chills (9%), asthenia (9%), diaphoresis (9%), malaise (7%), trunk pain (6%).

➤*Miscellaneous:* Adverse experiences related to intravenous administration included injection site reactions (9%) (ie, redness, swelling, pain), thrombosis (2%), phlebitis (2%) and a broken catheter (1%). These appear to be related to the infusion procedure and/or indwelling catheter, rather than the medication or the vehicle.

From day 15 to the last follow-up visit, the only events reported by greater than or equal to 5% of patients were fatigue (11%), rash (10%), headache (7%), cough (7%), and malaise (5%).

➤*Postmarketing reports:*

CNS – Neurological toxicity; however, severe neurotoxicity has been reported rarely following treatment with standard cladribine dosing regimens.

Dermatologic – Urticaria, hypereosinophilia. In isolated cases Stevens-Johnson and toxic epidermal necrolysis have been reported in patients who were receiving or had recently been treated with other medications (eg, allopurinol or antibiotics) known to cause these syndromes.

Hematologic – Bone marrow suppression with prolonged pancytopenia, including some reports of aplastic anemia; hemolytic anemia, which was reported in patients with lymphoid malignancies, occurring within the first few weeks following treatment.

Hepatic – Reversible, generally mild increases in bilirubin and transaminases.

Immunologic – Opportunistic infections have occurred in the acute phase of treatment due to the immunosuppression mediated by cladribine.

Respiratory – Pulmonary interstitial infiltrates; in most cases, an infectious etiology was identified.

Overdosage

High doses of cladribine have been associated with: irreversible neurologic toxicity (paraparesis/quadriparesis), acute nephrotoxicity, and severe bone marrow suppression resulting in neutropenia, anemia and thrombocytopenia. There is no known specific antidote to overdosage. Treatment of overdosage consists of discontinuation of cladribine, careful observation and appropriate supportive measures. It is not known whether the drug can be removed from the circulation by dialysis or hemofiltration.

FLUDARABINE PHOSPHATE

Rx	**Fludarabine Phosphate** (Sicor)	**Injection**: 25 mg/mL	Preservative free. In single-dose vials.[a]
Rx	**Fludara** (Berlex)	**Powder for Injection, lyophilized**: 50 mg	In single-dose vials.[b]

[a] With 25 mg/mL mannitol and sodium hydroxide.

[b] With 50 mg mannitol and sodium hydroxide.

FLUDARABINE PHOSPHATE — INJECTION

WARNING

Fludarabine phosphate should be administered under the supervision of a qualified physician experienced in the use of antineoplastic therapy. Fludarabine phosphate can severely suppress bone marrow function. When used at high doses in dose-ranging studies in patients with acute leukemia, fludarabine was associated with severe neurologic effects, including blindness, coma, and death. This severe central nervous system toxicity occurred in 36% of patients treated with doses ≈ 4 times > (96 mg/m²/day for 5 to 7 days) the recommended dose. Similar severe central nervous system toxicity has been rarely (≤ 0.2%) reported in patients treated at doses in the range of the dose recommended for chronic lymphocytic leukemia.

Instances of life-threatening and sometimes fatal autoimmune hemolytic anemia have been reported to occur after 1 or more cycles of treatment with fludarabine. Patients undergoing treatment with fludarabine phosphate should be evaluated and closely monitored for hemolysis.

In a clinical investigation using fludarabine phosphate for injection in combination with pentostatin (dexoxycoformycin) for the treatment of refractory chronic lymphocytic leukemia (CLL), there was an unacceptably high incidence of fatal pulmonary toxicity. Therefore, the use of fludarabine phosphate in combination with pentostatin is not recommended.

Indications

➤*B-cell chronic lymphocytic leukemia:* For the treatment of patients with B-cell chronic lymphocytic leukemia (CLL) who have not responded to or whose disease has progressed during treatment with at least 1 standard alkylating-agent containing regimen. The safety and effectiveness of fludarabine in previously untreated or non-refractory patients with CLL have not been established.

➤*Unlabeled uses:* Treatment of non-Hodgkin lymphoma; may be used in combination therapy for the treatment of primary resistant or relapsing acute myelogenous leukemia (AML), acute lymphoblastic leukemia (ALL), and secondary AML.

Administration and Dosage

➤*Approved by the FDA:* April 1991.

➤*Usual dose:* 25 mg/m² administered intravenously over a period of approximately 30 minutes daily for 5 consecutive days. Each 5 day course of treatment should commence every 28 days. Dosage may be decreased or delayed based on evidence of hematologic or nonhematologic toxicity. Physicians should consider delaying or discontinuing the drug if neurotoxicity occurs.

Special risk – A number of clinical settings may predispose to increased toxicity from fludarabine. These include advanced age, renal insufficiency, and bone marrow impairment. Such patients should be monitored closely for excessive toxicity and the dose modified accordingly.

Duration – The optimal duration of treatment has not been clearly established. It is recommended that 3 additional cycles of fludarabine be administered following the achievement of a maximal response and then the drug should be discontinued.

➤*Preparation of solutions:* Fludarabine phosphate should be prepared for parenteral use by aseptically adding Sterile Water for Injection USP. When reconstituted with 2 mL of Sterile Water for Injection, USP, the solid cake should fully dissolve in 15 seconds or less; each mL of the resulting solution will contain 25 mg of fludarabine phosphate, 25 mg of mannitol, and sodium hydroxide to adjust the pH to 7.7. The pH range for the final product is 7.2 to 8.2. In clinical studies, the product has been diluted in 100 cc or 125 cc of 5% Dextrose Injection USP or 0.9% Sodium Chloride USP.

Reconstituted fludarabine phosphate contains no antimicrobial preservative and thus should be used within 8 hours of reconstitution. Care must be taken to assure the sterility of prepared solutions. Parenteral drug products should be inspected visually for particulate matter and discoloration prior to administration.

FLUDARABINE PHOSPHATE — INJECTION

➤*Handling and disposal:* Caution should be exercised in the handling and preparation of fludarabine solution. The use of latex gloves and safety glasses is recommended to avoid exposure in case of breakage of the vial or other accidental spillage. If the solution contacts the skin or mucous membranes, wash thoroughly with soap and water; rinse eyes thoroughly with plain water. Avoid exposure by inhalation or by direct contact of the skin or mucous membranes.

➤*Storage/Stability:* Store under refrigeration, between 2° to 8°C (36° to 46°F).

Actions

➤*Pharmacology:* Fludarabine phosphate is rapidly dephosphorylated to 2-fluoro-ara-A and then phosphorylated intracellularly by deoxycytidine kinase to the active triphosphate, 2-fluoro-ara-ATP. This metabolite appears to act by inhibiting DNA polymerase alpha, ribonucleotide reductase, and DNA primase, thus inhibiting DNA synthesis. The mechanism of action of this antimetabolite is not completely characterized and may be multi-faceted.

➤*Pharmacokinetics:* Phase I studies in humans have demonstrated that fludarabine phosphate is rapidly converted to the active metabolite, 2-fluoro-ara-A, within minutes after intravenous infusion. Consequently, clinical pharmacology studies have focused on 2-fluoro-ara-A pharmacokinetics. In a study with 4 patients treated with 25 mg/m^2/day for 5 days, the half-life of 2-fluoro-ara-A was approximately 10 hours. The mean total plasma clearance was 8.9 L/hr/m^2 and the mean volume of distribution was 98 L/m^2. Approximately 23% of the dose was excreted in the urine as unchanged 2-fluoro-ara-A. The mean C_{max} after the day 1 dose was 0.57 mcg/mL and after the day 5 dose was 0.54 mcg/mL. No information is available on pharmacokinetic parameters, other than C_{max}, following the day 5 dose of 25 mg/m^2. Total body clearance of 2-fluoro-ara-A has been shown to be inversely correlated with serum creatinine, suggesting renal elimination of the compound.

A correlation was noted between the degree of absolute granulocyte count nadir and increased area under the concentration time curve (AUC).

Contraindications

Hypersensitivity to this drug or its components.

Warnings

➤*Dose-dependent toxicity:* There are clear dose dependent toxic effects seen with fludarabine phosphate. Dose levels ≈ 4 times > (96 mg/m^2/day for 5 to 7 days) that recommended for CLL (25 mg/m^2/day for 5 days) were associated with a syndrome characterized by delayed blindness, coma, and death. Symptoms appeared from 21 to 60 days following the last dose. Thirteen of 36 patients (36%) who received fludarabine at high doses (96 mg/m^2/day for 5 to 7 days) developed this severe neurotoxicity. This syndrome has been reported rarely in patients treated with doses in the range of the recommended CLL dose of 25 mg/m^2/day for 5 days every 28 days. The effect of chronic administration of fludarabine phosphate on the central nervous system is unknown, however, patients have received the recommended dose for up to 15 courses of therapy.

➤*Hematologic effects:* Severe bone marrow suppression, notably anemia, thrombocytopenia, and neutropenia has been reported in patients treated with fludarabine. In a phase I study in solid tumor patients, the median time to nadir counts was 13 days (range, 3 to 25 days) for granulocytes and 16 days (range, 2 to 32) for platelets. Most patients had hematologic impairment at baseline either as a result of disease or as a result of prior myelosuppressive therapy. Cumulative myelosuppression may be seen. While chemotherapy-induced myelosuppression is often reversible, administration of fludarabine requires careful hematologic monitoring.

Instances of life-threatening and sometimes fatal autoimmune hemolytic anemia have been reported to occur after 1 or more cycles of treatment with fludarabine in patients with or without a history of autoimmune hemolytic anemia or a positive Coombs' test and who may or may not be in remission from their disease. Steroids may or may not be effective in controlling these hemolytic episodes. The majority of patients rechallenged with fludarabine phosphate developed a recurrence in the hemolytic process. The mechanism(s) which predispose patients to the development of this complication has not been identified. Patients undergoing treatment with fludarabine phosphate should be evaluated and closely monitored for hemolysis.

Transfusion-associated graft-versus-host disease has been observed rarely after transfusion of non-irradiated blood in fludarabine treated patients. Consideration should, therefore, be given to the use of irradiated blood products in those patients requiring transfusions while undergoing treatment with fludarabine.

➤*Pulmonary toxicity:* In a clinical investigation using fludarabine phosphate in combination with pentostatin (deoxycoformycin) for the treatment of refractory chronic lymphocytic leukemia (CLL), there was an unacceptably high incidence of fatal pulmonary toxicity. Therefore, the use of fludarabine phosphate in combination with pentostatin is not recommended.

➤*Fatalities:* Of the 133 CLL patients in the 2 trials, there were 29 fatalities during study. Approximately 50% of the fatalities were due to infection and 25% due to progressive disease.

➤*Renal function impairment:* There are inadequate data on dosing of patients with renal insufficiency. Fludarabine phosphate must be administered cautiously in patients with renal insufficiency. The total body clearance of 2-fluoro-ara-A has been shown to be inversely correlated with serum creatinine, suggesting renal elimination of the compound.

➤*Mutagenesis:* Fludarabine phosphate has been shown to be nonmutagenic to several strains of *Salmonella typhimurium*, including TA-98, TA-100, TA-1535, and TA-1537. In addition, fludarabine phosphate was nonmutagenic to Chinese hamster ovary (CHO) cells at the hypoxanthine-guaninephosphoribosyltransferase (HGPRT) locus under both activated and non-activated metabolic conditions. Chromosomal aberrations were observed in an in vitro assay using CHO cells under metabolically activated conditions. Fludarabine phosphate was determined to cause increased sister chromatid exchanges using an in vitro sister chromatid exchange (SCE) assay under both metabolically activated and non-activated conditions. In addition, fludarabine phosphate has also been shown to be mutagenic as indicated by an increase in the number of micronucleated erthrocytes in the in vivo mouse micronucleus test at doses up to 1000 mg/kg.

➤*Fertility impairment:* Studies in mice, rats and dogs have demonstrated dose-related adverse effects on the male reproductive system. Observations consisted of a decrease in mean testicular weights in mice and rats with a trend toward decreased testicular weights in dogs and degeneration and necrosis of spermatogenic epithelium of the testes in mice, rats and dogs. The possible adverse effects on fertility in humans have not been adequately evaluated.

➤*Pregnancy: Category D.* Fludarabine phosphate may cause fetal harm when administered to a pregnant woman. Fludarabine phosphate was teratogenic in rats and in rabbits. Fludarabine phosphate was administered intravenously at doses of 0, 1, 10 or 30 mg/kg/day to pregnant rats on days 6 to 15 of gestation. At 10 and 30 mg/kg/day in rats, there was an increased incidence of various skeletal malformations. Fludarabine phosphate was administered intravenously at doses of 0, 1, 5 or 8 mg/kg/day to pregnant rabbits on days 6 to 15 of gestation. Dose-related teratogenic effects manifested by external deformities and skeletal malformations were observed in the rabbits at 5 and 8 mg/kg/day. Drug-related deaths or toxic effects on maternal and fetal weights were not observed. There are no adequate and well-controlled studies in pregnant women.

If fludarabine is used during pregnancy, or if the patient becomes pregnant while taking this drug, the patient should be apprised of the potential hazard to the fetus. Women of childbearing potential should be advised to avoid becoming pregnant.

➤*Lactation:* It is not known whether this drug is excreted in human milk. Because many drugs are excreted in human milk and because of the potential for serious adverse reactions in nursing infants from fludarabine, a decision should be made to discontinue nursing or discontinue the drug, taking into account the importance of the drug for the mother.

➤*Children:* The safety and effectiveness of fludarabine phosphate in children have not been established.

Precautions

➤*Monitoring:* During treatment, the patient's hematologic profile (particularly neutrophils and platelets) should be monitored regularly to determine the degree of hematopoietic suppression.

Hematologic toxicity – Fludarabine phosphate is a potent antineoplastic agent with potentially significant toxic side effects. Patients undergoing therapy should be closely observed for signs of hematologic and nonhematologic toxicity. Periodic assessment of peripheral blood counts is recommended to detect the development of anemia, neutropenia, and thrombocytopenia.

➤*Tumor lysis syndrome:* Tumor lysis syndrome associated with fludarabine treatment has been reported in CLL patients with large tumor burdens. Since fludarabine injection can induce a response as early as the first week of treatment, precautions should be taken in those patients at risk of developing this complication.

Drug Interactions

➤*Pentostatin:* See Warnings for more information.

Adverse Reactions

The most common adverse events include myelosuppression (neutropenia, thrombocytopenia, and anemia), fever and chills, infection, and nausea and vomiting. Other commonly reported events include malaise, fatigue, anorexia, and weakness. Serious opportunistic infections have occurred in CLL patients treated with fludarabine phosphate. The most frequently reported adverse events and those reactions which are more clearly related to the drug are arranged below according to body system. More than 3000 patients received fludarabine phospate in studies of other leukemias, lymphomas, and other solid tumors. The spectrum of adverse effects reported in these studies was consistent with the data below.

➤*Cardiovascular:* Edema has been frequently reported. One patient developed a pericardial effusion possibly related to treatment with fludarabine. No other severe cardiovascular events were considered to be drug related.

➤*CNS:* Objective weakness, agitation, confusion, visual disturbances, and coma have occurred in CLL patients treated with fludarabine phosphate at the recommended dose. Peripheral neuropathy has been observed in patients treated with fludarabine phosphate and 1 case of wrist-drop was reported.

➤*Dermatologic:* Skin toxicity, consisting primarily of skin rashes, has been reported in patients treated with fludarabine phosphate. The following data are derived from the 133 patients with CLL who received fludarabine in the MDAH and SWOG studies.

➤*GI:* Gastrointestinal disturbances such as nausea and vomiting, anorexia, diarrhea, stomatitis, and gastrointestinal bleeding have been reported in patients treated with fludarabine phosphate.

FLUDARABINE PHOSPHATE — INJECTION

➤*GU:* Rare cases of hemorrhagic cystitis have been reported in patients treated with fludarabine phosphate.

➤*Hematologic:* Hematologic events (neutropenia, thrombocytopenia, or anemia) were reported in the majority of CLL patients treated with fludarabine. During fludarabine treatment of 133 patients with CLL, the absolute neutrophil count decreased to < 500/mm^3 in 59% of patients, hemoglobin decreased from pretreatment values by at least 2 grams percent in 60%, and platelet count decreased from pretreatment values by at least 50% in 55%. Myelosuppression may be severe and cumulative. Bone marrow fibrosis occurred in 1 CLL patient treated with fludarabine phosphate.

See Warnings for more information.

➤*Metabolic:* Tumor lysis syndrome has been reported in CLL patients treated with fludarabine phosphate. This complication may include hyperuricemia, hyperphosphatemia, hypocalcemia, metabolic acidosis, hyperkalemia, hematuria, urate crystalluria, and renal failure. The onset of this syndrome may be heralded by flank pain and hematuria.

➤*Pulmonary:* Pneumonia, a frequent manifestation of infection in CLL patients, occurred in 16% and 22% of those treated with fludarabine phosphate in the MDAH and SWOG studies, respectively. Pulmonary hypersensitivity reactions to fludarabine characterized by dyspnea, cough, and interstitial pulmonary infiltrate have been observed.

➤*Adverse reactions derived from MDAH and SWOG studies:* Data in the following table are derived from the 133 patients with CLL who received fludarabine phosphate for injection in the MDAH and SWOG studies.

Percent of CLL patients reporting non-hematologic adverse reactions

Body system/Adverse reaction	MDAH (n = 101)	SWOG (n = 32)
Any adverse reaction	88%	91%
Cardiovascular	12%	38%
Edema	8%	19%
Angina	0%	6%
Congestive heart failure	0%	3%
Arrhythmia	0%	3%
Supraventricular tachycardia	0%	3%
Myocardial infarction	0%	3%
Deep venous thrombosis	1%	3%
Phlebitis	1%	3%
Transient ischemic attack	1%	0%
Aneurysm	1%	0%
Cerebrovascular accident	0%	3%
CNS	21%	69%
Weakness	9%	65%
Paresthesia	4%	12%
Headache	3%	0%
Visual disturbance	3%	15%
Hearing loss	2%	6%
Sleep disorder	1%	3%
Depression	1%	0%
Cerebellar syndromes	1%	0%
Impaired mentation	1%	0%
Dermatologic	17%	18%
Rash	15%	15%
Pruritus	1%	3%
Seborrhea	1%	0%
GI	46%	63%
Nausea/vomiting	36%	31%
Diarrhea	15%	13%
Anorexia	7%	34%
Stomatitis	9%	0%
GI bleeding	3%	13%
Esophagitis	3%	0%
Mucositis	2%	0%
Liver failure	1%	0%
Abnormal liver function test	1%	3%
Cholelithiasis	0%	3%
Constipation	1%	3%
Dysphagia	1%	0%
GU	12%	22%
Dysuria	4%	3%
Urinary infection	2%	15%
Hematuria	2%	3%
Renal failure	1%	0%
Abnormal renal function test	1%	0%
Proteinuria	1%	0%
Hesitancy	0%	3%
Musculoskeletal	7%	16%
Myalgia	4%	16%
Osteoporosis	2%	0%
Arthralgia	1%	0%
Tumor lysis syndrome	1%	0%
Respiratory	35%	69%
Cough	10%	44%
Pneumonia	16%	22%
Dyspnea	9%	22%
Sinusitis	5%	0%
Pharyngitis	0%	9%
Upper respiratory tract infection	2%	16%
Allergic pneumonitis	0%	6%
Epistaxis	1%	0%
Hemoptysis	1%	6%
Bronchitis	1%	0%
Hypoxia	1%	0%
Miscellaneous	72%	84%
Fever	60%	69%
Chills	11%	19%
Fatigue	10%	38%
Infection	33%	44%
Pain	20%	22%
Malaise	8%	6%
Diaphoresis	1%	13%
Alopecia	0%	3%
Anaphylaxis	1%	0%
Hemorrhage	1%	0%
Hyperglycemia	1%	6%
Dehydration	1%	0%

Overdosage

➤*Symptoms:* High doses of fludarabine phosphate have been associated with an irreversible central nervous system toxicity characterized by delayed blindness, coma, and death. High doses are also associated with severe thrombocytopenia and neutropenia due to bone marrow suppression.

➤*Treatment:* There is no known specific antidote for fludarabine phosphate overdosage. Treatment consists of drug discontinuation and supportive therapy.

MERCAPTOPURINE (6-Mercaptopurine; 6-MP)

Rx	**Mercaptopurine** (Par)	**Tablets**: 50 mg	Lactose. (P02). Lt. yellow to off-white, diamond shape, scored. In 60s.
Rx	**Purinethol** (GlaxoSmithKline)		(Purinethol O4A). Off-white, scored. In 25s and 250s.

MERCAPTOPURINE — ORAL

WARNING

Mercaptopurine is a potent drug. It should not be used unless a diagnosis of acute lymphatic leukemia has been adequately established, and the responsible physician is knowledgeable in assessing response to chemotherapy.

Indications

➤*Acute lymphatic leukemia:* For remission induction and maintenance therapy of acute lymphatic leukemia. The response to this agent depends upon the particular subclassification of acute lymphatic leukemia and the age of the patient (pediatric patient or adult).

Given as a single agent for remission induction, mercaptopurine induces complete remission in approximately 25% of pediatric patients and approximately 10% of adults. However, reliance upon mercaptopurine alone is not justified for initial remission induction of acute lymphatic leukemia, since combination chemotherapy with vincristine, prednisone, and L-asparaginase results in more frequent complete remission induction than with mercaptopurine alone or in combination. The duration of complete remission induced in acute lymphatic leukemia is so brief without the use of maintenance therapy that some form of drug therapy is considered essential. Mercaptopurine, as a single agent, is capable of significantly prolonging complete remission duration; however, combination therapy has produced remission duration longer than that achieved with mercaptopurine alone.

➤*Acute myelogenous (and acute myelomonocytic) leukemia:* As a single agent, mercaptopurine will induce complete remission in approximately 10% of pediatric patients and adults with acute myelogenous leukemia or its subclassifications. These results are inferior to those achieved with combination chemotherapy employing optimum treatment schedules.

Administration and Dosage

➤*Induction therapy:* The dosage which will be tolerated and effective varies from patient to patient, and, therefore, careful titration is necessary to obtain the optimum therapeutic effect without incurring excessive, unintended toxicity. The usual initial dosage for pediatric patients and adults is 2.5 mg/kg of body weight per day (100 to 200 mg in the average adult and 50 mg in an average 5-year-old child). Pediatric patients with acute leukemia have tolerated this dose without difficulty in most cases; it may be continued daily for several weeks or more in some patients. If, after 4 weeks at this dosage, there is no clinical improvement and no definite evidence of leukocyte or platelet depression, the dosage may be increased up to 5 mg/kg daily. A dosage of 2.5 mg/kg/day may result in a rapid fall in leukocyte count within 1 to 2 weeks in some adults with acute lymphatic leukemia and high total leukocyte counts.

The total daily dosage may be given at 1 time. It is calculated to the nearest multiple of 25 mg. The dosage of mercaptopurine should be reduced to one-third to one-fourth of the usual dose if allopurinol is given concurrently. Because the drug may have a delayed action, it should be discontinued at the first sign of an abnormally large or rapid fall in the leukocyte or platelet count. If subsequently the leukocyte count or platelet count remains constant for 2 or 3 days, or rises, treatment may be resumed.

➤*Maintenance therapy:* Once a complete hematologic remission is obtained, maintenance therapy is considered essential. Maintenance doses will vary from patient to patient. A usual daily maintenance dose of mercaptopurine is 1.5 to 2.5 mg/kg/day as a single dose. It is to be emphasized that in pediatric patients with acute lymphatic leukemia in remission, superior results have been obtained when mercaptopurine has been combined with other agents (most frequently with methotrexate) for remission maintenance. Mercaptopurine should rarely be relied upon as a single agent for the maintenance of remissions induced in acute leukemia.

➤*Storage/Stability:* Store at 15° to 25°C (59° to 77°F) in a dry place.

Actions

➤*Pharmacology:* Mercaptopurine competes with hypoxanthine and guanine for the enzyme hypoxanthine-guanine phosphoribosyltransferase (HGPRTase) and is itself converted to thioinosinic acid (TIMP). This intracellular nucleotide inhibits several reactions involving inosinic acid (IMP), including the conversion of IMP to xanthylic acid (XMP) and the conversion of IMP to adenylic acid (AMP) via adenylosuccinate (SAMP). In addition, 6-methylthioinosinate (MTIMP) is formed by the methylation of TIMP. Both TIMP and MTIMP have been reported to inhibit glutamine-5-phosphoribosylpyrophosphate amidotransferase, the first enzyme unique to the de novo pathway for purine ribonucleotide synthesis.

Experiments indicate that radiolabeled mercaptopurine may be recovered from the DNA in the form of deoxythioguanosine. Some mercaptopurine is converted to nucleotide derivatives of 6-thioguanine (6-TG) by the sequential actions of inosinate (IMP) dehydrogenase and xanthylate (XMP) aminase, converting TIMP to thioguanylic acid (TGMP).

Animal tumors that are resistant to mercaptopurine often have lost the ability to convert mercaptopurine to TIMP. However, it is clear that resistance to mercaptopurine may be acquired by other means as well, particularly in human leukemias.

➤*Pharmacokinetics:*

Absorption – Clinical studies have shown that the absorption of an oral dose of mercaptopurine in humans is incomplete and variable, averaging ≈ 50% of the administered dose. The factors influencing absorption are unknown.

Distribution – IV administration of an investigational preparation of mercaptopurine revealed a plasma half-disappearance time of 21 minutes in pediatric patients and 47 minutes in adults. The volume of distribution usually exceeded that of the total body water.

There is negligible entry of mercaptopurine into cerebrospinal fluid.

Plasma protein binding averages 19% over the concentration range 10 to 50 mcg/mL (a concentration only achieved by IV administration of mercaptopurine at doses exceeding 5 to 10 mg/kg).

Metabolism/Excretion – Following the oral administration of ^{35}S-6-mercaptopurine in 1 subject, a total of 46% of the dose could be accounted for in the urine (as parent drug and metabolites) in the first 24 hours. Metabolites of mercaptopurine were found in urine within the first 2 hours after administration. Radioactivity (in the form of sulfate) could be found in the urine for weeks afterwards. Monitoring of plasma levels of mercaptopurine during therapy is of questionable value. There is technical difficulty in determining plasma concentrations which are seldom greater than 1 to 2 mcg/mL after a therapeutic oral dose. More significantly, mercaptopurine enters rapidly into the anabolic and catabolic pathways for purines, and the active intracellular metabolites have appreciably longer half-lives than the parent drug. The biochemical effects of a single dose of mercaptopurine are evident long after the parent drug has disappeared from plasma. Because of this rapid metabolism of mercaptopurine to active intracellular derivatives, hemodialysis would not be expected to appreciably reduce toxicity of the drug. There is no known pharmacologic antagonist to the biochemical actions of mercaptopurine in vivo.

Contraindications

Mercaptopurine should not be used unless a diagnosis of acute lymphatic leukemia has been adequately established and the responsible physician is knowledgeable in assessing response to chemotherapy.

Mercaptopurine should not be used in patients whose disease has demonstrated prior resistance to this drug. In animals and humans, there is usually complete cross-resistance between mercaptopurine and thioguanine.

Warnings

➤*Bone marrow toxicity:* The most consistent, dose-related toxicity is bone marrow suppression. This may be manifest by anemia, leukopenia, thrombocytopenia, or any combination of these. Any of these findings may also reflect progression of the underlying disease. Since mercaptopurine may have a delayed effect, it is important to withdraw the medication temporarily at the first sign of an abnormally large fall in any of the formed elements of the blood.

There are rare individuals with an inherited deficiency of the enzyme thiopurine methyltransferase (TPMT) who may be unusually sensitive to the myelosuppressive effects of mercaptopurine and prone to developing rapid bone marrow suppression following the initiation of treatment. Substantial dosage reductions may be required to avoid the development of life-threatening bone marrow suppression in these patients. This toxicity may be more profound in patients treated with concomitant allopurinol (see Drug Interactions).

➤*Immunosuppression:* Mercaptopurine recipients may manifest decreased cellular hypersensitivities and impaired allograft rejection. Induction of immunity to infectious agents or vaccines will be subnormal in these patients; the degree of immunosuppression will depend on antigen dose and temporal relationship to drug. This immunosuppressive effect should be carefully considered with regard to intercurrent infections and risk of subsequent neoplasia.

➤*Renal function impairment:* It is probably advisable to start with smaller dosages in patients with impaired renal function, since the latter might result in slower elimination of the drug and metabolites and a greater cumulative effect.

➤*Hepatic function impairment:* Mercaptopurine is heptotoxic in animals and humans. A small number of deaths have been reported which may have been attributed to hepatic necrosis due to administration of mercaptopurine. Hepatic injury can occur with any dosage, but seems to occur with more frequency when doses of 2.5 mg/kg/day are exceeded. The histologic pattern of mercaptopurine hepatotoxicity includes features of both intrahepatic cholestasis and parenchymal cell necrosis, either of which may predominate. It is not clear how much of the hepatic damage is due to direct toxicity from the drug and how much may be due to a hypersensitivity reaction. In some patients jaundice has cleared following withdrawal of mercaptopurine and reappeared with its reintroduction.

Monitoring of serum transaminase levels, alkaline phosphatase, and bilirubin levels may allow early detection of hepatotoxicity. It is advisable to monitor these liver function tests at weekly intervals when first beginning therapy and at monthly intervals thereafter. Liver function tests may be advisable more frequently in patients who are receiving mercaptopurine with other hepatotoxic drugs or with known preexisting liver disease.

MERCAPTOPURINE — ORAL

The concomitant administration of mercaptopurine with other hepatotoxic agents requires especially careful clinical and biochemical monitoring of hepatic function. Combination therapy involving mercaptopurine with other drugs not felt to be hepatotoxic should nevertheless be approached with caution. The combination of mercaptopurine with doxorubicin was reported to be hepatotoxic in 19 of 20 patients undergoing remission-induction therapy for leukemia resistant to previous therapy.

The hepatotoxicity has been associated in some cases with anorexia, diarrhea, jaundice, and ascites. Hepatic encephalopathy has occurred.

The onset of clinical jaundice, hepatomegaly, or anorexia with tenderness in the right hypochondrium are immediate indications for withholding mercaptopurine until the exact etiology can be identified. Likewise, any evidence of deterioration in liver function studies, toxic hepatitis, or biliary stasis should prompt discontinuation of the drug and a search for an etiology of the hepatotoxicity.

➤*Carcinogenesis:* Carcinogenic potential exists in humans, but the extent of the risk is unknown.

➤*Mutagenesis:* Mercaptopurine causes chromosomal aberrations in animals and humans and induces dominant-lethal mutations in male mice.

➤*Fertility impairment:* In mice, surviving female offspring of mothers who received chronic low doses of mercaptopurine during pregnancy were found sterile, or if they became pregnant, had smaller litters and more dead fetuses as compared to control animals.

➤*Pregnancy: Category D.* Mercaptopurine can cause fetal harm when administered to a pregnant woman. Women receiving mercaptopurine in the first trimester of pregnancy have an increased incidence of abortion; the risk of malformation in offspring surviving first trimester exposure is not accurately known. In a series of 28 women receiving mercaptopurine after the first trimester of pregnancy, 3 mothers died undelivered, 1 delivered a stillborn child, and 1 aborted; there were no cases of macroscopically abnormal fetuses. Since such experience cannot exclude the possibility of fetal damage, mercaptopurine should be used during pregnancy only if the benefit clearly justifies the possible risk to the fetus, and particular caution should be given to the use of mercaptopurine in the first trimester of pregnancy.

There are no adequate and well-controlled studies in pregnant women. If this drug is used during pregnancy or if the patient becomes pregnant while taking the drug, the patient should be apprised of the potential hazard to the fetus. Women of childbearing potential should be advised to avoid becoming pregnant.

➤*Lactation:* It is not known whether this drug is excreted in human milk. Because many drugs are excreted in human milk, and because of the potential for serious adverse reactions in nursing infants from mercaptopurine, a decision should be made whether to discontinue nursing or to discontinue the drug, taking into account the importance of the drug to the mother.

➤*Children:* See Administration and Dosage.

Precautions

➤*Monitoring:* It is recommended that evaluation of the hemoglobin or hematocrit, total white blood cell count and differential count, and quantitative platelet count be obtained weekly while the patient is on therapy with mercaptopurine. In cases where the cause of fluctuations in the formed elements in the peripheral blood is obscure, bone marrow examination may be useful for the evaluation of marrow status. The decision to increase, decrease, continue, or discontinue a given dosage of mercaptopurine must be based not only on the absolute hematologic values, but also upon the rapidity with which changes are occurring. In many instances, particularly during the induction phase of acute leukemia, complete blood counts will need to be done more frequently than once weekly in order to evaluate the effect of the therapy.

➤*Hematologic:* The most frequent, serious, toxic effect of mercaptopurine is myelosuppression, resulting in leukopenia, thrombocytopenia, and anemia. These toxic effects are often unavoidable during the induction phase of adult acute leukemia if remission induction is to be successful. Whether or not these manifestations demand modification or cessation of dosage depends both upon the response of the underlying disease and a careful consideration of supportive facilities (granulocyte and platelet transfusions) which may be available. Life-threatening infections and bleeding have been observed as a consequence of mercaptopurine-induced granulocytopenia and thrombocytopenia. Severe hematologic toxicity may require supportive therapy with platelet transfusions for bleeding, and antibiotics and granulocyte transfusions if sepsis is documented.

If it is not the intent to deliberately induce bone marrow hypoplasia, it is important to discontinue the drug temporarily at the first evidence of an abnormally large fall in white blood cell count, platelet count, or hemoglobin concentration. In many patients with severe depression of the formed elements of the blood due to mercaptopurine, the bone marrow appears hypoplastic on aspiration or biopsy, whereas in other cases it may appear normocellular. The qualitative changes in the erythroid elements toward the megaloblastic series, characteristically seen with the folic acid antagonists and some other antimetabolites, are not seen with this drug.

Drug Interactions

➤*Thioguanine:* There is usually complete cross-resistance between mercaptopurine and thioguanine.

Mercaptopurine Drug Interactions

Precipitant drug	Object drug[a]		Description
Allopurinol	Mercaptopurine	↑	When administered concomitantly with mercaptopurine, reduce mercaptopurine to ⅓ to ¼ the usual dose. Failure to observe this dosage reduction will delay catabolism of mercaptopurine and increase likelihood of severe toxicity.
Trimethroprim-sulfamethoxazole			When coadministered with mercaptopurine, enhanced marrow suppression has occurred.

[a] ↑ = Object drug increased.

Adverse Reactions

➤*Dermatologic:* Dermatologic reactions can occur as a consequence of disease. The administration of mercaptopurine has been associated with skin rashes and hyperpigmentation.

➤*GI:* Intestinal ulceration has been reported. Nausea, vomiting, and anorexia are uncommon during initial administration. Mild diarrhea and sprue-like symptoms have been noted occasionally, but it is difficult at present to attribute these to the medication. Oral lesions are rarely seen, and when they occur they resemble thrush rather than antifolic ulcerations.

An increased risk of pancreatitis may be associated with the investigational use of mercaptopurine in inflammatory bowel disease.

➤*Hematologic:* See Warnings for more information.

➤*Renal:* Hyperuricemia may occur in patients receiving mercaptopurine as a consequence of rapid cell lysis accompanying the antineoplastic effect. Adverse effects can be minimized by increased hydration, urine alkalinization, and the prophylactic administration of a xanthine oxidase inhibitor such as allopurinol. The dosage of mercaptopurine should be reduced to one third to one quarter of the usual dose if allopurinol is given concurrently.

➤*Miscellaneous:* Drug fever has been very rarely reported with mercaptopurine. Before attributing fever to mercaptopurine, every attempt should be made to exclude more common causes of pyrexia, such as sepsis, in patients with acute leukemia.

Overdosage

➤*Symptoms:* Signs and symptoms of overdosage may be immediate (eg, anorexia, nausea, vomiting, diarrhea); or delayed (eg, myelosuppression, liver dysfunction, gastroenteritis). The oral LD_{50} of mercaptopurine was determined to be 480 mg/kg in the mouse and 425 mg/kg in the rat.

➤*Treatment:* There is no known pharmacologic antagonist of mercaptopurine. The drug should be discontinued immediately if unintended toxicity occurs during treatment. If a patient is seen immediately following an accidental overdosage of the drug, it may be useful to induce emesis.

Dialysis cannot be expected to clear mercaptopurine. Hemodialysis is thought to be of marginal use due to the rapid intracellular incorporation of mercaptopurine into active metabolites with long persistence.

Patient Information

Patients should be informed that the major toxicities of mercaptopurine are related to myelosuppression, hepatotoxicity, and GI toxicity. Patients should never be allowed to take the drug without medical supervision and should be advised to consult their physician if they experience fever, sore throat, jaundice, nausea, vomiting, signs of local infection, bleeding from any site, or symptoms suggestive of anemia. Women of childbearing potential should be advised to avoid becoming pregnant.

PENTOSTATIN (2′-deoxycoformycin; DCF)

Rx	**Nipent** (SuperGen)	**Powder for injection:** 10 mg/vial	50 mg mannitol/vial. In single-dose vials.

PENTOSTATIN — INJECTION

WARNING

Pentostatin should be administered under the supervision of a physician qualified and experienced in the use of cancer chemotherapeutic agents. The use of higher doses than those specified (see Administration and Dosage) is not recommended. Dose-limiting severe renal, liver, pulmonary, and CNS toxicities occurred in Phase 1 studies that used pentostatin at higher doses (20 to 50 mg/m^2 in divided doses over 5 days) than recommended.

In a clinical investigation in patients with refractory chronic lymphocytic leukemia using pentostatin at the recommended dose in combination with fludarabine phosphate, 4 of 6 patients entered in the study had severe or fatal pulmonary toxicity. The use of pentostatin in combination with fludarabine phosphate is not recommended.

Indications

➤*Hairy-cell leukemia:* Single-agent treatment for both untreated and alpha-interferon-refractory hairy-cell leukemia patients with active disease as defined by clinically significant anemia, neutropenia, thrombocytopenia, or disease-related symptoms.

➤*Unlabeled uses:* Treatment of prolymphocytic leukemia or cutaneous T-cell lymphoma; palliative therapy of chronic lymphocytic leukemia, refractory acute lymphocytic leukemia, mycosis fungoides.

Administration and Dosage

➤*Approved by the FDA:* October 11, 1991.

➤*Hydration:* It is recommended that patients receive hydration with 500 to 1000 mL of 5% Dextrose in 0.5 Normal Saline or equivalent before pentostatin administration. An additional 500 mL of 5% Dextrose or equivalent should be administered after pentostatin is given.

➤*Usual dosage:* 4 mg/m^2 every other week. Pentostatin may be administered intravenously by bolus injection or diluted in a larger volume and given over 20 to 30 minutes. (See Preparation of Intravenous Solution.) Higher doses are not recommended.

➤*Duration of therapy:* The optimal duration of treatment has not been determined. In the absence of major toxicity and with observed continuing improvement, the patient should be treated until a complete response has been achieved. Although not established as required, the administration of two additional doses has been recommended following the achievement of a complete response.

➤*Response to treatment:* All patients receiving pentostatin at 6 months should be assessed for response to treatment. If the patient has not achieved a complete or partial response, treatment with pentostatin should be discontinued.

If the patient has achieved a partial response, pentostatin treatment should be continued in an effort to achieve a complete response. At any time thereafter that a complete response is achieved, 2 additional doses of pentostatin are recommended. Pentostatin treatment should then be stopped. If the best response to treatment at the end of 12 months is a partial response, it is recommended that treatment with pentostatin be stopped.

➤*Withholding dose / discontinuation:* Withholding or discontinuation of individual doses may be needed when severe adverse reactions occur. Drug treatment should be withheld in patients with severe rash, and withheld or discontinued in patients showing evidence of nervous system toxicity.

Pentostatin treatment should be withheld in patients with active infection occurring during the treatment but may be resumed when the infection is controlled.

Patients who have elevated serum creatinine should have their dose withheld and a creatinine clearance determined. There are insufficient data to recommend a starting or a subsequent dose for patients with impaired renal function (creatinine clearance less than 60 mL/min).

➤*Renal function impairment:* Patients with impaired renal function should be treated only when the potential benefit justifies the potential risk. Two patients with impaired renal function (creatinine clearances 50 to 60 mL/min) achieved complete response without unusual adverse events when treated with 2 mg/m^2. No dosage reduction is recommended at the start of therapy with pentostatin in patients with anemia, neutropenia, or thrombocytopenia. In addition, dosage reductions are not recommended during treatment in patients with anemia and thrombocytopenia if patients can be otherwise supported hematologically. Pentostatin should be temporarily withheld if the absolute neutrophil count falls during treatment below 200 cells/mm^3 in a patient who had an initial neutrophil count greater than 500 cells/mm^3 and may be resumed when the count returns to predose levels.

➤*Preparation of intravenous solution:*

1.) Procedures for proper handling and disposal of anticancer drugs should be followed. Several guidelines on this subject have been published. There is no general agreement that all of the procedures recommended in the guidelines are necessary or appropriate. Spills and wastes should be treated with a 5% sodium hypochlorite solution prior to disposal.
2.) Protective clothing including polyethylene gloves must be worn.
3.) Transfer 5 mL of Sterile Water for Injection USP to the vial containing pentostatin and mix thoroughly to obtain complete dissolution of a solution yielding 2 mg/mL. Parenteral drug products should be inspected visually for particulate matter and discoloration prior to administration.
4.) Pentostatin may be given intravenously by bolus injection or diluted in a larger volume (25 to 50 mL) with 5% Dextrose Injection USP or 0.9% Sodium Chloride Injection USP. Dilution of the entire contents of a reconstituted vial with 25 mL or 50 mL provides a pentostatin concentration of 0.33 mg/mL or 0.18 mg/mL, respectively, for the diluted solutions.
5.) Pentostatin solution when diluted for infusion with 5% Dextrose Injection USP or 0.9% Sodium Chloride Injection USP does not interact with PVC infusion containers or administration sets at concentrations of 0.18 mg/mL to 0.33 mg/mL.

➤*Storage / Stability:* Pentostatin vials are stable at refrigerated storage temperature 2° to 8°C (36° to 46°F) for the period stated on the package. Vials reconstituted or reconstituted and further diluted as directed may be stored at room temperature and ambient light but should be used within 8 hours because pentostatin contains no preservatives.

Actions

➤*Pharmacology:* Pentostatin is a potent transition state inhibitor of the enzyme adenosine deaminase (ADA). The greatest activity of ADA is found in cells of the lymphoid system with T-cells having higher activity than B-cells and T-cell malignancies higher ADA activity than B-cell malignancies. Pentostatin inhibition of ADA, particularly in the presence of adenosine or deoxyadenosine, leads to cytoxicity, and this is believed to be due to elevated intracellular levels of dATP which can block DNA synthesis through inhibition of ribonucleotide reductase. Pentostatin can also inhibit RNA synthesis as well as cause increased DNA damage. In addition to elevated dATP, these mechanisms may also contribute to the overall cytotoxic effect of pentostatin. The precise mechanism of pentostatin's antitumor effect, however, in hairy-cell leukemia is not known.

➤*Pharmacokinetics:*

Special populations –

Renal function impairment: A positive correlation was observed between pentostatin clearance and creatinine clearance (Ccr) in patients with creatinine clearance values ranging from 60 mL/min to 130 mL/min. Pentostatin half-life in patients with renal impairment (Ccr less than 50 mL/min, n = 2) was 18 hours, which was much longer than that observed in patients with normal renal function (Ccr greater than 60 mL/min, n = 14), about 6 hours.

Following a single dose of 4 mg/m^2 of pentostatin infused over 5 minutes, the distribution half-life was 11 minutes, the mean terminal half-life was 5.7 hours, the mean plasma clearance was 68 mL/min/m^2, and approximately 90% of the dose was excreted in the urine as unchanged pentostatin and/or metabolites as measured by adenosine deaminase inhibitory activity. The plasma protein binding of pentostatin is low, approximately 4%.

Contraindications

Hypersensitivity to pentostatin.

Warnings

➤*Myelosuppression:* Patients with hairy-cell leukemia may experience myelosuppression primarily during the first few courses of treatment. Patients with infections prior to pentostatin treatment have in some cases developed worsening of their condition leading to death, whereas others have achieved complete response. Patients with infection should be treated only when the potential benefit of treatment justifies the potential risk to the patient. Efforts should be made to control the infection before treatment is initiated or resumed.

In patients with progressive hairy-cell leukemia, the initial courses of pentostatin treatment were associated with worsening of neutropenia. Therefore, frequent monitoring of complete blood counts during this time is necessary. If severe neutropenia continues beyond the initial cycles, patients should be evaluated for disease status, including a bone marrow examination.

➤*Rashes:* Rashes, occasionally severe, were commonly reported and may worsen with continued treatment. Withholding of treatment may be required. (See Administration and Dosage.)

➤*Combination therapy:* Acute pulmonary edema and hypotension, leading to death, have been reported in the literature in patients treated with pentostatin in combination with carmustine, etoposide and high dose cyclophosphamide as part of the ablative regimen for bone marrow transplant.

➤*Renal function impairment:*

Toxicity – Renal toxicity was observed at higher doses in early studies; however, in patients treated at the recommended dose, elevations in serum creatinine were usually minor and reversible. There were some patients who began treatment with normal renal function who had evidence of mild to moderate toxicity at a final assessment. (See Administration and Dosage.)

➤*Mutagenesis:* When tested with strain TA-100, a repeatable statistically significant response trend was observed with and without metabolic activation. The response was 2.1 to 2.2 fold higher than the background at 10 mg/plate, the maximum possible drug concentration. Formulated pentostatin was clastogenic in the in vivo mouse bone marrow micronucleus assay at 20, 120, and 240 mg/kg.

PENTOSTATIN — INJECTION

➤*Fertility impairment:* No fertility studies have been conducted in animals; however, in a 5-day intravenous toxicity study in dogs, mild seminiferous tubular degeneration was observed with doses of 1 and 4 mg/kg. The possible adverse effects on fertility in humans have not been determined.

➤*Pregnancy: Category D.* Pentostatin can cause fetal harm when administered to a pregnant woman. Pentostatin was administered intravenously at doses of 0, 0.01, 0.1, or 0.75 mg/kg/day (0, 0.06, 0.6, and 4.5 mg/m^2) to pregnant rats on days 6 through 15 of gestation. Drug-related maternal toxicity occurred at doses of 0.1 and 0.75 mg/kg/day (0.6 and 4.5 mg/m^2). Teratogenic effects were observed at 0.75 mg/kg/day (4.5 mg/m^2) manifested by increased incidence of various skeletal malformations. In a dose range-finding study, pentostatin was administered intravenously to rats at doses of 0, 0.05, 0.1, 0.5, 0.75, or 1 mg/kg/day (0, 0.3, 0.6, 3, 4.5, 6 mg/m^2), on days 6 through 15 of gestation. Fetal malformations that were observed were an omphalocele at 0.05 mg/kg (0.3 mg/m^2), gastroschisis at 0.75 mg/kg and 1 mg/kg (4.5 and 6 mg/m^2), and a flexure defect of the hind limbs at 0.75 mg/kg (4.5 mg/m^2). Pentostatin was also shown to be teratogenic in mice when administered as a single 2 mg/kg (6 mg/m^2) intraperitoneal injection on day 7 of gestation. Pentostatin was not teratogenic in rabbits when administered intravenously on days 6 through 18 of gestation at doses of 0, 0.005, 0.01, or 0.02 mg/kg/day (0, 0.015, 0.03, or 0.06 mg/m^2); however maternal toxicity, abortions, early deliveries, and deaths occurred in all drug-treated groups. There are no adequate and well-controlled studies in pregnant women. If pentostatin is used during pregnancy, or if the patient becomes pregnant while taking (receiving) this drug, the patient should be apprised of the potential hazard to the fetus. Women of childbearing potential receiving pentostatin should be advised to avoid becoming pregnant.

➤*Lactation:* It is not known whether pentostatin is excreted in human milk. Because many drugs are excreted in human milk, and because of the potential for serious adverse reactions in nursing infants from pentostatin, a decision should be made whether to discontinue nursing or discontinue the drug, taking into account the importance of pentostatin to the mother.

➤*Children:* Safety and effectiveness in children or adolescents have not been established.

Precautions

➤*Monitoring:* Therapy with pentostatin requires regular patient observation and monitoring of hematologic parameters and blood chemistry values. If severe adverse reactions occur, the drug should be withheld (see Administration and Dosage), and appropriate corrective measures should be taken according to the clinical judgment of the physician.

Prior to initiating therapy with pentostatin, renal function should be assessed with a serum creatinine and/or a creatinine clearance assay (see Pharmacology and Administration and Dosage). Complete blood counts and serum creatinine should be performed before each dose of pentostatin and at other appropriate periods during therapy (see Administration and Dosage). Severe neutropenia has been observed following the early courses of treatment with pentostatin and therefore frequent monitoring of complete blood counts is recommended during this time. If hematologic parameters do not improve with subsequent courses, patients should be evaluated for disease status, including a bone marrow examination. Periodic monitoring of the peripheral blood for hairy cells should be performed to assess the response to treatment.

In addition, bone marrow aspirates and biopsies may be required at 2 to 3 month intervals to assess the response to treatment.

➤*Lab test abnormalities:* Elevations in liver function tests occurred during treatment with pentostatin and were generally reversible.

Drug Interactions

➤*Allopurinol:* Allopurinol and pentostatin are both associated with skin rashes. Based on clinical studies in 25 refractory patients who received both pentostatin and allopurinol, the combined use of pentostatin and allopurinol did not appear to produce a higher incidence of skin rashes than observed with pentostatin alone. There has been a report of one patient who received both drugs and experienced a hypersensitivity vasculitis that resulted in death. It was unclear whether this adverse event and subsequent death resulted from the drug combination.

➤*Vidarabine:* Biochemical studies have demonstrated that pentostatin enhances the effects of vidarabine, a purine nucleoside with antiviral activity. The combined use of vidarabine and pentostatin may result in an increase in adverse reactions associated with each drug. The therapeutic benefit of the drug combination has not been established.

➤*Fludarabine:* See the Warning box for more information.

➤*Carmustine / Etoposide / Cyclophosphamide:* See Warnings for more information.

Adverse Reactions

Adverse Reactions for Pentostatin When Used as Front-line and IFN-Refractory Therapy (%)

All adverse reactions[a]	Frontline, treated with pentostatin (n = 180)	Frontline, treated with IFN (n = 176)	IFN-refractory, treated with pentostatin (n = 197)
Nausea/vomiting	63%	22%	53%[b]
Fever	46%	59%	42%
Rash	43%	30%	26%
Fatigue	42%	55%	29%
Leukopenia	22%	15%	60%
Pruritus	21%	6%	10%
Coughing/increased cough	20%	15%	17%
Myalgia	19%	36%	11%
Chills	19%	34%	11%
Headache	17%	29%	13%
Diarrhea	17%	17%	15%
Abdominal pain	16%	15%	4%
Anorexia	13%	10%	16%
Upper respiratory tract infection	13%	8%	16%
Asthenia	12%	13%	10%
Stomatitis	12%	7%	5%
Rhinitis	11%	15%	10%
Dyspnea	11%	13%	8%
Anemia	8%	5%	35%
Pain	8%	19%	20%
Pharyngitis	8%	11%	10%
Sweating/increased sweating	8%	21%	10%
Viral infection	8%	17%	NR*
Infection	7%[c]	2%[c]	36%
Arthralgia	6%	14%	3%
Thrombocytopenia	6%	6%	32%
Skin disorder	4%	5%	17%
Allergic reaction	2%	1%	11%
Hepatic disorder/elevated liver function tests[d]	2%	2%	19%
Neurologic disorder, CNS/ CNS toxicity	1%	NR*	11%
Lung disorder/disease	NR*	1%	12%
Nausea	NR*	NR*	22%
Genitourinary disorder	NR*	NR*	15%

* Not reported.
[a] Occurring in > 10% of patients, in any group, regardless of drug association.
[b] Includes only nausea with vomiting.
[c] These figures represent only unspecified infections. Refer to infection table.
[d] Elevated liver enzymes and liver disorder for SWOG.

Adverse Reactions in the SWOG study (%)

Type of infection	Frontline, treated with pentostatin (n = 180)	Frontline, treated with IFN (n = 176)
Upper respiratory tract infection	13%	8%
Rhinitis	11%	15%
Herpes zoster	8%	1%
Pharyngitis	8%	11%
Viral infection	8%	17%
Infection (unspecified)	7%	2%
Sinusitis	6%	4%
Cellulitis	6%	3%
Bacterial infection	5%	4%
Pneumonia	5%	7%
Conjunctivitis	4%	2%
Furunculosis	4%	< 1%
Herpes simplex	4%	1%
Bronchitis	3%	2%
Sepsis	3%	2%
Urinary tract infection	3%	3%
Abscess, skin	2%	4%
Moniliasis, oral	2%	< 1%

PENTOSTATIN — INJECTION

Adverse Reactions in the SWOG study (%)		
Type of infection	Frontline, treated with pentostatin (n = 180)	Frontline, treated with IFN (n = 176)
Mycotic infection, skin	< 1%	3%
Osteomyelitis	1%	0%

➤*The drug relatedness of the adverse events listed below cannot be excluded. The following adverse events occurred in 3% to 10% of pentostatin-treated patients in the initial phase of the SWOG study:*

Cardiovascular – Hemorrhage, hypotension.

CNS – Confusion, dizziness, insomnia, paresthesia, somnolence.

Dermatologic – Skin dry, urticaria.

GI – Dental abnormalities, dyspepsia, flatulence, gingivitis.

Hematologic / Lymphatic – Agranulocytosis.

Lab test abnormalities – Elevated creatinine.

Musculoskeletal – Arthralgia.

Psychiatric – Anxiety, depression, nervousness.

Respiratory – Asthma.

Miscellaneous – Chest pain, death, face edema, peripheral edema.

➤*The remaining adverse events which occurred in less than 3% of pentostatin-treated patients during the initial phase of the SWOG study:*

Cardiovascular – Angina pectoris, arrhythmia, A-V block, bradycardia, extrasystoles ventricular, heart arrest, heart failure, hypertension, pericardial effusion, phlebitis, pulmonary embolus, sinus arrest, tachycardia, thrombophlebitis (deep), vasculitis.

CNS – Amnesia, ataxia, convulsions, dreaming abnormal, dysarthria, encephalitis, hyperkinesia, meningism, neuralgia, neuritis, neuropathy, paralysis, syncope, twitching, vertigo.

Dermatologic – Acne, alopecia, eczema, petechial rash, photosensitivity reaction.

GI – Constipation, dysphagia, glossitis, ileus.

GU – Amenorrhea, breast lump, impotence, kidney function abnormal, nephropathy, renal failure, renal insufficiency, renal stone.

Hematologic / Lymphatic – Acute leukemia, hemolytic anemia, aplastic anemia.

Lab test abnormalities – Hypercalcemia, hyponatremia.

Musculoskeletal – Arthritis, gout.

Psychiatric – Decrease/loss of libido, emotional liability, hallucination, hostility, neurosis, thinking abnormal.

Respiratory – Bronchospasm, larynx edema.

Special senses – Amblyopia, deafness, earache, eyes dry, labyrinthitis, lacrimation disorder, nonreactive eye, photophobia, retinopathy, tinnitus, unusual taste, vision abnormal, watery eyes.

Miscellaneous – Flu-like symptoms, hangover effect, neoplasm. One patient with hairy-cell leukemia treated with pentostatin during another clinical study developed unilateral uveitis with vision loss.

Nineteen (5%) patients withdrew from the Phase 3 SWOG 8691 study because of adverse events; 9 during initial pentostatin treatment, 4 during pentostatin crossover, 5 during initial IFN treatment, and 1 during both initial IFN treatment and pentostatin crossover. In the Phase 2 studies in IFN-refractory hairy-cell leukemia, 11% of patients withdrew from treatment with pentostatin due to an adverse event.

Overdosage

No specific antidote for pentostatin overdose is known. Pentostatin administered at higher doses (20 to 50 mg/m^2 in divided doses over 5 days) than recommended was associated with deaths due to severe renal, hepatic, pulmonary, and CNS toxicity. In case of overdose, management would include general supportive measures through any period of toxicity that occurs.

Patient Information

Patients should be advised of the signs and symptoms of adverse events associated with pentostatin therapy (see Adverse Reactions).

THIOGUANINE (TG; 6-Thioguanine)

Rx	**Tabloid** (GlaxoSmithKline)	**Tablets:** 40 mg	Lactose. (Wellcome U3B). Greenish yellow, scored. In 25s.

THIOGUANINE — ORAL

Indications

➤*Acute nonlymphocytic leukemias:* For remission induction and remission consolidation treatment of acute nonlymphocytic leukemias. However, it is not recommended for use during maintenance therapy or similar long-term continuous treatments because of the high risk of liver toxicity.

The response to this agent depends upon the age of the patient (younger patients faring better than older) and whether thioguanine is used in previously treated or previously untreated patients. Reliance upon thioguanine alone is seldom justified for initial remission induction of acute nonlymphocytic leukemias because combination chemotherapy including thioguanine results in more frequent remission induction and longer duration of remission than thioguanine alone.

➤*Other neoplasms:* Thioguanine is not effective in chronic lymphocytic leukemia, Hodgkin lymphoma, multiple myeloma, or solid tumors. Although thioguanine is one of several agents with activity in the treatment of the chronic phase of chronic myelogenous leukemia, more objective responses are observed with busulfan, and therefore busulfan is usually regarded as the preferred drug.

➤*Unlabeled uses:* Chronic myelogenous leukemia; psoriasis; second-line treatment for ulcerative colitis and Crohn disease.

Administration and Dosage

➤*Approved by the FDA:* January 18, 1966.

➤*Dosage:* On those occasions when single-agent chemotherapy with thioguanine may be appropriate, the usual initial dosage for pediatric patients and adults is approximately 2 mg/kg of body weight per day. If, after 4 weeks on this dosage, there is no clinical improvement and no leukocyte or platelet depression, the dosage may be cautiously increased to 3 mg/kg/day. The total daily dose may be given at one time.

➤*Thiopurine methyltransferase (TPMT) deficiency:* See Warnings for more information.

➤*Concomitant therapy:* The dosage of thioguanine used does not depend on whether or not the patient is receiving allopurinol; this is in contradistinction to the dosage reduction that is mandatory when mercaptopurine or azathioprine is given simultaneously with allopurinol.

➤*Storage / Stability:* Store at 15° to 25°C (59° to 77°F) in a dry place.

Actions

➤*Pharmacology:* Thioguanine is one of a large series of purine analogues that interferes with nucleic acid biosynthesis, and has been found active against selected human neoplastic diseases.

Thioguanine competes with hypoxanthine and guanine for the enzyme hypoxanthine-guanine phosphoribosyltransferase (HGPRTase) and is itself converted to 6-thioguanylic acid (TGMP). This nucleotide reaches high intracellular concentrations at therapeutic doses. TGMP interferes at several points with the synthesis of guanine nucleotides. It inhibits de novo purine biosynthesis by pseudo-feedback inhibition of glutamine-5-phosphoribosylpyrophosphate amidotransferase, the first enzyme unique to the de novo pathway for purine ribonucleotide synthesis. TGMP also inhibits the conversion of inosinic acid (IMP) to xanthylic acid (XMP) by competition for the enzyme IMP dehydrogenase. At one time, TGMP was felt to be a significant inhibitor of ATP:GMP phosphotransferase (guanylate kinase), but recent results have shown this not to be so.

Thioguanylic acid is further converted to the di- and triphosphates, thioguanosine diphosphate (TGDP) and thioguanosine triphosphate (TGTP) (as well as their 2′-deoxyribosyl analogues), by the same enzymes that metabolize guanine nucleotides. Thioguanine nucleotides are incorporated into the RNA and the DNA by phosphodiester linkages, and it has been argued that incorporation of such fraudulent bases contributes to the cytotoxicity of thioguanine.

Thus, thioguanine has multiple metabolic effects and at present it is not possible to designate 1 major site of action. Its tumor inhibitory properties may be caused by 1 or more of its effects on feedback inhibition of de novo purine synthesis, inhibition of purine nucleotide interconversions, or incorporation into the DNA and the RNA. The net consequence of its actions is a sequential blockade of the synthesis and utilization of the purine nucleotides.

In some animal tumors, resistance to the effect of thioguanine correlates with the loss of HGPRTase activity and the resulting inability to convert thioguanine to thioguanylic acid. However, other resistance mechanisms, such as increased catabolism of TGMP by a nonspecific phosphatase, may be operative. Although not invariable, it is usual to find cross-resistance between thioguanine and its close analogue, mercaptopurine.

➤*Pharmacokinetics:*

Absorption – Clinical studies have shown that the absorption of an oral dose of thioguanine in humans is incomplete and variable, averaging approximately 30% of the administered dose (range, 14% to 46%). Following oral administration of ^{35}S-6-thioguanine, total plasma radioactivity reached a maximum at 8 hours and declined slowly thereafter. Parent drug represented only a very small fraction of the total plasma radioactivity at any time, being virtually undetectable throughout the period of measurements.

Distribution – Intravenous administration of ^{35}S-6-thioguanine disclosed a median plasma half-disappearance time of 80 minutes (range, 25 to 240 minutes) when the compound was given in single doses of 65 to 300 mg/m^2. Although initial plasma levels of thioguanine did correlate with the dose level, there was no correlation between the plasma half-disappearance time and the dose.

Thioguanine is incorporated into the DNA and the RNA of human bone marrow cells. Studies with IV ^{35}S-6-thioguanine have shown that the amount of thioguanine incorporated into nucleic acids is more than 100 times higher after 5 daily doses than after a single dose. With the 5-dose schedule, from

THIOGUANINE — ORAL

one half to virtually all of the guanine in the residual DNA was replaced by thioguanine. Tissue distribution studies of ^{35}S-6-thioguanine in mice showed only traces of radioactivity in brain after oral administration. No measurements have been made of thioguanine concentrations in human cerebrospinal fluid (CSF), but observations on tissue distribution in animals, together with the lack of CNS penetration by the closely related compound, mercaptopurine, suggest that thioguanine does not reach therapeutic concentrations in the CSF.

Metabolism – Monitoring of plasma levels of thioguanine during therapy is of questionable value. There is technical difficulty in determining plasma concentrations, which are seldom greater than 1 to 2 mcg/mL after a therapeutic oral dose. More significantly, thioguanine enters rapidly into the anabolic and catabolic pathways for purines, and the active intracellular metabolites have appreciably longer half-lives than the parent drug. The biochemical effects of a single dose of thioguanine are evident long after the parent drug has disappeared from plasma. Because of this rapid metabolism of thioguanine to active intracellular derivatives, hemodialysis would not be expected to appreciably reduce toxicity of the drug.

The catabolism of thioguanine and its metabolites is complex and shows significant differences between humans and mice. In both humans and mice, after oral administration of ^{35}S-6-thioguanine, urine contains virtually no detectable intact thioguanine. While deamination and subsequent oxidation to thiouric acid occurs only to a small extent in humans, it is the main pathway in mice. The product of deamination by guanase, 6-thioxanthine is inactive, having negligible antitumor activity. This pathway of thioguanine inactivation is not dependent on the action of xanthine oxidase, and an inhibitor of that enzyme (eg, allopurinol) will not block the detoxification of thioguanine even though the inactive 6-thioxanthine is normally further oxidized by xanthine oxidase to thiouric acid before it is eliminated. In humans, methylation of thioguanine is much more extensive than in the mouse. The product of methylation, 2-amino-6-methylthiopurine, is also substantially less active and less toxic than thioguanine, and its formation is likewise unaffected by the presence of allopurinol. Appreciable amounts of inorganic sulfate are also found in both murine and human urine, presumably arising from further metabolism of the methylated derivatives.

Excretion – The oral administration of radiolabeled thioguanine revealed only trace quantities of parent drug in the urine. However, a methylated metabolite, 2-amino-6-methylthiopurine (MTG), appeared very early, rose to a maximum 6 to 8 hours after drug administration, and was still being excreted after 12 to 22 hours. Radiolabeled sulfate appeared somewhat later than MTG but was the principal metabolite after 8 hours. Thiouric acid and some unidentified products were found in the urine in small amounts.

Contraindications

Prior resistance to this drug. In animals and humans, there is usually complete cross-resistance between mercaptopurine and thioguanine.

Warnings

➤*Hepatic toxicity:* Thioguanine is not recommended for maintenance therapy or similar long-term continuous treatments because of the high risk of liver toxicity associated with vascular endothelial damage. This liver toxicity has been observed in a high proportion of children receiving thioguanine as part of maintenance therapy for acute lymphoblastic leukemia and in other conditions associated with continuous use of thioguanine. This liver toxicity is particularly prevalent in men. Liver toxicity usually presents as the clinical syndrome of hepatic veno-occlusive disease (hyperbilirubinemia, tender hepatomegaly, weight gain caused by fluid retention, and ascites) or with signs of portal hypertension (splenomegaly, thrombocytopenia, esophageal varices). Histopathological features associated with this toxicity include hepatoportal sclerosis, nodular regenerative hyperplasia, peliosis hepatitis, and periportal fibrosis.

Discontinue thioguanine therapy in patients with evidence of liver toxicity because reversal of signs and symptoms of liver toxicity have been reported upon withdrawal.

A few cases of jaundice have been reported in patients with leukemia receiving thioguanine. Among these were 2 adult men and 4 children with acute myelogenous leukemia and a man with acute lymphocytic leukemia who developed hepatic veno-occlusive disease while receiving chemotherapy for their leukemia. Six patients had received cytarabine prior to treatment with thioguanine, and some were receiving other chemotherapy in addition to thioguanine when they became symptomatic. While hepatic veno-occlusive disease has not been reported in patients treated with thioguanine alone, it is recommended that thioguanine be withheld if there is evidence of toxic hepatitis or biliary stasis, and that appropriate clinical and laboratory investigations be initiated to establish the etiology of the hepatic dysfunction. Deterioration in liver function studies during thioguanine therapy should prompt discontinuation of treatment and a search for an explanation of the hepatotoxicity.

Carefully monitor patients. Early indications of liver toxicity are signs associated with portal hypertension, such as thrombocytopenia out of proportion with neutropenia and splenomegaly. Elevations of liver enzymes have also been reported in association with liver toxicity but do not always occur.

➤*Bone marrow suppression:* The most consistent, dose-related toxicity is bone marrow suppression. This may be manifested by anemia, leukopenia, thrombocytopenia, or any combination of these. Any one of these findings also may reflect progression of the underlying disease. Because thioguanine may have a delayed effect, it is important to withdraw the medication temporarily at the first sign of an abnormally large fall in any of the formed elements of the blood.

There are individuals with an inherited deficiency of the TPMT who may be unusually sensitive to the myelosuppressive effects of thioguanine and prone to developing rapid bone marrow suppression following initiation of treatment. Substantial dose reductions may be required to avoid the development of life-threatening bone marrow suppression in these patients. Be aware that some laboratories offer testing for TPMT deficiency. Because bone marrow suppression may be associated with factors other than TPMT deficiency, TPMT testing may not identify all patients at risk for severe toxicity. Therefore, close monitoring of clinical and hematologic parameters is important. Bone marrow suppression could be exacerbated by coadministration with drugs that inhibit TPMT, such as olsalazine, mesalazine, and sulfasalazine.

Myelosuppression is often unavoidable during the induction phase of adult acute nonlymphocytic leukemias if remission induction is to be successful. Whether or not this demands modification or cessation of dosage depends upon the response of the underlying disease and a careful consideration of supportive facilities (granulocyte and platelet transfusions) that may be available. Life-threatening infections and bleeding have been observed as consequences of thioguanine-induced granulocytopenia and thrombocytopenia.

See Precautions for more information.

➤*Carcinogenesis:* In view of its action on cellular DNA, thioguanine is potentially carcinogenic; give consideration to the theoretical risk of carcinogenesis when thioguanine is administered.

➤*Mutagenesis:* In view of its action on cellular DNA, thioguanine is potentially mutagenic.

➤*Elderly:* Clinical studies of thioguanine did not include sufficient numbers of subjects 65 years of age and older to determine whether they respond differently from younger subjects. Other reported clinical experience has not identified differences in responses between the elderly and younger patients. In general, dose selection for an elderly patient should be cautious, usually starting at the low end of the dosing range, reflecting the greater frequency of decreased hepatic, renal, or cardiac function, and of concomitant disease or other drug therapy.

➤*Pregnancy: Category D.* Drugs such as thioguanine are potential mutagens and teratogens. Thioguanine may cause fetal harm when administered to a pregnant woman. Thioguanine has been shown to be teratogenic in rats when given in doses 5 times the human dose. When given to the rat on the fourth and fifth days of gestation, 13% of surviving placentas did not contain fetuses, and 19% of offspring were malformed or stunted. The malformations noted included generalized edema, cranial defects, and general skeletal hypoplasia, hydrocephalus, ventral hernia, situs inversus, and incomplete development of the limbs. There are no adequate and well-controlled studies in pregnant women. If this drug is used during pregnancy, or if the patient becomes pregnant while taking the drug, apprise the patient of the potential hazard to the fetus. Advise women of childbearing potential to avoid becoming pregnant.

➤*Lactation:* It is not known whether this drug is excreted in human milk. Because of the potential for tumorigenicity shown for thioguanine, decide whether to discontinue breast-feeding or to discontinue the drug, taking into account the importance of the drug to the mother.

➤*Children:* Ninety-six (59%) of 163 pediatric patients with previously untreated acute nonlymphocytic leukemia obtained complete remission with a multiple-drug protocol including thioguanine, prednisone, cytarabine, cyclophosphamide, and vincristine. Remission was maintained with daily thioguanine, 4-day pulses of cytarabine and cyclophosphamide, and a single dose of vincristine every 28 days. The median duration of remission was 11.5 months.

Precautions

➤*Monitoring:* See Warnings for more information.

It is advisable to monitor liver function tests (serum transaminases, alkaline phosphatase, bilirubin) at weekly intervals when first beginning therapy and at monthly intervals thereafter. It may be advisable to perform liver function tests more frequently in patients with known preexisting liver disease or in patients who are receiving thioguanine and other hepatotoxic drugs. Instruct patients to discontinue thioguanine immediately if clinical jaundice is detected.

It is recommended that evaluation of the hemoglobin concentration or hematocrit, total WBC count and differential count, and quantitative platelet count be obtained frequently while the patient is on thioguanine therapy. In cases where the cause of fluctuations in the formed elements in the peripheral blood is obscure, bone marrow examination may be useful for the evaluation of marrow status. Base the decision to increase, decrease, continue, or discontinue a given dosage of thioguanine not only on the absolute hematologic values, but also upon the rapidity with which changes are occurring. In many instances, particularly during the induction phase of acute leukemia, complete blood counts will need to be done more frequently in order to evaluate the effect of the therapy. The dosage of thioguanine may need to be reduced when this agent is combined with other drugs whose primary toxicity is myelosuppression.

➤*Immunization:* Avoid administration of live vaccines to immunocompromised patients.

➤*Other toxicities:* Although the primary toxicity of thioguanine is myelosuppression, other toxicities have occasionally been observed, particularly when thioguanine is used in combination with other cancer chemotherapeutic agents.

Drug Interactions

➤*Aminosalicylate derivatives:* Because there is in vitro evidence that aminosalicylate derivatives (eg, olsalazine, mesalazine, sulfasalazine)

THIOGUANINE — ORAL

inhibit the TPMT enzyme, administer them with caution to patients receiving concurrent thioguanine therapy.

➤*Mercaptopurine:* There is usually complete cross-resistance between mercaptopurine and thioguanine.

Adverse Reactions

➤*GI:* Less frequent adverse reactions include nausea, vomiting, anorexia, and stomatitis. Intestinal necrosis and perforation have been reported in patients who received multiple-drug chemotherapy including thioguanine.

➤*Hematologic:* The most frequent adverse reaction to thioguanine is myelosuppression. The induction of complete remission of acute myelogenous leukemia usually requires combination chemotherapy in dosages that produce marrow hypoplasia. Because consolidation and maintenance of remission are also affected by multiple-drug regimens whose component agents cause myelosuppression, pancytopenia is observed in nearly all patients. Adjust dosages and schedules to prevent life-threatening cytopenias whenever these adverse reactions are observed.

➤*Hepatic:* See Warnings for more information.

Liver toxicity during short-term cyclical therapy presents as veno-occlusive disease. Reversal of signs and symptoms of this liver toxicity has been reported upon withdrawal of short-term or long-term continuous therapy.

Centrilobular hepatic necrosis has been reported in a few cases; however, the reports are confounded by the use of high doses of thioguanine, other chemotherapeutic agents, and oral contraceptives and chronic alcohol abuse.

➤*Metabolic:* Hyperuricemia frequently occurs in patients receiving thioguanine as a consequence of rapid cell lysis accompanying the antineoplastic effect. Adverse reactions can be minimized by increased hydration, urine alkalinization, and the prophylactic administration of a xanthine oxidase inhibitor such as allopurinol. Unlike mercaptopurine and azathioprine, thioguanine may be continued in the usual dosage when allopurinol is used conjointly to inhibit uric acid formation.

Overdosage

➤*Symptoms:* Signs and symptoms of overdosage may be immediate, such as nausea, vomiting, malaise, hypotension, and diaphoresis; or delayed, such as myelosuppression and azotemia. The oral LD_{50} of thioguanine was determined to be 823 mg/kg ± 50.73 mg/kg and 740 mg/kg ± 45.24 mg/kg for male and female rats, respectively. Symptoms of overdosage may occur after a single dose of as little as thioguanine 2 to 3 mg/kg. As much as 35 mg/kg has been given in a single oral dose with reversible myelosuppression observed.

➤*Treatment:* There is no known pharmacologic antagonist of thioguanine. Immediately discontinue the drug if unintended toxicity occurs during treatment. Severe hematologic toxicity may require supportive therapy with platelet transfusions for bleeding, and granulocyte transfusions and antibiotics if sepsis is documented. It is not known whether thioguanine is dialyzable. Hemodialysis is thought to be of marginal use because of the rapid intracellular incorporation of thioguanine into active metabolites with long persistence.

Patient Information

Inform patients that the major toxicities of thioguanine are related to myelosuppression, hepatotoxicity, and GI toxicity. Never allow patients to take the drug without medical supervision and advise them to consult their physicians if they experience fever, sore throat, jaundice, nausea, vomiting, signs of local infection, bleeding from any site, or symptoms suggestive of anemia. Advise women of childbearing potential to avoid becoming pregnant.

ALLOPURINOL

Rx	**Allopurinol** (Various, eg, Boots, Geneva, Major, Mylan, Parmed, Vangard)	**Tablets:** 100 mg	In 100s, 500s, 1000s, and UD 100s.
Rx	**Zyloprim** (GlaxoWellcome)		Lactose. (Zyloprim 100). White, scored. In 100s.
Rx	**Allopurinol** (Various, eg, Boots, Geneva, Major, Mylan, Parmed, Vangard)	**Tablets:** 300 mg	In 100s, 500s, 1000s, and UD 100s.
Rx	**Zyloprim** (GlaxoWellcome)		Lactose. (Zyloprim 300). Peach, scored. In 100s and 500s.
Rx	**Allopurinol Sodium** (Bedford Labs)	**Power for injection, lyophilized:** 500 mg	Preservative free. In 30 mL vials with rubber stoppers.
Rx	**Aloprim** (Nabi)		Preservative free. In 30 ml vials with rubber stoppers.

ALLOPURINOL

For more complete prescribing information on tablets, see the Allopurinol monograph in the Agents for Gout section.

Indications

➤*Leukemia/Lymphoma/Solid tumor malignancies:*

Injection – For the management of patients with leukemia, lymphoma, and solid tumor malignancies who are receiving cancer therapy that causes elevations of serum and urinary uric acid levels and who cannot tolerate oral therapy.

Tablets – Management of patients with leukemia, lymphoma, and malignancies receiving therapy that causes elevations of serum and urinary uric acid. Discontinue allopurinol when the potential for overproduction of uric acid is no longer present. For more complete prescribing information on tablets, see the Allopurinol monograph in the Agents for Gout section.

Administration and Dosage

➤*Injection:*

Children and adults – The dosage of allopurinol sodium for injection to lower serum uric acid to normal or near-normal varies according to disease severity. The amount and frequency of dosage for maintaining the serum uric acid just within the normal range is best determined by using the serum uric acid level as an index. In adults, doses > 600 mg/day did not appear to be more effective. The recommended daily dose of allopurinol sodium for injection is as follows:

Recommended Daily Dose	
Adult	200 to 400 mg/m²/day Maximum 600 mg/day
Child	Starting dose 200 mg/m²/day

Hydration – A fluid intake sufficient to yield a daily urinary output of ≥ 2 L in adults and the maintenance of a neutral or, preferably, slightly alkaline urine is desirable.

Impaired renal function – Reduce the dose of allopurinol sodium for injection in patients with impaired renal function to avoid accumulation of allopurinol and its metabolites:

Recommended Daily Dose for Impaired Renal Function	
Ccr	Recommended daily dose
10 to 20 ml/min	200 mg/day
3 to 10 ml/min	100 mg/day
< 3 ml/min	100 mg/day at extended intervals

Administration – In adults and children, the daily dose can be given as a single infusion or in equally divided infusions at 6-, 8-, or 12-hour intervals at the recommended final concentration of ≤ 6 mg/ml (see Preparation of Solution). The rate of infusion depends on the volume of infusate. Whenever possible, initiate therapy with allopurinol sodium for injection 24 to 48 hours before the start of chemotherapy known to cause tumor lysis (including adrenocorticosteroids). Do not mix allopurinol sodium for injection with or administer through the same IV port with agents that are incompatible in solution with allopurinol sodium for injection (see IV incompatibilities).

Preparation of solution – Allopurinol sodium for injection must be reconstituted and diluted. Dissolve the contents of each 30 ml vial with 25 ml of Sterile Water for Injection. Reconstitution yields a clear, almost colorless solution with no more than a slight opalescence. This concentration solution has a pH of 11.1 to 11.8. Dilute it to the desired concentration with 0.9% Sodium Chloride Injection or 5% Dextrose for Injection. Do not use sodium bicarbonate-containing solutions. A final concentration of ≤ 6 mg/ml is recommended. Begin administration within 10 hours after reconstitution.

IV incompatibilities: Drugs that are physically incompatible in a solution with allopurinol sodium for injection include the following: Amikacin sulfate, amphotericin B, carmustine, cefotaxime sodium, chlorpromazine HCl, cimetidine HCl, clindamycin phosphate, cytarabine, dacarbazine, daunorubicin HCl, diphenhydramine HCl, doxorubicin HCl, doxycycline hyclate, droperidol, floxuridine, gentamicin sulfate, haloperidol lactate, hydroxyzine HCl, idarubicin HCl, imipenem-cilastatin sodium, mechlorethamine HCl, meperidine HCl, metoclopramide HCl, methylprednisolone sodium succinate, minocycline HCl, nalbuphine HCl, netilmicin sulfate, ondansetron HCl, prochlorperazine edisylate, promethazine HCl, sodium bicarbonate, streptozocin, tobramycin sulfate, vinorelbine tartrate.

➤*Tablets:*

Prevention of uric acid nephropathy during vigorous therapy of neoplastic disease – 600 to 800 mg daily for 2 to 3 days with a high fluid intake. (For more complete prescribing information on tablets, see the Allopurinol monograph in the Agents for Gout section.)

ALLOPURINOL

➤*Storage/Stability:*

Powder for injection – Store unreconstituted powder at 25°C (77°F). Excursions permitted to 15° to 30°C (59° to 86°F). Store the reconstituted solution at 20° to 25°C (68° to 77°F). Do not refrigerate the reconstituted and/or diluted product.

Tablets – Store at 15° to 25°C (59° to 77°F) in a dry place, and protect from light.

Actions

➤*Pharmacology:* Allopurinol acts on purine catabolism without disrupting the biosynthesis of purines. It reduces the production of uric acid by inhibiting the biochemical reactions immediately preceding its formation. The degree of this decrease is dose-dependent.

Allopurinol is a structural analog of the natural purine base, hypoxanthine. It is an inhibitor of xanthine oxidase, the enzyme responsible for the conversion of hypoxanthine to xanthine and of xanthine to uric acid, the end product of purine metabolism in humans. Allopurinol is metabolized to the corresponding xanthine analog, oxypurinol (alloxanthine), which also is an inhibitor of xanthine oxidase.

Reutilization of both hypoxanthine and xanthine for nucleotide and nucleic acid synthesis is markedly enhanced when their oxidations are inhibited by allopurinol and oxypurinol. However, this reutilization does not disrupt normal nucleic acid anabolism because feedback inhibition is an integral part of purine biosynthesis. As a result of xanthine oxidase inhibition, the serum concentration of hypoxanthine plus xanthine in patients receiving allopurinol for treatment of hyperuricemia is usually in the range of 0.3 to 0.4 mg/dl compared with a normal level of ≈ 0.15 mg/dl. A maximum of 0.9 mg/dl of these oxypurines has been reported when the serum urate was lowered to < 2 mg/dl by high doses of allopurinol. These values are far below the saturation levels, at which point their precipitation would be expected to occur (> 7 mg/dl).

The renal clearance of hypoxanthine and xanthine is ≥ 10 times greater than that of uric acid. The increased xanthine and hypoxanthine in the urine have not been accompanied by problems of nephrolithiasis. There are isolated case reports of xanthine crystalluria in patients who were treated with oral allopurinol. The action of oral allopurinol differs from that of uricosuric agents, which lower the serum uric acid level by increasing urinary excretion of uric acid. Allopurinol reduces both the serum and urinary uric acid levels by inhibiting the formation of uric acid. The use of allopurinol to block the formation of urates avoids the hazard of increased renal excretion of uric acid posed by uricosuric drugs.

➤*Pharmacokinetics:* Following IV administration in 6 healthy male and female subjects, allopurinol was rapidly eliminated from the systemic circulation primarily via oxidative metabolism to oxypurinol, with no detectable plasma concentration of allopurinol after 5 hours post-dosing. Approximately 12% of the allopurinol IV dose was excreted unchanged, 76% excreted as oxypurinol, and the remaining dose excreted as riboside conjugates in the urine. The rapid conversion of allopurinol to oxypurinol was not significantly different after repeated allopurinol dosing. Oxypurinol was present in systemic circulation in much higher concentrations and for a much longer period than allopurinol; thus, it is generally believed the pharmacological action of allopurinol is mediated via oxypurinol. Oxypurinol was primarily eliminated unchanged in urine by glomerular filtration and tubular reabsorption, with a net renal clearance of ≈ 30 ml/min.

To compare the pharmacokinetics of allopurinol and oxypurinol between IV and oral administration of allopurinol sodium for injection, a well-controlled, 4-way crossover study was conducted in 16 healthy male volunteers. Allopurinol sodium for injection was administered via an IV infusion over 30 minutes. Pharmacokinetic parameter estimates of allopurinol (mean ± S.D.) following single IV and oral administration of allopurinol sodium for injection are summarized as follows:

Administration of Allopurinol Sodium for Injection				
Allopurinol parameters	100 mg IV	300 mg IV	100 mg PO (n = 7)	300 mg PO
C_{max} (mcg/ml)	1.58	5.12	0.53	1.35
T_{max} (hr)	0.5	0.5	1	1.67
$T_{1/2}$ (hr)	1	1.21	0.08	1.32
$AUC_{0-\infty}$ (hr•mcg/ml)	1.99	7.1	1.03	3.69
CL (ml/min/kg)	12.2	9.94		
V_{ss} (L/kg)	0.84	0.87		
$F_{absolute}$ (%)[a]			48.8	52.7

[a] Absolute bioavailability.

Oxypurinol was measurable in the plasma within 10 to 15 minutes following the administration of allopurinol sodium for injection. Pharmacokinetic parameter estimates of oxypurinol following IV and oral administration of allopurinol sodium for injection are shown below:

Administration of Allopurinol Sodium for Injection				
Oxypurinol parameters	100 mg IV	300 mg IV	100 mg PO	300 mg PO
C_{max} (mcg/ml)	2.2	6.18	2.36	6.36
T_{max} (hr)	3.89	4.16	3.1	4.13
$T_{1/2}$ (hr)	24.1	23.5	24.9	23.7
$AUC_{0-\infty}$ (hr•mcg/ml)	80	231	83	245
$F_{relative}$ (%)[a]			107	108

[a] Relative bioavailability.

In general, the ratio of the area under the plasma concentration vs time curve ($AUC_{0-\infty}$) between oxypurinol and allopurinol was in the magnitude of 30 to 40. The C_{max} and $AUC_{0-\infty}$ for both allopurinol and oxypurinol following IV administration of allopurinol sodium for injection were dose-proportional in the dose range of 100 to 300 mg. The half-life of allopurinol and oxypurinol was not influenced by the route of allopurinol sodium for injection administration. Oral and IV administration of allopurinol sodium for injection at equal doses produced nearly superimposable oxypurinol plasma concentration vs time profiles, and the relative bioavailability of oxypurinol, ($F_{relative}$) was ≈ 100%. Thus, the pharmacokinetics and plasma profiles of oxypurinol, the major pharmacological components derived from allopurinol, are similar after IV and oral administration of allopurinol sodium for injection.

Contraindications

Patients who previously have developed a severe reaction to allopurinol.

Warnings

➤*Hepatotoxicity:* A few cases of reversible clinical hepatotoxicity have been noted in patients taking oral allopurinol, and in some patients asymptomatic rises in serum alkaline phosphatase or serum transaminase have been observed. If anorexia, weight loss, or pruritus develop in patients on allopurinol, include an evaluation of liver function as part of their diagnostic workup. In patients with preexisting liver disease, periodic liver function tests are recommended during the early stages of therapy.

➤*Hypersensitivity reactions:* Discontinue allopurinol at the first appearance of skin rash or other signs that may indicate an allergic reaction. In some instances with oral allopurinol, a skin rash may be followed by more severe hypersensitivity reactions such as exfoliative, urticarial, and purpuric lesions as well as Stevens-Johnson syndrome (erythema multiforme exudativum), and/or generalized vasculitis, irreversible hepatotoxicity and, on rare occasions, death.

➤*Renal function impairment:* The occurrence of hypersensitivity reactions to allopurinol may be increased in patients with decreased renal function receiving thiazides and allopurinol concurrently. Administer such combinations with caution in patients with decreased renal function.

A few patients with preexisting renal disease or poor urate clearance have shown a rise in BUN during allopurinol administration, although a decrease in BUN has also been observed. In patients with hyperuricemia due to malignancy, the vast majority of changes in renal function are attributable to the underlying malignancy rather than to therapy with allopurinol. Concurrent conditions such as multiple myeloma and congestive myocardial disease were present among those patients whose renal function deteriorated after allopurinol was begun. Renal failure is rarely associated with hypersensitivity reactions to allopurinol.

See Administration and Dosage for more information.

➤*Elderly:* Clinical studies of allopurinol sodium for injection did not include sufficient numbers of patients ≥ 65 years of age to determine whether they respond differently than younger patients. Other reported clinical experience has not identified differences in responses between the elderly and younger patients. In general, start at the low end of the dosing range when selecting a dose for the elderly.

➤*Pregnancy: Category C.* There is a published report in pregnant mice that single intraperitoneal doses of 50 or 100 mg/kg (≈ ⅓ or ¾ the human dose on a mg/m^2 basis) of allopurinol on gestation days 10 or 13 produced significant increases in fetal deaths and teratogenic effects (cleft palate, harelip, and digital defects). It is uncertain whether these findings represented a fetal effect or an effect secondary to maternal toxicity. There are, however, no adequate or well-controlled studies in pregnant women. Because animal reproduction studies are not always predictive of human response, use this drug during pregnancy only if the potential benefit justifies the potential risk to the fetus. Experience with allopurinol during human pregnancy has been limited partly because women of reproductive age rarely require treatment with allopurinol. Two unpublished reports and one published paper describe women giving birth to normal offspring after receiving oral allopurinol during pregnancy. There have been no pregnancies reported in patients receiving allopurinol sodium for injection, but it is assumed that the same risks would apply.

➤*Lactation:* Allopurinol and oxypurinol have been found in the milk of a mother who was receiving allopurinol. Because the effect of allopurinol on the nursing infant is unknown, exercise caution when allopurinol is administered to a nursing woman.

➤*Children:* Clinical data are available on ≈ 200 children treated with allopurinol sodium for injection. The efficacy and safety profile observed in this patient population were similar to that observed in adults (see Indications and Administration and Dosage).

Precautions

➤*Monitoring:* The correct dosage and schedule for maintaining the serum uric acid within the normal range is best determined by using the serum uric acid as an index. In patients with pre-existing liver disease, periodic liver function tests are recommended during the early stages of therapy (see Warnings). Allopurinol and its primary active metabolite, oxypurinol, are eliminated by the kidneys; therefore, changes in renal function have a profound effect on dosage. In patients with decreased renal function, or who have concurrent illnesses that can affect renal function such as hypertension and diabetes mellitus, periodic laboratory parameters of renal function, particularly BUN and serum creatinine or creatinine clearance, should be performed and the patient's allopurinol dosage reassessed. Assess prothrombin time periodically in patients receiving dicumarol who are given allopurinol.

ALLOPURINOL

➤*Fluid intake:* See Administration and Dosage for more information.

➤*Bone marrow suppression:* Bone marrow suppression has been reported in patients receiving allopurinol; however, most of these patients were receiving concomitant medications with the known potential to cause such an effect. The suppression has occurred from as early as 6 weeks to as long as 6 years after the initiation of allopurinol therapy.

➤*Hazardous tasks:* Because of the occasional occurrence of drowsiness, alert patients to the need for caution when engaging in activities where alertness is mandatory.

Drug Interactions

Allopurinol Drug Interactions

Precipitant drug	Object drug[a]		Description
Uricosuric agents	Allopurinol	↑	Because the excretion of oxypurinol is similar to that of urate, uricosuric agents, which increase the excretion of urate, are also likely to increase the excretion of oxypurinol. As a result, the concomitant administration of uricosuric agents decreases the inhibition of xanthine oxidase by oxypurinol and increases the urinary excretion of uric acid.
Allopurinol	Ampicillin/ Amoxicillin	↑	An increase in the frequency of skin rash has been reported among patients receiving ampicillin or amoxicillin concurrently with allopurinol compared with patients who are not receiving both drugs. The cause of this reaction has not been established.
Allopurinol	Chlorpropamide	↑	The half-life of chlorpropamide in the plasma may be prolonged by allopurinol, because allopurinol and chlorpropamide may compete for excretion in the renal tubule. The risk of hypoglycemia secondary to this mechanism may be increased if allopurinol and chlorpropamide are given concomitantly in the presence of renal insufficiency.
Allopurinol	Cyclosporine	↑	Reports indicate that cyclosporine levels may be increased during concomitant treatment with allopurinol sodium for injection. Monitor cyclosporine levels, and adjust cyclosporine dosage when these drugs are co-administered.
Allopurinol	Cytotoxic agents	↑	Enhanced bone marrow suppression by cyclophosphamide and other cytotoxic agents has been reported among patients with neoplastic disease, except leukemia, in the presence of allopurinol. However, in a well-controlled study of patients with lymphoma on combination therapy, allopurinol did not increase the marrow toxicity of patients treated with cyclophosphamide, doxorubicin, bleomycin, procarbazine, or mechlorethamine.
Allopurinol	Dicumarol	↑	It has been reported that allopurinol prolongs the half-life of the anticoagulant, dicumarol. Consequently, reassess prothrombin time periodically in patients receiving both drugs. The clinical basis of this drug interaction has not been established.
Allopurinol	Mercaptopurine/ Azathioprine	↑	Allopurinol inhibits the enzymatic oxidation of mercaptopurine and azathioprine to 6-thiouric acid (inactive). This results in increased levels of the active drug. Therefore, the concomitant administration of 300 to 600 mg of oral allopurinol per day will require a reduction in dose to approximately one-third to one-fourth of the usual dose of mercaptopurine or azathioprine. Make subsequent adjustment of doses of mercaptopurine or azathioprine on the basis of therapeutic response and the appearance of toxic effects.

[a] ↑ = Object drug increased.

Adverse Reactions

In an uncontrolled, compassionate plea protocol, 125 of 1378 patients reported a total of 301 adverse reactions while receiving allopurinol sodium for injection. Most of the patients had advanced malignancies or serious underlying diseases and were taking multiple concomitant medications. Side effects directly attributable to allopurinol sodium for injection were reported in 19 patients. Fifteen of these adverse experiences were allergic in nature (rash, eosinophilia, local injection site reaction). One adverse experience of severe diarrhea and one indicidence of nausea were also reported as being possibly attributable to allopurinol sodium for injection. Two patients had serious adverse experiences (decreased renal function and generalized seizure) reported as being possibly attributable to allopurinol sodium for injection.

A listing of the adverse reactions regardless of causality reported from clinical trials follows:

➤*Cardiovascular:* Bradycardia, cardiorespiratory arrest, cardiovascular disorder, decreased venous pressure, ECG abnormality, flushing, headache, heart failure, hemorrhage, hypertension, hypotension, pulmonary embolus, septic shock, stroke, thrombophlebitis, ventricular fibrillation (less than 1%).

➤*CNS:* Agitation, cerebral infarction, coma, dystonia, mental status changes, myoclonus, paralysis, seizure, status epilepticus, tremor, twitching (less than 1%).

➤*Dermatologic:* Rash (1.5%); local injection site reaction, pruritus, urticaria (less than 1%).

➤*GI:* Nausea (1.3%); vomiting (1.2%); diarrhea, GI bleeding, splenomegaly, hepatomegaly, intestinal obstruction, flatulence, constipation, proctitis (less than 1%).

➤*GU:* Renal failure/insufficiency (1.2%); hematuria, increased creatinine, kidney function abnormality, oliguria, urinary tract infection (less than 1%).

➤*Hematologic:* Anemia, bone marrow suppression, disseminated intravascular coagulation, ecchymosis, eosinophilia, leukopenia, marrow aplasia, neutropenia, pancytopenia, thrombocytopenia (less than 1%).

➤*Hepatic:* Hepatomegaly, hyperbilirubinemia, liver failure, jaundice (less than 1%).

➤*Hypersensitivity:* See Warnings for more information.

➤*Metabolic:* Edema, electrolyte abnormality, glycosuria, hypercalcemia, hyperglycemia, hyperkalemia, hypernatremia, hyperphosphatemia, hyperuricemia, hypocalcemia, hypokalemia, hypomagnesemia, hyponatremia, lactic acidosis, metabolic acidosis, water intoxication (less than 1%).

➤*Respiratory:* Apnea, ARDS, respiratory failure/insufficiency, increased respiration rate (less than 1%).

➤*Miscellaneous:* Alopecia, blast crisis, cellulitis, chills, diaphoresis, enlarged abdomen, fever, hypervolemia, hypotonia, infection, mucositis/pharyngitis, pain, sepsis, tumor lysis syndrome, arthralgia (less than 1%).

Overdosage

Massive overdosing or acute poisoning by allopurinol sodium for injection has not been reported. In mice, the minimal lethal dose is 45 mg/kg given IV or 500 mg/kg orally (≈ ⅓ or 4 times the usual human dose on a mg/m^2 basis). Hypoactivity was observed with these doses. In rats, the minimum lethal dose is 100 mg/kg IV and 5000 mg/kg orally (≈ 1.5 and 75 times the usual human dose on a mg/m^2 basis). In the management of overdosage, there is no specific antidote for allopurinol sodium for injection. There has been no clinical experience in the management of a patient who has taken massive amounts of allopurinol. Both allopurinol and oxypurinol are dialyzable; however, the usefulness of hemodialysis or peritoneal dialysis in the management of an overdose of allopurinol sodium for injection is unknown.

RASBURICASE

Rx	**Elitek** (Sanofi-Synthelabo)	**Powder for injection, lyophilized:** 1.5 mg/vial	10.6 mg mannitol. In single-use vials with 1 mL amps of diluent.

RASBURICASE — INJECTION

WARNING

Anaphylaxis – Rasburicase may cause severe hypersensitivity reactions including anaphylaxis. Rasburicase should be immediately and permanently discontinued in any patient developing clinical evidence of a serious hypersensitivity reaction. Signs and symptoms of these reactions include chest pain, dyspnea, hypotension and/or urticaria.

Hemolysis – Rasburicase administered to patients with glucose-6-phosphate dehydrogenase (G6PD) deficiency can cause severe hemolysis. It is recommended that patients at higher risk for G6PD deficiency (eg, patients of African or Mediterranean ancestry) be screened prior to starting rasburicase therapy. Rasburicase is contraindicated in patients with G6PD deficiency because hydrogen peroxide is one of the major by-products of the conversion of uric acid to allantoin. In clinical studies, 2 patients developed severe hemolytic reactions [National Cancer Institute Common Toxicity Criteria (NCI CTC) grade 3 and 4] within 2 to 4 days of the start of rasburicase. G6PD deficiency was subsequently identified in one of these patients. Rasburicase administration should be immediately and permanently discontinued in any patient developing hemolysis, and appropriate patient monitoring and support measures initiated (eg, transfusion support).

Methemoglobinemia – Rasburicase use has been associated with methemoglobinemia. In clinical studies, methemoglobinemia has been reported in 2 patients receiving rasburicase. Both patients developed serious hypoxemia requiring intervention with the appropriate medical support measures. It is not known whether patients with deficiency of cytochrome b_5 reductase (formerly known as methemoglobin reductase) or of other enzymes with antioxidant activity are at increased risk for methemoglobinemia or hemolytic anemia. Rasburicase administration should be immediately and permanently discontinued in any patient identified as having developed methemoglobinemia, and appropriate monitoring and support measures (eg, transfusion support, methylene-blue administration) implemented.

Interference with uric acid measurements – At room temperature, rasburicase causes enzymatic degradation of the uric acid in blood/plasma/serum samples potentially resulting in spuriously low plasma uric acid assay readings. The following special sample handling procedure must be followed to avoid ex vivo uric acid degradation.

Uric acid must be analyzed in plasma. Blood must be collected into prechilled tubes containing heparin anticoagulant. Samples must be immediately immersed in an ice water bath. Plasma samples must be prepared by centrifugation in a pre-cooled centrifuge (4°C). Finally, the plasma must be maintained in an ice water bath and analyzed for uric acid within four hours of collection.

Indications

➤*Hyperuricemia:* For the initial management of plasma uric acid levels in pediatric patients with leukemia, lymphoma, and solid tumor malignancies who are receiving anti-cancer therapy expected to result in tumor lysis and subsequent elevation of plasma uric acid.

➤*Unlabeled uses:* Prevent or reduce chemotherapy-induced tumor lysis syndrome and elevated plasma uric acid concentrations in adults with leukemia, lymphoma, or solid tumors.

Administration and Dosage

➤*Approved by the FDA:* July 16, 2002

➤*Dosage:* 0.15 or 0.2 mg/kg as a single daily dose for 5 days. Because the safety and effectiveness of other schedules have not been established, dosing beyond 5 days or administration of more than 1 course of rasburicase is not recommended. Chemotherapy should be initiated 4 to 24 hours after the first dose of rasburicase. Do not administer as a bolus infusion. Rasburicase should be administered as an intravenous infusion over 30 minutes.

➤*Reconstitution:* Determine the number of vials of rasburicase needed to achieve the proper dosage, based on the individual patient's weight and the dose per kilogram. Rasburicase must be reconstituted in the diluent provided. Add 1 mL of the provided reconstitution solution (diluent) to each vial of rasburicase and mix by swirling very gently. Do not shake or vortex. Parenteral drug products should be inspected visually for particulate matter and discoloration prior to administration, and discarded if particulate matter is visible or if product is discolored.

➤*Dilution and administration:* Using aseptic technique and syringes of appropriate volume, remove the predetermined dose of rasburicase from the reconstituted vials and inject into an infusion bag containing the appropriate volume of 0.9% sterile sodium chloride, to achieve a final total volume of 50 mL. This final solution for injection is to be infused over 30 minutes. No filters should be used for the infusion.

The reconstituted rasburicase contains no preservatives and must be administered within 24 hours of reconstitution. The reconstituted or diluted solution can be stored up to 24 hours at 2° to 8°C (36° to 46°F). Discard any unused product.

Rasburicase should be infused through a different line than that used for the infusion of other concomitant medications. If use of a separate line is not possible, the line should be flushed with at least 15 mL of saline solution prior to and after infusion with rasburicase.

➤*Storage/Stability:* The lyophilized drug product and the diluent for reconstitution should be stored at 2° to 8°C (36° to 46°F). Do not freeze. Protect from light.

Actions

➤*Pharmacology:* In humans, uric acid is the final step in the catabolic pathway of purines. The rapid increase of plasma uric acid levels is one of the main elements of tumor lysis syndrome, which may be seen shortly following the initiation of treatment of hematological malignancies, especially in children.

Rasburicase rapidly catalyzes enzymatic oxidation of an inactive and soluble metabolite (allantoin), which is readily excreted by the kidneys, thereby permitting optimal treatment of the patient's cancer.

Rasburicase is only active at the end of the purine catabolic pathway.

➤*Pharmacokinetics:* Pharmacokinetics of rasburicase were evaluated in 2 studies that enrolled patients with lymphoid leukemia (B and T cell), non-Hodgkin's lymphoma (including Burkitt's lymphoma) or acute myelogenous leukemia. rasburicase exposure, as measured by $AUC_{0\text{-}24\,hr}$ and C_{max}, tended to increase linearly with doses over a limited dose range (0.15 to 0.2 mg/kg). The overall elimination half-life was 18 hours. No accumulation of rasburicase was observed between days 1 and 5 of dosing. Rasburicase mean volume of distribution was 110 to 127 mL/kg in pediatric patients. There are insufficient data to characterize pharmacokinetics in adult patients.

Contraindications

Deficiency in glucose-6-phosphatase dehydrogenase (G6PD); history of anaphylaxis or hypersensitivity reactions, hemolytic reactions, or methemoglobinemia reactions to rasburicase or any of the excipients.

Warnings

➤*Anaphylaxis:* See the Warning box for more information.

➤*Hemolysis:* See the Warning box for more information.

➤*Methemoglobinemia:* See the Warning box for more information.

➤*Pregnancy: Category C.* Animal reproduction studies have not been conducted with rasburicase. It is also not known whether rasburicase can cause fetal harm when administered to a pregnant woman or can affect reproduction capacity. Rasburicase should be given to a pregnant woman only if clearly needed.

➤*Lactation:* It is not known whether this drug is excreted in human milk. Because many drugs are excreted in human milk and because of the potential for serious adverse reactions in nursing infants, a decision should be made whether to discontinue nursing or to discontinue rasburicase, taking into account the importance of the drug to the mother.

➤*Children:* The safety and efficacy of rasburicase were studied in 246 pediatric patients ranging in age from 1 month to 17 years. There were an insufficient number of patients in the 0 to 6 months age group (n = 7) to determine whether they respond differently from older children. These patients were pooled into the less than 2 years of age group (n = 24). Children less than 2 years of age had a higher mean uric acid $AUC_{0\text{ to }96\,hr}$ than those age 2 to 17 years (150 ± SE 16 mg•hr/dL vs 108 ± SE 4 mg•hr/dL, respectively). In addition, the data suggest that children less than 2 years of age had a lower rate of success at achieving maintenance uric acid concentration by 48 hours [83% (95% CI: 62 to 95) vs. 93% (95% CI: 89 to 95), respectively]. Children less than 2 years old also experienced more toxicity. The following adverse events were observed more frequently in children less than 2 years of age compared to those age 2 to 17 years respectively: Vomiting (75% vs. 55%), diarrhea (63% vs 20%), fever (50% vs 38%), and rash (38% vs 10%).

Precautions

➤*Hydration:* Patients on rasburicase should receive IV hydration according to standard medical practice for the management of plasma uric acid in patients at risk for tumor lysis syndrome.

Drug Interactions

➤*Drug/Lab test interactions:* At room temperature, rasburicase causes enzymatic degradation of the uric acid in blood/plasma/serum samples potentially resulting in spuriously low plasma uric acid assay readings. The following special sample handling procedure must be followed to avoid ex vivo uric acid degradation.

See the Warning box for more information.

Adverse Reactions

Among the 703 patients for whom serious adverse reactions were assessed, the most serious adverse reactions caused by rasburicase were allergic reactions including anaphylaxis (less than 1%), rash (1 %), hemolysis (less than 1%), and methemoglobinemia (less than 1%). The commonly observed serious adverse reactions were fever (5%), neutropenia with fever (4%), respiratory distress (3%), sepsis (3%), neutropenia (2%), and mucositis (2%). The following additional serious adverse reactions were observed in less than or

RASBURICASE — INJECTION

equal to 1% of patients regardless of causality: Acute renal failure, arrhythmia, cardiac failure, cardiac arrest, cellulitis, cerebrovascular disorder, chest pain, convulsions, cyanosis, diarrhea, dehydration, hot flushes, ileus, infection, intestinal obstruction, hemorrhage, myocardial infarction, paresthesia, pancytopenia, pneumonia, pulmonary edema, pulmonary hypertension, retinal hemorrhage, rigors, thrombosis, and thrombophlebitis.

Among the 347 patients for whom all adverse reactions regardless of severity were assessed, the most frequently observed adverse reactions (incidence greater than or equal to 10%) were vomiting (50%), fever (46%), nausea (27%), headache (26%), abdominal pain (20%), constipation (20%), diarrhea (20%), mucositis (15%), and rash (13%). In Study 1, an active control study, the following adverse events occurred more frequently in rasburicase-treated subjects than allopurinol-treated subjects: Vomiting, fever, nausea, diarrhea, and headache. Although the incidence of rash was similar in the 2 arms, severe rash (NCI CTC, Grade 3 or 4) was reported only in 1 rasburicase-treated patient.

➤*Immunogenicity:* Rasburicase is immunogenic in healthy volunteers, and can elicit antibodies that inhibit the activity of rasburicase in vitro. Signs and symptoms of these reactions include chest pain, dyspnea, hypotension and/or urticaria.

In a study of 28 healthy volunteers, the incidence of antibody responses to either a single dose or to 5 daily doses was assessed. Binding antibodies to rasburicase were detected by ELISA in 17/28 (61%) volunteers and neutralizing antibodies were detected in 18/28 (64%) volunteers. Time to detection of antibodies ranged from 1 to 6 weeks after rasburicase exposure. In 2 subjects with extended follow-up, antibodies persisted for 333 and 494 days.

The incidence of antibody responses in patients with hematologic malignancy has not been adequately assessed. In clinical trials of patients with hematologic malignancies, 24 of the 218 patients tested (11%) developed antibodies by day 28 following rasburicase administration. However, this is not a reliable estimate of the true incidence of antibody responses in patients with hematologic malignancies, because the data from the healthy volunteer study indicate that antibody may not be detectable until some time point beyond day 28.

The incidence of antibody responses detected is highly dependent on the sensitivity and specificity of the assay, which have not been fully evaluated. Additionally, the observed incidence of antibody positivity in an assay may be influenced by several factors, including serum sampling, timing and methodology, concomitant medications, and underlying disease. For these reasons, comparison of the incidence of antibodies to rasburicase with the incidence of antibodies to other products may be misleading.

Overdosage

No cases of overdosage with rasburicase have been reported. The maximum dose of rasburicase that has been administered as a single dose is 0.2 mg/kg; the maximum daily dose that has been administered is 0.4 mg/kg/day. According to the mechanism of action of rasburicase, an overdose will lead to low or undetectable plasma uric acid concentration, which has no known clinical consequences. Patients suspected of receiving an overdose should be monitored, and general supportive measures should be initiated as no specific antidote for rasburicase has been identified.

CLOFARABINE

Rx	**Clolar** (Genzyme Corporation)	**Solution for injection:** 1 mg/mL	Preservative free. In 20 mL vials.

CLOFARABINE — INTRAVENOUS INFUSION

Indications

➤*Acute lymphoblastic leukemia (ALL):* For the treatment of patients 1 to 21 years of age with relapsed or refractory acute lymphoblastic leukemia after at least 2 prior regimens. This use is based on the induction of complete responses. Randomized trials demonstrating increased survival or other clinical benefit have not been conducted.

➤*Unlabeled uses:* Treatment of other relapsed or refractory leukemias including acute myelocytic leukemia, myelodysplastic syndrome, and chronic myeloid leukemia in blast phase.

Administration and Dosage

➤*Approved by the FDA:* December 28, 2004.

➤*Recommended dose:* 52 mg/m^2 administered by (intravenous) IV infusion over 2 hours daily for 5 consecutive days. Treatment cycles are repeated following recovery or return to baseline organ function, approximately every 2 to 6 weeks. The dosage is based on the patients body surface area (BSA), calculated using the actual height and weight before the start of each cycle. To prevent drug incompatibilities, do not administer any other medications through the same IV line.

Preparation for administration – Filter clofarabine through a sterile 0.2 mcm syringe filter and then further dilute per instructions below with 5% dextrose injection or 0.9% sodium chloride injection prior to IV infusion.

Prevention of adverse events – Give continuous IV fluids throughout the 5 days of clofarabine administration to reduce the effects of tumor lysis and other adverse events. The use of prophylactic steroids (eg, hydrocortisone 100 mg/m^2 on days 1 through 3) may be of benefit in preventing signs or symptoms of systemic inflammatory response syndrome (SIRS) or capillary leak (eg, hypotension). If patients show early signs or symptoms of SIRS or capillary leak (eg, hypotension), immediately discontinue clofarabine administration and provide appropriate supportive measures.

Monitoring of toxicities – See Precautions for more information.

➤*Storage/Stability:* Vials containing undiluted clofarabine should be stored at 25 °C (77°F); excursions permitted to 15 to 30°C (59 to 86°F).

Filter clofarabine through a sterile 0.2 mcm syringe filter and then further dilute with 5% dextrose injection or 0.9% sodium chloride injection prior to IV infusion. The resulting admixture may be stored at room temperature but must be used within 24 hours of preparation.

Actions

➤*Pharmacology:* Clofarabine is sequentially metabolized intracellularly to the 5′-monophosphate metabolite by deoxycytidine kinase and mono- and di-phosphokinases to the active 5′-triphosphate metabolite. Clofarabine has high affinity for the activating phosphorylating enzyme, deoxycytidine kinase, equal to or greater than that of the natural substrate, deoxycytidine. Clofarabine inhibits DNA synthesis by decreasing cellular deoxynucleotide triphosphate pools through an inhibitory action on ribonucleotide reductase, and by terminating DNA chain elongation and inhibiting repair through incorporation into the DNA chain by competitive inhibition of DNA polymerases. The affinity of clofarabine triphosphate for these enzymes is similar to or greater than that of deoxyadenosine triphosphate. In preclinical models, clofarabine has demonstrated the ability to inhibit DNA repair by incorporation into the DNA chain during the repair process. Clofarabine 5′-triphosphate also disrupts the integrity of mitochondrial membrane, leading to the release of the pro-apoptotic mitochondrial proteins, cytochrome C and apoptosis-inducing factor, leading to programmed cell death.

Clofarabine is cytotoxic to rapidly proliferating and quiescent cancer cell types in vitro.

➤*Pharmacokinetics:*

Absorption/Distribution – The population pharmacokinetics of clofarabine were studied in 40 pediatric patients 2 to 19 years of age (21 males/19 females) with relapsed or refractory ALL or AML. At the given 52 mg/m^2 dose, similar concentrations were obtained over a wide range of BSAs. Clofarabine was 47% bound to plasma proteins, predominantly to albumin. Based on noncompartmental analysis, volume of distribution at steady-state was estimated to be 172 L/m^2.

Metabolism/Excretion – Based on noncompartmental analysis, systemic clearance was estimated to be 28.8 L/h/m^2. The terminal half-life was estimated to be 5.2 hours.

Based on 24-hour urine collections in the pediatric studies, 49% to 60% of the dose is excreted in the urine unchanged. In vitro studies using isolated human hepatocytes indicate very limited metabolism (0.2%); therefore, the pathways of nonrenal elimination remain unknown.

Contraindications

None.

Warnings

➤*Administration:* Administer clofarabine under the supervision of a qualified physician experienced in the use of antineoplastic therapy.

➤*Bone marrow suppression:* Anticipate suppression of bone marrow function. This is usually reversible and appears to be dose dependent. The use of clofarabine is likely to increase the risk of infection, including severe sepsis, as a result of bone marrow suppression.

Severe bone marrow suppression, including neutropenia, anemia, and thrombocytopenia, has been observed in patients treated with clofarabine. At initiation of treatment, most patients in the clinical studies had hematological impairment as a manifestation of leukemia. Because of the preexisting immunocompromised condition of these patients and prolonged neutropenia that can result from treatment with clofarabine, patients are at increased risk for severe opportunistic infections.

➤*Tumor lysis syndrome and other adverse events:* Administration of clofarabine results in a rapid reduction in peripheral leukemia cells. For this reason, evaluate patients undergoing treatment with clofarabine and monitor for signs and symptoms of tumor lysis syndrome, as well as signs and symptoms of cytokine release (eg, tachypnea, tachycardia, hypotension, pulmonary edema) that could develop into SIRS/capillary leak syndrome, and organ dysfunction. Physicians are encouraged to give continuous IV fluids throughout the 5 days of clofarabine administration to reduce the effects of tumor lysis and other adverse events. Administer allopurinol if hyperuricemia is expected. Discontinue clofarabine immediately in the event of clinically significant signs or symptoms of SIRS or capillary leak syndrome, either of which can be fatal, and consider use of steroids, diuretics, and albumin. Clofarabine can be re-instituted when the patient is stable, generally at a lower dose.

➤*Renal/Hepatic function impairment:* Clofarabine has not been studied in patients with hepatic or renal dysfunction. Use with caution in this patient population.

➤*Mutagenesis:* Clofarabine showed clastogenic activity in the in vitro mammalian cell chromosome aberration assay (CHO cells) and in the in vivo rat micronucleus assay. It did not show evidence of mutagenic activity in the bacterial mutation assay (Ames test).

CLOFARABINE — INTRAVENOUS INFUSION

➤*Fertility impairment:* Studies in mice, rats, and dogs have demonstrated dose-related adverse effects on male reproductive organs. Seminiferous tubule and testicular degeneration and atrophy were reported in male mice receiving intraperitoneal doses of 3 mg/kg/day (9 mg/m²/day, approximately 17% of clinical recommended dose on a mg/m² basis). The testes of rats receiving 25 mg/kg/day (150 mg/m²/day, approximately 3 times the recommended clinical dose on a mg/m² basis) in a 6-month IV study had bilateral degeneration of the seminiferous epithelium with retained spermatids and atrophy of interstitial cells. In a 6-month IV dog study, cell degeneration of the epididymis and degeneration of the seminiferous epithelium in the testes were observed in dogs receiving 0.375 mg/kg/day (7.5 mg/m²/day, approximately 14% of the clinical recommended dose on a mg/m² basis). Ovarian atrophy or degeneration and uterine mucosal apoptosis were observed in female mice at 75 mg/kg/day (225 mg/m²/day, approximately 4-fold the recommended human dose on a mg/m² basis), the only dose administered to female mice. The effect on human fertility is unknown.

➤*Pregnancy:* *Category D.* Clofarabine may cause fetal harm when administered to a pregnant woman. Clofarabine was teratogenic in rats and rabbits. Developmental toxicity (reduced fetal body weight and increased postimplantation loss) and increased incidences of malformations and variations (gross external, soft tissue, skeletal and retarded ossification) were observed in rats receiving 54 mg/m²/day (approximately equivalent to the recommended clinical dose on a mg/m² basis), and in rabbits receiving 12 mg/m²/day (approximately 23% of the recommended clinical dose on a mg/m² basis).

There are no adequate and well-controlled studies in pregnant women using clofarabine. If this drug is used during pregnancy, or if the patient becomes pregnant while taking this drug, apprise the patient of the potential hazard to the fetus.

Advise women of childbearing potential to avoid becoming pregnant while receiving treatment with clofarabine.

➤*Lactation:* It is not known whether clofarabine or its metabolites are excreted in human milk. Because of the potential for tumorigenicity shown for clofarabine in animal studies and the potential for serious adverse reactions, women treated with clofarabine should not breastfeed.

Precautions

➤*Monitoring:* Obtain complete blood counts and platelet counts at regular intervals during clofarabine therapy, and more frequently in patients who develop cytopenias. In addition, frequently monitor liver and kidney function during the 5 days of clofarabine administration.

Careful hematological monitoring during therapy is important. Assess hepatic and renal function prior to and during treatment with clofarabine because of clofarabine's predominant renal excretion and because the liver is a target organ for clofarabine toxicity. Closely monitor the respiratory status and blood pressure during clofarabine infusion.

➤*Adults:* Safety and efficacy have not been established in adults. One study was performed in highly refractory and/or relapsed adult patients with hematologic malignancies. The phase 2 dose of clofarabine was determined to be 40 mg/m²/day administered as a 1- to 2-hour IV infusion daily for 5 days every 28 days.

Adverse Reactions

The most common adverse effects after clofarabine treatment, regardless of causality, were GI tract symptoms, including vomiting, nausea, and diarrhea; hematologic effects, including anemia, leukopenia, thrombocytopenia, neutropenia, and febrile neutropenia; and infection.

Clofarabine Adverse Events (≥ 10% Overall)

	Clofarabine 52 mg/m² (N = 96)					
	Total		Grade 3		Grade 4	
Adverse Reaction[a]	N	%	n	%	n	%
Cardiovascular						
Flushing	17	18	–	–	–	–
Hypertension NOS[b]	11	11	4	4	–	–
Hypotension NOS	28	29	12	13	7	7
Tachycardia NOS	33	34	6	6	–	–
CNS						
Anxiety NEC[c]	21	22	2	2	–	–
Depression NEC	11	11	1	1	–	–
Dizziness (excluding vertigo)	15	16	–	–	–	–
Headache NOS	44	46	4	4	–	–
Irritability	11	11	1	1	–	–
Somnolence	10	10	1	1	–	–
Tremor NEC	10	10	–	–	–	–
Dermatologic						
Contusion	11	11	1	1	–	–
Dermatitis NOS	39	41	7	7	–	–
Dry skin	10	10	1	1	–	–
Erythema NEC	17	18	–	–	–	–
Palmar-plantar erythrodysesthesia syndrome	12	13	4	4	–	–
Petechiae	28	29	7	7	–	–
Pruritus NOS	45	47	1	1	–	–
GI						
Abdominal pain NOS	35	36	7	7	–	–
Constipation	20	21	–	–	–	–
Diarrhea NOS	51	53	10	10	–	–
Gingival bleeding	14	15	7	7	1	1
Nausea	72	75	14	15	1	1
Sore throat NOS	13	14	–	–	–	–
Vomiting NOS	80	83	8	8	1	1
GU						
Hematuria	16	17	2	2	–	–
Hematologic/Lymphatic						
Febrile neutropenia	55	57	51	53	3	3
Neutropenia	10	10	3	3	7	7
Transfusion reaction	10	10	3	3	–	–
Hepatic						
Hepatomegaly	14	15	8	8	–	–
Jaundice NOS	14	15	2	2	–	–
Metabolic/Nutrition						
Anorexia	30	31	5	5	7	7
Appetite decreased NOS	11	11	–	–	–	–
Edema NOS	19	20	1	1	2	2
Weight decreased	10	10	1	1	–	–
Musculoskeletal						
Arthralgia	11	11	3	3	–	–
Back pain	12	13	3	3	–	–
Myalgia	13	14	–	–	–	–
Pain in limb	28	29	5	5	–	–
Respiratory						
Cough	18	19	–	–	–	–
Dyspnea NOS	12	13	4	4	2	2
Epistaxis	30	31	14	15	–	–
Pleural effusion	10	10	3	3	2	2
Pneumonia NOS	10	10	5	5	2	2
Respiratory distress	13	14	6	6	5	5
Miscellaneous						
Bacteremia	10	10	10	10	–	–
Cellulitis	11	11	9	9	–	–
Fatigue	35	36	3	3	1	1
Herpes simplex	11	11	6	6	–	–
Injection site pain	13	14	1	1	–	–
Lethargy	11	11	–	–	–	–
Mucosal inflammation NOS	17	18	3	3	–	–
Oral candidiasis	12	13	2	2	–	–
Pain NOS	18	19	6	6	1	1
Pyrexia	39	41	15	16	–	–
Rigors	36	38	3	3	–	–
Sepsis NOS	14	15	7	7	7	7
Staphylococcal infection NOS	12	13	10	10	–	–

[a] Patients with more than one occurrence of the same preferred term are counted only once. Grade 4 includes deaths (Grade 5).
[b] Not otherwise specified.
[c] Not elsewhere classified.

CLOFARABINE — INTRAVENOUS INFUSION

➤*Cardiovascular:* The most frequently reported cardiac disorder was tachycardia (34%), which was, however, already present in 27.4% of patients at study entry. Most of the cardiac adverse events were reported in the first 2 cycles.

Pericardial effusion was a frequent finding in these patients on posttreatment studies, (19/55 [35%]). The effusion was almost always minimal to small and in no cases had hemodynamic significance.

Left ventricular systolic dysfunction (LVSD) was also noted. Fifteen out of fifty-five patients (15/55 [27%]) had some evidence of LVSD after study entry. In most cases where subsequent follow-up data were available, the LVSD appeared to be transient. The exact etiology for the LVSD is unclear because of previous therapy or serious concurrent illness.

➤*Hepatic:* Hepatobiliary toxicities were frequently observed in pediatric patients during treatment with clofarabine. Grade 3 or 4 elevated AST occurred in 38% of patients and grade 3 or 4 elevated ALT occurred in 44% of patients. Grade 3 or 4 elevated bilirubin occurred in 15% of patients, with 2 cases of grade 4 hyperbilirubinemia resulting in treatment discontinuation.

For patients with follow-up data, elevations in AST and ALT were transient and typically of less than 2 weeks duration. The majority of AST and ALT elevations occurred within 1 week of clofarabine administration and returned to baseline or grade 2 or below within several days. Although less common, elevations in bilirubin appeared to be more persistent. Where follow-up data are available, the median time to recovery from grade 3 and grade 4 elevations in bilirubin to grade 2 or below was 6 days.

➤*Infection:* At baseline 47% of the patients had 1 or more concurrent infections. A total of 85% of patients experienced at least 1 infection after clofarabine treatment, including fungal, viral, and bacterial infections.

➤*Renal:* The most prevalent renal toxicity was elevated creatinine. Grade 3 or 4 elevated creatinine occurred in 6% of patients. Nephrotoxic medications, tumor lysis, and tumor lysis with hyperuricemia may contribute to renal toxicity.

➤*SIRS/Capillary leak syndrome:* Capillary leak syndrome or SIRS (signs and symptoms of cytokine release, [eg, tachypnea, tachycardia, hypotension, pulmonary edema]) occurred in 4 pediatric patients overall (3 ALL, 1 AML). Several patients developed rapid onset of respiratory distress, hypotension, capillary leak (pleural and pericardial effusions), and multiorgan failure. Close monitoring for this syndrome and early intervention are recommended. The use of prophylactic steroids (eg, 100 mg/m^2 hydrocortisone on days 1 through 3) may be of benefit in preventing signs or symptoms of SIRS or capillary leak. Health care providers should be alert to early indications of this syndrome and should immediately discontinue clofarabine administration if they occur and provide appropriate supportive measures. After the patient is stabilized and organ function has returned to baseline, retreatment with clofarabine can be considered at a lower dose.

Overdosage

There were no known overdoses of clofarabine. The highest daily dose administered to a human to date (on a mg/m^2 basis) has been 70 mg/m^2/day for 5 days (2 pediatric ALL patients). The toxicities included in these 2 patients included grade 4 hyperbilirubinemia, grade 2 and 3 vomiting, and grade 3 maculopapular rash.

Patient Information

Patients receiving clofarabine may experience vomiting and diarrhea; therefore, advise them regarding appropriate measures to avoid dehydration. Instruct patients to seek medical advice if they experience symptoms of dizziness, lightheadedness, fainting spells, or decreased urine output. Stop clofarabine administration if the patient develops hypotension for any reason during the 5 days of administration. If hypotension is transient and resolves without pharmacological intervention, clofarabine treatment can be re-instituted, generally at a lower dose.

Because clofarabine is excreted primarily by the kidneys, avoid drugs with known renal toxicity during the 5 days of clofarabine administration. In addition, because the liver is a known target organ for clofarabine toxicity, avoid concomitant use of medications known to induce hepatic toxicity. Closely monitor patients taking medications known to affect blood pressure or cardiac function during administration of clofarabine.

Advise all patients to use effective contraceptive measures to prevent pregnancy. Advise female patients to avoid breastfeeding during treatment with clofarabine.

ANTIMITOTIC AGENTS

Vinca Alkaloids

VINBLASTINE SULFATE (VLB)

Rx	**Vinblastine Sulfate** (Various, eg, Cetus, VHA Supply)	**Powder for injection:** 10 mg	In vials.
Rx	**Velban** (Lilly)		In vials.
Rx	**Vinblastine Sulfate** (Various, eg, Quad)	**Injection:** 1 mg/ml	In 10 and 25 ml vials.[1]

[1] With 0.9% benzyl alcohol.

VINBLASTINE SULFATE (VLB) — INJECTION

WARNING

It is extremely important the needle be properly positioned in the vein before this product is injected. If leakage into surrounding tissue should occur during IV administration of vinblastine sulfate, it may cause considerable irritation. Immediately discontinue the injection, and introduce any remaining portion of the dose into another vein. Local injection of hyaluronidase and the application of moderate heat to the area of leakage will help disperse the drug and may minimize the discomfort and the possibility of cellulitis.

Fatal if given intrathecally. For IV use only.

Indications

Palliative treatment of the following:

➤*Frequently responsive malignancies:* Generalized Hodgkin's disease (stages III and IV, Ann Arbor modification of Rye staging system), lymphocytic lymphoma (nodular and diffuse, poorly and well differentiated); histiocytic lymphoma; mycosis fungoides (advanced stages); advanced testicular carcinoma; Kaposi's sarcoma and Letterer-Siwe disease (histiocytosis X).

➤*Less frequently responsive malignancies:* Choriocarcinoma resistant to other chemotherapy; breast cancer unresponsive to endocrine surgery and hormonal therapy.

➤*Multiple drug protocols:* Vinblastine, effective as a single agent, is usually administered with other antineoplastics. Combination therapy enhances therapeutic effect without additive toxicity when agents with different dose-limiting toxicities and mechanisms of action are selected.

➤*Hodgkin's disease:* Vinblastine used as a single agent; advanced Hodgkin's disease also has been successfully treated with multiple-drug regimens that included vinblastine.

➤*Advanced testicular germinal-cell cancers (embryonal carcinoma, teratocarcinoma, and choriocarcinoma):* Advanced testicular germinal-cell cancers are sensitive to vinblastine alone, but better clinical results are achieved with combination therapy. Vinblastine enhances the effect of bleomycin if given 6 to 8 hours prior to bleomycin administration; this schedule permits more cells to be arrested during metaphase, the stage in which bleomycin is active.

➤*Unlabeled uses:* Treatment of non-small cell lung carcinoma; bladder cancer; refractory idiopathic thrombocytopenic purpura.

Administration and Dosage

Leukopenic responses vary following therapy. For this reason, do not administer drug more than once weekly. Initiate therapy for adults with a single IV dose of 3.7 mg/m^2 of body surface. Thereafter, measure WBC counts to determine patient's sensitivity. A 50% dose reduction is recommended for patients having a direct serum bilirubin value > 3 mg/dlL. Because metabolism and excretion are primarily hepatic, no modification is recommended for patients with impaired renal function.

Incremental Vinblastine Dosage (Weekly Intervals)

	Adult dose (mg/m^2)	Pediatric dose (mg/m^2)
First dose	3.7	2.5
Second dose	5.5	3.75
Third dose	7.4	5
Fourth dose	9.25	6.25
Fifth dose	11.1	7.5

Use the same increments until a maximum dose not exceeding 18.5 mg/m^2 for adults and 12.5 mg/m^2 for children is reached. Do not increase dose after WBC count is reduced to ≈ 3000 cells/mm^3. For most adults the weekly dosage range is 5.5 to 7.4 mg/m^2.

➤*Maintenance therapy:* When the dose produces the above degree of leukopenia, administer a dose one increment smaller at weekly intervals for maintenance. Even though 7 days have elapsed, do not give the next dose until the WBC count has returned to at least 4000/mm^3. In some cases, oncolytic activity may be encountered before leukopenic effect but do not increase the size of subsequent doses.

Duration of maintenance therapy varies according to the disease and the combination of antineoplastics used. Prolonged chemotherapy for maintaining remission involves several risks: Life-threatening infections, sterility, secondary cancers through suppression of immune surveillance. In some disorders, survival following complete remission may not be as prolonged as that achieved with shorter periods of maintenance therapy. Conversely, failure to provide maintenance therapy may lead to unnecessary relapse; com-

VINBLASTINE SULFATE (VLB) — INJECTION

plete remission in patients with testicular cancer, unless maintained for at least 2 years, often results in early relapse.

➤*Administration:* Inject into either the tubing of a running IV infusion or directly into a vein over 1 minute. To prevent cellulitis or phlebitis, secure the needle within the vein so that no solution extravasates. To further minimize extravasation, rinse syringe and needle with venous blood before withdrawal of needle. Do not dilute the dose in large volumes of diluent (ie, 100 to 250 mL) or give IV for prolonged periods (≥ 30 min), because this often results in vein irritation and increases the chance of extravasation.

Because of the enhanced possibility of thrombosis, do not inject solution into an extremity in which circulation is impaired or potentially impaired by conditions such as compressing or invading neoplasm, phlebitis, or varicosity.

➤*Preparation (powder for injection):* Add 10 mL of Bacteriostatic Sodium Chloride Injection (preserved with phenol or benzyl alcohol) to the vial for a concentration of 1 mg/mL. The drug dissolves instantly to give a clear solution. A preservative-containing solvent is unnecessary if unused portions are discarded immediately.

➤*Compatibility:* Do not dilute with solvents that raise or lower the pH of the resulting solution from between 3.5 and 5. Make solutions with either Normal Saline or 0.9% Sodium Chloride Injection (each with or without preservative) and do not combine in the same container with any other chemical.

➤*Storage/Stability:* After reconstitution and removal of a portion from the vial, refrigerate the remainder for 28 days without loss of potency. Refrigerate unopened vials at 2° to 8°C (36° to 46°F).

Actions

➤*Pharmacology:* Vinblastine sulfate, an alkaloid extracted from Vinca rosea Linn, interferes with metabolic pathways of amino acids leading from glutamic acid to the citric acid cycle and urea. Studies have demonstrated a stathmokinetic effect and various atypical mitotic figures. However, therapeutic responses are not fully explained by the cytologic changes, because these changes are sometimes observed clinically and experimentally in the absence of any oncolytic effects.

Vinblastine has an effect on cell energy production required for mitosis and interferes with nucleic acid synthesis. In vitro, the drug arrests growing cells in metaphase.

Reversal of the antitumor effect by glutamic acid or tryptophan has occurred.

➤*Pharmacokinetics:*

Absorption/Distribution – Similar to vincristine, vinblastine undergoes rapid distribution and extensive tissue binding following IV injection. Vinblastine also localizes in platelets and leukocyte fractions of whole blood.

Metabolism/Excretion – Vinblastine is partially metabolized to deacetyl vinblastine, which is more active than the parent drug. Plasma decline follows a triphasic pattern. The initial, middle, and terminal half-lives are 3.7 minutes, 1.6 hours and 24.8 hours, respectively. Toxicity may be increased if liver disease is present.

Vinblastine is metabolized by the hepatic P450 3A cytochromes, and the major route of excretion may be through the biliary system.

Contraindications

Leukopenia; presence of bacterial infection (infections must be under control prior to initiating therapy); significant granulocytopenia unless it is a result of the disease being treated.

Warnings

➤*For IV use only:* The intrathecal administration of vinblastine has resulted in death. Label syringes containing this product "Vinblastine Sulfate for Intravenous Use Only."

Extemporaneously prepared syringes containing this product must be packaged in an overwrap that is labeled "Do Not Remove Covering Until Moment of Injection. Fatal if Given Intrathecally. For Intravenous Use Only."

➤*Hematologic effects:* Leukopenia is expected; leukocyte count is an important guide to therapy. In general, the larger the dose, the more profound and longer lasting the leukopenia will be. If the WBC count returns to normal after drug induced leukopenia, the white cell producing mechanism is not permanently depressed. Usually, WBC count has completely returned to normal after virtual disappearance of white cells from peripheral blood. The nadir in WBC count occurs 5 to 10 days after the last dose of drug is given. Recovery of the WBC count is fairly rapid and usually complete within 7 to 14 days. With smaller doses employed for maintenance therapy, leukopenia may not occur.

Although the thrombocyte count ordinarily is not significantly lowered by therapy, recently impaired bone marrow by prior therapy with radiation or with other oncolytic drugs may show thrombocytopenia (< 200,000 platelets/mm^3). When other chemotherapy or radiation has not been previously employed, thrombocytopenia is rare, even when vinblastine may be causing significant leukopenia. Rapid recovery (within a few days) from thrombocytopenia is the rule.

The effect on red blood cell count and hemoglobin is usually insignificant in the absence of other therapy; however, patients with malignant disease may exhibit anemia in the absence of any therapy.

If leukopenia (< 2000 WBC/mm^3) occurs following a dose of this drug, carefully watch the patient for evidence of infection until a safe WBC count has returned.

When cachexia or ulcerated skin surface occurs, a more profound leukopenic response may occur; avoid use in older persons suffering from these conditions.

In patients with malignant cell infiltration of bone marrow, leukocyte and platelet counts have sometimes fallen precipitously after moderate doses, making further use of the drug inadvisable.

Leukopenia (granulocytopenia) may reach dangerously low levels following use of the higher recommended doses. Follow recommended dosage technique. Stomatitis and neurologic toxicity, although not common or permanent, can be disabling.

➤*Hepatic function impairment:* See Administration and Dosage for more information.

➤*Fertility impairment:* Aspermia has been reported. Amenorrhea has occurred in some patients treated with a combination of an alkylating agent, procarbazine, prednisone and vinblastine. Its occurrence was related to the total dose of these agents. Recovery of menses was frequent. The same combination of drugs given to male patients produced azoospermia; if spermatogenesis did return, it was not likely to do so with less than 2 years of unmaintained remission.

➤*Pregnancy: Category D.* Information is very limited. Animal studies suggest teratogenicity may occur. Animals given the drug early in pregnancy suffered resorption of the conceptus; surviving fetuses demonstrated gross deformities. There are no adequate and well controlled studies in pregnant women, but the drug can cause fetal harm. If the drug is used during pregnancy, or if the patient becomes pregnant while receiving this drug, apprise her of the potential hazard to the fetus. Advise women of childbearing potential to avoid becoming pregnant.

➤*Lactation:* It is not known whether this drug is excreted in breast milk. Because of the potential for serious adverse reactions in nursing infants, decide whether to discontinue nursing or to discontinue the drug, taking into account the importance of the drug to the mother.

Precautions

➤*Long-term use:* Using small amounts of drug daily for long periods is not advised, even though the resulting total weekly dose may be similar to that recommended. Strict adherence to the recommended dosage schedule is very important. When amounts equal to several times the recommended weekly dosage were given in 7 daily installments for long periods, convulsions, severe and permanent CNS damage and death occurred.

➤*Avoid eye contamination:* Severe irritation or corneal ulceration (if the drug was delivered under pressure) may result. Thoroughly wash the eye with water immediately.

➤*Pulmonary reactions:* Acute shortness of breath and severe bronchospasm have occurred following use of vinca alkaloids. These reactions occur most frequently when the vinca alkaloid is used with mitomycin. Onset may be within minutes or several hours after the vinca is injected and may occur up to 2 weeks after the dose of mitomycin. (See Drug Interactions.)

➤*Benzyl alcohol:* Benzyl alcohol, contained in some of these products as a preservative, has been associated with a fatal "gasping syndrome" in premature infants.

Drug Interactions

Vinblastine Drug Interactions

Precipitant drug	Object drug*		Description
Vinblastine	Mitomycin	↑	Acute shortness of breath and severe bronchospasm have occurred following use of vinca alkaloids in patients who had previously or simultaneously received mitomycin. Onset may be within minutes or several hours after the vinca alkaloid is injected and may occur up to 2 weeks after the dose of mitomycin.
Vinblastine	Phenytoin	↓	Combination chemotherapy (including vinblastine) may reduce phenytoin plasma levels and increase seizure activity. Adjust the dosage based on serial blood level monitoring.
Erythromycin	Vinblastine	↑	May cause toxicity of vinblastine. Severe myalgia, neutropenia and constipation have been reported.
Agents that inhibit the cytochrome P450 pathway	Vinblastine	↑	Vinblastine is metabolized by the P450 3A enzyme. Use caution when coadministering drugs that inhibit P450 enzymes.

* ↑ = Object drug increased. ↓ = Object drug decreased.

Adverse Reactions

Incidence of adverse reactions is dose-related. Except for epilation, leukopenia and neurologic side effects, adverse reactions have not usually persisted for longer than 24 hours. Neurologic side effects are not common; when they occur, they often last for more than 24 hours. Leukopenia, the most common adverse reaction, is usually the dose-limiting factor.

VINBLASTINE SULFATE (VLB) — INJECTION

➤*Cardiovascular:* Hypertension. Cases of unexpected myocardial infarction and cerebrovascular accidents have occurred in patients undergoing combination chemotherapy with vinblastine, bleomycin and cisplatin.

➤*CNS:* Numbness of digits; paresthesias; peripheral neuritis; mental depression; loss of deep tendon reflexes; headache; convulsions.

➤*Dermatologic:* Alopecia is common. Total epilation infrequently develops. In some cases, hair regrows during maintenance therapy. A single case of light sensitivity has been associated with this drug.

➤*GI:* Nausea and vomiting (may be controlled by antiemetics); pharyngitis; vesiculation of the mouth; ileus; diarrhea; constipation; anorexia; abdominal pain; rectal bleeding; hemorrhagic enterocolitis; bleeding from an old peptic ulcer.

➤*Hematologic:* Leukopenia (granulocytopenia), anemia, thrombocytopenia (myelosuppression). See Warnings.

➤*Miscellaneous:* Malaise; weakness; dizziness; pain in tumor site; bone and jaw pain. The syndrome of inappropriate secretion of antidiuretic hormone has occurred with higher than recommended doses.

Extravasation during IV injection may lead to cellulitis and phlebitis; sloughing may occur (see Administration and Dosage).

There are isolated reports of Raynaud's phenomenon occurring in patients with testicular carcinoma treated with bleomycin, cisplatin and vinblastine sulfate. It is unknown whether the cause was the disease, the drugs or a combination of these.

Overdosage

➤*Symptoms:* Side effects are dose-related. After an overdose, expected exaggerated effects. In addition, neurotoxicity similar to that with vincristine may occur.

➤*Treatment:* Supportive care should include prevention of side effects that result from the syndrome of inappropriate secretion of antidiuretic hormone (ie, restriction of the volume of daily fluid intake to that of the urine output plus insensible loss and perhaps use of a diuretic affecting the function of the loop of Henle and the distal tubule); administration of an anticonvulsant; prevention of ileus; monitoring the cardiovascular system; and determining daily blood counts for guidance in transfusion requirements and assessing the risk of infection. The major effect of excessive doses will be myelosuppression, which may be life-threatening. There is no information regarding the effectiveness of dialysis nor of cholestyramine for the treatment of overdosage.

In the dry state, the drug is irregularly and unpredictably absorbed from the GI tract following oral administration. Absorption of the solution has not been studied. If vinblastine is swallowed, oral activated charcoal in a water slurry may be given along with a cathartic. The use of cholestyramine in this situation has not been reported.

Patient Information

Immediately report sore throat, fever, chills or sore mouth to the physician.

The following may occur: Alopecia, jaw pain, pain in the organs containing tumor tissue, nausea and vomiting. Scalp hair will regrow to its pretreatment extent, even with continued treatment. Report any other serious medical event to the physician.

Avoid constipation.

VINCRISTINE SULFATE (VCR; LCR)

Rx	**Vincristine Sulfate** (Various, eg, Quad, VHA Supply)	**Injection:** 1 mg/ml	In 1, 2 and 5 ml vials.
Rx	**Vincasar PFS** (Gensia Sicor)		In 1, 2, 5 ml flip-top vials.[1]

[1] With 100 mg mannitol. Refrigerate.

VINCRISTINE SULFATE (VCR; LCR) — INTRAVENOUS

WARNING

It is extremely important that the IV needle or catheter be properly positioned before injection. Leakage into surrounding tissue may cause considerable irritation.

This preparation is for IV use only. Intrathecal use usually results in death.

Indications

➤*Acute leukemia:* For acute leukemia.

➤*Combination therapy:* Combination therapy in Hodgkin's disease, non-Hodgkin's malignant lymphomas (lymphocytic, mixed-cell, histiocytic, undifferentiated, nodular and diffuse types), rhabdomyosarcoma, neuroblastoma and Wilms' tumor.

➤*Unlabeled uses:* Vincristine has been used in the treatment of idiopathic thrombocytopenic purpura, Kaposi's sarcoma, breast cancer, bladder cancer, small cell lung carcinoma, brain tumors, multiple myeloma, chronic lymphocytic and myelocytic leukemias, and autoimmune hemolytic anemia..

Administration and Dosage

Cautiously calculate and administer dose; overdosage may be serious or fatal.

Administer IV only, at weekly intervals. Inject solution either directly into a vein or into the tubing of a running IV infusion. Injection may be completed in about 1 minute.

➤*Adults:* 1.4 mg/m^2.

➤*Children:* 2 mg/m^2. For children weighing ≤ 10 kg or having a body surface area < 1 m^2, give 0.05 mg/kg once a week.

➤*Hepatic function impairment:* A 50% reduction in the dose is recommended for patients having a direct serum bilirubin value > 3 mg/dl.

➤*Extravasation:* Properly position needle in vein before injecting. Leakage into surrounding tissue may cause considerable irritation. Discontinue immediately; finish dose in another vein. Locally inject hyaluronidase; apply moderate heat to the area to disperse drug and minimize discomfort and possibility of cellulitis.

➤*Compatibility:* Do not dilute in solutions that raise or lower the pH outside the range of 3.5 to 5.5. Do not mix with anything other than normal saline or glucose in water.

Actions

➤*Pharmacology:* Vincristine sulfate is an alkaloid obtained from the periwinkle (Vinca rosea Linn). Mode of action is unknown. In vitro, it arrests mitotic division at metaphase. Antineoplastic effects are related to interference with intracellular tubulin function. It reversibly binds to microtubule and spindle proteins in the S phase.

➤*Pharmacokinetics:*

Absorption/Distribution – Within 15 to 30 minutes following IV administration, > 90% of the drug is distributed from blood into tissue where it remains tightly, but not irreversibly, bound. Penetration across the blood-brain barrier is poor.

Metabolism/Excretion – Studies in cancer patients show a triphasic serum decay pattern following rapid IV injection. Initial, middle and terminal half-lives are 5 min, 2.3 hrs and 85 hrs, respectively; the range of the terminal half-life is 19 to 155 hrs. The liver is the major excretory organ; ≈ 80% of a dose appears in feces and 10% to 20% in urine. Hepatic dysfunction may alter elimination kinetics and augment toxicity.

Contraindications

Do not give to patients with demyelinating form of Charcot-Marie-Tooth syndrome.

Warnings

➤*Administer IV only:* See the Warning box for more information.

➤*Hypersensitivity reactions:* Hypersensitivity temporally related to vincristine therapy, has occurred. Refer to Management of Acute Hypersensitivity Reactions. See Adverse Reactions.

➤*Carcinogenesis:* Patients who received vincristine with anticancer drugs known to be carcinogenic have developed secondary malignancies. Vincristine's contributing role in this development has not been determined.

➤*Fertility impairment:* Laboratory tests failed to conclusively demonstrate mutagenicity. Reports of both males and females who received multiple agent chemotherapy that included vincristine indicate azoospermia and amenorrhea can occur in postpubertal patients. Recovery occurred many months after chemotherapy completion in some. It is much less likely to cause permanent azoospermia and amenorrhea in prepubertal patients.

➤*Pregnancy: Category D.* Vincristine can cause fetal harm when administered to a pregnant woman. In several animal species, it induces teratogenic effects and embryolethality with doses that are nontoxic to the mother. There are no adequate and well controlled studies in pregnant women. If this drug is used during pregnancy or if the patient becomes pregnant while receiving it, apprise her of the potential hazard to the fetus. Advise women of childbearing potential to avoid becoming pregnant.

➤*Lactation:* It is not known whether this drug is excreted in breast milk. Because of the potential for serious adverse reactions in nursing infants, decide whether to discontinue nursing or the drug, taking into account importance of the drug to the mother.

Precautions

➤*Monitoring:* Dose-limiting clinical toxicity is manifested as neurotoxicity; clinical evaluation (history, physical examination) is necessary to detect need for dosage modification. Following vincristine, some patients may have a fall in WBC or platelet counts, particularly when previous therapy or the disease has reduced bone marrow function. Perform complete blood count before each dose. Acute serum uric acid elevation may occur during induction of remission in acute leukemia; thus determine such levels frequently during the first 3 to 4 treatment weeks or take appropriate measures to prevent uric acid nephropathy.

➤*Acute uric acid nephropathy:* Acute uric acid nephropathy has occurred.

➤*CNS leukemia:* CNS leukemia has occurred in patients undergoing otherwise successful therapy with vincristine. If CNS leukemia is diagnosed, additional agents may be required, since this drug does not adequately cross the blood-brain barrier.

VINCRISTINE SULFATE (VCR; LCR) — INTRAVENOUS

➤*Leukopenia or complicating infection:* In the presence of these conditions, administration of the next dose warrants careful consideration.

➤*Neuromuscular disease:* Pay particular attention to dosage and neurological side effects if administered to patients with preexisting neuromuscular disease or when other neurotoxic drugs are used.

➤*Eye contamination:* Eye contamination should be avoided with concentrations used clinically. If accidental contamination occurs, severe irritation (or, if drug was delivered under pressure, even corneal ulceration) may result. Wash eyes immediately and thoroughly.

➤*Pulmonary reactions:* Acute shortness of breath and severe bronchospasm have followed administration of vinca alkaloids, most frequently when the drug was used with mitomycin-C. The onset may be within minutes or several hours after the vinca is injected and may occur up to 2 weeks following the dose of mitomycin.

➤*Concomitant radiation therapy:* Do not give to patients receiving radiation therapy through ports that include the liver.

Drug Interactions

Vincristine Drug Interactions

Precipitant drug	Object drug*		Description
Vincristine	Digoxin	↓	Combination chemotherapy (including vincristine) may decrease digoxin plasma levels and renal excretion.
L-asparaginase	Vincristine	↑	Administering L-asparaginase first may reduce hepatic clearance of vincristine. Give vincristine 12 to 24 hrs before L-asparaginase to minimize toxicity.
Mitomycin	Vincristine	↑	Acute pulmonary reactions may occur (see Precautions).
Vincristine	Phenytoin	↓	Combination chemotherapy (including vincristine) may reduce phenytoin plasma levels, requiring increased dosage to maintain therapeutic plasma levels.

* ↑ = Object drug increased. ↓ = Object drug decreased.

Adverse Reactions

Adverse reactions are generally reversible and dose-related. With single weekly doses, leukopenia, neuritic pain, and constipation may occur and are usually of short duration (ie, < 7 days). When dosage is reduced, reactions may lessen or disappear. They seem to increase when the drug is given in divided doses. Other adverse reactions, such as hair loss, sensory loss, paresthesia, difficulty in walking, slapping gait, loss of deep tendon reflexes, and muscle wasting may persist for at least as long as therapy is continued. Generalized sensorimotor dysfunction may become progressively more severe with continued treatment. Neuromuscular difficulties usually disappear by the sixth week after treatment is discontinued, but they may persist for prolonged periods in some patients. Hair regrowth may occur while maintenance therapy continues.

SIADH – The syndrome of inappropriate antidiuretic hormone secretion (SIADH), including high urinary sodium excretion in the presence of hyponatremia, occurs rarely. Renal or adrenal disease, hypotension, dehydration, azotemia, and clinical edema are absent. With fluid deprivation, hyponatremia and renal sodium loss improve.

➤*CNS:* Loss of deep-tendon reflexes, ataxia, footdrop, and paralysis have been seen with continued use. Cranial nerve manifestations, including isolated paresis or paralysis of muscles may occur; extraocular and laryngeal muscles are most commonly involved. Severe pain may occur in the jaw, pharynx, parotid gland, bones, back, and limbs. Myalgias have occurred. Reduced intestinal motility results in constipation. Convulsions, often with hypertension, have occurred in a few patients. Convulsions followed by coma have been seen in children. Frequently, there is a sequence in the development of neuropathy: Initially, sensory impairment and paresthesias, then neuritic pain may appear and later, motor difficulties. Neurotoxicity is dose-related and cumulative to where therapy must be stopped after a cumulative dose of 30 to 50 mg. It is reversible upon discontinuation, but recovery may take several months.

In one study, the administration of glutamic acid (500 mg 3 times daily) decreased the neurotoxicity induced by vincristine.

➤*GI:* Oral ulceration; abdominal cramps; nausea; vomiting; diarrhea; anorexia; intestinal necrosis or perforation.

Constipation – Constipation may take the form of upper colon impaction, and, on examination, the rectum may be empty. Colicky abdominal pain may accompany an empty rectum. A flat film of the abdomen demonstrates this condition. Cases respond to high enemas and laxatives. Use routine prophylaxis for constipation.

Paralytic ileus – Paralytic ileus that mimics the "surgical abdomen" may occur, particularly in young children. The ileus will reverse itself upon temporary discontinuation of vincristine and with symptomatic care.

➤*GU:* Polyuria; dysuria; urinary retention due to bladder atony. Discontinue other drugs known to cause urinary retention (particularly in the elderly), if possible, for the first few days following administration.

➤*Hematologic:* Serious bone marrow depression (usually not dose-limiting); anemia; leukopenia; thrombocytopenia. Thrombocytopenia, if present when therapy is begun, may improve before the appearance of marrow remission.

➤*Hypersensitivity:* Rare cases of allergic type reactions, such as anaphylaxis, rash and edema, that are temporally related to vincristine therapy have occurred in patients receiving vincristine as a part of multi-drug chemotherapy regimens (see Warnings).

➤*Ophthalmic:* Optic atrophy with blindness; transient cortical blindness; ptosis; diplopia; photophobia.

➤*Pulmonary:* See Precautions for more information.

➤*Miscellaneous:* Hyper- or hypotension; weight loss; fever; alopecia; rash; headache.

Overdosage

➤*Symptoms:* Side effects are dose-related. After an overdose, expect exaggerated side effects. In children < 13 years of age, death has occurred after doses 10 times those recommended; severe symptoms may occur with 3 to 4 mg/m^2. Adults may experience severe symptoms after single doses ≥ 3 mg/m^2.

➤*Treatment:* Supportive care should include prevention of side effects resulting from SIADH (eg, fluid intake restriction; perhaps a diuretic affecting function of Henle's loop and distal tubule); phenobarbital (anticonvulsant); enemas or cathartics to prevent ileus (in some instances, GI tract decompression may be necessary); monitor cardiovascular system; determine daily blood counts to guide transfusion requirements.

Folinic acid, 100 mg IV every 3 hours for 24 hours, then every 6 hours for at least 48 hours, may help treat overdose. Folinic acid does not eliminate the need for supportive measures.

Most of an IV dose is excreted into the bile after rapid tissue binding. Hemodialysis is not likely to be helpful. Patients with liver disease sufficient to decrease biliary excretion may experience increased severity of side effects.

VINORELBINE TARTRATE

Rx	**Vinorelbine Tartrate** (GensiaSicor)	**Injection:** 10 mg/ml	In 1 and 5 mL vials.
Rx	**Navelbine** (GlaxoSmithKline)		Preservative free. In 1 and 5 mL single-use vials.

VINORELBINE TARTRATE — INJECTION

WARNING

Vinorelbine tartrate injection should be administered under the supervision of a physician experienced in the use of cancer chemotherapeutic agents. This product is for IV use only. Intrathecal administration of other vinca alkaloids has resulted in death. Syringes containing this product should be labeled "Warning — for IV use only. Fatal if given intrathecally."

Severe granulocytopenia resulting in increased susceptibility to infection may occur. Granulocyte counts should be greater than or equal to 1000 $cells/mm^3$ prior to the administration of vinorelbine tartrate. The dosage should be adjusted according to complete blood counts with differentials obtained on the day of treatment.

Caution – It is extremely important that the intravenous needle or catheter be properly positioned before vinorelbine tartrate is injected. Administration of vinorelbine tartrate may result in extravasation causing local tissue necrosis or thrombophlebitis.

Indications

➤*Non-small cell lung cancer:* As a single agent or in combination with cisplatin for the first-line treatment of ambulatory patients with unresectable, advanced nonsmall cell lung cancer (NSCLC). In patients with stage IV NSCLC, vinorelbine tartrate is indicated as a single agent or in combination with cisplatin. In stage III NSCLC, vinorelbine tartrate is indicated in combination with cisplatin.

➤*Unlabeled uses:* Metastatic breast cancer; carcinoma of the uterine cervix; desmoid tumors and fibromatosis; advanced Kaposi's sarcoma; ovarian cancer; cervical cancer; Hodgkin lymphoma; non-Hodgkin lymphoma.

Administration and Dosage

➤*Approved by the FDA:* December 23, 1994.

➤*Single-agent vinorelbine tartrate:* 30 mg/m^2 administered weekly. The recommended method of administration is an intravenous injection over 6 to 10 minutes. In controlled trials, single-agent vinorelbine tartrate was given weekly until progression or dose-limiting toxicity.

VINORELBINE TARTRATE — INJECTION

Vinorelbine tartrate in combination with cisplatin – Vinorelbine tartrate may be administered weekly at a dose of 25 mg/m^2 in combination with cisplatin given every 4 weeks at a dose of 100 mg/m^2.

Blood counts should be checked weekly to determine whether dose reductions of vinorelbine tartrate or cisplatin are necessary. In the SWOG study, most patients required a 50% dose reduction of vinorelbine tartrate at day 15 of each cycle and a 50% dose reduction of cisplatin by cycle 3.

Vinorelbine tartrate may also be administered weekly at a dose of 30 mg/m^2 in combination with cisplatin, given on days 1 and 29, then every 6 weeks at a dose of 120 mg/m^2.

➤*Hematologic toxicity:* Granulocyte counts should be greater than or equal to 1000 cells/mm^3 prior to the administration of vinorelbine tartrate. Adjustments in the dosage of vinorelbine tartrate should be based on granulocyte counts obtained on the day of treatment according to the table below:

Dose Adjustments Based on Granulocyte Counts	
Granulocytes on day of treatment (cells/mm^3)	Percentage of starting dose of vinorelbine tartrate injection
≥ 1,500	100%
1,000 to 1,499	50%
< 1,000	Do not administer. Repeat granulocyte count in 1 week. If 3 consecutive weekly doses are held because granulocyte count is < 1,000 cells/mm^3, discontinue vinorelbine tartrate.
Note: For patients who, during treatment with vinorelbine tartrate, experienced fever or sepsis while granulocytopenic or had 2 consecutive weekly doses held due to granulocytopenia, subsequent doses of vinorelbine tartrate should be:	
≥ 1,500	75%
1,000 to 1,499	37.5%
< 1,000	See above

➤*Hepatic insufficiency:* Vinorelbine tartrate should be administered with caution to patients with hepatic insufficiency. In patients who develop hyperbilirubinemia during treatment with vinorelbine tartrate, the dose should be adjusted for total bilirubin according to the table below:

Dose modification based on total bilirubin	
Total bilirubin (mg/dL)	Percentage of starting dose of vinorelbine tartrate
≤ 2	100%
2.1 to 3	50%
> 3	25%

➤*Concurrent hematologic toxicity and hepatic insufficiency:* In patients with both hematologic toxicity and hepatic insufficiency, the lower of the doses based on the corresponding starting dose of vinorelbine determined from information above should be administered

➤*Neurotoxicity:* If grade greater than or equal to 2 neurotoxicity develops, vinorelbine should be discontinued.

➤*Administration precautions:* Vinorelbine tartrate must be administered intravenously. It is extremely important that the intravenous needle or catheter be properly positioned before any vinorelbine tartrate is injected. Leakage into surrounding tissue during intravenous administration of vinorelbine tartrate may cause considerable irritation, local tissue necrosis, or thrombophlebitis. If extravasation occurs, the injection should be discontinued immediately, and any remaining portion of the dose should then be introduced into another vein. Since there are no established guidelines for the treatment of extravasation injuries with vinorelbine tartrate, institutional guidelines may be used. The ONS Chemotherapy Guidelines provide additional recommendations for the prevention of extravasation injuries.

As with other toxic compounds, caution should be exercised in handling and preparing the solution of vinorelbine tartrate. Skin reactions may occur with accidental exposure. The use of gloves is recommended. If the solution of vinorelbine tartrate contacts the skin or mucosa, immediately wash the skin or mucosa thoroughly with soap and water. Severe irritation of the eye has been reported with accidental contamination of the eye with another vinca alkaloid. If this happens with vinorelbine tartrate, the eye should be flushed with water immediately and thoroughly.

➤*Preparation for administration:* Vinorelbine tartrate injection must be diluted in either a syringe or IV bag using 1 of the recommended solutions. The diluted vinorelbine tartrate should be administered over 6 to 10 minutes into the side port of a free-flowing IV closest to the IV bag followed by flushing with at least 75 to 125 mL of 1 of the solutions. Diluted vinorelbine tartrate may be used for up to 24 hours under normal room light when stored in polypropylene syringes or polyvinyl chloride bags at 5° to 30°C (41° to 86°F).

Syringe – The calculated dose of vinorelbine tartrate should be diluted to a concentration between 1.5 and 3 mg/mL. The following solutions may be used for dilution: 5% dextrose injection, 0.9% sodium chloride injection.

IV bag – The calculated dose of vinorelbine tartrate should be diluted to a concentration between 0.5 and 2 mg/mL. The following solutions may be used for dilution: 5% dextrose injection, 0.9% sodium chloride injection, 0.45% sodium chloride injection, 5% dextrose and 0.45% sodium chloride injection, Ringer's injection, lactated Ringer's injection.

➤*Storage/Stability:* Unopened vials of vinorelbine tartrate are stable until the date indicated on the package when stored under refrigeration at 2° to 8°C (36° to 46°F) and protected from light in the carton. Unopened vials of vinorelbine tartrate are stable at temperatures up to 25°C (77°F) for up to 72 hours. This product should not be frozen. Store the vials under refrigeration at 2° to 8°C (36° to 46°F) in the carton. Protect from light. Do not freeze.

Actions

➤*Pharmacology:* Vinorelbine is a vinca alkaloid that interferes with microtubule assembly. The vinca alkaloids are structurally similar compounds comprised of 2 multiringed units, vindoline and catharanthine. Unlike other vinca alkaloids, the catharanthine unit is the site of structural modification for vinorelbine. The antitumor activity of vinorelbine is thought to be due primarily to inhibition of mitosis at metaphase through its interaction with tubulin. Like other vinca alkaloids, vinorelbine may also interfere with: 1) amino acid, cyclic AMP, and glutathione metabolism, 2) calmodulin-dependent Ca^{++}-transport ATPase activity, 3) cellular respiration, and 4) nucleic acid and lipid biosynthesis. In intact tectal plates from mouse embryos, vinorelbine, vincristine, and vinblastine inhibited mitotic microtubule formation at the same concentration (2 mcM), inducing a blockade of cells at metaphase. Vincristine produced depolymerization of axonal microtubules at 5 mcM, but vinblastine and vinorelbine did not have this effect until concentrations of 30 mcM and 40 mcM, respectively. These data suggest relative selectivity of vinorelbine for mitotic microtubules.

➤*Pharmacokinetics:* The pharmacokinetics of vinorelbine were studied in 49 patients who received doses of 30 mg/m^2 in 4 clinical trials. Doses were administered by 15- to 20-minute constant-rate infusions. Following intravenous administration, vinorelbine concentration in plasma decays in a triphasic manner. The initial rapid decline primarily represents distribution of drug to peripheral compartments followed by metabolism and excretion of the drug during subsequent phases. The prolonged terminal phase is due to relatively slow efflux of vinorelbine from peripheral compartments. The terminal phase half-life averages 27.7 to 43.6 hours and the mean plasma clearance ranges from 0.97 to 1.26 L/hr per kg. Steady-state volume of distribution (V_{ss}) values range from 25.4 to 40.1 L/kg.

Vinorelbine demonstrated high binding to human platelets and lymphocytes. The free fraction was approximately 0.11 in pooled human plasma over a concentration range of 234 to 1169 ng/mL. The binding to plasma constituents in cancer patients ranged from 79.6% to 91.2%. Vinorelbine binding was not altered in the presence of cisplatin, 5-fluorouracil, or doxorubicin.

Vinorelbine undergoes substantial hepatic elimination in humans, with large amounts recovered in feces after intravenous administration to humans. Two metabolites of vinorelbine have been identified in human blood, plasma, and urine; vinorelbine N-oxide and deacetylvinorelbine. Deacetylvinorelbine has been demonstrated to be the primary metabolite of vinorelbine in humans, and has been shown to possess antitumor activity similar to vinorelbine. Therapeutic doses of vinorelbine (30 mg/m^2) yield very small, if any, quantifiable levels of either metabolite in blood or urine. The metabolism of vinca alkaloids has been shown to be mediated by hepatic cytochrome P450 isoenzymes in the CYP3A subfamily. This metabolic pathway may be impaired in patients with hepatic dysfunction or who are taking concomitant potent inhibitors of these isoenzymes. The effects of renal or hepatic dysfunction on the disposition of vinorelbine have not been assessed, but based on experience with other anticancer vinca alkaloids, dose adjustments are recommended for patients with impaired hepatic function.

The disposition of radiolabeled vinorelbine given intravenously was studied in a limited number of patients. Approximately 18% of the administered dose was recovered in the urine and 46% in the feces. Incomplete recovery in humans is consistent with results in animals where recovery is incomplete, even after prolonged sampling times. A separate study of the urinary excretion of vinorelbine using specific chromatographic analytical methodology showed that 10.9% ± 0.7% of a 30 mg/m^2 intravenous dose was excreted unchanged in the urine. Although the pharmacokinetics of vinorelbine are not influenced by the concurrent administration of cisplatin, the incidence of granulocytopenia with vinorelbine tartrate used in combination with cisplatin is significantly higher than with single-agent vinorelbine tartrate.

Contraindications

Pretreatment granulocyte counts less than 1000 cells/mm^3.

Warnings

➤*Myelosuppression:* Patients treated with vinorelbine tartrate should be frequently monitored for myelosuppression both during and after therapy. Granulocytopenia is dose-limiting. Granulocyte nadirs occur between 7 and 10 days after dosing with granulocyte count recovery usually within the following 7 to 14 days. Complete blood counts with differentials should be performed and results reviewed prior to administering each dose of vinorelbine tartrate. Vinorelbine tartrate should not be administered to patients with granulocyte counts less than 1000 cells/mm^3. Patients developing severe granulocytopenia should be monitored carefully for evidence of infection or fever. Patients with a granulocyte count of greater than or equal to 1500 cells/mm^3 on treatment days should receive 100% starting dose of vinorelbine. Patients with a granulocyte count of 1000 to 1499 cells/mm^3 on treatment days should receive 50% starting dose of vinorelbine. Patients with a granulocyte count less than 1000 cells/mm^3 on treatment days should not receive vinorelbine; repeat the granulocyte count in 1 week and if 3 consecutive weekly doses are held because of the granulocyte less than 1000 cells/mm^3, discontinue vinorelbine.

VINORELBINE TARTRATE — INJECTION

➤*Pulmonary toxicity:* Reported cases of interstitial pulmonary changes and acute respiratory distress syndrome (ARDS), most of which were fatal, occurred in patients treated with single-agent vinorelbine tartrate. The mean time to onset of these symptoms after vinorelbine administration was 1 week (range 3 to 8 days). Patients with alterations in their baseline pulmonary symptoms or with new onset of dyspnea, cough, hypoxia, or other symptoms should be evaluated promptly.

➤*Hepatic function impairment:* See Administration and Dosage for more information.

➤*Mutagenesis:* Vinorelbine has been shown to affect chromosome number and possibly structure in vivo (polyploidy in bone marrow cells from Chinese hamsters and a positive micronucleus test in mice). It was not mutagenic in the Ames test and gave inconclusive results in the mouse lymphoma TK Locus assay. The significance of these or other short-term test results for human risk is unknown.

➤*Fertility impairment:* Vinorelbine did not affect fertility to a statistically significant extent when administered to rats on either a once-weekly (9 mg/m^2, approximately one third the human dose) or alternate-day schedule (4.2 mg/m^2, approximately one seventh the human dose) prior to and during mating. However, biweekly administration for 13 or 26 weeks in the rat at 2.1 and 7.2 mg/m^2 (approximately one fifteenth and one fourth the human dose) resulted in decreased spermatogenesis and prostate/seminal vesicle secretion.

➤*Elderly:* Of the total number of patients in North American clinical studies of IV vinorelbine tartrate, approximately one third were 65 years of age or greater. No overall differences in effectiveness or safety were observed between these patients and younger patients. Other reported clinical experience has not identified differences in responses between the elderly and younger patients, but greater sensitivity of some older individuals cannot be ruled out.

➤*Pregnancy: Category D.* Vinorelbine tartrate may cause fetal harm if administered to a pregnant woman. A single dose of vinorelbine has been shown to be embryo- or fetotoxic in mice and rabbits at doses of 9 mg/m^2 and 5.5 mg/m^2, respectively (one third and one sixth the human dose). At nonmaternotoxic doses, fetal weight was reduced and ossification was delayed. There are no studies in pregnant women. If vinorelbine tartrate is used during pregnancy, or if the patient becomes pregnant while receiving this drug, the patient should be apprised of the potential hazard to the fetus. Women of childbearing potential should be advised to avoid becoming pregnant during therapy with vinorelbine tartrate.

➤*Lactation:* It is not known whether the drug is excreted in human milk. Because many drugs are excreted in human milk and because of the potential for serious adverse reactions in nursing infants from vinorelbine tartrate, it is recommended that nursing be discontinued in women who are receiving therapy with vinorelbine tartrate.

➤*Children:* Safety and effectiveness in pediatric patients have not been established. Data from a single-arm study in 46 patients with recurrent solid malignant tumors, including rhabdomyosarcoma/undifferentiated sarcoma, neuroblastoma, and CNS tumors, at doses similar to those used in adults, showed no meaningful clinical activity. Toxicities were similar to those reported in adults.

Precautions

➤*Monitoring:* Patients with a history or preexisting neuropathy, regardless of etiology, should be monitored for new or worsening signs and symptoms of neuropathy while receiving vinorelbine tartrate.

➤*Discontinuation:* Most drug-related adverse events of vinorelbine tartrate are reversible. If severe adverse events occur, vinorelbine tartrate should be reduced in dosage or discontinued and appropriate corrective measures taken. Reinstitution of therapy with vinorelbine tartrate should be carried out with caution and alertness as to possible recurrence of toxicity.

➤*Bone marrow:* Vinorelbine tartrate should be used with extreme caution in patients whose bone marrow reserve may have been compromised by prior irradiation or chemotherapy, or whose marrow function is recovering from the effects of previous chemotherapy.

➤*Prior radiation therapy:* Administration to patients with prior radiation therapy may result in radiation recall reactions.

➤*Bronchospasm:* Acute shortness of breath and severe bronchospasm have been reported infrequently, following the administration of vinorelbine tartrate and other vinca alkaloids, most commonly when the vinca alkaloid was used in combination with mitomycin. These adverse events may require treatment with supplemental oxygen, bronchodilators, or corticosteroids, particularly when there is preexisting pulmonary dysfunction.

➤*Pulmonary toxicity:* See Warnings for more information.

➤*GI:* Vinorelbine tartrate has been reported to cause severe constipation (eg, grade 3 to 4), paralytic ileus, intestinal obstruction, necrosis, or perforation. Some events have been fatal.

➤*Eye contact:* Care must be taken to avoid contamination of the eye with concentrations of vinorelbine tartrate used clinically. Severe irritation of the eye has been reported with accidental exposure to another vinca alkaloid. If exposure occurs, the eye should immediately be thoroughly flushed with water.

➤*Lab test abnormalities:* Since dose-limiting clinical toxicity is the result of depression of the white blood cell count, it is imperative that complete blood counts with differentials be obtained and reviewed on the day of treatment prior to each dose of vinorelbine tartrate.

Drug Interactions

➤*P-450 enzymes:* Caution should be exercised in patients concurrently taking drugs known to inhibit drug metabolism by hepatic cytochrome P450 isoenzymes in the CYP3A subfamily, or in patients with hepatic dysfunction. Concurrent administration of vinorelbine tartrate with an inhibitor of this metabolic pathway may cause an earlier onset or an increased severity of side effects.

Vinorelbine Drug Interactions

Precipitant drug	Object drug*		Description
Cisplatin	Vinorelbine	↑	Although the pharmacokinetics of vinorelbine are not influenced by the concurrent administration of cisplatin, the incidence of granulocytopenia with vinorelbine used in combination with cisplatin is significantly higher than with single-agent vinorelbine.
Mitomycin	Vinorelbine	↑	Acute pulmonary reactions have been reported with vinorelbine and other anticancer vinca alkaloids used in conjunction with mitomycin.
Paclitaxel	Vinorelbine	↑	Monitor for signs and symptoms of neuropathy for patients who receive vinorelbine and paclitaxel, either concomitantly or sequentially.

* ↑ = Object drug increased.

Adverse Reactions

Summary of Adverse Reactions in 365 Patients Receiving Single-agent Vinorelbine Tartrate[a,b]

Adverse reaction	All patients (n = 365)	NSCLC (n = 143)
Bone marrow		
Granulocytopenia < 2000 cells/mm^3	90%	80%
Granulocytopenia < 500 cells/mm^3	36%	29%
Leukopenia < 4000 cells/mm^3	92%	81%
Leukopenia < 1000 cells/mm^3	15%	12%
Thrombocytopenia < 100,000 cells/mm^3	5%	4%
Thrombocytopenia < 50,000 cells/mm^3	1%	1%
Anemia < 11 g/dL	83%	77%
Anemia < 8 g/dL	9%	1%
Hospitalizations due to granulocytopenic complications	9%	8%

[a] None of the reported toxicities were influenced by age. Grade based on modified criteria from the National Cancer Institute.
[b] Patients with NSCLC had not received prior chemotherapy. The majority of the remaining patients had received prior chemotherapy.

Vinorelbine Tartrate Injection Adverse Reactions (%)

	All grades		Grade 3		Grade 4	
Adverse reaction	All patients	NSCLC	All patients	NSCLC	All patients	NSCLC
Clinical chemistry elevations, total bilirubin (n = 351)	13%	9%	4%	3%	3%	2%
AST (n = 346)	67%	54%	5%	2%	1%	1%
GI						
Nausea	44%	34%	2%	1%	0%	0%
Vomiting	20%	15%	2%	1%	0%	0%
Constipation	35%	29%	3%	2%	0%	0%
Diarrhea	17%	13%	1%	1%	0%	0%
Peripheral neuropathy[a]	25%	20%	1%	1%	< 1%	0%
Dyspnea	7%	3%	2%	2%	1%	0%
Alopecia	12%	12%	≤ 1%	1%	0%	0%
Miscellaneous						
Asthenia	36%	27%	7%	5%	0%	0%
Injection site reactions	28%	38%	2%	5%	0%	0%
Injection site pain	16%	13%	2%	1%	0%	0%
Phlebitis	7%	10%	< 1%	1%	0%	0%

[a] Incidence of paresthesia plus hypesthesia.

VINORELBINE TARTRATE — INJECTION

➤*Cardiovascular:* Chest pain was reported in 5% of patients. Most reports of chest pain were in patients who had either a history of cardiovascular disease or tumor within the chest. There have been rare reports of myocardial infarction.

➤*CNS:* Loss of deep tendon reflexes occurred in less than 5% of patients. The development of severe peripheral neuropathy was infrequent (1%) and generally reversible.

➤*Dermatologic:* Like other anticancer vinca alkaloids, vinorelbine tartrate is a moderate vesicant. Injection site reactions, including erythema, pain at injection site, and vein discoloration occurred in approximately one third of patients; 5% were severe. Chemical phlebitis along the vein proximal to the site of injection was reported in 10% of patients.

➤*GI:* Prophylactic administration of antiemetics was not routine in patients treated with single-agent vinorelbine tartrate. Due to the low incidence of severe nausea and vomiting with single-agent vinorelbine tartrate, the use of serotonin antagonists is generally not required.

➤*Hematologic:* Granulocytopenia was the major dose-limiting toxicity with vinorelbine tartrate. Dose adjustments are required for hematologic toxicity and hepatic insufficiency. Granulocytopenia was generally reversible and not cumulative over time. Granulocyte nadirs occurred 7 to 10 days after the dose, with granulocyte recovery usually within the following 7 to 14 days. Granulocytopenia resulted in hospitalizations for fever and/or sepsis in 8% of patients. Septic deaths occurred in approximately 1% of patients. Prophylactic hematologic growth factors have not been routinely used with vinorelbine tartrate. If medically necessary, growth factors may be administered at recommended doses no earlier than 24 hours after the administration of cytotoxic chemotherapy. Growth factors should not be administered in the period 24 hours before the administration of chemotherapy.

Whole blood or packed red blood cells were administered to 18% of patients who received vinorelbine tartrate.

➤*Hepatic:* Transient elevations of liver enzymes were reported without clinical symptoms.

➤*Pulmonary:* Shortness of breath was reported in 3% of patients; it was severe in 2%. Interstitial pulmonary changes were documented.

➤*Miscellaneous:* Fatigue occurred in 27% of patients. It was usually mild or moderate but tended to increase with cumulative dosing. Other toxicities that have been reported in less than 5% of patients include jaw pain, myalgia, arthralgia, and rash. Hemorrhagic cystitis and the syndrome of inappropriate ADH secretion were each reported in less than 1% of patients.

➤*Postmarketing:*

Cardiovascular – Hypertension, hypotension, vasodilation, tachycardia, and pulmonary edema have been reported.

CNS – Peripheral neurotoxicities such as, but not limited to, muscle weakness and disturbance of gait, have been observed in patients with and without prior symptoms. There may be increased potential for neurotoxicity in patients with preexisting neuropathy, regardless of etiology, who receive vinorelbine tartrate. Vestibular and auditory deficits have been observed with vinorelbine tartrate, usually when used in combination with cisplatin.

Dermatologic – Injection site reactions, including localized rash and urticaria, blister formation, and skin sloughing have been observed in clinical practice. Some of these reactions may be delayed in appearance.

GI – Dysphagia, mucositis, and pancreatitis have been reported.

Hematologic – Thromboembolic events including pulmonary embolus and deep venous thrombosis have been reported primarily in seriously ill and debilitated patients with known predisposing risk factors for these events.

Hypersensitivity – Systemic allergic reactions reported as anaphylaxis, pruritus, urticaria, and angioedema; flushing; and radiation recall events such as dermatitis and esophagitis have been reported.

Musculoskeletal – Headache has been reported, with and without other musculoskeletal aches and pains.

Pulmonary – Pneumonia has been reported.

Miscellaneous – Pain in tumor-containing tissue, back pain, and abdominal pain have been reported. Electrolyte abnormalities, including hyponatremia with or without the syndrome of inappropriate ADH secretion, have been reported in seriously ill and debilitated patients.

Overdosage

There is no known antidote for overdoses of vinorelbine tartrate. Overdoses involving quantities up to 10 times the recommended dose (30 mg/m^2) have been reported. The toxicities described were consistent with the adverse reactions, including paralytic ileus, stomatitis, and esophagitis. Bone marrow aplasia, sepsis, and paresis have also been reported. Fatalities have occurred following overdose of vinorelbine tartrate. If overdosage occurs, general supportive measures together with appropriate blood transfusions, growth factors, and antibiotics should be instituted as deemed necessary by the physician.

Patient Information

Patients should be informed that the major acute toxicities of vinorelbine tartrate are related to bone marrow toxicity, specifically granulocytopenia with increased susceptibility to infection. They should be advised to report fever or chills immediately. Women of childbearing potential should be advised to avoid becoming pregnant during treatment.

Patients should be advised to contact their physician if they experience increased shortness of breath, cough, or other new pulmonary symptoms, or if they experience symptoms of abdominal pain or constipation.

PACLITAXEL

Rx	**Paclitaxel** (SuperGen)	**Injection:** 6 mg/mL	In 5 and 16.7 mL multi-dose vials.[a]
Rx	**Taxol** (Bristol-Myers Squibb)		In 5, 16.7, and 50 mL multi-dose vials.[a]
Rx	**Onxol** (Zenith Goldline Pharmaceuticals)		In 5, 25, and 50 mL multi-dose vials.[b]
Rx	**Abraxane** (Abraxis Oncology)	**Powder for injection, lyophilized (albumin-bound):** 100 mg	In single-use vials.[c]

[a] With 527 mg/mL polyoxyethylated castor oil (*Cremophor EL*) and 49.7% dehydrated alcohol.
[b] With 527 mg/mL polyoxyl 35 castor oil and 49.7% dehydrated alcohol.
[c] With 900 mg human albumin.

PACLITAXEL — INJECTION

WARNING

Administer paclitaxel under the supervision of a health care provider experienced in the use of cancer chemotherapeutic agents. Appropriate management of complications is possible only when adequate diagnostic and treatment facilities are readily available.

Paclitaxel injection – Do not give paclitaxel therapy to patients with solid tumors who have baseline neutrophil counts of less than 1,500 cells/mm^3, and do not give to patients with AIDS-related Kaposi sarcoma if the baseline neutrophil count is less than 1,000 cells/mm^3. In order to monitor the occurrence of bone marrow suppression, primarily neutropenia, which may be severe and result in infection, perform frequent peripheral blood cell counts on all patients receiving paclitaxel.

Anaphylaxis and severe hypersensitivity reactions characterized by dyspnea and hypotension requiring treatment, angioedema, and generalized urticaria have occurred in 2% to 4% of patients receiving paclitaxel in clinical trials. Fatal reactions have occurred in patients despite premedication. Pretreat all patients with corticosteroids, diphenhydramine, and H_2 antagonists. Do not rechallenge patients who experience severe hypersensitivity reactions to paclitaxel with the drug.

Abraxane – Do not give paclitaxel therapy to patients with metastatic breast cancer who have baseline neutrophil counts of less than 1,500 cells/mm^3. In order to monitor the occurrence of bone marrow suppression, primarily neutropenia, which may be severe and result in infection, perform frequent peripheral blood cell counts on all patients receiving paclitaxel.

WARNING (cont.)

An albumin form of paclitaxel may substantially affect a drug's functional properties relative to those of drug in solution. Do not substitute for or with other paclitaxel formulations.

Indications

➤*Taxol*:

Ovarian cancer – As first-line and subsequent therapy for the treatment of advanced carcinoma of the ovary. As first-line therapy, paclitaxel is indicated in combination with cisplatin.

Breast cancer – Adjuvant treatment of node-positive breast cancer administered sequentially to standard doxorubicin-containing combination chemotherapy. In the clinical trial, there was an overall favorable effect on disease-free and overall survival in the total population of patients with receptor-positive and receptor-negative tumors, but the benefit has been specifically demonstrated by available data (median follow-up, 30 months) only in the patients with estrogen and progesterone receptor-negative tumors.

Indicated for the treatment of breast cancer after failure of combination chemotherapy for metastatic disease or relapse within 6 months of adjuvant chemotherapy. Previous therapy should have included an anthracycline unless clinically contraindicated.

Non-small cell lung cancer (NSCLC) – In combination with cisplatin, for the first-line treatment of NSCLC in patients who are not candidates for potentially curative surgery or radiation therapy.

AIDS-related Kaposi sarcoma – For the second-line treatment of AIDS-related Kaposi sarcoma.

PACLITAXEL — INJECTION

➤*Onxol:*

Ovarian cancer – As subsequent therapy for the treatment of advanced carcinoma of the ovary.

Breast cancer – For the treatment of breast cancer after failure of combination chemotherapy for metastatic disease or relapse within 6 months of adjuvant chemotherapy. Previous therapy should have included an anthracycline unless clinically contraindicated.

➤*Abraxane:*

Breast cancer – For the treatment of breast cancer after failure of combination chemotherapy for metastatic disease or relapse within 6 months of adjuvant chemotherapy. Previous therapy should have included an anthracycline unless clinically contraindicated.

➤*Unlabeled uses:* Squamous cell head and neck cancer, small-cell lung cancer, bladder cancer, endometrial cancer, esophageal cancer, prostate cancer, gastric cancer, testicular cancer, and germ cell tumors. Paclitaxel has also been used for refractory leukemia and recurrent Wilms tumor in children.

Administration and Dosage

➤*Approved by the FDA:* December 29, 1992.

➤*Preparation:* Prior to infusion, dilute paclitaxel concentrate in 0.9% sodium chloride injection; 5% dextrose injection, USP; 5% dextrose and 0.9% sodium chloride injection; or 5% dextrose in Ringer's injection to a final concentration of 0.3 to 1.2 mg/mL. The solutions are physically and chemically stable for up to 27 hours at ambient temperature (approximately 25°C; 77°F) and room lighting conditions. Inspect parenteral drug products visually for particulate matter and discoloration prior to administration whenever solution and container permit.

Upon preparation, solutions may show haziness, which is attributed to the formulation vehicle. No significant losses in potency have been noted following simulated delivery of the solution through IV tubing containing an in-line (0.22 micron) filter. The use of an in-line (0.22 micron) filter is not recommended with *Abraxane*.

➤*Recommended dose:*

Taxol –

Ovarian cancer:

1.) For previously untreated patients with carcinoma of the ovary, 1 of the following recommended regimens may be given every 3 weeks. In selecting the appropriate regimen, consider differences in toxicities.
   a.) Paclitaxel 175 mg/m^2 administered intravenously (IV) over 3 hours followed by cisplatin 75 mg/m^2.
   b.) Paclitaxel 135 mg/m^2 administered IV over 24 hours followed by cisplatin 75 mg/m^2.
2.) In patients previously treated with chemotherapy for carcinoma of the ovary, paclitaxel has been used at several doses and schedules; however, the optimal regimen is not yet clear. The recommended regimen is paclitaxel 135 or 175 mg/m^2 administered IV over 3 hours every 3 weeks.

Breast cancer:

1.) For the adjuvant treatment of node-positive breast cancer, the recommended regimen is paclitaxel 175 mg/m^2 IV over 3 hours every 3 weeks for 4 courses administered sequentially to doxorubicin-containing combination chemotherapy. The clinical trial used 4 courses of doxorubicin and cyclophosphamide.
2.) After failure of initial chemotherapy for metastatic disease or relapse within 6 months of adjuvant chemotherapy, paclitaxel 175 mg/m^2 administered IV over 3 hours every 3 weeks has been shown to be effective.

NSCLC: Given every 3 weeks, paclitaxel 135 mg/m^2 is administered IV over 24 hours followed by cisplatin 75 mg/m^2.

Repeated course: For the therapy of patients with solid tumors (ovary, breast, and NSCLC), do not repeat courses of *Taxol* until neutrophil count is at least 1,500 cells/mm^3 and the platelet count is at least 100,000 cells/mm^3.

AIDS-related Kaposi sarcoma: Do not give *Taxol* to patients with AIDS-related Kaposi sarcoma if the baseline or subsequent neutrophil count is less than 1,000 cells/mm^3. Paclitaxel 135 mg/m^2 given IV over 3 hours every 3 weeks or at a dose of 100 mg/m^2 given IV over 3 hours every 2 weeks is recommended (dose intensity 45 to 50 mg/m^2/week). In the 2 clinical trials evaluating these schedules, the former schedule (135 mg/m^2 every 3 weeks) was more toxic than the latter. In addition, all patients with low performance status were treated with the latter schedule (100 mg/m^2 every 2 weeks).

Based upon the immunosuppression in patients with advanced HIV disease, the following modifications are recommended in these patients:

1.) Reduce the dose of dexamethasone (as 1 of the 3 premedication drugs) to 10 mg orally (instead of 20 mg orally).
2.) Initiate or repeat treatment with paclitaxel only if the neutrophil count is at least 1,000 cells/mm^3.
3.) Reduce the dose of subsequent courses of paclitaxel 20% for patients who experience severe neutropenia (neutrophil less than 500 cells/mm^3 for a week or longer).
4.) Initiate concomitant hematopoietic growth factor (G-CSF) as clinically indicated.

• *Hepatic function impairment* – Patients with hepatic impairment may be at increased risk of toxicity, particularly grade 3 to 4 myelosuppression. Recommendations for dosage adjustment for the first course of therapy are shown in the table below for 3- and 24-hour infusions. Base further dose reduction in subsequent courses on individual tolerance. Monitor patients closely for the development of profound myelosuppression.

Paclitaxel Dosing Recommendations in Patients with Hepatic Impairment Based on Clinical Trial Data[a]

Transaminase levels		Bilirubin levels[b]	Recommended paclitaxel dose[c]
24-hour infusion			
< 2 × ULN[d]	and	≤ 1.5 mg/dL	135 mg/m^2
2 to < 10 × ULN	and	≤ 1.5 mg/dL	100 mg/m^2
< 10 × ULN	and	1.6 to 7.5 mg/dL	50 mg/m^2
≥ 10 × ULN	or	> 7.5 mg/dL	Not recommended
3-hour infusion			
< 10 × ULN	and	≤ 1.25 × ULN	175 mg/m^2
< 10 × ULN	and	1.26 to 2 × ULN	135 mg/m^2
< 10 × ULN	and	2.01 to 5 × ULN	90 mg/m^2
≥ 10 × ULN	or	> 5 × ULN	Not recommended

[a] These recommendations are based on doses for patients without hepatic impairment of 135 mg/m^2 over 24 hours or 175 mg/m^2 over 3 hours; data are not available to make dose adjustment recommendations for other regimens (eg, for AIDS-related Kaposi sarcoma).
[b] Differences in criteria for bilirubin levels between the 3- and 24-hour infusion are caused by differences in clinical trial design.
[c] Dose recommendations are for the first course of therapy; base further dose reduction in subsequent courses on individual tolerance.
[d] ULN = Upper limit normal.

Onxol –

Ovarian cancer: In patients previously treated with chemotherapy for carcinoma of the ovary, paclitaxel has been used at several doses and schedules; however, the optimal regimen is not yet clear. The recommended regimen is paclitaxel 135 or 175 mg/m^2 administered IV over 3 hours every 3 weeks.

Breast cancer: After failure of initial chemotherapy for metastatic disease or relapse within 6 months of adjuvant chemotherapy, paclitaxel 175 mg/m^2 administered IV over 3 hours every 3 weeks has been shown to be effective.

• *Repeat courses* – For therapy of patients with solid tumors (ovary and breast), do not repeat courses of paclitaxel until the neutrophil count is at least 1,500 cells/mm^3 and the platelet count is at least 100,000 cells/mm^3.

Abraxane – After failure of combination chemotherapy for metastatic breast cancer or relapse within 6 months of adjuvant chemotherapy, the recommended regimen for paclitaxel protein-bound particles is 260 mg/m^2 administered IV over 30 minutes every 3 weeks.

Dose reduction –

Taxol/Onxol: In patients who experience severe neutropenia (neutrophil counts less than 500 cells/mm^3 for 1 week or longer) or severe peripheral neuropathy during paclitaxel injection therapy, reduce the dosage 20% for subsequent courses of paclitaxel. The incidence of neurotoxicity and the severity of neutropenia increase with dose.

Abraxane: In patients who experience severe neutropenia (neutrophil counts less than 500 cells/mm^3 for 1 week or longer) or severe sensory neuropathy during paclitaxel protein-bound particles therapy, reduce the dosage to 220 mg/m^2 for subsequent courses of paclitaxel protein-bound particles. For recurrence of severe neutropenia or severe sensory neuropathy, make an additional dose reduction to 180 mg/m^2. For grade 3 sensory neuropathy, hold treatment until resolution to grade 1 or 2, followed by a dose reduction for all subsequent courses of paclitaxel protein-bound particles.

➤*Administration:* Given the possibility of extravasation, it is advisable to closely monitor the infusion site for possible infiltration during drug administration. A specific treatment for extravasation reactions is unknown.

Taxol/Onxol – Administer paclitaxel through an in-line filter with a microporous membrane not more than 0.22 microns. Use of filter devices, such as *IVEX-2* filters that incorporate short inlet and outlet PVC-coated tubing, has not resulted in significant leaching of (di-[2-ethylhexyl]phthalate) DEHP.

Do not use the *Chemo Dispensing Pin* device or similar devices with spikes with vials of paclitaxel because they can cause the stopper to collapse, resulting in loss of sterile integrity of the paclitaxel solution.

Premedication: Premedicate all patients prior to paclitaxel administration to prevent severe hypersensitivity reactions. Such premedication may consist of oral dexamethasone 20 mg administered approximately 12 and 6 hours before paclitaxel, diphenhydramine (or its equivalent) 50 mg IV 30 to 60 minutes prior to paclitaxel, and cimetidine 300 mg or ranitidine 50 mg IV 30 to 60 minutes before paclitaxel.

PVC equipment: Contact of the undiluted paclitaxel concentrate with plasticized PVC equipment or devices used to prepare solutions for infusion is not recommended. Data collected for the presence of the extractable plasticizer di-(2-ethylhexyl)phthalate (DEHP) show that levels increase with time and concentration when dilutions are prepared in polyvinyl chloride (PVC) containers. In order to minimize patient exposure to the plasticizer DEHP, which may be leached from PVC infusion bags or sets, store diluted paclitaxel solutions in bottles (glass, polypropylene) or plastic bags (polypropylene, polyolefin) and administer through polyethylene-lined administration sets.

Abraxane – Paclitaxel protein-bound particles are supplied as a sterile lyophilized powder for reconstitution before use. To avoid errors, read entire preparation instructions prior to reconstitution.

1.) Aseptically reconstitute each vial by injecting 20 mL of 0.9% sodium chloride injection.
2.) Slowly inject the 20 mL of 0.9% sodium chloride injection over a minimum of 1 minute, using the sterile syringe to direct the solution flow onto the inside wall of the vial.
3.) Do not inject the 0.9% sodium chloride injection directly onto the lyophilized cake because this will result in foaming.

PACLITAXEL — INJECTION

4.) Once the injection is complete, allow the vial to sit for a minimum of 5 minutes to ensure proper wetting of the lyophilized cake/powder.
5.) Gently swirl and/or invert the vial slowly for at least 2 minutes until complete dissolution of any cake/powder occurs. Avoid generation of foam.
6.) If foaming or clumping occurs, stand solution for at least 15 minutes until foam subsides.

Each milliliter of the reconstituted formulation will contain paclitaxel 5 mg/mL.

Calculate the exact total dosing volume of 5 mg/mL suspension required for the patient:

Dosing volume (mL) = total dose (mg) ÷ 5 (mg/mL).

The reconstituted sample should be milky and homogenous without visible particulates. If particulates or settling are visible, gently invert the vial again to ensure complete resuspension prior to use.

PVC equipment: Inject the appropriate amount of reconstituted paclitaxel into an empty, sterile, PVC-type IV bag. The use of specialized DEHP-free solution containers or administration sets is not necessary to prepare or administer infusions of paclitaxel protein-bound particles. The use of an in-line filter is not recommended.

Powder: Reconstitute each vial by slowly (over a minimum of 1 minute) injecting 20 mL of 0.9% sodium chloride injection, using the sterile syringe to direct the solution flow onto the inside wall of the vial. Do not inject the 0.9% sodium chloride injection directly onto the lyophilized cake as this will result in foaming. Allow the vial to sit for a minimum of 5 minutes to ensure proper wetting of the lyophilized cake/powder. Gently swirl and/or invert the vial slowly for at least 2 minutes until complete dissolution of any cake/powder occurs. Avoid generation of foam. If foaming or clumping occurs, stand solution for at least 15 minutes until foam subsides. Each mL of the reconstituted formulation will contain 5 mg/mL paclitaxel. the reconstituted sample should be milky and homogenous without visible particulates. If particulates or settling are visible, gently invert the vial again to ensure complete resuspension prior to use. Inject the appropriate amount of reconstituted *Abraxane* into an empty, sterile, polyvinyl chloride type IV bag. The use of an in-line filter is not recommended.

Premedication: No premedication to prevent hypersensitivity reactions for *Abraxane* is required.

➤*Admixture compatibility:* One study indicates compatibility in 5% dextrose injection or normal saline at 0.1 and 1 mg/mL concentrations, at 4°, 22°, or 32°C (39.2°, 71.6°, or 89.6°F) for 3 days. Small, needlelike crystals form after 3 days.

Another study showed admixtures of paclitaxel 0.3 and 1.2 mg/mL with carboplatin 2 mg/mL in normal saline injection or 5% dextrose injection were stable for at least 24 hours at 4°, 23°, and 32°C (39.2°, 71.6°, or 89.6°F). Paclitaxel 0.2 mg/mL mixed with cisplatin 0.2 mg/mL in normal saline injection showed unacceptable cisplatin loss in 24 hours. Utility time of paclitaxel mixed with carboplatin or cisplatin is limited due to paclitaxel microcrystalline precipitation and decomposition of carboplatin and cisplatin.

Paclitaxel 0.3 or 1.2 mg/mL combined with doxorubicin 200 mcg/mL in normal saline injection or 5% dextrose injection was found to be stable for at least 24 hours at temperatures of 4°, 23°, and 32°C (39.2°, 71.6°, or 89.6°F). Microcrystalline precipitation of paclitaxel developed within 3 days.

➤*Storage / Stability:*

Taxol/Onxol – Store between 20° to 25°C (68° to 77°F) in the original package. Upon refrigeration, components in the paclitaxel vial may precipitate, but will redissolve upon reaching room temperature with little or no agitation. There is no impact on product quality under these circumstances. If the solution remains cloudy or if an insoluble precipitate is noted, discard the vial. Solutions for infusion prepared as recommended are stable at ambient temperature (approximately 25°C; 77°F) and lighting conditions for up to 27 hours.

Abraxane: Store between 20° to 25°C (68° to 77°F) in the original package. Use reconstituted paclitaxel protein-bound particles immediately; may be refrigerated at 2° to 8°C (36° to 46°F) for a maximum of 8 hours if necessary. If not used immediately, replace each vial of reconstituted suspension in the original carton to protect it from bright light. Discard any unused portion. Neither freezing nor refrigeration adversely affects the stability of the product. Some settling of the reconstituted suspension may occur. Ensure complete resuspension by mild agitation before use. Discard the reconstituted suspension if precipitates are observed. The suspension for infusion prepared as recommended in an infusion bag is stable at ambient temperature (approximately 25°C; 77°F) and lighting conditions for up to 8 hours.

Actions

➤*Pharmacology:* Paclitaxel is a novel antimicrotubule agent that promotes the assembly of microtubules from tubulin dimers and stabilizes microtubules by preventing depolymerization. This stability results in the inhibition of the normal dynamic reorganization of the microtubule network that is essential for vital interphase and mitotic cellular functions. Paclitaxel induces abnormal arrays or "bundles" of microtubules throughout the cell cycle and multiple asters of microtubules during mitosis.

➤*Pharmacokinetics:*

Absorption / Distribution – Following IV administration of paclitaxel, paclitaxel plasma concentrations declined in a biphasic manner. The initial rapid decline represents distribution to the peripheral compartment and elimination of the drug. The later phase is due, in part, to a relatively slow efflux of paclitaxel from the peripheral compartment.

It appeared that with the 24-hour infusion of paclitaxel, a 30% increase in dose (135 mg/m² versus 175 mg/m²) increased the maximum plasma concentration (C_{max}) by 87%, whereas the area under the plasma concentration-time curve [$AUC_{(0-\infty)}$] remained proportional. However, with a 3-hour infusion for a 30% increase in dose, the C_{max} and $AUC_{(0-\infty)}$ were increased by 68% and 89%, respectively. The mean apparent volume of distribution at steady state with the 24-hour infusion of paclitaxel ranged from 227 to 688 L/m², indicating extensive extravascular distribution or tissue binding of paclitaxel.

The pharmacokinetics of paclitaxel also were evaluated in adult cancer patients who received single doses of 15 to 135 mg/m² given by 1-hour infusions (n = 15), 30 to 275 mg/m² given by 6-hour infusions (n = 36), and 200 to 275 mg/m² given by 24-hour infusions (n = 54) in phase 1 and 2 studies. Values for total body clearance (CL_T) and volume of distribution were consistent with the findings in the phase 3 study. The pharmacokinetics of paclitaxel in patients with AIDS-related Kaposi sarcoma have not been studied.

In vitro studies of binding to human serum proteins using paclitaxel concentrations ranging from 0.1 to 50 mcg/mL indicate that between 89% to 98% of drug is bound; the presence of cimetidine, ranitidine, dexamethasone, or diphenhydramine did not affect protein binding of paclitaxel.

Metabolism – In vitro studies with human liver microsomes and tissue slices showed that paclitaxel was metabolized primarily to 6α-hydroxypaclitaxel by the cytochrome P-450 isozyme CYP2C8; and to 2 minor metabolites, 3′-p-hydroxypaclitaxel and 6α, 3′-p-dihydroxypaclitaxel, by CYP3A4. In vitro, the metabolism of paclitaxel to 6α-hydroxypaclitaxel was inhibited by a number of agents (eg, ketoconazole, verapamil, diazepam, quinidine, dexamethasone, cyclosporine, teniposide, etoposide, and vincristine), but the concentrations used exceeded those found in vivo following normal therapeutic doses. Testosterone, 17α-ethinyl estradiol, retinoic acid, and quercetin, a specific inhibitor of CYP2C8, also inhibited the formation of 6α-hydroxypaclitaxel in vitro. The pharmacokinetics of paclitaxel may also be altered in vivo as a result of interactions with compounds that are substrates, inducers, or inhibitors of CYP2C8 or CYP3A4.

Excretion – After IV administration of 15 to 275 mg/m² doses of paclitaxel as 1-, 6-, or 24-hour infusions, mean values for cumulative urinary recovery of unchanged drug ranged from 1.3% to 12.6% of the dose, indicating extensive nonrenal clearance. In 5 patients administered a 225 or 250 mg/m² dose of radiolabeled paclitaxel as a 3-hour infusion, a mean of 71% of the radioactivity was excreted in the feces in 120 hours, and 14% was recovered in the urine. Total recovery of radioactivity ranged from 56% to 101% of the dose. Paclitaxel represented a mean of 5% of the administered radioactivity recovered in the feces, while metabolites, primarily 6α-hydroxypaclitaxel, accounted for the balance.

Special populations –

Hepatic function impairment: The disposition and toxicity of a paclitaxel 3-hour infusion were evaluated in 35 patients with varying degrees of hepatic function. Relative to patients with normal bilirubin, plasma paclitaxel exposure in patients with abnormal serum bilirubin less than or equal to 2 times ULN administered 175 mg/m² was increased, but with no apparent increase in the frequency or severity of toxicity. In 5 patients with serum total bilirubin greater than 2 times ULN, there was a statistically nonsignificant higher incidence of severe myelosuppression, even at a reduced dose (110 mg/m²), but no observed increase in plasma exposure.

Summary of Paclitaxel Pharmacokinetic Parameters (Mean Values)[a]

Dose (mg/m²)	Infusion duration (h)	Patients (n)	C_{max} (ng/mL)	$AUC_{(0-\infty)}$ (ng•h/mL)	t½ (h)	CL_T (L/h/m²)
135	24	2	195	6,300	52.7	21.7
175	24	4	365	7,993	15.7	23.8
135	3	7	2,170	7,952	13.1	17.7
175	3	5	3,650	15,007	20.2	12.2

[a] C_{max}, $AUC_{(0-\infty)}$, and CL_T.

Abraxane –

Absorption / Distribution: The pharmacokinetics of total paclitaxel following 30- and 180-minute infusions of paclitaxel protein-bound particles at dose levels of 80 to 375 mg/m² were determined in clinical studies. Following IV administration of paclitaxel protein-bound particles, paclitaxel plasma concentrations declined in a biphasic manner, the initial rapid decline representing distribution to the peripheral compartment and the slower second phase representing drug elimination. The terminal half-life was approximately 27 hours.

The drug exposure (AUCs) was dose proportional over 80 to 375 mg/m² and the pharmacokinetics of paclitaxel for paclitaxel protein-bound particles were independent of the duration of administration. At the recommended paclitaxel protein-bound particles clinical dose, 260 mg/m², the mean maximum concentration of paclitaxel, which occurred at the end of the infusion, was 18,741 ng/mL. The mean total clearance was 15 L/h/m². The mean volume of distribution was 632 L/m²; the large volume of distribution indicates extensive extravascular distribution and/or tissue binding of paclitaxel.

In vitro studies of binding to human serum proteins using paclitaxel concentrations ranging from 0.1 to 50 mcg/mL indicate that between 89% to 98% of drug is bound; the presence of cimetidine, ranitidine, dexamethasone, or diphenhydramine did not affect protein binding of paclitaxel.

The pharmacokinetic data of paclitaxel protein-bound particles 260 mg/m² administered over 30 minutes was compared with the pharmacokinetics of paclitaxel 175 mg/m² injection over 3 hours. The clearance of paclitaxel protein-bound particles was larger (43%) than the clearance of paclitaxel injection, and the volume of distribution of paclitaxel protein-bound par-

PACLITAXEL — INJECTION

ticles was also higher (53%). Differences in C_{max} and C_{max} corrected for dose reflected differences in total dose and rate of infusion. There were no differences in terminal half-lives.

Metabolism: In vitro studies with human liver microsomes and tissue slices showed that paclitaxel was metabolized primarily to 6α-hydroxypaclitaxel by the cytochrome P-450 isozyme CYP2C8; and to 2 minor metabolites, 3′-p-hydroxypaclitaxel and 6α, 3′-p-dihydroxypaclitaxel, by CYP3A4. In vitro, the metabolism of paclitaxel to 6α-hydroxypaclitaxel was inhibited by a number of agents (eg, ketoconazole, verapamil, diazepam, quinidine, dexamethasone, cyclosporine, teniposide, etoposide, vincristine), but the concentrations used exceeded those found in vivo following normal therapeutic doses. Testosterone, 17α-ethinyl estradiol, retinoic acid, and quercetin, a specific inhibitor of CYP2C8, also inhibited the formation of 6α-hydroxypaclitaxel in vitro. The pharmacokinetics of paclitaxel also may be altered in vivo as a result of interactions with compounds that are substrates, inducers, or inhibitors of CYP2C8 or CYP3A4. The effect of renal or hepatic dysfunction on the disposition of paclitaxel protein-bound particles have not been investigated.

Excretion: After a 30-minute infusion of 260 mg/m² doses of paclitaxel protein-bound particles, the mean values for cumulative urinary recovery of unchanged drug (4%) indicated extensive nonrenal clearance. Less than 1% of the total administered dose was excreted in urine as the metabolites 6α-hydroxypaclitaxel and 3′-*p*-hydroxypaclitaxel. Fecal excretion was approximately 20% of the total dose administered.

Contraindications

➤*Taxol/Onxol*: Paclitaxel is contraindicated in patients who have a history of hypersensitivity reactions with paclitaxel or other drugs formulated in polyoxyethylated castor oil (*Cremophor EL*).

See the Warning box for more information.

➤*Abraxane*: See the Warning box for more information.

Warnings

➤*Bone marrow suppression:* Bone marrow suppression (primarily neutropenia) is dose dependent and is a dose-limiting toxicity. Neutrophil nadirs occurred at a median of 11 days. Do not administer paclitaxel to patients with baseline neutrophil counts of less than 1,500 cells/mm³ (less than 1,000 cells/mm³ for patients with Kaposi's sarcoma). Institute frequent monitoring of blood counts during paclitaxel treatment. Do not retreat patients with subsequent cycles of paclitaxel until neutrophils recover to a level greater than 1,500 cells/mm³ (greater than 1,000 cells/mm³ for patients with Kaposi sarcoma) and platelets recover to a level greater than 100,000 cells/mm³.

➤*Cardiac effects:*

Taxol/Onxol – Severe conduction abnormalities have been documented in less than 1% of patients during paclitaxel therapy and in some cases requiring pacemaker placement. If patients develop significant conduction abnormalities during paclitaxel infusion, administer appropriate therapy and perform continuous cardiac monitoring during subsequent therapy with paclitaxel.

Hypotension, bradycardia, and hypertension have been observed during administration of paclitaxel, but generally do not require treatment. Occasionally paclitaxel infusions must be interrupted or discontinued because of initial or recurrent hypertension. Frequent vital sign monitoring, particularly during the first hour of paclitaxel infusion, is recommended. Continuous cardiac monitoring is not required except for patients with serious conduction abnormalities.

➤*Albumin (human):*

Abraxane – Paclitaxel protein-bound particles contains albumin (human), a derivative of human blood. Based on effective donor screening and product manufacturing processes, it carries an extremely remote risk for transmission of viral disease. A theoretical risk for transmission of Creutzfeldt-Jakob disease also is considered extremely remote. No cases of transmission of viral diseases or Creutzfeldt-Jakob disease have ever been identified for albumin.

➤*Use in men:* Advise men not to father a child while receiving treatment with paclitaxel.

➤*Hypersensitivity reactions:*

Taxol/Onxol – See the Warning box for more information.

Do not treat patients with a history of severe hypersensitivity reactions to products containing polyoxyethylated castor oil (eg, cyclosporin for injection concentrate and teniposide for injection concentrate) with paclitaxel. Minor symptoms, such as flushing, skin reactions, dyspnea, hypotension, or tachycardia, do not require interruption of therapy. However, severe reactions, such as hypotension requiring treatment, dyspnea requiring bronchodilators, angioedema, or generalized urticaria, require immediate discontinuation of paclitaxel and aggressive symptomatic therapy. Do not rechallenge patients who have developed severe hypersensitivity reactions with paclitaxel.

Abraxane – See Administration and Dosage for more information.

➤*Hepatic function impairment:*

Taxol – See Actions for more information.

Onxol – There is evidence that the toxicity of paclitaxel is enhanced in patients with elevated liver enzymes. Exercise caution when administering paclitaxel to patients with moderate to severe hepatic impairment and consider dose adjustments.

➤*Mutagenesis:* Paclitaxel has been shown to be clastogenic in vitro (chromosome aberrations in human lymphocytes) and in vivo (micronucleus test in mice). Paclitaxel was not mutagenic in the Ames test or the Chinese hamster ovary/hypoxanthine guanine phosphoribosyltransferase (CHO/HGPRT) gene mutation assay.

➤*Fertility impairment:*

Taxol/Onxol: Administration of paclitaxel prior to and during mating produced impairment of fertility in male and female rats at dosages equal to or greater than 1 mg/kg/day (about 0.04 times the daily maximum recommended human dosage on a mg/m² basis). At this dose, paclitaxel caused reduced fertility and reproductive indices, and increased embryotoxicity and fetotoxicity.

Abraxane: Administration of paclitaxel protein-bound particles to male rats at 42 mg/m² on a weekly basis (approximately 16% of the daily maximum recommended human exposure on a mg/m² basis) for 11 weeks prior to mating with untreated female rats resulted in significantly reduced fertility accompanied by decreased pregnancy rates and increased loss of embryos in mated females. A low incidence of skeletal and soft tissue fetal anomalies was also observed at dosages of 3 and 12 mg/m²/week in this study (approximately 1% to 5% of the daily maximum recommended human exposure on a mg/m² basis). Testicular atrophy/degeneration also has been observed in single-dose toxicology studies in rodents administered paclitaxel protein-bound particles at 54 mg/m² and dogs administered 175 mg/m².

➤*Elderly:*

Taxol – Of 2,228 patients who received paclitaxel in 8 clinical studies evaluating its safety and effectiveness in the treatment of advanced ovarian cancer, breast carcinoma, or NSCLC, and 1,570 patients who were randomized to receive paclitaxel in the adjuvant breast cancer study, 649 patients (17%) were 65 years of age or older and 49 patients (1%) were 75 years of age or older. In most studies, severe myelosuppression was more frequent in elderly patients; in some studies, severe neuropathy was more common in elderly patients. In 2 clinical studies in NSCLC, the elderly patients treated with paclitaxel had a higher incidence of cardiovascular events. Estimates of efficacy appeared similar in elderly patients and in younger patients; however, comparative efficacy cannot be determined with confidence because of the small number of elderly patients studied. In a study of first-line treatment with ovarian cancer, elderly patients had a lower median survival than younger patients, but no other efficacy parameters favored the younger group. The table below presents the incidences of grade IV neutropenia and severe neuropathy in clinical studies according to age.

Selected Adverse Reactions in Elderly Patients Receiving Paclitaxel Injection in Clinical Studies

Indication (study/regimen)	Patients [n/total (%)]			
	Neutropenia (grade 4) Age (years)		Peripheral neuropathy (grades 3/4) Age (years)	
	≥ 65	< 65	≥ 65	< 65
Ovarian cancer				
Intergroup first-line/ T175/3 c75[a]	34/83 (41%)	78/252 (31%)	24/84 (29%)[b,c]	46/255 (18%)[c]
GOG-111 first-line/ T135/24 c75[a]	48/61 (79%)	106/129 (82%)	3/62 (5%)	2/134 (1%)
Phase 3 second-line/ T175/3[d]	5/19 (26%)	21/76 (28%)	1/19 (5%)	0/76 (0%)
Phase 3 second-line/ T175/24[d]	21/25 (84%)	57/79 (72%)	0/25 (0%)	2/80 (3%)
Phase 3 second-line/ T135/3[d]	4/16 (25%)	10/81 (12%)	0/17 (0%)	0/81 (0%)
Phase 3 second-line/ T135/24[d]	17/22 (77%)	53/83 (64%)	0/22 (0%)	0/83 (0%)
Phase 3 second-line pooled	47/82 (57%)[b]	141/319 (44%)	1/83 (1%)	2/320 (1%)
Adjuvant breast cancer				
Intergroup/ AC followed by T[e]	56/102 (55%)	734/1468 (50%)	5/102 (5%)[f]	46/1468 (3%)[f]
Phase 3/T175/3[d]	7/24 (29%)	56/200 (28%)	3/25 (12%)	12/204 (6%)
Phase 3/T135/3[d]	7/20 (35%)	37/207 (18%)	0/20 (0%)	6/209 (3%)

PACLITAXEL — INJECTION

Selected Adverse Reactions in Elderly Patients Receiving Paclitaxel Injection in Clinical Studies				
	Patients [n/total (%)]			
Indication (study/regimen)	Neutropenia (grade 4) Age (years)		Peripheral neuropathy (grades 3/4) Age (years)	
	≥ 65	< 65	≥ 65	< 65
NSCLC				
ECOG/T135/24 c75[a]	58/71 (82%)	86/124 (69%)	9/71 (13%)[g]	16/124 (13%)[g]
Phase 3/T175/3 c80[a]	37/89 (42%)[b]	56/267 (21%)	11/91 (12%)[b]	11/271 (4%)

[a] Paclitaxel dose in mg/m²/infusion duration in hours; cisplatin doses in mg/m².
[b] $P < 0.05$.
[c] Peripheral neuropathy was included within the neurotoxicity category in the Intergroup First-Line Ovarian Cancer study.
[d] Paclitaxel dose in mg/m²/infusion duration in hours.
[e] Paclitaxel (T) following 4 courses of doxorubicin and cyclophosphamide (AC) at a dose of 175 mg/m² every 3 hours every 3 weeks for 4 courses.
[f] Peripheral neuropathy reported as neurosensory toxicity in the Intergroup Adjuvant Breast Cancer study.
[g] Peripheral neuropathy reported as neurosensory toxicity in the ECOG NSCLC study.

➤*Pregnancy: Category D.*

Taxol/Onxol – Paclitaxel can cause fetal harm when administered to a pregnant woman. Administration of paclitaxel during the period of organogenesis to rabbits at dosages of 3 mg/kg/day (about 0.2 times the daily maximum recommended human dosage on a mg/m² basis) caused embryo- and fetotoxicity, as indicated by intrauterine mortality, increased resorptions, and increased fetal deaths. Maternal toxicity also was observed at this dosage. No teratogenic effects were observed at 1 mg/kg/day (about 1/15 the daily maximum recommended human dosage on a mg/m² basis); teratogenic potential could not be assessed at higher doses because of extensive fetal mortality.

Abraxane – Paclitaxel protein-bound particles can cause fetal harm when administered to a pregnant woman. Administration of paclitaxel protein-bound particles to rats on gestation days 7 to 17 at dose of 6 mg/m² (approximately 2% of the daily maximum recommended human dose on a mg/m² basis) caused embryo- and fetotoxicity, as indicated by intrauterine mortality, increased resorptions (up to 5-fold), reduced numbers of litters and live fetuses, reduction in fetal body weight, and increase in fetal anomalies. Fetal anomalies included soft tissue and skeletal malformations, such as eye bulge, folded retina, microphthalmia, and dilation of brain ventricles. A lower incidence of soft tissue and skeletal malformations also was exhibited at 3 mg/m² (approximately 1% of the daily maximum recommended human dose on a mg/m² basis).

There are no adequate and well-controlled studies in pregnant women. If paclitaxel is used during pregnancy, or if the patient becomes pregnant while receiving this drug, apprise the patient of the potential hazard to the fetus. Advise women of childbearing potential to avoid becoming pregnant while receiving paclitaxel treatment.

➤*Lactation:* It is not known whether paclitaxel is excreted in human milk. Following IV administration of C^{14}-labeled paclitaxel to rats on days 9 to 10 postpartum, concentrations of radioactivity in milk were higher than in plasma and declined in parallel with the plasma concentrations. Because many drugs are excreted in human milk and because of the potential for serious adverse reactions in nursing infants, it is recommended that breastfeeding be discontinued when receiving paclitaxel therapy.

➤*Children:* The safety and efficacy of paclitaxel in pediatric patients have not been established.

Taxol/Onxol – There have been reports of CNS toxicity (rarely associated with death) in a clinical trial in pediatric patients in which paclitaxel was infused IV over 3 hours at doses ranging from 350 to 420 mg/m². The toxicity is most likely attributable to the high dose of the ethanol component of the paclitaxel vehicle given over a short infusion time. The use of concomitant antihistamines may intensify this effect. Although a direct effect of the paclitaxel itself cannot be discounted, consider the high doses used in this study (over twice the recommended adult dosage) in assessing the safety of paclitaxel for use in this population.

Precautions

➤*Monitoring:* Do not administer paclitaxel therapy to patients with baseline neutrophil counts of less than 1,500 cells/mm³. In order to monitor the occurrence of myelotoxicity, it is recommended that frequent peripheral blood cell counts be performed on all patients receiving paclitaxel. Do not retreat patients with subsequent cycles of paclitaxel until neutrophils recover to a level greater than 1,500 cells/mm³ and platelets recover to a level greater than 100,000 cells/mm³. In the case of severe neutropenia (less than 500 cells/mm³ for 7 days or more) during a course of paclitaxel therapy (*Taxol* or *Onxol*), a 20% reduction in dose for subsequent courses of therapy is recommended. For patients with advanced HIV disease and poor-risk AIDS-related Kaposi sarcoma, paclitaxel (*Taxol*), at the recommended dose for this disease, can be initiated and repeated if the neutrophil count is at least 1,000 cells/mm³.

In patients who experience severe neutropenia (neutrophil counts less than 500 cells/mm³ for a week or longer) or severe sensory neuropathy during *Abraxane* therapy, reduce the dose to 220 mg/m² for subsequent courses of *Abraxane*. For recurrence of severe neutropenia or severe sensory neuropathy, additionally reduce the dose to 180 mg/m². For grade 3 sensory neuropathy, hold treatment until resolution to grade 1 or 2, followed by a dose reduction for all subsequent courses of *Abraxane*.

➤*PVC equipment/devices:*
Taxol/Onxol – See Administration and Dosage for more information.

➤*CNS:*
Taxol/Onxol – Although the occurrence of peripheral neuropathy is frequent, the development of severe symptomatology is unusual and requires a dose reduction of 20% for all subsequent courses of paclitaxel.

Paclitaxel contains dehydrated alcohol 396 mg/mL; consider possible CNS and other effects of alcohol. There have been reports of CNS toxicity (rarely associated with death) in a clinical trial in pediatric patients in which paclitaxel was infused IV over 3 hours at doses ranging from 350 to 420 mg/m². The toxicity is most likely attributable to the high dose of the ethanol component of the paclitaxel vehicle given over a short infusion time. The use of concomitant antihistamines may intensify this effect. Although a direct effect of the paclitaxel itself cannot be discounted, consider the high doses used in this study (over twice the recommended adult dose) in assessing the safety of paclitaxel for use in this population.

Abraxane – Sensory neuropathy occurs frequently with paclitaxel protein-bound particles. The occurrence of grade 1 or 2 sensory neuropathy generally does not require dose modification. If grade 3 sensory neuropathy develops, withhold treatment until resolution to grade 1 or 2 followed by a dose reduction for all subsequent courses of paclitaxel protein-bound particles.

➤*Injection-site reactions:*
Taxol/Onxol – Injection site reactions, including reactions secondary to extravasation, were usually mild and consisted of erythema, tenderness, skin discoloration, or swelling at the injection site. These reactions have been observed more frequently with the 24-hour infusion than with the 3-hour infusion. Recurrence of skin reactions at a site of previous extravasation following administration of paclitaxel at a different site ("recall") has been reported rarely.

Rare reports of more severe events, such as phlebitis, cellulitis, induration, skin exfoliation, necrosis, and fibrosis, have been received as part of the continuing surveillance of paclitaxel safety. In some cases, the onset of the injection site reaction occurred during a prolonged infusion or was delayed by a week to 10 days.

A specific treatment for extravasation reactions is unknown at this time. Given the possibility of extravasation, closely monitor the infusion site for possible infiltration during drug administration.

Abraxane – Injection-site reactions occur infrequently with paclitaxel protein-bound particles and were mild in the randomized clinical trial. Given the possibility of extravasation, closely monitor the infusion site for possible infiltration during drug administration.

Drug Interactions

Paclitaxel Drug Interactions			
Precipitant drug	Object drug*		Description
Cisplatin	Paclitaxel	⬆	In a phase 1 trial using escalating doses of paclitaxel (110 to 200 mg/m²) and cisplatin (50 or 75 mg/m²) given as sequential infusions, myelosuppression was more profound when paclitaxel was given after cisplatin than with paclitaxel before cisplatin. Data demonstrated a decrease in paclitaxel clearance of approximately 33% when paclitaxel was administered following cisplatin.
CYP2C8 inhibitors (eg, 17α-ethinylestradiol, diazepam, doxorubicin, felodipine, ketoconazole, midazolam, retinoic acid)	Paclitaxel	⬆	Metabolism of paclitaxel may be decreased through the inhibition of CYP2C8 by any of these drugs.
CYP3A4 inducers (eg, carbamazepine, phenobarbital)	Paclitaxel	⬇	Coadministration of either of these drugs may induce the metabolism of paclitaxel through the cytochrome CYP3A4 isoenzyme.
CYP3A4 inhibitors (eg, cyclosporin, doxorubicin, felodipine, ketoconazole)	Paclitaxel	⬆	Metabolism of paclitaxel may be decreased through the inhibition of CYP3A4 by any of these drugs.

PACLITAXEL — INJECTION

Paclitaxel Drug Interactions			
Precipitant drug	Object drug*		Description
Paclitaxel	Doxorubicin	↑	Doxorubicin and its active metabolite doxorubicinol may be increased when coadministered with paclitaxel.

* ↑ = Object drug increased. ↓ = Object drug decreased.

Adverse Reactions

➤*Pooled analysis of adverse reactions from single-agent studies: Taxol/Onxol* – Data in the following table are based on the experience of 812 patients (493 with ovarian cancer and 319 with breast cancer) enrolled in 10 studies who received single-agent paclitaxel. Two hundred seventy-five patients were treated in 8 phase 2 studies with paclitaxel doses ranging from 135 to 300 mg/m² administered over 24 hours (in 4 of these studies, G-CSF was administered as hematopoietic support). Three hundred one patients were treated in the randomized phase 3 ovarian cancer study that compared 2 doses (135 or 175 mg/m²) and 2 schedules (3 or 24 hours) of paclitaxel. Two hundred and thirty-six patients with breast carcinoma received paclitaxel (135 or 175 mg/m²) administered over 3 hours in a controlled study.

Summary[a] of Adverse Reactions in Patients with Solid Tumors Receiving Single-Agent Paclitaxel (%)	
Adverse reactions	Patients (N = 812)
Cardiovascular	
Abnormal electrocardiogram (ECG)	
All patients	23%
Patients with normal baseline (n = 559)	14%
Vital sign changes[b]	
Bradycardia (n = 537)	3%
Hypotension (n = 532)	12%
Significant cardiovascular events	1%
CNS	
Peripheral neuropathy	
Any symptoms	60%
Severe symptoms[c]	3%
Dermatologic	
Alopecia	87%
GI	
Diarrhea	38%
Mucositis	31%
Nausea/Vomiting	52%
Hematologic	
Anemia hemoglobin < 11 g/dL	78%
Anemia hemoglobin < 8 g/dL	16%
Bleeding	14%
Leukopenia < 4,000/mm³	90%
Leukopenia < 1,000/mm³	17%
Neutropenia < 2,000/mm³	90%
Neutropenia < 500/mm³	52%
Platelet transfusions	2%
Red cell transfusions	25%
Thrombocytopenia < 100,000/mm³	20%
Thrombocytopenia < 50,000/mm³	7%
Hepatic[d]	
Alkaline phosphatase elevations (n = 575)	22%
AST elevations (n = 591)	19%
Bilirubin elevations (n = 765)	7%
Hypersensitivity[e]	
All	41%
Severe[c]	2%
Musculoskeletal	
Myalgia/arthralgia	
Any symptoms	60%
Severe symptoms[c]	8%
Miscellaneous	
Infections	30%
Injection site reaction	13%

[a] Based on worst course analysis.
[b] During the first 3 hours of infusion.
[c] Severe reactions are defined as at least grade 3 toxicity.
[d] Patients with normal baseline and on study data
[e] All patients received premedication.

➤*Disease-specific adverse reactions: first-line ovary cancer in combination:*

Taxol – For the 1,084 patients who were evaluable for safety in the phase 3 first-line ovary combination therapy studies, the following table shows the incidence of important adverse reactions. For both studies, the analysis of safety was based on all courses of therapy (6 courses for the GOG-111 study and up to 9 courses for the Intergroup study.

Frequency[a] of Important Adverse Reactions in the Phase 3 First-Line Ovarian Cancer Studies (%)				
	Intergroup		GOG-111	
Adverse reactions	Paclitaxel 175 mg/m² over 3 hours followed by cisplatin 75 mg/m² (n = 339)	Cyclophosphamide 750 mg/m² followed by cisplatin 75 mg/m² (n = 336)	Paclitaxel 135 mg/m² over 24 hours followed by cisplatin 75 mg/m² (n = 196)	Cyclophosphamide 750 mg/m² followed by cisplatin 75 mg/m² (n = 213)
CNS				
Neurotoxicity[b]				
Any symptoms	87%[c]	52%[c]	25%	20%
Severe symptoms[d]	21%[c]	2%[c]	3%[c]	0%[c]
Dermatologic				
Alopecia				
Any symptoms	96%[c]	89%[c]	55%[c]	37%[c]
Severe symptoms	51%[c]	21%[c]	6%	8%
GI				
Diarrhea				
Any symptoms	37%[c]	29%[c]	16%[c]	8%[c]
Severe symptoms[d]	2%	3%	4%	1%
Nausea/Vomiting				
Any symptoms	88%	93%	65%	69%
Severe symptoms[d]	18%	24%	10%	11%
Hematologic				
Anemia hemoglobin < 11 g/dL[e]	96%	97%	88%	86%
Anemia hemoglobin < 8 g/dL	3%[c]	8%[c]	13%	9%
Febrile neutropenia	4%	7%	15%[c]	4%[c]

PACLITAXEL — INJECTION

Frequency[a] of Important Adverse Reactions in the Phase 3 First-Line Ovarian Cancer Studies (%)

Adverse reactions	Intergroup: Paclitaxel 175 mg/m^2 over 3 hours followed by cisplatin 75 mg/m^2 (n = 339)	Intergroup: Cyclophosphamide 750 mg/m^2 followed by cisplatin 75 mg/m^2 (n = 336)	GOG-111: Paclitaxel 135 mg/m^2 over 24 hours followed by cisplatin 75 mg/m^2 (n = 196)	GOG-111: Cyclophosphamide 750 mg/m^2 followed by cisplatin 75 mg/m^2 (n = 213)
Neutropenia < 2,000/mm^3	91%[c]	95%[c]	96%	92%
Neutropenia < 500/mm^3	33%[c]	43%[c]	81%[c]	58%[c]
Thrombocytopenia < 100,000/mm^3[f]	21%[c]	33%[c]	26%	30%
Thrombocytopenia < 50,000/mm^3	3%[c]	7%[c]	10%	9%
All	11%[c]	6%[c]	8%[c,f]	1%[c,g]
Severe[d]	1%	1%	3%[c,f]	[c,g]
Musculoskeletal				
Myalgia/Arthralgia				
Any symptoms	60%[c]	27%[c]	9%[c]	2%[c]
Severe symptoms[d]	6%[c]	1%[c]	1%	0%
Miscellaneous				
Asthenia				
Any symptoms	NC[h]	NC	17%[c]	10%[c]
Severe symptoms[d]	NC	NC	1%	1%
Infections	25%	27%	21%	15%

[a] Based on worst course analysis.
[b] In the GOG-111 study, neurotoxicity was collected as peripheral neuropathy and in the Intergroup study, neurotoxicity was collected as either neuromotor or neurosensory symptoms.
[c] $P < 0.05$ by Fisher exact test.
[d] Severe reactions are defined as at least grade 3 toxicity.
[e] Less hemoglobin than 12 g/dL in the Intergroup study.
[f] Less than 130,000/mm^3 in the Intergroup study.
[g] All patients received premedication.
[h] NC = not collected.

➤*Second-line ovarian cancer:*

Taxol/Onxol – For the 403 patients who received single-agent paclitaxel in the phase 3 second-line ovarian cancer study, the following table shows the incidence of important adverse reactions.

Frequency[a] of Important Adverse Reactions in the Phase 3 Second-Line Ovarian Cancer Study (%)

Adverse reactions	Paclitaxel 175 mg/m^2 over 3 hours (n = 95)	Paclitaxel 175 mg/m^2 over 24 hours (n = 105)	Paclitaxel 135 mg/m^2 over 3 hours (n = 98)	Paclitaxel 135 mg/m^2 over 24 hours (n = 105)
CNS				
Peripheral neuropathy				
Any symptoms	63%	60%	55%	42%
Severe symptoms[b]	1%	2%	0%	0%
GI				
Mucositis				
Any symptoms	17%	35%	21%	25%
Severe symptoms[b]	0%	3%	0%	2%
Hematologic				
Anemia hemoglobin < 11 g/dL	84%	90%	68%	88%
Anemia hemoglobin < 8 g/dL	11%	12%	6%	10%
Neutropenia < 2,000/mm^3	78%	98%	78%	98%
Neutropenia < 500/mm^3	27%	75%	14%	67%
Thrombocytopenia < 100,000/mm^3	4%	18%	8%	6%
Thrombocytopenia < 50,000/mm^3	1%	7%	2%	1%
Hypersensitivity[c]				
All	41%	45%	38%	45%
Severe[b]	2%	0%	2%	1%
Miscellaneous				
Infections	26%	29%	20%	18%

[a] Based on worst course analysis.
[b] Severe reactions are defined as at least grade 3 toxicity.
[c] All patients received premedication.

Myelosuppression was dose and schedule related, with the schedule effect being more prominent. The development of severe hypersensitivity reactions was rare, 1% of the patients and 0.2% of the courses overall. There was no apparent dose or schedule effect seen for the hypersensitivity reactions. Peripheral neuropathy was clearly dose-related, but schedule did not appear to affect the incidence.

➤*Adjuvant breast cancer:*

Taxol – For the phase 3 adjuvant breast cancer study, the following table shows the incidence of important severe adverse reactions for the 3,121 patients (total population) who were evaluable for safety as well as for a group of 325 patients (early population) who, per the study protocol, were monitored more intensively than other patients.

Frequency[a] of Important Severe[b] Adverse Reactions in the Phase 3 Adjuvant Breast Cancer Study (%)

Adverse reactions	Early population: Cyclophosphamide plus doxorubicin[c] (n = 166)	Early population: Cyclophosphamide plus doxorubicin[c] followed by paclitaxel[d] (n = 159)	Total population: Cyclophosphamide plus doxorubicin[c] (n = 1,551)	Total population: Cyclophosphamide plus doxorubicin[c] followed by paclitaxel[d] (n = 1,570)
CNS				
Neuromotor toxicity	1%	1%	< 1%	1%
Neurosensory toxicity	-	3%	< 1%	3%
GI				
Mucositis	13%	4%	6%	5%
Nausea/Vomiting	13%	18%	8%	9%
Hematologic[e]				
Anemia hemoglobin < 8 g/dL	17%	21%	8%	8%

PACLITAXEL — INJECTION

Frequency[a] of Important Severe[b] Adverse Reactions in the Phase 3 Adjuvant Breast Cancer Study (%)

Adverse reactions	Early population		Total population	
	Cyclophosphamide plus doxorubicin[c] (n = 166)	Cyclophosphamide plus doxorubicin[c] followed by paclitaxel[d] (n = 159)	Cyclophosphamide plus doxorubicin[c] (n = 1,551)	Cyclophosphamide plus doxorubicin[c] followed by paclitaxel[d] (n = 1,570)
Cardiovascular	1%	2%	1%	2%
Fever without infection	-	3%	< 1%	1%
Hypersensitivity[f]	1%	4%	1%	2%
Neutropenia < 500/mm³	79%	76%	48%	50%
Thrombocytopenia < 50,000/mm³	27%	25%	11%	11%
Musculoskeletal				
Myalgia/Arthralgia	-	2%	< 1%	2%
Miscellaneous				
Infections	6%	14%	5%	6%

[a] Based on worst course analysis.
[b] Severe reactions are defined as at least grade 3 toxicity.
[c] Patients received 600 mg/m² cyclophosphamide and doxorubicin (AC) at doses of either 60 mg/m², 75 mg/m², or 90 mg/m² (with prophylactic G-CSF support and ciprofloxacin), every 3 weeks for 4 courses.
[d] Paclitaxel (T) following 4 courses of AC at a dose of 175 mg/m² over 3 hours every 3 weeks for 4 courses.
[e] The incidence of febrile neutropenia was not reported in this study.
[f] All patients were to receive premedication.

The incidence of an adverse reaction for the total population likely represents an underestimation of the actual incidence given that safety data were collected differently based on enrollment cohort. However, because safety data were collected consistently across regimens, the safety of the sequential addition of paclitaxel injection following AC therapy may be compared with AC therapy alone. Compared with patients who received AC alone, patients who received AC followed by paclitaxel experienced grade 3/4 neurosensory toxicity, grade 3/4 myalgia/arthralgia, grade 3/4 neurologic pain (5% vs 1%), grade 3/4 flu-like symptoms (5% vs 3%), and grade 3/4 hyperglycemia (3% vs 1%). During the additional 4 courses of treatment with paclitaxel, 2 deaths (0.1%) were attributed to treatment. During paclitaxel treatment, grade 4 neutropenia was reported in 15% of patients, grade 2/3 neurosensory toxicity in 15%, grade 2/3 myalgias in 23%, and alopecia in 46%.

The incidences of severe hematologic toxicities, infections, mucositis, and cardiovascular reactions increased with higher doses of doxorubicin.

➤*Breast cancer after failure of initial chemotherapy:*

Taxol/Onxol – For the 458 patients who received single-agent paclitaxel in the phase 3 breast cancer study, the following table shows the incidence of important adverse reactions by treatment arm (each arm was administered by a 3-hour infusion).

Frequency[a] of Important Adverse Reactions in the Phase 3 Study of Breast Cancer After Failure of Initial Chemotherapy or Within 6 Months of Adjuvant Chemotherapy (%)

Adverse reactions	Paclitaxel 175 mg/m² over 3 hours (n = 229)	Paclitaxel 135 mg/m² over 3 hours (n = 229)
CNS		
Peripheral neuropathy		
Any symptoms	70%	46%
Severe symptoms[b]	7%	3%
GI		
Mucositis		
Any symptoms	23%	17%
Severe symptoms[b]	3%	< 1%
Hematologic		
Anemia hemoglobin < 11 g/dL	55%	47%
Anemia hemoglobin < 8 g/dL	4%	2%
Febrile neutropenia	2%	2%
Neutropenia < 2,000/mm³	90%	81%
Neutropenia < 500/mm³	28%	19%
Thrombocytopenia < 100,000/mm³	11%	7%
Thrombocytopenia < 50,000/mm³	3%	2%
Hypersensitivity[c]		
All	36%	31%
Severe[b]	0%	< 1%
Miscellaneous		
Infections	23%	15%

[a] Based on worst course analysis.
[b] Severe reactions are defined as at least grade 3 toxicity.
[c] All patients received premedication.

Myelosuppression and peripheral neuropathy were dose related. There was 1 severe hypersensitivity reaction observed at the dose of 135 mg/m².

➤*First-line NSCLC in combination:*

Taxol – In the ECOG study, patients were randomized to either paclitaxel (T) 135 mg/m² as a 24-hour infusion in combination with cisplatin (c) 75 mg/m², paclitaxel (T) 250 mg/m² as a 24-hour infusion in combination with cisplatin (c) 75 mg/m² with G-CSF support, or cisplatin (c) 75 mg/m² on day 1, followed by etoposide (VP) 100 mg/m² on days 1, 2, and 3 (control).

Frequency[a] of Important Adverse Reactions in the Phase 3 Study for First-Line NSCLC (%)

Adverse reactions	Paclitaxel 135 mg/m² over 24 hours with cisplatin 75 mg/m² (n = 195)	Paclitaxel 250 mg/m² over 24 hours with cisplatin 75 mg/m² with G-CSF support (n = 197)	Cisplatin 75 mg/m² on day 1 followed by etoposide 100 mg/m² on days 1, 2, 3[b] (n = 196)
Cardiovascular			
Any symptoms	33%	39%	24%
Severe symptoms[c]	13%	12%	8%
CNS			
Neuromotor toxicity			
Any symptoms	37%	47%	44%
Severe symptoms[c]	6%	12%	7%
Neurosensory toxicity			
Any symptoms	48%	61%	25%
Severe symptoms[c]	13%	28%[d]	8%
GI			
Mucositis			
Any symptoms	18%	28%	16%
Severe symptoms[c]	1%	4%	2%
Nausea/Vomiting			
Any symptoms	85%	87%	81%
Severe symptoms[c]	27%	29%	22%
Hematologic			
Anemia hemoglobin < normal	94%	96%	95%
Anemia hemoglobin < 8 g/dL	22%	19%	28%
Neutropenia < 2000/mm³	89%	86%	84%
Neutropenia < 500/mm³	74%[d]	65%	55%
Thrombocytopenia < normal	48%	68%	62%
Thrombocytopenia < 50,000/mm³	6%	12%	16%
Hypersensitivity[e]			
All	16%	27%	13%
Severe[c]	1%	4%[d]	1%
Musculoskeletal			
Arthralgia/Myalgia			

PACLITAXEL — INJECTION

Frequency[a] of Important Adverse Reactions in the Phase 3 Study for First-Line NSCLC (%)

Adverse reactions	Paclitaxel 135 mg/m² over 24 hours with cisplatin 75 mg/m² (n = 195)	Paclitaxel 250 mg/m² over 24 hours with cisplatin 75 mg/m² with G-CSF support (n = 197)	Cisplatin 75 mg/m² on day 1 followed by etoposide 100 mg/m² on days 1, 2, 3[b] (n = 196)
Any symptoms	21%[d]	42%[d]	9%
Severe symptoms[c]	3%	11%	1%
Miscellaneous			
Infections	38%	31%	35%

[a] Based on worst course analysis.
[b] Etoposide (VP) dose in mg/m² was administered IV on days 1, 2, and 3; cisplatin dose in mg/m².
[c] Severe reactions are defined as at least grade 3 toxicity.
[d] $P < 0.05$.
[e] All patients received premedication.

Toxicity was generally more severe in the high-dose paclitaxel treatment arm (paclitaxel 250 mg/cisplatin 75 mg) than in the low-dose paclitaxel arm (paclitaxel 135 mg/cisplatin 75 mg). Compared with the cisplatin/etoposide arm, patients in the low-dose paclitaxel arm experienced more arthralgia/myalgia of any grade and more severe neutropenia. The incidence of febrile neutropenia was not reported in this study.

Kaposi sarcoma –

Taxol: The following table shows the frequency of important adverse reactions in the 85 patients with Kaposi sarcoma treated with 2 different single-agent paclitaxel regimens.

Frequency[a] of Important Adverse Reactions in the AIDS-Related Kaposi Sarcoma Studies (%)

Adverse reactions	Study CA139-174 Paclitaxel 135 mg/m² over 3 hours every 3 weeks (n = 29)	Study CA139-281 Paclitaxel 100 mg/m² over 3 hours every 2 weeks (n = 56)
Cardiovascular		
Bradycardia	3%	-
Hypotension	17%	9%
CNS		
Peripheral neuropathy		
Any	79%	46%
Severe[b]	10%	2%
GI		
Diarrhea	90%	73%
Mucositis	45%	20%
Nausea/Vomiting	69%	70%
Hematologic		
Anemia hemoglobin < 11 g/dL	86%	73%
Anemia hemoglobin < 8 g/dL	34%	25%
Febrile neutropenia	55%	9%
Neutropenia < 2,000/mm³	100%	95%
Neutropenia < 500/mm³	76%	35%
Thrombocytopenia < 100,000/mm³	52%	27%
Thrombocytopenia < 50,000/mm³	17%	5%
Hypersensitivity[c]		
All	14%	9%
Musculoskeletal		
Myalgia/Arthralgia		
Any	93%	48%
Severe[b]	14%	16%
Opportunistic infection		
Any	76%	54%
Candidiasis, esophageal	7%	9%
Cryptosporidiosis	7%	7%
Cryptococcal meningitis	3%	2%
Cytomegalovirus	45%	27%
Herpes simplex	38%	11%
Leukoencephalopathy	-	2%
Mycobacterium avium intracellulare	24%	4%
Pneumocystis carinii	14%	21%
Renal (creatinine elevation)		
Any	34%	18%
Severe[b]	7%	5%
Discontinuation for drug toxicity	7%	16%

[a] Based on worst course analysis.
[b] Severe reactions are defined as at least grade 3 toxicity.
[c] All patients received premedication.

As demonstrated previously, toxicity was more pronounced in the study utilizing paclitaxel at a dose of 135 mg/m² every 3 weeks than in the study utilizing paclitaxel at a dose of 100 mg/m² every 2 weeks. Notably, severe neutropenia (76% vs 35%), febrile neutropenia (55% vs 9%), and opportunistic infections (76% vs 54%) were more common with the former dose and schedule. Take into account the differences between the 2 studies with respect to dose escalation and use of hematopoietic growth factors, as described previously. Note also that only 26% of the 85 patients in these studies received concomitant treatment with protease inhibitors, whose effect on paclitaxel metabolism has not yet been studied.

➤*Abraxane*: The following table shows the frequency of important adverse reactions in the randomized comparative trial for the patients who received either single-agent *Abraxane* or paclitaxel injection for the treatment of metastatic breast cancer.

Frequency[a] of Important Treatment Emergent Adverse Reactions in the Randomized Study on an Every-3-Weeks Schedule (%)

Adverse reactions	Paclitaxel protein-bound particles 260 mg/m² over 30 minutes (n = 229)	Paclitaxel injection 175 mg/m² over 3 hours[b] (n = 225)
Cardiovascular		
Abnormal ECG		
All patients	60%	52%
Patients with normal baseline	35%	30%
Vital sign changes[c]		
Bradycardia	< 1%	< 1%
Hypotension	5%	5%
Severe cardiovascular events[d]	3%	4%
CNS		
Sensory neuropathy		
Any symptoms	71%	56%
Severe symptoms[d]	10%	2%
Dermatologic		
Alopecia	90%	94%
GI		
Diarrhea		
Any symptoms	26%	15%
Severe symptoms[d]	< 1%	1%
Mucositis		
Any symptoms	7%	7%
Severe symptoms[d]	< 1%	0%
Nausea		
Any symptoms	30%	21%
Severe symptoms[d]	3%	< 1%
Vomiting		
Any symptoms	18%	9%
Severe symptoms[d]	4%	1%
Hematologic		
Anemia		
Bleeding	2%	2%
Febrile neutropenia	2%	1%

PACLITAXEL — INJECTION

Frequency[a] of Important Treatment Emergent Adverse Reactions in the Randomized Study on an Every-3-Weeks Schedule (%)		
Adverse reactions	Paclitaxel protein-bound particles 260 mg/m² over 30 minutes (n = 229)	Paclitaxel injection 175 mg/m² over 3 hours[b] (n = 225)
Hemoglobin		
< 11 g/L	33%	25%
< 8 g/L	1%	< 1%
Neutropenia		
< 2,000/mm³	80%	82%
< 500/mm³	9%	22%
Thrombocytopenia		
< 100,000/mm³	2%	3%
< 50,000/mm³	< 1%	1%
Hepatic (patients with normal baseline)		
Alkaline phosphatase elevations	36%	31%
AST elevations	39%	32%
Bilirubin elevations	7%	7%
Hypersensitivity[c]		
All	4%	12%
Severe[d]	0%	2%
Musculoskeletal		
Myalgia/arthralgia		
Any symptoms	44%	49%
Severe symptoms[d]	8%	4%
Respiratory		
Cough	6%	6%
Dyspnea	12%	9%
Miscellaneous		
Asthenia		
Any symptoms	47%	38%
Severe symptoms[d]	8%	3%
Fluid retention/Edema		
Any symptoms	10%	8%
Severe symptoms[d]	0%	< 1%
Infections	24%	20%
Injection site reaction	1%	1%

[a] Based on worst grade.
[b] Paclitaxel injection patients received premedication.
[c] During study drug dosing.
[d] Severe events are defined as at least grade 3 toxicity.
[e] Includes treatment-related events related to hypersensitivity (eg, flushing, dyspnea, chest pain, hypotension) that began on a day of dosing.

Miscellaneous – Myelosuppression and sensory neuropathy were dose related.

➤*Adverse reactions by body system:*

Cardiovascular –

Taxol/Onxol: Hypotension during the first 3 hours of infusion occurred in 12% of all patients and 3% of all courses administered. Bradycardia during the first 3 hours of infusion occurred in 3% of all patients and 1% of all courses. In the phase 3 second-line ovarian study, neither dose nor schedule had an effect on the frequency of hypotension and bradycardia. These vital sign changes most often caused no symptoms and required neither specific therapy nor treatment discontinuation. The frequency of hypotension and bradycardia were not influenced by prior anthracycline therapy.

Significant cardiovascular reactions, possibly related to single-agent paclitaxel, occurred in approximately 1% of all patients. These reactions included syncope, rhythm abnormalities, hypertension, and venous thrombosis. One of the patients with syncope treated with paclitaxel at 175 mg/m² over 24 hours had progressive hypotension and died. The arrhythmias included asymptomatic ventricular tachycardia, bigeminy, and complete atrioventricular block requiring pacemaker placement.

ECG abnormalities were common among patients at baseline. ECG abnormalities on study did not usually result in symptoms, were not dose-limiting, and required no intervention. ECG abnormalities were noted in 23% of all patients. Among patients with a normal ECG prior to study entry, 14% of all patients developed an abnormal tracing while on study. The most frequently reported ECG modifications were nonspecific repolarization abnormalities, sinus bradycardia, sinus tachycardia, and premature beats. Among patients with normal ECGs at baseline, prior therapy with anthracyclines did not influence the frequency of ECG abnormalities.

Cases of myocardial infarction have been reported rarely. Congestive heart failure has been reported typically in patients who have received other chemotherapy, notably anthracyclines.

Rare reports of atrial fibrillation and supraventricular tachycardia have been received as part of the continuing surveillance of paclitaxel safety.

Taxol: Among patients with NSCLC treated with paclitaxel in combination with cisplatin in the phase 3 study, significant cardiovascular reactions occurred in 12% to 13%. This apparent increase in cardiovascular reactions is possibly caused by an increase in cardiovascular risk factors in patients with lung cancer.

Abraxane: Hypotension during the 30-minute infusion occurred in 5% of patients in the randomized metastatic breast cancer trial. Bradycardia, during the 30-minute infusion, occurred in less than 1% of patients. These vital sign changes most often caused no symptoms and required neither specific therapy nor treatment discontinuation.

Severe cardiovascular events, possibly related to single-agent paclitaxel protein-bound particles, occurred in approximately 3% of patients in the randomized trial. These events included chest pain, cardiac arrest, supraventricular tachycardia, edema, thrombosis, pulmonary thromboembolism, pulmonary emboli, and hypertension. Cases of cerebrovascular attacks (strokes) and transient ischemic attacks have been reported rarely.

ECG abnormalities were common among patients at baseline. ECG abnormalities on study did not usually result in symptoms, were not dose-limiting, and required no intervention. ECG abnormalities were noted in 60% of all patients in the metastatic breast cancer randomized trial. Among patients with a normal ECG prior to study entry, 35% of all patients developed an abnormal tracing while on study. The most frequently reported ECG modifications were nonspecific repolarization abnormalities, sinus bradycardia, and sinus tachycardia.

CNS –

Taxol/Onxol: The frequency and severity of neurologic manifestations were dose-dependent but were not influenced by infusion duration. Peripheral neuropathy was observed in 60% of all patients (3% severe) and in 52% (2% severe) of the patients without preexisting neuropathy.

The frequency of peripheral neuropathy increased with cumulative dose. Neurologic symptoms were observed in 27% of the patients after the first course of treatment and in 34% to 51% from course 2 to 10.

Peripheral neuropathy was the cause of paclitaxel discontinuation in 1% of all patients. Sensory symptoms have usually improved or resolved within several months of paclitaxel discontinuation. The incidence of neurologic symptoms did not increase in the subset of patients previously treated with cisplatin. Preexisting neuropathies resulting from prior therapies are not a contraindication for paclitaxel therapy.

Other than peripheral neuropathy, serious neurologic reactions following paclitaxel administration have been rare (less than 1%) and have included grand mal seizures, syncope, ataxia, and neuroencephalopathy.

Rare reports of autonomic neuropathy, resulting in paralytic ileus, have been received as part of the continuing surveillance of paclitaxel safety. Optic nerve or visual disturbances (scintillating scotomata) have also been reported, particularly in patients who have received higher doses than those recommended. These effects generally have been reversible. However, rare reports of abnormal visual in the literature evoked potentials in patients have suggested persistent optic nerve damage.

Taxol: The assessment of neurologic toxicity was conducted differently among the studies as evident from the data reported in each individual study (see previous tables). Moreover, the frequency and severity of neurologic manifestations were influenced by prior and/or concomitant therapy with neurotoxic agents.

In the Intergroup first-line ovarian cancer study, neurotoxicity included reports of neuromotor and neurosensory events. The regimen with *Taxol* 175 mg/m² given by 3-hour infusion plus cisplatin 75 mg/m² resulted in a greater incidence and severity of neurotoxicity than the regimen containing cyclophosphamide and cisplatin, 87% (21% severe) versus 52% (2% severe), respectively. The duration of grade 3 or 4 neurotoxicity cannot be determined with precision for the Intergroup study because the resolution dates of adverse reactions were not collected in the case report forms for this trial and complete follow-up documentation was available only in a minority of these patients. In the GOG first-line ovarian cancer study, neurotoxicity was reported as peripheral neuropathy. The regimen with *Taxol* 135 mg/m² injection given by 24-hour infusion plus cisplatin 75 mg/m² resulted in an incidence of neurotoxicity that was similar to the regimen containing cyclophosphamide plus cisplatin, 25% (3% severe) versus 20% (0% severe), respectively. Cross-study comparison of neurotoxicity in the Intergroup and GOG trials suggests that when *Taxol* is given in combination with cisplatin 75 mg/m², the incidence of severe neurotoxicity is more common at a *Taxol* dose of 175 mg/m² given by 3-hour infusion (21%) than at a dose of 135 mg/m² given by 24-hour infusion (3%).

In patients with NSCLC, administration of paclitaxel followed by cisplatin resulted in greater incidence of severe neurotoxicity compared with the incidence in patients with ovarian or breast cancer treated with single-agent paclitaxel. Severe neurosensory symptoms were noted in 13% of NSCLC patients receiving paclitaxel 135 mg/m² by 24-hour infusion followed by cisplatin 75 mg/m² and 8% of NSCLC patients receiving cisplatin/etoposide.

Abraxane: The frequency and severity of neurologic manifestations were influenced by prior and/or concomitant therapy with neurotoxic agents.

In general, the frequency and severity of neurologic manifestation were dose-dependent in patients receiving single-agent paclitaxel protein-bound particles. In the randomized trial, sensory neuropathy was observed in 71% of patients (10% severe) in the paclitaxel protein-bound particles arm and in 56% of patients (2% severe) in the paclitaxel injection arm. The frequency of sensory neuropathy increased with cumulative dose. Sensory neuropathy

PACLITAXEL — INJECTION

was the cause of paclitaxel protein-bound particles discontinuation in 7/229 (3%) patients in the randomized trail. In the randomized comparative study, 24 patients (10%) treated with paclitaxel protein-bound particles developed grade 3 peripheral neuropathy; of these patients, 14 had documented improvement after a median of 22 days; 10 patients resumed treatment at a reduced dose of paclitaxel protein-bound particles and 2 discontinued because of peripheral neuropathy. Of the 10 patients without documented improvement, 4 discontinued the study because of peripheral neuropathy.

No incidences of grade 4 sensory neuropathies were reported in the clinical trial. Only 1 incident of motor neuropathy (grade 1) was observed in either arm of the controlled trial.

Reports of autonomic neuropathy, resulting in paralytic ileus, have been received as part of the continuing surveillance of paclitaxel injection safety.

Dermatologic –

Taxol/Onxol: Alopecia was observed in almost all (87%) of the patients. Transient skin changes caused by paclitaxel-related hypersensitivity reactions have been observed, but no other skin toxicities were significantly associated with paclitaxel administration. Nail changes (changes in pigmentation or discoloration of nail bed) were uncommon (2%). Edema was reported in 21% of all patients (17% of those without baseline edema); only 1% had severe edema and none of these patients required treatment discontinuation. Edema was most commonly focal and disease-related. Edema was observed in 5% of all courses for patients with normal baseline and did not increase with time on study.

Rare reports of skin abnormalities related to radiation recall as well as reports of maculopapular rash and pruritus have been received as part of the continuing surveillance of paclitaxel safety.

Abraxane: Alopecia was observed in almost all of the patients. Nail changes (changes in pigmentation or discoloration of nail bed) were uncommon. Edema (fluid retention) was infrequent (10% of randomized trial patients); no patients had severe edema.

GI –

Taxol/Onxol: Nausea/Vomiting, diarrhea, and mucositis were reported by 52%, 38%, and 31% of all patients, respectively. These manifestations were usually mild to moderate. Mucositis was schedule dependent and occurred more frequently with the 24-hour than with the 3-hour infusion.

Rare reports of intestinal obstruction, intestinal perforation, pancreatitis, ischemic colitis, and dehydration have been received as part of the continuing surveillance of paclitaxel safety. Rare reports of neutropenic enterocolitis (typhlitis), despite the coadministration of G-CSF, were observed in patients treated with paclitaxel alone and in combination with other chemotherapeutic agents.

Taxol: In patients with poor-risk AIDS-related Kaposi sarcoma, nausea/vomiting, diarrhea, and mucositis were reported by 69%, 79%, and 28% of patients, respectively. One third of patients with Kaposi sarcoma complained of diarrhea prior to study start.

In the first-line, phase 3 ovarian cancer studies, the incidence of nausea and vomiting when paclitaxel injection was administered in combination with cisplatin appeared to be greater compared with the database for single-agent paclitaxel in ovarian and breast cancer. In addition, diarrhea of any grade was reported more frequently compared with the control arm, but there was no difference for severe diarrhea in these studies.

Abraxane: Nausea/Vomiting, diarrhea, and mucositis were reported by 33%, 27%, and 7% of paclitaxel protein-bound particles treated patients in the randomized trial.

Rare reports of intestinal obstruction, intestinal perforation, pancreatitis, and ischemic colitis have been received as part of the continuing surveillance of paclitaxel injection safety and may occur following paclitaxel protein-bound particles treatment. Rare reports of neutropenic enterocolitis (typhlitis), despite the coadministration of G-CSF, were observed in patients treated with paclitaxel injection alone and in combination with other chemotherapeutic agents.

Hematologic –

Taxol/Onxol: Bone marrow suppression was the major dose-limiting toxicity of paclitaxel. Neutropenia, the most important hematologic toxicity, was dose-dependent, schedule-dependent, and generally rapidly reversible. Among patients treated in the phase 3 second-line ovarian study with a 3-hour infusion, neutrophil counts declined below 500 cells/mm^3 in 14% of the patients treated with a dose of 135 mg/m^2 compared with 27% at a dose of 175 mg/m^2 ($P = 0.05$). In the same study, severe neutropenia (less than 500 cells/mm^3) was more frequent with the 24-hour than with the 3-hour infusion; infusion duration had a greater impact on myelosuppression than dose. Neutropenia did not appear to increase with cumulative exposure and did not appear to be more frequent nor more severe for patients previously treated with radiation therapy.

Fever was frequent (12% of all treatment courses). Infectious episodes occurred in 30% of all patients and 9% of all courses; these episodes were fatal in 1% of all patients, and included sepsis, pneumonia, and peritonitis. In the phase 3, second-line ovarian study, infectious episodes were reported in 20% and 26% of the patients treated with a dose of 135 or 175 mg/m^2 given as 3-hour infusions, respectively. Urinary tract infections and upper respiratory tract infections were the most frequently reported infectious complications.

Thrombocytopenia was uncommon and almost never severe (less than 50,000 cells/mm^3). Twenty percent of the patients experienced a drop in their platelet count below 100,000 cells/mm^3 at least once while on treatment; 7% had a platelet count less than 50,000 cells/mm^3 at the time of their worst nadir. Bleeding episodes were reported in 4% of all courses and by 14% of all patients. Most of the hemorrhagic episodes were localized, and the frequency of these reactions was unrelated to the paclitaxel injection dose and schedule. In the phase 3, second-line ovarian study, bleeding episodes were reported in 10% of the patients; no patients treated with the 3-hour infusion received platelet transfusions.

Anemia (hemoglobin less than 11 g/dL) was observed in 78% of all patients and was severe (hemoglobin less than 8 g/dL) in 16% of the cases. No consistent relationship between dose or schedule and the frequency of anemia was observed. Among all patients with normal baseline hemoglobin, 69% became anemic on study but only 7% had severe anemia. Red cell transfusions were required in 25% of all patients and in 12% of those with normal baseline hemoglobin levels.

Taxol: In the study where paclitaxel was administered to patients with ovarian cancer at a dose of 135 mg/m^2 over 24 hours in combination with cisplatin versus the control arm of cyclophosphamide plus cisplatin, the incidences of grade 4 neutropenia and of febrile neutropenia were significantly greater in the paclitaxel plus cisplatin arm than in the control arm. Grade 4 neutropenia occurred in 81% on the paclitaxel plus cisplatin arm versus 58% on the cyclophosphamide plus cisplatin arm, and febrile neutropenia occurred in 15% and 4% respectively. On the paclitaxel/cisplatin arm, there were 35 out of 1,074 (3%) courses with fever in which grade 4 neutropenia was reported at some time during the course. When paclitaxel followed by cisplatin was administered to patients with advanced NSCLC in the ECOG study, the incidences of grade 4 neutropenia were 74% (paclitaxel 135 mg/m^2 over 24 hours followed by cisplatin) and 65% (paclitaxel 250 mg/m^2 over 24 hours followed by cisplatin and G-CSF) compared with 55% in patients who received cisplatin/etoposide.

In the immunosuppressed patient population with advanced HIV disease and poor-risk AIDS-related Kaposi sarcoma, 61% of the patients reported at least 1 opportunistic infection. The use of supportive therapy, including G-CSF, is recommended for patients who have experienced severe neutropenia.

In the adjuvant breast cancer trial, the incidence of severe thrombocytopenia and platelet transfusions increased with higher doses of doxorubicin.

Abraxane: Neutropenia, the most important hematologic toxicity, was dose dependent and reversible. Among patients with metastatic breast cancer in the randomized trial, neutrophil counts declined below 500 cells/mm^3 (grade 4) in 9% of the patients treated with a dose of 260 mg/m^2 compared with 22% in patients receiving paclitaxel injection at a dose of 175 mg/m^2.

In the randomized, metastatic breast cancer study, infectious episodes were reported in 24% of the patients treated with a dose of 260 mg/m^2 given as a 30-minute infusion. Oral candidiasis, respiratory tract infections, and pneumonia were the most frequently reported infectious complications. Febrile neutropenia was reported in 2% of patients in the paclitaxel protein-bound particles arm and 1% of patients in the paclitaxel injection arm.

Thrombocytopenia was uncommon. In the randomized, metastatic breast cancer study, bleeding episodes were reported in 2% of the patients in each treatment arm.

Anemia (hemoglobin less than 11 g/dL) was observed in 33% in the randomized trial and was severe (hemoglobin less than 8 g/dL) in 1% of the cases. Among all patients with normal baseline hemoglobin, 31% became anemic on study and 1% had severe anemia.

Hepatic – Rare reports of hepatic necrosis and hepatic encephalopathy leading to death have been received as part of the continuing surveillance of paclitaxel injection safety and may occur following paclitaxel protein-bound particles treatment.

Taxol/Onxol: No relationship was observed between liver function abnormalities and either dose or schedule of paclitaxel administration. Among patients with normal baseline liver function 7%, 22%, and 19% had elevations in bilirubin, alkaline phosphatase, and AST, respectively. Prolonged exposure to paclitaxel was not associated with cumulative hepatic toxicity.

Abraxane: Among patients with normal baseline liver function 7%, 36%, and 39% had elevations in bilirubin, alkaline phosphatase, and AST, respectively. Grade 3 or 4 elevations in gamma-glutamyltransferase (GGT) were reported for 14% of patients treated with paclitaxel protein-bound particles and 10% of patients treated with paclitaxel injection in the randomized trial.

Hypersensitivity –

Taxol/Onxol: All patients received premedication prior to paclitaxel. The frequency and severity of hypersensitivity reactions were not affected by the dose or schedule of paclitaxel administration. Premedicate all patients prior to paclitaxel administration in order to prevent severe hypersensitivity reactions. Such premedication may consist of dexamethasone 20 mg orally administered approximately 12 and 6 hours before paclitaxel, diphenhydramine (or its equivalent) 50 mg IV 30 to 60 minutes prior to paclitaxel, and cimetidine 300 mg or ranitidine 50 mg IV 30 to 60 minutes before paclitaxel. In the phase 3 second-line ovarian study, the 3-hour infusion was not associated with a greater increase in hypersensitivity reactions when compared with the 24-hour infusion. Hypersensitivity reactions were observed in 20% of all courses and in 41% of all patients. These reactions were severe in less than 2% of the patients and 1% of the courses. No severe reactions were observed after course 3 and severe symptoms occurred generally within the first hour of paclitaxel infusion. The most frequent symptoms observed during these severe reactions were dyspnea, flushing, chest pain, and tachycardia.

The minor hypersensitivity reactions consisted mostly of flushing (28%), rash (12%), hypotension (4%), dyspnea (2%), tachycardia (2%), and hypertension (1%). The frequency of hypersensitivity reactions remained relatively stable during the entire treatment period. Rare reports of chills and reports of back pain in association with hypersensitivity reactions have been received as part of the continuing surveillance of paclitaxel safety.

Local – Injection site reactions, including reactions secondary to extravasation, were usually mild and consisted of erythema, tenderness, skin discoloration, or swelling at the injection site. These reactions have been observed more frequently with the 24-hour infusion than with the 3-hour infusion. Recur-

PACLITAXEL — INJECTION

rence of skin reactions at a site of previous extravasation following administration of paclitaxel at a different site ("recall") has been reported rarely.

Rare reports of more severe reactions, such as phlebitis, cellulitis, induration, skin exfoliation, necrosis, and fibrosis, have been received as part of the continuing surveillance of paclitaxel safety. In some cases the onset of the injection site reaction either occurred during a prolonged infusion or was delayed by a week to 10 days.

A specific treatment for extravasation reactions is unknown at this time. Given the possibility of extravasation, it is advisable to closely monitor the infusion site for possible infiltration during drug administration.

Musculoskeletal –

Taxol/Onxol: There was no consistent relationship between dose or schedule of paclitaxel and the frequency or severity of arthralgia/myalgia. Sixty percent of all patients treated experienced arthralgia/myalgia; 8% experienced severe symptoms. The symptoms were usually transient, occurred 2 or 3 days after paclitaxel administration, and resolved within a few days. The frequency and severity of musculoskeletal symptoms remained unchanged throughout the treatment period.

Abraxane: Forty-four percent of patients treated in the randomized trial experienced arthralgia/myalgia; 8% experienced severe symptoms. The symptoms were usually transient, occurred 2 or 3 days after paclitaxel protein-bound particles administration, and resolved within a few days.

Ophthalmic –

Abraxane: Ocular/Visual disturbances occurred in 13% of all patients (n = 366) treated with paclitaxel protein-bound particles in single arm and randomized trials and 1% were severe. The severe cases (keratitis and blurred vision) were reported in patients in a single arm study who received higher doses that those recommended (300 or 375 mg/m^2). These effects generally have been reversible. However, rare reports in the literature of abnormal visual evoked potentials in patients treated with paclitaxel injection have suggested persistent optic nerve damage.

Renal –

Taxol: Among the patients treated for Kaposi sarcoma with paclitaxel, 5 patients had renal toxicity of grade 3 or 4 severity. One patient with suspected HIV nephropathy of grade 4 severity had to discontinue therapy. The other 4 patients had renal insufficiency with reversible elevations of serum creatinine.

Abraxane: Overall 11% of patients experienced creatinine elevation; 1% was severe. No discontinuations, dose reductions, or dose delays were caused by renal toxicities.

Respiratory –

Taxol/Onxol: Rare reports of interstitial pneumonia, lung fibrosis, and pulmonary embolism have been received as part of the continuing surveillance of paclitaxel safety. Rare reports of radiation pneumonitis have been received in patients receiving concurrent radiotherapy.

Abraxane: Reports of dyspnea (12%) and cough (6%) were reported after treatment with paclitaxel protein-bound particles in the randomized trial. Rare reports (less than 1%) of pneumothorax were reported after treatment with paclitaxel protein-bound particles. There is no experience with the use of paclitaxel protein-bound particles with concurrent radiotherapy.

Miscellaneous –

Taxol: Reports of asthenia and malaise have been received as part of the continuing surveillance of paclitaxel safety. In the phase 3 trial of paclitaxel 135 mg/m^2 over 24 hours in combination with cisplatin as first-line therapy of ovarian cancer, asthenia was reported in 17% of the patients, significantly greater than the 10% incidence observed in the control arm of cyclophosphamide/cisplatin.

Abraxane: Asthenia was reported in 47% of patients (8% severe) treated with paclitaxel protein-bound particles in the randomized trial. Asthenia included reports of asthenia, fatigue, weakness, lethargy, and malaise.

Rare cases of cardiac ischemia/infarction and thrombosis/embolism, possibly related to paclitaxel protein-bound particles treatment, have been reported.

The following rare adverse reactions have been reported as part of the continuing surveillance of paclitaxel injection safety and may occur following paclitaxel protein-bound particles treatment: skin abnormalities related to radiation recall, as well as reports of maculopapular rash, Stevens-Johnson syndrome, toxic epidermal necrolysis, conjunctivitis, and increased lacrimation.

Postmarketing:

• *Taxol* – Postmarketing reports of ototoxicity (hearing loss and tinnitus) have been received.

Rare reports of conjunctivitis and increased lacrimation have been received as part of the continuing surveillance of paclitaxel injection safety.

Accidental exposure: No reports of accidental exposure to paclitaxel protein-bound particles have been received. However, upon inhalation of paclitaxel injection, dyspnea, chest pain, burning eyes, sore throat, and nausea have been reported. Following topical exposure, reactions have included tingling, burning, and redness.

Overdosage

➤*Symptoms:* The primary anticipated complications of overdosage would consist of bone marrow suppression, sensory neurotoxicity, and mucositis. Overdoses in pediatric patients may be associated with acute ethanol toxicity. There have been reports of CNS toxicity (rarely associated with death) in a clinical trial in pediatric patients in which paclitaxel was infused IV over 3 hours at doses ranging from 350 to 420 mg/m^2. The toxicity is most likely attributable to the high dose of the ethanol component of the paclitaxel vehicle given over a short infusion time. The use of concomitant antihistamines may intensify this effect. Although a direct effect of the paclitaxel itself cannot be discounted, the high doses used in this study (over twice the recommended adult dosage) must be considered in assessing the safety of paclitaxel for use in this population.

➤*Treatment:* There is no known antidote for paclitaxel overdosage.

DOCETAXEL

Rx	**Taxotere** (Aventis)	**Injection**: 20 mg per 0.5 mL	Polysorbate 80.[a] In single-dose vials with 1.5 mL diluent.[b]
		80 mg per 2 mL	Polysorbate 80.[a] In single-dose vials with 6 mL diluent.[b]

[a] Polysorbate 80 1,040 mg/mL.

[b] Contains 13% ethanol in water for injection.

DOCETAXEL — INJECTION

WARNING

Administer docetaxel under the supervision of a qualified health care provider experienced in the use of antineoplastic agents. Appropriate management of complications is possible only when adequate diagnostic and treatment facilities are readily available.

The incidence of treatment-related mortality associated with docetaxel therapy is increased in patients with abnormal liver function, patients receiving higher doses, and patients with non-small cell lung cancer (NSCLC) and a history of treatment with platinum-based chemotherapy who receive docetaxel as a single agent at a dose of 100 mg/m^2.

Hepatic function impairment – Generally, do not give docetaxel to patients with bilirubin greater than the upper limit of normal (ULN), or patients with AST and/or ALT greater than 1.5 times ULN concomitant with alkaline phosphatase greater than 2.5 times ULN. Patients with elevations of bilirubin or abnormalities of transaminase concurrent with alkaline phosphatase are at increased risk for the development of grade 4 neutropenia, febrile neutropenia, infections, severe thrombocytopenia, severe stomatitis, severe skin toxicity, and toxic death. Patients with isolated elevations of transaminase greater than 1.5 times ULN also had a higher rate of febrile neutropenia grade 4, but did not have an increased incidence of toxic death. Obtain and review bilirubin, AST or ALT, and alkaline phosphatase values prior to each cycle of docetaxel therapy.

Neutropenia – Do not give docetaxel therapy to patients with neutrophil counts of less than 1,500 cells/mm^3. In order to monitor the occurrence of neutropenia, which may be severe and result in infection, perform frequent blood cell counts on all patients receiving docetaxel.

Hypersensitivity – Severe hypersensitivity reactions characterized by hypotension and/or bronchospasm, or generalized rash/erythema occurred in 2.2% (2/92) of patients who received the recommended 3-day dexamethasone premedication. Hypersensitivity reactions requiring discontinuation of the docetaxel infusion were reported in 5 patients who did not receive premedication. These reactions resolved after discontinuation of the infusion and the administration of appropriate therapy. Do not give docetaxel to patients who have a history of severe hypersensitivity reactions to docetaxel or to other drugs formulated with polysorbate 80.

Fluid retention – Severe fluid retention occurred in 6.5% (6/92) of patients despite use of a 3-day dexamethasone premedication regimen. It was characterized by 1 or more of the following reactions: poorly tolerated peripheral edema, generalized edema, pleural effusion requiring urgent drainage, dyspnea at rest, cardiac tamponade, or pronounced abdominal distention (due to ascites). Premedicate patients with oral corticosteroids prior to each docetaxel administration to reduce the incidence and severity of fluid retention. Closely monitor patients with preexisting effusions from the first dose for the possible exacerbation of the effusions.

Indications

➤*Breast cancer:* Docetaxel is indicated for the treatment of patients with locally advanced or metastatic breast cancer after failure of prior chemotherapy.

Docetaxel in combination with doxorubicin and cyclophosphamide is indicated for the adjuvant treatment of patients with operable node-positive breast cancer.

➤*NSCLC:* Docetaxel is indicated as a single agent for the treatment of patients with locally advanced or metastatic NSCLC after failure of prior platinum-based chemotherapy.

DOCETAXEL — INJECTION

Docetaxel in combination with cisplatin is indicated for the treatment of patients with unresectable, locally advanced or metastatic NSCLC who have not previously received chemotherapy for this condition.

➤*Prostate cancer:* Docetaxel in combination with prednisone is indicated for the treatment of patients with androgen independent (hormone-refractory) metastatic prostate cancer.

➤*Unlabeled uses:* Gastric cancer, head and neck cancer, ovarian cancer, urothelial cancer, small cell lung cancer, melanoma, soft tissue sarcomas, esophageal cancer.

Administration and Dosage

➤*Approved by the FDA:* May 14, 1996.

➤*Breast cancer:* The recommended dosage of docetaxel is 60 to 100 mg/m² administered intravenously (IV) over 1 hour every 3 weeks.

In the adjuvant treatment of operable node-positive breast cancer, the recommended docetaxel dosage is 75 mg/m² administered 1 hour after doxorubicin 50 mg/m² and cyclophosphamide 500 mg/m² every 3 weeks for 6 courses. Prophylactic granulocyte colony-stimulating factor (G-CSF) may be used to mitigate the risk of hematological toxicities.

➤*NSCLC:* For treatment after failure of prior platinum-based chemotherapy, docetaxel was evaluated as monotherapy, and the recommended dosage of docetaxel is 75 mg/m² administered IV over 1 hour every 3 weeks. A dose of 100 mg/m² in patients previously treated with chemotherapy was associated with increased hematologic toxicity, infection, and treatment-related mortality in randomized, controlled trials.

For chemotherapy-naïve patients, docetaxel was evaluated in combination with cisplatin. The recommended dosage of docetaxel is 75 mg/m² administered IV over 1 hour immediately followed by cisplatin 75 mg/m² over 30 to 60 minutes every 3 weeks.

➤*Prostate cancer:* For androgen-independent metastatic prostate cancer, the recommended dosage of docetaxel is 75 mg/m² every 3 weeks as a 1-hour infusion. Prednisone 5 mg orally twice daily is administered continuously.

➤*Premedication regimen:* Premedicate all patients with oral corticosteroids, such as dexamethasone 16 mg/day (eg, 8 mg 2 times a day), for 3 days starting 1 day prior to docetaxel administration in order to reduce the incidence and severity of fluid retention as well as the severity of hypersensitivity reactions.

Prostate cancer – For androgen-independent metastatic prostate cancer, given the concurrent use of prednisone, the recommended premedication regimen is dexamethasone 8 mg orally at 12 hours, 3 hours, and 1 hour before the docetaxel infusion. Severe hypersensitivity reactions characterized by hypotension or bronchospasm, or generalized rash/erythema occurred in 2.2% (2/92) of patients who received the recommended 3-day dexamethasone premedication.

➤*Dosage adjustments during treatment:*

Breast cancer – Adjust dose from 100 to 75 mg/m² in patients who are dosed initially at 100 mg/m² and experience either febrile neutropenia, neutrophils less than 500 cells/mm³ for more than 1 week, or severe or cumulative cutaneous reactions during docetaxel therapy. If the patient continues to experience these reactions, either decrease the dosage from 75 to 55 mg/m² or discontinue treatment. Conversely, patients who are dosed initially at 60 mg/m² and who do not experience febrile neutropenia, neutrophils less than 500 cells/mm³ for more than 1 week, severe or cumulative cutaneous reactions, or severe peripheral neuropathy during docetaxel therapy may tolerate higher doses. Discontinue docetaxel treatment in patients who develop greater than grade 3 peripheral neuropathy.

Combination therapy with docetaxel in the adjuvant treatment of breast cancer – Administer docetaxel in combination with doxorubicin and cyclophosphamide when the neutrophil count is 1,500 cells/mm³ or more. Give G-CSF in all subsequent cycles to patients who experience febrile neutropenia. Keep patients who continue to experience this reaction on G-CSF and reduce their docetaxel dose to 60 mg/m². Reduce the dosage of docetaxel from 75 to 60 mg/m² in patients who experience severe or cumulative cutaneous reactions or moderate neurosensory signs and/or symptoms during docetaxel therapy. If the patient continues to experience these reactions at 60 mg/m², discontinue treatment.

NSCLC –

Monotherapy with docetaxel for NSCLC treatment after failure of prior platinum-based chemotherapy: Until resolution of toxicity, withhold treatment in patients who are dosed initially at 75 mg/m² and experience either febrile neutropenia, neutrophils less than 500 cells/mm³ for more than 1 week, severe or cumulative cutaneous reactions, or other grade 3/4 nonhematological toxicities during docetaxel treatments, and then resume at 55 mg/m². Discontinue docetaxel treatment in patients who develop grade 3 or higher peripheral neuropathy.

Combination therapy with docetaxel for chemotherapy-naïve NSCLC: For patients who are dosed initially at docetaxel 75 mg/m² in combination with cisplatin, and whose nadir of platelet count during the previous course of therapy is less than 25,000 cells/mm³, patients who experience febrile neutropenia, and patients with serious nonhematologic toxicities, reduce the docetaxel dosage in subsequent cycles to 65 mg/m². In patients who require a further dose reduction, a dose of 50 mg/m² is recommended. For cisplatin dosage adjustments, see cisplatin monograph.

Combination therapy with docetaxel for androgen-independent metastatic prostate cancer – Administer docetaxel when the neutrophil count is 1,500 cells/mm³ or more. In patients who experience either febrile neutropenia, neutrophils less than 500 cells/mm³ for more than 1 week, severe or cumulative cutaneous reactions, or moderate neurosensory signs and/or symptoms during docetaxel therapy, reduce the dosage of docetaxel from 75 to 60 mg/m². If the patient continues to experience these reactions at 60 mg/m², discontinue treatment.

➤*Hepatic function impairment:* See the Warning box for more information.

➤*Preparation of solution:*

Equipment – Contact of the docetaxel concentrate with plasticized polyvinyl chloride (PVC) equipment or devices used to prepare solutions for infusion is not recommended. In order to minimize patient exposure to the plasticizer diethylhexyl phthalate (DEHP), which may be leached from PVC infusion bags or sets, store diluted docetaxel solution in bottles (glass, polypropylene) or plastic bags (polypropylene, polyolefin) and administer through polyethylene-lined administration sets. Docetaxel for injection concentrate requires 2 dilutions prior to administration. Please use the following preparation instructions.

Overfill of solution – Both the docetaxel for injection concentrate and the diluent vials contain an overfill to compensate for liquid loss during preparation. This overfill ensures that after dilution with the entire contents of the accompanying diluent, there is an initial diluted solution containing docetaxel 10 mg/mL.

The following table provides the fill range of the diluent, approximate extractable volume of diluent when the entire contents of the diluent vial are withdrawn, and concentration of the initial diluted solution for docetaxel 20 and 80 mg.

Preparation of Docetaxel Solutions

Product	Diluent 13% (w/w) ethanol in water for injection fill range (mL)	Approximate extractable volume of diluent when entire contents are withdrawn (mL)	Concentration of the initial diluted solution (docetaxel mg/mL)
Docetaxel 20 mg per 0.5 mL	1.88 to 2.08 mL	1.8 mL	10 mg/mL
Docetaxel 80 mg per 2 mL	6.96 to 7.7 mL	7.1 mL	10 mg/mL

Preparation of the initial diluted solution:

1.) Store docetaxel vials between 2° and 25°C (36° and 77°F). If the vials are stored under refrigeration, allow the appropriate number of vials of docetaxel injection concentrate and diluent (13% ethanol in water for injection) vials to stand at room temperature for approximately 5 minutes.
2.) Aseptically withdraw the entire contents of the appropriate diluent vial (approximately 1.8 mL for docetaxel 20 mg and approximately 7.1 mL for docetaxel 80 mg) into a syringe by partially inverting the vial, and transfer it to the vial of docetaxel for injection concentrate. If the procedure is followed as described, an initial diluted solution of docetaxel 10 mg/mL will result.
3.) Mix the initial diluted solution vial by repeated inversions for at least 45 seconds to ensure full mixture of the concentrate and diluent. Do not shake.
4.) The initial diluted docetaxel solution (docetaxel 10 mg/mL) should be clear; however, there may be some foam on top of the solution due to the polysorbate 80. Allow the solution to stand for a few minutes to allow any foam to dissipate. It is not required that all foam dissipate prior to continuing the preparation process. The initial diluted solution may be used immediately or stored either in the refrigerator or at room temperature for a maximum of 8 hours.

Preparation of the final dilution for infusion:

1.) Aseptically withdraw the required amount of initial diluted docetaxel solution (docetaxel 10 mg/mL) with a calibrated syringe and inject into a 250 mL infusion bag or bottle of either 0.9% sodium chloride solution or 5% dextrose solution to produce a final concentration of 0.3 to 0.74 mg/mL. If a dose greater than 200 mg of docetaxel is required, use a larger volume of the infusion vehicle so that a concentration of docetaxel 0.74 mg/mL is not exceeded.
2.) Thoroughly mix the infusion by manual rotation.
3.) As with all parenteral products, visually inspect docetaxel for particulate matter or discoloration prior to administration whenever the solution and container permit. If the docetaxel for injection initial diluted solution or final dilution for infusion is not clear or appears to have precipitation, discard the dilution.

Administer the final docetaxel solution for infusion IV as a 1-hour infusion under ambient room temperature and lighting conditions.

➤*Storage/Stability:*

Stability – Docetaxel infusion solution, if stored between 2° and 25°C (36° and 77°F) is stable for 4 hours. Use fully prepared docetaxel infusion solution (in either 0.9% sodium chloride solution or 5% dextrose solution) within 4 hours (including the 1 hour IV administration). The initial diluted solution may be used immediately or stored either in the refrigerator or at room temperature for a maximum of 8 hours.

Storage – Store between 2° and 25°C (36° and 77°F). Retain in the original package to protect from bright light. Freezing does not adversely affect the product.

Actions

➤*Pharmacology:* Docetaxel is an antineoplastic agent that acts by disrupting the microtubular network in cells that is essential for mitotic and

DOCETAXEL — INJECTION

interphase cellular functions. Docetaxel binds to free tubulin and promotes the assembly of tubulin into stable microtubules while simultaneously inhibiting their disassembly. This leads to the production of microtubule bundles without normal function and to the stabilization of microtubules, which results in the inhibition of mitosis in cells. Docetaxel's binding to microtubules does not alter the number of protofilaments in the bound microtubules, a feature that differs from most spindle poisons currently in clinical use.

➤*Pharmacokinetics:*

Absorption/Distribution – The pharmacokinetics of docetaxel have been evaluated in cancer patients after administration of 20 to 115 mg/m^2 in phase 1 studies. The area under the curve (AUC) was dose proportional following doses of 70 to 115 mg/m^2 with infusion times of 1 to 2 hours.

Mean value for steady-state volume of distribution was 113 L.

In vitro studies showed that docetaxel is about 94% protein bound, mainly to α_1-acid glycoprotein, albumin, and lipoproteins. In 3 cancer patients, the in vitro binding to plasma proteins was found to be approximately 97%. Dexamethasone does not affect the protein binding of docetaxel.

Excretion – Clearance of docetaxel in combination therapy with cisplatin was similar to that previously observed following monotherapy with docetaxel. The pharmacokinetic profile of cisplatin in combination therapy with docetaxel was similar to that observed with cisplatin alone.

A study of ^{14}C-docetaxel was conducted in 3 cancer patients. Docetaxel was eliminated in both the urine and feces following oxidative metabolism of the tert-butyl ester group, but fecal excretion was the main elimination route. Within 7 days, urinary and fecal excretion accounted for approximately 6% and 75% of the administered radioactivity, respectively. About 80% of the radioactivity recovered in feces is excreted during the first 48 hours as 1 major and 3 minor metabolites with very small amounts (less than 8%) of unchanged drug.

Docetaxel's pharmacokinetic profile is consistent with a 3-compartment pharmacokinetic model, with half-lives for the α, β, and γ phases of 4 minutes, 36 minutes, and 11.1 hours, respectively. The initial rapid decline represents distribution to the peripheral compartments and the late (terminal) phase is due, in part, to a relatively slow efflux of docetaxel from the peripheral compartment. Mean value for total body clearance was 21 L/h/m^2.

Special populations –

Hepatic function impairment: In patients with clinical chemistry data suggestive of mild to moderate liver function impairment (AST or ALT greater than 1.5 times the ULN concomitant with alkaline phosphatase greater than 2.5 times ULN), total body clearance was lowered by an average of 27%, resulting in a 38% increase in systemic exposure (AUC). This average, however, includes a substantial range and there is, at present, no measurement that would allow recommendation for dose adjustment in such patients. Generally, do not treat patients with combined abnormalities of transaminase and alkaline phosphatase with docetaxel.

Contraindications

Docetaxel is contraindicated in patients who have a history of severe hypersensitivity reactions to docetaxel or to other drugs formulated with polysorbate 80.

See the Warning box for more information.

Warnings

➤*Toxic deaths:*

Breast cancer – Docetaxel administered at 100 mg/m^2 was associated with deaths considered possibly or probably related to treatment in 2% (19/965) of metastatic breast cancer patients, both previously treated and untreated, with normal baseline liver function and in 11.5% (7/61) of patients with various tumor types who had abnormal baseline liver function (AST and/or ALT greater than 1.5 times ULN together with alkaline phosphatase greater than 2.5 times ULN). Among patients dosed at 60 mg/m^2, mortality related to treatment occurred in 0.6% (3/481) of patients with normal liver function, and in 3 of 7 patients with abnormal liver function. Approximately half of these deaths occurred during the first cycle. Sepsis accounted for the majority of the deaths.

NSCLC – Docetaxel administered at a dose 100 mg/m^2 in patients with locally advanced or metastatic NSCLC who had a history of platinum-based chemotherapy was associated with increased treatment-related mortality (14% and 5% in 2 randomized, controlled studies). There were 2.8% treatment-related deaths among the 176 patients treated at the 75 mg/m^2 dose in the randomized trials. Among patients who experienced treatment-related mortality at the 75 mg/m^2 dose level, 3 of 5 patients had a performance status of 2 at study entry.

➤*Premedication regimen:* See Administration and Dosage for more information.

➤*Hematologic effects:* Neutropenia (less than 2,000 neutrophils/mm^3) occurs in virtually all patients given 60 to 100 mg/m^2 of docetaxel and grade 4 neutropenia (less than 500 cells/mm^3) occurs in 85% of patients given 100 mg/m^2 and 75% of patients given 60 mg/m^2. Frequent monitoring of blood cell counts is, therefore, essential so that dose can be adjusted. Do not administer docetaxel to patients with neutrophils less than 1,500 cells/mm^3.

Febrile neutropenia occurred in about 12% of patients given 100 mg/m^2 but was very uncommon in patients given 60 mg/m^2. Hematologic responses, febrile reactions and infections, and rates of septic death for different regimens are dose related.

Three breast cancer patients with severe liver impairment (bilirubin greater than 1.7 times ULN) developed fatal GI bleeding associated with severe drug-induced thrombocytopenia.

➤*Fluid retention:* See the Warning box for more information.

➤*Acute myeloid leukemia (AML):* Treatment-related AML has occurred in patients given anthracyclines and/or cyclophosphamide, including use in adjuvant therapy for breast cancer. In the adjuvant breast cancer trial, AML occurred in 3 of 744 patients who received docetaxel, doxorubicin, and cyclophosphamide and in 1 of 736 patients who received fluorouracil, doxorubicin, and cyclophosphamide.

➤*Hypersensitivity reactions:* See the Warning box for more information.

➤*Hepatic function impairment:* See the Warning box for more information.

➤*Mutagenesis:* Docetaxel has been shown to be clastogenic in the in vitro chromosome aberration test in Chinese hamster ovary (CHO)-K$_1$ cells and in the in vivo micronucleus test in the mouse, but it did not induce mutagenicity in the Ames test or the CHO/hypoxanthine guanine phosphoribosyltransferase (HGPRT) gene mutation assays.

➤*Fertility impairment:* Docetaxel produced no impairment of fertility in rats when administered in multiple IV doses of up to 0.3 mg/kg (about 1/50 the recommended human dose on a mg/m^2 basis), but decreased testicular weights were reported. This correlates with findings of a 10-cycle toxicity study (dosing once every 21 days for 6 months) in rats and dogs in which testicular atrophy or degeneration was observed at IV doses of 5 mg/kg in rats and 0.375 mg/kg in dogs (about ⅓ and 1/15 the recommended human dose on a mg/m^2 basis, respectively). An increased frequency of dosing in rats produced similar effects at lower dose levels.

➤*Elderly:* In general, dose selection for an elderly patient should be cautious, reflecting the greater frequency of decreased hepatic, renal, or cardiac function and of concomitant disease or other drug therapy in elderly patients.

➤*Pregnancy:* *Category D.* Docetaxel can cause fetal harm when administered to pregnant women. Studies in both rats and rabbits at dosages greater than or equal to 0.3 and 0.03 mg/kg/day, respectively (about 1/50 and 1/300 the daily maximum recommended human dose on a mg/m^2 basis), administered during the period of organogenesis, have shown that docetaxel is embryotoxic and fetotoxic (characterized by intrauterine mortality, increased resorption, reduced fetal weight, and fetal ossification delay). These dosages also caused maternal toxicity.

There are no adequate and well-controlled studies in pregnant women using docetaxel. If docetaxel is used during pregnancy, or if the patient becomes pregnant while receiving this drug, apprise the patient of the potential hazard to the fetus or potential risk for loss of the pregnancy. Advise women of childbearing potential to avoid becoming pregnant during therapy with docetaxel.

➤*Lactation:* It is not known whether docetaxel is excreted in human milk. Because many drugs are excreted in human milk, and because of the potential for serious adverse reactions in breast-feeding infants from docetaxel, advise mothers to discontinue breast-feeding prior to taking the drug.

➤*Children:* The safety and efficacy of docetaxel in children younger than 16 years of age have not been established.

Precautions

➤*Monitoring:*

Hematologic effects – In order to monitor the occurrence of myelotoxicity, perform frequent peripheral blood cell counts on all patients receiving docetaxel. Do not retreat patients with subsequent cycles of docetaxel until neutrophils recover to a level greater than 1,500 cells/mm^3 and platelets recover to a level greater than 100,000 cells/mm^3.

A 25% reduction in the dose of docetaxel is recommended during subsequent cycles following severe neutropenia (less than 500 cells/mm^3) lasting 7 days or more, febrile neutropenia, or a grade 4 infection in a docetaxel cycle.

Hepatic function impairment – Obtain bilirubin, AST or ALT, and alkaline phosphatase values prior to each cycle of docetaxel therapy.

Responding patients may not experience an improvement in performance status on therapy and may experience worsening. The relationship between changes in performance status, response to therapy, and treatment-related adverse reactions has not been established.

➤*Cutaneous:* See Adverse Reactions for more information.

➤*Fluid retention:* When fluid retention occurs, peripheral edema usually starts in the lower extremities and may become generalized with a median weight gain of 2 kg.

For more information, see the Warning box.

➤*Neurologic:* Severe neurosensory symptoms (paresthesia, dysesthesia, pain) were observed in 5.5% (53/965) of metastatic breast cancer patients, and resulted in treatment discontinuation in 6.1%. When these symptoms occur, adjust dosage. If symptoms persist, discontinue treatment. Patients who experienced neurotoxicity in clinical trials and for whom follow-up information on the complete resolution of the event was available had spontaneous reversal of symptoms with a median of 9 weeks from onset (range, 0 to 106 weeks). Severe peripheral motor neuropathy mainly manifested as distal extremity weakness occurred in 4.4% (42/965).

➤*Asthenia:* Severe asthenia has been reported in 14.9% (144/965) of metastatic breast cancer patients but has led to treatment discontinuation in only 1.8%. Symptoms of fatigue and weakness may last a few days up to sev-

DOCETAXEL — INJECTION

eral weeks and may be associated with deterioration of performance status in patients with progressive disease.

Drug Interactions

➤*Cytochrome P-450 system:* In vitro studies have shown that the metabolism of docetaxel may be modified by the coadministration of compounds that induce, inhibit, or are metabolized by cytochrome P-450 3A4 (ie, cyclosporine, terfenadine, ketoconazole, erythromycin, troleandomycin). Exercise caution with these drugs when treating patients receiving docetaxel as there is a potential for a significant interaction.

Adverse Reactions

➤*Monotherapy with docetaxel for locally advanced or metastatic breast cancer after failure of prior chemotherapy:*

Docetaxel 100 mg/m² –

Adverse Reactions in Patients Receiving Docetaxel at 100 mg/m²			
Adverse reaction	All tumor types normal LFTs[a] (n = 2,045)	All tumor types elevated LFTs[b] (n = 61)	Breast cancer normal LFTs[c] (n = 965)
CNS			
Asthenia (any)	61.8%	52.5%	66.3%
Asthenia (severe)	12.8%	24.6%	14.9%
Neurosensory (any)	49.3%	34.4%	58.3%
Neurosensory (severe)	4.3%	0%	5.5%
Dermatologic			
Alopecia	75.8%	62.3%	74.2%
Cutaneous (any)	47.6%	54.1%	47%
Cutaneous (severe)	4.8%	9.8%	5.2%
Nail changes (any)	30.6%	23%	40.5%
Nail changes (severe)	2.5%	4.9%	3.7%
GI			
Diarrhea	38.7%	32.8%	42.6%
Nausea	38.8%	37.7%	42.1%
Severe diarrhea	4.7%	4.9%	5.5%
Stomatitis (any)	41.7%	49.2%	51.7%
Stomatitis (severe)	5.5%	13%	7.4%
Vomiting	22.3%	23%	23.4%
Hematologic			
Anemia < 8 g/dL	8.8%	31.1%	7.7%
Anemia < 11 g/dL	90.4%	91.8%	93.6%
Febrile neutropenia[c]	11%	26.2%	12.3%
Leukopenia < 1,000 cells/mm³	31.6%	46.6%	43.7%
Leukopenia < 4,000 cells/mm³	95.6%	98.3%	98.6%
Neutropenia < 500 cells/mm³	75.4%	87.5%	85.9%
Neutropenia < 2,000 cells/mm³	95.5%	96.4%	98.5%
Thrombocytopenia < 100,000 cells/mm³	8%	24.6%	9.2%
Hypersensitivity			
Regardless of premedication (any)	21%	19.7%	17.6%
Regardless of premedication (severe)	4.2%	9.8%	2.6%
With 3-day premedication	(n = 92)	(n = 3)	(n = 92)
Any	15.2%	33.3%	15.2%
Severe	2.2%	0%	2.2%
Metabolic			
Fluid retention:			
Regardless of premedication (any)	47%	39.3%	59.7%
Regardless of premedication (severe)	6.9%	8.2%	8.9%
With 3-day premedication	(n = 92)	(n = 3)	(n = 92)
Any	64.1%	66.7%	64.1%
Severe	6.5%	33.3%	6.5%
Musculoskeletal			
Arthralgia	9.2%	6.6%	8.2%
Myalgia (any)	18.9%	16.4%	21.1%
Myalgia (severe)	1.5%	1.6%	1.8%
Miscellaneous			
Fever in absence of infection (any)	31.2%	41%	35.1%
Fever in absence of infection (severe)	2.1%	8.2%	2.2%
Infections (any)	21.6%	32.8%	22.2%
Infections (severe)	6.1%	16.4%	6.4%
Infusion-site reactions	4.4%	3.3%	4%
Nonseptic death	0.6%	6.6%	0.6%
Septic death	1.6%	4.9%	1.4%

[a] Normal baseline LFTs: transaminases less than or equal to 1.5 times ULN or alkaline phosphatase less than or equal to 2.5 times ULN or isolated elevations or transaminases or alkaline phosphatase up to 5 times ULN.
[b] Elevated baseline LFTs: AST and/or ALT greater than 1.5 times ULN concurrent with alkaline phosphatase greater than 2.5 times ULN.
[c] Febrile neutropenia: absolute neutrophil count grade 4 with fever greater than 38°C (100.4°F) with IV antibiotics and/or hospitalization.

Cardiovascular – Hypotension occurred in 2.8% of patients with solid tumors; 1.2% required treatment. Clinically meaningful reactions such as heart failure, sinus tachycardia, atrial flutter, dysrhythmia, unstable angina, pulmonary edema, and hypertension occurred rarely. Seven of 86 (8.1%) metastatic breast cancer patients receiving docetaxel 100 mg/m² in a randomized trial and who had serial left ventricular ejection fraction (LVEF) assessed developed deterioration of LVEF by greater than or equal to 10% associated with a drop below the institutional lower limit of normal.

CNS – See Precautions for more information.

Dermatologic – Localized erythema of the extremities with edema followed by desquamation has been observed. In case of severe skin toxicity, an adjustment in dosage is recommended. The discontinuation rate due to skin toxicity was 1.6% (15/965) for metastatic breast cancer patients. Among 92 breast cancer patients premedicated with 3-day corticosteroids, there were no cases of severe skin toxicity reported and no patient discontinued docetaxel due to skin toxicity. Reversible cutaneous reactions characterized by a rash including localized eruptions, mainly on the feet or hands, but also on the arms, face, or thorax, usually associated with pruritus, have been observed. Eruptions generally occurred within 1 week after docetaxel infusion, recovered before the next infusion, and were not disabling.

Severe nail disorders were characterized by hypo- or hyperpigmentation, and occasionally by onycholysis (in 0.8% of patients with solid tumors) and pain.

GI – GI reactions (nausea, vomiting or diarrhea) were generally mild to moderate. Severe reactions occurred in 3% to 5% of patients with solid tumors and to a similar extent among metastatic breast cancer patients. The incidence of severe reactions was 1% or less for the 92 breast cancer patients premedicated with 3-day corticosteroids.

Severe stomatitis occurred in 5.5% of patients with solid tumors, 7.4% of patients with metastatic breast cancer, and 1.1% of the 92 breast cancer patients premedicated with 3-day corticosteroids.

Hematologic – Reversible marrow suppression was the major dose-limiting toxicity of docetaxel. The median time to nadir was 7 days, while the median duration of severe neutropenia (less than 500 cells/mm³) was 7 days. Among 2,045 patients with solid tumors and normal baseline LFTs, severe neutropenia occurred in 75.4% and lasted for more than 7 days in 2.9% of cycles.

Febrile neutropenia (less than 500 cells/mm³ with fever greater than 38°C [100.4°F] with IV antibiotics and/or hospitalization) occurred in 11% of patients with solid tumors, 12.3% of patients with metastatic breast cancer, and 9.8% of 92 breast cancer patients premedicated with 3-day corticosteroids.

Severe infectious episodes occurred in 6.1% of patients with solid tumors, 6.4% of patients with metastatic breast cancer, and 5.4% of 92 breast cancer patients premedicated with 3-day corticosteroids.

Thrombocytopenia (less than 100,000 cells/mm³) associated with fatal GI hemorrhage has been reported.

Hepatic – In patients with normal LFTs at baseline, bilirubin values greater than the ULN occurred in 8.9% of patients. Increases in AST or ALT greater than 1.5 times the ULN, or alkaline phosphatase greater than 2.5 times ULN, were observed in 18.9% and 7.3% of patients, respectively. While on docetaxel, increases in AST and/or ALT greater than 1.5 times ULN concomitant with alkaline phosphatase greater than 2.5 times ULN occurred in 4.3% of patients with normal LFTs at baseline (whether these changes were related to the drug or underlying disease has not been established).

Hypersensitivity – See the Warning box for more information.

Minor reactions, including flushing, rash with or without pruritus, chest tightness, back pain, dyspnea, drug fever, or chills, have been reported and resolved after discontinuing the infusion and appropriate therapy.

Local – Infusion-site reactions were generally mild and consisted of hyperpigmentation, inflammation, redness or dryness of the skin, phlebitis, extravasation, or swelling of the vein.

Metabolic –

Fluid retention: See the Warning box for more information.

DOCETAXEL — INJECTION

➤*Adjuvant treatment of breast cancer:*

Adverse Reactions in Patients Receiving Docetaxel in Combination with Doxorubicin and Cyclophosphamide (TAX 316)

Adverse reaction	Docetaxel 75 mg/m² plus doxorubicin 50 mg/m² plus cyclophosphamide 500 mg/m² (TAC) (n = 744)		Fluorouracil 500 mg/m² plus doxorubicin 50 mg/m² plus cyclophosphamide 500 mg/m² (FAC) (n = 736)	
	Any	Grade 3/4	Any	Grade 3/4
Cardiovascular				
Cardiac dysrhythmias	7.9%	0.3%	6%	0.3%
Hypotension	2.6%	0%	1.1%	0.1%
Phlebitis	1.2%	0%	0.8%	0%
Syncope	1.6%	0.5%	1.2%	0.3%
Vasodilation	27%	1.1%	21.2%	0.5%
CNS				
Asthenia	80.8%	11.2%	71.2%	5.6%
Neurocerebellar	2.4%	0.1%	2%	0
Neurocortical	5.1%	0.5%	6.4%	0.7%
Neuropathy motor	3.8%	0.1%	2.2%	0
Neuropathy sensory	25.5%	0	10.2%	0
Dermatologic				
Alopecia	97.8%	NA[a]	97.1%	NA[a]
Nail disorders	18.5%	0.4%	14.4%	0.1%
Skin toxicity	26.5%	0.8%	17.7%	0.4%
GI				
Abdominal pain	10.9%	0.7%	5.3%	0
Anorexia	21.6%	2.2%	17.7%	1.2%
Constipation	33.9%	1.1%	31.8%	1.4%
Diarrhea	35.2%	3.8%	27.9%	1.8%
Nausea	80.5%	5.1%	88%	9.5%
Stomatitis	69.4%	7.1%	52.9%	2%
Taste perversion	27.8%	0.7%	15.1%	0
Vomiting	44.5%	4.3%	59.2%	7.3%
GU				
Amenorrhea	61.7%	NA[a]	52.4%	NA[a]
Hematologic				
Anemia	91.5%	4.3%	71.7%	1.6%
Febrile neutropenia	24.7%	NA[a]	2.5%	NA[a]
Neutropenia	71.4%	65.5%	82%	49.3%
Neutropenic infection	12.1%	NA[a]	6.3%	NA[a]
Thrombocytopenia	39.4%	2%	27.7%	1.2%
Hypersensitivity				
Hypersensitivity reactions	13.4%	1.3%	3.7%	0.1%
Metabolic/Nutritional				
Fluid retention[b]	35.1%	0.9%	14.7%	0.1%
Peripheral edema	26.9%	0.4%	7.3%	0
Weight gain	12.9%	0.3%	8.6%	0.3%
Musculoskeletal				
Arthralgia	19.4%	0.5%	9%	0.3%
Myalgia	26.7%	0.8%	9.9%	0
Ophthalmic				
Conjunctivitis	5.1%	0.3%	6.0%	0.1%
Lacrimation disorder	11.3%	0.1%	7.1%	0
Respiratory				
Cough	13.7%	0	9.8%	0.1%
Miscellaneous				
Fever in absence of infection	46.5%	1.3%	17.1%	0
Infection	39.4%	3.9%	36.3%	2.2%
Lymphedema	4.4%	0	1.2%	0

[a] NA = not applicable.
[b] COSTART term and grading system for reactions related to treatment.

Of the 744 patients treated with TAC, 36.3% experienced severe treatment-emergent adverse reactions compared with 26.6% of the 736 patients treated with FAC. Dose reductions due to hematologic toxicity occurred in 1% of cycles in the TAC arm vs 0.1% of cycles in the FAC arm. Six percent of patients treated with TAC discontinued treatment due to adverse reactions, compared with 1.1% treated with FAC; fever in the absence of infection and allergy being the most common reasons for withdrawal among TAC-treated patients. Two patients died in each arm within 30 days of their last study treatment; 1 death per arm was attributed to study drugs.

GI – In addition to GI reactions reflected in the preceding table, 7 patients in the TAC arm were reported to have colitis/enteritis/large intestine perforation vs 1 patient in the FAC arm. Five of the 7 TAC-treated patients required treatment discontinuation; no deaths due to these reactions occurred.

Cardiovascular – More cardiovascular reactions were reported in the TAC arm vs the FAC arm; dysrhythmias, all grades (7.9% vs 6%); hypotension, all grades (2.6% vs 1.1%); and congestive heart failure (1.6% vs 0.5%). One patient in each arm died due to heart failure.

Miscellaneous –

Fever and infection: Fever in the absence of infection was seen in 46.5% of TAC-treated patients and in 17.1% of FAC-treated patients. Grade 3/4 fever in the absence of infection was seen in 1.3% and 0% of TAC- and FAC-treated patients, respectively. Infection was seen in 39.4% of TAC-treated patients compared with 36.3% of FAC-treated patients. Grade 3/4 infection was seen in 3.9% and 2.2% of TAC-treated and FAC-treated patients, respectively. There were no septic deaths in either treatment arm.

AML: See Warnings for more information.

➤*Treatment of NSCLC:*

Docetaxel Adverse Reactions in NSCLC Patients

Adverse reaction	Previously treated with platinum-based chemotherapy[a]			Chemotherapy-naive	
	Docetaxel 75 mg/m² (n = 176)	Best supportive care (n = 49)	Vinorelbine/ifosfamide (n = 119)	Docetaxel 75 mg/m² plus cisplatin 75 mg/m² (n = 406)	Vinorelbine 25 mg/m² plus cisplatin 100 mg/m² (n = 396)
CNS					
Asthenia (any)[b]	52.8%	57.1%	53.8%	74	75
Asthenia (severe or life-threatening)[b]	18.2%	38.8%	22.7%	12	14
Neuromotor (any)	15.9%	8.2%	10.1%	19	17
Neuromotor (grade 3/4)	4.5%	6.1%	3.4%	3	6
Neurosensory (any)	23.3%	14.3%	28.6%	47	42
Neurosensory (grade 3/4)	1.7%	6.1%	5%	4	4
Dermatologic					
Alopecia (any)	56.3%	34.7%	49.6%	75	42
Alopecia (grade 3)	—	—	—	< 1	0
Dermatologic (any)	19.9%	6.1%	16.8%	—	—
Dermatologic (grade 3/4)	0.6%	2%	0.8%	—	—
Nail disorder (any)[b]	11.4%	0%	1.7%	14	< 1
Nail disorder (severe)[b]	1.1%	0%	0%	< 1	0
Skin (any)	—	—	—	16	14
Skin (grade 3/4)	—	—	—	< 1	1
GI					
Anorexia (any)[b]	—	—	—	42	40
Anorexia (severe or life-threatening)[b]	—	—	—	5	5

DOCETAXEL — INJECTION

Docetaxel Adverse Reactions in NSCLC Patients

	Previously treated with platinum-based chemotherapy[a]			Chemotherapy-naive	
Adverse reaction	Docetaxel 75 mg/m² (n = 176)	Best supportive care (n = 49)	Vinorelbine/ifosfamide (n = 119)	Docetaxel 75 mg/m² plus cisplatin 75 mg/m² (n = 406)	Vinorelbine 25 mg/m² plus cisplatin 100 mg/m² (n = 396)
Diarrhea (any)	22.7%	6.1%	11.8%	47	25
Diarrhea (grade 3/4)	2.8%	0%	4.2%	7	3
Nausea (any)	33.5%	30.6%	31.1%	72	76
Nausea (grade 3/4)	5.1%	4.1%	7.6%	10	17
Stomatitis (any)	26.1%	6.1%	7.6%	24	21
Stomatitis (grade 3/4)	1.7%	0%	0.8%	2	1
Taste perversion (any)	5.7%	0%	0%	—	—
Taste perversion (severe)[b]	0.6%	0%	0%	—	—
Vomiting (any)	21.6%	26.5%	21.8%	55	61
Vomiting (grade 3/4)	2.8%	2%	5.9%	8	16
Hematologic					
Anemia (any)	91%	55.1%	90.8%	89	94
Anemia (grade 3/4)	9.1%	12.2%	14.3%	7	25
Febrile neutropenia[c]	6.3%	NA[d]	0.8%	5	5
Leukopenia (any)	83.5%	6.1%	89.1%	—	—
Leukopenia (grade 3/4)	49.4%	0%	42.9%	—	—
Neutropenia (any)	84.1%	14.3%	83.2%	91	90
Neutropenia (grade 3/4)	65.3%	12.2%	57.1%	74	78
Thrombocytopenia (any)	8%	0%	7.6%	15	15
Thrombocytopenia (grade 3/4)	2.8%	0%	1.7%	3	4
Hypersensitivity					
Hypersensitivity reactions (any)[e]	5.7%	0%	0.8%	12	4
Hypersensitivity reactions (grade 3/4)[e]	2.8%	0%	0%	3	< 1
Metabolic/Nutritional					
Fluid retention (any)[b]	33.5%	ND[f]	22.7%	54	42
Fluid retention (severe or life-threatening)[b]	2.8%	ND[f]	3.4%	2	2
Peripheral edema (any)	—	—	—	34	18
Peripheral edema (severe or life-threatening)	—	—	—	< 1	< 1
Weight gain (any)	—	—	—	15	9
Weight gain (severe or life-threatening)	—	—	—	< 1	< 1
Musculoskeletal					
Arthralgia (any)	3.4%	2%	1.7%	—	—
Arthralgia (severe)[b]	0%	0%	0.8%	—	—
Myalgia (any)[b]	6.3%	0%	2.5%	18	12
Myalgia (severe)[b]	0%	0%	0%	< 1	< 1
Respiratory					
Pleural effusion (any)	—	—	—	23	22
Pleural effusion (severe or life-threatening)	—	—	—	2	2
Pulmonary (any)	40.9%	49%	45.4%	—	—
Pulmonary (grade 3/4)	21%	28.6%	18.5%	—	—
Miscellaneous					
Fever in absence of infection (any)	—	—	—	33	29
Fever in absence of infection (grade 3/4)	—	—	—	< 1	1
Infection (any)	33.5%	28.6%	30.3%	35	37
Infection (grade 3/4)	10.2%	6.1%	9.2%	8	8
Treatment-related mortality	2.8%	NA[d]	3.4%	—	—

[a] Normal baseline LFTs: transaminases less than or equal to 1.5 times ULN or alkaline phosphatase less than or equal to 2.5 times ULN or isolated elevations of transaminases or alkaline phosphatase up to 5 times ULN.
[b] COSTART term and grading system.
[c] Febrile neutropenia: ANC grade 4 with fever greater than 38°C (100.4°F) with IV antibiotics or hospitalization.
[d] NA = Not applicable.
[e] ND = Not done.
[f] Replaces NCI term "Allergy."

Deaths within 30 days of last study treatment occurred in 31 patients (7.6%) in the docetaxel plus cisplatin arm and 37 patients (9.3%) in the vinorelbine plus cisplatin arm. Deaths within 30 days of last study treatment attributed to study drug occurred in 9 patients (2.2%) in the docetaxel plus cisplatin arm and 8 patients (2%) in the vinorelbine plus cisplatin arm.

The second comparison in the study, vinorelbine plus cisplatin vs docetaxel plus carboplatin (which did not demonstrate a superior survival associated with docetaxel) demonstrated a higher incidence of thrombocytopenia, diarrhea, fluid retention, hypersensitivity reactions, skin toxicity, alopecia, and nail changes on the docetaxel plus carboplatin arm, while a higher incidence

DOCETAXEL — INJECTION

of anemia, neurosensory toxicity, nausea, vomiting, anorexia, and asthenia was observed on the vinorelbine plus cisplatin arm.

➤*Combination therapy with docetaxel in patients with prostate cancer:*

Adverse Reactions in Patients with Prostate Cancer Who Received Docetaxel in Combination with Prednisone (TAX327)

Adverse reaction	Docetaxel 75 mg/m^2 every 3 weeks plus prednisone 5 mg twice daily (n = 332)		Mitoxantrone 12 mg/m^2 every 3 weeks plus prednisone 5 mg twice daily (n = 335)	
	Any	Grade 3/4	Any	Grade 3/4
Cardiovascular				
Cardiac left ventricular function	9.6%	0.3%	22.1%	1.2%
CNS				
Fatigue	53.3%	4.5%	34.6%	5.1%
Neuropathy motor	7.2%	1.5%	3%	0.9%
Neuropathy sensory	30.4%	1.8%	7.2%	0.3%
Dermatologic				
Alopecia	65.1%	NA	12.8%	NA
Nail changes	29.5%	0	7.5%	0
Rash/Desquamation	6%	0.3%	3.3%	0.6%
GI				
Anorexia	16.6%	1.2%	14.3%	0.3%
Diarrhea	31.6%	2.1%	9.6%	1.2%
Nausea	41%	2.7%	35.5%	1.5%
Stomatitis/Pharyngitis	19.6%	0.9%	8.4%	0
Taste disturbance	18.4%	0	6.6%	0
Vomiting	16.9 %	1.5%	14%	1.5%
Hematologic				
Anemia	66.5%	4.9%	57.8%	1.8%
Febrile neutropenia	2.7%	NA	1.8%	NA
Neutropenia	40.9%	32%	48.2%	21.7%
Thrombocytopenia	3.4%	0.6%	7.8%	1.2%
Hypersensitivity				
Allergic reactions	8.4%	0.6%	0.6%	0
Metabolic/Nutritional				
Fluid retention[a]	24.4%	0.6%	4.5%	0.3%
Peripheral edema[a]	18.1%	0.3%	1.5%	0
Weight gain[a]	7.5%	0.3%	3%	0
Musculoskeletal				
Arthralgia	8.1%	0.6%	5.1%	1.2%
Myalgia	14.5%	0.3%	12.8%	0.9%
Respiratory				
Cough	12.3%	0	7.8%	0
Dyspnea	15.1%	2.7%	8.7%	0.9%
Epistaxis	5.7%	0.3%	1.8%	0
Miscellaneous				
Infection	32.2%	5.7%	20.3%	4.2%
Tearing	9.9%	0.6%	1.5%	0

[a] Related to treatment.

➤*Postmarketing experiences:* The following adverse reactions have been identified from clinical trials or postmarketing surveillance. Because they are reported from a population of unknown size, precise estimates of frequency cannot be made:

Cardiovascular – Atrial fibrillation, chest pain, electrocardiogram (ECG) abnormalities, deep vein thrombosis, myocardial infarction, pulmonary embolism, syncope, tachycardia, thrombophlebitis.

CNS – Confusion, rare cases of seizures or transient loss of consciousness have been observed, sometimes appearing during the infusion of the drug.

Dermatologic – Rare cases of bullous eruption, such as erythema multiforme or Stevens-Johnson syndrome. Multiple factors may have contributed to the development of these effects.

GI – Abdominal pain, anorexia, colitis, constipation, duodenal ulcer, esophagitis, GI hemorrhage, GI perforation, ileus, intestinal obstruction, ischemic colitis, and neutropenic enterocolitis and dehydration as a consequence to GI reactions have been reported.

Hematologic – Bleeding episodes.

Hepatic – Rare cases of hepatitis have been reported.

Ophthalmic – Conjunctivitis, lacrimation, or lacrimation with or without conjunctivitis. Excessive tearing that may be attributable to lacrimal duct obstruction has been reported.

Rare cases of transient visual disturbances (flashes, flashing lights, scotomata) typically occurring during drug infusion and in association with hypersensitivity reactions have been reported. These were reversible upon discontinuation of the infusion.

Renal – Renal insufficiency.

Respiratory – Acute pulmonary edema, acute respiratory distress syndrome, dyspnea, interstitial pneumonia. Pulmonary fibrosis has been rarely reported.

Miscellaneous – Diffuse pain, radiation recall phenomenon.

Overdosage

➤*Symptoms:* There were 2 reports of overdose. One patient received 150 mg/m^2 and the other received 200 mg/m^2 as 1-hour infusions. Both patients experienced severe neutropenia, mild asthenia, cutaneous reactions, and mild paresthesia, and recovered without incident.

In mice, lethality was observed following single IV doses that were greater than or equal to 154 mg/kg (about 4.5 times the recommended human dose on a mg/m^2 basis); neurotoxicity associated with paralysis, nonextension of hind limbs, and myelin degeneration was observed in mice at 48 mg/kg (about 1.5 times the recommended human dose on a mg/m^2 basis). In male and female rats, lethality was observed at a dose of 20 mg/kg (comparable to the recommended human dose on a mg/m^2 basis) and was associated with abnormal mitosis and necrosis of multiple organs.

➤*Treatment:* There is no known antidote for docetaxel overdosage. In case of overdosage, keep the patient in a specialized unit where vital functions can be closely monitored. Anticipated complications of overdosage include bone marrow suppression, peripheral neurotoxicity, and mucositis. Give patients therapeutic G-CSF as soon as possible after discovery of overdose. Take other appropriate symptomatic measures as needed.

Patient Information

Inform patients that side effects associated with docetaxel may include low white blood cell count, hair loss, fatigue, fluid retention, numbness, mouth irritation, cutaneous changes, nausea, and diarrhea.

Inform patients that the health care provider may prescribe other medications, including a corticosteroid such as dexamethasone, that help to avoid or lessen some of the side effects of treatment.

Inform patients that if they have a fever over 100°F, to call their health care provider immediately. Other symptoms of infection, such as sore throat, cough, or burning sensation while urinating also should be reported.

Advise patients to tell their health care provider immediately if they feel a warm sensation, tightness in the chest, difficulty in breathing, or itching during or shortly after treatment.

Inform patients to alert their health care provider if there are any signs of fluid retention (ie, swelling of the feet or hands, increased weight).

Advise patients to tell their health care provider if they feel prolonged fatigue during the course of treatment.

Patients receiving docetaxel may develop a red, blotchy rash. This usually occurs on the feet and hands but may also appear on the arms, face, or body. If it occurs, the rash generally appears within the week after docetaxel treatment and usually disappears after a week or two. Advise patients to inform their health care provider if this occurs.

Some patients receiving docetaxel experience numbness, tingling, or burning sensations in their fingers and/or toes.

Advise patients that changes in the color of the nails may occur. Occasionally, nails become soft and tender. In rare cases, nails may fall off.

EPIPODOPHYLLOTOXINS

Podophyllotoxin Derivatives

WARNING

Severe myelosuppression – Severe myelosuppression with resulting infection or bleeding may occur.

Hypersensitivity reactions – Hypersensitivity reactions, including anaphylaxis-like symptoms, may occur with initial dosing or at repeated exposure to teniposide. Epinephrine, with or without corticosteroids and antihistamines, has been used to alleviate symptoms.

Indications

➤*Etoposide:*

Refractory testicular tumors – Refractory testicular tumors in combination with other chemotherapeutic agents in patients who have received surgery, chemotherapy and radiotherapy. Adequate data on the use of oral etoposide are not available.

Small cell lung cancer – Small cell lung cancer in combination with other agents as first line treatment.

➤*Teniposide:* In combination with other approved anticancer agents for induction therapy in patients with refractory childhood acute lymphoblastic leukemia (ALL). Available under a Treatment IND since 1988 for relapsed or refractory ALL.

➤*Unlabeled uses:*

Etoposide – Etoposide has been used alone or in combination in acute nonlymphocytic leukemias (monocytic), Hodgkin's disease, non-Hodgkin's lymphomas, Kaposi's sarcoma and neuroblastoma. Other tumors with a response rate of 5% to 20% to etoposide as a single agent include: Choriocarcinoma; rhabdomyosarcoma; hepatocellular carcinoma; epithelial ovarian, non-small and small cell lung, testicular, gastric, endometrial and breast cancers; acute lymphocytic leukemia; soft tissue sarcoma.

Actions

➤*Pharmacology:* These drugs are semisynthetic derivatives of podophyllotoxin.

Etoposide – Its main effect appears to be at the G_2 portion of the cell cycle. Two dose-dependent responses occur: At high concentrations (≥ 10 mcg/ml), lysis of cells entering mitosis is seen; at low concentrations (0.3 to 10 mcg/ml), cells are inhibited from entering prophase. The predominant macromolecular effect appears to be DNA synthesis inhibition.

Teniposide – Teniposide is a phase-specific cytotoxic drug, acting in the late S or early G_2 phase of the cell cycle, thus preventing cells from entering mitosis. Teniposide causes dose-dependent single- and double-stranded breaks in DNA and DNA:protein cross-links. The mechanism of action appears to be related to the inhibition of type II topoisomerase activity since teniposide does not intercalate into DNA or bind strongly to DNA. The cytotoxic effects of teniposide are related to the relative number of double-stranded DNA breaks produced in cells, which are a reflection of the stabilization of a topoisomerase II-DNA intermediate. Teniposide has a broad spectrum of in vivo antitumor activity against murine tumors, including hematologic malignancies and various solid tumors. Notably, it is active against sublines of certain murine leukemias with acquired resistance to cisplatin, doxorubicin, amsacrine, daunorubicin, mitoxantrone or vincristine.

➤*Pharmacokinetics:*

Absorption/Distribution –

Various Pharmacokinetic Parameters for Etoposide and Teniposide

Parameter	Etoposide	Teniposide
Total body clearance (ml/min)	33-48	10.3
Terminal half-life (hrs)	4-11	5
Volume of distribution (L)	18-29	3-11 (children) 8-44 (adults)
Protein binding (%)	97	> 99
Elimination	Renal (35%) and nonrenal (ie, mostly metabolism, ≤ 6% bile)	Renal (44%) and fecal (≤ 10%)
Excreted unchanged in urine (%)	< 50	4-12

Etoposide: The mean oral bioavailability is approximately 50% (range, 25% to 75%). There is no evidence of a first-pass effect for etoposide. On IV administration, the disposition of etoposide is a biphasic process with a distribution half-life of about 1.5 hours. The areas under the plasma concentration-time curves (AUC) and maximum plasma concentration (C_{max}) values increase linearly with dose. Etoposide does not accumulate in the plasma following daily administration of 100 mg/m^2 for 4 to 5 days. After either IV infusion or oral administration, C_{max} and AUC values exhibit marked intra- and intersubject variability. These values for oral etoposide consistently fall in the same range as the C_{max} and AUC values for an IV dose of half the size of the oral dose.

Although detectable in CSF and intracerebral tumors, the concentrations are lower than in extracerebral tumors and plasma. Concentrations are higher in normal lung than in lung metastases and are similar in primary tumors and normal tissues of the myometrium. An inverse relationship between plasma albumin levels and renal clearance is found in children.

Metabolism/Excretion – The major urinary metabolite is the hydroxy acid. Glucuronide or sulfate conjugates of etoposide are excreted in human urine and represent 5% to 22% of the dose.

In adults, total body clearance is correlated with creatinine clearance, serum albumin concentration and nonrenal clearance. In children, elevated serum ALT levels are associated with reduced drug total body clearance. Prior use of cisplatin may also result in a decrease of etoposide total body clearance in children. The pharmacokinetic characteristics of teniposide differ from those of etoposide. Teniposide is more extensively bound to plasma proteins and its cellular uptake is greater. Teniposide also has a lower systemic clearance, a longer elimination half-life and is excreted in the urine as parent drug to a lesser extent than etoposide.

Teniposide – Plasma drug levels decline biexponentially following IV infusion in children. In adults, plasma levels increase linearly with dose. Drug accumulation did not occur after daily administration for 3 days. In children, C_{max} after infusions of 137 to 203 mg/m^2 over a period of 1 to 2 hours exceeded 40 mcg/ml; by 20 to 24 hours after infusion plasma levels were generally < 2 mcg/ml.

The blood-brain barrier appears to limit diffusion of teniposide into the brain, although in a study in patients with brain tumors, CSF levels were higher than in patients without brain tumors.

Contraindications

Hypersensitivity to etoposide, teniposide or *Cremophor EL* (polyoxyethylated castor oil, present in the teniposide preparation).

Warnings

➤*Myelosuppression:* Observe patients for myelosuppression during and after therapy. Dose-limiting bone marrow suppression is the most significant toxicity.

Laboratory studies – Perform at the start of therapy and prior to each subsequent dose: Platelet count, hemoglobin, white blood cell count and differential. A platelet count < 50,000/mm^3 or an absolute neutrophil count < 500/mm^3 is an indication to withhold further therapy until the blood counts have sufficiently recovered.

➤*Anaphylaxis:* Anaphylaxis manifested by chills, fever, tachycardia, bronchospasm, dyspnea, facial flushing, hypertension or hypotension may occur (etoposide, 0.7% to 2%; teniposide, ≈ 5%). The reactions usually respond to cessation of infusion and institution of appropriate therapy. Refer to Management of Acute Hypersensitivity Reactions.

This reaction may occur with the first dose of teniposide and may be life threatening if not treated promptly with antihistamines, corticosteroids, epinephrine, IV fluids and other supportive measures as clinically indicated. The exact cause of these reactions is unknown; they may be due to the polyoxyethylated castor oil component of the vehicle or to teniposide itself. The incidence appears to be increased in patients with brain tumors and neuroblastoma. Patients who have experienced prior hypersensitivity reactions to teniposide are at risk for recurrence of symptoms and should only be retreated if the antileukemic benefit already demonstrated clearly outweighs the risk of a probable hypersensitivity reaction for that patient. When a decision is made to retreat a patient, pretreat with corticosteroids and antihistamines and carefully observe during and after the infusion. To date, there is no evidence to suggest cross-sensitization between teniposide and etoposide.

➤*Hypotension:* Administer by slow IV infusion (30 to 60 minutes or longer) since hypotension may occur with rapid IV injection. With teniposide, it may also be due to a direct effect of the polyoxyethylated castor oil component. If hypotension occurs, stop infusion and give fluids or other supportive therapy, as appropriate. When restarting infusion, use a slower rate.

➤*Benzyl alcohol:* Teniposide contains benzyl alcohol, which has been associated with a fatal "gasping" syndrome in premature infants.

➤*CNS depression:* Acute CNS depression and hypotension have occurred in patients receiving investigational infusions of high-dose teniposide who were pretreated with antiemetic drugs. The depressant effects of the antiemetic agents and the alcohol content of the teniposide formulation may place patients receiving higher than recommended doses at risk for CNS depression.

➤*Down's syndrome patients:* Patients with both Down's syndrome and leukemia may be especially sensitive to myelosuppressive chemotherapy; therefore, reduce initial dosing with teniposide in these patients. It is suggested that the first course be given at half the usual dose. Subsequent courses may be administered at higher dosages depending on the degree of myelosuppression and mucositis encountered in earlier courses in an individual patient.

➤*Hepatic function impairment:* There appears to be some association between an increase in serum alkaline phosphatase or gamma glutamyltranspeptidase and a decrease in plasma clearance of teniposide. Therefore, exercise caution if teniposide is administered to patients with hepatic dysfunction. In children, elevated serum ALT levels are associated with reduced drug total body clearance of etoposide.

➤*Carcinogenesis:* These agents are possible carcinogens. Mutagenic and genotoxic potential has been established in mammalian cells.

Children with ALL in remission who received maintenance therapy with teniposide at weekly or twice weekly doses (plus other chemotherapeutic agents) had a relative risk of developing secondary acute nonlymphocytic leukemia (ANLL) approximately 12 times that of patients treated according to other less intensive schedules. A short course of teniposide for remission-induction or consolidation therapy was not associated with an increased risk of secondary ANLL, but the number of patients assessed was small. The potential benefit must be weighed on a case by case basis against the potential risk of the induction of a secondary leukemia.

➤*Pregnancy: Category D.* Etoposide and teniposide may cause fetal harm. They are teratogenic and embryotoxic in animals. There are no adequate and well controlled studies in pregnant women. If used during pregnancy, or if the patient becomes pregnant while receiving this drug, apprise her of the potential hazard to the fetus. Advise women of childbearing potential to avoid becoming pregnant.

➤*Lactation:* It is not known whether this drug is excreted in breast milk. Because of the potential for serious adverse reactions in nursing infants, decide whether to discontinue nursing or the drug, accounting for the importance of the drug to the mother.

➤*Children:* Safety and efficacy for use of etoposide in children have not been established. Teniposide is indicated for use in children.

Precautions

➤*Monitoring:* In addition to hematologic tests, carefully monitor renal and hepatic function tests prior to and during therapy.

Drug Interactions

Etoposide/Teniposide Drug Interactions			
Precipitant drug	Object drug[a]		Description
Etoposide	Warfarin	↑	Prolongation of the prothrombin time may occur.
Teniposide	Methotrexate	↑	Plasma clearance of methotrexate may be slightly increased. In vitro, increased intracellular levels were observed.
Sodium salicylate Sulfamethizole Tolbutamide	Teniposide	↑	Teniposide was displaced from protein-binding sites by these agents to a small but significant extent. Because of the extremely high binding of teniposide to plasma proteins, these small decreases in binding could cause substantial increases in free drug levels, resulting in potentiation of toxicity.

[a] ↑ = Object drug increased.

Adverse Reactions

Most adverse reactions are reversible if detected early. If severe reactions occur, reduce or discontinue dosage and institute corrective measures. Reinstitute therapy with caution, consider further need for the drug and be alert to recurrence of toxicity.

Etoposide/Teniposide Adverse Reactions (%)		
Adverse reaction	Etoposide	Teniposide
Cardiovascular		
Hypotension[a]	1-2	2
Hypertension	✓[c]	—[d]
Dermatologic		
Alopecia (reversible)[b]	≤ 66	9
Rash	✓	3
Pigmentation	✓	—
Pruritus	✓	—
Radiation recall dermatitis	one report	—
GI		
Mucositis	—	76
Nausea/Vomiting	31-43	29
Anorexia	10-13	—
Diarrhea	1-13	33
Abdominal pain	≤ 2	—
Stomatitis	1-6	—
Hepatic dysfunction/toxicity	≤ 3	< 1
Dysphagia	✓	—
Constipation	✓	—
Hematologic		
Myelosuppression, nonspecified	✓	75
Leukopenia (WBC/mm^3)		
< 4000	60-91	—
< 3000	—	89
< 1000	3-17	—
Neutropenia (ANC/mm^3)		
< 2000	—	95
Thrombocytopenia (platelets/mm^3)		
< 100,000	22-41	85
< 50,000	1-20	—
Anemia	≤ 33	88
Miscellaneous		
Hypersensitivity/Anaphylactic reactions[a]	0.7-2 (< 1 oral)	≈ 5
Peripheral neurotoxicity	1-2	< 1
Aftertaste	✓	—
Fever	✓	3
Transient cortical blindness	✓	—
Infection	—	12
Bleeding	—	5
Renal dysfunction	—	< 1
Metabolic abnormalities	—	< 1

[a] See Warnings.
[b] Sometimes progressing to total baldness.
[c] ✓ = Adverse reaction observed, incidence not reported.
[d] — = Adverse reaction not reported.

Overdosage

➤*Symptoms:* The anticipated complications of overdosage are secondary to bone marrow suppression.

➤*Treatment:* There is no known antidote for overdosage. Treatment should consist of supportive care including blood products and antibiotics as indicated.

Patient Information

Contraceptive measures are recommended during treatment.

Notify physician of any of these: Fever; chills; rapid heartbeat; difficult breathing.

ETOPOSIDE (VP-16-213)

Rx	**VePesid** (Bristol-Myers Oncology)	**Capsules:** 50 mg	Sorbitol. (Bristol 3091). Pink. In blisterpack 20s.
Rx	**Etoposide** (Various, eg, Pharmachemie B.V.)	**Injection:** 20 mg/ml	In 5, 12.5 and 25 ml vials.[a]
Rx	**VePesid** (Bristol-Myers Oncology)		In 5 ml vials.[b]
Rx	**Toposar** (Gensia Sicor)		In 5, 10 and 25 ml.[c]
Rx	**Etopophos** (Bristol-Myers Oncology)	**Powder for Injection, lyophilized:** 100 mg	In single dose vials.

[a] May contain alcohol, benzyl alcohol, 80 mg polysorbate 80, polyethylene glycol or citric acid.
[b] With 30 mg/ml benzyl alcohol, 80 mg polysorbate 80, 650 mg polyethylene glycol 300, 30.5% alcohol.
[c] With 30 mg/ml benzyl alcohol, 30.5% alcohol.

ETOPOSIDE — ORAL

For complete and comparative prescribing information, refer to the Podophyllotoxin Derivatives group monograph.

WARNING

Etoposide should be administered under the supervision of a qualified physician experienced in the use of cancer chemotherapeutic agents. Severe myelosuppression with resulting infection or bleeding may occur.

Indications

➤*Small cell lung cancer:* In combination with other approved chemotherapeutic agents, as first-line treatment in patients with small cell lung cancer.

➤*Unlabeled uses:* Treatment of bladder carcinoma, lymphomas, leukemias, Ewing sarcoma, Kaposi sarcoma, brain tumors, gestational trophoblastic tumors, ovarian germ cell tumors, rhabdomyosarcomas, Wilms tumor, bone marrow transplantation.

Administration and Dosage

➤*Approved by the FDA:* December 30, 1986.

➤*Small cell lung cancer:* 2 times the IV dose rounded to the nearest 50 mg.

The dosage, by either route, should be modified to take into account the myelosuppressive effects of other drugs in the combination or the effects of prior x-ray therapy or chemotherapy which may have compromised bone marrow reserve.

➤*Administration precautions:* As with other potentially toxic compounds, caution should be exercised in handling and preparing the solution of etoposide. Skin reactions associated with accidental exposure to etoposide may occur. The use of gloves is recommended. If etoposide solution contacts the skin or mucosa, immediately and thoroughly wash the skin with soap and water and flush the mucosa with water.

➤*Renal function impairment:* The following initial dose modification should be considered based on measured creatinine clearance:

Etoposide in Renal Function Impairment		
Measured creatinine clearance	> 50 mL/min	15 to 50 mL/min
Etoposide	100% of dose	75% of dose

Subsequent etoposide dosing should be based on patient tolerance and clinical effect.

Data are not available in patients with creatinine clearances < 15 mL/min and further dose reduction should be considered in these patients.

➤*Storage / Stability:* Capsules are to be stored under refrigeration 2° to 8°C (36° to 46°F). Do not freeze. The capsules are stable for 24 months under such refrigeration conditions. Dispense in child-resistant containers.

ETOPOSIDE — INJECTION

For complete and comparative prescribing information, refer to the Podophyllotoxin Derivatives group monograph.

WARNING

Etoposide injection should be administered under the supervision of a qualified physician experienced in the use of cancer chemotherapeutic agents. Severe myelosuppression with resulting infection or bleeding may occur.

Indications

➤*Refractory testicular tumors:* In combination therapy with other approved chemotherapeutic agents, in patients with refractory testicular tumors who have already received appropriate surgical, chemotherapeutic and radiotherapeutic therapy.

➤*Small cell lung cancer:* In combination with other approved chemotherapeutic agents, as first-line treatment in patients with small cell lung cancer.

➤*Unlabeled uses:* Treatment of bladder carcinoma, lymphomas, leukemias, Ewing sarcoma, Kaposi sarcoma, brain tumors, gestational trophoblastic tumors, ovarian germ cell tumors, rhabdomyosarcomas, Wilms tumor, bone marrow transplantation.

Administration and Dosage

➤*Approved by the FDA:* 1983.

➤*Note:* Plastic devices made of acrylic or ABS (a polymer composed of acrylonitrile, butadiene and styrene) have been reported to crack and leak when used with undiluted etoposide injection.

➤*Refractory testicular tumors:* The usual dose of etoposide in testicular cancer in combination with other approved chemotherapeutic agents ranges from 50 to 100 mg/m^2/day on days 1 through 5 to 100 mg/m^2/day on days 1, 3, and 5.

➤*Small cell lung cancer:* In small cell lung cancer, the etoposide dose in combination with other approved chemotherapeutic drugs ranges from 35 mg/m^2/day for 4 days to 50 mg/m^2/day for 5 days.

Chemotherapy courses are repeated at 3- to 4-week intervals after adequate recovery from any toxicity.

The dosage should be modified to take into account the myelosuppressive effects of other drugs in the combination or the effects of prior x-ray therapy or chemotherapy which may have compromised bone marrow reserve.

➤*Administration precautions:* As with other potentially toxic compounds, caution should be exercised in handling and preparing the solution of etoposide. Skin reactions associated with accidental exposure to etoposide may occur. The use of gloves is recommended. If etoposide solution contacts the skin or mucosa, immediately and thoroughly wash the skin with soap and water and flush the mucosa with water.

➤*Renal function impairment:* The following initial dose modification should be considered based on measured creatinine clearance:

Etoposide Injection in Renal Function Impairment		
Measured creatinine clearance	> 50 mL/min	15 to 50 mL/min
Etoposide	100% of dose	75% of dose

Subsequent etoposide dosing should be based on patient tolerance and clinical effect.

Data are not available in patients with creatinine clearances less than 15 mL/min and further dose reduction should be considered in these patients.

➤*Preparation for intravenous administration:* Etoposide must be diluted prior to use with either 5% Dextrose Injection, or 0.9% Sodium Chloride Injection, to give a final concentration of 0.2 to 0.4 mg/mL. If solutions are prepared at concentrations above 0.4 mg/mL, precipitation may occur. Hypotension following rapid intravenous administration has been reported; hence, it is recommended that the etoposide solution be administered over a 30- to 60-minute period. A longer duration of administration may be used if the volume of fluid to be infused is a concern. Etoposide should not be given by rapid intravenous injection.

➤*Storage/Stability:* Store at 15° to 30°C (59° to 86°F).

Stability – Unopened vials of etoposide are stable for 24 months at room temperature (25°C; 77°F). Vials diluted as recommended to a concentration of 0.2 or 0.4 mg/mL are stable for 96 and 24 hours, respectively, at room temperature (25°C; 77°F) under normal room fluorescent lights in both glass and plastic containers.

ETOPOSIDE PHOSPHATE — INJECTION

For complete and comparative prescribing information, refer to the Podophyllotoxin Derivatives group monograph.

WARNING

Etoposide phosphate for injection should be administered under the supervision of a qualified physician experienced in the use of cancer chemotherapeutic agents. Severe myelosuppression with resulting infection or bleeding may occur.

Indications

➤*Refractory testicular tumors:* In combination therapy with other approved chemotherapeutic agents in patients with refractory testicular tumors who have already received appropriate surgical, chemotherapeutic, and radiotherapeutic therapy.

➤*Small cell lung cancer:* In combination with other approved chemotherapeutic agents as first-line treatment in patients with small cell lung cancer.

➤*Unlabeled uses:* Treatment of bladder carcinoma, lymphomas, leukemias, Ewing sarcoma, Kaposi sarcoma, brain tumors, gestational trophoblastic tumors, ovarian germ cell tumors, rhabdomyosarcomas, Wilms tumor, bone marrow transplantation.

Administration and Dosage

➤*Approved by the FDA:* 1983.

➤*Refractory testicular tumors:* The usual dose of etoposide for injection in testicular cancer in combination with other approved chemotherapeutic agents ranges from 50 to 100 mg/m^2/day on days 1 through 5 to 100 mg/m^2/day on days 1, 3, and 5. Equivalent doses of etoposide phosphate for injection should be used.

➤*Small cell lung cancer:* In small cell lung cancer, the etoposide for injection dose in combination with other approved chemotherapeutic drugs ranges from 35 mg/m^2/day for 4 days to 50 mg/m^2/day for 5 days. Equivalent doses of etoposide phosphate should be used.

Etoposide phosphate solutions may be administered at infusion rates from 5 to 210 minutes. Chemotherapy courses are repeated at 3 to 4 week intervals after adequate recovery from any toxicity.

➤*Dosage modification:* The dosage should be modified to take into account the myelosuppressive effect of other drugs in the combination or the effects of prior x-ray therapy or chemotherapy which may have compromised bone marrow reserve.

➤*Administration precautions:* As with other potentially toxic compounds, caution should be exercised in handling and preparing the solution of etoposide phosphate. Skin reactions associated with accidental exposure to etoposide phosphate may occur. The use of gloves is recommended. If etoposide phosphate solution contacts the skin or mucosa, immediately and thoroughly wash the skin with soap and water and flush the mucosa with water.

➤*Preparation for intravenous administration:* Prior to use, the content of each vial must be reconstituted with Sterile Water for Injection, USP; 5% Dextrose Injection, USP; 0.9% Sodium Chloride Injection, USP; Sterile Bacteriostatic Water for Injection with Benzyl Alcohol; or Bacteriostatic Sodium Chloride for Injection with Benzyl Alcohol to a concentration equivalent to 20 mg/mL or 10 mg/mL etoposide (22.7 mg/mL or 11.4 mg/mL etoposide phosphate, respectively). Use the quantity of diluent shown below to reconstitute the product.

Vial strength	Volume of diluent	Final concentration
100 mg	5 mL	20 mg/mL
	10 mL	10 mg/mL

Following reconstitution, etoposide phosphate can be further diluted to concentrations as low as 0.1 mg/mL etoposide with either 5% Dextrose Injection, USP or 0.9% Sodium Chloride Injection.

➤*Renal function impairment:* The following initial dose modification should be considered based on measured creatinine clearance:

Etoposide Phosphate Injection in Renal Function Impairment		
Measured creatinine clearance	> 50 mL/min	15 to 50 mL/min
Etoposide	100% of dose	75% of dose

Subsequent etoposide dosing should be based on patient tolerance and clinical effect. Equivalent dose adjustments of etoposide phosphate should be used.

Data are not available in patients with creatinine clearances < 15 mL/min and further dose reduction should be considered in these patients.

➤*Storage/Stability:* Store the unopened vials under refrigeration 2° to 8°C (36° to 46°F). Retain in original package to protect from light.

Stability – Unopened vials of etoposide phosphate for injection are stable until the date indicated on the package when stored under refrigeration 2° to 8°C (36° to 46°F) in the original package. When reconstituted as directed, etoposide phosphate solutions can be stored in glass or plastic containers under refrigeration 2° to 8°C (36° to 46°F) for 7 days; at controlled room temperature 20° to 25°C (68° to 77°F) for 24 hours following reconstitution with Sterile Water for Injection, USP, 5% Dextrose Injection, USP, or 0.9% Sodium Chloride Injection, USP; or at controlled room temperature 20° to 25°C (68° to 77°F) for 48 hours following reconstitution with Sterile Bacteriostatic Water for Injection with Benzyl Alcohol or Bacteriostatic Sodium Chloride for Injection with Benzyl Alcohol. Etoposide phosphate solutions further diluted as directed can be stored under refrigeration 2° to 8°C (36° to 46°F) or at controlled room temperature 20° to 25°C (68° to 77°F) for 24 hours.

Podophyllotoxin Derivatives

TENIPOSIDE (VM-26)

Rx	**Vumon** (Bristol-Myers Oncology)	**Injection:**[a] 50 mg (10 mg/ml)	In 5 ml amps.[b]

[a] Must be diluted prior to administration.

[b] With 30 mg benzyl alcohol and 500 mg *Cremophor EL* (polyoxyethylated castor oil) per ml, with 42.7% dehydrated alcohol.

TENIPOSIDE — INJECTION

For complete and comparative prescribing information, refer to the Podophyllotoxin Derivatives group monograph.

WARNING

Teniposide for injection concentrate is a cytotoxic drug, which should be administered under the supervision of a qualified physician experienced in the use of cancer chemotherapeutic agents. Appropriate management of therapy and complications is possible only when adequate treatment facilities are readily available.

Severe myelosuppression with resulting infection or bleeding may occur. Hypersensitivity reactions, including anaphylaxis-like symptoms, may occur with initial dosing or at repeated exposure to teniposide. Epinephrine, with or without corticosteroids and antihistamines has been employed to alleviate hypersensitivity reaction symptoms.

Indications

➤*Acute lymphoblastic leukemia:* In combination with other approved anticancer agents for induction therapy in patients with refractory childhood acute lymphoblastic leukemia (ALL).

➤*Unlabeled uses:* Treatment of adult acute lymphocytic leukemia; non-Hodgkin lymphoma.

Administration and Dosage

➤*Approved by the FDA:* July 14,1992.

➤*Note:* Contact of undiluted teniposide with plastic equipment or devices used to prepare solutions for infusion may result in softening or cracking and possible drug product leakage. This effect has not been reported with diluted solutions of teniposide.

In order to prevent extraction of the plasticizer DEHP [di(2- ethylhexyl)phtalate], solutions of teniposide should be prepared in non-DEHP-containing LVP containers such as glass or polyolefin plastic bags or containers.

Teniposide solutions should be administered with non-DEHP-containing IV-administration sets.

➤*Dosage:* In 1 study, childhood acute lymphoblastic leukemia (ALL) patients failing induction therapy with a cytarabine-containing regimen were treated with the combination of teniposide 165 mg/m^2 and cytarabine 300 mg/m^2 IV, twice weekly for 8 to 9 doses. In another study, patients with childhood ALL refractory to vincristine/prednisone-containing regimens were treated with the combination of teniposide 250 mg/m^2 and vincristine 1.5 mg/m^2 IV, weekly for 4 to 8 weeks and prednisone 40 mg/m^2 orally for 28 days.

➤*Renal / Hepatic function impairment:* Adequate data in patients with hepatic insufficiency or renal insufficiency are lacking, but dose adjustments may be necessary for patients with significant renal or hepatic impairment.

➤*Preparation for IV administration:* Teniposide must be diluted with either 5% Dextrose Injection, USP, or 0.9% Sodium Chloride Injection, USP, to give final teniposide concentrations of 0.1 mg/mL, 0.2 mg/mL, 0.4 mg/mL or 1 mg/mL. Solutions prepared in 5% Dextrose Injection, USP, or 0.9% Sodium Chloride Injection, USP, at teniposide concentrations of 0.1 mg/mL, 0.2 mg/mL or 0.4 mg/mL are stable at room temperature for up to 24 hours after preparation. Teniposide solutions prepared at a final teniposide concentration of 1 mg/mL should be administered within 4 hours of preparation to reduce the potential for precipitation. Refrigeration of teniposide solutions is not recommended. Stability and use times are identical in glass and plastic parenteral solution containers.

Although solutions are chemically stable under the conditions indicated, precipitation of teniposide may occur at the recommended concentrations, especially if the diluted solution is subjected to more agitation than is recommended to prepare the drug solution for parenteral administration. In addition, storage time prior to administration should be minimized and care should be taken to avoid contact of the diluted solution with other drugs or fluids. Parenteral drug products should be inspected visually for particulate matter and discoloration prior to administration whenever solution and container permit. Precipitation has been reported during 24-hour infusions of teniposide diluted to teniposide concentrations of 0.1 to 0.2 mg/mL, resulting in occlusion of central venous access catheters in several patients. Heparin solution can cause precipitation of teniposide, therefore, the administration apparatus should be flushed thoroughly with 5% Dextrose Injection or 0.9% Sodium Chloride Injection, USP, before and after administration of teniposide.

➤*Administration:* Hypotension has been reported following rapid IV administration; it is recommended that the teniposide solution be administered over at least a 30- to 60-minute period. Teniposide should not be given by rapid IV injection.

In a 24-hour study under simulated conditions of actual use of the product relative to dilution strength, diluent and administration rates, dilutions at 0.1 to 1 mg/mL were chemically stable for at least 24 hours. Data collected for the presence of the extractable DEHP [di(2-ethylhexyl)phtalate] from PVC containers show that levels increased with time and concentration of the solutions. The data appeared similar for 0.9% Sodium Chloride Injection, USP, and 5% Dextrose Injection, USP. Consequently, the use of PVC containers is not recommended.

Similarly, the use of non-DEHP IV-administration sets is recommended. Lipid administration sets or low DEHP-containing nitroglycerin sets will keep patients' exposure to DEHP at low levels and are suitable for use. The diluted solutions are chemically and physically compatible with the recommended IV-administration sets and LVP containers for up to 24 hours at ambient room temperature and lighting conditions. Because of the potential for precipitation, compatibility with other drugs, infusion materials or IV pumps cannot be ensured.

➤*Patients with Down's syndrome:* Patients with both Down's syndrome and leukemia may be especially sensitive to myelosuppressive chemotherapy; therefore, initial dosing with teniposide should be reduced in these patients. It is suggested that the first course of teniposide should be given at half the usual dose. Subsequent courses may be administered at higher dosages depending on the degree of myelosuppression and mucositis encountered in earlier courses in an individual patient.

➤*Storage / Stability:* Store the unopened ampules under refrigeration (2° to 8°C; 36° to 46°F). Retain in original package to protect from light.

ANTIBIOTICS

Anthracyclines

DAUNORUBICIN HYDROCHLORIDE

Rx	**Daunorubicin HCl for Injection** (Various, eg, Abbott, Bedford)	**Injection:** 5 mg/ml (equivalent to 5.34 mg daunorubicin HCl)[a]	Preservative-free. In 4 and 10 ml single-use vials.
Rx	**Daunorubicin HCl** (Various, eg, Abbott, Gensia Sicor)	**Powder for Injection, lyophilized:** 21.4 mg (equivalent to 20 mg daunorubicin)	100 mg mannitol. In 10 ml single-dose vials.
Rx	**Cerubidine** (Bedford)		100 mg mannitol. In single-dose vials.
Rx	**Daunorubicin HCl** (Various, eg, Abbott, Gensia Sicor)	**Powder for Injection, lyophilized:** 53.5 mg (equivalent to 50 mg daunorubicin)	250 mg mannitol. In 20 ml single-dose vials.

[a] 9 mg NaCl.

DAUNORUBICIN HYDROCHLORIDE — INJECTION

WARNING

Give daunorubicin into a rapidly flowing IV infusion. Do not administer IM or SC. Severe local tissue necrosis will result if extravasation occurs.

Myocardial toxicity, in its most severe form, as potentially fatal congestive heart failure, may occur when total cumulative dosage exceeds 400 to 550 mg/m^2 in adults, 300 mg/m^2 in children older than 2 years of age, or 10 mg/kg in children younger than 2 years of age. This may occur during therapy or several months to years after therapy.

It is recommended that daunorubicin be administered only by physicians who are experienced in leukemia chemotherapy and in facilities with laboratory and supportive resources adequate to monitor drug tolerance and protect and maintain a patient compromised by drug toxicity.

The physician and institution must be capable of responding rapidly and completely to severe hemorrhagic conditions or overwhelming infection.

Severe myelosuppression occurs when used in therapeutic doses; this may lead to infection or hemorrhage.

Reduce dosage in patients with impaired hepatic or renal function.

Indications

➤*Acute nonlymphocytic/lymphocytic leukemia:* In combination with other approved anticancer drugs, for remission induction in acute nonlymphocytic leukemia (myelogenous, monocytic, erythroid) of adults and for remission induction in acute lymphocytic leukemia of children and adults.

➤*Unlabeled uses:* Treatment of chronic myelogenous leukemia; Kaposi sarcoma.

Administration and Dosage

For IV use only.

To eradicate the leukemic cells and induce a complete remission, a profound suppression of bone marrow is usually required. Evaluation of both the peripheral blood and bone marrow are mandatory in the formulation of treatment plans.

➤*Adult acute nonlymphocytic leukemia:*

Patients younger than 60 years of age – Daunorubicin 45 mg/m^2/day IV on days 1, 2, and 3 of the first course and on days 1 and 2 of subsequent courses and cytosine arabinoside 100 mg/m^2/day IV infusion daily for 7 days for the first course and for 5 days for subsequent courses.

Patients 60 years of age and older – Daunorubicin 30 mg/m^2/day IV on days 1, 2, and 3 of the first course and on days 1 and 2 of subsequent courses and cytosine arabinoside 100 mg/m^2/day IV infusion daily for 7 days for the first course and for 5 days for subsequent courses. This daunorubicin dose reduction is based on a single study and may not be appropriate if optimal supportive care is available.

Attaining a normal appearing bone marrow may require ≤ 3 courses of induction therapy. Evaluate bone marrow following recovery from the previous induction course to determine the need for a further course of induction treatment.

➤*Pediatric acute lymphocytic leukemia:* Daunorubicin 25 mg/m^2 IV on day 1 every week, vincristine 1.5 mg/m^2 IV on day 1 every week, oral prednisone 40 mg/m^2/day. Generally, complete remission will be obtained with 4 courses of therapy; however, if after 4 courses the patient is in partial remission, an additional 1 or, if necessary, 2 courses may be given in an effort to obtain a complete remission.

In children younger than 2 years of age or less than 0.5 m^2 body surface area, calculate dosage on the basis of weight (mg/kg) instead of body surface area.

➤*Adult acute lymphocytic leukemia:* Daunorubicin 45 mg/m^2/day IV on days 1, 2, and 3 and vincristine 2 mg IV on days 1, 8, and 15; prednisone 40 mg/m^2/day orally on days 1 through 22, then tapered between days 22 to 29; L-asparaginase 500 IU/kg/day × 10 days IV on days 22 through 32.

➤*Hepatic or renal function impairment:* Reduce dosage.

Daunorubicin HCl Dosage in Hepatic or Renal Function Impairment (%)		
Serum bilirubin	Serum creatinine	Dose reduction
1.2 to 3.0 mg	—	25
> 3 mg	—	50
—	> 3 mg	50

➤*Preparation/Storage of solution:* Reconstitute vial contents with 4 ml Sterile Water for Injection to prepare a solution of 5 mg of daunorubicin activity per ml. Withdraw the desired dose into a syringe containing 10 to 15 ml of normal saline; inject into the tubing or sidearm of a rapidly flowing IV infusion of 5% glucose or normal saline solution.

➤*IV admixture compatibilities/incompatibilities:* Do not mix with other drugs or heparin.

➤*Storage/Stability:* Store unopened vials in refrigerator, 2° to 8°C (36° to 46°F). Store prepared solution for infusion at room temperature, 15° to 30°C (59° to 86°F) for up to 24 hours. Contains no preservative. Discard unused portion. Protect from light.

Actions

➤*Pharmacology:* Daunorubicin has antimitotic and cytotoxic activity through a number of proposed mechanisms of action. It forms complexes with DNA by intercalation between base pairs. It inhibits topoisomerase II activity by stabilizing the DNA-topoisomerase II complex, preventing the religation portion of the ligation-religation reaction that topoisomerase II catalyzes. Single-strand and double-strand DNA breaks result. Daunorubicin may also inhibit polymerase activity, affect regulation of gene expression, and produce free radical damage to DNA.

➤*Pharmacokinetics:*

Absorption/Distribution – Following IV injection, daunorubicin undergoes rapid tissue uptake and concentration. It does not cross the blood-brain barrier. Plasma and tissue protein binding is rapid and extensive; highest concentrations occur in the spleen, kidneys, liver, lungs, and heart.

Metabolism/Excretion – Daunorubicin is extensively metabolized in the liver and other tissues, mainly by cytoplasmic aldo-keto reductases, producing daunorubicinol, the major metabolite, which has antineoplastic activity. Approximately 40% of the drug in the plasma is present as daunorubicinol within 30 minutes and 60% in 4 hours after a dose of daunorubicin. Further metabolism via reduction cleavage of the glycosidic bond, 4-O demethylation and conjugation with both sulfate and glucuronide have been demonstrated. Terminal half-lives for daunorubicin and daunorubicinol are 18.5 and 26.7 hours, respectively. About 25% is eliminated in active form by urinary excretion and 40% by biliary excretion.

Contraindications

Hypersensitivity to daunorubicin or any component of the product.

Warnings

➤*Previous cumulative dose:* Do not use in patients who have previously received the recommended maximum cumulative dose of either doxorubicin or daunorubicin.

➤*Bone marrow suppression:* Bone marrow suppression will occur in all patients given a therapeutic dose of this drug. Do not start therapy in patients with preexisting drug-induced bone marrow suppression unless the benefit from such treatment warrants the risk. Persistent, severe myelosuppression may result in superinfection or hemorrhage.

➤*Cardiotoxicity:* Preexisting heart disease or previous doxorubicin therapy are cofactors of increased risk of cardiotoxicity; weigh benefit-to-risk ratio before starting therapy. Give attention to the drug's potential cardiac toxicity, particularly in infants and children.

In adults, at total cumulative doses less than 550 mg/m^2, acute CHF is seldom encountered. However, rare instances of pericarditis-myocarditis, not dose-related, have occurred. At cumulative doses more than 550 mg/m^2, there is an increased incidence of CHF. This limit appears lower (400 mg/m^2) in patients receiving radiation therapy that encompassed the heart. In infants and children, there is a greater susceptibility to anthracycline-induced cardiotoxicity compared with adults, which is more clearly dose-related. However, there is little risk for children older than 2 years of age below a cumulative dose of 300 mg/m^2 or in children younger than 2 years of age (or less than 0.5 m^2 body surface area) below a cumulative dose of 10 mg/kg. Furthermore, the total dose given to children and adults should take into account any previous or concomitant therapy with other potentially cardiotoxic agents or related compounds such as doxorubicin.

There is no reliable method for predicting patients who will develop acute CHF; certain ECG changes and a decrease in the systolic injection fraction from pretreatment baseline may aid in recognizing those patients at greatest risk. A decrease of at least 30% in limb lead QRS voltage has been associated with significant risk of drug-induced cardiomyopathy. Perform an ECG or determine systolic ejection fraction before each course. If one or the other of these predictive parameters occurs, weigh the benefit of continued therapy against the risk of producing cardiac damage.

➤*Secondary leukemias:* There have been reports of secondary leukemias in patients exposed to topoisomerase II inhibitors when used in combination with other antineoplastic agents or radiation therapy.

➤*Extravasation at injection site:* Extravasation at injection site can cause severe local tissue necrosis. Stop the injection immediately. For management see the Antineoplastics Introduction

➤*Renal/Hepatic function impairment:* Hepatic and renal function impairment can enhance toxicity; assess hepatic and renal function prior to therapy.

➤*Carcinogenesis:* Daunorubicin injected SC into mice caused fibrosarcomas to develop at the injection site. In male rats administered daunorubicin 3 times weekly for 6 months at 1/70 the recommended human dose on a body surface area basis, peritoneal sarcomas were found at 18 months. A single IV dose of daunorubicin administered to rats at 1.6-fold the recommended human dose on a body surface basis caused mammary adenocarcinomas to appear at 1 year.

➤*Mutagenesis:* Daunorubicin was mutagenic in vitro (Ames assay, V79 hamster cell assay), and clastogenic in vitro (CCRFCEM human lymphoblasts) and in vivo (SCE assay in mouse bone marrow) tests.

➤*Fertility impairment:* In male dogs, at a daily dose of 0.25 mg/kg administered IV, testicular atrophy was noted at autopsy. Histologic examination revealed total aplasia of the spermatocyte series in the seminiferous tubules with complete aspermatogenesis.

➤*Pregnancy: Category D.* Due to its teratogenic potential, daunorubicin can cause fetal harm if administered to a pregnant woman. An increased incidence of fetal abnormalities (parieto-occipital cranioschisis, umbilical hernias, or rachischisis) and abortions occurred in rabbits at doses of 0.05 mg/kg/day or approximately 1/100 of the highest recommended human dose on a body-surface-area basis. Decreases in fetal birth weight and post-

DAUNORUBICIN HYDROCHLORIDE — INJECTION

delivery growth rate were observed in mice. There are no adequate and well-controlled studies in pregnant women. Advise women of childbearing potential to avoid becoming pregnant.

➤*Lactation:* It is not known whether this drug is excreted in breast milk. Due to the potential for serious adverse reactions in nursing infants from daunorubicin, advise mothers to discontinue nursing during daunorubicin therapy.

Precautions

➤*Monitoring:* Observe patient closely and monitor chemical and laboratory tests extensively. Evaluate cardiac, renal, and hepatic function prior to each course of treatment.

➤*Urine discoloration:* Urine discoloration (red) may occur transiently; advise patient appropriately.

➤*Infections:* Control any systemic infection before beginning therapy.

➤*Hyperuricemia:* Hyperuricemia may be induced secondary to rapid lysis of leukemic cells. As a precaution, administer allopurinol prior to initiating antileukemic therapy. Monitor serum uric acid levels; initiate therapy if hyperuricemia develops.

Drug Interactions

Daunorubicin HCl Drug Interactions			
Precipitant drug	Object drug[a]		Description
Cyclophosphamide	Daunorubicin	↑	Cyclophosphamide used concurrently with daunorubicin may result in increased cardiotoxicity.
Myelosuppressive agents	Daunorubicin	↑	Dosage reduction of daunorubicin may be required when used concurrently with other myelosuppressive agents.
Hepatotoxic medications (eg, methotrexate)	Daunorubicin	↑	Hepatotoxic medications, such as high-dose methotrexate, may impair liver function and increase the risk of toxicity.

[a] ↑ = Object drug increased.

Adverse Reactions

Dose-limiting toxicity includes myelosuppression and cardiotoxicity (see Warnings).

➤*Dermatologic:* Reversible alopecia; rash; contact dermatitis; urticaria.

➤*GI:* Acute nausea and vomiting (usually mild). Antiemetic therapy may help. Mucositis may occur 3 to 7 days after administration. Diarrhea and abdominal pain occur occasionally.

➤*Local:* If extravasation occurs, tissue necrolysis, severe cellulitis, thrombophlebitis, or painful induration can result at the site.

➤*Miscellaneous:* Rarely, anaphylactoid reactions, fever, and chills can occur. Hyperuricemia may occur, especially in patients with leukemia; monitor serum uric levels.

DAUNORUBICIN CITRATE LIPOSOMAL

Rx	**DaunoXome** (Gilead Sciences)	**Injection:** 2 mg/mL (equivalent to 50 mg daunorubicin base)	In single-use vials and single-unit packs.

DAUNORUBICIN CITRATE LIPOSOMAL — INJECTION

WARNING

Monitor cardiac function regularly in patients receiving liposomal daunorubicin because of the potential risk for cardiac toxicity and congestive heart failure (CHF). Cardiac monitoring is especially advised in those patients who have received prior anthracyclines, have had preexisting cardiac disease, or who have had prior radiotherapy encompassing the heart. Severe myelosuppression may occur.

Administer liposomal daunorubicin only under the supervision of a physician who is experienced in the use of cancer chemotherapeutic agents.

Reduce dosage in patients with impaired hepatic function (see Administration and Dosage).

A triad of back pain, flushing, and chest tightness has been reported in 13.8% of the patients (16/116) treated with liposomal daunorubicin in the phase 3 clinical trial, and in 2.7% of treatment cycles (27/994). This triad generally occurs during the first 5 minutes of the infusion, subsides with interruption of the infusion, and generally does not recur if the infusion is then resumed at a slower rate.

Indications

➤*Advanced HIV-associated Kaposi sarcoma:* As first-line cytotoxic therapy for advanced HIV-associated Kaposi sarcoma.

Administration and Dosage

➤*Approved by the FDA:* April 8, 1996.

Administer IV over a 60-minute period at a dose of 40 mg/m^2, with doses repeated every 2 weeks. Continue treatment until there is evidence of progressive disease (eg, based on best response achieved; new visceral sites of involvement or progression of visceral disease; development of 10 or more new cutaneous lesions or a 25% increase in the number of lesions compared with baseline; a change in the character of at least 25% of all previously counted flat lesions to raised; increase in surface area of the indicator lesions) or until other intercurrent complications of HIV disease preclude continuation of therapy.

Repeat blood counts prior to each dose and withhold therapy if the absolute granulocyte count is less than 750 cells/mm^3.

➤*Hepatic or renal function impairment:* Reduce dosage.

Liposomal Daunorubicin Dosage in Hepatic or Renal Function Impairment		
Serum bilirubin	Serum creatinine	Recommended dose
1.2 to 3 mg/dL	—	¾ normal dose
> 3 mg/dL	> 3 mg/dL	½ normal dose

➤*Preparation:* Dilute liposomal daunorubicin 1:1 with 5% dextrose injection before administration. Do not use an in-line filter for IV infusion. Do not mix liposomal daunorubicin with other drugs.

The recommended concentration after dilution is 1 mg daunorubicin/mL of solution.

➤*Storage/Stability:* Refrigerate at 2° to 8°C (36° to 46°F). If not used immediately, store reconstituted solution for a maximum of 6 hours under refrigeration. Do not freeze. Protect from light.

Actions

➤*Pharmacology:* Liposomal daunorubicin contains an aqueous solution of the citrate salt of daunorubicin encapsulated within lipid vesicles (liposomes) composed of a lipid bilayer of distearoylphosphatidylcholine and cholesterol (2:1 molar ratio). Daunorubicin is an anthracycline antibiotic with antineoplastic activity originally obtained from *Streptomyces peucetius*. It may also be isolated from *Streptomyces coeruleorubidus*. Daunorubicin has a 4-ring anthracycline moiety linked by a glycosidic bond to daunosamine, an amino sugar.

Liposomal daunorubicin is a liposomal preparation of daunorubicin formulated to maximize the selectivity of daunorubicin for solid tumors in situ. In the circulation, the liposomal daunorubicin formulation helps to protect the entrapped daunorubicin from chemical and enzymatic degradation, minimizes protein binding, and generally decreases uptake by normal (nonreticuloendothelial system) tissues. The specific mechanism by which liposomal daunorubicin is able to deliver daunorubicin to solid tumors in situ is not known. However, it is believed to be a function of increased permeability of the tumor neovasculature to some particles in the size range of liposomal daunorubicin. Once within the tumor environment, daunorubicin is released over time, enabling it to exert its antineoplastic activity.

➤*Pharmacokinetics:*

Absorption/Distribution –

Liposomal Daunorubicin Pharmacokinetic Parameters		
Parameters (units)	Daunorubicin citrate liposomal (n = 30)	Conventional daunorubicin (n = 4)
Plasma clearance (mL/min)	17.3 ± 6.1	236 ± 181[a]
Volume of distribution (L)	6.4 ± 1.5	1006 ± 622
Distribution half-life (h)	4.41 ± 2.33	0.77 ± 0.3
Elimination half-life (h)	4.4 (apparent)	55.4 ± 13.7

[a] Calculated.

The plasma pharmacokinetics of liposomal daunorubicin differ significantly from conventional daunorubicin HCl. The differences in the volume of distribution and clearance result in a higher daunorubicin exposure (in terms of AUC) from liposomal daunorubicin than with conventional daunorubicin HCl. The apparent elimination half-life of liposomal daunorubicin is far shorter than that of daunorubicin HCl, and probably represents a distribution half-life. Preclinical biodistribution data in animals suggest that liposomal daunorubicin crosses the normal blood-brain barrier, however, it is unknown if this occurs in humans.

Metabolism – Daunorubicinol, the major active metabolite of daunorubicin, was detected at low levels in the plasma.

DAUNORUBICIN CITRATE LIPOSOMAL — INJECTION

Contraindications

Hypersensitivity reaction to previous doses of liposomal daunorubicin or to any of its constituents.

Warnings

➤*Myelosuppression:* The primary toxicity of liposomal daunorubicin is myelosuppression, especially of the granulocytic series, which may be severe and associated with fever and may result in infection. Effects on the platelets and erythroid series are much less marked. Careful hematologic monitoring is required. Because patients with HIV infection are immunocompromised, carefully observe patients for evidence of intercurrent or opportunistic infections.

➤*Potential cardiac toxicity:* Give special attention to the potential cardiac toxicity of liposomal daunorubicin. Although there is no reliable means of predicting CHF, cardiomyopathy induced by anthracyclines is usually associated with a decrease of the left ventricular ejection fraction (LVEF). Evaluate cardiac function in each patient by means of a history and physical examination before each course of liposomal daunorubicin, and perform determination of LVEF at total cumulative doses of liposomal daunorubicin 320 mg/m^2 and every 160 mg/m^2 thereafter.

Patients who have received prior therapy with anthracyclines (doxorubicin greater than 300 mg/m^2 or equivalent), have preexisting cardiac disease, or have received previous radiotherapy encompassing the heart may be less "cardiac" tolerant to treatment with liposomal daunorubicin. Therefore, monitor LVEF at cumulative liposomal daunorubicin doses prior to therapy and every 160 mg/m^2 of liposomal daunorubicin.

In patients with Kaposi sarcoma, CHF has been reported in 1 patient at a cumulative dose of 340 mg/m^2 of liposomal daunorubicin. In 8 Kaposi sarcoma patients, LVEF decreases were reported at cumulative doses ranging from 200 to 2100 mg/m^2 (median dose 320 mg/m^2) of liposomal daunorubicin. In clinical studies in malignancies other than Kaposi sarcoma treated with doses of liposomal daunorubicin greater than the recommended dose of 40 mg/m^2, CHF has been reported at a cumulative dose as low as 200 mg/m^2 of liposomal daunorubicin; 7 patients have been reported with LVEF decreases. The proportion of patients at risk for cardiotoxicity is unknown because the denominator is uncertain since there were several instances of missing repeat cardiac evaluations.

➤*Back pain, flushing, and chest tightness:* See the Warning box for more information.

➤*Extravasation at injection site:* Conventional daunorubicin has been associated with local tissue necrosis at the site of drug extravasation. Although grade 3 to 4 injection-site inflammation was reported in 2 patients treated with liposomal daunorubicin, no instances of local tissue necrosis were observed with extravasation. Take care to ensure there is no extravasation of the drug when liposomal daunorubicin is administered.

➤*Hepatic function impairment:* See Administration and Dosage for more information.

➤*Carcinogenesis:* A high incidence of mammary tumors was observed approximately 120 days after a single IV dose of 12.5 mg/kg daunorubicin in rats (approximately 2 times the human dose on a mg/m^2 basis).

➤*Mutagenesis:* Daunorubicin was mutagenic in in vitro tests and clastogenic in in vitro and in vivo tests.

➤*Fertility impairment:* Daunorubicin IV doses of 0.25 mg/kg/day (approximately 8 times the human dose on a mg/m^2 basis) in male dogs caused testicular atrophy and total aplasia of spermatocytes in the seminiferous tubules.

➤*Pregnancy: Category D.* Liposomal daunorubicin can cause fetal harm when administered to a pregnant woman. If liposomal daunorubicin is used during pregnancy or if the patient becomes pregnant while taking liposomal daunorubicin, warn the patient of the potential hazard to the fetus.

➤*Children:* Safety and efficacy in children have not been established.

Adverse Reactions

Adverse Reactions of Liposomal Daunorubicin Compared with ABV (%)

	Liposomal daunorubicin (n = 116)		ABV (n = 111)	
Adverse reaction	Mild/Moderate	Severe	Mild/Moderate	Severe
CNS				
Depression	7	3	6	-
Dizziness	8	-	9	-
Fatigue	43	6	44	7
Headache	22	3	23	2
Insomnia	6	-	14	-
Malaise	9	1	11	1
Neuropathy	12	1	38	3
Dermatologic				
Alopecia	8	-	36	-
Pruritus	7	-	14	-
GI				
Abdominal pain	20	3	23	4
Anorexia	21	2	26	2
Constipation	7	-	18	-
Diarrhea	34	4	29	6
Nausea	51	3	45	5
Stomatitis	9	1	8	-
Vomiting	20	3	26	2
Musculoskeletal				
Arthralgia	7	-	6	-
Back pain	16	-	8	-
Myalgia	7	-	12	-
Rigors	19	-	23	-
Respiratory				
Cough	26	2	19	-
Dyspnea	23	3	17	3
Rhinitis	12	-	6	-
Sinusitis	8	-	5	1
Miscellaneous				
Abnormal vision	3	2	3	-
Allergic reaction	21	3	19	2
Chest pain	9	1	7	-
Edema	9	2	8	1
Fever	42	5	49	5
Influenza-like symptoms	5	-	5	-
Sweating, increased	12	2	12	-
Tenesmus	4	1	1	-

Summary of Important Safety Data (Liposomal Daunorubicin vs ABV)

	Daunorubicin citrate liposomal (n = 116)	ABV (n = 111)
Neutropenia (less than 1000 cells/mm^3)	36%	35%
Neutropenia (less than 500 cells/mm^3)	15%	5%
Opportunistic infections/illnesses	40%	27%
Median time to first opportunistic infections/illnesses	214 days	412 days[b]
Number of cases with absolute reduction in ejection fraction of 20% to 25%	3	1
Number of cases removed from therapy because of cardiac causes[a]	2	0
Alopecia (all grades)	8%	36%[c]
Neuropathy (all grades)	13%	41%[c]

[a] The denominator is uncertain because there were several instances of missing repeat cardiac evaluations.
[b] $P = 0.21$.
[c] $P < 0.001$.

➤*Cardiovascular:* Angina pectoris; atrial fibrillation; cardiac arrest; hot flushes; hypertension; myocardial infarction; palpitation; pericardial effusion; pericardial tamponade; pulmonary hypertension; sinus tachycardia; supraventricular tachycardia; syncope; tachycardia; ventricular extrasystoles (5% or less).

➤*CNS:* Abnormal gait; abnormal thinking; amnesia; anxiety; ataxia; confusion; convulsions; emotional lability; hallucinations; hyperkinesia; hypertonia; meningitis; somnolence; tremors (5% or less).

➤*Dermatologic:* Dry skin; folliculitis; seborrhea (5% or less).

➤*GI:* Dry mouth; dysphagia; gastritis; GI hemorrhage; gingival bleeding; hemorrhoids; hepatomegaly; melena; tooth caries (5% or less).

➤*GU:* Dysuria; nocturia; polyuria (5% or less).

➤*Respiratory:* Hemoptysis; hiccups; increased sputum; pulmonary infiltration (5% or less).

➤*Special senses:* Conjunctivitis; deafness; earache; eye pain; taste perversion; tinnitus (5% or less).

➤*Miscellaneous:* Dehydration; increased appetite; injection-site inflammation; lymphadenopathy; splenomegaly; thirst (5% or less).

Overdosage

Symptoms of acute overdosage are increased severities of the observed dose-limiting toxicities of therapeutic doses, myelosuppression (especially granulocytopenia), fatigue, nausea, and vomiting.

Patient Information

Advise patients that this medicine will be prepared and administered by a health care provider in a medical setting.

DAUNORUBICIN CITRATE LIPOSOMAL — INJECTION

Advise patients that lab tests will be required to monitor therapy. Instruct patients to be sure to keep appointments.

Advise patients not to take any otc or prescription medications or dietary supplements without talking with their health care provider.

Advise patients to avoid becoming pregnant during therapy.

DOXORUBICIN, CONVENTIONAL

Rx	**Doxorubicin HCl** (Bedford Labs)	**Powder for Injection (lyophilized)**: 10 mg	50 mg lactose. In single-dose flip-top vials.
Rx	**Adriamycin RDF** (Pharmacia & Upjohn)		In single-dose vials.[b] *Rapid dissolution formula.*
Rx	**Doxorubicin HCl** (Bedford Labs)	**Powder for Injection (lyophilized)**: 20 mg	100 mg lactose. In single-dose flip-top vials.
Rx	**Adriamycin RDF** (Pharmacia & Upjohn)		In single-dose vials.[b] *Rapid dissolution formula.*
Rx	**Doxorubicin HCl** (Bedford Labs)	**Powder for Injection (lyophilized)**: 50 mg	250 mg lactose. In single-dose flip-top vials.
Rx	**Adriamycin RDF** (Pharmacia & Upjohn)		In single-dose vials.[b] *Rapid dissolution formula.*
Rx	**Adriamycin RDF** (Pharmacia & Upjohn)	**Powder for Injection (lyophilized)**: 150 mg[a]	In single-dose vials.[b] *Rapid dissolution formula.*
Rx	**Doxorubicin HCl** (Bedford Labs)	**Injection, aqueous:** 2 mg/ml	0.9% NaCl, hydrochloric acid. In 5, 10, 25, and 100 ml vials.
Rx	**Adriamycin PFS** (Pharmacia & Upjohn)	**Injection:** 2 mg/ml	Preservative-free. In 5, 10, 25, and 37.5 ml single-dose vials and 100 ml multi-dose vials.

[a] Multiple-dose vial.

[b] With methylparaben and 50, 100, 250, and 750 mg lactose, respectively.

DOXORUBICIN HYDROCHLORIDE — INJECTION

Note: The following monograph pertains to the conventional form of doxorubicin only. For complete prescribing information for the liposomal form of doxorubicin, refer to the Doxorubicin, Liposomal monograph.

WARNING

Severe local tissue necrosis will occur if there is extravasation during administration. On IV administration of doxorubicin, extravasation may occur, with or without an accompanying burning or stinging sensation, even if blood returns well on aspiration of the infusion needle. If any signs or symptoms of extravasation have occurred, the injection or infusion should be immediately terminated and restarted in another vein. If extravasation is suspected, intermittent application of ice to the site for 15 minutes 4 times daily for 3 days may be useful. The benefit of local administration of drugs has not been clearly established. Because of the progressive nature of extravasation reactions, close observation and plastic surgery consultation is recommended. Blistering, ulceration or persistent pain are indications for wide excision surgery, followed by split-thickness skin grafting.

Doxorubicin must not be given by the IM or SC route.

Myocardial toxicity manifested in its most severe form by potentially fatal congestive heart failure may occur either during therapy or months to years after termination of therapy. The probability of developing impaired myocardial function based on a combined index of signs, symptoms, and decline in left ventricular ejection fraction (LVEF) is estimated to be 1% to 2% at a total cumulative dose of 300 mg/m^2 of doxorubicin, 3% to 5% at a dose of 400 mg/m^2, 5% to 8% at 450 mg/m^2, and 6% to 20% at 500 mg/m^2. The risk of developing CHF increases rapidly with increasing total cumulative doses of doxorubicin in excess of 450 mg/m^2. This toxicity may occur at lower cumulative doses in patients with prior mediastinal irradiation or on concurrent cyclophosphamide therapy or with preexisting heart disease. Pediatric patients are at increased risk for developing delayed cardiotoxicity.

Dosage should be reduced in patients with impaired hepatic function.

Severe myelosuppression may occur.

Doxorubicin should be administered only under the supervision of a physician who is experienced in the use of cancer chemotherapeutic agents.

Indications

➤*Disseminated neoplastic conditions:* Doxorubicin HCl has been used successfully to produce regression in disseminated neoplastic conditions such as acute lymphoblastic leukemia, acute myeloblastic leukemia, Wilms' tumor, neuroblastoma, soft tissue and bone sarcomas, breast carcinoma, ovarian carcinoma, transitional cell bladder carcinoma, thyroid carcinoma, gastric carcinoma, Hodgkin's disease, malignant lymphoma and bronchogenic carcinoma in which the small cell histologic type is the most responsive compared to other cell types.

➤*Unlabeled uses:* Treatment of refractory multiple myeloma; endometrial, islet cell, and lung cancers, AIDS-related Kaposi sarcoma.

Administration and Dosage

➤*Approved by the FDA:* May 20, 1985.

➤*Extravasation:* See the Warning box for more information.

➤*Recommended dosage schedule:* The most commonly used dose schedule when used as a single agent is 60 to 75 mg/m^2 as a single IV injection and is administered at 21-day intervals. The lower dosage should be given to patients with inadequate marrow reserves due to old age, or prior therapy, or neoplastic marrow infiltration. Doxorubicin HCl has been used concurrently with other approved chemotherapeutic agents. Evidence is available that in some types of neoplastic disease combination chemotherapy is superior to single agents. The benefits and risks of such therapy continue to be elucidated. When used in combination with other chemotherapy drugs, the most commonly used dosage of doxorubicin is 40 to 60 mg/m^2 given as a single IV injection every 21 to 28 days. Doxorubicin dosage must be reduced in case of hyperbilirubinemia as follows:

Plasma bilirubin concentration (mg/dL)	Dosage reduction (%)
1.2 to 3	50
3.1 to 5	75

➤*Reconstitution directions:* Doxorubicin HCl powder 10 mg, 20 mg, 50 mg, and 150 mg vials should be reconstituted with 5 mL, 10 mL, 25 mL, and 75 mL, respectively, of Sodium Chloride Injection, USP (0.9%), to give a final concentration of 2 mg/mL of doxorubicin HCl. An appropriate volume of air should be withdrawn from the vial during reconstitution to avoid excessive pressure buildup. Bacteriostatic diluents are not recommended.

After adding the diluent, the vial should be shaken and the contents allowed to dissolve. The reconstituted solution is stable for 7 days at room temperature and under normal room light (100 foot candles) and 15 days under refrigeration (2° to 8°C; 36° to 46°F). It should be protected from exposure to sunlight. Discard any of the unused solution from the 10 mg, 20 mg, and 50 mg single-dose vials. Unused solutions of the multiple-dose vial remaining beyond the recommended storage times should be discarded.

➤*IV infusion:* It is recommended that doxorubicin HCl be slowly administered into the tubing of a freely running IV infusion of Sodium Chloride Injection, USP, or 5% Dextrose Injection, USP. The tubing should be attached to a *Butterfly* needle and inserted, preferably into a large vein. If possible, avoid veins over joints or in extremities with compromised venous or lymphatic drainage. The rate of administration is dependent on the size of the vein and the dosage. However, the dose should be administered in not less than 3 to 5 minutes. Local erythematous streaking along the vein as well as facial flushing may be indicative of too rapid an administration. A burning or stinging sensation may be indicative of perivenous infiltration, and the infusion should be immediately terminated and restarted in another vein. Perivenous infiltration may occur painlessly.

➤*IV incompatibilities:* Doxorubicin should not be mixed with heparin or fluorouracil, since it has been reported that these drugs are incompatible to the extent that a precipitate may form. Until specific compatibility data are available, it is not recommended that doxorubicin be mixed with other drugs. Parenteral drug products should be inspected visually for particulate matter and discoloration prior to administration, whenever solution and container permit.

➤*Handling and disposal:* Skin reactions associated with doxorubicin have been reported. Skin accidentally exposed to doxorubicin should be rinsed copiously with soap and warm water, and if the eyes are involved, standard irrigation techniques should be used immediately. The use of goggles, gloves, and protective gowns is recommended during preparation and administration of the drug. Procedures for proper handling and disposal of anticancer drugs should be considered. Several guidelines on this subject have been published. There is no general agreement that all the procedures recommended in the guidelines are necessary or appropriate.

Caregivers of pediatric patients receiving doxorubicin should be counseled to take precautions (such as wearing latex gloves) to prevent contact with the patient's urine and other body fluids for at least 5 days after each treatment.

➤*Storage/Stability:*

Powder – Store at controlled room temperature, 15° to 30°C (59° to 86°F). Protect from light. Retain in carton until time of use. Contains no preservative. Discard unused portion.

Solution – Store refrigerated at 2° to 8°C (36° to 46°F). Protect from light. Retain in carton until time of use. Discard unused portion.

Reconstituted solution stability – After adding the diluent, the vial should be shaken and the contents allowed to dissolve. The reconstituted solution is stable for 7 days at room temperature and under normal room light (100 foot candles) and 15 days under refrigeration (2° to 8°C; 36° to 46°F). It should be protected from exposure to sunlight. Discard any unused solution from the 10 mg, 20 mg and 50 mg single-dose vials. Unused solutions of the multiple-dose vial remaining beyond the recommended storage times should be discarded.

Actions

➤*Pharmacology:* The cytotoxic effect of doxorubicin on malignant cells and its toxic effects on various organs are thought to be related to nucleotide

DOXORUBICIN HYDROCHLORIDE — INJECTION

base intercalation and cell membrane lipid-binding activities of doxorubicin. Intercalation inhibits nucleotide replication and action of DNA and RNA polymerases. The interaction of doxorubicin with topoisomerase II to form DNA-cleavable complexes appears to be an important mechanism of doxorubicin cytocidal activity. Doxorubicin cellular membrane-binding may effect a variety of cellular functions. Enzymatic electron reduction of doxorubicin by a variety of oxidases, reductases and dehydrogenases generate highly reactive species including the hydroxyl-free radical OH•. Free radical formation has been implicated in doxorubicin cardiotoxicity by means of Cu (II) and Fe (III) reduction at the cellular level. Cells treated with doxorubicin have been shown to manifest the characteristic morphologic changes associated with apoptosis or programmed cell death. Doxorubicin-induced apoptosis may be an integral component of the cellular mechanism of action relating to therapeutic effects, toxicities, or both.

Animal studies have shown activity in a spectrum of experimental tumors, immunosuppression, carcinogenic properties in rodents, induction of a variety of toxic effects, including delayed and progressive cardiac toxicity, myelosuppression in all species and atrophy to testes in rats and dogs.

➤*Pharmacokinetics:*

Absorption/Distribution – Pharmacokinetic studies, determined in patients with various types of tumors undergoing either single or multiagent therapy have shown that doxorubicin follows a multiphasic disposition after IV injection.

The initial distributive half-life of approximately 5 minutes suggests rapid tissue uptake of doxorubicin, while its slow elimination from tissues is reflected by a terminal half-life of 20 to 48 hours. Steady-state distribution volumes exceed 20 to 30 L/kg and are indicative of extensive drug uptake into tissues.

Metabolism/Excretion – Plasma clearance is in the range of 8 to 20 mL/min/kg and is predominately by metabolism and biliary excretion. Approximately 40% of the dose appears in the bile in 5 days, while only 5% to 12% of the drug and its metabolites appear in the urine during the same time period. Binding of doxorubicin and its major metabolite, doxorubicinol to plasma proteins is about 74% to 76% and is independent of plasma concentration of doxorubicin up to 2 mcM. Enzymatic reduction at the 7 position and cleavage of the daunosamine sugar yields aglycones which are accompanied by free radical formation, the local production of which may contribute to the cardiotoxic activity of doxorubicin. Disposition of doxorubicinol (DOX-OL) in patients is formation rate limited. The terminal half-life of DOX-OL is similar to doxorubicin. The relative exposure of DOX-OL, compared to doxorubicin ranges between 0.4 to 0.6. In urine, less than 3% of the dose was recovered as DOX-OL over 7 days.

Contraindications

Doxorubicin therapy should not be started in patients who have marked myelosuppression induced by previous treatment with other antitumor agents or by radiotherapy. Doxorubicin treatment is contraindicated in patients who received previous treatment with complete cumulative doses of doxorubicin, daunorubicin, idarubicin, or other anthracyclines and anthracenes.

This medication is contraindicated in patients with a history of hypersensitivity reactions to conventional or liposomal doxorubicin or their components.

Warnings

➤*Cardiac toxicity:* Special attention must be given to the cardiotoxicity induced by doxorubicin. Irreversible myocardial toxicity, manifested in its most severe form by life-threatening or fatal congestive heart failure, may occur either during therapy or months to years after termination of therapy. The probability of developing impaired myocardial function, based on a combined index of signs, symptoms and decline in left ventricular ejection fraction (LVEF) is estimated to be 1% to 2% at a total cumulative dose of 300 mg/m^2 of doxorubicin, 3% to 5% at a dose of 400 mg/m^2, 5% to 8% at a dose of 450 mg/m^2 and 6% to 20% at a dose of 500 mg/m^2 given in a schedule of a bolus injection once every 3 weeks. In a retrospective review by Von Hoff et al, the probability of developing congestive heart failure (CHF) was reported to be 5/168 (3%) at a cumulative dose of 430 mg/m^2 of doxorubicin, 8/110 (7%) at 575 mg/m^2 and 3/14 (21%) at 728 mg/m^2. The cumulative incidence of CHF was 2.2%. In a prospective study of doxorubicin in combination with cyclophosphamide, fluorouracil or vincristine in patients with breast cancer or small cell lung cancer, the cumulative incidence of CHF was 5% to 6%. The probability of CHF at various cumulative doses of doxorubicin was 1.5% at 300 mg/m^2, 4.9% at 400 mg/m^2, 7.7% at 450 mg/m^2 and 20.5% at 500 mg/m^2.

Cardiotoxicity may occur at lower doses in patients with prior mediastinal irradiation, concurrent cyclophosphamide therapy exposure at an early age and advanced age. Data also suggest that preexisting heart disease is a cofactor for increased risk of doxorubicin cardiotoxicity. In such cases, cardiac toxicity may occur at doses lower than the respective recommended cumulative dose of doxorubicin. Studies have suggested that concomitant administration of doxorubicin and calcium channel entry blockers may increase the risk of doxorubicin cardiotoxicity. The total dose of doxorubicin administered to the individual patient should also take into account previous or concomitant therapy with related compounds such as daunorubicin, idarubicin and mitoxantrone. Cardiomyopathy or congestive heart failure may be encountered several months or years after discontinuation of doxorubicin therapy.

Treatment of doxorubicin-induced CHF includes the use of digitalis, diuretics, after load reducers such as angiotensin I-converting enzyme (ACE) inhibitors, low salt diet, and bed rest. Such intervention may relieve symptoms and improve the functional status of the patient.

➤*Monitoring of cardiac function:* See Precautions for more information.

➤*Hematologic monitoring:* See Precautions for more information.

➤*Concurrent chemotherapy:* See Drug Interactions for more information.

➤*Necrotizing colitis:* Necrotizing colitis manifested by typhlitis (cecal inflammation), bloody stools and severe and sometimes fatal infections have been associated with a combination of doxorubicin given by IV push daily for 3 days and cytarabine given by continuous infusion daily for 7 or more days.

➤*Extravasation:* See the Warning box for more information.

➤*Hepatic function impairment:* Since metabolism and excretion of doxorubicin occurs predominantly by the hepatobiliary route, toxicity to recommended doses of doxorubicin can be enhanced by hepatic impairment; therefore, prior to the individual dosing, evaluation of hepatic function is recommended using conventional laboratory tests such as AST, ALT, alkaline phosphatase and bilirubin.

➤*Mutagenesis:* Doxorubicin and related compounds have been shown to have mutagenic and carcinogenic properties when tested in experimental models (including bacterial systems, mammalian cells in culture, and female Sprague-Dawley rats).

➤*Fertility impairment:* The possible adverse effect on fertility in males and females in humans or experimental animals have not been adequately evaluated. Testicular atrophy was observed in rats and dogs. A variant of chemotherapy-related acute nonlymphocytic leukemia has been reported to occur infrequently a few years after multiple drug treatment of some neoplasms, which sometimes included doxorubicin. The exact role of doxorubicin has not been elucidated. Pediatric patients treated with doxorubicin or other topoisomerase II inhibitors are at increased risk for developing acute myelogenous leukemia and other neoplasms. The extent of increased risk associated with doxorubicin has not been precisely quantified.

➤*Pregnancy:* *Category D.* Safe use of doxorubicin in pregnancy has not been established. Doxorubicin is embryotoxic and teratogenic in rats and embryotoxic and abortifacient in rabbits. There are no adequate and well-controlled studies in pregnant women. If doxorubicin is to be used during pregnancy, or if the patient becomes pregnant during therapy, the patient should be apprised of the potential hazard to the fetus. Women of childbearing age should be advised to avoid becoming pregnant.

➤*Lactation:* Because of the potential for serious adverse reactions in nursing infants from doxorubicin, mothers should be advised to discontinue nursing during doxorubicin therapy.

➤*Children:* Pediatric patients are at increased risk for developing delayed cardiotoxicity. Follow-up cardiac evaluations are recommended periodically to monitor for this delayed cardiotoxicity. Doxorubicin, as a component of intensive chemotherapy regimens administered to pediatric patients, may contribute to prepubertal growth failure. It may also contribute to gonadal impairment, which is usually temporary.

The risk of congestive heart failure and other acute manifestations of doxorubicin cardiotoxicity in pediatric patients may be as much or lower than in adults. Pediatric patients appear to be at particular risk for developing delayed cardiac toxicity in that doxorubicin induced cardiomyopathy impairs myocardial growth as pediatric patients mature, subsequently leading to possible development of congestive heart failure during early adulthood. As many as 40% of pediatric patients may have subclinical cardiac dysfunction and 5% to 10% of pediatric patients may develop congestive heart failure on long-term follow-up. This late cardiac toxicity may be related to the dose of doxorubicin. The longer the length of follow-up the greater the increase in the detection rate.

Precautions

➤*Monitoring:* Initial treatment with doxorubicin requires observation of the patient and periodic monitoring of complete blood counts, hepatic function tests, and radionuclide left ventricular ejection fraction. Like other cytotoxic drugs, doxorubicin may induce "tumor lysis syndrome" and hyperuricemia in patients with rapidly growing tumors. Appropriate supportive and pharmacologic measures may prevent or alleviate this complication.

Monitoring of cardiac function – In adult patients severe cardiac toxicity may occur precipitously without antecedent ECG changes. Cardiomyopathy induced by anthracyclines is usually associated with very characteristic histopathologic changes on an endomyocardial biopsy (EM biopsy), and a decrease of LVEF, as measured by multigated radionuclide angiography (MUGA scans) or echocardiogram (ECHO), from pretreatment baseline values. However, it has not been demonstrated that monitoring of the ejection fraction will predict when individual patients are approaching their maximally tolerated cumulative dose of doxorubicin. Cardiac function should be carefully monitored during treatment to minimize the risk of cardiac toxicity. A baseline cardiac evaluation with an ECG, LVEF, or an echocardiogram (ECHO) is recommended especially in patients with risk factors for increased cardiac toxicity (preexisting heart disease, mediastinal irradiation, or concurrent cyclophosphamide therapy). Subsequent evaluations should be obtained at a cumulative dose of doxorubicin of at least 400 mg/m^2 and periodically thereafter during the course of therapy. Pediatric patients are at increased risk for developing delayed cardiotoxicity following doxorubicin administration and therefore a follow-up cardiac evaluation is recommended periodically to monitor for this delayed cardiotoxicity.

In adults, a 10% decline in LVEF to below the lower limit of normal or an absolute LVEF of 45%, or a 20% decline in LVEF at any level is indicative of deterioration in cardiac function. In pediatric patients, deterioration in cardiac function during or after the completion of therapy with doxorubicin is indicated by a drop in fractional shortening (FS) by an absolute value of greater than or equal to 10 percentile units or below 29%, and a decline in LVEF of 10 percentile units or an LVEF below 55%. In general, if test results indicate deterioration in cardiac function associated with doxorubicin, the

DOXORUBICIN HYDROCHLORIDE — INJECTION

benefit of continued therapy should be carefully evaluated against the risk of producing irreversible cardiac damage.

Acute life-threatening arrhythmias have been reported to occur during or within a few hours after doxorubicin administration.

Hematologic monitoring – There is a high incidence of bone-marrow depression, primarily of leukocytes, requiring careful hematologic monitoring. With the recommended dose schedule, leukopenia is usually transient, reaching its nadir 10 to 14 days after treatment with recovery usually occurring by the 21st day. White blood counts as low as 1000/mm^3 are to be expected during treatment with appropriate doses of doxorubicin. Red blood cell and platelet levels should also be monitored since they may also be depressed. Hematologic toxicity may require dose reduction or suspension or delay of doxorubicin therapy. Persistent severe myelosuppression may result in superinfection or hemorrhage.

Doxorubicin is not an antimicrobial agent.

Drug Interactions

➤*Concurrent chemotherapy:* Doxorubicin may potentiate the toxicity of other anticancer therapies. Exacerbation of cyclophosphamide-induced hemorrhagic cystitis and enhancement of the hepatotoxicity of 6-mercaptopurine have been reported. Radiation-induced toxicity to the myocardium, mucosae, skin and liver have been reported to be increased by the administration of doxorubicin. Pediatric patients receiving concomitant doxorubicin and actinomycin-D have manifested acute "recall" pneumonitis at variable times after local radiation therapy.

Literature reports have also described the following drug interactions: Phenobarbital increases the elimination of doxorubicin, phenytoin levels may be decreased by doxorubicin, streptozocin may inhibit hepatic metabolism of doxorubicin, and administration of live vaccines to immunosuppressed patients including those undergoing cytotoxic chemotherapy may be hazardous.

Doxorubicin Drug Interactions

Precipitant drug	Object drug[a]		Description
Cyclosporine	Doxorubicin	↑	The addition of cyclosporine to doxorubicin may result in increases in AUC for doxorubicin and doxorubicinol possibly because of a decrease in clearance of parent drug and a decrease in metabolism of doxorubicinol. Literature reports suggest that adding cyclosporine to doxorubicin results in more profound and prolonged hematologic toxicity than doxorubicin alone. Coma or seizures have also been described.
Paclitaxel	Doxorubicin	↑	Two published studies report that initial administration of paclitaxel infused over 24 hours followed by doxorubicin administered over 48 hours resulted in a significant decrease in doxorubicin clearance with more profound neutropenic and stomatitis episodes than the reverse sequence of administration.
Phenobarbital	Doxorubicin	↓	Phenobarbital increases doxorubicin elimination.
Progesterone	Doxorubicin	↑	In a published study, progesterone was given IV to patients with advanced malignancies (ECOG PS < 2) at high doses (up to 10 g over 24 hours) concomitantly with a fixed doxorubicin dose (60 mg/m^2) via bolus. Enhanced doxorubicin-induced neutropenia and thrombocytopenia were observed.
Streptozocin	Doxorubicin	↑	Streptozocin may inhibit hepatic metabolism of doxorubicin.
Verapamil	Doxorubicin	↑	A study of the effects of verapamil on the acute toxicity of doxorubicin in mice revealed higher initial peak concentrations of doxorubicin in the heart with a higher incidence and severity of degenerative changes in cardiac tissue resulting in shorter survival.

Doxorubicin Drug Interactions

Precipitant drug	Object drug[a]		Description
Doxorubicin	Actinomycin-D	↑	Pediatric patients receiving concomitant doxorubicin and actinomycin-D have manifested acute "recall" pneumonitis at variable times after local radiation therapy.
Doxorubicin	Cyclophosphamide Mercaptopurine	↑	Exacerbation of cyclophosphamide-induced hemorrhagic cystitis and enhancement of 6-mercaptopurine have occurred.
Doxorubicin	Digoxin	↓	Serum levels may be decreased by combination chemotherapy (including doxorubicin). Digitoxin and digoxin capsules do not appear to be affected.
Doxorubicin	Phenytoin	↓	Phenytoin levels may be decreased by doxorubicin.
Doxorubicin	Radiation	↑	Radiation-induced toxicity to the myocardium, mucosa, skin, and liver have been increased by doxorubicin administration.

[a] ↑ = Object drug increased. ↓ = Object drug decreased.

Adverse Reactions

➤*CNS:*

Neurological – Peripheral neurotoxicity in the form of local-regional sensory or motor disturbances have been reported in patients treated intra-arterially with doxorubicin, mostly in combination with cisplatin. Animal studies have demonstrated seizures and coma in rodents and dogs treated with intracarotid doxorubicin. Seizures and coma have been reported in patients treated with doxorubicin in combination with cisplatin or vincristine.

➤*Dermatologic:* Reversible complete alopecia occurs in most cases. Hyperpigmentation of nailbeds and dermal crease, primarily in pediatric patients, and onycholysis have been reported in a few cases. Recall of skin reaction due to prior radiotherapy has occurred with doxorubicin administration.

➤*GI:* Acute nausea and vomiting occurs frequently and may be severe. This may be alleviated by antiemetic therapy. Mucositis (stomatitis and esophagitis) may occur 5 to 10 days after administration. The effect may be severe leading to ulceration and represents a site of origin for severe infections. The dosage regimen consisting of administration of doxorubicin on 3 successive days results in greater incidence and severity of mucositis. Ulceration and necrosis of the colon, especially the cecum, may occur leading to bleeding or severe infections which can be fatal. This reaction has been reported in patients with acute nonlymphocytic leukemia treated with a 3-day course of doxorubicin combined with cytarabine. Anorexia and diarrhea have been occasionally reported.

➤*Hematologic:* The occurrence of secondary acute myeloid leukemia with or without a preleukemic phase has been reported rarely in patients concurrently treated with doxorubicin in association with DNA-damaging antineoplastic agents. Such cases could have a short (1 to 3 years) latency period. Pediatric patients are also at risk of developing secondary acute myeloid leukemia.

➤*Hypersensitivity:* Fever, chills and urticaria have been reported occasionally. Anaphylaxis may occur. A case of apparent cross-sensitivity to lincomycin has been reported.

➤*Local:* Severe cellulitis, vesication and tissue necrosis will occur if extravasation of doxorubicin occurs during administration. Erythematous streaking along the vein proximal to the site of injection had been reported. A burning or stinging sensation may be indicative of perivenous infiltration, and the infusion should be immediately terminated and restarted in another vein. Perivenous infiltration may occur painlessly.

Phlebosclerosis has been reported especially when small veins are used or a single vein is used for repeated administration. Facial flushing may occur if the injection is given too rapidly.

➤*Miscellaneous:* Conjunctivitis and lacrimation occur rarely.

Overdosage

Acute overdosage with doxorubicin enhances the toxic effect of mucositis, leukopenia and thrombocytopenia. Treatment of acute overdosage consists of treatment of the severely myelosuppressed patient with hospitalization, antimicrobials, platelet transfusions and symptomatic treatment of mucositis. Use of hemopoietic growth factor (G-CSF, GM-CSF) may be considered.

The 150 mg doxorubicin HCl powder and the 75 mL and 100 mL (2 mg/mL) doxorubicin HCl solution vials are packaged as multiple-dose vials and caution should be exercised to prevent inadvertent overdosage.

Cumulative dosage with doxorubicin increases the risk of cardiomyopathy and resultant congestive heart failure. Treatment consists of vigorous management of congestive heart failure with digitalis preparations, diuretics, and afterload reducers such as ACE inhibitors.

DOXORUBICIN HYDROCHLORIDE — INJECTION

Patient Information

Doxorubicin HCl imparts a red coloration to the urine for 1 to 2 days after administration, and patients should be advised to expect this during active therapy.

DOXORUBICIN, LIPOSOMAL

Rx	**Doxil** (Ortho Biotech)	**Solution for injection**: 20 mg (liposomal)[a]	Sucrose. In 10 mL single-use vials.
		50 mg (liposomal)[a]	Sucrose. In 30 mL single-use vials.

[a] Requires dilution.

DOXORUBICIN HYDROCHLORIDE LIPOSOME — INJECTION

Note: The following monograph pertains to the liposomal form of doxorubicin only. For conventional prescribing information, refer to the Doxorubicin, Conventional monograph.

WARNING

Myocardial damage may lead to congestive heart failure (CHF) and may be encountered as the total cumulative dose of doxorubicin approaches 550 mg/m². The use of liposomal doxorubicin may lead to cardiac toxicity. In a large clinical study in patients with advanced breast cancer, 250 patients received liposomal doxorubicin at a starting dose of 50 mg/m² every 4 weeks. At all cumulative anthracycline doses between 450 to 500 mg/m² or between 500 to 550 mg/m², the risk of cardiac toxicity for patients treated with liposomal doxorubicin was 11%. Include prior use of other anthracyclines or anthracenediones in calculations of total cumulative dosage. Cardiac toxicity also may occur at lower cumulative doses in patients with prior mediastinal irradiation or those who are receiving concurrent cyclophosphamide therapy.

Acute infusion-related reactions including, but not limited to, flushing, shortness of breath, facial swelling, headache, chills, back pain, tightness in the chest or throat, and/or hypotension have occurred in up to 10% of patients treated with liposomal doxorubicin. In most patients, these reactions resolve over the course of several hours to a day once the infusion is terminated. In some patients, the reaction has resolved with slowing of the infusion rate. Serious and sometimes life-threatening or fatal allergic/anaphylactoid-like infusion reactions have been reported. Medications to treat such reactions, as well as emergency equipment, should be available for immediate use. Administer liposomal doxorubicin at an initial rate of 1 mg/min to minimize the risk of infusion reactions.

Severe myelosuppression may occur.

Reduce dosage in patients with impaired hepatic function.

Accidental substitution of liposomal doxorubicin for conventional doxorubicin has resulted in severe side effects. Do not substitute liposomal doxorubicin for conventional doxorubicin on a mg-per-mg basis.

Liposomal doxorubicin should be administered only under the supervision of a health care provider experienced in the use of cancer chemotherapeutic agents.

Indications

➤*AIDS-related Kaposi sarcoma (KS):* For the treatment of AIDS-related KS in patients with disease that has progressed on prior combination chemotherapy or in patients who are intolerant to such therapy.

The treatment of patients with AIDS-related KS is based on objective tumor response rates. No results are available from controlled trials that demonstrate a clinical benefit resulting from this treatment, such as improvement in disease-related symptoms or increased survival.

➤*Ovarian cancer:* For the treatment of patients with ovarian cancer whose disease has progressed or recurred after platinum-based chemotherapy.

➤*Unlabeled uses:* Treatment of refractory metastatic breast cancer.

Administration and Dosage

➤*Approved by the FDA:* November 17, 1995.

➤*AIDS-related KS:* Liposomal doxorubicin should be administered intravenously (IV) at a dose of 20 mg/m² (doxorubicin equivalent). An initial rate of 1 mg/min should be used to minimize the risk of infusion-related reactions. If no infusion-related adverse reactions are observed, the infusion rate should be increased to complete the administration of the drug over 1 hour. The dose should be repeated once every 3 weeks, for as long as patients respond satisfactorily and tolerate treatment.

➤*Ovarian cancer:* Liposomal doxorubicin should be administered IV at a dose of 50 mg/m² (doxorubicin equivalent) at an initial rate of 1 mg/min to minimize the risk of infusion reactions. If no infusion-related adverse reactions are observed, the rate of infusion can be increased to complete administration of the drug over 1 hour. The patient should be dosed once every 4 weeks, for as long as the patient does not progress, shows no evidence of cardiotoxicity, and continues to tolerate treatment. A minimum of 4 courses is recommended because the median time to response in clinical trials was 4 months. To manage adverse reactions, such as hand-foot syndrome (HFS), stomatitis, or hematologic toxicity, the doses may be delayed or reduced. Pretreatment with or concomitant use of antiemetics should be considered.

➤*Extravasation:* Liposomal doxorubicin should be considered an irritant, and precautions should be taken to avoid extravasation. With IV administration of liposomal doxorubicin, extravasation may occur with or without an accompanying stinging or burning sensation, even if blood returns well on aspiration of the infusion needle. If any signs or symptoms of extravasation have occurred, the infusion should be terminated immediately and restarted in another vein. The application of ice over the site of extravasation for approximately 30 minutes may be helpful in alleviating the local reaction. Liposomal doxorubicin must not be given by the intramuscular (IM) or subcutaneous route.

➤*Dose modification guidelines:* Liposomal doxorubicin exhibits nonlinear pharmacokinetics at 50 mg/m²; therefore, dose adjustments may result in a nonproportional greater change in plasma concentration and exposure to the drug.

Patients should be carefully monitored for toxicity. Adverse reactions, such as HFS, hematologic toxicities, and stomatitis may be managed by dose delays and adjustments. Following the first appearance of a grade 2 or higher adverse reaction, the dosing should be adjusted or delayed as described in the following tables. Once the dose has been reduced, it should not be increased at a later time.

Liposomal Doxorubicin Dose Modification for HFS

Toxicity grade	Symptoms	Dose adjustment
1	Mild erythema, swelling, or desquamation not interfering with daily activities	Redose unless patient has experienced previous grade 3 or 4 HFS. If so, delay up to 2 weeks and decrease dose by 25%. Return to original dosing interval.
2	Erythema, desquamation, or swelling interfering with, but not precluding, normal physical activities; small blisters or ulcerations less than 2 cm in diameter	Delay dosing up to 2 weeks or until resolved to grade 0 to 1. If after 2 weeks there is no resolution, liposomal doxorubicin should be discontinued. If resolved to grade 0 to 1 within 2 weeks, and there was no prior grade 3 to 4 HFS, continue treatment at previous dose and return to original dosing interval. If patient experienced previous grade 3 or 4 toxicity, continue treatment with a 25% dose reduction and return to original dosing interval.
3	Blistering, ulceration, or swelling interfering with walking or normal daily activities; cannot wear regular clothing	Delay dosing up to 2 weeks or until resolved to grade 0 to 1. Decrease dose by 25% and return to original dosing interval. If after 2 weeks there is no resolution, liposomal doxorubicin should be discontinued.
4	Diffuse or local process causing infectious complications, or a bedridden state or hospitalization	Delay dosing up to 2 weeks or until resolved to grade 0 to 1. Decrease dose by 25% and return to original dosing interval. If after 2 weeks there is no resolution, liposomal doxorubicin should be discontinued.

Liposomal Doxorubicin Dose Modification for Hematological Toxicity

Grade	ANC[a]	Platelets	Modification
1	1,500 to 1,900	75,000 to 150,000	Resume treatment with no dose reduction.
2	1,000 to < 1,500	50,000 to < 75,000	Wait until ANC ≥ 1,500 and platelets ≥ 75,000; redose with no dose reduction.
3	500 to 999	25,000 to < 50,000	Wait until ANC ≥ 1,500 and platelets ≥ 75,000; redose with no dose reduction.
4	< 500	< 25,000	Wait until ANC ≥ 1,500 and platelets ≥ 75,000; redose at 25% dose reduction or continue full dose with cytokine support.

[a] ANC = absolute neutrophil count.

DOXORUBICIN HYDROCHLORIDE LIPOSOME — INJECTION

Liposomal Doxorubicin Dose Modification for Stomatitis		
Toxicity grade	Symptoms	Dose adjustment
1	Painless ulcers, erythema, or mild soreness	Redose unless patient has experienced previous grade 3 or 4 toxicity. If so, delay up to 2 weeks and decrease dose by 25%. Return to original dosing interval.
2	Painful erythema, edema, or ulcers, but can eat	Delay dosing up to 2 weeks or until resolved to grade 0 to 1. If after 2 weeks there is no resolution, liposomal doxorubicin should be discontinued. If resolved to grade 0 to 1 within 2 weeks, and there was no prior grade 3 or 4 stomatitis, continue treatment at previous dose and return to original dosing interval. If patient experienced previous grade 3 or 4 toxicity, continue treatment with a 25% dose reduction and return to original dosing interval.
3	Painful erythema, edema, or ulcers, and cannot eat	Delay dosing up to 2 weeks or until resolved to grade 0 to 1. Decrease dose by 25% and return to original dosing interval. If after 2 weeks there is no resolution, liposomal doxorubicin should be discontinued.
4	Requires parenteral or enteral support	Delay dosing up to 2 weeks or until resolved to grade 0 to 1. Decrease dose by 25% and return to liposomal doxorubicin original dosing interval. If after 2 weeks there is no resolution, liposomal doxorubicin should be discontinued.

➤*Administration:* Do not administer as a bolus injection or an undiluted solution. Rapid infusion may increase the risk of infusion-related reactions.

➤*Hepatic function impairment:* Limited clinical experience exists in treating hepatically impaired patients with liposomal doxorubicin. Based on experience with doxorubicin, it is recommended that liposomal doxorubicin dosage be reduced if the bilirubin is elevated as follows: serum bilirubin 1.2 to 3 mg/dL, give half the normal dose; serum bilirubin greater than 3 mg/dL, give one fourth the normal dose.

➤*Dilution:* Each 10 mL vial contains doxorubicin 20 mg at a concentration of 2 mg/mL.

Each 30 mL vial contains doxorubicin 50 mg at a concentration of 2 mg/mL.

Liposomal doxorubicin up to 90 mg must be diluted in 250 mL of 5% dextrose injection prior to administration. Doses exceeding 90 mg should be diluted in 500 mL of 5% dextrose injection prior to administration. Aseptic technique must be strictly observed because no preservative or bacteriostatic agent is present in liposomal doxorubicin.

In-line filters – Do not use with in-line filters.

Rapid infusion – Rapid flushing of the infusion line should be avoided.

➤*IV compatibilities/incompatibilities:* Until specific compatibility data are available, it is not recommended that liposomal doxorubicin be mixed with other drugs.

➤*Storage/Stability:* Refrigerate unopened vials of liposomal doxorubicin at 2° to 8°C (36° to 46°F). Diluted liposomal doxorubicin should be refrigerated at 2° to 8°C (36° to 46°F) and administered within 24 hours. Avoid freezing. Prolonged freezing may adversely affect liposomal drug products; however, short-term freezing (less than 1 month) does not appear to have a deleterious effect on liposomal doxorubicin.

Actions

➤*Pharmacology:* The active ingredient of liposomal doxorubicin is doxorubicin. The mechanism of action of doxorubicin is thought to be related to its ability to bind DNA and inhibit nucleic acid synthesis. Cell structure studies have demonstrated rapid cell penetration and perinuclear chromatin binding, rapid inhibition of mitotic activity and nucleic acid synthesis, and induction of mutagenesis and chromosomal aberrations.

Liposomal doxorubicin is doxorubicin encapsulated in long-circulating *STEALTH* liposomes. Liposomes are microscopic vesicles composed of a phospholipid bilayer that are capable of encapsulating active drugs. The *STEALTH* liposomes of liposomal doxorubicin are formulated with surface-bound methoxypolyethylene glycol (MPEG), a process often referred to as pegylation, to protect liposomes from detection by the mononuclear phagocyte system (MPS) and to increase blood circulation time.

STEALTH liposomes have a half-life of approximately 55 hours in humans. They are stable in blood, and direct measurement of liposomal doxorubicin shows that at least 90% of the drug (the assay used cannot quantify less than 5% to 10% free doxorubicin) remains liposome-encapsulated during circulation.

It is hypothesized that because of their small size (approximately 100 nm) and persistence in the circulation, the pegylated liposomal doxorubicin liposomes are able to penetrate the altered and often compromised vasculature of tumors. This hypothesis is supported by studies using colloidal gold-containing *STEALTH* liposomes, which can be visualized microscopically. Evidence of penetration of *STEALTH* liposomes from blood vessels and their entry and accumulation in tumors has been seen in mice with C-26 colon carcinoma tumors and in transgenic mice with KS-like lesions. Once the *STEALTH* liposomes distribute to the tissue compartment, the encapsulated doxorubicin becomes available. The exact mechanism of release is not understood.

➤*Pharmacokinetics:*

Absorption – The plasma pharmacokinetics of liposomal doxorubicin were evaluated in 42 patients with AIDS-related KS who received single doses of 10 or 20 mg/m^2 administered by a 30-minute infusion. Twenty-three of these patients received single doses of both 10 and 20 mg/m^2 with a 3-week washout period between doses. The pharmacokinetic parameter values of liposomal doxorubicin, given for total doxorubicin (mostly liposomally bound), are presented in following table.

Pharmacokinetic Parameters of Liposomal Doxorubicin in Patients With AIDS-Related KS (N = 23)		
	Dose	
Parameter (units)	10 mg/m^2	20 mg/m^2
Peak plasma concentration (mcg/mL)	4.12 ± 0.215	8.34 ± 0.49
Plasma clearance (L/h/m^2)	0.056 ± 0.01	0.041 ± 0.004
Steady-state volume of distribution (L/m^2)	2.83 ± 0.145	2.72 ± 0.12
AUC (mcg•h/mL)	277 ± 32.9	590 ± 58.7
First phase (λ_1) half-life (h)	4.7 ± 1.1	5.2 ± 1.4
Second phase (λ_2) half-life (h)	52.3 ± 5.6	55 ± 4.8

Liposomal doxorubicin displayed linear pharmacokinetics over the range of 10 to 20 mg/m^2. Disposition occurred in 2 phases after liposomal doxorubicin administration, with a relatively short first phase (approximately 5 hours) and a prolonged second phase (approximately 55 hours) that accounted for the majority of the area under the curve (AUC).

The pharmacokinetics of liposomal doxorubicin at a 50 mg/m^2 dose is reported to be nonlinear. At this dose, the elimination half-life of liposomal doxorubicin is expected to be longer and the clearance lower compared with a 20 mg/m^2 dose. The exposure (AUC) is thus expected to be more than proportional at a 50 mg/m^2 dose when compared with the lower doses.

Distribution – In contrast to the pharmacokinetics of doxorubicin, which displays a large volume of distribution ranging from 700 to 1,100 L/m^2, the small steady-state volume of distribution of liposomal doxorubicin shows that liposomal doxorubicin is confined mostly to the vascular fluid volume. Plasma protein binding of liposomal doxorubicin has not been determined; the plasma protein binding of doxorubicin is approximately 70%.

Metabolism – Doxorubicinol, the major metabolite of doxorubicin, was detected at very low levels (range, 0.8 to 26.2 ng/mL) in the plasma of patients who received liposomal doxorubicin 10 or 20 mg/m^2.

Excretion – The plasma clearance of liposomal doxorubicin was slow, with a mean clearance value of 0.041 L/h/m^2 at a dose of 20 mg/m^2. This is in contrast to doxorubicin, which displays a plasma clearance value ranging from 24 to 35 L/h/m^2.

Because of its slower clearance, the AUC of liposomal doxorubicin, primarily representing the circulation of liposome-encapsulated doxorubicin, is approximately 2 to 3 orders of magnitude larger than the AUC for a similar dose of conventional doxorubicin as reported in the literature.

Contraindications

Hypersensitivity to a conventional formulation of doxorubicin or the components of liposomal doxorubicin; breast-feeding mothers.

Warnings

➤*Cardiac toxicity:* Give special attention to the myocardial damage that may be associated with cumulative doses of doxorubicin. Acute left ventricular failure may occur with doxorubicin, particularly in patients who have received a total cumulative dosage of doxorubicin exceeding the currently recommended limit of 550 mg/m^2. Lower (400 mg/m^2) doses appear to cause heart failure in patients who have received radiotherapy to the mediastinal area or concomitant therapy with other potentially cardiotoxic agents, such as cyclophosphamide.

Observe caution in patients who have received other anthracyclines; the total dose of doxorubicin given should take into account any previous or concomitant therapy with other anthracyclines or related compounds. CHF or cardiomyopathy may be encountered after discontinuation of anthracycline therapy. Administer liposomal doxorubicin to patients with a history of cardiovascular disease only when the potential benefit of treatment outweighs the risk.

Carefully monitor cardiac function in patients treated with liposomal doxorubicin. The most definitive test for anthracycline myocardial injury is endomyocardial biopsy. Other methods, such as echocardiography or multigated radionuclide scans, have been used to monitor cardiac function during anthracycline therapy. Employ any of these methods to monitor potential cardiac toxicity in patients treated with liposomal doxorubicin. If these test results indicate possible cardiac injury associated with liposomal doxorubicin therapy, carefully weigh the benefit of continued therapy against the risk of myocardial injury.

See the Warning box for more information.

➤*Myelosuppression:* In patients with relapsed ovarian cancer, myelosuppression was generally moderate and reversible. In the 3 single-arm studies, anemia was the most common hematologic adverse reaction (52.6%), fol-

DOXORUBICIN HYDROCHLORIDE LIPOSOME — INJECTION

lowed by leukopenia (white blood cells [WBC] less than 4,000/mm^3; 42.2%), thrombocytopenia (24.2%), and neutropenia (ANC less than 1,000/mm^3; 19%). In the randomized study, anemia was the most common hematologic adverse reaction (40.2%), followed by leukopenia (WBC less than 4,000/mm^3; 36.8%), neutropenia (ANC less than 1,000/mm^3; 35.1%), and thrombocytopenia (13%).

In patients with relapsed ovarian cancer, 4.6% received granulocyte colony-stimulating factor (G-CSF) or granulocyte-macrophage colony-stimulating factor (GM-CSF) to support their blood counts.

For patients with AIDS-related KS who often present with baseline myelosuppression because of such factors as HIV disease or concomitant medications, myelosuppression appears to be the dose-limiting adverse reaction at the recommended dose of 20 mg/m^2. Leukopenia is the most common adverse reaction experienced in this population; anemia and thrombocytopenia also can be expected. Sepsis occurred in 5% of patients; for 0.7% of patients the reaction was considered possibly or probably related to liposomal doxorubicin. Eleven patients (1.6%) discontinued the study because of bone marrow suppression or neutropenia.

In all patients, because of the potential for bone marrow suppression, careful hematologic monitoring is required during use of liposomal doxorubicin, including WBC, neutrophil, platelet counts, and hemoglobin/hematocrit. With the recommended dosage schedule, leukopenia is usually transient. Hematologic toxicity may require dose reduction or delay or suspension of liposomal doxorubicin therapy. Persistent severe myelosuppression may result in superinfection, neutropenic fever, or hemorrhage. Development of sepsis in the setting of neutropenia has resulted in discontinuation of treatment and, in rare cases, death.

Liposomal doxorubicin may potentiate the toxicity of other anticancer therapies. In particular, hematologic toxicity may be more severe when liposomal doxorubicin is administered in combination with other agents that cause bone marrow suppression.

➤*Infusion reactions:* Acute infusion-related reactions were reported in 7.1% of patients treated with liposomal doxorubicin in the randomized ovarian cancer study. These reactions were characterized by 1 or more of the following symptoms: apnea, asthma, back pain, bronchospasm, chest pain, chills, cyanosis, facial swelling, fever, flushing, headache, hypotension, pruritus, rash, shortness of breath, syncope, tachycardia, and tightness in the chest and throat. In most patients, these reactions resolve over the course of several hours to a day once the infusion is terminated. In some patients, the reaction resolved when the rate of infusion was slowed. In this study, 2 patients treated with liposomal doxorubicin (0.8%) discontinued because of infusion-related reactions. In clinical studies, 6 patients with AIDS-related KS (0.9%) and 13 (1.7%) solid tumor patients discontinued liposomal doxorubicin therapy because of infusion-related reactions.

Serious and sometimes life-threatening or fatal allergic/anaphylactoid-like infusion reactions have been reported. Medications to treat such reactions, as well as emergency equipment, should be available for immediate use.

The majority of infusion-related reactions occurred during the first infusion. Similar reactions have not been reported with conventional doxorubicin; they presumably represent a reaction to the liposomal doxorubicin liposomes or one of its surface components.

The initial rate of infusion should be 1 mg/min to help minimize the risk of infusion reactions.

➤*HFS:* In the randomized study, 50.6% of patients treated with liposomal doxorubicin at 50 mg/m^2 every 4 weeks experienced HFS (developed palmar-plantar skin eruptions characterized by swelling, pain, erythema, and for some patients, desquamation of the skin on the hands and the feet), with 23.8% of the patients reporting HFS grade 3 or 4 events. Ten subjects (4.2%) discontinued treatment because of HFS or other skin toxicity.

Among 705 patients with AIDS-related KS treated with liposomal doxorubicin at 20 mg/m^2, 24 (3.4%) developed HFS, with 3 (0.9%) discontinuing.

HFS was generally seen after 2 or 3 cycles of treatment but may occur earlier. In most patients, the reaction is mild and resolves in 1 to 2 weeks so that prolonged delay of therapy need not occur. However, dose modification may be required to manage HFS. The reaction can be severe and debilitating in some patients and may require discontinuation of treatment.

➤*Toxicity potentiation:* The doxorubicin in liposomal doxorubicin may potentiate the toxicity of other anticancer therapies. Exacerbation of cyclophosphamide-induced hemorrhagic cystitis and enhancement of the hepatotoxicity of 6-mercaptopurine have been reported with the conventional formulation of doxorubicin. Radiation-induced toxicity to the myocardium, mucosae, skin, and liver have been reported to be increased by the administration of doxorubicin.

➤*Extravasation:* See Administration and Dosage for more information.

➤*Hepatic function impairment:* See Administration and Dosage for more information.

➤*Mutagenesis:* Although no studies have been conducted with liposomal doxorubicin, doxorubicin and related compounds have been shown to have mutagenic properties when tested in experimental models.

➤*Fertility impairment:* The possible adverse effects on fertility in males and females in humans or experimental animals have not been adequately evaluated. However, liposomal doxorubicin resulted in mild to moderate ovarian and testicular atrophy in mice after a single dose of 36 mg/kg (about twice the 50 mg/m^2 human dose on a mg/m^2 basis). Decreased testicular weights and hypospermia were present in rats after repeat dosages 0.25 mg/kg/day or greater (about 1/30 the 50 mg/m^2 human dose on a mg/m^2 basis), and diffuse degeneration of the seminiferous tubules and a marked decrease in spermatogenesis were observed in dogs after repeat dosages of 1 mg/kg/day (about one half the 50 mg/m^2 human dose on a mg/m^2 basis).

➤*Pregnancy: Category D.* Liposomal doxorubicin can cause fetal harm when administered to a pregnant woman. Liposomal doxorubicin is embryotoxic at dosages of 1 mg/kg/day in rats and is embryotoxic and abortifacient at 0.5 mg/kg/day in rabbits (both dosages are about one eighth the 50 mg/m^2 human dose on a mg/m^2 basis). Embryotoxicity was characterized by increased embryo-fetal deaths and reduced live litter sizes.

There are no adequate and well-controlled studies in pregnant women. If liposomal doxorubicin is to be used during pregnancy, or if the patient becomes pregnant during therapy, apprise the patient of the potential hazard to the fetus. If pregnancy occurs in the first few months following treatment with liposomal doxorubicin, consider the prolonged half-life of the drug. Advise women of childbearing potential to avoid pregnancy.

➤*Lactation:* It is not known whether this drug is excreted in human milk. Because many drugs, including anthracyclines, are excreted in human milk and because of the potential for serious adverse reactions in breast-feeding infants from liposomal doxorubicin, mothers should discontinue breast-feeding prior to taking this drug.

➤*Children:* The safety and efficacy of liposomal doxorubicin in pediatric patients have not been established.

Precautions

➤*Monitoring:* Patients receiving therapy with liposomal doxorubicin should be monitored by a health care provider experienced in the use of cancer chemotherapeutic agents. Most adverse reactions are manageable with dose reductions or delays.

Obtain complete blood cell counts, including platelet counts, frequently and, at a minimum, prior to each dose of liposomal doxorubicin.

Prior to liposomal doxorubicin administration, evaluation of hepatic function is recommended using conventional clinical laboratory tests such as AST, ALT, alkaline phosphatase, and bilirubin.

➤*Radiation therapy:* Recall of a skin reaction due to prior radiotherapy has occurred with liposomal doxorubicin administration.

Drug Interactions

Conventional Doxorubicin Drug Interactions

Precipitant drug	Object drug[a]		Description
Phenobarbital	Doxorubicin	⬇	Phenobarbital increases doxorubicin elimination.
Doxorubicin	Digoxin	⬇	Serum levels may be decreased by combination chemotherapy (including doxorubicin). Digitoxin and digoxin capsules do not appear to be affected.
Doxorubicin	Quinolones Ciprofloxacin	⬇	The antimicrobial effect of quinolones may be decreased.
Doxorubicin	Radiation	⬆	Radiation-induced toxicity to the myocardium, mucosa, skin, and liver have been increased by doxorubicin administration.

[a] ⬆ = Object drug increased. ⬇ = Object drug decreased.

Adverse Reactions

➤*Ovarian cancer:*

Liposomal Doxorubicin Hematology Data Reported in Patients with Ovarian Cancer

Adverse reaction	Liposomal doxorubicin patients (n = 239)	Topotecan patients (n = 235)
Neutropenia		
500 to < 1,000/mm^3	19 (7.9%)	33 (14%)
< 500/mm^3	10 (4.2%)	146 (62.1%)
Anemia		
6.5 to < 8 g/dL	13 (5.4%)	59 (25.1%)
< 6.5 g/dL	1 (0.4%)	10 (4.3%)
Thrombocytopenia		
10,000 to < 50,000/mm^3	3 (1.3%)	40 (17%)
< 10,000/mm^3	0 (0%)	40 (17%)

DOXORUBICIN HYDROCHLORIDE LIPOSOME — INJECTION

Ovarian Cancer Nonhematologic Adverse Reactions with Liposomal Doxorubicin (≥ 10%)

Adverse reaction	Liposomal doxorubicin (n = 239)		Topotecan (n = 235)	
	All grades	Grades 3 to 4	All grades	Grades 3 to 4
CNS				
Asthenia	40.2%	7.1%	51.5%	8.1%
Dizziness	4.2%	0%	10.2%	0%
Headache	10.5%	0.8%	14.9%	0%
Paresthesia	10%	0%	8.9%	0%
Dermatologic				
Alopecia	19.2%	NA[a]	52.3%	NA[a]
HFS	50.6%	23.8%	0.9%	0%
Rash	28.5%	4.2%	12.3%	0.4%
GI				
Abdominal pain	33.5%	10.4%	37.9%	9.8%
Anorexia	20.1%	2.5%	21.7%	1.3%
Constipation	30.1%	2.5%	45.5%	5.6%
Diarrhea	20.9%	2.5%	34.9%	4.2%
Dyspepsia	12.1%	0.8%	14%	0%
Intestinal obstruction	11.3%	9.6%	11.1%	9%
Nausea	46%	5.4%	63%	8.1%
Stomatitis	41.4%	8.3%	15.3%	0.4%
Vomiting	32.6%	7.9%	43.8%	9.8%
Metabolic/Nutritional				
Peripheral edema	11.3%	2.1%	17.4%	2.6%
Respiratory				
Cough increased	9.6%	0%	11.5%	0%
Dyspnea	15.1%	4.1%	23.4%	4.3%
Pharyngitis	15.9%	0%	17.9%	0.4%
Miscellaneous				
Back pain	11.7%	1.7%	10.2%	0.9%
Fever	21.3%	0.8%	30.6%	5.5%
Infection	11.7%	2.1%	6.4%	0.9%
Mucous membrane disorder	14.2%	3.8%	3.4%	0%
Pain	20.9%	2.1%	17%	1.7%

[a] NA = not applicable.

The following additional adverse reactions (not in table; incidence 1% to 10%) were observed in patients with ovarian cancer with doses administered every 4 weeks; only reactions considered at least possibly drug related by investigators are included.

Cardiovascular – Cardiac arrest, deep thrombophlebitis, hypotension, pallor, tachycardia, vasodilation.

CNS – Agitation, anxiety, confusion, depression, dizziness, hypertonia, insomnia, neuralgia, neuropathy, peripheral neuritis, somnolence, vertigo.

Dermatologic – Acne, dry skin, exfoliative dermatitis, fungal dermatitis, furunculosis, herpes simplex, herpes zoster, maculopapular rash, pruritus, skin discoloration, sweating, vesiculobullous rash.

GI – Abdomen enlarged, ascites, dry mouth, dysphagia, esophagitis, flatulence, gingivitis, ileus, mouth ulceration, oral moniliasis, rectal bleeding.

GU – Cystitis, dysuria, hematuria, leukorrhea, pelvic pain, urinary frequency, urinary incontinence, urinary tract infection, urinary urgency, vaginal bleeding, vaginal moniliasis.

Hematologic/Lymphatic – Ecchymosis.

Metabolic/Nutritional – Cachexia, dehydration, edema, hyperbilirubinemia, hypercalcemia, hyperglycemia, hypokalemia, hyponatremia, weight loss.

Musculoskeletal – Arthralgia, myalgia, pathological fracture.

Respiratory – Apnea, epistaxis, pleural effusion, pneumonia, rhinitis, sinusitis.

Special senses – Conjunctivitis, dry eyes, ear pain, taste perversion.

➤*AIDS-related KS:*

Liposomal Doxorubicin Hematology Data Reported in Patients with AIDS-Related KS

Adverse reaction	Patients with refractory or intolerant AIDS-related KS (n = 74)	Total patients with AIDS-related KS (n = 720)
Neutropenia		
< 1,000/mm^3	34 (45.9%)	352 (48.9%)
< 500/mm^3	8 (10.8%)	96 (13.3%)
Anemia		
< 10 g/dL	43 (58.1%)	399 (55.4%)
< 8 g/dL	12 (16.2%)	131 (18.2%)
Thrombocytopenia		
< 150,000/mm^3	45 (60.8%)	439 (60.9%)
< 25,000/mm^3	1 (1.4%)	30 (4.2%)

Liposomal Doxorubicin Nonhematologic Adverse Reactions Reported in Patients with AIDS-Related KS (≥ 5%)

Adverse reaction	Patients with refractory or intolerant AIDS-related KS (n = 77)	Total patients with AIDS-related KS (n = 705)
GI		
Diarrhea	4 (5.2%)	55 (7.8%)
Nausea	14 (18.2%)	119 (16.9%)
Stomatitis	4 (5.2%)	48 (6.8%)
Vomiting	6 (7.8%)	55 (7.8%)
Miscellaneous		
Alkaline phosphatase increase	1 (1.3%)	55 (7.8%)
Alopecia	7 (9.1%)	63 (8.9%)
Asthenia	5 (6.5%)	70 (9.9%)
Fever	6 (7.8%)	64 (9.1%)
Hypochromic anemia	4 (5.2%)	69 (9.8%)
Oral moniliasis	1 (1.3%)	39 (5.5%)

The following additional (not in table) adverse reactions were observed in patients with AIDS-related KS; only reactions considered at least possibly drug related by investigators are included.

Cardiovascular – Chest pain, hypotension, tachycardia (1% to 5%); bundle branch block, cardiomegaly, cardiomyopathy, CHF, heart arrest, hemorrhage, palpitation, pericardial effusion, syncope, thrombophlebitis, thrombosis, ventricular arrhythmia (less than 1%).

CNS – Chills, dizziness, emotional lability, headache, somnolence (1% to 5%); acute brain syndrome, anxiety, confusion, convulsion, depression, hemiplegia, hypertonia, hypokinesia, hypothermia, hypotonia, insomnia, migraine, neuropathy, paresthesia, peripheral neuritis, vertigo (less than 1%).

Dermatologic – Herpes simplex, itching, rash (1% to 5%); cutaneous moniliasis, erythema multiforme, erythema nodosum, exfoliative dermatitis, furunculosis, herpes zoster, maculopapular rash, psoriasis, pustular rash, skin discoloration, skin necrosis, skin ulcer, urticaria, vesiculobullous rash (less than 1%).

Endocrine – Diabetes mellitus (less than 1%).

GI – Abdominal pain, anorexia, aphthous stomatitis, constipation, dysphagia, glossitis, mouth ulceration (1% to 5%); cholestatic jaundice, colitis, dyspepsia, esophageal ulcer, esophagitis, fecal impaction, gastritis, GI hemorrhage, gingivitis, increased appetite, jaundice, leukoplakia of mouth, pancreatitis, sclerosing cholangitis, tenesmus, ulcerative proctitis, ulcerative stomatitis (less than 1%).

GU – Balanitis, cystitis, dysuria, genital edema, glycosuria, hematuria, kidney failure (less than 1%).

Hematologic – Hemolysis, increased prothrombin time (1% to 5%); eosinophilia, lymphadenopathy, lymphangitis, lymphedema, petechia, thromboplastin decrease (less than 1%).

Hepatic – Hepatic failure, hepatitis, hepatosplenomegaly (less than 1%).

Metabolic/Nutritional – Hyperbilirubinemia, hyperglycemia, hypocalcemia, ALT increase, weight loss (1% to 5%); creatinine increase, dehydration, edema, face edema, hypercalcemia, hyperkalemia, hyperlipemia, hypernatremia, hyperuricemia, hypoglycemia, hypokalemia, hypolipemia, hypomagnesemia, hyponatremia, hypophosphatemia, hypoproteinemia, ketosis, lactic dehydrogenase increase, serum urea nitrogen (BUN) increase, weight gain (less than 1%).

Musculoskeletal – Arthralgia, bone pain, myalgia, myositis (less than 1%).

DOXORUBICIN HYDROCHLORIDE LIPOSOME — INJECTION

Respiratory – Dyspnea, pneumonia (1% to 5%); asthma, bronchitis, cough increase, hyperventilation, pharyngitis, pleural effusion, pneumothorax, rhinitis, sinusitis (less than 1%).

Special senses – Retinitis (1% to 5%(; abnormal vision, blindness, conjunctivitis, eye pain, optic neuritis, otitis media, taste perversion, tinnitus, visual field defect (less than 1%).

Miscellaneous – Albuminuria, allergic reaction, back pain, infection (1% to 5%); abscess, ascites, cellulitis, cryptococcosis, flu syndrome, injection-site hemorrhage, injection-site pain, moniliasis, radiation injury, sepsis (less than 1%).

Overdosage

➤*Symptoms:* Acute overdosage with doxorubicin causes increases in mucositis, leukopenia, and thrombocytopenia.

➤*Treatment:* Treatment of acute overdosage consists of treatment of the severely myelosuppressed patient with hospitalization, antibiotics, platelet and granulocyte transfusions, and symptomatic treatment of mucositis.

Patient Information

Inform patients and patients' caregivers of the expected adverse effects of liposomal doxorubicin, particularly HFS, stomatitis, and neutropenia and related complications of neutropenic fever, infection, and sepsis.

Instruct patients who experience tingling or burning, redness, flaking, bothersome swelling, small blisters, or small sores on the palms of their hands or soles of their feet (symptoms of HFS) to notify their health care provider.

Instruct patients who experience painful redness, swelling, or sores in the mouth (symptoms of stomatitis) to notify their health care provider.

Instruct patients who develop neutropenia and a fever of 38°C (100.5°F) or higher to notify their health care provider.

Instruct patients who develop nausea, vomiting, tiredness, weakness, rash, or mild hair loss to notify their health care provider.

Following its administration, liposomal doxorubicin may impart a reddish orange color to the urine and other body fluids. This nontoxic reaction is due to the color of the product and will dissipate as the drug is eliminated from the body.

EPIRUBICIN HYDROCHLORIDE

Rx	**Ellence** (Pharmacia & Upjohn)	**Injection:** 2 mg/mL	Preservative-free. In 25 and 100 mL single-use vials.

EPIRUBICIN HYDROCHLORIDE — INJECTION

WARNING

Severe local tissue necrosis will occur if there is extravasation during administration. It is recommended that epirubicin HCl be slowly administered into the tubing of a freely running intravenous infusion usually between 3 and 20 minutes depending upon dosage and volume of the infusion solution. If possible, veins over joints or in extremities with compromised venous or lymphatic drainage should be avoided. A burning or stinging sensation may be indicative of perivenous infiltration, and the infusion should be immediately terminated and restarted in another vein. Perivenous infiltration may occur without causing pain. Epirubicin must not be given by the intramuscular or subcutaneous route.

Myocardial toxicity, manifested in its most severe form by potentially fatal congestive heart failure (CHF), may occur either during therapy with epirubicin or months to years after termination of therapy. The probability of developing clinically evident CHF is estimated as approximately 0.9% at a cumulative dose of 550 mg/m^2, 1.6% at 700 mg/m^2, and 3.3% at 900 mg/m^2. In the adjuvant treatment of breast cancer, the maximum cumulative dose used in clinical trials was 720 mg/m^2. The risk of developing CHF increases rapidly with increasing total cumulative doses of epirubicin in excess of 900 mg/m^2; this cumulative dose should only be exceeded with extreme caution. Active or dormant cardiovascular disease, prior or concomitant radiotherapy to the mediastinal/pericardial area, previous therapy with other anthracyclines or anthracenediones, or concomitant use of other cardiotoxic drugs may increase the risk of cardiac toxicity. Cardiac toxicity with epirubicin may occur at lower cumulative doses whether or not cardiac risk factors are present.

Secondary acute myelogenous leukemia (AML) has been reported in patients with breast cancer treated with anthracyclines, including epirubicin. The occurrence of refractory secondary leukemia is more common when such drugs are given in combination with DNA-damaging antineoplastic agents, when patients have been heavily pretreated with cytotoxic drugs, or when doses of anthracyclines have been escalated. The cumulative risk of developing treatment-related AML, in 3844 patients with breast cancer who received adjuvant treatment with epirubicin-containing regimens, was estimated as 0.2% at 3 years and 0.8% at 5 years.

Dosage should be reduced in patients with impaired hepatic function. Definitive recommendation regarding use of epirubicin HCl in patients with hepatic dysfunction are not available because patients with hepatic abnormalities were excluded from participation in adjuvant trials of FEC-100/CEF-120 therapy. In patients with elevated serum AST or serum total bilirubin concentrations, the following dose reductions were recommended in clinical trials, although few patients experienced hepatic impairment:
- Bilirubin 1.2 to 3 mg/dL or AST 2 to 4 times upper limit of normal: ½ of recommended starting dose.
- Bilirubin greater than 3 mg/dL or AST greater than 4 times upper limit of normal: ¼ of recommended starting dose.

Severe myelosuppression may occur.

Epirubicin should be administered only under the supervision of a physician who is experienced in the use of cancer chemotherapeutic agents.

Indications

➤*Breast cancer:* Epirubicin HCl injection is indicated as a component of adjuvant therapy in patients with evidence of axillary node tumor involvement following resection of primary breast cancer.

➤*Unlabeled uses:* In combination with other chemotherapeutic agents for the treatment of various forms of cancer such as advanced esophageal cancer (epirubicin plus cisplatin and 5-fluorouracil), small cell lung cancer, non-small cell lung cancer, Hodgkin lymphoma, and non-Hodgkin lymphoma.

Administration and Dosage

➤*Approved by the FDA:* September 15, 1999.

Epirubicin HCl injection is administered to patients by intravenous infusion. Epirubicin HCl is given in repeated 3- to 4-week cycles. The total dose of epirubicin HCl may be given on day 1 of each cycle or divided equally and given on days 1 and 8 of each cycle. The recommended dosages of epirubicin HCl are as follows:

➤*Starting doses:* The recommended starting dose of epirubicin HCl is 100 to 120 mg/m^2. The following regimens were used in the trials supporting use of epirubicin HCl as a component of adjuvant therapy in patients with axillary-node positive breast cancer:

Epirubicin Regimens in Adjuvant Therapy		
CEF-120	Cyclophosphamide	75 mg/m^2 orally days 1 to 14
	Epirubicin	60 mg/m^2 IV ays 1, 8
	5-flourouracil (repeated every 28 days for 6 cycles)	500 mg/m^2 IV days 1, 8
FEC-100*	5-fluorouracil	500 mg/m^2
	Epirubicin	100 mg/m^2
	Cyclophosphamide	500 mg/m^2

* All drugs were administered intravenously on day 1 and repeated every 21 days for 6 cycles.

Concurrent antibiotics – Patients administered the 120 mg/m^2 regimen of epirubicin HCl also received prophylactic antibiotic therapy with trimethoprim-sulfamethoxazole or a fluoroquinolone.

Bone marrow dysfunction – Consideration should be given to administration of lower starting doses (75 to 90 mg/m^2) for heavily pretreated patients, patients with preexisting bone marrow depression, or in the presence of neoplastic bone marrow infiltration.

Hepatic dysfunction – See the Warning box for more information.

Renal function impairment – While no specific dose recommendation can be made based on the limited available data in patients with renal impairment, lower doses should be considered in patients with severe renal impairment (serum creatinine greater than 5 mg/dL).

➤*Dose modifications:* Dosage adjustments after the first treatment cycle should be made based on hematologic and nonhematologic toxicities. Patients experiencing during treatment cycle nadir platelet counts less than 50,000/mm^3, absolute neutrophil counts (ANC) less than 250/mm^3, neutropenic fever, or grades 3/4 nonhematologic toxicity should have the day 1 dose in subsequent cycles reduced to 75% of the day 1 dose given in the current cycle. Day 1 chemotherapy in subsequent courses of treatment should be delayed until platelet counts are greater than or equal to 100,000/mm^3, ANC greater than or equal to 1500/mm^3, and nonhematologic toxicities have recovered to less than or equal to grade 1.

For patients receiving a divided dose of epirubicin HCl (day 1 and day 8), the day 8 dose should be 75% of day 1 if platelet counts are 75,000 to 100,000/mm^3 and ANC is 1000 to 1499/mm^3. If day 8 platelet counts are less than 75,000/mm^3, ANC less than 1000/mm^3, or grade 3/4 nonhematologic toxicity has occurred, the day 8 dose should be omitted.

➤*Preparation and administration precautions:*

Protective measures –
- Personnel should be trained in appropriate techniques for reconstitution and handling.
- Pregnant staff should be excluded from working with this drug.

EPIRUBICIN HYDROCHLORIDE — INJECTION

- Personnel handling epirubicin HCl should wear protective clothing: Goggles, gowns and disposable gloves and masks.
- A designated area should be defined for syringe preparation (preferably under a laminar flow system), with the work surface protected by disposable, plastic-backed, absorbent paper.
- All items used for reconstitution, administration or cleaning (including gloves) should be placed in high-risk, waste-disposal bags for high temperature incineration.

Spillage or leakage should be treated with dilute sodium hypochlorite (1% available chlorine) solution, preferably by soaking, and then water. All contaminated and cleaning materials should be placed in high-risk, waste-disposal bags for incineration. Accidental contact with the skin or eyes should be treated immediately by copious lavage with water, or soap and water, or sodium bicarbonate solution; however, do not abrade the skin by using a scrub brush. Medical attention should be sought. Always wash hands after removing gloves.

Incompatibilities – Prolonged contact with any solution of an alkaline pH should be avoided as it will result in hydrolysis of the drug. Epirubicin HCl should not be mixed with heparin or fluorouracil due to chemical incompatibility that may lead to precipitation.

Epirubicin HCl can be used in combination with other antitumor agents, but it is not recommended that it be mixed with other drugs in the same syringe.

➤*Preparation of infusion solution:* Epirubicin HCl is provided as a preservative-free, ready-to-use solution.

Epirubicin HCl should be administered into the tubing of a freely flowing intravenous infusion (0.9% sodium chloride or 5% glucose solution). The usual infusion time ranges between 3 and 20 minutes depending upon dosage and volume of the infusion solution. This technique is intended to minimize the risk of thrombosis or perivenous extravasation, which could lead to severe cellulitis, vesication, or tissue necrosis. A direct push injection is not recommended due to the risk of extravasation, which may occur even in the presence of adequate blood return upon needle aspiration. Venous sclerosis may result from injection into small vessels or repeated injections into the same vein. Epirubicin HCl should be used within 24 hours of first penetration of the rubber stopper. Discard any unused solution.

➤*Storage/Stability:* Store refrigerated between 2° and 8°C (36° and 46°F). Do not freeze. Protect from light. Discard unused portion.

Actions

➤*Pharmacology:* Epirubicin is an anthracycline cytotoxic agent. Although it is known that anthracyclines can interfere with a number of biochemical and biological functions within eukaryotic cells, the precise mechanisms of epirubicin's cytotoxic and/or antiproliferative properties have not been completely elucidated.

Epirubicin forms a complex with DNA by intercalation of its planar rings between nucleotide base pairs, with consequent inhibition of nucleic acid (DNA and RNA) and protein synthesis. Such intercalation triggers DNA cleavage by topoisomerase II, resulting in cytocidal activity. Epirubicin also inhibits DNA helicase activity, preventing the enzymatic separation of double-stranded DNA and interfering with replication and transcription. Epirubicin is also involved in oxidation/reduction reactions by generating cytotoxic free radicals. The antiproliferative and cytotoxic activity of epirubicin is thought to result from these or other possible mechanisms.

Epirubicin is cytotoxic in vitro to a variety of established murine and human cell lines and primary cultures of human tumors. It is also active in vivo against a variety of murine tumors and human xenografts in athymic mice, including breast tumors.

➤*Pharmacokinetics:*

Absorption – Epirubicin pharmacokinetics are linear over the dose range of 60 to 150 mg/m² and plasma clearance is not affected by the duration of infusion or administration schedule. Pharmacokinetic parameters for epirubicin following 6- to 10-minute, single-dose intravenous infusions of epirubicin at doses of 60 to 150 mg/m² in patients with solid tumors are shown in the table below. The plasma concentration declined in a triphasic manner with mean half-lives for the alpha, beta, and gamma phases of about 3 minutes, 2.5 hours, and 33 hours, respectively.

Summary of Mean Pharmacokinetic Parameters in Patients[1] with Solid Tumors Receiving IV Epirubicin 60 to 150 mg/m²

Dose[2] (mg/m²)	C_{max}[3] (mcg/mL)	AUC[4] (mcg•hr/mL)	$t_{½}$[5] (hours)	CL[6] (L/hour)	V_{ss}[7] (L/kg)
60	5.7 ± 1.6	1.6 ± 0.2	35.3 ± 9	65 ± 8	21 ± 2
75	5.3 ± 1.5	1.7 ± 0.3	32.1 ± 5	83 ± 14	27 ± 11
120	9 ± 3.5	3.4 ± 0.7	33.7 ± 4	65 ± 13	23 ± 7
150	9.3 ± 2.9	4.2 ± 0.8	31.1 ± 6	69 ± 13	21 ± 7

[1] Advanced solid tumor cancers, primarily of the lung.
[2] N = 6 patients per dose level.
[3] Plasma concentration at the end of 6- to 10-minute infusion.
[4] Area under the plasma concentration curve.
[5] Half-life of terminal phase.
[6] Plasma clearance.
[7] Steady-state volume of distribution.

Distribution – Following intravenous administration, epirubicin is rapidly and widely distributed into the tissues. Binding of epirubicin to plasma proteins, predominantly albumin, is about 77% and is not affected by drug concentration. Epirubicin also appears to concentrate in red blood cells; whole blood concentrations are approximately twice those of plasma.

Metabolism – Epirubicin is extensively and rapidly metabolized by the liver and is also metabolized by other organs and cells, including red blood cells. Four main metabolic routes have been identified:

1.) Reduction of the C-13 keto-group with the formation of the 13(S)-dihydro derivative, epirubicinol.
2.) Conjugation of both the unchanged drug and epirubicinol with glucuronic acid.
3.) Loss of the amino sugar moiety through a hydrolytic process with the formation of the doxorubicin and doxorubicinol aglycones.
4.) Loss of the amino sugar moiety through a redox process with the formation of the 7-deoxy-doxorubicin aglycone and 7-deoxy-doxorubicinol aglycone. Epirubicinol has in vitro cytotoxic activity one-tenth that of epirubicin. As plasma levels of epirubicinol are lower than those of the unchanged drug, they are unlikely to reach in vivo concentrations sufficient for cytotoxicity. No significant activity or toxicity has been reported for the other metabolites.

Excretion – Epirubicin and its major metabolites are eliminated through biliary excretion and, to a lesser extent, by urinary excretion. Mass-balance data from one patient found about 60% of the total radioactive dose in feces (34%) and urine (27%). These data are consistent with those from 3 patients with extrahepatic obstruction and percutaneous drainage, in whom approximately 35% and 20% of the administered dose were recovered as epirubicin or its major metabolites in bile and urine, respectively, in the 4 days after treatment.

Special populations –

Renal function impairment: No significant alterations in the pharmacokinetics of epirubicin or its major metabolite, epirubicinol, have been observed in patients with serum creatinine less than 5 mg/dL. A 50% reduction in plasma clearance was reported in 4 patients with serum creatinine greater than or equal to 5 mg/dL. Patients on dialysis have not been studied.

Hepatic function impairment: Epirubicin is eliminated by both hepatic metabolism and biliary excretion and clearance is reduced in patients with hepatic dysfunction. In a study of the effect of hepatic dysfunction, patients with solid tumors were classified into 3 groups. Patients in group 1 (n = 22) had serum AST levels above the upper limit of normal (median, 93 IU/L) and normal serum bilirubin levels (median, 0.5 mg/dL) and were given epirubicin doses of 12.5 to 90 mg/m². Patients in group 2 had alterations in both serum AST (median, 175 IU/L) and bilirubin levels (median, 2.7 mg/dL) and were treated with an epirubicin dose of 25 mg/m² (n = 8). Their pharmacokinetics were compared to those of patients with normal serum AST and bilirubin values, who received epirubicin doses of 12.5 to 120 mg/m². The median plasma clearance of epirubicin was decreased compared to patients with normal hepatic function by about 30% in patients in group 1 and by 50% in patients in group 2. Patients with more severe hepatic impairment have not been evaluated. Definitive recommendation regarding use of epirubicin HCl in patients with hepatic dysfunction are not available because patients with hepatic abnormalities were excluded from participation in adjuvant trials of FEC-100/CEF-120 therapy. In patients with elevated serum AST or serum total bilirubin concentrations, the following dose reductions were recommended in clinical trials, although few patients experienced hepatic impairment:

- Bilirubin 1.2 to 3 mg/dL or AST 2 to 4 times upper limit of normal: ½ of recommended starting dose.
- Bilirubin greater than 3 mg/dL or AST greater than 4 times upper limit of normal: ¼ of recommended starting dose.

Age: A population analysis of plasma data from 36 cancer patients (13 males and 23 females, 20 to 73 years) showed that age affects plasma clearance of epirubicin in female patients. The predicted plasma clearance for a female patient of 70 years of age was about 35% lower than that for a female patient of 25 years of age. An insufficient number of males greater than 50 years of age were included in the study to draw conclusions about age-related alterations in clearance in males. Although a lower epirubicin starting dose does not appear necessary in elderly female patients, and was not used in clinical trials, particular care should be taken in monitoring toxicity when epirubicin is administered to female patients greater than 70 years of age.

Contraindications

Baseline neutrophil count less than 1500 cells/mm³; severe myocardial insufficiency, recent myocardial infarction, severe arrhythmias; previous treatment with anthracyclines up to the maximum cumulative dose; hypersensitivity to epirubicin, other anthracyclines, or anthracenediones; or severe hepatic dysfunction.

Warnings

➤*Administration:* Epirubicin HCl injection should be administered only under the supervision of qualified physicians experienced in the use of cytotoxic therapy. Before beginning treatment with epirubicin, patients should recover from acute toxicities (eg, stomatitis, neutropenia, thrombocytopenia, and generalized infections) of prior cytotoxic treatment. Also, initial treatment with epirubicin HCl should be preceded by a careful baseline assessment of blood counts; serum levels of total bilirubin, AST, and creatinine; and cardiac function as measured by left ventricular ejection function (LVEF). Patients should be carefully monitored during treatment for possible clinical complications due to myelosuppression. Supportive care may be necessary for the treatment of severe neutropenia and severe infectious complications. Monitoring for potential cardiotoxicity is also important, especially with greater cumulative exposure to epirubicin.

➤*Hematologic toxicity:* A dose-dependent, reversible leukopenia and/or neutropenia is the predominant manifestation of hematologic toxicity associated with epirubicin and represents the most common acute dose-limiting toxicity of this drug. In most cases, the white blood cell (WBC) nadir is

EPIRUBICIN HYDROCHLORIDE — INJECTION

reached 10 to 14 days from drug administration. Leukopenia/neutropenia is usually transient, with WBC and neutrophil counts generally returning to normal values by day 21 after drug administration. As with other cytotoxic agents, epirubicin HCl at the recommended dose in combination with cyclophosphamide and fluorouracil can produce severe leukopenia and neutropenia. Severe thrombocytopenia and anemia may also occur. Clinical consequences of severe myelosuppression include fever, infection, septicemia, septic shock, hemorrhage, tissue hypoxia, symptomatic anemia, or death. If myelosuppressive complications occur, appropriate supportive measures (eg, intravenous antibiotics, colony-stimulating factors, transfusions) may be required. Myelosuppression requires careful monitoring. Total and differential WBC, red blood cell (RBC), and platelet counts should be assessed before and during each cycle of therapy with epirubicin HCl.

➤*Cardiac function:* Cardiotoxicity is a known risk of anthracycline treatment. Anthracycline-induced cardiac toxicity may be manifested by early (or acute) or late (delayed) events. Early cardiac toxicity of epirubicin consists mainly of sinus tachycardia or ECG abnormalities such as non-specific ST-T wave changes, but tachyarrhythmias, including premature ventricular contractions and ventricular tachycardia, bradycardia, as well as atrioventricular and bundle-branch block have also been reported. These effects do not usually predict subsequent development of delayed cardiotoxicity, are rarely of clinical importance, and are generally not considered an indication for the suspension of epirubicin treatment. Delayed cardiac toxicity results from a characteristic cardiomyopathy that is manifested by reduced LVEF and/or signs and symptoms of congestive heart failure (CHF) (eg, tachycardia, dyspnea, pulmonary edema, dependent edema, hepatomegaly, ascites, pleural effusion, gallop rhythm). Life-threatening CHF is the most severe form of anthracycline-induced cardiomyopathy. This toxicity appears to be dependent on the cumulative dose of epirubicin HCl and represents the cumulative dose-limiting toxicity of the drug. If it occurs, delayed cardiotoxicity usually develops late in the course of therapy with epirubicin HCl or within 2 to 3 months after completion of treatment, but later events (several months to years after treatment termination) have been reported.

Given the risk of cardiomyopathy, a cumulative dose of 900 mg/m^2 epirubicin HCl should be exceeded only with extreme caution. Risk factors (active or dormant cardiovascular disease, prior or concomitant radiotherapy to the mediastinal/pericardial area, previous therapy with other anthracyclines or anthracenediones, concomitant use of other drugs with the ability to suppress cardiac contractility) may increase the risk of cardiac toxicity. Although not formally tested, it is probable that the toxicity of epirubicin and other anthracyclines or anthracenediones is additive. Cardiac toxicity with epirubicin HCl may occur at lower cumulative doses whether or not cardiac risk factors are present.

Although endomyocardial biopsy is recognized as the most sensitive diagnostic tool to detect anthracycline-induced cardiomyopathy, this invasive examination is not practically performed on a routine basis. Electrocardiogram (ECG) changes such as dysrhythmias, a reduction of the QRS voltage, or a prolongation beyond normal limits of the systolic time interval may be indicative of anthracycline-induced cardiomyopathy, but ECG is not a sensitive or specific method for following anthracycline-related cardiotoxicity. The risk of serious cardiac impairment may be decreased through regular monitoring of LVEF during the course of treatment with prompt discontinuation of epirubicin HCl at the first sign of impaired function. The preferred method for repeated assessment of cardiac function is evaluation of LVEF measured by multi-gated radionuclide angiography (MUGA) or echocardiography (ECHO). A baseline cardiac evaluation with an ECG and a MUGA scan or an ECHO is recommended, especially in patients with risk factors for increased cardiac toxicity. Repeated MUGA or ECHO determinations of LVEF should be performed, particularly with higher, cumulative anthracycline doses. The technique used for assessment should be consistent through follow-up. In patients with risk factors, particularly prior anthracycline or anthracenedione use, the monitoring of cardiac function must be particularly strict and the risk-benefit of continuing treatment with epirubicin HCl in patients with impaired cardiac function must be carefully evaluated.

➤*Secondary leukemia:* The occurrence of secondary acute myelogenous leukemia, with or without a preleukemic phase, has been reported in patients treated with anthracyclines. Secondary leukemia is more common when such drugs are given in combination with DNA-damaging antineoplastic agents, when patients have been heavily pretreated with cytotoxic drugs, or when doses of the anthracyclines have been escalated. These leukemias can have a short 1- to 3-year latency period. An analysis of 3844 patients who received adjuvant treatment with epirubicin in controlled clinical trials, showed a cumulative risk of secondary acute myelogenous leukemia of about 0.2% (approximately 95% CI: 0.05 to 0.4) at 3 years and approximately 0.8% (approximately 95% CI: 0.3 to 1.2) at 5 years. Epirubicin HCl is mutagenic, clastogenic, and carcinogenic in animals.

➤*Tumor lysis syndrome:* As with other cytotoxic agents, epirubicin HCl may induce hyperuricemia as a consequence of the extensive purine catabolism that accompanies drug-induced rapid lysis of highly chemosensitive neoplastic cells (tumor lysis syndrome). Other metabolic abnormalities may also occur. While not generally a problem in patients with breast cancer, physicians should consider the potential for tumor lysis syndrome in potentially susceptible patients and should consider monitoring serum uric acid, potassium, calcium phosphate, and creatinine immediately after initial chemotherapy administration. Hydration, urine alkalinization, and prophylaxis with allopurinol to prevent hyperuricemia may minimize potential complications of tumor lysis syndrome.

➤*Renal function impairment:* See Administration and Dosage for more information.

➤*Hepatic function impairment:* See the Warning box for more information.

➤*Carcinogenesis:* Treatment-related acute myelogenous leukemia has been reported in women treated with epirubicin-based adjuvant chemotherapy regimens. Conventional long-term animal studies to evaluate the carcinogenic potential of epirubicin have not been conducted, but intravenous administration of a single 3.6 mg/kg epirubicin dose to female rats (approximately 0.2 times the maximum recommended human dose on a body surface area basis) approximately doubled the incidence of mammary tumors (primarily fibroadenomas) observed at 1 year. Administration of 0.5 mg/kg epirubicin intravenously to rats (approximately 0.025 times the maximum recommended human dose on a body surface area basis) every 3 weeks for 10 doses increased the incidence of subcutaneous fibromas in males over an 18-month observation period. In addition, subcutaneous administration of 0.75 or 1 mg/kg/day (approximately 0.015 times the maximum recommended human dose on a body surface area basis) to newborn rats for 4 days on both the first and tenth day after birth for a total of 8 doses increased the incidence of animals with tumors compared to controls during a 24-month observation period.

➤*Mutagenesis:* Epirubicin was mutagenic in vitro to bacteria (Ames test) either in the presence or absence of metabolic activation and to mammalian cells (HGPRT assay in V79 Chinese hamster lung fibroblasts) in the absence but not in the presence of metabolic activation. Epirubicin was clastogenic in vitro (chromosome aberrations in human lymphocytes) both in the presence and absence of metabolic activation and was also clastogenic in vivo (chromosome aberration in mouse bone marrow).

➤*Fertility impairment:* In fertility studies in rats, males were given epirubicin daily for 9 weeks and mated with females that were given epirubicin daily for 2 weeks prior to mating and through day 7 of gestation. When 0.3 mg/kg/day (approximately 0.015 times the maximum recommended human single dose on a body surface area basis) was administered to both sexes, no pregnancies resulted. No effects on mating behavior or fertility were observed at 0.1 mg/kg/day, but male rats had atrophy of the testes and epididymis, and reduced spermatogenesis. The 0.1 mg/kg/day dose also caused embryolethality. An increased incidence of fetal growth retardation was observed in these studies at 0.03 mg/kg/day (approximately 0.0015 times the maximum recommended human single dose on a body surface area basis). Multiple-daily doses of epirubicin to rabbits and dogs also caused atrophy of male reproductive organs. Single 20.5 and 12 mg/kg doses of intravenous epirubicin caused testicular atrophy in mice and rats, respectively (both approximately 0.5 times the maximum recommended human dose on a body surface area basis). A single dose of 16.7 mg/kg epirubicin caused uterine atrophy in rats.

Although experimental data are not available, epirubicin HCl could induce chromosomal damage in human spermatozoa due to its genotoxic potential. Men undergoing treatment with epirubicin HCl should use effective contraceptive methods. Epirubicin HCl may cause irreversible amenorrhea (premature menopause) in premenopausal women.

➤*Elderly:* Although a lower starting dose of epirubicin HCl was not used in trials in elderly female patients, particular care should be taken in monitoring toxicity when epirubicin HCl is administered to female patients greater than or equal to 70 years of age.

➤*Pregnancy:* *Category D.* Epirubicin HCl may cause fetal harm when administered to a pregnant woman. Administration of 0.8 mg/kg/day intravenously of epirubicin to rats (about 0.04 times the maximum recommended single human dose on a body surface area basis) during days 5 to 15 of gestation was embryotoxic (increased resorptions and postimplantation loss) and caused fetal growth retardation (decreased body weight), but was not teratogenic up to this dose. Administration of 2 mg/kg/day intravenously of epirubicin to rats (approximately 0.1 times the maximum recommended single human dose on a body surface area basis) on days 9 and 10 of gestation was embryotoxic (increased late resorptions, postimplantation losses, and dead fetuses; and decreased live fetuses), retarded fetal growth (decreased body weight), and caused decreased placental weight. This dose was also teratogenic, causing numerous external (anal atresia, misshapen tail, abnormal genital tubercle), visceral (primarily gastrointestinal, urinary, and cardiovascular systems), and skeletal (deformed long bones and girdles, rib abnormalities, irregular spinal ossification) malformations. Administration of intravenous epirubicin to rabbits at doses up to 0.2 mg/kg/day (approximately 0.02 times the maximum recommended single human dose on a body surface area basis) during days 6 to 18 of gestation was not embryotoxic or teratogenic, but a maternally toxic dose of 0.32 mg/kg/day increased abortions and delayed ossification. Administration of a maternally toxic intravenous dose of 1 mg/kg/day epirubicin to rabbits (approximately 0.1 times the maximum recommended single human dose on a body surface area basis) on days 10 to 12 of gestation induced abortion, but no other signs of embryofetal toxicity or teratogenicity were observed. When doses up to 0.5 mg/kg/day epirubicin were administered to rat dams from day 17 of gestation to day 21 after delivery (approximately 0.025 times the maximum recommended single human dose on a body surface area basis), no permanent changes were observed in the development, functional activity, behavior, or reproductive performance of the offspring.

There are no adequate and well-controlled studies in pregnant women. Two pregnancies have been reported in women taking epirubicin. A 34-year-old woman, 28 weeks pregnant at her diagnosis of breast cancer, was treated with cyclophosphamide and epirubicin every 3 weeks for 3 cycles. She received the last dose at 34 weeks of pregnancy and delivered a healthy baby at 35 weeks. A second 34-year-old woman with breast cancer metastatic to the liver was randomized to FEC-50 but was removed from study because of pregnancy. She experienced a spontaneous abortion. If epirubicin is used during pregnancy, or if the patient becomes pregnant while taking this drug, the patient should be apprised of the potential hazard to the fetus. Women of childbearing potential should be advised to avoid becoming pregnant.

EPIRUBICIN HYDROCHLORIDE — INJECTION

➤*Lactation:* Epirubicin was excreted into the milk of rats treated with 0.5 mg/kg/day of epirubicin during peri- and postnatal periods. It is not known whether epirubicin is excreted in human milk. Because many drugs, including other anthracyclines, are excreted in human milk and because of the potential for serious adverse reactions in nursing infants from epirubicin, mothers should discontinue nursing prior to taking this drug.

➤*Children:* The safety and effectiveness of epirubicin in pediatric patients have not been established in adequate and well-controlled clinical trials. Pediatric patients may be at greater risk for anthracycline-induced acute manifestations of cardiotoxicity and for chronic CHF.

Precautions

➤*Monitoring:* Blood counts, including absolute neutrophil counts and liver function should be assessed before and during each cycle of therapy with epirubicin. Repeated evaluations of LVEF should be performed during therapy.

➤*Injection-site reactions:* Epirubicin HCl injection is administered by intravenous infusion. Venous sclerosis may result from an injection into a small vessel or from repeated injections into the same vein. Extravasation of epirubicin during the infusion may cause local pain, severe tissue lesions (vesication, severe cellulitis) and necrosis. It is recommended that epirubicin HCl be slowly administered into the tubing of a freely running intravenous infusion usually between 3 and 20 minutes depending upon dosage and volume of the infusion solution. If possible, veins over joints or in extremities with compromised venous or lymphatic drainage should be avoided. A burning or stinging sensation may be indicative of perivenous infiltration, and the infusion should be immediately terminated and restarted in another vein. Perivenous infiltration may occur without causing pain.

Facial flushing, as well as local erythematous streaking along the vein, may be indicative of excessively rapid administration. It may precede local phlebitis or thrombophlebitis.

➤*Prophylactic antibiotics:* Patients administered the 120 mg/m^2 regimen of epirubicin HCl as a component of combination chemotherapy should also receive prophylactic antibiotic therapy with trimethoprim-sulfamethoxazole or a fluoroquinolone.

➤*Antiemetics:* Epirubicin is emetigenic. Antiemetics may reduce nausea and vomiting; prophylactic use of antiemetics should be considered before administration of epirubicin HCl, particularly when given in conjunction with other emetigenic drugs.

➤*Inflammatory recall reactions:* As with other anthracyclines, administration of epirubicin HCl after previous radiation therapy may induce an inflammatory recall reaction at the site of the irradiation.

➤*Thrombophlebitis/Thromboembolism:* As with other cytotoxic agents, thrombophlebitis and thromboembolic phenomena, including pulmonary embolism (in some cases fatal) have been coincidentally reported with the use of epirubicin.

Drug Interactions

➤*Cytotoxic drugs:* Epirubicin HCl when used in combination with other cytotoxic drugs may show on-treatment additive toxicity, especially hematologic and gastrointestinal effects.

➤*Cardioactive compounds:* Concomitant use of epirubicin HCl with other cardioactive compounds that could cause heart failure (eg, calcium channel blockers) requires close monitoring of cardiac function throughout treatment.

➤*Radiation therapy:* There are few data regarding the coadministration of radiation therapy and epirubicin. In adjuvant trials of epirubicin-containing CEF-120 or FEC-100 chemotherapies, breast irradiation was delayed until after chemotherapy was completed. This practice resulted in no apparent increase in local breast cancer recurrence relative to published accounts in the literature. A small number of patients received epirubicin-based chemotherapy concomitantly with radiation therapy but had chemotherapy interrupted in order to avoid potential overlapping toxicities. It is likely that use of epirubicin with radiotherapy may sensitize tissues to the cytotoxic actions of irradiation. Administration of epirubicin HCl after previous radiation therapy may induce an inflammatory recall reaction at the site of the irradiation.

➤*Cimetidine:* Cimetidine increased the AUC of epirubicin by 50%. Cimetidine treatment should be stopped during treatment with epirubicin.

Adverse Reactions

➤*Delayed reactions:* The table below describes the incidence of delayed adverse reactions in patients participating in the MA-5 and GFEA-05 trials.

Long-Term Adverse Reactions in Patients with Early Breast Cancer (%)

Adverse reaction	FEC-100/CEF-120 (n = 620)	FEC-50 (n = 280)	CMF (n = 360)
Cardiac toxicity			
Asymptomatic drops in LVEF	1.8%	1.4%	0.8%
CHF	1.5%	0.4%	0.3%
Leukemia			
AML	0.8%	0%	0.3%

Two cases of acute lymphoid leukemia (ALL) were also observed in patients receiving epirubicin. However, an association between anthracyclines such as epirubicin and ALL has not been clearly established.

➤*Overview of acute and delayed toxicities:*

Cardiovascular – See Warnings for more information.

Dermatologic – Alopecia occurs frequently, but is usually reversible, with hair regrowth occurring within 2 to 3 months from the termination of therapy. Flushes, skin and nail hyperpigmentation, photosensitivity, and hypersensitivity to irradiated skin (radiation-recall reaction) have been observed. Urticaria and anaphylaxis have been reported in patients treated with epirubicin; signs and symptoms of these reactions may vary from skin rash and pruritus to fever, chills, and shock.

GI – A dose-dependent mucositis (mainly oral stomatitis, less often esophagitis) may occur in patients treated with epirubicin. Clinical manifestations of mucositis may include a pain or burning sensation, erythema, erosions, ulcerations, bleeding, or infections. Mucositis generally appears early after drug administration and, if severe, may progress over a few days to mucosal ulcerations; most patients recover from this adverse event by the third week of therapy. Hyperpigmentation of the oral mucosa may also occur.

Nausea, vomiting, and occasionally diarrhea and abdominal pain can also occur. Severe vomiting and diarrhea may produce dehydration. Antiemetics may reduce nausea and vomiting; prophylactic use of antiemetics should be considered before therapy, particularly if epirubicin is given in conjunction with other emetigenic drugs.

Hematologic – See Warnings for more information.

Local – Venous sclerosis may result from an injection into a small vessel or from repeated injections into the same vein. Extravasation of epirubicin during the infusion may cause local pain, severe tissue lesions (vesication, severe cellulitis) and necrosis.

Secondary leukemia – See Warnings for more information.

Overdosage

➤*Symptoms:* A 36-year-old man with non-Hodgkin's lymphoma received a daily 95 mg/m^2 dose of epirubicin HCl injection for 5 consecutive days. Five days later, he developed bone marrow aplasia, grade 4 mucositis, and gastrointestinal bleeding. No signs of acute cardiac toxicity were observed. He was treated with antibiotics, colony-stimulating factors, and antifungal agents, and recovered completely. A 63-year-old women with breast cancer and liver metastasis received a single 320 mg/m^2 dose of epirubicin HCl. She was hospitalized with hyperthermia and developed multiple organ failure (respiratory and renal), with lactic acidosis, increased lactate dehydrogenase, and anuria. Death occurred within 24 hours after administration of epirubicin HCl. Additional instances of administration of doses higher than recommended have been reported at doses ranging from 150 to 250 mg/m^2. The observed adverse reactions in these patients were qualitatively similar to known toxicities of epirubicin. Most of the patients recovered with appropriate supportive care.

➤*Treatment:* If an overdose occurs, supportive treatment (including antibiotic therapy, blood and platelet transfusions, colony-stimulating factors, and intensive care as needed) should be provided until the recovery of toxicities. Delayed CHF has been observed months after anthracycline administration. Patients must be observed carefully over time for signs of CHF and provided with appropriate supportive therapy.

Patient Information

Patients should be informed of the expected adverse effects of epirubicin, including gastrointestinal symptoms (nausea, vomiting, diarrhea, and stomatitis) and potential neutropenic complications.

Patients should consult their physicians if vomiting, dehydration, fever, evidence of infection, symptoms of CHF, or injection-site pain occurs following therapy with epirubicin HCl. Patients should be informed that they will almost certainly develop alopecia.

Patients should be advised that their urine may appear red for 1 to 2 days after administration of epirubicin HCl and that they should not be alarmed.

Patients should understand that there is a risk of irreversible myocardial damage associated with treatment with epirubicin HCl, as well as a risk of treatment-related leukemia.

Because epirubicin may induce chromosomal damage in sperm, men undergoing treatment with epirubicin HCl should use effective contraceptive methods.

Women treated with epirubicin HCl may develop irreversible amenorrhea, or premature menopause.

IDARUBICIN HYDROCHLORIDE

Rx	**Idarubicin HCl** (GensiaSicor)	**Injection:** 1 mg/mL	Preservative-free. In 5, 10, and 20 mL single-use vials.
Rx	**Idamycin PFS** (Pfizer)		Preservative-free. In 5, 10, and 20 mL single-use vials.

IDARUBICIN HYDROCHLORIDE — INJECTION

WARNING

Idarubicin HCl should be given slowly into a freely flowing IV infusion; it must never be given IM or SC. Severe local tissue necrosis can occur if there is extravasation during administration.

As is the case with other anthracyclines, the use of idarubicin HCl can cause myocardial toxicity leading to congestive heart failure. Cardiac toxicity is more common in patients who have received prior anthracyclines or who have preexisting cardiac disease.

As is usual with antileukemic agents, severe myelosuppression occurs when idarubicin HCl is used at effective therapeutic doses.

It is recommended that idarubicin HCl be administered only under the supervision of a physician who is experienced in leukemia chemotherapy and in facilities with laboratory and supportive resources adequate to monitor drug tolerance and protect and maintain a patient compromised by drug toxicity. The physician and institution must be capable of responding rapidly and completely to severe hemorrhagic conditions or overwhelming infection.

Dosage should be reduced in patients with impaired hepatic or renal function. In patients with hepatic or renal impairment, a dose reduction of idarubicin HCl should be considered. Idarubicin HCl should not be administered if the bilirubin level exceeds 5 mg/dL.

Indications

➤*Acute myeloid leukemia:* In combination with other approved antileukemic drugs for the treatment of acute myeloid leukemia (AML) in adults. This includes French-American-British (FAB) classifications M1 through M7.

Administration and Dosage

➤*Approved by the FDA:* September 27, 1990.

➤*Induction therapy in adult patients with AML:* Idarubicin HCl 12 mg/m^2 daily for 3 days by slow (10 to 15 minute) IV injection in combination with cytarabine. The cytarabine may be given as 100 mg/m^2 daily by continuous infusion for 7 days or as cytarabine 25 mg/m^2 IV bolus followed by cytarabine 200 mg/m^2 daily for 5 days continuous infusion. In patients with unequivocal evidence of leukemia after the first induction course, a second course may be administered. Administration of the second course should be delayed in patients who experience severe mucositis, until recovery from this toxicity has occurred, and a dose reduction of 25% is recommended. In patients with hepatic or renal impairment, a dose reduction of idarubicin HCl should be considered. Idarubicin HCl should not be administered if the bilirubin level exceeds 5 mg/dL.

➤*Preparation of solution:* Idarubicin HCl 5 mg, 10 mg and 20 mg vials should be reconstituted with 5 mL, 10 mL and 20 mL, respectively, of Water for Injection to give a final concentration of 1 mg/mL of idarubicin HCl. Bacteriostatic diluents are not recommended. The reconstituted solution is hypotonic, and the recommended administration procedure via a freely flowing IV infusion must be followed.

The vial contents are under a negative pressure to minimize aerosol formation during reconstitution; therefore, particular care should be taken when the needle is inserted. Inhalation of any aerosol produced during reconstitution must be avoided.

Reconstituted solutions are physically and chemically stable for 72 hours (3 days) under refrigeration (2° to 8°C; 36° to 46°F) and at controlled room temperature, (15° to 30°C; 59° to 86°F). Discard unused solutions in an appropriate manner (see below).

➤*Extravasation:* Care in the administration of idarubicin HCl will reduce the chance of perivenous infiltration. It may also decrease the chance of local reactions such as urticaria and erythematous streaking. During IV administration of idarubicin HCl extravasation may occur with or without an accompanying stinging or burning sensation even if blood returns well on aspiration of the infusion needle. If any signs or symptoms of extravasation have occurred, the injection or infusion should be immediately terminated and restarted in another vein. If it is known or suspected that SC extravasation has occurred, it is recommended that intermittent ice packs (½ hour immediately, then ½ hour 4 times per day for 3 days) be placed over the area of extravasation and that the affected extremity be elevated. Because of the progressive nature of extravasation reactions, the area of injection should be frequently examined and plastic surgery consultation obtained early if there is any sign of a local reaction such as pain, erythema, edema or vesication. If ulceration begins or there is severe persistent pain at the site of extravasation, early wide excision of the involved area should be considered.

➤*Administration:* Idarubicin HCl should be administered slowly (over 10 to 15 minutes) into the tubing of a freely running IV infusion of Sodium Chloride Injection (0.9%) or 5% Dextrose Injection. The tubing should be attached to a butterfly needle or other suitable device and inserted preferably into a large vein.

➤*Incompatibility:* Unless specific compatibility data are available, idarubicin HCl should not be mixed with other drugs. Precipitation occurs with heparin. Prolonged contact with any solution of an alkaline pH will result in degradation of the drug.

➤*Storage/Stability:* Store at controlled room temperature, 15° to 30°C (59° to 86°F), and protect from light.

Preservative-free injection – Store under refrigeration 2° to 8°C (36° to 46°F), and protect from light. Retain in carton until the time of use.

Actions

➤*Pharmacology:* Idarubicin HCl is a DNA-intercalating analog of daunorubicin which has an inhibitory effect on nucleic acid synthesis and interacts with the enzyme topoisomerase II. The absence of a methoxy group at position 4 of the anthracycline structure gives the compound a high lipophilicity which results in an increased rate of cellular uptake compared with other anthracyclines.

➤*Pharmacokinetics:*

Absorption – Pharmacokinetic studies have been performed in adult leukemia patients with normal renal and hepatic function following IV administration of 10 to 12 mg/m^2 of idarubicin daily for 3 to 4 days as a single agent or combined with cytarabine. The plasma concentrations of idarubicin are best described by a 2 or 3 compartment open model.

Distribution – The disposition profile shows a rapid distributive phase with a very high volume of distribution presumably reflecting extensive tissue binding. Studies of cellular (nucleated blood and bone marrow cells) drug concentrations in leukemia patients have shown that peak cellular idarubicin concentrations are reached a few minutes after injection. Concentrations of idarubicin and idarubicinol in nucleated blood and bone marrow cells are greater than 100 times the plasma concentrations. Idarubicin disappearance rates in plasma and cells were comparable with a terminal half-life of about 15 hours. The terminal half-life of idarubicinol in cells was about 72 hours. The extent of drug and metabolic accumulation predicted in leukemia patients for days 2 and 3 of dosing, based on the mean plasma levels and half-life obtained after the first dose, is 1.7- and 2.3-fold, respectively, and suggests no change in kinetics following a daily × 3 regimen. The percentages of idarubicin and idarubicinol bound to human plasma proteins averaged 97% and 94%, respectively, at concentrations similar to maximum plasma levels obtained in the pharmacokinetic studies. The binding is concentration independent. The plasma clearance is twice the expected hepatic plasma flow indicating extensive extrahepatic metabolism.

Metabolism – The primary active metabolite formed is idarubicinol. As idarubicinol has cytotoxic activity, it presumably contributes to the effects of idarubicin.

Excretion – The elimination rate of idarubicin from plasma is slow with an estimated mean terminal half-life of 22 hours (range, 4 to 48 hours) when used as a single agent and 20 hours (range, 7 to 38 hours) when used in combination with cytarabine. The elimination of the primary active metabolite, idarubicin, is considerably slower than that of the parent drug with an estimated mean terminal half-life that exceeds 45 hours; hence, its plasma levels are sustained for a period greater than 8 days. The drug is eliminated predominately by biliary and to a lesser extent by renal excretion, mostly in the form of idarubicinol.

Special populations –
Renal function impairment: See Warnings for more information.
Hepatic function impairment: See Warnings for more information.

Warnings

➤*Bone marrow suppression:* Idarubicin HCl is a potent bone marrow suppressant. Idarubicin HCl should not be given to patients with preexisting bone marrow suppression induced by previous drug therapy or radiotherapy unless the benefit warrants the risk.

➤*Severe myelosuppression:* Severe myelosuppression will occur in all patients given a therapeutic dose of this agent for induction, consolidation or maintenance. Careful hematologic monitoring is required. Deaths due to infection or bleeding have been reported during the period of severe myelosuppression. Facilities with laboratory and supportive resources adequate to monitor drug tolerability and protect and maintain a patient compromised by drug toxicity should be available. It must be possible to treat rapidly and completely a severe hemorrhagic condition or a severe infection.

➤*Cardiotoxicity:* Preexisting heart disease and previous therapy with anthracyclines at high cumulative doses or other potentially cardiotoxic agents are cofactors for increased risk of idarubicin-induced cardiac toxicity and the benefit to risk ratio of idarubicin therapy in such patients should be weighed before starting treatment with idarubicin HCl.

Myocardial toxicity as manifested by potentially fatal congestive heart failure, acute life-threatening arrhythmias or other cardiomyopathies may occur following therapy with idarubicin HCl. Appropriate therapeutic measures for the management of congestive heart failure or arrhythmias are indicated.

IDARUBICIN HYDROCHLORIDE — INJECTION

Cardiac function should be carefully monitored during treatment in order to minimize the risk of cardiac toxicity of the type described for other anthracycline compounds. The risk of such myocardial toxicity may be higher following concomitant or previous radiation to the mediastinal-pericardial area or in patients with anemia, bone marrow depression, infections, leukemic pericarditis or myocarditis. While there are no reliable means for predicting congestive heart failure, cardiomyopathy induced by anthracyclines is usually associated with a decrease of the left ventricular ejection fraction (LVEF) from pretreatment baseline values.

➤*Renal/Hepatic function impairment:* Since hepatic or renal function impairment can affect the disposition of idarubicin HCl, liver and kidney function should be evaluated with conventional clinical laboratory tests (using serum bilirubin and serum creatinine as indicators) prior to and during treatment. In a number of phase III clinical trials, treatment was not given if bilirubin or creatinine serum levels exceeded 2 mg/dL. However, in 1 phase III trial, patients with bilirubin levels between 2.6 mg/dL and 5 mg/dL received the anthracycline with a 50% reduction in dose. Dose reduction of idarubicin HCl should be considered if the bilirubin or creatinine levels are above the normal range (greater than 5 mg/dL).

➤*Carcinogenesis:* Formal long-term carcinogenicity studies have not been conducted with idarubicin. Idarubicin and related compounds have been shown to have carcinogenic properties when tested in experimental models (including bacterial systems, mammalian cells in culture and female Sprague-Dawley rats).

➤*Mutagenesis:* Idarubicin and related compounds have been shown to have mutagenic properties when tested in experimental models (including bacterial systems, mammalian cells in culture and female Sprague-Dawley rats).

➤*Fertility impairment:* In male dogs given 1.8 mg/m^2/day 3 times a week (about one-seventh the weekly human dose on a mg/m^2 basis) for 13 weeks, or 3 times the human dose, testicular atrophy was observed with inhibition of spermatogenesis and sperm maturation with few or no mature sperm. These effects were not readily reversed after a recovery of 8 weeks.

➤*Elderly:* Patients over 60 years of age who were undergoing induction therapy experienced congestive heart failure, serious arrhythmias, chest pain, MI, and asymptomatic declines in LVEF more frequently than younger patients.

➤*Pregnancy: Category D.* Idarubicin was embryotoxic and teratogenic in the rat at a dose of 1.2 mg/m^2/day or one-tenth the human dose, which was nontoxic to dams, idarubicin was embryotoxic but not teratogenic in the rabbit even at a dose of 2.4 mg/m^2/day or two-tenths the human dose, which was toxic to dams.

There is no conclusive information about idarubicin adversely affecting human fertility or causing teratogenesis. There has been 1 report of a fetal fatality after maternal exposure to idarubicin during the second trimester.

There are no adequate and well-controlled studies in pregnant women. If idarubicin HCl is to be used during pregnancy, or if the patient becomes pregnant during therapy, the patient should be apprised of the potential hazard to the fetus. Women of childbearing potential should be advised to avoid pregnancy.

➤*Lactation:* It is not known whether this drug is excreted in human milk. Because many drugs are excreted in human milk and because of the potential for serious adverse reactions in nursing infants from idarubicin, mothers should discontinue nursing prior to taking this drug.

➤*Children:* Safety and effectiveness in children have not been established.

Precautions

➤*Monitoring:* Frequent complete blood counts and monitoring of hepatic and renal function tests are recommended.

Therapy with idarubicin HCl requires close observation of the patient and careful laboratory monitoring. Hyperuricemia secondary to rapid lysis of leukemic cells may be induced. Appropriate measures must be taken to prevent hyperuricemia and to control any systemic infection before beginning therapy.

➤*Extravasation:* See Administration and Dosage for more information.

Adverse Reactions

Idarubicin Induction Phase Adverse Reactions (%)

Adverse reactions	IDR (n = 110)	DNR (n = 118)
Infection	95%	97%
Nausea/vomiting	82%	80%
Hair loss	77%	72%
Abdominal cramps/diarrhea	73%	68%
Hemorrhage	63%	65%
Mucositis	50%	55%
Dermatologic	46%	40%
Mental status	41%	34%
Pulmonary (clinical)	39%	39%
Fever (not elsewhere classified)	26%	28%
Headache	20%	24%
Cardiac (clinical)	16%	24%
Neurologic (peripheral nerves)	7%	9%
Pulmonary allergy	2%	4%
Seizure	4%	5%
Cerebellar	4%	4%

The duration of aplasia and incidence of mucositis were greater on the IDR arm than the DNR arm, especially during consolidation in some US controlled trials.

➤*Cardiovascular:* Congestive heart failure (frequently attributed to fluid overload), serious arrhythmias including atrial fibrillation, chest pain, MI and asymptomatic declines in LVEF have been reported in patients undergoing induction therapy for AML. Myocardial insufficiency and arrhythmias were usually reversible and occurred in the setting of sepsis, anemia and aggressive IV fluid administration. The events were reported more frequently in patients greater than 60 years of age and in those with preexisting cardiac disease.

➤*Dermatologic:* Alopecia was reported frequently and dermatologic reactions including generalized rash, urticaria and a bullous erythrodermatous rash of the palms and soles have occurred. The dermatologic reactions were usually attributed to concomitant antibiotic therapy. Recall of skin reaction due to prior radiotherapy has occurred with idarubicin HCl injection administration.

➤*GI:* Nausea or vomiting, mucositis, abdominal pain and diarrhea were reported frequently, but were severe (equivalent to WHO grade 4) in less than 5% of patients. Severe enterocolitis with perforation has been reported rarely. The risk of perforation may be increased by instrumental intervention. The possibility of perforation should be considered in patients who develop severe abdominal pain and appropriate steps for diagnosis and management should be taken.

➤*Hepatic:* Changes in hepatic function tests have been observed. These changes were usually transient and occurred in the setting of sepsis and while patients were receiving potentially hepatotoxic antibiotics and antifungal agents. Severe changes in hepatic function (equivalent to WHO grade 4) occurred in less than 5% of patients.

➤*Immunologic:* Severe myelosuppression is the major toxicity associated with idarubicin HCl therapy, but this effect of the drug is required in order to eradicate the leukemic clone. During the period of myelosuppression, patients are at risk of developing infection and bleeding which may be life-threatening or fatal.

➤*Local:* Local reactions including hives at the injection site have been reported.

➤*Renal:* Changes in renal function tests have been observed. These changes were usually transient and occurred in the setting of sepsis and while patients were receiving potentially nephrotoxic antibiotics and antifungal agents. Severe changes in renal function (equivalent to WHO grade 4) occurred in no more than 1% of patients. Severe changes in renal function (equivalent to WHO grade 4) occurred in no more than 1% of patients.

Overdosage

➤*Symptoms:* Two cases of fatal overdosage in patients receiving therapy for AML have been reported. The doses were 135 mg/m^2 over 3 days and 45 mg/m^2 of idarubicin and 90 mg/m^2 of daunorubicin over a 3-day period.

It is anticipated that overdosage with idarubicin will result in severe and prolonged myelosuppression and possibly in increased severity of GI toxicity. Adequate supportive care including platelet transfusions, antibiotics and symptomatic treatment of mucositis is required. The effect of acute overdose on cardiac function is not fully known, but severe arrhythmia occurred in 1 of the 2 patients exposed. It is anticipated that very high doses of idarubicin may cause acute cardiac toxicity and may be associated with a higher incidence of delayed cardiac failure.

➤*Treatment:* There is no known antidote to idarubicin HCl injection.

Disposition studies with idarubicin in patients undergoing dialysis have not been carried out. The profound multicompartment behavior, extensive extravascular distribution and tissue binding, coupled with the low unbound fraction available in the plasma pool make it unlikely that therapeutic efficacy or toxicity would be altered by conventional peritoneal or hemodialysis.

BLEOMYCIN SULFATE (BLM)

Rx	**Bleomycin** (Various, eg, Bedford Laboratories, Gensia Sicor)	**Powder for injection:** 15 units[a]	In vials.
		30 units[a]	In vials.
Rx	**Blenoxane** (Bristol-Myers Oncology)	**Powder for injection:** 15 units[a]	In vials.
		30 units[a]	In vials.

[a] A unit of bleomycin is equal to the formerly used milligram activity.

BLEOMYCIN SULFATE — INJECTION

WARNING

It is recommended that bleomycin for injection be administered under the supervision of a qualified physician experienced in the use of cancer chemotherapeutic agents. Appropriate management of therapy and complications is possible only when adequate diagnostic and treatment facilities are readily available.

Pulmonary fibrosis is the most severe toxicity associated with bleomycin. The most frequent presentation is pneumonitis occasionally progressing to pulmonary fibrosis. Its occurrence is higher in elderly patients and in those receiving greater than 400 units total dose, but pulmonary toxicity has been observed in young patients and those treated with low doses.

A severe idiosyncratic reaction consisting of hypotension, mental confusion, fever, chills, and wheezing has been reported in approximately 1% of lymphoma patients treated with bleomycin.

Indications

Bleomycin for injection should be considered a palliative treatment. It has been shown to be useful in the management of the following neoplasms either as a single agent or in proven combinations with other approved chemotherapeutic agents:

➤*Squamous cell carcinoma:* Head and neck (including mouth, tongue, tonsil, nasopharynx, oropharynx, sinus, palate, lip, buccal mucosa, gingiva, epiglottis, skin, larynx), penis, cervix, and vulva. The response to bleomycin is poorer in patients with head and neck cancer previously irradiated.

➤*Lymphomas:* Hodgkin's disease, non-Hodgkin's lymphoma.

➤*Testicular carcinoma:* Embryonal cell, choriocarcinoma, and teratocarcinoma.

➤*Unlabeled uses:* Treatment of mycosis fungoides; osteosarcoma; AIDS-related Kaposi sarcoma. Has been used in children for palliative treatment of lymphomas; testicular carcinoma; germ cell tumors; sclerosis of pleural effusions.

Administration and Dosage

➤*Initial doses:* Because of the possibility of an anaphylactoid reaction, lymphoma patients should be treated with 2 units or less of bleomycin for injection for the first 2 doses. If no acute reaction occurs, then the regular dosage schedule may be followed.

➤*Squamous cell carcinoma, non-Hodgkin's lymphoma, testicular carcinoma:* The following dose schedule is recommended: 0.25 to 0.5 U/kg (10 to 20 U/m^2) given intravenously, intramuscularly, or subcutaneously weekly or twice weekly.

➤*Hodgkin's disease:* The following dose schedule is recommended: 0.25 to 0.5 U/kg (10 to 20 U/m^2) given intravenously, intramuscularly, or subcutaneously weekly or twice weekly. After a 50% response, a maintenance dose of 1 unit daily or 5 units weekly intravenously or intramuscularly should be given.

➤*Dosage over 400 U/day:* Pulmonary toxicity of bleomycin appears to be dose related with a striking increase when the total dose is over 400 U. Total doses over 400 U should be given with great caution.

➤*Note:* When bleomycin is used in combination with other antineoplastic agents, pulmonary toxicities may occur at lower doses.

Improvement of Hodgkin's disease and testicular tumors is prompt and noted within 2 weeks. If no improvement is seen by this time, improvement is unlikely. Squamous cell cancers respond more slowly, sometimes requiring as long as 3 weeks before any improvement is noted.

➤*Administration:* Bleomycin may be given by the intravenous, intramuscular, or subcutaneous routes.

Preparation of solutions –

Intramuscular or subcutaneous: The bleomycin 15 units vial should be reconstituted with 1 to 5 mL of sterile water for injection, sodium chloride for injection, 0.9%, or sterile bacteriostatic water for injection. The bleomycin 30 units vial should be reconstituted with 2 to 10 mL of the above diluents.

Intravenous: The bleomycin 15 units or 30 units vial should be dissolved in 5 mL or 10 mL, respectively, of sodium chloride for injection, 0.9%, and administered slowly over a period of 10 minutes.

➤*Storage/Stability:* The sterile powder is stable under refrigeration (2° to 8°C; 36° to 46°F) and should not be used after the expiration date is reached.

Bleomycin is stable for 24 hours at room temperature in Sodium Chloride Injection.

Admixture incompatibilities – Bleomycin should not be reconstituted or diluted with D_5W or other dextrose containing diluents. When reconstituted in D_5W and analyzed by HPLC, bleomycin demonstrates a loss of A_2 and B_2 potency that does not occur when bleomycin is reconstituted in 0.9% sodium chloride.

Actions

➤*Pharmacology:* Although the exact mechanism of action of bleomycin is unknown, available evidence would seem to indicate that the main mode of action is the inhibition of DNA synthesis with some evidence of lesser inhibition of RNA and protein synthesis.

➤*Pharmacokinetics:*

Absorption/Distribution – Following IV administration, bleomycin has a rapid initial distribution half-life of 10 to 20 minutes. IM injection produces peak blood levels in 30 to 60 minutes that are approximately one-third of those produced IV.

Metabolism/Excretion – In patients with normal renal function, 60% to 70% of an administered dose is recovered in the urine as active bleomycin. In patients with a creatinine clearance of greater than 35 mL/min, the serum or plasma terminal elimination half-life of bleomycin is approximately 115 minutes. In patients with a creatinine clearance of less than 35 mL/min, the plasma or serum terminal elimination half-life increases exponentially as the creatinine clearance decreases.

Special populations –

Renal function impairment: It was reported that patients with moderately severe renal failure excreted less than 20% of the dose in the urine. This result would suggest that severe renal impairment could lead to accumulation of the drug in blood.

Contraindications

Bleomycin for injection is contraindicated in patients who have demonstrated a hypersensitive or an idiosyncratic reaction to it.

Warnings

➤*Observation:* Patients receiving bleomycin for injection must be observed carefully and frequently during and after therapy. It should be used with extreme caution in patients with significant impairment of renal function or compromised pulmonary function.

➤*Pulmonary toxicities:* Pulmonary toxicities occur in 10% of treated patients. In approximately 1%, the nonspecific pneumonitis induced by bleomycin progresses to pulmonary fibrosis, and death. Although this is age and dose related, the toxicity is unpredictable. Frequent roentgenograms are recommended.

➤*Hypersensitivity reactions:* See the Warning box for more information.

➤*Renal/Hepatic function impairment:* Bleomycin clearance may be reduced in patients with impaired renal function. No guidelines have been established for dose adjustments, but bleomycin should be used with extreme caution in patients with significant renal impairment.

Renal or hepatic toxicity, beginning as a deterioration in renal or liver function tests, have been reported infrequently. These toxicities may occur, however, at any time after initiation of therapy.

➤*Carcinogenesis:* The carcinogenic potential of bleomycin in humans is unknown. A study in F344-type male rats demonstrated an increased incidence of nodular hyperplasia after induced lung carcinogenesis by nitrosamines, followed by treatment with bleomycin. In another study where the drug was administered to rats by subcutaneous injection at 0.35 mg/kg weekly (3.82 units/m^2 weekly or about 30% at the recommended human dose), necropsy findings included dose related injection site fibrosarcomas as well as various renal tumors.

➤*Mutagenesis:* Bleomycin has been shown to be mutagenic both in vitro and in vivo.

➤*Pregnancy: Category D.*

Teratogenic – Bleomycin can cause fetal harm when administered to a pregnant woman. It has been shown to be teratogenic in rats. Administration of intraperitoneal doses of 1.5 mg/kg/day to rats (about 1.6 times the recommended human dose on a unit/m^2 basis) on days 6 to 15 of gestation caused skeletal malformations, shortened innominate artery and hydroureter. Bleomycin is abortifacient but not teratogenic in rabbits, at IV doses of 1.2 mg/kg/day (about 2.4 times the recommended human dose on a unit/m^2 basis) given on gestation days 6 to 18.

There have been no studies in pregnant women. If bleomycin is used during pregnancy, or if the patient becomes pregnant while receiving this drug, the patient should be apprised of the potential hazard to the fetus. Women of childbearing potential should be advised to avoid becoming pregnant during therapy with bleomycin.

➤*Lactation:* It is not known whether the drug is excreted in human milk. Because many drugs are excreted in human milk and because of the potential for serious adverse reactions in nursing infants, it is recommended that nursing be discontinued by women receiving bleomycin therapy.

➤*Children:* Safety and effectiveness of bleomycin in pediatric patients have not been established.

BLEOMYCIN SULFATE — INJECTION

Drug Interactions

Bleomycin Drug Interactions			
Precipitant drug	Object drug[a]		Description
Bleomycin	Digoxin	⬇	Digoxin serum levels may be decreased by combination chemotherapy (including bleomycin). Digoxin capsules do not appear to be affected. Monitor patients for signs of reduction in pharmacologic effect (eg, deteriorating heart failure). Increase digoxin dose if necessary; serum level monitoring may facilitate tailoring dosage.
Bleomycin	Phenytoin	⬇	Phenytoin serum concentrations may be decreased by combination chemotherapy. Monitor serum phenytoin levels and adjust the phenytoin dosage appropriately. IV phenytoin may be useful.
Oxygen	Bleomycin	⬆	Risk for pulmonary toxicity is increased (see Warnings).
Bleomycin	Oxygen		

[a] ⬆ = Object drug increased. ⬇ = Object drug decreased.

Adverse Reactions

➤*Allergic:* See the Warning box for more information.

➤*Cardiovascular:* Vascular toxicities coincident with the use of bleomycin in combination with other antineoplastic agents have been reported rarely. The reactions are clinically heterogeneous and may include myocardial infarction, cerebrovascular accident, thrombotic microangiopathy (HUS) or cerebral arteritis. Various mechanisms have been proposed for these vascular complications. There are also reports of Raynaud's phenomenon occurring in patients treated with bleomycin in combination with vinblastine with or without cisplatin or, in a few cases, with bleomycin as a single agent. It is currently unknown if the cause of Raynaud's phenomenon in these cases is the disease, underlying vascular compromise, bleomycin, vinblastine, hypomagnesemia, or a combination of any of these factors.

➤*Dermatologic:* These are the most frequent side effects, being reported in approximately 50% of treated patients. These consist of erythema, rash, striae, vesiculation, hyperpigmentation, and tenderness of the skin. Hyperkeratosis, nail changes, alopecia, pruritus, and stomatitis have also been reported. It was necessary to discontinue bleomycin therapy in 2% of treated patients because of these toxicities.

Skin toxicity is a relatively late manifestation usually developing in the second and third week of treatment after 150 to 200 units of bleomycin have been administered and appears to be related to the cumulative dose.

Scleroderma-like skin changes have also been reported as part of postmarketing surveillance.

➤*Pulmonary:* This is potentially the most serious side effect, occurring in approximately 10% of patients treated with bleomycin for injection. The most frequent presentation is pneumonitis occasionally progressing to pulmonary fibrosis. Approximately 1% of patients treated have died of pulmonary fibrosis. Pulmonary toxicity is both dose and age related, being more common in patients over 70 years of age and in those receiving over 400 units total dose. This toxicity, however, is unpredictable and has been seen occasionally in young patients receiving low doses.

Because of lack of specificity of the clinical syndrome, the identification of patients with pulmonary toxicity due to bleomycin has been extremely difficult. The earliest symptom associated with bleomycin pulmonary toxicity is dyspnea. The earliest sign is fine rales.

Radiographically, bleomycin-induced pneumonitis produces nonspecific patchy opacities, usually of the lower lung fields. The most common changes in pulmonary function tests are a decrease in total lung volume and a decrease in vital capacity. However, these changes are not predictive of the development of pulmonary fibrosis.

The microscopic tissue changes due to bleomycin toxicity include bronchiolar squamous metaplasia, reactive macrophages, atypical alveolar epithelial cells, fibrinous edema, and interstitial fibrosis. The acute stage may involve capillary changes and subsequent fibrinous exudation into alveoli producing a change similar to hyaline membrane formation and progressing to a diffuse interstitial fibrosis resembling the Hamman-Rich syndrome. These microscopic findings are nonspecific (eg, similar changes are seen in radiation pneumonitis and pneumocystic pneumonitis).

To monitor the onset of pulmonary toxicity, roentgenograms of the chest should be taken every 1 to 2 weeks. If pulmonary changes are noted, treatment should be discontinued until it can be determined if they are drug related. Recent studies have suggested that sequential measurement of the pulmonary diffusion capacity for carbon monoxide (DL_{CO}) during treatment with bleomycin may be an indicator of subclinical pulmonary toxicity. It is recommended that the DL_{CO} be monitored monthly if it is to be employed to detect pulmonary toxicities, and thus the drug should be discontinued when the DL_{CO} falls below 30% to 35% of the pretreatment value.

Because of bleomycin's sensitization of lung tissue, patients who have received bleomycin are at greater risk of developing pulmonary toxicity when oxygen is administered in surgery. While long exposure to very high oxygen concentrations is a known cause of lung damage, after bleomycin administration, lung damage can occur at lower concentrations that are usually considered safe. Suggestive preventive measures are:

1.) Maintain FIO_2 at concentrations approximating that of room air (25%) during surgery and the postoperative period.
2.) Monitor carefully fluid replacement, focusing more on colloid administration rather than crystalloid.

Sudden onset of an acute chest pain syndrome suggestive of pleuropericarditis has been rarely reported during bleomycin infusions. Although each patient must be individually evaluated, further courses of bleomycin do not appear to be contraindicated.

➤*Miscellaneous:* Malaise was also reported as part of postmarketing surveillance.

Fever, chills, and vomiting were frequently reported side effects. Anorexia and weight loss are common and may persist long after termination of this medication. Pain at tumor site, phlebitis, and other local reactions were reported infrequently.

DACTINOMYCIN (Actinomycin D; ACT)

Rx	**Cosmegen** (Merck)	**Powder for injection, lyophilized:** 500 mcg	In vials.[a]

[a] With mannitol 20 mg.

DACTINOMYCIN — INJECTION

WARNING

Dactinomycin should be administered only under the supervision of a physician who is experienced in the use of cancer chemotherapeutic agents.

This drug is highly toxic and both powder and solution must be handled and administered with care. Inhalation of dust or vapors and contact with skin or mucous membranes, especially those of the eyes, must be avoided. Avoid exposure during pregnancy. Due to the toxic properties of dactinomycin (eg, corrosivity, carcinogenicity, mutagenicity, teratogenicity), special handling procedures should be reviewed prior to handling and followed diligently.

Dactinomycin is extremely corrosive to soft tissue. If extravasation occurs during IV use, severe damage to soft tissues will occur. In at least one instance, this has led to contracture of the arms.

Indications

➤*Wilm's tumor, rhabdomyosarcoma, Ewing's sarcoma, nonseminomatous testicular cancer:* As part of a combination chemotherapy and/or multi-modality treatment regimen for the treatment of Wilms' tumor, childhood rhabdomyosarcoma, Ewing's sarcoma and metastatic, nonseminomatous testicular cancer.

➤*Gestational trophoblastic neoplasia:* As a single agent or as part of a combination chemotherapy regimen for the treatment of gestational trophoblastic neoplasia.

➤*Solid malignancies:* As a component of regional perfusion for the palliative and/or adjunctive treatment of locally recurrent or locoregional solid malignancies.

➤*Unlabeled uses:* Treatment of osteosarcoma; malignant melanoma; Paget disease of the bone.

Administration and Dosage

Not for oral administration. Toxic reactions due to dactinomycin are frequent and may be severe, thus limiting in many instances the amount that may be administered. However, the severity of toxicity varies markedly and is only partly dependent on the dose employed.

➤*IV use:* The dosage of dactinomycin varies depending on the tolerance of the patient, the size, and location of the neoplasm, and the use of other forms of therapy. It may be necessary to decrease the usual dosages suggested below when other chemotherapy or radiation therapy is used concomitantly or has been used previously.

The dosage for dactinomycin is calculated in micrograms (mcg). The dose intensity per 2-week cycle adults or children should not exceed 15 mcg/kg/day or 400 to 600 mcg/m²/day IV for 5 days. Calculation of the dosage for obese or edematous patients should be performed on the basis of surface area in an effort to more closely relate dosage to lean body mass.

A wide variety of single agent and combination chemotherapy regimens with dactinomycin may be employed. Because chemotherapeutic regimens are constantly changing, dosing and administration should be performed under the direct supervision of physicians familiar with current oncologic practices and new advances in therapy. The following suggested regimens are based upon a review of current literature concerning therapy with dactinomycin and are on a per cycle basis.

DACTINOMYCIN — INJECTION

Wilms' tumor, childhood rhabdomyosarcoma and Ewing's sarcoma – Regimens of 15 mcg/kg intravenously daily for 5 days administered in various combinations and schedules with other chemotherapeutic agents have been utilized in the treatment of Wilms' tumor, rhabdomyosarcoma and Ewing's sarcoma.

Metastatic nonseminomatous testicular cancer – 1000 mcg/m^2 intravenously on Day 1 as part of a combination regimen with cyclophosphamide, bleomycin, vinblastine, and cisplatin.

Gestational trophoblastic neoplasia – 12 mcg/kg intravenously daily for 5 days as a single agent.

500 mcg intravenously on Days 1 and 2 as part of a combination regimen with etoposide, methotrexate, folinic acid, vincristine, cyclophosphamide and cisplatin.

Regional perfusion in locally recurrent and locoregional solid malignancies – The dosage schedules and the technique itself vary from one investigator to another; the published literature, therefore, should be consulted for details. In general, the following doses are suggested:
50 mcg (0.05 mg) per kilogram of body weight for lower extremity or pelvis.
35 mcg (0.035 mg) per kilogram of body weight for upper extremity.

Reduced doses – It may be advisable to use lower doses in obese patients, or when previous chemotherapy or radiation therapy has been employed.

Preparation of solution for IV administration – This drug is highly toxic and both powder and solution must be handled and administered with care. Since dactinomycin is extremely corrosive to soft tissues, it is intended for intravenous use. Inhalation of dust or vapors and contact with skin or mucous membranes, especially those of the eyes, must be avoided. Appropriate protective equipment should be worn when handling dactinomycin. Should accidental eye contact occur, copious irrigation for at least 15 minutes with water, normal saline or a balanced salt ophthalmic irrigating solution should be instituted immediately, followed by prompt ophthalmologic consultation. Should accidental skin contact occur, the affected part must be irrigated immediately with copious amounts of water for at least 15 minutes while removing contaminated clothing and shoes. Medical attention should be sought immediately. Contaminated clothing should be destroyed and shoes cleaned thoroughly before reuse.

Reconstitute dactinomycin by adding 1.1 mL of sterile water for injection (without preservative) using aseptic precautions. The resulting solution of dactinomycin will contain approximately 500 mcg (0.5 mg) per mL.

Once reconstituted, the solution of dactinomycin can be added to infusion solutions of dextrose injection 5% or sodium chloride injection either directly or to the tubing of a running IV infusion.

Although reconstituted dactinomycin is chemically stable, the product does not contain a preservative and accidental microbial contamination might result. Any unused portion should be discarded. Use of water containing preservatives (benzyl alcohol or parabens) to reconstitute dactinomycin injection, results in the formation of a precipitate.

Partial removal of dactinomycin from IV solutions by cellulose ester membrane filters used in some IV in-line filters has been reported.

Since dactinomycin is extremely corrosive to soft tissue, precautions for materials of this nature should be observed.

If the drug is given directly into the vein without the use of an infusion, the "two-needle technique" should be used. Reconstitute and withdraw the calculated dose from the vial with one sterile needle. Use another sterile needle for direct injection into the vein.

Discard any unused portion of the dactinomycin solution.

Management of extravasation – Care in the administration of dactinomycin will reduce the chance of perivenous infiltration. It may also decrease the chance of local reactions such as urticaria and erythematous streaking. On intravenous administration of dactinomycin, extravasation may occur with or without an accompanying burning or stinging sensation, even if blood returns well on aspiration of the infusion needle. If any signs or symptoms of extravasation have occurred, the injection or infusion should be immediately terminated and restarted in another vein. If extravasation is suspected, intermittent application of ice to the site for 15 minutes 4 times daily for 3 days may be useful. The benefit of local administration of drugs has not been clearly established. Because of the progressive nature of extravasation reactions, close observation and plastic surgery consultation is recommended. Blistering, ulceration and/or persistent pain are indications for wide excision surgery, followed by split-thickness skin grafting.

➤*Storage/Stability:* Store at 25°C (77°F); excursions permitted to 15° to 30°C (59° to 86°F). Protect from light and humidity.

Actions

➤*Pharmacology:* Generally, the actinomycins exert an inhibitory effect on gram-positive and gram-negative bacteria and on some fungi. However, the toxic properties of the actinomycins (including dactinomycin) in relation to antibacterial activity are such as to preclude their use as antibiotics in the treatment of infectious diseases.

Because the actinomycins are cytotoxic, they have an antineoplastic effect that has been demonstrated in experimental animals with various types of tumor implant. This cytotoxic action is the basis for their use in the palliative treatment of certain types of cancer. Dactinomycin is believed to produce its cytotoxic effects by binding DNA and inhibiting RNA synthesis.

Dactinomycin anchors into a purine-pyrimidine (DNA) base pair by intercalation, inhibiting messenger RNA synthesis. Although maximal cell-kill is noted in G^1 phase, the cytotoxic action is primarily cell cycle nonspecific. Activity proliferating cells are more sensitive.

➤*Pharmacokinetics:* Very little active drug can be detected in circulating blood 2 minutes after IV injection.Results of a study in patients with malignant melanoma indicate that dactinomycin (^{3}H actinomycin D) is minimally metabolized, is concentrated in nucleated cells, and does not penetrate the blood-brain barrier. Approximately 30% of the dose was recovered in urine and feces in 1 week. The terminal plasma half-life for radioactivity was approximately 36 hours.

Contraindications

Dactinomycin should not be given at or about the time of infection with chickenpox or herpes zoster because of the risk of severe generalized disease which may result in death.

Warnings

➤*Carcinogenesis:* Reports indicate an increased incidence of second primary tumors (including leukemia) following treatment with radiation and antineoplastic agents, such as dactinomycin. Multi-modal therapy creates the need for careful, long-term observation of cancer survivors.

The International Agency on Research on Cancer has judged that dactinomycin is a positive carcinogen in animals. Local sarcomas were produced in mice and rats after repeated subcutaneous or intraperitoneal injection. Mesenchymal tumors occurred in male F344 rats given intraperitoneal injections of 50 mcg/kg, 2 to 5 times per week for 18 weeks. The first tumor appeared at 23 weeks.

➤*Mutagenesis:* Dactinomycin has been shown to be mutagenic in a number of test systems in vitro and in vivo including human fibroblasts and leukocytes, and HELA cells. DNA damage and cytogenetic effects have been demonstrated in the mouse and the rat.

➤*Elderly:* Clinical studies of dactinomycin did not include sufficient numbers of subjects aged 65 and over to determine whether they respond differently from younger subjects. Other reported clinical experience has not identified differences in responses between the elderly and younger patients. However, a published meta-analysis of all studies performed by the Eastern Cooperative Oncology Group (ECOG) over a 13-year period suggests that administration of dactinomycin to elderly patients may be associated with an increased risk of myelosuppression compared to younger patients. In general, dose selection for an elderly patient should be cautious, usually starting at the low end of the dosing range, reflecting the greater frequency of decreased hepatic, renal, or cardiac function, and of concomitant disease or other drug therapy.

➤*Pregnancy:* *Category D.* Dactinomycin may cause fetal harm when administered to a pregnant woman. Dactinomycin has been shown to cause malformations and embryotoxicity in rat, rabbit, and hamster when given in doses of 50 to 100 mcg/kg (approximately 0.5 to 2 times the maximum recommended daily human dose on a body surface area basis). If this drug is used during pregnancy, or if the patient becomes pregnant while receiving this drug, the patient should be apprised of the potential hazard to the fetus. Women of childbearing potential must be warned to avoid becoming pregnant.

➤*Lactation:* It is not known whether this drug is excreted in human milk. Because many drugs are excreted in human milk and because of the potential for serious adverse reactions in nursing infants from dactinomycin, a decision should be made whether to discontinue nursing or to discontinue the drug, taking into account the importance of the drug to the mother.

➤*Children:* The greater frequency of toxic effects of dactinomycin in infants suggests that this drug should be given to infants only over the age of 6 to 12 months.

Precautions

➤*Monitoring:* Many abnormalities of renal, hepatic, and bone marrow function have been reported in patients with neoplastic diseases receiving dactinomycin. Renal, hepatic, and bone marrow functions should be assessed frequently.

➤*Highly toxic:* This drug is highly toxic and both powder and solution must be handled and administered with care. Since dactinomycin is extremely corrosive to soft tissues, it is intended for intravenous use.

If extravasations occurs, immediately discontinue the infusion. Apply cold compresses to the area. Local infiltration with an injectable corticosteroid may lessen the local reaction. Dilute the drug by infusing saline injection through the line into the infiltrated area.

Inhalation of dust or vapors and contact with skin or mucous membranes, especially those of the eyes, must be avoided. Appropriate protective equipment should be worn when handling dactinomycin. Should accidental eye contact occur, copious irrigation for at least 15 minutes with water, normal saline or a balanced salt ophthalmic irrigating solution should be instituted immediately, followed by prompt ophthalmologic consultation. Should accidental skin contact occur, the affected part must be irrigated immediately with copious amounts of water for at least 15 minutes, while removing contaminated clothing and shoes. Medical attention should be sought immediately. Contaminated clothing should be destroyed and shoes cleaned thoroughly before reuse.

➤*Toxicities:* As with all antineoplastic agents, dactinomycin is a toxic drug and very careful and frequent observation of the patient for adverse reactions is necessary. These reactions may involve any tissue of the body, most commonly the hematopoietic system resulting in myelosuppression. The possibility of an anaphylactoid reaction should be borne in mind.

It is extremely important to observe the patient daily for toxic side effects when combination chemotherapy is employed, since a full course of therapy occasionally is not tolerated. If stomatitis, diarrhea, or severe hematopoietic depression appear during therapy, these drugs should be discontinued until the patient has recovered.

DACTINOMYCIN — INJECTION

➤*Radiation therapy:* An increased incidence of gastrointestinal toxicity and marrow suppression has been reported with combined therapy incorporating dactinomycin and radiation. Moreover, the normal skin, as well as the buccal and pharyngeal mucosa, may show early erythema. A smaller than usual radiation dose administered in combination with dactinomycin causes erythema and vesiculation, which progress more rapidly through the stages of tanning and desquamation. Healing may occur in 4 to 6 weeks rather than 2 to 3 months. Erythema from previous radiation therapy may be reactivated by dactinomycin alone, even when radiotherapy was administered many months earlier, and especially when the interval between the 2 forms of therapy is brief. This potentiation of radiation effect represents a special problem when the radiotherapy involves the mucous membrane. When irradiation is directed toward the nasopharynx, the combination may produce severe oropharyngeal mucositis. Severe reactions may ensue if high doses of both dactinomycin and radiation therapy are used or if the patient is particularly sensitive to such combined therapy.

Particular caution is necessary when administering dactinomycin within 2 months of irradiation for the treatment of right-sided Wilms' tumor, since hepatomegaly and elevated AST levels have been noted. In general, dactinomycin should not be concomitantly administered with radiotherapy in the treatment of Wilms' tumor unless the benefit outweighs the risk.

➤*Regional perfusion therapy:* Complications of the perfusion technique are related mainly to the amount of drug that escapes into the systemic circulation and may consist of hematopoietic depression, absorption of toxic products from massive destruction of neoplastic tissue, increased susceptibility to infection, impaired wound healing, and superficial ulceration of the gastric mucosa. Other side effects may include edema of the extremity involved, damage to soft tissues of the perfused area, and (potentially) venous thrombosis.

Drug Interactions

➤*Drug/Lab test interactions:* Dactinomycin may interfere with bioassay procedures for the determination of antibacterial drug levels.

Adverse Reactions

Toxic effects (except nausea and vomiting) usually do not become apparent until 2 to 4 days after a course of therapy is stopped, and may not be maximal before 1 to 2 weeks have elapsed. Deaths have been reported. However, adverse reactions are usually reversible on discontinuance of therapy. They include the following:

➤*Dermatologic:* Alopecia; skin eruptions; acne; flare-up of erythema or increased pigmentation of previously irradiated skin. Dactinomycin is extremely corrosive. If extravasation occurs during IV use, severe damage to soft tissues will occur. In at least one instance, this has led to contracture of the arms. Epidermolysis, erythema, and edema, at times severe, have been reported with regional limb perfusion.

➤*GI:* Anorexia; nausea; vomiting; abdominal pain; diarrhea; gastrointestinal ulceration; liver toxicity including ascites; hepatomegaly; hepatic veno-occlusive disease; hepatitis; and liver function test abnormalities. Nausea and vomiting, which occur early during the first few hours after administration, may be alleviated by giving antiemetics. Cheilitis; dysphagia; esophagitis; ulcerative stomatitis; pharyngitis.

➤*Hematologic:* Anemia, even to the point of aplastic anemia; agranulocytosis; leukopenia; thrombopenia; pancytopenia; reticulopenia. Platelet and white cell counts should be performed frequently daily to detect severe hemopoietic depression. If either count markedly decreases, the drug should be withheld to allow marrow recovery. This often takes up to 3 weeks.

➤*Pulmonary:* Pneumonitis.

➤*Miscellaneous:* Malaise; fatigue; lethargy; fever; myalgia; proctitis; hypocalcemia, growth retardation, infection.

Overdosage

Dactinomycin was lethal to mice and rats at intravenous doses of 700 and 500 mcg/kg, respectively (approximately 3.8 and 5.4 times the maximum recommended daily human dose on a body surface area basis, respectively). The oral LD_{50} of dactinomycin is 7.8 mg/kg and 7.2 mg/kg in the mouse and rat, respectively.

MITOMYCIN (Mitomycin-C; MTC)

Rx	**Mitomycin** (Various, eg, American Pharmaceutical Partners, Bedford)	**Powder for Injection**: 5 mg	10 mg mannitol. In vials.
Rx	**Mutamycin** (Bristol-Myers Oncology)		10 mg mannitol. In vials.
Rx	**Mitomycin** (Various, eg, American Pharmaceutical Partners, Bedford)	**Powder for Injection**: 20 mg	40 mg mannitol. In vials.
Rx	**Mutamycin** (Bristol-Myers Oncology)		40 mg mannitol. In vials.
Rx	**Mitomycin** (Various, eg, American Pharmaceutical Partners, Bedford)	**Powder for Injection**: 40 mg	80 mg mannitol. In vials.
Rx	**Mutamycin** (Bristol-Myers Oncology)		80 mg mannitol. In vials.

MITOMYCIN — INJECTION

WARNING

Mitomycin should be administered under the supervision of a qualified physician experienced in the use of cancer chemotherapeutic agents. Appropriate management of therapy and complications is possible only when adequate diagnostic and treatment facilities are readily available.

Bone marrow suppression, notably thrombocytopenia and leukopenia, which may contribute to overwhelming infections in an already compromised patient, is the most common and severe of the toxic effects of mitomycin.

Hemolytic uremic syndrome (HUS), a serious complication of chemotherapy, consisting primarily of microangiopathic hemolytic anemia, thrombocytopenia, and irreversible renal failure has been reported in patients receiving systemic mitomycin. The syndrome may occur at any time during systemic therapy with mitomycin as a single agent or in combination with other cytotoxic drugs; however, most cases occur at doses greater than or equal to 60 mg of mitomycin. Blood product transfusion may exacerbate the symptoms associated with this syndrome.

The incidence of the syndrome has not been defined.

Indications

➤*Disseminated adenocarcinoma of the stomach or pancreas:* Mitomycin for injection is not recommended as single-agent, primary therapy. It has been shown to be useful in the therapy of disseminated adenocarcinoma of the stomach or pancreas in proven combinations with other approved chemotherapeutic agents and as palliative treatment when other modalities have failed. Mitomycin is not recommended to replace appropriate surgery or radiotherapy.

➤*Unlabeled uses:* Mitomycin has been given by the intravesical route for the management of superficial bladder cancer. Mitomycin as an ophthalmic solution appears beneficial as an adjunct to surgical excision in primary or recurrent pterygia.

Treatment of colorectal cancer, breast cancer, squamous cell carcinoma of head and neck, lungs or cervix.

Administration and Dosage

➤*Approved by the FDA:* March 10, 1988.

Mitomycin should be given intravenously only, using care to avoid extravasation of the compound. If extravasation occurs, cellulitis, ulceration, and slough may result.

➤*Reconstitution:* Each vial contains either mitomycin 5 mg and hydroxypropyl β cyclodextrin (HPβCD) 2 g. To administer, add Sterile Water for Injection, 8.5 mL. Shake to dissolve. If product does not dissolve immediately, allow to stand at room temperature until solution is obtained.

➤*Repeat doses:* Repeat doses of mitomycin have only been evaluated at a dose of 15 mg/m^2. After full hematological recovery (see guide to dosage adjustment) from any previous chemotherapy, the following dosage schedule may be used at 6- to 8-week intervals: 15 mg/m^2 intravenously as a single dose via a functioning intravenous catheter.

➤*Dosage adjustment:* Because of cumulative myelosuppression, patients should be fully reevaluated after each course of mitomycin, and the dose reduced if the patient has experienced any toxicities. Doses greater than 20 mg/m^2 have not been shown to be more effective, and are more toxic than lower doses.

The following schedule is suggested as a guide to dosage adjustment:

Nadir After Prior Dose		
Leukocytes/mm^3	Platelets/mm^3	Percentage of prior dose to be given
> 4000	> 100,000	100%
3000 to 3999	75,000 to 99,999	100%
2000 to 2999	25,000 to 74,999	70%
< 2000	< 25,000	50%

No repeat dosage should be given until leukocyte count has returned to 4000/mm^3 and platelet count to 100,000/mm^3.

➤*Concurrent myelosuppressive agents:* When mitomycin is used in combination with other myelosuppressive agents, the doses should be adjusted accordingly. If the disease continues to progress after 2 courses of mitomycin, the drug should be stopped since chances of response are minimal.

➤*Storage/Stability:*

Unreconstituted – Store dry powder at controlled room temperature 15° to 30°C (59° to 86°F) and protect from light. Dry powder is stable for the lot life indicated on the package.

MITOMYCIN — INJECTION

Reconstituted – Reconstituted with Sterile Water for Injection to a concentration of 0.5 mg per mL, the reconstituted mitomycin should be used within 24 hours. Protect from light.

Diluted – Diluted in various IV fluids at room temperature, to a concentration of 40 mcg/mL:

Dilution Stability	
IV fluid	Stability
5% Dextrose Injection	No more than 4 hours
0.9% Sodium Chloride Injection	No more than 48 hours
Sodium Lactate Injection	No more than 24 hours

The combination of mitomycin (5 mg to 15 mg) and heparin (1000 units to 10,000 units) in 30 mL of 0.9% Sodium Chloride Injection is stable for 72 hours at room temperature.

Store dry powder at room temperature 15° to 30°C (59° to 86°F), protected from light. Avoid excessive heat, over 40°C (104°F). Protect reconstituted solution from light. Store solution under refrigeration 2° to 8°C (36° to 46°F), discard after 14 days. If unrefrigerated, discard after 7 days.

Actions

➤*Pharmacology:* Mitomycin selectively inhibits the synthesis of deoxyribonucleic acid (DNA). The guanine and cytosine content correlates with the degree of mitomycin-induced cross-linking. At high concentrations of the drug, cellular RNA and protein synthesis are also suppressed.

➤*Pharmacokinetics:*

Absorption / Distribution – *Mitozytrex* was found bioequivalent to mitomycin in an open-label randomized crossover study in cancer patients who received single doses (15 mg/m^2 by a 30-minute infusion) of each formulation. In another open-label study, sequential cycles of mitomycin showed similar pharmacokinetics to mitomycin when administered every 6 weeks (15 mg/m^2 by a 30-minute infusion). The maximal serum concentration of mitomycin ranged from 0.38 to 1.89 mcg/mL after a 30-minute infusion of 15 mg/m^2 mitomycin. The disposition of mitomycin is biphasic with a mean terminal half life of 46 minutes.

Metabolism – In humans, mitomycin is rapidly cleared from the serum after intravenous administration. Time required to reduce the serum concentration by 50% after a 30 mg bolus injection is 17 minutes. After injection of 30 mg, 20 mg, or 10 mg IV, the maximal serum concentrations were 2.4 mcg/mL, 1.7 mcg/mL, and 0.52 mcg/mL, respectively. Clearance is effected primarily by metabolism in the liver, but metabolism occurs in other tissues as well. The rate of clearance is inversely proportional to the maximal serum concentration because, it is thought, of saturation of the degradative pathways.

Excretion – Approximately 10% of a dose of mitomycin is excreted unchanged in the urine. Since metabolic pathways are saturated at relatively low doses, the percentage of a dose excreted in urine increases with increasing dose. In children, excretion of intravenously administered mitomycin is similar.

Approximately 80% to 90% of HPβCD, the solubilizing agent in mitomycin, is eliminated through the kidneys, and greater than 93% is excreted unchanged in the urine within 12 hours after dosing.

Special populations –
Renal function impairment: See Warnings for more information.

Contraindications

Hypersensitivity or idiosyncratic reaction to mitomycin; thrombocytopenia, coagulation disorder, or an increase in bleeding tendency due to other causes.

Warnings

➤*Bone marrow suppression:* The use of mitomycin results in a high incidence of bone marrow suppression, particularly thrombocytopenia and leukopenia. Therefore, the following studies should be obtained repeatedly during therapy and for at least 8 weeks following therapy: Platelet count, white blood cell count, differential, and hemoglobin. The occurrence of a platelet count below 100,000/mm^3 or a WBC below 4000/mm^3 or a progressive decline in either is an indication to withhold further therapy until blood counts have recovered above these levels.

Patients should be advised of the potential toxicity of this drug, particularly bone marrow suppression. Deaths have been reported due to septicemia as a result of leukopenia due to the drug.

➤*Pulmonary toxicity:* This has occurred infrequently but can be severe and may be life threatening. Dyspnea with a nonproductive cough and radiographic evidence of pulmonary infiltrates may be indicative of mitomycin-induced pulmonary toxicity. If other etiologies are eliminated, mitomycin therapy should be discontinued. Steroids have been employed as treatment of this toxicity, but the therapeutic value has not been determined.

Acute shortness of breath and severe bronchospasm have been reported following the administration of vinca alkaloids in patients who had previously or simultaneously received mitomycin. The onset of this acute respiratory distress occurred within minutes to hours after the vinca alkaloid injection. The total number of doses for each drug has varied considerably. Bronchodilators, steroids or oxygen have produced symptomatic relief.

A few cases of adult respiratory distress syndrome have been reported in patients receiving mitomycin in combination with other chemotherapy and maintained at FIO_2 concentrations greater than 50% perioperatively. Therefore, caution should be exercised using only enough oxygen to provide adequate arterial saturation since oxygen itself is toxic to the lungs. Careful attention should be paid to fluid balance and overhydration should be avoided.

➤*Hemolytic uremic syndrome (HUS):* This serious complication of chemotherapy, consisting primarily of microangiopathic hemolytic anemia (hematocrit less than or equal to 25%), thrombocytopenia (less than or equal to 100,000/mm^3, and irreversible renal failure (serum creatinine greater than or equal to 1.6 mg/dL) has been reported in patients receiving systemic mitomycin. Microangiopathic hemolysis with fragmented red blood cells on peripheral blood smears has occurred in 98% of patients with the syndrome. Other less frequent complications of the syndrome may include pulmonary edema (65%), neurologic abnormalities (16%), and hypertension. Exacerbation of the symptoms associated with HUS has been reported in some patients receiving blood product transfusions. A high mortality rate (52%) has been associated with this syndrome.

The syndrome may occur at any time during systemic therapy with mitomycin as a single agent or in combination with other cytotoxic drugs. Less frequently, HUS has also been reported in patients receiving combinations of cytotoxic drugs not including mitomycin. Of 83 patients studied, 72 developed the syndrome at total doses exceeding 60 mg of mitomycin. Consequently, patients receiving greater than or equal to 60 mg of mitomycin should be monitored closely for unexplained anemia with fragmented cells on peripheral blood smear, thrombocytopenia, and decreased renal function.

➤*Cardiac toxicity:* Congestive heart failure, often treated effectively with diuretics and cardiac glycosides, has rarely been reported. Almost all patients who experienced this side effect had received prior doxorubicin therapy.

➤*Bladder toxicity:* Bladder fibrosis/contraction has been reported with intravesical administration of mitomycin (not an approved route of administration), which in rare cases has required cystectomy. The safety of intravesical administration of mitomycin and its HPβCD excipient has not been studied. Evidence of bladder toxicities have been observed following parenteral administration of the HPβCD excipient of mitomycin as single and repeat doses equal to or greater than 0.15 g/m^2 and 0.5 g/m^2 in rodents and dogs, respectively (about 1⁄60 and 1⁄20 the amount of HPβCD administered per recommended human intravenous dose of mitomycin on a mg/m^2 basis). Findings included edema, inflammation, cellular inclusions and bladder stones associated with metaplasia; findings persisted at least 3 months following dosing.

➤*Renal function impairment:* Patients receiving mitomycin should be observed for evidence of renal toxicity. Mitomycin should not be given to patients with a serum creatinine greater than 1.7 mg/dL.

Renal toxicity – Two percent (2%) of 1281 patients demonstrated a statistically significant rise in creatinine. There appeared to be no correlation between total dose administered or duration of therapy and the degree of renal impairment. In a study where a single intravenous dose of 200 mg of HPβCD was given to subjects with severe renal impairment (creatinine clearance less than or equal to 19 mL/min), clearance of HPβCD was reduced 6-fold compared to subjects with normal renal function.

➤*Carcinogenesis:* Mitomycin contains the excipient HPβCD, which produced pancreatic adenocarcinomas in a rat carcinogenicity study. These findings were not observed in a similar mouse carcinogenicity study. The clinical relevance of these findings is unclear.

Mitomycin is carcinogenic in mice and rats. Three different strains of mice administered intraperitoneal mitomycin at 0.2 mcg/mouse (about 1.6 times the recommended human dose on a mg/m^2 basis) twice weekly for 35 doses exhibited increases in undifferentiated sarcomas by study week 40. Likewise, subcutaneous administration of mitomycin produced undifferentiated sarcomas in 2 of 4 mouse strains tested. Following bladder installation in rats, mitomycin produced bladder papillomas and dysplasia.

HPβCD is carcinogenic in rats. A conventional carcinogenesis study at doses of 500 to 5000mg/kg/day HPβCD (about 1⁄3rd to 3 times the amount of HPβCD per recommended human dose of mitomycin on a mg/m^2 basis) administered in the feed for 25 months revealed a significant increase in the incidence of hyperplasia and adenoma and adenocarcinoma of the exocrine pancreas. Similar findings were not observed in the untreated control group and are not reported in historical controls. Development of these tumors may theoretically be related to a mitogenic action of cholecystokinin. A significant trend was also observed in adenocarcinoma of the large intestine and mammary gland of rats of this same study administered 5000 mg/kg/day HPβCD (about 3 times the amount of HPβCD per recommended human dose of mitomycin on a mg/m^2 basis). These findings were not observed in mice administered the same doses of HPβCD for 22 to 23 months. The clinical relevance of these findings is unclear.

➤*Mutagenesis:* Mitomycin is a known mutagen and clastogen. Mitomycin has been shown to be positive in the Ames bacterial mutation assay, chromosomal aberrations assays in mice, Chinese hamsters and human lymphocytes, unscheduled DNA synthesis assay in human lymphocytes, micronucleus test in mice and human lymphocytes and somatic mutation and recombination assays in *Drosophila melanogaster*.

➤*Fertility impairment:* Intraperitoneal administration of mitomycin to male mice in a single dose of 5mg/kg (about equal to the recommended human dose on a mg/m^2 basis) or 1 mg/kg (about 1⁄5 the recommended human dose on a mg/m^2 basis) for 5 days significantly decreased sperm production, sperm count and sperm motility and resulted in reduced pregnancy rates and an increased frequency of malformations. Doses of 2 and 4 mg/kg/day administered intravenously to female mice (about 2⁄5 and 4⁄5 the recommended human dose on a mg/m^2 basis) inhibited fertilization and implantation.

➤*Elderly:* Clinical studies of mitomycin did not include sufficient numbers of subjects aged 65 and over to determine whether they tolerate the drug

MITOMYCIN — INJECTION

differently than younger subjects. In general, elderly patients should be treated with caution due to the greater frequency of decreased hepatic, renal, or cardiac function, and concomitant disease or other drug therapy.

➤*Pregnancy: Category D.* Mitomycin can cause fetal harm when administered to a pregnant woman. If mitomycin is used during pregnancy, or if the patient becomes pregnant while receiving this drug, the patient should be apprised of the potential hazard to the fetus or potential risk for loss of the pregnancy.

Studies in both mice and rats at mitomycin doses equal to or greater than 0.5 mg/kg/day (about 1⁄10 and 1⁄5, respectively, of the recommended human dose on a mg/m^2 basis), administered intraperitoneally during the period of organogenesis showed a significant decrease in number of live fetuses; mitomycin was lethal to dams at 2 mg/kg/day (about 4⁄10's the recommended human dose on a mg/m^2 basis) in mice. Evidence of fetotoxicity, including delayed fetal development (eg, depressed fetal body weights, incomplete ossification), fetal external anomalies (eg, exencephaly, club foot, cleft palate, maldirection of digits, kinked tail), and neonatal anomalies (hydronephrosis, retarded development of reproductive organs) was observed in mice and rats administered doses equal to or greater than 0.05 mg/kg/day (about 1⁄100 and 1⁄50, respectively, of the recommended human dose on a mg/m^2 basis). In a separate study, mitomycin was administered to pregnant female mice; offspring exhibited significantly retarded reproductive tract development.

In 2 separate studies, HPβCD, the excipient for mitomycin, was fetotoxic (decreased number of live fetuses, depressed fetal body weight, incomplete ossification) in rats dosed by gavage and intravenously at doses equal to or greater than 50 and 250mg/kg/day, respectively (about 1⁄30 and 1⁄6 the amount of HPβCD administered per recommended human dose of mitomycin on a mg/m^2 basis).

➤*Lactation:* It is not known if mitomycin is excreted in human milk. Because many drugs are excreted in human milk and because of the potential for serious adverse reactions in nursing infants from mitomycin, it is recommended that nursing be discontinued when receiving mitomycin therapy.

➤*Children:* Safety and effectiveness in pediatric patients have not been established.

Precautions

➤*Monitoring:* Patients being treated with mitomycin must be observed carefully and frequently during and after therapy.

Patients receiving mitomycin should be observed for evidence of renal toxicity. Mitomycin should not be given to patients with a serum creatinine greater than 1.7 mg/dL.

Nephrotoxicity, including irreversible renal necrosis, was observed in rodents and non-rodents following parenteral administration of HPβCD, the excipient contained in mitomycin. This nephrotoxicity appeared to be the result of the accumulation and recrystallization of HPβCD in the proximal tubules of the kidney.

As severe renal impairment prolongs the elimination rate of HPβCD, mitomycin should not be used in patients with severe renal dysfunction (creatinine clearance less than 30 mL/min).

➤*Bladder toxicity:* See Warnings for more information.

Adverse Reactions

➤*Bone marrow toxicity:* This was the most common and most serious toxicity, occurring in 605 of 937 patients (64.4%) treated with mitomycin. Thrombocytopenia or leukopenia may occur anytime within 8 weeks after onset of therapy with an average time of 4 weeks. Recovery after cessation of therapy was within 10 weeks. About 25% of the leukopenic or thrombocytopenic episodes did not recover. Mitomycin produces cumulative myelosuppression.

➤*Integument and mucous membrane toxicity:* This has occurred in approximately 4% of patients treated with mitomycin. Cellulitis at the injection site has been reported and is occasionally severe. Stomatitis and alopecia also occur frequently. Rashes are rarely reported. The most important dermatological problem with this drug, however, is the necrosis and consequent sloughing of tissue which results if the drug is extravasated during injection. Extravasation may occur with or without an accompanying stinging or burning sensation and even if there is adequate blood return when the injection needle is aspirated. There have been reports of delayed erythema or ulceration occurring either at or distant from the injection site, weeks to months after mitomycin, even when no obvious evidence of extravasation was observed during administration. Skin grafting has been required in some of the cases.

➤*Renal toxicity:* See Warnings for more information.

➤*Pulmonary toxicity:* See Warnings for more information.

➤*Hemolytic uremic syndrome (HUS):* See Warnings for more information.

➤*Cardiac toxicity:* See Warnings for more information.

➤*Acute side effects due to mitomycin:* Fever, anorexia, nausea, and vomiting. They occurred in about 14% of 1281 patients.

➤*Other:* Headache, blurring of vision, confusion, drowsiness, syncope, fatigue, edema, thrombophlebitis, hematemesis, diarrhea, and pain. These did not appear to be dose related and were not unequivocally drug related. They may have been due to the primary or metastatic disease processes. Malaise and asthenia have been reported as part of postmarketing surveillance. Bladder fibrosis/contraction has been reported with intravesical administration (not an approved route of administration). The safety of intravesical administration of mitomycin and its HPβCD excipient has not been studied.

HORMONES

Androgens

TESTOLACTONE

c-iii	**Teslac** (Bristol-Myers Squibb)	**Tablets:** 50 mg	Lactose. (690). White, biconvex. In 100s.

TESTOLACTONE — ORAL

This is an abbreviated monograph. For complete and comparative information on Androgens, see the group monograph in the Endocrine/Metabolic chapter.

Indications

➤*Breast cancer:* As adjunctive therapy in the palliative treatment of advanced or disseminated breast cancer in postmenopausal women when hormonal therapy is indicated. It may also be used in women who were diagnosed as having had disseminated breast carcinoma when premenopausal, in whom ovarian function has been subsequently terminated.

Administration and Dosage

The recommended oral dose is 250 mg 4 times daily. In order to evaluate the response, therapy with testolactone should be continued for a minimum of 3 months unless there is active progression of the disease.

➤*Storage/Stability:* Store at room temperature 25°C (77°F).

Actions

➤*Pharmacology:* Although the precise mechanism by which testolactone produces its clinical antineoplastic effects has not been established, its principal action is reported to be inhibition of steroid aromatase activity and consequent reduction in estrone synthesis from adrenal androstenedione, the major source of estrogen in postmenopausal women. Based on in vitro studies, the aromatase inhibition may be noncompetitive and irreversible. This phenomenon may account for the persistence of testolactone's effect on estrogen synthesis after drug withdrawal.

➤*Pharmacokinetics:*

Absorption – Testolactone is well absorbed from the GI tract.

Metabolism/Excretion – Testolactone is metabolized to several derivatives in the liver, all of which preserve the lactone D-ring. These metabolites, as well as some unmetabolized drug, are excreted in the urine. Additional pharmacokinetic data in humans are unavailable.

Contraindications

Breast cancer in men; hypersensitivity to the drug.

Warnings

➤*Elderly:* Insufficient data from clinical studies of testolactone are available for patients 65 years of age and older to determine whether they respond differently than younger patients. Other reported clinical experience has not identified differences in responses between elderly and younger patients. In general, caution should be exercised when prescribing to elderly patients, reflecting the greater frequency of decreased hepatic, renal, or cardiac function, and of concomitant disease or other drug therapy.

Testolactone and its metabolites appear to be substantially excreted by the kidney, and the risk of toxic reactions to this drug may be greater in patients with impaired renal function. Because elderly patients are more likely to have decreased renal function, care should be taken in dose selection, and it may be useful to monitor renal function.

➤*Pregnancy: Category C.* In rats, testolactone has been shown to produce increased fetal mortality, increased abnormal fetal development, and increased mortality in growing pups when given at doses 5 to 15 times the recommended human dose. In rabbits, no teratologic effects were observed at doses 2.5 to 7.5 times the recommended human dose. There are no adequate and well-controlled studies in pregnant women. Testolactone is intended for use only in postmenopausal women and should not be used during pregnancy.

➤*Lactation:* It is not known whether this drug is excreted in human milk. Because many drugs are excreted in human milk, a decision should be made whether or not to discontinue nursing.

➤*Children:* Safety and efficacy in children have not been established.

Precautions

➤*Monitoring:* Plasma calcium levels should be routinely determined in any patient receiving therapy for mammary cancer, particularly during peri-

TESTOLACTONE — ORAL

ods of active remission of bony metastases. If hypercalcemia occurs, appropriate measures should be instituted.

➤*Drug abuse and dependence:* Testolactone is classified as a controlled substance under the Anabolic Steroids Control Act of 1990 and has been assigned to schedule III.

Drug Interactions

➤*Anticoagulants:* When administered concurrently, testolactone may increase the effects of oral anticoagulants; monitor and adjust anticoagulant dosage accordingly.

➤*Drug/Lab test interactions:* Physiologic effects of testolactone may result in decreased estradiol concentrations with radioimmunoassays for estradiol, increased plasma calcium concentrations, and increased 24-hour urinary excretion of creatine and 17-ketosteroids.

Adverse Reactions

Certain signs and symptoms have been reported in association with the use of this drug but, in these instances, it is often impossible to determine the relationship of the underlying disease and drug administration to the reported reaction. Such reactions include maculopapular erythema, increase in blood pressure, paresthesia, malaise, aches and edema of the extremities, glossitis, anorexia, and nausea and vomiting. Alopecia alone and with associated nail growth disturbance have been reported rarely; these side effects subsided without interruption of treatment.

Overdosage

There have been no reports of acute overdosage.

Patient Information

The physician should be consulted regarding missed doses. Notify the physician if adverse reactions occur or become more pronounced.

Contraceptive measures are recommended during treatment.

BICALUTAMIDE

Rx	**Casodex** (AstraZeneca)	**Tablets:** 50 mg	Lactose. (CDX50 Casodex). White. Film-coated. In 30s, 100s, and UD 30s.

BICALUTAMIDE — ORAL

Indications

➤*Prostate cancer:* For use in combination therapy with a luteinizing hormone-releasing hormone (LHRH) analog for the treatment of Stage D_2 metastatic carcinoma of the prostate.

Administration and Dosage

➤*Approved by the FDA:* October 4, 1995.

The recommended dose for bicalutamide therapy, in combination with an LHRH analog, is one 50 mg tablet once daily (morning or evening), with or without food. It is recommended that bicalutamide be taken at the same time each day. Treatment with bicalutamide should be started at the same time as treatment with an LHRH analog.

➤*Storage/Stability:* Store at controlled room temperature, 20° to 25°C (68° to 77°F).

Actions

➤*Pharmacology:* Bicalutamide is a nonsteroidal antiandrogen. It competitively inhibits the action of androgens by binding to cytosol androgen receptors in the target tissue. Prostatic carcinoma is known to be androgen sensitive and responds to treatment that counteracts the effect of androgen and/or removes the source of androgen.

➤*Pharmacokinetics:*

Absorption – Bicalutamide is well absorbed following oral administration, although the absolute bioavailability is unknown. Coadministration of bicalutamide with food has no clinically significant effect on rate or extent of absorption.

Distribution – Bicalutamide is highly protein-bound (96%).

Metabolism/Excretion – Bicalutamide undergoes stereospecific metabolism. The S (inactive) isomer is metabolized primarily by glucuronidation. The R (active) isomer also undergoes glucuronidation but is predominantly oxidized to an inactive metabolite followed by glucuronidation. Both the parent and metabolite glucuronides are eliminated in the urine and feces. The S-enantiomer is rapidly cleared relative to the R-enantiomer, with the R-enantiomer accounting for about 99% of total steady-state plasma levels.

Bicalutamide Pharmacokinetic Parameters

Parameter	Mean	Standard deviation
Healthy males (n = 30)		
Apparent oral clearance (L/h)	0.32	0.103
Single dose peak concentration (mcg/mL)	0.768	0.178
Single dose time to peak concentration (h)	31.3	14.6
Half-life (days)	5.8	2.29
Patients with prostate cancer (n = 40)		
C_{ss}[a] (mcg/mL)	8.939	3.504

[a] C_{ss} = Mean steady-state concentration.

Contraindications

Hypersensitivity reaction to the drug or any of the tablet's components.

Bicalutamide has no indication for women, and should not be used in this population, particularly for nonserious or nonlife-threatening conditions. Further, bicalutamide should not be used by women who are or may become pregnant. If this drug is used during pregnancy, or if the patient becomes pregnant while taking this drug, the patient should be apprised of the potential hazard to the fetus. Bicalutamide may cause fetal harm when administered to pregnant women. The male offspring of rats receiving doses of 10 mg/kg/day (plasma drug concentrations in rats equal to approximately ⅔ human therapeutic concentrations (based on a maximum dose of 50 mg/day of bicalutamide for an average 70 kg patient) and above were observed to have reduced anogenital distance and hypospadias in reproductive toxicology studies. These pharmacological effects have been observed with other antiandrogens. No other teratogenic effects were observed in rabbits receiving doses up to 200 mg/kg/day (approximately ⅓ human therapeutic concentrations based on a maximum dose of 50 mg/day of bicalutamide for an average 70 kg patient) or rats receiving doses up to 250 mg/kg/day (approximately 2 times human therapeutic concentrations (based on a maximum dose of 50 mg/day of bicalutamide for an average 70 kg patient).

Warnings

➤*Hepatic function impairment:* Rare cases of death or hospitalization due to severe liver injury have been reported postmarketing in association with the use of bicalutamide. Hepatotoxicity in these reports generally occurred within the first 3 to 4 months of treatment. Hepatitis or marked increases in liver enzymes leading to drug discontinuation occurred in approximately 1% of bicalutamide patients in controlled clinical trials.

Bicalutamide should be used with caution in patients with moderate-to-severe hepatic impairment. Bicalutamide is extensively metabolized by the liver. Limited data in subjects with severe hepatic impairment suggest that excretion of bicalutamide may be delayed and could lead to further accumulation. Periodic liver function tests should be considered for hepatically impaired patients on long-term therapy.

➤*Carcinogenesis:* Two-year oral carcinogenicity studies were conducted in both male and female rats and mice at doses of 5, 15 or 75 mg/kg/day of bicalutamide. A variety of tumor target organ effects were identified and were attributed to the antiandrogenicity of bicalutamide, namely, testicular benign interstitial (Leydig) cell tumors in male rats at all dose levels (the steady-state plasma concentration with the 5 mg/kg/day dose is approximately ⅔ human therapeutic concentrations based on a maximum dose of 50 mg/day of bicalutamide for an average 70 kg patient and uterine adenocarcinoma in female rats at 75 mg/kg/day (approximately 1.5 times the human therapeutic concentrations based on a maximum dose of 50 mg/day of bicalutamide for an average 70 kg patient). There is no evidence of Leydig cell hyperplasia in patients; uterine tumors are not relevant to the indicated patient population.

➤*Fertility impairment:* Administration of bicalutamide may lead to inhibition of spermatogenesis. The long-term effects of bicalutamide on male fertility have not been studied.

➤*Pregnancy: Category X.*

See Contraindications for more information.

➤*Lactation:* Bicalutamide is not indicated for use in women. It is not known whether this drug is excreted in human milk. Because many drugs are excreted in human milk, caution should be exercised when bicalutamide is administered to a nursing woman.

➤*Children:* Safety and efficacy of bicalutamide in pediatric patients have not been established.

Precautions

➤*Monitoring:* Serum transaminase levels should be measured prior to starting treatment with bicalutamide, at regular intervals for the first 4 months of treatment, and periodically thereafter. If clinical symptoms or signs suggestive of liver dysfunction occur (eg, nausea, vomiting, abdominal pain, fatigue, anorexia, "flu-like" symptoms, dark urine, jaundice, right upper quadrant tenderness), the serum transaminases, in particular the serum ALT, should be measured immediately. If at any time a patient has jaundice, or their ALT rises above 2 times the upper limit of normal, bicalutamide should be immediately discontinued with close follow-up of liver function.

Regular assessments of serum prostate-specific antigen (PSA) may be helpful in monitoring the patient's response. If PSA levels rise during bicalutamide therapy, the patient should be evaluated for clinical progression. For patients who have objective progression of disease together with an elevated PSA, a treatment-free period of antiandrogen, while continuing the LHRH analog, may be considered.

BICALUTAMIDE — ORAL

Drug Interactions

➤*Anticoagulants:* In vitro studies have shown bicalutamide can displace coumarin anticoagulants, such as warfarin, from their protein-binding sites. It is recommended that if bicalutamide is started in patients already receiving coumarin anticoagulants, prothrombin times should be closely monitored and adjustment of the anticoagulant dose may be necessary.

Adverse Reactions

In patients with advanced prostate cancer treated with bicalutamide in combination with an LHRH analog, the most frequent adverse reaction was hot flashes (53%).

Bicalutamide Adverse Reactions (≥ 5%)		
Adverse reaction	Bicalutamide plus LHRH analog (n = 401)	Flutamide plus LHRH analog (n = 407)
Miscellaneous		
General pain	142 (35%)	127 (31%)
Back pain	102 (25%)	105 (26%)
Asthenia	89 (22%)	87 (21%)
Pelvic pain	85 (21%)	70 (17%)
Infection	71 (18%)	57 (14%)
Abdominal pain	46 (11%)	46 (11%)
Chest pain	34 (8%)	34 (8%)
Headache	29 (7%)	27 (7%)
Flu syndrome	28 (7%)	30 (7%)
Cardiovascular		
Hot flashes	211 (53%)	217 (53%)
Hypertension	34 (8%)	29 (7%)
GI		
Constipation	87 (22%)	69 (17%)
Nausea	62 (15%)	58 (14%)
Diarrhea	49 (12%)	107 (26%)
Increased liver enzyme test[a]	30 (7%)	46 (11%)
Dyspepsia	30 (7%)	23 (6%)
Flatulence	26 (6%)	22 (5%)
Anorexia	25 (6%)	29 (7%)
Vomiting	24 (6%)	32 (8%)
Hematologic/lymphatic		
Anemia[b]	45 (11%)	53 (13%)
Metabolic/nutritional		
Peripheral edema	53 (13%)	42 (10%)
Weight loss	30 (7%)	39 (10%)
Hyperglycemia	26 (6%)	27 (7%)
Increased alkaline phosphatase	22 (5%)	24 (6%)
Weight gain	22 (5%)	18 (4%)
Musculoskeletal		
Bone pain	37 (9%)	43 (11%)
Myasthenia	27 (7%)	19 (5%)
Arthritis	21 (5%)	29 (7%)
Pathological fracture	17 (4%)	32 (8%)
CNS		
Dizziness	41 (10%)	35 (9%)
Paresthesia	31 (8%)	40 (10%)
Insomnia	27 (7%)	39 (10%)
Anxiety	20 (5%)	9 (2%)
Depression	16 (4%)	33 (8%)
Respiratory		
Dyspnea	51 (13%)	32 (8%)
Increased cough	33 (8%)	24 (6%)
Pharyngitis	32 (8%)	23 (6%)
Bronchitis	24 (6%)	22 (3%)
Pneumonia	18 (4%)	19 (5%)
Rhinitis	15 (4%)	22 (5%)
Dermatologic		
Rash	35 (9%)	30 (7%)
Sweating	25 (6%)	20 (5%)
GU		
Nocturia	49 (12%)	55 (14%)
Hematuria	48 (12%)	26 (6%)
Urinary tract infection	35 (9%)	36 (9%)
Gynecomastia	36 (9%)	30 (7%)
Impotence	27 (7%)	35 (9%)
Breast pain	23 (6%)	15 (4%)
Urinary frequency	23 (6%)	29 (7%)
Urinary retention	20 (5%)	14 (3%)
Impaired urination	19 (5%)	15 (4%)
Urinary incontinence	15 (4%)	32 (8%)

[a] Increased liver enzyme test includes increases in AST, ALT or both.
[b] Anemia includes anemia, hypochromic- and iron deficiency anemia.

➤*Other adverse reactions (greater than or equal to 2%, but less than 5%):*

Cardiovascular – Angina pectoris; congestive heart failure; myocardial infarct; heart arrest; coronary artery disorder; syncope.

CNS – Hypertonia; confusion; somnolence; libido decreased; neuropathy; nervousness.

Dermatologic – Dry skin; alopecia; pruritus; herpes zoster; skin carcinoma; skin disorder.

GI – Melena; rectal hemorrhage; dry mouth; dysphagia; GI disorder; periodontal abscess; GI carcinoma.

GU – Dysuria; urinary urgency; hydronephrosis; urinary tract disorder. In clinical trials with bicalutamide as a single agent for prostate cancer, gynecomastia and breast pain have been reported in up to 38% and 39% of patients, respectively.

Lab test abnormalities – Laboratory abnormalities including elevated AST, ALT, bilirubin, blood urea nitrogen (BUN), and creatinine and decreased hemoglobin and white cell count have been reported in both bicalutamide-LHRH analog treated and flutamide-LHRH analog-treated patients.

Metabolic / Nutritional – Edema; increased BUN; increased creatinine; dehydration; gout; hypercholesteremia.

Musculoskeletal – Myalgia; leg cramps.

Respiratory – Lung disorder; asthma; epistaxis; sinusitis.

Special senses – Cataract specified.

Miscellaneous – Neoplasm; neck pain; fever; chills; sepsis; hernia; cyst.

➤*Postmarketing experience:* Rare cases of interstitial pneumonitis and pulmonary fibrosis have been reported with bicalutamide.

Overdosage

➤*Symptoms:* Long-term clinical trials have been conducted with dosages up to 200 mg of bicalutamide daily and these dosages have been well tolerated. A single dose of bicalutamide that results in symptoms of an overdose considered to be life-threatening has not been established.

➤*Treatment:* There is no specific antidote; treatment of an overdose should be symptomatic.

In the management of an overdose with bicalutamide, vomiting may be induced if the patient is alert. It should be remembered that, in this patient population, multiple drugs may have been taken. Dialysis is not likely to be helpful since bicalutamide is highly protein bound and is extensively metabolized. General supportive care, including frequent monitoring of vital signs and close observation of the patient, is indicated.

Patient Information

Patients should be informed that therapy with bicalutamide and the LHRH analog should be initiated concomitantly, and that they should not interrupt or stop taking these medications without consulting their physician. Treatment with bicalutamide should be started at the same time as treatment with an LHRH analog.

FLUTAMIDE

Rx	**Flutamide** (Eon, Ivax, Zenith Goldline)	**Capsules:** 125 mg	May contain lactose. In 100s, 180s, 500s, and UD 100s.

FLUTAMIDE — ORAL

WARNING

Hepatic injury – There have been postmarketing reports of hospitalization and rarely death due to liver failure in patients taking flutamide. Evidence of hepatic injury included elevated serum transaminase levels, jaundice, hepatic encephalopathy and death related to acute hepatic failure. The hepatic injury was reversible after discontinuation of therapy in some patients. Approximately half of the reported cases occurred within the initial 3 months of treatment with flutamide.

Serum transaminase levels should be measured prior to starting treatment with flutamide. Flutamide is not recommended in patients whose ALT values exceed twice the upper limit of normal. Serum transaminase levels should then be measured monthly for the first 4 months of therapy, and periodically thereafter. Liver function tests also should be obtained at the first signs and symptoms suggestive of liver dysfunction (eg, nausea, vomiting, abdominal pain, fatigue, anorexia, "flu-like" symptoms, hyperbilirubinuria, jaundice, right upper quadrant tenderness). If at any time, a patient has jaundice, or their ALT rises above 2 times the upper limit of normal, flutamide should be immediately discontinued with close follow-up of liver function tests until resolution.

Indications

➤*Prostatic carcinoma:* For use in combination with LHRH-agonists for the management of locally confined Stage B_2-C and Stage D_2 metastatic carcinoma of the prostate.

Stage B_2-C prostatic carcinoma – Treatment with flutamide capsules and the goserelin acetate implant should start 8 weeks prior to initiating radiation therapy and continue during radiation therapy.

Stage D_2 metastatic carcinoma – To achieve benefit from treatment, flutamide capsules should be initiated with the LHRH-agonist and continued until progression.

➤*Unlabeled uses:* Treatment of hirsutism in women.

Administration and Dosage

➤*Approved by the FDA:* January 27, 1989.

The recommended dosage is 2 capsules 3 times a day at 8-hour intervals for a total daily dose of 750 mg.

➤*Storage/Stability:* Dispense with a child-resistant closure in a tight, light-resistant container as defined in the USP/NF. Store at 25°C (77°F); excursions permitted to 15° to 30°C (59° to 86°F).

Actions

➤*Pharmacology:* In animal studies, flutamide demonstrates potent antiandrogenic effects. It exerts its antiandrogenic action by inhibiting androgen uptake or by inhibiting nuclear binding of androgen in target tissues or both. Prostatic carcinoma is known to be androgen sensitive and responds to treatment that counteracts the effect of androgen or removes the source of androgen, (eg, castration). Elevations of plasma testosterone and estradiol levels have been noted following flutamide administration.

➤*Pharmacokinetics:*

Absorption – Analysis of plasma, urine, and feces following a single oral 200 mg dose of tritium-labeled flutamide to human volunteers showed that the drug is rapidly and completely absorbed. Following a single 250 mg oral dose to healthy adult volunteers, the biologically active alpha-hydroxylated metabolite reaches maximum plasma concentrations in about 2 hours, indicating that it is rapidly formed from flutamide. Food has no effect on the bioavailability of flutamide.

Distribution – In male rats administered an oral 5 mg/kg dose of ^{14}C-flutamide, neither flutamide nor any of its metabolites is preferentially accumulated in any tissue except the prostate. Total drug levels were highest 6 hours after drug administration in all tissues. Levels declined at roughly similar rates to low levels at 18 hours. Flutamide, in vivo, at steady-state plasma concentrations of 24 to 78 ng/mL, is 94% to 96% bound to plasma proteins. The active metabolite of flutamide, in vivo, at steady-state plasma concentrations of 1556 to 2284 ng/mL, is 92% to 94% bound to plasma proteins.

The major metabolite was present at higher concentrations than flutamide in all tissues studied. Following a single 250 mg oral dose to healthy adult volunteers, low plasma concentrations of flutamide were detected. The plasma half-life for the alpha-hydroxylated metabolite of flutamide is approximately 6 hours.

Metabolism – The composition of plasma radioactivity, following a single 200 mg oral dose of tritium-labeled flutamide to healthy adult volunteers, showed that flutamide is rapidly and extensively metabolized, with flutamide comprising only 2.5% of plasma radioactivity 1 hour after administration. At least 6 metabolites have been identified in plasma. The major plasma metabolite is a biologically active alpha-hydroxylated derivative which accounts for 23% of the plasma tritium 1 hour after drug administration. The major urinary metabolite is 2-amino-5-nitro-4-(trifluoromethyl)phenol.

Excretion – Flutamide and its metabolites are excreted mainly in the urine with only 4.2% of a single dose excreted in the feces over 72 hours.

Contraindications

Hypersensitivity to flutamide or any component of this preparation; severe hepatic impairment (baseline hepatic enzymes should be evaluated prior to treatment).

Warnings

➤*Use in women:* Flutamide capsules are for use only in men. This product has no indication for women, and should not be used in this population, particularly for non-serious or non-life-threatening conditions.

➤*Fetal toxicity:* Flutamide may cause fetal harm when administered to a pregnant woman (see Pregnancy).

➤*Aniline toxicity:* One metabolite of flutamide is 4-nitro-3-fluoromethylaniline. Several toxicities consistent with aniline exposure, including methemoglobinemia, hemolytic anemia and cholestatic jaundice have been observed in both animals and humans after flutamide administration. In patients susceptible to aniline toxicity (eg, persons with glucose-6-phosphate dehydrogenase deficiency, hemoglobin M disease and smokers), monitoring of methemoglobin levels should be considered.

➤*Hepatic function impairment:* See Warning Box.

➤*Carcinogenesis:* In a 1-year dietary study in male rats, interstitial cell adenomas of the testes were present in 49% to 75% of all treated rats (daily doses of 10, 30, and 50 mg/kg/day were administered). These produced plasma C_{max} values that are 1-, 2- to 3-, and 4-fold, respectively, those associated with therapeutic doses in humans. In male rats similarly dosed for 1 year, tumors were still present after 1 year of a drug-free period, but the incidences were 43% to 47%.

➤*Mutagenesis:* Flutamide did not demonstrate DNA-modifying activity in the Ames *Salmonella*/microsome mutagenesis assay. Dominant lethal tests in rats were negative. Reduced sperm counts were observed during a 6-week study of flutamide monotherapy in healthy human volunteers. Flutamide did not affect estrous cycles or interfere with the mating behavior of male and female rats when the drug was administered at 25 and 75 mg/kg/day prior to mating. Males treated with 150 mg/kg/day (30 times the minimum effective antiandrogenic dose) failed to mate; mating behavior returned to normal after dosing was stopped. Conception rates were decreased in all dosing groups. Suppression of spermatogenesis was observed in rats dosed for 52 weeks at approximately 3, 8, or 17 times the human dose and in dogs dosed for 78 weeks at 1.4, 2.3, and 3.7 times the human dose.

➤*Pregnancy: Category D.* There was decreased 24-hour survival in the offspring of pregnant rats treated with flutamide at doses of 30, 100 or 200 mg/kg/day (approximately 3, 9 and 19 times the human dose). A slight increase in minor variations in the development of the sternebrae and vertebrae was seen in fetuses of rats treated with 2 higher doses. Feminization of the male rats also occurred at the 2 higher dose levels. There was a decreased survival rate in the offspring of rabbits receiving the highest dose (15 mg/kg/day, equal 1.4 times the human dose).

Precautions

➤*Monitoring:* Regular assessment of serum prostate specific antigen (PSA) may be helpful in monitoring the patient's response. If PSA levels rise significantly and consistently during flutamide therapy, the patient should be evaluated for clinical progression. For patients who have objective progression of disease together with an elevated PSA, a treatment period free of antiandrogen while continuing the LHRH analogue may be considered.

Drug Interactions

➤*Anticoagulants:* Increases in prothrombin time have been noted in patients receiving long-term warfarin therapy after flutamide was initiated. Therefore close monitoring of prothrombin time is recommended, and adjustment of the anticoagulant dose may be necessary when flutamide capsules are administered concomitantly with warfarin.

Adverse Reactions

Gynecomastia – In clinical trials, gynecomastia occurred in 9% of patients receiving flutamide together with medical castration.

➤*Stage B_2-C prostatic carcinoma:*

Flutamide Adverse Reactions During Acute Radiation Therapy (%)

Adverse reaction	Goserelin acetate implant and flutamide and radiation (n = 231)	Radiation only (n = 235)
Rectum/large bowel	80%	76%
Bladder	58%	60%
Skin	37%	37%

FLUTAMIDE — ORAL

Flutamide Adverse Reactions During Late Radiation Phase (%)		
Adverse reaction	Goserelin acetate implant and flutamide and radiation (n = 231)	Radiation only (n = 235)
Diarrhea	36%	40%
Cystitits	16%	16%
Rectal bleeding	14%	20%
Proctitis	8%	8%
Hematuria	7%	12%

Additional adverse event data were collected for the combination therapy with radiation group over both the hormonal treatment and hormonal treatment plus radiation phases of the study. Adverse experiences occurring in more than 5% of patients in this group, over both parts of the study, were hot flashes (46%), diarrhea (40%), nausea (9%), and skin rash (8%).

➤*Stage D_2 metastatic carcinoma:* The following adverse experiences were reported during a multicenter clinical trial comparing flutamide and LHRH agonist vs placebo and LHRH agonist.

Flutamide Adverse Reactions (%)		
Adverse reaction	Flutamide and LHRH agonist (n = 294)	Placebo and LHRH agonist (n = 285)
Hot flashes	61%	57%
Loss of libido	36%	31%
Impotence	33%	29%
Diarrhea	12%	4%
Nausea/vomiting	11%	10%
Gynecomastia	9%	11%
Other	7%	9%
Other GI	6%	4%

As shown in the table, for both treatment groups, the most frequently occurring adverse experiences (hot flashes, impotence, loss of libido) were those known to be associated with low serum androgen levels and known to occur with LHRH agonists alone.

The only notable difference was the higher incidence of diarrhea in the flutamide and LHRH agonist group (12%), which was severe in 5% as opposed to the placebo and LHRH agonist (4%), which was severe in less than 1%.

➤*Additional adverse reactions:*

Cardiovascular – Hypertension in 1% of patients.

CNS – Drowsiness, confusion, depression, anxiety, or nervousness occurred in 1% of patients.

GI – Anorexia 4%, and other GI disorders occurred in 6% of patients.

Hematologic – Anemia occurred in 6%, leukopenia in 3%, and thrombocytopenia in 1% of patients.

Hepatic – Hepatitis and jaundice in less than 1% of patients.

Lab test abnormalities – Laboratory abnormalities including elevated AST, ALT, bilirubin values, SGGT, blood urea nitrogen (BUN), and serum creatinine have been reported.

Local – Irritation at the injection site and rash occurred in 3% of patients.

Miscellaneous – Edema occurred in 4%, GU and neuromuscular symptoms in 2%, and pulmonary symptoms in less than 1% of patients. Malignant breast neoplasms have occurred rarely in male patients being treated with flutamide.

Postmarketing: In addition, the following spontaneous adverse experiences have been reported during the marketing of flutamide: Hemolytic anemia, macrocytic anemia, methemoglobinemia, sulfhemoglobinemia, photosensitivity reactions (including erythema, ulceration, bullous eruptions, and epidermal necrolysis), and urine discoloration. The urine was noted to change to an amber or yellow-green appearance which can be attributed to the flutamide or its metabolites. Also reported were cholestatic jaundice, hepatic encephalopathy, and hepatic necrosis. The hepatic conditions were often reversible after discontinuing therapy; however, there have been reports of death following severe hepatic injury associated with use of flutamide.

Overdosage

➤*Symptoms:* In animal studies with flutamide alone, signs of overdose included hypoactivity, piloerection, slow respiration, ataxia, or lacrimation, anorexia, tranquilization, emesis, and methemoglobinemia.

Clinical trials have been conducted with flutamide in doses up to 1500 mg/day for periods up to 30 weeks with no serious adverse effects reported. Those adverse reactions reported included gynecomastia, breast tenderness, and some increases in AST. The single dose of flutamide ordinarily associated with symptoms of overdose or considered to be life-threatening has not been established.

➤*Treatment:* Flutamide is highly protein bound and is not cleared by hemodialysis. As in the management of overdosage with any drug, it should be borne in mind that multiple agents may have been taken. If vomiting does not occur spontaneously, it should be induced if the patient is alert. General supportive care, including frequent monitoring of the vital signs and close observation of the patient, is indicated.

Patient Information

Patients should be informed that flutamide capsules and the drug used for medical castration should be administered concomitantly, and that they should not interrupt their dosing or stop taking these medications without consulting their physician.

NILUTAMIDE

Rx	**Nilandron** (Aventis)	**Tablets:** 50 mg	Lactose. (168). White, biconvex. In 90s.
		150 mg	Lactose. (168D). White, biconvex. In 30s.

NILUTAMIDE — ORAL

Indications

➤*Metastatic prostate cancer:* For use in combination with surgical castration for the treatment of metastatic prostate cancer (stage D_2). For maximum benefit, nilutamide treatment must begin on the same day as or on the day after surgical castration.

➤*Unlabeled uses:* Treatment of metastatic prostate cancer alone or in combination with luteinizing hormone-releasing hormone (LHRH) agonists.

Administration and Dosage

➤*Approved by the FDA:* September 19, 1996.

The recommended dosage is 300 mg once a day for 30 days, followed thereafter by 150 mg once a day. Can be taken with or without food.

➤*Storage/Stability:* Store at 25°C (77°F); excursions permitted between 15° and 30°C (59° to 86°F [see USP controlled room temperature]). Protect from light.

Actions

➤*Pharmacology:* Prostate cancer is known to be androgen-sensitive and responds to androgen ablation. In animal studies, nilutamide has demonstrated antiandrogenic activity without other hormonal (ie, estrogen, progesterone, mineralocorticoid, glucocorticoid) effects. In vitro, nilutamide blocks the effects of testosterone at the androgen receptor level. In vivo, nilutamide interacts with the androgen receptor and prevents the normal androgenic response.

➤*Pharmacokinetics:*

Absorption – Analysis of blood, urine, and feces samples following a single oral 150 mg dose of (^{14}C-nilutamide in patients with metastatic prostate cancer showed that the drug is rapidly and completely absorbed and that it yields high and persistent plasma concentrations. In a 2-way crossover bioavailability study between a single nilutamide 150 mg tablet and 3 nilutamide 50 mg tablets, it was found that the 2 treatments were bioequivalent.

Distribution – After absorption of the drug, there is a detectable distribution phase. There is moderate binding of the drug to plasma proteins and low binding to erythrocytes. The binding is nonsaturable except in the case of alpha-1-glycoprotein, which makes a minor contribution to the total concentration of proteins in the plasma. The results of binding studies do not indicate any effects that would cause nonlinear pharmacokinetics.

Metabolism – The results of a human metabolism study using ^{14}C-radiolabeled tablets show that nilutamide is extensively metabolized, and less than 2% of the drug is excreted unchanged in urine after 5 days. Five (5) metabolites have been isolated from human urine. Two (2) metabolites display an asymmetric center, due to oxidation of a methyl group, resulting in the formation of D- and L-isomers. One of the metabolites was shown, in vitro, to possess 25% to 50% of the pharmacological activity of the parent drug, and the D-isomer of the active metabolite showed equal or greater potency compared to the L-isomer. However, the pharmacokinetics and the pharmacodynamics of the metabolites have not been fully investigated.

Excretion – The majority (62%) of orally administered (^{14}C)-nilutamide is eliminated in the urine during the first 120 hours after a single 150 mg dose. Fecal elimination is negligible, ranging from 1.4% to 7% of the dose after 4 to 5 days. Excretion of radioactivity in urine likely continues beyond 5 days. The mean elimination half-life of nilutamide determined in studies in which subjects received a single dose of 100 to 300 mg ranged from 38 to 59.1 hours, with most values between 41 and 49 hours. The elimination of at least 1 metabolite is generally longer than that of unchanged nilutamide (59 to 126 hours). During multiple dosing of 3 times 50 mg twice a day, steady state was reached within 2 to 4 weeks for most patients, and mean steady state AUC_{0-12} was 110% higher than the $AUC_{0-\infty}$ obtained from the first dose of 3 times 50 mg. These data and in vitro metabolism data suggest that, upon multiple dosing, metabolic enzyme inhibition may occur for this drug.

Contraindications

Severe hepatic impairment (baseline hepatic enzymes should be evaluated prior to treatment); severe respiratory insufficiency; hypersensitivity to nilutamide or any component of this preparation.

NILUTAMIDE — ORAL

Warnings

➤*Interstitial pneumonitis:* Interstitial pneumonitis has been reported in 2% of patients in controlled clinical trials in patients exposed to nilutamide. A small study in Japanese subjects showed that 8 of 47 patients (17%) developed interstitial pneumonitis. Reports of interstitial changes including pulmonary fibrosis that led to hospitalization and death have been reported rarely postmarketing. Symptoms included exertional dyspnea, cough, chest pain, and fever. X-rays showed interstitial or alveolo-interstitial changes, and pulmonary function tests revealed a restrictive pattern with decreased DLco. Most cases occurred within the first 3 months of treatment with nilutamide, and most reversed with discontinuation of therapy.

A routine chest x-ray should be performed prior to initiating treatment with nilutamide. Baseline pulmonary function tests may be considered. Patients should be instructed to report any new or worsening shortness of breath that they experience while on nilutamide. If symptoms occur, nilutamide should be immediately discontinued until it can be determined if the symptoms are drug related.

➤*Use in women:* Nilutamide has no indication for women, and should not be used in this population, particularly for nonserious or nonlife-threatening conditions.

➤*Aplastic anemia:* Foreign postmarketing surveillance has revealed isolated cases of aplastic anemia in which a causal relationship with nilutamide could not be ascertained.

➤*Hepatic function impairment:*

Hepatitis – Rare cases of death or hospitalization due to severe liver injury have been reported postmarketing in association with the use of nilutamide. Hepatotoxicity in these reports generally occurred within the first 3 to 4 months of treatment. Hepatitis or marked increases in liver enzymes leading to drug discontinuation occurred in 1% of nilutamide patients in controlled clinical trials.

Serum transaminase levels should be measured prior to starting treatment with nilutamide, at regular intervals for the first 4 months of treatment, and periodically thereafter. Liver function tests should also be obtained at the first sign or symptom suggestive of liver dysfunction (eg, nausea, vomiting, abdominal pain, fatigue, anorexia, "flu-like" symptoms, dark urine, jaundice, right upper quadrant tenderness). If at any time, a patient has jaundice, or their ALT rises above 2 times the upper limit of normal, nilutamide should be immediately discontinued with close follow-up of liver function tests until resolution.

➤*Carcinogenesis:* Administration of nilutamide to rats for 18 months at doses of 0, 5, 15, or 45 mg/kg/day produced benign Leydig-cell tumors in 35% of the high-dose male rats (AUC exposures in high-dose rats were approximately 1 to 2 times human AUC exposures with therapeutic doses). The increased incidence of Leydig-cell tumors is secondary to elevated luteinizing hormone (LH) concentrations resulting from loss of feedback inhibition at the pituitary. Elevated LH and testosterone concentrations are not observed in castrated men receiving nilutamide. Nilutamide had no effect on the incidence, size, or time of onset of any spontaneous tumor in rats.

➤*Pregnancy: Category C.* Animal reproduction studies have not been conducted with nilutamide. It is also not known whether nilutamide can cause fetal harm when administered to a pregnant woman or can affect reproductive capacity. Nilutamide should be given to a pregnant woman only if clearly needed.

➤*Children:* Safety and efficacy in pediatric patients have not been determined.

Drug Interactions

➤*CYP450 isoenzymes:* In vitro, nilutamide has been shown to inhibit the activity of liver cytochrome P450 isoenzymes and, therefore, may reduce the metabolism of compounds requiring these systems.

➤*Vitamin K antagonists/phenytoin/theophylline:* Consequently, drugs with a low therapeutic margin, such as vitamin K antagonists, phenytoin, and theophylline, could have a delayed elimination and increases in their serum half-life leading to a toxic level. The dosage of these drugs or others with a similar metabolism may need to be modified if they are administered concomitantly with nilutamide. For example, when vitamin K antagonists are administered concomitantly with nilutamide, prothrombin time should be carefully monitored and, if necessary, the dosage of vitamin K antagonists should be reduced.

Adverse Reactions

Nilutamide Adverse Reactions (%)

Adverse reaction	Nilutamide and surgical castration (n = 225)	Placebo and surgical castration (n = 232)
Cardiovascular		
Hypertension	5.3%	2.6%
GI		
Nausea	9.8%	6%
Constipation	7.1%	3.9%
Endocrine		
Hot flushes	28.4%	22.4%
Metabolic/Nutritional		
Increased AST	8%	3.9%
Increased ALT	7.6%	4.3%
CNS		
Dizziness	7.1%	3.4%
Respiratory		
Dyspnea	6.2%	7.3%
Special senses		
Impaired adaptation to dark	12.9%	1.3%
Abnormal vision	6.7%	1.7%
GU		
Urinary tract infection	8%	9.1%

Nilutamide Adverse Reactions (> 5%)

Adverse reactions	Nilutamide and leuprolide (n = 209)	Placebo and leuprolide (n = 202)
Miscellaneous		
Pain	26.8%	27.7%
Headache	13.9%	10.4%
Asthenia	19.1%	20.8%
Back pain	11.5%	16.8%
Abdominal pain	10%	5.4%
Chest pain	7.2%	4.5%
Flu syndrome	7.2%	3%
Fever	5.3%	6.4%
Cardiovascular		
Hypertension	9.1%	9.9%
GI		
Nausea	23.9%	8.4%
Constipation	19.6%	16.8%
Anorexia	11%	6.4%
Dyspepsia	6.7%	4.5%
Vomiting	5.7%	4%
Endocrine		
Hot flushes	66.5%	59.4%
Impotence	11%	12.9%
Libido decreased	11%	4.5%
Hematologic/Lymphatic		
Anemia	7.2%	6.4%
Metabolic/Nutritional		
Increased AST	12.9%	13.9%
Peripheral edema	12.4%	17.3%
Increased ALT	9.1%	8.9%
Musculoskeletal		
Bone pain	6.2%	5%
CNS		
Insomnia	16.3%	15.8%
Dizziness	10%	11.4%
Depression	8.6%	7.4%
Hypesthesia	5.3%	2%
Respiratory		
Dyspnea	10.5%	7.4%
Upper respiratory tract infection	8.1%	10.9%
Pneumonia	5.3%	3.5%
Dermatologic		
Sweating	6.2%	3%
Body hair loss	5.7%	0.5%

NILUTAMIDE — ORAL

Nilutamide Adverse Reactions (> 5%)		
Adverse reactions	Nilutamide and leuprolide (n = 209)	Placebo and leuprolide (n = 202)
Dry skin	5.3%	2.5%
Rash	5.3%	4%
Special senses		
Impaired adaptation to dark	56.9%	5.4%
Chromatopsia	8.6%	0%
Impaired adaptation to light	7.7%	1%
Abnormal vision	6.2%	4.5%
GU		
Testicular atrophy	16.3%	12.4%
Gynecomastia	10.5%	11.9%
Urinary tract infection	8.6%	21.3%
Hematuria	8.1%	7.9%
Urinary tract disorder	7.2%	10.4%
Nocturia	6.7%	6.4%

Some frequently occurring adverse experiences (eg, hot flushes, impotence, and decreased libido) are known to be associated with low serum androgen levels and known to occur with medical or surgical castration alone. Notable was the higher incidence of visual disturbances (variously described as impaired adaptation to darkness, abnormal vision, and colored vision), which led to treatment discontinuation in 1% to 2% of patients.

Interstitial pneumonitis – Interstitial pneumonitis occurred in one (less than 1%) patient receiving nilutamide in combination with surgical castration and in 7 patients (3%) receiving nilutamide in combination with leuprolide and 1 patient receiving placebo in combination with leuprolide. Overall, it has been reported in 2% of patients receiving nilutamide. This included a report of interstitial pneumonitis in 8 of 47 patients (17%) in a small study performed in Japan. In addition, the following adverse experiences were reported in 2% to 5% of patients treated with nilutamide in combination with leuprolide or orchiectomy:

➤*Cardiovascular:* Angina (2%), heart failure (3%), syncope (2%).

➤*CNS:* Dry mouth (2%), nervousness (2%), paresthesia (3%).

➤*Dermatologic:* Pruritus (2%).

➤*GI:* Diarrhea (2%), GI disorder (2%), GI hemorrhage (2%), melena (2%).

➤*Lab test abnormalities:* Increased haptoglobin (2%), leukopenia (3%), alkaline phosphatase increased (3%), increased blood urea nitrogen (BUN) (2%), creatinine increased (2%), hyperglycemia (4%).

➤*Metabolic/Nutritional:* Alcohol intolerance (5%), edema (2%), weight loss (2%).

➤*Musculoskeletal:* Arthritis (2%).

➤*Respiratory:* Increased cough (2%), interstitial lung disease (2%), lung disorder (4%), rhinitis (2%).

➤*Special senses:* Cataract (2%), photophobia (2%).

➤*Miscellaneous:* Malaise (2%).

Overdosage

➤*Symptoms:* One case of massive overdosage has been published. A 79-year-old man attempted suicide by ingesting 13 g of nilutamide (ie, 43 times the maximum recommended dose). Despite immediate gastric lavage and oral administration of activated charcoal, plasma nilutamide levels peaked at 6 times the normal range 2 hours after ingestion. There were no clinical signs or symptoms or changes in parameters such as transaminases or chest x-ray. Maintenance treatment (150 mg/day) was resumed 30 days later.

In repeated-dose tolerance studies, doses of 600 mg/day and 900 mg/day were administered to 9 and 4 patients, respectively. The ingestion of these doses was associated with GI disorders, including nausea and vomiting, malaise, headache, and dizziness. In addition, a transient elevation in hepatic enzyme levels was noted in 1 patient.

➤*Treatment:* Since nilutamide is protein bound, dialysis may not be useful as treatment for overdose. As in the management of overdosage with any drug, it should be borne in mind that multiple agents may have been taken. If vomiting does not occur spontaneously, it should be induced if the patient is alert. General supportive care, including frequent monitoring of the vital signs and close observation of the patient, is indicated.

Patient Information

Patients should be informed that nilutamide tablets should be started on the day of, or on the day after, surgical castration. They should also be informed that they should not interrupt their dosing of nilutamide or stop taking this medication without consulting their physicians.

Because of the possibility of interstitial pneumonitis, patients should also be told to report immediately any dyspnea or aggravation of preexisting dyspnea.

Because of the possibility of hepatitis, patients should be told to consult with their physicians should nausea, vomiting, abdominal pain, or jaundice occur.

Because of the possibility of an intolerance to alcohol (eg, facial flushes, malaise, hypotension) following ingestion of nilutamide, it is recommended that intake of alcoholic beverages be avoided by patients who experience this reaction. This effect has been reported in about 5% of patients treated with nilutamide.

In clinical trials, 13% of 57% of patients receiving nilutamide reported a delay in adaptation to dark, ranging from seconds to a few minutes, when passing from a lighted area to a dark area. This effect sometimes does not abate as drug treatment is continued. Patients who experience this effect should be cautioned about driving at night or through tunnels. This effect can be alleviated by the wearing of tinted glasses.

Progestins

MEGESTROL ACETATE

Megestrol acetate is also available as a suspension for appetite enhancement in AIDS patients; refer to the monograph in the Endocrine and Metabolic Agents chapter. For complete and comparative prescribing information, see the Progestins group monograph in the Endocrine/Metabolic chapter.

MEDROXYPROGESTERONE ACETATE

For complete and comparative prescribing information, see the Progestins group monograph in the Endocrine/Metabolic chapter and the Medroxyprogesterone injection monograph in the Contraceptive Hormones group monograph.

Antiestrogens

TAMOXIFEN CITRATE

Rx	**Tamoxifen Citrate** (Various, eg, Barr, Ivax, Mylan, Roxane, Teva)	**Tablets:** 10 mg (as base)	In 60s, 180s, 500s, 1,000s, and UD 100s.
Rx	**Nolvadex** (AstraZeneca)		(NOLVADEX 600). White. In 60s.
Rx	**Tamoxifen Citrate** (Various, eg, Barr, Ivax, Mylan, Roxane, Teva)	**Tablets:** 20 mg (as base)	In 30s, 90s, 100s, 500s, 1,000s, and UD 100s.
Rx	**Nolvadex** (AstraZeneca)		(NOLVADEX 604). White. In 30s.
Rx sf	**Soltamox** (Savient)	**Oral solution:** 10 mg per 5 mL (15.2 mg as tamoxifen citrate)	Ethanol, sorbitol. Licorice and aniseed flavors. In 150 mL.

TAMOXIFEN CITRATE — ORAL

WARNING

For women with ductal carcinoma in situ (DCIS) and women at high risk for breast cancer – Serious and life-threatening events associated with tamoxifen in the risk-reduction setting (women at high risk for cancer and women with DCIS) include uterine malignancies, stroke, and pulmonary embolism (PE). Incidence rates for these events were estimated from the National Surgical Adjuvant Breast and Bowel Project (NSABP) P-1 trial. Uterine malignancies consist of both endometrial adenocarcinoma (incidence rate per 1,000 women years of 2.2 for tamoxifen versus 0.71 for placebo) and uterine sarcoma (incidence rate per 1,000 women years of 0.17 for tamoxifen versus 0.4 for placebo). (Updated long-term follow-up data [median length of follow-up is 6.9 years] from NSABP P-1 study.)

For stroke, the incidence rate per 1,000 women years was 1.43 for tamoxifen versus 1 for placebo. For PE, the incidence rate per 1,000 women years was 0.75 for tamoxifen versus 0.25 for placebo.

Some of the strokes, PE, and uterine malignancies were fatal.

Discuss the potential benefits versus the potential risks of these serious events with women at high risk of breast cancer and with women with DCIS considering tamoxifen to reduce their risks of developing breast cancer.

The benefits of tamoxifen outweigh its risks in women already diagnosed with breast cancer.

Indications

➤*Adjuvant treatment of breast cancer:* For the treatment of node-positive breast cancer in postmenopausal women following total mastectomy or segmental mastectomy, axillary dissection, and breast irradiation. In some tamoxifen adjuvant studies, most of the benefit to date has been in the subgroup with 4 or more positive axillary nodes.

For the treatment of axillary node-negative breast cancer in women following total mastectomy or segmental mastectomy, axillary dissection, and breast irradiation.

The ER- and progesterone-receptor values may help to predict whether adjuvant tamoxifen therapy is likely to be beneficial.

Tamoxifen reduces the occurrence of contralateral breast cancer in patients receiving adjuvant tamoxifen therapy for breast cancer.

➤*DCIS:* In women with DCIS, following breast surgery and radiation, tamoxifen is indicated to reduce the risk of invasive breast cancer. Base the decisions regarding therapy with tamoxifen for the reduction in breast cancer incidence upon an individual assessment of the benefits and risks of tamoxifen therapy.

Current data from clinical trials support 5 years of adjuvant tamoxifen therapy for patients with breast cancer.

➤*Metastatic breast cancer:* Effective in the treatment of metastatic breast cancer in women and men. In premenopausal women with metastatic breast cancer, tamoxifen is an alternative to oophorectomy or ovarian irradiation. Available evidence indicates that patients whose tumors are estrogen receptor (ER) positive are more likely to benefit from tamoxifen therapy.

➤*Reduction of breast cancer incidence in high-risk women:* To reduce the incidence of breast cancer in women at high risk for breast cancer. This effect was shown in a study of 5 years planned duration, with a median follow-up of 4.2 years. Twenty-five percent of the participants received the drug for 5 years. The longer-term effects are not known. In this study, there was no impact of tamoxifen on overall or breast cancer–related mortality.

Tamoxifen is indicated only for high-risk women. "High risk" is defined as women at least 35 years of age with a 5-year predicted risk of breast cancer greater than or equal to 1.67%, as calculated by the Gail model.

Examples of combinations of factors predicting a 5-year risk greater than or equal to 1.67% are the following:

35 years of age or older and any of the following combination of factors –
- one first-degree relative with a history of breast cancer, 2 or more benign biopsies, and a history of a breast biopsy showing atypical hyperplasia
- at least 2 first-degree relatives with a history of breast cancer and a personal history of at least 1 breast biopsy
- lobular cancer in situ (LCIS)

40 years of age or older and any of the following combination of factors –
- one first-degree relative with a history of breast cancer, 2 or more benign biopsies, age at first live birth 25 years or older, and age at menarche 11 years or younger
- at least 2 first-degree relatives with a history of breast cancer and age at first live birth 19 years or younger.
- one first-degree relative with a history of breast cancer and a personal history of a breast biopsy showing atypical hyperplasia

45 years of age or older and any of the following combination of factors –
- at least 2 first-degree relatives with a history of breast cancer and age at first live birth 24 years or younger.
- one first-degree relative with a history of breast cancer with a history of a benign breast biopsy, age at menarche 11 years or younger, and age at first live birth 20 years or older.

50 years of age or older and any of the following combination of factors –
- at least 2 first-degree relatives with a history of breast cancer
- history of 1 breast biopsy showing atypical hyperplasia, age at first live birth 30 years or older, and age at menarche 11 years or younger
- history of at least 2 breast biopsies with a history of atypical hyperplasia, and age at first live birth 30 years or older

55 years of age or older and any of the following combination of factors –
- one first-degree relative with a history of breast cancer with a personal history of a benign breast biopsy and age at menarche 11 years or younger
- history of at least 2 breast biopsies with a history of atypical hyperplasia and age at first live birth 20 years or older

60 years of age or older and the following –
- five-year predicted risk of breast cancer greater than or equal to 1.67%, as calculated by the Gail model

For women whose risk factors are not described in the preceding examples, the Gail model is necessary to estimate absolute breast cancer risk. Health care providers can obtain a Gail model risk assessment tool by calling 1-800-544-2007.

There are no data available regarding the effect of tamoxifen on breast cancer incidence in women with inherited mutations (BRCA1, BRCA2) to be able to make specific recommendations on the efficacy of tamoxifen in these patients.

After an assessment of the risk of developing breast cancer, base the decision regarding therapy with tamoxifen for the reduction in breast cancer incidence upon an individual assessment of the benefits and risks. In the NSABP P-1 trial, tamoxifen treatment lowered the risk of developing breast cancer during the follow-up period of the trial but did not eliminate breast cancer risk.

➤*Unlabeled uses:* Ovulation stimulation in specially selected anovulatory women desiring pregnancy, mainly those with amenorrhea or oligomenorrhea who were previously taking oral contraceptives; management and treatment of some types of mastalgia (eg, cyclical); malignant carcinoid tumor and carcinoid syndrome; migraine associated with menstruation; metastatic malignant melanoma; oligozoospermia; McCune-Albright syndrome in female pediatric patients (in combination with other agents); metastatic melanoma; desmoid tumors; symptomatic gynecomastia (10 to 40 mg/day).

Administration and Dosage

➤*Approved by the FDA:* December 10, 1985.

➤*Breast cancer:* 20 to 40 mg; dosages greater than 20 mg/day should be given in divided doses (morning and evening). A 20 mg dose of tamoxifen oral solution is administered as 10 mL (equivalent to 2 teaspoons).

In 3 single-agent adjuvant studies in women, 1 tamoxifen 10 mg tablet was administered 2 (Eastern Cooperative Oncology Group [ECOG] and tamoxifen adjuvant trial organization [NATO]) or 3 (Toronto) times a day for 2 years. In the NSABP B-14 adjuvant study in women with node-negative breast cancer, 1 tamoxifen 10 mg tablet was given twice a day for at least 5 years. Results of the B-14 study suggest that continuation of therapy beyond 5 years does not provide additional benefit. In the Early Breast Cancer Trialists' Collaborative Group (EBCTCG) 1995 overview, the reduction in recurrence and mortality was greater in those studies that used tamoxifen for approximately 5 years than in those that used tamoxifen for a shorter period of therapy. There was no indication that dosages greater than 20 mg/day were more effective. Current data from clinical trials support 5 years of adjuvant tamoxifen therapy for patients with breast cancer.

➤*DCIS:* 20 mg/day for 5 years.

➤*Reduction of breast cancer incidence in high-risk women:* 20 mg/day for 5 years; there are no data to support the use of tamoxifen for other than for 5 years.

➤*Storage/Stability:*

Tablets – Store at room temperature, 20° to 25°C (68° to 77°F). Keep in a well-closed, light-resistant container. Keep out of the reach of children.

Oral solution – Do not store above 25°C (77°F). Store in the original package in order to protect from light. Use within 3 months of opening. Do not freeze or refrigerate.

Actions

➤*Pharmacology:* Tamoxifen is a nonsteroidal agent that has demonstrated potent antiestrogenic properties in animal test systems. The antiestrogenic effects may be related to its ability to compete with estrogen for binding sites in target tissues such as breast. Tamoxifen inhibits the induction of rat mammary carcinoma induced by dimethylbenzanthracene (DMBA) and causes the regression of already established DMBA-induced

TAMOXIFEN CITRATE — ORAL

tumors. In this rat model, tamoxifen appears to exert its antitumor effects by binding the estrogen receptors.

In cytosols derived from human breast adenocarcinomas, tamoxifen competes with estradiol for ER protein.

➤*Pharmacokinetics:*

Absorption/Distribution –

Tablets: Following a single, oral dose of tamoxifen 20 mg, an average peak plasma concentration (C_{max}) of 40 ng/mL (range, 35 to 45 ng/mL) occurred approximately 5 hours after dosing. The decline in plasma concentrations of tamoxifen is biphasic, with a terminal elimination half-life of about 5 to 7 days. The average C_{max} of N-desmethyl tamoxifen is 15 ng/mL (range, 10 to 20 ng/mL). Chronic administration of tamoxifen 10 mg given twice daily for 3 months to patients results in average steady-state plasma concentrations of 120 ng/mL (range, 67 to 183 ng/mL) for tamoxifen and 336 ng/mL (range, 148 to 654 ng/mL) for N-desmethyl tamoxifen. The average steady-state plasma concentrations (C_{ss}) of tamoxifen and N-desmethyl tamoxifen after administration of tamoxifen 20 mg once daily for 3 months are 122 ng/mL (range, 71 to 183 ng/mL) and 353 ng/mL (range, 152 to 706 ng/mL), respectively. After initiation of therapy, C_{ss} for tamoxifen are achieved in about 4 weeks, and C_{ss} for N-desmethyl tamoxifen are achieved in about 8 weeks, suggesting a half-life of approximately 14 days for this metabolite. In a steady-state, crossover study of tamoxifen 10 mg tablets given twice a day versus a tamoxifen 20 mg tablet given once daily, the tamoxifen 20 mg tablet was bioequivalent to the tamoxifen 10 mg tablets.

Oral solution: A pharmacokinetic study was performed in healthy peri- and postmenopausal women to evaluate the bioavailability of tamoxifen oral solution (n = 30) in comparison with the commercially available tamoxifen tablets (n = 33) under fasting conditions. A third arm evaluated the effect of food on tamoxifen oral solution (n = 16 evaluable). The rate and extent of absorption of tamoxifen oral solution was found to be bioequivalent to that of tamoxifen tablets under fasting conditions.

• *Effect of food* – In the food effect arm, the C_{max} and area under the curve (AUC) were comparable to the fasting group. Time to maximum concentration was slightly longer in the fed group. There was no difference in bioavailability of tamoxifen oral solution between fed and fasting states, and therefore tamoxifen oral solution can be given without regard to meals.

Metabolism – Tamoxifen is extensively metabolized after oral administration. N-desmethyl tamoxifen is the major metabolite found in patients' plasma. The biological activity of N-desmethyl tamoxifen appears to be similar to that of tamoxifen. Four-hydroxytamoxifen and a side chain primary alcohol derivative of tamoxifen have been identified as minor metabolites in plasma. Tamoxifen is a substrate of cytochrome P-450 3A, 2C9, and 2D6, and an inhibitor of P-glycoprotein.

Excretion – Studies in women receiving 20 mg of ^{14}C (radiolabeled) tamoxifen have shown that approximately 65% of the administered dose was excreted from the body over a period of 2 weeks, with fecal excretion as the primary route of elimination. The drug is excreted mainly as polar conjugates, with unchanged drug and unconjugated metabolites accounting for less than 30% of the total fecal radioactivity.

Special populations –

Children: In pediatric patients, an average $C_{ss,\ max}$ and AUC were of 187 ng/mL and 4,110 ng h/mL, respectively, and $C_{ss,\ max}$ occurred approximately 8 hours after dosing. Clearance (CL/F) as body weight adjusted in female pediatric patients was approximately 2.3-fold higher than in female breast cancer patients. In the youngest cohort of female pediatric patients (2 to 6 years of age), CL/F was 2.6-fold higher; in the oldest cohort (7 to 10.9 years of age), CL/F was approximately 1.9-fold higher. Exposure to N-desmethyl tamoxifen was comparable between the pediatric and adult patients. The safety and efficacy of tamoxifen for girls 2 to 10 years of age with McCune-Albright syndrome and precocious puberty have not been studied beyond 1 year of treatment. The long-term effects of tamoxifen therapy in girls have not been established. In adults treated with tamoxifen, an increase in incidence of uterine malignancies, stroke, and PE has been noted.

The use of tamoxifen oral solution in pediatric patients has not been evaluated.

Contraindications

Known hypersensitivity to the drug or any of its ingredients.

➤*Reduction of breast cancer incidence in high-risk women:* In women who require concomitant coumarin-type anticoagulant therapy or in women with a history of deep vein thrombosis (DVT) or PE.

Warnings

➤*Hypercalcemia:* As with other additive hormonal therapy (estrogens and androgens), hypercalcemia has been reported in some breast cancer patients with bone metastases within a few weeks of starting treatment with tamoxifen. If hypercalcemia does occur, take appropriate measures and, if severe, discontinue tamoxifen.

➤*Uterus (endometrial cancer) and uterine sarcoma effects:* An increased incidence of uterine malignancies has been reported in association with tamoxifen treatment. The underlying mechanism is unknown, but may be related to the estrogen-like effect of tamoxifen. Most uterine malignancies seen in association with tamoxifen are classified as adenocarcinoma of the endometrium. However, rare uterine sarcomas, including malignant mixed mullerian tumors, have also been reported. Uterine sarcoma is generally associated with a higher International Federation of Gynecology and Obstetrics (FIGO) stage (III/IV) at diagnosis, poorer prognosis, and shorter survival. Uterine sarcoma has been reported to occur more frequently among long-term users (greater than or equal to 2 years) of tamoxifen than nonusers. Some of the uterine malignancies (endometrial carcinoma or uterine sarcoma) have been fatal.

In the NSABP P-1 trial, among participants randomized to tamoxifen, there was a statistically significant increase in the incidence of endometrial cancer: 33 cases of invasive endometrial cancer compared with 14 cases among participants randomized to placebo (relative risk [RR], 2.48; 95% confidence interval [CI], 1.27 to 4.92). The 33 cases in participants receiving tamoxifen were FIGO stage I, including 20 IA, 12 IB, and 1 IC endometrial adenocarcinomas. In participants randomized to placebo, 13 were FIGO stage 1 (8 IA and 5 IB) and 1 was FIGO stage IV. Five women on tamoxifen and 1 on placebo received postoperative radiation therapy in addition to surgery. This increase was observed primarily among women at least 50 years of age at the time of randomization (26 cases of invasive endometrial cancer, compared with 6 cases among participants randomized to placebo (RR, 4.5; 95% CI, 1.78 to 13.16). Among women 49 years of age or younger at the time of randomization, there were 7 cases of invasive endometrial cancer, compared with 8 cases among participants randomized to placebo (RR, 0.94; 95% CI, 0.28 to 2.89). If age at the time of diagnosis is considered, there were 4 cases of endometrial cancer among participants 49 years of age or younger randomized to tamoxifen compared with 2 among participants randomized to placebo (RR, 2.21; 95% CI, 0.4 to 12). For women 50 years of age or older at the time of diagnosis, there were 29 cases among participants randomized to tamoxifen compared with 12 among women on placebo (RR, 2.5; 95% CI, 1.3 to 4.9). The risk ratios were similar in the 2 groups, although fewer events occurred in younger women. Most (29 of 33 cases in the tamoxifen group) endometrial cancers were diagnosed in symptomatic women, although 5 of 33 cases in the tamoxifen group occurred in asymptomatic women. Among women receiving tamoxifen, the events appeared between 1 and 61 months (average, 32 months) from the start of treatment.

In an updated review of long-term data (median length of total follow-up is 6.9 years, including blind follow-up) on 8,306 women with an intact uterus at randomization in the NSABP P-1 risk reduction trial, the incidence of both adenocarcinomas and rare uterine sarcomas was increased in women taking tamoxifen. During blinded follow-up, there were 36 cases of FIGO stage I endometrial adenocarcinoma (22 were FIGO stage IA, 13 IB, and 1 IC) in women receiving tamoxifen and 15 cases in women receiving placebo (14 were FIGO stage I [9 IA and 5 IB], and 1 case was FIGO stage IV). Of the patients receiving tamoxifen who developed endometrial cancer, 1 with stage IA and 4 with stage IB cancers received radiation therapy. In the placebo group, 1 patient with FIGO stage 1B cancer received radiation therapy and the patient with FIGO stage IVB cancer received chemotherapy and hormonal therapy. During total follow-up, endometrial adenocarcinoma was reported in 53 women randomized to tamoxifen (30 cases of FIGO stage IA, 20 were stage IB, 1 was stage IC, and 2 were stage IIIC) and 17 women randomized to placebo (9 cases were FIGO stage IA, 6 were stage IB, 1 was stage IIIC, and 1 was stage IVB) (incidence per 1,000 women-years of 2.2 and 0.71, respectively). Some patients received postoperative radiation therapy in addition to surgery. Uterine sarcomas were reported in 4 women randomized to tamoxifen (1 was FIGO IA, 1 was FIGO IB, 1 was FIGO IIA, and 1 was FIGO IIIC) and 1 patient randomized to placebo (FIGO 1A) (incidence per 1,000 women-years of 0.17 and 0.04, respectively). Of the patients randomized to tamoxifen, the FIGO IA and IB cases were a malignant mixed mullerian tumor (MMMT) and sarcoma, respectively; the FIGO II was an MMMT; and the FIGO III was a sarcoma; and the 1 patient randomized to placebo had an MMMT. A similar increased incidence in endometrial adenocarcinoma and uterine sarcoma was observed among women receiving tamoxifen in 5 other NSABP clinical trials.

Promptly evaluate any patient receiving or who has previously received tamoxifen who reports abnormal vaginal bleeding. Perform annual gynecological exams on patients receiving or who have previously received tamoxifen, and they should be advised to promptly inform their health care provider if they experience any abnormal gynecological symptoms (eg, menstrual irregularities, abnormal vaginal bleeding, changes in vaginal discharge, pelvic pain or pressure).

In the P-1 trial, endometrial sampling did not alter the endometrial cancer detection rate compared with women who did not undergo endometrial sampling (0.6% with sampling, 0.5% without sampling) for women with an intact uterus. There are no data to suggest that routine endometrial sampling in asymptomatic women taking tamoxifen to reduce the incidence of breast cancer would be beneficial.

Nonmalignant effects on the uterus – An increased incidence of endometrial changes including hyperplasia and polyps have been reported in association with tamoxifen treatment. The incidence and pattern of this increase suggest that the underlying mechanism is related to the estrogenic properties of tamoxifen.

There have been a few reports of endometriosis and uterine fibroids in women receiving tamoxifen. The underlying mechanism may be due to the partial estrogenic effect of tamoxifen. Ovarian cysts have also been observed in a small number of premenopausal patients with advanced breast cancer who have been treated with tamoxifen.

Tamoxifen has been reported to cause menstrual irregularity or amenorrhea.

➤*Thromboembolic effects:* There is evidence of an increased incidence of thromboembolic events, including DVT and PE, during tamoxifen therapy. When tamoxifen is coadministered with chemotherapy, there may be a further increase in the incidence of thromboembolic effects. For treatment of breast cancer, carefully consider the risks and benefits of tamoxifen in women with a history of thromboembolic events.

Data from the NSABP P-1 trial show that participants receiving tamoxifen without a history of PE had a statistically significant increase in PE (18, tamoxifen; 6, placebo; RR, 3.01; 95% CI, 1.15 to 9.27). Three of the PE, all in the tamoxifen arm, were fatal. Eighty-seven percent of the cases of PE occurred in women at least 50 years of age at randomization. Among women receiving tamoxifen, the events appeared between 2 and 60 months (average, 27 months) from start of treatment.

TAMOXIFEN CITRATE — ORAL

In this same population, a nonstatistically significant increase in DVT was seen in the tamoxifen group (30, tamoxifen; 19, placebo; RR, 1.59; 95% CI, 0.86 to 2.98). The same increase in RR was seen in women 49 years of age or younger and in women 50 years of age or older, although fewer events occurred in younger women. Women with thromboembolic events were at risk for a second related event (7 out of 25 women on placebo, 5 out of 48 women on tamoxifen) and were at risk for complications of the event and its treatment (0 out of 25 on placebo, 4 out of 48 on tamoxifen). Among women receiving tamoxifen, DVT events occurred between 2 and 57 months (average, 19 months) from the start of treatment.

There was a nonstatistically significant increase in stroke among patients randomized to tamoxifen (24, placebo; 34, tamoxifen; RR, 1.42; 95% CI, 0.82 to 2.51). Six of the 24 strokes in the placebo group were considered hemorrhagic in origin, and 10 of the 34 strokes in the tamoxifen group were categorized as hemorrhagic. Seventeen of the 34 strokes in the tamoxifen group were considered occlusive, and 7 were considered to be of unknown etiology. Fourteen of the 24 strokes on the placebo arm were reported to be occlusive and 4 of unknown etiology. Among these strokes, 3 strokes in the placebo group and 4 strokes in the tamoxifen group were fatal. Eighty-eight percent of the strokes occurred in women 50 years of age or older at the time of randomization. Among women receiving tamoxifen, the events occurred between 1 and 63 months (average, 30 months) from the start of treatment.

➤*Ophthalmic effects:* Ocular disturbances, including corneal changes, decrement in color perception, retinal vein thrombosis, and retinopathy have been reported in patients receiving tamoxifen. An increased incidence of cataracts and the need for cataract surgery have been reported in patients receiving tamoxifen.

In the NSABP P-1 trial, an increased risk of borderline significance of developing cataracts among those women without cataracts at baseline (540, tamoxifen; 483, placebo; RR, 1.13; 95% CI, 1 to 1.28) was observed. Among these same women, tamoxifen was associated with an increased risk of having cataract surgery (101, tamoxifen; 63, placebo; RR, 1.62; 95% CI, 1.18 to 2.22). Among all women on the trial (with or without cataracts at baseline), tamoxifen was associated with an increased risk of having cataract surgery (201, tamoxifen; 129, placebo; RR, 1.58; 95% CI, 1.26 to 1.97). Eye examinations were not required during the study. No other conclusions regarding noncataract ophthalmic events can be made.

➤*Hepatic effects:*

Liver cancer – In the Swedish trial using adjuvant tamoxifen 40 mg/day for 2 to 5 years, 3 cases of liver cancer have been reported in the tamoxifen-treated group versus 1 case in the observation group. In other clinical trials evaluating tamoxifen, no cases of liver cancer have been reported to date.

One case of liver cancer was reported in NSABP P-1 in a participant randomized to tamoxifen.

Nonmalignant effects – Tamoxifen has been associated with changes in liver enzyme levels, and on rare occasions, a spectrum of more severe liver abnormalities including fatty liver, cholestasis, hepatitis, and hepatic necrosis. A few of these serious cases included fatalities. In most reported cases, the relationship to tamoxifen is uncertain. However, some positive rechallenges and dechallenges have been reported.

In the NSABP P-1 trial, few grade 3 to 4 changes in liver function (AST, ALT, bilirubin, alkaline phosphatase) were observed (10 on placebo, 6 on tamoxifen). Serum lipids were not systematically collected.

➤*Carcinogenesis:* A conventional carcinogenesis study in rats at dosages of 5, 20, and 35 mg/kg/day (about 1-, 3-, and 7-fold the daily maximum recommended human dosage [MRHD] on a mg/m^2 basis) administered by oral gavage for up to 2 years revealed a significant increase in hepatocellular carcinoma at all doses. The incidence of these tumors was significantly greater among rats administered 20 or 35 mg/kg/day (69%) compared with those administered 5 mg/kg/day (14%). In a separate study, rats were administered tamoxifen 45 mg/kg/day (about 9-fold the daily MRHD on a mg/m^2 basis); hepatocellular neoplasia was exhibited at 3 to 6 months.

Granulosa cell ovarian tumors and interstitial cell testicular tumors were observed in 2 separate mouse studies. The mice were administered the trans and racemic forms of tamoxifen for 13 to 15 months at dosages of 5, 20, and 50 mg/kg/day (about 0.5-, 2-, and 5-fold the daily MRHD on a mg/m^2 basis).

Other cancers: A number of second primary tumors, occurring at sites other than the endometrium, have been reported following the treatment of breast cancer with tamoxifen in clinical trials. Data from the NSABP B-14 and P-1 studies show no increase in other (nonuterine) cancers among patients receiving tamoxifen. Whether an increased risk for other (nonuterine) cancers is associated with tamoxifen is still uncertain and continues to be evaluated.

➤*Mutagenesis:* No genotoxic potential was found in a conventional battery of in vivo and in vitro tests with pro- and eukaryotic test systems with drug-metabolizing systems. However, increased levels of deoxyribonucleic acid (DNA) adducts were observed by ^{32}P postlabeling in DNA from rat liver and cultured human lymphocytes. Tamoxifen has also been found to increase levels of micronucleus formation in vitro in human lymphoblastoid cell line (MCL-5). Based on these findings, tamoxifen is genotoxic in rodent and human MCL-5 cells.

➤*Fertility impairment:* Tamoxifen produced impairment of fertility and conception in female rats at dosages of 0.04 mg/kg/day (about 0.01-fold the daily MRHD on a mg/m^2 basis) when dosed for 2 weeks prior to mating through day 7 of pregnancy. At this dose, fertility and reproductive indices were markedly reduced with total fetal mortality. Fetal mortality was also increased at dosages of 0.16 mg/kg/day (about 0.03-fold the daily MRHD on a mg/m^2 basis) when female rats were dosed from days 7 to 17 of pregnancy. Tamoxifen produced abortion, premature delivery, and fetal death in rabbits administered dosages greater than or equal to 0.125 mg/kg/day (about 0.05-fold the daily MRHD on a mg/m^2 basis). There were no teratogenic changes in either rats or rabbits.

➤*Pregnancy: Category D.* Tamoxifen may cause fetal harm when administered to a pregnant woman. Advise women not to become pregnant while taking tamoxifen or within 2 months of discontinuing tamoxifen and to use barrier or nonhormonal contraceptive measures if sexually active. Tamoxifen does not cause infertility, even in the presence of menstrual irregularity. Effects on reproductive functions are expected from the antiestrogenic properties of the drug. In reproductive studies in rats at dose levels equal to or below the human dose, nonteratogenic developmental skeletal changes were seen and were found reversible. In addition, in fertility studies in rats and in teratology studies in rabbits using doses at or below those used in humans, a lower incidence of embryo implantation and a higher incidence of fetal death or retarded in utero growth were observed, with slower learning behavior in some rat pups when compared with historical controls. Several pregnant marmosets were dosed with 10 mg/kg/day (about 2-fold the daily MRHD on a mg/m^2 basis) during organogenesis or in the last half of pregnancy. No deformations were seen and, although the dose was high enough to terminate pregnancy in some animals, those that did maintain pregnancy showed no evidence of teratogenic malformations.

In rodent models of fetal reproductive tract development, tamoxifen (at dosages 0.002- to 2.4-fold the MRHD on a mg/m^2 basis) caused changes in both sexes that are similar to those caused by estradiol, ethinylestradiol, and diethylstilbestrol. Although the clinical relevance of these changes is unknown, some of these changes, especially vaginal adenosis, are similar to those seen in young women who were exposed to diethylstilbestrol in utero and who have a 1 in 1,000 risk of developing clear cell adenocarcinoma of the vagina or cervix. To date, in utero exposure to tamoxifen has not been shown to cause vaginal adenosis or clear cell adenocarcinoma of the vagina or cervix in young women. However, only a small number of young women have been exposed to tamoxifen in utero, and a smaller number have been followed long enough (to 15 to 20 years of age) to determine whether vaginal or cervical neoplasia could occur as a result of this exposure.

There are no adequate and well-controlled trials of tamoxifen in pregnant women. There have been a small number of reports of vaginal bleeding, spontaneous abortions, birth defects, and fetal deaths in pregnant women. If this drug is used during pregnancy, or the patient becomes pregnant while taking this drug, or within approximately 2 months after discontinuing therapy, inform the patient of the potential risks to the fetus, including the potential long-term risk of a diethylstilbestrol-like syndrome.

Reduction of breast cancer incidence in high-risk women – For sexually active women of childbearing potential, initiate tamoxifen therapy during menstruation. In women with menstrual irregularity, a negative chorionic gonadotropin immediately prior to the initiation of therapy is sufficient.

Women who are pregnant or who plan to become pregnant should not take tamoxifen to reduce their risk of breast cancer. Effective nonhormonal contraception must be used by all premenopausal women taking tamoxifen if they are sexually active. Tamoxifen does not cause infertility, even in the presence of menstrual irregularity. For sexually active women of childbearing potential, initiate tamoxifen therapy during menstruation. In women with menstrual irregularity, a negative chorionic gonadotropin immediately prior to the initiation of therapy is sufficient.

➤*Lactation:* It is not known whether this drug is excreted in human milk. Because many drugs are excreted in human milk and because of the potential for serious adverse reactions in breast-feeding infants from tamoxifen, decide whether to discontinue breast-feeding or the drug, taking into account the importance of the drug to the mother.

Tamoxifen has been reported to inhibit lactation. Two placebo-controlled studies in over 150 women have shown that tamoxifen significantly inhibits early postpartum milk production. In both studies tamoxifen was administered within 24 hours of delivery for between 5 and 18 days. The effect of tamoxifen on established milk production is not known.

There are no data that address whether tamoxifen is excreted into human milk. If excreted, there are no data regarding the effects of tamoxifen in breast milk on the breast-fed infant or breast-fed animals. However, direct neonatal exposure of tamoxifen to mice and rats (not via breast milk) produced (1) reproduction tract lesions in female rodents (similar to those seen in humans after intrauterine exposure to diethylstilbestrol) and (2) functional defects of the reproductive tract in male rodents such as testicular atrophy and arrest of spermatogenesis.

Because of the potential for serious adverse reactions in breast-feeding infants from tamoxifen, women taking tamoxifen should not breast-feed.

➤*Children:* The safety and efficacy of tamoxifen for girls 2 to 10 years of age with McCune-Albright syndrome and precocious puberty have not been studied beyond 1 year of treatment. The long-term effects of tamoxifen therapy for girls have not been established. In adults treated with tamoxifen, an increase in incidence of uterine malignancies, stroke, and PE has been noted.

Precautions

➤*Monitoring:* Perform periodic complete blood cell counts, including platelet counts and periodic liver function tests.

Instruct women who are taking or having previously taken tamoxifen to seek prompt medical attention for new breast lumps, vaginal bleeding, gynecologic symptoms (eg, menstrual irregularities, changes in vaginal discharge, pelvic pain or pressure), symptoms of leg swelling or tenderness,

TAMOXIFEN CITRATE — ORAL

unexplained shortness of breath, or changes in vision. Women should inform all health care providers, regardless of the reason for evaluation, that they take tamoxifen.

Women taking tamoxifen to reduce the incidence of breast cancer should have a breast examination, a mammogram, and a gynecologic examination prior to the initiation of therapy. These studies should be repeated at regular intervals while on therapy, in keeping with good medical practice. Women taking tamoxifen as adjuvant breast cancer therapy should follow the same monitoring procedures as women taking tamoxifen for the reduction in the incidence of breast cancer. Women taking tamoxifen as treatment for metastatic breast cancer should review this monitoring plan with their health care provider and select the appropriate modalities and schedule of evaluation.

➤*Reduction of invasive breast cancer and DCIS in women with DCIS:* Women with DCIS treated with lumpectomy and radiation therapy who are considering tamoxifen to reduce the incidence of a second breast cancer event should assess the risks and benefits of therapy, since treatment with tamoxifen decreased the incidence of invasive breast cancer but has not been shown to affect survival.

➤*Reduction of breast cancer incidence in high-risk women:* Women who are at high risk for breast cancer can consider taking tamoxifen therapy to reduce the incidence of breast cancer. Whether the benefits of treatment are considered to outweigh the risks depends on a woman's personal health history and how she weighs the benefits and risks. Tamoxifen therapy to reduce the incidence of breast cancer may therefore not be appropriate for all women at high risk for breast cancer. Women who are considering tamoxifen therapy should consult their health care provider for an assessment of the potential benefits and risks prior to starting therapy for reduction in breast cancer incidence. Women should understand that tamoxifen reduces the incidence of breast cancer but may not eliminate risk. Tamoxifen decreased the incidence of small ER-positive tumors but did not alter the incidence of ER-negative tumors or larger tumors. In women with breast cancer who are at high risk of developing a second breast cancer, treatment with about 5 years of tamoxifen reduced the annual incidence rate of a second breast cancer by approximately 50%.

➤*Lab test abnormalities:* Decreases in platelet counts, usually to 50,000 to 100,000/mm^3, infrequently lower, have been occasionally reported in patients taking tamoxifen for breast cancer. In patients with significant thrombocytopenia, rare hemorrhagic episodes have occurred, but it is uncertain if these episodes are due to tamoxifen therapy. Leukopenia has been observed, sometimes in association with anemia or thrombocytopenia. There have been rare reports of neutropenia and pancytopenia in patients receiving tamoxifen; this can sometimes be severe.

In the NSABP P-1 trial, 6 women on tamoxifen and 2 on placebo experienced grade 3 to 4 drops in platelet counts (less than or equal to 50,000/mm^3).

Drug Interactions

➤*Rifampin/aminoglute thimide:* Tamoxifen and N-desmethyl tamoxifen plasma concentrations have been shown to be reduced when coadministered with rifampin or aminoglutethimide. Induction of CYP3A4-mediated metabolism is considered to be the mechanism by which these reductions occur; other CYP3A4-inducing agents have not been studied to confirm this effect.

Rifampin induced the metabolism of tamoxifen and significantly reduced the plasma concentrations of tamoxifen in 10 patients. Aminoglutethimide reduces tamoxifen and N-desmethyl tamoxifen plasma concentrations.

➤*Medroxyprogesterone:* Medroxyprogesterone reduces plasma concentrations of N-desmethyl, but not tamoxifen.

Tamoxifen Drug Interactions

Precipitant drug	Object drug[a]		Description
Aminoglutethimide	Tamoxifen	⬇	Aminoglutethimide reduces tamoxifen and N-desmethyl tamoxifen plasma concentrations.
Bromocriptine	Tamoxifen	⬆	Bromocriptine may elevate serum tamoxifen and N-desmethyl tamoxifen levels.
Cytotoxic agents	Tamoxifen	⬆	The risk of thromboembolic events increases with coadministration.
Medroxyprogesterone	Tamoxifen	⬇	Medroxyprogesterone reduces plasma concentrations of N-desmethyl tamoxifen (metabolite) but not tamoxifen.
Phenobarbital	Tamoxifen	⬇	One patient receiving tamoxifen with concomitant phenobarbital exhibited a steady-state serum level of tamoxifen lower than that observed for other patients (ie, 26 ng/mL vs mean value of 122 ng/mL). The clinical significance of this is unknown.
Rifamycins	Tamoxifen	⬇	Plasma concentrations of tamoxifen may be reduced. Rifampin reduced tamoxifen AUC and C_{max} by 86% and 55%, respectively. It may be necessary to increase the tamoxifen dose during coadministration.
Tamoxifen	Anticoagulants	⬆	The hypoprothrombinemic effect may be increased by concurrent tamoxifen. Carefully monitor prothrombin time.
Tamoxifen	Letrozole	⬇	Tamoxifen reduced plasma letrozole concentrations by 37% when these drugs were coadministered.

[a] ⬆ = Object drug increased. ⬇ = Object drug decreased.

➤*Drug/Lab test interactions:* During postmarketing surveillance, thyroxine elevations were reported for a few postmenopausal patients, which may be explained by increases in thyroid-binding globulin. These elevations were not accompanied by clinical hyperthyroidism.

Variations in the karyopyknotic index on vaginal smears and various degrees of estrogen effect on Pap smears have been infrequently seen in postmenopausal patients given tamoxifen.

In the postmarketing experience with tamoxifen, infrequent cases of hyperlipidemias have been reported. Periodic monitoring of plasma triglycerides and cholesterol may be indicated in patients with preexisting hyperlipidemias.

Adverse Reactions

Adverse reactions to tamoxifen are relatively mild and rarely severe enough to require discontinuation of treatment in breast cancer patients.

Continued clinical studies have resulted in further information that better indicates the incidence of adverse reactions with tamoxifen as compared with placebo.

In one single-dose pharmacokinetic study in healthy peri- and postmenopausal female volunteers, throat irritation was reported by 3 of 60 evaluable subjects (5%) in the tamoxifen oral solution groups while none of the subjects in the tamoxifen reference group reported this reaction. All reactions were mild and occurred within an hour after dosing. All reactions were resolved within 24 hours.

➤*Metastatic breast cancer:* Increased bone and tumor pain and local disease flare have occurred, which are sometimes associated with a good tumor response. Patients with increased bone pain may require additional analgesics. Patients with soft tissue disease may have sudden increases in the size of preexisting lesions, sometimes associated with marked erythema within and surrounding the lesions or the development of new lesions. When they occur, the bone pain or disease flare are seen shortly after starting tamoxifen and generally subside rapidly.

In patients treated with tamoxifen for metastatic breast cancer, the most frequent adverse reaction to tamoxifen is hot flashes.

Other adverse reactions which are seen infrequently are hypercalcemia, peripheral edema, distaste for food, pruritus vulvae, depression, dizziness, light-headedness, headache, hair thinning or partial hair loss, and vaginal dryness.

➤*Premenopausal women:* The following table summarizes the incidence of adverse reactions reported at a frequency of greater than or equal to 2% from clinical trials (Ingle, Pritchard, Buchanan) that compared tamoxifen therapy with ovarian ablation in premenopausal patients with metastatic breast cancer.

Tamoxifen Adverse Reactions Vs Ovarian Ablation (≥ 2%)

Adverse reaction[a]	Tamoxifen (all effects) n = 104	Ovarian ablation (all effects) n = 100
CNS		
Depression	2%	2%
Fatigue	4%	1%
Dermatologic		
Flush	33%	46%
GI		
Abdominal cramps	1%	2%
Anorexia	1%	2%
Nausea	5%	4%
GU		
Altered menses	13%	5%
Amenorrhea	16%	69%
Menstrual disorder	6%	4%
Oligomenorrhea	9%	1%
Ovarian cyst(s)	3%	2%
Musculoskeletal		
Bone pain	6%	6%
Musculoskeletal pain	3%	0%

TAMOXIFEN CITRATE — ORAL

Tamoxifen Adverse Reactions Vs Ovarian Ablation (≥ 2%)		
Adverse reaction[a]	Tamoxifen (all effects) n = 104	Ovarian ablation (all effects) n = 100
Respiratory		
Cough/coughing	4%	1%
Miscellaneous		
Edema	4%	1%
Pain	3%	4%

[a] Some women had more than 1 adverse reaction.

➤*Male breast cancer:* Tamoxifen is well tolerated in men with breast cancer. Reports from the literature and case reports suggest that the safety profile of tamoxifen in men is similar to that seen in women. Loss of libido and impotence have resulted in discontinuation of tamoxifen therapy in male patients. Also, in oligospermic men treated with tamoxifen, luteinizing hormone, follicle-stimulating hormone, testosterone, and estrogen levels were elevated. No significant clinical changes were reported.

➤*Adjuvant breast cancer:* In the NSABP B-14 study, women with axillary node–negative breast cancer were randomized to 5 years of tamoxifen 20 mg/day or placebo following primary surgery. The reported adverse reactions are given in the following table (mean follow-up of approximately 6.8 years), showing adverse reactions more common on tamoxifen than on placebo. The incidence of hot flashes (64% vs 48%), vaginal discharge (30% vs 15%), and irregular menses (25% vs 19%) were higher with tamoxifen compared with placebo. All other adverse reactions occurred with similar frequency in the 2 treatment groups, with the exception of thrombotic events, a higher incidence was seen in tamoxifen-treated patients (through 5 years, 1.7% vs 0.4%). Two of the patients treated with tamoxifen who had thrombotic events died.

Tamoxifen Adverse Reaction in NSABP B-14 Study		
Adverse reaction	Tamoxifen (n = 1,422)	Placebo (n = 1,437)
Cardiovascular		
DVT	0.8%	0.2%
Dermatologic		
Skin changes	19%	15%
GI		
Nausea	26%	24%
GU		
Irregular menses	25%	19%
Vaginal discharge	30%	15%
Hematologic		
Thrombocytopenia[a]	2%	1%
Hepatic		
Increased AST	5%	3%
Increased bilirubin	2%	1%
Renal		
Increased creatinine	2%	1%
Respiratory		
PE	0.5%	0.2%
Miscellaneous		
Fluid retention	32%	30%
Hot flashes	64%	48%
Superficial phlebitis	0.4%	0%
Weight loss (> 5%)	23%	18%

[a] Defined as a platelet count of less than 100,000/mm^3.

In the ECOG adjuvant breast cancer trial, tamoxifen or placebo was administered for 2 years to women following mastectomy. When compared with placebo, tamoxifen showed a significantly higher incidence of hot flashes (19% vs 8% for placebo). The incidence of all other adverse reactions was similar in the 2 treatment groups with the exception of thrombocytopenia where the incidence for tamoxifen was 10% versus 3% for placebo, an observation of borderline statistical significance. In other adjuvant studies, Toronto and NATO, women received either tamoxifen or no therapy. In the Toronto study, hot flashes were observed in 29% of patients for tamoxifen versus 1% in the untreated group. In the NATO trial, hot flashes and vaginal bleeding were reported in 2.8%, and 2% of women, respectively, for tamoxifen versus 0.2% for each in the untreated group.

➤*DCIS:* The type and frequency of adverse reactions in the NSABP B-24 trial were consistent with those observed in the other adjuvant trials conducted with tamoxifen.

➤*Reduction in breast cancer incidence in high-risk women:*

NSABP-1 trial – In the NSABP P-1 trial, there was an increase in 5 serious adverse reactions in the tamoxifen group: endometrial cancer (33 cases in the tamoxifen group vs 14 in the placebo group), PE (18 cases in the tamoxifen group vs 6 in the placebo group), DVT (30 cases in the tamoxifen group vs 19 in the placebo group), stroke (34 cases in the tamoxifen group vs 24 in the placebo group), cataract formation (540 cases in the tamoxifen group vs 483 in the placebo group), and cataract surgery (101 cases in the tamoxifen group vs 63 in the placebo group).

The following table presents the adverse reactions observed in NSABP P-1 by treatment arm. Only adverse reactions more common on tamoxifen than on placebo are shown.

Tamoxifen Adverse Reactions in NSABP P-1 Trial		
Adverse reactions	Tamoxifen (n = 6,681)	Placebo (n = 6,707)
Self-reported symptoms	n = 6,441 [a]	n = 6,469 [a]
Hot flashes	80%	68%
Vaginal bleeding	23%	22%
Vaginal discharges	55%	35%
Laboratory test abnormalities	n = 6,520 [b]	n = 6,535 [b]
Platelets decreased	0.7%	0.3%

[a] Number with quality of life questionnaires.
[b] Number with treatment follow-up questionnaires.

Tamoxifen Adverse Reactions in NSABP P-1 Trial		
Adverse reaction	n = 6,492 [a]	n = 6,484 [a]
CNS		
Mood	11.6%	10.8%
Dermatologic		
Alopecia	5.2%	4.4%
Skin	5.6%	4.7%
GI		
Constipation	4.4%	3.2%
Miscellaneous		
Allergy	2.5%	2.1%
Infection/sepsis	6%	5.1%

[a] Number with adverse drug reaction forms.

In the NSABP P-1 trial, 15% and 9.7% of participants receiving tamoxifen and placebo therapy, respectively, withdrew from the trial for medical reasons. The medical reasons for withdrawal from tamoxifen and placebo therapy, respectively, were hot flashes (3.1% vs 1.5%) and vaginal discharge (0.5% vs 0.1%).

In the NSABP P-1 trial, 8.7% and 9.6% of participants receiving tamoxifen and placebo therapy, respectively, withdrew for nonmedical reasons. On the NSABP P-1 trial, hot flashes of any severity occurred in 68% of women on placebo and in 80% of women on tamoxifen. Severe hot flashes occurred in 28% of women on placebo and 45% of women on tamoxifen. Vaginal discharge occurred in 35% and 55% of women on placebo and tamoxifen, respectively, and was severe in 4.5% and 12.3%, respectively. There was no difference in the incidence of vaginal bleeding between treatment arms.

➤*Pediatric patients:*

McCune-Albright syndrome: Mean uterine volume increased after 6 months of treatment and doubled at the end of the 1-year study. A causal relationship has not been established; however, as an increase in the incidence of endometrial adenocarcinoma and uterine sarcoma has been noted in adults treated with tamoxifen, continued monitoring of McCune-Albright patients treated with tamoxifen for long-term effects is recommended. The safety and efficacy of tamoxifen for girls 2 to 10 years of age with McCune-Albright syndrome and precocious puberty have not been studied beyond 1 year of treatment. The long-term effects of tamoxifen therapy in girls have not been established.

➤*Postmarketing:*

Miscellaneous – Less frequently reported adverse reactions are vaginal bleeding, vaginal discharge, menstrual irregularities, skin rash, and headaches. Usually these have not been of sufficient severity to require dosage reduction or discontinuation of treatment. Very rare reports of erythema multiforme, Stevens-Johnson syndrome, bullous pemphigoid, interstitial pneumonitis, and rare reports of hypersensitivity reactions including angioedema have been reported with tamoxifen therapy. In some of these cases, the time to onset was more than 1 year. Rarely, elevation of serum triglyceride levels, in some cases with pancreatitis, may be associated with the use of tamoxifen.

Overdosage

➤*Symptoms:* Signs observed at the highest doses following studies to determine the median lethal dose in animals were respiratory difficulties and convulsions.

Acute overdosage in humans has not been reported. In a study of advanced metastatic cancer patients that specifically determined the maximum tolerated dose of tamoxifen in evaluating the use of very high doses to reverse multidrug resistance, acute neurotoxicity manifested by tremor, hyperreflexia, unsteady gait, and dizziness were noted. These symptoms occurred within 3 to 5 days of beginning tamoxifen and cleared within 2 to 5 days after stopping therapy. No permanent neurologic toxicity was noted. One patient experienced a seizure several days after tamoxifen was discontinued and neurotoxic symptoms had resolved. The causal relationship of the seizure to tamoxifen therapy is unknown. Doses given in these patients were all greater than 400 mg/m^2 loading dose, followed by maintenance doses of 150 mg/m^2 of tamoxifen given twice a day.

In the same study, prolongation of the QT interval on the electrocardiogram was noted when patients were given doses greater than 250 mg/m^2 loading dose, followed by maintenance doses of 80 mg/m^2 of tamoxifen given twice a

TAMOXIFEN CITRATE — ORAL

day. For a woman with a body surface area of 1.5 m^2, the minimal loading dose and maintenance doses given at which neurological symptoms and QT changes occurred were at least 6-fold higher in respect to the maximum recommended dose.

➤*Treatment:* No specific treatment for overdosage is known; treatment must be symptomatic.

Patient Information

Advise patients that tamoxifen reduces the incidence of breast cancer but may not eliminate risk. Instruct patients on the benefits of tamoxifen versus the risk.

Women with DCIS treated with lupectomy and radiation therapy who are considering tamoxifen to reduce the incidence of a second breast cancer event should assess the risks and benefits of therapy because treatment with tamoxifen decreased the incidence of invasive breast cancer but has not been shown to affect survival.

Advise women who are receiving or who have previously received tamoxifen to have regular gynecologic examinations and promptly inform their health care provider of menstrual irregularities, abnormal vaginal bleeding, change in vaginal discharge, or pelvic pain or pressure.

Women who are pregnant or who plan to become pregnant should not take tamoxifen to reduce the risk of breast cancer. Effective nonhormonal contraception must be used by all premenopausal women taking tamoxifen and for approximately 2 months after discontinuing therapy if they are sexually active. Tamoxifen does not cause infertility, even in the presence of menstrual irregularity. For sexually active women of childbearing potential, initiate tamoxifen therapy during menstruation. In women with menstrual irregularity, a negative chorionic gonadotropin immediately prior to the initiation of therapy is sufficient.

Advise patients to notify their health care provider of pain/swelling/tenderness of legs, unexplained shortness of breath, changes in vision, new breast lumps, vaginal bleeding, or gynecologic symptoms (eg, menstrual irregularites, changes in vaginal discharge, pelvic pain or pressure).

TOREMIFENE CITRATE

Rx	**Fareston** (Shire)	**Tablets:** 60 mg	Lactose. (TO 60). White. In 30s and 100s.

TOREMIFENE CITRATE — ORAL

Indications

➤*Breast cancer:* For the treatment of metastatic breast cancer in postmenopausal women with estrogen-receptor positive or unknown tumors.

Administration and Dosage

➤*Approved by the FDA:* May 30, 1997.

The dosage of toremifene citrate is 60 mg, once daily, orally. Treatment is generally continued until disease progression is observed.

➤*Storage/Stability:* Store at 25°C (77°F); excursions permitted to 15° to 30°C (59° to 86°F). Protect from heat and light.

Actions

➤*Pharmacology:* Toremifene is a nonsteroidal triphenylethylene derivative. Toremifene binds to estrogen receptors and may exert estrogenic, antiestrogenic, or both activities, depending upon the duration of treatment, animal species, gender, target organ, or endpoint selected. In general, however, nonsteroidal triphenylethylene derivatives are predominantly antiestrogenic in rats and humans and estrogenic in mice. In rats, toremifene causes regression of established dimethylbenzanthracene (DMBA)-induced mammary tumors. The antitumor effect of toremifene in breast cancer is believed to be mainly due to its antiestrogenic effects (ie, its ability to compete with estrogen for binding sites in the cancer, blocking the growth-stimulating effects of estrogen in the tumor).

Toremifene causes a decrease in the estradiol-induced vaginal cornification index in some postmenopausal women, indicative of its antiestrogenic activity. Toremifene also has estrogenic activity as shown by decreases in serum gonadotropin concentration (follicle-stimulating hormone and luteinizing hormone).

➤*Pharmacokinetics:*

Absorption/Distribution – Toremifene is well absorbed after oral administration and absorption is not influenced by food. Peak plasma concentrations are obtained within 3 hours. Toremifene displays linear pharmacokinetics after single oral doses of 10 to 680 mg. After multiple dosing, dose proportionality was observed for doses of 10 to 400 mg. Steady-state concentrations were reached in about 4 to 6 weeks. Toremifene has an apparent volume of distribution of 580 L and binds extensively (greater than 99.5%) to serum proteins, mainly to albumin.

The plasma concentration time profile of toremifene declines biexponentially after absorption with a mean distribution half-life of about 4 hours and an elimination half-life of about 5 days.

Metabolism/Excretion – Elimination half-lives of major metabolites, N-demethyltoremifene and (deaminohydroxy) toremifene were 6 and 4 days, respectively. Mean total clearance of toremifene was approximately 5 L/hr.

Toremifene is extensively metabolized, principally by CYP3A4 to N-demethyltoremifene, which is also antiestrogenic but with weak in vivo antitumor potency. Serum concentrations of N-demethyltoremifene are 2 to 4 times higher than toremifene at steady state. Toremifene is eliminated as metabolites predominantly in the feces, with about 10% excreted in the urine during a 1-week period. Elimination of toremifene is slow, in part because of enterohepatic circulation.

Special populations –

Hepatic function impairment: The mean elimination half-life of toremifene was increased by less than 2-fold in 10 patients with hepatic impairment (cirrhosis or fibrosis) compared to subjects with healthy hepatic function. The pharmacokinetics of N-demethyltoremifene were unchanged in these patients. Ten patients on anticonvulsants (phenobarbital, clonazepam, phenytoin, and carbamazepine) showed a 2-fold increase in clearance and a decrease in the elimination half-life of toremifene.

Elderly: The pharmacokinetics of toremifene were studied in 10 healthy young males and 10 elderly females following a single 120 mg dose under testing conditions. Increases in the elimination half-life (4.2 vs 7.2 days) and the volume of distribution (457 vs 627 L) of toremifene were seen in the elderly females without any change in clearance or AUC.

Contraindications

Hypersensitivity to the drug.

Warnings

➤*Hypercalcemia and tumor flare:* As with other antiestrogens, hypercalcemia and tumor flare have been reported in some breast cancer patients with bone metastases during the first weeks of treatment with toremifene citrate. Tumor flare is a syndrome of diffuse musculoskeletal pain and erythema with increased size of tumor lesions that later regress. It is often accompanied by hypercalcemia. Tumor flare does not imply failure of treatment or represent tumor progression. If hypercalcemia occurs, appropriate measures should be instituted and if hypercalcemia is severe, discontinue toremifene citrate treatment.

➤*Tumorigenicity:* Since most toremifene trials have been conducted in patients with metastatic disease, adequate data on the potential endometrial tumorigenicity of long-term treatment with toremifene citrate are not available. Endometrial hyperplasia has been reported. Some patients treated with toremifene citrate have developed endometrial cancer, but circumstances (short duration of treatment or prior antiestrogen treatment of premalignant conditions) make it difficult to establish the role of toremifene citrate.

➤*Carcinogenesis:* Studies in mice at doses of 1 to 30 mg/kg/day (about 1/15 to 2 times the daily maximum recommended human dose on a mg/m^2 basis) for up to 2 years revealed increased incidence of ovarian and testicular tumors, and increased incidence of osteoma and osteosarcoma. The significance of the mouse findings is uncertain because of the different rate of estrogens in mice and the estrogenic effect of toremifene in mice. An increased incidence of ovarian and testicular tumors in mice has also been observed with other human antiestrogenic agents that have primarily estrogenic activity in mice.

➤*Fertility impairment:* Toremifene produced impairment of fertility and conception in male and female rats at doses greater than or equal to 25 and 0.14 mg/kg/day, respectively (about 3.5 times and 1/50 the daily maximum recommended human dose on a mg/m^2 basis). At these doses, sperm counts, fertility index, and conception rate were reduced in males with atrophy of seminal vesicles and prostate. In females, fertility and reproductive indices were markedly reduced with increased pre- and post-implantation loss. In addition, offspring of treated rats exhibited depressed reproductive indices. Toremifene produced ovarian atrophy in dogs administered doses greater than or equal to 3 mg/kg/day (about 1.5 times the daily maximum recommended human dose on a mg/m^2 basis) for 16 weeks. Cystic ovaries and reduction in endometrial stromal cellularity were observed in monkeys at doses greater than or equal to 1 mg/kg/day (about 1/4 the daily maximum recommended human dose on a mg/m^2 basis) for 52 weeks.

➤*Pregnancy: Category D.* Toremifene citrate may cause fetal harm when administered to pregnant women. Studies in rats at doses greater than or equal to 1 mg/kg/day (about 1/4 the daily maximum recommended human dose on a mg/m^2 basis) administered during the period of organogenesis, have shown that toremifene is embryotoxic and fetotoxic, as indicated by intrauterine mortality, increased resorption, reduced fetal weight, and fetal anomalies, including malformation of limbs, incomplete ossification, misshapen bones, ribs/spine anomalies, hydroureter, hydronephrosis, testicular displacement, and subcutaneous edema. Fetal anomalies may have been a consequence of maternal toxicity. Toremifene has been shown to cross the placenta and accumulate in the rodent fetus.

Embryotoxicity and fetotoxicity were observed in rabbits at doses greater than or equal to 1.25 mg/kg/day and 2.5 mg/kg/day, respectively (about 1/3 and 2/3 the daily maximum recommended human dose on a mg/m^2 basis); fetal anomalies included incomplete ossification and anencephaly.

There are no studies in pregnant women. If toremifene citrate is used during pregnancy, or if the patient becomes pregnant while receiving this drug, apprise the patient of the potential hazard to the fetus or potential risk for loss of the pregnancy.

➤*Lactation:* Toremifene has been shown to be excreted in the milk of lactating rats. It is not known if this drug is excreted in human milk.

➤*Children:* There is no indication for use of toremifene in children.

TOREMIFENE CITRATE — ORAL

Precautions

➤*Monitoring:* Periodic complete blood counts, calcium levels, and liver function tests should be obtained.

Patients with bone metastases should be monitored closely for hypercalcemia during the first weeks of treatment. Leukopenia and thrombocytopenia have been reported rarely; leukocyte and platelet counts should be monitored when using toremifene citrate in patients with leukopenia and thrombocytopenia.

➤*Thromboembolic disease/pre-existing endometiral hyperplasia:* Patients with a history of thromboembolic diseases should generally not be treated with toremifene citrate. In general, patients with preexisting endometrial hyperplasia should not be given long-term toremifene citrate treatment.

Drug Interactions

➤*Thiazide diuretics:* Drugs that decrease renal calcium excretion (eg, thiazide diuretics) may increase the risk of hypercalcemia in patients receiving toremifene citrate.

➤*Anticoagulants:* There is a known interaction between antiestrogenic compounds of the triphenylethylene derivative class and coumarin-type anticoagulants (eg, warfarin), leading to an increased prothrombin time. When concomitant use of anticoagulants with toremifene citrate is necessary, careful monitoring of the prothrombin time is recommended.

➤*CYP450 isoenzymes:* Cytochrome P450 3A4 enzyme inducers, such as phenobarbital, phenytoin, and carbamazepine, increase the rate of toremifene metabolism, lowering the steady-state concentration in serum. Metabolism of toremifene may be inhibited by drugs known to inhibit the CYP3A4-6 enzymes. Examples of such drugs are ketoconazole and similar antimycotics as well as erythromycin and similar macrolides. This interaction has not been studied and its clinical relevance is uncertain.

Adverse Reactions

Adverse drug reactions are principally due to the antiestrogenic hormonal actions of toremifene citrate and typically occur at the beginning of treatment.

Toremifene Citrate Adverse Reactions in the North American Study (%)

Adverse reaction	FAR60 (n = 221)	TAM20 (n = 215)
Dizziness	9%	7%
Edema	5%	5%
Hot flashes	35%	30%
Nausea	14%	15%
Sweating	20%	17%
Vaginal bleeding	2%	4%
Vaginal discharge	13%	16%
Vomiting	4%	2%

Approximately 1% of patients receiving toremifene citrate (n = 592) in the 3 controlled studies discontinued treatment as a result of adverse events (nausea and vomiting, fatigue, thrombophlebitis, depression, lethargy, anorexia, ischemic attack, arthritis, pulmonary embolism, and myocardial infarction).

Toremifene Citrate Adverse Events in 3 Controlled Studies (%)

	North American				Eastern European				Nordic			
Adverse events	FAR60 (n = 221)		TAM20 (n = 215)		FAR60 (n = 157)		TAM40 (n = 149)		FAR60 (n = 214)		TAM40 (n = 201)	
Cardiovascular												
Angina pectoris	*		—		1	(< 1)	*		1	(< 1)	2	(1)
Arrhythmia	*		—		—		*		3	(1.5)	1	(< 1)
Cardiac failure	2	(1)	1	(< 1)	—		1	(< 1)	2	(1)	3	(1.5)
Myocardial infarction	2	(1)	3	(1.5)	1	(< 1)	2	(1)	—		1	(< 1)
*Elevated liver tests***												
Alkaline phosphatase	41	(19)	24	(11)	16	(10)	13	(9)	18	(8)	31	(15)
AST	11	(5)	4	(2)	30	(19)	22	(15)	32	(15)	35	(17)
Bilirubin	3	(1.5)	4	(2)	2	(1)	1	(< 1)	2	(1)	3	(1.5)
Hypercalcemia	6	(3)	6	(3)	1	(< 1)	—		—		—	
*Ocular**												
Abnormal vision/diplopia	*		—		—		*		3	(1.5)	—	
Abnormal visual fields	8	(4)	10	(5)	*		*		—		1	(< 1)
Cataracts	22	(10)	16	(7.5)	—		*		—		5	(3)
Corneal keratopathy	4	(2)	2	(1)	—		*		—		—	
Dry eyes	20	(9)	16	(7.5)	—		—		—		*	
Glaucoma	3	(1.5)	2	(1)	1	(< 1)	—		—		1	(< 1)
Thromboembolic												
CVA/TIA	1	(< 1)	—		—		1	(< 1)	4	(2)	4	(2)
Pulmonary embolism	4	(2)	2	(1)	1	(< 1)	—		*		1	(< 1)
Thrombophlebitis	—		2	(1)	1	(< 1)	1	(< 1)	4	(2)	3	(1.5)
Thrombosis	—		1	(< 1)	1	(< 1)	—		3	(1.5)	4	(2)

* Most of the ocular abnormalities were observed in the North American study in which on-study and biannual ophthalmic examinations were performed. No cases of retinopathy were observed in any arm.

** Elevated defined as follows: North American study; AST greater than 100 Units/L; alkaline phosphatase greater than 200 Units/L; bilirubin greater than 2 mg/dL. Eastern European and Nordic studies; AST, alkaline phosphatase, and bilirubin - WHO Grade 1 (1.25 times the upper limit of normal).

Other adverse events of unclear causal relationship to toremifene citrate included leukopenia and thrombocytopenia, skin discoloration or dermatitis, constipation, dyspnea, paresis, tremor, vertigo, pruritus, anorexia, reversible corneal opacity (corneal verticulata), asthenia, alopecia, depression, jaundice, and rigors.

In the 200 and 240 mg toremifene citrate-dose arms, the incidence of AST elevation and nausea was higher. Approximately 4% of patients were withdrawn for toxicity from the high-dose toremifene citrate-treatment arms. Reasons for withdrawal included hypercalcemia, abnormal liver function tests, and 1 case each of toxic hepatitis, depression, dizziness, incoordination, ataxia, blurry vision, diffuse dermatitis, and a constellation of symptoms consisting of nausea, sweating, and tremor.

Overdosage

Lethality was observed in rats following single oral doses that were greater than or equal to 1,000 mg/kg (about 150 times the recommended human dose on a mg/m^2 basis) and was associated with gastric atony/dilatation leading to interference with digestion and adrenal enlargement.

➤*Symptoms:* Vertigo, headache, and dizziness were observed in healthy volunteer studies at a daily dose of 680 mg for 5 days. The symptoms occurred in 2 of the 5 subjects during the third day of the treatment and disappeared within 2 days of discontinuation of the drug. No immediate concomitant changes in any measured clinical chemistry parameters were found. In a study in postmenopausal breast cancer patients, toremifene 400 mg/m^2/day caused dose-limiting nausea, vomiting, and dizziness, as well as reversible hallucinations and ataxia in one patient.

Theoretically, overdose may be manifested as an increase of antiestrogenic effects, such as hot flashes; estrogenic effects, such as vaginal bleeding; or nervous system disorders, such as vertigo, dizziness, ataxia, and nausea.

➤*Treatment:* There is no specific antidote and the treatment is symptomatic.

Patient Information

Vaginal bleeding has been reported in patients using toremifene citrate. Inform patients about this and instruct them to contact their physicians if such bleeding occurs.

Inform patients with bone metastases about the typical signs and symptoms of hypercalcemia and instruct them to contact their physicians for further assessment if such signs or symptoms occur.

FULVESTRANT

Rx	**Faslodex** (AstraZeneca)	**Injection:** 50 mg/mL	Alcohol, benzyl alcohol, castor oil. In 5 mL or two 2.5 mL prefilled syringes.

FULVESTRANT — INJECTION

Indications

➤*Breast cancer:* For the treatment of hormone receptor-positive metastatic breast cancer in postmenopausal women with disease progression following antiestrogen therapy.

Administration and Dosage

➤*Approved by the FDA:* April 25, 2002.

➤*Adults:* 250 mg administered intramuscularly into the buttock at intervals of 1 month as either a single 5 mL injection or 2 concurrent 2.5 mL injections. The injection should be administered slowly.

➤*Preparation/Administration:*

1.) Remove glass syringe barrel from tray and check that it is not damaged.
2.) Remove perforated patient record label from syringe.
3.) Peel open the safety needle outer packaging. For complete instructions refer below to the "Directions for use of safety needle."
4.) Break the seal of the white plastic cover on the syringe luer connector to remove the cover with the attached rubber tip cap .
5.) Twist to lock the needle to the luer connector.
6.) Remove needle sheath.
7.) Remove excess gas from the syringe (a small gas bubble may remain).
8.) Administer intramuscularly slowly in the buttock.
9.) Immediately activate needle protection device upon withdrawal from patient by pushing lever arm completely forward until needle tip is fully covered.
10.) Visually confirm that the lever arm has fully advanced and the needle tip is covered. If unable to activate, discard immediately into an approved sharps collector.
11.) Repeat steps 1 through 10 for second syringe.

For the 2 × 2.5 mL syringe package only, both syringes must be administered to receive the 250 mg recommended monthly dose.

➤*Safety needle instructions:*

Caution concerning the safety needle – To help avoid HIV (AIDS), HBV (Hepatitis), and other infectious diseases due to accidental needlesticks, contaminated needles should not be recapped or removed, unless there is no alternative or that such action is required by a specific medical procedure.

Warning concerning the safety needle – Do not autoclave the safety needle before use. Hands must remain behind the needle at all times during use and disposal.

Directions for use of the safety needle – Peel apart packaging of the safety needle, break the seal of the white plastic cover on the syringe luer connector and attach the safety needle to the luer lock of the syringe by twisting.

Transport filled syringe to point of administration.

Pull shield straight off needle to avoid damaging needle point.

Administer injection following package instruction.

For user convenience, the needle 'bevel up' position is orientated to the lever arm.

Immediately activate needle protection device upon withdrawal from patient by pushing lever arm completely forward until needle tip is fully covered.

Visually confirm that the lever arm has fully advanced and the needle tip is covered. If unable to activate, discard immediately into an approved sharps collector.

Activation of the protective mechanism may cause minimal splatter of fluid that may remain on the needle after injection.

For greatest safety, use a one-handed technique and activate away from self and others.

➤*Storage/Stability:* Refrigerate, 2° to 8°C (36° to 46°F). Store in the original package.

Actions

➤*Pharmacology:* Many breast cancers have estrogen receptors (ER), and the growth of these tumors can be stimulated by estrogen. Fulvestrant is an estrogen receptor antagonist that binds to the estrogen receptor in a competitive manner with affinity comparable to that of estradiol. Fulvestrant downregulates the ER protein in human breast cancer cells.

In a clinical study in postmenopausal women with primary breast cancer treated with single doses of fulvestrant 15 to 22 days prior to surgery, there was evidence of increasing down regulation of ER with increasing dose. This was associated with a dose-related decrease in the expression of the progesterone receptor (PgR), an estrogen-regulated protein. These effects on the ER pathway were also associated with a decrease in Ki67 labeling index, a marker of cell proliferation.

In vitro studies demonstrated that fulvestrant is a reversible inhibitor of the growth of tamoxifen-resistant, as well as estrogen-sensitive human breast cancer (MCF-7) cell lines. In in vivo tumor studies, fulvestrant delayed the establishment of tumors from xenografts of human breast cancer MCF-7 cells in nude mice. Fulvestrant inhibited the growth of established MCF-7 xenografts and of tamoxifen-resistant breast tumor xenografts. Fulvestrant-resistant breast tumor xenografts may also be cross-resistant to tamoxifen.

Fulvestrant showed no agonist-type effects in in vivo uterotropic assays in immature or ovariectomized mice and rats. In in vivo studies in immature rats and ovariectomized monkeys, fulvestrant blocked the uterotrophic action of estradiol. In postmenopausal women, the absence of changes in plasma concentrations of FSH and LH in response to fulvestrant treatment (250 mg monthly) suggests no peripheral steroidal effects.

➤*Pharmacokinetics:*

Absorption – Following IV administration, fulvestrant is rapidly cleared at a rate approximating hepatic blood flow (about 10.5 mL plasma/min/kg). After an IM injection plasma concentrations are maximal at about 7 days and are maintained over a period of at least 1 month, with trough concentration about one-third of C_{max}. The apparent half-life was about 40 days. After administration of 250 mg of fulvestrant intramuscularly every month, plasma levels approach steady-state after 3 to 6 doses, with an average 2.5-fold increase in plasma AUC compared to single dose AUC and trough levels about equal to the single dose C_{max}.

Fulvestrant Pharmacokinetic Parameters in Postmenopausal Advanced Breast Cancer Patients after IM Administration of a 250 mg dose (mean ± SD)					
	C_{max} (ng/mL)	C_{min} (ng/mL)	AUC (ng•d/mL)	t½ (days)	CL (mL/min)
Single dose	8.5 ± 5.4	2.6 ± 1.1	131 ± 62	40 ± 11	690 ± 226
Multidose steady state	15.8 ± 2.4	7.4 ± 1.7	328 ± 48		

Distribution – Fulvestrant was subject to extensive and rapid distribution. The apparent volume of distribution at steady state was approximately 3 to 5 L/kg. This suggests that distribution is largely extravascular. Fulvestrant was highly (99%) bound to plasma proteins; very low density lipoprotein (VLDL), low density lipoprotein (LDL) and high density lipoprotein (HDL) fractions appear to be the major binding components. The role of sex hormone-binding globulin, if any, could not be determined.

Metabolism – Biotransformation and disposition of fulvestrant in humans have been determined following IM and IV administration of ^{14}C-labeled fulvestrant. Metabolism of fulvestrant appears to involve combinations of a number of possible biotransformation pathways analogous to those of endogenous steroids, including oxidation, aromatic hydroxylation, conjugation with glucuronic acid and/or sulphate at the 2, 3 and 17 positions of the steroid nucleus, and oxidation of the side chain sulphoxide. Identified metabolites are either less active or exhibit similar activity to fulvestrant in antiestrogen models. Studies using human liver preparations and recombinant human enzymes indicate that cytochrome P450 3A4 (CYP 3A4) is the only P450 isoenzyme involved in the oxidation of fulvestrant; however, the relative contribution of P450 and non-P450 routes in vivo is unknown.

Excretion – Fulvestrant was rapidly cleared by the hepatobiliary route with excretion primarily via the feces (approximately 90%). Renal elimination was negligible (less than 1%).

Contraindications

Pregnant women; hypersensitivity to the drug or to any of its components.

Warnings

Because fulvestrant is administered intramuscularly, it should not be used in patients with bleeding diatheses, thrombocytopenia or patients on anticoagulants.

➤*Carcinogenesis:* A two-year carcinogenesis study was conducted in female and male rats, at IM doses of 15 mg/kg/30 days, 10 mg/rat/30 days and 10 mg/rat/15 days. These doses correspond to approximately 1-, 3-, and 5-fold (in females) and 1.3-, 1.3-, and 1.6-fold (in males) the systemic exposure [$AUC_{0\text{-}30\ days}$] achieved in women receiving the recommended dose of 250 mg/month. An increased incidence of benign ovarian granulosa cell tumors and testicular Leydig cell tumors was evident, in females dosed at 10 mg/rat/15 days and males dosed at 15 mg/rat/30 days, respectively. Induction of such tumors is consistent with the pharmacology-related endocrine feedback alterations in gonadotropin levels caused by an antiestrogen.

➤*Fertility impairment:* In female rats, fulvestrant administered at doses greater than or equal to 0.01 mg/kg/day (approximately one-hundredth of the human recommended dose based on BSA for 2 weeks prior to and for 1 week following mating, caused a reduction in fertility and embryonic survival. No adverse effects on female fertility and embryonic survival were evident in female animals dosed at 0.001 mg/kg/day (approximately one-thousandth of the human dose based on BSA). Restoration of female fertility to values similar to controls was evident following a 29-day withdrawal period after dosing at 2 mg/kg/day (twice the human dose based on BSA). The effects of fulvestrant on the fertility of female rats appear to be consistent with its antiestrogenic activity. The potential effects of fulvestrant on the fertility of male animals were not studied but in a 6-month toxicology study, male rats treated with IM doses of 15 mg/kg/30 days, 10 mg/rat/30 days, or 10 mg/rat/15 days fulvestrant showed a loss of spermatozoa from the seminiferous tubules, seminiferous tubular atrophy, and degenerative changes in the epididymides. Changes in the testes and epididymides had not recovered 20 weeks after cessation of dosing. These fulvestrant doses correspond to approximately 2-, 3-, and 3-fold the systemic exposure [$AUC_{0\text{-}30\ days}$] achieved in women.

FULVESTRANT — INJECTION

➤*Pregnancy: Category D.* Women of childbearing potential should be advised not to become pregnant while receiving fulvestrant. Fulvestrant can cause fetal harm when administered to a pregnant woman and has been shown to cross the placenta following single IM doses in rats and in rabbits. In studies in the pregnant rat, IM doses of fulvestrant 100 times lower than the maximum recommended human dose (based on BSA), caused an increased incidence of fetal abnormalities and death. Similarly, rabbits failed to maintain pregnancy and the fetuses showed an increased incidence of skeletal variations when fulvestrant was administered at one-half the recommended human dose (based on BSA).

There are no studies in pregnant women using fulvestrant. If fulvestrant is used during pregnancy or if the patient becomes pregnant while receiving this drug, the patient should be apprised of the potential hazard to the fetus, or potential risk for loss of the pregnancy.

➤*Lactation:* Fulvestrant is found in rat milk at levels significantly higher (approximately 12-fold) than plasma after administration of 2 mg/kg. Drug exposure in rodent pups from fulvestrant-treated lactating dams was estimated as 10% of the administered dose. It is not known if fulvestrant is excreted in human milk. Because many drugs are excreted in human milk, and because of the potential for serious adverse reactions from fulvestrant in nursing infants, a decision should be made whether to discontinue nursing or to discontinue the drug taking into account the importance of the drug to the mother.

➤*Children:* Safety and efficacy have not been established.

Precautions

➤*Childbearing women:* Before starting treatment with fulvestrant, pregnancy must be excluded.

See Warnings for more information.

Adverse Reactions

The most commonly reported adverse experiences in the fulvestrant and anastrozole treatment groups, regardless of the investigator's assessment of causality, were GI symptoms (including nausea, vomiting, constipation, diarrhea and abdominal pain), headache, back pain, vasodilatation (hot flushes), and pharyngitis.

Fulvestrant Adverse Reactions (≥ 5%)

Adverse reaction[1]	Fulvestrant 250 mg (n = 423)	Anastrozole 1 mg (n = 423)
Miscellaneous	68.3%	67.6%
Asthenia	22.7%	27%
Pain	18.9%	20.3%
Headache	15.4%	16.8%
Back pain	14.4%	13.2%
Abdominal pain	11.8%	11.6%
Injection site pain[2]	10.9%	6.6%
Pelvic pain	9.9%	9%
Chest pain	7.1%	5%
Flu syndrome	7.1%	6.4%
Fever	6.4%	6.4%
Accidental injury	4.5%	5.7%
Cardiovascular system	30.3%	27.9%
Vasodilatation	17.7%	17.3%
Digestive system	51.5%	48%
Nausea	26%	25.3%
Vomiting	13%	11.8%
Constipation	12.5%	10.6%
Diarrhea	12.3%	12.8%
Anorexia	9%	10.9%
Hemic/lymphatic systems	13.7%	13.5%
Anemia	4.5%	5.%
Metabolic/nutritional disorders	18.2%	17.7%
Peripheral edema	9%	10.2%
Musculoskeletal system	25.5%	27.9%
Bone pain	15.8%	13.7%
Arthritis	2.8%	6.1%
CNS	34.3%	33.8%
Dizziness	6.9%	6.6%
Insomnia	6.9%	8.5%
Paresthesia	6.4%	7.6%
Depression	5.7%	6.9%
Anxiety	5%	3.8%
Respiratory system	38.5%	33.6%
Pharyngitis	16.1%	11.6%
Dyspnea	14.9%	12.3%
Cough increased	10.4%	10.4%
Dermatologic system	22.2%	23.4%
Rash	7.3%	8%
Sweating	5%	5.2%
GU system	18.2%	14.9%
Urinary tract infection	6.1%	3.5%

[1] A patient may have more than one adverse event.
[2] All patients on fulvestrant received injections, but only those anastrozole patients who were in the North American study received placebo injections.

Other adverse events reported as drug-related and seen infrequently (less than 1%) include thromboembolic phenomena, myalgia, vertigo, and leukopenia.

➤*GU:* Vaginal bleeding has been reported infrequently (less than 1%), mainly in patients during the first 6 weeks after changing from existing hormonal therapy to treatment with fulvestrant. If bleeding persists, further evaluation should be considered.

➤*Local:* Injection site reactions with mild transient pain and inflammation were seen with fulvestrant and occurred in 7% of patients (1% of treatments) given the single 5 mL injection (European Trial) and in 27% of patients (4.6% of treatments) given the 2 × 2.5 mL injections (North American Trial).

Overdosage

Animal studies have shown no effects other than those related directly or indirectly to antiestrogen activity with IM doses of fulvestrant higher than the recommended human dose. There is no clinical experience with overdosage in humans. No adverse effects were seen in healthy male and female volunteers who received IV fulvestrant, which resulted in peak plasma concentrations at the end of the infusion, that were approximately 10 to 15 times those seen after IM injection.

HISTRELIN ACETATE

Rx	**Vantas** (Valeras)	**Implant:** 50 mg	In carton with implantation kit.

HISTRELIN — IMPLANT

Indications

➤*Advanced prostate cancer:* For the palliative treatment of advanced prostate cancer.

Administration and Dosage

➤*Approved by the FDA:* October 12, 2004.

➤*Recommended dosage:* 1 implant for 12 months. Each implant contains 50 mg histrelin acetate. The implant is inserted subcutaneously in the inner aspect of the upper arm and provides continuous release of histrelin for 12 months of hormonal therapy.

Histrelin implant must be removed after 12 months of therapy. At the time an implant is removed, another implant may be inserted to continue therapy.

➤*Storage / Stability:* Upon receipt, refrigerate the small carton containing the amber plastic pouch and glass vial (with the implant inside) until the day of insertion. Store the implant refrigerated, 2° to 8°C (36° to 46°F), in the unopened glass vial with the 1.8% sterile sodium chloride solution, overwrapped in the amber plastic pouch and carton. Protect from light. Do not freeze.

Actions

➤*Pharmacology:* Histrelin, an LH-RH agonist, acts as a potent inhibitor of gonadotropin secretion when given continuously in therapeutic doses. Both animal and human studies indicate that following an initial stimulatory phase, chronic, subcutaneous administration of histrelin desensitizes responsiveness of the pituitary gonadotropin which, in turn, causes a reduction in testicular steroidogenesis.

In humans, administration of histrelin acetate results in an initial increase in circulating levels of luteinizing hormone (LH) and follicle-stimulating

HISTRELIN — IMPLANT

hormone (FSH), leading to a transient increase in concentration of gonadal steroids (testosterone and dihydrotestosterone in males). However, continuous administration of histrelin results in decreased levels of LH and FSH. In males, testosterone is reduced to castrate levels. These decreases occur within 2 to 4 weeks after initiation of treatment.

The histrelin implant is designed to provide continuous subcutaneous release of histrelin at a nominal rate of 50 to 60 mcg/day over 12 months.

➤*Pharmacokinetics:*

Absorption – Following subcutaneous insertion of 1 histrelin 50 mg implant in advanced prostate cancer patients (n = 17), peak serum concentrations of 1.1 ± 0.375 ng/mL (mean ± SD) occurred at a median of 12 hours. Continuous subcutaneous release was evident, as serum levels were sustained throughout the 52-week dosing period. The mean serum histrelin concentration at the end of the 52-week treatment duration was 0.13 ± 0.065 ng/mL. When histrelin serum concentrations were measured following a second implant inserted after 52 weeks, the observed serum concentrations over 8 weeks following the second implant were comparable to the same period following the first implant. The average rate of subcutaneous drug release from 41 implants assayed for residual drug content was 56.7 ± 7.71 mcg/day over the 52-week dosing period. The relative bioavailability for the histrelin implant in prostate cancer patients with normal renal and hepatic function compared with a subcutaneous bolus dose in healthy male volunteers was 92%. Serum histrelin concentrations were proportional to dose after 1, 2, or 4 histrelin 50 mg implants (50, 100, or 200 mg histrelin) in 42 prostate cancer patients.

Distribution – The apparent volume of distribution of histrelin following a subcutaneous bolus dose (500 mcg) in healthy volunteers was 58.4 ± 7.86 L. The fraction of drug unbound in plasma measured in vitro was 29.5% ± 8.9% (mean ± SD).

Metabolism – An in vitro drug metabolism study using human hepatocytes identified a single histrelin metabolite resulting from C-terminal dealkylation. Peptide fragments resulting from hydrolysis also are likely metabolites. Following a subcutaneous bolus dose in healthy volunteers, the apparent clearance of histrelin was 179 ± 37.8 mL/min (mean ± SD) and the terminal half-life was 3.92 ± 1.01 hours (mean ± SD). The apparent clearance following a histrelin 50 mg implant in 17 prostate cancer patients was 174 ± 56.5 mL/min (mean ± SD).

Contraindications

Hypersensitivity to GnRH, GnRH agonist analogs, or any of the components in histrelin implant. Anaphylactic reactions to synthetic LH-RH or LH-RH agonist analogs have been reported in the literature.

Histrelin is contraindicated in women and in pediatric patients and was not studied in these patient populations. Moreover, histrelin can cause fetal harm when administered to a pregnant woman.

Warnings

➤*Worsening of signs and symptoms:* Histrelin, like other LH-RH agonists, causes a transient increase in serum concentrations of testosterone during the first week of treatment. Patients may experience worsening of symptoms or onset of new symptoms, including bone pain, neuropathy, hematuria, or ureteral or bladder outlet obstruction. Cases of ureteral obstruction and spinal cord compression, which may contribute to paralysis with or without fatal complications, have been reported with LH-RH agonists. If spinal cord compression or renal impairment develops, institute standard treatment of these complications.

➤*Carcinogenesis:* Carcinogenicity studies were conducted in rats for 2 years at dosages of 5, 25, or 150 mcg/kg/day (up to 15 times the human dosage) and in mice for 18 months at dosages of 20, 200, or 2,000 mcg/kg/day (up to 200 times the human dosage). As seen with other LH-RH agonists, histrelin acetate injection administration was associated with an increase in tumors of hormonally responsive tissues. There was a significant increase in pituitary adenomas in rats. There was an increase in pancreatic islet-cell adenomas in treated female rats and a non-dose-related increase in testicular Leydig cell tumors (highest incidence in the low-dose group). In mice, there was significant increase in mammary-gland adenocarcinomas in all treated females. In addition, there were increases in stomach papillomas in male rats given high doses, and an increase in histiocytic sarcomas in female mice at the highest dose.

➤*Fertility impairment:* Fertility studies have been conducted in rats and monkeys given subcutaneous daily doses of histrelin up to 180 mcg/kg for 6 months, and full reversibility of fertility suppression was demonstrated. The development and reproductive performance of offspring from parents treated with histrelin has not been investigated.

➤*Pregnancy:* Category X. Major fetal abnormalities were observed in rabbits but not in rats after administration of histrelin throughout gestation. There were increased fetal mortality and decreased fetal weights in rats and rabbits. The effects on fetal mortality are expected consequences of the alterations in hormonal levels brought about by this drug. The possibility exists that spontaneous abortion may occur.

➤*Children:* Histrelin is contraindicated in children and was not studied in children.

Precautions

➤*Monitoring:* Monitor response to histrelin by measuring serum concentrations of testosterone and PSA periodically, especially if the anticipated clinical or biochemical response to treatment has not been achieved.

Results of testosterone determinations are dependent on assay methodology. It is advisable to be aware of the type and precision of the assay methodology to make appropriate clinical and therapeutic decisions.

Closely observe patients with metastatic vertebral lesions and/or urinary tract obstruction during the first few weeks of therapy.

➤*Administration and removal:* Implant insertion is a surgical procedure. Carefully adhere to the recommended insertion and removal procedures to minimize the potential for complications and implant expulsion. In addition, instruct patients to refrain from wetting the arm for 24 hours and from heavy lifting or strenuous exertion of the inserted arm for 7 days after implant insertion.

In all clinical trials combined, an implant was not recovered in 8 patients. For 2 of these, serum testosterone rose above castrate level and the implant was neither palpable nor visualized with ultrasound. These 2 implants were believed to have been extruded without appreciation by the patients. In the other 6, serum testosterone remained below the castrate level, but the implant was not palpable. No further diagnostic tests were conducted. One of these patients underwent in-clinic surgical exploration that did not locate the implant. Based upon these findings, it is important to know that histrelin implant is not radio-opaque and, therefore, will not be visible through x-ray. However, if the implant is difficult to locate by palpation, ultrasound and CT scan may be used.

Drug Interactions

➤*Drug/Lab test interactions:* Therapy with histrelin results in suppression of the pituitary-gonadal system. Results of diagnostic tests of pituitary gonadotropic and gonadal functions conducted during and after histrelin therapy may be affected.

Adverse Reactions

Histrelin implant, like other LH-RH analogs, caused a transient increase in serum testosterone concentrations during the first week of treatment. Therefore, potential exacerbations of signs and symptoms of the disease during the first few weeks of treatment are of concern in patients with vertebral metastases and/or urinary obstruction or hematuria. If these conditions are aggravated, it may lead to neurological problems such as weakness and/or paresthesia of the lower limbs or worsening of urinary symptoms.

➤*Local:* In the first 12 months after initial insertion of the implants, an implant extruded through the incision site in 8 of 171 patients in the clinical trials.

In the pivotal study (Study 301), a detailed evaluation for implant-site reactions was conducted. Of the 138 patients in the study, 19 (13.8%) patients experienced local or insertion-site reactions. All local site reactions were reported as mild in severity. The majority were associated with initial insertion or removal and insertion of a new implant, and began and resolved within the first 2 weeks following implant insertion. Reactions persisted in 4 (2.8%) patients. An additional 4 (2.8%) patients developed application-site reactions after the first 2 weeks following insertion.

Local reactions after implant insertion included bruising (7.2%) and pain/soreness/tenderness (3.6%). Other, less frequently reported reactions included erythema (2.8%) and swelling (0.7%). In this study, 2 patients had events described as local infections/inflammations, one that resolved after treatment with oral antibiotics and the other without treatment.

Local reactions following insertion of a subsequent implant were comparable to those seen after initial insertion. The following possibly or probably related systemic adverse reactions occurred during clinical trials of up to 24 months of treatment with histrelin implant, and were reported in 2% or more of patients (see the following table).

Histrelin Adverse Reactions (≥ 2%)

Adverse reaction	Number (%)
Cardiovascular	
Hot flashes[a]	112 (65.5%)
CNS	
Headache	5 (2.9%)
Insomnia	5 (2.9%)
Libido decreased[a]	4 (2.3%)
Dermatologic	
Implant-site reaction	10 (5.8%)
GI	
Constipation	6 (3.5%)
GU	
Erectile dysfunction[a]	6 (3.5%)
Gynecomastia[a]	7 (4.1%)
Renal impairment[b]	8 (4.7%)
Testicular atrophy[a]	9 (5.3%)
Miscellaneous	
Fatigue	17 (9.9%)
Weight increased	4 (2.3%)

[a] Expected pharmacological consequences of testosterone suppression.
[b] Five of the 8 patients had a single occurrence of mild renal impairment (defined as Ccr 30 mL/min to less than 60 mL/min), which returned to a normal range by the next visit.

HISTRELIN — IMPLANT

Hot flashes were the most common adverse reaction reported (65.5%). In terms of severity, 2.3% of patients reported severe hot flashes, 25.4 % of patients reported moderate hot flashes, and 37.7% reported mild hot flashes. In addition, the following possibly or probably related systemic adverse reactions were reported by less than 2% of patients using histrelin implant in clinical studies.

➤*Cardiovascular:* Flushing, hematoma, palpitations, ventricular extrasystoles.

➤*CNS:* Depression, dizziness, irritability, tremor.

➤*Dermatologic:* Contusion, hypotrichosis, night sweats, pruritus, sweating increased.

➤*GI:* Abdominal discomfort, nausea.

➤*GU:* Breast pain, breast tenderness, calculus renal, dysuria, genital pruritus male, gynecomastia aggravated, hematuria aggravated, renal failure aggravated, sexual dysfunction, urinary frequency, urinary frequency aggravated, urinary retention.

➤*Hematologic:* Anemia.

➤*Hepatic:* Hepatic disorder.

➤*Lab test abnormalities:* Aspartate aminotransferase increased, blood glucose increased, blood lactate dehydrogenase increased, blood testosterone increased, Ccr decreased, prostatic acid phosphatase increased.

➤*Metabolic/Nutritional:* Appetite increased, fluid retention, food craving, hypercalcemia, hypercholesterolemia.

➤*Musculoskeletal:* Arthralgia, back pain, back pain aggravated, bone pain, muscle twitching, myalgia, neck pain, pain in limb.

➤*Respiratory:* Dyspnea exertional.

➤*Miscellaneous:* Feeling cold, lethargy, malaise, pain, pain exacerbated, peripheral edema, stent occlusion, weakness, weight decreased.

Decreased bone density has been reported in the medical literature in men who have had orchiectomy or have been treated with an LH-RH agonist analog. It can be anticipated that long periods of medical castration in men will have effects on bone density.

Overdosage

Histrelin injection of up to 200 mcg/kg (rats, rabbits) or 2,000 mcg/kg (mice) resulted in no systemic toxicity. This represents 20 to 200 times the maximal recommended human dosage of 10 mcg/kg/day. Adverse reaction profiles were similar in patients receiving 1, 2, or 4 histrelin implants.

LEUPROLIDE ACETATE

Rx	**Leuprolide Acetate Injection** (Various, eg, Bedford Laboratories)	**Injection:** 5 mg/mL	In 2.8 mL multiple-dose vials.[a]
Rx	**Lupron** (TAP Pharm)		In 2.8 mL multiple-dose vials.[a]
Rx	**Lupron for Pediatric Use** (TAP Pharm)		In 2.8 mL multiple-dose vials.[a]
Rx	**Eligard** (Sanofi-Synthelabo	**Powder for Injection, lyophilized:** 7.5 mg	In single-use kits with a 2-syringe mixing system and 20-gauge, ½-inch needle.
Rx	**Eligard** (Sanofi-Synthelabo	**Injection:** 22.5 mg (3-month depot)	In single-use kits with a 2-syringe mixing system and 20-gauge, ½-inch needle.
		30 mg (4-month depot)	In single-use kit with 2-syringe mixing system and syringe containing *Atrigel.*
		45 mg (6-month depot)	In single-use kit with 2-syringe mixing system and syringe containing *Atrigel.*
Rx	**Lupron Depot** (TAP Pharm)	**Microspheres for Injection, lyophilized:**[b] 3.75 mg	Mannitol. Preservative free. In single kits, multi-packs, and prefilled dual-chamber syringe.
		7.5 mg	Mannitol. Preservative free. In single kits, multi-packs, and prefilled dual-chamber syringe.
Rx	**Lupron Depot-Ped** (TAP Pharm)	**Microspheres for Injection, lyophilized:**[b] 7.5 mg	Mannitol. Preservative free. In single-dose kit and pre-filled dual-chamber syringe.
		11.25 mg	Mannitol. Preservative free. In single-dose kit and pre-filled dual-chamber syringe.
		15 mg	Mannitol. Preservative free. In single-dose kit and pre-filled dual-chamber syringe.
Rx	**Lupron Depot - 3 Month** (TAP Pharm)	**Microspheres for Injection, lyophilized:**[b] 11.25 mg	Mannitol. Preservative free. In single-use kit containing 11.25 mg vial leuprolide with 1.5 mL diluent and in pre-filled dual-chamber syringes.
		22.5 mg	Mannitol. Preservative free. In single-use kit containing 22.5 mg vial leuprolide with 1.5 mL diluent and in pre-filled dual-chamber syringes.
Rx	**Lupron Depot - 4 Month** (TAP Pharm)	**Microspheres for Injection, lyophilized:**[b] 30 mg	Mannitol. Preservative free. In single-use kit containing 30 mg vial leuprolide with 1.5 mL diluent and in pre-filled dual-chamber syringes.
Rx	**Viadur** (ALZA Corporation)	**Implant:** 72 mg	In single-dose kit.

[a] With 9 mg/mL benzyl alcohol as preservative and sodium chloride.

[b] Listed as total dose; vials are combined to provide proper strength.

LEUPROLIDE ACETATE — INJECTION

Indications

➤*Advanced prostatic cancer (injection, implant, or depot 7.5, 22.5, 30, and 45 mg):* Palliative treatment of advanced prostatic cancer that offers an alternative when orchiectomy or estrogen administration are not indicated or are unacceptable to the patient.

➤*Endometriosis (depot 3.75 and 11.25 mg):* Management of endometriosis, including pain relief and reduction of endometriotic lesions. Experience is limited to women ≥ 18 years of age treated for ≤ 6 months.

➤*Uterine leiomyomata (fibroids) (depot 3.75 and 11.25 mg):* Concomitantly with iron therapy for the preoperative hematologic improvement of patients with anemia caused by uterine leiomyomata. Experience with leuprolide depot in females has been limited to women ≥ 18 years of age and treated for ≤ 6 months.

➤*Central precocious puberty (CPP) (pediatric injection or Depot-Ped):* Treatment of children with CPP.

➤*Unlabeled uses:* Treatment of breast cancer, ovarian carcinoma.

Administration and Dosage

➤*Depot:* Because of different release characteristics, a fractional dose of the 3-, 4-, or 6-month depot formulation is not equivalent to the same dose of the monthly formulation and should not be given. Do not use needles smaller than 22-gauge. Reconstitute only with diluent provided.

➤*Injection:* Vary the injection site periodically. Use the syringes provided in the kit; if alternate syringes are needed, use insulin syringes.

➤*Advanced prostate cancer:*

Injection – 1 mg daily given subcutaneously.

Depot – 7.5 mg monthly, 22.5 mg every 3 months (84 days), 30 mg every 4 months (16 weeks), or 45 mg every 6 months.

Lupron: Administer IM.

Eligard: Administer subcutaneously.

➤*Endometriosis (depot only):* 3.75 mg IM monthly or 11.25 mg IM every 3 months.

Recommended duration is 6 months. Retreatment cannot be recommended since safety data are not available. If the symptoms of endometriosis recur after a course of therapy and further treatment is contemplated, it is recommended that bone density be assessed before retreatment begins to ensure that values are within normal limits.

➤*Uterine leiomyomata (depot only):* 3.75 mg IM monthly or one 11.25 mg IM injection with concomitant iron therapy.

LEUPROLIDE ACETATE — INJECTION

11.25 mg is indicated only for women for whom 3 months of hormonal suppression is deemed necessary.

The clinician may wish to consider a 1-month trial period of iron alone, because some patients may respond to iron alone.

Recommended duration of therapy is ≤ 3 months. The symptoms associated with uterine leiomyomata will recur following discontinuation of therapy. If additional treatment is contemplated, assess bone density prior to initiation of therapy to ensure that values are within normal limits.

➤*CPP:* Individualize dosage based on a mg/kg ratio of drug to body weight. Younger children require higher doses on a mg/kg ratio.

Injection – May be administered by a patient/parent or health care professional. Recommended starting dose is 50 mcg/kg/day as a single subcutaneous injection. If total downregulation is not achieved, titrate upward by 10 mcg/kg/day, which will be considered the maintenance dose.

Depot-Ped (7.5, 11.25, and 15 mg) – Must be administered under physician supervision. Recommended starting dose is 0.3 mg/kg/4 weeks (minimum, 7.5 mg) as a single IM injection. Determine the starting dose as follows:

Leuprolide Depot Starting Dose for CPP	
Weight (kg)	Dose (mg)
≤ 25	7.5
more than 25 to 37.5	11.25
more than 37.5	15

If total downregulation is not achieved, titrate upward in 3.75 mg increments every 4 weeks, which will be considered the maintenance dose.

Injection / Depot – After 1 to 2 months of initiating therapy or changing doses, monitor with a GnRH stimulation test, sex steroids, and Tanner staging to confirm downregulation. Monitor measurements of bone age for advancement every 6 to 12 months. Titrate the dose upwards until no progression of the condition is noted either clinically or by lab parameters. The first dose to result in adequate downregulation can probably be maintained for duration of therapy in most children. However, there are insufficient data to guide dosage adjustment as patients move into higher weight categories. Verify adequate downregulation in patients whose weight has increased significantly while on therapy. Vary the injection site periodically. Consider discontinuation of therapy before 11 years of age in females and before 12 years of age in males.

➤*Depot preparation:*

Single use kit – For a single IM injection, reconstitute the lyophilized microspheres with diluent provided. Using a 22-gauge needle, withdraw appropriate amount of diluent from amp (1 or 1.5 mL); inject into vial. Shake well to obtain uniform suspension. It will appear milky. Withdraw entire contents into syringe and inject immediately.

Prefilled dual-chamber syringe – See prescribing information. The suspension will appear milky. If the microspheres (particles) adhere to the stopper, tap the syringe against your finger. Remove the needle guard and advance the plunger to expel air from the syringe. Inject the entire contents of the syringe IM (*Lupron*) or subcutaneously (*Eligard*) as you would for a normal injection. The suspension settles very quickly following reconstitution; therefore, it is preferable to mix and use immediately. Reshake suspension if settling occurs.

➤*Storage / Stability:*

Injection – Store below room temperature (25°C; 77°F). Avoid freezing. Protect from light; store vial in carton until use.

Depot –

Lupron: Store at 25°C (77°F); excursions permitted to 15° to 30°C (59° to 86°F). The product does not contain a preservative; therefore, discard if not used immediately.

Eligard: Store at 2° to 3°C (35.6° to 46.4°F). Once mixed, the product must be administered within 30 minutes.

Actions

➤*Pharmacology:* Leuprolide, an LH-RH and GnRH agonist, acts as a potent inhibitor of gonadotropin secretion when given continuously in therapeutic doses. Animal and human studies indicate that following an initial stimulation, chronic administration of leuprolide results in suppression of ovarian and testicular steroidogenesis. This effect is reversible upon discontinuation of drug therapy. Administration of leuprolide has resulted in inhibition of the growth of certain hormone-dependent tumors (prostatic tumors in Noble and Dunning male rats and DMBA-induced mammary tumors in female rats) as well as atrophy of the reproductive organs.

In humans, administration of leuprolide results in an initial increase in circulating levels of luteinizing hormone (LH) and follicle-stimulating hormone (FSH), leading to a transient increase in levels of the gonadal steroids (testosterone and dihydrotestosterone in males, and estrone and estradiol in premenopausal females). However, continuous administration of leuprolide results in decreased levels of LH and FSH in all patients; in males, testosterone is reduced to castrate levels or to below the castrate threshold (less than or equal to 50 ng/dL). These decreases occur within 2 to 4 weeks after initiation of treatment.

➤*Pharmacokinetics:*

Absorption – In adults, bioavailability by subcutaneous administration is comparable to that by IV administration.

Daily injection: Leuprolide is not active when given orally. Leuprolide acetate has a plasma half-life of approximately 3 hours. The metabolism, distribution, and excretion of leuprolide in humans have not been determined. A pharmacokinetic study of leuprolide in children has not been performed.

7.5 mg (monthly) injection: The pharmacokinetics/pharmacodynamics was observed during 3 once-monthly injections (7.5 mg) in 20 patients with advanced carcinoma of the prostate.Mean serum leuprolide concentrations following the initial injection rose to 25.3 ng/mL (C_{max}) at approximately 5 hours after injection. After the initial increase following each injection, serum concentrations remained relatively constant (0.28 to 2 ng/mL). There was no evidence of significant accumulation during repeated dosing. Nondetectable leuprolide plasma concentrations have been observed during chronic leuprolide 7.5 mg administration, but testosterone levels were maintained at castrate levels.

22.5 mg (3-month) injection: The pharmacokinetics/pharmacodynamics was observed during 2 injections every 3 months (leuprolide 22.5 mg) in 22 patients with advanced carcinoma of the prostate. Mean serum leuprolide concentrations rose to 127 ng/mL and 107 ng/mL at approximately 5 hours following the initial and second injections, respectively. After the initial increase following each injection, serum leuprolide concentrations remained relatively constant (0.2 to 2 ng/mL). There was no evidence of significant accumulation during repeated dosing. Nondetectable leuprolide plasma concentrations have been observed during chronic leuprolide 22.5 mg administration, but testosterone levels were maintained at castrate levels.

30 mg (4-month) injection: The pharmacokinetics/pharmacodynamics was observed during injections administered initially and at 4 months (leuprolide 30 mg) in 24 patients with advanced carcinoma of the prostate. Mean serum leuprolide concentrations following the initial injection rose rapidly to 150 ng/mL (C_{max}) at approximately 3.3 hours after injection. After the initial increase following each injection, mean serum concentrations remained relatively constant (0.1 to 1 ng/mL). There was no evidence of significant accumulation during repeated dosing. Nondetectable leuprolide plasma concentrations have been occasionally observed during leuprolide 30 mg administration, but testosterone levels were maintained at castrate levels.

3.75 mg (monthly) depot suspension: A single dose of leuprolide 3.75 mg depot suspension was administered by IM injection to healthy female volunteers. The absorption of leuprolide was characterized by an initial increase in plasma concentration, with peak concentration ranging from 4.6 to 10.2 ng/mL at 4 hours postdosing. However, intact leuprolide and an inactive metabolite could not be distinguished by the assay used in the study. Following the initial rise, leuprolide concentrations started to plateau within 2 days after dosing and remained relatively stable for about 4 to 5 weeks with plasma concentrations of about 0.3 ng/mL.

7.5 mg (monthly) depot suspension and pediatric formulations: Following a single leuprolide 7.5 mg depot suspension injection to adult patients, mean peak leuprolide plasma concentration was almost 20 ng/mL at 4 hours and then declined to 0.36 ng/mL at 4 weeks. However, intact leuprolide and an inactive major metabolite could not be distinguished by the assay which was employed in the study. Nondetectable leuprolide plasma concentrations have been observed during chronic leuprolide 7.5 mg depot suspension administration, but testosterone levels appear to be maintained at castrate levels.

11.25 mg (3-month) depot suspension: Following a single injection of the 3-month formulation of leuprolide for 11.25 mg (3-month) depot suspension in female subjects, a mean plasma leuprolide concentration of 36.3 ng/mL was observed at 4 hours. Leuprolide appeared to be released at a constant rate following the onset of steady-state levels during the third week after dosing, and mean levels then declined gradually to near the lower limit of detection by 12 weeks. The mean (± standard deviation) leuprolide concentration from 3 to 12 weeks was 0.23 ± 0.09 ng/mL. However, intact leuprolide and an inactive major metabolite could not be distinguished by the assay which was employed in the study. The initial burst, followed by the rapid decline to a steady-state level, was similar to the release pattern seen with the monthly formulation.

22.5 mg (3-month) depot suspension: Following a single injection of the 3-month formulation of leuprolide 22.5 mg (3-month) depot suspension in patients, mean peak plasma leuprolide concentration of 48.9 ng/mL was observed at 4 hours and then declined to 0.67 ng/mL at 12 weeks. Leuprolide appeared to be released at a constant rate following the onset of steady-state levels during the third week after dosing, providing steady plasma concentrations through the 12-week dosing interval. However, intact leuprolide and an inactive major metabolite could not be distinguished by the assay which was employed in the study. Detectable levels of leuprolide were present at all measurement points in all patients. The initial burst, followed by the rapid decline to a steady-state level, was similar to the release pattern seen with the monthly formulation.

30 mg (4-month) depot suspension: Following a single injection of leuprolide 30 mg (4-month) depot suspension in 16 orchiectomized prostate cancer patients, mean plasma leuprolide concentration of 59.3 ng/mL was observed at 4 hours, and the mean concentration then declined to 0.3 ng/mL at 16 weeks. The mean plasma concentration of leuprolide from weeks 3.5 to 16 was 0.44 ± 0.2 ng/mL (range 0.2 to 1.06). Leuprolide appeared to be released at a constant rate following the onset of steady-state levels during the fourth week after dosing, providing steady plasma concentrations throughout the 16-week dosing interval. However, intact leuprolide and an inactive major metabolite could not be distinguished by the assay which was employed in the study. The initial burst, followed by the rapid decline to a steady-state level, was similar to the release pattern seen with the other depot formulations.

Distribution – The mean steady-state volume of distribution of leuprolide following IV bolus administration to healthy male volunteers was 27 L. In vitro binding to human plasma proteins ranged from 43% to 49%.

Metabolism –

7.5 mg (monthly) injection, 22.5 mg (3-month), 30 mg (4-month): In healthy male volunteers, a 1 mg bolus of leuprolide administered IV revealed that the mean systemic clearance was 8.34 L/hr, with a terminal elimination half-life of approximately 3 hours based on a 2-compartment model.

LEUPROLIDE ACETATE — INJECTION

No drug metabolism study was conducted with leuprolide 7.5 mg, 22.5 mg (3-month), or 30 mg (4-month) injections. Upon administration with different leuprolide formulations, the major metabolite of leuprolide is a pentapeptide (M-1) metabolite.

Daily pediatric injection and pediatric depot suspensions, 3.75 (monthly) depot suspension, 7.5 mg (monthly) depot suspension, 11.25 mg (3-month) depot suspension, 22.5 mg (3-month) depot suspension, 30 mg (4-month) depot suspension: In healthy male volunteers, a 1 mg bolus of leuprolide administered IV revealed that the mean systemic clearance was 7.6 L/hr, with a terminal elimination half-life of approximately 3 hours based on a 2-compartment model.

In a pharmacokinetic/pharmacodynamic study of endometriosis patients, IM 3.75 mg (monthly) leuprolide depot suspension (n = 15) every 4 weeks or IM 11.25 mg (3-month) depot suspension (n = 19) every 12 weeks was administered for 24 weeks. There was no statistically significant difference in changes of serum estradiol concentration from baseline between the 2 treatment groups.

M-I plasma concentrations measured in 5 prostate cancer patients reached maximum concentration 2 to 6 hours after dosing and were approximately 6% of the peak parent drug concentration. One week after dosing, mean plasma M-I concentrations were approximately 20% of mean leuprolide concentrations.

Excretion – Following administration of leuprolide for depot suspension 3.75 mg to 3 patients, less than 5% of the dose was recovered as parent and M-I metabolite in the urine.

7.5 mg (monthly), 22.5 mg (3–month), 30 mg (4-month) injections: No drug excretion study was conducted with leuprolide 7.5 mg (monthly), 22.5 mg (3-month), or 30 mg (4-month) injections.

Contraindications

Hypersensitivity to GnRH, GnRH agonist analogs, or any of the components in the various formulations of leuprolide for injection. Reports of anaphylactic reactions to synthetic GnRH or GnRH agonist analogs have been reported in the medical literature.

Leuprolide is contraindicated in women with undiagnosed abnormal vaginal bleeding.

All doses of leuprolide injections and depot suspensions are contraindicated in women who are or may become pregnant while receiving the drug. Leuprolide may cause fetal harm when administered to a pregnant woman. Major fetal abnormalities were observed in rabbits but not in rats after administration of leuprolide throughout gestation. There was increased fetal mortality and decreased fetal weights in rats and rabbits. The effects on fetal mortality are expected consequences of the alterations in hormonal levels brought about by this drug. Therefore, the possibility exists that spontaneous abortion may occur if the drug is administered during pregnancy. If this drug is used during pregnancy, or if the patient becomes pregnant while taking this drug, apprise the patient of the potential hazard to the fetus.

Leuprolide is contraindicated in women who are breastfeeding.

➤*7.5 mg (monthly), 22.5 mg (3-month), 30 mg (4-month) injections:* Leuprolide 7.5 mg (monthly), 22.5 mg (3-month), and 30 mg (4-month) injections are contraindicated in women and in pediatric patients and were not studied in women or children.

Warnings

➤*Worsening of symptoms:*

Central precocious puberty – During the early phase of therapy, gonadotropins and sex steroids rise above baseline because of the natural stimulatory effect of the drug. Therefore, an increase in clinical signs and symptoms may be observed.

Noncompliance with drug regimen or inadequate dosing may result in inadequate control of the pubertal process. The consequences of poor control include the return of pubertal signs such as menses, breast development, and testicular growth. The long-term consequences of inadequate control of gonadal steroid secretion are unknown, but may include a further compromise of adult stature.

Advanced prostatic cancer – Initially, leuprolide, like other LH-RH agonists, causes transient increases in serum levels of testosterone to approximately 50% above baseline during the first week of treatment. Isolated cases of worsening of signs and symptoms during the first weeks of treatment have been reported with LH-RH analogs. Transient worsening of symptoms, or the occurrence of additional signs and symptoms of prostate cancer, may occasionally develop during the first few weeks of leuprolide treatment, including bone pain, neuropathy, hematuria, or bladder outlet obstruction. As with other LH-RH agonists, isolated cases of ureteral obstruction and spinal cord compression have been observed, which may contribute to paralysis, with or without fatal complications.

For patients at risk, the physician may consider initiating therapy with daily leuprolide injection for the first 2 weeks to facilitate withdrawal of treatment if that is considered necessary.

If spinal cord compression or renal impairment develops, institute standard treatment of these complications.

Endometriosis and uterine leiomyomata – Safe use of leuprolide in pregnancy has not been established clinically. Before starting treatment with leuprolide depot suspensions, pregnancy must be excluded.

When used at the recommended dose and dosing interval, leuprolide 3.75 mg (monthly) depot suspension and 11.25 mg (3-month) depot suspension usually inhibit ovulation and stop menstruation. Contraception is not ensured, however, by taking leuprolide. Therefore, patients should use nonhormonal methods of contraception. Advise patients to see their physicians if they believe they may be pregnant. If a patient becomes pregnant during treatment, the drug must be discontinued, and the patient must be apprised of the potential risk to the fetus.

During the early phase of therapy, sex steroids temporarily rise above baseline because of the physiologic effect of the drug. Therefore, an increase in clinical signs and symptoms may be observed during the initial days of therapy, but these will dissipate with continued therapy.

➤*Hypersensitivity reactions:* Patients with known allergies to benzyl alcohol, an ingredient of the vehicle of leuprolide daily injection and daily pediatric injection, may present symptoms of hypersensitivity, usually local, in the form of erythema and induration at the injection site.

Symptoms consistent with an anaphylactoid or asthmatic process have been rarely reported postmarketing.

➤*Renal function impairment:* If renal impairment develops, institute standard treatment of this complication.

➤*Carcinogenesis:* Two-year carcinogenicity studies were conducted in rats and mice. In rats, a dose-related increase of benign pituitary hyperplasia and benign pituitary adenomas was noted at 24 months when the drug was administered subcutaneously at high daily doses (0.6 to 4 mg/kg). There was a significant but not dose-related increase of pancreatic islet-cell adenomas in females and of testicular interstitial cell adenomas in males (highest incidence in the low-dose group). In mice, no leuprolide-induced tumors or pituitary abnormalities were observed at a dose as high as 60 mg/kg for 2 years. Adult patients have been treated with leuprolide for up to 3 years with doses as high as 10 mg/day and for 2 years with doses as high as 20 mg/day without demonstrable pituitary abnormalities.

➤*Pregnancy: Category X.*

See Contraindications for more information.

➤*Lactation:* It is not known whether leuprolide is excreted in human milk. Because many drugs are excreted in human milk, and because the effects of leuprolide on lactation or the breastfed child have not been determined, leuprolide should not be used by nursing mothers.

➤*Children:* The safety and effectiveness of leuprolide, apart from the pediatric formulations for the treatment of central precocious puberty, have not been established in pediatric patients. See the labeling for the pediatric formulations for their safety and effectiveness in children with central precocious puberty.

3.75 (monthly) and 11.25 mg (3-month) depot suspension – Experience with leuprolide 3.75 monthly depot suspension for the treatment of endometriosis has been limited to women 18 years of age and older.

7.5 mg (monthly), 22.5 mg (3-month), and 30 mg (4-month) injections – Leuprolide 7.5 mg (monthly), 22.5 mg (3-month), and 30 mg (4-month) injections are contraindicated in pediatric patients and were not studied in children.

Precautions

➤*Monitoring:*

Central precocious puberty –

Pediatric formulations: Monitor response to leuprolide pediatric formulations 1 to 2 months after the start of therapy with a GnRH stimulation test and sex steroid levels. Perform measurement of bone age for advancement every 6 to 12 months.

Sex steroids may increase or rise above prepubertal levels if the dose is inadequate. Once a therapeutic dose has been established, gonadotropin and sex steroid levels will decline to prepubertal levels.

Advanced prostatic cancer – Closely observe patients with metastatic vertebral lesions or with urinary tract obstruction during the first few weeks of therapy.

Monitor response to leuprolide by measuring serum levels of testosterone, as well as prostate-specific antigen and prostatic acid phosphatase.

7.5 mg (monthly) injection and depot suspension and 22.5 mg (3-month) injection and depot suspension, 30 mg (4-month) injection and depot suspension – Transient increases in prostatic acid phosphatase levels may occur sometime early in treatment. However, by the fourth week, the elevated levels can be expected to decrease to values at or near baseline.

Results of testosterone determinations are dependent on assay methodology. It is advisable to be aware of the type and precision of the assay methodology to make appropriate clinical and therapeutic decisions.

3.75 mg (monthly) depot suspension –

Endometriosis: During early clinical trials with leuprolide 3.75 mg monthly depot suspension for endometriosis, regular laboratory monitoring revealed that AST levels were more than twice the upper limit of normal in only 1 patient. There was no clinical or other laboratory evidence of abnormal liver function.

In 2 other clinical trials, 6 of 191 patients receiving leuprolide 3.75 mg monthly depot suspension plus norethindrone acetate 5 mg daily for up to 12 months developed an elevated (at least twice the upper limit of normal) ALT or gamma-glutamyl-transferase (GGT). Five of the 6 increases were observed beyond 6 months of treatment. None was associated with elevated bilirubin concentration.

Triglycerides were increased above the upper limit of normal in 12% of the endometriosis patients who received leuprolide 3.75 mg monthly depot suspension.

LEUPROLIDE ACETATE — INJECTION

Uterine leiomyomata (fibroids): In clinical trials with leuprolide 3.75 mg monthly depot suspension for uterine leiomyomata, five (3%) patients had a post-treatment transaminase value that was at least twice the baseline value and above the upper limit of the normal range. None of the laboratory increases was associated with clinical symptoms.

Lipids: Of those endometriosis and uterine fibroid patients whose pretreatment cholesterol values were in the normal range, mean change following therapy was +16 mg/dL to +17 mg/dL in endometriosis patients and +11 mg/dL to +29 mg/dL in uterine fibroid patients. In the endometriosis-treated patients, increases from the pretreatment values were statistically significant (*P* less than 0.03).

Chemistry: Slight to moderate mean increases were noted for glucose, uric acid, blood urea nitrogen, creatinine, total protein, albumin, bilirubin, alkaline phosphatase, LDH, calcium, and phosphorus. None of these increases was clinically significant.

Drug Interactions

➤*Drug/Lab test interactions:* Administration of leuprolide in therapeutic doses results in suppression of the pituitary-gonadal system. Normal function is usually restored within 4 to 12 weeks after treatment is discontinued. Therefore, diagnostic tests of pituitary gonadotropic and gonadal functions conducted during treatment and for up to 3 months after discontinuation of leuprolide or leuprolide depot suspensions may be misleading.

Adverse Reactions

➤*Central precocious puberty (CPP):* Potential exacerbation of signs and symptoms during the first few weeks of treatment is a concern in patients with rapidly advancing central precocious puberty.

Leuprolide Adverse Reactions in Children With CPP (≥ 2%)

Adverse reaction	Patients (n = 395)	(%)
Dermatologic		
Acne/seborrhea	7	2%
Injection site reactions, including abscess	21	5%
Rash, including erythema multiforme	8	2%
GU		
Vaginitis/bleeding/discharge	7	2%
Miscellaneous		
General pain	7	2%

In those same studies, the following adverse reactions were reported in less than 2% of the patients.

Cardiovascular – Syncope, vasodilation.

CNS – Emotional lability, nervousness, personality disorder, somnolence.

Dermatologic – Alopecia, skin striae.

Endocrine – Accelerated sexual maturity.

GI – Dysphagia, gingivitis, nausea/vomiting.

GU – Cervix disorder, gynecomastia/breast disorders, urinary incontinence.

Metabolic/Nutritional – Peripheral edema, weight gain.

Respiratory – Epistaxis.

Miscellaneous – Body odor, fever, headache, infection.

➤*CPP (postmarketing):* Symptoms consistent with an anaphylactoid or asthmatic process have been rarely (incidence rate of about 0.002%) reported. Rash, urticaria, and photosensitivity reactions have also been reported.

Cardiovascular – Hypotension, pulmonary embolism.

CNS – Peripheral neuropathy, spinal fracture/paralysis.

Dermatologic – Hair growth.

GU – Prostate pain.

Hematologic/Lymphatic – Decreased white blood cells.

Hepatic – Hepatic dysfunction.

Local – Localized reactions, including induration and abscess, have been reported at the site of injection.

Musculoskeletal – Tenosynovitis-like symptoms.

Respiratory – Respiratory disorders.

Special senses – Hearing disorder.

Miscellaneous – Hard nodule in throat, weight gain, increased uric acid. Symptoms consistent with fibromyalgia (eg, joint and muscle pain, headaches, sleep disorders, GI distress, shortness of breath) have been reported individually and collectively.

Changes in bone density – Decreased bone density has been reported in the medical literature in men who have had orchiectomy or who have been treated with an LH-RH agonist analog. In a clinical trial, 25 men with prostate cancer, 12 of whom had been treated previously with leuprolide for at least 6 months, underwent bone density studies as a result of pain. The leuprolide-treated group had lower bone density scores than the nontreated control group. The effects on bone density in children are unknown.

➤*Advanced prostate cancer (daily injection):* In the majority of patients, testosterone levels increased above baseline during the first week, declining thereafter to baseline levels or below by the end of the second week of treatment. This transient increase was occasionally associated with a temporary worsening of signs and symptoms, usually manifested by an increase in bone pain. In a few cases, a temporary worsening of existing hematuria and urinary tract obstruction occurred during the first week. Temporary weakness and paresthesia of the lower limbs have been reported in a few cases.

Potential exacerbations of signs and symptoms during the first few weeks of treatment is a concern in patients with vertebral metastases or urinary obstruction which, if aggravated, may lead to neurological problems or increase the obstruction.

Leuprolide Adverse Reactions (≥ 5%)

Adverse reaction	Leuprolide (n = 98)	DES (n = 101)
Cardiovascular		
Congestive heart failure	1	5
ECG changes/ischemia	19	22
High blood pressure	8	5
Murmur	3	8
Peripheral edema	12	30
Phlebitis/thrombosis	2	10
CNS/peripheral nervous system		
Dizziness/lightheadedness	5	7
General pain	13	13
Headache	7	4
Insomnia/sleep disorders	7	5
Dermatologic		
Dermatitis	5	8
Endocrine		
Decreased testicular size[a]	7	11
Gynecomastia/breast tenderness or pain[a]	7	63
Hot flashes[a]	55	12
Impotence[a]	4	12
GI		
Anorexia	6	5
Constipation	7	9
Nausea/vomiting	5	17
GU		
Frequency/urgency	6	8
Hematuria	6	4
Urinary tract infection	3	7
Hematologic-lymphatic		
Anemia	5	5
Musculoskeletal		
Bone pain	5	2
Myalgia	3	9
Respiratory		
Dyspnea	2	8
Sinus congestion	5	6
Miscellaneous		
Asthenia	10	10

[a] Physiologic effect of decreased testosterone.

In this same study, the following adverse reactions were reported in less than 5% of the patients on leuprolide:

Cardiovascular – Angina, cardiac arrhythmias, myocardial infarction, pulmonary emboli.

CNS – Anxiety, blurred vision, lethargy, memory disorder, mood swings, nervousness, numbness, paresthesia, peripheral neuropathy, syncope/blackouts.

Dermatologic – Carcinoma of skin/ear, dry skin, ecchymosis, hair loss, itching, local skin reactions, pigmentation, skin lesions.

Endocrine – Decreased libido, thyroid enlargement.

GI – Diarrhea, dysphagia, gastrointestinal bleeding, gastrointestinal disturbance, peptic ulcer, rectal polyps.

GU – Bladder spasms, dysuria, incontinence, testicular pain, urinary obstruction.

Musculoskeletal – Joint pain.

Ophthalmic – Swelling (temporal bone).

Respiratory – Cough, pleural rub, pneumonia, pulmonary fibrosis.

LEUPROLIDE ACETATE — INJECTION

Special senses – Taste disorders.

Miscellaneous – Depression, diabetes, fatigue, fever/chills. hypoglycemia, increased BUN, increased calcium, increased creatinine, infection/inflammation.

➤*Advanced prostate cancer (additional adverse reactions reported with leuprolide daily injection during other clinical trials or during postmarketing surveillance):*

Cardiovascular – Hypotension, transient ischemic attack/stroke.

CNS – Hearing disorder, peripheral neuropathy, spinal fracture/paralysis.

Dermatologic – Hair growth.

Endocrine – Increased libido.

GU – Penile swelling, prostate pain.

Hepatic – Hepatic dysfunction.

Hematologic/Lymphatic – Decreased WBC, hemoptysis.

Musculoskeletal – Ankylosing spondylosis, pelvic fibrosis.

Respiratory – Pulmonary infiltrate, respiratory disorders.

Miscellaneous – Hypoproteinemia, hard nodule in throat, increased uric acid, weight gain.

➤*Advanced prostate cancer (7.5 mg [monthly] injection):* See Warnings for more information.

In Study AGL9904, 120 patients were dosed with leuprolide 7.5 mg for up to 6 months, and injection sites were closely monitored. In all, 716 injections of leuprolide 7.5 mg (monthly) injection were administered. Transient burning/stinging was reported following 248 (34.6%) injections, with the majority (84%) of these events reported as mild. Pain was reported following 4.3% of study injections (18.3% of patients) and was generally reported as brief in duration and mild in intensity.

Erythema was reported following 2.6% of injections (12.5% of patients). These events were all reported as mild and generally resolved within a few days postinjection. Mild bruising was reported following 2.5% of injections (11.7% of patients). Pruritus, induration, and ulceration was reported following 1.4% (11 patients), 0.4% (3 patients), and 0.1% (1 patient) of study injections, respectively.

Adverse Reactions with Leuprolide 7.5 mg for ≤ 6 months in Study AGL9904 (≥ 2%)

Body system	Adverse event	Patients (n = 120)
Cardiovascular	Hot flashes/sweats[a]	68 (56.7%)
GI	Gastroenteritis/colitis	3 (2.5%)
GU	Atrophy of testes[a]	6 (5%)
Miscellaneous	Malaise and fatigue	21 (17.5%)
	Dizziness	4 (3.3%)

[a] Expected pharmacological consequences of testosterone suppression. In the patient populations studied, a total of 86 hot flashes/sweats adverse events were reported in 70 patients. Of these, 71 events (83%) were mild; 14 (16%) were moderate; 1 (1%) were severe.

Adverse Reactions Reported by Surgically Castrated Patients Treated with a Single-Dose of Leuprolide 7.5 mg in Study AGL9802 (≥ 2%)

Body system	Adverse event	Number (n = 8)
Cardiovascular	Hot flashes/sweats[a]	2 (25%)

[a] Expected pharmacological consequences of testosterone suppression. In the patient populations studied, a total of 86 hot flashes/sweats adverse events were reported in 70 patients. Of these, 71 events (83%) were mild; 14 (16%) were moderate; 1 (1%) were severe.

In addition, the following possibly or probably related systemic adverse events were reported by less than 2% of the patients using leuprolide 7.5 mg (monthly) injection in clinical studies.

CNS – Depression, disturbance of smell and taste, vertigo.

Dermatologic – Alopecia.

GI – Constipation, flatulence.

GU – Breast soreness, decreased libido†, gynecomastia, impotence†, testicular soreness.

Hematologic – Decreased red blood cell count, hematocrit and hemoglobin.

Metabolic – Weight gain.

Musculoskeletal – Backache, joint pain, tremor.

Miscellaneous – Insomnia, sweating, syncope.

Changes in bone density (7.5 mg [monthly] injection) – Decreased bone density has been reported in the medical literature in men who have had orchiectomy or who have been treated with an LH-RH agonist analog. It can be anticipated that long periods of medical castration in men will have effects on bone density.

➤*Advanced prostate cancer (22.5 mg [3-month] injection):* See Warnings for more information.

In Study AGL9909, 117 patients were dosed with leuprolide 22.5 mg (3-month) injection every 3 months for up to 6 months, and injection sites were closely monitored. In all, 230 injections of leuprolide 22.5 mg (3-month) injection were administered. Transient burning/stinging was reported following 50 injections (21.7%), with the majority (86%) of these events reported as mild. Pain was reported following 3.5% of study injections (6% of patients) and was generally reported as brief in duration and mild in intensity.

Erythema was reported following 2 injections (0.9% of study injections, 1.7% of patients). One of the reports characterized the erythema as mild and resolved within 7 days. The other was moderate and resolved within 15 days. Neither patient experienced erythema at multiple injections. Mild bruising was reported following 4 injections (1.7% of study injections, 3.4% of patients). Mild pruritus was reported following 1 injection (0.4% of study injections, 0.9% of patients).

Adverse Events Reported by Patients Treated with Leuprolide 22.5 mg (3-Month) Injection for ≤ 6 months; Study AGL9909 (≥ 2%)

Body system	Adverse event	Number (n = 117)
Cardiovascular		
Vascular disorders	Hot flashes/sweats[a]	66 (56.4%)
Dermatologic	Pruritus	3 (2.6%)
GI	Nausea	4 (3.4%)
GU	Urinary frequency	3 (2.6%)
Musculoskeletal	Arthralgia	4 (3.4%)
Miscellaneous	Fatigue	7 (6%)

[a] Expected pharmacological consequence of testosterone suppression. In the patient population studied, a total of 84 hot flashes/sweats events were reported in 66 patients. Of these, 73 events (87%) were described as mild; 11 (13%) as moderate; none were severe.

In addition, the following possibly or probably related systemic adverse events were reported by less than 2% of the patients using leuprolide 22.5 mg (3-month) injection in the clinical study.

Cardiovascular –
Vascular: Hypertension, hypotension.

Dermatologic – Clamminess, increased sweating††, night sweats††.

GI – Dyspepsia.

GU – Breast tenderness††, gynecomastia††, impotence††, testicular atrophy††, testicular pain.

Renal – Bladder spasm, blood in urine, difficulties with urination, pain on urination, scanty urination, and urinary retention.

Miscellaneous – Lethargy, rigors, weakness.

Changes in bone density (22.5 mg [3-month] injection) – Decreased bone density has been reported in the medical literature in men who have had orchiectomy or who have been treated with an LH-RH agonist analog. It can be anticipated that long periods of medical castration in men will have effects on bone density.

➤*Advanced prostate cancer (30 mg [4-month] injection):* See Warnings for more information.

In Study AGL0001, 90 patients were dosed with leuprolide 30 mg (4-month) every 4 months for up to 8 months, and injection sites were closely monitored. In all, 175 injections of leuprolide 30 mg (4-month) injection were administered. Transient burning/stinging was reported at the injection site following 35 (20%) injections, with all (100%) of these events reported as mild. Pain was reported following 2.3% of study injections (3.3% of patients) and was generally reported as mild in intensity. A single event reported as moderate pain resolved within 2 minutes, and all 3 mild pain events resolved within several days. Erythema was reported following 1.1% of injections (2.2% of patients). These events were all reported as mild and generally resolved within a few days postinjection.

Adverse Events Reported by Patients Treated with Leuprolide 30 mg (4-Month) Injection for up to 8 Months in Study AGL0001 (≥ 2%)

Body system	Adverse event	Number (N = 90)
Cardiovascular	Hot flashes[a]	66 (73.3%)
CNS	Dizziness	4 (4.4%)
Dermatologic	Alopecia	2 (2.2%)
	Clamminess[a]	
	Night sweats[a]	3 (3.3%)

† Expected pharmacological consequences of testosterone suppression. In the patient populations studied, a total of 86 hot flashes/sweats adverse events were reported in 70 patients. Of these, 71 events (83%) were mild; 14 (16%) were moderate; 1 (1%) were severe.

†† Expected pharmacological consequence of testosterone suppression. In the patient population studied, a total of 84 hot flashes/sweats events were reported in 66 patients. Of these, 73 events (87%) were described as mild; 11 (13%) as moderate; none was severe.

LEUPROLIDE ACETATE — INJECTION

Adverse Events Reported by Patients Treated with Leuprolide 30 mg (4-Month) Injection for up to 8 Months in Study AGL0001 (≥ 2%)		
Body system	Adverse event	Number (N = 90)
GI	Nausea	2 (2.2%)
GU	Gynecomastia[a]	2 (2.2%)
	Testicular atrophy[*]	4 (4.4%)
	Testicular pain	2 (2.2%)
Musculoskeletal	Myalgia	2 (2.2%)
Ronal/Urinary	Nocturia	2 (2.2%)
	Urinary frequency	2 (2.2%)
Miscellaneous	Fatigue	12 (13.3%)

[a] Expected pharmacological consequences of testosterone suppression. In the patient population studied, a total of 75 hot flash adverse events were reported in 66 patients. Of these, 57 events (76%) were mild; 16 (21%) were moderate; 2 (3%) were severe.

In addition, the following possibly or probably related systemic adverse events were reported by 1.1% of patients using leuprolide 30 mg (4-month) injection in the clinical study.

GU – Breast enlargement†, erectile dysfunction†, reduced penis size.

Musculoskeletal – Limb pain, muscle atrophy.

Psychiatric – Depression, insomnia.

Renal – Incontinence, urinary urgency.

Miscellaneous – Lethargy.

Changes in bone density (30 mg [4-month] injection) – Decreased bone density has been reported in the medical literature in men who have had orchiectomy or who have been treated with an LH-RH agonist analog. It can be anticipated that long periods of medical castration in men will have effects on bone density.

➤*Advanced prostate cancer (7.5 mg [monthly] depot formulation):* See Warnings for more information.

Leuprolide 7.5 mg (Monthly) Depot Suspension		
	(n = 56)	(%)
Cardiovascular		
Hot flashes/sweats[a]	32	(57.1%)
CNS		
Decreased libido[a]	3	(5.4%)
GI		
GI disorders	8	(14.3%)
GU		
Impotence[a]	3	(5.4%)
Testicular atrophy[a]	3	(5.4%)
Urinary disorder	7	(12.5%)
Metabolic/nutritional		
Edema	8	(14.3%)
Respiratory		
Respiratory disorder	6	(10.7%)
Miscellaneous		
General pain	13	(23.2%)
Infection	3	(5.4%)

[a] Due to the expected physiologic effect of decreased testosterone levels.

In the same study, the following adverse reactions were reported in less than 5% of the patients on leuprolide 7.5 mg (monthly) depot suspension.

Cardiovascular – Angina, congestive heart failure.

CNS – Agitation, insomnia/sleep disorders, neuromuscular disorders.

Dermatologic – Hair disorder, skin reaction.

GI – Anorexia, dysphagia, eructation, peptic ulcer.

GU – Balanitis, breast enlargement, urinary tract infection.

Hematologic/Lymphatic – Ecchymosis.

Lab test abnormalities – Abnormalities of certain parameters were observed, but their relationship to drug treatment are difficult to assess in this population. The following were recorded in greater than or equal to 5% of patients at final visit: Decreased albumin, decreased hemoglobin/hematocrit, decreased prostatic acid phosphatase, decreased total protein, decreased urine-specific gravity, hyperglycemia, hyperuricemia, increased BUN, increased creatinine, increased liver function tests (AST, LDH), increased phosphorus, increased platelets, increased prostatic acid phosphatase, increased total cholesterol, increased urine-specific gravity, leukopenia.

Musculoskeletal – Myalgia.

Respiratory – Emphysema, hemoptysis, increased sputum, lung edema.

Miscellaneous – Asthenia, cellulitis, fever, headache, injection-site reaction, neoplasm.

➤*Advanced prostate cancer (postmarketing, 7.5 mg [monthly] depot suspension):* Symptoms consistent with an anaphylactoid or asthmatic process have been rarely (incidence rate of about 0.002%) reported. Rash, urticaria, and photosensitivity reactions have also been reported.

Localized reactions, including induration and abscess have been reported at the site of injection.

Symptoms consistent with a fibromyalgia (eg, joint and muscle pain, headaches, sleep disorders, GI distress, and shortness of breath) have been reported individually and collectively.

Cardiovascular – Hypotension, pulmonary embolism.

CNS – Peripheral neuropathy, spinal fracture/paralysis.

GU – Prostate pain.

Hematologic/Lymphatic – Decreased white blood cells.

Musculoskeletal – Tenosynovitis-like symptoms.

Changes in bone density (7.5 mg [monthly] depot suspension) – Decreased bone density has been reported in the medical literature in men who have had orchiectomy or who have been treated with an LH-RH agonist analog. In a clinical trial, 25 men with prostate cancer, 12 of whom had been treated previously with leuprolide for at least 6 months, underwent bone density scans as a result of pain. The leuprolide-treated group had lower bone density scores than the nontreated control group. It can be anticipated that long periods of medical castration in men will have effects on bone density.

➤*Advanced prostate cancer (22.5 mg [3-month] depot suspension):* See Warnings for more information.

Leuprolide 22.5 mg (3-month) Depot Suspension		
Adverse reaction	n = 94	(%)
Cardiovascular		
Hot flashes/sweats[a]	55	(58.5%)
Central/peripheral nervous system		
Dizziness/vertigo	6	(6.4%)
Insomnia/sleep disorders	8	(8.5%)
Neuromuscular disorders	9	(9.6%)
Dermatologic		
Skin reaction	8	(8.5%)
GI		
GI disorders	15	(16%)
GU		
Testicular atrophy[a]	19	(20.2%)
Urinary disorders	14	(14.9%)
Musculoskeletal		
Joint disorders	11	(11.7%)
Respiratory		
Respiratory disorders	6	(6.4%)
Miscellaneous		
Asthenia	7	(7.4%)
General pain	25	(26.6%)
Headache	6	(6.4%)
Injection site reaction	13	(13.8%)

[a] Physiologic effect of decreased testosterone.

In these same studies, the following adverse reactions were reported in less than 5% of the patients on leuprolide for depot suspension 22.5 mg (3-month).

Cardiovascular – Arrhythmia, bradycardia, heart failure, hypertension, hypotension, varicose vein.

CNS – Anxiety, delusions, depression, hypesthesia, decreased libido (physiologic effect of decreased testosterone), nervousness, paresthesia.

GI – Anorexia, duodenal ulcer, increased appetite, thirst/dry mouth.

GU – Gynecomastia, impotence (physiologic effect of decreased testosterone), penis disorders, testis disorders.

Hematologic/Lymphatic – Anemia, lymphedema.

Lab test abnormalities – Abnormalities of certain parameters were observed, but are difficult to assess in this population. The following were recorded in greater than or equal to 5% of patients: Increased BUN, hyperglycemia, hyperlipidemia (total cholesterol, LDL cholesterol, triglycerides), hyperphosphatemia, abnormal liver function tests, increased PT, increased

† Expected pharmacological consequences of testosterone suppression. In the patient population studied, a total of 75 hot flash adverse events were reported in 66 patients. Of these, 57 events (76%) were mild; 16 (21%) were moderate; 2 (3%) were severe.

LEUPROLIDE ACETATE — INJECTION

PTT. Additional laboratory abnormalities reported were decreased platelets, decreased potassium, and increased WBC.

Metabolic/Nutritional – Dehydration, edema.

Respiratory – Epistaxis, pharyngitis, pleural effusion, pneumonia.

Special senses – Abnormal vision, amblyopia, dry eyes, tinnitus.

Miscellaneous – Enlarged abdomen, fever.

➤*Advanced prostate cancer (postmarketing, 22.5 [3-month] depot suspension):* Symptoms consistent with an anaphylactoid or asthmatic process have been reported rarely (incidence rate of about 0.002%). Rash, urticaria, and photosensitivity reactions have also been reported.

Localized reactions, including induration and abscess, have been reported at the site of injection.

Symptoms consistent with fibromyalgia (eg, joint and muscle pain, headaches, sleep disorders, GI distress, and shortness of breath) have been reported individually and collectively.

Cardiovascular – Hypotension, pulmonary embolism.

CNS – Peripheral neuropathy, spinal fracture/paralysis.

GU – Prostate pain.

Hematologic/Lymphatic – Decreased white blood cells.

Musculoskeletal – Tenosynovitis-like symptoms.

➤*Advanced prostate cancer (30 mg, [4-month] depot suspension):* See Warnings for more information.

Adverse Reactions Reported in Patients Regardless of Causality (Leuprolide for depot suspension 30 mg [4-month]) (≥ 5%)

	Nonorchiectomized (n = 49) Study 013		Orchiectomized (n = 24) Study 012	
Adverse reaction	n	(%)	n	(%)
Cardiovascular				
Hot flashes/sweats[a]	23	(46.9%)	2	(8.3%)
CNS				
Dizziness/vertigo	3	(6.1%)	2	(8.3%)
Neuromuscular disorders	3	(6.1%)	1	(4.2%)
Paresthesia	4	(8.2%)	1	(4.2%)
Dermatologic				
Skin reaction	6	(12.2%)	0	(0%)
GI				
GI disorders	5	(10.2%)	3	(12.5%)
GU				
Urinary disorders	5	(10.2%)	4	(16.7%)
Metabolic/Nutritional				
Dehydration	4	(8.2%)	0	(0%)
Edema	4	(8.2%)	5	(20.8%)
Musculoskeletal				
Joint disorder	8	(16.3%)	1	(4.2%)
Myalgia	4	(8.2%)	0	(0%)
Respiratory				
Respiratory disorder	4	(8.2%)	1	(4.2%)
Miscellaneous				
Asthenia	6	(12.2%)	1	(4.2%)
Flu syndrome	6	(12.2%)	0	(0%)
General pain	16	(32.7%)	1	(4.2%)
Headache	5	(10.2%)	1	(4.2%)
Injection-site reaction	4	(8.2%)	9	(37.5%)

[a] Due to the expected physiologic effects of decreased testosterone levels.

In these same studies, the following adverse reactions were reported in less than 5% of the patients on leuprolide 30 mg (4–month) depot suspension.

Cardiovascular – Atrial fibrillation, deep thrombophlebitis, hypertension.

CNS – Abnormal thinking, amnesia, confusion, convulsion, dementia, depression, insomnia/sleep disorders, libido decreased (due to the expected physiologic effects of decreased testosterone levels), neuropathy, paralysis.

Dermatologic – Herpes zoster, melanosis.

GI – Anorexia, eructation, gastrointestinal hemorrhage, gingivitis, gum hemorrhage, hepatomegaly, increased appetite, intestinal obstruction, periodontal abscess.

GU – Bladder carcinoma, epididymitis, impotence (due to the expected physiologic effects of decreased testosterone levels), prostate disorder, testicular atrophy (due to the expected physiologic effects of decreased testosterone levels), urinary incontinence, urinary tract infection.

Hematologic/Lymphatic – Lymphadenopathy.

Lab test abnormalities – Abnormalities of certain parameters were observed, but their relationship to drug treatment are difficult to assess in this population. The following were recorded in greater than or equal to 5% of patients: Decreased bicarbonate, decreased hemoglobin/hematocrit/RBC, hyperlipidemia (total cholesterol, LDL cholesterol, triglycerides), decreased HDL cholesterol, eosinophilia, increased glucose, increased liver function tests (ALT, AST, GGTP, LDH), increased phosphorus. Additional laboratory abnormalities were reported: Increased BUN and PT, leukopenia, thrombocytopenia, uricaciduria.

Metabolic/Nutritional – Abnormal healing, hypoxia, weight loss.

Musculoskeletal – Leg cramps, pathological fracture, ptosis.

Respiratory – Asthma, bronchitis, hiccup, lung disorder, sinusitis, voice alteration.

Miscellaneous – Abscess, accidental injury, allergic reaction, cyst, fever, generalized edema, hernia, neck pain, neoplasm.

➤*Postmarketing advanced prostate cancer (30 mg [4-month] depot suspension):* Symptoms consistent with an anaphylactoid or asthmatic process have been rarely (incidence rate of about 0.002%) reported. Rash, urticaria, and photosensitivity reactions have also been reported.

Localized reactions, including induration and abscess, have been reported at the site of injection.

Symptoms consistent with fibromyalgia (eg, joint and muscle pain, headaches, sleep disorders, GI distress, and shortness of breath) have been reported individually and collectively.

Cardiovascular – Hypotension, pulmonary embolism.

CNS – Peripheral neuropathy, spinal fracture/paralysis.

GU – Prostate pain.

Hematologic/Lymphatic – Decreased white blood cells.

Musculoskeletal – Tenosynovitis-like symptoms.

Changes in bone density (22.5 mg [3-month] and 30 mg [4-month] depot suspensions) – Decreased bone density has been reported in the medical literature in men who have had orchiectomies or who have been treated with LH-RH agonist analogs. In a clinical trial, 25 men with prostate cancer, 12 of whom had been treated previously with leuprolide for at least 6 months, underwent bone density studies as a result of pain. The leuprolide-treated group had lower bone density scores than the nontreated control group. It can be anticipated that long periods of medical castration in men will have effects on bone density.

➤*Endometriosis (3.75 mg [monthly] depot suspension):* Estradiol levels may increase during the first weeks following the initial injection, but then decline to menopausal levels. This transient increase in estradiol can be associated with a temporary worsening of signs and symptoms.

As would be expected with a drug that lowers serum estradiol levels, the most frequently reported adverse reactions were those related to hypoestrogenism.

In controlled studies for endometriosis comparing leuprolide for depot suspension 3.75 mg monthly and danazol (800 mg/day) or placebo, adverse reactions included the following:

Cardiovascular – Palpitations, syncope, tachycardia.

CNS – Anxiety (possible effect of decreased estrogen), delusions, memory disorder, personality disorder.

Dermatologic – Alopecia, ecchymosis, hair disorder.

GI – Appetite changes, dry mouth, thirst.

GU – Dysuria (possible effect of decreased estrogen), lactation.

Miscellaneous – Lymphadenopathy, ophthalmologic disorders (possible effect of decreased estrogen).

Potentially drug-related adverse events observed in at least 5% of patients in any treatment group during the first 6 months of treatment in the add-back clinical studies (3.75 mg [monthly] depot suspension) – The following table lists the potentially drug-related adverse events observed in at least 5% of patients in any treatment group during the first 6 months of treatment in the add–back clinical studies.

Treatment-related Adverse Events Occurring in ≥ 5% of Patients

	Controlled study				Open-label study	
	LD-only[a] (n = 51)		LD/N[b] (n = 55)		LD/N[b] (n = 136)	
Adverse events	n	(%)	n	(%)	n	(%)
Any adverse event	50	(98%)	53	(96%)	126	(93%)
Cardiovascular						
Hot flashes/sweats	50	(98%)	48	(87%)	78	(57%)
CNS						
Anxiety	3	(6%)	0	(0%)	11	(8%)
Depression/emotional lability	16	(31%)	15	(27%)	46	(34%)
Dizziness/vertigo	8	(16%)	6	(11%)	10	(7%)
Insomnia/sleep disorder	16	(31%)	7	(13%)	20	(15%)
Libido changes	5	(10%)	2	(4%)	10	(7%)
Memory disorder	3	(6%)	1	(2%)	6	(4%)

LEUPROLIDE ACETATE — INJECTION

Treatment-related Adverse Events Occurring in ≥ 5% of Patients						
	Controlled study				Open-label study	
	LD-only[a] (n = 51)		LD/N[b] (n = 55)		LD/N[b] (n = 136)	
Adverse events	n	(%)	n	(%)	n	(%)
Nervousness	4	(8%)	2	(4%)	15	(11%)
Neuromuscular disorder	1	(2%)	5	(9%)	4	(3%)
Dermatologic						
Alopecia	0	(0%)	5	(9%)	4	(3%)
Androgen-like effects	2	(4%)	3	(5%)	24	(18%)
Skin/mucous membrane reaction	2	(4%)	5	(9%)	15	(11%)
GI						
Altered bowel function	7	(14%)	8	(15%)	14	(10%)
Changes in appetite	2	(4%)	0	(0%)	8	(6%)
GI disturbance	2	(4%)	4	(7%)	6	(4%)
Nausea/vomiting	13	(25%)	16	(29%)	17	(13%)
GU						
Breast changes/pain/ tenderness	3	(6%)	7	(13%)	11	(8%)
Menstrual disorders	1	(2%)	0	(0%)	7	(5%)
Vaginitis	10	(20%)	8	(15%)	11	(8%)
Metabolic/Nutritional						
Edema	0	(0%)	5	(9%)	9	(7%)
Weight changes	6	(12%)	7	(13%)	6	(4%)
Miscellaneous						
Asthenia	9	(18%)	10	(18%)	15	(11%)
Headache/migraine	33	(65%)	28	(51%)	63	(46%)
Injection site reaction	1	(2%)	5	(9%)	4	(3%)
Pain	12	(24%)	16	(29%)	29	(21%)

[a] LD-only = leuprolide 3.75 mg (monthly) depot suspension.
[b] LD/N = leuprolide 3.75 mg plus norethindrone acetate 5 mg.

In the controlled clinical trial, 50 of 51 (98%) patients in the LD group and 48 of 55 (87%) patients in the LD/N group reported experiencing hot flashes on 1 or more occasions during treatment. During month 6 of treatment, 32 of 37 (86%) patients in the LD group and 22 of 38 (58%) patients in the LD/N group reported having experienced hot flashes. The mean number of days on which hot flashes were reported during this month of treatment was 19 and 7 in the LD and LD/N treatment groups, respectively. The mean maximum number of hot flashes in a day during this month of treatment was 5.8 and 1.9 in the LD and LD/N treatment groups, respectively.

➤*Uterine leiomyomata (fibroids) (3.75 mg [monthly] depot suspension):*

Adverse Reactions Observed in Patients and Thought to be Potentially Related to Drug (more than 5%)				
	Leuprolide 3.75 mg monthly depot suspension		Placebo	
Adverse reaction	(n = 166)	(%)	(n = 163)	(%)
Cardiovascular				
Hot flashes/sweats[a]	121	(72.9%)	29	(17.8%)
CNS				
Depression/emotional lability[a]	18	(10.8%)	7	(4.3%)
GU				
Vaginitis[a]	19	(11.4%)	3	(1.8%)
Metabolic/Nutritional				
Edema	9	(5.4%)	2	(1.2%)
Musculoskeletal				
Joint disorder[a]	13	(7.8%)	5	(3.1%)
Miscellaneous				
Asthenia	14	(8.4%)	8	(4.9%)
General pain	14	(8.4%)	10	(6.1%)
Headache[a]	43	(25.9%)	29	(17.8%)

[a] Possible effect of decreased estrogen.

Symptoms reported in less than 5% of patients included:

Cardiovascular – Tachycardia.

CNS – Anxiety, decreased libido (possible effect of decreased estrogen), dizziness, insomnia, nervousness (possible effect of decreased estrogen), neuromuscular disorders (possible effect of decreased estrogen), paresthesias.

Dermatologic – Androgen-like effects, nail disorder, skin reactions.

GI – Appetite changes, dry mouth, GI disturbances, nausea/vomiting.

GU – Breast changes (possible effect of decreased estrogen), menstrual disorders.

Metabolic / Nutritional – Weight changes.

Musculoskeletal – Myalgia.

Respiratory – Rhinitis.

Special senses – Conjunctivitis, taste perversion.

Miscellaneous – Body odor, flu syndrome, injection-site reactions.

In 1 controlled clinical trial, patients received a higher dose (7.5 mg) of leuprolide for depot suspension. Events seen with this dose that were thought to be potentially related to drug and were not seen at the lower dose included palpitations, syncope, glossitis, ecchymosis, hypesthesia, confusion, lactation, pyelonephritis, and urinary disorders. Generally, a higher incidence of hypoestrogenic effects was observed at the higher dose.

Changes in bone density (3.75 mg [monthly] and 11.25 mg [3-month] depot suspensions) – In controlled clinical studies, patients with endometriosis (6 months of therapy) or uterine fibroids (3 months of therapy) were treated with leuprolide 3.75 mg monthly depot suspension. In endometriosis patients, vertebral bone density as measured by dual energy x-ray absorptiometry (DEXA) decreased by an average of 3.2% at 6 months compared with the pretreatment value. Clinical studies demonstrate that concurrent hormonal therapy (norethindrone acetate 5 mg daily) and calcium supplementation is effective in significantly reducing the loss of bone mineral density that occurs with leuprolide treatment, without compromising the efficacy of leuprolide in relieving symptoms of endometriosis.

Leuprolide 3.75 mg (monthly) depot suspension plus norethindrone acetate 5 mg daily was evaluated in 2 clinical trials. The results from this regimen were similar in both studies. Leuprolide 3.75 mg (monthly) depot suspension was used as a control group in 1 study. The bone mineral density data of the lumbar spine from these 2 studies are presented in the following table:

Mean Percent Change from Baseline in Bone Mineral Density of Lumbar Spine						
	Leuprolide 3.75 mg monthly depot suspension		Leuprolide 3.75 mg monthly depot suspension plus norethindrone acetate 5 mg daily			
	Controlled study		Controlled study		Open-label study	
	n	Change	n	Change	n	Change
Week 24[a]	41	−3.2%	42	−0.3%	115	−0.2%
Week 52[b]	29	−6.3%	32	−1%	84	−1.1%

[a] Includes on-treatment measurements that fell within 2 to 252 days after the first day of treatment.
[b] Includes on-treatment measurements greater than 252 days after the first days of treatment.

In the phase IV 6-month pharmacokinetic/pharmacodynamic study in endometriosis patients who were treated with leuprolide 3.75 mg (monthly) depot suspension or leuprolide 11.25 mg (3-month) depot suspension, vertebral bone density measured by DEXA decreased compared with baseline by an average of 3% and 2.8% at 6 months for the 2 groups, respectively.

When leuprolide 3.75 mg (monthly) depot suspension was administered for 3 months in uterine fibroid patients, vertebral trabecular bone mineral density as assessed by quantitative digital radiography (QDR) revealed a mean decrease of 2.7% compared with baseline. Six months after discontinuation of therapy, a trend toward recovery was observed. Use of leuprolide 3.75 mg (monthly) depot suspension for longer than 3 months (uterine fibroids) or 6 months (endometriosis) or in the presence of other known risk factors for decreased bone mineral content may cause additional bone loss and is not recommended.

➤*Endometriosis and uterine leiomyomata, fibroids (changes in laboratory values during treatment, 3.75 mg [monthly] depot suspension):*

Plasma enzymes –

Endometriosis: During early clinical trials with leuprolide 3.75 mg monthly depot suspension for endometriosis, regular laboratory monitoring revealed that AST levels were more than twice the upper limit of normal in only 1 patient. There was no clinical or other laboratory evidence of abnormal liver function.

In 2 other clinical trials, 6 of 191 patients receiving leuprolide 3.75 mg (monthly) depot suspension plus norethindrone acetate 5 mg daily for up to 12 months developed an elevated (at least twice the upper limit of normal) ALT or gamma-glutamyl-transferase (GGT). Five of the 6 increases were observed beyond 6 months of treatment. None was associated with elevated bilirubin concentration.

Uterine leiomyomata (fibroids): In clinical trials with leuprolide 3.75 mg (monthly) depot suspension for uterine leiomyomata, five (3%) patients had a post-treatment transaminase value that was at least twice the baseline value and above the upper limit of the normal range. None of the laboratory increases was associated with clinical symptoms.

➤*Endometriosis and uterine leiomyomata, fibroids (3.75 mg [monthly] depot suspension):*

Lipids –

Endometriosis: Triglycerides were increased above the upper limit of normal in 12% of the endometriosis patients who received leuprolide 3.75 mg (monthly) depot suspension and in 32% of the subjects receiving leuprolide 11.25 mg (3-month) depot suspension.

LEUPROLIDE ACETATE — INJECTION

Of those endometriosis and uterine fibroid patients whose pretreatment cholesterol values were in the normal range, mean change following therapy was +16 mg/dL to +17 mg/dL in endometriosis patients and +11 mg/dL to +29 mg/dL in uterine fibroid patients. In the endometriosis-treated patients, increases from the pretreatment values were statistically significant (*P* less than 0.03). There was essentially no increase in the LDL/HDL ratio in patients from either population receiving leuprolide 3.75 mg (monthly) depot suspension.

In 2 other clinical trials, leuprolide 3.75 mg (monthly) depot suspension plus norethindrone acetate 5 mg daily were evaluated for 12 months of treatment. Leuprolide 3.75 mg (monthly) depot suspension was used as a control group in 1 study. Percent changes from baseline for serum lipids and percentages of patients with serum lipid values outside of the normal range in the 2 studies are summarized in the following tables:

Serum Lipids: Mean Percent Changes from Baseline Values at Treatment Week 24

	Leuprolide		Leuprolide plus norethindrone acetate 5 mg daily			
	Baseline value[a]	Week 24 (% change)	Baseline value[a]	Week 24 (% change)	Baseline value[a]	Week 24 (% change)
Total cholesterol	170.5	9.2%	179.3	0.2%	181.2	2.8%
HDL cholesterol	52.4	7.4%	51.8	−18.8%	51	−14.6%
LDL cholesterol	96.6	10.9%	101.5	14.1%	109.1	13.1%
LDL/HDL ratio	2[b]	5%	2.1[b]	43.4%	2.3[b]	39.4%
Triglycerides	107.8	17.5%	130.2	9.5%	105.4	13.8%

[a] mg/dL.
[b] ratio.

Changes from baseline tended to be greater at week 52. After treatment, mean serum lipid levels from patients with follow-up data returned to pretreatment values.

Percentage of Patients with Serum Lipid Values Outside of the Normal Range

	Leuprolide		Leuprolide plus norethindrone acetate 5 mg daily			
	Controlled study (n = 39)		Controlled study (n = 41)		Open-label study (n = 117)	
	Week 0	Week 24[a]	Week 0	Week 24[a]	Week 0	Week 24[a]
Total cholesterol (> 240 mg/dL)	15%	23%	15%	20%	6%	7%
HDL cholesterol (< 40 mg/dL)	15%	10%	15%	44%	15%	41%
LDL cholesterol (> 160 mg/dL)	0%	8%	5%	7%	9%	11%
LDL/HDL ratio (> 4)	0%	3%	2%	15%	7%	21%
Triglycerides (> 200 mg/dL)	13%	13%	12%	10%	5%	9%

[a] Includes all patients regardless of baseline value.

Low HDL cholesterol (less than 40 mg/dL) and elevated LDL cholesterol (greater than 160 mg/dL) are recognized risk factors for cardiovascular disease. The long-term significance of the observed treatment-related changes in serum lipids in women with endometriosis is unknown. Therefore, consider assessment of cardiovascular risk factors prior to initiation of concurrent treatment with leuprolide 3.75 mg (monthly) depot suspension and norethindrone acetate.

• *Chemistry* – Slight-to-moderate mean increases were noted for glucose, uric acid, blood urea nitrogen, creatinine, total protein, albumin, bilirubin, alkaline phosphatase, LDH, calcium, and phosphorus. None of these increases were clinically significant. In the hormonal add-back studies, leuprolide 11.25 mg (3-month) depot suspension in combination with norethindrone acetate was associated with elevations of GGT and ALT in 6% to 7% of patients.

Uterine leiomyomata (fibroids): In patients receiving leuprolide 3.75 mg monthly depot suspension, mean changes in cholesterol (+11 mg/dL to +29 mg/dL), LDL cholesterol (+8 mg/dL to +22 mg/dL), HDL cholesterol (0 to +6 mg/dL), and the LDL/HDL ratio (−0.1 to +0.5) were observed across studies. In the 1 study in which triglycerides were determined, the mean increase from baseline was 32 mg/dL.

➤*Endometriosis and uterine leiomyomata (fibroids) (3.75 mg [monthly] depot suspension):*

Other changes –

Endometriosis: The following changes were seen in approximately 5% to 8% of patients. In the earlier comparative studies, leuprolide 3.75 mg (monthly) depot suspension was associated with elevations of LDH and phosphorus, and decreases in WBC counts. Danazol therapy was associated with increases in hematocrit, platelet count, and LDH. In the hormonal add-back studies leuprolide 3.75 mg (monthly) depot suspension in combination with norethindrone acetate was associated with elevations of GGT and ALT.

Uterine leiomyomata (fibroids):

• *Hematology* – In leuprolide 3.75 mg (monthly) depot suspension-treated patients, although there were statistically significant mean decreases in platelet counts from baseline to final visit, the last mean platelet counts were within the normal range. Decreases in total WBC count and neutrophils were observed, but were not clinically significant.

• *Chemistry* – Slight to moderate mean increases were noted for glucose, uric acid, BUN, creatinine, total protein, albumin, bilirubin, alkaline phosphatase, LDH, calcium, and phosphorus. None of these increases were clinically significant.

➤*Endometriosis and uterine leiomyomata (postmarketing, 3.75 mg [monthly] and 11.25 mg [3-month]depot suspensions):* During postmarketing surveillance, the following adverse events were reported. Like other drugs in this class, mood swings, including depression, have been reported as a physiologic effect of decreased sex steroids. There have been rare reports of suicidal ideation and attempt. Many, but not all, of these patients had histories of depression or other psychiatric illness. Counsel patients on the possibility of development or worsening of depression during treatment with leuprolide.

Symptoms consistent with an anaphylactoid or asthmatic process have been rarely reported. Rash, urticaria, and photosensitivity reactions have also been reported.

Localized reactions, including induration and abscess, have been reported at the site of injection.

Symptoms consistent with fibromyalgia (eg, joint and muscle pain, headaches, sleep disorder, GI distress, and shortness of breath) have been reported individually and collectively. Other events reported are as follows:

Cardiovascular – Hypotension, pulmonary embolism.

CNS – Peripheral neuropathy, spinal fracture/paralysis.

GU – Prostate pain.

Hematologic / Lymphatic – Decreased white blood cells.

Musculoskeletal – Tenosynovitis-like symptoms.

➤*Endometriosis and uterine fibroids (11.25 mg [3-month] depot suspension):* The monthly formulation of leuprolide 3.75 mg depot suspension was utilized in controlled clinical trials that studied the drug in 166 endometriosis and 166 uterine fibroids patients. Adverse events reported in greater than or equal to 5% of patients in either of these populations and thought to be potentially related to the drug are noted in the following table.

Adverse Reactions Reported to be Causally Related to Drug (≥ 5%)

	Endometriosis (2 studies)						Uterine fibroids (4 studies)			
	Leuprolide 3.75 mg depot suspension (n = 166)		Danazol (n = 136)		Placebo (n = 31)		Leuprolide 3.75 mg depot suspension (n = 166)		Placebo (n = 163)	
Adverse reaction	n	(%)	n	(%)	n	(%)	n	(%)	n	(%)
Cardiovascular										
Hot flashes/sweats[a]	139	(84%)	77	(57%)	9	(29%)	121	(72.9%)	29	(17.8%)
CNS										
Decreased libido[a]	19	(11%)	6	(4%)	0	(0%)	3	(1.8%)	0	(0%)
Depression/emotional lability[a]	36	(22%)	27	(20%)	1	(3%)	18	(10.8%)	7	(4.3%)
Dizziness	19	(11%)	4	(3%)	0	(0%)	3	(1.8%)	6	(3.7%)

LEUPROLIDE ACETATE — INJECTION

Adverse Reactions Reported to be Causally Related to Drug (≥ 5%)

	Endometriosis (2 studies)						Uterine fibroids (4 studies)			
	Leuprolide 3.75 mg depot suspension (n = 166)		Danazol (n = 136)		Placebo (n = 31)		Leuprolide 3.75 mg depot suspension (n = 166)		Placebo (n = 163)	
Adverse reaction	n	(%)	n	(%)	n	(%)	n	(%)	n	(%)
Nervousness[a]	8	(5%)	11	(8%)	0	(0%)	8	(4.8%)	1	(0.6%)
Neuromuscular disorders[a]	11	(7%)	17	(13%)	0	(0%)	3	(1.8%)	0	(0%)
Paresthesias	12	(7%)	11	(8%)	0	(0%)	2	(1.2%)	1	(0.6%)
Dermatologic										
Skin reactions	17	(10%)	20	(15%)	1	(3%)	5	(3%)	2	(1.2%)
Endocrine										
Acne	17	(10%)	27	(20%)	0	(0%)	0	(0%)	0	(0%)
Hirsutism	2	(1%)	9	(7%)	1	(3%)	1	(0.6%)	0	(0%)
GI										
Nausea/vomiting	21	(13%)	17	(13%)	1	(3%)	8	(4.8%)	6	(3.7%)
GI disturbances[a]	11	(7%)	8	(6%)	1	(3%)	5	(3%)	2	(1.2%)
GU										
Breast changes/tenderness/pain[a]	10	(6%)	12	(9%)	0	(0%)	3	(1.8%)	7	(4.3%)
Vaginitis[a]	46	(28%)	23	(17%)	0	(0%)	19	(11.4%)	3	(1.8%)
Metabolic/Nutritional										
Edema	12	(7%)	17	(13%)	1	(3%)	9	(5.4%)	2	(1.2%)
Weight gain/loss	22	(13%)	36	(26%)	0	(0%)	5	(3%)	2	(1.2%)
Musculoskeletal										
Joint disorder[a]	14	(8%)	11	(8%)	0	(0%)	13	(7.8%)	5	(3.1%)
Myalgia[a]	1	(1%)	7	(5%)	0	(0%)	1	(0.6%)	0	(0%)
Miscellaneous										
Asthenia	5	(3%)	9	(7%)	0	(0%)	14	(8.4%)	8	(4.9%)
General pain	31	(19%)	22	(16%)	1	(3%)	14	(8.4%)	10	(6.1%)
Headache[a]	53	(32%)	30	(22%)	2	(6%)	43	(25.9%)	29	(17.8%)

[a] Physiologic effect of the drug.

In these same studies, symptoms reported in less than 5% of patients included:

Cardiovascular – Palpitations, syncope, tachycardia.

CNS – Anxiety (physiologic effect of the drug), delusions, insomnia/sleep disorders (physiologic effect of the drug), memory disorder, personality disorder.

Dermatologic – Alopecia, hair disorder, nail disorder.

Endocrine – Androgen-like effects.

GI – Appetite changes, dry mouth, thirst.

GU – Dysuria (physiologic effect of the drug), lactation, menstrual disorders.

Hematologic / Lymphatic – Ecchymosis, lymphadenopathy.

Respiratory – Rhinitis.

Special senses – Conjunctivitis, ophthalmologic disorders (physiologic effect of the drug), taste perversion.

Miscellaneous – Body odor, flu syndrome, injection site reactions. In 1 controlled clinical trial utilizing the monthly formulation of leuprolide for depot suspension, patients diagnosed with uterine fibroids received a higher dose (7.5 mg) of leuprolide for depot suspension. Events seen with this dose that were thought to be potentially related to drug and were not seen at the lower dose included glossitis, hypesthesia, lactation, pyelonephritis, and urinary disorders. Generally, a higher incidence of hypoestrogenic effects was observed at the higher dose.

In a pharmacokinetic trial involving 20 healthy female subjects receiving leuprolide 11.25 mg (3-month) depot suspension a few adverse events were reported with this formulation that were not reported previously. These included face edema, agitation, laryngitis, and ear pain.

The following table lists the potentially drug-related adverse events observed in at least 5% of patients in any treatment group, during the first 6 months of treatment in the add-back clinical studies, in which patients were treated with monthly leuprolide 3.75 mg (monthly) depot suspension with or without norethindrone acetate cotreatment.

Treatment-related Adverse Events Occurring in ≥ 5% of Patients

	Controlled study		Open-label study
	Leuprolide 3.75 mg monthly depot suspension[a] (n = 51)	Leuprolide 3.75 mg monthly depot suspension/ norethindrone acetate[b] (n = 55)	Leuprolide 3.75 mg monthly depot suspension[b]/ norethindrone acetate (n = 136)
Adverse events	n (%)	n (%)	n (%)
Any adverse event	50 (98%)	53 (96%)	126 (93%)
Cardiovascular			
Hot flashes/sweats	50 (98%)	48 (87%)	78 (57%)
CNS			
Anxiety	3 (6%)	0 (0%)	11 (8%)
Depression/ emotional lability	16 (31%)	15 (27%)	46 (34%)
Dizziness/vertigo	8 (16%)	6 (11%)	10 (7%)
Insomnia/ sleep disorder	16 (31%)	7 (13%)	20 (15%)
Libido changes	5 (10%)	2 (4%)	10 (7%)
Memory disorder	3 (6%)	1 (2%)	6 (4%)
Nervousness	4 (8%)	2 (4%)	15 (11%)
Neuromuscular disorder	1 (2%)	5 (9%)	4 (3%)
Dermatologic			
Alopecia	0 (0%)	5 (9%)	4 (3%)
Androgen-like effects	2 (4%)	3 (5%)	24 (18%)
Skin/mucous membrane reaction	2 (4%)	5 (9%)	15 (11%)

LEUPROLIDE ACETATE — INJECTION

Treatment-related Adverse Events Occurring in ≥ 5% of Patients			
	Controlled study		Open-label study
	Leuprolide 3.75 mg monthly depot suspension[a] (n = 51)	Leuprolide 3.75 mg monthly depot suspension/ norethindrone acetate[b] (n = 55)	Leuprolide 3.75 mg monthly depot suspension[b]/ norethindrone acetate (n = 136)
Adverse events	n (%)	n (%)	n (%)
GI			
Altered bowel function	7 (14%)	8 (15%)	14 (10%)
Changes in appetite	2 (4%)	0 (0%)	8 (6%)
GI disturbance	2 (4%)	4 (7%)	6 (4%)
Nausea/vomiting	13 (25%)	16 (29%)	17 (13%)
GU			
Breast changes/ pain/tenderness	3 (6%)	7 (13%)	11 (8%)
Menstrual disorders	1 (2%)	0 (0%)	7 (5%)
Vaginitis	10 (20%)	8 (15%)	11 (8%)
Metabolic/Nutritional			
Edema	0 (0%)	5 (9%)	9 (7%)
Weight changes	6 (12%)	7 (13%)	6 (4%)
Miscellaneous			
Asthenia	9 (18%)	10 (18%)	15 (11%)
Headache/migraine	33 (65%)	28 (51%)	63 (46%)
Injection-site reaction	1 (2%)	5 (9%)	4 (3%)
Pain	12 (24%)	16 (29%)	29 (21%)

[a] Leuprolide acetate 3.75 mg (monthly) depot suspension.
[b] Leuprolide acetate/norethindrone acetate 3.75 mg (monthly) depot suspension plus norethindrone acetate 5 mg.

In the controlled clinical trial, 50 of 51 (98%) patients in the leuprolide 3.75 mg monthly depot suspension and 48 of 55 (87%) patients in the leuprolide 3.75 mg (monthly) depot suspension plus norethindrone acetate 5 mg daily reported experiencing hot flashes on 1 or more occasions during treatment. During month 6 of treatment, 32 of 37 (86%) patients in the leuprolide depot suspension group and 22 of 38 (58%) patients in the leuprolide 3.75 mg (monthly) depot suspension plus norethindrone acetate group reported having experienced hot flashes. The mean number of days on which hot flashes were reported during this month of treatment was 19 and 7 in the leuprolide depot suspension group and the leuprolide depot suspension plus norethindrone acetate treatment groups, respectively. The mean maximum number of hot flashes in a day during this month of treatment was 5.8 and 1.9 in the leuprolide depot suspension group and the leuprolide depot suspension plus norethindrone acetate treatment groups, respectively.

➤*Endometriosis and uterine leiomyomata (changes in laboratory values during treatment, 11.25 mg [3-month] depot suspension):*

Liver enzymes – Three percent of uterine fibroid patients treated with 3.75 mg monthly depot suspension manifested posttreatment transaminase values that were at least twice the baseline value and above the upper limit of normal range. None of the laboratory increases was associated with clinical symptoms.

Lipids – Triglycerides were increased above the upper limit of normal in 12% of the endometriosis patients who received leuprolide 3.75 mg (monthly) depot suspension and in 32% of the subjects receiving leuprolide 11.25 mg (3-month) depot suspension.

Of those endometriosis and uterine fibroid patients whose pretreatment cholesterol values were in the normal range, mean change following therapy was + 16 mg/dL to + 17 mg/dL in endometriosis patients and +11 mg/dL to +29 mg/dL in uterine fibroid patients. In the endometriosis-treated patients, increases from the pretreatment values were statistically significant (P less than 0.03). There was essentially no increase in the LDL/HDL ratio in patients from either population receiving leuprolide 3.75 mg (monthly) suspension.

Overdosage

In rats, subcutaneous administration of 125 to 500 times the recommended human pediatric dose, expressed on a per body weight basis, resulted in dyspnea, decreased activity, and local irritation at the injection site. There is no evidence at present that there is a clinical counterpart of this phenomenon.

In early clinical trials using daily subcutaneous leuprolide in adult patients, doses as high as 20 mg/day for up to 2 years caused no adverse effects differing from those observed with the 1 mg/day dose.

LEUPROLIDE ACETATE — IMPLANT

Indications

➤*Advanced prostatic cancer:* Palliative treatment of advanced prostatic cancer that offers an alternative when orchiectomy or estrogen administration are not indicated or are unacceptable to the patient.

Administration and Dosage

➤*Advanced prostate cancer:* One implant every 12 months. Each implant contains 65 mg leuprolide. The implant is inserted SC in the inner aspect of the upper arm and provides the continuous release of leuprolide for 12 months of hormonal therapy.

Leuprolide acetate implant must be removed after 12 months of therapy. At the time an implant is removed, another implant may be inserted to continue therapy.

➤*Storage/Stability:* Store at 25°C (77°F); excursions permitted to 15° to 30°C (59° to 86°F).

Actions

➤*Pharmacology:* Leuprolide acetate, an LHRH agonist, acts as a potent inhibitor of gonadotropin secretion when given continuously and in therapeutic doses. Animal and human studies indicate that after an initial stimulation, chronic administration of leuprolide acetate results in suppression of ovarian and testicular steroidogenesis.

In humans, administration of leuprolide acetate results in an initial increase in circulating levels of luteinizing hormone (LH) and follicle-stimulating hormone (FSH), leading to a transient increase in concentrations of gonadal steroids (testosterone and dihydrotestosterone in males, and estrone and estradiol in premenopausal females). However, continuous administration of leuprolide acetate results in decreased levels of LH and FSH. In males, testosterone is reduced to castrate levels. These decreases occur within 2 to 4 weeks after initiation of treatment.

One leuprolide acetate implant nominally delivers 120 mcg of leuprolide acetate per day over 12 months. Leuprolide acetate is not active when given orally.

➤*Pharmacokinetics:*

Absorption – After insertion of leuprolide acetate implant, mean serum leuprolide concentrations were 16.9 ng/mL at 4 hours and 2.4 ng/mL at 24 hours. Thereafter, leuprolide was released at a constant rate. Mean serum leuprolide concentrations were maintained at 0.9 ng/mL (0.3 to 3.1 ng/mL; SD = ± 0.4) for 12 months. Upon removal and insertion of a new leuprolide acetate implant at 12 months, steady-state serum leuprolide concentrations were maintained.

Distribution – The mean steady-state volume of distribution of leuprolide following 1 mg IV bolus administration to healthy male volunteers was 27 L. In vitro binding to human plasma proteins ranged from 43% to 49%.

Metabolism – In healthy male volunteers administered a 1 mg IV bolus of leuprolide, the mean systemic clearance was 8.34 L/hr, with a terminal elimination half-life of approximately 3 hours, based on a 2-compartment model. A pentapeptide (M-1) is the major leuprolide metabolite upon administration with different leuprolide acetate formulations. No drug metabolism study was conducted with leuprolide acetate implant.

Contraindications

Hypersensitivity to GnRH, GnRH agonist analogs, or any of the components in leuprolide acetate implant. Anaphylactic reactions to synthetic GnRH or GnRH agonist analogs have been reported in the literature.

Leuprolide acetate implant is contraindicated in women and in pediatric patients and was not studied in women or children. Moreover, leuprolide acetate can cause fetal harm when administered to a pregnant woman. Major fetal abnormalities were observed in rabbits but not in rats after administration of leuprolide acetate throughout gestation. There were increased fetal mortality and decreased fetal weights in rats and rabbits. The effects on fetal mortality are expected consequences of the alterations in hormonal levels brought about by this drug. The possibility exists that spontaneous abortion may occur.

Warnings

➤*Worsening of symptoms:* Leuprolide acetate implant, like other LHRH agonists, causes a transient increase in serum concentrations of testosterone during the first week of treatment. Patients may experience worsening of symptoms or onset of new symptoms, including bone pain, neuropathy, hematuria, or ureteral or bladder outlet obstruction.

➤*Ureteral obstruction/spinal cord compression:* Cases of ureteral obstruction and spinal cord compression, which may contribute to paralysis with or without fatal complications, have been reported with LHRH agonists. If spinal cord compression or renal impairment develops, standard treatment of these complications should be instituted.

➤*Carcinogenesis:* Two-year carcinogenicity studies were conducted in rats and mice. In rats, dose-related increases of benign pituitary hyperplasia and benign pituitary adenomas were noted at 24 months when the drug was administered SC at high daily doses (4 to 24 mg/m^2, 50 to 300 times the daily human exposure based on body surface area). There were significant but not dose-related increases of pancreatic islet-cell adenomas in females and of testicular interstitial cell adenomas in males (highest incidence in the low dose group). In mice no pituitary abnormalities were observed at up to 180 mg/m^2 (over 2000 times the daily human exposure based on body surface area) for 2 years.

LEUPROLIDE ACETATE — IMPLANT

➤*Pregnancy: Category X.*

See Contraindications for more information.

➤*Children:* Leuprolide acetate implant is contraindicated in pediatric patients and was not studied in children.

Precautions

➤*Monitoring:* Response to leuprolide acetate implant should be monitored by measuring serum concentrations of testosterone and prostate-specific antigen periodically.

Patients with metastatic vertebral lesions or with urinary tract obstruction should be closely observed during the first few weeks of therapy.

➤*MRI procedures:* The titanium alloy reservoir of leuprolide acetate implant is nonferromagnetic and is not affected by magnetic resonance imaging (MRI). Slight image distortion around leuprolide acetate implant may occur during MRI procedures.

Drug Interactions

➤*Drug/Lab test interactions:* Therapy with leuprolide results in suppression of the pituitary-gonadal system. Results of diagnostic tests of pituitary gonadotropic and gonadal functions conducted during and after leuprolide therapy may be affected.

Adverse Reactions

See Warnings for more information.

Leuprolide Implant Adverse Reactions (≥ 2%)

Adverse reaction	Number	(%)
Cardiovascular		
Vasodilation (hot flashes)[a]	89	67.9%
CNS		
Depression	7	5.3%
Dermatologic		
Sweating[a]	7	5.3%
Alopecia	3	2.3%
GI		
Diarrhea	3	2.3%
GU		
Gynecomastia/breast enlargement[a]	9	6.9%
Nocturia	5	3.8%
Urinary frequency	5	3.8%
Testis atrophy or pain[a]	5	3.8%
Breast pain[a]	4	3.1%
Impotence[a]	3	2.3%
Hematologic/Lymphatic		
Ecchymosis	6	4.6%
Anemia	3	2.3%
Metabolic/Nutritional		
Peripheral edema	4	3.1%
Weight gain	3	2.3%
Respiratory		
Dyspnea	3	2.3%
Miscellaneous		
Asthenia	10	7.6%
Headache	6	4.6%
Extremity pain	4	3.1%

[a] Expected pharmacologic consequence of testosterone suppression.

In addition, the following possibly or probably related systemic adverse events were reported by less than 2% of patients using leuprolide acetate implant in clinical studies.

➤*CNS:* Dizziness, insomnia, paresthesia, amnesia, anxiety.

➤*Dermatologic:* Pruritus, rash, hirsutism.

➤*GI:* Constipation, nausea.

➤*GU:* Urinary urgency, prostatic disorder, urinary tract infection, dysuria, urinary incontinence, urinary retention.

➤*Hematologic:* Iron deficiency anemia.

➤*Local:* Local reactions after initial insertion of a single implant included bruising (34.6%) and burning (5.6%). Other, less frequently reported reactions included pulling, pressure, itching, erythema, pain, edema, and bleeding.

In 2 clinical trials, 4 patients had local infection/inflammations that resolved after treatment with oral antibiotics.

Local reactions following insertion of a subsequent implant were comparable to those seen after initial insertion.

In the first 12 months after initial insertion of the implant(s), an implant extruded through the incision site in 3 of 131 patients.

The majority of local reactions associated with initial insertion or removal and insertion of a new implant began and resolved within the first 2 weeks. Reactions persisted in 9.3% of patients; 10.3% of patients developed application-site reactions after the first 2 weeks following insertion.

➤*Metabolic:* Edema, weight loss.

➤*Musculoskeletal:* Bone pain, arthritis.

Changes in bone density – Decreased bone density has been reported in the medical literature in men who have had orchiectomy or who have been treated with an LHRH agonist analog. In a clinical trial, 25 men with prostate cancer, 12 of whom had been treated previously with leuprolide acetate for at least 6 months, underwent bone density studies as a result of pain. The leuprolide-treated group had lower bone density scores than the nontreated control group. It can be anticipated that long periods of medical castration in men will have effects on bone density.

➤*Miscellaneous:* General pain, chills, abdominal pain, malaise, dry mucous membranes.

Overdosage

In clinical trials using daily SC leuprolide acetate in patients with prostate cancer, doses as high as 20 mg/day for up to 2 years caused no adverse effects differing from those observed with the 1 mg/day dose. The adverse event profiles were similar in patients receiving 1 or 2 leuprolide acetate implants.

GOSERELIN ACETATE

Rx	**Zoladex** (AstraZeneca)	**Implant:** 3.6 mg	In preloaded syringes (16-gauge needle).
		10.8 mg	In preloaded syringes (14-gauge needle).

GOSERELIN ACETATE — IMPLANT

Indications

➤*Advanced breast cancer (3.6 mg only):* For use in the palliative treatment of advanced breast cancer in pre- and postmenopausal women.

The estrogen and progesterone receptor values may help to predict whether goserelin therapy is likely to be beneficial.

➤*Endometrial thinning (3.6 mg only):* For use as an endometrial-thinning agent prior to endometrial ablation for dysfunctional uterine bleeding.

➤*Endometriosis (3.6 mg only):* For the management of endometriosis, including pain relief and reduction of endometriotic lesions for the duration of therapy. Experience with goserelin for the management of endometriosis has been limited to women 18 years of age and older treated for 6 months.

➤*Prostatic carcinoma:* In the palliative treatment of advanced carcinoma of the prostate.

➤*Stage B2 to C prostatic carcinoma:* For use in combination with flutamide for the management of locally confined stage T2b to T4 (stage B2-C) carcinoma of the prostate. Treatment with goserelin and flutamide should start 8 weeks prior to initiating radiation therapy and continue during radiation therapy.

Administration and Dosage

➤*Approved by the FDA:* December 29, 1989.

➤*Monthly (3.6 mg) implant:* Administer 3.6 mg goserelin subcutaneously every 28 days into the anterior abdominal wall below the navel line using an aseptic technique under the supervision of a physician.

While the delay of a few days is permissible, make every effort to adhere to the 28-day schedule.

➤*3-Month (10.8 mg) implant:* Administer 10.8 mg goserelin subcutaneously every 12 weeks into the upper abdominal wall using an aseptic technique under the supervision of a physician.

While a delay of a few days is permissible, make every effort to adhere to the 12-week schedule.

➤*Advanced breast cancer (3.6 mg only):* For the management of advanced breast cancer, goserelin is intended for long-term administration unless clinically inappropriate.

➤*Endometrial thinning (3.6 mg only):* For use as an endometrial-thinning agent prior to endometrial ablation, the dosing recommendation is 1 or 2 depots (with each depot given 4 weeks apart). When 1 depot is admin-

GOSERELIN ACETATE — IMPLANT

istered, perform surgery at 4 weeks. When 2 depots are administered, perform surgery within 2 to 4 weeks following administration of the second depot.

➤*Endometriosis (3.6 mg only):* For the management of endometriosis, the recommended duration of administration is 6 months.

Retreatment cannot be recommended for the management of endometriosis because safety data for retreatment are not available. If the symptoms of endometriosis recur after a course of therapy, and further treatment with goserelin is contemplated, consider monitoring bone mineral density. Clinical studies suggest the addition of hormone replacement therapy (estrogens and/or progestins) to goserelin is effective in reducing the bone mineral loss that occurs with goserelin alone without compromising the efficacy of goserelin in relieving the symptoms of endometriosis. The addition of hormone replacement therapy also may reduce the occurrence of vasomotor symptoms and vaginal dryness associated with hypoestrogenism. The optimal drugs, dose, and duration of treatment have not been established.

➤*Prostatic carcinoma:* For the management of advanced prostate cancer, goserelin is intended for long-term administration unless clinically inappropriate.

➤*Stage B2 to C prostatic carcinoma:* When goserelin is given in combination with radiotherapy and flutamide for patients with stage T2b to T4 (stage B2 to C) prostatic carcinoma, start treatment 8 weeks prior to initiating radiotherapy and continue during radiation therapy. Administer a treatment regimen using one 3.6 mg goserelin depot 8 weeks before radiotherapy, followed in 28 days by one 10.8 mg goserelin depot. Alternatively, 4 injections of 3.6 mg depot can be administered at 28-day intervals, 2 depots preceding and 2 during radiotherapy.

➤*Women:* The 10.8 mg goserelin implant is not indicated in women as the data are insufficient to support reliable suppression of serum estradiol. For female patients requiring treatment with goserelin, refer to the use of the 3.6 mg goserelin implant below.

➤*Storage/Stability:* The unit is sterile and comes in a sealed, light- and moisture-proof, aluminum foil laminate pouch containing a desiccant capsule. Store at room temperature (do not exceed 25°C; 77°F).

Actions

➤*Pharmacology:* Goserelin is a synthetic decapeptide analogue of LHRH. Goserelin acts as a potent inhibitor of pituitary gonadotropin secretion when administered in the biodegradable formulation.

Following initial administration in males, goserelin causes an initial increase in serum-luteinizing hormone (LH) and follicle-stimulating hormone (FSH) levels with subsequent increases in serum levels of testosterone. Chronic administration of goserelin leads to sustained suppression of pituitary gonadotropins, and serum levels of testosterone consequently fall into the range normally seen in surgically castrated men approximately 2 to 4 weeks after initiation of therapy. This leads to accessory sex organ regression.

In animal and in vitro studies, administration of goserelin resulted in the regression or inhibition of growth of the hormonally sensitive dimethylbenzanthracene (DMBA)-induced rat mammary tumor and Dunning R3327 prostate tumor.

In clinical trials using 3.6 mg goserelin with follow-up of more than 2 years, suppression of serum testosterone to castrate levels has been maintained for the duration of therapy.

In women, a similar down-regulation of the pituitary gland by chronic exposure to goserelin leads to suppression of gonadotropin secretion, a decrease in serum estradiol to levels consistent with the postmenopausal state, and would be expected to lead to a reduction of ovarian size and function, reduction in the size of the uterus and mammary gland, as well as a regression of sex hormone-responsive tumors, if present. Serum estradiol is suppressed to levels similar to those observed in postmenopausal women within 3 weeks following initial administration; however, after suppression was attained, isolated elevations of estradiol were seen in 10% of the patients enrolled in clinical trials. Serum LH and FSH are suppressed to follicular phase levels within 4 weeks after initial administration of drug and are usually maintained at that range with continued use of goserelin. In 5% or less of women treated with goserelin, FSH and LH levels may not be suppressed to follicular phase levels on day 28 post treatment with use of a single 3.6 mg depot injection. In certain individuals, suppression of any of these hormones to such levels may not be achieved with goserelin. Estradiol, LH, and FSH levels return to pretreatment values within 12 weeks following the last implant administration in all but rare cases.

➤*Pharmacokinetics:*

Absorption –

3.6 mg: The absorption of radiolabeled drug was rapid, and the peak blood radioactivity levels occurred between 0.5 and 1 hour after dosing. The mean (± standard deviation) pharmacokinetic parameter estimates of goserelin after administration of 3.6 mg depot for 2 months in males (n = 7) and females (n = 7) are presented in the following table.

Goserelin Pharmacokinetic Parameters for the 3.6 mg Depot

Parameters (units)	Men (n = 7)	Women (n = 7)
Peak plasma concentration (ng/mL)	2.84 ± 1.81	1.46 ± 0.82
Time to peak concentration (days)	12 to 15	8 to 22

Goserelin Pharmacokinetic Parameters for the 3.6 mg Depot

Parameters (units)	Men (n = 7)	Women (n = 7)
AUC (0 to 28 days) (ng•hr/mL)	27.8 ± 15.3	18.5 ± 10.3
Systemic clearance (mL/min)	110.5 ± 47.5	163.9 ± 71
Apparent volume of distribution (L)[1]	44.1 ± 13.6	20.3 ± 4.1
Elimination half-life (h)[1]	4.2 ± 1.1	2.3 ± 0.6

[1] The apparent volume of distribution and the elimination half-life were determined after subcutaneous administration of 250 mcg aqueous solution of goserelin.

Goserelin is released from the depot at a much slower rate initially for the first 8 days, and then there is more rapid and continuous release for the remainder of the 28-day dosing period. Despite the change in the releasing rate of goserelin, administration of goserelin every 28 days resulted in testosterone levels that were suppressed to and maintained in the range normally seen in surgically castrated men.

10.8 mg: The pharmacokinetics of goserelin have been determined in healthy male volunteers and patients. In healthy males, radiolabeled goserelin was administered as a single 250 mcg (aqueous solution) dose by the subcutaneous route. The absorption of radiolabeled drug was rapid, and the peak blood radioactivity levels occurred between 0.5 and 1 hour after dosing.

The overall pharmacokinetic profile of goserelin following administration of a 10.8 mg goserelin depot to patients with prostate cancer was determined. The initial release of goserelin from the depot was relatively rapid resulting in a peak concentration at 2 hours after dosing. From day 4 until the end of the 12-week dosing interval, the sustained release of goserelin from the depot produced reasonably stable systemic exposure. Mean (standard deviation) pharmacokinetic data are presented below. There is no clinically significant accumulation of goserelin following administration of 4 depots administered at 12-week intervals. Pharmacokinetic data were obtained using an RIA method, which has been shown to be specific for goserelin in the presence of its metabolites.

Goserelin Pharmacokinetic Parameters for the 10.8 mg Depot

Parameter	n	Mean	(SD)[2]	95% CI[3] Lower	95% CI[3] Upper
Systemic clearance (mL/min)	41	121	(42.4)	108	134
C_{max} (ng/mL)	41	8.85	(2.83)	7.96	9.74
T_{max} (hr)	41	1.8	(0.34)	1.7	1.92
C_{min} (ng/mL)	44	0.37	(0.21)	0.3	0.43
Elimination half-life (hr)[1]	7	4.16	(1.12)	3.12	5.2

[1] Determined after subcutaneous administration of 250 mcg aqueous solution of goserelin.
[2] Standard deviation.
[3] 95% confidence interval.

Serum goserelin concentrations in prostate cancer patients administered three 3.6 mg depots followed by one 10.8 mg depot are displayed below. The profiles for both formulations are primarily dependent upon the rate of drug release from the depots. For the 3.6 mg depot, mean concentrations gradually rise to reach a peak of about 3 ng/mL at around 15 days after administration and then decline to approximately 0.5 ng/mL by the end of the treatment period. For the 10.8 mg depot, mean concentrations increase to reach a peak of about 8 ng/mL within the first 24 hours and then decline rapidly up to day 4. Thereafter, mean concentrations remain relatively stable in the range of about 0.3 to 1 ng/mL up to the end of the treatment period.

Administration of four 10.8 mg goserelin depots to patients with prostate cancer resulted in testosterone levels that were suppressed to and maintained within the range normally observed in surgically castrated men (0 to 1.73 nmol/L or 0 to 50 ng/dL), over the dosing interval in approximately 91% (145 out of 160) of patients studied. In 6 of 15 patients that escaped from castrate range, serum testosterone levels were maintained below 2 nmol/L (58 ng/dL), and in only 1 of the 15 patients did the depot completely fail to maintain serum testosterone levels to within the castrate range over a 336-day period (4 depot injections). In the 8 additional patients, a transient escape was followed 14 days later by a level within the castrate range.

Distribution –

3.6 mg: The apparent volumes of distribution determined after subcutaneous administration of 250 mcg aqueous solution of goserelin were 44.1 and 20.3 L for males and females, respectively. The plasma protein binding of goserelin obtained from one sample was found to be 27.3%.

10.8 mg: The apparent volume of distribution determined after subcutaneous administration of 250 mcg aqueous solution of goserelin was 44.1 ± 13.6 L for healthy males. The plasma protein binding of goserelin was found to be 27%.

Metabolism – Metabolism of goserelin, by hydrolysis of the C-terminal amino acids, is the major clearance mechanism. The major circulating component in serum appeared to be 1 to 7 fragment, and the major component present in urine of 1 healthy male volunteer was 5 to 10 fragment. The metabolism of goserelin in humans yields a similar but narrow profile of

GOSERELIN ACETATE — IMPLANT

metabolites to that found in other species. All metabolites found in humans also have been found in toxicology species.

Excretion – Clearance of goserelin following subcutaneous administration of a radiolabeled solution of goserelin was very rapid and occurred via a combination of hepatic and urinary excretion. More than 90% of a subcutaneous radiolabeled solution formulation dose of goserelin was excreted in urine. Approximately 20% of the dose recovered in urine was accounted for by unchanged goserelin.

Special populations –

Body weight: A decline of approximately 1% to 2.5% in the AUC after administration of a 10.8 mg depot was observed with a kg increase in body weight. In obese patients who have not responded clinically, closely monitor testosterone levels.

Contraindications

Hypersensitivity to LHRH, LHRH agonist analogues, or any of the components in goserelin; women who are breastfeeding; women being treated for endometriosis or endometrial thinning who are or may become pregnant while receiving the drug. Goserelin can cause fetal harm when administered to a pregnant woman. Effects on reproductive function, as a result of antigonadotrophic properties of the drug, are expected to occur on chronic administration.

Effective nonhormonal contraception must be used by all premenopausal women during goserelin therapy and for 12 weeks following discontinuation of therapy. There are no adequate and well-controlled studies in pregnant women using goserelin. If this drug is used during pregnancy, or if the patient being treated for endometriosis or endometrial thinning becomes pregnant while taking this drug, apprise the patient of the potential hazard to the fetus or potential risk for loss of the pregnancy. Advise women of childbearing potential to avoid becoming pregnant.

The 10.8 mg goserelin implant is not indicated in women as the data are insufficient to support reliable suppression of serum estradiol.

Goserelin is contraindicated in women who are or may become pregnant while receiving the drug. In studies in rats and rabbits, goserelin increased preimplantation loss, resorptions, and abortions. In rats and dogs, goserelin suppressed ovarian function, decreased ovarian weight and size, and led to atrophic changes in secondary sex organs. Further evidence suggests that fertility was reduced in female rats that became pregnant after goserelin was stopped. These effects are an expected consequence of the hormonal alterations produced by goserelin in humans. If a patient becomes pregnant during treatment, the drug must be discontinued and the patient must be apprised of the potential risk for loss of the pregnancy because of possible hormonal imbalance as a result of the expected pharmacologic action of goserelin treatment. In animal studies, there was no evidence that goserelin possessed the potential to cause teratogenicity in rabbits; however, in rats the incidence of umbilical hernia was significantly increased with treatment.

Warnings

➤*Prostate and breast cancer:* Initially, goserelin, like other LHRH agonists, causes transient increases in serum levels of testosterone in men with prostate cancer, and estrogen in women with breast cancer. Transient worsening of symptoms or the occurrence of additional signs and symptoms of prostate or breast cancer, may occasionally develop during the first few weeks of goserelin treatment. A small number of patients may experience a temporary increase in bone pain, which can be managed symptomatically. As with other LHRH agonists, isolated cases of ureteral obstruction and spinal cord compression have been observed. If spinal cord compression or renal impairment develops, institute standard treatment of these complications. For extreme cases in prostate cancer patients, consider an immediate orchiectomy.

As with other LHRH agonists or hormonal therapies (eg, antiestrogens, estrogens), hypercalcemia has been reported in some prostate and breast cancer patients with bone metastases after starting treatment with goserelin. If hypercalcemia does occur, initiate appropriate treatment measures.

➤*Hypersensitivity reactions:* Hypersensitivity, antibody formation and acute anaphylactic reactions have been reported with LHRH agonist analogues.

➤*Carcinogenesis:* Subcutaneous implant of goserelin in male and female rats once every 4 weeks for 1 year and recovery for 23 weeks at doses of about 80 and 150 mcg/kg (males) and 50 and 100 mcg/kg (females) daily (about 3 to 9 times the recommended human dose on a mg/m^2 basis) resulted in an increased incidence of pituitary adenomas. An increased incidence of pituitary adenomas also was observed following subcutaneous implant of goserelin in rats at similar dose levels for a period of 72 weeks in males and 101 weeks in females. The relevance of the rat pituitary adenomas to humans has not been established. Subcutaneous implants of goserelin every 3 weeks for 2 years delivered to mice at doses of up to 2,400 mcg/kg/day (about 70 times the recommended human dose on a mg/m^2 basis) resulted in an increased incidence of histiocytic sarcoma of the vertebral column and femur.

➤*Fertility impairment:* Administration of goserelin led to changes that were consistent with gonadal suppression in both male and female rats as a result of its endocrine action. In male rats administered 500 to 1,000 mcg/kg/day (about 30 to 60 times the recommended human dose on a mg/m^2 basis), a decrease in weight and atrophic histological changes were observed in the testes, epididymis, seminal vesicle, and prostate gland with complete suppression of spermatogenesis. In female rats administered 50 to 1,000 mcg/kg/day (about 3 to 60 times the recommended human dose on a mg/m^2 basis), suppression of ovarian function led to decreased size and weight of ovaries and secondary sex organs; follicular development was arrested at the antral stage and the corpora lutea were reduced in size and number. Except for the testes, almost complete histologic reversal of these effects in males and females was observed several weeks after dosing was stopped; however, fertility and general reproductive performance were reduced in those that became pregnant after goserelin was discontinued. Fertile matings occurred within 2 weeks after cessation of dosing, even though total recovery of reproductive function may not have occurred before mating took place; and, the ovulation rate, the corresponding implantation rate, and number of live fetuses were reduced.

➤*Pregnancy: Category D* (breast cancer); *Category X* (endometriosis, endometrial thinning; 10.8 mg strength).

See Contraindications for more information.

There are no adequate and well-controlled studies in pregnant women using goserelin. Advise women of childbearing potential to avoid becoming pregnant.

➤*Lactation:* Goserelin has been shown to be excreted in the milk of lactating rats. It is not known if this drug is excreted in human milk. Because many drugs are excreted in human milk and there is a potential for serious adverse reactions in nursing infants of mothers receiving goserelin, mothers should discontinue nursing prior to taking the drug.

See Contraindications for more information.

➤*Children:* Safety and efficacy have not been established.

Precautions

➤*Antibody formation:* Of 115 women worldwide treated with 3.6 mg goserelin and tested for development of binding to goserelin following treatment with goserelin, 1 patient showed low-titer binding to goserelin. On further testing of this patient's plasma obtained following treatment, her goserelin binding component was found not to be precipitated with rabbit antihuman immunoglobulin polyvalent sera. These findings suggest the possibility of antibody formation.

➤*Endometrial ablation:* The pharmacologic action of goserelin on the uterus and cervix may cause an increase in cervical resistance. Therefore, exercise caution when dilating the cervix for endometrial ablation.

Drug Interactions

➤*Drug/Lab test interactions:* Administration of goserelin in therapeutic doses results in suppression of the pituitary-gonadal system. Because of this suppression, diagnostic tests of pituitary-gonadotropic and gonadal functions conducted during treatment and until resumption of menses may show results which are misleading. Normal function is usually restored within 12 weeks after treatment is discontinued.

Adverse Reactions

➤*Hypersensitivity:* Rarely, hypersensitivity reactions (including urticaria and anaphylaxis) have been reported in patients receiving goserelin.

➤*Hypocalcemia:* As with other endocrine therapies, hypercalcemia (increased calcium) has rarely been reported in cancer patients with bone metastases following initiation of treatment with goserelin or other LHRH agonists.

➤*Hypotension/Hypertension:* Changes in blood pressure, manifested as hypotension or hypertension, have been occasionally observed in patients administered goserelin. The changes are usually transient, resolving either during continued therapy or after cessation of therapy with goserelin. Rarely, such changes have been sufficient to require medical intervention including withdrawal of treatment from goserelin.

➤*Pituitary apoplexy:* As with other agents in this class, very rare cases of pituitary apoplexy have been reported following initial administration.

➤*Postmarketing:* There have been postmarketing reports of osteoporosis, decreased bone mineral density, and bony fracture in men treated with goserelin for prostate cancer.

➤*Men - Prostatic carcinoma:* Goserelin has been found to be generally well tolerated in clinical trials. Adverse reactions reported in these trials were rarely severe enough to result in the patients' withdrawal from goserelin treatment. As seen with other hormonal therapies, the most commonly observed adverse reactions during goserelin therapy were caused by the expected physiological effects from decreased testosterone levels. These included hot flashes, sexual dysfunction, and decreased erections.

Initially, goserelin, like other LHRH agonists, causes transient increases in serum levels of testosterone. A small percentage of patients experienced a temporary worsening of signs and symptoms, usually manifested by an increase in cancer-related pain which was managed symptomatically. Isolated cases of exacerbation of disease symptoms, either ureteral obstruction or spinal cord compression, occurred at similar rates in controlled clinical trials with both goserelin and orchiectomy. The relationship of these reactions to therapy is uncertain.

Two controlled clinical trials using 10.8 mg goserelin vs 3.6 mg goserelin were conducted. During a comparative phase, patients were randomized to receive either a single 10.8 mg implant or 3 consecutive 3.6 mg implants every 4 weeks over weeks 0 to 12. During this phase, the only adverse reaction reported in greater than 5% of patients was hot flashes, with an incidence of 47% in the 10.8 mg goserelin group and 48% in the 3.6 mg goserelin group.

From weeks 12 to 48, all patients were treated with a 10.8 mg implant every 12 weeks. During this noncomparative phase, the following adverse reactions were reported in greater than 5% of patients:

GOSERELIN ACETATE — IMPLANT

Goserelin 10.8 mg Adverse Reactions in Patients with Prostatic Carcinoma (%)	
Adverse reaction	Goserelin 10.8 mg (n = 157)
Asthenia	5%
Bone pain	6%
Gynecomastia	8%
Hot flashes	64%
Pain (general)	14%
Pelvic pain	6%

➤*Goserelin vs orchiectomy:*

Adverse Reactions of Goserelin 3.6 mg versus Orchiectomy (%)		
Adverse reaction	Goserelin (n = 242)	Orchiectomy (n = 254)
Anorexia	5%	2%
Chronic obstructive pulmonary disease	5%	3%
Complications of surgery	0%	18%[1]
CHF	5%	1%
Decreased erections	18%	16%
Dizziness	5%	4%
Edema	7%	8%
Hot flashes	62%	53%
Insomnia	5%	1%
Lethargy	8%	4%
Lower urinary tract symptoms	13%	8%
Nausea	5%	2%
Pain (worsened in the first 30 days)	8%	3%
Rash	6%	1%
Sexual dysfunction	21%	15%
Sweating	6%	4%
Upper respiratory tract infection	7%	2%

[1] Complications related to surgery were reported in 18% of the orchiectomy patients, while only 3% of goserelin patients reported adverse reactions at the injection site. The surgical complications included scrotal infections (5.9%), groin pain (4.7%), wound seepage (3.1%), scrotal hematoma (2.8%), incisional discomfort (1.6%), and skin necrosis (1.2%).

➤*The following adverse reactions were reported in greater than 1%, but less than 5% of patients treated with 10.8 mg goserelin implant every 12 weeks. Some of these are commonly reported in elderly patients:*

Cardiovascular – Angina pectoris, cerebral ischemia, cerebrovascular accident, heart failure, pulmonary embolus, varicose veins.

CNS – Dizziness, headache, paresthesia.

Dermatologic – Herpes simplex, pruritus.

Endocrine – Diabetes mellitus.

GI – Abdominal pain, diarrhea, hematemesis.

GU – Bladder neoplasm, breast pain, hematuria, impotence, urinary frequency, urinary incontinence, urinary tract disorder, urinary tract infection, urination impaired, urinary retention.

Hematologic – Anemia.

Metabolic – Peripheral edema.

Respiratory – Cough increased, dyspnea, pneumonia.

Miscellaneous – Back pain, flu syndrome, sepsis, aggravation reaction.

➤*Men - Stage B2 to C prostatic carcinoma:* Treatment with goserelin and flutamide did not add substantially to the toxicity of radiation treatment alone. The following adverse reactions were reported during a multicenter clinical trial comparing goserelin + flutamide + radiation vs radiation alone. The most frequently reported (greater than 5%) adverse reactions are listed below.

Adverse Reactions During Acute Radiation Therapy (%)		
Adverse reaction	Flutamide + goserelin + radiation (n = 231)	Radiation only (n = 235)
Bladder	58%	60%
Rectum/large bowel	80%	76%
Skin	37%	37%

Adverse Reactions During Late Radiation Therapy (%)		
Adverse reaction	Flutamide + goserelin + radiation (n = 231)	Radiation only (n = 235)
Cystitis	16%	16%
Diarrhea	36%	40%
Hematuria	7%	12%
Proctitis	8%	8%
Rectal bleeding	14%	20%

Additional adverse reaction data were collected for the combination therapy with radiation group over both the hormonal treatment and hormonal treatment plus radiation phases of the study. Adverse reactions occurring in more than 5% of patients in this group, over both parts of the study, were hot flashes (46%), diarrhea (40%), nausea (9%), and skin rash (8%).

Lab test abnormalities –

Plasma enzymes: Elevation of liver enzymes (ALT, AST) have been reported in female patients exposed to 3.6 mg goserelin (representing less than 1% of all patients). There was no other evidence of abnormal liver function. Causality between these changes and goserelin have not been established.

Lipids: In a controlled trial in females, 3.6 mg goserelin therapy resulted in a minor, but statistically significant effect on serum lipids. In patients treated for endometriosis at 6 months following initiation of therapy, danazol treatment resulted in a mean increase in LDL cholesterol of 33.3 mg/dL and a decrease in HDL cholesterol of 21.3 mg/dL compared with increases of 21.3 and 2.7 mg/dL in LDL cholesterol and HDL cholesterol, respectively, for goserelin-treated patients. Triglycerides increased by 8 mg/dL in goserelin-treated patients compared with a decrease of 8.9 mg/dL in danazol-treated patients.

In patients treated for endometriosis, goserelin increased total cholesterol and LDL cholesterol during 6 months of treatment. However, goserelin therapy resulted in HDL cholesterol levels which were significantly higher relative to danazol therapy. At the end of 6 months of treatment, HDL cholesterol fractions (HDL_2 and HDL_3) were decreased by 13.5 and 7.7 mg/dL, respectively, for danazol-treated patients compared with treatment increases of 1.9 and 0.8 mg/dL, respectively, for goserelin-treated patients.

➤*Women:* As would be expected with a drug that results in hypoestrogenism, the most frequently reported adverse reactions were those related to this effect.

As with other LHRH agonists, there have been reports of ovarian cyst formation and, when 3.6 mg goserelin is used in combination with gonadotropins, of ovarian hyperstimulation syndrome (OHSS).

Endometriosis –

Goserelin Adverse Reactions (%)		
Adverse reaction	Goserelin (n = 411)	Danazol (n = 207)
Abdominal pain	7%	7%
Acne	42%	55%
Application site reaction	6%	0%
Asthenia	11%	13%
Back pain	7%	13%
Breast atrophy	33%	42%
Breast enlargement	18%	15%
Breast pain	7%	4%
Decreased libido	61%	44%
Depression	54%	48%
Dizziness	6%	4%
Dyspareunia	14%	5%
Emotional lability	60%	56%
Flu syndrome	5%	5%
Hair disorders	4%	11%
Headache	75%	63%
Hirsutism	7%	15%
Hot flashes	96%	67%
Hypertonia	1%	10%
Increased appetite	2%	5%
Increased libido	12%	19%
Infection	13%	11%
Insomnia	11%	4%
Leg cramps	2%	6%
Myalgia	3%	11%
Nausea	8%	14%
Nervousness	3%	5%
Pain	17%	16%
Pelvic symptoms	18%	23%

GOSERELIN ACETATE — IMPLANT

Goserelin Adverse Reactions (%)		
Adverse reaction	Goserelin (n = 411)	Danazol (n = 207)
Peripheral edema	21%	34%
Pharyngitis	5%	2%
Pruritus	2%	6%
Seborrhea	26%	52%
Sweating	45%	30%
Vaginitis	75%	43%
Voice alterations	3%	8%
Weight gain	3%	23%

➤*The following adverse reactions not already listed above were reported at a frequency of 1% or greater, regardless of causality, in goserelin-treated women from all clinical trials:*

Cardiovascular – Hemorrhage, hypertension, migraine, palpitations, tachycardia.

CNS – Anxiety, paresthesia, somnolence, abnormal thinking.

Dermatologic – Alopecia, dry skin, rash, skin discoloration.

GI – Constipation, diarrhea, dry mouth, dyspepsia, flatulence.

GU – Dysmenorrhea, urinary frequency, urinary tract infection, vaginal hemorrhage.

Hematologic – Ecchymosis.

Metabolic/Nutritional – Edema.

Musculoskeletal – Arthralgia, joint disorder.

Respiratory – Bronchitis, increased cough, epistaxis, rhinitis, sinusitis.

Special senses – Amblyopia, dry eyes.

Miscellaneous – Allergic reaction, chest pain, fever, malaise, anorexia.

➤*Hormone replacement therapy:* Clinical studies suggest the addition of hormone replacement therapy (estrogens and/or progestins) to goserelin may decrease the occurrence of vasomotor symptoms and vaginal dryness associated with hypoestrogenism without compromising the efficacy of goserelin in relieving pelvic symptoms. The optimal drugs, dose, and duration of treatment have not been established.

➤*Changes in bone mineral density:* After 6 months of goserelin treatment, 109 female patients treated with goserelin showed an average 4.3% decrease of vertebral trabecular bone mineral density (BMD) as compared with pretreatment values. BMD was measured by dual-photon absorptiometry or dual energy x-ray absorptiometry. Sixty-six of these patients were assessed for BMD loss 6 months after the completion (posttherapy) of the 6-month therapy period. Data from these patients showed an average 2.4% BMD loss compared with pretreatment values. Twenty-eight of the 109 patients were assessed for BMD at 12 months posttherapy. Data from these patients showed an average decrease of 2.5% in BMD compared with pretreatment values. These data suggest a possibility of partial reversibility. Clinical studies suggest the addition of hormone replacement therapy (estrogens and/or progestins) to goserelin is effective in reducing the bone mineral loss which occurs with goserelin alone without compromising the efficacy of goserelin in relieving the symptoms of endometriosis. The optimal drugs, dose, and duration of treatment have not been established.

➤*Breast cancer:* The adverse reaction profile for women with advanced breast cancer treated with goserelin is consistent with the profile described above for women treated with goserelin for endometriosis. In a controlled clinical trial (SWOG-8692) comparing goserelin with oophorectomy in premenopausal and perimenopausal women with advanced breast cancer, the following reactions were reported at a frequency of 5% or greater in either treatment group regardless of causality.

Goserelin Adverse Reactions (%)		
Adverse reaction	Goserelin (n = 57)	Oophorectomy (n = 55)
Edema	5%	0%
Hot flashes	70%	47%
Malaise/fatigue/lethargy	5%	2%
Nausea	11%	7%
Tumor flare	23%	4%
Vomiting	4%	7%

In the phase 2 clinical trial program in 333 pre- and perimenopausal women with advanced breast cancer, hot flashes were reported in 75.9% of patients and decreased libido was noted in 47.7% of patients. These 2 adverse reactions reflect the pharmacological actions of goserelin.

Injection site reactions were reported in less than 1% of patients.

➤*Endometrial thinning:* The following adverse reactions were reported at a frequency of 5% or greater in premenopausal women presenting with dysfunctional uterine bleeding in Trial 0022 for endometrial thinning. These results indicate that headache, hot flushes, and sweating were more common in the goserelin group than in the placebo group.

Goserelin Adverse Reactions (≥ 5%)		
Adverse reaction	Goserelin 3.6 mg (n = 180)	Placebo (n = 177)
Miscellaneous		
Back pain	4%	7%
Pelvic pain	9%	6%
Cardiovascular		
Hypertension	6%	2%
Migraine	7%	4%
Vasodilatation	57%	18%
GI		
Abdominal pain	11%	10%
Nausea	5%	6%
CNS		
Depression	3%	7%
Headache	32%	22%
Nervousness	5%	3%
Respiratory		
Pharyngitis	6%	9%
Sinusitis	3%	6%
Dermatologic		
Sweating	16%	5%
GU		
Dysmenorrhea	7%	9%
Menorrhagia	4%	5%
Uterine hemorrhage	6%	4%
Vaginitis	1%	6%
Vulvovaginitis	5%	1%

Overdosage

The pharmacologic properties of goserelin and its mode of administration make accidental or intentional overdosage unlikely. There is no experience of overdosage from clinical trials. Animal studies indicate that no increased pharmacologic effect occurred at higher doses or more frequent administration. Subcutaneous doses of the drug as high as 1 mg/kg/day in rats and dogs did not produce any nonendocrine related sequelae; this dose is greater than 400 times that proposed for human use. If overdosage occurs, it should be managed symptomatically.

Patient Information

➤*Men:* Carefully consider the use of goserelin in patients at particular risk of developing ureteral obstruction or spinal cord compression and closely monitor the patients during the first month of therapy. Patients with ureteral obstruction or spinal cord compression should have appropriate treatment prior to initiation of goserelin therapy.

➤*Women:* Since menstruation should stop with effective doses of goserelin, the patient should notify her physician if regular menstruation persists. Patients missing 1 or more successive doses of goserelin may experience breakthrough menstrual bleeding.

Do not prescribe goserelin if the patient is pregnant, breastfeeding, lactating, has nondiagnosed abnormal vaginal bleeding, or is allergic to any of the components of goserelin.

Use of goserelin in pregnancy is contraindicated in women being treated for endometriosis or endometrial thinning. Therefore, a nonhormonal method of contraception should be used during treatment. Advise patients that if they miss 1 or more successive doses of goserelin, breakthrough menstrual bleeding or ovulation may occur with the potential for conception. If a patient becomes pregnant during treatment for endometriosis or endometrial thinning, discontinue goserelin treatment and advise the patient on the possible risks to the pregnancy and fetus. In studies in rats and rabbits, 10.8 mg goserelin increased preimplantation loss, resorptions, and abortions. In rats and dogs, 10.8 mg goserelin suppressed ovarian function, decreased ovarian weight and size, and led to atrophic changes in secondary sex organs. Further evidence suggests that fertility was reduced in female rats that became pregnant after goserelin was stopped. These effects are an expected consequence of the hormonal alterations produced by goserelin in humans. In animal studies, there was no evidence that goserelin possessed the potential to cause teratogenicity in rabbits; however, in rats, the incidence of umbilical hernia was significantly increased with treatment.

Those adverse reactions occurring most frequently in clinical studies with goserelin are associated with hypoestrogenism; of these, the most frequently reported are hot flashes (flushes), headaches, vaginal dryness, emotional lability, change in libido, depression, sweating and change in breast size. Clinical studies in endometriosis suggest the addition of hormone replacement therapy (estrogens and/or progestins) to goserelin may decrease the occurrence of vasomotor symptoms and vaginal dryness associated with hypoestrogenism without compromising the efficacy of goserelin in relieving pelvic symptoms. The optimal drugs, dose, and duration of treatment have not been established.

GOSERELIN ACETATE — IMPLANT

As with other LHRH agonist analogues, treatment with goserelin induces a hypoestrogenic state which results in a loss of bone mineral density (BMD) over the course of treatment, some of which may not be reversible. In patients with a history of prior treatment that may have resulted in bone mineral density loss or in patients with major risk factors for decreased bone mineral density, such as chronic alcohol abuse or tobacco abuse, significant family history of osteoporosis, or chronic use of drugs that can reduce bone density such as anticonvulsants and corticosteroids, goserelin therapy may pose an additional risk. In these patients, the risks and benefits must be weighed carefully before therapy with goserelin is instituted. Clinical studies suggest the addition of hormone replacement therapy (estrogens and/or progestins) to goserelin is effective in reducing the bone mineral loss which occurs with goserelin alone. The optimal drugs, dose, and duration of treatment have not been established.

Currently, there are no clinical data on the effects of retreatment or treatment of benign gynecological conditions with goserelin for periods in excess of 6 months.

As with other hormonal interventions that disrupt the pituitary-gonadal axis, some patients may have delayed return to menses. The rare patient, however, may experience persistent amenorrhea.

TRIPTORELIN PAMOATE

Rx	**Trelstar Depot** (Pharmacia)	**Microgranules for injection, lyophilized:** Equivalent to 3.75 mg triptorelin peptide base	Mannitol. In single-dose vials.
Rx	**Trelstar LA** (Pharmacia)	**Microgranules for injection, lyophilized:** Equivalent to 11.25 mg triptorelin peptide base	Mannitol. In single-dose vials.

TRIPTORELIN PAMOATE — INJECTION

Indications

➤*Advanced prostate cancer:* As palliative treatment of advanced prostate cancer. They offer an alternative treatment for prostate cancer when orchiectomy or estrogen administration are either not indicated or unacceptable to the patient.

➤*Unlabeled uses:* Treatment of ovarian cancer, pancreatic carcinoma, endometriosis, hyperandrogenism, growth hormone deficiency, in vitro fertilization, uterine leiomyomata.

Administration and Dosage

➤*Approved by the FDA:* June 15, 2000.

➤*Triptorelin depot injection:* 3.75 mg incorporated in a depot formulation and administered monthly as a single intramuscular (IM) injection.

Dosage adjustments – Patients with renal or hepatic impairment showed 2- to 4-fold higher exposure than young healthy males. The clinical consequences of this increase, as well as the potential need for dose adjustment, is unknown.

➤*Triptorelin long-acting injection:* 11.25 mg incorporated in a long-acting formulation administered every 84 days as a single IM injection administered in either buttock.

➤*Reconstitution of depot and long-acting injections:* Reconstitute the lyophilized microgranules in sterile water. Do not use any other diluent. Reconstitute in accordance with the following:

1.) Using a syringe fitted with a sterile 20-gauge needle, withdraw 2 mL sterile water for injection, and, after removing the flip-off seal from the vial, inject into the vial.
2.) Shake well to thoroughly disperse particles to obtain a uniform suspension. The suspension will appear milky.
3.) Withdraw the entire contents of the reconstituted suspension into the syringe and inject it immediately.
4.) For the triptorelin long-acting injection, inject the patient in either buttock with the contents of the syringe.

Discard the suspension if not used immediately after reconstitution.

➤*Storage/Stability:* Store at 20° to 25°C (68° to 77°F); excursions permitted to 15° to 30°C (59° to 86°F). Do not freeze.

Actions

➤*Pharmacology:* Triptorelin is a potent inhibitor of gonadotropin secretion when given continuously and in therapeutic doses. Following the first administration, there is a transient surge in circulating levels of luteinizing hormone (LH), follicle-stimulating hormone (FSH), testosterone, and estradiol. After chronic and continuous administration, usually 2 to 4 weeks after initiation of therapy, a sustained decrease in LH and FSH secretion and marked reduction of testicular and ovarian steroidogenesis is observed. In men, a reduction of serum testosterone concentration to a level typically seen in surgically castrated men is obtained. Consequently, tissues and functions that depend on these hormones for maintenance become quiescent. These effects are usually reversible after cessation of therapy.

Triptorelin depot injection – Following a single IM injection of triptorelin depot injection to healthy male volunteers, serum testosterone levels first increased, peaking on day 4, and thereafter declined to low levels by week 4. Similar testosterone profiles were observed in patients with advanced prostate cancer, when injected with triptorelin injection. In healthy volunteers, testosterone serum levels returned to near baseline by week 8.

Triptorelin long-acting injection – Following a single IM injection of triptorelin long-acting injection to men with advanced prostate cancer, serum testosterone levels first increased, peaking on days 2 to 3, and thereafter declined to low levels by weeks 3 to 4.

➤*Pharmacokinetics:*

Absorption – Triptorelin is not active when given orally.

Triptorelin depot injection: IM injection of the depot formulation provides plasma concentrations of triptorelin over a period of 1 month. The pharmacokinetic parameters following a single IM injection of 3.75 mg of triptorelin depot injection to 20 healthy male volunteers are listed in the following table. The plasma concentrations declined to 0.084 ng/mL at 4 weeks.

Triptorelin Pharmacokinetic Parameters Following IM Administration of Triptorelin Depot Injection to Healthy Male Volunteers

Dose (number of subjects)	C_{max} (ng/mL)	T_{max} (h)	$AUC_{0\text{-}28d}$ (h•ng/mL)	F (%)[a] (number of days)
3.75 mg (n = 20)	28.43 ± 7.31[b]	1 (1 to 3)[c]	223.15 ± 46.96[b]	83 (28 d)

[a] Computed as the mean AUC of the study divided by the mean area under the curve (AUC) of healthy volunteers corrected for dose where AUC = 36.1 h•ng/mL and 500 mcg intravenous (IV) bolus dose of triptorelin was administered.
[b] Mean ± SD.
[c] Median (range).

Triptorelin long-acting injection: The pharmacokinetic parameters following a single IM injection of 11.25 mg of triptorelin long-acting injection to 13 patients with prostate cancer are listed in the following table. Triptorelin did not accumulate over 9 months of treatment.

Triptorelin Pharmacokinetic Parameters (Mean ± SD) Following IM Administration of Triptorelin Long-Acting Injection to Patients with Prostate Cancer

Dose (number of subjects)	C_{max} (0 to 85 d) (ng/mL)	T_{max} (1 to 85 d) (h)	$AUC_{(1\ to\ 85\ d)}$ (h•ng/mL)
11.25 mg (n = 13)	38.5 ± 10.5	2.9 ± 1.3	2,268 ± 444.6

Distribution – The volume of distribution following an IV bolus dose of 0.5 mg of triptorelin peptide was 30 to 33 L in healthy male volunteers. There is no evidence that triptorelin, at clinically relevant concentrations, binds to plasma proteins.

Results of pharmacokinetic investigations conducted in healthy men indicate that after IV bolus administration, triptorelin is distributed and eliminated according to a 3-compartment model, and corresponding half-lives are approximately 6 minutes, 45 minutes, and 3 hours.

Metabolism – The metabolism of triptorelin in humans is unknown, but is unlikely to involve hepatic microsomal enzymes (cytochrome P-450). However, the effect of triptorelin on the activity of other drug-metabolizing enzymes is unknown. Thus far, no metabolites of triptorelin have been identified. Pharmacokinetic data suggest that C-terminal fragments produced by tissue degradation are either completely degraded in the tissues, or rapidly degraded in plasma, or cleared by the kidneys.

Excretion – Triptorelin is eliminated by both the liver and the kidneys. Following IV administration of 0.5 mg triptorelin peptide to 6 healthy male volunteers with a creatinine clearance of 149.9 mL/min, 41.7% of the dose was excreted in urine as intact peptide with a total triptorelin clearance of 211.9 mL/min. This percentage increased to 62.3% in patients with liver disease who have a lower creatinine clearance (89.9 mL/min). It has also been observed that the nonrenal clearance of triptorelin (patient anuric, Ccr = 0) was 76.2 mL/min, thus indicating that the nonrenal elimination of triptorelin is mainly dependent on the liver.

Special populations –

Renal function impairment: After an IV injection of 0.5 mg triptorelin peptide, the 2 distribution half-lives were unaffected by renal impairment, but renal impairment led to a decrease in total triptorelin clearance proportional to the decrease in creatinine clearance as well as an increase in volume of distribution and, consequently, an increase in elimination half-life. The decrease in triptorelin clearance was more pronounced in subjects with liver insufficiency, but the half-life was prolonged similarly in subjects with renal impairment, since the volume of distribution was only minimally increased. Patients with renal impairment had 2- to 4-fold higher exposure (AUC) values than young healthy males.

Hepatic function impairment: After an IV injection of 0.5 mg triptorelin peptide, the 2 distribution half-lives were unaffected by hepatic impairment. Patients with hepatic impairment had 2- to 4-fold higher exposure (AUC) values than young healthy men.

TRIPTORELIN PAMOATE — INJECTION

Triptorelin Pharmacokinetic Parameters						
Group	C_{max} (ng/mL)	AUC_{inf} (h•ng/mL)	Cl_p (mL/min)	Cl_{renal} (mL/min)	$t_{½}$ (h)	Ccr (mL/min)
6 healthy men	48.2 ± 11.8	36.1 ± 5.8	211.9 ± 31.6	90.6 ± 35.3	2.81 ± 1.21	149.9 ± 7.3
6 men with moderate renal impairment	45.6 ± 20.5	69.9 ± 24.6	120 ± 45	23.3 ± 17.6	6.56 ± 1.25	39.7 ± 22.5
6 men with severe renal impairment	46.5 ± 14	88 ± 18.4	88.6 ± 19.7	4.3 ± 2.9	7.65 ± 1.25	8.9 ± 6
6 men with liver disease	54.1 ± 5.3	131.9 ± 18.1	57.8 ± 8	35.9 ± 5	7.58 ± 1.17	89.9 ± 15.1

Contraindications

Hypersensitivities to triptorelin or any other component of the product, other LHRH agonists, or LHRH. Three postmarketing reports of anaphylactic shock and 7 postmarketing reports of angioedema related to triptorelin administration have been reported since 1986.

Triptorelin injections are contraindicated in women who are or may become pregnant while receiving the drug. Triptorelin injections may cause fetal harm when administered to pregnant women.

Warnings

➤*Worsening of signs and symptoms:* Initially, triptorelin, like other LHRH agonists, causes a transient increase in serum testosterone levels. As a result, isolated cases of worsening of signs and symptoms of prostate cancer during the first weeks of treatment have been reported with LHRH agonists. Patients may experience worsening of symptoms or onset of new symptoms, including bone pain, neuropathy, hematuria, or urethral or bladder outlet obstruction. Cases of spinal cord compression, which may contribute to paralysis with or without fatal complications, have been reported with LHRH agonists.

If spinal cord compression develops, institute standard treatment of these complications, and, in extreme cases, consider an immediate orchiectomy.

➤*Hypersensitivity reactions:* Do not administer triptorelin injections to individuals who are hypersensitive to triptorelin, to other LHRH agonists, or to LHRH. Rare reports of anaphylactic shock and angioedema related to triptorelin administration have been reported. In the event of a hypersensitivity reaction, immediately discontinue therapy with triptorelin injection and administer the appropriate supportive and symptomatic care.

➤*Renal function impairment:* If renal impairment develops, institute standard treatment of this complication, and, in extreme cases, consider an immediate orchiectomy.

➤*Carcinogenesis:* In rats, doses of 120, 600, and 3,000 mcg/kg given every 28 days (approximately 0.3, 2, and 8 times the recommended human therapeutic dose based on body surface area) resulted in increased mortality with a drug treatment period of 13 to 19 months. The incidence of benign and malignant pituitary tumors and histiosarcomas were increased in a dose-related manner. No oncogenic effect was observed in mice administered triptorelin for 18 months at doses up to 6,000 mcg/kg every 28 days (approximately 8 times the human therapeutic dose based on body surface area).

➤*Pregnancy: Category X.* See Contraindications for more information.

Triptorelin injections are contraindicated in women who are or may become pregnant while receiving the drug. Studies in pregnant rats administered triptorelin at doses of 2, 10, and 100 mcg/kg/day (approximately equivalent to 0.2, 0.8, and 8 times the recommended human therapeutic dose based on body surface area) during the period of organogenesis displayed maternal toxicity and embryotoxicity, but no fetotoxicity or teratogenicity. Similarly, no teratogenic effects were observed when mice were administered doses of 2, 20, and 200 mcg/kg/day (approximately equivalent to 0.1, 0.7, and 7 times the recommended human therapeutic dose based on body surface area). If this drug is used during pregnancy or if the patient becomes pregnant while taking this drug, apprise the patient of the potential hazard to the fetus.

➤*Lactation:* It is not known whether triptorelin injections are excreted in human milk. Because many drugs are excreted in human milk, and because the effects of triptorelin injections on lactation and/or the breast-fed child have not been determined, breast-feeding mothers should not use triptorelin injections.

➤*Children:* Triptorelin injections have not been studied in pediatric patients and are not indicated for use in pediatric patients.

Precautions

➤*Monitoring:* Monitor response to triptorelin depot injection by measuring serum levels of testosterone and prostate-specific antigen. Measure testosterone levels immediately prior to or immediately after dosing.

Closely observe patients with metastatic vertebral lesions and/or with upper or lower urinary tract obstruction during the first few weeks of therapy. Hypersensitivity and anaphylactic reactions have been reported with triptorelin as with other LHRH agonists.

Drug Interactions

➤*Hyperprolactinemic drugs:* No drug-drug interaction studies involving triptorelin have been conducted. In the absence of relevant data and as a precaution, do not prescribe hyperprolactinemic drugs concomitantly with triptorelin depot injection since hyperprolactinemia reduces the number of pituitary GnRH receptors.

➤*Drug/Lab test interactions:* Chronic or continuous administration of triptorelin in therapeutic doses results in suppression of the pituitary-gonadal axis. Diagnostic tests of the pituitary-gonadal function conducted during treatment and after cessation of therapy may therefore be misleading.

Adverse Reactions

In the majority of patients, testosterone levels increased above baseline during the first week following the initial injection, declining thereafter to baseline levels or below by the end of the second week of treatment. The transient increase in testosterone levels may be associated with temporary worsening of disease signs and symptoms, including bone pain, hematuria, and bladder outlet obstruction. Isolated cases of spinal cord compression with weakness or paralysis of the lower extremities have occurred.

In a controlled, comparative clinical trial, the following adverse reactions were reported to have a possible or probable relationship to therapy as ascribed by the treating physician in 1% or more of the patients receiving triptorelin. Often, causality is difficult to assess in patients with metastatic prostate cancer. Reactions considered not drug related are excluded.

Triptorelin depot injection –

Triptorelin Adverse Reactions (≥ 1%)		
Adverse reaction	Triptorelin (n = 140)	
Cardiovascular		
Hypertension	5	3.6%
CNS/peripheral		
Dizziness	2	1.4%
Headache	7	5%
Dermatologic		
Pruritus	2	1.4%
GI		
Diarrhea	2	1.4%
Vomiting	3	2.1%
GU		
Urinary retention	2	1.4%
Urinary tract infection	2	1.4%
Hematologic (red blood cell disorders)		
Anemia	2	1.4%
Local		
Injection-site pain	5	3.6%
Musculoskeletal		
Skeletal pain	17	12.1%
Psychiatric		
Emotional lability	2	1.4%
Impotence[a]	10	7.1%
Insomnia	3	2.1%
Miscellaneous		
Fatigue	3	2.1%
Hot flushes[a]	82	58.6%
Leg pain	3	2.1%
Pain	3	2.1%

[a] Expected pharmacologic consequences of testosterone suppression.

Triptorelin long-acting injection –

Triptorelin Long-Acting Injection Adverse Reactions (≥ 1%)		
Adverse reaction	Triptorelin long-acting injection (n = 174)	
Cardiovascular		
Dependent edema	4	2.3%
Hypertension	7	4%
CNS/peripheral		
Dizziness	5	2.9%
Headache	12	6.9%

Gonadotropin-Releasing Hormone Analog

TRIPTORELIN PAMOATE — INJECTION

Triptorelin Long-Acting Injection Adverse Reactions (≥ 1%)		
Adverse reaction	Triptorelin long-acting injection (n = 174)	
Leg cramps	3	1.7%
Dermatologic		
Rash	3	1.7%
GI		
Abdominal pain	2	1.1%
Constipation	3	1.7%
Diarrhea	2	1.1%
Dyspepsia	3	1.7%
Nausea	5	2.9%
GU		
Breast pain	4	2.3%
Dysuria	8	4.6%
Gynecomastia	3	1.7%
Urinary retention	2	1.1%
Hepatic		
Abnormal hepatic function	2	1.1%
Local		
Injection-site pain	7	4%
Metabolic/Nutritional		
Edema in legs	11	6.3%
Increased alkaline phosphatase	3	1.7%
Musculoskeletal		
Arthralgia	4	2.3%
Myalgia	2	1.1%
Skeletal pain	23	13.2%
Psychiatric		
Anorexia	3	1.7%
Decreased libido[a]	4	2.3%
Impotence[a]	4	2.3%
Insomnia	3	1.7%
Respiratory		
Coughing	3	1.7%
Dyspnea	2	1.1%
Pharyngitis	2	1.1%
Ophthalmic		
Conjunctivitis	2	1.1%
Eye pain	2	1.1%
Miscellaneous		
Asthenia	2	1.1%
Back pain	5	2.9%
Chest pain	3	1.7%
Fatigue	4	2.3%
Hot flushes[a]	127	73%
Leg pain	9	5.2%
Pain	6	3.4%
Peripheral edema	2	1.1%

[a] Expected pharmacological consequences of testosterone suppression.

➤*Lab test abnormalities:*

Triptorelin long-acting injection – The following abnormalities in laboratory values not present at baseline were observed in 10% or more of patients at the day 253 visit: decreased hemoglobin and RBC count and increased glucose, BUN, AST, ALT, and alkaline phosphatase. The relationship of these changes to drug treatment is difficult to assess in this population.

Overdosage

The pharmacological properties of triptorelin and its mode of administration make accidental or intentional overdosage unlikely. There were no reported overdoses in clinical trials. In single-dose toxicity studies in mice and rats, the subcutaneous LD_{50} of triptorelin was 400 mg/kg in mice and 250 mg/kg in rats, approximately 7,000 and 4,000 times, respectively, the usual human dose. If overdosage occurs, however, discontinue therapy immediately and administer the appropriate supportive and symptomatic treatment.

Aromatase Inhibitors

ANASTROZOLE

Rx	**Arimidex** (AstraZeneca)	**Tablets:** 1 mg	Lactose. (A/Adx 1). White. Film-coated. In 30s.

ANASTROZOLE — ORAL

Indications

➤*Breast cancer:* For adjuvant treatment of postmenopausal women with hormone receptor positive early breast cancer.

For the first-line treatment of postmenopausal women with hormone receptor positive or hormone receptor unknown locally advanced or metastatic breast cancer.

For the treatment of advanced breast cancer in postmenopausal women with disease progression following tamoxifen therapy.

Patients with estrogen receptor-negative disease and patients who did not respond to previous tamoxifen therapy rarely responded to anastrozole.

➤*Unlabeled uses:* Male infertility.

Administration and Dosage

➤*Approved by the FDA:* December 27, 1995.

➤*Recommended dosage:* 1 mg once a day. For patients with advanced breast cancer, anastrozole should be continued until tumor progression.

➤*Duration of therapy:* For adjuvant treatment of early breast cancer in postmenopausal women, the optimal duration of therapy is unknown. The median duration of therapy at the time of data analysis was 31 months; the ongoing ATAC trial is planned for 5 years of treatment.

➤*Storage/Stability:* Store at controlled room temperature, 20° to 25°C (68° to 77°F).

Actions

➤*Pharmacology:* Many breast cancers have estrogen receptors and growth of these tumors can be stimulated by estrogen. In postmenopausal women, the principal source of circulating estrogen (primarily estradiol) is conversion of adrenally generated androstenedione to estrone by aromatase in peripheral tissues, such as adipose tissue, with further conversion of estrone to estradiol. Many breast cancers also contain aromatase; the importance of tumor-generated estrogens is uncertain.

Anastrozole is a potent and selective nonsteroidal aromatase inhibitor. It significantly lowers serum estradiol concentrations and has no detectable effect on formation of adrenal corticosteroids or aldosterone.

➤*Pharmacokinetics:*

Metabolism/Excretion – Studies in postmenopausal women demonstrated that anastrozole is extensively metabolized with about 10% of the dose excreted in the urine as unchanged drug within 72 hours of dosing, and the remainder (about 60% of the dose) is excreted in urine as metabolites. Metabolism of anastrozole occurs by N-dealkylation, hydroxylation and glucuronidation. Three metabolites of anastrozole have been identified in human plasma and urine. The known metabolites are triazole, a glucuronide conjugate of hydroxy-anastrozole, and a glucuronide of anastrozole itself. Several minor (less than 5% of the radioactive dose) metabolites have not been identified.

Special populations –

Renal function impairment: Anastrozole pharmacokinetics have been investigated in subjects with renal insufficiency. Anastrozole renal clearance decreased proportionally with creatinine clearance and was approximately 50% lower in volunteers with severe renal impairment (creatinine clearance less than 30 mL/min/1.73 m^2) compared to controls. Since only about 10% of anastrozole is excreted unchanged in the urine, the reduction in renal clearance did not influence the total body clearance.

Hepatic function impairment: Hepatic metabolism accounts for approximately 85% of anastrozole elimination. Anastrozole pharmacokinetics have been investigated in subjects with hepatic cirrhosis related to alcohol abuse. The apparent oral clearance (CL/F) of anastrozole was approximately 30% lower in subjects with stable hepatic cirrhosis than in control subjects with normal liver function. However, plasma anastrozole concentrations in the subjects with hepatic cirrhosis were within the range of concentrations seen in healthy subjects across all clinical trials, so that no dosage adjustment is needed.

Contraindications

Hypersensitivity reaction to the drug or to any of the excipients.

Warnings

➤*Carcinogenesis:* A conventional carcinogenesis study in rats at doses of 1 to 25 mg/kg/day (about 10 to 243 times the daily maximum recommended

ANASTROZOLE — ORAL

human dose on a mg/m^2 basis) administered by oral gavage for up to 2 years revealed an increase in the incidence of hepatocellular adenoma and carcinoma and uterine stromal polyps in females and thyroid adenoma in males at the high dose. A dose-related increase was observed in the incidence of ovarian and uterine hyperplasia in females. At 25 mg/kg/day, plasma $AUC_{0\text{-}24\,hr}$ levels in rats were 110 to 125 times higher than the level exhibited in postmenopausal volunteers at the recommended dose. A separate carcinogenicity study in mice at oral doses of 5 to 50 mg/kg/day (about 24 to 243 times the daily maximum recommended human dose on a mg/m^2 basis) for up to 2 years produced an increase in the incidence of benign ovarian stromal, epithelial and granulosa cell tumors at all dose levels. A dose-related increase in the incidence of ovarian hyperplasia was also observed in female mice. These ovarian changes are considered to be rodent-specific effects of aromatase inhibition and are of questionable significance to humans. The incidence of lymphosarcoma was increased in males and females at the high dose. At 50 mg/kg/day, plasma AUC levels in mice were 35 to 40 times higher than the level exhibited in postmenopausal volunteers at the recommended dose.

➤*Fertility impairment:* Oral administration of anastrozole to female rats (from 2 weeks before mating to pregnancy day 7) produced significant incidence of infertility and reduced numbers of viable pregnancies at 1 mg/kg/day (about 10 times the recommended human dose on a mg/m^2 basis and 9 times higher than the $AUC_{0\text{-}24\,hr}$ found in postmenopausal volunteers at the recommended dose). Preimplantation loss of ova or fetus was increased at doses equal to or greater than 0.02 mg/kg/day (about one-fifth the recommended human dose on a mg/m^2 basis). Recovery of fertility was observed following a 5-week nondosing period which followed 3 weeks of dosing. It is not known whether these effects observed in female rats are indicative of impaired fertility in humans.

➤*Pregnancy: Category D.* Anastrozole can cause fetal harm when administered to a pregnant woman. Anastrozole has been found to cross the placenta following oral administration of 0.1 mg/kg in rats and rabbits (about 1 and 1.9 times the recommended human dose, respectively, on a mg/m^2 basis). Studies in both rats and rabbits at doses equal to or greater than 0.1 and 0.02 mg/kg/day, respectively (about 1 and ⅓, respectively, the recommended human dose on a mg/m^2 basis), administered during the period of organogenesis showed that anastrozole increased pregnancy loss (increased pre- or postimplantation loss, increased resorption, and decreased numbers of live fetuses); effects were dose related in rats. Placental weights were significantly increased in rats at doses of 0.1 mg/kg/day or more.

Evidence of fetotoxicity, including delayed fetal development (ie, incomplete ossification and depressed fetal body weights), was observed in rats administered doses of 1 mg/kg/day (which produced plasma anastrozole $C_{ss\,max}$ and $AUC_{0\text{-}24\,hr}$ that were 19 times and 9 times higher than the respective values found in healthy postmenopausal humans at the recommended dose). There was no evidence of teratogenicity in rats administered doses up to 1 mg/kg/day. In rabbits, anastrozole caused pregnancy failure at doses equal to or greater than 1 mg/kg/day (about 16 times the recommended human dose on a mg/m^2 basis); there was no evidence of teratogenicity in rabbits administered 0.2 mg/kg/day (about 3 times the recommended human dose on a mg/m^2 basis).

There are no adequate and well-controlled studies in pregnant women using anastrozole. If anastrozole is used during pregnancy, or if the patient becomes pregnant while receiving this drug, the patient should be apprised of the potential hazard to the fetus or potential risk for loss of the pregnancy.

➤*Lactation:* It is not known if anastrozole is excreted in human milk. Because many drugs are excreted in human milk, caution should be exercised when anastrozole is administered to a nursing woman.

➤*Children:* The safety and efficacy of anastrozole in pediatric patients have not been established.

Precautions

➤*Pregnancy:* See Warnings for more information.

➤*Lab test abnormalities:* During the ATAC trial, more patients receiving anastrozole were reported to have an elevated serum cholesterol compared to patients receiving tamoxifen (7% versus 3%, respectively).

Adverse Reactions

➤*Adjuvant therapy:*

Anastrozole Adverse Reactions (≥ 5%)

Adverse reaction*	Anastrozole 1 mg (n = 3092)	Tamoxifen 20 mg (n = 3093)	Anastrozole 1 mg plus tamoxifen 20 mg (n = 3098)
Miscellaneous			
Asthenia	512 (17%)	491 (16%)	468 (15%)
Pain	461 (15%)	435 (14%)	407 (13%)
Back pain	256 (8%)	255 (8%)	258(8%)
Headache	277 (9%)	216 (7%)	214 (7%)
Abdominal pain	227 (7%)	228 (7%)	219 (7%)
Infection	223 (7%)	225 (7%)	211 (7%)
Accidental injury	221 (7%)	221 (7%)	226 (7%)
Flu syndrome	154 (5%)	170 (5%)	170 (5%)
Chest pain	164 (5%)	122 (4%)	152 (5%)
Cardiovascular			
Vasodilatation	1082 (35%)	1246 (40%)	1261 41%)
Hypertension	292 (9%)	252 (8%)	270 (9%)
GI			
Nausea	307 (10%)	298 (10%)	324 (10%)
Constipation	201 (7%)	214 (7%)	232 (7%)
Diarrhea	227 (7%)	186 (6%)	193 (6%)
Dyspepsia	166 (5%)	137 (4%)	156 (5%)
GI disorder	155 (5%)	122 (4%)	127 (4%)
Hematologic/Lymphatic			
Lymphoedema	267 (9%)	299 (10%)	296 (10%)
Metabolic			
Peripheral edema	255 (8%)	275 (9%)	281 (9%)
Weight gain	253 (8%)	250 (8%)	264 (9%)
Hypercholesteremia	210 (7%)	79 (3%)	72 (2%)
Musculoskeletal			
Arthritis	431 (14%)	344 (11%)	364 (12%)
Arthralgia	390 (13%)	251 (8%)	265 (9%)
Osteoporosis	229 (7%)	161 (5%)	174 (6%)
Fracture	219 (7%)	137 (4%)	178 (6%)
Bone pain	165 (5%)	149 (5%)	143 (5%)
Arthrosis	179 (6%)	136 (4%)	119 (4%)
CNS			
Depression	348 (11%)	341 (11%)	342 (11%)
Insomnia	266 (9%)	245 (8%)	227 (7%)
Dizziness	198 (6%)	207 (7%)	190 (6%)
Anxiety	168 (5%)	157 (5%)	140 (5%)
Paraesthesia	195 (6%)	116 (4%)	120 (4%)
Respiratory			
Pharyngitis	376 (12%)	359 (12%)	350 (11%)
Increased cough	212 (7%)	237 (8%)	203 (7%)
Dyspnea	186 (6%)	185 (6%)	175 (6%)
Dermatologic			
Rash	300 (10%)	331 (11%)	326 (11%)
Sweating	121 (4%)	165 (5%)	142 (5%)
GU			
Leukorrhea	75 (2%)	265 (9%)	277 (9%)
Urinary tract infection	192 (6%)	252 (8%)	228 (7%)
Breast pain	205 (7%)	136 (4%)	182 (6%)
Vulvovaginitis	180 (6%)	134 (4%)	134 (4%)

* A patient may have had more than 1 adverse reaction, including more than 1 adverse reaction in the same body system.

Nonpathologic fractures were reported more frequently in the anastrozole-treated patients (219 [7%]) than in the tamoxifen-treated patients (137 [4%]).

Certain adverse reactions and combinations of adverse reactions were prospectively specified for analysis, based on the known pharmacologic properties and side effect profiles of the 2 drugs (see table below). Patients receiving anastrozole had an increase in musculoskeletal events and fractures (including fractures of the spine, hip and wrist) compared with patients receiving tamoxifen. Patients receiving anastrozole had a decrease in hot flashes, vaginal bleeding, vaginal discharge, endometrial cancer, venous thromboembolic events (including deep venous thrombosis), and ischemic cerebrovascular events compared with patients receiving tamoxifen.

Number of Patients with Prespecified Adverse Reaction in ATAC Trial (%)

Adverse reactions	Anastrozole (n = 3092) (%)	Tamoxifen (n = 3093) (%)	Odds - ratio	95% CI
All fractures	224 (7%)	145 (5%)	1.59	1.28 to 1.97
Fractures of spine, hip, wrist	89 (3%)	62 (2%)	1.45	1.04 to 2.04
Musculoskeletal disorders[1]	940 (30%)	737 (24%)	1.41	1.28 to 1.55

ANASTROZOLE — ORAL

Number of Patients with Prespecified Adverse Reaction in ATAC Trial (%)				
Adverse reactions	Anastrozole (n = 3092) (%)	Tamoxifen (n = 3093) (%)	Odds - ratio	95% CI
Ischemic cardiovascular disease	92 (3%)	74 (2%)	1.25	0.91 to 1.72
Asthenia	513 (17%)	491 (16%)	1.05	0.93 to 1.2
Nausea and vomiting	348 (11%)	342 (11%)	1.02	0.88 to 1.19
Mood disturbances	521 (17%)	511 (17%)	1.02	0.90 to 1.16
Cataracts	128 (4%)	140 (5%)	0.91	0.71 to 1.17
Hot flashes	1082 (35%)	1246 (40%)	0.8	0.73 to 0.87
Venous thromboembolic events	73 (2%)	120 (4%)	0.6	0.44 to 0.81
Deep venous thromboembolic events	40 (1%)	60 (2%)	0.66	0.43 to 1
Ischemic cerebrovascular event	40 (1%)	74 (2%)	0.53	0.35 to 0.8
Vaginal bleeding	147 (5%)	270 (9%)	0.52	0.42 to 0.64
Vaginal discharge	94 (3%)	378 (12%)	0.23	0.18 to 0.28
Endometrial cancer	3 (0.1%)	15 (0.5%)	0.2	0.04 to 0.7

[1] Refers to joint symptoms, including arthritis, arthrosis, and arthralgia.

Angina pectoris was reported more frequently in the anastrozole-treated patients (52 [1.7%]) than in the tamoxifen-treated patients (30 [1.0%]); the incidence of MI was comparable (anastrozole 24 patients [0.8%]; tamoxifen 25 patients [0.8%]. Preliminary results from the ATAC trial bone substudy demonstrated that patients receiving anastrozole had a mean decrease in both lumbar spine and total hip bone mineral density (BMD) compared to baseline. Patients receiving tamoxifen had a mean increase in both lumbar spine and total hip BMD compared to baseline.

➤*First-line therapy:*

Anastrozole Adverse Reactions (≥ 5%)		
Adverse reaction[a]	Anastrozole (n = 506)	Tamoxifen (n = 511)
Miscellaneous		
Asthenia	83 (16%)	81 (16%)
Pain	70 (14%)	73 (14%)
Back pain	60 (12%)	68 (13%)
Headache	47 (9%)	40 (8%)
Abdominal pain	40 (8%)	38 (7%)
Chest pain	37 (7%)	37 (7%)
Flu syndrome	35 (7%)	30 (6%)
Pelvic pain	23 (5%)	30 (6%)
Cardiovascular		
Vasodilation	128 (25%)	106 (21%)
Hypertension	25 (5%)	36 (7%)
GI		
Nausea	94 (19%)	106 (21%)
Constipation	47 (9%)	66 (13%)
Diarrhea	40 (8%)	33 (6%)
Vomiting	38 (8%)	36 (7%)
Anorexia	26 (5%)	46 (9%)
Metabolic/Nutritional		
Peripheral edema	51 (10%)	41 (8%)
Musculoskeletal		
Bone pain	54 (11%)	52 (10%)
CNS		
Dizziness	30 (6%)	22 (4%)
Insomnia	30 (6%)	38 (7%)
Depression	23 (5%)	32 (6%)
Hypertonia	16 (3%)	26 (5%)
Respiratory		
Cough increased	55 (11%)	52 (10%)
Dyspnea	51 (10%)	47 (9%)
Pharyngitis	49 (10%)	68 (13%)
Dermatologic		
Rash	38 (8%)	34 (8%)
GU		
Leukorrhea	9 (2%)	31 (6%)

[a] A patient may have had more than 1 adverse reaction.

Adverse Reactions Reported with Anastrozole and Tamoxifen (%)		
Adverse reactions	Anastrozole 1 mg (n = 506)	Tamoxifen 20 mg (n = 511)
Depression	23 (5%)	32 (6%)
Tumor flare	15 (3%)	18 (4%)
Thromboembolic disease[a]	18 (4%)	33 (6%)
Venous thromboembolic disease[b]	5	15
Coronary and cerebral thromboembolic disease[c]	13	19
GI disturbance	170 (34%)	196 (38%)
Hot flushes	134 (26%)	118 (23%)
Vaginal dryness	9 (2%)	3 (1%)
Lethargy	6 (1%)	15 (3%)
Vaginal bleeding	5 (1%)	11 (2%)
Weight gain	11 (2%)	8 (2%)

[a] A patient may have had more than 1 adverse reaction.
[b] Includes pulmonary embolus, thrombophlebitis, retinal vein thrombosis.
[c] Includes MI, myocardial ischemia, angina pectoris, cerebrovascular accident, cerebral ischemia, and cerebral infarct.

Despite the lack of estrogenic activity for anastrozole, there was no increase in MI or fracture when compared with tamoxifen.

➤*Second-line therapy:*

Anastrozole Adverse Reactions (%)[a]			
Adverse reaction	Anastrozole 1 mg (n = 262)	Anastrozole 10 mg (n = 246)	Megestrol acetate 160 mg (n = 253)
Asthenia	42 (16%)	33 (13%)	47 (19%)
Nausea	41 (16%)	48 (20%)	28 (11%)
Headache	34 (13%)	44 (18%)	24 (9%)
Hot flushes	32 (12%)	29 (11%)	21 (8%)
Pain	28 (11%)	38 (15%)	29 (11%)
Back pain	28 (11%)	26 (11%)	19 (8%)
Dyspnea	24 (9%)	27 (11%)	53 (21%)
Vomiting	24 (9%)	26 (11%)	16 (6%)
Cough increased	22 (8%)	18 (7%)	19 (8%)
Diarrhea	22 (8%)	18 (7%)	7 (3%)
Constipation	18 (7%)	18 (7%)	21 (8%)
Abdominal pain	18 7%)	14 (6%)	18 (7%)
Anorexia	18 (7%)	19 (8%)	11 (4%)
Bone pain	17 (6%)	26 (12%)	19 (8%)
Pharyngitis	16 (6%)	23 (9%)	15 (6%)
Dizziness	16 (6%)	12 (5%)	15 (6%)
Rash	15 (6%)	15 (6%)	19 (8%)
Dry mouth	15 (6%)	11 (4%)	13 (5%)
Peripheral edema	14 (5%)	21 (9%)	28 (11%)
Pelvic pain	14 (5%)	17 (7%)	13 (5%)
Depression	14 (5%)	6 (2%)	5 (2%)
Chest pain	13 (5%)	18 (7%)	13 (5%)
Paresthesia	12 (5%)	15 (6%)	9 (4%)
Vaginal hemorrhage	6 (2%)	4 (2%)	13 (5%)
Weight gain	4 (2%)	9 (4%)	30 (12%)
Sweating	4 (2%)	3 (1%)	16 (6%)
Increased appetite	0 (0%)	1 (0%)	13 (5%)

[a] A patient may have more than 1 adverse reaction.

ANASTROZOLE — ORAL

➤*Other less frequent (2% to 5%) adverse reactions:* Other less frequent (2% to 5%) adverse reactions reported in patients receiving anastrozole 1 mg in either Trial 0004 or Trial 0005 are listed below. These adverse reactions are listed by body system and are in order of decreasing frequency within each body system regardless of assessed causality.

Cardiovascular – Hypertension; thrombophlebitis.

CNS – Somnolence; confusion; insomnia; anxiety; nervousness.

Dermatologic – Hair thinning; pruritus.

GU – Urinary tract infection; breast pain.

Hematologic – Anemia; leukopenia.

Hepatic – GGT increased; AST increased; ALT increased.

Metabolic/Nutritional – Alkaline phosphatase increased; weight loss.

Mean serum total cholesterol levels increased by 0.5 mmol/L among patients receiving anastrozole. Increases in LDL cholesterol have been shown to contribute to these changes.

Musculoskeletal – Myalgia; arthralgia; pathological fracture.

Miscellaneous – Flu syndrome; fever; neck pain; malaise; accidental injury; infection.

Respiratory – Sinusitis; bronchitis; rhinitis.

➤*Adverse reactions related to 1 or both of the therapies:* The incidences of the following adverse reaction groups potentially causally related to 1 or both of the therapies because of their pharmacology, were statistically analyzed: Weight gain, edema, thromboembolic disease, GI disturbance, hot flushes, and vaginal dryness. These 6 groups, and the adverse reactions captured in the groups, were prospectively defined. The results are shown in the table below.

Number and Percentage of Patients Reporting Adverse Reactions Related to One or Both Therapies (%)

Adverse reaction group	Anastrozole 1 mg (n = 262)	Anastrozole 10 mg (n = 246)	Megestrol acetate 160 mg (n = 253)
GI disturbance	77 (29%)	81 (33%)	54 (21%)
Hot flushes	33 (13%)	29 (12%)	35 (14%)
Edema	19 (7%)	28 (11%)	35 (14%)
Thromboembolic disease	9 (3%)	4 (2%)	12 (5%)
Vaginal dryness	5 (2%)	3 (1%)	2 (1%)
Weight gain	4 (2%)	10 (4%)	30 (12%)

More patients treated with megestrol acetate reported weight gain as an adverse reaction compared to patients treated with anastrozole 1 mg ($P < 0.0001$). Other differences were not statistically significant.

Weight gain – An examination of the magnitude of change in weight in all patients was also conducted. Thirty-four percent (87 out of 253) of the patients treated with megestrol acetate experienced weight gain of 5% or more and 11% (27 out of 253) of the patients treated with megestrol acetate experienced weight gain of 10% or more. Among patients treated with anastrozole 1 mg, 13% (33 out of 262) experienced weight gain of 5% or more and 3% (6 out of 262) experienced weight gain of 10% or more. On average, this 5% to 10% weight gain represented between 6 and 12 lbs.

Vaginal bleeding – Vaginal bleeding has been reported infrequently, mainly in patients during the first few weeks after changing from existing hormonal therapy to treatment with anastrozole. If bleeding persists, further evaluation should be considered.

Joint pain/stiffness – During clinical trials and postmarketing experience joint pain/stiffness has been reported in association with the use of anastrozole.

Rash – Anastrozole may also be associated with rash, including very rare cases of mucocutaneous disorders such as erythema multiforme and Stevens-Johnson syndrome.

Overdosage

Clinical trials have been conducted with anastrozole, up to 60 mg in a single dose given to healthy male volunteers and up to 10 mg daily given to postmenopausal women with advanced breast cancer; these dosages were well tolerated. A single dose of anastrozole that results in life-threatening symptoms has not been established. In rats, lethality was observed after single oral doses that were greater than 100 mg/kg (about 800 times the recommended human dose on a mg/m^2 basis) and was associated with severe irritation to the stomach (necrosis, gastritis, ulceration, and hemorrhage).

In an oral acute toxicity study in the dog the median lethal dose was greater than 45 mg/kg/day.

➤*Treatment:* There is no specific antidote to overdosage and treatment must be symptomatic. In the management of an overdose, consider that multiple agents may have been taken. Vomiting may be induced if the patient is alert. Dialysis may be helpful because anastrozole is not highly protein bound. General supportive care, including frequent monitoring of vital signs and close observation of the patient, is indicated.

LETROZOLE

Rx	**Femara** (Novartis)	**Tablets:** 2.5 mg	Lactose. (FV CG). Dark yellow. Film-coated. In 30s.

LETROZOLE — ORAL

Indications

➤*Adjuvant treatment of early breast cancer:* For the adjuvant treatment of postmenopausal women with hormone receptor-positive early breast cancer. The efficacy of letrozole in early breast cancer is based on an analysis of disease-free survival in patients treated for a median of 24 months and followed for a median of 26 months. Follow-up analyses will determine long-term outcomes for both safety and efficacy.

➤*Advanced or metastatic breast cancer:* For first-line treatment of postmenopausal women with hormone receptor–positive or hormone receptor–unknown locally advanced or metastatic breast cancer. Letrozole is indicated for the treatment of advanced breast cancer in postmenopausal women with disease progression following antiestrogen therapy.

➤*Extended adjuvant treatment of early breast cancer:* For the extended adjuvant treatment of early breast cancer in postmenopausal women who have received 5 years of adjuvant tamoxifen therapy. The efficacy of letrozole in extended adjuvant treatment of early breast cancer is based on an analysis of disease-free survival in patients treated for a median of 24 months. Further data is required to determine a long-term outcome.

➤*Unlabeled uses:* For ovulation stimulation to improve the chances of pregnancy.

Administration and Dosage

➤*Approved by the FDA:* July 30, 1997.

➤*Adults:* The recommended dosage of letrozole is 2.5 mg administered once daily, without regard to meals. Patients treated with letrozole do not require glucocorticoid or mineralocorticoid replacement therapy.

➤*Duration:* In patients with advanced disease, continue treatment with letrozole until tumor progression is evident. In the extended adjuvant setting, the optimal treatment duration with letrozole is not known. The planned duration of treatment in the study was 5 years. However, at the time of the analysis, the median treatment duration was 24 months; 25% of patients were treated for at least 3 years, and less than 1% of patients were treated for the planned duration of 5 years. The median duration of follow-up was 28 months. Treatment should be discontinued at tumor relapse.

In the adjuvant setting, the optimal duration of treatment with letrozole is unknown. The planned duration of treatment in the study is 5 years. However, at the time of analysis, the median duration of treatment was 24 months, median duration of follow-up was 26 months, and 16% of the patients had been treated for 5 years. Treatment should be discontinued at relapse.

➤*Hepatic function impairment:* No dosage adjustment is recommended for patients with mild to moderate hepatic impairment, although letrozole blood concentrations were increased modestly in subjects with moderate hepatic impairment caused by cirrhosis. Reduce the dosage of letrozole in patients with cirrhosis and severe hepatic dysfunction by 50%. The recommended dosage of letrozole for such patients is 2.5 mg administered every other day. The effect of hepatic impairment on letrozole exposure in noncirrhotic cancer patients with elevated bilirubin levels has not been determined.

➤*Storage/Stability:* Store at 25°C (77°F); excursions permitted to 15° to 30°C (59° to 86°F).

Actions

➤*Pharmacology:* The growth of some cancers of the breast is stimulated or maintained by estrogens. Treatment of breast cancer thought to be hormonally responsive (ie, estrogen and/or progesterone receptor-positive or receptor-unknown) has included a variety of efforts to decrease estrogen levels (eg, ovariectomy, adrenalectomy, hypophysectomy) or inhibit estrogen effects (eg, antiestrogens, progestational agents). These interventions lead to decreased tumor mass or delayed progression of tumor growth in some women.

In postmenopausal women, estrogens are derived mainly from the action of the aromatase enzyme, which converts adrenal androgens (primarily androstenedione and testosterone) to estrone and estradiol. The suppression of estrogen biosynthesis in peripheral tissues, and in the cancer tissue itself, can be achieved by specifically inhibiting the aromatase enzyme.

Letrozole is a nonsteroidal competitive inhibitor of the aromatase enzyme system; it inhibits the conversion of androgens to estrogens. In adult nontumor- and tumor-bearing female animals, letrozole is as effective as an ovariectomy in reducing uterine weight, elevating serum luteinizing hormone (LH), and causing the regression of estrogen-dependent tumors. In

LETROZOLE — ORAL

contrast to ovariectomy, treatment with letrozole does not lead to an increase in serum follicle-stimulating hormone (FSH). Letrozole selectively inhibits gonadal steroidogenesis but has no significant effect on adrenal mineralocorticoid or glucocorticoid synthesis.

Letrozole inhibits the aromatase enzyme by competitively binding to the heme of the cytochrome P-450 subunit of the enzyme, resulting in a reduction of estrogen biosynthesis in all tissues. Treatment of women with letrozole significantly lowers serum estrone, estradiol, and estrone sulfate, and has not been shown to significantly affect adrenal corticosteroid synthesis, aldosterone synthesis, or synthesis of thyroid hormones.

Pharmacodynamics – In postmenopausal patients with advanced breast cancer, daily doses of letrozole 0.1 to 5 mg suppressed plasma concentrations of estradiol, estrone, and estrone sulfate by 75% to 95% from baseline, with maximal suppression achieved within 2 to 3 days. Suppression is dose-related, with doses greater than or equal to 0.5 mg giving many values of estrone and estrone sulfate that were below the limit of detection in the assays. Estrogen suppression was maintained throughout treatment in all patients treated at greater than or equal to 0.5 mg.

Letrozole is highly specific in inhibiting aromatase activity. There is no impairment of adrenal steroidogenesis. No clinically relevant changes were found in the plasma concentrations of cortisol, aldosterone, 11-deoxycortisol, 17-hydroxy-progesterone, corticotropin (ACTH), or in plasma renin activity among postmenopausal patients treated with a daily doses of letrozole 0.1 to 5 mg. The ACTH stimulation test, performed after 6 and 12 weeks of treatment with daily doses of 0.1, 0.25, 0.5, 1, 2.5, and 5 mg, did not indicate any attenuation of aldosterone or cortisol production. Glucocorticoid or mineralocorticoid supplementation therefore is not necessary.

No changes were noted in plasma concentrations of androgens (androstenedione and testosterone) among healthy postmenopausal women after single doses of letrozole 0.1, 0.5, and 2.5 mg, or in plasma concentrations of androstenedione among postmenopausal patients treated with daily dosages of 0.1 to 5 mg. This indicates that the blockade of estrogen biosynthesis does not lead to accumulation of androgenic precursors. Plasma levels of LH and FSH were not affected by letrozole in patients, nor was thyroid function as evaluated by thyrotropin (TSH) levels, triiodothyronine (T_3) uptake, and thyroxine (T_4) levels.

➤*Pharmacokinetics:*

Absorption/Distribution – Letrozole is absorbed rapidly and completely from the GI tract, and absorption is not affected by food. Steady-state plasma concentration after daily 2.5 mg dosing is reached in 2 to 6 weeks. Plasma concentrations at steady state are 1.5 to 2 times higher than predicted from the concentrations measured after a single dose, indicating a slight nonlinearity in the pharmacokinetics upon daily administration of letrozole 2.5 mg. These steady-state levels are maintained over extended periods, however, and continuous accumulation of letrozole does not occur. Letrozole is weakly protein bound and has a large volume of distribution (approximately 1.9 L/kg).

Metabolism/Excretion – Metabolism to a pharmacologically inactive carbinol metabolite (4,4′-methanol-bisbenzonitrile) and renal excretion of the glucuronide conjugate of this metabolite is the major pathway of letrozole clearance. About 90% of radiolabeled letrozole is recovered in urine. Of the radiolabel recovered in urine, at least 75% was the glucuronide of the carbinol metabolite, approximately 9% was 2 unidentified metabolites, and 6% was unchanged letrozole.

In human microsomes with specific CYP isozyme activity, CYP3A4 metabolized letrozole to the carbinol metabolite while CYP2A6 formed both this metabolite and its ketone analog. In human liver microsomes, letrozole strongly inhibited CYP2A6 and moderately inhibited CYP2C19.

Letrozole's terminal elimination half-life is about 2 days.

Special populations –

Hepatic function impairment: In a study of subjects with mild to moderate nonmetastatic hepatic dysfunction (eg, cirrhosis, Child-Pugh class A and B), the mean area under the curve (AUC) values of the volunteers with moderate hepatic impairment were 37% higher than in healthy subjects, but still within the range seen in subjects without impaired function. In a pharmacokinetics study, subjects with liver cirrhosis and severe hepatic impairment (Child-Pugh class C, which included bilirubins about 2 to 11 times the upper limit of normal [ULN] with minimal to severe ascites) had 2-fold increases in exposure (AUC) and 47% reduction in systemic clearance. Breast cancer patients with severe hepatic impairment are thus expected to be exposed to higher levels of letrozole than patients with normal liver function receiving similar doses of this drug.

Contraindications

Hypersensitivity to letrozole or any of its excipients.

Warnings

➤*Hepatic function impairment:* Patients with cirrhosis and severe hepatic dysfunction who were dosed with letrozole 2.5 mg experienced approximately twice the exposure to letrozole as healthy volunteers with normal liver function. Therefore, a dosage reduction is recommended for this patient population. The effect of hepatic impairment on letrozole exposure in cancer patients with elevated bilirubin levels has not been determined.

➤*Carcinogenesis:* A conventional carcinogenesis study in mice at dosages of 0.6 to 60 mg/kg/day (about 1 to 100 times the daily maximum recommended human dose [MRHD] on a mg/m^2 basis) administered by oral gavage for up to 2 years revealed a dose-related increase in the incidence of benign ovarian stromal tumors. The incidence of combined hepatocellular adenoma and carcinoma showed a significant trend in females when the high-dosage group was excluded because of low survival. In a separate study, plasma $AUC_{0\text{-}12h}$ levels in mice at 60 mg/kg/day were 55 times higher than the $AUC_{0\text{-}24h}$ level in breast cancer patients at the recommended dose. The carcinogenicity study in rats at oral dosages of 0.1 to 10 mg/kg/day (about 0.4 to 40 times the daily MRHD on a mg/m^2 basis) for up to 2 years also produced an increase in the incidence of benign ovarian stromal tumors at 10 mg/kg/day. Ovarian hyperplasia was observed in females at dosages greater than or equal to 0.1 mg/kg/day. At 10 mg/kg/day, plasma $AUC_{0\text{-}24h}$ levels in rats were 80 times higher than the level in breast cancer patients at the recommended dose.

➤*Mutagenesis:* Letrozole was not mutagenic in in vitro tests (Ames and *Escherichia coli* bacterial tests), but was observed to be a potential clastogen in in vitro assays (CHO K1 and CCL 61 Chinese hamster ovary cells). Letrozole was not clastogenic in vivo (micronucleus test in rats).

➤*Fertility impairment:* Studies to investigate the effect of letrozole on fertility have not been conducted; however, repeated dosing caused sexual inactivity in females and atrophy of the reproductive tract in males and females at doses of 0.6, 0.1, and 0.03 mg/kg in mice, rats, and dogs, respectively (about 1, 0.4, and 0.4 the daily MRHD on a mg/m^2 basis, respectively).

➤*Elderly:* The median age of patients in all studies of first- and second-line treatment for metastatic breast cancer was 64 to 65 years of age. About one third of the patients were 70 years of age and older. In the first-line study, patients 70 years of age and older experienced longer time to tumor progression and higher response rates than patients younger than 70 years of age.

For the extended adjuvant setting, more than 5,100 postmenopausal women were enrolled in the clinical study. In total, 41% of patients were 65 years of age and older at enrollment, while 12% were 75 years of age and older. No overall differences in safety or efficacy were observed between these older and younger patients, and other reported clinical experience has not identified differences in responses between the elderly and younger patients, but greater sensitivity of some older individuals cannot be ruled out.

In the adjuvant setting, more than 8,000 postmenopausal women were enrolled in the clinical study. In total, 36% of patients were 65 years of age or older at enrollment, while 12% were 75 years of age or older. More adverse reactions were generally reported in elderly patients irrespective of study treatment allocation. However, in comparison with tamoxifen, no overall differences with regard to the safety and efficacy profiles were observed between elderly and younger patients.

➤*Pregnancy: Category D.* Letrozole may cause fetal harm when administered to pregnant women. Studies in rats at doses greater than or equal to 0.003 mg/kg (about 1/100 the daily MRHD on a mg/m^2 basis) administered during the period of organogenesis, have shown that letrozole is embryotoxic and fetotoxic, as indicated by intrauterine mortality, increased resorption, increased postimplantation loss, decreased numbers of live fetuses, and fetal anomalies, including absence and shortening of renal papilla, dilation of ureter, edema, and incomplete ossification of frontal skull, and metatarsals. Letrozole was teratogenic in rats. A 0.03 mg/kg dose (about 1/10 the daily MRHD on a mg/m^2 basis) caused fetal domed head and cervical/centrum vertebral fusion.

Letrozole is embryotoxic at doses greater than or equal to 0.002 mg/kg and fetotoxic when administered to rabbits at 0.02 mg/kg (about 1/100,000 and 1/10,000 the daily MRHD on a mg/m^2 basis, respectively). Fetal anomalies included incomplete ossification of the skull, sternebrae, and fore- and hindlegs.

There are no studies in pregnant women. Letrozole is indicated for postmenopausal women. If there is exposure to letrozole during pregnancy, apprise the patient of the potential hazard to the fetus and the potential risk for miscarriage.

➤*Lactation:* It is not known if letrozole is excreted in human milk. Because many drugs are excreted in human milk, exercise caution when letrozole is administered to a breast-feeding woman.

➤*Children:* The safety and efficacy in children have not been established.

Precautions

➤*Monitoring:* Consider monitoring bone mineral density (BMD).

➤*Lab test abnormalities:* No dose-related effect of letrozole on any hematologic or clinical chemistry parameter was evident. Moderate decreases in lymphocyte counts, of uncertain clinical significance, were observed in some patients receiving letrozole 2.5 mg. This depression was transient in about half of those affected. Two patients on letrozole developed thrombocytopenia; relationship to the study drug was unclear. Patient withdrawal because of laboratory abnormalities, whether related to study treatment or not, was infrequent.

Increases in AST, ALT, and gamma glutamyltransferase greater than or equal to 5 times the ULN and of bilirubin greater than or equal to 1.5 times the ULN were most often associated with metastatic disease in the liver. About 3% of study participants receiving letrozole had abnormalities in liver chemistries not associated with documented metastases; these abnormalities may have been related to study drug therapy.

In the megestrol comparative study, approximately 8% of patients treated with megestrol had abnormalities in liver chemistries that were not associated with documented liver metastases; in the aminoglutethimide study, about 10% of aminoglutethimide-treated patients had abnormalities in liver chemistries not associated with hepatic metastases.

In the adjuvant setting, an increase in total cholesterol (generally nonfasting) in patients who had baseline values of total serum cholesterol within the normal range, and then subsequently had an increase in total serum cholesterol of 1.5 ULN was 173/3,203 (5.4%) on letrozole versus 40/3,224

LETROZOLE — ORAL

(1.2%) on tamoxifen. Lipid-lowering medications were used by 18% of patients on letrozole and 12% on tamoxifen.

Bone effects – In the extended adjuvant setting, preliminary results (median duration of follow-up was 20 months) from the bone substudy (calcium 500 mg and vitamin D 400 units/day mandatory; biphosphonates not allowed) demonstrated that at 2 years the mean decrease compared with baseline in hip BMD in letrozole patients was 3% versus 0.4% for placebo ($P = 0.048$). The mean decrease from baseline BMD results for the lumbar spine at 2 years was letrozole 4.6% and placebo 2.2% ($P = 0.069$). Consider monitoring BMD.

➤*Hazardous tasks:* This medicine may cause dizziness, fatigue, and somnolence. Use caution while driving or performing other tasks that require alertness, coordination, or physical dexterity.

Drug Interactions

➤*Tamoxifen:* Coadministration of letrozole and tamoxifen 20 mg daily resulted in a reduction of letrozole plasma levels by 38% on average. Clinical experience in the second-line breast cancer pivotal trials indicates that the therapeutic effect of letrozole therapy is not impaired if letrozole is administered immediately after tamoxifen.

Adverse Reactions

Letrozole was generally well tolerated across all studies in first- and second-line metastatic breast cancer, adjuvant treatment, as well as extended adjuvant treatment in women who have received prior adjuvant tamoxifen treatment. Generally, the observed adverse reactions were mild or moderate in nature.

➤*Adjuvant treatment of early breast cancer in postmenopausal women:* The median duration of adjuvant treatment was 24 months and the median duration of follow-up for safety was 26 months for patients receiving letrozole and tamoxifen.

Certain adverse reactions were prospectively specified for analysis, based on the known pharmacologic properties and side effects of the 2 drugs.

Adverse reactions were analyzed irrespective of whether a symptom was present or absent at baseline. Most adverse reactions reported (82%) were grade 1 or 2 applying the National Cancer Institute Common Toxicity Criteria (NCI-CTC) version 2.0. The following table describes adverse reactions (grades 1 through 4) irrespective of relationship to study treatment in the adjuvant BIG 1-98 trial (safety population, during treatment or within 30 days of stopping treatment).

Letrozole Adverse Reactions (Grades 1 through 4)

Adverse reaction	Grades 1 through 4		Grades 3 through 4	
	Letrozole (n = 3,975)	Tamoxifen (n = 3,988)	Letrozole (n = 3,975)	Tamoxifen (n = 3,988)
Cardiovascular				
Angina	27 (0.7%)	24 (0.6%)	17 (0.4%)	7 (0.2%)
Cerebrovascular/ Transient ischemic attack	44 (1.1%)	41 (1%)	43 (1.1%)	40 (1%)
Myocardial infarction	17 (0.4%)	14 (0.4%)	15 (0.4%)	11 (0.3%)
Other cardiovascular	261 (6.6%)	248 (6.2%)	97 (2.4%)	71 (1.8%)
Thromboembolic event	44 (1.1%)	109 (2.7%)	29 (0.7%)	79 (2%)
CNS				
Dizziness/light-headedness	96 (2.4%)	110 (2.8%)	1 (< 0.1%)	8 (0.2%)
Fatigue (lethargy, malaise, asthenia)	333 (8.4%)	345 (8.7%)	9 (0.2%)	9 (0.2%)
Headache	141 (3.5%)	126 (3.2%)	12 (0.3%)	6 (0.2%)
GI				
Constipation	59 (1.5%)	95 (2.4%)	4 (0.1%)	1 (< 0.1%)
Nausea	378 (9.5%)	416 (10.4%)	6 (0.2%)	10 (0.3%)
Vomiting	109 (2.7%)	106 (2.7%)	6 (0.2%)	8 (0.2%)
GU				
Endometrial cancer[a]	7/3,089 (0.2%)	12/3,157 (0.4%)		
Endometrial proliferation disorders	10 (0.3%)	71 (1.8%)	1 (< 0.1%)	12 (0.3%)
Other endometrial disorders	3 (< 0.1%)	4 (0.1%)	0	1 (< 0.1%)
Vaginal bleeding	177 (4.5%)	411 (10.3%)	2 (< 0.1%)	7 (0.2%)
Vaginal irritation	139 (3.5%)	122 (3.1%)	6 (0.2%)	3 (< 0.1%)

Letrozole Adverse Reactions (Grades 1 through 4)

Adverse reaction	Grades 1 through 4		Grades 3 through 4	
	Letrozole (n = 3,975)	Tamoxifen (n = 3,988)	Letrozole (n = 3,975)	Tamoxifen (n = 3,988)
Metabolic				
Edema	286 (7.2%)	287 (7.2%)	5 (0.1%)	2 (< 0.1%)
Weight increase	425 (10.7%)	515 (12.9%)	21 (0.5%)	44 (1.1%)
Musculoskeletal				
Arthralgia/arthritis	840 (21.1%)	535 (13.4%)	88 (2.2%)	49 (1.2%)
Bone fractures	223 (5.6%)	158 (4%)	76 (1.9%)	45 (1.1%)
Myalgia	255 (6.4%)	243 (6.1%)	26 (0.7%)	17 (0.4%)
Osteoporosis	79 (2%)	44 (1.1%)	6 (0.2%)	7 (0.2%)
Miscellaneous				
Hot flashes/flushes	1,338 (33.7%)	1,515 (38%)	0	0
Night sweats	561 (14.1%)	654 (16.4%)	0	0
Second malignancies[b]	76/4,003 (1.9%)	96/4,007 (2.4%)		

[a] Based on safety population excluding patients who had undergone hysterectomy; time frame is any time after randomization; no CTC grades collected (yes/no response).
[b] Based on the intent-to-treat population; time frame is any time after randomization; no CTC grades collected (yes/no response).

When considering all grades, a higher incidence of reactions was seen for letrozole regarding fractures (5.7% vs 4%), myocardial infarctions (0.6% vs 0.4%), and arthralgia (21.2% vs 13.5%) (letrozole vs tamoxifen, respectively). A higher incidence was seen for tamoxifen regarding thromboembolic reactions (1.2% vs 2.8%), endometrial cancer (0.2% vs 0.4%), and endometrial proliferative disorders (0.3% vs 1.8%) (letrozole vs tamoxifen, respectively).

➤*Extended adjuvant treatment of early breast cancer in postmenopausal women:* The median duration of extended adjuvant treatment was 24 months, and the median duration of follow-up for safety was 28 months for patients receiving letrozole and placebo.

The following table describes the adverse reactions occurring at a frequency of at least 5% in any treatment group during treatment. Most adverse reactions reported were grade 1 and grade 2 based on the NCI-CTC version 2.0. In the extended adjuvant setting, the reported drug-related adverse reactions that were significantly different from placebo were arthralgia/arthritis, hot flashes, and myalgia.

Letrozole Adverse Reactions

Adverse reaction	Number (%) of patients with grade 1 to 4 adverse reaction		Number (%) of patients with grade 3 to 4 adverse reaction	
	Letrozole (n = 2,563)	Placebo (n = 2,573)	Letrozole (n = 2,563)	Placebo (n = 2,573)
CNS	863 (33.7%)	819 (31.8%)	65 (2.5%)	58 (2.3%)
Asthenia	862 (33.6%)	826 (32.1%)	16 (0.6%)	7 (0.3%)
Dizziness	363 (14.2%	342 (13.3%)	9 (0.4%)	6 (0.2%)
Headache	516 (20.1%)	508 (19.7%)	18 (0.7%)	17 (0.7%)
Insomnia	149 (5.8%)	120 (4.7%)	2 (< 0.1%)	2 (< 0.1%)
Psychiatric disorders	320 (12.5%)	276 (10.7%)	21 (0.8%)	16 (0.6%)
Dermatologic	830 (32.4%)	787 (30.6%)	17 (0.7%)	16 (0.6%)
Increased sweating	619 (24.2%)	577 (22.4%)	1 (< 0.1%)	0
GI	725 (28.3%)	731 (28.4%)	43 (1.7%)	42 (1.6%)
Constipation	290 (11.3%)	304 (11.8%)	6 (0.2%)	2 (< 0.1%)
Diarrhea NOS[a]	128 (5%)	143 (5.6%)	12 (0.5%)	8 (0.3%)
Nausea	221 (8.6%)	212 (8.2%)	3 (0.1%)	10 (0.4%)
GU	303 (11.8%)	357 (13.9%)	9 (0.4%)	8 (0.3%)
Vaginal hemorrhage	123 (4.8%)	171 (6.6%)	2 (< 0.1%)	5 (0.2%)
Vulvovaginal dryness	137 (5.3%)	127 (4.9%)	0	0

LETROZOLE — ORAL

Letrozole Adverse Reactions				
	Number (%) of patients with grade 1 to 4 adverse reaction		Number (%) of patients with grade 3 to 4 adverse reaction	
Adverse reaction	Letrozole (n = 2,563)	Placebo (n = 2,573)	Letrozole (n = 2,563)	Placebo (n = 2,573)
Musculoskeletal	978 (38.2%)	836 (32.5%)	71 (2.8%)	50 (1.9%)
Arthralgia	565 (22%)	465 (18.1%)	25 (1%)	20 (0.8%)
Arthritis NOS[a]	173 (6.7%)	124 (4.8%)	10 (0.4%)	5 (0.2%)
Back pain	129 (5%)	112 (4.4%)	8 (0.3%)	7 (0.3%)
Myalgia	171 (6.7%)	122 (4.7%)	8 (0.3%)	6 (0.2%)
Vascular disorders	1,375 (53.6%)	1,230 (47.8%)	59 (2.3%)	74 (2.9%)
Metabolic	551 (21.5%)	537 (20.9%)	24 (0.9%)	32 (1.2%)
Edema NOS[a]	471 (18.4%)	416 (16.2%)	4 (0.2%)	3 (0.1%)
Hypercholesterolemia	401 (15.6%)	398 (15.5%)	2 (< 0.1%)	5 (0.2%)
Respiratory	279 (10.9%)	260 (10.1%)	30 (1.2%)	28 (1.1%)
Dyspnea	140 (5.5%)	137 (5.3%)	21 (0.8%)	18 (0.7%)
Miscellaneous	1,154 (45%)	1,090 (42.4%)	30 (1.2%)	28 (1.1%)
Any adverse reaction	2,232 (87.1%)	2,174 (84.5%)	419 (16.3%)	389 (15.1%)
Flushing	1,273 (49.7%)	1,114 (43.3%)	3 (0.1%)	0
Infections and infestations	166 (6.5%)	163 (6.3%)	40 (1.6%)	33 (1.3%)
Investigations	184 (7.2%)	147 (5.7%)	13 (0.5%)	13 (0.5%)
Renal disorders	130 (5.1%)	100 (3.9%)	12 (0.5%)	6 (0.2%)

[a] NOS = not otherwise specified.

The duration of follow-up for both the main clinical study and the bone study were insufficient to assess fracture risk associated with long-term use of letrozole. Based on a median follow-up of patients for 28 months, the incidence of clinical fractures from the core randomized study in patients who received letrozole was 5.9% (152) and placebo was 5.5% (142). The incidence of self-reported osteoporosis was higher in patients who received letrozole 6.9% (176) than in patients who received placebo 5.5% (141). Bisphosphonates were administered to 21.1% of the patients who received letrozole and 18.7% of the patients who received placebo.

Preliminary results (median duration of follow-up was 20 months) from the bone substudy (calcium 500 mg and vitamin D 400 units/day mandatory; biphosphonates not allowed) demonstrated that at 2 years the mean decrease compared with baseline in hip BMD in letrozole patients was 3% versus 0.4% for placebo. The mean decrease from baseline BMD results for the lumbar spine at 2 years were letrozole 4.6% and placebo 2.2%.

The incidence of cardiovascular ischemic events from the core randomized study was comparable between patients who received letrozole 6.8% (175) and placebo 6.5% (167).

Preliminary results (median duration of follow-up was 30 months) from the lipid substudy did not show significant differences between the letrozole and placebo groups. The high:low-density lipoprotein ratio decreased after the first 6 months of therapy, but the decrease was similar in both groups, and no statistically significant differences were detected.

A patient-reported measure that captures treatment impact on important symptoms associated with estrogen deficiency demonstrated a difference in favor of placebo for vasomotor and sexual symptom domains.

➤*First-line breast cancer:* A total of 455 patients was treated for a median time of exposure of 11 months. The incidence of adverse reactions was similar for letrozole and tamoxifen. The most frequently reported adverse reactions were arthralgia, back pain, bone pain, dyspnea, hot flushes, and nausea. Discontinuations for adverse reactions other than progression of tumor occurred in 10 of 455 (2%) of patients on letrozole and in 15 of 455 (3%) patients on tamoxifen.

Adverse reactions, regardless of relationship to study drug, that were reported in at least 5% of the patients treated with letrozole 2.5 mg or tamoxifen 20 mg in the first-line treatment study are shown in the following table.

Letrozole Adverse Reactions (> 5%)		
Adverse reaction	Letrozole 2.5 mg (n = 455)	Tamoxifen 20 mg (n = 455)
Cardiovascular		
Hypertension	8%	4%
CNS		
Fatigue	13%	13%
Headache NOS	8%	7%
Insomnia	7%	4%
Weakness	6%	4%
GI		
Anorexia	4%	6%
Constipation	10%	11%
Diarrhea	8%	4%
Nausea	17%	17%
Vomiting	7%	8%
GU		
Urinary tract infection NOS	6%	3%
Metabolic		
Decreased weight	7%	5%
Peripheral edema	5%	6%
Musculoskeletal		
Arthralgia	16%	15%
Back pain	18%	19%
Bone pain	22%	21%
Limb pain	10%	8%
Respiratory		
Chest wall pain	6%	6%
Cough	13%	13%
Dyspnea	18%	17%
Miscellaneous		
Breast pain	7%	7%
Chest pain	8%	9%
Hot flushes	19%	16%
Influenza	6%	4%
Pain NOS	5%	7%
Postmastectomy lymphedema	7%	7%

Less frequent (less than 2%) adverse reactions –

CV: Angina, coronary heart disease, myocardial infarction, myocardial ischemia, portal vein thrombosis, pulmonary embolism, thrombophlebitis, thrombotic or hemorrhagic strokes, transient ischemic attacks, venous thrombosis.

CNS: Development of hemiparesis.

➤*Second-line breast cancer:* Letrozole was generally well tolerated in 2 controlled, clinical trials.

Study discontinuations in the megestrol comparison study for adverse reactions other than progression of tumor occurred in 5 of 188 (2.7%) patients on letrozole 0.5 mg, in 4 of 174 (2.3%) patients on letrozole 2.5 mg, and in 15 of 190 (7.9%) patients on megestrol. There were fewer thromboembolic events at both letrozole doses than on the megestrol acetate arm (0.6% vs 4.7%). There also was less vaginal bleeding (0.3% vs 3.2%) on letrozole than on megestrol. In the aminoglutethimide comparison study, discontinuations for reasons other than progression occurred in 6 of 193 (3.1%) patients on letrozole 0.5 mg, 7 of 185 (3.8%) patients on letrozole 2.5 mg, and 7 of 178 (3.9%) patients on aminoglutethimide.

Comparisons of the incidence of adverse reactions revealed no significant differences between the high- and low-dose letrozole groups in either study. Most of the adverse reactions observed in all treatment groups were mild to moderate in severity, and it was generally not possible to distinguish adverse reactions caused by treatment from the consequences of the patient's metastatic breast cancer, the effects of estrogen deprivation, or intercurrent illness.

Adverse reactions, regardless of relationship to study drug, that were reported in at least 5% of the patients treated with letrozole 0.5 mg, letrozole 2.5 mg, megestrol, or aminoglutethimide in the 2 controlled trials are shown in the following table.

LETROZOLE — ORAL

Letrozole Adverse Reactions (> 5%)				
Adverse reaction	Pooled letrozole 2.5 mg (n = 359)	Pooled letrozole 0.5 mg (n = 380)	Megestrol 160 mg (n = 189)	Aminoglutethimide 500 mg (n = 178)
Cardiovascular				
Hypertension	5%	7%	5%	6%
CNS				
Asthenia	4%	5%	4%	5%
Dizziness	3%	5%	7%	3%
Fatigue	8%	6%	11%	3%
Headache	9%	12%	9%	7%
Somnolence	3%	2%	2%	9%
Dermatologic				
Pruritus	1%	2%	5%	3%
Rash [a]	5%	4%	3%	12%
GI				
Abdominal pain	6%	5%	9%	8%
Anorexia	5%	3%	5%	5%
Constipation	6%	7%	9%	7%
Diarrhea	6%	5%	3%	4%
Dyspepsia	3%	4%	6%	5%
Nausea	13%	15%	9%	14%
Vomiting	7%	7%	5%	9%
Metabolic				
Hypercholesterolemia	3%	3%	0%	6%
Peripheral edema[b]	5%	5%	8%	3%
Weight increase	2%	2%	9%	3%
Musculoskeletal				
Arthralgia	8%	8%	8%	3%
Musculoskeletal pain[c]	21%	22%	30%	14%
Respiratory				
Coughing	6%	5%	7%	5%
Dyspnea	7%	9%	16%	5%
Miscellaneous				
Chest pain	6%	3%	7%	3%
Hot flushes	6%	5%	4%	3%
Viral infection	6%	5%	6%	3%

[a] Includes rash, erythematous rash, maculopapular rash, psoriaform rash, vesicular rash.
[b] Includes peripheral edema, leg edema, dependent edema, edema.
[c] Includes musculoskeletal pain, skeletal pain, back pain, arm pain, leg pain.

Other less frequent (less than 5%) adverse reactions considered consequential and reported in at least 3 patients treated with letrozole included alopecia, anxiety, depression, fracture, hypercalcemia, increased sweating, pleural effusion, and vertigo.

➤*Postmarketing:* Cases of blurred vision and increased hepatic enzymes have been reported in less than 1% since market introduction.

Overdosage

➤*Symptoms:* Isolated cases of letrozole overdose have been reported. In these instances, the highest single dose ingested was 62.5 mg or 25 tablets. No serious adverse reactions were reported in these cases. In single-dose studies the highest dose used was 30 mg, which was well tolerated; in multiple-dose trials, the largest dose of 10 mg was well tolerated.

Lethality was observed in mice and rats following single oral doses that were greater than or equal to 2,000 mg/kg (approximately 4,000 to 8,000 times the daily MRHD on a mg/m^2 basis); death was associated with reduced motor activity, ataxia, and dyspnea. Lethality was observed in cats following single intravenous doses that were greater than or equal to 10 mg/kg (approximately 50 times the daily MRHD on a mg/m^2 basis); death was preceded by depressed blood pressure and arrhythmias.

➤*Treatment:* Because of the limited data available, no firm recommendations for treatment can be made. However, emesis could be induced if the patient is alert. In general, supportive care and frequent monitoring of vital signs are appropriate.

Patient Information

Advise patients to tell their health care provider or pharmacist if any of the following occurs: severe allergic reactions (rash; hives; difficulty breathing; tightness in the chest; swelling of the mouth, face, lips, or tongue), shortness of breath.

Advise patients to take this medicine with a small glass of water at about the same time each day, with or without meals.

Advise patients that this medicine may cause dizziness and drowsiness. Patients should use caution while driving or performing other tasks that require alertness, coordination, or physical dexterity.

EXEMESTANE

Rx	**Aromasin** (Pharmacia & Upjohn)	**Tablets:** 25 mg	Mannitol, methylparaben, polyvinyl alcohol. (7663). Off-white to gray. Biconvex. In 30s.

EXEMESTANE — ORAL

Indications

➤*Breast cancer:* For the treatment of advanced breast cancer in postmenopausal women whose disease has progressed following tamoxifen therapy.

➤*Unlabeled uses:* Prevention of prostate carcinogenesis.

Administration and Dosage

➤*Approved by the FDA:* October 21, 1999.

The recommended dose of exemestane tablets is 25 mg once daily after a meal. Treatment with exemestane should continue until tumor progression is evident.

➤*Storage/Stability:* Store at 25°C (77°F); excursions permitted to 15° to 30°C (59° to 86°F) (see USP controlled room temperature).

Actions

➤*Pharmacology:* Breast cancer cell growth may be estrogen-dependent. Exemestane is the principal enzyme that converts androgens to estrogens both in pre- and postmenopausal women. While the main source of estrogen (primarily estradiol) is the ovary in premenopausal women, the principal source of circulating estrogens in postmenopausal women is from conversion of adrenal and ovarian androgens (androstenedione and testosterone) to estrogens (estrone and estradiol) by the aromatase enzyme in peripheral tissues. Estrogen deprivation through aromatase inhibition is an effective and selective treatment for some postmenopausal patients with hormone-dependent breast cancer.

Exemestane is an irreversible, steroidal aromatase inactivator, structurally related to the natural substrate androstenedione. It acts as a false substrate for the aromatase enzyme, and is processed to an intermediate that binds irreversibly to the active site of the enzyme causing its inactivation, an effect also known as "suicide inhibition." Exemestane significantly lowers circulating estrogen concentrations in postmenopausal women, but has no detectable effect on adrenal biosynthesis of corticosteroids or aldosterone. Exemestane has no effect on other enzymes involved in the steroidogenic pathway up to a concentration at least 600 times higher than that inhibiting the aromatase enzyme.

➤*Pharmacokinetics:*

Absorption – Following oral administration to healthy postmenopausal women, exemestane is rapidly absorbed. After maximum plasma concentration is reached, levels decline polyexponentially with a mean terminal half-life of about 24 hours. Exemestane is extensively distributed and is cleared from the systemic circulation primarily by metabolism. The pharmacokinetics of exemestane are dose proportional after single (10 to 200 mg) or repeated oral doses (0.5 to 50 mg). Following repeated daily doses of exemestane 25 mg, plasma concentrations of unchanged drug are similar to levels measured after a single dose.

Pharmacokinetic parameters in postmenopausal women with advanced breast cancer following single or repeated doses have been compared with those in healthy, postmenopausal women. Exemestane appeared to be more rapidly absorbed in the women with breast cancer than in the healthy women, with a mean t_{max} of 1.2 hours in the women with breast cancer and 2.9 hours in the healthy women. After repeated dosing, the average oral clearance in women with advanced breast cancer was 45% lower than the oral clearance in healthy postmenopausal women, with corresponding higher systemic exposure. Mean AUC values following repeated doses in women with breast cancer (75.4 ng•hr/mL) were about twice those in healthy women (41.4 ng•hr/mL).

Following oral administration of radiolabeled exemestane, at least 42% of radioactivity was absorbed from the gastrointestinal tract. Exemestane plasma levels increased by approximately 40% after a high-fat breakfast.

Distribution – Exemestane is distributed extensively into tissues. Exemestane is 90% bound to plasma proteins and the fraction bound is independent of the total concentration. Albumin and α_1-acid glycoprotein both contribute to the binding. The distribution of exemestane and its metabolites into blood cells is negligible.

Metabolism/Excretion – Following administration of radiolabeled exemestane to healthy postmenopausal women, the cumulative amounts of

EXEMESTANE — ORAL

radioactivity excreted in urine and feces were similar (42 ± 3% in urine and 42 ± 6% in feces over a 1-week collection period). The amount of drug excreted unchanged in urine was less than 1% of the dose.

Exemestane is extensively metabolized, with levels of the unchanged drug in plasma accounting for less than 10% of the total radioactivity. The initial steps in the metabolism of exemestane are oxidation of the methylene group in position 6 and reduction of the 17-keto group with subsequent formation of many secondary metabolites. Each metabolite accounts only for a limited amount of drug-related material. The metabolites are inactive or inhibit aromatase with decreased potency compared with the parent drug. One metabolite may have androgenic activity. Studies using human liver preparations indicate that cytochrome P450 3A4 (CYP3A4) is the principal isoenzyme involved in the oxidation of exemestane.

Special populations –

Renal function impairment: See Warnings for more information.

Hepatic function impairment: See Warnings for more information.

Contraindications

Hypersensitivity to the drug or to any of the excipients.

Warnings

➤*Renal function impairment:* The AUC of exemestane after a single 25 mg dose was approximately 3 times higher in subjects with moderate or severe renal insufficiency (creatinine clearance < 35 mL/min/1.73 m^2) compared with the AUC in healthy volunteers. The safety of chronic dosing in patients with moderate or severe renal impairment has not been studied. Based on experience with exemestane at repeated doses up to 200 mg daily that demonstrated a moderate increase in non-life threatening adverse events, dosage adjustment does not appear to be necessary.

➤*Hepatic function impairment:* The pharmacokinetics of exemestane have been investigated in subjects with moderate or severe hepatic insufficiency (Childs-Pugh class B or C). Following a single 25 mg oral dose, the AUC of exemestane was approximately 3 times higher than that observed in healthy volunteers. The safety of chronic dosing in patients with moderate or severe hepatic impairment has not been studied. Based on experience with exemestane at repeated doses up to 200 mg daily that demonstrated a moderate increase in non-life threatening adverse events, dosage adjustment does not appear to be necessary.

➤*Mutagenesis:* Exemestane was not mutagenic in bacteria (Ames test) or mammalian cells (V79 Chinese hamster lung cells). Exemestane was clastogenic in human lymphocytes in vitro without metabolic activation but was not clastogenic in vivo (micronucleus assay in mouse bone marrow). Exemestane did not increase unscheduled DNA synthesis in rat hepatocytes.

➤*Fertility impairment:* Untreated female rats showed reduced fertility when mated to males treated with 500 mg/kg/day exemestane (≈ 200 times the recommended human dose on a mg/m^2 basis) for 63 days prior to and during cohabitation. Exemestane given to female rats 14 days prior to mating and through day 15 or 20 of gestation increased the placental weights at 4 mg/kg/day (≈ 1.5 times the human dose on a mg/m^2 basis). Exemestane showed no effects on female fertility parameters (eg, ovarian function, mating behavior, conception rate) in rats given doses up to 20 mg/kg/day (≈ 8 times the human dose on a mg/m^2 basis), but mean litter size was decreased at this dose. In general toxicology studies, changes in the ovary, including hyperplasia, an increase in ovarian cysts and a decrease in corpora lutea were observed with variable frequency in mice, rats and dogs at doses that ranged from 3 to 20 times the human dose on a mg/m^2 basis.

➤*Pregnancy: Category D.* Exemestane tablets may cause fetal harm when administered to a pregnant woman. Radioactivity related to ^{14}C-exemestane crossed the placenta of rats following oral administration of 1 mg/kg exemestane. The concentration of exemestane and its metabolites was approximately equivalent in maternal and fetal blood. When rats were administered exemestane from 14 days prior to mating until either days 15 or 20 of gestation, and resuming for the 21 days of lactation, an increase in placental weight was seen at 4 mg/kg/day (≈ 1.5 times the recommended human daily dose on a mg/m^2 basis). Prolonged gestation and abnormal or difficult labor was observed at doses ≥ 20 mg/kg/day. Increased resorption, reduced number of live fetuses, decreased fetal weight, and retarded ossification were also observed at these doses. No malformations were noted when exemestane was administered to pregnant rats during the organogenesis period at doses up to 810 mg/kg/day (≈ 320 times the recommended human dose on a mg/m^2 basis). Daily doses of exemestane, given to rabbits during organogenesis caused a decrease in placental weight at 90 mg/kg/day (≈ 70 times the recommended human daily dose on a mg/m^2 basis). Abortions, an increase in resorptions, and a reduction in fetal body weight were seen at 270 mg/kg/day. There was no increase in the incidence of malformations in rabbits at doses up to 270 mg/kg/day (≈ 210 times the recommended human dose on a mg/m^2 basis).

There are no studies in pregnant women using exemestane. Exemestane is indicated for postmenopausal women. If there is exposure to exemestane during pregnancy, the patient should be apprised of the potential hazard to the fetus and potential risk for loss of the pregnancy.

➤*Lactation:* Exemestane is only indicated in postmenopausal women. However, radioactivity related to exemestane appeared in rat milk within 15 minutes of oral administration of radiolabeled exemestane. Concentrations of exemestane and its metabolites were approximately equivalent in the milk and plasma of rats for 24 hours after a single oral dose of 1 mg/kg ^{14}C-exemestane. It is not known whether exemestane is excreted in human milk. Because many drugs are excreted in human milk, caution should be exercised if a nursing woman is inadvertently exposed to exemestane.

➤*Children:* The safety and effectiveness of exemestane in pediatric patients have not been established.

Precautions

➤*Premenopausal women:* Exemestane tablets should not be administered to premenopausal women. Exemestane should not be coadministered with estrogen-containing agents as these could interfere with its pharmacologic action.

➤*Lab test abnormalities:* Approximately 20% of patients receiving exemestane in clinical studies experienced common toxicity criteria (CTC) grade 3 or 4 lymphocytopenia. Of these patients, 89% had a preexisting lower grade lymphopenia. Forty percent of patients either recovered or improved to a lesser severity while on treatment. Patients did not have a significant increase in viral infections, and no opportunistic infections were observed. Elevations of serum levels of AST, ALT, alkaline phosphatase, and gamma glutamyl transferase > 5 times the upper value of the healthy range (ie, ≥ CTC grade 3) have been rarely reported but appear mostly attributable to the underlying presence of liver or bone metastases. In the comparative study, CTC grade 3 or 4 elevation of gamma glutamyl transferase without documented evidence of liver metastasis was reported in 2.7% of patients treated with exemestane and in 1.8% of patients treated with megestrol acetate.

Adverse Reactions

A total of 1058 patients were treated with exemestane 25 mg once daily in the clinical trials program. Exemestane was generally well tolerated, and adverse events were usually mild to moderate. Only 1 death was considered possibly related to treatment with exemestane; an 80-year-old woman with known coronary artery disease had a myocardial infarction with multiple organ failure after 9 weeks on study treatment. In the clinical trials program, only 3% of the patients discontinued treatment with exemestane because of adverse events, mainly within the first 10 weeks of treatment; late discontinuations because of adverse events were uncommon (0.3%).

In the comparative study, adverse reactions were assessed for 358 patients treated with exemestane and 400 patients treated with megestrol acetate. Fewer patients receiving exemestane discontinued treatment because of adverse events than those treated with megestrol acetate (2% vs 5%). Adverse events that were considered drug related or of indeterminate cause included hot flashes (13% vs 5%), nausea (9% vs 5%), fatigue (8% vs 10%), increased sweating (4% vs 8%), and increased appetite (3% vs 6%). The proportion of patients experiencing an excessive weight gain (> 10% of their baseline weight) was significantly higher with megestrol acetate than with exemestane (17% versus 8%). The data below shows the adverse events of all CTC grades, regardless of causality, reported in 5% or greater of patients in the study treated either with exemestane or megestrol acetate.

Exemestane Adverse Reactions (≥ 5%)

Adverse reaction	Exemestane 25 mg once daily (n = 358)	Megestrol acetate 40 mg 4 times/day (n = 400)
Autonomic nervous system		
Increased sweating	6	9
Miscellaneous		
Fatigue	22	29
Hot flashes	13	6
Pain	13	13
Influenza-like symptoms	6	5
Edema (includes edema, peripheral edema, leg edema)	7	6
Cardiovascular		
Hypertension	5	6
CNS		
Depression	13	9
Insomnia	11	9
Anxiety	10	11
Dizziness	8	6
Headache	8	7
GI		
Nausea	18	12
Vomiting	7	4
Abdominal pain	6	11
Anorexia	6	5
Constipation	5	8
Diarrhea	4	5
Increased appetite	3	6
Respiratory		
Dyspnea	10	15
Coughing	6	7

* Graded according to Common Toxicity Criteria.

➤*Less frequent adverse events (from 2% to 5%):* Less frequent adverse events of any cause (from 2% to 5%) reported in the comparative study for

EXEMESTANE — ORAL

patients receiving exemestane 25 mg once daily were fever, generalized weakness, paresthesia, pathological fracture; bronchitis, sinusitis, rash, itching, urinary tract infection, and lymphedema.

➤*Additional adverse events:* Additional adverse events of any cause observed in the overall clinical trials program (n = 1058) in 5% or greater of patients treated with exemestane 25 mg once daily but not in the comparative study included the following: Pain at tumor sites (8%), asthenia (6%), and fever (5%). Adverse events of any cause reported in 2% to 5% of all patients treated with exemestane 25 mg in the overall clinical trials program but not in the comparative study included the following: Chest pain, hypoesthesia, confusion, dyspepsia, arthralgia, back pain, skeletal pain, infection, upper respiratory tract infection, pharyngitis, rhinitis, and alopecia.

Overdosage

Clinical trials have been conducted with exemestane given as a single dose to healthy female volunteers at doses as high as 800 mg and daily for 12 weeks to postmenopausal women with advanced breast cancer at doses as high as 600 mg. These dosages were well tolerated. There is no specific antidote to overdosage and treatment must be symptomatic. General supportive care, including frequent monitoring of vital signs and close observation of the patient, is indicated.

A male child (age unknown) accidentally ingested a 25 mg tablet of exemestane. The initial physical examination was normal, but blood tests performed 1 hour after ingestion indicated leucocytosis (WBC 25,000/mm^3 with 90% neutrophils). Blood tests were repeated 4 days after the incident and were healthy. No treatment was given.

In mice, mortality was observed after a single oral dose of exemestane of 3200 mg/kg, the lowest dose tested (about 640 times the recommended human dose on a mg/m^2 basis). In rats and dogs, mortality was observed after single oral doses of exemestane of 5000 mg/kg (about 2000 times the recommended human dose on a mg/m^2 basis) and 3000 mg/kg (about 4000 times the recommended human dose on a mg/m^2 basis), respectively.

Convulsions were observed after single doses of exemestane of 400 mg/kg and 3000 mg/kg in mice and dogs ($\approx$ 80 and 4000 times the recommended human dose on a mg/m^2 basis), respectively.

ENZYMES

ASPARAGINASE

Rx	**Elspar** (Merck)	**Powder for Injection, lyophilized:** 10,000 IU	80 mg mannitol. Preservative free. In 10 ml vials.

ASPARAGINASE — INJECTION

WARNING

It is recommended that asparaginase be administered to patients only in a hospital setting under the supervision of a physician who is qualified by training and experience to administer cancer chemotherapeutic agents, because of the possibility of severe reactions, including anaphylaxis and sudden death. The physician must be prepared to treat anaphylaxis at each administration of the drug.

In the treatment of each patient the physician must weigh carefully the possibility of achieving therapeutic benefit versus the risk of toxicity. The following data should be thoroughly reviewed before administering the compound.

Indications

➤*Acute lymphocytic leukemia:* Therapy of patients with acute lymphocytic leukemia. This agent is useful primarily in combination with other chemotherapeutic agents in the induction of remissions of the disease in pediatric patients. Asparaginase should not be used as the sole induction agent unless combination therapy is deemed inappropriate. Asparaginase is not recommended for maintenance therapy.

Administration and Dosage

As a component of selected multiple agent induction regimens, asparaginase may be administered by either the intravenous or the intramuscular route. When administered intravenously, this enzyme should be given over a period of not less than thirty minutes through the side arm of an already running infusion of Sodium Chloride Injection or Dextrose Injection 5% (D_5W). Asparaginase has little tendency to cause phlebitis when given intravenously. Anaphylactic reactions require the immediate use of epinephrine, oxygen, and intravenous steroids.

When administering asparaginase intramuscularly, the volume at a single injection site should be limited to 2 ml. If a volume greater than 2 ml is to be administered, two injection sites should be used.

Unfavorable interactions of asparaginase with some antitumor agents have been demonstrated. It is recommended therefore, that asparaginase be used in combination regimens only by physicians familiar with the benefits and risks of a given regimen. During the period of its inhibition of protein synthesis and cell replication, asparaginase may interfere with the action of drugs such as methotrexate which require cell replication for their lethal effect. Asparaginase may interfere with the enzymatic detoxification of other drugs, particularly in the liver.

➤*Recommended induction regimens:* When using chemotherapeutic agents in combination for the induction of remissions in patients with acute lymphocytic leukemia, regimens are sought which provide maximum chance of success while avoiding excessive cumulative toxicity or negative drug interactions.

One of the following combination regimens incorporating asparaginase is recommended for acute lymphocytic leukemia in children.

In the regimens below, Day 1 is considered to be the first day of therapy.

Regimen I –

Prednisone: 40 mg/m^2 of body surface area per day orally in three divided doses for 15 days, followed by tapering of the dosage as follows:

20 mg/m^2 for 2 days, 10 mg/m^2 for 2 days, 5 mg/m^2 for 2 days, 2.5 mg/m^2 for 2 days and then discontinue.

Vincristine sulfate: 2 mg/m^2 of body surface area intravenously once weekly on days 1, 8, and 15 of the treatment period. The maximum single dose should not exceed 2.0 mg.

Asparaginase : 1,000 IU/kg/day intravenously for 10 successive days beginning on Day 22 of the treatment period.

Regimen II – Prednisone 40 mg/m^2 of body surface area per day orally in 3 divided doses for 28 days (the total daily dose should be to the nearest 2.5 mg), following which the dosage of prednisone should be discontinued gradually over a 14 day period.

Vincristine sulfate – 1.5 mg/m^2 of body surface area intravenously weekly for 4 doses, on days 1, 8, 15, and 22 of the treatment period. The maximum single dose should not exceed 2.0 mg.

Asparaginase – 6,000 IU/m^2 of body surface area intramuscularly on days 4, 7, 10, 13, 16, 19, 22, 25, and 28 of the treatment period. When a remission is obtained with either of the above regimens, appropriate maintenance therapy must be instituted. Asparaginase should not be used as part of a maintenance regimen. The above regimens do not preclude a need for special therapy directed toward the prevention of central nervous system leukemia.

It should be noted that asparaginase has been used in combination regimens other than those recommended above. It is important to keep in mind that asparaginase administered intravenously concurrently with or immediately before a course of vincristine and prednisone may be associated with increased toxicity. Physicians using a given regimen should be thoroughly familiar with its benefits and risks. Clinical data are insufficient for a recommendation concerning the use of combination regimens in adults. Asparaginase toxicity is reported to be greater in adults than in pediatric patients.

Use of asparaginase as the sole induction agent should be undertaken only in an unusual situation when a combined regimen is inappropriate because of toxicity or other specific patient-related factors, or in cases refractory to other therapy. When asparaginase is to be used as the sole induction agent for pediatric patients or adults, the recommended dosage regimen is 200 IU/kg/day intravenously for 28 days. When complete remissions were obtained with this regimen, they were of short duration, 1 to 3 months. Asparaginase has been used as the sole induction agent in other regimens. Physicians using a given regimen should be thoroughly familiar with its benefits and risks.

Patients undergoing induction therapy must be carefully monitored and the therapeutic regimen adjusted according to response and toxicity.

Such adjustments should always involve decreasing dosages of one or more agents or discontinuation depending on the degree of toxicity. Patients who have received a course of asparaginase, if re-treated, have an increased risk of hypersensitivity reactions. Therefore, re-treatment should be undertaken only when the benefit of such therapy is weighed against the increased risk.

➤*Intradermal Skin Test:* Because of the occurrence of allergic reactions, an intradermal skin test should be performed prior to the initial administration of asparaginase and when asparaginase is given after an interval of a week or more has elapsed between doses. The skin test solution may be prepared as follows: Reconstitute the contents of a 10,000 IU vial with 5.0 ml of diluent. From this solution (2,000 IU/ml) withdraw 0.1 ml and inject it into another vial containing 9.9 ml of diluent, yielding a skin test solution of approximately 20.0 IU/ml. Use 0.1 ml of this solution (about 2.0 IU) for the intradermal skin test. The skin test site should be observed for at least one hour for the appearance of a wheal or erythema either of which indicates a positive reaction. An allergic reaction even to the skin test dose in certain sensitized individuals may rarely occur.

A negative skin test reaction does not preclude the possibility of the development of an allergic reaction.

➤*Desensitization:* Desensitization should be performed before administering the first dose of asparaginase on initiation of therapy in positive reactors, and on re-treatment of any patient in whom such therapy is deemed necessary after carefully weighing the increased risk of hypersensitivity reactions. Rapid desensitization of the patient may be attempted with progressively increasing amounts of intravenously administered asparaginase provided adequate precautions are taken to treat an acute allergic reaction should it occur. One reported schedule begins with a total of 1 IU given intravenously and doubles the dose every 10 minutes, provided no reaction has occurred, until the accumulated total amount given equals the planned doses for that day.

ASPARAGINASE — INJECTION

For convenience the following information is included to calculate the number of doses necessary to reach the patient's total dose for that day.

Asparaginase Dosing Based on Total Daily Requirements		
Injection number[a]	Dose (IU)	Accumulated total dose (IU)
1	1	1
2	2	3
3	4	7
4	8	15
5	16	31
6	32	63
7	64	127
8	128	255
9	256	511
10	512	1023
11	1024	2047
12	2048	4095
13	4096	8191
14	8192	16,383
15	16,384	32,767
16	32,768	65,535
17	65,536	131,071
18	131,072	262,143

[a] For example: A patient weighing 20 kg who is to receive 200 IU/kg (total dose 4000 IU) would receive injections 1 through 12 during desensitization.

➤*Directions for reconstitution:*

For intravenous use – Reconstitute with Sterile Water for Injection or with Sodium Chloride Injection. The volume recommended for reconstitution is 5 ml for the 10,000 unit vials. Ordinary shaking during reconstitution does not inactivate the enzyme. This solution may be used for direct intravenous administration within an 8 hour period following restoration. For administration by infusion, solutions should be diluted with the isotonic solutions, Sodium Chloride Injection or Dextrose Injection 5%. These solutions should be infused within 8 hours and only if clear.

Occasionally, a very small number of gelatinous fiber-like particles may develop on standing. Filtration through a 5.0 micron filter during administration will remove the particles with no resultant loss in potency. Some loss of potency has been observed with the use of a 0.2 micron filter.

For intramuscular use – When asparaginase is administered intramuscularly according to the schedule cited in the induction regimen, reconstitution is carried out by adding 2 ml Sodium Chloride Injection to the 10,000 unit vial. The resulting solution should be used within 8 hours and only if clear.

➤*Storage/Stability:* Store at 2° to 8°C (36° to 46°F). Asparaginase does not contain a preservative. Unused, reconstituted solution should be stored at 2° to 8°C (36 to 46°F) and discarded after 8 hours, or sooner if it becomes cloudy.

Actions

➤*Pharmacology:* In a significant number of patients with acute leukemia, particularly lymphocytic, the malignant cells are dependent on an exogenous source of asparagine for survival. Normal cells, however, are able to synthesize asparagine and thus are affected less by the rapid depletion produced by treatment with the enzyme asparaginase. This is a unique approach to therapy based on a metabolic defect in asparagine synthesis of some malignant cells. Asparagine, derived from *Escherichia coli*, is effective in inducing remissions in some patients with acute lymphocytic leukemia.

Administration of asparaginase hydrolyzes serum asparagine to nonfunctional aspartic acid and ammonia, depriving tumor cells of a required amino acid. Tumor cell proliferation is blocked due to interruption of asparagine-dependent protein synthesis. The inhibitory activity is maximal in the postmitotic (G_1) phase of the cell cycle.

➤*Pharmacokinetics:*

Metabolism – In a study in patients with metastatic cancer and leukemia, initial plasma levels of L-asparaginase following intravenous administration were correlated to dose. Daily administration resulted in a cumulative increase in plasma levels. Plasma half-life varied from 8 to 30 hours; it did not appear to be influenced by dosage, either single or repetitive, and could not be correlated with age, sex, surface area, renal or hepatic function, diagnosis or extent of disease. Apparent volume of distribution was approximately 70%-80% of estimated plasma volume. There was some slow movement of asparaginase from vascular to extravascular, extracellular space. L-asparaginase was detected in the lymph. Cerebrospinal fluid levels were less than 1% of concurrent plasma levels. Only trace amounts appeared in the urine.

In a study in which patients with leukemia and metastatic cancer received intramuscular L-asparaginase, peak plasma levels of asparaginase were reached 14 to 24 hours after dosing. Plasma half-life was 39 to 49 hours. No asparaginase was detected in the urine.

Contraindications

Previous anaphylactic reactions to asparaginase; history of pancreatitis. Acute hemorrhagic pancreatitis, in some instances fatal, has been reported following asparaginase administration.

Warnings

➤*Allergic reactions:* Allergic reactions to asparaginase are frequent and may occur during the primary course of therapy. They are not completely predictable on the basis of the intradermal skin test. Anaphylaxis and death have occurred even in a hospital setting with experienced observers.

➤*Re-treatment:* Once a patient has received asparaginase as part of a treatment regimen, retreatment with this agent at a later time is associated with increased risk of hypersensitivity reactions. In patients found by skin testing to be hypersensitive to asparaginase, and in any patient who has received a previous course of therapy with asparaginase, therapy with this agent should be instituted or reinstituted only after successful desensitization, and then only if in the judgement of the physician the possible benefit is greater than the increased risk. Desensitization itself may be hazardous. (See Administration and Dosage.)

➤*Special risk:* In view of the unpredictability of the adverse reactions to asparaginase, it is recommended that this product be used in a hospital setting. Asparaginase has an adverse effect on liver function in the majority of patients. Therapy with asparaginase may increase pre-existing liver impairment caused by prior therapy or the underlying disease. Because of this there is a possibility that asparaginase may increase the toxicity of other medications.

➤*Carcinogenesis:* The intraperitoneal injection of 2500 IU/kg/day for 4 days in newborn Swiss mice resulted in a small increase in pulmonary adenomas; lymphatic leukemia was not increased.

➤*Pregnancy: Category C.* In mice and rats asparaginase has been shown to retard the weight gain of mothers and fetuses when given in doses of more than 1000 IU/kg (the recommended human dose). Resorptions, gross abnormalities and skeletal abnormalities were observed. The intravenous administration of 50 or 100 IU/kg (one-twentieth or one-tenth of the human dose) to pregnant rabbits on Day 8 and 9 of gestation resulted in dose dependent embryotoxicity and gross abnormalities. There are no adequate and well-controlled studies in pregnant women. Asparaginase should be used during pregnancy only if the potential benefit justifies the potential risk to the fetus.

➤*Lactation:* It is not known whether this drug is secreted in human milk. Because many drugs are secreted in human milk and because of the potential for serious adverse reactions in nursing infants from asparaginase, a decision should be made whether to discontinue nursing or to discontinue the drug, taking into account the importance of the drug to the mother.

➤*Children:* Asparaginase toxicity is reported to be greater in adults than in pediatric patients.

Precautions

➤*Accidental contact:* This drug may be a contact irritant and both powder and solution must be handled and administered with care. Inhalation of dust or vapors and contact with skin or mucous membranes, especially those of the eyes, must be avoided. In case of contact, wash with copious amounts of water for at least 15 minutes.

➤*Immunosuppression:* Asparaginase has been reported to have immunosuppressive activity in animal experiments. Accordingly, the possibility that use of the drug in man may predispose to infection should be considered.

➤*Lab test abnormalities:* The fall in circulating lymphoblasts often is quite marked; normal or below normal leukocyte counts are noted frequently within the first several days after initiating therapy. This may be accompanied by a marked rise in serum uric acid. The possible development of uric acid nephropathy should be borne in mind. Appropriate preventive measures should be taken, eg, allopurinol, increased fluid intake, alkalization of urine. As a guide to the effects of therapy, the patient's peripheral blood count and bone marrow should be monitored frequently.

Frequent serum amylase determinations should be obtained to detect early evidence of pancreatitis. If pancreatitis occurs, therapy should be stopped and not reinstituted.

Blood sugar should be monitored during therapy with asparaginase because hyperglycemia may occur.

Drug Interactions

➤*Antitumor agents:* Unfavorable interactions of asparaginase with some antitumor agents have been demonstrated. It is recommended therefore, that asparaginase be used in combination regimens only by physicians familiar with the benefits and risks of a given regimen. During the period of its inhibition of protein synthesis and cell replication, asparaginase may interfere with the action of drugs such as methotrexate which require cell replication for their lethal effect. Asparaginase may interfere with the enzymatic detoxification of other drugs, particularly in the liver.

ASPARAGINASE — INJECTION

Asparaginase Drug Interactions			
Precipitant drug	Object drug[a]		Description
Asparaginase	Methotrexate	⬇	Asparaginase may diminish or abolish methotrexate's effect on malignant cells; this effect persists as long as plasma asparagine levels are suppressed. Do not use methotrexate with, or following asparaginase, while asparagine levels are below normal.
Vincristine and prednisone	Asparaginase	⬆	IV administration of asparaginase concurrently with or immediately before a course of these drugs may be associated with increased toxicity.

[a] ⬆ = Object drug increased. ⬇ = Object drug decreased.

➤*Drug/Lab test interactions:* L-asparaginase has been reported to interfere with the interpretation of thyroid function tests by producing a rapid and marked reduction in serum concentrations of thyroxine-binding globulin within 2 days after the first dose. Serum concentrations of thyroxine-binding globulin returned to pretreatment values within 4 weeks of the last dose of L-asparaginase.

The intravenous administration of calcium gluconate alleviated or prevented the adverse effects.

Adverse Reactions

➤*Bone marrow suppression:* Rarely, transient bone marrow depression has been observed, as evidenced by a delay in return of hemoglobin or hematocrit levels to normal in patients undergoing hematologic remission of leukemia.

Marked leukopenia has been reported.

➤*CNS:* Some patients have shown central nervous system effects consisting of depression, somnolence, fatigue, coma, confusion, agitation, and hallucinations varying from mild to severe. Rarely, a Parkinson-like syndrome has occurred, with tremor and a progressive increase in muscular tone. These side effects usually have reversed spontaneously after treatment was stopped. Therapy with asparaginase is associated with an increase in blood ammonia during the conversion of asparagine to aspartic acid by the enzyme. No clear correlation exists between the degree of elevation of blood ammonia levels and the appearance of CNS changes. Chills, fever, nausea, vomiting, anorexia, abdominal cramps, weight loss, headache, and irritability may occur and usually are mild.

➤*Hematologic:* In addition to hypofibrinogenemia, depression of various other clotting factors has been reported. Most marked has been a decrease in plasma levels of factors V and VIII with a variable decrease in factors VII and IX. A decrease in circulating platelets has occurred in low incidence which, together with the increased levels of fibrin degradation products in the serum, may indicate development of a consumption coagulopathy. Bleeding has been a problem in only a minority of patients with demonstrable coagulopathy. However, intracranial hemorrhage and fatal bleeding associated with low fibrinogen levels have been reported. Increased fibrinolytic activity, apparently compensatory in nature, also has occurred.

➤*Hepatic:* A variety of liver function abnormalities have been reported, including elevations of AST, ALT, alkaline phosphatase, bilirubin (direct and indirect), and depression of serum albumin, cholesterol (total and esters), and plasma fibrinogen. Increases and decreases of total lipids have occurred. Marked hypoalbuminemia associated with peripheral edema has been reported. However, these abnormalities usually are reversible on discontinuance of therapy and some reversal may occur during the course of therapy. Fatty changes in the liver have been documented by biopsy. Malabsorption syndrome has been reported.

➤*Hyperglycemia:* Hyperglycemia with glucosuria and polyuria has been reported in low incidence. Serum and urine acetone usually have been absent or negligible in these patients; this syndrome thus resembles hyperosmolar, nonketotic, hyperglycemia induced by a variety of other agents. This complication usually responds to discontinuance of asparaginase, judicious use of intravenous fluid, and insulin, but may be fatal on occasion.

➤*Hypersensitivity:* Allergic reactions, including skin rashes, urticaria, arthralgia, respiratory distress, and acute anaphylaxis have been reported. (See Warnings.) Acute reactions have occurred in the absence of a positive skin test and during continued maintenance of therapeutic serum levels of asparaginase.

In pediatric patients with advanced leukemia, a lower incidence of anaphylaxis has been reported with intramuscular administration, although there was a higher incidence of milder hypersensitivity reactions than with intravenous administration.

Fatal hyperthermia has been reported.

➤*Pancreatitis:* Pancreatitis, sometimes fulminant and fatal, has occurred during or following therapy with asparaginase.

➤*Renal:* Azotemia, usually pre-renal, occurs frequently. Acute renal shut down and fatal renal insufficiency have been reported during treatment. Proteinuria has occurred infrequently.

Overdosage

The acute intravenous LD_{50} of asparagine for mice was about 500,000 IU/kg and for rabbits about 22,000 IU/kg.

PEGASPARGASE (PEG-L-asparaginase)

Rx	**Oncaspar** (Enzon)	**Injection:** 750 IU/ml in a phosphate buffered saline solution	Preservative free. In single-use vials.

PEGASPARGASE (PEG-L-ASPARAGINASE) — INJECTION

Indications

➤*Acute lymphoblastic leukemia:* For patients with acute lymphoblastic leukemia who require L-asparaginase in their treatment regimen, but have developed hypersensitivity to the native forms of L-asparaginase.

Pegaspargase is generally used in combination with other chemotherapeutic agents, such as vincristine, methotrexate, cytarabine, daunorubicin, and doxorubicin. Use of pegaspargase as a single agent should only be undertaken when multi-agent chemotherapy is judged to be inappropriate for the patient.

Administration and Dosage

➤*Approved by the FDA:* February 1, 1994.

➤*Recommended dose:* As a component of selected multiple agent regimens, the recommended dose of pegaspargase is 2500 IU/m^2 every 14 days by the intramuscular route of administration.

➤*Children:* The safety and effectiveness of pegaspargase have been established in patients with known previous hypersensitivity to L-asparaginase whose ages ranged from 1 to 21 years old. The recommended dose of pegaspargase for children with a body surface area greater than or equal to 0.6 m^2 is 2500 IU/m^2 administered every 14 days. The recommended dose of pegaspargase for children with a body surface area less than 0.6 m^2 is 82.5 IU/kg administered every 14 days.

➤*Administration:* When administering pegaspargase intramuscularly, the volume at a single injection site should be limited to 2 mL. If the volume to be administered is greater than 2 mL, multiple injection sites should be used.

➤*Hypersensitivity reactions:* See Warnings for more information.

➤*Monotherapy:* Use of pegaspargase as the sole induction agent should be undertaken only in an unusual situation when a combined regimen, which uses other chemotherapeutic agents such as vincristine, methotrexate, cytarabine, daunorubicin, or doxorubicin, is inappropriate because of toxicity or other specific patient-related factors, or in patients refractory to other therapy. When pegaspargase is to be used as the sole induction agent, the recommended dosage regimen is also 2500 IU/m^2 every 14 days.

➤*Maintenance therapy:* When a remission is obtained, appropriate maintenance therapy may be instituted. Pegaspargase may be used as part of a maintenance regimen.

➤*Storage / Stability:* Avoid excessive agitation. Do not shake. Keep refrigerated at 2° to 8°C (36° to 46°F). Do not use if stored at room temperature for more than 48 hours. Do not freeze. Do not use product if it is known to have been frozen. Freezing destroys activity, which cannot be detected visually.

Actions

➤*Pharmacology:* Leukemic cells are unable to synthesize asparagine due to a lack of asparagine synthetase and are dependent on an exogenous source of asparagine for survival. Rapid depletion of asparagine which results from treatment with the enzyme L-asparaginase, kills the leukemic cells. Normal cells, however, are less affected by the rapid depletion due to their ability to synthesize asparagine. This is an approach to therapy based on a specific metabolic defect in some leukemic cells which do not produce asparagine synthetase.

Contraindications

History of pancreatitis; significant hemorrhagic events associated with prior L-asparaginase therapy; previous serious allergic reactions, such as generalized urticaria, bronchospasm, laryngeal edema, hypotension, or other unacceptable adverse reactions to pegaspargase.

Warnings

➤*Hypersensitivity reactions:* Especially in patients with known hypersensitivity to the other forms of L-asparaginase, hypersensitivity reactions to pegaspargase, including life-threatening anaphylaxis, may occur during therapy. As a routine precaution, patients should be kept under observation for 1 hour with resuscitation equipment and other agents necessary to treat anaphylaxis (epinephrine, oxygen, intravenous steroids) available.

➤*Pregnancy:* *Category C.* Animal reproduction studies have not been conducted with pegaspargase. It is also not known whether pegaspargase can cause fetal harm when administered to a pregnant woman or can affect reproduction capacity. Pegaspargase should be given to a pregnant woman only if clearly needed.

PEGASPARGASE (PEG-L-ASPARAGINASE) — INJECTION

➤*Lactation:* It is not known whether pegaspargase is excreted in human milk. Because many drugs are excreted in human milk and because of the potential for serious adverse reactions due to pegaspargase in nursing infants, a decision should be made whether to discontinue nursing or discontinue the drug, taking into account the importance of the drug to the mother.

Precautions

➤*Monitoring:* A fall in circulating lymphoblasts is often noted after initiating therapy. This may be accompanied by a marked rise in serum uric acid. As a guide to the effects of therapy, the patient's peripheral blood count and bone marrow should be monitored.

Frequent serum amylase determinations should be obtained to detect early evidence of pancreatitis. Pegaspargase is contraindicated in patients with pancreatitis or a history of pancreatitis. Blood sugar should be monitored during therapy with pegaspargase because hyperglycemia may occur. When using pegaspargase in conjunction with hepatotoxic chemotherapy, patients should be monitored for liver dysfunction.

This drug may be a contact irritant, and the solution must be handled and administered with care. Gloves are recommended. Inhalation of vapors and contact with skin or mucous membranes, especially those of the eyes, must be avoided. In case of contact, wash with copious amounts of water for at least 15 minutes. Anaphylactic reactions require the immediate use of epinephrine, oxygen, intravenous steroids, and antihistamines. Patients taking pegaspargase are at higher than usual risk for bleeding problems, especially with simultaneous use of other drugs that have anticoagulant properties, such as aspirin, nonsteroidal anti-inflammatories coumadin, heparin, and dipyridamole. Pegaspargase may have immunosuppressive activity. Therefore, it is possible that use of the drug in patients may predispose the patient to infection. Severe hepatic and central nervous system toxicity following multi-agent chemotherapy that includes pegaspargase may occur. Caution appears warranted when treating patients with pegaspargase given in combination with hepatotoxic agents, particularly when liver dysfunction is present.

Patients undergoing pegaspargase therapy must be carefully monitored and the therapeutic regimen adjusted according to response and toxicity. Physicians using a given treatment regimen incorporating pegaspargase should be thoroughly familiar with its benefits and risks.

➤*Lab test abnormalities:* Pegaspargase may affect a number of plasma proteins; therefore, monitoring of fibrinogen, PT, and PTT may be indicated.

Drug Interactions

➤*Concurrent drug therapy:* Unfavorable interactions of L-asparaginase with some antitumor agents have been demonstrated. It is recommended, therefore, that pegaspargase be used in combination regimens only by physicians familiar with the benefits and risks of a given regimen. Depletion of serum proteins by pegaspargase may increase the toxicity of other drugs which are protein bound. Additionally, during the period of its inhibition of protein synthesis and cell replication, pegaspargase may interfere with the action of drugs such as methotrexate, which require cell replication for their lethal effects. Pegaspargase may interfere with the enzymatic detoxification of other drugs, particularly in the liver. Physicians using a given treatment regimen should be thoroughly familiar with its benefits and risks.

➤*Anticoagulation agents:* Imbalances in coagulation factors have been noted with the use of pegaspargase predisposing to bleeding or thrombosis. Caution should be used when administering any concurrent anticoagulant therapy, such as coumadin, heparin, dipyridamole, aspirin, or nonsteroidal anti-inflammatories.

Adverse Reactions

Excluding hypersensitivity reactions, the most frequently occurring known L-asparaginase related toxicities and adverse experiences reported for the 174 patients in clinical studies were chemical hepatotoxicities and coagulopathies, the majority of which did not result in any significant clinical events. The incidence of significant clinical events included clinical pancreatitis (1%), hyperglycemia requiring insulin therapy (3%), and thrombosis (4%).

➤*Adverse reactions reported most frequently (greater than 5%):* Allergic reactions (which may have included rash, erythema, edema, pain, fever, chills, urticaria, dyspnea, or bronchospasm), SGPT increase, nausea or vomiting, fever, and malaise.

➤*Adverse reactions reported occasionally (greater than 1% but less than 5%):* Anaphylactic reactions, dyspnea, injection site hypersensitivity, lip edema, rash, urticaria, abdominal pain, chills, pain in the extremities, hypotension, tachycardia, thrombosis, anorexia, diarrhea, jaundice, abnormal liver function test, decreased anticoagulant effect, disseminated intravascular coagulation, decreased fibrinogen, hemolytic anemia, leukopenia, pancytopenia, thrombocytopenia, increased thromboplastin, injection site pain, injection site reaction, bilirubinemia, hyperglycemia, hyperuricemia, hypoglycemia, hypoproteinemia, peripheral edema, increased SGOT, arthralgia, myalgia, convulsion, headache, night sweats, and paresthesia.

➤*Adverse reactions reported rarely (less than 1%):* Bronchospasm, petechial rash, face edema, lesional edema, sepsis, septic shock, chest pain, endocarditis, hypertension, constipation, flatulence, gastrointestinal pain, hepatomegaly, increased appetite, liver fatty deposits, coagulation disorder, increased coagulation time, decreased platelet count, purpura, increased amylase, edema, excessive thirst, hyperammonemia, hyponatremia, weight loss, bone pain, joint disorder, confusion, dizziness, emotional lability, somnolence, increased cough, epistaxis, upper respiratory tract infection, erythema simplex, pruritus, hematuria, increased urinary frequency, and abnormal kidney function.

➤*The following pegaspargase related adverse reactions have been observed in patients with hematologic malignancies:*

Cardiovascular – Chest pain, subacute bacterial endocarditis, hypertension, severe hypotension, and tachycardia have occurred.

CNS – Status epilepticus and temporal lobe seizures, somnolence, coma, malaise, mental status changes, dizziness, emotional lability, headache, lip numbness, finger paresthesia, mood changes, night sweats, and a Parkinson-like syndrome have occurred. Mild to severe confusion, disorientation, and paresthesia have also occurred. These side effects usually have reversed spontaneously after treatment was stopped.

Dermatologic – Itching, alopecia, fever blister, purpura, hand whiteness and fungal changes, nail whiteness and ridging, erythema simplex, jaundice, and petechial rash have occurred.

Endocrine – Pancreatitis, sometimes fulminant and fatal, has occurred. Increased serum amylase and lipase have also occurred.

GI – Anorexia, constipation, decreased appetite, diarrhea, indigestion, flatulence, gas, gastrointestinal pain, mucositis, hepatomegaly, elevated gamma-glutamyltranspeptidase, increased appetite, mouth tenderness, severe colitis, and nausea or vomiting have been observed.

Hematologic – Hypofibrinogenemia, prolonged prothrombin times, prolonged partial thromboplastin times, and decreased antithrombin III have been observed. Superficial and deep venous thrombosis, sagittal sinus thrombosis, venous catheter thrombosis, and atrial thrombosis have occurred. Leukopenia, agranulocytosis, pancytopenia, thrombocytopenia, disseminated intravascular coagulation, severe hemolytic anemia, and anemia have been observed. Clinical hemorrhage, which may be fatal; easy bruisability, and ecchymosis have also been observed.

Hepatic – A variety of liver function abnormalities have been observed, including elevations of SGOT, SGPT, and bilirubin (direct and indirect). Jaundice, ascites, and hypoalbuminemia, which may be associated with peripheral edema, have been observed. These abnormalities usually are reversible on discontinuance of therapy, and some reversal may occur during the course of therapy. Fatty changes in the liver and liver failure have occurred.

Hypersensitivity – A variety of hypersensitivity reactions have occurred. These reactions may be acute or delayed, and include acute anaphylaxis, bronchospasm, dyspnea, urticaria, arthralgia, erythema, induration, edema, pain, tenderness, hives, swelling, lip edema, chills, fever, and skin rashes. Pegaspargase is also contraindicated in patients who have had previous serious allergic reactions, such as generalized urticaria, bronchospasm, laryngeal edema, hypotension, or other unacceptable adverse reactions to pegaspargase. As a routine precaution, patients should be kept under observation for 1 hour with resuscitation equipment and other agents necessary to treat anaphylaxis (epinephrine, oxygen, intravenous steroids) available.

Metabolic – Mild to severe hyperglycemia has been observed in low incidence, and usually responds to discontinuation of pegaspargase and the judicious use of intravenous fluid and insulin. Hypoglycemia, increased thirst and hyponatremia, uric acid nephropathy, hyperuricemia, hypoproteinemia, and peripheral edema have also been observed. Hypoalbuminemia, proteinuria, weight loss, and metabolic acidosis have occurred. Therapy with pegaspargase is associated with an increase in blood ammonia during the conversion of L-asparagine to aspartic acid by the enzyme.

Musculoskeletal – Diffuse and local musculoskeletal pain, arthralgia, joint stiffness, and cramps have occurred.

Renal – Increased BUN, increased creatinine, urinary frequency, hematuria due to thrombopenia, severe hemorrhagic cystitis, renal dysfunction, and renal failure have been observed.

Respiratory – Cough, epistaxis, severe bronchospasm, and upper respiratory tract infection have been observed.

Miscellaneous – Localized edema, injection site reactions (including pain, swelling, or redness), malaise, infection, sepsis, fatigue, and septic shock may occur.

Overdosage

Three patients received 10,000 IU/m^2 of pegaspargase as an intravenous infusion. One patient experienced a slight increase in liver enzymes. A second patient developed a rash 10 minutes after the start of the infusion, which was controlled with the administration of an antihistamine and by slowing down the infusion rate. A third patient did not experience any adverse reactions.

Patient Information

Patients should be informed of the possibility of hypersensitivity reactions, including immediate anaphylaxis, to pegaspargase Patients taking pegaspargase are at higher than usual risk for bleeding problems. Patients should be instructed that the simultaneous use of pegaspargase with other drugs that may increase the risk of bleeding should be avoided aspirin, NSAIDS, coumadin, heparin, and dipyridamole. Pegaspargase may affect the ability of the liver to function normally in some patients. Therapy with pegaspargase may increase the toxicity of other medications. Depletion of serum proteins by pegaspargase may increase the toxicity of other drugs which are protein bound. Additionally, during the period of its inhibition of protein synthesis and cell replication, pegaspargase may interfere with the action of drugs such as methotrexate, which require cell replication for their lethal effects. Pegaspargase may interfere with the enzymatic detoxification of other drugs, particularly in the liver. Pegaspargase may have immunosuppressive activity. Therefore, it is possible that use of the drug in patients may predispose the patient to infection. Patients should notify their physicians of any adverse reactions that occur.

CHROMIC PHOSPHATE P 32

Rx	**Phosphocol P 32** (Mallinckrodt)	**Suspension**: 15 mCi with a concentration of up to 5 mCi/ml and specific activity of up to 5 mCi/mg at time of standardization.	In 10 ml vials.[a]

[a] With 2% benzyl alcohol, NaCl and sodium acetate.

CHROMIC PHOSPHATE P 32 — INTRAPERITONEAL/INTRAPLEURAL

Indications

➤*Peritoneal/Pleural effusions caused by metastatic cancer:* For the treatment of peritoneal or pleural effusions caused by metastatic disease, and may be injected interstitially for the treatment of cancer.

Administration and Dosage

The suggested dose range employed in the average patient (70 kg) is as follows:

➤*Intraperitoneal instillation:* 370 to 740 mBq (10 to 20 mCi).

➤*Intrapleural instillation:* 222 to 444 mBq (6 to 12 mCi).

Doses for interstitial use should be based on estimated gram weight of tumor, about 3.7 to 18.5 MBq/g (0.1 to 0.5 mCi/g).

The patient dose should be measured by a suitable radioactivity calibration system immediately prior to administration.

➤*Physical characteristics:* Phosphorus P 32 decays by beta emission, with a physical half-life of 14.3 days. The mean energy of the beta particle is 695 keV (see the following information):

Principal radiation emission data – Principal radiation emission data for chromic phosphate P 32 is as follows: Radiation type, Beta-1; mean percent disintegration, 100%; and mean energy (keV), 694.9.

The range of the phosphorus P 32 beta particle, which has a maximum energy of 1.71 MeV, is 2.8 mm of aluminum.

To correct for physical decay of this radionuclide, the percentages that remain at selected time intervals before and after the day of calibration are shown in the following information.

Physical decay chart; phosphorus P 32, half-life 14.3 days – For phosphorus P 32, with a half-life of 14.3 days, the fraction remaining is as follows: Day −15, 2.07; day −10, 1.62; day −5, 1.28; day −2, 1.1; day −1, 1.05; day 0 (calibration day), 1; day 1, 0.953.

Day 2, 0.908; day 5, 0.785; day 10, 0.616; day 15, 0.483; day 20, 0.379; day 25, 0.297; day 30, 0.233; day 35, 0.183; day 40, 0.144; day 45, 0.113; day 50, 0.089; day 55, 0.07; day 60, 0.055; and day 65, 0.043.

➤*Radiation dosimetry:* The effective half-life of phosphorus P 32 is considered to be equal to its physical half-life, with a residence time of 495 hours.

The radiation dose from a uniformly distributed concentration of 37 kilobecquerels (1 microcurie) per gram within a 16 g prostate is estimated to be equivalent to about 7.3 grays (730 rads). The paragraph below shows the estimated radiation doses to the prostate and the pleural or peritoneal surfaces of an average patient (70 kg) from a dose of 740 megabecquerels (20 millicuries) of phosphorus P 32.

In comparison to the distribution in the prostate, the distribution of phosphorus P 32 on the pleural and peritoneal surfaces is nonuniform, with great extremes in local doses. To obtain an estimate of the average dose, the surface area of the pleural and peritoneal cavities can be assumed to amount to 4000 and 5000 cm^2, respectively. The estimated radiation doses to an average patient (70 kg) with 90% retention of a dose of 740 megabecquerels (20 millicuries) of phosphorus P 32 distributed uniformly over these areas are shown below. The decreases of the averaged radiation doses at various tissue depths away from the surfaces of the pleural and peritoneal cavities are also tabulated.

Estimated radiation doses – Estimated radiation doses to pleural, peritoneal, and prostate surfaces for an average (70 kg) patient from a 740 mBq (20 mCi) dose of phosphorus P 32 are as follows:

With depth in tissue of 0.004 cm and dose rate (for surface deposition of 37 kBq (1 mcCi)/cm^2) of 10.2 rads/hr (102 mGy/hr), 23,000 rads (230 grays) to pleural surface, 18,000 rads (180 grays) to peritoneal surface, and 910,000 rads (9100 grays) to prostate surface.

With depth in tissue of 0.008 cm and dose rate of 8.58 rads/hr (85.8 mGy/hr), 19,000 rads (190 grays) to pleural surface and 15,000 rads (150 grays) to peritoneal surface.

With depth in tissue of 0.012 cm and dose rate of 7.61 rads/hr (76.1 mGy/hr), 17,000 rads (170 grays) to pleural surface and 14,000 rads (140 grays) to peritoneal surface.

With depth in tissue of 0.016 cm and dose rate of 6.91 rads/hr (69.1 mGy/hr), 15,000 rads (150 grays) to pleural surface and 12,000 rads (120 grays) to peritoneal surface.

With depth in tissue of 0.02 cm and dose rate of 6.36 rads/hr (63.6 mGy/hr), 14,000 rads (140 grays) to pleural surface and 11,000 rads (110 grays) to peritoneal surface.

With depth in tissue of 0.1 cm and dose rate of 2.41 rads/hr (24.1 mGy/hr), 5400 rads (54 grays) to pleural surface and 4300 rads (43 grays) to peritoneal surface.

With depth in tissue of 0.2 cm and dose rate of 0.94 rads/hr (9.4 mGy/hr), 2100 rads (21 grays) to pleural surface and 1700 rads (17 grays) to peritoneal surface.

➤*Storage/Stability:* Store at controlled room temperature 20° to 25°C (68° to 77°F).

Actions

➤*Pharmacology:* Local irradiation by beta emission.

Contraindications

Chromic phosphate P 32 therapy should not be used in the presence of ulcerative tumors.

Administration should not be made in exposed cavities or where there is evidence of loculation, unless the extent of loculation is determined.

Warnings

Chromic phosphate P 32 is not for intravascular use.

➤*Pregnancy:* This radiopharmaceutical should not be administered to patients who are pregnant, unless the therapeutic benefits outweigh the potential hazards.

➤*Lactation:* This radiopharmaceutical should not be administered to patients who are experiencing lactation, unless the therapeutic benefits outweigh the potential hazards.

➤*Children:* Safety and efficacy in pediatric patients have not been established.

Precautions

➤*Intracavity installation:* Careful intracavitary instillation is required to avoid placing the dose of chromic phosphate P 32 into intrapleural or intraperitoneal loculations, bowel lumen or into the body wall. Intestinal fibrosis or necrosis and chronic fibrosis of the body wall have been reported to result from unrecognized misplacement of the therapeutic agent.

➤*Large tumor masses:* The presence of large tumor masses indicates the need for other forms of treatment. However, when other forms of treatment fail to control the effusion, chromic phosphate P 32 may be useful. In bloody effusion, treatment may be less effective.

Adverse Reactions

Untoward effects may be associated with use of chromic phosphate P 32. These include transitory radiation sickness, bone marrow depression, pleuritis, peritonitis, nausea and abdominal cramping. Radiation damage may occur if accidentally injected interstitially or into a loculation.

SODIUM IODIDE I 131

Rx	**Iodotope** (Bracco Diagnostics)	**Capsules**: Radioactivity ranging from 1 to 50 mCi per capsule at time of calibration	Blue/bluff
		Oral solution: Radioactivity concentration of 7.05 mCi/ml at time of calibration	1 mg/ml EDTA. In vials containing ≈ 7, 14, 28, 70 or 106 mCi at time of calibration.
Rx	**Sodium Iodide I 131** (Mallinckrodt)	**Capsules**: Radioactivity ranging from 0.75 to 100 mCi per capsule.	Various strengths.
		Oral solution: Radioactivity ranging from 3.5 to 150 mCi/vial.	0.1% sodium bisulfite and 0.2% EDTA. In vials.

SODIUM IODIDE I 131 — ORAL

Sodium Iodide I 131 is also used for treatment of hyperthyroidism. Refer to the Antithyroid Agents group monograph in the Endocrine/Metabolic chapter.

Indications

➤*Diagnostic capsules:* For use in performance of the radioactive iodide (RAI) uptake test to evaluate thyroid function. Diagnostic doses may also be employed in localizing metastases associated with thyroid malignancies.

➤*Therapeutic capsules and oral solution:* For the treatment of hyperthyroidism and selected cases of carcinoma of the thyroid. Palliative effects may be seen in patients with papillary or follicular carcinoma of the thyroid. Stimulation of radioiodide uptake may be achieved by the administration of thyrotropin. (Radioiodide will not be taken up by giant cell and spindle cell carcinoma of the thyroid nor by amyloid solid carcinomas.)

SODIUM IODIDE I 131 — ORAL

Administration and Dosage

➤*Diagnostic capsules:* The suggested oral dosage ranges employed in the average patient (70 kg) for diagnostic procedures for thyroid function are as follows:

Thyroid uptake – 0.185 to 0.555 megabecquerels (5 to 15 microcuries).

Scintiscanning – 1.85 to 3.7 megabecquerels (50 to 100 microcuries).

Localization of extra-thyroidal metastases – 37 megabecquerels (1000 microcuries).

Waterproof gloves should be used during the entire handling and administration procedure.

The patient dose should be measured by a suitable radioactivity calibration system immediately prior to administration.

Radiation dosimetry – The estimated absorbed radiation doses to an average (70 kg) euthyroid (normal functioning thyroid) patient from an oral dose of 3.7 megabecquerels (100 microcuries) of iodine I 131 are shown in the following table:

Absorbed Radiation Doses for 3.7 megabecquerels (100 microcuries)

	Thyroid uptake					
	5%		15%		25%	
Tissue	mGy	rads	mGy	rads	mGy	rads
Thyroid	260	26	800	80	1300	130
Stomach wall	1.7	0.17	1.6	0.16	1.4	0.14
Red marrow	0.14	0.014	.20	0.02	0.26	0.026
Liver	0.2	0.02	0.35	0.035	0.48	0.048
Testes	0.08	0.008	0.09	0.009	0.09	0.009
Ovaries	0.14	0.014	0.14	0.014	0.14	0.014
Total body	0.24	0.024	0.47	0.047	0.71	0.071

➤*Therapeutic capsules and oral solution:* Antithyroid therapy of a severely hyperthyroid patient is usually discontinued 3 to 4 days before administration of radioiodide.

For hyperthyroidism, the usual dose range is 148 to 370 megabecquerels (4 to 10 millicuries). Toxic nodular goiter and other special situations will require the use of larger doses.

For thyroid carcinoma, 1850 megabecquerels (50 millicuries) is the usual dose for ablation of normal thyroid tissue, and 3700 to 5550 megabecquerels (100 to 150 millicuries) is the usual subsequent therapeutic dose.

Waterproof gloves should be used during the entire handling and administration procedure. Maintain adequate shielding during the life of the product.

The patient dose should be measured by a suitable radioactivity calibration system immediately prior to administration.

Radiation dosimetry – The estimated absorbed radiation doses to an average (70 kg) euthyroid (normal functioning thyroid) patient from an oral dose of iodine-131 in both milligrays per megabecquerel and rads per millicurie are shown in the following table:

Absorbed Radiation Doses

	Thyroid uptake					
	5%		15%		25%	
Tissue	mGy/MBq	rads/mCi	mGy/MBq	rads/mCi	mGy/MBq	rads/mCI
Thyroid	70.3	260	216.2	800	351.4	1300
Stomach wall	0.459	1.7	0.432	1.6	0.378	1.4
Red marrow	0.038	0.14	0.054	0.2	0.07	0.26
Liver	0.054	0.2	0.095	0.35	0.13	0.48
Testes	0.023	0.084	0.023	0.085	0.024	0.088
Ovaries	0.038	0.14	0.038	0.14	0.038	0.14
Total body	0.065	0.24	0.127	0.47	0.192	0.71

➤*Storage/Stability:* Sodium iodide I 131 diagnostic capsules, therapeutic capsules and therapeutic oral solution should be stored at controlled room temperature at 20° to 25°C (68° to 77°F).

Storage and disposal of sodium iodide I 131 diagnostic capsules, therapeutic capsules and therapeutic oral solution should be controlled in a manner that is in compliance with the appropriate regulations of the government agency authorized to license the use of this radionuclide.

The US Nuclear Regulatory Commission has approved distribution of this radiopharmaceutical to persons licensed to use byproduct material listed in Section 35.100, and to persons who hold an equivalent license by an agreement state.

Actions

➤*Pharmacokinetics:*

Absorption/Distribution – Sodium iodide is readily absorbed from the GI tract. Following absorption, the iodide is distributed primarily within the extracellular fluid of the body.

Sodium iodide I 131 therapeutic capsules and oral solution: About 90% of local irradiation is the result of beta radiation and 10% is the result of gamma radiation.

Physical characteristics (diagnostic use and therapeutic use): Iodine I-131 decays by beta and associated gamma emissions with a physical half-life of 8.04 days. The principle beta emissions and gamma photons are listed in the following table:

Principal Radiation Emission Data

Radiation	Mean % per disintegration	Energy (keV)
Beta-1	2.12	69.4 Avg
Beta-3	7.36	96.6 Avg
Beta-4	89.3	191.6 Avg
Gamma-7	6.05	284.3
Gamma-14	81.2	364.5
Gamma-17	7.26	637

External radiation (diagnostic use and therapeutic use): The specific gamma ray constant for iodine I-131 is 2.27 R/hr-mCi at 1 cm. The first half-value thickness of lead (Pb) for iodine I-131 is 0.24 cm. A range of values for the relative attenuation of the radiation emitted by this radionuclide that results from interposition of various thicknesses of Pb is shown in the information below. For example, the use of 4.6 cm of Pb will decrease the external radiation exposure by a factor of about 1000.

Radiation Attenuation by Lead Shielding

Shield thickness (Pb), cm	Coefficient of attenuation
0.24	0.5
0.95	10^{-1}
2.6	10^{-2}
4.6	10^{-3}
6.5	10^{-4}

To correct for physical decay of this radionuclide, the fractions that remain at selected time intervals after the date of calibration are shown in the following table:

Physical Decay Chart, Iodine I 131, Half-life 8.04 days

Days	Fraction remaining	Days	Fraction remaining
0*	1	16	0.252
1	0.917	17	0.231
2	0.842	18	0.212
3	0.772	19	0.194
4	0.708	20	0.178
5	0.65	21	0.164
6	0.596	22	0.15
7	0.547	23	0.138
8	0.502	24	0.126
9	0.46	25	0.116
10	0.422	26	0.106
11	0.387	27	0.098
12	0.355	28	0.089
13	0.326	29	0.082
14	0.299	30	0.075
15	0.274		

* Calibration day.

Metabolism/Excretion – It is concentrated and organified by the thyroid, and trapped but not organified by the stomach and salivary glands. It is also promptly excreted by the kidneys.

Contraindications

Vomiting and diarrhea represent contraindications to the use of radioiodide.

Therapeutic doses of sodium iodide I 131 may cause fetal harm when administered to a pregnant woman. Therapeutic doses of sodium iodide I 131 are contraindicated in women who are or may become pregnant. If this drug is used during pregnancy, or if the patient becomes pregnant while taking this drug, the patient should be apprised of the potential hazards to the fetus.

Warnings

➤*Pregnancy: Category C* (diagnostic capsules) and *Category X* (therapeutic capsules and oral solution).

Diagnostic capsules – Animal reproduction studies have not been conducted with sodium iodide I 131 diagnostic capsules. It is also not known whether sodium iodide I 131 diagnostic capsules can cause fetal harm when administered to a pregnant woman or can affect reproduction capacity. Sodium iodide I 131 diagnostic capsules should be given to a pregnant woman only if clearly needed.

SODIUM IODIDE I 131 — ORAL

Childbearing women – Ideally, examinations using radiopharmaceutical drug products (especially those elective in nature) of women of childbearing capability should be performed during the first 10 days following the onset of menses.

Therapeutic capsules and oral solution – See Contraindications for more information.

Radioiodide therapy in women of childbearing capability should only be performed when appropriate contraceptive measures have been taken or when pregnancy testing is negative.

➤*Lactation:* Radioiodine is excreted in human milk during lactation. Therefore, formula feedings should be substituted for breast milk.

➤*Children:*

Diagnostic capsules – Safety and efficacy in pediatric patients have not been established.

Therapeutic capsules and oral solution – Sodium iodide I 131 is not usually used for treatment of hyperthyroidism in patients under 30 years of age.

Precautions

➤*Radiographic contrast media:* The uptake of radioiodide will be affected by recent intake of stable iodine in any form, or by the use of thyroid, antithyroid and certain other drugs. Accordingly, the patient should be questioned carefully regarding previous medication and procedures involving radiographic contrast media.

➤*Expiration date:* The expiration date is not later than 1 month after the calibration date. The calibration date and the expiration date are stated on the container label.

➤*Sulfite sensitivity:*

Therapeutic oral solution – Some of these products may contain sodium bisulfite, a sulfite that may cause allergic-type reactions, including anaphylactic symptoms and life-threatening or less severe asthmatic episodes in certain susceptible people. The overall prevalence of sulfite sensitivity in the general population is unknown and probably low. Sulfite sensitivity is seen more frequently in asthmatic than in nonasthmatic people.

Adverse Reactions

Diagnostic capsules – Although rare, reactions associated with the administration of iodine-containing radiopharmaceuticals for diagnostic use include, in decreasing order of frequency, nausea, vomiting, chest pain, tachycardia, itching skin, rash and hives.

➤*Therapeutic capsules and oral solution:* Although rare, reactions have been reported following the administration of iodine-containing radiopharmaceuticals, including, in decreasing order of frequency, nausea, vomiting, chest pain, tachycardia, itching skin, rash, and hives. Depression of the hematopoietic system may occur when large doses are employed. Such potential side effects include radiation sickness, increase in clinical symptoms, bone marrow depression, acute leukemia, anemia, chromosomal abnormalities, acute thyroid crisis, blood dyscrasia, leukopenia, thrombocytopenia, and death.

SODIUM PHOSPHATE P 32

Rx	**Sodium Phosphate P 32** (Mallinckrodt)	**Injection:** 0.67 mCi/ml	5 mCi per vial.

SODIUM PHOSPHATE P 32 — INJECTION

Indications

➤*Polycythemia vera/Chronic myelocytic leukemia/Chronic lymphocytic leukemia:* For the treatment of polycythemia vera, and it is effective for the treatment of chronic myelocytic leukemia and chronic lymphocytic leukemia. Sodium phosphate P 32 is also used in palliative treatment of selected patients with multiple areas of skeletal metastases.

Administration and Dosage

The patient dose should be measured by a suitable radioactivity calibration system immediately prior to administration.

Oral administration of high-specific-activity sodium phosphate P 32 in the fasting state may equal intravenous administration.

➤*Handling:* Waterproof gloves should be used during the entire handling and administration procedure.

Maintain adequate shielding during the life of the product and use a sterile, shielded syringe for withdrawing and injecting the drug.

➤*Polycythemia vera:* For polycythemia vera, intravenous dosages from 37 to 296 MBq (1 to 8 mCi) are given depending upon the stage of disease and size of the patient. Repeat doses must be adjusted to individual needs.

➤*Chronic leukemia:* For chronic leukemia, the individual dose is 222 to 555 MBq (6 to 15 mCi), usually administered with concomitant hormone manipulation.

➤*Storage/Stability:* Store at controlled room temperature 20° to 25°C (68° to 77°F).

Actions

➤*Pharmacology:* Phosphorus is necessary to metabolic and proliferative activity of cells. Radioactive phosphorus concentrates to a very high degree in rapidly proliferating tissue.

➤*Pharmacokinetics:*

External radiation – The range of the phosphorus P 32 beta particle, which has a maximum energy of 1.71 MeV, is 2.8 mm of aluminum.

To correct for physical decay of this radionuclide, the fractions remaining at selected time intervals before and after the day of calibration are shown as follows.

With a half-life of 14.3 days, the fraction remaining following the specified number of days after the day of calibration is: 1 day, 0.953; 2 days, 0.908; 5 days, 0.785; 10 days, 0.616; 15 days, 0.483; 20 days, 0.379; 25 days, 0.297; 30 days, 0.233; 35 days, 0.183; 40 days, 0.144; 45 days, 0.113; 50 days, 0.089; 55 days, 0.07; 60 days, 0.055.

Radiation dosimetry – The estimated absorbed radiation doses to an average patient (70 kg) following intravenous administration of 555 megabequerels (15 millicuries) of sodium phosphate P 32 are shown as follows. The skeleton will receive 9.45 grays (945 rads), the liver 0.93 grays (93 rads); the spleen 1.10 grays (110 rads), the brain 0.45 grays (45 rads); the testes 0.15 grays (15 rads), the ovaries 0.12 grays (12 rads), and the total body 1.50 grays (150 rads).

Contraindications

Sodium phosphate P 32 should not be used as a part of sequential treatment with a chemotherapeutic agent.

In polycythemia vera, sodium phosphate P 32 should not be administered when the leukocyte count is below $5000/mm^3$, or a platelet count is below $150{,}000/mm^3$.

In chronic myelocytic leukemia, sodium phosphate P 32 should not be administered when the leukocyte count is below $20{,}000/mm^3$.

For treatment of bone metastases it is usually not administered when the leukocyte count is below $5000/mm^3$, and platelet count is below $100{,}000/mm^3$.

Warnings

➤*Intracavitary use:* This radiopharmaceutical should not be administered for intracavitary use.

➤*Hemopoietic system:* Overdose of sodium phosphate P 32 may produce serious effects on the hemopoietic system. The blood and bone marrow should be carefully monitored at regular intervals.

➤*Retinoblastomas:* Sodium phosphate P 32 ordinarily does not localize in retinoblastomas.

➤*Pregnancy: Category C.* Animal reproduction studies have not been conducted with sodium phosphate P 32. It is also not known whether sodium phosphate P 32 can cause fetal harm when administered to a pregnant woman or can affect reproductive capacity. Sodium phosphate P 32 should be given to a pregnant woman only if clearly needed.

Ideally, examinations using radiopharmaceuticals, especially those elective in nature, of a woman of childbearing capability should be performed during the first few (approximately 10) days following the onset of menses.

➤*Lactation:* It is not known whether this drug is excreted in human milk. As a general rule, nursing should not be undertaken when a patient is being given sodium phosphate P 32.

➤*Children:* Safety and effectiveness in pediatric patients have not been established.

Adverse Reactions

None known.

STRONTIUM-89 CHLORIDE

Rx	**Metastron** (Medi-Physics/Amersham)	**Injection:** 148 MBq, 4 mCi (10.9 to 22.6 mg/ml)	Preservative free. In 10 ml vials with Water for Injection.

STRONTIUM-89 CHLORIDE — INJECTION

Indications

➤*Bone pain due to skeletal metastases:* For the relief of bone pain in patients with painful skeletal metastases.

Administration and Dosage

➤*Approved by the FDA:* June 19, 1993.

➤*Recommended dose:* The recommended dose of strontium-89 chloride is 148 megabecquerels (MBq), 4 mCi, administered by slow IV injection (1 to 2 minutes). Alternatively, a dose of 1.5 to 2.2 MBq/kg, 40 to 60 μCi/kg body weight may be used.

➤*Repeat doses:* Repeated administrations of strontium-89 chloride should be based on an individual patient's response to therapy, current symptoms, and hematologic status, and are generally not recommended at intervals of fewer than 90 days.

The patient dose should be measured by a suitable radioactivity calibration system immediately prior to administration.

➤*Radiation dosimetry:* The estimated radiation dose that would be delivered over time by the IV injection of 37 MBq, 1 mCi of strontium-89 to a healthy adult is given in the information below. Data are taken from the *ICRP* publication "Radiation Dose to Patients from Radiopharmaceuticals"- *ICRP* #53, Vol. 18, No. 1 to 4; 171, Pergamon Press, 1988.

Strontium-89 Dosimetry

Organ	mGy/MBq	rad/mCi
Bone surface	17	63
Red bone marrow	11	40.7
Lower bowel wall	4.7	17.4
Bladder wall	1.3	4.8
Testes	0.8	2.9
Ovaries	0.8	2.9
Uterine wall	0.8	2.9
Kidneys	0.8	2.9

When blastic osseous metastases are present, significantly enhanced localization of the radiopharmaceutical will occur with correspondingly higher doses to the metastases compared with normal bones and other organs.

The radiation dose hazard in handling strontium-89 chloride injection during dose dispensing and administration is similar to that from phosphorus-32. The beta emission has a range in water of about 8 mm (max) and in glass of about 3 mm, but the bremsstrahlung radiation may augment the contact dose.

Measured values of the dose on the surface of the unshielded vial are about 65 mR/min/mCi.

It is recommended that the vial be kept inside its transportation shield whenever possible.

➤*Storage/Stability:* The vial and its contents should be stored inside its transportation container at room temperature (15° to 25°C; 59° to 77°F).

The calibration date (for radioactivity content) and expiration date are quoted on the vial label. The expiration date will be 28 days after calibration. Stability studies have shown no change in any of the product characteristics monitored during routine product quality control over the period from manufacture to expiration.

Actions

➤*Pharmacology:* Following IV injection, soluble strontium compounds behave like their calcium analogs, clearing rapidly from the blood and selectively localizing in bone mineral. Uptake of strontium by bone occurs preferentially in sites of active osteogenesis; thus, primary bone tumors and areas of metastatic involvement (blastic lesions) can accumulate significantly greater concentrations of strontium than surrounding normal bone.

Strontium-89 chloride is retained in metastatic bone lesions much longer than in normal bone, where turnover is about 14 days. In patients with extensive skeletal metastases, well over half of the injected dose is retained in the bones.

Strontium-89 is a pure beta emitter, and strontium-89 chloride selectively irradiates sites of primary and metastatic bone involvement with minimal irradiation of soft tissues distant from the bone lesions. (The maximum range in tissue is 8 mm; maximum energy is 1.463 MeV).

➤*Pharmacokinetics:*

Absorption/Distribution –

Physical characteristics: Strontium-89 decays by beta emission, with a physical half-life of 50.5 days. The maximum beta energy is 1.463 MeV (100%). The maximum range of beta- from strontium-89 in tissue is approximately 8 mm.

Radioactive decay factors to be applied to the stated value for radioactive concentration at calibration, when calculating injection volumes at the time of administration, are given in the following table:

Decay of Strontium-89

Day*	Factor
−24	1.39
−22	1.35
−20	1.32
−18	1.28
−16	1.25
−14	1.21
−12	1.18
−10	1.15
−8	1.12
−6	1.09
−4	1.06
−2	1.03
0 = calibration	1
+6	0.92
+8	0.9
+10	0.87
+12	0.85
+14	0.83
+16	0
+18	0.78
+20	0.76
+22	0.74
+24	0.72
+26	0.7
+28	0.68

* Days before (−) or after (+) the calibration date stated on the vial.

Excretion – Excretion pathways are two-thirds urinary and one-third fecal in patients with bone metastases. Urinary excretion is higher in people without bone lesions. Urinary excretion is greatest in the first 2 days following injection.

Contraindications

None known.

Warnings

➤*Hematologic toxicity:* Use of strontium-89 chloride in patients with evidence of seriously compromised bone marrow from previous therapy or disease infiltration is not recommended unless the potential benefit of the treatment outweighs its risks. Bone marrow toxicity is to be expected following the administration of strontium-89 chloride, particularly white blood cells and platelets. The extent of toxicity is variable. It is recommended that the patient's peripheral blood cell counts be monitored at least once every other week. Typically, platelets will be depressed by about 30% compared to preadministration levels. The nadir of platelet depression in most patients is found between 12 and 16 weeks following administration of strontium-89 chloride. White blood cells are usually depressed to a varying extent compared to preadministration levels. Thereafter, recovery occurs slowly, typically reaching preadministration levels 6 months after treatment unless the patient's disease or additional therapy intervenes.

➤*Repeat administration:* In considering repeat administration of strontium-89 chloride, the patient's hematologic response to the initial dose, current platelet level and other evidence of marrow depletion should be carefully evaluated.

Verification of dose and patient identification is necessary prior to administration because strontium-89 chloride delivers a relatively high dose of radioactivity.

➤*Renal function impairment:* Strontium-89 chloride is excreted primarily by the kidneys. In patients with renal dysfunction, the possible risks of administering strontium-89 chloride should be weighed against the possible benefits.

➤*Carcinogenesis:* Data from a repetitive-dose animal study suggests that strontium-89 chloride is a potential carcinogen. Thirty-three (33) of 40 rats injected with strontium-89 chloride in 10 consecutive monthly doses of either 250 or 350 μCi/kg developed malignant bone tumors after a latency period of approximately 9 months. No neoplasia was observed in the control animals. Treatment with strontium-89 chloride should be restricted to patients with well-documented metastatic bone disease.

➤*Pregnancy: Category D.* Strontium-89 chloride may cause fetal harm when administered to a pregnant woman. There are no adequate and well-controlled studies in pregnant women. If this drug is used during pregnancy,

STRONTIUM-89 CHLORIDE — INJECTION

or if the patient becomes pregnant while receiving this drug, the patient should be apprised of the potential hazard to the fetus. Women of childbearing potential should be advised to avoid becoming pregnant.

➤*Lactation:* Because strontium acts as a calcium analog, secretion of strontium-89 chloride into human milk is likely. It is recommended that nursing be discontinued by mothers about to receive IV strontium-89 chloride. It is not known whether this drug is excreted in human milk.

➤*Children:* Safety and efficacy in children below the age of 18 years have not been established.

Precautions

➤*Short-life expectancy:* In view of the delayed onset of pain relief, typically 7 to 20 days postinjection, administration of strontium-89 chloride to patients with very short life expectancy is not recommended.

➤*Rapid administration:* A calcium-like flushing sensation has been observed in patients following a rapid (less than 30 second injection) administration.

➤*Incontinence:* Special precautions, such as urinary catheterization, should be taken following administration to patients who are incontinent to minimize the risk of radioactive contamination of clothing, bed linen and the patient's environment.

➤*Special risk:* Strontium-89 chloride is not indicated for use in patients with cancer not involving bone. Strontium-89 chloride should be used with caution in patients with platelet counts below 60,000 and white cell counts below 2400.

Adverse Reactions

➤*Fatal septicemia:* A single case of fatal septicemia following leukopenia was reported during clinical trials. Most severe reactions of marrow toxicity can be managed by conventional means.

➤*Other adverse reactions:* A small number of patients have reported a transient increase in bone pain at 36 to 72 hours after injection. This is usually mild and self-limiting, and controllable with analgesics. A single patient reported chills and fever 12 hours after injection without long-term sequelae.

Patient Information

The patient may feel a slight increase in pain for 2 or 3 days beginning 2 or 3 days after injection. The physician may suggest a temporary increase in the dose of pain medication until the pain is under control. After about 1 or 2 weeks, the pain should begin to diminish.

The patient can eat and drink normally and there is no need to avoid alcohol or caffeine unless already advised to do so. The physician may want to carry out periodic, routine blood tests.

Advise patients to tell any health practitioner who is giving them medical treatment that they have received strontium-89.

During the first week after injection, strontium-89 will be present in the blood and urine. It is therefore important to consider the following common sense precautions for 1 week: where a normal toilet is available, use in preference to a urinal. Flush the toilet twice. Wipe up any spilled urine with a tissue and flush it away. Always wash hands after using the toilet. Immediately wash any linen or clothes that become stained with urine or blood. Wash them separately from other clothes and rinse thoroughly. If any urine collection device is used, follow instructions on its use. Wash away any spilled blood if a cut occurs.

In many people who receive strontium-89, the effect lasts for several months. If pain returns, consult the physician.

SAMARIUM SM 153 LEXIDRONAM

Rx	**Quadramet** (Du Pont Pharma)	**Injection:** 1850 MBq/ml (50 mCi/ml) at calibration	Frozen, single-dose 10 ml vials. In 2 ml fill (3700 MBq) and 3 ml fill (5550 MBq).

SAMARIUM SM 153 LEXIDRONAM — INJECTION

Indications

➤*Pain due to osteoblastic metastatic bone lesions:* For relief of pain in patients with confirmed osteoblastic metastatic bone lesions that enhance on radionuclide bone scan.

Administration and Dosage

➤*Approved by the FDA:* March 28, 1997.

➤*Recommended dose:* 1 mCi/kg, administered intravenously over a period of 1 minute through a secure in-dwelling catheter and followed with a saline flush. Dose adjustment in patients at the extremes of weight have not been studied. Caution should be exercised when determining the dose in very thin or very obese patients.

The dose should be measured by a suitable radioactivity calibration system, such as a radioisotope dose calibrator, immediately before administration.

The dose of radioactivity to be administered and the patient should be verified before administering samarium SM 153 lexidronam. Patients should not be released until their radioactivity levels and exposure rates comply with federal and local regulations.

➤*Fluid intake:* The patient should ingest (or receive by IV administration) a minimum of 500 mL (2 cups) of fluids prior to injection and should void as often as possible after injection to minimize radiation exposure to the bladder.

➤*Admixture incompatibilities:* Samarium SM 153 lexidronam contains calcium and may be incompatible with solutions that contain molecules that can complex with and form calcium precipitates.

Samarium SM 153 lexidronam should not be diluted or mixed with other solutions.

➤*Thawing:* Thaw at room temperature before administration and use within 8 hours of thawing.

➤*Radiation dosimetry:* The estimated absorbed radiation doses to an average 70 kg adult patient from an IV injection of samarium SM 153 lexidronam are shown below. The dosimetry estimates were based on clinical biodistribution studies using methods developed for radiation dose calculations by the Medical Internal Radiation Dose (MIRD) Committee of the Society of Nuclear Medicine.

Radiation exposure is based on a urinary voiding interval of 4.8 hours. Radiation dose estimates for bone and marrow assume that radioactivity is deposited on bone surfaces, as noted in autoradiograms of biopsy bone samples in 7 patients who received samarium SM 153 lexidronam. Although electron emissions from ^{153}Sm are abundant, with energies up to 810 keV, rapid blood clearance of samarium SM 153 lexidronam and low energy and abundant photon emissions generally result in low radiation doses to those parts of the body where the complex does not localize.

When blastic osseous lesions are present, significantly enhanced localization of the radiopharmaceutical will occur, with correspondingly higher doses to the lesions compared with normal bones and other organs.

The following are the radiation absorbed doses by target organ for a 70 kg adult, each of the values are expressed as Rad/mCi (and mGy/MBq): Bone surfaces: 25 (6.76); red marrow: 5.7 (1.54); urinary bladder wall: 3.6 (0.097); kidneys: 0.065 (0.018); whole body: 0.04 (0.011); lower large intestine: 0.037 (0.01); ovaries: 0.032 (0.0086); muscle: 0.028 (0.0076); small intestine: 0.023 (0.0062); upper large intestine: 0.02 (0.0054); testes: 0.02 (0.0054); liver: 0.019 (0.0051); spleen: 0.018 (0.0049); stomach: 0.015 (0.0041).

➤*Storage/Stability:* Store frozen at −10° to −20°C (14° to −4°F) in a lead shielded container.

Storage and disposal of samarium SM 153 lexidronam should be controlled in a manner that complies with the appropriate regulations of the government agency authorized to license the use of this radionuclide.

Actions

➤*Pharmacology:* Samarium (Samarium Sm-153 EDTMP) has an affinity for bone and concentrates in areas of bone turnover in association with hydroxyapatite. In clinical studies employing planar imaging techniques, more samarium accumulates in osteoblastic lesions than in normal bone with a lesion-to-normal bone ratio of approximately 5. The mechanism of action of samarium in relieving the pain of bone metastases is not known.

➤*Pharmacokinetics:*

Absorption – The greater the number of metastatic lesions, the more skeletal uptake of Sm-153 radioactivity. The relationship between skeletal uptake and the size of the metastatic lesions has not been studied. The total skeletal uptake of radioactivity was 65.5% ± 15.5% of the injected dose in 453 patients with metastatic lesions from a variety of primary malignancies. In a study of 22 patients with a wide range in the number of metastatic sites, the percentage of the injected dose (% ID) taken up by bone ranged from 56.3% in a patient with 5 metastatic lesions to 76.7% in a patient with 52 metastatic lesions. If the number of metastatic lesions is fixed, over the range 0.1 to 3 mCi/kg, the percent ID taken up by bone is the same regardless of the dose.

Distribution – Human protein binding has not been studied; however, in dog, rat and bovine studies, less than 0.5% of samarium-153 EDTMP is bound to protein. At physiologic pH, greater than 90% of the complex is present as $^{153}Sm[EDTMP]^{-5}$, and less than 10% as $^{153}SmH[EDTMP]^{-4}$. The octanol/water partition coefficient is less than 10^{-5}.

Metabolism – The complex formed by samarium and EDTMP is excreted as an intact, single species that consists of 1 atom of the Sm-153 and 1 molecule of the EDTMP, as shown by an analysis of urine samples from patients (n = 5) administered samarium Sm-153 EDTMP. Metabolic products of samarium Sm-153 EDTMP were not detected in humans.

Excretion – For samarium, calculations of the percent ID detected in the whole body, urine and blood were corrected for radionuclide decay. The clearance of activity through the urine is expressed as the cumulated activity excreted. The whole body retention is the simple reciprocal of the cumulated urine activity. (See Absorption).

Urine: Samarium Sm-153 EDTMP radioactivity was excreted in the urine after intravenous injection. During the first 6 hours, 34.5% (± 15.5%) was

SAMARIUM SM 153 LEXIDRONAM — INJECTION

excreted. Overall, the greater the number of metastatic lesions, the less radioactivity was excreted.

Blood: Clearance of radioactivity from the blood demonstrated biexponential kinetics after intravenous injection in 19 patients (10 men, 9 women) with a variety of primary cancers that were metastatic to bone. Over the first 30 minutes, the radioactivity (mean ± SD) in the blood decreased to 15% (± 8%) of the injected dose with a t ½ of 5.5 min (±1.1 min). After 30 minutes, the radioactivity cleared from the blood more slowly with a t½ of 65.4 min (± 9.6 min). Less than 1% of the dose injected remained in the blood 5 hours after injection.

Contraindications

Hypersensitivity to EDTMP or similar phosphonate compounds.

Warnings

➤*Bone marrow suppression:* Samarium causes bone marrow suppression. In clinical trials, white blood cell counts and platelet counts decreased to a nadir of approximately 40% to 50% of baseline in 123 (95%) of patients within 3 to 5 weeks after samarium, and tended to return to pretreatment levels by 8 weeks. The grade of marrow toxicity is as follows.

In the clinical trials of samarium (1 mCi/kg), the number of patients who experienced marrow toxicity was assessed using the toxicity grade based on the National Cancer Institute criteria. Normal levels according to this criteria is a hemoglobin count greater than 10 g/dL, leucocyte count greater than or equal to 4 x 103/mcL, and a platelet count greater than or equal to 150,000/mcL. For the hemoglobin count, the number (and percent) of patients, as assessed by toxicity grade, for the placebo group (n = 85) and samarium group (n = 185), respectively, is as follows: Toxicity grade 0 to 2: 78 (92%) vs 162 (88%); toxicity grade 3: 6 (7%) vs 20 (11%); and toxicity grade 4: 1 (1%) vs 3 (2%). For the leucocyte count, the number (and percent) of patients, as assessed by toxicity grade, for the placebo group (n = 85) and samarium group (n = 184), respectively, is as follows: Toxicity grade 0-2: 85 (100%) vs. 169 (92%); toxicity grade 3: 0 vs. 15 (8%); and toxicity grade 4: 0 vs. 0. For the platelet count, the number (and percent) of patients, as assessed by toxicity grade, for the placebo group (n = 85) and samarium group (n = 185), respectively, is as follows: Toxicity grade 0 to 2: 85 (100%) vs. 173 (94%); toxicity grade 3: 0 vs 10 (5%); and toxicity grade 4: 0 vs 2 (1%).

Before samarium is administered, consideration should be given to the patient's current clinical and hematologic status and bone marrow response history to treatment with myelotoxic agents. Metastatic prostate and other cancers can be associated with disseminated intravascular coagulation (DIC); caution should be exercised in treating cancer patients whose platelet counts are falling or who have other clinical or laboratory findings suggesting DIC. Because of the unknown potential for additive effects on bone marrow, samarium should not be given concurrently with chemotherapy or external beam radiation therapy unless the clinical benefits outweigh the risks. Use of samarium in patients with evidence of compromised bone marrow reserve from previous therapy or disease involvement is not recommended unless the potential benefits of the treatment outweigh the risks. Blood counts should be monitored weekly for at least 8 weeks, or until recovery of adequate bone marrow function.

➤*Pregnancy: Category D.* As with other radiopharmaceutical drugs, samarium can cause fetal harm when administered to a pregnant woman. Adequate and well controlled studies have not been conducted in animals or pregnant women. Women of childbearing age should have a negative pregnancy test before administration of samarium. If this drug is used during pregnancy, or if a patient becomes pregnant after taking this drug, the patient should be apprised of the potential hazard to the fetus. Women of childbearing potential should be advised to avoid becoming pregnant soon after receiving samarium. Men and women patients should be advised to use an effective method of contraception after the administration of samarium.

➤*Lactation:* It is not known whether samarium is excreted in human milk. Because of the potential for serious adverse reactions in nursing infants from samarium, a decision should be made whether to continue nursing or to administer the drug. If samarium is administered, formula feedings should be substituted for breastfeedings.

➤*Children:* Safety and effectiveness in pediatric patients below the age of 16 years have not been established.

Precautions

➤*Monitoring:* Because concomitant hydration is recommended to promote the urinary excretion of samarium, appropriate monitoring and consideration of additional supportive treatment should be used in patients with a history of congestive heart failure or renal insufficiency.

Because of the potential for bone marrow suppression, beginning 2 weeks after samarium administration, blood counts should be monitored weekly for at least 8 weeks, or until recovery of adequate bone marrow function.

➤*Hypocalcemia:* In a subset of 31 patients who had serum calcium monitored during the first 2 hours after samarium infusion, a clear pattern of calcium change was not identified. However, 10 (32%) patients had at least 1 serum calcium level that was below normal (7.16 to 8.28). The extent to which samarium-153 EDTMP is related to this hypocalcemia is not known. Caution should be exercised when administering samarium to patients at risk for developing hypocalcemia.

➤*Skeletal:* Spinal cord compression frequently occurs in patients with known metastases to the cervical, thoracic or lumbar spine. In clinical studies of samarium, spinal cord compression was reported in 7% of patients who received placebo and in 8.3% of patients who received 1 mCi/kg samarium. Samarium is not indicated for treatment of spinal cord compression. Samarium administration for pain relief of metastatic bone cancer does not prevent the development of spinal cord compression. When there is a clinical suspicion of spinal cord compression, appropriate diagnostic and therapeutic measures must be taken immediately to avoid permanent disability.

➤*ECG changes:* EDTMP is a chelating agent. Although the chelating effects have not been evaluated thoroughly in humans, dogs that received non-radioactive samarium EDTMP (6 times the human dose based on body weight, 3 times based on surface area) developed a variety of electrocardiographic (ECG) changes (with or without the presence of hypocalcemia). The causal relationship between the hypocalcemia and ECG changes has not been studied. Whether samarium causes electrocardiographic changes or arrhythmias in humans has not been studied. Caution and appropriate monitoring should be given when administering samarium to patients.

➤*Bone marrow suppression:* This drug should be used with caution in patients with compromised bone marrow reserves. Samarium causes bone marrow suppression. In clinical trials, white blood cell counts and platelet counts decreased to a nadir of approximately 40% to 50% of baseline in 123 (95%) of patients within 3 to 5 weeks after samarium, and tended to return to pretreatment levels by 8 weeks.

➤*Incontinence:* Special precautions, such as bladder catheterization, should be taken with incontinent patients to minimize the risk of radioactive contamination of clothing, bed linen, and the patient's environment. Urinary excretion of radioactivity occurs over about 12 hours (with 35% occurring during the first 6 hours). Studies have not been done on the use of samarium in patients with renal impairment.

Drug Interactions

➤*Chemotherapy/Radiation:* The potential for additive bone marrow toxicity of samarium with chemotherapy or external beam radiation has not been studied. Samarium should not be given concurrently with chemotherapy or external beam radiation therapy unless the benefit outweighs the risks. Samarium should not be given after either of these treatments until there has been time for adequate marrow recovery. Drug-drug interaction studies have not been made.

Adverse Reactions

Of these patients, 472 (83%) had at least 1 adverse reaction. In a subgroup of 399 patients who received samarium 1 mCi/kg, there were 23 deaths and 46 serious adverse reactions. The deaths occurred an average of 67 days (9 to 130) after samarium. Serious reactions occurred an average of 46 days (1 - 118) after samarium. Although most of the patient deaths and serious adverse reactions appear to be related to the underlying disease, the relationship of end stage disease, marrow invasion by cancer cells, previous myelotoxic treatment and samarium toxicity can not be easily distinguished. In clinical studies, 2 patients with rapidly progressive prostate cancer developed thrombocytopenia and died 4 weeks after receiving samarium. One (1) of the patients showed evidence of disseminated intravascular coagulation (DIC); the other patient experienced a fatal cerebrovascular accident, with a suspicion of DIC. The relationship of the DIC to the bone marrow suppressive effect of samarium is not known. Marrow toxicity occurred in 277 (47%) patients.

In controlled studies, 7% of patients receiving 1 mCi/kg samarium (as compared to 6% of patients receiving placebo) reported a transient increase in bone pain shortly after injection (flare reaction). This was usually mild, self-limiting, and responded to analgesics.

Samarium Adverse Reactions in People Who Received Samarium or Placebo in Controlled Clinical Trials (≥ 1 %)

Adverse reactions	Placebo (n = 90)	Samarium 1 mCi/kg (n = 199)
Patients with any adverse reaction	72 (80%)	169 (85%)
Body as a whole	56 (62%)	100 (50%)
Pain flare reaction	5 (5.6%)	14 (7%)
Cardiovascular	19 (21%)	32 (16%)
Arrhythmias	2 (2.2%)	10 (5%)
Chest pain	4 (4.4%)	8 (4%)
Hypertension	0	6 (3%)
Hypotension	2 (2.2%)	4 (2%)
Digestive	44 (49%)	82 (41%)
Abdominal pain	7 (7.8%)	12 (6%)
Diarrhea	3 (3.3%)	12 (6%)
Nausea and/or vomiting	37 (41.1%)	65 (32.7%)
Hematologic and lymphatic	12 (13%)	54 (27%)
Coagulation disorder	0	3 (1.5%)
Hemoglobin decreased	21 (23.3%)	81 (40.7%)
Leukopenia	6 (6.7%)	118 (59.3%)
Lymphadenopathy	0	4 (2%)
Thrombocytopenia	8 (8.9%)	138 (69.3%)
Any bleeding manifestations*	8 (8.9%)	32 (16.1%)
Ecchymosis	1 (1.1%)	3 (3%)
Epistaxis	1 (1.1%)	4 (2%)

SAMARIUM SM 153 LEXIDRONAM — INJECTION

Samarium Adverse Reactions in People Who Received Samarium or Placebo in Controlled Clinical Trials (≥ 1 %)		
Adverse reactions	Placebo (n = 90)	Samarium 1 mCi/kg (n = 199)
Hematuria	3 (3.3%)	10 (5%)
Infection	10 (11.1%)	34 (17.1%)
Fever and/or chills	10 (11.1%)	17 (8.5%)
Infection, not specified	4 (4.4%)	14 (7%)
Oral moniliasis	1 (1.1%)	4 (2%)
Pneumonia	1 (1.1%)	3 (1.5%)
Musculoskeletal	28 (31%)	55 (27%)
Myasthenia	8 (8.9%)	13 (6.5%)
Pathologic fracture	2 (2.2%)	5 (2.5%)
Nervous	39 (43%)	59 (30%)
Dizziness	1 (1.1%)	8 (4%)
Paresthesia	7 (7.8%)	4 (2%)
Spinal cord compression	5 (5.5%)	13 (6.5%)
Cerebrovascular accident/stroke	0	2 (1%)
Respiratory	24 (27%)	35 (18%)
Bronchitis/cough increased	2 (2.2%)	8 (4%)
Special senses	11 (12%)	11 (6%)
Skin and appendages	17 (19%)	13 (7%)
Purpura	0	2 (1%)
Rash	2 (2.2%)	2 (1%)

* Includes hemorrhage (gastrointestinal, ocular) reported in < 1%.

In an additional 200 patients who received samarium in uncontrolled clinical trials, adverse events that were reported at a rate of greater than or equal to 1% were similar except for 9 (4.5%) patients who had agranulocytosis. Other selected adverse events that were reported in less than 1% of the patients who received samarium 1 mCi/kg in any clinical trial include alopecia, angina, congestive heart failure, sinus bradycardia, and vasodilation.

Overdosage

Overdosage with samarium has not been reported. An antidote for samarium overdosage is not known. The anticipated complications of overdosage would likely be secondary to bone marrow suppression from the radioactivity of ^{153}Sm, or secondary to hypocalcemia and cardiac arrhythmias related to the EDTMP.

Patient Information

Patients who receive samarium should be advised that for several hours following administration, radioactivity will be present in excreted urine. To help protect themselves and others in their environment, precautions need to be taken for 12 hours following administration. Whenever possible, a toilet should be used, rather than a urinal, and the toilet should be flushed several times after each use. Spilled urine should be cleaned up completely and patients should wash their hands thoroughly. If blood or urine gets onto clothing, the clothing should be washed separately, or stored for 1 to 2 weeks to allow for decay of the ^{153}Sm.

Some patients have reported a transient increase in bone pain shortly after injection (flare reaction). This is usually mild and self-limiting and occurs within 72 hours of injection. Such reactions are usually responsive to analgesics.

Patients who respond to samarium might begin to notice the onset of pain relief 1 week after samarium. Maximal pain relief generally occurs at 3 to 4 weeks after injection of samarium. Patients who experience a reduction in pain may be encouraged to decrease their use of opioid analgesics.

PLATINUM COORDINATION COMPLEX

CARBOPLATIN

Rx	**Carboplatin** (Various, eg, Bedford Labs, Mayne)	**Injection**: 10 mg/mL	In 5, 15, and 45 mL single-use vials.
Rx	**Paraplatin** (Bristol-Myers Squibb Oncology)		In 5 mL, 15 mL, and 45 mL single-dose vials.
Rx	**Carboplatin** (Baxter)	**Powder for injection, lyophilized**: 50 mg	Mannitol. In single-dose vials.
Rx	**Paraplatin** (Bristol-Myers Squibb Oncology)		Mannitol. In single-dose vials.
Rx	**Carboplatin** (Baxter)	150 mg	Mannitol. In single-dose vials.
Rx	**Paraplatin** (Bristol-Myers Squibb Oncology)		Mannitol. In single-dose vials.
Rx	**Carboplatin** (Baxter)	450 mg	Mannitol. In single-dose vials.
Rx	**Paraplatin** (Bristol-Myers Squibb Oncology)		Mannitol. In single-dose vials.

CARBOPLATIN — INJECTION

WARNING

Carboplatin should be administered under the supervision of a qualified physician experienced in the use of cancer chemotherapeutic agents. Appropriate management of therapy and complications is possible only when adequate treatment facilities are readily available.

Bone marrow suppression is dose related and may be severe, resulting in infection or bleeding. Anemia may be cumulative and may require transfusion support. Vomiting is another frequent drug-related side effect.

Anaphylactic-like reactions to carboplatin have been reported and may occur within minutes of carboplatin administration. Epinephrine, corticosteroids, and antihistamines have been employed to alleviate symptoms.

Indications

➤*Advanced ovarian carcinoma:* For the initial treatment of advanced ovarian carcinoma in established combination with other approved chemotherapeutic agents.

Carboplatin is indicated for the palliative treatment of patients with ovarian carcinoma recurrent after prior chemotherapy, including patients who have been previously treated with cisplatin.

➤*Unlabeled uses:* As a single agent in previously treated and untreated patients with small cell lung cancer and non-small cell lung cancer, but is most effective when combined with other agents (eg, etoposide); alone or in combination (usually with fluorouracil) in the treatment of advanced or recurrent squamous cell carcinoma of the head and neck; advanced endometrial cancer, in relapsed and refractory acute leukemia and for seminoma of testicular cancer.

Administration and Dosage

➤*Approved by the FDA:* March 3, 1989.

➤*Aluminum:* Aluminum reacts with carboplatin causing precipitate formation and loss of potency; therefore, needles or intravenous sets containing aluminum parts that may come in contact with the drug must not be used for the preparation or administration of carboplatin.

➤*Single agent therapy:* Carboplatin, as a single agent, has been shown to be effective in patients with recurrent ovarian carcinoma at a dosage of 360 mg/m^2 IV on day 1 every 4 weeks (alternately, see Formula dosing). In general, however, single intermittent courses of carboplatin should not be repeated until the neutrophil count is at least 2000 and the platelet count is at least 100,000.

➤*Combination therapy with cyclophosphamide:* In the chemotherapy of advanced ovarian cancer, an effective combination for previously untreated patients consists of:

Carboplatin 300 mg/m^2 IV on day 1 every 4 weeks for 6 cycles (alternately, see Formula dosing).

Cyclophosphamide 600 mg/m^2 IV on day 1 every 4 weeks for 6 cycles. For directions regarding the use and administration of cyclophosphamide, please refer to its package insert.

Intermittent courses of carboplatin in combination with cyclophosphamide should not be repeated until the neutrophil count is at least 2000 and the platelet count is at least 100,000.

➤*Dose adjustment recommendations:* Pretreatment platelet count and performance status are important prognostic factors for severity of myelosuppression in previously treated patients.

Suggested Dose Adjustments for Single Agent or Combination Therapy		
Platelets	Neutrophils	Adjusted dose* (from prior course)
> 100,000	> 2000	125%
50 to 100,000	500 to 2000	No adjustment
< 50,000	< 500	75%

* Percentages apply to carboplatin injection as a single agent or to both carboplatin and cyclophosphamide in combination. In the controlled studies, dosages were also adjusted at a lower level (50% to 60%) for severe myelosuppression. Escalations above 125% were not recommended for these studies.

CARBOPLATIN — INJECTION

Carboplatin is usually administered by an infusion lasting 15 minutes or longer. No pre- or post-treatment hydration or forced diuresis is required.

➤*Renal function impairment:* Patients with creatinine clearance values below 60 mL/min are at increased risk of severe bone marrow suppression. In renally impaired patients who received single agent carboplatin therapy, the incidence of severe leukopenia, neutropenia, or thrombocytopenia has been about 25% when the dosage modifications below have been used.

Dosage Modifications in Renal Function Impairment	
Baseline creatinine clearance	Recommended dose on Day 1
41 to 59 mL/min	250 mg/m^2
16 to 40 mL/min	200 mg/m^2

The data available for patients with severely impaired kidney function (creatinine clearance below 15 mL/min) are too limited to permit a recommendation for treatment.

Subsequent dosages – These dosing recommendations apply to the initial course of treatment. Subsequent dosages should be adjusted according to the patient's tolerance based on the degree of bone marrow suppression.

➤*Formula dosing:* Another approach for determining the initial dose of carboplatin is the use of mathematical formulae, which are based on a patient's preexisting renal function or renal function and desired platelet nadir. Renal excretion is the major route of elimination for carboplatin. The use of dosing formulae, as compared to empirical dose calculation based on body surface area, allows compensation for patient variations in pretreatment renal function that might otherwise result in either underdosing (in patients with above average renal function) or overdosing (in patients with impaired renal function).

A simple formula for calculating dosage, based upon a patient's glomerular filtration rate (GFR in mL/min) and carboplatin target area under the concentration vs time curve (AUC in mg/mL•min), has been proposed by Calvert. In these studies, GFR was measured by ^{51}Cr-EDTA clearance.

Calvert Formula for Carboplatin Dosing
Total dose (mg) = (target AUC) × (GFR + 25)
Note: With the Calvert formula, the total dose of carboplatin is calculated in mg, not mg/m^2

The target AUC of 4 to 6 mg/mL•min using single agent carboplatin appears to provide the most appropriate dose range in previously treated patients. This study also showed a trend between the AUC of single agent carboplatin administered to previously treated patients and the likelihood of developing toxicity.

Actual Toxicity in Previously Treated Patients (%)		
AUC (mg/mL•min)	Grade 3 or 4 thrombocytopenia	Grade 3 or 4 leukopenia
4 to 5	16%	13%
6 to 7	33%	34%

➤*Geriatric dosing:* Because renal function is often decreased in elderly patients, formula dosing of carboplatin based on estimates of GFR should be used in elderly patients to provide predictable plasma carboplatin AUCs and thereby minimize the risk of toxicity.

➤*Preparation of intravenous solutions:* Carboplatin injection is a premixed aqueous solution of 10 mg/mL carboplatin.

Carboplatin can be further diluted to concentrations as low as 0.5 mg/mL with 5% Dextrose in Water (D_5W) or 0.9% Sodium Chloride Injection, USP.

When prepared as directed, carboplatin solutions are stable for 8 hours at room temperature (25°C; 77°F). Since no antibacterial preservative is contained in the formulation, it is recommended that carboplatin solutions be discarded 8 hours after dilution.

➤*Storage/Stability:* Store at 25°C (77°F); excursions permitted from 15° to 30°C (59° to 86°F). Protect from light.

Actions

➤*Pharmacology:* Carboplatin, like cisplatin, produces predominantly interstrand DNA cross-links rather than DNA-protein cross-links. This effect is apparently cell-cycle nonspecific. The aquation of carboplatin, which is thought to produce the active species, occurs at a slower rate than in the case of cisplatin. Despite this difference, it appears that both carboplatin and cisplatin induce equal numbers of drug-DNA cross-links, causing equivalent lesions and biological effects. The differences in potencies for carboplatin and cisplatin appear to be directly related to the difference in aquation rates.

➤*Pharmacokinetics:*

Absorption/Distribution – Carboplatin is not bound to plasma proteins. No significant quantities of protein-free, ultrafilterable platinum-containing species other than carboplatin are present in plasma. However, platinum from carboplatin becomes irreversibly bound to plasma proteins and is slowly eliminated with a minimum half-life of 5 days.

Metabolism/Excretion – The major route of elimination of carboplatin is renal excretion. Patients with creatinine clearances of approximately 60 mL/min or greater excrete 65% of the dose in the urine within 12 hours and 71% of the dose within 24 hours. All of the platinum in the 24-hour urine is present as carboplatin. Only 3% to 5% of the administered platinum is excreted in the urine between 24 and 96 hours. There are insufficient data to determine whether biliary excretion occurs.

Special populations –

Renal function impairment: In patients with creatinine clearances below 60 mL/min the total body and renal clearances of carboplatin decrease as the creatinine clearance decreases. Carboplatin dosages should therefore be reduced in these patients.

In patients with creatinine clearances of about 60 mL/min or greater, plasma levels of intact carboplatin decay in a biphasic manner after a 30-minute intravenous infusion of 300 to 500 mg/m^2 of carboplatin. The initial plasma half-life (alpha) was found to be 1.1 to 2 hours (n = 6), and the postdistribution plasma half-life (beta) was found to be 2.6 to 5.9 hours (n = 6). The total body clearance, apparent volume of distribution and mean residence time for carboplatin are 4.4 L/hour, 16 L and 3.5 hours, respectively. The C_{max} values and areas under the plasma concentration vs time curves from 0 to infinity (AUC inf) increase linearly with dose, although the increase was slightly more than dose proportional. Carboplatin, therefore, exhibits linear pharmacokinetics over the dosing range studied (300 to 500 mg/m^2).

The primary determinant of carboplatin clearance is glomerular filtration rate (GFR) and this parameter of renal function is often decreased in elderly patients. Dosing formulas incorporating estimates of GFR to provide predictable carboplatin plasma AUCs should be used in elderly patients to minimize the risk of toxicity.

Contraindications

Severe allergic reactions to cisplatin or other platinum-containing compounds, or mannitol; severe bone marrow depression or significant bleeding.

Warnings

➤*Bone marrow suppression:* Bone marrow suppression (leukopenia, neutropenia, and thrombocytopenia) is dose-dependent and is also the dose-limiting toxicity. Peripheral blood counts should be frequently monitored during carboplatin treatment and, when appropriate, until recovery is achieved. Median nadir occurs at day 21 in patients receiving single-agent carboplatin.By day 28, 90% of patients have platelet counts greater than 100,000/mm^3; 74% have neutrophil counts greater than 2,000/mm^3; 67% have leukocyte counts greater than 4,000/mm^3. In general, single intermittent courses of carboplatin should not be repeated until leukocyte, neutrophil, and platelet counts have recovered.

Since anemia is cumulative, transfusions may be needed during treatment with carboplatin, particularly in patients receiving prolonged therapy.

Bone marrow suppression is increased in patients who have received prior therapy, especially regimens including cisplatin. Marrow suppression is also increased in patients with impaired kidney function. Initial carboplatin dosages in these patients should be appropriately reduced and blood counts should be carefully monitored between courses. The use of carboplatin in combination with other bone marrow suppressing therapies must be carefully managed with respect to dosage and timing in order to minimize additive effects.

➤*Toxicity:* Carboplatin has limited nephrotoxic potential, but concomitant treatment with aminoglycosides has resulted in increased renal or audiologic toxicity, and caution must be exercised when a patient receives both drugs. Clinically significant hearing loss has been reported to occur in pediatric patients when carboplatin was administered at higher than recommended doses in combination with other ototoxic agents.

➤*Emesis:* Carboplatin can induce emesis, which can be more severe in patients previously receiving emetogenic therapy. The incidence and intensity of emesis have been reduced by using premedication with antiemetics. Although no conclusive efficacy data exist with the following schedules of carboplatin, lengthening the duration of single intravenous administration to 24 hours or dividing the total dose over 5 consecutive daily pulse doses has resulted in reduced emesis.

➤*Peripheral neurotoxicity:* Although peripheral neurotoxicity is infrequent, its incidence is increased in patients greater than 65 years of age and in patients previously treated with cisplatin. Preexisting cisplatin-induced neurotoxicity does not worsen in about 70% of the patients receiving carboplatin as secondary treatment.

➤*Ophthalmic:* Loss of vision, which can be complete for light and colors, has been reported after the use of carboplatin for injection with doses higher than those recommended. Vision appears to recover totally or to a significant extent within weeks of stopping these high doses.

➤*Allergic reactions:* As in the case of other platinum coordination compounds, allergic reactions to carboplatin have been reported. These may occur within minutes of administration and should be managed with appropriate supportive therapy. There is increased risk of allergic reactions including anaphylaxis in patients previously exposed to platinum therapy. Carboplatin is contraindicated in patients with a history of severe allergic reactions to cisplatin or other platinum-containing compounds.

➤*Lab test abnormalities:* See Adverse Reactions for more information.

➤*Mutagenesis:* Carboplatin has been shown to be mutagenic both in vitro and in vivo.

➤*Elderly:* Of the 789 patients in initial treatment combination therapy studies (NCIC and SWOG), 395 patients were treated with carboplatin in combination with cyclophosphamide. Of these, 141 were over 65 years of age and 22 were 75 years of age or older. In these trials, age was not a prognostic factor for survival. In terms of safety, elderly patients treated with carboplatin were more likely to develop severe thrombocytopenia than younger patients. In a combined database of 1,942 patients (414 were greater than or

CARBOPLATIN — INJECTION

equal to 65 years of age) that received single-agent carboplatin for different tumor types, a similar incidence of adverse events was seen in patients 65 years and older and in patients less than 65. Other reported clinical experience has not identified differences in responses between elderly and younger patients, but greater sensitivity of some older individuals cannot be ruled out. Because renal function is often decreased in the elderly, renal function should be considered in the selection of carboplatin dosage.

➤*Pregnancy: Category D.* Carboplatin may cause fetal harm when administered to a pregnant woman. Carboplatin has been shown to be embryotoxic and teratogenic in rats. There are no adequate and well-controlled studies in pregnant women. If this drug is used during pregnancy, or if the patient becomes pregnant while receiving this drug, the patient should be apprised of the potential hazard to the fetus. Women of childbearing potential should be advised to avoid becoming pregnant.

➤*Lactation:* It is not known whether carboplatin is excreted in human milk. Because there is a possibility of toxicity in nursing infants secondary to carboplatin treatment of the mother, it is recommended that breastfeeding be discontinued if the mother is treated with carboplatin.

➤*Children:* Safety and effectiveness in children have not been established.

Precautions

➤*Aluminum:* See Administration and Dosage for more information.

Drug Interactions

Carboplatin Drug Interactions			
Precipitant drug	Object drug[a]		Description
Aminoglycosides	Carboplatin	↑	Coadministration has resulted in increased renal and/or audiologic toxicity. Use with caution.
Carboplatin	Aminoglycosides	↑	
Carboplatin	Phenytoin	↓	Serum concentrations of phenytoin may be decreased, resulting in a loss of therapeutic effect. Monitor phenytoin levels and adjust dose appropriately.
Carboplatin	Warfarin	↑	The anticoagulant effect of warfarin may be increased. Monitor coagulation parameters and adjust warfarin as needed.

[a] ↑ = Object drug increased. ↓ = Object drug decreased.

Adverse Reactions

➤*Allergic:* Hypersensitivity to carboplatin has occurred in 2% of the patients and may occur within minutes of administration; manage with appropriate supportive therapy. These allergic reactions have been similar in nature and severity to those reported with other platinum-containing compounds, ie, rash, urticaria, erythema, pruritus, and rarely bronchospasm and hypotension. Anaphylactic reactions have been reported as part of postmarketing surveillance. These reactions have been successfully managed with standard epinephrine, corticosteroid, and antihistamine therapy.

➤*CNS:* Peripheral neuropathies have been observed in 4% of the patients receiving carboplatin (6% of pretreated ovarian cancer patients) with mild paresthesias occurring most frequently. Carboplatin therapy produces significantly fewer and less severe neurologic side effects than does therapy with cisplatin. However, patients greater than 65 years of age or previously treated with cisplatin appear to have an increased risk (10%) for peripheral neuropathies. In 70% of the patients with preexisting cisplatin-induced peripheral neurotoxicity, there was no worsening of symptoms during therapy with carboplatin. Clinical ototoxicity and other sensory abnormalities such as visual disturbances and change in taste have been reported in only 1% of the patients. Central nervous system symptoms have been reported in 5% of the patients and appear to be most often related to the use of antiemetics.

Although the overall incidence of peripheral neurologic side effects induced by carboplatin is low, prolonged treatment, particularly in cisplatin pretreated patients, may result in cumulative neurotoxicity.

➤*Electrolyte disturbance:* The incidences of abnormally decreased serum electrolyte values reported were as follows: Sodium, 29%; potassium, 20%; calcium, 22%; and magnesium, 29%; (47%, 28%, 31%, and 43%, respectively, in pretreated ovarian cancer patients). Electrolyte supplementation was not routinely administered concomitantly with carboplatin, and these electrolyte abnormalities were rarely associated with symptoms.

➤*GI:* Vomiting occurs in 65% of the patients (81% of previously treated ovarian cancer patients) and in about one-third of these patients it is severe. Carboplatin, as a single agent or in combination, is significantly less emetogenic than cisplatin; however, patients previously treated with emetogenic agents, especially cisplatin, appear to be more prone to vomiting. Nausea alone occurs in an additional 10% to 15% of patients. Both nausea and vomiting usually cease within 24 hours of treatment and are often responsive to antiemetic measures. Although no conclusive efficacy data exist with the following schedules, prolonged administration of carboplatin, either by continuous 24-hour infusion or by daily pulse doses given for 5 consecutive days, was associated with less severe vomiting than the single dose intermittent schedule. Emesis was increased when carboplatin was used in combination with other emetogenic compounds. Other gastrointestinal effects observed frequently were pain in 17% of the patients; diarrhea in 6%; and constipation also in 6%.

➤*Hematologic:* Bone marrow suppression is the dose-limiting toxicity of carboplatin. Thrombocytopenia with platelet counts below 50,000/mm^3 occurs in 25% of the patients (35% of pretreated ovarian cancer patients); neutropenia with granulocyte counts below 1,000/mm^3 occurs in 16% of the patients (21% of pretreated ovarian cancer patients); leukopenia with WBC counts below 2,000/mm^3 occurs in 15% of the patients (26% of pretreated ovarian cancer patients). The nadir usually occurs about day 21 in patients receiving single-agent therapy. By day 28, 90% of patients have platelet counts above 100,000/mm^3; 74% have neutrophil counts above 2,000/mm^3; 67% have leukocyte counts above 4,000/mm^3.

Marrow suppression is usually more severe in patients with impaired kidney function. Patients with poor performance status have also experienced a higher incidence of severe leukopenia and thrombocytopenia.

The hematologic effects, although usually reversible, have resulted in infectious or hemorrhagic complications in 5% of the patients treated with carboplatin for injection, with drug related death occurring in less than 1% of the patients. Fever has also been reported in patients with neutropenia.

Anemia with hemoglobin less than 11 g/dL has been observed in 71% of the patients who started therapy with a baseline above that value. The incidence of anemia increases with increasing exposure to carboplatin. Transfusions have been administered to 26% of the patients treated with carboplatin (44% of previously treated ovarian cancer patients).

Bone marrow depression may be more severe when carboplatin is combined with other bone marrow suppressing drugs or with radiotherapy.

➤*Hepatic:* The incidences of abnormal liver function tests in patients with normal baseline values were reported as follows: Total bilirubin, 5%; AST, 15%; and alkaline phosphatase, 24% (5%, 19%, and 37%, respectively, in pretreated ovarian cancer patients). These abnormalities have generally been mild and reversible in about one-half of the cases, although the role of metastatic tumor in the liver may complicate the assessment in many patients. In a limited series of patients receiving very high dosages of carboplatin and autologous bone marrow transplantation, severe abnormalities of liver function tests were reported.

➤*Local:* Injection site reactions, including redness, swelling, and pain have been reported during postmarketing surveillance. Necrosis associated with extravasation has also been reported.

➤*Lab test abnormalities:* High dosages of carboplatin (greater than 4 times the recommended dose) have resulted in severe abnormalities of liver function tests. Total bilirubin, AST, and alkaline phosphatase abnormalities have generally been mild and reversible in approximately 50% of the cases.

➤*Renal:* Renal toxicity is limited, but concomitant treatment with aminoglycosides has resulted in increased renal or audiologic toxicity. Exercise caution when a patient receives both drugs. Development of abnormal renal function test results is uncommon, despite the fact that carboplatin, unlike cisplatin, has usually been administered without high-volume fluid hydration or forced diuresis. The incidences of abnormal renal function tests reported are 6% for serum creatinine and 14% for blood urea nitrogen (10% and 22%, respectively, in pretreated ovarian cancer patients). Most of these reported abnormalities have been mild and about one-half of them were reversible.

Creatinine clearance has proven to be the most sensitive measure of kidney function in patients receiving carboplatin, and it appears to be the most useful test for correlating drug clearance and bone marrow suppression. Twenty-seven percent (27%) of the patients who had a baseline value of 60 mL/min or more demonstrated a reduction below this value during carboplatin therapy.

➤*Miscellaneous:* Pain and asthenia were the most frequently reported miscellaneous adverse effects; their relationship to the tumor and to anemia was likely. Alopecia was reported (3%). Cardiovascular, respiratory, genitourinary, and mucosal side effects have occurred in 6% or less of the patients. Cardiovascular events (cardiac failure, embolism, cerebrovascular accidents) were fatal in less than 1% of the patients and did not appear to be related to chemotherapy. Cancer-associated hemolytic uremic syndrome has been reported rarely.

Malaise, anorexia, and hypertension have been reported as part of postmarketing surveillance.

Carboplatin Adverse Reactions in Patients with Ovarian Cancer (%)			
Adverse reactions		First line combination therapy*	Second line single agent therapy**
Bone marrow			
Thrombocytopenia	< 100,000/mm^3	66%	62%
	< 50,000/mm^3	33%	35%
Neutropenia	< 2000 cells/mm^3	96%	67%
	< 1000 cells/mm^3	82%	21%
Leukopenia	< 4000 cells/mm^3	97%	85%
	< 2000 cells/mm^3	71%	26%
Anemia	< 11 g/dL	90%	90%
	< 8 g/dL	14%	21%

CARBOPLATIN — INJECTION

Carboplatin Adverse Reactions in Patients with Ovarian Cancer (%)		
Adverse reactions	First line combination therapy*	Second line single agent therapy**
Infections	16%	5%
Bleeding	8%	5%
Transfusions	35%	44%
GI		
Nausea and vomiting	93%	92%
Vomiting	83%	81%
Other GI side effects	46%	21%
Neurologic		
Peripheral neuropathies	15%	6%
Ototoxicity	12%	1%
Other sensory side effects	5%	1%
Central neurotoxicity	26%	5%
Renal		
Serum creatinine elevations	6%	10%
Blood urea elevations	17%	22%
Hepatic		
Bilirubin elevations	5%	5%
AST elevations	20%	19%
Alkaline phosphatase elevations	29%	37%
Electrolytes loss		
Sodium	10%	47%
Potassium	16%	28%
Calcium	16%	31%
Magnesium	61%	43%
Other side effects		
Pain	44%	23%
Asthenia	41%	11%
Cardiovascular	19%	6%
Respiratory	10%	6%
Allergic	11%	2%
GU	10%	2%
Alopecia	49%	2%
Mucositis	8%	1%

* Use with cyclophosphamide for initial treatment of ovarian cancer: Data are based on the experience of 393 patients with ovarian cancer (regardless of baseline status) who received initial combination therapy with carboplatin and cyclophosphamide in 2 randomized controlled studies conducted by SWOG and NCIC.Combination with cyclophosphamide as well as duration of treatment may be responsible for the differences that can be noted in the adverse experiences table.

** Single agent use for the secondary treatment of ovarian cancer: Data are based on the experience of 553 patients with previously treated ovarian carcinoma (regardless of baseline status) who received single-agent carboplatin.

Overdosage

There is no known antidote for carboplatin overdosage. The anticipated complications of overdosage would be secondary to bone marrow suppression or hepatic toxicity.

CISPLATIN (CDDP)

Rx	**Cisplatin** (Various, eg, Abbott, American Pharmaceutical, Bedford Labs)	**Injection:** 1 mg/mL	In 50, 100, and 200 ml multi-dose vials.

CISPLATIN (CDDP) — INJECTION

WARNING

Cisplatin should be administered under the supervision of a qualified physician experienced in the use of cancer chemotherapeutic agents. Appropriate management of therapy and complications is possible only when adequate diagnostic and treatment facilities are readily available.

Cumulative renal toxicity – Cumulative renal toxicity associated with cisplatin is severe (see Warnings). Other major dose-related toxicities are myelosuppression, nausea, and vomiting.

Ototoxicity – Ototoxicity, which may be more pronounced in children, and is manifested by tinnitus or loss of high frequency hearing and, occasionally, deafness, is significant.

Anaphylactic-like reactions – Anaphylactic-like reactions have occurred (see Warnings). Facial edema, bronchoconstriction, tachycardia, and hypotension may occur within minutes of cisplatin administration. Epinephrine, corticosteroids, and antihistamines have been effectively employed to alleviate symptoms (see Warnings and Adverse Reactions).

Exercise caution to prevent inadvertent cisplatin overdose. Doses > 100 mg/m^2/cycle once every 3 to 4 weeks are rarely used. Care must be taken to avoid inadvertent cisplatin overdose due to confusion with carboplatin or prescribing practices that fail to differentiate daily doses from total dose per cycle.

Indications

➤*Metastatic testicular tumors:* In combination therapy in patients who have received appropriate surgical or radiotherapeutic procedures.

➤*Metastatic ovarian tumors:* In combination therapy (eg, cyclophosphamide) in patients who have received appropriate surgical or radiotherapeutic procedures. Cisplatin, as a single agent, is indicated as secondary therapy in patients refractory to standard chemotherapy who have not previously received cisplatin.

➤*Advanced bladder cancer:* As a single agent for patients with transitional cell bladder cancer no longer amenable to local treatments (eg, surgery or radiotherapy).

➤*Unlabeled uses:* Treatment of squamous cell carcinoma of the head and neck, cervix; lung carcinomas; osteogenic sarcoma; brain tumors; advanced esophageal, adrenal cortex, breast, endometrial, and liver carcinoma; bone marrow transplantation.

Administration and Dosage

For IV use only. Administer by IV infusion over 6 to 8 hours.

Note to pharmacist: Exercise caution to prevent inadvertent cisplatin overdosage. Please call prescriber if dose > 100 mg/m^2 per cycle. Aluminum and flip-off seal of vial have been imprinted with the following statement: Call Dr. if dose > 100 mg/m^2/cycle.

➤*Metastatic testicular tumors:* The usual cisplatin dose in combination with other approved chemotherapeutic agents is 20 mg/m^2/day IV for 5 days/cycle.

➤*Metastatic ovarian tumors:* In combination with cyclophosphamide:

Cisplatin – 75 to 100 mg/m^2 IV/cycle once every 4 weeks.

Cyclophosphamide – 600 mg/m^2 IV once every 4 weeks (Day 1).

In combination therapy, administer cisplatin and cyclophosphamide sequentially.

Administer cisplatin as a single agent at a dose of 100 mg/m^2 IV/cycle once every 4 weeks.

➤*Advanced bladder cancer:* Administer as a single agent. Give 50 to 70 mg/m^2 IV/cycle once every 3 to 4 weeks, depending on prior radiation therapy or chemotherapy. For heavily pretreated patients, give an initial dose of 50 mg/m^2/cycle repeated every 4 weeks.

➤*Repeat courses:* Do not give a repeat course until the serum creatinine is < 1.5 mg/dl or the BUN is < 25 mg/dl or until circulating blood elements are at an acceptable level (platelets ≥ 100,000/mm^3, WBC ≥ 4000/mm^3). Do not give subsequent doses until an audiometric analysis indicates that auditory acuity is within normal limits.

➤*Note:* Do not use needles or IV sets containing aluminum parts for preparation or administration. Aluminum reacts with cisplatin, causing precipitation and a loss of potency.

➤*Hydration:* Perform pretreatment hydration with 1 to 2 L fluid infused for 8 to 12 hours prior to dose. Then dilute the drug in 2 L of 5% Dextrose in ½ or ⅓ Normal Saline containing 37.5 g mannitol and infuse over 6 to 8 hours. If diluted solution is not to be used within 6 hours, protect from light. Do not dilute cisplatin in just 5% Dextrose Injection. Maintain adequate hydration and urinary output during the following 24 hours.

➤*Admixture compatibility:* Cisplatin and fluorouracil admixtures are stable in 0.9% Normal Saline for 1 hour.

➤*Storage/Stability:* Store at 15° to 25°C. Protect unopened container from light. Do not refrigerate. The cisplatin remaining in the amber vial following initial entry is stable for 28 days protected from light or for 7 days under fluorescent room light.

Actions

➤*Pharmacology:* Cisplatin is an inorganic heavy metal coordination complex containing a central atom of platinum surrounded by 2 chloride atoms and 2 ammonia molecules in the cis position. The antitumor effect of cisplatin has been correlated with binding to DNA, production of intrastrand crosslinks and formation of DNA adducts.

CISPLATIN (CDDP) — INJECTION

➤*Pharmacokinetics:*

Absorption/Distribution – Plasma concentrations of the parent compound, cisplatin, have a half-life of ≈ 20 to 30 minutes; the total body clearance and volume of distribution at steady-state are ≈ 15 L/hr/m² and ≈ 11 L/m², respectively. The ratios of cisplatin to total free platinum in the plasma vary considerably between patients and range from 0.5 to 1.1. Cisplatin does not undergo binding to plasma proteins; however, platinum is 90% bound to several plasma proteins including albumin, transferrin, and gamma globulin. The albumin-platinum complexes do not dissociate significantly and are slowly eliminated with a minimum half-life of ≥ 5 days.

Maximum red blood cell concentrations of platinum are reached within 90 to 150 minutes and have a terminal half-life of 36 to 47 days. Concentrations of platinum are highest in liver, prostate, and kidney, somewhat lower in bladder, muscle, testicle, pancreas, and spleen, and lowest in bowel, adrenal, heart, lung, cerebrum, and cerebellum. Platinum is present in tissues for as long as 180 days after the last administration.

Metabolism/Excretion – 90% of the drug is removed by renal mechanisms whereas < 10% is removed by biliary excretion. The parent compound, cisplatin, is excreted in the urine and accounts for 13% to 17% of the administered dose excreted within 1 hour of administration. The renal clearance of cisplatin and platinum exceed creatinine clearance, indicating active secretion by the kidney. The mean renal clearance of cisplatin is 50 to 62 ml/min/m²; platinum clearance is non-linear, variable, and dependent on dose, urine flow rate, and individual variability of active secretion and possible tubular reabsorption. Approximately 10% to 40% of the administered platinum is excreted in the urine within 24 hours with a mean of 35% to 51% excreted in the urine over 5 days.

Contraindications

Preexisting renal impairment; myelosuppression; hearing impairment; history of allergic reactions to cisplatin or other platinum-containing compounds.

Warnings

➤*Renal toxicity:* Dose-related and cumulative renal insufficiency is the major dose-limiting toxicity. Renal toxicity has been noted in 28% to 36% of patients treated with a single dose of 50 mg/m². First noted during the second week after a dose, it is manifested by elevations in BUN and creatinine, serum uric acid, or a decrease in creatinine clearance. Renal toxicity becomes more prolonged and severe with repeated courses of the drug. Renal function must return to normal before another dose can be given.

Amifostine can be used to reduce cumulative renal toxicity in patients with advanced ovarian cancer receiving repeated cisplatin administration.

Impairment of renal function is associated with renal tubular damage. The administration of cisplatin using a 6- to 8-hour infusion with IV hydration and mannitol has been used to reduce nephrotoxicity. However, renal toxicity can still occur (see Precautions).

➤*Ototoxicity:* Ototoxicity has occurred in ≤ 31% of patients given a single 50 mg/m² dose. It is manifested by tinnitus or hearing loss in the high frequency range (4000 to 8000 Hz); decreased ability to hear normal conversational tones occurs occasionally. Ototoxic effects may be more severe in children. Hearing loss can be unilateral or bilateral and is more frequent and severe with repeated doses. Ototoxicity may be enhanced with prior or simultaneous cranial irradiation. It is unclear whether ototoxicity is reversible. Ototoxic effects may be related to the peak plasma concentration of cisplatin. Because ototoxicity of cisplatin is cumulative, carefully perform audiometry before starting therapy and prior to subsequent doses. Vestibular toxicity has occurred. Deafness after the initial dose of cisplatin has been reported rarely.

Ototoxicity may become more severe in patients being treated with other drugs with nephrotoxic potential.

➤*Hematologic:* Myelosuppression occurs in 25% to 30% of patients treated with cisplatin. The nadirs in circulating platelets and leukocytes occur between days 18 and 23 (range, 7.5 to 45); most patients recover by day 39 (range, 13 to 62). Leukopenia and thrombocytopenia are more pronounced at doses > 50 mg/m². Anemia (decrease of 2 g hemoglobin/dL) occurs at the same frequency and with the same timing as leukopenia and thrombocytopenia. Fever and infection also have been reported in patients with neutropenia.

In addition to anemia secondary to myelosuppression, a Coombs' positive hemolytic anemia has been reported. In the presence of cisplatin hemolytic anemia, a further course of treatment may be accompanied by increased hemolysis and this risk should be weighed by the treating physician.

The development of acute leukemia coincident with the use of cisplatin has rarely been reported in humans. In these reports, cisplatin was generally given in combination with other leukemogenic agents.

➤*Hepatotoxicity:* Transient elevations of liver enzymes, especially AST, as well as bilirubin, have been reported to be associated with cisplatin administration at the recommended doses.

➤*Vascular toxicities:* Vascular toxicities coincident with use of cisplatin in combination with other antineoplastic agents have occurred rarely. The events are clinically heterogeneous and may include MI, cerebrovascular accident, thrombotic microangiopathy, or cerebral arteritis. Various mechanisms have been proposed for these vascular complications. There are also reports of Raynaud's phenomenon occurring in patients treated with the combination of bleomycin and vinblastine with or without cisplatin. Hypomagnesemia developing coincident with use of cisplatin may be an added, although not essential, factor associated with this event. However, it is currently unknown if the cause of Raynaud's phenomenon in these cases is the disease, underlying vascular compromise, bleomycin, vinblastine, hypomagnesemia, or a combination of any of these factors.

➤*Hyperuricemia:* Hyperuricemia occurs at approximately the same frequency as increases in BUN and serum creatinine. It is more pronounced after doses > 50 mg/m², and peak uric acid levels generally occur 3 to 5 days after the dose. Allopurinol therapy is effective.

➤*Electrolyte disturbance:* Hypomagnesemia, hypocalcemia, hyponatremia, hypokalemia, and hypophosphatemia have occurred and are probably related to renal tubular damage. Tetany has occasionally occurred in those patients with hypocalcemia and hypomagnesemia. Generally, normal serum electrolyte levels are restored by administering supplemental electrolytes and discontinuing cisplatin.

Increased plasma iron levels and inappropriate antidiuretic hormone syndrome also have occurred.

➤*Ophthalmic effects:* Optic neuritis, papilledema, and cerebral blindness have occurred infrequently in patients receiving standard recommended cisplatin doses. Improvement or total recovery usually occurs after drug discontinuation. Steroids with or without mannitol have been used; however, efficacy has not been established.

Blurred vision and altered color perception have occurred after the use of regimens with higher doses or greater dose frequencies than those recommended. The altered color perception manifests as a loss of color discrimination, particularly in the blue-yellow axis. The only finding on funduscopic exam is irregular retinal pigmentation of the macular area.

➤*Neuropathies:* Neurotoxicity, usually characterized by peripheral neuropathy, has occurred. Severe neuropathies have occurred in patients receiving higher doses of cisplatin or greater dose frequencies than those recommended or after prolonged therapy (4 to 7 months); however, neurologic symptoms have been reported to occur after a single dose. Although symptoms and signs of cisplatin neuropathy usually develop during treatment, symptoms of neuropathy may begin 3 to 8 weeks after the last dose of cisplatin (rare). These neuropathies may be irreversible and are seen as paresthesias in a stocking-glove distribution, areflexia, and loss of proprioception and vibratory sensation. Loss of motor function also has occurred. Discontinue therapy when symptoms are first observed. Neuropathy may progress further even after stopping treatment. Preliminary evidence suggests peripheral neuropathy may be irreversible in some patients.

➤*High/Cumulative doses:* Muscle cramps, defined as localized, painful, involuntary skeletal muscle contractions of sudden onset and short duration, have occurred and were usually associated in patients receiving a relatively high cumulative dose of cisplatin and with a relatively advanced symptomatic stage of peripheral neuropathy.

➤*Hypersensitivity reactions:* Anaphylactic-like reactions have occurred. Facial edema, wheezing, tachycardia, and hypotension may occur within minutes of use in patients with prior drug exposure. Symptoms are alleviated by use of epinephrine, corticosteroids, and antihistamines. Refer to Management of Acute Hypersensitivity Reactions.

➤*Mutagenesis:* The drug is mutagenic in bacteria and produces chromosome aberrations in animal cell tissue cultures.

➤*Pregnancy: Category D.* Of 7 reported pregnancy cases, 1 infant developed profound leukopenia with neutropenia, which resolved after 10 days. The mother had developed profound neutropenia just prior to delivery. By 12 weeks of age, the child was developing normally, except for moderate bilateral hearing loss. Advise patients to avoid becoming pregnant.

➤*Lactation:* Cisplatin has been reported to be found in breast milk; patients receiving cisplatin should not breastfeed.

➤*Children:* Safety and efficacy in children have not been established.

Precautions

➤*Monitoring:* Monitor peripheral blood counts weekly and liver function periodically. Measure serum creatinine, BUN, creatinine clearance, magnesium, sodium, calcium, and potassium levels prior to initiating therapy and prior to each subsequent course. Do not give more frequently than once every 3 to 4 weeks at the recommended dosage. Perform neurologic and auditory examinations regularly. Carefully perform audiometry before starting therapy and prior to subsequent doses.

➤*GI:* Marked nausea and vomiting occur in almost all patients and are occasionally so severe that the drug must be discontinued. Nausea and vomiting usually begin 1 to 4 hours after treatment and last up to 24 hours; nausea and anorexia may persist for up to 1 week after treatment. Metoclopramide in high doses has been used in the prophylaxis of vomiting associated with cisplatin therapy. Delayed nausea and vomiting (beginning or persisting ≥ 24 hours after chemotherapy) has occurred in patients attaining complete emetic control on the day of therapy.

Drug Interactions

Cisplatin Drug Interactions

Precipitant drug	Object drug[a]		Description
Aminoglycosides	Cisplatin	⬆	Cisplatin produces cumulative nephrotoxicity that is potentiated by aminoglycosides (see Warnings).
Loop diuretics	Cisplatin	⬆	Concomitant use of loop diuretics and cisplatin may produce additive ototoxicity (see Warnings).

CISPLATIN (CDDP) — INJECTION

Cisplatin Drug Interactions			
Precipitant drug	Object drug[a]		Description
Cisplatin	Phenytoin	↓	Combination chemotherapy (including cisplatin) may reduce phenytoin plasma levels.

[a] ↑ = Object drug increased. ↓ = Object drug decreased.

Adverse Reactions

➤*CNS:* Peripheral neuropathies; seizures; dorsal column myelopathy; malaise; Lhermitte's sign; autonomic neuropathy (see Warnings).

➤*Dermatologic:* Local soft tissue toxicity has rarely been reported following extravasation of cisplatin. Severity of the local tissue toxicity appears to be related to the concentration of the cisplatin solution. Infusion of solutions with a cisplatin concentration > 0.5 mg/mL may result in tissue cellulitis, fibrosis, and necrosis.

➤*Electrolyte disturbance:* Hypomagnesemia; hypocalcemia; hyponatremia; hypokalemia; hypophosphatemia; increased plasma iron levels; antidiuretic hormone syndrome (see Warnings).

➤*GI:* Nausea, vomiting, anorexia (see Precautions); diarrhea; loss of taste.

➤*Hematologic:* Myelosuppression (25% to 30%); leukopenia; thrombocytopenia; anemia (see Warnings).

➤*Ophthalmic:* Optic neuritis, papilledema, cerebral blindness (infrequent); blurred vision; altered color perception (see Warnings).

➤*Renal:* Renal insufficiency, renal tubular damage (see Warnings).

➤*Special senses:* Tinnitus, high frequency hearing loss, vestibular toxicity (see Warnings).

➤*Miscellaneous:* Vascular toxicities (rare); hyperuricemia, ototoxicity, anaphylactic-like reactions (see Warnings); elevated AST; alopecia; asthenia.

Infrequent – Cardiac abnormalities; hiccups; rash; elevated serum amylase.

Overdosage

➤*Symptoms:* Exercise caution to prevent inadvertent overdosage with cisplatin. Acute overdosage with this drug may result in kidney failure, liver failure, deafness, ocular toxicity (including detachment of the retina), significant myelosuppression, intractable nausea and vomiting, or neuritis. In addition, death can occur following overdosage.

➤*Treatment:* No proven antidotes have been established for cisplatin overdosage. Hemodialysis, even when initiated 4 hours after the overdosage, appears to have little effect on removing platinum from the body because of cisplatin's rapid and high degree of protein binding. Management of overdosage should include general supportive measures to sustain the patient through any period of toxicity that may occur. Refer to General Management of Acute Overdosage.

OXALIPLATIN

Rx	Eloxatin (Sanofi-Synthelabo)	Injection: 50 mg	Preservative free. In single-use vials.
		100 mg	Preservative free. In single-use vials.

OXALIPLATIN — INJECTION

WARNING

Administer oxaliplatin under the supervision of a qualified health care provider experienced in the use of cancer chemotherapeutic agents. Appropriate management of therapy and complications is possible only when adequate diagnostic and treatment facilities are readily available.

Anaphylactic-like reactions to oxaliplatin have been reported, and may occur within minutes of administration. Epinephrine, corticosteroids, and antihistamines have been employed to alleviate symptoms.

Indications

➤*Adjuvant treatment of stage III colon cancer:* In combination with infusional 5-fluorouracil/leucovorin for adjuvant treatment of stage III colon cancer patients who have undergone complete resection of the primary tumor.

➤*Advanced carcinoma of the colon or rectum:* In combination with infusional 5-fluorouracil/leucovorin for the treatment of advanced carcinoma of the colon or rectum.

➤*Unlabeled uses:* Treatment of relapsed or refractory non-Hodgkin lymphoma; treatment of advanced ovarian cancer.

Administration and Dosage

➤*Approved by the FDA:* August 9, 2002.

➤*Adjuvant treatment in stage III colon cancer:* Recommended for a total of 6 months (ie, 12 cycles, every 2 weeks), according to the dose schedule for previously treated patients with advanced colorectal cancer.

➤*Advanced colorectal cancer (previously untreated and previously treated patients):*

- Day 1: oxaliplatin 85 mg/m^2 intravenous (IV) infusion in 5% dextrose in water (D5W) 250 to 500 mL and leucovorin 200 mg/m^2 IV infusion in D5W both given over 120 minutes at the same time in separate bags using a Y-line, followed by 5-fluorouracil 400 mg/m^2 IV bolus given over 2 to 4 minutes, followed by 5-fluorouracil 600 mg/m^2 IV infusion in D5W 500 mL (recommended) as a 22-hour continuous infusion.
- Day 2: leucovorin 200 mg/m^2 IV infusion over 120 minutes, followed by 5-fluorouracil 400 mg/m^2 IV bolus given over 2 to 4 minutes, followed by 5-fluorouracil 600 mg/m^2 IV infusion in D5W 500 mL (recommended) as a 22-hour continuous infusion.

Repeat cycle every 2 weeks.

Premedication – Premedication with antiemetics, including 5-HT$_3$ blockers with or without dexamethasone, is recommended.

Dose modification – Prior to subsequent therapy cycles, patients should be evaluated for clinical toxicities and laboratory tests. Prolongation of infusion time for oxaliplatin from 2 to 6 hours decreases the maximum drug concentration (C_{max}) by an estimated 32% and may mitigate acute toxicities. The infusion times for infusional 5-fluorouracil and leucovorin do not need to be changed.

➤*Adjuvant therapy in stage III colon cancer:* For patients who experience persistent grade 2 neurosensory events that do not resolve, a dose reduction of oxaliplatin to 75 mg/m^2 should be considered. For patients with persistent grade 3 neurosensory events, discontinuing therapy should be considered. The infusional 5-fluorouracil/leucovorin regimen need not be altered.

A dose reduction of oxaliplatin to 75 mg/m^2 and infusional 5-fluorouracil to 300 mg/m^2 bolus and 500 mg/m^2 22-hour infusion is recommended for patients after recovery from grade 3/4 GI (despite prophylactic treatment) or grade 4 neutropenia or grade 3/4 thrombocytopenia. The next dose should be delayed until neutrophils are 1.5 × 10^9/L or more and platelets are 75 × 10^9/L or more.

➤*Advanced colorectal cancer (previously untreated and previously treated patients):* For patients who experience persistent grade 2 neurosensory events that do not resolve, a dose reduction of oxaliplatin to 65 mg/m^2 should be considered. For patients with persistent grade 3 neurosensory events, discontinuing therapy should be considered. The 5-fluorouracil/leucovorin regimen need not be altered.

A dose reduction of oxaliplatin to 65 mg/m^2 and 5-fluorouracil by 20% (300 mg/m^2 and 500 mg/m^2 22-hour infusion) is recommended for patients after recovery from grade 3/4 GI (despite prophylactic treatment), grade 4 neutropenia, or grade 3/4 thrombocytopenia. The next dose should be delayed until: neutrophils are greater than or equal to 1.5 × 10^9/L and platelets are greater than or equal to 75 × 10^9/L.

➤*Preparation for administration:* Do not freeze and protect the concentrated solution from light. A final dilution must never be performed with a sodium chloride solution or other chloride-containing solutions. The solution must be further diluted in an infusion solution of 250 to 500 mL of 5% dextrose injection.

Incompatibilities – Oxaliplatin is incompatible in solution with alkaline medications or media (such as basic solutions of 5-fluorouracil) and must not be mixed with these or administered simultaneously through the same infusion line. The infusion line should be flushed with D5W prior to administration of any concomitant medications.

Needles or IV administration sets containing aluminum parts that may come in contact with oxaliplatin should not be used for the preparation or mixing of the drug. Aluminum has been reported to cause degradation of platinum compounds.

➤*Storage/Stability:* Store at 25°C (77°F); excursions permitted to 15° to 30°C (59° to 86°F). Do not freeze and protect from light (keep in original outer carton). After dilution with 250 to 500 mL of 5% dextrose injection, the shelf life is 6 hours at room temperature (20° to 25°C [68° to 77°F]) or up to 24 hours under refrigeration (2° to 8°C [36° to 46°F]). After final dilution, protection from light is not required.

Actions

➤*Pharmacology:* Oxaliplatin undergoes nonenzymatic conversion in physiologic solutions to active derivatives via displacement of the labile oxalate ligand. Several transient reactive species are formed, including monoaquo and diaquo diaminocyclohexane (DACH) platinum, which covalently bind with macromolecules. Both inter- and intrastrand Pt-deoxyribonucleic acid (DNA) crosslinks are formed. Crosslinks are formed between the N7 positions of 2 adjacent guanines (GG), adjacent adenine-guanines (AG), and guanines separated by an intervening nucleotide (GNG). These crosslinks inhibit DNA replication and transcription. Cytotoxicity is cell-cycle nonspecific.

In vivo studies have shown antitumor activity of oxaliplatin against colon carcinoma. In combination with 5-fluorouracil, oxaliplatin exhibits in vitro and in vivo antiproliferative activity greater than either compound alone in several tumor models (HT29 [colon], GR [mammary], and L1210 [leukemia]).

OXALIPLATIN — INJECTION

➤*Pharmacokinetics:*

Absorption / Distribution – The reactive oxaliplatin derivatives are present as a fraction of the unbound platinum in plasma ultrafiltrate. The decline of ultrafilterable platinum levels following oxaliplatin administration is triphasic, characterized by 2 relatively short distribution phases ($t_{½\alpha}$: 0.43 hours and $t_{½\beta}$: 16.8 hours) and a long terminal elimination phase ($t_{½\gamma}$: 391 hours). Pharmacokinetic parameters obtained after a single 2-hour IV infusion of oxaliplatin at a dose of 85 mg/m^2 expressed as an ultrafilterable platinum were a C_{max} of 0.814 mcg/mL and a volume of distribution of 440 L.

Interpatient and intrapatient variability in ultrafilterable platinum exposure (area under the curve [AUC $_{0-48h}$]) assessed over 3 cycles was moderate to low (23% and 6%, respectively). A pharmacodynamic relationship between platinum ultrafiltrate level and clinical safety and efficacy has not been established.

At the end of a 2-hour infusion of oxaliplatin, approximately 15% of the administered platinum is present in the systemic circulation. The remaining 85% is rapidly distributed into tissues or eliminated in the urine. In patients, plasma protein binding of platinum is irreversible and is greater than 90%. The main binding proteins are albumin and gamma-globulins. Platinum also binds irreversibly and accumulates (approximately 2-fold) in erythrocytes, where it appears to have no relevant activity. No platinum accumulation was observed in plasma ultrafiltrate following 85 mg/m^2 every 2 weeks.

Metabolism – Oxaliplatin undergoes rapid and extensive nonenzymatic biotransformation. There is no evidence of cytochrome P-450–mediated metabolism in vitro.

Up to 17 platinum-containing derivatives have been observed in plasma ultrafiltrate samples from patients, including several cytotoxic species (monochloro DACH platinum, dichloro DACH platinum, and monoaquo and diaquo DACH platinum) and a number of noncytotoxic, conjugated species.

Excretion – The major route of platinum elimination is renal excretion. At 5 days after a single 2-hour infusion of oxaliplatin, urinary elimination accounted for about 54% of the platinum eliminated, with fecal excretion accounting for only about 2%. Platinum was cleared from plasma at a rate (10 to 17 L/h) that was similar to or exceeded the average human glomerular filtration rate (GFR; 7.5 L/h). There was no significant effect of gender on the clearance of ultrafilterable platinum. The renal clearance of ultrafilterable platinum is significantly correlated with GFR.

Special populations –

Renal function impairment: The AUC $_{0-48h}$ of platinum in the plasma ultrafiltrate increases as renal function decreases. The AUC $_{0-48h}$ of platinum in patients with mild (creatinine clearance [Ccr] 50 to 80 mL/min), moderate (Ccr 30 to less than 50 mL/min), and severe renal (Ccr less than 30 mL/min) function impairment is increased by about 60%, 140%, and 190%, respectively, compared with patients with normal renal function (Ccr greater than 80 mL/min).

Contraindications

History of known allergy to oxaliplatin or other platinum compounds.

Warnings

➤*Hypersensitivity reactions:* As in the case for other platinum compounds, hypersensitivity and anaphylactic/anaphylactoid reactions to oxaliplatin have been reported. These allergic reactions were similar in nature and severity to those reported with other platinum-containing compounds (ie, rash, urticaria, erythema, pruritus; bronchospasm, hypotension [rare]). These reactions occur within minutes of administration; manage with appropriate supportive therapy. Drug-related deaths associated with platinum compounds from this reaction have been reported.

➤*Renal function impairment:* The safety and efficacy of the combination of oxaliplatin and 5-fluorouracil/leucovorin in patients with renal impairment have not been evaluated. Use caution with the combination of oxaliplatin and 5-fluorouracil/leucovorin in patients with preexisting renal impairment because the primary route of platinum elimination is renal. Clearance of ultrafilterable platinum is decreased in patients with mild, moderate, and severe renal impairment. A pharmacodynamic relationship between platinum ultrafiltrate levels and clinical safety and efficacy has not been established.

➤*Mutagenesis:* Oxaliplatin was not mutagenic to bacteria (Ames test) but was mutagenic to mammalian cells in vitro (L5178Y mouse lymphoma assay). Oxaliplatin was clastogenic in vitro (chromosome aberration in human lymphocytes) and in vivo (mouse bone marrow micronucleus assay).

➤*Fertility impairment:* In a fertility study, male rats were given oxaliplatin at 0, 0.5, 1, or 2 mg/kg/day for 5 days every 21 days for a total of 3 cycles prior to mating with females that received 2 cycles of oxaliplatin on the same schedule. A dosage of 2 mg/kg/day (less than 1/7 the recommended human dose on a body surface area basis) did not affect pregnancy rate, but caused developmental mortality (increased early resorptions, decreased live fetuses, decreased live births) and delayed growth (decreased fetal weight).

Testicular damage, characterized by degeneration, hypoplasia, and atrophy, was observed in dogs administered oxaliplatin at 0.75 mg/kg/day for 5 days every 28 days for 3 cycles. A no-effect level was not identified. This daily dose is approximately 1/6 the recommended human dose on a body surface area basis.

➤*Elderly:* See Adverse Reactions for more information.

➤*Pregnancy:* *Category D.* Oxaliplatin may cause fetal harm when administered to a pregnant woman. Pregnant rats were administered oxaliplatin 1 mg/kg/day (less than 1/10 the recommended human dose based on body surface area) during gestation days 1 to 5 (preimplantation), 6 to 10, or 11 to 16 (during organogenesis). Oxaliplatin caused developmental mortality (increased early resorptions) when administered on days 6 to 10 and 11 to 16 and adversely affected fetal growth (decreased fetal weight, delayed ossification) when administered on days 6 to 10. If this drug is used during pregnancy or if the patient becomes pregnant while taking this drug, apprise the patient of the potential hazard to the fetus. Advise women of childbearing potential to avoid becoming pregnant while receiving treatment with oxaliplatin.

➤*Lactation:* It is not known whether oxaliplatin or its derivatives are excreted in human milk. Because many drugs are excreted in human milk and because of the potential for serious adverse reactions in breast-feeding infants from oxaliplatin, decide whether to discontinue breast-feeding or delay the use of the drug, taking into account the importance of the drug to the mother.

➤*Children:* The safety and efficacy of oxaliplatin in children have not been established.

Precautions

➤*Monitoring:* Standard monitoring of the white blood cell count with differential, hemoglobin, platelet count, and blood chemistries (including ALT, AST, bilirubin, creatinine) is recommended before each oxaliplatin cycle. Patients receiving oxaliplatin plus 5-fluorouracil/leucovorin and requiring oral anticoagulants may require closer monitoring.

➤*Administration:* See the Warning box for more information.

➤*Hepatotoxicity:* Hepatotoxicity, as evidenced in the adjuvant study by increase in transaminases (57% vs 34%) and alkaline phosphatase (42% vs 20%), was observed more commonly in the oxaliplatin combination arm. The incidence of increased bilirubin was similar on both arms. Changes noted on liver biopsies include: peliosis, nodular regenerative hyperplasia or sinusoidal alterations, perisinusoidal fibrosis, and veno-occlusive lesions. Consider hepatic vascular disorders and, if appropriate, investigate in case of abnormal liver function test results or portal hypertension that cannot be explained by liver metastases.

➤*Neuropathy:*

Stage II or III colon cancer – See Adverse Reactions for more information.

Advanced colorectal cancer (previously untreated and previously treated patients) – See Adverse Reactions for more information.

➤*Pulmonary toxicity:* Oxaliplatin has been associated with pulmonary fibrosis (less than 1% of study patients), which may be fatal. The combined incidence of cough and dyspnea was 7.4% (any grade) and less than 1% (grade 3) with no grade 4 events in the oxaliplatin plus infusional 5-fluorouracil/leucovorin arm compared with 4.5% (any grade) and no grade 3 and 0.1% grade 4 events in the infusional 5-fluorouracil/leucovorin alone arm in adjuvant colon cancer patients. In this study, 1 patient died from eosinophil pneumonia in the oxaliplatin combination arm. The combined incidence of cough, dyspnea, and hypoxia was 43% (any grade) and 7% (grade 3 and 4) in the oxaliplatin plus 5-fluorouracil/leucovorin arm compared with 32% (any grade) and 5% (grade 3 and 4) in the irinotecan plus 5-fluorouracil/leucovorin arm of unknown duration for patients with previously untreated colorectal cancer. In case of unexplained respiratory symptoms such as nonproductive cough, dyspnea, crackles, or radiological pulmonary infiltrates, discontinue oxaliplatin until further pulmonary investigation excludes interstitial lung disease or pulmonary fibrosis.

Drug Interactions

➤*Anticoagulants:* There have been reports while in study and from postmarketing surveillance of prolonged prothrombin time and international normalized ratio (INR) occasionally associated with hemorrhage in patients who received oxaliplatin plus 5-fluorouracil/leucovorin while on anticoagulants.

➤*5-fluorouracil / leucovorin:* No pharmacokinetic interaction between oxaliplatin 85 mg/m^2 and 5-fluorouracil/leucovorin has been observed in patients treated every 2 weeks. Increases of 5-fluorouracil/leucovorin plasma concentrations by approximately 20% have been observed with doses of 130 mg/m^2 oxaliplatin dosed every 3 weeks.

➤*Nephrotoxic drugs:* Because platinum-containing species are eliminated primarily through the kidney, clearance of these products may be decreased by coadministration of potentially nephrotoxic compounds; although, this has not been specifically studied.

Adverse Reactions

The most common adverse reactions in patients with stage II or III colon cancer receiving adjuvant therapy were anemia, diarrhea, emesis, fatigue, increase in transaminases and alkaline phosphatase, nausea, neutropenia, peripheral sensory neuropathy, stomatitis, and thrombocytopenia. The most common adverse reactions in previously untreated and treated patients were diarrhea, emesis, fatigue, nausea, neutropenia, and peripheral sensory neuropathies.

➤*Combination adjuvant therapy with oxaliplatin and infusional 5-fluorouracil / leucovorin in patients with stage II or III colon cancer:* One thousand one hundred eight patients with stage II or III colon cancer who had undergone complete resection of the primary tumor have been treated in a clinical study with oxaliplatin in combination with infusional 5-fluorouracil/leucovorin. The incidence of grade 3 or 4 adverse reactions was 70% in the oxaliplatin combination arm and 31% on the infusional 5-fluorouracil/leucovorin arm. The adverse reactions in this trial are shown in the following tables. Discontinuation of treatment due to adverse reactions occurred in 15% of the patients receiving oxaliplatin and infusional

OXALIPLATIN — INJECTION

5-fluorouracil/leucovorin. Both 5-fluorouracil/leucovorin and oxaliplatin are associated with GI or hematologic adverse reactions. When oxaliplatin is administered in combination with infusional 5-fluorouracil/leucovorin, the incidence of these reactions is increased.

The incidence of death within 28 days of last treatment, regardless of causality, was 0.5% (n = 6) in the oxaliplatin combination and infusional 5-fluorouracil/leucovorin arms, respectively. Deaths within 60 days from initiation of therapy were 0.3% (n = 3) in the oxaliplatin combination and infusional 5-fluorouracil/leucovorin arms, respectively. On the oxaliplatin combination arm, 3 deaths were due to sepsis/neutropenic sepsis, 2 from intracerebral bleeding, and 1 from eosinophilic pneumonia. On the 5-fluorouracil/leucovorin arm, 1 death was due to suicide, 2 from Stevens-Johnson syndrome (1 patient also had sepsis), 1 unknown cause, 1 anoxic cerebral infarction, and 1 probable abdominal aorta rupture.

Oxaliplatin Adverse Reactions (≥ 5%)

Adverse reaction	Oxaliplatin + 5-fluorouracil/ leucovorin (n = 1,108) All grades	Grade 3/4	5-fluorouracil/ leucovorin (n = 1,111) All grades	Grades 3/4
Any event	100%	70%	99%	31%
CNS				
Fatigue	44%	4%	38%	1%
Overall peripheral sensory neuropathy	92%	12%	16%	< 1%
Dermatologic				
Skin disorder	32%	2%	36%	2%
GI				
Abdominal pain	18%	1%	17%	2%
Anorexia	13%	1%	8%	< 1%
Diarrhea	56%	11%	48%	7%
Nausea	74%	5%	61%	2%
Stomatitis	42%	3%	40%	2%
Vomiting	47%	6%	24%	1%
Miscellaneous				
Allergic reaction	10%	3%	2%	< 1%
Fever	27%	1%	12%	1%
Infection	25%	4%	25%	3%
Injection site reaction[a]	11%	3%	10%	3%

[a] Includes thrombosis related to the catheter.

Oxaliplatin Adverse Reactions (≥ 5%)

Adverse reaction	Oxaliplatin + 5-fluorouracil/ leucovorin (n = 1,108) All grades	5-fluorouracil/ leucovorin (n = 1,111) All grades
CNS		
Headache	7%	5%
Sensory disturbance	8%	1%
Dermatologic		
Alopecia	30%	28%
GI		
Constipation	22%	19%
Dyspepsia	8%	5%
Taste perversion	12%	8%
Metabolic/Nutritional		
Phosphate alkaline increased	42%	20%
Weight increase	10%	10%
Respiratory		
Dyspnea	5%	3%
Epistaxis	16%	12%
Rhinitis	6%	8%
Special senses		
Conjunctivitis	9%	15%
Lacrimation abnormal	4%	12%
Miscellaneous		
Pain	5%	5%

Although specific reactions can vary, the overall frequency of adverse reactions was similar in men and women and in patients younger than 65 years of age and 65 years of age and older. However, the following grade 3/4 reactions were more common in women: diarrhea, fatigue, granulocytopenia, nausea, and vomiting. In patients 65 years of age and older, the incidence of grade 3/4 diarrhea and granulocytopenia was higher than in younger patients. Insufficient subgroup sizes prevented analysis of safety by race. The following additional adverse reactions were reported in 2% or more and less than 5% of the patients in the oxaliplatin and infusional 5-fluorouracil/leucovorin combination arm: coughing, leukopenia, pain, weight decrease.

Patients previously untreated for advanced colorectal cancer – Both 5-fluorouracil and oxaliplatin are associated with GI and hematologic adverse reactions. When oxaliplatin is administered in combination with 5-fluorouracil, the incidence of these reactions is increased.

The incidence of death within 30 days of treatment in the previously untreated advanced colorectal cancer study, regardless of causality, was 3% with the oxaliplatin and 5-fluorouracil/leucovorin combination, 5% with irinotecan plus 5-fluorouracil/leucovorin, and 3% with oxaliplatin plus irinotecan. Deaths within 60 days from initiation of therapy were 2.3% with the oxaliplatin and 5-fluorouracil/leucovorin combination, 5.1% with irinotecan plus 5-fluorouracil/leucovorin, and 3.1% with oxaliplatin plus irinotecan.

Oxaliplatin Adverse Reactions (≥ 5%)

Adverse reaction	Oxaliplatin + 5-fluorouracil/ leucovorin (n = 259) All grades	Grade 3/4	Irinotecan + 5-fluorouracil/ leucovorin (n = 256) All grades	Grade 3/4	Oxaliplatin + irinotecan (n= 258) All grades	Grade 3/4
Any reaction	99%	82%	98%	70%	99%	76%
Cardiovascular						
Hypotension	5%	3%	6%	3%	4%	3%
Thrombosis	6%	5%	6%	6%	3%	3%
CNS						
Fatigue	70%	7%	58%	11%	66%	16%
Neuralgia	5%	0%	0%	0%	2%	1%
Neuro NOS[a]	1%	0%	1%	0%	1%	0%
Neurosensory	12%	1%	2%	0%	9%	1%
Overall neuropathy	82%	19%	18%	2%	69%	7%
Paresthesias	77%	18%	16%	2%	62%	6%
Pharyngolaryngeal dysesthesias	38%	2%	1%	0%	28%	1%
Dermatologic						
Skin reaction, hand/foot	7%	1%	2%	1%	1%	0%
GI						
Abdominal pain	29%	8%	31%	7%	39%	10%
Anorexia	35%	2%	25%	4%	27%	5%
Constipation	32%	4%	27%	2%	21%	2%
Diarrhea	56%	12%	65%	29%	76%	25%
Diarrhea-colostomy	13%	2%	16%	7%	16%	3%
GI NOS[a]	5%	2%	4%	2%	3%	2%
Nausea	71%	6%	67%	15%	83%	19%
Stomatitis	38%	0%	25%	1%	19%	1%
Vomiting	41%	4%	43%	13%	64%	23%
GU						
Urinary frequency	5%	1%	2%	1%	3%	1%
Hematologic						
Febrile neutropenia	4%	4%	15%	14%	12%	11%
Lymphopenia	6%	2%	4%	1%	5%	2%
Metabolic/Nutritional						
Dehydration	9%	5%	16%	11%	14%	7%
Hyperglycemia	14%	2%	11%	3%	12%	3%
Hypoalbuminemia	8%	0%	5%	2%	9%	1%
Hypokalemia	11%	3%	7%	4%	6%	2%
Hyponatremia	8%	2%	7%	4%	4%	1%
Musculoskeletal						
Myalgia	14%	2%	6%	0%	9%	2%
Respiratory						
Cough	35%	1%	25%	2%	17%	1%
Dyspnea	18%	7%	14%	3%	11%	2%
Special senses						
Abnormal vision	5%	0%	2%	1%	6%	1%

OXALIPLATIN — INJECTION

Oxaliplatin Adverse Reactions (≥ 5%)						
	Oxaliplatin + 5-fluorouracil/ leucovorin (n = 259)		Irinotecan + 5-fluorouracil/ leucovorin (n = 256)		Oxaliplatin + irinotecan (n= 258)	
Adverse reaction	All grades	Grade 3/4	All grades	Grade 3/4	All grades	Grade 3/4
Miscellaneous						
Hiccups	5%	1%	2%	0%	3%	2%
Hypersensitivity	12%	2%	5%	0%	6%	1%
Infection, ANC	8%	8%	12%	11%	9%	8%
Infection, no ANC	10%	4%	5%	1%	7%	2%
Injection-site reaction	6%	0%	1%	0%	4%	1%
Pain	7%	1%	5%	1%	6%	1%

[a] NOS = not otherwise specified.

Oxaliplatin Adverse Reactions (≥ 5%)			
	Oxaliplatin + 5-fluorouracil/ leucovorin (n = 259)	Irinotecan + 5-fluorouracil/ leucovorin (n = 256)	Oxaliplatin + irinotecan (n =258)
Adverse reactions	All grades	All grades	All grades
CNS			
Anxiety	5%	2%	0%
Depression	9%	5%	7%
Dizziness	8%	6%	10%
Headache	13%	6%	9%
Insomnia	13%	9%	11%
Dermatologic			
Alopecia	38%	44%	67%
Dry skin	6%	2%	5%
Flushing	7%	2%	5%
Pruritus	6%	4%	2%
Rash	11%	4%	7%
Sweating	5%	6%	12%
GI			
Dyspepsia	12%	7%	5%
Dysphasia	5%	3%	3%
Flatulence	9%	6%	5%
Mouth dryness	5%	2%	3%
Taste perversion	14%	6%	8%
Metabolic/Nutritional			
Edema	15%	13%	10%
Elevated creatinine	4%	4%	5%
Hypocalcemia	7%	5%	4%
Weight loss	11%	9%	11%
Respiratory			
Epistaxis	10%	2%	2%
Rhinitis, allergic	10%	6%	6%
Special senses			
Tearing	9%	1%	2%
Miscellaneous			
Arthralgia	5%	5%	8%
Fever, no ANC	16%	9%	9%
Rigors	8%	2%	7%

Adverse reactions were similar in men and women and in patients younger than 65 years of age and 65 years of age and older, but older patients may have been more susceptible to dehydration, diarrhea, hypokalemia, leukopenia, fatigue, and syncope. The following additional adverse reactions, at least possibly related to treatment and potentially important, were reported in greater than or equal to 2% and less than 5% of the patients in the oxaliplatin and infusional 5-fluorouracil/leucovorin combination arm: bone pain, catheter infection, chest pain, dysuria, hypertension, hypoxia, metabolic, nail changes, pigmentation changes, pneumonitis, prothrombin time, pulmonary, rectal bleeding, rectal pain, syncope, unknown infection, urticaria, and vertigo.

Advanced colorectal cancer (previously treated patients) – Thirteen percent of patients in the oxaliplatin and 5-fluorouracil/leucovorin combination arm and 18% in the 5-fluorouracil/leucovorin arm of the previously treated study had to discontinue treatment because of adverse reactions related to GI or hematologic adverse reactions or neuropathies. Both 5-fluorouracil and oxaliplatin are associated with GI and hematologic adverse reactions. When oxaliplatin is administered in combination with 5-fluorouracil, the incidence of these reactions is increased.

The incidence of death within 30 days of treatment in the previously treated study, regardless of causality, was 5% with the oxaliplatin and 5-fluorouracil/leucovorin combination, 8% with oxaliplatin alone, and 7% with 5-fluorouracil/leucovorin. Of the 7 deaths that occurred on the oxaliplatin and 5-fluorouracil/leucovorin combination arm within 30 days of stopping treatment, 3 may have been treatment related, associated with GI bleeding or dehydration.

Oxaliplatin Adverse Reactions (≥ 5%)						
	5-fluorouracil/ leucovorin (n = 142)		Oxaliplatin (n = 153)		Oxaliplatin + 5-fluorouracil/ leucovorin (n = 150)	
Adverse reaction	All grades	Grade 3/4	All grades	Grade 3/4	All grades	Grade 3/4
Any reaction	98%	41%	100%	46%	99%	73%
Cardiovascular						
Thromboembolism	4%	2%	2%	1%	9%	8%
CNS						
Acute neuropathy	10%	0%	65%	5%	56%	2%
Fatigue	52%	6%	61%	9%	68%	7%
Neuropathy	17%	0%	76%	7%	74%	7%
Persistent neuropathy	9%	0%	43%	3%	48%	6%
GI						
Abdominal pain	31%	5%	31%	7%	33%	4%
Anorexia	20%	1%	20%	2%	29%	3%
Diarrhea	44%	3%	46%	4%	67%	11%
Gastroesophageal reflux	3%	0%	1%	0%	5%	2%
Nausea	59%	4%	64%	4%	65%	11%
Stomatitis	32%	3%	14%	0%	37%	3%
Vomiting	27%	4%	37%	4%	40%	9%
Hematologic						
Febrile neutropenia	1%	1%	0%	0%	6%	6%
Metabolic/Nutritional						
Dehydration	6%	4%	5%	3%	8%	3%
Edema	13%	1%	10%	1%	15%	1%
Hypokalemia	3%	1%	3%	2%	9%	4%
Musculoskeletal						
Back pain	16%	4%	11%	0%	19%	3%
Respiratory						
Coughing	9%	0%	11%	0%	19%	1%
Dyspnea	11%	2%	13%	7%	20%	4%
Miscellaneous						
Chest pain	4%	1%	5%	1%	8%	1%
Fever	23%	1%	25%	1%	29%	1%
Injection-site reaction	5%	1%	9%	0%	10%	3%
Pain	9%	3%	14%	3%	15%	2%

Oxaliplatin Adverse Reactions (≥ 5%)			
	5-fluorouracil/ leucovorin (n =142)	Oxaliplatin (n = 153)	Oxaliplatin + 5-fluorouracil/ leucovorin (n =150)
Adverse reactions	All grades	All grades	All grades
CNS			
Dizziness	8%	7%	13%
Headache	8%	13%	17%
Insomnia	4%	11%	9%
Dermatologic			
Alopecia	3%	3%	7%
Flushing	2%	3%	10%
Hand-foot syndrome	13%	1%	11%
Rash	5%	5%	9%

OXALIPLATIN — INJECTION

Oxaliplatin Adverse Reactions (≥ 5%)

Adverse reactions	5-fluorouracil/ leucovorin (n =142) All grades	Oxaliplatin (n = 153) All grades	Oxaliplatin + 5-fluorouracil/ leucovorin (n =150) All grades
GI			
Constipation	23%	31%	32%
Dyspepsia	10%	7%	14%
Flatulence	6%	3%	5%
Mucositis	10%	2%	7%
Taste perversion	1%	5%	13%
GU			
Dysuria	1%	1%	6%
Hematuria	4%	0%	6%
Metabolic/Nutritional			
Peripheral edema	11%	5%	10%
Respiratory			
Epistaxis	1%	2%	9%
Hiccups	0%	2%	5%
Pharyngitis	10%	2%	9%
Rhinitis	4%	6%	15%
Upper respiratory tract infection	4%	7%	10%
Special senses			
Abnormal lacrimation	6%	1%	7%
Miscellaneous			
Allergic reaction	1%	3%	10%
Arthralgia	10%	7%	10%
Rigors	6%	9%	7%

Adverse reactions were similar in men and women and in patients younger than 65 years of age and 65 years of age and older, but older patients may have been more susceptible to dehydration, diarrhea, hypokalemia, and fatigue. The following additional adverse reactions, at least possibly related to treatment and potentially important, were reported in 2% or more and less than 5% of the patients in the oxaliplatin and 5-fluorouracil/leucovorin combination arm: abnormal micturition frequency, anxiety, ascites, ataxia, conjunctivitis, depression, dry mouth, dry skin, enlarged abdomen, erythematous rash, gingivitis, hemoptysis, hemorrhoids, hot flashes, increased sweating, intestinal obstruction, involuntary muscle contractions, melena, muscle weakness, myalgia, nervousness, pneumonia, proctitis, pruritus, purpura, rectal hemorrhage, somnolence, tachycardia, tenesmus, urinary incontinence, vaginal hemorrhage, weight decrease.

Cardiovascular – The incidence of thromboembolic events in adjuvant patients with colon cancer was 6% (1.8% grade 3/4) in the infusional 5-fluorouracil/leucovorin arm and 6% (1.2% grade 3/4) in the oxaliplatin and infusional 5-fluorouracil/leucovorin combined arm, respectively. The incidence was 6% and 9% of the patients previously untreated for advanced colorectal cancer and previously treated patients in the oxaliplatin and infusional 5-fluorouracil/leucovorin combination arm, respectively.

CNS – Peripheral sensory neuropathy was reported in adjuvant patients treated with the oxaliplatin combination with a frequency of 92% (all grades) and 13% (grade 3), and by 18 months of follow-up, 21% of patients had persistent peripheral sensory neuropathy (all grades). In these patients, the median cycle of onset for grade 3 peripheral sensory neuropathy was 9. In patients previously untreated for advanced colorectal cancer, neuropathy was reported in 82% (all grades) and 19% (grade 3/4), and in the previously treated patients in 74% (all grades) and 7% (grade 3/4 events). Oxaliplatin is consistently associated with 2 types of peripheral neuropathy. In the previously treated patients, the incidence of overall and grade 3/4 persistent peripheral neuropathy was 48% and 6%, respectively. The majority of the patients (80%) that developed grade 3 persistent neuropathy progressed from prior grade 1 or 2 events. The median number of cycles administered on the oxaliplatin with infusional 5-fluorouracil/leucovorin combination arm was 6.

Dermatologic – Oxaliplatin did not increase the incidence of alopecia compared with infusional 5-fluorouracil/leucovorin alone. No complete alopecia was reported. The incidence of grade 3/4 skin disorders was 2% in both the oxaliplatin plus infusional 5-fluorouracil/leucovorin and the infusional 5-fluorouracil/leucovorin alone arms in the adjuvant colon cancer patients. The incidence of hand-foot syndrome in patients previously untreated for advanced colorectal cancer was 2% in the irinotecan plus 5-fluorouracil/leucovorin arm and 7% in the oxaliplatin and 5-fluorouracil/leucovorin combination arm. The incidence of hand-foot syndrome in previously treated patients was 13% in the 5-fluorouracil/leucovorin arm and 11% in the oxaliplatin and 5-fluorouracil/leucovorin combination arm.

GI – In patients receiving the combination of oxaliplatin plus infusional 5-fluorouracil/leucovorin for adjuvant treatment for colon cancer, the incidence of grade 3/4 nausea and vomiting was greater than those receiving infusional 5-fluorouracil/leucovorin alone. In patients previously untreated for advanced colorectal cancer receiving the combination of oxaliplatin and 5-fluorouracil/leucovorin, the incidence of grade 3 and 4 vomiting and diarrhea was less compared with irinotecan plus 5-fluorouracil/leucovorin controls. In previously treated patients receiving the combination of oxaliplatin and 5-fluorouracil/leucovorin, the incidence of grade 3 and 4 nausea, vomiting, diarrhea, and mucositis/stomatitis increased compared with 5-fluorouracil/leucovorin controls.

The incidence of GI adverse reactions in the previously untreated and previously treated patients appears to be similar across cycles. Premedication with antiemetics, including 5-HT_3 blockers, is recommended. Diarrhea and mucositis may be exacerbated by the addition of oxaliplatin to 5-fluorouracil/leucovorin; manage with appropriate supportive care. Because cold temperature can exacerbate acute neurological symptoms, avoid using ice (mucositis prophylaxis) during the infusion of oxaliplatin.

Hematologic –

Oxaliplatin Adverse Hematologic Reactions in Patients with Stage II or III Colon Cancer Receiving Adjuvant Therapy (≥ 5% of Patients)

Hematologic adverse reaction	Oxaliplatin + 5-fluorouracil/ leucovorin (n = 1,108) All grades	Grade 3/4	5-fluorouracil/ leucovorin (n = 1,111) All grades	Grade 3/4
Anemia	76%	1%	67%	< 1%
Neutropenia	79%	41%	40%	5%
Thrombocytopenia	77%	2%	19%	< 1%

Oxaliplatin Adverse Hematologic Reactions in Patients Previously Untreated for Advanced Colorectal Cancer (≥ 5% of Patients)

Hematologic adverse reaction	Oxaliplatin + 5-fluorouracil/ leucovorin (n = 259) All grades	Grade 3/4	Irinotecan + 5-fluorouracil/ leucovorin (n = 256) All grades	Grade 3/4	Oxaliplatin + irinotecan (n = 258) All grades	Grade 3/4
Anemia	27%	3%	28%	4%	25%	3%
Leukopenia	85%	20%	84%	23%	76%	24%
Neutropenia	81%	53%	77%	44%	71%	36%
Thrombocytopenia	71%	5%	26%	2%	44%	4%

Adverse Hematologic Experiences in Previously Treated Patients (≥ 5% of patients)

Hematologic adverse reactions	5-fluorouracil/ leucovorin (N = 142) All grades (%)	Grade 3/4 (%)	Oxaliplatin (N = 153) All grades (%)	Grade 3/4 (%)	Oxaliplatin + 5-fluorouracil/ leucovorin (n = 150) All grades (%)	Grade 3/4 (%)
Anemia	68%	2%	64%	1%	81%	2%
Leukopenia	34%	1%	13%	0%	76%	19%
Neutropenia	25%	5%	7%	0%	73%	44%
Thrombocytopenia	20%	0%	30%	3%	64%	4%

Thrombocytopenia: Thrombocytopenia was frequently reported with the combination of oxaliplatin and infusional 5-fluorouracil/leucovorin. The incidence of all hemorrhagic events in the adjuvant and previously treated patients was higher in the oxaliplatin combination arm compared with the infusional 5-fluorouracil/leucovorin arm. These events included GI bleeding, hematuria, and epistaxis. In the adjuvant trial, 2 patients died from intracerebral hemorrhages.

The incidence of grade 3/4 thrombocytopenia was 2% in adjuvant patients with colon cancer. In patients treated for advanced colorectal cancer, the incidence of grade 3/4 thrombocytopenia was 3% to 5%, and the incidence of these events was greater for the combination of oxaliplatin and 5-fluorouracil/leucovorin over the irinotecan plus 5-fluorouracil/leucovorin or 5-fluorouracil/leucovorin control groups. Grade 3/4 GI bleeding was reported in 0.2% of adjuvant patients receiving oxaliplatin and 5-fluorouracil/leucovorin. In the previously untreated patients, the incidence of epistaxis was 10% in the oxaliplatin and 5-fluorouracil/leucovorin arm, and 2% and 1%, respectively, in the irinotecan plus 5-fluorouracil/leucovorin or irinotecan plus oxaliplatin arms.

Neutropenia: Neutropenia was frequently observed with the combination of oxaliplatin and 5-fluorouracil/leucovorin, with grade 3 and 4 events reported in 29% and 12% of adjuvant patients with colon cancer, respectively. In the adjuvant trial, 3 patients died from sepsis/neutropenic sepsis. Grade 3 and 4 events were reported in 35% and 18% of the patients previ-

OXALIPLATIN — INJECTION

ously untreated for advanced colorectal cancer, respectively. Grade 3 and 4 events were reported in 27% and 17% of previously treated patients, respectively. In adjuvant patients, the incidence of either febrile neutropenia (0.7%) or documented infection with concomitant grade 3/4 neutropenia (1.1%) was 1.8% in the oxaliplatin and 5-fluorouracil/leucovorin arm. The incidence of febrile neutropenia in the patients previously untreated for advanced colorectal cancer was 15% (3% of cycles) in the irinotecan plus 5-fluorouracil/leucovorin arm and 4% (less than 1% of cycles) in the oxaliplatin and 5-fluorouracil/leucovorin combination arm. Additionally, in this same population, infection with grade 3 or 4 neutropenia was 12% in the irinotecan plus 5-fluorouracil/leucovorin, and 8% in the oxaliplatin and 5-fluorouracil/leucovorin combination. The incidence of febrile neutropenia in the previously treated patients was 1% in the 5-fluorouracil/leucovorin arm and 6% (less than 1% of cycles) in the oxaliplatin and 5-fluorouracil/leucovorin combination arm.

Hepatic –

Oxaliplatin Adverse Hepatic Reactions in Patients with Stage II or III Colon Cancer Receiving Adjuvant Therapy (≥ 5% of Patients)

Hepatic adverse reaction	Oxaliplatin + 5-fluorouracil/leucovorin (n = 1,108) All grades	Grade 3/4	5-fluorouracil/leucovorin (n = 1,111) All grades	Grade 3/4
Alkaline phosphatase increased	42%	< 1%	20%	< 1%
Bilirubinemia	20%	4%	20%	5%
Increase in transaminases	57%	2%	34%	1%

Oxaliplatin Adverse Hepatic Lab Test Abnormalities in Patients Previously Untreated for Advanced Colorectal Cancer (≥ 5% of Patients)

Hepatic lab test abnormalities	Oxaliplatin + 5-fluorouracil/leucovorin (n = 259) All grades	Grade 3/4	Irinotecan + 5-fluorouracil/leucovorin (n = 256) All grades	Grade 3/4	Oxaliplatin + irinotecan (n = 258) All grades	Grade 3/4
Alkaline phosphatase	16%	0%	8%	0%	14%	2%
ALT	6%	1%	2%	0%	5%	2%
AST	17%	1%	2%	1%	11%	1%
Total bilirubin	6%	1%	3%	1%	3%	2%

Adverse Hepatic Clinical Chemistry Experience in Previously Treated Patients (≥ 5% of Patients)

Clinical chemistry	5-fluorouracil/leucovorin (N = 142) All grades	Grade 3/4	Oxaliplatin (N = 153) All grades	Grade 3/4	Oxaliplatin + 5-fluorouracil/leucovorin (n = 150) All grades	Grade 3/4
ALT	28%	3%	36%	1%	31%	0%
AST	39%	2%	54%	4%	47%	0%
Total bilirubin	22%	6%	13%	5%	13%	1%

Hypersensitivity – Grade 3/4 hypersensitivity to oxaliplatin has been observed in 2% to 3% of colon cancer patients. These allergic reactions, which can be fatal, can occur at any cycle, and were similar in nature and severity to those reported with other platinum-containing compounds (eg, erythema, pruritus, rash, urticaria; bronchospasm, hypotension [rare]). The symptoms associated with hypersensitivity reactions reported in the previously untreated patients were bronchospasm, chest pains, diaphoresis, diarrhea associated with oxaliplatin infusion, disorientation, flushing of the face, hypotension, pruritus, shortness of breath, syncope, and urticaria. These reactions are usually managed with standard epinephrine, corticosteroid, or antihistamine therapy and may require discontinuation of therapy.

Lab test abnormalities –

Thromboembolism: The incidence of thromboembolic events in adjuvant patients with colon cancer was 6% (1.8% grade 3/4) in the infusional 5-fluorouracil/leucovorin arm and 6% (1.2% grade 3/4) in the oxaliplatin and infusional 5-fluorouracil/leucovorin combined arm, respectively. The incidence was 6% and 9% of the patients previously untreated for advanced colorectal cancer and previously treated in the oxaliplatin and 5-fluorouracil/leucovorin combination arm, respectively.

Local – Extravasation may result in local pain and inflammation that may be severe and lead to complications, including necrosis. Injection-site reaction, including redness, swelling, and pain have been reported.

Renal – About 5% to 10% of patients in all groups had some degree of elevation of serum creatinine. The incidence of grade 3/4 elevations in serum creatinine in the oxaliplatin and infusional 5-fluorouracil/leucovorin combination arm was 1% in the previously treated patients. Serum creatinine measurements were not reported in the adjuvant trial.

Respiratory – Pulmonary oxaliplatin has been associated with pulmonary fibrosis. One patient treated with the oxaliplatin combination regimen in the adjuvant trial died from eosinophilic pneumonia.

➤*Postmarketing:*

CNS – Cranial nerve palsies, dysarthria, fasciculations, Lhermitte sign, loss of deep tendon reflexes.

GI – Colitis (including *Clostridium difficile* diarrhea), ileus, intestinal obstruction, pancreatitis, severe diarrhea/vomiting resulting in hypokalemia.

Hematologic – Hemolytic uremic syndrome, immuno-allergic hemolytic anemia, immuno-allergic thrombocytopenia, prolongation of prothrombin time and of INR in patients receiving anticoagulants.

Hepatic – Perisinusoidal fibrosis (which, rarely, may progress), veno-occlusive disease of liver (also known as sinusoidal obstruction syndrome).

Respiratory – Pulmonary fibrosis, other interstitial lung diseases.

Special senses – Deafness, decrease of visual acuity, optic neuritis, visual field disturbance.

Miscellaneous – Anaphylactic shock, angioedema, metabolic acidosis.

Overdosage

➤*Symptoms:* There have been 5 oxaliplatin overdoses reported. One patient received two 130 mg/m^2 doses of oxaliplatin (cumulative dose of 260 mg/m^2) within a 24-hour period. The patient experienced grade 4 thrombocytopenia (less than 25,000/mm^3) without any bleeding, which resolved. Two other patients were mistakenly administered oxaliplatin instead of carboplatin. One patient received a total oxaliplatin dose of 500 mg and the other received 650 mg. The first patient experienced dyspnea, wheezing, paresthesia, profuse vomiting, and chest pain on the day of administration. She developed respiratory failure and severe bradycardia, and subsequently did not respond to resuscitation efforts. The other patient also experienced dyspnea, wheezing, paresthesia, and vomiting. Her symptoms resolved with supportive care. Another patient who was mistakenly administered a 700 mg dose experienced rapid onset of dysesthesia. Inpatient supportive care was given, including hydration, electrolyte support, and platelet transfusion. Recovery occurred 15 days after the overdose. The last patient received an overdose of oxaliplatin at 360 mg instead of 120 mg over a 1-hour infusion by mistake. At the end of the infusion, the patient experienced 2 episodes of vomiting, laryngospasm, and paresthesia. The patient fully recovered from the laryngospasm within half an hour. At the time of reporting, 1 hour after onset of the event, the patient was recovering from paresthesia. In addition to thrombocytopenia, the anticipated complications of an oxaliplatin overdose include myelosuppression, nausea, vomiting, diarrhea, and neurotoxicity.

➤*Treatment:* There is no known antidote for oxaliplatin overdose. Monitor patients suspected of receiving an overdose and administer supportive treatment.

Patient Information

Inform patients and patient caregivers of the expected side effects of oxaliplatin, particularly its neurologic effects, both the acute, reversible effects and the persistent neurosensory toxicity. Inform patients that the acute neurosensory toxicity may be precipitated or exacerbated by exposure to cold or cold objects. Instruct patients to avoid cold drinks and the use of ice, and to cover exposed skin prior to exposure to cold temperature or cold objects.

Adequately inform patients of the risk of low blood cell counts and instruct them to contact their health care provider immediately if fever, particularly if associated with persistent diarrhea, or evidence of infection develop.

Instruct patients to contact their health care provider if persistent vomiting, diarrhea, signs of dehydration, coughing, breathing difficulties, or signs of allergic reaction occur.

ANTHRACENEDIONE

MITOXANTRONE HYDROCHLORIDE

Rx	**Novantrone** (Serono)	**Injection:** 2 mg mitoxantrone free base per ml	Preservative free. In 10, 12.5, and 15 ml multi-dose vials.[a]

[a] With 0.8% NaCl, 0.005% sodium acetate, and 0.046% acetic acid.

MITOXANTRONE HYDROCHLORIDE — INJECTION

WARNING

Mitoxantrone for injection concentrate should be administered under the supervision of a physician experienced in the use of cytotoxic chemotherapy agents.

Mitoxantrone should be given slowly into a freely flowing intravenous (IV) infusion. It must never be given subcutaneously, intramuscularly (IM), or intra-arterially. Severe local tissue damage may occur if there is extravasation during administration.

Not for intrathecal use. Severe injury with permanent sequelae can result from intrathecal administration.

Except for the treatment of acute nonlymphocytic leukemia (ANLL), mitoxantrone therapy generally should not be given to patients with baseline neutrophil counts of less than 1,500 cells/mm^3. In order to monitor the occurrence of bone marrow suppression, primarily neutropenia, which may be severe and result in infection, it is recommended that frequent peripheral blood cell counts be performed on all patients receiving mitoxantrone.

Use of mitoxantrone has been associated with cardiotoxicity. Cardiotoxicity can occur at any time during mitoxantrone therapy, and the risk increases with cumulative dose. Congestive heart failure (CHF), potentially fatal, may occur either during therapy with mitoxantrone or months to years after termination of therapy. All patients should be carefully assessed for cardiac signs and symptoms by history and physical examination prior to start of mitoxantrone therapy. Baseline evaluation of left ventricular ejection fraction (LVEF) by echocardiogram or multigated radionuclide angiography (MUGA) should be performed. Multiple sclerosis (MS) patients with baseline LVEF less than 50% should not be treated with mitoxantrone. LVEF should be reevaluated by echocardiogram or MUGA prior to each dose administered to patients with MS. Additional doses of mitoxantrone should not be administered to MS patients who have experienced either a drop in LVEF to below 50% or a clinically significant reduction in LVEF during mitoxantrone therapy. Patients with MS should not receive a cumulative dose greater than 140 mg/m^2. In cancer patients, the risk of symptomatic CHF was estimated to be 2.6% for patients receiving up to a cumulative dose of 140 mg/m^2. Presence or history of cardiovascular disease, prior or concomitant radiotherapy to the mediastinal/pericardial area, previous therapy with other anthracyclines or anthracenediones, or concomitant use of other cardiotoxic drugs may increase the risk of cardiac toxicity. Cardiac toxicity with mitoxantrone may occur whether or not cardiac risk factors are present.

Secondary acute myelogenous leukemia (AML) has been reported in MS and cancer patients treated with mitoxantrone. In a cohort of mitoxantrone treated MS patients followed for varying periods of time, an elevated leukemia risk of 0.25% (2/802) has been observed. Postmarketing cases of secondary AML have also been reported. In 1,774 patients with breast cancer who received mitoxantrone concomitantly with other cytotoxic agents and radiotherapy, the cumulative risk of developing treatment-related AML was estimated as 1.1% and 1.6% at 5 and 10 years, respectively. Secondary AML has been reported in cancer patients treated with anthracyclines. Mitoxantrone is an anthracenedione, a related drug.

The occurrence of refractory secondary leukemia is more common when anthracyclines are given in combination with DNA-damaging antineoplastic agents, when patients have been heavily pretreated with cytotoxic drugs, or when doses of anthracyclines have been escalated.

Indications

➤*ANLL:* In combination with other approved drug(s), is indicated in the initial therapy of ANLL in adults. This category includes myelogenous, promyelocytic, monocytic, and erythroid acute leukemias.

➤*MS:* For reducing neurologic disability and/or the frequency of clinical relapses in patients with secondary (chronic) progressive, progressive relapsing, or worsening relapsing-remitting MS (ie, patients whose neurologic status is significantly abnormal between relapses). Mitoxantrone is not indicated in the treatment of patients with primary progressive MS.

The clinical patterns of MS in the studies were characterized as follows: secondary progressive and progressive relapsing disease were characterized by gradual increasing disability with or without superimposed clinical relapses, and worsening relapsing-remitting disease was characterized by clinical relapses, resulting in a stepwise worsening of disability.

➤*Prostate cancer:* In combination with corticosteroids, as initial chemotherapy for the treatment of patients with pain related to advanced hormone-refractory prostate cancer.

➤*Unlabeled uses:* Treatment of breast cancer, non-Hodgkin's lymphoma, autologous bone marrow transplantation.

Administration and Dosage

➤*Approved by the FDA:* December 23, 1987.

➤*MS:* 12 mg/m^2 given as a short (approximately 5 to 15 minutes) IV infusion every 3 months.

LVEF should be evaluated by echocardiogram or MUGA prior to administration of the initial dose of mitoxantrone and all subsequent doses. In addition, LVEF evaluations are recommended if signs or symptoms of CHF develop at any time during treatment with mitoxantrone. Mitoxantrone should not be administered to MS patients with an LVEF less than 50%, with a clinically significant reduction in LVEF, or to those who have received a cumulative lifetime dose of greater than or equal to 140 mg/m^2.

➤*Prostate cancer:* 12 to 14 mg/m^2 given as a short IV infusion every 21 days.

➤*ANLL:*

Adults – Induction therapy, the recommended dosage is 12 mg/m^2 of mitoxantrone daily on days 1 to 3 given as an IV infusion, and 100 mg/m^2 of cytarabine for 7 days given as a continuous 24-hour infusion on days 1 to 7.

Most complete remissions will occur following the initial course of induction therapy. In the event of an incomplete antileukemic response, a second induction course may be given. Mitoxantrone should be given for 2 days and cytarabine for 5 days using the same daily dosage levels.

If severe or life-threatening nonhematologic toxicity is observed during the first induction course, the second induction course should be withheld until toxicity resolves.

Consolidation therapy – 12 mg/m^2 of mitoxantrone given by IV infusion daily on days 1 and 2 and cytarabine, 100 mg/m^2 for 5 days given as a continuous 24-hour infusion on days 1 to 5. The first course was given approximately 6 weeks after the final induction course, the second was generally administered 4 weeks after the first. Severe myelosuppression occurred.

➤*Preparation:* Mitoxantrone concentrate must be diluted prior to use. Parenteral drug products should be inspected visually for particulate matter and discoloration prior to administration whenever solution and container permit.

The dose of mitoxantrone should be diluted to at least 50 mL with either 0.9% sodium chloride injection or 5% dextrose injection. Mitoxantrone may be further diluted into dextrose 5% in water, normal saline, or dextrose 5% with normal saline and use immediately. Do not freeze.

Administration – The diluted solution should be introduced slowly into the tubing as a freely running IV infusion of 0.9% sodium chloride injection or 5% dextrose injection over a period of not less than 3 minutes. The tubing should be attached to a butterfly needle or other suitable device and inserted preferably into a large vein. If possible, avoid veins over joints or in extremities with compromised venous or lymphatic drainage. Mitoxantrone should not be administered subcutaneously.

Avoid contact of mitoxantrone with the skin, mucous membranes, or eyes. Skin accidentally exposed to mitoxantrone should be rinsed copiously with warm water and, if the eyes are involved, standard irrigation techniques should be used immediately. The use of goggles, gloves, and protective gowns is recommended during preparation and administration of the drug.

Extravasation – Care in the administration of mitoxantrone will reduce the chance of extravasation. If any signs or symptoms of extravasation have occurred, including burning, pain, pruritus, erythema, swelling, blue discoloration, or ulceration, the injection or infusion should be immediately terminated and restarted in another vein. During IV administration of mitoxantrone, extravasation may occur with or without an accompanying stinging or burning sensation, even if blood returns well on aspiration of the infusion needle. If it is known or suspected that subcutaneous extravasation has occurred, it is recommended that intermittent ice packs be placed over the area of extravasation and that the affected extremity be elevated. Because of the progressive nature of extravasation reactions, the area of injection should be frequently examined and surgery consultation obtained early if there is any sign of a local reaction.

IV incompatibility – Mitoxantrone should not be mixed in the same infusion as heparin since a precipitate may form. Because specific compatibility data are not available, it is recommended that mitoxantrone not be mixed in the same infusion with other drugs.

➤*Storage/Stability:* Store between 15° to 25°C (59° to 77°F). Do not freeze.

Unused infusion solutions should be discarded immediately in an appropriate fashion. In the case of multidose use, after penetration of the stopper, the remaining portion of the undiluted mitoxantrone concentrate should be stored not longer than 7 days between 15° to 25°C (59° to 77°F) or 14 days under refrigeration. Contains no preservative.

Actions

➤*Pharmacology:* Mitoxantrone, a deoxyribonucleic acid (DNA)-reactive agent that intercalates into DNA through hydrogen bonding, causes crosslinks and strand breaks. Mitoxantrone also interferes with ribonucleic acid (RNA) and is a potent inhibitor of topoisomerase II, an enzyme responsible for uncoiling and repairing damaged DNA. It has a cytocidal effect on both proliferating and nonproliferating cultured human cells, suggesting lack of cell cycle phase specificity.

Mitoxantrone has been shown in vitro to inhibit B-cell, T-cell, and macrophage proliferation and impair antigen presentation, as well as the secretion of interferon gamma, TNFα, and IL-2.

➤*Pharmacokinetics:*

Absorption/Distribution – Pharmacokinetic studies have not been performed in humans receiving multiple daily dosing. Distribution to tissues is extensive; steady-state volume of distribution exceeds 1,000 L/m^2. Tissue concentrations of mitoxantrone appear to exceed those in the blood during the terminal elimination phase. In the monkey, distribution to the brain, spinal cord, eye, and spinal fluid is low.

In patients administered 15 to 90 mg/m^2 of mitoxantrone IV, there is a linear relationship between dose and the area under the plasma concentration-time curve (AUC).

MITOXANTRONE HYDROCHLORIDE — INJECTION

Mitoxantrone is 78% bound to plasma proteins in the observed concentration range of 26 to 455 ng/mL. This binding is independent of concentration and is not affected by the presence of phenytoin, doxorubicin, methotrexate, prednisone, prednisolone, heparin, or aspirin.

Metabolism / Excretion – Mitoxantrone is excreted in urine and feces as either unchanged or as inactive metabolites. In human studies, 11% and 25% of the dose were recovered in urine and feces, respectively, as either parent drug or metabolite during the 5-day period following drug administration. Of the material recovered in the urine, 65% is unchanged drug. The remaining 35% is comprised primarily of a mono- and a dicarboxylic acid derivative and their glucuronide conjugates. The pathways leading to metabolism of mitoxantrone have not been elucidated.

Pharmacokinetics of mitoxantrone in patients following a single IV administration of mitoxantrone can be characterized by a 3-compartment model. The mean alpha half-life of mitoxantrone is 6 to 12 minutes, the mean beta half-life is 1.1 to 3.1 hours and the mean gamma (terminal or elimination) half-life is 23 to 215 hours (median approximately 75 hours).

Special populations –

Hepatic function impairment: Mitoxantrone clearance is reduced by hepatic impairment. Patients with severe hepatic dysfunction (bilirubin greater than 3.4 mg/dL) have an AUC more than 3 times greater than that of patients with healthy hepatic function receiving the same dose.

Patients with MS who have hepatic impairment should ordinarily not be treated with mitoxantrone. Treat other patients with hepatic impairment with caution, and dosage adjustment may be required.

Elderly: In elderly patients with breast cancer, the systematic mitoxantrone clearance was 21.3 L/h/m^2, compared with 28.3 L/h/m^2 and 16.2 L/h/m^2 for nonelderly patients with nasopharyngeal carcinoma and malignant lymphoma, respectively.

Contraindications

Patients who have demonstrated prior hypersensitivity to it.

Warnings

➤*Myelosuppression:* When mitoxantrone is used in high doses (greater than 14 mg/m^2/day × 3 days) such as indicated for the treatment of leukemia, severe myelosuppression will occur. Therefore, it is recommended that mitoxantrone be administered only by physicians experienced in the chemotherapy of this disease. Laboratory and supportive services must be available for hematologic and chemistry monitoring and adjunctive therapies, including antibiotics. Blood and blood products must be available to support patients during the expected period of medullary hypoplasia and severe myelosuppression. Give particular care to ensuring full hematologic recovery before undertaking consolidation therapy (if this treatment is used) and monitor patients closely during this phase. Mitoxantrone administered at any dose can cause myelosuppression.

Patients with preexisting myelosuppression as the result of prior drug therapy should not receive mitoxantrone unless it is felt that the possible benefit from such treatment warrants the risk of further medullary suppression.

➤*Hepatic function impairment:* Do not ordinarily treat patients with MS who have hepatic impairment with mitoxantrone. Administer mitoxantrone with caution to other patients with hepatic impairment. In patients with severe hepatic impairment, the AUC is more than 3 times greater than the value observed in patients with healthy hepatic function.

➤*Administration:* Safety for use by routes other than IV administration has not been established. Mitoxantrone is not indicated for subcutaneous, IM, or intra-arterial injection. There have been reports of local/regional neuropathy, some irreversible, following intra-arterial injection.

Mitoxantrone must not be given by intrathecal injection. There have been reports of neuropathy and neurotoxicity, both central and peripheral, following intrathecal injection. These reports have included seizures leading to coma and severe neurologic sequelae, and paralysis with bowel and bladder dysfunction.

➤*Acute leukemia / myelodysplasia:* Topoisomerase II inhibitors, including mitoxantrone, have been associated with the development of secondary AML and myelosuppression.

➤*Cardiac effects:* Because of the possible danger of cardiac effects in patients previously treated with daunorubicin or doxorubicin, determine the benefit-to-risk ratio of mitoxantrone therapy in such patients before starting therapy.

Functional cardiac changes including decreases in LVEF and irreversible CHF can occur with mitoxantrone. Cardiac toxicity may be more common in patients with prior treatment with anthracyclines, prior mediastinal radiotherapy, or with preexisting cardiovascular disease. Such patients should have regular cardiac monitoring of LVEF from the initiation of therapy.

Cancer patients who received cumulative doses of 140 mg/m^2 either alone or in combination with other chemotherapeutic agents had a cumulative 2.6% probability of clinical CHF. In comparative oncology trials, the overall cumulative probability rate of moderate or severe decreases in LVEF at this dose was 13%.

MS – Changes in cardiac function may occur in patients with MS treated with mitoxantrone. In 1 controlled trial (study 1), 2 patients (2%) of 127 receiving mitoxantrone, 1 receiving a 5 mg/m^2 dose and the other receiving a 12 mg/m^2 dose, had LVEF values that decreased to below 50%. An additional patient receiving 12 mg/m^2, who did not have LVEF measured, had a decrease in another echocardiographic measurement of ventricular function (fractional shortening) that led to discontinuation from the trial. There were no reports of CHF in either controlled trial.

Evaluation of LVEF (by echocardiogram or MUGA) is recommended prior to administration of the initial dose of mitoxantrone. Do not treat MS patients with a baseline LVEF of less than 50% with mitoxantrone. Subsequent LVEF evaluations are recommended if signs or symptoms of CHF develop, and prior to all doses administered to MS patients. Do not administer mitoxantrone to MS patients with an LVEF less than 50%, with a clinically significant reduction in LVEF, or to those who have received a cumulative lifetime dose of greater than 140 mg/m^2.

Leukemia – Acute CHF may occasionally occur in patients treated with mitoxantrone for ANLL. In first-line comparative trials of mitoxantrone and cytarabine vs daunorubicin and cytarabine in adult patients with previously untreated ANLL, therapy was associated with CHF in 6.5% of patients on each arm. A causal relationship between drug therapy and cardiac effects is difficult to establish in this setting since myocardial function is frequently depressed by the anemia, fever and infection, and hemorrhage which often accompany the underlying disease.

Hormone-refractory prostate cancer – Functional cardiac changes such as decreases in LVEF and CHF may occur in patients with hormone-refractory prostate cancer treated with mitoxantrone. In a randomized comparative trial of mitoxantrone plus low-dose prednisone vs low-dose prednisone, 7 of 128 patients (5.5%) treated with mitoxantrone had a cardiac event defined as any decrease in LVEF below the normal range, CHF (n = 3), or myocardial ischemia. Two patients had a history of cardiac disease. The total mitoxantrone dose administered to patients with cardiac effects ranged from greater than 48 to 212 mg/m^2.

Among 112 patients evaluable for safety on the mitoxantrone and hydrocortisone arm of the CALGB trial, 18 patients (19%) had a reduction in cardiac function, 5 patients (5%) had cardiac ischemia, and 2 patients (2%) experienced pulmonary edema. The range of total mitoxantrone doses administered to these patients is not available.

➤*Secondary leukemia:* See the Warning box for more information.

➤*Carcinogenesis:* IV treatment of rats and mice, once every 21 days for 24 months, with mitoxantrone resulted in an increased incidence of fibroma and external auditory canal tumors in rats at a dose of 0.03 mg/kg (0.02-fold the recommended human dose, on a mg/m^2 basis), and hepatocellular adenoma in male mice at a dose of 0.1 mg/kg (0.03-fold the recommended human dose, on a mg/m^2 basis).

IV treatment of rats, once every 21 days for 12 months with mitoxantrone resulted in an increased incidence of external auditory canal tumors in rats at a dose of 0.3 mg/kg (0.15-fold the recommended human dose, on a mg/m^2 basis).

➤*Mutagenesis:* Mitoxantrone was clastogenic in the in vivo rat bone marrow assay. Mitoxantrone was also clastogenic in 2 in vitro assays; it induced DNA damage in primary rat hepatocytes and sister chromatid exchanges in Chinese hamster ovary cells. Mitoxantrone was mutagenic in bacterial and mammalian test systems (Ames/*Salmonella* and *E. coli* and L5178Y TK ± mouse lymphoma).

➤*Elderly:*

Hormone-refractory prostate cancer – One hundred forty-six patients 65 years of age and older and 52 younger patients (less than 65 years of age) have been treated with mitoxantrone in controlled clinical studies. These studies did not include sufficient numbers of younger patients to determine whether they respond differently from older patients. However, greater sensitivity of some older individuals cannot be ruled out.

ANLL – Although definitive studies with mitoxantrone have not been performed in geriatric patients with ANLL, toxicity may be more frequent in the elderly. Elderly patients are more likely to have age-related comorbidities due to disease or disease therapy.

➤*Pregnancy:* *Category D*. Mitoxantrone may cause fetal harm when administered to a pregnant woman. Advise women of childbearing potential to avoid becoming pregnant. Mitoxantrone is considered a potential human teratogen because of its mechanism of action and the developmental effects demonstrated by related agents. Treatment of pregnant rats during the organogenesis period of gestation was associated with fetal growth retardation at doses greater than 0.1 mg/kg/day (0.01 times the recommended human dose on a mg/m^2 basis). When pregnant rabbits were treated during organogenesis, an increased incidence of premature delivery was observed at doses greater than or equal to 0.1 mg/kg/day (0.01 times the recommended human dose on a mg/m^2 basis). No teratogenic effects were observed in these studies, but the maximum doses tested were well below the recommended human dose (0.02 and 0.05 times in rats and rabbits, respectively, on a mg/m^2 basis). There are no adequate and well-controlled studies in pregnant women. Women with multiple sclerosis who are biologically capable of becoming pregnant should have a pregnancy test prior to each dose, the results should be known prior to administration of the drug. If this drug is used during pregnancy or if the patient becomes pregnant while taking this drug, apprise the patient of the potential risk to the fetus.

➤*Lactation:* Mitoxantrone is excreted in human milk and significant concentrations (18 ng/mL) have been reported for 28 days after the last administration. Because of the potential for serious adverse reactions in infants from mitoxantrone, discontinue breast-feeding before starting treatment.

➤*Children:* Safety and efficacy in pediatric patients have not been established.

Precautions

➤*Monitoring:* Accompany therapy with mitoxantrone by close and frequent monitoring of hematologic and chemical laboratory parameters, as well as frequent patient observation.

MITOXANTRONE HYDROCHLORIDE — INJECTION

In leukemia treatment, hyperuricemia may occur as a result of rapid lysis of tumor cells by mitoxantrone. Monitor serum uric acid levels and institute hypouricemic therapy prior to the initiation of antileukemic therapy.

Obtain a complete blood count, including platelets, prior to each course of mitoxantrone and in the event that signs and symptoms of infection develop. Generally, do not administer mitoxantrone to multiple sclerosis patients with neutrophil counts less than 1,500 cells/mm^3. Perform liver function tests prior to each course of therapy. Mitoxantrone therapy in MS patients with abnormal liver function tests is not recommended because mitoxantrone clearance is reduced by hepatic impairment and no laboratory measurement can predict drug clearance and dose adjustments.

Carefully assess all patients for cardiac signs and symptoms by history and physical examination prior to start of therapy. Perform baseline evaluation of LVEF by echocardiogram or MUGA. Reevaluate LVEF prior to each dose administered to patients with MS.

Women with MS who are biologically capable of becoming pregnant, even if they are using birth control, should have a pregnancy test, and the results should be known, before receiving each dose of mitoxantrone.

➤*Systemic infections:* Treat systemic infections concomitantly with or just prior to commencing therapy with mitoxantrone.

Drug Interactions

➤*CYP450 system:* In vitro drug interaction studies have demonstrated that mitoxantrone did not inhibit CYP450 1A2, 2A6, 2C9, 2C19, 2D6, 2E1, and 3A4 across a broad concentration range. The results of in vitro induction studies are inconclusive, but suggest that mitoxantrone is a weak inducer of CYP450 2E1 activity.

Pharmacokinetic studies of the interaction of mitoxantrone with concomitantly administered medications have not been performed. The pathways leading to the metabolism of mitoxantrone have not been elucidated. To date, postmarketing experience has not revealed any significant drug interactions in patients who have received mitoxantrone for treatment of cancer. Information on drug interactions in patients with MS is limited.

➤*Corticosteroids:* Following concurrent administration of mitoxantrone with corticosteroids, no evidence of drug interactions has been observed.

Adverse Reactions

➤*MS:* Mitoxantrone has been administered to 149 patients with MS in 2 randomized clinical trials, including 21 patients who received mitoxantrone in combination with corticosteroids.

In study 1, the proportion of patients who discontinued treatment due to adverse reaction was 9.7% (n = 6) in the 12 mg/m^2 mitoxantrone arm (leukopenia, depression, decreased LV function, bone pain and emesis, renal failure, and 1 discontinuation to prevent future complications from repeated urinary tract infections) compared with 3.1% (n = 2) in the placebo arm (hepatitis and myocardial infarction). The following clinical adverse reactions were significantly more frequent in the mitoxantrone groups: nausea, alopecia, urinary tract infection, and menstrual disorders, including amenorrhea.

The table below summarizes clinical adverse reactions of all intensities occurring in greater than or equal to 5% of patients in either dose group of mitoxantrone and that were numerically greater on drug than on placebo in study 1. The majority of these events were of mild-to-moderate intensity, and nausea was the only adverse reaction that occurred with severe intensity in more than 1 patient (3 patients [5%] in the 12 mg/m^2 group). Of note, alopecia consisted of mild hair thinning.

Two of the 127 patients treated with mitoxantrone in study 1 had decreased LVEF to below 50% at some point during the 2 years of treatment. An additional patient receiving 12 mg/m^2 did not have LVEF measured, but had another echocardiographic measure of ventricular function (fractional shortening) that led to discontinuation from the study.

Mitoxantrone Adverse Reactions (≥ 5%)

Study 1			
Adverse reaction	Placebo (n = 64)	5 mg/m^2 mitoxantrone (n = 65)	12 mg/m^2 mitoxantrone (n = 62)
Cardiovascular			
Arrhythmia	8%	6%	18%
ECG abnormal	3%	5%	11%
CNS			
Headache	5%	6%	6%
Dermatologic			
Alopecia	31%	38%	61%
GI			
Constipation	6%	14%	10%
Diarrhea	11%	25%	16%
Nausea	20%	55%	76%
Stomatitis	8%	15%	19%
GU			
Amenorrhea[a]	3%	28%	43%
Menstrual disorder[a]	26%	51%	61%
Urine abnormal	6%	5%	11%
Urinary tract infection	13%	29%	32%
Respiratory			
Sinusitis	2%	3%	6%
Upper respiratory tract infection	52%	51%	53%
Miscellaneous			
Back pain	5%	6%	8%

[a] Percentage of female patients.

The proportion of patients experiencing any infection during study 1 was 67% for the placebo group, 85% for the 5 mg/m^2 group, and 81% for the 12 mg/m^2 group. However, few of these infections required hospitalization; 1 placebo patient (tonsillitis), three 5 mg/m^2 patients (enteritis, urinary tract infection, viral infection), and four 12 mg/m^2 patients (tonsillitis, urinary tract infection [2], endometritis).

Mitoxantrone Lab Test Abnormalities (≥ 5%)[a]

Study 1			
Reaction	Placebo (n = 64)	5 mg/m^2 mitoxantrone (n = 65)	12 mg/m^2 mitoxantrone (n = 62)
Leukopenia[b]	0%	9%	19%
Gamma-GT increased	3%	3%	15%
AST increased	8%	9%	8%
Granulocytopenia[c]	2%	6%	6%
Anemia	2%	9%	6%
ALT increased	3%	6%	5%

[a] Assessed using World Health Organization (WHO) toxicity criteria.
[b] Less than 4,000 cells/mm^3.
[c] Less than 2,000 cells/mm^3.

In study 2, mitoxantrone was administered once a month. Clinical adverse reactions most frequently reported in the mitoxantrone group included amenorrhea (53% of female patients), alopecia (33% of patients), nausea (29% of patients), and asthenia (24% of patients). The tables below respectively summarize adverse reactions and laboratory abnormalities occurring in greater than 5% of patients in the mitoxantrone group and numerically more frequent than in the control group.

Mitoxantrone Adverse Reactions (≥ 5%)[a]

Study 2		
Adverse reaction	Methylprednisolone (n = 21)	Mitoxantrone and methylprednisolone (n = 21)
Dermatologic		
Alopecia	0	33%
Cutaneous mycosis	0	10%
GI		
Aphthosis	0	10%
Gastralgia/ stomach burn/ epigastric pain	5%	14%
Nausea	0	29%
GU		
Amenorrhea[b]	0	53%
Menorrhagia[b]	0	7%
Respiratory		
Pharyngitis/ throat infection	5%	19%
Rhinitis	0	10%
Miscellaneous		
Asthenia	0	24%

[a] Assessed using National Cancer Institute (NCI) common toxicity criteria.
[b] Percentage of female patients.

Mitoxantrone Lab Test Abnormalities (≥ 5%)[a]

Study 2		
Adverse reaction	Methylprednisolone (n = 21)	Mitoxantrone and methylprednisolone (n = 21)
WBC low[b]	14%	100%
ANC low[c]	10%	100%
Lymphocytes low	43%	95%
Hemoglobin low	48%	43%

MITOXANTRONE HYDROCHLORIDE — INJECTION

Mitoxantrone Lab Test Abnormalities (≥ 5%)[a]		
Study 2		
Adverse reaction	Methylprednisolone (n = 21)	Mitoxantrone and methylprednisolone (n = 21)
Platelets low[d]	0%	33%
AST high	5%	15%
ALT high	10%	15%
Glucose high	5%	10%
Potassium low	0%	10%

[a] Assessed using National Cancer Institute (NCI) common toxicity criteria.
[b] Less than 4,000 cells/mm^3.
[c] Less than 1,500 cells/mm^3.
[d] Less than 100,000 cells/mm^3.

Leukopenia and neutropenia were reported in the mitoxantrone plus methylprednisolone group (see the preceding table). Neutropenia occurred within 3 weeks after mitoxantrone administration and was always reversible. Only mild-to-moderate intensity infections were reported in 9 of 21 patients in the mitoxantrone plus methylprednisolone group and in 3 of 21 patients in the methylprednisolone group; none of these required hospitalization. There was no difference among treatment groups in the incidence or severity of hemorrhagic events. There were no withdrawals from study 2 for safety reasons.

➤*Leukemia:* Mitoxantrone has been studied in approximately 600 patients with ANLL. The following table represents the adverse reaction experience in the large US comparative study of mitoxantrone + cytarabine vs daunorubicin + cytarabine. Experience in the large international study was similar. A much wider experience in a variety of other tumor types revealed no additional important reactions other than cardiomyopathy. It should be appreciated that the listed adverse reaction categories include overlapping clinical symptoms related to the same condition (eg, dyspnea, cough, and pneumonia). In addition, the listed adverse reactions cannot all necessarily be attributed to chemotherapy as it is often impossible to distinguish effects of the drug and effects of the underlying disease. It is clear, however, that the combination of mitoxantrone + cytarabine was responsible for nausea and vomiting, alopecia, mucositis/stomatitis, and myelosuppression.

The following table summarizes adverse reactions occurring in patients treated with mitoxantrone + cytarabine in comparison with those who received daunorubicin + cytarabine for therapy of ANLL in a large multicenter randomized prospective US trial.

Adverse reactions are presented as major categories and selected examples of clinically significant subcategories.

Mitoxantrone Adverse Reactions in ANLL patients				
	Induction % patients entering induction		Consolidation % patients entering induction	
Adverse reaction	Mitoxantrone (n = 102)	Daunorubicin (n = 102)	Mitoxantrone (n = 55)	Daunorubicin (n = 49)
Cardiovascular	26%	28%	11%	24%
Arrhythmias	3%	3%	4%	4%
Bleeding	37%	41%	20%	6%
CHF	5%	6%	0	0
CNS	30%	30%	34%	35%
Headache	10%	9%	13%	8%
Seizures	4%	4%	2%	8%
Dermatologic				
Alopecia	37%	40%	22%	16%
GI	16%	12%	2%	2%
Abdominal pain	15%	9%	9%	4%
Diarrhea	47%	47%	18%	8%
Gastrointestinal	88%	85%	58%	51%
Mucositis/ stomatitis	29%	33%	18%	8%
Nausea/ vomiting	72%	67%	31%	31%
Petechiae/ ecchymoses	7%	9%	11%	2%
GU				
Renal failure	8%	6%	0	2%
Hepatic	10%	11%	14%	2%
Jaundice	3%	8%	7%	0
Respiratory				
Cough	13%	9%	9%	2%
Dyspnea	18%	20%	6%	0
Pulmonary	43%	43%	24%	14%
Special senses				
Conjunctivitis	5%	1%	0	0
Eye	7%	6%	2%	4%
Miscellaneous				
Fever	78%	71%	24%	18%
Fungal infections	15%	13%	9%	6%
Infections	66%	73%	60%	43%
Pneumonia	9%	7%	9%	0
Sepsis	34%	36%	31%	18%
UTI	7%	2%	7%	2%

➤*Hormone-refractory prostate cancer:* Detailed safety information is available for a total of 353 patients with hormone-refractory prostate cancer treated with mitoxantrone, including 274 patients who received mitoxantrone in combination with corticosteroids.

Mitoxantrone Adverse Reactions (≥ 5%)		
Trial CCI-NOV22		
Adverse reaction	Mitoxantrone and prednisone (n = 80)	Prednisone (n = 81)
Cardiovascular		
Decreased LVEF	5%	0
CNS		
Anxiety/depression	5%	3%
Fatigue	39%	14%
Dermatologic		
Alopecia	29%	0
Skin infection	5%	3%
GI		
Anorexia	25%	6%
Constipation	16%	14%
Dyspepsia	5%	6%
Emesis	9%	5%
Mucositis	10%	0
Nausea	61%	35%
Respiratory		
Cough	5%	0
Dyspnea	11%	5%
Miscellaneous		
Anemia	5%	3%
Blurred vision	3%	5%
Edema	10%	4%
Fever	6%	3%
Hemorrhage/bruise	6%	1%
Nail bed changes	11%	0
Pain	8%	9%
Systemic infection	10%	7%
UTI	9%	4%

Mitoxantrone Adverse Reactions (≥ 5%)		
Trial CALGB 9182		
Adverse reaction	Mitoxantrone and hydrocortisone (n = 112)	Hydrocortisone (n = 113)
Cardiovascular		
Cardiac dysrhythmia	7%	3%
Cardiac function	18%	0
Cardiac ischemia	5%	1%
Hypertension	4%	5%
CNS		
Malaise/fatigue	34%	14%
Neuro/mood	6%	2%
Neuro/motor	7%	3%
Other neurologic	11%	5%
Dermatologic		
Alopecia	20%	1%
Skin	6%	4%
Sweats	9%	2%
GI		
Anorexia	22%	14%
Diarrhea	14%	4%
Nausea	26%	8%
Neuro/constipation	7%	2%

MITOXANTRONE HYDROCHLORIDE — INJECTION

Mitoxantrone Adverse Reactions (≥ 5%)		
Trial CALGB 9182		
Adverse reaction	Mitoxantrone and hydrocortisone (n = 112)	Hydrocortisone (n = 113)
Other GI	14%	11%
Stomatitis	8%	1%
Vomiting	11%	5%
Weight gain	14%	15%
Weight loss	17%	12%
GU		
BUN	22%	20%
Creatinine	13%	10%
Hematuria	11%	6%
Impotence/libido	7%	3%
Other kidney/ bladder	5%	3%
Proteinuria	6%	3%
Sterility	5%	3%
Hematologic		
Decreased hemo- globin	75%	39%
Decreased WBC	87%	4%
Granulocytes/bands	79%	3%
Hemorrhage	5%	3%
Lymphocytes	72%	25%
Platelets	39%	7%
Hepatic		
Alkaline phospha- tase	37%	38%
Other liver	8%	8%
Transaminase	20%	14%
Metabolic		
Edema	30%	14%
Hyperglycemia	31%	30%
Hypocalcemia	10%	5%
Hypokalemia	7%	4%
Hyponatremia	9%	3%
Other endocrine	6%	4%
Respiratory		
Dyspnea	15%	8%
Other pulmonary	5%	3%
Miscellaneous		
Chills	5%	0
Fever in absence of infection	14%	6%
Infection	17%	4%
Myalgias/arthralgias	5%	3%
Pain	41%	39%

➤*General:*

Cardiovascular – CHF, tachycardia, EKG changes including arrhythmias, chest pain and asymptomatic decreases in left ventricular ejection fraction have occurred.

GI – Nausea and vomiting occurred acutely in most patients and may have contributed to reports of dehydration, but were generally mild to moderate and could be controlled through the use of antiemetics. Stomatitis/mucositis occurred within 1 week of therapy.

Hematologic – Topoisomerase II inhibitors, including mitoxantrone, in combination with other antineoplastic agents, have been associated with the development of acute leukemia.

Leukemia: Myelosuppression is rapid in onset and is consistent with the requirement to produce significant marrow hypoplasia in order to achieve a response in acute leukemia. The incidences of infection and bleeding seen in the US trial are consistent with those reported for other standard induction regimens.

Hormone-refractory prostate cancer: In a randomized study where dose escalation was required for nadir neutrophil counts greater than 1000/mm^3, grade 4 neutropenia (ANC less than 500/mm^3) was observed in 54% of patients treated with mitoxantrone + low-dose prednisone. In a separate randomized trial where patients were treated with 14 mg/m^2, grade 4 neutropenia in 23% of patients treated with mitoxantrone plus hydrocortisone was observed. Neutropenic fever/infection occurred in 11% and 10% of patients receiving mitoxantrone plus corticosteroids, respectively, on the 2 trials. Platelets less than 50,000/mm^3 were noted in 4% and 3% of patients receiving mitoxantrone plus corticosteroids on these trials, and there was 1 patient death on mitoxantrone plus hydrocortisone due to intracranial hemorrhage after a fall.

Hypersensitivity – Hypotension, urticaria, dyspnea and rashes have been reported occasionally. Anaphylaxis/anaphylactoid reactions have been reported rarely.

Pulmonary – Interstitial pneumonitis has been reported in cancer patients receiving combination chemotherapy that included mitoxantrone.

Miscellaneous – Extravasation at the infusion site has been reported, which may result in erythema, swelling, pain, burning, and/or blue discoloration of the skin. Extravasation can result in tissue necrosis with resultant need for debridement and skin grafting. Phlebitis has also been reported at the site of infusion.

Overdosage

➤*Symptoms:* Accidental overdoses have been reported. Four patients receiving 140 to 180 mg/m^2 as a single bolus injection died as a result of severe leukopenia with infection.

➤*Treatment:* There is no known specific antidote for mitoxantrone. Hematologic support and antimicrobial therapy may be required during prolonged periods of severe myelosuppression.

Although patients with severe renal failure have not been studied, mitoxantrone is extensively tissue bound and it is unlikely that the therapeutic effect or toxicity would be mitigated by peritoneal or hemodialysis.

Patient Information

Mitoxantrone may impart a blue-green color to the urine for 24 hours after administration; advise patients to expect this during therapy. Bluish discoloration of the sclera may also occur. Advise patients of the signs and symptoms of myelosuppression.

Provide patients with MS with the patient information section at the time that the decision is made to treat with mitoxantrone and prior to and in close temporal proximity to each treatment. In addition, the physician should discuss the issues addressed in the patient information section with the patient.

SUBSTITUTED UREAS

HYDROXYUREA

Rx	**Droxia** (Bristol-Myers Squibb Oncology)	**Capsules:** 200 mg	Lactose. (Droxia 6335). Blue-green. In 60s.
		300 mg	Lactose. (Droxia 6336). Purple. In 60s.
		400 mg	Lactose. (Droxia 6337). Reddish-orange. In 60s.
Rx	**Hydroxyurea** (Various, eg, Barr, Major, Par, Roxane)	**Capsules:** 500 mg	In 100s and UD 100s.
Rx	**Hydrea** (Bristol-Myers Squibb)		Lactose. (Hydrea 830). Green and pink. In 100s.

HYDROXYUREA — ORAL

Indications

➤*Droxia*: To reduce the frequency of painful crises and to reduce the need for blood transfusions in adult patients with sickle cell anemia with recurrent moderate to severe painful crises (generally at least 3 during the preceding 12 months).

➤*Hydrea*: Significant tumor response to *Hydrea* (**hydroxyurea** capsules, USP) has been demonstrated in melanoma, resistant chronic myelocytic leukemia, and recurrent, metastatic, or inoperable carcinoma of the ovary.

Hydroxyurea used concomitantly with irradiation therapy is intended for use in the local control of primary squamous cell (epidermoid) carcinomas of the head and neck, excluding the lip.

➤*Unlabeled uses:* Treatment of cervical carcinoma, polycythemia vera, essential thrombocytosis. In combination with radiation therapy, used as a radiation sensitizer in brain tumors, cervical cancer, and head and neck cancer.

Thrombocythemia – To reduce platelet count and prevent thrombosis in high-risk patients with essential thrombocythemia (approximately 15 mg/kg/day).

HIV – Potential antiviral activity of hydroxyurea may be enhanced by didanosine.

Psoriasis – Management of refractory psoriasis (0.5 to 1.5 g daily).

Administration and Dosage

➤*Approved by the FDA:* February 25, 1998.

➤*Droxia:* Dosage should be based on the patient's actual or ideal weight, whichever is less. The initial dose of *Droxia* is 15 mg/kg/day as a single dose. The patient's blood count must be monitored every 2 weeks (see Warnings).

HYDROXYUREA — ORAL

If blood counts are in an acceptable range, the dose may be increased by 5 mg/kg/day every 12 weeks until a maximum tolerated dose (the highest dose that does not produce toxic blood counts over 24 consecutive weeks), or 35 mg/kg/day, is reached.

If blood counts are between the acceptable range and toxic (see parameters for acceptable and toxic below) the dose is not increased.

If blood counts are considered toxic, *Droxia* should be discontinued until hematologic recovery. Treatment may then be resumed after reducing the dose by 2.5 mg/kg/day from the dose associated with hematologic toxicity. *Droxia* may then be titrated up or down, every 12 weeks in 2.5 mg/kg/day increments, until the patient is at a stable dose that does not result in hematologic toxicity for 24 weeks. Any dosage on which a patient develops hematologic toxicity twice should not be tried again.

Acceptable ranges – Neutrophils at least 2500 cells/mm^3, platelets at least 95,000/mm^3, hemoglobin more than 5.3 g/dL, and reticulocytes at least 95,000/mm^3, if the hemoglobin concentration is less than 9 g/dL.

Toxic – Neutrophils less than 2000 cells/mm^3, platelets less than 80,000/mm^3, hemoglobin less than 4.5 g/dL, and reticulocytes less than 80,000/mm^3, if the hemoglobin concentration is less than 9 g/dL.

➤*Hydrea*: Because of the rarity of melanoma, resistant chronic myelocytic leukemia, carcinoma of the ovary, and carcinomas of the head and neck in pediatric patients, dosage regimens have not been established.

All dosage should be based on the patient's actual or ideal weight, whichever is less. Concurrent use of *Hydrea* with other myelosuppressive agents may require adjustment of dosages.

Solid tumors –

Intermittent therapy: 80 mg/kg administered orally as a single dose every third day.

Continuous therapy: 20 to 30 mg/kg administered orally as a single-dose daily.

Concomitant therapy with irradiation: Carcinoma of the head and neck, 80 mg/kg administered orally as a single dose every third day. Administration of hydroxyurea should begin at least 7 days before initiation of irradiation and continued during radiotherapy as well as indefinitely afterwards provided that the patient may be kept under adequate observation and evidences no unusual or severe reactions.

Resistant chronic myelocytic leukemia – Until the intermittent therapy regimen has been evaluated, continuous therapy (20 to 30 mg/kg administered orally as a single dose daily) is recommended.

An adequate trial period for determining the antineoplastic effectiveness of hydroxyurea is 6 weeks of therapy. When there is regression in tumor size or arrest in tumor growth, therapy should be continued indefinitely. Therapy should be interrupted if the white blood cell count drops below 2500/mm^3, or the platelet count below 100,000/mm^3. In these cases, the counts should be reevaluated after 3 days, and therapy resumed when the counts return to acceptable levels. Since the hematopoietic rebound is prompt, it is usually necessary to omit only a few doses. If prompt rebound has not occurred during combined *Hydrea* and irradiation therapy, irradiation may also be interrupted. However, the need for postponement of irradiation has been rare; radiotherapy has usually been continued using the recommended dosage and technique. Severe anemia, if it occurs, should be corrected without interrupting hydroxyurea therapy. Because hematopoiesis may be compromised by extensive irradiation or by other antineoplastic agents, it is recommended that hydroxyurea be administered cautiously to patients who have recently received extensive radiation therapy or chemotherapy with other cytotoxic drugs.

Pain or discomfort from inflammation of the mucous membranes at the irradiated site (mucositis) is usually controlled by measures such as topical anesthetics and orally administered analgesics. If the reaction is severe, hydroxyurea therapy may be temporarily interrupted; if it is extremely severe, irradiation dosage may, in addition, be temporarily postponed. However, it has rarely been necessary to terminate these therapies.

Severe gastric distress (eg, nausea, vomiting, and anorexia) resulting from combined therapy may usually be controlled by temporary interruption of hydroxyurea administration.

➤*Renal insufficiency:* There are no data that support specific guidance for dosage adjustment in patients with renal impairment. As renal excretion is a pathway of elimination, consideration should be given to decreasing the dosage of hydroxyurea in patients with renal impairment. Close monitoring of hematologic parameters is advised in these patients.

➤*Storage/Stability:* Store at 25°C (77°F); excursions permitted to 15° to 30°C (59° to 86°F) [see USP controlled room temperature]. Keep tightly closed.

Actions

➤*Pharmacology:* Various studies support the hypothesis that hydroxyurea causes an immediate inhibition of DNA synthesis by acting as a ribonucleotide reductase inhibitor, without interfering with the synthesis of ribonucleic acid or of protein.

Droxia – The precise mechanism by which hydroxyurea produces its cytotoxic and cytoreductive effects is not known. The mechanisms by which *Droxia* produces its beneficial effects in patients with sickle cell anemia (SCA) are uncertain. Known pharmacologic effects of *Droxia* that may contribute to its beneficial effects include increasing hemoglobin F levels in RBCs, decreasing neutrophils, increasing the water content of RBCs, increasing deformability of sickled cells, and altering the adhesion of RBCs to endothelium.

Hydrea – The precise mechanism by which *Hydrea* produces its antineoplastic effects cannot, at present, be described. Three mechanisms of action have been postulated for the increased effectiveness of concomitant use of hydroxyurea therapy with irradiation on squamous cell (epidermoid) carcinomas of the head and neck. In vitro studies utilizing Chinese hamster cells suggest the following: *Hydrea* is lethal to normally radioresistant S-stage cells; *Hydrea* holds other cells of the cell cycle in the G1 or pre-DNA synthesis stage where they are most susceptible to the effects of irradiation; the third mechanism of action has been theorized on the basis of in vitro studies of HeLa cells: it appears that hydroxyurea, by inhibition of DNA synthesis, hinders the normal repair process of cells damaged but not killed by irradiation, thereby decreasing their survival rate; RNA and protein syntheses have shown no alteration.

➤*Pharmacokinetics:*

Absorption – Hydroxyurea is readily absorbed after oral administration. Peak plasma levels are reached in 1 to 4 hours after an oral dose. With increasing doses, disproportionately greater mean peak plasma concentrations and AUCs are observed.

Distribution – Hydroxyurea distributes rapidly and widely in the body with an estimated volume of distribution approximating total body water.

Plasma to ascites fluid ratios range from 2:1 to 7.5:1. Hydroxyurea concentrates in leukocytes and erythrocytes.

Metabolism – Up to 50% of an oral dose undergoes conversion through metabolic pathways that are not fully characterized. In 1 minor pathway, hydroxyurea may be degraded by urease found in intestinal bacteria. Acetohydroxamic acid was found in the serum of 3 leukemic patients receiving hydroxyurea and may be formed from hydroxylamine resulting from action of urease on hydroxyurea.

Excretion – Excretion of hydroxyurea in humans is a nonlinear process occurring through 2 pathways. One is saturable, probably hepatic metabolism; the other is first-order renal excretion. In adults with SCA, mean cumulative urinary hydroxyurea excretion was 62% of the administered dose at 8 hours.

Special populations –

Renal function impairment: See Administration and Dosage for more information.

Contraindications

Hypersensitivity to hydroxyurea or any other component of its formulation.

➤*Hydrea*: *Hydrea* is contraindicated in patients with marked bone marrow depression (ie, leukopenia [less than 2500 WBC] or thrombocytopenia [less than 100,000]) or severe anemia.

Warnings

➤*Bone marrow suppression:*

Droxia – *Droxia* is a cytotoxic and myelosuppressive agent. *Droxia* should not be given if bone marrow function is markedly depressed, as indicated by neutrophils less than 2,000 cells/mm^3; a platelet count less than 80,000/mm^3; a hemoglobin level less than 4.5 g/dL; or reticulocytes less than 80,000/mm^3 when the hemoglobin concentration is less than 9 g/dL. Neutropenia is generally the first and most common manifestation of hematologic suppression (see Administration and Dosage, *Droxia*). Thrombocytopenia and anemia occur less often, and are seldom seen without a preceding leukopenia. Recovery from myelosuppression is usually rapid when therapy is interrupted. *Droxia* causes macrocytosis, which may mask the incidental development of folic acid deficiency. Prophylactic administration of folic acid is recommended.

Hydrea – Treatment with hydroxyurea should not be initiated if bone marrow function is markedly depressed (see Contraindications). Bone marrow suppression may occur, and leukopenia is generally its first and most common manifestation. Thrombocytopenia and anemia occur less often, and are seldom seen without a preceding leukopenia. However, the recovery from myelosuppression is rapid when therapy is interrupted. It should be borne in mind that bone marrow depression is more likely in patients who have previously received radiotherapy or cytotoxic cancer chemotherapeutic agents; hydroxyurea should be used cautiously in such patients.

Patients who have received irradiation therapy in the past may have an exacerbation of postirradiation erythema.

Severe anemia must be corrected before initiating therapy with hydroxyurea.

Erythrocytic abnormalities: Megaloblastic erythropoiesis, which is self-limiting, is often seen early in the course of *Hydrea* therapy. The morphologic change resembles pernicious anemia, but is not related to vitamin B_{12} or folic acid deficiency. Hydroxyurea may also delay plasma iron clearance and reduce the rate of iron utilization by erythrocytes, but it does not appear to alter the red blood cell survival time.

In patients receiving long-term hydroxyurea for myeloproliferative disorders, such as polycythemia vera and thrombocythemia, secondary leukemia has been reported. It is unknown whether this leukemogenic effect is secondary to hydroxyurea or associated with the patients' underlying disease.

➤*Fatal and nonfatal pancreatitis in HIV-infected patients:* Fatal and nonfatal pancreatitis have occurred in HIV-infected patients during therapy with hydroxyurea and didanosine, with or without stavudine. Hepatotoxicity and hepatic failure resulting in death have been reported during postmarketing surveillance in HIV-infected patients treated with hydroxyurea and other antiretroviral agents. Fatal hepatic events were reported most often in patients treated with the combination of hydroxyurea, didanosine, and stavudine. Peripheral neuropathy, which was severe in some cases,

HYDROXYUREA — ORAL

has been reported in HIV-infected patients receiving hydroxyurea in combination with antiretroviral agents, including didanosine, with or without stavudine.

➤*Renal function impairment:* Hydroxyurea should be used with caution in patients with renal dysfunction (see Administration and Dosage).

➤*Carcinogenesis:* (See Warning Box.) Hydroxyurea is genotoxic in a wide range of test systems and is thus presumed to be a human carcinogen. In patients receiving long-term hydroxyurea for myeloproliferative disorders, such as polycythemia vera and thrombocythemia, secondary leukemia has been reported. It is unknown whether this leukemogenic effect is secondary to hydroxyurea or is associated with the patients' underlying disease. Skin cancer has also been reported in patients receiving long-term hydroxyurea.

➤*Mutagenesis:* Hydroxyurea is mutagenic in vitro to bacteria, fungi, protozoa, and mammalian cells. Hydroxyurea is clastogenic in vitro (hamster cells, human lymphoblasts) and in vivo (SCE assay in rodents, mouse micronucleus assay). Hydroxyurea causes the transformation of rodent embryo cells to a tumorigenic phenotype.

➤*Fertility impairment:* Hydroxyurea administered to male rats at 60 mg/kg/day (approximately 0.3 times the maximum recommended human daily dose on a mg/m^2 basis) produced testicular atrophy, decreased spermatogenesis, and significantly reduced their ability to impregnate females.

➤*Elderly:*

Hydrea – Elderly patients may be more sensitive to the effects of hydroxyurea, and may require a lower dose regimen.

➤*Pregnancy: Category D.* Drugs that affect DNA synthesis, such as hydroxyurea, may be potential mutagenic agents. The physician should carefully consider this possibility before administering this drug to male or female patients who may contemplate conception.

Hydroxyurea can cause fetal harm when administered to a pregnant woman. Hydroxyurea has been demonstrated to be a potent teratogen in a wide variety of animal models, including mice, hamsters, cats, miniature swine, dogs and monkeys at doses within 1-fold of the human dose given on a mg/m^2 basis. Hydroxyurea is embryotoxic and causes fetal malformations (partially ossified cranial bones, absence of eye sockets, hydrocephaly, bipartite sternebrae, missing lumbar vertebrae) at 180 mg/kg/day (approximately 0.8 times the maximum recommended human daily dose on a mg/m^2 basis) in rats and at 30 mg/kg/day (approximately 0.3 times the maximum recommended human daily dose on a mg/m^2 basis) in rabbits. Embryotoxicity was characterized by decreased fetal viability, reduced live litter sizes, and developmental delays. Hydroxyurea crosses the placenta. Single doses of 375 mg/kg or more (approximately 1.7 times the maximum recommended human daily dose on a mg/m^2 basis) to rats caused growth retardation and impaired learning ability. There are no adequate and well-controlled studies in pregnant women. If this drug is used during pregnancy or if the patient becomes pregnant while taking this drug, the patient should be apprised of the potential harm to the fetus. Women of childbearing potential should be advised to avoid becoming pregnant.

➤*Lactation:* Hydroxyurea is excreted in human milk. Because of the potential for serious adverse reactions with hydroxyurea, a decision should be made either to discontinue nursing or to discontinue the drug, taking into account the importance of the drug to the mother.

➤*Children:* Safety and effectiveness in pediatric patients have not been established.

Precautions

➤*Monitoring:* Therapy with hydroxyurea requires close supervision.

➤*Droxia*: Some patients treated at the recommended initial dose of 15 mg/kg/day have experienced severe or life-threatening myelosuppression, requiring interruption of treatment and dose reduction. The hematologic status of the patient as well as kidney and liver function should be determined prior to, and repeatedly during, treatment. Treatment should be interrupted if neutrophil levels fall to less than 2000/mm^3; platelets fall to less than 80,000/mm^3; hemoglobin declines to less than 4.5 g/dL; or if reticulocytes fall less than 80,000/mm^3 when the hemoglobin concentration is less than 9 g/dL. Following recovery, treatment may be resumed at lower doses (see Administration and Dosage).

Patients must be able to follow directions regarding drug administration and their monitoring and care.

➤*Hydrea*: The complete status of the blood, including bone marrow examination, if indicated, as well as kidney function and liver function should be determined prior to, and repeatedly during, treatment. The determination of the hemoglobin level, total leukocyte counts, and platelet counts should be performed at least once a week throughout the course of hydroxyurea therapy. If the white blood cell count decreases to less than 2500/mm^3, or the platelet count to less than 100,000/mm^3, therapy should be interrupted until the values rise significantly toward normal levels. Severe anemia, if it occurs, should be managed without interrupting hydroxyurea therapy.

Hydroxyurea is not indicated for the treatment of HIV infection; however, if HIV-infected patients are treated with hydroxyurea, and in particular, in combination with didanosine or stavudine, close monitoring for signs and symptoms of pancreatitis and hepatotoxicity is recommended. Patients who develop signs and symptoms of pancreatitis or hepatotoxicity should permanently discontinue therapy with hydroxyurea (see Warnings and Adverse Reactions).

Drug Interactions

➤*Hydrea*: Concurrent use of *Hydrea* and other myelosuppressive agents or radiation therapy may increase the likelihood of bone marrow depression or other adverse events (see Warnings and Adverse Reactions).

Uricosuric agents – Because hydroxyurea may raise the serum uric acid level, dosage adjustment of uricosuric medication may be necessary.

Adverse Reactions

➤*Adverse reactions:* Adverse reactions associated with the use of hydroxyurea, in the treatment of neoplastic diseases, in addition to hematologic effects include the following:

CNS – Neurological disturbances have occurred extremely rarely and were limited to headache, dizziness, disorientation, hallucinations, and convulsions.

Large doses may produce moderate drowsiness.

Dermatologic – Maculopapular rash, skin ulceration, dermatomyositis-like skin changes, peripheral erythema and facial erythema. Hyperpigmentation, atrophy of skin and nails, scaling, and violet papules have been observed in some patients after several years of long-term daily maintenance therapy with hydroxyurea. Skin cancer has been reported.

GI – Stomatitis, anorexia, nausea, vomiting, diarrhea, and constipation.

GU – Dysuria and alopecia occur very rarely.

Hematologic –

Hydrea: Adverse reactions have been primarily bone marrow depression (leukopenia, anemia, and occasionally thrombocytopenia).

Lab test abnormalities – Abnormal BSP retention has been reported.

Elevation of hepatic enzymes have also been reported.

Renal – Hydroxyurea occasionally may cause temporary impairment of renal tubular function accompanied by elevations in serum uric acid, BUN, and creatinine levels.

Miscellaneous – Fever, chills, malaise, edema, asthenia.

➤*Acute pulmonary reactions:*

Respiratory – The association of hydroxyurea with the development of acute pulmonary reactions consisting of diffuse pulmonary infiltrates, fever and dyspnea has been rarely reported. Pulmonary fibrosis also has been reported rarely.

➤*Fatal and nonfatal pancreatitis and hepatotoxicity:* Fatal and nonfatal pancreatitis and hepatotoxicity, and severe peripheral neuropathy have been reported in HIV-infected patients who received hydroxyurea in combination with antiretroviral agents, in particular, didanosine plus stavudine. Patients treated with hydroxyurea in combination with didanosine, stavudine, and indinavir in study ACTG 5025 showed a median decline in CD4 cells of approximately 100/mm^3 (see Warnings and Precautions).

➤*Droxia*:

Sickle cell anemia – In patients treated for sickle cell anemia in the Multicenter Study of Hydroxyurea in Sickle Cell Anemia, the most common adverse reactions were hematologic, with neutropenia, and low reticulocyte and platelet levels necessitating temporary cessation in almost all patients. Hematologic recovery usually occurred in two weeks.

Nonhematologic events that possibly were associated with treatment include hair loss, skin rash, fever, gastrointestinal disturbances, weight gain, bleeding, and parvovirus B-19 infection; however, these nonhematologic events occurred with similar frequencies in the hydroxyurea and placebo treatment groups. Melanonychia has also been reported in patients receiving *Droxia* for SCA.

➤*Hydrea*:

Irradiation therapy – Adverse reactions observed with combined *Hydrea* and irradiation therapy are similar to those reported with the use of hydroxyurea or radiation treatment alone. These effects primarily include bone marrow depression (anemia and leukopenia), gastric irritation, and mucositis. Almost all patients receiving an adequate course of combined hydroxyurea and irradiation therapy will demonstrate concurrent leukopenia. Platelet depression (less than 100,000 cells/mm^3) has occurred rarely and only in the presence of marked leukopenia. *Hydrea* may potentiate some adverse reactions usually seen with irradiation alone, such as gastric distress and mucositis.

Overdosage

➤*Animal pharmacology and toxicology with Hydrea*: The oral LD_{50} of hydroxyurea is 7330 mg/kg in mice and 5780 mg/kg in rats, given as a single dose.

In subacute and chronic toxicity studies in the rat, the most consistent pathological findings were an apparent dose-related mild to moderate bone marrow hypoplasia as well as pulmonary congestion and mottling of the lungs. At the highest dosage levels (1260 mg/kg/day for 37 days then 2520 mg/kg/day for 40 days), testicular atrophy with absence of spermatogenesis occurred; in several animals, hepatic cell damage with fatty metamorphosis was noted. In the dog, mild to marked bone marrow depression was a consistent finding except at the lower dosage levels. Additionally, at the higher dose levels (140 to 420 mg or 140 to 1260 mg/kg/week given 3 or 7 days weekly for 12 weeks), growth retardation, slightly increased blood glucose values, and hemosiderosis of the liver or spleen were found; reversible spermatogenic arrest was noted. In the monkey, bone marrow depression, lymphoid atrophy of the spleen, and degenerative changes in the epithelium of the small and large intestines were found. At the higher, often

HYDROXYUREA — ORAL

lethal, doses (400 to 800 mg/kg/day for 7 to 15 days), hemorrhage and congestion were found in the lungs, brain, and urinary tract. Cardiovascular effects (changes in heart rate, blood pressure, orthostatic hypotension, EKG changes) and hematological changes (slight hemolysis, slight methemoglobinemia) were observed in some species of laboratory animals at doses exceeding clinical levels.

➤*Symptoms:* Acute mucocutaneous toxicity has been reported in patients receiving hydroxyurea at dosages several times the therapeutic dose. Soreness, violet erythema, edema on palms and soles followed by scaling of hands and feet, severe generalized hyperpigmentation of the skin, and stomatitis have been observed.

METHYLHYDRAZINE DERIVATIVES

PROCARBAZINE HYDROCHLORIDE (N-Methylhydrazine; MIH)

Rx	**Matulane** (Sigma-Tau)	**Capsules:** 50 mg	Talc, mannitol, parabens. (Matulane Sigma-Tau). Ivory. In 100s.

PROCARBAZINE HYDROCHLORIDE — ORAL

WARNING

It is recommended that procarbazine hydrochloride be given only by or under the supervision of a physician experienced in the use of potent antineoplastic drugs. Adequate clinical and laboratory facilities should be available to patients for proper monitoring of treatment.

Indications

➤*Hodgkin's disease:* Procarbazine hydrochloride is indicated for use in combination with other anticancer drugs for the treatment of Stage III and IV Hodgkin's disease. Procarbazine hydrochloride is used as part of the MOPP (nitrogen mustard, vincristine, procarbazine, prednisone) regimen.

➤*Unlabeled uses:* Treatment of non-Hodgkin lymphoma, brain tumors, small cell lung cancer, melanoma, mycosis fungoides, and multiple myeloma.

Administration and Dosage

➤*Approved by the FDA:* July 26, 1969.

The following doses are for administration of the drug as a single agent. When used in combination with other anticancer drugs, the procarbazine hydrochloride dose should be appropriately reduced (eg, in the MOPP regimen, the procarbazine hydrochloride dose is 100 mg/m^2 daily for 14 days). All dosages are based on the patient's actual weight. However, the estimated lean body mass (dry weight) is used if the patient is obese or if there has been a spurious weight gain due to edema, ascites or other forms of abnormal fluid retention.

➤*Adults:* To minimize the nausea and vomiting experienced by a high percentage of patients beginning procarbazine hydrochloride therapy, single or divided doses of 2 to 4 mg/kg/day for the first week are recommended. Daily dosage should then be maintained at 4 to 6 mg/kg/day until maximum response is obtained or until the white blood count falls below 4000/cmm or the platelets fall below 100,000/cmm. When maximum response is obtained, the dose may be maintained at 1 to 2 mg/kg/day. Upon evidence of hematologic or other toxicity, the drug should be discontinued until there has been satisfactory recovery. Prompt cessation of therapy is recommended if any one of the following occurs:

- CNS signs or symptoms such as paresthesias, neuropathies or confusion.
- Leukopenia (white blood count under 4000).
- Thrombocytopenia (platelets under 100,000).
- Hypersensitivity reaction.
- Stomatitis (the first small ulceration or persistent spot soreness around the oral cavity is a signal for cessation of therapy).
- Diarrhea (frequent bowel movements or watery stools).
- Hemorrhage or bleeding tendencies. After toxic side effects have subsided, therapy may then be resumed at the discretion of the physician, based on clinical evaluation and appropriate laboratory studies, at a dosage of 1 to 2 mg/kg/day.

➤*Pediatric patients:* Very close clinical monitoring is mandatory. Undue toxicity, evidenced by tremors, coma and convulsions, has occurred in a few cases. Dosage, therefore, should be individualized. The following dosage schedule is provided as a guideline only.

Fifty (50) mg per square meter of body surface per day is recommended for the first week. Dosage should then be maintained at 100 mg per square meter of body surface per day until maximum response is obtained or until leukopenia or thrombocytopenia occurs. When maximum response is attained, the dose may be maintained at 50 mg per square meter of body surface per day. Upon evidence of hematologic or other toxicity, the drug should be discontinued until there has been satisfactory recovery, based on clinical evaluation and appropriate laboratory tests. After toxic side effects have subsided, therapy may then be resumed.

Actions

➤*Pharmacology:* The precise mode of cytotoxic action of procarbazine has not been clearly defined. There is evidence that the drug may act by inhibition of protein, RNA and DNA synthesis. Studies have suggested that procarbazine may inhibit transmethylation of methyl groups of methionine into t-RNA. The absence of functional t-RNA could cause the cessation of protein synthesis and consequently DNA and RNA synthesis. In addition, procarbazine may directly damage DNA. Hydrogen peroxide, formed during the auto-oxidation of the drug, may attack protein sulfhydryl groups contained in residual protein which is tightly bound to DNA.

➤*Pharmacokinetics:*

Absorption – Procarbazine is rapidly and completely absorbed. Following oral administration of 30 mg of ^{14}C-labeled procarbazine, maximum peak plasma radioactive concentrations were reached within 60 minutes.

Distribution – Procarbazine crosses the blood-brain barrier and rapidly equilibrates between plasma and cerebrospinal fluid after oral administration.

Metabolism – Procarbazine is metabolized primarily in the liver and kidneys. The drug appears to be auto-oxidized to the azo derivative with the release of hydrogen peroxide. The azo derivative isomerizes to the hydrazone, and following hydrolysis splits into a benzylaldehyde derivative and methylhydrazine. The methylhydrazine is further degraded to CO_2 and CH_4 and possibly hydrazine, whereas the aldehyde is oxidized to N-isopropylterephthalamic acid, which is excreted in the urine.

Excretion – After intravenous injection, the plasma half-life of procarbazine is approximately 10 minutes. Approximately 70% of the radioactivity is excreted in the urine as N-isopropylterephthalamic acid within 24 hours following both oral and intravenous administration of ^{14}C-labeled procarbazine.

Contraindications

Procarbazine hydrochloride is contraindicated in patients with known hypersensitivity to the drug or inadequate marrow reserve as demonstrated by bone marrow aspiration. Due consideration of this possible state should be given to each patient who has leukopenia, thrombocytopenia or anemia.

Warnings

➤*Drug/Food warnings:* To minimize CNS depression and possible potentiation, barbiturates, antihistamines, narcotics, hypotensive agents or phenothiazines should be used with caution. Ethyl alcohol should not be used since there may be a disulfiram-like reaction. Because procarbazine hydrochloride exhibits some monoamine oxidase inhibitory activity, sympathomimetic drugs, tricyclic antidepressant drugs (eg, amitriptyline HCl, imipramine HCl) and other drugs and foods with known high tyramine content, such as wine, yogurt, ripe cheese and bananas, should be avoided. A further phenomenon of toxicity common to many hydrazine derivatives is hemolysis and the appearance of Heinz-Ehrlich inclusion bodies in erythrocytes.

➤*Renal/Hepatic function impairment:* Undue toxicity may occur if procarbazine hydrochloride is used in patients with impairment of renal and/or hepatic function. When appropriate, hospitalization for the initial course of treatment should be considered.

➤*Carcinogenesis:* The carcinogenicity of procarbazine hydrochloride in mice, rats and monkeys has been reported in a considerable number of studies. Instances of a second nonlymphoid malignancy, including lung cancer and acute myelocytic leukemia, have been reported in patients with Hodgkin's disease treated with procarbazine in combination with other chemotherapy and/or radiation. The risks of secondary lung cancer from treatment appear to be multiplied by tobacco use. The International Agency for Research on Cancer (IARC) considers that there is "sufficient evidence" for the human carcinogenicity of procarbazine hydrochloride when it is given in intensive regimens which include other antineoplastic agents but that there is inadequate evidence of carcinogenicity in humans given procarbazine hydrochloride alone.

➤*Mutagenesis:* Procarbazine hydrochloride has been shown to be mutagenic in a variety of bacterial and mammalian test systems.

➤*Fertility impairment:* Azoospermia and antifertility effects associated with procarbazine hydrochloride administration in combination with other chemotherapeutic agents for treating Hodgkin's disease have been reported in human clinical studies. Since these patients received multicombination therapy, it is difficult to determine to what extent procarbazine hydrochloride alone was involved in the male germ-cell damage. The usual Segment I fertility/reproduction studies in laboratory animals have not been carried out with procarbazine hydrochloride. However, compounds which inhibit DNA, RNA and/or protein synthesis might be expected to have adverse effects on gametogenesis. Unscheduled DNA synthesis in the testis of rabbits and decreased fertility in male mice treated with procarbazine hydrochloride have been reported.

➤*Pregnancy: Category D.*

Teratogenic – Procarbazine hydrochloride can cause fetal harm when administered to a pregnant woman. While there are no adequate and well-controlled studies with procarbazine hydrochloride in pregnant women, there are case reports of malformations in the offspring of women who were exposed to procarbazine hydrochloride in combination with other antineoplastic agents during pregnancy. Procarbazine hydrochloride should be used during pregnancy only if the potential benefit justifies the potential risk to

PROCARBAZINE HYDROCHLORIDE — ORAL

the fetus. If this drug is used during pregnancy, or if the patient becomes pregnant while taking this drug, the patient should be apprised of the potential hazard to the fetus. Women of childbearing potential should be advised to avoid becoming pregnant. Procarbazine hydrochloride is teratogenic in the rat when given at doses approximately 4 to 13 times the maximum recommended human therapeutic dose of 6 mg/kg/day.

Nonteratogenic – Procarbazine hydrochloride has not been adequately studied in animals for its effects on peri- and postnatal development. However, neurogenic tumors were noted in the offspring of rats given intravenous injections of 125 mg/kg of procarbazine hydrochloride on day 22 of gestation. Compounds which inhibit DNA, RNA and protein synthesis might be expected to have adverse effects on peri- and postnatal development.

➤*Lactation:* It is not known whether procarbazine hydrochloride is excreted in human milk. Because of the potential for tumorigenicity shown for procarbazine hydrochloride in animal studies, mothers should not nurse while receiving this drug.

➤*Children:* Undue toxicity, evidenced by tremors, coma and convulsions, has occurred in a few cases. Dosage, therefore, should be individualized. All dosages are based on the patient's actual weight. However, the estimated lean body mass (dry weight) is used if the patient is obese or if there has been a spurious weight gain due to edema, ascites or other forms of abnormal fluid retention. Very close clinical monitoring is mandatory.

Precautions

➤*Monitoring:* Baseline laboratory data should be obtained prior to initiation of therapy. The hematologic status as indicated by hemoglobin, hematocrit, white blood count (WBC), differential, reticulocytes and platelets should be monitored closely, at least every 3 or 4 days.

Hepatic and renal evaluation are indicated prior to beginning therapy. Urinalysis, transaminase, alkaline phosphatase and blood urea nitrogen tests should be repeated at least weekly.

➤*Prior radiation/chemotherapy:* If radiation or a chemotherapeutic agent known to have marrow-depressant activity has been used, an interval of 1 month or longer without such therapy is recommended before starting treatment with procarbazine hydrochloride. The length of this interval may also be determined by evidence of bone marrow recovery based on successive bone marrow studies.

➤*Discontinuation:* Prompt cessation of therapy is recommended if any one of the following occurs: CNS signs or symptoms such as paresthesias, neuropathies, or confusion; leukopenia (white blood count under 4,000); thrombocytopenia (platelets under 100,000); hypersensitivity reaction; stomatitis (the first small ulceration or persistent spot soreness around the oral cavity is a signal for cessation of therapy); diarrhea (frequent bowel movements or watery stools); hemorrhage or bleeding tendencies.

➤*Bone marrow depression:* Bone marrow depression often occurs 2 to 8 weeks after the start of treatment. If leukopenia occurs, hospitalization of the patient may be needed for appropriate treatment to prevent systemic infection.

Drug Interactions

Procarbazine Drug Interactions

Precipitant drug	Object drug*		Description
Procarbazine	CNS depressants (ie, narcotics, hypotensive agents, phenothiazines, antihistamines, barbiturates, sedatives)	↑	Concomitant use may result in depressant effects on the CNS (ie, respiratory depression).
Procarbazine	Ethanol	↑	Concomitant ingestion has resulted in a disulfiram-like reaction (ie, flushing of the face).
Procarbazine	Methotrexate	↑	The nephrotoxicity of methotrexate may be increased; consider an interval of ≥ 72 hours between administration of the final dose of procarbazine and the initiation of a high-dose methotrexate infusion.
Procarbazine	Sympathomimetics (eg, ephedrine, epinephrine)	↑	May cause an abrupt increase in blood pressure, resulting in a potentially fatal hypertensive crisis.
Procarbazine	Tricyclic antidepressants (eg, amitriptyline, imipramine)	↑	Severe toxic and fatal reactions including excitability, fluctuations in blood pressure, convulsions, and coma may occur. However, some studies report uneventful concurrent use with MAOIs.
Procarbazine	Radiation or other chemotherapy	↑	If radiation or other chemotherapy known to have marrow depressant activity has been used, wait ≥ 1 month before starting procarbazine. Interval length may also be determined by evidence of bone marrow recovery based on successive bone marrow studies.

* ↑ = Object drug increased. ↓ = Object drug decreased.

Adverse Reactions

Leukopenia, anemia and thrombopenia occur frequently. Nausea and vomiting are the most commonly reported side effects.

Other adverse reactions are:

➤*Allergic:* Generalized allergic reactions.

➤*Cardiovascular:* Hypotension, tachycardia, syncope.

➤*CNS:* Coma, convulsions, neuropathy, ataxia, paresthesia, nystagmus, diminished reflexes, falling, foot drop, headache, dizziness, unsteadiness.

➤*Dermatologic:* Herpes, dermatitis, pruritus, alopecia, hyperpigmentation, rash, urticaria, flushing.

➤*Endocrine:* Gynecomastia in prepubertal and early pubertal boys.

➤*GI:* Hepatic dysfunction, jaundice, stomatitis, hematemesis, melena, diarrhea, dysphagia, anorexia, abdominal pain, constipation, dry mouth.

➤*GU:* Hematuria, urinary frequency, nocturia.

➤*Hematologic:* Pancytopenia, eosinophilia, hemolytic anemia, bleeding tendencies such as petechiae, purpura, epistaxis and hemoptysis.

➤*Musculoskeletal:* Pain, including myalgia and arthralgia; tremors.

➤*Ophthalmic:* Retinal hemorrhage, papilledema, photophobia, diplopia, inability to focus.

➤*Psychiatric:* Hallucinations, depression, apprehension, nervousness, confusion, nightmares.

➤*Respiratory:* Pneumonitis, pleural effusion, cough.

➤*Miscellaneous:* Intercurrent infections, hearing loss, pyrexia, diaphoresis, lethargy, weakness, fatigue, edema, chills, insomnia, slurred speech, hoarseness, drowsiness.

Second nonlymphoid malignancies (including lung cancer, acute myelocytic leukemia and malignant myelosclerosis) and azoospermia have been reported in patients with Hodgkin's disease treated with procarbazine in combination with other chemotherapy and/or radiation. The risks of secondary lung cancer from treatment appear to be multiplied by tobacco use.

Overdosage

The major manifestations of overdosage with procarbazine hydrochloride would be anticipated to be nausea, vomiting, enteritis, diarrhea, hypotension, tremors, convulsions and coma. Treatment should consist of either the administration of an emetic or gastric lavage. General supportive measures such as intravenous fluids are advised. Since the major toxicity of procarbazine hydrochloride is hematologic and hepatic, patients should have frequent complete blood counts and liver function tests throughout their period of recovery and for a minimum of 2 weeks thereafter. Should abnormalities appear in any of these determinations, appropriate measures for correction and stabilization should be immediately undertaken.

The estimated mean lethal dose of procarbazine hydrochloride in laboratory animals varied from approximately 150 mg/kg in rabbits to 1300 mg/kg in mice.

Patient Information

Patients should be warned not to drink alcoholic beverages while on procarbazine hydrochloride therapy since there may be an disulfiram-like reaction. They should also be cautioned to avoid foods with known high tyramine content such as wine, yogurt, ripe cheese and bananas. Over-the-counter drug preparations which contain antihistamines or sympathomimetic drugs should also be avoided. Patients taking procarbazine hydrochloride should also be warned against the use of prescription drugs without the knowledge and consent of their physician. Patients should be advised to discontinue tobacco use.

TEMOZOLOMIDE

Rx	Temodar (Schering)	Capsules: 5 mg	Lactose. In 5s and 20s.
		20 mg	Lactose. In 5s and 20s.
		100 mg	Lactose. In 5s and 20s.
		250 mg	Lactose. In 5s and 20s.

TEMOZOLOMIDE — ORAL

Indications

➤*Glioblastoma multiforme:* For the treatment of adult patients with newly diagnosed glioblastoma multiforme concomitantly with radiotherapy and then as maintenance treatment.

➤*Anaplastic astrocytoma:* For the treatment of adult patients with refractory anaplastic astrocytoma (ie, patients who have experienced disease progression on a drug regimen containing a nitrosourea and procarbazine).

➤*Unlabeled uses:* Metastatic melanoma.

Administration and Dosage

➤*Approved by the FDA:* August 11, 1999.

Dosage of temozolomide capsules must be adjusted according to nadir neutrophil and platelet counts in the previous cycle and the neutrophil and platelet counts at the time of initiating the next cycle.

For temozolomide dosage calculations based on body surface area (BSA) and for suggested capsule combinations on a daily dose, see the tables in the following section.

➤*Glioblastoma multiforme:*

Concomitant phase – Temozolomide is administered orally at 75 mg/m^2 daily for 42 days concomitant with focal radiotherapy (60 Gy administered in 30 fractions) followed by maintenance temozolomide for 6 cycles. Focal radiotherapy includes the tumor bed or resection site with a 2 to 3 cm margin. No dose reductions are recommended during the concomitant phase; however, dose interruptions or discontinuation may occur based on toxicity. Continue the temozolomide dose throughout the 42-day concomitant period up to 49 days if all of the following conditions are met: absolute neutrophil count (ANC) greater than or equal to 1.5 × 10^9/L, platelet count greater than or equal to 100 × 10^9/L, common toxicity criteria (CTC) nonhematological toxicity less than or equal to grade 1 (except for alopecia, nausea, vomiting). During treatment, obtain a complete blood cell count (CBC) weekly. Interrupt or discontinue temozolomide dosing during the concomitant phase according to the hematological and nonhematological toxicity criteria as noted in the following table. *Pneumocystis carinii* pneumonia (PCP) prophylaxis is required during the coadministration of temozolomide and radiotherapy; continue in patients who develop lymphocytopenia until recovery from lymphocytopenia (CTC grade less than or equal to 1).

Temozolomide Dosing Interruption or Discontinuation During Concomitant Radiotherapy

Toxicity	Temozolomide interruption[a]	Temozolomide discontinuation
ANC	≥ 0.5 and < 1.5 × 10^9/L	< 0.5 × 10^9/L
Platelet count	≥ 10 and < 100 × 10^9/L	< 10 × 10^9/L
CTC nonhematological toxicity (except for alopecia, nausea, vomiting)	CTC grade 2	CTC grade 3 or 4

[a] Treatment with concomitant temozolomide could be continued when all of the following conditions were met: ANC greater than or equal to 1.5 × 10^9/L, platelet count greater than or equal to 100 × 10^9/L, CTC nonhematological toxicity less than or equal to grade 1 (except for alopecia, nausea, vomiting).

Maintenance phase cycle 1 – Four weeks after completing the temozolomide plus radiotherapy phase, temozolomide is administered for an additional 6 cycles of maintenance treatment. Dosage in cycle 1 (maintenance) is 150 mg/m^2 once daily for 5 days followed by 23 days without treatment.

Cycles 2 to 6 – At the start of cycle 2, the dose is escalated to 200 mg/m^2 if the CTC nonhematologic toxicity for cycle 1 is less than or equal to grade 2 (except for alopecia, nausea, and vomiting), ANC is greater than or equal to 1.5 × 10^9/L, and the platelet count is greater than or equal to 100 × 10^9/L. The dosage remains at 200 mg/m^2/day for the first 5 days of each subsequent cycle, except if toxicity occurs. If the dose is not escalated at cycle 2, escalation should not be done in subsequent cycles.

Dose reduction or discontinuation during maintenance – During treatment, obtain a CBC on day 22 (21 days after the first dose of temozolomide) or within 48 hours of that day and weekly until the ANC is above 1.5 × 10^9/L (1,500/mcL), and the platelet count exceeds 100 × 10^9/L (100,000/mcL). Do not start the next cycle of temozolomide until the ANC and platelet count exceed these levels. Base dose reductions during the next cycle on the lowest blood counts and worst nonhematologic toxicity during the previous cycle. Apply dose reductions or discontinuations during the maintenance phase according to the following tables.

Temozolomide Dose Levels for Maintenance Treatment

Dose level	Dose (mg/m^2/day)	Remarks
−1	100	Reduction for prior toxicity
0	150	Dose during cycle 1
1	200	Dose during cycles 2 to 6 in absence of toxicity

Temozolomide Dose Reduction or Discontinuation During Maintenance Treatment

Toxicity	Reduce temozolomide by 1 dose level[a]	Discontinue temozolomide
ANC	< 1 × 10^9/L	[b]
Platelet count	< 50 × 10^9/L	[b]
CTC nonhematological toxicity (except for alopecia, nausea, vomiting)	CTC grade 3	CTC grade 4[b]

[a] Temozolomide dose levels are listed in the previous table.
[b] Temozolomide is to be discontinued if dose reduction to less than 100 mg/m^2 is required or if the same grade 3 nonhematological toxicity (except for alopecia, nausea, vomiting) recurs after dose reduction.

➤*Anaplastic astrocytoma:* For adults, the initial dosage is 150 mg/m^2 orally once daily for 5 consecutive days per 28-day treatment cycle. For adult patients, if the nadir and day of dosing (day 29, day 1 of next cycle) ANC are greater than or equal to 1.5 × 10^9/L (1,500/mcL) and the nadir and day 29, day 1 of next cycle platelet counts are greater than or equal to 100 × 10^9/L (100,000/mcL), the temozolomide dose may be increased to 200 mg/m^2/day for 5 consecutive days per 28-day treatment cycle. During treatment, obtain a complete blood cell count on day 22 (21 days after the first dose) or within 48 hours of that day, and weekly until the ANC is above 1.5 × 10^9/L (1,500/mcL) and the platelet count exceeds 100 × 10^9/L (100,000 mcL). Do not start the next cycle of temozolomide until the ANC and platelet count exceed these levels. If the ANC falls to less than 1 × 10^9/L (1,000/mcL) or the platelet count is less than 50 × 10^9/L (50,000/mcL) during any cycle, reduce the next cycle by 50 mg/m^2, but not below 100 mg/m^2, the lowest recommended dose. Temozolomide therapy can be continued until disease progression. In the clinical trial, treatment could be continued for a maximum of 2 years, but the optimum duration of therapy is not known.

Daily Dose Calculations of Temozolomide by BSA

Total BSA (m^2)	75 mg/m^2 (mg daily)	150 mg/m^2 (mg daily)	200 mg/m^2 (mg daily)
1	75	150	200
1.1	82.5	165	220
1.2	90	180	240
1.3	97.5	195	260
1.4	105	210	280
1.5	112.5	225	300
1.6	120	240	320
1.7	127.5	255	340
1.8	135	270	360
1.9	142.5	285	380
2	150	300	400
2.1	157.5	315	420
2.2	165	330	440
2.3	172.5	345	460
2.4	180	360	480
2.5	187.5	375	500

Suggested Temozolomide Capsule Combinations Based on Daily Dose

Total daily dose (mg)	Number of daily capsules by strength (mg)			
	250	100	20	5
75	0	0	3	3
82.5	0	0	4	0
90	0	0	4	2
97.5	0	1	0	0

TEMOZOLOMIDE — ORAL

Suggested Temozolomide Capsule Combinations Based on Daily Dose				
	Number of daily capsules by strength (mg)			
Total daily dose (mg)	250	100	20	5
105	0	1	0	1
112.5	0	1	0	2
120	0	1	1	0
127.5	0	1	1	1
135	0	1	1	3
142.5	0	1	2	0
150	0	1	2	2
157.5	0	1	3	0
165	0	1	3	1
172.5	0	1	3	2
180	0	1	4	0
187.5	0	1	4	1
195	0	1	4	3
200	0	2	0	0
210	0	2	0	2
220	0	2	1	0
225	0	2	1	1
240	0	2	2	0
255	1	0	0	1
260	1	0	0	2
270	1	0	1	0
280	1	0	1	2
285	1	0	1	3
300	0	3	0	0
315	0	3	0	3
320	0	3	1	0
330	1	0	4	0
340	0	3	2	0
345	0	3	2	1
360	0	3	3	0
375	1	1	1	1
380	1	1	1	2
400	0	4	0	0
420	0	4	1	0
440	0	4	2	0
460	1	2	0	2
480	1	2	1	2
500	2	0	0	0

Administration – In clinical trials, temozolomide was administered under fasting and nonfasting conditions; however, absorption is affected by food, and consistency of administration with respect to food is recommended. There are no dietary restrictions with temozolomide. To reduce nausea and vomiting, take temozolomide on an empty stomach. Bedtime administration may be advised. Antiemetic therapy may be administered prior to and/or following administration of temozolomide capsules.

Advise patients not to open or chew temozolomide capsules. Patients should swallow them whole with a glass of water.

➤*Handling and disposal:* Temozolomide causes the rapid appearance of malignant tumors in rats. Do not open capsules. If capsules are accidentally opened or damaged, take rigorous precautions with the capsule contents to avoid inhalation or contact with the skin or mucous membranes. Consider procedures for proper handling and disposal of anticancer drugs. Several guidelines on this subject have been published. There is no general agreement that all of the procedures recommended in the guidelines are necessary or appropriate.

➤*Storage/Stability:* Store at 25°C (77°F); excursions permitted to 15° to 30°C (59° to 86°F).

Actions

➤*Pharmacology:* Temozolomide is not directly active but undergoes rapid nonenzymatic conversion at physiologic pH to the reactive compound MTIC. The cytotoxicity of MTIC is thought to be caused primarily by alkylation of deoxyribonucleic acid (DNA). Alkylation (methylation) occurs mainly at the O^6 and N^7 positions of guanine.

➤*Pharmacokinetics:*

Absorption – Temozolomide is absorbed rapidly and completely after oral administration; peak plasma concentrations occur in 1 hour. Food reduces the rate and extent of temozolomide absorption. Mean peak plasma concentration and AUC decreased by 32% and 9%, respectively, and T_{max} increased 2-fold (1.1 to 2.25 hours) when temozolomide was administered after a modified high-fat breakfast.

Distribution – Temozolomide has a mean apparent volume of distribution of 0.4 L/kg (% coefficient of variation = 13%). It is weakly bound to human plasma proteins; the mean percent bound of drug-related total radioactivity is 15%.

Metabolism – Temozolomide is hydrolyzed spontaneously at physiologic pH to the active species, MTIC and to temozolomide acid metabolite. MTIC is further hydrolyzed to 5-amino-imidazole-4-carboxamide (AIC), which is known to be an intermediate in purine and nucleic acid biosynthesis and to methylhydrazine, which is believed to be the active alkylating species. Cytochrome P-450 enzymes play only a minor role in the metabolism of temozolomide and MTIC. Relative to the AUC of temozolomide, the exposure to MTIC and AIC is 2.4% and 23%, respectively.

Excretion – Temozolomide is eliminated rapidly with a mean elimination half-life of 1.8 hours and exhibits linear kinetics over the therapeutic dosing range. About 38% of the administered temozolomide total radioactive dose is recovered over 7 days; 37.7% in urine and 0.8% in feces. The majority of the recovery of radioactivity in urine is as unchanged temozolomide (5.6%), AIC (12%), temozolomide acid metabolite (2.3%), and unidentified polar metabolite(s) (17%). Overall clearance of temozolomide is approximately 5.5 L/h/m^2.

Special populations –

Gender: Population pharmacokinetic analysis indicates that women have an approximate 5% lower clearance (adjusted for BSA) for temozolomide than men. Women have higher incidences of grade 4 neutropenia and thrombocytopenia in the first cycle of therapy than men.

Contraindications

Hypersensitivity reaction to temozolomide or any of its components; also contraindicated in patients who have a history of hypersensitivity to dacarbazine because both drugs are metabolized to MTIC.

Warnings

➤*Myelosuppression:* Patients treated with temozolomide may experience myelosuppression. Prior to dosing, patients must have an ANC greater than or equal to 1.5×10^9/L and a platelet count greater than or equal to 100×10^9/L. Obtain a CBC on day 22 (21 days after the first dose) or within 48 hours of that day, and weekly until the ANC is above 1.5×10^9/L and platelet count exceeds 100×10^9/L. Geriatric patients and women have been shown in clinical trials to have a higher risk of developing myelosuppression.

Very rare cases of myelodysplastic syndrome and secondary malignancies, including myeloid leukemia, have also been observed.

PCP – Prophylaxis against PCP is required for all patients receiving concomitant temozolomide and radiotherapy for the 42-day regimen.

There may be a higher occurrence of PCP when temozolomide is administered during a longer dosing regimen. However, closely observe all patients receiving temozolomide, particularly patients receiving steroids, for the development of PCP regardless of the regimen.

➤*Renal/Hepatic function impairment:* Exercise caution when temozolomide is administered to patients with severe hepatic or renal impairment.

➤*Carcinogenesis:* Standard carcinogenicity studies were not conducted with temozolomide. In rats treated with 200 mg/m^2 temozolomide (equivalent to the maximum recommended daily human dose) on 5 consecutive days every 28 days for 3 cycles, mammary carcinomas were found in both males and females. With 6 cycles of treatment at 25, 50, and 125 mg/m^2 (approximately 1/8 to one-half the maximum recommended daily human dose), mammary carcinomas were observed at all doses and fibrosarcomas of the heart, eye, seminal vesicles, salivary glands, abdominal cavity, uterus, and prostate; carcinoma of the seminal vesicles, schwannoma of the heart, optic nerve, and harderian gland; and adenomas of the skin, lung, pituitary, and thyroid were observed at the high dose.

➤*Mutagenesis:* Temozolomide was mutagenic in vitro in bacteria (Ames assay) and clastogenic in mammalian cells (human peripheral blood lymphocyte assays).

➤*Fertility impairment:* Reproductive function studies have not been conducted with temozolomide. However, multicycle toxicology studies in rats and dogs have demonstrated testicular toxicity (syncytial cells/immature sperm, testicular atrophy) at doses of 50 mg/m^2 in rats and 125 mg/m^2 in dogs (¼ and ⅝, respectively, of the maximum recommended human dose on a body surface area basis).

➤*Elderly:* In the anaplastic astrocytoma study population, patient 70 years of age or older had a higher incidence of grade 4 neutropenia and grade 4 thrombocytopenia (2/8; 25%, $P = 0.31$ and 2/10; 20%, $P = 0.09$, respectively) in the first cycle of therapy than patients younger than 70 years of age.

➤*Pregnancy: Category D.* Temozolomide may cause fetal harm when administered to a pregnant woman. Five consecutive days of oral administration of 75 mg/m^2/day in rats and 150 mg/m^2/day in rabbits during the period of organogenesis (⅜ and three-fourths the maximum recommended human dose, respectively) caused numerous malformations of the external organs, soft tissues, and skeleton in both species. Dosages of 150 mg/m^2/day in rats and rabbits also caused embryolethality as indicated by increased resorptions. There are no adequate and well-controlled studies in pregnant women. If this drug is used during pregnancy, or if the patient becomes pregnant while taking this drug, apprise the patient of the potential hazard to the fetus. Advise women of childbearing potential to avoid becoming pregnant during therapy with temozolomide.

TEMOZOLOMIDE — ORAL

➤*Lactation:* It is not known whether this drug is excreted in human milk. Because many drugs are excreted in human milk and because of the potential for serious adverse reactions in breast-feeding infants from temozolomide, patients receiving temozolomide should discontinue breast-feeding.

➤*Children:* Temozolomide efficacy in children has not been demonstrated. Temozolomide capsules have been studied in 2 open-label phase 2 studies in pediatric patients (3 to 18 years of age) at a dose of 160 to 200 mg/m^2 daily for 5 days every 28 days. In 1 trial, 29 patients with recurrent brain stem glioma and 34 patients with recurrent high-grade astrocytoma were enrolled. All patients had failed surgery and radiation therapy, while 31% also failed chemotherapy. In a second phase 2 open-label study conducted by the Children's Oncology Group (COG), 122 patients were enrolled, including medulloblastoma/primitive neuroectodermal tumors (PNET) (29), high-grade astrocytoma (23), low-grade astrocytoma (22), brain stem glioma (16), ependymoma (14), other CNS tumors (9), and non-CNS tumors (9). The temozolomide toxicity profile in children is similar to adults.

Precautions

➤*Monitoring:* For the concomitant treatment phase with radiotherapy, obtain a CBC weekly.

For the 28-day treatment cycles, obtain a CBC on day 22 (21 days after the first dose). Perform blood counts weekly until recovery if the ANC falls below 1.5 × 10^9/L and the platelet count falls below 100 × 10^9/L.

For patients with refractory anaplastic astrocytoma, during treatment, obtain a complete blood cell count on day 22 (21 days after the first dose) or within 48 hours of that day, and weekly until the ANC is above 1.5 × 10^9/L (1,500/mcL), and the platelet count exceeds 100 × 10^9/L (100,000/mcL).

Drug Interactions

➤*Valproic acid:* Administration of valproic acid decreases oral clearance of temozolomide by about 5%. The clinical implication of this effect is not known.

➤*Drug/Food interactions:* Food reduces the rate and extent of temozolomide absorption. Mean peak plasma concentration and area under the curve (AUC) decreased by 32% and 9%, respectively, and T_{max} increased 2-fold (from 1.1 to 2.25 hours) when temozolomide was administered after a modified high-fat breakfast.

Adverse Reactions

➤*Glioblastoma multiforme:* During the concomitant phase (temozolomide plus radiotherapy), adverse reactions, including thrombocytopenia, nausea, vomiting, anorexia, and constipation, were more frequent in the temozolomide plus radiotherapy arm. The incidence of other adverse reactions was comparable in the 2 arms. The most common adverse reactions across the cumulative temozolomide experience were alopecia, anorexia, constipation, headache, nausea, and vomiting (see the following table). Forty-nine percent of patients treated with temozolomide reported 1 or more severe or life-threatening events, most commonly fatigue (13%), convulsions (6%), headache (5%), and thrombocytopenia (5%). Overall, the pattern of events during the maintenance phase was consistent with the known safety profile of temozolomide.

Temozolomide Adverse Reactions (≥ 5%)

	Concomitant phase				Maintenance phase	
	Radiotherapy alone (n = 285)		Radiotherapy plus temozolomide (n = 288)[a]		Temozolomide (n = 224)	
Adverse reactions	All reactions	Grade ≥ 3	All reactions	Grade ≥ 3	All reactions	Grade ≥ 3
Subjects reporting any adverse reaction	258 (91%)	74 (26%)	266 (92%)	80 (28%)	206 (92%)	82 (37%)
CNS						
Confusion	12 (4%)	6 (2%)	11 (4%)	4 (1%)	12 (5%)	4 (2%)
Convulsions	20 (7%)	9 (3%)	17 (6%)	10 (3%)	25 (11%)	7 (3%)
Dizziness	10 (4%)	0	12 (4%)	2 (1%)	12 (5%)	0
Fatigue	139 (49%)	15 (5%)	156 (54%)	19 (7%)	137 (61%)	20 (9%)
Headache	49 (17%)	11 (4%)	56 (19%)	5 (2%)	51 (23%)	9 (4%)
Insomnia	9 (3%)	1 (< 1%)	14 (5%)	0	9 (4%)	0
Memory impairment	12 (4%)	1 (< 1%)	8 (3%)	1 (< 1%)	16 (7%)	4 (2%)
Weakness	9 (3%)	3 (1%)	10 (3%)	5 (2%)	16 (7%)	4 (2%)
Dermatologic						
Alopecia	179 (63%)	0	199 (69%)	0	124 (55%)	0
Dry skin	6 (2%)	0	7 (2%)	0	11 (5%)	1 (< 1%)
Erythema	15 (5%)	0	14 (5%)	0	2 (1%)	0
Pruritus	4 (1%)	0	11 (4%)	0	11 (5%)	0
Rash	42 (15%)	0	56 (19%)	3 (1%)	29 (13%)	3 (1%)
GI						
Abdominal pain	2 (1%)	0	7 (2%)	1 (< 1%)	11 (5%)	1 (< 1%)
Anorexia	25 (9%)	1 (< 1%)	56 (19%)	2 (1%)	61 (27%)	3 (1%)
Constipation	18 (6%)	0	53 (18%)	3 (1%)	49 (22%)	0
Diarrhea	9 (3%)	0	18 (6%)	0	23 (10%)	2 (1%)
Nausea	45 (16%)	1 (< 1%)	105 (36%)	2 (1%)	110 (49%)	3 (1%)
Stomatitis	14 (5%)	1 (< 1%)	19 (7%)	0	20 (9%)	3 (1%)
Vomiting	16 (6%)	1 (< 1%)	57 (20%)	1 (< 1%)	66 (29%)	4 (2%)
Hypersensitivity						
Allergic reaction	7 (2%)	1 (< 1%)	13 (5%)	0	6 (3%)	0
Respiratory						
Coughing	3 (1%)	0	15 (5%)	2 (1%)	19 (8%)	1 (< 1%)
Dyspnea	9 (3%)	4 (1%)	11 (4%)	5 (2%)	12 (5%)	1 (< 1%)
Special senses						
Blurred vision	25 (9%)	4 (1%)	26 (9%)	2 (1%)	17 (8%)	0
Taste perversion	6 (2%)	0	18 (6%)	0	11 (5%)	0
Miscellaneous						
Arthralgia	2 (1%)	0	7 (2%)	1 (< 1%)	14 (6%)	0
Radiation injury NOS[b]	11 (4%)	1 (< 1%)	20 (7%)	0	5 (2%)	0
Thrombocytopenia	3 (1%)	0	11 (4%)	8 (3%)	19 (8%)	8 (4%)

[a] One patient who was randomized to radiotherapy-only arm received radiotherapy plus temozolomide.Grade 5 (fatal) adverse reactions are included in the grade greater than or equal to 3 column.
[b] NOS = not otherwise specified.

➤*Myelosuppression:* Myelosuppression (neutropenia and thrombocytopenia), which are known dose-limiting toxicities for most cytotoxic agents, including temozolomide, were observed. When laboratory abnormalities and adverse reactions were combined, grade 3 or 4 neutrophil abnormalities, including neutropenic events, were observed in 8% of the patients and grade 3 or 4 platelet abnormalities, including thrombocytopenic events, were observed in 14% of the patients treated with temozolomide.

➤*Anaplastic astrocytoma:* The following tables show the incidence of adverse reactions in the 158 patients in the anaplastic astrocytoma study for whom data are available. In the absence of a control group, it is not clear in many cases whether these events should be attributed to temozolomide or the patients' underlying conditions, but nausea, vomiting, fatigue, and hematologic effects appear to be clearly drug related. The most frequently occurring side effects were fatigue, headache, nausea, and vomiting. The adverse reactions were usually National Cancer Institute (NCI) CTC grade 1 or 2 (mild to moderate in severity) and were self-limiting, with nausea and vomiting readily controlled with antiemetics. The incidence of severe nausea and vomiting (CTC grade 3 or 4) was 10% and 6%, respectively. Myelosuppression (thrombocytopenia and neutropenia) was the dose-limiting adverse reaction. It usually occurred within the first few cycles of therapy and was not cumulative.

Myelosuppression occurred late in the treatment cycle and returned to normal, on average, within 14 days of nadir counts. The median nadirs occurred at 26 days for platelets (range, 21 to 40 days) and 28 days for neutrophils (range, 1 to 44 days). Only 14% (22 of 158) of patients had a neutrophil nadir and 20% (32 of 158) of patients had a platelet nadir which may have delayed the start of the next cycle. Less than 10% of patients required hospitalization, blood transfusion, or discontinuation of therapy because of myelosuppression.

In clinical trial experience with 110 to 111 women and 169 to 174 men (depending on measurements), there were higher rates of grade 4 neutropenia (ANC less than 500 cells/mcL) and thrombocytopenia (less than 20,000 cells/mcL) in women than men in the first cycle of therapy (12% vs 5% and 9% vs 3%, respectively).

In the entire safety database for which hematologic data exist (N = 932), 7% (4 of 61) and 9.5% (6 of 63) of patients over 70 years of age experienced grade

TEMOZOLOMIDE — ORAL

4 neutropenia or thrombocytopenia in the first cycle, respectively. For patients 70 years of age and younger, 7% (62 of 871) and 5.5% (48 of 879) experienced grade 4 neutropenia or thrombocytopenia in the first cycle, respectively. Pancytopenia, leukopenia, and anemia also have been reported.

Temozolomide Adverse Reactions (≥ 5%)		
Adverse reaction	All reactions (N = 158)	Grade 3/4 (N = 158)
Any adverse reaction	153 (97%)	79 (50%)
CNS		
Abnormal coordination	17 (11%)	2 (1%)
Abnormal gait	9 (6%)	1 (1%)
Amnesia	16 (10%)	6 (4%)
Anxiety	11 (7%)	1 (1%)
Asthenia	20 (13%)	9 (6%)
Ataxia	12 (8%)	3 (2%)
Confusion	8 (5%)	0
Convulsions	36 (23%)	8 (5%)
Depression	10 (6%)	0
Dizziness	19 (12%)	1 (1%)
Fatigue	54 (34%)	7 (4%)
Headache	65 (41%)	10 (6%)
Hemiparesis	29 (18%)	10 (6%)
Insomnia	16 (10%)	0
Local convulsions	9 (6%)	0
Paresis	13 (8%)	4 (3%)
Paresthesia	15 (9%)	1 (1%)
Somnolence	15 (9%)	5 (3%)
Dermatologic		
Pruritus	12 (8%)	2 (1%)
Rash	13 (8%)	0
GI		
Abdominal pain	14 (9%)	2 (1%)
Anorexia	14 (9%)	1 (1%)
Constipation	52 (33%)	1 (1%)
Diarrhea	25 (16%)	3 (2%)
Dysphasia	11 (7%)	1 (1%)
Nausea	84 (53%)	16 (10%)
Vomiting	66 (42%)	10 (6%)
GU		
Breast pain, female	4 (6%)	
Micturition increased frequency	9 (6%)	0
Urinary incontinence	13 (8%)	3 (2%)
Urinary tract infection	12 (8%)	0
Metabolic/Nutritional		
Peripheral edema	17 (11%)	1 (1%)
Weight increase	8 (5%)	0
Ophthalmic		
Abnormal vision[a]	8 (5%)	
Diplopia	8 (5%)	0
Respiratory		
Coughing	8 (5%)	0
Pharyngitis	12 (8%)	0
Sinusitis	10 (6%)	0
Upper respiratory tract infection	13 (8%)	0
Miscellaneous		
Adrenal hypercorticism	13 (8%)	0
Back pain	12 (8%)	4 (3%)
Fever	21 (13%)	3 (2%)
Myalgia	8 (5%)	
Viral infection	17 (11%)	0

[a] Blurred vision, visual deficit, vision changes, vision troubles.

➤*Hematologic:*

Temozolomide Adverse Hematologic Effects (Grade 3 to 4)		
	Temozolomide[a]	
Hemoglobin	7/158	(4%)
Lymphopenia	83/152	(55%)
Neutrophils	20/142	(14%)
Platelets	29/156	(19%)
WBC[b]	18/158	(11%)

[a] Change from grade 0 to 2 at baseline to grade 3 or 4 during treatment.
[b] WBC = white blood cell.

➤*Postmarketing:* In addition, the following spontaneous adverse reactions have been reported during the marketing surveillance of temozolomide capsules; allergic reactions, including rare cases of anaphylaxis. Rare cases of erythema multiforme have been reported, which resolved after discontinuation of temozolomide and, in some cases, recurred upon rechallenge. Rare cases of opportunistic infections, including *P. carinii* pneumonia have also been reported.

➤*Adverse reactions in children:* Temozolomide efficacy in children has not been demonstrated. Temozolomide capsules have been studied in 2 open-label phase 2 studies in pediatric patients (3 to 18 years of age) at a dosage of 160 to 200 mg/m^2/day for 5 days every 28 days. In 1 trial, 29 patients with recurrent brain stem glioma and 34 patients with recurrent high-grade astrocytoma were enrolled. All patients had failed surgery and radiation therapy, while 31% also failed chemotherapy. In a second phase 2 open-label study conducted by the COG, 122 patients were enrolled, including medulloblastoma/PNET (29), high-grade astrocytoma (23), low-grade astrocytoma (22), brain stem glioma (16), ependymoma (14), other CNS tumors (9), and non-CNS tumors (9). The temozolomide toxicity profile in children is similar to adults. The following table shows the adverse reactions in 122 children in the COG phase 2 study.

Temozolomide Adverse Reactions in Pediatric Cooperative Group Trial (≥ 10%)[a]		
Body system/ organ class adverse reaction	All reactions (n = 122)	Grade 3/4 (n = 122)
Subjects reporting an adverse reaction	107 (88%)	69 (57%)
CNS		
Central cerebral CNS cortex	22 (18%)	13 (11%)
GI		
Nausea	56 (46%)	5 (4%)
Vomiting	62 (51%)	4 (3%)
Hematologic		
Decreased hemoglobin	62 (51%)	7 (6%)
Decreased WBC	71 (58%)	21 (17%)
Lymphopenia	73 (60%)	48 (39%)
Neutropenia	62 (51%)	24 (20%)
Thrombocytopenia	71 (58%)	31 (25%)

[a] These various tumors included the following: PNET-medulloblastoma, glioblastoma, low-grade astrocytoma, brain stem tumor, ependymoma, mixed glioma, oligodendroglioma, neuroblastoma, Ewing sarcoma, pineoblastoma, alveolar soft-part sarcoma, neurofibrosarcoma, optic glioma, and osteosarcoma.

Overdosage

➤*Symptoms:* Doses of 500, 750, 1,000, and 1,250 mg/m^2 (total dose per cycle over 5 days) have been evaluated clinically in patients. Dose-limiting toxicity was hematologic and was reported with any dose but is expected to be more severe at higher doses. An overdose of 2,000 mg/day for 5 days was taken by 1 patient, and the adverse reactions reported were pancytopenia, pyrexia, multiorgan failure, and death. There are reports of patients who have taken more than 5 days of treatment (up to 64 days) with adverse reactions reported, including bone marrow suppression, which in some cases was severe and prolonged, and infections, which resulted in death.

➤*Treatment:* In the event of an overdose, hematologic evaluation is needed. Provide supportive measures as necessary.

Patient Information

In clinical trials, nausea and vomiting were among the most frequently occurring adverse reactions. These were usually either self-limiting or readily controlled with standard antiemetic therapy. Swallow capsules whole with a full glass of water. Do not open or chew capsules. If capsules are accidentally opened or damaged, take rigorous precautions with the capsule contents to avoid inhalation or contact with the skin or mucous membranes. Keep the medication away from children and pets.

AMIFOSTINE

Rx	**Ethyol** (MedImmune Oncology)	**Powder for Injection, lyophilized:** 500 mg (anhydrous basis)	In 10 ml single-use vials.

AMIFOSTINE — INJECTION

Indications

➤*Renal toxicity:* Reduction of cumulative renal toxicity associated with repeated administration of cisplatin in patients with advanced ovarian cancer or non-small cell lung cancer.

➤*Xerostomia:* Reduction of the incidence of moderate-to-severe xerostomia in patients undergoing postoperative radiation treatment for head and neck cancer, where the radiation port includes a substantial portion of the parotid glands.

➤*Unlabeled uses:* To prevent or reduce cisplatin-induced neurotoxicity and cyclophosphamide-induced granulocytopenia; prevent or reduce toxicity of radiation therapy to other areas; reduce toxicity of paclitaxel.

Administration and Dosage

➤*Reduction of cumulative renal toxicity with chemotherapy:* Recommended starting dose is 910 mg/m^2 administered once daily as a 15-minute IV infusion, starting 30 minutes prior to chemotherapy. The 15-minute infusion is better tolerated than more extended infusions.

Adequately hydrate patients prior to amifostine infusion, and keep them in a supine position during the infusion. Monitor blood pressure every 5 minutes during the infusion and thereafter as clinically indicated.

Interrupt the infusion of amifostine if the systolic blood pressure decreases significantly from the baseline value as listed in the guideline below.

Guideline for Interrupting Amifostine Infusion Due to Decrease in Systolic Blood Pressure

	Baseline Systolic Blood Pressure (mm Hg)				
	< 100	100 to 119	120 to 139	140 to 179	≥ 180
Decrease in systolic blood pressure during infusion of amifostine (mmHg)	20	25	30	40	50

If hypotension requiring interruption of therapy occurs, place patients in either the Trendelenburg or supine position and administer a Normal Saline solution using a separate IV line. If the blood pressure returns to normal within 5 minutes and the patient is asymptomatic, the infusion may be restarted so that the full dose of amifostine may be administered. If the full dose of amifostine cannot be administered, the dose of amifostine for subsequent cycles should be 740 mg/m^2.

It is recommended that antiemetic medication, including dexamethasone 20 mg IV and a serotonin $5HT_3$ receptor antagonist, be administered prior to and in conjunction with amifostine. Additional antiemetics may be required based on the chemotherapy drugs concomitantly administered.

➤*Reduction of moderate-to-severe xerostomia from radiation of the head and neck:* 200 mg/m^2 administered once daily as a 3-minute IV infusion 15 to 30 minutes prior to standard fraction radiation therapy (1.8 to 2 Gy).

Adequately hydrate patients prior to amifostine infusion. Monitor blood pressure before and immediately after the infusion and as clinically indicated.

Administer antiemetic medication prior to and in conjunction with amifostine. Oral $5HT_3$ receptor antagonists, alone or in combination with other antiemetics, have been used effectively in the radiotherapy setting.

➤*Reconstitution:* Reconstitute with 9.7 ml of 0.9% Sodium Chloride Injection.

➤*Admixture incompatibility:* The compatibility of amifostine with solutions other than 0.9% Sodium Chloride for Injection, or sodium chloride solutions with other additives, has not been studied and is not recommended. The use of other solutions is not recommended.

➤*Storage / Stability:* Store the lyophilized dosage form at controlled room temperature (20° to 25°C; 68° to 77°F). The reconstituted solution is chemically stable for up to 5 hours at room temperature (≈ 25°C; 77°F) or up to 24 hours under refrigeration (2° to 8°C; 36° to 46°F).

Actions

➤*Pharmacology:* Amifostine is an organic thiophosphate cytoprotective agent. This pro-drug is dephosphorylated by alkaline phosphatase in tissues to a pharmacologically active free thiol metabolite that can reduce the renal toxicity of cisplatin and for the reduction of the toxic effects of radiation on normal oral tissues. The ability to differentially protect normal tissues is attributed to the higher capillary alkaline phosphatase activity, higher pH, and better vascularity of normal tissues relative to tumor tissue. The result is a more rapid generation of the active thiol metabolite as well as a higher rate constant for uptake into cells. The higher concentration of the thiol metabolite in normal tissues is thus available to bind to, and thereby detoxify, reactive metabolites of cisplatin. The thiol metabolites also scavenge reactive oxygen species generated by exposure to cisplatin or radiation.

➤*Pharmacokinetics:* Amifostine is rapidly cleared from the plasma with a distribution half-life of less than 1 minute and an elimination half-life of approximately 8 minutes. Less than 10% of amifostine remains in the plasma 6 minutes after drug administration. Amifostine is rapidly metabolized to an active free thiol metabolite. A disulfide metabolite is produced subsequently and is less active than the free thiol. After a 10-second bolus dose of amifostine 150 mg/m^2, renal excretion of the parent drug and its 2 metabolites was low during the hour following drug administration, averaging 0.69%, 2.64%, and 2.22% of the administered dose for the parent, thiol, and disulfide, respectively. Measurable levels of the free thiol metabolite have been found in bone marrow cells 5 to 8 minutes after IV infusion of amifostine.

Contraindications

Sensitivity to aminothiol compounds.

Warnings

➤*Hypersensitivity:* Allergic manifestations including anaphylaxis and severe cutaneous reactions have been associated rarely with amifostine administration. Serious cutaneous hypersensitivity reactions have included erythema multiforme, Stevens-Johnson syndrome, toxic epidermal necrolysis, toxoderma and exfoliative dermatitis, which have been reported more frequently when amifostine is used as a radioprotectant (see Adverse Reactions). Some of these reactions have been fatal or have required hospitalization and/or discontinuance of therapy. Patients should be carefully monitored prior to, during, and after amifostine administration.

In case of severe acute allergic reactions, amifostine should be immediately and permanently discontinued. Epinephrine and other appropriate measures should be available for treatment of serious allergic events such as anaphylaxis. Amifostine should also be permanently discontinued for serious or severe cutaneous reactions or for cutaneous reactions associated with fever or other constitutional symptoms not known to be due to another etiology. Amifostine should be withheld and dermatologic consultation and biopsy considered for cutaneous reactions or mucosal lesions of unknown etiology appearing outside of the injection site or radiation port and for erythematous, edematous, or bullous lesions on the palms of the hand or soles of the feet. Reinitiation of amifostine should be at the physician's discretion based on medical judgment and appropriate dermatologic evaluation.

➤*Effectiveness of the cytotoxic regimen:* Limited data are available on the preservation of antitumor efficacy when amifostine is administered prior to cisplatin therapy in settings other than advanced ovarian cancer or non-small cell lung cancer. Although some animal data suggest interference is possible, in most tumor models, the antitumor effects of chemotherapy are not altered by amifostine. Amifostine, therefore, should not be used in patients receiving chemotherapy for malignancies in which chemotherapy can produce a significant survival benefit or cure (eg, certain malignancies of germ cell origin), except in the context of a clinical study.

➤*Effectiveness of radiotherapy:* Do not administer amifostine in patients receiving definitive radiotherapy, except during a clinical trial, due to insufficient data to exclude a tumor-protective effect in this setting. Amifostine was studied only with standard fractionated radiotherapy and when at least 75% of both parotid glands were exposed to radiation. Amifostine's effects on the incidence of xerostomia, on toxicity in the setting of combined chemotherapy and radiotherapy, and in the setting of accelerated and hyperfractionated therapy have not been systematically studied.

➤*Hypotension:* In a randomized study of patients with ovarian cancer given 910 mg/m^2 amifostine prior to chemotherapy, transient hypotension occurred in 62% of patients treated. Mean time of onset was 14 minutes into the infusion; mean duration was 6 minutes. In some cases, the infusion had to be prematurely terminated because of a more pronounced drop in systolic pressure. In general, blood pressure returns to normal within 5 to 15 minutes. Fewer than 3% of patients discontinued amifostine because of blood pressure reductions. In the randomized study of patients with head and neck cancer given amifostine at a dose of 200 mg/m^2 prior to radiotherapy, hypotension was observed in 15% of patients treated.

Patients who are hypotensive or dehydrated should not receive amifostine. Patients receiving amifostine at doses recommended for chemotherapy should have antihypertensive therapy interrupted 24 hours preceding administration of amifostine. Patients receiving amifostine at doses recommended for chemotherapy who are taking antihypertensive therapy that cannot be stopped for 24 hours preceding amifostine treatment also should not receive amifostine. Adequately hydrate patients prior to amifostine infusion, and keep in a supine position during the infusion. Monitor blood pressure every 5 minutes during the infusion, and thereafter as clinically indicated. It is important that the duration of the 910 mg/m^2 infusion not exceed 15 minutes, as administration as a longer infusion is associated with a higher incidence of side effects. Monitor blood pressure at least before and immediately after infusions with durations < 5 minutes, and thereafter as clinically indicated. If hypotension occurs, place patient in the Trendelenburg position and give an infusion of normal saline using a separate IV line. During and after amifostine infusion, take care to monitor the blood pressure of patients whose antihypertensive medication has been interrupted since hypertension may be exacerbated by discontinuation of antihypertensive medication and other causes such as IV hydration. Guidelines for interrupting and restarting amifostine infusion if a decrease in systolic blood pressure occurs are in Administration and Dosage. Hypotension may occur during or shortly after amifostine infusion, despite adequate hydration and positioning of the patient. Hypotension has been reported to be associated with dyspnea, apnea, hypoxia, and in rare cases seizures, unconsciousness, respiratory arrest, and renal failure.

AMIFOSTINE — INJECTION

➤*Nausea and vomiting:* Administer antiemetic medication prior to and in conjunction with amifostine. When amifostine is administered with highly emetogenic chemotherapy, carefully monitor the fluid balance of the patient.

➤*Hypocalcemia:* Monitor serum calcium levels in patients at risk of hypocalcemia, such as those with nephrotic syndrome or patients receiving multiple doses. If necessary, administer calcium supplements.

➤*Elderly:* Dose selection for an elderly patient should be cautious, reflecting the greater frequency of decreased hepatic, renal, or cardiac function and of concomitant disease or other drug therapy in elderly patients.

➤*Pregnancy: Category C.* Amifostine is embryotoxic in rabbits at doses of 50 mg/kg, approximately 60% of the recommended dose in humans on a body surface area basis. There are no adequate and well-controlled studies in pregnant women. Do not use during pregnancy unless the potential benefit justifies the potential risk to the fetus.

➤*Lactation:* No information is available on the excretion of amifostine or its metabolites into breast milk. Discontinue breastfeeding if treating with amifostine.

➤*Children:* Safety and efficacy have not been established.

Precautions

➤*Monitoring:* Monitor serum calcium levels in patients at risk of hypocalcemia, such as those with nephrotic syndrome or patients receiving multiple doses of amifostine. When used prior to chemotherapy, monitor blood pressure every 5 minutes during the infusion and thereafter as clinically indicated. When used prior to radiation therapy, monitor blood pressure at least before and immediately after the infusion and thereafter as clinically indicated.

➤*Special risk:* Safety has not been established in elderly patients, or patients with preexisting cardiovascular or cerebrovascular conditions such as ischemic heart disease, arrhythmias, CHF, or history of stroke or transient ischemic attacks. Use amifostine with particular care in these and other patients in whom the common amifostine adverse effects of nausea/vomiting and hypotension may be more likely to have serious consequences.

Drug Interactions

➤*Antihypertensives:* Give special consideration to amifostine administration in patients receiving antihypertensive medications or other drugs that could cause or potentiate hypotension.

Adverse Reactions

➤*Cardiovascular:* Hypotension, usually brief systolic and diastolic, has been associated with one or more of the following adverse events: Apnea, dyspnea, hypoxia, tachycardia, bradycardia, extrasystoles, chest pain, myocardial ischemia, and convulsion. Rare cases of renal failure, MI, respiratory and cardiac arrest have been observed during or after hypotension (see Warnings).

Rare cases of arrhythmias such as atrial fibrillation/flutter and supraventricular tachycardia have been reported. These are sometimes associated with hypotension or allergic reactions.

Transient hypertension and exacerbations of pre-existing hypertension have been observed rarely after amifostine administration.

➤*GI:* Nausea and/or vomiting occur frequently after amifostine infusion and may be severe. In the ovarian cancer randomized study, the incidence of severe nausea/vomiting on day 1 of cyclophosphamide-cisplatin chemotherapy was 10% in patients who did not receive amifostine and 19% in patients who did receive amifostine. In the randomized study of patients with head and neck cancer, the incidence of severe nausea/vomiting was 8% in patients who received amifostine and 1% in patients who did not receive amifostine.

➤*Hypersensitivity:* Hypotension; fever; chills/rigors; dyspnea; cutaneous eruptions; urticaria; hypoxia; laryngeal edema; chest tightness; cardiac arrest. Other skin reactions including erythema multiforme, and in rare cases, Stevens-Johnson syndrome and toxic epidermal necrolysis, have been reported. There have been rare reports of anaphylactoid reactions.

➤*Miscellaneous:* Hypocalcemia (< 1%; see Warnings); hypotension (see Warnings); short-term, reversible loss of consciousness, seizures, syncope (rare); flushing/feeling of warmth; chills/feeling of coldness; fever; dizziness; somnolence; hiccoughs; sneezing.

Overdosage

In clinical trials, the maximum single dose of amifostine was 1300 mg/m^2. Children have received single doses of up to 2700 mg/m^2. At the higher doses, anxiety and reversible urinary retention occurred. Administration of amifostine at 2 and 4 hours after the initial dose has not led to increased nausea and vomiting or hypotension. The most likely symptom of overdosage is hypotension; manage by infusion of normal saline and other supportive measures as clinically indicated.

DEXRAZOXANE

Rx	**Dexrazoxane** (Bedford)	**Powder for Injection, lyophilized**: 250 mg (10 mg/mL reconstituted)	In single-use vials with 25 mL vial sodium lactate injection.
Rx	**Zinecard** (Pfizer)		In single-use vials with 25 mL vial sodium lactate injection.
Rx	**Dexrazoxane** (Bedford)	**Powder for Injection, lyophilized**: 500 mg (10 mg/mL reconstituted)	In single-use vials with 50 mL vial sodium lactate injection.
Rx	**Zinecard** (Pfizer)		In single-use vials with 50 mL vial sodium lactate injection.

DEXRAZOXANE — INJECTION

Indications

➤*Cardiomyopathy associated with doxorubicin use:* Dexrazoxane is indicated for reducing the incidence and severity of cardiomyopathy associated with doxorubicin administration in women with metastatic breast cancer who have received a cumulative doxorubicin dose of 300 mg/m^2 and who will continue to receive doxorubicin therapy to maintain tumor control. It is not recommended for use with the initiation of doxorubicin therapy. Doxorubicin should not be given prior to the intravenous injection of dexrazoxane.

➤*Unlabeled uses:* Cardioprotectant for other anthracyclines (epirubicin).

Administration and Dosage

➤*Approved by the FDA:* May 26, 1995.

The recommended dosage ratio of dexrazoxane:doxorubicin is 10:1 (eg, 500 mg/m^2 dexrazoxane:50 mg/m^2 doxorubicin).

➤*Renal function impairment:* In patients with moderate to severe renal dysfunction (creatinine clearance values less than 40 mL/min), the recommended dosage ratio of dexrazoxane:doxorubicin is 5:1 (e.g., 250 mg/m^{2}dexrazoxane:50 mg/m^2 doxorubicin).

➤*Hepatic function impairment:* Since a doxorubicin dose reduction is recommended in the presence of hyperbilirubinemia, the dexrazoxane dosage should be proportionately reduced (maintaining the 10:1 ratio) in patients with hepatic impairment.

➤*Preparation/administration:* Dexrazoxane must be reconstituted with 0.167 Molar (M/6) Sodium Lactate Injection, USP, to give a concentration of 10 mg dexrazoxane for each mL of sodium lactate. The reconstituted solution should be given by slow IV push or rapid drip intravenous infusion from a bag. After completing the infusion of dexrazoxane, and prior to a total elapsed time of 30 minutes (from the beginning of the dexrazoxane infusion), the intravenous injection of doxorubicin should be given.

The reconstituted dexrazoxane solution may be diluted with either 0.9% Sodium Chloride Injection, USP or 5% Dextrose Injection, USP to a concentration range of 1.3 to 5 mg/mL in IV infusion bags.

➤*Admixture incompatibility:* Dexrazoxane should not be mixed with other drugs.

➤*Storage/Stability:* Store at 25°C (77°F); excursions permitted to 15° to 30°C (59° to 86°F) [see USP controlled room temperature]. Reconstituted solutions of dexrazoxane are stable for 6 hours at controlled room temperature or under refrigeration, 2° to 8°C (36° to 46°F). Discard unused solutions.

Actions

➤*Pharmacology:* The mechanism by which dexrazoxane exerts its cardioprotective activity is not fully understood. Dexrazoxane is a cyclic derivative of EDTA that readily penetrates cell membranes. Results of laboratory studies suggest that dexrazoxane is converted intracellularly to a ring-opened chelating agent that interferes with iron-mediated free radical generation thought to be responsible, in part, for anthracycline-induced cardiomyopathy.

➤*Pharmacokinetics:*

Special populations –

Hepatic function impairment: The pharmacokinetics of dexrazoxane have not been evaluated in patients with hepatic impairment. The dexrazoxane dose is dependent upon the dose of doxorubicin. Since a doxorubicin dose reduction is recommended in the presence of hyperbilirubinemia, the dexrazoxane dosage is proportionately reduced in patients with hepatic impairment. The pharmacokinetics of dexrazoxane have been studied in advanced cancer patients with normal renal and hepatic function. Generally, the pharmacokinetics of dexrazoxane can be adequately described by a 2-compartment open model with first-order elimination. Dexrazoxane has been administered as a 15 minute infusion over a dose range of 60 to 900 mg/m^2 with 60 mg/m^2 of doxorubicin, and at a fixed dose of 500 mg/m^2 with 50 mg/m^2 doxorubicin. The disposition kinetics of dexrazoxane are dose-independent, as shown by linear relationship between the area under plasma concentration-time curves and administered doses ranging from 60 to 900 mg/m^2. The mean peak plasma concentration of dexrazoxane was 36.5 mcg/mL at the end of the 15 minute infusion of a 500 mg/m^2 dose of dexrazoxane administered 15 to 30 minutes prior to the 50 mg/m^2 doxorubicin dose.

DEXRAZOXANE — INJECTION

Summary of mean (% CV[a]) dexrazoxane pharmacokinetic parameters at a dosage ratio of 10:1 of dexrazoxane: doxorubicin						
Dose doxorubicin (mg/m^2)	Dose dexrazoxane (mg/m^2)	Number of subjects	Elimination half-life (hours)	Plasma clearance ($L/hr/m^2$)	Renal clearance ($L/hr/m^2$)	[b]Volume of distribution (L/m^2)
50	500	10	2.5 (16)	7.88 (18)	3.35 (36)	22.4 (22)
60	600	5	2.1 (29)	6.25 (31)	-	22 (55)

[a] Coefficient of variation.
[b] Steady-state volume of distribution.

Following a rapid distributive phase (approximately 0.2 to 0.3 hours), dexrazoxane reaches postdistributive equilibrium within 2 to 4 hours. The estimated steady-state volume of distribution of dexrazoxane suggests its distribution primarily in the total body water (25 L/m^2). The mean systemic clearance and steady-state volume of distribution of dexrazoxane in 2 Asian female patients at 500 mg/m ^{2} dexrazoxane along with 50 mg/m^2 doxorubicin were 15.15 $L/h/m^2$ and 36.27 L/m^2, respectively, but their elimination half-life and renal clearance of dexrazoxane were similar to those of the 10 Caucasian patients from the same study. Qualitative metabolism studies with dexrazoxane have confirmed the presence of unchanged drug, a diacid-diamide cleavage product, and 2 monoacid-monoamide ring products in the urine of animals and man. The metabolite levels were not measured in the pharmacokinetic studies.

Urinary excretion plays an important role in the elimination of dexrazoxane. Forty-two percent (42%) of the 500 mg/m^2 dose of dexrazoxane was excreted in the urine.

Protein binding – In vitro studies have shown that dexrazoxane is not bound to plasma proteins.

Contraindications

Dexrazoxane should not be used with chemotherapy regimens that do not contain an anthracycline.

Warnings

➤*Myelosuppression:* Dexrazoxane may add to the myelosuppression caused by chemotherapeutic agents.

➤*Antitumor interference:* There is some evidence that the use of dexrazoxane concurrently with the initiation of fluorouracil, doxorubicin, and cyclophosphamide (FAC) therapy interferes with the antitumor efficacy of the regimen, and this use is not recommended. In the largest of 3 breast cancer trials, patients who received dexrazoxane starting with their first cycle of FAC therapy had a lower response rate (48% versus 63%; P = 0.007) and shorter time to progression than patients who did not receive dexrazoxane. Therefore, dexrazoxane should only be used in those patients who have received a cumulative doxorubicin dose of 300 mg/m^2 and are continuing with doxorubicin therapy.

➤*Anthracycline-induced cardiac toxicity:* Although clinical studies have shown that patients receiving FAC with dexrazoxane may receive a higher cumulative dose of doxorubicin before experiencing cardiac toxicity than patients receiving FAC without dexrazoxane, the use of dexrazoxane in patients who have already received a cumulative dose of doxorubicin of 300 mg/m^2 without dexrazoxane, does not eliminate the potential for anthracycline-induced cardiac toxicity. Therefore, cardiac function should be carefully monitored.

➤*Renal / Hepatic function impairment:* See Administration and Dosage for more information.

➤*Carcinogenesis:* Secondary malignancies (primarily acute myeloid leukemia) have been reported in patients treated chronically with oral razoxane. Razoxane is the racemic mixture, of which dexrazoxane is the S(+)-enantiomer. In these patients, the total cumulative dose of razoxane ranged from 26 to 480 g and the duration of treatment was from 42 to 319 weeks. One case of T-cell lymphoma, a case of B-cell lymphoma and 6 to 8 cases of cutaneous basal cell or squamous cell carcinoma have also been reported in patients treated with razoxane.

➤*Mutagenesis:* Dexrazoxane was not mutagenic in the Ames test but was found to be clastogenic to human lymphocytes in vitro and to mouse bone marrow erythrocytes in vivo (micronucleus test).

➤*Fertility impairment:* The possible adverse effects of dexrazoxane on the fertility of humans and experimental animals, male or female, have not been adequately studied. Testicular atrophy was seen with dexrazoxane administration at doses as low as 30 mg/kg weekly for 6 weeks in rats (⅓ the human dose on a mg/m^2 basis) and as low as 20 mg/kg weekly for 13 weeks in dogs (approximately equal to the human dose on a mg/m^2 basis).

➤*Elderly:* In general, elderly patients should be treated with caution due to the greater frequency of decreased hepatic, renal, or cardiac function, and concomitant disease or other drug therapy.

➤*Pregnancy: Category C.* Dexrazoxane was maternotoxic at doses of 2 mg/kg (1/40 the human dose on a mg/m^2 basis) and embryotoxic and teratogenic at 8 mg/kg (approximately 1/10 the human dose on a mg/m^2 basis) when given daily to pregnant rats during the period of organogenesis. Teratogenic effects in the rat included imperforate anus, microphthalmia, and anophthalmia. In offspring allowed to develop to maturity, fertility was impaired in the male and female rats treated in utero during organogenesis at 8 mg/kg. In rabbits, doses of 5 mg/kg (approximately 1/10 the human dose on a mg/m^2 basis) daily during the period of organogenesis were maternotoxic and dosages of 20 mg/kg (½ the human dose on a mg/m^2 basis) were embryotoxic and teratogenic. Teratogenic effects in the rabbit included several skeletal malformations such as short tail, rib and thoracic malformations, and soft tissue variations including subcutaneous, eye, and cardiac hemorrhagic areas, as well as agenesis of the gallbladder and of the intermediate lobe of the lung. There are no adequate and well-controlled studies in pregnant women. Dexrazoxane should be used during pregnancy only if the potential benefit justifies the potential risk to the fetus.

➤*Lactation:* It is not known whether dexrazoxane is excreted in human milk. Because many drugs are excreted in human milk and because of the potential for serious adverse reactions in nursing infants exposed to dexrazoxane, mothers should be advised to discontinue nursing during dexrazoxane therapy.

➤*Children:* Safety and efficacy of dexrazoxane in children have not been established.

Precautions

➤*Monitoring:* As dexrazoxane will always be used with cytotoxic drugs, patients should be monitored closely. While the myelosuppressive effects of dexrazoxane at the recommended dose are mild, additive effects upon the myelosuppressive activity of chemotherapeutic agents may occur.

➤*Lab test abnormalities:* As dexrazoxane may add to the myelosuppressive effects of cytotoxic drugs, frequent complete blood counts are recommended. Patients receiving FAC with dexrazoxane experienced more severe leukopenia, granulocytopenia, and thrombocytopenia at nadir than patients receiving FAC without dexrazoxane, but recovery counts were similar for the 2 groups of patients.

Adverse Reactions

Dexrazoxane at a dose of 500 mg/m^2 has been administered in combination with FAC in randomized, placebo-controlled, double-blind studies to patients with metastatic breast cancer. The dose of doxorubicin was 50 mg/m^2 in each of the trials. Courses were repeated every 3 weeks, provided recovery from toxicity had occurred. The table below lists the incidence of adverse reactions for patients receiving FAC with either dexrazoxane or placebo in the breast cancer studies. Adverse reactions occurring during courses 1 through 6 are listed for patients receiving dexrazoxane or placebo with FAC beginning with their first course of therapy. Adverse reactions occurring at course 7 and beyond for patients who received placebo with FAC during the first 6 courses and who then received either dexrazoxane or placebo with FAC are also listed.

Percentage (%) of Breast Cancer Patients with Adverse Reactions				
	FAC + dexrazoxane		FAC + placebo	
Adverse reaction	Courses 1 - 6 (n = 413)	Courses ≥ 7 (n = 102)	Courses 1 - 6 (n = 458)	Courses ≥ 7 (n = 99)
Alopecia	94	100	97	98
Nausea	77	51	84	60
Vomiting	59	42	72	49
Fatigue/malaise	61	48	58	55
Anorexia	42	27	47	38
Stomatitis	34	26	41	28
Fever	34	22	29	18
Infection	23	19	18	21
Diarrhea	21	14	24	7
Pain on injection	12	13	3	0
Sepsis	17	12	14	9
Neurotoxicity	17	10	13	5
Streaking/erythema	5	4	4	2
Phlebitis	6	3	3	5
Esophagitis	6	3	7	4
Dysphagia	8	0	10	5
Hemorrhage	2	3	2	1
Extravasation	1	3	1	2
Urticaria	2	2	2	0
Recall skin reaction	1	1	2	0

The adverse reactions listed above are likely attributable to the FAC regimen with the exception of pain on injection that was observed mainly on the dexrazoxane arm.

➤*Hematologic:* Patients receiving FAC with dexrazoxane experienced more severe leukopenia, granulocytopenia, and thrombocytopenia at nadir than patients receiving FAC without dexrazoxane, but recovery counts were similar for the 2 groups of patients.

DEXRAZOXANE — INJECTION

➤*Lab test abnormalities:* Some patients receiving FAC plus dexrazoxane or FAC plus placebo experienced marked abnormalities in hepatic or renal function tests, but the frequency and severity of abnormalities in bilirubin, alkaline phosphatase, BUN, and creatinine were similar for patients receiving FAC with or without dexrazoxane.

Overdosage

There have been no instances of drug overdose in clinical studies.

The maximum dose administered during the cardioprotective trials was 1000 mg/m^2 every 3 weeks.

Disposition studies with dexrazoxane have not been conducted in cancer patients undergoing dialysis, but retention of a significant dose fraction (greater than 0.4) of the unchanged drug in the plasma pool, minimal tissue partitioning or binding, and availability of greater than 90% of the systemic drug levels in the unbound form suggest that it could be removed using conventional peritoneal or hemodialysis.

There is no known antidote for dexrazoxane. Instances of suspected overdose should be managed with good supportive care until resolution of myelosuppression and related conditions is complete. Management of overdose should include treatment of infections, fluid regulation, and maintenance of nutritional requirements.

MESNA

Rx	**Mesna** (Baxter)	**Tablets:** 400 mg	Lactose. (M4). White, oblong, scored. Film coated. In 10 blisters.
Rx	**Mesnex** (Bristol-Myers Squibb)		Lactose, simethicone. (M4). White, oblong, scored. Film coated. In 10 blisters.
Rx	**Mesna** (Various, eg, American Pharmaceutical Partners, Baxter)	**Injection:** 100 mg/mL	With 0.25 mg/mL EDTA. In 10 mL multidose vials.[a]
Rx	**Mesnex** (Bristol-Myers Squibb)		With 0.25 mg/mL EDTA. In 10 mL multidose vials.[a]

[a] With 10.4 mg benzyl alcohol as a preservative.

MESNA — ORAL

Indications

➤*Ifosfamide-induced hemorrhagic cystitis:* As a prophylactic agent in reducing the incidence of ifosfamide-induced hemorrhagic cystitis.

Administration and Dosage

➤*Approved by the FDA:* December 30, 1988.

For the prophylaxis of ifosfamide-induced hemorrhagic cystitis, mesna tablets may be given on a fractionated dosing schedule of 3 bolus IV injections or a single bolus injection followed by 2 oral administrations of mesna tablets as outlined below.

➤*IV and oral dosing:* Mesna injection is given as IV bolus injections in a dosage equal to 20% of the ifosfamide dosage (w/w) at the time of ifosfamide administration. Mesna tablets are given orally in a dosage equal to 40% of the ifosfamide dose 2 and 6 hours after each dose of ifosfamide. The total daily dose of mesna is 100% of the ifosfamide dose.

Recommended Mesna Injection Dosing Schedule

	0 hours	2 hours	6 hours
Ifosamide	1.2 g/m^2		
Mesna injection	240 mg/m^2		
Mesna tablets		480 mg/m^2	480 mg/m^2

Patients who vomit within 2 hours of taking oral mesna should repeat the dose or receive IV mesna. The efficacy and safety of this ratio of IV and oral mesna has not been established as being effective for daily doses of ifosfamide higher than 2 g/m^2.

The dosing schedule should be repeated on each day that ifosfamide is administered. When the dosage of ifosfamide is adjusted (either increased or decreased), the ratio of mesna to ifosfamide should be maintained.

➤*Storage/Stability:* Store at controlled room temperature 20° to 25°C (68° to 77°F).

Actions

➤*Pharmacology:* Mesna was developed as a prophylactic agent to reduce the risk of hemorrhagic cystitis induced by ifosfamide.

Analogous to the physiological cysteine-cystine system, mesna is rapidly oxidized to its major metabolite, mesna disulfide (dimesna). Mesna disulfide remains in the intravascular compartment and is rapidly eliminated by the kidneys.

In the kidney, the mesna disulfide is reduced to the free thiol compound, mesna, which reacts chemically with the urotoxic ifosfamide metabolites (acrolein and 4-hydroxy-ifosfamide) resulting in their detoxification. The first step in the detoxification process is the binding of mesna to 4-hydroxy-ifosfamide forming a nonurotoxic 4-sulfoethylthioifosfamide. Mesna also binds to the double bonds of acrolein and to other urotoxic metabolites.

In multiple human xenograft or rodent tumor model studies of limited scope, using IV or intraperitoneal (IP) routes of administration, mesna, in combination with ifosfamide (at dose ratios of up to 20-fold as single or multiple courses), failed to demonstrate interference with antitumor efficacy.

➤*Pharmacokinetics:*

Absorption/Distribution –

IV-oral-oral regimen: The half-life of mesna ranged from 1.2 to 8.3 hours after administration of IV plus oral doses of mesna, as recommended in Administration and Dosage. The urinary bioavailability of oral mesna ranged from 45% to 79% of IV mesna. Food does not affect the urinary availability of orally administered mesna. Approximately 18% to 26% of the combined IV and oral mesna dose appears as free mesna in the urine. When compared to IV mesna, the IV plus oral dosing regimen increases systemic exposures (150%) and provides more sustained excretion of mesna in the urine over a 24-hour period. Approximately 5% of the mesna dose is excreted during the 12- to 24-hour interval, as compared to negligible amounts in patients given the IV regimen. The fraction of the administered dose of mesna excreted in the urine is independent of dose. Protein binding of mesna is in a moderate range (69% to 75%).

Metabolism/Excretion – At doses of 2 to 4 g/m^2, the terminal elimination half-life of ifosfamide is about 4 to 8 hours. As a result, in order to maintain adequate levels of mesna in the urinary bladder during the course of elimination of the urotoxic ifosfamide metabolites, repeated doses of mesna are required.

Contraindications

Hypersensitivity to mesna or other thiol compounds.

Warnings

➤*Usage:* Mesna has been developed as an agent to reduce the risk of ifosfamide-induced hemorrhagic cystitis. It will not prevent or alleviate any of the other adverse reactions or toxicities associated with ifosfamide therapy.

➤*Hematuria:* Mesna does not prevent hemorrhagic cystitis in all patients. Up to 6% of patients treated with mesna have developed hematuria (greater than 50 RBC/hpf or World Health Organization [WHO] grade 2 and above). As a result, a morning specimen of urine should be examined for the presence of hematuria (microscopic evidence of red blood cells) each day prior to ifosfamide therapy. If hematuria develops when mesna is given with ifosfamide according to the recommended dosage schedule, depending on the severity of the hematuria, dosage reductions or discontinuation of ifosfamide therapy may be initiated.

In order to reduce the risk of hematuria, mesna must be administered with each dose of ifosfamide as outlined in Administration and Dosage. Mesna is not effective in reducing the risk of hematuria due to other pathological conditions such as thrombocytopenia.

➤*Hypersensitivity reactions:* Allergic reactions to mesna ranging from mild hypersensitivity to systemic anaphylactic reactions have been reported. Patients with autoimmune disorders who were treated with cyclophosphamide and mesna appeared to have a higher incidence of allergic reactions. The majority of these patients received mesna orally.

➤*Elderly:* In general, dose selection for an elderly patient should be cautious, reflecting the greater frequency of decreased hepatic, renal, or cardiac function, and of concomitant disease or other drug therapy. However, the ratio of ifosfamide to mesna should remain unchanged.

➤*Pregnancy: Category B.* There are no adequate and well-controlled studies in pregnant women. Because animal reproductive studies are not always predictive of human response, this drug should be used during pregnancy only if clearly needed.

➤*Lactation:* It is not known whether mesna or dimesna is excreted in human milk. Because many drugs are excreted in human milk and because of the potential for adverse reactions in nursing infants from mesna, a decision should be made whether to discontinue nursing or discontinue the drug, taking into account the importance of the drug to the mother.

➤*Children:* Safety and efficacy of mesna tablets in pediatric patients have not been established.

Drug Interactions

➤*Drug/Lab test interactions:* A false-positive test for urinary ketones may arise in patients treated with mesna. In this test, a red-violet color develops which, with the addition of glacial acetic acid, will return to violet.

Adverse Reactions

The most frequently reported side effects (observed in 2 or more patients) for patients receiving single doses of mesna IV were headache, injection-site reactions, flushing, dizziness, nausea, vomiting, somnolence, diarrhea, anorexia, fever, pharyngitis, hyperaesthesia, influenza-like symptoms, and coughing. Among patients who received a single 1200 mg dose as an oral solution, rigors, back pain, rash, conjunctivitis, and arthralgia were also reported. In 2 phase 1 multiple-dose studies where patients received mesna tablets alone or IV mesna followed by repeated doses of mesna tablets, flatu-

MESNA — ORAL

lence and rhinitis were reported. In addition, constipation was reported by patients who had received repeated doses of IV mesna.

Incidence of Adverse Reactions and Incidence of Most Frequently Reported Adverse Reactions in Controlled Studies (%)		
Mesna regimen	IV-IV-IV (N = 119)	IV-oral-oral (N = 119)
Incidence of adverse reactions	101 (84.9%)	106 (89.1%)
Nausea	65 (54.6%)	64 (53.8%)
Vomiting	35 (29.4%)	45 (37.8%)
Constipation	28 (23.5%)	21 (17.6%)
Leukopenia	25 (21%)	21 (17.6%)
Fatigue	24 (20.2%)	24 (20.2%)
Fever	24 (20.2%)	18 (15.1%)
Anorexia	21 (17.6%)	19 (16%)
Thrombocytopenia	21 (17.6%)	16 (13.4%)
Anemia	20 (16.8%)	21 (17.6%)
Granulocytopenia	16 (13.4%)	15 (12.6%)
Asthenia	15 (12.6%)	21 (17.6%)
Abdominal pain	14 (11.8%)	18 (15.1%)
Alopecia	12 (10.1%)	13 (10.9%)
Dyspnea	11 (9.2%)	11 (9.2%)
Chest pain	10 (8.4%)	9 (7.6%)
Hypokalemia	10 (8.4%)	11 (9.2%)
Diarrhea	9 (7.6%)	17 (14.3%)
Dizziness	9 (7.6%)	5 (4.2%)
Headache	9 (7.6%)	13 (10.9%)
Pain	9 (7.6%)	10 (8.4%)
Increased sweating	9 (7.6%)	2 (1.7%)
Back pain	8 (6.7%)	6 (5%)
Hematuria *	8 (6.7%)	7 (5.9%)
Injection-site reaction	8 (6.7%)	10 (8.4%)
Edema	8 (6.7%)	9 (7.6%)
Peripheral edema	8 (6.7%)	8 (6.7%)
Somnolence	8 (6.7%)	12 (10.1%)
Anxiety	7 (5.9%)	4 (3.4%)
Confusion	7 (5.9%)	6 (5%)
Face edema	6 (5%)	5 (4.2%)
Insomnia	6 (5%)	11 (9.2%)
Coughing	5 (4.2%)	10 (8.4%)
Dyspepsia	4 (3.4%)	6 (5%)
Hypotension	4 (3.4%)	6 (5%)
Pallor	4 (3.4%)	6 (5%)
Dehydration	3 (2.5%)	7 (5.9%)
Pneumonia	2 (1.7%)	8 (6.7%)
Tachycardia	1 (0.8%)	7 (5.9%)
Flushing	1 (0.8%)	6 (5.0%)

* All grades.

➤*Postmarketing surveillance:* Allergic reactions, decreased platelet counts associated with allergic reactions, hypertension, hypotension, increased heart rate, increased liver enzymes, injection site reactions (including pain and erythema), limb pain, malaise, myalgia, ST-segment elevation, tachycardia, and tachypnea have been reported as part of postmarketing surveillance.

Overdosage

➤*Symptoms:* Oral doses of 6.1 and 4.3 g/kg were lethal to mice and rats, respectively. These doses are approximately 15 and 22 times the maximum recommended human dose on a body surface area basis. Death was preceded by diarrhea, tremor, convulsions, dyspnea, and cyanosis.

➤*Treatment:* There is no known antidote for mesna.

Patient Information

It is important for the patient to drink at least a quart (4 cups) of liquid a day whenever taking mesna.

A small number of patients who take mesna get blood in their urine (hematuria). Therefore, laboratory testing of the urine will be perfomed by the health care provider each day of mesna therapy. The laboratory test can find low levels of blood in the urine that undetectable by viewing.

If the patient's urine has turned a pink or red color, contact the health care provider as soon as possible. Certain prescription medicines and foods, such as red beets, may also cause urine to change color. A laboratory test of urine will show if the source of the color is due to one of these causes or hematuria.

Mesna tablets should be taken at the exact times advised by the health care provider. If a dose is missed, it should be taken as soon as possible and the health care provider should be contacted for more instructions. The dose should not be doubled to make up for the missed dose.

Mesna should not be taken if the patient has had an allergic reaction to mesna or other medicines that contain sulfur.

Before beginning treatment with mesna, the patient should check with the health care provider regarding the following:

- Pregnancy. The patient and health care provider should discuss if mesna is the right therapy.
- Breast-feeding. The health care provider may advise the patient to stop breast-feeding or not to use mesna.
- Autoimmune disorders (eg, rheumatoid arthritis, systemic lupus erythematosis [SLE], or nephritis [a type of kidney problem]). The patient may be more likely to get an allergic reaction from mesna.

Mesna should be taken at the exact times in the exact amounts instructed by the health care provider. If the first dose is IV and the other doses are oral, the patient will get the IV dose at the same time as the ifosfamide. Tablets should be taken 2 and 6 hours after the ifosfamide.

The dose of mesna depends on the amount of the ifosfamide dose. Advise patients to pay careful attention to the number of tablets the health care provider instructs them to take. Half tablets for the dose may be required. Each tablet has a groove in the middle that makes it easy to break the tablets in half.

The most common side effects reported for mesna tablets are headache; digestive symptoms such as nausea, vomiting, diarrhea, stomach pain, and low or no appetite; flu-like symptoms including dizziness, flushing, and fever; sensitive skin; sleepiness; coughing; sore throat; cold-like symptoms; injection site reactions. Some patients may get allergic reactions, rash, constipation, paleness, fluid retention, and decreased blood pressure. These are not all the possible side effects of mesna. For a complete list, consult the health care provider.

If there is suspicion that someone may have taken more than the prescribed dose of mesna, contact the local poison control center or emergency room right away.

Store mesna tablets in a cool, dry place protected from excess moisture and heat. If possible, it should not be stored in the kitchen or bathroom. Any unused portion should be thrown away after the expiration date.

MESNA — INJECTION

Indications

➤*Ifosfamide-induced hemorrhagic cystitis:* Mesna has been shown to be effective as a prophylactic agent in reducing the incidence of ifosfamide-induced hemorrhagic cystitis.

➤*Unlabeled uses:* Mesna may be useful in reducing the incidence of cyclophosphamide-induced hemorrhagic cystitis.

Administration and Dosage

➤*Approved by the FDA:* December 30, 1988.

For the prophylaxis of ifosfamide-induced hemorrhagic cystitis, mesna may be given on a fractionated dosing schedule of 3 bolus intravenous (IV) injections or a single bolus injection followed by 2 oral administrations of mesna tablets as outlined

➤*IV and oral dosing:* Mesna injection is given as IV bolus injections in a dosage equal to 20% of the ifosfamide dosage (w/w) at the time of ifosfamide administration. Mesna tablets are given orally in a dosage equal to 40% of the ifosfamide dose 2 and 6 hours after each dose of ifosfamide. The total daily dose of mesna is 100% of the ifosfamide dose.

Recommended Mesna Dosing Schedule (IV and Oral Dosing)			
	0 hours	2 hours	6 hours
Ifosfamide	1.2 g/m^2	-	-
Mesna injection	240 mg/m^2	-	-
Mesna tablets	-	480 mg/m^2	480 mg/m^2

Patients who vomit within 2 hours of taking oral mesna should repeat the dose or receive IV mesna. The efficacy and safety of this ratio of IV and oral mesna has not been established as being effective for daily doses of ifosfamide higher than 2 g/m^2.

➤*IV schedule:* Mesna is given as IV bolus injections in a dosage equal to 20% of the ifosfamide dosage (w/w) at the time of ifosfamide administration and 4 and 8 hours after each dose of ifosfamide. The total daily dose of mesna is 60% of the ifosfamide dose.

Recommended Mesna and Ifosfamide Dosing			
	0 hours	4 hours	8 hours
Ifosfamide	1.2 g/m^2	-	-
Mesna	240 mg/m^2	240 mg/m^2	240 mg/m^2

MESNA — INJECTION

In order to maintain adequate protection, this dosing schedule should be repeated on each day that ifosfamide is administered. When the dosage of ifosfamide is adjusted (either increased or decreased), the ratio of mesna to ifosamide should be maintained. When exposed to oxygen, mesna is oxidized to the disulfide, dimesna. As a result, if the ampules are used, any unused mesna remaining in the ampules after dosing should be discarded and new ampules used for each administration.

➤*Preparation of IV solutions / stability:* The mesna multidose vials may be stored and used for up to 8 days.

For IV administration the drug can be diluted by adding the contents of a mesna injection ampule to any of the following fluids obtaining final concentrations of 20 mg mesna/mL fluid: 5% Dextrose Injection; 5% Dextrose and 0.2% Sodium Chloride Injection; 5% Dextrose and 0.33% Sodium Chloride Injection 5% Dextrose and 0.45% Sodium Chloride Injection; 0.92% Sodium Chloride Injection; Lactated Ringer's Injection.

For example, 1 mL of mesna multidose vial 100 mg/mL may be added to 4 mL, or 1 ampule of mesna injection 200 mg/2 mL may be added to 8 mL of any of the solutions listed above to create a final concentration of 20 mg mesna/mL fluid.

Diluted solutions are chemically and physically stable for 24 hours at 25°C (77°F).

Mesna is not compatible with cisplatin or carboplatin.

➤*Storage / Stability:* Store at controlled room temperature 20° to 25°C (68° to 77°F).

The mesna multidose vials may be stored and used for up to 8 days.

Diluted solutions are chemically and physically stable for 24 hours at 25°C (77°F).

Actions

➤*Pharmacology:* Mesna was developed as a prophylactic agent to prevent the hemorrhagic cystitis induced by ifosfamide. Analogous to the physiological cysteine-cystine system, following IV administration, mesna is rapidly oxidized to its only metabolite, mesna disulfide (dimesna). Mesna disulfide remains in the intravascular compartment and is rapidly eliminated by the kidneys.

In the kidney, the mesna disulfide is reduced to the free thiol compound, mesna, which reacts chemically with the urotoxic ifosfamide metabolites (acrolein and 4-hydroxy-ifosfamide) resulting in their detoxification. The first step in the detoxification process is the binding of mesna to 4-hydroxy-ifosfamide forming a nonurotoxic 4-sulfoethylthioifosfamide. Mesna also binds to the double bonds of acrolein and other urotoxic metabolites.

In multiple human xenograft or rodent tumor model studies of limited scope, using IV or intraperitoneal (IP) routes of administration, mesna in combination with ifosfamide (at dose ratios of up to 20-fold as single or multiple courses) failed to demonstrate interference with antitumor efficacy.

➤*Pharmacokinetics:* At doses of 2 to 4 g/m^2, the terminal elimination half-life of ifosfamide is about 4 to 8 hours. As a result, in order to maintain adequate levels of mesna in the urinary bladder during the course of elimination of the urotoxic ifosfamide metabolites, repeated doses of mesna are required.

IV-IV-IV regimen – After IV administration of an 800 mg dose the half-lives of mesna and dimesna in the blood are 0.36 hours and 1.17 hours, respectively. Approximately 32% and 33% of the administered dose was eliminated in the urine in 24 hours as mesna and dimesna, respectively. The majority of the dose recovered was eliminated within 4 hours. Mesna has a volume of distribution of 0.652 L/kg and a plasma clearance of 1.23 L/kg/hr.

IV-oral-oral regimen – The half-life of mesna ranged from 1.2 to 8.3 hours after administration of the recommended IV plus oral doses of mesna. The urinary bioavailability of oral mesna ranged from 45% to 79% of IV administered mesna. Food does not affect the urinary availability of orally administered mesna. Approximately 18% to 26% of the combined IV and oral mesna dose appears as free mesna in the urine. When compared to IV administered mesna, the IV plus oral dosing regimen increases systemic exposures (150%) and provides more sustained excretion of mesna in the urine over a 24 hour period. Approximately 5% of the mesna dose is excreted during the 12- to 24-hour interval, as compared to negligible amounts in patients given the IV regimen. The fraction of the administered dose of mesna excreted in the urine is independent of dose. Protein binding of mesna is in a moderate range (69% to 75%).

Contraindications

Hypersensitivity to mesna or other thiol compounds.

Warnings

➤*Usage:* Mesna has been developed as an agent to prevent ifosfamide-induced hemorrhagic cystitis. It will not prevent or alleviate any of the other adverse reactions or toxicities associated with ifosfamide therapy.

➤*Hematuria:* Mesna does not prevent hemorrhagic cystitis in all patients. Up to 6% of patients treated with mesna have developed hematuria (greater than 50 red blood cells/high powered field or WHO grade 2 and above). As a result, a morning specimen of urine should be examined for the presence of hematuria (red blood cells) each day prior to ifosfamide therapy. If hematuria develops when mesna is given with ifosfamide according to the recommended dosage schedule, depending on the severity of the hematuria, dosage reductions or discontinuation of ifosfamide therapy may be initiated.

In order to reduce the risk of hematuria, mesna must be administered with each dose of ifosfamide as outlined: Mesna injection is given as IV bolus injections in a dosage equal to 20% of the ifosfamide dosage (w/w) at the time of ifosfamide administration. Mesna tablets are given orally in a dosage equal to 40% of the ifosfamide dose 2 and 6 hours after each dose of ifosfamide. The total daily dose of mesna is 100% of the ifosfamide dose. Mesna is not effective in reducing the risk of hematuria due to other pathological conditions such as thrombocytopenia.

➤*Hypersensitivity reactions:* Allergic reactions to mesna ranging from mild hypersensitivity to systemic anaphylactic reactions have been reported. Patients with autoimmune disorders who were treated with cyclophosphamide and mesna appeared to have a higher incidence of allergic reactions. The majority of these patients received mesna orally.

➤*Elderly:* Clinical studies of mesna did not include sufficient numbers of subjects aged 65 and over to determine whether they respond differently from younger subjects. In general, dose selection for an elderly patient should be cautious, reflecting the greater frequency of decreased hepatic, renal, or cardiac function, and of concomitant disease or other drug therapy. However, the ratio of ifosfamide to mesna should remain unchanged.

➤*Pregnancy: Category B.* There are no adequate and well-controlled studies in pregnant women. Because animal reproductive studies are not always predictive of human response, this drug should be used during pregnancy only if clearly needed.

➤*Lactation:* It is not known whether mesna or dimesna is excreted in human milk. Because many drugs are excreted in human milk and because of the potential for adverse reactions in nursing infants, from mesna, a decision should be made whether to discontinue nursing or discontinue the drug, taking into account the importance of the drug to the mother.

➤*Children:* Because of the benzyl alcohol content, the multidose vial should not be used in neonates or infants and should be used with caution in older pediatric patients.

Precautions

➤*Monitoring:* Healthcare providers should advise patients taking mesna to drink at least a quart of liquid a day. Patients should be informed to report if their urine has turned a pink or red color, if they vomit within 2 hours of taking oral mesna, or if they miss a dose of oral mesna.

➤*Lab test abnormalities:* A false-positive test for urinary ketones may arise in patients treated with mesna injection. In this test, a red-violet color develops which, with the addition of glacial acetic acid, will return to violet.

Adverse Reactions

The most frequently reported side effects (observed in 2 or more patients) for patients receiving single doses of mesna IV were headache, injection site reactions, flushing, dizziness, nausea, vomiting, somnolence, diarrhea, anorexia, fever, pharyngitis, hyperaesthesia, influenza-like symptoms, and coughing. Among patients who received a single 1200 mg dose as an oral solution, rigors, back pain, rash, conjunctivitis, and arthralgia were also reported. In 2 phase I multiple-dose studies where patients received mesna tablets alone or IV mesna followed by repeated doses of mesna tablets, flatulence and rhinitis were reported. In addition, constipation was reported by patients who had received repeated doses of IV mesna.

In phase I studies in which IV bolus doses of 0.8 to 1.6 g/m^2 mesna were administered as single or 3 repeated doses to a total of 10 patients, a bad taste in the mouth (100%) and soft stools (70%) were reported. At IV and oral bolus doses of 2.4 g/m^2 which are approximately 10 times the recommended clinical doses (0.24 g/m^2) headache (50%), fatigue (33%), nausea (33%), diarrhea (83%), limb pain (50%), hypotension (17%) and allergy (17%) have also been reported in the 6 patients who participated in this study.

In controlled clinical studies, adverse reactions which can be reasonably associated with mesna were vomiting, diarrhea and nausea.

Incidence of Adverse Events and Incidence of Most Frequently Reported Adverse Events in Controlled Studies (%)

Mesna regimen	IV-IV-IV (N = 119)	IV-oral-oral (N = 119)
Incidence of AEs	101 (84.9%)	106 (89.1%)
Nausea	65 (54.6%)	64 (53.8%)
Vomiting	35 (29.4%)	45 (37.8%)
Constipation	28 (23.5%)	21 (17.6%)
Leukopenia	25 (21%)	21 (17.6%)
Fatigue	24 (20.2%)	24 (20.2%)
Fever	24 (20.2%)	18 (15.1%)
Anorexia	21 (17.6%)	19 (16%)
Thrombocytopenia	21 (17.6%)	16 (13.4%)
Anemia	20 (16.8%)	21 (17.6%)
Granulocytopenia	16 (13.4%)	15 (12.6%)
Asthenia	15 (12.6%)	21 (17.6%)
Abdominal pain	14 (11.8%)	18 (15.1%)
Alopecia	12 (10.1%)	13 (10.9%)
Dyspnea	11 (9.2%)	11 (9.2%)
Chest pain	10 (8.4%)	9 (7.6%)
Hypokalemia	10 (8.4%)	11 (9.2%)
Diarrhea	9 (7.6%)	17 (14.3%)

MESNA — INJECTION

Incidence of Adverse Events and Incidence of Most Frequently Reported Adverse Events in Controlled Studies (%)		
Mesna regimen	IV-IV-IV (N = 119)	IV-oral-oral (N = 119)
Incidence of AEs	101 (84.9%)	106 (89.1%)
Dizziness	9 (7.6%)	5 (4.2%)
Headache	9 (7.6%)	13 (10.9%)
Pain	9 (7.6%)	10 (8.4%)
Sweating increased	9 (7.6%)	2 (1.7%)
Back pain	8 (6.7%)	6 (5%)
Hematuria*	8 (6.7%)	7 (5.9%)
Injection site reaction	8 (6.7%)	10 (8.4%)
Edema	8 (6.7%)	9 (7.6%)
Peripheral edema	8 (6.7%)	8 (6.7%)
Somnolence	8 (6.7%)	12 (10.1%)
Anxiety	7 (5.9%)	4 (3.4%)
Confusion	7 (5.9%)	6 (5%)
Face edema	6 (5%)	5 (4.2%)
Insomnia	6 (5%)	11 (9.2%)
Coughing	5 (4.2%)	10 (8.4%)
Dyspepsia	4 (3.4%)	6 (5%)
Hypotension	4 (3.4%)	6 (5%)
Pallor	4 (3.4%)	6 (5%)
Dehydration	3 (2.5%)	7 (5.9%)
Pneumonia	2 (1.7%)	8 (6.7%)
Tachycardia	1 (0.8%)	7 (5.9%)
Flushing	1 (0.8%)	6 (5%)

* All grades.

➤*Postmarketing surveillance:* Allergic reactions, decreased platelet counts associated with allergic reactions, hypertension, hypotension, increased heart rate, increased liver enzymes, injection site reactions (including pain and erythema), limb pain, malaise, myalgia, ST-segment elevation, tachycardia, and tachypnea have been reported as part of post-marketing surveillance.

Overdosage

There is no known antidote for mesna.

Oral doses of 6.1 and 4.3 g/kg were lethal to mice and rats, respectively. These doses are approximately 15 and 22 times the maximum recommended human dose on a body surface area basis. Death was preceded by diarrhea, tremor, convulsions, dyspnea, and cyanosis.

Patient Information

It is important for the patient to drink at least a quart (4 cups) of liquid a day whenever taking mesna.

A small number of patients taking mesna get blood in their urine (hematuria). Therefore, laboratory testing of the urine will be performed by the health care provider each day of mesna therapy. The laboratory test can find low levels of blood in the urine undetectable by viewing.

If the patient's urine has turned a pink or red color, contact the health care provider as soon as possible. Certain prescription medicines and foods, such as red beets, may also cause the urine to change color. A laboratory test of your urine will show if the source of the color is due to one of these causes or hematuria.

Mesna injection should be stored in a cool, dry place protected from excess moisture and heat. If possible, it should not be stored in the kitchen or bathroom. Any unused portion should be thrown away after the expiration date.

DNA DEMETHYLATION AGENTS

AZACITIDINE

Rx	**Vidaza** (Pharmion)	**Powder for injection, lyophilized:** 100 mg	100 mg mannitol. In single-use vials.

AZACITIDINE — INJECTION

Indications

➤*Myelodysplastic syndrome (MOS) subtypes:* Azacitidine is indicated for the treatment of patients with the following myelodysplastic syndrome (MDS) subtypes: Refractory anemia (RA) or refractory anemia with ringed sideroblasts (RARS) (if accompanied by neutropenia or thrombocytopenia or requiring transfusions), refractory anemia with excess blasts (RAEB), refractory anemia with excess blasts in transformation (RAEB-T), and chronic myelomonocytic leukemia (CMMoL).

➤*Unlabeled uses:* Treatment of refractory acute lymphocytic leukemia; refractory acute myelogenous leukemia.

Administration and Dosage

➤*Approved by the FDA:* May 19, 2004.

The recommended starting dose is 75 mg/m^2 subcutaneously, administered daily for 7 days, every 4 weeks. Premedicate patients for nausea and vomiting. The dose may be increased to 100 mg/m^2 if no beneficial effect is seen after 2 treatment cycles and if no toxicity other than nausea and vomiting has occurred. It is recommended that patients be treated for a minimum of 4 cycles. However, complete or partial response may require more than 4 treatment cycles. Treatment may be continued as long as the patient continues to benefit.

Monitor patients for hematologic response and renal toxicities. Dosage delay or reduction as described below may be necessary.

➤*Dosage adjustment based on hematology laboratory values:* For patients with baseline (start of treatment) WBC greater than or equal to 3 × 10^9/L, ANC greater than or equal to 1.5 × 10^9/L, and platelets greater than or equal to 75 × 10^9/L, adjust the dose as follows, based on nadir counts for any given cycle:

Nadir counts		% dose in the next course
ANC (x 10^9/L)	Platelets (x 10^9/L)	
< 0.5	< 25	50%
0.5 to 1.5	25 to 50	67%
> 1.5	> 50	100%

For patients whose baseline counts are WBC less than 3 x 10^9/L, ANC less than 1.5 x10^9/L, or platelets less than 75 x10^9/L, base dose adjustments on nadir counts and bone marrow biopsy cellularity at the time of the nadir as noted below, unless there is clear improvement in differentiation (percentage of mature granulocytes is higher and ANC is higher than at onset of that course) at the time of the next cycle, in which case the dose of the current treatment should be continued.

WBC or platelet nadir % decrease in counts from baseline	Bone Marrow Biopsy Cellularity at Time of Nadir (%)		
	30 to 60	15 to 30	< 15
	% dose in the next course		
50 to 75	100	50	33
> 75	75	50	33

If a nadir as defined in the table above has occurred, give the next course of treatment 28 days after the start of the preceding course, provided that both the WBC and the platelet counts are greater than 25% above the nadir and rising. If a greater than 25% increase above the nadir is not seen by day 28, reassess counts every 7 days. If a 25% increase is not seen by day 42, then treat the patient with 50% of the scheduled dose.

➤*Dosage adjustment based on renal function and serum electrolytes:* If unexplained reductions in serum bicarbonate levels to less than 20 mEq/L occur, reduce the dosage by 50% on the next course. Similarly, if unexplained elevations of BUN or serum creatinine occur, delay the next cycle until values return to normal or baseline and reduce the dose by 50% on the next treatment course.

➤*Use in the Elderly:* See Warnings for more information.

➤*Preparation of azacitidine:* Reconstitute azacitidine aseptically with 4 mL sterile water for injection. Inject the diluent slowly into the vial. Invert the vial 2 to 3 times, and gently rotate until a uniform suspension is achieved. The suspension will be cloudy. The resulting suspension will contain azacitidine 25 mg/mL.

➤*Preparation for immediate administration:* Divide doses greater than 4 mL equally into 2 syringes. The product may be held at room temperature for up to 1 hour, but must be administered within 1 hour after reconstitution.

➤*Preparation for delayed administration:* The reconstituted product may be kept in the vial or drawn into a syringe. Divide doses greater than 4 mL equally into 2 syringes. The product must be refrigerated immediately, and may be held under refrigerated conditions (2° to 8°C, 36° to 46°F) for up to 8 hours. After removal from refrigerated conditions, the suspension may be allowed to equilibrate to room temperature for up to 30 minutes prior to administration.

AZACITIDINE — INJECTION

Administration – To provide a homogeneous suspension, the contents of the syringe must be resuspended by inverting the syringe 2 to 3 times and gently rolling the syringe between the palms for 30 seconds immediately prior to administration.

Azacitidine is administered subcutaneously. Divide doses greater than 4 mL equally into 2 syringes and inject into 2 separate sites. Rotate sites for each injection (thigh, abdomen, or upper arm). Give new injections at least 1 inch from an old site and never into areas were the site is tender, bruised, red, or hard.

➤*Storage/Stability:* Store unreconstituted vials at 25°C (77°F); excursions permitted to 15° to 30°C (59° to 86°F).

Stability – Reconstituted azacitidine may be stored for up to 1 hour at 25°C (77°F) or for up to 8 hours between 2° and 8°C (36° and 46°F). The azacitidine vial is for single use and does not contain any preservatives. Discard unused portions of each vial properly. See Handling and disposal. Do not save any unused portions for later administration.

Actions

➤*Pharmacology:* Azacitidine is believed to exert its antineoplastic effects by causing hypomethylation of DNA and direct cytotoxicity on abnormal hematopoietic cells in the bone marrow. The concentration of azacitidine required for maximum inhibition of DNA methylation in vitro does not cause major suppression of DNA synthesis. Hypomethylation may restore normal function to genes that are critical for differentiation and proliferation. The cytotoxic effects of azacitidine cause the death of rapidly dividing cells, including cancer cells that are no longer responsive to normal growth control mechanisms. Nonproliferating cells are relatively insensitive to azacitidine.

➤*Pharmacokinetics:*

Absorption/Distribution – The pharmacokinetics of azacitidine were studied in six MDS patients following a single 75 mg/m^2 subcutaneous dose and a single 75 mg/m^2 IV dose. Azacitidine is rapidly absorbed after subcutaneous administration; the peak plasma azacitidine concentration of 750 ± 403 ng/mL occurred in 0.5 hour. The bioavailability of subcutaneous azacitidine relative to IV azacitidine is approximately 89%, based on area under the curve. Mean volume of distribution following IV dosing is 76 ± 26 L. Mean apparent subcutaneous clearance is 167 ± 49 L/hour, and mean half-life after subcutaneous administration is 41 ± 8 minutes.

Metabolism/Excretion – An in vitro study of azacitidine incubation in human liver fractions indicated that azacitidine may be metabolized by the liver.

Published studies indicate that urinary excretion is the primary route of elimination of azacitidine and its metabolites. Following IV administration of radioactive azacitidine to 5 cancer patients, the cumulative urinary excretion was 85% of the radioactive dose. Fecal excretion accounted for less than 1% of administered radioactivity over 3 days. Mean excretion of radioactivity in urine following subcutaneous administration of ^{14}C-azacitidine was 50%. The mean elimination half-lives of total radioactivity (azacitidine and its metabolites) were similar after IV and subcutaneous administrations, about 4 hours.

Special populations – The effects of renal or hepatic impairment, gender, age, or race on the pharmacokinetics of azacitidine have not been studied. Renal abnormalities ranging from elevated serum creatinine to renal failure and death have been reported rarely in patients treated with IV azacitidine in combination with other chemotherapeutic agents for non-MDS conditions. In addition, renal tubular acidosis, defined as a fall in serum bicarbonate to less than 20 mEq/L in association with an alkaline urine and hypokalemia (serum potassium less than 3 mEq/L) developed in 5 patients with CML treated with azacitidine and etoposide. If unexplained reductions in serum bicarbonate less than 20 mEq/L or elevations of BUN or serum creatinine occur, reduce the dosage or hold as described previously. Azacitidine is contraindicated in patients with advanced malignant hepatic tumors. Because azacitidine is potentially hepatotoxic in patients with severe preexisting hepatic impairment, caution is needed in patients with liver disease. Patients with extensive tumor burden due to metastatic disease have been rarely reported to experience progressive hepatic coma and death during azacitidine treatment, especially in such patients with baseline albumin less than 30 g/L. Azacitidine is contraindicated in patients with advanced malignant hepatic tumors.

Contraindications

Azacitidine is contraindicated in patients with known hypersensitivities to azacitidine or mannitol. Azacitidine is also contraindicated in patients with advanced malignant hepatic tumors (see Precautions).

Warnings

➤*Use in men:* Advise men not to father a child while receiving treatment with azacitidine (see Fertility impairment).

➤*Renal function impairment:* Safety and efficacy of azacitidine in patients with renal impairment have not been studied, as these patients were excluded from the clinical trials.

Closely monitor patients with renal impairment for toxicity since azacitidine and its metabolites are primarily excreted by the kidneys.

See Actions for more information.

➤*Hepatic function impairment:* Safety and efficacy of azacitidine in patients with hepatic impairment have not been studied, as these patients were excluded from the clinical trials.

See Actions for more information.

➤*Carcinogenesis:* The potential carcinogenicity of azacitidine was evaluated in mice and rats. Azacitidine induced tumors of the hematopoietic system in female mice at 2.2 mg/kg (6.6 mg/m^2, approximately 8% the recommended human daily dose on a mg/m^2 basis) administered intraperitoneally 3 times per week for 52 weeks. An increased incidence of tumors in the lymphoreticular system, lung, mammary gland, and skin was seen in mice treated with azacitidine intraperitoneally at 2 mg/kg (6 mg/m^2, approximately 8% the recommended human daily dose on a mg/m^2 basis) once a week for 50 weeks. A tumorigenicity study in rats dosed twice weekly at 15 or 60 mg/m^2 (approximately 20% to 80% the recommended human daily dose on a mg/m^2 basis) revealed an increased incidence of testicular tumors compared with controls.

➤*Mutagenesis:* The mutagenic and clastogenic potential of azacitidine was tested in in vitro bacterial systems *Salmonella typhimurium* strains TA100 and several strains of *trpE8*, *Escherichia coli* strains WP14 Pro, WP3103P, WP3104P, and CC103; in in vitro forward gene mutation assay in mouse lymphoma cells and human lymphoblast cells; and in an in vitro micronucleus assay in mouse L5178Y lymphoma cells and Syrian hamster embryo cells. Azacitidine was mutagenic in bacterial and mammalian cell systems. The clastogenic effect of azacitidine was shown by the induction of micronuclei in L5178Y mouse cells and Syrian hamster embryo cells.

➤*Fertility impairment:* Administration of azacitidine to male mice at 9.9 mg/m^2 (approximately 9% the recommended human daily dose on a mg/m^2 basis) daily for 3 days prior to mating with untreated female mice resulted in decreased fertility and loss of offspring during subsequent embryonic and postnatal development. Treatment of male rats 3 times/week for 11 or 16 weeks at doses of 15 to 30 mg/m^2 (approximately 20% to 40%, the recommended human daily dose on a mg/m^2 basis) resulted in decreased weight of the testes and epididymides, and decreased sperm counts accompanied by decreased pregnancy rates and increased loss of embryos in mated females. In a related study, male rats treated for 16 weeks at 24 mg/m^2 resulted in an increase in abnormal embryos in mated females when examined on day 2 of gestation.

➤*Elderly:* Azacitidine and its metabolites are known to be substantially excreted by the kidney, and the risk of toxic reactions to this drug may be greater in patients with impaired renal function. Because elderly patients are more likely to have decreased renal function, it may be useful to monitor renal function.

➤*Pregnancy:* *Category D.*

Teratogenic – Azacitidine may cause fetal harm when administered to a pregnant woman. Early embryotoxicity studies in mice revealed a 44% frequency of intrauterine embryonal death (increased resorption) after a single intraperitoneal injection of 6 mg/m^2 (approximately 8% of the recommended human daily dose on a mg/m^2 basis) azacitidine on gestation day 10. Developmental abnormalities in the brain have been detected in mice given azacitidine on or before gestation day 15 at doses of approximately 3 to 12 mg/m^2 (approximately 4% to 16% the recommended human daily dose on a mg/m^2 basis).

In rats, azacitidine was clearly embryotoxic when given intraperitoneally on gestation days 4 to 8 (postimplantation) at a dose of 6 mg/m^2 (approximately 8% of the recommended human daily dose on a mg/m^2 basis), although treatment in the preimplantation period (on gestation days 1 to 3) had no adverse effect on the embryos. Azacitidine caused multiple fetal abnormalities in rats after a single intraperitoneal dose of 3 to 12 mg/m^2 (approximately 8% the recommended human daily dose on a mg/m^2 basis) given on gestation day 9, 10, 11, or 12. In this study azacitidine caused fetal death when administered at 3 to 12 mg/m^2 on gestation days 9 and 10; average live animals per litter was reduced to 9% of control at the highest dose on gestation day 9. Fetal anomalies included CNS anomalies (exencephaly/encephalocele), limb anomalies (micromelia, club foot, syndactyly, oligodactyly), and others (micrognathia, gastroschisis, edema, and rib abnormalities).

There are no adequate and well-controlled studies in pregnant women using azacitidine. If this drug is used during pregnancy, or if the patient becomes pregnant while taking this drug, apprise the patient of the potential hazard to the fetus.

Advise women of childbearing potential to avoid becoming pregnant while receiving treatment with azacitidine.

➤*Lactation:* It is not known whether azacitidine or its metabolites are excreted in human milk. Because of the potential for tumorigenicity shown for azacitidine in animal studies and the potential for serious adverse reactions, women treated with azacitidine should not nurse.

➤*Children:* Safety and efficacy in pediatric patients have not been established.

Precautions

➤*Monitoring:* Perform complete blood counts should be performed as needed to monitor response and toxicity, but at a minimum, prior to each cycle. Obtain liver chemistries and serum creatinine prior to initiation of therapy.

Treatment with azacitidine is associated with neutropenia and thrombocytopenia. Perform complete blood counts as needed to monitor response and toxicity, but at a minimum, prior to each dosing cycle. After administration of the recommended dosage for the first cycle, reduce or delay dosage for subsequent cycles based on nadir counts and hematologic response.

Closely monitor patients with renal impairment for toxicity since azacitidine and its metabolites are primarily excreted by the kidneys.

➤*MOS:* Safety and effectiveness of azacitidine in patients with MDS have not been studied, as these patients were excluded from the clinical trials.

AZACITIDINE — INJECTION

Drug Interactions

➤*Concurrent chemotherapy:* Renal abnormalities ranging from elevated serum creatinine to renal failure and death have been reported rarely in patients treated with IV azacitidine in combination with other chemotherapeutic agents for non-MDS conditions. In addition, renal tubular acidosis, defined as a fall in serum bicarbonate to less than 20 mEq/L in association with an alkaline urine and hypokalemia (serum potassium less than 3 mEq/L) developed in 5 patients with CML treated with azacitidine and etoposide. If unexplained reductions in serum bicarbonate less than 20 mEq/L or elevations of BUN or serum creatinine occur, reduce or hold the dosage.

Adverse Reactions

➤*Adverse reactions described in other labeling sections:* Elevated serum creatinine, hepatic coma, hypokalemia, neutropenia, thrombocytopenia, renal failure, renal tubular acidosis.

➤*Most commonly occurring adverse reactions (subcutaneous route):* Anemia, constipation, diarrhea, ecchymosis, fatigue, injection-site erythema, leukopenia, nausea, neutropenia, pyrexia, thrombocytopenia, vomiting.

➤*Adverse reactions most frequently (greater than 2%) resulting in clinical intervention (subcutaneous route):*

Discontinuation – Leukopenia (5%), thrombocytopenia (3.6%), neutropenia (2.7%).

Dose held – Leukopenia (4.5%), neutropenia (4.5%), febrile neutropenia (2.7%).

Dose reduced – Leukopenia (4.5%), neutropenia (4.1%), thrombocytopenia (3.2%).

➤*Discussion of adverse reactions information:*

Most Frequently Observed Adverse Events with Azacitidine (≥ 5%)[a]

Preferred term[b]	All azacitidine (n = 220)[c]	Observation (n = 92)[d]
At least 1 TEAE	219 (99.5%)	89 (96.7%)
Abdominal pain	34 (15.5%)	12 (13%)
Abdominal pain, upper	23 (10.5%)	3 (3.3%)
Abdominal tenderness	26 (11.8%)	1 (1.1%)
Abdominal distension	13 (5.9%)	4 (4.3%)
Aggravated anemia	12 (5.5%)	5 (5.4%)
Aggravated fatigue	28 (12.7%)	4 (4.3%)
Anemia	153 (69.5%)	59 (64.1%)
Anorexia	45 (20.5%)	6 (6.5%)
Anxiety	29 (13.2%)	3 (3.3%)
Arthralgia	49 (22.3%)	3 (3.3%)
Atelectasis	11 (5%)	2 (2.2%)
Back pain	41 (18.6%)	7 (7.6%)
Cardiac murmur	22 (10%)	8 (8.7%)
Cellulitis	18 (8.2%)	4 (4.3%)
Chest pain	36 (16.4%)	5 (5.4%)
Chest wall pain	11 (5%)	0
Constipation	74 (33.6%)	6 (6.5%)
Contusion	41 (18.6%)	9 (9.8%)
Cough	65 (29.5%)	14 (15.2%)
Decreased appetite	28 (12.7%)	8 (8.7%)
Decreased breath sounds	17 (7.7%)	1 (1.1%)
Decreased weight	35 (15.9%)	10 (10.9%)
Depression	26 (11.8%)	7 (7.6%)
Diarrhea	80 (36.4%)	13 (14.1%)
Dizziness	41 (18.6%)	5 (5.4%)
Dry skin	11 (5%)	1 (1.1%)
Dyspepsia	15 (6.8%)	4 (4.3%)
Dysphagia	11 (5%)	2 (2.2%)
Dyspnea	64 (29.1%)	11 (12%)
Dysuria	18 (8.2%)	2 (2.2%)
Ecchymosis	67 (30.5%)	14 (15.2%)
Epistaxis	36 (16.4%)	9 (9.8%)
Erythema	37 (16.8%)	4 (4.3%)
Exacerbated dyspnea	11 (5%)	3 (3.3%)
Exertional dyspnea	31 (14.1%)	15 (16.3%)
Fatigue	79 (35.9%)	23 (25%)
Febrile neutropenia	36 (16.4%)	4 (4.3%)
Gingival bleeding	21 (9.5%)	4 (4.3%)
Headache	48 (21.8%)	10 (10.9%)
Hematoma	19 (8.6%)	0
Hemorrhoids	15 (6.8%)	1 (1.1%)
Herpes simplex	20 (9.1%)	5 (5.4%)
Hypoesthesia	11 (5%)	1 (1.1%)
Hypokalemia	28 (12.7%)	12 (13%)
Hypotension	15 (6.8%)	2 (2.2%)
Increased sweating	23 (10.5%)	2 (2.2%)
Injection site bruising	31 (14.1%)	0
Injection site erythema	77 (35%)	0
Injection site granuloma	11 (5%)	0
Injection site pain	50 (22.7%)	0
Injection site pigmentation changes	11 (5%)	0
Injection site pruritus	15 (6.8%)	0
Injection site reaction	30 (13.6%)	0
Injection site swelling	11 (5%)	0
Insomnia	24 (10.9%)	4 (4.3%)
Lethargy	17 (7.7%)	2 (2.2%)
Leukopenia	106 (48.2%)	27 (29.3%)
Loose stools	12 (5.5%)	0
Lung crackles	23 (10.5%)	8 (8.7%)
Lymphadenopathy	21 (9.5%)	3 (3.3%)
Malaise	24 (10.9%)	1 (1.1%)
Mouth hemorrhage	11 (5%)	1 (1.1%)
Muscle cramps	13 (5.9%)	3 (3.3%)
Myalgia	35 (15.9%)	2 (2.2%)
Nasal congestion	12 (5.5%)	1 (1.1%)
Nasopharyngitis	32 (14.5%)	3 (3.3%)
Nausea	155 (70.5%)	16 (17.4%)
Neutropenia	71 (32.3%)	10 (10.9%)
Night sweats	19 (8.6%)	3 (3.3%)
Oral mucosal petechiae	17 (7.7%)	3 (3.3%)
Pain	24 (10.9%)	3 (3.3%)
Pain in limb	44 (20%)	5 (5.4%)
Pallor	34 (15.5%)	7 (7.6%)
Peripheral edema	41 (18.6%)	10 (10.9%)
Peripheral swelling	16 (7.3%)	5 (5.4%)
Petechiae	52 (23.6%)	8 (8.7%)
Pharyngitis	44 (20%)	7 (7.6%)
Pitting edema	32 (14.5%)	9 (9.8%)
Pleural effusion	14 (6.4%)	6 (6.5%)
Pneumonia	24 (10.9%)	5 (5.4%)
Postnasal drip	13 (5.9%)	3 (3.3%)
Post procedural hemorrhage	13 (5.9%)	1 (1.1%)
Post procedural pain	11 (5%)	2 (2.2%)
Productive cough	25 (11.4%)	4 (4.3%)
Pruritus	27 (12.3%)	11 (12%)
Pyrexia	114 (51.8%)	28 (30.4%)
Rales	19 (8.6%)	8 (8.7%)
Rash	31 (14.1%)	9 (9.8%)
Rhinorrhea	22 (10%)	2 (2.2%)
Rhonchi	13 (5.9%)	2 (2.2%)
Rigors	56 (25.5%)	10 (10.9%)
Sinusitis	11 (5%)	3 (3.3%)
Skin lesion	32 (14.5%)	8 (8.7%)
Skin nodule	11 (5%)	1 (1.1%)
Stomatitis	17 (7.7%)	0
Syncope	13 (5.9%)	5 (5.4%)
Tachycardia	19 (8.6%)	6 (6.5%)

AZACITIDINE — INJECTION

Most Frequently Observed Adverse Events with Azacitidine (≥ 5%)[a]		
Preferred term[b]	All azacitidine (n = 220)[c]	Observation (n = 92)[d]
Thrombocytopenia	144 (65.5%)	42 (45.7%)
Tongue ulceration	11 (5%)	2 (2.2%)
Transfusion reaction	15 (6.8%)	0
Upper respiratory tract infection	28 (12.7%)	4 (4.3%)
Urinary tract infection	17 (7.7%)	5 (5.4%)
Urticaria	13 (5.9%)	1 (1.1%)
Vomiting	119 (54.1%)	5 (5.4%)
Weakness	64 (29.1%)	19 (20.7%)
Wheezing	19 (8.6%)	2 (2.2%)

[a] Mean azacitidine exposure = 11.4 months. Mean time in observation arm = 6.1 months.
[b] Multiple reports of the same preferred terms for a patient are only counted once within each treatment group.
[c] Includes events from all patients exposed to azacitidine, including patients after crossing over from observation.
[d] Includes events from observation period only; excludes any events after crossover to azacitidine.

Nausea, vomiting, diarrhea, and constipation all tended to increase in incidence with increasing doses of azacitidine. Nausea, vomiting, injection site erythema, constipation, rigors, petechiae, injection-site pain, dizziness, injection-site bruising, anxiety, hypokalemia, insomnia, epistaxis, and rales tended to be more pronounced during the first 1 to 2 cycles of subcutaneous azacitidine treatment compared with later cycles of treatment. There did not appear to be any adverse events that increased in frequency over the course of treatment. There did not appear to be any relevant differences in adverse events by gender.

In clinical studies of either subcutaneous or IV azacitidine, the following serious treatment-related adverse events occurring at a rate of less than 5% (not described in the previous table) were reported:

Cardiovascular – Atrial fibrillation, cardiac failure, cardiac failure congestive, cardio-respiratory arrest, congestive cardiomyopathy.
Vascular disorders: Orthostatic hypotension.

CNS – Convulsions, intracranial hemorrhage.

Dermatologic – Pyoderma gangrenosum, pruritic rash, skin induration.

GI – Diverticulitis, gastrointestinal hemorrhage, melena, perirectal abscess.

GU – Hematuria, loin pain.

Hematologic/Lymphatic – Agranulocytosis, bone marrow depression, splenomegaly.

Hepatic – Cholecystitis.

Hypersensitivity – Anaphylactic shock, hypersensitivity.

Metabolic/Nutritional – Dehydration.

Musculoskeletal – Aggravated bone pain, muscle weakness, neck pain.

Psychiatric – Confusion.

Systemic – Leukemia cutis.

Renal – Renal failure.

Respiratory – Hemoptysis, lung infiltration, pneumonitis, respiratory distress.

Miscellaneous – Catheter site hemorrhage, general physical health deterioration, systemic inflammatory response syndrome.
Infections and infestations: Limb abscess, bacterial infection, blastomycosis, injection site infection, *Klebsiella* sepsis, pharyngitis streptococcal, pneumonia *Klebsiella*, sepsis, staphylococcal bacteremia, staphylococcal infection, toxoplasmosis.
Surgical and medical procedures: Cholecystectomy.

Overdosage

➤*Symptoms:* One case of overdose with azacitidine was reported during clinical trials. A patient experienced diarrhea, nausea, and vomiting after receiving a single IV dose of approximately 290 mg/m^2, almost 4 times the recommended starting dose. The events resolved without sequelae, and the correct dose was resumed the following day.

➤*Treatment:* In the event of overdosage, monitor the patient with appropriate blood counts and receive supportive treatment, as necessary. There is no known specific antidote for azacitidine overdosage.

Patient Information

Patients should inform their physicians about any underlying liver or renal disease.

Advise women of childbearing potential to avoid becoming pregnant while receiving treatment with azacitidine.

Advise men not to father children while receiving treatment with azacitidine.

NELARABINE

Rx	**Arranon** (GlaxoSmithKline)	**Injection:** 250 mg (5 mg/mL)	Sodium chloride 4.5 mg/mL. In 50 mL vials.

NELARABINE — INJECTION

WARNING

Administer nelarabine under the supervision of a physician experienced in the use of cancer chemotherapeutic agents. This product is for intravenous (IV) use only.

Neurologic events – Severe neurologic events have been reported with the use of nelarabine. These events have included the following: altered mental states including severe somnolence, CNS effects including convulsions, and peripheral neuropathy ranging from numbness and paresthesias to motor weakness and paralysis. There have also been reports of events associated with demyelination and ascending peripheral neuropathies similar in appearance to Guillain-Barré syndrome.

Full recovery from these events has not always occurred with cessation of therapy with nelarabine. Close monitoring for neurologic events is strongly recommended; discontinue nelarabine for neurologic events of National Cancer Institute (NCI) Common Toxicity Criteria grade 2 or greater.

Indications

➤*Leukemia/lymphoma:* Nelarabine is indicated for the treatment of patients with T-cell acute lymphoblastic leukemia and T-cell lymphoblastic lymphoma whose disease has not responded to or has relapsed following treatment with at least 2 chemotherapy regimens. This use is based on the induction of complete responses. Randomized trials demonstrating increased survival or other clinical benefit have not been conducted.

Administration and Dosage

➤*Approved by the FDA:* October 28, 2005.

➤*Dosage:*

Adults – The recommended adult dose of nelarabine is 1,500 mg/m^2 administered IV over 2 hours on days 1, 3, and 5 repeated every 21 days. Nelarabine is administered undiluted.

Children – The recommended pediatric dose of nelarabine is 650 mg/m^2 administered IV over 1 hour daily for 5 consecutive days, repeated every 21 days. Nelarabine is administered undiluted.

➤*Duration of therapy:* The recommended duration of treatment for adult and pediatric patients has not been clearly established. In clinical trials, treatment was generally continued until there was evidence of disease progression, the patient experienced unacceptable toxicity, the patient became a candidate for bone marrow transplant, or the patient no longer continued to benefit from treatment.

➤*Preparation for administration:* Nelarabine is not diluted prior to administration. The appropriate dose of nelarabine is transferred into polyvinylchloride (PVC) infusion bags or glass containers and administered as a 2-hour infusion in adult patients and as a 1-hour infusion in pediatric patients.

➤*Supportive care:* Appropriate measures (eg, hydration, urine alkalinization, prophylaxis with allopurinol) must be taken to prevent hyperuricemia of tumor lysis syndrome.

➤*Discontinuation:* Nelarabine should be discontinued for neurologic events of NCI Common Toxicity Criteria grade 2 or greater. Dosage may be delayed for other toxicity including hematologic toxicity.

➤*Storage/Stability:* Store at 25°C (77°F); excursions permitted to 15° to 30°C (59° to 86°F).

Nelarabine is stable in PVC infusion bags and glass containers for up to 8 hours at up to 30°C (86°F).

Actions

➤*Pharmacology:* Nelarabine is a pro-drug of the deoxyguanosine analog 9-β-D-arabinofuranosylguanine (ara-G). Nelarabine is demethylated by adenosine deaminase (ADA) to ara-G, mono-phosphorylated by deoxyguanosine kinase and deoxycytidine kinase, and subsequently converted to the active 5 -triphosphate, ara-GTP. Accumulation of ara-GTP in leukemic blasts allows for incorporation into deoxyribonucleic acid (DNA), leading to inhibition of DNA synthesis and cell death. Other mechanisms may contribute to the cytotoxic and systemic toxicity of nelarabine.

➤*Pharmacokinetics:*

Absorption – Plasma ara-G C_{max} values generally occurred at the end of the nelarabine infusion and were generally higher than nelarabine C_{max} values, suggesting rapid and extensive conversion of nelarabine to ara-G. Mean plasma nelarabine and ara-G C_{max} values were 5 ± 3 mcg/mL and 31.4 ± 5.6 mcg/mL, respectively, after a 1,500 mg/m^2 nelarabine dose infused over 2 hours in adult patients. Exposure to ara-G area under the curve (AUC) is 37 times higher than that for nelarabine on day 1 after nelarabine IV infusion of 1,500 mg/m^2 dose (162 ± 49 mcg•h/mL vs 4.4 ±2.2 mcg•h/mL, respectively). Comparable C_{max} and AUC were obtained for nelarabine between days 1 and 5 at the proposed nelarabine adult dosage of 1,500 mg/m^2, indicating that the pharmacokinetics of nelarabine after multiple dosing

NELARABINE — INJECTION

are predictable from single dosing. There are not enough data for ara-G to make a comparison between day 1 and day 5. After a nelarabine adult dosage of 1,500 mg/m², a mean intracellular C_{max} for ara-GTP appeared within 3 to 25 hours on day 1. Exposure (AUC) to intracellular ara-GTP was 532 times higher than that for nelarabine and 14 times higher than that for ara-G (2,339 ± 2,628 mcg•h/mL vs 4.4 ± 2.2 mcg•h/mL and 162 ± 49 mcg•h/mL, respectively).

Distribution – Nelarabine and ara-G are extensively distributed throughout the body. Specifically, for nelarabine, V_{ss} values were 197 ± 216 L/m² and 213 ± 358 L/m² in adult and pediatric patients, respectively. For ara-G, V_{ss}/F values were 50 ± 24 L/m² and 33 ± 9.3 L/m² in adult and pediatric patients, respectively.

Nelarabine and ara-G are not substantially bound to human plasma proteins (less than 25%) in vitro, and binding is independent of nelarabine or ara-G concentrations up to 600 mcM.

Metabolism – The principal route of metabolism for nelarabine is O-demethylation by ADA to form ara-G, which undergoes hydrolysis to form guanine. In addition, some nelarabine is hydrolyzed to form methylguanine, which is O-demethylated to form guanine. Guanine is N-deaminated to form xanthine, which is further oxidized to yield uric acid. Ring opening of uric acid followed by further oxidation results in the formation of allantoin.

Excretion – Pharmacokinetic studies in adult patients with refractory leukemia or lymphoma have demonstrated that nelarabine and ara-G are rapidly eliminated from plasma with a half-life of approximately 30 minutes and 3 hours, respectively, after a 1,500 mg/m² nelarabine dose.

Combined phase 1 pharmacokinetic data at nelarabine doses of 104 to 2,900 mg/m² indicate that the mean clearance (CL) of nelarabine is about 30% higher in children than in adult patients (259 ± 409 L/h/m² vs 197 ± 189 L/h/m², respectively) (n = 66 adults, n = 22 children) on day 1. The apparent clearance of ara-G (CL/F) is comparable between the 2 groups (10.5 ± 4.5 L/h/m² in adult patients and 11.3 ± 4.2 L/h/m² in children) on day 1.

Nelarabine and ara-G are partially eliminated by the kidneys. Mean urinary excretion of nelarabine and ara-G was 6.6% ± 4.7% and 27% ±15% of the administered dose, respectively, in 28 adult patients over the 24 hours after nelarabine infusion on day 1. Renal clearance averaged 24 ± 23 L/h for nelarabine and 6.2 ± 5 L/h for ara-G in 21 adult patients.

Special populations –

Children: No pharmacokinetic data are available in children at the once-daily 650 mg/m² nelarabine dosage. Combined phase 1 pharmacokinetic data at nelarabine doses of 104 to 2,900 mg/m² indicate that the mean clearance (CL) of nelarabine is about 30% higher in children than in adult patients (259 ± 409 L/h/m² vs 197 ±189 L/h/m², respectively) (n = 66 adults, n = 22 children) on day 1. The apparent clearance of ara-G (CL/F) is comparable between the 2 groups (10.5 ± 4.5 L/h/m² in adult patients and 11.3 ± 4.2 L/h/m² in children) on day 1.

Nelarabine and ara-G are extensively distributed throughout the body. Specifically, for nelarabine, V_{ss} values were 197 ± 216 L/m² and 213 ± 358 L/m² in adult and pediatric patients, respectively. For ara-G, V_{ss}/F values were 50 ± 24 L/m² and 33 ± 9.3 L/m² in adult and pediatric patients, respectively.

Contraindications

Nelarabine is contraindicated in patients who have a history of hypersensitivity to nelarabine or any other components of nelarabine.

Warnings

➤*Administration:* See the Warning box for more information.

➤*Neurologic effects:* Nelarabine is a potent antineoplastic agent with potentially significant toxic side effects. Neurotoxicity is the dose-limiting toxicity of nelarabine. Closely observe patients undergoing therapy with nelarabine for signs and symptoms of neurologic toxicity.

Common signs and symptoms of nelarabine-related neurotoxicity include somnolence, confusion, convulsions, ataxia, paraesthesia, and hypesthesia. Severe neurologic toxicity can manifest as coma, status epilepticus, craniospinal demyelination, or ascending neuropathy similar in presentation to Guillain-Barré syndrome.

Patients treated previously or concurrently with intrathecal chemotherapy or previously with craniospinal irradiation may be at increased risk for neurologic adverse reactions.

➤*Renal function impairment:* Ara-G clearance decreased as renal function decreased. Because the risk of adverse reactions to this drug may be greater in patients with severe renal function impairment (Ccr less than 30 mL/min), closely monitor patients for toxicities when treated with nelarabine.

➤*Hepatic function impairment:* The influence of hepatic function impairment on the pharmacokinetics of nelarabine has not been evaluated. Because the risk of adverse reactions to this drug may be greater in patients with severe hepatic function impairment (bilirubin greater than 3 mg/dL), closely monitor these patients for toxicities when treated with nelarabine

➤*Mutagenesis:* Nelarabine was mutagenic when tested in vitro in L5178Y/TK mouse lymphoma cells with and without metabolic activation.

➤*Elderly:* Clinical studies of nelarabine did not include sufficient numbers of patients aged 65 years and over to determine whether they respond differently from younger patients. In an exploratory analysis, increasing age, especially 65 years of age and older, appeared to be associated with increased rates of neurologic adverse reactions.

Decreased renal function, which may be more common in the elderly, may reduce ara-G clearance.

➤*Pregnancy: Category D.* Nelarabine may cause fetal harm when administered to a pregnant woman. There are no studies of nelarabine in pregnant women. When compared with controls, nelarabine administration during the period of organogenesis caused increased incidences of fetal malformations, anomalies, and variations in rabbits at doses greater than or equal to 360 mg/m²/day (8-hour IV infusion; approximately one-fourth the adult dose compared on a mg/m² basis), which was the lowest dose tested. Cleft palate was seen in rabbits given 3,600 mg/m²/day (approximately 2-fold the adult dose), absent pollices (digits) in rabbits given greater than or equal to 1,200 mg/m²/day (approximately three-fourths the adult dose), while absent gallbladder, absent accessory lung lobes, fused or extra sternebrae, and delayed ossification was seen at all doses. Maternal body weight gain and fetal body weights were reduced in rabbits given 3,600 mg/m²/day (approximately 2-fold the adult dose), but could not account for the increased incidence of malformations seen at this or lower administered doses. If this drug is used during pregnancy, or if the patient becomes pregnant while taking this drug, warn the patient of the potential hazard to the fetus. Advise women of childbearing potential to avoid becoming pregnant while receiving treatment with nelarabine.

➤*Lactation:* It is not known whether nelarabine or ara-G are excreted in human milk. Because many drugs are excreted in human milk and because of the potential for serious adverse reactions in breast-feeding infants from nelarabine, discontinue breast-feeding in women who are receiving therapy with nelarabine.

➤*Children:* The safety and efficacy of nelarabine in children were studied in a clinical trial conducted by the Children's Oncology Group (COG P9673). This study included patients 21 years of age and younger, who had relapsed or refractory T-cell acute lymphoblastic leukemia (T-ALL) or T-cell lymphoblastic lymphoma (T-LBL). Eighty-four patients, 39 of whom had received 2 or more prior induction regimens, were treated with 650 mg/m²/day of nelarabine administered IV over 1 hour daily for 5 consecutive days, repeated every 21 days (see the following table). Patients who experienced signs or symptoms of grade 2 or greater neurologic toxicity on therapy were to be discontinued from further therapy with nelarabine.

Pediatric Clinical Study—Patient Allocation	
Patient population	N
Patients treated at 650 mg/m²/day × 5 days every 21 days	84
Patients with T-ALL or T-LBL with 2 or more prior induction treated at 650 mg/m²/day × 5 days every 21 days	39
Patients with T-ALL or T-LBL with 1 prior induction treated at 650 mg/m²/day × 5 days every 21 days	31

The 84 patients ranged in age from 2.5 to 21.7 years (overall mean, 11.9 years); 52% were 3 to 12 years of age, and most were male (74%) and white (62%). The majority (77%) of patients had a diagnosis of T-ALL.

Complete response in this study was defined as bone marrow blast counts less than or equal to 5%, no other evidence of disease, and full recovery of peripheral blood counts. Complete response without full hematologic recovery was also assessed as a meaningful outcome in this heavily pretreated population. Duration of response is reported from date of response to date of relapse, and may include subsequent stem cell transplant. Efficacy results are presented in the following table.

Efficacy Results in Patients 21 Years of Age and Younger at Diagnosis with ≥2 Prior Inductions Treated with 650 mg/m² of Nelarabine Administered IV Over 1 Hour Daily for 5 Consecutive Days, Repeated Every 21 Days	
	N = 39
CR[a] plus CR[b] % (n) [95% C]	23% (9) [11%, 39%]
CR[a] % (n) [95% CI]	13% (5) [4%, 27%]
CR[b] % (n) [95% CI]	10% (4) [3%, 24%]
Duration of CR[a] plus CR[b] (range in weeks)[c]	3.3 to 9.3
Median overall survival (weeks) [95% CI]	13.1 [8.7, 17.4]

[a] CR = complete response.
[b] CR = complete response without hematologic recovery.
[c] Does not include 5 patients who were transplanted or had subsequent systemic chemotherapy (duration of response in these 5 patients was 4.7 to 42.1 weeks).

The mean number of days on therapy was 46 days (range, 7 to 129 days). Median time to complete response plus complete response without hematologic recovery was 3.4 weeks (95% CI, 3 to 3.7).

Precautions

➤*Monitoring:* Leukopenia, thrombocytopenia, anemia, and neutropenia, including febrile neutropenia have been associated with nelarabine therapy. Regularly monitor complete blood counts, including platelets.

➤*IV hydration:* Patients receiving nelarabine should receive IV hydration according to standard medical practice for the management of hyperuricemia in patients at risk for tumor lysis syndrome. Consider the use of allopurinol in patients at risk of hyperuricemia.

➤*Immunocompromised patients:* Avoid administration of live vaccines to immunocompromised patients.

➤*Hazardous tasks:* Because patients receiving nelarabine therapy may experience somnolence, caution them about operating hazardous machinery, including automobiles.

NELARABINE — INJECTION

Adverse Reactions

The most common adverse reactions in children, regardless of causality, were hematologic disorders (eg, anemia, leukopenia, neutropenia, thrombocytopenia). Of the nonhematologic adverse reactions in children, the most frequent reactions reported were headache, increased transaminase levels, decreased blood potassium, decreased blood albumin, increased blood bilirubin, and vomiting.

The most common adverse reactions in adults, regardless of causality, were fatigue, GI disorders (eg, constipation, diarrhea, nausea, vomiting), hematologic disorders (eg, anemia, neutropenia, thrombocytopenia), respiratory disorders (eg, cough, dyspnea), nervous system disorders (eg, somnolence, dizziness), and pyrexia.

Nelarabine Adverse Reactions in Children (≥ 5%)

Adverse reaction	Percentage of patients: 650 mg/m²; n = 84		
	Toxicity grade		
	Grade 3	Grade 4+[a]	All grades
GI			
Vomiting	0%	0%	10%
Hematologic/Lymphatic			
Anemia	45%	10%	95%
Leukopenia	14%	7%	38%
Neutropenia	17%	62%	94%
Thrombocytopenia	27%	32%	88%
Hepatic			
Blood albumin decreased	5%	1%	10%
Blood bilirubin increased	7%	2%	10%
Transaminases increased	4%	0%	12%
Lab test abnormalities			
Blood calcium decreased	1%	1%	8%
Blood creatinine increased	0%	0%	6%
Blood glucose decreased	4%	0%	6%
Blood magnesium decreased	2%	0%	6%
Blood potassium decreased	4%	2%	11%
Miscellaneous			
Asthenia	1%	0%	6%
Infection	2%	1%	5%

[a] Grade 4+ = Grade 4 and Grade 5.

➤*Fatal events:* Three patients had a fatal event. Fatal events included the following: neutropenia and pyrexia (n = 1), status epilepticus/seizure (n = 1), and fungal pneumonia (n = 1). The status epilepticus was thought to be related to treatment with nelarabine. All other fatal events were unrelated to treatment with nelarabine.

Nelarabine Adverse Reactions in Adult Patients (≥ 5%)

Adverse reaction	Percentage of patients; n= 103		
	Toxicity grade		
	Grade 3	Grade 4+[a]	All grades
Cardiovascular			
Hypotension	1%	1%	8%
Sinus tachycardia	1%	0%	8%
CNS			
Abnormal gait	0%	0%	6%
Asthenia	0%	1%	17%
Confusional state	2%	0%	8%
Depression	1%	0%	6%
Fatigue	10%	2%	50%
Insomnia	0%	0%	7%
Rigors	0%	0%	8%
Dermatologic			
Petechiae	2%	0%	12%
GI			
Abdominal distension	0%	0%	6%
Abdominal pain	1%	0%	9%
Anorexia	0%	0%	9%
Constipation	1%	0%	21%
Diarrhea	1%	0%	22%
Nausea	0%	0%	41%
Stomatitis	1%	0%	8%
Vomiting	1%	0%	22%
Hematologic/ Lymphatic			
Anemia	20%	14%	99%
Febrile neutropenia	9%	1%	12%
Neutropenia	14%	49%	81%
Thrombocytopenia	37%	22%	86%
Hepatic			
AST increased	1%	1%	6%
Metabolic/Nutritional			
Dehydration	3%	1%	7%
Edema	0%	0%	11%
Edema, peripheral	0%	0%	15%
Hyperglycemia	1%	0%	6%
Musculoskeletal			
Arthralgia	1%	0%	9%
Back pain	0%	0%	8%
Muscular weakness	5%	0%	8%
Myalgia	1%	0%	13%
Pain in extremity	1%	0%	7%
Respiratory			
Cough	0%	0%	25%
Dyspnea	4%	2%	20%
Dyspnea, exertional	0%	0%	7%
Epistaxis	0%	0%	8%
Pleural effusion	5%	1%	10%
Pneumonia	4%	1%	8%
Sinusitis	1%	0%	7%
Wheezing	0%	0%	5%
Miscellaneous			
Chest pain	0%	0%	5%
Chest pain, Non-cardiac	0%	1%	5%
Infection	2%	1%	9%
Pain	3%	0%	11%
Pyrexia	5%	0%	23%

[a] Grade 4+ = Grade 4 and Grade 5.

➤*Fatal events:* Five patients had a fatal event. Fatal events included the following: hypotension (n = 1), respiratory arrest (n = 1), pleural effusion/pneumothorax (n = 1), pneumonia (n = 1), and cerebral hemorrhage/coma/leukoencephalopathy (n = 1). The cerebral hemorrhage/coma/leukoencephalopathy was thought to be related to treatment with nelarabine. All other fatal events were unrelated to treatment with nelarabine.

➤*Other adverse reactions:* Blurred vision was also reported in 4% of adult patients.

There was a single report of biopsy-confirmed progressive multifocal leukoencephalopathy in the adult patient population.

CNS – Nervous system events, regardless of drug relationship, were reported for 64% of patients across the phase 1 and phase 2 studies.

Children: The most common neurologic adverse reactions (greater than or equal to 2%), regardless of causality, including all grades (NCI Common Toxicity Criteria) are shown in the following table for children.

Nelarabine Neurologic Adverse Reactions (≥ 2%) in Children

Neurologic adverse reaction	Percentage of patients; n = 84				
	Grade 1	Grade 2	Grade 3	Grade 4+[a]	All grades
Ataxia	1%	0	1%	0	2%
Headache	8%	2%	4%	2%	17%
Hypesthesia	1%	1%	4%	0	6%
Motor dysfunction	1%	1%	1%	0	4%
Nervous system disorder	1%	2%	0	0	4%
Paresthesia	0	2%	1%	0	4%
Peripheral neurologic disorders, any event	1%	4%	7%	0	12%
Peripheral motor neuropathy	1%	0	2%	0	4%
Peripheral neuropathy	0	4%	2%	0	6%
Peripheral sensory neuropathy	0	0	6%	0	6%
Somnolence	1%	4%	1%	1%	7%
Seizures	0	0	0	6%	6%
Convulsions	0	0	0	3%	4%
Generalized tonic-clonic convulsions	0	0	0	1%	1%
Status epilepticus	0	0	0	1%	1%
Tremor	1%	2%	0	0	4%

[a] Grade 4+ = Grade 4 and Grade 5.

Fatal events: One patient had a fatal neurologic event, status epilepticus. This event was thought to be related to treatment with nelarabine.

Other neurologic events: The other grade 3 event in children, regardless of causality, was hypertonia reported in 1 patient (1%). The additional grade 4+ events, regardless of causality, were third nerve paralysis, and sixth

NELARABINE — INJECTION

nerve paralysis, each reported in 1 patient (1%). The other neurologic adverse reactions, regardless of causality, reported as grade 1, 2, or unknown in children were dysarthria, encephalopathy, hydrocephalus, hyporeflexia, lethargy, mental impairment, paralysis, and sensory loss, each reported in 1 patient (1%).

Adults: The most common neurologic adverse reactions (greater than or equal to 2%), regardless of causality, including all grades (NCI Common Toxicity Criteria) are shown for adult patients in the following table.

Nelarabine Neurologic Adverse Reactions (≥ 2%) in Adult Patients					
Neurologic adverse reaction	Percentage of patients; n = 103				
	Grade 1	Grade 2	Grade 3	Grade 4	All grades
Amnesia	2%	1%	0	0	3%
Ataxia	1%	6%	2%	0	9%
Balance disorder	1%	1%	0	0	2%
Depressed level of consciousness	4%	1%	0	1%	6%
Dizziness	14%	8%	0	0	21%
Dysgeusia	2%	1%	0	0	3%
Headache	11%	3%	1%	0	15%
Hypesthesia	5%	10%	2%	0	17%
Paresthesia	11%	4%	0	0	15%
Peripheral neurologic disorders, any event	8%	12%	2%	0	21%
Neuropathy	0	4%	0	0	4%
Peripheral motor neuropathy	3%	3%	1%	0	7%
Peripheral neuropathy	2%	2%	1%	0	5%
Peripheral sensory neuropathy	7%	6%	0	0	13%
Sensory loss	0	2%	0	0	2%
Somnolence	20%	3%	0	0	23%
Tremor	2%	3%	0	0	5%

- *Fatal events* – One patient had a fatal neurologic reaction, cerebral hemorrhage/coma/leukoencephalopathy. This reaction was thought to be related to treatment with nelarabine.
- *Other neurologic adverse events* – Most nervous system events in the adult patients were evaluated as grade 1 or 2. The additional grade 3 events in adult patients, regardless of causality, were aphasia, convulsion, hemiparesis, and loss of consciousness, each reported in 1 patient (1%). The additional grade 4 events, regardless of causality, were cerebral hemorrhage, coma, intracranial hemorrhage, leukoencephalopathy, and metabolic encephalopathy, each reported in 1 patient (1%).

The other neurologic adverse reactions, regardless of causality, reported as grade 1, 2, or unknown in adult patients were abnormal coordination, burning sensation, disturbance in attention, dysarthria, hyporeflexia, neuropathic pain, nystagmus, peroneal nerve palsy, sciatica, sensory disturbance, sinus headache, and speech disorder, each reported in 1 patient (1%).

There have also been reports of events associated with demyelination and ascending peripheral neuropathies similar in appearance to Guillain-Barré syndrome.

Overdosage

➤*Symptoms:* It is anticipated that overdosage would result in severe neurotoxicity (possibly including paralysis, coma), myelosuppression, and potentially death.

Nelarabine has been administered in clinical trials up to a dose of 2,900 mg/m^2 on days 1, 3, and 5 to two adult patients. At a dose of 2,200 mg/m^2 given on days 1, 3, and 5 every 21 days, 2 patients developed a significant grade 3 ascending sensory neuropathy. Magnetic resonance imaging (MRI) evaluations of the 2 patients demonstrated findings consistent with a demyelinating process in the cervical spine.

A single IV dose of 4,800 mg/m^2 was lethal in monkeys, and was associated with CNS signs, including reduced/shallow respiration, reduced reflexes, and flaccid muscle tone.

➤*Treatment:* There is no known antidote for overdoses of nelarabine. In the event of overdose, provide supportive care consistent with good clinical practice.

Patient Information

Because patients receiving nelarabine therapy may experience somnolence, caution them about operating hazardous machinery, including automobiles.

Instruct patients to contact their physician if they experience new or worsening symptoms of peripheral neuropathy. These signs and symptoms include the following: tingling or numbness in fingers, hands, toes, or feet; difficulty with the fine motor coordination tasks such as buttoning clothing; unsteadiness while walking; weakness arising from a low chair; weakness in climbing stairs; increased tripping while walking over uneven surfaces.

Instruct patients that seizures have been known to occur in patients who receive nelarabine. If a seizure occurs, promptly inform the physician administering nelarabine.

Patients who develop fever or signs of infection while on therapy should notify their physician promptly.

Advise patients to use effective contraceptive measures to prevent pregnancy and to avoid breast-feeding during treatment with nelarabine.

DECITABINE

Rx	**Dacogen** (MGI Pharma)	**Powder for injection, lyophilized:** 50 mg	In single-dose vials.

DECITABINE — INJECTION

Indications

➤*Myelodysplastic syndromes (MDS):* For treatment of patients with MDS, including previously treated and untreated, de novo and secondary MDS of all French-American-British (FAB) subtypes (refractory anemia, refractory anemia with ringed sideroblasts, refractory anemia with excess blasts, refractory anemia with excess blasts in transformation, and chronic myelomonocytic leukemia) and intermediate-1, intermediate-2, and high-risk International Prognostic Scoring System (IPSS) groups.

Administration and Dosage

➤*Approved by the FDA:* May 2, 2006.

➤*First treatment cycle:* 15 mg/m^2 administered by continuous intravenous (IV) infusion over 3 hours, repeated every 8 hours for 3 days. Patients may be premedicated with standard antiemetic therapy.

➤*Subsequent treatment cycles:* The above cycle should be repeated every 6 weeks. It is recommended that patients be treated for a minimum of 4 cycles; however, a complete or partial response may take longer than 4 cycles. Treatment may be continued as long as the patient continues to benefit.

➤*Dose adjustment or delay:*

Hematological toxicities – If hematologic recovery (absolute neutrophil count [ANC] at least 1,000/mcL and platelets at least 50,000/mcL) from a previous decitabine treatment cycle requires more than 6 weeks, then the next cycle of decitabine therapy should be delayed and dosing temporarily reduced by following this algorithm:

- Recovery requiring more than 6, but less than 8 weeks — Decitabine dosing to be delayed for up to 2 weeks and the dose temporarily reduced to 11 mg/m^2 every 8 hours (33 mg/m^2/day, 99 mg/m^2/cycle) upon restarting therapy.
- Recovery requiring more than 8, but less than 10 weeks — Patient should be assessed for disease progression (by bone marrow aspirates); in the absence of progression, the decitabine dose should be delayed up to 2 more weeks and the dose reduced to 11 mg/m^2 every 8 hours (33 mg/m^2/day, 99 mg/m^2/cycle) upon restarting therapy, then maintained or increased in subsequent cycles as clinically indicated.

Nonhematological toxicities – If any of the following nonhematologic toxicities are present, decitabine treatment should not be restarted until the toxicity is resolved: (1) serum creatinine at least 2 mg/dL; (2) ALT, total bilirubin at least 2 times the upper limit of normal; and (3) active or uncontrolled infection.

➤*Preparation for administration:* Decitabine is a cytotoxic drug and, as with other potentially toxic compounds, caution should be exercised when handling and preparing decitabine.

Decitabine should be aseptically reconstituted with 10 mL sterile water for injection; upon reconstitution, each mL contains approximately 5 mg of decitabine at pH 6.7 to 7.3. Immediately after reconstitution, the solution should be further diluted with 0.9% sodium chloride injection, 5% dextrose injection, or Ringer's lactate injection to a final drug concentration of 0.1 to 1 mg/mL. Unless used within 15 minutes of reconstitution, the diluted solution must be prepared using cold (2° to 8°C) infusion fluids and stored at 2° to 8° C (36° to 46°F) for up to a maximum of 7 hours until administration.

➤*Handling and disposal:* Procedures for proper handling and disposal of antineoplastic drugs should be applied.

➤*Storage/Stability:* Store vials at 25°C (77°F); excursions are permitted to 15° to 30°C (59° to 86°F). Unless used within 15 minutes of reconstitution, the diluted solution must be prepared using cold (2° to 8°C) infusion fluids and stored at 2° to 8°C (36° to 46°F) for up to a maximum of 7 hours until administration.

Actions

➤*Pharmacology:* Decitabine is believed to exert its antineoplastic effects after phosphorylation and direct incorporation into deoxyribonucleic acid (DNA) and inhibition of DNA methyltransferase, causing hypomethylation of DNA and cellular differentiation or apoptosis. Decitabine inhibits DNA methylation in vitro, which is achieved at concentrations that do not cause major suppression of DNA synthesis. Decitabine-induced hypomethylation in neoplastic cells may restore normal function to genes that are critical for the control of cellular differentiation and proliferation. In rapidly dividing cells, the cytotoxicity of decitabine also may be attributed to the formation of covalent adducts between DNA methyltransferase and decitabine incorporated into DNA. Nonproliferating cells are relatively insensitive to decitabine.

DECITABINE — INJECTION

➤*Pharmacokinetics:*

Absorption/Distribution – No information is available on the pharmacokinetics of decitabine at the indicated dose of 15 mg/m². Patients with advanced solid tumors received a 72-hour infusion of decitabine at 20 to 30 mg/m²/day. Decitabine pharmacokinetics were characterized by a biphasic disposition. Plasma protein binding of decitabine is negligible (less than 1%).

Metabolism/Excretion – The total body clearance (mean ± standard deviation [SD]) was 124 ± 19 L/h/m², and the terminal phase elimination half-life was 0.51 ± 0.31 hour. The exact route of elimination and metabolic fate of decitabine is not known in humans. One of the pathways of elimination of decitabine appears to be deamination by cytidine deaminase found principally in the liver but also in granulocytes, intestinal epithelium, and whole blood.

Contraindications

Hypersensitivity to decitabine.

Warnings

➤*Use in men:* Advise men not to father a child while receiving treatment with decitabine and for 2 months afterwards.

➤*Renal/Hepatic function impairment:* There are no data on the use of decitabine in patients with renal or hepatic dysfunction; therefore, use decitabine with caution in these patients. While metabolism is extensive, the cytochrome P-450 system does not appear to be involved. In clinical trials, decitabine was not administered to patients with serum creatinine less than 2 mg/dL, transaminase greater than 2 times normal, or serum bilirubin less than 1.5 mg/dL.

➤*Mutagenesis:* The mutagenic potential of decitabine was tested in several in vitro and in vivo systems. Decitabine increased mutation frequency in L5178Y mouse lymphoma cells, and mutations were produced in an *Escherichia coli* lac-I transgene in colonic DNA of decitabine-treated mice. Decitabine caused chromosomal rearrangements in larvae of fruit flies.

➤*Fertility impairment:* The effect of decitabine on postnatal development and reproductive capacity was evaluated in mice administered a single 3 mg/m² intraperitoneal (IP) injection (approximately 7% the recommended daily clinical dose) on day 10 of gestation. Body weights of males and females exposed in utero to decitabine were significantly reduced relative to controls at all postnatal time points. No consistent effect on fertility was seen when female mice exposed in utero were mated to untreated males. Untreated females mated to males exposed in utero showed decreased fertility at 3 and 5 months of age (36% and 0% pregnancy rate, respectively). In male mice given IP injections of decitabine 0.15, 0.3, or 0.45 mg/m² (approximately 0.3% to 1% the recommended clinical dose) 3 times a week for 7 weeks, decitabine did not affect survival, body weight gain, or hematological measures (hemoglobin and white blood cell counts). Testes weights were reduced, abnormal histology was observed and significant decreases in sperm number were found at doses 0.3 mg/m² or more. In females mated to males dosed with 0.3 mg/m² or more decitabine, pregnancy rate was reduced and preimplantation loss was significantly increased.

➤*Pregnancy: Category D.*

Teratogenic – Decitabine may cause fetal harm when administered to a pregnant woman. The developmental toxicity of decitabine was examined in mice exposed to single IP injections (0, 0.9, and 3 mg/m², approximately 2% and 7% of the recommended daily clinical dose, respectively) over gestation days 8, 9, 10, or 11. No maternal toxicity was observed but reduced fetal survival was observed after treatment at 3 mg/m² and decreased fetal weight was observed at both dose levels. The 3 mg/m² dose elicited characteristic fetal defects for each treatment day, including supernumerary ribs (both dose levels), fused vertebrae and ribs, cleft palate, vertebral defects, hindlimb defects, and digital defects of fore- and hind limbs. In rats given a single IP injection of 2.4, 3.6, or 6 mg/m² (approximately 5%, 8%, or 13% the daily recommended clinical dose, respectively) on gestation days 9 to 12, no maternal toxicity was observed. No live fetuses were seen at any dose when decitabine was injected on gestation day 9. A significant decrease in fetal survival and reduced fetal weight at doses greater than 3.6 mg/m² was seen when decitabine was given on gestation day 10. Increased incidences of vertebral and rib anomalies were seen at all dose levels, and induction of exophthalmia, exencephaly, and cleft palate were observed at 6 mg/m². Increased incidence of foredigit defects was seen in fetuses at doses greater than 3.6 mg/m². Reduced size and ossification of long bones of the fore- and hindlimb were noted at 6 mg/m².

There are no adequate and well-controlled studies in pregnant women using decitabine. Advise women of childbearing potential to avoid becoming pregnant while receiving treatment with decitabine. If this drug is used during pregnancy, or if the patient becomes pregnant while taking this drug, inform the patient of the potential hazard to the fetus.

➤*Lactation:* It is not known whether decitabine or its metabolites are excreted in human milk. Because many drugs are excreted in human milk, and because of the potential for serious adverse reactions from decitabine in breast-feeding infants, decide whether to discontinue the drug, taking into account the importance of the drug to the mother.

➤*Children:* The safety and efficacy in children have not been established.

Precautions

➤*Monitoring:* Perform complete blood counts and platelet counts as needed to monitor response and toxicity, but at a minimum, prior to each cycle. Obtain liver chemistries and serum creatinine prior to initiation of treatment.

➤*Hematologic toxicity:* Treatment with decitabine is associated with neutropenia and thrombocytopenia. Perform complete blood and platelet counts as needed to monitor response and toxicity, but at a minimum, prior to each dosing cycle. After administration of the recommended dosage for the first cycle, adjust dosage for subsequent cycles as described in Administration and Dosage. Consider the need for early institution of growth factors and/or antimicrobial agents for the prevention or treatment of infections in patients with MDS. Myelosuppression and worsening neutropenia may occur more frequently in the first or second treatment cycles, and may not necessarily indicate progression of underlying MDS.

Adverse Reactions

➤*Most commonly occurring adverse reactions:* Anemia, constipation, cough, diarrhea, fatigue, hyperglycemia, nausea, neutropenia, petechiae, pyrexia, and thrombocytopenia.

➤*Adverse reactions most frequently (at least 1%) resulting in clinical intervention in the phase 3 trial in the decitabine arm:*

Discontinuation – Abnormal liver function tests, cardio-respiratory arrest, increased blood bilirubin, intracranial hemorrhage, *Mycobacterium avium* complex infection, neutropenia, pneumonia, thrombocytopenia.

Dose delayed – Atrial fibrillation, central-line infection, febrile neutropenia, neutropenia, pulmonary edema.

Dose reduced – Anemia, depression, edema, lethargy, neutropenia, pharyngitis, tachycardia, thrombocytopenia.

➤*Other adverse reactions:* Decitabine was studied in 2 single-arm, phase 2 studies (N = 66, N = 98) and 1 controlled phase 3 (supportive care) study (n = 83 exposed to decitabine). The following data reflect exposure to decitabine in 83 patients in the phase 3 MDS trial. In the phase 3 trial, patients received 15 mg/m² IV every 8 hours for 3 days every 6 weeks. The median number of decitabine cycles was 3 (range, 0 to 9).

The following table presents all adverse reactions regardless of causality occurring in at least 5% of patients in the decitabine group and at a rate greater than supportive care.

Decitabine Adverse Reactions Reported (≥ 5% of Patients in the Decitabine Group and at a Rate Greater Than Supportive Care)

Adverse reaction	Decitabine (n = 83)	Supportive care (n = 81)
Cardiovascular		
Cardiac murmur NOS[a]	13 (16%)	9 (11%)
Hypotension NOS	5 (6%)	4 (5%)
CNS		
Anxiety	9 (11%)	8 (10%)
Confusional state	10 (12%)	3 (4%)
Dizziness	15 (18%)	10 (12%)
Headache	23 (28%)	11 (14%)
Hypesthesia	9 (11%)	1 (1%)
Insomnia	23 (28%)	11 (14%)
Dermatologic		
Alopecia	7 (8%)	1 (1%)
Ecchymosis	18 (22%)	12 (15%)
Erythema	12 (14%)	5 (6%)
Pallor	19 (23%)	10 (12%)
Petechiae	32 (39%)	13 (16%)
Pruritis	9 (11%)	2 (2%)
Rash NOS	16 (19%)	7 (9%)
Skin lesion NOS	9 (11%)	3 (4%)
Swelling face	5 (6%)	0 (0%)
Urticaria NOS	5 (6%)	1 (1%)
GI		
Abdominal distension	4 (5%)	1 (1%)
Abdominal pain NOS	12 (14%)	5 (6%)
Abdominal pain upper	4 (5%)	1 (1%)
Anorexia	13 (16%)	8 (10%)
Appetite decreased NOS	13 (16%)	12 (15%)
Ascites	8 (10%)	2 (2%)
Constipation	29 (35%)	11 (14%)
Diarrhea NOS	28 (34%)	13 (16%)
Dyspepsia	10 (12%)	1 (1%)
Dysphagia	5 (6%)	2 (2%)
Gastroesophageal reflux disease	4 (5%)	0 (0%)
Glossodynia	4 (5%)	0 (0%)
Gingival bleeding	7 (8%)	5 (6%)
Hemorrhoids	7 (8%)	3 (4%)

DECITABINE — INJECTION

Adverse reaction	Decitabine (n = 83)	Supportive care (n = 81)
Lip ulceration	4 (5%)	3 (4%)
Loose stools	6 (7%)	3 (4%)
Nausea	35 (42%)	13 (16%)
Oral mucosal petechiae	11 (13%)	4 (5%)
Oral soft tissue disorder NOS	5 (6%)	1 (1%)
Stomatitis	10 (12%)	5 (6%)
Tongue ulceration	6 (7%)	2 (2%)
Vomiting NOS	21 (25%)	7 (9%)
GU		
Dysuria	5 (6%)	3 (4%)
Urinary frequency	4 (5%)	1 (1%)
Urinary tract infection NOS	6 (7%)	1 (1%)
Hematologic/Lymphatic		
Anemia NOS	68 (82%)	60 (74%)
Febrile neutropenia	24 (29%)	5 (6%)
Hematoma NOS	4 (5%)	3 (4%)
Leukopenia NOS	23 (28%)	11 (14%)
Lymphadenopathy	10 (12%)	6 (7%)
Neutropenia	75 (90%)	58 (72%)
Thrombocythemia	4 (5%)	1 (1%)
Thrombocytopenia	74 (89%)	64 (79%)
Lab test abnormalities		
AST increased	8 (10%)	7 (9%)
Blood albumin decreased	6 (7%)	0 (0%)
Blood alkaline phosphatase NOS increased	9 (11%)	7 (9%)
Blood bicarbonate decreased	4 (5%)	1 (1%)
Blood bicarbonate increased	5 (6%)	1 (1%)
Blood bilirubin decreased	4 (5%)	1 (1%)
Blood chloride decreased	5 (6%)	1 (1%)
Blood lactate dehydrogenase increased	7 (8%)	5 (6%)
Blood urea increased	8 (10%)	1 (1%)
Protein total decreased	4 (5%)	3 (4%)
Metabolic/Nutritional		
Dehydration	5 (6%)	4 (5%)
Edema NOS	15 (18%)	5 (6%)
Edema peripheral	21 (25%)	13 (16%)
Hyperbilirubinemia	12 (14%)	4 (5%)
Hyperglycemia NOS	27 (33%)	16 (20%)
Hyperkalemia	11 (13%)	3 (4%)
Hypoalbuminemia	20 (24%)	14 (17%)
Hypokalemia	18 (22%)	10 (12%)
Hypomagnesemia	20 (24%)	6 (7%)
Hyponatremia	16 (19%)	13 (16%)
Musculoskeletal		
Arthralgia	17 (20%)	8 (10%)
Back pain	14 (17%)	5 (6%)
Chest wall pain	6 (7%)	1 (1%)
Musculoskeletal discomfort	5 (6%)	0 (0%)
Myalgia	4 (5%)	1 (1%)
Pain in limb	16 (19%)	8 (10%)
Respiratory		
Breath sounds decreased	8 (10%)	7 (9%)
Cough	33 (40%)	25 (31%)
Crackles lung	12 (14%)	1 (1%)
Hypoxia	8 (10%)	4 (5%)
Pharyngitis	13 (16%)	6 (7%)
Pneumonia NOS	18 (22%)	11 (14%)
Postnasal drip	4 (5%)	2 (2%)
Pulmonary edema NOS	5 (6%)	0 (0%)
Rales	7 (8%)	2 (2%)
Special senses		
Vision blurred	5 (6%)	0 (0%)
Miscellaneous		
Abrasion NOS	4 (5%)	1 (1%)
Bacteremia	4 (5%)	0 (0%)
Candidal infection NOS	8 (10%)	1 (1%)
Catheter-related infection	7 (8%)	0 (0%)
Catheter site erythema	4 (5%)	1 (1%)
Catheter site pain	4 (5%)	0 (0%)
Cellulitis	10 (12%)	6 (7%)
Chest discomfort	6 (7%)	3 (4%)
Crepitations NOS	4 (5%)	1 (1%)
Fall	7 (8%)	3 (4%)
Injection site swelling	4 (5%)	0 (0%)
Intermittent pyrexia	5 (6%)	3 (4%)
Lethargy	10 (12%)	3 (4%)
Malaise	4 (5%)	1 (1%)
Oral candidiasis	5 (6%)	2 (2%)
Pain NOS	11 (13%)	5 (6%)
Pyrexia	44 (53%)	23 (28%)
Rigors	18 (22%)	14 (17%)
Tenderness NOS	9 (11%)	0 (0%)
Transfusion reaction	6 (7%)	3 (4%)
Sinusitis NOS	4 (5%)	2 (2%)
Staphylococcal infection	6 (7%)	0 (0%)

Table title: Decitabine Adverse Reactions Reported (≥ 5% of Patients in the Decitabine Group and at a Rate Greater Than Supportive Care)

[a] NOS = not otherwise specified.

In the phase 3 trial, the highest incidence of grade 3 or 4 adverse reactions in the decitabine arm were neutropenia (87%), thrombocytopenia (85%), febrile neutropenia (23%), and leukopenia (22%). Bone marrow suppression was the most frequent cause of dose reduction, delay, and discontinuation. Six patients had fatal reactions associated with their underlying disease and myelosuppression (anemia, neutropenia, and thrombocytopenia) that were considered at least possibly related to drug treatment. Of the 83 decitabine-treated patients, 8 permanently discontinued therapy for adverse reactions; compared with 1 of 81 patients in the supportive care arm.

Serious adverse reactions that occurred in patients receiving decitabine regardless of causality, not previously reported in the previous table include the following.

Cardiovascular – Atrial fibrillation, cardiomyopathy, cardiorespiratory arrest, congestive cardiac failure, myocardial infarction, supraventricular tachycardia.

CNS – Intracranial hemorrhage, mental status changes.

GI – Gingival pain, upper GI hemorrhage.

GU – Renal failure, urethral hemorrhage.

Hematologic / Lymphatic – Myelosuppression, splenomegaly.

Hypersensitivity – Hypersensitivity (anaphylactic reaction) to decitabine has been reported in a phase 2 trial.

Respiratory – Bronchopulmonary aspergillosis, dyspnea, hemoptysis, lung infiltration, pseudomonal lung infection, pulmonary mass, pulmonary embolism, respiratory arrest, respiratory tract infection, upper respiratory tract infection.

Miscellaneous – Asthenia, catheter site hemorrhage, chest pain, cholecystitis, fungal infection, mucosal inflammation, *Mycobacterium avium* complex infection, peridiverticular abscess, postprocedural hemorrhage, postprocedural pain, sepsis.

Overdosage

➤*Symptoms:* Higher doses are associated with increased myelosuppression, including prolonged neutropenia and thrombocytopenia.

➤*Treatment:* There is no known antidote for overdosage with decitabine. Take standard supportive measures in the event of an overdose.

Patient Information

Advise patients to inform their health care provider about any underlying liver or kidney disease.

Advise women of childbearing potential to avoid becoming pregnant while receiving treatment with decitabine.

DECITABINE — INJECTION

Advise men not to father a child while receiving treatment with decitabine, and for 2 months afterwards.

DNA TOPOISOMERASE INHIBITORS

IRINOTECAN HYDROCHLORIDE

Rx	**Camptosar** (Pharmacia)	**Injection:** 20 mg/mL	45 mg sorbitol. In 2 and 5 mL vials.

IRINOTECAN HYDROCHLORIDE— INJECTION

WARNING

Administer irinotecan under the supervision of a physician who is experienced in the use of cancer chemotherapeutic agents. Appropriate management of complications is possible only when adequate diagnostic and treatment facilities are readily available.

Irinotecan can induce both early and late forms of diarrhea that appear to be mediated by different mechanisms. Both forms of diarrhea may be severe. Early diarrhea (occurring during or shortly after infusion of irinotecan) may be accompanied by chlolinergic symptoms of rhinitis, increased salivation, miosis, lacrimation, diaphoresis, flushing, and intestinal hyperperistalsis that can cause abdominal cramping. Early diarrhea and other cholinergic symptoms may be prevented or ameliorated by atropine (see Warnings). Late diarrhea (generally occurring more than 24 hours after administration of irinotecan) can be life-threatening because it may be prolonged and may lead to dehydration, electrolyte imbalance, or sepsis. Treat late diarrhea promptly with loperamide. Carefully monitor patients with diarrhea and give fluid and electrolyte replacement if they become dehydrated, or antibiotic therapy if they develop ileus, fever, or severe neutropenia (see Warnings). Interrupt administration of irinotecan and reduce subsequent doses if severe diarrhea occurs (see Administration and Dosage).

Severe myelosuppression may occur (see Warnings).

Indications

➤*Metastatic carcinoma of the colon or rectum:* First-line therapy in combination with 5-fluorouracil (5-FU) and leucovorin for patients with metastatic colon or rectal carcinomas.

It is also indicated for the treatment of metastatic carcinoma of the colon or rectum in patients whose disease has recurred or progressed following initial 5-FU-based therapy.

Administration and Dosage

➤*Approved by the FDA:* June 14, 1996.

➤*Combination agent dosage schedules:*

Irinotecan Dosage Regimens and Dose Modifications[a]

Starting dose and modified dose levels (mg/m²)				
		Starting dose	Dose level 1	Dose level 2
Regimen 1 6-week course with bolus 5-FU/LV (next course begins on day 43)	Irinotecan[b]	125	100	75
	LV[c]	20	20	20
	5-FU[c]	500	400	300
Regimen 2 6-week course with infusional 5-FU/LV (next course begins on day 43)	Irinotecan[d]	180	150	120
	LV[e]	200	200	200
	5-FU bolus[f]	400	320	240
	5-FU infusion[g,h]	600	480	360

[a] Dose reductions beyond dose level 2 by decrements of ≈ 20% may be warranted for patients continuing to experience toxicity. If intolerable toxicity does not develop, treatment with additional courses may be continued indefinitely as long as patients continue to experience clinical benefit.
[b] IV over 90 minutes day 1, 8, 15, 22.
[c] IV bolus day 1, 8, 15, 22.
[d] IV over 90 minutes day 1, 15, 29.
[e] IV over 2 hours day 1, 2, 15, 16, 29, 30.
[f] IV bolus day 1, 2, 15, 16, 29, 30.
[g] Infusion follows bolus administration.
[h] IV over 22 hours day 1, 2, 15, 16, 29, 30.

Do not begin a new course of therapy until the granulocyte count has recovered to greater than or equal to 1500/mm³ and the platelet count has recovered to greater than or equal to 100,000/mm³ and treatment-related diarrhea is fully resolved. Delay treatment 1 to 2 weeks to allow for recovery from treatment-related toxicities. If the patient has not recovered after a 2-week delay, consider discontinuing therapy.

Irinotecan Recommended Dose Modifications

Toxicity NCI CTC grade[a] (value)	During a course of therapy	At the start of subsequent courses of therapy[b]
No toxicity	Maintain dose level	Maintain dose level
Neutropenia		
1 (1500 to 1999/mm³)	Maintain dose level	Maintain dose level
2 (1000 to 1499/mm³)	↓ 1 dose level	Maintain dose level
3 (500 to 999/mm³)	Omit dose until resolved to ≤ grade 2, then ↓ 1 dose level	↓ 1 dose level
4 (< 500/mm³)	Omit dose until resolved to ≤ grade 2, then ↓ 2 dose levels	↓ 2 dose levels
Neutropenic fever	Omit dose until resolved, then ↓ 2 dose levels	
Other hematologic toxicities	Dose modifications for leukopenia or thrombocytopenia during a cycle of therapy and at the start of subsequent cycles of therapy are also based on NCI toxicity criteria and are the same as recommended for neutropenia above.	
Diarrhea		
1 (2 to 3 stools/day pretreatment)	Delay dose until resolved to baseline, then give same dose	Maintain dose level
2 (4 to 6 stools/day pretreatment)	Omit dose until resolved at baseline, then ↓ 1 dose level	Maintain dose level
3 (7 to 9 stools/day pretreatment)	Omit dose until resolved to baseline, then ↓ 1 dose level	↓ 1 dose level
4 (≥ 10 stools/day pretreatment)	Omit dose until resolved to baseline, then ↓ 2 dose levels	↓ 2 dose levels
Other nonhematologic toxicities[c]		
Grade 1 toxicity	Maintain dose level	Maintain dose level
Grade 2 toxicity	Omit dose until resolved to ≤ grade 1, then ↓ 1 dose level	Maintain dose level
Grade 3 toxicity	Omit dose until resolved to ≤ grade 2, then ↓ 1 dose level	↓ 1 dose level
Grade 4 toxicity	Omit dose until resolved to ≤ grade 2, then ↓ 2 dose levels	↓ 2 dose levels
	For mucositis/stomatitis, decrease only 5-FU, not irinotecan	*For mucositis/stomatitis, decrease only 5-FU, not irinotecan*

* ↓ = decrease
[a] National Cancer Institute Common Toxicity Criteria (NCI CTC).
[b] Relative to the starting dose used in the previous course.
[c] Excludes alopecia, anorexia, and asthenia.

➤*Single-agent dosage schedules:*

Irinotecan Regimens and Dose Modifications

	Starting dose and modified dose levels (mg/m²)		
	Starting dose	Dose level 1	Dose level 2
Weekly regimen[a,b,c]	125	100	75
Once every 3-week regimen[c,d,e]	350	300	250

[a] Subsequent doses may be adjusted as high as 150 mg/m² or to as low as 50 mg/m² in 25 to 50 mg/m² decrements depending upon individual patient tolerance.
[b] IV over 90 minutes day 1, 8, 15, 22 then 2-week rest.
[c] If intolerable toxicity does not develop, treatment with additional courses may be continued indefinitely as long as patients continue to experience clinical benefit.
[d] Subsequent doses may be adjusted as low as 200 mg/m² in 50 mg/m² decrements depending upon individual patient tolerance.
[e] IV over 90 minutes once every 3 weeks.

Do not begin a new course of therapy until the granulocyte count has recovered to at least 1500/mm³ and the platelet count has recovered to at least 100,000/mm³ and treatment-related diarrhea is fully resolved. Delay treatment 1 to 2 weeks to allow for recovery from treatment-related toxicities. If the patient has not recovered after a 2-week delay, consider discontinuing irinotecan.

IRINOTECAN HYDROCHLORIDE— INJECTION

Irinotecan Recommended Dose Modifications[a]

Worst toxicity NCI grade[b] (value)	During a course of therapy: Weekly	At the start of the next course of therapy (after adequate recovery) compared with the starting dose in the previous course[a]: Weekly	At the start of the next course: Once every 3 weeks
No toxicity	Maintain dose level	↑ 25 mg/m² up to a maximum dose of 150 mg/m²	Maintain dose level
Neutropenia			
1 (1500 to 1999/mm³)	Maintain dose level	Maintain dose level	Maintain dose level
2 (1000 to 1499/mm³)	↓ 25 mg/m²	Maintain dose level	Maintain dose level
3 (500 to 999/mm³)	Omit dose, then ↓ 25 mg/m² when resolved to ≤ grade 2	↓ 25 mg/m²	↓ 50 mg/m²
4 (< 500/mm³)	Omit dose, then ↓ 50 mg/m² when resolved to ≤ grade 2	↓ 50 mg/m²	↓ 50 mg/m²
Neutropenic fever	Omit dose until resolved, then ↓ 50 mg/m² when resolved	↓ 50 mg/m²	↓ 50 mg/m²
Other hematologic toxicities	Dose modifications for leukopenia, thrombocytopenia, and anemia during a cycle of therapy and at the start of subsequent cycles of therapy are also based on NCI toxicity criteria and are the same as recommended for neutropenia above.		
Diarrhea			
1 (2 to 3 stools/day pretreatment)	Maintain dose level	Maintain dose level	Maintain dose level
2 (4 to 6 stools/day pretreatment)	↓ 25 mg/m²	Maintain dose level	Maintain dose level
3 (7 to 9 stools/day pretreatment)	Omit dose, then ↓ 25 mg/m² when resolved to ≤ grade 2	↓ 25 mg/m²	↓ 50 mg/m²
4 (≥ 10 stools/day pretreatment)	Omit dose, then ↓ 50 mg/m² when resolved to ≤ grade 2	↓ 50 mg/m²	↓ 50 mg/m²
Other nonhematologic toxicities[c]			
Grade 1 toxicity	Maintain dose level	Maintain dose level	Maintain dose level
Grade 2 toxicity	↓ 25 mg/m²	↓ 25 mg/m²	↓ 50 mg/m²
Grade 3 toxicity	Omit dose, then ↓ 25 mg/m² when resolved to ≤ grade 2	↓ 25 mg/m²	↓ 50 mg/m²
Grade 4 toxicity	Omit dose, then ↓ 50 mg/m² when resolved to ≤ grade 2	↓ 50 mg/m²	↓ 50 mg/m²

* ↓ = decrease ↑ = increase
[a] All dose modifications should be based on the worst preceding toxicity.
[b] National Cancer Institute Common Toxicity Criteria (NCI CTC).
[c] Excludes alopecia, anorexia, and asthenia.

Premedicating patients with antiemetic agents is recommended.

➤*Preparation:* Dilute in 5% Dextrose Injection (preferred) or 0.9% Sodium Chloride Injection to a final concentration of 0.12 to 2.8 mg/mL. As with other potentially toxic anticancer agents, exercise care in the handling and preparation of infusion solutions prepared from irinotecan injection. The use of gloves is recommended. If a solution of irinotecan contacts the skin, wash the skin immediately and thoroughly with soap and water. If irinotecan contacts the mucous membranes, flush thoroughly with water. Several published guidelines for handling and disposal of anticancer agents are available.

➤*Storage/Stability:* The solution is physically and chemically stable for up to 24 hours at room temperature (approximately 25°C) and in ambient fluorescent lighting. Solutions diluted in 5% Dextrose Injection, refrigerated (approximately 2° to 8°C; 36° to 46°F), and protected from light are physically and chemically stable for 48 hours. Refrigeration of admixtures using 0.9% Sodium Chloride Injection is not recommended because of a low and sporadic incidence of visible particulates. Freezing irinotecan and admixtures of irinotecan may result in precipitation of the drug and should be avoided. Because of possible microbial contamination during dilution, use the admixture prepared with 5% Dextrose Injection within 24 hours if refrigerated (2° to 8°C; 36° to 46°F). In the case of admixtures prepared with 5% Dextrose Injection or Sodium Chloride Injection, use the solutions within 6 hours if kept at room temperature (15° to 30°C; 59° to 86°F).

Do not add other drugs to the infusion solution. Visually inspect parenteral drug products for particulate matter and discoloration prior to administration whenever solution and container permit.

Store vials at controlled room temperature (15° to 30°C; 59° to 86°F). Protect from light. It is recommended that the vial (and backing/plastic blister remain in the carton until the time of use.

Actions

➤*Pharmacology:* Irinotecan is a derivative of camptothecin. Camptothecins interact specifically with the enzyme topoisomerase I, which relieves torsional strain in DNA by inducing reversible single-strand breaks. Irinotecan and its active metabolite SN-38 bind to the topoisomerase I-DNA complex and prevent religation of these single-strand breaks. Current research suggests that the cytotoxicity of irinotecan is due to double-strand DNA damage produced during DNA synthesis when replication enzymes interact with the ternary complex formed by topoisomerase I, DNA, and either irinotecan or SN-38. Mammalian cells cannot efficiently repair these double-strand breaks.

In vitro cytotoxicity assays show that the potency of SN-38 relative to irinotecan varies from 2- to 2000-fold. Thus, the precise contribution of SN-38 to the activity of irinotecan is unknown.

➤*Pharmacokinetics:*

Absorption/Distribution – Over the dose range of 50 to 350 mg/m², the AUC of irinotecan increases linearly with dose; the AUC of SN-38 increases less than proportionally with dose. Maximum concentrations of the active metabolite SN-38 are generally seen within 1 hour following the end of a 90-minute infusion of irinotecan.

Irinotecan exhibits moderate plasma protein binding (30% to 68%). SN-38 is highly bound to human plasma proteins (approximately 95%). The plasma protein to which irinotecan and SN 38 predominantly binds is albumin.

Metabolism/Excretion – The metabolic conversion of irinotecan to the active metabolite SN-38 is mediated by carboxylesterase enzymes and primarily occurs in the liver. SN-38 subsequently undergoes conjugation to form a glucuronide metabolite. SN-38 glucuronide had 1/50 to 1/100 the activity of SN-38 in cytotoxicity assays using 2 cell lines in vitro. The disposition of irinotecan has not been fully elucidated in humans. The urinary excretion of irinotecan is 11% to 20%; SN-38, less than 1%; and SN-38 glucuronide, 3%. The cumulative biliary and urinary excretion of irinotecan and its metabolites (SN-38 and SN-38 glucuronide) over a period of 48 hours following irinotecan administration in 2 patients ranged from approximately 25% (100 mg/m²) to 50% (300 mg/m²).

Mean Irinotecan and SN-38 Pharmacokinetic Parameters in Patients with Solid Tumors

Dose (mg/m²)	Irinotecan C_{max} (ng/mL)	Irinotecan AUC_{0-24}[a] (ng•h/mL)	Irinotecan t½ (h)	Irinotecan V_Z[b] (L/m²)	Irinotecan CL (L/h/m²)	SN-38 C_{max} (ng/mL)	SN-38 AUC_{0-24} (ng•h/mL)	SN-38 t½ (h)
125 (N = 64)	1660	10,200	5.8[c]	110	13.3	26.3	229	10.4[c]
340 (N = 6)	3392	20,604	11.7[d]	234	13.9	56	474	21[d]

[a] AUC_{0-24} = Area under the plasma concentration-time curve from time 0 to 24 hours after the end of the 90-minute infusion.
[b] V_Z = Volume of distribution of terminal elimination phase.
[c] Plasma specimens collected for 24 hours following the end of the 90-minute infusion.
[d] Plasma specimens collected for 48 hours following the end of the 90-minute infusion. Because of the longer collection period, these values provide a more accurate reflection of the terminal elimination half-lives of irinotecan and SN-38.

Elderly – The terminal half-life of irinotecan was 6 hours in patients who were 65 years of age or older and 5.5 hours in patients younger than 65 years of age. Dose-normalized AUC_{0-24} for SN-38 in patients who were at least 65 years of age was 11% higher than in patients younger than 65 years of age. No change in the starting dose is recommended for geriatric patients receiving the weekly dosage schedule of irinotecan.

Contraindications

Hypersensitivity to irinotecan.

Warnings

➤*Toxic deaths:* Do not use in combination with the Mayo Clinic regimen of 5-FU/LV (administration for 4 to 5 consecutive days every 4 weeks) because of reports of increased toxicity, including toxic deaths. Use irinotecan as recommended.

In patients receiving either irinotecan/5-FU/LV or 5-FU/LV in the clinical trials, higher rates of hospitalization, neutropenic fever, thromboembolism, first-cycle treatment discontinuation, and early deaths were observed in patients with a baseline performance status of 2 than in patients with a baseline performance status of 0 or 1.

➤*Diarrhea:* Irinotecan injection can induce early and late forms of diarrhea that appear to be mediated by different mechanisms. Early diarrhea (occurring during or shortly after irinotecan administration) is cholinergic in nature. It is usually transient and only infrequently severe. It may be accompanied by symptoms of rhinitis, increased salivation, miosis, lacrimation, diaphoresis, flushing, and intestinal hyperperistalsis that can cause abdominal cramping. Early diarrhea may be prevented or ameliorated by atropine.

Late diarrhea (generally occurring more than 24 hours after administration of irinotecan) can be life-threatening because it may be prolonged and may

IRINOTECAN HYDROCHLORIDE— INJECTION

lead to dehydration, electrolyte imbalance, or sepsis. Treat late diarrhea promptly with loperamide. Carefully monitor patients with diarrhea; give fluid and electrolyte replacement if they become dehydrated and antibiotic support if they develop ileus, fever, or severe neutropenia. After the first treatment, delay subsequent weekly chemotherapy treatments in patients until return of pretreatment bowel function for at least 24 hours without need for antidiarrhea medication. If grade 2, 3, or 4 late diarrhea occurs, decrease subsequent doses of irinotecan within the current cycle (see Administration and Dosage).

➤*Irradiation:* Patients who have previously received pelvic/abdominal irradiation are at an increased risk of severe myelosuppression following irinotecan administration. The concurrent administration of irinotecan with irradiation has not been adequately studied and is not recommended.

➤*Neutropenia:* Deaths caused by sepsis following severe neutropenia have been reported in patients treated with irinotecan. Manage neutropenic complications promptly with antibiotic support. Temporarily discontinue therapy during a cycle of therapy if neutropenic fever occurs or if the absolute neutrophil count drops below 1500/mm^3. After the patient recovers to an absolute neutrophil count greater than or equal to 1500/mm^3, reduce subsequent doses of irinotecan depending upon the level of neutropenia observed. Routine administration of a colony-stimulating factor (CSF) is not necessary, but physicians may consider CSF use in patients experiencing significant neutropenia.

➤*Thromboembolism:* Thromboembolic events have been observed in patients receiving irinotecan-containing regimens; the specific cause of these events has not been determined.

➤*Orthostatic hypotension:* Dizziness sometimes may represent symptomatic evidence of orthostatic hypotension in patients with dehydration.

➤*Colitis / Ileus:* Cases of colitis complicated by ulceration, bleeding, ileus, and infection have been observed. Give patients experiencing ileus prompt antibiotic support.

➤*Hypersensitivity reactions:* Hypersensitivity reactions including severe anaphylactic or anaphylactoid reactions have been observed.

➤*Renal function impairment:* Rare cases of renal impairment and acute renal failure have been identified, usually in patients who became volume depleted from severe vomiting or diarrhea.

➤*Elderly:* Closely monitor patients older than 65 years of age because of a greater risk of late diarrhea in this population. The starting dose of irinotecan in patients 70 years of age and older for the once-every-3-week-dosage schedule should be 300 mg/m^2.

➤*Pregnancy: Category D.* Irinotecan may cause fetal harm when administered to a pregnant woman. There are no adequate and well-controlled studies in pregnant women. If the drug is used during pregnancy, or if the patient becomes pregnant while receiving the drug, apprise the patient of the potential hazard to the fetus. Advise women of childbearing potential to avoid becoming pregnant while receiving treatment with irinotecan.

➤*Lactation:* Because many drugs are excreted in breast milk and because of the potential for serious adverse reactions in nursing infants, discontinue nursing when receiving therapy with irinotecan.

➤*Children:* The safety and efficacy of irinotecan in children have not been established.

Precautions

➤*Monitoring:* Monitor the white blood cell count with differential, hemoglobin, and platelet count before each irinotecan dose.

➤*Extravasation:* Irinotecan is administered by IV infusion. Take care to avoid extravasation and monitor the infusion site for signs of inflammation. If extravasation occurs, flush the site with sterile water and apply ice.

➤*Premedication with antiemetics:* Irinotecan is emetogenic. It is recommended that patients receive premedication with antiemetic agents. In clinical studies, the majority of patients received 10 mg dexamethasone given in conjunction with another type of antiemetic agent, such as a 5-HT$_3$ blocker (eg, ondansetron, granisetron). Give antiemetic agents on the day of treatment, starting at least 30 minutes before administration of irinotecan. Consider providing patients with an antiemetic regimen (eg, prochlorperazine) for subsequent use as needed.

➤*Special risk:* In clinical trials of the weekly dosage schedule, it has been noted that patients with modestly elevated baseline serum total bilirubin levels (1 to 2 mg/dL) have had a significantly greater likelihood of experiencing first-course grade 3 or 4 neutropenia than those with bilirubin levels that were less than 1 mg/dL. Patients with abnormal glucuronidation of bilirubin, such as those with Gilbert's syndrome, may also be at greater risk of myelosuppression when receiving therapy with irinotecan. An association between baseline bilirubin elevations and an increased risk of late diarrhea has not been observed in studies of the weekly dosage schedule.

Drug Interactions

Irinotecan Drug Interactions

Precipitant drug	Object drug*		Description
Antineoplastics	Irinotecan	↑	The adverse effects of irinotecan, such as myelosuppression and diarrhea, would be expected to be exacerbated by other antineoplastic agents having similar adverse effects.
Dexamethasone	Irinotecan	↑	Lymphocytopenia has been reported in patients receiving irinotecan, and it is possible that the administration of dexamethasone as antiemetic prophylaxis may have enhanced the likelihood of this effect. Hyperglycemia also has been reported in patients receiving irinotecan. It is probable that dexamethasone given as emetic prophylaxis contributed to hyperglycemia in some patients.
Laxatives	Irinotecan	↑	It would be expected that laxative use during therapy with irinotecan would worsen the incidence or severity of diarrhea, but this has not been studied.
Prochlorperazine	Irinotecan	↑	The incidence of akathisia in clinical trials was greater (8.5%) when prochlorperazine was administered on the same day as irinotecan than when these drugs were given on separate days (1.3%). However, the 8.5% incidence of akathisia is within the range reported for use of prochlorperazine when given as a premedication for other chemotherapeutics.
Irinotecan	Diuretics	↑	In view of the potential risk of dehydration secondary to vomiting and diarrhea induced by irinotecan, the physician may wish to withhold diuretics during dosing with irinotecan and during periods of active vomiting or diarrhea.

* ↑ = Object drug increased.

Adverse Reactions

➤*First-line combination therapy:*

Death – In Study I, 49 patients died within 30 days of study treatment: 21 received irinotecan in combination with 5-FU/LV, 15 received 5-FU/LV alone, and 13 received irinotecan alone. Deaths potentially related to treatment occurred in 2 patients who received irinotecan in combination with 5-FU/LV (2 neutropenic fever/sepsis), 3 patients who received 5-FU/LV alone (1 neutropenic fever/sepsis, 1 CNS bleeding during thrombocytopenia, 1 unknown), and 2 patients who received irinotecan alone (2 neutropenic fever).

Discontinuations because of adverse events were reported for 17 patients who received irinotecan in combination with 5-FU/LV, 14 patients who received 5-FU/LV alone, and 26 patients received irinotecan alone.

Study 1: Patients Experiencing Adverse Reactions in Combination Therapies (%)[a]

	Irinotecan + bolus 5-FU/LV weekly × 4 every 6 wks (N = 225)		Bolus 5-FU/LV daily × 5 every 4 wks (N = 219)		Irinotecan weekly × 4 every 6 wks (N = 223)	
Adverse reaction	Grade 1-4	3 & 4	1-4	3 & 4	1-4	3 & 4
Total adverse reactions	100	53.3	100	45.7	99.6	45.7
Cardiovascular						
Vasodilation	9.3	0.9	5	0	9	0
Hypotension	5.8	1.3	2.3	0.5	5.8	1.7
Thromboembolic events[b]	9.3	-	11.4	-	5.4	-
CNS						
Dizziness	23.1	1.3	16.4	0	21.1	1.8
Somnolence	12.4	1.8	4.6	1.8	9.4	1.3
Confusion	7.1	1.8	4.1	0	2.7	0

IRINOTECAN HYDROCHLORIDE— INJECTION

Study 1: Patients Experiencing Adverse Reactions in Combination Therapies (%)[a]

Adverse reaction	Irinotecan + bolus 5-FU/LV weekly × 4 every 6 wks (N = 225) Grade 1-4	3 & 4	Bolus 5-FU/LV daily × 5 every 4 wks (N = 219) 1-4	3 & 4	Irinotecan weekly × 4 every 6 wks (N = 223) 1-4	3 & 4
Dermatologic						
Exfoliative dermatitis	0.9	0	3.2	0.5	0	0
Rash	19.1	0	26.5	0.9	14.3	0.4
Alopecia[c]	43.1	-	26.5		46.1	
GI						
Diarrhea						
Late	84.9	22.7	69.4	13.2	83	31
grade 3	-	15.1	-	5.9	-	18.4
grade 4	-	7.6	-	7.3	-	12.6
Early	45.8	4.9	31.5	1.4	43	6.7
Nausea	79.1	15.6	67.6	8.2	81.6	16.1
Abdominal pain	63.1	14.6	50.2	11.5	67.7	13
Vomiting	60.4	9.7	46.1	4.1	62.8	12.1
Anorexia	34.2	5.8	42	3.7	43.9	7.2
Constipation	41.3	3.1	31.5	1.8	32.3	0.4
Mucositis	32.4	2.2	76.3	16.9	29.6	2.2
Hematologic						
Neutropenia	96.9	53.8	98.6	66.7	96.4	31.4
grade 3	-	29.8	-	23.7	-	19.3
grade 4	-	24	-	42.5		12.1
Leukopenia	96.9	37.8	98.6	23.3	96.4	21.5
Anemia	96.9	8.4	98.6	5.5	96.9	4.5
Neutropenic fever	-	7.1	-	14.6	-	5.8
Thrombocytopenia	96	2.6	98.6	2.7	96	1.7
Neutropenic infection	-	1.8	-	0	-	2.2
Respiratory						
Dyspnea	27.6	6.3	16	0.5	22	2.2
Cough	26.7	1.3	18.3	0	20.2	0.4
Pneumonia	6.2	2.7	1.4	1	3.6	1.3
Miscellaneous						
Increased bilirubin	87.6	7.1	92.2	8.2	83.9	7.2
Asthenia	70.2	19.5	64.4	11.9	69.1	13.9
Pain	30.7	3.1	26.9	3.6	22.9	2.2
Fever	42.2	1.7	32.4	3.6	43.5	0.4
Infection	22.2	0	16	1.4	13.9	0.4

[a] Severity of adverse events based on NCI CTC.
[b] Includes angina pectoris, arterial thrombosis, cerebral infarct, cerebrovascular accident, deep thrombophlebitis, embolus lower extremity, heart arrest, MI, myocardial ischemia, peripheral vascular disorder, pulmonary embolus, sudden death, thrombophlebitis, thrombosis, vascular disorder.
[c] Complete hair loss = grade 2.

In Study 2, 10 patients died within 30 days of last study treatment: 6 received irinotecan in combination with 5-FU/LV and 4 received 5-FU/LV alone. There was 1 potentially treatment-related death that occurred in a patient who received irinotecan in combination with 5-FU/LV (0.7%, neutropenic sepsis). Deaths from any cause within 60 days of first study treatment were reported for 3 patients who received irinotecan in combination with 5-FU/LV and 2 patients who received 5-FU/LV alone. Discontinuations because of adverse events were reported for 9 patients who received irinotecan in combination with 5-FU/LV and 1 patient who received 5-FU/LV alone.

The most clinically significant adverse events for patients receiving irinotecan-based therapy were diarrhea, nausea, vomiting, neutropenia, and alopecia. In Study I, grade 4 neutropenia, neutropenic fever (defined as grade 2 fever and grade 4 neutropenia), and mucositis were observed less often with weekly irinotecan/5-FU/LV than with monthly administration of 5-FU/LV.

Study 2: Patients Experiencing Clinically Relevant Adverse Reactions in Combination Therapies (%)[a]

Adverse reaction	Irinotecan + 5-FU/LV infusional days 1 and 2 every 2 wks (N = 145) Grade 1-4	3 & 4	5-FU/LV infusional days 1 and 2 every 2 wks (N = 143) 1-4	3 & 4
Total adverse reactions	100	72.4	100	39.2
Cardiovascular				
Hypotension	3.4	1.4	0.7	0
Thromboembolic events[b]	11.7	-	5.6	-
Dermatologic				
Hand and foot syndrome	10.3	0.7	12.6	0.7
Cutaneous signs	17.2	0.7	20.3	0
Alopecia[c]	56.6	-	16.8	-
GI				
Diarrhea				
Late	72.4	14.4	44.8	6.3
grade 3	-	10.3	-	4.2
grade 4	-	4.1	-	2.1
Cholinergic syndrome[d]	28.3	1.4	0.7	0
Nausea	66.9	2.1	55.2	3.5
Abdominal pain	17.2	2.1	16.8	0.7
Vomiting	44.8	3.5	32.2	2.8
Anorexia	35.2	2.1	18.9	0.7
Constipation	30.3	0.7	25.2	1.4
Mucositis	40	4.1	28.7	2.8
Hematologic				
Neutropenia	82.5	46.2	47.9	13.4
grade 3	-	36.4	-	12.7
grade 4	-	9.8	-	0.7
Leukopenia	81.3	17.4	42	3.5
Anemia	97.2	2.1	90.9	2.1
Neutropenic fever	-	3.4	-	0.7
Thrombocytopenia	32.6	0	32.2	0
Neutropenic infection	-	2.1	-	0
Miscellaneous				
Asthenia	57.9	9	48.3	4.2
Dyspnea	9.7	1.4	4.9	0
Fever	22.1	0.7	25.9	0.7
Increased bilirubin	19.1	3.5	35.9	10.6
Infection	35.9	7.6	33.6	3.5
Pain	64.1	9.7	61.5	8.4

[a] Severity of adverse events based on NCI CTC.
[b] Includes angina pectoris, arterial thrombosis, cerebral infarct, cerebrovascular accident, deep thrombophlebitis, embolus lower extremity, heart arrest, MI, myocardial ischemia, peripheral vascular disorder, pulmonary embolus, sudden death, thrombophlebitis, thrombosis, vascular disorder.
[c] Complete hair loss = grade 2.
[d] Includes rhinitis, increased salivation, miosis, lacrimation, diaphoresis, flushing, abdominal cramping or diarrhea (occurring during or shortly after infusion of irinotecan).

➤*Second-line single-agent therapy:*
Weekly dosage schedule:

Adverse Reactions Occurring in > 10% of Previously Treated Irinotecan Patients with Metastatic Carcinoma of the Colon or Rectum (N = 304)[a]

Adverse reaction	% of patients reporting Grade 1-4	Grade 3 & 4
CNS		
Insomnia	19	0
Dizziness	15	0
Dermatologic		
Alopecia	60	na[b]
Sweating	16	0
Rash	13	1
GI		
Diarrhea (late)[c]	88	31
7 to 9 stools/day (grade 3)	-	16
≥ 10 stools/day (grade 4)	-	14
Nausea	86	17
Vomiting	67	12
Anorexia	55	6
Diarrhea (early)[d]	51	8
Constipation	30	2
Flatulence	12	0
Stomatitis	12	1
Dyspepsia	10	0
Hematologic		
Leukopenia	63	28
Anemia	60	7
Neutropenia	54	26
500 to < 1000/mm^3 (grade 3)	-	15
< 500/mm^3 (grade 4)	-	12
Metabolic/Nutritional		
Decreased body weight	30	1
Dehydration	15	4
Increased alkaline phosphatase	13	4

IRINOTECAN HYDROCHLORIDE— INJECTION

Adverse Reactions Occurring in > 10% of Previously Treated Irinotecan Patients with Metastatic Carcinoma of the Colon or Rectum (N = 304)[a]

	% of patients reporting	
Adverse reaction	Grade 1-4	Grade 3 & 4
Increased AST	10	1
Respiratory		
Dyspnea	22	4
Increased coughing	17	0
Rhinitis	16	0
Miscellaneous		
Asthenia	76	12
Abdominal cramping/pain	57	16
Fever	45	1
Pain	24	2
Headache	17	1
Back pain	14	2
Chills	14	0
Minor infections[d]	14	0
Vasodilation (flushing)	11	0
Edema	10	1
Abdominal enlargement	10	0

[a] Severity of adverse events of adverse events based on NCI CTC.
[b] Not applicable: Complete hair loss = NCI grade 2.
[c] Occurring > 24 hours after irinotecan administration.
[d] Occurring ≤ 24 hours after irinotecan administration.
[e] Primarily upper respiratory tract infections.

Once-every-3-week dosage schedule:

Patients Experiencing Grade 3 and 4 Adverse Reactions (%)[a]

	Study 1		Study 2	
Adverse reaction	Irinotecan N = 189	BSC[b] N = 90	Irinotecan N = 127	5-FU N = 129
Total grade 3/4 adverse reactions	79	67	69	54
Cardiovascular[c]	9	3	4	2
CNS[d]	12	13	9	4
Dermatologic				
Hand and foot syndrome	0	0	0	5
Cutaneous signs[e]	2	0	1	3
GI				
Diarrhea	22	6	22	11
Vomiting	14	8	14	5
Nausea	14	3	11	4
Abdominal pain	14	16	9	8
Constipation	10	8	8	6
Anorexia	5	7	6	4
Mucositis	2	1	2	5
Hematologic				
Leukopenia/ Neutropenia	22	0	14	2
Anemia	7	6	6	3
Hemorrhage	5	3	1	3
Thrombocytopenia	1	0	4	2
Infection				
Without grade 3/4 neutropenia	8	3	1	4
With grade 3/4 neutropenia	1	0	2	0
Fever				
Without grade 3/4 neutropenia	2	1	2	0
With grade 3/4 neutropenia	2	0	4	2
Respiratory[f]	10	8	5	7
Other[g]	32	28	12	14

Patients Experiencing Grade 3 and 4 Adverse Reactions (%)[a]

	Study 1		Study 2	
Adverse reaction	Irinotecan N = 189	BSC[b] N = 90	Irinotecan N = 127	5-FU N = 129
Miscellaneous				
Pain	19	22	17	13
Asthenia	15	19	13	12
Hepatic[h]	9	7	9	6

[a] Severity of adverse events based on NCI CTC.
[b] Best supportive care.
[c] Includes events such as dysrhythmias, ischemia, and mechanical cardiac dysfunction.
[d] Includes events such as somnolence.
[e] Includes events such as rash.
[f] Includes events such as dyspnea and cough.
[g] Includes events such as accidental injury, hepatomegaly, syncope, vertigo, and weight loss.
[h] Includes events such as ascites and jaundice.

➤*Cardiovascular:* Flushing may occur during administration. Bradycardia also may occur but has not required intervention. These effects have been attributed to the cholinergic syndrome sometimes observed during or shortly after infusion. Thromboembolic events have been observed in patients receiving irinotecan; the specific cause of these events has not been determined.

➤*Dermatologic:* Alopecia; rash.

➤*Hematologic:* Serious thrombocytopenia was uncommon. Neutropenic fever (concurrent NCI grade 4 neutropenia and fever of grade 2 or greater; 3%); NCI grade 3 or 4 anemia (7%); blood transfusions (10%). The frequency of grade 3 and 4 neutropenia was significantly higher in patients who received previous pelvic/abdominal irradiation than in those who had not received irradiation (48% vs 24%).

➤*Hepatic:* NCI grade 3 or 4 liver enzyme abnormalities (fewer than 10%). These events occurred in patients with known hepatic metastases.

➤*Respiratory:* Severe pulmonary events were infrequent; NCI grade 3 or 4 dyspnea was reported in 4% of patients. Over half of the patients with dyspnea had lung metastases; the extent to which malignant pulmonary involvement or other pre-existing lung disease may have contributed to dyspnea in these patients is unknown.

➤*Postmarketing:* The following events have been identified during postmarketing use of irinotecan in clinical practice. Cases of colitis complicated by ulceration, bleeding, ileus, or infection have been observed. There have been rare cases of renal impairment and acute renal failure, generally in patients who became infected or volume depleted from severe GI toxicities. Hypersensitivity reactions, including severe anaphylactic or anaphylactoid reactions, also have been observed (see Warnings).

Overdosage

Single doses of up to 750 mg/m^2 of irinotecan have been given. The adverse events in these patients were similar to those reported with the recommended dose and regimen. There is no known antidote for overdosage of irinotecan. Institute maximum supportive care to prevent dehydration caused by diarrhea and to treat any infectious complications.

Patient Information

Inform patients and caregivers of the expected toxic effects of irinotecan, particularly of its GI complications, such as nausea, vomiting, abdominal cramping, diarrhea, and infection. Instruct each patient to have loperamide readily available and to begin treatment for late diarrhea (generally occurring more than 24 hours after administration) at the first episode of poorly formed or loose stools or the earliest onset of bowel movements more frequent than normally expected for the patient. One dosage regimen for loperamide used in clinical trials consisted of the following (Note: This dosage regimen exceeds the usual dosage recommendations for loperamide): 4 mg at the first onset of late diarrhea and then 2 mg every 2 hours until the patient is diarrhea-free for at least 12 hours. During the night, the patient may take 4 mg loperamide every 4 hours. Premedication with loperamide is not recommended.

Avoid the use of drugs with laxative properties because of the potential for exacerbation of diarrhea. Advise patients to contact their physician to discuss any laxative use.

Instruct patients to consult their physician if any of the following occur: Diarrhea for the first time during treatment; black or bloody stools; symptoms of dehydration, such as lightheadedness, dizziness, or faintness; inability to take fluids by mouth because of nausea or vomiting; inability to get diarrhea under control within 24 hours; or fever or evidence of infection.

Patients should be alerted to the possibility of alopecia.

TOPOTECAN HYDROCHLORIDE

Rx	**Hycamtin** (GlaxoSmithKline)	**Powder for injection, lyophilized:** 4 mg (as base)	48 mg mannitol. In single-dose vials.

TOPOTECAN HYDROCHLORIDE — INJECTION

WARNING

Administer topotecan for injection under the supervision of a health care provider experienced in the use of cancer chemotherapeutic agents. Appropriate management of complications is possible only when adequate diagnostic and treatment facilities are readily available.

Do not give therapy with topotecan to patients with baseline neutrophil counts of less than 1,500 cells/mm^3. In order to monitor the occurrence of bone-marrow suppression, primarily neutropenia, which may be severe and result in infection and death, perform frequent peripheral blood cell counts on all patients receiving topotecan.

Indications

➤*Cervical cancer (in combination with cisplatin):* For the treatment of stage IV-B, recurrent, or persistent carcinoma of the cervix that is not amenable to curative treatment with surgery and/or radiation therapy.

➤*Ovarian cancer and small cell lung cancer:* For the treatment of the following: metastatic carcinoma of the ovary after failure of initial or subsequent chemotherapy; small cell lung cancer–sensitive disease after failure of first-line chemotherapy. In clinical studies submitted to support approval, sensitive disease was defined as disease responding to chemotherapy but subsequently progressing at least 60 days (in the phase 3 study) or at least 90 days (in the phase 2 studies) after chemotherapy.

➤*Unlabeled uses:* Treatment of non-small cell lung cancer.

Administration and Dosage

➤*Approved by the FDA:* May 28, 1996.

➤*Cervical cancer:* Prior to administration of the first course of topotecan, patients must have a baseline absolute neutrophil count of greater than 1,500 cells/mm^3 and a platelet count of greater than 100,000 cells/mm^3. The recommended dose of topotecan is 0.75 mg/m^2 by intravenous (IV) infusion over 30 minutes daily on days 1, 2, and 3; followed by cisplatin 50 mg/m^2 by IV infusion on day 1 repeated every 21 days (a 21-day course).

Dosage adjustments for subsequent courses of topotecan in combination with cisplatin are specific for each drug.

In the event of severe febrile neutropenia (defined as less than 1,000 cells/mm^3 with temperature of 38°C [100.4°F]), the dose of topotecan should be reduced by 20% to 0.6 mg/m^2 for subsequent courses. Doses of topotecan should be similarly reduced (by 20% to 0.6 mg/m^2) if the platelet count falls below 10,000 cells/mm^3. Alternatively, in the event of severe febrile neutropenia, G-CSF may be administered following the subsequent course (before resorting to dose reduction) starting from day 4 of the course (24 hours after completion of administration of topotecan). If febrile neutropenia occurs despite the use of G-CSF, the dose of topotecan should be reduced by another 20% to 0.45 mg/m^2 for subsequent courses.

See the cisplatin monograph for cisplatin administration and hydration guidelines and for cisplatin dosage adjustment in the event of hematologic toxicity.

➤*Ovarian cancer and small cell lung cancer:* Prior to administration of the first course of topotecan, patients must have a baseline neutrophil count of greater than 1,500 cells/mm^3 and a platelet count of greater than 100,000 cells/mm^3. The recommended dosage of topotecan is 1.5 mg/m^2 by IV infusion over 30 minutes daily for 5 consecutive days, starting on day 1 of a 21-day course. In the absence of tumor progression, a minimum of 4 courses is recommended because tumor response may be delayed. The median time to response in 3 ovarian clinical trials was 9 to 12 weeks, and median time to response in 4 small cell lung cancer trials was 5 to 7 weeks. In the event of severe neutropenia during any course, reduce the dose by 0.25 mg/m^2 (to 1.25 mg/m^2) for subsequent courses. Doses should be similarly reduced if the platelet count falls below 25,000 cells/mm^3. Alternatively, in the event of severe neutropenia, granulocyte colony-stimulating factor (G-CSF) may be administered following the subsequent course (before resorting to dose reduction) starting from day 6 of the course (24 hours after completion of topotecan administration).

➤*Adjustment of dose in special populations:*

Renal function impairment – No dosage adjustment appears to be required for treating patients with mild renal function impairment (creatinine clearance [Ccr] 40 to 60 mL/min). Dosage adjustment to 0.75 mg/m^2 is recommended for patients with moderate renal function impairment (Ccr 20 to 39 mL/min.). Insufficient data are available in patients with severe renal function impairment to provide a dosage recommendation.

Topotecan in combination with cisplatin for the treatment of cervical cancer should only be initiated in patients with serum creatinine less than or equal to 1.5 mg/dL. In the clinical trial, cisplatin was discontinued for a serum creatinine greater than 1.5 mg/dL. Insufficient data are available regarding continuing monotherapy with topotecan after cisplatin discontinuation in patients with cervical cancer.

➤*Preparation for administration:* Topotecan is a cytotoxic anticancer drug. As with other potentially toxic compounds, prepare topotecan under a vertical laminar flow hood while wearing gloves and protective clothing. If topotecan solution contacts the skin, wash the skin immediately and thoroughly with soap and water. If topotecan contacts mucous membranes, flush thoroughly with water.

Preparation for IV administration – Each topotecan 4 mg vial is reconstituted with 4 mL of sterile water for injection. Then the appropriate volume of the reconstituted solution is diluted in either 0.9% sodium chloride IV infusion or 5% dextrose IV infusion prior to administration.

Because the lyophilized dosage form contains no antibacterial preservative, use the reconstituted product immediately.

➤*Storage/Stability:* Unopened vials of topotecan are stable until the date indicated on the package when stored between 20° and 25°C (68° and 77°F) and protected from light in the original package. Because the vials contain no preservative, use the contents immediately after reconstitution.

Reconstituted vials of topotecan diluted for infusion are stable at approximately 20° to 25°C (68° to 77°F) and ambient lighting conditions for 24 hours.

Store the vials protected from light in the original cartons at controlled room temperature between 20° and 25°C (68° and 77°F).

Actions

➤*Pharmacology:* Topoisomerase I relieves torsional strain in DNA by inducing reversible single-strand breaks. Topotecan binds to the topoisomerase I-DNA complex and prevents religation of these single-strand breaks. The cytotoxicity of topotecan is thought to be due to double-strand DNA damage produced during DNA synthesis when replication enzymes interact with the ternary complex formed by topotecan, topoisomerase I and DNA. Mammalian cells cannot efficiently repair these double-strand breaks.

➤*Pharmacokinetics:*

Absorption/Distribution – The pharmacokinetics of topotecan have been evaluated in cancer patients following doses of 0.5 to 1.5 mg/m^2 administered as a 30-minute infusion. Topotecan exhibits multiexponential pharmacokinetics with a terminal half-life of 2 to 3 hours. Total exposure (AUC) is approximately dose-proportional. Binding of topotecan to plasma proteins is approximately 35%.

Metabolism/Excretion – Topotecan undergoes a reversible, pH-dependent hydrolysis of its lactone moiety; it is the lactone form that is pharmacologically active. At pH less than or equal to 4, the lactone is exclusively present, whereas the ring-opened hydroxy-acid form predominates at physiologic pH. In vitro studies in human liver microsomes indicate that metabolism of topotecan to a N-demethylated metabolite represents a minor metabolic pathway.

In humans, about 30% of the dose is excreted in the urine and renal clearance is an important determinant of topotecan elimination.

Special populations –

Renal function impairment: In patients with mild renal impairment (Ccr 40 to 60 mL/min), topotecan plasma clearance was decreased to about 67% of the value in patients with healthy renal function. In patients with moderate renal impairment (Ccr 20 to 39 mL/min), topotecan plasma clearance was reduced to about 34% of the value in control patients, with an increase in half-life. Mean half-life, estimated in 3 renally impaired patients, was about 5 hours. Dosage adjustment is recommended for these patients. No dosage adjustment appears to be required for treating patients with mild renal impairment (Ccr 40 to 60 mL/min). Dosage adjustment to 0.75 mg/m^2 is recommended for patients with moderate renal impairment (Ccr 20 to 39 mL/min.). Insufficient data are available in patients with severe renal impairment to provide a dosage recommendation.

Hepatic function impairment: Plasma clearance in patients with hepatic impairment (serum bilirubin levels between 1.7 and 15 mg/dL) was decreased to about 67% of the value in patients without hepatic impairment. Topotecan half-life increased slightly, from 2 hours to 2.5 hours, but these hepatically impaired patients tolerated the usual recommended topotecan dosage regimen. No dosage adjustment appears to be required for treating patients with impaired hepatic function (plasma bilirubin greater than 1.5 to less than 10 mg/dL).

Elderly: See Warnings for more information.

Gender: The overall mean topotecan plasma clearance in male patients was approximately 24% higher than in female patients, largely reflecting difference in body size.

Contraindications

Topotecan is contraindicated in patients who have a history of hypersensitivity reactions to topotecan or to any of its ingredients. Do not use topotecan in patients who are pregnant or breastfeeding, or in those with severe bone marrow depression.

Warnings

➤*Hematologic:* Bone marrow suppression (primarily neutropenia) is the dose-limiting toxicity of topotecan. Neutropenia is not cumulative over time. The following data on myelosuppression with topotecan are based on the combined experience of 879 patients with metastatic ovarian cancer or small cell lung cancer.

➤*Neutropenia:* Grade 4 neutropenia (less than 500 cells/mm^3) was most common during course 1 of treatment (60% of patients) and occurred in 39% of all courses, with a median duration of 7 days. The nadir neutrophil count occurred at a median of 12 days. Therapy-related sepsis or febrile neutropenia occurred in 23% of patients and sepsis was fatal in 1%.

TOPOTECAN HYDROCHLORIDE — INJECTION

➤*Thrombocytopenia:* Grade 4 thrombocytopenia (less than 25,000/mm^3) occurred in 27% of patients and in 9% of courses, with a median duration of 5 days and platelet nadir at a median of 15 days. Platelet transfusions were given to 15% of patients in 4% of courses.

➤*Anemia:* Grade 3 or 4 anemia (less than 8 g/dL) occurred in 37% of patients and in 14% of courses. Median nadir was at day 15. Transfusions were needed in 52% of patients in 22% of courses.

In ovarian cancer, the overall treatment-related death rate was 1%. In the comparative study in small cell lung cancer, however, the treatment-related death rates were 5% for topotecan and 4% for CAV.

➤*Monitoring of bone marrow function:* Administer topotecan only in patients with adequate bone marrow reserves, including baseline neutrophil count of at least 1,500 cells/mm^3 and platelet count at least 100,000/mm^3. Frequent monitoring of peripheral blood cell counts should be instituted during treatment with topotecan. Patients should not be treated with subsequent courses of topotecan until neutrophils recover to greater than 1,000 cells/mm^3, platelets recover to greater than 100,000 cells/mm^3 and hemoglobin levels recover to 9 g/dL (with transfusion if necessary). Severe myelotoxicity has been reported when topotecan is used in combination with cisplatin. In a reported study on concomitant administration of cisplatin 50 mg/m^2 and topotecan at a dose of 1.25 mg/m^2/day × 5 days, 1 of 3 patients had severe neutropenia for 12 days and a second patient died with neutropenic sepsis. There are no adequate data to define a safe and effective regimen for topotecan and cisplatin in combination.

➤*Carcinogenesis:* Carcinogenicity testing of topotecan has not been performed. Topotecan, however, is known to be genotoxic to mammalian cells and is a probable carcinogen.

➤*Mutagenesis:* Topotecan was mutagenic to L5178Y mouse lymphoma cells and clastogenic to cultured human lymphocytes with and without metabolic activation. It was also clastogenic to mouse bone marrow. Topotecan did not cause mutations in bacterial cells.

➤*Elderly:* Of the 879 patients with metastatic ovarian cancer or small cell lung cancer in clinical studies of topotecan, 32% (n = 281) were 65 years and older, while 3.8% (n = 33) were 75 years of age and older. No overall differences in effectiveness or safety were observed between these patients and younger adult patients. Other reported clinical experience has not identified differences in responses between the elderly and younger adult patients, but greater sensitivity of some older individuals cannot be ruled out.

This drug is known to be substantially excreted by the kidney, and the risk of toxic reactions to this drug may be greater in patients with impaired renal function. Because elderly patients are more likely to have decreased renal function, care should be taken in dose selection, and it may be useful to monitor renal function.

➤*Pregnancy: Category D.* Topotecan may cause fetal harm when administered to a pregnant woman. The effects of topotecan on pregnant women have not been studied. If topotecan is used during a patient's pregnancy, or if a patient becomes pregnant while taking topotecan, warn her of the potential hazard to the fetus. Warn fecund women to avoid becoming pregnant. In rabbits, a dose of 0.1 mg/kg/day (about equal to the clinical dose on a mg/m^2 basis) given on days 6 through 20 of gestation caused maternal toxicity, embryolethality, and reduced fetal body weight. In the rat, a dose of 0.23 mg/kg/day (about equal to the clinical dose on a mg/m^2 basis) given for 14 days before mating through gestation day 6 caused fetal resorption, microphthalmia, preimplant loss, and mild maternal toxicity. A dose of 0.1 mg/kg/day (about half the clinical dose on a mg/m^2 basis) given to rats on days 6 through 17 of gestation caused an increase in postimplantation mortality. This dose also caused an increase in total fetal malformations. The most frequent malformations were of the eye (microphthalmia, anophthalmia, rosette formation of the retina, coloboma of the retina, ectopic orbit), brain (dilated lateral and third ventricles), skull, and vertebrae.

➤*Lactation:* It is not known whether the drug is excreted in human milk. Discontinue breastfeeding in women who are receiving topotecan.

➤*Children:* Safety and efficacy in pediatric patients have not been established.

Precautions

➤*Monitoring:* See Warnings for more information.

➤*Extravasation:* Inadvertent extravasation with topotecan has been associated with mild local reactions such as erythema and bruising.

➤*Hazardous tasks:* As with other chemotherapeutic agents, topotecan may cause asthenia or fatigue; if these symptoms occur, observe caution when driving or operating machinery.

Drug Interactions

Topotecan Drug Interactions

Precipitant drug	Object drug*		Description
Cisplatin	Topotecan	↑	Myelosuppression is more severe when topotecan is given in combination with cisplatin. There are no adequate data to define a safe and effective regimen for topotecan and cisplatin in combination. Coadministration of a platinum agent on day 1 of topotecan dosing required lower doses of each agent compared with coadministration on day 5 of the topotecan dosing schedule. Greater myelosuppression also is likely to be seen when topotecan is used in combination with other cytotoxic agents, thereby necessitating a dose reduction.
Filgrastim (G-CSF)	Topotecan	↑	Coadministration can prolong the duration of neutropenia. If G-CSF is used, do not initiate until day 6 of the course of therapy, 24 hours after completion of treatment with topotecan.

* ↑ = Object drug increased.

Adverse Reactions

Data in the following section are based on the combined experience of 453 patients with metastatic ovarian carcinoma and 426 patients with small cell lung cancer treated with topotecan. The first section lists the principal hematologic toxicities followed by the nonhematologic toxicities occurring in at least 15% of patients.

Summary of Hematologic Adverse Reactions in Patients Receiving Topotecan (%)

Hematologic adverse reactions	Patients (n = 879)	Courses (n = 4,124)
Neutropenia		
< 1,500 cells/mm^3	97%	81%
< 500 cells/mm ^{3}	78%	39%
Leukopenia		
< 3,000 cells/mm^3	97%	80%
< 1,000 cells/mm^3	32%	11%
Thrombocytopenia		
< 75,000/mm^3	69%	42%
< 25,000/mm^3	27%	9%
Anemia		
< 10 g/dL	89%	71%
< 8 g/dL	37%	14%
Sepsis or fever/infection with grade 4 neutropenia	23%	7%
Platelet transfusions	15%	4%
RBC transfusions	52%	22%

Summary on Nonhematologic Adverse Reactions in Patients Receiving Topotecan (%)

Nonhematologic adverse reactions	All grades		Grade 3		Grade 4	
	Patients (n = 879)	Courses (n = 4,124)	Patients (n = 879)	Courses (n = 4,124)	Patients (n = 879)	Courses (n = 4,124)
CNS						
Headache	18%	7%	1%	< 1%	< 1%	0%
Dermatologic						
Alopecia	49%	54%	NA	NA	NA	NA
Rash[b]	16%	6%	1%	< 1%	0%	0%
GI						
Abdominal pain	22%	10%	2%	1%	2%	< 1%
Anorexia	19%	9%	2%	1%	< 1%	< 1%
Constipation	29%	15%	2%	1%	1%	< 1%
Diarrhea	32%	14%	3%	1%	1%	< 1%
Nausea	64%	42%	7%	2%	1%	< 1%
Stomatitis	18%	8%	1%	< 1%	< 1%	< 1%
Vomiting	45%	22%	4%	1%	1%	< 1%

TOPOTECAN HYDROCHLORIDE — INJECTION

Summary on Nonhematologic Adverse Reactions in Patients Receiving Topotecan (%)						
Nonhematologic adverse reactions	All grades		Grade 3		Grade 4	
	Patients (n = 879)	Courses (n = 4,124)	Patients (n = 879)	Courses (n = 4,124)	Patients (n = 879)	Courses (n = 4,124)
Respiratory						
Coughing	15%	7%	1%	< 1%	0%	0%
Dyspnea	22%	11%	5%	2%	3%	1%
Miscellaneous						
Asthenia	25%	13%	4%	1%	2%	< 1%
Fatigue	29%	22%	5%	2%	0%	0%
Fever	28%	11%	1%	< 1%	< 1%	< 1%
Pain[a]	23%	11%	2%	1%	1%	< 1%

[a] Pain includes body pain, back pain and skeletal pain.
[b] Rash also includes pruritus, rash erythematous, urticaria, dermatitis, bullous eruption, and rash maculopapular.

➤*Other adverse reactions in clinical trials:* Premedications were not routinely used in these clinical trials.

CNS – Headache (18% of patients) was the most frequently reported neurologic toxicity. Paresthesia occurred in 7% of patients but was generally grade 1.

Dermatologic – Total alopecia (grade 2) occurred in 31% of patients.

GI – The incidence of nausea was 64% (8% grade 3 or 4) and vomiting occurred in 45% (6% grade 3 or 4) of patients (see the preceding table). The prophylactic use of antiemetics was not routine in patients treated with topotecan. Thirty-two percent (32%) of patients had diarrhea (4% grade 3 or 4), 29% constipation (2% grade 3 or 4) and 22% had abnormal pain (4% grade 3 or 4). Grade 3 or 4 abdominal pain was 6% in ovarian cancer patients and 2% in small cell lung cancer patients.

Hematologic –

Neutropenia: Grade 4 neutropenia (less than 500 cells/mm^3) was most common during course 1 of treatment (60% of patients) and occurred in 39% of all courses, with a median duration of 7 days. The nadir neutrophil count occurred at a median of 12 days. Therapy-related sepsis or febrile neutropenia occurred in 23% of patients and sepsis was fatal in 1%.

Thrombocytopenia: Grade 4 thrombocytopenia (less than 25,000/mm^3) occurred in 27% of patients and in 9% of courses, with a median duration of 5 days and platelet nadir at a median of 15 days. Platelet transfusions were given to 15% of patients in 4% of courses.

Anemia: Grade 3 or 4 anemia (less than 8 g/dL) occurred in 37% of patients and in 14% of courses. Median nadir was at day 15. Transfusions were needed in 52% of patients in 22% of courses.

In ovarian cancer, the overall treatment-related death rate was 1%. In the comparative study in small cell lung cancer, however, the treatment-related death rates were 5% for topotecan and 4% for CAV.

Hepatic – Grade 1 transient elevations in hepatic enzymes occurred in 8% of patients. Greater elevations, grade 3 or 4, occurred in 4%. Grade 3 or 4 elevated bilirubin occurred in less than 2% of patients.

Respiratory – The incidence of grade 3 or 4 dyspnea was 4% in ovarian cancer patients and 12% in small cell lung cancer patients.

➤*Topotecan/paclitaxel comparator trial:* The table below shows the grade 3 or 4 hematologic and major nonhematologic adverse reactions in the topotecan/paclitaxel comparator trial in ovarian cancer.

Comparative Toxicity Profiles for Ovarian Cancer Patients Randomized to Receive Topotecan or Paclitaxel (%)				
	Topotecan		Paclitaxel	
Adverse reaction	Patients (n = 112)	Courses (n = 597)	Patients (n = 114)	Courses (n = 589)
Hematologic grade 3 or 4				
Death related to sepsis	2%	NA	0%	NA
Documented sepsis	5%	1%	2%	< 1%
Fever/grade 4 neutropenia	23%	6%	4%	1%
Grade 3 or 4 anemia (Hgb < 8 g/dL)	41%	16%	6%	2%
Grade 4 neutropenia (< 500 cells/mL)	80%	36%	21%	9%
Grade 4 thrombocytopenia (< 25,000 platelets/mL)	27%	10%	3%	< 1%
Nonhematologic grade 3 or 4 *Constitutional*				
Anorexia	4%	1%	0%	0%
Dyspnea	6%	2%	5%	1%
Fatigue	7%	2%	6%	2%
Malaise	2%	< 1%	2%	< 1%
Dermatologic				
Rash[b]	0%	0%	1%	< 1%
GI				
Abdominal pain	5%	1%	4%	1%
Constipation	5%	1%	0%	0%
Diarrhea	6%	2%	1%	< 1%
Intestinal obstruction	5%	1%	4%	1%
Nausea	10%	3%	2%	< 1%
Stomatitis	1%	< 1%	1%	< 1%
Vomiting	10%	2%	3%	< 1%
Neuromuscular				
Arthralgia	1%	< 1%	3%	< 1%
Asthenia	5%	2%	3%	1%
Chest pain	2%	< 1%	1%	< 1%
Headache	1%	< 1%	2%	1%
Myalgia	0%	0%	3%	2%
Pain[a]	5%	1%	7%	2%
Hepatic				
Increased hepatic enzymes[c]	1%	< 1%	1%	< 1%

[a] Pain includes body pain, skeletal pain and back pain.
[b] Rash also includes pruritus, rash erythematous, urticaria, dermatitis, bullous eruption and rash maculopapular.
[c] Increased hepatic enzymes includes increased AST, increased ALT, and increased hepatic enzymes.

Premedications were not routinely used in patients randomized to topotecan, while patients receiving paclitaxel received routine pretreatment with corticosteroids, diphenhydramine, and histamine receptor type 2 blockers.

➤*Topotecan/CAV comparator trial:* The table below shows the grade 3 or 4 hematologic and major nonhematologic adverse reactions in the topotecan/CAV comparator trial in small cell lung cancer.

Comparative Toxicity Profiles for Small Cell Lung Cancer Patients Randomized to Receive Topotecan or CAV (%)				
	Topotecan		CAV	
Adverse reaction	Patients (n = 107)	Courses (n = 446)	Patients (n = 104)	Courses (n = 359)
Hematologic grade 3 or 4				
Death related to sepsis	3%	NA	1%	NA
Documented sepsis	5%	1%	5%	1%
Fever/grade 4 neutropenia	28%	9%	26%	13%
Grade 3 or 4 anemia (Hgb < 8 g/dL)	42%	18%	20%	7%
Grade 4 neutropenia (< 500 cells/mL)	70%	38%	72%	51%
Grade 4 thrombocytopenia (< 25,000 platelets/mL)	29%	10%	5%	1%
Nonhematologic grade 3 or 4 *Constitutional*				
Anorexia	3%	1%	4%	2%
Dyspnea	9%	5%	14%	7%
Fatigue	6%	4%	10%	3%
Dermatologic				
Rash[b]	1%	< 1%	1%	< 1%
GI				
Abdominal pain	6%	1%	4%	2%
Constipation	1%	< 1%	0%	0%
Diarrhea	1%	< 1%	0%	0%
Nausea	8%	2%	6%	2%
Stomatitis	2%	< 1%	1%	< 1%
Vomiting	3%	< 1%	3%	1%
Hepatic				
Increased hepatic enzymes[c]	1%	< 1%	0%	0%
Neuromuscular				
Asthenia	9%	4%	7%	2%
Headache	0%	0%	2%	< 1%
Pain[a]	5%	2%	7%	4%

TOPOTECAN HYDROCHLORIDE — INJECTION

Comparative Toxicity Profiles for Small Cell Lung Cancer Patients Randomized to Receive Topotecan or CAV (%)				
	Topotecan		CAV	
Adverse reaction	Patients (n = 107)	Courses (n = 446)	Patients (n = 104)	Courses (n = 359)
Respiratory				
Coughing	2%	1%	0%	0%
Pneumonia	8%	2%	6%	2%

[a] Pain includes body pain, skeletal pain, and back pain.
[b] Rash also includes pruritus, rash erythematous, urticaria, dermatitis, bullous eruption, and rash maculopapular.
[c] Increased hepatic enzymes includes increased AST, increased ALT, and increased hepatic enzymes.

Premedications were not routinely used in patients randomized to topotecan, while patients receiving CAV received routine pretreatment with corticosteroids, diphenhydramine, and histamine receptor type 2 blockers.

➤*Postmarketing reports of adverse reactions:* Reports of adverse reactions in patients taking topotecan received after market introduction, which are not listed above, include the following:

Dermatologic –
Rare: Severe dermatitis, severe pruritus.

Hematologic – Severe bleeding (in association with thrombocytopenia).

Miscellaneous –
Infrequent: Allergic manifestations.
Rare: Anaphylactoid reactions, angioedema.

Overdosage

➤*Symptoms:* The primary anticipated complication of overdosage would consist of bone marrow suppression.

One patient on a single-dose regimen of 17.5 mg/m^2 given on day 1 of a 21-day cycle had received a single dose of 35 mg/m^2. This patient experienced severe neutropenia (nadir of 320/mm^3) 14 days later but recovered without incident.

The LD_{10} in mice receiving single IV infusions of topotecan was 75 mg/m^2 (95% CI: 47 to 97).

➤*Treatment:* There is no known antidote for overdosage with topotecan.

Patient Information

As with other chemotherapeutic agents, topotecan may cause asthenia or fatigue; if these symptoms occur, observe caution when driving or operating machinery.

BIOLOGICAL RESPONSE MODIFIERS

ALDESLEUKIN (Interleukin-2; IL-2)

Rx	**Proleukin** (Chiron)	**Powder for injection, lyophilized:** 22 x 10^6 IU/vial (18 million IU [1.1 mg] per mL when reconstituted)	Preservative-free. In single-use vials.[a]

[a] With 50 mg mannitol, 0.18 mg sodium dodecyl sulfate, and 0.17 mg monobasic and 0.89 mg dibasic sodium phosphate.

ALDESLEUKIN — INJECTION

WARNING

Restrict therapy with aldesleukin for injection to patients with normal cardiac and pulmonary functions as defined by thallium stress testing and formal pulmonary function testing. Use extreme caution in patients with a normal thallium stress test and a normal pulmonary function test who have a history of cardiac or pulmonary disease.

Administer aldesleukin in a hospital setting under the supervision of a qualified physician experienced in the use of anticancer agents. An intensive care facility and specialists skilled in cardiopulmonary or intensive care medicine must be available.

Aldesleukin administration has been associated with capillary leak syndrome (CLS) which is characterized by a loss of vascular tone and extravasation of plasma proteins and fluid into the extravascular space. CLS results in hypotension and reduced organ perfusion which may be severe and can result in death. CLS may be associated with cardiac arrhythmias (supraventricular and ventricular), angina, myocardial infarction, respiratory insufficiency requiring intubation, gastrointestinal bleeding or infarction, renal insufficiency, edema, and mental status changes.

Aldesleukin treatment is associated with impaired neutrophil function (reduced chemotaxis) and with an increased risk of disseminated infection, including sepsis and bacterial endocarditis. Consequently, preexisting bacterial infections should be adequately treated prior to initiation of aldesleukin therapy. Patients with indwelling central lines are particularly at risk for infection with gram-positive microorganisms. Antibiotic prophylaxis with oxacillin, nafcillin, ciprofloxacin, or vancomycin has been associated with a reduced incidence of staphylococcal infections.

Withhold aldesleukin administration in patients developing moderate to severe lethargy or somnolence; continued administration may result in coma.

Indications

➤*Metastatic renal cell carcinoma:* For the treatment of adults with metastatic renal cell carcinoma (metastatic RCC).

➤*Metastatic melanoma:* For the treatment of adults with metastatic melanoma.

➤*Patient selection:* Careful patient selection is mandatory prior to the administration of aldesleukin.

Evaluation of clinical studies to date reveals that patients with more favorable ECOG performance status (ECOG PS 0) at treatment initiation respond better to aldesleukin, with a higher response rate and lower toxicity. Therefore, selection of patients for treatment should include assessment of performance status.

Experience in patients with ECOG PS greater than 1 is extremely limited.

➤*Unlabeled uses:* May be beneficial when used in combination with highly active antiretroviral therapy (HAART) in the treatment of HIV patients; in combination for treatment of cutaneous T-cell lymphoma; treatment of colorectal cancer, non-Hodgkin lymphoma, acute myelogenous leukemia (AML), after autologous bone marrow transplantation (ABMT).

Administration and Dosage

➤*Approved by the FDA:* May 5, 1992.

The recommended aldesleukin for injection treatment regimen is administered by a 15-minute IV infusion every 8 hours. Before initiating treatment, carefully review the entire monograph, particularly regarding patient selection, possible serious adverse events, patient monitoring, and withholding dosage. The following schedule has been used to treat adult patients with metastatic renal cell carcinoma (metastatic RCC) or metastatic melanoma. Each course of treatment consists of two 5-day treatment cycles separated by a rest period.

600,000 units/kg (0.037 mg/kg) dose administered every 8 hours by a 15-minute IV infusion for a maximum of 14 doses. Following 9 days of rest, the schedule is repeated for another 14 doses, for a maximum of 28 doses per course, as tolerated. During clinical trials, doses were frequently withheld for toxicity. Metastatic RCC patients treated with this schedule received a median of 20 of the 28 doses during the first course of therapy. Metastatic melanoma patients received a median of 18 doses during the first course of therapy.

➤*Retreatment:* Evaluate patients for response approximately 4 weeks after completion of a course of therapy and again immediately prior to the scheduled start of the next treatment course. Give additional courses of treatment to patients only if there is some tumor shrinkage following the last course and retreatment is not contraindicated. Separate each treatment course by a rest period of at least 7 weeks from the date of hospital discharge.

➤*Dose modifications:* Accomplish dose modification for toxicity by withholding or interrupting a dose rather than reducing the dose to be given. Decisions to stop, hold, or restart aldesleukin therapy must be made after a global assessment of the patient. With this in mind, use the following guidelines.

Hold doses and restart according to the following table:

Body system	Hold dose for	Subsequent doses may be given if
Cardiovascular	Atrial fibrillation, supraventricular tachycardia, or bradycardia that requires treatment or is recurrent or persistent.	Patient is asymptomatic with full recovery to normal sinus rhythm.
	Systolic BP < 90 mm Hg with increasing requirements for pressors.	Systolic BP is ≥ 90 mm Hg and stable or improving requirements for pressors.
	Any ECG change consistent with MI, ischemia, or myocarditis with or without chest pain or suspicion of cardiac ischemia.	Patient is asymptomatic, MI and myocarditis have been ruled out, clinical suspicion of angina is low, and there is no evidence of ventricular hypokinesia.
CNS	Mental status changes, including moderate confusion or agitation.	Mental status changes completely resolved.

ALDESLEUKIN — INJECTION

Body system	Hold dose for	Subsequent doses may be given if
Dermatologic	Bullous dermatitis or marked worsening of preexisting skin condition, avoid topical steroid therapy.	Resolution of all signs of bullous dermatitis occurs.
GI	Signs of hepatic failure including encephalopathy, increasing ascites, liver pain, and hypoglycemia.	All signs of hepatic failure have resolved.[a]
	Stool guaiac repeatedly > 3 to 4+.	Stool guaiac negative.
GU	Serum creatinine > 4.5 mg/dL or a serum creatinine of ≥ 4 mg/dL in the presence of severe volume overload, acidosis, or hyperkalemia.	Serum creatinine is < 4 mg/dL and fluid and electrolyte status is stable.
	Persistent oliguria, urine output of < 10 mL/hr for 16 to 24 hours with rising serum creatinine.	Urine output is > 10 mL/hr with a decrease of serum creatinine of > 1.5 mg/dL or normalization of serum creatinine.
Respiratory	O_2 saturation < 90%	O_2 saturation > 90%
Miscellaneous	Sepsis syndrome, patient is clinically unstable.	Sepsis syndrome has resolved, patient is clinically stable, infection is under treatment.

[a] Discontinue all further treatment for that course. Initiate a new course of treatment, if warranted, no sooner than 7 weeks after cessation of adverse event and hospital discharge.

➤*Reconstitution and dilution directions:* Reconstitution and dilution procedures other than those recommended may alter the delivery or pharmacology of aldesleukin, and thus should be avoided.

1.) Aldesleukin is a sterile, white to off-white, preservative-free, lyophilized powder suitable for IV infusion upon reconstitution and dilution. Each vial contains 22 million units (1.3 mg) of aldesleukin and should be reconstituted aseptically with 1.2 mL of Sterile Water for Injection. When reconstituted as directed, each mL contains 18 million units (1.1 mg) of aldesleukin. The resulting solution should be a clear, colorless to slightly yellow liquid. The vial is for single use only. Discard any unused portion.
2.) During reconstitution, direct the Sterile Water for Injection at the side of the vial and gently swirl the contents to avoid excess foaming. Do not shake.
3.) The dose of aldesleukin, reconstituted with Sterile Water for Injection (without preservative) should be diluted aseptically in 50 mL of 5% Dextrose Injection (D5W) and infused over a 15-minute period. In cases where the total dose of aldesleukin is 1.5 mg or less (eg, a patient with a body weight of less than 40 kg), dilute the dose of aldesleukin in a smaller volume of D5W. Concentrations of aldesleukin below 30 mcg/mL and above 70 mcg/mL have shown increased variability in drug delivery. Avoid dilution and delivery of aldesleukin outside of this concentration range.
4.) Glass bottles and plastic (polyvinyl chloride) bags have been used in clinical trials with comparable results. It is recommended that plastic bags be used as the dilution container since experimental studies suggest that use of plastic containers results in more consistent drug delivery. Do not use in-line filters when administering aldesleukin.
5.) Before and after reconstitution and dilution, store in a refrigerator at 2° to 8°C (36° to 46°F). Do not freeze. Administer aldesleukin within 48 hours of reconstitution. Bring the solution to room temperature prior to infusion in the patient.
6.) Avoid reconstitution or dilution with Bacteriostatic Water for Injection or 0.9% sodium chloride injection because of increased aggregation. Do not coadminister aldesleukin with other drugs in the same container.
7.) Visually inspect parenteral drugs products for particulate matter and discoloration prior to administration, whenever solution and container permit.

➤*Storage/Stability:* Store vials of lyophilized aldesleukin in a refrigerator at 2° to 8°C (36° to 46°F). Protect from light. Store in carton until time of use.

Reconstituted or diluted aldesleukin is stable for up to 48 hours at refrigerated and room temperatures, 2° to 25°C (36° to 77°F). However, since this product contains no preservative, store the reconstituted and diluted solutions in the refrigerator.

Actions

➤*Pharmacology:* Aldesleukin has been shown to possess the biological activities of human native interleukin-2. In vitro studies performed on human cell lines demonstrate the immunoregulatory properties of aldesleukin, including:

1.) Enhancement of lymphocyte mitogenesis and stimulation of long-term growth of human interleukin-2 dependent cell lines.
2.) Enhancement of lymphocyte cytotoxicity.
3.) Induction of killer cell (lymphokine-activated [LAK] and natural [NK]) activity.
4.) Induction of interferon-gamma production.

The in vivo administration of aldesleukin in animals and humans produces multiple immunological effects in a dose-dependent manner. These effects include activation of cellular immunity with profound lymphocytosis, eosinophilia, and thrombocytopenia, and the production of cytokines including tumor necrosis factor, IL-1, and gamma interferon. In vivo experiments in murine tumor models have shown inhibition of tumor growth. The exact mechanism by which aldesleukin mediates its antitumor activity in animals and humans is unknown.

➤*Pharmacokinetics:*

Absorption/Distribution – Aldesleukin exists as biologically active, noncovalently bound microaggregates with an average size of 27 recombinant interleukin-2 molecules. The solubilizing agent, sodium dodecyl sulfate, may have an effect on the kinetic properties of this product.

The pharmacokinetic profile of aldesleukin is characterized by high plasma concentrations following a short IV infusion, rapid distribution into the extravascular space and elimination from the body by metabolism in the kidneys with little or no bioactive protein excreted in the urine. Studies of IV aldesleukin in sheep and humans indicate that upon completion of infusion, approximately 30% of the administered dose is detectable in plasma. This finding is consistent with studies in rats using radiolabeled aldesleukin, which demonstrate a rapid (less than 1 minute) uptake of the majority of the label into the lungs, liver, kidney, and spleen.

The serum half-life ($t_{½}$) curves of aldesleukin remaining in the plasma are derived from studies done in 52 cancer patients following a 5-minute IV infusion. These patients were shown to have a distribution and elimination $t_{½}$ of 13 and 85 minutes, respectively.

Metabolism/Excretion – Following the initial rapid organ distribution, the primary route of clearance of circulating aldesleukin is the kidney. In humans and animals, aldesleukin is cleared from the circulation by both glomerular filtration and peritubular extraction in the kidney. This dual mechanism for delivery of aldesleukin to the proximal tubule may account for the preservation of clearance in patients with rising serum creatinine values. Greater than 80% of the amount of aldesleukin distributed to plasma, cleared from the circulation and presented to the kidney is metabolized to amino acids in the cells lining the proximal convoluted tubules. In humans, the mean clearance rate in cancer patients is 268 mL/min.

The relatively rapid clearance of aldesleukin has led to dosage schedules characterized by frequent, short infusions. Observed serum levels are proportional to the dose of aldesleukin.

Immunogenicity – 57 of 77 (74%) metastatic renal cell carcinoma patients treated with an every 8-hour aldesleukin regimen and 33 of 50 (66%) metastatic melanoma patients treated with a variety of IV regimens developed low titers of nonneutralizing antialdesleukin antibodies. Neutralizing antibodies were not detected in this group of patients, but have been detected in 1 of 106 (less than 1%) patients treated with IV aldesleukin using a wide variety of schedules and doses. The clinical significance of antialdesleukin antibodies is unknown.

Contraindications

History of hypersensitivity to interleukin-2 or any component of the aldesleukin formulation; abnormal thallium stress test or abnormal pulmonary function tests; organ allografts. Retreatment with aldesleukin is contraindicated in patients who have experienced the following drug-related toxicities while receiving an earlier course of therapy: sustained ventricular tachycardia (greater than or equal to 5 beats); cardiac arrhythmias not controlled or unresponsive to management; chest pain with ECG changes, consistent with angina or myocardial infarction; cardiac tamponade; intubation for greater than 72 hours; renal failure requiring dialysis greater than 72 hours; coma or toxic psychosis lasting greater than 48 hours; repetitive or difficult to control seizures; bowel ischemia/perforation; GI bleeding requiring surgery.

Warnings

➤*Severe adverse events:* Because of the severe adverse events which generally accompany aldesleukin therapy at the recommended dosages, perform thorough clinical evaluation to identify patients with significant cardiac, pulmonary, renal, hepatic, or CNS impairment in whom aldesleukin is contraindicated. Patients with normal cardiovascular, pulmonary, hepatic, and CNS function may experience serious, life-threatening, or fatal adverse events. Adverse events are frequent, often serious, and sometimes fatal.

Should adverse events, which require dose modification occur, withhold dosage rather than reduce it.

➤*Exacerbation of pre-existing diseases:* Aldesleukin has been associated with exacerbation of preexisting or initial presentation of autoimmune disease and inflammatory disorders. Exacerbation of Crohn's disease, scleroderma, thyroiditis, inflammatory arthritis, diabetes mellitus, oculobulbar myasthenia gravis, crescentic IgA glomerulonephritis, cholecystitis, cerebral vasculitis, Stevens-Johnson syndrome, and bullous pemphigoid has been reported following treatment with IL-2.

All patients should have thorough evaluation and treatment of CNS metastases and have a negative scan prior to receiving aldesleukin therapy. New neurologic signs, symptoms, and anatomic lesions following aldesleukin therapy have been reported in patients without evidence of CNS metastases. Clinical manifestations included changes in mental status, speech difficulties, cortical blindness, limb or gait ataxia, hallucinations, agitation, obtundation, and coma. Radiological findings included multiple and, less

ALDESLEUKIN — INJECTION

commonly, single cortical lesions on MRI and evidence of demyelination. Neurologic signs and symptoms associated with aldesleukin therapy usually improve after discontinuation of aldesleukin therapy; however, there are reports of permanent neurologic defects. One case of possible cerebral vasculitis, responsive to dexamethasone, has been reported. In patients with known seizure disorders, exercise extreme caution as aldesleukin may cause seizures.

➤*Hypersensitivity reactions:* Hypersensitivity reactions have been reported in patients receiving combination regimens containing sequential high-dose aldesleukin and antineoplastic agents, specifically, dacarbazine, cis-platinum, tamoxifen, and interferon-alfa. These reactions consisted of erythema, pruritus, and hypotension and occurred within hours of administration of chemotherapy. These events required medical intervention in some patients.

➤*Renal/Hepatic function impairment:* Kidney and liver function are impaired during aldesleukin treatment. Use of concomitant nephrotoxic or hepatotoxic medications may further increase toxicity to the kidney or liver. Serum creatinine should be less than or equal to 1.5 mg/dL prior to initiation of aldesleukin treatment.

➤*Fertility impairment:* There have been no studies conducted assessing the effect of aldesleukin on fertility. It is recommended that this drug not be administered to fertile persons of either gender not practicing effective contraception.

➤*Elderly:* Aldesleukin is known to be substantially excreted by the kidney, and the risk of toxic reactions to this drug may be greater in patients with impaired renal function. The pattern of organ system toxicity and the proportion of patients with severe toxicities by organ system were generally similar in patients 65 and older and younger patients. There was a trend, however, towards an increased incidence of severe urogenital toxicities and dyspnea in the older patients.

➤*Pregnancy: Category C.* Aldesleukin has been shown to have embryolethal effects in rats when given in doses at 27 to 36 times the human dose (scaled by body weight). Significant maternal toxicities were observed in pregnant rats administered aldesleukin by IV injection at doses 2.1 to 36 times higher than the human dose during critical period of organogenesis. No evidence of teratogenicity was observed other than that attributed to maternal toxicity. There are no adequate well-controlled studies of aldesleukin in pregnant women. Use aldesleukin during pregnancy only if the potential benefit justifies the potential risk to the fetus.

➤*Lactation:* It is not known whether this drug is excreted in human milk. Because many drugs are excreted in human milk and because of the potential for serious adverse reactions in nursing infants from aldesleukin, a decision should be made whether to discontinue nursing or to discontinue the drug, taking into account the importance of the drug to the mother.

➤*Children:* Safety and effectiveness in children younger than 18 years of age have not been established.

Precautions

➤*Monitoring:* Daily monitoring during therapy with aldesleukin should include vital signs (temperature, pulse, blood pressure, and respiration rate), weight, and fluid intake and output. In a patient with a decreased systolic blood pressure, especially less than 90 mm Hg, conduct constant cardiac rhythm monitoring. If an abnormal complex or rhythm is seen, perform an ECG. Take vital signs in these hypotensive patients hourly.

The following clinical evaluations are recommended for all patients, prior to beginning treatment and then daily during drug administration: standard hematologic tests, including CBC, differential and platelet counts; blood chemistries, including electrolytes, renal and hepatic function tests; chest x-rays.

➤*Capillary leak syndrome (CLS):* Patients should have normal cardiac, pulmonary, hepatic, and CNS function at the start of therapy. CLS begins immediately after aldesleukin treatment starts and is marked by increased capillary permeability to protein and fluids and reduced vascular tone. In most patients, this results in a concomitant drop in mean arterial blood pressure within 2 to 12 hours after the start of treatment. With continued therapy, clinically significant hypotension (defined as systolic blood pressure below 90 mm Hg or a 20 mm Hg drop from baseline systolic pressure) and hypoperfusion will occur. In addition, extravasation of protein and fluids into the extravascular space will lead to the formation of edema and creation of new effusions.

Medical management of CLS begins with careful monitoring of the patient's fluid and organ perfusion status. This is achieved by frequent determination of blood pressure and pulse, and by monitoring organ function, which includes assessment of mental status and urine output. Hypovolemia is assessed by catheterization and central pressure monitoring.

Fluid status – Flexibility in fluid and pressor management is essential for maintaining organ perfusion and blood pressure. Consequently, use extreme caution in treating patients with fixed requirements for large volumes of fluid (eg, patients with hypercalcemia). Administration of IV fluids, either colloids or crystalloids is recommended for treatment of hypovolemia. Correction of hypovolemia may require large volumes of IV fluids but caution is required because unrestrained fluid administration may exacerbate problems associated with edema formation or effusions. With extravascular fluid accumulation, edema is common and ascites, pleural or pericardial effusions may develop. Management of these events depends on a careful balancing of the effects of fluid shifts so that neither the consequences of hypovolemia (eg, impaired organ perfusion) nor the consequences of fluid accumulations (eg, pulmonary edema) exceed the patient's tolerance.

Dopamine – Clinical experience has shown that early administration of dopamine (1 to 5 mcg/kg/min) to patients manifesting capillary leak syndrome, before the onset of hypotension, can help to maintain organ perfusion particularly to the kidney and thus preserve urine output. Carefully monitor weight and urine output. If organ perfusion and blood pressure are not sustained by dopamine therapy, clinical investigators have increased the dose of dopamine to 6 to 10 mcg/kg/min or have added phenylephrine hydrochloride (1 to 5 mcg/kg/min) to low-dose dopamine. Prolonged use of pressors, either in combination or as individual agents, at relatively high doses, may be associated with cardiac rhythm disturbances. If there has been excessive weight gain or edema formation, particularly if associated with shortness of breath from pulmonary congestion, use of diuretics, once blood pressure has normalized, has been shown to hasten recovery. Note: Prior to the use of any product mentioned, the physician should refer to the package insert for the respective product.

Withhold aldesleukin treatment for failure to maintain organ perfusion as demonstrated by altered mental status, reduced urine output, a fall in the systolic blood pressure below 90 mm Hg, or onset of cardiac arrhythmias. Recovery from CLS begins soon after cessation of aldesleukin therapy. Usually, within a few hours, the blood pressure rises, organ perfusion is restored and reabsorption of extravasated fluid and protein begins.

CNS toxicity – Mental status changes including irritability, confusion, or depression which occur while receiving aldesleukin may be indicators of bacteremia or early bacterial sepsis, hypoperfusion, occult CNS malignancy, or direct aldesleukin-induced CNS toxicity. Alterations in mental status due solely to aldesleukin therapy may progress for several days before recovery begins. Rarely, patients have sustained permanent neurologic deficits.

Exacerbation of pre-existing diseases – Exacerbation of preexisting autoimmune disease or initial presentation of autoimmune and inflammatory disorders has been reported following aldesleukin alone or in combination with interferon. Hypothyroidism, sometimes preceded by hyperthyroidism, has been reported following aldesleukin treatment. Some of these patients required thyroid replacement therapy. Changes in thyroid function may be a manifestation of autoimmunity. Onset of symptomatic hyperglycemia or diabetes mellitus has been reported during aldesleukin therapy.

Transplant patients – Aldesleukin enhancement of cellular immune function may increase the risk of allograft rejection in transplant patients.

Pulmonary – All patients should have baseline pulmonary function tests with arterial blood gases. Document adequate pulmonary function (FEV_1 greater than 2 L or greater than or equal to 75% of predicted for height and age) prior to initiating therapy.

During treatment, monitor pulmonary function on a regular basis by clinical examination, assessment of vital signs, and pulse oximetry. Further assess patients with dyspnea or clinical signs of respiratory impairment (tachypnea or rales) with arterial blood gas determination. Repeat these tests as often as clinically indicated.

Stress thallium study – Screen all patients with a stress thallium study. Document normal ejection fraction and unimpaired wall motion. If a thallium stress test suggests minor wall motion abnormalities, further testing is suggested to exclude significant coronary artery disease.

Cardiac – Assess cardiac function daily by clinical examination and assessment of vital signs. Further assess patients with signs or symptoms of chest pain, murmurs, gallops, irregular rhythm or palpitations with an ECG examination and cardiac enzyme evaluation. Evidence of myocardial injury, including findings compatible with myocardial infarction or myocarditis, has been reported. Ventricular hypokinesia due to myocarditis may be persistent for several months. If there is evidence of cardiac ischemia or congestive heart failure, hold aldesleukin therapy, and perform a repeat thallium study.

Drug Interactions

➤*Current chemotherapy:* Hypersensitivity reactions have been reported in patients receiving combination regimens containing sequential high-dose aldesleukin and antineoplastic agents, specifically, dacarbazine, cisplatinum, tamoxifen and interferon-alfa. These reactions consisted of erythema, pruritus, and hypotension and occurred within hours of administration of chemotherapy. These events required medical intervention in some patients.

➤*Interferon-alfa:* Myocardial injury, including myocardial infarction, myocarditis, ventricular hypokinesia, and severe rhabdomyolysis appear to be increased in patients receiving aldesleukin and interferon-alfa concurrently.

Exacerbation or the initial presentation of a number of autoimmune and inflammatory disorders has been observed following concurrent use of interferon-alfa and aldesleukin, including crescentic IgA glomerulonephritis, oculo-bulbar myasthenia gravis, inflammatory arthritis, thyroiditis, bullous pemphigoid, and Stevens-Johnson syndrome.

➤*Iodinated contrast media:* A review of the literature revealed that 12.6% (range 11% to 28%) of 501 patients treated with various interleukin-2 containing regimens who were subsequently administered radiographic iodinated contrast media experienced acute, atypical adverse reactions. The onset of symptoms usually occurred within hours (most commonly 1 to 4 hours) following the administration of contrast media. These reactions include fever, chills, nausea, vomiting, pruritus, rash, diarrhea, hypotension, edema, and oliguria. Some clinicians have noted that these reactions resemble the immediate side effects caused by interleukin-2 administration; however, the cause of contrast reactions after interleukin-2 therapy is unknown. Most events were reported to occur when contrast media was

ALDESLEUKIN — INJECTION

given within 4 weeks after the last dose of interleukin-2. These events were also reported to occur when contrast media was given several months after interleukin-2 treatment.

Aldesleukin Drug Interactions

Precipitant drug	Object drug*		Description
Antihypertensives	Aldesleukin	↑	Antihypertensives may potentiate the hypotension seen with aldesleukin.
Corticosteroids	Aldesleukin	↓	Although glucocorticoids reduce the side effects of aldesleukin, coadministration may reduce the antitumor effectiveness of aldesleukin; avoid concurrent use.
Cardiotoxic agents (eg, doxorubicin)	Aldesleukin	↑	Increased toxicity in these organ systems may occur during coadministration.
Hepatotoxic agents (eg, methotrexate, asparaginase)			
Myelotoxic agents (eg, cytotoxic chemotherapy)			
Nephrotoxic agents (eg, aminoglycosides, indomethacin)			
Aldesleukin	Protease inhibitors (eg, indinavir)	↑	Protease concentrations may be elevated, increasing risk of toxicity. May need to adjust the dose of indinavir when aldesleukin is initiated or stopped.
Aldesleukin	Psychotropic agents (eg, narcotics, analgesics, sedatives, antiemetics, tranquilizers)	↔	Aldesleukin may affect CNS function. Therefore, interactions could occur following coadministration of these agents.

* ↑ = Object drug increased. ↓ = Object drug decreased.
↔ = Undetermined clinical effect.

Adverse Reactions

The rate of drug-related deaths in the 255 metastatic RCC patients who received single-agent aldesleukin was 4% (11 of 255); the rate of drug-related deaths in the 270 metastatic melanoma patients who received single-agent aldesleukin was 2% (6 of 270).

Adverse Events Occurring in Patients Treated with Aldesleukin (≥ 10%)

Body system/Adverse reactions	Patients (n = 525)
Cardiovascular	
Arrhythmia	10%
Cardiovascular disorder[a]	11%
Hypotension	71%
Supraventricular tachycardia	12%
Tachycardia	23%
Vasodilation	13%
CNS	
Anxiety	12%
Confusion	34%
Dizziness	11%
Somnolence	22%
Dermatologic	
Exfoliative dermatitis	18%
Pruritus	24%
Rash	42%
GI	
Anorexia	20%
Diarrhea	67%
Nausea	35%
Nausea and vomiting	19%
Stomatitis	22%
Vomiting	50%
GU	
Oliguria	63%
Hemic/Lymphatic	
Anemia	29%
Leukopenia	16%
Thrombocytopenia	37%
Metabolic/Nutritional	
Acidosis	12%
Alkaline phosphatase increase	10%
AST increase	23%
Bilirubinemia	40%
Creatinine increase	33%
Edema	15%
Hypoglycemia	11%
Hypomagnesemia	12%
Peripheral edema	28%
Weight gain	16%
Respiratory	
Cough increase	11%
Dyspnea	43%
Lung disorder[b]	24%
Respiratory tract disorder[c]	11%
Rhinitis	10%
Miscellaneous	
Abdominal pain	11%
Asthenia	23%
Chills	52%
Enlarged abdomen	10%
Fever	29%
Infection	13%
Malaise	27%
Pain	12%

[a] Cardiovascular disorder: Fluctuations in blood pressure, asymptomatic ECG changes, CHF.
[b] Lung disorder: Physical findings associated with pulmonary congestion, rales, rhonchi.
[c] Respiratory disorder: ARDS, CXR infiltrates, unspecified pulmonary changes.

Life-threatening (Grade 4) Adverse Events (%)

Body system/Adverse reaction	Patients (n = 525)
Cardiovascular	
Cardiovascular disorder[a]	7 (1%)
Heart arrest	4 (1%)
Hypotension	15 (3%)
Myocardial infarction	7 (1%)
Supraventricular tachycardia	3 (1%)
Ventricular tachycardia	5 (1%)
CNS	
Coma	8 (2%)
Confusion	5 (1%)
Psychosis	7 (1%)
Stupor	3 (1%)
GI	
Diarrhea	10 (2%)
Vomiting	7 (1%)
GU	
Acute kidney failure	3 (1%)
Anuria	25 (5%)
Oliguria	33 (6%)
Hemic/Lymphatic	
Coagulation disorder[b]	4 (1%)
Thrombocytopenia	5 (1%)

ALDESLEUKIN — INJECTION

Life-threatening (Grade 4) Adverse Events (%)	
Body system/Adverse reaction	Patients (n = 525)
Metabolic/Nutritional	
Acidosis	4 (1%)
AST increase	3 (1%)
Bilirubinemia	13 (2%)
Creatinine increase	5 (1%)
Respiratory	
Apnea	5 (1%)
Dyspnea	5 (1%)
Respiratory tract disorder[c]	14 (3%)
Miscellaneous	
Fever	5 (1%)
Infection	7 (1%)
Sepsis	6 (1%)

[a] Cardiovascular disorder: Fluctuations in blood pressure.
[b] Coagulation disorder: Intravascular coagulopathy.
[c] Respiratory disorder: ARDS, respiratory failure, intubation.

The following life-threatening (grade 4) events were reported by less than 1% of the 525 patients: Hypothermia; shock; bradycardia; ventricular extrasystoles; myocardial ischemia; syncope; hemorrhage; atrial arrhythmia; phlebitis; AV block second degree; endocarditis; pericardial effusion; peripheral gangrene; thrombosis; coronary artery disorder; stomatitis; nausea and vomiting; liver function tests abnormal; gastrointestinal hemorrhage; hematemesis; bloody diarrhea; gastrointestinal disorder; intestinal perforation; pancreatitis; anemia; leukopenia; leukocytosis; hypocalcemia; alkaline phosphatase increase; BUN increase; hyperuricemia; NPN increase; respiratory acidosis; somnolence; agitation; neuropathy; paranoid reaction; convulsion; grand mal convulsion; delirium; asthma; lung edema; hyperventilation; hypoxia; hemoptysis; hypoventilation; pneumothorax; mydriasis; pupillary disorder; kidney function abnormal; kidney failure; acute tubular necrosis.

➤*Serious adverse reactions:* In an additional population of greater than 1,800 patients treated with aldesleukin-based regimens using a variety of doses and schedules (eg, subcutaneous, continuous infusion, administration with LAK cells) the following serious adverse events were reported: Duodenal ulceration; bowel necrosis; myocarditis; supraventricular tachycardia; permanent or transient blindness secondary to optic neuritis; transient ischemic attacks; meningitis; cerebral edema; pericarditis; allergic interstitial nephritis; tracheoesophageal fistula.

➤*Fatal adverse reactions:* In the same clinical population, the following fatal events each occurred with a frequency of less than 1%: Malignant hyperthermia; cardiac arrest; myocardial infarction; pulmonary emboli; stroke; intestinal perforation; liver or renal failure; severe depression leading to suicide; pulmonary edema; respiratory arrest; respiratory failure. In patients with both metastatic RCC and metastatic melanoma, those with ECOG PS of 1 or higher had a higher treatment-related mortality and serious adverse events.

➤*Permanent sequelae:* Most adverse reactions are self-limiting and, usually, but not invariably, reverse or improve within 2 or 3 days of discontinuation of therapy. Examples of adverse reactions with permanent sequelae include myocardial infarction, bowel perforation/infarction, and gangrene.

➤*Postmarketing:* In postmarketing experience, the following serious adverse events have been reported in a variety of treatment regimens that include interleukin-2: Anaphylaxis; cellulitis; injection-site necrosis; retroperitoneal hemorrhage; cardiomyopathy; cerebral hemorrhage; fatal endocarditis; hypertension; cholecystitis; colitis; gastritis; hepatitis; hepatosplenomegaly; intestinal obstruction; hyperthyroidism; neutropenia; myopathy; myositis; rhabdomyolysis; cerebral lesions; encephalopathy; extrapyramidal syndrome; insomnia; neuralgia; neuritis; neuropathy (demyelination); urticaria; pneumonia (bacterial, fungal, viral).

➤*Exacerbation of pre-exisitng diseases:* Exacerbation or initial presentation of a number of autoimmune and inflammatory disorders have been reported. Persistent but nonprogressive vitiligo has been observed in malignant melanoma patients treated with interleukin-2. Synergistic, additive and novel toxicities have been reported with aldesleukin used in combination with other drugs. Novel toxicities include delayed adverse reactions to iodinated contrast media and hypersensitivity reactions to antineoplastic agents.

➤*Concurrent therapy:* Experience has shown the following concomitant medications to be useful in the management of patients on aldesleukin therapy:

1.) Standard antipyretic therapy, including nonsteroidal anti-inflammatories (NSAIDs), started immediately prior to aldesleukin to reduce fever. Monitor renal function, as some NSAIDs may cause synergistic nephrotoxicity.
2.) Meperidine used to control the rigors associated with fever.
3.) H_2 antagonists given for prophylaxis of gastrointestinal irritation and bleeding.
4.) Antiemetics and antidiarrheals used as needed to treat other gastrointestinal side effects. Generally these medications were discontinued 12 hours after the last dose of aldesleukin.

➤*Other:* Patients with indwelling central lines have a higher risk of infection with gram-positive organisms. A reduced incidence of staphylococcal infections in aldesleukin studies has been associated with the use of antibiotic prophylaxis which includes the use of oxacillin, nafcillin, ciprofloxacin, or vancomycin. Hydroxyzine or diphenhydramine has been used to control symptoms from pruritic rashes and continued until resolution of pruritus. Apply topical creams and ointments as needed for skin manifestations. Avoid preparations containing a steroid (eg, hydrocortisone). Note: Prior to the use of any product mentioned, the physician should refer to drug monograph for the respective product.

Overdosage

➤*Symptoms:* Side effects following the use of aldesleukin appear to be dose related. Exceeding the recommended dose has been associated with a more rapid onset of expected dose-limiting toxicities.

➤*Treatment:* Monitor symptoms that persist after cessation of aldesleukin, and treat supportively. Life-threatening toxicities may be ameliorated by the IV administration of dexamethasone, which may also result in loss of the therapeutic effects of aldesleukin.

BCG, INTRAVESICAL

Rx	**TICE BCG** (Organon)	**Powder for suspension, lyophilized:** 1 to 8 x 10^8 CFU (equivalent to ≈ 50 mg wet weight)	Lactose. Preservative free. In ≈ 50 mg vial.
Rx	**TheraCys** (Aventis Pasteur)	**Powder for suspension, lyophilized:** 10.5 ± 8.7 x 10^8 CFU (equivalent to ≈ 81 mg dry weight)	MSG. In 81 mg vial with 3 ml diluent vial.

BCG LIVE — INTRAVESICAL

BCG vaccines for tuberculosis prevention are discussed in the Biologic and Immunologics section.

WARNING

Tice BCG and *TheraCys* contain live, attenuated mycobacteria. Because of the potential risk for transmission, they should be prepared, handled, and disposed of as a biohazardous material (see Precautions and Administration and Dosage).

BCG infections have been reported in healthcare workers, primarily from exposures resulting from accidental needle sticks or skin lacerations during the preparation of BCG for administration. Nosocomial infections have been reported in patients, including immunosuppressed patients, receiving parenteral drugs that were prepared in areas in which BCG was reconstituted. BCG is capable of dissemination when administered by the intravesical route, and serious infections, including fatal infections, have been reported in patients receiving intravesical BCG (see Warnings, Precautions, and Adverse Reactions).

Indications

➤*Carcinoma in situ (CIS) / Ta or T1 papillary tumors:* For the treatment and prophylaxis of carcinoma in situ (CIS) of the urinary bladder, and for the prophylaxis of primary or recurrent stage Ta or T1 papillary tumors following transurethral resection (TUR). *Tice BCG* and *TheraCys* are not recommended for stage TaG1 papillary tumors, unless they are judged to be at high risk of tumor recurrence.

BCG live is not indicated for papillary tumors of stages higher than T1 nor as an immunizing agent for the prevention of tuberculosis.

➤*Unlabeled uses:* Local control of accessible tumor.

Administration and Dosage

Do not inject subcutaneously or intravenously.

➤*Tice BCG:* The dose for the intravesical treatment of carcinoma in situ and for the prophylaxis of recurrent papillary tumors consists of 1 vial of *Tice BCG* suspended in 50 mL preservative-free saline.

➤*TheraCys:* One dose of *TheraCys* (BCG live [intravesical]) consists of the intravesical instillation of 81 mg (dry weight) BCG. This dose is prepared by reconstituting the vial containing freeze-dried BCG with the contents of the vial containing diluent. The vial of reconstituted *TheraCys* is further diluted in 50 mL of sterile, preservative-free saline, for a total of 53 mL instillation volume (see reconstitution instructions).

A urethral catheter is inserted into the bladder under aseptic conditions, the bladder is drained, and then 53 mL suspension of *TheraCys* is instilled slowly by gravity, following which the catheter is withdrawn.

The patient retains the suspension for as long as possible for a total of up to 2 hours. During the first 15 minutes following instillation, the patient

BCG LIVE — INTRAVESICAL

should lie prone. Thereafter, the patient is allowed to be up. At the end of 2 hours, all patients should void in a seated position for safety reasons. Patients should be instructed to maintain adequate hydration.

➤*Preparation of agents:* The preparation of the *Tice BCG* cake and *TheraCys* powder should be done using aseptic technique. To avoid cross-contamination, parenteral drugs should not be prepared in areas where BCG cake and powder have been prepared. A separate area for the preparation of the BCG cake and powder is recommended. All equipment, supplies and receptacles in contact with BCG cake and powder should be handled and disposed of as biohazardous. The pharmacist or individual responsible for mixing the agent should wear gloves and eye protection, and take precautions to avoid contact of BCG cake and powder with broken skin. If the preparation cannot be performed in a biocontainment hood, then a mask and gown may be worn to avoid inhalation of BCG cake and powder organisms and inadvertent exposure to broken skin.

Tice BCG – Draw 1 mL of sterile, preservative-free saline (0.9% Sodium Chloride Injection USP) at 4° to 25°C (39.2° to 77°F), into a small syringe (eg, 3 mL) and add to 1 vial of *Tice BCG* to resuspend. Gently swirl the vial until a homogenous suspension is obtained. Avoid forceful agitation which may cause clumping of the mycobacteria.

Dispense the cloudy *Tice BCG* suspension into the top end of a catheter-tip syringe which contains 49 mL of saline diluent, bringing the total volume to 50 mL. To mix, gently rotate the syringe. The suspended *Tice BCG* should be used immediately after preparation. Discard after 2 hours.

Note: Do not filter the contents of the *Tice BCG* vial. Precautions should be taken to avoid exposing the *Tice BCG* cake to direct sunlight. Bacteriostatic solutions must be avoided. In addition, use only sterile preservative-free saline, 0.9% Sodium Chloride Injection USP, as diluent.

TheraCys – *TheraCys* should not be handled by persons with an immunologic deficiency.

Do not remove the rubber stopper from the vial.

Apply a sterile piece of cotton moistened with a suitable antiseptic to the surface of the rubber stoppers of the vial of diluent and vial of *TheraCys*. Reconstitute the freeze-dried material with the total 3 mL volume of diluent. Shake the vial gently until a fine, even suspension results. Avoid foaming since this will prevent withdrawal of the proper dose. Withdraw the entire contents (≈ 3 mL) of the reconstituted material into the syringe.

TheraCys should be reconstituted only with the diluent provided to ensure proper dispersion of the organisms.

The reconstituted material from the vial (1 dose) is further diluted in an additional 50 mL of sterile, preservative-free saline to a final volume of 53 mL for intravesical instillation.

TheraCys should be used immediately after reconstitution. However, if there is an unavoidable delay between reconstitution and administration, this delay must not exceed 2 hours. Any reconstituted product which exhibits flocculation or clumping that cannot be dispersed with gentle shaking should not be used.

➤*Treatment schedule:*

Tice BCG – Allow 7 to 14 days to elapse after bladder biopsy before *Tice BCG* is administered. Patients should not drink fluids for 4 hours before treatment and should empty their bladder prior to *Tice BCG* administration. The reconstituted *Tice BCG* is instilled into the bladder by gravity flow via the catheter. Do not depress plunger and force the flow of the *Tice BCG*. The *Tice BCG* is retained in the bladder 2 hours and then voided. Patients unable to retain the suspension for 2 hours should be allowed to void sooner, if necessary.

While the *Tice BCG* is retained in the bladder, the patient should ideally be repositioned from left side to right side and also should lie upon the back and the abdomen, changing these positions every 15 minutes to maximize bladder surface exposure to the agent.

A standard treatment schedule consists of 1 intravesical instillation per week for 6 weeks. This schedule may be repeated once if tumor remission has not been achieved and if the clinical circumstances warrant. Thereafter, intravesical *Tice BCG* administration should continue at approximately monthly intervals for at least 6 to 12 months. There are no data to support the interchangeability of BCG live products.

TheraCys – Intravesical treatment of the urinary bladder should begin 7 to 14 days after biopsy or transurethral resection, and consists of induction and maintenance therapy. For the induction therapy, 1 dose of *TheraCys* is administered each week for 6 consecutive weeks. Induction therapy should be followed by maintenance therapy, consisting of 1 dose given 3, 6, 12, 18, and 24 months following the initial dose.

➤*Storage/Stability:*

Tice BCG cake – The intact vials of *Tice BCG* should be stored refrigerated at 2° to 8°C (36° to 46°F).

This agent contains live bacteria and should be protected from direct sunlight. The product should not be used after the expiration date printed on the label.

TheraCys powder – *TheraCys* and the accompanying diluent should be kept in a refrigerator at a temperature between 2° to 8°C (36° to 46°F). It should not be used after the expiration date marked on the vial, otherwise it may be inactive.

At no time should the freeze-dried *TheraCys* be exposed to sunlight, direct or indirect. Exposure to artificial light should be kept to a minimum.

Latex – See Warnings for more information.

Actions

➤*Pharmacology:* *Tice BCG* and *TheraCys* promote a local acute inflammatory and sub-acute granulomatous reaction with macrophage and lymphocyte infiltration in the urothelium and lamina propria of the urinary bladder. The exact mechanism of action is unknown, but the anti-tumor effect appears to be T-lymphocyte-dependent.

Contraindications

Immunosuppressed patients or persons with congenital or acquired immune deficiencies, whether due to concurrent disease (eg, AIDS, leukemia, lymphoma), cancer therapy (eg, cytotoxic drugs, radiation), or immunosuppressive therapy (eg, corticosteroids).

Treatment should be postponed until resolution of a concurrent febrile illness, urinary tract infection, or gross hematuria. Seven to fourteen days should elapse before BCG is administered following biopsy, TUR, or traumatic catheterization.

Tice BCG and *TheraCys* should not be administered to persons with active tuberculosis. Active tuberculosis should be ruled out in individuals who are PPD-positive before starting treatment with *Tice BCG* and *TheraCys*.

Warnings

➤*Tuberculosis:* See Indications for more information.

➤*Infectious complications:* *Tice BCG* and *TheraCys* are infectious agents. Physicians using these products should be familiar with the literature on the prevention and treatment of BCG-related complications, and should be prepared in such emergencies to contact an infectious disease specialist with experience in treating the infectious complications of intravesical BCG. The treatment of the infectious complications of BCG requires long-term antibiotic therapy. Special culture media are required for mycobacteria, and physicians administering intravesical BCG or those caring for these patients should have these media readily available.

➤*Management of serious BCG complications:* Acute, localized irritative toxicities of *Tice BCG* and *TheraCys* may be accompanied by systemic manifestations, consistent with a "flu-like" syndrome. Systemic adverse effects of 1 to 2 days duration such as malaise, fever, and chills often reflect hypersensitivity reactions. However, symptoms such as fever of ≥ 38.5°C (101.3°F), or acute localized inflammation such as epididymitis, prostatitis, or orchitis persisting longer than 2 to 3 days suggest active infection, and evaluation for serious infectious complications should be considered.

In patients who develop persistent fever or experience an acute febrile illness, consistent with BCG infection, two or more antimycobacterial agents should be administered while diagnostic evaluation, including cultures, is conducted. BCG treatment should be discontinued. Negative cultures do not necessarily rule out infection. Physicians using this product should be familiar with the literature on prevention, diagnosis, and treatment of BCG-related complications, and when appropriate, should consult an infectious disease specialist or other physician with experience in the diagnosis and treatment of mycobacterial infections. *Tice BCG* and *TheraCys* are sensitive to the most commonly used antituberculous agents (isoniazid, rifampin, and ethambutol).

➤*Elderly:* Of the total number of subjects in clinical studies of *Tice BCG*, the average age was 66 years old. No overall difference in safety or effectiveness was observed between older and younger subjects. Other reported clinical experience has not identified differences in responses between elderly and younger patients, but greater sensitivity of some older individual to BCG cannot be ruled out.

➤*Pregnancy:* *Category C.*

Teratogenic – Animal reproduction studies have not been conducted with *Tice BCG* and *TheraCys*. It is also not known whether *Tice BCG* and *TheraCys* can cause fetal harm when administered to a pregnant woman or can affect reproduction capacity. *Tice BCG* and *TheraCys* should be given to pregnant woman only if clearly needed. Women should be advised not to become pregnant while on therapy.

➤*Lactation:* It is not known whether *Tice BCG* and *TheraCys* are excreted in human milk. Because many drugs are excreted in human milk and because of the potential for serious adverse reactions in nursing infants from *Tice BCG* and *TheraCys*, a decision should be made whether to discontinue nursing or to discontinue the drug, taking into account the importance of the drug to the mother.

➤*Children:* Safety and effectiveness of *Tice BCG* and *TheraCys* for the treatment of superficial bladder cancer in pediatric patients have not been established.

Precautions

➤*Monitoring:* Deaths have been reported as a result of systemic BCG infection and sepsis. Patients should be monitored for the presence of symptoms and signs of toxicity after each intravesical treatment. Febrile episodes with flu-like symptoms lasting more than 72 hours, fever ≥ 39.4°C (103°F), systemic manifestations increasing in intensity with repeated instillations, or persistent abnormalities of liver function tests suggest systemic BCG infection and may require anti-tuberculous therapy (see Adverse Reactions). Local symptoms (prostatitis, epididymitis, orchitis) lasting more than 2 to 3 days may also suggest active infection (see Warnings, Management of serious BCG complications).

Tice BCG and *TheraCys* contain live mycobacteria and should be prepared and handled using aseptic technique (see Administration and Dosage, Preparation of agent). BCG infections have been reported in healthcare workers preparing BCG for administration. Needle stick injuries should be avoided during the handling and mixing of *Tice BCG* and *TheraCys*. Noso-

BCG LIVE — INTRAVESICAL

comial infections have been reported in patients, and immunosuppressed patients, receiving parenteral drugs which were prepared in areas in which BCG was prepared.

BCG is capable of dissemination when administered by intravesical route and serious reactions, including fatal infections, have been reported in patients receiving intravesical BCG. Care should be taken not to traumatize the urinary tract or to introduce contaminants into the urinary system. Seven to fourteen days should elapse before *Tice BCG* and *TheraCys* are administered following TUR, biopsy, or traumatic catheterization.

➤*HIV:* *Tice BCG* and *TheraCys* should be administered with caution to persons in groups at high risk for HIV infection.

➤*Concurrent infections:* Intravesical instillations of BCG should be postponed during treatment with antibiotics, since antimicrobial therapy may interfere with the effectiveness of *Tice BCG* and *TheraCys*. *Tice BCG* and *TheraCys* should not be used in individuals with concurrent infections.

➤*Bleeding mucosa:* Instillation of *Tice BCG* and *TheraCys* into a patient with an actively bleeding mucosa may promote systemic BCG infection. Treatment should be postponed for at least 1 week following transurethral resection, biopsy, truamatic catheterization, or gross hematuria.

➤*Small bladder:* Small bladder capacity has been associated with increased risk of severe local reactions and should be considered in deciding to use *Tice BCG* and *TheraCys* therapy.

➤*Immunosuppression:* For patients with a condition that may in the future require mandatory immunosuppression (eg, awaiting an organ transplant, myasthenia gravis) the decision to treat with *TheraCys* should by considered carefully.

➤*Aneurysms/Prosthetic devices:* BCG infection of aneurysms and prosthetic devices (including arterial grafts, cardiac devices, and artificial joints) have been reported following intravesical administration of BCG. The risk of these ectopic BCG infections has not been determined, but is considered to be very small. The benefits of BCG therapy must be carefully weighed against the posibility of an ectopic BCG infection in patients with preexisting arterial aneurysms or prosthetic devices of any kind.

➤*Latex:* The stopper of the vial for *TheraCys* contains natural rubber latex which may cause allergic reactions.

➤*Lab test abnormalities:* The use of *Tice BCG* and *TheraCys* may cause tuberculin sensitivity. It is advisable to determine the tuberculin reactivity of patients receiving *Tice BCG* and *TheraCys* by PPD skin testing before treatment is initiated.

Drug Interactions

➤*Immunosuppressants/Bone marrow depressants/Radiation/Antibiotics/Antituberculosis drugs:* Drug combinations containing immunosuppressants or bone marrow depressants or radiation interfere with the development of the immune response and should not be used in combination with *Tice BCG* and *TheraCys*. Antimicrobial therapy for other infections may interfere with the effectiveness of *Tice BCG* and *TheraCys*. There are no data to suggest that the acute, local urinary tract toxicity common with BCG is due to mycobacterial infection and antituberculosis drugs (eg, isoniazid) should not be used to prevent or treat the local, irritative toxicities of *Tice BCG* and *TheraCys*.

See Precautions for more information.

Adverse Reactions

➤*Bladder irritability:* Symptoms of bladder irritability, related to the inflammatory response induced, are reported in approximately 50% to 60% of patients receiving *Tice BCG* and *TheraCys*. The symptoms typically begin 4 to 6 hours after instillation and last 24 to 72 hours. The irritative side effects are usually seen following the third instillation, and tend to increase in severity after each administration.

The irritative bladder adverse effects can usually be managed symptomatically with products such as pyridium, propantheline bromide, oxybutynin chloride, and acetaminophen. The mechanism of action of the irritative side effects has not been firmly established, but is most consistent with an immunological mechanism. There is no evidence that dose reduction or antituberculous drug therapy can prevent or lessen the irritative toxicity of *Tice BCG* and *TheraCys*.

➤*Hypersensitivity:* Flu-like symptoms (malaise, fever, and chills) which may accompany the localized, irritative toxicities often reflect hypersensitivity reactions which can be treated symptomatically. Antihistamines have also been used.

➤*Serious infections:* Although uncommon, serious infectious complications of intravesical BCG have been reported. The most serious infectious complication of BCG is disseminated sepsis with associated mortality. In addition, *M. bovis* infections have been reported in lung, liver, bone, bone marrow, kidney, regional lymph nodes, and prostate in patients who have received intravesical BCG. Some male genitourinary tract infections (orchitis/epididymitis) have been resistant to multiple drug antituberculous therapy and required orchiectomy.

If a patient develops persistent fever or experiences an acute febrile illness consistent with BCG infection, BCG treatment should be discontinued and the patient immediately evaluated and treated for systemic infection (see Warnings).

➤*TheraCys:* Ocular symptoms (including uveitis, conjunctivitis, iritis, keratitis, granulomatous choreoretinitis) alone, or in combination with joint symptoms (arthritis or arthralgia), urinary symptoms or skin rash, have been reported following administration of intravesical BCG. The risk appears to be elevated among patients who are positive for HLA-B27.

➤*Summary of adverse effects seen in 674 patients with superficial bladder cancer, including 153 with carcinoma in situ for Tice BCG:*

Adverse Reactions in Patients with Superficial Bladder Cancer (%)		
Adverse event	Number of patients	Overall (grade ≥ 3)
Dysuria	401	60% (11%)
Urinary frequency	272	40% (7%)
Flu-like syndrome	224	33% (9%)
Hematuria	175	26% (7%)
Fever	134	20% (8%)
Malaise/fatigue	50	7% (0)
Cystitis	40	6% (2%)
Urgency	39	6% (1%)
Nocturia	30	5% (1%)
Cramps/pain	27	4% (1%)
Rigors	22	3% (1%)
Nausea/vomiting	20	3% (< 1%)
Arthritis/myalgia	18	3% (< 1%)
Headache/dizziness	16	2% (0)
Urinary incontinance	16	2% (0)
Anorexia/weight loss	15	2% (< 1%)
Urinary debris	15	2% (< 1%)
Allergy	14	2% (< 1%)
Cardiac (unclassified)	13	2% (1%)
Genital inflammation/abscess	12	2% (< 1%)
Respiratory (unclassified)	11	2% (< 1%)
Urinary tract infection	10	2% (1%)
Abdominal pain	10	2% (1%)

➤*Adverse events reported in ≤ 1% for Tice BCG:* The following adverse events were reported in ≤ 1% of patients:

Miscellaneous – Anemia, BCG sepsis, coagulopathy, contracted bladder, diarrhea, epididymitis/prostatitis, hepatic granuloma, hepatitis, leukopenia, neurologic (unclassified), orchitis, pneumonitis, pyuria, rash, thrombocytopenia, urethritis, and urinary obstruction.

➤*Tice BCG:* In SWOG study 8795, toxicity evaluations were available on a total of 222 *Tice BCG*-treated patients and 220 mitomycin C-treated patients. Direct bladder toxicity (cramps, dysuria, frequency, urgency, hematuria, hemorrhagic cystitis, or incontinence) was seen more often with *Tice BCG*, with 356 events compared to 234 events for mitomycin C. Grade ≤ 2 toxicity was seen significantly more frequently following *Tice BCG* treatment (p = 0.003). No life-threatening toxicity was seen in either arm. Systemic toxicity with *Tice BCG* was markedly increased compared to that of mitomycin C, with 181 events for *Tice BCG* live compared to 80 for mitomycin C. The frequency of toxicity was increased in all grades, particularly for grades 2 and 3. The most common complaints were malaise, fatigue and lethargy, fever, and abdominal pain. Thirty-two *Tice BCG* live patients were reported to have been treated with isoniazid. Five *Tice BCG* patients had liver enzyme elevation, including 2 with grade 3 elevations. Eighteen of the 222 (8.1%) *Tice BCG* live patients failed to complete the prescribed protocol compared to 6.2% in the mitomycin C group.

Most Common Adverse Reaction in SWOG Study 8795*				
	Tice BCG (n = 222)		Mitomcyin C (n = 220)	
Adverse event	All grades	Grade ≥ 3	All grades	Grade ≥ 3
Dysuria	115 (52%)	6 (3%)	77 (35%)	5 (2%)
Urgency/frequency	112 (50%)	5 (2%)	63 (29%)	7 (3%)
Hematuria	85 (38%)	6 (3%)	56 (25%)	5 (2%)
Flu-like symptoms	54 (24%)	1 (< 1%)	29 (13%)	0
Fever	37 (17%)	1 (< 1%)	7 (3%)	0
Pain (not specified)	37 (17%)	4 (2%)	22 (10%)	1 (< 1%)
Hemorrhagic cystitis	19 (9%)	3 (1%)	10 (5%)	0
Chills	19 (9%)	0	2	(1%) 0
Bladder cramps	18 (8%)	0	9 (4%)	0
Nausea	16 (7%)	0	12 (5%)	0
Incontinence	8 (4%)	0	3 (1%)	0
Myalgia/arthralgia	7 (3%)	0	0	0
Diaphoresis	7 (3%)	0	1 (< 1%)	0
Rash	6 (3%)	1 (< 1%)	16 (7%)	2 (1%)

* The adverse reaction profile of *Tice BCG* was similar in the Nijmegen study.

BCG LIVE — INTRAVESICAL

➤*TheraCys:*

SWOG Study 8216 - Toxicity	
Adverse event	Percent of patients overall (grade ≥ 3)
Dysuria	52% (4%)
Urinary frequency	40% (2%)
Malaise	40% (2%)
Hematuria	39% (7%)
Fever (> 38°C; 100.4°F)	38% (3%)
Chills	34% (3%)
Cystitis	29% (0%)
Anemia	21% (0%)
Urinary tract infection	18% (1%)
Urgency	18% (0%)
Nausea/vomiting	16% (0%)
Anorexia	11% (0%)
Renal toxicity (NOS)	10% (2%)
Genital pain	10% (0%)
Arthralgia/myalgia	7% (1%)
Urinary incontinence	6% (0%)
Cramps/pain	6% (0%)
Diarrhea	6% (0%)
Contracted bladder	5% (0%)
Leukopenia	5% (0%)
Coagulopathy	3% (0%)
Abdominal pain	3% (0%)
Liver involvement	3% (0%)
Systemic infection	3% (0%)
Pulmonary infection	3% (0%)
Cardiac (unclassified)	3% (0%)
Headache	2% (0%)
Skin rash	2% (0%)

➤*Adverse reactions reported in ≤ 1% of TheraCys patients:* The following adverse events were reported in ≤ 1% of *TheraCys* patients: Tissue in urine, local infection, constipation, dizziness, fatigue, thrombocytopenia, and flank pain. In this study, local irritative symptoms were more common with *TheraCys* than with doxorubicin; however, grade ≥ 3 irritative toxicity was similiar, occuring in approximately 2% to 7% of patients. Systemic symptoms (eg, fever, chills, malaise) were also more common with *TheraCys*. Overall, grade ≥ 3 toxicities were seen in 26 patients (23%) treated with *TheraCys* and 25 patients (21%) treated with doxorubicin. "Systemic infection" was reported to occur in 3 patients treated with *TheraCys* (1 grade 2 and 2 grade 3) and 1 patient treated with doxorubicin (grade 2). In 4 patients, treatment was discontinued because of toxicity (2 with irritative symptoms, 1 with severe hematuria, and 1 with possible BCG infection). In addition, 6 patients refused further treatment because of severe local toxicity or chills. Six of these 10 patients received *TheraCys*. The information below compares the common adverse events reported in SWOG study 8216.

➤*Comparative toxicity for TheraCys:*

SWOG Study 8216 - Comparative Toxicity				
	TheraCys (n = 112)		Doxorubicin (n = 119)	
Adverse event	All grades	Grade ≥ 3	All grades	Grade ≥ 3
Dysuria	58 (52%)	4 (4%)	48 (40%)	7 (6%)
Frequency	45 (40%)	2 (2%)	34 (29%)	5 (4%)
Malaise	45 (40%)	2 (2%)	17 (14%)	0
Hematuria	44 (39%)	8 (7%)	33 (28%)	8 (7%)
Fever (> 38°C; 100.4°F)	43 (38%)	3 (3%)	11 (9%)	0
Chills	38 (34%)	3 (3%)	7 (6%)	0
Cystitis	33 (29%)	0	23 (19%)	1 (< 1%)
Urgency	20 (18%)	1 (< 1%)	14 (12%)	3 (2%)
Nausea/vomiting	18 (16%)	0	10 (8%)	1 (< 1%)
Bladder cramps/pain	7 (6%)	0	6 (5%)	2 (1%)

Overdosage

Overdosage occurs if more than 1 vial of *Tice BCG* and *TheraCys* are administered per instillation. The patient should be closely monitored for signs of active local or systemic BCG infection. For acute local or systemic reactions suggesting active infection, an infectious disease specialist experienced in BCG complications should be consulted.

Patient Information

Tice BCG and *TheraCys* are retained in the bladder for 2 hours and then voided. Patients should void while seated in order to avoid splashing of urine. For the 6 hours after treatment, urine voided should be disinfected for 15 minutes with an equal volume of household bleach before flushing. Patients should be instructed to increase fluid intake in order to flush the bladder in the hours following BCG treatment. Patients may experience burning with the first void after treatment.

Patients should be attentive to side effects, such as fever, chills, malaise, flu-like symptoms, or increased fatigue. If the patient experiences severe urinary side effects, such as burning or pain on urination, urgency, frequency of urination, blood in urine, or other symptoms such as joint pain, cough, or skin rash, the physician should be notified.

DENILEUKIN DIFTITOX

Rx	**Ontak** (Ligand Pharmaceuticals)	**Solution for Injection, frozen:** 150 mcg/ml	EDTA. In single-use vials.

DENILEUKIN DIFTITOX — INJECTION

WARNING

Only physicians experienced in the use of antineoplastic therapy and management of patients with cancer should use denileukin diftitox. Patients treated with denileukin diftitox must be managed in a facility equipped and staffed for cardiopulmonary resuscitation and where the patient can be closely monitored for an appropriate period based on his or her health status.

Indications

➤*T-cell lymphoma:* For the treatment of patients with persistent or recurrent cutaneous T-cell lymphoma whose malignant cells express the CD25 component of the IL-2 receptor. Prior to administration of this product, the patient's malignant cells should be tested for CD25 expression. A testing service for the assay of CD25 on skin biopsy samples is available. For information on this service call 800-964-5836. The safety and efficacy of denileukin diftitox in patients with CTCL whose malignant cells do not express the CD25 component of the IL-2 receptor have not been examined.

➤*Unlabeled uses:* Treatment of chronic lymphocytic leukemia refractory to fludarabine; non-Hodgkin lymphoma.

Administration and Dosage

➤*Approved by the FDA:* February 5, 1999.

Denileukin diftitox is for IV use only. The recommended treatment regimen (one treatment cycle) is 9 or 18 mcg/kg/day administered intravenously for 5 consecutive days every 21 days. Denileukin diftitox should be infused over at least 15 minutes. If infusional adverse reactions occur, the infusion should be discontinued or the rate should be reduced depending on the severity of the reaction. There is no clinical experience with prolonged infusion times (greater than 80 minutes).

➤*Duration of therapy:* The optimal duration of therapy has not been determined; however, only 2% (1/51) of patients who did not demonstrate at least a 25% decrease in tumor burden prior to the fourth course of treatment subsequently responded.

➤*Special handling:*
- Denileukin diftitox must be brought to room temperature, up to 25°C (77°F), before preparing the dose. The vials may be thawed in the refrigerator at 2° to 8°C (36° to 46°F) for not more than 24 hours or at room temperature for 1 to 2 hours. Denileukin diftitox must not be heated.
- The solution in the vial may be mixed by gentle swirling; do not vigorously shake the denileukin diftitox solution.
- After thawing, a haze may be visible. This haze should clear when the solution is at room temperature.
- Denileukin diftitox solution must not be used unless the solution is clear, colorless and without visible particulate matter.
- Denileukin diftitox must not be refrozen.

➤*Preparation and administration:*
- Use appropriate aseptic technique in dilution and administration of denileukin diftitox.
- Prepare and hold diluted denileukin diftitox in plastic syringes or soft plastic IV bags. Do not use a glass container because adsorption to glass may occur in the dilute state.
- The concentration of denileukin diftitox must be at least 15 mcg/mL during all steps in the preparation of the solution for IV infusion. This is best accomplished by withdrawing the calculated dose from the vial(s) and injecting it into an empty IV infusion bag. For each 1 mL of denileukin diftitox from the vial(s), no more than 9 mL of sterile saline without preservative should then be added to the IV bag.

DENILEUKIN DIFTITOX — INJECTION

- The denileukin diftitox dose should be infused over at least 15 minutes.
- Denileukin diftitox should not be administered as a bolus injection.
- Do not physically mix denileukin diftitox with other drugs.
- Do not administer denileukin diftitox through an in-line filter.
- Prepared solutions of denileukin diftitox should be administered within 6 hours, using a syringe pump or IV infusion bag.
- Unused portions of denileukin diftitox should be discarded immediately.

➤*Storage / Stability:* Store frozen at or below −10°C (14°F).

Actions

➤*Pharmacology:* Denileukin diftitox is a fusion protein designed to direct the cytocidal action of diphtheria toxin to cells which express the IL-2 receptor. The human IL-2 receptor exists in 3 forms, low (CD25), intermediate (CD122/CD132) and high (CD25/CD122/CD132) affinity. The high affinity form of this receptor is usually found only on activated T lymphocytes, activated β lymphocytes and activated macrophages. Malignant cells expressing 1 or more of the subunits of the IL-2 receptor are found in certain leukemias and lymphomas including cutaneous T-cell lymphoma (CTCL). Ex vivo studies suggest that denileukin diftitox interacts with the high affinity IL-2 receptor on the cell surface and inhibits cellular protein synthesis, resulting in cell death within hours.

➤*Pharmacokinetics:*

Distribution – The biodistribution and excretion of radiolabeled denileukin diftitox were evaluated over 48 hours in rats. The liver and kidneys were the primary sites of distribution and accumulation of radiolabeled material outside of the vasculature.

Metabolism / Excretion – Denileukin diftitox was metabolized by proteolytic degradation. Excreted material was less than 25% of the total injected dose and consisted of low molecular weight breakdown products. Pharmacokinetic parameters associated with denileukin diftitox were determined over a range of doses (3 to 31 mcg/kg/day) in patients with lymphoma. Denileukin diftitox was administered as an IV infusion following the schedule used in the clinical trials. Following the first dose, denileukin diftitox displayed 2-compartment behavior with a distribution phase (half-life approximately 2 to 5 minutes) and a terminal phase (half-life approximately 70 to 80 minutes). Systemic exposure was variable but proportional to dose. Clearance was approximately 1.5 to 2 mL/min/kg and the volume of distribution was similar to that of circulating blood (0.06 to 0.08 L/kg). No accumulation was evident between the first and fifth doses. Development of antibodies to denileukin diftitox has been shown to significantly impact clearance rates. Gender, age, and race were introduced into a multivariate analysis with various pharmacokinetic parameters. The limited available data revealed no statistical relationships between these variables.

Contraindications

Hypersensitivity to denileukin diftitox or any of its components: Diphtheria toxin, interleukin-2, or excipients.

Warnings

➤*Vascular leak syndrome:* This syndrome, characterized by 2 or more of the following 3 symptoms (hypotension, edema, hypoalbuminemia) was reported in 27% (38/143) of patients in the clinical studies. Six percent (8/143) of patients were hospitalized for the management of these symptoms. The onset of symptoms in patients with vascular leak syndrome was delayed, usually occurring within the first 2 weeks of infusion and may persist or worsen after the cessation of denileukin diftitox. Cases of vascular (capillary) leak with a fatal outcome have been reported. Special caution should be taken in patients with preexisting cardiovascular disease. Two patients, both of whom had known or suspected preexisting coronary artery disease, sustained acute myocardial infarctions while on study.

Weight, edema, blood pressure and serum albumin levels should be carefully monitored on an outpatient basis. This syndrome is usually self-limited and treatment should be used only if clinically indicated. The type of treatment will depend on whether edema or hypotension is the primary clinical problem. Preexisting low serum albumin levels appear to predict and may predispose patients to the syndrome. Eighty-three percent (118/143) of patients with lymphoma experienced hypoalbuminemia, which was considered moderate or severe in 17% (20/118) of the affected patients. For most patients, the nadir for hypoalbuminemia occurs 1 to 2 weeks after denileukin diftitox administration. Serum albumin levels should be monitored prior to the initiation of each treatment course. Administration of denileukin diftitox should be delayed until serum albumin levels are at least 3 g/dL.

➤*Hypersensitivity reactions:* Acute hypersensitivity reactions were reported in 98 of 143 patients (69%) during or within 24 hours of denileukin diftitox infusion; approximately half of the events occurred on the first day of dosing regardless of the treatment cycle. The constellation of symptoms included 1 or more of the following, defined as the incidence (%) in these 98 patients: Hypotension (50%), back pain (30%), dyspnea (28%), vasodilation (28%), rash (25%), chest pain or tightness (24%), tachycardia (12%), dysphagia or laryngismus (5%), syncope (3%), allergic reaction (1%) or anaphylaxis (1%). These events were severe in 2% of patients. Death during infusion has been reported. Management consists of interruption or a decrease in the rate of infusion (depending on the severity of the reaction); 3% of infusions were terminated prematurely and reduction in rate occurred in 4% of the infusions during the clinical trials. The administration of IV antihistamines, corticosteroids, and epinephrine may also be required; 2 subjects received epinephrine and 18 (13%) received systemic corticosteroids in the clinical studies. These drugs and resuscitative equipment should be readily available during denileukin diftitox administration.

➤*Elderly:* 49% (35/71) of the patients enrolled in the randomized two dose study were greater than or equal to 65 years of age, and those patients had response rates similar to those seen in younger patients. The following adverse events (regardless of causality) tended to be more frequent and/or more severe in lymphoma patients who were greater than or equal to 65 years of age: Anorexia, hypotension, anemia, confusion, rash, nausea or vomiting.

➤*Pregnancy: Category C.* Animal reproduction studies have not been conducted with denileukin diftitox. It is also not known whether denileukin diftitox can cause fetal harm when administered to a pregnant woman or affect reproductive capacity. Denileukin diftitox should be given to a pregnant woman only if clearly needed.

➤*Lactation:* It is not known whether this drug is excreted in human milk. Because many drugs are excreted in human milk, and because of the potential for serious adverse reactions in nursing infants, patients receiving denileukin diftitox should discontinue nursing.

➤*Children:* Safety and effectiveness in pediatric patients have not been established.

Precautions

➤*Monitoring:* Prior to administration of this product, the patient's malignant cells should be tested for CD25 expression. A testing service for the assay of CD25 on skin biopsy samples is available. For information on this service call 800-964-5836.

A complete blood count and a blood chemistry panel, including liver and renal function and serum albumin levels, should be performed prior to initiation of denileukin diftitox treatment and weekly during therapy.

Hypoalbuminemia – Eighty-three percent (118/143) of patients with lymphoma experienced hypoalbuminemia, which was considered moderate or severe in 17% (20/118) of the affected patients. For most patients, the nadir for hypoalbuminemia occurs 1 to 2 weeks after denileukin diftitox administration. Serum albumin levels should be monitored prior to the initiation of each treatment course. Administration of denileukin diftitox should be delayed until serum albumin levels are at least 3 g/dL.

➤*Infection:* Patients should be monitored carefully for infection since patients with CTCL have a predisposition to cutaneous infection. Also, the binding of denileukin diftitox to activated lymphocytes and macrophages can lead to cell death and may impair immune function in patients.

➤*Immunogenicity:* The immunogenicity data reflect the percentage of patients whose test results were considered positive for antibody to denileukin diftitox in ELISA assays and in a functional cellular assay. These results are highly dependent on the sensitivity and the specificity of the assays. Additionally, the observed incidence of the antibody positivity may be influenced by several factors, including sample handling, concomitant medication, and underlying disease. For these reasons, the comparison of the incidence of antibodies to denileukin diftitox with the incidence of antibodies to other products may be misleading. Patients who develop a hypersensitivity to denileukin diftitox may have allergic or hypersensitivity reactions to other products produced in *E. coli* expression systems and to vaccines against diphtheria.

An immune response to denileukin diftitox was assessed using 2 enzyme-linked immunoassays (ELISA), 1 measuring reactivity directed against the intact DAB_{389}IL-2 and the other against the IL-2 portion of the protein. An additional in vitro cell-based assay that measured the ability of antibodies in serum to protect a human IL-2R-expressing cell line from toxicity by DAB_{389}IL-2, was used to detect the presence of antibodies which inhibited functional activity. A total of 131 patients were assessed for an immune response by ELISA prior to treatment. Of these, 51 patients (39%) had antibodies to the intact fusion protein and 24 (18%) had antibodies that were directed against the IL-2 portion of the molecule. Among the 60 patients assessed prior to treatment, 27 (45%) had evidence of an immune response inhibiting activity in the cellular assay. After 1 cycle of treatment, 76% of the patients tested had an antibody response against DAB_{389}IL-2 and 35% against the IL-2 portion by ELISA; 73% of patients had a positive immune response in the cellular assay. After 3 cycles of treatment, 97% of patients tested had an immune response to DAB_{389}IL-2 in both the ELISA and the cellular assay.

The development of antibodies was correlated with a significant increase (2- to 3-fold) in clearance. The increased clearance resulted in a decrease in mean systemic exposure of approximately 75%. The presence of antibodies did not correlate with risk of immediate hypersensitivity-type infusional adverse events.

Adverse Reactions

All patients experienced one or more adverse events. Twenty-one percent of patients required hospitalization for drug-related adverse events; the most common reasons were evaluation of fever, management of vascular leak syndrome or dehydration secondary to gastrointestinal toxicity. Five percent of clinical adverse reactions were severe or life-threatening. The occurrence of adverse events tended to diminish in frequency after the first 2 courses, possibly related to antibody development.

DENILEUKIN DIFTITOX — INJECTION

Adverse Reactions Occurring in Lymphoma Patients (≥ 5%) patients			
Body system	Combined term	All grades (n = 143) (%)	Grades 3 and 4 (n = 143) (%)
Miscellaneous	Chills/fever	116 (81%)	31 (22%)
	Asthenia	95 (66%)	31 (22%)
	Infection	69 (48%)	34 (24%)
	Pain	69 (48%)	19 (13%)
	Headache	37 (26%)	5 (3%)
	Chest pain	34 (24%)	8 (6%)
	Flu-like syndrome	11 (8%)	0
	Injection site reaction	11 (8%)	1 (1%)
Cardiovascular	Hypotension	52 (36%)	11 (8%)
	Vasodilation	31 (22%)	1 (1%)
	Tachycardia	17 (12%)	2 (1)%
	Thrombotic events	10 (7%)	6 (4%)
	Hypertension	9 (6%)	0
	Arrhythmia	8 (6%)	5 (3%)
GI	Nausea/vomiting	91 (64%)	20 (14%)
	Anorexia	51 (36%)	12 (8%)
	Diarrhea	42 (29%)	5 (3%)
	Constipation	13 (9%)	2 (1%)
	Dyspepsia	10 (7%)	0
	Dysphagia	9 (6%)	2 (1%)
Hematologic/ Lymphatic	Anemia	26 (18%)	9 (6%)
	Thrombocytopenia	12 (8%)	3 (2%)
	Leukopenia	9 (6%)	4 (3%)
Metabolic/ Nutritional	Hypoalbuminemia	118 (83%)	20 (14%)
	Transaminase increase	87 (61%)	22 (15%)
	Edema	67 (47%)	22 (15%)
	Hypocalcemia	24 (17%)	4 (3%)
	Weight decrease	20 (14%)	6 (4%)
	Dehydration	13 (9%)	10 (7%)
	Hypokalemia	9 (6%)	0
Musculoskeletal	Myalgia	25 (17%)	3 (2%)
	Arthralgia	11 (8%)	2 (1%)
CNS	Dizziness	31 (22%)	1 (1%)
	Paresthesia	19 (13%)	2 (1%)
	Nervousness	16 (11%)	2 (1%)
	Confusion	11 (8%)	8 (6%)
	Insomnia	13 (9%)	4 (3%)
Respiratory	Dyspnea	42 (29%)	20 (14%)
	Cough increase	37 (26%)	3 (2%)
	Pharyngitis	25 (17%)	0
	Rhinitis	19 (13%)	2 (1%)
	Lung disorder	11 (8%)	0
Dermatologic	Rash	48 (34%)	18 (13%)
	Pruritus	29 (20%)	5 (3%)
	Sweating	15 (10%)	1 (1%)
GU	Hematuria	15 (10%)	5 (3%)
	Albuminuria	14 (10%)	1 (1%)
	Pyuria	14 (10%)	1 (1%)
	Creatinine increase	10 (7%)	1 (1%)

➤*Cardiovascular:* Two patients, both of whom had known or suspected preexisting coronary artery disease, sustained acute myocardial infarctions while on study. Ten additional patients (7%) experienced thrombotic events. Two patients with progressive disease and multiple medical problems experienced deep vein thrombosis. Another patient sustained a deep vein thrombosis and pulmonary embolus during hospitalization for management of congestive heart failure and vascular leak syndrome. One patient with a history of severe peripheral vascular disease sustained an arterial thrombosis. Six patients experienced less severe superficial thrombophlebitis. Thrombotic events were also observed in preclinical animal studies.

➤*Dermatologic:* Generalized maculopapular, petechial, vesicular bullous, urticarial or eczematous with both acute and delayed onset, have been reported in 34% (48/143) of patients. Antihistamines may be effective in relieving the symptoms, but more severe rashes may require the use of topical or oral corticosteroids.

➤*GI:* Diarrhea was reported in 29% (42/143) of the study population. The onset of diarrhea may be delayed and the duration can be prolonged. Dehydration, usually concurrent with vomiting or anorexia, occurred in 9% (13/143) of the patients. The majority of transient hepatic transaminase elevations occurred during the first course of denileukin diftitox, were self-limited and resolved within 2 weeks.

➤*Hematologic:* See Precautions for more information.

➤*Hypersensitivity:* See Warnings for more information.

➤*Miscellaneous:*

Vascular leak syndrome – See Warnings for more information.

Infectious complications – Infections of various types were reported by 48% (69/143) of the study population, of which 23% (16/69) were considered severe. Six of the 143 patients (4%) discontinued denileukin diftitox therapy because of infections.

Decreased lymphocyte counts (less than 900 cells/mcL) occurred in 34% of lymphoma patients. In general, lymphocyte counts dropped during the dosing period (days 1 to 5) and then returned to normal by day 15. Smaller changes and more rapid recoveries were observed with subsequent courses.

Infusion-associated reactions – There are two distinct clinical syndromes associated with denileukin diftitox infusion, an acute hypersensitivity-type symptom complex and a flu-like symptom complex. Overall, 69% of patients had infusion-related, hypersensitivity-type symptoms; for additional information, see Hypersensitivity above. A flu-like syndrome was experienced by 91% of patients within several hours to days after denileukin diftitox infusion. The symptom complex consists of one or more of the following: Fever or chills (81%), asthenia (66%), digestive (64%), myalgias (17%) and arthralgias (8%). In the majority of patients, these symptoms were mild to moderate and responded to treatment with antipyretics or antiemetics. Antipyretics or antiemetics were used to relieve flu-like symptoms; however, the usefulness of these agents in ameliorating these toxicities or as prophylactic agents to decrease the incidence of the acute, flu-like toxicities has not been prospectively studied.

➤*Infrequent serious adverse events:* The following serious adverse events occurred at an incidence of less than 5%: Pancreatitis, acute renal insufficiency, microscopic hematuria, hyperthyroidism and hypothyroidism.

Overdosage

There is no clinical experience with accidental denileukin diftitox overdosage and no known antidote. At a dose of 31 mcg/kg/day, the dose-limiting toxicities were moderate-to-severe nausea, vomiting, fever, chills or persistent asthenia. Doses greater than 31 mcg/kg/day have not been evaluated in humans. If overdose occurs, hepatic and renal function and overall fluid balance should be closely monitored.

RETINOIDS

TRETINOIN (ALL-TRANS-RETINOIC ACID)

Rx	**Vesanoid** (Roche)	**Capsules:** 10 mg	(Vesanoid 10 Roche). Orange-yellow/reddish brown. In 100s.

TRETINOIN (all-trans retinoic acid) — ORAL

WARNING

Experienced health care provider and institution – Patients with acute promyelocytic leukemia (APL) are at high risk in general and can have severe adverse reactions to tretinoin. Therefore, administer tretinoin only to patients with APL under the strict supervision of a health care provider who is experienced in the management of patients with acute leukemia, and in a facility with laboratory and supportive services sufficient to monitor drug tolerance and protect and maintain a patient compromised by drug toxicity, including respiratory compromise. Use of tretinoin requires that the health care provider conclude the possible benefit to the patient outweighs the following known adverse reactions in therapy.

Retinoic acid-APL syndrome – Approximately 25% of patients with APL treated with tretinoin have experienced the retinoic acid-APL (RA-APL) syndrome, characterized by fever, dyspnea, acute respiratory distress, weight gain, radiographic pulmonary infiltrates, pleural and pericardial effusions, edema, and hepatic, renal, and multiorgan failure. This syndrome occasionally has been accompanied by impaired myocardial contractility and episodic hypotension. It has been observed with or without concomitant leukocytosis. Endotracheal intubation and mechanical ventilation have been required in some cases due to progressive hypoxemia, and several patients have expired with multiorgan failure. The syndrome generally occurs during the first month of treatment, with some cases reported following the first dose of tretinoin.

The management of the syndrome has not been defined rigorously, but high-dose steroids given at the first suspicion of the RA-APL syndrome appear to reduce morbidity and mortality. At the first signs suggestive of the syndrome (eg, unexplained fever, dyspnea and/or weight gain, abnormal chest auscultatory findings, radiographic abnormalities), initiate high-dose steroids (dexamethasone 10 mg intravenous [IV] administered every 12 hours for 3 days or until the resolution of symptoms) immediately, irrespective of the leukocyte count. The majority of patients do not require termination of tretinoin therapy during treatment of the RA-APL syndrome. However, in cases of moderate and severe RA-APL syndrome, consider temporary interruption of tretinoin therapy.

Leukocytosis – During tretinoin treatment, approximately 40% of patients will develop rapidly evolving leukocytosis. Patients who present with high white blood cell (WBC) at diagnosis (more than 5×10^9/L) have an increased risk of a further rapid increase in WBC counts. Rapidly evolving leukocytosis is associated with a higher risk of life-threatening complications.

If signs and symptoms of the RA-APL syndrome are present together with leukocytosis, immediately initiate treatment with high-dose steroids. Some investigators routinely add chemotherapy to tretinoin treatment in the case of patients presenting with a WBC count of more than 5×10^9/L or in the case of a rapid increase in WBC count for patients leukopenic at start of treatment, and have reported a lower incidence of the RA-APL syndrome. Consider adding full-dose chemotherapy (including an anthracycline if not contraindicated) to tretinoin therapy on day 1 or 2 for patients presenting with a WBC count of more than 5×10^9/L; immediately add for patients presenting with a WBC count of less than 5×10^9/L, if the WBC count reaches greater than or equal to 6×10^9/L by day 5, greater than or equal to 10×10^9/L by day 10, or greater than or equal to 15×10^9/L by day 28.

Teratogenic effects –

Pregnancy (Category D): There is a high risk that a severely deformed infant will result if tretinoin is administered during pregnancy. If, nonetheless, it is determined that tretinoin represents the best available treatment for a pregnant woman or a woman of childbearing potential, it must be assured that the patient has received full information and warnings of the risk to the fetus if she were to be pregnant and of the risk of possible contraception failure. Instruct the patient to use 2 reliable forms of contraception simultaneously during therapy and for 1 month following discontinuation of therapy, and emphasize the need for using dual contraception, unless abstinence is the chosen method.

Within 1 week prior to the institution of tretinoin therapy, collect blood or urine from the patient for a serum or urine pregnancy test with a sensitivity of at least 50 milliunits/mL. When possible, delay tretinoin therapy until a negative result from this test is obtained. When a delay is not possible, place the patient on 2 reliable forms of contraception. Repeat pregnancy testing and contraception counseling monthly throughout the period of tretinoin treatment.

Indications

➤*Induction of remission:* Tretinoin capsules are indicated for the induction of remission in patients with APL, French-American-British (FAB) classification M3 (including the M3 variant), characterized by the presence of the t(15;17) translocation and/or the presence of the PML/RARα gene, who are refractory to, or who have relapsed from, anthracycline chemotherapy, or for whom anthracycline-based chemotherapy is contraindicated. Tretinoin is for the induction of remission only. The optimal consolidation or maintenance regimens have not been defined, but all patients should receive an accepted form of remission consolidation and/or maintenance therapy for APL after completion of induction therapy with tretinoin.

➤*Unlabeled uses:* Maintain remission of acute promyelocytic leukemia.

Administration and Dosage

➤*Approved by the FDA:* November 22, 1995.

The recommended dose is 45 mg/m²/day administered as 2 evenly divided doses until complete remission is documented. Discontinue therapy 30 days after achievement of complete remission or after 90 days of treatment, whichever occurs first.

If, after initiation of treatment of tretinoin, the presence of the t(15;17) translocation is not confirmed by cytogenetics and/or by polymerase chain reaction studies and the patient has not responded to tretinoin, consider alternative therapy appropriate for acute myelogenous leukemia.

Tretinoin is for the induction of remission only. Optimal consolidation or maintenance regimens have not been determined. Therefore, all patients should receive a standard consolidation and/or maintenance chemotherapy regimen for APL after induction therapy with tretinoin, unless otherwise contraindicated.

➤*Storage/Stability:* Store at 15° to 30°C (59° to 86°F). Protect from light.

Actions

➤*Pharmacology:* Tretinoin is not a cytolytic agent, but, instead, it induces cytodifferentiation and decreased proliferation of APL cells in culture and in vivo. In APL patients, tretinoin treatment produces an initial maturation of the primitive promyelocytes derived from the leukemic clone, followed by a repopulation of the bone marrow and peripheral blood by normal, polyclonal hematopoietic cells in patients achieving complete remission (CR). The exact mechanism of action of tretinoin in APL is unknown.

➤*Pharmacokinetics:*

Absorption – Tretinoin activity primarily is caused by the parent drug. In human pharmacokinetics studies, an orally administered drug was well absorbed into the systemic circulation. A single 45 mg/m² (approximately 80 mg) oral dose to APL patients resulted in a mean ± SD peak tretinoin concentration of 347 ± 266 ng/mL. Time to reach peak concentration was between 1 and 2 hours.

Plasma tretinoin concentrations decrease on average to one third of their day 1 values during 1 week of continuous therapy. Mean ± SD peak tretinoin concentrations decreased from 394 ± 89 to 138 ± 139 ng/mL, while area under the curve (AUC) values decreased from 537 ± 191 ng•h/mL to 249 ± 185 ng•h/mL during 45 mg/m ² daily dosing in 7 APL patients. Increasing the dose to "correct" for this change has not increased response.

Distribution – The apparent volume of distribution of tretinoin has not been determined. Tretinoin is more than 95% bound in plasma, predominately to albumin. Plasma protein binding remains constant over the concentration range of 10 to 500 ng/mL.

Metabolism – Tretinoin metabolites have been identified in plasma and urine. Cytochrome P-450 enzymes have been implicated in the oxidative metabolism of tretinoin. Metabolites include 13-cis retinoic acid, 4-oxo trans retinoic acid, 4-oxo cis retinoic acid, and 4-oxo trans retinoic acid glucuronide. In APL patients, daily administration of a 45 mg/m² dose of tretinoin resulted in an approximately 10-fold increase in the urinary excretion of 4-oxo trans retinoic acid glucuronide after 2 to 6 weeks of continuous dosing, when compared with baseline values. There is evidence that tretinoin induces its own metabolism.

Excretion – Approximately two thirds of the administered radiolabeled dose was recovered in the urine. The terminal elimination half-life of tretinoin following initial dosing is 0.5 to 2 hours in patients with APL. Studies with radiolabeled drug have demonstrated that after the oral administration of 2.75 and 50 mg doses of tretinoin, more than 90% of the radioactivity was recovered in the urine and feces. Based upon data from 3 subjects, approximately 63% of radioactivity was recovered in the urine within 72 hours, and 31% appeared in the feces within 6 days.

Drug-drug interactions – In 13 patients who received daily doses of tretinoin for 4 consecutive weeks, administration of ketoconazole (400 to 1,200 mg oral dose) 1 hour prior to the administration of the tretinoin dose on day 29 led to a 72% increase (218 ± 224 vs 375 ± 285 ng•h/mL) in tretinoin mean plasma AUC. The precise cytochrome P-450 enzymes involved in these interactions have not been specified; CYP 3A4, 2C8, and 2E have been implicated in various preliminary reports.

Contraindications

Hypersensitivity to tretinoin, any of its components, or other retinoids. Do not give tretinoin to patients who are sensitive to parabens, which are used as preservatives in the gelatin capsule.

Warnings

➤*Patients without the t(15;17) translocation:* Initiation of therapy with tretinoin may be based on the morphological diagnosis of APL. Seek confirmation of the diagnosis of APL by detection of the t(15;17) genetic marker by cytogenetic studies. If these are negative, seek PML/RARα fusion using molecular diagnostic techniques. The response rate of other AML subtypes to tretinoin has not been demonstrated; therefore, consider alternative treatment for patients who lack the genetic marker.

➤*RA-APL syndrome:* In up to 25% of patients with APL treated with tretinoin, RA-APL syndrome occurs, which can be fatal.

See the Warning box for more information.

➤*Leukocytosis:* See the Warning box for more information.

➤*Pseudotumor cerebri:* Retinoids, including tretinoin, have been associated with pseudotumor cerebri (benign intracranial hypertension), especially in children. The concomitant use of other agents known to cause pseudotumor cerebri/intracranial hypertension, such as tetracyclines, might increase the risk of this condition. Early signs and symptoms of pseudotu-

TRETINOIN (all-trans retinoic acid) — ORAL

mor cerebri include papilledema, headache, nausea, vomiting, and visual disturbances. Evaluate patients with these symptoms for pseudotumor cerebri, and, if present, institute appropriate care in concert with neurological assessment.

➤*Lipids:* Up to 60% of patients experienced hypercholesterolemia and/or hypertriglyceridemia, which was reversible upon completion of treatment. The clinical consequences of temporary elevation of triglycerides and cholesterol are unknown, but venous thrombosis and myocardial infarction (MI) have been reported in patients who ordinarily are at low risk for such complications.

➤*Carcinogenesis:* No long-term carcinogenicity studies with tretinoin have been conducted. In short-term carcinogenicity studies, tretinoin at a dosage of 30 mg/kg/day (about 2 times the human dosage on a mg/m^2 basis) was shown to increase the rate of diethylnitrosamine (DEN)-induced mouse liver adenomas and carcinomas.

➤*Mutagenesis:* Tretinoin was negative when tested in the Ames and Chinese hamster V79 cell HGPRT assays for mutagenicity. A 2-fold increase in the sister chromatid exchange has been demonstrated in human diploid fibroblasts, but other chromosome aberration assays, including an in vitro assay in human peripheral lymphocytes and an in vivo mouse micronucleus assay, did not show a clastogenic or aneuploidogenic effect.

➤*Fertility impairment:* Adverse reactions on fertility and reproductive performance were not observed in studies conducted in rats at dosages up to 5 mg/kg/day (approximately two thirds) the human dosage on a mg/m^2 basis). In a 6-week toxicology study in dogs, minimal to marked testicular degeneration, with increased numbers of immature spermatozoa, were observed at 10 mg/kg/day (about 4 times the equivalent human dosage in mg/m^2).

➤*Elderly:* Of the total number of subjects in clinical studies of tretinoin, 21.4% were 60 years of age and older. No overall differences in safety or efficacy were observed between these subjects and younger subjects, and other reported clinical experience has not identified differences in responses between the elderly and younger patients, but greater sensitivity of some older individuals cannot be ruled out.

➤*Pregnancy: Category D.* Tretinoin has teratogenic and embryotoxic effects in mice, rats, hamsters, rabbits, and pigtail monkeys, and may be expected to cause fetal harm when administered to a pregnant woman. Tretinoin causes fetal resorptions and a decrease in live fetuses in all animals studied. Gross external, soft tissue, and skeletal alterations occurred at dosages greater than 0.7 mg/kg/day in mice, 2 mg/kg/day in rats, 7 mg/kg/day in hamsters, and at a dosage of 10 mg/kg/day (the only dosage tested) in pigtail monkeys (about 1/20, 1/4, and 1/2, and 4 times the human dosage, respectively, on a mg/m^2 basis).

There are no adequate and well-controlled studies in pregnant women. Although experience with humans administered tretinoin is extremely limited, increased spontaneous abortions and major human fetal abnormalities related to the use of other retinoids have been documented in humans. Reported defects include abnormalities of the CNS, musculoskeletal system, external ear, eye, thymus, and great vessels; facial dysmorphia; cleft palate; and parathyroid hormone deficiency. Some of these abnormalities were fatal. Cases of intelligence quotient scores less than 85, with or without obvious CNS abnormalities, also have been reported. All fetuses exposed during pregnancy can be affected and, at the present time, there is no antepartum means of determining which fetuses are and are not affected.

Effective contraception must be used by all women during tretinoin therapy and for 1 month following discontinuation of therapy. Microdosed progesterone preparations (ie, minipill) may be an inadequate method of contraception during treatment with tretinoin. Contraception must be used even when there is a history of infertility or menopause, unless a hysterectomy has been performed. Whenever contraception is required, it is recommended that 2 reliable forms of contraception be used simultaneously, unless abstinence is the chosen method. If pregnancy does occur during treatment, the health care provider and patient should discuss the desirability of continuing or terminating the pregnancy.

➤*Lactation:* It is not known whether this drug is excreted in human milk. Because many drugs are excreted in human milk, and because of the potential for serious adverse reactions from tretinoin in breast-feeding infants, advise mothers to discontinue breastfeeding prior to taking this drug.

➤*Children:* There are limited clinical data on the pediatric use of tretinoin. Of 15 children (range, 1 to 16 years of age) treated with tretinoin, the incidence of complete remission was 67%. Safety and efficacy in children younger than 1 year of age have not been established. Some children experienced severe headache and pseudotumor cerebri, requiring analgesic treatment and lumbar puncture for relief. Increased caution is recommended in the treatment of children. Consider dose reduction for children experiencing serious and/or intolerable toxicity; however, the efficacy and safety of tretinoin at dosages less than 45 mg/m^2/day have not been evaluated in the pediatric population.

Precautions

➤*Monitoring:* Frequently monitor the patient's hematologic profile, coagulation profile, liver function test results, and triglyceride and cholesterol levels.

➤*Thrombosis:* There is a risk of thrombosis (venous and arterial) that may involve any organ system during the first month of treatment. Therefore, exercise caution when treating patients with the combination of tretinoin and antifibrinolytic agents, such as tranexamic acid, aminocaproic acid, or aprotinin.

➤*Toxic adverse reactions:* Tretinoin has potentially significant toxic adverse reactions in APL patients. Closely observe patients undergoing therapy for signs of respiratory compromise and/or leukocytosis. Maintain supportive care appropriate for APL patients (eg, prophylaxis for bleeding, prompt therapy for infection) during therapy with tretinoin.

➤*Lab test abnormalities:* Elevated liver function test results occur in 50% to 60% of patients during treatment. Carefully monitor liver function test results during treatment and give consideration to a temporary withdrawal of tretinoin if test results reach greater than 5 times the upper limit of normal values. However, the majority of these abnormalities resolve without interruption of tretinoin or after completion of treatment.

➤*Hazardous tasks:* The ability to drive or operate machinery might be impaired in patients treated with tretinoin, particularly if they are experiencing dizziness or severe headache.

Drug Interactions

➤*CYP-450 system:* As tretinoin is metabolized by the hepatic P-450 system, there is a potential for alteration of pharmacokinetic parameters in patients coadministered medications that also are inducers or inhibitors of this system. Medications that generally induce hepatic P-450 enzymes include rifampin, glucocorticoids, phenobarbital, and pentobarbital. Medications that generally inhibit hepatic P-450 enzymes include ketoconazole, cimetidine, erythromycin, verapamil, diltiazem, and cyclosporine. To date there are no data to suggest that coadministration with these medications increases or decreases either efficacy or toxicity of tretinoin.

Tretinoin Drug Interactions

Precipitant drug	Object drug*		Description
Ketoconazole	Tretinoin	↑	In 13 patients given ketoconazole 400 to 1,200 mg 1 hour prior to tretinoin, a 72% increase in tretinoin mean plasma AUC occurred.
Tretinoin	Tetracyclines	↑	Coadministration of tretinoin and agents known to cause pseudotumor cerebri/intracranial hypertension, such as tetracyclines, may increase the risk of this condition.
Tetracyclines	Tretinoin		
Tretinoin	Vitamin A	↑	As with other retinoids, tretinoin must not be administered in combination with vitamin A because symptoms of hypervitaminosis A could be aggravated.
Antifibrinolytic agents (eg, tranexamic acid, aminocaproic acid, aprotinin)	Tretinoin	↑	Cases of fatal thrombotic complications have been reported rarely in patients coadministered tretinoin and antifibrinolytic agents. Use with caution.

* ↑ = Object drug increased

➤*Agents known to cause pseudotumor cerebri/intracranial hypertension (such as tetracyclines):* Tretinoin may cause pseudotumor cerebri/intracranial hypertension. Coadministration of tretinoin and agents also known to cause pseudotumor cerebri/intracranial hypertension might increase the risk of this condition.

➤*Vitamin A:* As with other retinoids, do not administer tretinoin in combination with vitamin A because symptoms of hypervitaminosis A could be aggravated.

➤*Antifibrinolytic agents:* Cases of fatal thrombotic complications have been reported rarely in patients concomitantly treated with tretinoin and antifibrinolytic agents (eg, tranexamic acid, aminocaproic acid, aprotinin). Therefore, exercise caution when administering tretinoin concomitantly with these agents.

➤*Drug/Food interactions:* No data on the effect of food on the absorption of tretinoin are available. The absorption of retinoids as a class is enhanced when taken concurrently with food.

Adverse Reactions

Virtually all patients experience some drug-related toxicity, especially headache, fever, weakness, and fatigue. These adverse reactions seldom are permanent or irreversible, nor do they usually require interruption of therapy. Some of the adverse reactions are common in patients with APL, including hemorrhage, infections, GI hemorrhage, disseminated intravascular coagulation, pneumonia, septicemia, and cerebral hemorrhage. Respiratory system disorders were reported commonly in APL patients administered tretinoin. The majority of these reactions are symptoms of the RA-APL syndrome. The following describes the adverse reactions that were observed in patients treated with tretinoin, regardless of drug relationship.

➤*Cardiovascular:* Arrhythmias and flushing (23%); hypotension (14%); hypertension and phlebitis (11%); cardiac failure (6%); cardiac arrest, enlarged heart, heart murmur, ischemia, MI, myocarditis, pericarditis, pulmonary hypertension, secondary cardiomyopathy, and stroke (3%); thrombosis (venous and arterial) involving various sites (eg, cerebrovascular accident, MI, renal infarct) (rare).

➤*CNS:* Dizziness (20%); anxiety, paresthesia (17%); depression, insomnia, (14%); confusion (11%); agitation, cerebral hemorrhage, intracranial hypertension (9%); hallucination (6%); abnormal gait, agnosia, aphasia, asterixis, cerebellar disorders, cerebellar edema, CNS depression, coma, convulsions, dementia, dysarthria, encephalopathy, facial paralysis, forgetfulness,

TRETINOIN (all-trans retinoic acid) — ORAL

hemiplegia, hyporeflexia, hypotaxia, leg weakness, neurologic reaction, no light reflex, slow speech, somnolence, spinal cord disorder, tremor, unconsciousness (3%).

➤*Dermatologic:* Cellulitis (8%); pallor (6%); genital ulceration; vasculitis (predominantly involving the skin) (rare).

➤*GI:* GI hemorrhage (34%); abdominal pain (31%); other GI disorders (26%); diarrhea (23%); constipation, anorexia (17%); dyspepsia (14%); abdominal distention (11%); hepatosplenomegaly (9%); hepatitis, ulcer, unspecified liver disorder (3%).

➤*GU:* Renal impairment (11%); dysuria (9%); acute renal failure, enlarged prostate, micturition frequency, renal tubular necrosis (3%).

➤*Hematologic/Lymphatic:* Hemorrhage (60%); disseminated intravascular coagulation (26%); lymph disorders (6%); thrombocytosis (rare).

➤*Metabolic:* Peripheral edema (52%); edema (29%); weight increase (23%); weight decrease (17%); face edema, fluid imbalance (6%).

➤*Respiratory:* Upper respiratory tract disorders (63%); dyspnea (60%); respiratory insufficiency (26%); pleural effusion (20%); expiratory wheezing, pneumonia, rales (14%), lower respiratory tract disorders (9%); pulmonary infiltration (6%); bronchial asthma, larynx edema, pulmonary edema, unspecified pulmonary disease (3%).

➤*Special senses:* Earache or feeling of fullness in the ears (23%); hearing loss and other unspecified auricular disorders (6%); irreversible hearing loss (less than 1%).

➤*Miscellaneous:* Malaise (66%); shivering (63%); infections (58%); pain (37%); chest discomfort (32%); injection-site reactions (17%); myalgia (14%); flank pain (9%); acidosis, ascites, hypothermia (3%).

Isolated cases of basophilia, erythema nodosum, hypercalcemia, hyperhistaminemia, myositis, organomegaly, pancreatitis, and Sweet syndrome have been reported.

RA-APL syndrome – See the Warning box for more information.

Typical retinoid toxicity – The most frequently reported adverse reactions were similar to those described in patients taking high doses of vitamin A and included the following: headache (86%); fever (83%); skin/mucous membrane dryness, bone pain (77%); nausea/vomiting (57%); rash (54%); mucositis (26%); pruritus, increased sweating (20%); visual disturbances, ocular disorders (17%); alopecia and skin changes (14%); changed visual acuity (6%); bone inflammation and visual field defects (3%).

Overdosage

➤*Symptoms:* There has been no experience with acute overdosage in humans. The maximal tolerated dosage in patients with myelodysplastic syndrome or solid tumors was 195 mg/m²/day. The maximal tolerated dosage in children was lower at 60 mg/m²/day. Overdosage with other retinoids has been associated with transient headache, facial flushing, cheilosis, abdominal pain, dizziness, and ataxia. These symptoms quickly have resolved without apparent residual effects.

➤*Treatment:* There is no specific treatment in the case of an overdose; however, it is important the patient be treated in a special hematological unit.

REXINOIDS

BEXAROTENE

Rx	**Targretin** (Ligand Pharm.)	**Capsules, soft gelatin:** 75 mg	(Targretin). Off-white, oblong. In 100s.

BEXAROTENE — ORAL

Bexarotene is also available as a gel for cutaneous T-cell lymphoma (CTCL) lesions; refer to the monograph in the Dermatologic Agents chapter.

WARNING

Bexarotene capsules are a member of the retinoid class of drugs that is associated with birth defects in humans. Bexarotene capsules also caused birth defects when administered orally to pregnant rats. Bexarotene capsules must not be administered to a pregnant woman.

Indications

➤*Ta: Cutaneous T-cell lymphoma (CTCL):* Bexarotene capsules are indicated for the treatment of cutaneous manifestations of CTCL in patients who are refractory to at least 1 prior systemic therapy.

Administration and Dosage

➤*Approved by the FDA:* December 29, 1999.

➤*Initial dose:* The recommended initial dose of bexarotene capsules is 300 mg/m²/day (see table below). Bexarotene capsules should be taken as a single oral daily dose with a meal.

Bexarotene Capsule Initial Dose Calculation According to Body Surface Area

Initial dose level (300 mg/m²/day)		
Body surface area (m²)	Total daily dose (mg/day)	Number of 75 mg bexarotene capsules
0.88 to 1.12	300	4
1.13 to 1.37	375	5
1.38 to 1.62	450	6
1.63 to 1.87	525	7
1.88 to 2.12	600	8
2.13 to 2.37	675	9
2.38 to 2.62	750	10

➤*Women of childbearing potential:* See Contraindications for more information.

➤*Dose modification guidelines:* The 300 mg/m²/day dose level of bexarotene capsules may be adjusted to 200 mg/m²/day then to 100 mg/m²/day, or temporarily suspended, if necessitated by toxicity. When toxicity is controlled, doses may be carefully readjusted upward. If there is no tumor response after 8 weeks of treatment and if the initial dose of 300 mg/m²/day is well tolerated, the dose may be escalated to 400 mg/m²/day with careful monitoring.

➤*Duration of therapy:* In clinical trials in CTCL, bexarotene capsules were administered for up to 97 weeks.

Bexarotene capsules should be continued as long as the patient is deriving benefit.

➤*Storage/Stability:* Store at 2° to 25°C (36° to 77°F). Avoid exposing to high temperatures and humidity after the bottle is opened. Protect from light.

Actions

➤*Pharmacology:* Bexarotene selectively binds and activates retinoid X receptor subtypes (RXRα, RXRβ, RXRγ). RXRs can form heterodimers with various receptor partners such as RARs, vitamin D receptor, thyroid receptor, and peroxisome proliferator activator receptors (PPARs). Once activated, these receptors function as transcription factors that regulate the expression of genes that control cellular differentiation and proliferation. Bexarotene inhibits the growth in vitro of some tumor cell lines of hematopoietic and squamous cell origin. It also induces tumor regression in vivo in some animal models. The exact mechanism of action of bexarotene in the treatment of CTCL is unknown.

➤*Pharmacokinetics:*

Absorption/Distribution – After oral administration of bexarotene capsules, bexarotene is absorbed with a t_{max} of about 2 hours. Terminal half-life of bexarotene is about 7 hours. Studies in patients with advanced malignancies show approximate single dose linearity within the therapeutic range and low accumulation with multiple doses. Plasma bexarotene AUC and C_{max} values resulting from a 75 to 300 mg dose were 35% and 48% higher, respectively, after a fat-containing meal than after a glucose solution. Bexarotene is highly bound (greater than 99%) to plasma proteins. The plasma proteins to which bexarotene binds have not been elucidated, and the ability of bexarotene to displace drugs bound to plasma proteins and the ability of drugs to displace bexarotene binding have not been studied. The uptake of bexarotene by organs or tissues has not been evaluated.

Metabolism – Four bexarotene metabolites have been identified in plasma: 6- and 7-hydroxy-bexarotene and 6- and 7-oxo-bexarotene. In vitro studies suggest that cytochrome P450 3A4 is the major cytochrome P450 responsible for formation of the oxidative metabolites and that the oxidative metabolites may be glucuronidated. The oxidative metabolites are active in in vitro assays of retinoid receptor activation, but the relative contribution of the parent and any metabolites to the efficacy and safety of bexarotene capsules is unknown.

Excretion – The renal elimination of bexarotene and its metabolites was examined in patients with type 2 diabetes mellitus. Neither bexarotene nor its metabolites were excreted in urine in appreciable amounts. Bexarotene is thought to be eliminated primarily through the hepatobiliary system.

Special populations –
Renal function impairment: See Warnings for more information.
Hepatic function impairment: See Warnings for more information.

Contraindications

Bexarotene capsules are contraindicated in patients with a known hypersensitivity to bexarotene or other components of the product.

➤*Pregnancy:* Bexarotene capsules may cause fetal harm when administered to a pregnant woman. Bexarotene capsules must not be given to a pregnant woman or a woman who intends to become pregnant. If a woman becomes pregnant while taking bexarotene capsules, the capsules must be stopped immediately and the woman given appropriate counseling.

Bexarotene caused malformations when administered orally to pregnant rats during days 7 to 17 of gestation. Developmental abnormalities included incomplete ossification at 4 mg/kg/day and cleft palate, depressed eye bulge/microphthalmia, and small ears at 16 mg/kg/day. The plasma AUC of bexarotene in rats at 4 mg/kg/day is approximately one third the AUC in humans at the recommended daily dose. At doses greater than 10 mg/kg/day,

BEXAROTENE — ORAL

bexarotene caused developmental mortality. The no effect dose for fetal effects in rats was 1 mg/kg/day (producing an AUC approximately one sixth of the AUC at the recommended human daily dose).

Women of childbearing potential should be advised to avoid becoming pregnant when bexarotene capsules are used. The possibility that a woman of childbearing potential is pregnant at the time therapy is instituted should be considered. A negative pregnancy test (eg, serum beta-human chorionic gonadotropin [beta-HCG]) with a sensitivity of at least 50 mIU/L should be obtained within 1 week prior to bexarotene capsules therapy, and the pregnancy test must be repeated at monthly intervals while the patient remains on bexarotene capsules. Effective contraception must be used for 1 month prior to the initiation of therapy, during therapy and for at least 1 month following discontinuation of therapy; it is recommended that 2 reliable forms of contraception be used simultaneously unless abstinence is the chosen method. Bexarotene can potentially induce metabolic enzymes and thereby theoretically reduce the plasma concentrations of hormonal contraceptives. Thus, if treatment with bexarotene capsules is intended in a woman with childbearing potential, it is strongly recommended that 1 of the 2 reliable forms of contraception should be nonhormonal. Male patients with sexual partners who are pregnant, possibly pregnant, or who could become pregnant must use condoms during sexual intercourse while taking bexarotene capsules and for at least 1 month after the last dose of drug. Bexarotene capsules therapy should be initiated on the second or third day of a normal menstrual period. No more than a 1 month supply of bexarotene capsules should be given to the patient so that the results of pregnancy testing can be assessed and counseling regarding avoidance of pregnancy and birth defects can be reinforced.

Warnings

➤*Lipid abnormalities:* Bexarotene capsules induce major lipid abnormalities in most patients. These must be monitored and treated during long-term therapy. About 70% of patients with CTCL who received an initial dose of greater than or equal to 300 mg/m²/day of bexarotene capsules had fasting triglyceride levels greater than 2.5 times the upper limit of normal. About 55% had values over 800 mg/dL with a median of about 1200 mg/dL in those patients. Cholesterol elevations above 300 mg/dL occurred in approximately 60% and 75% of patients with CTCL who received an initial dose of 300 mg/m²/day or greater than 300 mg/m²/day, respectively. Decreases in high density lipoprotein (HDL) cholesterol to less than 25 mg/dL were seen in about 55% and 90% of patients receiving an initial dose of 300 mg/m²/day or greater than 300 mg/m²/day, respectively, of bexarotene capsules. The effects on triglycerides, HDL cholesterol, and total cholesterol were reversible with cessation of therapy, and could generally be mitigated by dose reduction or concomitant antilipemic therapy.

Fasting blood lipid determinations should be performed before bexarotene capsules therapy is initiated and weekly until the lipid response to bexarotene capsules is established, which usually occurs within 2 to 4 weeks, and at 8 week intervals thereafter. Fasting triglycerides should be normal or normalized with appropriate intervention prior to initiating bexarotene capsules therapy. Attempts should be made to maintain triglyceride levels below 400 mg/dL to reduce the risk of clinical sequelae. If fasting triglycerides are elevated or become elevated during treatment, antilipemic therapy should be instituted, and if necessary, the dose of bexarotene capsules reduced or suspended. In the 300 mg/m²/day initial dose group, 60% of patients were given lipid lowering drugs. Atorvastatin was used in 48% (73/152) of patients with CTCL. Because of a potential drug-drug interaction, gemfibrozil is not recommended for use with bexarotene capsules.

➤*Pancreatitis:* Acute pancreatitis has been reported in 4 patients with CTCL and in 6 patients with non-CTCL cancers treated with bexarotene capsules; the cases were associated with marked elevations of fasting serum triglycerides, the lowest being 770 mg/dL in 1 patient. One patient with advanced non-CTCL cancer died of pancreatitis. Patients with CTCL who have risk factors for pancreatitis (eg, prior pancreatitis, uncontrolled hyperlipidemia, excessive alcohol consumption, uncontrolled diabetes mellitus, biliary tract disease, and medications known to increase triglyceride levels or to be associated with pancreatic toxicity) should generally not be treated with bexarotene capsules.

➤*Liver function test abnormalities:* For patients with CTCL receiving an initial dose of 300 mg/m²/day of bexarotene capsules, elevations in liver function tests (LFTs) have been observed in 5% (AST), 2% (ALT), and 0% (bilirubin). In contrast, with an initial dose greater than 300 mg/m²/day of bexarotene capsules, the incidence of LFT elevations was higher at 7% (AST), 9% (ALT), and 6% (bilirubin). Two patients developed cholestasis, including 1 patient who died of liver failure. In clinical trials, elevation of LFTs resolved within 1 month in 80% of patients following a decrease in dose or discontinuation of therapy. Baseline LFTs should be obtained, and LFTs should be carefully monitored after 1, 2, and 4 weeks of treatment initiation, and if stable, at least every 8 weeks thereafter during treatment. Consideration should be given to a suspension or discontinuation of bexarotene capsules if test results reach greater than 3 times the upper limit of normal values for AST, ALT, or bilirubin.

➤*Thyroid axis alterations:* Bexarotene capsules induce biochemical evidence of or clinical hypothyroidism in about half of all patients treated, causing a reversible reduction in thyroid hormone (total thyroxine [total T_4]) and thyroid-stimulating hormone (TSH) levels. The incidence of decreases in TSH and total T_4 were about 60% and 45%, respectively, in patients with CTCL receiving an initial dose of 300 mg/m²/day. Hypothyroidism was reported as an adverse event in 29% of patients. Treatment with thyroid hormone supplements should be considered in patients with laboratory evidence of hypothyroidism. In the 300 mg/m²/day initial dose group, 37% of patients were treated with thyroid hormone replacement. Baseline thyroid function tests should be obtained and patients monitored during treatment.

➤*Leukopenia:* A total of 18% of patients with CTCL receiving an initial dose of 300 mg/m²/day of bexarotene capsules had reversible leukopenia in the range of 1000 to less than 3000 WBC/mm³. Patients receiving an initial dose greater than 300 mg/m²/day of bexarotene capsules had an incidence of leukopenia of 43%. No patient with CTCL treated with bexarotene capsules developed leukopenia of less than 1000 WBC/mm³. The time to onset of leukopenia was generally 4 to 8 weeks. The leukopenia observed in most patients was explained by neutropenia. In the 300 mg/m²/day initial dose group, the incidence of NCI grade 3 and grade 4 neutropenia, respectively, was 12% and 4%. The leukopenia and neutropenia experienced during bexarotene capsules therapy resolved after dose reduction or discontinuation of treatment, on average within 30 days in 93% of the patients with CTCL and 82% of patients with non-CTCL cancers. Leukopenia and neutropenia were rarely associated with severe sequelae or serious adverse events. Determination of WBC with differential should be obtained at baseline and periodically during treatment.

➤*Cataracts:* Posterior subcapsular cataracts were observed in preclinical toxicity studies in rats and dogs administered bexarotene daily for 6 months. In 15 of 79 patients who had serial slit lamp examinations, new cataracts or worsening of previous cataracts were found. Because of the high prevalence and rate of cataract formation in older patient populations, the relationship of bexarotene capsules and cataracts cannot be determined in the absence of an appropriate control group. Patients treated with bexarotene capsules who experience visual difficulties should have an appropriate ophthalmologic evaluation.

➤*Hypersensitivity reactions:* Bexarotene capsules should be used with caution in patients with a known hypersensitivity to retinoids. Clinical instances of cross-reactivity have not been noted.

➤*Renal function impairment:* No formal studies have been conducted with bexarotene capsules in patients with renal insufficiency. Urinary elimination of bexarotene and its known metabolites is a minor excretory pathway for bexarotene (less than 1% of administered dose), but because renal insufficiency can result in significant protein binding changes, and bexarotene is greater than 99% protein bound, pharmacokinetics may be altered in patients with renal insufficiency.

➤*Hepatic function impairment:* No specific studies have been conducted with bexarotene capsules in patients with hepatic insufficiency. Because less than 1% of the dose is excreted in the urine unchanged and there is in vitro evidence of extensive hepatic contribution to bexarotene elimination, hepatic impairment would be expected to lead to greatly decreased clearance. Bexarotene capsules should be used only with great caution in this population.

➤*Fertility impairment:* No formal fertility studies were conducted with bexarotene. Bexarotene caused testicular degeneration when oral doses of 1.5 mg/kg/day were given to dogs for 91 days (producing an AUC of approximately ⅕ the AUC at the recommended human daily dose).

➤*Elderly:* Of the total patients with CTCL in clinical studies of bexarotene capsules, 64% were 60 years or older, while 33% were 70 years or older. No overall differences in safety were observed between patients 70 years or older and younger patients, but greater sensitivity of some older individuals to bexarotene capsules cannot be ruled out. Responses to bexarotene capsules were observed across all age group decades, without preference for any individual age group decade.

➤*Pregnancy:* Category X.

See Contraindications for more information.

➤*Lactation:* It is not known whether bexarotene is excreted in human milk. Because many drugs are excreted in human milk and because of the potential for serious adverse reactions in nursing infants from bexarotene, a decision should be made whether to discontinue nursing or to discontinue the drug, taking into account the importance of the drug to the mother.

➤*Children:* Safety and effectiveness in pediatric patients have not been established.

Precautions

➤*Monitoring:* Blood lipid determinations should be performed before bexarotene capsules are given. Fasting triglycerides should be normal or normalized with appropriate intervention prior to therapy. Hyperlipidemia usually occurs within the initial 2 to 4 weeks. Therefore, weekly lipid determinations are recommended during this interval. Subsequently, in patients not hyperlipidemic, determinations can be performed less frequently.

A white blood cell count with differential should be obtained at baseline and periodically during treatment. Baseline liver function tests should be obtained and should be carefully monitored after 1, 2, and 4 weeks of treatment initiation, and if stable, periodically thereafter during treatment. Baseline thyroid function tests should be obtained and then monitored during treatment as indicated.

➤*Vitamin A supplementation:* In clinical studies, patients were advised to limit vitamin A intake to less than or equal to 15,000 IU/day. Because of the relationship of bexarotene to vitamin A, patients should be advised to limit vitamin A supplements to avoid potential additive toxic effects.

➤*Special risk:*

Diabetes mellitus – Caution should be used when administering bexarotene capsules in patients using insulin, agents enhancing insulin secretion (eg, sulfonylureas), or insulin-sensitizers (eg, troglitazone). Based on the mechanism of action, bexarotene capsules could enhance the action of these agents, resulting in hypoglycemia. Hypoglycemia has not been associated with the use of bexarotene capsules as monotherapy.

BEXAROTENE — ORAL

➤*Photosensitivity:* Retinoids as a class have been associated with photosensitivity. In vitro assays indicate that bexarotene is a potential photosensitizing agent. Mild phototoxicity manifested as sunburn and skin sensitivity to sunlight was observed in patients who were exposed to direct sunlight while receiving bexarotene capsules. Patients should be advised to minimize exposure to sunlight and artificial ultraviolet light while receiving bexarotene capsules.

Drug Interactions

Bexarotene Drug Interactions			
Precipitant drug	Object drug*		Description
CYP450 inducers (eg, rifampin, phenytoin, phenobarbital)	Bexarotene	↓	On the basis of bexarotene metabolism, cytochrome P450 3A4 inducers may reduce plasma bexarotene concentrations.
CYP450 inhibitors (eg, ketoconazole, itraconazole, erythromycin, grapefruit juice)	Bexarotene	↑	On the basis of bexarotene metabolism, cytochrome P450 3A4 inhibitors may increase plasma bexarotene concentrations.
Gemfibrozil	Bexarotene	↑	Coadministration of bexarotene and gemfibrozil resulted in substantial increases in plasma concentrations of bexarotene. Concomitant administration of gemfibrozil with bexarotene is not recommended.
Vitamin A	Bexarotene	↑	Bexarotene is a member of the retinoids. Limit vitamin A supplements to avoid potential additive toxic effects (≤ 15,000 IU/day; see Precautions).
Bexarotene	Vitamin A		
Bexarotene	Antidiabetic agents	↑	Bexarotene may enhance antidiabetic agents, resulting in hypoglycemia (see Precautions).
Bexarotene	Tamoxifen	↓	Coadministration of bexarotene capsules and tamoxifen in women with breast cancer who were progressing on tamoxifen resulted in a modest decrease in plasma tamoxifen concentrations, possibly through an induction of cytochrome P450 3A4.
Bexarotene	Oral contraceptives	↓	Bexarotene can potentially induce metabolic enzymes and thereby theoretically reduce plasma concentrations of hormonal contraceptives. It is strongly recommended that 2 reliable forms of contraception be used concurrently, 1 of which should be nonhormonal.

* ↑ = Object drug increased. ↓ = Object drug decreased.

➤*Drug/Lab test interactions:* CA125 assay values in patients with ovarian cancer may be increased by bexarotene capsule therapy.

➤*Drug/Food interactions:* In all clinical trials, patients were instructed to take bexarotene capsules with or immediately following a meal. In one clinical study, plasma bexarotene AUC and C_{max} values were substantially higher following a fat-containing meal versus those following the administration of a glucose solution. Because safety and efficacy data are based upon administration with food, it is recommended that bexarotene capsules be administered with food.

Adverse Reactions

The safety of bexarotene capsules has been evaluated in clinical studies of 152 patients with CTCL who received bexarotene capsules for up to 97 weeks and in 352 patients in other studies. The mean duration of therapy for the 152 patients with CTCL was 166 days. The most common adverse events reported with an incidence of at least 10% in patients with CTCL treated at an initial dose of 300 mg/m²/day of bexarotene capsules are shown below. The events at least possibly related to treatment are lipid abnormalities (elevated triglycerides, elevated total and LDL cholesterol and decreased HDL cholesterol), hypothyroidism, headache, asthenia, rash, leukopenia, anemia, nausea, infection, peripheral edema, abdominal pain, and dry skin. Most adverse events occurred at a higher incidence in patients treated at starting doses of greater than 300 mg/m²/day (see table).

Adverse events leading to dose reduction or study drug discontinuation in at least 2 patients were hyperlipemia, neutropenia/leukopenia, diarrhea, fatigue/lethargy, hypothyroidism, headache, liver function test abnormalities, rash, pancreatitis, nausea, anemia, allergic reaction, muscle spasm, pneumonia, and confusion.

The moderately severe (NCI grade 3) and severe (NCI grade 4) adverse events reported in 2 or more patients with CTCL treated at an initial dose of 300 mg/m²/day of bexarotene capsules were hypertriglyceridemia, pruritus, headache, peripheral edema, leukopenia, rash, and hypercholesterolemia. Most of these moderately severe or severe adverse events occurred at a higher rate in patients treated at starting doses of greater than 300 mg/m²/day than in patients treated at a starting dose of 300 mg/m²/day.

In patients with CTCL receiving an initial dose of 300 mg/m²/day, the incidence of NCI grade 3 or 4 elevations in triglycerides and total cholesterol was 28% and 25%, respectively. In contrast, in patients with CTCL receiving greater than 300 mg/m²/day, the incidence of NCI Grade 3 or 4 elevated triglycerides and total cholesterol was 45% and 45%, respectively. Other grade 3 and 4 laboratory abnormalities are shown below.

In addition to the 152 patients enrolled in the 2 CTCL studies, 352 patients received bexarotene capsules as monotherapy for various advanced malignancies at doses from 5 mg/m²/day to 1000 mg/m²/day. The common adverse events (incidence greater than 10%) were similar to those seen in patients with CTCL.

In the 504 patients (CTCL and non-CTCL) who received bexarotene capsules as monotherapy, drug-related serious adverse events that were fatal, in 1 patient each, were acute pancreatitis, subdural hematoma, and liver failure.

In the patients with CTCL receiving an initial dose of 300 mg/m²/day of bexarotene capsules, adverse events reported at an incidence of less than 10% and not included in other sections or discussed in other parts of labeling and possibly related to treatment were as follows:

➤*Cardiovascular:* Hemorrhage, hypertension, angina pectoris, right heart failure, syncope, and tachycardia.

➤*CNS:* Depression, agitation, ataxia, cerebrovascular accident, confusion, dizziness, hyperesthesia, hypesthesia, and neuropathy.

➤*Dermatologic:* Skin ulcer, acne, alopecia, skin nodule, maculopapular rash, pustular rash, serous drainage, and vesicular bullous rash.

➤*GI:* Constipation, dry mouth, flatulence, colitis, dyspepsia, cheilitis, gastroenteritis, and melena.

➤*GU:* Albuminuria, hematuria, urinary incontinence, urinary tract infection, urinary urgency, dysuria, kidney function abnormal, and breast pain.

➤*Hematologic/Lymphatic:* Eosinophilia, thrombocythemia, coagulation time increased, lymphocytosis, and thrombocytopenia.

➤*Metabolic/Nutritional:* LDH increased, creatinine increased, hypoproteinemia, hyperglycemia, weight decreased, weight increased, and amylase increased.

➤*Musculoskeletal:* Arthralgia, myalgia, bone pain, myasthenia, and arthrosis.

➤*Respiratory:* Pharyngitis, rhinitis, dyspnea, pleural effusion, bronchitis, cough increased, lung edema, hemoptysis, and hypoxia.

➤*Special senses:* Dry eyes, conjunctivitis, ear pain, blepharitis, corneal lesion, keratitis, otitis externa, and visual field defect.

➤*Miscellaneous:* Chills, cellulitis, chest pain, sepsis, gingivitis, liver failure, and monilia.

➤*Adverse reactions with incidence greater than or equal to 10% in CTCL trials:*

Adverse Reactions in CTL Trials (≥ 10%)		
	Initial assigned dose group	
Body system/Adverse reaction[1,2]	300 mg/m²/day (n = 84)	> 300 mg/m²/day (n = 53)
Metabolic/Nutritional		
Hyperlipidemia	66 (78.6%)	42 (79.2%)
Hypercholesteremia	27 (32.1%)	33 (62.3%)
Lactic dehydrogenase increased	6 (7.1%)	7 (13.2%)
Miscellaneous		
Headache	25 (29.8%)	22 (41.5%)
Asthenia	17 (20.2%)	24 (45.3%)
Infection	11 (13.1%)	12 (22.6%)
Abdominal pain	9 (10.7%)	2 (3.8%)
Chills	8 (9.5%)	7 (13.2%)
Fever	4 (4.8%)	9 (17%)
Flu syndrome	3 (3.6%)	7 (13.2%)
Back pain	2 (2.4%)	6 (11.3%)
Infection, bacterial	1 (1.2%)	7 (13.2%)
Endocrine		
Hypothyroidism	24 (28.6%)	28 (52.8%)
Dermatologic		
Rash	14 (16.7%)	12 (22.6%)
Dry skin	9 (10.7%)	5 (9.4%)
Exfoliative dermatitis	8 (9.5%)	15 (28.3%)

BEXAROTENE — ORAL

Adverse Reactions in CTL Trials (≥ 10%)		
	Initial assigned dose group	
Body system/Adverse reaction[1,2]	300 mg/m²/day (n = 84)	> 300 mg/m²/day (n = 53)
Alopecia	3 (3.6%)	6 (11.3%)
Hematologic/Lymphatic		
Leukopenia	14 (16.7%)	25 (47.2%)
Anemia	5 (6%)	13 (24.5%)
Hypochromic anemia	3 (3.6%)	7 (13.2%)
GI		
Nausea	13 (15.5%)	4 (7.5%)
Diarrhea	6 (7.1%)	22 (41.5%)
Vomiting	3 (3.6%)	7 (13.2%)
Anorexia	2 (2.4%)	12 (22.6%)
Cardiovascular		
Peripheral edema	11 (13.1%)	6 (11.3%)
CNS		
Insomnia	4 (4.8%)	6 (11.3%)

[1] Preferred English term coded according to Ligand-modified COSTART 5 Dictionary.
[2] Patients are counted at most once in each adverse reaction category.

➤*Incidence of moderately severe and severe adverse reactions reported in at least 2 patients (CTCL trials):*

Incidence of Moderately Severe and Severe Adverse Reactions Reported in ≥ 2 Patients (CTCL trials) (%)				
	Initial assigned dose group			
	300 mg/m²/day (n = 84)		> 300 mg/m²/day (n = 53)	
Body system/Adverse reaction[1,2]	Moderate/ Severe	Severe	Moderate/ Severe	Severe
Miscellaneous				
Asthenia	1 (1.2%)	0	11 (20.8%)	0
Headache	3 (3.6%)	0	5 (9.4%)	1 (1.9%)
Infection, bacterial	1 (1.2%)	0	0	2 (3.8%)
Cardiovascular				
Peripheral edema	2 (2.4%)	1 (1.2%)	0	0
GI				
Anorexia	0	0	3 (5.7%)	0
Diarrhea	1 (1.2%)	1 (1.2%)	2 (3.8%)	1 (1.9%)
Pancreatitis	1 (1.2%)	0	3 (5.7%)	0
Vomiting	0	0	2 (3.8%)	0
Endocrine				
Hypothyroidism	1 (1.2%)	1 (1.2%)	2 (3.8%)	0
Hematologic/Lymphatic				
Leukopenia	3 (3.6%)	0	6 (11.3%)	1 (1.9%)
Metabolic/Nutritional				
Bilirubinemia	0	1 (1.2%)	2 (3.8%)	0
Hypercholesteremia	2 (2.4%)	0	5 (9.4%)	0
Hyperlipemia	16 (19%)	6 (7.1%)	17 (32.1%)	5 (9.4%)
AST increased	0	0	2 (3.8%)	0
ALT increased	0	0	2 (3.8%)	0
Respiratory				
Pneumonia	0	0	2 (3.8%)	2 (3.8%)
Dermatologic				
Exfoliative dermatitis	0	1 (1.2%)	3 (5.7%)	1 (1.9%)
Rash	1 (1.2%)	2 (2.4%)	1 (1.9%)	0

[1] Preferred English term coded according to Ligand-modified COSTART 5 Dictionary.
[2] Patients are counted at most once in each adverse reaction category. Patients are classified by the highest severity within each row.

➤*Treatment-emergent abnormal laboratory values in CTCL trials:*

Treatment-Emergent Abnormal Laboratory Values in CTCL Trials (%)				
	Initial assigned dose			
	300 mg/m²/day (n = 83)[1]		> 300 mg/m²/day (n = 53)[1]	
Analyte	Grade 3[2]	Grade 4[2]	Grade 3	Grade 4
Triglycerides[3]	21.3%	6.7%	31.8%	13.6%
Total cholesterol[3]	18.7%	6.7%	15.9%	29.5%
Alkaline phosphatase	1.2%	0	0	1.9%
Hyperglycemia	1.2%	0	5.7%	0
Hypocalcemia	1.2%	0	0	0
Hyponatremia	1.2%	0	0.4%	0
ALT	1.2%	0	1.9%	1.9%
Hyperkalemia	0	0	1.9%	0
Hypernatremia	0	1.2%	0	0
AST	0	0	1.9%	1.9%
Total bilirubin	0	0	0	1.9%
ANC	12%	3.6%	18.9%	7.5%
ALC	7.2%	0	15.1%	0
WBC	3.6%	0	11.3%	0
Hemoglobin	0	0	1.9%	0

[1] Number of patients with at least 1 analyte value post-baseline.
[2] Adapted from NCI Common Toxicity Criteria, grade 3 and 4, Version 2.0. Patients are considered to have had a grade 3 or 4 value if either of the following occurred: Value becomes grade 3 or 4 during the study or value is abnormal at baseline and worsens to grade 3 or 4 on study, including all values beyond study drug discontinuation, as defined in data handling conventions.
[3] The denominator used to calculate the incidence rates for fasting total cholesterol and triglycerides were n = 75 for the 300 mg/m²/day initial dose group and n = 44 for the greater than 300 mg/m²/day initial dose group.

Overdosage

Doses up to 1000 mg/m²/day of bexarotene capsules have been administered in short-term studies in patients with advanced cancer without acute toxic effects. Single doses of 1500 mg/kg and 720 mg/kg were tolerated without significant toxicity in rats and dogs, respectively. These doses are approximately 30 and 50 times, respectively, the recommended human dose on a mg/m² basis.

No clinical experience with an overdose of bexarotene capsules has been reported. Any overdose with bexarotene capsules should be treated with supportive care for the signs and symptoms exhibited by the patient.

Patient Information

Bexarotene capsules can cause major damage to a fetus. Pregnancy must be avoided in patients receiving bexarotene capsules. The health care provider should be contacted immediately if pregnancy is suspected while taking bexarotene capsules and until 1 month after discontinuing bexarotene capsules. For women of childbearing potential, pregnancy tests are required within 1 week before starting bexarotene capsule therapy and monthly while taking bexarotene capsules, confirming absence of pregnancy. Effective contraception (birth control) is required continuously starting 1 month before beginning treatment with bexarotene capsules until 1 month after discontinuing bexarotene capsules. It is strongly recommended that 2 reliable forms of contraception be used together. At least 1 of these 2 forms of contraception should include condoms, diaphragms, cervical caps, IUDs, or spermicides. If the patient is a man and has a partner who is pregnant or capable of becoming pregnant, he should discuss with the partner the precautions that should be taken.

The most common side effect is an increase in blood lipids (fats in the blood). Periodic blood tests will be needed to determine blood levels of lipids, including triglycerides and cholesterol. Medication may be needed to control high fat levels in the blood.

Another common side effect is underactive thyroid. The symptoms of underactive thyroid may be difficult to detect because they may develop very gradually and may be very mild. For example, a patient may begin to always feel tired, low on energy, or unusually cold all the time. A thyroid hormone medication is readily available to fully control these temporary symptoms, so the health care provider should be contacted early if the patient begins to experience any of these symptoms. Periodic blood tests will be needed to detect this.

The patient should not take bexarotene capsules if allergic to the medicine.

The patient should discuss the following conditions with the health care provider (if applicable) before starting to take this medicine: pregnancy or possibility of pregnancy, pancreatitis, breast-feeding, taking gemfibrozil (a medication to reduce high triglyceride and cholesterol levels in the blood), taking tamoxifen.

Because vitamin A in large doses may cause some side effects that are similar to those seen in patients taking bexarotene capsules, advise the patient not take more than the recommended daily dietary allowance of vitamin A (4,000 to 5,000 IU). If taking vitamins, instruct patient to check the label to see how much vitamin A they contain. If unsure, advise patient to ask the health care provider or pharmacist.

BEXAROTENE — ORAL

Skin may become more sensitive to sunlight while taking this medicine. Advise patient to minimize exposure to sunlight and to not use a sunlamp.

Advise patient to always take bexarotene capsules as instructed (ie, taking prescribed number of capsules each day; taking the daily dose of bexarotene capsules all at once; taking the dose once each day with or immediately following a meal. For example, a patient may take the daily amount of bexarotene capsules with the evening meal).

Capsules should be swallowed whole; not chewed or dissolved in liquid or in the mouth. Depending on the health and condition of the patient, the health care provider may change the daily dose (the number of capsules taken) during treatment.

If a dose is missed, advise the patient to take it as soon as possible with food. However, if it is nearing time for the next dose, instruct patient to skip the missed dose and continue the dose schedule as before and not double the dose.

If too many bexarotene capsules are taken or someone else accidentally takes the medicine, instruct patients to contact their health care provider, emergency room, or the nearest hospital immediately.

Although some patients see improvement within the first several weeks of bexarotene capsule treatment, most patients require several months or more of treatment to improve CTCL. The health care provider should determine how long to take bexarotene capsules and when treatment may be stopped.

As an infrequent side effect of bexarotene capsule treatment, pancreatitis (inflamed pancreas) may occur. Symptoms of pancreatitis include persistent nausea, vomiting, and abdominal or back pain. If the patient develops any of these symptoms while taking bexarotene capsules, contact the health care provider immediately.

Store capsules in a dry place in a closed container, away from light and heat, at room temperature. The capsules should not be used after the expiration date printed on the bottle. Keep this medicine out of the reach and sight of children. If bexarotene capsules are broken or leaking, advise patients not to touch the capsules or the contents and notify the pharmacist immediately. Should the contents of a broken capsule get on the skin, instruct patient to immediately wash the area with soap and water and notify the health care provider.

MONOCLONAL ANTIBODIES

RITUXIMAB

Rx	**Rituxan** (Biogen Idec/Genentech)	**Injection:** 10 mg/mL	Preservative free. Contains 0.7 mg/mL polysorbate 80. In 10 and 50 mL single-use vials.

RITUXIMAB — INJECTION

WARNING

Fatal infusion reactions – Deaths within 24 hours of infusion have been reported. These fatal reactions followed an infusion reaction complex which included hypoxia, pulmonary infiltrates, adult respiratory distress syndrome, myocardial infarction, ventricular fibrillation or cardiogenic shock. Approximately 80% of fatal infusion reactions occurred in association with the first infusion. Signs and symptoms of severe infusion reactions may include hypotension, angioedema, hypoxia or bronchospasm, and may require interruption of rituximab administration. The most severe manifestations and sequelae include pulmonary infiltrates, acute respiratory distress syndrome, MI, ventricular fibrillation, and cardiogenic shock. In the reported cases, the following factors were more frequently associated with fatal outcomes: Female gender, pulmonary infiltrates, and chronic lymphocytic leukemia or mantle cell lymphoma.

Patients who develop severe infusion reactions should have rituximab infusion discontinued and receive medical treatment.

Tumor lysis syndrome (TLS) – Rapid reduction in tumor volume followed by acute renal failure, hyperkalemia, hypocalcemia, hyperuricemia, or hyperphosphatasemia, has been reported within 12 to 24 hours after the first rituximab infusion. Rare instances of fatal outcome have been reported in the setting of TLS following treatment with rituximab. The risks of TLS appear to be higher in patients with high numbers of circulating malignant cells (greater than or equal to 25,000/mm^3) or high tumor burden. Prophylaxis for TLS should be considered for patients at high risk. Correction of electrolytes abnormalities, monitoring of renal function and fluid balance, and supportive care, including dialysis, should be initiated as indicated. Following complete resolution of the complications of TLS, rituximab has been tolerated when readministered in conjunction with prophylactic therapy for TLS in a limited number of cases.

Severe mucocutaneous reactions – Severe mucocutaneous reactions, some with fatal outcome, have been reported in association with rituximab treatment. Mucocutaneous reactions, some with fatal outcome, have been reported in patients treated with rituximab. These reports include paraneoplastic pemphigus (an uncommon disorder which is a manifestation of the patient's underlying malignancy), Stevens-Johnson syndrome, lichenoid dermatitis, vesiculobullous dermatitis, and toxic epidermal necrolysis. The onset of the reaction in the reported cases has varied from 1 to 13 weeks following rituximab exposure. Patients experiencing a severe mucocutaneous reaction should not receive any further infusions and seek prompt medical evaluation. Skin biopsy may help to distinguish among different mucocutaneous reactions and guide subsequent treatment. The safety of readministration of rituximab to patients with any of these mucocutaneous reactions has not been determined.

Indications

➤*Non-Hodgkin's lymphoma (NHL):* For the treatment of patients with relapsed or refractory, low-grade or follicular, CD20 positive, B-cell NHL.

Rituximab is indicated for the first-line treatment of diffuse large B-cell, CD20-positive, NHL in combination with CHOP or other anthracycline-based chemotherapy regimens.

Administration and Dosage

➤*Approved by the FDA:* November 26, 1997.

➤*Relapsed or refractory, low-grade or follicular, CD20-positive, B-cell, NHL:*

Initial therapy – Rituximab is given at 375 mg/m^2 IV infusion once weekly for 4 or 8 doses.

Patients who subsequently develop progressive disease may be safely retreated with rituximab 375 mg/m^2 IV infusion once weekly for 4 doses. Currently there are limited data concerning more than 2 courses.

➤*Diffuse large B-cell NHL:* Rituximab is given at 375 mg/m^2 IV infusion given on Day 1 of each cycle of chemotherapy for up to 8 infusions.

➤*Rituximab as a component of ibritumomab tiuxetan therapeutic regimen:* As a required component of the ibritumomab tiuxetan therapeutic regimen, rituximab 250 mg/m^2 should be infused within 4 hours prior to the administration of Indium-111-(In-111-) ibritumomab tiuxetan and within 4 hours prior to the administration of Yttrium-90-(Y-90-) ibritumomab tiuxetan. Administration of rituximab and In-111-ibritumomab tiuxetan should precede rituximab and Y-90-ibritumomab tiuxetan by 7 to 9 days. Refer to the ibritumomab tiuxetan monograph for full prescribing information regarding the ibritumomab tiuxetan therapeutic regimen.

➤*Preparation for administration:* Use appropriate aseptic technique. Withdraw the necessary amount of rituximab and dilute to a final concentration of 1 to 4 mg/mL into an infusion bag containing either 0.9% Sodium Chloride, or 5% Dextrose in Water. Gently invert the bag to mix the solution. Discard any unused portion left in the vial. Parenteral drug products should be inspected visually for particulate matter and discoloration prior to administration.

Rituximab solutions for infusion are stable at 2° to 8°C (36° to 46° F) for 24 hours. Rituximab solutions for infusion have been shown to be stable for an additional 24 hours at room temperature. However, since rituximab solutions do not contain a preservative, diluted solutions should be stored refrigerated (2° to 8°C; 36° to 46°F).

➤*Administration:* Do not administer as an IV push or bolus. Rituximab may be administered in an outpatient setting. Rituximab should be administered intravenously at an initial rate of 50 mg/h.

Hypersensitivity reactions – Hypersensitivity reactions may occur. Rituximab infusion should be interrupted for severe reactions and can be resumed at a 50% reduction in rate (eg, from 100 mg/hr to 50 mg/hr) when symptoms have completely resolved. Treatment of these symptoms with diphenhydramine and acetaminophen is recommended; additional treatment with bronchodilators or IV saline may be indicated. In most cases, patients who have experienced non-life-threatening reactions have been able to complete the full course of therapy. Medications for the treatment of hypersensitivity reactions (eg, epinephrine, antihistamines, and corticosteroids) should be available for immediate use in the event of a reaction during administration. Premedication consisting of acetaminophen and diphenhydramine should be considered before each infusion of rituximab. Premedication may attenuate infusion reactions. Since transient hypotension may occur during rituximab infusion, consideration should be given to withholding antihypertensive medications 12 hours prior to rituximab infusion.

First infusion – The rituximab solution for infusion should be administered intravenously at an initial rate of 50 mg/hr. Rituximab should not be mixed or diluted with other drugs. If hypersensitivity or infusion-related events do not occur, escalate the infusion rate in 50 mg/hr increments every 30 minutes, to a maximum of 400 mg/hr. If hypersensitivity (non-IgE-mediated) or an infusion-related event develops, the infusion should be temporarily slowed or interrupted. The infusion can continue at one-half the previous rate upon improvement of patient symptoms.

Subsequent infusions – If the patient tolerated the first infusion well, subsequent rituximab infusions can be administered at an initial rate of 100 mg/hr, and increased by 100 mg/hr increments at 30-minute intervals, to a maximum of 400 mg/hr as tolerated. If the patient did not tolerate the first infusion well, follow the guidelines under First infusion.

➤*Admixture incompatibilities:* It should not be mixed or diluted with other drugs. No incompatibilities between rituximab and polyvinylchloride or polyethylene bags have been observed.

RITUXIMAB — INJECTION

➤*Storage / Stability:* Rituximab vials are stable at 2° to 8°C (36° to 46°F). Do not use beyond expiration date stamped on carton. Rituximab vials should be protected from direct sunlight. Rituximab solutions for infusion are stable at 2° to 8°C (36° to 46° F) for 24 hours. Rituximab solutions for infusion have been shown to be stable for an additional 24 hours at room temperature. However, since rituximab solutions do not contain a preservative, diluted solutions should be stored refrigerated (2° to 8°C; 36° to 46°F). No incompatibilities between rituximab and polyvinylchloride or polyethylene bags have been observed.

Actions

➤*Pharmacology:* Rituximab binds specifically to the antigen CD20 (human B-lymphocyte-restricted differentiation antigen, Bp35), a hydrophobic transmembrane protein with a molecular weight of approximately 35 kD located on pre-B and mature B lymphocytes. The antigen is also expressed on greater than 90% of B-cell non-Hodgkin's lymphomas (NHL) but is not found on hematopoietic stem cells, pro-B cells, normal plasma cells or other normal tissues. CD20 regulates an early step(s) in the activation process for cell cycle initiation and differentiation, and possibly functions as a calcium ion channel. CD20 is not shed from the cell surface and does not internalize upon antibody binding. Free CD20 antigen is not found in the circulation.

The Fab domain of rituximab binds to the CD20 antigen on B lymphocytes, and the Fc domain recruits immune effector functions to mediate B-cell lysis in vitro. Possible mechanisms of cell lysis include complement-dependent cytotoxicity (CDC) and antibody-dependent cell mediated cytotoxicity (ADCC). The antibody has been shown to induce apoptosis in the DHL-4 human B-cell lymphoma line.

Normal tissue cross-reactivity – Rituximab binding was observed on lymphoid cells in the thymus, the white pulp of the spleen, and a majority of B lymphocytes in peripheral blood and lymph nodes. Little or no binding was observed in the nonlymphoid tissues examined.

➤*Pharmacokinetics:* In patients given single doses at 10, 50, 100, 250 or 500 mg/m^2 as an IV infusion, serum levels and the half-life of rituximab were proportional to dose. In 14 patients given 375 mg/m^2 as an IV infusion for 4 weekly doses, the mean serum half-life was 76.3 hours (range, 31.5 to 152.6 hours) after the first infusion and 205.8 hours (range, 83.9 to 407 hours) after the fourth infusion. The wide range of half-lives may reflect the variable tumor burden among patients and the changes in CD20 positive (normal and malignant) B-cell populations upon repeated administrations.

Rituximab at a dose of 375 mg/m^2 was administered as an IV infusion at weekly intervals for 4 doses to 203 patients naive to rituximab. The mean C_{max} following the fourth infusion was 486 mcg/mL (range, 77.5 to 996.6 mcg/mL). The peak and trough serum levels of rituximab were inversely correlated with baseline values for the number of circulating CD20 positive B cells and measures of disease burden. Median steady-state serum levels were higher for responders compared with nonresponders; however, no difference was found in the rate of elimination as measured by serum half-life. Serum levels were higher in patients with International Working Formulation (IWF) subtypes B, C, and D as compared with those with subtype A. Rituximab was detectable in the serum of patients 3 to 6 months after completion of treatment.

Rituximab at a dose of 375 mg/m^2 was administered as an IV infusion at weekly intervals for 8 doses to 37 patients. The mean C_{max} after 8 infusions was 550 mcg/mL (range, 171 to 1177 mcg/mL). The mean C_{max} increased with each successive infusion through the eighth infusion.

The pharmacokinetic profile of rituximab when administered as 6 infusions of 375 mg/m^2 in combination with 6 cycles of CHOP chemotherapy was similar to that seen with rituximab alone.

Administration of rituximab resulted in a rapid and sustained depletion of circulating and tissue-based B cells. Lymph node biopsies performed 14 days after therapy showed a decrease in the percentage of B cells in 7 of 8 patients who had received single doses of rituximab greater than or equal to 100 mg/m^2. Among the 166 patients in the pivotal study, circulating B cells (measured as CD19-positive cells) were depleted within the first 3 doses with sustained depletion for up to 6 to 9 months posttreatment in 83% of patients. Of the responding patients assessed (n = 80), 1% failed to show significant depletion of CD19-positive cells after the third infusion of rituximab as compared to 19% of the nonresponding patients. B-cell recovery began at approximately 6 months following completion of treatment. Median B-cell levels returned to normal by 12 months following completion of treatment.

There were sustained and statistically significant reductions in both IgM and IgG serum levels observed from 5 through 11 months following rituximab administration. However, only 14% of patients had reductions in IgM and/or IgG serum levels, resulting in values below the normal range.

Contraindications

Known anaphylaxis or IgE-mediated hypersensitivity to murine proteins or to any component of this product.

Warnings

➤*Severe infusion reactions:* Rituximab has caused severe infusion reactions. In some cases, these reactions were fatal. These severe reactions typically occurred during the first infusion with time to onset of 30 to 120 minutes. Signs and symptoms of severe infusion reactions may include hypotension, angioedema, hypoxia or bronchospasm, and may require interruption of rituximab administration. The most severe manifestations and sequelae include pulmonary infiltrates, acute respiratory distress syndrome, MI, ventricular fibrillation, and cardiogenic shock. In the reported cases, the following factors were more frequently associated with fatal outcomes: Female gender, pulmonary infiltrates, and chronic lymphocytic leukemia or mantle cell lymphoma.

Management of severe infusion reactions – The rituximab infusion should be interrupted for severe reactions and supportive care measures instituted as medically indicated (eg, IV fluids, vasopressors, oxygen, bronchodilators, diphenhydramine, and acetaminophen). In most cases, the infusion can be resumed at a 50% reduction in rate (eg, from 100 mg/hr to 50 mg/hr) when symptoms have completely resolved. Patients requiring close monitoring during first and all subsequent infusions include those with preexisting cardiac and pulmonary conditions, those with prior clinically significant cardiopulmonary adverse events and those with high numbers of circulating malignant cells (greater than or equal to 25,000/mm^3) with or without evidence of high tumor burden.

➤*Tumor lysis syndrome (TLS):* Rapid reduction in tumor volume followed by acute renal failure, hyperkalemia, hypocalcemia, hyperuricemia, or hyperphosphatasemia, has been reported within 12 to 24 hours after the first rituximab infusion. Rare instances of fatal outcome have been reported in the setting of TLS following treatment with rituximab. The risks of TLS appear to be higher in patients with high numbers of circulating malignant cells (greater than or equal to 25,000/mm^3) or high tumor burden. Prophylaxis for TLS should be considered for patients at high risk. Correction of electrolytes abnormalities, monitoring of renal function and fluid balance, and supportive care, including dialysis, should be initiated as indicated. Following complete resolution of the complications of TLS, rituximab has been tolerated when readministered in conjunction with prophylactic therapy for TLS in a limited number of cases.

➤*Cardiovascular:* Infusions should be discontinued in the event of serious or life-threatening cardiac arrhythmias. Patients who develop clinically significant arrhythmias should undergo cardiac monitoring during and after subsequent infusions of rituximab. Patients with preexisting cardiac conditions including arrhythmias and angina have had recurrences of these events during rituximab therapy and should be monitored throughout the infusion and immediate postinfusion period.

➤*Severe mucocutaneous reactions:* Mucocutaneous reactions, some with fatal outcome, have been reported in patients treated with rituximab. These reports include paraneoplastic pemphigus (an uncommon disorder which is a manifestation of the patient's underlying malignancy), Stevens-Johnson syndrome, lichenoid dermatitis, vesiculobullous dermatitis, and toxic epidermal necrolysis. The onset of the reaction in the reported cases has varied from 1 to 13 weeks following rituximab exposure. Patients experiencing a severe mucocutaneous reaction should not receive any further infusions and seek prompt medical evaluation. Skin biopsy may help to distinguish among different mucocutaneous reactions and guide subsequent treatment. The safety of readministration of rituximab to patients with any of these mucocutaneous reactions has not been determined.

➤*Renal toxicity:* Rituximab administration has been associated with severe renal toxicity including acute renal failure requiring dialysis and in some cases, has led to a fatal outcome. Renal toxicity has occurred in patients with high numbers of circulating malignant cells (greater than 25,000/mm^3) or high tumor burden who experience tumor lysis syndrome (see Tumor lysis syndrome) and in patients administered concomitant cisplatin therapy during clinical trials. The combination of cisplatin and rituximab is not an approved treatment regimen. If this combination is used in clinical trials extreme caution should be exercised; patients should be monitored closely for signs of renal failure. Discontinuation of rituximab should be considered for those with rising serum creatinine or oliguria.

➤*Hypersensitivity reactions:* Rituximab is associated with hypersensitivity reactions (non-IgE-mediated reactions) which may respond to adjustments in the infusion rate and in medical management. Hypotension, bronchospasm, and angioedema have occurred in association with rituximab infusion (see above). Rituximab infusion should be interrupted for severe reactions and can be resumed at a 50% reduction in rate (eg, from 100 mg/hr to 50 mg/hr) when symptoms have completely resolved. Treatment of these symptoms with diphenhydramine and acetaminophen is recommended; additional treatment with bronchodilators or IV saline may be indicated. In most cases, patients who have experienced non-life-threatening reactions have been able to complete the full course of therapy. Medications for the treatment of hypersensitivity reactions (eg, epinephrine, antihistamines, and corticosteroids) should be available for immediate use in the event of a reaction during administration.

➤*Elderly:* Among the 331 patients enrolled in clinical studies of single agent rituximab, 24% were 65 to 75 years old and 5% were 75 years old and older. The overall response rates were higher in older (age greater than or equal to 65 years) vs younger (age less than 65 years) patients (52% vs 44%, respectively). However, the median duration of response, based on Kaplan-Meier estimates, was shorter in older vs younger patients: 10.1 months (range, 1.9 to 36.5+) vs 11.4 months (range, 2.1 to 42.1+), respectively. This shorter duration of response was not statistically significant. Adverse reactions, including incidence, severity and type of adverse reaction were similar between older and younger patients.

➤*Pregnancy:* *Category C* Individuals of childbearing potential should use effective contraceptive methods during treatment and for up to 12 months following rituximab therapy..

Animal reproduction studies have not been conducted with rituximab. It is not known whether rituximab can cause fetal harm when administered to a pregnant woman or whether it can affect reproductive capacity. Human IgG is known to pass the placental barrier, and thus may potentially cause fetal B-cell depletion; therefore, rituximab should be given to a pregnant woman only if clearly needed.

RITUXIMAB — INJECTION

➤*Lactation:* It is not known whether rituximab is excreted in human milk. Because human IgG is excreted in human milk and the potential for absorption and immunosuppression in the infant is unknown, women should be advised to discontinue nursing until circulating drug levels are no longer detectable. The half-life of rituximab varies.

➤*Children:* The safety and effectiveness of rituximab in pediatric patients have not been established.

Precautions

➤*Monitoring:* Because rituximab targets all CD20-positive B lymphocytes, malignant and nonmalignant, complete blood counts (CBC) and platelet counts should be obtained at regular intervals during rituximab therapy and more frequently in patients who develop cytopenias. Grade 3 and 4 cytopenias were reported in 12% of patients treated with rituximab; these include: Lymphopenia (40%), neutropenia (6%), leukopenia (4%), anemia (3%), and thrombocytopenia (2%). The median duration of lymphopenia was 14 days (range, 1 to 588 days) and of neutropenia was 13 days (range, 2 to 116 days). A single occurrence of transient aplastic anemia (pure red cell aplasia) and 2 occurrences of hemolytic anemia following rituximab therapy were reported. In addition, there have been rare postmarketing reports of prolonged pancytopenia and marrow hypoplasia. The duration of cytopenias caused by rituximab can extend well beyond the treatment period.

➤*Human antichimeric antibody (HACA) formation:* HACA was detected in 4 of 356 patients and 3 had an objective clinical response. The data reflect the percentage of patients whose test results were considered positive for antibodies to rituximab using an enzyme-linked immunosorbant assay (limit of detection = 7 ng/mL). The observed incidence of antibody positivity in an assay is highly dependent on the sensitivity and specificity of the assay and may be influenced by several factors including sample handling, concomitant medications, and underlying disease. For these reasons, comparison of the incidence of antibodies to rituximab with the incidence of antibodies to other products may be misleading.

➤*Immunization:* The safety of immunization with live viral vaccines following rituximab therapy has not been studied. The ability to generate a primary or anamnestic humoral response to any vaccine has also not been studied.

Drug Interactions

There have been no formal drug interaction studies performed with rituximab. However, renal toxicity was seen with this drug in combination with cisplatin in clinical trials. The combination of cisplatin and rituximab is not an approved treatment regimen. If this combination is used in clinical trials extreme caution should be exercised; patients should be monitored closely for signs of renal failure.

Adverse Reactions

The most serious adverse reactions caused by rituximab include infusion reactions, tumor lysis syndrome, mucocutaneous reactions, hypersensitivity reactions, cardiac arrhythmias and angina, and renal failure. Infusion reactions and lymphopenia are the most commonly occurring adverse reactions.

Where specific percentages are noted, these data are based on 356 patients treated in nonrandomized, single-arm studies of rituximab administered as a single agent. Most patients received rituximab 375 mg/m^2 weekly for 4 doses. These include 39 patients with bulky disease (lesions greater than or equal to 10 cm) and 60 patients who received more than 1 course of rituximab. Thirty-seven (37) patients received 375 mg/m^2 for 8 doses and 25 patients received doses other than 375 mg/m^2 for 4 doses and up to 500 mg/m^2 single dose in the Phase 1 setting. Adverse events of greater severity are referred to as "Grade 3 and 4 events" defined by the commonly used National Cancer Institute Common Toxicity Criteria.

Incidence of adverse events ≥ 5% of patients in clinical trials (n = 356) (adverse events were followed for a period of 12 months following rituximab therapy)

	All grades (%)	Grade 3 and 4 (%)
Adverse reactions	99%	57%
Miscellaneous	86%	10%
Fever	53%	1%
Chills	33%	3%
Infection	31%	4%
Pain	12%	1%
Back pain	10%	1%
Throat irritation	9%	0%
Flushing	5%	0%
Cardiovascular	25%	3%
Hypotension	10%	1%
Hypertension	6%	1%
GI	37%	2%
Nausea	23%	1%
Abdominal pain	14%	1%
Diarrhea	10%	1%
Vomiting	10%	1%
Hemic/lymphatic	67%	48%
Lymphopenia	48%	40%
Leukopenia	14%	4%
Neutropenia	14%	6%
Thrombocytopenia	12%	2%
Anemia	8%	3%
Metabolic/nutritional	38%	3%
Angioedema	11%	1%
Hyperglycemia	9%	1%
Peripheral edema	8%	0%
LDH increase	7%	0%
Musculoskeletal	26%	3%
Myalgia	10%	1%
Arthralgia	10%	1%
CNS	32%	1%
Dizziness	10%	1%
Asthenia	26%	1%
Headache	19%	1%
Anxiety	5%	1%
Respiratory	38%	4%
Increased cough	13%	1%
Rhinitis	12%	1%
Bronchospasm	8%	1%
Dyspnea	7%	1%
Sinusitis	6%	0%
Dermatologic	44%	2%
Night sweats	15%	1%
Rash	15%	1%
Pruritus	14%	1%
Urticaria	8%	1%

➤*Risk factors associated with increased rates of adverse events:* Administration of rituximab weekly for 8 doses resulted in higher rates of Grade 3 and 4 adverse events overall (70%) compared with administration weekly for 4 doses (57%). The incidence of Grade 3 or 4 adverse events was similar in patients retreated with rituximab compared with initial treatment (58% and 57%, respectively). The incidence of the following clinically significant adverse events was higher in patients with bulky disease (lesions greater than or equal to 10 cm) (n = 39) versus patients with lesions less than 10 cm (n = 195); abdominal pain, anemia, dyspnea, hypotension, and neutropenia.

➤*Infusion reactions:* Mild to moderate infusion reactions consisting of fever and chills/rigors occurred in the majority of patients during the first rituximab infusion. Other frequent infusion reaction symptoms included nausea, pruritus, angioedema, asthenia, hypotension, headache, bronchospasm, throat irritation, rhinitis, urticaria, rash, vomiting, myalgia, dizziness, and hypertension. These reactions generally occurred within 30 to 120 minutes of beginning the first infusion, and resolved with slowing or interruption of the rituximab infusion and with supportive care (diphenhydramine, acetaminophen, IV saline, and vasopressors). In an analysis of data from 356 patients with relapsed or refractory, low-grade NHL who received 4 (n = 319) or 8 (n = 37) weekly infusions of rituximab, the incidence of infusion reactions was highest during the first infusion (77%) and decreased with each subsequent infusion (30% with fourth infusion and 14% with eighth infusion).

➤*Infectious events:* Rituximab induced B-cell depletion in 70% to 80% of patients and was associated with decreased serum immunoglobulins in a minority of patients; the lymphopenia lasted a median of 14 days (range, 1 to 588 days). Infectious events occurred in 31% of patients: 19% of patients had bacterial infections, 10% had viral infections, 1% had fungal infections, and 6% were unknown infections. Incidence is not additive because a single patient may have had more than 1 type of infection. Serious infectious events (Grade 3 or 4), including sepsis, occurred in 2% of patients.

➤*Cardiovascular:* Grade 3 or 4 cardiac-related events include hypotension. Rare, fatal cardiac failure with symptomatic onset weeks after rituximab has also been reported. Patients who develop clinically significant cardiopulmonary events should have rituximab infusion discontinued.

➤*Hematologic:* Grade 3 and 4 cytopenias were reported in 12% of patients treated with rituximab; these include: Lymphopenia (40%), neutropenia (6%), leukopenia (4%), anemia (3%), and thrombocytopenia (2%). The median duration of lymphopenia was 14 days (range, 1 to 588 days) and of neutropenia was 13 days (range, 2 to 116 days). A single occurrence of transient aplastic anemia (pure red cell aplasia) and 2 occurrences of hemolytic

RITUXIMAB — INJECTION

anemia following rituximab therapy were reported. In addition, there have been rare postmarketing reports of prolonged pancytopenia and marrow hypoplasia.

➤*Immunologic:* Immune/autoimmune events have been reported, including uveitis, optic neuritis in a patient with systemic vasculitis, pleuritis in a patient with a lupus-like syndrome, serum sickness with polyarticular arthritis, and vasculitis with rash.

➤*Pulmonary:* One-hundred and thirty-five (135) patients (38%) experienced pulmonary events. The most common respiratory system adverse events experienced were increased cough, rhinitis, bronchospasm, dyspnea, and sinusitis. Three (3) pulmonary events have been reported in temporal association with rituximab infusion as a single agent: Acute bronchospasm, acute pneumonitis presenting 1 to 4 weeks post-rituximab infusion, and bronchiolitis obliterans. One case of bronchiolitis obliterans was associated with progressive pulmonary symptoms and culminated in death several months following the last rituximab infusion. The safety of resumption or continued administration of rituximab in patients with pneumonitis or bronchiolitis obliterans is unknown.

➤*Less commonly observed events:* In clinical trials, less than 5% but greater than 1% of the patients experienced the following events regardless of causality assessment: Agitation, anorexia, arthritis, conjunctivitis, depression, dyspepsia, edema, hyperkinesia, hypertonia, hypesthesia, hypoglycemia, injection site pain, insomnia, lacrimation disorder, malaise, nervousness, neuritis, neuropathy, paresthesia, somnolence, vertigo, weight decrease.

Overdosage

There has been no experience with overdosage in human clinical trials. Single doses of up to 500 mg/m^2 have been given in controlled clinical trials.

IBRITUMOMAB TIUXETAN

Rx	**Zevalin** (Biogen Idec)	**Injection**: 3.2 mg	Preservative free. In 2 mL vials. In In-111 ibritumomab tiuxetan and Y-90 ibritumomab tiuxetan kits with 50 mM sodium acetate vial, formulation buffer vial, reaction vial, and identification labels.[a]

[a] The Indium-111 (In-111) Chloride Sterile Solution must be ordered separately from Amersham Health Inc. or Mallinckrodt, Inc. at the time the In-111 ibritumomab tiuxetan kit is ordered. The Yttrium-90 (Y-90) Chloride Sterile Solution will be shipped directly from MDS Nordion upon placement of an order for the Y-90 ibritumomab tiuxetan kit.

IBRITUMOMAB TIUXETAN — INJECTION

WARNING

Fatal infusion reactions – Deaths have occurred within 24 hours of rituximab infusion, an essential component of the ibritumomab tiuxetan therapeutic regimen. These fatalities were associated with an infusion reaction symptom complex that included hypoxia, pulmonary infiltrates, acute respiratory distress syndrome, MI, ventricular fibrillation, or cardiogenic shock. Approximately 80% of fatal infusion reactions occurred in association with the first rituximab infusion (see Warnings and Adverse Reactions). Discontinue rituximab, In-111 ibritumomab tiuxetan, and Y-90 ibritumomab tiuxetan infusions in patients who develop severe infusion reactions and give medical treatment.

Prolonged and severe cytopenias – Y-90 ibritumomab tiuxetan administration results in severe and prolonged cytopenias in most patients. Do not administer the ibritumomab tiuxetan therapeutic regimen to patients with ≥ 25% lymphoma marrow involvement or impaired bone marrow reserve (see Adverse Reactions).

Dosing – The prescribed, measured, and administered dose of Y-90 ibritumomab tiuxetan should not exceed the absolute maximum allowable dose of 32 mCi (1184 MBq).

Do not administer Y-90 ibritumomab tiuxetan to patients with altered biodistribution as determined by imaging with In-111 ibritumomab tiuxetan.

In-111 ibritumomab tiuxetan and Y-90 ibritumomab tiuxetan are radiopharmaceuticals and should be used only by physicians and other professionals qualified by training and experienced in the safe use and handling of radionuclides.

Indications

➤*Non-Hodgkin's lymphoma (NHL):* As part of the ibritumomab tiuxetan therapeutic regimen for the treatment of patients with relapsed or refractory low-grade, follicular, or transformed B-cell NHL, including patients with rituximab-refractory follicular NHL.

Administration and Dosage

➤*Approved by the FDA:* February 19, 2002.

➤*Rituximab administration:* Note that the dose of rituximab was lower when used as part of the ibritumomab tiuxetan therapeutic regimen, as compared with the dose of rituximab when used as a single agent. Do not administer rituximab as an IV push or bolus. Hypersensitivity reactions may occur (see Warnings). Consider premedication, consisting of acetaminophen and diphenhydramine, before each rituximab infusion.

➤*Dose modification:* Reduce the Y-90 ibritumomab tiuxetan dose to 0.3 mCi/kg (11.1 MBq/kg) for patients with a baseline platelet count between 100,000 and 149,000 cells/mm^3.

➤*Radionuclides:* Two separate and distinctly labeled kits are ordered for the preparation of a single dose each of In-111 ibritumomab tiuxetan and Y-90 ibritumomab tiuxetan. In-111 ibritumomab tiuxetan and Y-90 ibritumomab tiuxetan are radiopharmaceuticals and should be used only by physicians and other professionals qualified by training and experienced in the safe use and handling of radionuclides. Changing the ratio of any of the reactants in the radiolabeling process may adversely impact therapeutic results. In-111 ibritumomab tiuxetan and Y-90 ibritumomab tiuxetan should not be used in the absence of the rituximab predose.

➤*Ibritumomab tiuxetan therapeutic regimen administration:*

Step 1 –

First rituximab infusion: Administer rituximab at a dose of 250 mg/m^2 IV at an initial rate of 50 mg/hr. Do not mix or dilute rituximab with other drugs. If hypersensitivity or infusion-related events do not occur, escalate the infusion rate in 50 mg/hr increments every 30 minutes, to a maximum of 400 mg/hr. If hypersensitivity or an infusion-related event develops, temporarily slow or interrupt the infusion (see Warnings). The infusion can continue at 50% the previous rate upon improvement of patient symptoms.

In-111 ibritumomab tiuxetan injection: Within 4 hours following completion of the rituximab dose, 5 mCi (1.6 mg total antibody dose) of In-111 ibritumomab tiuxetan is injected IV over a period of 10 minutes.

Assess biodistribution:

First image 2 to 24 hours after In-111 ibritumomab tiuxetan;
Second image 48 to 72 hours after In-111 ibritumomab tiuxetan.
Optional: Third image 90 to 120 hours after In-111 ibritumomab tiuxetan.
If biodistribution is not acceptable, do not proceed.

Step 2 – Step 2 of the ibritumomab tiuxetan therapeutic regimen is initiated 7 to 9 days following Step 1 instructions.

Second rituximab infusion: Rituximab at a dose of 250 mg/m^2 is administered IV at an initial rate of 100 mg/hr (50 mg/hr if infusion-related events were documented during the first rituximab administration) and increased by 100 mg/hr increments at 30-minute intervals, to a maximum of 400 mg/hr, as tolerated.

Y-90 ibritumomab tiuxetan injection: Within 4 hours following completion of the rituximab dose, Y-90 ibritumomab tiuxetan at a dose of 0.4 mCi/kg (14.8 MBq/kg) actual body weight for patients with a platelet count > 150,000 cells/mm^3, and 0.3 mCi/kg (11.1 MBq/kg) actual body weight for patients with a platelet count of 100,000 to 149,000 cells/mm^3 is injected IV over a period of 10 minutes. Take precautions to avoid extravasation. Establish a free-flowing IV line prior to Y-90 ibritumomab tiuxetan injection. Close monitoring for evidence of extravasation during the injection of Y-90 ibritumomab tiuxetan is required. If any signs or symptoms of extravasation have occurred, immediately terminate the infusion and restart in another vein. The prescribed, measured, and administered dose of Y-90 ibritumomab tiuxetan must not exceed the absolute maximum allowable dose of 32 mCi (1184 MBq), regardless of the patient's body weight. Do not give Y-90 ibritumomab tiuxetan to patients with a platelet count < 100,000/mm^3 (see Warnings).

See manufacturer's product labeling for product preparation instructions.

➤*Storage/Stability:* Store at 2° to 8°C (36° to 46°F). Do not freeze.

Actions

➤*Pharmacology:* Ibritumomab tiuxetan is the immunoconjugate resulting from a stable thiourea covalent bond between the monoclonal antibody ibritumomab and the linker-chelator tiuxetan. This linker-chelator provides a high affinity, conformationally restricted chelation site for Indium-111 or Yttrium-90. The approximate molecular weight of ibritumomab tiuxetan is 148 kD.

The antibody moiety of ibritumomab tiuxetan is ibritumomab, a murine IgG_1 kappa monoclonal antibody directed against the CD20 antigen, which is found on the surface of normal and malignant B lymphocytes. Ibritumomab is produced in Chinese hamster ovary cells and is composed of 2 murine gamma 1 heavy chains of 445 amino acids each and 2 kappa light chains of 213 amino acids each.

Ibritumomab, like rituximab, induces apoptosis in CD20+ B-cell lines in vitro. The chelate tiuxetan, which tightly binds In-111 or Y-90, is covalently linked to the amino groups of exposed lysines and arginines contained within the antibody. The beta emission from Y-90 induces cellular damage by the formation of free radicals in the target and neighboring cells.

Ibritumomab tiuxetan binding was observed in vitro on lymphoid cells of the bone marrow, lymph node, thymus, red and white pulp of the spleen, and lymphoid follicles of the tonsil, as well as lymphoid nodules of other organs such as the large and small intestines. Binding was not observed on the non-lymphoid tissues or gonadal tissues.

➤*Pharmacokinetics:* In pharmacokinetic studies of patients receiving the ibritumomab tiuxetan therapeutic regimen, the mean effective half-life of Y-90 activity in blood was 30 hours, and the mean area under the fraction of injected activity (FIA) vs time curve in blood was 39 hours. Over 7 days, a median of 7.2% of the injected activity was excreted in urine.

In clinical studies, administration of the ibritumomab tiuxetan therapeutic regimen resulted in sustained depletion of circulating B cells. At 4 weeks, the median number of circulating B cells was 0 (range, 0 to 1084 cells/mm^3). B-cell recovery began at ≈ 12 weeks following treatment, and the median

IBRITUMOMAB TIUXETAN — INJECTION

level of B cells was within the normal range (32 to 341 cells/mm^3) by 9 months after treatment. Median serum levels of IgG and IgA remained within the normal range throughout the period of B-cell depletion. Median IgM serum levels dropped below normal (median, 49 mg/dL; range, 13 to 3990 mg/dL) after treatment and recovered to normal values by 6-month posttherapy.

Contraindications

Patients with known Type I hypersensitivity or anaphylactic reactions to murine proteins or to any component of this product, including rituximab, yttrium chloride, and indium chloride.

Warnings

➤*Altered biodistribution:* Do not administer Y-90 ibritumomab tiuxetan to patients with altered biodistribution of In-111 ibritumomab tiuxetan. The expected biodistribution of In-111 ibritumomab tiuxetan includes easily detectable uptake in the blood pool areas on the first day image, with less activity in the blood pool areas on the second or third day image; moderately high to high uptake in healthy liver and spleen during the first day and the second or third day image; and moderately low or very low uptake in healthy kidneys, urinary bladder, and healthy bowel on the first day image and the second or third day image. Altered biodistribution of In-111 ibritumomab tiuxetan can be characterized by diffuse uptake in normal lung more intense than the cardiac blood pool on the first day image or more intense than the liver on the second or third day image; kidneys with greater intensity than the liver on the posterior view of the second or third day image; or intense areas of uptake throughout the healthy bowel comparable to uptake by the liver on the second or third day images.

➤*Severe infusion reactions:* The ibritumomab tiuxetan therapeutic regimen may cause severe, and potentially fatal, infusion reactions. These severe reactions typically occur during the first rituximab infusion with time to onset of 30 to 120 minutes. Signs and symptoms of severe infusion reaction may include hypotension, angioedema, hypoxia, or bronchospasm, and may require interruption of rituximab, In-111 ibritumomab tiuxetan, or Y-90 ibritumomab tiuxetan administration. The most severe manifestations and sequelae may include pulmonary infiltrates, acute respiratory distress syndrome, MI, ventricular fibrillation, and cardiogenic shock.

Because the ibritumomab tiuxetan therapeutic regimen includes the use of rituximab, also see prescribing information for rituximab (*Rituxan*).

➤*Hematologic toxicity:* The most common severe adverse reactions reported with the ibritumomab tiuxetan therapeutic regimen were thrombocytopenia (61% of patients with platelet counts < 50,000 cells/mm^3) and neutropenia (57% of patients with absolute neutrophil count [ANC] < 1000 cells/mm^3) in patients with ≥ 150,000 platelets/mm^3 prior to treatment. Both incidences of severe thrombocytopenia and neutropenia increased to 78% and 74% for patients with mild thrombocytopenia at baseline (platelet count of 100,000 to 149,000 cells/mm^3). For all patients, the median time to nadir was 7 to 9 weeks and the median duration of cytopenias was 22 to 35 days. In < 5% of cases, patients experienced severe cytopenia that extended beyond the prospectively defined protocol treatment period of 12 weeks following administration of the ibritumomab tiuxetan therapeutic regimen. Some of these patients eventually recovered from cytopenia, while others experienced progressive disease, received further anticancer therapy, or died of their lymphoma without having recovered from cytopenia. The cytopenias may have influenced subsequent treatment decisions.

Hemorrhage, including fatal cerebral hemorrhage, and severe infections have occurred in a minority of patients in clinical studies. Careful monitoring for and management of cytopenias and their complications (eg, febrile neutropenia, hemorrhage) for up to 3 months after use of the ibritumomab tiuxetan therapeutic regimen are necessary. Exercise caution in treating patients with drugs that interfere with platelet function or coagulation following the ibritumomab tiuxetan therapeutic regimen and closely monitor patients receiving such agents.

Do not administer the ibritumomab tiuxetan therapeutic regimen to patients with ≥ 25% lymphoma marrow involvement or impaired bone marrow reserve (eg, prior myeloablative therapies; platelet count < 100,000 cells/mm^3; neutrophil count < 1500 cells/mm^3; hypocellular bone marrow [≤ 15% cellularity or marked reduction in bone marrow precursors]) or to patients with a history of failed stem cell collection.

➤*Viral diseases:* This product contains albumin, a derivative of human blood. Based on effective donor screening and product manufacturing processes, it carries an extremely remote risk for transmission of viral diseases. A theoretical risk for transmission of Creutzfeldt-Jakob disease (CJD) also is considered extremely remote. No cases of transmission of viral disease or CJD have ever been identified for albumin.

➤*Hypersensitivity reactions:* Anaphylactic and other hypersensitivity reactions have been reported following the IV administration of proteins to patients. Medications for the treatment of hypersensitivity reactions (eg, epinephrine, antihistamines, corticosteroids) should be available for immediate use in the event of an allergic reaction during administration of ibritumomab tiuxetan. Screen patients who have received murine proteins for human antimouse antibodies (HAMA). Patients with evidence of HAMA have not been studied and may be at increased risk of allergic or serious hypersensitivity reactions during ibritumomab tiuxetan therapeutic regimen administrations.

➤*Carcinogenesis:* Radiation is a potential carcinogen and mutagen. The ibritumomab tiuxetan therapeutic regimen results in a significant radiation dose to the testes. There is a potential risk that the ibritumomab tiuxetan therapeutic regimen could cause toxic effects on the male and female gonads. Effective contraception should be used during treatment and for up to 12 months following the ibritumomab tiuxetan therapeutic regimen.

➤*Elderly:* No overall differences in safety or efficacy were observed between these subjects and younger subjects, but greater sensitivity of some older individuals cannot be ruled out.

➤*Pregnancy: Category D.* Y-90 ibritumomab tiuxetan can cause fetal harm when administered to a pregnant woman. There are no adequate and well-controlled studies in pregnant women. If this drug is used during pregnancy, or if the patient becomes pregnant while receiving this drug, apprise the patient of the potential hazard to the fetus. Advise women of childbearing age to avoid becoming pregnant.

➤*Lactation:* It is not known whether ibritumomab tiuxetan is excreted in human milk. Because human IgG is excreted in human milk and the potential for ibritumomab tiuxetan exposure in the infant is unknown, advise women to discontinue nursing and substitute formula feedings for breast feedings (see Pharmacology).

➤*Children:* The safety and efficacy of the ibritumomab tiuxetan therapeutic regimen in children have not been established.

Precautions

➤*Monitoring:* Obtain CBC and platelet counts weekly following the ibritumomab tiuxetan therapeutic regimen and until levels recover. Monitor CBC and platelet counts more frequently in patients who develop severe cytopenia, or as clinically indicated.

➤*Radionuclide precautions:* The contents of the ibritumomab tiuxetan kit are not radioactive. However, during and after radiolabeling ibritumomab tiuxetan with In-111 or Y-90, take care to minimize radiation exposure to patients and to medical personnel, consistent with institutional good radiation safety practices and patient management procedures.

➤*Immunization:* The safety of immunization with live viral vaccines following the ibritumomab tiuxetan therapeutic regimen has not been studied. Also, the ability of patients who received the ibritumomab tiuxetan therapeutic regimen to generate a primary or anamnestic humoral response to any vaccine has not been studied.

➤*Secondary malignancies:* A total of 2% of patients developed secondary malignancies following the ibritumomab tiuxetan therapeutic regimen. One patient developed a Grade 1 meningioma, 3 developed acute myelogenous leukemia, and 2 developed a myelodysplastic syndrome. The onset of a second cancer was 8 to 34 months following the ibritumomab tiuxetan therapeutic regimen and 4 to 14 years following the patients' diagnosis of NHL.

➤*Immunogenicity:* Of 211 patients who received the ibritumomab tiuxetan therapeutic regimen in clinical trials and who were followed for 90 days, there were 8 (3.8%) patients with evidence of HAMA (n = 5) or human antichimeric antibody (HACA) (n = 4) at any time during the course of the study. Two patients had low titers of HAMA prior to initiation of the ibritumomab tiuxetan therapeutic regimen; 1 remained positive without an increase in titer while the other had a negative titer posttreatment. Three patients had evidence of HACA responses prior to initiation of the ibritumomab tiuxetan; 1 had a marked increase in HACA titer while the other 2 had negative titers posttreatment. Of the 3 patients who had negative HAMA or HACA titers prior to the ibritumomab tiuxetan therapeutic regimen, 2 developed HAMA in absence of HACA titers, and 1 had HAMA and HACA positive titers posttreatment. Evidence of immunogenicity may be masked in patients who are lymphopenic. There has not been adequate evaluation of HAMA and HACA at delayed timepoints, concurrent with the recovery from lymphopenia at 6 to 12 months, to establish whether masking of the immunogenicity at early timepoints occurs. The data reflects the percentage of patients whose test results were considered positive for antibodies to ibritumomab or rituximab using kinetic enzyme immunoassays to ibritumomab or rituximab. The observed incidence of antibody positivity in an assay is highly dependent on the sensitivity and specificity of the assay and may be influenced by several factors including sample handling and concomitant medications. Comparisons of the incidence of HAMA/HACA to the ibritumomab tiuxetan therapeutic regimen with the incidence of antibodies to other products may be misleading.

Drug Interactions

No formal drug interaction studies have been performed with ibritumomab tiuxetan. Because of the frequent occurrence of severe and prolonged thrombocytopenia, weigh the potential benefits of medications that interfere with platelet function or anticoagulation against the potential increased risks of bleeding and hemorrhage. Patients receiving medications that interfere with platelet function or coagulation should have more frequent laboratory monitoring for thrombocytopenia. In addition, the transfusion practices for such patients may need to be modified given the increased risk of bleeding.

Adverse Reactions

The most serious adverse reactions caused by the ibritumomab tiuxetan therapeutic regimen include the following: Infections (predominantly bacterial in origin), allergic reactions (bronchospasm and angioedema), and hemorrhage while thrombocytopenic (resulting in deaths). In addition, patients who have received the ibritumomab tiuxetan therapeutic regimen have developed myeloid malignancies and dysplasias. Fatal infusion reactions have occurred following the infusion of rituximab.

The most common toxicities reported were the following: Neutropenia, thrombocytopenia, anemia, GI symptoms (eg, nausea, vomiting, abdominal pain, diarrhea), increased cough, dyspnea, dizziness, arthralgia, anorexia, anxiety, and ecchymosis. Hematologic toxicity was often severe and prolonged, whereas most nonhematologic toxicity was mild in severity. The following table lists adverse events that occurred in ≥ 5% of patients. The

IBRITUMOMAB TIUXETAN — INJECTION

second table is a more detailed description of the incidence and duration of hematologic toxicities, according to baseline platelet count (as an indicator of bone marrow reserve).

Incidence of Adverse Reactions in ≥ 5% of Patients Receiving the Ibritumomab Tiuxetan Therapeutic Regimen (n = 349)[a]

Adverse reaction	All grades	Grade 3/4
Any adverse event	99	89
Cardiovascular	17	3
Hypotension	6	1
CNS	27	2
Headache	12	1
Dizziness	10	< 1
Insomnia	5	0
Dermatologic	28	1
Pruritus	9	< 1
Rash	8	< 1
Flushing	6	0
GI	48	3
Nausea	31	1
Abdominal pain	16	3
Vomiting	12	0
Throat irritation	10	0
Diarrhea	9	< 1
Anorexia	8	0
Abdominal enlargement	5	0
Constipation	5	0
GU	6	< 1
Hematologic/Lymphatic	98	86
Thrombocytopenia	95	63
Neutropenia	77	60
Anemia	61	17
Ecchymosis	7	< 1
Metabolic/Nutritional	23	3
Peripheral edema	8	1
Angioedema	5	< 1
Musculoskeletal	18	1
Arthralgia	7	1
Myalgia	7	< 1
Respiratory	36	3
Dyspnea	14	2
Increased cough	10	0
Rhinitis	6	0
Bronchospasm	5	0
Special senses	7	< 1
Miscellaneous		
Asthenia	43	3
Infection	29	5
Chills	24	< 1
Fever	17	1
Pain	13	1
Back pain	8	1

[a] Adverse events were followed for a period of 12 weeks following the first rituximab infusion of the ibritumomab tiuxetan therapeutic regimen.Note: All adverse events are included, regardless of relationship.

The following adverse events (except for those noted in the above table) occurred in between 1% and 4% of patients during the treatment period: Urticaria, anxiety, dyspepsia, sweats (4%); petechia, epistaxis (3%); allergic reaction, melena (2%).

Severe or life-threatening adverse events occurred in 1% to 5% of patients (except for those noted in the above table) consisted of pancytopenia (2%); allergic reactions, GI hemorrhage, melena, tumor pain, apnea (1%). The following severe or life-threatening events occurred in ≤ 1% of patients: Angioedema, tachycardia, urticaria, arthritis, lung edema, pulmonary embolus, encephalopathy, hematemesis, subdural hematoma, vaginal hemorrhage.

➤*Hematologic:* Hematologic toxicity was the most frequently observed adverse event in clinical trials. The following table presents the incidence and duration of severe hematologic toxicity for patients with normal baseline platelet count (≥ 150,000 cells/mm^3) treated with the ibritumomab tiuxetan therapeutic regimen and patients with mild thrombocytopenia (platelet count 100,000 to 149,000 cells/mm^3) at baseline who were treated with a modified ibritumomab tiuxetan therapeutic regimen that included a lower specific activity Y-90 ibritumomab tiuxetan dose at 0.3 mCi/kg (11.1 MBq/kg).

Ibritumomab Tiuxetan Severe Hematologic Toxicity

	Ibritumomab tiuxetan therapeutic regimen using 0.4 mCi/kg Y-90 dose (14.8 MBq/kg)	Modified ibritumomab tiuxetan therapeutic regimen using 0.3 mCi/kg Y-90 dose (11.1 MBq/kg)
ANC		
Median nadir (cells/mm^3)	800	600
Per patient incidence ANC < 1000 cells/mm^3	57%	74%
Per patient incidence ANC < 500 cells/mm^3	30%	35%
Median duration (days)[a] ANC < 1000 cells/mm^3	22	29
Platelets		
Median nadir (cells/mm^3)	41,000	24,000
Per patient incidence Platelets < 50,000 cells/mm^3	61%	78%
Per patient incidence Platelets < 10,000 cells/mm^3	10%	14%
Median duration (days)[b] Platelets < 50,000 cells/mm^3	24	35

[a] Median duration of neutropenia for patients with ANC < 1000 cells/mm^3 (date from last laboratory value showing ANC ≥ 1000 cells/mm^3 to date of first laboratory value following nadir showing ANC ≥ 1000 cells/mm^3, censored at initiation of next treatment or death).

[b] Median duration of thrombocytopenia for patients with platelets < 50,000 cells/mm^3 (date from last laboratory value showing platelet count ≥ 50,000 cells/mm^3 to date of first laboratory value following nadir showing platelet count ≥ 50,000 cells/mm^3, censored at initiation of next treatment or death).

Median time to ANC nadir was 62 days, to platelet nadir was 53 days, and to hemoglobin nadir was 68 days. Information on growth factor use and platelet transfusions is based on 211 patients for whom data were collected. Filgrastim was given to 13% of patients and erythropoietin to 8%. Platelet transfusions were given to 22% of patients and red blood cell transfusions to 20%.

➤*Miscellaneous:*

Infectious events – During the first 3 months after initiating the ibritumomab tiuxetan therapeutic regimen, 29% of patients developed infections. Three percent of patients developed serious infections comprising urinary tract infection, febrile neutropenia, sepsis, pneumonia, cellulitis, colitis, diarrhea, osteomyelitis, and upper respiratory tract infection. Life-threatening infections were reported for 2% of patients that included sepsis, empyema, pneumonia, febrile neutropenia, fever, and biliary stent-associated cholangitis. During follow-up from 3 months to 4 years after the start of treatment with ibritumomab tiuxetan, 6% of patients developed infections. Two percent of patients had serious infections comprising urinary tract infection, bacterial or viral pneumonia, febrile neutropenia, perihilar infiltrate, pericarditis, and IV drug-associated viral hepatitis. One percent of patients had life-threatening infections that included bacterial pneumonia, respiratory disease, and sepsis.

Overdosage

Doses as high as 0.52 mCi/kg (19.2 MBq/kg) of Y-90 ibritumomab tiuxetan were administered in ibritumomab tiuxetan therapeutic regimen clinical trials and severe hematological toxicities were observed. No fatalities or second organ injury resulting from overdosage administrations were documented. However, single doses up to 50 mCi (1850 MBq) of Y-90 ibritumomab tiuxetan and multiple doses of 20 mCi (740 MBq) followed by 40 mCi (1480 MBq) of Y-90 ibritumomab tiuxetan were studied in a limited number of subjects. In these trials, some patients required autologous stem cell support to manage hematological toxicity.

CETUXIMAB

Rx	**Erbitux** (Bristol-Myers Squibb)	**Injection:** 2 mg/mL	Preservative-free. In single-use 50 mL vial.[a]

[a] With 1.88 mg/mL sodium phosphate dibasic heptahydrate and 0.42 mg/mL sodium phosphate monobasic monohydrate.

CETUXIMAB — INJECTION

WARNING

Infusion reactions – Severe infusion reactions occurred with the administration of cetuximab in approximately 3% of patients, rarely with fatal outcome (less than 1 in 1,000). Approximately 90% of severe infusion reactions were associated with the first infusion of cetuximab. Severe infusion reactions are characterized by rapid onset of airway obstruction (bronchospasm, stridor, hoarseness), urticaria, and hypotension. Severe infusion reactions require immediate interruption of the cetuximab infusion and permanent discontinuation from further treatment.

Cardiopulmonary arrest – Cardiopulmonary arrest and/or sudden death occurred in 2% (4/208) of patients with squamous cell carcinoma of the head and neck treated with radiation therapy and cetuximab as compared to none of 212 patients treated with radiation therapy alone. Fatal events occurred within 1 to 43 days after the last cetuximab treatment. Cetuximab in combination with radiation therapy should be used with caution in head and neck cancer patients with known coronary artery disease, congestive heart failure, and arrhythmias. Although the etiology of these events is unknown, close monitoring of serum electrolytes, including serum magnesium, potassium, and calcium, during and after cetuximab therapy is recommended.

Indications

➤*Head and neck cancer:* Cetuximab, in combination with radiation therapy, is indicated for the treatment of locally or regionally advanced squamous cell carcinoma of the head and neck.

Cetuximab as a single agent is indicated for the treatment of patients with recurrent or metastatic squamous cell carcinoma of the head and neck for whom prior platinum-based therapy has failed.

➤*Colorectal cancer:* Cetuximab, used in combination with irinotecan, is indicated for the treatment of epidermal growth factor receptor (EGFR)-expressing, metastatic colorectal carcinoma in patients who are refractory to irinotecan-based chemotherapy.

Cetuximab administered as a single agent is indicated for the treatment of EGFR-expressing, metastatic colorectal carcinoma in patients who are intolerant to irinotecan-based chemotherapy.

Administration and Dosage

➤*Approved by the FDA:* February 12, 2004.

➤*Squamous cell carcinoma of the head and neck:* The recommended dose of cetuximab, in combination with radiation therapy, is 400 mg/m^2 as an initial loading dose (first infusion) administered as a 120 minute IV infusion (maximum infusion rate 5 mL/min) one week prior to initiation of a course of radiation therapy. The recommended weekly maintenance dose (all other infusions) is 250 mg/m^2 infused over 60 minutes (maximum infusion rate 5 mL/min) weekly for the duration of radiation therapy (6–7 weeks). In clinical studies, cetuximab was administered 1 hour prior to radiation therapy.

The recommended dosing regimen for single-agent cetuximab in the treatment of recurrent or metastatic squamous cell carcinoma of the head and neck is a 400 mg/m^2 initial dose followed by 250 mg/m^2 weekly until disease progression or unacceptable toxicity.

➤*Colorectal cancer:* The recommended dose of cetuximab, in combination with irinotecan or as monotherapy, is 400 mg/m^2 as an initial loading dose (first infusion) administered as a 120 minute IV infusion (maximum infusion rate 5 mL/min). The recommended weekly maintenance dose (all other infusions) is 250 mg/m^2 infused over 60 minutes (maximum infusion rate 5 mL/min).

➤*Premedication:* Premedication with an H_1 antagonist (eg, 50 mg of IV diphenhydramine) is recommended.

➤*Dose modifications:*

Infusion reactions – If the patient experiences a mild or moderate (Grade 1 or 2) infusion reaction, permanently reduce the infusion rate by 50%. Appropriate medical resources for the treatment of severe infusion reactions should be available during cetuximab infusions.

Immediately and permanently discontinue cetuximab in patients who experience severe (Grade 3 or 4) infusion reactions.

Dermatologic toxicity and related disorders – If a patient experiences severe acneform rash, make treatment adjustments according to the table below. In patients with mild and moderate skin toxicity, continue treatment without dose modification.

Cetuximab Dose Modification Guidelines

Severe acneform rash	Cetuximab	Outcome	Cetuximab dose modification
First occurrence	Delay infusion 1 to 2 weeks	Improvement	Continue at 250 mg/m^2
		No improvement	Discontinue cetuximab
Second occurrence	Delay infusion 1 to 2 weeks	Improvement	Reduce dose to 200 mg/m^2
		No improvement	Discontinue cetuximab
Third occurrence	Delay infusion 1 to 2 weeks	Improvement	Reduce dose to 150 mg/m^2
		No improvement	Discontinue cetuximab
Fourth occurrence	Discontinue cetuximab		

➤*Preparation for administration:* Do not administer cetuximab as an IV push or bolus.

Administer cetuximab with the use of a low protein binding 0.22-micrometer in-line filter.

Cetuximab is supplied as a 50 mL, single-use vial containing 100 mg of cetuximab at a concentration of 2 mg/mL in phosphate buffered saline. The solution should be clear and colorless and may contain a small amount of easily visible, white, amorphous, cetuximab particulates. Do not shake or dilute.

Cetuximab can be administered via infusion pump or syringe pump.

Infusion pump –
- Draw up the volume of a vial using a sterile syringe attached to an appropriate needle (a vented spike or other appropriate transfer device may be used).
- Fill cetuximab into a sterile evacuated container or bag such as glass containers, polyolefin bags (eg, *Baxter Intravia*), ethylene vinyl acetate bags (eg, *Baxter Clintec*), DEHP plasticized PVC bags (eg, *Abbott Lifecare*), or PVC bags.
- Repeat procedure until the calculated volume has been put into the container. Use a new needle for each vial.
- Administer through a low protein binding 0.22-micrometer in-line filter (placed as proximal to the patient as practical).
- Affix the infusion line, and prime it with cetuximab before starting the infusion.
- Maximum infusion rate should not exceed 5 mL/min.
- Use 0.9% saline solution to flush line at the end of infusion.

Syringe pump –
- Draw up the volume of a vial using a sterile syringe attached to an appropriate needle (a vented spike may be used).
- Place the syringe into the syringe driver of a syringe pump and set the rate.
- Administer through a low protein binding 0.22-micrometer in-line filter rated for syringe pump use (placed as proximal to the patient as practical).
- Connect up the infusion line and start the infusion after priming the line with cetuximab.
- Repeat procedure until the calculated volume has been infused.
- Use a new needle and filter for each vial.
- Maximum infusion rate should not exceed 5 mL/min.
- Use 0.9% saline solution to flush line at the end of infusion.

Cetuximab should be piggybacked to the patient's infusion line.

Following the cetuximab infusion, a 1-hour observation period is recommended.

➤*Storage/Stability:* Store vials under refrigeration at 2° to 8°C (36° to 46°F). Do not freeze. Increased particulate formation may occur at temperatures at or below 0°C (32°F). This product contains no preservatives. Preparations of cetuximab in infusion containers are chemically and physically stable for up to 12 hours at 2° to 8°C (36° to 46°F) and up to 8 hours at controlled room temperature (20° to 25°C; 68° to 77°F). Discard any remaining solution in the infusion container after 8 hours at controlled room temperature or after 12 hours at 2° to 8°C (36° to 46°F). Discard any unused portion of the vial.

Actions

➤*Pharmacology:* Cetuximab binds specifically to the epidermal growth factor receptor (EGFR, HER1, c-ErbB-1) on both normal and tumor cells, and competitively inhibits the binding of epidermal growth factor (EGF) and other ligands, such as transforming growth factor-alpha. Binding of cetuximab to the EGFR blocks phosphorylation and activation of receptor-associated kinases, resulting in inhibition of cell growth, induction of apoptosis, and decreased matrix metalloproteinase and vascular endothelial growth factor production. The EGFR is a transmembrane glycoprotein that is a member of a subfamily of type I receptor tyrosine kinases including EGFR (HER1), HER2, HER3, and HER4. The EGFR is constitutively expressed in many normal epithelial tissues, including the skin and hair follicle. Over-expression of EGFR is also detected in many human cancers including those of the colon and rectum.

In vitro assays and in vivo animal studies have shown that cetuximab inhibits the growth and survival of tumor cells that over-express the EGFR. No antitumor effects of cetuximab were observed in human tumor xenografts lacking EGFR expression. The addition of cetuximab to irinotecan or irinotecan plus 5-fluorouracil in animal studies resulted in an increase in antitumor effects compared to chemotherapy alone.

CETUXIMAB — INJECTION

➤*Pharmacokinetics:*

Absorption/Distribution – Cetuximab administered as monotherapy or in combination with concomitant chemotherapy or radiotherapy exhibits nonlinear pharmacokinetics. The area under the concentration time curve (AUC) increased in a greater than dose proportional manner as the dose increased from 20 to 400 mg/m^2. Cetuximab clearance (CL) decreased from 0.08 to 0.02 L/hr/m^2 as the dose increased from 20 to 200 mg/m^2, and at doses greater than 200 mg/m^2, it appeared to plateau. The volume of the distribution (Vd) for cetuximab appeared to be independent of dose and approximated the vascular space of 2 to 3 L/m^2.

Metabolism/Excretion – Following a 2-hour infusion of 400 mg/m^2 of cetuximab, the maximum mean serum concentration (C_{max}) was 184 mcg/mL (range 92 to 327 mcg/mL) and the mean elimination half-life was 97 hours (range 41 to 213 hours). A 1-hour infusion of 250 mg/m^2 produced a mean C_{max} of 140 mcg/mL (range 120 to 170 mcg/mL). Following the recommended dose regimen (400 mg/m^2 initial dose and 250 mg/m^2 weekly dose), cetuximab concentrations reached steady-state levels by the third weekly infusion with mean peak and trough concentrations across studies ranging from 168 to 235 and 41 to 85 mcg/mL, respectively. The mean half-life was 114 hours (range 75 to 188 hours).

Special populations –

Gender: Female patients had a 25% lower intrinsic cetuximab clearance than male patients. Similar efficacy and safety were observed for female and male patients in the clinical trials; therefore, dose modification based on gender is not necessary. None of the other covariates explored appeared to have an impact on cetuximab pharmacokinetics.

Contraindications

None.

Warnings

➤*Infusion reactions:* Severe infusion reactions occurred with the administration of cetuximab in approximately 3% (17/633) of patients, rarely with fatal outcome (less than 1 in 1,000). Approximately 90% of severe infusion reactions were associated with the first infusion of cetuximab despite the use of prophylactic antihistamines. These reactions were characterized by the rapid onset of airway obstruction (bronchospasm, stridor, hoarseness), urticaria, or hypotension. Exercise caution with every cetuximab infusion, as there were patients who experienced their first severe infusion reaction during later infusions.

Severe infusion reactions require the immediate interruption of cetuximab therapy and permanent discontinuation from further treatment. Appropriate medical therapy including epinephrine, corticosteroids, intravenous antihistamines, bronchodilators, and oxygen should be available for use in the treatment of such reactions. Carefully observe patients until the complete resolution of all signs and symptoms.

In clinical trials, mild to moderate infusion reactions were managed by slowing the infusion rate of cetuximab and by continued use of antihistamine medications (eg, diphenhydramine) in subsequent doses.

➤*Pulmonary toxicity:* Interstitial lung disease was reported in 3 of 633 (less than 0.5%) patients with advanced colorectal cancer receiving cetuximab. Interstitial pneumonitis with noncardiogenic pulmonary edema resulting in death was reported in 1 case. Two patients had preexisting fibrotic lung disease and experienced an acute exacerbation of their disease while receiving cetuximab in combination with irinotecan. In the clinical investigational program, an additional case of interstitial pneumonitis was reported in a patient with head and neck cancer treated with cetuximab and cisplatin. The onset of symptoms occurred between the fourth and eleventh doses of treatment in all reported cases.

In the event of acute onset or worsening pulmonary symptoms, interrupt therapy and initiate a prompt investigation of these symptoms. If interstitial lung disease is confirmed, discontinue cetuximab and treat the patient appropriately.

➤*Dermatologic toxicity:* In cynomolgus monkeys, cetuximab, when administered at doses of approximately 0.4 to 4 times the weekly human exposure (based on total body surface area), resulted in dermatologic findings, including inflammation at the injection site and desquamation of the external integument. At the highest dose level, the epithelial mucosa of the nasal passage, esophagus, and tongue were similarly affected, and degenerative changes in the renal tubular epithelium occurred. Deaths due to sepsis were observed in 50% (5/10) of the animals at the highest dose level beginning after approximately 13 weeks of treatment.

In clinical studies of cetuximab, dermatologic toxicities, including acneform rash, skin drying and fissuring, and inflammatory and infectious sequelae (eg, blepharitis, cheilitis, cellulitis, cyst) were reported. In patients with advanced colorectal cancer, acneform rash was reported in 88% (560/633) of all treated patients, and was severe (Grade 3 or 4) in 12% (79/633) of these patients. Subsequent to the development of severe dermatologic toxicities, complications including *S. aureus* sepsis and abscesses requiring incision and drainage were reported.

Monitor patients developing dermatologic toxicities while receiving cetuximab for the development of inflammatory or infectious sequelae, and initiate appropriate treatment of these symptoms. Institute dose modifications of any future cetuximab infusions in case of severe acneform rash. Consider treatment with topical or oral antibiotics; topical corticosteroids are not recommended.

➤*Hypersensitivity reactions:* Use with caution in patients with known hypersensitivity to cetuximab, murine proteins, or any component of this product.

➤*Fertility impairment:* A 39-week toxicity study in cynomolgus monkeys receiving 0.4 to 4 times the human dose of cetuximab (based on total body surface area) revealed a tendency for impairment of menstrual cycling in treated female monkeys, including increased incidences of irregularity or absence of cycles, when compared to control animals, and beginning from week 25 of treatment and continuing through the 6-week recovery period. Serum testosterone levels and analysis of sperm counts, viability, and motility were not remarkably different between cetuximab-treated and control male monkeys. It is not known if cetuximab can impair fertility in humans.

➤*Elderly:* Of the 633 patients who received cetuximab with irinotecan or cetuximab monotherapy in 4 advanced colorectal cancer studies, 206 patients (33%) were 65 years of age or older. No overall differences in safety or efficacy were observed between these patients and younger patients.

➤*Pregnancy: Category C.* Animal reproduction studies have not been conducted with cetuximab. However, the EGFR has been implicated in the control of prenatal development and may be essential for normal organogenesis, proliferation, and differentiation in the developing embryo. In addition, human IgG1 is known to cross the placental barrier; therefore cetuximab has the potential to be transmitted from the mother to the developing fetus. It is not known whether cetuximab can cause fetal harm when administered to a pregnant woman or whether cetuximab can affect reproductive capacity. There are no adequate and well-controlled studies of cetuximab in pregnant women. Give to a pregnant woman, or any woman not employing adequate contraception only if the potential benefit justifies the potential risk to the fetus. Counsel all patients regarding the potential risk of cetuximab treatment to the developing fetus prior to initiation of therapy. If the patient becomes pregnant while receiving this drug, apprise her of the potential hazard to the fetus or the potential risk for loss of the pregnancy.

➤*Lactation:* It is not known whether cetuximab is secreted in human milk. Because human IgG1 is secreted in human milk, the potential for absorption and harm to the infant after ingestion is unknown. Based on the mean half-life of cetuximab after multiple dosing of 114 hours [range 75 to 188 hours], advise women to discontinue nursing during treatment with cetuximab and for 60 days following the last dose of cetuximab.

➤*Children:* The safety and effectiveness of cetuximab in pediatric patients have not been established.

Precautions

➤*EGF receptor testing:* Patients enrolled in the clinical studies were required to have immunohistochemical evidence of positive EGFR expression using the *DakoCytomation EGFR pharmDx* test kit. Perform assessment for EGFR expression by laboratories with demonstrated proficiency in the specific technology being utilized. Improper assay performance, including use of suboptimally fixed tissue, failure to utilize specified reagents, deviation from specific assay instructions, and failure to include appropriate controls for assay validation, can lead to unreliable results. Refer to the *DakoCytomation* test kit package insert for full instructions on assay performance.

➤*Immunogenicity:* As with all therapeutic proteins, there is potential for immunogenicity. Potential immunogenic responses to cetuximab were assessed using either a double antigen radiometric assay or an enzyme-linked immunosorbant assay. Due to limitations in assay performance and sampling timing, the incidence of antibody development in patients receiving cetuximab has not been adequately determined. The incidence of antibodies to cetuximab was measured by collecting and analyzing serum pre-study, prior to selected infusions and during treatment followup. Patients were considered evaluable if they had a negative pretreatment sample and a posttreatment sample. Nonneutralizing anti-cetuximab antibodies were detected in 5% (28 of 530) of evaluable patients. In patients positive for anti-cetuximab antibody, the median time to onset was 44 days (range 8 to 281 days). Although the number of sero-positive patients is limited, there does not appear to be any relationship between the appearance of antibodies to cetuximab and the safety or antitumor activity of the molecule.

The observed incidence of anti-cetuximab antibody responses may be influenced by the low sensitivity of available assays, inadequate to reliably detect lower antibody titers. Other factors which might influence the incidence of anti-cetuximab antibody response include sample handling, timing of sample collection, concomitant medications, and underlying disease. For these reasons, comparison of the incidence of antibodies to cetuximab with the incidence of antibodies to other products may be misleading.

➤*Photosensitivity:* Patients should wear sunscreen and hats and limit sun exposure while receiving cetuximab as sunlight can exacerbate any skin reactions that may occur.

Drug Interactions

None known.

Adverse Reactions

Except where indicated, the data described below reflect exposure to cetuximab in 633 patients with advanced metastatic colorectal cancer. Cetuximab was studied in combination with irinotecan (n = 354) or as monotherapy (n = 279). Patients receiving cetuximab plus irinotecan received a median of 12 doses (with 88/354 [25%] treated for over 6 months), and patients receiving cetuximab monotherapy received a median of 7 doses (with 26/279 [9%] treated for over 6 months). The population had a median age of 59 and was 60% male and 91% white. The range of dosing for patients receiving cetuximab plus irinotecan was 1 to 84 infusions, and the range of dosing for patients receiving cetuximab monotherapy was 1 to 63 infusions.

The most serious adverse reactions associated with cetuximab were:

- Infusion reaction (3%).
- Dermatologic toxicity (1%).

CETUXIMAB — INJECTION

- Interstitial lung disease (0.5%).
- Fever (5%).
- Sepsis (3%).
- Kidney failure (2%).
- Pulmonary embolus (1%).
- Dehydration (5%) in patients receiving cetuximab plus irinotecan, 2% in patients receiving cetuximab monotherapy.
- Diarrhea (6%) in patients receiving cetuximab plus irinotecan, 0% in patients receiving cetuximab monotherapy.

Thirty-seven (10%) patients receiving cetuximab plus irinotecan and 14 (5%) patients receiving cetuximab monotherapy discontinued treatment primarily because of adverse events.

The most common adverse events seen in 354 patients receiving cetuximab plus irinotecan were acneform rash (88%), asthenia/malaise (73%), diarrhea (72%), nausea (55%), abdominal pain (45%), and vomiting (41%).

The most common adverse events seen in 279 patients receiving cetuximab monotherapy were acneform rash (90%), asthenia/malaise (49%), fever (33%), nausea (29%), constipation (28%), and diarrhea (28%).

Incidence of Adverse Events (≥ 10%) in Patients with Advanced Colorectal Carcinoma

Body system preferred term[1]	Cetuximab plus irinotecan (n = 354) Grades 1 to 4	Cetuximab plus irinotecan (n = 354) Grades 3 and 4	Cetuximab monotherapy (n = 279) Grades 1 to 4	Cetuximab monotherapy (n = 279) Grades 3 and 4
	% of patients			
Body as a whole				
Abdominal pain	45%	8%	25%	7%
Asthenia/malaise[2]	73%	16%	49%	10%
Back pain	16%	3%	11%	3%
Fever[3]	34%	4%	33%	0%
Headache	14%	2%	25%	3%
Infection	16%	1%	11%	1%
Infusion reaction[4]	19%	3%	25%	2%
Pain	23%	6%	19%	5%
GI				
Anorexia	36%	4%	25%	3%
Constipation	30%	2%	28%	1%
Diarrhea	72%	22%	28%	2%
Dyspepsia	14%	0%	7%	0%
Nausea	55%	6%	29%	2%
Stomatitis	26%	2%	11%	< 1%
Vomiting	41%	7%	25%	3%
Hematic/lymphatic				
Anemia	16%	5%	10%	4%
Leukopenia	25%	17%	1%	0%
Metabolic/nutritional				
Dehydration	15%	6%	9%	2%
Peripheral edema	16%	1%	10%	< 1%
Weight loss	21%	0%	9%	1%
CNS				
Depression	10%	0%	9%	0%
Insomnia	12%	0%	10%	< 1%
Respiratory				
Dyspnea[3]	23%	2%	20%	7%
Increased cough	20%	0%	10%	1%
Skin/appendages				
Acneform rash[5]	88%	14%	90%	10%
Alopecia	21%	0%	5%	0%
Conjunctivitis	14%	1%	7%	< 1%
Nail disorder	12%	< 1%	16%	< 1%
Pruritus	10%	1%	10%	< 1%
Skin disorder	15%	1%	5%	0%

[1] Adverse events that occurred (toxicity Grades 1 through 4) in greater than or equal to 10% of patients with refractory colorectal carcinoma treated with cetuximab plus irinotecan or in greater than or equal to 10% of patients with refractory colorectal carcinoma treated with cetuximab monotherapy.
[2] Asthenia/malaise is defined as any event described as "asthenia", "malaise", or "somnolence".
[3] Includes cases reported as infusion reaction.
[4] Infusion reaction is defined as any event described at any time during the clinical study as "allergic reaction" or "anaphylactoid reaction", or any event occurring on the first day of dosing described as "allergic reaction", "anaphylactoid reaction", "fever", "chills", "chills and fever", or "dyspnea".
[5] Acneform rash is defined as any event described as "acne", "rash", "maculopapular rash", "pustular rash", "dry skin", or "exfoliative dermatitis".

➤*Infusion reactions:* In clinical trials, severe, potentially fatal infusion reactions were reported. These events include the rapid onset of airway obstruction (bronchospasm, stridor, hoarseness), urticaria, or hypotension. In studies in advanced colorectal cancer, severe infusion reactions were observed in 3% of patients receiving cetuximab plus irinotecan and 2% of patients receiving cetuximab monotherapy. Grade 1 and 2 infusion reactions, including chills, fever, and dyspnea usually occurring on the first day of initial dosing, were observed in 16% of patients receiving cetuximab plus irinotecan and 23% of patients receiving cetuximab monotherapy.

In the clinical studies described above, a 20 mg test dose was administered IV over 10 minutes prior to the loading dose to all patients. The test dose did not reliably identify patients at risk for severe allergic reactions.

➤*Dermatologic toxicity and related disorders:* Non-suppurative acneform rash described as "acne", "rash", "maculopapular rash", "pustular rash", "dry skin", or "exfoliative dermatitis" was observed in patients receiving cetuximab plus irinotecan or cetuximab monotherapy. One or more of the dermatological adverse events were reported in 88% (14% Grade 3) of patients receiving cetuximab plus irinotecan and in 90% (10% Grade 3) of patients receiving cetuximab monotherapy. Acneform rash most commonly occurred on the face, upper chest, and back, but could extend to the extremities and was characterized by multiple follicular- or pustular-appearing lesions. Skin drying and fissuring were common in some instances, and were associated with inflammatory and infectious sequelae (eg, blepharitis, cellulitis, cyst). Two cases of *S. aureus* sepsis were reported. The onset of acneform rash was generally within the first 2 weeks of therapy. Although in a majority of the patients the event resolved following cessation of treatment, in nearly half of the cases, the event continued beyond 28 days.

A related nail disorder, occurring in 14% of patients (0.3% Grade 3), was characterized as a paronychial inflammation with associated swelling of the lateral nail folds of the toes and fingers, with the great toes and thumbs as the most commonly affected digits.

➤*Use with radiation therapy:* In a study of 21 patients with locally advanced squamous cell cancer of the head and neck, patients treated with cetuximab, cisplatin, and radiation had a 95% incidence of rash (19% Grade 3). The incidence and severity of cutaneous reactions with combined modality therapy appears to be additive, particularly within the radiation port. The addition of radiation to cetuximab therapy in patients with colorectal cancer should be done with appropriate caution.

Overdosage

Single doses of cetuximab higher than 500 mg/m^2 have not been tested. There is no experience with overdosage in human clinical trials.

BEVACIZUMAB

Rx	**Avastin** (Genentech)	**Injection:** 25 mg/mL	Preservative-free. In single-use 4 and 16 mL vials.

BEVACIZUMAB — INJECTION

WARNING

GI perforations/Wound-healing complications – Bevacizumab administration can result in the development of GI perforation and wound dehiscence, in some instances resulting in fatality. GI perforation, sometimes associated with intraabdominal abscess, occurred throughout treatment with bevacizumab (ie, was not correlated to duration of exposure). The incidence of GI perforation in patients receiving bolus irinotecan/5-fluorouracil/leucovorin (IFL)with bevacizumab was 2%. The typical presentation was reported as abdominal pain associated with symptoms such as constipation and vomiting. Include GI perforation in the differential diagnosis of patients who present with abdominal pain on bevacizumab. Permanently discontinue bevacizumab therapy in patients with GI perforation or wound dehiscence requiring medical intervention. The appropriate interval between termination of bevacizumab and subsequent elective surgery required to avoid the risks of impaired wound healing/wound dehiscence has not been determined.

Hemorrhage – Serious, and in some cases fatal, hemoptysis has occurred in patients with non-small cell lung cancer treated with chemotherapy and bevacizumab. In a small study, the incidence of serious or fatal hemoptysis was 31% in patients with squamous histology and 4% in patients with adenocarcinoma receiving bevacizumab as compared with no cases in patients treated with chemotherapy alone. Patients with recent hemoptysis should not receive bevacizumab.

Indications

➤*Colon or rectum metastatic carcinoma:* Bevacizumab, used in combination with intravenous (IV) 5-fluorouracil-based chemotherapy, is indicated for first-line treatment of patients with metastatic carcinoma of the colon or rectum.

➤*Unlabeled uses:* Metastatic renal cell carcinoma; in combination with carboplatin and paclitaxel to treat non-small cell lung cancer.

Administration and Dosage

➤*Approved by the FDA:* February 26, 2004.

The recommended dosage of bevacizumab is 5 mg/kg given once every 14 days as an IV infusion until disease progression is detected.

Do not initiate bevacizumab therapy for at least 28 days following major surgery. The surgical incision should be fully healed prior to initiation of bevacizumab.

➤*Dose modifications:* There are no recommended dose reductions for the use of bevacizumab. If needed, either discontinue or temporarily suspend bevacizumab as described in the following paragraphs.

Permanently discontinue bevacizumab in patients who develop GI perforation, wound dehiscence requiring medical intervention, serious bleeding, a severe arterial thromboembolic event, nephrotic syndrome, or hypertensive crisis.

Temporary suspension of bevacizumab is recommended in patients with evidence of moderate to severe proteinuria pending further evaluation and in patients with severe hypertension that is not controlled with medical management. The risk of continuation or temporary suspension of bevacizumab in patients with moderate to severe proteinuria is unknown.

Suspend bevacizumab at least several weeks prior to elective surgery. Do not resume bevacizumab until the surgical incision is fully healed.

➤*Preparation for administration:* Bevacizumab should be diluted for infusion by a health care provider using aseptic technique. Withdraw the necessary amount of bevacizumab for a dose of 5 mg/kg and dilute in a total volume of 100 mL of 0.9% sodium chloride injection. Discard any unused portion left in a vial, as the product contains no preservatives. Visually inspect parenteral drug products for particulate matter and discoloration prior to administration.

Admixture incompatibility – No incompatibilities between bevacizumab and polyvinylchloride or polyolefin bags have been observed. Do not administer or mix bevacizumab infusions with dextrose solutions.

➤*Administration:* Do not administer as an IV push or bolus. Deliver the initial bevacizumab dose over 90 minutes as an IV infusion following chemotherapy. If the first infusion is well tolerated, the second infusion may be administered over 60 minutes. If the 60-minute infusion is well tolerated, all subsequent infusions may be administered over 30 minutes.

➤*Storage/Stability:* Bevacizumab vials must be refrigerated at 2° to 8°C (36° to 46°F). Protect bevacizumab vials from light. Store in the original carton until time of use. Do not freeze. Do not shake. Diluted bevacizumab solutions for infusion may be stored at 2° to 8°C (36° to 46°F) for up to 8 hours.

Actions

➤*Pharmacology:* Bevacizumab binds VEGF and prevents the interaction of VEGF to its receptors (Flt-1 and KDR) on the surface of endothelial cells. The interaction of VEGF with its receptors leads to endothelial cell proliferation and new blood vessel formation in in vitro models of angiogenesis. Administration of bevacizumab to xenotransplant models of colon cancer in nude (athymic) mice caused reduction of microvascular growth and inhibition of metastatic disease progression.

➤*Pharmacokinetics:*

Absorption/Distribution – The pharmacokinetic profile of bevacizumab was assessed using an assay that measures total serum bevacizumab concentrations (ie, the assay did not distinguish between free bevacizumab and bevacizumab bound to VEGF ligand). Based on a population pharmacokinetic analysis of 491 patients who received 1 to 20 mg/kg of bevacizumab weekly, every 2 weeks or every 3 weeks, the estimated half-life of bevacizumab was approximately 20 days (range, 11 to 50 days). The predicted time to reach steady state was 100 days. The accumulation ratio following a dose of 10 mg/kg of bevacizumab every 2 weeks was 2.8.

Metabolism/Excretion – The clearance of bevacizumab varied by body weight, gender, and tumor burden. After correcting for body weight, men had a higher bevacizumab clearance (0.262 L/day vs 0.207 L/day) and a larger V_c (3.25 L vs 2.66 L) than women. Patients with higher tumor burden (at or above median value of tumor surface area) had a higher bevacizumab clearance (0.249 L/day vs 0.199 L/day) than patients with tumor burdens below the median. In a randomized study of 813 patients (study 1), there was no evidence of lesser efficacy (hazard ratio for overall survival) in men or patients with higher tumor burden treated with bevacizumab as compared with women and patients with low tumor burden. The relationship between bevacizumab exposure and clinical outcomes has not been explored.

Contraindications

None known.

Warnings

➤*GI perforations/Wound-healing complications:* GI perforation and wound dehiscence, complicated by intraabdominal abscesses, occurred at an increased incidence in patients receiving bevacizumab as compared with controls. Bevacizumab has also been shown to impair wound healing in preclinical animal models.

In study 1, 1 of 396 (0.3%) patients receiving bolus-IFL plus placebo, 6 of 392 (2%) patients receiving bolus-IFL plus bevacizumab, and 4 of 109 (4%) patients receiving 5-fluorouracil/leucovorin plus bevacizumab developed GI perforation, in some instances with fatal outcome. These episodes occurred with or without intraabdominal abscesses and at various time points during treatment. The typical presentation was reported as abdominal pain associated with symptoms such as constipation and vomiting.

In addition, 2 of 396 (0.5%) patients receiving bolus-IFL plus placebo, 4 of 392 (1%) patients receiving bolus-IFL plus bevacizumab, and 1 of 109 (1%) patients receiving 5-fluorouracil/leucovorin plus bevacizumab developed a wound dehiscence during study treatment.

The appropriate interval between surgery and subsequent initiation of bevacizumab required to avoid the risks of impaired wound healing has not been determined. In study 1, the clinical protocol did not permit initiation of bevacizumab for at least 28 days following surgery. There was 1 patient (among 501 patients receiving bevacizumab on study 1) in whom an anastomotic dehiscence occurred when bevacizumab was initiated per protocol. In this patient, the interval between surgery and initiation of bevacizumab was greater than 2 months.

Similarly, the appropriate interval between termination of bevacizumab and subsequent elective surgery required to avoid the risks of impaired wound healing has not been determined. In study 1, 39 patients who were receiving bolus-IFL plus bevacizumab underwent surgery following bevacizumab therapy and, of these patients, 6 (15%) had wound healing/bleeding complications. In the same study, 25 patients in the bolus-IFL arm underwent surgery and, of these patients, 1 of 25 (4%) had wound healing/bleeding complications. The longest interval between last dose of study drug and dehiscence was 56 days; this occurred in a patient on the bolus-IFL plus bevacizumab arm. The interval between termination of bevacizumab and subsequent elective surgery should take into consideration the calculated half-life of bevacizumab (approximately 20 days).

Discontinue bevacizumab therapy in patients with GI perforation or wound dehiscence requiring medical intervention.

➤*Hemorrhage:* Two distinct patterns of bleeding have occurred in patients receiving bevacizumab. The first is minor hemorrhage, most commonly grade 1 epistaxis. The second is serious, and in some cases fatal, hemorrhagic events. Serious hemorrhagic events occurred primarily in patients with non-small cell lung cancer, an indication for which bevacizumab is not approved. In a randomized study in patients with non-small cell lung cancer receiving chemotherapy with or without bevacizumab, 4 of 13 (31%) bevacizumab-treated patients with squamous cell histology and 2 of 53 (4%) bevacizumab-treated patients with non-squamous histology experienced life-threatening or fatal pulmonary hemorrhage as compared with none of the 32 (0%) patients receiving chemotherapy alone. Of the patients experiencing events of life-threatening pulmonary hemorrhage, many had cavitation and/or necrosis of the tumor, either preexisting or developing during bevacizumab therapy. These serious hemorrhagic events occurred suddenly and presented as major or massive hemoptysis.

The risk of CNS bleeding in patients with CNS metastases receiving bevacizumab has not been evaluated because these patients were excluded from the manufacturer-sponsored studies following development of CNS hemorrhage in a patient with a CNS metastasis in phase 1 studies.

BEVACIZUMAB — INJECTION

Other serious bleeding events reported in patients receiving bevacizumab were uncommon and included GI hemorrhage, subarachnoid hemorrhage, and hemorrhagic stroke.

Patients with serious hemorrhage (ie, requiring medical intervention) should have bevacizumab treatment discontinued and receive aggressive medical management. Patients with recent hemoptysis should not receive bevacizumab.

➤*Arterial thromboembolic events:* Arterial thromboembolic events occurred at a higher incidence in patients receiving bevacizumab in combination with chemotherapy as compared with those receiving chemotherapy alone. Arterial thromboembolic events included cerebral infarction, transient ischemic attacks (TIAs), myocardial infarction (MI), angina, and a variety of other arterial thromboembolic events. These events were fatal in some instances.

In an exploratory analysis pooling the data from 5 randomized, controlled clinical trials involving 1,745 patients, the overall incidence of arterial thromboembolic events was increased (4.4% vs 1.9%) among the 963 patients treated with bevacizumab in combination with chemotherapy as compared with 782 patients treated with chemotherapy alone. Fatal outcomes from arterial thromboembolic events occurred in 7 of 963 patients (0.7%) who were treated with bevacizumab in combination with chemotherapy, compared with 3 of 782 patients (0.4%) who were treated with chemotherapy alone. The incidences of both cerebrovascular arterial events (1.9% vs 0.5%) and cardiovascular arterial events (2.1% vs 1%) were increased in patients receiving bevacizumab. In addition, there was a correlation between age (65 years and older) and the increase in risk of thromboembolic events.

The safety of resumption of bevacizumab therapy after resolution of an arterial thromboembolic event has not been studied. Permanently discontinue bevacizumab therapy in patients who experience a severe arterial thromboembolic event during treatment.

➤*Hypertension:* The incidence of hypertension and severe hypertension was increased in patients receiving bevacizumab in study 1 (see the following table).

Incidence of Hypertension and Severe Hypertension in Study 1			
	Arm 1 IFL + placebo (n = 394)	Arm 2 IFL + bevacizumab (n = 392)	Arm 3 5-fluorouracil/ leucovorin + bevacizumab (n = 109)
Hypertension[a] (> 150/100 mm Hg)	43%	60%	67%
Severe hypertension[a] (> 200/110 mm Hg)	2%	7%	10%

[a] This includes patients with either a systolic or diastolic reading greater than the cutoff value on one or more occasions.

Among patients with severe hypertension in the bevacizumab arms, slightly over half the patients (51%) had a diastolic reading greater than 110 associated with a systolic reading less than 200.

Medication classes used for management of patients with grade 3 hypertension receiving bevacizumab included angiotensin-converting enzyme inhibitors, beta-blockers, diuretics, and calcium channel blockers. Four months after discontinuation of therapy, persistent hypertension was present in 18 of 26 patients who received bolus-IFL plus bevacizumab and 8 of 10 patients who received bolus-IFL plus placebo.

Across pooled clinical studies (n = 1,032), development or worsening of hypertension resulted in hospitalization or discontinuation of bevacizumab in 17 patients. Four of these 17 patients developed hypertensive encephalopathy. Severe hypertension was complicated by subarachnoid hemorrhage in 1 patient.

In the postmarketing experience, acute increases in blood pressure associated with initial or subsequent infusions of bevacizumab have been reported. Some cases were serious and associated with clinical sequelae.

Permanently discontinue bevacizumab in patients with hypertensive crisis. Temporary suspension is recommended in patients with severe hypertension that is not controlled with medical management.

➤*Proteinuria:* In study 1, both the incidence and severity of proteinuria (defined as a urine dipstick reading of 1+ or greater) was increased in patients receiving bevacizumab as compared with those receiving bolus-IFL plus placebo. Urinary dipstick readings of 2+ or greater occurred in 14% of patients receiving bolus-IFL plus placebo, 17% receiving bolus-IFL plus bevacizumab, and in 28% receiving 5-fluorouracil/leucovorin plus bevacizumab. Twenty-four-hour urine collections were obtained in patients with new onset or worsening proteinuria. None of the 118 patients receiving bolus-IFL plus placebo, 3 of 158 patients (2%) receiving bolus-IFL plus bevacizumab, and 2 of 50 (4%) patients receiving 5-fluorouracil/leucovorin plus bevacizumab who had a 24-hour collection experienced National Cancer Institute-Common Toxicity Criteria (NCI-CTC) grade 3 proteinuria (greater than 3.5 g protein per 24 hours).

In a dose-ranging, placebo-controlled, randomized study of bevacizumab in patients with metastatic renal cell carcinoma, an indication for which bevacizumab is not approved, 24-hour urine collections were obtained in approximately half the patients enrolled. Among patients in whom 24-hour urine collections were obtained, 4 of 19 (21%) patients receiving bevacizumab at 10 mg/kg every 2 weeks, 2 of 14 (14%) receiving bevacizumab at 3 mg/kg every 2 weeks, and none of the 15 placebo patients experienced NCI-CTC grade 3 proteinuria (greater than 3.5 g protein per 24 hours).

Nephrotic syndrome occurred in 5 of 1,032 (0.5%) patients receiving bevacizumab in the manufacturer-sponsored studies. One patient died and 1 required dialysis. In 3 patients, proteinuria decreased in severity several months after discontinuation of bevacizumab. No patient had normalization of urinary protein levels (by 24-hour urine) following discontinuation of bevacizumab.

Discontinue bevacizumab in patients with nephrotic syndrome. The safety of continued bevacizumab treatment in patients with moderate to severe proteinuria has not been evaluated. In most clinical studies, bevacizumab was interrupted for greater than or equal to 2 g of proteinuria per 24 hours and resumed when proteinuria was less than 2 g per 24 hours. Regularly monitor patients with moderate to severe proteinuria based on 24-hour collections until improvement and/or resolution is observed.

➤*Congestive heart failure:* Congestive heart failure (CHF), defined as NCI-CTC grade 2 to 4 left ventricular dysfunction, was reported in 22 of 1,032 (2%) patients receiving bevacizumab in the manufacturer-sponsored studies. Congestive heart failure occurred in 6 of 44 (14%) patients receiving bevacizumab and concurrent anthracyclines. Congestive heart failure occurred in 13 of 299 (4%) patients who received prior anthracyclines and/or left chest wall irradiation. In a controlled study, the incidence was higher in patients receiving bevacizumab plus chemotherapy as compared with patients receiving chemotherapy alone. The safety of continuation or resumption of bevacizumab in patients with cardiac dysfunction has not been studied.

➤*Hypersensitivity reactions:* Use bevacizumab with caution in patients with known hypersensitivity to bevacizumab or any component of this drug product.

➤*Fertility impairment:* Bevacizumab may impair fertility. Dose-related decreases in ovarian and uterine weights, endometrial proliferation, number of menstrual cycles, and arrested follicular development or absent corpora lutea were observed in female cynomolgus monkeys treated with 10 or 50 mg/kg of bevacizumab for 13 or 26 weeks. Following a 4- or 12-week recovery period, which examined only the high-dose group, trends suggestive of reversibility were noted in the 2 females for each regimen that were assigned to recover. After the 12-week recovery period, follicular maturation arrest was no longer observed, but ovarian weights were still moderately decreased. Reduced endometrial proliferation was no longer observed at the 12-week recovery time point, but uterine weight decreases were still notable, corpora lutea were absent in 1 out of 2 animals, and the number of menstrual cycles remained reduced (67%).

➤*Elderly:* In study 1, NCI-CTC grade 3 to 4 adverse reactions were collected in all patients receiving study drug (396 bolus-IFL plus placebo, 392 bolus-IFL plus bevacizumab, 109 5-fluorouracil/leucovorin plus bevacizumab), while NCI-CTC grade 1 and 2 adverse reactions were collected in a subset of 309 patients. There were insufficient numbers of patients 65 years of age and older in the subset in which grade 1 to 4 adverse reactions were collected to determine whether the overall adverse reaction profile was different in the elderly as compared with younger patients. Among the 392 patients receiving bolus-IFL plus bevacizumab, 126 were at least 65 years of age. Severe adverse reactions that occurred at a higher incidence (greater than or equal to 2%) in the elderly when compared with those younger than 65 years of age were asthenia, sepsis, deep thrombophlebitis, hypertension, hypotension, myocardial infarction, CHF, diarrhea, constipation, anorexia, leukopenia, anemia, dehydration, hypokalemia, and hyponatremia. The effect of bevacizumab on overall survival was similar in elderly patients as compared with younger patients.

Of the 742 patients enrolled in the manufacturer-sponsored clinical studies in which all adverse reactions were captured, 212 (29%) were 65 years of age or older and 43 (6%) were 75 years of age or older. Adverse reactions of any severity that occurred at a higher incidence in the elderly as compared with younger patients, in addition to those described above, were dyspepsia, GI hemorrhage, edema, epistaxis, increased cough, and voice alteration.

In an exploratory, pooled analysis of 1,745 patients treated in 5 randomized, controlled studies, there were 618 (35%) patients 65 years of age or older and 1,127 patients younger than 65 years of age. The overall incidence of arterial thromboembolic events was increased in all patients receiving bevacizumab with chemotherapy as compared with those receiving chemotherapy alone, regardless of age. However, the increase in arterial thromboembolic events incidence was greater in patients older than 65 years of age (8.5% vs 2.9%) as compared with those younger than 65 years of age (2.1% vs 1.4%)

➤*Pregnancy: Category C.* Bevacizumab has been shown to be teratogenic in rabbits when administered in doses that are 2-fold greater than the recommended human dose on a mg/kg basis. Observed effects included decreases in maternal and fetal body weights, an increased number of fetal resorptions, and an increased incidence of specific gross and skeletal fetal alterations. Adverse fetal outcomes were observed at all doses tested.

Angiogenesis is critical to fetal development and the inhibition of angiogenesis following administration of bevacizumab is likely to result in adverse effects on pregnancy. There are no adequate and well-controlled studies in pregnant women. Use bevacizumab during pregnancy or in any woman not employing adequate contraception only if the potential benefit justifies the potential risk to the fetus. Counsel all patients regarding the potential risk of bevacizumab to the developing fetus prior to initiation of therapy. If the patient becomes pregnant while receiving bevacizumab, apprise her of the potential hazard to the fetus or the potential risk of loss of pregnancy. Also counsel patients who discontinue bevacizumab concerning the prolonged exposure following discontinuation of therapy (half-life of approximately 20 days) and the possible effects of bevacizumab on fetal development.

BEVACIZUMAB — INJECTION

➤*Lactation:* It is not known whether bevacizumab is secreted in human milk. Because human IgG1 is secreted into human milk, the potential for absorption and harm to the infant after ingestion is unknown. Advise women to discontinue breast-feeding during treatment with bevacizumab and for a prolonged period following the use of bevacizumab, taking into account the half-life of the product, approximately 20 days (range, 11 to 50 days).

➤*Children:* The safety and efficacy of bevacizumab in pediatric patients have not been studied. However, physeal dysplasia was observed in juvenile cynomolgus monkeys with open growth plates treated for 4 weeks with doses that were less than the recommended human dose based on mg/kg and exposure. The incidence and severity of physeal dysplasia were dose-related and were at least partially reversible upon cessation of treatment.

Precautions

➤*Monitoring:* Conduct blood pressure monitoring every 2 to 3 weeks during treatment with bevacizumab. Patients who develop hypertension on bevacizumab may require blood pressure monitoring at more frequent intervals. Patients with bevacizumab-induced or -exacerbated hypertension who discontinue bevacizumab should continue to have their blood pressure monitored at regular intervals.

Monitor patients receiving bevacizumab for the development or worsening of proteinuria with serial urinalyses. Patients with a 2+ or greater urine dipstick reading should undergo further assessment (eg, a 24-hour urine collection).

➤*Infusion reactions:* In clinical studies, infusion reactions with the first dose of bevacizumab were uncommon (less than 3%), and severe reactions occurred in 0.2% of patients. Infusion reactions reported in the clinical trials and postmarketing experience include hypertension, hypertensive crises associated with neurologic signs and symptoms, wheezing, oxygen desaturation, grade 3 hypersensitivity, chest pain, headaches, rigors, and diaphoresis. Adequate information on rechallenge is not available. Interrupt bevacizumab infusion and administer appropriate medical therapy in all patients with severe infusion reactions.

There are no data regarding the most appropriate method of identification of patients who may safely be retreated with bevacizumab after experiencing a severe infusion reaction.

➤*Surgery:* Do not initiate bevacizumab therapy for at least 28 days following major surgery. The surgical incision should be fully healed prior to initiation of bevacizumab. Because of the potential for impaired wound healing, suspend bevacizumab prior to elective surgery. The appropriate interval between the last dose of bevacizumab and elective surgery is unknown; however, the half-life of bevacizumab is estimated to be 20 days and the interval chosen should take into consideration the half-life of the drug.

➤*Cardiovascular disease:* Patients were excluded from participation in bevacizumab clinical trials if, in the previous year, they had experienced clinically significant cardiovascular disease. In an exploratory analysis pooling the data from 5 randomized, placebo-controlled, clinical trials conducted in patients without a recent history of clinically significant cardiovascular disease, the overall incidence of arterial thromboembolic events, the incidence of fatal arterial thromboembolic events, and the incidence of cardiovascular thromboembolic events were increased in patients receiving bevacizumab plus chemotherapy as compared with bevacizumab alone.

➤*Immunogenicity:* As with all therapeutic proteins, there is a potential for immunogenicity. The incidence of antibody development in patients receiving bevacizumab has not been adequately determined because the assay sensitivity was inadequate to reliably detect lower titers. Enzyme-linked immunosorbent assays (ELISAs) were performed on sera from approximately 500 patients treated with bevacizumab, primarily in combination with chemotherapy. High titer human anti-bevacizumab antibodies were not detected.

Immunogenicity data are highly dependent on the sensitivity and specificity of the assay. Additionally, the observed incidence of antibody positivity in an assay may be influenced by several factors, including sample handling, timing of sample collection, concomitant medications, and underlying disease. For these reasons, comparison of the incidence of antibodies to bevacizumab with the incidence of antibodies to other products may be misleading.

Drug Interactions

➤*Irinotecan:* No formal drug interaction studies with antineoplastic agents have been conducted. In Study 1, patients with colorectal cancer were given irinotecan/5-fluorouracil/leucovorin (bolus-IFL) with or without bevacizumab. Irinotecan concentrations were similar in patients receiving bolus-IFL alone and in combination with bevacizumab. The concentrations of SN38, the active metabolite of irinotecan, were on average 33% higher in patients receiving bolus-IFL in combination with bevacizumab when compared with bolus-IFL alone. In Study 1, patients receiving bolus-IFL plus bevacizumab had a higher incidence of grade 3 to 4 diarrhea and neutropenia. Because of high interpatient variability and limited sampling, the extent of the increase in SN38 levels in patients receiving concurrent irinotecan and bevacizumab is uncertain.

Adverse Reactions

The most serious adverse reactions associated with bevacizumab were GI perforations/wound-healing complications, hemorrhage, arterial thromboembolic events, hypertensive crises, nephrotic syndrome, CHF.

The most common severe (NCI-CTC grade 3 to 4) adverse reactions among 1,032 patients receiving bevacizumab in the manufacturer-sponsored studies were asthenia, pain, hypertension, diarrhea, and leukopenia.

The most common adverse reactions of any severity among the 742 patients receiving bevacizumab in the manufacturer-sponsored studies were asthenia, pain, abdominal pain, headache, hypertension, diarrhea, nausea, vomiting, anorexia, stomatitis, constipation, upper respiratory infection, epistaxis, dyspnea, exfoliative dermatitis, and proteinuria.

In pooled safety data, 1,032 patients with metastatic colorectal cancer (n = 568) and with other cancers (n = 464) received bevacizumab either as a single agent (n = 157) or in combination with chemotherapy (n = 875) in the manufacturer-sponsored clinical trials. All adverse reactions were collected in 742 of the 1,032 patients; for the remaining 290, all NCI-CTC grade 3 and 4 adverse reactions and only selected grade 1 and 2 adverse reactions (hypertension, proteinuria, thromboembolic events) were collected. Adverse reactions across all the manufacturer-sponsored studies were used to further characterize specific adverse reactions.

Comparative data on adverse reactions, except where indicated, are limited to study 1, a randomized, active-controlled study in 897 patients receiving initial treatment for metastatic colorectal cancer. All NCI-CTC grade 3 and 4 adverse reactions and selected grade 1 and 2 adverse reactions (hypertension, proteinuria, thromboembolic events) were reported for the overall study population. In Study 1, the median age was 60 years, 60% were men, 78% had colon primary lesion, and 29% had prior adjuvant or neoadjuvant chemotherapy. The median duration of exposure to bevacizumab in study 1 was 8 months in arm 2 and 7 months in arm 3. All adverse reactions, including all NCI-CTC grade 1 and 2 adverse reactions, were reported in a subset of 309 patients. The baseline entry characteristics in the 309 patient safety subset were similar to the overall study population and well-balanced across the 3 study arms.

NCI-CTC Grade 3 and 4 Adverse Reactions in Study 1 (Occurring at Higher Incidence [≥ 2%] in Bevacizumab vs Control)

	Arm 1 IFL + placebo (n = 396)	Arm 2 IFL + bevacizumab (n = 392)
Grade 3 to 4 reactions	295 (74%)	340 (87%)
Cardiovascular		
Deep vein thrombosis	19 (5%)	34 (9%)
Hypertension	10 (2%)	46 (12%)
Intraabdominal thrombosis	5 (1%)	13 (3%)
GI		
Abdominal pain	20 (5%)	32 (8%)
Constipation	9 (2%)	14 (4%)
Diarrhea	99 (25%)	133 (34%)
Hematologic/Lymphatic		
Leukopenia	122 (31%)	145 (37%)
Neutropenia[a]	41 (14%)	58 (21%)
Miscellaneous		
Asthenia	28 (7%)	38 (10%)
Pain	21 (5%)	30 (8%)
Syncope	4 (1%)	11 (3%)

[a] Central laboratories were collected on days 1 and 21 of each cycle. Neutrophil counts are available in 303 patients in arm 1 and 276 in arm 2.

NCI-CTC Grade 1 to 4 Adverse Reactions in Study 1 Subset (Occurring at Higher Incidence [≥ 5%] in Bevacizumab vs Control)

Adverse reaction	Arm 1 IFL + placebo (n = 98)	Arm 2 IFL + bevacizumab (n = 102)	Arm 3 5-fluorouracil/ leucovorin + bevacizumab (n = 109)
Cardiovascular			
Deep vein thrombosis	3 (3%)	9 (9%)	6 (6%)
Hypertension	14 (14%)	23 (23%)	37 (34%)
Hypotension	7 (7%)	15 (15%)	8 (7%)
Pain	54 (55%)	62 (61%)	67 (62%)
CNS			
Abnormal gait	0 (0%)	1 (1%)	5 (5%)
Confusion	1 (1%)	1 (1%)	6 (6%)
Dizziness	20 (20%)	27 (26%)	21 (19%)
Headache	19 (19%)	27 (26%)	30 (26%)
Dermatologic			
Alopecia	25 (26%)	33 (32%)	6 (6%)
Dry skin	7 (7%)	7 (7%)	22 (20%)
Exfoliative dermatitis	3 (3%)	3 (3%)	21 (19%)
Nail disorder	3 (3%)	2 (2%)	9 (8%)
Skin discoloration	3 (3%)	2 (2%)	17 (16%)
Skin ulcer	1 (1%)	6 (6%)	7 (6%)

BEVACIZUMAB — INJECTION

NCI-CTC Grade 1 to 4 Adverse Reactions in Study 1 Subset (Occurring at Higher Incidence [≥ 5%] in Bevacizumab vs Control)			
Adverse reaction	Arm 1 IFL + placebo (n = 98)	Arm 2 IFL + bevacizumab (n = 102)	Arm 3 5-fluorouracil/ leucovorin + bevacizumab (n = 109)
GI			
Abdominal pain	54 (55%)	62 (61%)	55 (50%)
Anorexia	29 (30%)	44 (43%)	38 (35%)
Colitis	1 (1%)	6 (6%)	1 (1%)
Constipation	28 (29%)	41 (40%)	32 (29%)
Dry mouth	2 (2%)	7 (7%)	4 (4%)
Dyspepsia	15 (15%)	25 (24%)	19 (17%)
Flatulence	10 (10%)	11 (11%)	21 (19%)
GI hemorrhage	6 (6%)	25 (24%)	21 (19%)
Stomatitis	18 (18%)	33 (32%)	33 (30%)
Vomiting	46 (47%)	53 (52%)	51 (47%)
GU			
Proteinuria	24 (24%)	37 (36%)	39 (36%)
Urinary frequency/ urgency	1 (1%)	3 (3%)	6 (6%)
Metabolic/Nutritional			
Bilirubinemia	0 (0%)	1 (1%)	7 (6%)
Hypokalemia	11 (11%)	12 (12%)	18 (16%)
Weight loss	10 (10%)	15 (15%)	18 (16%)
Respiratory			
Dyspnea	15 (15%)	26 (26%)	27 (25%)
Epistaxis	10 (10%)	36 (35%)	35 (32%)
Upper respiratory tract infection	38 (39%)	48 (47%)	44 (40%)
Voice alteration	2 (2%)	9 (9%)	6 (6%)
Special senses			
Excess lacrimation	2 (2%)	6 (6%)	20 (18%)
Taste disorder	9 (9%)	14 (14%)	23 (21%)
Miscellaneous			
Asthenia	68 (70%)	75 (74%)	80 (73%)
Myalgia	7 (7%)	8 (8%)	16 (15%)
Thrombocytopenia	0 (0%)	5 (5%)	5 (5%)

➤*Mucocutaneous hemorrhage:* In study 1, both serious and non-serious hemorrhagic events occurred at a higher incidence in patients receiving bevacizumab. In the 309 patients in which grade 1 to 4 adverse reactions were collected, epistaxis was common and reported in 35% of patients receiving bolus-IFL plus bevacizumab compared with 10% of patients receiving bolus-IFL plus placebo. These reactions were generally mild in severity (NCI-CTC grade 1) and resolved without medical intervention. Other mild to moderate hemorrhagic events reported more frequently in patients receiving bolus-IFL plus bevacizumab when compared with those receiving bolus-IFL plus placebo included GI hemorrhage (24% vs 6%), minor gum bleeding (2% vs 0%), and vaginal hemorrhage (4% vs 2%).

➤*Venous thromboembolic events:* In study 1, 15.1% of patients receiving bolus-IFL plus bevacizumab and 13.6% of patients receiving bolus-IFL plus placebo experienced a grade 3 to 4 thromboembolic event. The incidence of the following grade 3 and 4 thromboembolic events was higher in patients receiving bolus-IFL plus bevacizumab as compared with patients receiving bolus-IFL plus placebo: deep venous thrombosis (34 vs 19 patients), and intraabdominal venous thrombosis (10 vs 5 patients). The incidence of pulmonary embolism was higher in patients receiving bolus-IFL plus placebo (16 vs 20 patients).

In study 1, 53 of 392 (14%) patients who received bolus-IFL plus bevacizumab and 30 of 396 (8%) patients who received bolus-IFL plus placebo had a thromboembolic event and received full-dose warfarin. Two patients in each treatment arm (4 total) developed bleeding complications. In the 2 patients treated with full-dose warfarin and bevacizumab, these events were associated with marked elevations in their INR. Eleven of 53 (21%) patients receiving bolus-IFL plus bevacizumab and 1 of 30 (3%) patients receiving bolus-IFL developed an additional thromboembolic event.

➤*Other serious adverse reactions:* The following other serious adverse reactions are considered unusual in cancer patients receiving cytotoxic chemotherapy and occurred in at least 1 subject treated with bevacizumab in clinical studies:

GI – Anastomotic ulceration, intestinal necrosis, intestinal obstruction, mesenteric venous occlusion.

GU – Ureteral stricture.

Hematologic / Lymphatic – Pancytopenia.

Metabolic / Nutritional – Hyponatremia.

Miscellaneous – Polyserositis.

Overdosage

The maximum tolerated dose of bevacizumab has not been determined. The highest dose tested in humans (20 mg/kg IV) was associated with headache in 9 of 16 patients and with severe headache in 3 of 16 patients.

TRASTUZUMAB

Rx	**Herceptin** (Genentech)	**Powder for injection, lyophilized:** 440 mg	Vial: Preservative free. Diluent: 20 mL vial of bacteriostatic water for injection with 1.1% benzyl alcohol.

TRASTUZUMAB — INJECTION

WARNING

Cardiomyopathy – Trastuzumab administration can result in the development of ventricular dysfunction and congestive heart failure. Left ventricular function should be evaluated in all patients prior to and during treatment with trastuzumab. Discontinuation of trastuzumab treatment should be strongly considered in patients who develop a clinically significant decrease in left ventricular function. The incidence and severity of cardiac dysfunction was particularly high in patients who received trastuzumab in combination with anthracyclines and cyclophosphamide.

Hypersensitivity reactions including anaphylaxis, infusion reactions, and pulmonary events – Trastuzumab administration can result in severe hypersensitivity reactions (including anaphylaxis), infusion reactions, and pulmonary events. Rarely, these have been fatal. In most cases, symptoms occurred during or within 24 hours of administration of trastuzumab. Trastuzumab infusion should be interrupted for patients experiencing dyspnea or clinically significant hypotension. Patients should be monitored until signs and symptoms completely resolve. Discontinuation of trastuzumab treatment should be strongly considered for patients who develop anaphylaxis, angioedema, or acute respiratory distress syndrome.

Indications

➤*Breast cancer:* Trastuzumab as a single agent is indicated for the treatment of patients with metastatic breast cancer whose tumors overexpress the human epidermal growth factor receptor 2 (HER2) protein and who have received 1 or more chemotherapy regimens for their metastatic disease. Trastuzumab in combination with paclitaxel is indicated for treatment of patients with metastatic breast cancer whose tumors overexpress the HER2 protein and who have not received chemotherapy for their metastatic disease. Trastuzumab should be used in patients whose tumors have been evaluated with an assay validated to predict HER2 protein overexpression.

Administration and Dosage

➤*Approved by the FDA:* September 25, 1998.

➤*Usual dose:* The recommended initial loading dose is 4 mg/kg trastuzumab administered as a 90-minute infusion. The recommended weekly maintenance dose is 2 mg/kg trastuzumab and can be administered as a 30-minute infusion if the initial loading dose was well tolerated. Trastuzumab may be administered in an outpatient setting. Trastuzumab is to be diluted in saline for IV infusion. Do not administer as an IV push or bolus.

➤*Preparation for administration:* The diluent provided has been formulated to maintain the stability and sterility of trastuzumab for up to 28 days. Other diluents have not been shown to contain effective preservatives for trastuzumab. Each vial of trastuzumab should be reconstituted with 20 mL of Bacteriostatic Water for Injection, 1.1% benzyl alcohol preserved, as supplied, to yield a multi-dose solution containing 21 mg/mL trastuzumab. Immediately upon reconstitution with Bacteriostatic Water for Injection, the vial of trastuzumab must be labeled in the area marked "Do not use after:" with the future date that is 28 days from the date of reconstitution.

If the patient has known hypersensitivity to benzyl alcohol, trastuzumab must be reconstituted with Sterile Water for Injection. Trastuzumab which has been reconstituted with Sterile Water for Injection must be used immediately and any unused portion discarded. Use of other reconstitution diluents should be avoided.

TRASTUZUMAB — INJECTION

Shaking the reconstituted trastuzumab or causing excessive foaming during the addition of diluent may result in problems with dissolution and the amount of trastuzumab that can be withdrawn from the vial.

Use appropriate aseptic technique when performing the following reconstitution steps:

1.) Using a sterile syringe, slowly inject 20 mL of the diluent into the vial containing the lyophilized cake of trastuzumab. The stream of diluent should be directed into the lyophilized cake.
2.) Swirl the vial gently to aid reconstitution. Trastuzumab may be sensitive to shear-induced stress (eg, agitation or rapid expulsion from a syringe). Do not shake.
3.) Slight foaming of the product upon reconstitution is not unusual. Allow the vial to stand undisturbed for approximately 5 minutes. The solution should be essentially free of visible particulates, clear to slightly opalescent, and colorless to pale yellow.

Determine the number in mg of trastuzumab needed, based on a loading dose of 4 mg trastuzumab/kg body weight or a maintenance dose of 2 mg trastuzumab/kg body weight. Calculate the volume of 21 mg/mL trastuzumab solution and withdraw this amount from the vial and add it to an infusion bag containing 250 mL of 0.9% sodium chloride injection. Dextrose (5%) solution should not be used. Gently invert the bag to mix the solution. The reconstituted preparation results in a colorless to pale yellow transparent solution.

➤*Administration:* Treatment may be administered in an outpatient setting by administration of a 4 mg/kg trastuzumab loading dose by IV infusion over 90 minutes. Do not administer as an IV push or bolus. Patients should be observed for fever and chills or other infusion-associated symptoms. Rarely, these have been fatal. In most cases, symptoms occurred during or within 24 hours of administration of trastuzumab. Trastuzumab infusion should be interrupted for patients experiencing dyspnea or clinically significant hypotension. Patients should be monitored until signs and symptoms completely resolve. Other signs or symptoms may include nausea, vomiting, pain (in some cases at tumor sites), rigors, headache, dizziness, dyspnea, hypotension, rash, and asthenia. If prior infusions are well tolerated, subsequent weekly doses of 2 mg/kg trastuzumab may be administered over 30 minutes.

➤*Admixture incompatibility:* Trastuzumab should not be mixed or diluted with other drugs. Trastuzumab infusions should not be administered or mixed with dextrose solutions.

➤*Storage / Stability:* Vials of trastuzumab are stable at 2° to 8°C (36° to 46°F) prior to reconstitution. Do not use beyond the expiration date stamped on the vial. A vial of trastuzumab reconstituted with Bacteriostatic Water for Injection, as supplied, is stable for 28 days after reconstitution when stored refrigerated at 2° to 8°C (36° to 46°F), and the solution is preserved for multiple use. Discard any remaining multi-dose reconstituted solution after 28 days. If unpreserved Sterile Water for Injection (not supplied) is used, the reconstituted trastuzumab solution should be used immediately and any unused portion must be discarded. Do not freeze trastuzumab that has been reconstituted.

Solution of trastuzumab for infusion diluted in polyvinylchloride or polyethylene bags containing 0.9% sodium chloride injection may be stored at 2° to 8°C (36° to 46°F) for up to 24 hours prior to use. Diluted trastuzumab has been shown to be stable for up to 24 hours at room temperature (2° to 25°C; 36° to 77°F). However, since diluted trastuzumab contains no effective preservative, the reconstituted and diluted solution should be stored refrigerated (2° to 8°C; 36° to 46°F).

Actions

➤*Pharmacology:* The HER2 (or c-erbB2) proto-oncogene encodes a transmembrane receptor protein of 185 kDa, which is structurally related to the epidermal growth factor receptor. HER2 protein overexpression is observed in 25% to 30% of primary breast cancers. HER2 protein overexpression can be determined using an immunohistochemistry (IHC) and gene amplification can be determined using fluorescence in situ hybridization (FISH) of fixed tumor blocks. In referenced studies where trastuzumab use was not studied, approximately 96% to 98% of biopsy specimens that were found to have protein overexpression also had gene amplification and 100% of those with gene amplification also had protein overexpression. The precision of the determination of protein overexpression or gene amplification, however, may vary depending on the sensitivity and specificity of the particular assay and assay procedures used. Improper assay performance, including use of suboptimally fixed tissue, failure to utilize specified reagents, deviation from specific assay instructions, and failure to include appropriate controls for assay validation, can lead to unreliable results. When compared to the referenced studies noted above, the correlation between detectable protein overexpression using IHC and detectable gene amplification using FISH was not as high in the studies of trastuzumab clinical trial specimens.

Trastuzumab has been shown, in both in vitro assays and in animals, to inhibit the proliferation of human tumor cells that overexpress HER2.

Trastuzumab is a mediator of antibody-dependent cellular cytotoxicity (ADCC). In vitro, trastuzumab-mediated ADCC has been shown to be preferentially exerted on HER2 overexpressing cancer cells compared with cancer cells that do not overexpress HER2.

➤*Pharmacokinetics:* The pharmacokinetics of trastuzumab were studied in breast cancer patients with metastatic disease. Short duration IV infusions of 10 to 500 mg once weekly demonstrated dose-dependent pharmacokinetics. Mean half-life increased and clearance decreased with increasing dose level. The half-life averaged 1.7 and 12 days at the 10 and 500 mg dose levels, respectively. Trastuzumab's volume of distribution was approximately that of serum volume (44 mL/kg). At the highest weekly dose studied (500 mg), mean peak serum concentrations were 377 mcg/mL.

In studies using a loading dose of 4 mg/kg followed by a weekly maintenance dose of 2 mg/kg, a mean half-life of 5.8 days (range, 1 to 32 days) was observed.

Between weeks 16 and 32, trastuzumab serum concentrations reached a steady-state with a mean trough and peak concentrations of approximately 79 mcg/mL and 123 mcg/mL, respectively.

Detectable concentrations of the circulating extracellular domain of the HER2 receptor (shed antigen) are found in the serum of some patients with HER2 overexpressing tumors. Determination of shed antigen in baseline serum samples revealed that 64% (286 of 447) of patients had detectable shed antigen, which ranged as high as 1,880 ng/mL (median, 11 ng/mL). Patients with higher baseline shed antigen levels were more likely to have lower serum trough concentrations. However, with weekly dosing, most patients with elevated shed antigen levels achieved target serum concentrations of trastuzumab by week 6.

Contraindications

None known.

Warnings

➤*Cardiotoxicity:* Signs and symptoms of cardiac dysfunction, such as dyspnea, increased cough, paroxysmal nocturnal dyspnea, peripheral edema, S_3 gallop, or reduced ejection fraction, have been observed in patients treated with trastuzumab. Congestive heart failure associated with trastuzumab therapy may be severe and has been associated with disabling cardiac failure, death, and mural thrombosis leading to stroke.

Candidates for treatment with trastuzumab should undergo thorough baseline cardiac assessment including history and physical exam and one or more of the following: EKG, echocardiogram, and MUGA scan. There are no data regarding the most appropriate method of evaluation for the identification of patients at risk for developing cardiotoxicity. Monitoring may not identify all patients who will develop cardiac dysfunction.

Extreme caution should be exercised in treating patients with preexisting cardiac dysfunction.

Patients receiving trastuzumab should undergo frequent monitoring for deteriorating cardiac function.

The probability of cardiac dysfunction was highest in patients who received trastuzumab concurrently with anthracyclines. The data suggest that advanced age may increase the probability of cardiac dysfunction.

Preexisting cardiac disease or prior cardiotoxic therapy (eg, anthracycline or radiation therapy to the chest) may decrease the ability to tolerate trastuzumab therapy; however, the data are not adequate to evaluate the correlation between trastuzumab-induced cardiotoxicity and these factors.

Discontinuation of trastuzumab therapy should be strongly considered in patients who develop clinically significant congestive heart failure. In the clinical trials, most patients with cardiac dysfunction responded to appropriate medical therapy often including discontinuation of trastuzumab. The safety of continuation or resumption of trastuzumab in patients who have previously experienced cardiac toxicity has not been studied. There are insufficient data regarding discontinuation of trastuzumab therapy in patients with asymptomatic decreases in ejection fraction; such patients should be closely monitored for evidence of clinical deterioration.

➤*Infusion reactions:* In the postmarketing setting, rare occurrences of severe infusion reactions leading to a fatal outcome have been associated with the use of trastuzumab.

In clinical trials, infusion reactions consisted of a symptom complex characterized by fever and chills, and on occasion included nausea, vomiting, pain (in some cases at tumor sites), headache, dizziness, dyspnea, hypotension, rash, and asthenia. These reactions were usually mild to moderate in severity.

However, in postmarketing reports, more severe adverse reactions to trastuzumab infusion were observed and included bronchospasm, hypoxia, and severe hypotension. These severe reactions were usually associated with the initial infusion of trastuzumab and generally occurred during or immediately following the infusion. However, the onset and clinical course were variable. For some patients, symptoms progressively worsened and led to further pulmonary complications. In other patients with acute onset of signs and symptoms, initial improvement was followed by clinical deterioration. Delayed post-infusion events with rapid clinical deterioration have also been reported. Rarely, severe infusion reactions culminated in death within hours or up to 1 week following an infusion.

Some severe reactions have been treated successfully with interruption of the trastuzumab infusion and administration of supportive therapy including oxygen, IV fluids, beta agonists, and corticosteroids.

There are no data regarding the most appropriate method of identification of patients who may safely be retreated with trastuzumab after experiencing a severe infusion reaction. Trastuzumab has been readministered to some patients who fully recovered from the previous severe reaction. Prior to readministration of trastuzumab, the majority of these patients were prophylactically treated with premedication including antihistamines or corticosteroids. While some of these patients tolerated retreatment, others had severe reactions again despite the use of prophylactic premedications.

➤*Exacerbation of chemotherapy-induced neutropenia:* In randomized, controlled clinical trials designed to assess the impact of the addition of trastuzumab on chemotherapy, the per-patient incidences of moderate to severe neutropenia and of febrile neutropenia were higher in patients receiving trastuzumab in combination with myelosuppressive chemotherapy as compared to those who received chemotherapy alone. In the postmarket-

TRASTUZUMAB — INJECTION

ing setting, deaths due to sepsis in patients with severe neutropenia have been reported in patients receiving trastuzumab and myelosuppressive chemotherapy, although in controlled clinical trials (pre- and postmarketing), the incidence of septic deaths was not significantly increased. The pathophysiologic basis for exacerbation of neutropenia has not been determined; the effect of trastuzumab on the pharmacokinetics of chemotherapeutic agents has not been fully evaluated.

➤*Pulmonary events:* Severe pulmonary events leading to death have been reported rarely with the use of trastuzumab in the postmarketing setting. Signs, symptoms, and clinical findings include dyspnea, pulmonary infiltrates, pleural effusions, non-cardiogenic pulmonary edema, pulmonary insufficiency and hypoxia, and acute respiratory distress syndrome. These events may or may not occur as sequelae of infusion reactions (see Infusion reactions above). Patients with symptomatic intrinsic lung disease or with extensive tumor involvement of the lungs, resulting in dyspnea at rest, may be at greater risk of severe reactions.

Other severe events reported rarely in the postmarketing setting include pneumonitis and pulmonary fibrosis.

➤*Hypersensitivity reactions:* Severe hypersensitivity reactions have been infrequently reported in patients treated with trastuzumab. Signs and symptoms include anaphylaxis, urticaria, bronchospasm, angioedema, or hypotension. In some cases, the reactions have been fatal. The onset of symptoms generally occurred during an infusion, but there have also been reports of symptoms onset after the completion of an infusion. Reactions were most commonly reported in association with the initial infusion.

Trastuzumab infusion should be interrupted in all patients with severe hypersensitivity reactions. In the event of a hypersensitivity reaction, appropriate medical therapy should be administered, which may include epinephrine, corticosteroids, diphenhydramine, bronchodilators, and oxygen. Patients should be evaluated and carefully monitored until complete resolution of signs and symptoms.

There are no data regarding the most appropriate method of identification of patients who may safely be retreated with trastuzumab after experiencing a severe hypersensitivity reaction. Trastuzumab has been readministered to some patients who fully recovered from a previous severe reaction. Prior to readministration of trastuzumab, the majority of these patients were prophylactically treated with premedication including antihistamines or corticosteroids. While some of these patients tolerated retreatment, others had severe reactions again despite the use of prophylactic premedications.

➤*Elderly:* Trastuzumab has been administered to 133 patients who were 65 years of age or over. The risk of cardiac dysfunction may be increased in geriatric patients. The reported clinical experience is not adequate to determine whether older patients respond differently from younger patients.

➤*Pregnancy: Category B.* Reproduction studies have been conducted in cynomolgus monkeys at doses up to 25 times the weekly human maintenance dose of 2 mg/kg trastuzumab and have revealed no evidence of impaired fertility or harm to the fetus. However, HER2 protein expression is high in many embryonic tissues including cardiac and neural tissues; in mutant mice lacking HER2, embryos died in early gestation. Placental transfer of trastuzumab during the early (days 20 to 50 of gestation) and late (days 120 to 150 of gestation) fetal development period was observed. There are, however, no adequate and well-controlled studies in pregnant women. Because animal reproduction studies are not always predictive of human response, this drug should be used during pregnancy only if clearly needed.

➤*Lactation:* A study conducted in lactating cynomolgus monkeys at doses 25 times the weekly human maintenance dose of 2 mg/kg trastuzumab demonstrated that trastuzumab is secreted in the milk. The presence of trastuzumab in the serum of infant monkeys was not associated with any adverse effects on their growth or development from birth to 3 months of age. It is not known whether trastuzumab is excreted in human milk. Because human IgG is excreted in human milk, and the potential for absorption and harm to the infant is unknown, women should be advised to discontinue nursing during trastuzumab therapy and for 6 months after the last dose of trastuzumab.

➤*Children:* The safety and effectiveness of trastuzumab in pediatric patients have not been established.

Precautions

➤*Special risk:* Trastuzumab therapy should be used with caution in patients with known hypersensitivity to trastuzumab, Chinese hamster ovary cell proteins, or any component of this product.

Drug Interactions

➤*Paclitaxel:* There have been no formal drug interaction studies performed with trastuzumab in humans. Administration of paclitaxel in combination with trastuzumab resulted in a 2-fold decrease in trastuzumab clearance in a nonhuman primate study and in a 1.5-fold increase in trastuzumab serum levels in clinical studies.

➤*Benzyl alcohol:* For patients with a known hypersensitivity to benzyl alcohol (the preservative in Bacteriostatic Water for Injection), reconstitute trastuzumab with Sterile Water for Injection. Discard the Sterile Water for Injection reconstituted trastuzumab vial following a single use.

Adverse Reactions

The most serious adverse reactions caused by trastuzumab include cardiomyopathy, hypersensitivity reactions including anaphylaxis, infusion reactions, pulmonary events, and exacerbation of chemotherapy-induced neutropenia. The most common adverse reactions associated with trastuzumab use are fever, diarrhea, infections, chills, increased cough, headache, rash and insomnia.

Cardiac failure/dysfunction – See Warnings for more information.

Anemia and leukopenia – In a randomized, controlled trial, the per-patient incidences of anemia (30% vs 21%) and leukopenia (53% vs 37%) were higher in patients receiving trastuzumab in combination with chemotherapy as compared to those receiving chemotherapy alone. The majority of these cytopenic events were mild or moderate in intensity, reversible, and none resulted in discontinuation of therapy with trastuzumab.

In a randomized, controlled trial conducted in the postmarketing setting, there were also increased incidences of NCI-CTC Grade 3/4 neutropenia (32% [29/92] vs 22% [21/94]) and of febrile neutropenia (23% [21/91] vs 17% [16/94]) in patients randomized to trastuzumab in combination with mylosuppressive chemotherapy as compared to chemotherapy alone.

Hematologic toxicity is infrequent following administration of trastuzumab as a single agent, with an incidence of Grade III toxicities for WBC, platelets, hemoglobin all less than 1%. No Grade IV toxicities were observed.

Diarrhea – Of patients treated with trastuzumab as a single agent, 25% experienced diarrhea. An increased incidence of diarrhea, primarily mild to moderate in severity, was observed in patients receiving trastuzumab in combination with chemotherapy.

Infection – In a randomized, controlled trial, the incidence of infections, primarily mild upper respiratory tract infections of minor clinical significance or catheter infections, was higher (46% vs 30%) in patients receiving trastuzumab in combination with chemotherapy as compared to those receiving chemotherapy alone.

In a randomized, controlled trial conducted in the postmarketing setting, the reported incidence of febrile neutropenia was higher (23% [21/92] vs 17% [16/94] in patients receiving trastuzumab in combination with mylosuppressive chemotherapy as compared to chemotherapy alone.

In the postmarketing setting there have also been reports of febrile neutropenia and infection with neutropenia culminating in death associated with the use of trastuzumab and myelosuppressive chemotherapy.

Infusion reactions – During the first infusion with trastuzumab, a symptom complex most commonly consisting of chills or fever was observed in about 40% of patients. The symptoms were usually mild to moderate in severity and were treated with acetaminophen, diphenhydramine, and meperidine (with or without reduction in the rate of trastuzumab infusion). Trastuzumab discontinuation was infrequent. Other signs or symptoms may include nausea, vomiting, pain (in some cases at tumor sites), rigors, headache, dizziness, dyspnea, hypotension, elevated blood pressure, rash, and asthenia. The symptoms occurred infrequently with subsequent trastuzumab infusions.

Hypersensitivity reactions including anaphylaxis –

Pulmonary events: In the postmarketing setting, severe hypersensitivity reactions (including anaphylaxis), infusion reactions, and pulmonary adverse events have been reported. These reactions include anaphylaxis, angioedema, bronchospasm, hypotension, hypoxia, dyspnea, pulmonary infiltrates, pleural effusions, non-cardiogenic pulmonary edema, and acute respiratory distress syndrome.

Glomerulopathy: In the postmarketing setting, rare cases of nephrotic syndrome with pathologic evidence of glomerulopathy have been reported. The time to onset ranged from 4 months to approximately 18 months from initiation of trastuzumab therapy. Pathologic findings included membranous glomerulonephritis, focal glomerulosclerosis and fibrillary glomerulonephritis. Complications included volume overload and congestive heart failure.

Adverse Reactions Occurring in Patients at Increased Incidence in Trastuzumab: a Randomized Study (≥ 5%)

Adverse reaction	Single agent (n = 352)	Trastuzumab + Paclitaxel (n = 91)	Paclitaxel (n = 95)	Trastuzumab + AC (n = 143)	AC Alone (n = 135)
Cardiovascular					
Congestive heart failure	7%	11%	1%	28%	7%
Tachycardia	5%	12%	4%	10%	5%
CNS					
Depression	6%	12%	13%	20%	12%
Dizziness	13%	22%	24%	24%	18%
Insomnia	14%	25%	13%	29%	15%
Neuropathy	1%	13%	5%	4%	4%
Paresthesia	9%	48%	39%	17%	11%
Peripheral neuritis	2%	23%	16%	2%	2%
Dermatologic					
Acne	2%	11%	3%	3%	< 1%
Herpes simplex	2%	12%	3%	7%	9%
Rash	18%	38%	18%	27%	17%

TRASTUZUMAB — INJECTION

Adverse Reactions Occurring in Patients at Increased Incidence in Trastuzumab: a Randomized Study (≥ 5%)					
Adverse reaction	Single agent (n = 352)	Trastuzumab + Paclitaxel (n = 91)	Paclitaxel (n = 95)	Trastuzumab + AC (n = 143)	AC Alone (n = 135)
GI					
Anorexia	14%	24%	16%	31%	26%
Diarrhea	25%	45%	29%	45%	26%
Nausea	33%	51%	9%	76%	77%
Nausea and vomiting	8%	14%	11%	18%	9%
Vomiting	23%	37%	28%	53%	49%
GU					
Urinary tract infection	5%	18%	14%	13%	7%
Hematologic/Lymphatic					
Anemia	4%	14%	9%	36%	26%
Leukopenia	3%	24%	17%	52%	34%
Metabolic					
Edema	8%	10%	8%	11%	5%
Peripheral edema	10%	22%	20%	20%	17%
Musculoskeletal					
Arthralgia	6%	37%	21%	8%	9%
Bone pain	7%	24%	18%	7%	7%
Respiratory					
Cough increased	26%	41%	22%	43%	29%
Dyspnea	22%	27%	26%	42%	25%
Pharyngitis	12%	22%	14%	30%	18%
Rhinitis	14%	22%	5%	22%	16%
Sinusitis	9%	21%	7%	13%	6%
Miscellaneous					
Abdominal pain	22%	34%	22%	23%	18%
Accidental injury	6%	13%	3%	9%	4%
Allergic reaction	3%	8%	2%	4%	2%
Asthenia	42%	62%	57%	54%	55%
Back pain	22%	34%	30%	27%	15%
Chills	32%	41%	4%	35%	11%
Fever	36%	49%	23%	56%	34%
Flu syndrome	10%	12%	5%	12%	6%
Headache	26%	36%	28%	44%	31%
Infection	20%	47%	27%	47%	31%
Pain	47%	61%	62%	57%	42%

➤*Other serious adverse reactions.* The following other serious adverse reactions occurred in at least 1 of the 958 patients treated with trastuzumab in clinical studies:

Cardiovascular – Vascular thrombosis, pericardial effusion, heart arrest, hypotension, syncope, hemorrhage, shock, arrhythmia.

CNS – Convulsion, ataxia, confusion, manic reaction.

Dermatologic – Herpes zoster, skin ulceration.

Endocrine – Hypothyroidism.

GI – Hepatic failure, gastroenteritis, hematemesis, ileus, intestinal obstruction, colitis, esophageal ulcer, stomatitis, pancreatitis, hepatitis.

GU – Hydronephrosis, kidney failure, cervical cancer, hematuria, hemorrhagic cystitis, pyelonephritis.

Hematologic – Pancytopenia, acute leukemia, coagulation disorder, lymphangitis.

Metabolic – Hypercalcemia, hypomagnesemia, hyponatremia, hypoglycemia, growth retardation, weight loss.

Musculoskeletal – Pathological fractures, bone necrosis, myopathy.

Respiratory – Apnea, pneumothorax, asthma, hypoxia, laryngitis.

Miscellaneous – Cellulitis, anaphylactoid reaction, ascites, hydrocephalus, radiation injury, deafness, amblyopia.

➤*Immunogenicity:* Of 903 patients who have been evaluated, human anti-human antibody (HAHA) to trastuzumab was detected in 1 patient, who had no allergic manifestations.

The data reflect the percentage of patients whose test results were considered positive for antibodies to trastuzumab in the HAHA assay for trastuzumab, and are highly dependent on the sensitivity and specificity of the assay. Additionally, the observed incidence of antibody positivity in an assay may be influenced by several factors including sample handling, timing of sample collection, concomitant medications, and underlying disease. For these reasons, comparison of the incidence of antibodies to trastuzumab with the incidence of antibodies to other products may be misleading.

Overdosage

There is no experience with overdosage in human clinical trials. Single doses greater than 500 mg have not been tested.

GEMTUZUMAB OZOGAMICIN

Rx	**Mylotarg** (Wyeth-Ayerst)	**Powder for injection, lyophilized:** 5 mg	Preservative free. NaCl, mono/dibasic sodium phosphate. In single 20 ml vials.

GEMTUZUMAB OZOGAMICIN — INJECTION

WARNING

Administer gemtuzumab ozogamicin under the supervision of doctors experienced in the treatment of acute leukemia and in facilities equipped to monitor and treat leukemia patients.

There are no controlled trials demonstrating efficacy and safety using gemtuzumab ozogamicin in combination with other chemotherapeutic agents. Therefore, use gemtuzumab ozogamicin only as single agent chemotherapy and not in combination chemotherapy regimens outside clinical trials.

Severe myelosuppression occurs when gemtuzumab ozogamicin is used at recommended doses.

Hypersensitivity reactions, including anaphylaxis, infusion reactions, and pulmonary events – Gemtuzumab ozogamicin administration can result in severe hypersensitivity reactions (including anaphylaxis), and other infusion-related reactions that may include severe pulmonary events. Infrequently, hypersensitivity reactions and pulmonary events have been fatal. In most cases, infusion-related symptoms occurred during the infusion or within 24 hours of administration of gemtuzumab ozogamicin and resolved. Interrupt gemtuzumab ozogamicin infusion for patients experiencing dyspnea or clinically significant hypotension. Monitor patients until signs and symptoms completely resolve. Strongly consider discontinuation of gemtuzumab ozogamicin treatment for patients who develop anaphylaxis, pulmonary edema, or acute respiratory distress syndrome. Because patients with high peripheral blast counts may be at greater risk for pulmonary events and tumor lysis syndrome, consider leukoreduction with hydroxyurea or leukapheresis to reduce the peripheral white count to below 30,000/mcL before administration of gemtuzumab ozogamicin.

WARNING (cont.)

Hepatotoxicity – Hepatotoxicity, including severe hepatic veno-occlusive disease (VOD), has been reported in association with the use of gemtuzumab ozogamicin as a single agent, as part of a combination chemotherapy regimen, and in patients without a history of liver disease or hematopoietic stem-cell transplant (HSCT). Patients who receive gemtuzumab ozogamicin either before or after HSCT, patients with underlying hepatic disease or abnormal liver function, and patients receiving gemtuzumab ozogamicin in combinations with other chemotherapy are at increased risk for developing VOD, including severe VOD. Death from liver failure and from VOD has been reported in patients who received gemtuzumab ozogamicin. Monitor patients carefully for symptoms of hepatotoxicity, particularly VOD. These symptoms can include rapid weight gain, right upper quadrant pain, hepatomegaly, ascites, and elevations in bilirubin and/or liver enzymes. However, careful monitoring may not identify all patients at risk or prevent the complications of hepatotoxicity.

Indications

➤*Acute myeloid leukemia:* For the treatment of patients with CD33-positive acute myeloid leukemia in first relapse who are 60 years of age and older and who are not considered candidates for other cytotoxic chemotherapy. Safety and efficacy in patients with poor performance status and organ dysfunction have not been established.

Administration and Dosage

➤*Approved by the FDA:* May 18, 2000.

GEMTUZUMAB OZOGAMICIN — INJECTION

The recommended dose of gemtuzumab ozogamicin is 9 mg/m^2, administered as a 2-hour intravenous (IV) infusion. Consider leukoreduction with hydroxyurea or leukapheresis to reduce the peripheral white blood count to below 30,000/mcL prior to administration of gemtuzumab ozogamicin. Appropriate measures (eg, hydration and allopurinol) must be taken to prevent hyperuricemia. Give patients the following prophylactic medications 1 hour before gemtuzumab ozogamicin administration: diphenhydramine 50 mg orally and acetaminophen 650 to 1,000 mg orally; thereafter, 2 additional doses of acetaminophen 650 to 1,000 mg orally, 1 dose every 4 hours as needed. Monitor vital signs during infusion and for 4 hours following infusion. The recommended treatment course with gemtuzumab ozogamicin is a total of 2 doses with 14 days between the doses. Full recovery from hematologic toxicities is not a requirement for administration of the second dose.

➤*Premedication:* Methylprednisolone given prior to gemtuzumab infusion may ameliorate infusion-related symptoms.

➤*Hepatic impairment:* See Warnings for more information.

➤*Instructions for reconstitution:* The drug product is light sensitive and must be protected from direct and indirect sunlight and unshielded fluorescent light during the preparation and administration of the infusion. All preparation should take place in a biologic safety hood with the fluorescent light off. Prior to reconstitution, allow drug vials to come to room temperature. Reconstitute the contents of each vial with 5 mL sterile water for injection using sterile syringes. Gently swirl each vial. Inspect each vial for complete solution and for particulate. The final concentration of drug in the vial is 1 mg/mL. While in the vial, the reconstituted drug may be stored refrigerated (2° to 8°C; 36° to 46°F) and protected from light for up to 8 hours.

➤*Instructions for dilution:* Withdraw the desired volume from each vial and inject into a 100 mL IV bag of 0.9% sodium chloride injection. Place the 100 mL IV bag into an ultraviolet (UV) protectant bag. Use the resulting drug solution in the IV bag immediately.

➤*Administration:* Do not administer as an IV push or bolus.

Once the reconstituted gemtuzumab ozogamicin is diluted into the IV bag containing normal saline, infuse the resulting solution over a 2-hour period. A separate IV line equipped with a low protein-binding 1.2 micron terminal filter must be used for administration of the drug. Gemtuzumab ozogamicin may be given peripherally or through a central line. Give premedication, consisting of acetaminophen and diphenhydramine, before each infusion to reduce the incidence of a postinfusion symptom complex. These symptoms generally occurred after the end of the 2-hour IV infusion and resolved after 2 to 4 hours with a supportive therapy of acetaminophen, diphenhydramine, and IV fluids. Fewer infusion-related reactions were observed after the second dose.

➤*Storage/Stability:* Store refrigerated (2° to 8°C; 36° to 46°F) and protected from light.

Visually inspect gemtuzumab ozogamicin for particulate matter and discoloration, following reconstitution and prior to administration. Protect from light and use an UV protective bag over the IV bag during infusion. Consider procedures for handling and disposal of anticancer drugs. Several guidelines on this subject have been published.

Actions

➤*Pharmacology:* Gemtuzumab ozogamicin binds to the CD33 antigen. This antigen is expressed on the surface of leukemic blasts in greater than 80% of patients with acute myeloid leukemia (AML). CD33 is also expressed on normal and leukemic myeloid colony-forming cells, including leukemic clonogenic precursors, but it is not expressed on pluripotent hematopoietic stem cells or on nonhematopoietic cells.

Gemtuzumab ozogamicin is directed against the CD33 antigen expressed by hematopoietic cells. Binding of the anti-CD33 antibody portion of gemtuzumab ozogamicin with the CD33 antigen results in the formation of a complex that is internalized. Upon internalization, the calicheamicin derivative is released inside the lysosomes of the myeloid cell. The released calicheamicin derivative binds to DNA in the minor groove resulting in DNA double strand breaks and cell death.

Gemtuzumab ozogamicin is cytotoxic to the CD33 positive HL-60 human leukemia cell line. Gemtuzumab ozogamicin produces significant inhibition of colony formation in cultures of adult leukemic bone marrow cells. The cytotoxic effect on normal myeloid precursors leads to substantial myelosuppression, but this is reversible because pluripotent hematopoietic stem cells are spared. In preclinical animal studies, gemtuzumab ozogamicin demonstrates antitumor effects in the HL-60 human promyelocytic leukemia xenograft tumor in athymic mice.

➤*Pharmacokinetics:* After administration of the first recommended 9 mg/m^2 dose of gemtuzumab ozogamicin, given as a 2-hour infusion, the elimination half lives of total and unconjugated calicheamicin were about 41 and 143 hours, respectively. After the second 9 mg/m^2 dose, the half-life of total calicheamicin was increased to about 64 hours and the area under the concentration-time curve (AUC) was about twice that in the first dose period. The AUC for the unconjugated calicheamicin increased 30% after the second dose.

Patients, especially patients previously treated with HSCT, have an underlying risk of VOD. The AUC of total calicheamicin was correlated with additional risk of hepatomegaly and the risk of VOD. There is no evidence that reducing gemtuzumab ozogamicin dose will reduce the underlying risk of VOD. Metabolic studies indicate hydrolytic release of the calicheamicin derivative from gemtuzumab ozogamicin. Many metabolites of this derivative were found after in vitro incubation of gemtuzumab ozogamicin in human liver microsomes and cytosol, and in HL-60 promyelocytic leukemia cells. Metabolic studies characterizing the possible isozymes involved in the metabolic pathway of gemtuzumab ozogamicin have not been performed.

Contraindications

Hypersensitivity to gemtuzumab ozogamicin or any of its components: anti-CD33 antibody (hP67.6), calicheamicin derivatives, or inactive ingredients.

Warnings

➤*Myelosuppression:* Severe myelosuppression will occur in all patients given the recommended dose of this agent. Careful hematologic monitoring is required. Treat systemic infections.

➤*Pulmonary events:* Severe pulmonary events leading to death have been reported infrequently with the use of gemtuzumab ozogamicin in the postmarketing setting. Signs, symptoms, and clinical findings include dyspnea, pulmonary infiltrates, pleural effusions, noncardiogenic pulmonary edema, pulmonary impairment and hypoxia, and acute respiratory distress syndrome. These events occur as sequelae of infusion reactions; patients with WBC counts greater than or equal to 30,000/mcL may be at increased risk. Consider leukoreduction with hydroxyurea or leukapheresis to reduce the peripheral white count to below 30,000/mcL prior to administration of gemtuzumab ozogamicin. Patients with symptomatic intrinsic lung disease may also be at greater risk of severe pulmonary reactions.

➤*Tumor lysis syndrome (TLS):* TLS may be a consequence of leukemia treatment with any chemotherapeutic agent including gemtuzumab ozogamicin. Renal failure secondary to TLS has been reported in association with the use of gemtuzumab ozogamicin. Appropriate measures (eg, hydration, allopurinol) must be taken to prevent hyperuricemia. Consider leukoreduction with hydroxyurea or leukapheresis to reduce the peripheral white blood count to less than 30,000/mcL prior to administration of gemtuzumab ozogamicin.

➤*Hepatotoxicity:* See the Warning box for more information.

➤*Hypersensitivity reactions:*

Hypersensitivity reactions including anaphylaxis, infusion reactions, pulmonary events – See the Warning box for more information.

Infusion reactions – Gemtuzumab ozogamicin can produce a postinfusion symptom complex of fever and chills, and, less commonly, hypotension and dyspnea that may occur during the first 24 hours after administration. Grade 3 or 4 nonhematologic infusion-related adverse events included chills, fever, hypotension, hypertension, hyperglycemia, hypoxia, and dyspnea. Most patients received the following prophylactic medications before administration: diphenhydramine 50 mg orally and acetaminophen 650 mg to 1,000 mg orally; thereafter, 2 additional doses of acetaminophen 650 mg to 1,000 mg orally, 1 dose every 4 hours as needed. Monitor vital signs during infusion and for the 4 hours following infusion.

In clinical studies, these symptoms generally occurred after the end of the 2-hour IV infusion and resolved after 2 to 4 hours with a supportive therapy of acetaminophen, diphenhydramine, and IV fluids. Fewer infusion-related events were observed after the second dose.

➤*Hepatic function impairment:* Gemtuzumab ozogamicin has not been studied in patients with bilirubin greater than 2 mg/dL. Exercise extra caution when administering gemtuzumab ozogamicin to patients with hepatic impairment.

➤*Mutagenesis:* Gemtuzumab ozogamicin was clastogenic in the mouse in vivo micronucleus test. This positive result is consistent with the known ability of calicheamicin to cause double-stranded breaks in DNA.

➤*Fertility impairment:* Gemtuzumab ozogamicin adversely affected male, but not female, fertility in rats. Following daily administration of gemtuzumab ozogamicin to male rats for 28 days at doses of 0.02 to 0.16 mg/kg/day (approximately 0.01 to 0.11 times the human dose on a mg/m^2 basis), gemtuzumab ozogamicin caused the following: decreased fertility rates, epididymal sperm counts, and sperm motility; increased incidence of sperm abnormalities; and microscopic evidence of decreased spermatogonia and spermatocyte count. These findings did not resolve following a 9-week recovery period.

➤*Pregnancy: Category D.* Gemtuzumab ozogamicin may cause fetal harm when administered to a pregnant woman. Daily treatment of pregnant rats with gemtuzumab ozogamicin during organogenesis caused dose-related decreases in fetal weight in association with dose-related decreases in fetal skeletal ossification beginning at 0.025 mg/kg/day. Doses of 0.06 mg/kg/day (approximately 0.04 times the recommended human single dose on a mg/m^2 basis) produced increased embryo-fetal mortality (increased numbers of resorptions and decreased numbers of live fetuses per litter). Gross external, visceral, and skeletal alterations at the 0.06 mg/kg/day dose level included digital malformations (ectrodactyly, brachydactyly) in 1 or both hind feet, absence of the aortic arch, wavy ribs, anomalies of the long bones in the forelimb(s) (short/thick humerus, misshapen radius and ulna, and short/thick ulna), misshapen scapula, absence of vertebral centrum, and fused sternebrae. This dose was also associated with maternal toxicity (decreased weight gain, decreased food consumption). There are no adequate and well-controlled studies in pregnant women. If gemtuzumab ozogamicin is used in pregnancy, or if the patient becomes pregnant while taking it, apprise the patient of the potential hazard to the fetus. Advise women of childbearing potential to avoid becoming pregnant while receiving treatment with gemtuzumab ozogamicin.

➤*Lactation:* It is not known if gemtuzumab ozogamicin is excreted in human milk. Because many drugs, including immunoglobulins, are excreted in human milk, and because of the potential for serious adverse reactions in breast-feeding infants from gemtuzumab ozogamicin, make a decision whether to discontinue breast-feeding or to discontinue the drug, taking into account the importance of the drug to the mother.

➤*Children:* The safety and efficacy of gemtuzumab ozogamicin for injection in children have not been studied.

GEMTUZUMAB OZOGAMICIN — INJECTION

Precautions

➤*Monitoring:* Electrolytes, tests of hepatic function, complete blood counts (CBCs) and platelet counts should be monitored during gemtuzumab ozogamicin therapy.

See Administration and Dosage for more information.

➤*Treatment by experienced physicians:* See the Warning box for more information.

Adverse Reactions

➤*Acute infusion-related events:*

Number and Percentage of Patients Reported to Have Acute Infusion-Related Adverse Events (n = 277) (%)		
Adverse event	Any severity	Grade 3 or 4
Chills	183 (66%)	21 (8%)
Dyspnea	73 (26%)	4 (1%)
Fever	227 (82%)	17 (6%)
Headache	102 (37%)	2 (< 1%)
Hyperglycemia	29 (10%)	3 (1%)
Hypertension	43 (16%)	5 (2%)
Hypotension	55 (20%)	12 (4%)
Hypoxia	15 (5%)	4 (1%)
Nausea	188 (68%)	8 (3%)
Vomiting	162 (58%)	3 (1%)

Fever and chills were commonly reported despite prophylactic treatment with acetaminophen and antihistamines. Generally, these symptoms occurred at the end of the 2-hour infusion and resolved after 2 to 4 hours with supportive therapy including acetaminophen, diphenhydramine, and IV fluids. These events all occurred on the same day as gemtuzumab ozogamicin infusion. Fewer infusion-related events were observed after the second dose. Methylprednisolone given prior to gemtuzumab ozogamicin infusion may ameliorate infusion-related symptoms.

➤*Antibody formation:* Antibodies to gemtuzumab ozogamicin were not detected in any of the 277 patients, including the 20 patients who received more than 1 course of study drug, in the phase 2 clinical studies. Two patients in a phase 1 study developed antibody titers against the calicheamicin/calicheamicin-linker portion of gemtuzumab ozogamicin after 3 doses. One patient experienced transient fever, hypotension, and dyspnea; the other patient had no clinical symptoms. No patient developed antibody responses to the hP67.6 antibody portion of gemtuzumab ozogamicin.

➤*Myelosuppression:* See the Warning box for more information.

➤*Neutropenia:* During the treatment phase, 267 of 272 (98%) patients experienced grade 3 or grade 4 neutropenia. For all patients, the median times to ANC recovery at 500/mcL for the CR and CRp patients were 40 and 43 days, respectively.

➤*Anemia, thrombocytopenia:* During the treatment phase, 143 of 276 (52%) patients experienced grade 3 or grade 4 anemia and 272 of 276 (99%) patients experienced grade 3 or grade 4 thrombocytopenia.

Median Time to Recovery of Platelet Counts for All CR and CRp Patients (Days)				
	CR		CRp	
Platelet levels	< 60 years of age	≥ 60 years of age	< 60 years of age	≥ 60 years of age
> 25,000/mcL	35	38	39	75
50,000/mcL	42	40	56	100

Median Time to Recovery of Platelet Counts for All CR and CRp Patients (Days)				
	CR		CRp	
Platelet levels	< 60 years of age	≥ 60 years of age	< 60 years of age	≥ 60 years of age
75,000/mcL	48	42	122	NA[a]
100,000/mcL	56	50	NA[a]	NA[a]

[a] NA = Not available.

➤*Infection:* During the treatment phase, 84 of 277 (30%) patients experienced grade 3 or grade 4 infections, including opportunistic infections. The most frequent grade 3 or grade 4 infection-related treatment-emergent adverse events were sepsis (17%), pneumonia (8%), shock (4%), infection (3%), stomatitis (2%), and herpes simplex (2%).

➤*Bleeding:* During the treatment phase, 36 of 277 (13%) patients experienced grade 3 or grade 4 bleeding. The most common bleeding events for all patients were epistaxis (3%), cerebral hemorrhage (2%), intracranial hemorrhage (1%), melena (1%), petechiae (1%), hematuria (1%), and disseminated intravascular coagulation (1%).

A greater proportion of NR patients (15%) experienced NCI grade 3 or 4 bleeding events compared with OR patients (7%). Among CR patients, 1 grade 3 bleeding event, epistaxis, was experienced. Bleeding events occurred in 1 of 35 CR patients and 4 of 36 CRp patients.

➤*Transfusions:* During the treatment phase, more transfusions were required in the NR and CRp patients compared with the CRs (see table below):

Number of Transfusions by Response Group				
Transfusions	All patients (n = 277)	CR (n = 35)	CRp (n = 36)	NR (n = 206)
Platelet transfusions				
Mean (SD)	NA	6.8 (7)	23.7 (67)	15.7 (20)
(95% CI)[a]	NA	(5.6, 8)	(12.5, 34.9)	(14.3, 17.1)
RBC transfusions				
Mean (SD)	NA	2.9 (3)	5.4 (4)	8.1 (22)
(95% CI)	NA	(2.4, 3.4)	(4.7, 10.1)	(8, 8.2)

[a] Calculated - mean ± se where se = sd/sqr(n).

➤*Mucositis:* A total of 69 of 277 (25%) patients were reported to have a treatment-emergent adverse event consistent with oral mucositis or stomatitis. During the treatment phase, 9 of 277 (3%) patients experienced grade 3 or 4 stomatitis/mucositis after the first dose.

➤*Hepatotoxicity:* In clinical studies, 80 of 274 (29%) patients experienced grade 3 or grade 4 hyperbilirubinemia. Twenty-six of 274 (9%) patients experienced grade 3 or grade 4 abnormalities in levels of ALT, and 49 of 274 (18%) patients experienced grade 3 or grade 4 abnormalities in levels of AST. One patient died with liver failure in the setting of tumor lysis syndrome and multisystem organ failure 22 days after treatment. Another patient died after an episode of persistent jaundice and hepatosplenomegaly 156 days after treatment. Ascites, an event that can be associated with liver damage, was observed in 8 patients. Abnormalities of liver function were often transient and reversible.

VOD – A total of 299 courses of gemtuzumab ozogamicin were administered in 277 relapsed patients and 16 episodes of VOD (in 15 patients) were identified (16/299, 5%). The incidence of VOD in patients treated with gemtuzumab ozogamicin who had no prior or subsequent HSCT was 1%. The risk of developing VOD was 20% for patients with a history of HSCT prior to gemtuzumab ozogamicin administration. In patients who received HSCT after gemtuzumab ozogamicin administration, the risk of developing VOD was 15%. (See table below). In the 15 patients that developed VOD, 9 patients had fatal VOD or ongoing VOD at the time of death:

Incidence of VOD Reported by Treatment Groups						
	Number of courses of gemtuzumab ozogamicin	Number of episodes of VOD	Incidence of VOD (episodes per courses)	Number of patients in classification	Number of patients with VOD	Incidence of VOD (in patients)
Gemtuzumab total	299	16	5%	277	15	5%
Gemtuzumab only	215	2	1%	200	2	1%
HSCT with gemtuzumab (total)[a]	84	14	17%	77	13	17%
HSCT prior to gemtuzumab[b,c]	30	6	20%	27	6	22%
HSCT following gemtuzumab	54	8	15%	52	8	15%

[a] Three patients are included in more than one HSCT category.
[b] Two patients with a pretrial history of HSCT each received HSCT after gemtuzumab ozogamicin.
[c] One patient received gemtuzumab ozogamicin followed by HSCT and then received a second course of gemtuzumab ozogamicin. This patient developed VOD after HSCT and again after the second course of gemtuzumab ozogamicin.

➤*Skin:* Pruritus was reported in 18 of 277 (6%) patients, while rash occurred in 51 of 277 (18%) patients. Cutaneous herpes simplex was reported in 59 of 277 (21%) patients. No patient experienced alopecia.

➤*Early mortality in clinical studies:* The overall mortality rate within 28 days of last dose was 16% (44 of 277). The mortality rate was 14% (17 of 120) for patients who were younger than 60 years of age, and 17% (27/157) for patients who were at least 60 years of age.

➤*Retreatment events:* Twenty patients received additional courses of gemtuzumab ozogamicin in the studies. One patient received a total of 4 courses of treatment.

➤*Dose relationship for adverse events:* Dose-relationship data were generated from a small dose-escalation study. The most common clinical adverse event observed in this study was an infusion-related symptom complex of fever and chills. In general, the severity of fever, but not chills,

GEMTUZUMAB OZOGAMICIN — INJECTION

increased as the dose level increased. Only 1 dose level of gemtuzumab ozogamicin was studied in the phase 2 clinical trials in relapsed AML.

➤*Treatment-emergent adverse events:*

Commonly Reported (≥ 10%) Treatment-emergent Adverse Events by Age Group: Number (%) of Patients			
Body system/ Adverse reaction	≥ 60 years of age (n = 157)	< 60 years of age (n = 120)	Any age (n = 277)
Any adverse event	157 (100%)	119 (99%)	276 (100%)
Cardiovascular			
Hemorrhage	14 (9%)	16 (13%)	30 (11%)
Hypertension	27 (17%)	16 (13%)	43 (16%)
Hypotension	28 (18%)	27 (23%)	55 (20%)
Tachycardia	17 (11%)	11 (9%)	28 (10%)
CNS			
Anxiety	15 (10%)	8 (7%)	23 (8%)
Depression	15 (10%)	9 (8%)	24 (9%)
Dizziness	15 (10%)	18 (15%)	33 (12%)
Insomnia	17 (11%)	16 (13%)	33 (12%)
Dermatologic			
Herpes simplex	29 (18%)	30 (25%)	59 (21%)
Pruritus	6 (4%)	12 (10%)	18 (6%)
Rash	29 (18%)	22 (18%)	51 (18%)
GI			
Abdominal pain	41 (26%)	47 (39%)	88 (32%)
Anorexia	43 (27%)	26 (22%)	69 (25%)
Constipation	36 (23%)	27 (23%)	63 (23%)
Diarrhea	47 (30%)	43 (36%)	90 (32%)
Dyspepsia	13 (8%)	15 (13%)	28 (10%)
Gum hemorrhage	8 (5%)	17 (14%)	25 (9%)
Nausea	99 (63%)	89 (74%)	188 (68%)
Stomatitis	34 (22%)	35 (29%)	69 (25%)
Vomiting	83 (53%)	79 (66%)	162 (58%)
GU			
Metrorrhagia	1 (2%)	6 (10%)	7 (3%)
Vaginal hemorrhage	3 (5%)	9 (15%)	12 (4%)
Hematologic/Lymphatic			
Anemia	34 (22%)	26 (22%)	60 (22%)
Ecchymosis	17 (11%)	11 (9%)	28 (10%)
Leukopenia	67 (43%)	62 (52%)	129 (47%)
Petechiae	30 (19%)	24 (20%)	54 (19%)
Thrombocytopenia	77 (49%)	62 (52%)	139 (50%)
Hepatic			
Liver function tests abnormal	31 (20%)	35 (29%)	66 (24%)
Metabolic/Nutritional			
Alkaline phosphatase increased	15 (10%)	6 (5%)	21 (8%)
Bilirubinemia	18 (11%)	15 (13%)	33 (12%)
Hyperglycemia	17 (11%)	12 (10%)	29 (10%)
Hypocalcemia	15 (10%)	14 (12%)	29 (10%)
Hypokalemia	38 (24%)	35 (29%)	73 (26%)
Hypomagnesemia	4 (3%)	12 (10%)	16 (6%)
Hypophosphatemia	9 (6%)	12 (10%)	21 (8%)
Lactic dehydrogenase increased	28 (18%)	17 (14%)	45 (16%)
Peripheral edema	30 (19%)	10 (8%)	40 (14%)
Musculoskeletal			
Myalgia	5 (3%)	13 (11%)	18 (6%)
Respiratory			
Cough increased	28 (18%)	19 (16%)	47 (17%)
Dyspnea	41 (26%)	32 (27%)	73 (26%)
Epistaxis	37 (24%)	41 (34%)	78 (28%)
Pharyngitis	16 (10)	17 (14%)	33 (12%)
Pneumonia	20 (13)	15 (13%)	35 (13%)
Pulmonary physical finding	13 (8%)	12 (10%)	25 (9%)
Rhinitis	11 (7%)	12 (10%)	23 (8%)
Miscellaneous			
Asthenia	56 (36%)	44 (37%)	100 (36%)
Back pain	19 (12%)	19 (16%)	38 (14%)
Chills	101 (64%)	82 (68%)	183 (66%)
Fever	122 (78%)	105 (88%)	227 (82%)
Headache	42 (27%)	60 (50%)	102 (37%)
Infection	16 (10%)	10 (8%)	26 (9%)
Local reaction to procedure	27 (17%)	33 (28%)	60 (22%)
Neutropenic fever	30 (19%)	18 (15%)	48 (17%)
Pain	28 (18%)	21 (18%)	49 (18%)
Sepsis	40 (25%)	33 (28%)	73 (26%)

Number of Patients Reporting NCI[a] Grade 3 or 4 Treatment-emergent Adverse Events During Part I by Age Group (≥ 10%)			
Body system/ Adverse event	≥ 60 years of age (n = 157)	< 60 years of age (n = 120)	Any age (n = 277)
Any adverse event	138 (88%)	112 (93%)	250 (90%)
Hematologic/Lymphatic			
Anemia	19 (12%)	19 (16%)	38 (14%)
Leukopenia	67 (43%)	60 (50%)	127 (46%)
Thrombocytopenia	75 (48%)	61 (51%)	136 (49%)
Hepatic			
Liver function tests abnormal	11 (7%)	12 (10%)	23 (8%)
Respiratory			
Dyspnea	15 (10%)	8 (7%)	23 (8%)
Miscellaneous			
Chills	17 (11%)	9 (8%)	26 (9%)
Fever	20 (13%)	16 (13%)	36 (13%)
Sepsis	23 (15%)	24 (20%)	47 (17%)

[a] NCI = National Cancer Institute.

Number of Patients with Laboratory Test Results of Grade 3 or 4 Severity (%[a] [b])			
	Efficacy and safety studies grades 3 to 4		
	≥ 60 years of age (n = 157)	< 60 years of age (n = 120)	All patients (n = 277)
Hematologic			
Hemoglobin	79/157 (50%)	64/119 (54%)	143/276 (52%)
Lymphocytes	144/155 (93%)	111/117 (95%)	255/272 (94%)
Partial thromboplastin time	1/66 (2%)	1/61 (2%)	2/127 (2%)
Platelet count	155/157 (99%)	117/119 (98%)	272/276 (99%)
Prothrombin time	2/35 (6%)	4/34 (12%)	6/69 (9%)
Total neutrophils, absolute	152/155 (98%)	115/117 (98%)	267/272 (98%)
WBC	149/157 (95%)	117/119 (98%)	266/276 (96%)
Nonhematologic			
Alkaline phosphatase	4/156 (3%)	7/118 (6%)	11/274 (4%)
ALT	12/156 (8%)	14/118 (12%)	26/274 (9%)
AST	25/156 (16%)	24/118 (20%)	49/274 (18%)
Calcium (hypo/hyper)	14/157 (9%)	21/119 (18%)	35/276 (13%)
Creatinine	1/157 (< 1%)	4/119 (3%)	5/276 (2%)
Glucose (hypo/hyper)	19/155 (12%)	13/119 (11%)	32/274 (12%)
Total bilirubin	45/156 (29%)	35/118 (30%)	80/274 (29%)

[a] Percentage is based on the number of patients receiving a particular laboratory test during the study as is indicated for each test.
[b] Severity as defined by NCI common toxicity scale version 1.

➤*Postmarketing:* In postmarketing experience and other clinical trials, additional cases of VOD have been reported, some in association with the use of other chemotherapeutic agents, underlying hepatic disease/abnormal liver function, or a history of prior or subsequent HSCT. Renal failure sec-

GEMTUZUMAB OZOGAMICIN — INJECTION

ondary to TLS, hypersensitivity reactions, anaphylaxis, pulmonary events, and GI hemorrhage have also been reported in association with the use of gemtuzumab ozogamicin for injection.

Overdosage

No cases of overdose with gemtuzumab ozogamicin were reported in clinical experience. Single doses greater than 9 mg/m^2 in adults were not tested. When a single dose of gemtuzumab ozogamicin was administered to animals, mortality was observed in rats at the dose of 2 mg/kg (approximately 1.3 times the recommended human dose on a mg/m^2 basis), and in male monkeys at the dose of 4.5 mg/kg (approximately 6 times the recommended human dose on a mg/m^2 basis).

➤*Treatment:* Follow general supportive measures in case of overdose. Carefully monitor blood pressure and blood counts. Gemtuzumab ozogamicin is not dialyzable.

ALEMTUZUMAB

Rx	**Campath** (Berlex)	**Solution for injection:** 30 mg/mL	Sodium chloride 8 mg, dibasic sodium phosphate 1.44 mg, potassium chloride 0.2 mg, monobasic potassium phosphate 0.2 mg, polysorbate 80 0.1 mg, EDTA 0.0187 mg. Preservative free. In single use vials.

ALEMTUZUMAB — INJECTION

WARNING

Administer alemtuzumab under the supervision of a health care provider experienced in the use of antineoplastic therapy.

Hematologic toxicity – Serious and, in rare instances, fatal pancytopenia/marrow hypoplasia, autoimmune idiopathic thrombocytopenia, and autoimmune hemolytic anemia have occurred in patients receiving alemtuzumab therapy. Do not administer single doses of alemtuzumab greater than 30 mg or cumulative doses greater than 90 mg/week because these doses are associated with a higher incidence of pancytopenia.

Infusion reactions – Alemtuzumab can result in serious and, in some cases, fatal infusion reactions. Carefully monitor patients during infusions and discontinue alemtuzumab if indicated. Gradual escalation to the recommended maintenance dose is required at the initiation of therapy and after interruption of therapy for at least 7 days.

Infections / Opportunistic infections – Serious, sometimes fatal, bacterial, viral, fungal, and protozoan infections have been reported in patients receiving alemtuzumab therapy. Prophylaxis directed against *Pneumocystis carinii* pneumonia and herpes virus infections has been shown to decrease, but not eliminate, the occurrence of these infections.

Indications

➤*B-cell chronic lymphocytic leukemia (B-CLL):* For the treatment of B-CLL in patients who have been treated with alkylating agents and who have failed fludarabine therapy.

➤*Unlabeled uses:* Treatment of rheumatoid arthritis; multiple sclerosis.

Administration and Dosage

➤*Approved by the FDA:* May 7, 2001.

➤*Dosing schedule:* Initiate alemtuzumab therapy at a dosage of 3 mg/day administered as a 2-hour IV infusion. When the alemtuzumab 3 mg/day dosage is tolerated (eg, infusion-related toxicities are less than or equal to grade 2), escalate the daily dose to 10 mg and continue until tolerated. When the 10 mg dose is tolerated, the maintenance dosage of alemtuzumab 30 mg may be initiated. The maintenance dosage of alemtuzumab is 30 mg/day administered 3 times/week on alternate days (ie, Monday, Wednesday, and Friday) for up to 12 weeks. In most patients, escalation to 30 mg can be accomplished in 3 to 7 days. Dose escalation to the recommended maintenance dosage of 30 mg/day administered 3 times/week is required. Do not administer single doses of alemtuzumab greater than 30 mg or cumulative weekly doses of greater than 90 mg because higher doses are associated with an increased incidence of pancytopenia.

➤*Premedication:* Give premedication prior to the first dose, at dose escalations, and as clinically indicated. The premedication used in clinical studies was diphenhydramine 50 mg and acetaminophen 650 mg administered 30 minutes prior to alemtuzumab infusion. In cases in which severe infusion-related reactions occurred, treatment with hydrocortisone 200 mg was used in decreasing the infusion-related reactions.

Give patients anti-infective prophylaxis to minimize the risks of serious opportunistic infections. The anti-infective regimen used in study 1 consisted of trimethoprim/sulfamethoxazole double strength twice daily 3 times/week and famciclovir or equivalent 250 mg twice daily upon initiation of alemtuzumab therapy. Continue prophylaxis for 2 months after completion of alemtuzumab therapy or until the CD4$^+$ count is greater than or equal to 200 cells/mcL, whichever occurs later.

➤*Dose modification and reinitiation of therapy:* Discontinue alemtuzumab therapy during serious infection, serious hematologic toxicity, or other serious toxicity until the event resolves. Permanently discontinue alemtuzumab therapy if evidence of autoimmune anemia or thrombocytopenia appears. The following table includes recommendations for dose modification for severe neutropenia or thrombocytopenia.

Alemtuzumab Dose Modification and Reinitiation of Therapy for Hematologic Toxicity

Hematologic toxicity	Dose modification and reinitiation of therapy
For first occurrence of absolute neutrophil count (ANC) < 250/mcL and/or platelet count ≤ 25,000/mcL	Withhold alemtuzumab therapy. When the ANC is ≥ 500/mcL and the platelet count is ≥ 50,000/mcL, resume alemtuzumab therapy at the same dose. If the delay between dosing is ≥ 7 days, initiate therapy at alemtuzumab 3 mg and escalate to 10 mg and then 30 mg as tolerated.
For second occurrence of ANC < 250/mcL and/or platelet count ≤ 25,000/mcL	Withhold alemtuzumab therapy. When the ANC is ≥ 500/mcL and the platelet count is ≥ 50,000/mcL, resume alemtuzumab therapy at 10 mg. If the delay between dosing is ≥ 7 days, initiate alemtuzumab therapy at 3 mg and escalate to 10 mg only.
For third occurrence of ANC < 250/mcL and/or platelet count ≤ 25,000/mcL	Discontinue alemtuzumab therapy permanently.
For a decrease of ANC and/or platelet count to ≤ 50% of the baseline value in patients initiating therapy with a baseline ANC ≤ 500/mcL and/or baseline platelet count ≤ 25,000/mcL	Withhold alemtuzumab therapy. When the ANC and/or platelet count returns to baseline value(s), resume alemtuzumab therapy. If the delay between dosing is ≥ 7 days, initiate therapy at alemtuzumab 3 mg and escalate to 10 mg and then to 30 mg as tolerated.

➤*Administration:* Administer alemtuzumab IV only. Administer the infusion over a 2-hour period. Do not administer as an IV push or bolus.

➤*Preparation for administration:* Withdraw the necessary amount of alemtuzumab from the vial into a syringe. To prepare the 3 mg dose, withdraw 0.1 mL into a 1 mL syringe calibrated in increments of 0.1 mL. To prepare the 10 mg dose, withdraw 0.33 mL into a 1 mL syringe calibrated in increments of 0.1 mL. To prepare the 30 mg dose, withdraw 1 mL in either a 1 or 3 mL syringe calibrated in 0.1 mL increments.

Inject into 100 mL sterile 0.9% sodium chloride or 5% dextrose in water. Gently invert the bag to mix the solution. Discard syringe. Use alemtuzumab within 8 hours after dilution.

The vial contains no preservatives and is intended for single use only. Discard vial including any unused portion after withdrawal of dose.

➤*Incompatibilities:* Do not add or simultaneously infuse other drug substances through the same IV line.

➤*Storage / Stability:* Store alemtuzumab vials at 2° to 8°C (36° to 46°F) and protect from direct sunlight. Do not freeze. Discard if vial has been frozen. Use alemtuzumab within 8 hours after dilution. Alemtuzumab contains no preservatives and is intended for single use only. Alemtuzumab solutions may be stored at room temperature (15° to 30°C; 59° to 86°F) or refrigerated. Protect from light.

Actions

➤*Pharmacology:* Alemtuzumab binds to CD52, a nonmodulating antigen that is present on the surface of essentially all B and T lymphocytes, a majority of monocytes, macrophages, and NK cells, and a subpopulation of granulocytes. Analysis of samples collected from multiple volunteers has not identified CD52 expression on erythrocytes or hematopoietic stem cells. The proposed mechanism of action is antibody-dependent lysis of leukemic cells following cell surface binding. Alemtuzumab-1H Fab binding was observed in lymphoid tissues and the mononuclear phagocyte system. A proportion of bone marrow cells, including some CD34$^+$ cells, express variable levels of

ALEMTUZUMAB — INJECTION

CD52. Significant binding also was observed in the skin and male reproductive tract (epididymis, sperm, seminal vesicle). Mature spermatozoa stain for CD52, but neither spermatogenic cells nor immature spermatozoa show evidence of staining.

➤*Pharmacokinetics:*

Absorption/Distribution – Alemtuzumab pharmacokinetics were characterized in a study of 30 alemtuzumab-naive patients with B-CLL who had failed previous therapy with purine analogs. Alemtuzumab was administered as a 2-hour IV infusion, at the recommended dosing schedule, starting at 3 mg and increasing to 30 mg 3 times/week for up to 12 weeks. Alemtuzumab pharmacokinetics displayed nonlinear elimination kinetics. After the last 30 mg dose, the mean volume of distribution at steady state was 0.18 L/kg (range, 0.1 to 0.4 L/kg). Systemic clearance decreased with repeated administration because of decreased receptor-mediated clearance (ie, loss of CD52 receptors in the periphery). After 12 weeks of dosing, patients exhibited a 7-fold increase in mean area under the curve (AUC).

Excretion – Mean half-life was 11 hours (range, 2 to 32 hours) after the first 30 mg dose and was 6 days (range, 1 to 14 days) after the last 30 mg dose.

Contraindications

Alemtuzumab is contraindicated in patients who have active systemic infections, underlying immunodeficiency (eg, seropositive for HIV), or known type I hypersensitivity or anaphylactic reactions to alemtuzumab or to any of its components.

Warnings

➤*Infusion-related reactions:* Alemtuzumab has been associated with infusion-related reactions, including hypotension, rigors, fever, shortness of breath, bronchospasm, chills, and rash. In postmarketing reports, the following serious infusion-related reactions were reported: syncope, pulmonary infiltrates, acute respiratory distress syndrome (ARDS), respiratory arrest, cardiac arrhythmias, myocardial infarction (MI), and cardiac arrest. The cardiac adverse reactions have resulted in death in some cases. In order to ameliorate or avoid infusion-related reactions, premedicate patients with an oral antihistamine and acetaminophen prior to dosing and monitor closely for infusion-related adverse reactions. In addition, initiate alemtuzumab at a low dose, with gradual escalation to the effective dose. Careful monitoring of blood pressure and hypotensive symptoms is recommended, especially in patients with ischemic heart disease and in patients on antihypertensive medications. If therapy is interrupted for 7 days or more, reinstitute alemtuzumab with gradual dose escalation.

➤*Immunosuppression/Opportunistic infections:* Alemtuzumab induces profound lymphopenia. A variety of opportunistic infections have been reported in patients receiving alemtuzumab therapy. If a serious infection occurs, interrupt alemtuzumab therapy; it may be reinitiated following the resolution of the infection.

See the Warning box for more information.

Anti-infective prophylaxis is recommended upon initiation of therapy and for a minimum of 2 months following the last dose of alemtuzumab or until $CD4^+$ counts are greater than or equal to 200 cells/mcL. The median time to recovery of $CD4^+$ counts to greater than or equal to 200 cells/mcL was 2 months; however, full recovery (to baseline) of $CD4^+$ and $CD8^+$ counts may take longer than 12 months.

Because of the potential for graft vs host disease in severely lymphopenic patients, irradiation of any blood products administered prior to recovery from lymphopenia is recommended.

➤*Hematologic toxicity:* Severe, prolonged, and, in rare instances, fatal myelosuppression has occurred in patients with leukemia and lymphoma receiving alemtuzumab. Bone marrow aplasia and hypoplasia were observed in the clinical studies at the recommended dose. The incidence of these complications increased with doses above the recommended dose. In addition, severe and fatal autoimmune anemia and thrombocytopenia were observed in patients with CLL. Discontinue alemtuzumab for severe hematologic toxicity or in any patient with evidence of autoimmune hematologic toxicity. Following resolution of transient, nonimmune myelosuppression, alemtuzumab may be reinitiated with caution. There is no information on the safety of resumption of alemtuzumab in patients with autoimmune cytopenias or marrow aplasia.

➤*Pregnancy: Category C.* Animal reproduction studies have not been conducted with alemtuzumab. It is not known whether alemtuzumab can affect reproductive capacity or cause fetal harm when administered to a pregnant woman. However, human IgG is known to cross the placental barrier, and, therefore, alemtuzumab may cross the placental barrier and cause fetal B and T lymphocyte depletion. Give alemtuzumab to a pregnant woman only if clearly needed.

➤*Lactation:* Excretion of alemtuzumab in human breast milk has not been studied. Because many drugs, including human IgG, are excreted in human milk, discontinue breast-feeding during treatment and for at least 3 months following the last dose of alemtuzumab.

➤*Children:* The safety and efficacy of alemtuzumab in children have not been established.

Precautions

➤*Monitoring:* Obtain complete blood cell counts (CBC) and platelet counts at weekly intervals during alemtuzumab therapy and more frequently if worsening anemia, neutropenia, or thrombocytopenia is observed on therapy. Assess $CD4^+$ counts after treatment until recovery to greater than or equal to 200 cells/mcL. Careful monitoring of blood pressure and hypotensive symptoms is recommended, especially in patients with ischemic heart disease or those on antihypertensive medications.

➤*Immunization:* Do not immunize patients who have recently received alemtuzumab with live viral vaccines because of their immunosuppression. The safety of immunization with live viral vaccines following alemtuzumab therapy has not been studied. The ability to generate a primary or anamnestic humoral response to any vaccine following alemtuzumab therapy has not been studied.

➤*Immunogenicity:* Four (1.9%) of 211 patients evaluated for development of an immune response were found to have antibodies to alemtuzumab. The data reflect the percentage of patients whose test results were considered positive for antibody to alemtuzumab in a kinetic enzyme immunoassay, and are highly dependent on the sensitivity and specificity of the assay. The observed incidence of antibody positivity may be influenced by several additional factors, including sample handling, concomitant medications, and underlying disease. For these reasons, comparison of the incidence of antibodies to alemtuzumab with the incidence of antibodies to other products may be misleading. Patients who develop hypersensitivity to alemtuzumab may have allergic or hypersensitivity reactions to other monoclonal antibodies.

Drug Interactions

➤*Drug/Lab test interactions:* An immune response to alemtuzumab may interfere with subsequent diagnostic serum tests that utilize antibodies.

Adverse Reactions

Alemtuzumab Adverse Reactions in the B-CLL Study Population During Treatment or Within 30 Days (> 5%)

	B-CLL studies (N = 149)	
Adverse reactions	Any grade	Grade 3 or 4
Cardiovascular		
Hypertension	11%	2%
Hypotension	32%	5%
Tachycardia, supraventricular tachycardia	11%	3%
CNS		
Depression	7%	1%
Dizziness	12%	1%
Dysesthesia	15%	—
Fatigue	34%	5%
Headache	24%	1%
Insomnia	10%	—
Myalgias	11%	—
Somnolence	5%	1%
Tremor	7%	—
Dermatologic		
Pruritus	24%	1%
Rash, maculopapular rash, erythematous rash	40%	3%
Sweating increased	19%	1%
Urticaria	30%	5%
GI		
Abdominal pain	11%	2%
Anorexia	20%	3%
Constipation	9%	1%
Diarrhea	22%	1%
Dyspepsia	10%	—
Nausea	54%	2%
Stomatitis, ulcerative stomatitis, mucositis	14%	1%
Vomiting	41%	4%
Hematologic/Lymphatic		
Epistaxis	7%	1%
Pancytopenia	5%	3%
Purpura	8%	—
Red blood cell (RBC) disorders: anemia	80%	38%
Thrombocytopenia	72%	50%
White blood cell (WBC) disorders: neutropenia	85%	64%
Respiratory		
Bronchitis, pneumonitis	21%	13%
Bronchospasm	9%	2%
Cough	25%	2%

ALEMTUZUMAB — INJECTION

Alemtuzumab Adverse Reactions in the B-CLL Study Population During Treatment or Within 30 Days (> 5%)

	B-CLL studies (N = 149)	
Adverse reactions	Any grade	Grade 3 or 4
Dyspnea	26%	9%
Pharyngitis	12%	—
Pneumonia	16%	10%
Rhinitis	7%	—
Miscellaneous		
Asthenia	13%	4%
Back pain	10%	3%
Chest pain	10%	1%
Edema, peripheral edema	13%	1%
Fever	85%	19%
Herpes simplex	11%	1%
Infection (other viral or unidentified)	7%	1%
Malaise	9%	1%
Moniliasis	8%	1%
Pain, skeletal pain	24%	2%
Rigors	86%	16%
Sepsis	15%	10%
Temperature change sensation	5%	—

➤*Infusion-related adverse reactions:* Infusion-related adverse reactions resulted in discontinuation of alemtuzumab therapy in 6% of the patients enrolled in study 1. The most commonly reported infusion-related adverse reactions in this study included rigors (89%), drug-related fever (83%), nausea (47%), vomiting (33%), and hypotension (15%). Other frequently reported infusion-related reactions include the following: rash (30%); fatigue, urticaria (22%); dyspnea (17%); pruritus (14%); headache, diarrhea (13%). Similar types of adverse reactions were reported in the supporting studies. Acute infusion-related reactions were most common during the first week of therapy. In postmarketing reports, the following serious infusion-related reactions have been reported: ARDS, cardiac arrest, cardiac arrhythmias, MI, pulmonary infiltrates, respiratory arrest, and syncope. The cardiac adverse reactions have resulted in death in some cases. Acetaminophen, antiemetics, antihistamines, corticosteroids, and meperidine, as well as incremental dose escalation, were used to prevent or ameliorate infusion-related reactions.

➤*Infections:* In study 1, all patients were required to receive antiherpes and anti-*P. carinii* prophylaxis and were followed for infections for 6 months. Forty (43%) of 93 patients experienced 59 infections (1 or more infections per patient) related to alemtuzumab during treatment or within 6 months of the last dose. Of these, 34 (37%) patients experienced 42 infections that were of grade 3 or 4 severity; 11 (18%) were fatal. Fifty-five percent of the grade 3 or 4 infections occurred during treatment or within 30 days of last dose. In addition, 1 or more episodes of febrile neutropenia (ANC 500 cells/mcL or less) were reported in 10% of patients.

The following types of infections were reported in study 1: grade 3 or 4 sepsis in 12% of patients with 1 fatality, grade 3 or 4 pneumonia in 15% with 5 fatalities, and opportunistic infections in 17% with 4 fatalities. *Candida* infections were reported in 5% of patients; cytomegalovirus infections in 8% (4% of grade 3 or 4 severity); aspergillosis in 2%, with fatal aspergillosis in 1%; fatal mucormycosis in 2%; fatal cryptococcal pneumonia in 1%; *Listeria monocytogenes* meningitis in 1%; disseminated herpes zoster in 1%; grade 3 herpes simplex in 2%; torulopsis pneumonia in 1%. *P. carinii* pneumonia occurred in 1 (1%) patient who discontinued *P. carinii* pneumonia prophylaxis.

In studies 2 and 3, in which antiherpes and anti-*P. carinii* pneumonia prophylaxis was optional, 37 (66%) patients had 47 infections while on or after receiving alemtuzumab therapy. In addition to the opportunistic infections reported, the following types of related reactions were observed on these studies: interstitial pneumonitis of unknown etiology and progressive multifocal leukoencephalopathy.

➤*Hematologic adverse reactions:*

Pancytopenia/Marrow hypoplasia – Alemtuzumab therapy was permanently discontinued in 6 (6%) patients because of pancytopenia/marrow hypoplasia. Two (2%) cases of pancytopenia/marrow hypoplasia were fatal.

Anemia – Forty-four (47%) patients had 1 or more episodes of new onset NCI-CTC grade 3 or 4 anemia. Sixty-two (67%) patients required RBC transfusions. In addition, erythropoietin use was reported in 19 (20%) patients. Autoimmune hemolytic anemia secondary to alemtuzumab therapy was reported in 1% of patients. Positive Coomb's test without hemolysis was reported in 2%.

Neutropenia – Sixty-five (70%) patients had 1 or more episodes of NCI-CTC grade 3 or 4 neutropenia. Median duration of grade 3 or 4 neutropenia was 28 days (range, 2 to 165 days).

Thrombocytopenia – Forty-eight (52%) patients had 1 or more episodes of new onset grade 3 or 4 thrombocytopenia. Median duration of thrombocytopenia was 21 days (range, 2 to 165 days). Thirty-five (38%) patients required platelet transfusions for management of thrombocytopenia. Autoimmune thrombocytopenia was reported in 2% of patients with 1 fatal case of alemtuzumab-related autoimmune thrombocytopenia.

Lymphopenia – The median $CD4^+$ count was 2 cells/mcL at 4 weeks after initiation of alemtuzumab therapy, 207 cells/mcL at 2 months after discontinuation of alemtuzumab therapy, and 470 cells/mcL 6 months after discontinuation. The pattern of change in median $CD8^+$ lymphocyte counts was similar to that of $CD4^+$ cells. In some patients treated with alemtuzumab, $CD4^+$ and $CD8^+$ lymphocyte counts had not returned to baseline levels at longer than 1 year after therapy.

➤*Serious adverse reactions:*

Cardiovascular – Angina pectoris, atrial fibrillation, cardiac arrest, cardiac failure, cerebral hemorrhage, cerebrovascular disorder, coronary artery disorder, cyanosis, deep vein thrombosis, increased capillary fragility, intracranial hemorrhage, MI, pericarditis, pulmonary embolism, subarachnoid hemorrhage, syncope, thrombophlebitis, ventricular arrhythmia, ventricular tachycardia.

CNS – Abnormal gait, abnormal thinking, apathy, aphasia, coma, confusion, grand mal convulsions, hallucinations, meningitis, nervousness, paralysis.

Dermatologic – Angioedema, bullous eruption, cellulitis, purpuric rash.

Endocrine – Hyperthyroidism.

GI – Biliary pain, colitis, duodenal ulcer, esophagitis, gastroenteritis, GI hemorrhage, gingivitis, hematemesis, hemorrhoids, hepatic failure, hepatocellular damage, hyperbilirubinemia, hypoalbuminemia, intestinal obstruction, intestinal perforation, melena, pancreatitis, paralytic ileus, peptic ulcer, peritonitis, pseudomembranous colitis.

GU – Abnormal renal function, acute renal failure, anuria, cervical dysplasia, facial edema, hematuria, toxic nephropathy, ureteric obstruction, urinary retention, urinary tract infection.

Hematologic/Lymphatic – Agranulocytosis, aplasia, coagulation disorder, decreased haptoglobin, disseminated intravascular coagulation, hematoma, hemolysis, hemolytic anemia, lymphadenopathy, marrow depression, splenic infarction, splenomegaly, thrombocythemia.

Metabolic/Nutritional – Acidosis, aggravated diabetes mellitus, dehydration, fluid overload, hyperglycemia, hyperkalemia, hypoglycemia, hypokalemia, hyponatremia, increased alkaline phosphatase, respiratory alkalosis.

Musculoskeletal – Arthritis or worsening arthritis, arthropathy, bone fracture, muscle atrophy, muscle weakness, myositis, osteomyelitis, polymyositis.

Respiratory – Asthma, bronchitis, chronic obstructive pulmonary disease, hemoptysis, hypoxia, pleural effusion, pleurisy, pneumothorax, pulmonary edema, pulmonary fibrosis, pulmonary infiltration, respiratory depression, respiratory insufficiency, sinusitis, stridor, throat tightness.

Special senses – Decreased hearing, endophthalmitis, otitis media, taste loss.

Miscellaneous – Abscess, allergic reactions, anaphylactoid reaction, ascites, bacterial infection, herpes zoster infection, hypovolemia, influenza-like syndrome, malignant lymphoma, malignant testicular neoplasm, mouth edema, neutropenic fever, *P. carinii* infection, plasma cell dyscrasia, prostatic cancer, secondary leukemia, squamous cell carcinoma, transformation to aggressive lymphoma, transformation to prolymphocytic leukemia, tuberculosis infection, viral infection.

Postmarketing: Additional adverse reactions have been identified during postmarketing use of alemtuzumab. Because these reactions are reported voluntarily from a population of uncertain size, it is not always possible to reliably estimate their frequency or establish a causal relationship to alemtuzumab exposure. Decisions to include these reactions in labeling are typically based on 1 or more of the following factors: seriousness of the reaction, frequency of the reporting, or strength of causal connection to alemtuzumab.

The following serious adverse reactions were identified in postmarketing reports: Goodpasture syndrome, Graves disease, Guillain-Barré syndrome, optic neuropathy, and serum sickness, tumor lysis syndrome.

Overdosage

➤*Symptoms:* Initial doses of alemtuzumab of greater than 3 mg are not well tolerated. One patient who received 80 mg as an initial dose by IV infusion experienced acute bronchospasm, cough, and shortness of breath, followed by anuria and death. A review of the case suggested that tumor lysis syndrome may have played a role.

Do not administer single doses of alemtuzumab greater than 30 mg or a cumulative weekly dose greater than 90 mg, as higher doses have been associated with a higher incidence of pancytopenia.

➤*Treatment:* There is no known specific antidote for alemtuzumab overdosage. Treatment consists of drug discontinuation and supportive therapy.

Patient Information

Serious infections, blood disorders, and infusion reactions (eg, chills, fever, rash, rigid muscles, shortness of breath, tightness in the throat) have occurred from the use of this medicine.

Instruct patients to tell their health care provider or pharmacist if any of the following occurs: change in body temperature, changes in heart rhythm, chest pain, chills, diarrhea, fainting, fever, giant hives, hives, infection, itching, interrupted breathing, mouth sores, nausea, paralysis, purple patches under the skin, rash, rigid muscles, shortness of breath, stomach pain, swelling of the mouth, tightness in the lungs, unusual bleeding or bruising, urination problems, vomiting.

ALEMTUZUMAB — INJECTION

It may be necessary to take certain medications (eg, acetaminophen, antibiotics) before receiving this medicine to avoid infection or other side effects.

Advise patients they should not receive live viral vaccines if they have recently taken this medicine.

Advise women of childbearing potential and men of reproductive potential to use effective birth control methods while receiving this medication and for at least 6 months after therapy.

Instruct women to stop breast-feeding while receiving this medicine and for at least 3 months after receiving the last dose of this medicine.

This medicine may cause dizziness or drowsiness. Advise patients to use caution while driving or performing other tasks requiring alertness, coordination, or physical dexterity.

TOSITUMOMAB AND IODINE ^{131}I-TOSITUMOMAB

Rx	**Bexxar Dosimetric Packaging**[a] (Corixa/GlaxoSmithKline)		A carton containing 2 single-use 225 mg vials and 1 single–use 35 mg vial of tositumomab. A package containing a single-use vial of ^{131}I-tositumomab.
Rx	**Tositumomab** (McKesson Biosciences)	**Injection**: 14 mg/mL	10% (w/v) maltose. Preservative-free. In 35 and 225 mg single-use vials.
Rx	**Iodine ^{131}I-Tositumomab**[b] (MDS Nordion[c])	**Injection**: 0.1 mg/mL (0.61 mCi/mL at calibration)	Preservative-free. Single-use vials.[d]
Rx	**Bexxar Therapeutic Packaging**[a] (Corixa/GlaxoSmithKline)		A carton containing 2 single-use 225 mg vials and 1 single-use 35 mg vial of tositumomab. A package containing 1 or 2 single-use vials of ^{131}I-tositumomab.
Rx	**Tositumomab** (McKesson Biosciences)	**Injection**: 14 mg/mL	10% (w/v) maltose. Preservative-free. In 35 and 225 mg single-use vials.
Rx	**Iodine ^{131}I-Tositumomab**[b] (MDS Nordion[c])	**Injection**: 1.1 mg/mL (5.6 mCi/mL at calibration)	Preservative-free. Single-use vials.[e]

[a] The components are shipped from separate sites; when ordering, ensure that the components are scheduled to arrive on the same day. The components are shipped only to individuals who are participating in the certification program.
[b] Refer to the product specification sheet for the lot specific protein concentration, activity concentration, total activity, and expiration date.
[c] MDS Nortion, 447 March Road, Ottawa, ON K2K 1X8, Canada; (613) 592-2790, (800) 267-6211.
[d] Contains 5% to 6% povidone, 1 to 2 mg/mL maltose, 0.85 to 0.95 mg/mL sodium chloride, and 0.9 to 1.3 mg/mL ascorbic acid.
[e] Contains 5% to 6% povidone, 9 to 15 mg/mL maltose, 0.85 to 0.95 mg/mL sodium chloride, and 0.9 to 1.3 mg/mL ascorbic acid.

TOSITUMOMAB AND IODINE ^{131}I-TOSITUMOMAB — INJECTION

WARNING

Hypersensitivity reactions, including anaphylaxis – Medications for the treatment of severe hypersensitivity reactions should be available for immediate use.

Prolonged and severe cytopenias – The majority of patients who received therapy experienced severe thrombocytopenia and neutropenia. Do not administer the therapeutic regimen to patients with more than 25% lymphoma marrow involvement and/or impaired bone marrow reserve.

Pregnancy – Category X. Tositumomab/^{131}I-tositumomab can cause fetal harm when administered to a pregnant woman.

Special requirements – Tositumomab/^{131}I-tositumomab contains a radioactive component and should be administered only by physicians and other health care professionals qualified by training in the safe use and handling of therapeutic radionuclides. The therapeutic regimen should be administered only by physicians who are in the process of being or have been certified by Corixa Corporation in dose calculation and administration of the therapeutic regimen.

Indications

➤*Non-Hodgkin lymphoma (NHL):* For the treatment of patients with CD20 positive, follicular NHL, with and without transformation, whose disease is refractory to rituximab and has relapsed following chemotherapy. This regimen is not indicated for the initial treatment of patients with CD20 positive NHL.

Administration and Dosage

➤*Approved by the FDA:* June 27, 2003.

The therapeutic regimen is intended as a single course of treatment. The safety of multiple courses of this drug complex, or combination of this complex with other forms of irradiation or chemotherapy have not been evaluated.

The therapeutic regimen consists of 4 components administered in 2 discrete steps: The dosimetric step, followed 7 to 14 days later by a therapeutic step. The safety of the therapeutic regimen was established only in the setting of patients receiving thyroid blocking agents and premedication to ameliorate/prevent infusion reactions. The therapeutic regimen is administered via an IV tubing set with an in-line 0.22 micron filter. The same IV tubing set and filter must be used throughout the entire dosimetric or therapeutic step. A change in filter can result in loss of drug.

➤*Dosimetric step:* Administer tositumomab 450 mg IV in 50 mL 0.9% sodium chloride over 60 minutes. Reduce the rate of infusion by 50% for mild to moderate infusional toxicity; interrupt infusion for severe infusional toxicity. After complete resolution of severe infusional toxicity, infusion may be resumed with a 50% reduction in the rate of infusion.

^{131}I-tositumomab (containing 5 mCi ^{131}I and 35 mg tositumomab) IV in 30 mL 0.9% sodium chloride over 20 minutes. Reduce the rate of infusion by 50% for mild to moderate infusional toxicity; interrupt infusion for severe infusional toxicity. After complete resolution of severe infusional toxicity, infusion may be resumed with a 50% reduction in the rate of infusion.

➤*Therapeutic step:* Do not administer the therapeutic step if biodistribution is altered.

Administer tositumomab 450 mg IV in 50 mL 0.9% sodium chloride over 60 minutes. Reduce the rate of infusion by 50% for mild to moderate infusional toxicity; interrupt infusion for severe infusional toxicity. After complete resolution of severe infusional toxicity, infusion may be resumed with a 50% reduction in the rate of infusion.

For ^{131}I-tositumomab, reduce the rate of infusion by 50% for mild to moderate infusional toxicity; interrupt infusion for severe infusional toxicity. After complete resolution of severe infusional toxicity, infusion may be resumed with a 50% reduction in the rate of infusion.

- In patients with 150,000 platelets/mm^3 or more, the recommended dose is the activity of ^{131}I calculated to deliver 75 cGy total body irradiation and 35 mg tositumomab, administered IV over 20 minutes.
- In patients with NCI grade 1 thrombocytopenia (platelet counts = 100,000 but less than 150,000 platelets/mm^3), the recommended dose is the activity of ^{131}I calculated to deliver 65 cGy total body irradiation and 35 mg tositumomab, administered IV over 20 minutes.

➤*Premedication:* The safety of the therapeutic regimen was established in studies in which all patients received the following concurrent medications.

➤*Thyroid protective agents:* Saturated solution of potassium iodide (SSKI) 4 drops orally, 3 times daily; Lugol's solution 20 drops orally, 3 times daily; or potassium iodide tablets 130 mg orally, every day. Initiate thyroid protective agents at least 24 hours prior to administration of the ^{131}I-tositumomab dosimetric dose and continue until 2 weeks after administration of the ^{131}I-tositumomab therapeutic dose.

Do not administer the dosimetric dose of ^{131}I-tositumomab to patients if they have not yet received at least 3 doses of SSKI, 3 doses of Lugol's solution, or 1 dose of 130 mg potassium iodide tablets (at least 24 hours prior to the dosimetric dose).

➤*Ameliorate/prevent infusion reactions:* Acetaminophen 650 mg orally and diphenhydramine 50 mg orally, 30 minutes prior to administration of tositumomab in the dosimetric and therapeutic steps.

➤*Preparation of therapeutic regimen and dosimetric step:* See manufacturer's product labeling for product specific preparation instructions.

➤*Storage/Stability:*

Tositumomab – Refrigerate vials of tositumomab at 2° to 8°C (36° to 46°F) prior to dilution. Protect from strong light. Do not shake. Do not freeze. Discard any unused portions left in the vial. Solutions of diluted tositumomab are stable for up to 24 hours when refrigerated at 2° to 8°C (36° to 46°F) and for up to 8 hours at room temperature. It is recommended that the diluted solution be refrigerated at 2° to 8°C (36° to 46°F) prior to administration because it does not contain preservatives. Any unused portion must be discarded. Do not freeze solutions of diluted tositumomab.

^{131}I-tositumomab – Store frozen in the original lead pots. Store in a freezer at a temperature of −20°C (−4°F) or below until it is removed for thawing prior to administration.

Thawed dosimetric and therapeutic doses of ^{131}I-tositumomab are stable for up to 8 hours at 2° to 8°C (36° to 46°F) or at room temperature. Solution of ^{131}I-tositumomab diluted for infusion contains no preservatives; store refrigerated at 2° to 8°C (36° to 46°F) prior to administration, do not freeze. Any unused portion must be discarded.

Actions

➤*Pharmacology:* The tositumomab/^{131}I-tositumomab complex is an antineoplastic radioimmunotherapeutic monoclonal antibody-based regimen composed of the monoclonal antibody, tositumomab, and the radiolabeled monoclonal antibody, ^{131}I-tositumomab.

TOSITUMOMAB AND IODINE ^{131}I-TOSITUMOMAB — INJECTION

Tositumomab is a murine IgG_{2a} lambda monoclonal antibody that binds specifically to the CD20 antigen. This antigen is a transmembrane phosphoprotein expressed on pre-B lymphocytes and at higher density on mature B lymphocytes. The antigen is also expressed on more than 90% of B-cell NHL. The recognition epitope for tositumomab is found within the extracellular domain of the CD20 antigen. CD20 does not shed from the cell surface and does not internalize following antibody binding.

Possible mechanisms of action include induction of apoptosis, complement-dependent cytotoxicity (CDC), and antibody-dependent cellular cytotoxicity (ADCC) mediated by the antibody. Additionally, cell death is associated with ionizing radiation from the radioisotope.

➤*Pharmacokinetics:* The median blood clearance following administration of 485 mg tositumomab in 110 patients with NHL was 68.2 mg/h. Patients with high tumor burden, splenomegaly, or bone marrow involvement were noted to have a faster clearance, shorter terminal half-life, and larger volume of distribution. The total body clearance, as measured by total body gamma camera counts, was dependent on the same factors noted for blood clearance.

^{131}I decays with beta and gamma emissions with a physical half-life of 8.04 days. Elimination of ^{131}I occurs by decay and excretion in the urine. Urine was collected for 49 dosimetric doses. After 5 days, the whole body clearance was 67% of the injected dose. Ninety-eight percent of the clearance was accounted for in the urine.

In clinical studies, administration of the therapeutic regimen resulted in sustained depletion of circulating CD20 positive cells. One of them was conducted in chemotherapy-naïve patients and 1 in heavily pretreated patients. At 7 weeks, the median number of circulating CD20 positive cells was 0. Lymphocyte recovery began at approximately 12 weeks following treatment. Among patients who had CD20 positive cell counts recorded at baseline and at 6 months, 14% chemotherapy naïve patients had CD20 positive cell counts below normal limits at 6 months, and 32% of heavily pretreated patients had CD20 positive cell counts below normal limits at 6 months. There was no consistent effect of the therapeutic regimen on posttreatment serum IgG, IgA, or IgM levels.

Contraindications

Known hypersensitivity to murine proteins or any other component of the therapeutic regimen.

Warnings

➤*Prolonged and severe cytopenias:* The most common adverse reactions associated with the therapeutic regimen were severe or life-threatening cytopenias (NCI CTC grade 3 or 4) with 71% of the 230 patients enrolled in clinical studies experiencing grade 3 or 4 cytopenias. These consisted primarily of grade 3 or 4 thrombocytopenia (53%) and grade 3 or 4 neutropenia (63%). The time to nadir was 4 to 7 weeks, and the duration of cytopenias was approximately 30 days. Thrombocytopenia, neutropenia, and anemia persisted for more than 90 days following administration of the tositumomab-iodine drug complex in 7%, 7%, and 5% of the patients, respectively. Due to the variable onset of cytopenias, obtain complete blood counts weekly for 10 to 12 weeks. The sequelae of severe cytopenias were commonly observed in clinical studies and included infections (45%), hemorrhage (12%), a requirement for growth factors (12% G- or GM-CSF; 7% epoetin alfa) and blood product support (15% platelet transfusions; 16% red blood cell transfusions).

The safety of the therapeutic regimen has not been established in patients with more than 25% lymphoma marrow involvement, platelet count less than 100,000 cells/mm^3, or neutrophil count less than 1500 cells/mm^3.

➤*Secondary malignancies:* Myelodysplastic syndrome (MDS) and/or acute leukemia were reported in 8% of patients enrolled in the clinical studies and 2% of patients included in expanded access programs. The median time to development of MDS/leukemia was 27 months following treatment; however, the cumulative rate continues to increase. Additional malignancies were also reported in 52 of the 995 patients enrolled in clinical studies. Approximately half of these were nonmelanomatous skin cancers. The remainder, which occurred in 2 or more patients, included breast, lung, bladder, head and neck cancer, colon cancer, and melanoma, in order of decreasing incidence.

➤*Hypothyroidism:* Therapy may result in hypothyroidism. Initiate thyroid-blocking medications at least 24 hours before receiving the dosimetric dose, and continue until 14 days after the therapeutic dose. All patients must receive thyroid blocking agents; do not administer this therapeutic regimen for any patient who is unable to tolerate thyroid blocking agents. Evaluate patients for signs and symptoms of hypothyroidism and screen for biochemical evidence of hypothyroidism annually.

➤*Hypersensitivity reactions:* Hypersensitivity reactions, including anaphylaxis, were reported during and following administration of the this therapeutic regimen. Medications for the treatment of hypersensitivity reactions (eg, epinephrine, antihistamines, and corticosteroids) should be available for immediate use in the event of an allergic reaction. Screen patients who have received murine proteins for human antimouse antibodies (HAMA). Patients who are positive for HAMA may be at increased risk of anaphylaxis and serious hypersensitivity reactions during administration of the therapeutic regimen.

➤*Renal function impairment:* ^{131}I-tositumomab and ^{131}I are excreted primarily by the kidneys. Impaired renal function may decrease the rate of excretion of the radiolabeled iodine and increase patient exposure to the radioactive component of the therapeutic regimen. There are no data regarding the safety of administration of the therapeutic regimen in patients with impaired renal function.

➤*Carcinogenesis:* Radiation is a potential carcinogen. Administration of this therapeutic regimen results in delivery of a significant radiation dose to the testes. There is a potential risk that the drug complex may cause toxic effects on the male and female gonads.

➤*Elderly:* Across all studies, the overall response rate was lower in patients 65 years of age and older (41% vs 61%), and the duration of responses were shorter (10 months vs 16 months). The duration of severe hematologic toxicity was longer in those 65 years of age and older as compared to patients younger than 65 years of age. Due to limited experience, greater sensitivity of some older individuals cannot be ruled out.

➤*Pregnancy: Category X.* ^{131}I-tositumomab (a component of the therapeutic regimen) is contraindicated for use in women who are pregnant. ^{131}I may cause harm to the fetal thyroid gland when administered to pregnant women. Review of the literature has shown that transplacental passage of radioiodide may cause severe, and possibly irreversible, hypothyroidism in neonates. While there are no adequate and well-controlled studies of this drug complex in pregnant animals or humans, defer use of therapy in women of childbearing age until the possibility of pregnancy has been ruled out. If the patient becomes pregnant while being treated with the drug complex, apprise the patient of the potential hazard to the fetus. Use effective contraceptive methods during treatment and for 12 months following administration.

➤*Lactation:* Radioiodine is excreted in breast milk and may reach concentrations equal to or greater than maternal plasma concentrations. Immunoglobulins are also known to be excreted in breast milk. The absorption potential and potential for adverse effects of the monoclonal antibody component (tositumomab) in the infant are not known. Therefore, substitute formula feedings for breastfeedings before starting treatment. Advise women to discontinue nursing.

➤*Children:* The safety and efficacy of the therapeutic regimen in children have not been established.

Precautions

➤*Monitoring:* Obtain a complete blood count (CBC) with differential and platelet count prior to, and at least weekly following administration of the therapeutic regimen. Continue weekly monitoring of blood counts for a minimum of 10 weeks or, if persistent, until severe cytopenias have completely resolved. More frequent monitoring is indicated in patients with evidence of moderate or more severe cytopenias. Monitor thyroid stimulating hormone (TSH) level before treatment and annually thereafter. Measure serum creatinine levels immediately prior to administration of the therapeutic regimen.

➤*Radionuclide:* ^{131}I-tositumomab is radioactive. To minimize exposure of medical personnel and other patients, exercise caution by staying consistent with the institutional radiation safety practices and applicable federal guidelines.

➤*Immunization:* The safety of immunization with live viral vaccines following administration of the therapeutic regimen has not been studied. The ability of patients who have received this therapeutic regimen to generate a primary or anamnestic humoral response to any vaccine has not been studied.

➤*Immunogenicity:* Administration of this therapeutic regimen may result in the development of human antimurine antibodies (HAMA). The presence of HAMA may affect the accuracy of the results of in vitro and in vivo diagnostic tests and may affect the toxicity profile and efficacy of therapeutic agents that rely on murine antibody technology. Patients who are HAMA positive may be at increased risk for serious allergic reactions and other side effects if they undergo in vivo diagnostic testing or treatment with murine monoclonal antibodies.

Drug Interactions

No formal drug interaction studies have been performed. Due to the frequent occurrence of severe and prolonged thrombocytopenia, weigh the potential benefits of medications that interfere with platelet function and/or anticoagulation against the potential increased risk of bleeding and hemorrhage.

Adverse Reactions

The most serious adverse reactions observed in the clinical trials were severe and prolonged cytopenias and the sequelae of cytopenias which included infections (sepsis) and hemorrhage in thrombocytopenic patients, allergic reactions (bronchospasm and angioedema), secondary leukemia and myelodysplasia (see Warnings).

The most common adverse reactions occurring in the clinical trials included neutropenia, thrombocytopenia, and anemia that are both prolonged and severe. Less common but severe adverse reactions included pneumonia, pleural effusion, and dehydration.

Nonhematologic Adverse Reactions in 5% or more of Patients Treated with Tositumomab/^{131}I-Tositumomab (N = 230) (%)

Adverse reaction	All Grades (96%)	Grade 3/4 (48%)
Cardiovascular		
Hypotension	7	1
Vasodilation	5	0
CNS		
Dizziness	5	0
Headache	16	0

TOSITUMOMAB AND IODINE ^{131}I-TOSITUMOMAB — INJECTION

Nonhematologic Adverse Reactions in 5% or more of Patients Treated with Tositumomab/^{131}I-Tositumomab (N = 230) (%)

Adverse reaction	All Grades (96%)	Grade 3/4 (48%)
Somnolence	5	0
Dermatologic		
Rash	17	< 1
Pruritus	10	0
Sweating	8	< 1
GI		
Abdominal pain	15	3
Anorexia	14	0
Constipation	6	1
Diarrhea	12	0
Dyspepsia	6	< 1
Nausea	36	3
Vomiting	15	1
Metabolic		
Peripheral edema	9	0
Weight loss	6	< 1
Musculoskeletal		
Arthralgia	10	1
Myalgia	13	< 1
Respiratory		
Cough increased	21	1
Dyspnea	11	3
Pharyngitis	12	0
Pneumonia	6	0
Rhinitis	10	0
Miscellaneous		
Asthenia	46	2
Back pain	8	1
Chest pain	7	0
Chills	18	1
Fever	37	2
Hypothyroidism	7	0
Infection[a]	21	< 1
Neck pain	6	1
Pain	19	1

[a] "Infection includes" a subset of infections (eg, upper respiratory infection, pneumonia, and sepsis).

Tositumomab/^{131}I-Tositumomab Hematologic Toxicity[a] (N = 230)

Endpoint	Values
Platelets	
Median nadir (cells/mm^3)	43,000
Per patient incidence[a] platelets < 50,000/mm^3	53%
Median[b] duration of platelets < 50,000/mm^3 (days)	32
Grade 3/4 without recovery to Grade 2	7%
Per patient incidence[c] platelets < 25,000/mm^3	21%
ANC	
Median nadir (cells/mm^3)	690
Per patient incidence[a] ANC < 1000 cells/mm^3	63%
Median[b] duration of ANC < 1000 cells/mm^3 (days)	31
Grade 3/4 without recovery to Grade 2	7%
Per patient incidence[c] ANC < 500 cells/mm^3	25%
Hemoglobin	
Median nadir (g/dL)	10
Per patient incidence[a] < 8 g/dL	29%
Median[b] duration of hemoglobin < 8 g/dL (days)	23
Grade 3/4 without recovery to Grade 2	5%
Per patient incidence[c] hemoglobin < 6.5 g/dL	5%

[a] Grade 3/4 toxicity was assumed if patient was missing 2 or more weeks of hematology data between weeks 5 and 9.
[b] Duration of Grade 3/4 of 1000+ days (censored) was assumed for those patients with undocumented Grade 3/4 and no hematologic data on or after week 9.
[c] Grade 4 toxicity was assumed if patient had documented Grade 3 toxicity and was missing 2 or more weeks of hematology data between weeks 5 and 9.

➤*Hematologic:* Hematologic toxicity was the most frequently observed adverse event in clinical trials with the therapeutic regimen. Twenty-seven percent of the patients received 1 or more hematologic supportive care measures following the therapeutic dose. Twelve percent received G-CSF; 7% received epoetin alfa; 15% received platelet transfusions; 16% received packed red blood cell transfusions. Twelve percent of patients experienced hemorrhagic events; the majority were mild to moderate.

➤*Infections:* Forty-five percent of patients experienced 1 or more adverse events possibly related to infection. The majority were viral (eg, rhinitis, pharyngitis, flu symptoms, or herpes) or other minor infections. Eight percent of patients experienced infections that were considered serious because the patient was hospitalized to manage the infection. Documented infections included pneumonia, bacteremia, septicemia, bronchitis, and skin infections.

➤*Hypersensitivity:* Six percent experienced 1 or more of the following adverse events: Allergic reaction, face edema, injection site hypersensitivity, anaphylactoid reaction, laryngismus, and serum sickness.

➤*GI toxicity:* Thirty-eight percent of patients experienced 1 or more of the following GI adverse events: Nausea, emesis, abdominal pain, and diarrhea. These events were temporally related to the infusion of the antibody. Nausea, vomiting, and abdominal pain were often reported within days of infusion, whereas diarrhea was generally reported days to weeks after infusion.

➤*Infusional toxicity:* Symptoms, including fever, rigors or chills, sweating, hypotension, dyspnea, bronchospasm, and nausea have been reported during or within 48 hours of infusion. Twenty-nine percent of patients reported fever, rigors/chills, or sweating within 14 days following the dosimetric dose. Infusional toxicities were managed by slowing and/or temporarily interrupting the infusion. Symptomatic management was required in more severe cases.

➤*Delayed adverse reactions:*

Secondary leukemia and myelodysplastic syndrome (MDS) – There were 32 new cases of MDS/secondary leukemia reported among 3.2% of patients included in clinical studies.

Secondary malignancies – There were 52 reports of second malignancies, excluding secondary leukemias. The most common included nonmelanomatous skin cancers, breast, lung, bladder, and head and neck cancers. Some of these events included recurrence of an earlier diagnosis of cancer.

Hypothyroidism – Twelve percent of the patients included from the clinical studies had an elevated TSH level (8%) or no TSH level obtained (4%) prior to treatment. The overall incidence of hypothyroidism was 14%. New events have been observed up to 72 months post treatment.

Immunogenicity – Of the 220 patients who were seronegative prior to treatment, 99.5% had at least 1 posttreatment HAMA value obtained. Eleven percent seroconverted to HAMA positivity. The median time to development of HAMA was 6 months. In a study of 77 patients who were chemotherapy naïve, the incidence of conversion to HAMA seropositivity was 70%, with a median time to development of HAMA of 27 days.

Overdosage

The maximum dose of the tositumomab/^{131}I-tositumomab therapeutic regimen that was administered in clinical trials was 88 cGy. Three patients were treated with a total body dose of 85 cGy of iodine ^{131}I-tositumomab in a dose escalation study. Two of the 3 patients developed Grade 4 toxicity of 5 weeks duration with subsequent recovery. In addition, accidental overdose of the therapeutic regimen occurred in 1 patient at total body doses of 88 cGy. The patient developed Grade 3 hematologic toxicity of 18 days duration. Monitor patients who receive an accidental overdose of ^{131}I-tositumomab closely for cytopenias and radiation-related toxicity. The effectiveness of hematopoietic stem cell transplantation as a supportive care measure for marrow injury has not been studied; however, the timing of such support should take into account the pharmacokinetics of the therapeutic regimen and decay rate of the ^{131}I in order to minimize the possibility of irradiation of infused hematopoietic stem cells.

Patient Information

Inform patients that they will have a radioactive material in their body for several days upon their release from the hospital or clinic.

After discharge, provide patients with both oral and written instructions for minimizing exposure of family members, friends, and the general public.

Assess the pregnancy status of women of childbearing potential, and advise these women of the potential risks to the fetus. Instruct women who are breastfeeding to discontinue breastfeeding.

Advise patients of the potential risk of toxic effects on the male and female gonads following the therapeutic regimen, and instruct patients to use effective contraceptive methods during treatment and for 12 months following the administration of the therapeutic regimen.

Inform patients of the risks of hypothyroidism, and advise them of the importance of compliance with thyroid blocking agents and the need for lifelong monitoring.

Inform patients of the risks of cytopenias and symptoms associated with cytopenia and the need for frequent monitoring.

Inform patients that certain antineoplastic agents used in the treatment of malignancy have been associated with the development of MDS, secondary leukemia, and solid tumors.

IMATINIB MESYLATE

Rx	**Gleevec** (Novartis)	**Tablets**: 100 mg (as base)	(NVR SA). Very dark yellow to brownish-orange, scored. Film-coated. In 100s.
		400 mg (as base)	(NVR SL). Very dark yellow to brownish-orange, oval. Film-coated. In 30s.

IMATINIB MESYLATE — ORAL

Indications

➤*Chronic myeloid leukemia (CML):* Imatinib is indicated for the treatment of newly diagnosed adult patients with Philadelphia chromosome-positive chronic myeloid leukemia (CML) in chronic phase. Follow-up is limited.

Imatinib is also indicated for the treatment of patients with Philadelphia chromosome-positive (Ph+) CML in blast crisis, accelerated phase, or in chronic phase after failure of interferon alpha therapy. Imatinib is also indicated for the treatment of pediatric patients with Ph+ chronic phase CML whose disease has recurred after stem-cell transplant or who are resistant to interferon alpha therapy. There are no controlled trials demonstrating a clinical benefit, such as improvement in disease-related symptoms or increased survival.

➤*GI stromal tumors:* Imatinib is also indicated for the treatment of patients with Kit (CD117)-positive unresectable or metastatic malignant GI stromal tumors (GIST). The effectiveness of imatinib in GIST is based on objective response rate. There are no controlled trials demonstrating a clinical benefit, such as improvement in disease-related symptoms or increased survival.

Administration and Dosage

➤*Approved by the FDA:* May 10, 2001.

Therapy should be initiated by a physician experienced in the treatment of patients with chronic myeloid leukemia or GI stromal tumors (GIST).

➤*Recommended dosage:* The recommended dosage of imatinib is 400 mg/day for adult patients in chronic phase CML and 600 mg/day for patients in accelerated phase or blast crisis. The recommended imatinib dosage is 260 mg/m²/day for children with Ph+ chronic phase CML recurrent after stem-cell transplant or who are resistant to interferon alpha therapy. The recommended dosage of imatinib is 400 mg/day or 600 mg/day for adult patients with unresectable or metastatic, malignant GIST.

The prescribed dose should be administered orally, with a meal and a large glass of water. Doses of 400 mg or 600 mg should be administered once daily, whereas a dose of 800 mg should be administered as 400 mg twice a day.

➤*Children:* In children, imatinib treatment can be given as a once-daily dose or, alternatively, the daily dose may be split into 2, once in the morning and once in the evening. There is no experience with imatinib treatment in children under 3 years of age.

For patients unable to swallow the film-coated tablets, the tablets may be dispersed in a glass of water or apple juice. The required number of tablets should be placed in the appropriate volume of beverage (approximately 50 mL for a 100 mg tablet, and 200 mL for a 400 mg tablet) and stirred with a spoon. The suspension should be administered immediately after complete disintegration of the tablet(s).

➤*Duration of therapy:* Treatment may be continued as long as there is no evidence of progressive disease or unacceptable toxicity.

➤*Dose increase:* In CML, a dose increase from 400 to 600 mg in adult patients with chronic phase disease, or from 600 to 800 mg (given as 400 mg twice daily) in adult patients in accelerated phase or blast crisis may be considered in the absence of severe adverse drug reaction and severe non-leukemia-related neutropenia or thrombocytopenia in the following circumstances: Disease progression (at any time); failure to achieve a satisfactory hematologic response after at least 3 months of treatment; failure to achieve a cytogenetic response after 6 to 12 months of treatment; loss of a previously achieved hematologic or cytogenetic response. In children with chronic phase CML, daily doses can be increased under circumstances similar to those leading to an increase in adult chronic phase disease, from 260 mg/m²/day to 340 mg/m²/day, as clinically indicated.

➤*Concurrent CYP3A4 inducers:* Dosage of imatinib should be increased by at least 50%, and clinical response should be carefully monitored, in patients receiving imatinib with a potent CYP3A4 inducer such as rifampin or phenytoin.

➤*Iron:* For daily dosing of 800 mg and above, dosing should be accomplished using the 400 mg tablet to reduce exposure to iron. Patients at a total dose of 1,200 mg daily may have an increased susceptibility to excess iron. If routine blood sampling indicates sustained increases in iron levels, attempts to lower other sources of iron exposure should be undertaken.

➤*Dose adjustment for hepatotoxicity and other nonhematologic adverse reactions:* If a severe nonhematologic adverse reaction develops (such as severe hepatotoxicity or severe fluid retention), imatinib should be withheld until the event has resolved. Thereafter, treatment can be resumed as appropriate, depending on the initial severity of the event.

If elevations in bilirubin greater than 3 × institutional upper limit of normal (IULN) or in liver transaminases greater than 5 × IULN occur, imatinib should be withheld until bilirubin levels have returned to a less than 1.5 × IULN and transaminase levels to less than 2.5 × IULN. In adults, treatment with imatinib may then be continued at a reduced daily dose (ie, 400 to 300 mg or 600 to 400 mg). In children, daily doses can be reduced under the same circumstances from 260 mg/m²/day to 200 mg/m²/day or from 340 mg/m²/day to 260 mg/m²/day, respectively.

➤*Dose adjustment for hematologic adverse reactions:* Dose reduction or treatment interruptions for severe neutropenia and thrombocytopenia are recommended as indicated in the following table:

Dosage Adjustments for Neutropenia and Thrombocytopenia		
Chronic phase CML (starting dose 400 mg[1]) or GIST (starting dose either 400 mg or 600 mg)	ANC < 1 × 10^9/L and/or platelets < 50 × 10^9/L	Stop imatinib until ANC ≥ 1.5 × 10^9/L and platelets ≥ 75 × 10^9/L. Resume treatment with imatinib at the original starting dose of 400 mg[1] or 600 mg. If recurrence of ANC < 1 × 10^9/L and/or platelets < 50 × 10^9/L, repeat step 1 and resume imatinib at a reduced dose (300 mg[2] if starting dose was 400 mg[1], 400 mg if starting dose was 600 mg).
Accelerated phase CML and blast crisis (starting dose 600 mg)	[3]ANC < 0.5 × 10^9/L and/or platelets < 10 × 10^9/L	Check if cytopenia is related to leukemia (marrow aspirate or biopsy). If cytopenia is unrelated to leukemia, reduce dose of imatinib to 400 mg. If cytopenia persists 2 weeks, reduce further to 300 mg. If cytopenia persists 4 weeks and is still unrelated to leukemia, stop imatinib until ANC ≥ 1 × 10^9/L and platelets ≥ 20 × 10^9/L and then resume treatment at 300 mg.

[1] Or 260 mg/m² in children.
[2] Or 200 mg/m² in children.
[3] Occurring after at least 1 month of treatment.

➤*Storage/Stability:* Store at 25°C (77°F); excursions permitted to 15° to 30°C (59° to 86°F). Protect from moisture.

Dispense in a tight container.

Actions

➤*Pharmacology:* Imatinib is a protein-tyrosine kinase inhibitor that inhibits the Bcr-Abl tyrosine kinase, the constitutive abnormal tyrosine kinase created by the Philadelphia chromosome abnormality in CML. It inhibits proliferation and induces apoptosis in Bcr-Abl-positive cell lines as well as fresh leukemic cells from Philadelphia chromosome positive chronic myeloid leukemia. In colony formation assays using ex vivo peripheral blood and bone marrow samples, imatinib shows inhibition of Bcr-Abl positive colonies from CML patients.

In vivo, it inhibits tumor growth of Bcr-Abl transfected murine myeloid cells as well as Bcr-Abl-positive leukemia lines derived from CML patients in blast crisis.

Imatinib is also an inhibitor of the receptor tyrosine kinases for platelet-derived growth factor (PDGF) and stem-cell factor (SCF), c-kit, and inhibits PDGF- and SCF-mediated cellular events. In vitro, imatinib inhibits proliferation and induces apoptosis in GIST cells, which express an activating c-kit mutation.

➤*Pharmacokinetics:*

Absorption/Distribution – The pharmacokinetics of imatinib have been evaluated in studies in healthy subjects and in population pharmacokinetic studies in over 900 patients. Imatinib is well absorbed after oral administration, with C_{max} achieved within 2 to 4 hours postdose. Mean absolute bioavailability is 98%. Following oral administration in healthy volunteers, the elimination half-lives of imatinib and its major active metabolite, the N-desmethyl derivative, were approximately 18 and 40 hours, respectively. Mean imatinib AUC increases proportionally, with increasing doses ranging

IMATINIB MESYLATE — ORAL

from 25 mg to 1,000 mg. There is no significant change in the pharmacokinetics of imatinib on repeated dosing, and accumulation is 1.5- to 2.5-fold at steady state when imatinib is dosed once daily. At clinically relevant concentrations of imatinib, binding to plasma proteins in in vitro experiments is approximately 95%, mostly to albumin and α_1-acid glycoprotein.

Metabolism/Excretion – CYP3A4 is the major enzyme responsible for metabolism of imatinib. Other cytochrome P450 enzymes, such as CYP1A2, CYP2D6, CYP2C9, and CYP2C19, play a minor role in its metabolism. The main circulating active metabolite in humans is the N-demethylated piperazine derivative, formed predominantly by CYP3A4. It shows in vitro potency similar to the parent imatinib. The plasma AUC for this metabolite is about 15% of the AUC for imatinib. The plasma-protein binding of the N-demethylated metabolite CGP71588 is similar to that of the parent compound.

Elimination is predominately in the feces, mostly as metabolites. Based on the recovery of compound(s) after an oral ^{14}C-labeled dose of imatinib, approximately 81% of the dose was eliminated within 7 days, in feces (68% of dose) and urine (13% of dose). Unchanged imatinib accounted for 25% of the dose (5% urine, 20% feces), the remainder being metabolites.

Typically, clearance of imatinib in a 50-year-old patient weighing 50 kg is expected to be 8 L/hr, while for a 50-year-old patient weighing 100 kg the clearance will increase to 14 L/hr. However, the interpatient variability of 40% in clearance does not warrant initial dose adjustment based on body weight or age but indicates the need for close monitoring for treatment-related toxicity.

Contraindications

Use of imatinib is contraindicated in patients with hypersensitivity to imatinib or to any other component of imatinib.

Warnings

➤*Hepatic function impairment:*

Hepatotoxicity – See Precautions for more information.

➤*Mutagenesis:* Positive genotoxic effects were obtained for imatinib in an in vitro mammalian cell assay (Chinese hamster ovary) for clastogenicity (chromosome aberrations) in the presence of metabolic activation. Two intermediates of the manufacturing process, which are also present in the final product, are positive for mutagenesis in the Ames assay. One of these intermediates was also positive in the mouse lymphoma assay. Imatinib was not genotoxic when tested in an in vitro bacterial cell assay (Ames test), an in vitro mammalian cell assay (mouse lymphoma) and an in vivo rat micronucleus assay.

➤*Fertility impairment:* In a study of fertility, in male rats dosed for 70 days prior to mating, testicular and epididymal weights and percent motile sperm were decreased at 60 mg/kg, approximately three-fourths the maximum clinical dose of 800 mg/day, based on body surface area. This was not seen at doses less than or equal to 20 mg/kg (one-fourth the maximum human dose of 800 mg). When female rats were dosed 14 days prior to mating and through to gestational day 6, there was no effect on mating or on number of pregnant females.

In female rats dosed with imatinib at 45 mg/kg (approximately one-half the maximum human dose of 800 mg, based on body surface area) from gestational day 6 until the end of lactation, red vaginal discharge was noted on either gestational day 14 or 15.

➤*Pregnancy: Category D.* Women of childbearing potential should be advised to avoid becoming pregnant.

Imatinib was teratogenic in rats when administered during organogenesis at doses greater than or equal to 100 mg/kg, approximately equal to the maximum clinical dose of 800 mg/day (based on body surface area). Teratogenic effects included exencephaly or encephalocele, absent/reduced frontal and absent parietal bones. Female rats administered doses greater than or equal to 45 mg/kg (approximately one-half the maximum human dose of 800 mg/day, based on body surface area) also experienced significant postimplantation loss as evidenced by either early fetal resorption or stillbirths, nonviable pups, and early pup mortality between postpartum days 0 and 4. At doses higher than 100 mg/kg, total fetal loss was noted in all animals. These effects were not seen at doses less than or equal to 30 mg/kg (one-third the maximum human dose of 800 mg).

Male and female rats were exposed in utero to a maternal imatinib dose of 45 mg/kg (approximately one-half the maximum human dose of 800 mg) from day 6 of gestation and through milk during the lactation period. These animals then received no imatinib exposure for nearly 2 months. Body weights were reduced from birth until terminal sacrifice in these rats. Although fertility was not affected, fetal loss was seen when these male and female animals were then mated.

There are no adequate and well-controlled studies in pregnant women. If imatinib is used during pregnancy, or if the patient becomes pregnant while taking (receiving) imatinib, the patient should be apprised of the potential hazard to the fetus.

➤*Lactation:* It is not known whether imatinib or its metabolites are excreted in human milk. However, in lactating female rats administered 100 mg/kg, a dose approximately equal to the maximum clinical dose of 800 mg/day based on body surface area, imatinib and its metabolites were extensively excreted in milk. Concentration in milk was approximately 3-fold higher than in plasma. It is estimated that approximately 1.5% of a maternal dose is excreted into milk, which is equivalent to a dose to the infant of 30% the maternal dose per unit body weight. Because many drugs are excreted in human milk and because of the potential for serious adverse reactions in nursing infants, women should be advised against breastfeeding while taking imatinib.

➤*Children:* Imatinib safety and efficacy have been demonstrated only in children with Ph+ chronic phase CML with recurrence after stem-cell transplantation or resistance to interferon alpha therapy. There are no data in children under 3 years of age.

Precautions

➤*Monitoring:*

Hematologic toxicity – Treatment with imatinib is often associated with anemia, neutropenia or thrombocytopenia. Complete blood counts should be performed weekly for the first month, biweekly for the second month, and periodically thereafter as clinically indicated (for example every 2 to 3 months). The occurrence of these cytopenias is dependent on the stage of disease and is more frequent in patients with accelerated phase CML or blast crisis than in patients with chronic phase CML.

Hepatotoxicity – Hepatotoxicity, occasionally severe, may occur with imatinib. Liver function (transaminases, bilirubin, and alkaline phosphatase) should be monitored before initiation of treatment and monthly or as clinically indicated. Laboratory abnormalities should be managed with interruption or dose reduction of the treatment with imatinib. Patients with hepatic impairment should be closely monitored because exposure to imatinib may be increased. As there are no clinical studies of imatinib in patients with impaired liver function, no specific advice concerning initial dosing adjustment can be given.

➤*Dermatologic toxicities:* Bullous dermatologic reactions, including erythema multiforme and Stevens-Johnson syndrome, have been reported with use of imatinib. In some cases reported during postmarketing surveillance, a recurrent dermatologic reaction was observed upon rechallenge. Several foreign postmarketing reports have described cases in which patients tolerated the reintroduction of imatinib therapy after resolution or improvement of the bullous reaction. In these instances, imatinib was resumed at a dose lower than that at which the reaction occurred and some patients also received concomitant treatment with corticosteroids or antihistamines.

➤*Fluid retention and edema:* Imatinib is often associated with edema and occasionally serious fluid retention. Patients should be weighed and monitored regularly for signs and symptoms of fluid retention. An unexpected rapid weight gain should be carefully investigated and appropriate treatment provided. The probability of edema was increased with higher imatinib dose and age greater than 65 years in the CML studies. Severe superficial edema was reported in 0.9% of newly diagnosed CML patients taking imatinib, and in 2% to 6% of other adult CML patients taking imatinib. In addition, other severe fluid retention (eg, pleural effusion, pericardial effusion, pulmonary edema, ascites) events were reported in 2% to 6% of other adult CML patients taking imatinib. Severe superficial edema and severe fluid retention (pleural effusion, pulmonary edema and ascites) were reported in 1% to 6% of patients taking imatinib for GIST.

There have been postmarketing reports, including fatalities, of cardiac tamponade, cerebral edema, increased intracranial pressure, and papilledema in patients treated with CML treated with imatinib.

➤*GI irritation:* Imatinib is sometimes associated with GI irritation. Imatinib should be taken with food and a large glass of water to minimize this problem.

➤*Hemorrhage:* In the newly diagnosed CML trial, 0.7% of patients had grade 3/4 hemorrhage. In the GIST clinical trial, 7 patients (5%), 4 in the 600 mg dose group and 3 in the 400 mg dose group, had a total of 8 events of CTC grade 3/4: GI bleeds (3 patients), intratumoral bleeds (3 patients), or both (1 patient). GI tumor sites may have been the source of GI bleeds.

➤*Toxicities from long-term use:* It is important to consider potential toxicities suggested by animal studies, specifically, liver and kidney toxicity and immunosuppression. Severe liver toxicity was observed in dogs treated for 2 weeks, with elevated liver enzymes, hepatocellular necrosis, bile duct necrosis, and bile duct hyperplasia. Renal toxicity was observed in monkeys treated for 2 weeks, with focal mineralization and dilation of the renal tubules and tubular nephrosis. Increased BUN and creatinine were observed in several of these animals. An increased rate of opportunistic infections was observed with chronic imatinib treatment in laboratory animal studies. In a 39-week monkey study, treatment with imatinib resulted in worsening of normally suppressed malarial infections in these animals. Lymphopenia was observed in animals (as in humans).

IMATINIB MESYLATE — ORAL

Drug Interactions

Imatinib Drug Interactions			
Precipitant drug	Object drug*		Description
Acetaminophen	Imatinib	↑	Increased risk of hepatoxicity may occur. There has been 1 report of fatal hepatic failure with coadministration.
Imatinib	Acetaminophen		
Inducers of CYP3A4 (eg, carbamazepine, dexamethasone, phenobarbital, phenytoin, rifampin, St. John's wort)	Imatinib	↓	Substances that induce CYP3A4 activity may increase metabolism and decrease imatinib plasma concentrations. Coadministration of multiple doses of rifampin and a single dose of imatinib increased imatinib clearance by 3.8-fold, which significantly decreased the mean C_{max} and $AUC_{(0-\infty)}$. When rifampin or other CYP3A4 inducers are indicated with imatinib, consider other therapeutic agents with less enzyme induction potential.
Inhibitors of CYP3A4 (eg, clarithromycin, erythromycin, itraconazole, ketoconazole)	Imatinib	↑	Substances that inhibit the CYP3A4 isoenzyme activity may decrease metabolism and increase imatinib concentrations. Concomitant administration with a single dose of ketoconazole resulted in an increase in the mean AUC and C_{max} of 26% and 40%, respectively, of imatinib.
Imatinib	Certain HMG-CoA reductase inhibitors (eg, simvastatin) Dihydropyridine calcium channel blockers Oral contraceptives (ie, ethinyl estradiol) Triazolobenzodiazepines	↑	Imatinib will increase plasma concentrations of other CYP3A4 metabolized drugs. Coadministration of simvastatin and imatinib resulted in an increase in the mean C_{max} and AUC of simvastatin by 2- and 3.5-fold, respectively.
Imatinib	Cyclosporine Pimozide	↑	Particular caution is recommended when administering imatinib with CYP3A4 substrates that have a narrow therapeutic window.
Imatinib	Warfarin	↑	Because warfarin is metabolized by CYP2C9 and CYP3A4, patients who require anticoagulation should receive low molecular weight or standard heparin.

* ↑ = Object drug increased. ↓ = Object drug decreased. ↔ = Undetermined clinical effect.

Adverse Reactions

➤*Chronic myeloid leukemia (CML):* The majority of imatinib-treated patients experienced adverse reactions at some time. Most events were of mild-to-moderate grade, but drug was discontinued for drug-related adverse events in 4% of patients in chronic phase, 5% in accelerated phase and 5% in blast crisis.

The most frequently reported drug-related adverse events were edema, nausea and vomiting, muscle cramps, musculoskeletal pain, pain, diarrhea, and rash (see tables below for newly diagnosed CML and for other CML patients). Edema was most frequently periorbital or in lower limbs and was managed with diuretics, other supportive measures, or by reducing the dose of imatinib. The frequency of severe edema was 0.9% to 6%.

A variety of adverse reactions represent local or general fluid retention including pleural effusion, ascites, pulmonary edema and rapid weight gain with or without superficial edema. These events appear to be dose related, were more common in the blast crisis and accelerated phase studies (where the dose was 600 mg/day), and are more common in the elderly. These events were usually managed by interrupting imatinib treatment and with diuretics or other appropriate supportive care measures. However, a few of these events may be serious or life threatening, and 1 patient with blast crisis died with pleural effusion, congestive heart failure, and renal failure.

Adverse Reactions Reported in Newly Diagnosed CML Clinical Trial (≥ 10% of All Patients) (%)[1]

Preferred term	All grades		CTC grades 3/4	
	Imatinib (n = 551)	Interferon alfa plus cytarabine (n = 533)	Imatinib (n = 551)	Interferon alfa plus cytarabine (n = 533)
Abdominal pain	23.4%	22.9%	2%	3.6%
Cough	12.5%	21.6%	0.2%	0.6%
Diarrhea	30.3%	40.9%	1.3%	3.2%
Dizziness	13.2%	23.1%	0.5%	3.4%
Dyspepsia	15.1%	9%	0%	0.8%
Fatigue	30.7%	64.7%	1.1%	24%
Fluid retention	54.1%	10.1%	0.9%	0.9%
Headache	28.5%	41.8%	0.4%	3.2%
Hemorrhage	18.9%	19.9%	0.7%	1.3%
Insomnia	11.4%	18.4%	0%	2.3%
Joint pain	26.7%	38.3%	2.2%	6.8%
Muscle cramps	35.4%	9.9%	1.1%	0.2%
Musculoskeletal pain	33.6%	40.5%	2.7%	7.7%
Myalgia	20.9%	38.6%	1.5%	8.1%
Nasopharyngitis	19.2%	7.7%	0%	0.2%
Nausea	42.5%	60.8%	0.4%	5.1%
Other fluid retention events	3.4%	1.5%	0%	0.6%
Pharyngolaryngeal pain	14.2%	11.4%	0.2%	0%
Pyrexia	11.8%	38.6%	0.5%	2.8%
Rash	31.9%	25%	2%	2.1%
Superficial edema	53.2%	8.8%	0.9%	0.4%
Upper respiratory tract infection	12.5%	7.9%	0.2%	0.4%
Vomiting	14.7%	26.6%	0.9%	3.4%
Weight increased	11.6%	1.5%	0.7%	0.2%

[1] All adverse events occurring in greater than or equal to 10% of patients are listed regardless of suspected relationship to treatment.

Adverse Reactions Reported in Other CML Clinical Trials (≥ 10% of All Patients in Any Trial) (%)[1]

Preferred term	Myeloid blast crisis (n = 260)		Accelerated phase (n = 235)		Chronic phase, interferon alfa failure (n = 532)	
	All grades	Grade 3/4	All grades	Grade 3/4	All grades	Grade 3/4
Abdominal pain	30%	6%	33%	4%	32%	1%
Anorexia	14%	2%	17%	2%	7%	0%
Anxiety	8%	0.8%	12%	0%	8%	0.4%
Arthralgia	25%	5%	34%	6%	40%	1%
Asthenia	18%	5%	21%	5%	15%	0.2%
Chest pain	7%	2%	10%	0.4%	11%	0.8%
CNS hemorrhage	9%	7%	3%	3%	2%	1%
Constipation	16%	2%	16%	0.9%	9%	0.4%
Cough	14%	0.8%	27%	0.9%	20%	0%
Diarrhea	43%	4%	57%	5%	48%	3%
Dizziness	12%	0.4%	13%	0%	16%	0.2%
Dyspepsia	12%	0%	22%	0%	27%	0%
Dyspnea	15%	4%	21%	7%	12%	0.9%
Fatigue	30%	4%	46%	4%	48%	1%
Fluid retention	72%	11%	76%	6%	69%	4%
GI hemorrhage	8%	4%	6%	5%	2%	0.4%
Headache	27%	5%	32%	2%	36%	0.6%
Hemorrhage	53%	19%	49%	11%	30%	2%
Hypokalemia	13%	4%	9%	2%	6%	0.8%
Influenza	0.8%	0.4%	6%	0%	11%	0.2%
Insomnia	10%	0%	14%	0%	14%	0.2%
Liver toxicity	10%	5%	12%	6%	6%	3%
Muscle cramps	28%	1%	47%	0.4%	62%	2%
Musculoskeletal pain	42%	9%	49%	9%	38%	2%
Myalgia	9%	0%	24%	2%	27%	0.2%

IMATINIB MESYLATE — ORAL

Adverse Reactions Reported in Other CML Clinical Trials (≥ 10% of All Patients in Any Trial) (%)[1]

Preferred term	Myeloid blast crisis (n = 260) All grades	Myeloid blast crisis (n = 260) Grade 3/4	Accelerated phase (n = 235) All grades	Accelerated phase (n = 235) Grade 3/4	Chronic phase, interferon alfa failure (n = 532) All grades	Chronic phase, interferon alfa failure (n = 532) Grade 3/4
Nasopharyngitis	10%	0%	17%	0%	22%	0.2%
Nausea	71%	5%	73%	5%	63%	3%
Night sweats	13%	0.8%	17%	1%	14%	0.2%
Other fluid retention events[2]	22%	6%	15%	4%	7%	2%
Pharyngitis	10%	0%	12%	0%	15%	0%
Pneumonia	13%	7%	10%	7%	4%	1%
Pruritus	8%	1%	14%	0.9%	14%	0.8%
Pyrexia	41%	7%	41%	8%	21%	2%
Rigors	10%	0%	12%	0.4%	10%	0%
Sinusitis	4%	0.4%	11%	0.4%	9%	0.4%
Skin rash	36%	5%	47%	5%	47%	3%
Superficial edema	66%	6%	74%	3%	67%	2%
Upper respiratory tract infection	3%	0%	12%	0.4%	19%	0%
Vomiting	54%	4%	58%	3%	36%	2%
Weight increased	5%	1%	17%	5%	32%	7%

[1] All adverse reactions occurring in greater than or equal to 10% are listed regardless of suspected relationship to treatment.
[2] Other fluid retention events include pleural effusion, ascites, pulmonary edema, pericardial effusion, anasarca, aggravated edema, and fluid retention not otherwise specified.

Hematologic – Cytopenias, and particularly neutropenia and thrombocytopenia, were a consistent finding in all studies, with a higher frequency at doses greater than or equal to 750 mg (phase I study). However, the occurrence of cytopenias was also dependent on the stage of the disease.

In patients with newly diagnosed CML, cytopenias were less frequent than in the other CML patients (see tables below). The frequency of grade 3 or 4 neutropenia and thrombocytopenia between 2- and 3-fold higher in blast crisis and accelerated phase compared to chronic phase (see tables below). The median duration of the neutropenic and thrombocytopenic episodes varied from 2 to 3 weeks, and from 2 to 4 weeks, respectively. These events can usually be managed with either a reduction of the dose or an interruption of treatment with imatinib, but, in rare cases, require permanent discontinuation of treatment.

Hepatic – Severe elevation of transaminases or bilirubin occurred in 3% to 6% and were usually managed with dose reduction or interruption (the median duration of these episodes was approximately 1 week). Treatment was discontinued permanently because of liver laboratory abnormalities in less than 1% of patients. However, 1 patient, who was taking acetaminophen regularly for fever, died of acute liver failure.

➤*Adverse reactions in pediatric population:* The overall safety profile of pediatric patients treated with imatinib in 39 children studied was similar to that found in studies with adult patients, except that musculoskeletal pain was less frequent (20.5%), and peripheral edema was not reported.

➤*Adverse effects in other subpopulations:* In older patients (greater than or equal to 65 years old), with the exception of edema, where it was more frequent, there was no evidence of an increase in the incidence or severity of adverse events. In women there was an increase in the frequency of neutropenia, as well as grade 1/2 superficial edema, headache, nausea, rigors, vomiting, rash and fatigue. No differences were seen related to race but the subsets were too small for proper evaluation.

➤*Lab test abnormalities:*

Laboratory Abnormalities in Newly Diagnosed CML Trial (%)

CTC Grades	Imatinib (n = 551) Grade 3	Imatinib (n = 551) Grade 4	Interferon alfa plus cytarabine (n = 533) Grade 3	Interferon alfa plus cytarabine (n = 533) Grade 4
Biochemistry parameters				
Elevated alkaline phosphatase	0.2%	0%	0.8%	0%
Elevated ALT	3.1%	0.4%	5.6%	0%
Elevated AST	2.9%	0.2%	3.8%	0.4%
Elevated bilirubin	0.2%	0.5%	0.2%	0%
Elevated creatinine	0%	0%	0.4%	0%
Hematology parameters				
Anemia	2.7%	0.4%	4.1%	0.2%
Neutropenia*	11.4%	2.2%	20.3%	4.3%
Thrombocytopenia*	6.9%	0.2%	15.8%	0.6%

* $P < 0.001$ (difference in grade 3 plus 4 abnormalities between the 2 treatment groups).

Lab Abnormalities in Other CML Clinical Trials (%)

CTC grades*	Myeloid blast crisis (n = 260); 600 mg (n = 223); 400 mg (n = 37) Grade 3	Grade 4	Accelerated phase (n = 235); 600 mg (n = 158); 400 mg (n = 77) Grade 3	Grade 4	Chronic phase, interferon alfa failure (n = 532) 400 mg Grade 3	Grade 4
Biochemistry parameters						
Elevated alkaline phosphatase	4.6%	0%	5.5%	0.4%	0.2%	0%
Elevated ALT	2.3%	0.4%	4.3%	0%	2.1%	0%
Elevated AST	1.9%	0%	3%	0%	2.3%	0%
Elevated bilirubin	3.8%	0%	2.1%	0%	0.6%	0%
Elevated creatinine	1.5%	0%	1.3%	0%	0.2%	0%
Hematology parameters						
Anemia	42%	11%	34%	7%	6%	1%
Neutropenia	16%	48%	23%	36%	27%	9%
Thrombocytopenia	30%	33%	31%	13%	21%	< 1%

* CTC grades are as follows: Neutropenia (grade 3 greater than or equal to 0.5 to 1×10^9/L, grade 4 less than 0.5×10^9/L), thrombocytopenia (grade 3 greater than or equal to 10 to 50×10^9/L, grade 4 less than 10×10^9/L), anemia (hemoglobin greater than or equal to 65 to 80 g/L, grade 4 less than 65 g/L), elevated creatinine (grade 3 greater than 3 to 6 × upper limit normal range [ULN], grade 4 greater than 6 × ULN), elevated bilirubin (grade 3 greater than 3 to 10 × ULN, grade 4 greater than 10 × ULN), elevated alkaline phosphatase (grade 3 greater than 5 to 20 × ULN, grade 4 greater than 20 × ULN), elevated AST or ALT (grade 3 greater than 5 to 20 × ULN, grade 4 greater than 20 × ULN).

➤*Gastrointestinal stromal tumors:* The majority of imatinib-treated patients experienced adverse reactions at some time. The most frequently reported adverse reactions were edema, nausea, diarrhea, abdominal pain, muscle cramps, fatigue and rash. Most events were of mild-to-moderate severity. Drug was discontinued for adverse reactions in 6 patients (8%) in both dose levels studied. Superficial edema, most frequently periorbital or lower extremity edema, was managed with diuretics, other supportive measures, or by reducing the dose of imatinib. Severe (CTC grade 3/4) superficial edema was observed in 3 patients (2%), including face edema in 1 patient. Grade 3/4 pleural effusion or ascites was observed in 3 patients (2%).

Adverse reactions, regardless of relationship to study drug, that were reported in at least 10% of the patients treated with imatinib are shown in the table below. No major differences were seen in the severity of adverse reactions between the 400 mg or 600 mg treatment groups, although overall incidence of diarrhea, muscle cramps, headache, dermatitis, and edema was somewhat higher in the 600 mg treatment group.

Adverse Reactions Reported in GIST Trial (≥ 10% of All Patients at Either Dose) (%)[1]

Preferred term	All CTC grades Initial dose 400 mg/day (n = 73)	All CTC grades Initial dose 600 mg/day (n = 74)	CTC grade 3/4 Initial dose 400 mg/day (n = 73)	CTC grade 3/4 Initial dose 600 mg/day (n = 74)
Abdominal pain	37%	37%	7%	3%
Any hemorrhage	18%	19%	5%	8%
Back pain	11%	10%	1%	0%
Cerebral hemorrhage	1%	0%	1%	0%
Diarrhea	56%	60%	1%	4%
Fatigue	33%	38%	1%	0%
Flatulence	16%	23%	0%	0%
Fluid retention	71%	76%	6%	3%
GI tract hemorrhage	6%	4%	4%	1%
Headache	25%	35%	0%	0%
Increased lacrimation	6%	11%	0%	0%
Insomnia	11%	11%	0%	0%
Muscle cramps	30%	41%	0%	0%
Musculoskeletal pain	19%	11%	3%	0%
Nasopharyngitis	12%	14%	0%	0%
Nausea	53%	56%	3%	3%
Pleural effusion or ascites	6%	4%	1%	3%
Pyrexia	12%	5%	0%	0%
Skin rash	26%	38%	3%	3%
Superficial edema	71%	76%	4%	0%
Taste disturbance	1%	14%	0%	0%
Tumor hemorrhage	1%	4%	1%	4%
Upper respiratory tract infection	6%	11%	0%	0%
Vomiting	22%	23%	1%	3%

[1] All adverse reactions occurring in greater than or equal to 10% of patients are listed regardless of suspected relationship to treatment.

IMATINIB MESYLATE — ORAL

Laboratory Abnormalities in GIST Trial (%)				
	400 mg (n = 73)		600 mg (n = 74)	
CTC grades*	Grade 3	Grade 4	Grade 3	Grade 4
Biochemistry parameters				
Elevated alkaline phosphatase	0%	0%	1%	0%
Elevated ALT	3%	0%	4%	0%
Elevated AST	3%	0%	1%	1%
Elevated bilirubin	1%	0%	1%	3%
Elevated creatinine	0%	1%	3%	0%
Reduced albumin	3%	0%	4%	0%
Hematology parameters				
Anemia	3%	0%	4%	1%
Neutropenia	3%	3%	5%	4%
Thrombocytopenia	0%	0%	1%	0%

* CTC grades are as follows: Neutropenia (grade 3 greater than or equal to 0.5 to 1 × 10^9/L, grade 4 less than 0.5 × 10^9/L), thrombocytopenia (grade 3 greater than or equal to 10 to 50 × 10^9/L, grade 4 less than 10 × 10^9/L, anemia (grade 3 greater than or equal to 65 to 80 g/L, grade 4 less than 65 g/L), elevated creatinine (grade 3 greater than 3 to 6 × ULN, grade 4 greater than 6 × ULN), elevated bilirubin (grade 3 greater than 3 to 10 × ULN, grade 4 greater than 10 × ULN), elevated alkaline phosphatase, ALT or AST (grade 3 greater than 5 to 20 × ULN, grade 4 greater than 20 × ULN), albumin (grade 3 less than 20 g/L).

➤*Additional data from multiple clinical trials:* The following less common (estimated 1% to 10%), infrequent (estimated 0.1% to 1%), and rare (estimated less than 0.1%) adverse events have been reported during clinical trials of imatinib. These events are included based on clinical relevance.

Cardiovascular –
Infrequent: Cardiac failure, tachycardia, hypertension, hypotension, flushing, peripheral coldness.
Rare: Pericarditis.
Vascular disorders:
• *Rare* – Thrombosis/embolism.

CNS –
Less common: Paresthesia.
Infrequent: Depression, anxiety, syncope, peripheral neuropathy, somnolence, migraine, memory impairment.
Rare: Increased intracranial pressure, cerebral edema (including fatalities), confusion, convulsions.

Dermatologic –
Less common: Dry skin, alopecia.
Infrequent: Exfoliative dermatitis, bullous eruption, nail disorder, skin pigmentation changes, photosensitivity reaction, purpura, psoriasis.
Rare: Vesicular rash, Stevens-Johnson syndrome, acute generalized exanthematous pustulosis.

GI –
Less common: Abdominal distension, gastroesophageal reflux, mouth ulceration.
Infrequent: Gastric ulcer, gastroenteritis, gastritis.
Rare: Colitis, ileus/intestinal obstruction, pancreatitis.

GU –
Infrequent: Breast enlargement, menorrhagia, sexual dysfunction.

Hematologic –
Infrequent: Pancytopenia.
Rare: Aplastic anemia.

Hypersensitivity –
Rare: Angioedema.

Lab test abnormalities –
Infrequent: Blood CPK increased, blood LDH increased.

Metabolic/Nutritional –
Infrequent: Hypophosphatemia, dehydration, gout, appetite disturbances, weight decreased.
Rare: Hyperkalemia, hyponatremia.

Musculoskeletal –
Less common: Joint swelling.
Infrequent: Sciatica, joint and muscle stiffness.

Renal –
Infrequent: Renal failure, urinary frequency, hematuria.

Respiratory –
Rare: Interstitial pneumonitis, pulmonary fibrosis.

Special senses –
Less common: Conjunctivitis, vision blurred.
Infrequent: Conjunctival hemorrhage, dry eye, vertigo, tinnitus.
Rare: Macular edema, papilledema, retinal hemorrhage, glaucoma, vitreous hemorrhage.

Miscellaneous –
General disorders and administration site conditions:
• *Rare* – Tumor necrosis.
Infections:
• *Infrequent* – Sepsis, herpes simplex, herpes zoster.

Overdosage

Experience with doses greater than 800 mg is limited.

An oral dose of 1,200 mg/m²/day, approximately 2.5 times the human dose of 800 mg, based on body surface area, was not lethal to rats following 14 days of administration. A dose of 3,600 mg/m²/day, approximately 7.5 times the human dose of 800 mg, was lethal to rats after 7 to 10 administrations, due to general deterioration of the animals with secondary degenerative histological changes in many tissues.

➤*Treatment:* In the event of overdosage, the patient should be observed and appropriate supportive treatment given.

SUNITINIB MALATE

Rx	Sutent (Pfizer)	**Capsules:** 12.5 mg (as base)	(Pfizer STN 12.5 mg). Orange. In 30s.
		25 mg (as base)	(Pfizer STN 25 mg). Caramel/Orange. In 30s.
		50 mg (as base)	(Pfizer STN 50 mg). Caramel. In 30s.

SUNITINIB MALATE — ORAL

Indications

➤*GI stromal tumor (GIST):* For the treatment of GIST after disease progression on or intolerance to imatinib.

➤*Advanced renal cell carcinoma (RCC):* For the treatment of advanced RCC.

Approval for advanced RCC is based on partial response rates and duration of responses. There are no randomized trials of sunitinib demonstrating clinical benefit, such as increased survival or improvement in disease-related symptoms in RCC.

Administration and Dosage

➤*Approved by the FDA:* January 26, 2006.

➤*Recommended dose:* The recommended dose for GIST and advanced RCC is one 50 mg oral dose taken once daily on a schedule of 4 weeks on treatment followed by 2 weeks off. It may be taken with or without food.

➤*Dose modification:* Dose increase or reduction of 12.5 mg increments is recommended based on individual safety and tolerability.

➤*Concomitant therapy:* Selection of an alternative concomitant medication with no or minimal enzyme induction potential is recommended. A dosage increase for sunitinib to a maximum of 87.5 mg daily should be considered if sunitinib must be coadministered with a CYP3A4 inducer. If dose is increased, the patient should be monitored carefully for toxicity.

Selection of an alternative concomitant medication with no or minimal enzyme inhibition potential is recommended. A dosage reduction for sunitinib to a minimum of 37.5 mg daily should be considered if sunitinib must be coadministered with a strong CYP3A4 inhibitors. If dosage is increased, monitor carefully for toxicity.

➤*Storage/Stability:* Store at 25°C (77°F); excursions are permitted to 15° to 30°C (59° to 86°F).

Actions

➤*Pharmacology:* Sunitinib is a small molecule that inhibits multiple receptor tyrosine kinases (RTKs), some of which are implicated in tumor growth, pathologic angiogenesis, and metastatic progression of cancer. Sunitinib was evaluated for its inhibitory activity against a variety of kinases (greater than 80 kinases) and was identified as an inhibitor of platelet-derived growth factor receptors (PDGFRα and PDGFRβ), vascular endothelial growth factor receptors (VEGFR1, VEGFR2, and VEGFR3), stem cell factor receptor (KIT), fms-like tyrosine kinase-3, colony stimulating factor receptor type 1, and the glial cell-line derived neurotrophic factor receptor (RET). Sunitinib inhibition of the activity of these RTKs has been demonstrated in biochemical and cellular assays, and inhibition of function has been demonstrated in cell proliferation assays. The primary metabolite exhibits similar potency compared with sunitinib in biochemical and cellular assays.

Sunitinib inhibited the phosphorylation of multiple RTKs (PDGFRβ, VEGFR2, KIT) in tumor xenografts expressing RTK targets in vivo and demonstrated inhibition of tumor growth or tumor regression and/or inhibited metastases in some experimental models of cancer. Sunitinib demonstrated the ability to inhibit growth of tumor cells expressing dysregulated target RTKs (PDGFR, RET, or KIT) in vitro and to inhibit PDGFRβ and VEGFR2-dependent tumor angiogenesis in vivo.

➤*Pharmacokinetics:*

Absorption – The pharmacokinetics of sunitinib have been evaluated in 135 healthy volunteers and in 266 patients with solid tumors.

The pharmacokinetics were similar in healthy volunteers and in the solid tumor patient populations tested, including patients with GIST and metastatic RCC (MRCC).

SUNITINIB MALATE — ORAL

Maximum plasma concentrations (C_{max}) of sunitinib are generally observed between 6 and 12 hours (time to maximum concentration) following oral administration. Food has no effect on the bioavailability of sunitinib. Sunitinib may be taken with or without food.

Distribution – Binding of sunitinib and its primary metabolite to human plasma protein in vitro was 95% and 90%, respectively, with no concentration dependence in the range of 100 to 4,000 ng/mL. The apparent volume of distribution for sunitinib was 2,230 L. In the dosing range of 25 to 100 mg, the area under the plasma concentration-time curve (AUC) and C_{max} increase proportionately with dose.

Metabolism/Excretion – Sunitinib is metabolized primarily by the cytochrome P–450 enzyme, CYP3A4, to produce its primary active metabolite, which is further metabolized by CYP3A4. The primary active metabolite comprises 23% to 37% of the total exposure. Elimination is primarily via feces. In a human mass balance study of ^{14}C sunitinib, 61% of the dose was eliminated in feces, with renal elimination accounting for 16% of the administered dose. Sunitinib and its primary active metabolite were the major drug-related compounds identified in plasma, urine, and feces, representing 91.5%, 86.4%, and 73.8% of radioactivity in pooled samples, respectively. Minor metabolites were identified in urine and feces but generally not found in plasma. Total oral clearance ranged from 34 to 62 L/h with an interpatient variability of 40%.

Following administration of a single oral dose in healthy volunteers, the terminal half-lives of sunitinib and its primary active metabolite are approximately 40 to 60 hours and 80 to 110 hours, respectively. With repeated daily administration, sunitinib accumulates 3- to 4-fold while the primary metabolite accumulates 7- to 10-fold. Steady-state concentrations of sunitinib and its primary active metabolite are achieved within 10 to 14 days. By day 14, combined plasma concentrations of sunitinib and its active metabolite ranged from 62.9 to 101 ng/mL. No significant changes in the pharmacokinetics of sunitinib or the primary active metabolite were observed with repeated daily administration or with repeated cycles in the dosing regimens tested.

Contraindications

Hypersensitivity to sunitinib or to any other component of the product.

Warnings

➤*Fertility impairment:* Effects on the female reproductive system were identified in a 3-month repeat dose monkey study (2, 6, 12 mg/kg/day), where ovarian changes (decreased follicular development) were noted at 12 mg/kg/day (approximately 5.1 times the AUC in patients administered the RDD), in which uterine changes (endometrial atrophy) were noted at greater than or equal to 2 mg/kg/day (approximately 0.4 times the AUC in patients administered the recommended daily dose [RDD]). With the addition of vaginal atrophy, the uterine and ovarian effects were reproduced at 6 mg/kg/day in the 9-month monkey study (0.3, 1.5, and 6 mg/kg/day administered daily for 28 days followed by a 14 day respite; the 6 mg/kg dose produced a mean AUC that was approximately 0.8 times the AUC in patients administered the RDD). A no-effect level was not identified in the 3 month study; 1.5 mg/kg/day represents a no–effect level in monkeys administered sunitinib for 9 months.

Although fertility was not affected in rats, sunitinib may impair fertility in humans. In female rats, no fertility effects were observed at dosages of less than or equal to 5 mg/kg/day ([0.5, 1.5, 5 mg/kg/day] administered for 21 days up to gestational day 7. The 5 mg/kg dose produced an AUC that was approximately 5 times the AUC in patients administered the RDD); however, significant embryolethality was observed at the 5 mg/kg dose. No reproductive effects were observed in male rats dosed (1, 3, or 10 mg/kg/day) for 58 days prior to mating with untreated females. Fertility, copulation, conception indices, and sperm evaluation (morphology, concentration, and motility) were unaffected by sunitinib at dosages less than or equal to 10 mg/kg/day (the 10 mg/kg/day dosage produced a mean AUC that was approximately 25.8 times the AUC in patients administered the RDD).

➤*Elderly:* Of the 450 patients with solid tumors reported from clinical studies of sunitinib, 115 (25.6%) were 65 years of age and older. No overall differences in safety or efficacy were observed between younger and older patients.

➤*Pregnancy: Category D.* Sunitinib was evaluated in pregnant rats (0.3, 1.5, 3, 5 mg/kg/day) and rabbits (0.5, 1, 5, 20 mg/kg/day) for effects on the embryo. Significant increases in the incidence of embryolethality and structural abnormalities were observed in rats at the dosage of 5 mg/kg/day (approximately 5.5 times the systemic exposure in patients administered the RDD). Significantly increased embryolethality was observed in rabbits at 5 mg/kg/day while developmental effects were observed at greater than or equal to 1 mg/kg/day (approximately 0.3 times the AUC in patients administered the RDD of 50 mg/day). Developmental effects consisted of fetal skeletal malformations of the ribs and vertebrae in rats. In rabbits, cleft lip was observed at 1 mg/kg/day, and cleft lip and cleft palate were observed at 5 mg/kg/day (approximately 2.7 times the AUC in patients administered the RDD). Neither fetal loss nor malformations were observed in rats dosed at less than or equal to 3 mg/kg/day (approximately 2.3 times the AUC in patients administered the RDD).

As angiogenesis is a critical component of embryonic and fetal development, inhibition of angiogenesis following administration of sunitinib should be expected to result in adverse effects on pregnancy. There are no adequate and well-controlled studies of sunitinib in pregnant women. If the drug is used during pregnancy, or if the patient becomes pregnant while receiving this drug, apprise the patient of the potential hazard to the fetus. Advise women of childbearing potential to avoid becoming pregnant while receiving treatment with sunitinib.

➤*Lactation:* Sunitinib and/or its metabolites are excreted in rat milk. In lactating female rats administered 15 mg/kg, sunitinib and its metabolites were extensively excreted in milk at concentrations up to 12-fold higher than in plasma. It is not known whether sunitinib or its primary active metabolite are excreted in human milk. Because drugs are commonly excreted in human milk and because of the potential for serious adverse reactions in breast-feeding infants, advise women against breast-feeding while taking sunitinib.

➤*Children:* The safety and efficacy of sunitinib in children have not been studied in clinical trials.

Precautions

➤*Monitoring:* Perform complete blood counts (CBCs) with platelet count and serum chemistries including phosphate at the beginning of each treatment cycle for patients receiving treatment with sunitinib .

Monitor for clinical signs and symptoms of congestive heart failure (CHF). Consider baseline and periodic evaluations of left ventricular ejection fraction (LVEF). Monitor for hypertension and myelosuppression regularly. Monitor for adrenal insufficiency in patients who experience stress such as trauma, surgery, or severe infection. Monitor thyroid function in patients with symptoms suggestive of hypothyroidism.

➤*Left ventricular dysfunction:* In the 2 MRCC studies, 25 patients (15%) had decreases in LVEF to below the lower limit of normal (LLN). In GIST study A, 22 patients (11%) on sunitinib and 3 patients (3%) on placebo had treatment-emergent LVEF values below the LLN. Nine of 22 GIST patients on sunitinib with LVEF changes recovered without intervention. Five patients had documented LVEF recovery following intervention (dose reduction, 1 patient; addition of antihypertensive or diuretic medications, 4 patients). Six patients went off study without documented recovery. Additionally, 3 patients (1%) on sunitinib had grade 3 reductions in left ventricular systolic function to LVEF less than 40%; 2 of these patients died without receiving further study drug. No GIST patients on placebo had grade 3 decreased LVEF. In GIST study A, 1 patient (less than 1%) on sunitinib and 1 patient (1%) on placebo died of diagnosed heart failure; 2 patients (1%) on sunitinib and 2 patients (2%) on placebo died of treatment-emergent cardiac arrest.

Patients who presented with cardiac events within 12 months prior to sunitinib administration, such as myocardial infarction (including severe/unstable angina), coronary/peripheral artery bypass graft, symptomatic CHF, cerebrovascular accident or transient ischemic attack, or pulmonary embolism were excluded from sunitinib clinical studies. It is unknown whether patients with these concomitant conditions may be at a higher risk of developing drug-related left ventricular dysfunction. Weigh this risk against the potential benefits of the drug. Carefully monitor these patients for clinical signs and symptoms of CHF while receiving sunitinib. Consider baseline and periodic evaluations of LVEF, while the patient is receiving sunitinib. Also consider a baseline evaluation of ejection fraction, in patients without cardiac risk factors.

In the presence of clinical manifestations of CHF, discontinuation of sunitinib is recommended. Interrupt and/or reduced the dose of sunitinib in patients without clinical evidence of CHF but with an ejection fraction less than 50% and greater than 20% below baseline.

➤*Hemorrhagic events:* Bleeding events occurred in 44 of 169 patients (26%) receiving sunitinib for MRCC and 37 of 202 patients (18%) receiving sunitinib in GIST study A, compared with 17 of 102 patients (17%) receiving placebo. Epistaxis was the most common hemorrhagic adverse reaction reported. Less common bleeding reactions in MRCC or GIST patients included rectal, gingival, upper GI, genital, and wound bleeding. Most reactions in MRCC patients were grade 1 or 2; there was one grade 3 reaction (bleeding foot wound). In GIST study A, 14 of 202 patients (7%) receiving sunitinib and 9 of 102 patients (9%) on placebo had grade 3 or 4 bleeding reactions. In addition, 1 patient in study A taking placebo had a fatal GI bleeding reaction during cycle 2.

Tumor-related hemorrhage has been observed in patients treated with sunitinib. These reactions may occur suddenly, and, in the case of pulmonary tumors, may present as severe and life–threatening hemoptysis or pulmonary hemorrhage. Fatal pulmonary hemorrhage occurred in 2 patients receiving sunitinib on a clinical trial of patients with metastatic non-small cell lung cancer (NSCLC). Both patients had squamous cell histology. Sunitinib is not approved for use in patients with NSCLC. Treatment-emergent grade 3 and 4 tumor hemorrhage occurred in 5 of 202 patients (3%) with GIST receiving sunitinib on study A. Tumor hemorrhages were observed as early as cycle 1 and as late as cycle 6. One of these 5 patients received no further drug following tumor hemorrhage. None of the other 4 patients discontinued treatment or experienced dose delay because of to tumor hemorrhage. No patients with GIST in the study A placebo arm were observed to undergo intratumoral hemorrhage. Tumor hemorrhage has not been observed in patients with MRCC. Clinical assessment of these reactions should include serial CBCs and physical examinations.

➤*GI effects:* Serious, sometimes fatal GI complications including GI perforation, have occurred rarely in patients with intra-abdominal malignancies treated with sunitinib.

➤*Hypertension:* Hypertension (all grades) was reported in 48 of 169 MRCC patients (28%), 31 of 202 GIST patients on sunitinib (15%), and 11 of 102 GIST patients on placebo (11%). Grade 3 hypertension was reported in 10 MRCC patients (6%), 9 GIST patients on sunitinib (4%), and none of the GIST patients on placebo. No grade 4 hypertension was reported. Sunitinib dosing was reduced or temporarily delayed for hypertension in 6 of 169 MRCC patients (4%) and none of the patients in GIST study A. No patients were discontinued from treatment with sunitinib because of to systemic hypertension. Severe hypertension (greater than 200 mm Hg systolic or

SUNITINIB MALATE — ORAL

110 mm Hg diastolic) occurred in 10 of 169 MRCC patients (6%), 8/202 GIST patients on sunitinib (4%), and 1 of 102 GIST patients on placebo (1%).

Monitor patients for hypertension and treat as needed with standard antihypertensive therapy. In cases of severe hypertension, temporary suspension of sunitinib is recommended until hypertension is controlled.

➤*Adrenal function:* Adrenal toxicity was noted in nonclinical repeat—dose studies of 14 days to 9 months in rats and monkeys at plasma exposures as low as 0.7 times the AUC observed in clinical studies. Histological changes of the adrenal gland were characterized as hemorrhage, necrosis, congestion, hypertrophy, and inflammation. In clinical studies, computerized tomography/magnetic resonance imaging obtained in 336 patients after exposure to one or more cycles of sunitinib demonstrated no evidence of adrenal hemorrhage or necrosis. Corticotropin (ACTH) stimulation testing was performed in approximately 400 patients across multiple clinical trials of sunitinib. Among patients with normal baseline ACTH stimulation testing, 1 patient developed consistently abnormal test results during treatment that are unexplained and may be related to treatment with sunitinib. Eleven additional patients with normal baseline testing had abnormalities in the final test performed, with peak cortisol levels of 12 to 16.4 mcg/dL (normal is greater than 18 mcg/dL) following stimulation. None of these patients were reported to have clinical evidence of adrenal insufficiency.

Drug Interactions

➤*CYP-450 system:* In vitro studies in human liver microsomes and hepatocytes of the activity of CYP isoforms CYP1A2, CYP2A6, CYP2B6, CYP2C8, CYP2C9, CYP2C19, CYP2D6, CYP2E1, CYP3A4/5, and CYP4A9/11 indicate that sunitinib and its primary active metabolite are unlikely to have any clinically relevant drug-drug interactions with drugs that may be metabolized by these enzymes.

➤*CYP3A4 inducers:* Coadministration of sunitinib with inducers of the CYP3A4 family (eg, dexamethasone, carbamazepine, phenobarbital, phenytoin, rifabutin, rifampin, rifapentine, St. John's wort) may decrease sunitinib concentrations.

Coadministration of sunitinib with the strong CYP3A4 inducer, rifampin, resulted in a 23% and 46% reduction in the combined (sunitinib plus primary active metabolite) C_{max} and AUC $_{0-\infty}$ values, respectively, after a single dose of sunitinib in healthy volunteers.

St. John's wort may decrease sunitinib plasma concentrations unpredictably. Patients receiving sunitinib should not take St. John's wort concomitantly.

Selection of an alternative concomitant medication with no or minimal enzyme induction potential is recommended. Consider a dosage increase for sunitinib to a maximum of 87.5 mg daily if sunitinib must be coadministered with a CYP3A4 inducer. If dose is increased, carefully monitor the patient carefully for toxicity.

➤*CYP3A4 inhibitors:* Coadministration of sunitinib with strong inhibitors of the CYP3A4 family (eg, atazanavir, clarithromycin, indinavir, itraconazole, ketoconazole, nefazodone, nelfinavir, ritonavir, saquinavir, telithromycin, voriconazole) may increase sunitinib concentrations.

Coadministration of sunitinib with the strong CYP3A4 inhibitor, ketoconazole, resulted in 49% and 51% increases in the combined (sunitinib plus primary active metabolite) C_{max} and $AUC_{0-\infty}$ values, respectively, after a single dose of sunitinib in healthy volunteers.

Selection of an alternative concomitant medication with no or minimal enzyme inhibition potential is recommended. Consider a dosage reduction for sunitinib to a minimum of 37.5 mg daily if sunitinib must be coadministered with a strong CYP3A4 inhibitors. If dosage is increased, monitor carefully for toxicity.

➤*Drug/Food interactions:* Grapefruit may increase plasma concentrations of sunitinib.

Adverse Reactions

➤*GIST study A:* Median duration of blinded study treatment was 2 cycles for patients on sunitinib (mean, 3; range, 1 to 9) and 1 cycle (mean, 1.8; range, 1 to 6) for patients on placebo. Dose reductions occurred in 23 patients (11%) on sunitinib and none on placebo. Dose interruptions occurred in 59 patients (29%) on sunitinib and 31 patients (30%) on placebo. The rates of treatment–emergent, nonfatal adverse reactions resulting in permanent discontinuation were 7% and 6% in the sunitinib and placebo groups, respectively.

Most treatment-emergent adverse reactions in both study arms were grade 1 or 2 in severity. Grade 3 or 4 treatment-emergent adverse reactions were reported in 56% versus 51% of patients on sunitinib versus placebo, respectively. Diarrhea, hypertension, bleeding, mucositis, skin abnormalities, and altered taste were more common in patients receiving sunitinib. The following table compares the incidence of common (greater than 10%) treatment-emergent adverse reactions for patients receiving sunitinib versus those on placebo.

Sunitinib Adverse Reactions (at Least 10% of GIST Patients)[a]

Adverse reactions	Sunitinib (n = 202)		Placebo (n = 102)	
	All grades	Grade 3/4[b]	All grades	Grade 3/4[c]
Any		114 (56%)		52 (51%)
CNS				
Fatigue	84 (42%)	17 (8%)	48 (47%)	8 (8%)
Cardiovascular				
Hypertension	31 (15%)	9 (4%)	11 (11%)	0
CNS				
Headache	26 (13%)	3 (2%)	23 (23%)	0
Dermatologic				
Hand-foot syndrome	28 (14%)	9 (4%)	10 (10%)	3 (3%)
Rash	28 (14%)	2 (1%)	9 (9%)	0
Skin discoloration	61 (30%)	0	23 (23%)	0
GI				
Altered taste[d]	42 (21%)	0	12 (12%)	0
Anorexia	67 (33%)	1 (1%)	30 (29%)	5 (5%)
Diarrhea	81 (40%)	9 (4%)	27 (27%)	0
Nausea	63 (31%)	3 (2%)	33 (32%)	5 (5%)
Mucositis/Stomatitis	58 (29%)	2 (1%)	18 (18%)	2 (2%)
Vomiting	49 (24%)	4 (2%)	24 (24%)	3 (3%)
Constipation	41 (20%)	0	14 (14%)	2 (2%)
Abdominal pain[e]	67 (33%)	22 (11%)	39 (38%)	12 (12%)
Musculoskeletal				
Arthralgia	24 (12%)	2 (1%)	16 (16%)	0
Back pain	23 (11%)	2 (1%)	16 (16%)	4 (4%)
Myalgia/Limb pain	28 (14%)	1 (1%)	9 (9%)	1 (1%)
Respiratory				
Dyspnea	20 (10%)	0	19 (19%)	3 (3%)
Cough	17 (8%)	0	13 (13%)	0
Miscellaneous				
Asthenia	45 (22%)	10 (5%)	11 (11%)	3 (3%)
Fever	36 (18%)	3 (2%)	17 (17%)	1 (1%)
Bleeding, all sites	37 (18%)	14 (7%)	17 (17%)	9 (9%)

[a] Common Toxicity Criteria for Adverse reactions (CTCAE), Version 3.0
[b] Grade 4 adverse reactions in patient on sunitinib included abdominal pain (2%) and bleeding (2%).
[c] Grade 4 adverse reactions in patients on placebo included bone pain (1%), mucositis (1%), vomiting (1%), back pain (1%), fatigue (3%), and abdominal pain (3%).
[d] Includes decreased appetite
[e] Includes abdominal quadrant, gastric, hypochondrial, abdominal, flank, and cancer-related pain

➤*Other adverse reactions:* Oral pain other than mucositis/stomatitis occurred in 12 patients (6%) on sunitinib versus 3 (3%) on placebo. Hair color changes occurred in 15 patients (7%) on sunitinib versus 4 (4%) on placebo. Alopecia was observed in 10 patients (5%) on sunitinib versus 2 (2%) on placebo.

Lab test abnormalities –

Sunitinib Laboratory Abnormalities (10% or More of GIST Patients)[a]

Laboratory test	Sunitinib (n = 202)		Placebo (n = 102)	
	All grades	Grade 3/4[b]	All grades	Grade 3/4[c]
Any		68 (34%)		22 (22%)
AST/ALT	78 (39%)	3 (2%)	23 (23%)	1 (1%)
Alkaline phosphatase	48 (24%)	7 (4%)	21 (21%)	4 (4%)
Total bilirubin	32 (16%)	2 (1%)	8 (8%)	0
Indirect bilirubin	20 (10%)	0	4 (4%)	0
Amylase	35 (17%)	10 (5%)	12 (12%)	3 (3%)
Lipase	50 (25%)	20 (10%)	17 (17%)	7 (7%)
Decreased LVEF	21 (10%)	2 (1%)	3 (3%)	0
Creatinine	25 (12%)	1 (1%)	7 (7%)	0
Hypokalemia	24 (12%)	1 (1%)	4 (4%)	0
Hypernatremia	20 (10%)	0	4 (4%)	1 (1%)
Uric acid	31 (15%)	16 (8%)	16 (16%)	8 (8%)
Neutropenia	107 (53%)	20 (10%)	4 (4%)	0
Lymphopenia	76 (38%)	0	16 (16%)	0

SUNITINIB MALATE — ORAL

Sunitinib Laboratory Abnormalities (10% or More of GIST Patients)[a]

Laboratory test	Sunitinib (n = 202)		Placebo (n = 102)	
	All grades	Grade 3/4[b]	All grades	Grade 3/4[c]
Anemia	52 (26%)	6 (3%)	22 (22%)	2 (2%)
Thrombocytopenia	76 (38%)	10 (5%)	4 (4%)	0

[a] CTCAE, Version 3.0
[b] Grade 4 adverse reactions in patients on sunitinib included thrombocytopenia (1%), alkaline phosphatase (1%), creatinine (1%), hypokalemia (1%), lipase (2%), neutropenia (2%), and anemia (2%).
[c] Grade 4 adverse reactions in patients on placebo included amylase (1%), lipase (1%), anemia (2%), and thrombocytopenia (1%)

Grade 3 or 4 treatment-emergent laboratory abnormalities were observed in 68 (34%) versus 22 (22%) patients on sunitinib and placebo, respectively. Elevated liver function tests, pancreatic enzymes, and creatinine were more common in patients treated with sunitinib than placebo. Decreased LVEF and myelosuppression were also more common with sunitinib treatment. Treatment-emergent electrolyte disturbances of all types were more common in patients on sunitinib than on placebo, including hyperkalemia (6% vs 4%), hypokalemia (12% vs 4%), hypernatremia (10% vs 4%), hyponatremia (6% vs 1%), and hypophosphatemia (9% vs 0%). Three sunitinib patients (1.5%) had grade 3 hypophosphatemia. Acquired hypothyroidism was noted in 8 patients (4%) on sunitinib versus 1 (1%) on placebo.

➤*MRCC studies:* The data described in the following table reflect exposure to sunitinib in 169 patients with MRCC enrolled in studies 1 and 2. The median duration of treatment was 5.5 months (range, 0.8 to 11.2) for study 1 and 7.7 months (range, 0.2 to 16.1) for study 2. Dose interruptions occurred in 48 patients (45%) on study 1 and 45 patients (71%) on study 2; 1 or more dose reductions occurred in 23 patients (22%) on study 1 and 22 patients (35%) on study 2. The following table summarizes treatment emergent adverse reactions for at least 10 % of all patients with MRCC who received at least one 50 mg dose of sunitinib. Hematology laboratory abnormalities are presented separately, in the second table that follows.

Sunitinib Adverse Reactions (at Least 10% MRCC Patients)[a]

Adverse reaction	MRCC (n = 169)	
	All grades	Grade 3[b]
Any	169 (100%)	123 (73%)
Cardiovascular		
Edema, peripheral	28 (17%)	1 (1%)
Hypertension	48 (28%)	10 (6%)
CNS		
Fatigue	125 (74%)	19 (11%)
Headache	43 (25%)	2 (1%)
Dizziness	27 (16%)	3 (2%)
Dermatologic		
Alopecia	20 (12%)	0
Dry skin	29 (17%)	0
Hair color changes	29 (17%)	0
Hand-foot syndrome	21 (12%)	5 (3%)
Rash	64 (38%)	1 (1%)
Skin discoloration	55 (33%)	0
GI		
Abdominal pain	34 (20%)	5 (3%)
Altered taste	73 (43%)	0
Anorexia	53 (31%)	1 (1%)
Constipation	57 (34%)	1 (1%)
Diarrhea	93 (55%)	8 (5%)
Dyspepsia	77 (46%)	1 (1%)
Flatulence	24 (14%)	0
Glossodynia	25 (15%)	0
Mucositis/Stomatitis	90 (53%)	4 (2%)
Nausea	92 (54%)	7 (4%)
Vomiting	63 (37%)	7 (4%)
Metabolic/Nutritional		
Dehydration	19 (11%)	5 (3%)
Musculoskeletal		
Arthralgia	48 (28%)	2 (1%)
Back pain	29 (17%)	1 (1%)
Myalgia	29 (17%)	1 (1%)
Pain in limb	31 (18%)	1 (1%)
Respiratory		
Cough	29 (17%)	1 (1%)
Dyspnea	47 (28%)	8 (5%)
Miscellaneous		
Bleeding, all sites	44 (26%)	1 (1%)
Fever	26 (15%)	2 (1%)

[a] CTCAE, Version 3.0
[b] There were no grade 4 adverse reactions among the reactions reported with a greater than or equal to 10% incidence in the MRCC population.

➤*Other adverse reactions:*

Lab test abnormalities – Other significant adverse reactions occurring in MRCC patients receiving sunitinib included peripheral neuropathy (10%), appetite disturbance (9%), blistering of the skin (7%), periorbital edema (7%) and increased lacrimation (6%).

Sunitinib Laboratory Abnormalities in MRCC Patients[a]

Laboratory test	Unit	MRCC (n = 169)		
		Grade 3	Grade 4	Total (grade 3 and 4)
Hematology		54 (32%)	4 (2%)	58 (34%)
Anemia	g/L	9 (5%)	3 (2%)	12 (7%)
Leukopenia	10^9/L	12 (7%)	0	12 (7%)
Lymphopenia	10^9/L	33 (20%)	2 (1%)	35 (21%)
Neutropenia	10^9/L	21 (12%)	1 (1%)	22 (13%)
Thrombocytopenia	10^9/L	5 (3%)	0	5 (3%)

[a] CTCAE, Version 3.0

Common treatment-emergent grade 3 and 4 chemistry laboratory abnormalities in the MRCC studies included increased lipase (16%), increased amylase (5%), hypophosphatemia (10%), and hyperuricemia (10%).

➤*Cardiovascular:* Two patients with MRCC experienced grade 3 myocardial ischemia, 1 had grade 2 "cardiovascular toxicity" reported as an adverse reaction and 1 patient experienced a fatal myocardial infarction while on treatment.

Data from nonclinical (in vitro and in vivo) studies indicate that sunitinib has the potential to inhibit the cardiac action potential repolarization process (eg, prolongation of QT interval). In GIST study A, 23 patients (11%) on sunitinib versus 12 (12%) on placebo had observed QT prolongation greater than 20 milliseconds from baseline. No consistent, clinically significant QTc prolongation has been observed in completed clinical studies.

Four patients (2%) on the 2 MRCC studies had venous thromboembolic reactions reported; 2 patients with pulmonary embolism (both grade 4) and 2 patients with deep venous thrombosis (DVT) (both grade 3). Dose interruption occurred in one of these cases. Seven patients (3%) on sunitinib and none on placebo in GIST study A experienced venous thromboembolic reactions; 5 of the 7 were grade 3 DVTs, and 2 were grade 1 or 2. Four of these 7 GIST patients discontinued treatment following first observation of DVT.

➤*Endocrine:* Hypothyroidism was reported as an adverse reaction in 7 patients (4%) across the 2 MRCC studies. Additionally, thyrotropin TSH elevations were reported in 4 patients (2%). Overall, 7% of the MRCC population had either clinical or laboratory evidence of treatment-emergent hypothyroidism. Treatment-emergent acquired hypothyroidism was noted in 8 GIST patients (4%) on sunitinib versus 1 (1%) on placebo.

Patients with symptoms suggestive of hypothyroidism should have laboratory monitoring of thyroid function performed and be treated as per standard medical practice.

➤*CNS:* In clinical studies of sunitinib , seizures have been observed in subjects with radiological evidence of brain metastases. In addition, there have been rare (less than 1%) reports of subjects presenting with seizures and radiological evidence of reversible posterior leukoencephalopathy syndrome (RPLS). None of these subjects had a fatal outcome to the reaction. Patients with seizures and signs/symptoms consistent with RPLS, such as hypertension, headache, decreased alertness, altered mental functioning, and visual loss, including cortical blindness, should be controlled with medical management including control of hypertension. Temporary suspension of sunitinib is recommended; following resolution, treatment may be resumed at the discretion of the treating health care provider.

➤*Hematologic/Lymphatic:* Grade 3 and 4 neutropenia were reported in 21 (13%) and 1 (1%) patients with MRCC, 19 (9%) and 3 (2%) patients with GIST on sunitinib, respectively. In study A, 1 patient each in the sunitinib and placebo groups had febrile neutropenia. Grade 3 and 4 thrombocytopenia was reported in 5 (3%) and zero patients with MRCC, 7 (4%) and 1 (1%) patients with GIST on sunitinib, respectively. No GIST patients receiving placebo experienced either grade 3 or 4 neutropenia or thrombocytopenia. The rates of dose reductions and delays for hematologic abnormalities were 4% and 2% for neutropenia, 2% and 0% for anemia, and 1% and 1% for thrombocytopenia for MRCC and GIST patients, respectively. One MRCC patient with an adverse reaction report of grade 4 thrombocytopenia discontinued treatment.

SUNITINIB MALATE — ORAL

Regularly monitor patients receiving sunitinib for myelosuppression.

➤*Miscellaneous:* Grade 3 and 4 increases in serum lipase were observed in 23 (14%) and 4 (2%), respectively, of 169 patients receiving sunitinib for MRCC. Grade 3 and 4 increases in serum amylase were observed in 8 (5%) and 1 (1%) MRCC patients, respectively. Increases in lipase levels were transient and were generally not accompanied by signs or symptoms of pancreatitis in subjects with either MRCC or GIST. Pancreatitis has been observed rarely (less than 1%) in patients receiving sunitinib for GIST or MRCC. If symptoms of pancreatitis are present, discontinue sunitinib and provide appropriate supportive care.

Overdosage

➤*Symptoms:* In nonclinical studies mortality was observed following as few as 5 daily doses of 500 mg/kg (3,000 mg/m^2) in rats. At this dose, signs of toxicity included impaired muscle coordination, head shakes, hypoactivity, ocular discharge, piloerection, and GI distress. Mortality and similar signs of toxicity were observed at lower doses when administered for longer durations.

➤*Treatment:* Treatment of overdose with sunitinib should consist of general supportive measures. There is no specific antidote for overdosage with sunitinib . If indicated, achieve elimination of unabsorbed drug by emesis or gastric lavage.

Patient Information

Advise patients of aGI disorders such as diarrhea, nausea, stomatitis, dyspepsia, and vomiting were the most commonly reported GI reactions occurring in patients who received sunitinib. Supportive care for GI adverse reactions requiring treatment may include antiemetic or antidiarrheal medication.

Advise patients that possible skin discoloration is due to the drug color (yellow), which occurs in approximately one third of patients. Advise patients that depigmentation of the hair or skin may occur during treatment with sunitinib. Other possible dermatologic effects may include dryness, thickness or cracking of skin, blister, or rash on the palms of the hands and soles of the feet.

Advise patients that other commonly reported adverse reactions include fatigue, high blood pressure, bleeding, swelling, mouth pain/irritation, and taste disturbance.

Advise patients to inform their health care providers of all concomitant medications, including nonprescription medications and dietary supplements.

EPIDERMAL GROWTH FACTOR RECEPTOR INHIBITORS

GEFITINIB

Rx	**Iressa** (AstraZeneca)	**Tablets:** 250 mg	Lactose. (IRESSA 250). Brown. Film-coated. In 30s.

GEFITINIB — ORAL

Indications

➤*Non-small cell lung cancer:* As monotherapy for the treatment of patients with locally advanced or metastatic non-small cell lung cancer after failure of both platinum-based and docetaxel chemotherapies.

Results from 2 large, controlled, randomized trials in first-line treatment of non-small cell lung cancer showed no benefit from adding gefitinib to doublet, platinum-based chemotherapy. Therefore, gefitinib is not indicated for use in this setting.

➤*Unlabeled uses:* Treatment of squamous cell head and neck cancer.

Administration and Dosage

➤*Approved by the FDA:* May 5, 2003.

The recommended daily dose of gefitinib is one 250 mg tablet with or without food. Higher doses do not give a better response and cause increased toxicity.

➤*Dosage adjustment:* Patients with poorly tolerated diarrhea (sometimes associated with dehydration) or skin adverse drug reactions may be successfully managed by providing a brief (up to 14 days) therapy interruption followed by reinstatement of the 250 mg daily dose.

In the event of acute onset or worsening of pulmonary symptoms (dyspnea, cough, fever), gefitinib therapy should be interrupted and a prompt investigation of these symptoms should occur and appropriate treatment initiated. If interstitial lung disease is confirmed, gefitinib should be discontinued and the patient treated appropriately. Cases of interstitial lung disease (ILD) have been observed in patients receiving gefitinib at an overall incidence of about 1%. Approximately ⅓ of the cases have been fatal. The reported incidence of ILD was about 2% in the Japanese postmarketing experience, about 0.3% in approximately 23,000 patients treated with gefitinib in a US expanded access program and about 1% in the studies of first-line use in NSCLC (but with similar rates in both treatment and placebo groups). Reports have described the adverse reaction as interstitial pneumonia, pneumonitis and alveolitis. Patients often present with the acute onset of dyspnea, sometimes associated with cough or low-grade fever, often becoming severe within a short time and requiring hospitalization. ILD has occurred in patients who have received prior radiation therapy (31% of reported cases), prior chemotherapy (57% of reported patients), and no previous therapy (12% of reported cases). Patients with concurrent idiopathic pulmonary fibrosis whose condition worsens while receiving gefitinib have been observed to have an increased mortality compared to those without concurrent idiopathic pulmonary fibrosis.

Patients who develop onset of new eye symptoms such as pain should be medically evaluated and managed appropriately, including gefitinib therapy interruption and removal of an aberrant eyelash if present. After symptoms and eye changes have resolved, the decision should be made concerning reinstatement of the 250 mg daily dose. In patients receiving gefitinib therapy, there were reports of eye pain and corneal erosion/ulcer, sometimes in association with aberrant eyelash growth.

Concurrent rifampin/phenytoin – In patients receiving a potent CYP3A4 inducer such as rifampin or phenytoin, a dose increase to 500 mg daily should be considered in the absence of severe adverse drug reaction, and clinical response and adverse reactions should be carefully monitored.

➤*Storage/Stability:* Store at controlled room temperature 20° to 25°C (68° to 77°F).

Actions

➤*Pharmacology:* The mechanism of the clinical antitumor action of gefitinib is not fully characterized. Gefitinib inhibits the intracellular phosphorylation of numerous tyrosine kinases associated with transmembrane cell surface receptors, including the tyrosine kinases associated with the epidermal growth factor receptor (EGFR-TK). EGFR is expressed on the cell surface of many normal cells and cancer cells. No clinical studies have been performed that demonstrate a correlation between EGFR receptor expression and response to gefitinib.

➤*Pharmacokinetics:*

Absorption/Distribution – Gefitinib is absorbed slowly after oral administration with mean bioavailability of 60%. Elimination is by metabolism (primarily CYP3A4) and excretion in feces. The elimination half-life is about 48 hours. Daily oral administration of gefitinib to cancer patients resulted in a 2-fold accumulation compared to single dose administration. Steady state plasma concentrations are achieved within 10 days.

Gefitinib is slowly absorbed, with peak plasma levels occurring 3 to 7 hours after dosing and mean oral bioavailability of 60%. Bioavailability is not significantly altered by food. Gefitinib is extensively distributed throughout the body with a mean steady state volume of distribution of 1400 L following intravenous administration. In vitro binding of gefitinib to human plasma proteins (serum albumin and α 1-acid glycoprotein) is 90% and is independent of drug concentrations.

Metabolism/Excretion – Gefitinib undergoes extensive hepatic metabolism in humans, predominantly by CYP3A4. Three sites of biotransformation have been identified: Metabolism of the N-propoxymorpholino-group, demethylation of the methoxy-substituent on the quinazoline, and oxidative defluorination of the halogenated phenyl group.

Five metabolites were identified in human plasma. Only O-desmethyl gefitinib has exposure comparable to gefitinib. Although this metabolite has similar EGFR-TK activity to gefitinib in the isolated enzyme assay, it had only 1/14 of the potency of gefitinib in 1 of the cell-based assays.

Gefitinib is cleared primarily by the liver, with total plasma clearance and elimination half-life values of 595 mL/min and 48 hours, respectively, after intravenous administration. Excretion is predominantly via the feces (86%), with renal elimination of drug and metabolites accounting for less than 4% of the administered dose.

Contraindications

Severe hypersensitivity to gefitinib or any other component of gefitinib.

Warnings

➤*Pulmonary toxicity:* Cases of interstitial lung disease (ILD) have been observed in patients receiving gefitinib at an overall incidence of about 1%. Approximately ⅓ of the cases have been fatal. The reported incidence of ILD was about 2% in the Japanese postmarketing experience, about 0.3% in approximately 23,000 patients treated with gefitinib in a US expanded access program and about 1% in the studies of first-line use in NSCLC (but with similar rates in both treatment and placebo groups). Reports have described the adverse reaction as interstitial pneumonia, pneumonitis and alveolitis. Patients often present with the acute onset of dyspnea, sometimes associated with cough or low-grade fever, often becoming severe within a short time and requiring hospitalization. ILD has occurred in patients who have received prior radiation therapy (31% of reported cases), prior chemotherapy (57% of reported patients), and no previous therapy (12% of reported cases). Patients with concurrent idiopathic pulmonary fibrosis whose condition worsens while receiving gefitinib have been observed to have an increased mortality compared to those without concurrent idiopathic pulmonary fibrosis.

In the event of acute onset or worsening of pulmonary symptoms (dyspnea, cough, fever), gefitinib therapy should be interrupted and a prompt investigation of these symptoms should occur. If interstitial lung disease is confirmed, gefitinib should be discontinued and the patient treated appropriately.

GEFITINIB — ORAL

➤*Renal function impairment:* The effect of severe renal impairment on the pharmacokinetics of gefitinib is not known. Patients with severe renal impairment should be treated with caution when given gefitinib.

➤*Hepatic function impairment:* In vitro and in vivo evidence suggest that gefitinib is cleared primarily by the liver. Therefore, gefitinib exposure may be increased in patients with hepatic dysfunction. In patients with liver metastases and moderately to severely elevated biochemical liver abnormalities, however, gefitinib pharmacokinetics were similar to the pharmacokinetics of individuals without liver abnormalities. The influence of non-cancer related hepatic impairment on the pharmacokinetics of gefitinib has not been evaluated.

➤*Pregnancy: Category D.* Gefitinib may cause fetal harm when administered to a pregnant woman. A single dose study in rats showed that gefitinib crosses the placenta after an oral dose of 5 mg/kg (30 mg/m^2, about ⅕ the recommended human dose on a mg/m^2 basis). When pregnant rats were treated with 5 mg/kg from the beginning of organogenesis to the end of weaning gave birth, there was a reduction in the number of offspring born alive. This effect was more severe at 20 mg/kg and was accompanied by high neonatal mortality soon after parturition. In this study a dose of 1 mg/kg caused no adverse effects.

In rabbits, a dose of 20 mg/kg/day (240 mg/m^2, about twice the recommended dose in humans on a mg/m^2 basis) caused reduced fetal weight.

There are no adequate and well-controlled studies in pregnant women using gefitinib. If gefitinib is used during pregnancy or if the patient becomes pregnant while receiving this drug, she should be apprised of the potential hazard to the fetus or potential risk for loss of the pregnancy.

➤*Lactation:* It is not known whether gefitinib is excreted in human milk. Following oral administration of carbon-14 labeled gefitinib to rats 14 days postpartum, concentrations of radioactivity in milk were higher than in blood. Levels of gefitinib and its metabolites were 11- to 19-fold higher in milk than in blood, after oral exposure of lactating rats to a dose of 5 mg/kg. Because many drugs are excreted in human milk and because of the potential for serious adverse reactions in nursing infants, women should be advised against breastfeeding while receiving gefitinib therapy.

➤*Children:* Safety and effectiveness of gefitinib in pediatric patients have not been studied.

Precautions

➤*Monitoring:* Asymptomatic increases in liver transaminases have been observed in gefitinib treated patients; therefore, periodic liver function (transaminases, bilirubin, and alkaline phosphatase) testing should be considered. Discontinuation of gefitinib should be considered if changes are severe.

Drug Interactions

Gefitinib Drug Interactions

Precipitant drug	Object drug*		Description
CYP3A4 inducers (eg, rifampin, phenytoin)	Gefitinib	⬇	The plasma concentration of gefitinib is decreased due to an increase in its metabolism. Coadministration with rifampin caused a decrease in gefitinib AUC by 85%. Consider a dose increase of gefitinib if coadministered with a potent CYP3A4 inducer (see Administration and Dosage).
CYP3A4 inhibitors (eg, ketoconazole, itraconazole)	Gefitinib	⬆	Potent CYP3A4 inhibitors decrease gefitinib metabolism and increase its plasma concentrations. Coadministration with itraconazole increased gefitinib AUC by 88%. Use with caution.
H_2 antagonist (eg, ranitidine, cimetidine) Sodium bicarbonate	Gefitinib	⬇	Drugs that cause significant sustained elevations in gastric pH may reduce plasma concentrations of gefitinib and may reduce efficacy.
Gefitinib	Metoprolol	⬆	Exposure to metoprolol, a substrate of CYP2D6, was increased by 30% when given with gefitinib.
Gefitinib	Warfarin	⬆	INR elevations and/or bleeding events have been reported in some patients taking warfarin while on gefitinib therapy. Monitor PT or INR regularly.

* ⬆ = Object drug increased. ⬇ = Object drug decreased.

Adverse Reactions

Drug-related Adverse Reactions (≥ 5%)

Drug-related adverse reaction[a]	250 mg/day (n = 102)	500 mg/day (n = 114)
Diarrhea	49 (48%)	76 (67%)
Rash	44 (43%)	61 (54%)
Acne	25 (25%)	37 (33%)
Dry skin	13 (13%)	30 (26%)
Nausea	13 (13%)	20 (18%)
Vomiting	12 (12%)	10 (9%)
Pruritus	8 (8%)	10 (9%)
Anorexia	7 (7%)	11 (10%)
Asthenia	6 (6%)	5 (4%)
Weight loss	3 (3%)	6 (5%)

[a] A patient may have had more than 1 drug-related adverse reaction.

The table below provides drug-related adverse reactions with an incidence of greater than or equal to 5% by CTC grade for the patients who received the 250 mg/day dose of gefitinib monotherapy for treatment of NSCLC. Only 2% of patients stopped therapy due to an adverse drug reaction (ADR). The onset of these ADRs occurred within the first month of therapy.

Drug-related Adverse Reactions at 250 mg Dose by Worst CTC Grade (n = 102) (≥ 5%)

Adverse reaction	All grades	CTC grade 1	CTC grade 2	CTC grade 3	CTC grade 4
Diarrhea	48%	41%	6%	1%	0%
Rash	43%	39%	4%	0%	0%
Acne	25%	19%	6%	0%	0%
Dry skin	13%	12%	1%	0%	0%
Nausea	13%	7%	5%	1%	0%
Vomiting	12%	9%	2%	1%	0%
Pruritus	8%	7%	1%	0%	0%
Anorexia	7%	3%	4%	0%	0%
Asthenia	6%	2%	2%	1%	1%

➤*Other adverse reactions:* Other adverse reactions reported at an incidence of less than 5% in patients who received either 250 mg or 500 mg as monotherapy for treatment of NSCLC (along with their frequency at the 250 mg recommended dose) include the following: Peripheral edema (2%), amblyopia (2%), dyspnea (2%), conjunctivitis (1%), vesiculobullous rash (1%), and mouth ulceration (1%).

In patients receiving gefitinib therapy, there were reports of eye pain and corneal erosion/ulcer, sometimes in association with aberrant eyelash growth. There were also rare reports of pancreatitis and very rare reports of corneal membrane sloughing, ocular ischemia/hemorrhage, toxic epidermal necrolysis, erythema multiforme, and allergic reactions, including angioedema and urticaria.

➤*Hematologic:* See Drug Interactions for more information.

➤*Cardiac:* Data from nonclinical (in vitro and in vivo) studies indicate that gefitinib has the potential to inhibit the cardiac action potential repolarization process (eg, QT interval). The clinical relevance of these findings is unknown.

➤*Interstitial lung disease:* Cases of interstitial lung disease (ILD) have been observed in patients receiving gefitinib at an overall incidence of about 1%. Approximately ⅓ of the cases have been fatal. The reported incidence of ILD was about 2% in the Japanese postmarketing experience, about 0.3% in approximately 23,000 patients treated with gefitinib in a US expanded access program and about 1% in the studies of first-line use in NSCLC (but with similar rates in both treatment and placebo groups). Reports have described the adverse reaction as interstitial pneumonia, pneumonitis and alveolitis. Patients often present with the acute onset of dyspnea, sometimes associated with cough or low-grade fever, often becoming severe within a short time and requiring hospitalization. ILD has occurred in patients who have received prior radiation therapy (31% of reported cases), prior chemotherapy (57% of reported patients), and no previous therapy (12% of reported cases). Patients with concurrent idiopathic pulmonary fibrosis whose condition worsens while receiving gefitinib have been observed to have an increased mortality compared to those without concurrent idiopathic pulmonary fibrosis.

In the reaction of acute onset or worsening of pulmonary symptoms (dyspnea, cough, fever), gefitinib therapy should be interrupted and a prompt investigation of these symptoms should occur. If interstitial lung disease is confirmed, gefitinib should be discontinued and the patient treated appropriately.

Overdosage

The acute toxicity of gefitinib up to 500 mg in clinical studies has been low. In non-clinical studies, a single dose of 12,000 mg/m^2 (about 80 times the recommended clinical dose on a mg/m^2 basis) was lethal to rats. Half this dose caused no mortality in mice.

GEFITINIB — ORAL

➤*Treatment:* There is no specific treatment for an gefitinib overdose and possible symptoms of overdose are not established. However, in Phase 1 clinical trials, a limited number of patients were treated with daily doses of up to 1000 mg. An increase in frequency and severity of some adverse reactions was observed, mainly diarrhea and skin rash. Adverse reactions associated with overdose should be treated symptomatically; in particular, severe diarrhea should be managed appropriately.

Patient Information

Advise patients to seek medical advice promptly if they develop the following: severe or persistent diarrhea, nausea, anorexia, or vomiting, as these have sometimes been associated with dehydration; an onset or worsening of pulmonary symptoms (ie, shortness of breath or cough); an eye irritation; any other new symptom.

Advise women of childbearing potential to avoid becoming pregnant.

ERLOTINIB

Rx	**Tarceva** (Genentech Inc.)	**Tablets:** 25 mg	Lactose. (T 25). White. Film-coated. In 30s.
		100 mg	Lactose. (T 100). White. Film-coated. In 30s.
		150 mg	Lactose. (T 150). White. Film-coated. In 30s.

ERLOTINIB — ORAL

Indications

➤*Nonsmall cell lung cancer (NSCLC):* Erlotinib monotherapy is indicated for the treatment of patients with locally advanced or metastatic NSCLC after failure of at least 1 prior chemotherapy regimen.

➤*Pancreatic cancer:* Erlotinib in combination with gemcitabine is indicated for the first-line treatment of patients with locally advanced, unresectable, or metastatic pancreatic cancer.

➤*Unlabeled uses:* Treatment of squamous cell head and neck cancer.

Administration and Dosage

➤*Approved by the FDA:* November 18, 2004.

➤*NSCLC:* The recommended daily dose is 150 mg taken at least 1 hour before or 2 hours after the ingestion of food. Continue treatment until disease progression or unacceptable toxicity occurs. There is no evidence that treatment beyond progression is beneficial.

➤*Pancreatic cancer:* The recommended daily dose is 100 mg taken at least 1 hour before or 2 hours after the ingestion of food, in combination with gemcitabine. Continue treatment until disease progression or unacceptable toxicity occurs.

➤*Dose modifications:* When dose reduction is necessary, reduce the erlotinib dose in 50 mg decrements.

Pulmonary symptoms – In patients who develop an acute onset of new or progressive pulmonary symptoms, such as dyspnea, cough, or fever, interrupt treatment with erlotinib pending diagnostic evaluation. If interstitial lung disease (ILD) is diagnosed, discontinue erlotinib and institute appropriate treatment as necessary.

Diarrhea / Skin reactions – Diarrhea can usually be managed with loperamide. Patients with severe diarrhea who are unresponsive to loperamide or who become dehydrated may require dose reduction or temporary interruption of therapy. Patients with severe skin reactions also may require dose reduction or temporary interruption of therapy.

Concomitant medications – In patients who are being concomitantly treated with a strong CYP3A4 inhibitor (eg, atazanavir, clarithromycin, indinavir, itraconazole, ketoconazole, nefazodone, nelfinavir, ritonavir, saquinavir, telithromycin, troleandomycin, voriconazole), consider a dose reduction if severe adverse reactions occur.

Pretreatment with the CYP3A4-inducer rifampin decreased erlotinib area under the curve (AUC) by approximately two thirds. Consider alternate treatments lacking CYP3A4-inducing activity. If an alternative treatment is unavailable, consider an erlotinib dose greater than 150 mg. If the erlotinib dose is adjusted upward, the dose will need to be reduced upon discontinuation of rifampin or other inducers. Other CYP3A4 inducers include, but are not limited to, rifabutin, rifapentine, phenytoin, carbamazepine, phenobarbital, and St. John's wort. Avoid these, too, if possible.

➤*Hepatic function impairment:* Erlotinib is eliminated by hepatic metabolism and biliary excretion. Therefore, use caution when administering erlotinib to patients with hepatic function impairment. Consider dose reduction or interruption of erlotinib if severe adverse reactions occur.

➤*Storage / Stability:* Store at 25°C (77°F); excursions permitted to 15° to 30°C (59° to 86°F).

Actions

➤*Pharmacology:* The mechanism of clinical antitumor action of erlotinib is not fully characterized. Erlotinib inhibits the intracellular phosphorylation of tyrosine kinase associated with the epidermal growth factor receptor (EGFR). Specificity of inhibition with regard to other tyrosine kinase receptors has not been fully characterized. EGFR is expressed on the cell surface of normal cells and cancer cells.

➤*Pharmacokinetics:*

Absorption / Distribution – Erlotinib is approximately 60% absorbed after oral administration and its bioavailability is substantially increased by food to almost 100%.

Bioavailability of erlotinib following an erlotinib 150 mg oral dose is approximately 60% and peak plasma levels occur 4 hours after dosing.

Following absorption, erlotinib is approximately 93% protein-bound to albumin and alpha-$_1$ acid glycoprotein (AAG). Erlotinib has an apparent volume of distribution of 232 L.

Metabolism / Excretion – The half-life of erlotinib is approximately 36 hours, and it is cleared predominantly by CYP3A4 metabolism.

In vitro assays of CYP450 metabolism showed that erlotinib is metabolized primarily by CYP3A4 and, to a lesser extent, CYP1A2 and the extrahepatic isoform CYP1A1. Following a 100 mg oral dose, 91% of the dose was recovered: 83% in feces (1% of the dose as intact parent) and 8% in urine (0.3% of the dose as intact parent).

A population pharmacokinetic analysis in 591 patients receiving single-agent erlotinib showed a median half-life of 36.2 hours. Time to reach steady-state plasma concentration would, therefore, be 7 to 8 days. No significant relationships of clearance to patient age, body weight, or gender were observed. Smokers had a 24% higher rate of erlotinib clearance.

A second population pharmacokinetic analysis was conducted that incorporated erlotinib data from 204 pancreatic cancer patients who received erlotinib plus gemcitabine. This analysis demonstrated that covariates affecting erlotinib clearance in patients from the pancreatic study were very similar to those seen in the prior single-agent pharmacokinetic analysis. No new covariate effects were identified. Coadministration of gemcitabine had no effect on erlotinib plasma clearance.

Contraindications

None known.

Warnings

➤*Pulmonary effects:* There have been infrequent reports of serious ILD-like events, including fatalities, in patients receiving erlotinib for treatment of NSCLC, pancreatic cancer, or other advanced solid tumors. In the randomized, single-agent NSCLC study, the incidence of ILD-like events (0.8%) was the same in both the placebo and erlotinib groups. In the pancreatic cancer study, the incidence of ILD-like events was 2.5% in the erlotinib plus gemcitabine group vs 0.4% in the placebo plus gemcitabine group.

The overall incidence of ILD-like events in approximately 4,900 erlotinib-treated patients from all studies (including uncontrolled studies and studies with concurrent chemotherapy) was approximately 0.7%. Reported diagnoses in patients suspected of having ILD-like events included acute respiratory distress syndrome, hypersensitivity pneumonitis, ILD, interstitial pneumonia, lung infiltration, obliterative bronchiolitis, pneumonitis, pulmonary fibrosis, and radiation pneumonitis. Symptoms started from 5 days to more than 9 months (median, 39 days) after initiating erlotinib therapy. In the lung cancer trials, most of the cases were associated with confounding or contributing factors, such as concomitant/prior chemotherapy, prior radiotherapy, preexisting parenchymal lung disease, metastatic lung disease, or pulmonary infections.

In the event of acute onset of new or progressive, unexplained pulmonary symptoms, such as dyspnea, cough, and fever, interrupt erlotinib therapy pending diagnostic evaluation. If ILD is diagnosed, discontinue erlotinib and institute appropriate treatment as necessary.

➤*Cardiovascular effects:*

Myocardial infarction / Ischemia – In the pancreatic carcinoma trial, 6 patients (incidence of 2.3%) in the erlotinib/gemcitabine group developed myocardial infarction/ischemia. One of these patients died because of myocardial infarction. In comparison, 3 patients in the placebo/gemcitabine group developed myocardial infarction (incidence, 1.2%) and 1 died because of myocardial infarction.

Cerebrovascular accident – In the pancreatic carcinoma trial, 6 patients in the erlotinib/gemcitabine group developed cerebrovascular accidents (incidence, 2.3%). One of these was hemorrhagic and was the only fatal event. In comparison, in the placebo/gemcitabine group, there were no cerebrovascular accidents.

➤*Hematologic effects:* In the pancreatic carcinoma trial, 2 patients in the erlotinib/gemcitabine group developed microangiopathic hemolytic anemia with thrombocytopenia (incidence: 0.8%). Both patients received erlotinib and gemcitabine concurrently. In comparison, in the placebo/gemcitabine group, there were no cases of microangiopathic hemolytic anemia with thrombocytopenia.

➤*Hepatic function impairment:* In vitro and in vivo evidence suggests that erlotinib is cleared primarily by the liver. Therefore, erlotinib exposure may be increased in patients with hepatic dysfunction.

➤*Elderly:* Of the total number of patients participating in the randomized NSCLC trial, 62% were younger than 65 years of age, and 38% were 65 years of age or older. The survival benefit was maintained across both age groups. In the pancreatic cancer study, 53% of patients were younger than

ERLOTINIB — ORAL

65 years of age and 47% were 65 years of age and older. No meaningful differences in safety or pharmacokinetics were observed between younger and older patients in either study. Therefore, no dosage adjustments are recommended in elderly patients.

➤*Pregnancy: Category D.* Erlotinib has been shown to cause maternal toxicity with associated embryo/fetal lethality and abortion in rabbits when given at doses that result in plasma drug concentrations of approximately 3 times those in humans (AUCs at 150 mg daily dose). When given during the period of organogenesis to achieve plasma drug concentrations approximately equal to those in humans, based on AUC, there was no increased incidence of embryo/fetal lethality or abortion in rabbits or rats. However, female rats treated with erlotinib 30 mg/m^2/day or 60 mg/m^2/day (0.3 or 0.7 times the clinical dose, on a mg/m^2 basis) prior to mating through the first week of pregnancy had an increase in early resorptions that resulted in a decrease in the number of live fetuses.

No teratogenic effects were observed in rabbits or rats.

There are no adequate and well-controlled studies in pregnant women using erlotinib. Advise women of childbearing potential to avoid pregnancy while on erlotinib. Adequate contraceptive methods should be used during therapy, and for at least 2 weeks after completing therapy. Only continue treatment in pregnant women if the potential benefit to the mother outweighs the risk to the fetus. If erlotinib is used during pregnancy, apprise the patient of the potential hazard to the fetus or potential risk for loss of the pregnancy.

➤*Lactation:* It is not known whether erlotinib is excreted in human milk. Because many drugs are excreted in human milk and because the effects of erlotinib on infants have not been studied, advise women against breastfeeding while receiving erlotinib therapy.

➤*Children:* The safety and efficacy of erlotinib in pediatric patients have not been studied.

Precautions

➤*Monitoring:* Perform periodic liver function tests in erlotinib-treated patients. Regularly monitor patients taking erlotinib and warfarin or other coumarin-derivative anticoagulants for changes in prothrombin time or INR.

➤*Hepatic effects:* Asymptomatic increases in liver transaminases have been observed in erlotinib-treated patients; therefore, consider periodic liver function testing (transaminases, bilirubin, and alkaline phosphatase). Consider dose reduction or interruption of erlotinib if changes in liver function are severe.

Drug Interactions

Erlotinib (Oral) Drug Interactions

Precipitant drug	Object drug[a]		Description
CYP3A4 inhibitors (eg, ketoconazole, atazanavir, clarithromycin, indinavir, itraconazole, nefazodone, nelfinavir, ritonavir, saquinavir, telithromycin, troleandomycin, voriconazole)	Erlotinib	↑	Potent CYP3A4 inhibitors decrease erlotinib metabolism and increase its plasma concentration. Coadministration with ketoconazole increased erlotinib AUC by two thirds. Use with caution.
CYP3A4 inducers (eg, rifampin, phenytoin, carbamazepine, phenobarbital)	Erlotinib	↓	The plasma concentration of erlotinib is decreased because of an increase in its metabolism. Coadministration with rifampin increased erlotinib clearance 3-fold and reduced AUC two thirds. Consider a dose increase of erlotinib if coadministered with a potent CYP3A4 inducer (see Administration and Dosage).
St. John's wort	Erlotinib	↓	Erlotinib plasma concentrations may be reduced, decreasing the therapeutic effects.
Erlotinib	Warfarin	↑	INR elevations and infrequent reports of bleeding, including GI and non-GI bleeding, have been reported during warfarin coadministration. Monitor for changes in prothrombin time or INR.

[a] ↑ = Object drug increased. ↓ = Object drug decreased.

Adverse Reactions

Safety evaluation of erlotinib is based on 856 cancer patients who received erlotinib as monotherapy, 308 patients who received erlotinib 100 or 150 mg plus gemcitabine, and 1,228 patients who received erlotinib concurrently with other chemotherapies.

There have been reports of serious events, including fatalities, in patients receiving erlotinib for treatment of NSCLC, pancreatic cancer, or other advanced solid tumors.

➤*NSCLC:* Adverse reactions, regardless of causality, that occurred in at least 10% of patients treated with single-agent erlotinib at 150 mg and at least 3% more often than in the placebo group in the randomized trial of patients with NSCLC are summarized by National Cancer Institute – Common Toxicity Criteria (NCI-CTC; version 2.0) Grade in the following table.

The most common adverse reactions in patients receiving single-agent erlotinib 150 mg were rash and diarrhea. Grade 3/4 rash and diarrhea occurred in 9% and 6%, respectively, in erlotinib-treated patients. Rash and diarrhea each resulted in study discontinuation in 1% of erlotinib-treated patients. Six percent and 1% of patients needed dose reduction for rash and diarrhea, respectively. The median time to onset of rash was 8 days, and the median time to onset of diarrhea was 12 days.

Adverse Reactions Occurring in Single-Agent–Erlotinib-Treated NSCLC Patients (≥ 10%)

NCI-CTC grade	Erlotinib 150 mg (n = 485)			Placebo (n = 242)		
	Any grade	Grade 3	Grade 4	Any grade	Grade 3	Grade 4
MedDRA[a] preferred term						
Dermatologic						
Dry skin	12%	0%	0%	4%	0%	0%
Pruritus	13%	< 1%	0%	5%	0%	0%
Rash	75%	8%	< 1%	17%	0%	0%
GI						
Abdominal pain	11%	2%	< 1%	7%	1%	< 1%
Anorexia	52%	8%	1%	38%	5%	< 1%
Diarrhea	54%	6%	< 1%	18%	< 1%	0%
Nausea	33%	3%	0%	24%	2%	0%
Stomatitis	17%	< 1%	0%	3%	0%	0%
Vomiting	23%	2%	< 1%	19%	2%	0%
Ophthalmic						
Conjunctivitis	12%	< 1%	0%	2%	< 1%	0%
Keratoconjunctivitis sicca	12%	0%	0%	3%	0%	0%
Respiratory						
Cough	33%	4%	0%	29%	2%	0%
Dyspnea	41%	17%	11%	35%	15%	11%
Miscellaneous						
Fatigue	52%	14%	4%	45%	16%	4%
Infection	24%	4%	0%	15%	2%	0%

[a] MedDRA = Medical Dictionary for Regulatory Activities.

Liver function test abnormalities (including elevated ALT, AST, and bilirubin) were observed in patients receiving single-agent erlotinib 150 mg. These elevations were mainly transient or associated with liver metastases. Grade 2 (more than 2.5 to 5 times the upper limit of normal [ULN]) ALT elevations occurred in 4% and less than 1% of erlotinib- and placebo-treated patients, respectively. Grade 3 (more than 5 to 20 times the ULN) elevations were not observed in erlotinib-treated patients. Consider dose reduction or interruption of erlotinib if changes in liver function are severe.

➤*Pancreatic cancer:* Adverse reactions, regardless of causality, that occurred in at least 10% of patients treated with erlotinib 100 mg plus gemcitabine in the randomized trial of patients with pancreatic cancer are summarized by NCI-CTC (version 2.0) grade in Table 6.

The most common adverse reactions in pancreatic cancer patients receiving erlotinib 100 mg plus gemcitabine were fatigue, rash, nausea, anorexia, and diarrhea. In the erlotinib plus gemcitabine arm, grade 3/4 rash and diarrhea were each reported in 5% of erlotinib plus gemcitabine-treated patients. The median time to onset of rash and diarrhea was 10 and 15 days, respectively. Rash and diarrhea each resulted in dose reductions in 2% of patients, and resulted in study discontinuation in up to 1% of patients receiving erlotinib plus gemcitabine. The 150 mg cohort was associated with a higher rate of certain class-specific adverse reactions, including rash, and required more frequent dose reductions or interruptions.

Adverse Reactions in Erlotinib-Treated Pancreatic Cancer Patients: Erlotinib 100 mg Cohort (≥ 10%)

NCI-CTC grade	Erlotinib + Gemcitabine 1,000 mg/m^2 IV (n = 259)			Placebo + Gemcitabine 1,000 mg/m^2 IV (n = 256)		
	Any grade	Grade 3	Grade 4	Any grade	Grade 3	Grade 4
CNS						
Anxiety	13%	1%	0%	11%	< 1%	0%
Depression	19%	2%	0%	14%	< 1%	0%
Dizziness	15%	< 1%	0%	13%	0%	< 1%

ERLOTINIB — ORAL

Adverse Reactions in Erlotinib-Treated Pancreatic Cancer Patients: Erlotinib 100 mg Cohort (≥ 10%)						
	Erlotinib + Gemcitabine 1,000 mg/m² IV (n = 259)			Placebo + Gemcitabine 1,000 mg/m² IV (n = 256)		
NCI-CTC grade	Any grade	Grade 3	Grade 4	Any grade	Grade 3	Grade 4
Fatigue	73%	14	2%	70%	13%	2%
Headache	15%	< 1%	0%	10%	0%	0%
Insomnia	15%	< 1%	0%	16%	< 1%	0%
Neuropathy	13%	1%	< 1%	10%	< 1%	0%
Rigors	12%	0%	0%	9%	0%	0%
Dermatologic						
Alopecia	14%	0%	0%	11%	0%	0%
Rash	69%	5%	0%	30%	1%	0%
GI						
Abdominal pain	46%	9%	< 1%	45%	12%	< 1%
Anorexia	52%	6%	< 1%	52%	5%	< 1%
Constipation	31%	3%	1%	34%	5%	1%
Diarrhea	48%	5%	< 1%	36%	2%	0%
Dyspepsia	17%	< 1%	0%	13%	< 1%	0%
Flatulence	13%	0%	0%	9%	< 1%	0%
Nausea	60%	7%	0%	58%	7%	0%
Stomatitis	22%	< 1%	0%	12%	0%	0%
Vomiting	42%	7%	< 1%	41%	4%	< 1%
Weight decreased	39%	2%	0%	29%	< 1%	0%
Musculoskeletal						
Bone pain	25%	4%	< 1%	23%	2%	0%
Myalgia	21%	1%	0%	20%	< 1%	0%
Respiratory						
Cough	16%	0%	0%	11%	0%	0%
Dyspnea	24%	5%	< 1%	23%	5%	0%
Miscellaneous						
Edema	37%	3%	< 1%	36%	2%	< 1%
Infection[a]	39%	13%	3%	30%	9%	2%
Pyrexia	36%	3%	0%	30%	4%	0%

[a] Includes all MedDRA preferred terms in the Infections and Infestations System Organ Class.

Severe adverse reactions (at least grade 3 NCI-CTC) in the erlotinib plus gemcitabine group with incidences less than 5% included syncope, arrhythmias, ileus, pancreatitis, hemolytic anemia including microangiopathic hemolytic anemia with thrombocytopenia, myocardial infarction/ischemia, cerebrovascular accidents including cerebral hemorrhage, and renal insufficiency.

Deep vein thrombosis (DVT) – In the pancreatic carcinoma trial, 10 patients in the erlotinib/gemcitabine group developed DVT (incidence: 3.9%). In comparison, 3 patients in the placebo/gemcitabine group developed DVT (incidence: 1.2%). The overall incidence of grade 3 or 4 thrombotic events, including DVT, was similar in the 2 treatment arms: 11% for erlotinib plus gemcitabine and 9% for placebo plus gemcitabine.

Hematologic – No differences in grade 3 or 4 hematologic laboratory toxicities were detected between the erlotinib plus gemcitabine group, compared with the placebo plus gemcitabine group.

Lab test abnormalities – Liver function test abnormalities (including elevated ALT, AST, and bilirubin) have been observed following the administration of erlotinib plus gemcitabine in patients with pancreatic cancer. The following table displays the most severe NCI-CTC grade of liver function abnormalities that developed. Consider dose reduction or interruption of erlotinib if changes in liver function are severe.

Liver Function Test Abnormalities (Most Severe NCI-CTC grade) in Pancreatic Cancer Patients: Erlotinib 100 mg Cohort						
	Erlotinib + Gemcitabine 1,000 mg/m² IV (n = 259)			Placebo + Gemcitabine 1,000 mg/m² IV (n = 256)		
NCI-CTC grade	Grade 2	Grade 3	Grade 4	Grade 2	Grade 3	Grade 4
Bilirubin	17%	10%	< 1%	11%	10%	3%
ALT	31%	13%	< 1%	22%	9%	0%
AST	24%	10%	< 1%	19%	9%	0%

➤*NSCLC and pancreatic cancer:* During the NSCLC and the combination pancreatic cancer trials, infrequent cases of GI bleeding have been reported in clinical studies, some associated with warfarin coadministration and some with nonsteroidal anti-inflammatory drug (NSAID) coadministration. These adverse reactions were reported as peptic ulcer bleeding (gastritis, gastroduodenal ulcers), hematemesis, hematochezia, melena, and hemorrhage from possible colitis. Cases of grade 1 epistaxis were also reported in the single-agent NSCLC and the pancreatic cancer clinical trials.

NCI-CTC grade 3 conjunctivitis and keratitis have been reported infrequently in patients receiving erlotinib therapy in the NSCLC and pancreatic cancer clinical trials. Corneal ulcerations also may occur.

Overdosage

➤*Symptoms:* Single oral doses of erlotinib up to 1,000 mg in healthy subjects and up to 1,600 mg in cancer patients have been tolerated. Repeated twice-daily doses of 200 mg single-agent erlotinib in healthy subjects were poorly tolerated after only a few days of dosing. Based on the data from these studies, an unacceptable incidence of severe adverse reactions, such as diarrhea, rash, and liver transaminase elevation, may occur above the recommended dose of 150 mg daily.

➤*Treatment:* In case of suspected overdose, withhold erlotinib and institute symptomatic treatment.

Patient Information

Advise patients to seek medical advice promptly if the following signs or symptoms occur: anorexia, nausea, severe or persistent diarrhea, or vomiting; eye irritation; onset or worsening of unexplained shortness of breath or cough.

Advise women of childbearing potential to avoid becoming pregnant while taking erlotinib. Adequate contraceptive methods should be used during therapy and for at least 2 weeks after completing therapy.

PROTEASOME INHIBITORS

BORTEZOMIB

Rx	**Velcade** (Millennium)	**Powder for injection, lyophilized:** 3.5 mg	35 mg mannitol. Preservative-free. Single-dose vials.

BORTEZOMIB — INJECTION

Indications

➤*Multiple myeloma:* For the treatment of multiple myeloma patients who have received at least 2 prior therapies and have demonstrated disease progression on the last therapy.

Administration and Dosage

➤*Approved by the FDA:* May 13, 2003.

➤*Recommended dose:* The recommended dose of bortezomib for injection is 1.3 mg/m²/dose administered as a bolus intravenous injection twice weekly for 2 weeks (days 1, 4, 8, and 11) followed by a 10-day rest period (days 12 to 21).

This 3-week period is considered a treatment cycle. At least 72 hours should elapse between consecutive doses of bortezomib for injection.

➤*Dose modification and reinitiation of therapy:* Bortezomib injection therapy should be withheld at the onset of any grade 3 non-hematological or grade 4 hematological toxicities excluding neuropathy as discussed below. Once the symptoms of the toxicity have resolved, bortezomib injection therapy may be reinitiated at a 25% reduced dose (1.3 mg/m²/dose reduced to 1 mg/m²/dose; 1 mg/m²/dose reduced to 0.7 mg/m²/dose). The following information contains the recommended dose modification for the management of patients who experience bortezomib-related neuropathic pain or peripheral sensory neuropathy (see data below). Patients with preexisting severe neuropathy should be treated with bortezomib only after careful risk/benefit assessment.

Recommended dose modification for bortezomib-related neuropathic pain or peripheral sensory neuropathy –

In patients with grade 1 (paresthesias or loss of reflexes) without pain or loss of function, no modification of dose or regimen is required.

In patients with grade 1 with pain or grade 2 (interfering with function but not with activities of daily living), reduce the dose of bortezomib to 1 mg/m².

In patients with grade 2 with pain or grade 3 (interfering with activities of daily living), withhold the bortezomib therapy until toxicity resolves. When toxicity resolves reinitiate with a reduced dose of bortezomib at 0.7 mg/m² and change the treatment schedule to once per week.

In patients with grade 4 (permanent sensory loss that interferes with function), discontinue bortezomib.

BORTEZOMIB — INJECTION

➤*Administration precautions:* Caution should be used during handling and preparation. Proper aseptic technique should be used. Use of gloves and other protective clothing to prevent skin contact is recommended. In clinical trials, local skin irritation was reported in 5% of patients, but extravasation of bortezomib for injection was not associated with tissue damage.

➤*Preparation for administration:* Prior to use, the contents of each vial must be reconstituted with 3.5 mL of normal (0.9%) saline, Sodium Chloride Injection. The reconstituted product should be a clear and colorless solution.

➤*Storage / Stability:* Unopened vials may be stored at controlled room temperature 25°C (77°F); excursions permitted from 15° to 30°C (59° to 86°F). Retain in original package to protect from light.

Bortezomib for injection contains no antimicrobial preservative. When reconstituted as directed, bortezomib for injection may be stored at 25°C (77°F); excursions permitted from 15° to 30°C (59° to 86°F). Reconstituted bortezomib for injection should be administered within 8 hours of preparation. The reconstituted material may be stored in the original vial or the syringe prior to administration. The product may be stored for up to 3 hours in a syringe; however, total storage time for the reconstituted material must not exceed 8 hours when exposed to normal indoor lighting.

Actions

➤*Pharmacology:* Bortezomib is a reversible inhibitor of the chymotrypsin-like activity of the 26S proteasome in mammalian cells. The 26S proteasome is a large protein complex that degrades ubiquitinated proteins. The ubiquitin-proteasome pathway plays an essential role in regulating the intracellular concentration of specific proteins, thereby maintaining homeostasis within cells. Inhibition of the 26S proteasome prevents this targeted proteolysis which can affect multiple signaling cascades within the cell. This disruption of normal homeostatic mechanisms can lead to cell death. Experiments have demonstrated that bortezomib is cytotoxic to a variety of cancer cell types in vitro. Bortezomib causes a delay in tumor growth in vivo in non-clinical tumor models, including multiple myeloma.

➤*Pharmacokinetics:*

Absorption – Following intravenous administration of a 1.3 mg/m^2 dose, the median estimated maximum plasma concentration of bortezomib was 509 ng/mL (range = 109 to 1300 ng/mL) in 8 patients with multiple myeloma and creatinine clearance values ranging from 31 to 169 mL/min. The mean elimination half-life of bortezomib after first dose ranged from 9 to 15 hours at doses ranging from 1.45 to 2 mg/m^2 in patients with advanced malignancies. The pharmacokinetics of bortezomib as a single agent have not been fully characterized at the recommended dose in multiple myeloma patients.

Distribution – The distribution volume of bortezomib as a single agent was not assessed at the recommended dose in patients with multiple myeloma. The binding of bortezomib to human plasma proteins averaged 83% over the concentration range of 100 to 1000 ng/mL.

Metabolism – In vitro studies with human liver microsomes and human cDNA-expressed cytochrome P450 isozymes indicate that bortezomib is primarily oxidatively metabolized via cytochrome P450 enzymes, 3A4, 2D6, 2C19, 2C9, and 1A2. The major metabolic pathway is deboronation to form 2 deboronated metabolites that subsequently undergo hydroxylation to several metabolites. Deboronated-bortezomib metabolites are inactive as 26S proteasome inhibitors. Pooled plasma data from 8 patients at 10 minutes and 30 minutes after dosing indicate that the plasma levels of metabolites are low compared to the parent drug.

Contraindications

Hypersensitivity to bortezomib, boron, or mannitol.

Warnings

➤*Administration:* Bortezomib for injection should be administered under the supervision of a physician experienced in the use of antineoplastic therapy.

➤*Renal function impairment:* No clinical information is available on the use of bortezomib for injection in patients with creatinine clearance values less than 13 mL/min and patients on hemodialysis. These patients should be closely monitored for toxicities when treated with bortezomib for injection.

➤*Hepatic function impairment:* Bortezomib is metabolized by liver enzymes and bortezomib's clearance may decrease in patients with hepatic impairment. These patients should be closely monitored for toxicities when treated with bortezomib for injection.

➤*Mutagenesis:* Bortezomib showed clastogenic activity (structural chromosomal aberrations) in the in vitro chromosomal aberration assay using Chinese hamster ovary cells. Bortezomib was not genotoxic when tested in the in vitro mutagenicity assay (Ames test) and in vivo micronucleus assay in mice.

➤*Fertility impairment:* Fertility studies with bortezomib were not performed but evaluation of reproductive tissues has been performed in the general toxicity studies. In the 6-month rat toxicity study, degenerative effects in the ovary were observed at doses greater than or equal to 0.3 mg/m^2 (one-fourth of the recommended clinical dose), and degenerative changes in the testes occurred at 1.2 mg/m^2. Bortezomib for injection could have a potential effect on either male or female fertility.

➤*Elderly:* Of the 202 patients enrolled, 35% were 65 years of age or older. Nineteen percent (19%) of patients aged 65 years or older experienced responses versus 32% in patients under the age of 65 years. Across the 256 patients analyzed for safety, the incidence of grade 3 or 4 events reported was 74%, 80%, and 85% for patients less than or equal to 50 years, 51 to 65 years, and greater than 65 years, respectively.

➤*Pregnancy: Category D.* Women of childbearing potential should avoid becoming pregnant while being treated with bortezomib for injection.

Pregnant rabbits given bortezomib during organogenesis at a dose of 0.05mg/kg (0.6 mg/m^2) experienced significant post-implantation loss and decreased number of live fetuses. Live fetuses from these litters also showed significant decreases in fetal weight. The dose is approximately 0.5 times the clinical dose of 1.3 mg/m^2 based on body surface area.

No placental transfer studies have been conducted with bortezomib. There are no adequate and well-controlled studies in pregnant women. If bortezomib for injection is used during pregnancy, or if the patient becomes pregnant while receiving this drug, the patient should be apprised of the potential hazard to the fetus.

➤*Lactation:* It is not known whether bortezomib is excreted in human milk. Because many drugs are excreted in human milk and because of the potential for serious adverse reactions in nursing infants from bortezomib for injection, women should be advised against breastfeeding while being treated with bortezomib for injection.

➤*Children:* The safety and effectiveness of bortezomib for injection in children have not been established.

Precautions

➤*Peripheral neuropathy:* Bortezomib for injection treatment causes a peripheral neuropathy that is predominantly sensory, although cases of mixed sensori-motor neuropathy have also been reported. Patients with pre-existing symptoms (numbness, pain or a burning feeling in the feet or hands) or signs of peripheral neuropathy may experience worsening during treatment with bortezomib for injection. Patients should be monitored for symptoms of neuropathy, such as a burning sensation, hyperesthesia, hypesthesia, paresthesia, discomfort or neuropathic pain. Patients experiencing new or worsening peripheral neuropathy may require change in the dose and schedule of bortezomib for injection. Limited follow-up data regarding the outcome of peripheral neuropathy are available. Of the patients who experienced treatment emergent neuropathy more than 70% had previously been treated with neurotoxic agents and more than 80% of these patients had signs or symptoms of peripheral neuropathy at baseline.

See Administration and Dosage for more information.

➤*Hypotension:* Bortezomib for injection treatment can cause orthostatic/postural hypotension in about 12% of patients. These events are observed throughout therapy. Caution should be used when treating patients with a history of syncope, patients receiving medications known to be associated with hypotension, and patients who are dehydrated. Management of orthostatic/postural hypotension may include adjustment of antihypertensive medications, hydration, or administration of mineralocorticoids.

➤*Gastrointestinal adverse reactions:* Bortezomib for injection treatment can cause nausea, diarrhea, constipation, and vomiting sometimes requiring use of antiemetics and antidiarrheals. Fluid and electrolyte replacement should be administered to prevent dehydration.

➤*Thrombocytopenia:* Thrombocytopenia, which occurred in about 40% of patients throughout therapy, was maximal at day 11 and usually recovered by the next cycle. Complete blood counts including platelet counts should be frequently monitored throughout treatment. Onset is most common in cycles 1 and 2 but can continue throughout therapy. There have been reports of gastrointestinal and intracerebral hemorrhage in association with bortezomib for injection induced thrombocytopenia. Bortezomib for injection treatment may be temporarily discontinued if patients experience grade 4 thrombocytopenia. Bortezomib for injection may be reinitiated at a reduced dose after resolution of thrombocytopenia. Bortezomib injection therapy should be withheld at the onset of any grade 3 non-hematological or grade 4 hematological toxicities excluding neuropathy. Once the symptoms of the toxicity have resolved, bortezomib injection therapy may be reinitiated at a 25% reduced dose (1.3 mg/m^2/dose reduced to 1 mg/m^2/dose; 1 mg/m^2/dose reduced to 0.7 mg/m^2/dose).

Drug Interactions

Bortezomib Drug Interactions

Precipitant drug	Object drug*		Description
CYP450 inducers or inhibitors	Bortezomib	↑↓	Bortezomib is a substrate for cytochrome P450 3A4, 2D6, 2C19, 2C9, and 1A2. Closely monitor patients for toxicities or reduced efficacy when bortezomib is coadministered with drugs that are inducers/inhibitors of cytochrome P450 3A4.
Bortezomib	CYP450 2C19 substrates	↑	Bortezomib may inhibit 2C19 isoenzyme activity and increase exposure to drugs that are substrates for this isoenzyme.
Bortezomib	Oral hypoglycemic agents	↑↓	Coadministration has resulted in hypo- and hyperglycemia. Closely monitor blood glucose levels and adjust dose of antidiabetic medication if necessary.

* ↑ = Object drug increased. ↓ = Object drug decreased.

BORTEZOMIB — INJECTION

Adverse Reactions

The most commonly reported adverse reactions were asthenic conditions (including fatigue, malaise and weakness) (65%), nausea (64%), diarrhea (51%), appetite decreased (including anorexia) (43%), constipation (43%), thrombocytopenia (43%), peripheral neuropathy (including peripheral sensory neuropathy and peripheral neuropathy aggravated) (37%), pyrexia (36%), vomiting (36%), and anemia (32%). Fourteen percent (14%) of patients experienced at least 1 episode of grade 4 toxicity, with the most common toxicity being thrombocytopenia (3%) and neutropenia (3%).

➤*Serious adverse reactions:* Serious adverse events are defined as any event, regardless of causality that: Results in death, is life-threatening, requires hospitalization or prolongs a current hospitalization, results in a significant disability or is deemed to be an important medical event. A total of 113 (50%) of the 228 patients experienced serious adverse reactions during the studies. The most commonly reported serious adverse reactions included pyrexia (7%), pneumonia (7%), diarrhea (6%), vomiting (5%), dehydration (5%), and nausea (4%).

Adverse reactions thought by the investigator to be drug-related and leading to discontinuation occurred in 18% of patients. The reasons for discontinuation included peripheral neuropathy (5%), thrombocytopenia (4%), diarrhea (2%), and fatigue (2%).

Two deaths were reported and considered by the investigator to be possibly related to study drug: 1 case of cardiopulmonary arrest and 1 case of respiratory failure.

In the single-arm studies conducted, it is often not possible to distinguish adverse reactions that are drug-caused and those that reflect the patient's underlying disease. See discussion of specific adverse reactions following the table below.

Most Commonly Reported Adverse Reactions (≥ 10% overall)

	All patients (n = 228)		
Adverse reaction	All reactions	Grade 3 reactions	Grade 4 reactions
Asthenic conditions	149 (65%)	42 (18%)	1 (< 1%)
Nausea	145 (64%)	13 (6%)	0
Diarrhea	116 (51%)	16 (7%)	2 (< 1%)
Decreased appetite	99 (43%)	6(3%)	0
Constipation	97 (43%)	5 (2%)	0
Thrombocytopenia	97 (43%)	61 (27%)	7 (3%)
Peripheral neuropathy	84 (37%)	31 (14%)	0
Pyrexia	82 (36%)	9 (4%)	0
Vomiting	82 (36%)	16 (7%)	1 (< 1%)
Anemia	74 (32%)	21 (9%)	0
Headache	63 (28%)	8 (4%)	0
Insomnia	62 (27%)	3 (1%)	0
Arthralgia	60 (26%)	11 (5%)	0
Pain in limb	59 (26%)	16 (7%)	0
Edema	58 (25%)	3 (1%)	0
Neutropenia	55 (24%)	30 (13%)	6 (3%)
Paresthesia and dysesthesia	53 (23%)	6 (3%)	0
Dyspnea	50 (22%)	7 (3%)	1 (< 1%)
Dizziness (excluding vertigo)	48 (21%)	3 (1%)	0
Rash	47 (21%)	1 (< 1%)	0
Dehydration	42 (18%)	15 (7%)	0
Upper respiratory tract infection	41 (18%)	0	0
Cough	39 (17%)	1 (< 1%)	0
Bone pain	33 (14%)	5 (2%)	0
Anxiety	32 (14%)	0	0
Myalgia	32 (14%)	5 (2%)	0
Back pain	31 (14%)	9 (4%)	0
Muscle cramps	31 (14%)	1 (< 1%)	0
Dyspepsia	30 (13%)	0	0
Abdominal pain	29 (13%)	5 (2%)	0
Dysgeusia	29 (13%)	1 (< 1%)	0
Hypotension	27 (12%)	8 (4%)	0
Rigors	27 (12%)	1 (< 1%)	0
Herpes zoster	26 (11%)	2 (< 1%)	0
Pruritus	26 (11%)	0	0
Vision blurred	25 (11%)	1 (< 1%)	0
Pneumonia	23 (10%)	12 (5%)	0

➤*Asthenic conditions (fatigue, malaise, weakness):* Asthenia was reported in 65% of patients and was predominantly reported as grade 1 or 2. The first onset of fatigue was most often reported during the first and second cycles of therapy. Asthenia was grade 3 for 18% of patients. Two percent (2%) of patients discontinued treatment due to fatigue.

➤*Gastrointestinal reactions:* The majority of patients experienced gastrointestinal adverse reactions during the studies, including nausea, diarrhea, constipation, and vomiting. Grade 3 or 4 GI reactions occurred in 21% of patients and were considered serious in 13% of patients. Vomiting and diarrhea each were of grade 3 severity in 7% of patients and were grade 4 in less than 1%. Five percent (5%) of patients discontinued due to gastrointestinal reactions. Appetite decreased (anorexia) was reported as an adverse reaction for 43% of patients. The incidence of grade 3 decreased appetite was 3%.

➤*Thrombocytopenia:* Thrombocytopenia was reported during treatment with bortezomib for injection for 43% of patients. The thrombocytopenia was characterized by a dose related decrease in platelet count during the bortezomib for injection dosing period (days 1 to 11) with a return to base line in platelet count during the rest period (days 12 to 21) in each treatment cycle. Thrombocytopenia was grade 3 or 4 in intensity for 27% and 3% respectively of patients. Four percent (4%) of patients discontinued bortezomib for injection treatment due to thrombocytopenia of any grade.

➤*Peripheral sensory neuropathy:* Events reported as peripheral neuropathy, peripheral sensory neuropathy, and peripheral neuropathy aggravated occurred in 37% of patients. Peripheral neuropathy was grade 3 for 14% of patients with no grade 4 events. New onset or worsening of existing neuropathy was noted throughout the cycles of treatment. Six percent (6%) of patients discontinued bortezomib for injection due to neuropathy. More than 80% of all study patients had signs or symptoms of peripheral neuropathy at baseline evaluation. The incidence of grade 3 neuropathy was 5% (2 of 41 patients) in patients without baseline neuropathy. Symptoms may improve or return to baseline in some patients upon discontinuation of bortezomib for injection. The complete time-course of this toxicity has not been fully characterized.

➤*Pyrexia:* Pyrexia (greater than 38°C; 100.4°F) was reported as an adverse reaction for 36% of patients and was assessed as grade 3 in 4% of patients.

➤*Neutropenia:* Neutropenia occurred in 24% of patients and was grade 3 in 13% and grade 4 in 3%. The incidence of febrile neutropenia was less than 1%.

➤*Hypotension:* Hypotension (including reports of orthostatic hypotension) was reported in 12% of patients. Most reactions were grade 1 or 2 in severity. Grade 3 hypotension occurred in 4% of patients; no patient experienced grade 4 hypotension. Patients developing orthostatic hypotension did not have evidence of orthostatic hypotension at study entry; half had preexisting hypertension and one-third had evidence of peripheral neuropathy. Doses of antihypertensive medications may need to be adjusted in patients receiving bortezomib for injection. Four percent (4%) of patients experienced hypotension, including orthostatic hypotension, and had a concurrent syncopal event.

➤*Serious adverse reactions from clinical studies:*

Cardiovascular – Atrial fibrillation aggravated, atrial flutter, cardiac amyloidosis, cardiac arrest, cardiac failure congestive, myocardial ischemia, myocardial infarction, pericardial effusion, pulmonary edema, ventricular tachycardia. Cerebrovascular accident, deep venous thrombosis, peripheral embolism, pulmonary embolism.

CNS – Ataxia, coma, dizziness, dysarthria, dysautonomia, cranial palsy, grand mal convulsion, hemorrhagic stroke, motor dysfunction, spinal cord compression, transient ischemic attack.

GI – Ascites, dysphagia, fecal impaction, gastritis hemorrhagic, gastrointestinal hemorrhage, hematemesis, ileus paralytic, large intestinal obstruction, paralytic intestinal obstruction, small intestinal obstruction, large intestinal perforation, stomatitis, melena, pancreatitis acute.

GU – Bladder spasm, hematuria urinary incontinence, urinary retention.

Hematologic / Lymphatic – Disseminated intravascular coagulation.

Hepatic – Hyperbilirubinemia, portal vein thrombosis.

Metabolic / Nutritional – Hypocalcemia, hyperuricemia, hypokalemia, hyponatremia, tumor lysis syndrome.

Psychiatric – Agitation, confusion, psychotic disorder, suicidal ideation.

Renal – Renal calculus, bilateral hydronephrosis, acute and chronic renal failure, proliferative glomerular nephritis.

Respiratory – Acute respiratory distress syndrome, atelectasis, chronic obstructive airways disease exacerbated, dysphagia, dyspnea, dyspnea exertional, epistaxis, hemoptysis, hypoxia, lung infiltration, pleural effusion, pneumonitis, respiratory distress, respiratory failure.

➤*Miscellaneous:* Anaphylactic reaction, drug hypersensitivity, immune complex mediated hypersensitivity. Bacteremia, skeletal fracture, subdural hematoma.

Overdosage

Cardiovascular safety pharmacology studies in monkeys show that lethal IV doses are associated with decreases in blood pressure, increases in heart rate, increases in contractility, and ultimately terminal hypotension. In monkeys, doses of 3 mg/m^2 and greater (approximately twice the recommended clinical dose) resulted in progressive hypotension starting at 1 hour and progressing to death by 12 to 14 hours following drug administration.

No cases of overdosage with bortezomib for injection were reported during clinical trials. Single doses of up to 2 mg/m^2 per week have been administered in adults.

BORTEZOMIB — INJECTION

➤*Treatment:* In the event of overdosage, patient's vital signs should be monitored and appropriate supportive care should be given to maintain blood pressure and body temperature. Management of orthostatic/postural hypotension may include adjustment of antihypertensive medications, hydration, or administration of mineralocorticoids.

There is no known specific antidote for bortezomib for injection overdosage.

Patient Information

Because bortezomib for injection may be associated with fatigue, dizziness, syncope, orthostatic/postural hypotension, diplopia or blurred vision, patients should be cautious when operating machinery, including automobiles.

Patients should be advised to use effective contraceptive measures to prevent pregnancy and to avoid breast feeding during treatment with bortezomib for injection.

Because patients receiving bortezomib for injection therapy may experience vomiting or diarrhea, patients should be advised regarding appropriate measures to avoid dehydration. Patients should be instructed to seek medical advice if they experience symptoms of dizziness, light headedness, or fainting spells.

Patients should be advised to drink plenty of fluids.

Patients should be cautioned about the use of concomitant medications that may be associated with peripheral neuropathy (eg, amiodarne, antivirals, isoniazid, nitrofurantoin, statins), or with a decrease in blood pressure.

Patients should be instructed to contact their physician if they experience new or worsening symptoms of peripheral neuropathy. Patients with preexisting symptoms (numbness, pain or a burning feeling in the feet or hands) or signs of peripheral neuropathy may experience worsening during treatment with bortezomib for injection. Patients should be monitored for symptoms of neuropathy, such as a burning sensation, hyperesthesia, hypesthesia, paresthesia, discomfort or neuropathic pain.

Patients should contact their physicians if they experience numbness, pain, or burning feelings in the feet and hands.

MULTIKINASE INHIBITOR

SORAFENIB

Rx	**Nexavar** (Bayer Pharmaceutical)	**Tablets:** 200 mg	(200). Red. Film coated. In 120s.

SORAFENIB — ORAL

Indications

➤*Advanced renal cell carcinoma:* For the treatment of patients with advanced renal cell carcinoma.

Administration and Dosage

➤*Approved by the FDA:* December 20, 2005.

➤*Recommended dose:* The recommended daily dose of sorafenib is 400 mg (two 200 mg tablets) taken twice daily, without food (at least 1 hour before or 2 hours after eating). Treatment should continue until the patient is no longer clinically benefiting from therapy or until unacceptable toxicity occurs.

➤*Dosage adjustment:* Management of suspected adverse drug reactions may require temporary interruption and/or dose reduction of sorafenib therapy. When dose reduction is necessary, the sorafenib dose may be reduced to 400 mg once daily. If additional dose reduction is required, sorafenib may be reduced to a single 400 mg dose every other day.

Suggested Sorafenib Dose Modifications for Skin Toxicity

Skin toxicity grade	Occurrence	Suggested dose modification
Grade 1: Numbness, dysesthesia, paresthesia, tingling, painless swelling, erythema, or discomfort of the hands or feet that does not disrupt normal activities	Any occurrence	Continue treatment and consider topical therapy for symptomatic relief.
Grade 2: Painful erythema and swelling of the hands or feet and/or discomfort affecting normal activities	First occurrence	Continue treatment and consider topical therapy for symptomatic relief. If no improvement within 7 days, see below.
	No improvement within 7 days or second or third occurrence	Interrupt treatment until toxicity resolves to grade 0 to 1. When resuming treatment, decrease dose by one dose level (400 mg daily or 400 mg every other day).
	Fourth occurrence	Discontinue sorafenib.
Grade 3: Moist desquamation, ulceration, blistering, or severe pain of the hands or feet, or severe discomfort that causes inability to work or perform activities of daily living	First or second occurrence	Interrupt treatment until toxicity resolves to grade 0 to 1. When resuming treatment, decrease dose by one dose level (400 mg daily or 400 mg every other day).
	Third occurrence	Discontinue sorafenib.

➤*Storage/Stability:* Store at 25°C (77°F). Excursions permitted to 15° to 30°C (59° to 86°F). Store in a dry place.

Actions

➤*Pharmacology:* Sorafenib is a multikinase inhibitor that decreases tumor cell proliferation in vitro. Sorafenib inhibited tumor growth of the murine renal cell carcinoma (RENCA) and several other human tumor xenografts in athymic mice. A reduction in tumor angiogenesis was seen in some tumor xenograft models. Sorafenib was shown to interact with multiple intracellular (CRAF, BRAF and mutant BRAF) and cell surface kinases (kinase tyrosine [KIT], 3' fluoro-2', 3'-dideoxythymidine fluorothymidine [FLT-3], vascular endothelial growth factor receptor [VEGFR]-2, VEGFR-3, and platelet-derived growth factor receptor [PDGFR]-β). Several of these kinases are thought to be involved in angiogenesis.

➤*Pharmacokinetics:*

Absorption/Distribution – After administration of sorafenib tablets, the mean relative bioavailability is 38% to 49% when compared with an oral solution. Multiple dosing of sorafenib for 7 days resulted in 2.5- to 7-fold accumulation compared with single dose administration. steady state plasma sorafenib concentrations are achieved within 7 days, with a peak-to-trough ratio of mean concentrations of less than 2.

Following oral administration, sorafenib reaches plasma level in approximately 3 hours. When given with a moderate-fat meal, bioavailability was similar to that in the fasted state. With a high-fat meal, sorafenib bioavailability was reduced by 29% compared with administration in the fasted state. It is recommended that sorafenib be administered without food (at least 1 hour before or 2 hours after eating).

Mean maximum effective plasma concentration (C_{max}) and area under the plasma concentration time curve (AUC) increased less than proportionally beyond doses of 400 mg administered orally twice daily.

In vitro binding to sorafenib to human plasma proteins is 99.5%.

Metabolism/Excretion – Sorafenib is metabolized primarily in the liver, undergoing oxidative metabolism, mediated by CYP3A4, as well as glucuronidation mediated by UGT1A9.

Sorafenib accounts for approximately 70% to 85% of the circulating analytes in plasma at steady state. Eight metabolites of sorafenib have been identified, of which 5 have been detected in plasma. The main circulating metabolite of sorafenib in plasma, the pyridine N-oxide, shows in vitro potency similar to that of sorafenib. This metabolite comprises approximately 9% to 16% of circulating analytes at steady state.

Following oral administration of a 100 mg dose of a solution formulation of sorafenib, 96% of the dose was recovered within 14 days, with 77% of the dose excreted in feces and 19% of the dose excreted in urine as glucuronidated metabolites. Unchanged sorafenib, accounting for 51% of the dose, was found in feces but not in urine.

The mean elimination half-life of sorafenib is approximately 25 to 48 hours.

Special populations –

Race: Limited pharmacokinetic data on sorafenib 400 mg twice daily in a study in Japanese patients (N = 6) showed a 45% lower systemic exposure (mean steady state AUC) as compared with pooled phase 1 pharmacokinetic data in white patients (n = 25). The clinical significance of this finding is not known.

Contraindications

Sorafenib is contraindicated in patients with known severe hypersensitivity to sorafenib or any other component of sorafenib.

Warnings

➤*Mutagenesis:* Sorafenib was clastogenic when tested in an in vitro mammalian cell assay (Chinese hamster ovary) in the presence of metabolic activation. Sorafenib was not mutagenic in the in vitro Ames bacterial cell assay or clastogenic in and in vivo mouse micronucleus assay. One intermediate in the manufacturing process, which is also present in the final drug substance (less than 0.15%), was positive for mutagenesis in an in vitro bacterial cell assay (Ames test) when tested independently.

➤*Fertility impairment:* No specific studies with sorafenib have been conducted in animals to evaluate the effect on fertility. However, results from the repeat-dose toxicity studies suggest there is a potential for sorafenib to impair reproductive performance and fertility. Multiple adverse reactions were observed in male and female reproductive organs, with the rat being more susceptible than mice or dogs. Typical changes in rats consisted of testicular atrophy or degeneration, degeneration of epididymis, prostate, and seminal vesicles, central necrosis of the corpora lutea, and arrested follicular development. Sorafenib-related effects on the reproductive organs of rats were manifested at daily oral doses of 30 mg/m^2 or more (approximately 0.5 times the AUC in cancer patients at the recommended human dose). Dogs showed tubular degeneration in the testes at 600 mg/m^2/day (approximately 0.3 times the AUC at the recommended human dose) and oligospermia at 1,200 mg/m^2/day of sorafenib.

Adequate contraception should be used during therapy and for at least 2 weeks after completing therapy.

➤*Elderly:* In total, 32% of renal cell carcinoma patients treated with sorafenib were 65 years of age or older, and 4% were 75 years of age and older. No differences in safety or efficacy were observed between older and younger patients, and other reported clinical experience has not identified differences in responses between the elderly and younger patients, but greater sensitivity of some older individuals cannot be ruled out.

➤*Pregnancy: Category D.* In rats and rabbits, sorafenib has been shown to be teratogenic and to induce embryo-fetal toxicity (including increased postimplantation loss, resorptions, skeletal retardations, and retarded fetal weight). The effects occurred at dosages considerably below the recommended human dosage of 400 mg twice daily (approximately 500 mg/m^2/day on a body surface area basis). Adverse intrauterine development effects were seen at dosages at or above1.2 mg/m^2/day in rats and 3.6 mg/m^2/day in rabbits (approximately 0.008 times the AUC seen in cancer patients at the recommended human dose). A no observed adverse effect level (NOAEL) was not defined for either species because lower doses were not tested.

Based on the proposed mechanism of multikinase inhibition and multiple adverse reactions seen in animals at exposure levels significantly below the clinical dose, sorafenib should be assumed to cause fetal harm when administered to a pregnant woman. If this drug is used during pregnancy, or if the patient becomes pregnant while taking this drug, apprise the patient of the potential hazard to the fetus.

There are no adequate and well-controlled studies in pregnant women using sorafenib. Advise women of childbearing potential to avoid becoming pregnant while on sorafenib. Use sorafenib during pregnancy only if the potential benefits justify the potential risks to the fetus.

➤*Lactation:* It is not known whether sorafenib is excreted in human milk. Following administration of ^{14}C-sorafenib to lactating Wistar rats, approximately 27% of the radioactivity was secreted into the milk. The milk to plasma AUC ratio was approximately 5:1.

Because many drugs are excreted in human milk and because the effects of sorafenib on infants have not been studied, advise women against breastfeeding while receiving sorafenib.

➤*Children:* The safety and efficacy of sorafenib in children have not been studied.

Precautions

➤*Dermatologic toxicities:* Hand-foot skin reaction and rash represent the most common adverse reactions attributed to sorafenib. Analysis of cumulative event rates from study 1 suggest that rash and hand-foot skin reactions are usually Common Terminology Criteria for Adverse Events (CTCAE) grade 1 and 2 and generally appear during the first 6 weeks of treatment with sorafenib. Management of dermatologic toxicities may include topical therapies for symptomatic relief, temporary treatment interruption, and/or dose modification of sorafenib, or in severe or persistent cases, permanent discontinuation of sorafenib. Permanent discontinuation of therapy because of hand-foot skin reaction occurred in 3 of 451 sorafenib patients.

➤*Hypertension:* In study 1, treatment-emergent hypertension was reported in approximately 16.9% of sorafenib-treated patients and 1.8% of patients in the placebo group. Hypertension was usually mild to moderate, occurred early in the course of treatment, and was managed with standard antihypertensive therapy. Monitor blood pressure weekly during the first 6 weeks of sorafenib therapy and monitor and treat thereafter, if required, in accordance with standard medical practice. In cases of severe or persistent hypertension, despite institution of antihypertensive therapy, consider temporary or permanent discontinuation of sorafenib. Permanent discontinuation because of hypertension occurred in 1 of 451 sorafenib patients.

➤*Hemorrhage:* An increased risk of bleeding may occur after sorafenib administration. In study 1, bleeding regardless of causality was reported in 15.3% of patients in the sorafenib group and 8.2% of patients in the placebo group. The incidence of CTCAE grade 3 and 4 bleeding events was 2% and 0%, respectively, in sorafenib patients, and 1.3% and 0.2%, respectively, in placebo patients. There was one fatal hemorrhage in each treatment group in study 1. If any bleeding event necessitates medical intervention, consider permanent discontinuation of sorafenib.

➤*Cardiac effects:* In study 1, the incidence of treatment-emergent cardiac ischemia/infarction events was higher in the sorafenib group (2.9%) compared with the placebo group (0.4%). Patients with unstable coronary artery disease or recent myocardial infarction were excluded from this study. Consider temporary or permanent discontinuation of sorafenib in patients who develop cardiac ischemia and/or infarction.

➤*Race:* See Actions for more information.

➤*Wound healing complications:* No formal studies of the effect of sorafenib on wound healing have been conducted. Temporary interruption of sorafenib therapy is recommended in patients undergoing major surgical procedures. There is limited clinical experience regarding the timing of reinitiation of sorafenib therapy following major surgical intervention. Therefore, base the decision to resume sorafenib therapy following a major surgical intervention on clinical judgment of adequate wound healing.

Drug Interactions

➤*UGT1A1 system:* Caution is recommended when administering sorafenib with compounds that are metabolized/eliminated predominantly by the UGT1A1 pathway (eg, irinotecan).

➤*Doxorubicin:* Concomitant treatment with sorafenib resulted in a 21% increase in the AUC of doxorubicin. Caution is recommended when administering doxorubicin with sorafenib.

➤*Warfarin:* Infrequent bleeding events or elevations in the international normalized ratio (INR) have been reported in some patients taking warfarin while on sorafenib therapy. Regularly monitor patients taking concomitant warfarin for changes in prothrombin time, INR, or clinical bleeding episodes.

➤*CYP450 system:* Sorafenib inhibits CYP2B6 and CYP2C8 in vitro with K_i values of 6 and 1-2 micromolars, respectively. Systemic exposure to substrates of CYP2B6 and CYP2C8 is expected to increase when coadministered with sorafenib. Caution is recommended when administering substrates of CYP2B6 and CYP2C8 with sorafenib.

There is no clinical information on the effect of CYP3A4 inducers on the pharmacokinetics sorafenib. Substances that are inducers of CYP3A4 activity (eg, carbamazepine, dexamethasone, phenobarbital, phenytoin, rifampin, St. John's wort) are expected to increase metabolism of sorafenib and thus decrease sorafenib concentrations.

➤*Other antineoplastic agents:* In clinical studies, sorafenib has been administered with a variety of other antineoplastic agents at their commonly used dosing regimens, including gemcitabine, oxaliplatin, doxorubicin, and irinotecan. Sorafenib had no effect on the pharmacokinetics of gemcitabine or oxaliplatin. Concomitant treatment with sorafenib resulted in a 21% increase in the AUC of doxorubicin. When administered with irinotecan, whose active metabolite SN-38 is further metabolized by the UGT1A1 pathway, there was a 67% to 120% increase in the AUC of SN-38 and a 26% to 42% increase in the AUC of irinotecan. The clinical significance of these findings is unknown.

➤*Drug/Food interactions:* See Actions for more information.

Adverse Reactions

The following table shows the percentage of patients experiencing treatment-emergent adverse reactions that were reported in at least 10% of patients who received sorafenib in study 1. CTCAE grade 3 treatment-emergent adverse reactions were reported in 31% of patients receiving sorafenib compared with 22% of patients receiving placebo. CTCAE grade 4 treatment-emergent adverse reactions were reported in 7% of patients receiving sorafenib compared with 6% of patients receiving placebo.

Sorafenib Adverse Reactions (≥ 10%)

	Sorafenib n =451			Placebo n =451		
Adverse Reaction	All grades	Grade 3	Grade 4	All grades	Grade 3	Grade 4
Any reaction	95%	31%	7%	86%	22%	6%
Cardiovascular						
Hypertension	17%	3%	< 1%	2%	< 1%	0%
CNS						
Neuropathy–sensory	13%	< 1%	0%	6%	< 1%	0%
Pain, headache	10%	< 1%	0%	6%	< 1%	0%
Dermatological						
Alopecia	27%	< 1%	0%	3%	0%	0%
Dry skin	11%	0%	0%	4%	0%	0%
Hand-foot skin reaction	30%	6%	0%	7%	0%	0%
Pruritus	19%	< 1%	0%	6%	0%	0%
Rash/desquamation	40%	< 1%	0%	16%	< 1%	0%
GI						
Anorexia	16%	< 1%	0%	13%	1%	0%
Constipation	15%	< 1%	0%	11%	< 1%	0%
Diarrhea	43%	2%	0%	13%	< 1%	0%
Nausea	23%	< 1%	0%	19%	< 1%	0%
Pain, abdomen	11%	2%	0%	9%	2%	0%
Vomiting	16%	< 1%	0%	12%	1%	0%
Hematologic						
Hemorrhage—all sites	15%	2%	0%	8%	1%	< 1%
Respiratory						
Cough	13%	< 1%	0%	14%	< 1%	0%
Dyspnea	14%	3%	< 1%	12%	2%	< 1%
Miscellaneous						
Fatigue	37%	5%	< 1%	28%	3%	< 1%
Pain, joint	10%	2%	0%	6%	< 1%	0%
Weight loss	10%	< 1%	0%	6%	0%	0%

The rate of adverse reactions (including reactions associated with progressive disease) resulting in permanent discontinuation was similar in both the sorafenib and placebo groups (10% of sorafenib patients and 8% of placebo patients).

SORAFENIB — ORAL

➤*Lab test abnormalities:* Hypophosphatemia was a common laboratory finding, observed in 45% of sorafenib-treated patients compared with 11% of placebo patients. CTCAE grade 3 hypophosphatemia (1 to 2 mg/dL) occurred in 13% of sorafenib-treated patients and 3% of patients in the placebo group. There were no cases of CTCAE grade 4 hypophosphatemia (less than 1 mg/dL) reported in either sorafenib or placebo patients. The etiology of hypophosphatemia associated with sorafenib is not known.

Elevated lipase was observed in 41% of patients treated with sorafenib compared with 30% of patients in the placebo group. CTCAE grade 3 or 4 lipase elevations occurred in 12% of patients in the sorafenib group compared with 7% of patients in the placebo group. Elevated amylase was observed in 30% of patient treated with sorafenib compared with 23% of patients in the placebo group. CTCAE grade 3 or 4 amylase elevations were reported in 1% of patients in the sorafenib group compared with 3% of patients in the placebo group. Many of the lipase and amylase elevations were transient, and in the majority of cases sorafenib treatment was not interrupted. Clinical pancreatitis was reported in 3 of 451 sorafenib-treated patients (one CTCAE grade 2 and two grade 4) and 1 of 451 patients (CTCAE grade 2) in the placebo group.

Lymphopenia was observed in 23% of sorafenib-treated patients and 13% of placebo patients. CTCAE grade 3 or 4 lymphopenia was reported in 13% of sorafenib-treated patients and 7% of placebo patients. Neutropenia was observed in 18% of sorafenib-treated patients and 10% of placebo patients. CTCAE grade 3 or 4 neutropenia was reported in 5% of sorafenib-treated patients and 2% of placebo patients.

Anemia was observed in 44% of sorafenib-treated patients and 49% of placebo patients. CTCAE grade 3 or 4 anemia was reported in 2% of sorafenib-patients and 4% of placebo patients.

Thrombocytopenia was observed in 12% of sorafenib-treated patients and 5% of placebo patients. CTCAE grade 3 or 4 thrombocytopenia was reported in 1% of sorafenib-treated patients and 0% of placebo patients.

Safety was also assessed in phase 2 study pool comprised of 638 sorafenib-treated patients, including 202 patients with renal cell carcinoma, 137 patients with hepatocellular carcinoma, and 299 patients with other cancers. The most common drug-related adverse reactions reported in sorafenib-treated patients in this pool were rash (38%), diarrhea (37%), hand-foot skin reaction (35%), and fatigue (33%). The respective rates of CTC (v 2.0) grade 3 and 4 drug-related adverse reactions in sorafenib-treated patients were 37% and 3%, respectively.

➤*Additional drug-related adverse reactions and laboratory abnormalities:*

Cardiovascular – Hypertensive crisis, myocardial ischemia and/or infarction (0.1% to less than 1%).

CNS – Depression (1% to less than 10%). Tinnitus (0.1% to less than 1%).

Dermatologic – Erythema (10% or greater). Acne, exfoliative dermatitis, flushing (1% to less than 10%). Eczema, erythema multiform, folliculitis, (0.1% to less than 1%).

GI – Increased amylase, increased lipase, (10% or greater). Dyspepsia, dysphagia, mucositis, stomatitis (including dry mouth and glossodynia), (1% to less than 10%). Gastritis, gastrointestinal reflux, pancreatitis, (0.1% to less than 1%).

Note that elevations in lipase are very common (41%, see Lab test abnormalities); do not make a diagnosis of pancreatitis solely on the basis of abnormal laboratory values.

GU – Erectile dysfunction (1% to less than 10%). Gynecomastia (0.1% to less than 1%).

Hematologic – Leukopenia, lymphopenia (10% or greater). Anemia, neutropenia, thrombocytopenia (1% to less than 10%). INR abnormal (0.1% to less than 1%).

Hypersensitivity – Hypersensitivity reactions (including skin reactions and urticaria) (0.1% to less than 1%).

Metabolic/Nutritional – Hypophosphatemia (10% or greater). Transient increases in transaminases (1% to less than 10%). Dehydration, hyponatremia, hypothyroidism, increased bilirubin (including jaundice), transient increases in alkaline phosphatase (0.1% to less than 1%).

Musculoskeletal – Arthralgia, myalgia (1% to less than 10%).

Respiratory – Hoarseness (1% to less than 10%). Rhinorrhea (0.1% to less than 1%).

Miscellaneous – Asthenia, pain (including mouth pain, bone pain, and muscle pain) (10% or greater). Decreased appetite, influenza-like illness, pyrexia (1% to less than 10%). Infection (0.1% to less than 1%).

Additional reactions – In addition, the following medically significant adverse reactions were reported infrequently during clinical trials of sorafenib: acute renal failure, arrhythmia, cardiac failure, cerebral hemorrhage, transient ischemic attack, thromboembolism. For these reactions, the causal relationship to sorafenib has not been established.

Overdosage

➤*Symptoms:* The highest dosage of sorafenib studied clinically is 800 mg twice daily. The adverse reactions observed at this dosage were primarily diarrhea and dermatologic events. No information is available on symptoms of acute overdose in animals because of the saturation of absorption in oral acute toxicity studies conducted in animals.

➤*Treatment:* There is no specific treatment for sorafenib overdose. In cases of suspected overdose, withhold sorafenib and institute supportive care.

Patient Information

Inform female patients that sorafenib may cause birth defects or fetal loss and that they should not become pregnant during treatment with sorafenib and for at least 2 weeks after stopping treatment. Counsel male and female patients to use effective birth control during treatment with sorafenib and for at least 2 weeks after stopping treatment. Also advise female patients against breast-feeding while receiving sorafenib.

Advise patients of the possible occurrence of hand-foot skin reaction and rash during sorafenib treatment and appropriate countermeasures. Inform patients that hypertension may develop during sorafenib treatment, especially during the first 6 weeks of therapy, and to monitor blood pressure regularly during treatment.

Inform patients that sorafenib may increase the risk of bleeding and that they should promptly report any episodes of bleeding.

Discuss with patients that cardiac ischemia and/or infarction has been reported during sorafenib treatment, and that they should immediately report any episodes of chest pain or other symptoms of cardiac ischemia and/or infarction.

MISCELLANEOUS ANTINEOPLASTICS

PORFIMER SODIUM

Rx	**Photofrin** (Axican Scandipharm)	**Cake or powder for injection (freeze-dried):** 75 mg	Preservative-free. In vials.

PORFIMER SODIUM — INJECTION

Indications

➤*Esophageal cancer:* Palliation of patients with completely obstructing esophageal cancer, or of patients with partially obstructing esophageal cancer who, in the opinion of their physician, cannot be satisfactorily treated with Nd:YAG laser therapy.

➤*Endobronchial nonsmall cell lung cancer (NSCLC):* The reduction of obstruction and palliation of symptoms in patients with completely or partially obstructing endobronchial NSCLC.

Microinvasive endobronchial NSCLC – The treatment of microinvasive endobronchial NSCLC in patients for whom surgery and radiotherapy are not indicated.

Barrett's esophagus – Ablation of high-grade dysplasia in Barrett's esophagus patients who do not undergo esophagectomy.

➤*Unlabeled uses:* For treatment of AIDS-related cutaneous Kaposi sarcoma, primary or recurrent basal cell carcinoma, and squamous cell carcinoma.

Administration and Dosage

➤*Approved by the FDA:* December 27, 1995.

Photodynamic therapy with porfimer sodium is a 2-stage process requiring administration of both drug and light. The first stage of PDT is the IV injection of porfimer sodium at 2 mg/kg. Illumination with laser light 40 to 50 hours following injection with porfimer sodium constitutes the second stage of therapy. A second laser light application may be given 96 to 120 hours after injection, preceded by gentle debridement of residual tumor (see Administration of laser light). In clinical studies of esophageal and endobronchial cancers, debridement via endoscopy was required 2 days after the initial light application. Standard endoscopic techniques are used for light administration and debridement. Practitioners should be fully familiar with the patient's condition and trained in the safe and efficacious treatment of esophageal or endobronchial cancer, or high-grade dysplasia in Barrett's esophagus using photodynamic therapy with porfimer sodium and associated light delivery devices.

➤*Esophageal/Endobronchial cancer:* For the treatment of esophageal and endobronchial cancer, patients may receive a second course of PDT a minimum of 30 days after the initial therapy; up to 3 courses of PDT (each separated by a minimum of 30 days) can be given. Before each course of treatment, patients with esophageal cancer should be evaluated for the presence of a tracheoesophageal or bronchoesophageal fistula. Porfimer sodium is contraindicated in the presence of these conditions. In patients with endobronchial lesions who have recently undergone radiotherapy, sufficient time (approximately 4 weeks) should be allowed between the therapies to ensure that the acute inflammation produced by radiotherapy has subsided prior to PDT. Patients with endobronchial lesions must be closely monitored between the laser light therapy and the mandatory debridement bronchoscopy for any evidence of respiratory distress. Inflammation, mucositis, and necrotic debris may cause obstruction of the airway. If respiratory distress occurs, the physician should be prepared to carry out immediate bronchoscopy to remove secretions and debris to open the airway. All patients should be evaluated for the possibility that the tumor may be eroding into a major blood vessel. Porfimer sodium is also contraindicated in the presence of this condition.

PORFIMER SODIUM — INJECTION

➤*Barrett's esophagus:* For the ablation of high-grade dysplasia in Barrett's esophagus, patients may receive an additional course of PDT at a minimum of 90 days after the initial therapy; up to 3 courses of PDT (each injection separated by a minimum of 90 days) can be given to a previously treated segment which still shows high-grade dysplasia, low-grade dysplasia, or Barrett's metaplasia, or to a new segment if the initial Barrett's segment was greater than 7 cm in length. Both residual and additional segments may be treated in the same light session(s) provided that the total length of the segments treated with the balloon/diffuser combination is not greater than 7 cm. In the case of a previously treated esophageal segment, if it has not sufficiently healed and/or histological assessment of biopsies is not clear, the subsequent course of PDT may be delayed for an additional 1 to 2 months.

➤*Administration:* Porfimer sodium should be administered as a single slow IV injection over 3 to 5 minutes at 2 mg/kg body weight. Reconstitute each vial of porfimer sodium with 31.8 mL of either 5% Dextrose Injection or 0.9% Sodium Chloride Injection, resulting in a final concentration of 2.5 mg/mL. Shake well until dissolved. Do not mix porfimer sodium with other drugs in the same solution. Porfimer sodium, reconstituted with 5% Dextrose Injection or with 0.9% Sodium Chloride Injection, has a pH in the range of 7 to 8. Porfimer sodium has been formulated with an overage to deliver the 75 mg labeled quantity. The reconstituted product should be protected from bright light and used immediately. Reconstituted porfimer sodium is an opaque solution, in which detection of particulate matter by visual inspection is extremely difficult. Reconstituted porfimer sodium, however, like all parenteral drug products, should be inspected visually for particulate matter and discoloration prior to administration whenever solution and container permit.

Extravasation – Precautions should be taken to prevent extravasation at the injection site. If extravasation occurs, care must be taken to protect the area from light. There is no known benefit from injecting the extravasation site with another substance.

➤*Storage/Stability:* Porfimer sodium freeze dried cake or powder should be stored at controlled room temperature 20° to 25°C (68° to 77°F).

Spills and disposal – Spills of porfimer sodium should be wiped up with a damp cloth. Skin and eye contact should be avoided due to the potential for photosensitivity reactions upon exposure to light; use of rubber gloves and eye protection is recommended. All contaminated materials should be disposed of in a polyethylene bag in a manner consistent with local regulations.

Accidental exposure – Porfimer sodium is neither a primary ocular irritant nor a primary dermal irritant. However, because of its potential to induce photosensitivity, porfimer sodium might be an eye and skin irritant in the presence of bright light. It is important to avoid contact with the eyes and skin during preparation and administration. As with therapeutic overdosage, any overexposed person must be protected from bright light.

Actions

➤*Pharmacology:* The cytotoxic and antitumor actions of porfimer sodium are light and oxygen dependent. PDT with porfimer sodium is a 2-stage process. The first stage is the IV injection of porfimer sodium. Clearance from a variety of tissues occurs over 40 to 72 hours, but tumors, skin, and organs of the reticuloendothelial system (including liver and spleen) retain porfimer sodium for a longer period. Illumination with 630 nm wavelength laser light constitutes the second stage of therapy. Tumor selectivity in treatment occurs through a combination of selective retention of porfimer sodium and selective delivery of light. Cellular damage caused by porfimer sodium PDT is a consequence of the propagation of radical reactions. Radical initiation may occur after porfimer sodium absorbs light to form a porphyrin excited state. Spin transfer from porfimer sodium to molecular oxygen may then generate singlet oxygen. Subsequent radical reactions can form superoxide and hydroxyl radicals. Tumor death also occurs through ischemic necrosis secondary to vascular occlusion that appears to be partly mediated by thromboxane A_2 release. The laser treatment induces a photochemical, not a thermal, effect. The necrotic reaction and associated inflammatory responses may evolve over several days.

➤*Pharmacokinetics:*

Absorption/Distribution – Following a 2 mg/kg dose of porfimer sodium to 4 male cancer patients, the average peak plasma concentration was 15 ± 3 mcg/mL, the elimination half-life was 250 ± 285 hours, the steady-state volume of distribution was 0.49 ± 0.28 L/kg, and the total plasma clearance was 0.051 ± 0.035 mL/min/kg. The mean plasma concentration at 48 hours was 2.6 ± 0.4 mcg/mL. The influence of impaired hepatic function on porfimer sodium disposition has not been evaluated.

Porfimer sodium was approximately 90% protein bound in human serum, studied in vitro. The binding was independent of concentration over the concentration range of 20 to 100 mcg/mL.

Special populations –

Gender: The pharmacokinetics of porfimer sodium was also studied in 24 healthy subjects (12 men and 12 women) who received a single dose of 2 mg/kg porfimer sodium given via the intravenous route. The serum decay was biexponential, with a slow distribution phase and a very long elimination phase. The elimination half-life was 415 ± 104 hours (17 ± 4.3 days). C_{max} was determined to be 40 ± 11.6 mcg/mL and AUC_{inf} was 2400 ± 552 mcg•hr/mL. Women had a lower C_{max} and a higher AUC. The clinical significance of these differences is unknown. T_{max} was approximately 1.5 hours in women and 0.17 hours in men. At the time of intended photoactivation 40 to 50 hours after injection, the pharmacokinetic profiles of porfimer sodium in men and women were similar.

Contraindications

Porfimer sodium is contraindicated in patients with porphyria or in patients with known allergies to porphyrins.

PDT is contraindicated in patients with an existing tracheoesophageal or bronchoesophageal fistula.

PDT is contraindicated in patients with tumors eroding into a major blood vessel.

Photodynamic therapy is not suitable for emergency treatment of patients with severe acute respiratory distress caused by an obstructing endobronchial lesion because 40 to 50 hours are required between injection with porfimer sodium and laser light treatment.

Photodynamic therapy is not suitable for patients with esophageal or gastric varices, or patients with esophageal ulcers greater than 1 cm in diameter.

Warnings

➤*Photosensitivity:* All patients who receive porfimer sodium will be photosensitive and must observe precautions to avoid exposure of skin and eyes to direct sunlight or bright indoor light (from examination lamps, including dental lamps, operating room lamps, unshaded light bulbs at close proximity) for at least 30 days. Some patients may remain photosensitive for greater than or equal to 90 days. The photosensitivity is due to residual drug, which will be present in all parts of the skin. Exposure of the skin to ambient indoor light is, however, beneficial because the remaining drug will be inactivated gradually and safely through a photobleaching reaction. Therefore, patients should not stay in a darkened room during this period and should be encouraged to expose their skin to ambient indoor light. The level of photosensitivity will vary for different areas of the body, depending on the extent of previous exposure to light. Before exposing any area of skin to direct sunlight or bright indoor light, the patient should test it for residual photosensitivity. A small area of skin should be exposed to sunlight for 10 minutes. If no photosensitivity reaction (erythema, edema, blistering) occurs within 24 hours, the patient can gradually resume normal outdoor activities, initially continuing to exercise caution and gradually allowing increased exposure. If some photosensitivity reaction occurs with the limited skin test, the patient should continue precautions for another 2 weeks before retesting.

The tissue around the eyes may be more sensitive, and therefore, it is not recommended that the face be used for testing. If patients travel to a different geographical area with greater sunshine, they should retest their level of photosensitivity.

Conventional UV (ultraviolet) sunscreens are of no value in protecting against photosensitivity reactions because photoactivation is caused by visible light.

➤*Esophageal cancer:* If the esophageal tumor is eroding into the trachea or bronchial tree, the likelihood of tracheoesophageal or bronchoesophageal fistula resulting from treatment is sufficiently high that PDT is not recommended.

Patients with esophageal varices should be treated with extreme caution. Light should not be given directly to the variceal area because of the high risk of bleeding.

➤*Endobronchial cancer:* Patients should be assessed for the possibility that a tumor may be eroding into a pulmonary blood vessel. Porfimer sodium is contraindicated in the presence of this condition. Patients at high risk for fatal massive hemoptysis (FMH) include those with large, centrally located tumors, those with cavitating tumors, or those with extensive tumor extrinsic to the bronchus.

Fistula – If the endobronchial tumor invades deeply into the bronchial wall, the possibility exists for fistula formation upon resolution of tumor.

Treatment-induced inflammation – PDT should be used with extreme caution for endobronchial tumors in locations where treatment-induced inflammation could obstruct the main airway (eg, long or circumferential tumors of the trachea, tumors of the carina that involve both mainstem bronchi circumferentially, or circumferential tumors in the mainstem bronchus in patients with prior pneumonectomy).

➤*High-grade dysplasia (HGD) in Barrett's esophagus:* The long-term effect of PDT on HGD in BE is unknown. There is always a risk of leaving cancerous cells behind or leaving residual abnormal epithelium beneath the new squamous cell epithelium; these facts emphasize the risk of overlooking cancer in such patients and the need for rigorous continuing surveillance despite the endoscopic appearance of complete squamous cell reepithelialization. It is recommended that endoscopic biopsy surveillance be conducted every 3 months, until 4 consecutive negative evaluations for HGD have been recorded; further follow-up may be scheduled every 6 to 12 months, as per judgment of physicians. The follow-up period of the pivotal study at the time of analysis was a minimum of 2 years (ranging from 2 to 3.6 years).

➤*Carcinogenesis:* No long-term studies have been conducted to evaluate the carcinogenic potential of porfimer sodium. In vitro, porfimer sodium PDT did not cause mutations in the Ames test, nor did it cause chromosome aberrations or mutations (HGPRT locus) in Chinese hamster ovary (CHO) cells. Porfimer sodium caused less than 2-fold, but significant, increases in sister chromatid exchange in CHO cells irradiated with visible light and a 3-fold increase in Chinese hamster lung fibroblasts irradiated with near UV light. Porfimer sodium PDT caused an increase in thymidine kinase mutants and DNA-protein cross-links in mouse L5178Y cells, but not mouse LYR83 cells. Porfimer sodium PDT caused a light-dose dependent increase in DNA-strand breaks in malignant human cervical carcinoma cells, but not in normal cells.

PORFIMER SODIUM — INJECTION

➤*Fertility impairment:* Porfimer sodium given to male and female rats intravenously, at 4 mg/kg/day (0.32 times the clinical dose on a mg/m² basis) before conception and through day 7 of pregnancy caused no impairment of fertility. In this study, long-term dosing with porfimer sodium caused discoloration of testes and ovaries and hypertrophy of the testes. Porfimer sodium also caused decreased body weight in the parent rats.

➤*Pregnancy:* *Category C.* There are no adequate and well-controlled studies in pregnant women. Porfimer sodium should be used during pregnancy only if the potential benefit justifies the potential risk to the fetus.

Women of childbearing potential should practice an effective method of contraception during therapy.

Porfimer sodium given to rat dams during fetal organogenesis intravenously at 8 mg/kg/day (0.64 times the clinical dose on a mg/m² basis) for 10 days caused no major malformations or developmental changes. This dose caused maternal and fetal toxicity resulting in increased resorptions, decreased litter size, delayed ossification, and reduced fetal weight. Porfimer sodium caused no major malformations when given to rabbits intravenously during organogenesis at 4 mg/kg/day (0.65 times the clinical dose on a mg/m² basis) for 13 days. This dose caused maternal toxicity resulting in increased resorptions, decreased litter size, and reduced fetal body weight.

Porfimer sodium given to rats during late pregnancy through lactation intravenously at 4 mg/kg/day (0.32 times the clinical dose on a mg/m² basis) for at least 42 days caused a reversible decrease in growth of offspring. Parturition was unaffected.

➤*Lactation:* It is not known whether this drug is excreted in human milk. Because many drugs are excreted in human milk and because of the potential for serious adverse reactions in nursing infants from porfimer sodium, women receiving porfimer sodium must not breastfeed.

➤*Children:* Safety and efficacy in children have not been established.

Precautions

➤*Ocular sensitivity:* Ocular discomfort, commonly described as sensitivity to sun, bright lights, or car headlights, has been reported in patients who received porfimer sodium. For 30 days, when outdoors, patients should wear dark sunglasses, which have an average white light transmittance of less than 4%.

➤*Before or after radiotherapy:* If PDT is to be used before or after radiotherapy, sufficient time should be allotted between the 2 therapies to ensure that the inflammatory response produced by the first treatment has subsided before commencing the second treatment. The inflammatory response from PDT will depend on tumor size and extent of surrounding normal tissue that receives light. It is recommended that 2 to 4 weeks be allowed after PDT before commencing radiotherapy. Similarly, if PDT is to be given after radiotherapy, the acute inflammatory reaction from radiotherapy usually subsides within 4 weeks after completing radiotherapy, after which PDT may be given.

➤*Chest pain:* As a result of PDT treatment, patients may complain of substernal chest pain because of inflammatory responses within the area of treatment. Such pain may be of sufficient intensity to warrant the short-term prescription of opiate analgesics.

➤*Respiratory distress:* Patients with endobronchial lesions must be closely monitored between the laser light therapy and the mandatory debridement bronchoscopy for any evidence of respiratory distress. Inflammation, mucositis, and necrotic debris may cause obstruction of the airway. If respiratory distress occurs, the physician should be prepared to carry out immediate bronchoscopy to remove secretions and debris to open the airway.

➤*Esophageal strictures:* Esophageal strictures as a result of PDT of HGD in BE are common adverse events. An esophageal stricture was defined as a fixed lumen narrowing with solid food dysphagia and requiring dilation.

Regardless of the indication, esophageal strictures were reported in 122 of the 318 (38%) patients enrolled in the three clinical studies. Overall, esophageal strictures occurred within six months following PDT and were manageable through dilations. Multiple dilations of esophageal strictures may be required, as shown in the table below. Special care should be taken during dilation to avoid perforation of the esophagus.

Esophageal Dilations in Patients with Treatment-Related Strictures

Number of dilations	Number of patients with strictures (n = 122)	Patients with strictures (%)
1 to 2 dilations	38	31%
3 to 5 dilations	33	27%
6 to 10 dilations	26	21%
> 10 dilations	25	20%

A high proportion of patients who developed an esophageal stricture received a nodule pretreatment prior to developing the event (49%) and/or had a mucosal segment treated twice, Therefore, nodule pretreatment and retreating the same mucosal segment more than once may influence the risk of developing an esophageal stricture.

Prior to initiating treatment with porfimer sodium PDT, the diagnosis of high-grade dysplasia in Barrett's esophagus should be confirmed by an expert GI pathologist. Photodynamic therapy with porfimer sodium should be applied by physicians trained in the endoscopic use of PDT with porfimer sodium, and only in those facilities properly equipped for the procedure.

➤*Avoidance of pregnancy:* See Warnings for more information.

➤*Photosensitivity:* See Warnings for more information.

Drug Interactions

➤*Photosensitizing agents:* There have been no formal interaction studies of porfimer sodium and any other drugs. However, it is possible that concomitant use of other photosensitizing agents (eg, tetracyclines, sulfonamides, phenothiazines, sulfonylurea hypoglycemic agents, thiazide diuretics, griseofulvin, fluoroquinolones) could increase the photosensitivity reaction.

➤*Miscellaneous:* Porfimer sodium PDT causes direct intracellular damage by initiating radical chain reactions that damage intracellular membranes and mitochondria. Tissue damage also results from ischemia secondary to vasoconstriction, platelet activation and aggregation, and clotting. Research in animals and in cell culture has suggested that many drugs could influence the effects of PDT, possible examples of which are described below. There are no human data that support or rebut these possibilities.

Compounds that quench active oxygen species or scavenge radicals, such as dimethyl sulfoxide, beta carotene, ethanol, formate, and mannitol would be expected to decrease PDT activity. Preclinical data also suggest that tissue ischemia, allopurinol, calcium channel blockers, and some prostaglandin synthesis inhibitors could interfere with porfimer sodium PDT. Drugs that decrease clotting, vasoconstriction, or platelet aggregation (eg, thromboxane A_2 inhibitors, could decrease the efficacy of PDT.

Glucocorticoid hormones given before or concomitant with PDT may decrease the efficacy of the treatment.

Adverse Reactions

Systemically induced effects associated with PDT with porfimer sodium consist of photosensitivity and mild constipation. All patients who receive porfimer sodium will be photosensitive and must observe precautions to avoid sunlight and bright indoor light. Photosensitivity reactions occurred in approximately 20% of cancer patients and in 68% of high-grade dysplasia (HGD) in Barrett's esophagus (BE) patients treated with porfimer sodium. Typically, these reactions were mostly mild-to-moderate erythema but they also included swelling, itching, burning sensation, feeling hot, or blisters. In a single study of 24 healthy subjects, some evidence of photosensitivity reactions occurred in all subjects. Other less common skin manifestations were also reported in areas where photosensitivity reactions had occurred, such as increased hair growth, skin discoloration, skin nodules, increased wrinkles and increased skin fragility. These manifestations may be attributable to a pseudoporphyria state (temporary drug-induced cutaneous porphyria).

Most toxicities associated with this therapy are local effects seen in the region of illumination and occasionally in surrounding tissues. The local adverse reactions are characteristic of an inflammatory response induced by the photodynamic effect.

➤*Esophageal carcinoma:*

Adverse Reactions Reported in Patients [a] with Obstructing Esophageal Cancer (≥ 5%)

Body system/Adverse reaction	Number of patients (n = 88)	
Patients with ≥ 1 adverse reaction	84	(95%)
CNS		
Hypertension	5	(6%)
Hypotension	6	(7%)
Miscellaneous		
Asthenia	5	(6%)
Back pain	10	(11%)
Chest pain	19	(22%)
Chest pain (substernal)	4	(5%)
Edema (generalized)	4	(5%)
Edema (peripheral)	6	(7%)
Fever	27	(31%)
Pain	19	(22%)
Surgical complication	4	(5%)
Cardiovascular		
Cardiac failure	6	(7%)
GI		
Abdominal pain	18	(20%)
Constipation	21	(24%)
Diarrhea	4	(5%)
Dyspepsia	5	(6%)
Dysphagia	9	(10%)
Eructation	4	(5%)
Esophageal edema	7	(8%)
Esophageal tumor bleeding	7	(8%)
Esophageal stricture	5	(6%)
Esophagitis	4	(5%)
Hematemesis	7	(8%)

PORFIMER SODIUM — INJECTION

Adverse Reactions Reported in Patients [a] with Obstructing Esophageal Cancer (≥ 5%)

Body system/Adverse reaction	Number of patients (n = 88)	
Melena	4	(5%)
Nausea	21	(24%)
Vomiting	15	(17%)
Heart rate/rhythm		
Atrial fibrillation	9	(10%)
Tachycardia	5	(6%)
Motabolic/Nutritional		
Dehydration	6	(7%)
Weight decrease	8	(9%)
Psychiatric		
Anorexia	7	(8%)
Anxiety	6	(7%)
Confusion	7	(8%)
Insomnia	12	(14%)
Hematologic		
Anemia	28	(32%)
Resistance mechanism		
Moniliasis	8	(9%)
Respiratory		
Coughing	6	(7%)
Dyspnea	18	(20%)
Pharyngitis	10	(11%)
Pleural effusion	28	(32%)
Pneumonia	16	(18%)
Respiratory insufficiency	9	(10%)
Tracheoesophageal fistula	5	(6%)
Dermatologic		
Photosensitivity reaction	17	(19%)
GU		
Urinary tract infection	6	(7%)

[a] Based on adverse reactions reported at any time during the entire period of follow-up.

Location of the tumor was a prognostic factor for 3 adverse reactions: Upper-third of the esophagus (esophageal edema), middle-third (atrial fibrillation), and lower-third, the most vascular region (anemia). Also, patients with large tumors (greater than 10 cm) were more likely to experience anemia. Two of 17 patients with complete esophageal obstruction from tumor experienced esophageal perforations, which were considered to be possibly treatment associated; these perforations occurred during subsequent endoscopies.

Serious and other notable adverse reactions observed in less than 5% of PDT-treated patients with obstructing esophageal cancer in the clinical studies include the following; their relationship to therapy is uncertain. The temporal relationship of some GI, cardiovascular, and respiratory events to the administration of light was suggestive of mediastinal inflammation in some patients.

Cardiovascular – Angina pectoris, bradycardia, MI, sick sinus syndrome, and supraventricular tachycardia.

GI – Esophageal perforation, gastric ulcer, ileus, jaundice, and peritonitis have occurred.

Ophthalmic – Abnormal vision, diplopia, eye pain, and photophobia have been reported.

Respiratory – Bronchitis, bronchospasm, laryngotracheal edema, pneumonitis, pulmonary hemorrhage, pulmonary edema, respiratory failure, and stridor have occurred.

Miscellaneous – Sepsis has been reported occasionally.

➤*Obstructing endobronchial cancer:*

Adverse Reactions Reported in Patients with Obstructing Endobronchial Cancers (≥ 5%)

Body system/ Adverse reaction	Within 30 days of treatment		Entire follow-up period[a]	
	PDT (n = 86)	Nd:YAG (n = 86)	PDT (n = 86)	Nd:YAG (n = 86)
Patients with ≥ 1 adverse reaction	43 (50%)	33 (38%)	62 (72%)	48 (56%)
Miscellaneous				
Back pain	3 (3%)	1 (1%)	3 (3%)	5 (6%)
Chest pain	6 (7%)	6 (7%)	7 (8%)	8 (9%)
Edema (peripheral)	3 (3%)	3 (3%)	4 (5%)	3 (3%)
Fever	7 (8%)	7 (8%)	14 (16%)	8 (9%)
Pain	1 (1%)	4 (5%)	4 (5%)	8 (9%)
CNS				
Dysphonia	3 (3%)	2 (2%)	4 (5%)	2 (2%)
GI				
Constipation	4 (5%)	1 (1%)	4 (5%)	2 (2%)
Dyspepsia	1 (1%)	4 (5%)	2 (2%)	5 (6%)
Psychiatric				
Anxiety	3 (3%)	0	5 (6%)	0
Insomnia	4 (5%)	2 (2%)	4 (5%)	3 (4%)
Respiratory				
Bronchitis	9 (10%)	2 (2%)	9 (10%)	2 (2%)
Coughing	5 (6%)	8 (9%)	13 (15%)	11 (13%)
Dyspnea	15 (17%)	7 (8%)	26 (30%)	13 (15%)
Hemoptysis	6 (7%)	5 (6%)	14 (16%)	7 (8%)
Pleural effusion	0	0	4 (5%)	1 (1%)
Pneumonia	5 (6%)	4 (5%)	10 (12%)	5 (6%)
Pneumothorax	0	0	0	4 (5%)
Respiratory insufficiency	0	0	5 (6%)	1 (1%)
Sputum increased	4 (5%)	5 (6%)	7 (8%)	6 (7%)
Dermatologic				
Photosensitivity reaction	16 (19%)	0	18 (21%)	0

[a] The follow-up was 33% longer for the PDT group than for the Nd:YAG group, introducing a bias against PDT when adverse reactions are compared for the entire follow-up period.

Transient inflammatory reactions in PDT-treated patients occur in approximately 10% of patients and manifest as fever, bronchitis, chest pain, and dyspnea. The incidences of bronchitis and dyspnea were higher with PDT than with Nd:YAG. Most cases of bronchitis occurred within 1 week of treatment and all but one were mild or moderate in intensity. The reactions usually resolved within 10 days with antibiotic therapy. Treatment-related worsening of dyspnea is generally transient and self-limiting. Debridement of the treated area is mandatory to remove exudate and necrotic tissue. Life-threatening respiratory insufficiency likely due to therapy occurred in 3% of PDT-treated patients and 2% of Nd:YAG-treated patients. Patients with endobronchial lesions must be closely monitored between the laser light therapy and the mandatory debridement bronchoscopy for any evidence of respiratory distress. Inflammation, mucositis, and necrotic debris may cause obstruction of the airway. If respiratory distress occurs, the physician should be prepared to carry out immediate bronchoscopy to remove secretions and debris to open the airway.

There was a trend toward a higher rate of fatal hemoptysis (FMH) occurring on the PDT arm (10%) vs the Nd:YAG arm (5%); however, the rate of FMH occurring within 30 days of treatment was the same for PDT and Nd:YAG (4% total reactions, 3% treatment-associated reactions). Patients who have received radiation therapy have a higher incidence of FMH after treatment with PDT and after other forms of local therapy than patients who have not received radiation therapy, but analyses suggest that this increased risk may be due to associated prognostic factors such as having a centrally located tumor. The incidence of FMH in patients previously treated with radiotherapy was 21% (6/29) in the PDT group and 10% (3/29) in the Nd:YAG group. In patients with no prior radiotherapy, the overall incidence of FMH was less than 1%. Characteristics of patients at high risk for FMH are patients with tumors eroding into a major blood vessel, or with a tracheoesophageal or bronchoesophageal fistula.

Other serious or notable adverse reactions were observed in less than 5% of PDT-treated patients with endobronchial cancer; their relationship to therapy is uncertain. In the respiratory system, pulmonary thrombosis, pulmonary embolism, and lung abscess have occurred. Cardiac failure, sepsis and possible cerebrovascular accident have also been reported in 1 patient each.

➤*Superficial endobronchial tumors:*

Adverse Reactions Reported in Patients [a] with Superficial Endobronchial Tumors (≥ 5%)

Adverse reaction	Number of patients (n = 90)	
Patients with ≥ 1 adverse reaction	44	(49%)
Photosensitivity reaction	20	(22%)

PORFIMER SODIUM — INJECTION

Adverse Reactions Reported in Patients [a] with Superficial Endobronchial Tumors (≥ 5%)

Adverse reaction	Number of patients (n = 90)	
Coughing	8	(9%)
Dyspnea	6	(7%)
Edema	16	(18%)
Exudate	20	(22%)
Obstruction	19	(21%)
Stricture	10	(11%)
Ulceration	8	(9%)

[a] Based on adverse reactions reported at any time during the entire period of follow-up.

In patients with superficial endobronchial tumors, 44 of 90 patients (49%) experienced an adverse reaction, two-thirds of which were related to the respiratory system. The most common reaction to therapy was a mucositis reaction in one-fifth of the patients that manifested as edema, exudate, and obstruction. The obstruction (mucus plug) is easily removed with suction or forceps. Mucositis can be minimized by avoiding exposure of normal tissue to excessive light. PDT should be used with extreme caution for endobronchial tumors in locations where treatment-induced inflammation could obstruct the main airway (eg, long or circumferential tumors of the trachea, tumors of the carina that involve both mainstem bronchi circumferentially, or circumferential tumors in the mainstem bronchus in patients with prior pneumonectomy). Three patients experienced life-threatening dyspnea: 1 was given a double dose of light, 1 was treated concurrently in both mainstem bronchi, and the other had prior pneumonectomy and was treated in the sole remaining main airway. Stent placement was required in 3% of the patients due to endobronchial stricture. Fatal hemoptysis occurred within 30 days of treatment in 1 patient with superficial tumors (1%).

➤*High-grade dysplasia (HGD) in Barrett's esophagus (BE):*

Treatment-Emergent Adverse Events Reported in Patients Treated with Porfimer Sodium PDT in the Clinical Trials on High-Grade Dysplasia in Barrett's Esophagus[a] (≥ 5%)

Body system/ Adverse event*	Treatment groups: HGD[a] porfimer sodium PDT + OM (n = 219)	HGD[b] OM Only (n = 69)	Other[c] porfimer sodium PDT (n = 99)	Total porfimer sodium PDT (n = 318)
Patients with ≥1 adverse event	217 (99%)	51 (74%)	99 (100%)	316 (99%)
GI	180 (82%)	25 (36%)	87 (88%)	267 (84%)
Nausea	61 (28%)	5 (7%)	63 (64%)	124 (39%)
Esophageal stricture[d]	85 (39%)	0	37 (37%)	122 (38%)
Vomiting	72 (33%)	4 (6%)	35 (35%)	107 (34%)
Dysphagia	50 (23%)	1 (1%)	27 (27%)	77 (24%)
Esophageal narrowing[e]	60 (27%)	4 (6%)	16 (16%)	76 (24%)
Constipation	45 (21%)	5 (7%)	9 (9%)	54 (17%)
Abdominal pain (upper, lower, NOS)	32 (15%)	4 (6%)	8 (8%)	40 (12%)
Diarrhea	22 (10%)	7 (10%)	6 (6%)	28 (9%)
Esophageal pain	15 (7%)	0	9 (9%)	24 (8%)
Hiccup	18 (8%)	0	1 (1%)	19 (6%)
Dyspepsia	12 (5%)	3 (4%)	6 (6%)	18 (6%)
Odynophagia	13 (6%)	0	4 (4%)	17 (5%)
Eructation	11 (5%)	0	4 (4%)	15 (5%)
Miscellaneous	135 (62%)	17 (25%)	66 (67%)	201 (63%)
Chest pain	71 (32%)	8 (12%)	40 (40%)	111 (35%)
Pyrexia	47 (21%)	3 (4%)	13 (13%)	60 (19%)
Chest discomfort	14 (6%)	1 (1%)	21 (21%)	35 (11%)
Pain	17 (8%)	2 (3%)	7 (7%)	24 (8%)
Fatigue	13 (6%)	2 (3%)	0	13 (4%)
Dermatologic	120 (55%)	8 (12%)	29 (29%)	149 (47%)
Photosensitivity reaction	101 (46%)	0	16 (16%)	117 (37%)
Rash	14 (6%)	3 (4%)	7 (7%)	21 (7%)
Pruritus	13 (6%)	1 (1%)	1 (1%)	14 (4%)
Respiratory	67 (31%)	21 (30%)	22 (22%)	89 (28%)
Pleural effusion	25 (11%)	0	15 (15%)	40 (13%)
Dyspnea	16 (7%)	3 (4%)	4 (4%)	20 (6%)

[a] Includes all HGD patients in the safety population from PHO BAR 01 (n = 133), TCSC 93-07 (n = 44), and TCSC 96-01 (n = 42).
[b] Includes all HGD patients in the safety population from PHO BAR 01 (n = 69).
[c] Includes patients with Barrett's metaplasia, indefinite dysplasia, LGD, and adenocarcinoma at baseline in the Safety population from TCSC 93-07 (n = 55) and TCSC 96-01 (n = 44).
[d] In the controlled clinical trial, an esophageal stricture was defined as a fixed lumen narrowing with solid food dysphagia which required dilations. In the uncontrolled clinical trials, an esophageal stricture was defined as any dilated esophageal narrowing.
[e] An esophageal narrowing was defined as an undilated esophageal stenosis.
* Note: Adverse events classified using MedDRA 5.0 dictionary except esophageal strictures/narrowing.

Treatment-Emergent Adverse Events Reported in Patients Treated with Porfimer Sodium PDT in the Clinical Trials on High-Grade Dysplasia in Barrett's Esophagus (≥ 5%)

Body system/ Adverse event*	Treatment groups: HGD[a] porfimer sodium PDT + OM (n = 219)	HGD[b] OM Only (n = 69)	Other[c] porfimer sodium PDT (n = 99)	Total porfimer sodium PDT (n = 318)
Infections and infestations	58 (26%)	22 (32%)	8 (8%)	66 (21%)
Sinusitis	11 (5%)	3 (4%)	2 (2%)	13 (4%)
Bronchitis	10 (5%)	3 (4%)	2 (2%)	12 (4%)
Metabolic/Nutritional	53 (24%)	9 (13%)	16 (16%)	69 (22%)
Dehydration	24 (11%)	2 (3%)	8 (8%)	32 (10%)
Anorexia	6 (3%)	2 (3%)	8 (8%)	14 (4%)
CNS	51 (23%)	14 (20%)	11 (11%)	62 (19%)
Headache	17 (8%)	6 (9%)	2 (2%)	19 (6%)
Miscellaneous	42 (19%)	10 (14%)	19 (19%)	61 (19%)
Post procedural pain	16 (7%)	1 (1%)	14 (14%)	30 (9%)
Sunburn	8 (4%)	0	6 (6%)	14 (4%)
Musculoskeletal	46 (21%)	18 (26%)	9 (9%)	55 (17%)
Back pain	15 (7%)	4 (6%)	1 (1%)	16 (5%)
Arthralgia	10 (5%)	6 (9%)	1 (1%)	11 (3%)
Investigations	41 (19%)	5 (7%)	14 (14%)	55 (17%)
Weight decreased	17 (8%)	2 (3%)	3 (3%)	20 (6%)
Body temperature increased	8 (4%)	0	8 (8%)	16 (5%)
Psychiatric	37 (17%)	8 (12%)	4 (4%)	41 (13%)
Insomnia	11 (5%)	3 (4%)	1 (1%)	12 (4%)
Depression	10 (5%)	3 (4%)	0	10 (3%)
Anxiety	10 (5%)	1 (1%)	0	10 (3%)
Cardiovascular	25 (11%)	6 (9%)	4 (4%)	29 (9%)
Hypertension	10 (5%)	1 (1%)	0	10 (3%)

[a] Includes all HGD patients in the safety population from PHO BAR 01 (n = 133), TCSC 93-07 (n = 44), and TCSC 96-01 n = 42).
[b] Includes all HGD patients in the safety population from PHO BAR 01 (n = 69)
[c] Includes patients with Barrett's metaplasia, indefinite dysplasia, LGD, and adenocarcinoma at baseline in the Safety population from TCSC 93-07 (n = 55) and TCSC 96-01 (n = 44)
* Note: Adverse events classified using MedDRA 5.0 dictionary except esophageal strictures/narrowing.

In the porfimer sodium PDT + OM group, severe treatment-associated adverse events included chest pain of non-cardiac origin, dysphagia, nausea, vomiting, regurgitation, and heartburn. The severity of these symptoms decreased within 4 to 6 weeks following treatment.

The majority of the photosensitivity reactions occurred within 90 days following porfimer sodium injection and was of mild (69%) or moderate (24%) intensity. Almost all (98%) of the photosensitivity reactions were considered to be associated with treatment. Fourteen (10%) patients reported severe reactions, all of which resolved. The typical reaction was described as skin disorder, sunburn or rash, and affected mostly the face, hands, and neck. Associated symptoms and signs were swelling, pruritus, erythema, blisters, itching, burning sensation, and feeling of heat.

PORFIMER SODIUM — INJECTION

The majority of esophageal stenosis and strictures reported in the porfimer sodium PDT + OM group were of mild (55%) or moderate (37%) intensity, while approximately 8% were of severe intensity. The majority of esophageal strictures were reported during course 2 of treatment. All esophageal strictures were considered to be associated with treatment. Most esophageal strictures were manageable through dilations.

➤*Lab test abnormalities:* In patients with esophageal cancer, PDT with porfimer sodium may result in anemia due to tumor bleeding. No significant effects were observed for other parameters or in patients with endobronchial carcinoma or with high-grade dysplasia in Barrett's esophagus.

Overdosage

There is no information on overdosage situations involving porfimer sodium. Higher than recommended drug doses of two 2 mg/kg doses given 2 days apart (10 patients) and three 2 mg/kg doses given within 2 weeks (1 patient), were tolerated without notable adverse reactions. Effects of overdosage on the duration of photosensitivity are unknown. Laser treatment should not be given if an overdose of porfimer sodium is administered. In the event of an overdose, patients should protect their eyes and skin from direct sunlight or bright indoor lights for 30 days. At this time, patients should test for residual photosensitivity. Porfimer sodium is not dialyzable.

➤*Overdose of laser light following porfimer sodium injection:* Light doses of 2 to 3 times the recommended dose have been administered to a few patients with superficial endobronchial tumors. One patient experienced life-threatening dyspnea and the others had no notable complications. Increased symptoms and damage to normal tissue might be expected following an overdose of light.

There is no information on overdose of laser light following porfimer sodium injection in patients with esophageal cancer or in patients with high-grade dysplasia in Barrett's esophagus.

Patient Information

Advise patients that this medicine will be prepared and administered by a healthcare provider in a medical setting.

Advise patients to contact a doctor if they experience severe chest pain, difficulty breathing, or abnormal blood loss.

Inform patients this drug will cause sensitivity to the sun, bright lights, or car headlights. For 30 days, they should avoid exposure of skin and eyes to direct sunlight from skylights or undraped windows or bright indoor light.

Instruct patients to test skin for sensitivity before exposing skin to bright indoor light or direct sunlight. To test the skin, expose a small skin area to sunlight for 10 minutes. If no sensitivity reactions (eg, rash, swelling, blistering) occur within 24 hours, gradually resume normal outdoor activities.

If patients must go out during daylight hours, instruct them to cover the skin as much as possible (long-sleeved shirts, slacks, gloves, socks) and wear dark sunglasses even on cloudy days or when in a car.

Contraceptive measures (birth control) are recommended during treatment to avoid birth defects. Instruct patients to inform their doctors if they are pregnant, become pregnant, are planning to become pregnant, or if they are breastfeeding.

Inform patients that lab tests may be required to monitor treatment and that they should keep their appointments.

MITOTANE (o,p'-DDD)

Rx	**Lysodren** (Bristol-Myers Squibb Oncology)	**Tablets:** 500 mg	Scored. In 100s.

MITOTANE — ORAL

WARNING

Mitotane should be administered under the supervision of a qualified physician experienced in the uses of cancer chemotherapeutic agents. Mitotane should be temporarily discontinued immediately following shock or severe trauma since adrenal suppression is its prime action. Exogenous steroids should be administered in such circumstances, since the depressed adrenal may not immediately start to secrete steroids.

Indications

➤*Adrenal cortical carcinoma:* Mitotane is indicated in the treatment of inoperable adrenal cortical carcinoma of both functional and nonfunctional types.

➤*Unlabeled uses:* Treatment of Cushing syndrome secondary to pituitary disorders.

Administration and Dosage

➤*Recommended dosage:* The recommended treatment schedule is to start the patient at 2 to 6 g of mitotane per day in divided doses, either 3 or 4 times a day. Doses are usually increased incrementally to 9 to 10 g/day. If severe side effects appear, the dose should be reduced until the maximum tolerated dose is achieved. If the patient can tolerate higher doses and improved clinical response appears possible, the dose should be increased until adverse reactions interfere. Experience has shown that the maximum tolerated dose (MTD) will vary from 2 to 16 g/day, but has usually been 9 to 10 g/day. The highest dose used in the studies to date were 18 to 19 g/day.

Treatment should be instituted in the hospital until a stable dosage regimen is achieved.

➤*Duration of therapy:* Treatment should be continued as long as clinical benefits are observed. Maintenance of clinical status or slowing of growth of metastatic lesions can be considered clinical benefits if they can clearly be shown to have occurred.

If no clinical benefits are observed after 3 months at the maximum tolerated dose, the case would generally be considered a clinical failure. However, 10% of the patients who showed a measurable response required more than 3 months at the MTD. Early diagnosis and prompt institution of treatment improve the probability of a positive clinical response. Clinical effectiveness can be shown by reduction in tumor mass; reduction in pain, weakness or anorexia; and reduction of symptoms and signs due to excessive steroid production.

A number of patients have been treated intermittently with treatment being restarted when severe symptoms have reappeared. Patients often do not respond after the third or fourth such course. Experience accumulated to date suggests that continuous treatment with the maximum possible dosage of mitotane is the best approach.

➤*Storage/Stability:* Tablets may be stored at room temperature (15° to 30°C; 59° to 86°F).

Actions

➤*Pharmacology:* Mitotane can best be described as an adrenal cytotoxic agent, although it can cause adrenal inhibition, apparently without cellular destruction. Its biochemical mechanism of action is unknown. Data are available to suggest that the drug modifies the peripheral metabolism of steroids as well as directly suppressing the adrenal cortex. The administration of mitotane alters the extra-adrenal metabolism of cortisol in man; leading to a reduction in measurable 17-hydroxy corticosteroids, even though plasma levels of corticosteroids do not fall. The drug apparently causes increased formation of 6-β-hydroxyl cortisol.

➤*Pharmacokinetics:*

Absorption – Data in adrenal carcinoma patients indicate that about 40% of oral mitotane is absorbed.

Distribution – A variable amount of metabolite (1% to 17%) is excreted in the bile and the balance is apparently stored in the tissues. Autopsy data have provided evidence that mitotane is found in most tissues of the body; however, fat tissues are the primary site of storage.

Metabolism/Excretion – Approximately 10% of administered dose is recovered in the urine as a water-soluble metabolite. No unchanged mitotane has been found in urine or bile. Following discontinuation of mitotane, the plasma terminal half-life has ranged from 18 to 159 days. In most patients blood levels become undetectable after 6 to 9 weeks.

Contraindications

Mitotane should not be given to individuals who have demonstrated a previous hypersensitivity to it.

Warnings

➤*Adrenal insufficiency:* Adrenal insufficiency may develop in patients treated with mitotane, and adrenal steroid replacement should be considered for these patients.

A substantial percentage of the patients treated show signs of adrenal insufficiency. It therefore appears necessary to watch for and institute steroid replacement in those patients. However, some investigators have recommended that steroid replacement therapy be administered concomitantly with mitotane. It has been shown that the metabolism of exogenous steroids is modified and consequently somewhat higher doses than normal replacement therapy may be required.

➤*Liver function impairment:* Mitotane should be administered with care to patients with liver disease other than metastatic lesions from the adrenal cortex, since the metabolism of mitotane may be interfered with and the drug may accumulate.

➤*Hypersensitivity reactions:* Mitotane should be temporarily discontinued immediately following shock or severe trauma, since adrenal suppression is its prime action. Exogenous steroids should be administered in such circumstances, since the depressed adrenal may not immediately start to secrete steroids.

➤*Pregnancy: Category C.* Animal reproduction studies have not been conducted with mitotane. It is also not known whether mitotane can cause fetal harm when administered to a pregnant woman or can affect reproduction capacity. Mitotane should be given to a pregnant woman only if clearly needed.

➤*Lactation:* It is not known whether this drug is excreted in human milk. Because many drugs are excreted in human milk and because of the potential for adverse reactions in nursing infants from mitotane, a decision should be made whether to discontinue nursing or to discontinue the drug, taking into account the importance of the drug to the mother.

➤*Children:* Safety and efficacy in children have not been established.

MITOTANE — ORAL

Precautions

➤*Special risk:* All possible tumor tissues should be surgically removed from large metastatic masses before mitotane administration is instituted. This is necessary to minimize the possibility of infarction and hemorrhage in the tumor due to a rapid cytotoxic effect of the drug.

Long-term continuous administration of high doses of mitotane may lead to brain damage and impairment of function. Behavioral and neurological assessments should be made at regular intervals when continuous mitotane treatment exceeds 2 years.

➤*Hazardous tasks:* Since sedation, lethargy, vertigo, and other CNS side effects can occur, ambulatory patients should be cautioned about driving, operating machinery, and other hazardous pursuits requiring mental and physical alertness.

Drug Interactions

Mitotane Drug Interactions

Precipitant drug	Object drug*		Description
Mitotane	Corticosteroids	⬇	Corticosteroid metabolism may be altered by mitotane; higher dosages may be required.
Mitotane	Warfarin	⬇	The metabolism of warfarin may be accelerated by the mechanism of hepatic microsomal enzyme induction, leading to an increase in dosage requirements of warfarin. Monitor patients for a change in anticoagulant dosage requirements when administering mitotane to patients on coumarin-type anticoagulants.
Spironolactone	Mitotane	⬇	Adrenolytic effects of mitotane may be blocked by spironolactone; observe for diminished clinical signs of mitotane; consider discontinuation of spironolactone.

* ⬇ = Object drug decreased.

Adverse Reactions

➤*CNS:* Central nervous system side effects occur in 40% of the patients. These consist primarily of depression as manifested by lethargy and somnolence (25%), and dizziness or vertigo (15%).

➤*Dermatologic:* Skin toxicity has been observed in about 15% of the cases. These skin changes consist primarily of transient skin rashes which do not seem to be dose related. In some instances, this side effect subsided while the patients were maintained on the drug without a change of dose.

➤*GI:* Gastrointestinal disturbances, which consist of anorexia, nausea or vomiting, and in some cases diarrhea, occur in about 80% of the patients.

➤*Infrequently occurring side effects:* Infrequently occurring side effects include:

Cardiovascular – Hypertension, orthostatic hypotension, and flushing.

GU – Hematuria, hemorrhagic cystitis, and albuminuria.

Ophthalmic – Visual blurring, diplopia, lens opacity, toxic retinopathy.

Miscellaneous – Generalized aching, hyperpyrexia, and lowered protein bound iodine (PBI).

Overdosage

No proven antidotes have been established for mitotane overdosage.

ARSENIC TRIOXIDE

Rx	**Trisenox** (Cell Therapeutics, Inc.)	**Injection:** 1 mg/1 ml	Preservative-free. In 10s.

ARSENIC TRIOXIDE — INJECTION

WARNING

Experienced physician and institution – Arsenic trioxide injection should be administered under the supervision of a physician who is experienced in the management of patients with acute leukemia.

APL differentiation syndrome – Some patients with acute promyelocytic leukemia (APL) treated with arsenic trioxide have experienced symptoms similar to a syndrome called the retinoic-acid-acute promyelocytic leukemia (RA-APL) or APL differentiation syndrome, characterized by fever, dyspnea, weight gain, pulmonary infiltrates and pleural or pericardial effusions, with or without leukocytosis. This syndrome can be fatal. The management of the syndrome has not been fully studied, but high-dose steroids have been used at the first suspicion of the APL differentiation syndrome and appear to mitigate signs and symptoms. At the first signs that could suggest the syndrome (unexplained fever, dyspnea or weight gain, abnormal chest auscultatory findings or radiographic abnormalities), high-dose steroids (dexamethasone 10 mg intravenously twice a day) should be immediately initiated, irrespective of the leukocyte count, and continued for at least 3 days or longer until signs and symptoms have abated. The majority of patients do not require termination of arsenic trioxide therapy during treatment of the APL differentiation syndrome.

ECG abnormalities – Arsenic trioxide can cause QT interval prolongation and complete atrioventricular block. QT prolongation can lead to a torsade de pointes-type ventricular arrhythmia, which can be fatal. The risk of torsade de pointes is related to the extent of QT prolongation, concomitant administration of QT prolonging drugs, a history of torsade de pointes, preexisting QT interval prolongation, congestive heart failure, administration of potassium-wasting diuretics, or other conditions that result in hypokalemia or hypomagnesemia. One patient (also receiving amphotericin B) had torsade de pointes during induction therapy for relapsed APL with arsenic trioxide.

ECG and electrolyte monitoring recommendations – Prior to initiating therapy with arsenic trioxide, a 12-lead ECG should be performed and serum electrolytes (potassium, calcium, and magnesium) and creatinine should be assessed; preexisting electrolyte abnormalities should be corrected and, if possible, drugs that are known to prolong the QT interval should be discontinued. For QTc > 500 msec, corrective measures should be completed and the QTc reassessed with serial ECGs prior to considering using arsenic trioxide. During therapy with arsenic trioxide, potassium concentrations should be kept above 4 mEq/dL and magnesium concentrations should be kept above 1.8 mg/dL. Patients who reach an absolute QT interval value > 500 msec should be reassessed and immediate action should be taken to correct concomitant risk factors, if any, while the risk/benefit of continuing versus suspending arsenic trioxide therapy should be considered. If syncope, rapid or irregular heartbeat develops, the patient should be hospitalized for monitoring, serum electrolytes should be assessed, arsenic trioxide therapy should be temporarily discontinued until the QTc interval regresses to below 460 msec,

WARNING (cont.)

electrolyte abnormalities are corrected, and the syncope and irregular heartbeat cease. There are no data on the effect of arsenic trioxide on the QTc interval during the infusion.

Indications

➤*Acute promyelocytic leukemia (APL):* Arsenic trioxide is indicated for induction of remission and consolidation in patients with acute promyelocytic leukemia (APL) who are refractory to, or have relapsed from, retinoid and anthracycline chemotherapy, and whose APL is characterized by the presence of the t(15;17) translocation or PML/RAR-alpha gene expression.

Administration and Dosage

➤*Approved by the FDA:* September 25, 2000.

➤*Dilution:* Arsenic trioxide should be diluted with 100 to 250 mL 5% Dextrose Injection, USP or 0.9% Sodium Chloride Injection, USP, using proper aseptic technique, immediately after withdrawal from the ampule. The arsenic trioxide ampule is single-use and does not contain any preservatives. Unused portions of each ampule should be discarded properly. Do not save any unused portions for later administration. Do not mix arsenic trioxide with other medications.

➤*Administration:* Arsenic trioxide should not be administered intravenously over 1 to 2 hours. The infusion duration may be extended up to 4 hours if acute vasomotor reactions are observed. A central venous catheter is not required.

➤*Dosing regimen:* Arsenic trioxide is recommended to be given according to the following schedule:

Induction treatment schedule – Arsenic trioxide should be administered intravenously at a dose of 0.15 mg/kg daily until bone marrow remission. Total induction dose should not exceed 60 doses.

Consolidation treatment schedule – Consolidation treatment should begin 3 to 6 weeks after completion of induction therapy. Arsenic trioxide should be administered intravenously at a dose of 0.15 mg/kg daily for 25 doses over a period up to 5 weeks.

➤*Storage/Stability:* Store at 25°C (77°F); excursions permitted to 15° to 30°C (59° to 86°F). Do not freeze. Do not use beyond expiration date printed on the label.

After dilution, arsenic trioxide is chemically and physically stable when stored for 24 hours at room temperature and 48 hours when refrigerated.

Actions

➤*Pharmacology:* The mechanism of action of arsenic trioxide is not completely understood. Arsenic trioxide causes morphological changes and DNA fragmentation characteristic of apoptosis in NB4 human promyelocytic leukemia cells in vitro. Arsenic trioxide also causes damage or degradation of the fusion protein PML-RAR alpha.

ARSENIC TRIOXIDE — INJECTION

➤*Pharmacokinetics:*

Metabolism – The metabolism of arsenic trioxide involves reduction of pentavalent arsenic to trivalent arsenic by arsenate reductase and methylation of trivalent arsenic to monomethylarsonic acid and monomethylarsonic acid to dimethylarsinic acid by methyltransferases. The main site of methylation reactions appears to be the liver. Arsenic is stored mainly in liver, kidney, heart, lung, hair and nails.

Excretion – Disposition of arsenic following intravenous administration has not been studied. Trivalent arsenic is mostly methylated in humans and excreted in urine.

The pharmacokinetics of trivalent arsenic, the active species of arsenic trioxide, have not been characterized.

Contraindications

Arsenic trioxide is contraindicated in patients who are hypersensitive to arsenic.

Warnings

See Warning Box.

➤*APL differentiation syndrome (see Warning Box):* Nine of 40 patients with APL treated with arsenic trioxide, at a dose of 0.15 mg/kg, experienced the APL differentiation syndrome (see Warning Box and Adverse Reactions).

➤*Hyperleukocytosis:* Treatment with arsenic trioxide has been associated with the development of hyperleukocytosis ($\geq 10 \times 10^3$/mcL) in 20 of 40 patients. A relationship did not exist between baseline WBC counts and development of hyperleukocytosis nor baseline WBC counts and peak WBC counts. Hyperleukocytosis was not treated with additional chemotherapy. WBC counts during consolidation were not as high as during induction treatment.

➤*QT prolongation (see Warning Box):* QT/QTc prolongation should be expected during treatment with arsenic trioxide and torsade de pointes as well as complete heart block has been reported. Over 460 ECG tracings from 40 patients with refractory or relapsed APL treated with arsenic trioxide were evaluated for QTc prolongation. Sixteen of 40 patients (40%) had at least one ECG tracing with a QTc interval greater than 500 msec. Prolongation of the QTc was observed between 1 and 5 weeks after arsenic trioxide infusion, and then returned towards baseline by the end of 8 weeks after arsenic trioxide infusion. In these ECG evaluations, women did not experience more pronounced QT prolongation than men, and there was no correlation with age.

➤*Complete AV block:* Complete AV block has been reported with arsenic trioxide in the published literature including a case of a patient with APL.

➤*Renal/Hepatic function impairment:* Safety and effectiveness of arsenic trioxide in patients with renal and hepatic impairment have not been studied. Particular caution is needed in patients with renal failure receiving arsenic trioxide, as renal excretion is the main route of elimination of arsenic.

➤*Carcinogenesis:* Carcinogenicity studies have not been conducted with arsenic trioxide by intravenous administration. Arsenic trioxide is a human carcinogen.

➤*Mutagenesis:* Arsenic trioxide and trivalent arsenite salts have not been demonstrated to be mutagenic to bacteria, yeast or mammalian cells. Arsenite salts are clastogenic in vitro (human fibroblasts, human lymphocytes, Chinese hamster ovary cells, Chinese hamster V79 lung cells). Trivalent arsenic produced an increase in the incidence of chromosome aberrations and micronuclei in bone marrow cells of mice.

➤*Pregnancy: Category D.* Arsenic trioxide may cause fetal harm when administered to a pregnant woman. Studies in pregnant mice, rats, hamsters, and primates have shown that inorganic arsenicals cross the placental barrier when given orally or by injection. The reproductive toxicity of arsenic trioxide has been studied in a limited manner. An increase in resorptions, neural-tube defects, anophthalmia and microphthalmia were observed in rats administered 10 mg/kg of arsenic trioxide on gestation day 9 (approximately 10 times the recommended human daily dose on a mg/m^2 basis). Similar findings occurred in mice administered a 10 mg/kg dose of a related trivalent arsenic, sodium arsenite, (approximately 5 times the projected human dose on a mg/m^2 basis) on gestation days 6, 7, 8 or 9. Intravenous injection of 2 mg/kg sodium arsenite (approximately equivalent to the projected human daily dose on a mg/m^2 basis) on gestation day 7 (the lowest dose tested) resulted in neural-tube defects in hamsters.

There are no studies in pregnant women using arsenic trioxide. If this drug is used during pregnancy or if the patient becomes pregnant while taking this drug, the patient should be apprised of the potential harm to the fetus. One patient who became pregnant while receiving arsenic trioxide had a miscarriage. Women of childbearing potential should be advised to avoid becoming pregnant.

➤*Lactation:* Arsenic is excreted in human milk. Because of the potential for serious adverse reactions in nursing infants from arsenic trioxide, a decision should be made whether to discontinue nursing or to discontinue the drug, taking into account the importance of the drug to the mother.

➤*Children:* There are limited clinical data on the pediatric use of arsenic trioxide. Of 5 patients below the age of 18 years (range 5 to 16 years) treated with arsenic trioxide, at the recommended dose of 0.15 mg/kg/day, 3 achieved a complete response.

Safety and effectiveness in pediatric patients below the age of 5 years have not been studied.

Precautions

➤*Monitoring:* The patient's electrolyte, hematologic and coagulation profiles should be monitored at least twice weekly, and more frequently for clinically unstable patients during the induction phase and at least weekly during the consolidation phase. ECGs should be obtained weekly, and more frequently for clinically unstable patients, during induction and consolidation.

Drug Interactions

➤*Antiarrhythmics/Thioridazine:* No formal assessments of pharmacokinetic drug-drug interactions between arsenic trioxide and other agents have been conducted. Caution is advised when arsenic trioxide is coadministered with other medications that can prolong the QT interval (eg certain antiarrhythmics or thioridazine) or lead to electrolyte abnormalities (such as diuretics or amphotericin B).

Adverse Reactions

Safety information was available for 52 patients with relapsed or refractory APL who participated in clinical trials of arsenic trioxide. Forty patients in the pPhase 2 study received the recommended dose of 0.15 mg/kg of which 29 completed both induction and consolidation treatment cycles. An additional 12 patients with relapsed or refractory APL received doses generally similar to the recommended dose. Most patients experienced some drug-related toxicity, most commonly leukocytosis, gastrointestinal (nausea, vomiting, diarrhea, and abdominal pain), fatigue, edema, hyperglycemia, dyspnea, cough, rash or itching, headaches, and dizziness. These adverse effects have not been observed to be permanent or irreversible nor do they usually require interruption of therapy.

Serious adverse events (SAEs), grade 3 or 4 according to version 2 of the NCI Common Toxicity Criteria, were common. Those SAEs attributed to arsenic trioxide in the Phase 2 study of 40 patients with refractory or relapsed APL included APL differentiation syndrome (n = 3), hyperleukocytosis (n = 3), QTc interval ≥ 500 msec (n = 16, 1 with torsade de pointes), atrial dysrhythmias (n = 2), and hyperglycemia (n = 2).

➤*Adverse events (any grade) occurring in ≥ 5% of 40 patients with APL who received arsenic trioxide at a dose of 0.15 mg/kg/day:*

Adverse Events (any grade) Occurring in Patients with APL Who Received Arsenic Trioxide (≥ 5%)				
System organ class/ Adverse Event	All adverse events, any grade		Grade 3 and 4 events	
	n	%	n	%
Miscellaneous				
Fatigue	25	63	2	5
Pyrexia (Fever)	25	63	2	5
Edema - nonspecific	16	40		
Rigors	15	38		
Chest pain	10	25	2	5
Injection site pain	8	20		
Pain - nonspecific	6	15	1	3
Injection site erythema	5	13		
Injection site edema	4	10		
Weakness	4	10	2	5
Hemorrhage	3	8		
Weight gain	5	13		
Weight loss	3	8		
Drug hypersensitivity	2	5	1	3
GI				
Nausea	30	75		
Anorexia	9	23		
Appetite decreased	6	15		
Diarrhea	21	53		
Vomiting	23	58		
Abdominal pain (lower and upper)	23	58	4	10
Sore throat	14	40		
Constipation	11	28	1	3
Loose stools	4	10		
Dyspepsia	4	10		
Oral blistering	3	8		
Fecal incontinence	3	8		
GI hemorrhage	3	8		
Dry mouth	3	8		
Abdominal tenderness	3	8		
Diarrhea hemorrhagic	3	8		
Abdominal distension	3	8		

ARSENIC TRIOXIDE — INJECTION

Adverse Events (any grade) Occurring in Patients with APL Who Received Arsenic Trioxide (≥ 5%)

System organ class/ Adverse Event	All adverse events, any grade		Grade 3 and 4 events	
	n	%	n	%
Metabolic/Nutritional				
Hypokalemia	20	50	5	13
Hypomagnesemia	18	45	5	13
Hyperglycemia	18	45	5	13
ALT increased	8	20	2	5
Hyperkalemia	7	18	2	5
AST increased	5	13	1	3
Hypocalcemia	4	10		
Hypoglycemia	3	8		
Acidosis	2	5		
CNS				
Headache	24	60	1	3
Insomnia	17	43	1	3
Paresthesia	13	33	2	5
Dizziness (excluding vertigo)	9	23		
Tremor	5	13		
Convulsion	3	8	2	5
Somnolence	3	8		
Coma	2	5	2	5
Respiratory				
Cough	26	65		
Dyspnea	21	53	4	10
Epistaxis	10	25		
Hypoxia	9	23	4	10
Pleural effusion	8	20	1	3
Post nasal drip	5	13		
Wheezing	5	13		
Decreased breath sounds	4	10		
Crepitations	4	10		
Rales	4	10		
Hemoptysis	3	8		
Tachypnea	3	8		
Rhonchi	3	8		
Dermatologic				
Dermatitis	17	43		
Pruritus	13	33	1	2
Ecchymosis	8	20		
Dry Skin	6	11		
Erythema- nonspecific	5	11		
Increased sweating	5	11		
Facial edema	3	8		
Night sweats	3	8		
Petechiae	3	8		
Hyperpigmentation	3	8		
Non specific skin lesions	3	8		
Urticaria	3	8		
Local exfoliation	2	5		
Eyelid edema	2	5		
Cardiovascular				
Tachycardia	22	55		
ECG QT corrected interval prolonged > 500 msec	16	38		
Palpitations	4	10		
ECG abnormal other than QT interval prolongation	3	11		
Hypotension	10	25	2	5
Flushing	4	10		
Hypertension	4	10		
Pallor	4	10		
Infections and infestations				
Sinusitis	8	20		
Herpes simplex	5	13		
Upper respiratory tract infection	5	13	1	3
Bacterial infection- nonspecific	3	8	1	3
Herpes zoster	3	8		
Nasopharyngitis	2	5		
Oral candidiasis	2	5		
Sepsis	2	5	2	5
Musculoskeletal				
Arthralgia	13	33	3	8
Myalgia	10	25	2	5
Bone pain	9	23	4	10
Back pain	7	18	1	3
Neck pain	5	13		
Pain in limb	5	13	2	5
Hematologic				
Leukocytosis	20	50	1	3
Anemia	8	14	2	5
Thrombocytopenia	7	19	5	12
Febrile neutropenia	5	13	3	8
Neutropenia	4	10	4	10
Disseminated intravascular coagulation	3	8	3	8
Lymphadenopathy	3	8		
Psychiatric				
Anxiety	12	30		
Depression	8	20		
Agitation	2	5		
Confusion	2	5		
Special senses				
Eye irritation	4	10		
Blurred vision	4	10		
Dry eye	3	8		
Painful red eye	2	5		
Earache	3	8		
Tinnitus	2	5		
GU				
Renal failure	3	8	1	3
Renal impairment	3	8		
Oliguria	2	5		
Incontinence	2	5		
Vaginal hemorrhage	5	13		
Intermenstrual bleeding	3	8		

Overdosage

If symptoms suggestive of serious acute arsenic toxicity (eg, convulsions, muscle weakness and confusion) appear, arsenic trioxide should be immediately discontinued and chelation therapy should be considered. A conventional protocol for acute arsenic intoxication includes dimercaprol administered at a dose of 3 mg/kg intramuscularly every 4 hours until immediate life-threatening toxicity has subsided. Thereafter, penicillamine at a dose of 250 mg orally, up to a maximum frequency of 4 times per day (≤ 1 g day), may be given.

TALC POWDER, STERILE

Rx	**Sclerosol** (Bryan)	**Aerosol:** 4 g talc	CFC-12. In single-use aluminum canister with 2 delivery tubes of 15 and 25 cm.
	Sterile Talc Powder (Bryan)	**Powder:** 5 g talc	In 100 mL glass bottle.

STERILE TALC POWDER

Indications

➤*Malignant pleural effusions:* Sterile talc powder, administered intrapleurally via chest tube, is indicated as a sclerosing agent to decrease the recurrence of malignant pleural effusions in symptomatic patients.

➤*Unlabeled uses:* Treatment of benign pleural effusions, pneumothorax, and malignant pericardial effusions.

Administration and Dosage

Sterile talc powder should be administered after adequate drainage of the effusion. The success of the pleurodesis appears to be related to the completeness of the drainage of the pleural fluid, as well as the full re-expansion of the lung, both of which will promote symphysis of the pleural surfaces.

The recommended dose is 5 g, dissolved in 50 to 100 mL Sodium Chloride Injection. Although the optimal dose for effective pleurodesis is unknown, 5 g was the dose most frequently reported in the published literature.

➤*Talc preparation:* Prepare the talc slurry using aseptic technique in an appropriate laminar flow hood. Remove talc container from packaging. Remove protective flip-off seal.

Each brown bottle contains 5 g of sterilized talc powder. To dispense the contents:

1.) Using a 16 gauge needle attached to a 60 mL *LuerLok* syringe, measure and draw up 50 mL of Sodium Chloride Injection. Vent the talc bottle using a needle. Slowly inject the 50 mL of Sodium Chloride Injection into the bottle. For doses more than 5 g, repeat this procedure with a second bottle.

2.) Swirl the bottle(s) to disperse the talc powder and continue swirling to avoid settling of the talc in the slurry. Each bottle will contain 5 g sterile talc powder dispersed in 50 mL of Sodium Chloride Injection.

3.) Divide the content of each bottle into two 60 mL irrigation syringes by withdrawing 25 mL of the slurry into each syringe with continuous swirling. QS each syringe with Sodium Chloride Injection to a total volume of 50 mL in each syringe. Draw air into each syringe to the 60 mL mark to serve as a headspace for mixing prior to administration.

4.) When appropriately labeled, each syringe contains 2.5 g of sterile talc in 50 mL of Sodium Chloride Injection with an air headspace of 10 mL. Once the slurry has been made, use within 12 hours or discard and prepare fresh slurry. Label the syringes appropriately noting the expiration date and time, with the statement "For pleurodesis only, Not for IV administration," the identity of the patient intended to receive this material and a cautionary statement to shake well before use.

5.) Prior to administration, completely and continuously agitate the syringes to evenly redisperse the talc and avoid settlement. Immediately prior to administration, vent the 10 mL air headspace from each syringe.

6.) Attach the adapter and place a syringe tip on the adapter. Maintain continuous agitation of the syringes.

Notice – Shake well before installation. Each 25 mL of prepared slurry in the syringe contains 1.25 g of talc. Not for IV administration.

➤*Administration:* Administer the talc slurry through the chest tube by gently applying pressure to syringe plunger and empty the contents of the syringe into the chest cavity. After application, discard the empty syringe according to general hospital procedures. After the talc slurry has been administered through the chest tube into the pleural cavity, the chest tube may be flushed with 10 to 25 mL sodium chloride solution to ensure that the complete dose of talc is delivered.

Following introduction of the talc slurry, the chest drainage tube is clamped, and the patient is asked to move, at 20- to 30-minute intervals, from supine to alternating decubitus positions, so that over a period of about 2 hours the talc is distributed within the chest cavity. Recent evidence suggests that this step may not be necessary.

At the end of this period, the chest drainage tube is unclamped, and the excess saline is removed by the routine continual external suction on the tube.

➤*Storage/Stability:* Store at room temperature (18° to 25°C [64.4° to 77°F]). Protect against sunlight.

Actions

➤*Pharmacology:* The therapeutic action of talc instilled into the pleural cavity is believed to result from induction of an inflammatory reaction. This reaction promotes adherence of the visceral and parietal pleura, obliterating the pleural space and preventing reaccumulation of pleural fluid.

The extent of systemic absorption of talc after intrapleural administration has not been adequately studied. Systemic exposure could be affected by the integrity of the pleural surface, and therefore could be increased if talc is administered immediately following lung resection or biopsy.

Contraindications

None known.

Warnings

➤*Pregnancy:* *Category B.* An oral administration study has been performed in the rabbit at 900 mg/kg. Approximately 5 fold higher than a human dose on mg/m^2 basis, and has revealed no evidence of teratogenicity due to talc. There are, however, no adequate and well-controlled studies in pregnant women. Because animal reproduction studies are not always predictive of human response, this drug should not be used during pregnancy unless the benefit outweighs the risk.

➤*Children:* The safety and efficacy of sterile talc powder in pediatric patients have not been established.

Precautions

➤*Future procedures:* The possibility of the future diagnostic and therapeutic procedures involving the hemithorax to be treated must be considered prior to administering sterile talc powder. Sclerosis of the pleural space may preclude subsequent diagnostic procedures of the pleura on the treated side. Talc sclerosis may complicate or preclude future ipsilateral lung resective surgery, including pneumonectomy for transplantation purposes.

➤*Use in potentially curable disease:* Talc has no known antineoplastic activity and should not be used alone for potentially curable malignancies where systemic therapy would be more appropriate (eg, a malignant effusion secondary to a potentially curable lymphoma).

➤*Pulmonary complications:* Acute pneumonitis and acute respiratory distress syndrome (ARDS) have been reported in association with intrapleural talc administration. Three of the case reports of ARDS have occurred after treatment with a relatively large talc dose (10 g) administered via intrapleural chest tube instillation. One patient died 1 month post treatment and 2 patients recovered without further sequelae.

Adverse Reactions

Intrathoracic administration of talc slurry has been described in medical literature reports involving more than 2,000 patients. Patients with malignant pleural effusions were treated with talc via poudrage or slurry. In general, with respect to reported adverse experiences, it is difficult to distinguish the effects of talc from the effects of the procedure(s) associated with its administration. The most often reported adverse experiences to intrapleurally administered talc were fever and pain.

➤*Cardiovascular:* Complications reported included tachycardia, myocardial infarction, hypotension, hypovolemia, and asystolic arrest.

➤*Respiratory:* Complications reported include hypoxemia, dyspnea, unilateral pulmonary edema, pneumonia, ARDS, bronchopleural fistula, hemoptysis and pulmonary emboli.

➤*Miscellaneous:*

Infection – Complications reported include empyema.

Delivery procedure – Adverse reactions due to the delivery procedure and the chest tube may include pain, infection at the site of thoracostomy or thoracoscopy, localized bleeding, and subcutaneous emphysema.

Chronic toxicity – Since patients in clinical studies had a limited life expectancy, data on chronic toxicity are limited.

Overdosage

No definite relationship between dose and toxicity has been established. Excessive talc may be partially removed with saline lavage.

The following is a list of available diagnostic aids for professional office use or for use by patients at home (when noted). Those tests requiring special equipment and used primarily by commercial laboratories are not included. For complete information on specific uses, directions and characteristics of these products, consult the manufacturers' package literature.

ACETONE (Ketone) TESTS

To detect the presence of ketones.

Acetest (Bayer Corp)	**Reagent tablets** for urine, whole blood, serum or plasma tests	In 100s.
Chemstrip K (Boehringer Mannheim)	**Reagent strips** for urine tests	In 25s.
Ketostix (Bayer Corp)[1]	**Reagent strips** for urine tests	In 50s, 100s and UD 20s.
KetoCare (Home Diagnostics)	**Reagent strips** for urine tests	In 50s.

[1] For use by patient at home.

ALBUMIN TESTS

To detect the presence of protein.

Albustix (Bayer Corp)	**Reagent strips** for urine tests	In 100s.
Chemstrip Micral (Boehringer Mannheim)	**Reagent strips** for urine tests	In 30s.

BACTERIURIA TESTS

To detect nitrate, nitrite, uropathogens, total bacterial or gram-negative bacterial counts.

Microstix-3 (Bayer Corp)	**Reagent strips** for urine tests	In test kits containing 25 reagent strips, 25 incubation pouches and 25 ID labels.
Uricult (LifeSign LLC)	**Culture paddles** for urine tests	In 10s.
Isocult for Bacteriuria (Remel)	**Culture paddles** for urine tests	In 12s.
UTI Urinary Tract Infection Urine Test Strips (Consumers Choice Systems)	**Test strips** for urine tests	In 6 strips and 6 cups.

BILIRUBIN TESTS

To detect the presence of bilirubin.

Ictotest (Bayer Corp)	**Reagent tablets** for urine tests	In 100s.

BLOOD UREA NITROGEN TESTS

To estimate amounts of urea nitrogen.

Azostix (Bayer Corp)	**Reagent strips** for whole blood tests	In 25s.

CANDIDA TESTS

To detect *Candida albicans.*

Isocult for ***Candida*** (Remel)	**Culture paddles** for vaginal specimen tests	In 4s.
CandidaSure (LifeSign LLC)	**Reagent slides** for vaginal specimen tests	In kits containing 20 slides.

CHLAMYDIA TRACHOMATIS TESTS

To detect and identify *Chlamydia trachomatis.*

Chlamydiazyme (Abbott)	**Reagent kit** for enzyme immunoassay	In kits containing 100 and 500 tests.
MicroTrak *Chlamydia Trachomatis* (Syva)	**Slide tests** for urogenital, rectal, conjunctival or nasopharyngeal specimens	In kits containing 60 tests.
Amplicor (Roche Diagnostics Systems)	**Reagent kit** for endocervical, male urethral and male urine specimens	In kits containing 10, 96 and 100 tests.
Sure Cell Chlamydia (Kodak)	**Reagent kit** for endocervical, urethral, male urine or ocular specimens	In kits containing 10, 25 and 100 tests.
Clearview Chlamydia (Wampole)	**Color-label immunoassay** for endocervical specimens	In 20s.

CHOLESTEROL TESTS

To estimate cholesterol levels. For use by patient at home.

Advanced Care Cholesterol Test (Johnson & Johnson)	**Cassette** for blood test	In kits containing test cassette, result chart, lancet, gauze pad, adhesive bandage, instruction booklet and question and answer booklet.

COLOR ALLERGY SCREENING TESTS

For determination of immunoglobulin E.

CAST (Biomerica)	**Reagent sticks** for serum tests	In kits containing reagent sticks for 25 tests.

CRYPTOCOCCAL ANTIGEN TESTS

For the qualitative or quantitative determination of *Cryptococcus neoformans* antigen.

Crypto-LA (Wampole)	**Slide tests** for CSF and serum	In 70s.

DRUGS OF ABUSE TESTS

For detecting drugs of abuse (marijuana, cocaine, amphetamine, methamphetamine, phencyclidine, codeine, morphine, and heroin).

otc	**Dr. Brown's Home Drug Testing System** (Personal Health and Hygiene)	**Collection kit:** 1 urine specimen collection kit	In 1s.

GASTROINTESTINAL TESTS

For determination of GI disorders.

Entero-Test (HDC Corp)	**String capsules** for collection of duodenal fluid	In packages containing 25 capsules, pH sticks and color charts.
Entero-Test Pediatric Capsules (HDC Corp)	**String capsules** for collection of duodenal fluid	In packages containing 25 capsules, pH sticks and color charts.
Gastro-Test (HDC Corp)	**String capsules** for collection of stomach acid	In packages containing 25 capsules, pH sticks and color charts.
Pathway Anti-c-KIT (9.7) Primary Antibody (Ventana[a])	**Kit** for detection of c-KIT protein in GI stromal tumors	In kits containing reagents. For use on *Ventana Automated Slide Stainers.*
Pyloriset (LifeSign LLC)	**Reagent kit** for serum test	In kits containing 20 latex reagents, positive and negative controls, dilution buffers, mixing sticks and test cards.

[a] Ventana Medical Systems, Inc., 1910 Innovation Park Drive, Tucson, AZ; (800) 227-2155.

BLOOD GLUCOSE METERS

Product & Distributor[a]	Compatible test strips	Alternate test sites	Required blood volume
Accu-Chek Active (Roche Diagnostic)	*Accu-Chek Active*	Yes	1 mcL
Accu-Chek Advantage (Roche Diagnostic)	*Accu-Chek Comfort Curve*	No	4 mcL
Accu-Chek Compact (Roche Diagnostic)[b]	*Accu-Chek Compact Test Drum*	Yes	1.5 mcL
Accu-Chek Complete (Roche Diagnostic)	*Accu-Chek Comfort Curve*	No	4 mcL
Accu-Chek Voicemate (Roche Diagnostic)[c]	*Accu-Chek Comfort Curve*	No	4 mcL
Ascensia BREEZE (Bayer HealthCare)[d]	*Ascensia AutoDisc*	Yes	2.5 to 3.5 mcL
Ascensia CONTOUR (Bayer HealthCare)	*Ascensia Microfil*	Yes	0.6 mcL
Ascensia DEX 2 (Bayer HealthCare)[d]	*Ascensia AutoDisc*	Yes	2.5 to 3.5 mcL
Ascensia ELITE (Bayer HealthCare)	*Ascensia ELITE*	Yes	2 mcL
Ascensia ELITE XL (Bayer HealthCare)	*Ascensia ELITE*	Yes	2 mcL
BD Logic (Becton, Dickinson and Company)	*BD*	No	0.3 mcL
FreeStyle (TheraSense)	*FreeStyle*	Yes	0.3 mcL
FreeStyle Flash (TheraSense)	*FreeStyle*	Yes	0.3 mcL
InDuo (Novo Nordisk Pharmaceuticals)[e]	*OneTouch Ultra*	Yes	1 mcL
OneTouch Basic (Lifescan)	*OneTouch*	No	10 mcL
OneTouch FastTake (Lifescan)[f]	*OneTouch FastTake*	Yes	1.5 mcL
OneTouch SureStep (Lifescan)	*OneTouch SureStep*	No	10 mcL
OneTouch Ultra (Lifescan)	*OneTouch Ultra*	Yes	1 mcL
OneTouch UltraSmart (Lifescan)	*OneTouch Ultra*	Yes	1 mcL
Precision Q•I•D (MediSense)	*Precision Q•I•D*	No	3.5 mcL
Precision Sof-Tact (MediSense)	*Precision Sof-Tact*	Yes	2 to 3 mcL
Precision Xtra (MediSense)[g]	*Precision Xtra*	No	3.5 mcL
Prestige IQ (Home Diagnostics)	*Prestige Smart System*	No	7 mcL
Prestige TrueTrack Smart System (Home Diagnostics)	*TrueTrack*	No	1 mcL

[a] Products listed are representative of currently available and widely distributed brands. Similar products, including regional and private label brands, may also exist.
[b] Uses drum instead of individual test strips.
[c] Audio features for people with visual impairments.
[d] Uses disc, not strips.
[e] Also an insulin delivery system.
[f] Available through mail order only.
[g] Also measures ketones.

GLUCOSE, BLOOD TESTS[a]

To determine blood glucose levels. For use by patient at home.

Accu-Chek Active (Roche Diagnostic)	**Reagent strips** for blood tests	In 10s, 25s, 50s, and 100s for use with *Accu-Chek Active* blood glucose meter.
Accu-Chek Comfort Curve (Roche Diagnostic)		In 10s and 50s for use with *Accu-Chek Advantage* and *Accu-Chek Complete* meters, and with the *AccuData GTS Plus/GTS, Accu-Chek HG,* and *Accu-Chek Inform Systems.*
Accu-Chek Compact (Roche Diagnostics)		In 17s/1 drum for use with *Accu-Chek Compact* blood glucose meter.
Accu-Chek Instant Glucose (Roche Diagnostic)		In 25s, 50s, and 100s for use with *Glucometer 3, Glucometer QA,* and *Glucometer M+* blood glucose meters.
Ascensia AutoDisc (Bayer HealthCare)		In 10 discs/100 test strips for use with *Ascensia Glucometer DEX 2, Ascensia Breeze,* and *Glucometer DEX* blood glucose meters.
Ascensia Elite (Bayer HealthCare)		In 25s , 50s, and 100s for use with *Ascensia Elite* and *Ascensia Elite XL* blood glucose meters.
Ascensia Microfil (Bayer HealthCare)		In 50s and 100s for use with *Ascensia CONTOUR* blood glucose meter.
BD Test Strips (Becton, Dickinson and Company)		In 50s for use with *BD Logic* and *BD Latitude* blood glucose monitoring systems.
Freestyle Test Strips (TheraSense)		In 25s, 50s, and 100s for use with *FreeStyle* and *Freestyle Flash* blood glucose meters.
OneTouch Test Strips (Lifescan)		In 25s, 50s, and 100s for use with *OneTouch Basic Meter, OneTouch Profile,* and *OneTouch II* blood glucose meters.
OneTouch Ultra Test Strips (Lifescan)		In 25s, 50s, and 100s for use with *OneTouch Ultra Brand, OneTouch Ultra Smart Brand,* and *InDuo Brand* blood glucose meters.
OneTouch FastTake Test Strips (Lifescan)		In 50s and 100s for use with *FastTake* blood glucose meter.
OneTouch SureStep Test Strips (Lifescan)		In 50s and 100s for use with *OneTouch SureStep* blood glucose meter.
Precision Q•I•D (MediSense)		For use with *Precision Q•I•D* blood glucose monitor, *Precision Q•I•D* pen, *MediSense 2* card and pen blood glucose monitors, and the *Companion 2* card and pen blood glucose monitors.
Precision Sof-Tact (MediSense)		For use with the *MediSense Precision Sof-Tact* and *MediSense Sof-Tact Diabetes Management System.*
Precision Xtra (MediSense)		For use with the *Precision Xtra* blood glucose meters.
Prestige Smart System (Home Diagnostics)		In 50s for use with products featuring the *Prestige IQ Smart System* logo.
True Track Test (Home Diagnostics)		In 50s and 100s for use with meters featuring the *True Track Smart System* logo.

[a] Products listed are representative of currently available and widely distributed brands. Similar products, including regional and private label brands, may also exist.

GLUCOSE, URINE TESTS

To measure glucose in urine. For use by patient at home.

Clinitest (Bayer Corp)	**Reagent tablets** for urine tests	In 36s and 100s with color charts and sets containing 36 tablets, 1 test tube, 1 dropper and color chart.
Chemstrip bG (Boehringer Mannheim)	**Reagent strips** for urine tests	In 100s.
Chemstrip uG (Boehringer Mannheim)		In 100s.
Clinistix (Bayer Corp)		In 50s.
Diastix (Bayer Corp)		In 50s and 100s.

GONORRHEA TESTS

Used as a presumptive test for *Neisseria gonorrhoeae.*

Biocult-GC (Orion Diagnostica)	**Culture paddles** for endocervical, oropharyngeal, anterior urethra or anal cultures	In kits containing vials, CO_2-generating tablets, swabs, reagent and specimen ID labels.
Gonozyme Diagnostic (Abbott)	**Reagent kit** for urogenital swab specimens	In test kits containing reagent, reaction trays, assay tubes with identifying racks and cover seals for 100 tests.
LCx Assay (Abbott)	**Reagent kit** in endocervical, male urethral and urine swab specimens.	In kits containing swabs, vials and reagent for 100 tests.
Isocult for *Neisseria gonorrhoeae* (Remel)	**Culture paddles** for endocervical, rectal and urethral cultures	In test kits containing culture tubes, CO_2-generating tablets, reagent and information sheet for 12 tests.
MicroTrak *Neisseria gonorrhoeae* Culture Confirmation Test (Syva)	**Reagent kit** for endocervical, urethral, rectal, conjunctival and pharyngeal cultures	In test kits containing reagent, reconstitution diluent and mounting fluid for 85 tests.

H. PYLORI TESTS

For use in the detection of gastric urease as an aid in the diagnosis of *H. pylori* infection in the human stomach. The test utilizes a liquid scintillation counter for the measurement of $^{14}CO_2$ in breath samples.

PYtest (Tri-Med Specialties, Inc.)	**Capsules** 14c urea	Clear, gelatin. In UD packages of 1s, 10s, and 100s. In *PYtest Kit* containing a capsule and breath collection equipment.

HEMATOCRIT/HEMOGLOBIN TESTS

To determine hematocrit/hemoglobin measurement.

Stat-Crit (Wampole)	**Electrode device** for blood samples	In 120s for use with *STAT-CRIT* instrument kit.

HEMOGLOBIN, GLYCATED (HbA_{1c}) TESTS

In diabetes (Type 1 or 2) for the quantitative measurement of glycated hemoglobin levels.

A1cNow (Metrika)	**Kit** for blood samples	In 1-pack test kit with monitor, lancets, and dilution kit and in 10-pack professional use kits.
Choice DM (Bristol-Myers Squibb)		In 1 single-use test kit.

HUMAN IMMUNODEFICIENCY VIRUS (HIV) TESTS

For the detection of HIV.

HIV-1 LA Recombigen HIV-1 Latex Agglutination Test (Cambridge Biotech)	**Reagent kit** for blood, serum, plasma or capillary sample tests	In kits containing vial, diluent, card, and transfer loop for 100 tests.
HIVAB HIV-1 EIA (Abbott)	**Reagent kit** for serum or plasma tests	In kits containing reagents for 100 tests.
HIVAG-1 (Abbott)	**Reagent kit** for serum or plasma tests	In kits containing reagents for 100 tests.
Amplicor HIV-1 Monitor (Roche)	**Reagent kit** for plasma HIV-1 tests	In kits containing reagents for 24 tests.
Confide (Direct Access Diagnostics)	**Reagent kit** for HIV blood tests	In kit containing materials to draw blood sample, a test card, and a protective mailer for 1 test.
OraQuick Advance Rapid HIV-1/2 Antibody Test (OraSure Technologies)	**In vitro immunoassay** for qualitative detection of antibodies to human immunodeficiency virus types 1 or 2 in oral fluid, whole blood, or plasma	In kits containing test device, absorbent packet, developer solution vial, test stands, and specimen collection loops for 25 or 100 tests.
HIVAB HIV-1/HIV-2 (rDNA) EIA (Abbott)	**In vitro enzyme immunoassay** for qualitative detection of antibodies to human immunodeficiency viruses type 1 or type 2 in human serum or plasma	In 100, 1,000, and 5,000 test kits.
OraSure (Epitope)[a]	**Reagent kit** for oral fluid tests	In kit containing collection pad, vial, and reagent for 1 test.
OraSure HIV-1 (Epitope)	**Collection kit** for oral specimen collection	In kit containing cotton fiber on stick with collection vial.

[a] For use by patient at home.

LANCET DEVICES

Product & Distributor[a]	Description
Ascensia MICROLET VACULANCE[b] (Bayer HealthCare)	**Device**: 4 depth settings, vacuum action.
Gentle-Lance (Futura Medical Corporation)	**Device**: 5 depth settings.
Ascensia MICROLET (Bayer HealthCare)	**Device**: 5 depth settings, spring-loaded.
Accu-Chek SoftTouch (Roche Diagnostics)	**Device**: 5 depth settings, dial.
auto-Lancet (Palco Laboratories)	**Device**: 5 depth settings, dial.
auto-Lancet Mini (Palco Laboratories)	**Device**: 5 depth settings, dial.
BD Lancet Device (Becton, Dickinson and Company)	**Device**: 6 depth settings, spring-loaded.
OneTouch UltraSoft[b] (Lifescan)	**Device**: 7 depth settings, dial.
Penlet Plus (Lifescan)	**Device**: 7 depth settings, dial.
Autolet Impression[b] (Owen Mumford)	**Device**: 7 depth settings, dial, force adjustment.
Accu-Chek Softclix[b] (Roche Diagnostics)	**Device**: 11 depth settings (0.8 to 2.3 mm), spring-loaded, dial.
Accu-Chek Safe-T-Pro[c] (Roche Diagnostics)	**Device**: 1.8 mm; 21-gauge needle.
Safe-T-Lance Plus[c] (Futura Medical Corporation)	**Device**: 1.8 mm; 18-, 21-, and 25-gauge needle.
Unistik 2[c] (Owen Mumford)	**Device**: 2.4 and 3 mm; 26-gauge needle.
Vitalet Pro[c] (Medical Plastic Devices, Inc.)	**Device**: 2.4 and 3 mm.

[a] Products listed are representative of currently available and widely distributed brands. Similar products, including regional and private label brands, may also exist.

[b] Can be used on alternate test sites.

[c] Single-time use lancets

LANCET NEEDLES

Product & Distributor[a]	Description
BD Ultra-Fine 33 (Becton, Dickinson and Company)	**Needle**: 33-gauge
BD Ultra-Fine II (Becton, Dickinson and Company)	**Needle**: 30-gauge
Sunmark Super Thin Lancets (McKesson)	
Accu-Chek Softclix (Roche Diagnostic)	**Needle**: 28-gauge
Accu-Chek SoftTouch (Roche Diagnostic)	
Ascensia MICROLET (Bayer)	
Cleanlet (Gainor)	
EZ-Lets Thin (Palco Laboratories)	
Gentle-Let (general purpose) (Futura Medical Corporation)	
MediSense Thin Lancets (MediSense)	
OneTouch UltraSoft (Lifescan)	
Unilet ComforTouch (Boca Medical)	
Unilet GP Ultralite (Boca Medical)	
EZ-Lets Thin (Palco Laboratories)	**Needle**: 26-gauge
Gentle-Let (general purpose) (Futura Medical Corporation)	
Vitalet (Medical Plastic Devices, Inc.)	
Cleanlet (Gainor)	**Needle**: 25-gauge
OneTouch FinePoint (Lifescan)	

LANCET NEEDLES

Product & Distributor[a]	Description
EZ-Lets (Palco Laboratories)	**Needle**: 23-gauge
Gentle-Let (general purpose) (Futura Medical Corporation)	
Gentle-Let (safety style) (Futura Medical Corporation)	
Unilet GP Superlite (Boca Medical)	
Unilet Superlite (Boca Medical)	
Vitalet (Medical Plastic Devices, Inc.)	
EZ-Lets (Palco Laboratories)	**Needle**: 21-gauge
Gentle-Let (general purpose) (Futura Medical Corporation)	
Gentle-Let (safety style) (Futura Medical Corporation)	
Unilet (Boca Medical)	
Unilet GP (Boca Medical)	

[a] Products listed are representative of currently available and widely distributed brands. Similar products, including regional and private label brands, may also exist.

MONONUCLEOSIS TESTS

For qualitative and quantitative identification of heterophilic antibodies for the diagnosis of infectious mononucleosis.

Mono-Diff (Wampole)	**Reagent kit** for serum or plasma tests	In kits containing reagent, absorbent I and II, positive control serum, calibrated capillary tubes and bulbs, disposable stirrers and disposable card slides for 20 tests.
Mono-Latex (Wampole)	**Reagent kit** for serum or plasma tests	In kits containing reagent latex, positive control, negative control, capillary tubes and bulbs, black glass slide and disposable stirrers for 20 and 50 tests.
Mono-Plus (Wampole)	**Reagent kit** for serum or plasma tests	In kits containing *micro-plus* test devices and *mono-plus* developer solution for 30 tests.
Monospot (Meridian Diagnostics)	**Slide test** for serum or plasma	In kits containing reagents I and II, indicator cells, positive and negative control serum, glass slide, microcapillary pipettes, rubber bulbs, plastic pipettes and wooden applicators for 20 tests.
Monosticon Dri-Dot (Organon Teknika)	**Slide test** for serum, plasma or whole blood tests	In kits containing test slides, positive and negative I.M. serum controls, dropper bottle and *dispenstirs* for 25 and 100 tests.
Mono-Test (Wampole)	**Slide test** for serum or plasma	In kits containing reagent, positive and negative control serums, calibrated capillary tubes and bulbs, glass slides, disposable stirrers and card slides for 40 and 100 tests.
Quantaffirm (Organon Teknika)	**Reagent kit** for serum tests	In test kits containing vials and reagent for 4 tests.

OCCULT BLOOD SCREENING TESTS

To detect occult blood.

ColoCare (Helena Labs)[1]	**Kit** for fecal specimens	In kits containing 3 tests.
ColoScreen (Helena Labs)	**Slide tests** for fecal specimens	In kits containing slides, monitors, tape, developer, specimen applicators and mailing envelopes for 100 tests.
EZ Detect (Biomerica)[1]	**Kit** for fecal specimens	In kits containing 5 test tissues, control and control card for 48 tests.
Hemoccult II Dispensapak (SmithKline Diagnostics)[1]	**Slide tests** for fecal specimens	In kits containing slides, applicators and developer for 100 tests.
Hemoccult II Dispensapak Plus (SmithKline Diagnostics)[1]	**Slide tests** for fecal specimens	In kits containing slides, sample collection tissues, applicators and mailing pouch for 40 tests.
Hemoccult II (SmithKline Diagnostics)	**Slide tests** for fecal specimens	In kits containing developer and applicators for 102 and 1020 tests.
Hemoccult Slides (SmithKline Diagnostics)	**Slide tests** for fecal specimens	In kits containing developer and applicators for 100 and 1000 tests.
Hemoccult Tape (SmithKline Diagnostics)	**Tape** for fecal specimens	In kits containing tape dispenser and developer for 100 tests.
Hemoccult SENSA (SmithKline Diagnostics)	**Slide tests** for fecal specimens	In 100s and 1000s with developer and applicators.
Hemoccult II SENSA (SmithKline Diagnostics)	**Slide tests** for fecal specimens	In kits containing slides, tissues, applicators and mailing pouches for 40 tests.
HemeSelect Reagent (SmithKline Diagnostics)	**Reagent kit** for fecal specimens	In kits containing vials, diluent, Hb positive control, microtiter plate and droppers for 40 tests. *For use with HemeSelect Sample Collection Kit.*
HemeSelect Collection (SmithKline Diagnostics)[1]	**Collection kit** for fecal specimens	In kits containing sample collection card, applicator, self-sealing sample bag and instructions. *For use with the HemeSelect Reagent Kit.*
Hema-Chek (Bayer Corp)[1]	**Slide tests** for fecal specimens	In kits containing slide pak, developer, control and applicator sticks for 100 and 300 tests.
Hematest (Bayer Corp)	**Reagent tablets** for fecal specimens	In packages containing reagent tablets and filter paper for 100 tests.
Hemastix (Bayer Corp)	**Reagent strips** for urine specimens	In 50s.
Gastroccult (SmithKline Diagnostics)	**Slide tests** for gastric specimens	In kits containing slides, developer and applicators for 40 tests.

[1] For use by patient at home.

OVULATION TESTS

To measure luteinizing hormone for prediction of ovulation.

Answer Ovulation (Carter Wallace)[a]	**Kit** for urine tests	In kits containing test sticks for 5 tests.
First Response Ovulation Predictor (Carter Wallace)[a]	**Kit** for urine tests	In kits containing test sticks for 5 tests.
Clearblue Easy (Unipath Diagnostic)[a]	**Kit** for urine tests	In kits containing test sticks for 7 tests.

[a] For use by patient at home.

PREGNANCY TESTS

To detect the presence of human chorionic gonadotropin.

Advance (Ortho)[1]	**Stick** for urine test	In 1s.
Answer One-Step Pregnancy Test (Carter Wallace)[1]	**Stick** for urine test	In 1s.
Answer Plus (Carter Wallace)[1]	**Kit** for urine test	In kits containing urine collection cup, filter dropper, vial, test well, test tray and tube for 1 test.
Answer Quick & Simple (Carter Wallace)[1]	**Kit** for urine test	In kits containing dropper, tube and color key for 2 tests.
Conceive Pregnancy (Quidel)[1]	**Kit** for urine test	In kits containing tape cassette, dropper, plastic cup for 1 and 2 tests.
Clearblue Easy (Whitehall)[1]	**Stick** for urine test	In 1s.
e.p.t. Quick Stick (Parke-Davis)[1]	**Stick** for urine test	In 1s.
Fact Plus (Ortho)[1]	**Kit** for urine test	In kits containing test disk, urine collection cup and urine dropper.
First Response (Carter Wallace)[1]	**Stick** for urine test	In 1s.
Fortel Midstream (Biomerica)	**Stick** for urine test	In 1s.
Fortel Plus (Biomerica)[1]	**Kit** for urine test	In kits containing urine collection cup, test device, dropper and absorbent packet.
One Step Midstream (Biocare International)[1]	**Stick** for urine test	In 1s.
Midstream Pregnancy Test Kit (Goldline)	**Kit** for urine test	In 1s.
Pregnosis (Roche)[1]	**Slide tests** for urine	In kits containing reagents, droppers, pipettes, applicator stick and slide for 50 and 200 tests.
Nimbus Quick Strip (Biomerica)[1]	**Test strips** for urine	In 25s.
RapidVue (Quidel)[1]	**Kit** for urine test	In kits containing cup, dropper and test cassette.
QTest (Quidel)[1]	**Stick** for urine test	In kits containing vial, test stick, reagent, developer and solution for 1 test.
UCG Slide (Wampole)	**Slide tests** for urine	In kits containing latex reagent, antibody reagent, slide stirrers and plastic cup for 30, 100, 300 and 1000 tests.
Abbott TestPack hCG-Urine Plus (Abbott)	**Kit** for urine test	In kits containing reaction dish and transfer pipette. In 20s.
Nimbus (Biomerica)	**Kit** for urine test	In kits containing tube, conjugate and pipettes for 25, 50 and 100 tests.
Nimbus Plus (Biomerica)	**Kit** for urine test	In kits containing test devices and droppers for 25 tests.
Unistep hCG (Orion Diagnostica)	**Kit** for urine test	In kits containing hCG reaction packs and droppers for 25 and 50 tests.
QuickVue (Quidel)	**Cassettes** for urine test	In kits containing test cassettes and pipettes 25 and 75 tests.
SureCell Pregnancy (Kodak)	**Kit** for urine test	In kits containing reagents for 10, 25 and 100 tests.
SureCell hCG-Urine Test (Kodak)	**Kit** for urine test	In 10s, 25s and 100s.
UCG Beta-Slide Monoclonal II (Wampole)	**Slide tests** for urine	In kits containing slide test and reagent for 50, 100 and 300 tests.

[1] For use by patient at home.

RHEUMATOID FACTOR TEST

To detect rheumatoid factor in blood.

Rheumatex (Wampole)	**Slide tests** for blood	In kits containing reagents and slides for 100 and 200 tests.
Rheumaton (Wampole)	**Slide tests** for serum or synovial fluid	In kits containing reagent, positive and negative control, tubes, bulbs and slides for 20, 50 and 150 tests.

SICKLE CELL TEST

To detect hemoglobin S.

Sickledex (Ortho)	**Kit** for blood tests	In kits containing reagents and solution for 12 and 100 tests.

STAPHYLOCOCCUS TEST

To determine the presence of *Staphylococcus aureus*.

Isocult for *Staphylococcus aureus* (Remel)	**Culture paddles** for exudate	In kits containing reagents for 12 tests.

STREPTOCOCCI TESTS

To detect beta-hemolytic group A streptococci, group B streptococci, streptococcal pharyngitis, antibodies to DNase-B, *Streptococcus pneumoniae* and streptococcal extracellular antigens.

Sure Cell Streptococci (Kodak)	**Kit** for the detection of group A streptococcal antigen from throat swabs and blood	In kits containing test cells, extraction blocks, reagents, dye solutions, filter and swabs for 25 and 100 tests.
Culturette 10 Minute Group A Strep ID (Becton Dickinson)	**Slide test** for the detection of group A streptococcal antigen from throat swabs	In kits containing reagents and test slides for 55 and 200 tests.
Isocult for *Streptococcal pharyngitis* (Remel)	**Culture paddles** for the detection of streptococcal pharyngitis from throat swabs	In kits culture paddles and reagents for 12 tests.
Respiracult-Strep (LifeSign LLC)	**Culture paddles** for the detection of group A beta-hemolytic streptococci from throat and nasopharyngeal sources	In kits containing reagents and culture paddles for 25 and 50 tests.
Streptonase-B (Wampole)	**Kit** for the detection of antibodies to DNase-B in serum	In kits containing reagents and tubes for 10 tests.
Test Pack (Abbott)	**Kit** for the detection of group A streptococci from throat specimens	In kits containing reagents, extraction tubes and swabs for 40 and 80 tests.
Bactigen B Streptococcus-CS (Wampole)	**Slide tests** for the detection of group B streptococcus antigen from vaginal and cervical swabs	In kits containing reagents, slides, droppers and stirrers for 48 tests.
Streptozyme (Wampole)	**Slide tests** for the detection of streptococcal extracellular antigens in blood, plasma and serum	In kits containing reagents, tubes, positive and negative control serum, bulbs and slides for 15, 50 and 150 tests.
Detect-A-Strep (Antibodies Inc.)	**Slide tests** for the detection of streptococcal antigen from throat swabs	In kits containing reagents and test plates for 6 tests.

TOXOPLASMOSIS TEST

To detect the presence of *Toxoplasma gondii* in blood.

TPM Test (Wampole)	**Kit** for blood test	In kits including reagents for 120 tests.

VIRUS TESTS

To detect human T-Lymphotropic type 1, HSV-1, HSV-2, herpes, rotavirus, rubella and C-reactive protein.

Human T-Lymphotropic Virus Type I EIA (Abbott)	**Reagent kit** for serum or plasma tests	In kits containing reagents, vials and reaction trays for 100 tests.
MicroTrak HSV 1/HSV 2 Culture Identification/Typing Test (Syva)	**Culture test** for tissue	1 test per kit.
MicroTrak HSV1/HSV2 Direct Specimen Identification/Typing Test (Syva)	**Slide test** for external lesions	In kits containing reagent for 60 tests.
Sure Cell Herpes (Kodak)	**Reagent kit** for genital, rectal, oral or dermal swabs	In 10s and 25s.
Rubazyme for Rubella (Abbott)	**Reagent kit** for serum test	In kits containing reagents and diluent for 1 and 5 tests.
Virogen Herpes (Wampole)	**Slide test** for the detection of herpes simplex virus antigens directly from lesions or cell culture	In kits containing reagents, stirrers, slides and slide covers for 100 tests.
Virogen Rotatest for Rotavirus (Wampole)	**Slide test** for fecal specimens	In kits containing reagents, extraction buffer and slides for 50 tests.
Immunex C-Reactive Protein (Wampole)	**Kit** for blood tests	In kits containing reagents and slides for 100 tests.
Impact Rubella (Wampole)	**Slide test** for serum	In kits containing reagents and slides for 100, 500 and 5000 tests.

COMBINATION TESTS

To detect a multiplicity of conditions, including *Haemophilus influenzae* type b, *Neisseria meningitidis* serogroups A/B/C/Y/W135, *Streptococcus pneumoniae, Salmonella, Shigella, N. gonorrhoeae, T. vaginalis* and *Candida*.

Bactigen Meningitis Panel (Wampole)	**Slide test** for cerebrospinal fluid, serum, urine and blood	In 54s.
Bactigen *Salmonella-Shigella* (Wampole)	**Slide test** for cultures	In kits containing reagents, dispenser cannulae, droppers, slides and stirrers for 96 tests.
Isocult for *N. gonorrhoeae* and *Candida* (Remel)	**Culture test** for endocervical rectal, urethral, pharyngeal and vaginal specimens	In 12s.
Isocult for *T. vaginalis* and *Candida* (Remel)	**Culture test** for vaginal and urethral cultures	In kits containing culture tubes and reagents for 12 tests.

SODIUM AND pH URINE TEST

Used for the quantitative detection of Na and pH in urine and for the qualitative detection of bladder tumor associated antigen in urine.

BTA stat Test (Polymedco, Inc.)	**Kit** for bladder cancer test	In kits containing 30 foil packages with a BTA stat device, disposable dropper, and disposable desiccant pouch.

MULTIPLE URINE TEST PRODUCTS

To make simultaneous determinations of two or more urine tests.

Product & Distributor	Glucose	Protein	pH	Blood	Ketones	Bilirubin	Urobilinogen	Nitrite	Leukocytes	How Supplied
Chemstrip 2 GP (Boehringer Mannheim)	X	X								In 100s.
Uristix (Bayer Corp)	X	X								In 100s.
Combistix (Bayer Corp)	X	X	X							In 100s.
Hema-Combistix (Bayer Corp)	X	X	X	X						In 100s.
Uristix 4 (Bayer Corp)	X	X						X	X	In 100s.
Chemstrip 4 the OB (Boehringer Mannheim)	X	X		X					X	In 100s.
Chemstrip uGK (Boehringer Mannheim)	X				X					In 50s.
Keto-Diastix (Bayer Corp)	X				X					In 50s and 100s.
Chemstrip 6 (Boehringer Mannheim)	X	X	X	X	X				X	In 100s.
Labstix (Bayer Corp)	X	X	X	X	X					In 100s.
Bili-Labstix (Bayer Corp)	X	X	X	X	X	X				In 100s.
Chemstrip 7 (Boehringer Mannheim)	X	X	X	X	X	X			X	In 100s.
Multistix (Bayer Corp)	X	X	X	X	X	X	X			In 100s.
Multistix SG[1] (Bayer Corp)	X	X	X	X	X	X	X			In 100s.
Multistix 7 (Bayer Corp)	X	X	X	X	X			X	X	In 100s.
Multistix 8 SG[1] (Bayer Corp)	X	X	X	X	X			X	X	In 100s.
Chemstrip 8 (Boehringer Mannheim)	X	X	X	X	X	X	X		X	In 100s.
N-Multistix (Bayer Corp)	X	X	X	X	X	X	X	X		In 100s.
N-Multistix SG[1] (Bayer Corp)	X	X	X	X	X	X	X	X		In 100s.
Multistix 9 SG[1] (Bayer Corp)	X	X	X	X	X	X		X	X	In 100s.
Multistix 10 SG[1] (Bayer Corp)	X	X	X	X	X	X	X	X	X	In 100s.
Chemstrip 10 With SG[1] (Boehringer Mannheim)	X	X	X	X	X	X	X	X	X	In 100s.
Chemstrip 9 (Boehringer Mannheim)	X	X	X	X	X	X	X	X	X	In 100s.

MULTIPLE URINE TEST PRODUCTS

Product & Distributor	Glucose	Protein	pH	Blood	Ketones	Bilirubin	Urobilinogen	Nitrite	Leukocytes	How Supplied
Multistix 9 (Bayer Corp)	X	X	X	X	X	X	X	X	X	In 100s.
Chemstrip 2 LN (Boehringer Mannheim)								X	X	In 100s.
Multistix 2 (Bayer Corp)								X	X	In 100s.
Biotel Kidney (Biotel)		X		X						In 12s.

[1] Also tests specific gravity.

IN VIVO DIAGNOSTIC AIDS

The following is a list of available diagnostic aids for professional office use or for use by patients at home (when noted). Those tests requiring special equipment and used primarily by commercial laboratories are not included. For complete information on specific uses, directions and characteristics of these products, consult the manufacturers' package literature.

AMINOHIPPURATE SODIUM (PAH)

For the estimation of renal plasma flow and to measure the functional capacity of the renal tubular secretory mechanism.

Rx	**Aminohippurate Sodium** (Merck)	**Injection:** 20% aqueous solution	In 10 ml vials.

AMINOHIPPURATE SODIUM — INJECTION

Indications

➤*Renal function studies:* Estimation of effective renal plasma flow (ERPF). Measurement of the functional capacity of the renal tubular secretory mechanism.

HYSTEROSCOPY FLUID

For use with the hysteroscope as an aid in distending the uterine cavity and in irrigating and visualizing its surfaces.

Rx	**Hyskon** (Pharmacia & Upjohn)	**Solution:** 32% w/v dextran 70 in 10% w/v dextrose	In 100 and 250 ml.

INDIGOTINDISULFONATE SODIUM

For localizing ureteral orifices during cystoscopy and ureteral catheterization.

Rx	**Indigo Carmine** (American Regent)	**Solution ampules for injection:** 0.8% aqueous solution	In 5 ml amps.

INDIGOTINDISULFONATE SODIUM — INJECTION

Indications

➤*Localized ureteral orifices:* Originally employed as a kidney function test, the chief application of indigotindisulfonate at present is localizing ureteral orifices during cystoscopy and ureteral catheterization.

INDOCYANINE GREEN

Rx	**IC-Green** (Akorn)	**Powder for Injection:** 25 mg	In vials with 10 mL amps of aqueous solvent. In 6s.
Rx	**Cardio-Green** (Becton Dickinson)	**Powder**	In 25 and 50 mg vials with solvent.

INDOCYANINE GREEN — INJECTION

Indications

➤*Angiography:* For ophthalmic angiography.

➤*In vivo diagnostics:* For determining cardiac output, hepatic function, and liver blood flow.

Administration and Dosage

➤*Indicator-dilution studies:* Indocyanine green permits recording of the indicator-dilution curves for both diagnostic and research purpose independently of fluctuations in oxygen saturation. In the performance of dye dilution curves, a known amount of dye is usually injected as a single bolus as rapidly as possible via a cardiac catheter into selected sites in the vascular system. A recording instrument (oximeter or densitometer) is attached to a needle or catheter for sampling of the dye-blood mixture from a systemic arterial sampling site.

Under sterile conditions, dissolve the indocyanine green powder with the aqueous solvent provided for this product, and use the solution within 10 hours after it is prepared. If a precipitate is present, discard the solution. The amount of solvent to be used can be calculated from the dosage form that follows. It is recommended that the syringe used for injection of the dye be rinsed with this diluent. Use isotonic saline to flush the residual dye from the cardiac catheter into the circulation to avoid hemolysis. With the exception of the rinsing of the dye injection syringe, saline is used in all other parts of the catheterization procedure.

This matter of rinsing the dye syringe with distilled water may not be critical, since it is known that an amount of sodium chloride sufficient to make an isotonic solution may be added to dye that has first been dissolved in distilled water. This procedure has been used for constant-rate injection techniques without precipitation of the dye.

Usual Doses of Indocyanine Green Used for Dilution	
Adults	5 mg
Children	2.5 mg
Infants	1.25 mg

These doses of the dye are usually injected in a mL volume. An average of 5 dilution curves are required in the performance of a diagnostic cardiac catheterization. Keep the total dose of dye injected below 2 mg/kg.

➤*Hepatic function studies:* Due to its absorption spectrum, changing concentrations of sterile indocyanine green in the blood can be monitored by ear densitometry or by obtaining blood specimens at timed intervals. The technique for both methods is as follows.

Study the patient in a fasting, basal state. Weigh the patient and calculate the dosage on the basis of 0.5 mg/kg of body weight.

Under sterile conditions, dissolve the indocyanine green powder with the aqueous solvent provided. Add exactly 5 mL aqueous solvent to the 25 mg vial or add exactly 10 mL aqueous solvent to the 50 mg vial, giving 5 mg of dye per mL of solution.

Inject the correct amount of dye into the lumen of an arm vein as rapidly as possible, without allowing the dye to escape outside the vein. (If the photometric method is used, prior to injecting indocyanine green, withdraw 6 mL venous blood from the patient's arm for serum blank and standard curve construction, and through the same needle, inject the correct amount of dye.)

Ear densitometry – Ear oximetry has also been used and makes it possible to monitor the appearance and disappearance of indocyanine green without the necessity of withdrawal and spectrophotometric analysis of blood samples for calibration. An ear densitometer that has a compensatory photoelectric cell to correct for changes in blood volume and hematocrit, and a detection photocell that registers levels has been described. This device permits simultaneous measurement of cardiac output, blood volume, and hepatic clearance of indocyanine green and was found to provide a reliable index of plasma removal kinetics after single injections or continuous intrusions of indocyanine green. This technique was employed in newborn infants, healthy adults, and in children and adults with liver disease. The normal subject has a removal rate of 18% to 24% per minute. Due to the absence of extra-hepatic removal, indocyanine green was found to be ideally suited for serial study of severe chronic liver disease and to provide a stable measurement of hepatic blood flow. In larger doses, indocyanine green has proven to be particularly valuable in detecting drug-induced alterations of hepatic function and in the detection of mild liver injury.

INDOCYANINE GREEN — INJECTION

Photometric method –

Percentage retention: A single 20-minute sample (withdrawn from a vein in the opposite arm to that injected) is allowed to clot, centrifuged, and its optical density is determined at 805 nm using the patient's normal serum as the blank. Dye concentration is read from the curve above. A single 20-minute sample of serum in healthy subjects should contain no more than 4% of the initial concentration of the dye. The use of percentage retention is less accurate than percentage disappearance rate, but provides reproducible results. Hemolysis does not interfere with a reading.

Determination using disappearance rate of dye: To calculate the percentage disappearance rate, obtain samples at 5, 10, 15 and 20 minutes after injecting the dye. Prepare the sample as in the previous section and measure the optical densities at 805 nm, using the patient's normal serum as the blank. The indocyanine green concentration in each timed specimen can be determined by using the concentration curve illustrated. Plot values on semilogarithmic paper.

Read specimens containing indocyanine green at the same temperature because its optical density is influenced by temperature variations.

Normal values: Percentage disappearance rate in healthy subjects is 18% to 24% per minute. Normal biological half-time is 2.5 to 3 minutes.

➤*Ophthalmic angiography studies:* The excitation and emission spectra and the absorption spectra of indocyanine green make it useful in ophthalmic angiography. The peak absorption and emission of indocyanine green lie in a region (800 to 850 nm) where transmission of energy by the pigment epithelium is more efficient than in the region of visible light energy. Indocyanine green also has the property of being nearly 98% bound to blood protein, and therefore, excessive dye extravasation does not take place in the highly fenestrated choroidal vasculature. It is, therefore, useful in both absorption and fluorescence infrared angiography of the choroidal vasculature when using appropriate filters and film in a fundus camera.

Dosages up to 40 mg indocyanine green dye in 2 mL of aqueous solvent have been found to give optimal angiograms, depending on the imaging equipment and technique used. The antecubital vein injected indocyanine green dye bolus should immediately be followed by a 5 mL bolus of normal saline.

Clinically, angiograms of uniformly good quality can be assured only after taking care to optimize the contributions of all possible factors, such as patient cooperation and dye injection. The foregoing injection regimen is designed to provide delivery of a spatially limited dye bolus of optimal concentration to the choroidal vasculature following IV injection.

➤*Storage / Stability:* Indocyanine green is unstable in aqueous solution and must be used within 10 hours. However, the dye is stable in plasma and whole blood so that samples obtained in discontinuous sampling techniques may be read hours later. Use sterile techniques in handling the dye solution and in the performance of the dilution curves.

Indocyanine green powder may cling to the vial or lump together because it is freeze-dried in the vials. This is not due to the presence of water; the moisture content is carefully controlled.

Actions

➤*Pharmacology:* Indocyanine green is a sterile, water soluble, tricarbocyanine dye with a peak spectral absorption at 800 to 810 nm in blood plasma or blood. Indocyanine green contains not more than 5% sodium iodide.

Indocyanine green permits recording of indicator-dilution curves for both diagnostic and research purposes independently of fluctuations in oxygen saturation. In the performance of dye dilution curves, a known amount of dye is usually injected as a single bolus as rapidly as possible via a cardiac catheter into selected sites in the vascular system. A recording instrument (oximeter or densitometer) is attached to a needle or catheter for sampling of the blood-dye mixture from a systemic arterial sampling site.

The peak absorption and emission of indocyanine green lie in a region (800 to 850 nm) where transmission of energy by the pigment epithelium is more efficient than in the region of visible light energy. Because indocyanine green is also nearly 98% bound to blood protein, excessive dye extravasation does not take place in the highly fenestrated choroidal vasculature. It is, therefore, useful in absorption and fluorescence infrared angiography of the choroidal vasculature when using appropriate filters and film in a fundus camera.

➤*Pharmacokinetics:* Following intravenous injection, indocyanine green is rapidly bound to plasma protein, of which albumin is the principle carrier (95%). Indocyanine green undergoes no significant extrahepatic or enterohepatic circulation; simultaneous arterial and venous blood estimations have shown negligible renal, peripheral, lung, or cerebro-spinal uptake of the dye. Indocyanine green is taken up from the plasma almost exclusively by the hepatic parenchymal cells and is secreted entirely into the bile. After biliary obstruction, the dye appears in the hepatic lymph, independently of the bile, suggesting that the biliary mucosa is sufficiently intact to prevent diffusion of the dye, but allow diffusion of bilirubin. These characteristics make indocyanine green a helpful index of hepatic function.

Contraindications

Indocyanine green contains sodium iodide; use with caution in patients who have a history of allergy to iodides.

Warnings

➤*Compatibility:* Use the aqueous solvent provided for this product, pH 5.5 to 6.5, which is especially prepared sterile water for injection, to dissolve indocyanine green because there have been reports of incompatibility with some commercially available water for injection.

➤*Hypersensitivity reactions:* Two anaphylactic deaths have been reported following indocyanine green administration during cardiac catheterization. One of these was in a patient with a history of sensitivity to penicillin and sulfa drugs.

➤*Pregnancy: Category C.* Animal reproduction studies have not been conducted with indocyanine green. It is also not known whether indocyanine green can cause fetal harm when administered to a pregnant woman or can affect reproduction capacity. Give indocyanine green to a pregnant woman only if clearly indicated.

➤*Lactation:* It is not known whether this drug is excreted in human milk. Because many drugs are excreted in human milk, exercise caution when indocyanine green is administered to a nursing woman.

Precautions

➤*Indocyanine green powder and solution:* Indocyanine green is unstable in aqueous solution and must be used within 10 hours. However, the dye is stable in plasma and whole blood so that samples obtained in discontinuous sampling techniques may be read hours later. Use sterile techniques in handling the dye solution as well as in the performance of the dilution curves.

Indocyanine green powder may cling to the vial or lump together because it is freeze-dried in the vials. This is not due to the presence of water; the moisture content is carefully controlled.

The plasma fractional disappearance rate at the recommended 0.5 mg/kg dose has been reported to be significantly greater in women than in men, although there was no significant difference in the calculated value for clearance.

Radioactive iodine uptake studies should not be performed for at least a week following the use of indocyanine green.

Drug Interactions

➤*Drug / Lab test interactions:* Heparin preparations containing sodium bisulfite reduce the absorption peak of indocyanine green in blood and, therefore, should not be used as an anticoagulant for the collection of samples for analysis.

Adverse Reactions

➤*Hypersensitivity:* Anaphylactic or urticarial reactions have been reported in patients with or without history of allergy to iodides. If such reactions occur, administer treatment with the appropriate agents (eg, epinephrine, antihistamines, corticosteroids).

Overdosage

There are no data available describing the signs, symptoms, or laboratory findings accompanying overdosage. The LD_{50} after IV administration ranges between 60 and 80 mg/kg in mice, 50 and 70 mg/kg in rats, and 50 and 80 mg/kg in rabbits.

INULIN

For measurement of glomerular filtration rate (GFR).

Rx	**Inulin Injection** (Iso-Tex Diagnostics)	**Injection:** 100 mg per ml	In 50 ml vials.[1]

[1] With 0.9% Sodium Chloride in Water for Injection.

INULIN — INJECTION

Indications

➤*Renal function studies:* For measurement of glomerular filtration rate.

MANNITOL

See the Mannitol monograph in the Renal and Genitourinary Agents chapter.

SODIUM IODIDE I^{123}

Rx	**Sodium Iodide I-123** (Mallinckrodt Medical)	**Capsules:** 3.7 MBq	Sucrose. Red/white. In 1s, 3s, and 5s.
		7.4 MBq	Sucrose. Green/white. In 1s, 3s, and 5s.

SODIUM IODIDE I-123 — ORAL

Indications

➤*Thyroid function studies:* As a diagnostic procedure in evaluating thyroid function or morphology.

Administration and Dosage

➤*Approved by the FDA:* May 27, 1982.

The recommended oral dose for the average patient (70 kg) is 3.7 to 14.8 megabecquerels (MBq) (100 to 400 µCi). The lower part of the dosage range, 3.7 MBq (100 µCi), is recommended for uptake studies alone, and the higher part, 14.8 MBq (400 µCi), for thyroid imaging. The determination of I-123 concentration in the thyroid gland may be initiated at 6 hours after administering the dose and should be measured in accordance with standardized procedures.

The patient dose should be measured by a suitable radioactivity calibration system immediately prior to administration. The capsules can be utilized up to 30 hours after calibration time and date. Thereafter, discard the capsules in accordance with standard safety procedures. The user should wear waterproof gloves at all times when handling the capsules or container.

➤*Storage/Stability:* The contents of the vial are radioactive, and adequate shielding and handling precautions must be maintained. Dispense and preserve capsules in tightly closed containers that are adequately shielded. Store at controlled room temperature, 20° to 25°C (68° to 77°F). Storage and disposal of sodium iodide I-123 capsules should be controlled in a manner that is in compliance with the appropriate regulations of the government agency authorized to license the use of this radionuclide.

Actions

➤*Pharmacokinetics:*

Absorption/Distribution – Sodium iodide I-123 is readily absorbed from the upper GI tract. Following absorption, the iodide is distributed primarily within the extracellular fluid of the body.

The fraction of the administered dose which is accumulated in the thyroid gland may be a measure of thyroid function in the absence of unusually high or low iodine intake or administration of certain drugs which influence iodine accumulation by the thyroid gland. Accordingly, the patient should be questioned carefully regarding previous medications or procedures involving radiographic media. Healthy subjects can accumulate approximately 10% to 50% of the administered iodine dose in the thyroid gland, however, the normal and abnormal ranges are established by individual physician's criteria. The mapping (imaging) of sodium iodide I-123 distribution in the thyroid gland may provide useful information concerning thyroid anatomy and definition of normal or abnormal functioning of tissue within the gland.

Excretion – Sodium iodide I-123 is trapped and organically bound by the thyroid and concentrated by the stomach, choroid plexus and salivary glands. It is excreted by the kidneys.

Contraindications

No known contraindications.

Warnings

➤*Pregnancy: Category C.* Animal reproduction studies have not been conducted with this drug. It is also not known whether sodium iodide I-123 can cause fetal harm when administered to a pregnant woman or can affect reproductive capacity. Sodium iodide I-123 should be given to a pregnant woman only if clearly needed.

Ideally, examinations using radiopharmaceuticals, especially those elective in nature, in women of childbearing capability should be performed during the first few (approximately 10) days following the onset of menses.

➤*Lactation:* Since I-123 is excreted in human milk, formula feeding should be substituted for breastfeeding if the agent must be administered to the mother during lactation.

➤*Children:* Safety and efficacy in pediatric patients have not been established.

Precautions

➤*Radioactivity:* The contents of the capsule are radioactive. Adequate shielding of the preparation must be maintained at all times.

➤*Administration:* The prescribed sodium iodide I-123 dose should be administered as soon as practical from the time of receipt of product (ie, as close to calibration time as possible), in order to minimize the fraction of radiation exposure due to the relative increase of radionuclidic contaminants with time.

➤*Handle with care:* Sodium iodide I-123, as well as other radioactive drugs, must be handled with care and appropriate safety measures should be used to minimize radiation exposure to clinical personnel. Care should also be taken to minimize radiation exposure to the patient consistent with proper patient management.

Radiopharmaceuticals should be used only by physicians who are qualified by training and experience in the safe use and handling of radionuclides, and whose experience and training have been approved by the appropriate government agency authorized to license the use of radionuclides.

Adverse Reactions

Although rare, reactions associated with the administration of sodium iodide isotopes for diagnostic use include, in decreasing order of frequency, nausea, vomiting, chest pain, tachycardia, itching skin, rash and hives.

THYROTROPIN ALFA

Rx	**Thyrogen** (Genzyme)	**Powder for injection, lyophilized:** 1.1 mg thyrotropin alfa (≥ 4 IU)/vial	Kit of two 1.1 mg single-use vials of thyrotropin alfa and two 10 mL vials of diluent.[1]

[1] 36 mg mannitol, 5.1 mg sodium phosphate, 2.4 mg NaCl.

THYROTROPIN ALFA — INJECTION

Indications

➤*Adjunctive diagnostic tool for serum thyroglobulin (Tg) testing:* For use as an adjunctive diagnostic tool for serum Tg testing with or without radioiodine imaging in the follow-up of patients with well-differentiated thyroid cancer.

Other potential clinical uses – May be used in patients with an undetectable Tg on thyroid hormone suppressive therapy to exclude the diagnosis of residual or recurrent thyroid cancer.

May be used in patients requiring serum Tg testing and radioiodine imaging who are unwilling to undergo thyroid hormone withdrawal testing and whose treating physician believes that use of a less sensitive test is justified.

May be used in patients who are either unable to mount an adequate endogenous thyroid stimulating hormone (TSH) response to thyroid hormone withdrawal or in whom withdrawal is medically contraindicated.

It is not recommended to stimulate radioiodine uptake for the purposes of ablative radiotherapy of thyroid cancer.

Administration and Dosage

➤*Approved by the FDA:* November 30, 1998.

Administer thyrotropin alfa IM only. Do not administer IV.

After reconstitution with 1.2 mL Sterile Water for Injection, administer a 1 mL solution (0.9 mg thyrotropin alfa) by IM injection to the buttock. Reconstitute the powder immediately prior to use with 1.2 mL of the diluent provided.

➤*Usual dose:* 0.9 mg IM may be administered every 24 hours for 2 doses or every 72 hours for 3 doses.

➤*Adjunctive thyroid testing:* For radioiodine imaging, administer radioiodine 24 hours following the final thyrotropin alfa injection. Perform scanning 48 hours after radioiodine administration (72 hours after the final injection of thyrotropin alfa).

For serum Tg testing, obtain the serum sample 72 hours after the final injection of thyrotropin alfa.

➤*Storage/Stability:* Store at 2° to 8°C (36° to 46°F). If necessary, the reconstituted solution can be stored for up to 24 hours between 2° to 8°C (36° to 46°F), while avoiding microbial contamination.

After reconstitution with the accompanying Sterile Water for Injection visually inspect each vial for particulate matter or discoloration before use. Do not use any vial exhibiting particulate matter or discoloration.

Do not use after the expiration date on the vial. Protect from light.

Actions

➤*Pharmacology:* Thyrotropin alfa (recombinant human thyroid stimulating hormone) is a heterodimeric glycoprotein produced by recombinant DNA technology. It has comparable biochemical properties to the human pituitary TSH. Binding of thyrotropin alfa to TSH receptors on normal thyroid epithelial cells or on well-differentiated thyroid cancer tissue stimulates iodine uptake and organification, and synthesis and secretion of thyroglobulin (Tg), triiodothyronine (T_3), and thyroxine (T_4).

➤*Pharmacokinetics:* The pharmacokinetics of thyrotropin alfa were studied in 16 patients with well-differentiated thyroid cancer given a single 0.9 mg IM dose. Mean peak concentrations of ≈ 116 mU/L were reached between 3 and 24 hours after injection (median of 10 hours). The mean apparent elimination half-life was ≈ 25 hours. The organ(s) of TSH clear-

THYROTROPIN ALFA — INJECTION

ance in humans have not been identified, but studies of pituitary-derived TSH suggest the involvement of the liver and kidneys.

Warnings

➤*Pregnancy: Category C.* It is not known whether thyrotropin alfa can cause fetal harm when administered to a pregnant woman or can affect reproductive capacity. Give thyrotropin alfa to a pregnant woman only if clearly needed.

➤*Lactation:* It is not known whether the drug is excreted in human milk. Because many drugs are excreted in milk, exercise caution when administering thyrotropin alfa to a breast-feeding woman.

➤*Children:* Safety and efficacy in pediatric patients younger than 16 years of age have not been established.

Precautions

➤*Diagnosis:* Even when thyrotropin alfa-stimulated Tg testing is performed in combination with radioiodine imaging, there remains a meaningful risk of missing a diagnosis of thyroid cancer or of underestimating the extent of disease. Therefore, thyroid hormone withdrawal Tg testing with radioiodine imaging remains the standard diagnostic modality to assess the presence, location, and extent of thyroid cancer.

A newly detectable Tg level or a Tg level rising over time after thyrotropin alfa, or a high index of suspicion of metastatic disease, even in the setting of a negative or low-stage thyrotropin alfa radioiodine scan, should prompt further evaluation such as thyroid hormone withdrawal to definitively establish the location and extent of thyroid cancer. On the other hand, none of the 31 patients studied with undetectable thyrotropin alfa Tg levels (less than 2.5 ng/mL) had metastatic disease. Therefore, an undetectable thyrotropin alfa Tg level suggests the absence of clinically significant disease.

➤*Thyroglobulin antibodies:* Tg antibodies may confound the Tg assay and render Tg levels uninterpretable. Therefore, in such cases, even with a negative or low-stage thyrotropin alfa radioiodine scan, give consideration to evaluating patients further with, for example, a confirmatory thyroid hormone withdrawal scan to determine the location and extent of thyroid cancer.

➤*Previous treatment with bovine TSH:* Exercise caution when thyrotropin alfa is administered to patients who have been previously treated with bovine TSH and, in particular, to those patients who have experienced hypersensitivity reactions to bovine TSH.

➤*Special risk:* Thyrotropin alfa is known to cause a transient but significant rise in serum thyroid hormone concentration. Therefore, exercise caution in patients with a known history of heart disease and with significant residual thyroid tissue.

Adverse Reactions

Thyrotropin Alfa Adverse Events (≥ 1%)

Adverse reaction	n = 381
CNS	
Headache	7.3
Dizziness	1.6
Paresthesia	1.6
GI	
Nausea	10.5
Vomiting	2.1
Nausea and vomiting	1.3
Miscellaneous	
Asthenia	3.4
Chills	1
Fever	1
Flu syndrome	1

Post-marketing –

Hypersensitivity: There have been several reports of hypersensitivity reactions consisting of urticaria, rash, pruritus, and flushing. However, in clinical trials no patients have developed antibodies to thyrotropin alfa, either after single or repeated (27 patients) use of the product.

Four patients out of 55 (7.3%) with CNS metastases who were followed in a special treatment protocol experienced acute hemiplegia, hemiparesis, or pain 1 to 3 days after thyrotropin alfa administration. The symptoms were attributed to local edema or focal hemorrhage at the site of the cerebral or spinal cord metastases. In addition, 1 case each of acute visual loss and of dysphagia secondary to laryngeal edema, requiring tracheotomy, have been reported 24 hours after thyrotropin alfa administration in patients with metastases to the optic nerve and paratracheal areas, respectively. Pretreatment with corticosteroids may be considered under such circumstances.

A 77-year-old nonthyroidectomized patient with a history of heart disease and spinal metastases who received 4 thyrotropin alfa injections over 6 days in a special treatment protocol experienced a fatal MI 24 hours after he received the last thyrotropin alfa injection. The event was likely related to thyrotropin alfa-induced hyperthyroidism.

Overdosage

➤*Symptoms:* There has been no reported experience of overdose in humans. However, in clinical trials, 3 patients experienced symptoms after receiving thyrotropin alfa doses higher than those recommended. Two patients had nausea after a 2.7 mg IM dose, and in 1 of these patients, the event was accompanied by weakness, dizziness, and headache. Another patient experienced nausea, vomiting, and hot flashes after a 3.6 mg IM dose.

In addition, 1 patient experienced symptoms after receiving thyrotropin alfa IV. This patient received 0.3 mg thyrotropin alfa as a single IV bolus and 15 minutes later experienced severe nausea, vomiting, diaphoresis, hypotension (BP decreased from 115/66 mmHg to 81/44 mmHg), and tachycardia (pulse increased from 75 to 117 bpm).

GONADORELIN HYDROCHLORIDE

Rx	**Factrel** (Wyeth-Ayerst)	**Powder for injection, lyophilized:** 100 mcg (as hydrochloride)/vial.[1]	With 2 mL sterile diluent.[2]
		500 mcg (as hydrochloride)/vial.[1]	

[1] With 100 mg lactose.

[2] With 2% benzyl alcohol.

GONADORELIN HYDROCHLORIDE — INJECTION

Indications

➤*Gonadorelin test:* Evaluating the functional capacity and response of the gonadotropes of anterior pituitary. This single-injection test does not measure pituitary gonadotropic reserve, for which more prolonged or repeated administration may be required. The LH response is useful in testing patients with suspected gonadotropin deficiency, whether due to the hypothalamus alone or in combination with anterior pituitary failure. Gonadorelin hydrochloride is also indicated for evaluating residual gonadotropic function of the pituitary following removal of a pituitary tumor by surgery or irradiation. In clinical studies to date, however, the single-injection test has not been useful in differentiating pituitary disorders from hypothalamic disorders. The gonadorelin hydrochloride test can be performed concomitantly with other posttreatment evaluations. The results of the gonadorelin hydrochloride test complement the clinical examination and other laboratory tests used to confirm or substantiate hypogonadotropic hypogonadism.

Administration and Dosage

➤*Approved by the FDA:* September 30, 1982.

➤*Adults:* 100 mcg dose, subcutaneously or intravenously. In females for whom the phase of the menstrual cycle can be established, the test should be performed in the early follicular phase (days 1 to 7).

➤*Test methodology:* To determine the status of the gonadotropin secretory capacity of the anterior pituitary, a test procedure requiring 7 venous blood samples for LH is recommended.

➤*Interpretation of test results:* Interpretation of the LH response to gonadorelin hydrochloride requires an understanding of the hypothalamic-pituitary physiology, knowledge of the clinical status of the individual patient, and familiarity with the normal ranges and the standards used in the laboratory performing the LH assays.

In cases where there is a blunted or borderline response, the gonadorelin hydrochloride test should be repeated.

The gonadorelin hydrochloride test complements the clinical assessment of patients with a variety of endocrine disorders involving the hypothalamic-pituitary axis. In cases where there is a normal response, it indicates the presence of functional pituitary gonadotropes. The single-injection test does not determine the pathophysiological cause for the subnormal response and does not measure pituitary gonadotropic reserve.

Preparation of solution – Reconstitute 100 mcg vial with 1 mL and the 500 mcg vial with 2 mL of accompanying diluent. Prepare immediately before use. After reconstitution, store at room temperature (approximately 25°C; approximately 77°F); use within 1 day. Discard unused solution and diluent.

➤*Storage/Stability:* Store at room temperature (approximately 25°C; approximately 77°F). After reconstitution, store at room temperature and use within 1 day. Discard unused solution and diluent.

Actions

➤*Pharmacokinetics:* Gonadorelin hydrochloride is a synthetic luteinizing hormone-releasing hormone (LH-RH), also referred to as gonadotropin-releasing hormone (GnRH), and has been shown to have gonadotropin-releasing effects upon the anterior pituitary. The range for normal baseline LH levels, as determined from the literature, is 5 to 25 mIU/mL in postpubertal males, and postpubertal and premenopausal females. The standard used is the Second International Reference Preparation-HMC. This range may not correspond in each laboratory performing the assay, since the concentration of LH in normal individuals varies with different assay methods.

Contraindications

Hypersensitivity to gonadorelin hydrochloride or any of the components.

Warnings

➤*Hypersensitivity reactions:* Although allergic and hypersensitivity reactions have been observed with other polypeptide hormones, and rarely with multiple doses of gonadorelin hydrochloride, to date no such reactions have been reported following the administration of a single 100 mcg dose of gonadorelin hydrochloride.

➤*Mutagenesis:* Repetitive, high doses of gonadorelin hydrochloride may cause luteolysis and inhibition of spermatogenesis.

➤*Pregnancy: Category B.* There are no adequate and well-controlled studies in pregnant women. Because animal reproduction studies are not always predictive of human response, this drug should be used during pregnancy only if clearly needed.

Appropriate precautions should be taken because the effects of LH-RH on the fetus and developing offspring have not been adequately evaluated.

➤*Lactation:* It is not known whether this drug is excreted in human milk. Because many drugs are excreted in human milk, caution should be exercised when gonadorelin hydrochloride is administered to a breast-feeding woman.

➤*Children:* Safety and effectiveness in pediatric patients have not been established.

Precautions

➤*Antibody formation:* Antibody formation has been reported rarely after chronic administration of large doses of gonadorelin hydrochloride.

Drug Interactions

➤*Androgens, estrogens, progestins, or glucocorticoids:* The gonadorelin hydrochloride test should be conducted in the absence of other drugs which directly affect the pituitary secretion of the gonadotropins. These would include a variety of preparations which contain androgens, estrogens, progestins, or glucocorticoids.

➤*Levodopa and spirondactone:* The gonadotropin levels may be transiently elevated by spironolactone and minimally elevated by levodopa.

➤*Digoxin and oral contraceptives:* The gonadotropin levels may be suppressed by oral contraceptives and digoxin.

➤*Phenothiazines and dopamine antagonists:* The response to gonadorelin hydrochloride may be blunted by phenothiazines and dopamine antagonists which cause a rise in prolactin.

Adverse Reactions

➤*Cardiovascular:* Flushing.

➤*CNS:* Headache, lightheadedness.

➤*Dermatologic:* Local swelling, occasionally with pain and pruritus at the injection site may occur following subcutaneous administration; local and generalized skin rash have been noted after chronic subcutaneous administration.

➤*GI:* Nausea, abdominal discomfort.

➤*Hypersensitivity:* Rare instances of hypersensitivity reaction (bronchospasm, tachycardia, flushing, urticaria, induration at injection site) and anaphylactic reactions have been reported following multiple-dose administration.

➤*Miscellaneous:* There has been a report of pituitary apoplexy and sudden blindness following gonadotropin-releasing hormone administration to a patient with a gonadotropin-secreting adenoma.

Overdosage

➤*Symptoms:* Gonadorelin hydrochloride has been administered parenterally in doses up to 3 mg twice daily for 28 days without any signs or symptoms of overdosage.

➤*Treatment:* In case of overdosage or idiosyncrasy, symptomatic treatment should be administered as required.

TOLBUTAMIDE SODIUM

Rx	**Orinase Diagnostic** (Pharmacia)	**Powder for Injection:** 1 g (as sodium)/vial	In vials.

TOLBUTAMIDE SODIUM — INJECTION

Indications

➤*Diagnostic aid:* As an aid in the diagnosis of pancreatic islet cell adenoma.

Administration and Dosage

➤*Fajans test:*

1.) The patient should receive a high carbohydrate diet of 150 to 300 g daily for at least 3 days prior to the test.
2.) On morning of test, after an overnight fast, withdraw a fasting blood specimen.
3.) Inject entire volume (20 mL) of tolbutamide sodium solution by IV at a constant rate over a 2- to 3-minute period.
4.) Withdraw blood specimens at the following intervals (in minutes) after the midpoint of the injection: 20, 30, 45, 60, 90, 120, 150, and 180. Of greater significance than the magnitude of blood glucose fall in these patients is the persistence of the hypoglycemia for 3 hours after the administration of tolbutamide sodium. The determination of serum insulin levels before, and at 10, 20, and 30 minutes after the IV administration of the drug as described below, provides a specific and safer test for insulinoma. It also permits the performance of the test in the presence of moderate fasting hypoglycemia, since interpretation is not based on the decline of the blood glucose.

TOLBUTAMIDE SODIUM — INJECTION

5.) Blood glucose determinations are made by the true glucose procedures. The procedure is terminated with a feeding of readily assimilable carbohydrate or breakfast.

Interpretation of results –

Healthy subjects: A decrease to a blood glucose of 38% to 79% of the fasting level may be expected. At 90 to 120 minutes a level of from 78% to 100% of initial level may be seen. Similar responses are to be found in patients with functional hyperinsulinism.

Insulinoma patients: Minimum blood glucose levels of 17% to 50% of fasting values are seen. In the 90- to 180-minute interval, levels are in the range of 40% to 64%. Some patients with liver disease may show the same type of blood glucose response as do patients with insulinomas. Therefore, appropriate laboratory and clinical tests must be employed to distinguish between these 2 conditions.

Use with serum insulin determination in insulinoma patients – If a method of assay for serum insulin is available, the test for insulinoma may be made shorter and more specific.

The determination of serum insulin levels before, and at 10, 20, and 30 minutes after the IV administration of the drug described above, provides a specific and safer test for insulinoma, and permits the performance of the test in the presence of moderate fasting hypoglycemia, since interpretation is not based on the decline of the blood glucose. The test may be terminated after the 30-minute specimen by the feeding of carbohydrate as described above.

➤*Storage/Stability:* Store unreconstituted product at controlled room temperature 20° to 25°C (68° to 77°F). Use immediately after reconstitution (within 1 hour) but only if solution is complete and clear.

Actions

➤*Pharmacology:* The prompt decrease in blood glucose in healthy individuals is associated with a prompt increase in serum insulin levels, as determined by immunoassay, which rise from a fasting mean value of 19 mcU/mL to a peak mean value of approximately 40 mcU/mL (range, 27 to 89) 20 minutes after injection. In patients with functioning islet cell adenoma, tolbutamide sodium has a marked and prolonged blood glucose lowering effect associated with an excessive, prompt rise in serum insulin (118 to 1055 mcU/mL), resulting in a marked and prolonged blood glucose effect.

It will be noted that the administration of 1 g of tolbutamide sodium to healthy subjects results in a rapid fall in blood glucose levels for 30 to 45 minutes, followed by a secondary rise of the blood glucose concentration into the normal range in the ensuing 90 to 180 minutes. The initial hypoglycemia results from the rapid release of insulin from the pancreatic beta cells, while the secondary rise is due to activation of counter-regulatory factors. In contrast, patients with insulinomas were found to exhibit tolbutamide-induced blood glucose decreases of greater magnitude than healthy persons. Of greater significance than the magnitude of blood glucose fall in these patients is the persistence of the hypoglycemia for 3 hours after the administration of tolbutamide sodium. It is this phenomenon of persistent tolbutamide-induced hypoglycemia for 3 hours rather than degree of blood glucose decrease that is of importance in the diagnosis of pancreatic islet cell adenomas. False-positive responses have been observed in a few patients with liver disease, alcohol hypoglycemia, idiopathic hypoglycemia of infancy, severe under nutrition, azotemia, sarcoma, and other extrapancreatic insulin-producing tumors.

Contraindications

Children; previous allergy to tolbutamide or related sulfonylureas.

Warnings

➤*Hypoglycemia:* Severe hypoglycemic symptoms may develop during the test, particularly in patients with fasting blood glucose levels in the hypoglycemic range. If they occur, the test should be terminated immediately by intravenously injecting 12.5 to 25 g of glucose in a 25% to 50% solution.

➤*Hypersensitivity reactions:* As with all intravenous injections, epinephrine and other resuscitative drugs should be at hand to administer in the event of anaphylaxis.

➤*Renal/Hepatic function impairment:* Severe and prolonged hypoglycemia following oral administration of tolbutamide has been reported in patients suffering from severe liver disease and severe renal disease.

➤*Pregnancy: Category C.*

Teratogenic – Tolbutamide sodium has been shown to be teratogenic in rats given doses 25 to 100 times the human dose. In some studies, pregnant rats given high doses of tolbutamide have shown increased mortality in offspring and ocular and bony abnormalities. Repeat studies in other species (rabbits) have not demonstrated a teratogenic effect. There are no adequate and well-controlled studies in pregnant women. Tolbutamide sodium is not recommended for the treatment of pregnant diabetic patients. Serious consideration should also be given to the possible hazards of the use of tolbutamide sodium in women of childbearing age and potential who might become pregnant while using the drug.

Nonteratogenic – Prolonged severe hypoglycemia (4 to 10 days) has been reported in neonates born to mothers who were receiving a sulfonylurea drug at the time of delivery. This has been reported more frequently with the use of agents with prolonged half lives. Use of the drug in pregnant patients is not recommended.

➤*Lactation:* Tolbutamide is excreted in small amounts in the breast milk of breast-feeding mothers. Because of the potential for serious adverse reactions in breast-feeding infants, a decision should be made whether to discontinue breast-feeding or to discontinue the drug, taking into account the importance of the drug to the mother.

➤*Children:* Because of the lack of data to establish ideal dosage and the inability to interpret results, use of tolbutamide sodium is not recommended in children.

Precautions

➤*Test-dose-induced hypoglycemic symptoms:* It is essential that only a true glucose procedure (Somogyi-Nelson, Modified Folin-Wu, AutoAnalyzer, or glucose oxidase) be used to determine blood glucose in order to eliminate highly variable amounts of nonglucose-reducing substances as a major source of error.

Although the hypoglycemic symptoms produced by this test dose are usually not severe, certain nondiabetics may develop moderate to severe symptoms. To avoid this occurrence, the diagnostic test should be terminated by the oral administration of carbohydrate immediately after the 30-minute blood sample has been withdrawn.

Because hypoglycemia of considerable magnitude can occur in certain nondiabetics, it would be wise to routinely terminate each test immediately upon withdrawal of the 30-minute blood sample by the oral administration of carbohydrate, especially in the testing of persons with atherosclerosis.

Drug Interactions

➤*Other drugs that potentiate hypoglycemia:* Certain drugs may potentiate the hypoglycemic action of tolbutamide. These include dicumarol, phenyramidol, salicylates, sulfonamides, oxyphenbutazone, phenylbutazone, probenecid, monoamine oxidase inhibitors, beta-adrenergic blocking agents, and chloramphenicol. There is a danger of both increased or prolonged hypoglycemia if these drugs are used together.

➤*Salicylates, sulfonamides, oxyphenbutazone, phenylbutazone, probenecid, and MAOIs:* Concomitant ingestion of salicylates, sulfonamides, oxyphenbutazone, phenylbutazone, probenecid, and monoamine oxidase inhibitors (MAOIs) may interfere with results of a tolbutamide tolerance test.

➤*Beta-adrenergic blocking agents:* Response to tolbutamide is diminished in patients on therapy with beta-adrenergic blocking agents.

➤*Drug/Lab test interactions:* On very rare occasions, urine containing the tolbutamide metabolite may give a false-positive reaction for albumin by the usual test (acidification after boiling) since this procedure causes the metabolite to precipitate as flocculent particles. This problem may be circumvented by the use of bromphenol reagent strips.

Adverse Reactions

➤*Local:* Rarely a patient may experience a mild pain in the shoulder or slight burning sensation along the course of an arm vein during the IV injection. Such pain which lasts no more than 2 to 3 minutes, is attributed to venospasm and may be obviated by administering the test solution over a period of no less than 2, preferably, 3 minutes.

Thrombophlebitis with thrombosis – Thrombophlebitis with thrombosis of the injected vein has been found to occur in a small percentage of patients (0.8% to 2.4%). This is usually painless, detectable only by careful palpation and may not appear for 1 or 2 weeks after injection. No sequelae have been noted. The vein gradually shrinks or recanalizes.

Overdosage

➤*Symptoms:* Overdosage of sulfonylureas, including tolbutamide sodium, will produce symptoms of hypoglycemia. The symptoms produced may be mild, consisting only of sweating, trembling, weakness, fatigue, nervousness, hunger, or nausea. They may be more severe, including lethargy, confusion, stupor, loss of consciousness, or coma. Seizures may occur with marked hypoglycemia. In these cases, laboratory evaluation will reveal a low blood glucose level.

The dose of medication that may cause hypoglycemia in humans is variable. In some individuals, usual therapeutic doses have been known to cause symptomatic hypoglycemia.

➤*Treatment:* Mild symptoms of hypoglycemia without loss of consciousness should be treated aggressively with oral glucose and appropriate adjustment in drug dosage and meal patterns. Monitoring should continue until such time as the patient is out of danger. Severe hypoglycemic reactions with coma, seizure, or other neurological impairment are rare, but constitute medical emergencies and require immediate hospitalization. If hypoglycemic coma is suspected or diagnosed, the patient should be given a rapid IV injection of concentrated (50%) dextrose solution. This can be repeated as needed. This should be followed by a continuous infusion of a more dilute (10%) dextrose solution at a rate which will maintain the blood glucose level above 100 mg/dL. Patients should be closely monitored in the hospital for a minimum of 24 to 48 hours, since hypoglycemia may recur after apparent clinical recovery.

Overdosage with sulfonylurea drugs has not been reported to be responsive to either peritoneal dialysis or hemodialysis. The experience, however, is quite limited.

METHACHOLINE CHLORIDE

Rx	**Provocholine** (Methapharm)	**Solution for inhalation (after reconstitution of powder):** 100 mg per 5 ml	In 5 ml vials.

METHACHOLINE CHLORIDE — INHALATION

WARNING

Methacholine chloride powder for inhalation is a bronchoconstrictor agent for diagnostic purposes only and should not be used as a therapeutic agent. Methacholine chloride powder for inhalation challenge should be performed only under the supervision of a physician trained in and thoroughly familiar with all aspects of the technique of methacholine challenge, all contraindications, warnings and precautions, and the management of respiratory distress.

Emergency equipment and medication should be immediately available to treat acute respiratory distress.

Methacholine chloride powder for inhalation should be administered only by inhalation. Severe bronchoconstriction and reduction in respiratory function can result from the administration of methacholine chloride powder for inhalation. Patients with severe hyperreactivity of the airways can experience bronchoconstriction at a dosage as low as 0.025 mg/mL (0.125 cumulative units). If severe bronchoconstriction occurs, it should be reversed immediately by the administration of a rapid-acting inhaled bronchodilator agent (beta-agonist). Because of the potential for severe bronchoconstriction, provocholine (methacholine chloride powder for inhalation) challenge should not be performed in any patient with clinically apparent asthma, wheezing, or very low baseline pulmonary function tests (eg, FEV^1 less than 1 to 1.5 L or less than 70% of the predicted values). Please consult standard nomograms for predicted values.

Indications

➤*Bronchial airway hyperreactivity:* For the diagnosis of bronchial airway hyperreactivity in subjects who do not have clinically apparent asthma.

Administration and Dosage

Before methacholine chloride powder for inhalation challenge is begun, baseline pulmonary function tests must be performed. A subject to be challenged must have an FEV_1 of at least 70% of the predicted value.

The target level for a positive challenge is a 20% reduction in the FEV_1 compared with the baseline value after inhalation of the control sodium chloride solution. This target value should be calculated and recorded before methacholine chloride powder for inhalation challenge is started.

➤*Dilutions:* (Note: Do not inhale powder. Do not handle this material if you have asthma or hay fever.) All dilutions should be made with 0.9% sodium chloride injection containing 0.4% phenol (pH 7) using sterile, empty USP Type I borosilicate glass vials. After adding the sodium chloride solution, shake each vial to obtain a clear solution.

Dilution sequence for single patient testing		
Vials		Concentrations
A	Add 4 mL of 0.9% sodium chloride injection containing 0.4% phenol (pH 7) to the 20 mL vial containing 100 mg of methacholine chloride powder for inhalation. This is vial A.	25 mg/mL
B	Remove 1 mL from vial A, transfer to another vial and add 1.5 mL of 0.9% sodium chloride injection containing 0.4% phenol (pH 7). This is vial B.	10 mg/mL
C	Remove 1 mL from vial A, transfer to another vial and add 9 mL of 0.9% sodium chloride injection containing 0.4% phenol (pH 7). This is vial C.	2.5 mg/mL
D	Remove 1 mL from vial C, transfer to another vial and add 9 mL of 0.9% sodium chloride injection containing 0.4% phenol (pH 7). This is vial D.	0.25 mg/mL
E	Remove 1 mL from vial D, transfer to another vial and add 9 mL of 0.9% sodium chloride injection containing 0.4% phenol (pH 7). This is vial E. Vial E must be prepared on the day of challenge	0.025 mg/mL

A sterile bacterial-retentive filter (porosity 0.22 mcm should be used when transferring a solution from each vial (at least 2 mL) to a nebulizer.

➤*Procedure:* The challenge is performed by giving a subject ascending serial concentrations of methacholine chloride powder for inhalation. At each concentration, 5 breaths are administered by a nebulizer that permits intermittent delivery time of 0.6 seconds by a breath-actuated timing device (dosimeter).

At each of 5 inhalations of a serial concentration, the subject begins at functional residual capacity (FRC) and slowly and completely inhales the dose delivered. Within 5 minutes, FEV_1 values are determined. The procedure ends either when there is a 20% or greater reduction in the FEV_1 compared with the baseline sodium chloride solution value (ie, a positive response) or if 188.88 total cumulative units has been administered (see data below) and the FEV_1 has been reduced by 14% or less (ie, a negative response). If there is a reduction of 15% to 19% in the FEV_1 compared with baseline, either the challenge may be repeated at that concentration or a higher concentration may be given a long as the dosage administered does not result in total cumulative units exceeding 188.88.

The following is a suggested schedule for the administration of methacholine chloride powder for inhalation challenge. Cumulative units are calculated by multiplying the number of breaths by the concentration administered. Total cumulative units is the sum of cumulative units for each concentration administered.

Serial concentration	Number of breaths	Cumulative units per concentration	Total cumulative units
0.025 mg/mL	5	0.125	0.125
0.25 mg/mL	5	1.25	1.375
2.5 mg/mL	5	12.5	13.88
10 mg/mL	5	50	63.88
25 mg/mL	5	125	188.88

An inhaled beta agonist may be administered after methacholine chloride powder for inhalation challenge to expedite the return of the FEV_1 to baseline and to relieve the discomfort of the subject. Most patients revert to healthy pulmonary function within 5 minutes following bronchodilators or within 30 to 45 minutes without any bronchodilator.

➤*Storage/Stability:* Store the powder at 15° to 30°C (59° to 86°F). Refrigerate the reconstituted solutions (dilutions A to D) at 2° to 8°C (36° to 46°F) for not more than 2 weeks, then discard the vials. Freezing does not affect the stability of dilutions A through D. Dilution E must be prepared on the day of the challenge.

Actions

➤*Pharmacology:* Methacholine chloride is the β-methyl homolog of acetylcholine and differs from the latter primarily in its greater duration and selectivity of action. Bronchial smooth muscle contains significant parasympathetic (cholinergic) innervation.

Bronchoconstriction occurs when the vagus nerve is stimulated and acetylcholine is released from the nerve endings. Muscle constriction is essentially confined to the local site of release because acetylcholine is rapidly inactivated by acetylcholinesterase.

Compared with acetylcholine, methacholine chloride is more slowly hydrolyzed by acetylcholinesterase and is almost totally resistant to inactivation by nonspecific cholinesterase or pseudocholinesterase.

When a sodium chloride solution containing methacholine chloride is inhaled, subjects with asthma are markedly more sensitive to methacholine-induced bronchoconstriction than are healthy subjects. This difference in response is the pharmacologic basis for the methacholine chloride powder for inhalation diagnostic challenge. However, it should be recognized that methacholine challenge may occasionally be positive after influenza, upper respiratory tract infections or immunizations. In very young or very old patients, or in patients with chronic lung disease (cystic fibrosis, sarcoidosis, tuberculosis, chronic obstructive pulmonary disease). The challenge may also be positive in patients with allergic rhinitis without asthma, in smokers, in patients after exposure to air pollutants, or in patients who have had or will in the future develop asthma.

Contraindications

Known hypersensitivity to this drug or to other parasympathomimetic agents; repeated administration of methacholine other than on the day of challenge with increasing doses; patients receiving any beta-adrenergic blocking agent because in such patients responses to methacholine can be exaggerated or prolonged, and may not respond as readily to treatment (see Warning Box).

Warnings

➤*Pregnancy: Category C.* Animal reproduction studies have not been conducted with methacholine chloride. It is not known whether methacholine chloride can cause fetal harm when administered to a pregnant patient or affect reproductive capacity. Methacholine chloride should be given to a pregnant woman only if clearly needed.

In females of childbearing potential, the inhalation challenge for methacholine chloride powder for inhalation should be performed either within 10 days following the onset of menses or within 2 weeks of a negative pregnancy test.

➤*Lactation:* The inhalation challenge for methacholine chloride powder for inhalation should not be administered to a breast-feeding mother since it is not known whether methacholine chloride when inhaled is excreted in breast milk.

➤*Children:* The safety and efficacy of methacholine chloride powder for inhalation in the inhalation challenge have not been established in children below the age of 5 years.

Precautions

➤*Special risk:* Administration of methacholine chloride powder for inhalation to patients with epilepsy, cardiovascular disease accompanied by bradycardia, vagotonia, peptic ulcer disease, thyroid disease, urinary tract obstruction or other condition that could be adversely affected by a cholin-

METHACHOLINE CHLORIDE — INHALATION

ergic agent should be undertaken only if the physician feels benefit to the individual outweighs the potential risks.

Adverse Reactions

➤*Inhalation:* Adverse reactions associated with 153 inhaled methacholine chloride challenges include 1 occurrence each of headache, throat irritation, lightheadedness and itching.

➤*Oral or injection:* Methacholine chloride powder for inhalation is to be administered only by inhalation. When administered orally or by injection, methacholine chloride is reported to be associated with nausea and vomiting, substernal pain or pressure, hypotension, fainting and transient complete heart block (see Overdosage).

Overdosage

➤*Symptoms:* Methacholine chloride powder for inhalation is to be administered only by inhalation. When administered orally or by injection, overdosage with methacholine chloride can result in a syncopal reaction, with cardiac arrest and loss of consciousness.

➤*Treatment:* Serious toxic reactions should be treated with 0.5 mg to 1 mg of atropine sulfate, administered IM or IV.

Patient Information

1.) Patients should be instructed regarding symptoms that may occur as a result of the test and how such symptoms can be managed.
2.) A female patient should inform her physician if she is pregnant, or the date of her last onset of menses, or the date and result of her last pregnancy test (see Warnings, Pregnancy).

Gastrointestinal Function Tests

SECRETIN

Rx	**SecreFlo** (Repligen)	**Powder for injection, lyophilized:** 16 mcg of purified secretin	In vials.[1]

[1] With 20 mg mannitol, 15 mg L-cysteine.

SECRETIN — INJECTION

Indications

➤*Pancreatic secretin stimulation:* For the stimulation of pancreatic secretions, including bicarbonate, to aid in the diagnosis of pancreatic exocrine dysfunction.

For the stimulation of pancreatic secretions to facilitate the identification of the ampulla of Vater and accessory papilla during endoscopic retrograde cholangiopancreatography (ERCP).

Gastrin secretion stimulation – For the stimulation of gastrin secretion to aid in the diagnosis of gastrinoma.

Administration and Dosage

➤*Approved by the FDA:* April 4, 2002.

➤*Preparation for administration:* Dissolve the contents of the vial of secretin injection in 8 mL of sodium chloride injection to yield a concentration of 2 mcg/mL. Shake vigorously to ensure dissolution. Use immediately after reconstitution. Discard any unused portion after reconstitution.

➤*Dosage:*

To stimulate pancreatic secretions, including bicarbonate, to aid in the diagnosis of exocrine pancreas dysfunction – 0.2 mcg/kg body weight by IV injection over 1 minute.

Stimulation of gastrin secretion to aid in the diagnosis of gastrinoma: – 0.4 mcg/kg body weight by IV injection over 1 minute.

Facilitation of the identification of the ampulla of Vater and accessory papilla during ERCP to aid in the cannulation of the pancreatic ducts: – 0.2 mcg/kg body weight by IV injection over 1 minute.

➤*Administration:*

To stimulate pancreatic secretions, including bicarbonate, to aid in the diagnosis of exocrine pancreas dysfunction – A radiopaque, double-lumen tube is passed through the mouth following a 12- to 15-hour fast. Under fluoroscopic control, the opening of the proximal lumen of the tube is placed in the gastric antrum and the opening of the distal lumen just beyond the papilla of Vater. The positioning of the tube must be confirmed and the tube secured prior to secretin injection testing. Intermittent negative pressure of 25 to 40 mm Hg is applied to both lumens and maintained throughout the test. When duodenal contents have a pH of greater than or equal to 6, a baseline sample of duodenal fluids is collected for a 10 minute period. A test dose of secretin injection 0.2 mcg (0.1 mL) is injected IV to test of possible allergies. After 1 minute, if there are no untoward reactions, secretin injection at a dose of 0.2 mcg/kg of body weight is injected IV over 1 minute. Duodenal fluid is collected for 60 minutes thereafter. The aspirate is divided into 4 collection periods of 15 minutes each. The duodenal lumen of the tube is cleared with an injection of air after collection of each sample. Wide variation in volume of the aspirate is indicative of incomplete aspiration. Each sample of duodenal fluid is to be chilled and subsequently analyzed for volume and bicarbonate concentration. Exocrine pancreas dysfunction typically associated with chronic pancreatitis is indicated if the peak bicarbonate concentration for any sample is less than 80 mEq/L.

Stimulation of gastrin to aid in the diagnosis of gastrinoma – The patient should have fasted for at least 12 hours prior to beginning the test. Before injecting secretin, 2 blood samples are drawn for determination of fasting serum gastrin levels (baseline values). Subsequently, a test dose of secretin injection 0.2 mcg (0.1 mL) is injected IV, to test for possible allergies. If no untoward reactions, 0.4 mcg/kg of secretin injection is administered IV over 1 minute; postinjection blood samples are collected after 1, 2, 5, 10, and 30 minutes for determination of serum gastrin concentrations. Gastrinoma is strongly suspected in patients who show an increase in serum gastrin concentration of more than 110 pg/mL over basal levels on any of the postinjection samples.

Facilitation of the identification of the ampulla of Vater and accessory papilla during ERCP – When difficulty is encountered by the endoscopist in identifying the ampulla of Vater or in identifying the accessory papilla in patients with pancreas divisum, administration of secretin at a dose of 0.2 mcg/kg of body weight IV over 1 minute will result in visible excretion of pancreatic fluids from the orifices of these papillae enabling their identification and facilitating cannulation.

➤*Storage/Stability:* The unreconstituted product should be stored at −20°C (−4°F) (freezer).

Actions

➤*Pharmacology:* The primary action of secretin injection is to increase the volume and bicarbonate content of secreted pancreatic juices. The standard unit of activity used for secretin injection is the clinical unit defined by Jorpes & Mutt in 1966. In the validated cat bioassay, which was used to define and quantitate the biological activity of secretin and as the release test for the biologically derived porcine secretin product, secretin demonstrates a potency of approximately 5,000 clinical units per milligram of peptide as opposed to 3,000 clinical units per mg for biologically derived porcine secretin. As a pure peptide drug product, secretin dosing is expressed by weight in micrograms. The relationship of micrograms of secretin to biological activity is 0.2 mcg = 1 clinical unit.

➤*Pharmacokinetics:*

Absorption – The pharmacokinetic profile for secretin injection was evaluated in 12 healthy subjects. After IV bolus administration of 0.4 mcg/kg, secretin concentration rapidly declines to baseline secretin levels within 60 to 90 minutes in most of the healthy volunteers studied.

Excretion – The elimination half-life of secretin is 27 minutes. The clearance of secretin is 487 ± 136 mL/minute and the volume of distribution is about 2 L.

Contraindications

Do not administer secretin injection to patients with acute pancreatitis until the acute episode has subsided.

Warnings

➤*Hypersensitivity reactions:* Because of a potential allergic reaction to secretin injection, give patients an IV test dose of 0.2 mcg (0.1 mL). If no allergic reaction is noted after 1 minute, the recommended dose for the specific indication may be injected slowly over 1 minute. A test dose is especially important in patients with a history of atopic allergy and/or asthma. Appropriate measures for the treatment of acute hypersensitivity reactions should be immediately available. No allergic reactions were observed after the test dose or full dose of secretin injection in over 981 patients.

➤*Elderly:* Among the 981 patients who have received secretin injection in clinical trials, 16% were 65 years of age or older and 11% were 75 years of age or older. Dosing was identical to the overall population of patients. No overall differences in safety, pharmacological response, or diagnostic efficacy were observed between these subjects and younger subjects, and other reported clinical experience has not identified differences in responses between the elderly and the younger patients; however, greater sensitivity of some older individuals cannot be ruled out.

➤*Pregnancy: Category C.* Animal reproduction studies have not been conducted with secretin injection. It is also not known whether secretin injection can cause fetal harm when administered to a pregnant woman or can affect reproduction capacity. Give secretin to a pregnant woman only if clearly needed.

➤*Lactation:* It is not known whether secretin injection is excreted in human milk. Because many drugs are excreted in human milk, exercise caution when secretin injection is administered to a breast-feeding woman.

➤*Children:* Safety and efficacy in pediatric patients have not been established.

Precautions

➤*Special risk:* Patients who have undergone vagotomy, are receiving anticholinergic agents at the time of secretin stimulation testing, or who have inflammatory bowel disease may be hyporesponsive to secretin stimulation. This response does not indicate pancreatic disease. A greater than normal

SECRETIN — INJECTION

volume response to secretin stimulation, which may mask coexisting pancreatic disease, is occasionally encountered in patients with alcoholic or other liver disease.

Drug Interactions

➤*Anticholinergics:* The concomitant use of anticholinergic agents may make patients hyporesponsive (ie, may produce a false positive result).

Adverse Reactions

Adverse Reactions	
	Secretin injection (n = 981)
Reaction	Incidence (patients)
Abdominal cramps	2% (2)
Abdominal discomfort	7% (7)
Bleeding (sphincterectomy)	6% (6)
Bleeding (upper GI 2° to endoscopic abrasion)	2% (2)
Bloating	1% (1)
Bradycardia (mild)	2% (2)
Burning in stomach	3% (2)
Decreased blood pressure	6% (5)
Diaphoresis	6% (4)
Diarrhea	1% (1)
Endoscopic perforation of pancreatic duct	2% (2)
Fatigue	1% (1)
Fever	1% (1)
Flushing	6% (5)

Adverse Reactions	
	Secretin injection (n = 981)
Reaction	Incidence (patients)
Headache	2% (2)
Hot sensation	1% (1)
Hunger pangs	1% (1)
Leukocytoplastic vasculitis	1% (1)
Light-headedness	3% (2)
Nausea	8% (8)
Numbness/Tingling in extremities	2% (1)
Pallor	1% (1)
Possible seizure	1% (1)
Abdominal rash	1% (1)
Thready pulse	1% (1)
Transient low O_2 saturation	1% (1)
Transient respiratory distress	2% (2)
Urticaria 2° contrast material (prior to secretin injection administration)	1% (1)
Vomiting	1% (1)
Total patients with adverse reactions	73% (7.4%)

Overdosage

A single IV 20 mcg/kg secretin injection dose was not lethal to mice or rabbits.

SIMETHICONE-COATED CELLULOSE

Rx	**SonoRx** (Bracco Diagnostics)	**Oral suspension:** 7.5 mg/mL simethicone-coated cellulose	Fructose. Orange flavor. In 400 mL single-dose glass bottles.

SIMETHICONE-COATED CELLULOSE — ORAL

Indications

➤*Diagnostic ultrasound imaging agent:* An orally administered gas shadowing reduction agent used to enhance the delineation of upper abdominal anatomy in conjunction with ultrasound imaging. Simethicone-coated cellulose suspension (SCCS) is not indicated as a therapeutic antiflatuence or GI motility agent.

Administration and Dosage

➤*Approved by the FDA:* October 29, 1998.

The recommended dose of SCCS is 400 mL administered orally over 15 minutes. Take after fasting for at least 4 hours.

➤*Imaging:* Begin abdominal ultrasound imaging within 10 minutes after completing the ingestion of SCCS.

➤*Drug preparation:* Prior to administration, invert the container of SCCS and shake vigorously to resuspend any material that has settled. Let the suspension stand unopened for 2 minutes before administration to the patient to allow excess air to escape.

➤*Storage/Stability:* Store at controlled room temperature 20° to 25°C (68° to 77°F). Do not freeze.

Actions

➤*Pharmacology:* SCCS is an aqueous suspension diagnostic ultrasound imaging agent that consists of 22-micron cellulose fibers coated with 0.25% simethicone and is intended for oral administration. SCCS, when resuspended, acts locally within the GI tract to adsorb and disperse gas within the bowel lumen.

➤*Pharmacokinetics:*

Metabolism – Metabolic studies of simethicone coated cellulose were not conducted. Cellulose is not metabolized by humans.

Excretion – The cellulose component of SCCS is eliminated in the feces.The kinetics of SCCS were evaluated in a vehicle control study of 10 healthy volunteers; 7 received SCCS, 3 received the control. Silicon measurements in the blood and urine were monitored as the surrogate marker for simethicone. Silicon was measured over 5 days before dosing, and at 15 and 30 minutes, and 1, 2, 3, 6, 10, 15, 24, and 48 hours after dosing. In these subjects, the concentrations of silicon detected in the blood (6.04 to 7.47 mcg/mL) in 2 of the SCCS treated subjects before SCCS were similar to those detected in the blood after SCCS (5.61 to 11.42 mcg/mL).

The other 5 SCCS-treated subjects did not have silicon detected in the blood before SCCS, and 2 of the 5 had levels of silicon detected after SCCS; however, these levels were similar to those subjects who had silicon detected in the blood before and after SCCS. Urine levels of silicon in all subjects were similar before and after SCCS. The silicon levels in the blood and urine before and after the control were similar to those before and after SCCS.

Special populations – The pharmacokinetics and rate of fecal elimination was studied in 15 patients with impaired bowel motility or impaired bowel mucosa. Of these patients, 12 received SCCS and 3 received the vehicle. In these patients, the detection of silicon, as a surrogate marker for simethicone, in the blood and urine was similar to that of the healthy volunteers reported in the preceding pharmacokinetics section.

As in the healthy volunteers, the cellulose component of SCCS was eliminated in feces. Based on the fraction of ingested fiber that was eliminated in feces following the administration of SCCS, the rate of fecal elimination of cellulose appears to be lower in the patients with impaired bowel motility or impaired bowel mucosa than in the healthy volunteers.

Contraindications

Known or suspected intestinal perforation and obstruction (see Warnings); allergy to its active or inactive ingredients.

Warnings

➤*Aspiration:* The ingestion of SCCS may cause vomiting that could be associated with aspiration. Of the 385 patients or healthy volunteers who received SCCS, nausea was reported in 3.4% and vomiting in 2.1%. Patients who have a tracheoesophageal fistula may aspirate. Take precautions to avoid aspiration.

➤*Peritoneal tissues:* The effects of SCCS on human peritoneal tissues have not been studied. In rats, throughout a 3-month study observation period, after the intraperitoneal injection of SCCS at the lowest test dose of 5 mL/kg, capsular granulomatous inflammation of the spleen, liver, and kidneys, and apparent accumulation of cellulose in the red pulp of the spleen and glomeruli of the kidneys were observed. The effects of SCCS on human peritoneal tissues are not known.

➤*Pregnancy: Category B.* Adequate and well-controlled clinical studies have not been conducted in pregnant women. Use in pregnancy only if essential.

➤*Lactation:* Studies have not been conducted to determine whether SCCS is excreted in breast milk. Exercise caution when administering to a breast-feeding woman.

➤*Children:* Safety and efficacy in children have not been established. Dose adjustments for the capacity of the upper GI tract have not been studied.

SIMETHICONE-COATED CELLULOSE — ORAL

Precautions

➤*GI effects:* SCCS is associated with nausea, vomiting, and abdominal pain. In patients who have these symptoms before the ingestion of SCCS, the symptoms could increase in severity. This could confound the ability to distinguish adverse effects of SCCS from the signs and symptoms of obstruction or perforation and from any preexisting conditions.

Patients who have a current or recent history of hiatal hernia, esophageal reflux, nausea, vomiting, or abdominal pain may not be able to tolerate SCCS. Studies have not been conducted in these patients.

➤*Fluid shifts/intake:* Give SCCS with caution to patients who cannot tolerate large fluid shifts and who are on specific fluid intake requirements.

Adverse Reactions

Of the 448 subjects evaluated, 18% who received SCCS and 12% who received a control agent reported at least 1 adverse event. Of the subjects who received SCCS, at least 1 adverse event was reported in 19% of patients and 8% of healthy volunteers. Deaths or serious adverse events were not reported during the study observation period.

The most frequently reported adverse events were associated with the digestive system. Diarrhea was reported in 5.5%, nausea in 3.4%, and vomiting in 2.1% of subjects who received SCCS. Orange-colored stools may occur.

Simethicone Coated Cellulose Suspension Adverse Reactions (> 0.5%)

Adverse reaction	SCCS control (n = 385)	Control agent (n = 138)
GI		
Diarrhea	5.5	2.9
Dyspepsia	0.5	1.4
Eructation	1	0.7
Flatulence	0.5	0
Nausea	3.4	0.7
Vomiting	2.1	0
Respiratory		
Pharyngitis	0.5	0
Rhinitis	0.5	0
Miscellaneous		
Abdominal pain	2.1	0.7

Simethicone Coated Cellulose Suspension Adverse Reactions (> 0.5%)

Adverse reaction	SCCS control (n = 385)	Control agent (n = 138)
Back pain	1	0.7
Chest pain	0.8	0.7
Chills	0.5	0
Ear pain	0.5	0
Headache	1.8	0.7
Rash	0.5	0

The following additional adverse events were reported in less than 0.5% of people who received SCCS:

➤*Cardiovascular:* Bradycardia; hematoma; hypertension; pallor; palpitations; tachycardia.

➤*CNS:* Hypertonia; somnolence.

➤*GI:* Dysphagia; dry mouth; melena.

➤*Hematologic/Lymphatic:* Ecchymosis; lymphadenopathy.

➤*Respiratory:* Epistaxis; pneumothorax; sinusitis.

➤*Miscellaneous:* Asthenia; fever; malaise; neck pain; pelvic pain; pain; hypoglycemia; dysuria.

Patient Information

Instruct patients who are candidates to receive SCCS to inform the physician if they are pregnant or breastfeeding.

Inform patients of the following:

SCCS is prescribed for delineation of abdominal anatomy during ultrasound imaging.

- SCCS can cause nausea, vomiting, diarrhea, abdominal pain, or other GI discomfort.
- For most patients, complete elimination of SCCS occurs within 24 to 48 hours following administration.
- Feces may appear orange-colored until SCCS is completely eliminated.

Ask patients if they are able to drink approximately 400 mL (14 oz or 1 pt) over a 15-minute period. Ask patients if they have a hiatal hernia or problems with regurgitation when they lie on their backs after eating.

SINCALIDE

Rx	**Kinevac** (Bracco Diagnostics)	**Powder for injection, lyophilized:** 5 mcg/vial for reconstitution (1 mcg/mL when reconstituted)	In vials.

SINCALIDE — INJECTION

Indications

➤*Gallbladder contraction stimulation:* To stimulate gallbladder contraction, as may be assessed by contrast agent cholecystography or ultrasonography, or to obtain by duodenal aspiration a sample of concentrated bile for analysis of cholesterol, bile salts, phospholipids, and crystals.

➤*Pancreatic secretion stimulation:* To stimulate pancreatic secretion (especially in conjunction with secretin) prior to obtaining a duodenal aspirate for analysis of enzyme activity, composition, and cytology.

➤*Barium meal transit time acceleration:* To accelerate the transit of a barium meal through the small bowel, thereby decreasing the time and extent of radiation associated with fluoroscopy and X-ray examination of the intestinal tract.

Administration and Dosage

➤*Contraction of the gallbladder:* 0.02 mcg/kg (1.4 mcg/70 kg) injected IV over 30 to 60 seconds; if satisfactory gallbladder contraction does not occur in 15 minutes, a second dose (0.04 mcg/kg) may be given. To reduce the intestinal side effects, an IV infusion may be prepared at a dose of 0.12 mcg/kg in 100 mL of Sodium Chloride Injection and given at a rate of 2 mL/min; alternatively, an IM dose of 0.1 mcg/kg may be given. When sincalide is used in cholecystography, roentgenograms are usually taken at 5-minute intervals after the injection. For visualization of the cystic duct, it may be necessary to take roentgenograms at 1-minute intervals during the first 5 minutes after the injection.

➤*Barium meal transit time acceleration:* To accelerate the transit time of a barium meal through the small bowel, administer sincalide after the barium meal is beyond the proximal jejunum. (Sincalide, like cholecystoidnin, may cause pyloric contraction.) The recommended dose is 0.04 mcg/kg sincalide (2.8 mcg/70 kg) injected IV over a 30- to 60-second interval; if satisfactory transit of the barium meal has not occurred in 30 minutes, a second dose of 0.04 mcg/kg sincalide may be administered. For reduction of side effects, a 30-minute IV infusion of sincalide (0.12 mcg/kg [8.4 mcg/70 kg] diluted to approximately 100 mL with Sodium Chloride Injection) may be administered.

➤*Pancreatic secretion stimulation:* Secretin dose of 0.25 units/kg is infused IV over 60 minutes. Thirty minutes after initiating secretin, give a separate IV infusion of sincalide at a total dose of 0.02 mcg/kg over 30 minutes. For example, the total dose for a 70 kg patient is 1.4 mcg sincalide; therefore, dilute 1.4 mL reconstituted sincalide solution to 30 mL with Sodium Chloride Injection and administer at a rate of 1 mL/min.

➤*Preparation of solution:* To reconstitute, add 5 mL Sterile Water for Injection to the vial; make any additional dilution with 0.9% Sodium Chloride for Injection. The solution may be kept at room temperature. Use within 24 hours after reconstitution; discard any unused portion.

➤*Storage/Stability:* Store at room temperature 15° to 30° C (59° to 86° F) prior to reconstitution.

Actions

➤*Pharmacology:* Sincalide IV substantially reduces gallbladder size by causing it to contract. The evacuation of bile that results is similar to the physiological response to endogenous cholecystokinin. Bolus IV administration causes a prompt contraction of the gallbladder that becomes maximal in 5 to 15 minutes, as compared with the stimulus of a fatty meal, which causes a progressive contraction that becomes maximal after approximately 40 minutes. Generally, a 40% reduction in radiographic area of the gallbladder is satisfactory, although some patients will show area reduction of 60% to 70%.

Like cholecystokinin, sincalide stimulates pancreatic secretion; concurrent administration with secretin increases the volume of pancreatic secretion and the output of bicarbonate and protein (enzymes) by the gland. This combined effect of secretin and sincalide permits the assessment of specific pancreatic function through measurement and analysis of the duodenal aspirate. The parameters determined are the following: Volume of the secretion; bicarbonate concentration; amylase content (which parallels the content of trypsin and total protein).

Cholecystokinin and sincalide stimulate intestinal motility and may cause pyloric contraction, which retards gastric emptying.

Contraindications

Hypersensitivity to sincalide; intestinal obstruction.

Warnings

➤*Pregnancy:* *Category B.* There are no adequate and well-controlled studies in pregnant women. Because animal reproduction studies are not always predictive of human response, use this drug during pregnancy only if clearly needed.

SINCALIDE — INJECTION

Do not administer sincalide to pregnant women near term because of its effect on smooth muscle; the possibility of prematurely inducing labor exists.

➤*Lactation:* It is not known whether this drug is excreted in human milk. Because many drugs are excreted in human milk, exercise caution when sincalide is administered to a breast-feeding woman.

➤*Children:* The safety for use in children has not been established.

Precautions

➤*Gallbladder stones:* Stimulation of gallbladder contraction in patients with small gallbladder stones may lead to the evacuation of the stones, resulting in their lodging in the cystic duct or in the common bile duct. The risk is minimal because sincalide, when given as directed, does not ordinarily cause complete contraction of the gallbladder.

Adverse Reactions

➤*Most frequent:* Reactions to sincailde are generally mild and of short duration. The most frequent adverse reactions were abdominal discomfort or pain, and nausea; rapid IV injection of 0.04 mcg/kg sincalide expectably causes transient abdominal cramping. These phenomena are usually manifestations of the physiologic action of the drug, including delayed gastric emptying and increased intestinal motility. These reactions occurred in approximately 20% of patients; they are not to be construed as necessarily indicating an abnormality of the biliary tract unless there is other clinical or radiologic evidence of disease.

The incidence of other adverse reactions, including vomiting, flushing, sweating, rash, hypotension, hypertension, shortness of breath, urge to defecate, headache, diarrhea, sneezing, and numbness was less than 1%; dizziness was reported in approximately 2% of patients. These manifestations are usually lessened by slower injection rate.

Overdosage

➤*Symptoms:* GI symptoms (abdominal cramps, nausea, vomiting, and diarrhea) should be expected. Hypotension with dizziness or fainting might also occur. Starting with single bolus IV injection comparable with the human dose of 0.4 mg/kg, sincalide caused hypotension and bradycardia in dogs. Higher doses injected once or repeatedly in dogs caused syncope and ECG changes in addition. These effects were attributed to sincalide-induced vagal stimulation in that all were prevented by pretreatment with atropine or bilateral vagotomy.

➤*Treatment:* Treat overdosage symptoms symptomatically over a short duration.

DIPYRIDAMOLE

Rx	**Dipyridamole** (Various, eg, American Pharm., Bedford, ESI Lederle)	**Injection**: 5 mg/ml[1]	In 2 and 10 ml vials.

[1] With 50 mg polyethylene glycol 600 and 2 mg tartaric acid.

DIPYRIDAMOLE — INJECTION

Dipyridamole oral is used as an antiplatelet agent. Refer to the individual monograph in the Hematologic Agents chapter.

Indications

➤*Diagnostic aid:* As an alternative to exercise in thallium-201 myocardial perfusion imaging for the evaluation of coronary artery disease in patients who cannot exercise adequately.

Administration and Dosage

➤*Approved by the FDA:* December 13, 1990.

➤*Dosage:* The dose of IV dipyridamole as an adjunct to thallium-201 myocardial perfusion imaging should be adjusted according to the weight of the patient. The recommended dose is 0.142 mg/kg/min (0.57 mg/kg total) infused over 4 minutes. Although the maximum tolerated dose has not been determined, clinical experience suggests that a total dose beyond 60 mg is not needed for any patient.

➤*Preparation/administration:* Prior to IV administration, dipyridamole injection should be diluted in at least a 1:2 ratio with 0.45% sodium chloride injection, 0.9% sodium chloride injection, or 5% dextrose injection for a total volume of approximately 20 to 50 mL. Infusion of undiluted dipyridamole may cause local irritation.

Thallium-201 should be injected within 5 minutes following the 4-minute infusion of dipyridamole.

➤*Admixture incompatibility:* Do not mix dipyridamole injection with other drugs in the same syringe or infusion container.

➤*Storage/Stability:* Store between 15° to 25°C (59° to 77°F). Avoid freezing. Protect from light. Retain in carton until time of use. Discard unused portion.

Actions

➤*Pharmacology:* In a study of 10 patients with angiographically normal or minimally stenosed (less than 25% luminal diameter narrowing) coronary vessels, dipyridamole injection in a dose of 0.56 mg/kg infused over 4 minutes resulted in an average fivefold increase in coronary blood flow velocity compared to resting coronary flow velocity (range 3.8 to 7 times resting velocity). The mean time to peak flow velocity was 6.5 minutes from the start of the 4-minute infusion (range 2.5 to 8.7 minutes). Cardiovascular responses to the IV administration of dipyridamole when given to patients in the supine position include a mild but significant increase in heart rate of approximately 20% and mild but significant decreases in both systolic and diastolic blood pressure of approximately 2% to 8%, with vital signs returning to baseline values in approximately 30 minutes.

Dipyridamole is a coronary vasodilator. The mechanism of vasodilation has not been fully elucidated, but may result from inhibition of uptake of adenosine, an important mediator of coronary vasodilation. The vasodilatory effects of dipyridamole are abolished by administration of the adenosine receptor antagonist theophylline.

How dipyridamole-induced vasodilation leads to abnormalities in thallium-201 distribution and ventricular function is also uncertain but presumably represents a "steal" phenomenon in which relatively intact vessels dilate, and sustain enhanced flow, leaving reduced pressure and flow across areas of hemodynamically important coronary vascular constriction.

➤*Pharmacokinetics:*

Absorption/Distribution – Plasma dipyridamole concentrations decline in a triexponential fashion following IV infusion of dipyridamole with half-lives averaging 3 to 12 minutes, 33 to 62 minutes, and 11.6 to 15 hours. Two minutes following a 0.568 mg/kg dose of IV dipyridamole administered as a 4–minute IV infusion, the mean dipyridamole serum concentration is 4.6 ± 1.3 mcg/mL. The average plasma protein binding of dipyridamole is approximately 99%, primarily to α_1-glycoprotein. The average total body clearance is 2.3 to 3.5 mL/min/kg, with an apparent volume of distribution at steady state of 1 to 2.5 L/kg and a central apparent volume of 3 to 5 L.

Metabolism/Excretion – Dipyridamole is metabolized in the liver to the glucuronic acid conjugate and excreted with the bile.

Contraindications

Hypersensitivity to dipyridamole.

Warnings

➤*Cardiotoxicity and bronchospasm:* Serious adverse reactions associated with the administration of IV dipyridamole have included cardiac death, fatal and non-fatal myocardial infarction, ventricular fibrillation, symptomatic ventricular tachycardia, stroke, transient cerebral ischemia, seizures, anaphylactoid reaction and bronchospasm. There have been reported cases of asystole, sinus node arrest, sinus node depression and conduction block. Patients with abnormalities of cardiac impulse formation/conduction or severe coronary artery disease may be at increased risk for these events.

In a study of 3911 patients given IV dipyridamole as an adjunct to thallium-201 myocardial perfusion imaging, 2 types of serious adverse events were reported: 1) four cases of myocardial infarction (0.1%), 2 fatal (0.05%); and 2 non-fatal (0.05%); and 2) six cases of severe bronchospasm (0.2%). Although the incidence of these serious adverse events was small (0.3%, 10 of 3911), the potential clinical information to be gained through use of IV dipyridamole thallium-201 imaging must be weighed against the risk to the patient. The sensitivity of the dipyridamole test (true positive dipyridamole divided by the total number of patients with positive angiography) was about 85%. The specificity (true negative divided by the number of patients with negative angiograms) was about 50%. Patients with a history of unstable angina may be at a greater risk for severe myocardial ischemia. Patients with a history of asthma may be at a greater risk for bronchospasm during IV dipyridamole use.

When thallium-201 myocardial perfusion imaging is performed with IV dipyridamole, parenteral aminophylline should be readily available for relieving adverse events such as bronchospasm or chest pain. Vital signs should be monitored during, and for 10 to 15 minutes following, the IV infusion of dipyridamole and an electrocardiographic tracing should be obtained using at least 1 chest lead. Should severe chest pain or bronchospasm occur, parenteral aminophylline may be administered by slow IV injection (50 to 100 mg over 30 to 60 seconds) in doses ranging from 50 to 250 mg. In the case of severe hypotension, the patient should be placed in a supine position with the head tilted down if necessary, before administration of parenteral aminophylline. If 250 mg of aminophylline does not relieve chest pain symptoms within a few minutes, sublingual nitroglycerin may be administered. If chest pain continues despite use of aminophylline and nitroglycerin, the possibility of myocardial infarction should be considered. If the clinical condition of a patient with an adverse event permits a 1 minute delay in the administration of parenteral aminophylline, thallium-201 may be injected and allowed to circulate for 1 minute before the injection of aminophylline. This will allow initial thallium-201 perfusion imaging to be performed before reversal of the pharmacologic effects of IV dipyridamole on the coronary circulation.

➤*Myasthenia gravis:* Myasthenia gravis patients receiving therapy with cholinesterase inhibitors may experience worsening of their disease in the presence of dipyridamole.

➤*Fertility impairment:* A significant reduction in number of corpora lutea with consequent reduction in implantations and live fetuses was, however, observed at 1250 mg/kg/day.

➤*Pregnancy: Category B.* There are no adequate and well controlled studies in pregnant women. Because animal reproduction studies are not always predictive of human responses, this drug should be used during pregnancy only if clearly needed.

➤*Lactation:* Dipyridamole is excreted in human milk.

➤*Children:* Safety and effectiveness in the pediatric population have not been established.

Drug Interactions

➤*Xanthine derivatives:* Oral maintenance theophylline and other xanthine derivatives such as caffeine may abolish the coronary vasodilatation induced by IV dipyridamole administration. This could lead to a false negative thallium-201 imaging result.

Adverse Reactions

➤*Serious reactions:* See Warnings for more information.

➤*Most frequent:* In the study of 3911 patients, the most frequent adverse reactions were: chest pain/angina pectoris (19.7%), electrocardiographic changes (most commonly ST-T changes) (15.9%), headache (12.2%), and dizziness (11.8%).

Adverse reactions occurring in > 1% of patients

Adverse reaction	Incidence (%) of drug-related adverse reactions
Blood pressure lability	1.6%
Chest pain/angina pectoris	19.7%
Dizziness	11.8%
Dyspnea	2.6%
Electrocardiographic abnormalities/extrasystoles	5.2%
Electrocardiographic abnormalities/ST-T changes	7.5%
Electrocardiographic abnormalities/tachycardia	3.2%
Fatigue	1.2%
Flushing	3.4%
Headache	12.2%
Hypertension	1.5%
Hypotension	4.6%
Nausea	4.6%
Paresthesia	1.3%
Unspecified pain	2.6%

DIPYRIDAMOLE — INJECTION

➤*Cardiovascular:* Electrocardiographic abnormalities unspecified (0.8%), arrhythmia unspecified (0.6%), palpitation (0.3%), ventricular tachycardia (0.2%), bradycardia (0.2%), myocardial infarction (0.1%), AV block (0.1%), syncope (0.1%), orthostatic hypotension (0.1%), atrial fibrillation (0.1%), supraventricular tachycardia (0.1%), ventricular arrhythmia unspecified (0.03%), heart block unspecified (0.03%), cardiomyopathy (0.03%), edema (0.03%).

➤*CNS:* Hypesthesia (0.5%), hypertonia (0.3%), nervousness/anxiety (0.2%), tremor (0.1%), abnormal coordination (0.03%), somnolence (0.03%), dysphonia (0.03%), migraine (0.03%), vertigo (0.03%).

➤*GI:* Dyspepsia (1.0%), dry mouth (0.8%), abdominal pain (0.7%), flatulence (0.6%), vomiting (0.4%), eructation (0.1%), dysphagia (0.03%), tenesmus (0.03%), appetite increased (0.03%).

➤*Respiratory:* Pharyngitis (0.3%), bronchospasm (0.2%; parenteral aminophylline should be readily available), hyperventilation (0.1%), rhinitis (0.1%), coughing (0.03%), pleural pain (0.03%).

➤*Miscellaneous:* Myalgia (0.9%), back pain (0.6%), injection site reaction unspecified (0.4%), diaphoresis (0.4%), asthenia (0.3%), malaise (0.3%), arthralgia (0.3%), injection site pain (0.1%), rigor (0.1%), earache (0.1%), tinnitus (0.1%), vision abnormalities unspecified (0.1%), dysgeusia (0.1%), thirst (0.03%), depersonalization (0.03%), eye pain (0.03%), renal pain (0.03%), perineal pain (0.03%), breast pain (0.03%), intermittent claudication (0.03%), leg cramping (0.03%).

➤*Postmarketing:* there have been rare reports of allergic reaction including urticaria, pruritus, dermatitis and rash.

Overdosage

No cases of overdosage in humans have been reported. It is unlikely that overdosage will occur because of the nature of use (ie, single IV administration in controlled settings).

SERMORELIN ACETATE

Rx	**Geref** (Serono Labs)	**Powder for Injection, lyophilized:** 50 mcg (as the acetate)[1]	In amps with 2 ml of 0.9% Sodium Chloride Injection as a diluent in vials.

[1] With 5 mg mannitol, 0.66 mg monobasic sodium phosphate and 0.04 mg dibasic sodium phosphate; may contain up to 1% albumin (Human).

SERMORELIN ACETATE — INJECTION

Indications

➤*Growth hormone deficiency:* For the treatment of idiopathic growth hormone deficiency in children with growth failure. Most of these short, slowly growing children retain pituitary responsiveness to growth hormone releasing hormone.

➤*Pituitary gland evaluation:* For evaluating the ability of the somatotroph of the pituitary gland to secrete growth hormone (GH).

Administration and Dosage

➤*Approved by the FDA:* December 28, 1990.

➤*Growth hormone deficiency:* 0.03 mg (30 mcg) per kg of body weight once daily at bedtime by SC injection. SC injection sites should be periodically rotated.

Treatment with sermorelin acetate for injection should be discontinued when the epiphyses are fused. Patients who fail to respond adequately while on sermorelin acetate therapy should be evaluated to determine the cause of unresponsiveness.

Height should be assessed at least every 6 months during treatment. During sermorelin acetate therapy, care should be taken to ensure that the child continues to grow at a rate consistent with the child's age and stage of development, and treatment with sermorelin acetate should be reevaluated if the response is inadequate. Treatment with growth hormone should be considered for children with a poor or waning response to sermorelin acetate.

Preparation for administration –

After determining the appropriate patient dose, reconstitute each vial of sermorelin acetate for injection with 0.5 to 1 mL of Sodium Chloride Injection, USP.

➤*Pituitary gland evaluation:* Sermorelin acetate diagnostic dosage should be individualized for each patient according to his/her weight. It is recommended that sermorelin acetate diagnostic be administered in a single intravenous dose of 1 mcg/kg body weight in the morning following an overnight fast.

Children (or subjects less than 50 kg) –

1.) Reconstitute the contents of one 50 mcg ampule of sermorelin acetate diagnostic with a minimum of 0.5 mL of the accompanying sterile diluent.
2.) Venous blood samples for growth hormone determinations should be drawn 15 minutes before and immediately prior to sermorelin acetate diagnostic administration.
3.) Administer a bolus of 1 mcg/kg body weight sermorelin acetate diagnostic intravenously followed by a 3 mL normal saline flush.
4.) Draw venous blood samples for growth hormone determinations at 15, 30, 45, and 60 minutes after sermorelin acetate diagnostic administration.

Adults (or subjects more than 50 kg) –

1.) Determine the number of ampules needed, based on a dose of 1 mcg/kg body weight.
2.) Reconstitute the contents of each ampule with a minimum of 0.5 mL of the accompanying sterile diluent.
3.) Follow steps 2 to 4 above.

Parenteral drug products should be inspected visually for particulate matter and discoloration prior to administration, whenever solution and container permit. The drug should be discarded if not dissolved or if the reconstituted solution is cloudy or discolored.

➤*Storage/Stability:* Vials of sermorelin acetate for injection should be stored refrigerated between 2° to 8°C (36° to 46°F) before reconstitution. After reconstitution with Sodium Chloride Injection, USP, sermorelin should be administered immediately. Discard unused material.

Sermorelin diagnostic – Lyophilized product should be refrigerated (2° to 8°C; 36° to 46°F), use immediately after reconstitution.

Actions

➤*Pharmacology:* Sermorelin acetate for injection increases plasma growth hormone (GH) concentration by stimulating the pituitary gland to release GH. Sermorelin acetate is similar to the native hormone (GRF [1-44]-NH_2) in its ability to stimulate GH secretion in humans.

Diagnostic use – Sermorelin increases plasma growth hormone (GH) concentrations by direct stimulation of the pituitary gland to release GH. Because baseline GH levels are generally very low (less than 4 ng/mL), provocative tests may be useful in determining the functional GH-secreting capability of the pituitary somatotroph. Adults and children with normal responses to standard provocative tests of GH secretion were used to define the range of normal plasma GH-level responses to sermorelin acetate diagnostic. It was found that the absolute peak GH level following sermorelin acetate diagnostic infusion and the time elapsed from infusion to that peak are appropriate measures to evaluate the response to GH infusion. Doses of sermorelin acetate diagnostic used in children and adults in these studies ranged from 0.3 to 6.06 mcg/kg with a majority of patients receiving 1 mcg/kg. Based on these studies and published reports, 1 mcg/kg was chosen as the recommended dose for diagnostic purposes.

➤*Pharmacokinetics:*

Absorption – In SC administration of 2 mg sermorelin to 12 healthy volunteers, peak concentrations of sermorelin were reached in 5 to 20 minutes. The mean absolute bioavailability after SC administration is about 6%.

Distribution – After IV administration of 0.25 to 1 mg sermorelin acetate to 12 healthy volunteers, the mean volume of distribution ranged between 23.7 to 25.8 L.

Excretion – Sermorelin is rapidly cleared from the circulation, with clearance values in adults ranging between 2.4 to 2.8 L/min. The half-life of sermorelin acetate is short, 11 to 12 minutes after either IV or SC administration.

Contraindications

Known sensitivity to sermorelin or any of the excipients.

Warnings

➤*GH deficiency:* A normal plasma GH response to sermorelin acetate diagnostic demonstrates that the somatotroph is intact. However, a normal response does not exclude GH deficiency because this deficiency is frequently the result of hypothalamic dysfunction in the presence of an intact somatotroph. The sermorelin acetate diagnostic stimulation test is most easily interpreted when there is a subnormal response to conventional provocative testing and a normal response to sermorelin acetate diagnostic. Such findings suggest that hypothalamic dysfunction is the cause for the growth hormone deficiency. When both conventional and sermorelin acetate diagnostic testing result in subnormal GH responses, the site of dysfunction cannot be determined with certainty because some patients with GH deficiency due to hypothalamic dysfunction require repeated sermorelin acetate diagnostic administration before demonstrating a normal response.

➤*Acromegaly:* The sermorelin acetate diagnostic test has not been found useful in the diagnosis of acromegaly.

➤*Hypersensitivity reactions:* Although hypersensitivity reactions have been observed with other polypeptide hormones, to date no such reactions have been reported following the administration of a single dose of sermorelin acetate diagnostic. Antibody formation has been reported in humans after chronic subcutaneous administration of large doses of sermorelin (see Adverse Reactions).

As with the administration of any peptide, local or systemic allergic reactions may occur. Parents/Patients should be informed that such reactions are possible and that prompt medical attention should be sought if allergic reactions occur.

➤*Pregnancy: Category C.* During teratology studies sermorelin acetate produced minor variations in fetuses of rats and rabbits when given at a dose of 0.5 mg/kg/day. This dose is approximately 3 and 6 times (88 and 176 times for sermorelin acetate diagnostic) the daily human dose calculated on a body surface area (mg/m^2) basis, for rats and rabbits, respectively.

SERMORELIN ACETATE — INJECTION

There are no adequate and well-controlled studies in pregnant women. Sermorelin acetate should be used during pregnancy only if the potential benefit justifies the potential risk to the fetus.

➤*Lactation:* It is not known whether sermorelin acetate is excreted in human milk. Because many drugs are excreted in human milk, caution should be exercised when sermorelin acetate is administered to a breastfeeding woman.

Precautions

➤*Monitoring:* The growth response of children treated with sermorelin acetate should be evaluated on a periodic basis and children with a poor or waning response should be considered for treatment with growth hormone. The effect of sermorelin acetate therapy beyond 1 year and on final adult height remains to be determined.

Bone age should be monitored periodically during sermorelin acetate administration, especially in patients who are pubertal and/or receiving concomitant thyroid replacement therapy. Under these circumstances, epiphyseal maturation may progress rapidly.

➤*Subnormal GH response:* Obesity, hyperglycemia, and elevated plasma fatty acids generally are associated with subnormal GH responses to sermorelin acetate diagnostic.

➤*Hypothyroidism:* In clinical studies, the incidence of hypothyroidism during sermorelin acetate therapy was 6.5%. In the largest clinical study, 8 of 110 enrolled patients were on thyroid replacement therapy prior to sermorelin acetate therapy and an additional 5 after initiating therapy. Untreated hypothyroidism can jeopardize the response to sermorelin acetate. Therefore, thyroid hormone determinations should be performed before the initiation and throughout the duration of sermorelin acetate therapy. Thyroid hormone replacement therapy should be initiated when indicated.

➤*Intracranial lesions:* Patients with growth hormone deficiency secondary to an intracranial lesion were not studied in clinical trials. It is not recommended that such patients be treated with sermorelin acetate.

➤*Lab test abnormalities:* Serum levels of inorganic phosphorus, alkaline phosphatase, GH and IGF-I may increase with sermorelin acetate therapy.

Drug Interactions

➤*Glucocorticoids:* Concomitant glucocorticoid therapy may inhibit the response to sermorelin acetate.

➤*Interactions with the diagnostic test:* The sermorelin acetate diagnostic test should not be conducted in the presence of drugs that directly affect the pituitary secretion of somatotropin. These include preparations that contain or release somatostatin, insulin, glucocorticoids, or cyclooxygenase inhibitors such as aspirin or indomethacin. Somatotropin levels may be transiently elevated by clonidine, levodopa, and insulin-induced hypoglycemia. Response to sermorelin acetate diagnostic may be blunted in patients who are receiving muscarinic antagonists (atropine) or who are hypothyroid or being treated with antithyroid medication such as propylthiouracil. Exogenous growth hormone therapy should be discontinued at least 1 week before administering the sermorelin acetate diagnostic test.

Adverse Reactions

➤*Growth hormone deficiency:*

Antibody formation – A large proportion of patients develop anti-GRF antibodies at least once during treatment with sermorelin acetate for injection. The significance of these antibodies is not clear and often a positive test at one growth assessment will become negative by the next assessment. The presence of antibodies does not appear to affect growth or appear to be related to a specific adverse reaction profile. No generalized allergic reactions to sermorelin acetate have been reported. The most common treatment-related adverse event (occurring in about 1 patient in 6) is local injection reaction characterized by pain, swelling or redness. Of 350 patients exposed to sermorelin acetate in clinical trials, 3 discontinued therapy due to injection reactions. Other treatment-related adverse events had individual occurrence rates of less than 1% and include headache, flushing, dysphagia, dizziness, hyperactivity, somnolence, and urticaria.

➤*Diagnostic use:* The following adverse reactions have been reported following sermorelin administration:

Antibody formation – Approximately 1 in 4 patients given repeated doses of 1 or more of the 3 forms of GRH (1-29, 1-40, and 1-44) has developed antibodies to GRH. The clinical significance of these antibodies is unknown. One patient who developed antibodies to GRH (1-44) also experienced an allergic reaction described as severe redness, swelling, and urticaria at the injection sites. No long-lasting effects from this reaction were reported. No symptomatic allergic reactions to GRH (1-29) have been reported.

GI – Nausea, vomiting, dysgeusia.

Local – Injection site pain, redness and/or swelling at injection site.

Miscellaneous – Transient warmth or flushing of the face, headache, paleness, tightness in the chest.

Overdosage

➤*Symptoms:* Changes of heart rate and blood pressure have been reported with the various GRH peptides in IV doses exceeding 10 mcg/kg. Cardiovascular collapse is a conceivable, but as of yet, unreported, complication of overdosage with GRH (1-29).

Patient Information

Patients being treated with sermorelin acetate or their parents should be informed of the potential benefits and risks associated with treatment. If home use is determined to be desirable by the physician, instructions on appropriate use should be given, including a review of the contents of this section of the monograph. This information is intended to aid in the safe and effective administration of the medication. It is not a disclosure of all possible adverse or intended effects.

If home use is prescribed, a puncture resistant container for the disposal of used syringes and needles should be recommended to the patient. Patients or parents should be thoroughly instructed in the importance of proper disposal and cautioned against any reuse of needles and syringes.

ADENOSINE

Rx	**Adenoscan** (Fujisawa)	**Injection:** 3 mg/ml	Preservative-free. In 30 ml single-dose vials.

ADENOSINE — INJECTION

For information on the use of adenosine as an antiarrhythmic agent, refer to the monograph in the Cardiovascular Agents chapter.

Indications

➤*Diagnostic aid:* Adjunct to thallium-201 myocardial perfusion scintigraphy in patients unable to exercise adequately.

Administration and Dosage

➤*Approved by the FDA:* Adenosine (diagnostic aid) approved May 1995.

For intravenous infusion only. The safety and efficacy of adenosine administered by the intracoronary route have not been established.

Adenosine should be given as a continuous peripheral intravenous infusion.

The recommended intravenous dose for adults is 140 mcg/kg/min infused for six minutes (total dose of 0.84 mg/kg).

The required dose of thallium-201 should be injected at the midpoint of the adenosine infusion (i.e., after the first three minutes of adenosine). Thallium-201 is physically compatible with adenosine and may be injected directly into the adenosine infusion set.

The injection should be as close to the venous access as possible to prevent an inadvertent increase in the dose of adenosine (the contents of the IV tubing) being administered.

➤*Infusion guidelines:* The following adenosine infusion rate guide may be used to determine the appropriate infusion rate corrected for total body weight:

45 kg (99 lbs.) Infusion rate is 2.1 ml/min.

50 kg (110 lbs.) Infusion rate is 2.3 ml/min

55 kg (121 lbs.) Infusion rate is 2.6 ml/min.

60 kg (132 lbs.) Infusion rate is 2.8 ml/min.

65 kg (143 lbs.) Infusion rate is 3.0 ml/min.

70 kg (154 lbs.) Infusion rate is 3.3 ml/min.

75 kg (165 lbs.) Infusion rate is 3.5 ml/min.

80 kg (176 lbs.) Infusion rate is 3.8 ml/min.

85 kg (187 lbs.) Infusion rate is 4.0 ml/min.

90 (198 lbs.) Infusion rate is 4.2 ml/min.

This guide was derived from the following general formula:

$$\frac{0.140\ (\text{mg/kg/min}) \times \text{total body weight (kg)}}{\text{Adenosine concentration (3 mg/ml)}} = \text{infusion rate (ml/min)}$$

➤*Storage/Stability:* Store at controlled room temperature 15° to 30°C (59° to 86°F). Do not refrigerate as crystallization may occur. If crystallization has occurred, dissolve crystals by warming to room temperature. The solution must be clear at the time of use. Contains no preservative. Discard unused protion.

Actions

➤*Pharmacology:* Adenosine is a potent vasodilator in most vascular beds, except in renal afferent arterioles and hepatic veins where it produces vasoconstriction. Adenosine is thought to exert its pharmacological effects through activation of purine receptors (cell-surface A_1 and A_2 adenosine receptors). Although the exact mechanism by which adenosine receptor activation relaxes vascular smooth muscle is not known, there is evidence to support both inhibition of the slow inward calcium current reducing calcium uptake, and activation of adenylate cyclase through A_2 receptors in smooth muscle cells. Adenosine may also lessen vascular tone by modulating sympathetic neurotransmission. The intracellular uptake of adenosine is mediated by a specific transmembrane nucleoside transport system. Once inside the cell, adenosine is rapidly phosphorylated by adenosine kinase to adenosine monophosphate, or deaminated by adenosine deaminase to inosine. These intracellular metabolites of adenosine are not vasoactive.

Myocardial uptake of thallium-201 is directly proportional to coronary blood flow. Since adenosine significantly increases blood flow in normal coronary arteries with little or no increase in stenotic arteries, adenosine causes relatively less thallium-201 uptake in vascular territories supplied by stenotic coronary arteries i.e., a greater difference is seen after adenosine between areas served by normal and areas served by stenotic vessels than is seen prior to adenosine.

ADENOSINE — INJECTION

Hemodynamics – Adenosine produces a direct negative chronotropic, dromotropic, and inotropic effect on the heart, presumably due to A_1-receptor agonism, and produces peripheral vasodilation, presumably due to A_2-receptor agonism. The net effect of adenosine in humans is typically a mild to moderate reduction in systolic, diastolic and mean arterial blood pressure associated with a reflex increase in heart rate. Rarely, significant hypotension and tachycardia have been observed.

➤*Pharmacokinetics:* Intravenously administered adenosine is rapidly cleared from the circulation via cellular uptake, primarily by erythrocytes and vascular endothelial cells. This process involves a specific transmembrane nucleoside carrier system that is reversible, nonconcentrative, and bidirectionally symmetrical. Intracellular adenosine is rapidly metabolized either via phosphorylation to adenosine monophosphate by adenosine kinase, or via deamination to inosine by adenosine deaminase in the cytosol. Since adenosine kinase has a lower K_m and V_{max} than adenosine deaminase, deamination plays a significant role only when cytosolic adenosine saturates the phosphorylation pathway. Inosine formed by deamination of adenosine can leave the cell intact or can be degraded to hypoxanthine, xanthine, and ultimately uric acid. Adenosine monophosphate formed by phosphorylation of adenosine is incorporated into the high-energy phosphate pool. While extracellular adenosine is primarily cleared by cellular uptake with a half-life of less than 10 seconds in whole blood, excessive amounts may be deaminated by an ecto-form of adenosine deaminase. As adenosine requires no hepatic or renal function for its activation or inactivation, hepatic and renal failure would not be expected to alter its effectiveness or tolerability.

Contraindications

Second- or third-degree AV block (except in patients with a functioning artificial pacemaker); sinus node disease, such as sick sinus syndrome or symptomatic bradycardia (except in patients with a functioning artificial pacemaker); known or suspected bronchoconstrictive or bronchospastic lung disease (e.g., asthma); known hypersensitivity to adenosine.

Warnings

➤*Cardiac effects:* Fatal cardiac arrest, sustained ventricular tachycardia (requiring resuscitation), and non-fatal myocardial infarction have been reported coincident with adenosine infusion. Patients with unstable angina may be at greater risk. Appropriate resuscitative measures should be available.

Sinoatrial and Atrioventricular Nodal Block – Adenosine exerts a direct depressant effect on the SA and AV nodes and has the potential to cause first-, second- or third-degree AV block, or sinus bradycardia. Approximately 6.3% of patients develop AV block with adenosine, including first-degree (2.9%), second-degree (2.6%) and third-degree (0.8%) heart block. All episodes of AV block have been asymptomatic, transient, and did not require intervention. Adenosine can cause sinus bradycardia. Adenosine should be used with caution in patients with pre-existing first-degree AV block or bundle branch block and should be avoided in patients with high-grade AV block or sinus node dysfunction (except in patients with a functioning artificial pacemaker). Adenosine should be discontinued in any patient who develops persistent or symptomatic high-grade AV block. Sinus pause has been rarely observed with adenosine infusions.

Hypotension – Adenosine is a potent peripheral vasodilator and can cause significant hypotension. Patients with an intact baroreceptor reflex mechanism are able to maintain blood pressure and tissue perfusion in response to Adenosine by increasing heart rate and cardiac output. However, Adenosine should be used with caution in patients with autonomic dysfunction, stenotic valvular heart disease, pericarditis or pericardial effusions, stenotic carotid artery disease with cerebrovascular insufficiency, or uncorrected hypovolemia, due to the risk of hypotensive complications in these patients. Adenosine should be discontinued in any patient who develops persistent or symptomatic hypotension.

Hypertension: Increases in systolic and diastolic pressure have been observed (as great as 140 mm Hg systolic in one case) concomitant with Adenosine infusion; most increases resolved spontaneously within several minutes, but in some cases, hypertension lasted for several hours.

➤*Bronchoconstriction:* Adenosine is a respiratory stimulant (probably through activation of carotid body chemoreceptors) and intravenous administration in man has been shown to increase minute ventilation (Ve) and reduce arterial PCO_2 causing respiratory alkalosis. Approximately 28% of patients experience breathlessness (dyspnea) or an urge to breathe deeply with adenosine. These respiratory complaints are transient and only rarely require intervention.

Adenosine administered by inhalation has been reported to cause bronchoconstriction in asthmatic patients, presumably due to mast cell degranulation and histamine release. These effects have not been observed in normal subjects. Adenosine has been administered to a limited number of patients with asthma and mild to moderate exacerbation of their symptoms has been reported. Respiratory compromise has occurred during adenosine infusion in patients with obstructive pulmonary disease. Adenosine should be used with caution in patients with obstructive lung disease not associated with bronchoconstriction (e.g., emphysema, bronchitis, etc.) and should be avoided in patients with bronchoconstriction or bronchospasm (e.g., asthma). Adenosine should be discontinued in any patient who develops severe respiratory difficulties.

Drug Interactions

➤*Dipyridamole:* The vasoactive effects of adenosine are potentiated by nucleoside transport inhibitors, such as dipyridamole. Thus, smaller doses of adenosine may be effective in the presence of dipyridamole. The safety and efficacy of adenosine in the presence of dipyridamole has not been systematically evaluated.

Whenever possible, drugs that might inhibit or augment the effects of adenosine should be withheld for at least five half-lives prior to the use of adenosine.

Adenosine Drug Interactions

Precipitant drug	Object drug*		Description
Cardioactive agents	Adenosine	⬆	Because of the potential for additive or synergistic depressant effects on the SA and AV nodes, use with caution in the presence of these agents.
Methylxanthines (eg, caffeine and theophylline)	Adenosine	⬇	The vasoactive effect of adenosine is inhibited by adenosine receptor antagonists, such as methylxanthines.

* ⬆ = Object drug increased. ⬇ = Object drug decreased.

Adverse Reactions

The following reactions with an incidence of at least 1% were reported with intravenous adenosine among 1421 patients enrolled in controlled and uncontrolled U.S. clinical trials. Despite the short half-life of adenosine, 10.6% of the side effects occurred not with the infusion of adenosine but several hours after the infusion terminated. Also, 8.4% of the side effects that began coincident with the infusion persisted for up to 24 hours after the infusion was complete. In many cases, it is not possible to know whether these late adverse events are the result of adenosine infusion.

➤*Cardiovascular:* Flushing (44%); chest discomfort (40%); ST segment depression (3%); first-degree AV block (3%); second-degree AV block (3%); hypotension (2%); arrhythmias (1%); nonfatal myocardial infarction; life-threatening ventricular arrhythmia; third-degree AV block; bradycardia; palpitation; sinus exit block; sinus pause; sweating; T-wave changes, hypertension (systolic blood pressure more than 200 mm Hg).

➤*CNS:* Headache (18%); lightheadedness/dizziness (12%); nervousness (2%); drowsiness; emotional instability; tremors.

➤*GU:* Vaginal pressure; urgency.

➤*Respiratory:* Dyspnea or urge to breathe deeply (28%); cough.

➤*Special senses:* Blurred vision; dry mouth; ear discomfort; metallic taste; nasal congestion; scotomas; tongue discomfort.

➤*Miscellaneous:* Throat, neck, or jaw discomfort (15%); gastrointestinal discomfort (13%); upper extremity discomfort (4%); paresthesia (2%); back discomfort; lower extremity discomfort; weakness.

Note: Adverse reactions without any numerals or percentages are equal to less than 1%.

Overdosage

➤*Symptoms:* The half-life of adenosine is less than 10 seconds and side effects of adenosine (when they occur) usually resolve quickly when the infusion is discontinued, although delayed or persistent effects have been observed.

➤*Treatment:* Treatment of any prolonged adverse effects should be individualized and be directed toward the specific effect. Methylxanthines, such as caffeine and theophylline, are competitive adenosine receptor antagonists and theophylline has been used to effectively terminate persistent side effects. In controlled U.S. clinical trials, theophylline (50 to 125 mg slow intravenous injection) was needed to abort adenosine side effects in less than 2% of patients.

Refer to general management of acute overdosage.

ARGININE HYDROCHLORIDE

Rx	**R-Gene 10** (Pharmacia & Upjohn)	**Injection:** 10% arginine hydrochloride (950 mOsmol/L)	With 47.5 mEq chloride ion per 100 ml. In 300 ml.

ARGININE HYDROCHLORIDE — INJECTION

Indications

➤*Diagnostic aid:* As an IV stimulant to the pituitary for the release of human growth hormone (HGH) in patients where the measurement of pituitary reserve for HGH can be of diagnostic usefulness. It can be used as a diagnostic aid in such conditions as panhypopituitarism, pituitary dwarfism, chromophobe adenoma, postsurgical craniopharyngioma, hypophysectomy, pituitary trauma, acromegaly, gigantism, and problems of growth and stature.

Administration and Dosage

➤*Adults:* 300 mL (30 g) IV.

➤*Children:* 5 mL (0.5 g) per kg of body weight IV.

➤*Test procedure:* The IV infusion of arginine hydrochloride is a part of the test for measurement of pituitary reserve of human growth hormone and, for successful administration of the test, clinical conditions and procedures should be as follows:

ARGININE HYDROCHLORIDE — INJECTION

1.) The test should be scheduled in the morning following a normal night's sleep, and an overnight fast should continue through the test period.
2.) Patients must be placed at bed rest for at least 30 minutes before the infusion begins. Care should be taken to minimize apprehension and distress. This is particularly important in children.
3.) Arginine hydrochloride injection should be infused through an indwelling needle or soft catheter placed in an antecubital vein or other suitable vein. Blood samples should be taken by venipuncture from the contra-lateral arm.
4.) A desirable schedule for drawing blood samples is at −30, 0, 30, 60, 90, 120 and 150 minutes.
5.) Arginine hydrochloride should be infused beginning at zero time at a uniform rate which will permit the recommended dose to be administered in 30 minutes.
6.) Blood samples should be promptly centrifuged and the plasma stored at −20°C (−4°F) until assayed by one of the published radioimmunoassay procedures.
7.) Diagnostic test results showing a deficiency of pituitary reserve for HGH should be confirmed by a second test with arginine hydrochloride, or one may elect to confirm with the insulin hypoglycemia test. A waiting period of 1 day is advised between tests.

➤*Storage/Stability:* Avoid excessive heat. Store at room temperature 25°C (77°F); however, brief exposure up to 40°C (104°F) does not adversely affect the product. Solution that has been frozen must not be used.

Actions

➤*Pharmacology:* IV infusion of arginine hydrochloride often induces a pronounced rise in the plasma level of HGH in subjects with intact pituitary function. This rise is usually diminished or absent in patients with impairment of this function.

Expected plasma levels of HGH in ng/mL		
Patient	Control range	Range of peak response to arginine
Healthy	0 to 6	10 to 30
Pituitary deficient	0 to 4	0 to 10

These ranges are based on the mean values of plasma HGH levels calculated from the data of several clinical investigators and reflect their experiences with various methods of radioimmunoassay. Upon gaining experience with this diagnostic test, each clinician will establish his own ranges for control and peak levels of HGH.

L-arginine is a normal metabolite in animals and man and has a low order of toxicity.

Contraindications

Highly allergic tendencies.

Warnings

➤*Deficiency of pituitary reserve for HGH:* If the insulin hypoglycemia test has indicated a deficiency of pituitary reserve for HGH, a test with arginine hydrochloride is advisable to confirm the negative response. This can be done after a waiting period of 1 day. As patients may not respond to 10% arginine hydrochloride injection during the first test, the unresponsive patient should be tested again to confirm the negative result. A second test can be performed after a waiting period of 1 day. Some patients who respond to arginine hydrochloride do not respond to insulin and vice versa. The rate of false-positive responses for arginine hydrochloride is approximately 32%, and the rate of false-negatives is approximately 27%.

➤*IV administration:* Arginine hydrochloride should always be administered by IV injection because of its hypertonicity. Arginine hydrochloride is a hypertonic (950 mOsmol/L) and acidic (average pH of 5.6) solution that can irritate tissues. Care should be used to insure administration of arginine hydrochloride through a patent catheter within a patent vein.

➤*Diagnostic aid:* Arginine hydrochloride is a diagnostic aid and is not intended for therapeutic use.

➤*Hypersensitivity reactions:* A suitable antihistaminic drug should be available in the event that an allergic reaction occurs.

➤*Renal function impairment:* The arginine in arginine hydrochloride can be metabolized resulting in nitrogen-containing products for excretion. The effect of an acute amino acid or nitrogen burden upon patients with impairment of renal function should be considered when arginine hydrochloride is to be administered.

➤*Pregnancy: Category B.* There have been no adequate or well-controlled studies for the use of arginine hydrochloride in pregnant women. Because animal reproduction studies are not always predictive of human response, this drug should not be used during pregnancy.

➤*Lactation:* It is not known whether IV administration of arginine hydrochloride could result in significant quantities of arginine in breast milk. Systemically administered amino acids are secreted into breast milk in quantities not likely to have a deleterious effect on the infant. Nevertheless, caution should be exercised when arginine hydrochloride is to be administered to breast-feeding women.

➤*Children:* There have been 2 reports of possible overdosage of arginine hydrochloride in children. Extreme caution must be exercised when infusing arginine hydrochloride into pediatric patients. Overdosage of arginine hydrochloride in pediatric patients can result in hyperchloremic metabolic acidosis, cerebral edema, or possibly death.

Precautions

➤*Excessive infusion rates:* Excessive rates of infusion may result in local irritation and in flushing, nausea, or vomiting. Inadequate dosing or prolongation of the infusion period may diminish the stimulus to the pituitary and nullify the test.

➤*Chloride content:* The chloride content of arginine hydrochloride is 47.5 mEq per 100 mL of solution, and the effect of infusing this amount of chloride into patients with electrolyte imbalance should be evaluated before the test is undertaken.

➤*Growth hormone levels:* The basal and post stimulation levels of growth hormone are elevated in patients who are pregnant or are taking oral contraceptives.

Adverse Reactions

➤*Allergic:* One patient had an allergic reaction which was manifested as a confluent macular rash with reddening and swelling of the hands and face. The rash subsided rapidly after the infusion was terminated and 50 mg of diphenhydramine were administered.

➤*Cardiovascular:* One patient with a history of acrocyanosis had an exacerbation of this condition following infusion of arginine hydrochloride.

➤*Hematologic:* One patient had an apparent decrease in platelet count from 150,000 to 60,000.

➤*Miscellaneous:* Nonspecific side effects consisting of nausea, vomiting, headache, flushing, numbness and local venous irritation were reported in approximately 3% of the patients.

Overdosage

➤*Symptoms:* An overdosage may cause a transient metabolic acidosis with hyperventilation. The acidosis will be compensated and the base deficit will return to normal following completion of the infusion.

➤*Treatment:* If the condition persists, the deficit should be determined and corrected by a calculated dose of an alkalizing agent.

CORTICORELIN OVINE TRIFLUTATE

Rx	**Acthrel** (Ferring)	**Cake, lyophilized:** 100 mcg corticorelin ovine (as trifluoroacetate)[1]	In 5 ml single-dose vials with diluent.

[1] With 0.88 mg ascorbic acid, 10 mg lactose and 26 mg cysteine hydrochloride monohydrate.

CORTICORELIN OVINE TRIFLUTATE — INJECTION

Indications

➤*Cushing's syndrome, differential diagnosis:* Differentiating pituitary and ectopic production of ACTH in patients with ACTH-dependent Cushing's syndrome.

Administration and Dosage

➤*Approved by the FDA:* May 1996.

➤*Test Methodology:* To evaluate the status of the pituitary-adrenal axis in the differentiation of a pituitary source from an ectopic source of excessive ACTH secretion, a corticorelin test procedure requires a minimum of five blood samples.

Procedure –

1.) Venous blood samples should be drawn 15 minutes before and immediately prior to corticorelin administration. The ACTH baseline is obtained by averaging the values of the two samples.
2.) Administer corticorelin as an intravenous infusion over a 30- to 60-second interval at a dose of 1 mcg/kg body weight. Higher dosages are not recommended (see Precautions and Adverse Reactions).
3.) Draw venous blood samples at 15, 30, and 60 minutes after administration.

Cortisol determinations may be performed on the same blood samples for the same time points as outlined above. The blood sample handling precautions noted for ACTH should be followed for cortisol.

➤*Dosage:* A single intravenous dose of corticorelin at 1 mcg/kg is recommended for the testing of pituitary corticotropin function. A dose of 1 mcg/kg is the lowest dose that produces maximal cortisol responses and significant (though apparently sub-maximal) ACTH responses. Doses above 1 mcg/kg are not recommended. (See Precautions and Adverse Reactions)

If a repeat evaluation using the corticorelin stimulation test with corticorelin is needed, it is recommended that the repeat test be carried out at the same time of day as the original test because there are differences in basal levels and peak response levels following a.m. or p.m. administration to normal humans.

➤*Interpretation of Test Results:* The interpretation of the ACTH and cortisol responses following corticorelin administration requires a knowledge of the clinical status of the individual patient, understanding of hypothalamic-pituitary-adrenal physiology, and familiarity with the normal

CORTICORELIN OVINE TRIFLUTATE — INJECTION

hormonal ranges and the standards used by the laboratory that performs the ACTH and cortisol assays.

Cushing's Disease – The results of challenge with corticorelin injection have been reported in approximately 300 patients with Cushing's disease. Although the ACTH and cortisol responses were variable, a hyper-response to corticorelin was seen in a majority of patients, despite high basal cortisol levels. This response pattern indicates an impairment of the negative feedback of cortisol on the pituitary. Patients with pituitary-dependent Cushing's disease tested with corticorelin do not show the negative correlation between basal and stimulated levels of ACTH and cortisol that is found in normal subjects. A positive correlation between basal ACTH levels and maximum ACTH increments after corticorelin administration has been found in Cushing's disease patients.

Ectopic ACTH Secretion – Patients with Cushing's syndrome due to ectopic ACTH secretion (N=32) were found to have very high basal levels of ACTH and cortisol, which were not further stimulated by corticorelin. However, there have been rare instances of patients with ectopic sources of ACTH that have responded to the corticorelin test.

➤*Administration/Preparation:* Corticorelin is to be reconstituted aseptically with 2 ml of Sodium Chloride Injection, USP (0.9% sodium chloride), at the time of use by injecting 2 ml of the saline diluent into the lyophilized drug product cake. To avoid bubble formation, do not shake the vial; instead, roll the vial to dissolve the drug product. The sterile solution containing 50 mcg corticorelin/ml is then ready for injection by the intravenous route. The dosage to be administered is determined by the patient's weight (1 mcg corticorelin/kg). Some of the adverse effects can be reduced by administering the drug as an infusion over 30 seconds instead of as a bolus injection.

➤*Storage/Stability:* Refrigerate at 2°C to 8°C (36°F to 45°F) and protect from light. The reconstituted solution is stable up to 8 hours under refrigerated conditions. Discard unused reconstituted solution.

Actions

➤*Pharmacology:*

Pharmacodynamics – In normal subjects, intravenous administration of corticorelin results in a rapid and sustained increase of plasma ACTH levels and a near parallel increase of plasma cortisol. In addition, intravenous administration of corticorelin to normal subjects causes a concomitant and prolonged release of the related proopiomelanocortin peptides β- and γ-lipotropins (β- and γ-LPH) and β-endorphin (β-END). A number of dose-response studies have been performed on normal subjects using a range of corticorelin doses. In one study, doses of corticorelin ranging from 0.001 to 30 mcg/kg body weight were administered to 29 healthy volunteers. Blood samples were taken over a 2-hour period for determination of plasma ACTH and cortisol concentrations. There was a direct dose-dependent relationship that was more pronounced for ACTH than for cortisol. The threshold dose was 0.03 mcg/kg, the half-maximal dose was 0.3-1.0 mcg/kg and the maximally effective dose was 3-10 mcg/kg.

Baseline ACTH and cortisol levels are usually higher in the morning. Pooled ACTH values from normal unstressed subjects (n=119) were 25 ± 7 pg/ml in the a.m., and 10 ± 3 in the p.m., similar pooled cortisol values (n=170) were 11 ± 3 mcg/dl in the a.m. and 4 ± 2 mcg/dl in the p.m. The normal unstressed person has about seven to ten secretory episodes of ACTH each day. Most of them occur in the early morning hours and are responsible for the morning plasma cortisol surge. Insulin, plasma renin activity, prolactin, and growth hormone release are not affected by corticorelin administration in humans.

Continuous 24-hour infusion of corticorelin (0.5, 1.0, and 3.0 mcg/kg/hr) increased plasma ACTH concentrations to a plateau of 15-20 pg/ml by the third hour and urinary-free cortisol reaches 173 ± 43 mcg/dl by 24 hours, comparable to those levels observed in patients with major depression, but less than levels noted in Cushing's disease. Continuous infusion did not abolish the circadian rhythm of plasma ACTH and cortisol, but did appear to desensitize the corticotroph. Intermittent doses of corticorelin (25 mcg every 4 hours for 72 hours), however, continued to elicit the expected ACTH and cortisol responses.

Intravenous administration of 1 mcg/kg corticorelin in combination with 10 pressor units intramuscular vasopressin had a synergistic effect on ACTH and a less marked synergistic effect on cortisol secretion.

➤*Pharmacokinetics:* Plasma ACTH levels in normal subjects increased 2 minutes after injection of corticorelin doses of ≥0.3 mcg/kg and reached peak levels after 10-15 minutes. Plasma cortisol levels increased within 10 minutes and reached peak levels at 30 to 60 minutes. As the dose of corticorelin was increased, the rises in plasma ACTH and cortisol were more sustained, showing a biphasic response with a second lower peak at 2-3 hours after injection. Similar results were found in another study using 0.3, 3.0, and 30 mcg/kg doses. The duration of mean plasma ACTH increase after injection of 0.3, 3.0, and 30 mcg/kg was 4, 7, and 8 hours, respectively. The effect on plasma cortisol was similar, but more prolonged. Because there are differences in basal levels and peak response levels following a.m. or p.m. administration, it is recommended that subsequent evaluations in the same patient using the corticorelin stimulation test be carried out at the same time of day as the original evaluation.

Following a single intravenous injection of 1 mcg/kg of corticorelin to normal men, the disappearance of immunoreactive corticorelin (IR-corticorelin) from plasma follows a biexponential decay curve. Plasma half-lives for IR-corticorelin are 11.6 ± 1.5 minutes (mean ± SE) for the fast component and 73 ± 8 minutes for the slow component. The mean volume of distribution for IR-corticorelin is 6.2 ± 0.5 L with an approximate metabolic clearance rate of 95 ± 11 L/m^2/day. Graded intravenous doses of corticorelin (0.01, 0.03, 0.1, 0.3, 1, 3, 10, 30 mcg/kg) produced a linear increase in plasma IR-corticorelin. Corticorelin does not appear to be bound specifically by a circulating plasma protein.

Warnings

➤*Pregnancy: Category C.* Animal reproduction studies have not been conducted with corticorelin. It is also not known whether corticorelin can cause fetal harm when administered to a pregnant woman or can affect reproductive capacity. Corticorelin should be given to a pregnant woman only if clearly needed.

➤*Lactation:* It is not known whether corticorelin is secreted in human milk. Because many drugs are excreted in human milk, caution should be exercised when corticorelin is administered to a breast-feeding woman.

➤*Children:* Only a few tests have been performed on children. Dosages were 1 mcg/kg body weight. Patient studies have involved only children with multiple hypothalamic and/or pituitary hormone deficiencies, or tumors. Only two studies with normal pediatric subjects have been conducted. No differences in response to the corticorelin test have been reported in the children studied.

Precautions

➤*Dose dependent effects:* The severity of adverse effects to a corticorelin injection appear to be dose-dependent. Dosages above 1 mcg/kg are not recommended. While few adverse effects have been observed at the 1 mcg/kg or 100 mcg dose, higher doses have been associated with transient tachycardia, decreased blood pressure, loss of consciousness, and asystole (see Adverse Reactions). These symptoms can be substantially reduced by administering the drug as a 30-second intravenous infusion instead of a bolus injection.

Drug Interactions

➤*Dexamethasone:* The plasma ACTH response to corticorelin injection is inhibited or blunted in normal subjects pretreated with dexamethasone.

➤*Heparin:* The use of a heparin solution to maintain IV cannula patency during the corticorelin test is not recommended. A possible interaction between corticorelin and heparin may have been responsible for a major hypotensive reaction that occurred after corticorelin administration. (See Adverse Reactions.)

Adverse Reactions

Adverse effects reported with 1 mcg/kg or 100 mcg/patient include flushing of the face, neck, and upper chest (16%: 45/276), beginning almost immediately and lasting 3 to 5 minutes. Recipients have also reported an urge to take a deep breath (6%: 3/49), which occurs with a timing similar to, but less frequently than, that of flushing. Higher doses (≥3 mcg/kg) are associated with more prolonged flushing, tachycardia, hypotension, dyspnea, and chest compression or tightness. In addition, at doses of ≥ 5 mcg/kg, significant increases in heart rate and decreases in blood pressure were observed. The cardiovascular effects occurred 2-3 minutes after injection and lasted for 30-60 minutes. The facial flushing was more prolonged, lasting up to 4 hours in some subjects. All signs and symptoms could be reduced by administering the drug as a 30-second infusion instead of by bolus injection.

Overdosage

➤*Symptoms:* Symptoms of overdose include severe facial flushing, cardiovascular changes, and dyspnea.

➤*Treatment:* In the event of toxic overdose (see Adverse Reactions), adverse effects should be treated symptomatically.

METYRAPONE

Rx	**Metopirone** (Novartis)	**Capsules:** 250 mg	(CIBA LN) Soft gelatin. White to yellowish white. Oblong. In 18s.

METYRAPONE — ORAL

Indications

➤*Diagnostic aid:* For testing hypothalamic-pituitary adrenocorticotropic hormone (ACTH) function.

Administration and Dosage

➤*Approved by the FDA:* January 25, 1962.

➤*Single-dose short test:* This test, usually given on an outpatient basis, determines plasma 11-desoxycortisol or ACTH levels after a single dose of metyrapone. The patient is given 30 mg/kg (maximum 3 g metyrapone) at midnight with yogurt or milk. The same dose is recommended in children. The blood sample for the assay is taken early the following morning (7:30 to 8 am). The plasma should be frozen as soon as possible. The patient is then given a prophylactic dose of 50 mg cortisone acetate.

Interpretation – Normal values will depend on the method used to determine ACTH and 11-desoxycortisol levels. An intact ACTH reserve is generally indicated by an increase in plasma ACTH to at least 44 pmol/L (200 ng/L) or by an increase in 11-desoxycortisol to over 0.2 mcmol/L (70 mcg/L). Patients with suspected adrenocortical insufficiency should be hospitalized overnight as a precautionary measure.

➤*Multiple-dose test:*

Day 1 –

Control period: Collect 24-hour urine for measurement of 17-hydroxycorticosteroids (17-OHCS) or 17-ketogenic steroids (17-KGS).

METYRAPONE — ORAL

Day 2 –

ACTH test to determine the ability of adrenals to respond: Standard ACTH test such as infusion of 50 units ACTH over 8 hours and measurement of 24-hour urinary steroids. If results indicate adequate response, the metyrapone test may proceed.

Day 3 to 4 – Rest period.

Day 5 –

Administration of metyrapone: Recommended with milk or snack.

Adults – 750 mg orally, every 4 hours for 6 doses. A single dose is approximately equivalent to 15 mg/kg.

Children – 15 mg/kg orally every 4 hours for 6 doses. A minimal single dose of 250 mg is recommended.

Day 6 –

After administration of metyrapone: Determination of 24-hour urinary steroids for effect.

Interpretation –

ACTH test: The normal 24-hour urinary excretion of 17-OHCS ranges from 3 to 12 mg. Following continuous IV infusion of 50 units ACTH over a period of 8 hours, 17-OHCS excretion increases to 15 to 45 mg per 24 hours.

➤*Metyrapone:*

Normal response – In patients with a normally functioning pituitary, administration of metyrapone is followed by a 2- to 4-fold increase of 17-OHCS excretion or doubling of 17-KGS excretion.

Subnormal response – Subnormal response in patients without adrenal insufficiency is indicative of some degree of impairment of pituitary function, either panhypopituitarism or partial hypopituitarism (limited pituitary reserve).

Panhypopituitarism: Panhypopituitarism is readily diagnosed by the classical clinical and chemical evidences of hypogonadism, hypothyroidism, and hypoadrenocorticism. These patients usually have subnormal basal urinary steroid levels. Depending upon the duration of the disease and degree of adrenal atrophy, they may fail to respond to exogenous ACTH in the normal manner. Administration of metyrapone is not essential in the diagnosis, but if given, it will not induce an appreciable increase in urinary steroids.

Partial hypopituitarism: Partial hypopituitarism or limited pituitary reserve is the more difficult diagnosis as these patients do not present the classical signs and symptoms of hypopituitarism. Measurements of target organ functions often are normal under basal conditions. The response to exogenous ACTH is usually normal, producing the expected rise of urinary steroids (17-OHCS or 17-KGS).

The response, however, to metyrapone is subnormal; that is, no significant increase in 17-OHCS or 17-KGS excretion occurs.

This failure to respond to metyrapone may be interpreted as evidence of impaired pituitary-adrenal reserve. In view of the normal response to exogenous ACTH, the failure to respond to metyrapone is inferred to be related to a defect in the CNS-pituitary mechanisms which normally regulate ACTH secretions. Presumably the ACTH secreting mechanisms of these individuals are already working at their maximal rates to meet everyday conditions and possess limited "reserve" capacities to secrete additional ACTH either in response to stress or to decreased cortisol levels occurring as a result of metyrapone administration.

Subnormal response in patients with Cushing's syndrome is suggestive of either autonomous adrenal tumors that suppress the ACTH-releasing capacity of the pituitary or nonendocrine ACTH-secreting tumors.

Excessive response – An excessive excretion of 17-OHCS or 17-KGS after administration of metyrapone is suggestive of Cushing's syndrome associated with adrenal hyperplasia. These patients have an elevated excretion of urinary corticosteroids under basal conditions and will often, but not invariably, show a "supernormal" response to ACTH and also to metyrapone, excreting more than 35 mg per 24 hours of either 17-OHCS or 17-KGS.

➤*Storage/Stability:* Do not store above 30°C (86°F). Protect from moisture and heat. Dispense in tight container (USP).

Actions

➤*Pharmacology:* The pharmacological effect of metyrapone is to reduce cortisol and corticosterone production by inhibiting the 11-β-hydroxylation reaction in the adrenal cortex. Removal of the strong inhibitory feedback mechanism exerted by cortisol results in an increase in ACTH production by the pituitary. With continued blockade of the enzymatic steps leading to production of cortisol and corticosterone, there is a marked increase in adrenocortical secretion of their immediate precursors, 11-desoxycortisol and desoxycorticosterone, which are weak suppressors of ACTH release, and a corresponding elevation of these steroids in the plasma and of their metabolites in the urine. These metabolites are readily determined by measuring urinary 17-OHCS or 17-KGS. Because of these actions, metyrapone is used as a diagnostic test, with urinary 17-OHCS measured as an index of pituitary ACTH responsiveness. Metyrapone may also suppress biosynthesis of aldosterone, resulting in a mild natriuresis.

The response to metyrapone does not occur immediately. Following oral administration, peak steroid excretion occurs during the subsequent 24-hour period.

➤*Pharmacokinetics:*

Absorption – Metyrapone is absorbed rapidly and well when administered orally as prescribed. Peak plasma concentrations are usually reached 1 hour after administration. After administration of 750 mg, mean peak plasma concentrations are 3.7 mcg/mL, falling to 0.5 mcg/mL 4 hours after administration. Following a single 2000 mg dose, mean peak plasma concentrations of metyrapone in plasma are 7.3 mcg/mL.

Metabolism – The major biotransformation is reduction of the ketone to metyrapol, an active alcohol metabolite. Eight hours after a single oral dose, the ratio of metyrapone to metyrapol in the plasma is 1:1.5. Metyrapone and metyrapol are both conjugated with glucuronide.

Excretion – Metyrapone is rapidly eliminated from the plasma. The mean ± SD terminal elimination half-life is 1.9 ± 0.7 hours. Metyrapol takes about twice as long as metyrapone to be eliminated from the plasma. After administration of 4.5 g metyrapone (750 mg every 4 hours), an average of 5.3% of the dose was excreted in the urine in the form of metyrapone (9.2% free and 90.8% as glucuronide) and 38.5% in the form of metyrapol (8.1% free and 91.9% as glucuronide) within 72 hours after the first dose was given.

Contraindications

Adrenal cortical insufficiency, or hypersensitivity to metyrapone or to any of its excipients.

Warnings

➤*Acute adrenal insufficiency:* Metyrapone may induce acute adrenal insufficiency in patients with reduced adrenal secretory capacity.

➤*Pregnancy:* *Category C.* A subnormal response to metyrapone may occur in pregnant women. Animal reproduction studies have not been conducted with metyrapone. The metyrapone test was administered to 20 pregnant women in their second and third trimester of pregnancy, and evidence was found that the fetal pituitary responded to the enzymatic block. It is not known if metyrapone can affect reproduction capacity. Metyrapone should be given to a pregnant woman only if clearly needed.

➤*Lactation:* It is not known whether this drug is excreted in human milk. Because many drugs are excreted in human milk, caution should be exercised when metyrapone is administered to a breast-feeding woman.

Precautions

➤*Response to adrenals:* Ability of adrenals to respond to exogenous ACTH should be demonstrated before metyrapone is employed as a test.

➤*Hypo-/Hyperthyroidism:* In the presence of hypo- or hyperthyroidism, response to the metyrapone test may be subnormal.

➤*Hazardous tasks:* Since metyrapone may cause dizziness and sedation, patients should exercise caution when driving or operating machinery.

Drug Interactions

➤*Corticosteroids:* Drugs affecting pituitary or adrenocortical function, including all corticosteroid therapy, must be discontinued prior to and during testing with metyrapone.

➤*Phenytoin:* The metabolism of metyrapone is accelerated by phenytoin; therefore, results of the test may be inaccurate in patients taking phenytoin within 2 weeks before.

➤*Estrogens:* A subnormal response may occur in patients on estrogen therapy.

➤*Acetaminophen:* Metyrapone inhibits the glucuronidation of acetaminophen and could possibly potentiate acetaminophen toxicity.

Adverse Reactions

➤*CNS:* Headache, dizziness, sedation.

➤*Dermatologic:* Allergic rash.

➤*GI:* Nausea, vomiting, abdominal discomfort or pain.

➤*Hematologic:* Rarely, decreased white blood cell count or bone marrow depression.

Overdosage

➤*Acute toxicity:* One case has been recorded in which a 6 year old girl died after 2 doses of metyrapone, 2 g.

➤*Symptoms:* The clinical picture of poisoning with metyrapone is characterized by gastrointestinal symptoms and by signs of acute adrenocortical insufficiency.

CV – Cardiac arrhythmias, hypotension, dehydration.

CNS – Anxiety, confusion, weakness, impairment of consciousness.

GI – Nausea, vomiting, epigastric pain, diarrhea.

Lab test abnormalities – Hyponatremia, hypochloremia, hyperkalemia.

In patients under treatment with insulin or oral antidiabetics, the signs and symptoms of acute poisoning with metyrapone may be aggravated or modified.

➤*Treatment:* There is no specific antidote. Besides general measures to eliminate the drug and reduce its absorption, a large dose of hydrocortisone should be administered at once, together with saline and glucose infusions. For a few days blood pressure and fluid and electrolyte balance should be monitored.

CAPROMAB PENDETIDE — INJECTION

Rx	**ProstaScint** (Cytogen)	**Kit:** Each contains 0.5 mg capromab pendetide/ml of sodium phosphate buffered saline and 1 vial of 82 mg sodium acetate in 2 ml Sterile Water for Injection	Preservative free. Includes 1 sterile 0.22 mcm *Millex GV filter,* prescribing information, and 2 identification labels.

Indications

➤*Prostate cancer:* As a diagnostic imaging agent in newly-diagnosed patients with biopsy-proven prostate cancer, thought to be clinically-localized after standard diagnostic evaluation (eg, chest x-ray, bone scan, CT scan, or MRI), who are at high risk for pelvic lymph node metastases. It is not indicated in patients who are not at high risk.

➤*Post-prostatectomy patients:* As a diagnostic imaging agent in post-prostatectomy patients with a rising PSA and a negative or equivocal standard metastatic evaluation in whom there is a high clinical suspicion of occult metastatic disease. The imagine performance following radiation therapy has not been studied.

Consider the information provided by capromab in conjunction with other diagnostic information. Confirm scans that are positive for metastatic disease histologically in patients who are otherwise candidates for surgery or radiation therapy unless medically contraindicated. Do not use scans that are negative for metastatic disease in lieu of histological confirmation.

It is not indicated as a screening tool for carcinoma of the prostate nor for readministration for assessment of response to treatment.

Administration and Dosage

The patient dose of the radiolabel must be measured in a dose calibrator prior to administration.

The recommended dose of capromab pendetide is 0.5 mg radiolabeled with 5 mCi of Indium In 111 chloride. Each dose is IV administered over 5 minutes. Do not mix with any other medication during its administration. Indium In 111 capromab may be readministered following infiltration or a technically inadequate scan; however, it is not indicated for readministration for assessment of response to treatment.

Each kit is a unit dose package. After radiolabeling with Indium In 111, administer the entire Indium In 111 capromab dose to the patient. Reducing the dose of Indium In 111, unlabeled capromab, or Indium In 111 capromab may adversely impact imaging results and is, therefore, not recommended. Inspect parenteral drug products visually for particulate matter and discoloration prior to administration whenever solution and container permit.

For further dosing information, see kit instructions.

IN VIVO DIAGNOSTIC BIOLOGICALS

CANDIDA ALBICANS SKIN TEST ANTIGEN

Rx	**Candin** (Allermed)	**Injection:** Prepared from the culture filtrate and cells of two strains of *Candida albicans.*	In 1 ml multidose vial.

CANDIDA ALBICANS SKIN TEST ANTIGEN — INJECTION

Indications

➤*Reduced cellular hypersensitivity:* For use as a recall antigen for detecting delayed-type hypersensitivity (DTH) by intracutaneous (intradermal) testing. The product may be useful in evaluating the cellular immune response in patients suspected of having reduced cellular hypersensitivity. Because some persons with normal cellular immunity are not hypersensitive to *Candida albicans,* a response rate less than 100% to the antigen is to be expected in healthy individuals. Therefore, the concurrent use of other licensed DTH skin test antigens is recommended.

➤*HIV:* Antigens of *C. albicans* are useful in the assessment of diminished cellular immunity in persons infected with HIV. Responses to DTH antigens have prognostic value in patients with cancer. Because HIV infection can modify the DTH response to tuberculin, it is advisable to skin test HIV-infected patients at high risk of tuberculosis with antigens in addition to tuberculin, to assess their competency to react to tuberculin. (See Warnings.)

Administration and Dosage

➤*Approved by the FDA:* November 27, 1995.

➤*Test method: C. albicans* skin test antigen is administered intradermally, on the volar surface of the forearm or on the outer aspect of the upper arm. The test dose is 0.1 ml. Cleanse the skin with 70% alcohol before applying the skin test. (See Precautions.)

➤*Interpretation:* A positive DTH reaction consists of induration ≥ 5 mm. The time required for the induration response to reach maximum intensity varies with the individual. The reaction usually begins within 24 hours and peaks between 24 and 48 hours. Read the skin test after 48 hours by visually inspecting the test site and palpating the indurated area. Measure across two diameters. Report the mean of the longest and midpoint diameters of the indurated area as the DTH response. For example, a reaction that is 10 mm (longest diameter) by 8 mm (midpoint orthogonal diameter) has a sum of 18 mm and a mean of 9 mm. The DTH response is therefore 9 mm.

➤*Storage / Stability:* Store between 2° to 8°C (35° to 46°F). Do not freeze.

Actions

➤*Pharmacology:* The potency of *C. albicans* is measured by dose-response skin tests in healthy adults. The procedure involves concurrent (side-by-side) testing of production lots with an internal reference (IR), using sensitive adults who have been previously screened and qualified to serve as test subjects. The induration response at 48 hours elicited by 0.1 ml of a production lot is measured and compared to the response elicited by 0.1 ml of the IR. The test is satisfactory if the potency of the production lot does not differ more than ± 20% from the potency of the IR, when analyzed by the paired t-test.

Cellular or DTH can be assessed by intracutaneous testing with bacterial, viral and fungal antigens to which most healthy persons are sensitized. A positive skin test denotes prior antigenic exposure, T-cell competency and an intact inflammatory response. The reaction usually peaks 48 hours after antigen is introduced into the skin and is manifest as induration at the test site.

Recall antigens may be useful in evaluating DTH by eliciting positive induration reactions 48 to 72 hours after intracutaneous administration. Except for mumps skin test antigen, most commonly used recall antigens were developed for other purposes, and the size of the reaction elicited may not be directly related to cellular immunity because of variability in antigen source and dose and skin test administration and measurement techniques. Useful antigens are those which elicit a reaction size greater than 5 mm in more than 50% of healthy individuals. The combination of results from skin testing with more than one antigen should result in detection of DTH in at least 95% of healthy subjects.

The inflammatory response associated with the DTH reaction is characterized by an infiltration of lymphocytes and macrophages at the site of antigen deposition. Specific cell types that appear to play a major role in the DTH response include CD4+ and CD8+ T-lymphocytes which leave the recirculating lymphocyte pool in response to exogenous antigen. Both CD4+ and CD8+ lymphocytes have been recovered from DTH reactions elicited by *Candida* antigen.

Contraindications

History of a previous unacceptable adverse reaction to this antigen or to a similar product (eg, extreme hypersensitivity or allergy).

Warnings

➤*Type I allergy:* The product should not be used to diagnose or treat Type I allergy to *C. albicans.*

➤*Immunodeficiency:* Immunodeficiency states, such as advanced HIV infection or cancer, can modify the DTH response to tuberculin. It may be advisable to skin test patients at high risk of tuberculosis with antigens in addition to tuberculin to confirm the patient's state of cellular immunity.

➤*Local reactions:* Usually subside within hours or days after administration of the skin test. In some patients, skin discoloration may persist for several weeks. Local reactions may be treated with a cold compress and topical steroids. Severe loval reactions may require additional measures as appropriate.

In persons with a bleeding tendency, bruising and non-specific induration may occur due to the trauma of the skin test.

➤*Systemic reactions to C. albicans:* Systemic reactions to *C. albicans* have not been observed. However, all foreign antigens have the remote possibility of causing type I anaphylaxis and even death when injected intradermally. Systemic reactions usually occur within 30 minutes after the injection of antigen.

➤*Hypersensitivity reactions:* As has been observed with other, unstandardized antigens used for DTH skin testing, it is possible that some patients may have exquisite immediate hypersensitivity to *C. albicans.* These reactions are characterized by the presence of an edematous hive surrounded by a zone of erythema. They occur ≈ 15 to 20 minutes after the intradermal injection of the antigen. The size of the immediate reaction varies depending on the sensitivity of the individual. Immediate hypersensitivity reactions have been reported in 17% to 22% of patients, with erythema of 10 to 24 mm in diameter, and in another 5% to 13% of patients, with erythema of 5 to 9 mm. When using this product, have available the facilities and medications necessary to treat all potential local and systemic side effects. Refer to Management of Acute Hypersensitivity Reactions.

➤*Elderly: C. albicans* has not been adequately studied in elderly patients. However, the DTH response to *C. albicans* may be diminished in elderly patients, since the aging process is known to alter cell-mediated immunity.

CANDIDA ALBICANS SKIN TEST ANTIGEN — INJECTION

➤*Pregnancy:* *Category C.* It is not known whether *C. albicans* can cause fetal harm when administered to a pregnant woman or can affect reproduction capacity. Give to pregnant women only if clearly needed. Problems in pregnancy are unlikely.

➤*Lactation:* It is not known whether *C. albicans* is excreted in breast milk. Problems in breastfeeding are unlikely.

➤*Children:* The safety and efficacy in children has not been established.

Precautions

➤*Route of administration:* Inject the antigen intradermally as superficially as possible causing a distinct, sharply defined bleb at the skin test site. An unreliable reaction may result if the product is injected subcutaneously. It must not be given IV. Do not inject into a blood vessel.

Drug Interactions

➤*Corticosteroids:* Pharmacologic doses of corticosteroids may variably suppress the DTH skin test response after 2 weeks of therapy. The mechanism of suppression is believed to involve a decrease in monocytes and lymphocytes, particularly T-cells. The skin test response usually returns to the pretreatment level within several weeks after steroid therapy is discontinued.

Adverse Reactions

➤*Systemic:* Sneezing; coughing; itching; shortness of breath; abdominal cramps; vomiting; diarrhea; tachycardia; hypotension; respiratory failure. Progression of the delayed reaction to vesiculation, necrosis and ulceration is possible (see Warnings).

➤*Local:* Redness; swelling; bruising; pruritus; excoriation; discoloration of the skin; rash; vesiculation; bullae dermal exfoliation, cellulitis (severe). (See Warnings.)

COCCIDIOIDIN

Rx	**BioCox** (Iatric)	**Injection**: 1:100 w/v	0.01% thimerosal. Mycelial derivative. In 1 ml 10-test multidose vial.
	Spherulin (ALK)		0.01% thimerosal. Spherule derivative. In 1 ml 10-test multidose vial.
Rx	**BioCox** (Iatric)	**Injection**: 1:10 w/v	0.01% thimerosal. Mycelial derivative. In 10-test multidose vial.
	Spherulin (ALK)		0.01% thimerosal. Spherule derivative. In 10-test multidose vial.

COCCIDIOIDIN — INJECTION

Indications

➤*Coccidioidomycosis, diagnosis:* For detection of delayed hypersensitivity to *Coccidioides immitis*. Serves as an aid in the diagnosis of coccidioidomycosis. The skin test is a valuable diagnostic tool to differentiate coccidioidomycosis from the common cold, influenza and other mycotic or bacterial infections (eg, blastomycosis, histoplasmosis, tuberculosis, sarcoidosis).

➤*Unlabeled uses:* In endemic areas (eg, the southwestern US), coccidioidin may be a useful addition to anergy skin-test panels to assess competence of recipients' cell-mediated immunity, but use of mycelial coccidioidin may obscure the results of other fungal assays.

Administration and Dosage

➤*Test method:* Inject 0.1 ml of a 1:100 dilution intradermally on the flexor surface of the forearm. Use a weaker 1:1,000 or 1:10,000 dilution if erythema nodosum is evident.

Perform the 1:10 dilution skin test only on persons nonreactive to the 1:100 dilution.

➤*Interpretation:* Consider the following points in interpretation: (1) A positive reaction may cause a transitory rise in titer of complement fixation antibody to histoplasma antigens, but not to coccidioidin; (2) coccidioidin may elicit skin test cross-reactions in individuals infected with *Histoplasma*, *Blastomyces* and possibly other fungi; (3) coccidioidin may boost level of skin sensitivity to coccidioidin in already sensitive individuals; (4) the skin test may be negative in severe forms of disease (anergy) or when prolonged periods of time have passed since infection.

Positive reaction – Induration of ≥ 5 mm. Erythema without induration is considered negative. Read tests both at 24 and 48 hours because some reactions may fade after 36 hours. A positive test reaction indicates present or past infection with *Coccidioides immitis*.

Negative reaction – A negative test (less than 5 mm in duration) means the individual has not been sensitized to coccidioidin or has lost sensitivity.

➤*Storage/Stability:* Store at 2° to 8°C (36° to 46°F). Discard if frozen. Product can tolerate 14 days at room temperature. Refrigerate dilutions after compounding and discard within 24 hours.

Actions

➤*Pharmacology:* Positive skin tests result from activation of sensitized T-lymphocytes, a delayed-hypersensitivity reaction involving cellular immunity. Coccidioidin deposited in the skin reacts with sensitized lymphocytes, causing the release of mediators that induce the inflammatory, edematous reaction recognized as a positive reaction. The reaction depends on the person having been previously sensitized to coccidioidin.

Spherule-derived coccidioidin may detect significantly more infected persons than mycelium-derived coccidioidin. Nonetheless, 50% false-negative rates have occurred in patients with disseminated disease. Coccidioidin tests are highly specific, implying that few healthy test recipients will test falsely positive. Mycelium- and spherule-derived products are probably equally specific.

Contraindications

Hypersensitivity to thimerosal; patients with erythema nodosum.

Warnings

➤*Immunodeficiency:* Persons receiving immunosuppressive therapy or with other immunodeficiencies (especially those involving cell-mediated immunity) may have a diminished skin-test response to this and other diagnostic antigens.

➤*Hypersensitivity reactions:* Because of the possibility of an immediate systemic allergic reaction, observe the patient for 15 minutes after the injection. Have epinephrine available in case an acute hypersensitivity reaction occurs. See also Management of Acute Hypersensitivity Reactions.

➤*Pregnancy:* *Category C.* Use only if clearly needed. It is unlikely that coccidioidin crosses the placenta.

➤*Lactation:* It is not likely that coccidioidin is excreted in breast milk.

➤*Children:* Safety and efficacy of mycelial coccidioidin have not been specifically established in children, but spherule-derived coccidioidin is safe and effective in children, including those younger than 5 years of age.

Drug Interactions

Coccidioidin Drug Interactions

Precipitant drug	Object drug[a]		Description
Immunosuppressants	Coccidioidin	↑	Reactivity to any delayed-hypersensitivity test may be suppressed in persons receiving corticosteroids or other immunosuppressive drugs, or in persons who were recently immunized with live virus vaccines (eg, measles, mumps, rubella, poliovirus). If delayed-hypersensitivity skin testing is indicated, perform it either preceding or simultaneous with immunization or 4 to 6 weeks after immunization.
Cimetidine	Coccidioidin	↑	Several weeks of cimetidine therapy may augment or enhance delayed-hypersensitivity responses to skin test antigens, although this effect was not consistently observed. The effect may be mediated through cimetidine binding to suppressor T-lymphocytes.

[a] ↑ = Object drug increased.

➤*Drug/Lab test interactions:* A positive reaction to *BioCox* may cause a rise in titers of complement-fixing antibodies against *Emmonsiella capsulata* (*Histoplasma capsulatum*) and coccidioidin. Unlike *BioCox*, *Spherulin* does not induce humoral antibodies nor does it affect complement-fixation titers for either histoplasmosis or coccidioidomycosis. Either coccidioidin may boost existing hypersensitivity in recipients, manifested after a subsequent test.

Adverse Reactions

➤*Local:* An occasional patient may develop an immediate local wheal reaction. Occasionally, large local reactions may lead to vesiculation, local tissue necrosis and scar formation.

➤*Systemic:* Patients with great sensitivity may rarely develop a systemic reaction consisting of fever or erythema nodosum. There are no reports that skin testing can cause a recrudescence of the disease.

HISTAMINE PHOSPHATE

Rx	**Histatrol** (Center Laboratories)	**Scratch/Prick**: 1 mg/ml histamine base as the phosphate (2.75 mg/ml histamine phosphate)	Glycerin 50% w/v, 0.4% phenol. In 5 ml vials.
		Multi-Test: 1 mg/ml histamine base as the phosphate	Glycerin 50% w/v. In 5 ml vials.
		Intradermal: 0.1 mg/ml histamine base as the phosphate (0.275 mg/ml histamine phosphate)	Glycerin free. 0.4% phenol. In 5 ml vials.

HISTAMINE PHOSPHATE — INTRADERMAL

Indications

➤*Allergenic skin testing:* For use as a positive control in evaluation of allergenic skin testing.

Administration and Dosage

➤*Interpretation:* The patient's response is based on the size of erythema (degree of redness) and size of wheal (smooth, slightly elevated area) which appear after 15 to 20 minutes.

Prick, puncture, and scratch testing – Use histamine base 1 mg/ml (histamine phosphate 2.75 mg/ml) to give a positive reaction. In a large population, the NHANES II survey reports a mean (average of length and width) wheal of 4.4 mm and a mean erythema of 18.4 mm. Interpret all positive reactions against an appropriate negative control.

Intradermal skin testing – Use histamine base 0.1 mg/ml (histamine phosphate 0.275 mg/ml) or 0.01 mg/ml to give a positive reaction. In 2 successive years of testing, the Committee on Standardization of the American College of Allergy reported positive reactions at histamine base doses ≥ 0.01 mg/ml. Mean sum of diameter (sum of length and width) of wheals were ≈ 14 mm and sum of erythema was ≈ 52 mm following 0.01 ml intradermal doses of 0.01 mg/ml histamine base. When 0.01 ml of 0.1 mg/ml histamine base was injected, the sum of crossed diameters of wheal ranged from 15 to 20 mm and the sum of crossed diameters of erythema ranged from 60 to 80 mm. The available 0.1 mg/ml concentration must be diluted to achieve this dose. Interpret all positive reactions against an appropriate negative control.

➤*Storage / Stability:* Refrigerate and protect vials from light.

Actions

➤*Pharmacology:* Histamine acts as a potent vasodilator when released from mast cells during an allergic reaction. It is largely responsible for the immediate skin test reaction of a sensitive patient when challenged with an offending allergen.

Contraindications

Do not inject histamine into individuals with hypotension, severe hypertension, or severe cardiac, pulmonary, or renal disease.

Warnings

➤*Intracutaneous testing:* Use caution in intracutaneous testing to avoid injection into a venule or capillary.

➤*Bronchial disease:* Small doses by any route of administration may precipitate asthma in patients with bronchial disease.

➤*Hypersensitivity reactions:* Epinephrine injection (1:1000) and injectable antihistamines should be available for immediate use in the event the patient exhibits a severe response. A tourniquet can be applied above the test site to slow absorption if a severe response occurs.

➤*Pregnancy: Category C.* There are no adequate and well-controlled studies in pregnant women. However, based on histamine's known ability to contract uterine muscle, avoid exposure or repeated doses. Use histamine phosphate during pregnancy only if the potential benefit justifies the potential risk to the fetus or mother.

➤*Children:* Histamine solutions for percutaneous testing have been given safely in infants and young children. Therefore, anticipate small skin test reactions in children < 6 years of age. Safety and efficacy for intracutaneous testing in children < 6 years of age have not been established.

Drug Interactions

➤*Antiallergic drugs:* In the period of 24 hours prior to testing, the patient should not have taken any antiallergic drugs. The pharmacologic action of such agents interferes with the skin test response.

Adverse Reactions

Following the injection of large doses of histamine, systemic reactions may include flushing, dizziness, headache, bronchial constriction, urticaria, asthma, marked hypertension or hypotension, abdominal cramps, vomiting, metallic taste, and local or generalized allergic manifestations.

Overdosage

➤*Symptoms:* A large SC dose of histamine phosphate may cause severe occipital headache, blurred vision, anginal pain, a rapid drop in blood pressure, and cyanosis of the face.

➤*Treatment:* Give epinephrine injection SC or IM in case of emergency due to severe reactions (see Warnings). An antihistamine preparation may be given IM to ameliorate systemic reaction to overdose.

HISTOPLASMIN

Rx	**Histoplasmin, Diluted** (Parke-Davis)	**Injection**: 1:100 w/v (P-D) or v/v (ALK). Standardized sterile filtrate from cultures of *Histoplasma capsulatum*	0.5% phenol, polysorbate 80. Mycelial derivative. In 1 ml, 10 test multidose vials.
Rx	**Histolyn-CYL** (ALK Labs)		0.4% phenol, polysorbate 80, human serum albumin. Controlled yeast lysate. In 1.3 ml multidose vials.

HISTOPLASMIN — INJECTION

Indications

➤*Histoplasmosis, diagnosis:* An aid in the diagnosis of histoplasmosis and the differentiation of possible histoplasmosis from coccidioidomycosis, sarcoidosis and other mycotic or bacterial infections and in the interpretation of roentgenographic plates showing pulmonary infiltration and calcification.

➤*Unlabeled uses:* In endemic areas (eg, the Ohio and Mississippi River valleys), histoplasmin may be a useful addition to anergy skin test panels to assess competence of recipients' cell-mediated immunity, but use of mycelial histoplasmin may obscure the results of other fungal assays.

Administration and Dosage

➤*Test method:* The skin test is performed by injecting 0.1 mL intradermally into the flexor surface of the forearm. The site of injection is first cleansed with 70% alcohol and allowed to dry. A tuberculin syringe (one that has not been used for tuberculin) and a 26 g × ⅜" or 27 g × ½" needle is used. If injections are correctly made, a small bleb will rise over the needle point. The reactions should be read in a well-lighted room 48 to 72 hours after injection.

➤*Interpretation of reaction:* The reaction should be described and measured in terms of mm of induration and degree of reaction (from slight induration to vesiculation and necrosis). In many studies reported in the literature a reaction of 5 mm or greater induration is considered to be positive. In case of doubt, and if clinically indicated, the test should be repeated but only after obtaining serum for antibody titer.

Positive reaction – A positive histoplasmin reaction may be indicative of a past infection or a mild, subacute or chronic infection with *Histoplasma capsulatum* or immunologically related organisms, such as *Blastomyces* or *Coccidioides* species. It may also denote improvement in cases of serious illness of symptomatic histoplasmosis that previously may have been histoplasmin-negative.

Differential diagnosis – Histoplasmin is of little value in diagnosing acute fulminating infections because a negative reaction usually occurs in such cases. In mild infections, repeatedly negative reactions may suggest the exclusion of *Histoplasma* as the causative agent. It is advised that the tuberculin test be employed in conjunction with histoplasmin in order to exclude the possibility of tuberculosis. The histoplasmin skin test sometimes causes elevation of serum antibody titers to histoplasmin.

One study employed 3 criteria to distinguish lesions associated with histoplasmin sensitivity from those due to other causes. These are: the individual has skin sensitivity to histoplasmin but not tuberculin; lesions must persist for 2 months (to exclude transient pneumonic lesions); and laboratory and clinical examinations to exclude tuberculosis, Boeck's sarcoid, coccidioidosis, Hodgkins' disease, etc. These criteria might be helpful in the interpretation of roentgenographic findings.

➤*Storage / Stability:* Store at temperature between 2° and 8°C (36° and 46°F).

Actions

➤*Pharmacology:* The sterile culture filtrates of *Histoplasma capsulatum* are grown on liquid synthetic medium.

The histoplasmin test is based on the fact that infection with *Histoplasma capsulatum* produces sensitivity to certain antigens. The reaction to intracutaneously injected histoplasmin reflects a delayed (cellular) hypersensitivity reaction. Clinically, a delayed hypersensitivity reaction to histoplasmin is nearly always a manifestation of previous infection with *Histoplasma capsulatum* or a variety of other mycotic or bacterial infections.

Contraindications

Known histoplasmin positive reactors because of the severity of reactions (eg, vesiculation, ulceration, or necrosis) that may occur at the test site in very highly sensitive individuals.

HISTOPLASMIN — INJECTION

Warnings

➤*Hypersensitivity reactions:* As with any biological product, epinephrine should be immediately available in case an anaphylactoid or acute hypersensitivity reaction occurs.

➤*Pregnancy: Category C.* Animal reproduction studies have not been conducted with histoplasmin. It is also not known whether histoplasmin can cause fetal harm when administered to a pregnant woman or can affect the reproduction capacity. Histoplasmin should be given to a pregnant woman only if clearly needed.

➤*Children:* Safety and effectiveness in pediatric patients have not been established.

Precautions

➤*Local reactions:* Doses greater than that recommended may produce severe erythema and induration followed by necrosis and ulceration that may last for several weeks.

➤*Administration:* Inject intradermally only. A separate sterile syringe and needle should be used for each individual patient to prevent transmission of hepatitis B virus and other infectious agents from one person to another.

➤*Serological studies:* If serological studies are clinically indicated, the blood sample should preferably be drawn prior to administering the skin test. If the sample is not obtained prior to skin testing, it may be obtained within 48 to 96 hours following the skin test injection. After the aforementioned time period, a rise in titer, as associated with a positive skin test, may occur.

Drug Interactions

Histoplasmin Drug Interactions

Precipitant drug	Object drug[a]		Description
Cimetidine	Histoplasmin	↑	Several weeks of cimetidine therapy may augment or enhance delayed-hypersensitivity responses to skin test antigens, although this effect was not consistently observed. The effect may be mediated through cimetidine binding to suppressor T-lymphocytes.
Immunosuppressants Vaccines, virus	Histoplasmin	↓	Reactivity to any delayed-hypersensitivity test may be suppressed in persons receiving corticosteroids or other immunosuppressive drugs, or in persons who were recently immunized with live virus vaccines (eg, measles, mumps, rubella, poliovirus). If delayed-hypersensitivity skin testing is indicated, perform it either preceding or simultaneously with immunization or 4 to 6 weeks after immunization.

[a] ↑ = Object drug increased. ↓ = Object drug decreased.

Adverse Reactions

➤*Hypersensitivity:* Hypersensitivity reactions such as urticaria, shortness of breath and excessive perspiration may occur.

➤*Local:* In highly sensitive individuals, strongly positive reactions including vesiculation, ulceration or necrosis may occur at the test site and may result in scarring. Cold packs or topical steroid preparations may be employed for symptomatic relief of the associated pain, pruritus and discomfort.

MUMPS SKIN TEST ANTIGEN (MSTA)

Rx	**MSTA** (Pasteur-Mérieux Connaught)	**Injection:** 40 complement-fixing units/ml	0.012 M glycine, < 1:8,000 formaldehyde solution, and 1:10,000 thimerosal. In 1 ml vials (10 tests).

MUMPS SKIN TEST ANTIGEN (MSTA) — INJECTION

Indications

➤*Delayed hypersensitivity to mumps:* For detection of delayed hypersensitivity to mumps antigens and assessment of cell-mediated immunity. Because most of the population (except the very young) have had contact or infection with mumps virus, they usually demonstrate a delayed cutaneous hypersensitivity to mumps skin test antigen if an adequate cellular immune system exists; 67% to 90% of healthy adults demonstrate a delayed hypersensitivity reaction.

Administration and Dosage

Must be given intradermally. If it is injected SC, no reaction or an unreliable reaction may occur.

➤*Test method:* Shake vial well before withdrawing each dose. Inject 0.1 ml intradermally on the inner surface of the forearm after suitable preparation of the skin. Examine the reaction in 48 to 72 hours.

➤*Interpretation:* Positive reaction consists of a mean diameter of induration ≥ 5 mm (ie, the average of the longest width and the longest length). A positive test implies previous antigenic exposure and, indirectly, T-lymphocyte competence and an intact inflammatory response, and confirms the integrity of the cellular immune response.

➤*Negative reaction:* If the test has been given correctly, it probably indicates either anergy or nonsensitivity.

➤*Pseudopositive reactions:* May develop in persons sensitive to egg protein.

➤*Storage/Stability:* Store between 2° and 8°C (36° to 46°F). Discard if frozen. Product can tolerate ≤ 4 days at ≤ 37°C (100°F). Do not freeze.

Actions

➤*Pharmacology:* Positive skin tests result from activation of sensitized T-lymphocytes, a delayed-hypersensitivity reaction involving cellular immunity. MSTA deposited in the skin reacts with sensitized lymphocytes, causing the release of mediators that induce the inflammatory, edematous reaction recognized as a positive reaction. The reaction depends on the person having been previously sensitized to mumps.

When used to assess delayed hypersensitivity reactivity in a group of 90 cancer patients, MSTA was essentially 100% sensitive (as confirmed by reaction to at least 1 other delayed hypersensitivity test antigen), implying that no immunocompetent test recipients would test falsely negative.

Contraindications

Generally, do not administer this product to anyone with a history of hypersensitivity, especially anaphylactic reactions, to eggs, egg products, or thimerosal.

Warnings

➤*Immunodeficiency:* Persons receiving immunosuppressive therapy or with other immunodeficiencies (especially those involving cell-mediated immunity) may have a diminished skin-test response to this and other diagnostic antigens. Tuberculosis, bacterial or viral infection, malnutrition, malignancy, and immunosuppression may suppress skin-test responsiveness.

➤*Hypersensitivity reactions:* Mumps skin test antigen is propagated in eggs and also contains thimerosal as a preservative. Do not administer to anyone with a history of hypersensitivity (allergy) to eggs, egg products, or thimerosal. Epinephrine injection (1:1000) must be immediately available to combat unexpected anaphylactic or other allergic reactions. See also Management of Acute Hypersensitivity Reactions.

➤*Elderly:* Skin-test responsiveness may be delayed or reduced in magnitude in older people.

➤*Pregnancy: Category C.* It is unlikely that MSTA crosses the placenta. It is not known whether MSTA can cause fetal harm when administered to a pregnant woman or can affect reproductive capacity. Give to a pregnant woman only if clearly needed.

➤*Lactation:* It is unlikely that MSTA is excreted into breast milk. It is not known whether this drug is excreted in human milk. Exercise caution when MSTA is administered to a nursing women.

➤*Children:* Safety and efficacy in children have not been established.

Precautions

➤*Mumps:* MSTA was initially used to determine susceptibility to mumps. It is no longer considered effective for identifying immunity to mumps virus infection. Safety and efficacy have not been established in young adults who have been immunized with live mumps vaccine.

MUMPS SKIN TEST ANTIGEN (MSTA) — INJECTION

Drug Interactions

Mumps Skin-Test Antigen Drug Interactions

Precipitant drug	Object drug[a]		Description
Cimetidine	MSTA	↑	Several weeks of cimetidine therapy may augment or enhance delayed hypersensitivity responses to skin-test antigens, although this effect was not consistently observed. The effect may be mediated through cimetidine binding to suppressor T-lymphocytes.
Immunosuppressants	MSTA	↓	Reactivity to any delayed hypersensitivity test may be suppressed in people receiving corticosteroids or other immunosuppressive drugs, or in people who were recently immunized with live virus vaccines (eg, measles, mumps, rubella, poliovirus). If delayed hypersensitivity skin testing is indicated, perform it either preceding or simultaneously with immunization, or 4 to 6 weeks after immunization.
Vaccines, viral	MSTA		

[a] ↑ = Object drug increased. ↓ = Object drug decreased.

Adverse Reactions

Local reactions may include tenderness, pruritus, vesiculation, and rash. Sloughing, necrosis, abscess formation, or regional lymphadenopathy may be associated with unusually large delayed hypersensitivity reactions. Adverse reactions may include nausea, anorexia, headache, unsteadiness, drowsiness, sweating, sensation of warmth, and lymphadenopathy.

Skin Test Antigens, Multiple

ALLERGEN PATCH TESTING

Rx	**T.R.U.E. Test** (GlaxoWellcome)	Allergen-containing patches. In multipack cartons (5s).

ALLERGEN PATCH TEST — INTRADERMAL

For additional information, refer to the Skin Test Antigens, Multiple Introduction.

Indications

➤*Contact dermatitis:* Primarily as an aid in the diagnosis of allergic contact dermatitis in patients whose histories suggest sensitivity to ≥ 1 of the substances included on the test panels. May also be used adjunctively to evaluate other eczemas (atopic, seborrheic, venous, palmar, and plantar hyperkeratotic eczema, vesiculosis, or neurodermatitis) and other dermatologic diseases that do not heal, such as leg ulcers and psoriasis, to determine whether there may be a contact hypersensitivity component.

Administration and Dosage

The test is best applied on the upper part of the back. Apply to healthy skin that is free of acne, scars, dermatitis, or any other condition that may interfere with interpretation of test results. Discontinue use of topical steroids on the test site or oral steroids (equivalent to 15 mg prednisolone) for ≥ 2 weeks prior to testing. Topical steroids on nontest areas may be appropriate. Instruct patients to avoid extreme physical activity or mechanical action that may result in reduced adhesion or loss of patch test material. Avoid getting the area around the patch wet. Minimize exposure to the sun in order to prevent a sun-induced skin reaction that may interfere with interpretation of test results. Older patients may exhibit an increased frequency of cutaneous allergies.

➤*Application:* Apply patches taken directly from the refrigerator or allow them to come to room temperature (15 to 20 minutes) prior to application. Remove protective plastic covering from test panel 1.1. Position the allergen patch test on the upper left side of the patient's back (≈ 5 cm from the midline) so that #1 allergen is in the upper left corner. Avoid applying on the margin of the scapula; smooth outward toward the edges. With a medical marking pen, indicate on the skin the location of the 2 notches on the panel.

Repeat the process with test panel 2.1 on the upper right side of the patient's back so that #13 allergen is in the upper left corner. Have the patient wear the patch test for a minimum of 48 hours.

➤*Interpretation:* A positive test reaction should meet the criteria for an allergic reaction (papular or vesicular erythema and infiltration).

The reaction should be read at 72 to 96 hours, when allergic reactions are fully developed and mild irritant reactions have faded. If reading at 48 hours is considered, another reading at 72 to 96 hours is recommended. Advise patients to report reactions occurring after 7 days to detect potential sensitizations. Note that p-phenylenediamine may turn the patch test area black on some patients. This is because the allergen is a dye and does not represent an allergic reaction. Discoloration may remain for approximately ≤ 2 weeks.

Neomycin sulfate and p-phenylenediamine sometimes cause reactions that may not appear until 4 or 5 days (or later) after the application. Instruct patients to report this. An additional office visit will verify a late reaction.

False negatives – False-negative results may be caused by insufficient patch contact with the skin, sensitization to a substance not present in the test panel, or premature evaluation of the test.

False positives – A false-positive result may occur when an irritant reaction (patchy follicular or homogeneous erythema without infiltration) cannot be differentiated from an allergic reaction. If an irritant reaction cannot be distinguished, a retest may be considered in a few weeks or months.

A test reaction that appears 7 days or later with no preceding reaction may be a sign of contact sensitization.

Dermatitis flare up may occur in some patients. Excited skin syndrome (angry back) consists of a hyperreactive state of the skin in which false-positive patch test reactions concur with dermatitis at a distant body site or with adjacent strong positive skin test reactions. On rare occasions, it may be necessary to remove the test strip from the patient because of severe itching or burning sensations.

Evaluate test results carefully in patients with multiple, positive, concomitant patch test results. To determine false positives, retesting at a later date may be considered.

➤*Storage/Stability:* Store between 2° and 8°C (36° and 46°F).

Actions

➤*Pharmacology:* A positive response to the patch test is a classical delayed cell-mediated hypersensitivity reaction (type IV), which normally appears within 9 to 96 hours after exposure.

Following primary contact, an allergen penetrates the skin and binds covalently or noncovalently to epidermal Langerhans cells. The processed allergen is presented to helper T-lymphocytes, resulting in the release of lymphokines, including interleukin 2. Interleukin 2 stimulates the production of other lymphocytes, chemotactic factors that recruit macrophages, basophils, eosinophils, and migration inhibitory factor, all which induce macrophages to remain at the reaction site. The resulting inflammation produces a papular, vesicular, or bullous response with erythema and itching at the site of application.

The allergens in allergen patch test were selected from those substances that have been widely reported to induce allergic contact dermatitis. They represent ≈ 80% of the most common allergens. Nickel sulfate normally induces the greatest number of positive patch test responses when screening prospective patients. The frequency of positive responses to the various allergens can change depending upon the specific patient population as well as occupational and environmental influences. The epidemiology of allergic contact dermatitis and the frequency of positive patch test reactions to various causative allergens have been the subject of several extensive studies.

Contraindications

The minor amount of allergen on each allergen patch test patch that penetrates the skin will rarely induce a flare-up of dermatitis. In the case of extensive ongoing contact dermatitis, however, the test should not be applied since it may provoke an intensified reaction on both the present and previously affected sites and may also cause a false-positive test result.

Warnings

➤*Hypersensitivity reactions:* The use of allergen patch test in patients with a known history of severe systemic or local reactions to any of the allergen components or inactive substances included in the allergen patch test panels should be carefully evaluated before application.

Patients should be warned that itching and burning sensations are common occurrences with patch testing and may be severe in extremely sensitive patients. The use of medication may be considered necessary to relieve these itching or burning sensations.

Sensitization to a substance included on the test panel may occur with patch testing but is extremely rare. A test reaction that appears 7 days or later with no preceding reaction may be a sign of contact sensitization.

Dermatitis flare-up may occur in some patients.

Occasionally, hyperpigmentation of the test site occurs during healing. Healing with or without medication normally takes place within 5 days to 2 weeks, although reactions in some individuals may persist longer.

ALLERGEN PATCH TEST — INTRADERMAL

Extremely sensitive patients may exhibit extreme (+++) reactions that may be bullous or ulcerative with pronounced erythema, infiltration, and coalescing vesicles.

Excited skin syndrome (angry back) is a state of hyper-reactivity induced by a dermatitis on other parts of the body or by a strong positive skin-test reaction.

Therefore, test results should be evaluated carefully in patients with multiple, positive, concomitant patch test results. To determine which reactions are false positives, retesting at a later date may be considered.

The safety and efficacy of repetitive testing with allergen patch test is unknown. Sensitization or increased reactivity to one or more of the allergens may occur. The benefits of repeat testing should therefore be carefully evaluated against the possible risks.

On rare occasions, it may be necessary to remove the test strip from the patient because of severe itching or burning sensations. One patient taking part in the clinical studies removed the test tape after 24 hours because of severe itching.

➤*Carcinogenesis:* Formaldehyde is a known carcinogen. Nickel refinery dust, nickel sulfite, and formaldehyde are known carcinogens. Nickel sulfate, potassium dichromate, cobalt dichloride, epoxy resin, and thiuram mix are suspected carcinogens. The potential effects of using very low concentrations of these substances for single or multiple applications are currently unknown. The following components of allergen patch test have been reviewed as part of the Cosmetic Ingredient Review and found to be safe or safe with qualifications: Those found to be safe are hydroxypropyl cellulose, methylcellulose, wool alcohols, paraben mix, Quaternium-15, and p-Phenylenediamine and those found to be safe with qualifications are N-phenyl-p-phenylenediamine, Cl+ Me− isothiazolinone, and formaldehyde.

➤*Elderly:* More frequent patch test responses can be expected in geriatric patients. While no conclusive explanation is available, older patients may exhibit an increased frequency of cutaneous allergies.

➤*Pregnancy: Category C.* Animal reproduction studies have not been conducted with allergen patch test. It is also not known whether allergen patch test can cause fetal harm when administered to pregnant women or whether it can affect reproduction capacity. Allergen patch test should be applied to pregnant women only if clearly needed.

➤*Lactation:* No studies have been performed to evaluate absorption of allergen patch test allergens in nursing mothers. It is not known if allergen patch test allergens appear in human milk. Because many drugs are excreted in human milk, caution should be exercised when allergen patch test is administered to a nursing woman.

➤*Children:* The safety and effectiveness of allergen patch test in children have not been established.

Precautions

➤*Patch testing during the summer months:* Allergen patch test may be applied throughout the year. However, during the summer months, excessive sweating is to be avoided in order to maintain sufficient adhesion to the skin. In addition, exposure to the sun should be minimized in order to prevent a sun-induced skin reaction that may interfere with interpretation of test results.

➤*Patch application:* See Administration and Dosage for more information.

➤*Severe patch test reaction:* If a severe patch test reaction develops, the patient may be treated with a topical corticosteroid or, in rare cases, with a systemic corticosteroid.

Adverse Reactions

Sensitization – In some cases, allergenic responses may be delayed in onset. One type of delayed reaction is a sensitization, which is not well defined in the literature but is described as a positive reaction observed at 10 to 14 days after application or later and at 2 to 4 days after the test is repeated. The positive reaction should meet the criteria for an allergic reaction (papular or vesicular erythema and infiltration) in order to distinguish between a false-positive result and a sensitization.

Delayed reactions – In clinical studies conducted with allergen patch test, there have been 3 reports of delayed reactions occurring at 21 days or later. None of these patients were retested to verify a sensitization reaction. There is enough data for only 2 of these patients to indicate probable sensitization. For more details of these reactions, refer to summaries of studies No. 3 and No. 4 in the Clinical Pharmacology section.

Other adverse reactions – There are reports of other adverse reactions associated with patch testing. These include keloids, sarcoid infiltrates, vitiligo spots, edema, crusting, and sensitization.

➤*Adverse reactions reported during patient follow-up:*

Adverse reactions reported during patient follow-up[1]					
	Number of events reported				
Reaction reported	Study 1 (n = 33)[2]	Study 2 (n = 102)[3]	Study 3 (n = 104)[3]	Study 4 (n = 32)[2]	Nickel use (n = 31)[2]
Erythema	2	2	27	2	
Hyperpigmentation	9	2	8	6	8
Pruritus	3	1	27	2	
Scarring			2		
Urticaria					1
Delayed reaction (allergen known)			1[4]		
Delayed reaction (allergen unknown)		2	2		
Sensitization (potential)			1[5]		
Sensitization (probable)			1[6]	1[7]	

[1] Patient follow-up was either via telephone or an office visit; time of follow-up ranged from 4 to 80 days after testing.
[2] Number of patients with positive test results who took part in clinical follow-up.
[3] Number of total patients who took part in the clinical follow-up.
[4] Neomycin sulfate.
[5] Wool alcohols.
[6] p-tert Butylphenol formaldehyde resin.
[7] Cl+Me− isothiazolinone.

➤*Incidences of itching and burning events:* The table below shows itching and burning events from the 5 clinical studies described in Clinical trials. A number of patients in the study groups were prescribed medication to either promote healing or to relieve itching or burning sensations. Itching and burning sensations are commonly associated with patch testing. Treatment may be required and the more severe reactions can be expected to require longer times to heal.

In addition, the adhesive tape may also cause an irritation at the test site. Reports of tape irritation are infrequent, usually mild in nature, and self-limiting in clinical studies conducted with allergen patch test, though no data was collected in these studies beyond a day 21 safety visit. In the nickel use test study and in a Panel 2 clinical study (study no. 2), problems with tape adhesion were observed. Twenty-four percent and 11%, respectively, of the patients in these studies reported poor tape adhesion. (See Clinical Pharmacology section for complete descriptions of these studies.) In both studies, the problem was subsequently attributed to the lot of adhesive tape used to produce the clinical test samples. No adhesion problems have been reported in other studies.

Incidences of itching and burning sensations reported by the patients at the time of patch test removal					
	Number of events reported				
Event reported	Study 1 (n = 128)*	Study 2 (n = 122)*	Study 3 (n = 122)*	Study 4 (n = 50)*	Nickel use (n = 50)*
Itching					
Mild	31	23	48	14	30
Moderate				2	
Strong	21	5	17		24
Burning sensations					
Mild	7	4	8	14	4
Moderate				2	
Strong	5	2	1		8
Total events	04	34	74	32	66

* Total number of patients in study.

Patient Information

Patients should be instructed to avoid extreme physical activity or mechanical action that may result in reduced adhesion or actual loss of patch test material. Use appropriate measures to avoid getting the area around the patch wet.

Patients should also be advised that a strong allergic response to one or more test allergens can be associated with significant itching, burning, erythema, and vesiculation. Patients who experience intense discomfort should contact their physician concerning possible removal of the test.

TUBERCULIN PURIFIED PROTEIN DERIVATIVE (Mantoux; PPD; Tuberculin skin test [TST])

Rx	**Aplisol** (Monarch)	**Injection:** 5 TU[a]/0.1 mL	In 1 mL (10 tests) and 5 mL (50 tests) vials.[b]
Rx	**Tubersol** (Aventis Pasteur)		In 1 mL (10 tests) and 5 mL (50 tests) vials.[c]

[a] TU = tuberculin units.
[b] With potassium and sodium phosphates, 0.35% phenol, and polysorbate 80.
[c] In isotonic phosphate buffer saline with 0.28% phenol and polysorbate 80.

TUBERCULIN PURIFIED PROTEIN DERIVATIVE (MANTOUX) — INJECTION

Indications

➤*Tuberculosis (TB) skin test:* An aid in the detection of infection with *Mycobacterium tuberculosis*.

Purified protein derivative (PPD) tuberculin may be used as an aid in the diagnosis of tuberculosis infection in persons with a history of BCG vaccination. HIV-infected individuals should receive tuberculin skin testing as recommended.

Administration and Dosage

In addition, it is essential that the physician or nurse record the test results in millimeters of induration, including 0, in the permanent medical record of each patient. This permanent medical record should contain the name of the product, date given, dose, manufacturer and lot number. Reporting results only as negative or positive is not satisfactory.

➤*The test:* The Mantoux test is performed by injecting intradermally, with a syringe and needle, 0.1 mL of tuberculin purified protein derivative (Mantoux). For the intradermal (Mantoux) tuberculin test, the dose is 5 US units (TU) per test dose of 0.1 mL.

Two-step testing should be performed on the initial testing if tuberculin testing will subsequently be conducted at regular intervals, for instance among healthcare workers. If the first test showed either no reaction or a small reaction, the second test should be performed 1 to 4 weeks later. Both tests should be read and recorded at 48 to 72 hours. Patients with a second tuberculin test (booster) response of 10 mm or more should be considered to have experienced past or old infection.

Persons who do not boost when given repeat tests at 1 week, but whose tuberculin reactions change to positive after 1 year, should be considered to have newly acquired tuberculosis infection and managed accordingly.

➤*Method of administration:*

1.) The preferred site of the test is the flexor (volar) surface of the forearm.
2.) The skin site is first cleansed with suitable germicide and should be dry prior to injection of the antigen.
3.) The recommended test dose (0.1 mL) of tuberculin PPD is administered with a 1 mL syringe calibrated in tenths and fitted with a short, one-quarter to one-half inch, 26- or 27-gauge needle.
4.) The rubber cap of the vial should be wiped with a suitable germicide and should be dry prior to needle insertion. The needle is then inserted gently through the cap, and 0.1 mL of tuberculin PPD is drawn into the syringe. Care should be taken to avoid injection of excess air with removal of each dose so as to not overpressurize the vial, thus causing possible seepage at the site of the puncture.
5.) The point of the needle is inserted into the epidermal (most superficial) layers of the skin with the needle bevel pointing upward. If the intradermal injection is performed properly, a definite pale bleb will rise at the needle point, about 10 mm (3/8 inch) in diameter. This bleb will disperse within minutes. No dressing is required.

In the event of an improperly performed injection (ie, no bleb formed), the test should be repeated immediately at another site.

➤*Interpretation:* The test should be read 48 to 72 hours after administration of tuberculin PPD. Sensitivity is indicated by induration only, and any erythema is disregarded. Distinctly palpable induration should be measured in millimeters transversely to the long axis of the forearm and recorded in millimeters.

Presence and size of necrosis and edema if present should also be recorded, although not used in the interpretation of the test.

Sensitivity to tuberculin may be the result of a previous infection with mycobacteria. This infection, likely due to *M. tuberculosis*, may have occurred years ago or may be of recent origin.

Positive reaction – An induration of greater than or equal to 5 mm is classified as positive for people who have human immunodeficiency virus (HIV) infection or risk factors for HIV infection but unknown HIV status; those who have had recent close contact (recent close contact implies either household or social contact or unprotected occupational exposure similar in intensity and duration to household contact) with persons who have active TB; or people who have fibrotic chest radiographs (consistent with healed TB).

An induration of greater than or equal to 10 mm is classified as positive in all persons who do not meet any of the criteria above but who have other risk factors for TB (high-risk group and high prevalence groups as defined by the CDC).

An induration of greater than or equal to 15 mm is classified as positive in persons who do not meet any of the above criteria.

Recent converters: Recent converters are defined on the basis of both size of induration and age of the person being tested:

- A greater than or equal to 10 mm increase within a 2-year period is classified as a recent conversion for persons younger than 35 years of age.
- A greater than or equal to 15 mm increase within a 2-year period is classified as a recent conversion for persons greater than or equal to 35 years of age.

Healthcare workers (HCWs): In general, the recommendations above should be followed when interpreting skin test results in HCWs. However, the prevalence of TB in the facility should be considered when choosing the appropriate cutpoint for defining a positive PPD reaction. In facilities where there is essentially no risk for exposure to *M. tuberculosis* (ie, minimal- or very low-risk facilities), an induration greater than or equal to 15 mm may be a suitable cutpoint for HCWs who have no other risk factors. In facilities where TB patients receive care, the cutpoint for HCWs with no other risk factors may be greater than or equal to 10 mm.

A recent conversion in an HCW should be defined generally as a greater than or equal to 10 mm increase in size of induration within a 2-year period. For HCWs who work in facilities where exposure to TB is very unlikely (eg, minimal-risk facilities), an increase of greater than or equal to 15 mm within a 2-year period may be more appropriate for defining a recent conversion because of the lower positive-predictive value of the test in such groups.

BCG vaccination: The possibility should be considered that the skin test sensitivity may also be due to a previous contact with atypical mycobacteria or previous Bacille Calmette-Guérin vaccine (BCG) vaccination.

BCG vaccination may produce a PPD reaction that cannot be distinguished reliably from a reaction caused by infection with *M. tuberculosis*. For a person who was vaccinated with BCG, the probability that a PPD reaction results from infection with *M. tuberculosis* increases as the size of the reaction increases, when the person is a contact of a person with TB, when the person's country of origin has a high prevalence of TB, and as the length of time between vaccination and PPD testing increases. For example, a PPD test reaction of 10 mm probably can be attributed to *M. tuberculosis* infection in an adult who was vaccinated with BCG as a child and who is from a country with high prevalence of TB.

Retesting: Induration of less than 15 mm in healthy persons is considered negative. An individual who does not show a positive reaction to 5 TU on the first test, but is suspected of being TB positive, may be retested with 5 TU.

Tuberculin negative – Any individual who does not show a positive reaction to an initial injection of 5 TU, or a second test with 5 TU may be considered as tuberculin negative.

An individual who is considered to be at a high risk for contacting tuberculosis, should have an annual PPD skin test.

False-negative reactions – False-negative tuberculin skin-test reactions have many potential causes. Nonresponsiveness to delayed-type hypersensitivity-inducing antigens like tuberculin is common among persons having impaired immunity (eg, HIV-infected persons). Delayed-type hypersensitivity can also be assessed with skin-test antigens such as tetanus toxoid, mumps, and Candida. Most healthy persons in the population are sensitized to these antigens. Anergy testing is usually not part of routine screening for TB infection.

All HIV-infected persons should be tuberculin tested. Those who are tuberculin-positive (greater than or equal to 5 mm) should be evaluated for TB disease and placed on appropriate curative or preventive therapy. Preventive therapy should be administered to tuberculin-positive, HIV-infected persons, regardless of age. If they are at high risk for TB, persons failing to react to tuberculin may be evaluated for anergy, although the lack of standardization of anergy testing practices should be considered.

Booster effect – Infection of an individual with tubercle bacilli or other mycobacteria results in a delayed hypersensitivity response to tuberculin which is demonstrated by the skin test. The delayed hypersensitivity response may gradually wane over a period of years. If a person receives a tuberculin test at this time (after several years) the response may be a reaction that is not significant. The stimulus of the test may boost or increase the size of the reaction to a second test, sometimes causing an apparent conversion or development of sensitivity.

Tuberculin reactivity may indicate prior infection or disease with *M. tuberculosis* and does not necessarily indicate the presence of active tuberculous disease. Individuals showing a tuberculin reaction should be further evaluated with other diagnostic procedures.

Those individuals giving a positive tuberculin reaction may or may not show evidence of tuberculosis disease. Chest x-ray examination and microbiological examination of the sputum in these cases are recommended as a means of determining the presence or absence of pulmonary tuberculosis.

➤*Storage/Stability:* Tuberculin PPD (Mantoux) should be stored between 2° and 8°C (35° and 46°F). Do not freeze. Discard product if exposed to freezing. Tuberculin solutions can be adversely affected by exposure to light. The product should be stored in the dark except when doses are actually being withdrawn from the vial.

A vial of tuberculin PPD which has been opened and in use for 1 month should be discarded because oxidation and degradation may have reduced the potency. Do not use after expiration date.

Actions

➤*Pharmacology:* Tuberculin PPD is indicated for the detection of a delayed hypersensitivity reaction to tuberculin as an aid in the detection of infection with *Mycobacterium tuberculosis*.

The reaction to intradermally injected tuberculin is a delayed (cellular) hypersensitivity reaction. The reaction which characteristically shows a delayed course, reaching its peak more than 48 to 72 hours after administration, consists of induration caused by cellular infiltration of lyphocytes.

TUBERCULIN PURIFIED PROTEIN DERIVATIVE (MANTOUX) — INJECTION

Clinically, a delayed hypersensitivity reaction to tuberculin is a manifestation of previous infection with *M. tuberculosis* or a variety of nontuberculosis bacteria. Sensitization may be induced by natural mycobacterial infection or by vaccination with BCG vaccine.

The sensitization following infection with mycobacteria occurs primarily in the regional lymph nodes. Small lymphocytes (T lymphocytes) proliferate in response to the antigenic stimulus to give rise to specifically sensitized lymphocytes. After several weeks, these lymphocytes enter the blood stream and circulate for long periods of time. Subsequent restimulation of these sensitized lymphocytes with the same or a similar antigen, such as the intradermal injection of tuberculin, evokes a local reaction caused by infiltration of these cells.

The tuberculin reaction is characterized by the early predominance of mononuclear cells (small- and medium-sized lymphocytes and monocytes). Only a small proportion of these cells appear to be lymphocytes sensitized to tuberculin. Most cells are brought into the reaction through the release of biologically active substances by sensitized lymphocytes. An increase in vascular permeability leading to erythema and edema also occurs in tuberculin reactions.

Characteristically, delayed hypersensitivity reactions to tuberculin begin at 5 to 6 hours, are maximal at 48 to 72 hours and subside over a period of days. Immediate hypersensitivity (allergic) reactions to tuberculin or to constituents of the diluent may also occur, but these allergic reactions have no diagnostic importance.

The repeated testing of uninfected persons does not sensitize them to tuberculin.

Contraindications

Allergy to any component of tuberculin purified protein derivative (Mantoux); an allergic reaction to a previous test of tuberculin purified protein derivative (Mantoux).

Tuberculin purified protein derivative (Mantoux) should not be administered to persons who previously experienced a severe reaction (eg, vesiculation, ulceration, necrosis) because of the severity of reactions that may occur at the test site.

Warnings

➤*SC injection:* Avoid injecting tuberculin PPD (Mantoux) SC. If this occurs, no local reaction will develop, and the test cannot be interpreted.

➤*False-negative reactions:* Not all infected persons will have a delayed hypersensitivity reaction to a tuberculin test. A large number of factors has been reported to cause a decreased ability to respond to the tuberculin test in the presence of tuberculous infection including viral infections (measles, mumps, chickenpox and HIV), live virus vaccinations (measles, mumps, rubella, oral polio and yellow fever), overwhelming tuberculosis, other bacterial infections, drugs (corticosteroids and many other immunosuppressive agents), and malignancy.

Anything that impairs or attenuates cell-mediated immunity (CMI) potentially can cause a false negative tuberculin reaction (viral infections, particularly HIV, live virus vaccines, severe protein malnutrition, lymphoma, leukemia, sarcoidosis, use of glucocorticosteroids and other immunosuppressant drugs).

➤*HIV infection:* Because in HIV-infected individuals, tuberculin skin-test results are less reliable as CD4 counts decline, screening should be completed as early as possible after HIV infection occurs. Those HIV-infected patients at high risk for continuing exposure to patients who have TB should be screened periodically for TB infection. If they have TB symptoms or if they are exposed to a patient who has pulmonary TB, HIV-infected persons should be evaluated promptly for TB. Because active disease can develop rapidly in HIV-infected persons, the highest priority for contact investigation should be given to persons potentially coinfected with HIV and TB.

➤*Active TB:* Tuberculin PPD (Mantoux) should be administered with caution, or not at all, in persons with documented active tuberculosis or documented treatment in the past because of the severity of reactions (eg, vesiculation, ulceration, necrosis) that may occur at the test site.

➤*Hypersensitivity reactions:* Characteristically, delayed hypersensitivity reactions to tuberculin begin at 5 to 6 hours, are maximal at 48 to 72 hours and subside over a period of days. Immediate hypersensitivity (allergic) reactions to tuberculin or to constituents of the diluent may also occur, but these allergic reactions have no diagnostic importance.

The possibility of allergic reactions in individuals sensitive to the components of the product should be borne in mind. Epinephrine hydrochloride solution (1:1000) should be readily available for use in case an anaphylactic or acute hypersensitivity reaction occurs.

➤*Carcinogenesis:* The product should not be used for extended treatment over a long period of time.

➤*Mutagenesis:* The product should not be used for extended treatment over a long period of time.

➤*Fertility impairment:* The product should not be used for extended treatment over a long period of time.

➤*Pregnancy: Category C.* Animal reproduction studies have not been conducted with tuberculin PPD (Mantoux). However, the Advisory Council for Elimination of Tuberculosis states that tuberculin skin testing is considered valid and safe throughout pregnancy. No teratogenic effects of testing during pregnancy have been documented.

The risk of unrecognized tuberculosis and the close postpartum contact between a mother with active disease and an infant leaves the infant in grave danger of tuberculosis and complications such as tuberculous meningitis. Therefore, the prescribing physician will want to consider if the potential benefits outweigh the possible risks for performing the tuberculin test on a pregnant woman or a woman of childbearing age, particularly in certain high-risk populations.

➤*Children:* There is no age contraindication to tuberculin skin testing of infants. Because their immune systems are immature, many infants less than 6 weeks of age who are infected with *M. tuberculosis* do not react to tuberculin tests. Older infants and children develop tuberculin sensitivity 6 weeks or more after initial infection. Very young children are at increased risk for active tuberculosis once infected; therefore, during contact investigations, priority with regard to skin testing and evaluation for preventive therapy should be given to infants and young children who have been exposed to persons with active tuberculosis. These children should receive preventive therapy if their reactions to a tuberculin skin test measure greater than or equal to 5 mm. A cutoff of 10 mm is appropriate for children where tuberculosis case rates are high. A cutoff of 15 mm is used for children with minimal risk exposure to tuberculosis.

Precautions

➤*Sterile techniques:* A separate, sterile syringe and needle must be used for each individual injection to prevent the possibility of transmission of viral hepatitis or other infectious agents from 1 person to another. There have been case reports of transmission of HIV and hepatitis by failure to scrupulously observe sterile technique. In particular, the same needle must never be used to reenter a multidose vial even when it is to be used on the same patient. This may lead to the contamination of the vial contents and infection of patients who subsequently receive product from the vial. Needles should not be recapped and should be disposed of according to applicable biohazard waste guidelines.

Failure to store and handle tuberculin purified protein derivative (Mantoux) as recommended will result in a loss of potency and potentially inaccurate test results.

➤*Administration:* Special care should be taken to ensure the product is given intradermally and on the volar aspect of the forearm. Do not administer IV, IM or SC.

➤*Patient history:* Before using this product, all appropriate precautions should be taken to prevent adverse reactions. This includes a review of the patient's history with respect to possible hypersensitivity to the product, determination of previous use of tuberculin purified protein derivative (Mantoux) and the presence of any contraindications to the test.

➤*Altered reactivity:* See Drug Interactions for more information.

➤*Positive tuberculin reaction:* Tuberculin reactivity may indicate prior infection or disease with *M. tuberculosis* and does not necessarily indicate the presence of active tuberculous disease. Individuals showing a tuberculin reaction should be further evaluated with other diagnostic procedures, such as x-ray examination of the chest and microbiological examination of the sputum.

Drug Interactions

➤*Corticosteroids or immunosuppressants:* Reactivity to the test may be depressed or suppressed for up to 6 weeks in individuals who are receiving corticosteroids or immunosuppressive agents.

➤*Live viral vaccines:* Reactivity to PPD may be temporarily depressed by certain live virus vaccines (measles, mumps, rubella, oral polio, yellow fever, and varicella). Therefore, if a tuberculin test is to be performed, it should be administered either before or simultaneously, at separate sites, with these vaccines in combined form or as separate antigens, or testing should be postponed for 4 to 6 weeks.

Adverse Reactions

➤*Local:*

Very rare – Vesiculation, ulceration or necrosis may appear at the test site in highly sensitive persons. Cold packs or topical steroid preparations may be employed for symptomatic relief of the associated pain, pruritus and discomfort.

Strongly positive reactions may result in scarring at the test site.

Uncommon – Immediate erythematous or other reactions may occur at the injection site. The reason(s) for these occurrences are presently unknown.

➤*Systemic:* There have been rare systemic allergic reactions reported that were manifested by immediate skin rash or generalized rash within 24 hours. Two of the reported cases had concurrent symptoms of upper respiratory stridor. These reactions were treated with epinephrine and steroids and resolved. No cause and effect was able to be established with a specific component of skin test.

Patient Information

The healthcare provider should instruct patients to report to the healthcare provider adverse reactions such as vesiculation, ulceration or necrosis which may appear at the test site in highly sensitive patients. The healthcare provider should also inform the patient that pain, pruritus and discomfort at the site may also occur.

The healthcare provider should inform the patient of the need to return for the reading of the test. Self-reading of the test has been shown to be unreliable.

The healthcare provider should inform the patient of the need to maintain a personal immunization record.

Indications

Consult individual monographs for specific indications.

Actions

➤*Pharmacology:* Radiopaque agents are usually grouped according to osmolality (high or low), structure (monomeric or dimeric ring structure), and ion tendency (nonionic or ionic).

High-osmolality contrast media (HOCM) have an osmolality in solution between 1,200 and 2,400 mOsm/kg H_2O and are ionic monomers.

Low-osmolality contrast media (LOCM) are classified as ionic dimers (ie, ioxaglate), nonionic monomers, or nonionic dimers. Because of lower toxicities, nonionic monomers are becoming the more preferred contrast media. Ioversol and iohexal are 2 of the newer nonionic monomers and are more hydrophilic, thus possibly producing less toxicity. The nonionic dimers are still mostly in the developmental stages, but they are of limited clinical use because of their viscosity approaching that of plasma. The osmolality of LOCM is ≈ 290 to 860 mOsm/kg H_2O. LOCM agents are generally more costly than HOCM agents, but are less toxic.

The most important characteristic of contrast media is the iodine content. The relatively high atomic weight of iodine contributes sufficient radiodensity for radiographic contrast with surrounding tissues. Barium, one of the noniodine-containing contrast media, is an insoluble material that, because of its density, provides a positive contrast during x-ray examination.

Paramagnetic agents – Paramagnetic agents enhance the use of magnetic resonance imaging (MRI). When administered in living organisms, these agents influence the longitudinal or spin-lattice time (T_1) and the transverse or spin-spin relaxation time (T_2). By lowering the T_1 and T_2 values in tissues that retain them, the signal intensity and the image contrast are enhanced upon exposure to a strong magnetic field.

Nonionic vs ionic agents – Iohexol, iopamidol, ioversol, and iodixanol are nonionic iodine contrast media. The other iodinated contrast media currently available are ionic. The nonionic compounds are more hydrophilic than ionic agents, resulting in decreased protein-binding and tissue-binding propensities. The nonionic media have a lower osmolality than the ionic contrast media (1 to 3 times the osmolality of human serum vs 5 to 8) and are associated with a lower incidence of adverse effects. The nonionic media are also associated with a lower incidence of anaphylactoid reactions.

Pharmacokinetic Parameters of IV Radiopaque Agents

Radiopaque agent	Osmolality ($mOsm/kg H_2O$)	Viscosity (cps)	
Ionic agents			
Diatrizoate meglumine 30%	633	1.94[a]	1.42[b]
Diatrizoate meglumine 60%	1415	6.17[a]	4.12[b]
Diatrizoate meglumine 66% and diatrizoate sodium 10% (*Hypaque-76*)	2016	-	9.0[b]
Diatrizoate meglumine 66% and diatrizoate sodium 10% (*MD-76 R*)	1551	16.4[a]	10.5[b]
Diatrizoate meglumine 66% and diatrizoate sodium 10% (*RenoCal-76*)	1870	15.0[a]	9.1[b]
Diatrizoate sodium 50%	1515	3.25[a]	2.34[b]
Iothalamate meglumine 30%	600	2.0[a]	1.5[b]
Iothalamate meglumine 43%	1000	3.0[a]	2.0[b]
Iothalamate meglumine 60%	1400	6.0[a]	4.0[b]
Ioxaglate meglumine 39.3% and ioxaglate sodium 19.6%	600	15.7[c]	7.5[b]
Nonionic agents			
Gadodiamide	789	2.0[c]	1.4[b]
Gadoteridol	630	2.0[c]	1.3[b]
Gadoversetamide	1110	3.1[c]	2.0[b]
Iodixanol 270	290	12.7[c]	6.3[b]
Iodixanol 320	290	26.6[c]	11.8[b]
Iohexol 140	322	2.3[c]	1.5[b]
Iohexol 180	408	3.1[c]	2.0[b]
Iohexol 240	520	5.8[c]	3.4[b]
Iohexol 300	672	11.8[c]	6.3[b]
Iohexol 350	844	20.4[c]	10.4[b]
Iopamidol 41%	413	3.3[c]	2.0[b]
Iopamidol 51%	524	5.1[c]	3.0[b]
Iopamidol 61%	616	8.8[b]	4.7[b]
Iopamidol 76%	796	20.9[c]	9.4[b]
Iopromide 150	328	2.3[c]	1.5[b]
Iopromide 240	483	4.9[c]	2.8[b]
Iopromide 300	607	9.2[c]	4.9[b]
Iopromide 370	774	22.0[c]	10.0[b]
Ioversol 34%	355	2.7[a]	1.9[b]
Ioversol 51%	502	4.6[a]	3.0[b]
Ioversol 64%	651	8.2[a]	5.5[b]
Ioversol 68%	702	9.9[a]	5.8[b]
Ioversol 74%	792	14.3[a]	9.0[b]
Paramagnetic agents			
Ferumoxides	340	-	-
Gadopentetate dimeglumine	1960	4.9[c]	2.9[b]

Pharmacokinetic Parameters of IV Radiopaque Agents

Radiopaque agent	Osmolality ($mOsm/kg H_2O$)	Viscosity (cps)	
Mangofodipir trisodium	298	-	0.8[b]

[a] Viscosity at 25°C.
[b] Viscosity at 37°C.
[c] Viscosity at 20°C.

Contraindications

Consult package inserts for individual contraindications.

➤*Barium sulfate:* Barium sulfate products are contraindicated in patients with known or suspected obstruction of the colon, known or suspected GI tract perforation, suspected tracheoesophageal fistula, obstructing lesions of the small intestine, pyloric stenosis, inflammation or neoplastic lesions of the rectum, recent rectal biopsy, or known hypersensitivity to barium sulfate formulations.

Do not use barium sulfate suspensions for infants with swallowing disorders or for newborns with complete duodenal or jejunal obstruction or when distal small bowel or colon obstruction is suspected. Barium sulfate suspension is not recommended for very small preterm infants and young babies requiring small volumes of contrast media or for infants and young children when there is a possibility of leakage from the GI tract, such as necrotizing enterocolitis, unexplained pneumoperitoneum, gasless abdomen, other bowel perforation, esophageal perforation, or postoperative anastomosea.

Known hypersensitivity or allergy to latex is a contraindication for the use of enema tips with latex retention cuffs. The use of retention cuff enema tip is not necessary or desirable in patients with normal sphincter tone. The presence of adequate sphincter tone can be judged by preliminary rectal digital examination.

Warnings

➤*Inadvertent intrathecal administration:* Serious adverse reactions have been reported because of the inadvertent intrathecal administration of iodinated contrast media that are not indicated for intrathecal use. These serious adverse reactions include death, convulsions, cerebral hemorrhage, coma, paralysis, arachnoiditis, acute renal failure, cardiac arrest, seizures, rhabdomyolysis, hyperthermia, and brain edema. Special attention must be given to ensure that the drug product is not administered intrathecally.

➤*Blood coagulation inhibition:* Nonionic iodinated contrast media inhibit blood coagulation in vitro less than ionic contrast media. Clotting has been reported when blood remains in contact with syringes containing nonionic contrast media.

➤*Thromboembolic events:* Serious, rarely fatal, thromboembolic events causing MI and stroke have been reported during angiographic procedures with ionic and nonionic contrast media. Therefore, meticulous IV administration technique is necessary, particularly during angiographic procedures, to minimize thromboembolic events. Numerous factors, including length of procedure, catheter and syringe material, underlying disease state, and concomitant medications may contribute to the development of thromboembolic events. For these reasons, meticulous angiographic techniques are recommended, including close attention to guidewire and catheter manipulation, use of manifold systems and 3-way stopcocks, frequent catheter flushing with heparinized saline solutions and minimizing the length of the procedures. The use of plastic syringes in place of glass syringes has been reported to decrease but not eliminate the likelihood of in vitro clotting.

➤*Cardiac shunts (perflutren):* Exercise extreme caution when considering administering activated perflutren in patients who have cardiac shunts.

➤*Pulmonary vascular diseases (perflutren):* Administer with caution in patients with chronic pulmonary vascular disease such as severe emphysema, pulmonary vasculitis, or other causes of reduced pulmonary vascular cross-sectional area.

➤*Neurologic sequelae:* Serious neurologic sequelae, including permanent paralysis, can occur following cerebral arteriography, selective spinal arteriography, and arteriography of vessels supplying the spinal cord. A cause-effect relationship to the contrast medium has not been established because the patients' preexisting condition and procedural technique are causative factors in themselves. Do not inject contrast media arterially following the administration of vasopressors because they strongly potentiate neurologic effects.

➤*Special risk patients:* Exercise caution in patients with severely impaired renal function, combined renal and hepatic disease, severe thyrotoxicosis, myelomatosis, or anuria, particularly when large doses are administered.

➤*Nephrotoxicity:* Toxicity ranges from transient tubular enzymuria to irreversible oliguric renal failure. Incidence is estimated at ≤ 1% in healthy patients, to 30% to 70% in patients with major risk factors such as preexisting renal insufficiency, diabetes, and conditions associated with decreased renal blood flow. Preventive measures include avoiding use of radiographic contrast media in high-risk patients, and using the smallest effective dose; also ensure adequate hydration before procedure and discontinue other nephrotoxic agents. Some experts recommend the use of LOCM.

➤*Pheochromocytoma:* Perform administration of radiopaque materials to patients known or suspected of having pheochromocytoma with extreme caution. If, in the opinion of the physician, the possible benefits of such procedures outweigh the considered risks, the procedures may be performed; however, keep the amount of radiopaque medium injected to an absolute minimum. Assess the blood pressure throughout the procedure, and have measures for treatment of a hypertensive crisis available.

➤*Sickle cell disease/Hyperthyroidism:* Contrast media may promote sickling in individuals who are homozygous for sickle cell disease when administered intravascularly. Reports of thyroid storm following the IV use of iodinated radiopaque agents in patients with hyperthyroidism or with an autonomously functioning thyroid nodule, suggest that this additional risk be evaluated in such patients before use of any contrast medium.

➤*Hyperthyroidism:* Cases of hyperthyroidism have been reported with the use of oral contrast media. Some of these patients reportedly had multinodular goiters, which may have been responsible for the increased hormone synthesis in response to excess iodine. Exercise caution when administering enteral GI radiopaque agents to hyperthyroid and euthyroid goiterous patients.

➤*Hypersensitivity reactions:* The risk of a reaction to a nonionic LOCM is estimated to be ≥ 5 times lower than with conventional agents. Risk factors for an immediate reaction include the following: Previous immediate reaction, environmental allergies (ie, food or hay fever), asthma, CHF, use of beta-blockers, current or previous use of interleukin-2, and high anxiety state. Most guidelines suggest the use of LOCM in those who have a history of previous reactions, asthma, allergies, or who have a history of cardiac dysfunction. Pretreatment regimens may include prednisone, diphenhydramine, with or without ephedrine.

Reports of delayed reactions have ranged from 2.1% to 31% and were mostly mild and required no specific treatment. The most common symptoms included headache, itching, rash, and urticaria, with most developing within 6 hours after administration. Those patients who have been treated with interleukin-2 may have a higher tendency to delayed reactions. Refer to Management of Acute Hypersensitivity Reactions.

Patient Information

➤*Oral and rectal iodinated agents:* Take all medication with water after a fat-free dinner the evening before the test. Thereafter, take only water until the test is completed.

Inform physician of pregnancy or allergy to iodine, any foods, or x-ray materials.

These agents may cause mild and transient abdominal cramping, nausea, vomiting, diarrhea, skin rashes, itching, heartburn, dizziness, or headache.

Consult physician if thyroid tests are planned; iodine may interfere.

➤*Parenteral iodinated agents:* Prior to these procedures, notify physician if any of the following conditions exist: Pregnancy; diabetes; multiple myeloma; pheochromocytoma; homozygous sickle cell disease; thyroid disease; allergy to any drugs or food; reactions to previous injections of dyes used for x-ray procedures. Also notify physician if taking any other medications, including *otc* drugs or natural products.

These agents are to be given only by personnel experienced in their use, and only in facilities with proper equipment to deal with possible untoward effects.

GI Contrast Agents (Iodinated)

DIATRIZOATE SODIUM (59.87% iodine)

Rx	**Hypaque Sodium** (Nycomed)	**Powder:** 600 mg iodine/g	In 10 g bottles and 250 g cans with measuring spoon.[a]

[a] With polysorbate 80.

DIATRIZOATE SODIUM — ORAL

For complete and comparative prescribing information, refer to product package labeling.

Indications

➤*Radiographic examination:* For radiographic examination of the GI tract following oral administration.

DIATRIZOATE SODIUM — RECTAL

For complete and comparative prescribing information, refer to product package labeling.

Indications

➤*Radiographic examination:* For radiographic examination of the GI tract following rectal administration.

DIATRIZOATE MEGLUMINE 66% and DIATRIZOATE SODIUM 10% (36.7% iodine)

Rx	**Gastrografin** (Bracco Diagnostics)	**Solution:** 660 mg diatrizoate meglumine, 100 mg diatrizoate sodium, and 367 mg iodine/mL	Lemon flavor. In 120 mL bottles.[a]

[a] With EDTA, polysorbate 80, saccharin, simethicone.

DIATRIZOATE MEGLUMINE 66% and DIATRIZOATE SODIUM 10% (36.7% iodine) — ORAL

For complete and comparative prescribing information, refer to product package labeling.

Indications

Radiographic examination of segments of the GI tract and for computed tomography.

GI Contrast Agents (Miscellaneous)

BARIUM SULFATE

Rx	**Bar-test** (Glenwood)	**Tablet:** 650 mg	In 100s.
Rx	**Baro-cat** (Mallinckrodt)	**Suspension:** 1.5%	Pineapple-banana flavor. In 300, 900, and 1900 mL bottles.[a]
Rx	**Prepcat** (Mallinckrodt)		Strawberry flavor. In 450 mL bottles.[a]
Rx	**Bear•E•Yum CT** (Mallinckrodt)		In 200 and 1900 mL bottles.[a]
Rx	**Cheetah** (Mallinckrodt)	**Suspension:** 2.2%	In 250, 450, 900, and 1900 mL bottles.[b]
Rx	**Medescan** (Mallinckrodt)	**Suspension:** 2.3%	In 250, 450, and 1900 mL bottles.[c]
Rx	**Enecat CT** (Mallinckrodt)	**Concentrated suspension:** 5%	In 110 mL with 480 mL bottle for dilution with flexible tubing, clamp, and enema tip.[a]
Rx	**Tomocat** (Mallinckrodt)		Strawberry flavor. In 145 mL with 480 mL bottle for dilution, 225 mL with 1000 mL bottle for dilution, and enema kit in 110 mL with 480 mL bottle for dilution with flexible tubing, clamp, and enema tip.[a]
Rx	**Entrobar** (Mallinckrodt)	**Suspension:** 50%	In 500 mL with or without kit.[d]
Rx	**Liquid Barosperse** (Mallinckrodt)	**Suspension:** 60%	Vanilla flavor. In 355 and 1900 mL bottles.[d]
Rx	**Bear•E•Yum GI** (Mallinckrodt)		In 200 mL.[d]
Rx	**HD 85** (Mallinckrodt)	**Suspension:** 85%	Raspberry flavor. In 150 and 450 mL kits and 1900 mL bottles.[e]
Rx	**Imager ac** (Mallinckrodt)	**Suspension:** 100%	In 650 mL bottles with enema tip-tubing assemblies with kit and 1900 mL bottles.[f]
Rx	**Flo-Coat** (Mallinckrodt)		In 1850 mL bottles.[d]
Rx	**Medebar Plus** (Mallinckrodt)		In 1900 mL bottles and 650 mL bottles with enema tip-tubing assemblies.[d]
Rx	**Epi-C** (Mallinckrodt)	**Suspension:** 150%	Spearmint flavor. In 450 mL bottles.[d]
Rx	**Liqui-Coat HD** (Mallinckrodt)	**Suspension:** 210%	Vanilla-raspberry flavor. In UD 150 mL bottles.[b]

GI Contrast Agents (Miscellaneous)

BARIUM SULFATE

Rx	**Barobag** (Mallinckrodt)	**Powder for suspension:** 95%	Vanilla flavor. In UD 225 and 900 g bottles, and 340 and 454 g enema kits, and 25 lb bulk.[d]
Rx	**Barosperse** (Mallinckrodt)		Cherry flavor. In UD 180 and 1200 g bottles and 25 lb container.[a]
Rx	**Tonopaque** (Mallinckrodt)		In 340 and 454 g kits.[d]
Rx	**Baricon** (Mallinckrodt)	**Powder for suspension:** 98%	Lemon-vanilla flavor. In UD 340 g.[g]
Rx	**Enhancer** (Mallinckrodt)		Lemon-vanilla flavor. In UD 312 g.[g]
Rx	**HD 200 Plus** (Mallinckrodt)		Strawberry flavor. In UD 312 g.[g]
Rx	**Intropaste** (Mallinckrodt)	**Paste:** 70%	In 454 g tubes.[h]
Rx	**Anatrast** (Mallinckrodt)	**Paste:** 100%	In 500 g tubes and enema tip assemblies.[i]

[a] With simethicone, sorbitol.
[b] With simethicone, sorbitol, saccharin, sodium benzoate.
[c] With sorbitol, saccharin, sodium benzoate.
[d] With simethicone.
[e] With simethicone, saccharin.
[f] With simethicone, sorbitol, sodium benzoate.
[g] With simethicone, sorbitol, sucrose.
[h] With simethicone, sorbitol, saccharin, parabens.
[i] With simethicone, sorbitol, parabens.

BARIUM SULFATE — ORAL

For complete prescribing information, refer to product package labeling.

Indications

➤*Paste:* For use as a contrast medium during x-ray examination of the esophagus.

➤*95%, 85%, 60%, 2.3%, 2.2%, 1.5% (adult use), and 1.5% (pediatric use) suspensions:* For use as a contrast medium in x-ray diagnosis or for computed tomography of the GI tract.

➤*210% suspension:* For use as a contrast medium in double contrast stomach examinations.

➤*85% suspension:* May be administered without dilution for double contrast colon examinations. Aqueous dilutions of barium sulfate 85% suspension may be given orally for esophageal swallow, filled stomach, or enteroclysis procedures. Barium sulfate 85% suspension is also contained in the *EneSet* 2 colon examination kit.

➤*60% suspension:* Barium sulfate 60% suspension may be administered without dilution for esophageal swallow or filled stomach examinations.

➤*50% suspension:* For use in small bowel contrast x-ray examinations.

➤*Tablets:* For use as an intact-shaped Roentgen contrast medium in esophagoscopy.

BARIUM SULFATE — RECTAL

For complete prescribing information, refer to product package labeling.

Indications

➤*5% concentrated suspension enema:* For use as a diagnostic aid for computed tomography of the GI tract.

➤*85%, 95%, and 100% suspension enemas:* For use as a contrast medium in x-ray diagnosis of the GI tract.

The 85% suspension may be administered without dilution for double contrast colon examinations. Aqueous dilutions of 85% suspension may be administered rectally for routine filled colon studies or given orally for esophageal swallow, filled stomach, or enteroclysis procedures.

The 100% suspension enema may be administered without dilution for double contrast colon, single contrast esophagus, small bowel, and enteroclysis examinations. Aqueous dilutions of barium sulfate 100% suspension enema may be used for single contrast stomach and single contrast colon examinations.

➤*97% powder for suspension enema:* For suspension enema is indicated for use as a contrast medium in filled colon examinations.

➤*100% rectal paste:* For use in defecography.

RADIOPAQUE POLYVINYL CHLORIDE

Rx	**Sitzmarks** (Konsyl)	**Capsules:** Contains 24 radiopaque rings (1 mm × 4.5 mm)	In 10s.

RADIOPAQUE POLYVINYL CHLORIDE — ORAL

For complete and comparative prescribing information, refer to product package labeling.

Indications

For adult patients with severe constipation who have otherwise negative GI evaluations.

SODIUM BICARBONATE AND TARTARIC ACID

Rx	**Baros** (Mallinckrodt)	**Granules:** 460 mg sodium bicarbonate and 420 mg tartaric acid/g	Simethicone. In 3 g plastic ampules.

SODIUM BICARBONATE AND TARTARIC ACID — ORAL

For complete and comparative prescribing information, refer to product package labeling.

Indications

For use in double-contrast examinations of the stomach.

Miscellaneous Agents

DIATRIZOATE MEGLUMINE

Rx	**Cystografin Dilute** (Bracco Diagnostics)	**Injection:** 180 mg diatrizoate meglumine and 85 mg iodine/mL	In 300 mL bottles with or without administration sets.[a]
Rx	**Cystografin** (Bracco Diagnostics)	**Injection:** 300 mg diatrizoate meglumine and 141 mg iodine/mL	In 100 mL fill in 200 mL and 300 mL fill in 400 mL.[a]
Rx	**Hypaque-Cysto** (Nycomed)		Preservative-free. In 100 mL in a pediatric 300 mL dilution bottle and 250 mL in a 500 mL dilution bottle.[a]
Rx	**Reno-30** (Bracco Diagnostics)		In 50 mL multiple-dose vials.[b]
Rx	**Reno-Dip** (Bracco Diagnostics)		In 300 mL bottles[a] with or without infusion set.
Rx	**Hypaque Meglumine 60%** (Nycomed)	**Injection:** 600 mg diatrizoate meglumine and 282 mg iodine/mL	In 50 and 100 mL vials, 150 mL fill in 200 mL bottles, and 200 mL fill in 200 mL bottles.[a]
Rx	**Reno-60** (Bracco Diagnostics)		In 10 and 50 mL vials, 100 mL bottles, and 150 mL bottles with and without infusion sets.[a]

[a] With EDTA.
[b] With EDTA and parabens.

Miscellaneous Agents

DIATRIZOATE MEGLUMINE — INJECTION

For complete prescribing information, refer to product package labeling.

WARNING

Not for intrathecal use.

For retrograde pyelography.

Not intended for intravascular injection.

Indications

➤*18%:* For retrograde cystourethrography.

➤*30%:*

Reno-30 – For retrograde or ascending pyelography. This procedure may be used if intravenous excretion urography is contraindicated and it is also useful in complementing other diagnostic information.

Reno-dip –

Drip infusion pyelography: For use in those patients in whom routine pyelography would not be expected to be, or has not been, satisfactory for diagnosis. It is not intended to replace retrograde pyelography where this procedure is indicated.

Computed tomography: For radiographic contrast enhancement in computed tomography (CT) of the brain and body. Contrast enhancement may be advantageous in delineating or ruling out disease in suspicious areas which may otherwise not have been satisfactorily visualized.

Lower extremity venography: For lower extremity venography.

➤*60%:* For excretory urography; cerebral angiography; peripheral arteriography; venography; operative, T-tube, or percutaneous transhepatic cholangiography; splenoportography; arthrography; discography; and contrast enhancement of computed tomographic head imaging.

DIATRIZOATE MEGLUMINE 52% and DIATRIZOATE SODIUM 8% (29.3% iodine)

Rx	**Renografin-60** (Bracco Diagnostics)	**Injection**: 520 mg diatrizoate meglumine, 80 mg diatrizoate sodium, and 292.5 mg iodine/mL	In 10 and 50 mL vials and 100 mL bottles.[a]

[a] With EDTA.

DIATRIZOATE MEGLUMINE 52% and DIATRIZOATE SODIUM 8% (29.3% iodine) — INJECTION

For complete prescribing information, refer to product package labeling.

Indications

Urography; angiography; arteriography; venography; cholangiography; splenoportography; arthrography; discography; computed tomography.

DIATRIZOATE MEGLUMINE 66% and DIATRIZOATE SODIUM 10% (37% iodine)

Rx	**Hypaque-76** (Nycomed)	**Injection**: 660 mg diatrizoate meglumine, 100 mg diatrizoate sodium, and 370 mg iodine/mL	In 50 mL vials, 200 mL bottles, and 100 and 150 mL in 200 mL dilution bottles.[a]
Rx	**MD-76 R** (Mallinckrodt)		In 50 mL vials, 100, 150, and 200 mL bottles, and 125 mL power injector syringes.[a]
Rx	**RenoCal-76** (Bracco Diagnostics)		In 50 mL vials, 100, 150, and 200 mL bottles.[a]

[a] With EDTA.

DIATRIZOATE MEGLUMINE 66% and DIATRIZOATE SODIUM 10% (37% iodine) — INJECTION

For complete prescribing information, refer to product package labeling.

Indications

Urography, aortography, angiocardiography, ventriculography, angiography, arteriography, computed tomography; nephrotomography (*RenoCal-76* only); venography (*Hypaque-76* only).

DIATRIZOATE MEGLUMINE 52.7% and IODIPAMIDE MEGLUMINE 26.8% (38% iodine)

Rx	**Sinografin** (Bracco Diagnostics)	**Injection**: 527 mg diatrizoate meglumine, 268 mg iodipamide meglumine, and 380 mg iodine/mL	In 10 mL vials.[a]

[a] With EDTA.

DIATRIZOATE MEGLUMINE 52.7% and IODIPAMIDE MEGLUMINE 26.8% (38% iodine) — INJECTION

For complete prescribing information, refer to product package labeling.

Indications

Hysterosalpingography.

DIATRIZOATE SODIUM 50% (30% iodine)

Rx	**Hypaque Sodium 50%** (Nycomed)	**Injection**: 500 mg diatrizoate sodium and 300 mg iodine/mL	In 50 mL vials.[a]

[a] With EDTA.

DIATRIZOATE SODIUM — INJECTION

For complete prescribing information, refer to product package labeling.

Indications

For excretory urography, cerebral and peripheral angiography, aortography, intraosseous venography, direct cholangiography, hysterosalpingography, splenoportography, and contrast enhancement of computed tomographic head imaging.

IOTHALAMATE MEGLUMINE

Rx	**Conray 30** (Mallinckrodt)	**Injection**: 300 mg iothalamate meglumine and 141 mg iodine/mL	In 50 mL vials and 150 and 300 mL bottles.[a]
Rx	**Conray 43** (Mallinckrodt)	**Injection**: 430 mg iothalamate meglumine and 202 mg iodine/mL	In 50 and 100 mL vials, 150, 200, and 250 mL bottles, and 50 mL prefilled syringes.[a]
Rx	**Conray** (Mallinckrodt)	**Injection**: 600 mg iothalamate meglumine and 282 mg iodine/mL	In 30, 50, and 100 mL vials, 100, 150, and 200 mL bottles, and 50 and 125 mL prefilled power injector syringes.[a]

[a] With EDTA.

IOTHALAMATE MEGLUMINE — INJECTION

For complete prescribing information, refer to product package labeling.

Indications

Not for intrathecal use.

➤*43% (Cysto)* (not for intravascular administration): Iothalamate injection (*Cysto*) 43% is indicated for use in retrograde cystography and cystourethrography. Iothalamate injection 43% is also indicated for use in retrograde pyelography.

➤*30%:* For use in IV infusion urography, contrast enhancement of computed tomographic (CT) brain images, and arterial digital subtraction angiography.

Miscellaneous Agents

IOTHALAMATE MEGLUMINE — INJECTION

➤*43% and 60%:*

43% (parenteral agent) –

Intravascular indications: For use in lower extremity venography, IV infusion urography, contrast enhancement of CT brain images, and arterial digital subtraction angiography.

Retrograde urographic indications: For use in retrograde cystography, cystourethrography, and retrograde pyelography.

60% – For use in excretory urography, cerebral angiography, peripheral arteriography, venography, arthrography, direct cholangiography, endoscopic retrograde cholangiopancreatography, contrast enhancement of CT brain images, cranial computerized angiotomography, IV digital subtraction angiography, and arterial digital subtraction angiography. Iothalamate injection 43% and 60% may also be used for enhancement of CT scans performed for detection and evaluation of lesions in the liver, pancreas, kidneys, abdominal aorta, mediastinum, abdominal cavity, and retroperitoneal space.

IOXAGLATE MEGLUMINE 39.3% and IOXAGLATE SODIUM 19.6% (32% iodine)

Rx	**Hexabrix** (Mallinckrodt)	**Injection:** 393 mg ioxaglate meglumine, 196 mg ioxaglate sodium, and 320 mg iodine/mL	In 20, 30, and 50 mL vials, 150 mL bottles, 75 mL fill in 150 mL bottles, 100 mL fill In 150 mL bottles, 200 mL fill in 250 mL bottles, and 125 mL power injector syringes, 50 mL fill in 125 mL power injector syringes, and 100 mL fill in 125 mL powder injector syringes.[a]

[a] With EDTA.

IOXAGLATE MEGLUMINE 39.3% and IOXAGLATE SODIUM 19.6% (32% iodine) — INJECTION

For complete prescribing information, refer to product package labeling.

Indications

Pediatric angiocardiography; arteriography; ventriculography; aortography; angiography; venography; phlebography; urography; computed tomography; arthrography; hysterosalpingography.

IODIPAMIDE MEGLUMINE 52% (25.7% iodine)

Rx	**Cholografin Meglumine** (Bracco Diagnostics)	**Injection:** 520 mg iodipamide meglumine and 257 mg iodine/mL	In 20 mL vials.[a]

[a] With EDTA.

IODIPAMIDE MEGLUMINE — INJECTION

For complete prescribing information, refer to product package labeling.

Indications

For intravenous (IV) cholangiography and cholecystography.

GADODIAMIDE

Rx	**Omniscan** (Nycomed)	**Injection:** 287 mg/mL	Preservative-free. In 10, 20, and 50 mL vials, 5 mL fill in 10 mL vials, 15 mL fill in 20 mL vials, 10 mL fill in 20 mL prefilled syringes, 15 mL fill in 20 mL prefilled syringes, and 20 mL prefilled syringes.

GADODIAMIDE — INJECTION

For complete prescribing information, refer to product package labeling.

Indications

➤*CNS:* For intravenous use in magnetic resonance imaging (MRI) to visualize lesions with abnormal vascularity (or those thought to cause abnormalities in the blood-brain barrier) in the brain (intracranial lesions), spine, and associated tissues.

➤*Body (intrathoracic [noncardiac], intra-abdominal, pelvic and retroperitoneal regions):* For intravenous administration to facilitate the visualization of lesions with abnormal vascularity within the thoracic (noncardiac), abdominal, pelvic cavities, and the retroperitoneal space.

GADOTERIDOL

Rx	**ProHance** (Bracco Diagnostics)	**Injection:** 279.3 mg/mL	Preservative-free. In 5 mL fill in 15 mL vials, 10, 15, and 20 mL fill in 30 mL vials, and 10 and 17 mL fill in 20 mL prefilled syringes.

GADOTERIDOL — INJECTION

For complete prescribing information, refer to product package labeling.

Indications

➤*Central nervous system:* For use in magnetic resonance imaging (MRI) in adults and children over 2 years of age to visualize lesions with abnormal vascularity in the brain (intracranial lesions), spine and associated tissues.

➤*Extracranial/extraspinal tissues:* For use in MRI in adults to visualize lesions in the head and neck.

GADOVERSETAMIDE

Rx	**OptiMARK** (Mallinckrodt)	**Injection:** 330.9 mg gadoversetamide	Preservative-free. In 50 mL bottles.

GADOVERSETAMIDE — INJECTION

For complete prescribing information, refer to product package labeling.

Indications

➤*CNS:* For use with MRI in patients with abnormal blood-brain barrier or abnormal vascularity of the brain, spine, and associated tissues.

➤*Hepatic:* For use with MRI to provide contrast enhancement and facilitate visualization of lesions with abnormal vascularity in the liver of patients who are highly suspect for liver structural abnormalities on computed tomography.

IODIXANOL

Rx	**Visipaque 270** (Nycomed)	**Injection:** 550 mg iodixanol and 270 mg iodine/mL	In 50 mL vials, 50, 100, and 200 mL bottles, 150 mL fill in 200 mL bottles, and 100, 150, and 200 mL flexible containers.[a]
Rx	**Visipaque 320** (Nycomed)	**Injection:** 652 mg iodixanol and 320 mg iodine/mL	In 50 mL vials, 50, 100, and 200 mL bottles, 150 mL fill in 200 mL bottles, and 100, 150, and 200 mL flexible containers.[a]

[a] With EDTA.

IODIXANOL — INJECTION

For complete prescribing information, refer to product package labeling.

WARNING

Not for intrathecal use.

Indications

➤*Intra-arterial:* Iodixanol injection (270 mgI/mL) is indicated for intra-arterial digital subtraction angiography.

Iodixanol injection (320 mgI/mL) is indicated for angiocardiography (left ventriculography and selective coronary arteriography), peripheral arteriography, visceral arteriography, and cerebral arteriography.

➤*IV:* Iodixanol injection (270 mgI/mL) is indicated for contrast enhanced computed tomography (CECT) imaging of the head and body, excretory urography, and peripheral venography.

Iodixanol injection (320 mgI/mL) is indicated for CECT imaging of the head and body, and excretory urography.

IOHEXOL

Rx	**Omnipaque 140** (Nycomed)	**Injection**: 302 mg iohexol equivalent to 140 mg iodine/mL	In 50 mL vials and bottles.[a]
Rx	**Omnipaque 240** (Nycomed)	**Injection**: 518 mg iohexol equivalent to 240 mg iodine/mL	In 10, 20, and 50 mL vials, 50 mL bottles, 100, 150, and 200 mL flexible containers, 50 mL prefilled syringes, 100 mL fill in 100 mL bottles, 150 mL fill in 200 mL bottles, and 200 mL fill in 200 mL bottles.[a]
Rx	**Omnipaque 300** (Nycomed)	**Injection**: 647 mg iohexol equivalent to 300 mg iodine/mL	In 10, 30, and 50 mL vials, 50 mL bottles, 100 and 150 mL flexible containers, 50 mL prefilled syringes, 75 mL fill in 100 mL bottles, 100 mL fill in 100 mL bottles, 125 mL fill in 200 mL bottles, 150 mL fill in 200 mL bottles, 125 mL fill in 150 mL flexible containers.[a]
Rx	**Omnipaque 350** (Nycomed)	**Injection**: 755 mg iohexol equivalent to 350 mg iodine/mL	In 50 mL vials, 50 mL bottles, 100, 150, and 200 mL flexible containers, 50 mL prefilled syringes, 75 mL fill in 100 mL bottles, 100 mL fill in 100 mL bottles, 125 mL fill in 200 mL bottles, 150 mL fill in 200 mL bottles, 200 mL fill in 200 mL bottles, 250 mL fill in 300 mL bottles, 125 mL fill in 150 mL flexible containers.[a]

[a] With EDTA.

IOHEXOL — INJECTION

For complete prescribing information, refer to product package labeling.

Indications

➤*Intrathecal:*

Adults – Iohexol 180, iohexol 240, and iohexol 300 are indicated for intrathecal administration in adults including myelography (lumbar, thoracic, cervical, total columnar) and in contrast enhancement for computerized tomography (myelography, cisternography, ventriculography).

Children – Iohexol 180 and iohexol 210 are indicated for intrathecal administration in children including myelography (lumbar, thoracic, cervical, total columnar) and in contrast enhancement for computerized tomography (myelography, cisternography).

➤*Intravascular:*

Angiocardiography –

Adults: Iohexol 350 is indicated in adults for angiocardiography (ventriculography, aortic root injections, and selective coronary arteriography).

Children: Iohexol 350 is indicated in children for angiocardiography (ventriculography, pulmonary arteriography, and venography, and studies of the collateral arteries).

Iohexol 300 at a concentration of 300 mgI/mL is indicated in children for angiocardiography (ventriculography).

Aortography and selective visceral arteriography –

Adults: Iohexol 300 at a concentration of 300 mgI/mL and iohexol 350 at a concentration of 350 mgI/mL are indicated in adults for use in aortography and selective visceral arteriography including studies of the aortic arch, ascending aorta, and abdominal aorta and its branches (celiac, mesenteric, renal, hepatic, and splenic arteries).

Children: Iohexol 350 at a concentration of 350 mgI/mL is indicated in children for use in aortography including studies of the aortic root, aortic arch, ascending and descending aorta.

Cerebral arteriography – Iohexol 300 at a concentration of 300 mgI/mL is indicated in adults for use in cerebral arteriography.

The degree of pain and flushing as the result of the use of iohexol 300 in cerebral arteriography is less than that seen with comparable injections of many contrast media.

Contrast enhanced computed tomography –

Adults: Iohexol 240 at a concentration of 240 mgI/mL, iohexol 300 at a concentration of 300 mgI/mL, and iohexol 350 at a concentration of 350 mgI/mL are indicated in adults for use in intravenous contrast enhanced computed tomographic head and body imaging by rapid injection or infusion technique.

Children: Iohexol 240 at a concentration of 240 mgI/mL and iohexol 300 at a concentration of 300 mgI/mL are indicated in children for use in intravenous contrast enhanced computed tomographic head imaging by rapid bolus injection.

Digital subtraction angiography –

Intravenous administration: Iohexol 350 at a concentration of 350 mgI/mL is indicated in adults for use in intravenous digital subtraction angiography (IVDSA) of the vessels of the head, neck, and abdominal, renal and peripheral vessels.

Peripheral angiography – Iohexol 300 at a concentration of 300 mgI/mL or iohexol 350 at a concentration of 350 mgI/mL is indicated in adults for use in peripheral arteriography. Iohexol 240 at a concentration of 240 mgI/mL or iohexol 300 at a concentration of 300 mgI/mL is indicated in adults for use in peripheral venography.

Excretory urography –

Adults: Iohexol 300 at a concentration of 300 mgI/mL or iohexol 350 at a concentration of 350 mgI/mL is indicated for use in adults in excretory urography to provide diagnostic contrast of the urinary tract.

Children: Iohexol 300 at a concentration of 300 mgI/mL is indicated in children for excretory urography (see Oral/body cavity, Voiding cystourethrography).

➤*Oral / body cavity:*

Oral use –

Adults: Iohexol 350 at a concentration of 350 mgI/mL is indicated in adults for use in oral pass-through examination of the gastrointestinal tract.

Iohexol diluted to concentrations from 6 mgI/mL to 9 mgI/mL administered orally in conjunction with iohexol 300 at a concentration of 300 mgI/mL administered intravenously is indicated in adults for use in contrast enhanced computed tomography of the abdomen.

Children – Iohexol 300 at a concentration of 300 mgI/mL administered orally or rectally is indicated in children for use in examination of the gastrointestinal tract.

Iohexol 240 at a concentration of 240 mgI/mL administered orally or rectally is indicated in children for use in examination of the gastrointestinal tract.

Iohexol 180 at a concentration of 180 mgI/mL administered orally or rectally is indicated in children for use in examination of the gastrointestinal tract.

Iohexol diluted to concentrations from 9 mgI/mL to 21 mgI/mL administered orally in conjunction with iohexol 240 at a concentration of 240 mgI/mL or iohexol 300 at a concentration of 300 mgI/mL administered intravenously is indicated in children for use in contrast enhanced computed tomography of the abdomen.

Voiding cystourethrography (VCU) – Iohexol diluted to concentrations from 50 mgI/mL to 100 mgI/mL is indicated in children for voiding cystourethrography. VCUs are often performed in conjunction with excretory urography.

Arthrography – Iohexol 240 at a concentration of 240 mgI/mL or iohexol 300 at a concentration of 300 mgI/mL or iohexol 350 at a concentration of 350 mgI/mL is indicated in radiography of the knee joint in adults, and iohexol 210 at a concentration of 210 mgI/mL or iohexol 240 at a concentration of 240 mgI/mL or iohexol 300 at a concentration of 300 mgI/mL is indicated in radiography of the shoulder joint in adults, and iohexol 300 at a concentration of 300 mgI/mL is indicated in radiography of the temporomandibular joint in adults. Arthrography may be helpful in the diagnosis of post-traumatic or degenerative joint diseases, synovial rupture, the visualization of communicating bursae or cysts, and in meniscography.

Endoscopic retrograde pancreatography (ERP) / endoscopic retrograde cholangiopancreatography (ERCP) – Iohexol 240 at a concentration of 240 mgI/mL is indicated in adults for use in ERP/ERCP.

Hysterosalpingography – Iohexol 240 at a concentration of 240 mgI/mL or iohexol 300 at a concentration of 300 mgI/mL is indicated in radiography of the internal group of adult female reproductive organs: Ovaries, fallopian tubes, uterus, and vagina. Hysterosalpingography is utilized as a diagnostic and therapeutic modality in the treatment of infertility and other abnormal gynecological conditions.

Herniography – Iohexol 240 at a concentration of 240 mgI/mL is indicated in adults for use in herniography.

IOPAMIDOL

Rx	**Isovue-200** (Bracco Diagnostics)	**Injection:** 408 mg iopamidol and 200 mg iodine/mL	In 50 mL vials, 100 mL bottles, and 200 mL bottles with infusion set.[a]
	Isovue-M 200 (Bracco Diagnostics)		In 10 and 20 mL vials.[a] *For intrathecal use.*
Rx	**Isovue-250** (Bracco Diagnostics)	**Injection:** 510 mg iopamidol and 250 mg iodine/mL	In 50 mL vials, 100, 150, and 200 mL bottles, 150 mL power injector syringes.[a]
Rx	**Isovue-300** (Bracco Diagnostics)	**Injection:** 612 mg iopamidol and 300 mg iodine/mL	In 30 and 50 mL vials, 75 and 100 mL bottles, 150 mL bottles with or without administration sets, 100 and 150 mL power injector syringes.[a]
Rx	**Isovue-M 300** (Bracco Diagnostics)		In 15 mL vials.[a] *For intrathecal use.*
Rx	**Isovue-370** (Bracco Diagnostics)	**Injection:** 755 mg iopamidol and 370 mg iodine/mL	In 20, 30, and 50 mL vials, 50, 75, 100, 125, 150, 175, and 200 mL bottles, 75 and 100 mL power injector syringes.[a]

[a] With EDTA.

IOPAMIDOL — INJECTION

For complete prescribing information, refer to product package labeling.

WARNING

Not for intrathecal use.

Indications

➤*Angiography:* For angiography throughout the cardiovascular system, including cerebral and peripheral arteriography, coronary arteriography and ventriculography, pediatric angiocardiography, selective visceral arteriography and aortography, peripheral venography (phlebography).

➤*Urography:* Adult and pediatric intravenous excretory urography.

➤*Computed tomography:* Intravenous adult and pediatric contrast enhancement of computed tomographic (CECT) head and body imaging.

IOPROMIDE

Rx	**Ultravist 150** (Berlex)	**Injection:** 311.70 mg iopromide and 150 mg iodine/mL	In 50 mL vials.[a]
Rx	**Ultravist 240** (Berlex)	**Injection:** 498.72 mg iopromide and 240 mg iodine/mL	In 50 and 100 mL vials and 200 mL fill in 250 mL vials.[a]
Rx	**Ultravist 300** (Berlex)	**Injection:** 623.4 mg iopromide and 300 mg iodine/mL	In 50, 100, and 150 mL vials.[a]
Rx	**Ultravist 370** (Berlex)	**Injection:** 768.86 mg iopromide and 370 mg iodine/mL	In 50, 100, and 150 mL vials, and 200 mL fill in 250 mL vials.[a]

[a] With EDTA.

IOPROMIDE INJECTION

For complete prescribing information, refer to product package labeling.

Indications

➤*Intra-arterial:* Iopromide injection (150 mg iodine/mL) is indicated for intra-arterial digital subtraction angiography (IA-DSA).

Iopromide injection (300 mg iodine/mL) is indicated for cerebral arteriography and peripheral arteriography.

Iopromide injection (370 mg iodine/mL) is indicated for coronary arteriography and left ventriculography, visceral angiography, and aortography.

➤*IV:* Iopromide injection (240 mg iodine/mL) is indicated for peripheral venography.

Iopromide injection (300 mg iodine/mL) is indicated for contrast-enhanced computed tomographic (CECT) imaging of the head and body, and excretory urography.

IOVERSOL

Rx	**Optiray 160** (Mallinckrodt)	**Injection:** 339 mg ioversol and 160 mg iodine/mL	In 50 and 100 mL bottles.[a]
Rx	**Optiray 240** (Mallinckrodt)	**Injection:** 509 mg ioversol and 240 mg iodine/mL	In 50, 100, and 150 mL bottles, 200 mL fill in 250 mL bottles, 50 mL hand-held syringes, and 125 mL power injector syringes.[a]
Rx	**Optiray 300** (Mallinckrodt)	**Injection:** 636 mg ioversol and 300 mg iodine/mL	In 50, 100, and 150 mL bottles, 200 mL fill in 250 mL bottles, 50 mL hand-held syringes, and 100 mL fill in 125 mL power injector syringes.[a]
Rx	**Optiray 320** (Mallinckrodt)	**Injection:** 678 mg ioversol and 320 mg iodine/mL	In 20 and 30 mL vials, 50, 100, and 150 mL bottles, 75 mL fill in 100 mL bottles, 200 mL fill in 250 mL bottles, 30 and 50 mL hand-held syringes, 50 mL fill in 125 mL power injector syringes, 75 mL fill in 125 mL power injector syringes, 100 mL fill in 125 mL power injector syringes, and 125 mL power injector syringes.[a]
Rx	**Optiray 350** (Mallinckrodt)	**Injection:** 741 mg ioversol and 350 mg iodine/mL	In 50, 100, and 150 mL bottles, 75 mL fill in 100 mL bottles, 200 mL fill in 250 mL bottles, 30 and 50 mL hand-held syringes, 50 mL fill in 125 mL power injector syringes, 75 mL fill in 125 mL power injector syringes, 100 mL fill in 125 mL power injector syringes, and 125 mL power injector syringes.[a]

[a] With EDTA.

IOVERSOL — INJECTION

For complete prescribing information, refer to product package labeling.

Indications

➤*74%:* Ioversol injection 74% is indicated in adults for peripheral and coronary arteriography and left ventriculography. Ioversol injection 74% is also indicated for contrast-enhanced, computed, tomographic imaging of the head and body, IV excretory urography, IV digital subtraction angiography and venography. Ioversol injection 74% is indicated in children for angiocardiography.

➤*68%:* Ioversol injection 68% is indicated in adults for angiography throughout the cardiovascular system. The uses include cerebral, coronary, peripheral, visceral and renal arteriography, venography, aortography, and left ventriculography. Ioversol injection 68% is also indicated for contrast-enhanced, computed, tomographic imaging of the head and body, and IV excretory urography.

Ioversol injection 68% is indicated in children for angiocardiography, contrast-enhanced, computed, tomographic imaging of the head and body, and IV excretory urography.

➤*64%:* Ioversol injection 64% is indicated for cerebral angiography and peripheral arteriography. Ioversol injection 64% is also indicated for contrast-enhanced, computed, tomographic imaging of the head and body, venography, and IV excretory urography.

➤*51%:* Ioversol injection 51% is indicated for cerebral angiography and venography. Ioversol injection 51% is also indicated for contrast-enhanced, computed, tomographic imaging of the head and body and IV excretory urography.

➤*34%:* Ioversol injection 34% is indicated for intra-arterial digital subtraction angiography (IA-DSA).

Miscellaneous Agents

FERUMOXIDES

Rx	**Feridex I.V.** (Berlex)	**Injectable solution:** 11.2 mg iron/mL (56 mg of iron/vial)	In 5 mL single-dose vials with administration filter.

FERUMOXIDES — INJECTION

For complete prescribing information, refer to product package labeling.

Indications

As an adjunct to MRI (in adult patients) to enhance the T2-weighted images used in the detection and evaluation of lesions of the liver that are associated with an alteration in the reticuloendothelial system.

GADOBENATE DIMEGLUMINE

Rx	**Multihance** (Bracco Diagnostics)	**Injection:** 529 mg/mL	Preservative free. In 5, 10, 15, and 20 mL single-dose vials.

GADOBENATE DIMEGLUMINE — INJECTION

For complete prescribing information, refer to the product package insert.

Indications

➤*CNS:* For intravenous use in magnetic resonance imaging of the CNS in adults to visualize lesions with abnormal blood brain barrier or abnormal vascularity of the brain, spine, and associated tissues.

GADOPENTETATE DIMEGLUMINE

Rx	**Magnevist** (Hospira)	**Injection:** 469.01 mg/mL	Preservative-free. In 100 mL pharmacy bulk packages.

GADOPENTETATE DIMEGLUMINE — INJECTION

For complete prescribing information, refer to product package labeling.

Indications

➤*CNS:* For use with magnetic resonance imaging (MRI) in adults, and pediatric patients ≥ 2 years of age to visualize lesions with abnormal vascularity in the brain (intracranial lesions), spine and associated tissues. Gadopentetate dimeglumine injection has been shown to facilitate visualization of intracranial lesions including but not limited to tumors.

➤*Extracranial/extraspinal tissues:* For use with MRI in adults and pediatric patients ≥ 2 years of age to facilitate the visualization of lesions with abnormal vascularity in the head and neck.

➤*Body:* For use in MRI in adults and pediatric patients ≥ 2 years of age to facilitate the visualization of lesions with abnormal vascularity in the body (excluding the heart).

MANGAFODIPIR TRISODIUM

Rx	**Teslascan** (Nycomed)	**Injection:** 37.9 mg (50 mcmol)/mL	Preservative-free. In 10 mL vials.

MANGAFODIPIR TRISODIUM — INJECTION

For complete prescribing information, refer to product package labeling.

Indications

➤*Adjunct to MRI:* For IV administration as an adjunct to MRI in patients to enhance the T_1-weighted images used in the detection, localization, characterization, and evaluation of lesions of the liver.

PERFLUTREN

Rx	**Definity** (Bristol-Myers Squibb)	**Injection:** 6.52 mg/mL octafluoropropane in lipid-coated microspheres	Preservative-free. In single-use 2 mL vials.[a]

[a] Requires activation with a *Vialmix* (not included).

PERFLUTREN — INJECTION

For complete prescribing information, refer to product package labeling.

Indications

To opacify the left ventricular chamber and to improve the delineation of the left ventricular endocardial border in patients with suboptimal echocardiography.

ISOSULFAN BLUE

Rx	**Lymphazurin 1%** (United States Surgical Corp.)	**Injection:** 10 mg/mL	Preservative-free. In 5 mL vials.

ISOSULFAN BLUE — INJECTION

For complete prescribing information, refer to product package labeling.

Indications

➤*Adjunct to lymphography:* Delineates the lymphatic vessels. It is an adjunct to lymphography (in primary and secondary lymphedema of the extremities; chyluria, chylous ascites or chylothorax; lymph node involvement by primary or secondary neoplasm; and lymph node response to therapeutic modalities) for visualization of the lymphatic system draining the region of injection.

PENTETREOTIDE

Rx	**OctreoScan** (Mallinckrodt)	**Kit:** 10 mcg pentetreotide and Indium In111 Chloride Sterile Solution	In 10 mL vials.

PENTETREOTIDE — INJECTION

For complete prescribing information, refer to product package labeling.

Indications

For the scintigraphic localization of primary and metastatic neuroendocrine tumors bearing somatostatin receptors.

Miscellaneous Agents

ETHIODIZED OIL (37% iodine)

Rx	**Ethiodol** (Savage)	**Injection:** 475 mg iodine/mL	In 10 mL amps.[a]

[a] With 1% poppyseed oil.

ETHIODIZED OIL — INJECTION

For complete prescribing information, refer to product package labeling.

Indications

➤*Hysterosalpinogography and lymphography:* For use as a radio-opaque medium for hysterosalpinogography and lymphography.

63The Orphan Drug Act defines an orphan drug as a drug or biological product for the diagnosis, treatment, or prevention of a rare disease or condition. A rare disease is one that affects fewer than 200,000 people in the United States or one that affects more than 200,000 people but for which there is no reasonable expectation that the cost of developing the drug and making it available will be recovered from sales of that drug in the United States.

The FDA Office of Orphan Products Development (OOPD) provides an information package that includes an overview of the FDA's orphan drug program, a brief description of the orphan products grant program, and a current list of designated orphan products. OOPD's information package also contains a directory sheet listing sources of information about the treatment of rare diseases, patient organizations, and availability of orphan drugs. Requests for the Rare Disease Information Directory or the entire orphan drugs information package may be made by contacting OOPD:

Office of Orphan Products Development
Food and Drug Administration, (HF-35)
5600 Fishers Lane
Rockville, MD 20857
(301) 827-3666 or (800) 300-7469; fax: (301) 443-4915
Internet: http://www.fda.gov/orphan/

Those agents that have been approved for marketing or whose specific indication has been approved for marketing are denoted with the footnote "a."

Orphan Drugs

Drug (*Trade name*)	Proposed use	Sponsor
40SD02	Chronic iron overload resulting from conventional transfusional treatment of beta-thalassemia major and sickle cell anemia	Biomedical Frontiers
90Y-hPAMA4 (*PAN-Cide*)	Pancreatic cancer	Immunomedics
166Ho-DOTMP	Multiple myeloma	NeoRx
506U78	Chronic lymphocytic leukemia	GlaxoSmithKline
A10 & AS2-1 antineoplaston (*A10 & AS2-1 antineoplaston*)	Brain stem glioma	Burzynski Research Institute
Abetimus	Lupus nephritis	La Jolla
ACA125	Epithelial ovarian cancer	Menarini Ricerche S.p.A
(+/-)-7-[3-(4-Acetyl-3-methoxy-2-propylphenoxy)propoxy]-3,4-dihydro-8-propyl-2H-1-benzopyran-2-2 carboxylic acid	Prevent serious adverse events associated with vascular leak syndrome caused by interleukin-2 therapy	Intarcia Therapeutics
N-Acetyl-sarcosyl-glycyl-L-valyl-D-alloisoleucyl-L-threonyl-L-norvaly-L-isoleucyl-L-arginyl-L-prolylethylaminde acetate	Soft tissue sarcoma	Abbott
N-Acetylcysteinate lysine (*Nacystelyn Dry Powder Inhaler*)	Cystic fibrosis	Galephar Pharmaceuticals Research
Acetylcysteine (*Acetadote*)	IV treatment for moderate to severe acetaminophen overdose[a]	Cumberland
(*Mucomyst/Mucomyst 10 IV*)		Bristol-Myers Squibb
N-Acetylcysteine	Acute liver failure	William M. Lee, MD, FACP University of Texas SW
N-Acetylprocainamide	Prevent life-threatening ventricular arrhythmias in patients with documented procainamide-induced lupus	NAPA of the Bahamas
(*Napa*)	Lower the defibrillation energy requirement sufficiently to allow automatic implantable cardioverter defibrillator therapy in patients who otherwise could not use the device	Medco Research
Acid sphingomyelinase	Niemann-Pick disease type B	Genzyme
Aconiazide	Tuberculosis	Lincoln Diagnostics
Adalimumab (*Humira*)	Juvenile rheumatoid arthritis	Abbott
Adeno-associated viral-based vector cystic fibrosis gene therapy	Cystic fibrosis	Targeted Genetics
Adeno-associated viral vector containing the gene for human coagulation Factor IX (*Coagulin-B*)	Intrahepatic and intramuscular treatment of moderate to severe hemophilia	Avigen
Adenosine	With BCNU (carmustine) in the treatment of brain tumors	Medco Research
S-Adenosylmethionine	AIDS-myelopathy	Alessandro Di Rocco, MD
Adenovirus-based vector Factor VIII complementary DNA to somatic cells (*MiniAdFVIII*)	Hemophilia A	GenStar Therapeutics
Adenovirus-mediated herpes simplex virus-thymidine kinase gene	With ganciclovir in the treatment of malignant glioma	Ark Therapeutics
Aerosolized pooled immune globulin	Respiratory syncytial virus lower respiratory tract disease	Pediatric
AI-RSA	Autoimmune uveitis	AutoImmune
Albendazole (*Albenza*)	Hydatid disease (cystic echinococcosis caused by *Echinococcus granulosus* larvae or alveolar echinococcosis caused by *E. multilocularis* larvae);[a] neurocysticercosis caused by *Taenia solium* as: 1) Chemotherapy of parenchymal, subarachnoidal, and racemose (cysts in spinal fluid) neurocysticercosis in symptomatic cases and 2) prophylaxis of epilepsy and other sequelae in asymptomatic neurocysticercosis[a]	SmithKline Beecham
Albuterol	Prevent paralysis caused by spinal cord injury	MotoGen
Aldesleukin (*Proleukin*)	Metastatic renal cell carcinoma[a]; metastatic melanoma[a]; primary immunodeficiency disease associated with T-cell defects; acute myelogenous leukemia; non-Hodgkin lymphoma	Chiron
Alemtuzumab (*Campath*)	Chronic lymphocytic leukemia[a]	Genzyme
Alendronate (*Fosamax*)	Osteogenesis imperfecta in pediatric patients 4 years of age and older	Merck
Alendronate disodium (*Fosamax*)	Bone manifestations of Gaucher disease	Richard J. Wenstrup, MD
Alglucerase injection (*Ceredase*)	Replacement therapy in Gaucher disease type I,[a] II, and III	Genzyme
Alitretinoin (*Panretin*)	Topical treatment of cutaneous lesions in AIDS-related Kaposi sarcoma[a]; acute promyelocytic leukemia	Ligand

Orphan Drugs

Drug (*Trade name*)	Proposed use	Sponsor
Allantoin (*Alwextin*)	Skin blistering and erosions associated with inherited epidermolysis bullosa	Alwyn
Allogeneic human retinal pigment epithelial cells on gelatin microcarriers (*Spheramine*)	Hoehn and Yahr stage III and IV Parkinson disease	Titan
Allogeneic peripheral blood mononuclear cells (sensitized against patient alloantigens by mixed lymphocyte culture) (*CYTOIMPLANT*)	Pancreatic cancer	Applied Immunotherapeutics
Allogeneic retinal epithelial cells transfected with plasmid vector expressing ciliary neurotrophic growth factor	Retinitis pigmentosa	Neurotech USA
Allogeneic T-cells cultured with anti-CD3 and IL-2; transduced with retroviral vector (SFCMM-3), expressing herpes simplex 1 virus-thymidine kinase (HSV-TK) and truncated low affinity nerve growth factor receptor; selected with anti-low affinity nerve growth factor	Immunotherapy for acceleration of T-cell reconstitution in patients undergoing allogeneic hematopoietic stem cell transplantation	MolMed S.p.A.
Allogeneic thymic tissue for transplantation, cultured, partially T-cell depleted	Therapy for primary immune deficiency resulting from athymia associated with complete DiGeorge syndrome	Duke University Medical Center
Allopurinol riboside	Chagas disease; cutaneous and visceral leishmaniasis	Burroughs Wellcome
Allopurinol sodium (*Aloprim for Injection*)	Ex-vivo preservation of cadaveric kidneys for transplantation	Burroughs Wellcome
	Management of patients with leukemia, lymphoma, and solid tumor malignancies who are receiving cancer therapy that causes elevations of serum and urinary uric acid levels and who cannot tolerate oral therapy[a]	Catalytica
17-Allylamino-17-demethoxygeldanamycin (17-AGG)	Multiple myeloma; chronic myelogenous leukemia	Kosan Biosciences
Alpha-1-acid glycoprotein	Tricyclic antidepressant poisoning; cocaine overdose	Bio Products Labs
Alpha-1-antitrypsin (recombinant DNA origin)	Supplementation therapy for alpha$_1$-antitrypsin deficiency in the ZZ phenotype population	Chiron
Alpha-galactosidase A (*CC-Galactosidase*)	Alpha-galactosidase A deficiency (Fabry disease)	David Calhoun, PhD
(*Fabrase*)	Fabry disease	Robert J. Desnick, MD
(*Replagal*)	Long-term enzyme replacement therapy for treatment of Fabry disease	Transkaryotic Therapies
Alpha-melanocyte stimulating hormone	Prevent and treat intrinsic acute renal failure caused by ischemia	National Institute of Diabetes, and Digestive and Kidney Diseases
Alpha$_1$-proteinase inhibitor (human) [API] (*ARC-API*)	Chronic inhalation therapy of individuals with congenital deficiency of alpha$_1$-proteinase inhibitor with demonstrable panacinar emphysema; cystic fibrosis	Kamada
(*Prolastin*)	Slow the progression of emphysema in alpha$_1$-antitrypsin deficient patients	Aventis Behring
	Replacement therapy in the alpha$_1$-proteinase inhibitor congenital deficiency state[a]	Bayer
Alprostadil	Severe peripheral arterial occlusive disease (critical limb ischemia) when other procedures, grafts, or angioplasty are not indicated	Schwarz Pharma
Alteplase (*Activase*)	Intraventricular hemorrhage associated with intracerebral hemorrhage	Daniel F. Hanley, MD
Altretamine (*Hexalen*)	Advanced ovarian adenocarcinoma[a]	Medimmune Oncology
Ambrisentan	Pulmonary arterial hypertension	Myogen
AMG 531	Immune thrombocytopenic purpura	Amgen
Amifostine (*Ethyol*)	Reduce the incidence of moderate to severe xerostomia in postoperative radiation treatment for head and neck cancer[a]; reduce the incidence and severity of toxicities associated with cisplatin administration; myelodysplastic syndromes; chemoprotective agent for the following: Cisplatin in metastatic melanoma, cisplatin in advanced ovarian carcinoma,[a] cyclophosphamide in advanced ovarian carcinoma	MedImmune Oncology
Amiloride hydrochloride solution for inhalation	Cystic fibrosis	GlaxoWellcome
N-[4-(4-Amino-2-ethyl-1H-imidazo[4,5-c]quinolin-1-yl)butyl]methanesulfonamide	Stages IIB through IV melanoma	3M
S(-)-3-[3-Amino-phthalimido]-glutaramide	Multiple myeloma	EntreMed
Aminocaproic acid (*Caprogel*)	Topical treatment of traumatic hyphema of the eye	Eastern Virginia Medical School
3-(4′Aminoisoindoline-1′-one)-1-piperidine-2,6-dione (CC-5013) (*Revimid*)	Multiple myeloma; myelodysplastic syndromes	Celgene
a-(3-Aminophthalimido) glutaramide (*Actimid*)	Multiple myeloma	Menarini Ricerche S.p.A.
Aminosalicylate sodium	Crohn disease	Syncom
Aminosalicylic acid (*Paser Granules*)	Tuberculosis infections[a]	Jacobus

Orphan Drugs

Drug (*Trade name*)	Proposed use	Sponsor
4-Aminosalicylic acid	Mild to moderate ulcerative colitis in patients intolerant to sulfasalazine	Warren Beeken, MD
(*Pamisyl*)		Parke-Davis
(*Rezipas*)		Squibb
Aminosidine (*Gabbromicina*)	Tuberculosis; *Mycobacterium avium* complex	Thomas P. Kanyok, PharmD
(*Paromomycin*)	Visceral leishmaniasis (kala-azar)	
	Visceral leishmaniasis	Institute for One World Health
Amiodarone (*Amio-Aqueous*)	Incessant ventricular tachycardia	Academic
Amiodarone hydrochloride (*Cordarone*)	Acute treatment and prophylaxis of life-threatening ventricular tachycardia or ventricular fibrillation[a]	Wyeth-Ayerst
Ammonium tetrathiomolybdate	Wilson disease	George J. Brewer, MD
Amphotericin B lipid complex (*Abelcet*)	Invasive protothecosis, sporotrichosis, coccidioidomycosis, zygomycosis, and candidiasis; invasive fungal infections[a]	Liposome
Amsacrine (*Amsidyl*)	Acute adult leukemia	Warner-Lambert
Anagrelide (*Agrylin*)	Polycythemia vera; essential thrombocythemia[a]; thrombocytosis in chronic myelogenous leukemia	Roberts
Ananain, comosain (*Vianain*)	Enzymatic debridement of severe burns	Genzyme
Anaritide acetate (*Auriculin*)	Acute renal failure; improvement of early renal allograft function following renal transplantation	Scios
Ancestim (*Stemgen*)	With filgrastim to decrease the number of phereses required to collect peripheral blood progenitor cells capable of providing rapid multilineage hematopoietic reconstitution following myelosuppressive or myeloablative therapy	Amgen
Ancrod (*Viprinex*)	Establish and maintain anticoagulation in heparin-intolerant patients undergoing cardiopulmonary bypass	Knoll
Angiotensin 1-7 (*MARstem*)	Neutropenia associated with autologous bone marrow transplantation; myelodysplastic syndrome	Maret
Anti-CD23 IgG1, kappa monoclonal antibody	Chronic lymphocytic leukemia	Biogen IDEC
Anti-CD45 monoclonal antibodies	Prevent acute graft rejection of human organ transplants	Baxter Healthcare
Anti-CEA sheep-human chimeric monoclonal antibody labeled w/iodine-131 (KAb201)	Pancreatic cancer	Xenova Biomedix
Anti-cytomegalovirus monoclonal antibodies	Prevent/Treat human cytomegalovirus infection in bone marrow and organ transplantation and in AIDS	Biomedical Research Institute
Anti-interferon-gamma Fab from goats	Immunologic corneal allograft rejection	Advanced Biotherapy
Anti pan T lymphocyte monoclonal antibody (*Anti-T Lymphocyte Immunotoxin Xmmly-h65-rta*)	In vivo treatment of bone marrow recipients to prevent graft rejection and graft versus host disease; ex vivo treatment to eliminate mature T-cells from potential bone marrow grafts	Xoma
Anti-tap-72 immunotoxin (*Xomazyme-791*)	Metastatic colorectal adenocarcinoma	Xoma
Anti-thymocyte globulin (rabbit) (*Thymoglobulin*)	Myelodysplastic syndrome (MDS)	Genzyme
Anti-thymocyte serum (*Nashville Rabbit Anti-thymocyte Serum*)	Allograft rejection, including solid organ (kidney, liver, heart, lung, pancreas) and bone marrow transplantation	Applied Medical Research
Antiangiogenic components extracted from marine cartilage (*Neovastat [AE-941]*)	Renal cell carcinoma	AEterna Zentaris
Antiepilepsirine	Drug-resistant generalized tonic-clonic epilepsy in children and adults	Children's Hospital, Columbus, OH
Antihemophilic factor (human) (*Alphanate*)	von Willebrand disease	Alpha Therapeutic
Antihemophilic factor (recombinant) (*Kogenate*)	Prophylaxis/Treatment of bleeding in hemophilia A[a] or for prophylaxis when surgery is required in these patients[a]	Bayer
(*ReFacto*)	Control/Prevent hemorrhagic episodes; for surgical prophylaxis in patients with hemophilia A (congenital factor VIII deficiency or classic hemophilia)	Genetics Institute
Antihemophilic factor/von Willebrand factor complex (human), dried, pasteurized (*Humate-P*)	Treat/Prevent bleeding in hemophilia A (classical hemophilia) in adult patients; treat spontaneous and trauma-induced bleeding episodes in severe von Willebrand disease, and in mild to moderate von Willebrand disease where use of desmopressin is known or suspected to be inadequate in adult and pediatric patients[a]	Aventis Behring
Antimelanoma antibody XMMME-001-DTPA 111 Indium (*Antimelanoma Antibody XMMME-001-DTPA 111 Indium*)	Diagnostic use in imaging systemic and nodal melanoma metastasis	Xoma
Antimelanoma antibody XMMME-001-RTA (*Antimelanoma Antibody XMMME-001-RTA*)	Stage III melanoma not amenable to surgical resection	Xoma
Antipyrine test	For use as an index of hepatic drug metabolizing capacity	Upsher-Smith

Orphan Drugs		
Drug (*Trade name*)	Proposed use	Sponsor
Antisense 20-mer phosphorothioate oligonucleotide [complementary to the coding region of R2 component of the human ribonucleotide reductase mRNA] (*GTI-2040*)	Renal cell carcinoma	Lorus Therapeutics
Antithrombin III (human) (*Antithrombin III human*)	Prevent/Arrest episodes of thrombosis in congenital AT-III deficiency and/or prevent the occurrence of thrombosis in patients with AT-III deficiency who have undergone trauma or who are about to undergo surgery or parturition	American National Red Cross
(*ATnativ*)	Hereditary antithrombin III deficiency in connection with surgical or obstetrical procedures or thromboembolism[a]	Pharmacia & Upjohn
(*Thrombate III*)	Replacement therapy in congenital deficiency of AT-III to prevent and treat thrombosis and pulmonary emboli[a]	Bayer
Antithrombin III (human) concentrate IV (*Kybernin P*)	Prophylaxis/Treatment of thromboembolic episodes in genetic AT-III deficiency	Aventis Behring
Antivenin Crotalidae polyvalent immune Fab (ovine) (*CroFab*)	Envenomations inflicted by North American crotalid snakes[a]	Protherics
Antivenin crotaline (pit-viper) equine immune F(ab)2 (*Antivipmyn*)	Envenomation by Crotaline snakes	Rare Disease Therapeutics
Antivenom (Crotalidae) purified (avian)	Envenomation by poisonous snakes belonging to the Crotalidae family	Ophidian
AP1903	Acute graft versus host disease in patients undergoing bone marrow transplantation	Ariad Gene Therapeutics
APL 400-020 V-Beta DNA vaccine	Cutaneous T-cell lymphoma	Wyeth-Lederle
Aplidin	Acute lymphoblastic leukemia	PharmaMar USA
Apomorphine	On-off fluctuations associated with late-stage Parkinson disease	Pentech
	Rescue treatment for early morning motor dysfunction in late-stage Parkinson disease	Scherer DDS
Apomorphine hydrochloride (*Apokyn*)	On-off fluctuations associated with late-stage Parkinson disease[a]	Mylan Bertek
Aprotinin (*Trasylol*)	Prophylaxis to reduce perioperative blood loss and the homologous blood transfusion requirement in patients undergoing cardiopulmonary bypass surgery in the course of repeat coronary artery bypass graft (CABG) surgery, and in selected cases of primary CABG surgery when the risk of bleeding is especially high (impaired hemostasis), or where transfusion is unavailable or unacceptable[a]	Bayer
Arcitumomab (*99m Tc-labeled CEA-Scan*)	Diagnosis and localization of primary, residual, recurrent, and metastatic medullary thyroid carcinoma	Immunomedics
Arginine butyrate	Beta-hemoglobinopathies and beta-thalassemia	Susan P. Perrine, MD
	Sickle cell disease and beta-thalassemia	Vertex
Arimoclomol	Amyotrophic lateral sclerosis	CytRx
Arsenic trioxide (*Trisenox*)	Acute promyelocytic leukemia[a]; chronic myeloid leukemia; multiple myeloma; myelodysplastic syndrome; acute myelocytic leukemia subtypes M0, M1, M2, M4, M5, M6, and M7; chronic lymphocytic leukemia; liver cancer; malignant glioma	Cell Therapeutics
Artesunate	Malaria	World Health Organization
As-101	AIDS	NPDC-AS101
AT1001	Fabry disease	Amicus Therapeutics
Atomoxetine hydrochloride (*Strattera*)	Tourette syndrome	Eli Lilly
Atovaquone (*Mepron*)	AIDS-associated *Pneumocystis carinii* pneumonia (PCP)[a]; prevent PCP in high-risk, HIV-infected patients (defined by a history of ≥ 1 episode of PCP and/or a peripheral CD4+ [T4 helper/inducer] lymphocyte count ≤ 200/mm^3)[a]; treat and suppress *Toxoplasma gondii* encephalitis; primary prophylaxis of HIV-infected people at high risk for developing *T. gondii* encephalitis	GlaxoSmithKline
Augmerosen (*Genasense*)	Multiple myeloma; acute myelocytic leukemia; chronic lymphocytic leukemia	Genta
Autologous antigen presenting cells pulsed with autologous tumor Ig idiotype (*Mylovenge*)	Multiple myeloma	Dendreon
Autologous dendritic cells pulsed with autologous glioblastoma multiforme acid-eluted tumor antigens (*DCVax-Brain*)	Glioblastoma multiforme	Northwest Biotherapeutics
Autologous DNP-conjugated tumor vaccine (*M-Vax*)	Adjuvant therapy in melanoma patients with surgically resectable lymph node metastasis (stage III and limited stage IV disease)	Avax Technologies
Autologous incubated macrophage	Improve the motor and sensory neurological outcome in acute cases of spinal cord injury	Proneuron Biotechnologies
Autologous tumor-derived gp96 heat shock protein-peptide complex (*Oncophage*)	Renal cell carcinoma; metastatic melanoma	Antigenics
Autolymphocyte therapy	Renal cell carcinoma	Cytogen
5-Aza-2′-deoxycytidine	Acute leukemia	SuperGen
Azacitadine (*Vidaza*)	Myelodysplastic syndromes[a]	Pharmion
Azathioprine (*Imuran*)	Oral manifestations of graft versus host disease	Oral Solutions

Orphan Drugs		
Drug (*Trade name*)	Proposed use	Sponsor
3′-Azido-2′,3′dideoxyuridine (*AZDU*)	AIDS	Berlex
Aztreonam	Inhalation therapy for control of gram-negative bacteria in the respiratory tract with cystic fibrosis	Corus Pharma
B lymphocyte stimulator (*BLyS*)	Common variable immunodeficiency	Human Genome Sciences
Bacitracin (*Altracin*)	Antibiotic-associated pseudomembranous enterocolitis caused by toxins A and B elaborated by *Clostridium difficile*	AL Labs
Baclofen (*Lioresal Intrathecal*)	Intractable spasticity caused by multiple sclerosis or spinal cord injury	Infusaid
	Intractable spasticity caused by spinal cord injury, multiple sclerosis, and other spinal diseases (eg, spinal ischemia, spinal tumor, transverse myelitis, cervical spondylosis, degenerative myelopathy)[a]; spasticity associated with cerebral palsy; dystonia	Medtronic
L-Baclofen	Trigeminal neuralgia	Gerhard Fromm, MD
(*Neuralgon*)	Trigeminal neuralgia; intractable spasticity from spinal cord injury or multiple sclerosis; intractable spasticity in children with cerebral palsy	Pharmascience
Basiliximab (*Simulect*)	Prophylaxis of solid organ rejection[a]	Novartis
Beclomethasone 17,21-dipropionate	Prevent GI graft versus host disease	Enteron
Beclomethasone dipropionate	Oral administration for intestinal graft versus host disease	Enteron
Benzoate and phenylacetate (*Ucephan*)	Adjunctive therapy to prevent/treat hyperammonemia in patients with urea cycle enzymopathy caused by carbamylphosphate synthetase, ornithine, transcarbamylase, or argininosuccinate synthetase deficiency[a]	Immunex
Benzoate/Phenylacetate (*Ammonul*)	Acute hyperammonemia and associated encephalopathy in patients with deficiencies in enzymes of the urea cycle[a]	Medicis
Benzophenone-3, octylmethyoxycinnamate, avobenzone, titanium dioxide, zinc oxide (*Total Block VL SPF 75*)	Prevent visible light-induced skin photosensitivity as a result of porfimer sodium photodynamic therapy	Fallien Cosmeceuticals
Benzydamine hydrochloride (*Tantum*)	Prophylactic treatment of oral mucositis resulting from radiation therapy for head and neck cancer	Angelini
Benzylpenicillin, benzylpenicilloic, benzylpenilloic acid (*Pre-Pen/MDM*)	Assess risk of penicillin administration when it is the preferred drug of choice in adult patients who have previously received penicillin and in adults who have a history of clinical penicillin sensitivity	Hollister-Stier
Beractant (*Survanta Intratracheal Suspension*)	Prevent/Treat neonatal respiratory distress syndrome[a]; for full-term newborns with respiratory failure caused by meconium aspiration syndrome, persistent pulmonary hypertension of the newborn, or pneumonia and sepsis	Ross
Beraprost	Pulmonary arterial hypertension associated with any New York Heart Association classification (class I, II, III, or IV)	United Therapeutics
Beta alethine (*Betathine*)	Multiple myeloma; metastatic melanoma	Dovetail Technologies
Betaine (*Cystadane*)	Homocystinuria[a]	Orphan Medical
Bethandidine sulfate	Prevent recurrence of primary ventricular fibrillation; treat primary ventricular fibrillation	Medco Research
Bevacizumab (*Avastin*)	Renal cell carcinoma; pancreatic cancer	Genentech
Bexarotene (*Targretin*)	Cutaneous manifestations of cutaneous T-cell lymphoma in patients who are refractory to ≥ 1 prior systemic therapy[a]	Ligand
Bifidobacterium longum infantis 35624	Pediatric Crohn disease	Alimentary Health
Bindarit	Lupus nephritis	Angelini
Bioartificial liver system utilizing xenogenic hepatocytes in a hollow fiber bioreactor cartridge (BAL)	In acute liver failure presenting with encephalopathy deteriorating beyond Parson grade 2	Excorp Medical
Bis(4-fluorophenyl)phenylacetamide	Sickle cell disease	ICAgen
1,2-Bis(methylsulfonyl)-1-(2-chloroethyl)-2-[(methylamino)carbonyl] hydrazine (*Cloretazine*)	Acute myelogenous leukemia	Vion
Bleomycin (*Blenoxane*)	Pancreatic cancer	Genetronics
Bleomycin sulfate (*Blenoxane*)	Malignant pleural effusion[a]	Bristol-Myers Squibb
BMY-45622	Ovarian cancer	Bristol-Myers Squibb
Bortezomib (*Velcade*)	Multiple myeloma[a]	Millennium
Bosentan (*Tracleer*)	Pulmonary arterial hypertension[a]	Actelion Life Sciences
Botulinum toxin type A	Synkinetic closure of the eyelid associated with VII cranial nerve aberrant regeneration	Botulinum Toxin Research
(*Botox*)	Blepharospasm and strabismus associated with dystonia in adults ≥ 12 years of age[a]; cervical dystonia[a]; dynamic muscle contracture in pediatric cerebral palsy	Allergan
(*Dysport*)	Spasmodic torticollis (cervical dystonia); dynamic muscle contractures in pediatric cerebral palsy; essential blepharospasm	Ipsen
Botulinum toxin type B (*Myobloc*)	Cervical dystonia[a]	Elan
Botulinum toxin type F	Spasmodic torticollis (cervical dystonia); essential blepharospasm	Ipsen

Orphan Drugs		
Drug (*Trade name*)	Proposed use	Sponsor
Botulism immune globulin (*BabyBIG*)	Infant botulism[a]	California Department of Health Services
Bovine colostrum	AIDS-related diarrhea	Donald Hastings, DVM
Bovine immunoglobulin concentrate, *Cryptosporidium parvum* (*Sporidin-G*)	Treatment and symptomatic relief of *Cryptosporidium parvum* infection of the GI tract in immunocompromised patients	GalaGen
Bovine whey protein concentrate (*Immuno-C*)	Cryptosporidiosis caused by *Cryptosporidium parvum* in the GI tract of patients who are immunodeficient/immunocompromised or immunocompetent	Biomune Systems
Branched chain amino acids	Amyotrophic lateral sclerosis	Mount Sinai Medical Center
Brimonidine (*Alphagan*)	Anterior ischemic optic neuropathy	Allergan
Bromhexine (*Bisolvon*)	Mild to moderate keratoconjunctivitis sicca in Sjogren syndrome	Boehringer Ingelheim
N-[4-Bromo-2-(1H-1,2,3,4-tetrazol-5-yl)phenyl]-N′-[3,5-bis(trifluoro-methyl)phenyl]urea	Sickle cell disease	NeuroSearch A/S
(1R,2S) 6-Bromo-alpha-[2-(dimethylamino)ethyl]-2-methoxy-alpha-(1-naphthyl)-beta-phenyl-3-quinoline ethanol	Pulmonary tuberculosis (active disease)	Tibotec
Broxuridine (*Broxine/Neomark*)	Radiation sensitizer in the treatment of primary brain tumors	NeoPharm
Bryostatin-1	With paclitaxel in the treatment of esophageal cancer	GPC Biotech
Buffered intrathecal electrolyte/dextrose injection (*Elliotts B Solution*)	As a diluent in intrathecal administration of methotrexate and cytarabine to prevent or treat meningeal leukemia and lymphocytic lymphoma[a]	Orphan Medical
Buffered ursodeoxycholic acid (*Ursocarb*)	Pruritus in patients with Alagille syndrome	Digestive Care
Buprenorphine hydrochloride (*Subutex*)	Opiate addictions in opiate users[a]	Reckitt Benckiser
Buprenorphine in combination with naloxone (*Suboxone*)	Opiate addiction in opiate users[a]	Reckitt Benckiser
Busulfan (*Busulfex*)	Preparative therapy in treating malignancies with bone marrow transplantation[a]	Protein Design Labs
(*Partaject*)	Preparative therapy for pediatric patients undergoing bone marrow transplantation	SuperGen
(*Spartaject*)	Preparative therapy for malignancies treated with bone marrow transplantation	Sparta
	Primary brain malignancies	SuperGen
(*Spartaject-Busulfan*)	Intrathecal therapy for neoplastic meningitis	SuperGen
1,5-(Butylimino)-1,5 dideoxy, D-glucitol	Fabry disease	Oxford GlycoSciences
2-0-Butyryl-1-0-octyl-myo-inositol 3,4,5,6-tetrakisphosphate	Cystic fibrosis	Inologic
Butyrylcholinesterase	Reduce and clear toxic blood levels of cocaine encountered during a drug overdose; postsurgical apnea	Shire
BW 12C	Sickle cell disease	Burroughs Wellcome
C-myb antisense oligodeoxynucleotide	Chronic myelogenous leukemia	Genta
C1 esterase inhibitor (human)	Prevent and treat angioedema caused by C1-esterase inhibitor deficiency	Alpha Therapeutic
	Angioedema	Lev
C1-esterase inhibitor, human, pasteurized (*Berinert P*)	Prevent and/or treat acute attacks of hereditary angioedema	Aventis Behring
C1-inhibitor (*C1-Inhibitor [human] Vapor Heated, Immuno*)	Acute attacks of angioedema; prevent acute attacks of angioedema, including short-term prophylaxis for patients requiring dental or other surgical procedures	Baxter Healthcare
Caffeine (*Cafcit*)	Apnea of prematurity[a]	OPR Development
Calcitonin-human for injection (*Cibacalcin*)	Symptomatic Paget disease (osteitis deformans)[a]	Novartis
Calcitonin-salmon nasal spray (*Miacalcin Nasal Spray*)	Symptomatic Paget disease (osteitis deformans)	Sandoz
Calcium acetate (*Phos-Lo*)	Hyperphosphatemia in end-stage renal disease	Pharmedic
	Hyperphosphatemia in end-stage renal failure[a]	Braintree
Calcium carbonate (*R & D Calcium Carbonate/600*)	Hyperphosphatemia in end-stage renal disease	R&D Labs
Calcium gluconate (*Calgonate*)	A wash for hydrofluoric acid spills on human skin	Calgonate
Calcium gluconate gel (*H-F Gel*)	Emergency topical treatment of hydrogen fluoride (hydrofluoric acid) burns	LTR
Calcium gluconate gel 2.5%	Emergency topical treatment of hydrogen fluoride (hydrofluoric acid) burns	Paddock
Calfactant (*Infasurf*)	Acute respiratory distress syndrome	ONY
Capsaicin	Painful HIV-associated neuropathy; erythromelalgia	NeurogesX

Orphan Drugs		
Drug (*Trade name*)	Proposed use	Sponsor
Carbamic acid,[[4-[[3-[[4-[1-(4-hydroxyphenyl)-1-methyl-ethyl] phenoxy]methyl]phenyl]methoxy] phenyl]iminomethyl]-,ethyl ester	Manage cystic fibrosis	Boehringer Ingelheim
Carbamylglutamic acid	N-acetylglutamate synthetase deficiency	Orphan Europe
Carbovir	AIDS and symptomatic HIV infection with CD4 count < 200/mm^3	GlaxoWellcome
3-Carboxy-2,3-dihydroxy-propionate 2-(3,5-dimethyl-1H-pyrrol-2-ylmethylene)-5-(1H-indol-2-yl)-3-methoxy-2H-pyrrolium	Chronic lymphocytic leukemia	Gemin X
Carboxypeptidase G2	Patients at risk of methotrexate toxicity	Protherics
Carmustine	Intracranial malignancies	Direct Therapeutics
Cascara sagrada fluid extract	Oral drug overdosage to speed lower bowel evacuation	Intramed
CD4 human truncated 369 AA polypeptide (*Soluble T4*)	AIDS	SmithKline Beecham
CD5-T lymphocyte immunotoxin (*Xomazyme-H65*)	Graft versus host disease and/or rejection in bone marrow transplant recipients	Xoma
CDP571	Crohn disease	Celltech Chiroscience
Cells produced using the Aastrom Replicelle System and SC-I Therapy Kit	For patients receiving high-dose chemotherapy who are unable to generate an acceptable dose of peripheral blood stem cells and have a sufficient bone marrow aspirate without morphological evidence of tumor	Aastrom Biosciences
Centruroides immune F(ab)2 (*Alacramyn*)	Scorpion envenomations requiring medical attention	Silanes Laboritories SA de CV
Ceramide trihexosidase/alpha-galactosidase A (*Fabrazyme*)	Fabry disease[a]	Genzyme
Cetiedil citrate injection	Sickle cell disease crisis	Baker Cummins
Cetuximab	Squamous cell cancer of the head and neck in patients who express epidermal growth factor receptor	ImClone Systems
Chenodeoxycholic acid (*Chenofalk*)	Cerebrotendinous xanthomatosis	Dr. Falk Pharma GmbH
Chenodiol (*Chenix*)	For patients with radiolucent stones in well-opacifying gallbladders, in whom elective surgery would be undertaken except for presence of increased surgical risk caused by systemic disease or age[a]	Solvay
Chimeric (human-murine) G250 IgG monoclonal antibody	Renal cell carcinoma	Wilex Biotechnology GmbH
Chimeric, humanized monoclonal antibody to *Staphylococcus*	Prophylaxis of *Staphylococcus epidermidis* sepsis in low birth weight (≤ 1,500 g) infants	Biosynexus
Chimeric M-T412 (human-murine) IgG monoclonal anti-CD4	Multiple sclerosis	Centocor
Chlorhexidine gluconate mouth rinse (*Peridex*)	Use in the amelioration of oral mucositis associated with cytoreductive therapy used in conditioning patients for bone marrow transplantation therapy	Procter & Gamble
(R)-N-[2-(6-Chloro-5-methoxy-1H-indol-3-yl)propyl]acetamide	Circadian rhythm sleep disorders in blind people with no light perception; neuroleptic-induced tardive dyskinesia in patients with schizophrenia	Phase 2 Discovery
2-Chloroethyl-3-sarcosinamide-1-nitrosourea (*Sarmustine*)	Malignant glioma	Pangene Lawrence Panasci, MD
Cholic acid (3 alpha, 7 alpha, 12 alpha trihydroxy 5-beta cholanolic acid) (*Falkochol*)	Inborn errors of cholesterol and bile acid synthesis and metabolism	Dr. Falk Pharma GmbH
Choline chloride (*Intrachol*)	Choline deficiency (specifically choline deficiency, hepatic steatosis, and cholestasis associated with long-term parenteral nutrition)	Orphan Medical
Chondrocyte-alginate gel suspension	Correct vesicoureteral reflux in the pediatric population	Curis
Chondroitinase	Patients undergoing vitrectomy	Bausch & Lomb
Ciliary neurotrophic factor	Amyotrophic lateral sclerosis	Regeneron
Ciliary neurotrophic factor, recombinant human	Motor neuron disease (including amyotrophic lateral sclerosis, progressive muscular atrophy, progressive bulbar palsy, and primary lateral sclerosis); spinal muscular atrophies	Syntex-Synergen Neuroscience
Cinacalcet (*Sensipar*)	Hypercalcemia in patients with parathyroid carcinoma[a]	Amgen
Cisplatin/Epinephrine (*IntraDose*)	Metastatic malignant melanoma; squamous cell carcinoma of the head and neck	Matrix
Citric acid, glucono-delta-lactone, and magnesium carbonate (*Renacidin Irrigation*)	Renal and bladder calculi of the apatite or struvite variety[a]	United-Guardian
Civamide (*Zucapsaicin*)	Postherpetic neuralgia of the trigeminal nerve	Winston
Cladribine (*Leustatin*)	Hairy cell leukemia[a]; chronic lymphocytic leukemia; non-Hodgkin lymphoma; acute myeloid leukemia	Johnson & Johnson
(*Mylinax*)	Chronic progressive multiple sclerosis	
Clindamycin (*Cleocin*)	Treat and prevent *Pneumocystis carinii* pneumonia associated with AIDS	Pharmacia & Upjohn, Pfizer
Clofarabine (*Clofarex*)	Acute lymphoblastic and myelogenous leukemia	Ilex Products
(*Clolar*)	Acute lymphoblastic leukemia[a]	Genzyme

Orphan Drugs		
Drug (*Trade name*)	Proposed use	Sponsor
Clofazimine (*Lamprene*)	Lepromatous leprosy, including dapsone-resistant lepromatous leprosy and lepromatous leprosy complicated by erythema nodosum leprosum[a]	Novartis
Clonazepam (*Klonopin*)	Hyperekplexia (startle disease)	Hoffmann-La Roche
Clonidine (*Duraclon*)	For continuous epidural administration as adjunctive therapy with intraspinal opiates for pain in cancer patients tolerant or unresponsive to intraspinal opiates[a]	Roxane
Clostridial collagenase	Advanced (involutional or residual stage) Dupuytren disease	L. Hurst, MD and M. Badalamente, PhD
Clotrimazole	Sickle cell disease	Carlo Brugnara, MD
Coagulation factor IX (*Mononine*)	Replacement treatment and prophylaxis of hemorrhagic complications of hemophilia B[a]	Armour
Coagulation factor IX (human) (*AlphaNine*)	Replacement therapy in hemophilia B for prevention and control of bleeding episodes and during surgery to correct defective hemostasis[a]	Alpha Therapeutic
Coagulation factor IX (recombinant) (*BeneFix*)	Hemophilia B[a]	Genetics Institute
Coagulation factor VIIa (recombinant) (*NovoSeven*)	Bleeding episodes in hemophilia A or B patients with inhibitors to Factor VIII or Factor IX[a]; prevent and treat bleeding episodes in Glanzmann thrombasthenia; prevent and treat bleeding episodes in hemophilia A or B with or without inhibitors; prevent and treat bleeding episodes in patients with acquired inhibitors to Factor VIII or IX; bleeding episodes in congenital Factor VII deficiency	Novo Nordisk
Coenzyme Q10	Huntington disease	Vitaline
Colchicine	Arrest the progression of neurologic disability caused by chronic progressive multiple sclerosis	Pharmacontrol
Colfosceril palmitate, cetyl alcohol, tyloxapol (*Exosurf*)	Adult respiratory distress syndrome	GlaxoSmithKline
(*Exosurf Neonatal for Intratracheal Suspension*)	Prevent hyaline membrane disease (respiratory distress syndrome) in infants born at ≤ 32 weeks gestation[a]; treat established hyaline membrane disease at all gestational ages[a]	GlaxoWellcome
Collagenase (lyophilized) for injection (*Plaquase*)	Peyronie disease	Advance Biofactures
Combretastatin A4 phosphate	Anaplastic thyroid cancer, medullary thyroid cancer, and stage VI papillary or follicular thyroid cancer	OXiGENE
Conjugate of human transferrin and a mutant diphtheria toxin (CRM 107) (*TransMID*)	Malignant tumors of the CNS	INTELLIgene Expressions
Conjugated bile acids (*COBARTin*)	Steatorrhea in short bowel syndrome	Jarrow Formulas
Corticorelin ovine triflutate (*Acthrel*)	To differentiate between pituitary and ectopic production of adrenocorticotropic hormone (ACTH) in ACTH-dependent Cushing syndrome[a]	Ferring
Corticotropin-releasing factor, human (*Xerecept*)	Peritumoral brain edema	Neurobiological Technologies
Coumarin (*Onkolox*)	Renal cell carcinoma	Drossapharm
Creatine (*Creapure*)	Amyotrophic lateral sclerosis	Avicena Group
Cromolyn sodium (*Gastrocrom*)	Mastocytosis[a]	Fisons
Cromolyn sodium 4% ophthalmic solution (*Opticrom 4% Ophthalmic Solution*)	Vernal keratoconjunctivitis[a]	Fisons
***Cryptosporidium* hyperimmune bovine colostrum IgG concentrate**	Diarrhea in AIDS patients caused by infection with *Cryptosporidium parvum*	ImmuCell
CT-2584 mesylate	Adult soft tissue sarcoma; malignant mesothelioma	Cell Therapeutics
CY-1503 (*Cylexin*)	Postischemic pulmonary reperfusion edema following surgical treatment for chronic thromboembolic pulmonary hypertension; for neonates and infants undergoing cardiopulmonary bypass during surgical repair of congenital heart lesions	Cytel
CY-1899	Chronic active hepatitis B infection in HLA-A2 positive patients	Cytel
(2Z)-2-Cyano-3-3hydroxy-N-[4-(trifluoromethyl)phenyl]-2-hepten-6-ynamide (*FK778*)	Prevent acute rejection following kidney, heart, and liver transplantation	Fujisawa Healthcare
8-Cyclopentyl 1,3-dipropylxanthine	Cystic fibrosis	SciClone
L-Cycloserine	Gaucher disease	Meir Lev, MD
Cyclosporin	Prophylaxis of organ rejection in patients receiving allogeneic lung transplant	Chiron
Cyclosporin A (*Cyclosporin*)	Amyotrophic lateral sclerosis and its variants	Maas BiolAB
Cyclosporine	Acute rejection in patients requiring allogeneic lung transplants	Chiron
Cyclosporine 2% ophthalmic ointment	Patients at high risk of graft rejection following penetrating keratoplasty; corneal melting syndromes of known or presumed immunologic etiopathogenesis, including Mooren ulcer	Allergan
Cyclosporine in combination with omega-3 polyunsaturated fatty acids	Prevent solid organ graft rejection	RTP Pharma
Cyclosporine ophthalmic (*Optimmune*)	Severe keratoconjunctivitis sicca associated with Sjogren syndrome	University of Georgia
Cyproterone acetate (*Androcur*)	Severe hirsutism	Berlex
Cysteamine (*Cystagon*)	Nephropathic cystinosis	Jess G. Thoene, MD
	Nephropathic cystinosis[a]	Mylan

Orphan Drugs

Drug (*Trade name*)	Proposed use	Sponsor
Cysteamine hydrochloride	Corneal cystine crystal accumulation in cystinosis patients	Sigma-Tau
L-Cysteine	Prevent and lessen photosensitivity in erythropoietic protoporphyria	Orphan Pharmaceuticals
Cystic fibrosis gene therapy	Cystic fibrosis	Genzyme
Cystic fibrosis Tr gene therapy (recombinant adenovirus) (*AdGVCFTR.10*)	Cystic fibrosis	GenVec
Cystic fibrosis transmembrane conductance regulator	Cystic fibrosis transmembrane conductance regulator protein replacement therapy in cystic fibrosis	Genzyme
Cystic fibrosis transmembrane conductance regulator gene	Cystic fibrosis	Genetic Therapy
Cytarabine liposomal (*DepoCyt*)	Neoplastic meningitis[a]	DepoTech
Cytomegalovirus immune globulin (human) (*CytoGam*)	Prevent or attenuate primary cytomegalovirus disease in immunosuppressed recipients of organ transplants[a]	MA Public Health Biological Labs
Cytomegalovirus immune globulin intravenous (human)	With ganciclovir sodium for the treatment of cytomegalovirus pneumonia in bone marrow transplant patients	Bayer
D-peptide of the sequence AKRHHGYKRKFH-NH2 (*PulmaDex*)	Cystic fibrosis	Demegen
Daclizumab (*Zenapax*)	Prevent acute renal allograft rejection[a]	Hoffmann-LaRoche
Dantrolene sodium (*Dantrium*)	Neuroleptic malignant syndrome	Norwich Eaton
Dapsone (*Dapsone*)	Prophylaxis of toxoplasmosis in severely immunocompromised patients with CD4 counts < 100; prophylaxis of *Pneumocystis carinii* pneumonia (PCP); with trimethoprim for treatment of PCP	Jacobus
Daunorubicin citrate liposome injection (*DaunoXome*)	Advanced HIV-associated Kaposi sarcoma[a]	NeXstar
DEAE-rebeccamycin	Bile duct tumors	Exelixis
(1S)-1-(9-Deazahypoxanthin-9-yl)-1, 4-dideoxy-1,4-imino-D-ribitol-hydrochloride	T-cell non-Hodgkin lymphoma; chronic lymphocytic leukemia and related leukemias to include prolymphocytic leukemia, adult T-cell leukemia, and hairy cell leukemia; acute lymphoblastic leukemia	BioCryst
Debrase (*Debridase*)	Debridement of acute, deep dermal burns in hospitalized patients	MediWound
Decitabine	Myelodysplastic syndromes; chronic myelogenous leukemia; sickle cell anemia	SuperGen
Deferasirox	Chronic iron overload in patients with transfusion-dependent anemias	Novartis
Deferiprone (*Ferriprox*)	Iron overload in patients with hematologic disorders requiring chronic transfusion therapy	Apotex Research
Deferitrin	Iron overload	Genzyme
Defibrotide	Thrombotic thrombocytopenic purpura	Crinos
	Hepatic veno-occlusive disease	Gentium SpA
Dehydroepiandrosterone (DHEA) (*Fidelin*)	Systemic lupus erythematosus (SLE) and reduction of steroid use in steroid-dependent SLE patients	Genelabs
	Replacement therapy in patients with adrenal insufficiency	Paladin Labs
Dehydroepiandrosterone sulfate sodium	To treat serious burns requiring hospitalization; to accelerate re-epithelialization of donor sites in those hospitalized burn patients who must undergo autologous skin grafting	Pharmadigm
Denileukin diftitox (*Ontak*)	Persistent or recurrent cutaneous T-cell lymphoma whose malignant cells express the CD25 component of the IL-2 receptor[a]	Ligand
2′-Deoxycytidine	Host-protective agent in acute myelogenous leukemia	Steven Grant, MD
1-Deoxygalactonojirimycin	Fabry disease	Amicus Therapeutics
Deoxyribose, phosphorothioate	Advanced malignant melanoma (stages II, III, and IV)	Genta
Depsipeptide	Cutaneous T-cell lymphoma	Gloucester
Desmoglein 3 synthetic peptide (PI-0824)	Pemphigus vulgaris	Peptimmune
Desmopressin acetate	Mild hemophilia A and von Willebrand disease[a]	Aventis Behring
2-0-Desulfated heparin (*Aeropin*)	Cystic fibrosis	Kennedy and Hoidal, MDs
Dexamethasone	Used in posterior segment drug delivery system in idiopathic intermediate uveitis	Allergan
Dexanabinol	For the attenuation or amelioration of the long-term neurological sequelae associated with moderate and severe traumatic brain injury	Pharmos
Dexrazoxane	Anthracycline extravasation during chemotherapy	Topo Target A/S
(*Zinecard*)	Prevent cardiomyopathy associated with doxorubicin administration[a]	Pharmacia & Upjohn
Dextran 1	Cystic fibrosis	BCY LifeSciences
Dextran 70 (*Dehydrex*)	Recurrent corneal erosion unresponsive to conventional therapy	Holles Labs
Dextran and deferoxamine (*Bio-Rescue*)	Acute iron poisoning	Biomedical Frontiers
Dextran sulfate (inhaled, aerosolized) (*Uendex*)	Adjunct in treating cystic fibrosis	Kennedy and Hoidal, MDs
Dextran sulfate sodium	AIDS	Ueno Fine Chemicals
DHA-paclitaxel (*Taxoprexin*)	Pancreatic cancer; metastatic malignant melanoma; adenocarcinoma of the stomach or lower esophagus	Luitpold

Orphan Drugs

Drug (*Trade name*)	Proposed use	Sponsor
3,4-Diaminopyridine	Lambert-Eaton myasthenic syndrome	Jacobus
Dianeal peritoneal dialysis solution with 1.1% amino acids (*Nutrineal [Peritoneal Dialysis Solution with 1.1% Amino Acid]*)	Nutritional supplement for malnourishment in patients undergoing continuous ambulatory peritoneal dialysis	Baxter Healthcare
Diazepam viscous solution for rectal administration	Manage selected, refractory patients with epilepsy on stable regimens of antiepileptic drugs who require intermittent use of diazepam to control bouts of increased seizure activity[a]	Xcel
Diaziquone	Primary brain malignancies (grade III and IV astrocytomas)	Warner-Lambert
4,5-Dibromorhodamine 123 (*Theralux Irradiation Device*)	Chronic myelogenous leukemia	Celmed BioSciences
2′-3′-Dideoxyadenosine	AIDS	National Cancer Institute
Dideoxyinosine	AIDS	Bristol-Myers Squibb
2-(3-Diethylaminopropyl)-8,8-dipropyl-2-azaspiro[4,5]decan dimaleate (*Atiprimod*)	Multiple myeloma and associated bone resorption	Callisto
Diethyldithiocarbamate (*Imuthiol*)	AIDS	Connaught
Diethylenetriaminepentaacetate (DPTA)	Known or suspected internal contamination with plutonium, americium, or curium to increase the rates of elimination	CIS-US
Diethylenetriaminepentaacetic acid (DTPA)	Known or suspected internal contamination with plutonium, americium, or curium to increase the rates of elimination[a]	Hameln Pharmaceuticals GmbH
Diethylnorspermine (DENSPM)	Hepatocellular carcinoma	Genzyme
Diferuloylmethane	Cystic fibrosis	Seer
Digitoxin	Soft tissue sarcomas; ovarian cancer	PrimeCyte
Digoxin immune FAB (ovine) (*Digibind*)	Potentially life-threatening digitalis intoxication in patients who are refractory to management by conventional therapy[a]	GlaxoWellcome
(*Digidote*)	Life-threatening acute cardiac glycoside intoxication manifested by conduction disorders, ectopic ventricular activity, and, in some cases, hyperkalemia	Boehringer Mannheim
N-(2,3-Dihydro-3,3-dimethyl-1H-indol-6-yl)-2-[(4-pyridinylmethyl) amino]-3-pyridinecarboxamide, phosphate (1:2)	GI stromal tumors	Amgen
5,6-Dihydro-5-azacytidine	Malignant mesothelioma	ILEX Oncology
Dihydrotestosterone (*Androgel-DHT*)	Weight loss in AIDS with HIV-associated wasting	Unimed
24,25 Dihydroxycholecalciferol	Uremic osteodystrophy	Lemmon
3-(3,5-Dimethyl-1H-2ylmethylene)-1, 3-dihydro-indol-2-one	Kaposi sarcoma; von Hippel-Lindau disease	Sugen
Dimethyl sulfoxide	Topical treatment to prevent soft tissue injury following extravasation of cytotoxic drugs; palmar-plantar-erythrodysesthesia syndrome	Cancer Technologies
	Increased intracranial pressure in patients with severe, closed-head injury (traumatic brain coma) for whom no other effective treatment is available	Pharma 21
	Cutaneous manifestations of scleroderma	Research Industries
Dipalmitoylphosphatidylcholine/ Phosphatidylglycerol (*ALEC*)	Prevent/Treat neonatal respiratory distress syndrome	Forum Products
Diphenylcyclopenone	Chronic severe forms of alopecia areata (alopecia totalis/alopecia universalis)	Lloyd E. King, Jr.
Disaccharide tripeptide glycerol dipalmitoyl (*Immther*)	Pulmonary and hepatic metastases in colorectal adenocarcinoma	ImmunoTherapeutics
Disodium clodronate	Hypercalcemia of malignancy	Discovery Experimental & Development
Disodium clodronate tetrahydrate (*Bonefos*)	Increased bone resorption caused by malignancy	Anthra
Disodium silibinin dihemisuccinate (*Legalon*)	Hepatic intoxication by *Amanita phalloides* (mushroom poisoning)	Pharmaquest
DMP 777	Therapeutic management of lung disease attributable to cystic fibrosis	DuPont
DNA-lipid complex (DMRIE/DOPE)/ plasmid vector (VCL-1102, Vical) expressing human interleukin-2 (*Leuvectin*)	Renal cell carcinoma	Vical
DNA plasmid vector expressing human IL-12 gene	Ovarian cancer	Expression Genetics
DNP-modified autologous tumor vaccine (*O-Vax*)	Adjuvant therapy for treating ovarian cancer	AVAX Technologies
Docosahexanoic acid-paclitaxel (*Taxoprexin*)	Hormone-refractory prostate cancer	Luitpold
1-(11-Dodecylamino-10-hydroxyundecyl)-3-7-dimethylxanthine hydrogen methanesulfonate	Hormone refractory prostate carcinoma	Cell Therapeutics
Doripenem	Bronchopulmonary infection in patients with cystic fibrosis who are colonized with *Pseudomonas aeruginosa* or *Burkholderia cepacia*	Peninsula
Dornase alfa (*Pulmozyme*)	Reduce mucous viscosity and enable the clearance of airway secretions in cystic fibrosis[a]	Genentech

Orphan Drugs		
Drug (*Trade name*)	Proposed use	Sponsor
Doxorubicin hydrochloride liposome injection (*Doxil*)	Multiple myeloma	Johnson & Johnson
Doxorubicin liposome (*Doxil*)	Ovarian cancer[a]	Alza
Dronabinol (*Marinol*)	Stimulate appetite and prevent weight loss in patients with a confirmed diagnosis of AIDS[a]	Unimed
Duramycin	Cystic fibrosis	MoliChem Medicines
Dynamine	Lambert-Eaton myasthenic syndrome; hereditary motor and sensory neuropathy type I (Charcot-Marie-Tooth disease)	Mayo Foundation
Eculizumab	Idiopathic membranous glomerular nephropathy; paroxysmal nocturnal hemoglobinuria	Alexion
Efaproxiral	Adjunct to whole brain radiation therapy to treat brain metastases in patients with breast cancer	Allos Therapeutics
Eflornithine hydrochloride (*Ornidyl*)	*Trypanosoma brucei* gambiense infection (sleeping sickness)[a]	Hoechst Marion Roussel
	Pneumocystis carinii pneumonia in AIDS	Marion Merrell Dow
Elcatonin	Intrathecal treatment of intractable pain	Innapharma
Enadoline hydrochloride	Severe head injury	Warner-Lambert
Encapsulated porcine islet preparation (*BetaRx*)	Patients with type 1 diabetes already on immunosuppression	VivoRx
Enisoprost	In organ transplantation to diminish the nephrotoxicity induced by cyclosporine; with cyclosporine in organ transplantation to reduce acute transplant rejection	G.D. Searle
Epidermal growth factor (human)	Acceleration of corneal epithelial regeneration and healing of stromal tissue in nonhealing corneal defects	Chiron Vision
	Promote cutaneous wound healing in extreme burn treatment protocols	Ethicon
Epirubicin (*Ellence*)	Breast cancer[a]	Pharmacia & Upjohn
Epoetin alfa	Myelodysplastic syndrome	Johnson & Johnson
(*Epogen*)	Anemia associated with end-stage renal disease[a] or HIV infection or treatment[a]	Amgen
(*Procrit*)	Anemia associated with end-stage renal disease; anemia of prematurity in preterm infants; HIV-associated anemia related to HIV infection or treatment	RW Johnson
Epoetin beta (*Marogen*)	Anemia associated with end-stage renal disease	Chugai-USA
Epoprostenol (*Cycloprostin*)	Replacement of heparin in patients requiring hemodialysis and who are at increased risk of hemorrhage	Upjohn
(*Flolan*)	Primary pulmonary hypertension[a]; secondary pulmonary hypertension caused by intrinsic precapillary pulmonary vascular disease[a]; replace heparin in patients requiring hemodialysis and who are at increased risk of hemorrhage	GlaxoSmithKline
Epratuzumab (*LymphoCIDE*)	Non-Hodgkin lymphoma	Immunomedics
Erlotinib hydrochloride (*Tarceva*)	Malignant gliomas	Genentech
Erwinia L-asparaginase	Alternative to *Escherichia coli* asparaginase in those situations where repeat courses of asparaginase therapy for acute lymphoblastic leukemia are required or when allergic reactions force the discontinuance of the *E. coli* preparation	Lyphomed
(*Erwinase*)	Acute lymphocytic leukemia	Porton International
Erythropoietin (recombinant human)	Anemia associated with end-stage renal disease	McDonnell Douglas
		Organon Teknika
Etanercept (*Enbrel*)	Reduce signs and symptoms of moderately to severely active polyarticular-course juvenile rheumatoid arthritis when there has been inadequate response to ≥ 1 disease-modifying antirheumatic drug[a]; Wegener granulomatosis	Immunex
Ethanolamine oleate (*Ethamolin*)	Prevent rebleeding of esophageal varices that have recently bled[a]	Block Drug
Ethinyl estradiol	Turner syndrome	Bio-Technology General
Ethiofos	A chemoprotective agent for cisplatin and cyclophosphamide in ovarian cancer	US Bioscience
(4S)-4-Ethyl-4-hydroxy-3, 14-dioxo-3,4,12,14-tetrahydro-1-H-pyrano[3',4':6,7]-indolizino-[1,2-b]-quinoline-11-carbaldehyde O-(tert-butyl)-(E)-oxime (*Gimatecan*)	Malignant glioma	Sigma-Tau Research
Ethyl eicosapentaenoate	Huntington disease	Laxdale
Etidronate disodium (*Didronel*)	Hypercalcemia of malignancy inadequately managed by dietary modification and/or oral hydration[a]	MGI Pharma
(*Didronel Intravenous Infusion*)	Prevent/Treat degenerative metabolic bone disease in patients who require long-term (≥ 6 months) total parenteral nutrition	
Etiocholanedione	Aplastic anemia; Prader-Willi syndrome	SuperGen
R-Etodolac	Chronic lymphocytic leukemia	Salmedix
Exemestane (*Aromasin*)	Advanced breast cancer in postmenopausal women whose disease has progressed following tamoxifen therapy[a]	Pharmacia & Upjohn
Exisulind	Suppress and control colonic adenomatous polyps in the inherited disease adenomatous polyposis coli	OSI
Factor XIII [A2] homodimer, recombinant DNA origin	Congenital Factor XIII deficiency; prophylaxis of bleeding associated with congenital Factor XIII deficiency	ZymoGenetics

Orphan Drugs		
Drug (*Trade name*)	Proposed use	Sponsor
Factor XIII concentrate (human) pasteurized (*Fibrogammin P*)	Congenital Factor XIII deficiency	Novo Nordisk
Factor XIII, recombinant	Congenital Factor XIII deficiency	Zymogenetics
Fampridine (*Neurelan*)	Relieve symptoms of multiple sclerosis; chronic, incomplete spinal cord injury	Acorda Therapeutics
Felbamate (*Felbatol*)	Lennox-Gastaut syndrome[a]	Wallace
Ferric hexacyanoferrate (II) (Prussian Blue)	Patients with known or suspected internal contamination with radioactive or nonradioactive cesium or thallium[a]	Degussa AG
FIAU	Adjunctive treatment of chronic active hepatitis B	Oclassen
Fibrinogen (human)	Control of bleeding and prophylactic treatment of patients deficient in fibrinogen	Alpha Therapeutics
Fibronectin (human plasma-derived)	For nonhealing corneal ulcers or epithelial defects unresponsive to conventional therapy and the underlying cause has been eliminated	Melville Biologics
Fibronectin (plasma-derived)	For nonhealing corneal ulcers or epithelial defects unresponsive to conventional therapy and for which any infectious cause of the defect has been eliminated	Chiron Vision
Filgrastim (*Neupogen*)	Severe chronic neutropenia (absolute neutrophil count < 500/mm^3)[a]; neutropenia associated with bone marrow transplants[a]; AIDS patients with cytomegalovirus retinitis being treated with ganciclovir; mobilization of peripheral blood progenitor cells for collection in patients who will receive myeloablative or myelosuppressive chemotherapy[a]; reduce duration of neutropenia, fever, antibiotic use, and hospitalization following induction and consolidation treatment for acute myeloid leukemia[a]; myelodysplastic syndrome	Amgen
Floxuridine, FUDR	Intraperitoneal treatment of gastric cancer	Franco Muggia, MD
Fludarabine phosphate (*Fludara*)	Treatment and management of non-Hodgkin lymphoma; chronic lymphocytic leukemia (CLL) including refractory CLL[a]	Berlex
Flumecinol (*Zixoryn*)	Hyperbilirubinemia in newborn infants unresponsive to phototherapy	Farmacon
Flunarizine (*Sibelium*)	Alternating hemiplegia	Janssen Research
Fluocinolone (*Retisert*)	Uveitis involving the posterior segment of the eye[a]	Bausch & Lomb
(3-[5-(2-Fluoro-phenyl)-[1,2,4]oxadiazole-3-yl]-benzoic acid	Cystic fibrosis resulting from a nonsense (premature stopcodon) mutation in the cystic fibrosis transmembrane conductance regulatory gene; muscular dystrophy resulting from premature stop mutations in the dystrophin gene	PTC Therapeutics
Fluorouracil	With interferon alpha-2a, recombinant, for advanced colorectal and esophageal carcinomas	Hoffmann-La Roche
	Glioblastoma multiforme	Ethypharm SA
(*Adrucil*)	With leucovorin for metastatic adenocarcinoma of the colon and rectum	Lederle
Fluoxetine (*Prozac*)	Autism	Eric Hollander, MD
Follitropin alfa, recombinant (*Gonal-F*)	Induction of spermatogenesis in men with primary and secondary hypogonadotropic hypogonadism in whom the cause of infertility is not caused by primary testicular failure[a]	Serono
Fomepizole (*Antizol*)	Methanol or ethylene glycol poisoning[a]	Orphan Medical
Fosphenytoin (*Cerebyx*)	Acute treatment of patients with status epilepticus of the grand mal type[a]	Warner-Lambert
Fructose-1,6-diphosphate (*Cordox*)	Painful vaso-occlusive episodes associated with sickle cell disease	Questcor
G17DT immunogen	Adenocarcinoma of the pancreas; gastric cancer	Aphton
Gabapentin (*Neurontin*)	Amyotrophic lateral sclerosis	Warner-Lambert
α-Galactosidase A (*Plant-Produced Human α-Galactosidase*)	Fabry disease	Large Scale Biology
Gallium nitrate injection (*Ganite*)	Hypercalcemia of malignancy[a]	Solopak
Galsulfase (*Naglazyme*)	Mucopolysaccharidosis type VI (Maroteaux-Lamy syndrome)[a]	BioMarin
Gamma hydroxybutyrate	Narcolepsy and auxiliary symptoms of cataplexy, sleep paralysis, hypnagogic hallucinations, and automatic behavior	Biocraft Labs
Gamma hydroxybutyric acid	Narcolepsy and auxiliary symptoms of cataplexy, sleep paralysis, hypnagogic hallucinations, and automatic behavior	Sigma Chemical
Gammalinolenic acid	Juvenile rheumatoid arthritis	Robert B. Zurier, MD
Ganaxolone	Infantile spasms	Purdue Pharma
Ganciclovir intravitreal implant (*Vitrasert Implant*)	Cytomegalovirus retinitis[a]	Bausch & Lomb Surgical, Chiron Vision
Ganciclovir sodium (*Cytovene*)	Cytomegalovirus retinitis in immunocompromised patients with AIDS[a]	Syntex
Gancyclovir	Severe human cytomegalovirus infections in specific immunosuppressed patient populations	Burroughs Wellcome
Gangliosides as sodium salts (*Cronassial*)	Retinitis pigmentosa	Fidia
Gavilimomab	Acute graft versus host disease	Abgenix
Gemtuzumab ozogamicin (*Mylotarg*)	CD33-positive acute myeloid leukemia[a]	Wyeth-Ayerst

Orphan Drugs		
Drug (*Trade name*)	Proposed use	Sponsor
Gene plasmid hVEGF165 driven by human cytomegalovirus, and [2,3-bis(oleoyl)propyl]trimethyl ammonium and dioleoyl phosphatidyl ethanolamine (*Trinam*)	Prevent complications caused by neointimal hyperplasia disease in certain vascular anastomoses	Ark Therapeutics
Gentamicin impregnated PMMA beads on surgical wire (*Septopal*)	Chronic osteomyelitis of posttraumatic, postoperative, or hematogenous origin	Lipha
Gentamicin liposome injection (*Maitec*)	Disseminated *Mycobacterium avium-intracellulare* infection	Liposome
Glatiramer acetate (*Copaxone*)	Multiple sclerosis[a]	Teva
Glatiramer acetate for injection (*Copaxone*)	Primary-progressive multiple sclerosis	Teva
Glutamine (*NutreStore*)	With human growth hormone in treating short bowel syndrome (nutrient malabsorption from the GI tract resulting from an inadequate absorptive surface)[a]	Nutritional Restart
L-Glutamine	Sickle cell disease	Emmaus Medical
L-Glutamyl-L-tryptophan	AIDS-related Kaposi sarcoma	Cytran
Glyceol	Decrease intracranial hypertension and/or alleviate cerebral edema in patients who may benefit from osmotherapy	Chugai
Glyceryl trioleate and glyceryl trierucate	Adrenoleukodystrophy	Hugo W. Moser, MD
Golimumab	Chronic sarcoidosis	Centocor
Gonadorelin acetate (*Lutrepulse*)	Ovulation induction in women with hypothalamic amenorrhea caused by a deficiency or absence in quantity or pulse pattern of endogenous GnRH secretion[a]	Ferring
Gossypol	Cancer of the adrenal cortex	Marcus M. Reidenberg, MD
Gp100 adenoviral gene therapy	Metastatic melanoma	Genzyme
Granulocyte macrophage-colony stimulating factor (*Leucomax*)	Neutropenia caused by hairy cell leukemia; neutropenia associated with bone marrow transplants; severe thermal injuries in patients with > 40% full or partial thickness burns; myelodysplastic syndrome; chronic lymphocytic leukemia to increase granulocyte count	Schering
Group B streptococcus immune globulin	Disseminated group B streptococcal infection in neonates	North American Biologicals
Growth hormone-releasing factor	Long-term treatment of children who have growth failure caused by a lack of adequate endogenous growth hormone secretion	Valeant
Guanethidine monosulfate (*Ismelin*)	Moderate to severe sympathetic reflex dystrophy and causalgia	Novartis
Guanfacine (*Tenex*)	Fragile X syndrome	Watson
Gusperimus (*Spanidin*)	Acute renal graft rejection episodes	Bristol-Myers Squibb
h5G1.1-mAb	Dermatomyositis	Alexion
Halofantrine (*Halfan*)	Mild to moderate acute malaria caused by susceptible strains of *Plasmodium falciparum* and *Plasmodium vivax*[a]	SmithKline Beecham
Halofuginone (*Stenorol*)	Systemic sclerosis	Collgard Biopharmaceuticals
Heme arginate (*Normosang*)	Symptomatic stage of acute porphyria; myelodysplastic syndromes	Orphan Europe
Hemin (*Panhematin*)	Amelioration of recurrent attacks of acute intermittent porphyria (AIP) temporarily related to the menstrual cycle in susceptible women and similar symptoms that occur in other patients with AIP, porphyria variegata, and hereditary coproporphyria[a]	Abbott
Hemin and zinc mesoporphyrin (*Hemex*)	Acute porphyric syndromes	Herbert L. Bonkovsky, MD
Heparin, oral unfractionated	Sickle cell disease	TRF Technologies
Hepatitis B immune globulin IV (human) (*Nabi-HB*)	Prophylaxis against hepatitis B virus reinfection in liver transplant patients	NABI
Hepatitis C virus immune globulin (human)	Prophylaxis of hepatitis C infection in liver transplant recipients	NABI
HepeX-B	Prevent hepatitis B virus reinfection in liver transplant patients	XTL Biopharmaceuticals
Herpes simplex virus gene	Primary and metastatic brain tumors	Genetic Therapy
Herpes simplex virus, genetically engineered (G207)	Malignant glioma	MediGene
Histamine (*Maxamine*)	Adjunctive to cytokine therapy in treatment of acute myeloid leukemia and malignant melanoma	Maxim
Histrelin	Treatment of acute intermittent porphyria, hereditary coproporphyria, and variegate porphyria	Karl E. Anderson, MD
Histrelin acetate (*Supprelin Injection*)	Central precocious puberty[a]	Roberts
HIV neutralizing antibodies (*Immupath*)	AIDS	Hemacare
HLA-B7/beta2M DNA lipid (DMRIE/DOPE) complex (*Allovectin-7*)	Invasive and metastatic melanoma (stages II, III, and IV)	Vical
Homoharringtonine	Chronic myelogenous leukemia	American BioScience
HPA-23	AIDS	Rhone-Poulenc Rorer
Hsp E7	Recurrent respiratory papillomatosis	StressGen Biotechnologies

Orphan Drugs		
Drug (*Trade name*)	Proposed use	Sponsor
Hu1D10, humanized, monoclonal antibody (*Remitogen*)	1D10+ B cell non-Hodgkin lymphoma	Protein Design Labs
Human acid precursor alpha-glucosidase, recombinant	Glycogen storage disease type II	Pharming/Genzyme
Human alpha 2,6 sialyltransferase adenoviral gene therapy	Invasive (malignant) brain and central nervous system tumors lacking alpha 2,6 sialyltransferase	Falk Center for Molecular Therapeutics
Human anti-CD30 monoclonal antibody	Hodgkin disease	Medarex
Human anti-CD4 monoclonal anti-body (*HuMax-CD4*)	Mycosis fungoides	Genmab A/S
Human anti-integrin receptor avb3/avb5 monoclonal antibody	High-risk stages II, III, and IV malignant melanoma	Centocor
Human anti-transforming growth factor-B1,2,3	Idiopathic pulmonary fibrosis	Genzyme
Human anti-transforming growth factor beta 1 monoclonal antibody	Systemic sclerosis	Genzyme
Human anti-tumor necrosis factor alpha monoclonal antibody	Uveitis of the posterior segment of noninfectious etiology, and uveitis of the anterior segment of noninfectious etiology and refractory to conventional therapy	Centocor
Human gammaglobulin	Juvenile rheumatoid arthritis; GI disturbances (eg, constipation, diarrhea, abdominal pain) associated with regression-onset autism in pediatric patients; idiopathic inflammatory myopathies	PediaMed
Human IgM monoclonal antibody (C-58) to cytomegalovirus (*Centovir*)	Cytomegalovirus infections in allogeneic bone marrow transplant patients; prophylaxis of cytomegalovirus infections in bone marrow transplant patients	Centocor
Human immunodeficiency virus immune globulin (*Hivig*)	AIDS; HIV-infected pregnant women and pediatric patients; infants of HIV-infected mothers	NABI
Human immunoglobulin (IgG1k) anti-CTLA-4 monoclonal antibody	High risk stages II, III, and IV melanoma	Medarex
Human monoclonal antibody against platelet-derived growth factor D	Slow the progression of IgA nephropathy and delay kidney failure in patients affected by the disease	CuraGen
Human T-lymphotropic virus type III Gp 160 antigens (*Vaxsyn HIV-1*)	AIDS	MicroGeneSys
Humanized anti-CD2 monoclonal antibody	Graft versus host disease	MedImmune
Humanized anti-human CD16 monoclonal antibody	Adult idiopathic thrombocytopenic purpura	Genzyme
Humanized anti-human CD2 MAb (*MEDI-507*)	Induction of donor-specific immunologic unresponsiveness resulting in prophylaxis of organ rejection without the need for chronic immunosuppressive therapy in allogeneic renal transplants	Biotransplant
Humanized anti-tac (*Zenapax*)	Prevent acute graft versus host disease following bone marrow transplantation	Hoffmann-La Roche
Humanized MAb (IDEC-131) to CD40L	Systemic lupus erythematosus	Biogen IDEC
Humanized monoclonal antibody against Shiga-like toxin II	Prevent the development of or to decrease the incidence and severity of hemolytic uremic syndrome and associated sequelae of Shiga-like toxin-producing *Escherichia coli*	Teijin America
Hyaluronic acid	Emphysema caused by alpha-1 antitrypsin deficiency	Exhale Therapeutics
Hydralazine	Severe intrapartum hypertension (diastolic blood pressure ≥ 110 or systolic blood pressure ≥ 160) associated with severe preeclampsia/eclampsia of pregnancy	Esp Pharma
Hydroxocobalamin (*Cyanokit*)	Acute cyanide poisoning	Orphan Medical EMD
Hydroxycobalamin/Sodium thiosulfate	Severe acute cyanide poisoning	Alan H. Hall, MD
6-Hydroxymethylacylfulvene	Histologically confirmed advanced or metastatic pancreatic cancer	MGI Pharma
N-[2-[(4-Hydroxyphenyl)amino]-3-pyridinyl]-4-methoxybenzenesulfonamide	Neuroblastoma	Abbott
L-5-Hydroxytryptophan	Tetrahydrobiopterin deficiency	Watson
Hydroxyurea (*Droxia*)	Sickle cell anemia as shown by the presence of hemoglobin S[a]	Bristol-Myers Squibb
Hypericin	Glioblastoma multiforme; cutaneous T-cell lymphoma	Nexell Therapeutics
I(131)-TM-601 (chlorotoxin)	Malignant glioma	TransMolecular
Ibritumomab tiuxetan (*Zevalin*)	B-cell non-Hodgkin lymphoma[a]	Biogen IDEC
Ibuprofen IV solution (*Salprofen*)	Prevent/Treat patent ductus arteriosus	Farmacon-IL
Icatibant	Angioedema	Jerini AG
Icatibant acetate	Burn patients hospitalized with burn-induced edema	Jerini AG
Icodextrin 7.5% with electrolytes peritoneal dialysis solution (*Extraneal [with 7.5% Icodextrin] Peritoneal Dialysis Solution*)	End-stage renal disease requiring peritoneal dialysis treatment[a]	Baxter Healthcare
Idarubicin (*Idamycin*)	Myelodysplastic syndromes; chronic myelogenous leukemia	Pharmacia & Upjohn

Orphan Drugs		
Drug (*Trade name*)	Proposed use	Sponsor
Idarubicin hydrochloride for injection (*Idamycin*)	Acute lymphoblastic leukemia in pediatric patients	Pharmacia & Upjohn
	Acute myelogenous leukemia (acute nonlymphocytic leukemia)[a]	Adria Labs
Idebenone (INN)	Cardiomyopathy associated with Friedreich ataxia	Santhera
IDN 6556	Undergoing solid organ transplantation	Idun
Idoxuridine	Nonparenchymatous sarcomas	NeoPharm
Iduronate-2-sulfatase	Long-term enzyme replacement therapy for mucopolysaccharidosis II (Hunter syndrome)	Transkaryotic Therapies
Ifosfamide (*Ifex*)	Testicular cancer[a]; bone sarcomas; soft tissue sarcomas	Bristol-Myers Squibb
IL-13-PE38QQR	Malignant glioma	NeoPharm
IL-4 pseudomonas toxin fusion protein (IL-4(38-37)-PE38KDEL)	Astrocytic glioma	Neurocrine Biosciences
Iloprost inhalation solution (*Ventavis*)	Pulmonary arterial hypertension[a]	CoTherix
Iloprost solution for infusion	Heparin-associated thrombocytopenia; Raynaud phenomenon secondary to systemic sclerosis	Berlex
Imatinib mesylate (*Gleevec*)	Chronic myelogenous leukemia[a]; GI stromal tumors[a]	Novartis
Imciromab pentetate (*Myoscint*)	To detect early necrosis as an indication of rejection of orthotopic cardiac transplants	Centocor
Imexon	Multiple myeloma; metastatic malignant melanoma; pancreatic adenocarcinoma	AmpliMed
Imiglucerase (*Cerezyme*)	Replacement therapy in patients with types 1, 2, and 3 Gaucher disease[a]	Genzyme
Immortalized human liver cells found in the extracorporeal liver assist device (*ELAD*)	Fulminant hepatic failure (acute liver failure)	Vital Therapies
Immune globulin (human) (*Gamunex*)	Chronic inflammatory demyelinating polyneuropathy	Bayer
Immune globulin (human) containing high titers of West Nile virus antibodies (*Omr-IgG-am 5% [WNV]*)	West Nile virus infection	OMRIX Biopharmaceuticals
Immune globulin intravenous (human) (*Carimune NF*)	Guillain-Barre syndrome	ZLB Bioplasma AG
(*Gamimune N*)	Infection prophylaxis in pediatric patients with HIV[a]	Bayer
(*Immuno, Iveegam*)	Acute myocarditis; polymyositis/dermatomyositis; juvenile rheumatoid arthritis	Immuno Clinical Research
Immune globulin subcutaneous (human) (*Vivaglobin P*)	Primary immune deficiency that are intolerant to immune globulin intravenous (IGIV) because of severe adverse events or poor venous access	Aventis Behring
Implitapide	Fredrickson type I or V hyperlipoproteinemia; homozygous familial hypercholesterolemia	Medical Research Labs International
Imported fire ant venom, allergenic extract	Skin testing for victims of fire ant stings to confirm fire ant sensitivity and, if positive, as immunotherapy for prevention of IgE-mediated anaphylactic reactions	ALK Labs
Indium In 111 altumomab pentetate (*Hybri-ceaker*)	Detect suspected and previously unidentified tumor foci of recurrent colorectal carcinoma	Hybritech
Indium In 111 murine monoclonal antibody FAB to myosin (*Myoscint*)	Aid in diagnosis of myocarditis	Centocor
^{111}Indium pentetreotide (*SomatoTher*)	Somatostatin receptor-positive neuroendocrine tumors	Louisiana State University Medical Center
Infliximab (*Remicade*)	Moderately to severely active Crohn disease for the reduction of the signs and symptoms in patients who have an inadequate response to conventional therapy[a]; fistulizing Crohn disease for the reduction in the number of draining enterocutaneous fistula(s)[a]; chronic sarcoidosis; giant cell arteritis; juvenile rheumatoid arthritis; Crohn disease and ulcerative colitis in pediatric (0 to 16 years of age) patients	Centocor
INGN 201 (*Advexin*)	Head and neck cancer	Introgen Therapeutics
INH-A00021 (*Veronate*)	Reduce (prevent) nosocomial bacteremia caused by staphylococci in very low birth weight infants	Inhibitex
Inolimomab (*Leukotac*)	Graft versus host disease	Opi
Inosine pranobex (*Isoprinosine*)	Subacute sclerosing panencephalitis	Newport
Interferon alfa-1b	Multiple myeloma	Ernest C. Borden
Interferon alfa-2a (recombinant) (*Roferon-A*)	AIDS-related Kaposi sarcoma[a]; renal cell carcinoma; with fluorouracil for esophageal carcinoma or advanced colorectal cancer; with teceleukin for metastatic renal cell carcinoma or metastatic malignant melanoma; chronic myelogenous leukemia[a]	Hoffmann-La Roche
Interferon alfa-2b (recombinant) (*Intron A*)	AIDS-related Kaposi sarcoma[a]; metastatic renal cell carcinoma; chronic myelogenous leukemia; laryngeal (respiratory) papillomatosis; acute hepatitis B; primary malignant brain tumors; invasive carcinoma of the cervix; carcinoma in situ of the urinary bladder; chronic delta hepatitis; ovarian carcinoma	Schering
Interferon alfa-n1 (*Wellferon*)	AIDS-related Kaposi sarcoma	Burroughs Wellcome
	Human papillomavirus in severe resistant/recurrent respiratory (laryngeal) papillomatosis	Glaxo Wellcome

Orphan Drugs		
Drug (*Trade name*)	Proposed use	Sponsor
Interferon beta-1a (recombinant human) (*Avonex*)	Acute non-A, non-B hepatitis; primary brain tumors; juvenile rheumatoid arthritis; multiple sclerosis[a]; pulmonary fibrosis	Biogen
(*r-HuIFN-beta*)	Systemically treat cutaneous T-cell lymphoma and cutaneous malignant melanoma; intralesional and/or systemically treat AIDS-related Kaposi sarcoma	Biogen
(*R-IFN-beta*)	Systemically treat metastatic renal cell carcinoma	Biogen
(*Rebif*)	Symptomatic patients with AIDS (including CD4 T-cell counts < 200 cells/mm^3); secondary progressive multiple sclerosis	Serono
Interferon beta-1b (recombinant human) (*Betaseron*)	Multiple sclerosis[a]	Berlex and Chiron
	AIDS	Berlex
Interferon gamma-1b (*Actimmune*)	Renal cell carcinoma	Genentech
	Chronic granulomatous disease[a]; delaying time to disease progression in patients with severe, malignant osteopetrosis[a]; idiopathic pulmonary fibrosis	InterMune
Interleukin-1 alpha, human recombinant	Hematopoietic potentiation in aplastic anemia; promotion of early engraftment in bone marrow transplantation	Immunex
Interleukin-1 receptor antagonist (human recombinant) (*Antril*)	Juvenile rheumatoid arthritis; prevent and treat graft versus host disease in transplant recipients	Amgen
Interleukin-1 Trap	CIAS1-associated periodic syndromes; Still disease, including juvenile rheumatoid arthritis and adult-onset Still disease	Regeneron
Interleukin-2 (*Teceleukin*)	Alone or with interferon alfa-2a for metastatic renal cell carcinoma; alone or with interferon alfa-2a for metastatic malignant melanoma	Hoffmann-La Roche
Interleukin-3 human (recombinant)	Promote erythropoiesis in Diamond-Blackfan anemia (congenital pure red cell aplasia)	Immunex
	Sequential administration with sargramostim to accelerate neutrophil and platelet recovery in patients undergoing autologous bone marrow transplantation for Hodgkin disease or non-Hodgkin lymphoma	Sandoz
Intraoral fluoride releasing system	Prevent dental caries caused by radiation-induced xerostomia in head and neck cancer	Digestive Care
Iobenguane sulfate I 131	Diagnostic adjunct in patients with pheochromocytoma[a]	University of Michigan
Iodine I 123 murine monoclonal antibody to alpha-fetoprotein	Detect hepatocellular carcinoma, and hepatoblastoma and alpha-fetoprotein-producing germ cell tumors	Immunomedics
Iodine I 123 murine monoclonal antibody to hCG	Detection of hCG-producing tumors (eg, germ cell, trophoblastic cell tumors)	Immunomedics
Iodine I 131 6B-iodomethyl-19-norcholesterol	Adrenal cortical imaging	David E. Kuhl, MD
Iodine I 131 bis(indium-diethylenetriaminepentaacetic acid)tyrosyllysine/hMN-14x m734 F(ab′)2 bispecific monoclonal antibody (*Pentacea*)	Small-cell lung cancer	IBC
Iodine I 131 Lym-1 monoclonal antibody	B-cell lymphoma	Lederle
Iodine I 131 murine monoclonal antibody IgG2a to B cell (*Immurait, LI-2-I-131*)	B-cell leukemia and B-cell lymphoma	Immunomedics
Iodine I 131 murine monoclonal antibody to alpha-fetoprotein	Hepatocellular carcinoma and hepatoblastoma; alpha-fetoprotein-producing germ cell tumors	Immunomedics
Iodine I 131 murine monoclonal antibody to hCG	hCG-producing tumors (eg, germ cell, trophoblastic cell tumors)	Immunomedics
Iodine I 131 radiolabeled chimeric MAb tumor necrosis treatment (TNT-1B) (*131IchTNT-1*)	Glioblastoma multiforme and anaplastic astrocytoma	Peregrine
Irofulven	Renal cell carcinoma; ovarian cancer	MGI Pharma
Iron(III)-hexacyanoferrate(II) (*Radiogardase*)	Known or suspected internal contamination with radioactive or nonradioactive cesium or thallium[a]	Heyl Chemisch
Isobutyramide	Sickle cell disease and beta-thalassemia	Alpha Therapeutics
(*Isobutyramide Oral Solution*)	Beta-hemoglobinopathies and beta-thalassemia syndromes	Susan P. Perrine, MD
Japanese encephalitis vaccine (live, attenuated)	Prevent Japanese encephalitis	Boran
Ketoconazole (*Nizoral*)	With cyclosporine A to diminish the nephrotoxicity induced by cyclosporine in organ transplantation	Pharmedic
Lactic acid (*Aphthaid*)	Severe aphthous stomatitis in severely, terminally immunocompromised patients	Frontier
Lactic acid bacteria (*Lactobacilli, Bifidobacteria,* and *Streptococcus* sp.)	Chronic active pouchitis; prevent disease relapse in patients with chronic pouchitis	VSL
Lactobin (*Lactobin*)	AIDS-associated diarrhea unresponsive to initial antidiarrheal therapy	Roxane
Lactoferrin alpha	Prevent and treat graft versus host disease	Agennix
Lamotrigine (*Lamictal*)	Lennox-Gastaut syndrome[a]	GlaxoWellcome
Lanreotide, somatostatin (*Ipstyl*)	Acromegaly	IPSEN
Laronidase (*Aldurazyme*)	Mucopolysaccharidosis-I[a]	BioMarin

Orphan Drugs

Drug (*Trade name*)	Proposed use	Sponsor
Latrodectus immune F(ab)2 (*Aracmyn*)	Black widow spider envenomations	Rare Disease Therapeutics
Leflunomide	Prevent acute and chronic rejection in patients with solid organ transplants	James W. Williams, MD
Lenalidomide (*Revimid*)	Myelodysplastic syndromes	Celgene
Lepirudin (*Refludan*)	Heparin-associated thrombocytopenia type II[a]	Hoechst Marion Roussel
Leucovorin (*Leucovorin calcium*)	With 5-fluorouracil for metastatic colorectal cancer[a]; rescue use after high-dose methotrexate therapy in treating osteosarcoma[a]	Immunex
L-Leucovorin (*Isovorin*)	With high-dose methotrexate in treating osteosarcoma; with 5-fluorouracil in the palliative treatment of metastatic adenocarcinoma of the colon and rectum	Targent
Leucovorin calcium (*Wellcovorin*)	With 5-fluorouracil for the treatment of metastatic colorectal cancer	GlaxoWellcome
Leupeptin	As an adjunct to microsurgical peripheral nerve repair	Neuromuscular Adjuncts
Leuprolide acetate (*Lupron Injection*)	Central precocious puberty[a]	Tap
Levocabastine hydrochloride ophthalmic suspension 0.05%	Vernal keratoconjunctivitis	Iolab
Levocarnitine (*Carnitor*)	Genetic carnitine deficiency[a]; primary and secondary carnitine deficiency of genetic origin[a]; pediatric cardiomyopathy; zidovudine-induced mitochondrial myopathy; manifestations of carnitine deficiency in patients with end-stage renal disease who require dialysis[a]; prevent and treat secondary carnitine deficiency in valproic acid toxicity	Sigma-Tau
Levodopa and carbidopa (*Duodopa*)	Late-stage Parkinson disease	Nouvel Pharma
Levomethadyl acetate hydrochloride (*ORLAAM*)	Heroin addiction suitable for maintenance on opiate agonists[a]	Biodevelopment
Liarozole	Congenital ichthyosis	Barrier Therapeutics
Lidocaine patch 5% (*Lidoderm Patch*)	Relieve allodynia (painful hypersensitivity) and chronic pain in postherpetic neuralgia[a]	Teikoku Pharma
Lintuzumab (*Zamyl*)	Acute myelogenous leukemia	Protein Design Labs
Liothyronine sodium injection (*Triostat*)	Myxedema coma/precoma[a]	SmithKline Beecham
Lipase, amylase, and protease (*TheraCLEC-Total*)	Pancreatic insufficiency	Altus Biologics
Lipid/DNA human cystic fibrosis gene	Cystic fibrosis	Genzyme
Liposomal amphotericin B (*AmBisome*)	Cryptococcal meningitis[a]; visceral leishmaniasis[a]; histoplasmosis	Fujisawa
Liposomal-cis-bis-neodecanoato-trans-R,R-1,2-diaminocyclohexane-Pt (II)	Malignant mesothelioma	Antigenics
Liposomal cyclosporin A (*Cyclospire*)	Aerosolized administration to prevent and treat lung allograft rejection and pulmonary rejection events associated with bone marrow transplantation	Vernon Knight, MD, Baylor College
Liposomal N-acetylglucosminyl-N-acetylmuramyl-L-ala-D-isoGln-L-ala-glycerolidpalmitoyl (*ImmTher*)	Osteosarcoma; Ewing sarcoma	Endorex
Liposomal nystatin (*Nyotran*)	Invasive fungal infections	University of Texas
Liposomal p-ethoxy growth receptor bound protein-2 antisense product	Chronic myelogenous leukemia	Interpath
Liposomal prostaglandin E1 injection	Acute respiratory distress syndrome	Liposome
Liposome encapsulated recombinant interleukin-2	Brain and CNS tumors; cancers of the kidney and renal pelvis	Biomira
Lisofylline	Patients undergoing induction therapy for acute myeloid leukemia	Cell Therapeutics
Lodoxamide tromethamine (*Alomide Ophthalmic Solution*)	Vernal keratoconjunctivitis[a]	Alcon
Loxoribine	Common variable immunodeficiency	RW Johnson
Lucinactant (*Surfaxin*)	Meconium aspiration syndrome in newborn infants; respiratory distress syndrome in premature infants; acute adult respiratory distress syndrome	Discovery Labs
Lysine acetylsalicylate injectable	Pain and fever secondary to sickle cell disease crisis	GD Searle
Mafenide acetate solution (*Sulfamylon solution*)	Adjunctive topical antimicrobial agent to control bacterial infection when used under moist dressings over meshed autografts on excised burn wounds[a]	Mylan
Mafosfamide	Neoplastic meningitis	Baxter Oncology GmbH
Mannitol (*Bronchitol*)	Facilitate clearance of mucus in patients with bronchiectasis and in patients with cystic fibrosis at risk for bronchiectasis	Pharmaxis
Mannopentaose phosphate sulfate	High-risk stages II, III, and IV melanoma	Progen Industries
Marijuana	HIV-associated wasting syndrome	Multidisciplinary Association for PsychedelicStudies
MART-1 adenoviral gene therapy for malignant melanoma	Metastatic melanoma	Genzyme
Matrix metalloproteinase inhibitor (*Galardin*)	Corneal ulcers	Glycomed
MaxAdFVIII	Hemophilia A	GenStar Therapeutics

Orphan Drugs		
Drug (*Trade name*)	Proposed use	Sponsor
Mazindol (*Sanorex*)	Duchenne muscular dystrophy	Platon J. Collipp, MD
Mecamylamine (*Inversine*)	Tourette syndrome	Targacept
Mecasermin	Growth hormone insufficiency syndrome	Tercica
(*Myotrophin*)	Amyotrophic lateral sclerosis	Cephalon
Mecasermin rinfabate (*SomatoKine*)	Growth hormone insensitivity syndrome (Laron syndrome)	Insmed
Meclorethamine or nitrogen mustard	Mycosis fungoides	Yaupon Therapeutics
Medroxyprogesterone acetate (*Hematrol*)	Immune thrombocytopenic purpura	InKine
Mefloquine hydrochloride (*Lariam*)	Acute malaria caused by *Plasmodium falciparum* and *Plasmodium vivax*[a]; prophylaxis of *P. falciparum* malaria resistant to other available drugs[a]	Hoffman-La Roche
(*Mephaquin*)	Prevent and treat chloroquine-resistant *Falciparum* malaria	Mepha AG
Megestrol acetate (*Megace*)	Anorexia, cachexia, or significant weight loss (≥ 10% of baseline body weight) with confirmed diagnosis of AIDS[a]	Bristol-Myers Squibb
Melanoma cell vaccine	Invasive melanoma	CancerVax
Melanoma peptide vaccine	HLA-A2+ patients with stage IIB, IIC, III, and IV malignant melanoma	Medarex
Melanoma vaccine (*Melacine*)	Stage III through IV melanoma	Ribi ImmunoChem Research
Melatonin	Circadian rhythm sleep disorders in blind people with no light perception	Robert Sack, MD
(*Circadin*)	Non-24-hour sleep-wake disorder in blind individuals without light perception	Neurim
Meloxicam (*Mobic*)	Juvenile rheumatoid arthritis	Boehringer Ingelheim
Melphalan (*Alkeran for Injection*)	For use in hyperthermic regional limb perfusion in treating metastatic melanoma of the extremity; treat patients with multiple myeloma for whom oral therapy is inappropriate[a]	GlaxoWellcome
Mepolizumab	First-line treatment in hypereosinophilic syndrome	GlaxoSmithKline
20-mer complementary to Akt mRNA	Stomach cancer	Rexahn
20-mer oligonucleotide complementary to Akt mRNA	Ovarian cancer; renal cell carcinoma; glioblastoma; pancreatic cancer	Rexahn
Meropenem (*Merrem IV*)	Manage acute pulmonary exacerbations in cystic fibrosis patients caused by respiratory tract infections with susceptible organisms	AstraZeneca
Mesna	Inhibition of the urotoxic effects induced by oxazaphosphorine compounds (eg, cyclophosphamide)	Asta Medica
(*Mesnex*)	As a prophylactic to reduce the incidence of ifosfamide-induced hemorrhagic cystitis[a]	Degussa
Methionine/L-methionine	AIDS myelopathy	Alessandro Di Rocco, MD, Beth Israel Medical Center
Methotrexate (*Rheumatrex*)	Juvenile rheumatoid arthritis	Wyeth-Ayerst
Methotrexate sodium (*Methotrexate*)	Osteogenic sarcoma[a]	Lederle
Methotrexate with laurocapram (*Methotrexate/Azone*)	Topical treatment of mycosis fungoides	Durham
Methoxsalen (*Uvadex*)	With the UVAR photopheresis system in treating graft versus host disease and diffuse systemic sclerosis; prevent acute rejection of cardiac allografts	Therakos
2-Methoxyestradiol (*Panzem*)	Multiple myeloma	EntreMed
(*Panzem NCD*)	Ovarian cancer	
5-Methyl-1-phenyl-2-(1H)-pyridone (CAS 53179-13-8) (*Pirfenidone*)	Idiopathic pulmonary fibrosis	InterMune
Methylbicyclone	Cystic fibrosis	Sucampo
(6R,S)5,10-Methylene-tetrahydrofolic acid (*CoFactor*)	With 5-fluorouracil for treating patients with pancreatic cancer	Adventrx
Methylnaltrexone	Chronic opioid-induced constipation unresponsive to conventional therapy	University of Chicago
Metreleptin	Metabolic disorders secondary to lipodystrophy; leptin deficiency secondary to generalized lipodystrophy and partial familial lipodystrophy	Amgen
Metronidazole (*Metrogel*)	Perioral dermatitis	Galderma Labs
Metronidazole (topical) (*Flagyl*)	Stage III and IV anaerobically infected decubitus ulcers	Searle
(*Metrogel*)	Acne rosacea[a]	Galderma Labs
Microbubble contrast agent (*Filmix Neurosonographic Contrast Agent*)	Intraoperative aid in the identification and localization of intracranial tumors	Cav-Con
Midodrine hydrochloride (*Amatine*)	Symptomatic orthostatic hypotension[a]	Schier Ridgewood FKA (Roberts)
Mifepristone (*Mifedren/Mifadren*)	Cushing syndrome secondary to ectopic adrenocorticotropic hormone secretion	HRA Pharma
Miglustat (*Zavesca*)	Gaucher disease[a]	Actelion

Orphan Drugs

Drug (*Trade name*)	Proposed use	Sponsor
Minocycline hydrochloride (*Minocin Intravenous*)	Chronic malignant pleural effusion	Lederle
Misoprostol (*GyMiso*)	Intrauterine fetal death, not accompanied by complete expulsion of the products of conception in the second and third trimesters of pregnancy	Gynuity Health Projects
Mitoguazone (*Apep*)	Diffuse non-Hodgkin lymphoma, including AIDS-related diffuse non-Hodgkin lymphoma	ILEX Oncology
Mitolactol	Adjuvant therapy in treating primary brain tumors; recurrent invasive or metastatic squamous carcinoma of the cervix	Biopharmaceutics
Mitomycin-C	Refractory glaucoma as an adjunct to ab externo glaucoma surgery	IOP
Mitoxantrone (*Novantrone*)	Progressive-relapsing multiple sclerosis[a]; secondary-progressive multiple sclerosis[a]	Immunex
	Hormone-refractory prostate cancer[a]	Serono
Mitoxantrone hydrochloride (*Novantrone*)	Acute myelogenous leukemia (acute nonlymphocytic leukemia)[a]	Lederle
MN14 monoclonal antibody to carcinoembryonic antigen (*Cea-Cide*)	Small-cell lung cancer; pancreatic cancer	Immunomedics
Modafinil (*Provigil*)	Excessive daytime sleepiness in narcolepsy[a]	Cephalon
Molgramostim (*Leucomax*)	Aplastic anemia; AIDS patients with neutropenia caused by the disease, zidovudine, or ganciclovir	Schering
Monarsen	Myasthenia gravis	Medica Venture Partners
Monoclonal Ab(murine) anti-idiotype melanoma-associated antigen (*Melimmune*)	Invasive cutaneous melanoma	IDEC
Monoclonal antibodies (murine or human) to B-cell lymphoma	B-cell lymphoma	IDEC
Monoclonal antibody 17-1a (*Panorex*)	Pancreatic cancer	Centocor
Monoclonal antibody-B43.13 (*Ovarex MAb-B43.13*)	Epithelial ovarian cancer	Unither
Monoclonal antibody for immunization against lupus nephritis	Lupus nephritis	VivoRx Autoimmune
5a8, Monoclonal antibody to CD4	Postexposure prophylaxis for occupational exposure to HIV	Biogen
Monoclonal antibody to cytomegalovirus (human)	Cytomegalovirus retinitis in AIDS; prophylaxis of cytomegalovirus disease in solid organ transplantation	Protein Design Labs
Monoclonal antibody to hepatitis B virus (human)	Prophylaxis of hepatitis B reinfection in liver transplantation secondary to end-stage chronic hepatitis B infection	Protein Design Labs
Monoclonal antiendotoxin antibody XMMEn-0e5	Gram-negative sepsis that has progressed to shock	Pfizer
Monoctanoin (*Moctanin*)	Dissolution of cholesterol gallstones retained in the common bile duct[a]	Ethitek
Monolaurin (*Glylorin*)	Congenital primary ichthyosis	GlaxoWellcome
Morphine sulfate concentrate (preservative free) (*Infumorph*)	In microinfusion devices for intraspinal administration for intractable chronic pain[a]	Elkins-Sinn
(9-[N-(3-Morpholinopropyl)-sulfonyl]-5,6-dihydro-5-oxo-11-H-indeno [1,2-c] isoquinoline methanesulfonic acid	Prevent postoperative complications of aortic aneurysm surgical repair	Inotek
Motexafin gadolinium (*Xcytrin*)	With whole brain radiation in treating brain metastases arising from solid tumors	Pharmacyclics
MTC-DOX for injection	Hepatocellular carcinoma	FeRx
Mucoid exopolysaccharide *Pseudomonas* hyperimmune globulin (*MEP IGIV*)	Prevent and treat pulmonary infections caused by *Pseudomonas aeruginosa* in cystic fibrosis	North American Biologicals
Multi-ligand somatostatin analogue	Functional gastroenteropancreatic neuroendocrine tumors (specifically, carcinoid, insulinoma, gastrinoma, somastatinoma, GRFoma, VIPoma, and glucagonoma)	Novartis
Multi-vitamin infusion (neonatal formula)	Establish and maintain total parenteral nutrition in very low birth-weight infants	Astra
Multi-vitamin infusion without vitamin K (*M.V.I.-12*)	Prevent vitamin deficiency and thromboembolic complications in people receiving home parenteral nutrition and warfarin-type anticoagulant therapy[a]	Mayne Pharma
Muramyltripeptide, phosphatidylethanolamine encased in multilamellar liposomes	Children and adolescent osteosarcoma	Immuno-Designed Molecules
Murine MAb (Lym-1) and Iodine I 131 radiolabeled murine MAb (Lym-1) to human B-cell lymphoma (*Oncolym*)	B-cell non-Hodgkin lymphoma	Peregrine
Murine MAb to polymorphic epithelial mucin, human milk fat globule 1 (*Theragyn*)	Adjunctive treatment for ovarian cancer	Antisoma plc
Mx-dnG1 or Rexin-G retroviral vector (*Rexin-G*)	Pancreatic cancer	Epeius Biotechnologies
***Mycobacterium avium* sensitin RS-10**	Used in diagnosing invasive *Mycobacterium avium* disease in immunocompetent individuals	Statens Seruminstitut

Orphan Drugs

Drug (*Trade name*)	Proposed use	Sponsor
Mycobacterium w immunomodulator, heat-killed (*CADI Mw*)	Adjunctive to multidrug therapy in managing multibacillary leprosy; active tuberculosis	CPL
Myelin	Multiple sclerosis	Autoimmune
Myo-inositol	Prevent retinopathy of prematurity in preterm infants at risk of developing the condition	Ross Products Division
Myristoylated recombinant SCR1-3 of human complement receptor type I (*APT070*)	Prevent delayed graft function in solid organ transplant	Inflazyme
Nafarelin acetate (*Synarel Nasal Solution*)	Central precocious puberty[a]	Syntex
Naltrexone hydrochloride (*Trexan*)	Blockade of the pharmacological effects of exogenous opioids as an adjunct to maintain opioid-free state in detoxified, formerly opioid-dependent individuals[a]	DuPont
Natural human lymphoblastoid interferon-alpha	Polycythemia vera; papillomavirus warts in the oral cavity of HIV-positive patients; Behcet disease	Amarillo Biosciences
NDROGE	Postanoxic intention myoclonus	Watson
Nebacumab (*Centoxin*)	Gram-negative bacteremia that has progressed to endotoxin shock	Centocor
Nelarabine	Acute lymphoblastic leukemia and lymphoblastic lymphoma	GlaxoSmithKline
Neurotrophin-1	Motor neuron disease/amyotrophic lateral sclerosis	Arthur Dale Ericsson, MD
NG-29 (*Somatrel*)	Diagnostic measure of the capacity of the pituitary gland to release growth hormone	Ferring Labs
Nifedipine	Interstitial cystitis	Jonathan Fleischmann, MD
Nimotuzumab	Glioma	YM Biosciences
Niprisan (*Hemoxin*)	Sickle cell disease	Xechem
Nitazoxanide (*Alinia*)	Intestinal giardiasis[a]; cryptosporidiosis[a]	Romark
(*Cryptaz*)	Intestinal amebiasis	
Nitisinone	Tyrosinemia type 1[a]; alkaptonuria	Swedish Orphan AB
Nitric oxide	Diagnose sarcoidosis	SensorMedics
(*INOmax*)	Persistent pulmonary hypertension in the newborn[a]; acute adult respiratory distress syndrome; reduce the risk of chronic lung disease in premature neonates	INO Therapeutics
9-Nitro-20-(S)-camptothecin (*Camvirex*)	Pancreatic cancer	SuperGen
	Pediatric HIV infection/AIDS	NovoMed
Nitroprusside	Prevent and treat cerebral vasospasm following subarachnoid hemorrhage	Jeffrey Evan Thomas, MD
Nolatrexed (*THYMITAQ*)	Hepatocellular carcinoma	EXIMIAS
Novel acting thrombolytic (NAT)	Peripheral arterial occlusion	Nuvelo
Nucleic acid aptamer binding to tumor cell nucleolin	Pancreatic cancer	Aptamera
NZ-1002	Enzyme replacement therapy in patients with all subtypes of mucopolysaccharidosis I	Novazyme
Oblimersen (*Genasense*)	Advanced malignant melanoma (stages II, III, and IV)	Genta
Octavalent *Pseudomonas aeruginosa* O-polysaccharide-toxin A conjugate (*Aerugen*)	Prevent *Pseudomonas aeruginosa* infections in cystic fibrosis	Berna Biotech
Octreotide (*Sandostatin LAR*)	Acromegaly[a]; severe diarrhea and flushing associated with malignant carcinoid tumors[a]; diarrhea associated with vasoactive intestinal peptide tumors (VIPoma)[a]	Novartis
Ofloxacin (*Ocuflox Ophthalmic Solution*)	Bacterial corneal ulcers[a]	Allergan
Oglufanide disodium	Ovarian cancer	Cytran
OM 401 (*Drepanol*)	Prophylactic treatment of sickle cell disease	Omex International
Omega-3 (n-3) polyunsaturated fatty acid (with all double bonds in the cis configuration)	Prevent organ graft rejection	Research Triangle
Omega-3 (n-3) polyunsaturated fatty acids (*Omacor*)	IgA nephropathy	Pronova Biocare, AS
Oncorad Ov103	Ovarian cancer	Cytogen
Oprelvekin (*Neumega*)	Prevent severe chemotherapy-induced thrombocytopenia[a]	Genetics Institute
Orgotein for injection	Familial amyotrophic lateral sclerosis associated with a mutation of the gene (on chromosome 21q) for copper, zinc superoxide dismutase	Oxis International
Oxaliplatin	Ovarian cancer	Debio Pharmaceuticals SA
Oxandrolone	Constitutional delay of growth and puberty	Bio-Technology General
(*Hepandrin*)	Moderate/Severe acute alcoholic hepatitis in the presence of moderate protein calorie malnutrition	
(*Oxandrin*)	Duchenne and Becker muscular dystrophy; adjunctive therapy for AIDS patients with HIV-wasting syndrome; short stature associated with Turner syndrome	
L-2-Oxothiazolidine-4-carboxylic acid (*Procysteine*)	Adult respiratory distress syndrome; amyotrophic lateral sclerosis	Transcend Therapeutics

Orphan Drugs		
Drug (*Trade name*)	Proposed use	Sponsor
Oxymorphone (*Numorphan H.P.*)	Relieve severe intractable pain in narcotic-tolerant patients	DuPont Merck
Oxypurinol	Hyperuricemia in patients intolerant to allopurinol	Cardiome Pharma
P1, P4-Di(uridine 5′-tetraphosphate), tetrasodium salt	Cystic fibrosis	Inspire
P1-(uridine 5′-)-p4-(2′-deoxycytidine 5′-) tetraphosphate, tetrasodium salt	Cystic fibrosis	Inspire
PA mAb (*Abthrax*)	Anthrax	Human Genome Sciences
Paclitaxel (*Paxene*)	AIDS-related Kaposi sarcoma	Baker Norton
(*Taxol*)[a]		Bristol-Myers Squibb
Paclitaxel (TOCOSOL)	Urothelial cancer	Sonus
Papain, trypsin, and chymotrypsin (*Wobe-Mugos*)	Multiple myeloma	Marlyn Nutraceuticals
Papaverine topical gel	Sexual dysfunction in spinal cord injury	Pharmedic
Parvovirus B19 (recombinant VP1 and VP2; *Spodoptera frugiperda* cells) vaccine (*MEDI-491*)	Prevent transient aplastic crisis in patients with sickle cell anemia	MedImmune
Patul-end	Patulous eustachian tube	Ear Foundation
PEG-glucocerebrosidase (*Lysodase*)	Chronic enzyme replacement therapy in Gaucher disease patients deficient in glucocerebrosidase	National Institute of Mental Health, NIH
PEG-interleukin-2	Primary immunodeficiencies associated with T-cell defects	Chiron
Pegademase bovine (*Adagen*)	Enzyme replacement for adenosine deaminase deficiency in patients with severe combined immunodeficiency[a]	Enzon
Pegaspargase (*Oncaspar*)	Acute lymphocytic leukemia[a]	Enzon
Peginterferon alfa-2a (*PEGASYS*)	Renal cell carcinoma; chronic myelogenous leukemia	Hoffmann-La Roche
Pegvisomant (*Somavert*)	Acromegaly[a]	Sensus
Pegylated arginine deiminase (*Hepacid*)	Hepatocellular carcinoma	Phoenix Pharmacologics
(*Melanocid*)	Invasive malignant melanoma	
Pegylated recombinant human megakaryocyte growth and development factor (*MEGAGEN*)	Reduce the period of thrombocytopenia in patients undergoing hematopoietic stem cell transplantation	Amgen
Peldesine	Cutaneous T-cell lymphoma	BioCryst
Pemetrexed disodium (*Alimta*)	Malignant pleural mesothelioma[a]	Eli Lilly
Pentamidine isethionate	Treat *Pneumocystis carinii* pneumonia	Aventis Behring
(*Nebupent*)	Prevent *Pneumocystis carinii* pneumonia in high-risk patients[a]	Fujisawa
(*Pentam 300*)	*Pneumocystis carinii* pneumonia[a]	
Pentamidine isethionate (inhalation) (*Pneumopent*)	Prevent *Pneumocystis carinii* pneumonia in high-risk patients	Fisons
Pentastarch (*Pentaspan*)	Adjunctive in leukapheresis to improve the harvesting and increase the yield of leukocytes by centrifugal means[a]	DuPont
Pentetate trisodium (*Diethylenetriaminepentaacetate*)	Known or suspected internal contamination with plutonium, americium, or curium	Heyl Chemisch
Pentosan polysulphate sodium (*Elmiron*)	Interstitial cystitis[a]	Alza
Pentostatin (*Nipent*)	Chronic lymphocytic leukemia; cutaneous T-cell lymphoma; peripheral T-cell lymphomas	SuperGen
Pentostatin for injection (*Nipent*)	Hairy cell leukemia[a]	SuperGen
Perflubron (*LiquiVent*)	Acute respiratory distress disease in adults	Alliance
Perfosfamide (*Pergamid*)	Ex vivo treatment of autologous bone marrow and subsequent reinfusion in acute myelogenous leukemia, also referred to as acute nonlymphocytic leukemia	Scios Nova
Pergolide (*Permax*)	Tourette syndrome	Floyd R. Sallee, MD, PhD
Phenylacetate	Adjunctive to surgery, radiation therapy, and chemotherapy for the treatment of patients with primary or recurrent malignant glioma	Elan Drug Delivery
Phenylalanine ammonia-lyase (*Phenylase*)	Hyperphenylalaninemia	Biomarin
Phenylbutyrate	Acute promyelocytic leukemia	Elan Drug Delivery
1,1′-[1,4-Phenylenebis(methylene)]-bis-1,4,8,11-tetraazacyclotetradecan	With filgrastim to improve the yield of progenitor cells in the apheresis product for subsequent stem cell transplantation following myelosuppressive or myeloablative chemotherapy	AnorMED
Phenylephrine	Ileal pouch anal anastomosis-related fecal incontinence	SLA Pharma
5,5′,5′′-[Phosphinothioylidyne-tris(imino-2,1-ethanediyl)]tris[5-methylchelidoninium]trihydroide hexahydrochloride	Pancreatic cancer	Now

Orphan Drugs		
Drug (*Trade name*)	Proposed use	Sponsor
Phosphocysteamine	Cystinosis	Medea Research Labs
Pilocarpine hydrochloride (*Salagen*)	Xerostomia induced by radiation therapy for head and neck cancer[a]; xerostomia and keratoconjunctivitis sicca in Sjogren syndrome[a]	MGI Pharma
Piracetam (*Nootropil*)	Myoclonus	UCB Pharma
Piritrexim isethionate	Infections caused by *Pneumocystis carinii, Toxoplasma gondii,* and *Mycobacterium avium-intracellulare*	Burroughs Wellcome
Plasmid DNA vector expressing cystic fibrosis transmembrane gene	Cystic fibrosis	Copernicus Therapeutics
Plitidepsin (*Aplidin*)	Multiple myeloma	PharmaMar
Polifeprosan 20 with carmustine (*Gliadel*)	Malignant glioma[a]	Guilford
Poloxamer 188 (*Flocor*)	Vasospasm in subarachnoid hemorrhage patients following surgical repair of a ruptured cerebral aneurysm; sickle cell crisis; severe burns requiring hospitalization	CytRx
Poloxamer 331 (*Protox*)	Initial therapy for toxoplasmosis in patients with AIDS	CytRx
Poly I: poly C12U (*Ampligen*)	AIDS; renal cell carcinoma; chronic fatigue syndrome; invasive metastatic melanoma (stage IIB, III, IV)	Hemispherx Biopharma
Polyethylene glycol-modified uricase (*Zurase*)	Tumor lysis syndrome in cancer patients undergoing chemotherapy; prophylaxis of hyperuricemia in cancer patients prone to develop tumor lysis syndrome during chemotherapy	Phoenix Pharmacologics
Polyethylene glycol (PEG)-uricase	Control the clinical consequences of hyperuricemia in patients with severe gout in whom conventional therapy is contraindicated or has been ineffective	Savient
Polyinosinic-polycytidilic acid (*Hiltonol*)	Orthopox virus infections	Oncovir
(*Poly-ICLC*)	Primary brain tumors; adjuvant to smallpox vaccination; flavivirus infections including those caused by West Nile, Japanese encephalitis, dengue, St. Louis encephalitis, yellow fever, Murray valley, and Banzai viruses	
Polymeric oxygen	Sickle cell anemia	Capmed
Porcine fetal neural dopaminergic cells and/or precursors aseptically prepared and coated with anti-MHC-1 Ab for intracerebral implantation (*NeuroCell-PD*)	Hoehn and Yahr stage IV and V Parkinson disease	Diacrin/Genzyme
Porcine fetal neural dopaminergic cells and/or precursors aseptically prepared for intracerebral implantation (*NeuroCell-PD*)	Hoehn and Yahr stage IV and V Parkinson disease	Diacrin/Genzyme
Porcine fetal neural gabaergic cells and/or precursors aseptically prepared and coated with anti-MHC-1 Ab for intracerebral implantation (*NeuroCell-HD*)	Huntington disease	Diacrin/Genzyme
Porcine fetal neural gabaergic cells and/or precursors aseptically prepared for intracerebral implantation for Huntington disease (*NeuroCell-HD*)	Huntington disease	Diacrin/Genzyme
Porcine Sertoli cells aseptically prepared for intracerebral co-implantation with fetal neural tissue (*N-Graft*)	Hoehn and Yahr stage IV and V Parkinson disease	Titan
Porfimer sodium (*Photofrin*)	Ablation of high-grade dysplasia in Barrett esophagus in patients who are not considered to be candidates for esophagectomy[a]; cholangiocarcinoma	Axcan Scandipharm
	Photodynamic therapy of patients with primary or recurrent obstructing (partially or completely) esophageal carcinoma[a]; photodynamic therapy of patients with transitional cell carcinoma in situ of the urinary bladder	QLT Phototherapeutics
Porfiromycin (*Promycin*)	Head, neck, and cervical cancer	Boehringer Ingelheim
Posaconazole (*Posoril*)	Zygomycosis	Schering
Potassium citrate (*Urocit-K*)	Prevent uric acid nephrolithiasis[a]; prevent calcium renal stones in patients with hypocitraturia[a]; avoid the complication of calcium stone formation in patients with uric lithiasis[a]	University of Texas Health Sciences Center, Dallas
Potassium citrate and citric acid	Dissolution and control of uric acid and cysteine calculi in the urinary tract	Willen Drug
Potassium iodide oral solution (*ThyroShield*)	Thyroid-blocking agent in pediatric patients exposed to radioactive iodine	Fleming
PR1 Vaccine	Myelodysplastic syndromes requiring therapy; acute myelogenous leukemia; chronic myelogenous leukemia	The Vaccine Company
Pr-122 (redox-phenytoin)	Emergency rescue treatment of status epilepticus, grand mal type	Pharmos
PR-225 (redox-acyclovir)	Herpes simplex encephalitis in AIDS	Pharmos
PR-239 (redox penicillin G)	AIDS-associated neurosyphilis	Pharmos
Pr-320 (molecusol-carbamazepine)	Emergency rescue treatment of status epilepticus, grand mal type	Pharmos
Pramiracetam sulfate	Manage cognitive dysfunction and enhance antidepressant activity with electroconvulsive therapy	Cambridge Neuroscience
Praziquantel	Neurocysticercosis	EM

Orphan Drugs		
Drug (*Trade name*)	Proposed use	Sponsor
Prednimustine (*Sterecyt*)	Malignant non-Hodgkin lymphomas	Pharmacia
Primaquine phosphate	With clindamycin hydrochloride in AIDS-associated *Pneumocystis carinii* pneumonia	Sanofi Winthrop
Progesterone	Establish and maintain pregnancy in women undergoing in vitro fertilization or embryo transfer procedures	Watson
Prostaglandin E1 enol ester (AS-013)	Fontaine stage IV chronic, critical limb ischemia	Mitsubishi Pharma
Prostaglandin E1 in lipid emulsion (*Lipo-PGE1*)	Ischemic ulceration of the lower limbs caused by peripheral arterial disease	Alpha Therapeutic
Protaxel	Ovarian cancer	Biophysica
Protein C concentrate (*Protein C Concentrate [Human] Vapor Heated, Immuno*)	Replacement therapy in patients with congenital or acquired protein C deficiency to prevent and treat warfarin-induced skin necrosis during oral anticoagulation; prevent and treat purpura fulminans in meningococcemia	Immuno Clinical Research
	Replacement therapy in congenital protein C deficiency to prevent and treat thrombosis, pulmonary emboli, and purpura fulminans	Baxter Healthcare
Protirelin	Prevent infant respiratory distress syndrome associated with prematurity	UCB Pharma
Protirelin injection	Amyotrophic lateral sclerosis	Abbott
Proxinium (*Proxinium*)	Ep-CAM-positive squamous cell carcinoma of the head and neck	Viventia Biotech
Pulmonary surfactant replacement	Prevent and treat infant respiratory distress syndrome	Scios Nova
Pulmonary surfactant replacement, porcine (*Curosurf*)	Prevent and treat respiratory distress syndrome in premature infants	Dey Labs
Purified extract of *Pseudomonas aeruginosa* (*ImmuDyn*)	Immune thrombocytopenic purpura when it is required to increase platelet counts	Able Labs
Purified type II collagen (*Colloral*)	Juvenile rheumatoid arthritis	AutoImmune
pVGI.1(VEGF2)	Thromboangiitis obliterans	Corautus Genetics
Pyruvate	Interstitial lung disease	Cellular Sciences
Quinacrine hydrochloride	Prevent recurrence of pneumothorax in high-risk patients	Lyphomed
Quinine sulfate	Malaria	Mutual
RII Retinamide	Myelodysplastic syndromes	Sparta
rAAV2-CB-hRPE65	Type II Leber congenital amaurosis	William Hauswirth, MD
Rasburicase (*Elitek*)	Malignancy-associated or chemotherapy-induced hyperuricemia[a]	Sanofi-Synthelabo
Recombinant adeno-associated virus alpha 1-antitrypsin vector (*rAAV-AAT*)	Alpha1-antitrypsin deficiency	Applied Genetic Technologies
Recombinant bactericidal/ permeability-increasing protein (*Neuprex*)	Severe meningococcal disease	Xoma
Recombinant glycine2-human glucagon-like peptide-2	Short bowel syndrome	NPS Allelix
Recombinant human acid alpha-glucosidase (*Myozyme*)	Glycogen storage disease type II	Genzyme
Recombinant human alpha-1 antitrypsin (rAAT)	Cystic fibrosis	Arriva
		PPL Therapeutics
	Delay progression of chronic obstructive pulmonary disease resulting from AAT deficiency-mediated emphysema and bronchiectasis	Baxter Healthcare
Recombinant human alpha-fetoprotein (rhAFP)	Myasthenia gravis	Merrimack
Recombinant human anti-GDF-8 (growth and differentiation factor-8) antibody	Duchenne and Becker muscular dystrophies	Wyeth
Recombinant human antithrombin III	Antithrombin III-dependent heparin resistance requiring anticoagulation	AT III
Recombinant human C1-esterase inhibitor	Prophylactic treatment of angioedema caused by hereditary or acquired C1-esterase inhibitor deficiency; acute attacks of angioedema caused by hereditary or acquired C1-esterase inhibitor deficiency	Pharming NV
Recombinant human CD4 immunoglobulin G	AIDS resulting from HIV-1 infection	Genentech
Recombinant human Clara Cell 10kDa protein	Prevent neonatal bronchopulmonary dysplasia in premature neonates with respiratory distress syndrome	Claragen
Recombinant human endostatin protein	Neuroendocrine tumors; metastatic melanoma	EntreMed
Recombinant human fibroblast growth factor-20	Radiation-induced oral mucositis	CuraGen
Recombinant human gelsolin	Respiratory symptoms of cystic fibrosis; acute and chronic respiratory symptoms of bronchiectasis	Biogen
Recombinant human highly phosphorylated acid alpha-glucosidase	Enzyme replacement therapy in patients with all subtypes of glycogen storage disease type II (GSDII, Pompe disease)	Novazyme
Recombinant human insulin-like growth factor-I	Postpoliomyelitis syndrome	Cephalon
(*IGF-1*)	Growth hormone receptor deficiency; antibody-mediated growth hormone resistance with isolated growth hormone deficiency Ia	Pharmacia & Upjohn

Orphan Drugs

Drug (*Trade name*)	Proposed use	Sponsor
(*PV802*)	Short-bowel syndrome as a result of resection of the small bowel or congenital dysfunction of the intestines	GroPep Pty
Recombinant human insulin-like growth factor-I/insulin-like growth factor binding protein-3	Major burns requiring hospitalization	Insmed
Recombinant human interleukin-12	Renal cell carcinoma	Genetics Institute
Recombinant human keratinocyte growth factor	Reduce the incidence and severity of radiation-induced xerostomia	Amgen
Recombinant human luteinizing hormone (*Luveris*)	With recombinant human follicle-stimulating hormone for women with chronic anovulation caused by hypogonadotropic hypogonadism[a]	Serono
Recombinant human monoclonal antibody to hsp90 (*Mycograb*)	Invasive candidiasis	NeuTec Pharma plc
Recombinant human nerve growth factor	HIV-associated sensory neuropathy	Genentech
Recombinant human neutrophil inhibitor (hNE)	Cystic fibrosis	Dyax
Recombinant human porphobilino-gen deaminase (*Porphozyme*)	Acute intermittent porphyria attacks	Zymmenex A/S
Recombinant human porphobilino-gen deaminase, erythropoetic form	Prevent acute intermittent porphyria attacks	Zymmenex A/S
Recombinant human relaxin	Progressive systemic sclerosis	Connetics
Recombinant human thrombopoietin	Accelerate platelet recovery in patients undergoing hematopoietic stem cell transplantation	Genentech
Recombinant humanized MAb 5c8	Prevent and treat Factor VIII/Factor IX inhibitors in hemophilia A or B; prevent rejection of solid organ transplants; prevent rejection of pancreatic islet cell transplants; immune thrombocytope-nic purpura; systemic lupus erythematosus	Biogen
Recombinant inhibitor of human plasma kallikrein	Angioedema	Dyax
Recombinant methionyl brain-derived neurotrophic factor	Amyotrophic lateral sclerosis	Amgen
Recombinant methionyl human stem cell factor	Primary bone marrow failure	Amgen
Recombinant retroviral vector-glucocerebrosidase	Enzyme replacement therapy for types I, II, or III Gaucher disease	Genetic Therapy
Recombinant secretory leucocyte protease inhibitor	Congenital alpha-1 antitrypsin deficiency; cystic fibrosis	Amgen
Recombinant soluble human CD4 (rCD4)	AIDS	Genentech
(*Receptin*)		Biogen
Recombinant T-cell receptor ligand	Multiple sclerosis patients who are HLA-DR2 positive and autoreactive to myelin oligodendro-cyte glycoprotein residues 35-55	Artielle Immuno Therapeutics
Recombinant urate oxidase	Prophylaxis of chemotherapy-induced hyperuricemia	Sanofi-Synthelabo
Recombinant vaccinia (human papillomavirus) (*TA-HPV*)	Cervical cancer	Xenova Research
Reduced L-glutathione (*Cachexon*)	AIDS-associated cachexia	Telluride
Remacemide (*Ecovia*)	Huntington disease	AstraZeneca
Repertaxin	Prevent delayed graft function in solid organ transplant	Dompe S.p.A.
Repository corticotropin or adreno-corticotropic hormone (*H.P. Acthar Gel*)	Infantile spasms	Questcor
Resiniferatoxin	Intractable pain at end-stage disease	Andrew J. Mannes, MD
Respiratory syncytial virus (RSV) immune globulin (human) (*Hypermune RSV*)	Respiratory syncytial virus lower respiratory tract infections in hospitalized infants and young children	MedImmune
(*Respigam*)	Prophylaxis of respiratory syncytial virus (RSV) lower respiratory tract infections in infants and young children at high risk of RSV disease[a]	MedImmune and MA Public Health Biologics
9-cis Retinoic acid (*Panretin*)	Prevent retinal detachment caused by proliferative vitreoretinopathy	Allergan
	Acute promyelocytic leukemia	Ligand
Retroviral gamma-c cDNA containing vector	X-linked severe combined immune deficiency disease	AVAX Technologies
Retroviral vector, R-GC and GC gene 1750	Gaucher disease	Genzyme
Reviparin sodium (*Clivarine*)	Deep vein thrombosis that may lead to pulmonary embolism in pediatric patients; long-term treatment of acute deep vein thrombosis with or without pulmonary embolism in pregnant patients	Abbott
RGG0853, E1A lipid complex	Ovarian cancer	Targeted Genetics
rh-microplasmin	Adjunct to surgery in cases of pediatric vitrectomy	ThromboGenics
rhIGF-I/rhIGFBP-3 (*SomatoKine*)	Extreme insulin-resistance syndromes (type A, Rabson-Mendenhall syndrome, leprechaunism, type B syndrome)	Insmed

Orphan Drugs		
Drug (*Trade name*)	Proposed use	Sponsor
Rho (D) immune globulin IV (human) (*WinRho SD*)	Immune thrombocytopenic purpura[a]	Rh Pharmaceuticals
rhuMAb VEGF (bevacizumab) (*Avastin*)	Renal cell carcinoma	Genentech
Ribavirin (*Rebetol*)	Chronic hepatitis C in pediatric patients[a]	Schering
(*Virazole*)	Hemorrhagic fever with renal syndrome	Valeant
Ricin (blocked) conjugated murine MCA (anti-B4)	B-cell leukemia and B-cell lymphoma; ex vivo purging of leukemic cells from the bone marrow of non-T-cell acute lymphocytic leukemia patients who are in complete remission	ImmunoGen
Ricin (blocked) conjugated murine MCA (anti-my9)	Myeloid leukemia, including acute myelogenous leukemia, and blast crisis of chronic myeloid leukemia; ex vivo treatment of autologous bone marrow and subsequent reinfusion in acute myelogenous leukemia	ImmunoGen
Ricin (blocked) conjugated murine MCA (n901)	Small-cell lung cancer	ImmunoGen
Ricin (blocked) conjugated murine monoclonal antibody (CD6)	Cutaneous T-cell lymphomas, acute T-cell leukemia-lymphoma, and related mature T-cell malignancies	ImmunoGen
Rifabutin	Disseminated *Mycobacterium avium* complex disease	Pfizer
(*Mycobutin*)	Prevent disseminated *Mycobacterium avium* complex disease in advanced HIV infection[a]	Adria Labs
Rifalazil	Pulmonary tuberculosis	PathoGenesis
Rifampin (*Rifadin IV*)	Antituberculosis treatment when oral doseform is not feasible[a]	Hoechst Marion Roussel
Rifampin, isoniazid, pyrazinamide (*Rifater*)	Short-course treatment of tuberculosis[a]	Hoechst Marion Roussel
Rifapentine (*Priftin*)	Pulmonary tuberculosis[a]; *Mycobacterium avium* complex (MAC) in patients with AIDS; prophylaxis of MAC in patients with AIDS and a CD4+ count ≤ 75/mm^3	Hoechst Marion Roussel
Rifaximin (*Normix*)	Hepatic encephalopathy	Salix
Riluzole (*Rilutek*)	Amyotrophic lateral sclerosis[a]; Huntington disease	Rhone-Poulenc Rorer
Rituximab (*Rituxan*)	Non-Hodgkin B-cell lymphoma[a]; chronic lymphocytic leukemia	Biogen IDEC
	Immune thrombocytopenic purpura	
Rofecoxib (*Vioxx*)	Juvenile rheumatoid arthritis	Merck
Roquinimex (*Linomide*)	Prolong time to relapse in leukemia patients who have undergone autologous bone marrow transplantation	Pharmacia & Upjohn
rSP-C lung surfactant (*Venticute*)	Adult respiratory distress syndrome	Byk Gulden
Rubitecan	HIV- and AIDS-infected pediatric patients	SuperGen
Rufinamide	Lennox-Gastaut syndrome	Eisai Medical Research
Sacrosidase (*Sucraid*)	Congenital sucrase-isomaltase deficiency[a]	Orphan Medical
Sargramostim (*Leukine*)	Neutropenia associated with bone marrow transplant, graft failure, and delay of engraftment and for promotion of early engraftment[a]; reduce neutropenia and leukopenia and decrease the incidence of death caused by infection in patients with acute myelogenous leukemia[a]	Immunex
Sarsasapogenin	Amyotrophic lateral sclerosis	Phytopharm plc
Satumomab pendetide (*OncoScint CR/OV*)	Detect ovarian carcinoma[a]	Cytogen
SB-408075	Pancreatic cancer	SmithKline Beecham
SC-1 monoclonal antibody	CD55 (sc-1) positive gastric tumors	H3 Pharma
SCH 58500	Primary ovarian cancer	Schering
Secalciferol (*Osteo-D*)	Familial hypophosphatemic rickets	Teva
Secretory leukocyte protease inhibitor	Bronchopulmonary dysplasia	Synergen
Selegiline hydrochloride (*Eldepryl*)	Adjuvant to levodopa and carbidopa in idiopathic Parkinson disease (paralysis agitans), postencephalitic parkinsonism, and symptomatic parkinsonism[a]	Somerset
Sermorelin acetate (*Geref*)	Idiopathic or organic growth hormone deficiency in children with growth failure[a]; adjunctive to gonadotropin in ovulation induction in anovulatory or oligo-ovulatory infertility after failure of clomiphene citrate or gonadotropin alone; AIDS-associated catabolism/weight loss	Serono
***Serratia marcescens* extract (polyribosomes)** (*Imuvert*)	Primary brain malignancies	Cell Technology
SGN-30 (anti-CD30 antibody)	CD30 positive T-cell lymphomas	Seattle Genetics
SGN-30 (anti-CD30 mAb)	Hodgkin disease	Seattle Genetics
SGN-40 (anti-CD40 antibody)	Multiple myeloma	Seattle Genetics
Short chain fatty acid enema (*Colomed*)	Chronic radiation proctitis	Richard I. Breuer, MD
Short chain fatty acid solution (*Colomed*)	Active phase of ulcerative colitis with involvement restricted to the left side of the colon	Richard I. Breuer, MD
Silver sulfadiazine and cerium nitrate (*Flammacerium*)	Prevent mortality in severely burned patients	Synthes
Siplizumab	T-cell lymphomas	Medimmune Oncology
Sitaxsentan sodium	Pulmonary arterial hypertension in the absence of chronic obstructive pulmonary disease or congestive heart failure	Encysive, L.P.

Orphan Drugs		
Drug (*Trade name*)	Proposed use	Sponsor
SK&F 110679	Long-term treatment of children who have growth failure caused by a lack of adequate endogenous growth hormone secretion	SmithKline Beecham
Sodium 1,3-propanedisulfonate	Secondary amyloidosis	Neurochem
Sodium aluminosilicate	Chronic hepatic encephalopathy	Framework Therapeutics
Sodium dichloroacetate	Congenital lactic acidosis	Peter W. Stacpoole, PhD, MD
		Questcor
	Lactic acidosis in severe malaria; homozygous familial hypercholesterolemia	Peter W. Stacpoole, PhD, MD
	Antidote in managing systemic monochloroacetic acid poisoning	EBD Group
(*Ceresine*)	Severe head injury	Questcor
Sodium monomercaptoundecahydro-closo-dodecaborate	With a thermal or epithermal neutron beam in boron nuclear capture therapy of glioblastoma multiforme	Theragenics
(*Borocell*)	In boron neutron capture therapy in glioblastoma multiforme	Neutron Technology & Neutron R&D Partner
Sodium Oxybate (*Xyrem*)	Narcolepsy[a]	Orphan Medical
Sodium phenylbutyrate	Adjunctive to surgery, radiation therapy, and chemotherapy for primary or recurrent malignant glioma	Elan Drug Delivery
(*Buphenyl*)	The following urea cycle disorders: Carbamylphosphate synthetase deficiency; ornithine transcarbamylase deficiency[a]; arginiosuccinic acid synthetase deficiency; sickling disorders including S-S, S-C, and S-thalassemia hemoglobinopathy	Medicis
Sodium pyruvate	Cystic fibrosis	Cellular Sciences
Sodium tetradecyl sulfate (*Sotradecol*)	Bleeding esophageal varices	Elkins-Sinn
Sodium thiosulfate	Prevent platinum-induced ototoxicity in pediatric patients	Adherex Technologies
Soluble complement receptor type 1	Prevent postcardiopulmonary bypass syndrome in children undergoing cardiopulmonary bypass	Avant Immunotherapeutics
Soluble recombinant human complement receptor type 1	Prevent and reduce adult respiratory distress syndrome	T Cell Sciences
Somatostatin	Bleeding esophageal varices	UCB
(*Zecnil*)	Adjunctive to nonoperative management of secreting cutaneous fistulas of the stomach, duodenum, small intestine (jejunum and ileum), or pancreas	Ferring Labs
Somatrem for injection (*Protropin*)	Long-term treatment of children with growth failure caused by lack of adequate endogenous growth hormone secretion[a]; short stature associated with Turner syndrome	Genentech
Somatropin (*Biotropin*)	Cachexia associated with AIDS	Bio-Technology General
(*Genotropin*)	Adults with growth hormone deficiency[a]	Pharmacia & Upjohn
(*Humatrope*)	Short stature associated with Turner syndrome[a]	Eli Lilly
(*Norditropin*)	Adjunctive in ovulation induction in women with infertility caused by hypogonadotropic hypogonadism or bilateral tubal occlusion or unexplained infertility who are undergoing in vivo or in vitro fertilization procedures; short stature associated with Turner syndrome	Novo Nordisk
(*Nutropin*)	Long-term treatment of children with growth failure caused by lack of adequate endogenous growth hormone secretion[a]	Genentech
(*Serostim*)	HIV-associated adipose redistribution syndrome	Serono
Somatropin for injection (*Humatrope*)	Long-term treatment of children who have growth failure caused by inadequate secretion of normal endogenous growth hormone[a]	Eli Lilly
(*Nutropin*)	Growth retardation associated with chronic renal failure[a]; short stature associated with Turner syndrome[a]; replacement therapy for growth hormone deficiency in adults after epiphyseal closure[a]	Genentech
(*Serostim*)	AIDS-associated catabolism/weight loss[a]	Serono
Somatropin (rDNA) (*Genotropin*)	Growth failure in children who were born small for gestational age[a]; short stature in patients with Prader-Willi syndrome[a]	Pharmacia & Upjohn
(*Nutropin Depot*)	Long-term treatment of children who have growth failure caused by a lack of adequate endogenous growth hormone secretion	Genentech
(*Saizen*)	Enhance nitrogen retention in hospitalized patients suffering from severe burns; idiopathic or organic growth hormone deficiency in children with growth failure	Serono
(*Zorbitive*)	Alone or with glutamine in short bowel syndrome[a]	Serono
Somatropin (rDNA) for injection (*Serostim*)	Children with AIDS-associated failure-to-thrive, including AIDS-associated wasting	Serono
Somatropin (rDNA origin) injection (*Norditropin*)	Growth failure in children caused by inadequate growth hormone secretion	Novo Nordisk
Sorafenib	Renal cell carcinoma	Bayer
Sorivudine (*BRAVAVIR*)	Herpes zoster (shingles) in immunocompromised patients	Bristol-Myers Squibb
Sotalol hydrochloride (*Betapace*)	Prevent and treat[a] life-threatening ventricular tachyarrhythmias	Berlex
Spiramycin (*Rovamycine*)	Symptomatic relief and parasitic cure of chronic cryptosporidiosis in immunodeficiency	Rhone-Poulenc Rorer
Squalamine lactate	Ovarian cancer refractory or resistant to standard chemotherapy	Genaera
SS1(dsFv)-PE38	Malignant mesothelioma; epithelial ovarian cancer	National Cancer Institute, NIH
ST1-RTA immunotoxin (SR 44163)	Prevent acute graft versus host disease in allogeneic bone marrow transplantation; treat B-chronic lymphocytic leukemia	Sanofi Winthrop

Orphan Drugs

Drug (*Trade name*)	Proposed use	Sponsor
***Staphylococcus aureus* immune globulin (human)** (*Altastaph*)	Prophylaxis against *Staphylococcus aureus* infections in low birth weight neonates	Nabi Biopharmaceuticals
Stem and progenitor cells derived from ex vivo expanded allogeneic umbilical cord blood (*StemEx*)	Hematopoietic support in patients with relapsed or refractory hematologic malignancies who are receiving high-dose therapy	Gamida Cell
SU101	Malignant glioma; ovarian cancer	Sugen
Suberoylanilide hydroxamic acid	Multiple myeloma; mesothelioma; T-cell non-Hodgkin lymphoma	Merck
Succimer (*Chemet*)	Prevent cystine kidney stones in patients with homozygous cystinuria who are prone to stone development; mercury intoxication	Sanofi Winthrop
(*Chemet capsules*)	Lead poisoning in children[a]	Bock Pharmacal
Sucralfate	Oral mucositis and stomatitis following radiation therapy for head and neck cancer	Fuisz Technologies
Sucralfate suspension	Oral complications of chemotherapy in bone marrow transplants; oral ulcerations and dysphagia in epidermolysis bullosa	Darby
Sulfadiazine	With pyrimethamine for *Toxoplasma gondii* encephalitis in patients with and without AIDS[a]	Eon
Sulfapyridine	Dermatitis herpetiformis	Jacobus
Superoxide dismutase (human)	Protect donor organ tissue from damage or injury mediated by oxygen-derived free radicals that are generated during the necessary periods of ischemia (hypoxia, anoxia) and especially reperfusion associated with the operative procedure	Pharmacia-Chiron Partnership
Superoxide dismutase (recombinant human) (*Oxsodrol*)	Prevent reperfusion injury to donor organ tissue	Bio-Technology General
Suramin (*Metaret*)	Hormone-refractory prostate cancer	Warner-Lambert
Surface active extract of saline lavage of bovine lungs (*Infasurf*)	Prevent and treat respiratory failure caused by pulmonary surfactant deficiency in preterm infants	ONY
Surfactant (human) (amniotic fluid derived) (*Human Surf*)	Prevent and treat neonatal respiratory distress syndrome	T. Allen Merritt, MD
Synsorb Pk	Verocytotoxogenic *Escherichia coli* infections	Synsorb Biotech
Synthetic human parathyroid hormone 1-34	Hypoparathyroidism	Orphan Pharmaceuticals
Synthetic human secretin	Evaluate exocrine pancreas function; obtaining desquamated pancreatic cells for cytopathologic examination in pancreatic carcinoma; diagnosing gastrinoma associated with Zollinger-Ellison syndrome; with diagnostic procedures for pancreatic disorders to increase pancreatic fluid secretion	ChiRhoClin
Synthetic porcine secretin	Evaluate exocrine pancreas function[a]; obtaining desquamated pancreatic cells for cytopathologic examination in pancreatic carcinoma; diagnosing gastrinoma associated with Zollinger-Ellison syndrome[a]; with diagnostic procedures for pancreatic disorders to increase pancreatic fluid secretion[a]	ChiRhoClin
T4 endonuclease V, liposome encapsulated	Prevent cutaneous neoplasms and other skin abnormalities in xeroderma pigmentosum	AGI Dermatics
T-cell depleted stem cell enriched cellular product from peripheral blood stem cells	Chronic granulomatous disease	Nexell Therapeutics
Tacrolimus (*Prograf*)	Prophylaxis of graft versus host disease	Fujisawa
TAK-603	Crohn disease	Tap Holdings
Talc powder, sterile (*Sclerosol Intrapleural Aerosol*)	Malignant pleural effusion[a]	Bryan
Talc, sterile (*Steritalc*)	Malignant pleural effusion; pneumothorax	Novatech SA
Technetium Tc99m anti-melanoma murine monoclonal antibody (*Oncotrac Melanoma Imaging Kit*)	Detect, by imaging, metastases of malignant melanoma	NeoRx
Technetium Tc99m murine monoclonal antibody (IgG2a) to B cell (*LymphoScan*)	Diagnostic imaging in evaluating the extent of disease in patients with histologically confirmed diagnosis of non-Hodgkin B-cell lymphoma, acute B-cell lymphoblastic leukemia (in children and adults), and chronic B-cell lymphocytic leukemia	Immunomedics
Technetium Tc99m murine monoclonal antibody to hCG (*Immuraid, hCG-Tc-99m*)	Detect human chorionic gonadotropin-producing tumors such as germ cell and trophoblastic cell tumors	Immunomedics
Technetium Tc99m murine monoclonal antibody to human AFP (*AFP-Scan*)	Detect alpha-fetoprotein-producing germ cell tumors; detect hepatocellular carcinoma and hepatoblastoma	Immunomedics
(*Immuraid*)	Detect hepatocellular carcinoma and hepatoblastoma	
Technetium Tc99m pterotetramide	Identification of ovarian carcinomas	Endocyte
Technetium Tc99m rh-Annexin V (*Apomate*)	Diagnosis or assessment of rejection status in heart, heart-lung, single lung, or bilateral lung transplants	Theseus Imaging
Temocillin sodium (*Negaban*)	Pulmonary infections caused by *Burkholderia cepacia*	Belpharma N.V.
Temoporfin (*Foscan*)	Palliative treatment of recurrent, refractory, or second primary squamous cell carcinomas of the head and neck considered to be incurable with surgery or radiotherapy	Scotia
Temozolomide (*Temodar*)	Advanced metastatic melanoma; malignant glioma[a]; recurrent malignant glioma[a]; newly diagnosed high-grade glioma	Schering-Plough
Temsirolimus	Renal cell carcinoma.	Wyeth

Orphan Drugs		
Drug (*Trade name*)	Proposed use	Sponsor
Teniposide (*Vumon for Injection*)	Refractory childhood acute lymphocytic leukemia[a]	Bristol-Myers Squibb
Teriparatide (*Parathar*)	Diagnostic agent for patients with clinical and laboratory evidence of hypocalcemia caused by hypoparathyroidism or pseudohypoparathyroidism	Rhone-Poulenc Rorer
	Idiopathic osteoporosis	Henri Beaufour Institute
Terlipressin (*Glypressin*)	Bleeding esophageal varices	Ferring Labs
Terlipressin (INN)	Hepatorenal syndrome	Orphan Therapeutics
Testosterone (*Androgel*)	Weight loss in AIDS patients with HIV-associated wasting	Unimed
(*TheraDerm Testosterone Transdermal System*)	Physiologic testosterone replacement in androgen-deficient, HIV-positive patients with an associated weight loss	Watson
Testosterone propionate ointment 2%	Vulvar dystrophies	Star
Testosterone sublingual	Constitutional delay of growth and puberty in boys	Bio-Technology General
Tetrabenazine	Moderate/Severe tardive dyskinesia; Huntington disease	Prestwick
Tetrahydrobiopterin	Hyperphenylalaninemia	Biomarin
Tetraiodothyroacetic acid	Suppression of thyroid-stimulating hormone in patients with well-differentiated cancer of the thyroid gland	Elliot Danforth Jr., MD
[5,10,15,20-Tetrakis(1,3-diethylimidazolium-2-yl)porphyrinato] manganese(III)pentachloride	Amyotrophic lateral sclerosis	Aeolus
Tezacitabine	Adenocarcinoma of the esophagus and stomach	Chiron
TGF(beta)2-specific phosphorothioate antisense oligodeoxynucleotide (*Oncomun*)	Malignant glioma	Antisense Pharma GmbH
Thalidomide	Treat and prevent recurrent aphthous ulcers in severely, terminally immunocompromised patients; treat and prevent graft versus host disease	Andrulis Research
	Clinical manifestations of mycobacterial infection caused by *Mycobacterium tuberculosis* and nontuberculous mycobacteria; primary brain malignancies; severe recurrent aphthous stomatitis in severely, terminally immunocompromised patients; Kaposi sarcoma	Celgene
	Treat and prevent graft versus host disease in bone marrow transplantation; treat and maintain reactional lepromatous leprosy	Pediatric
(*Synovir*)	HIV-associated wasting syndrome	Celgene
(*Thalomid*)	Erythema nodosum leprosum[a]; multiple myeloma; Crohn disease; myelodysplastic syndrome	Celgene
L-Threonine	Spasticity associated with familial spastic paraparesis	Interneuron
(*Threostat*)	Amyotrophic lateral sclerosis	Tyson & Associates
Thymalfasin (*Zadaxin*)	Chronic active hepatitis B; DiGeorge anomaly with immune defects; hepatocellular carcinoma	SciClone
Thymosin beta 4	Epidermolysis bullosa	RegeneRx Biopharmaceuticals
Thymoxamine hydrochloride	Reverse phenylephrine-induced mydriasis in patients who have narrow anterior angles and are at risk of developing an acute attack of angle-closure glaucoma following mydriasis	Iolab
Thyrotropin alfa (*Thyrogen*)	Well-differentiated papillary, follicular, or combined papillary/follicular carcinomas of the thyroid; adjunct in the diagnosis of thyroid cancer[a]	Genzyme
Tiapride	Tourette syndrome	Sanofi-Synthelabo
Tiazofurin (2-beta-D-ribofuranosyl-4-thiazolecarboxamide)	Chronic myelogenous leukemia	Ribapharm
Tin ethyl etiopurpurin	Prevent access graft disease in hemodialysis patients	Miravant Medical Technologies
Tinidazole (*Tindamax*)	Giardiasis[a]; amebiasis[a]	Presutti Labs
Tiopronin (*Thiola*)	Prevent cystine nephrolithiasis in patients with homozygous cystinuria[a]	Charles Y. C. Pak, MD
Tipifarnib (*Zarnestra*)	Acute myeloid leukemia	Johnson & Johnson
Tirapazamine	Head and neck cancer	Sanofi-Synthelabo
Tiratricol (*Triacana*)	With levothyroxine to suppress thyroid-stimulating hormone in patients with well-differentiated thyroid cancer who are intolerant to adequate doses of levothyroxine alone	Laphal Labs
Tizanidine hydrochloride (*Zanaflex*)	Spasticity associated with multiple sclerosis and spinal cord injury	Athena Neurosciences
Tobramycin (*Tobi*)	Bronchiectasis patients infected with *Pseudomonas aeruginosa*	Chiron
Tobramycin for inhalation (*TOBI*)	Bronchopulmonary infections of *Pseudomonas aeruginosa* in cystic fibrosis patients[a]	Pathogenesis
Tocophersolan oral solution (vitamin E-tpgs)	Vitamin E deficiency resulting from malabsorption caused by prolonged cholestatic hepatobiliary disease	Sterling Winthrop
Topiramate (*Topamax*)	Lennox-Gastaut syndrome[a]	Johnson & Johnson
Toralizumab	Immune thrombocytopenic purpura	Biogen IDEC
Toremifene (*Fareston*)	Hormonal therapy of metastatic breast carcinoma[a]; desmoid tumors	Orion
Tositumomab and iodine I 131 tositumomab (*Bexxar*)	Non-Hodgkin B-cell lymphoma[a]	GlaxoSmithKline

Orphan Drugs

Drug (*Trade name*)	Proposed use	Sponsor
Trabectedin (*Yondelis*)	Epithelial ovarian cancer; soft tissue sarcoma	Johnson & Johnson
Tramadol hydrochloride	Painful HIV-associated neuropathy	TheraQuest Biosciences
Tranexamic acid (*Cyklokapron*)	Patients with congenital coagulopathies who are undergoing surgical procedures (eg, dental extractions)[a]; undergoing prostatectomy where there is hemorrhage or risk of hemorrhage as a result of increased fibrinolysis or fibrinogenolysis; hereditary angioneurotic edema	Pharmacia
Tranilast (*Rizaben*)	Malignant glioma	Angiogen
Transforming growth factor-beta 2	Full-thickness macular holes	Celtrix
Transgenic human alpha 1 antitrypsin	Emphysema secondary to alpha 1 antitrypsin deficiency	PPL Therapeutics
Trastuzumab (*Herceptin*)	Pancreatic cancer that overexpresses p185HER2	Genentech
Treosulfan (*Ovastat*)	Ovarian cancer	Medac GmbH
Treprostinil (*Remodulin*)	Pulmonary arterial hypertension[a]	United Therapeutics
Tretinoin	Squamous metaplasia of the ocular surface epithelia (conjunctiva and/or cornea) with mucous deficiency and keratinization	Hannan Ophthalmic
(*ATRA-IV*)	Acute and chronic leukemia; T-cell non-Hodgkin lymphoma	Antigenics
(*Vesanoid*)	Acute promyelocytic leukemia[a]	Hoffmann-La Roche
Tri-antennary glycotripeptide derivative of 5-fluorodeoxyuridine monophosphate	Hepatocellular carcinoma	Cell Works
2′,3′,5′-Tri-o-acetyluridine	Mitochondrial disease	Repligen
Trientine hydrochloride (*Syprine*)	Wilson disease intolerant or inadequately responsive to penicillamine[a]	Merck
3,5,3′-Triiodothyroacetate	Well-differentiated papillary, follicular, or combined papillary/follicular carcinomas of the thyroid gland	Elliot Danforth Jr., MD
Trimetrexate glucuronate (*Neutrexin*)	Metastatic carcinoma of head and neck (buccal cavity, pharynx, larynx); metastatic colorectal adenocarcinoma; pancreatic adenocarcinoma; *Pneumocystis carinii* pneumonia in AIDS patients[a]; advanced non-small-cell carcinoma of the lung; metastatic osteogenic sarcoma	Medimmune Oncology
Triptorelin pamoate (*Decapeptyl Injection*)	Palliative treatment of advanced ovarian carcinoma of epithelial origin	Debio R.A.
Trisaccharides A and B (*Biosynject*)	Moderate to very severe clinical forms of transfusion reactions arising from ABO incompatible transfusions of blood, blood products, and blood derivatives; moderate to severe clinical forms of hemolytic disease in newborns arising from placental transfer of antibodies against blood groups A and B; ABO-incompatible solid organ transplantation including kidney, heart, liver, and pancreas; prevent ABO hemolytic reactions arising from ABO-incompatible bone marrow transplantation	Chembiomed
Trisodium citrate concentration (*Hemocitrate*)	Used in leukapheresis procedures	Hemotec Medical
Trisodium zinc diethylenetriamine-pentaacetate	Known or suspected internal contamination with plutonium, americium, or curium to increase the rate of elimination	CustomCare Pharmacy
Troxacitabine (*Troxatyl*)	Acute myeloid leukemia	Structural GenomiX
Tumor necrosis factor-binding protein I	Symptomatic AIDS patients including all patients with CD4 T-cell counts < 200 cells/mm^3	Serono
Tumor necrosis factor-binding protein II	Symptomatic AIDS patients including all patients with CD4 T-cell counts < 200 cells/mm^3	Serono
Tyloxapol (*Supervent*)	Cystic fibrosis	Kennedy and Hoidal, MDs
L-Tyrosine-L-serine-L-leucine (*CMS-024*)	Hepatocellular carcinoma	Pepharm R&D
Ubiquinol (*Ubi-Q-Nol, Li-Q-Nol*)	Huntington disease	Gel-Tec
Ubiquinol, coenzyme Q10, ubiquinone (*UBI-Q-NOL*)	Pediatric congestive heart failure	Gel-Tec
Ubiquinone (*Ubi-Q-Gel*)	Mitochondrial cytopathies	Gel-Tec
Unconjugated chimeric (human murine) G250 IgG monoclonal antibody	Renal cell carcinoma	Wilex Biotechnology GmbH
Uridine 5′-triphosphate	Cystic fibrosis; facilitate removal of lung secretions in primary ciliary dyskinesia	Inspire
Urofollitropin (*Fertinex*)	Initiate and reinitiate spermatogenesis in adult men with reproductive failure caused by hypothalamic or pituitary dysfunction; hypogonadotropic hypogonadism	Serono
(*Metrodin*)	Ovulation induction in patients with polycystic ovarian disease who have an elevated luteinizing hormone/follicle-stimulating hormone ratio and who have failed to respond to adequate clomiphene citrate therapy[a]	
Urogastrone	Accelerate corneal epithelial regeneration and heal stromal incisions from corneal transplant surgery	Chiron Vision
Ursodiol (*Actigall*)	Manage clinical signs and symptoms associated with primary biliary cirrhosis	Novartis
(*URSO*)	Primary biliary cirrhosis[a]	Axcan Pharma
Vaccinia immune globulin (human) intravenous	Severe complications from the smallpox vaccine[a]	DynPort Vaccine Company
(*CNJ-016*)	Complications of vaccinia vaccination	Cangene

Orphan Drugs		
Drug (*Trade name*)	Proposed use	Sponsor
Valine, isoleucine, and leucine (*VIL*)	Hyperphenylalaninemia	Leas Research Products
Valrubicin (*Valstar*)	Carcinoma in situ of the urinary bladder[a]	Anthra
Vapreotide (*Octastatin*)	GI and pancreatic fistulas; prevent early postoperative complications following pancreatic resection	Debiopharm S.A.
(*Sanvar*)	Acromegaly; symptomatic carcinoid tumors; esophageal variceal hemorrhage patients with portal hypertension	H3 Pharma
Vasoactive intestinal peptide	Pulmonary arterial hypertension	mondoBIOTECH Labs Anstalt
	Acute respiratory distress syndrome	Sami I. Said, MD
Vasoactive intestinal polypeptide	Acute esophageal food impaction	Research Triangle
Vigabatrin (*Sabril*)	Infantile spasms	Ovation
Viloxazine hydrochloride (*Catatrol*)	Narcolepsy; cataplexy	Stuart
Virulizin (*Virulizin*)	Pancreatic cancer	Lorus Therapeutics
Xenogeneic hepatocytes (*HepatAssist Liver Assist System*)	Severe liver failure	Circe Biomedical
Yttrium-90 radiolabeled humanized monoclonal anti-carcinoembryonic antigen IgG antibody (*Cea-Cide*)	Ovarian carcinoma	Immunomedics
Zalcitabine	AIDS	National Cancer Institute
(*Hivid*)	AIDS[a]	Hoffman-La Roche
Zidovudine (*Retrovir*)	AIDS[a]; AIDS-related complex[a]	GlaxoWellcome
Zinc acetate (*Galzin*)	Wilson disease[a]	Lemmon
Zoledronate (*Zometa, Zabel*)	Tumor-induced hypercalcemia[a]	Novartis

[a] Approved for marketing.

ABETIMUS SODIUM (*Riquent* by La Jolla Pharmaceutical) – An immunomodulator.

➤*Actions:*

Pharmacology – Abetimus is awaiting approval for the treatment of patients with systemic lupus erythematosus (SLE) at risk of renal disease. Autoantibodies against double-stranded DNA (anti-dsDNA) have been implicated in the pathogenesis of renal disease in patients with SLE. Increased levels of circulating anti-dsDNA often precede renal flares.

Abetimus is an immunomodulant designed to lower anti-dsDNA. Abetimus is a synthetic oligonucleotide conjugate with a molecular weight of approximately 54 kDaltons. It is composed of 4 double-stranded 20-mer oligonucleotides. Each oligonucleotide is attached through an aliphatic linker to a center, branched platform of triethylene glycol.

Abetimus reduces circulating anti-dsDNA by at least 2 mechanisms. It acutely depletes circulating anti-dsDNA by forming small, soluble complexes with the anti-dsDNA. It also acts by inducing highly selective B lymphocyte tolerance. This is done by cross linking anti-dsDNA receptors on B cells resulting in B cell anergy. The high-affinity autoantibodies produce the greatest response, but the affinity to abetimus declines with repeated administration.

Following IV administration in patients with SLE anti-dsDNA titers rapidly decline and remain below baseline for up to 4 weeks.

Pharmacokinetics – The plasma half-life of abetimus is approximately 1 hour.

Clinical trials – Abetimus was assessed in a phase 3, randomized, placebo-controlled study enrolling patients with SLE and an anti-dsDNA of 15 units/mL or greater. At baseline, at least 1 immunosuppressive agent was being used by 48% of patients in the abetimus group and 42% of patients in the placebo group; 83% of patients in both groups were on prednisone. Patients were randomized to receive 100 mg abetimus or placebo weekly for up to 22 months. Compared with placebo, abetimus was associated with a significant reduction in anti-dsDNA from baseline ($P = 0.0001$). Reductions in anti-dsDNA were correlated with increases in C3 ($P < 0.0001$). The intent-to-treat population consisted of patients with high-affinity anti-dsDNA (145 patients in the abetimus group and 153 patients in the placebo group). The incidence of renal flares did not differ in this analysis (12% on abetimus vs 16% on placebo), nor did the incidence of major SLE flares (24% on abetimus vs 31% on placebo). Use of high-dose corticosteroids and/or cyclophosphamide also was similar in the 2 groups (23% on abetimus and 24% on placebo). The median time to renal flare was 123 months in the abetimus group compared with 89 months in the placebo group. Subgroup analysis was performed with 43 of the patients with impaired renal function (serum creatinine of 1.5 mg/dL or greater at baseline; 20 patients in the abetimus group and 23 in the placebo group). Eight patients with impaired renal function experienced a renal flare (2 of 20 [10%] on abetimus and 6 of 23 [26%] on placebo). Among patients experiencing a sustained reduction in anti-dsDNA during this study, the incidence of renal flare was reduced. Renal flares occurred in 41 patients in this study, with 5 (12%) occurring in patients with sustained antibody reductions and 38 (88%) occurring in patients without sustained reductions. Abetimus appears most likely to reduce renal flares in SLE patients with a history of renal disease and impaired renal function and in those patients achieving sustained reductions in anti-dsDNA.

➤*Adverse Reactions:* Adverse events observed in abetimus clinical trials have been consistent with SLE. Adverse events occurred with similar frequency and were of similar type and severity in abetimus- and placebo-treated groups.

➤*Summary:* Abetimus is a unique therapy that may reduce the incidence of renal flares in patients with SLE. The greatest reduction in renal flares was observed in patients with a history of renal disease and impaired renal function and in patients achieving sustained reductions in anti-dsDNA titers. Additional data will be necessary to determine the optimal population to be treated with abetimus. An NDA was filed with the FDA in December 2004.

ACETORPHAN (by Laboratoire Bioproject, Paris, France) – An enkephalinase inhibitor.

➤*Actions:*

Pharmacology – Acetorphan is a lipophilic inhibitor of enkephalinase, a peptidase present in the GI tract and the CNS. By inhibiting enkephalinase, endogenous enkephalin concentrations increase, giving acetorphan varied therapeutic indications.

Acetorphan is used for symptomatic treatment of acute diarrhea in adults. Treatment should not last more than 7 days. Acetorphan administration does not obviate the need for hydration when relevant.

Pharmacokinetics – Available pharmacokinetic data in humans are limited to the dosing information included below.

Clinical trials – A double-blind, crossover design evaluated the ability of acetorphan to prevent diarrhea in patients receiving castor oil. Acetorphan was administered 45 minutes after the castor oil. Castor oil was selected to induce an experimental secretory diarrhea. Six subjects were studied. Prophylactic acetorphan significantly reduced the mean number of stools during the following 24 hours by 50% and the stool weight by 37%. No side effects other than nausea and discomfort, which were noted in all subjects, were reported.

One hundred ninety-nine patients randomly received acetorphan or placebo after being diagnosed with infectious diarrhea. Patients took 2 capsules (100 mg each) upon enrollment in the study and 1 capsule after each unformed stool for a maximum of 10 days. No other therapies were initiated during the trial with the exception of acetaminophen as needed. Patients receiving acetorphan experienced a significantly shorter duration of diarrhea. Of the patients still experiencing diarrhea on day 10, 7% received acetorphan, and 24% received placebo. Side effects were similar between the 2 groups.

One study compared the efficacy of acetorphan (100 mg 3 times/day) and loperamide (eg, *Imodium A-D*; 1.33 mg 3 times/day) in the treatment of infectious diarrhea. Therapy continued until resolution of diarrhea or for a maximum of 7 days. Thirty-seven patients received acetorphan, and 32 patients received loperamide. The mean duration of diarrhea did not differ between the 2 groups. However, abdominal distension and constipation were significantly more common in the loperamide group.

Another study compared the efficacy of acetorphan and clonidine (eg, *Catapres*) in suppressing opiate withdrawal symptoms. Nineteen heroin or synthetic opiate addicts were treated with 50 mg IV acetorphan twice daily or 0.075 mg clonidine 5 times/day; they displayed opioid withdrawal syndrome within 24 hours after a hospital admission. Changes in the overall Opiate Withdrawal Scale did not differ between the 2 groups; however, diarrhea and lacrimation were more improved in the acetorphan group. No side effects were noted in the acetorphan group; 1 clonidine patient experienced severe hypotension.

Published studies evaluating analgesic activity are only in the animal model. The potential for a new analgesic mechanism of action makes acetorphan a promising agent. Acetorphan has been shown to have minimal abuse potential and withdrawal is not precipitated upon abrupt discontinuation of the drug in animals.

Finally, a possible role in the treatment of gastroesophageal reflux disease (GERD) has been suggested based on the results of a study evaluating the drug's effects on the lower esophageal sphincter.

➤*Adverse Reactions:* No side effects significantly different from placebo have been identified in the clinical trials.

➤*Summary:* Acetorphan is not commercially available in the US, but it is available in France as 100 mg capsules. However, recent research suggests it will provide a novel antidiarrheal agent with minimal side effects. Several potential additional indications are currently being investigated, such as the treatment of opioid withdrawal, GERD, and analgesia.

AIDS DRUGS IN DEVELOPMENT

AIDS Drugs in Development			
Drug	Drug type	FDA status	Treatment sponsor
	Adipose redistribution syndrome		
Serostim[2] (somatropin [rDNA origin])	growth hormone	Phase II/III	Serono
	AIDS		
ACT (activated cellular therapy)	other	Phase II	Neoprobe
BMS-234475	nd[1]	Phase I	Bristol-Myers Squibb
Cytolin	nontoxid AIDS monoclonal antibody	Phase I/II	CytoDyn Inc.
MDX-240	virus-specific bispecific antibody	Phase I/II	Medarex Inc.
SPD 754	nd[1]	Phase I	Shire Pharmaceutical
SPD 756	nd[1]	Phase I	Shire Pharmaceutical
Tipranavir	protease inhibitor	Phase II	Boehringer-Ingelheim Pharmaceuticals
	Aphthous ulcers		
Thalomid (thalidomide)[2]	nd[1]	Phase III	Celgene
	Cachexia		
Testosterone[2]	anabolic steroid	Phase II	TheraTech
	CMV infection		
Benzimidavir (1263W94)	CMV-DNA inhibitor	Phase II	GlaxoSmithKline
T902611 (T611)	nd[1]	Phase I	Tularik
	CMV retinitis		
GW275175	CMV-DNA maturation inhibitor	Phase I	GlaxoSmithKline
	Dementia		
Memantine[2]	NMDA receptor antagonist/neuroprotective agent	Phase II	Neurobiological Technologies
	Diarrhea		
DiffGAM	nd[1]	Phase II	Immucell
Letrazurile	nd[1]	Phase II	Janssen Pharmaceutica
Synsorb CD (due to *Clostridium difficile*)	GI	Phase II	Synsorb Biotech
	Fungal infections		
FK463[1]	nd[1]	Phase III	Fujisawa
Oramed[1]	nd[1]	Phase II	Biosyn
Posaconazole[1] (oral triazole)	nd[1]	Phase III	Schering-Plough
	Hepatitis B co-infection		
Entecavir (BMS 200475)	nd[1]	Phase II	Bristol-Myers Squibb
	Herpes co-infection		
Forvade (cidofovir gel)	antiviral	Phase I/II completed	Gilead Sciences
ME-609 cream	nd[1]	Phase II completed	Medivir
	HIV infection		
AIDS vaccine	vaccine	Phase I	United Biomedical
Alferon N (interferon alfa-n3)[2] injection	nd[1]	Phase III	Interferon Sciences
ALVAC-E120TMG (vCP1521)	nd[1]	Phase II	Aventis Pasteur
ALVAC-MN120TMG (vCP205)	nd[1]	Phase I/II	Aventis Pasteur
Amdoxovir	nucleoside analog	Phase II	Gilead
Ampligen	nucleic acid	Phase II	HemispheRx Biopharma
Ancer 20 injection	nd[1]	Phase I	Zeria USA
Anticort[2] (procaine HCl)	nd[1]	Phase II completed	Samaritan
Aztec (zidovudine) controlled-release	antiviral	Phase III completed	Verex Pharmaceuticals
BAY 50-4798	nd[1]	Phase I	Bayer
Beta-L-Fd4C	nd[1]	Phase II	Achillion Pharmaceuticals
BMS-234475	second generation protease inhibitor	Phase II	Bristol-Myers Squibb
BMS 561390	NNRTI[3]	Phase II	Bristol-Myers Squibb
Calanolide A	NNRTI[3]	Phase I/II	Sarawak MediChem
CCR5	receptor antagonist	Phase I	Schering-Plough
Crixivan in *NanoCrystal* formulation (indinavir)	protease inhibitor	Phase II	NanoSystems LLC/Merck and Co. Inc.
CS-92	NRTI[4]	Phase I/II	Triangle Pharmaceuticals
Cytolin	nd[1]	Phase I/II	Amerimmune Pharmaceuticals
Epivir/lamivudine (once-daily dosing)	nd[1]	application submitted	GlaxoSmithKline
Epivir and *Ziagen* combination tablet	nd[1]	Phase III	GlaxoSmithKline
GEM 92	nd[1]	Phase I	Hybridon
HGP-30 and sargramostim[2]	nd[1]	Phase I	Cel-Sci Corp./Immunex Corp.
HGTV43	gene therapy	Phase I	Enzo Biochem
HIV Therapeutic	nd[1]	Phase I	United Biomedical

AIDS Drugs in Development			
Drug	Drug type	FDA status	Treatment sponsor
HIV-IT	nd[1]	Phase II	Chiron Viagene
IL-2	nd[1]	Phase I/II	Bayer
ISIS 5320	nd[1]	Phase I	Isis Pharmaceuticals, Inc.
L-708,906	integrase inhibitor	nd[1]	nd[1]
MIV-150	NNRTI[3]	Phase I	Chiron
MIV-310[2]	nd[1]	Phase II	Medivir
Multikine	immunotherapeutic agent	Phase I	Cel-Sci Corp.
PA-457	budding inhibitor	preclinical	Panacos Pharmaceuticals
Pro 542	recombinant fusion inhibitor	Phase II	Progenics/Genzyme Transgenics
Pro 2000 gel	antiviral agent/microbicide	Phase II	Interneuron
Proleukin[2] (aldesleukin) interleukin-2 (IL-2)	interleukin	Phase III	Chiron
Rev 123	nd[1]	Phase I/II	Novartis
S-1360 (GW810781)	integrase inhibitor	Phase II	GlaxoSmithKline
Savvy	vaginal gel microbicide and spermicide	Phase I/II	Biosyn
T-1249	fusion inhibitor	Phase I/II	Trimeris
TAT antagonist	antiviral	Phase I/II	Hoffman-LaRoche
Timunox (thymopentin)	immunomodulator	Phase III	Immunobiology Research Institute
Tipranavir	nonpeptidic protease inhibitor	Phase III	Boehringer-Ingelheim Pharmaceuticals
TM 114	protease inhibitor	Phase II	Tibotec
TMC125	NNRTI[3]	Phase II	Tibotec
TNX-355	anti-CD4 monoclonal antibody	Phase I	Tanox
Tucaresol (immunopotentiator)	immunomodulator/immunopotentiator	Phase II	GlaxoWellcome
Tumor necrosis factor (TNF)	antiviral	Phase I	Immunex
UK-427,857	entry inhibitor	Phase I	nd[1]
Ushercell	nd[1]	Phase I	Polydex
VX-175 (GW433908)	protease inhibitor	Phase III	Vertex Pharmaceuticals
VX-385	nd[1]	Phase I	Vertex Pharmaceuticals
WF10 OXO[2]	nd[1]	Phase III	Chemie
Zerit (stavudine) extended-release	nd[1]	application submitted	Bristol-Myers Squibb
HIV infection and AIDS			
Abavca/Perthon	plant derivative	Phase I/II	Advanced Plant Pharmaceuticals
Ampligen	nd[1]	Phase II/III	HemispheRx Biopharma
Capravirine	NNRTI[3]	Phase II	Agouron Pharmaceuticals
Emtriva and *Viread*	nd[1]	Research stage	Gilead
GS 4338	nd[1]	Research stage	Gilead
GS 7340	nd[1]	Phase I	Gilead
HE 2000	cellular energy regulators	Phase II	Hollis-Eden Pharmaceuticals
T-1249	peptide fusion inhibitor	Phase I/II	Trimeris
Tipranavir	protease inhibitor	Phase III	Boehringer-Ingelheim Pharmaceuticals
Zadaxin	nd[1]	Phase II	SciClone
HIV wasting			
Androderm[2]	testosterone replacement	Phase III	SmithKline Beecham
Androgel DHT (dihydrotestosterone gel)	steroid	Phase II	Unimed
Thalomid[2] (thalidomide)	TNF-alpha selective inhibitor	Phase III	Celgene
HPV co-infection			
Low-dose oral interferon alpha	nd[1]	Phase I	Atrix Laboratories
Multikine (leukocyte interleukin injection)	interleukin	Phase I	Cel-Sci Corp.
Veldona Lozenge (interferon alpha)	natural human interferon alpha	Phase III	Amarillo Biosciences
Kaposi sarcoma			
A-007	nd[1]	Phase I	Dekk-Tec
Panretin (alitretinoin) oral	retinoic acid	Phase II	Ligand Pharmaceuticals
BMS 275291	nd[1]	Phase I/II	National Cancer Institute
Cidofovir[2]	antiviral	Phase II completed	Gilead Sciences
Interleukin-12	interleukin	Phase III	National Cancer Institute
Metastat (4-dedimethysancycline)	matrix metallo proteinase inhibitor	Phase II	CollaGenex Pharmaceuticals
Panretin and interferon	nd[1]	Phase I/II	Ligand Pharmaceuticals
Paxene (paclitaxel), *Taxol*[2]	nd[1]	Phase III/Phase II/III	IVAX/National Cancer Institute
SU5416	angiogenesis inhibitor	Phase II completed	SUGEN

~ Bibliography Available on Request ~

AIDS Drugs in Development			
Drug	Drug type	FDA status	Treatment sponsor
Thalidomide[2]	cytokine-selective inhibitor	Phase II completed	National Cancer Institute
Virulizin	macrophage activator	Phase III	Imutec Pharma
Lymphomas			
Bryostatin	nd[1]	Phase I	National Cancer Institute
Proleukin[2] (aldesleukin, interleukin-2 [IL-2])	nd[1]	Phase II	National Cancer Institute
Rituxan (rituximab)	nd[1]	Phase II	National Cancer Institute/IDEC Pharmaceuticals
Virulizin	macrophage activator	Phase III	Imutec Pharma
Mycobacterial infection			
MiKasome (amikasin)	nd[1]	Phase II	NeXstar Pharmaceuticals
Mycobacterial avium complex			
Rifalazil (PA-1648)	rifampin derivative	Phase II	PathoGenesis
Non-Hodgkin lymphoma			
ATRA-IV (tretinoin)	liposomal all-transretinoic acid	Phase II	Aronex Pharmaceuticals
G3139	antisense compound	Phase I/II	Genta
LymphoCide	nd[1]	Phase III	Immunomedics
Proleukin[2] (aldesleukin, interleukin-2 [IL-2])	nd[1]	Phase II	National Cancer Institute
Rituxan (rituximab)	nd[1]	Phase II	National Cancer Institute/IDEC Pharmaceuticals
Pain			
DPI3290	nd[1]	Phase II	Ardent
Morphelan ROER (morphine sulfate rapid-onset extended-release)	nd[1]	application submitted	Elan Pharmaceuticals/Ligand Pharmaceuticals
Ziconotide	nd[1]	application submitted	Elan Pharmaceuticals
PCP infection			
Dapsone[2]	nd[1]	Phase III	Jacobus
Dapsone/pyrimethamine/folinic acid[2]	nd[1]	Phase III	Jacobus
Dapsone/trimethoprim[2]	nd[1]	Phase III	Jacobus
DB 289	nd[1]	Phase I	Immtech
Pediatric HIV			
Combivir[2] (zidovudine/lamivudine)	nucleoside analog reverse transcriptase inhibitor combination	nd[1]	GlaxoSmithKline
Crixivan[2] (indinavir)	protease inhibitor	nd[1]	Merck
Fortovase[2] (saquinavir)	protease inhibitor	nd[1]	Roche
HIV-1 immunogen	nd[1]	Phase I completed	Agouron Pharmaceuticals
Hivid[2] (zalcitabine, ddC)	NRTI[4]	nd[1]	Roche
Invirase[2] (saquinavir)	protease inhibitor	nd[1]	Roche
MKC-442	nd[1]	Phase II	Triangle Pharmaceuticals
Rescriptor[2] (delavirdine)	NNRTI[3]	Phase II	Pfizer
Viread (tenofovir disoproxil fumarate)	nucleoside analog reverse transcriptase inhibitor	Phase I	Gilead Sciences
Progressive multifocal leukoencephalopathy (PML)			
Topotecan (hycamtin)[1,2]	semi-synthetic derivative of camptothecin, toposiomerase I-inhibitor	Phase II completed	GlaxoSmithKline
Vaccines			
AIDS vaccine	multi-envelope HIV vaccine component	Phase I	St. Jude Children's Research Hospital
Aidsvax	vaccine	Phase III	VaxGen
ALVAC (vCP1452)	vaccine	Phase II	Aventis Pasteur
ALVAC (vCP1521)	vaccine	Phase II	Aventis Pasteur
Genevax-HIV/APL-400-003 (end/rev) facilitated DNA-based vaccine	vaccine	Phase I	Wyeth
Genevax-HIV/APL-400-047 (gag/pol) facilitated DNA-based vaccine	vaccine	Phase I	Wyeth
HIV vaccine	vaccine	Phase I	GlaxoSmithKline
HIV-1 peptide vaccine	vaccine	Phase I	National Cancer Institute
Remune	vaccine	Phase III	Immune Response
TBC-3B	vaccine, recombinant	Phase I	Therion Biologics

[1] nd = no data.
[2] Approved for other indications; refer to individual monographs.
[3] NNRTI = Non-nucleoside reverse transcriptase inhibitor.
[4] NRTI = Nucleoside reverse transcriptase inhibitor.

➤*Summary:* Acquired Immunodeficiency Syndrome (AIDS) is an immunodeficiency state caused by an infection with the human immunodeficiency virus, HIV. There are several drugs being studied for HIV, AIDS, and AIDS-related illnesses. Listed above are some antiviral, cytokine, immunomodulating drugs, and vaccines currently undergoing clinical trials.

~ Bibliography Available on Request ~

ALICAFORSEN (by ISIS) – An antisense inhibitor of ICAM-1

➤*Actions:*

Pharmacology – Alicaforsen is a 20-base antisense phosphorothioate oligodeoxynucleotide that selectively inhibits cytokine-induced intercellular adhesion molecule 1 (ICAM-1) expression in various human cells in vitro and in vivo. This drug is designed to hybridize to a sequence in the 3′ untranslated region of human ICAM-1 mRNA. The heterodimer formed by alicaforsen and mRNA serves as a substrate for mRNase H, an enzyme family that cleaves RNA in DNA-RNA heterodimers. In vitro, alicaforsen specifically reduces ICAM-1 mRNA thereby reducing ICAM-1 protein expression. A parenteral form of this drug is currently undergoing Phase 3 trials for treatment of Crohn disease. Phase 2 trials are being performed on an enema formulation for the treatment of ulcerative colitis and a topical preparation for psoriasis.

Pharmacokinetics – The metabolism and pharmacokinetics of alicaforsen have not been well defined, but it appears to follow a one-compartment model. Distribution into tissue is the primary route of clearance. Half-life, AUC, volume of distribution, C_{max}, and plasma clearance appear to be dose-dependent, indicating a saturable component to alicaforsen's distribution. Gender may also have an effect on kinetic profile of alicaforsen. In 1 study, men had plasma clearance rates up to 37% higher than women, resulting in a shorter half-life of 0.94 hours for 70 kg men vs 1.14 hours for 70 kg women. C_{max} and AUC values were higher in women than in men. Another study noted that men had a 20% higher plasma clearance of alicaforsen than women, resulting in lower AUC values in men versus women (55.5 µg.h/mL vs. 64.6 µg.h/mL). Volume of distribution might also be gender-dependent, which may be explained by differences in body fat composition since alicaforsen is poorly distributed into adipose tissue. Metabolism of alicaforsen was not altered by sex or exogenous estrogen therapy in 1 study.

Clinical trials

Crohn disease: Alicaforsen was compared with placebo in a randomized, controlled trial of 299 patients 14 to 80 years of age with steroid-dependent Crohn disease. Enrolled patients had moderately active disease (Crohn disease activity index [CDAI] 200 to 350) for at least 3 months prior to trial participation despite 10 to 40 mg of prednisone or equivalent with at least 1 unsuccessful steroid taper attempt within the previous 2 years and at study onset. Stable doses of aminosalicylates were allowed during the study, but immunosuppressants were excluded in the prior 4 weeks. Patients were stratified based on their current steroid dose (prednisone equivalent of 10 to 19 or 20 to 40 mg/day) and then randomized to receive placebo (n = 101) or 1 of 2 alicaforsen regimens, administered as 2 mg/kg IV infusions 3 times weekly for 2 (n = 99) or 4 weeks (n = 99). The maximum dose permitted was 200 mg. Baseline steroid doses were maintained in the high-dose stratum until day eight, at which time they were placed on prednisone 20 mg/day. The doses were then tapered by 2.5 mg/day/week as tolerated. Patients in the low-dose stratum were maintained on their baseline steroid doses and then placed on a taper regimen identical to the high-dose stratum to sustain dosage by study week with the high dose stratum. These patients were then placed on a taper regimen identical to the high dose group. At week 14, 64% of placebo patients and 78% of alicaforsen patients had successfully discontinued steroid therapy. The primary endpoint of steroid-free disease remission (CDAI less than 150, steroid dose = 0) was achieved by similar proportions of patients in each of the 3 treatment groups: 19.2% of the 2-week group, 21.2% of the 4-week group, and 18.8% of the placebo group. Patients with higher baseline steroid doses had a higher rate of steroid-free disease remission. Secondary endpoints, including decreased steroid doses and quality of life, were achieved by a similar number of patients in all 3 groups as well. Although not statistically significant, patients with higher alicaforsen AUC values had increased response rates, suggesting that alicaforsen may be effective if given at high enough doses.

In a double-blind, placebo-controlled trial, 20 patients 18 to 80 years of age with moderate Crohn disease (CDAI of 200 to 350) received 13 doses of alicaforsen or placebo over a 26-day period and were followed for an additional 5 months. At the conclusion of the treatment period, 7 of 15 alicaforsen patients (2 of 3 receiving 0.5 mg/kg, 1 of 3 receiving 1 mg/kg, and 4 of 9 receiving 2 mg/kg) were in remission vs 1 placebo patient. Five of the 7 alicaforsen-treated remitters were still in remission 6 months after therapy. Three of these patients were successfully weaned off of steroids and 1 was maintained at 10 mg/day. Mean corticosteroid doses decreased in alicaforsen patients throughout the study period, while placebo patients experienced increased steroid doses after the treatment period. Mean CDAI scores were not significantly different between the 3 groups throughout the study.

➤*Adverse Reactions:* Infusion-related reactions including fever/chills, nausea, vomiting, headaches, myalgia/arthralgia, increased diarrhea, and facial flushing were reported. Hypersensitivity reactions have occurred in a small number of study patients. Transient, clinically silent post-infusion aPTT prolongation has been noted in several trials.

➤*Summary:* Studies conducted to date, both in vitro and in vivo, suggest that alicaforsen is a novel agent with anti-inflammatory potential. Based on clinical trials, alicaforsen can reduce steroid requirements in patients with moderate Crohn disease and might induce disease remission in some patients. Alicaforsen appears to be well tolerated with a low incidence of side effects. Phase 3 trials were discontinued in 1999 due to lack of efficacy to support an NDA filing. ISIS reinstated Phase 3 studies in November 2001 and are ongoing at this time in the US, Europe, and Canada.

ALVIMOPAN (by Adolor/GlaxoSmithKline) – An opioid receptor antagonist

➤*Actions:*

Pharmacology – Alvimopan is a peripherally selective, mu opioid receptor antagonist used to reduce or prevent adverse GI side effects of opioid analgesics without reversing analgesia. The activation of peripheral receptors within the GI tract is particularly important because the magnitude of bowel dysfunction correlates more closely with opioid concentrations in the enteric nervous system than with concentrations in the CNS. When administered, opioids may delay gastric emptying, increase tone of GI smooth muscle, induce spasm and provoke colic, inhibit propulsive contractions, and decrease GI transit. These effects typically lead to constipation, bloating, nausea, vomiting, and abdominal distention.

Unlike other opioid antagonists, alvimopan is restricted in activity to the GI tract, therefore not antagonizing the desired central effects of analgesia. Other antagonists my reverse adverse effects of opioids on GI function, but these antagonists are centrally active, therefore antagonizing analgesia and precipitating symptoms of opioid withdrawal in morphine-dependent subjects.

Pharmacokinetics – Administered orally, alvimopan has very limited systemic absorption and a long duration of action. Because of its large size, alvimopan does not cross the blood-brain barrier and does not possess inherent prokinetic effects. No other data is available.

Clinical trials – Clinical trials have been performed to assess the effects of alvimopan on morphine-induced delay in GI transit, examine effects on morphine analgesia, and evaluate the length of recovery time of GI function after surgery.

In a double-blind, placebo-controlled, crossover trial, 14 patients were randomized to receive placebo plus IV saline, placebo plus 0.05 mg/kg IV morphine sulfate, or alvimopan plus 0.05 mg/kg IV morphine sulfate. Each participant received all 3 treatments in order to evaluate effects on GI transit time. IV morphine prolonged GI transit time from 69 to 103 minutes (P = 0.005). Oral administration of 2 mg alvimopan prevented the morphine-induced increase in GI transit (P = 0.004) and produced average transit times of 76 minutes.

A randomized, double-blind study enrolling 45 patients was performed to assess the effect of alvimopan on morphine analgesia. Patients were assigned to receive 4 mg oral alvimopan and 0.15 mg/kg IV morphine, oral placebo and 0.15 mg/kg IV morphine, or oral placebo and IV saline. Measurement included categorical pain scores, visual analog scale (VAS) pain score, pain relief scores, and pupil diameter. Results showed VAS scores to be significantly reduced by morphine with or without alvimopan, whereas IV saline solution did not affect VAS scores. Categorical pain and relief scores also showed significant analgesia with morphine that was unaffected by alvimopan. Morphine constricted pupil size whereas alvimopan did not affect pupil size. However, IV saline solution did not result in pupil constriction.

The effects of alvimopan on postoperative GI function and length of hospitalization were studied in patients undergoing major abdominal surgery. Seventy-nine patients were randomly given 1 mg alvimopan, 6 mg alvimopan, or identical placebo capsules. All patients received opioids for postoperative pain. Patients given the 6 mg alvimopan had significantly faster recovery of GI function than those given placebo. The median time to the first passage of flatus decreased from 70 to 49 hours (P = 0.03), the median time to first bowel movement decreased from 111 to 70 hours (P = 0.01), and discharge time decreased from 91 to 68 hours (P = 0.03). The 1 mg alvimopan group did not see such prominent improvements, indicating that dosing is a key factor in treatment.

➤*Summary:* Alvimopan is a novel medication shown to decrease GI side effects of opioid medications. Because activity is peripherally selective and does not cross the blood-brain barrier, these side effects can be reduced without compromising the effects of analgesia. This unique medication could play a significant role in treating adverse GI side effects from opioid medications, speeding recovery of bowel function after surgery, and shortening the duration of hospitalization. Optimal dosing and common side effects have not been established at this time. Alvimopan is currently in phase 3 clinical trials and an NDA is expected to be filed in 2003. Adolor and GlaxoSmithKline will jointly develop and market alvimopan.

AMSACRINE (*Amsidyl* by Parke-Davis) – A dye derivative for the treatment of acute leukemia and lymphoma

➤*Actions:*

Pharmacology – Amsacrine is an acridine dye derivative for the treatment of acute leukemia and lymphoma. It inhibits DNA synthesis by a mechanism similar to the anthracyclines, via intercalation with base pairs in the DNA molecule. The precise mechanism of action is not well understood; however, it is thought that amsacrine may also interact with cellular membranes and interfere with the enzyme topoisomerase II.

Pharmacokinetics – Amsacrine has demonstrated biphasic elimination characteristics. Its distribution half-life is 0.15 to 1.4 hours. The terminal half-life is 4.7 to 9 hours. Elimination is via hepatic metabolism and biliary excretion. More than 80% of an administered dose is excreted via the biliary route into the feces. Approximately 2% to 10% of the dose is excreted in the urine unchanged. Changes in hepatic function significantly reduce clearance and increase the elimination half-life. In patients with severe hepatic dysfunction, the elimination half-life is 17.2 hours. The major metabolite, which appears inactive, is an amsacrine-glutathione 5′ conjugate.

The volume of distribution is 1.7 to 2.6 L/kg. Amsacrine is highly plasma protein bound (96.4% to 97.7%), however, 2 hours after administration 50% plasma protein binding has also been reported. High levels of amsacrine have been found distributed in the gallbladder, kidney and lower levels in the lung, testes, muscle, fat, spleen, bladder, pancreas, colon, prostate, brain and cerebrospinal fluid.

Clinical trials –

Acute myelogenous leukemia (AML): Amsacrine and cytarabine were compared in 48 patients with AML in relapse. Patients were treated with either amsacrine 75 mg/m^2 daily for 7 days or high-dose cytarabine 3 g/m^2 every 12 hours for 6 days. Response rates in both groups were similar, with 3 of 23 amsacrine-treated patients and 3 of 25 cytarabine-treated patients achieving complete remission. All patients achieved remissions after only 1 course of therapy. Failures appeared to be primarily due to the inability to reduce the leukemic population (absolute drug resistance) or regrowth of leukemia (relative drug resistance), with over half the patients demonstrating drug resistance. Overall response rates with both agents were low. In another study, therapy with amsacrine administered as a continuous infusion at a dose of 90 mg/m^2/day for 5 days produced no complete responses in 21 patients with refractory or relapsed AML. Other studies have reported response rates of 15% to 29% for reinduction of complete remission.

Acute promyelocytic leukemia (APL): An amsacrine, cytarabine and thioguanine regimen was compared with a daunorubicin, cytarabine, thioguanine regimen in a small number of patients with APL. Complete remission was achieved in 7 of 7 patients receiving the amsacrine regimen and 5 of 9 patients receiving the daunorubicin regimen, suggesting amsacrine may effectively replace daunorubicin in some APL chemotherapy regimens.

Acute lymphoblastic leukemia (ALL): In patients with refractory or relapsed ALL, amsacrine alone was demonstrated to be as effective as a combination regimen with cytarabine and thioguanine. Complete remissions were achieved in 3 of 11 amsacrine-treated patients and 3 of 13 cytarabine-treated patients. Amsacrine plus high-dose cytarabine was also evaluated in ALL. As in other types of leukemia, this combination produced good remission rates but does not appear to impact long-term survival.

➤*Adverse Reactions:* Common adverse effects include myelosuppression, stomatitis/mucositis, nausea and vomiting, alopecia, phlebitis, diarrhea, hypersensitivity reactions, hepatoxicity, hyperbilirubinemia, hypoalbuminemia, mild hepatic dysfunction, elevations in alkaline phosphatase and transaminase levels, serious cardiac arrhythmias (ventricular tachycardia, supraventricular tachyarrhythmias), QT interval prolongation, hypokalemia, transient hypomagnesemia, acute myocardial necrosis, presented as an acute myocardial infarction, congestive heart failure, sudden death and seizures.

The most common adverse effects of the combination cytarabine and amsacrine regimens have included nausea and vomiting, ocular discomfort, mucositis, hepatic dysfunction, cutaneous erythremia and cerebellar dysfunction.

➤*Summary:* Amsacrine appears to be an active agent in the treatment of refractory/relapsed acute leukemia when administered alone or in combination with other chemotherapeutic agents, especially cytarabine. Amsacrine therapy has been demonstrated to improve the rate of complete remissions, but duration of survival has not been shown to improve. The role of amsacrine may be most effective in combination with other agents to induce remissions prior to bone marrow transplantation. An NDA has been filed with the FDA.

ANCESTIM (*Stemgen* by Amgen) – A hematopoietic growth factor

➤*Actions:*

Pharmacology – Ancestim is a recombinant human stem cell factor (SCF), also called *c-kit* ligand, Steel factor, and mast-cell growth factor. It exists as a soluble circulating glycoprotein and a membrane-bound molecule expressed on stromal cells in the bone marrow microenvironment. In combination with other cytokines, SCF induces proliferation and increases receptiveness to lineage commitment of primitive and mature hematopoietic progenitors. Administration of recombinant human SCF is associated with the mobilization of peripheral blood progenitor cells (PBPC). Ancestim alone is not sufficient to increase PBPC harvest to achieve hematapoietic recovery. When administered in combination with filgrastim (*Neupogen*), it synergistically increases the number of PBPCs in the peripheral blood. It also acts synergistically with other hematopoietic growth factors, including sargramostim (*Leukine*), erythropoietin (epoetin alfa; *Epogen*, *Procrit*), interleukin-3, interleukin-6, and interleukin-7.

Clinical trials –

Non-Hodgkin's lymphoma: In 38 patients with non-Hodgkin's lymphoma who were eligible for autologous transplantation, patients were treated with filgrastim alone or in combination with ancestim to mobilize PBPCs for 7 days, with apheresis performed on days 5 through 7. Three to 10 days after apheresis, patients began a 4-day regimen of high-dose chemotherapy and then received PBPC reinfusion and filgrastim until engraftment. Overall, the total mononuclear cell count, CD34+ cell content, granulocyte-macrophage colony-forming cells (GM-CFC) and burst-forming units-erythroid (BFU-E) per kg in the apheresis were similar in the 2 treatment groups.

Breast cancer: Breast cancer patients (n=215) having at least 1 prior cycle of cytotoxic chemotherapy at least 3 weeks before enrollment received either filgrastim alone (10 mcg/kg/day for 7 days) or in combination with ancestim 5 to 30 mcg/kg/day for 7, 10, or 13 days. Patients were then treated with high-dose chemotherapy followed by infusions of PBPCs on days 0 to 2 and filgrastim until absolute neutrophil count recovery. The median number of CD34+ cells collected was greater for patients treated with the combination. There were more CD34+ cells harvested in the groups receiving ancestim 20 and 25 mcg/kg/day 7-day treatment courses than with filgrastim alone.

The effects of ancestim plus filgrastim on PBPC harvest were compared with the effects of filgrastim alone in 62 patients with early-stage breast cancer. Concurrent therapy resulted in increased levels of PBPCs, which allowed for greater levels of PBPCs to be obtained by apheresis than with filgrastim alone. Pretreatment for several days with ancestim prior to initiation of filgrastim enhanced cell mobilization and allowed for collection of more cells than with concurrent ancestim plus filgrastim. Hematologic recovery following high-dose chemotherapy was rapid in each treatment group.

Multiple myeloma: In a study of patients with multiple myeloma, treatment with ancestim plus filgrastim was more effective than filgrastim alone for mobillizing PBPC. The combination therapy required fewer apheresis collections to achieve the target number of CD34+ cells.

Ovarian carcinoma: The effects of ancestim in PBPC mobilization and collection were evaluated in 48 patients with ovarian carcinoma. Forty-eight hours after chemotherapy, patients received filgrastim alone or with ancestim (5, 10, 15, or 20 mcg/kg/day). The combination of filgrastim plus ancestim 20 mcg/kg/day produced a 5.8-fold increase in long-term culture-initiating cells compared to the use of filgrastim alone. A 3-fold increase in CD34+ cells and up to a 64-fold increase in CD34+/33- cells were observed with the combination compared with the use of filgrastim alone.

➤*Adverse Reactions:* Injection site reactions including erythema, pruritus, swelling, and hyperpigmentation (> 80%); mild-to-moderate allergic reactions, including rash, respiratory symptoms (cough, hoarseness, laryngospasm), and itching (15%); urticaria; dermatographia; angioedema; hypotension. The major toxicity has been an anaphylactic-type reaction, which occurred in 33 of 564 patients studied; the reaction was severe, but not life-threatening, in 76% of those patients.

➤*Summary:* The administration of ancestim with filgrastim can increase mobilization and collection of PBPCs. Greater benefit may be achieved with the combination in patients who have received extensive chemotherapy. Ancestim should not be routinely used in all patients who will be undergoing PBPC collection. Additional studies are necessary to determine which patients may benefit from the effects of ancestim. Ancestim may offer an economic advantage if it allows for faster hematologic recovery, fewer days of growth factor administration, and fewer apheresis collections. The optimal dose has not been established. However, 1 large clinical trial demonstrated the optimal dose to be ancestim SC 20 mcg/kg/day plus filgrastim 10 mcg/kg/day, with daily apheresis beginning on day 5. Ancestim was recommended for approval by the FDA's Biological Response Modifiers Advisory Committee in July 1998.

ARTESUNATE (sponsored by the World Health Organization) – An antimalarial agent

➤*Actions:*

Pharmacology – Artesunate rectal capsules are undergoing FDA review for use in the emergency treatment of acute malaria in patients who cannot take medication by mouth and for whom parenteral treatment is not available. They are not to be used in settings where it is possible to provide immediate therapy with oral or parenteral antimalarials. Artesunate is a water-soluble derivative of artemisinin. Artemisinin is a sesquiterpene lactone endoperoxide isolated from the Chinese medicinal herb qinghao, *Artemisia annua* L. (sweet wormwood). Artesunate acts by increasing the oxidant stress on the plasmodia within the erythrocyte. Artesunate exerts this effect by increasing production of activated oxygen species (oxygen radicals) within the erythrocyte. Artesunate is highly active against *Plasmodium falciparum*, including multidrug-resistant strains; however, sensitivity has declined in regions where mefloquine resistance is prevalent. Artesunate also is highly active against *Plasmodium vivax*.

Pharmacokinetics – Artesunate is metabolized rapidly to an active metabolite dihydroartemisinin (DHA) by blood esterases and hepatic metabolism. The artesunate half-life is 2 to 3 minutes. From 25% to 72% of the total artesunate dose is converted to DHA. DHA is primarily excreted in the urine. The AUC of artesunate following oral administration is much lower than that achieved following rectal artesunate administration; however, the AUC of DHA is similar. Artesunate is 59% plasma protein bound; DHA is 43% plasma protein bound.

Clinical trials – Three pivotal studies were submitted to the FDA in which a single dose of rectal artesunate was administered during the first 24 hours of therapy and compared with a standard antimalarial regimen for 24 hours. These studies were performed in health care settings in Thailand, Malawi, and South Africa, and patients received full adjunctive therapy with fluid, transfusions, antipyretics, and anticonvulsants as needed. Two studies enrolled pediatric patients and 1 enrolled adults. Patients were treated with rectal artesunate 10 mg/kg as a single dose for the first 24 hours, or a regimen with a comparator agent (oral artesunate or parenteral quinine). In the study conducted in Thailand, patients received rectal or oral artesunate followed by oral artesunate plus mefloquine. In the studies conducted in Malawi and South Africa, patients received rectal artesunate or parenteral quinine, followed by oral sulfadoxine-pyrimethamine or parenteral quinine if unable to receive oral therapy. Parasitemia was the primary endpoint in these studies. At 24 hours, clinical success rates were similar in the patients receiving artesunate to those receiving the comparator agents. Parasitological success (parasite count less than or equal to 10% of baseline) was similar in the study comparing rectal and oral artesunate (73% and 71.4%), and much greater with artesunate in the studies comparing rectal artesunate with parenteral quinine (88% vs 13.6%, $P < 0.0001$, and 84.6% vs 25%, $P = 0.0034$). At 28 days, recrudescence or reinfection occurred in none of the evaluable patients in the study conducted in Thailand, 45.3% of artesunate-treated patients and 22.7% of quinine-treated patients in the study conducted in Malawi, and 8% of artesunate-treated patients and 25% of quinine-treated patients in the study conducted in South Africa. An FDA advisory committee recommended that additional studies large enough to detect a mortality benefit be conducted. An ongoing, double-blind, placebo-controlled field study currently is evaluating rectal artesunate administered according to the proposed indication in patients as young as 6 months of age. As of March 2002, a total of 3366 patients had been enrolled.

➤*Drug Interactions:* Artesunate alters the pharmacokinetics of mefloquine. When oral artesunate has been administered with oral mefloquine, the mefloquine peak concentration has been reduced, the clearance has been increased, and the volume of distribution has been expanded. In another study, administration of oral mefloquine on the third day of a 3-day oral artesunate regimen resulted in a 72% increase in mefloquine bioavailability compared with administration on day 1. Administration of mefloquine at the conclusion of artesunate administration may minimize the potential for interactions and also reduces the risk of vomiting associated with mefloquine.

➤*Adverse Reactions:* Adverse events occurring during rectal artesunate therapy have included abdominal pain, vomiting, diarrhea, and pruritus. The incidence and nature of adverse events observed in artesunate studies have been difficult to distinguish from the signs and symptoms of severe falciparum malaria.

➤*Summary:* Rectal artesunate offers an opportunity to initiate antimalarial therapy earlier in order to reduce malaria mortality. For the emergency treatment of malaria, the recommended dose is a single 10 mg/kg dose within the first 24 hours, followed by appropriate antimalarial therapy. Therapy with artesunate rectal capsules alone is not indicated for the therapy of malaria; supplemental oral or parenteral therapy must supplement the initial artesunate regimen. The results of ongoing studies should provide additional information on its effects on mortality in these at-risk populations. The available studies suggest artesunate therapy is useful in quickly lowering parasite counts. Rectal artesunate should be made widely available in those regions with endemic malaria and limited health care resources. The WHO submitted for approval of rectal artesunate suppositories under orphan drug status and with expedited review. In July 2002, an FDA advisory committee unanimously recommended accelerated approval.

ATRASENTAN (*Xinlay* by Abbott Laboratories) – A selective endothelin A receptor antagonist

➤*Actions:*

Pharmacology – Atrasentan is a highly potent and highly selective endothelin A (EtA) receptor antagonist. ETA receptors mediate the action of endothelin-1 (ET-1), an endothelial-cell-produced peptide that modulates apoptosis, nociception, and vasoconstriction and has been shown to induce mitosis in prostate cancer cell lines in vitro. Significantly elevated ET-1 levels have been found in metastatic prostate cancer. Additionally, ET-1 is a mitogen for osteoblasts, which are important in the common osteoblastic response of bone to metastatic prostate cancer. First in its class, atrasentan binds to ETA receptors, blocking the effects of excessive endogenous ET-1 in metastatic prostate tissue and on osteoblasts. A reduction of the proliferative effects in prostate and bone may delay the clinical progression of prostate cancer in men with hormone-refractory prostate cancer.

Pharmacokinetics – According to a phase 2 clinical trial, atrasentan is rapidly absorbed after oral administration with a time to maximum concentration ranging from 0.3 to 1.7 hours. In addition, the terminal half-life was approximately 26 hours, mean oral clearance was 21 L/h, and apparent volume of distribution was 790 L. This study also approximated atrasentan to be 98.8% bound to plasma proteins. Another study showed the pharmacokinetic profile to be dose proportional, with maximum concentration ranging between approximately 13 and 1,562 ng/mL for 2.5 to 95 mg doses, respectively, on day 28 of treatment.

Clinical trials – A phase 2, double-blind, randomized, placebo-controlled study consisting of 288 patients with hormone-refractory prostate cancer and evidence of metastatic disease evaluated the time to disease progression and the time to prostate-specific antigen (PSA) progression. Patients were randomized to receive either placebo or atrasentan 2.5 or 10 mg daily. Disease progression was defined as development of new lesions in bone or soft tissue, development of symptoms that required palliative opiate treatment, new disease-related symptoms requiring intervention (ie, chemotherapy radiation, surgery), or death. PSA progression was defined as an increase of greater than or equal to 50% over baseline. For 244 evaluable patients, the median time to disease progression was significantly prolonged in the 10 mg group compared with placebo (196 vs 129 days; $P = 0.021$). Using intent-to-treat analysis for all 288 patients, the median time to disease progression was prolonged in the 10 mg group vs placebo, but not significantly (183 vs 137 days; $P = 0.13$). The median time to PSA progression was twice as long in the 10 mg/day treatment arm compared with placebo (155 vs 71 days; $P = 0.002$). A separately published report of the same patient group focused on the changes of bone deposition and resorption markers and on bone scan index with atrasentan compared with placebo. This study reported 58% and 99% elevations from baseline in the bone deposition marker's total alkaline phosphatase and bone alkaline phosphatase, respectively, in the placebo group ($P < 0.001$), whereas the treatment group (10 mg/day) maintained stable levels. The treatment groups also demonstrated a slower progression in increasing bone resorption markers vs placebo. As measured by the bone scan index, a trend toward the slowing of the progression of metastatic bone lesions was found.

➤*Adverse Reactions:* Headache, rhinitis, and peripheral edema were the most common adverse reactions observed with low dosages (2.5 and 10 mg/day) of atrasentan therapy. These adverse reactions were mild to moderate and responded well to symptom-specific therapy when needed. Also reported were decreases in blood pressure and hemodilution. Dosages as high as 60 to 95 mg/day have been well tolerated; in 1 study, dose-limiting toxicity occurred at 75 mg/day, with patients experiencing severe hyponatremia and hypotension. Blood pressure may need to monitored while receiving atrasentan, perhaps necessitating adjustments of concomitant antihypertensive therapy. Until more data are available, use this agent with caution in patients with a history of heart failure.

➤*Summary:* Atrasentan is an investigational, oral, once-daily, nonhormonal, nonchemotherapy, anticancer agent that belongs to a class of compounds known as selective endothelin A receptor antagonists. It is currently being evaluated for use in metastatic hormone-refractive prostate cancer. Abbott's NDA submission in late December 2004 has been accepted for review by the FDA.

CARPROFEN (*Rimadyl* by Roche) – A nonsteroidal anti-inflammatory drug

➤*Actions:*

Pharmacology – Carprofen [(D,L)-6-chloro-alpha-methylcarbazole-2-acetic acid] is a member of the arylpropionic acid class of nonsteroidal anti-inflammatory drugs (NSAIDs), which includes ibuprofen (eg, *Motrin*), naproxen (eg, *Naprosyn*), and others. The drug also possesses analgesic and antipyretic activity.

Although the site and exact mechanism of action of the NSAIDs has not been fully elucidated, most investigators agree that these drugs owe their analgesic and anti-inflammatory activity, as well as their gastric irritant properties, to their ability to inhibit prostaglandin synthetase. Carprofen is considered to be a less potent inhibitor of prostaglandin biosynthesis than naproxen or ibuprofen and is only 1% to 4% as potent as indomethacin (eg, *Indocin*).

Considerable evidence suggests that the anti-inflammatory activity of carprofen is due primarily to the D-isomer; the L-isomer is only about one-seventh as potent.

Pharmacokinetics –

Absorption/Distribution: Carprofen is rapidly and extensively absorbed after oral administration. Peak concentrations of approximately 6 to 12 mcg/mL are achieved in 1 to 3 hours; absolute bioavailability is approximately 90%. Ingestion of food results in a slight reduction in the rate of absorption as well as the peak plasma concentration. However, the total amount of the drug absorbed is not reduced. Peak plasma concentrations may be higher in the elderly. Carprofen is highly protein bound (> 98%). In patients with osteoarthritis (OA) or rheumatoid arthritis (RA), the drug enters the synovial fluid rapidly, where it may achieve concentrations in excess of plasma concentrations.

Metabolism: Approximately 65% to 70% of an administered dose is metabolized by direct conjugation to an ester glucuronide. The elimination half-life ($t_{1/2}$) is between 13 to 25 hours. Despite the extensive hepatic metabolism, no difference has been observed in pharmacokinetics between cirrhotics and healthy volunteers. Thus, dosage adjustments are unnecessary in patients with renal or hepatic insufficiency.

Excretion: Most of an orally administered dose of carprofen (65% to 70%) is eliminated in the urine as the glucuronide metabolite; only 3% to 12% of a dose is excreted unchanged. The remainder of the drug is excreted in the feces after undergoing extensive enterohepatic recycling.

Clinical trials – Carprofen is effective in a variety of clinical settings including treatment of rheumatoid arthritis, osteoarthritis, ankylosing spondylitis, extra-articular inflammatory processes (eg, tendonitis, bursitis), acute pain syndromes (eg, dental and post-traumatic pain) and acute gouty arthritis. Dosages have ranged from 150 to 600 mg/day in 2 or 3 divided doses. The few available comparative studies have usually shown carprofen to be equal to, or superior to, aspirin up to 3600 mg/day. Comparisons with indomethacin 75 to 150 mg/day have usually shown the lower doses (up to 300 mg/day) of carprofen to be slightly less effective but better tolerated than indomethacin. Larger doses of carprofen (400 to 600 mg/day) have been used in the treatment of OA; however, the use of larger doses may not produce any additional response over lower doses.

➤*Adverse Reactions:*

Dermatologic – Cutaneous reactions such as eczema, skin rash, urticaria, and photosensitivity have occurred in 6% to 10% of patients.

GI – GI effects have occurred in approximately 15% of patients. Pain, nausea, heartburn, and dyspepsia are most common, while diarrhea is uncommon (approximately 1%). More serious GI side effects such as peptic ulceration are rare. Carprofen has been used along with antacids in patients with active peptic ulcer disease and has been well tolerated.

Hepatic enzyme elevation – Hepatic enzyme elevation occurred in 1.4% of patients in European trials and in as many as 14% of patients in large American trials. These enzyme elevations are usually asymptomatic.

Renal or urinary – Renal or urinary adverse reactions including urinary frequency, dysuria, burning, hematuria, nephritis, proteinuria, and acute renal failure occurred in 3.4% of 1521 patients in premarketing clinical trials.

➤*Summary:* Carprofen appears to be an effective NSAID that offers convenient twice daily dosing. Despite a low incidence of serious GI side effects, the drug does not appear superior to currently available agents.

Carprofen was approved by the FDA December 31, 1987. However, Roche has made a decision not to market carprofen at this time.

CELIPROLOL HCl (*Selecor* by Aventis) – A cardioselective beta-adrenergic blocking agent

➤*Actions:*

Pharmacology – Celiprolol is a third-generation, cardioselective, hydrophilic beta-adrenoreceptor blocking agent. It possesses weak vasodilating and bronchodilating effects attributed to partial, selective β_2-adrenoreceptor agonist activity and, possibly, direct papaverine-like smooth muscle relaxation. There is evidence for intrinsic sympathomimetic activity (ISA) at the β_2-receptor. The drug is devoid of membrane stabilizing activity (MSA, or quinidine-like effect). Weak alpha$_2$-antagonist properties also are present but are not considered clinically significant at therapeutic doses.

At therapeutic doses, celiprolol reduces heart rate and blood pressure. While the drug dose not generally produce any ECG changes, it can increase the AV nodal functional refractory period. Celiprolol does not appear to alter pulmonary function, nor inhibit bronchodilation induced by agents such as aminophylline (eg, *Phyllocontin*), albuterol (eg, *Proventil*), and ipratropium (*Atrovent*). Triglycerides, LDL cholesterol, and total cholesterol are decreased in some patients while HDL is increased; it appears that total lipid levels are not increased. A reduction in fibrinogen levels has occurred, which may be of some benefit in hypertensive patients with hypercoagulability.

Pharmacokinetics – Following oral administration, absorption is nonlinear and dose-dependent. Bioavailability ranges from 30% to 70% following a single 100 mg dose and averages 74% after a 400 mg dose. Single-dose bioavailability is reduced by chlorthalidone (eg, *Hygroton*), hydrochlorothiazide (eg, *Esidrix*), and theophylline (eg, *Theo-Dur*). Food also has reduced bioavailability in some studies, but data are conflicting. Peak plasma concentrations and pharmacodynamic activity are seen 2 to 4 hours after oral administration; pharmacodynamic activity persists for 24 hours. Protein binding is ≈ 25% and the drug follows a hydrophilic pattern of distribution.

Celiprolol is largely unmetabolized and is excreted unchanged in urine and feces. It does not undergo first-pass hepatic metabolism and there are no significant active metabolites. Approximately 15% (range, 3% to 22%) of an oral dose and 50% of an IV dose is recovered in the urine within 3 days, the rest being excreted in the feces. Steady-state concentrations are achieved after 2 to 3 days. The predominant mode of excretion of active drug is renal; renal dysfunction may cause a reduction in systemic clearance and the need for dose reduction. Bioavailability is decreased and the extent of renal elimination increased in patients with cirrhosis. The pharmacokinetics are not significantly different in the elderly. The elimination half-life averages 4 to 5 hours. Placental transfer averages 3% at steady state compared with 18% for propranolol (eg, *Inderal*) and 6% for atenolol (*Tenormin*).

Clinical trials – Celiprolol is a safe and effective drug for treatment of hypertension and angina. In doses of 200 to 500 mg once daily in the morning, celiprolol reduces blood pressure to comparable levels seen with other β-blockers, calcium blockers, and ACE inhibitors. In comparative trials in patients with mild to moderate hypertension, a 200 to 600 mg dose was similar in efficacy to 80 to 160 mg/day propranolol or 100 mg/day atenolol. In patients with angina, celiprolol 300 to 600 mg/day was as effective as propranolol 80 to 160 mg/day or atenolol 50 to 100 mg/day in improving exercise performance, reducing the number of angina attacks and nitroglycerin requirements, and increasing the time to, or reducing the degree of, ST segment depression. The addition of a diuretic to doses of 200 to 400 mg/day may be more effective at controlling blood pressure than the use of celiprolol monotherapy in doses of 300 to 600 mg/day.

➤*Adverse Reactions:* In a study of > 2300 patients, side effects were mild. GI symptoms (eg, nausea, abdominal discomfort, diarrhea), the most frequently reported complaints, were responsible for drug discontinuation in 13 patients. Cardiovascular symptoms included development of a modest degree of CHF, AV nodal block, and bradycardia. Other side effects included: Headache (6%); fatigue (4%); dizziness (3%); insomnia (1%); Raynaud's phenomenon; orthostatic hypotension; bronchial obstruction; tremor; rash; muscle cramps; impotence.

➤*Summary:* Celiprolol appears to be well tolerated and effective for the treatment of hypertension and angina. Its combination of cardioselectivity, β_2-agonist activity, hydrophilicity and long duration of action make it unique among currently available drugs in this class. Whether these properties will be useful in the myriad of other applications for which β-blockers have been used (eg, post-MI prophylaxis, migraine, selected arrhythmias) will require additional experience. Celiprolol is currently available in Europe.

CILAZAPRIL (*Inhibace* by Roche/Glaxo) – A non-sulfhydryl-containing ACE inhibitor

➤*Actions:*

Pharmacology – Cilazapril is a potent, structurally new, non-sulfhydryl-containing orally active angiotensin-converting enzyme (ACE) inhibitor prodrug under investigation for use in patients with hypertension and CHF. Following oral administration, cilazapril is de-esterified in the liver and other tissues to the active diacid form, cilazaprilat. Cilazaprilat is ≈ 10 times more potent than captopril (*Capoten*) and 5 times more potent than enalaprilat, the active form of enalapril (*Vasotec*).

ACE inhibitors block the enzymatic conversion of angiotensin I to the potent vasoconstrictor angiotensin II. While this inhibition also results in reduced metabolism of bradykinin, alterations in the prostaglandin system and reductions in plasma aldosterone and antidiuretic hormone, these responses do not appear to be responsible for the primary therapeutic effects of these agents. Blockade of angiotensin II production reduces supine and standing blood pressure in hypertensive patients. In patients with CHF, the vasodilatory response reduces afterload, leading to an increase in cardiac output. These beneficial responses may be facilitated by the responses mentioned above.

After administration of cilazapril, ACE activity, angiotensin II and plasma aldosterone concentrations, total peripheral resistance, blood pressure (systolic, diastolic, and mean), and the response to exogenous angiotension I are all reduced, while heart rate, baroreceptor reflex sensitivity, cardiovascular reflexes, and glomerular filtration rate are usually unchanged.

Pharmacokinetics – Cilazapril is rapidly absorbed after oral administration, with peak levels of the parent compound achieved at ≈ 1 hour. Conversion to cilazaprilat, the active form, is rapid and extensive, with peak levels attained at ≈ 1.8 hours with 57% absolute bioavailability of the active compound. In contrast to some other ACE inhibitors, the bioavailability is not significantly reduced by food. After single doses of 0.5, 1, 2.5, and 5 mg, peak plasma levels of cilazaprilat were 5.4, 12.4, 37.7, and 94.2 ng/mL, respectively, indicating that greater than proportional increases in the active compound are achieved over this dose range. The elimination of cilazaprilat is biphasic, with an initial half-life of 1 to 2 hours controlled by the rate of conversion to this active form, followed by a prolonged terminal elimination half-life of 30 to 50 hours. The volume of distribution is ≈ 20 L.

Clearance of cilazaprilat is almost exclusively renal. Patients with severe renal or hepatic impairment may require smaller or less frequent doses. One study suggests that hypertensive patients undergoing hemodialysis can be controlled on 0.5 mg cilazapril postdialysis. Presence of CHF or advanced age has not been shown to significantly alter pharmacokinetic parameters.

Clinical trials – Clinical trials in > 4500 hypertensive patients have evaluated the efficacy of cilazapril. Single daily doses of 2.5 to 5 mg are as effective as single daily doses of the following: 25 to 50 mg hydrochlorothiazide (HCTZ; eg, *Esidrix*); 50 to 100 mg atenolol (*Tenormin*); 80 to 160 mg sustained-release propranolol (eg, *Inderal LA*); and 10 to 20 mg enalapril. In patients with mild to moderate hypertension, a 5 mg cilazapril dose produces a maximal effect, which can be enhanced by the addition of 12.5 to 25 mg HCTZ. In patients with severe hypertension, including patients with left ventricular hypertrophy, the mean effective dose was 10 mg in combination with 12.5 to 25 mg HCTZ/day.

➤*Drug Interactions:* Indomethacin (eg, *Indocin*) considerably attenuates the antihypertensive activity of cilazapril. This attenuation was most pronounced when cilazapril was added to indomethacin, while the addition of indomethacin to a stable cilazapril regimen resulted in a degree of attenuation of effect, which was considered to be clinically insignificant. Thus, the significance of this interaction appears to be dependent on the order of drug administration.

➤*Adverse Reactions:* Cilazapril appears to be well tolerated. In controlled trials of cilazapril monotherapy in > 3500 patients, the most frequently reported side effects were: Headache (4.5%); dizziness (3.3%); fatigue (1.7%); cough (1.6%); chest pain (0.8%); rash, somnolence (0.6%). In patients ≥ 65 years of age, cough, dizziness, palpitations and somnolence occurred slightly more frequently than in younger patients. The addition of HCTZ in an additional 1000 patients resulted in a slightly higher incidence of dizziness, cough and somnolence, while the incidence of other side effects was comparable to cilazapril monotherapy.

➤*Summary:* Cilazapril is a long acting, potent ACE inhibitor. It appears to be well tolerated, while offering the advantage of once-daily dosing; this property may make it a useful addition to a class of drugs whose safety and efficacy continue to be confirmed in a variety of disease states. An NDA for cilazapril was filed in September 1989 for hypertension. Roche and Glaxo will comarket cilazapril as *Inhibace*. On August 13, 1992, the FDA classified cilazapril as "approvable".

CILOMILAST (*Ariflo* by GlaxoSmithKline) – A phosphodiesterase type-IV inhibitor

➤*Actions:*

Pharmacology – Cilomilast is under review for use in the maintenance of lung function in patients with COPD who are poorly responsive to albuterol. It also has been studied in the treatment of asthma. Cilomilast is an orally active phosphodiesterase (PDE) IV-specific inhibitor. It is more potent, but produces less emetogenic effects compared with previously developed oral PDE-IV inhibitors. (Theophylline is a non-selective PDE inhibitor.) PDE-IV is an enzyme that metabolizes cyclic 3',5'-adenosine monophosphate in inflammatory and immune cells, and in airway smooth muscle cells. Based on its mechanism, it was believed that cilomilast could produce bronchodilation and reduce inflammation in patients with airway disease. In vitro cilomilast produced suppression of eosinophils, neutrophils, basophils, and T-cells. Anti-inflammatory effects have been observed in vivo, as administration of cilomilast 15 mg twice daily for 12 weeks in patients with COPD was associated with reductions in CD8+ (P = 0.001) and CD68+ (P < 0.05) airway tissue inflammatory cells. Acute bronchodilatory effects were not observed, however, following single-dose administration of cilomilast 15 mg in patients with COPD.

Pharmacokinetics – Following oral administration on an empty stomach, the peak cilomilast levels are reached within 1 to 2 hours. Administration with food results in a delay in the time to peak of 2 to 4 hours and a reduction in the peak concentration by approximately 40%; however, overall extent of absorption (reflected by the AUC) is not altered by administration with food. Oral bioavailability is approximately 100%. Cilomilast is 99.5% plasma protein bound, primarily to albumin. The terminal elimination half-life of cilomilast is 6 to 8 hours. Cilomilast undergoes extensive hepatic metabolism via oxidation, acyl glucuronidation, and decyclopentylation, with subsequent glucuronidation or sulfation. The primary enzyme responsible for cilomilast metabolism is CYP2C8. Metabolites do not appear to contribute to the activity of cilomilast. Approximately 1% of the dose is excreted in the urine as unchanged cilomilast. Cilomilast is contraindicated in patients with severe hepatic impairment and should be used with caution in patients with mild or moderate hepatic impairment. Cilomilast plasma concentrations were unchanged in patients with renal impairment; however, reductions in protein binding and intrinsic clearance resulted in an increase in the AUC of unbound cilomilast and an increase in the elimination half-life.

Clinical trials – Cilomilast 15 mg twice daily was evaluated in 4 large, double-blind, placebo-controlled, 24-week studies enrolling patients with COPD. Enrolled patients were poorly responsive to inhaled albuterol, defined as an improvement in FEV_1 of 15% or less or 200 mL or less after albuterol administration. Patients using ipratropium at study enrollment could continue its use, and all patients received as-needed inhaled albuterol. Additional COPD medications were permitted for less than 14 days to treat COPD exacerbations. The primary outcomes were change from baseline in trough FEV_1 and in St. George's Respiratory Questionnaire score averaged over 24 weeks (a reduction in score reflects improvement in health status; a 4-point change is considered a clinically relevant change). Secondary outcomes included COPD exacerbations, forced vital capacity (FVC), exercise tolerance, postexercise breathlessness, and summary symptom score. In a combined analysis of 3 of the studies enrolling 2058 patients, the incidence of exacerbation-free survival was greater in the cilomilast-treated patients than the placebo-treated patients. During the 24-week studies, 58% of placebo-treated patients and 65.1% of cilomilast-treated patients experienced no exacerbations of any kind (P = 0.006), and 68.2% of placebo-treated patients and 75.7% of cilomilast-treated patients experienced no level 2 or 3 exacerbations (requiring physician treatment or hospitalization, P = 0.001). The pooled analysis of the 4 clinical trials (n = 2883) places the exacerbation-free rate (level 2 or 3 exacerbation, requiring physician treatment or hospitalization) at 72.3% with placebo and 75.7% with cilomilast therapy; relative risk of 0.88 (95% CI 0.75, 1.03; P = 0.1008).

➤*Drug Interactions:* Increased GI adverse effects were observed when erythromycin was administered concurrently with cilomilast. No pharmacokinetic interaction was observed. If erythromycin must be added to the cilomilast regimen, it should be done with caution and the patient monitored for GI adverse effects.

➤*Adverse Reactions:* The most frequently observed adverse reactions include nausea (16%), diarrhea (14%), abdominal pain (12%), vomiting (6%), dyspepsia (7%), and headache (8%). GI tolerance was improved when cilomilast was administered with food.

➤*Summary:* Cilomilast has some activity in COPD; however, further studies are necessary to better characterize its activity. The recommended dose is 15 mg twice daily, and it should be taken with food to improve GI tolerance. An NDA for cilomilast 15 mg tablets was filed in December 2002. In September 2003 the FDA's Pulmonary-Allergy Drugs Advisory Committee recommended that further long-term efficacy studies are necessary to recommend approval.

CISAPRIDE (*Propulsid* by Janssen) – Available through investigational limited access program

Indications

Cisapride was voluntarily withdrawn from the US market in July 2000 because of the risk of serious cardiac arrhythmias and death. This drug is available to licensed physicians in the US through an investigational limited access program within the following treatment protocols:

- *Adults*: Gastroesophageal reflux disease (GERD), gastroparesis, pseudo-obstruction, or severe chronic constipation refractory to standard therapy.
- *Pediatrics*: Refractory GERD or acute, life-threatening symptoms secondary to GERD, severe chronic constipation, and pseudo-obstruction unresponsive to appropriate therapy.
- *Neonates*: Enteral feeding intolerance.

To be enrolled in the investigational limited access program, patients must have failed all standard therapeutic modalities and have undergone an appropriate diagnostic evaluation, including radiologic examinations or endoscopy. In addition, physicians must perform a baseline screening assessment, including physical examination, laboratory tests, and ECG to screen for contraindicated risk factors. A physician evaluation (under the care of or by consultation with a gastroenterologist) and follow-up testing must be repeated at regular intervals according to the protocol.

Contraindications

Serious cardiac arrhythmias including ventricular tachycardia, ventricular fibrillation, torsades de pointes, and QT prolongation have been reported in patients taking cisapride with other drugs that inhibit cytochrome P450 3A4 or that prolong the QT interval. Some of these events have been fatal. Concomitant oral or IV administration of these drugs with cisapride is contraindicated. Cisapride is also contraindicated in patients with disorders that may predispose them to arrhythmias; patients in whom an increase in GI motility could be harmful (eg, in the presence of GI hemorrhage, mechanical obstruction, or perforation); and known hypersensitivity or intolerance to the drug.

➤*Drug Interactions:* Numerous drug classes and agents increase the risk of developing serious cardiac arrhythmias. Cisapride is contraindicated in patients taking certain macrolide antibiotics (eg, clarithromycin, erythomycin, troleandomycin), certain antifungals (eg, fluconazole, itraconazole, ketoconazole), protease inhibitors (eg, indinavir, ritonavir), phenothiazines (eg, proclorperazine, promethazine), class IA and class III antiarrhythmics (eg, quinidine, procainamide, sotalol), tricyclic antidepressants (eg, amitriptyline), certain antidepressants (eg, nefazodone, maprotiline), certain antipsychotic medications (eg, sertindole), bepridil, sparfloxacin, and grapefruit juice. Certain anticholinergic agents (eg, belladonna alkaloids, dicyclomine), oral anticoagulants, H_2-receptor antagonists, and diuretics (eg, furosemide, thiazides) also interact with cisapride. The preceding lists are not comprehensive.

➤*Adverse Reactions:* Serious cardiac arrhythmias including ventricular tachycardia, ventricular fibrillation, torsades de pointes, and QT prolongation have been reported in ongoing postmarketing surveillance. From July 1993 through May 1999, 341 such cases have been reported, including 80 fatalities. In ≈ 85% of these cases, the events occurred when cisapride was used in patients with known risk factors. In clinical trials, the following adverse experiences were reported in > 1% of patients treated with cisapride and at least as often on cisapride as on placebo: Headache, diarrhea, abdominal pain, nausea, constipation, flatulence, dyspepsia, rhinitis, sinusitis, coughing, viral infection, upper respiratory tract infection, pain, fever, urinary tract infection, micturition frequency, insomnia, anxiety, nervousness, rash, pruritus, arthralgia, abnormal vision, and vaginitis.

➤*Summary:* Cisapride is no longer commercially distributed in the US. Cisapride is available in the US only through an investigational limited access program.

Complete information on enrolling patients or receiving additonal information regarding the cisapride investigational limited access program sponsored by Janssen Pharmaceutica may be obtained by calling toll-free (877)795-4247.

CLOBAZAM (*Frisium* by Aventis) and NITRAZEPAM (*Mogadon* by Roche) – Two investigational benzodiazepines

➤*Actions:*

Pharmacology – Clobazam and nitrazepam are investigational benzodiazepine derivatives. The profile of these agents parallels those of approved benzodiazepines; subtle differences account for individual product distinction.

Clobazam: Clobazam is structurally and pharmacologically related to approved benzodiazepines. Antianxiety and anticonvulsant properties are similar to diazepam; the usual adult dose is 20 to 30 mg/day. Initially, clobazam is effective against all varieties of epilepsy; however, efficacy decreases within a few days to a few weeks in approximately one-third of patients. Success also has been demonstrated in cyclic exacerbations of epilepsy associated with menstruation. Clobazam is a weak hypnotic agent.

Nitrazepam: Nitrazepam has been widely used for many years in Europe and Canada as a sedative/hypnotic in doses of 2.5 to 10 mg, and in the management of myoclonic seizures of childhood epilepsy. Its structure and clinical effects are also analogous to other benzodiazepines.

Pharmacokinetics –

Clobazam: The pharmacokinetics are independent of dose and concentration. Oral clobazam is 87% absorbed. Concomitant administration with alcohol increases clobazam's bioavailability by 50%. Food may slow the rate but does not alter total absorption. Absorption is not influenced by age or sex. Clobazam is 85% bound to human serum protein; peak serum concentrations occur 1 to 4 hours after ingestion. It is metabolized via dealkylation and hydroxylation to a pharmacologically active metabolite, N-desmethylclobazam, and several inactive metabolites. The mean half-life of the unchanged drug is 18 hours, and up to 77 hours for metabolites. Clobazam is 81% to 97% excreted in the urine; accumulation is expected in impaired renal function.

Nitrazepam: Nitrazepam is 80% bioavailable following oral administration. Absorption is rapid: 0.5 to 5 hours to peak concentration; concomitant administration with food decreases peak levels by 30%. Nitrazepam is lipophilic and is widely distributed in the body; 10% to 15% is found in the cerebrospinal fluid; 85% to 90% is plasma protein bound. It crosses the placenta and is found in breast milk (50% and about 50% to 100% of maternal plasma concentration, respectively). Metabolism is extensive and excretion is urinary, primarily as inactive metabolites; only 1 is excreted as the unchanged drug. The elimination half-life is approximately 30 hours.

➤*Adverse Reactions:*

Clobazam – The most frequent (10% to 44%) side effects include: Drowsiness, hangover effects, dizziness, weakness, and lightheadedness. Less frequent (5% to 10%) adverse reactions include: Weight gain, orthostatic hypotension, syncope, headache, dry mouth, and incoordination.

Nitrazepam – The frequency of adverse reactions increases with age and dosage and parallels those of other benzodiazepines. The most common include: Fatigue, dizziness, lightheadedness, drowsiness, lethargy, mental confusion, staggering, ataxia, and falling. Nightmares, insomnia, agitation, rash, pruritus, headache, and GI disturbances also have been reported. The hangover effect is also common and may be a function of nitrazepam's long half-life.

➤*Summary:* Nitrazepam and clobazam appear to be safe and effective agents with antianxiety, anticonvulsant, and hypnotic properties. These agents have long elimination half-lives; this enhances the potential for drug accumulation and increases the potential for residual side effects. These agents are unlikely to replace established benzodiazepine derivatives; however, they may provide viable therapeutic alternatives.

CLOFAZIMINE (*Lamprene* by Novartis) – A leprosy agent

➤*Actions:*

Pharmacology – Beginning November 1, 2004, *Lamprene* (clofazimine) is available only on a limited access basis. Clofazimine is indicated for the treatment of lepromatous leprosy, including dapsone-resistant lepromatous leprosy and lepromatous leprosy complicated by erythema nodosum leprosum. Clofazimine exerts a slow bactericidal effect on *Mycobacterium leprae* (Hansen's bacillus). It inhibits mycobacterial growth and binds preferentially to mycobacterial DNA. The drug also exerts anti-inflammatory properties in controlling erythema nodosum leprosum reactions. Precise mechanism of action is unknown.

Pharmacokinetics – Absorption rate ranges from 45% to 62% after oral administration. Clofazimine is highly lipophilic and is deposited predominantly in fatty tissue and in the reticuloendothelial system. It is taken up by macrophages. Clofazimine crosses the human placenta (Pregnancy Category C) and is excreted in breast milk.

After ingestion of a single 300 mg dose, elimination of unchanged drug and its metabolites in urine in 24 hours was negligible. Clofazimine is retained in the human body for a long time. Half-life after repeated doses is estimated to be at least 70 days. Part of the drug recovered from feces may represent excretion via bile. A small amount is eliminated in sputum, sebum, and sweat.

➤*Drug Interactions:* Although not confirmed, dapsone may inhibit the anti-inflammatory activity of clofazimine. If leprosy-associated inflammatory reactions develop in patients being treated with dapsone and clofazimine, it is still advisable to continue treatment with both drugs.

➤*Adverse Reactions:* In general, clofazimine is well tolerated when administered in dosages of 100 mg/day or less. The most consistent adverse reactions are usually dose-related and reversible when the drug is discontinued. Severe abdominal symptoms have necessitated exploratory laparotomies in patients receiving clofazimine. Rare reports have included splenic infarction, bowel obstruction, and GI bleeding. Death has been reported following severe abdominal symptoms. Autopsies have revealed crystalline deposits of clofazimine in the intestinal mucosa, liver, gallbladder, bile, spleen, adrenals, subcutaneous fat, mesenteric lymph nodes, muscles, bone, and skin. Other common adverse reactions include the following: Pigmentation (pink to brownish black) in 75% to 100% of patients within a few weeks of treatment; ichthyosis, dryness (8% to 28%); rash, pruritus (1% to 5%); abdominal/epigastric pain, diarrhea, nausea, vomiting, GI intolerance (40% to 50%); conjunctival and corneal pigmentation caused by clofazimine crystal deposits; discolored urine, feces, sputum, or sweat.

➤*Summary:* Take clofazimine with meals. It should be used preferably in combination with one or more other antileprosy agents to prevent the emergence of drug resistance. For the treatment of dapsone-resistant leprosy, give clofazimine 100 mg/day in combination with one or more other antileprosy drugs for 3 years, followed by monotherapy with clofazimine 100 mg/day. Clinical improvement usually can be detected between the first and third months of treatment and is usually clearly evident by the sixth month. For the treatment of dapsone-sensitive multibacillary leprosy, combination therapy with 2 other antileprosy drugs is recommended. Give the triple-drug regimen for at least 2 years and continue, if possible, until negative skin smears are obtained. At this time, monotherapy with an appropriate antileprosy drug can be instituted. For the treatment of erythema nodosum leprosum, treatment depends on the severity of symptoms. In general, continue basic antileprosy treatment; if nerve injury or skin ulceration is threatened, give corticosteroids. Where prolonged corticosteroid therapy becomes necessary, clofazimine 100 to 200 mg/day for up to 3 months may be useful in eliminating or reducing corticosteroid requirements. Dosages greater than 200 mg/day are not recommended; taper dosage to 100 mg/day as quickly as possible after the reactive episode is controlled.

Clofazimine is only available to physicians enrolled as investigators under an Investigational New Drug (IND) held by National Hansen's Disease Programs, a unit of the US Health and Human Services. Physicians should call (225) 578-9861 for more information. In addition, clofazimine will be distributed via single patient INDs administered by the FDA for the treatment of multi-drug resistant tuberculosis (MDRTB). Requests for use of clofazimine for the treatment of MDRTB should be directed to the FDA at (301) 827-2127.

CONIVAPTAN (Yamanouchi Pharma America) – A Vasopressin Antagonist

➤*Actions:*

Pharmacology – An NDA has been filed for conivaptan hydrochloride for the treatment of hyponatremia. The drug also is being evaluated in phase 2 clinical trials as a potential treatment for heart failure. Hyponatremia can occur for various reasons (eg, ascites, liver cirrhosis, syndrome of inappropriate antidiuretic hormone [SIADH] secretion, heart failure, volume overload). Some of these are caused by a derangement in water handling and up-regulation of the vasopressin (antidiuretic hormone) system.

Conivaptan is an orally active benzazepine derivative of vasopressin. It is an antagonist of the V_{1A} and V_2 vasopressin receptors. Conivaptan is able to increase the excretion of free water by increasing urine output without increasing sodium output, thus normalizing the serum sodium concentrations. When vasopressin is released into the plasma, it stimulates 1 or all 3 vasopressin receptor subtypes: V_{1A}, V_2, and V_{1B}. The V_{1A} receptor is found in vascular smooth muscle, hepatocytes, and platelets. Stimulation of the V_{1A} receptor results in vasoconstriction, glycogenolysis, platelet aggregation, myocyte hypertrophy, anxiety, and stress. The V_{1B} receptor is found in the anterior pituitary, and stimulation of this receptor results in the release of adrenocorticotropin (ACTH). The V_2 receptor is located in the kidney, endothelium, and possibly other organs. Stimulation of the V_2 receptor results in vasodilation, release of Von Willebrand factor, and water retention. The effect of vasopressin on vascular contractility is dose dependent. At low concentrations it causes vasoconstriction and at higher concentrations it causes vasodilation. Thus, vasopressin antagonists could be useful in the treatment of liver cirrhosis, SIADH, and heart failure.

Pharmacokinetics – Conivaptan achieves peak plasma concentrations within 1 to 2 hours after oral administration. Peak plasma concentrations are 664 ng/mL after oral administration of 60 mg conivaptan hydrochloride. Its oral bioavailability is 44%. The terminal half-life of conivaptan is 5.6 hours and the Cl/F is 26 L/h following oral administration and 3.1 hours and 11 L/h following IV administration. The volume of distribution is 34 L.

Clinical trials – Minimal effectiveness data have been published on the use of conivaptan in the treatment of SIADH or heart failure. The majority of these available data are from short-term administration and reported only in abstract form.

IV administration of conivaptan hydrochloride for 3 days (20 to 30 mg on day 1 and 20 to 40 mg twice daily on days 2 and 3) was able to increase serum sodium, decrease urine osmolality, and increase free water clearance in 4 patients with SIADH and 4 patients with CHF. There was a small increase in the thirst index and no serious drug-related adverse events.

Single-dose IV administration of conivaptan (10, 20, or 40 mg) in patients with advanced heart failure produced reductions in pulmonary capillary wedge pressure, reductions in right atrial pressure, increases in urine output, increases in effective water clearance, and increases in free-water clearance without changing the cardiac index, systemic and pulmonary vascular resistance, blood pressure, or heart rate, and without potassium wasting.

The ADVANCE (A Dose evaluation of a Vasopressin Antagonist in CHF patients undergoing Exercise) trial is currently ongoing. This study is designed to use exercise time to reach 70% of peak oxygen consumption, other exercise parameters, and quality of life indicators in patients with heart failure treated with conivaptan or placebo.

These preliminary studies are suggestive that conivaptan may be useful in the treatment of patients with advanced heart failure and SIADH.

➤*Adverse Reactions:* Adverse effects reported with conivaptan therapy have included low blood pressure, lightheadedness, and constipation.

➤*Summary:* Conivaptan is the first orally active non-peptide designed to target the V_{1A} and V_2 vasopressin receptors. Conivaptan is able to increase the excretion of free water by increasing urine output without increasing the sodium output, thus normalizing the serum sodium concentration. Very little effectiveness data have been published on the use of conivaptan in the treatment of SIADH or heart failure. The majority of these data are from single-dose or short-term treatment studies reported only in abstract form. These preliminary studies are suggestive that conivaptan may be useful in the treatment of patients with advanced heart failure and SIADH. A New Drug Application for conivaptan was filed with the FDA in February 2004.

DALBAVANCIN (by Vicuron Pharmaceuticals) – A glycopeptide antibiotic

➤*Actions:*

Pharmacology – Dalbavancin is a semisynthetic glycopeptide antibiotic with activity against gram-positive aerobic and anaerobic bacteria. Dalbavancin has been submitted for FDA approval for the treatment of complicated skin and soft tissue infections caused by gram-positive bacteria, including methicillin-resistant *Staphylococcus aureus* (MRSA). It was developed via a chemical modification of a natural glycopeptide produced by *Nonomuria* species and is structurally related to teicoplanin. Dalbavancin interferes with the formation of the bacterial cell wall by binding to the terminal D-alanyl-D-alanine of nascent peptidoglycan chains. The glycopeptide-peptidoglycan chain complex then prevents transpeptidation and transglycosylation, thus interfering with cross-linking and polymerization. Dalbavancin shares the mechanism of other glycopeptides, but chemical modification has produced a compound with enhanced potency and a longer duration of action.

Pharmacokinetics – Dalbavancin steady-state concentrations were achieved by day 3 after administration of a loading dose and once-daily maintenance dose. The mean volume of distribution is 9.75 to 11.5 L. Dalbavancin is extensively (greater than 95%) plasma protein bound, primarily to albumin. The half-life of dalbavancin is 149 to 328 hours. Clearance is 0.0431 to 0.0473 L/h. About 34% of the dose is excreted renally, with 25% to 46% of the administered dose excreted in the urine unchanged. Urine concentrations remained above the level of quantification (0.5 mg/L) for 28 days after a single dose.

Clinical trials – Few clinical efficacy studies using dalbavancin have been published. Once-weekly dalbavancin was compared with a standard-of-care regimen in a multicenter, randomized, open-label study enrolling 62 patients with skin and soft tissue infections. Eligible infections included those involving deep soft tissue and/or requiring significant surgical intervention, such as a major abscess, infected ulcer, major burn, or deep and extensive cellulitis. Patients received dalbavancin 1,100 mg as a single intravenous (IV) infusion (20 patients) or 1,000 mg IV followed by 500 mg IV 1 week later (21 patients), or a prospectively defined standard-of-care regimen (21 patients). The standard-of-care regimen was determined by the investigator prior to randomization. Standard-of-care regimens included ceftriaxone alone or in combination (6 patients), cefazolin alone or in combination (4 patients), vancomycin alone or in combination (4 patients), piperacillin/tazobactam (3 patients), clindamycin alone (2 patients), linezolid alone (1 patient), and cephalexin alone (1 patient). If gram-negative or anaerobic coverage was necessary, aztreonam, ceftazidime, or metronidazole could be administered. *S. aureus* accounted for 83% of pathogens isolated. Gram-positive pathogens were isolated from 41 of 62 patients (66%). Clinical success at follow-up among clinically evaluable patients was 94.1% (16 of 17) among patients treated with 2 dalbavancin doses, 61.5% (8 of 13) treated with a single dalbavancin dose, and 76.2% (16 of 21) treated with a standard-of-care regimen. Among patients with MRSA, clinical success at follow-up was reported for 4 of 5 patients (80%) treated with 2 doses of dalbavancin, 3 of 6 patients (50%) treated with single-dose dalbavancin, and 1 of 2 patients (50%) treated with the comparator regimen. Microbiologic success among evaluable subjects with *S. aureus* isolated was 90% (9 of 10) for subjects treated with 2 doses of dalbavancin, 50% (5 of 10) for subjects treated with single-dose dalbavancin, and 60% (6 of 10) for subjects treated with the comparator agents. Tolerability of the 3 regimens was similar.

➤*Adverse Reactions:* Adverse reactions reported with dalbavancin therapy included pyrexia, headache, nausea, hypotension, hypokalemia, oral candidiasis, diarrhea, and constipation.

➤*Summary:* Dalbavancin will offer an additional agent for the treatment of infections caused by gram-positive organisms, especially MRSA and methicillin-resistant *S. epidermidis* (MRSE) infections. It is a novel antibiotic that offers once-weekly dosing, which could lead to pharmacoeconomic benefits. In February 2005, the FDA granted priority review status for dalbavancin for the treatment of complicated skin and soft tissue infections.

DOMPERIDONE (*Motilium* by Janssen Pharmaceutica) – An antiemetic

➤*Actions:*

Pharmacology – Acute nausea and vomiting induced by cytotoxic chemotherapy are frequent and serious toxicities distressful to cancer patients. Symptoms can be so pronounced and refractory that they interfere with therapeutic measures and patient nutrition. Available antiemetics block the chemoreceptor trigger zone (CTZ) (neuroleptics), sedate the vomiting centers (antihistamines), block afferent impulses at the vomiting center (anticholinergics), act peripherally and in the CNS (metoclopramide), or by less defined central mechanisms (cannabinoids). These agents are effective in most patients; however, side effects (eg, drowsiness, dry mouth, hypotension, extrapyramidal effects) are limitations. Domperidone, an investigational antiemetic, appears to act with minimum adverse effects.

Domperidone is chemically unrelated to the butyrophenones, phenothiazines, or metoclopramide; however, it shares pharmacological properties with these agents. In the medulla it produces a direct blocking effect of dopamine receptors in the CTZ. Like metoclopramide and haloperidol, domperidone is a peripheral dopamine antagonist; however, it contrasts in that it does not cross the blood-brain barrier and produce CNS effects. It selectively blocks peripheral dopamine receptors in the GI wall, thus enhancing normal synchronized GI peristalsis and motility in the proximal portion of the GI tract; it also may counteract anticholinergic-induced relaxation of the lower esophageal sphincter (LES).

Pharmacokinetics – Peak plasma levels are achieved within 30 minutes following IM or oral administration and between 1 to 4 hours after rectal administration. Approximately 40% of a dose is rapidly distributed into peripheral compartments. It is metabolized in the liver and eliminated in the urine, primarily as conjugates. Less than 1% appears in the urine as unchanged drug. Excretion is almost complete within 4 days. The duration of activity is between 2 and 4 hours following IV administration.

Clinical trials – The effectiveness of domperidone in the treatment of nausea and vomiting associated with cytotoxic chemotherapy has been evaluated. Several double-blind studies were conducted in patients with Hodgkin's disease. Domperidone 16 mg IV was preferred and superior to placebo; it was effective and well tolerated, and decreased the duration of nausea and vomiting by greater than ⅓ when injected 1 hour before the start of cytostatic treatment. Domperidone, 1 to 40 mg IV daily, was administered with chemotherapy infusion in 172 patients. Vomiting induced by agents considered to be moderate emetics (eg, cyclophosphamide, 5-fluorouracil, vinblastine) was reduced; however, patients with emesis induced by doxorubicin or mechlorethamine did not respond as well. The higher dosages of domperidone did not achieve a proportionally augmented response rate. In another study, 4 mg domperidone IV produced excellent or good response in 72% of patients receiving varied chemotherapy; poor responses occurred in patients receiving dacarbazine. When 12 mg domperidone IV was compared with 10 mg metoclopramide IV, both drugs produced a good or excellent response in 70% of patients; however, metoclopramide had a higher incidence of side effects. Domperidone 1 mg/kg IV or metoclopramide 0.5 mg/kg IV was used to prevent chemotherapy-induced nausea and vomiting in children. In the random crossover trial, domperidone decreased nausea and vomiting to a significantly greater extent than metoclopramide.

Domperidone has been compared favorably to cimetidine in 20 gastric ulcer patients; it also may have value in treating symptoms of gastroesophageal reflux and postoperative- or bromocriptine-induced nausea and vomiting.

➤*Adverse Reactions:* Domperidone does not appear to produce significant side effects or toxicities. Doses of 40 mg IV or 100 mg orally have not been reported to produce CNS or cardiovascular side effects, only facial flushing, headache, slight somnolence, and dry mouth. Unlike metoclopramide, domperidone does not cross the blood-brain barrier; therefore, the incidence of extrapyramidal or psychotropic effects should be low. Yet there have been isolated reports of idiosyncratic extrapyramidal reactions. Domperidone does not stimulate aldosterone secretion.

➤*Summary:* Domperidone selectively blocks peripheral dopamine receptors in the GI wall and in the CTZ. Its major advantage appears to be the lack of significant side effects; it may be an effective alternative to available antiemetics, including metoclopramide. Domperidone, like other antiemetics, produces variable effects on cytotoxic chemotherapy-induced nausea and vomiting, depending on the agent administered. There is limited or no data available comparing domperidone to more standard antiemetic agents other than metoclopramide. Domperidone was developed in Belgium by Janssen Pharmaceutica; it is available in Europe.

EFAPROXIRAL (by Allos Therapeutics, Inc.)

➤*Actions:*

Pharmacology – A New Drug Application for efaproxiral (RSR13) has been filed by Allos Therapeutics. They are seeking approval to market this agent as an adjunct to whole brain radiation therapy for the treatment of brain metastases in patients with breast cancer. Efaproxiral is a unique compound that appears to improve tumor radiation sensitivity. Efaproxiral is a synthetic allosteric modifier of hemoglobin. It is able to reduce hemoglobin oxygen-binding affinity, facilitating oxygen release and increasing tissue partial oxygen pressure. Efaproxiral binds to the central water cavity of the hemoglobin tetramer and stabilizes the deoxyhemoglobin state. This binding results in reduced hemoglobin-oxygen binding affinity and increased oxygen unloading to hypoxic tissues. The presence of oxygen within tumors is necessary for the effectiveness of radiation therapy, and hypoxic cells (eg, glioblastoma) tend to be resistant to radiation therapy. By increasing tumor oxygenation, efaproxiral enhances the efficacy of radiation therapy. It facilitates the release of oxygen from hemoglobin, increasing the level of oxygen within tumors and potentially sensitizing the hypoxic areas of tumors to radiation. Administration of efaproxiral with oxygen produces greater intratumor oxygen pressure than the administration of oxygen alone. Normal tissue should not become more sensitive to radiation therapy with the administration of oxygen or efaproxiral plus oxygen. Instead, only hypoxic cells should be sensitized by increasing oxygen delivery. So when the partial pressure of oxygen reaches 10 to 20 mm Hg, the tumor cells are fully radiosensitized.

Pharmacokinetics – Peak concentrations in plasma and red blood cells were 581 and 560 mcg/mL, respectively, at the end of the infusion and 20 and 14 mcg/mL, respectively, at trough (prior to the next infusion) with administration of a 100 mg/kg dose. In another pharmacokinetic study, end of infusion concentrations were 449 to 465 mcg/mL in plasma and 512 to 547 mcg/mL in red blood cells. The efaproxiral half-life is 3 to 4.5 hours. Reduced efaproxiral clearance has been observed in patients with renal dysfunction.

Clinical trials – Efaproxiral plus whole brain radiation therapy was compared with whole brain radiation therapy alone in a randomized, open-label, phase 3 study enrolling 538 patients with brain metastases. Patients in the efaproxiral group received 75 to 100 mg/kg/day efaproxiral IV plus supplemental oxygen followed by standard whole brain radiation therapy (30 Gy; 3 Gy/day for 10 days). The control group received standard whole brain radiation therapy plus supplemental oxygen. The primary study endpoint was the difference in overall survival between the 2 treatment groups. Median survival was slightly, but not significantly improved in the efaproxiral group (5.26 months vs 4.47 months; 17.6% improvement; $P = 0.17$). In a Cox multiple regression model, which adjusted for imbalances in prognostic factors between the 2 treatment groups, an advantage of efaproxiral was observed (hazard ratio 0.775, 95% Confidence Interval 0.639 to 0.941; $P = 0.01$). Among the subgroup of 414 patients with brain metastases from breast cancer and nonsmall cell lung cancer, a slight difference in favor of efaproxiral was also apparent (5.91 months vs 4.47 months; 32.4% improvement; $P = 0.12$). A difference between treatments was observed in the subgroup of 115 patients with brain metastases from breast cancer (60 patients in the efaproxiral group; 55 patients in the control group). Median survival was increased nearly 2-fold in patients with metastatic breast cancer who received efaproxiral compared with those who did not (8.67 months vs 4.57 months; $P = 0.006$). In the breast cancer subgroup, response to therapy was observed in 71.7% of patients in the efaproxiral group compared with 52.7% of patients in the control group ($P = 0.03$). Improvements in quality of life at 6 months (Karnofsky Performance Status, $P = 0.02$) and neurofunctional score ($P = 0.04$) also were observed in the breast cancer patients treated with efaproxiral.

➤*Adverse Reactions:* Hypoxia is the most frequent adverse effect. The Hypoxia is dose dependent and can be managed with supplemental oxygen. Other adverse effects observed in clinical studies included allergic rash, dizziness, fatigue, headache, hypotension, nausea, sepsis, transient creatinine increase, and vomiting.

➤*Summary:* Efaproxiral is a unique compound that appears to improve tumor radiation sensitivity. Clinical benefit was observed in a subgroup of patients with brain metastases from breast cancer treated with efaproxiral plus radiation therapy. Adverse effects appear manageable, although very limited tolerability information is available at this time. Efaproxiral is administered by central venous infusion to avoid the pain associated with its peripheral infusion. The FDA issued an approvable letter in June 2004.

EXISULIND (*Aptosyn* by Cell Pathways) – A selective apoptotic antineoplastic drug

➤*Actions:*

Pharmacology – Exisulind (sulindac sulphone) was being evaluated by the FDA for the treatment of familial adenomatous polyposis (FAP); the FDA notified Cell Pathways on September 22, 2000, that the drug was nonapprovable. Exisulind also is being evaluated for use in a number of other conditions, including Gardner's syndrome; sporadic colonic adenatomous polyps; Barrett's esophagus; prostate, breast, and lung cancer; and other solid tumors.

Pharmacokinetics – Exisulind reaches peak serum concentration within 2 to 2.5 hours after oral administration. The absorption half-life is 0.7 hours. Its elimination half-life ranges from 4.88 to 6.81 hours. The total body clearance of exisulind is 8.2 to 10.1 L/hr and its apparent volume of distribution is 58.8 to 69.3 L.

Clinical trials –

FAP: A phase I study was conducted in patients with FAP. All of the patients had undergone a subtotal colectomy ≥ 3 years prior to the study. In addition, each patient had to have ≥ 5 rectal polyps at the time of study enrollment. No NSAIDs were allowed for ≥ 2 weeks prior to the study and throughout the course of the study. Patients were treated with 200, 300, or 400 mg oral exisulind twice daily for ≥ 4 months. Dose escalation was allowed after a minimum of 2 weeks if toxicities did not occur. If toxicity occurred, it was possible to lower the dose of exisulind. Effectiveness and safety analysis included a sigmoidoscopic evaluation. The number of polyps in each rectal segment was counted and biopsies were obtained from normal-appearing mucosa in each segment. Twenty patients were enrolled in the study, but only 18 were evaluable. The number of polyps at baseline and after 1 month of therapy was similar in all treatment groups. No increase in polyp count occurred with the 300 and 400 mg twice daily dosing regimen after 4 to 6 months. However, the number of polyps increased in those patients treated with 200 mg twice daily after 4 to 6 months (> 50%).

A placebo-controlled study (n = 34) of patients with FAP was designed to show a difference in polyp formation rates in patients who historically formed between 10 and 40 new polyps per year. Patients were treated with 600 mg/day exisulind. The exisulind therapy resulted in a 53% reduction in the number of polyps formed compared with placebo after 1 year. Patients were then enrolled in an open-label extension study. At 6-month intervals, the number of rectal polyps was determined and removed. After 6 months of therapy, the original placebo-treated patients had a median reduction in polyps of 50%. Those previously treated with exisulind had an additional 50% reduction in polyp formation, which represented a 75% reduction over the 18-month observation period.

Other uses: Exisulind has shown promising results in mammary carcinogenesis and hepatocellular carcinoma in rat models or in vitro cell lines. Further studies will be necessary to determine if exisulind will be valuable in the treatment of mammary cancer.

A small phase I study (n = 18) was conducted to assess the safety and pharmacokinetics of exisulind in patients with FAP plus colonic adenomas. Three cohorts of 6 patients were treated with either 200, 300, or 400 mg exisulind twice daily for 6 months. Three of the patients in the 400 mg twice daily group had to have the medication discontinued or the dose reduced because of grade 2 or 3 hepatic toxicity and a fourth patient develped grade 1 hepatotoxicity. The number of polyps increased in the patients treated with 200 mg twice daily. The number of polyps in the 300 mg and 400/200 mg (patients started on 400 mg then reduced to 200 mg) groups remained stable with a regression in some polyps.

➤*Adverse Reactions:* The most common GI adverse reactions included nausea, vomiting, diarrhea, changes in the frequency or consistency of bowel movements, abdominal pain, and dyspepsia, and were found to be dose related. A dose-limiting hepatic toxicity occurred with the 400 mg twice daily regimen.

➤*Summary:* The adult dose of exisulind is 150 mg 4 times/day. Less frequent administration does not produce the same beneficial effects on polyp formation. The ability to decrease the number and size of polyps and cause regression in the colorectal adenomas with exisulind therapy is encouraging. However, it is still too early to determine if exisulind can replace, delay the need for, or limit the anatomical extent of proctocolectomy, and prevent the development of carcinoma. Until these data are available for review, exisulind (if approved) could only be considered an adjunct to the surgical management of the disease.

FEBUXOSTAT (by TAP Pharmaceutical Products Inc.) – A selective xanthine oxidase inhibitor

➤*Actions:*

Pharmacology – Febuxostat is an oral, non-purine, selective inhibitor of xanthine oxidase intended for the treatment of hyperuricemia in patients with chronic gout. Xanthine oxidase is an enzyme that catalyzes the conversion of hypoxanthine and xanthine to uric acid, the accumulation of which leads to uric crystal formation and tophaceous deposits. In vitro studies of febuxostat indicate it is an inhibitor for both the oxidized and reduced forms of xanthine oxidase leading to significant reductions in serum uric acid levels. Unlike purine-based antihyperuricemic agents, such as allopurinol, febuxostat does not interfere with a broad range of purine and pyrimidine metabolic reactions.

Pharmacokinetics – Time to maximum concentration of an orally administered dose of febuxostat is approximately 1 hour. Febuxostat is approximately 99% bound to albumin and has a steady state volume of distribution of 0.7 L/kg. Single-dose kinetics appear to be linear at doses of 10 to 120 mg with proportional increases in C_{max} and AUC after multiple oral doses. Febuxostat is primarily metabolized to an acylglucuronide metabolite and to active metabolites (67M-1, 67M-2 and 67M-4) via hepatobiliary conjugation. Less than 5% of orally administered drug is excreted unchanged in the urine.

Clinical trials – In a 28-day, multicenter, phase 2, double-blind, placebo controlled, dose response clinical trial, 153 patients with gout and hyperuricemia (serum uric acid levels of 8 mg/dL or more) were randomized to receive febuxostat 40, 80, or 120 mg or placebo once daily for 28 days. Patients also received colchicine prophylaxis (0.6 mg twice daily) for 14 days prior to and 14 days after randomization. The primary end point of this study was the efficacy of febuxostat in reducing serum uric acid concentrations to less then 6 mg/dL on day 28. Patients assigned to febuxostat treatment groups had significantly greater reductions in serum urate levels (50%, 59%, 91%, and 3% for febuxostat 40, 80, and 120 mg and placebo, respectively) compared to baseline by day 7, and maintained these levels throughout the remainder of the study (58%, 76%, 94%, and 0% for febuxostat 40, 80, and 120 mg and placebo, respectively). Patients with the highest serum urate baseline levels were less likely to achieve serum urate levels of 6 mg/dL or less taking 40 mg febuxostat compared to 80 or 120 mg. No significant differences were observed in treatment-related adverse events between febuxostat and placebo groups.

Results from an extended phase 2 trial and several phase 3 trials were presented at the 68th Annual Scientific Meeting of the American College of Rheumatology (San Antonio, TX; October 2004). Patients in the extended phase 2 trial receiving febuxostat 40, 80, or 120 mg for two years maintained reduced uric acid levels, with most patients (74% to 81%) having serum uric acid levels below 6 mg/dL at each visit and a mean reduction rate in serum uric acid level of 45% to 48% compared to baseline. Two phase 3 trials compared efficacy of febuxostat to allopurinol and reported greater reductions in serum uric acid levels in patients receiving febuxostat compared to allopurinol groups. An additional phase 3 trial reported dose-dependent reductions in serum uric acid levels with febuxostat 20 and 40 mg.

➤*Adverse Reactions:* Adverse events observed in the phase 2 and extended phase 2 trials were mild to moderate in severity with no trends indicating a dose-related relationship. Significant differences in adverse events were not observed between febuxostat and placebo. Reported adverse events included diarrhea, headache, GI disorder, abnormal liver function tests, increased creatinine levels, localized angioedema, and one patient that developed Guillain-Barré syndrome considered to be possibly related. Clinically significant changes in other laboratory parameters, vital signs, or ECG were not observed.

Phase 3 studies presented at the 68th Annual Scientific Meeting of the American College of Rheumatology reported similar adverse events between febuxostat, allopurinol, and placebo groups, with the most common adverse reactions being liver function test abnormalities, diarrhea, headache, nausea, gout flare, common cold syndrome, respiratory tract infection, nasopharyngitis, musculoskeletal, and connective tissue symptoms, joint-related signs and symptoms, increases from baseline in levels of C-reactive protein, creatine phosphokinase and triglycerides. The severities of these events were reported to be mild to moderate.

➤*Summary:* Febuxostat is a non-purine selective inhibitor of both oxidized and reduced forms of xanthine oxidase. Phase 2 and 3 trials indicate advantages over current antihyperuricemic therapy such as greater reduction of serum uric acid level for the treatment of gout. TAP Pharmaceuticals submitted an NDA for febuxostat in December 2004.

FENOTEROL HBr (*Berotec* by Boehringer Ingelheim) – A β_2 agonist

➤*Actions:*

Pharmacology – Fenoterol HBr is a β_2-adrenergic agonist undergoing investigation in the US as a bronchodilating agent. It has been available outside the US since the early 1970s as a metered dose inhaler (MDI), a solution for nebulization, a powder for inhalation, and an oral dosage form.

Stimulation of β_2-adrenoreceptors activates adenyl cyclase, which converts adenosine triphosphate into cAMP. Increased levels of cAMP inhibit mediator release and produce bronchodilation. Although controversial, an increase in mucociliary transport also may occur. In addition, β_2 stimulation causes vasodilation of peripheral blood vessels. This effect can result in a baroreceptor-mediated reflex-positive chronotropic response (increase in heart rate) and stimulation of skeletal muscle, leading to tremor. Fenoterol has greater β_2 selectivity than metaproterenol, but it is approximately equal in selectivity to albuterol and terbutaline. Bronchoselectivity is enhanced by administering fenoterol by inhalation; this allows for use of a lower dose to achieve a therapeutic effect and reduce dose-related side effects.

Usual therapeutic doses (200 to 400 mcg) of inhaled fenoterol do not significantly affect the cardiovascular system; however, marked cardiovascular effects have been observed after oral, SC, IM, or IV administration. Fenoterol prevents immediate antigen-induced bronchospasm but does not prevent delayed allergic reactions. A transient reduction in serum potassium levels (representing the uptake of potassium into the intracellular space) and an increase in serum glucose levels have been observed, but the clinical significance remains unclear.

Pharmacokinetics – Approximately 60% of an oral dose is absorbed, with peak plasma levels reached in 2 hours. After inhalation, fenoterol appears to undergo a 2-stage absorption process; the first stage is independent of dose, while the second is similar to that seen after oral administration. This is consistent with the observation that, when a drug is administered by inhalation, as much as 90% of the dose is swallowed. Fenoterol undergoes extensive first-pass metabolism. The half-life of total radioactive-labeled drug is 7 hours; however, this does not represent a true half-life for the parent compound. Although maximum effect of inhaled fenoterol is not achieved for 1 to 2 hours, 60% of the maximal response is seen within the first few minutes. The duration of action is ≈ 4 to 6 hours. However, because the lower therapeutic dose produces near maximal bronchodilatation, increasing the dose to near maximal effective concentrations will increase the duration of action without affecting the intensity of the peak response. After oral administration, < 2% of the dose is eliminated unchanged in the urine; the balance is excreted as acid conjugates in the urine and feces (40%).

Clinical trials – Clinical trials have established the efficacy of fenoterol for maintenance therapy in patients with moderate to severe asthma, therapy of chronic obstructive pulmonary disease (COPD), protection against exercise-induced asthma, and treatment of acute asthma attacks. It is difficult to evaluate many of the studies because they are single-dose studies, or because they do not compare equipotent doses when evaluated against albuterol and terbutaline. However, at equipotent doses (1 puff fenoterol [200 mcg/puff] = 2 puffs albuterol [100 mcg/puff] = 2 puffs terbutaline [250 mcg/puff]), there appears to be no clinically significant difference in duration of action, bronchoselectivity, or therapeutic efficacy among the 3 agents. The dose of fenoterol used to treat an acute asthma attack is 200 mcg (1 puff) repeated once in 5 minutes for children, and 1 to 3 puffs for adults. Maintenance therapy is 1 to 2 puffs 2 to 4 times/day for adults; give 1 puff twice daily to children. Increasing an inhaled dose of fenoterol to > 600 mcg (3 puffs) does not appear to increase the therapeutic response but may increase the incidence of side effects. In one study, an 800 mcg dose increased the heart rate 10% with a slow return to baseline over 2 hours. Although inhaled bronchodilators have many advantages, as many as 10% of the patients may not receive maximal therapeutic benefit due to improper MDI use.

➤*Adverse Reactions:* After inhalation of therapeutic doses of fenoterol, side effects are rare. After oral therapy, skeletal muscle tremor, tachycardia, palpitations and nervousness occur occasionally. Fenoterol is not recommended for use in patients with hyperthyroidism. Use with caution in patients with cardiovascular disease, diabetes mellitus, and hepatic or renal dysfunction.

➤*Summary:* Fenoterol by inhalation appears to be a safe and effective treatment for prophylaxis of exercise-induced bronchospasm, acute attacks of mild to moderate asthma, and maintenance therapy for chronic asthma or COPD. However, no apparent advantage of fenoterol over equipotent doses of the currently available β_2-selective agonists, albuterol or terbutaline, has yet been demonstrated. Further information on this product can be received from Boehringer Ingelheim Canada.

FENRETINIDE (by McNeil Pharmaceuticals) – A synthetic retinoid

➤*Actions:*

Pharmacology – Fenretinide (N-4-hydroxyphenylretinamide) is a synthetic retinoid currently under evaluation for use in prevention of breast, bladder, oral, and skin cancer. It does not act like other retinoids, because its activity does not correlate with cellular retinoic acid-binding proteins. However, it is believed that fenretinide is metabolized to an agent that competes for cellular retinoic acid-binding protein binding sites.

Pharmacokinetics – Peak levels are achieved in 3 to 9 hours following oral administration. Bioavailability is significantly increased by administration after a meal (189%), particularly after a high fat meal (200% to 300%). The elimination half-life is 17.4 to 27 hours. Fenretinide was present in very low amounts (at the limits of detectability) 50 days after discontinuation of treatment for 1 year with 200 mg/day. Levels were undetectable 6 days after the last dose following 1 month of treatment at that dose. After 5 years of continuous treatment, fenretinide concentrations were at the limits of detectability at 6 and 12 months after discontinuation, while levels of the metabolite were 5 times higher. Retinol concentrations returned to baseline after 1 month.

Clinical trials – The effects of fenretinide were evaluated in 149 women who received fenretinide for at least 4 years in a breast cancer chemoprevention trial. Evaluation was done by mammographies performed at baseline and then once a year. The results of mammographies after 4 years of fenretinide therapy reported no substantial changes in breast parenchymal patterns, except in 1 patient who demonstrated improvement (P2 to P1 Wolfe's classification). Preliminary studies are evaluating the effects of combination tamoxifen (eg, *Nolvadex*) and fenretinide in patients with previously untreated metastatic breast cancer.

One trial involved patients with previously untreated homogenous or nonhomogenous oral leukoplakias that had a benign postoperative histology following laser resection. Patients were randomized to receive fenretinide 200 mg/day for a maximum of 52 weeks (with a 3-day drug holiday at the end of each month) or no treatment. Of 153 patients in this study (74 treated with fenretinide and 79 in the control group), 19 patients had recurrences (9 in the control group and 10 in the fenretinide group), and 15 had new localizations (12 in the control group and 3 in the fenretinide group). The overall risk of recurrence and new localization was 6% in the fenretinide group and 30% in the control group.

Another report described the treatment of oral lichen planus (2 patients) and leukoplakias (6 patients) with topical fenretinide. Eight patients applied fenretinide twice daily by opening a 100 mg capsule and applying its contents to the affected sites after brushing teeth. Responses were apparent in all patients within 15 days. After 1 month of therapy, 2 patients had complete response and the other 6 had a > 75% response. No side effects were observed.

Results of a small study evaluating fenretinide effects on the outcomes of previously-resected superficial bladder cancer have been reported. Twelve patients were treated with fenretinide 200 mg/day and were compared with 17 non-randomized, untreated controls. The proportion of patients with DNA aneuploid stemlines in bladder washed cells decreased from 7 of 12 (58%) to 5 of 11 (45%) in the fenretinide group, but increased from 7 of 17 (41%) to 10 of 17 (59%) in the control group. Positive or suspicious cytologic examinations were present in 3 of 12 fenretinide-treated patients prior to therapy, but all reverted to normal. Positive or suspicious cytologic examinations increased from 4 of 17 to 6 of 17 during the study in the control group. These data suggest fenretinide may affect DNA content and abnormal cytology in patients with previously-resected superficial bladder cancer. Additional studies are necessary to further evaluate the effects of fenretinide in bladder cancer, including patients with previous bladder papillomas or transitional cell carcinoma.

It also has been suggested that fenretinide be evaluated as chemoprevention in patients with cervical dysplasia or previous basal cell or squamous cell actinic keratoses.

➤*Summary:* Insufficient information on the effects of fenretinide in cancer chemoprevention are available at this time. Fenretinide does appear to be better tolerated than currently-available retinoids under evaluation for cancer chemoprevention. Fenretinide is currently in phase III trials by McNeil.

FLUPIRTINE MALEATE – A nonnarcotic analgesic

➤*Actions:*

Pharmacology – Flupirtine maleate, a triaminopyridine derivative, is a nonnarcotic analgesic structurally unrelated to other analgesic agents. Although its exact mechanism of action is not known, flupirtine lacks affinity for any type of opiate receptor and therefore, has a mechanism that differs from the opiates. Flupirtine also appears to lack some of the side effects of the opiates including constipation, respiratory depression, withdrawal phenomena, development of tolerance, and abuse potential. It is suggested that flupirtine is a medium to strong analgesic; its duration of action is comparable with codeine, and it is up to 3 times as potent as codeine and propoxyphene (eg, *Darvon*), up to twice as potent as meperidine (eg, *Demerol*), and approximately 10 times as potent as acetaminophen (eg, *Tylenol*).

Pharmacokinetics – The pharmacokinetics of flupirtine have not been well defined. The drug appears to have linear kinetics. A dosage of 100 mg 3 times/day achieves average steady-state blood levels equivalent to the peak for a single 200 mg dose. In one study of 55 patients, the analgesic effect occurred within 45 minutes to 2 hours; the duration of action was 4 to 6 hours. The half-life of flupirtine appears to be 7 to 10 hours.

In 13 elderly patients receiving 100 mg flupirtine 3 times/day for 12 days, the mean elimination half-life was higher than in healthy young subjects (mean, 18.6 hours on day 12 vs 6.5 hours). This was associated with an increased maximum serum concentration and reduced clearance in the elderly subjects.

In 12 patients with renal impairment, the half-life of flupirtine was higher compared with healthy subjects (mean, 9.8 hours vs 6.5 hours) following a single oral 100 mg dose.

Flupirtine peak levels and area under the curve may be higher in patients with primary biliary cirrhosis. In a study of ten patients, flupirtine did not induce hepatic microsomal enzymes.

Clinical trials – Flupirtine is effective in the treatment of pain resulting from various procedures or conditions including episiotomy, cancer, and postoperative and dental pain. Dosages used have ranged from 100 to 600 mg/day; the most common dosages were 100 mg once daily or 100 mg 3 times/day. Capsules were used in most studies although the suppository form also was used. Analgesic efficacy of flupirtine was judged to be as effective as other analgesics used in the studies including acetaminophen, codeine, pentazocine (*Talwin NX*), oxycodone plus acetaminophen (eg, *Percocet*), naproxen (eg, *Naprosyn*), and diclofenac (*Voltaren*). Flupirtine appears to have no tolerance or addiction potential. In one study, the average number of capsules taken per month remained constant for 12 months, as did the analgesic effect.

Flupirtine significantly reduced seizure frequency in 8 of 9 patients with minimal side effects; however, because other derivatives of the drug may have greater activity, no further studies in the treatment of epilepsy are planned at this time.

➤*Adverse Reactions:* Flupirtine does not appear to share the common side effects of the opiates such as respiratory depression and constipation. The drug is generally well tolerated. In a study of 55 patients, the most common adverse effects were dizziness (11%), drowsiness (9% to 10%), pruritus (9%), and dry mouth (5%). Other side effects that occurred included: Pain in forehead; sensation of excessive fullness in stomach; muscular tremor; nausea; other GI disturbances (eg, vomiting, abdominal discomfort).

➤*Summary:* Flupirtine is a nonnarcotic analgesic that compares favorably in efficacy with other available analgesics. However, at this time, it offers no clear advantage over the nonsteroidal anti-inflammatory agents except perhaps in the GI and CNS side effect profile. It does offer an advantage over the opiates in side effect profile, abuse potential, withdrawal phenomena, and development of tolerance. The average dose appears to be 100 mg 1 to 3 times/day. It has been used in capsule and suppository formulations.

An NDA was filed for flupirtine by Carter-Wallace in April 1986. At one time, a 1989 approval was anticipated; however, there has been no recent projected approval date and Carter-Wallace is no longer interested in pursuing this product.

L-5-HYDROXYTRYPTOPHAN (L-5HTP)

➤*Indications:* L-5HTP in combination with carbidopa is effective in the therapy of post-anoxic intention myoclonus. In 41 patients, 65% experienced a 50% or more improvement. However, patients with intention myoclonus associated with head trauma and methyl bromide toxicity, progressive myoclonus epilepsy, essential myoclonus, and palatal myoclonus also show improvement. In addition, L-5HTP has shown some success in treating depression and in migraine prophylaxis.

➤*Administration and Dosage:* Begin with 25 mg L-5HTP 4 times/day; increase by 100 mg/day every 3 to 5 days if there are no significant side effects. If significant GI side effects develop, reduce the rate of increase to every 1 to 2 weeks. A reduction in myoclonus is usually first observed at 600 to 1000 mg/day (with carbidopa); the usual optimal dose of L-5HTP is between 1000 and 2000 mg/day in 4 divided doses.

➤*Actions:*

Pharmacology – L-5HTP is available as an "orphan" drug for the treatment of postanoxic intention myoclonus. Myoclonus is an uncommon neuromuscular movement disorder characterized by involuntary, irregular muscle contraction; it is associated with a variety of brain lesions. There is evidence that at least some of these disorders are related to brain neurotransmitter levels or function, specifically serotonin. L-5HTP is an aromatic amino acid, the immediate precursor of serotonin.

L-5HTP is administered with carbidopa (see individual monograph), a peripheral dopa-decarboxylase inhibitor that decreases the conversion of L-5HTP to serotonin in the extracerebral tissues. This permits the administration of lower doses of L-5HTP and reduces the peripheral GI side effects, such as diarrhea and nausea.

Pharmacokinetics – When administered orally with carbidopa (which produces a 5- to 15-fold increase in plasma L-5HTP), the systemic availability of L-5HTP is 47% to 84%; peak plasma concentrations of L-5HTP are reached at 1 to 3 hours. The biological half-life of L-5HTP, after pretreatment with carbidopa, is 2 to 7 hours. The major metabolic pathway of L-5HTP is decarboxylation to serotonin by L-aromatic amino acid decarboxylase; the highest activity is in the kidney, liver, and small intestine. However, carbidopa-decarboxylase inhibition is incomplete; this may account for the GI side effects.

➤*Contraindications:* L-5HTP/carbidopa is contraindicated in patients with renal disease, peptic ulcer, platelet disorders, scleroderma, and Parkinson's disease.

➤*Precautions:* Use L-5HTP/carbidopa with caution in patients with severe emotional or psychiatric disorders because of occasional mental side effects. Mental depression has improved in some patients.

➤*Drug Interactions:* Do not give monoamine oxidase inhibitors or reserpine concurrently with L-5HTP/carbidopa. Discontinue these drugs at least 2 weeks prior to initiating treatment with L-5HTP/carbidopa.

Discontinue tricyclic antidepressants with a major serotonin reuptake inhibition mechanism (ie, imipramine) prior to L-5HTP/carbidopa therapy. Also, avoid serotonin receptor antagonists like methysergide or cyproheptadine, which may reduce the therapeutic effects of L-5HTP/carbidopa.

Fenfluramine releases brain serotonin from serotonergic nerve terminals and may potentiate L-5HTP/carbidopa.

➤*Adverse Reactions:* The most common GI adverse effects include: Anorexia, nausea, diarrhea, and vomiting. These can usually be avoided or minimized by gradual increases of L-5HTP dosage; they rapidly disappear when the dose is reduced or discontinued. The diarrhea will respond to therapy with diphenoxylate; the other GI symptoms respond to treatment with prochlorperazine or trimethobenzamide. These side effects eventually disappear or diminish.

Other adverse effects include mental changes (ie, euphoria), which may progress to hypomania; restlessness; rapid speech; anxiety; insomnia; aggressiveness and agitation; mydriasis; lightheadedness; sleepiness; blurring of vision; bradycardia. Dyspnea, sometimes accompanied by hyperventilation and lightheadedness, is rare. L-5HTP/carbidopa might unmask subclinical scleroderma in patients with an abnormality in kynurenine metabolism.

➤*Overdosage:* Overdosage of L-5HTP/carbidopa can produce respiratory difficulties and hypotension.

INSULIN DETEMIR (by Novo Nordisk) – A long-acting insulin

➤*Actions:*

Pharmacology – Insulin detemir has been submitted to the FDA for approval as a treatment for patients with Type 1 diabetes mellitus or Type 2 diabetes mellitus who require basal (long-acting) insulin to control their hyperglycemia. Insulin detemir (Lys^{B29}-tetradecanoyl, des-(B30) human insulin; NN304) is a neutral, soluble insulin preparation in which the B29 lysine residue has been covalently bound to a 14-carbon fatty acid. The fatty acid extension facilitates the compounds ability to reservedly bind to albumin in the plasma, thereby prolonging the activity of insulin detemir by delaying its appearance in the interstitial fluid and delaying its action at insulin sensitive tissues.

The time-action profile of insulin detemir 0.15, 0.3, and 0.6 units/kg administered SC have been compared with that of NPH insulin 0.3 units/kg administered SC in 11 healthy volunteers. Peak insulin detemir concentrations were reached after 4 to 6 hours. A pronounced peak in metabolic effect was not observed with insulin detemir, in contrast with NPH insulin. Insulin detemir also demonstrated a slower onset of action. In a similar study, insulin detemir 0.3 and 0.6 units/kg also have been compared with NPH insulin 0.3 and 0.6 units/kg and placebo in 10 healthy volunteers. NPH insulin was more active at these doses than the equal doses of insulin detemir. As in the other study, insulin detemir was associated with a flatter activity profile. A similar crossover study has also been conducted comparing single doses of insulin detemir (0.1, 0.2, 0.4, 0.8, and 1.6 units/kg) and NPH insulin (0.3 units/kg) administered SC in 12 patients with Type 1 diabetes. While NPH insulin demonstrated peak activity around 6 to 8 hours, a flatter glucose infusion rate profile was observed for insulin detemir. The duration of action for the 0.4 unit/kg insulin detemir dose was 20 hours. In another study enrolling 6 patients with Type 1 diabetes, the peak action of insulin detemir was observed at 600 to 660 minutes after SC injection.

Pharmacokinetics – Insulin detemir is rapidly absorbed following SC administration, but slowly transported to the peripheral tissue. Insulin detemir is more than 98% bound to albumin in the plasma and more than 96% bound in the interstitial fluid. Only the free insulin detemir is available to cross the endothelial barrier. Peak plasma concentrations occur within 3 to 6 hours then decline to baseline within 24 hours. Maximal metabolic effect occurs within 6 to 11 hours after injection. The half-life of insulin detemir is 4 to 6 hours.

Clinical trials – Insulin detemir and NPH insulin were compared with a 6-month open-label study enrolling 747 patients with Type 1 diabetes. Patients were randomized 2:1 to therapy with insulin detemir or NPH insulin as basal insulin in conjunction with regular human insulin as bolus insulin. At baseline the mean age was 40.5 years, mean duration of diabetes was 16.9 years, mean body mass index was 25.2 kg/m^2, and mean HbA_{1C} was 8.35%. After 6 months glycemic control was similar (mean difference in HbA_{1C} [insulin detemir - NPH] was − 0.12% [95% CI − 0.25, 0.02]). Fasting plasma glucose levels were lower in patients treated with insulin detemir (−1.16 mmol/L, P = 0.001). The overall risk of hypoglycemia was similar in the 2 groups, although nocturnal hypoglycemia risk was 26% lower in patients receiving insulin detemir (P = 0.003). Patients lost a mean 0.2 kg in the insulin detemir group, but gained a mean of 0.4 kg in the NPH group after 6 months of therapy (baseline adjusted mean difference 0.5 kg, P = 0.003).

➤*Adverse Reactions:* Hypoglycemia is the most common adverse effect associated with insulin detemir therapy. SC injections of insulin detemir were well-tolerated.

➤*Summary:* Insulin detemir is a long-acting insulin formulation that will provide an alternative to NPH insulin and insulin glargine. Compared with NPH insulin, insulin detemir has a flat activity profile and does not produce peak insulin concentrations like that observed with NPH insulin. Comparisons with insulin glargine are not available. However, it appears that insulin detemir produces a similar type of flat activity profile as insulin glargine. Administer insulin detemir once or twice daily as a SC injection; however, insulin detemir is intended for once-daily SC administration at bedtime in most patients. The optimal dose and conversion factor for conversion from other long-acting insulin formulations have not been established. A New Drug Application was filed in December 2002 and an approvable letter was issued by the FDA in October 2003.

LACIDIPINE (*Lacipil* by GlaxoSmithKline) – A dihydropyridine calcium antagonist

➤*Actions:*

Pharmacology – Lacidipine, a 1,4 dihydropyridine calcium channel blocker, is a selective vasodilator that exerts little effect on myocardial contractility. The dose required to impair cardiac function is approximately 50 times greater than that needed for significant blood pressure reduction. Electrocardiographic studies indicate that it has no effect on SA node function or AV node conduction. Lacidipine effectively reduces blood pressure and decreases systemic vascular resistance by dilating peripheral and coronary arteries. This may lead to reflex tachycardia during the early stages of therapy. In addition to its cardiovascular effects, lacidipine has been shown in animal studies to have mild diuretic and natriuretic effects. In vitro studies also have demonstrated antioxidant activity and a possible tissue protective effect. As with other calcium channel blockers, there is some evidence to suggest activity toward inhibiting atherosclerosis. Lacidipine has been shown via a rat model to decrease infarct size following cerebral artery occlusion. The drug does not appear to affect carbohydrate or lipid metabolism.

Pharmacokinetics – Lacidipine is rapidly absorbed after oral administration and undergoes extensive first-pass metabolism. Virtually no parent drug is excreted in the urine or feces. Of the 2 primary metabolites, neither possesses pharmacologic activity. Due to the first-pass effect, the absolute bioavailability of lacidipine is < 20. Its high lipophilicity results in a prolonged pharmacologic effect, thus facilitating a single daily dose regimen. The elimination half-life ranges from 2 to 10 hours after a single dose, but increases to 12 to 15 hours at steady state. Plasma protein binding exceeds 90%. Volume of distribution after a single dose is ≈ 1 to 2 L/kg.

Metabolism of lacidipine is decreased in elderly patients and in those with liver impairment. The elimination of the drug appears to be unaffected by renal function.

Clinical trials – Dose titration studies involving over 400 patients with mild to moderate hypertension demonstrate a minimum response rate of 77%, as defined by the achievement of a diastolic blood pressure (DBP) ≤ 90 mmHg or a reduction in DBP of ≥ 15 mmHg. Doses of lacidipine ranged from 2 to 8 mg, administered once daily. One study treated 96 hypertensive patients with lacidipine, starting at a dose of 4 mg for 1 month. If DBP was not controlled after 1 month, the dose was increased to 8 mg. If DBP was not controlled after the second month, a beta blocker was added to the regimen. At 2 months, mean values for DBP and systolic blood pressure (SBP) dropped significantly. After 5 months, 87% of the patients were controlled: 63% on 4 mg, 21% on 8 mg, and 3% with combination therapy.

Studies have compared lacidipine 2 to 6 mg/day to hydrochlorothiazide (eg, *Esidrix*) 25 to 50 mg/day, atenolol (eg, *Tenormin*) 50 to 100 mg/day, sustained-release nifedipine (eg, *Procardia XL*) 20 to 40 mg twice daily and enalapril (*Vasotec*) 10 to 20 mg/day. In all cases, the differences in mean decrease for both SBP and DBP were not significantly different. In studies comparing lacidipine 4 mg/day to other long-acting dihydropyridine calcium antagonists, lacidipine showed greater antihypertensive effect than amlodipine (*Norvasc*) 10 mg/day and similar efficacy to that of isradipine 5 mg/day; further study is needed to clarify this issue.

➤*Adverse Reactions:* Adverse effects for lacidipine correspond to those expected for the dihydropyridine calcium antagonists, mostly due to the vasodilatory properties of these drugs: Headache (15%); flushing (10%); edema (8%); dizziness (6%); palpitations (5%); fatigue (4%); gastric irritation (3%). Generally, the side effects are mild and diminish over time. In most cases, they appear to be dose-related. Less common effects include paresthesia, impotence, and changes in liver function tests. The tolerability of lacidipine compares favorably to nifedipine; further study is needed to compare lacidipine with newer long-acting drugs in the class (eg, amlodipine).

➤*Summary:* Lacidipine appears to be a safe, effective agent for first-line treatment of mild to moderate hypertension. The recommended starting dose is 2 to 4 mg, titrated as needed up to 8 mg/day. Elderly patients and those with liver impairment should be started at 2 mg/day. Future clinical trials may elucidate additional beneficial effects of lacidipine and perhaps define new therapeutic roles for the drug.

Lacidipine is marketed as an antihypertensive drug in Europe by GlaxoSmithKline and other companies. It can be found under a variety of trade names, including *Lacipil*, *Viapres*, *Lacirex*, and *Motens*.

LEVOSIMENDAN (*Simdax* by Orion Pharma) – A calcium sensitizer

➤*Actions:*

Pharmacology – Levosimendan is a calcium sensitizer developed for the treatment of decompensated heart failure. It sensitizes troponin C to calcium and is dependent on calcium concentration. It increases the effects of calcium on cardiac myofilaments during systole when calcium concentration is increased. Normal diastolic relaxation occurs because of decreasing calcium concentration and sensitization. Levosimendan also opens ATP-sensitive potassium channels on vascular smooth muscle, causing coronary and systemic vasodilation. These dual mechanisms result in an increase in cardiac output without an increase in myocardial oxygen demand.

Pharmacokinetics – Levosimendan is well absorbed with a bioavailability of 85%; however, an oral formulation is not available. Approximately 97% of levosimendan is protein bound, mostly to albumin. The elimination half-life of levosimendan is 1 hour. Elimination is mainly by conjugation and excretion takes place in the urine and feces. A linear relationship is seen between the dose administered and the plasma concentration of levosimendan.

An active metabolite, OR-1896, is formed by acetylation and accounts for approximately 5% of the total plasma concentration of levosimendan. Peak concentration of OR-1896 is achieved 1 to 2 days after cessation of a 24-hour infusion of levosimendan. OR-1896 has a half-life of approximately 80 hours, and its pharmacologic effects may last for approximately 1 week. The duration of effect of levosimendan may be increased in rapid acetylators because of an increase in the formation of OR-1896. Levosimendan is not metabolized by cytochrome-P isoenzymes.

Renal dysfunction has little effect on levosimendan concentration but does prolong the half-life of OR-1896. The elimination half-life of levosimendan is slightly prolonged by liver cirrhosis; however, the effects on the production or metabolism of OR 1896 are unknown.

Clinical trials – A randomized, double-blind, dose-ranging study comparing levosimendan with placebo enrolled 504 patients with decompensated heart failure complicating acute myocardial infarction. The patients were randomized to receive either placebo or 1 of 4 dose regimens of levosimendan: 6 mcg/kg loading dose plus 0.1 mcg/kg/min continuous infusion; 12 mcg/kg loading dose plus 0.2 mcg/kg/min continuous infusion; 24 mcg/kg loading dose plus 0.2 mcg/kg/min continuous infusion; 24 mcg/kg loading dose plus 0.4 mcg/kg/min continuous infusion. The combined risk of death and worsening heart failure was lower for the 6-hour infusion compared with placebo (2% vs 5.9%, respectively; $P = 0.033$) and for 24 hours after the start of the infusion (4% vs 8.8%, respectively; $P = 0.044$). Sinus tachycardia was most common in the highest levosimendan dose group (5%). Myocardial rupture occurred more frequently with placebo than with levosimendan (3.9% vs 0.25%, respectively; $P = 0.027$).

A randomized, double-blind, double-dummy, parallel-group clinical trial comparing levosimendan with dobutamine enrolled 203 patients with low-output heart failure that required treatment with an IV inotropic agent. Patients were treated with either a loading dose of 24 mcg/kg levosimendan over 10 minutes followed by a continuous infusion of 0.1 mcg/kg/min levosimendan, or a continuous infusion of 5 mcg/kg/min dobutamine without a loading dose. At 24 hours, hemodynamic performance had improved in 28% of the levosimendan patients vs 15% of the dobutamine patients ($P = 0.022$). In the levosimendan group, 8% of the patients died within 31 days compared with 17% of the dobutamine group ($P = 0.049$). The most common adverse events seen with levosimendan use were headache or migraine (14%) and hypotension (9%). Rate and rhythm disorders and angina pectoris, chest pain, or myocardial ischemia occurred more frequently in the dobutamine group.

➤*Adverse Reactions:* The most common adverse reactions reported in clinical trials were headache, hypotension, and dizziness related to vasodilatory effects of levosimendan. Levosimendan was associated with tachycardia and ventricular extrasystoles in studies vs placebo. When compared with dobutamine, levosimendan was associated with increased incidence of headache and hypotension.

➤*Summary:* Studies conducted to date suggest that levosimendan is a unique positive inotropic agent for use in decompensated heart failure. Based on clinical data, levosimendan is more efficacious than dobutamine and appears to be associated with fewer adverse events. Levosimendan has been approved in several European countries. It is currently in phase 3 trials in the United States.

LOFEXIDINE HCl (by Britannia Pharmaceuticals Limited) – An α_2 adrenergic agonist for the treatment of opioid withdrawal symptoms

➤*Actions:*

Pharmacology – Lofexidine is a centrally acting α_2 adrenergic agonist. It is structurally related to clonidine, which has been used in the treatment of opiate withdrawal syndrome. Adrenergic agonists effectively suppress withdrawal symptoms, which may originate from adrenergic hyperactivity in the locus caeruleus.

Pharmacokinetics – Lofexidine exhibits a biphasic decline in plasma concentration. First phase half-life ranges from 1.3 to 3.7 hours; second phase half-life ranges from 9 to 18.3 hours.

Clinical trials – One randomized, double-blind study examined clinical response to methadone or lofexidine in treating 86 polydrug-abusing opiate addicts experiencing withdrawal. In this study, 42 patients received 0.6 mg lofexidine initially, increasing by 0.4 mg/day for 3 days. After the titration, patients were maintained on 2 mg/day for 3 days, followed by downward titration of 0.4 mg/day for 3 days. Investigators concluded that lofexidine and methadone are clinically equivalent with regard to overall treatment retention, although patients receiving lofexidine experienced more withdrawal symptoms than those receiving methadone.

Another randomized, double-blind study compared lofexidine with clonidine in treating 80 heroin addicts undergoing opiate withdrawal. Forty patients received four 0.2 mg lofexidine capsules during the first day of treatment. The investigator adjusted subsequent dosing based on evaluation of withdrawal symptoms and blood pressure. The maximum daily dose was 1.6 mg lofexidine. The results indicated that lofexidine and clonidine are equally effective in managing opiate withdrawal syndrome, and that fewer patients receiving lofexidine therapy experienced significant hypotension than patients in the clonidine group. Lofexidine therapy was withheld on 10.1% of patient-days due to hypotension, compared with 20.9% of patient-days during clonidine therapy.

This product is available in the United Kingdom. The recommended initial dose is 0.2 mg twice daily and may be increased by 0.2 to 0.4 mg/day to 2.4 mg maximum daily dose. Recommended duration of therapy is 7 to 10 days.

➤*Drug Interactions:* CNS depression associated with alcohol, barbiturates, and other sedatives may be enhanced with lofexidine administration. Lofexidine efficacy may be reduced with coadministration of tricyclic antidepressants.

➤*Adverse Reactions:* In clinical trials, the most common side effects associated with lofexidine therapy included dry mouth, dizziness, bradycardia, sedation, hypotension, lethargy, and headache. The risk of hypotension increases with increasing doses. Rebound hypertension may occur with sudden withdrawal. Avoid use of this agent in patients with cerebrovascular disease, ischemic heart disease, bradycardia, renal impairment, or history of depression.

➤*Summary:* The relief of acute opiate withdrawal syndrome is only one goal in a complex strategy for successful opiate addiction treatment. Effective therapy also must address social and psychological issues.

Adrenergic agonists have been studied for opiate withdrawal treatment for > 20 years and provide a nonnarcotic alternative for this use. Among agents in this class, lofexidine appears to be safer for withdrawal syndrome. Several small trials have been published that examine the use of lofexidine for suppression of opiate withdrawal symptoms; however, additional larger studies are needed. Lofexidine currently is being evaluated in phase III trials for this indication.

MILNACIPRAN (*Ixel* by Cypress Bioscience) – A serotonin norepinephrine reuptake inhibitor

➤*Actions:*

Pharmacology – Milnacipran is a cyclopropane derivative currently being considered for use in fibromyalgia and depression. It inhibits norepinephrine and serotonin reuptake at presynaptic sites. The drug does not interact with postsynaptic receptors, including adrenergic and muscarinic receptors, leading to significantly improved patient tolerance.

Pharmacokinetics – Milnacipran is rapidly and extensively absorbed from the GI tract with an absolute bioavailability of greater than 85%. Maximum plasma concentrations were observed in nearly 2 hours after administration, with indistinguishable profiles between IV or orally administered drug. The drug is excreted via active tubular secretion and the elimination half-life is 8 hours. Milnacipran has a low affinity for plasma proteins, binding only 13%. The main product of metabolism is the glucuronic acid conjugate and is present in plasma concentrations similar to the parent drug. Other metabolites are considered clinically insignificant. Cytochrome P450 enzymes are not implicated in the metabolism of milnacipran. The drug is not influenced by either age or liver insufficiency. Since the drug and its main metabolite are excreted via active tubular secretion, adjust the dose of milnacipran in patients with renal impairment.

Clinical trials – Milnacipran has been shown to be an effective antidepressant in controlled trials. The efficacy of milnacipran has been compared with both standard tricyclic antidepressants (imipramine, amitriptyline, clomipramine) and selective serotonin reuptake inhibitors (SSRIs) (fluoxetine, fluvoxamine). Studies comparing tricyclics and milnacipran have shown comparable efficacy. However, in a 26-week, double-blind, randomized, parallel study of 107 patients comparing clomipramine with milnacipran, milnacipran was shown to be inferior with respect to the rate of responders. The mean change in the Hamilton Depression Rating Scale (HAMD) score between the baseline and the last rating ranged from 23.7 to 12 in the milnacipran-treated patients and from 23.1 to 8 in the clomipramine-treated patients. In a 6-week, randomized, double-blind comparison of milnacipran with imipramine in 109 patients, milnacipran and imipramine were shown to be of equivalent efficacy. The reduction in HAMD scores was not significantly different. The mean change in score for the milnacipran group was 17.3 and 15.7 for the imipramine group. The overall reporting of adverse events was lower with milnacipran, while there were significantly more withdrawals from the imipramine group because of adverse events.

In a 6-week, randomized, parallel-group study comparing milnacipran with fluvoxamine in 113 patients, milnacipran was shown to be of superior efficacy with a decreased incidence of adverse events. The overall HAMD scores decreased by a mean of 62.1% for the milnacipran group and by 49.3% in the fluvoxamine group ($P = 0.05$).

A 12-week, phase 2 study of milnacipran for the treatment of fibromyalgia pain was completed in 125 patients. Patients who received milnacipran experienced statistical improvement in pain scores compared with those who received placebo. Other symptoms that showed statistical improvement were fatigue, mood, physical function, and patient global scores.

➤*Adverse Reactions:* Milnacipran has been shown to have a superior adverse event profile over tricyclic antidepressants and are generally better tolerated than the SSRIs. The most common adverse reactions experienced are abdominal pain, anxiety, constipation, dose-related nausea, dry mouth, dysuria, somnolence, tremor, and vertigo.

➤*Summary:* Milnacipran is a serotonin norepinephrine reuptake inhibitor that has been shown to be safe and effective for the treatment of depression. While being comparable in efficacy to the tricyclic antidepressants and superior in efficacy to the SSRIs, milnacipran is much less likely to cause adverse events. Milnacipran is currently undergoing phase 3 trials for use in the treatment of fibromyalgia syndrome, while being studied in preclinical trials for use in the treatment of irritable bowel syndrome.

~ Bibliography Available on Request ~

MURAGLITAZAR (*Pargluva* by Bristol-Myers Squibb) – A nonthiazolidinedione oxybenzylglycine dual alpha/gamma peroxisome proliferators-activated receptor (PPAR) agonist

➤*Actions:*

Pharmacology – Muraglitazar is a nonthiazolidinedione oxybenzylglycine dual alpha/gamma peroxisome proliferators-activated receptor (PPAR) agonist used in the treatment of patients with type 2 diabetes. In animal models, muraglitazar has been shown to prevent hyperglycemia and preserve pancreatic beta-cell function; reduce glucose, insulin, and lipid levels; reduce weight gain and adipocyte size; and increase basal metabolic rate.

Pharmacokinetics – Peak muraglitazar levels are reached within 1 to 6 hours following oral administration. The mean half-life ranges from 19 to 27 hours.

Clinical trials – Comparative trials with active control muraglitazar was compared with pioglitazone in a randomized, double-blind study enrolling 1,477 patients with type 2 diabetes inadequately controlled with diet and exercise. Patients received 1 of 5 doses of muraglitazar ranging from 0.5 to 20 mg or pioglitazone 15 mg once daily for 24 weeks. At 24 weeks, HbA_{1c} was reduced to 1.18% from 8.2% ($P < 0.0001$), and the fasting plasma glucose level was reduced 40 mg/dL in the patients treated with muraglitazar 5 mg ($P < 0.0001$). HbA_{1c} of 7% or less was achieved in 62% of patients treated with muraglitazar 5 mg (NNT = 6.7) and 47% treated with pioglitazone 15 mg. HbA_{1c} of 6.5% or less was achieved in 43% treated with muraglitazar 5 mg, compared with 26% of the patients treated with pioglitazone 15 mg. Lipid effects were assessed in 985 patients who completed the 24-week portion of the study and continued therapy for up to 2 years. Triglycerides were reduced 13.2% in the muraglitazar 1.5 mg group (75 patients), 22.4% in the muraglitazar 5 mg group (108 patients), and 12.3% of the patients in the pioglitazone group (65 patients). High-density lipoprotein (HDL) cholesterol was increased 17.2% in the muraglitazar 1.5 mg group, 28.9% in the muraglitazar 5 mg group, and 17.7% in the pioglitazone group. Non-HDL cholesterol was reduced 11.4% in the muraglitazar 1.5 mg group, 11.3% in the muraglitazar 5 mg group, and 8.8% in the pioglitazone group.

Muraglitazar was also compared with pioglitazone in a randomized, double-blind study enrolling 1,159 patients with type 2 diabetes inadequately controlled on metformin alone. Patients received muraglitazar 5 mg once daily or pioglitazone 30 mg once daily for 24 weeks while continuing metformin at a stable dose. Mean baseline HbA_{1c} was 8.1%. All analysis was conducted on the mean change from baseline; each was adjusted for baseline and used a last-observation-carried-forward technique for missing data. Mean daily metformin doses at baseline were 1,854 mg in the muraglitazar group and 1,851 mg in the pioglitazone group. After 24 weeks, HbA_{1c} was reduced 0.29% more in the muraglitazar group than the pioglitazone group (1.14% vs –0.85%, $P < 0.0001$). HbA_{1c} of less than 7% was achieved in 60% of muraglitazar-treated patients and 44% of pioglitazone-treated patients (NNT = 6.3). HbA_{1c} of less than 6.5% was achieved in 34% of patients treated with muraglitazar and 23% treated with pioglitazone. Adjusted mean fasting plasma glucose levels were also reduced to a greater extent in the muraglitazar group (–44 mg/dL vs –33 mg/dL). Edema occurred in 9.2% of patients in the muraglitazar group, compared with 7.2% of patients in the pioglitazone group. Mean weight gain was 1.4 kg in the muraglitazar group, compared with 0.6 kg in the pioglitazone group.

➤*Adverse Reactions:* Adverse reactions reported in clinical studies included hypoglycemia, weight gain, edema, and congestive heart failure.

➤*Summary:* Additional study results are necessary to determine the role of muraglitazar in the treatment of patients with type 2 diabetes; however, its effects on glucose and lipids are promising. The FDA issued an approvable letter for muraglitazar on October 18, 2005.

NITRENDIPINE (*Baypress* by Bayer) – A Type II calcium channel blocking agent

➤*Actions:*

Pharmacology – Nitrendipine is a 1,4-dihydropyridine derivative calcium entry blocker, structurally similar to nifedipine. It is further classified as a type II calcium antagonist because, at usual doses and concentrations, it is devoid of electrophysiologic effects but is a potent peripheral vasodilator. Relaxation of peripheral vascular smooth muscle occurs as a result of inhibition of calcium influx across cellular membranes.

Nitrendipine causes a decrease in systolic and diastolic blood pressure, primarily due to arteriolar dilation. Significant peripheral venodilation is unlikely, because postural hypotension is usually not seen. Reflex increases in heart rate, AV nodal conduction, and myocardial contractility occur frequently at therapeutic doses and may precipitate myocardial ischemia in patients with coronary artery disease. Plasma renin activity and catecholamine concentrations increase during therapy with nitrendipine; however, the fact that it reduces the pressor response to norepinephrine but affects no change in responses to angiotensin II may explain its greater effectiveness in the treatment of low-renin hypertension. Nitrendipine does not alter glomerular filtration rate (GFR), renal blood flow, or plasma aldosterone levels. A short-term, modest diuretic and natriuretic effect has been observed on initiation of therapy.

The dose/response relationship for this effect appears to be flat; a 10 mg dose produces maximum diuresis. It is unlikely that this has any therapeutic implications during long-term therapy. Preliminary data suggest that nitrendipine has no effect on blood glucose, total cholesterol, triglyceride, or uric acid levels.

Pharmacokinetics – Available pharmacokinetic data are based on experience with small numbers of patients using assays of varying sensitivity; data vary.

Nitrendipine appears to be well absorbed after oral administration. Peak serum concentrations are seen at 1 to 2 hours; peak effect is seen at approximately 4 hours. The distribution half-life ($t_{1/2}$-α) is approximately 1 hour. Beta elimination half-life ($t_{1/2}$-β) averages 8 to 11 hours. Nitrendipine is metabolized by the liver to an inactive pyridine analog and to several more polar metabolites that are excreted in the urine. Dosage adjustments appear to be necessary in patients with hepatic dysfunction, but specific guidelines are not established. A single-dose study in 16 patients with various degrees of renal dysfunction found no alterations in any kinetic parameters; dosage adjustments appear unnecessary in renal patients.

Clinical trials – Nitrendipine is effective in the treatment of mild to moderate hypertension (diastolic blood pressure 90 to 114 mmHg). Initial data suggest that the drug is particularly useful in low-renin hypertension, which accounts for 20% to 30% of the hypertensive population. Doses of 10 to 80 mg/day have been used, administered as a single dose or in 2 to 3 divided doses per day. Although a single daily dose will decrease blood pressure for 24 hours, most patients require twice-daily dosing for optimal blood pressure control. Due to reflex increases in heart rate and contractility, concomitant β-blocker therapy may be required in some patients. It has not been determined whether nitrendipine, like verapamil and nifedipine, tends to be more effective in older patients.

➤*Adverse Reactions:* Nitrendipine has a side effect profile similar to nifedipine. The side effect reported most frequently is headache. Fatigue, peripheral edema, flushing, palpitations, dizziness, polyuria, and mild elevations in liver function (in 2 patients) also have occurred.

➤*Summary:* Nitrendipine is a potent vasodilator that effectively reduces blood pressure when given 1 to 3 times/day. The drug appears most useful in low-renin hypertensives. Biochemical abnormalities common to other currently used antihypertensives (eg, hypokalemia, hyperglycemia, increased uric acid and lipids) are not seen with this class of drugs and may represent an advantage over β-blockers and diuretics. Although most patients will require twice-daily dosing, the only other available dihydropyridine (nifedipine) usually requires dosing 3 to 4 times/day.

A New Drug Application (NDA) is pending with the FDA for an antihypertensive indication. Nitrendipine will be comarketed by Miles and Roche; however, there are no plans to market nitrendipine at this time.

NXY-059 (*Cerovive* by AstraZeneca/Renovis) – A neuroprotectant

➤*Actions:*

Pharmacology – NXY-059 is in development as a neuroprotectant in patients with acute ischemic stroke (AIS). NXY-059 is a nitrone-based free radical trapping neuroprotectant that appears to reduce brain damage by neutralizing free radicals released during a stroke. Free radicals, which are generated rapidly in response to ischemia, trigger tissue oxidation, a major contributor to brain injury. Therefore, trapping these free radicals helps reduce neuronal injury, tissue damage, and ultimately stroke-related mortality and disability.

Pharmacokinetics – The steady-state concentration (C_{ss}) and area under the curve are linear relative to dose with approximately 93% of the C_{ss} reached in 4 hours. NXY-059 has a volume of distribution of approximately 16 L, and approximately 40% is protein bound. The elimination half-life in 48 healthy volunteers was approximately 2.6 hours, and the plasma clearance was approximately 7 L/h. Renal secretion accounted for over one third of renal clearance of the drug, while glomerular filtration accounted for the rest, with 82 to 89% being excreted unchanged in the urine. The terminal half-life in patients with moderate and severe renal impairment was 10 to 12 hours, potentially 5 times that of healthy adults. There appears to be a strong correlation between the clearance of NXY-059 and a patient's creatinine clearance (Ccr), thus dosing adjustments may be necessary in patients with renal impairment (Ccr less than 80 mL/min) in the elderly.

Clinical Trials – A multinational, multicenter, randomized, double-blind, placebo-controlled phase trial comparing NXY-059 with placebo enrolled 1,699 patients with acute ischemic stroke presenting within 6 hours of stroke onset. The patients were randomized to receive either placebo or NXY-059: 2,270 mg/h for 1 hour loading dose, followed by 480 to 960 mg/h for 71 hours. Patients receiving NXY-059 had significantly better scores on the primary outcome of disability as assessed on the Modified Rankin Scale (mRS) at 90 days ($P = 0.038$). Additional analysis of the data showed that 15.4% of the patients in the NXY-059 arm had an mRS score of 0, indicating no disability at 90 days, versus 11% of the 849 patients in the placebo arm ($P = 0.003$). However, on the National Institutes of Health Stroke Scale, NXY-059 did not significantly improve neurological function, and mortality was unaffected by treatment with NXY-059 compared with placebo ($P = 0.89$).

➤*Drug Interactions:* No drug interactions have been reported, but caution with NXY-059 is advised when using other medications that are renally cleared.

➤*Adverse Reactions:* The incidence and profile of adverse reactions were similar between groups. The most common adverse reactions occurring in both groups (5% or more) were pyrexia, constipation, headache, urinary tract infection, atrial fibrillation, hypertension, and hypokalemia. Symptomatic hemorrhage in patients treated with NXY-059 in combination with alteplase was lower than in patients treated with placebo and alteplase (2.5% vs 6.4%, respectively; $P = 0.036$). Asymptomatic hemorrhage occurred in 12.9% of patients who received alteplase and NXY-059, and in 20.9% of patients who received alteplase and placebo. Intracranial hemorrhage among patients not receiving thrombolysis was similar in both groups. This is noteworthy because current treatment options for AIS are unsafe for use in hemorrhagic stroke patients and require a computerized tomography scan prior to administration.

➤*Summary:* Available data suggest that NXY-059 may potentially provide a moderate benefit for most patients when used within 6 hours of the onset of a stroke. The optimal dosing method is the use of a loading dose followed by a continuous infusion, administered up to 6 hours after a stroke. The optimal dose has not yet been established, although clinical trials have administered NXY-059 as a 1 hour bolus of 2,270 mg followed by a maintenance dose of 480 to 960 mg per hour for 71 hours, with an aim of maintaining a target concentration of 260 mcmol/L. Although adverse reactions were similar to placebo, dosage adjustments may need to be made for patients with renal insufficiency and the elderly. SAINT II, an ongoing phase III trial, has a larger population and is expected to provide sufficient power to replicate the findings of SAINT I. In addition, the results of CHANT, a trial to assess the safety and tolerability of NXY-059 in acute intracerebral hemorrhage patients, found that there are comparable mortality rates (20% in each group) and stroke outcomes compared with placebo. A new drug application is expected to be filed with the FDA in the first half of 2007, pending positive results from SAINT II.

OMAPATRILAT (by Bristol-Myers Squibb) – A vasopeptidase inhibitor (VPI)

➤*Actions:*

Pharmacology – Omapatrilat is a vasopeptidase inhibitor (VPI) that simultaneously inhibits neural endopeptidase and angiotensin-converting enzyme. Oral administration of omapatrilat showed potent and long-lasting antihypertensive effects in low-, normal-, and high-renin animal models.

Omapatrilat has been shown to be a potent antihypertensive agent and to increase cardiac output, decrease left ventricular end-diastolic and peak systolic pressures, and decrease peripheral vascular resistance in patients with heart failure. The efficacy of omapatrilat suggests a utility in a broad range of patient types. The ability of vasopeptidase inhibition to lower arterial pressure, regardless of renin activation or sodium status, suggests a synergistic interplay between potentiation of the natriuretic peptide system (NPS) and inhibition of the renin-angiotensin-aldosterone system (RAAS).

Pharmacokinetics – Omapatrilat has an oral bioavailability of ≈ 30%, with a protein binding of 80%. It may be given with or without food, and it has a very large volume of distribution (1800 L), suggesting tissue penetration. The time to maximum concentration of an oral dose is ≈ 2 hours. Omapatrilat's effective half-life is 14 to 19 hours.

This drug is metabolized in the liver, forms disulphide bonds with endogenous thiols, and is extensively metabolized via amide hydrolysis, glucuronidation, S-oxidation, and S-methylation. There are no active metabolites of omapatrilat found in plasma. Approximately 80% of an IV dose and 64% of an oral dose were recovered in urine, with < 1% excreted as unchanged drug. Renal function does not appear to influence the disposition or excretion of omapatrilat and hemodialysis does not contribute to its clearance.

Biotransformation data based on in vivo and in vitro studies suggest that cytochrome P450 is not involved in the metabolism of omapatrilat. Several studies have shown that omapatrilat does not inhibit P450 isoenzymes CYP-1A2, CYP-3A4, CYP-2C19, CYP-2D6, and CYP-2C9. Omapatrilat has no known interaction with other medications.

Clinical trials – In a parallel, dose-finding, placebo-controlled trial, 174 patients with mild to moderate hypertension were divided into groups of ≈ 25 each and given daily doses of 1, 5, 12.5, 30, or 75 mg omapatrilat or placebo. The main efficacy end-point was the change from baseline in the average 24-hour ambulatory diastolic blood pressure on the last day of the double-blind treatment period. Omapatrilat produced dose-dependent decreases in the average 24-hour ambulatory blood pressure. Omapatrilat produced greater reductions in systolic blood pressure than diastolic pressure. Seven days after discontinuation of treatment, trough seated blood pressure was still decreased compared with baseline in all active drug groups. This may mean that rebound hypertension is unlikely with discontinuation or interruption of therapy. In patients ≥ 65 years of age, as well as in African-Americans, omapatrilat significantly reduced systolic and diastolic blood pressure. No changes in heart rate were associated with the antihypertensive effects of omapatrilat.

Another randomized, double-blind, multicenter trial of 369 patients with NYHA class II-IV heart failure evaluated the efficacy of omapatrilat 2.5, 5, 10, 20, or 40 mg/day for 12 weeks. Omapatrilat was administered once daily for 12 weeks; the first 190 patients received doses of 2.5, 5, or 10 mg, and the last 179 patients received doses of 2.5, 20, or 40 mg. Ejection fraction improved in a dose-dependent fashion and heart rate decreased with omapatrilat. Cardiac index remained unchanged while arterial pressure also decreased in a dose-related manner. The combined incidence of cointervention for heart failure, hospitalization, or death was 34% with 2.5 mg omapatrilat and 19% with 40 mg omapatrilat.

➤*Adverse Reactions:* Side effects were investigated in 1 clinical trial comparing omapatrilat with lisinopril in 573 patients with class II-IV CHF. More adverse events related to the GI tract (nausea, vomiting, constipation, and diarrhea), as well as neurological symptoms (eg, dizziness, vision disturbances, and hypotension) were noted with omapatrilat as compared with lisinopril.

In data submitted for the New Drug Application for omapatrilat, 44 instances of angioedema occurred among > 6000 patients, and 4 cases were severe enough to require intubation.

➤*Summary:* Omapatrilat represents a new class of pharmacologic agents that alter the balance of circulating and local humoral factors in favor of vasodilation. Omapatrilat offers the promise to be an important new advancement in the treatment of hypertension and heart failure. However, because of the instances of angioedema, additional studies are necessary to further define its place in therapy for efficacy and adverse effects. The FDA issued an approvable letter in 2002.

OXYPURINOL SODIUM (*Oxiprim* by Cardiome Pharma) – A xanthine oxidase inhibitor

➤*Actions:*

Pharmacology – Oxypurinol is indicated for the treatment of hyperuricemia in patients with symptomatic gout who are intolerant of allopurinol and have failed either rechallenge or desensitization with allopurinol. Oxypurinol is the active metabolite of allopurinol and is a xanthine oxidase inhibitor. The conversion of allopurinol to oxypurinol is catalyzed by the enzyme xanthine oxidase, and is associated with the generation of superoxide radicals that may contribute to some of the adverse reactions observed with allopurinol. It has been suggested that oxypurinol may be tolerated by some patients who are intolerant of allopurinol. Approximately 2% to 4% of patients treated with allopurinol develop a rash or other intolerance requiring discontinuation of therapy. Oxypurinol may be tolerated by approximately 70% of these patients, representing approximately 7,000 to 14,000 patients in the United States.

Pharmacokinetics – The relative bioavailability of oxypurinol is approximately 30% of allopurinol. Systemic availability is increased approximately 2-fold with administration of a high-fat meal. The plasma half-life of oxypurinol is 18 to 30 hours. With its longer half-life, oxypurinol is responsible for the maintenance of xanthine oxidase inhibition observed following once-daily allopurinol administration. Oxypurinol is not metabolized. Approximately 40% of the dose is eliminated renally. Oxypurinol is cleared by a standard 4-hour hemodialysis.

Clinical trials – Oxypurinol and allopurinol were compared in a randomized, double-blind, crossover study enrolling 99 male hyperuricemic patients (plasma uric acid greater than 7.5 mg/dL requiring treatment) with normal renal function (serum creatinine 1.5 mg/dL or less). Patients were randomized to receive allopurinol 300 mg or an equimolar amount of oxypurinol (384 mg) once daily in the morning for 10 or 14 days, followed by a crossover to the alternate therapy for 10 or 14 days. In the group treated with allopurinol, followed by oxypurinol (n = 51), mean plasma uric acid declined from 8.3 mg/dL at baseline to 5.4 mg/dL with allopurinol, then increased slightly to 5.7 mg/dL with oxypurinol. In the group treated with oxypurinol, followed by allopurinol (n = 48), mean plasma uric acid declined from 8.7 mg/dL at baseline to 6 mg/dL with oxypurinol, and then further declined to 5.6 mg/dL with allopurinol. The overall average reduction from baseline was 3 mg/dL with allopurinol and 2.6 mg/dL with oxypurinol ($P = 0.027$). The 90% confidence interval for the level of plasma uric acid with oxypurinol compared with the level achieved with allopurinol was 102.4% vs 110.6%, suggesting uric acid levels with an equimolar dose of oxypurinol will be higher than those achieved with allopurinol, but probably no more than 10% greater. The mean plasma oxypurinol concentration was 9.24 mcg/dL at the end of the allopurinol-treatment period and 9.9 mcg/dL at the end of the oxypurinol-treatment period (not significant). Hematocrit and leukocyte counts were reduced during oxypurinol treatment, but not during allopurinol treatment.

➤*Drug Interactions:* Drug interaction studies with oxypurinol have not been published. Drug interactions with oxypurinol are likely to be similar to those observed with allopurinol.

➤*Adverse Reactions:* Adverse reactions attributed to oxypurinol therapy in clinical trials include headache, nausea, and vomiting.

➤*Summary:* If approved, oxypurinol will offer an alternative for some patients with symptomatic gout who are unable to tolerate allopurinol therapy because of mild or moderate allergic-type reactions (including cutaneous, hepatic, renal, or hematologic reactions). Use of oxypurinol should be reserved for such patients. Oxypurinol has been available through a compassionate-use protocol for patients with allopurinol intolerance since 1966. The usual effective dosage of oxypurinol is 300 to 800 mg/day. Therapy should be initiated with a 100 mg dose and subsequently titrated in 100 mg increments weekly or every other week, as tolerated, until the target serum uric acid level is achieved or a maximum dosage of 800 mg/day is reached. Oxypurinol is contraindicated in patients with a history of severe hypersensitivity to oxypurinol or severe hypersensitivity reaction to allopurinol. A new drug application for oxypurinol was submitted to the FDA in December 2003 and accepted for priority review. The application was granted approvable status in June 2004, pending submission of additional clinical and manufacturing data.

PHENFORMIN – Available under IND exemption

Indications

May be used only in patients with adult-onset, nonketotic diabetics who meet all of the following criteria: In addition to elevated blood glucose, have symptoms such as polydipsia; symptoms are not controlled with diet and sulfonylureas or patient cannot take sulfonylureas because of nontolerance or allergy; symptoms are controlled by phenformin; there are no underlying risk factors that contraindicate the use; (a) his/her occupation is such that the risk of hypoglycemia from insulin would threaten his/her job or be a hazard to him/her or others, or (b) patient cannot take insulin because of disability and has no practical way to receive assistance.

Phenformin also is available under a separate IND for a dermatological condition called atrophie blanche or livedo vasculitis.

Contraindications

Although there is no absolute way to predict the population at risk for lactic acidosis, the following are recognized contraindications: Insulin-dependent diabetes; hypersensitivity to phenformin; renal disease with even mild degrees of impaired renal function; liver disease; history of lactic acidosis; alcohol abuse; any acute medical situation such as cardiovascular collapse (shock), CHF, MI, surgery or septicemia; disease states that may be associated with hypoxemia; complications of diabetes such as metabolic acidosis, coma, infection or gangrene; acute GI disturbances (vomiting or diarrhea), which are likely to result in dehydration and prerenal azotemia.

➤*Adverse Reactions:* Lactic acidosis in patients taking phenformin has been estimated to occur in 0.25 to 4 cases per 1000 phenformin treatment years. Lactic acidosis is characterized by elevated lactate levels, increased lactate-to-pyruvate ratio and decreased blood pH. In many of the reported cases, azotemia ranging from mild to severe was present.

Nausea, vomiting, hyperventilation, malaise, or abdominal pain may herald the onset of lactic acidosis. Instruct the patient to discontinue phenformin and notify the physician immediately if any of these symptoms occur.

Warn patients against using alcohol while receiving phenformin, because ethanol and phenformin potentiate the tendency of each to cause elevated blood lactate levels.

➤*Summary:* The biguanide hypoglycemic agent, phenformin, was removed from the US market on October 23, 1977, as a result of concern over the unacceptably high risk of lactic acidosis associated with its use. Phenformin is now available only through an Investigational New Drug (IND) Application, which must be filed with the US Food and Drug Administration. Use of phenformin is restricted to specific clearly defined situations and requires registration and reporting to the FDA. Complete information on use of phenformin, physician sponsor applications, patient consent forms, and request forms for ordering phenformin tablets or capsules are available from:

Center for Drug Evaluation and Research
Division of Metabolism and Endocrine
Drug Products (HFD-510)
Room 14-B-19
5600 Fishers Lane
Rockville, Maryland 20857
301-443-3510

Although phenformin has been removed from the market because of the potential for adverse effects, a select group of patients may require use of this agent. Careful patient selection is necessary to assure a reasonable risk-benefit ratio. Supplies of phenformin are available to practicing physicians from the FDA under an IND exemption.

~ Bibliography Available on Request ~

PINACIDIL (*Pindac* by Lilly) – An antihypertensive agent

➤*Actions:*

Pharmacology – Pinacidil is a vasodilator under investigation for use as an antihypertensive agent. Pinacidil acts at the level of the precapillary, arteriolar (resistance) vessels, causing direct relaxation of vascular smooth muscle. Its vasodilator effect is not altered by blockade of β-adrenergic, cholinergic, or histaminic receptors, or by the presence of prostaglandin inhibitors such as indomethacin.

When compared with other vasodilators with similar sites of action (eg, minoxidil [*Loniten*], guancydine, diazoxide [*Hyperstat*]), pinacidil, at comparable levels of blood pressure reduction, produces quantitatively identical increases in heart rate, reflex sympathetic mediated cardiac contractility, and cardiac output. However, when compared with hydralazine (another precapillary arteriolar vasodilator), pinacidil, at doses that produce equivalent reductions in total peripheral resistance, is a more potent blood pressure lowering agent. Because blood pressure is a function of the cardiac output multiplied by the total peripheral resistance, this difference may be explained by the fact that hydralazine appears to have a direct (as well as the indirect) cardiostimulatory effect that offsets some of the blood pressure reduction caused by vasodilation. As would be expected from their differing effects on cardiac output, pinacidil produces less of an increase in myocardial oxygen consumption than hydralazine.

Although an active metabolite has been identified, it does not appear to contribute significantly to the overall antihypertensive activity.

There is a linear correlation between pinacidil drug levels and the fall in mean blood pressure and total peripheral resistance; minimal therapeutic levels are 50 ng/mL.

Pharmacokinetics –

Absorption/Distribution: Available data are complicated by the fact that at least 2 different oral formulations have been used in clinical trials. However, in general, bioavailability approaches 100% after oral administration, with both peak serum levels and effect occurring at 1 hour. Coadministration of food does not alter bioavailability but slightly delays absorption. Approximately 60% of a dose is protein bound.

Metabolism/Excretion: Pinacidil is metabolized by the liver to a number of metabolites, the most significant being the active metabolite, pinacidil N-oxide. Within the first 24 hours, 55% to 60% of an administered dose appears in the urine as pinacidil or the N-oxide, 20% to 30% is excreted in the urine as other metabolites and 3% is recovered in the feces. The elimination half-life ($t_{1/2}$) varies between 1.5 to 3 hours. Average clearance values are 42 ± 5 L/hr.

Although exact dosage guidelines have not been established, patients with liver disease should have therapy initiated slowly, at low doses, and with careful blood pressure monitoring. Eight patients with chronic, stable cirrhosis showed a 50% reduction in clearance, prolongation of the half-life and a decrease in the percentage of parent compound converted to the N-oxide metabolite.

Clinical trials – Only a limited number of clinical studies, each involving only a few patients, have been published. This may reflect that pinacidil is not considered to be a first- or second-line drug in the stepped-care approach.

Pinacidil use has generally been confined to patients with moderate to severe hypertension. It is safe and effective, especially when added to a regimen of a diuretic and β-blocker in patients who failed the initial combination regimen. Pinacidil has been particularly effective in selected patients with renal impairment (dialysis and non-dialysis patients) with drug-resistant, non-volume dependent hypertension.

Although most studies have used doses of 10 to 100 mg twice daily, some clinicians feel that the drug may require 3 times/day dosing. The most effective dose range appears to be 12.5 or 25 mg twice daily.

➤*Adverse Reactions:* Pinacidil appears to be well tolerated. Only a few reports of mild side effects (eg, dizziness, headache, facial flushing) have been noted.

Edema has occurred in 23.5% to 45.2% of patients on doses of pinacidil alone of 25 to 50 mg. Concomitant diuretics may be required in most patients.

Two patients developed positive anti-nuclear antibody (ANA) titers while receiving pinacidil. Neither had clinical manifestations of a lupus-like syndrome, and a direct cause and effect relationship could not be linked to pinacidil; further studies are necessary to investigate the potential for pinacidil to cause a drug-induced lupus syndrome.

➤*Summary:* Pinacidil appears to be a promising alternative agent for the treatment of moderate to severe hypertension. However, further studies are needed to clarify the drug's optimal dosing schedule, long-term side effects, and optimal drug combinations.

The FDA's Cardio-Renal Drugs Advisory Committee recommended approval of pinacidil on May 28, 1987, with the stipulation that it be used concomitantly with diuretics. The drug was approved by the FDA in December 1989; however, Lilly has no plans to market pinacidil at this time.

PIRENZEPINE HCl (*Gastrozepine* by Boehringer Ingelheim) – An antiulcer agent

➤*Actions:*

Pharmacology – Pirenzepine is a tricyclic benzodiazepine antiulcer agent comparable to standard antiulcer agents such as cimetidine and ranitidine. However, its uniqueness and mechanism of action hinge on *selective* antimuscarinic activity for gastric acid secretory cells.

Pirenzepine selectively suppresses basal and stimulated acid and pepsin secretion with lesser effects on other muscarinic sites (eg, salivary secretion) compared with atropine and other classic anticholinergic agents. Controlled trials show that 50 mg, 2 to 3 times/day, inhibits acid secretion at least up to 4.5 hours after dosing. Higher doses inhibit esophageal and colonic motility and decrease lower esophageal sphincter pressure. Pirenzepine also may have cytoprotective effects; however, this is of questionable significance because it has little or no effect on gastric mucus and endogenous gastric prostaglandin production.

Pharmacokinetics – Pirenzepine is a hydrophilic molecule that has systemic bioavailability after oral dosing of 20% to 30%. Approximately 10% of the drug is protein bound. Little drug is found in the brain; brain to serum concentration is 1 to 10.

At least 80% is renally excreted unchanged. Most metabolites are of a desmethyl variety. The parent molecule has a half-life of about 10 hours.

These data indicate the potential for few CNS effects and the need to adjust dosage in patients with impaired renal function.

Clinical trials – Numerous short-term (1 to 6 weeks) studies have been conducted comparing pirenzepine with placebo and other antiulcer drugs in ulcer patients. In small doses (50 to 75 mg/day), duodenal ulcer healing percentages with pirenzepine are not superior to placebo. Doses of 100 to 150 mg/day produce healing in 70% to 90% of patients. Statistically significant symptomatic improvement (decreased antacid use and pain) occurs with both dosage levels.

Short-term double-blind studies comparing duodenal ulcer healing rates of pirenzepine (100 to 150 mg/day) and cimetidine (1 g/day) produced similar results (60% to 79% for pirenzepine and 53% to 85% for cimetidine). A single study comparing pirenzepine (100 mg/day) to cimetidine (1 g/day) and ranitidine (300 mg/day) found similar rates of ulcer healing. However, pirenzepine showed a slower effect on symptom disappearance.

Fewer studies have been conducted in patients with gastric ulcer. Double-blind studies comparing pirenzepine with placebo show a need to use adequate doses (100 to 150 mg/day). Pirenzepine and cimetidine have produced similar healing rates (50% vs 48%) in patients with gastric ulcer, but more studies are indicated.

Trials were performed comparing maintenance doses of pirenzepine (30 to 50 mg/day) to placebo and cimetidine (400 mg/day) in duodenal ulcer patients for 12 months. Results indicate statistically significant reductions in ulcer recurrences for active treatment groups vs placebo (24% recurrence in active treatment group vs 80 in placebo-treated patients). No difference was demonstrated in recurrence rates between pirenzepine and cimetidine patients.

Combined use of pirenzepine with ranitidine or cimetidine shows more effective inhibition of gastric acid secretion than with use of a single agent. Such combinations may be useful in peptic ulcer conditions resistant to single drug therapy and in the Zollinger-Ellison syndrome.

➤*Adverse Reactions:* Pirenzepine is well tolerated with few reported adverse effects. Dry mouth is the most common effect, but nausea, vomiting, diarrhea, constipation, increased appetite, anorexia, tiredness, and difficulty of accommodation have all occurred. Daily doses of less than 150 mg seem to significantly reduce the incidence of at least some of these problems.

➤*Summary:* In clinical studies, pirenzepine is equally effective as cimetidine in the treatment of peptic ulcer disease. Its low incidence of side effects and selective inhibition of muscarinic gastric acid secretion will make it a valuable addition to existing agents used to treat ulcers. Pirenzepine is currently available in some European countries; expected date of availability in the US is unknown. A New Drug Application is pending.

RAMOPLANIN (by Vicuron/Genome Therapeutics) – A glycolipodepsipeptide antibiotic

➤*Actions:*

Pharmacology – Ramoplanin is an oral, nonabsorbable glycolipodepsipeptide currently undergoing investigation in the United States for use as an antibiotic to prevent bloodstream infections caused by vancomycin-resistant enterococci (VRE) in patients who have GI colonization with VRE. Ramoplanin has a broad spectrum of activity and is bactericidal against many gram-positive aerobic and anaerobic bacteria, including vancomycin-resistant *Enterococcus faecium*, *Enterococcus faecalis*, and *Clostridium difficile*. It inhibits bacterial cell wall biosynthesis by interfering with peptidoglycan production. The N-acetylglucosaminyltransferase-catalyzed conversion of lipid intermediate I to lipid intermediate II, a step that occurs before the transglycosylation and transpeptidation reactions, is inhibited by ramoplanin. Ramoplanin's mechanism of action is distinct from that of glycopeptides – it does not complex with the D-Ala-D-Ala sequence of cell wall precursors.

Pharmacokinetics – Ramoplanin is not absorbed through the oral route and, therefore, is not absorbed into the bloodstream. Instead, ramoplanin remains in the GI tract where it exerts its bacteriocidal effects on VRE.

Clinical trials – The in vitro activity of ramoplanin was compared with that of teicoplanin, vancomycin (eg, *Vancocin*), linezolid (eg, *Zyvox*), and 5 other agents against 300 gram-positive and 54 gram-negative strains of intestinal anaerobes. Overall, ramoplanin had excellent activity against *C. difficile* and most gram-positive enteric anaerobes, including vancomycin-resistant strains but is largely inactive against gram-negative anaerobes.

In another trial, the in vitro activity of ramoplanin was compared with linezolid (*Zyvox*)-resistant and quinupristin/dalfopristin (*Synercid*)-resistant VRE. The MIC and killing curves of 7 linezolid-resistant and 2 quinupristin/dalfopristin-resistant VRE were evaluated against linezolid and quinupristin/dalfopristin susceptible VRE. Ramoplanin showed consistent in vitro activity (MIC of 0.125 to 0.25 mcg/mL) against VRE, including linezolid and quinupristin/dalfopristin-resistant isolates while time-kill curves demonstrated the bactericidal activity of ramoplanin against all 3 VRE in the study.

In vivo trials with ramoplanin that have been published to date are limited. In one randomized, double-blind, placebo-controlled study involving 68 patients, the safety and efficacy of oral ramoplanin was compared with placebo for the suppression of VRE in patients with asymptomatic GI colonization. Patients received either 100 mg ramoplanin, 400 mg ramoplanin, or placebo orally, twice daily for 7 days. The outcomes were accessed by comparing the proportion of people per group from whom VRE was not recovered in each active-drug treatment group with that in the placebo-treated group on days 7, 14, and 21 after treatment. By day 7, 90% of the patients treated with 400 mg ramoplanin had no detectable levels of VRE while all placebo-treated patients remained colonized. However, by day 21 (2 weeks after the end of therapy) only 29% of the patients treated with 400 mg ramoplanin remained free of detectable levels of VRE compared with 25% of placebo-treated patients.

A phase 2 study is underway to evaluate the safety and efficacy of ramoplanin for the treatment of *C. difficile*-associated diarrhea (CDAD). One in vivo study to date has evaluated the efficacy of ramoplanin against vancomycin (eg, *Vancocin*) and metronidazole (eg, *Flagyl*) for the prevention and treatment of CDAD in the hamster model. Hamsters were treated with a single SC injection of 100 mg/kg clindamycin (eg, *Cleocin*) and then received either 50 mg/kg ramoplanin or 50 mg/kg vancomycin once daily for 5 days. Another group of hamsters were treated with both clindamycin 100 mg/kg and *C. difficile* and then received either 25, 50, or 100 mg/kg ramoplanin, 25, 50, or 100 mg/kg vancomycin, or 100, 200, or 400 mg/kg metronidazole once daily for 5 days. Overall, treatment with ramoplanin showed higher survival rates than hamsters treated with vancomycin. Furthermore, high dose ramoplanin was superior to vancomycin at all doses in the clindamycin and *C. difficile*-induced colitis hamster model. Metronidazole showed no dose response and was the least effective agent.

➤*Adverse Reactions:* In the multiple dose study, ramoplanin was well tolerated and the occurrence of adverse events was similar across all treatment groups. Three patients developed diarrhea, 2 developed abdominal pain, 1 developed dyspepsia, 1 developed flatulence, and 1 developed nausea. Four deaths occurred during the 21-day study and an additional 8 patients died after completion of the study, but the investigators concluded the deaths to be directly related to the patients' underlying medical conditions and not to VRE infection nor to ramoplanin.

➤*Summary:* Ramoplanin has been given fast-track status from the FDA and appears to be a promising glycolipodepsipeptide antibiotic with a novel mechanism of action. Ramoplanin appears to be effective and well tolerated for the prevention of VRE bloodstream infections and is active against many gram-positive aerobic and anaerobic bacteria, including *C. difficile*. An NDA is not expected to be filed before spring/summer 2005.

REBOXETINE MESYLATE (*Vestra* by Pharmacia) – An antidepressant

➤*Actions:*

Pharmacology – Reboxetine is a selective norepinephrine reuptake inhibitor. It is chemically unrelated to the tricyclic or tetracyclic antidepressants, the monoamine oxidase inhibitors (MAOIs), or the selective serotonin reuptake inhibitors (SSRIs). It is an equimolar mixture of 2 enantiomers, but the (R,R)-enantiomer does not have any apparent pharmacologic effects. It has weak affinity for serotonin and dopamine and little affinity for muscarinic, histaminergic, or adrenergic receptors.

Pharmacokinetics – Peak plasma levels of reboxetine occur within 2 hours of oral administration. Administration of reboxetine with a high-fat meal results in a 2- to 3-hour delay in peak plasma concentrations, a small decrease in peak plasma concentrations (16.8%), and no change in the extent of absorption. The elimination half-life of reboxetine is 12 to 16 hours. The drug is extensively metabolized by the liver and excreted in the urine. Reboxetine is primarily metabolized by CYP 3A4 and not metabolized by cytochrome P450 2D6. It does not inhibit or induce the CYP 1A2, 2C9, 2C19, 2D6, 2E1, and 3A4 isoenzymes at therapeutic concentrations. Higher concentrations may inhibit CYP 3A4 and 2D6, but these concentrations are above those required for a therapeutic effect. The fraction excreted unchanged in the urine is 0.09. The pharmacokinetic values of reboxetine are similar in young, middle-aged, and elderly patients. However, patients ≥ 75 years of age may have an increased AUC and decreased plasma clearance. Decreased hepatic function can decrease the metabolic clearance of reboxetine, but it does not increase the systemic exposure to the drug. Patients with alcoholic liver disease have decreased clearance, increased half-life, and increased systemic exposure to the drug; therefore, a reduction in dose is warranted in patients with hepatic insufficiency. The clearance of reboxetine decreases with renal dysfunction, and the AUC is increased. Therefore, a dosage reduction may be necessary in patients with severe renal dysfunction.

➤*Drug Interactions:* Reboxetine has no effects on cytochrome P450 enzymes 1A2, 2C, 2D6, or 3A4 in therapeutic concentrations. Other antidepressants with no effects on these enzymes are bupropion (*Wellbutrin*), mirtazapine (*Remeron*), and venlafaxine (*Effexor*). Citalopram (*Celexa*), fluoxetine (*Prozac*), fluvoxamine (*Luvox*), nefazodone (*Serzone*), paroxetine (*Paxil*), and sertraline (*Zoloft*) inhibit at least 1 of these isoenzymes to some extent. Reboxetine is metabolized by the CYP 3A4 isoenzyme, so inhibitors (eg, ketoconazole [*Nizoral*], erythromycin [*E-mycin*]) and inducers (eg, rifampin [*Rifadin*], phenytoin [*Dilantin*]) of this isoenzyme may affect the metabolism of reboxetine. An interaction between reboxetine and MAOIs may occur because it has been reported with other antidepressants. To avoid this potential interaction, do not use reboxetine in combination with an MAOI within 7 days of initiating or 14 days of discontinuing therapy with an MAOI.

➤*Adverse Reactions:* Adverse effects reported with reboxetine therapy have included dry mouth, dizziness, headache, nausea, constipation, insomnia, somnolence, tremor, diaphoresis, urinary hesitancy or retention, agitation, anxiety, nervousness, tachycardia, and reduced blood pressure. Reboxetine has minimal effect on psychomotor and cognitive function compared with tricyclic antidepressants. Reboxetine plus ethanol does not adversely affect the cognitive function or psychomotor performance of the patient.

➤*Summary:* Like all newer antidepressant medications, reboxetine is better tolerated than the older tricyclic antidepressants. Reboxetine will offer clinicians an alternative agent for those patients who fail to respond to an SSRI or who are unable to tolerate a tricyclic antidepressant. Reboxetine also may be more effective in improving social functioning for some patients. The usual starting dosage of reboxetine was 4 mg twice daily. If necessary, the dose can be increased after 3 weeks. The dosages of reboxetine used in the clinical trials ranged from 4 to 12 mg/day. The drug is generally given in equally divided doses twice daily. The dosage used in elderly patients was 4 to 6 mg/day. The maximum recommended dosage in the US will be 10 mg/day. The starting dosage in patients with hepatic or renal dysfunction should be 2 mg twice daily; the maximum recommended dosage in these patients will be 6 mg/day. The safety and efficacy of reboxetine in children have not been established. Reboxetine is an effective antidepressant with efficacy and tolerability comparable with the other antidepressants.

REMOXIPRIDE (*Roxiam* by Astra/Merck) – An antipsychotic agent

➤*Actions:*

Pharmacology – Remoxipride, a substituted benzamide, is an atypical antipsychotic agent. It is a weak, but selective, dopamine-2 (D_2) receptor antagonist. D_2 receptors are thought to act in an inhibitory manner on adenylate cyclase, while dopamine-1 (D_1) receptors are associated with adenylate cyclase stimulation. The presynaptic dopamine "autoreceptors", which regulate the synthesis and release of dopamine, appear to be of the D_2 subtype. Many investigators have suggested that it is blockade of the D_2 receptor that mediates the clinical effects of most antipsychotic agents.

Remoxipride has a marked affinity for sigma receptors, which mediate opioid effects; clinical significance is unknown. There is a wide range between the dose that blocks apomorphine-induced hyperactivity and the dose that produces catalepsy, suggesting a favorable separation between the dose associated with antipsychotic effects and that producing extrapyramidal symptoms. The administration of remoxipride causes a significant, transient increase in prolactin release; however, prolonged administration (> 15 days) results in a reduction in this response.

Pharmacokinetics – Remoxipride is almost completely absorbed after oral administration with a bioavailability of 96% for both standard and controlled release (CR) formulations. There is no first-pass metabolism. Plasma levels peak within 1 to 2 hours after administration of standard formulations and within 2 to 6 hours after CR formulations and are linearly related to dose. Volume of distribution averages 0.5 to 0.7 L/kg. Protein binding averages 80%. CSF levels average 6% to 17% of total plasma levels. Breast milk concentrations are ≈ 30% of those in plasma.

Approximately 70% of an administered dose is metabolized in the liver to 6 inactive oxidized metabolites. Plasma concentrations of unchanged remoxipride are higher in slow debrisoquine metabolizers. Between 10% and 40% of an oral dose is excreted unchanged in the urine. Plasma elimination half-life averages 4 to 7 hours.

Remoxipride is a weak base (pKa 8.9). Urinary elimination is reduced and plasma half-life is prolonged in alkaline urine (pH 7.2). Conversely, acidification of urine (pH 5.2) results in increased urinary elimination and a reduction in half-life. Mean plasma concentrations are increased and the half-life is prolonged in the elderly, in patients with creatinine clearances < 25 mL/min, and in severe liver disease. Most investigators recommend initiating therapy with 50% the usual dose in the elderly.

Clinical trials – Remoxipride is an effective treatment for chronic schizophrenia and acute exacerbations of chronic schizophrenia. Improvement was documented in positive (eg, thought disturbances, hostility/suspiciousness, hallucinations, delusions) and negative (eg, emotional withdrawal, motor retardation) symptoms. In doses of 150 to 600 mg/day, remoxipride had similar antipsychotic efficacy to haloperidol (eg, *Haldol*) 5 to 45 mg/day and thioridazine (eg, *Mellaril*) 150 to 750 mg/day.

In most clinical trials, therapy was initiated with 300 mg/day. Patients responded to total daily doses of 300 to 450 mg/day (maximum dose, 600 mg/day) during initiation of therapy, and were tapered to usual maintenance doses of 150 to 300 mg/day. Dosage adjustments were made no more frequently than every 3 days and were based on patient response.

Remoxipride also may be effective in the treatment of acute mania.

➤*Adverse Reactions:* Remoxipride, like other atypical antipsychotic agents (eg, clozapine [*Clozaril*]), causes less frequent extrapyramidal symptoms (EPS) than the classic antipsychotic agents (eg, haloperidol). Long-term, comparative trials reported an EPS incidence of 2% to 15% and 7% to 27% in the remoxipride- and haloperidol-treated groups, respectively. Pooled data from 9 comparative trials with haloperidol also showed a lower incidence of insomnia, tiredness/drowsiness, difficulty in concentration, and dry mouth in the remoxipride-treated group. Although isolated reports of cardiovascular effects such as postural hypotension are documented, they are not considered to be clinically significant.

➤*Summary:* Available data suggests that remoxipride is a safe and effective treatment for schizophrenia. Its favorable side effect profile makes it an important therapeutic option for patients unable to tolerate traditional antipsychotic agents. Additional comparative and long-term studies are necessary to clarify its overall role in the treatment of schizophrenia and evaluate its potential to cause tardive dyskinesia.

An NDA for remoxipride was filed in December 1988. However, because of recent reports of aplastic anemia, including 1 death, in European patients, Astra/Merck notified investigators to discontinue use of the drug. The company has recommended restricting the use of the drug to patients who have failed other antipsychotics. The drug, which will be marketed as *Roxiam* by Astra/Merck, is currently available in the UK, Denmark, and Luxembourg. The NDA was withdrawn in December 1993.

RIMONABANT (*Acomplia* by Sanofi-Aventis) – A selective cannabinoid type 1 receptor blocker

➤*Actions:*

Pharmacology – Rimonabant is a neurokinin-3 antagonist and selective cannabinoid CB_1 receptor antagonist in the endocannabinoid system. By blocking activity at the CB_1 receptors, rimonabant may decrease the desire for excessive food intake as well as the desire to smoke. Rimonabant exhibits an increased affinity for the central cannabinoid receptor, CB_1, which is located in the brain and a variety of peripheral tissues, as compared to the CB_2 cannabinoid receptor, which is located in the immune system. Studies have shown that rimonabant has a 1,000-fold increased affinity for the CB_1 receptor over the CB_2 receptor. Rimonabant may have peripheral metabolic actions on the adipocytes, which may add to its ability to improve weight loss. Rimonabant has also been studied for effects on lipid and glucose metabolism, insulin resistance, and reduced intra-abdominal adiposity.

Pharmacokinetics – Rimonabant has shown an extended duration of action of at least 8 hours after oral administration.

Clinical trials – Rimonabant was assessed for its use in weight loss in a 1-year randomized, double-blind, placebo-controlled, parallel group, fixed dose, multicenter study utilizing 1,507 patients. Participants included in the study were men and women 18 years of age or older with a body mass index (BMI) of 30 kg/m^2 or greater, or a BMI greater than 27 kg/m^2 with treated or untreated hypertension or dyslipidemia. Patients were randomized to receive rimonabant 20 mg, rimonabant 5 mg, or placebo in a 2:2:1 ratio, respectively. Patients were also advised to decrease their daily caloric intake by 600 calories per day and were encouraged to increase physical activity. Weight loss was the primary end point, with change in waist circumference also being evaluated due to its relationship with cardiovascular and metabolic risk factors. Nine hundred twenty participants completed the 1-year study. The mean weight loss results at the end of the study are as follows: 3.6 kg for the placebo group, 4.8 kg for the rimonabant 5 mg group (P = 0.042 vs placebo), and 8.6 kg for the rimonabant 20 mg group ($P < 0.001$ vs placebo). The waist circumference also improved for all participants in the study. The placebo group decreased by 1.5 cm versus the rimonabant 5 mg group that decreased by 5.3 cm (P value not significant) and the rimonabant 20 mg group that decreased by 8.5 cm ($P < 0.001$). For participants in the rimonabant 20 mg group, the prevalence of metabolic syndrome decreased from 44.9% at the initiation of the study to 15.8% after 1 year ($P < 0.001$ vs placebo). Rimonabant appears to be effective in weight loss, but it is unknown if continuation of therapy is necessary to maintain the weight loss.

➤*Adverse Reactions:* Rimonabant has been well tolerated with few side effects being reported. In clinical trials involving rimonabant, nausea, dizziness, mood disorders, arthralgia, and diarrhea were the most commonly seen adverse effects. These adverse effects appear to be dose-related, mild to moderate in severity, and tended to resolve over time. Significant effects on vital signs or electrocardiogram have not been noted for rimonabant.

➤*Summary:* Rimonabant is a unique new medication that works on the endocannabinoid system and is being evaluated to aid in weight loss and smoking cessation. In clinical studies, rimonabant showed superior efficacy compared with placebo when it was evaluated for weight loss. Rimonabant has also been studied for use in smoking cessation and has been found to be very promising in helping patients stop smoking without the concern of weight gain. In June 2005, the FDA accepted for filing Sanofi-Aventis' NDA for rimonabant.

RITANSERIN (by Janssen) – A specific central serotonin S_2-antagonist

➤*Actions:*

Pharmacology – Ritanserin is a specific, long-acting central serotonin S_2-antagonist that does not affect norepinephrine, acetylcholine, or central dopamine antagonism, but does antagonize peripheral histamine. Ritanserin improves sleep quality, decreases fatigue, increases energy levels, improves depressed mood and anxiety and appears to lack abuse potential. Ritanserin 10 mg twice daily also improves neuroleptic-induced akathisia in patients resistant to traditional therapy (eg, anticholinergics, benzodiazepines, beta-blockers). These actions of ritanserin have caused researchers to investigate its effects in the treatment of anxiety, schizophrenia, alcoholism, drug abuse, depressive disorders, and Parkinsonism.

Pharmacokinetics – The oral bioavailability is about 75%. Following oral administration, very little drug is recovered unchanged in the urine after a 5 mg IV dose suggesting that it is extensively metabolized by the liver. In a study involving 9 healthy volunteers, peak plasma concentrations occurred within 2.39 hours after oral administration. Steady-state plasma concentrations are achieved within 1 week after initiating dosing and the half-life is ≈ 40 hours. Ritanserin is usually administered with or after a meal to decrease the incidence of transient side effects (eg, dizziness, tiredness, lightheadedness) that have been reported in 10% of patients.

Clinical trials – A trial involving 33 patients was conducted to determine the effectiveness of ritanserin in decreasing the negative symptoms in type II schizophrenia over a 6-week period. Patients initially received 10 mg ritanserin. Doses were increased by 10 mg increments to 30 mg as tolerated. The average total dose at the end of the study was 26 mg. Ritanserin significantly improved several negative symptoms such as facial expressions, global affective flattening, and relationships with friends and peers and also caused significant reductions in scores for emotional withdrawal and depressive mood compared with placebo. Three patients in the ritanserin group dropped out of the study because of lack of efficacy and one due to side effects (eg, unrest).

In another study, 9 patients with acute schizophrenia received 10 mg ritanserin twice daily for 4 weeks. Five of the nine patients experienced a 50% decrease in comprehensive psychological rating scale scores, and scores for negative symptoms also decreased significantly from baseline. No extrapyramidal side effects or akathisia that could be attributed to ritanserin were reported.

Several studies have examined the ability of ritanserin to affect the motor symptoms of Parkinson's disease. Initial studies demonstrated that ritanserin significantly reduced tremor. In contrast, 2 recent studies determined that ritanserin (range, 5 to 30 mg/day) had a positive effect on dyskinesias but not tremor.

Ritanserin's effect on dysthymia has been studied compared with placebo, amitriptyline (eg, *Elavil*), and imipramine (eg, *Tofranil*). Ritanserin was superior to placebo and equal to amitriptyline and imipramine for up to 8 weeks (n > 300).

Several studies have determined that ritanserin is effective in relieving anxiety, decreasing fatigue, and increasing energy in patients with generalized anxiety disorders compared with placebo, and 10 mg ritanserin appears to have equal efficacy to lorazepam (eg, *Ativan*). The antianxiety effects occurred after 2 to 4 weeks of treatment.

Ritanserin decreases craving for alcohol and cocaine. One study involving 39 patients concluded that 5 mg ritanserin decreased desire and craving for alcohol but did not change the amount of alcohol intake during 14 days of the study. Another small study (n = 5) suggested that patients receiving 10 mg ritanserin for 28 days not only had no desire to drink but also demonstrated improvement in mood. Several large scale double-blind studies that will include> 900 patients with various types of alcohol dependence are currently underway.

Slow wave sleep (SWS) patterns were significantly improved in several studies when ritanserin was given to patients with alcoholism and depressive disorders; one study found that ritanserin did not affect SWS in 12 depressed patients.

➤*Adverse Reactions:* Ritanserin appears to be well tolerated. Observed side effects in clinical trials were minimal, with 10% of patients reporting transient dizziness, tiredness, and lightheadedness.

➤*Summary:* Although ritanserin shows promise in the treatment of a variety of psychiatric illnesses including anxiety, schizophrenia, alcoholism, drug abuse, depressive disorders, and Parkinsonism, it is still undergoing clinical trials and has not been approved by the FDA. The dosing range used in the studies was from 5 to 30 mg/day in adults. Side effects are minimal and mild and there seems to be a lack of clinically significant changes in vital signs, laboratory values, ECGs, or mood evaluations. Research in the US has been discontinued.

ROTIGOTINE TRANSDERMAL SYSTEM (*Neupro* by Schwarz Pharma) – A dopamine receptor agonist

➤*Actions:*

Pharmacology – Rotigotine is a nonergot, selective D_2-dopamine receptor agonist being evaluated for the treatment of Parkinson disease and restless legs syndrome. It is a levorotatory enantiomer of a racemic aminotetraline compound.

Pharmacokinetics – Rotigotine has poor oral bioavailability (approximately 0.5% in rats) because of extensive first-pass metabolism via glucuronidation in the gut wall and liver, thus the reason for the transdermal delivery system. Following transdermal administration, rotigotine plasma concentrations are detectable in the systemic circulation within 2 to 3 hours after patch application and achieves peak concentrations 24 hours after application. Plasma concentrations increase linearly and are dose proportional. The terminal half-life of rotigotine is approximately 3.6 hours. Steady-state plasma concentrations are reached after 2 to 3 days of continuous daily applications.

Clinical trials – The rotigotine transdermal system was assessed in a multicenter, randomized, double-blind, placebo-controlled, dose-ranging study, enrolling 242 patients with early Parkinson disease who were not yet receiving dopaminergic therapy. Patients were randomized to therapy with patches containing rotigotine 4.5, 9, 13.5, or 18 mg, or placebo. The study consisted of a 4-week screening period with a 4- to 7-day placebo patch run-in period, a 4-week double-blind dose-titration period, a 7-week dose maintenance phase, a 1-week dose withdrawal phase, and a 2-week safety run-in period without study drug. Active patches contained rotigotine 4.5 mg and were identical to the placebo patches. All subjects were instructed to wear 4 patches containing various combinations of placebo and active patches to supply the randomized dose. Patches were applied once daily on rotating sites on the abdomen. All patients receiving rotigotine started therapy at 4.5 mg/day, with dosages adjusted weekly to reach the assigned dose. Initiation of the start of active drug was staggered so that all subjects reached their maintenance dose at the fourth week of the titration phase. Patients were permitted to take selegiline, amantadine, or anticholinergic agents if maintained at stable dosages for 28 days before baseline and throughout the study. The primary outcome was the change in the sum of the scores of the activities of daily living and motor components of the Unified Parkinson Disease Rating Scale (UPDRS) from baseline to the end of treatment. A dose-related improvement in the motor and activities of daily living UPDRS score from baseline to week 11 was observed for the 13.5 and 18 mg groups compared with placebo ($P < 0.01$). The mean change from baseline to week 11 in the combined motor and UPDRS-Activities of Daily Living (ADL) score was –0.29 with placebo, –1.2 with rotigotine 4.5 mg, –3.13 with rotigotine 9 mg, –5.09 with rotigotine 13.5 mg, and –5.3 with rotigotine 18 mg.

Transdermal rotigotine was also assessed in a multicenter, randomized, double-blind, placebo-controlled study including 63 patients with moderate to severe restless legs syndrome. Patients applied transdermal rotigotine 1.125, 2.25, or 4.5 mg (1.125 mg per 2.5 cm^2), or placebo daily for 1 week. The primary outcome was the total score on the International Restless Legs Syndrome Scale (IRLS). IRLS score improved by 10.5 points in the 1.125 mg group ($P = 0.41$), 12.3 points in the 2.25 mg group ($P = 0.18$), and 15.7 points in the 4.5 mg group ($P < 0.01$) compared with 8 points in the placebo group. Daytime symptoms improved with all rotigotine doses. Clinical Global Impression scores revealed improvement in the 4.5 mg group.

➤*Adverse Reactions:* Adverse reactions reported with rotigotine have included nausea, application site reactions, dizziness, insomnia, somnolence, vomiting, and fatigue. Nausea and vomiting occurred most frequently during the dose-titration phase. Application site reactions have ranged from mild to severe. Most reactions were mild to moderate, and largely consisted of erythema corresponding to the area of the removed patch. Itching and rash have also been reported. More severe reactions have included blistering and/or ulceration of the skin previously under the patch and the surrounding skin.

➤*Summary:* Rotigotine transdermal will offer a non-oral alternative to pramipexole and ropinirole for the therapy of Parkinson disease. The advantage of continuous delivery, with relatively stable blood concentrations, is theoretical and will need to be proven in a comparative clinical study before it can be considered an advantage over oral administration. A New Drug Application for rotigotine transdermal for the treatment of early Parkinson disease was submitted in January 2005. Rotigotine is also being evaluated for the treatment of restless legs syndrome, and a nasal spray formulation of rotigotine is being evaluated for the treatment of acute symptoms of Parkinson disease.

ROXATIDINE ACETATE (*Roxin* by Hoechst-Roussel) – An agent for peptic ulcers

➤*Actions:*

Pharmacology – Roxatidine acetate is a potent, selective, histamine H_2RA (H_2 receptor antagonist) that is structurally unrelated to cimetidine (eg, *Tagamet*) or ranitidine (eg, *Zantac*). Its potency is 3 to 6 times that of cimetidine and twice that of ranitidine. Basal gastric acid secretion is inhibited by > 90% 3 hours after a single 50 mg dose and by 86% 4 to 6 hours after a 75 mg dose. Unlike cimetidine, ranitidine, or famotidine (eg, *Pepcid*), roxatidine has a mucosal protective effect in animal models. It has no direct effect on serum gastrin levels (unlike cimetidine or ranitidine) and no antiandrogenic effect.

Pharmacokinetics – Roxatidine acetate is well absorbed with a bioavailability of > 95%. After administration, it is rapidly converted to roxatidine, its active metabolite, by esterases in the small intestine, plasma, and liver. The peak concentration occurs 3 hours after oral administration, with food and antacids having little or no clinical effect on its pharmacokinetics. Its volume of distribution is 3.2 L/kg after a single dose and 1.7 L/kg at steady state. Plasma protein binding is 6% to 7%. Elimination is primarily renal with 96% eliminated as roxatidine. The clearance is 21 to 29 L/hr and the half-life is 4 to 8 hours. Other than roxatidine, 9 other inactive metabolites have been identified. Because it is renally eliminated, the dose of roxatidine must be adjusted in patients with severe renal dysfunction.

The pharmacokinetic parameters of a single dose of 150 mg roxatidine were evaluated in 31 patients with varying degrees of renal dysfunction (control group, mild chronic renal failure [CRF], moderate CRF, severe CRF, or uremia). The half-life increased 12 hours in patients with uremia (Ccr < 7 mL/min), with the T_{max} doubling (2.08 hours vs 4.05 hours, respectively). In patients with renal failure, there can be an increase in half-life by 140% to 200% with peak plasma concentrations increasing by 50% to 70%. Data on the effects of hemodialysis are conflicting, ranging from no effect to a marked reduction in plasma concentration.

Clinical trials –

Duodenal ulcers (DU): 75 mg roxatidine twice daily is effective for the treatment of DU. Six-week healing rates were between 73% to 90%, with 8-week rates being between 87% to 95%.

The efficacy of roxatidine was evaluated in 356 patients with active DU in a multicenter, double-blind trial. Patients were randomized to receive roxatidine (150 mg at bedtime, n = 170) or placebo (n = 170) for 4 weeks; antacids were administered as needed for pain relief. Four-week ulcer healing rates were 68% for patients receiving roxatidine compared with 30% for placebo; roxatidine was also better at decreasing abdominal pain.

Roxatidine also is effective as maintenance therapy for the prevention of DU. In one trial, 105 patients with healed duodenal ulcers received 75 mg roxatidine at bedtime for 6 months as preventive therapy. Ulcer relapse rates were 18% after 3 months and 35% after 6 months. Relapse rates were higher in smokers. In another trial evaluating 372 patients with healed duodenal ulcers, cumulative ulcer relapse rates at 12 months were 35% for patients receiving roxatidine (75 mg at bedtime) vs 66% for placebo. Most patients who relapsed did so within 6 months. When patients relapsed, they were asymptomatic in 26% of patients receiving roxatidine vs 16% of patients receiving placebo. The study showed that roxatidine 75 mg at bedtime is effective as preventive therapy for DU.

Gastric ulcers (GU): In small, noncomparative trials in patients with gastric ulcers, 75 mg roxatidine twice daily had ulcer healing rates ranging from 77% to 96% at 8 weeks. In a double-blind, multicenter trial, patients with GU were randomized to receive 75 mg roxatidine twice daily (n = 172) or 150 mg at bedtime (n = 171). Both dosing regimens were found to produce symptomatic pain relief and to have comparable ulcer healing rates (84% and 86% at 8 weeks, respectively).

➤*Adverse Reactions:* The most common adverse effects are hypersensitivity reactions (rash), GI (diarrhea, constipation, nausea), or involve the CNS (headache, dizziness, fatigue).

➤*Summary:* Roxatidine acetate is a potent, selective H_2 receptor antagonist that is effective for treatment of and maintenance therapy for duodenal and gastric ulcers. It is generally well tolerated with the primary side effects involving the GI, cutaneous, or central nervous systems.

For the treatment of peptic ulcer disease, roxatidine should be dosed 75 mg twice daily or 150 mg at bedtime for 8 weeks. For prevention of DU or GU recurrence, the dose is 75 mg at bedtime. Decrease dose in patients with renal dysfunction; treatment doses of 75 mg once daily for a Ccr between 20 and 40 mL/min and 75 mg every other day for a CCr of < 20 ml/min have been suggested.

Hoechst-Roussel has filed an NDA for *Roxin*.

RUBOXISTAURIN (*Arxxant* by Eli Lilly and Company) – A protein kinase C beta inhibitor

➤*Actions:*

Pharmacology – Ruboxistaurin mesylate is a selective inhibitor of protein kinase C beta (PKC-β) 1 and 2 isoforms and is being evaluated for the treatment of diabetic retinopathy. Hyperglycemia-induced activation of PKC has been associated with causing damage and complications in the microvascular portion of the eye. PKC-β can be found in pancreatic islet cells and in the retina.

Pharmacokinetics – Ruboxistaurin is metabolized by cytochrome P–450 isoenzymes (primarily CYP3A4) to the active metabolite N-desmethyl-ruboxistaurin. Elimination of ruboxistaurin is mainly through the fecal/bilary route, and to a lesser degree through the renal pathway. Steady-state concentration is reached 7 to 21 days after twice-daily therapy. In dogs and rats, the half-life was found to be 2.5 to 4.3 hours and 5.7 to 10.7 hours, respectively.

Clinical Trials – Ruboxistaurin was compared with placebo in a multicenter, double-blind, randomized study enrolling 252 patients. Participants were men and women between 20 and 84 years of age with type 1 or type 2 diabetes and HbA_{1c} values of 5.1% to 13%. Subjects were randomized to 1 of 4 groups (placebo or ruboxistaurin 8, 16, or 32 mg/day) for 36 to 46 months. Exclusion criteria included history of significant heart disease within 6 months, significant hepatic or renal disease or anemia, hypertension (systolic blood pressure of at least 180 mm Hg or diastolic blood pressure of at least 105 mmHg), or major surgery within 3 months prior to the study. Subjects were required to meet certain ocular entry criteria for at least one eye based on the Early Treatment Diabetic Retinopathy Study (ETDRS). Ophthalmologic exams were executed at every visit during the study. The primary end point was progression of diabetic retinopathy, and secondary end points were moderate vision loss (MVL) and sustained MVL (SMVL). Results of the primary end point showed no statistically significant differences among groups for progression of diabetic retinopathy based on the ETDRS severity scale. However, for the secondary outcomes, rate of occurrence of MVL was lower in the ruboxistaurin 32 mg per day group compared with the placebo group. SMVL also showed benefit, with a lower percentage of patients with SMVL in the ruboxistaurin 32 mg per day group than in the placebo group.

➤*Drug Interactions:* Ruboxistaurin is a substrate of CYP3A4; coadministration with CYP3A4 inducers (eg, rifampin, carbamazepine, phenobarbital) or inhibitors (eg, ketoconazole) may alter the concentrations of ruboxistaurin and its metabolite N-desmethyl-ruboxistaurin.

➤*Adverse Reactions:* The most commonly reported adverse reactions from 2 clinical trials (PKC-DRS and PKC-DMES) that had an incidence of 1% or more and were statistically different among groups included coronary artery disease, diarrhea, flatulence, first degree atrioventricular block, asthma, nephropathy, proteinuria, hyperkeratosis, and dysuria. There were no serious adverse reactions reported.

➤*Summary:* Ruboxistaurin may reduce the risk of ocular complications in patients with diabetes. Ruboxistaurin was also evaluated for diabetic peripheral neuropathy, but no significant difference was found when compared with placebo. Eli Lilly plans to submit an NDA for ruboxistaurin for the treatment of diabetic retinopathy in early 2006.

RUFINAMIDE (by Eisai) – An anticonvulsant

➤*Actions:*

Pharmacology – An NDA has been submitted to the FDA for the use of rufinamide as adjunctive therapy for Lennox-Gastaut syndrome in children 4 years of age and older and as adjunctive therapy for partial-onset seizures with and without secondary generalization in adults and adolescents 12 years of age and older. Rufinamide is a triazole derivative, structurally distinct from other antiepileptic agents currently available. The exact mechanism of action for rufinamide is unknown. It is thought to work by limiting the firing of sodium-dependent action potentials in the neuron and providing a membrane-stabilizing effect.

Pharmacokinetics – Following oral administration, the T_{max} of rufinamide is approximately 3.4 to 8 hours with a 400 or 600 mg dose. Absorption is slower at higher doses. When administered with food, the peak concentration was increased about 100% and the AUC was increased 44%, compared with administration in the fasting state. Following a single 600 mg dose of rufinamide, the AUC was 57.2 mcg/mL when administered after an overnight fast and 81.7 mcg/mL after administration with a fat- and protein-rich breakfast ($P = 0.0001$). The T_{max} was reduced from 8 to 6 hours when administered with food. Rufinamide exhibits linear pharmacokinetics over the tested dosing range. The elimination half-life is 7 to 10 hours. Rufinamide undergoes extensive metabolism via hydrolysis. The major metabolite, an inactive carboxylic acid derivative (CGP 47292), accounts for 60% of the dose recovered in the urine. Less than 4% of the dose is eliminated unchanged in the urine.

Clinical trials –

Lennox-Gastaut syndrome: Rufinamide was assessed in a multicenter, randomized, double-blind, placebo-controlled study enrolling 138 patients between 4 and 30 years of age, with treatment-resistant Lennox-Gastaut syndrome. Following a 28-day baseline phase, patients entered a 14-day titration phase followed by a 70-day maintenance phase. Following study completion, all patients were permitted entry into an open-label extension phase. Patients were randomized to therapy with rufinamide (74 patients) or placebo (64 patients). The target rufinamide dosage was 45 mg/kg/day, administered in 2 divided doses. The median dosage at each visit was 1,800 mg/day in both groups, or 42 to 45 mg/kg/day. The median percent reduction in total seizure frequency per 28 days relative to baseline was 32.7% with rufinamide, compared with 11.7% with placebo ($P = 0.0015$). The median percent reduction in tonic-atonic seizure frequency per 28 days relative to baseline was 42.5% in the rufinamide group, compared with 1.4% in the placebo group ($P < 0.0001$). A 50% or greater reduction in frequency of tonic-atonic seizures was achieved in 42.5% of patients in the rufinamide group, compared with 16.7% of patients in the placebo group ($P = 0.002$; number needed to treat [NNT] = 3.9). Improvement in seizure frequency occurred in 53.4% of rufinamide-treated patients, compared with 30.6% of placebo-treated patients ($P = 0.0041$).

Partial seizures: Rufinamide as adjunctive therapy in adults with therapy-resistant partial seizures was assessed in a randomized, double-blind, placebo-controlled, 3-month study enrolling 313 patients between 16 and 72 years of age, had a minimum of 6 partial seizures during the 56-day baseline, and received 1 or 2 fixed-dose concomitant antiepileptic drugs during baseline and treatment. Patients were randomized to therapy with rufinamide 3,200 mg/day or placebo. Those treated with rufinamide had a 20.4% median reduction in partial seizure frequency from baseline, while placebo-treated patients had a 1.6% median increase ($P = 0.0158$). The rufinamide group also had more patients with a 50% or greater reduction in seizure frequency (specific results were not provided; $P = 0.0381$).

➤*Drug Interactions:* In vitro, rufinamide did not exhibit inhibitory activity on the cytochrome P450 isozymes CYP1A2, CYP2A6, CYP2C9, CYP2C19, CYP2D6, CYP2E1, CYP3A4/5, and CYP4A9/11. The rufinamide AUC and half-life were lower in patients treated with concomitant phenytoin or carbamazepine ($P < 0.001$), compared with patients on concomitant valproate. Administration of rufinamide 800 mg twice daily in healthy subjects stabilized on a norethindrone/ethinyl estradiol oral contraceptive (Ortho-Novum 1/35) resulted in a 22% (90% confidence interval [CI], 18% to 26%) reduction in the ethinyl estradiol AUC, a 33% (90% CI, 26% to 37%) reduction in the ethinyl estradiol peak concentration, a 14% (90% CI, 9% to 18%) reduction in norethindrone AUC, and an 18% (90% CI, 8% to 26%) reduction in norethindrone peak concentration.

➤*Adverse Reactions:* Rufinamide appears to have a wide therapeutic window. Adverse reactions seen with rufinamide, and at a higher frequency than with placebo, include headache, dizziness, fatigue, somnolence, nausea, vomiting, tremor, and diplopia. Adverse reactions have generally been described as occurring more commonly during dosage titration, transient, and mild to moderate in severity.

➤*Summary:* Limited data from clinical trials suggest rufinamide is effective in reducing seizure frequency when used as adjunctive therapy in Lennox-Gastaut syndrome and partial seizures. Additional adverse reaction and drug interaction information is necessary to determine its role compared with other adjunctive therapies. The NDA was submitted in September 2005. Rufinamide has been granted orphan drug status for the Lennox-Gastaut indication.

SERTINDOLE (*Serdolect* by Lundbeck A/S [Denmark]) – An antipsychotic agent

➤*Actions:*

Pharmacology – Sertindole is a new "atypical" antipsychotic agent with unique pharmacologic properties compared with traditional agents. The mechanism of action of sertindole is via its strong antagonism of dopamine D_2, serotonin 5-HT_2, and norepinephrine alpha$_1$ receptors. Sertindole appears to have low extrapyramidal symptoms (EPS) potential, does not cause anticholinergic side effects, does not inhibit cognitive functioning and has potent anxiolytic activity.

Pharmacokinetics –

Immunocompromised patients: Sertindole is slowly absorbed from the GI tract with a peak plasma concentration achieved after 8 to 10 hours. Following a single oral dose, the elimination half-life is approximately 60 hours, but there is great patient variability with 10% of subjects demonstrating half-lives > 100 hours after administration of a single dose. Due to sertindole's long half-life, steady-state concentrations are not reached until after 3 to 4 weeks. The long half-life of sertindole should allow for once-daily dosing. Sertindole is characterized by non-linear kinetics. Increasing the dose by 20% can increase plasma concentrations by approximately 40%. Sertindole is significantly bound to plasma proteins (> 99%), with only a small amount of the drug being renally excreted; therefore, sertindole will presumably not be eliminated by dialysis. In vitro studies have shown that sertindole is predominately metabolized by the hepatic cytochrome P450 3A4 isoform system and eliminated via the GI tract. Sertindole has 2 metabolites, norsertindole and Lu 28-092, but the activity of these metabolites has not been established.

Clinical trials – In 7 phase I trials, over 100 healthy patients received sertindole 0.5 to 32 mg as a single dose or in escalating dosing for up to 14 days. These studies demonstrated that, overall, sertindole was safe and well tolerated.

Three phase II studies examined the efficacy of sertindole in doses of 4 to 24 mg/day. The first was a pilot, double-blind, randomized, placebo-controlled, multi-center study designed to compare the efficacy of sertindole (n = 27) and placebo (n = 11) in patients diagnosed with schizophrenia or schizoaffective disorder. The study concluded that sertindole was effective in most patients at a dose of 16 or 20 mg/day and this therapy was associated with minimal adverse effects.

The second and third phase II studies were randomized, double-blind, multi-centered, and placebo-controlled with identical study designs except that each study had 4 different treatment groups: 8, 12, or 20 mg/day of sertindole or placebo in the second trial, and the third study had 4 or 12 mg/day sertindole, placebo, or 8 mg haloperidol (eg, *Haldol*) twice daily. All patients taking sertindole were titrated upwards starting with 4 mg/day and increasing by 4 mg every third day until the desired dose was reached. The titration phase lasted 12 days and the maintenance phase period was 28 days. Patients enrolled in both studies had to have a previous response to antipsychotic drugs. There were 205 patients enrolled in the second trial and 109 in the third; 153 patients completed at least 13% of the total 40 days of the second trial and were included in the final analysis (107 completed the entire study). Only the 20 mg sertindole group significantly improved in all efficacy parameters compared with placebo. Sertindole 20 mg was equally efficacious to haloperidol but caused fewer side effects.

In a long term, open-label study, sertindole 4 to 24 mg/day was administered to 170 patients for up to 2 years to determine its safety and efficacy. The mean exposure to sertindole was 121 days (range, 2 to 532 days) and the most common dose administered was 20 mg/day (33%).

➤*Adverse Reactions:* Adverse effects observed during phase I trials included lethargy, drowsiness, nasal congestion, sexual dysfunction, GI complaints, dizziness, lightheadedness, mild tremor, orthostatic hypotension, syncope, dystonia, postural hypotension, and cogwheel rigidity. No patients experienced EPS. The most common adverse effects experienced during phase II trials that occurred more often with sertindole 20 mg/day than with placebo included: Headache, nasal congestion (26%); dry ejaculation (17%); constipation, dizziness, somnolence (11%). Dry ejaculation was the only side effect that was found to be significantly greater than placebo ($P < 0.05$). Adverse effects experienced during the long-term study were similar, but incidence rates were higher.

➤*Summary:* Sertindole should provide an effective and safe alternative treatment when therapy with traditional antipsychotics have failed due to lack of efficacy or intolerable side effects. Additional trials are necessary to establish long-term safety, especially the incidence of tardive dyskinesia, and efficacy of sertindole. The drug, which will be available from Lundbeck A/S (Denmark), became "approvable" in 1998.

SITAGLIPTIN (*Januvia* by Merck) – A dipeptidyl peptidase-4 inhibitor

➤*Actions:*

Pharmacology – Sitagliptin is an orally active, selective dipeptidyl peptidase-4 (DPP-4) inhibitor for the treatment of type 2 diabetes mellitus (DM). Glucagon-like peptide 1 (GLP-1) is rapidly degraded by DPP-4, a serine protease. A DPP-4 inhibitor increases the half-life of active GLP-1 and prolongs the beneficial effects of the incretin hormone. GLP-1 is a glucose-dependent stimulator of insulin synthesis and secretion and inhibitor of glucagon release.

Pharmacokinetics – The time-to-peak sitagliptin concentration is 1 to 6 hours. Steady-state concentrations are reached within 2 days with twice-daily administration and 3 days with once-daily administration. The terminal elimination half-life ranges from 8 to 14 hours following single sitagliptin doses and 11 to 14 hours following multiple daily doses. Approximately 70% to 90% of the orally administered dose is excreted unchanged in the urine. Approximately 16% of the dose has been recovered as metabolites, and up to 10% has been recovered in the feces as unchanged drug. The sitagliptin area under the curve (AUC) was increased 1.6-fold in patients with mild renal impairment (creatinine clearance [Ccr] 50 to 80 mL/min), 2.3-fold in patients with moderate renal impairment (Ccr 30 to 50 mL/min), 3.8-fold in patients with severe renal impairment (Ccr less than 30 mL/min), and 4.5-fold in patients with end-stage renal disease compared with healthy subjects. Peak concentrations were increased 1.4- to 1.8-fold in patients with renal impairment. Dialysis removed approximately 13.5% of the dose.

Clinical Trials – Sitagliptin was assessed in a randomized, double-blind, placebo-controlled, dose-ranging study enrolling 552 patients 30 to 74 years of age with type 2 DM and a hemoglobin A_{1c} (HbA_{1c}) of 5.8% to 10.4%. Patients were randomized to receive placebo, sitagliptin 50 mg twice daily, or sitagliptin 25, 50, or 100 mg once daily for 12 weeks. Mean baseline HbA_{1c} ranged from 7.6% to 7.8% across treatment groups. After 12 weeks of therapy, placebo-subtracted HbA_{1c} ranged from −0.4% in the 25 mg once daily group to −0.6% in the 100 mg once daily group in last observation carried forward analysis, and from −0.4% to −0.7% in the per protocol analysis without data carried forward. Fasting plasma glucose increased 0.2 mg/dL in the placebo group but declined by 10.7 to 17 mg/dL in the active treatment groups. One hypoglycemic event was observed in each sitagliptin treatment group. No change in body weight was observed.

In a similar randomized, double-blind, placebo-controlled, dose-ranging study, sitagliptin was compared with glipizide in 743 patients 21 to 76 years of age with type 2 DM and an HbA_{1c} of 6.3% to 11%. Patients were randomized to receive placebo, glipizide 5 mg (titrated up to 10, 15, and then 20 mg per day), or sitagliptin 5, 12.5, 25, or 50 mg twice daily for 12 weeks. Mean baseline HbA_{1c} ranged from 7.8% to 7.9% across groups. After 12 weeks of therapy, placebo-subtracted differences in HbA_{1c} ranged from −0.4% to −0.8% in a dose-dependent manner for the sitagliptin groups, and −1% in the glipizide group. Fasting plasma glucose increased 7.9 mg/dL in the placebo group, dose-dependently decreased by 0.8 to 18.2 mg/dL in the sitagliptin groups, and decreased 24.8 mg/dL in the glipizide group. Weight change was not observed in the sitagliptin groups.

One or more hypoglycemic events occurred in 21 patients (17.1%) in the glipizide group, 2 patients in the placebo group, and 0 to 5 patients in the sitigliptin groups.

➤*Drug Interactions:* Administration of sitagliptin with cyclosporine, a potent p-glycoprotein inhibitor, was associated with a slight increase in sitagliptin peak concentration but not a significant increase in the sitagliptin AUC. Administration of sitagliptin with digoxin resulted in an 11% to 18% increase in digoxin AUC. This small increase in digoxin exposure is unlikely to be clinically important.

➤*Adverse Reactions:* Adverse reactions reported in clinical trials have included diarrhea, headache, joint pain, and symptoms associated with the common cold (eg, stuffy or runny nose, sore throat).

➤*Summary:* Sitagliptin is a new type of drug for the treatment of diabetes. It is an orally active, selective DPP-4 inhibitor. Sitagliptan results in improved glucose control without an increased risk of hypoglycemia. The NDA for sitagliptin was accepted in February 2006 and Merck expects FDA action by mid-October 2006.

SITAXSENTAN (*Thelin* by Encysive Pharmaceuticals) – An endothelin receptor antagonist

➤*Actions:*

Pharmacology – Sitaxsentan is an endothelin (ET) receptor antagonist with 6,500-fold greater selectivity for the ET_A receptor than the ET_B receptor. ET_A receptor activation facilitates sustained vasoconstriction and proliferation of vascular smooth muscle cells. ET_B receptors are believed to be primarily involved in clearance of ET, mainly in the vascular bed of the lungs and kidneys. Sitaxsentan is used for the treatment of pulmonary arterial hypertension (PAH).

Pharmacokinetics – Sitaxsentan is orally available. The half-life is 5 to 7 hours. Sitaxsentan elimination is not linear at a dose of 300 mg.

Clinical Trials – Sitaxsentan was evaluated in 2 phase 3 studies referred to as Sitaxsentan to Relieve Impaired Exercise (STRIDE). The STRIDE-1 study evaluated the efficacy of sitaxsentan in the treatment of patients with symptomatic PAH, despite treatment with anticoagulants, vasodilators, diuretics, cardiac glycosides, or supplemental oxygen, using a randomized, double-blind, placebo-controlled study design. Percent of predicted peak VO_2 increased 3.1% in the sitaxsentan 300 mg group compared with the placebo group ($P < 0.01$), but was unchanged in the 100 mg group. Six-minute walk distance after 12 weeks was significantly improved in both the sitaxsentan 100 and 300 mg groups. Pulmonary vascular resistance decreased from 1,025 to 805 dynes/sec/cm^{-5} with the 100 mg dose and from 946 to 753 dynes/sec/cm^{-5} with the 300 mg dose, compared with an increase from 911 to 960 dynes/sec/cm^{-5} in the placebo group. New York Heart Association functional class improved in 29% of patients in the 100 mg group and in 30% of patients in the 300 mg group, compared with 15% of patients in the placebo group.

The STRIDE-2 study was a randomized, double-blind, placebo-controlled study enrolling 248 patients in World Health Organization (WHO) functional classes II to IV with idiopathic PAH or PAH associated with connective tissue disease or a congenital heart defect. Patients received placebo, sitaxsentan 50 or 100 mg, or open-label bosentan therapy for 18 weeks. The placebo-subtracted treatment effect for 6-minute walk distance was 31.4 m ($P = 0.03$) for sitaxsentan 100 mg, 24.2 m (not significant) for sitaxsentan 50 mg, and 29.5 m ($P = 0.05$) for bosentan. WHO functional class improvement occurred in more patients in the sitaxsentan 100 mg group ($P = 0.04$).

➤*Drug Interactions:* Sitaxsentan is a potent inhibitor of CYP2C9, resulting in an increased international normalized ratio or prothrombin time when coadministered with warfarin. Reduce warfarin dose when sitaxsentan therapy is added. In the STRIDE-2 study, warfarin doses were reduced 80% on initiation of sitaxsentan therapy.

Sitaxsentan is also a moderate inhibitor of CYP2C19 and CYP3A4.

Coadministration of sitaxsentan with sildenafil is not expected to require dosage adjustments of either agent. With coadministration, sitaxsentan produced a slight increase in sildenafil peak concentration (18%) and area under the curve (28%). No effects were observed on the primary sildenafil metabolite and no change in blood pressure was observed. Sildenafil had no effect on sitaxsentan plasma concentrations.

➤*Adverse Reactions:* Adverse reactions observed most frequently in clinical trials included headache, peripheral edema, nausea, nasal congestion, dizziness, liver enzyme abnormalities, and reduced hemoglobin, all of which occurred more frequently with sitaxsentan than placebo.

➤*Summary:* Sitaxsentan offers an alternative to bosentan therapy. Sitaxsentan is dosed once daily, rather than twice daily like bosentan. In addition, it appears to be associated with a lower incidence of liver toxicity. Close monitoring will still be necessary, however, for hepatotoxicity and to reduce the possibility of exposure during pregnancy. An NDA was filed with the FDA in May 2005 and Encysive received an approvable letter on March 26, 2006.

TEICOPLANIN (*Targocid* by Aventis) – A glycopeptide antibiotic

➤*Actions:*

Pharmacology – Teicoplanin (teichomycin A2) is a glycopeptide antibiotic complex structurally related to vancomycin (eg, *Vancocin*). It has a similar spectrum of activity but a longer half-life, which allows less frequent dosing. It may be administered by IM and IV injection and brief (30 minute) infusion. Teicoplanin is a mixture of 6 closely related glycopeptide components designated as teicoplanin-A2 (1 through 5) and teicoplanin-A3. The components of the A2 complex account for 90% to 95% of teicoplanin. The drug interferes with cell wall synthesis in susceptible organisms by inhibiting peptidoglycan polymerization.

Like vancomycin, teicoplanin is active only against gram-positive organisms. It is bactericidal against most susceptible strains, with the possible exception of some coagulase-negative staphylococci (which may show reduced susceptibility), where it may be bacteriostatic. It has equivalent or superior activity (based on MIC data) to vancomycin against staphylococci, including both methicillin-sensitive and -resistant *S. aureus*, *S. epidermidis*, streptococci (including viridans group, and groups B, C, F, and G), enterococci, and many anaerobic gram-positive bacteria, including *Clostridium difficile*, *C. perfringens*, *Listeria monocytogenes*, and *Corynebacterium jeikeium*. Vancomycin-resistant enterococci may be resistant to teicoplanin.

Teicoplanin is usually synergistic with aminoglycosides and imipenem, and additive with rifampin (eg, *Rifadin*). A postantibiotic effect of 2.4 to 4.1 hours has been reported with both methicillin-sensitive and -resistant strains of *S. aureus*.

Pharmacokinetics – Like vancomycin, teicoplanin is minimally absorbed after oral administration; this route is acceptable only for the treatment of pseudomembranous colitis. Following IM administration of 3 mg/kg, peak levels of 5 to 7 mcg/mL are achieved at 2 to 4 hours; bioavailability is 90%. Peak serum levels after IV administration are dependent on the dose and the method of administration. Following administration of 3 mg/kg, peak levels after a 30-second injection or a 30-minute infusion average 53 and 20 mcg/mL, respectively. Trough (24 hour) levels are not influenced. The drug is widely distributed in most tissues and fluids (with the exception of the CSF), although the rate and extent varies. Volume of distribution (Vd) at steady state averages 0.6 to 0.8 L/kg. Protein binding is 90%.

The drug does not appear to undergo metabolism and is excreted in the urine almost entirely by glomerular filtration. The terminal elimination half-life averages 45 to 70 hours. In patients with renal dysfunction and the elderly, the elimination half-life is increased but the Vd is unchanged. Current dosing recommendations for renal impairment state that usual doses be given for the first 3 days. Thereafter, either the dose is reduced or the interval prolonged, based on the degree of renal insufficiency according to the following scheme: Creatinine clearance (Ccr) 40 to 60 mL/min, half the dose or twice the interval; Ccr < 40 mL/min, one-third the dose or triple the interval.

Clinical trials – Reported response rates by type of infection are: Skin and soft tissue (90%); septicemia, bone and joint (89%); endocarditis (83%); respiratory tract (77%). Other applications in which the drug has demonstrated efficacy include: Endocarditis prophylaxis in dental surgery; Hickman catheter and other indwelling device-related infections; neurosurgical shunt ventriculitis; chronic ambulatory peritoneal dialysis (CAPD)-related peritonitis (added to dialysate); surgical prophylaxis; presumed gram-positive infections in immunocompromised patients. The usual loading and maintenance doses of 6 mg/kg followed by 3 mg/kg/24 hours may need to be increased in children and in the treatment of *S. aureus* endocarditis and septicemia. A reduction in efficacy has been noted in diabetics, immunocompromised patients, and when foreign bodies are present.

➤*Adverse Reactions:* The overall incidence of side effects is 10.3%. Most commonly reported effects include: Non-specific complaints (fatigue, headache, diarrhea) (5.1%); injection-site intolerance (pain, redness, phlebitis) (3%); hypersensitivity skin reactions (pruritus, urticaria, maculopapular rash) (2.4%); hematologic abnormalities (eosinophilia, reversible neutropenia, increased platelet count) (2.2%); transient elevation of LFTs (1.7%); nephrotoxicity (0.35% to 0.6%); high-frequency hearing loss, which may be irreversible (0.28%); bronchospasm (0.2%); anaphylactoid reactions (0.07%). Teicoplanin does not appear to cause the dose or infusion rate-related histamine release associated with the "red man syndrome," as does vancomycin. Concomitant use of an aminoglycoside appears to increase the incidence of nephrotoxicity.

➤*Summary:* Teicoplanin appears to be a safe and effective alternative to vancomycin. Potential advantages appear to be the availability of IM administration, reduced infusion times, and volume requirements, the lack of infusion-related reactions and once daily dosing. The NDA for teicoplanin was filed in March 1991. The FDA has given the drug a "1A" priority review rating. Teicoplanin is currently available in 13 countries.

TEZOSENTAN (*Veletri* by Genentech) – A dual endothelin receptor antagonist

➤*Actions:*

Pharmacology – Tezosentan is a dual endothelin receptor antagonist that displays high affinity to endothelin-A and endothelin-B receptors. Endothelin is a potent vasoconstrictor and is responsible for increasing resistance in blood vessels. Because of its ability to block endothelin receptors and produce vasodilation, tezosentan is being studied for possible use in patients with acute heart failure, pulmonary edema, and hepatorenal syndrome.

Pharmacokinetics – Tezosentan is available in a parenteral dosage form only. Initial studies show that tezosentan most likely follows a standard 2-compartment model. One study demonstrates the half-lives of the 2 disposition phases to be approximately 6 minutes and 3.2 hours.

Tezosentan is metabolized in the liver and excreted almost exclusively in the bile. Less than 5% of the total dose is cleared renally. It has 1 metabolite that is formed by hydroxylation of the isopropyl side chain, and it is thought to be 10 times less potent than the parent compound. Therefore, it is currently considered to be clinically insignificant.

Clinical trials – Tezosentan is currently undergoing phase 3 clinical trials. Several studies have been performed and several others are currently ongoing. The randomized IV tezosentan (RITZ) trials have been completed with mixed outcomes. The initial trial RITZ-2 showed that tezosentan had a positive effect on cardiac index and pulmonary capillary wedge pressure (PCWP) in patients with acute heart failure. This double-blind study randomized 184 patients with NYHA III/IV heart failure to standard therapy plus placebo, 50 mg/h tezosentan, or 100 mg/h tezosentan. Cardiac index increased by approximately 0.4 L/min/m^2 in both tezosentan groups, which was significant compared with placebo (P < 0.0001). The patients' PCWP decreased by approximately 3.9 mm Hg in both tezosentan groups and was significant compared with placebo (P < 0.0001). However, later studies in the RITZ series showed that tezosentan produced no significant added benefit in improving clinical symptoms or mortality compared with the current standard of therapy in patients with acute heart failure. In addition, more patients in the tezosentan groups suffered from adverse effects in these trials. In the RITZ-1 trial, 669 patients with acute decompensated heart failure were randomized in a double-blind, placebo-controlled study. Three hundred thirty-eight patients were assigned to the standard treatment group plus placebo while 331 where assigned to the standard treatment plus 50 mg/h tezosentan group. Tezosentan did not produce significant improvement in dyspnea at 24 hours. In addition, tezosentan was unable to show significant improvement in time to death or worsening heart failure during the first 24 hours. The RITZ-4 trial evaluated the use of tezosentan in patients with acute heart failure associated with acute coronary syndrome. This double-blind, placebo-controlled study randomized 193 patients to receive standard therapy plus placebo or 25 mg/h tezosentan for 1 hour followed by 50 mg/h for 23 hours up to 48 hours. Improvement in the primary endpoint, which was a composite of death, worsening heart failure, recurrent ischemia, or recurrent or new MI within the first 72 hours of drug treatment was not significant (P = 0.52). Finally, the RITZ-5 trial evaluated the use of tezosentan in pulmonary edema. The primary endpoint was a change in SO_2 from baseline over the first hour. In this double-blind, placebo-controlled study, 84 patients were randomized to receive standard therapy plus placebo or 50 mg/h tezosentan for 30 minutes followed by a maintenance dose of 50 to 100 mg/h for a total of 24 hours. The conclusions for the primary endpoint did not show significant improvement in SO_2.

Researchers have hypothesized that an inappropriately high dose may be responsible for the significant adverse effects of tezosentan. The lack of improving clinical symptoms and mortality may be the result of patients responding well to conventional therapy, making it difficult to determine any additional effects of new therapy. Currently, tezosentan is undergoing morbidity and mortality trials in patients with acute heart failure (Veritas 1 and Veritas 2). The trials are expected to be concluded in the spring of 2005.

➤*Drug Interactions:* One study has shown that concomitant administration of tezosentan and cyclosporin may lead to increased exposure to tezosentan. The mechanism for this effect has not been completely elucidated but is thought to be related to the inhibition of transport proteins in the liver.

➤*Adverse Reactions:* In general, clinical studies investigating the use of tezosentan have shown that a nitrate-like headache was the most common adverse effect of tezosentan. Hypotension, dizziness, nausea, vomiting, and decreased renal function also were observed.

➤*Summary:* Tezosentan is a dual endothelin antagonist that has shown promising efficacy in increasing cardiac index and reducing pulmonary capillary wedge pressure. It has not shown significant improvement in clinical symptoms or mortality at the doses that have been selected in past phase 3 clinical trials. New morbidity and mortality studies are currently underway to evaluate its efficacy in the treatment of acute heart failure.

TIBOLONE (*Xyvion* by Organon) – A synthetic steroid

➤*Actions:*

Pharmacology – Tibolone is a synthetic steroid with weak estrogenic, progestogenic, and androgenic activity, structurally related to norethynodrel. It inhibits osteoclastic activity and increases trabecular and cortical bone mass in postmenopausal women. Compared with placebo, tibolone reduced serum alkaline phosphatase, osteocalcin, serum albumin, calcium, and phosphate concentrations, and suppressed the urinary calcium:creatinine and hydroxypyroline:creatinine ratios. In the endometrium, tibolone is transformed by 3β-hydroxysteroid dehydrogenase isomerase into the D-4 metabolite. This metabolite does not have estrogenic activity but does have intrinsic progestogenic activity, therefore not stimulating the endometrium. Tibolone therapy does not require an additional progestogen to protect the endometrium.

Pharmacokinetics – Tibolone given orally is rapidly absorbed, appearing in the plasma within 30 minutes and peaking in 4 hours. Metabolism is mainly in the liver and excretion occurs in the urine and feces. The elimination half-life is ≈ 45 hours.

Clinical trials – Tibolone was an effective synthetic steroid for the treatment of menopausal symptoms and the prevention of osteoporosis in controlled clinical trials. Its efficacy seems to be equivalent to combined hormone replacement therapy (HRT), with similar reductions in vasomotor symptoms and increased spinal bone mineral density. Tibolone also was reported to be effective in reducing vasomotor symptoms and bone loss when used as add-back therapy in patients undergoing therapy for endometriosis or uterine leiomyomata with gonadotropin-releasing hormone analog. Studies were also performed concerning tibolone and its effects on lipids. Tibolone reduced HDL-cholesterol and triglycerides to a greater extent than combined HRT, while producing an overall reduction in total cholesterol comparable with that of transdermal estradiol. Tibolone also has been studied to assess its effects on sexuality. Tibolone was associated with an increase in the frequency of sexual interest, frequency of orgasm, general sexual satisfaction, sexual responsiveness, and a reduction in the frequency of dyspareunia. The most commonly studied dosage has been 2.5 mg once daily, continuously.

➤*Adverse Reactions:* The most common side effects include edema, nausea, breast tenderness, vaginal spotting or bleeding, bloating, leg pain, headache, and weight gain. Although weight gain is reported as a side effect, tibolone has been demonstrated to prevent total body fat and lean muscle mass changes associated with menopause without weight changes in a small study. Bleeding occurs in 10% to 15% of women during the first month of treatment and ≈ 4% after 6 months of treatment. The rate of amenorrhea in one 6-year study was 90% after the first 6 months of therapy with tibolone and 91% in the control group. Breakthrough bleeding is more likely to occur in patients who are younger, recently menopausal, and with detectable estradiol levels. Weight gain, increased blood pressure, or impairment of glycemic control were not observed in a group of postmenopausal women with type 2 diabetes treated with tibolone 2.5 mg/day for 2 months. Similarly, a lack of effect on glucose tolerance was observed in another study enrolling healthy women.

➤*Summary:* Tibolone will offer an alternative for the treatment of menopausal symptoms and prevention of osteoporosis. Tibolone increases bone mineral density to an extent comparable with that achieved with estrogen replacement therapy. It has been associated with a high degree of amenorrhea, comparable with that achieved with combined continuous estrogen/progestogen regimens. Added weak androgenic activity may provide added benefits in some patients, although more data are necessary to evaluate this effect. The lipid profile, particularly the considerable drop in HDL-cholesterol, may limit its use, although therapy also has been associated with a significant drop in triglycerides, which may be beneficial in others. Tibolone is commercially available in Europe under the trade name *Livial.*

TIRILAZAD (*Freedox* by Upjohn) – A 21-aminosteroid antioxidant

➤*Actions:*

Pharmacology – Tirilazad mesylate is a 21-aminosteroid (also referred to as lazaroids) with distinct antioxidant properties. It does not manifest glucocorticoid activity. Tirilazad acts as a cytoprotective agent that oxidizes peroxyl radicals and stabilizes cell membranes. It also helps to preserve the membrane content of vitamin E (alphatocopherol), another important antioxidant. As a result of its ability to prevent lipid peroxidation in cell membranes, tirilazad promotes tissue survival in the vicinity of a CNS injury.

Because of the high content of polyunsaturated lipids in neuronal membranes, the CNS is particularly susceptible to the destructive effects of oxygen radicals. Tissue injury occurring during CNS trauma or a stroke increases oxygen radical production, which in turn leads to damaging lipid peroxidation reactions. Such oxygen radical-mediated processes appear to be involved in posttraumatic brain edema, spinal axonal degeneration and microvascular damage. The progressive secondary tissue destruction, which follows the precipitating event, may be amenable to therapy with antioxidants.

Pharmacokinetics – Tirilazad is administered in a citrate solution as an IV infusion over not > 30 minutes. It is a lipophilic substance that distributes extensively to tissue, with a volume of distribution of ≈ 1.7 L/kg. The drug appears to follow a multicompartment elimination pattern. Following a single dose, the half-life is ≈ 3.75 hours. However, upon multiple dosing, a terminal elimination half-life of 35 hours has been observed. Elimination occurs via hepatic metabolism. The clearance of tirilazad is roughly equal to hepatic plasma flow.

Clinical trials – In numerous neurological studies of animal models, tirilazad has shown distinct promise as a useful therapeutic agent for brain and spinal injury, aneurysmal subarachnoid hemorrhage (SAH), and stroke. Phase III clinical trials are currently being conducted in each of these areas.

The second National Acute Spinal Cord Injury Study (NASCIS 2) demonstrated that patients treated with high-dose methylprednisolone (eg, *Solu-Medrol*; 8 to 9 g/day) within 8 hours of injury, experienced significantly greater neurological improvement than those treated with placebo. The efficacy of methylprednisolone in slowing the progression of CNS damage is believed to be due to its antioxidant properties rather than its glucocorticoid activity. For this reason, in NASCIS 3 (an ongoing follow-up study), 1 of the 3 treatment arms involves 2 g methylprednisolone bolus, followed by 2.5 mg/kg tirilazad infusion every 6 hours for a total of 48 hours.

To date, most of the clinical efficacy trials conducted with tirilazad have studied its use in SAH. Upjohn has submitted 3 double-blind, randomized, placebo controlled study results to the FDA in support of an NDA for tirilazad in the treatment of SAH. However, an FDA committee determined that these studies did not confirm efficacy; 1 study showed an improvement in males, but this was not replicated in another study, and there were no differences in females.

Tirilazad and newer, more potent antioxidants also may be studied in other neurologic conditions in which peroxidative mechanisms have been implicated. These include Alzheimer's disease, Parkinson's disease, and multiple sclerosis.

➤*Adverse Reactions:* Tirilazad has been safe in elderly patients (≈ 66 years of age) with acute ischemic stroke at doses < 6 mg/kg/day for 3 days. In healthy volunteers, tirilazad had no effect on cerebral blood flow or oxygen metabolism. Studies have failed to show any significant glucocorticoid effect to be caused by the drug. Up to 50% of subjects in 1 study exhibited a moderate, transient increase in serum alanine transaminase. The most noted side effect has been mild to moderate pain at the injection site, occurring in 60% to 80% of patients.

Studies involving tirilazad and both nimodipine (*Nimotop*) and cimetidine (eg, *Tagamet*) have failed to identify a clinically significant drug interaction with either of those drugs.

➤*Summary:* Tirilazad is a potent antioxidant, similar in structure to other steroids, but without glucocorticoid activity. Because of its ability to prevent oxygen radical-mediated lipid peroxidation, it may prove to be useful in preventing progressive neuronal degeneration and associated complications following brain and spinal injury, SAH, and stroke.

Upjohn submitted a new drug application in June 1994 for tirilazad with the indication of SAH. Due to the lack of serious side effects that have been documented thus far, and the considerable potential benefit that this drug possesses as a therapeutic agent in areas greatly in need of new treatment modalities, approval is anticipated. However, on September 26, 1994, the FDA's Peripheral and Central Nervous System Drugs Advisory Committee decided that the studies for tirilazad did not confirm efficacy and that further studies would be necessary. A Treatment IND program was discussed as a possibility.

TROSPECTOMYCIN (*Spexil* by Upjohn) – An aminocyclitol antibiotic

➤*Actions:*

Pharmacology – Trospectomycin is a water soluble analog of spectinomycin (*Trobicin*) that is 8 to 10 times more potent and has a broader spectrum of activity. It has good gram-positive and gram-negative aerobic and anaerobic activity, including in vitro activity against *Staphylococci*, *Streptococci*, *Peptostreptococci*, *Peptococci*, *Haemophilus*, *Gardnerella*, *Neisseria*, *Bacteroides*, *Chlamydia*, *Mycoplasma*, and *Ureaplasma*. It has moderate activity against Enterobacteriaceae and no activity against *Pseudomonas*.

Trospectomycin acts by binding to the 30S component of the ribosome unit thereby inhibiting protein synthesis. It has a greater affinity for the 30S ribosome unit than spectinomycin and therefore has higher activity. Cross-resistance to spectinomycin has been observed in vitro.

Pharmacokinetics – Patients (n = 128) were randomized to receive trospectomycin (75 to 1000 mg) by IM injection or by 20 minute IV infusion. The IM product was 100% bioavailable. The mean peak plasma concentration and AUC were linear relative to dose, and the half-life was 2.1 hours. Serum concentrations were < 2 mcg/mL 12 hours post-dose, suggesting 2 to 3 times/day dosing as the MIC for most organisms is between 2 to 4 mcg/mL. In another trial, trospectomycin was administered by IV infusion. While almost no drug was found in the feces, 48% to 62% was recovered in the urine during the first 48 hours, suggesting that the drug is slowly released from tissues. The half-life of 2.18 hours did not change with increasing dose.

Clinical trials – The in vitro activity of trospectomycin was compared with that of amikacin (eg, *Amikin*), cephalothin (eg, *Keflin*), and vancomycin (eg, *Vancocin*) against 342 gram-positive organisms. Vancomycin was the most active agent overall, and trospectomycin was better than amikacin, especially for *Staphylococci* and *Streptococci*.

The activity of trospectomycin, clindamycin (eg, *Cleocin*), metronidazole (eg, *Flagyl*), imipenem (*Primaxin*), cefoxitin (*Mefoxin*), and piperacillin (*Pipracil*) was evaluated against 72 strains of *Bacteroides*. Trospectomycin had very good activity and was comparable with imipenem and metronidazole. Its activity was greater than that of piperacillin and cefoxitin. In another trial, trospectomycin was comparable with clindamycin and cefoxitin against *Bacteroides fragilis*, and there was no cross-resistance between the 3 drugs. Of the organisms tested, 90% to 100% were resistant to ampicillin (eg, *Polycillin*) and cefaclor (eg, *Ceclor*), and > 50% were resistant to doxycycline (eg, *Vibramycin*). None of the organisms tested were resistant to trospectomycin.

The effect of trospectomycin and several other antibiotics was evaluated against *Mycoplasma pneumoniae*, *M. hominis*, and *Ureaplasma urealyticum*. Trospectomycin and spectinomycin were equivalent to tetracycline (eg, *Achromycin*) against *M. pneumoniae* but less active against *M. hominis*. It was concluded that trospectomycin is active against *Mycoplasma*-induced respiratory or genital infections.

To date, published in vivo trials with trospectomycin are limited. The efficacy of a single 1 g IM dose was evaluated in 10 men with uncomplicated *C. trachomatis* urethritis. All were culture-positive at follow-up on days 4 to 8. On follow-up on days 21 to 28, 6 of the 8 men were still culture-positive. It was concluded that a single IM dose for the treatment of uncomplicated *C. trachomatis* urethritis is not effective.

➤*Adverse Reactions:* In one study, mild, transient and local reactions were seen in 20% of subjects receiving trospectomycin vs 22% with placebo; none of the reactions were thought to be drug-related. Overall, mild and transient side effects were seen in 32% of 64 subjects receiving trospectomycin; 12 had dizziness or lightheadedness and 17 who received > 600 mg had perioral/facial numbness. Results from a similar trial using IM injection were comparable.

In a multiple-dose trial involving 10 healthy males, trospectomycin caused significantly more pain at the injection site. There was also a significant increase in perioral paresthesias with increasing doses (especially at the 500 and 750 mg doses). Perioral paresthesias were mild and transient, were seen shortly after dosing and lasted about 1 to 2 hours. Tolerance did not develop over the 7 days of the study. Clinically significant orthostatic hypotension occurred after the first dose in patients receiving 500 or 750 mg but was not seen with subsequent dosing.

➤*Summary:* Trospectomycin is an injectable aminocyclitol aminoglycoside that is structurally related to spectinomycin. It has good gram-positive and gram-negative aerobic and anaerobic activity and may prove to be useful for the treatment of upper respiratory tract infections, bacterial vaginitis, pelvic inflammatory disease, and gonorrhea. Overall, it appears to be well tolerated and the major side effects are pain at the injection site and perioral paresthesias.

VALSPODAR (*Amdray* by Novartis) – A P-glycoprotein (P-gp) inhibitor

➤*Actions:*

Pharmacology – Valspodar (SDZ PSC 833), a cyclosporine analog, is employed in reversing classic multidrug resistance (MDR) to natural product-derived cytotoxic agents. MDR results from overexpression of the multidrug resistance gene (MDR-1) leading to overproduction of P-gp. P-gp is believed to function as a transmembrane efflux pump that prevents the intracellular accumulation of certain cytotoxic agents, such as anthracyclines, epidophyllotoxins, vinca alkaloids, and taxanes. Valspodar acts as a P-gp inhibitor, thus preventing drug resistance. In addition, valspodar is believed to influence clearance of some chemotherapeutic agents.

Pharmacokinetics – Valspodar is metabolized by cytochrome P450 3A. It can be administered by IV infusion or orally. The following 3 oral formulations have been tested: An oral solution, microemulsion oral solution, and microemulsion capsule. The microemulsion formulas have a greater bioavailability when compared with the conventional oral solution (≈ 54% and ≈ 52% for the microemulsion oral solution and capsule, respectively, as compared with ≈ 29% for the conventional oral solution). The microemulsion formulas also display a higher C_{max} and a lower t_{max} compared with the conventional oral solution.

Clinical trials – In a phase II study, researchers evaluating 2 regimens involving valspodar, mitoxantrone (*Novantrone*), and etoposide (eg, *VePesid*) for treatment of refractory and relapsed acute myelogenous leukemia (AML) concluded that their results of 32% of patients achieving complete remission appeared "encouraging." However, no comparison was made to a control or reference study. Additional studies are necessary.

➤*Drug Interactions:*

Digoxin (eg, Lanoxin) – Valspodar, given in a single oral dose to healthy subjects with steady-state levels of digoxin, increased digoxin AUC (in all of the subjects) and C_{max} (in 11 of the 12 subjects), while decreasing digoxin renal clearance (in 11 of the 12 subjects). Coadministration of digoxin and valspodar orally for 5 days in healthy subjects increased digoxin AUC (in all of the subjects) and C_{max} (in 11 of the 12 subjects), and decreased renal and nonrenal clearance of digoxin.

Paclitaxel (Taxol) – Valspodar slightly increases peak plasma levels and AUC of paclitaxel and significantly prolongs the paclitaxel elimination phase.

Etoposide – Valspodar decreased the clearance of etoposide by 57% when administered concomitantly.

➤*Adverse Reactions:* Valspodar lacks immunosuppressive and nephrotoxic qualities. Transient hyperbilirubinemia appears to be the most frequent adverse effect of valspodar among several studies. Reversible cerebellar ataxia also has been observed.

➤*Summary:* Valspodar is a P-gp inhibitor currently in phase III clinical studies for treatment of AML, decreasing chemotherapy resistance in relapsing multiple myeloma, and reducing drug resistance or inhibiting drug resistance development in ovarian cancer. Additional studies to demonstrate efficacy are warranted.

VESNARINONE (*Arkin-Z* by Otsuka) – An inotropic agent for CHF

➤*Actions:*

Pharmacology – Vesnarinone, a quinolinone derivative, is an oral inotropic agent with little to no effect on heart rate or myocardial oxygen consumption. The mechanism of action is largely unknown. It may be related to a slight inhibition of PDE III, which causes an increase in cyclic AMP and finally an increase in the inward calcium current. There is also a reduction in the potassium current.

In addition, vesnarinone inhibits the production and release of cytokines such as TNF-alpha, IL-1, IL-2, and IFN-gamma. This inhibition may relate directly to its efficacy as an inotropic agent. Increased concentrations of TNF-alpha are seen in patients with chronic heart failure. These increased concentrations depress myocardial contractility, alter muscle membrane potential, decrease blood pressure, and precipitate pulmonary edema. Therefore, reducing the concentration of TNF-alpha is beneficial in patients with heart failure.

Interestingly, vesnarinone also inhibits the replication of HIV-1 in peripheral blood lymphocytes and in chronically infected macrophages, suggesting that it may be useful in treating patients with HIV-1 disease.

Pharmacokinetics – The pharmacokinetic parameters of vesnarinone were evaluated in 21 healthy male volunteers in a 2-phase, nonblinded trial. In phase I, subjects received vesnarinone in a sequentially ascending single dose ranging from 7.5 to 240 mg. In phase II, 3 subjects received vesnarinone 30 mg/day for 15 days. The elimination half-life was 44.7 ± 1.2 hour and the clearance 0.284 ± 0.018 L/hr. The drug was fairly extensively metabolized, with only 11% to 27% (mean, 17.7%) being excreted unchanged in the urine. The authors concluded that elimination of vesnarinone is dose-dependent and that plasma concentrations are proportional to the dose administered.

Clinical trials – In 2 small, uncontrolled trials, vesnarinone was administered to a total of 20 patients with CHF; significant hemodynamic and functional improvement was seen. In a small, placebo controlled study, 8 patients with chronic, stable, moderate CHF received vesnarinone 60 mg/day or placebo for 4 to 8 weeks. Patients were then crossed over to the alternate treatment group. Symptomatic improvement was noted in 4 patients while receiving vesnarinone. In addition, vesnarinone caused an increase in contractility of the left ventricle. Mild to moderate dyspnea and fatigue on exertion was seen in all patients while receiving placebo. In 2 placebo-controlled, double-blind trials, a total of 159 patients with CHF were randomized to receive vesnarinone 60 mg/day or placebo for 12 weeks. In both trials, there was an improvement in the quality of life and a reduction in the severity or progression of heart failure in patients receiving vesnarinone.

The long-term use of vesnarinone was evaluated in a double-blind trial involving 477 patients with CHF. Patients were randomized to receive vesnarinone 60 mg/day or placebo for 6 months. Patients receiving vesnarinone experienced an improvement in their quality of life and a reduction in morbidity and mortality when compared with patients receiving placebo. In the initial design of this trial, patients also could be randomized to receive vesnarinone 120 mg/day. However, this treatment group was stopped after the first 253 patients had been enrolled because of a significant increase in mortality. These results suggest that vesnarinone may have a narrow therapeutic window.

➤*Adverse Reactions:* The primary side effect noted with vesnarinone use is reversible neutropenia seen in 2.5% of patients. Other reported side effects include: Reversible agranulocytosis; palpitations; dyspnea; gastric discomfort; nausea; headache; skin rash.

➤*Summary:* Vesnarinone is a new positive inotropic agent that appears to be effective in the management of CHF. Because of its unique mechanism of action involving inhibition of cytokines, vesnarinone may prove to be a useful alternative in the long-term management of this patient population. It appears to be well tolerated with the exception of the relatively high incidence of reversible neutropenia. Because of this potentially serious toxicity, the clinical utility of vesnarinone remains to be determined.

Although vesnarinone is currently available in Japan, all research ended in the US on July 31, 1996.

VIGABATRIN (*Sabril* by Aventis) – An anticonvulsant agent

➤*Actions:*

Pharmacology – Vigabatrin is a second generation antiepileptic that appears to exert its mechanism of action via increasing brain GABA levels by inhibition of GABA metabolism. These effects on GABA appear to be dose-related. Vigabatrin has an S(+)-enantiomer that inhibits GABA-T, whereas the R(-)-enantiomer has almost no effect. Vigabatrin's mechanism of action also may be attributed to its ability to decrease excitation-related amino acids, aspartate, glutamate, and glutamine concentrations in the brain, but these same changes do not occur in the CSF.

Pharmacokinetics – Although the exact bioavailability of vigabatrin is not known, following oral administration about 80% of the dose is recovered in the urine. In healthy volunteers, its absorption was rapid and peak plasma concentrations occurred within the first 2 hours. When vigabatrin was administered with food, its approximate bioavailability was 92% ± 11%. Vigabatrin has a volume of distribution of about 0.8 L/kg, is not bound to plasma proteins, and distributes into the CSF. The drug does not appear to be metabolized by the liver, or influence hepatic metabolism. The elimination half-life observed in 24 volunteers was ≈ 7 hours and does not appear to be significantly affected by single or multiple dosing, and appears to be similar in adults and children. Dosing adjustments may be necessary in patients with renal impairment (Ccr less than 60 mL/min) and in the elderly.

Clinical trials – When traditional antiepileptic therapies including add on treatments are used, up to 25% of patients still experience seizures. The studies examining the efficacy of vigabatrin as an antiepileptic medication were primarily add-on trials in patients with resistant epilepsy. Reductions in seizure frequency have been observed in patients with partial and complex partial seizures, but reductions have been observed less frequently with primary generalized seizures, and no reductions (and even worsening) of absence and myoclonic seizures. In a meta-analysis of 9 European trials, of the patients with complex partial seizures, 72% showed a > 25% decrease in seizure frequency over a 7- to 12-week period. When combining all clinical trials (including European studies) examining the efficacy of vigabatrin in treatment of resistant partial complex epilepsy, between 33% and 61% of patients experienced a > 50% reduction in seizure frequency at doses between 1 and 4 g/day.

The use of vigabatrin in doses ranging from 50 to 150 mg/kg/day also has been studied as add-on therapy in children with partial, generalized, Lennox-Gaustaut syndrome and West syndrome. Results appear similar to those in adults; children with partial seizures appeared to respond better with rates between 38% and 49% of patients experiencing between a 50% to 100% reduction in seizure frequency. Vigabatrin also has been examined in the use of intractable infantile spasms and was found to be effective in reducing spasms > 50% in 30 patients (71%), with complete relief of spasms in 16 patients (38%). Caution should be used in the interpretation of these results since great variability can occur with the incidence of infantile seizures over time.

➤*Drug Interactions:* One of the major advantages of vigabatrin is the fact that it does not appear to be metabolized by the liver, nor influence hepatic metabolism. Therefore, the typical drug interactions observed with traditional anticonvulsants are not seen with vigabatrin. However, vigabatrin was shown to decrease phenytoin (eg, *Dilantin*) levels by 20% to 30% in clinical trials. No mechanism of action could account for the decreased levels; therefore, phenytoin levels should be monitored if vigabatrin is added. Vigabatrin does not appear to interact with phenobarbital, primidone, carbamazepine (eg, *Tegretol*), or valproate (eg, *Depakene*) to any clinically significant degree.

➤*Adverse Reactions:* Vigabatrin appears to be well tolerated with minimal side effects and when they do occur, they are mild. In a trial of 254 patients who received vigabatrin from 12 months to > 2 years, up to 75% of patients reported no side effects. Data from pooled studies indicate that the most common side effects are: Somnolence; fatigue; irritability; dizziness; headache; depression; confusion; poor concentration; abdominal pain; anorexia (some trials have reported weight gain). In the studies involving children, the main side effects observed were agitation and insomnia, with a similar number of patients reporting a lack of side effects (79%).

➤*Summary:* Vigabatrin appears to be effective in the treatment of complex partial seizures, less effective for primary generalized seizures, and not effective (and may even worsen) absence and myoclonic seizures. The dosing range is from 1 to 4 g/day in adults, with 2 to 3 g appearing to be the most optimal, and a dose of 50 to 150 mg/kg/day in children. Side effects are minimal and mild and there seems to be a lack of clinically significant drug interactions, except that observed with phenytoin.

Vigabatrin is already available in Europe and Canada and has been deemed approvable in the US.

VILOXAZINE (*Catatrol* by AstraZeneca) – A bicyclic antidepressant

➤*Actions:*

Pharmacology – Viloxazine is a bicyclic antidepressant agent. It has noradrenergic reuptake blocking properties and acts, in part, as an amphetamine-like central stimulant. Overall sympathomimetic, sedative and anticholinergic activity is less than that seen with the tricyclic antidepressants (eg, imipramine [eg, *Tofranil*]). Conflicting data has been reported on the effects of viloxazine on the seizure threshold, with some reports indicating that seizure risk is greater, while others claiming it is less than that seen with traditional tricyclics. Rapid eye movement (REM) sleep and overall sleep time is markedly reduced with viloxazine. It does not appear to potentiate the effects of alcohol.

Pharmacokinetics – Viloxazine is rapidly and almost completely (85%) absorbed after oral administration in the small intestine. Peak blood levels occur 1 to 4 hours after ingestion; however, no correlation has been established between blood levels and clinical response. Volume of distribution averages 0.78 L/kg. The eliminiation half-life ranges from 2 to 5 hours. The drug is extensively metabolized by hydroxylation and oxidation to inactive metabolites in the liver. Only 12% to 15% of the parent compound is eliminated unchanged by the kidneys. In patients > 60 years of age, there appears to be a reduction in viloxazine clearance, possibly due to decreased hepatic metabolism. Specific dosage guidelines in the elderly and patients with hepatic dysfunction have not been established.

Clinical trials – Viloxazine was an effective antidepressant in controlled clinical trials of hospitalized and outpatient populations with depression. Its efficacy appears to be equivalent to imipramine, with a 60% response rate. Published trials have not examined whether efficacy rates vary with specific types of depression. Viloxazine also has been studied in small groups of patients with narcolepsy and cataplexy (a form of narcolepsy characterized by periods of momentary paralysis); this appears to be a potential target population. Fewer sleep attacks were reported during treatment.

➤*Drug Interactions:* Viloxazine decreases the elimination rate of theophylline (eg, *Theo-Dur*), carbamazepine (eg, *Tegretol*), and phenytoin (eg, *Dilantin*), possibly by competing for the same microsomal enzymes. When viloxazine was added to a stable regimen of these drugs, theophylline toxicity was reported (no levels available), carbamazepine levels increased by 55%, and those of its active metabolite by 16%, and phenytoin levels increased by an average of 36%.

➤*Adverse Reactions:* Nausea is the most commonly reported side effect, with an average incidence of 19%, but some studies have reported an incidence as high as 50%. Nausea progressing to vomiting was reported in 4.7% of patients. These effects may be minimized by initiating therapy with low doses accompanied by slow, upward dose titration. Headache is also commonly reported. Less frequently reported side effects include: Insomnia; taste disturbances; hypomania; mania; dizziness; tachycardia; ataxia; tremor; confusion; restlessness; dry mouth; constipation; drowsiness; difficult micturition; seizures. The anticholinergic-related side effects appear to occur less frequently than with the tricyclic agents.

➤*Summary:* Viloxazine is a safe and effective antidepressant with a somewhat different side effect profile than the tricyclic antidepressants, although it is most likely to be used in patients with narcolepsy or cataplexy. Available data has not established whether viloxazine has any advantages over currently available agents. Additional studies in specific populations of patients are needed to establish its place in therapy. Viloxazine currently has orphan drug status for the treatment of cataplexy and narcolepsy.

VINDESINE SULFATE (*Eldisine* by Lilly) – An antineoplastic

➤*Actions:*

Pharmacology – Vindesine sulfate (Lilly 99094, NSC-245467, DAVA, desacetyl vinblastine amide sulfate) is a synthetic vinca alkaloid derived from vinblastine sulfate, but more closely resembling the activity of vincristine.

A large number of studies support its utility in a diverse group of cancer types. Major and dose-limiting toxicities include myelosuppression and neurotoxicity.

The mechanism of vindesine's anticancer action is probably like that of the other vinca alkaloids; it is cell-cycle specific and blocks mitosis with metaphase arrest. Vinca alkaloids bind specifically to cellular microtubules of the mitotic apparatus and disrupt their function. This leads to inability of the dividing cell to correctly segregate chromosomes and ultimately, to cell death.

Pharmacokinetics – Vindesine sulfate appears to have similar pharmacokinetics to vincristine and vinblastine. The triphasic clearance profile of IV vindesine is summarized below:

IV Vindesine Clearance		
Phase	Half-life (minutes)	Volume of distribution (liters)
Alpha (α)	3 ± 1	5 ± 2
Beta (β)	99 ±45	58 ± 51
Gamma (γ)	1213 ± 493	598 ± 294

Elimination in the urine in the first 24 hours accounts for 13.2% of the total dose administered. The remainder is sequestered in the body or eliminated in the bile.

Clinical trials – Overall, vindesine demonstrates good activity in difficult-to-treat and refractory cancer types. Responses to vindesine in patients who have received vincristine or vinblastine therapy suggest a lack of cross-resistance between these agents. Doses have ranged from 3 to 4.5 mg/m^2 as an IV bolus every 1 to 2 weeks *or* 1 to 2 mg/m^2 /day for 2 to 10 days every 2 to 3 weeks. The results of clinical studies are summarized below:

Vindesine Clinical Studies				
		Response rate		
Cancer type	Number of patients treated	Range (%)	Average (%)	Complete number of patients
Colorectal	33	6	6	1
Esophageal	76	17 to 55	43	0
Leukemias	26	15 to 61	38	4
Lung	234	17 to 43	30	10
Lymphoma	61	34 to 50	41	4
Metastatic breast	120	0 to 28	18	0
Total	550	0 to 61	29	19

➤*Adverse Reactions:* Major dose-limiting toxicities include myelosuppression and neuropathy. The primary hematologic toxicity is leukopenia, which is reversible with dosage reduction or discontinuation. Anemia and thrombocytopenia occur but are rarely severe. Neurotoxicity appears to be a function of cumulative dose. Patients with hepatic dysfunction and those over 60 years of age may be at greater risk. Neurotoxic manifestations include peripheral paresthesia, decreased tendon reflexes, muscle weakness and myalgia, headache, parotid and jaw pain, constipation, and paralytic ileus.

Other side effects include: Nausea; vomiting; stomatitis; hoarseness; transient hepatic dysfunction; inappropriate antidiuretic hormone secretion; fever; skin rash; alopecia; local cellulitis. Vindesine sulfate is a potent vesicant; avoid extravasation into the SC tissues.

➤*Summary:* Vindesine sulfate is a vinca alkaloid that demonstrates promise for a wide variety of cancer types; however, its full extent of activity remains to be determined. Its major toxicities are similar to those of its family, myelotoxicity and neurotoxicity.

XIMELAGATRAN (*Exanta* by AstraZeneca Pharmaceuticals LP) – An Anticoagulant

➤*Actions:*

Pharmacology – Ximelagatran is an oral, direct, thrombin inhibitor being evaluated as an anticoagulant for prevention of stroke, as a consequence of atrial fibrillation, for primary and secondary prevention and treatment of a venous thromboembolic event (VTE) and for secondary prevention of post-MI. Ximelagatran, a small-molecule prodrug, is converted to its active form melagatran in vivo. Melagatran's anticoagulant effects are reversible and include inhibition of platelet activation and aggregation and reduction of fibrinolysis. Inhibition of circulating and clot-bound thrombin occurs via binding to the active site. Furthermore, this inhibition has been shown to decrease the amount of thrombin generation, most likely because of a reduction of thrombin-mediated positive feedback of the coagulation system.

Pharmacokinetics – Ximelagatran is rapidly absorbed and converted to melagatran postadministration. The bioavailability of melagatran is approximately 20%, peak levels are achieved within 2 hours, and its half-life ranges between 3 and 4 hours. The majority of melagatran is excreted unchanged via the kidney within 12 hours of administration.

Clinical trials – Several randomized, multicenter trials (Melagatran for thrombin inhibition in orthopedic surgery [METHRO], Expanded prophylaxis evaluation surgery study [EXPRESS], *Exanta* used to lessen thrombosis [EXULT]) to determine the efficacy and safety of ximelagatran for VTE prophylaxis in patients undergoing orthopedic hip or knee surgeries have been performed. Ximelagatran was compared with standard regimens of either warfarin or enoxaparin in these studies. A randomized, double-blind, multicenter, dose-finding study enrolling 443 patients evaluated ximelagatran for the prevention of VTE post-knee surgery. In this study, no significant difference was observed in the incidence of VTE between ximelagatran and enoxaparin. However, in a second randomized, double-blind, multicenter trial enrolling 1,557 patients designed to evaluate ximelagatran in the prevention of VTE post-hip surgery, ximelagatran exhibited a small but significantly higher incidence of VTE compared with enoxaparin (3.3%, 95% CI). Comparison for VTE prevention post-knee surgery in 3 different randomized, double-blind, multicenter trials enrolling a total of 4,337 patients showed ximelagatran to have comparable efficacy to warfarin at doses of 24 mg twice daily and higher efficacy at doses of 36 mg twice daily (EXULT A: 20.3% with ximelagatran vs 27.6% with warfarin, $P = 0.003$; EXULT B: 22.5% vs 31%, $P < 0.001$).

Thrombin inhibitor in venous thromboembolism (THRIVE) is a randomized, double-blind, multicenter trial enrolling 1,233 patients that evaluated the efficacy and safety of ximelagatran as compared with placebo in the extended secondary prevention of venous thromboembolism after 6 months of warfarin therapy. Over an 18-month follow-up, ximelagatran significantly reduced the recurrence rate of VTE (2.8% risk with ximelagatran vs 12.6% risk with placebo, $P < 0.001$) with continued reduction of risk over time.

The safety and efficacy of ximelagatran in prevention of stroke in patients with nonvalvular atrial fibrillation has been evaluated in randomized trials (stroke prevention using the oral direct thrombin inhibitor ximelagatran in patients with nonvalvular atrial fibrillation [SPORTIF]). A total of 7,329 participants randomized in SPORTIF III and IV trials had a diagnosis of atrial fibrillation plus at least 1 risk factor for stroke. Trial results have shown ximelagatran to have comparable efficacy to warfarin in prevention of stroke and systemic embolic events among high-risk patients.

A randomized, placebo-controlled, multicenter dose-finding study (Efficacy and safety of the oral direct thrombin inhibitor ximelagatran in patients with recent myocardial damage [ESTEEM]) to compare the effectiveness of ximelagatran with placebo for prevention of severe ischemia, nonfatal MI, and death in patients with history of a recent MI was performed. A total of 1,900 patients were randomized to receive 1 of 4 doses of oral ximelagatran twice daily or placebo for 6 months. All patients also received up to 160 mg of acetylsalicylic acid (ASA) once daily. Ximelagatran in combination with ASA was more effective than ASA alone when the composite endpoint of death, non-fatal MI, and severe recurrent ischemia were evaluated (12.7% vs 16.3%, respectively; $P = 0.036$). Additionally, incidence of major bleeding with ximelagatran was higher when compared with placebo (1.8% vs 0.9%, respectively).

➤*Adverse Reactions:* Ximelagatran has been associated with few adverse events in clinical trials. The incidence of bleeding is similar to that observed with warfarin or enoxaparin. Asymptomatic elevations of ALT have occurred at rates higher than those associated with warfarin; however, the elevated levels have spontaneously decreased with continued treatment or post-discontinuation of the drug.

➤*Summary:* Ximelagatran is an oral, direct, thrombin inhibitor that has proven effective in prevention of stroke as a consequence of atrial fibrillation in primary and secondary prevention and treatment of a VTE and in secondary prevention of post-MI. Its convenient route of oral administration and predictable pharmacokinetic and pharmacodynamic profile provide an advantage in its use over that of currently available anticoagulants; however, these benefits will most likely be weighed against its twice-daily dosing, higher cost, and incidence of hepatic effects. AstraZeneca Pharmaceuticals LP filed an NDA for ximelagatran in December 2003. Phase 3 trials are in progress. Ximelagatran is currently approved in France.

~ Bibliography Available on Request ~

FDA NEW DRUG CLASSIFICATION

The FDA developed an alpha-numeric drug classification to aid in the prioritization of a new drug review. The use of numbers identify the drug's chemical classification; letters identify the assessment of therapeutic potential or review priority. This system was revised in 1992. When the classification for a new drug is known, it is listed in parentheses following the approval date for the drug at the beginning of the Administration and Dosage section of the monograph.

FDA Classification System for Newly Approved Drugs

Chemical Ranking	
1 =	New chemical entity not previously marketed in US
2 =	New salt form of a drug currently on US market
3 =	New dosage formulation of a drug currently on US market
4 =	New combination of drugs already available in US
5 =	New manufacturer (ie, generic drug)
6 =	New indication for drug already approved
7 =	Marketed drug without an approved NDA (drugs marketed prior to 1938)
Therapeutic Potential/Review Priority	
A =	Represents significant therapeutic gain over drugs currently available *(replaced by "P" ranking in 1992)*
AA =	Represents important therapeutic gain for drugs indicated for AIDS
B =	Represents modest therapeutic advances in drug therapy *(replaced by "P" ranking in 1992)*
C =	Represents little or no therapeutic gain in drug class *(replaced by "S" ranking in 1992)*
E =	Drug used to treat life-threatening or severely debilitated patients
P =	Priority; represents a therapeutic gain or provides improved treatment over marketed drugs OR has modest advantages compared to marketed agents (this category was initiated in first quarter of 1992)
S =	Standard; has similar therapeutic properties when compared to marketed drugs (this category was initiated in the first quarter of 1992)

CONTROLLED SUBSTANCES

The Controlled Substances Act of 1970 regulates the manufacturing, distribution and dispensing of drugs that have abuse potential. The Drug Enforcement Administration (DEA) within the US Department of Justice is the chief federal agency responsible for enforcing the act.

➤*DEA Schedules:* Drugs under jurisdiction of the Controlled Substances Act are divided into five schedules based on their potential for abuse and physical and psychological dependence. All controlled substances listed in *Drug Facts and Comparisons®* are identified by schedule as follows:

Schedule I *(c-i):* High abuse potential and no accepted medical use (eg, heroin, marijuana, LSD).

Schedule II *(c-ii):* High abuse potential with severe dependence liability (eg, narcotics, amphetamines, dronabinol, some barbiturates).

Schedule III *(c-iii):* Less abuse potential than schedule II drugs and moderate dependence liability (eg, nonbarbiturate sedatives, nonamphetamine stimulants, limited amounts of certain narcotics).

Schedule IV *(c-iv):* Less abuse potential than schedule III drugs and limited dependence liability (eg, some sedatives, antianxiety agents, nonnarcotic analgesics).

Schedule V *(c-v):* Limited abuse potential. Primarily small amounts of narcotics (codeine) used as antitussives or antidiarrheals. Under federal law, limited quantities of certain *c-v* drugs may be purchased without a prescription directly from a pharmacist if allowed under state statutes. The purchaser must be at least 18 years of age and must furnish suitable identification. All such transactions must be recorded by the dispensing pharmacist.

➤*Registration:* Prescribing physicians and dispensing pharmacies must be registered with the DEA, PO Box 28083, Central Station, Washington, DC 20005.

➤*Inventory:* Separate records must be kept of purchases and dispensing of controlled substances. An inventory of controlled substances must be made every 2 years.

➤*Prescriptions:* Prescriptions for controlled substances must be written in ink and include: Date; name and address of the patient; name, address and DEA number of the physician. Oral prescriptions must be promptly committed to writing. Controlled substance prescriptions may not be dispensed or refilled more than 6 months after the date issued or be refilled more than five times. A written prescription signed by the physician is required for schedule II drugs. In case of emergency, oral prescriptions for schedule II substances may be filled; however, the physician must provide a signed prescription within 72 hours. Schedule II prescriptions cannot be refilled. A triplicate order form is necessary for the transfer of controlled substances in schedule II. Forms are available for the individual prescriber at no charge from the DEA.

➤*State Laws:* In many cases state laws are more restrictive than federal laws and therefore impose additional requirements (eg, triplicate prescription forms).

The rational use of any medication requires a risk versus benefit assessment. Among the myriad of risk factors which complicate this assessment, pregnancy is one of the most perplexing.

The FDA has established five categories to indicate the potential of a systemically absorbed drug for causing birth defects. The key differentiation among the categories rests upon the degree (reliability) of documentation and the risk vs benefit ratio. Pregnancy Category X is particularly notable in that if any data exists that may implicate a drug as a teratogen and the risk vs benefit ratio does not support use of the drug, the drug is contraindicated during pregnancy. These categories are summarized below:

FDA Pregnancy Categories

Pregnancy Category	Definition
A	Controlled studies show no risk. Adequate, well-controlled studies in pregnant women have failed to demonstrate risk to the fetus.
B	No evidence of risk in humans. Either animal findings show risk, but human findings do not; or if no adequate human studies have been done, animal findings are negative.
C	Risk cannot be ruled out. Human studies are lacking, and animal studies are either positive for fetal risk or lacking. However, potential benefits may justify the potential risks.
D	Positive evidence of risk. Investigational or post-marketing data show risk to the fetus. Nevertheless, potential benefits may outweigh the potential risks. If needed in a life-threatening situation or a serious disease, the drug may be acceptable if safer drugs cannot be used or are ineffective.
X	Contraindicated in pregnancy. Studies in animals or human, or investigational or post-marketing reports have shown fetal risk which clearly outweighs any possible benefit to the patient.

Regardless of the designated Pregnancy Category or presumed safety, no drug should be administered during pregnancy unless it is clearly needed and potential benefits outweigh potential hazards to the fetus.

ANTIHYPERTENSIVES

➤*Definition of hypertension:* Hypertension is defined as a systolic blood pressure (SBP) of greater than 140 mm Hg, diastolic blood pressure (DBP) of greater than 90 mm Hg, or the use of an antihypertensive medication. The classification of prehypertension recognizes the relationship between blood pressure (BP) and the risk of cardiovascular disease (CVD) events and calls for increased education of health care professionals and the public in order to reduce BP levels. Patients with SBP of 120 to 139 or a DBP of 80 to 89 should be considered prehypertensive and are at an increased risk for developing hypertension. These patients require health promoting lifestyle modifications to prevent CVD. In individuals 40 to 70 years of age, each elevation of 20 mm Hg in SBP or every 10 mm Hg in DBP doubles the risk of CVD across the entire BP range from 115/75 to 185/115 mm Hg. As a result, identifying and treating high BP decreases cardiovascular mortality and morbidity in these patients and protects against hypertension related complications of stroke, coronary events, heart failure, renal disease progression, progression to more severe hypertension, and all-cause mortality. In order to identify high-risk individuals, the following table presents the classification of adult BP.

Classification of BP for Adults ≥ 18 Years of Age[1]

Category	Systolic (mm Hg)		Diastolic (mm Hg)
Normal	< 120	and	< 80
Prehypertension[2]	120 to 139	or	80 to 89
Hypertension,[3] Stage 1	140 to 159	or	90 to 99
Hypertension,[3] Stage 2	≥ 160	or	≥ 100

[1] Not taking antihypertensive drugs and not acutely ill. When systolic and diastolic BPs fall into 2 different categories, select the higher category to classify the individual's BP status.
[2] Require health promoting lifestyle modifications to prevent CVD.
[3] Based on the average of ≥ 2 readings taken at each of ≥ 2 visits after an initial screening; also requires health promoting lifestyle modifications.

➤*BP measurement:* Measure BP in a standardized fashion using equipment that meets certification criteria.

- Seat patients in a chair with their backs supported and their arms bared and supported at heart level. Tell patients to refrain from smoking or ingesting caffeine during the 30 minutes preceding the measurement.
- Under special circumstances, measuring BP in the supine and standing positions may be indicated.
- Begin measurement after 5 minutes or more of rest.
- Use the appropriate cuff size to ensure accurate measurement. Make sure the bladder within the cuff encircles at least 80% of the arm. Many adults will require a large adult cuff.
- Take measurements preferably with a mercury sphygmomanometer; otherwise, a recently calibrated aneroid manometer or a validated electronic device can be used.
- Record SBP and DBP. The first appearance of sound (phase 1) is used to define SBP. The disappearance of sound (phase 5) is used to define DBP.
- Take the average of 2 or more readings separated by 2 minutes. If the first 2 readings differ by more than 5 mm Hg, obtain an average additional reading.

➤*Risk stratification:*

Major Cardiovascular Disease (CVD) Risk Factors
General
Hypertension
Cigarette smoking
Obesity (body mass index ≥ 30 kg/m^2)
Physical inactivity
Dyslipidemia
Diabetes mellitus
Microalbuminuria or estimated GFR < 60 mL/min
Age (> 55 years for men, > 65 years for women)
Family history of premature cardiovascular disease (women 65 years of age or men < 55 years of age)
Target organ damage
Heart disease
Left ventricular hypertrophy
Angina/prior MI
Heart failure
Prior coronary revascularization
Brain
Stroke or transient ischemic attack
Chronic kidney disease
Peripheral arterial disease
Retinopathy

Assess for Identifiable Causes of Hypertension
Sleep apnea
Drug induced/related
Chronic kidney disease
Primary aldosteronism
Renovascular disease
Cushing syndrome or steroid therapy
Pheochromocytoma
Coarctation of aorta
Thyroid/parathyroid disease

➤*Pharmacotherapy:* The use of pharmacologic agents to reduce BP has demonstrated decreases in cardiovascular morbidity and mortality protection against stroke, coronary events, heart failure, renal disease progression, progression to more severe hypertension, and all-cause mortality.

Goals of therapy: The ultimate goal is to reduce cardiovascular complications and renal morbidity and mortality. In patients 50 years of age or older, the primary focus should be on achieving the SBP goal, then the DBP goal will automatically fall into place. SBP and DBP treatment to targets of less than 140/90 mm Hg is associated with a decrease in CVD complications. In hypertensive diabetes or renal disease patients, the BP goal is less than 130/80 mm Hg.

Prevention and management: Reduction of morbidity and mortality may be attained by achieving and maintaining SBP 140 mm Hg or less and DBP 90 mm Hg or less if tolerated and controlling other modifiable risk factors for cardiovascular disease. This may be accomplished by lifestyle modification alone or with pharmacologic therapy.

Lifestyle modifications: Prescribe lifestyle modifications for all patients with prehypertension and hypertension.

- Lifestyle modifications offer the potential for preventing hypertension, lowering BP, and reducing other cardiovascular risk factors at little cost and with minimal risk. Strongly encourage patients to adopt these lifestyle modifications, particularly if they have additional risk factors for premature cardiovascular disease, such as dyslipidemia or diabetes mellitus. Even when lifestyle modifications alone are not adequate in controlling hypertension, they may reduce the number and dosage of antihypertensive medications needed to manage the condition.

Lifestyle Modifications for Hypertension Management[1,2]

Modification	Recommendation	Approximate SBP reduction
Weight loss	Maintain normal body weight index	5 to 20 mm Hg per 10 kg of weight loss
Institute DASH eating plan	Start a diet rich in vegetables, fruit, and low fat dietary products with a decreased content of saturated and total fat	8 to 14 mm Hg
Dietary sodium restriction	Reduce dietary sodium intake to 2.4 g sodium or 6 g sodium chloride	2 to 8 mm Hg
Limit alcohol consumption	Limit alcohol intake to less than 30 mL ethanol (eg, 720 mL beer, 300 mL wine, or 90 mL 80 proof whiskey) per day or 15 mL ethanol in women and lighter weight individuals	2 to 4 mm Hg
Physical activity	Regular aerobic activity at least 30 minutes/day on most days of the week.	4 to 9 mm Hg

[1] For overall cardiovascular risk, discontinue tobacco use.
[2] Effects of these modifications are time and dose dependent and may be enhanced for some individuals.

Considerations for individualizing drug therapy: The table below describes compelling indications that require certain antihypertensive drug classes for high-risk conditions. The drug selections for each compelling indication are based on favorable clinical data.

Compelling Indications for Individual Drug Classes

Compelling indication[1]	Recommended drug therapy[2]
Heart failure	Thiazide, BB, ACEI, ARB, ALDO ant
Post-MI	BB, ACEI, ALDO ant
High CVD risk	Thiazide, BB, ACEI, CCB
Diabetes	Thiazide, BB, ACEI, ARB, CCB
Chronic kidney disease	ACEI, ARB
Recurrent stroke prevention	Thiazide, ACEI

[1] Compelling indications for antihypertensive drugs are based on benefits from clinical study outcomes; the compelling indication is managed in parallel with the BP.
[2] BB = beta blocker; ACEI = angiotensin converting enzyme inhibitor; ARB = angiotensin receptor blocker; CCB = calcium channel blocker; ALDO ant = aldosterone antagonist.

ANTIHYPERTENSIVES

Initial drug therapy: When a decision has been made to begin antihypertensive therapy and there are no compelling indications for another type of drug, choose a thiazide-type diuretic, either alone or in combination with 1 of the other classes (eg, ACEI, ARB, BB, CCB). Numerous randomized controlled trials have shown a reduction in morbidity and mortality with these agents. The majority of patients who are hypertensive will require treatment with 2 or more antihypertensive medications in order to achieve their BP goals of less than 140/90 mm Hg or less than 130/80 mm Hg for patients with diabetes or chronic kidney disease. When BP is more than 20/10 mm Hg above goal BP, consider initiating therapy with 2 drugs, 1 of which is usually a thiazide-type diuretic, either as separate drugs or in fixed-dose combinations. Use caution and observe those patients at risk for orthostatic hypotension, such as diabetic patients and the elderly.

Follow-up recommendations: Once antihypertensive therapy is initiated, follow-ups at monthly intervals are necessary until BP goal is reached. Patients with stage 2 hypertension or with complicating comorbid conditions will require more frequent visits. Once BP is controlled and at goal, follow-up visits should take place at 3- to 6-month intervals. Comorbidities, such as heart failure and diabetes will also dictate the frequency of office visits and laboratory tests. Monitor serum potassium and creatinine levels at least once or twice per year. Consider low-dose aspirin therapy only once BP is controlled.

➤*Special patient populations:*

Race: Most black people are at greater risk for the development of high BP, type 2 diabetes, coronary heart disease, left ventricular hypertension, stroke, and end-stage renal disease; they will usually require combination antihypertensive therapy. As monotherapy, BBs, ARBs, and ACEIs may produce less BP lowering effects than thiazide diuretics and CCBs. Consider the following antihypertensive combinations: BB/diuretic, ACEI/diuretic, ACEI/CCB, or ARB/diuretic. For patients with uncomplicated hypertension, the target BP is less than 140/90 mm Hg, and for patients with high risk for cardiovascular events in association with type 2 diabetes or renal insufficiency, the target BP goal is less than 130/80 mm Hg. When prescribing ACEIs for black patients, it is important to note that there appears to be an increased risk for ACEI-associated angioedema and/or cough.

Resistant hypertension: Failure to reach BP goal in patients who followed proper treatment is known as resistant hypertension. Consider a consultation with a BP specialist if target BP cannot be achieved. See table for causes of resistant hypertension.

Causes of Resistant Hypertension
Improper BP measurement
Volume overload and pseudotolerance
Excess sodium intake
Volume retention from kidney disease
Inadequate diuretic therapy
Drug-induced or other causes
Nonadherence
Inadequate doses
Inappropriate combinations
Nonsteroidal anti-inflammatory drugs; cyclooxygenase 2 inhibitors
Cocaine, amphetamines, other illicit drugs
Sympathomimetics (decongestants, anoretics)
Oral contraceptives
Adrenal steroids
Cyclosporine and tacrolimus
Erythropoietin
Licorice (including some chewing tobacco)
Selected over the counter dietary supplements and medicines (eg, ephedra, ma haung, bitter orange)
Associated conditions
Obesity
Excess alcohol intake
Identifiable causes of hypertension

Hypertensive emergencies: Patients with marked BP elevations that also have acute target-organ damage (eg, encephalopathy, MI, unstable angina, pulmonary edema, eclampsia, stroke, head trauma, life-threatening arterial bleed, aortic dissection) require parenteral drug therapy and hospitalization. Patients with BP elevation without target-organ damage do not require hospitalization, but should receive immediate oral antihypertensive therapy while being carefully evaluated and monitored for precipitating causes or hypertension-induced heart or kidney disease.

Considerations for Individualizing Antihypertensive Drug Therapy[1]	
Indication	Drug therapy
May have favorable effects on comorbid conditions[2]	
Angina	Beta blockers, CCB
Atrial tachycardia and fibrillation	Beta blockers, CCB (non-DHP)
Cyclosporine-induced hypertension (caution with the dose of cyclosporine)	CCB
Diabetes mellitus (types 1 and 2) with proteinuria	ACE 1 (preferred), CCB
Diabetes mellitus (type 2)	Low-dose diuretics
Dyslipidemia	Alpha blockers
Essential tremor	Beta blockers (non-CS)
Heart failure	Carvedilol, losartan potassium
Hyperthyroidism	Beta blockers
Migraine	Beta blockers (non-CS), CCB (non-DHP)
MI	Diltiazem HCl, verapamil HCl
Osteoporosis	Thiazides
Preoperative hypertension	Beta blockers
Prostatism (BPH)	Alpha blockers
Renal insufficiency (caution in renovascular hypertension and creatinine ≥ 265.2 mmol/L [3 mg/dL])	ACEI
May have unfavorable effects on comorbid conditions[2,3]	
Bronchospastic disease	Beta blockers[4]
Depression	Beta blockers, central alpha agonists, reserpine[4]
Diabetes mellitus (types 1 and 2)	Beta blockers, high-dose diuretics
Dyslipidemia	Beta blockers (non-ISA), diuretics (high-dose)
Gout	Diuretics
2° or 3° heart block	Beta blockers,[4] CCB (non-DHP)[4]
Heart failure	Beta blockers (except carvedilol), CCB (except amlodipine besylate, felodipine)
Liver disease	Labetalol HCl, methyldopa[4]
Peripheral vascular disease	Beta blockers
Pregnancy	ACEI,[4] angiotensin II receptor blockers[4]
Renal insufficiency	Potassium-sparing agents
Renovascular disease	ACEI, angiotensin II receptor blockers

[1] ACEI= angiotensin-converting enzyme inhibitors; BPH = benign prostatic hyperplasia; CCB = calcium channel blocker; DHP = dihydropyridine; ISA = intrinsic sympathomimetic activity; MI = myocardial infarction; non-CS = noncardioselective.
[2] Conditions and drugs are listed in alphabetical order.
[3] These drugs may be used with special monitoring unless contraindicated.
[4] Contraindicated.

ALGORITHM FOR TREATMENT OF HYPERTENSION*

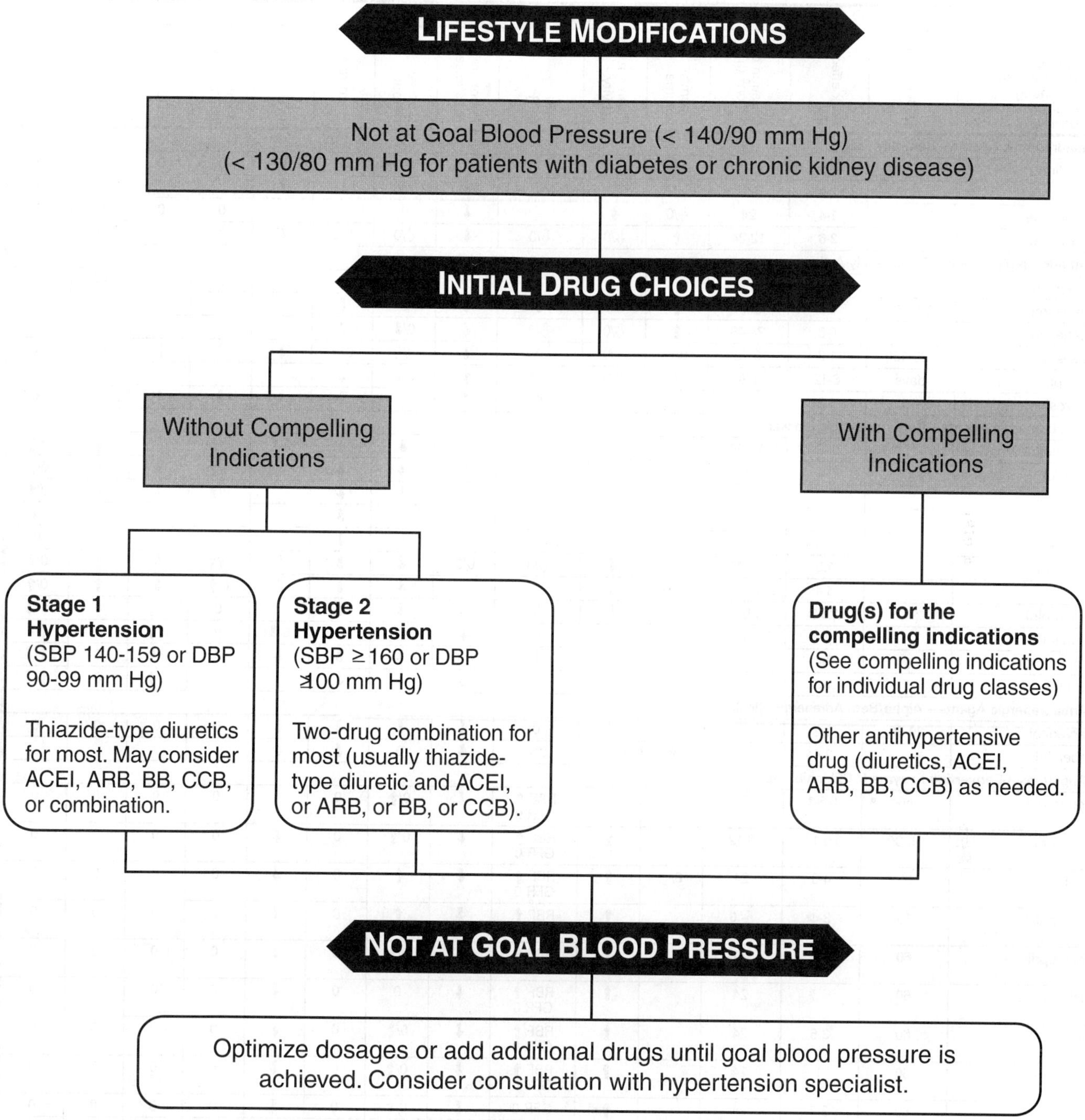

DBP, diastolic blood pressure; SBP, systolic blood pressure.
Drug abbreviations: ACEI, angiotensin converting enzyme inhibitor; ARB, angiotensin receptor blocker; BB, beta blocker; CCB, calcium channel blocker.

* *The Seventh Report of the Joint National Committee on Prevention, Detection, Evaluation, and Treatment of High Blood Pressure.* National Institutes of Health. May 2003.

ANTIHYPERTENSIVES

Agents used in hypertension therapy are listed in the following tables:

Pharmacological Effects of Antihypertensive Agents

↑ = increase ⇧ = slight increases 0 = no change ⇩ = slight decrease ↓ = decrease	Onset (min)	Peak effect[1] (h)	Duration of action[2] (h)	Plasma volume	Plasma renin activity	RBF GFR[3]	Peripheral resistance	Cardiac output	Heart rate	LVH	Total cholesterol	HDL	LDL	Triglycerides
Antiadrenergic Agents – Centrally Acting														
Clonidine	30-60	2-5	12-24	↑	⇩	⇩/0	↓	⇩/0	↓	↓	0	0	0	0
Guanabenz	60	2-4	6-12	0	↓	0	↓	0	↓	↓	0	0	0	0
Guanfacine		1-4	24	⇩/0	↓		↓	0	⇩	↓	0	0	0	0
Methyldopa	120	2-6	12-24	↑	⇩/0	⇩/0	↓	⇩/0	⇩/0	↓	0	0	0	0
Antiadrenergic Agents – Peripherally Acting														
Doxazosin		2-3								↓	↓	↑	0/↓	↓
Guanadrel	30-120	4-6	9-14	↑		0	↓	0	↓					
Guanethidine		6-8	24-48	↑	⇩/0	⇩/0	↓	0/↓	↓					
Prazosin	120-130	1-3	6-12	0/⇧	⇩/0	0	↓	0/⇧	0/⇧	↓	↓	↑	0/↑	↓
Reserpine	days	6-12	6-24	↑	⇩/0	⇩/0	↑	0/↓	↓					
Terazosin	15	1-2	12-24	0	0	0	↓	⇧	⇧	↓	↓	↑	0/↓	↓
Antiadrenergic Agents – Beta-Adrenergic Blockers														
Acebutolol		3-8	24-30				⇩	↓	↓	0/↓	0/↑	↓	↑	0/↑
Atenolol		2-4	24 +	⇩/0	↓	↓/0	0	↓	↓	↓	0/↑	↓	↑	0/↑
Betaxolol								↓	↓		0/↑	↓	↑	0/↑
Bisoprolol								↓	↓		0			0
Carteolol		1-3	24 +					↓	↓		0			0
Metoprolol		1.5	13-19	⇩/0	↓	⇩/0	0/↓	↓	↓	↓	0/↑	↓	↑	0/↑
Nadolol		3-4	17-24	⇩/0	↓	0	0	↓	↓	↓	0/↑	↓	↑	0/↑
Penbutolol		1.5-3	20 +		↓	⇩	0	↓	↓		0	0/↑	0	↑/↓
Pindolol		1	24 +		0	0	↓	⇩	⇩	0/↓	0	0/↑	0	↑/↓
Propranolol		2-4	8-12	⇩/0	↓	↓	⇩/0	↓	↓	↓	0	0/↑	0	↑/↓
Timolol		1-3	12	⇩/0	↓		0	↓	↓	↓	0	0/↑	0	↑/↓
Antiadrenergic Agents – Alpha/Beta-Adrenergic Blockers														
Carvedilol	30-60	1-2	> 15		↓	0	↓	↓	↓	↓	0	0	0	0
Labetalol		2-4	8-12	↑	↓	0/↑	↓	0	↓	↓				
Angiotensin-Converting Enzyme (ACE) Inhibitors														
Benazepril	60	0.5-1	24		↑	RBF ↑ GFR 0	↓	0/↑	0	↓	0	0	0	0
Captopril	15-30	0.5-1.5	6-12	⇧	↑	RBF ↑ GFR 0	↓	0/↑	0	↓	0	0	0	0
Enalapril	60	4-6	24	0/⇧	↑	RBF ↑ GFR 0	↓	↑	0	↓	0	0	0	0
Enalaprilat	15	3-4	≈ 6		↑	RBF ↑ GFR 0	↓	↑	0	↓	0	0	0	0
Fosinopril	60	≈ 3	24		↑	RBF ↑ GFR 0	↓	0/↑	0	↓	0	0	0	0
Lisinopril	60	≈ 7	24		↑	RBF ↑ GFR 0	↓	0	0	↓	0	0	0	0
Moexipril	60	3-6	24		↑	RBF ↑ GFR 0	↓	0/↑	0	↓	0	0	0	0
Quinapril	60	1	24		↑	RBF ↑ GFR 0	↓	0/↑	0	↓	0	0	0	0
Perindopril	60	3-7	24		↑	GFR 0	↓	0/↑	0	↓	0	0	0	0
Ramipril	60-120	1	24		↑	RBF ↑ GFR 0	↓	0/↑	0	↓	0	0	0	0
Trandolapril	120-240	6-8	24		↑	RBF ↑ GFR 0	↓	0/↑	0	↓	0	0	0	0
Angiotensin II Receptor Antagonists														
Candesartan	120-180	6-8	> 24	↓	↑	RBF ⇧ GFR 0	↓	↑	0	↓	0	0	0	0
Eprosartan	60-120	1-3	24	↓	↑	RBF ⇧ GFR 0	↓	↑	0	↓	0	0	0	0
Irbesartan	90-120	3-6	24	↓	↑	RBF ⇧[4] GFR 0	↓	↑	0	↓	0	0	0	0
Losartan	120-180	6	24	↓	↑	RBF ⇧[4] GFR 0	↓	↑	0	↓	0	0	0	0
Telmisartan	180	3-9	24	↓	↑	RBF ⇧[4] GFR 0	↓	↑	0	↓	0	0	0	0
Valsartan	120	6	24	↓	↑	RBF ⇧[4] GFR 0	↓	↑	0	↓	0	0	0	0
Olmesartan		1-2	24	↓	↑	RBF ⇧[4] GFR 0	↓	↑	0	↓	0	0	0	0

ANTIHYPERTENSIVES

Pharmacological Effects of Antihypertensive Agents

↑ = increase ⇧ = slight increases 0 = no change ⇩ = slight decrease ↓ = decrease	Onset (min)	Peak effect[1] (h)	Duration of action[2] (h)	Plasma volume	Plasma renin activity	RBF GFR[3]	Peripheral resistance	Cardiac output	Heart rate	LVH	Total cholesterol	HDL	LDL	Triglycerides
Calcium Channel Blocking Agents														
Amlodipine	gradual	6-12	> 24	0	0	↑	↓↓↓	0	0	↓	0	0	0	0
Diltiazem SR	30-60	6-11				0	↓	0-↑	↓-0	↓	0	0	0	0
Felodipine	120-300	2.5-5				0	↓↓↓	↑	↑	↓	0	0	0	0
Isradipine	120	1.5					↓↓↓	↑	↑/↓	↓	0	0	0	0
Nicardipine	20	0.5-2			⇧/↑	↑	↓	↑	↑	↓	0	0/⇧	0	0
Nifedipine SR	20	6				RBF↑ GFR ↑	↓↓↓	↑↑	↑	↓	0	0	0	0
Nisoldipine		1.5[5]			0		↓	⇧	⇧	↓	0	0	0	0
Verapamil	30	1-2.2			0/⇧	RBF↑ GFR ⇧	↓	↑/↓	↑/↓	↓	0	0/⇧	0	0
Diuretics														
Amiloride	120	6-10	24	↓	↑	0	↓	↓	0					
Loop diuretics	within 60	1-2	4-8	↓	↑	↑	↓	↓	0	0/↓	↑	0	↑	↑
Spironolactone	24-48 hr	48-72	48-72	↓	↑	0	↓	0	0					
Thiazides and derivatives	60-120	4-12	6-72	↓	↑	↓	↓	↓	0	0/↓	↑	0	↑	↑
Triamterene	2-4 hr	6-8	12-16											
Vasodilators														
Hydralazine	45	0.5-2	6-8	↑	↑	↑	↓	↑	↑	↑				
Minoxidil	30	2-3	24-72	↑	↑	0	↓	↑	↑	↑				
Agents For Pheochromocytoma														
Phentolamine	immed.		5-10 min	⇧	↑	↑	↓	0/↑	↑					
Phenoxy-benzamine	gradual	2-3	24 +	⇧	↑	↑	↓	↑	↓					
Metyrosine		6 +	2-3 days				↓		↓					
Agents For Hypertensive Emergencies/Urgencies														
Captopril[6]				⇧	↑	RBF ↑ GFR 0	↓	0/↑	0					
Clonidine	< 5			↑	⇩	⇩/0	↓	⇩/0	↓	↓				
Diazoxide	1-2	5 min	< 12	↑	↑	↑	↓	↑	↑					
Enalaprilat[6]					↑	RBF ↑ GFR 0	↓	↑	0					
Esmolol	1-2	5	10-20		0	0		↓	⇩					
Fenoldopam	5		30-60		↑	RBF⇧ GFR 0	⇩		⇧			NA		
Hydralazine	10-20		3-6											
Labetalol	5-10		3-6	↑	↓	0/↑	↓	0	↓					
Nicardipine (IV)	1-5		3-6		⇧/↑	⇧	↓	↑	↑					
Nitroglycerin (IV)[6]	immed.		tran-sient	0	0		↓	↑	↑					
Nitroprusside	0.5-1		3-5 min	↑	↑	0	↓	⇩	⇧					
Phentolamine[6]	1-2		3-10 min											
Miscellaneous Agents														
Tolazoline[6]							↓							
Eplerenone		1.5	> 24	↓	↑		↓		0	⇩	⇧			↑

[1] Peak clinical effect following a single oral dose, except where indicated.
[2] Duration of action is frequently dose-dependent.
[3] Renal blood flow and glomerular filtration rate.
[4] Experimental and small clinical studies indicate that angiotensin II receptor antagonists have effects on renal function similar to ACEIs.
[5] Immediate release; 6 to 12 hours for extended release.
[6] Unlabeled use.

H. PYLORI AGENTS

Helicobacter pylori is found in ≈ 100% of chronic active antral gastritis cases, 90% to 95% of duodenal ulcer patients, and 50% to 80% of gastric ulcer patients. The treatment of documented *H. pylori* infection in patients with confirmed peptic ulcer on first presentation or recurrence has been recommended by the National Institutes of Health in a 1994 Consensus Conference. Once *H. pylori* eradication has been achieved, reinfection rates are < 0.5% per year, and ulcer recurrence rates are dramatically reduced.

Numerous clinical trials have been done to determine the optimal regimen for *H. pylori* eradication, with cure rates ranging from ≈ 70% to 90%. There remains no gold standard of therapy to date. Base selection of the most appropriate therapy on consideration of treatment efficacy, cost, safety, drug-interaction potential, antibiotic resistance, tolerability, and convenience of administration. The FDA has approved 5 combination regimens for the treatment of *H. pylori* infection in patients with active duodenal ulcer. Studies have found that regimens consisting of a proton pump inhibitor (ie, lansoprazole or omeprazole) in conjunction with 2 antibiotics administered for 14 days are associated with cure rates that exceed 90%; this is in contrast to cure rates of 70% to 80% found with other regimens (eg, dual therapy, bismuth-based triple therapies).

Several studies have concluded that cure of *H. pylori* significantly reduces the risk of recurrent ulcer disease, obviating the need for continued maintenance therapy in patients with a history of uncomplicated disease. Make the decision to continue maintenance antisecretory therapy in patients with a history of complicated ulcer disease following successful *H. pylori* treatment on an individual basis.

The following is a brief description of the individual agents used in *H. pylori* eradication regimens and their role in eradication. Consult the individual drug monographs for complete prescribing information.

➤*Amoxicillin:* Amoxicillin works by inhibiting the synthesis of bacterial cell walls. It demonstrates topical activity and is stable in an acid environment but is most active at a neutral pH. *H. pylori* is very sensitive to amoxicillin in vitro and in vivo. Bacterial resistance to amoxicillin has not been reported. More common adverse effects include diarrhea, along with other GI effects, and hypersensitivity or allergic reactions. Take without regard to meals.

➤*Tetracycline:* This agent works by inhibiting bacterial protein synthesis. It acts topically and is active at a low pH. *H. pylori* is very sensitive to tetracycline. Bacterial resistance to tetracycline has not been reported. Adverse effects include diarrhea, along with other GI effects, esophageal ulcers, and photosensitivity reactions. Take on an empty stomach with plenty of water. Do not give simultaneously with dairy products (eg, milk, cheese), antacids, laxatives, or iron-containing products. If these agents are used, take them at least 2 hours before or after tetracycline.

➤*Metronidazole:* The exact mechanism of this agent is not well understood. It demonstrates selective toxicity to anaerobic or microaerophilic microorganisms and for anoxic or hypoxic cells. The drug diffuses into the cells and leads to the development of compounds that bind to DNA and inhibit synthesis, causing cell death. The activity of metronidazole is relatively independent of pH. Primary metronidazole resistance has been observed in 20% to 73% of *H. pylori* strains isolated and has been shown to significantly decrease *H. pylori* cure rates following treatment with a metronidazole-containing regimen. Adverse effects of metronidazole include metallic taste, nausea, peripheral neuropathy, and a disulfiram-type reaction manifested by flushing, nausea, tachycardia, vomiting, and other GI symptoms when used with alcohol. Metronidazole can be taken with food to minimize GI upset.

➤*Clarithromycin:* Clarithromycin is a macrolide antibiotic that inhibits bacterial protein synthesis. It is more acid-stable than erythromycin, better absorbed, and more effective against *H. pylori*. Resistance can develop when clarithromycin is used alone. It is generally < 8%. Adverse effects include abnormal taste, diarrhea, and nausea. Clarithromycin may be taken without regard to meals.

➤*Bismuth:* Bismuth compounds are topical compounds that disrupt the integrity of bacterial cell walls. The mechanism and role of bismuth in *H. pylori* eradication is multifactorial. Bismuth compounds are thought to lyse *H. pylori* near the gastric surface; prevent the adhesion of *H. pylori* to the gastric epithelium; inhibit its urease, phospholipase, and proteolytic activity; and decrease resistance development when used with antimicrobial agents such as metronidazole. Adverse effects of bismuth compounds may include a temporary and harmless darkening of the tongue and stool, diarrhea, and the potential for CNS toxicities when used in high doses. Take bismuth compounds without regard to meals.

➤*Antisecretory agents (H_2 antagonists, proton pump inhibitors):* Provide rapid symptom relief and accelerated ulcer healing when used with antimicrobial agents for *H. pylori* eradication. Proton pump inhibitors may have a direct effect on inhibiting the growth of *H. pylori* and also appear to have a synergistic effect when combined with antimicrobial agents.

➤*Eradication of H. pylori:*

Single antimicrobial agents: Monotherapy is not recommended because of the potential for the development of antimicrobial resistance.

Dual therapy:

- *Proton pump inhibitors plus amoxicillin* – Significant variation exists among numerous studies that have been conducted to date with eradication rates ranging from 30% to 80%. Therefore, dual therapy with these 2 agents is not recommended.
- *Proton pump inhibitors plus clarithromycin* – A number of studies have looked at the use of these agents in combination for *H. pylori* eradication, and the overall eradication appears to be ≈ 71%. Currently, the American College of Gastroenterology recommends adding a second antimicrobial agent to this regimen to enhance successful eradication.

Double antimicrobial therapy plus an antisecretory drug:

Regimens Used in the Eradication of *H. pylori*

Regimen	Dosing	Duration
Metronidazole + Clarithromycin + Omeprazole OR Lansoprazole	500 mg twice daily with meals 500 mg twice daily with meals 20 mg twice daily with meals 30 mg twice daily with meals	2 weeks
Amoxicillin + Clarithromycin + Omeprazole OR Lansoprazole	1 g twice daily with meals 500 mg twice daily with meals 20 mg twice daily before meals 30 mg twice daily with meals	2 weeks
Metronidazole + Omeprazole + Amoxicillin	500 mg twice daily with meals 20 mg twice daily before meals 1 g twice daily with meals	2 weeks

Triple-therapy regimens: These regimens have proved to be very effective in eradicating *H. pylori*. The primary disadvantage of these regimens is compliance because of the variety and number of medications used. Likewise, adverse effects are more common in patients taking these regimens compared with alternatives.

Regimens Used in the Eradication of *H. Pylori*

Regimen	Dosing	Duration
Bismuth subsalicylate +	525 mg 4 times/day with meals and at bedtime	2 weeks
Metronidazole +	250 mg 4 times/day with meals and at bedtime	1 week
Tetracycline +	500 mg 4 times/day	2 weeks
H_2-receptor antagonist	As directed[1]	2 weeks + additional 2 weeks
Bismuth subsalicylate +	525 mg 4 times/day with meals and at bedtime	2 weeks
Metronidazole +	500 mg 3 times/day with meals and at bedtime	2 weeks
Tetracycline +	500 mg 4 times/day	2 weeks
Omeprazole OR	20 mg/day before meals	2 weeks
Lansoprazole	30 mg/day	2 weeks
Ranitidine bismuth citrate +	400 mg 2 times/day with meals and at bedtime	2 weeks
Clarithromycin +	500 mg 2 times/day	2 weeks
Amoxicillin OR	1 g 2 times/day with meals and at bedtime	2 weeks
Metronidazole OR	500 mg 2 times/day with meals and at bedtime	2 weeks
Tetracycline	500 mg 2 times/day	2 weeks

[1] See individual monographs for dosing instructions.

Quadruple therapy regimens (2 antibiotics, bismuth, antisecretory agent): Like triple therapy regimens, these have proven to be effective in *H. pylori* eradication. The primary disadvantage of these regimens is compliance. In addition, because of the variety and number of medications used, adverse effects are more common in patients taking these regimens compared with alternatives.

H. PYLORI AGENTS

FDA-Approved Therapies for *H. pylori* Infection

Regimen	Dosing
Lansoprazole + Clarithromycin + Amoxicillin	30 mg 2 times daily for 10 to 14 days[1] 500 mg 2 times daily for 10 to 14 days[1] 1 g 2 times daily for 10 to 14 days[1]
Omeprazole + Clarithromycin + Amoxicillin	20 mg 2 times daily for 10 days 500 mg 2 times daily for 10 days 1 g 2 times daily for 10 days
Omeprazole + Clarithromycin Omeprazole	40 mg once daily for 2 weeks 500 mg 3 times daily for 2 weeks Follow by 20 mg once daily for additional 2 weeks
Ranitidine bismuth citrate + Clarithromycin Ranitidine bismuth citrate	400 mg 2 daily for 2 weeks 500 mg 3 times daily for 2 weeks Follow by 400 mg 2 times daily for additional 2 weeks
Bismuth subsalicylate + Metronidazole + Tetracycline + Histamine-2 (H_2)-receptor antagonist	525 mg 4 times daily for 2 weeks 250 mg 4 times daily for 2 weeks 500 mg 4 times daily for 2 weeks Dose as directed[2] for 2 weeks + additional 2 weeks
Lansoprazole + Amoxicillin	30 mg 3 times daily for 2 weeks 1 g 3 times daily for 2 weeks

[1] Therapy associated with ≥ 90% *H. pylori* eradication rate.
[2] See individual monographs for dosing instructions.

➤*Practice Guidelines from the American College of Gastroenterology:* In the 1996 Consensus Statement on Medical Treatment of Peptic Ulcer Disease, the American College of Gastroenterology does not recommend single-antibiotic combinations of either clarithromycin or amoxicillin with proton pump inhibitors because efficacy is < 70% (cure), and a high-dose, 2-week treatment period is required. The Consensus Statement recommends a two-antibiotic combination of clarithromycin, metronidazole or amoxicillin in regimens that do not employ a bismuth compound. In addition, the American College of Gastroenterology suggests adding either tetracycline or amoxicillin to the recently approved ranitidine-bismuth citrate-clarithromycin combination to enhance successful *H. pylori* eradication. Combining a proton pump inhibitor, either omeprazole or lansoprazole, with two antibiotics is thought to enhance effectiveness and allow for a shorter duration of treatment.

There are a number of factors that limit the effectiveness of regimens designed to eradicate *H. pylori*. The first, antibiotic resistance, is seen with metronidazole and clarithromycin but has not been reported with bismuth, amoxicillin or tetracycline. Because prior antibiotic exposure predicts drug resistance in individuals, take this factor into consideration when selecting a regimen. Although data are limited, studies have demonstrated that eradication of *H. pylori* is possible with metronidazole-containing regimens despite the presence of resistant organisms, but eradication rates are significantly lower. Alternatively, the American College of Gastroenterology suggests possible drug regimens to employ in cases of metronidazole resistance. These include bismuth, clarithromycin, and tetracycline or omeprazole, amoxicillin, and clarithromycin. On the other hand, clarithromycin resistance is more bothersome because resistant organisms do not respond favorably to clarithromycin-containing regimens.

Second, mild adverse effects (eg, diarrhea, metallic taste, black stools) do occur in ≈ 30% to 50% of patients. Therefore, shorter treatment periods in this group of patients may be better tolerated.

Finally, patient compliance is often a problem because of cumbersome regimens and adverse effects.

➤*Maintenance therapy with antisecretory agents:* Several studies have concluded that cure of *H. pylori* significantly reduces the risk of recurrent ulcer disease, obviating the need for continued maintenance therapy in patients with a history of uncomplicated disease. The decision to continue maintenance antisecretory therapy in patients with a history of complicated ulcer disease following successful *H. pylori* treatment should be made on an individual basis. Factors to be considered that may favor the continuation of antisecretory therapy include: The presence of comorbid illness or the use of medications (eg, NSAIDs, anticoagulant therapy) that may increase risk of recurrence or complications, and severity of the previous ulcer-related complications.

➤*Confirming successful eradication:* Confirming successful eradication is important in patients with a history of complicated or refractory ulcers but is controversial in those with uncomplicated ulcers who remain asymptomatic after therapy.

➤*Refractory ulcers in patients receiving antibiotic therapy for H. pylori eradication:* Refractory ulcers in patients receiving antibiotic therapy for *H. pylori* eradication is often due to failure to successfully eradicate *H. pylori* infection. Resistance patterns, as well as noncompliance, and concurrent NSAID use may play a role in refractory cases.

RABIES PROPHYLAXIS PRODUCTS

Although rabies rarely affects humans in the US, every year ≈ 16,000 to 39,000 people receive postexposure prophylaxis. Appropriate management depends on the interpretation of the risk of infection and the efficacy and risk of prophylactic treatment. There are 2 types of immunizing products: Vaccines and globulins. Use both types of products concurrently for rabies postexposure prophylaxis.

➤*Vaccines:* Vaccines induce an active immune response that requires about 7 to 10 days to develop, and usually persists for ≥ 2 years.

➤*Human Diploid Cell Rabies Vaccine (HDCV):* An inactivated virus vaccine prepared from fixed rabies virus grown in human diploid cell culture.

➤*Rabies Vaccine, Adsorbed (RVA):* A cell culture-derived vaccine prepared from the Kissling strain of rabies virus adapted to a diploid cell line of the fetal rhesus lung.

➤*Purified Chick Embryo Cell Vaccine (PCEC):* An inactivated virus, it is prepared from the fixed rabies virus strain Flury LEP grown in primary cultures of chicken fibroblasts.

Four formulations of 3 inactivated rabies vaccines are currently licensed for preexposure and postexposure prophylaxis in the US. When used as indicated, all 3 types of rabies vaccines are considered equally safe and efficacious. The potency of 1 dose is ≥ 2.5 IU per 1 ml of rabies virus antigen, which is the World Health Organization recommended standard. A full 1 ml dose can be used for both preexposure and postexposure prophylaxis. However, only the Imovax Rabies I.D. vaccine (HDCV) has been evaluated and approved by the FDA for the intradermal dose and route for preexposure vaccination. Therefore, do not use RVA and PCEC intradermally. Usually, an immunization series is initiated and completed with 1 vaccine product. No clinical studies have been conducted that document a change in efficacy or the frequency of adverse reactions when the series is completed with a second vaccine product.

➤*Globulins:* Globulins provide rapid passive immune protection that persists for a short time (half-life of about 21 days).

Rabies Immune Globulin, Human (RIG): Antirabies gamma globulin, concentrated from plasma of hyperimmunized human donors.

➤*Rationale of treatment:* Individually evaluate each possible rabies exposure. Consult local or state public health officials if questions arise about the need for prophylaxis. Consider the following factors before specific treatment is initiated:

Species of biting animal: Carnivorous animals (especially skunks, foxes, coyotes, raccoons, dogs and cats) and bats are more likely to be infective than other animals. Unless the animal is tested and shown not rabid, initiate postexposure prophylaxis upon bite or non-bite exposure to these animals. If treatment has been initiated and subsequent testing shows the exposing animal is not rabid, treatment can be discontinued.

Since the likelihood that a domestic dog or cat is infected with rabies varies from region to region, the need for postexposure prophylaxis also varies. Bites of rabbits, hares, squirrels, chipmunks, rats, mice, hamsters, guinea pigs, gerbils and other rodents are rarely found to be infected with rabies and have not been known to cause human rabies in the US. In these cases, consult state or local health departments before a decision is made to initiate postexposure antirabies prophylaxis.

Circumstances of biting incident: An unprovoked attack is more likely to mean that the animal is rabid. Bites inflicted during attempts to feed or handle an apparently healthy animal should generally be regarded as provoked.

Type of exposure: Rabies is transmitted by introducing the virus into open cuts or wounds in skin via mucous membranes. The likelihood of rabies infection varies with the nature and extent of the exposure.

- *Bite* – Any penetration of the skin by teeth.
- *Nonbite* – Scratches, abrasions, open wounds or mucous membranes contaminated with saliva or other potentially infectious material, such as brain tissue from a rabid animal. There have been two instances of airborne rabies acquired in laboratories and two probable airborne rabies cases acquired in one bat-infested cave.

Casual contact with a rabid animal, such as petting it (without a bite or nonbite exposure), is not an indication for prophylaxis.

The only documented cases of rabies due to human-to-human transmission occurred in 8 patients who received corneal transplants from persons who died of rabies undiagnosed at the time of death.

➤*Preexposure prophylaxis:* Preexposure immunization does not eliminate the need for prompt postexposure prophylaxis following an exposure; it only reduces the postexposure regimen.

Consider preexposure immunization for persons in high-risk groups: Veterinarians, animal handlers, certain laboratory workers and persons, especially children, spending time (eg, ≥ 1 month) in foreign countries where rabies is a constant threat. Also consider others whose vocational or avocational pursuits bring them into contact with potentially rabid dogs, cats, foxes, skunks or bats. Pre-exposure immunization of immunosuppressed persons is not recommended.

Preexposure prophylaxis is given for several reasons. First, it may provide protection to persons with inapparent exposure to rabies. Secondly, it may protect persons whose postexposure therapy might be expected to be delayed. Finally, although it does not eliminate the need for additional therapy after a rabies exposure, it simplifies therapy by eliminating the need for globulin and decreasing the number of doses of vaccine needed. This is of particular importance for persons at high risk of being exposed in countries where the available rabies immunizing products may carry a higher risk of adverse reactions.

Preexposure immunization: Preexposure immunization consists of 3 doses of HDCV, RVA, or PCEC 1 ml/dose, IM (ie, deltoid area), one each on days 0, 7 and 21 or 28. The intradermal dose is 0.1 ml in the deltoid area of either arm on days 0, 7 and 21 or 28. Administration of routine booster doses of vaccine depends on exposure risk category as noted below.

Criteria for Preexposure Immunization

Risk category	Nature of risk	Typical populations	Preexposure regimen
Continuous	Virus present continuously, often in high concentrations. Aerosol, bite or nonbite exposure possible. Specific exposures may go unrecognized.	Rabies research lab workers,[1] rabies biologics production workers.	Primary preexposure immunization course. Serology every 6 months. Booster immunization when antibody titer falls below acceptable level.[2]
Frequent	Exposure usually episodic, with source recognized or unrecognized. Aerosol, bite or nonbite exposure.	Rabies diagnostic lab workers,[1] spelunkers, veterinarians and staff and animal control and wildlife workers in rabies epizootic areas.	Primary preexposure immunization course. Serology every 2 years. Booster immunization when antibody titer falls below acceptable level.
Infrequent (greater than population-at-large)	Exposure nearly always episodic with source recognized. Bite or nonbite exposure.	Veterinarians and animal control wildlife workers in areas of low rabies endemicity. Travelers to foreign rabies epizootic areas. Veterinary students.	Primary preexposure immunization course. No routine booster immunization or serology.
Rare (population-at-large)	Exposure always episodic, or bite with source recognized.	US population-at-large, including individuals in rabies epi-zootic areas.	No preexposure immunization.

[1] Judgment of relative risk and extra monitoring of immunization status of laboratory workers is the responsibility of the laboratory supervisor (see US Department of Health and Human Services' *Biosafety in Microbiological and Biomedical Laboratories,*1984).

[2] Preexposure booster immunization consists of one dose of HDCV, PCEC, or RVA 1 ml/dose, IM or 0.1 ml ID day 0 only. Acceptable antibody level is 1:5 titer (complete inhibition in RFFIT at 1:5 dilution). Boost if titer falls below 1:5.

➤*Postexposure prophylaxis:*

Local wound treatment: Immediate and thorough washing of all bite wounds and scratches with soap and water is perhaps the most effective means of preventing rabies. Give tetanus and a virucidal agent such as povidone-iodine solution irrigation prophylaxis and control bacterial infection as indicated.

Immunization: Postexposure antirabies immunization should always include both passive immunization (preferably RIG) and vaccine, with one exception: Persons previously immunized with HDCV in recommended preexposure or postexposure regimens or with other types of vaccines and who have a documented adequate rabies antibody titer should receive only vaccine. The globulin/vaccine combination is recommended for both bite and nonbite exposures, regardless of the interval between exposure and treatment.

Treatment: Use the following recommendations as a guide in conjunction with knowledge of the circumstances of the situation. Consult public health officials with questions about the need for rabies prophylaxis.

Treatment Recommendations for Postexposure Rabies

Animal species	Condition of animal at time of attack	Treatment of exposed person[1]
Domestic: Dogs, cats and ferrets	Healthy & available for 10 days of observation	None, unless animal develops rabies[2]
	Rabid/suspected rabid	RIG and vaccine[3]
	Unknown (escaped)	Consult public health officials. If treatment is indicated, give RIG and vaccine[3]
Wild: Skunk, bat, fox, coyote, raccoon, bobcat and other carnivores	Regard as rabid unless proven negative by laboratory test[3]	Consider immediate vaccination[3]

RABIES PROPHYLAXIS PRODUCTS

Treatment Recommendations for Postexposure Rabies

Animal species	Condition of animal at time of attack	Treatment of exposed person[1]
Other: Livestock, rodents, rabbits and hares, large rodents and other mammals	Consider individually: Bites of squirrels, hamsters, guinea pigs, gerbils, chipmunks, rats, mice, other rodents, rabbits and hares almost never call for antirabies prophylaxis. Consult public health officials.	

[1] If treatment is indicated, administer both RIG and vaccine as soon as possible, regardless of the interval from exposure.
[2] Begin treatment with RIG and vaccine at first sign of rabies in biting domestic animals during the usual holding period of 10 days. Kill and test the symptomatic animal immediately.
[3] Kill and test animal as soon as possible. Holding for observation is not recommended. Discontinue vaccine if fluorescent antibody tests of animal are negative.

Treatment Schedule for Postexposure Rabies Prophylaxis

Vaccination status	Treatment[1]
Not previously vaccinated	*Local wound cleansing:* All postexposure treatment should begin with immediate, thorough cleansing of each wound with soap and water. If available, a virucidal agent such as povidone-iodine solution should be used to irrigate the wounds.
	Rabies immune globulin: Give 20 IU/kg. If anatomically feasible, infiltrate the full dose around the wound(s) and inject the balance IM at an anatomical site distant from vaccine administration. Do not give RIG through the same syringe or into the same anatomical site as rabies vaccine. Because RIG may partially suppress active induction of antirabies antibody, give no more than the recommended dose.
	Rabies vaccine: Give 1 ml IM in the deltoid area[2] on days 0, 3, 7, 14 and 28.
Previously vaccinated[3]	*Local wound cleansing:* All postexposure treatments begin with immediate, thorough cleansing of each wound with soap and water. If available, a virucidal agent such as povidone-iodine solution should be used to irrigate the wounds.
	Do not administer RIG.
	Rabies vaccine: Give 1 ml IM in the deltoid area on days 0 and 3.

[1] These regimens apply to all age groups, including children.
[2] The deltoid area is the only acceptable site of vaccination for adults and older children. For younger children, the outer aspect of the thigh may be used. Vaccine should never be administered in the gluteal area.
[3] Any person with a history of pre- or postexposure vaccination with HDCV, PCEC or RVA; or with both a history of vaccination with any other type of rabies vaccine and a documented history of antibody response to that vaccination.

Recommendations for Postexposure Immunization

2 doses of HDVC, 1 ml/dose, IM, one each on days 0 and 3.
RIG, 20 IU/kg. If anatomically feasible, infiltrate the full dose in the area around and into the wounds. Administer remaining volume IM at a distant site. Five doses of HDCV, RVA or PCEC, 1 ml/dose, IM, one each on days 0, 3, 7, 14 and 28.

➤*Passive immunization:* Administer RIG once at the beginning of antirabies therapy. If not given when vaccination was begun, RIG can be given through the seventh day after the first dose of vaccine. After that, RIG is not indicated, since an antibody response is presumed to have occurred. The recommended RIG dose is 20 IU/kg (≈ 9 IU/lb). If anatomically feasible, infiltrate the full dose in the area around and into the wound. Because RIG may partially suppress active production of antibody, do not exceed the recommended dose.

➤*Active immunization:* Administer the vaccine in conjunction with RIG on day 0. Give five 1 ml doses of the vaccine IM in the deltoid area. For children the anterolateral aspect of the thigh is also acceptable. Do not use gluteal area. Administer the first dose as soon as possible after the exposure; give an additional dose on each of days 3, 7, 14 and 28 after the first dose (day 0). WHO recommends a sixth dose at 90 days after the first dose. In unusual instances (eg, an immunosuppressed patient), serologic testing is indicated.

➤*Previously immunized persons:* When an immunized person who was vaccinated by the recommended regimen with HDCV, PCEC or RVA or who had previously demonstrated rabies antibody is exposed to rabies, that person should receive two doses of HDCV, PCEC or RVA 1 ml/dose, IM, one immediately and one 3 days later. If the person's immune status is not known, postexposure antirabies treatment may be necessary. If antibody can be demonstrated in a serum sample collected before vaccine is given, treatment can be discontinued after at least two doses of the vaccine.

Rapid intervention is essential to minimize morbidity and mortality in an acute toxic ingestion. Institute measures to prevent absorption and hasten elimination as soon as possible; however, symptomatic and supportive care takes precedence over other therapy. It is assumed that basic life support measures, (eg, cardiopulmonary resuscitation [CPR]) have been instituted. Specific antidotes are discussed in the overdosage section of individual or group monographs. The discussion below outlines procedures used in the management of acute overdosage of orally ingested systemic drugs.

ADVANCED LIFE SUPPORT MEASURES

➤*Adequate Airway:* Adequate Airway must be established and maintained, generally via oropharyngeal or endotracheal airways, cricothyrotomy or tracheostomy.

➤*Ventilation:* Ventilation may then be performed via mouth-to-mouth insufflation, hand-operated bag (ambu bag) or by mechanical ventilator.

➤*Circulation:* Circulation must be maintained.

- *Hypotension:* If hypotension/hypoperfusion occurs, place the patient in shock position (head lowered, feet elevated); specific therapy may include:

Establish IV access and initiate IV fluids (eg, 0.9% or 0.45% Saline, Lactated Ringer's, Dextrose). A maintenance flow rate is generally 100 to 200 ml/hour; individualize as necessary.

Plasma, plasma protein fractions, whole blood or plasma expanders may be required.

Severe hypotension may require judicious use of cardiovascular active agents. The most commonly recommended agents are dopamine, dobutamine and norepinephrine.

- *Arrhythmia* treatment is dictated by the offending drug.
- *Hypertension,* sometimes severe, may occur. (See Nitroprusside and Diazoxide, Parenteral in the Agents for Hypertensive Emergencies section.)

➤*Seizures:* Simple isolated seizures may require only observation and supportive care. Repetitive seizures or status epilepticus require therapy. Give IV diazepam or lorazepam followed by fosphenytoin and/or phenobarbital. Pancuronium may also be considered.

REDUCTION OF DRUG ABSORPTION

➤*Gastric emptying:* is generally recommended as soon as possible; however, this is generally not very effective unless employed within the first 1 to 2 hours after ingestion. Syrup of ipecac and gastric lavage are the two most commonly employed methods for gastric emptying.

- *Syrup of ipecac* is the method of choice outside the hospital. Do not induce vomiting if the medication is caustic or a petroleum or if the patient is in a coma or having seizures. Syrup of ipecac takes 20 to 30 minutes to work. Consider gastric lavage if response is needed immediately.
  - *6 months to 1 year* – 10 ml
  - *1 year to 12 years* – 15 ml
  - *> 12 years* – 30 ml

May be followed by a glass of water. A second dose may be given if results do not occur within 20 to 30 minutes.

- *Gastric lavage* is indicated in the comatose patient or for those in whom syrup of ipecac fails to produce emesis. Gastric lavage is immediate and does not have a delay reaction, and is preferred over forced emesis. Airway protection via endotracheal intubation is appropriate for the patient without a gag reflex or comatose patients. Position the patient on left side, face down and use a large bore tube. Instill warm water or saline 300 to 360 ml for adults. Avoid water for infants and children; use warm saline or 5% to 6% polyethylene glycol solution. Give until lavage solution becomes clear. Add charcoal before removing the tube.

➤*Adsorption:* Absorption, using activated charcoal alone or after completion of emesis or lavage, is indicated for virtually all significant toxic ingestions. It adsorbs a wide variety of toxins and there are no contraindications. However, it adsorbs many orally administered antidotes as well, so space dosage properly. Give an adult 50 to 100 g of activated charcoal mixed in 240 ml of water; the pediatric dose is 1 g/kg, or 25 to 50 g in 120 ml of water.

➤*Cathartics:* Cathertics increases the elimination of charcoal-poison complex. Generally using a saline or osmotic cathartic (eg, magnesium sulfate or citrate or sorbitol) with 3 ml/kg of a 35% to 75% solution of sorbitol has the most rapid effect.

➤*Whole bowel irrigation (WBI):* Whole bowel irrigation utilizes rapid administration of large volumes of lavage solutions, such as PEG. The dose is 4 to 6 L over 1 to 2 hours for adults and 0.5 L/hr for children. It may be most useful to remove iron tablets, sustained-release capsules or cocaine-containing condoms or balloons.

ELIMINATION OF ABSORBED DRUG

➤*Interruption of enterohepatic circulation:* Interruption of enterohepatic circulation by "gastric dialysis" uses scheduled doses of activated charcoal for 1 to 2 days. Gastric dialysis not only interrupts the enterohepatic cycle of some drugs, but also creates an osmotic gradient, drawing drug from the plasma back into the gastrointestinal lumen where it is bound by the charcoal and excreted in the feces.

➤*Diuresis:* Diuresis may be effective as identified in the individual drug monographs.

- *Forced diuresis* is occasionally useful. It may cause volume overload or electrolyte disturbances. Forced diuresis is useful for phenobarbital, bromides, lithium, salicylate or amphetamines overdoses. Do not use for tricyclic antidepressants, sedative-hypnotics or highly protein-bound medications. The most common agents employed are furosemide and osmotic diuretics with mannitol.
- *Alkaline diuresis* promotes elimination of weak acids (eg, barbiturates, salicylates) and is accomplished by the administration of IV sodium bicarbonate.
- *Acid diuresis* may be indicated in overdoses with weak bases (eg, amphetamines, fenfluramine, quinine) but use with caution in patients with renal or liver disease. It is usually accomplished with oral or IV ascorbic acid or ammonium chloride.

➤*Dialysis:* Dialysis is indicated in a minority of severe overdose cases. Drug factors that alter dialysis effectiveness include volume of distribution, drug compartmentalization, protein binding and lipid/water solubility.

- *Hemodialysis* may be used after an overdose and when the patient is having complications (eg, severe metabolic acidosis, electrolyte imbalances, renal failure).
- *Peritoneal dialysis* is even less effective than hemodialysis.
- *Charcoal hemoperfusion* is useful when a drug can be adsorbed by charcoal (eg, theophylline, barbiturates).

Poison Control Center: ________________

Consultation with a regional poison control center is highly recommended.

Type I hypersensitivity reactions (immediate hypersensitivity or anaphylaxis) are immunologic responses to a foreign antigen to which a patient has been previously sensitized. Anaphylactoid reactions are not immunologically mediated; however, symptoms and treatment are similar.

SIGNS AND SYMPTOMS

Acute hypersensitivity reactions typically begin within 1 to 30 minutes of exposure to the offending antigen. Tingling sensations and a generalized flush may proceed to a fullness in the throat, chest tightness or a "feeling of impending doom." Generalized urticaria and sweating are common. *Severe* reactions include life-threatening involvement of the airway and cardiovascular system.

TREATMENT

Appropriate and immediate treatment is imperative. The following general measures are commonly employed:

➤*Epinephrine:* 1:1000, 0.2 to 0.5 mg (0.2 to 0.5 ml) SC is the primary treatment. In children, administer 0.01 mg/kg or 0.1 mg. Doses may be repeated every 5 to 15 minutes if needed. A succession of small doses is more effective and less dangerous than a single large dose. Additionally, 0.1 mg may be introduced into an injection site where the offending drug was administered. If appropriate, the use of a tourniquet above the site of injection of the causative agent may slow its absorption and distribution. However, remove or loosen the tourniquet every 10 to 15 minutes to maintain circulation.

Epinephrine IV (generally indicated in the presence of hypotension) is often recommended in a 1:10,000 dilution, 0.3 to 0.5 mg over 5 minutes; repeat every 15 minutes, if necessary. In children, inject 0.1 to 0.2 mg or 0.01 mg/kg/dose over 5 minutes; repeat every 30 minutes.

A conservative IV epinephrine protocol includes 0.1 mg of a 1:100,000 dilution (0.1 mg of a 1:1000 dilution mixed in 10 ml normal saline) given over 5 to 10 minutes. If an IV infusion is necessary, administer at a rate of 1 to 4 mcg/min. In children, infuse 0.1 to 1.5 (maximum) mcg/kg/min.

Dilute epinephrine 1:10,000 may be administered through an endotracheal tube, if no other parenteral access is available, directly into the bronchial tree. It is rapidly absorbed there from the capillary bed of the lung.

➤*Airway:* Ensure a patent airway via endotracheal intubation or cricothyrotomy (ie, inferior laryngotomy, used prior to tracheotomy) and administer oxygen. Severe respiratory difficulty may respond to IV aminophylline or to other bronchodilators.

➤*Hypotension:* The patient should be recumbent with feet elevated. Depending upon the severity, consider the following measures:
- Establish a patent IV catheter in a suitable vein.
- Administer IV fluids (eg, Normal Saline, Lactated Ringer's).
- Administer plasma expanders.
- Administer cardioactive agents (see group and individual monographs). Commonly recommended agents include dopamine, dobutamine, norepinephrine and phenylephrine.

➤*Adjunctive therapy:* does not alter acute reactions, but may modify an ongoing or slow-onset process and shorten the course of the reaction.
- *Antihistamines: Diphenhydramine* – 50 to 100 mg IM or IV, continued orally at 5 mg/kg/day or 50 mg every 6 hours for 1 to 2 days. For children, give 5 mg/kg/day, maximum 300 mg/day.
  Chlorpheniramine: (adults, 10 to 20 mg; children, 5 to 10 mg) IM or slowly IV.
  Hydroxyzine: 10 to 25 mg orally or 25 to 50 mg IM 3 to 4 times daily.
- *Corticosteroids,* eg, hydrocortisone IV 100 to 1000 mg or equivalent, followed by 7 mg/kg/day IV or oral for 1 to 2 days. The role of corticosteroids is controversial.
- *H_2 antagonists: Cimetidine – Children,* 25 to 30 mg/kg/day IV in six divided doses; *adults,* 300 mg every 6 hours. *Ranitidine* – 50 mg IV over 3 to 5 minutes. May be of value in addition to H_1 antihistamines, although this opinion is not universally shared.

INTERNATIONAL SYSTEM OF UNITS

The *Système international d 'unités* (International System of Units) or *SI* is a modernized version of the metric system. The primary goal of the conversion to SI units is to revise the present confused measurement system and to improve test-result communications.

The SI has 7 basic units from which other units are derived:

Base Units of SI

Physical quantity	Base unit	SI symbol
length	meter	m
mass	kilogram	kg
time	second	s
amount of substance	mole	mol
thermodynamic temperature	kelvin	K
electric current	ampere	A
luminous intensity	candela	cd

Combinations of these base units can express any property, although, for simplicity, special names are given to some of these derived units.

Representative Derived Units

Derived unit	Name and symbol	Derivation from base units
area	square meter	m^2
volume	cubic meter	m^3
force	newton (N)	$kg{\bullet}m{\bullet}s^{-2}$
pressure	pascal (Pa)	$kg{\bullet}m^{-1}{\bullet}s^{-2}$ (N/m^2)
work, energy	joule (J)	$kg{\bullet}m^2{\bullet}s^{-2}$($N{\bullet}m$)
mass density	kilogram per cubic meter	kg/m^3
frequency	hertz (Hz)	1 $cycle/s^{-1}$
temperature degree	Celsius (°C)	°C = °K – 273.15
concentration		
mass	kilogram/liter	kg/L
substance	mole/liter	mol/L
molality	mole/kilogram	mol/kg
density	kilogram/liter	kg/L

Prefixes to the base unit are used in this system to form decimal multiples and submultiples. The preferred multiples and submultiples listed below change the quantity by increments of 10^3 or 10^{-3}. The exceptions to these recommended factors are within the middle rectangle.

Prefixes and Symbols for Decimal Multiples and Submultiples

Factor	Prefix	Symbol
10^{18}	exa	E
10^{15}	peta	P
10^{12}	tera	T
10^9	giga	G
10^6	mega	M
10^3	kilo	k
10^2	hecto	h
10^1	deka	da
10^{-1}	deci	d
10^{-2}	centi	c
10^{-3}	milli	m
10^{-6}	micro	μ
10^{-9}	nano	n
10^{-12}	pico	p
10^{-15}	femto	f
10^{-18}	atto	a

To convert drug concentrations to or from SI units:

Conversion factor (CF) $= \frac{1000}{\text{mol wt}}$

Conversion *to* SI units: μg/ml x CF = μmol/L

Conversion *from* SI units: μmol/L ÷ CF = μg/ml

NORMAL LABORATORY VALUES

In the following tables, normal reference values for commonly requested laboratory tests are listed in traditional units and in SI units. The tables are a guideline only. Values are method dependent and "normal values" may vary between laboratories.

Blood, Plasma or Serum

Determination	Reference Value: Conventional Units	Reference Value: SI Units
Ammonia (NH_3) – diffusion	20-120 mcg/dl	12-70 mcmol/L
Ammonia Nitrogen	15–45 μg/dl	11–32 μmol/L
Amylase	35-118 IU/L	0.58-1.97 mckat/L
Anion Gap (Na^+–[Cl^-+HCO_3^-]) (P)	7–16 mEq/L	7–16 mmol/L
Antinuclear antibodies	negative at 1:10 dilution of serum	negative at 1:10 dilution of serum
Antithrombin III (AT III)	80-120 U/dl	800-1200 U/L
Bicarbonate: Arterial Venous	21–28 mEq/L 22–29 mEq/L	21–28 mmol/L 22–29 mmol/L
Bilirubin: Conjugated (direct) Total	≤ 0.2 mg/dl 0.1-1 mg/dl	≤ 4 mcmol/L 2-18 mcmol/L
Calcitonin	< 100 pg/ml	< 100 ng/L
Calcium: Total Ionized	8.6-10.3 mg/dl 4.4-5.1 mg/dl	2.2-2.74 mmol/L 1-1.3 mmol/L
Carbon dioxide content (plasma)	21-32 mmol/L	21-32 mmol/L
Carcinoembryonic antigen	< 3 ng/ml	< 3 mcg/L
Chloride	95-110 mEq/L	95-110 mmol/L
Coagulation screen: Bleeding time Pothrombin time Partial thromboplastin time (activated) Protein C Protein S	 3-9.5 min 10-13 sec 22-37 sec 0.7-1.4 μ/ml 0.7-1.4 μ/ml	 180-570 sec 10-13 sec 22-37 sec 700-1400 U/ml 700-1400 U/ml
Copper, total	70-160 mcg/dl	11-25 mcmol/L
Corticotropin (ACTH adrenocorticotropic hormone) – 0800 hr	< 60 pg/ml	< 13.2 pmol/L
Cortisol: 0800 hr 1800 hr 2000 hr	5-30 mcg/dl 2-15 mcg/dl ≤ 50% of 0800 hr	138-810 nmol/L 50-410 nmol/L ≤ 50% of 0800 hr
Creatine kinase: Female Male	20-170 IU/L 30-220 IU/L	0.33-2.83 mckat/L 0.5-3.67 mckat/L
Creatine kinase isoenzymes, MB fraction	0-12 IU/L	0-0.2 mckat/L
Creatinine	0.5-1.7 mg/dl	44-150 mcmol/L
Fibrinogen (coagulation factor I)	150-360 mg/dl	1.5-3.6 g/L
Follicle-stimulating hormone (FSH): Female Midcycle Male	 2-13 mIU/ml 5-22 mIU/ml 1-8 mIU/ml	 2-13 IU/L 5-22 IU/L 1-8 IU/L
Glucose, fasting	65-115 mg/dl	3.6-6.3 mmol/L
Glucose Tolerance Test (Oral)	mg/dL Normal / Diabetic	mmol/L Normal / Diabetic
Fasting	70-105 / > 140	3.9-5.8 / > 7.8
60 min	120-170 / ≥ 200	6.7-9.4 / ≥11.1
90 min	100-140 / ≥ 200	5.6-7.8 / ≥ 11.1
120 min	70-120 / ≥ 140	3.9-6.7 / ≥ 7.8
(γ) - Glutamyltransferase (GGT): Male Female	9-50 units/L 8-40 units/L	9-50 units/L 8-40 units/L
Haptoglobin	44-303 mg/dl	0.44-3.03 g/L
Hematologic tests: Fibrinogen Hematocrit (Hct), female male Hemoglobin A_{1C} Hemoglobin (Hb), female male Leukocyte count (WBC) Erythrocyte count (RBC), female male Mean corpuscular volume (MCV) Mean corpuscular hemoglobin (MCH) Mean corpuscular hemoglobin concentrate (MCHC) Erythrocyte sedimentation rate (sedrate, ESR)	 200-400 mg/dl 36%-44.6% 40.7%-50.3% 5.3%-7.5% of total Hgb 12.1-15.3 g/dl 13.8-17.5 g/dl 3800-9800/mcl 3.5-5 × 10^6/mcl 4.3-5.9 × 10^6/mcl 80-97.6 mcm^3 27-33 pg/cell 33-36 g/dl ≤ 30 mm/hr	 2-4 g/L 0.36-0.446 fraction of 1 0.4-0.503 fraction of 1 0.053-0.075 121-153 g/L 138-175 g/L 3.8-9.8 x 10^9/L 3.5-5 x 10^{12}/L 4.3-5.9 x 10^{12}/L 80-97.6 fl 1.66-2.09 fmol/cell 20.3-22 mmol/L ≤ 30 mm/hr
Erythrocyte enzymes: Glucose-6-phosphate dehydroge nase (G-6-PD) Ferritin Folic acid: normal Platelet count Reticulocytes Vitamin B_{12}	250-5000 units/10^6 cells 10-383 ng/ml > 3.1-12.4 ng/ml 150-450 × 10^3/mcl 0.5%-1.5% of erythrocytes 223-1132 pg/ml	250-5000 mcunits/cell 23-862 pmol/L 7-28.1 nmol/L 150-450 × 10^9/L 0.005-0.015 165-835 pmol/L
Iron: Female Male	30-160 mcg/dl 45-160 mcg/dl	5.4-31.3 mcmol/L 8.1-31.3 mcmol/L
Iron binding capacity	220-420 mcg/dl	39.4-75.2 mcmol/L
Isocitrate Dehydrogenase	1.2-7 units/L	1.2-7 units/L

Blood, Plasma or Serum		
	Reference Value	
Determination	Conventional Units	SI Units
Isoenzymes		
Fraction 1	14%-26% of total	0.14-0.26 fraction of total
Fraction 2	29%-39% of total	0.29-0.39 fraction of total
Fraction 3	20%-26% of total	0.20-0.26 fraction of total
Fraction 4	8%-16% of total	0.08-0.16 fraction of total
Fraction 5	6%-16% of total	0.06-0.16 fraction of total
Lactate dehydrogenase	100-250 IU/L	1.67-4.17 mckat/L
Lactic acid (lactate)	6-19 mg/dl	0.7-2.1 mmol/L
Lead	≤ 50 mcg/dl	≤ 2.41 mcmol/L
Lipase	10-150 units/L	10-150 units/L
Lipids:		
Total Cholesterol		
Desirable	< 200 mg/dl	< 5.2 mmol/L
Borderline-high	200-239 mg/dl	< 5.2-6.2 mmol/L
High	> 239 mg/dl	> 6.2 mmol/L
LDL		
Desirable	< 130 mg/dl	< 3.36 mmol/L
Borderline-high	130-159 mg/dl	3.36-4.11 mmol/L
High	> 159 mg/dl	> 4.11 mmol/L
HDL (low)	< 35 mg/dl	< 0.91 mmol/L
Triglycerides		
Desirable	< 200 mg/dl	< 2.26 mmol/L
Borderline-high	200-400 mg/dl	2.26-4.52 mmol/L
High	400-1000 mg/dl	4.52-11.3 mmol/L
Very high	> 1000 mg/dl	> 11.3 mmol/L
Magnesium	1.3-2.2 mEq/L	0.65-1.1 mmol/L
Osmolality	280-300 mOsm/kg	280-300 mmol/kg
Oxygen saturation (arterial)	94%-100%	0.94-1 fraction of 1
PCO_2, arterial	35-45 mm Hg	4.7-6 kPa
pH, arterial	7.35-7.45	7.35-7.45
PO_2, arterial: Breathing room air[1]	80-105 mm Hg	10.6-14 kPa
On 100% O_2	> 500 mm Hg	
Phosphatase (acid), total at 37°C	0.13-0.63 IU/L	2.2-10.5 IU/L or 2.2-10.5 mckat/L
Phosphatase alkaline[2]	20-130 IU/L	20-130 IU/L or 0.33-2.17 mckat/L
Phosphorus, inorganic,[3] (phosphate)	2.5-5 mg/dl	0.8-1.6 mmol/L
Potassium	3.5-5 mEq/L	3.5-5 mmol/L
Progesterone		
Female	0.1-1.5 ng/ml	0.32-4.8 nmol/L
Follicular phase	0.1-1.5 ng/ml	0.32-4.8 nmol/L
Luteal phase	2.5-28 ng/ml	8-89 nmol/L
Male	< 0.5 ng/ml	< 1.6 nmol/L
Prolactin	1.4-24.2 ng/ml	1.4-24.2 mcg/L
Prostate specific antigen	0-4 ng/ml	0-4 ng/ml
Protein: Total	6-8 g/dl	60-80 g/L
Albumin	3.6-5 g/dl	36-50 g/L
Globulin	2.3-3.5 g/dl	23-35 g/L
Rheumatoid factor	< 60 IU/ml	< 60 kIU/L
Sodium	135-147 mEq/L	135-147 mmol/L
Testosterone: Female	6-86 ng/dl	0.21-3 nmol/L
Male	270-1070 ng/dl	9.3-37 nmol/L
Thyroid Hormone Function Tests:		
Thyroid-stimulating hormone (TSH)	0.35-6.2 mcU/ml	0.35-6.2 mU/L
Thyroxine-binding globulin capacity	10-26 mcg/dl	100-260 mcg/L
Total triiodothyronine (T_3)	75-220 ng/dl	1.2-3.4 nmol/L
Total thyroxine by RIA (T_4)	4-11 mcg/dl	51-142 nmol/L
T_3 resin uptake	25%-38%	0.25-0.38 fraction of 1
Transaminase, AST (aspartate aminotransferase, SGOT)	11-47 IU/L	0.18-0.78 mckat/L
Transaminase, ALT (alanine aminotrans ferase, SGPT)	7-53 IU/L	0.12-0.88 mckat/L
Transferrin	220-400 mg/dL	2.20-4.00 g/L
Urea nitrogen (BUN)	8-25 mg/dl	2.9-8.9 mmol/L
Uric acid	3-8 mg/dl	179-476 mcmol/L
Vitamin A (retinol)	15-60 mcg/dl	0.52-2.09 mcmol/L
Zinc	50-150 mcg/dl	7.7-23 mcmol/L

[1] Age dependent [2] Infants and adolescents up to 104 U/L [3] Infants in the first year up to 6 mg/dl

Urine		
	Reference Value	
Determination	Conventional Units	SI Units
Calcium[1]	50-250 mcg/day	1.25-6.25 mmol/day
Catecholamines: Epinephrine	< 20 mcg/day	< 109 nmol/day

Urine

Determination	Reference Value: Conventional Units	Reference Value: SI Units
Norepinephrine	< 100 mcg/day	< 590 nmol/day
Catecholamines, 24-hr	< 110 µg	< 650 nmol
Copper[1]	15-60 mcg/day	0.24-0.95 mcmol/day
Creatinine: Child	8-22 mg/kg	71-195 µmol/kg
Adolescent	8-30 mg/kg	71-265 µmol/kg
Female	0.6-1.5 g/day	5.3-13.3 mmol/day
Male	0.8-1.8 g/day	7.1-15.9 mmol/day
pH	4.5-8	4.5-8
Phosphate[1]	0.9-1.3 g/day	29-42 mmol/day
Potassium[1]	25-100 mEq/day	25-100 mmol/day
Protein		
Total	1-14 mg/dL	10-140 mg/L
At rest	50-80 mg/day	50-80 mg/day
Protein, quantitative	< 150 mg/day	< 0.15 g/day
Sodium[1]	100-250 mEq/day	100-250 mmol/day
Specific Gravity, random	1.002-1.030	1.002-1.030
Uric Acid, 24-hr	250-750 mg	1.48-4.43 mmol

[1] Diet dependent

Drug Levels†

Drug Class	Drug Determination	Reference Value: Conventional Units	Reference Value: SI Units
Aminoglycosides	Amikacin		
	(trough)	1-8 mcg/ml	1.7-13.7 mcmol/L
	(peak)	20-30 mcg/ml	34-51 mcmol/L
	Gentamicin		
	(trough)	0.5-2 mcg/ml	1-4.2 mcmol/L
	(peak)	6-10 mcg/ml	12.5-20.9 mcmol/L
	Kanamycin		
	(trough)	5-10 mcg/ml	nd
	(peak)	20-25 mcg/ml	nd
	Netilmicin		
	(trough)	0.5-2 mcg/ml	nd
	(peak)	6-10 mcg/ml	nd
	Streptomycin		
	(trough)	< 5 mcg/ml	nd
	(peak)	5-20 mcg/ml	nd
	Tobramycin		
	(trough)	0.5-2 mcg/ml	1.1-4.3 mcmol/L
	(peak)	5-20 mcg/ml	12.8-21.8 mcmol/L
Antiarrhythmics	Amiodarone	0.5-2.5 mcg/ml	1.5-4 mcmol/L
	Bretylium	0.5-1.5 mcg/ml	nd
	Digitoxin	9-25 mcg/L	11.8-32.8 nmol/L
	Digoxin	0.8-2 ng/ml	0.9-2.5 nmol/L
	Disopyramide	2-8 mcg/ml	6-18 mcmol/L
	Flecainide	0.2-1 mcg/ml	nd
	Lidocaine	1.5-6 mcg/ml	4.5-21.5 mcmol/L
	Mexiletine	0.5-2 mcg/ml	nd
	Procainamide	4-8 mcg/ml	17-34 mcmol/ml
	Propranolol	50-200 ng/ml	190-770 nmol/L
	Quinidine	2-6 mcg/ml	4.6-9.2 mcmol/L
	Tocainide	4-10 mcg/ml	nd
	Verapamil	0.08-0.3 mcg/ml	nd
Anti-convulsants	Carbamazepine	4-12 mcg/ml	17-51 mcmol/L
	Phenobarbital	10-40 mcg/ml	43-172 mcmol/L
	Phenytoin	10-20 mcg/ml	40-80 mcmol/L
	Primidone	4-12 mcg/ml	18-55 mcmol/L
	Valproic acid	40-100 mcg/ml	280-700 mcmol/L
Antidepressants	Amitriptyline	110-250 ng/ml[3]	500-900 nmol/L
	Amoxapine	200-500 ng/ml	nd
	Bupropion	25-100 ng/ml	nd
	Clomipramine	80-100 ng/ml	nd
	Desipramine	115-300 ng/ml	nd
	Doxepin	110-250 ng/ml[3]	nd
	Imipramine	225-350 ng/ml[3]	nd
	Maprotiline	200-300 ng/ml	nd
	Nortriptyline	50-150 ng/ml	nd
	Protriptyline	70-250 ng/ml	nd
	Trazodone	800-1600 ng/ml	nd

Drug Levels†

Drug Class	Drug Determination	Reference Value: Conventional Units	Reference Value: SI Units
Antipsychotics	Chlorpromazine	50-300 ng/ml	150-950 nmol/L
	Fluphenazine	0.13-2.8 ng/ml	nd
	Haloperidol	5-20 ng/ml	nd
	Perphenazine	0.8-1.2 ng/ml	nd
	Thiothixene	2-57 ng/ml	nd
Miscellaneous	Amantadine	300 ng/ml	nd
	Amrinone	3.7 mcg/ml	nd
	Chloramphenicol	10-20 mcg/ml	31-62 mcmol/L
	Cyclosporine[1]	250-800 ng/ml (whole blood, RIA) 50-300 ng/ml (plasma, RIA)	nd nd
	Ethanol[2]	0 mg/dl	0 mmol/L
	Hydralazine	100 ng/ml	nd
	Lithium	0.6-1.2 mEq/L	0.6-1.2 mmol/L
	Salicylate	100-300 mg/L	724-2172 mcmol/L
	Sulfonamide	5-15 mg/dl	nd
	Terbutaline	0.5-4.1 ng/ml	nd
	Theophylline	10-20 mcg/ml	55-110 mcmol/L
	Vancomycin		
	(trough)	5-15 ng/ml	nd
	(peak)	20-40 mcg/ml	nd

† The values given are generally accepted as desirable for treatment without toxicity for most patients. However, exceptions are not uncommon.
[1] 24 hour trough values [2] Toxic: 50-100 mg/dl (10.9-21.7 mmol/L) [3] Parent drug plus N-desmethyl metabolite
nd – No data available

Classification of Blood Pressure*

Category	Reference Value: Systolic (mm Hg)		Reference Value: Diastolic (mm Hg)
Optimal†	< 120	and	< 80
Normal	< 130	and	< 85
High-normal	130-139	or	85-89
Hypertension‡			
Stage 1	140-159	or	90-99
Stage 2	160-179	or	100-109
Stage 3	≥ 180	or	≥ 110

adopted from the Sixth Report of the Joint National Committee on Prevention, Detection, Evaluation, and Treatment of High Blood Pressure, National Institutes of Health

* For adults age 18 and older who are not taking antihypertensive drugs and not acutely ill. When systolic and diastolic blood pressures fall into different categories, the higher category should be selected to classify the individual's blood pressure status. In addition to classifying stages of hypertension on the basis of average blood pressure levels, clinicians should specify presence or absence of target organ disease and additional risk factors.

† Optimal blood pressure with respect to cardiovascular risk is below 120/88 mm Hg. However, unusually low readings should be evaluated for clinical significance.

‡ Based on the average of two or more readings taken at each of two or more visits after an initial screening.

To calculate milliequivalent weight: $mEq = \frac{\text{gram molecular weight/valence}}{1000}$

$mEq = \frac{mg}{\text{eq wt}}$ equivalent weight or eq wt = $\frac{\text{gram molecular weight}}{\text{valence}}$

Commonly used mEq weights			
Chloride	35.5 mg = 1 mEq	Magnesium	12 mg = 1 mEq
Sodium	23 mg = 1 mEq	Potassium	39 mg = 1 mEq
Calcium	20 mg = 1 mEq		

To convert temperature °C ↔ °F: $\frac{°C}{°F - 32} = \frac{5}{9}$ or $°C = \frac{5}{9}(°F - 32)$

$°F = 32 + \frac{9}{5}\,°C$

To calculate creatinine clearance (Ccr) from serum creatinine:

Male: $Ccr = \frac{\text{weight (kg)} \times (140 - \text{age})}{72 \times \text{serum creatinine (mg/dL)}}$

Female: $Ccr = 0.85 \times$ calculation for males

To calculate ideal body weight (kg):

Male = 50 kg + 2.3 kg (each inch > 5 ft)

Female = 45.5 kg + 2.3 kg (each inch > 5 ft)

To calculate body surface area (BSA) in adults and children:

1) *Dubois method:*

$SA\ (cm^2) = wt\ (kg)^{0.425} \times ht\ (cm)^{0.725} \times 71.84$

$SA\ (m^2) = K \times \sqrt[3]{wt^2}\ (kg)$ (common K value 0.1 for toddlers, 0.103 for neonates)

2) *Simplified method:*

$BSA\ (m^2) = \sqrt{\frac{\text{ht (cm)} \times \text{wt (kg)}}{3600}}$

To approximate surface area (m^2) of children from weight (kg):

Weight range (kg)	≈ Surface area (m^2)
1 to 5	(0.05 x kg) + 0.05
6 to 10	(0.04 x kg) + 0.10
11 to 20	(0.03 x kg) + 0.20
21 to 40	(0.02 x kg) + 0.40

Suggested Weights for Adults	
Height*	Weight in pounds†
4′10″	91-119
4′11″	94-124
5′0″	97-128
5′1″	101-132
5′2″	104-137
5′3″	107-141
5′4″	111-146
5′5″	114-150
5′6″	118-155
5′7″	121-160
5′8″	125-164
5′9″	129-169
5′10″	132-174
5′11″	136-179
6′0″	140-184
6′1″	144-189
6′2″	148-195
6′3″	152-200
6′4″	156-205
6′5″	160-211
6′6″	164-216

* Without shoes. † Without clothes.

The higher weights in the ranges generally apply to people with more muscle and bone. Source: Nutrition and Your Health: Dietary Guidelines for Americans, 4th ed, 1995. US Department of Agriculture, US Department of Health and Human Services. At press time, these new guidelines had not been officially released. It is possible some changes to this chart will occur.

➤*Standard Medical Abbreviations used in medical orders:*

Abbreviation	Meaning
≈	approximately equals
Δ	delta
ε	epsilon; molar absorption coefficient
Ω	omega; ohm
5-HIAA	5-hydroxyindoleacetic acid
5-HT	5-hydroxytryptamine (serotonin)
6-MP	6-mercaptopurine
17-OHCS	17-hydroxycorticosteroids
α	alpha
A	ampere(s)
Å	angstrom(s)
aa	of each (ana)
āā	of each (ana)
AA	Alcoholics Anonymous; amino acid
AACP	American Association of Clinical Pharmacy; American Association of Colleges of Pharmacy
AARP	American Association of Retired Persons
Ab	antibody
ABGs	arterial blood gases
abs feb	when fever is absent (*absente febre*)
ABVD	Adriamycin (doxorubicin), bleomycin, vinblastine, (and) dacarbazine
ac	before meals or food (*ante cibum*)
ACCP	American College of Clinical Pharmacy
ACD	acid-citrate-dextrose
ACE	angiotensin-converting enzyme
ACEI	angiotensin-converting enzyme inhibitor
ACh	acetylcholine
ACIP	Advisory Committee on Immunization Practices
ACLS	advanced cardiac life support
ACPE	American Council on Pharmaceutical Education
ACS	American Chemical Society
ACT	activated clotting time
ACTH	adrenocorticotropic hormone
ad to;	to; up to (*ad*)
a.d.	right ear (*aurio dextra*)
ADE	adverse drug experience
ADH	antidiuretic hormone
adhib	to be administered (*adhibendus*)
ad lib	as desired, at pleasure (*ad libitum*)
ADLs	activities of daily living
ADME	absorption, distribution, metabolism and elimination
admov	apply (*admove*)
ADP	adenosine diphosphate
ADR	adverse drug reaction
ADRRS	Adverse Drug Reaction Reporting System
ad sat	to saturation (*ad saturatum, ad saturandum*)
adst feb	when fever is present (*adstante febre*)
ad us.	ext for external use (*ad usum externum*)
adv	against (*adversum*)
aer	aerosol
Ag	antigen; silver (*argentum*)
agit. Ante us.	shake before using (*agita ante usum*)
agit. Bene	shake well (*agita bene*)
AHA	American Hospital Association
AID	artificial insemination donor
AIDS	acquired immunodeficiency syndrome
AJHP	*American Journal of Hospital Pharmacy*
al	left ear (*aurio laeva*)
ala	alanine
ALL	acute lymphocytic leukemia
ALT	alanine aminotransferase, serum (previously SGPT)
alt hor	every other hour (*alternis horis*)
A.M.	before noon; morning (*ante meridiem*)
AMA	American Medical Association
AML	acute myelogenous leukemia
AMP	adenosine monophosphate
ANA	antinuclear antibody(ies)
ANC	acid neutralizing capacity
ANDA	abbreviated new drug application
ANOVA	analysis of variance
ANUG	acute necrotizing ulcerative gingivitis
APA	antipernicious anemia (factor)
APAP	acetaminophen
APC	antigen presenting cell(s)
APhA	American Pharmaceutical Association
aPTT	activated partial thromboplastin time
aq	water (*aqua*)
aq. dest	distilled water (*aqua destillata*)
ARC	AIDS-related complex
ARDS	adult respiratory distress syndrome
ARF	acute renal failure
Arg	arginine
ARV	AIDS-related virus
as	left ear (*aurio sinister*)
ASHD	arteriosclerotic heart disease
ASHP	American Society of Hospital Pharmacists
Asn	asparagine
Asp	aspartic acid
AST	aspartate aminotransferase, serum (previously SGOT)
atm	standard atmosphere
ATN	acute tubular necrosis
ATP	adenosine triphosphate
ATPase	adenosine triphosphatase
ATPD	ambient temperature and pressure, saturated
at wt	atomic weight
au	each ear (*aures utrae*)
AU	gold (*aurum*)
AUC	area under the plasma concentration-time curve
AV	atrioventricular
A-V	arteriovenous; atrioventricular (block, bundle, conduction, dissociation, extrasystole)
AW	atomic weight
AWP	average wholesale price
ax.	axis
β	beta
BAC	blood-alcohol concentration
BADL	basic activities of daily life
BBB	blood brain barrier
BDZ	benzodiazepine
bib	drink (*bibe*)
bid	twice daily; two times a day (*bis in die*)
bm	bowel movement
BMR	basal metabolic rate
bp	boiling point
BP	blood pressure
BPH	benign prostatic hypertrophy
bpm	beats per minute
BSA	body surface area
BT	bleeding time
BUN	blood urea nitrogen
C	centigrade
C.	*clostridium*
c	gallon (*cong*)
c̄	with (*cum*)
°C	degrees Celsius

Abbreviation	Meaning
Ca	calcium
CA	cancer; carcinoma; cardiac arrest; chronologic age; croup-associated
CAD	coronary artery disease
Cal	Calorie (kilocalorie)
cAMP	cyclic adenosine monophosphate
caps	capsule (*capsula*)
CAS	Chemical Abstracts Service
CAT	computerized axial tomography
cath	catheterize
CBA	cost-benefit analysis
CBC	complete blood count
CC	chief complaint
cc	cubic centimeter
CCBs	calcium channel blockers
CCU	coronary care unit; critical care unit
CD4	T-helper lymphocytes and macrophages
CDC	Centers for Disease Control and Prevention
CEA	cost effectiveness analysis
CF	cystic fibrosis
CFC	chlorofluorocarbon
CFU	colony-forming units
CHD	coronary heart disease
CHF	congestive heart failure
Ci	curie
CK	creatinine kinase
Cl	chlorine
Cl_{cr}	creatinine clearance
cm	centimeter; cream
Cm	curium
cm^2	square centimeter(s)
cm^3	cubic centimeter
CMA	Certified Medical Assistant
CMC	carpometacarpal
CMI	cell-mediated immunity
CML	chronic myelocytic leukemia
C_{max}	maximum effective plasma concentration
C_{min}	minimum effective plasma concentration
CMT	Certified Medical Transcriptionist
CMV	cytomegalovirus I
CMVIG	cytomegalovirus immune globulin
CN	cranial nerve
CNM	Certified Nurse Midwife
CNS	central nervous system
CO	cardiac output
CO_2	carbon dioxide
CoA	coenzyme A
COG	center of gravity
comp	compound (*compositus*)
COMT	catecholamine-o-methyl transferase
cont rem	let the medicine be continued (*continuetur remedium*)
COPD	chronic obstructive pulmonary disease
CPAP	continuous positive airway pressure
CPK	creatine phosphokinase
CPR	cardiopulmonary resuscitation
CQI	continuous quality improvement
Cr	creatinine; chromium
CrCl	creatinine clearance
CRD	chronic respiratory disease
CRF	chronic renal failure
CRH	corticotropin-releasing hormone
crm	cream
CRNA	Certified Registered Nurse Anesthetist
C&S	culture and sensitivity
CSA	Controlled Substances Act; cyclosporin A
CSF	cerebrospinal fluid; colony-stimulating factors
CSP	cellulose sodium phosphate
ct	clotting time
CT	computerized tomography
CTZ	chemoreceptor trigger zone
cu	cubic
Cu	copper (*cuprum*)
CV	cardiovascular
CVA	cerebrovascular accident
CVP	central venous pressure
CXR	chest x-ray
cyl	cylinder; cylindrical (lens)
cys	cysteine
d	day (*dies*)
D5W	Dextrose 5% in Water Solution
D10W	Dextrose 10% in Water Solution
D&C	dilation and curettage; designation applied to dyes permitted for use in drugs and cosmetics
D&E	dilation and evacuation
DC	Doctor of Chiropractic
DDS	Doctor of Dental Surgery
DEA	Drug Enforcement Administration
deglut	swallow (*degluttiatur*)
DERM	dermatologic
det	give (*detur*)
DHHS	Department of Health and Human Services
DIC	disseminated intravascular coagulation
dieb alt	every other day (*diebus alternis*)
dil	dilute (*dilue*)
dim	one-half (*dimidius*)
dir prop	with proper direction (*directione propria*)
div in par aeq	divide into equal parts (*divide in partes aequales*)
DIS	drug information source
disp	dispense (*dispensa*)
div	divide
DJD	degenerative joint disease
DKA	diabetic ketoacidosis
dl	deciliter (100 ml)
DMD	Doctor of Dental Medicine
DMSO	dimethyl sulfoxide
DNA	deoxyribonucleic acid
DNR	do not resuscitate
DNS	Director of Nursing Service; Doctor of Nursing Services
DO	Doctor of Osteopathy
DOA	dead on arrival
DP	Doctor of Podiatry
DPH	Doctor of Public Health; Doctor of Public Hygiene
DPI	dry powder inhaler
DPM	Doctor of Physical Medicine; Doctor of Podiatric Medicine
DPS	disintegrations per second
DRG	diagnosis-related groups
DRI	Dietary Reference Intakes
drp	drop(s)
DrPh	Doctor of Public Health; Doctor of Public Hygiene
DRR	Drug Regimen Review
DT	delirium tremens
dtd	give of such a dose (*dentur tales doses*)
DTP	diphtheria, tetanus toxoids & pertussis vaccine
DTRs	deep tendon reflexes
DUB	dysfunctional uterine bleeding
DUE	Drug Usage Evaluations
DUR	Drug Utilization Review
dur dol	while pain lasts (*durante dolore*)
DVA	Department of Veterans Affairs
DVM	Doctor of Veterinary Medicine
DVT	deep venous thrombosis
E.	*Enterococcus; Escherichia*
EBV	Epstein-Barr virus

Abbreviation	Meaning
EC	enteric coated
ECG	electrocardiogram
ECT	electroconvulsive therapy
ed.	editor
ED	emergency department; effective dose
ED_{50}	median-effective dose
EDTA	ethylenediamine tetraacetic acid
EEG	electroencephalogram
EENT	eye, ear, nose, and throat
EF	ejection fraction
eg	for example (*exempli gratia*)
EIA	enzyme immunoassay
EKG	electrocardiogram
el	elixir
ELISA	enzyme-linked immunosorbent assay
elix	elixir
EMIT	enzyme-multiplied immunoassay test
emp	as directed
ENL	erythema nodosum leprosum
ENT	ear, nose, throat
EPA	Environmental Protection Agency
EPAP	expiratory positive airway pressure
EPO	erythropoietin
EPS	extrapyramidal syndrome (or symptoms)
ER	emergency room; estrogen receptor; extended release; endoplasmic reticulum
ESR	erythrocyte sedimentation rate; electron spin resonance
et	and
ET	via endotracheal tube
et al.	for 3 or more co-authors or co-workers (*et alii*)
ex aq	in water
ext rel	extended release
F	fluorine
f	make; let be made (*fac, fiat, fiant*)
°F	degrees Fahrenheit
Fab	fragment of immunoglobulin G involved in antigen binding
FAO	Food and Agriculture Organization
FAS	fetal alcohol syndrome
FBS	fasting blood sugar
FDA	Food and Drug Administration
FD&C	designation applied to dyes permitted for use in foods, drugs and cosmetics; Food, Drug and Cosmetic Act
Fe	iron (*ferrum*)
FEF	forced expiratory flow
FET	forced expiratory time
FEV_1	forced expiratory volume in 1 second
fl oz	fluid ounce(s)
Fru	fructose
FSH	follicle-stimulating hormone
ft	make; let be made (*fac, fiat, fiant*)
ft	foot (feet)
ft^2	square foot (feet)
FTC	Federal Trade Commission
FTI	free-thyroxine index
FUO	fever of unknown origin
FVC	forced vital capacity
γ	gamma
g	gram (*gramma*)
G-6-P	glucose-6-phosphate
G-6-PD	glucose-6-phosphate dehydrogenase
GABA	gamma-aminobutyric acid
Gal	galactose
gal	gallon
G-CSF	granulocyte colony-stimulating factor
GERD	gastroesophageal reflux disease
GFR	glomerular filtration rate
GGTP	gamma glutamyl transpeptidase
GH	growth hormone
GHRF	growth hormone-releasing factor
GHRH	growth hormone-releasing hormone
GI	gastrointestinal
GLC	gas-liquid chromatography
gln	glutamine
glu	glutamic acid; glutamyl
gly	glycine
Gm	gram (*gramma*)
gr	grain (*granum*)
grad	gradually (*gradatim*)
gran	granule(s)
GRAS	generally regarded as safe*
gtt	a drop (*gutta*)
GU	genitourinary
guttat	drop by drop (*guttatim*)
Gyn	gynecology
H.	*Haemophilus*; *Helicobacter*
h	hour (*hora*)
H_2	histamine 2
H_2O	water
HA	hyaluronic acid
Hb	hemoglobin
HbF	fetal hemoglobin
HBIG	hepatitis B immune specific globulin
HCFA	Health Care Financing Administration
HCG	human chorionic gonadotropin
HCl	hydrochloric acid
HCN	hydrogen cyanide
Hct	hematocrit
hd	bedtime (*hora decubitus*)
HDL	high-density lipoprotein
HEMA	hematologic
HEME	hematologic
hep	hepatic
HEPA	high efficiency particulate air
Hg	mercury (*hydragyrum*)
Hgb	hemoglobin
HGH	human pituitary growth hormone
Hib.	*Haemophilus influenzae*
His.	*Haemophilus influenzae* type b
HIV	human immunodeficiency virus
HLA	human leukocyte antigen
HMG-CoA	3-hydroxy-3-methylglutaryl coenzyme A
HMO	health maintenance organization
hor decub	at bedtime (*hora decubitus*)
hor som	at bedtime (*hora somni*)
HPA	hypothalamic-pituitary-adrenocortical (axis)
HPLC	high performance liquid chromatography
HPLC/MS	high performance liquid chromatography/mass spectrometry
HPMC	hydroxypropylmethylcellulose
HPV	human papillomavirus
HR	heart rate
hr	hour
hs	at bedtime (*hora somni*)
HSA	human serum albumin
HSV-1	herpes simplex virus type 1
HSV-2	herpes simplex virus type 2
Hz	hertz
I	iodine

Abbreviation	Meaning
IADL	instrumental activities of daily living
I/O	intake/output
IBW	ideal body weight
IC	intracoronary
ICD	International Classification of Diseases of the World Health Organization
ICF	intracellular fluid
ICP	intracranial pressure
ICU	intensive care unit
ID	intradermal; infective dose
IDDM	insulin-dependent diabetes mellitus (type 1 diabetes)
IDU	idoxuridine
IFN	interferon
Ig	immunoglobulin
IL	interleukin
Ile	isoleucine
IM	intramuscular
in	inch(es)
in^2	square inch(es)
IND	Investigational New Drug
in d	daily (*in dies*)
INDA	Investigational New Drug Application
Inh	inhaled
INH	isoniazid
Inhal	inhalation
Inj	injection
INR	International Normalizing Ratio
int cib	between meals (*inter cibos*)
IOP	intraocular pressure
IP	intraperitoneal(ly)
IPA	International Pharmaceutical Abstracts
IPPB	intermittent positive pressure breathing
IPV	poliovirus vaccine inactivated
IQ	intelligence quotient
ISA	intrinsic sympathomimetic activity
ISF	interstitial fluid
ISI	Institute for Scientific Information
ISO	International Organization for Standardization
IT	intrathecal(ly)
IU	international unit(s)
IUD	intrauterine device
IV	intravenous
IVF	intravascular fluid
IVP	intravenous piggyback
J	joule(s)
JCAH	Joint Commission on Accreditation of Hospitals
JCAHO	Joint Commission on Accreditation of Healthcare Organizations
K	potassium (*kalium*); kelvin
kcal	kilocalorie(s)
keV	kiloelectronvolt(s)
kg	kilogram
kJ	kilojoule(s)
Kleb.	*Klebsiella*
KVO	keep vein open
L	liter
L.	*Legionella*; *Listeria*
lb	pound
LBW	low body weight
LD	lethal dose
LD-50	a dose lethal to 50% of the specified animals or microorganisms
LDH	lactate dehydrogenase
LDL	low-density lipoprotein
LE	lupus erythematosus
Leu	leucine
LFT	liver function test
LH	luteinizing hormone
liq	liquid (*liquor*)
LM	Licentiate in Midwifery
LOC	level of consciousness
Lot	lotion
LPN	Licensed Practical Nurse
Lr	lawrencium
LSD	lysergic acid diethylamide
LTCF	long-term care facility
LTM	long-term memory
LUQ	left upper quadrant (of abdomen)
LVEDP	left ventricular end-diastolic pressure
LVET	left ventricular ejection time
LVF	left ventricular function
LVN	Licensed Visiting Nurse; Licensed Vocational Nurse
LVP	large-volume parenterals
Lw	former symbol for lawrencium (see Lr)
Lys	lysine
μm	micrometer
μg	microgram
m	meter
M	mix (*misce*)
M	molar (strength of a solution)
M.	*Moraxella*; *Mycobacterium*; *Mycoplasma*
m^2	square meter (of body surface area)
m^3	cubic meter(s)
MA	mental age
MAC	maximum allowable cost
MADD	Mothers Against Drunk Drivers
man pr	early morning; first thing in the morning (*mane primo*)
MAO	monoamine oxidase
MAOI	monoamine oxidase inhibitor
MAP	mean arterial pressure
max	maximum
MBC	minimum bactericidal concentration
MBD	minimal brain dysfunction
mcg	microgram
MCH	mean corpuscular hemoglobin
MCHC	mean corpuscular hemoglobin concentration
mCi	millicurie
MCT	medium-chain triglyceride
MCV	mean corpuscular volume
MD	Doctor of Medicine (*Medicinae Doctor*)
MDI	metered dose inhaler
m dict	as directed (*more dictor*)
MDR	minimum daily requirements
MEC	minimum effective concentration
MEDLARS	Medical Literature Analysis and Retrieval System
MEDLINE	National Library of Medicine medical database
mEq	milliequivalent
Met	methionine
MeV	megaelectronvolt(s)
Mg	magnesium
mg	milligram
MHC	major histocompatibility complex
MI	myocardial infarction
MIA	metabolite bacterial inhibition assay
MIC	minimum inhibitory concentration
MID	minimal infecting dose
min	minute
min.	minimum
MIP	maximum inspiratory pressure
mixt	a mixture (*mixtura*)
MJ	mejajoule(s)
ml	milliliter
mm	millimeter
mm^2	square millimeter(s)
mm^3	cubic millimeter(s)
mmHg	millimeters of mercury
mmol	millimole

Abbreviation	Meaning
MMR	measles, mumps and rubella virus vaccine, live
MMWR	*Morbidity and Mortality Weekly Report*
Mn	manganese
Mo	molybdenum
mo	month
mol	mole(s)
mor dict	in the manner stated (*more dicto*)
mor sol	as usual; as customary (*more solito*)
mOsm	milliosmole
MPH	Master of Public Health
MRI	magnetic resonance imaging
mRNA	messenger RNA
MS	mass spectrometry; mitral stenosis; multiple sclerosis
MW	molecular weight
N	normal (strength of a solution)
N.	*Neisseria*
Na	sodium (*natrium*)
NABP	National Association of Boards of Pharmacy
NABPLEX	National Association of Boards of Pharmacy Licensing Exam
NAD	nicotinamide-adenine dinucleotide phosphate
NADH	reduced form of nicotine adenine dinucleotide
NADP	nicotinamide-adenine dinucleotide phosphate
NADPH	nicotinamide-adenine dinucleotide phosphate (reduced form)
NAPA	*N*-acetyl procainamide
NARD	National Association of Retail Druggists - Now NCPA; National Assoc. of Community Pharmacists
nb	note well (*nota bene*)
nCi	nanocurie(s)
NCPA	National Assoc. of Community Pharmacists
ND	Doctor of Naturopathic Medicine
NDA	new drug application
NF	National Formulary
ng	nanogram
NG	nasogastric
NK	natural killer (cells); killer T cells
NIDDM	non-insulin dependent diabetes mellitus (type 2 diabetes)
NIH	National Institutes of Health
NLM	National Library of Medicine
nm	nanometer(s)
NMS	neuroleptic malignant syndrome
NMT	not more than (on prescriptions)
no	number (*numerus*)
noc	in the night (*nocturnal*)
noc maneq	at night and the morning (*nocte maneque*)
non rep	do not repeat; no refills (*non repetatur*)
NPN	nonprotein nitrogen
NPO	nothing by mouth
NS	normal saline (as in solution)
NSAIA	nonsteroidal anti-inflammatory agent
NSAID	nonsteroidal anti-inflammatory drug
NTD	neutral tube defect
O	a pint (*octarius*)
OB/GYN	obstetrics and gynecology
OBRA	Omnibus Budget Reconciliation Act of 1990
OBS	organic brain syndrome
OC	oral contraceptive
Oct	a pint (*octarius*)
od	right eye (*oculus dexter*)
OD	Doctor of Optometry; overdose
Oint	ointment
ol	left eye (*oculus laevus*)
omn hor	at every hour (*omni hora*)
Ophth	ophthalmic
os	left eye (*oculus sinister*)
OSHA	Occupational Safety and Health Administration
OT	occupational therapy
otc	over-the-counter (nonprescription)
OPV	oral poliovirus vaccine, live
ou	each eye (*oculo uterque*)
o/w	oil-in-water (emulsion)
oz	ounce
P	phosphorus
P	probability
P&T	pharmacy and therapeutics (committee)
Pa	pascal(s)
PA	Physician Assistant; Physician's Assistant
PABA	para-aminobenzoic acid
PAC	premature atrial contraction
$PaCO_2$	arterial plasma partial pressure of carbon dioxide
PAD	premature atrial depolarization
PAF	platelet-activating factor
PaO_2	partial alveolar oxygen
part aeq	equal parts/amounts (*partes aequales*)
part vic	in divided doses (*partitis vicibus*)
PAS	para-aminosalicylic acid
PAW	pulmonary arterial wedge
PAWP	pulmonary artery wedge pressure
Pb	lead (*plumbum*)
PBP	penicillin-binding protein
pc	after meals (*post cibum; post cibos*)
PCA	patient-controlled analgesia
pCO_2	plasma partial pressure of carbon dioxide
PCP	phencyclidine
PCR	polymerase chain reaction
PDGF	platelet-derived growth factor
PDLL	poorly differentiated lymphocytic lymphoma
PE	pulmonary embolism
PEEP	positive end expiratory pressure
PEG	polyethylene glycol
PERLA	pupils equal, react to light and accommodation
PET	positron emission tomography
pg	picogram(s)
PG	prostaglandin
PGA	prostaglandin A
PGB	prostaglandin B
PGE	prostaglandin E
PGF	prostaglandin F
pH	the negative logarithm of the hydrogen ion concentration
PharmD	Doctor of Pharmacy (*Pharmaciae Doctor*)
PhD	Doctor of Philosophy (*Philosophiae Doctor*)
Phe	phenylalanine
PhG	German Pharmacopeia (*Pharmacopoeia Germanica*)
PHS	Public Health Service
pKa	the negative logarithm of the dissociation constant
PKU	phenylketonuria
PMA	Pharmaceutical Manufacturers Association
PMN	polymorphonuclear leukocyte
PMR	patient medication record
PMS	premenstrual syndrome
PND	paroxysmal nocturnal dyspnea
po	by mouth; orally (*per os*)
pO_2	oxygen pressure (tension)

Abbreviation	Meaning
POR	problem-oriented medical record
POS	point of service
post cib	after meals (*post cibos*)
PPD	purified protein derivative of tuberculin
PPI	patient package insert
ppm	parts per million
PPO	preferred provider organization
pr	per rectum
Pr.	*Proteus*
prn	as needed; when required (*pro re nata*)
Pro	proline
pro rat. Aet.	According to patient's age (*pro ratione aetatis*)
Ps.	*Pseudomonas*
PSA	prostate-specific antigen
PSP	phenolsulfonphthalein
PSVT	paroxysmal supraventricular tachycardia
pt	pint
PT	prothrombin time; pharmacy and therapeutics; physical therapy
PTH	parathyroid hormone
PTT	partial thromboplastin time
PUD	peptic ulcer disease
pulv	a powder (*pulvis*)
PUVA	oral administration of psoralen and subsequent exposure to ultraviolet light of A wavelengths (UVA)
PVC	premature ventricular contraction; polyvinyl chloride
PVD	peripheral vascular disease; premature ventricular depolarizations
pwdr	powder
q	every
Q	volume of blood flow
QA	quality assurance
qad	every other day (*quoque alternis die*)
QC	quality control
qd	every day (*quaque die*)
qh	every hour (*quaque hora*)
q hr	every hour
qid	four times daily (*quarter in die*)
ql	as much as desired (*quantum libet*)
qod	every other day
q 2 hr	every 2 hours
qs	a sufficient quantity (*quantum sufficiat*)
qs	as much as is enough (*quantum satis*)
qs ad	a sufficient quantity to make
qt	quart
qv	as much as you wish (*quam volueris*)
R&D	research and development
RA	rheumatoid arthritis
RAI	radioactive iodine
RAS	renin-angiotensin system; reticular-activating system
RAST	radioallergosorbent test
RBC	red blood (cell) count
RDA	Recommended Dietary (Daily) Allowance
RDS	respiratory distress syndrome
RDW	red-cell distribution width
RE	reticuloendothelial
rem	radio equivalent man
REM	rapid eye movement
rep	let it be repeated (*repetatur*)
RES	reticuloendothelial system
RF	releasing factor
Rh	Rhesus (RH blood group)
RIA	radioimmunoassay
RN	Registered Nurse
RNA	ribonucleic acid
ROM	range of motion
RPh	registered pharmacist
rpm	revolutions per minute
rps	revolutions per second
RR	respiratory rate
RT$_3$U	total serum thyroxine concentration
RUL	right upper lobe (of lung)
RUQ	right upper quadrant (of abdomen)
Rx	prescription only; take; a recipe (*recipe*)
S.	*Salmonella*; *Serratia*
s	second
s	without (*sine*)
$\bar{s}$	without (*sine*)
S&S	signs and symptoms
S-A	sinoatrial
sa	according to art (*secundum artem*)
sat	saturated (*sataratus*)
Sb	antimony (*stibium*)
SBE	self breast examination; subacute bacterial endocarditis
SC	subcutaneous(ly)
S$_{cr}$	serum creatinine
SD	standard deviation; streptodornase
Se	selenium
sec	second
Ser	serine
sf	sugar free
SGGT	serum gamma-glutamyl transferase
SGOT	(see AST)
SGPT	(see ALT)
Sh.	*Shigella*
SIADH	syndrome of inappropriate secretion of antidiuretic hormone
SIDS	sudden infant death syndrome
Sig	label; let it be printed (*signa*)
SI units	International System of Units
SK	streptokinase
SL	sublingual(ly)
SLE	systemic lupus erythematosus
SMA	sequential multiple analysis
Sn	tin (*stannum*)
SNF	skilled nursing facility
sol	solution (*solutio*)
soln	solution
solv	dissolve
sp	species
SPECT	single photon emission computerized tomography
sp gr	specific gravity
SPF	sun protection factor
sq	square
SR	sedimentation rate; sustained-release
ss	one-half (*semis*)
$\bar{s}\bar{s}$	one-half (*semis*)
SSRI	selective serotonin reuptake inhibitors
Staph.	*Staphylococcus*
stat	immediately; at once (*statim*)
STM	short-term memory
STP	standard temperature and pressure
Str.	*Streptococcus*
STD	sexually transmitted disease
supp	suppository (*suppositorium*)
suppl	supplement(s)
susp	suspension
SV	stroke volume
syr	syrup (*syrupus*)
t$_{1/2}$	half-life
T$_3$	triiodothyronine
T$_4$	thyroxine
tab	tablet (*tabella*)
tal	such
tal dos	such doses

Abbreviation	Meaning
TB	tuberculosis
TBC	thyroxine-binding globulin
TBP	thyroxine-binding proteins
TBPA	thyroxine-binding pre-albumin
TBW	total body weight
TCA	tricyclic antidepressant
TD_{50}	median toxic dose
TEEC	transesophageal echocardiography
TEN	toxic epidermal necrolysis
TENS	transcutaneous electrical nerve stimulation
TG	total triglycerides
THC	tetrahydrocannabinol
Thr	threonine
TIA	transient ischemic attack
tid	three times daily (*ter in die*)
tbsp	tablespoonful
tinct	tincture
TLC	total lung capacity; thin layer chromatography
T_{max}	time to maximum concentration
TMJ	temporomandibular joint
TNF	tumor necrosis factor
TNM	tumor, node, metastasis (tumor staging)
top	topical(ly)
TOPV	trivalent oral polio vaccine
tPA	tissue plasminogen activator
TPN	total parenteral nutrition
TPR	temperature, pulse, respirations
TQM	total quality management
tr	tincture
trit	triturate (*tritura*)
tRNA	transfer RNA
Trp	tryptophan
TSA	tumor-specific antigens
TSH	thyroid-stimulating hormone
tsp	teaspoonful
TSS	toxic shock syndrome
TSTA	tumor-specific transplantation antigen
TT	thrombin time
TV	tidal volume
Tyr	tyrosine
U	unit
ud	as directed
UD	unit-dose package
UK	United Kingdom
ung	ointment (*unguentum*)
URI	upper respiratory infection
USAN	United States Adopted Name(s)
USP	*United States Pharmacopeia*
USPHS	United States Public Health Service
ut dict	as directed (*ut dictum*)
UTI	urinary tract infection
UVA	ultraviolet A wave
V	volt
VA	Veterans Administration
vag	vaginal(ly)
Val	valine
var	variety
VC	vital capacity
V_c	volume of distribution of the central compartment
V_d	volume of distribution (one compartment)
$V_{d\beta}$	volume of distribution of the β phase
V_{dss}	steady-state apparent volume of distribution
VHDL	very high density lipoprotein
VLDL	very low density lipoprotein
VMA	vanillylmandelic acid
vol	volume
VS	vital signs
v/v	volume in volume
v/w	volume in weight
wa	while awake
WBC	white blood (cell) count
WBCT	whole blood clotting time
WDLL	well-differentiated lymphocytic lymphoma
WFI	water for injection
WHO	World Health Organization
wk	week
WNL	within normal limits
w/o	water in oil
wt	weight
w/v	weight in volume
w/w	weight in weight
yo	years old
yr	year
ZE	Zollinger-Ellison
Zn	zinc

MANUFACTURER/DISTRIBUTOR ABBREVIATIONS

This listing includes only those manufacturers whose names are abbreviated in *Drug Facts and Comparisons®*. It is not a complete list of all manufacturers whose products are listed in this book.

B-D	Becton, Dickinson & Co.
B-I	Boehringer Ingelheim
B-Mannheim	Boehringer Mannheim
B-M Squibb	Bristol-Myers Squibb
Hickam	Dow B. Hickam
Inter. Ethical	International Ethical Labs
IMS	International Medication Systems
J & J	Johnson & Johnson
B-D	Becton, Dickinson & Co.
McNeil-CPC	McNeil Consumer Products Company
Mead-J	Mead Johnson Nutritional
Merck	Merck & Co.
P-D	Parke-Davis
PBH	PBH Wesley Jessen
P & G	Procter & Gamble
RPR	Rhone-Poulenc Rorer
B-D	Becton, Dickinson & Co.
Schwarz Pharma K-U	Schwarz Pharma Inc.
SK-Beecham, SKB	SmithKline Beecham
URL	United Research Labs
Warner-C	Warner Chilcott
Warner-L	Warner-Lambert
W-A	Wyeth-Ayerst

3M PERSONAL HEALTHCARE PRODS.
3M Center Bldg.
275-5W-01
St. Paul, MN 55133-3275
651-733-1110
800-364-3577
http://www.mmm.com

00089
3M PHARMACEUTICALS
3M Center
St. Paul, MN 55144-1000
888-364-3577
http://www.mmm.com

63801
7 OAKS PHARMACEUTICAL CORPORATION
161 Harry Stanley Dr.
Easely, SC 29640
864-850-1700
http://www.7oakspharma.com

93764
A & D MEDICAL
1555 McCandless Dr.
Milpitas, CA 95035
408-263-5333
888-726-9966
http://www.andmedical.com

66591
AAI PHARMA
2320 Scientific Park Dr.
Wilmington, NC 28405
910-254-7350
800-575-4224
http://www.aaipharma.com

60793
ABANA PHARMACEUTICALS, INC.
See King Pharmaceuticals, Inc.

ABBOTT DIABETES CARE
1420 Harbor Bay Pky., Ste. 290
Alameda, CA 94502
510-749-5400
888-298-4584 (Customer Service for Diabetes)
http://www.abbottdiabetescare.com

ABBOTT DIAGNOSTICS
100 Abbott Park Rd.
Abbott Park, IL 60064-6154
847-937-6100
800-323-9100
http://www.abbott.com

ABBOTT HOSPITAL PRODUCTS
See Hospira

00074
ABBOTT LABORATORIES PHARMACEUTICAL DIVISION
200 Abbott Park Rd.
Abbott Park, IL 60064-6400
847-937-6100
800-255-5162
http://www.abbott.com

ABRAXIS BIOSCIENCE, INC.
1501 E. Woodfield Rd.
Schaumberg, IL 60173-5837
888-386-1300
800-551-7176
http://www.abraxisbio.com

ACADEMIC PHARMACEUTICALS, INC.
25720 Saunders Road North
Lake Forest, IL 60045
847-735-1170

67404
ACCESS PHARMACEUTICALS
2600 Stemmons Fwy., Suite 176
Dallas, TX 75207-2107
214-905-5100
http://www.accesspharma.com

ACCUMED
2572 Brunswick Pike
Lawrenceville, NJ 08648
609-883-1818
http://www.accumed.org

00924
ACME UNITED CORP.
60 Round Tail Rd.
Fairfield, CT 06824
203-332-7330
800-835-2263
http://www.acmeunited.com

10144
ACORDA THERAPEUTICS
15 Skyline Dr.
Hawthorne, NY 10532
914-347-4300
http://www.acorda.com

ACTAVIS PHARMA
14 Commerce Drive
Cranford, NJ 07016
800-432-8534
http://www.purepac.com

66215
ACTELION PHARMACEUTICALS US, INC.
5000 Shoreline Ct., Suite 200
South San Francisco, CA 94080
650-624-6900
http://www.actelion.com

ACURA PHARMACEUTICALS, INC.
616 N. North Court
Palatine, IL 60067
847-705-7709
http://www.acurapharm.com

ACURA PHARMACEUTICALS TECHNOLOGIES
16235 State Rd. 17
Culver, IN 46511
574-842-3305
http://www.acurapharm.com

63824
ADAMS LABORATORIES, INC.
14801 Sovereign Road
Ft. Worth, TX 76155
817-786-1252
800-770-5270
http://www.adamslabs.com

ADRIA LABORATORIES
See Pfizer US Pharmaceutical Group.

ADVANCE BIOFACTURES CORP. (BIOSPECIFICS TECHNOLOGIES)
35 Wilbur Street
Lynbrook, NY 11563
516-593-7000
http://www.biospecifics.com

17714
ADVANCE PHARMACEUTICALS, INC.
2201-F 5th Ave.
Ronkonkoma, NY 11779
631-981-4600

10888
ADVANCED NUTRITIONAL TECHNOLOGY
6988 Sierra Ct.
Dublin, CA 94568
925-828-2128
800-624-6543
http://www.antlab.com

58790
ADVANCED VISION RESEARCH
660 Main St.
Woburn, MA 01801
781-932-8327
800-579-8327
http://www.theratears.com

11042
ADVANCIS PHARMACEUTICAL CORPORATION
20425 Seneca Meadows Pkwy.
Germantown, MD 20876
301-944-6600
http://www.advancispharm.com

66440
AERO PHARMACEUTICALS
3848 FAU Blvd., Ste 100
Boca Raton, FL 33431
561-208-2200
800-223-6837
http://www.aeropharmaceuticals.com

12539
A. G. MARIN PHARMACEUTICAL
1730 N.W. 79th Ave.
Miami, FL 33126
305-593-5333
800-241-4603

AGOURON PHARMACEUTICALS
See Pfizer US Pharmaceutical Group

A. H. ROBINS CONSUMER PRODUCTS
See Wyeth Consumer Health

A. H. ROBINS INC.
Five Giralda Farms
Madison, NJ 07940-0871
973-660-5500
800-322-3129
http://www.wyeth.com

38206
AID-PACK USA
See NutraMax Products

59196
AIRPHARMA
5370 College Park Blvd.
Overland Park, KS 66211
913-498-0700
800-262-9555
http://www.air-pharma.com

17478, 11098
AKORN, INC.
2500 Millbrook Dr.
Buffalo Grove, IL 60089
847-279-6100
http://www.akorn.com

41383
AKPHARMA, INC.
6840 Old Egg Harbor Rd.
Pleasantville, NJ 08232
609-645-6100
800-994-4711
http://www.akpharma.com

65162
AKYMA PHARMACEUTICALS
701 Columbia Avenue
Glasgow, KY 42141
270-629-2596
866-525-7270
http://www.akyma.com

68322
ALAMO PHARMACEUTICALS, LLC
8501 Wilshire Blvd.
Ste. 318
Beverly Hills, CA 90211-3119
310-859-7799
http://www.alamopharma.com

22400
ALBERTO CULVER
2525 Armitage Ave.
Melrose Park, IL 60160
708-450-3000
800-333-6666
http://www.alberto.com

20993
ALCON LABORATORIES, INC.
6201 South Freeway
Ft. Worth, TX 76134
817-293-0450
http://www.alconlabs.com

00065,08065
ALCON LABORATORIES, SURGICAL DIVISION
6201 South Freeway, S2-11
Ft. Worth, TX 76134
817-293-0450
800-862-5266

00065
ALCON LABORATORIES, VISION CARE
6201 South Freeway, T6-4
Ft. Worth, TX 76134
817-293-0450
800-862-5266

08514
ALIGN PHARMACEUTICALS
5625 Dillard Drive
Cary, NC 27511
919-398-6225
http://www.alignpharma.com

56121, 66177
ALIGON PHARMACEUTICALS
1860 County Rd. 95
Helena, AL 35080
205-663-0521
http://www.aligoninc.com

68611
ALIMERA SCIENCES
6120 Windward Pkwy.
Ste. 290
Alpharetta, GA 30005
678-990-5740
http://www.alimerasciences.com/

38697
ALK ABELLO
1700 Royston Lane
Round Rock, TX 78664
800-325-7354
http://www.alk-abello.us

A. L. LABS
See Alpharma USPD, Inc.

13279
ALLAN PHARMACEUTICAL
21 Radcliffe Dr.
Southampton, PA 18966
601-743-9706

ALLEN & HANBURYS
See GlaxoSmithKline

ALLENDALE PHARMACEUTICALS, INC.
73 Franklin Turnpike
Allendale, NJ 07401
212-813-2171
888-343-4499
http://www.allendalepharm.com

ALLERCREME
See Carme, Inc.

ALLERDERM LABORATORIES, INC.
3400 E. McDowell Road
Phoenix, AZ 85008
800-365-6868
http://www.allerderm.com

00023
ALLERGAN DERMATOLOGICS
2525 DuPont Drive
Irvine, CA 92715
800-433-8871
800-347-4500

11980
ALLERGAN, INC.
2525 DuPont Drive
Irvine, CA 92612-1599
714-246-4500
800-377-7790
http://www.allergan.com

ALLERGY LABORATORIES, INC.
PO Box 348
Oklahoma City, OK 73101-0348
405-235-1451
800-654-3971
http://www.allergylabs.com

49343
ALLERMED
7203 Convoy Ct.
San Diego, CA 92111-1020
858-292-1060
800-221-2748
http://www.allermed.com

ALLIANCE PHARMACEUTICAL CORP.
4660 LaJolla Village Dr.
San Diego, CA 92122
858-410-5200

08462
ALLIANCE TECH MEDICAL
19 W. 144 Milbrook Ct.
Downers Grove, IL 60516
817-326-3183
630-910-0993
800-848-8923
http://www.alliancetechmedical.com/

68188
ALLIANT PHARMACEUTICALS, INC.
333 North Pointe Center East
Alpharetta, GA 30004
770-817-4500

ALLIED PHARMACY
801 Stadium Drive
Arlington, TX 76011
817-226-5050

54569
ALLSCRIPTS, INC.
2401 Commerce Dr.
Libertyville, IL 60048-4464
847-680-3515
800-654-0889
http://www.allscripts.com

77379, 00311
ALMAY, INC.
1501 Williamsboro Street
Oxford, NC 27565
919-603-2953
800-992-5629
http://www.almay.com

ALPHA 1 BIOMEDICALS, INC.
See Arriva Pharmaceuticals, Inc.

49669
ALPHA THERAPEUTIC CORP.
See Grifols USA, Inc.

00228
ALPHARMA PUREPAC PHARMACEUTICALS
See Actavis Pharma

ALPHARMA USPD, INC.
333 Cassell Drive, Suite 3500
Baltimore, MD 21224-2654
410-298-1000
800-638-9096
http://www.alpharmaUSPD.com

59390
ALTAIRE PHARMACEUTICALS, INC.
311 West Lane
Aquebogue, NY 11931
631-722-5988
800-258-2471
http://www.otcdruggist.com

00168
ALTANA INC.
60 Baylis Road
Melville, NY 11747 2006
631-454-7677
800-645-9833
http://www.altana.com

00731
ALTO PHARMACEUTICALS, INC.
PO Box 271150
Tampa, FL 33688-1150
813-968-0522
800-330-2891
http://www.altopharm.com

72959
ALVA-AMCO PHARMACAL COMPANIES, INC.
7711 Merrimac Ave.
Niles, IL 60714
800-792-2582
http://www.alva-amco.com

17314
ALZA CORP.
1900 Charleston Road
Mountain View, CA 94039
650-564-5000
800-634-8977
http://www.alza.com

00187
AMARIN PHARMACEUTICALS
See Valeant Pharmaceuticals International

66870
AMBI PHARMACEUTICALS, INC.
16255-A Aviation Loop
Brooksville, FL 34604-6875
352-797-5227

10038
AMBIX LABORATORIES
55 West End Rd.
Totowa, NJ 07512
973-890-9002
http://www.ambixlabs.com

AMCON LABORATORIES
40 N. Rock Hill Road
St. Louis, MO 63119
314-961-5758
800-255-6161
http://www.amconlabs.com

61972
AMEND DRUG AND CHEMICAL CORPORATION
See Ruger Chemical Co.

AMERICAN DERMAL CORP.
See Sanofi-Aventis

62584
AMERICAN HEALTH PACKAGING
2550 John Glenn Avenue
Columbus, OH 43217
614-492-8177
800-707-4621
http://www.amerisourcebergen.com

00008
AMERICAN HOME PRODUCTS
See Wyeth Consumer Health

AMERICAN LECITHIN COMPANY
115 Hurley Road, Unit 2B
Oxford, CT 06478
203-262-7100
800-364-4416
http://www.americanlecithin.com

AMERICAN MEDICAL INDUSTRIES
330 E. Third Street
Dell Rapids, SD 57022-1918
605-428-5501

63323
AMERICAN PHARMACEUTICAL PARTNERS, INC.
1501 East Woodfield Rd.
Schaumburg, IL 60173-5837
847-969-2700
888-391-6300
http://www.appdrugs.com

52769
AMERICAN RED CROSS
2025 E Street, NW
Washington, DC 20006
202-303-4498
800-261-5772

00517
AMERICAN REGENT LABS., INC.
One Luitpold Drive
Shirley, NY 11967
631-924-4000
800-645-1706
http://www.americanregent.com

63921
AMERIDERM LABORATORIES, INC.
13 Kentucky Ave.
Paterson, NJ 07503
973-279-5100
800-455-7211
http://www.ameriderm.com

92961
AMERIFIT NUTRITION
166 Highland Park Dr.
Bloomfield, CT 06002
800-722-3476
http://www.amerifit.com

AMERIFIT PHARMA, INC.
11 State Street
Woburn, MA 01801
781-933-2020
800-536-8745
http://www.amerifit.com

62852
AMERILAB TECHNOLOGIES
2765 Niagara Lane North
Plymouth, MN 55447
763-525-1262
http://www.amerilabtech.com

AMERISOURCEBERGEN
1300 Morris Drive
Chesterbrook, PA 19087
610-727-7000
800-829-3132
http://www.amerisourcebergen.com

61470
AMERX HEALTH CARE CORP.
1300 S. Highland Ave.
Clearwater, FL 33756
727-443-0530
800-448-9599
http://www.amerigel.com

55513
AMGEN INC.
One Amgen Center Drive
Thousand Oaks, CA 91320
805-480-1299
800-772-6436
http://www.amgen.com

52152
AMIDE PHARMACEUTICALS, INC.
101 E. Main Street
Little Falls, NJ 07424
973-890-1440 Ext. 3059
http://www.amide.com

00548
AMPHASTAR PHARMACEUTICALS, INC.
11570 6th St.
Rancho Cucamonga, CA 91730
800-423-4136
http://www.amphastar.com

00402
AMSCO SCIENTIFIC
See Steris Corp.

66780
AMYLIN PHARMACEUTICALS
9360 Towne Centre Dr.
San Diego, CA 92121
858-552-2200
http://www.amylin.com

ANABOLIC INC.
17802 Gillette Ave.
Irvine, CA 92614
949-863-0340
800-445-6849
http://www.anaboliclabs.com

ANAQUEST
See Baxter Healthcare Corporation

19100
ANDREW JERGENS COMPANY
See Kao Brands Company

ANDRULIS PHARMACEUTICAL CORP.
11800 Baltimore Avenue
Beltsville, MD 20705-1561
301-419-2400

62022
ANDRX LABORATORIES, INC.
See First Horizon Pharmaceutical Corp.

62037
ANDRX PHARMACEUTICALS, INC.
8151 Peters Rd., 4th Floor
Plantation, FL 33324
954-382-7600
800-621-7143
http://www.andrx.com

ANGELINI PHARMACEUTICALS, INC.
50 Tice Blvd.
Woodcliff Lake, NJ 07677 7654
201-476-9000

70907, 14613, 71483
ANSELL HEALTHCARE, INC.
200 Schultz Drive
Red Bank, NJ 07701
732-345-5400
http://www.ansell.com

55948
ANTARES PHARMA
707 Eagleview Blvd.
Exton, PA 19341
610-458-6200
http://www.antarespharma.com

ANTIBODIES, INC.
PO Box 1560
Davis, CA 1560 95617
530-758-4400
800-824-8540
http://www.antibodiesinc.com

ANTIGENICS INC.
630 Fifth Avenue
New York, NY 10111
212-994-8200
http://www.antigenics.com

23601
APEX-CAREX HEALTHCARE PRODUCTS
7 West Kansas
Liberty, MO 64068
800-328-2935 (Apex)
800-526-8051 (Carex)
http://www.apex-carex.com

52380, 18407
APLICARE INC.
50 East Industrial Road
Branford, CT 06405
203-481-5000
800-760-3236
http://www.aplicare.com

60505
APOTEX CORP.
2400 N. Commerce Pkwy.
Westin, FL 33326
954-384-8007
800-706-5575
http://www.apotexcorp.com

60505
APOTEX USA
2400 N. Commerce Pkwy.
Westin, FL 33326
954-384-8007
800-706-5575
http://www.apotexcorp.com

25715
APOTHECARY PRODUCTS, INC.
11750 12th Avenue South
Burnsville, MN 55337
952-890-1940
800 328 2742
http://www.apothecaryproducts.com

APOTHECON, INC.
See Bristol-Myers Squibb Company

48723, 52925
APOTHECUS, INC.
220 Townsend Square
Oyster Bay, NY 11771
516-624-8200
800-227-2393
http://www.apothecus.com

A. P. PHARMA, INC.
123 Saginaw Dr.
Redwood City, CA 94063
650-366-2626
http://www.appharma.com

APPLIED ANALYTICAL INDUSTRIES
2320 Scientific Park Dr.
Wilmington, NC 28405
910-254-7000
800-575-4224
http://www.aaipharma.com

APPLIED BIOTECH, INC.
10237 Flanders Ct.
San Diego, CA 92121
858-587-6771
800-257-9525
http://www.abiapogent.com

92896
APPLIED DIABETES RESEARCH
1420 Valwood Pkwy.
Carrollton, TX 75006
972-241-1884
800-304-7293
http://www.applieddiabetes research.org

APPLIED GENETICS INC. DERMATICS
205 Buffalo Ave.
Freeport, NY 11520
516-868-9026
http://www.agiderm.com

13310
AR SCIENTIFIC
1100 Orthodox St.
Philadelphia, PA 19124
877-960-2400

74312
ARCO PHARMACEUTICALS, INC.
See Nature's Bounty

ARCOLA LABORATORIES
See Sanofi-Aventis

ARMOUR PHARMACEUTICAL
See ZLB Behring

ARRIVA PHARMACEUTICALS, INC.
2020 Challenger Dr.
Alameda, CA 94501
510-337-1250
http://www.arrivapharm.com

ARROW INTERNATIONAL CORP. HEADQUARTERS
2400 Bernville Rd.
Reading, PA 19605
610-378-0131
800-523-8446
http://www.arrowintl.com

12870
ARZOL
12 Norway Avenue, Suite 2
Keene, NH 03431
603-352-5242

65557
ASAFI PHARMACEUTICAL
PO Box 801764
Santa Clarita, CA 91380-1764
661-294-9509
http://www.asafi.com

99207
ASCENT PEDIATRICS, INC.
See Medicis Pharmaceutical Corp.

ASTELLAS
3 Parkway North
Deerfield, IL 60015
800-888-7704
http://www.us.astellas.com

00186
ASTRAZENECA LP
1800 Concord Pike
Wilmington, DE 19850
800-456-3669
http://www.AstraZeneca-us.com

59075
ATHENA NEUROSCIENCES, INC.
See Elan Pharmaceuticals

66813
ATHLON PHARMACEUTICALS, INC.
301 Snow Dr.
Birmingham, AL 35209
205-986-1111
http://www.athlonpharm.com

59702
ATLEY PHARMACEUTICALS, INC.
10511 Old Ridge Road
Ashland, VA 23005 2075
804-227-2250
http://www.atley.com

14629
AURIGA PHARMACEUTICALS
5555 Triangle Parkway
Norcross, GA 30092
678-282-1600

65862
AUROBINDO PHARMA USA, INC.
2615 Route 130 South
Cranbury, NJ 08512
866-850-2876

66887
AUXILIUM PHARMACEUTICALS, INC.
40 Valley Stream Pkwy.
Malvern, PA 19355
484-321-5900
http://www.auxilium.com

AVENTIS PHARMACEUTICALS
See Sanofi-Aventis

58914
AXCAN SCANDIPHARM
22 Inverness Center Pkwy.
Birmingham, AL 35242
205-991-8085
800-472-2634
http://www.axcanscandipharm.com

00264
B. BRAUN MEDICAL INC.
1601 Wallace Dr., Suite 150
Carrollton, TX 75006
800-854-6851
800-627-7867
http://www.bbraunusa.com

11414
BAKER CUMMINS DERMATOLOGICALS
See Ivax Pharmaceuticals, Inc.

11414
BAKER NORTON PHARMACEUTICALS
See Ivax Pharmaceuticals, Inc.

50770
BALLARD MEDICAL PRODUCTS (A DIVISION OF KIMBERLY-CLARK)
12050 South Lone Peak Parkway
Draper, UT 84020
801-572-6800
800-528-5591
http://www.kchealthcare.com

63162
BALLAY PHARMACEUTICALS, INC.
200 Stillwater
Wimberley, TX 78676
512-847-6458

BANNER PHARMACAPS
4125 Premier Dr.
High Point, NC 27265
336-812-8700
800-447-1140
http://www.banpharm.com

08011
BARD
See C. R. Bard

00555
BARR LABORATORIES, INC.
400 Chestnut Ridge Rd.
Woodcliff, NJ 07677
845-362-1100
800-222-0190
http://www.barrlabs.com

13478
BARRIER THERAPEUTICS
600 College Road East, Suite 3200
Princeton, NJ 08540-6697
609-945-1200
http://www.barriertherapeutics.com

10116
BARTOR PHARMACAL CO.
70 High Street
Rye, NY 10580
914-967-4219

00078
BASEL PHARMACEUTICALS
See Novartis Pharmaceuticals Corp.

BASF CORPORATION
100 Campus Drive
Florham Park, NJ 07932
973-245-6000
800-526-1072
http://www.basf.com/usa

00761, 07610
BASIC DRUGS & VITAMINS, INC.
300 Corporate Center Dr.
Vandalia, OH 45377

10119
BAUSCH & LOMB PERSONAL PRODUCTS DIVISION
1400 N. Goodman Street
Rochester, NY 14692
585-338-6000
800-344-8815
http://www.bausch.com

24208
BAUSCH & LOMB PHARMACEUTICALS
8500 Hidden River Pkwy.
Tampa, FL 33637
813-975-7770
800-323-0000
http://www.bausch.com

61772
BAUSCH & LOMB SURGICAL
180 Via Verde
San Dimas, CA 91773
800-338-2020
http://www.bausch.com

17191
BAXA CORPORATION
14445 Grasslands Dr.
Englewood, CO 80112-7062
303-690-4204
800-567-2292
http://www.baxa.com

10019, 60977
BAXTER HEALTHCARE CORPORATION
One Baxter Parkway
Deerfield, IL 60015
847-948-4710
800-422-9837
http://www.baxter.com

60977
BAXTER HEALTHCARE CORPORATION (ANESTHESIA CRITICAL CARE PHARMACEUTICALS)
95 Spring St.
New Providence, NJ 07974
908-286-7000
800-667-0959
http://www.baxter.com

00944
BAXTER HEALTHCARE CORPORATION (BAXTER BIOSCIENCE)
1 Baxter Way
Westlake Village, CA 91362
805-372-3000
800-422-9837
800-423-2090
http://www.baxter.com

00338
BAXTER HEALTHCARE CORPORATION (CLINTEC NUTRITION)
One Baxter Parkway
Deerfield, IL 60015
800-422-2751
http://www.nutriforum.com

00338
BAXTER HEALTHCARE CORPORATION (MEDICATION DELIVERY)
Route 120 and Wilson Rd.
Round Lake, IL 60073
847-948-4770
800-933-0303
http://www.baxter.com

64193
BAXTER HYLAND IMMUNO
See Baxter Healthcare Corporation (Baxter Bioscience)

60977
BAXTER PHARM. PRODS., INC. (BAXTER PPI)
See Baxter Healthcare Corporation (Anesthesia Critical Care Pharmaceuticals)

65044
BAYER ALLERGY PRODUCTS
See Hollister-Stier

BAYER CONSUMER CARE DIVISION
36 Columbia Rd.
Morristown, NJ 07962-1910
973-254-5000
800-331-4536
http://www.bayercare.com

00026
BAYER CORP.
100 Bayer Rd.
Pittsburgh, PA 15205-9741
412-777-2000
800-468-0894
http://www.bayer.com

00193
BAYER DIAGNOSTICS
511 Benedict Ave.
Tarrytown, NY 10591
877-229-3711
800-248-2637
http://www.bayerdiag.com

BD (BECTON DICKINSON & CO.)
One Becton Drive
Franklin Lakes, NJ 07417
201-847-6800
888-237-2762
http://www.bd.com

BD BIOSCIENCES
2350 Qume Drive
San Jose, CA 95131
877-232-8995
http://www.bdbiosciences.com

BD DIAGNOSTIC SYSTEMS & MEDICAL SUPPLIES
7 Loveton Circle
Sparks, MD 21152
800-675-0908
http://www.bd.com

00486
BEACH PRODUCTS
5220 S. Manhattan Ave.
Tampa, FL 33611
813-839-6565
800-322-8210

BECKMAN COULTER
4300 N. Harbor Blvd.
Fullerton, CA 92834-3100
800-742-2345
http://www.beckmancoulter.com

BECKMAN COULTER PRIMARY CARE DIAGNOSTICS
250 South Kraemer Blvd.
Brea, CA 92822-0550
714-993-5321
800-526-3821
http://www.beckmancoulter.com

BECTON DICKINSON MICROBIOLOGY SYSTEMS
7 Loveton Circle
Sparks, MD 21152
410-316-4000
800-638-8663
http://www.bd.com

55390
BEDFORD LABORATORIES
300 Northfield Road
Bedford, OH 44146
440-232-3320
800-521-5169
http://www.boehringer-ingelheim.com

BEIERSDORF, INC.
187 Danbury Rd.
Wilton, CT 06897
203-563-5800
800-233-2340
http://www.beiersdorf.com

24385
BERGEN BRUNSWIG DRUG CO.
See AmerisourceBergen

50419
BERLEX LABORATORIES, INC.
6 West Belt Rd.
Wayne, NJ 07470-6806
888-237-5394
http://www.berlex.com

58337
BERNA PRODUCTS CORP.
4216 Ponce de Leon Blvd.
Coral Gables, FL 33146
305-443-2900
800-533-5899
http://www.bernaproducts.com

BERTEK PHARMACEUTICALS, INC.
See Mylan Pharmaceuticals, Inc.

08515
BESTMED, LLC
311 Corporate Circle
Golden, CO 80401-5649
303-271-0300

53062
BETA DERMACEUTICALS
PO Box 691106
San Antonio, TX 78269-1106
210-349-9326
800-434-2382
http://www.beta-derm.com

00283
BEUTLICH PHARMACEUTICALS
1541 Shields Dr.
Waukegan, IL 60085
847-473-1100
800-238-8542
http://www.beutlich.com

00225
B. F. ASCHER AND CO.
15501 West 109th Street
Lenexa, KS 66219
913-888-1880
800-324-1880
http://www.bfascher.com

BI-COASTAL PHARMACEUTICAL CORP.
130 Maple Ave.
Red Bank, NJ 07701
732-530-6606
http://www.bicoastalpharm.com

53191
BIO-TECH PHARMACAL, INC.
PO Box 1992
Fayetteville, AR 72702
479-443-9148
800-345-1199
http://www.bio-tech-pharm.com

08216
BIOCORE MEDICAL TECHNOLOGIES
6030-M Marshelee Dr. #512
Elkridge, MA 21075
888-565-5243
888-689-5655
http://www.biocore.com

00093
BIOCRAFT LABORATORIES, INC.
See Teva Pharmaceuticals USA

BIOCRYST PHARMACEUTICALS, INC.
2190 Parkway Lake Drive
Birmingham, AL 35244
205-444-4600
http://www.biocryst.com

15594
BIOFILM, INC.
3225 Executive Ridge
Vista, CA 92081
760-727-9030
http://www.astroglide.com

59627.
BIOGEN
See Biogen Idec

59627
BIOGEN IDEC
14 Cambridge Center
Cambridge, MA 02142
617-679-2000
800-262-4363800-456-2255
http://www.biogenidec.com

BIOGENEX LABORATORIES
4600 Norris Canyon Road
San Ramon, CA 94583
925-275-0550
800-421-4149
http://www.biogenex.com

62436
BIOGLAN PHARMACEUTICALS
See Bradley Pharmaceutical

34061
BIOLIFE, LLC
1235 Tallevast Rd.
Sarasota, FL 34243
800-722-7559
http://www.biolife.com/

68135
BIOMARIN PHARMACEUTICAL INC.
105 Digital Way
Novato, CA 94949
415-506-6700
866-274-0606
http://www.biomarinpharm.com

BIOMEDICAL FRONTIERS, INC.
1095 10th Ave., S.E.
Minneapolis, MN 55414
612-378-0228

83059
BIOMERICA, INC.
1533 Monrovia Ave.
Newport Beach, CA 92663
949-645-2111
800-854-3002
http://www.biomerica.com

BIOMERIEUX
100 Rodolphe St.
Durham, NC 27712
630-628-6055
800-634-7656
http://www.biomerieux-usa.com

BIOMIRA USA, INC.
70 South Main Street
Cranbury, NJ 08512
780-490-2818
877-234-0444
http://www.biomira.com

17700
BIOMOLECULAR SCIENCES, INC.
13428 Maxella Avenue, Suite 285
Marina del Ray, CA 90292
818-804-5148
800-260-3587
http://biomolecularsciences.com

53110
BIONEXUS, LTD
30 Brown Road
Ithaca, NY 14850
607-266-9492
800-835-0869
http://www.bionxs.com

62086
BIONICHE PHARMA GROUP
231 Dundas Street East
Belleville, Ontario K8N 5J2
613-966-8058
800-265-5464
http://www.bioniche.com

59741
BIOPHARM LABS
2091 Hartel Street
Levittown, PA 19057
215-949-3711
http://www.bio-pharminc.com

BIOPURE CORP.
11 Hurley St.
Cambridge, MA 02141
617-234-6500
http://www.biopure.com

BIOSAFE TECHNOLOGIES
PO Box 1973
Denison, TX 75020
903-463-7321
877-828-4633
http://www.biosafetech.com

BIOSCRIP
10050 Crosstown Circle
Eden Prairie, MN 55344
952-979-3600
800-444-5951
http://www.bioscrip.com

BIOSPECIFICS TECHNOLOGIES CORP.
35 Wilbur St.
Lynbrook, NY 11563
516-593-7000
http://www.biospecifics.com

58023
BIOTROL INTERNATIONAL
13705 Shoreline Court East
Earth City, MO 63045
303-673-0341
800-822-8550
http://www.biotrol.com

64455
BIOVAIL PHARMACEUTICALS, INC.
700 Route 202-206 North
Bridgewater, NJ 08807
866-246-8245
http://www.biovail.com

BIRA CORP.
2525 Quicksilver
McDonald, PA 15057
724-796-1820

50289
BIRCHWOOD LABORATORIES, INC.
7900 Fuller Road
Eden Prairie, MN 55344
952-937-7900
800-328-6156
http://www.birchlabs.com

12136
BIRD PRODUCTS CORP.
1100 Bird Center Drive
Palm Springs, CA 92262
760-778-7200
800-232-7633
http://www.viasyscriticalcare.com

00165
BLAINE PHARMACEUTICALS
1717 Dixie Hwy., Suite 700
Ft. Wright, KY 41011
859-344-9600
800-633-9353
http://www.blainepharma.com

00154
BLAIR LABORATORIES
See Purdue Frederick Co.

50486
BLAIREX LABS, INC.
1600 Brian Drive
Columbus, IN 47201
812-378-1864
800-252-4739
http://www.blairex.com

51674
BLANSETT PHARMACAL CO., INC.
14 Parkstone Circle N.
North Little Rock, AR 72216
501-758-8635
800-816-9695
http://www.blansett.com

41388
BLISTEX INC.
1800 Swift Drive
Oak Brook, IL 60523
630-571-2870
800-837-1800
http://www.blistex.com

BLOCK DRUG CO., INC.
See GlaxoSmithKline Consumer Healthcare

BLUCO INC.
28350 Schoolcraft
Livonia, MI 48150
734-513-4500
http://www.blucoinc.com

08326, 43820, 00904
BOCA MEDICAL PRODUCTS
See Owen Mumford Inc.

64376
BOCA PHARMACAL, INC.
3550 NW 126th Ave.
Coral Springs, FL 33065
800-354-8460
http://www.bocamedicalproducts.com

00024
BOCK PHARMACAL CO.
See Sanofi Aventis

00597
BOEHRINGER INGELHEIM PHARMACEUTICALS, INC.
900 Ridgebury Road
Ridgefield, CT 06877-0368
203-798-9988
800-542-6257
http://www.boehringer-ingelheim.com

BOERICKE & TAFEL
See Nature's Way

00220
BOIRON LABORATORIES
98 C West Cochran St.
Simi Valley, CA 93065
610-325-7464
805-582-9091
http://www.boiron.com/index_en.asp

00725
BOLAR PHARMACEUTICALS
33 Ralph Avenue
Copiague, NY 11726-0030
516-842-8383
800-872-0159

50051
BONNE BELL
18519 Detroit Ave.
Lakewood, OH 44107
216-221-0800
800-321-1006
http://www.bonnebell.com

00074
BOOTS PHARMACEUTICALS, INC.
See Abbott Laboratories Pharmaceutical Division

BOTANICAL LABORATORIES
1441 West Smith Rd.
Ferndale, WA 98248
360-384-5656
800-232-4005
http://www.botlab.com

00270
BRACCO DIAGNOSTICS, INC.
107 College Road East
Princeton, NJ 08543
609-514-2200
877-272-2269
http://www.bracco.com

BRADLEY PHARMACEUTICAL
383 Rt. 46 West
Fairfield, NJ 07004
973-882-1505
800-929-9300
http://www.bradpharm.com

52268
BRAINTREE LABORATORIES, INC.
60 Columbian Street West
Braintree, MA 02185-0929
781-843-2202
800-874-6756
http://www.braintreelabs.com

00264
BRAUN MEDICAL, INC.
2525 McGaw Ave.
Irvine, CA 92663
610-266-6122
800-854-6851
http://www.bbraunusa.com

51991
BRECKENRIDGE PHARMACEUTICAL, INC.
1141 S. Rogers Circle, Suite 3
Boca Raton, FL 33487
561-443-3314
800-466-2700
http://www.bpirx.com

58659
BRIDGEPORT WHOLESALE PRODUCTS
2624 112th Street
Lakewood, WA 98499
425-656-0460

10914
BRIGHTON PHARMACEUTICALS
201 Shannon Oaks Circle, #200
Cary, NC 27511
919-654-7326

10007
BRIOSCHI
19-01 Pollitt Drive
Fair Lawn, NJ 07410
201-796-4226
http://www.brioschi-usa.com

00015
BRISTOL LABS
PO Box 4000
Princeton, NJ 08543-4000
609-252-4000
800-468-7746

BRISTOL-MYERS ONCOLOGY/VIROLOGY
PO Box 4500
Princeton, NJ 08543
609-897-2000
800-426-7644
http://www.bms.com

19810
BRISTOL-MYERS PRODUCTS (OTC/CONSUMER AFFAIRS)
See Novartis Pharmaceuticals Corp.

BRISTOL-MYERS SQUIBB COMPANY
PO Box 4500
Princeton, NJ 08543
609-897-2000
http://www.bms.com

63256.
BRYAN CORPORATION
Four Plympton Street
Woburn, MA 01801
781-935-0004
800-343-7711
http://www.bryancorp.com

BSN, JOBST
5825 Carnegie Blvd.
Charlotte, NC 28209
800-221-7573
http://www.jobst-usa.com

54396.
BTG PHARMACEUTICAL CORPORATION
See Savient Pharmaceuticals, Inc.

BURROUGHS WELLCOME CO.
See GlaxoSmithKline Consumer Healthcare

08237, 55559
CALGON VESTAL
See ConvaTec

00799
CALMOSEPTINE, INC.
16602 Burke Lane
Huntington Beach, CA 92647
800-800-3405
http://www.calmoseptineointment.com

81262
CALWOOD NUTRITIONALS, INC.
5331 Landing Rd.
Elkridge, MD 21075
410-796-5560
800-479-9942
http://www.calwoodnutritionals.com

CAMBREX BIOSCIENCE
One Meadowlands Plaza
East Rutherford, NJ 07073
207-594-3400
800-638-8174
http://www.cambrex.com

CAMBRIDGE NEUROSCIENCE
See Baxter Healthcare Corporation

43656
CAMBRIDGE NUTRACEUTICALS
See Baxter Healthcare Corporation (Clintec Nutrition)

38083
CAMPBELL LABS
See Chattem Consumer Products

08189
CAN-AM CARE CORP.
3780 Mansell Road
Alpharetta, GA 30022
678-795-3440
800-461-7448

CANGENE CORP.
155 Innovation Dr.
Winnipeg, Manitoba R3T 5Y3
204-275-4200

64543
CAPELLON PHARMACEUTICALS, LTD.
7509 Flagstone Street
Ft. Worth, TX 76118
817-595-5820
http://www.capellon.com

57664, 32247
CARACO PHARMACEUTICAL LABORATORIES LTD.
1150 Elijah McCoy Drive
Detroit, MI 48202
313-871-8400
800-818-4555
http://www.caraco.com

CARDINAL HEALTH
7000 Cardinal Place
Dublin, OH 43017
614-757-5000
800-234-8701
http://www.cardinal.com

83078
CARMA LABS, INC.
5801 West Airways Ave.
Franklin, WI 53132
414-421-7707
http://www.carma-labs.com

CARME, INC.
620 Airpark Rd.
Napa, CA 94558
707-226-3900
http://www.senetekplc.net

50000
CARNATION
See Nestle Infant Nutrition

00086
CARNRICK LABORATORIES
See Elan Pharmaceuticals

46287
CAROLINA MEDICAL PRODUCTS
8026 US 264 Alternate
Farmville, NC 27828
252-753-7111
800-227-6637
http://www.carolinamedical.com

53303
CARRINGTON
2001 Walnut Hill Lane
Irving, TX 75038
972-518-1300
800-527-5216
http://www.carringtonlabs.com

11411, 41140.
CARTER PRODUCTS
See Church & Dwight Co.

22600
CARTER-WALLACE
Half Acre Rd.
Cranbury, NJ 08512
212-339-5000
800-828-9032
http://www.astelin.com

00037
CARTER-WALLACE, INC
See Med Pointe Healthcare, Inc.

15370
CARWIN ASSOCIATES
180 St. Clair Shores Rd.
Cropwell, AL 35054
866-525-4566
http://www.carwinassoc.com/

C. B. FLEET CO., INC.
4615 Murray Place
Lynchburg, VA 24502
800-999-9711
http://www.cbfleet.com

18515
CCA INDUSTRIES, INC.
200 Murray Hill Pkwy.
East Rutherford, NJ 07073
800-524-2720
http://www.ccaindustries.com

64019
CEBERT PHARMACEUTICALS, INC.
1200 Corporate Dr., Suite 370
Birmingham, AL 35242
205-981-0201
800-211-0589
http://www.cebert.com

CELESTIAL SEASONINGS, INC.
4600 Sleepytime Dr.
Boulder, CO 80301
303-530-5300
800-525-0347
http://www.celestialseasonings.com

59572
CELGENE CORP.
86 Morris Ave.
Summit, NJ 07901
908-673-9000
888-423-5436
http://www.celgene.com

65231
CELL PATHWAYS
See OSI Pharmaceuticals

60553
CELL THERAPEUTICS
501 Elliott Ave. West
Seattle, WA 98119
206-282-7100
800-215-2355
http://www.ctiseattle.com

CELLEGY PHARMACEUTICALS, INC.
100 Marina Blvd.
Brisbane, CA 94005
650-616-2200
http://www.cellegy.com

CELLTECH PHARMACEUTICAL CO.
See UCB Pharmaceuticals, Inc.

CENTEON
See ZLB Behring

00268
CENTER LABORATORIES
See Alk-Abello

CENTERS FOR DISEASE CONTROL AND PREVENTION
1600 Clifton Rd. N.E.
Atlanta, GA 30333
404-639-3534
800-311-3435
http://www.cdc.gov

57894
CENTOCOR, INC.
800 Ridgeview Drive
Horsham, PA 19355
610-651-6000
800-457-6399
http://www.centocor.com

38083
CENTRAL PHARMACEUTICALS, INC.
See Schwarz Pharma

00436
CENTURY PHARMACEUTICALS, INC.
10377 Hague Road
Indianapolis, IN 46256-3399
317-849-4210
866-343-2576

63459
CEPHALON, INC.
145 Brandywine Pkwy.
West Chester, PA 19380
610-344-0200
800-782-3656
http://www.cephalon.com

00851
CERA PRODUCTS
9017 Mendenhall Court
Columbia, MD 21045
410-309-1000
888-237-2598
http://www.ceraproductsinc.com

CERENEX PHARMACEUTICALS
See GlaxoSmithKline

10223
CETYLITE INDUSTRIES, INC.
9051 River Road
Pennsauken, NJ 08110
865-665-6111
800-257-7740
http://www.cetylite.com

63868
CHAIN DRUG MARKETING ASSOCIATION, INC.
43157 W. Nine Mile Rd
Novi, MI 48376-0995
248-449-9300

CHARLES RIVER LABORATORIES INTERNATIONAL, INC.
251 Ballardvale St.
Wilmington, MA 01887-1000
978-658-6000
877-CRIVER1 (877-274-8371)
http://www.criver.com

54429
CHASE LABORATORIES
See Banner Pharmacaps

41167
CHATTEM CONSUMER PRODUCTS
1715 W. 38th Street
Chattanooga, TN 37409
423-821-4571
800-366-6833
http://www.chattem.com

CHESAPEAKE BIOLOGICAL LABS., INC.
1111 South Paca St.
Baltimore, MD 21230
410-843-5000
800-441-4225
http://www.cblinc.com

00521
CHESEBROUGH-PONDS USA, INC.
See Unilever Home and Personal Care USA

12462
CHESTER LABS
1900 Section Road
Cincinnati, OH 45237
513-458-3840
800-354-9709
http://www.chester-labs.com

CHEW-RITE CO.
265 S. Pioneer Blvd.
Springboro, OH 45066
937-746-5509

CHIESI PHARMACEUTICALS, INC.
9850 Key West Ave.
Rockville, MD 20850

CHILDREN'S HOSPITAL OF COLUMBUS
700 Children's Dr.
Columbus, OH 43205
614-722-2000
http://www.columbuschildrens.com

http://www.columbuschildrens.org

CHILTON LABS., INC.
299B Fairfield Ave.
Fairfield, NJ 07004
973-575-1992

53905
CHIRON THERAPEUTICS
4560 Horton Street
Emeryville, CA 94608-2916
510-655-8730
800-244-7668
http://www.chiron.com

61772
CHIRON VISION
See Bausch & Lomb Surgical

54993
CHRONIMED INC.
See Bioscrip

22600
CHURCH & DWIGHT CO.
469 N. Harrison St.
Princeton, NJ 08543
609-683-5900
800-833-9532
http://www.churchdwight.com

00067
CIBA CONSUMER
See Novartis Consumer Health

47113
CIBA VISION CORPORATION
11460 Johns Creek Parkway
Duluth, GA 30097
770-476-3937
http://www.cibavision.com

00078
CIBA-GEIGY PHARMACEUTICALS
See Novartis Pharmaceuticals Corp.

CIMA LABS
10000 Valley View Rd.
Eden Prairie, MN 55344
952-947-8700
http://www.cimalabs.com

52544
CIRCA PHARMACEUTICALS, INC.
See Watson Laboratories

CIRRUS HEALTHCARE PRODUCTS, L.L.C.
60 Main St.
Cold Spring Harbor, NY 11724
631-692-7600
800-327-6151
http://www.cirrushealthcare.com

CIS-US, INC.
10 DeAngelo Drive
Bedford, MA 01730
781-275-7120
800-221-7554
http://www.cisusinc.com

CITRA ANTICOAGULANTS
55 Messina Dr.
Braintree, MA 02814
781-848-2174
800-299-3411
http://www.citraanticoagulants.com

45802
CLAY-PARK LABS, INC.
1700 Bathgate Ave.
Bronx, NY 10457
718-901-2800
800-933-5550
http://www.claypark.com

55553
CLINT PHARMACEUTICALS
629 Shute Lane
Old Hickory, TN 37138
615-882-0042
800-677-5022
http://www.clintpharmaceuticals.com

CLOSURE MEDICAL CORP
See Johnson & Johnson

57145
CNS, INC.
7615 Smetana Lane
Eden Prairie, MN 55344
952-229-1500
http://www.cns.com

58826
COATS ALOE
2146 Merritt Dr.
Garland, TX 75041
972-278-9651
800-486-2563
http://www.coatsaloe.com

16252
COBALT LABORATORIES
24840 S. Tamiami Trail
Bonita Springs, FL 34134
239-390-0245

00126
COLGATE ORAL PHARMACEUTICALS
1302 Champion Circle
Carrollton, TX 75006
972-888-8300
800-821-2880
http://www.colgateprofessional.com

35000
COLGATE-PALMOLIVE CO.
300 Park Ave.
New York, NY 10022
212-310-2000
800-221-4607
http://www.colgate.com
http://www.colgateprofessional.com

64682, 27280
COLLAGENEX PHARMACEUTICALS, INC.
41 University Drive, Suite 200
Newtown, PA 18940
215-579-7388
888-339-5678
http://www.collagenex.com

COLOPLAST
1975 West Oak Circle
Marietta, GA 30062
800-533-0464
http://www.us.coloplast.com

COLORADO BIOLABS
404 Avenue M
Cozad, NE 69130
888-442-0067
http://www.coloradobiolabs.com

21406, 55056
COLUMBIA LABORATORIES, INC.
354 Eisenhower Pkwy. Plaza 1
Livingston, NJ 07039
973-994-3999
866-566-5636
http://www.columbialabs.com

11509
COMBE, INC.
1101 Westchester Ave.
White Plains, NY 10604
914-694-5454
800-873-7400
http://www.combe.com

COMPLIMED MEDICAL RESEARCH GROUP
1441 West Smith Road
Ferndale, WA 98248
360-384-5656
888-977-8008
http://www.complimed.com

CON-CISE CONTACT LENS CO.
14450 Doolittle Dr.
San Leandro, CA 94577
510-483-9400
800-772-3911
http://www.con-cise.com

CONAGRA FUNCTIONAL FOODS, INC.
11 ConAgra Drive
Omaha, NE 68102
888-828-4242
http://www.culturelle.com

74108
CONAIR INTERPLAX DIVISION
1 Cummings Point Rd.
Stamford, CT 06902
800-726-6247

20254
CONCORD LABORATORIES
140 New Dutch Lane
Fairfield, NJ 07004
973-227-6757

49281
CONNAUGHT LABS
See Sanofi Pasteur

63032
CONNETICS CORPORATION
3160 Porter Dr.
Palo Alto, CA 94303
650-843-2800
800-280-2879
http://www.connetics.com

00223
CONSOLIDATED MIDLAND CORP.
20 Main St.
Brewster, NY 10509
845-279-6108

97493
CONSUMERS CHOICE SYSTEMS, INC.
11445 Cronhill Dr.
Owings Mill, MD 21117
425-883-6310
800-479-5232
http://www.womanswellbeing.com

CONTINENTAL CONSUMER PRODUCTS
750 Standard Pkwy.
Auburn Hills, MI 48326
248-758-1817
800-542-5903

CONTINENTAL QUEST RESEARCH
1015 3rd Avenue S.W.
Carmel, IN 46032
317-843-2501
800-451-5773
http://www.continentalquest.com

10267
CONTRACT PHARMACAL CORP.
135 Adams Ave.
Hauppauge, NY 11788
631-231-4610
http://www.cpchealth.com

CONVATEC
PO Box 5254
Princeton, NJ 08543
908-904-2200
800-422-8811
http://www.convatec.com

63535
COOKE PHARMA, INC.
See Unither Pharma (United Therapeutics Corp)

59365
COOPER SURGICAL
95 Corporate Drive
Trumbull, CT 06611
203-601-5200
800-480-1985
http://www.coopersurgical.com

59426, 54027
COOPERVISION
370 Woodcliff Drive
Fairport, NY 14450
949-597-8130
800-538-7850
http://www.coopervision.com

00093
COPLEY PHARMACEUTICAL
See Teva Pharmaceuticals USA

63020
COR THERAPEUTICS, INC.
See Millennium Pharmaceuticals, Inc.

CORIXA
See GlaxoSmithKline

10122
CORNERSTONE BIOPHARMA INC.
2000 Regency Parkway
Cary, NC 27511
919-678-6611
888-466-6503
http://www.cornerstonebiopharma.com

10148
COTHERIX
5000 Shoreline Ct., Suite 101
South San Francisco, CA 94080
650-808-6500
877-483-6828
http://www.cotherix.com

COULTER CORP. (BECKMAN COULTER, INC.)
See Beckman Coulter

08011
C. R. BARD
730 Central Avenue
Murray Hill, NJ 07974
908-277-8000
800-526-4455
http://www.crbard.com

C. R. BARD, INC. UROLOGICAL DIVISION
8195 Industrial Blvd.
Covington, GA 30014
770-784-6100
800-526-4455
http://www.crbard.com

11025
CREATIVE MEDICAL CORPORATION
PR Road #172, KM 9.4
Cidra, PR 00739-1370
787-714-0100

15310
CREEKWOOD PHARMACEUTICAL
31 Inverness Center Pky., #270
Birmingham, AL 35242
732-292-2661

68734
CRITICAL THERAPEUTICS
60 Westview St.
Lexington, MA 02421
781-402-5700
http://www.criticaltherapeutics.com/

10486
C. S. DENT & CO DIVISION
See Grandpa Brands Company

67919
CUBIST PHARMACEUTICALS
65 Hayden Ave.
Lexington, MA 02421
781-860-8660
866-793-2786
http://www.cubist.com

00869
CUMBERLAND SWAN, INC.
One Swan Dr.
Smyrna, TN 37167-2099
615-459-8900
800-486-7926
http://www.cumberlandswan.com

66860
CURA PHARMACEUTICALS
542 Industrial Way West
Eatontown, NJ 07724

CURASCRIPT
250 Technology Park
Lake Mary, FL 32746
407-804-6700
800-892-9622
http://www.priorityhealthcare.com

55326
CURATEK PHARMACEUTICALS
See 3M Pharmaceuticals

65628
CUTIS PHARMA, INC.
100 Cummings Center
Beverly, MA 01915
978-867-1010
http://www.cutispharma.com

67159
CV THERAPEUTICS
3172 Porter Dr.
Palo Alto, CA 94304
650-384-8500
http://www.cvt.com/index2.html

CYANOTECH CORP.
73-4460 Queen Kaahamanu Hwy.
Kailua-Kona, HI 96740
808-326-1353
800-395-1353
http://www.cyanotech.com

53409
CYCLIN PHARMACEUTICALS INC.
1289 Deming Way
Madison, WI 53717
800-558-7046
http://www.womenshealth.com

08197
CYGNUS, INC.
400 Penobscot Drive
Redwood City, CA 94063
650-369-4300
http://www.cygn.com

54799
CYNACON/OCUSOFT
5311 Ave. N
Rosenberg, TX 77471
800-233-5469
http://www.ocusoft.com

60258
CYPRESS PHARMACEUTICAL, INC.
135 Industrial Blvd.
Madison, MS 39110
601-856-4393
800-856-4393
http://www.cypressrx.com

63004
CYPROS PHARMACEUTICAL CORP.
See Questcor Pharmaceuticals, Inc.

57902
CYTOGEN CORPORATION
650 College Rd. East
Princeton, NJ 08540
609-750-8200
800-833-3533
http://www.cytogen.com

23731
CYTOSOL LABORATORIES
55 Messina Drive
Braintree, MA 02184
781-848-9386
800-288-3858

61534
CYTOSOL OPTHALMICS
1325 William White Place, N.E.
Lenoir, NC 28645
828-758-2343
800-234-5166
http://www.cytosol.com

CYTRX CORP.
11726 San Vicente Blvd.
Los Angeles, CA 90049
310-826-5648
http://www.cytrx.com

65759, 10960
D & K HEALTHCARE RESOURCES
8235 Forsyth Blvd.
St. Louis, MO 63105-1659
314-727-3485
888-727-3485
http://www.dkwd.com

DADE BEHRING
1717 Deerfield Road
Deerfield, IL 60015
847-267-5300
800-241-0420
http://www.dadebehring.com

63395
DAIICHI PHARM. CORP.
11 Philips Parkway
Montvale, NJ 07645-1810
201-573-7000
877-324-4244
http://www.daiichius.com

00591, 52544
DANBURY PHARMACAL (WATSON LABORATORIES)
311 Bonnie Circle
Corona, CA 92880
951-493-5300
800-272-5525
http://www.watsonpharm.com

64875
DANCO LABS., LLC
PO Box 4816
New York, NY 10185
212-424-1950
877-432-7596

60793
DANIELS PHARMACEUTICALS, INC.
See King Pharmaceuticals, Inc.

58869
DARTMOUTH PHARMACEUTICALS
38 Church Ave.
Wareham, MA 02571
508-295-2200
800-414-3566
http://www.ilovemynails.com

68774
DAVA PHARMACEUTICALS
400 Kelby St.
Fort Lee, NJ 07024
201-947-7442

DAVOL, INC.
100 Sockanossett Crossroad
Cranston, RI 02920
401-463-7000
800-556-6275
http://www.davol.com

58865
DAWN PHARMACEUTICALS INC.
4555 W. Addison
Chicago, IL 60641
800-745-3296

52041
DAYTON LABORATORIES
See Propharma

DEGUSSA CORP.
379 Enterpace Parkway
Parsippany, NJ 07054
973-541-8000
877-273-2668
http://www.degussa.com

10310
DEL PHARMACEUTICALS
726 Reckson Plaza
Uniondale, NY 11553
516-844-2020
800-645-9888
http://www.dellabs.com

00316
DEL-RAY DERMATOLOGICALS
PO Box 1425
Johnson City, TN 37605
423-926-4413
800-877-8869
http://www.delrayderm.com

48532
DELMONT LABORATORIES, INC.
PO Box 269
Swarthmore, PA 19081
610-543-3365
800-562-5541
http://www.delmontlabs.info

53706
DELTA PHARMACEUTICALS
401 Western Lane
Irmo, SC 29063-7953
803-407-7733

DEN-MAT CORPORATION
2727 Skyway Dr.
Santa Maria, CA 93455
805-922-8491
800-433-6628

00295
DENISON PHARMACEUTICALS
60 Dunnell Lane
Pawtucket, RI 02860-5828 1305 02862
401-723-5500
http://www.hydrolatum.com

78112, 75137
(THE) DENOREX COMPANY
90 N. Broadway, Suite 301
Irvington, NY 10533
866-840-0011
http://www.denorex.com

DENTAL HERB CO.
1000 Holland Drive
Boca Raton, FL 33487
561-241-4262
800-747-4372
http://www.dentalherbcompany.com

13913
DEPOMED
1360 O'Brien Dr.
Menlo Park, CA 94025-1436
650-462-5900
http://www.depomedinc.com/

DEPOTECH CORP. (SKYEPHARMA)
10450 Science Center Dr.
San Diego, CA 92121
858-625-2424
http://www.skyepharma.com

25382
DERMA SCIENCE
214 Carnegie Center, Suite 100
Princeton, NJ 08540-6237
609-514-4744
800-825-4325
http://www.dermasciences.com

60974
DERMALOGIX PARTNERS
Scarsborough, ME 1510 04070
207-883-4103
800-753-0047
http://www.dermalogix.com

61924
DERMARITE
3 East 26th St.
Paterson, NJ 07513
973-569-9000
800-337-6296
http://www.dermarite.com

00066
DERMIK LABORATORIES, INC. (ARCOLA)
See Sanofi-Aventis

DEROYAL INDUSTRIES, INC.
200 DeBusk Lane
Powell, TN 37849
865-938-7828
888-938-7828
http://www.deroyal.com

65430
DEXGEN PHARMACEUTICALS, INC.
PO Box 675
Manasquan, NJ 08736
732-223-8811
877-339-4361
http://www.dexgen.com

49502
DEY LABORATORIES, INC.
2751 Napa Valley Corporate Dr.
Napa, CA 94558
707-224-3200
800-755-5560
http://www.deyinc.com

DFB PHARMACEUTICALS
3909 Hulen St.
Ft. Worth, TX 76107
800-441-8227
http://www.healthpoint.com
http://www.dfb.com

55887
DHS, INC.
250 Hembree Park Dr.
Roswell, GA 30076
770-751-1787
800-392-7717

17000
DIAL CORPORATION
15501 N. Dial Blvd.
Scottsdale, AZ 85260
480-754-3425
800-258-3425
http://www.dialcorp.com

DIAPHARMA GROUP, INC.
8948 Beckett Rd.
West Chester, OH 45069-2939
513-860-9324
800-526-5224
http://www.diapharma.com

50419.
DIATIDE, INC.
9 Delta Dr.
Londonderry, NH 03053
http://www.berlex.com/html/diatide.html

10331.
DICKINSON BRANDS, INC.
31 East High Street
East Hampton, CT 06424
860-267-2279
888-860-2279
http://www.witchhazel.com

59767
DIGESTIVE CARE INC.
1120 Win Dr.
Bethlehem, PA 18017-7059
610-882-5950
http://www.digestivecare.com

55392
DINNO PHARMACEUTICALS
PO Box 66106
Auburndale, MA 02466
617-645-5552

DISCOVERY LABORATORIES, INC.
2600 Kelly Road
Warrington, PA 18976-3622
215-488-9300
http://www.discoverylabs.com

DISCUS DENTAL INC.
8550 Higuera St.
Culver City, CA 90232
310-845-8600
800-422-9448
http://www.discusdental.com

68258
DISPENSING SOLUTIONS INC.
3000 West Warner Ave.
Santa Ana, CA 92704
714-437-0330
http://www.dispensingsolutionsinc.com

00777
DISTA PRODUCTS CO.
See Eli Lilly and Co.

DIXON-SHANE
See R & S Northeast

64455
DJ PHARMA, INC.
See Biovail Pharmaceuticals, Inc.

10337
DOAK DERMATOLOGICS
See Bradley Pharmaceutical

DONELL DERMEDEX
See Donell Inc.

DONELL INC.
Chrysler Building
New York, NY 10174
212-682-0666
800-324-7455
http://www.donellskin.com

51469
DOVER PHARMACEUTICAL, INC.
PO Box 809
Islington, MA 02090
781-821-5400
800-777-6847

00514
DOW HICKAM, INC.
See Mylan Pharmaceuticals, Inc.

DOW PHARMACEUTICAL SCIENCES
1330A Redwood Way
Petaluma, CA 94954-1169
707-793-2600
877-369-7476
http://www.dowpharm.com

55111
DR. REDDY'S LABORATORIES, INC.
200 Somerset Corporate Blvd.
Bridgewater, NJ 08807
908-203-4900
http://www.drreddys.com

64061
DREIR PHARMACEUTICALS, INC.
12502 E. Doubletree Ranch Rd.
Scottsdale, AZ 85259
480-607-3584
800-541-4044

52316
DSC LABORATORIES
1979 Latimer Dr.
Muskegon, MI 49442
231-777-3012
800-492-5988
http://www.dsclab.com

00217, 48878
DUNHALL PHARMACEUTICALS, INC.
See Omnii Pharmaceuticals

DUPONT PHARMACEUTICALS CO.
See Bristol-Myers Squibb Company

51285
DURAMED PHARMACEUTICALS
See Barr Laboratories, Inc.

02340
DUREX CONSUMER PRODUCTS
3585 Engineering Dr.
Norcross, GA 30092
770-582-2222
888-566-3468
http://www.durex.com

00145
DURHAM PHARMACAL CORP.
See Stiefel Laboratories, Inc.

67308
DUSA PHARMACEUTICALS, INC.
25 Upton Drive
Wilmington, MA 01887
978-657-7500
877-533-DUSA (877-533-3872)
http://www.dusapharma.com

55516
DYNA PHARM, INC.
P.O. Box 2141
Del Mar, CA 92014-2141

EAGLE VISION, INC.
8500 Wolf Lake Dr., Suite 110
Memphis, TN 38133
901-380-7000
800-222-7584
http://www.eaglevis.com

EASTMAN KODAK CO.
343 State St.
Rochester, NY 14650
585-724-4000
800-242-2424
http://www.kodak.com

EATON MEDICAL CORP.
1401 Heistan Place
Memphis, TN 38104
901-274-0000
800-253-5949
http://www.easyeyes.com

ECOLOGICAL FORMULAS, INC.
1061-B Shary Circle, Suite B
Concord, CA 94518
925-827-2636
800-888-4585
http://www.ecologicalformulas.net

38130
ECONO MED PHARMACEUTICALS
4305 Sartin Road
Burlington, NC 27217-7522
336-226-1091
800-327-6007

55053
ECONOLAB
See Breckenridge Pharmaceutical, Inc.

00095
ECR PHARMACEUTICALS
3969 Deep Rock Road
Richmond, VA 23233
804-527-1950
800-527-1955
http://www.ecrpharmaceuticals.com

00433
EDWARDS LIFESCIENCE
One Edwards Way
Irvine, CA 92614
800-424-3278
http://www.edwards.com

00485
EDWARDS PHARMACEUTICALS, INC.
111 Mulberry Street
Ripley, MS 38663
662-837-8182
800-543-9560

55806
EFFCON LABORATORIES
1165 Allgood Rd.
Marietta, GA 30062
770-579-3558
800-722-2428
http://www.effcon.com

00168
E. FOUGERA CO.
60 Baylis Rd
Melville, NY 11747 2006
631-454-7677
800-645-9833
http://www.fougera.com

62856
EISAI INC.
500 Frank W. Burr Blvd.
Glenpointe Centre West
Teaneck, NJ 07666
201-692-1100
http://www.eisai.com

59075
ELAN PHARMACEUTICALS
7475 Lusk Blvd.
San Diego, CA 92121
650-877-7496
800-859-8586888-638-7605
http://www.elan.com

ELANCO
2001 W. Main St.
Greenfield, IN 46140
317-277-3185
800-428-4441
http://www.elanco.com

00002
ELI LILLY AND CO.
Lilly Corporate Center
Indianapolis, IN 46285
317-276-2000
800-545-5979
http://www.lilly.com

EMD CHEMICALS, INC.
480 S. Democrat Road
Gibbstown, NJ 08027
856-423-6300
800-222-0342

64068
ENDIT LABORATORIES
PO Box 228
Shallotte, NC 28459 228
910-754-6856
http://www.endit.com

ENDO LABORATORIES, INC.
100 Endo Blvd.
Chadds Ford, PA 19317
800-892-6131
800-462-3636
http://www.endo.com

ENDURANCE PRODUCTS CO.
9914 S.W. Tigard St.
Tigard, OR 97223
503-639-9562
800-483-2532
http://www.endur.com

62333
ENVIRODERM PHARMACEUTICALS, INC.
154 West 131 Street
Los Angeles, CA 90061
310-768-0700
800-624-9659
http://www.enviroderm.com

57665
ENZON, INC.
685 Route 202/206
Bridgewater, NJ 08807
908-541-8600
http://www.enzon.com

00185
EON LABS MANUFACTURING, INC.
1999 Marcus Ave.
Lake Success, NY 11042
516-478-9700
800-526-0225
http://www.eonlabs.com

62942.
EPIEN MEDICAL
10225 Yellow Circle Dr.
Minneapolis, MN 55343
952-746-6770
888-884-4675
http://www.epien.com

E. R. SQUIBB & SONS, INC.
See Bristol-Myers Squibb Company

63475
ESCALON MEDICAL CORP.
565 East Swedesford Road
Wayne, PA 19087
618-688-6830
800-433-8197
http://www.escalonmed.com

67286
ESP PHARMA
2035 Lincoln Hwy., Suite 2150
Edison, NJ 08817
732-650-1377
866-437-7742
http://www.esppharm.com

15456
ESPRIT PHARMA
Two Tower Center Blvd.
East Brunswick, NJ 08816
732-828-9950
http://www.espritpharma.com

58177
ETHEX CORP.
10888 Metro Court
St. Louis, MO 63043-2413
314-567-3307
800-321-1705
http://www.ethex.com

63713
ETHICON, INC. (JOHNSON & JOHNSON)
US Route 22 West
Somerville, NJ 08876-0151
908-218-0707
800-255-2500
http://www.ethicon.com

ETI HOLDING
825 Challenger Drive
Green Bay, WI 54311
920-469-1313

EURAND AMERICA, INC.
845 Center Dr.
Vandalia, OH 45377
937-898-9669
http://www.eurand.com

66521
EVANS VACCINES LTD.
See Chiron Therapeutics

42700
EVENFLO COMPANY, INC.
707 Cross Road Ct.
Vandalia, OH 45377
937-415-3300
800-233-5921
http://www.evenflo.com

00642
EVERETT LABORATORIES, INC.
29 Spring St.
West Orange, NJ 07052
973-324-0795
800-964-9650
http://www.everettlabs.com

64125
EXCELLIUM PHARMACEUTICAL
3-G Oak Road
Fairfield, NJ 07004
973-276-9600

63807
EXCELSIOR MEDICAL CORPORATION
1923 Heck Ave.
Neptune, NJ 07753
732-776-7525
800-487-4276
http://www.excelsiormedical.com

60843
EYE CARE & CURE CORPORATION
1140 North Rosemont Blvd.
Tucson, AZ 85712
520-321-1262
800-486-6169
http://www.eyecareandcure.com

68782
EYETECH PHARMACEUTICALS
3 Times Square, 12th Floor
New York, NY 10036
212-824-3100
http://www.osieyetech.com

10361
E-Z-EM
1111 Marcus Ave., Suite LL26
Lake Success, NY 11042
516-333-8230
800-544-4624
http://www.ezem.com

58892
FALLENE
144 Ivy Lane
King of Prussia, PA 19406
610-337-9048
800-332-5536
http://www.fallene.com/

FARMACON, INC.
1071 Post Road East
Westport, CT 06880-5361
203-222-8801

60976
FARO PHARMACEUTICALS, INC.
See Cooper Surgical

61703
FAULDING USA
650 From Road
Paramus, NJ 07652
201-225-5500
877-328-5346
http://www.us.maynepharma.com

57464
(THE) F. C. STURTEVANT COMPANY
PO Box 607
Bronxville, NY 10708
914-337-5131
888-871-5661
http://www.columbiapowder.com

FDA
5600 Fishers Lane
Rockville, MD 20857-0001
301-827-1491
888-463-6332
http://www.fda.gov

11423
FEMALE HEALTH CO.
515 N. State St.
Chicago, IL 60610
312-595-9123
800-884-1601
http://www.femalehealthcompany.com

00496
FERNDALE LABORATORIES, INC.
780 West Eight Mile Road
Ferndale, MI 48220
248-548-0900
800-621-6003
http://www.ferndalelabs.com

31253, 08439
FERRARIS MEDICAL LTD.
1301 Courtesy Road
Louisville, CO 80027
http://www.ferrarismedical.com

55566
FERRING PHARMACEUTICALS INC.
400 Rella Blvd.
Suffern, NY 10901
888-337-7464
845-770-2600
http://www.ferringusa.com

FIBERTONE
See Marlyn Neutraceuticals, Inc.

59630
FIRST HORIZON PHARMACEUTICAL CORP.
6195 Shiloh Road
Alpharetta, GA 30005
770-442-9707
800-849-9707
http://www.firsthorizon.com

90891
FIRST QUALITY PRODUCTS
121 North Rd.
McElhattan, PA 17748
516-829-3030
800-227-3551
http://www.firstquality.com

FISHER SCIENTIFIC INTERNATIONAL
One Liberty Lane East
Hampton, NH 03842
603-926-5911
800-640-0640
http://www.fisherscientific.com

FISKE INDUSTRIES
50 Ramland Road
Orangeburg, NY 10962
845-398-3340
http://www.cosmeticsolutions.com

54323
FLANDERS, INC.
Charleston, SC 29416
843-571-3363
http://www.flandersbuttocksointment.com

00256
FLEMING & CO.
1733 Gilsinn Ln.
Fenton, MO 63026
636-343-5306
800-343-0164
http://www.flemingcompany.com

23185
FLENTS PRODUCTS COMPANY
11750 12th Ave. South
Burnsville, MN 55337-1295
800-328-2742
http://www.apothecaryproducts.com

FLEX-POWER
823 Gilman St.
Berkeley, CA 94710
510-527-9955
866-353-9769
http://www.flexpower.com

00288
FLUORITAB CORP.
1197 Lambert Dr.
Muskegon, MI 49441
231-755-9113

60762
FNC MEDICAL CORPORATION
6000 Leland St.
Ventura, CA 93003
805-644-7576
800-440-2888
http://www.fncmedical.com

00456
FOREST LABORATORIES IRELAND LTD
909 Third Ave.
New York, NY 10022
212-421-7850
800-947-5227
http://www.forestpharm.com

00456
FOREST LABORATORIES, INC.
909 Third Ave.
New York, NY 10022
212-421-7850
800-947-5227
800-678-1605
http://www.forestpharm.com

00456
FOREST PHARMACEUTICALS, INC.
13600 Shoreline Drive
St. Louis, MO 63045
314-493-7000
800-678-1605
http://www.forestpharm.com

64814
FORTE PHARMA
See Eon Labs Manufacturing, Inc.

00168
FOUGERA
60 Baylis Rd.
Melville, NY 11747 2006
631-454-7677
800-645-9833
http://www.fougera.com

FOURNIER PHARMA
4 Gatehall Dr.
Parsippany, NJ 07054
973-683-0024
http://www.fournierpharmacorp.com

58487
FREEDA VITAMINS, INC.
36 E. 41st Street
New York, NY 10017
212-685-4980
800-777-3737
http://www.freedavitamins.com

90816, 49230
FRESENIUS MEDICAL CARE NORTH AMERICA
95 Hayden Ave.
Lexington, MA 02420
781-402-9000
http://www.fmcna.com

13551
FSC LABORATORIES
4006 Beltline Rd., Suite 100
Addison, TX 75001
877-387-0021
http://www.fsclabs.com

FUISZ TECHNOLOGIES, LTD.
See Biovail Pharmaceuticals, Inc.

00713
G & W LABORATORIES
111 Coolidge Street
South Plainfield, NJ 07080-3895
908-753-2000
800-922-1038
http://www.gwlabs.com

00299
GALDERMA LABORATORIES, INC.
14501 N. Freeway
Ft. Worth, TX 76177
817-961-5000
800-582-8225
http://www.galdermausa.com

57284
GALEN PHARMA
22 Seagoe Industrial Estate
Craigavon, UK BT63-5UA
028-3833-4974
http://www.galen.co.uk

51552
GALLIPOT, INC.
2400 Pilot Knob Road
Mendota Heights, MN 55120
651-681-9517
800-423-6967
http://www.gallipot.com

GAMBRO, INC.
10810 W. Collins Ave.
Lakewood, CO 80215
800-232-6800
800-525-2623
http://www.gambro.com

57844
GATE PHARMACEUTICALS
1090 Horsham Rd.
North Wales, PA 19454
215-591-3000
800-292-4283
http://www.gatepharma.com

00407
GE HEALTHCARE
3000 N. Grandview Blvd.
Waukesha, WI 53188
262-544-3011
http://www.gehealthcare.com

00386
GEBAUER CO.
4444 East 153rd St.
Cleveland, OH 44128
216-581-3030
800-321-9348
http://www.gebauerco.com

50242
GENENTECH, INC.
1 DNA Way
South San Francisco, CA 94080-4990
650-225-1000
http://www.gene.com

GENERAL INJECTABLES & VACCINES
U.S. Hwy. 52 South
Bastian, VA 24314
276-688-4121
800-521-7468
http://www.glv.com

GENERAL NUTRITION INC.
300 6th Ave.
Pittsburgh, PA 15222
412-288-4600
888-462-2548
http://www.gnc.com

10139
GENERAMEDIX
150 Allen Rd.
Liberty Corner, NJ 07938
866-436-3721
http://www.generamedix.com/

GENESIS NUTRITION
1816 Wall St.
Florence, SC 29501
843-665-6928
800-451-7933
http://www.genesisnutrition.com

00398
GENESIS PHARMACEUTICALS
9 Campus Dr., 3rd Floor
Parsippany, NJ 07054
973-451-9020
800-459-8663

GENETIC THERAPY, INC.
938 Clopper Road
Gaithersburg, MD 20878
301-590-2626

00008
GENETICS INSTITUTE
87 Cambridge Park Dr.
Cambridge, MA 02140
617-876-1170
888-446-3344
http://www.genetics.com

00781
GENEVA PHARMACEUTICALS
See Sandoz Pharmaceuticals-Sandoz Consumer

15330
GENPHARM LP
150 Motor Parkway
Hauppauge, NY 11788
866-436-9155
http://www.genpharmusa.com

00703.
GENSIA SICOR PHARMACEUTICALS, INC.
19 Hughes
Irvine, CA 92618
949-455-4700
800-331-0124
http://www.gensiasicor.com

66657
GENTA INC.
Berkeley Heights, NJ 07922
888TO-GENTA

15014
GENTEX PHARMA LLC
805 Wellington Way
Madison, MS 39110
601-853-1835

GENVEC, INC.
65 W. Watkins Mill Rd.
Gaithersburg, MD 20878
240-632-5501
http://www.genvec.com

58468
GENZYME CORP.
500 Kendall St.
Cambridge, MA 02142
617-252-7500
800-326-7002
http://www.genzyme.com

63861
GENZYME TRANSPLANT
500 Kendall St.
Cambridge, MA 02142
617-252-7500
800-376-7002
http://www.genzyme.com

GEODESIC MEDITECH, INC.
2921 Sandy Pointe No. 3
Del Mar, CA 92014
858-692-0088
http://www.geodesicmeditech.com

72227
GERBER PRODUCTS COMPANY
445 State Street
Fremont, MI 49413-0001
231-928-2000
800-443-7237
http://www.gerber.com

57896
GERI-CARE PRODUCTS
250 Moonachie Ave.
Moonachie, NJ 07074-1897
201-440-0409
800-654-8322
http://www.geri-careproducts.com

54092
GERIATRIC PHARMACEUTICAL CORP.
See Shire US, Inc.

79277, 54162
GERITREX CORPORATION
144 Kingsbridge Road East
Mt. Vernon, NY 10550
914-668-4003
800-736-3437
http://www.geritrex.com

61958
GILEAD SCIENCES
333 Lakeside Drive
Foster City, CA 94404
650-574-3000
800-445-3235
http://www.gilead.com

GILLETTE ORAL CARE
Prudential Tower
Boston, MA 02199-8004
617-421-7000
http://www.gillette.com

47400
GILLETTE PERSONAL CARE
Prudential Tower
Boston, MA 02199-8004
617-421-7000
http://www.gillette.com

63218, 59366
GLADES PHARMACEUTICALS
6340 Sugarloaf Parkway
Duluth, GA 30097
866-436-0318
888-445-2337
http://www.glades.com

GLAXOSMITHKLINE
One Franklin Plaza
Philadelphia, PA 19102
888-825-5249
http://www.gsk.com

99929
GLAXOSMITHKLINE CONSUMER HEALTHCARE
1500 Littleton Rd.
Parsippany, NJ 07054
973-889-2100
800-245-1040
http://www.gsk.com

99929
GLAXOSMITHKLINE CONSUMER HEALTHCARE, L.P.
1000 GSK Dr.
Moon Township, PA 15108
412-200-4000
800-245-1040
http://www.gsk.com

GLAXOSMITHKLINE PHARM.
See GlaxoSmithKline

68462
GLENMARK PHARMACEUTICALS
750 Corporate Dr.
Mahwah, NJ 07430
201-684-8000
http://www.glenmarkpharma.com

41128, 00516
GLENWOOD, INC.
111 Cedar Land
Englewood, NJ 07631 5419
201-569-0050
800-542-0772
http://www.glenwood-llc.com

00115
GLOBAL PHARMACEUTICALS, INC.
30831 Huntwood Ave.
Hayward, CA 94544
510-476-2000
800-934-6729
http://www.globalphar.com

59618
GLOBAL SOURCE
5371 Hiatus Rd.
Sunrise, FL 33351
954-747-8977
800-662-7556
http://www.globalvitamin.com

58809
GM PHARMACEUTICAL
912 W. Randol Mill Rd.
Arlington, TX 76012-2564
817-303-3800

GML INDUSTRIES, LLC
See Biosafe Technologies

60429
GOLDEN STATE MEDICAL SUPPLY
1799 Eastman Ave
Ventura, CA 93003
805-477-9866
800-284-8633
http://www.gsms.us

GOLDLINE LABORATORIES, INC.
See Ivax Pharmaceuticals, Inc.

10481
GORDON LABORATORIES
6801 Ludlow Street
Upper Darby, PA 19082-2408
610-734-2011
800-356-7870
http://www.gordonlabs.com

12165
GRAHAM FIELD HEALTH PRODUCTS INC.
2935 Northeast Parkway
Atlanta, GA 30360
800-347-5678
http://www.grahamfield.com

10486
GRANDPA BRANDS COMPANY
1820 Airport Exchange Blvd.
Erlanger, KY 41018
859-647-0777
800-684-1468
http://www.grandpabrands.com

00034
GRAY PHARMACEUTICAL CO.
See Purdue Frederick Co.

51301
GREAT SOUTHERN LABORATORIES
10863 Rockley Road
Houston, TX 77099
281-530-3077
800-747-0783

GREEN TURTLE BAY VITAMIN CO.
56 High Street
Summit, NJ 07901
908-277-2240
800-887-8535
http://www.energywave.com

59762
GREENSTONE LIMITED
See Pfizer Consumer Health

22840
GREER LABORATORIES, INC.
PO Box 800
Lenoir, NC 28645
828-754-5327
800-378-3906
http://www.greerlabs.com

68516, 61953
GRIFOLS USA, INC.
2410 Lillyvale Ave.
Los Angeles, CA 90032-3514
888-474-3657
800-421-0008
http://www.grifolsusa.com

GUARDIAN DRUG COMPANY
2 Charles Court
Dayton, NJ 08810
609-860-2600
http://www.guardiandrug.com

00327
GUARDIAN LABORATORIES
230 Marcus Blvd.
Hauppauge, NY 11788
631-273-0900
800-645-5566
http://www.u-g.com

62750
GUM-TECH INDUSTRIES, INC.
See Matrixx Initiatives, Inc.

63955
GYNETICS
3371 US Highway 1
Lawrenceville, NJ 08648
609-919-1931

54765
GYNOPHARMA
50 Division Street
Somerville, NJ 08876

12164
HALOCARBON PRODUCTS CORPORATION
887 Kinderkamack Rd.
River Edge, NJ 07661
800-338-5803
http://www.halocarbon.com

17478
HAMELN PHARMACEUTICALS GMBH
See Akorn, Inc.

HARD TO FIND BRANDS, INC.
2525 Quicksilver
McDonald, PA 15057
724-796-0148
888-796-4832
http://www.hardtofindbrands.com

52512
HARMONY LABORATORIES
1109 S. Main St.
Landis, NC 28088
704-857-0707
800-245-6284
http://www.harmonylabs.com

HART HEALTH & SAFETY
Seattle, WA 98124
800-234-4278
http://www.harthealth.com

00904, 61147
HARVARD DRUG GROUP
31778 Enterprise Drive
Livonia, MI 48150
800-875-0123
http://www.harvardlink.com
http://www.harvarddrugs.com

67754
HARVEST PHARMACEUTICALS INC.
1881 Grove Ave.
Radford, VA 24141
540-633-7976
800-455-5525
http://www.harvest pharmaceuticals.com

HAUSER PHARMACEUTICAL INC.
4401 East U.S. Highway 30
Valparaiso, IN 46383
800-441-2309
http://www.hauserpharmaceutical.com

63717
HAWTHORN PHARMACEUTICALS INC.
135 Industrial Blvd.
Madison, MS 39110
601-856-4393
800-856-4393
http://www.cypressrx.com

HCD SALES
15424 N. Nebraska Ave.
Lutz, FL 33548 2439
813-978-3005
800-844-8345
http://www.hcdsales.com

HD SMITH
3063 Fiat Ave.
Springfield, IL 62703
866-232-1222
800-252-8090
http://www.hdsmith.com

HDC CORPORATION
628 Gibraltar Court
Milpitas, CA 95035
408-942-7340
800-227-8162
http://www.hdccorp.com

HEALTH ASURE, INC.
125 McPherson St.
Santa Cruz, CA 95060
831-420-2660
800-635-1233
http://www.healthasure.com

60569
HEALTH CARE PRODUCTS
369 Bayview Ave.
Amityville, NY 11701
631-789-8455
800-899-3116
http://www.diabeticproducts.com

79573
HEALTH ENTERPRISES
90 George Leven Dr.
N. Attelboro, MA 02760
508-695-0727
800-633-4243
http://www.healthenterprises.com

HEALTH PRODUCTS CORP.
1060 NepperHan
Yonkers, NY 10703
914-423-2900

HEALTHCARE DIRECT SERVICES
See HCD Sales

HEALTHFIRST CORP.
22316 70th Ave. West, Unit A
Mountlake, WA 98043-2184
425-771-5733
800-331-1984
http://www.healthfirst.com

00064
HEALTHPOINT MEDICAL
3909 Hulen St.
Fort Worth, TX 76107
800-441-8227
http://www.healthpoint.com

93595, 55966
HEALTHSTAR
145 Ricefield Lane
Hauppauge, NY 11788
631-273-2630

51800
HEARTLAND NEBULIZER SALES
140 N. 8th St., Suite 60
Lincoln, NE 83272
800-355-5312

50114
HEEL INC.
10421 Research Rd.
Albuquerque, NM 87123
514-353-4335
800-621-7644
http://www.Heel.com
http://www.Heel.ca

HELENA LABORATORIES
1530 Lindbergh
Beaumont, TX 77707
409-842-3714
800-231-5663
http://www.helena.com

HEMACARE CORP.
21101 Oxnard Street
Woodland Hills, CA 91367
818-226-1968
http://www.hemacare.com

HEMAGEN DIAGNOSTICS, INC.
9033 Red Branch Road
Columbia, MD 21045
443-367-5500
800-495-2180
http://www.hemagen.com

HEMISPHERX BIOPHARMA, INC.
One Penn Ctr., 1617 JFK Blvd.
Philadelphia, PA 19103
215-988-0080
http://www.hemispherx.net

HENRY SCHEIN, INC.
135 Duryea Rd.
Melville, NY 11747
631-843-5500
800-472-4346
http://www.henryschein.com

00023, 11980
HERBERT LABORATORIES
See Allergan Inc.

49730
HERCON LABORATORIES INC.
460 Park Avenue
New York, NY 10022
212-751-5600

50383
HI-TECH PHARMACAL CO. INC.
369 Bayview Ave.
Amityville, NY 11701
631-789-8228
800-262-9010
http://www.hitechpharm.com

28105
HILL DERMACEUTICALS, INC.
2650 S. Mellonville Ave.
Sanford, FL 32773
407-323-1187
800-344-5707
http://www.hillderm.com

10542
HILLESTAD PHARMACEUTICALS
178 U.S. Highway 51 North
Woodruff, WI 54568-1700
800-535-7742
http://www.hillestadlabs.com

HIMMEL NUTRITION
1926 10th Ave.
Suite 303
Lake Worth, FL 33461-3310
561-585-0070
800-535-3823
http://www.goliath.ecnext.com

17808
HIMMEL PHARMACEUTICALS, INC.
1926 10th Ave.
Suite 303
Lake Worth, FL 33461-3310
561-585-0070
800-535-3823
http://www.goliath.ecnext.com

46581
HISAMITSU AMERICA
3528 Torrance Blvd.
Torrance, CA 90503
310-540-1408
http://www.salonpas-usa.com

52959
H. J. HARKINS COMPANY, INC.
513 Sandydale Dr.
Nipomo, CA 93444
805-929-4060

00839
H. L. MOORE DRUG EXCHANGE, INC.
See Moore Medical Corp.

HOECHST-MARION ROUSSEL
See Sanofi-Aventis

95814
HOGIL PHARMACEUTICAL CORP.
237 Mamaroneck Ave., Ste. 303
White Plains, NY 10605
914-681-1800
http://www.hogil.com

HOLLES LABORATORIES, INC.
30 Forest Notch
Cohasset, MA 02025-1198
800-356-4015

65044
HOLLISTER-STIER
3525 N. Regal
Spokane, WA 9920
509-489-5656
800-962-1266
http://www.hollisterstier.com

83170
HOME ACCESS HEALTH CORPORATION
2401 West Hassell Rd.
Hoffman Estates, IL 60195
847-781-2500
800-448-8378
http://www.homeaccess.com

21292, 56151
HOME DIAGNOSTICS INC.
2400 NW 55th Ct.
Fort Lauderdale, FL 33309
954-677-9201
800-342-7226
http://www.homediagnostics.com

HONEYWELL HOMMED LLC
3400 Intertech Drive
Brookfield, WI 53045
262-783-5440
888-353-5440
http://www.hommed.com

60267
HOPE PHARMACEUTICALS
8260 E. Gelding Drive, #104
Scottsdale, AZ 85260
800-755-9595
http://www.hopepharm.com

60904
HORIZON PHARMACEUTICAL CORP.
See First Horizon Pharmaceutical Corp.

61678
HORMEL HEALTHLABS
3000 Tremont Rd.
Savannah, GA 31405
800-866-7757
http://www.hormelhealthlabs.com

66553
HOSPAK UNIT DOSE PRODUCTS
5910 Creekside Lane
Rockford, IL 61114
815-877-6480

00409
HOSPIRA
275 N. Field Dr.
Lake Forest, IL 60045
224-212-2000
877-946-7747
http://www.hospira.com

00591, 52544
HOUBA (HALSEY DRUG CO.)
See Acura Pharmaceuticals, Inc.

HOUBA/HALSEY DRUG CO.
See Acura Pharmaceuticals Technologies

00556
H R CENCI LABS
1415 Tuolumne Ave.
Fresno, CA 93706
209-237-3346

74312
HUDSON CORP.
90 Orville Drive
Bohemia, NY 11716
516-567-9500

44156
HUMANICARE INTERNATIONAL
9 Elkins Road
East Brunswick, NJ 08816
732-613-9000
800-631-5270
http://www.humanicare.com

03951, 00395
HUMCO HOLDING GROUP, INC.
7400 Alumax Dr.
Texarkana, TX 75501
903-831-7808
800-662-3435
http://www.humco.com

00219
HUMPHREYS PHARMACAL
31 East High St.
East Hampton, CT 06424
201-933-7744

00944
HYLAND THERAPEUTICS
See Baxter Healthcare Corporation (Baxter Bioscience)

08480
HYPOGUARD USA, INC.
7301 Ohms Lane
Edina, MN 55439
952-646-3200
952-646-3101
800-818-8877
http://www.hypoguard.com

00186
ICI PHARMACEUTICALS
See AstraZeneca LP

00187
ICN PHARMACEUTICALS
See Valeant Pharmaceuticals International

59627
IDEC PHARMACEUTICALS
See Biogen Idec

63861
ILEX ONCOLOGY INC.
See Genzyme Corp.

IMMUCELL CORP.
56 Evergreen Drive
Portland, ME 04103
207-878-2770
800-466-8235
http://www.immucell.com

54129
IMMUNO U.S., INC. (BAXTER HEALTHCARE CORP.)
See Baxter Healthcare Corporation

IMMUNOGEN
128 Sidney Street
Cambridge, MA 02139
617-995-2500
http://www.immunogen.com

IMMUNOMEDICS INC.
300 American Road
Morris Plains, NJ 07950
973-605-8200
http://www.immunomedics.com

28770
IMMUNOTEC RESEARCH LTD.
300 Joseph Carrier
Vandreuil-Dorion, QC J7V 5V5
450-424-9992
888-917-7779
http://www.immunotec.com

00115
IMPAX LABORATORIES, INC.
30831 Huntwood Ave.
Hayward, CA 95444
510-476-2000
http://www.impaxlabs.com

I. M. S., LTD.
See UCB Pharmaceuticals, Inc.

INAMED CORPORATION
5540 Ekwill Dr.
Santa Barbara, CA 93111
805-683-6761
800-722-2007
http://www.imamed.com

INDEVUS PHARMACEUTICALS, INC.
33 Hayden Ave.
Lexington, MA 02421
781-861-8444
800-370-4742
http://www.indevus.com

INFLABLOC PHARMACEUTICALS, INC.
2401 Foothill Dr.
Salt Lake City, UT 84109-1405
801-464-6100
866-440-7044
http://www.pharmadigm.com

61607, 66934
INKINE PHARMACEUTICAL COMPANY, INC.
See Salix Pharmaceuticals, Inc.

INNER HEALTH GROUP
6203 Woodlake Center
San Antonio, TX 78244
210-661-9257
800-381-4697
http://www.michaelshealth.com

INNOZEN, INC.
6429 Independence Ave.
Woodland Hills, CA 91367
818-593-4880
800-599-8892

INO THERAPEUTICS, INC.
6th State Route 173
Clinton, NJ 08809
908-238-6600
877-566-9466
http://www.inotherapeutics.com

08489
INPHARMA
101 Federal St., Suite 1900
Boston, MA 02110
877-241-8324

63736
INSIGHT PHARMACEUTICALS
Corporate Headquarters
4851 Lake Brook Drive
Glen Allen, VA 23060
804-565-3000
http://www.insmed.com

58441, 63252
INSOURCE
80 Summit View Ln.
Bastian, VA 24314-0009
276-688-0211
800-668-3452
http://www.insourceonline.com

INSPIRE PHARMACEUTICALS, INC.
4222 Emperor Blvd.
Durham, NC 27703
919-941-9777
877-800-4536
http://www.inspirepharm.com

08220
INTEGRA LIFESCIENCES
311 Enterprise Dr.
Plainsboro, NJ 08536
800-654-2873
http://www.integra-ls.com

08478, 64895
INTEGRA LIFESCIENCES CORP
311 Enterprise Dr.
Plainsboro, NJ 08536
800-654-2873
http://www.integra-ls.com

INTEGRATED THERAPEUTICS
See Integrative Therapeutics

88856
INTEGRATIVE HEALTH CONSULTING
655 Redwood Hwy., Suite 225
Mill Valley, CA 94941
415-381-7505
http://www.integrativehealthconsulting.com/

INTEGRATIVE THERAPEUTICS
9755 S.W. Commerce Circle
Wilsonville, OR 97070
800-917-3696
http://www.integrativeinc.com

10922
INTENDIS
340 Changebridge Rd.
Pine Brook, NJ 07058-9714
866-463-3634
http://www.intendis.com/scripts/en/index.php

INTERCHEM CORP.
120 Route 17 North
Paramus, NJ 07652
201-261-7333
800-261-7332
http://www.interchem.com

18968
INTERCURE, INC.
400 Kelby St.
Fort Lee, NJ 07024
201-720-7750
877-988-9388
http://www.intercure.com

54746
INTERFERON SCIENCES
See Hemispherx Biopharma, Inc.

INTERMAX PHARMACEUTICALS, INC.
228 Sherwood Ave.
Farmingdale, NY 11735
631-777-3318

64116
INTERMUNE PHARMACEUTICALS, INC.
3280 Bayshore Blvd.
Brisbane, CA 94005
415-466-2200
http://www.intermune.com

11584
INTERNATIONAL ETHICAL LABS
1021 Americo Miranda Avenue
Metropolitano, San Juan, PR 00921
787-765-3510
800-981-5068
http://www.intetlab.com

00665
INTERNATIONAL LABS
2350 31st St. South
St. Petersburg, FL 33712
727-327-4094
http://www.internationallabs.com

00548
INTERNATIONAL MEDICATION SYSTEMS, LTD.
1886 Santa Anita Avenue
South El Monte, CA 91733
909-908-9484
800-423-4136
http://www.ims-limited.com

INTERNEURON PHARMACEUTICALS, INC.
See Indevus Pharmaceuticals, Inc.

53746
INTERPHARM LTD.
99b Cobbold Rd.
Unit 1, Wellesden
London NW 109SL, UK
020-8830-0803
http://www.interpharm.co.uk

00814
INTERSTATE DRUG EXCHANGE
See Henry Schein, Inc.

INVERESK RESEARCH, INC.
See Charles River Laboratories International, Inc.

38396
INVERNESS MEDICAL INNOVATIONS
51 Sawyer Rd., Suite 200
Waltham, MA 02453-3448
781-647-3900
http://www.invernessmedical.com

00258
INWOOD LABORATORIES
See Forest Laboratories, Inc.

58768
IOLAB PHARMACEUTICALS
See Ciba Vision Corporation

61646
IOMED
See Iopharm

IOP, INC.
3184-B Airway Ave.
Costa Mesa, CA 92626
714-549-1185
800-535-3545
http://www.iopinc.com

61646
IOPHARM
7509 Flagstone St.
Ft. Worth, TX 76118
817-595-5820

54921
IPR PHARMACEUTICALS, INC.
Carolina, PR 00984
787-750-5353
800-477-6385

55688
IPSEN INC.
27 Maple
Milford, MA 01757
508-478-8900
http://www.ipsen.com

ISIS PHARMACEUTICALS
1896 Rutherford Rd.
Carlsbad, CA 92008
760-931-9200
http://www.isispharm.com

ISO-TEX DIAGNOSTICS, INC.
PO Box 909
Friendswood, TX 77546
281-482-1231
800-613-0600
http://www.isotexdiagnostics.com

67425
ISTA PHARMACEUTICALS
15295 Alton Parkway
Irvine, CA 92618
949-788-6000
http://www.istavision.com

IVAX CORPORATION
4400 Biscayne Blvd.
Miami, FL 33137
305-575-6000
800-327-4114
800-545-8800
http://www.ivaxpharmaceuticals.com

13613
IVAX DERMATOLOGICALS
4400 Biscayne Blvd., 11th Flr.
Miami, FL 33137
305-575-4312

IVAX PHARMACEUTICALS, INC.
4400 Biscayne Blvd.
Miami, FL 33137
305-575-6000
800-327-4114
http://www.ivaxpharmaceuticals.com

12126
IVY CORPORATION
299 Fairfield Ave.
Fairfield, NJ 07004
973-575-1990
800-443-8856

16837
J & J MERCK CONSUMER PHARM. CO.
7050 Camp Hill Road
Ft. Washington, PA 19034
215-273-7000
800-523-3484
http://www.jnj.com

49938
JACOBUS PHARMACEUTICAL CO.
37 Cleveland Lane
Princeton, NJ 08540
609-921-7447

10592
JAMOL LABS
13 Ackerman Ave.
Emerson, NJ 07630
201-262-6363

50458
JANSSEN PHARMACEUTICA
1125 Trenton-Harbourton Road
Titusville, NJ 08560
609-730-2000
800-526-7736
http://www.janssen.com

90011
JARROW FORMULAS
1824 S. Robertson Blvd.
Los Angeles, CA 90035
310-204-6936
800-726-0886
http://www.jarrow.com/

JAZZ PHARMACEUTICALS
3180 Porter Dr.
Palo Alto, CA 94304
650-496-3777
http://www.jazzpharmaceuticals.com

68968
JDS PHARMACEUTICALS
122 E. 42nd St., 41st Floor
New York, NY 10168
212-682-4420
http://www.jdspharma.com/

50564
JEROME STEVENS PHARMACEUTICALS, INC.
60 Da Vinci Drive
Bohemia, NY 11234
631-567-1113
800-325-9994

00304
J. J. BALAN, INC.
See HD Smith

25332
LEGERE PHARMACEUTICALS, INC.
7326 E. Evans Road
Scottsdale, AZ 85260
480-991-4033
800-528-3144

12496
LEHN & FINK
See Reckitt Benckiser Pharmaceuticals

05388, 74970, 74980, 59606, 54499
LEINER HEALTH PRODUCTS
901 E 233rd St.
Carson, CA 90745
310-835-8400
800-421-1168
http://www.leiner.com

10551
LEITNER PHARMACEUTICALS
340 Edgemont Ave., Ste. 300
Bristol, TN 37620
866-590-7600
http://www.leitnerpharm.net

00093
LEMMON CO.
See Teva Pharmaceuticals USA

08387
LIBERTY MEDICAL SUPPLY
10045 South Federal Hwy.
Port St. Lucie, FL 34952
http://www.libertymedical.com

00440
LIBERTY PHARMACEUTICAL
10045 South Federal Hwy.
Port St. Lucie, FL 34952
866-836-9936
800-615-0721
http://www.libertymedical.com

53885
LIFESCAN, INC.
1000 Gibraltar Dr.
Milpitas, CA 95035
800-227-8862
http://www.lifescan.com

LIFESIGN LLC
71 Veronica Ave.
Somerset, NJ 08875-0218
800-526-2125
http://www.lifesignmed.com

LIFESTYLE
1800 Route 34 North
Wall Township, NJ 07719
732-972-8585
800-622-7376
http://www.LifestyleCompany.com

64365
LIGAND PHARMACEUTICALS, INC.
10275 Science Center Drive
San Diego, CA 92121
858-550-7500
800-964-5836
http://www.ligand.com

LINCOLN DIAGNOSTICS
PO Box 1128
Decatur, IL 62525
217-877-2531
800-537-1336
http://www.lincolndiagnostics.com

05632
LINE ONE LABORATORIES
21230 Lassen St.
Chatsworth, CA 91311
818-886-2288
800-222-9848
http://www.lineonelabsusa.com

61799
LIPOSOME CO.
See Elan Pharmaceuticals

16110
LIVERITE PRODUCTS INC.
15405 Redhill Ave.
Tustin, CA 92780
888-425-5483
http://www.liverite.com

54859
LLORENS PHARMACEUTICAL
PO Box 720008
Miami, FL 33172
305-716-0595
866-595-5598
http://www.llorenspharm.com

00127
LOBANA LABORATORIES
1614 Industry Ave.
Park Rapids, MN 56470
218-732-2656
800-848-5637
http://www.lobanaproducts.com

34672
LOBOB LABORATORIES
1440 Atteberry Lane
San Jose, CA 95131-1410
408-432-0580
800-835-6262
http://www.loboblabs.com

55390
LOCH PHARMACEUTICALS
See Bedford Laboratories

09198
LOGAN PHARMACEUTICALS
7672 Montgomery Road
Suite 254
Cincinatti, OH 45236
859-344-1340
888-644-3478

08429
LOGIMEDIX
10407 N. Commerce Pkwy.
Miramar, FL 33025
800-821-0047
http://www.logimedix.com

61480
LOMA LUX LABORATORIES
PO Box 702418
Tulsa, OK 74170-2418
918-664-9882
800-316-9636
http://www.lomalux.com

71249
LOREAL SUNCARE RESEARCH
575 Fifth Avenue
New York, NY 10017
212-818-1500
800-322-2036
http://www.lorealusa.com

LOREAL USA
575 Fifth Ave.
New York, NY 10017
212-818-1500
http://www.lorealusa.com

00273
LORVIC CORP.
See Young Dental Mfg.

67754
LOTUS BIOCHEMICAL CORPORATION
See Harvest Pharmaceuticals Inc.

LSI AMERICA CORPORATION
4732 Twin Valley Dr.
Austin, TX 78731
800-720-5936
http://www.ondrox.com

LUITPOLD PHARMACEUTICALS, INC.
1 Luitpold Drive
Shirley, NY 11967
631-924-4000
800-645-1706
http://www.Luitpold.com

10892
LUNSCO
4657 Wurno Rd.
Pulaski, VA 24301
540-980-4358
800-264-8614

68180
LUPIN PHARMA
Harborplace Towers
Baltimore, MD 21202
410-576-2000
http://www.Lupin pharmaceuticals.com

LUYTIES PHARMACAL CO.
PO Box 8080
Richford, VT 63108
800-466-3672
http://www.1-800homeopathy.com

00374
LYNE LABORATORIES
10 Burke Drive
Brockton, MA 02301
508-583-8700
800-525-0450
http://www.lyne.com

LYPHO-MED
3 Pkwy. North
Deerfield, IL 60015-2548
708-317-8800
800-888-7704

58407
MAGNA PHARMACEUTICALS, INC.
11802 Brinley Ave., Suite 201
Louisville, KY 40243
888-206-5525
http://www.magnaweb.com

43292
MAGNO-HUMPHRIES LABORATORIES, INC.
8800 S.W. Commercial Street
Tigard, OR 97223
503-684-5464
http://www.magno-humphries.com

10705
MAJESTIC DRUG
996 Main Street, Route 42
South Fallsburg, NY 12779
845-436-0011
800-238-0220
http://www.majesticdrug.com

00904
MAJOR PHARMACEUTICALS, INC.
The Harvard Drug Group
Livonia, MI 48150
800-875-0123
http://www.harvardlink.com
http://www.harvarddrugs.com

10106
MALLINCKRODT BAKER, INC.
222 Red School Lane
Phillipsburg, NJ 08865
908-859-2151
800-582-2537
http://www.jtbaker.com

MALLINCKRODT CHEMICAL
2nd Street
Hazelwood, MO 63042
314-654-2000
800-325-8888
http://www.mallinckrodt.com

MALLINCKRODT INC.
675 McDonnell Blvd.
Hazelwood, MO 63042
314-654-2000
800-325-8888
http://www.mallinckrodt.com

10706
MANNE
Johns Island, SC 825 29455
843-768-4080
800-517-0228

12539
MARIN PHARMACEUTICALS
See A.G. Marin Pharmaceutical

MARION MERRELL DOW
See Sanofi-Aventis

10135
MARLEX PHARMACEUTICALS, INC.
50 McCullough Drive
New Castle, DE 19720
302-328-3355
http://www.marlexpharm.com

MARLIN INDUSTRIES
Grover City, CA 93483
805-473-2743
800-423-5926

12939
MARLOP PHARMACEUTICALS, INC.
230 Marshall St.
Elizabeth, NJ 07206
908-355-8854

MARLYN NUTRACEUTICALS, INC.
4404 E. Ellwood
Phoenix, AZ 85040
480-991-0200
888-766-4406
http://www.naturally.com

00682
MARNEL PHARMACEUTICALS, INC.
206 Luke Drive
Lafayette, LA 70506
337-232-1396
800-962-7635

00591, 52544
MARSAM PHARMACEUTICALS, INC.
See Watson Pharmaceuticals

52555
MARTEC PHARMACEUTICAL, INC.
1800 N. Topping Avenue
Kansas City, MO 64120
816-241-4144
800-822-6782
http://www.martec-kc.com

11845
MASON VITAMINS, INC.
5105 N.W. 159th Street
Miami Lakes, FL 33014
305-624-5557
888-860-5376
http://www.masonvitamins.com

14362
MASS. PUBLIC HEALTH BIO. LAB.
305 South Street
Jamaica Plains, MA 02130
617-983-6400

53905
MATRIX LABORATORIES, INC.
See Chiron Therapeutics

62750
MATRIXX INITIATIVES, INC.
4742 North 24th St.
Phoenix, AZ 85016
602-385-8888
800-808-4866
http://www.zicam.com

16169
MAYER LABORATORIES
646 Kennedy Street, Building C
Oakland, CA 94606
510-437-8989
800-426-6366
http://www.mayerlabs.com

61703
MAYNE PHARMA (USA) INC.
650 From Road
Paramus, NJ 07652
201-225-5500
866-594-8420
http://www.maynepharma.com/us

MAYO FOUNDATION
200 First Street Southwest
Rochester, MN 55905
507-284-2511
http://www.mayo.edu

00259
MAYRAND, INC.
See Merz Pharmaceuticals

00264
MCGAW, INC.
See B. Braun Medical Inc.

49072
MCGUFF PHARMACEUTICALS, INC.
2921 West MacArthur Blvd.
Santa Ana, CA 92704
714-918-7277
800-603-4795
http://www.mcguff.com

63739, 38703, 49348
MCKESSON DRUG CO.
One Post St.
San Francisco, CA 94101
415-983-8300
800-482-3784
http://www.mckesson.com

MCKESSON MEDICAL-SURGICAL
8741 Landmark Rd.
Richmond, VA 23228
804-264-7500
800-446-3008
http://www.mckgenmed.com

57935
MCNEIL CONSUMER & SPECIALTY PHARMACEUTICALS
7050 Camp Hill Road
Ft. Washington, PA 19034
215-273-7000
800-962-5357
http://www.tylenol.com

00045, 00062
MCNEIL PHARMACEUTICAL
See Ortho-McNeil Pharmaceutical

58605
MCR AMERICAN PHARMACEUTICALS
16255 Aviation Loop
Brooksville, FL 34604
352-754-8587
http://www.mcramerican.com

53014
MD PHARMACEUTICAL
3501 W. Garry Ave.
Santa Ana, CA 92704
714-751-5881

58607
ME PHARMACEUTICALS, INC.
2800 Southeast Pkwy.
Richmond, IN 47375
800-637-4276

MEAD JOHNSON LABORATORIES
See Bristol-Myers Squibb Company

MEAD JOHNSON NUTRITIONALS
2400 West Lloyd Expressway
Evansville, IN 47721-7189
812-429-5000
http://www.meadjohnson.com

00037
MED POINTE HEALTHCARE, INC.
265 Davidson Ave., Ste. 300
Somerset, NJ 08873-4120
732-564-2200
http://www.medpointepharma.com

53276
MED-CHEM PRODUCTS
160 New Boston St.
Woburn, MA 01801
781-932-5900
http://www.crbard.com

45565
MED-DERM PHARMACEUTICALS
See Del-Ray Dermatologicals

53978
MED-PRO, INC.
210 E. 4th Street
Lexington, NE 68850
308-324-4571
800-447-6060
http://www.med-pro-inc.com

MEDAREX, INC.
707 State Rd.
Princeton, NJ 08540
609-430-2880
http://www.medarex.com

11940
MEDCO LAB, INC.
5156 Richmond Road
Bedford Heights, OH 44146
216-292-7546
http://www.medcolabs.com

60793
MEDCO RESEARCH, INC.
See King Pharmaceuticals, Inc.

08212
MEDCON BIOLAB TECHNOLOGIES, INC.
50 Brigham Hill Rd.
Grafton, MA 01519-0196
508-839-4203
800-443-6332
http://www.ilexpaste.com

64253
MEDEFIL, INC
250 Windy Point Dr.
Glendale Heights, IL 60139
630-682-4600
http://www.medefil.com

MEDEGEN
10617 N. Hayden Rd.
Scottsdale, AZ 85260
901-867-2951
800-233-1987
http://www.medegen.com

MEDEVA PHARMACEUTICALS
See UCB Pharmaceuticals, Inc.

MEDI AID CORP.
See Baxa Corporation

00095
MEDI-PLEX PHARM., INC.
See ECR Pharmaceuticals

MEDICAL ACTION INDUSTRIES
800 Prime Place
Hauppauge, NY 11788
631-231-4600
800-645-7042
http://www.medical-action.com

26974
MEDICAL NUTRITION
10 West Forest Avenue
Englewood, NJ 07631
201-569-1188
800-221-0308
http://www.pbsnutrition.com

08271, 28465
MEDICAL PLASTIC DEVICES
161 Oneida Drive
Pointe Claire Quebec, Canada H9R1A9
514-694-9835
888-527-2842
http://www.medplas.com

00576
MEDICAL PRODUCTS PANAMERICANA
647 West Flagler Street
Miami, FL 33130
305-545-6524

65293
(THE) MEDICINES COMPANY
8 Campus Drive
Parsippany, NJ 07054
973-656-1616
800-388-1183
http://www.angiomax.com

99207
MEDICIS PHARMACEUTICAL CORP.
8125 North Hayden Rd.
Scottsdale, AZ 85258-2463
602-808-8800
800-550-5115
http://www.medicis.com

32671
MEDICORE INC.
2647 W. 81st Street
Hialeah, FL 33016
305-558-4000
800-327-8894
http://www.medicore.com

67150
MEDINICHE
167 Lamp & Lantern Village
Chesterfield, MO 63017
314-542-9539
800-711-4303
http://www.mediniche.com

47682
MEDIQUE PRODUCTS CO.
4159 Shoreline Dr.
St. Louis, MO 63045
314-344-1100
800-634-7680
http://www.greenguard.com

38779
MEDISCA INC.
661 Route 3, Unit C
Plattsburgh, NY 12901
518-561-0109
800-932-1039
http://www.medisca.com

MEDISENSE, INC.
See Abbott Diabetes Care

12418
MEDIX PHARMACEUTICALS AMERICAS, INC. (MPA)
See Johnson & Johnson Consumer Products Company

08327
MEDLINE INDUSTRIES
One Medline Place
Mundelein, IL 60060-4486
800-MEDLINE

MEDTECH LABORATORIES, INC.
3510 N. Lake Creek
Jackson, WY 83001
307-733-1680
800-443-4908
http://www.medtechinc.com

MEDTRONIC INC.
710 Medtronic Parkway
Minneapolis, MN 55432-5604
763-514-4000
800-328-2518
http://www.medtronic.com

66116
MEDVANTX, INC.
5810 Nancy Ridge Drive
San Diego, CA 92121
858-625-2990
http://www.medvantx.com

41250
MEIJER
2929 Walker Avenue N.W.
Grand Rapids, MI 49544
616-453-6711
http://www.meijer.com

13143
MELVILLE BIOLOGICS (PRECISION PHARMA SERVICES, INC.)
155 Duryea Rd.
Melville, NY 11747
631-752-7314
http://www.precisionpharma.com

MENICON AMERICA
1840 Gateway Drive
San Mateo, CA 94404
650-378-1424
800-636-4266
http://www.menicon.com

22200
MENNEN CO.
See Colgate-Palmolive Co.

42279
MENPER DISTRIBUTORS, INC.
6500 N.W. 35th Ave.
Miami, FL 33147-7508
305-836-0208
800-560-5223

10742
MENTHOLATUM CO., INC.
707 Sterling Drive
Orchard Park, NY 14127
716-677-2500
800-688-7660
http://www.mentholatum.com

81317
MENTOR UROLOGY
201 Mentor Drive
Santa Barbara, CA 93111
805-879-6000
800-525-0245
http://www.mentorcorp.com

00006
MERCK & CO.
PO Box 100
Whitehouse Station, NJ 08889-100
908-423-1000
http://www.merck.com

00006
MERCK HUMAN HEALTH (A DIVISION OF MERCK & CO.)
770 Sumneytown Pike
West Point, PA 19486
215-652-5000
800-672-6372
http://www.merck.com

62909
MERETEK DIAGNOSTICS, INC.
2655 Crescent Drive
Lafayette, CO 80026
720-479-6400
888-637-3835
http://www.meretek.com

00394
MERICON INDUSTRIES, INC.
8819 N. Pioneer Road
Peoria, IL 61615
309-693-2150
800-242-6464
http://www.mericon-industries.com

62991
MERIDIAN CHEMICAL & EQUIPMENT
1316 Commerce Dr.
Decatur, AL 35601
256-350-1297
800-239-5288
http://www.letcoinc.com

MERIDIAN MEDICAL TECHNOLOGIES
6350 Stevens Forest Rd.
Columbia, MD 21046
443-259-7800
800-638-8093
http://www.meridianmeds.com

30727
MERIT PHARMACEUTICALS
2611 San Fernando Road
Los Angeles, CA 90065
323-227-4831
800-696-3748
http://www.meritpharm.com

00259
MERZ PHARMACEUTICALS
PO Box 18806
Greensboro, NC 27419
336-856-2003
800-637-9872
http://www.merzusa.com

86560
MET-RX USA
90 Orville Dr.
Bohemia, NY 11716
800-556-3879
http://www.met-rx.com

64281
METHAPHARM, INC.
11772 West Sample Rd.
Coral Springs, FL 33065
954-341-0795
800-287-7686
http://www.methapharm.com

08368
METRIKA, INC.
510 Oakmead Pkwy.
Sunnyvale, CA 94085
408-524-2255
877-212-4968
http://www.AlcNow.com

58063
MGI PHARMA, INC.
5775 W. Old Shakopee Rd.
Bloomington, MN 55437
952-346-4700
800-562-5580
http://www.mgipharma.com

MICHIGAN DEPARTMENT OF HEALTH
201 Townsend St.
Lansing, MI 48913
517-373-3740

MICROGENESYS, INC.
See Protein Sciences Corp.

MICRON TECHNOLOGY, INC.
8000 S. Federal Way
Boise, ID 83707
208-368-4000
http://www.micron.com

15686
MIDLAND HEALTHCARE, LLC
1201 Douglas Ave.
Kansas City, KS 66103-1405
913-233-0054

68308
MIDLOTHIAN LABORATORIES
5323 Perimeter Parkway Ct.
Montgomery, AL 36116-5125
334-288-8661
800-344-8661

46672
MIKART, INC.
1750 Chattahoochee Ave.
Atlanta, GA 30318
404-351-4510
888-4MIKART
http://www.mikart.com

00026
MILES, INC.
See Bayer Corp.

00396
MILEX PRODUCTS, INC.
See Cooper Surgical

63020
MILLENNIUM PHARMACEUTICALS, INC.
40 Landsdowne St.
Cambridge, MA 02139
617-679-7000
800-390-5663
http://www.millennium.com

17204
MILLER PHARMACAL GROUP, INC.
350 Randy Road, Suite 2
Carol Stream, IL 60188-1831
630-871-9557
800-323-2935
http://www.millerpharmacal.com

53118
MILLGOOD LABORATORIES, INC.
250 D Arizona Ave.
PO Box 170159
Atlanta, GA 30317
404-377-6538

60307
MINRAD, INC.
847 Main St.
Buffalo, NY 14203
716-855-1068
800-832-3303
http://www.minrad.com

00485
MISEMER PHARMACEUTICALS, INC.
See Edwards Pharmaceuticals, Inc.

00178
MISSION PHARMACAL COMPANY
San Antonio, TX 78230-1355
210-696-8400
800-531-3333
http://www.missionpharmacal.com

MOLNLYCKE HEALTHCARE
826 Newtown-Yardley Road
Newtown, PA 18940
267-685-2000
800-882-4582
http://www.molnlycke.com

04351
MONAGHAN MEDICAL CORPORATION
5 Latour Avenue
Plattsburgh, NY 12901
518-561-7330
800-833-9653
http://www.monaghanmed.com

61570
MONARCH PHARMACEUTICALS
See King Pharmaceuticals

12162
MONTE SANO PHARMACEUTICALS
1406 Wellman Ave., NE
Huntsville, AL 35801-1934
256-518-2449

11868
MONTICELLO DRUG CO.
1604 Stockton Street
Jacksonville, FL 32204-4524
904-384-3666
800-735-0666
http://www.monticellocompanies.com

00839
MOORE MEDICAL CORP.
389 John Downey Dr.
New Britain, CT 06050
800-234-1464
http://www1.mooremedical.com

MOREPEN LABORATORIES LIMITED
Princeton Forrestal Village
Princeton, NJ 08540
609-987-1134
http://www.morepen.com

60432
MORTON GROVE PHARMACEUTICALS, INC.
6451 W. Main St.
Morton Grove, IL 60053
800-346-6854
http://www.mgp-online.com

MORTON INTERNATIONAL
100 Independence Mall West
Philadelphia, PA 19106
215-592-3000
http://www.rohmhaas.com

MORTON SALT
123 N. Wacker Dr.
Chicago, IL 60606
312-807-2000
http://www.mortonsalt.com

MOTHERSOY INTERNATIONAL, INC.
424 S. Kentucky Ave.
Evansville, IN 47714
812-424-5432
888-769-0769
http://www.mothersoy.com

MOVA PHARMACEUTICAL CORPORATION
Caguas, Puerto Rico 00725
787-746-8500
800-468-5201
http://www.movapharm.com

66977
MPM MEDICAL INC.
2301 Crown Ct.
Irving, TX 75038
972-893-4090
800-232-5512
http://www.mpmmedicalinc.com

00150
MURRAY DRUG CORP.
1103 Northwood Drive
Murray, KY 42071
270-753-6654

53489
MUTUAL PHARMACEUTICAL CO., INC.
1100 Orthodox Street
Philadelphia, PA 19124
215-288-6500
800-523-3684
http://www.urlmutual.com

00378
MYLAN PHARMACEUTICALS, INC.
781 Chestnut Ridge Road
Morgantown, WV 26504
304-599-2595
800-796-9526
http://www.mylan.com

59730
NABI
5800 Park of Commerce Blvd. NW
Boca Raton, FL 33487
561-989-5800
800-635-1766
http://www.nabi.com

57459
NASTECH PHARMACEUTICAL CO., INC.
3450 Monte Villa Parkway
Bothell, WA 98021
425-908-3600
http://www.nastech.com

08164
NATIONAL MEDICAL PRODUCTS, INC.
57 Parker Street
Irvine, CA 92618-1605
949-768-1147
http://www.jtip.com

54629
NATIONAL VITAMIN CO., INC.
2075 West Scranton Ave.
Porterville, CA 93257-8358
559-781-8871
800-538-5828
http://www.nationalvitamin.com

NATREN, INC.
3180 Willow Lane
Westlake Village, CA 91361
805-371-4737
800-992-3323
http://www.natren.com

47469
NATROL, INC.
21411 Prairie Street
Chatsworth, CA 91311
818-739-6000
800-262-8765
http://www.natrol.com

NATURALLY VITAMINS CO.
4404 E. Elwood
Phoenix, AZ 85040
602-991-0200
888-766-4406
http://www.naturallyvitamins.com

93265
NATURE'S BEST
550 N. Kingsbury St.
Chicago, IL 60610
312-245-2834
800-551-2544
http://www.naturesbestenzyme.com

74312
NATURE'S BOUNTY, INC.
90 Orville Drive
Bohemia, NY 11716
800-433-2990
http://www.naturesbounty.com

NATURE'S SUNSHINE PRODUCTS, INC.
75 East 1700 South
Provo, UT 84605
801-342-4300
800-223-8225
http://www.naturessunshine.com

NATURE'S WAY
1375 N. Mountain Springs Pkwy.
Springville, UT 84663
801-489-1500
800-926-8883
http://www.naturesway.com

74312
NBTY, INC.
See Nature's Bounty, Inc.

60242
NEIL LABS
55 Lake Drive
East Windsor, NJ 08520
609-448-5500
http://www.neillabs.com

72559
NELLSON NEUTRACEUTICAL
5801 Ayala Ave.
Irwindale, CA 91706
626-812-6522
800-869-1515

NEORX CORP.
300 Elliott Avenue West
Seattle, WA 98119
206-281-7001
http://www.neorx.com

58414
NEOSTRATA
307 College Road East
Princeton, NJ 08540
609-520-0715
800-225-9411
www.neostrata.com

59528
NEPHRO-TECH, INC.
PO Box 16106
Shawnee, KS 66203
785-883-4108
800-879-4755
http://www.nephrotech.com

00487
NEPHRON PHARMACEUTICALS CORP.
4121 S.W. 34th Street
Orlando, FL 32811
407-246-1389
800-433-4313
http://www.nephronpharm.com

NESTLE CLINICAL NUTRITION
800 N. Brand Blvd.
Glendale, CA 91203
847-317-2800
877-463-7853
http://www.nestleclinicalnutrition.com

NESTLE INFANT NUTRITION
Wilkes-Barre, PA 18703
800-284-9488
http://www.verybestbaby.com

62860
NEUREX PHARMACEUTICALS
See Elan Pharmaceuticals

NEUROGENESIS
120 Park Ave.
League City, TX 77573
800-345-8912
http://www.neurogenesis.com

NEUTRACEUTICAL SOLUTIONS, INC.
6704 Ranger Avenue
Corpus Christi, TX 78415
361-854-0755
800-856-7040
http://www.eliquidsolutions.com

10812
NEUTROGENA CORPORATION
5760 W. 96th Street
Los Angeles, CA 90045
310-642-1150
800-582-4048
http://www.neutrogena.com

NEUTRON TECHNOLOGY CORP.
See Micron Technology, Inc.

NEW WORLD TRADING CORP.
879 Spring Park Loop
Kissimmee, FL 34747
407-566-0608

10530
NEXCO PHARMA
PO Box 820023
Houston, TX 77282-0023
713-896-4949
http://www.nexcopharma.com

61958
NEXSTAR PHARMACEUTICALS, INC.
See Gilead Sciences

59016
NICHE PHARMACEUTICALS, INC.
209 N. Oak Street
Roanoke, TX 76262
817-491-2770
800-677-0355
http://www.niche-inc.com

12948
NITROMED
125 Spring St.
Lexington, MA 02421
781-266-4000
http://www.nitromed.com/index.asp

63044
NNODUM CORPORATION
1761 Tennessee Ave.
Cincinnati, OH 45229
513-861-2329
888-301-0457
http://www.zikspain.com

51801
NOMAX, INC.
40 North Rock Hill Road
St. Louis, MO 63119
314-961-2500
800-397-0012
http://www.nomax.com

NORAMCO INC.
1440 Olympic Dr.
Athens, GA 30601
706-353-4400
http://www.noramco.com

59730
NORTH AMERICAN BIOLOGICALS, INC.
See Nabi

62448
NORTH AMERICAN VACCINE, INC.
See Baxter Healthcare Corporation

92942
NORTHERN RESEARCH LABORATORIES, INC.
See Epien Medical

NOSTRUM PHARMACEUTICALS
505 Thornall Street
Edison, NJ 08837
732-635-0036
http://www.nostrumpharma.com

00702
NOVAPLUS
300 Decker Dr
Irvington, TX 75062
214-830-0000

00067.
NOVARTIS CONSUMER HEALTH
See Novartis Pharmaceuticals Corp.

00212, 41679
NOVARTIS MEDICAL NUTRITION
1600 Utica Ave., South
Minneapolis, MN 55416
952-848-6000
800-333-3785
http://www.novartisnutrition.com

58768
NOVARTIS OPHTHALMICS, INC.
See Novartis Pharmaceuticals Corp.

NOVARTIS PHARMA AG
See Novartis Pharmaceuticals Corp.

00078
NOVARTIS PHARMACEUTICALS CORP.
One Health Plaza
East Hanover, NJ 07936
862-778-8300
888-669-6682
http://www.pharma.us.novartis.com

66500
NOVAVAX, INC.
508 Lapp Road
Malvern, PA 19355
484-913-1200
800-340-2001
http://www.novavax.com

NOVEN PHARMACEUTICALS
11960 S.W. 144th Street
Miami, FL 33186
305-253-5099
888-253-5099
http://www.noven.com

00169, 59060
NOVO NORDISK PHARMACEUTICALS
100 College Rd. West
Princeton, NJ 08540
609-987-5800
800-727-6500
http://www.novonordisk-us.com

00093
NOVOPHARM USA, INC.
See Teva Pharmaceuticals USA

NU SKIN ENTERPRISES
One Nu Skin Plaza
Provo, UT 84601
801-345-1000
800-487-1000
http://www.nuskinenterprises.com

NUGYN, INC.
1633 County Highway One
Spring Lake Park, MN 55432
763-398-0108
877-774-1442
http://www.eros-therapy.com

55499
NUMARK LABORATORIES, INC.
164 Northfield Ave.
Edison, NJ 08818
732-417-1870
800-338-8079
http://www.numarklabs.com

NUTRACEA
1261 Hawk's Flight Court
El Dorado Hills, CA 95762
877-723-1700
http://www.nutracea.com

NUTRACEUTICAL SOLUTIONS
6704 Ranger Ave.
Corpus Christi, TX 78415
361-854-0755
800-856-7040
http://www.eliquidsolutions.com

55970
NUTRAMAX LABORATORIES, INC.
2208 Lakeside Blvd.
Edgewood, MD 21040
410-776-4000
800-925-5187
http://www.nutramaxlabs.com

NUTRAMAX PRODUCTS
51 Blackburn Dr.
Gloucester, MA 01930
978-282-1800
http://www.nutramax.com

NUTRI VENTION
6203 Woodlake Center
San Antonio, TX 78244
210-661-8589
800-390-7940

49735
NUTRICIA NORTH AMERICA
PO Box 117
Gaithersburg, MD 20884-0117
301-795-2300
800-636-2283
http://www.shsna.com

NUTRITION 21
4 Manhattanville Rd.
Purchase, NY 10577
914-701-4500
800-696-0860
http://www.nutrition21.com

00407
NYCOMED AMERSHAM
See GE Healthcare

11169
OAKHURST CO.
3000 Hempstead Turnpike
Levittown, NY 11756
516-731-5380
800-831-1135
http://www.oakhurst-medicine.com

55515, 80831.
OCLASSEN PHARMACEUTICALS, INC.
See Watson Pharmaceuticals

21406, 55056
O'CONNOR, INC.
See Columbia Laboratories, Inc.

67467
OCTAPHARMA USA, INC.
5885 Trinity Pkwy., Suite 350
Centerville, VA 20120
800-826-6905

65473
ODYSSEY PHARMACEUTICALS, INC.
72 Eaglerock Ave.
East Hanover, NJ 07932
877-427-9068
http://www.odysseypharm.com

51660
OHM LABORATORIES, INC.
1385 Livingston
New Brunswick, NJ 08902
877-646-5227
http://www.ohmlabs.com

OMNII ORAL PHARMACEUTICALS
1500 North Florida Mango Road
West Palm Beach, FL 33409
561-689-1140
800-445-3386
http://www.4oralcare.com

ONY, INC.
1576 Sweet Home Road
Amherst, NY 14228
716-636-9096
877-274-4669

11916, 64108
OPTICS LABORATORY, INC.
9480 Telstar Ave. #3
El Monte, CA 91731
626-350-1926
800-968-6788
http://www.opticslab.com

OPTIKEM INTERNATIONAL
2172 Jason Street
Denver, CO 80223
303-936-1136
800-525-1752

63369
OPTIMED CONTROLLED RELEASE LAB
2223 Killion Ave.
Seymour, IN 47274
812-524-0534

50520
OPTIMOX CORP.
PO Box 3378
Torrance, CA 90510-3378
310-618-9370
800-223-1601
http://www.optimox.com

00041
ORAL-B LABORATORIES
1 Gillette Park
South Boston, MA 02127-1096
800-566-7252
http://www.oral-b.com

65976
ORAPHARMA, INC.
732 Louis Dr.
Warminster, PA 18974
215-956-2200
866-273-7846
http://www.orapharma.com

ORASURE TECHNOLOGIES
220 East First St.
Bethlehem, PA 18015
610-882-1820
800-869-3535
http://www.orasure.com

ORGANOGENESIS INC.
150 Dan Rd.
Canton, MA 02021
781-575-0775
http://www.organogenesis.com

00052
ORGANON, INC.
56 Livingston Ave.
Roseland, NJ 07068
973-325-4500
800-631-1253
http://www.organon-usa.com

ORGANON TEKNIKA CORP.
See Biomerieux

62161
ORPHAN MEDICAL, INC.
See Jazz Pharmaceuticals

66607
ORPHAN PHARMACEUTICALS USA
See Rare Disease Therapeutics

ORTHO BIOTECH PRODUCTS, L.P.
430 Route 22 East
Bridgewater, NJ 08807-0914
908-541-4000
800-325-7504
http://www.orthobiotech.com

00562
ORTHO-CLINICAL DIAGNOSTICS
100 Indigo Creek Dr.
Rochester, NY 14626
800-828-6316
http://www.orthoclinical.com

00062
ORTHO-MCNEIL PHARMACEUTICAL
1000 Route 202 South
Raritan, NJ 08869
800-631-5273
800-526-7736
http://www.ortho-mcneil.com

ORTHO NEUTROGENA
199 Grandview Rd.
Skillman, NJ 08558
800-426-7762
http://www.orthoneutrogena.com

67707
OSCIENT PHARMACEUTICALS
1000 Winter
Waltham, MA 02451
781-398-2300
http://www.oscient.com

65231
OSI PHARMACEUTICALS
58 S. Service Rd.
Melville, NY 11747
631-962-2000
800-572-1932
http://www.osip.com

10244
OTIS CLAPP & SONS INC.
115 Shawmut Road
Canton, MA 02021
781-821-5400
800-777-5400
http://www.otisclapp.com

59148
OTSUKA AMERICA PHARMACEUTICAL, INC.
2440 Research Blvd.
Rockville, MD 20850
301-990-0030
800-562-3974
http://www.otsuka.com

67386
OVATION PHARMACEUTICALS, INC.
Four Parkway North
Deerfield, IL 60015
847-282-1000
888-514-5204
http://www.ovationpharma.com

08470, 08214
OWEN MUMFORD INC.
1755 West Oak Commons Ct.
Marietta, GA 30062
770-977-2226
800-421-6936
http://www.owenmumford.com

64803
OXFORD PHARMACEUTICAL SERVICES, INC.
1 US Highway 46 West
Totowa, NJ 07512
973-256-0600
http://www.oxfordpharm.com

OXIS INTERNATIONAL
323 B Vintage Park Dr.
Foster City, CA 94404
650-212-2568
800-547-3686
http://www.oxisresearch.com

P & S LABORATORIES, INC.
See Standard Homeopathic Co.

60758
PACIFIC PHARMA
Irvine, CA 92623
714-246-4600

16571
PACK PHARMACEUTICALS, LLC
1110 W. Lake Cook Rd.
Buffalo Grove, IL 60089
734-743-7007
800-821-5340
http://www.packpharma.com

00574
PADDOCK LABORATORIES
3940 Quebec Ave. North
Minneapolis, MN 55427
763-546-4676
800-328-5113
http://www.paddocklabs.com

38142
PAL MIDWEST LTD
1030 S. Main St.
Rockford, IL 61101-1418
815-965-2981

25294
PALCO LABS
360 El Pueblo Road, Suite 102
Scotts Valley, CA 95066
831-430-1600
800-346-4488
www.palcolabs.com

00516
PALISADES PHARMACEUTICALS, INC.
See Glenwood, Inc.

16477
PALMETTO PHARMACEUTICALS, INC.
2131 Woodruff Rd. Suite 2100 #315
Greenville, NC 29607
864- 313-9003

00525
PAMLAB, LLC
4099 Highway 190
Covington, LA 70433
985-893-4097
http://www.pamlab.com

PAN AMERICAN LABORATORIES
See Pamlab, LLC

49884
PAR PHARMACEUTICAL, INC.
300 Tice Blvd.
Woodcliff Lake, NJ 07667
201-802-4000
800-828-9393
http://www.parpharm.com

66758
PARENTA PHARMACEUTICALS, INC.
Three Southern Court
West Columbia, SC 29169
803-461-5500
800-892-3676
http://www.parentarx.com

PARKE-DAVIS - A PFIZER COMPANY
See Pfizer US Pharmaceutical Group

64029
PARKEDALE PHARMACEUTICALS
See King Pharmaceuticals, Inc.

00341
PARKER LABORATORIES, INC.
286 Eldridge Rd.
Fairfield, NJ 07004
973-276-9500
800-631-8888
http://www.parkerlabs.com

50930
PARNELL PHARMACEUTICALS, INC.
1525 Francisco Blvd
San Rafael, CA 94901
415-256-1800
800-457-4276
http://www.parnellpharm.com

49309
PARTHENON CO., INC.
3311 West 2400 South
Salt Lake City, UT 84119
801-972-5184
800-453-8898
http://www.parthenoninc.com

00418, 11098
PASADENA RESEARCH LABS
See Akorn, Inc.

10866
PASCAL CO., INC.
2929 N.E. Northup Way
Bellevue, WA 98004
425-827-4694
800-426-8051
http://www.pascaldental.com

PATHEON
7070 Mississauga Rd.
Mississauga, Ontario LN5 7J8
905-821-4001
888-728-4366
http://www.patheon.com

10147
PATRIOT PHARMACEUTICALS LLC
4060 Butler Pike
Plymouth Meeting, PA 19462
215-273-7676

PBI (PHARMACEUTICAL BASICS, INC.)
See Upsher-Smith Labs, Inc.

66213
PBM PHARMACEUTICALS
Linney House
Gordonsville, VA 22942
540-832-3282
800-485-9828
http://www.pbmproducts.com

55289
PD-RX PHARMACEUTICALS, INC.
727 North Ann Arbor
Oklahoma City, OK 73127
405-942-3040
800-299-7379
http://www.pdrx.com

66346
PEDIAMED PHARMACEUTICALS, INC.
7310 Turfway Rd., Suite 490
Florence, KY 41042
859-282-8582
866-543-6337
http://www.pediamedpharma.com

PEDIATRIC PHARMACEUTICALS
120 Wood Ave South, Suite 300
Iselin, NJ 08830
732-603-7708
http://www.pediatricpharm.com

00884
PEDINOL PHARMACAL, INC.
30 Banfi Plaza North
Farmingdale, NY 11735
631-293-9500
800-733-4665
http://www.pedinol.com

10974
PEGASUS LABORATORIES, INC.
8809 Ely Rd.
Pensacola, FL 32514
850-478-2770
http://www.pegasuslabs.com

25074
PENEDERM, INC.
See Mylan Pharmaceuticals, Inc.

13893
PENN LABORATORIES
130 Vintage Dr.
Huntsville, AL 35811
877-300-6153
http://www.pennlaboratories.com

60432
PENNEX PHARMACEUTICAL, INC.
See Morton Grove Pharmaceuticals, Inc.

PENTECH PHARMACEUTICALS, INC.
3315 Algonquin Road
Rolling Meadows, IL 60008
847-255-0303
http://www.pentechinc.com

00113
PERRIGO COMPANY
515 Eastern Ave.
Allegan, MI 49010
269-673-8451
800-719-9260
http://www.perrigo.com

00096
PERSON AND COVEY, INC.
616 Allen Ave.
Glendale, CA 91201
818-240-1030
800-423-2341
http://www.personandcovey.com

PERSONAL PRODUCTS COMPANY
199 Grandview Rd.
Skillman, NJ 08558
908-218-8625
800-582-6097
http://www.jnj.com

00927
PFEIFFER CO.
71 University Avenue SW
Atlanta, GA 30315
404-614-0255
800-342-6450
http://www.pfeifferpharmaceuticals.com

12547
PFIZER CONSUMER HEALTH
235 E. 42nd Street
New York, NY 10017
800-223-0182
http://www.pfizer.com

PFIZER US PHARMACEUTICAL GROUP
235 E. 42nd Street
New York, NY 10017
800-438-1985
888-474-3099
800-382-7219
http://www.pfizer.com

PHARMA FRONTIERS
2635 N. Crescent Ridge Dr.
The Woodlands, TX 77381
281-775-0609
http://www.pharmafrontier.com

62441
PHARMA MEDICA
966 Pantera Drive, Unit 31
Mississauga, Ontario L4W 2S1
905-624-9115
http://www.pharmamedica.com

52959
PHARMA PAC
513 Sandydale Drive
Nipomo, CA 93444
805-929-1333
800-841-5554
http://www.pharmapac.com

39822
PHARMA-TEK, INC.
See X-Gen Pharmaceuticals, Inc.

00121
PHARMACEUTICAL ASSOCIATES, INC.
201 Delaware St.
Greenville, SC 29605
864-277-7282
800-845-8210
http://www.pa-inc.net

PHARMACEUTICAL BASICS, INC.
See Upsher-Smith Labs, Inc.

51655
PHARMACEUTICAL CORP OF AMERICA (PCA)
6210 Technology Center Dr.
Indianapolis, IN 46278
317-616-4498
800-722-0772

21659
PHARMACEUTICAL LABS, INC.
See Neutraceutical Solutions, Inc.

45334
PHARMACEUTICAL SPECIALTIES, INC.
PO Box 6298
Rochester, MN 55903
507-288-8500
800-325-8232
http://www.psico.com

12547
PHARMACIA & UPJOHN CONSUMER HEALTHCARE (A DIVISION OF PFIZER)
See Pfizer Consumer Health

PHARMACIA CORP. (A DIVISION OF PFIZER)
See Pfizer US Pharmaceutical Group

63704
PHARMACIST PHARMACEUTICAL LLC
3229 Brandon Ave.
Roanoke, VA 24018
540-981-1004

00462
PHARMADERM
3237 Satellite Blvd.
Duluth, GA 30096
678-287-1500
866-337-6457
http://www.pharmaderm.com

55422, 65937
PHARMAKON LABS
6050 Jet Port Industrial Blvd.
Tampa, FL 33634
813-886-3216
800-888-4045
http://www.pharmakonlabs.com

15035
PHARMANEX
75 West Center Street
Provo, UT 84601
801-345-9800
http://www.pharmanex.com

51817
PHARMASCIENCE LAB
6111 Ave Royalmount
Montreal, Quebec H4P 2T4
514-340-9800
800-363-8805
http://www.pharmascience.com

48107
PHARMASSURE, INC.
200 Newbury Commons
Edders, PA 19319-9363
717-761-2633
http://www.gnc.com

31604, 78742
PHARMAVITE
PO Box 9606
Mission Hills, CA 91346-9606
818-221-6200
800-423-2405
http://www.pharmavite.com

53002
PHARMEDIX
3281 Whipple Rd.
Union City, CA 94587-1218
800-486-1811
http://www.pharmedixrx.com

66663
PHARMELLE
170 S. William Dillard Drive
Gilbert, AZ 85233
480-926-5369
877-577-2577
http://www.pharmelle.com

00813
PHARMICS, INC.
PO Box 27554
Salt Lake City, UT 84127-0554
801-966-4138
800-456-4138
http://www.pharmics.com

67211
PHARMION CORPORATION
2525 28th Street
Boulder, CO 80301
720-564-9100
866-742-7646
http://www.pharmion.com

54348
PHARMPAK, INC.
1221 Anderson Drive
San Rafael, CA 94901
415-455-9981
800-541-6315
http://www.pharmpakinc.com

PHOENIX LABORATORIES
200 Adams Blvd.
Farmingdale, NY 11735
516-822-1230

PHOTOMEDEX
147 Keystone Drive
Montgomeryville, PA 18936
215-619-3600
http://www.photomedex.com

54868
PHYSICIANS TOTAL CARE
5415 S. 125th East Avenue
Tulsa, OK 74146
918-254-2273
800-759-3650
http://www.physicianstotalcare.com

PHYTOPHARMICA, INC.
825 Challenger Dr.
Green Bay, WI 54311
920-469-1313
800-553-2370
http://www.enzy.com

60831
PIERRE FABRE PHARMACEUTICALS
9 Campus Dr.
Parsippany, NJ 07054
973-898-1042
http://www.pierre-fabre.com

PLAYTEX CO.
300 Nyala Farm Road
Wesport, CT 06880
800-222-0453
http://www.playtex.com

50111
PLIVA, INC.
72 Eagle Rock Ave.
East Hanover, NJ 07936
973-386-5566
800-922-0547
http://www.plivainc.com

41100, 11523
PLOUGH, INC.
See Schering-Plough Healthcare Products

37864
PLUS PHARMA
87 Modular Ave.
Commack, NY 11725
631-543-3334

50991
POLY PHARMACEUTICALS, INC.
200 N. Archusa Ave.
Quitman, MS 39355
601-776-3497
800-882-1041

POLYMEDICA CORPORATION
701 Edgewater
Wakefield, MA 01880
781-933-2020
800-886-4050
http://www.polymedica.com

POLYMEDICA PHARMACEUTICALS
See Amerifit Pharma, Inc.

47144
POLYMER TECHNOLOGY CORP.
100 Research Drive
Wilmington, MA 01887
978-658-6111
800-323-0000
http://www.polymer.com

08193
POLYMER TECHNOLOGY SYSTEMS (A DIVISION OF BAUSCH & LOMB)
100 Research Dr.
Wilmington, MA 01887
978-658-6111
800-323-0000
www.polymer.com

49963
PORTAL PHARMACEUTICAL
67E Mendez Vigo
Myaguez, PR 00680 126 00681
787-832-6645

55688
PORTON PRODUCT LIMITED
See Ipsen Inc.

POWDERJECT VACCINES
See Chiron Therapeutics

POYTHRESS
See ECR Pharmaceuticals

68158
PRAECIS PHARMACEUTICALS INCORPORATED
830 Winter St.
Waltham, MA 02451-1420
781-795-4100
http://www.praecis.com

66993
PRASCO LABORATORIES
7155 E. Kemper Rd.
Cincinnati, OH 45249
513-618-3333
866-525-0688
http://www.prasco.com

PRATT PHARMACEUTICALS
See Pfizer US Pharmaceutical Group

68094
PRECISION DOSE, INC.
722 Progressive Lane
South Beloit, IL 61080

75137
PRESTIGE BRANDS INTERNATIONAL
3510 N. Lake Creek Dr.
Wilson, WY 83014
914-524-6810
800-803-4471
http://www.prestigebrands.com

66378
PRESUTTI LABORATORIES
1685 Winetka Circle
Rolling Meadows, IL 60008
847-788-9192
http://www.presuttilabs.com

00684
PRIMEDICS LABORATORIES
14131 S. Avalon
Los Angeles, CA 90061
323-770-3005

68040
PRIMUS PHARMACEUTICALS, INC.
4725 N. Scottsdale Road
Scottsdale, AZ 85251
480-483-1410
http://www.primusrx.com

PRINCETON PHARM. PRODUCTS
See Bristol-Myers Squibb Company

PRIORITY HEALTHCARE
See Curascript

PROCTER & GAMBLE CO.
1 Procter & Gamble Plaza
Cincinnati, OH 45202-3314
513-983-1100
800-543-7270
http://www.pg.com

00149
PROCTER & GAMBLE PHARMACEUTICALS
8500 Governors Hill Dr.
Cincinnati, OH 45249
800-448-4878
http://www.pg.com

PROCYTE CORPORATION
8511 154th Avenue NE
Redmond, WA 98052-3557
425-869-1239
http://www.procyte.com

66869
PROETHIC PHARMACEUTICALS, INC.
5331 Perimeter Parkway Court
Montgomery, AL 36116
334-288-1288
http://www.proethic.com

66375
PROMEDICA LABS, INC.
209 McLean Blvd
Patterson, NJ 07504
973-925-1001

65483
PROMETHEUS LABORATORIES, INC.
5739 Pacific Center Boulevard
San Diego, CA 92121
858-824-0895
888-423-5227
http://www.prometheuslabs.com

67555
PRONOVA CORPORATION
7440 SW 59th Terrace, Suite 105
Miami, FL 33155
305-666-4831
866-703-3508
http://www.pronovacorp.com

50313
PROPHARMA
7760 N.W. 56th St.
Miami, FL 33166
305-592-9216
800-446-0255

65581
PROPST PHARMACEUTICALS
130 Vintage Dr.
Huntsville, AL 35811
256-704-6394

PROTEIN DESIGN LABS, INC.
34801 Campus Dr.
Fremont, CA 94555
510-574-1400
http://www.pdl.com

PROTEIN SCIENCES CORP.
1000 Research Pkwy.
Meriden, CT 06450
203-686-0800
800-488-7099
http://www.proteinsciences.com

PROTHERICS INC.
5214 Maryland Way
Brentwood, TN 37027
615-327-1027
888-327-1027
http://www.protherics.com

16241
PRX PHARM
See Par Pharmaceutical, Inc.

PSYCHEMEDICS CORP.
125 Nagog Park
Acton, MA 01720
978-206-8220
800-628-8073
http://www.psychemedics.com

65005
PTS LABORATORIES, INC.
8100 Secura Way
Santa Fe Springs, CA 90670
562-907-3607
http://www.ptsgeolabs.com

65005
PTS LABS INTERNATIONAL, INC.
4342 West 12th St.
Houston, TX 77055
713-680-2291
http://www.ptsgeolabs.com

00034
PURDUE FREDERICK CO.
One Stamford Forum
Stamford, CT 06901-3431
203-588-8000
800-877-5666
http://www.purduepharma.com

59011
PURDUE PHARMA
One Stamford Forum
201 Tresser Blvd.
Stamford, CT 06901
203-588-8000
800-877-5666
http://www.purduepharma.com

PURILENS, INC.
See Lifestyle

PURITANS PRIDE
1233 Montauk Highway
Oakdale, NY 11769-9001
800-645-9584
http://www.puritan.com

Q-PHARMA, INC.
2572 Brunswick Pike
Lawrenceville, NJ 08648
609-883-1818

QLT, INC.
887 Great Northern Way
Vancouver, British Columbia V5T 4T5
604-707-7000
800-663-5486
http://www.qltinc.com

QLT USA, Inc.
2579 Midpoint Drive
Ft. Collins, CO 80525
604-872-7881
800-663-5486
http://www.qlt-pdt.com

QUALICAPS, INC.
6505 Franz Warner Pkwy.
Whitsett, NC 27377
336-449-3900
800-227-7853
http://www.qualicaps.com

52917
QUALIS, INC
4600 Park Ave.
Des Moines, IA 50321-1237
515-243-3000

00603
QUALITEST PHARMACEUTICALS
130 Vintage Dr.
Huntsville, AL 35811
256-859-4011
800-444-4011

49999
QUALITY CARE PHARM, INC.
See Quality Care Products, LLC

49999
QUALITY CARE PRODUCTS, LLC
6061 Telegraph Road
Toledo, OH 43612
419-478-0441
http://www.qctmeds.com

63004
QUESTCOR PHARMACEUTICALS, INC.
3260 Whipple Rd.
Union City, CA 94587
510-400-0700
800-411-3065
http://www.questcor.com

QUIDEL CORP.
10165 McKellar Court
San Diego, CA 92121
858-552-1100
800-874-1517
http://www.quidel.com

61941
QUIGLEY CORP.
621 N. Shady Retreat Road
Doylestown, PA 18901
267-880-1100
http://www.quigley.com

54391
R & D LABORATORIES, INC.
See Watson Pharmaceuticals

17236
R & S NORTHEAST
256 Geiger Road
Philadelphia, PA 19115
215-673-7770
800-262-7770
http://www.rssalesllc.com

12830
R. A. MCNEIL COMPANY
1150 Latta Street
Chattanooga, TN 37406
423-493-9170
800-755-3038

RAINBOW LIGHT NUTRITIONAL SYSTEMS
125 McPherson St.
Santa Cruz, CA 95060
831-420-2660
800-635-1233

63304
RANBAXY PHARMACEUTICALS INC.
600 College Road East
Princeton, NJ 08540
609-720-9200
http://www.ranbaxy.com

RANDOB LABORATORIES, LTD.
PO Box 440
Cornwall, NY 12518
845-534-2197

66607
RARE DISEASE THERAPEUTICS
1101 Kermit Drive
Nashville, TN 37217
615-399-0700
http://www.raretx.com

12496
RECKITT BENCKISER PHARMACEUTICALS
10710 Midlothian Turnpike
Richmond, VA 23235
804-379-1090
800-444-7599

10952
RECSEI LABORATORIES
330 S. Kellogg, Bldg. M
Goleta, CA 93117-3875
805-964-2912

52380, 18407
REDI-PRODUCTS LABS, INC.
50 East Industrial Rd.
Branford, CT 06405
203-481-5000
800-760-3236

00091
REED & CARNRICK
See Schwarz Pharma

10956
REESE PHARMACEUTICAL CO., INC.
10617 Frank Ave.
Cleveland, OH 44106
800-321-7178
http://www.reesepharmaceutical.com

REGENERON PHARMACEUTICALS
777 Old Saw Mill River Road
Tarrytown, NY 10591
914-345-7400
http://www.regeneron.com

66779
REGENT LABS, INC.
700 W. Hillsboro Blvd #2-206
Deerfield Beach, FL 33441
800-872-1525
http://www.regentlabs.com

65726
RELIANT PHARMACEUTICALS
110 Allen Rd.
Liberty Corner, NJ 07938
908-580-1200
800-205-0180
http://www.reliantrx.com

REMEL, INC.
12076 Santa Fe Drive
Lenexa, KS 66215
800-255-6730
http://www.remel.com

67066
REPLIGEN CORP.
41 Seyon Street
Waltham, MA 02453
781-250-0111
800-622-2259
http://www.repligen.com

10961
REQUA, INC.
See W. F. Young, Inc.

00433
RESEARCH INDUSTRIES CORP.
See Edwards Lifescience

RESEARCH TRIANGLE INSTITUTE
PO Box 12194
Research Triangle Park, NC 27709
919-541-6000
http://www.rti.org

67492
RESICAL INC.
PO Box 489
Orchard Park, NY 14127
800-204-6434
http://www.resical.com/

60575
RESPA PHARMACEUTICALS, INC.
PO Box 88222
Carol Stream, IL
630-543-3333

08373
RESPIRONICS
1010 Murry Ridge Lane
Murrysville, PA 15668
724-387-4000
800-345-6443
http://www.respironics.com

00122
REXALL GROUP
See Rexall Sundown, Inc.

30768
REXALL SUNDOWN, INC.
851 Broken Sound Pkwy., NW
Boca Raton, FL 33487
561-241-9400
800-327-0908
http://www.rexallsundown.com

54092
REXAR PHARMACEUTICALS
396 Rockaway Ave.
PO Box 397
Valley Stream, NY 11582
516-561-7662

RH PHARMACEUTICALS, INC.
See Cangene Corp.

RHONE-POULENC RORER CONSUMER, INC.
See Sanofi-Aventis

RHONE-POULENC RORER PHARMACEUTICALS, INC.
See Sanofi-Aventis

RICHARDSON-VICKS, INC.
See Procter & Gamble Pharmaceuticals

RICHIE PHARMACAL, INC.
119 State Ave.
Glasgow, KY 42141
502-651-6159
800-627-0250
http://www.richiepharmacal.com

00115
RICHLYN LABORATORIES, INC.
See Global Pharmaceuticals, Inc.

54738
RICHMOND PHARMACEUTICALS
3510 Mayland Court
Richmond, VA 23233
804-270-4498

RICOLA USA, INC.
51 Gibraltar Drive
Morris Plains, NJ 07950
973-984-6811
http://www.ricolausa.com

54807
R. I. D, INC.
609 North Mednik Avenue
Los Angeles, CA 90022-1326
323-268-0635

R. I. J. PHARMACEUTICAL CORP.
40 Commercial Ave.
Middletown, NY 10941
845-692-5799
http://www.rijpharm.com

64980
RISING PHARM
411 Sette Drive, #N3
Paramus, NJ 07652
201-262-4200
http://www.risingpharma.com

68032
RIVER'S EDGE PHARMACEUTICAL
5400 Laurel Springs Pkwy.
Suwanee, GA 30024
770-886-3417

54092
ROBERTS PHARMACEUTICAL CORP.
See Shire US, Inc.

50924
ROCHE DIAGNOSTIC SYSTEMS, INC.
See Roche Laboratories

00004
ROCHE LABORATORIES
340 Kingsland Street
Nutley, NJ 07110-1199
973-235-5000
800-526-6367
http://www.rocheusa.com

66358
RODLEN LABORATORIES
100 Fairway Drive
Vernon Hills, IL 60061
847-362-8200

ROERIG
See Pfizer US Pharmaceutical Group

67546
ROMARK LABORATORIES
3000 Bayport Drive
Tampa, FL 33607
813-282-8544
http://www.romark.com

ROSEMONT PHARMACEUTICAL CORP.
See Upsher-Smith Labs, Inc.

70074
ROSS PRODUCTS DIVISION, ABBOTT LABS
625 Cleveland Ave
Columbus, OH 43215-1724
800-986-8510
http://www.ross.com

00054
ROXANE LABORATORIES, INC.
PO Box 16352
Columbus, OH 43216
800-962-8364
http://www.roxane.com

00591, 52544
ROYCE LABORATORIES, INC.
See Watson Laboratories

R. P. SCHERER CARDINAL HEALTH
14 Schoolhouse Road
Somerset, NJ 08873
732-537-6200
http://www.cardinal.com

00536
RUGBY LABS, INC.
1810 Peachtree Industrial Blvd
Duluth, GA 30097
951-493-5300
800-645-2158
http://www.watson.com

61972
RUGER CHEMICAL CO.
1515 W. Blanckey St.
Linden, NJ 07036
973-926-0331
800-274-7843
http://www.rugerchemical.com

66794, 08367
RX ELITE
1404 N. Main Street
Meridian, ID 83642
208-288-5550
800-414-1901
http://www.rxelite.com

59243
SAGE PHARMACEUTICALS
5408 Interstate Ave.
Shreveport, LA 71109
318-635-1594

53462, 08513
SAGE PRODUCTS
3909 Three Oaks Rd.
Cary, IL 60013
815-455-4700
800-323-2220
http://www.sageproducts.com/

65649
SALIX PHARMACEUTICALS, INC.
1700 Perimeter Park Dr.
Morrisville, NC 27560
919-862-1000
866-669-7597
http://www.salix.com

00067
SANDOZ CONSUMER
See Novartis Pharmaceuticals Corp.

00781, 00067
SANDOZ PHARMACEUTICALS - SANDOZ CONSUMER
506 Carnegie Center Dr.
Princeton, NJ 08540
609-627-8500
800-525-8747
http://www.us.sandoz.com

62053
SANGSTAT MEDICAL CORP.
See Genzyme Transplant

65597
SANKYO PHARMA
Two Hilton Court
Parsippany, NJ 07054
973-359-2600
877-472-6596
http://www.sankyopharma.com

00024
SANOFI-AVENTIS
300 Somerset Corporate Blvd.
Bridgewater, NJ 08807
800-207-8049
800-633-1610
908-243-6000
800-223-1062
http://www.sanofi-aventis.com/us

49281
SANOFI PASTEUR
Discovery Drive
Swiftwater, PA 18370
570-839-7187
800-822-2463
http://www.vaccineshoppe.com

SANOFI-SYNTHELABO, INC.
See Sanofi-Aventis

00024
SANOFI WINTHROP PHARMACEUTICALS
90 Park Ave.
New York, NY 10016
212-551-4000
800-446-6267
800-223-1062

68012
SANTARUS
10590 West Ocean Air Drive
Suite 200
San Diego, CA 92130
858-314-5701
http://www.santarus.com

65086
SANTEN, INC.
555 Gateway Rd.
Napa, CA 94558
707-254-1750
800-611-2011
http://www.santeninc.com

00281
SAVAGE LABORATORIES
60 Baylis Rd.
Melville, NY 11747 2006
631-454-9071
800-231-0206
http://www.savagelabs.com

54396
SAVIENT PHARMACEUTICALS, INC.
One Tower Center
East Brunswick, NJ 08816
732-418-9300
800-284-2480
http://www.savient.com

46500
S C JOHNSON
1525 Howe Street
Racine, WI 53403
262-260-2000
800-494-4855
http://www.scjohnson.com

SCANDINAVIAN FORMULAS, INC.
140 East Church St.
Sellersville, PA 18960
215-453-2507
800-688-2276
http://www.scandinavianformulas.com

SCHAFFER LABORATORIES
3128 Pacific Coast Hwy. #98
Torrance, CA 90505
310-325-4200
800-231-6725
http://www.schafferlabs.com

52544
SCHEIN PHARMACEUTICAL, INC.
See Watson Laboratories

00274
SCHERER LABORATORIES, INC.
2301 Ohio Dr. Suite 234
Plano, TX 75093
972-612-6225
800-449-8290

00085
SCHERING-PLOUGH CORP.
PO Box 599
Kenilworth, NJ 07033
908-298-4000
800-842-4090
http://www.sphcp.com

41000, 11523
SCHERING-PLOUGH HEALTHCARE PRODUCTS
2000 Galloping Hill Rd.
Kenilworth, NJ 07033-0533
908-298-4000
800-842-4090
http://www.sphcp.com

20525
SCHIFF NUTRITION INTERNATIONAL, INC.
2002 South 5070 West
Salt Lake City, UT 84104
801-975-5000
800-435-3948
http://www.schiffnutrition.com

00234, 02340
SCHMID PRODUCTS CO.
See Durex Consumer Products

41000, 11523
SCHOLL, INC.
See Schering-Plough Healthcare Products

00091
SCHWARZ PHARMA
PO Box 2038
Milwaukee, WI 53201
800-558-5114
http://www.schwarzusa.com

SCHWARZKOPF & DEP INC.
1063 McGaw Ave.
Irvine, CA 92614
800-326-2855
http://www.henkel.com

SCICLONE PHARMACEUTICALS, INC.
901 Mariner's Island Blvd.
San Mateo, CA 94404
650-358-3456
http://www.sciclone.com

66239
SCIENTIFIC LABORATORIES INC
9702 Philadelphia Way
Lanham, MD 20706
301-731-0098

65847
SCIOS INC.
6500 Paseo Padre Parkway
Fremont, CA 94555
510-248-2500
http://www.sciosinc.com

00372
SCOT-TUSSIN PHARMACAL, INC.
32 West Hamden Rd.
Cranston, RI 02920
401-942-8555
800-638-7268
http://www.scot-tussin.com

00905
SCS PHARMACEUTICALS
PO Box 5110
Chicago, IL 60680
800-323-1603
800-323-1603
http://www.monsanto.com

66424
SDA LABORATORIES
280 Railroad Ave.
Greenwich, CT 06830
203-861-0005

08471
SEA-BAND
15 Vernon Avenue, Unit 6
Newport, RI 02840-0991

SEARLE
See Pfizer US Pharmaceutical Group

15127
SELECT BRAND
3017 N. Midland Dr
Pine Bluff, AR 71603
870-535-3635

63402
SEPRACOR
84 Waterford Dr.
Marlborough, MA 01752
508-481-6700
800-245-5961
http://www.sepracor.com

SEPTODONT, INC.
245 C Quigley Blvd.
New Castle, DE 19720
302-328-1102
800-872-8305
http://www.septodontinc.com

17314
SEQUUS PHARMACEUTICALS, INC.
See Alza Corp.

50694
SERES LABORATORIES
3331-B Industrial Dr.
Santa Rosa, CA 95403
707-526-4526
http://www.sereslabs.com

44087
SERONO LABORATORIES, INC.
One Technology Place
Rockland, MA 02370
781-982-9000
800-283-8088
http://www.seronousa.com

11026
SEYER PHARMATEC, INC.
PO Box 9270
Cagus, PR 00725
787-728-7055
888-782-3585
http://www.spharmatec.com

SHAKLEE CORP.
4747 Willow Rd.
Pleasanton, CA 94588
925-924-2000
800-928-0327
http://www.shaklee.com

49813
SHEAR KERSHMAN LABS
701 Crown Industrial Court
Chesterfield, MO 63005
636-519-8900
http://www.shearkershman.com/

SHEFFIELD LABORATORIES
170 Broad St.
New London, CT 06320
860-442-4451
800-222-1087
http://www.sheffield-labs.com

12772
SHERWOOD
6 E.V. Hogan Drive
Hamlet, NC 28345
910-582-8800

17474, 08219
SHERWOOD DAVIS & GECK
See Kendall Health Care Products

SHIELD MANUFACTURING, INC.
425 Fillmore Ave
Tonawanda, NY 14150
716-694-7100
800-828-7669
http://www.shieldsports.com

54092
SHIRE US, INC.
725 Chesterbrook Blvd.
Wayne, PA 19087-5637
484-595-8800
800-828-2088
http://www.shire.com

49735
SHS NORTH AMERICA
See Nutricia North America

50111
SIDMAK LABORATORIES, INC.
See Pliva, Inc.

45749, 54482
SIGMA-TAU PHARMACEUTICALS
800 S. Frederick Avenue
Gaithersburg, MD 20877
301-948-1041
800-447-0169
http://www.sigmatau.com

54838
SILARX PHARMACEUTICALS, INC.
19 West Street
Spring Valley, NY 10977
845-352-4020
888-974-5279
http://www.silarx.com

53799, 94841
SIMILASAN
1745 Shea Center
Highlands Ranch, CO 80129
303-539-4060
800-240-9780
http://www.similsan.com

65880
SIRIUS LABORATORIES, INC.
100 Fairway Drive
Vernon Hills, IL 60061
847-968-2424
866-968-2425
http://www.siriuslabs.com

67402
SKINMEDICA, INC.
5909 Sea Lion Place
Carlsbad, CA 92010
760-448-3600
866-867-0110
http://www.skinmedica.com

SKYEPHARMA INC.
10 East 63rd St.
New York, NY 10021
212-753-5780
http://www.skyepharma.com

08436
SLIM FAST FOODS CO.
800 Sylvan Ave.
Engelwood Cliff, NJ 07632
561-833-9920
800-726-9866
http://www.slim-fast.com

SMITH & NEPHEW INC. ENDOSCOPY
150 Minuteman Rd.
Andover, MA 01810
978-749-1000
http://www.smith-nephew.com

08363
SMITH & NEPHEW ORTHO
1450 Brooks Rd.
Memphis, TN 38116
901-396-2121
800-821-5700
http://www.smith-nephew.com

40565, 50484
SMITH & NEPHEW WOUND MANAGEMENT
11775 Starkey Road
Largo, FL 33779
721-392-1261
800-876-1261
http://www.snwmd.com

58291
SNUVA, INC.
10323 W. Canterbury
West Chester, IL 60154-3503
708-725-3783
800-250-4258
http://www.snuva.com

SOLGAR CO., INC.
500 Willow Tree Road
Leonia, NJ 07605
201-944-2311
800-645-2246
http://www.solgar.com

10454
SOLSTICE NEUROSCIENCES
5 Great Valley Pkwy., Ste. 257
Malvern, PA 19355
650-243-4400
610-648-3835
http://www.solsticeneuro.com/

00032
SOLVAY PHARMACEUTICALS
901 Sawyer Road
Marietta, GA 30062-2224
770-578-9000
800-241-1643
http://www.solvay pharmaceuticals.com

61577
SOMBRA COSMETICS INC.
5951 Office Blvd. NE
Albuquerque, NM 87109
505-888-0288
800-225-3963

39506
SOMERSET PHARMACEUTICALS
2202 North West Shore Blvd.
Tampa, FL 33607
813-288-0040
800-892-8889
http://www.somersetpharm.com

45713, 61118
SOUTHWEST TECHNOLOGIES
1746 Levee Rd.
North Kansas City, KS 64116
816-221-2442
800-247-9951
http://www.elastogel.com

58016
SOUTHWOOD PHARMACEUTICALS
60 Empire Dr.
Lake Forest, CA 92630
800-442-4443
http://www.southwoodhealthcare.com

SOVEREIGN PHARMACEUTICALS
7590 Sand St.
Ft. Worth, TX 76118
817-284-0429
http://www.sovpharm.com

66530
SPEAR DERMATOLOGY PRODUCTS
1247 Sussex Turnpike
Randolph, NJ 07869
973-895-6447
http://www.speardermatology.com

38415
SPECIALTY MEDICAL SUPPLIES
3882 N.W. 124th St.
Coral Springs, FL 33065
954-752-5603
http://www.specialtymedical supplies.com

49452
SPECTRUM CHEMICAL MFG. CORP.
14422 S. San Pedro Street
Gardena, CA 90248-2027
310-516-8000
800-772-8786
http://www.spectrumchemical.com

38472
SPENCO MEDICAL CORPORATION
PO Box 2501
Waco, TX 76702
254-772-6000
800-877-3626
http://www.spenco.com

67336
TEAMM PHARMACEUTICALS, INC.
3000 Aerial Center Parkway
Morrisville, NC 27560
919-481-9020
866-481-9020
http://www.teammpharma.com

51879, 83626
TEC LABORATORIES, INC.
7100 Tec Labs Way SW
Albany, OR 97321
541-926-4577
800-482-4464
http://www.teclabsinc.com

TEL-TEST, INC.
PO Box 1421
Friendswood, TX 77549
281-482-2762
800-631-0600
http://www.tel-test.com

TELLURIDE PHARM. CORP.
300 Valley Rd.
Hillsborough, NJ 08844
908-369-1800
http://www.tellpharm.com

15054
TERCICA
2000 Sierra Point Parkway
Brisbane, CA 94005
650-624-4900
http://www.tercica.com/index.html

08418, 08970
TERUMO MEDICAL CORPORATION
2101 Cottontail Lane
Somerset, NJ 08873
732-302-4900
800-888-3786
http://www.terumomedical.com

TESTPAK, INC.
125 Algonquin Parkway
Whippany, NJ 07981
973-887-4440
http://www.testpak.com

TEVA MARION PARTNERS
901 East 104 St.
Kansas City, MO 64131
816-508-5000
800-221-4026
http://www.tevausa.com

00093
TEVA PHARMACEUTICALS USA
1090 Horsham Rd.
North Wales, PA 19454
215-591-3000
800-545-8800
http://www.tevausa.com

51672
THAMES PHARMACAL, INC.
See Taro Pharmaceuticals USA, Inc.

64011
THER-RX CORPORATION
2503 South Hanley Rd.
St. Louis, MO 63144
314-646-3700
877-567-7676
http://www.kvph.com

64067
THERAKOS, INC.
437 Creameryway
Exton, PA 19341
610-280-1000
http://www.therakos.com

THERAPEUTIC ANTIBODIES, INC.
See Protherics Inc.

THERASENSE
See Abbott Diabetes Care

11920
THOMPSON MEDICAL CO., INC.
See Chattem Consumer Products

49483
TIME-CAP LABS, INC.
7 Michael Avenue
Farmingdale, NY 11735
631-753-9090
http://www.timecaplabs.com

14654, 54023
TISHCON CORP.
30 New York Ave.
Westbury, NY 11590
516-333-3050
800-848-8442
http://www.tishcon.com

TOMS OF MAINE, INC.
302 Lafayette Center
Kennebunk, ME 04043
207-985-2944
800-367-8667
http://www.tomsofmaine.com

36800
TOPCO ASSOC. LLC
7711 Gross Point Rd.
Skokie, IL 60077
847-676-3030
888-423-0139
http://www.topco.com

58211
TOPIX PHARMACEUTICALS
5200 New Horizons Blvd.
North Amityville, NY 11701-1144
631-226-7979
800-445-2595

50201
TOWER LABORATORIES
8 Industrial Park Rd.
Centerbrook, CT 06409
860-737-2127
http://www.towerlabs.com

58433
TRANSDERMAL TECHNOLOGIES, INC.
1368 North Killian Drive
Lake Park, FL 33403
561-848-2345
800-282-5511
http://www.transdermal technologies.com

TRASK NUTRITION
163 Farrell Street
Somerset, NJ 08873
877-760-9258
800-579-3131
http://www.fibromalic.com

55654
TRI-MED LABORATORIES
68 Veronica Ave.
Somerset, NJ 08873
732-249-6363

TRI TECH LABORATORIES
1000 Robins Road
Lynchburg, VA 24504-3516
434-845-7073
http://www.tritechlabs.com

14290
TRIAX PHARMACEUTICALS
20 Commerce Dr., Suite 232
Cranford, NJ 07016-3599
973-433-3633
http://www.triaxpharma.com

13811
TRIGEN LABORATORIES, INC.
207 Kiley Dr.
Salisbury, MD 21802
410-860-8500
http://www.trigenlabs.com

TRIGEN LABS
See Jubilant Pharmaceuticals

61355
TRINITY TECHNOLOGIES
36 Washington Street
Wellesley, MA 02481
781-235-2223
http://www.trinitytechnologies.com

79511
TRITON CONSUMER PRODUCTS, INC.
561 West Golf Road
Arlington Heights, IL 60005-3904
847-228-7650
800-942-2009
http://www.mg217.com

10025
TROPICAL PHARMACAL
PO Box 813
Gurabo, PR 00778
787-737-8445

00463
TRUXTON
136 Harding Ave.
Bellmawr, NJ 08099
856-933-2333

TWEEZERMAN
2 Tri-Harbor Ct.
Port Washington, NY 11050
516-676-7772
800-645-3340
http://www.tweezerman.com

27434
TWINLAB CORP.
150 Motor Parkway
Hauppauge, NY 11788
631-467-3140
800-645-5626
http://www.twinlab.com

64915
TYLER, INC.
See Integrative Therapeutics

53335
TYSON NUTRACEUTICALS
3535 Lomita Blvd.
Torrance, CA 90505
310-325-5600
http://www.tysonnutraceuticals.com

00456
UAD LABORATORIES, INC.
See Forest Pharmaceuticals, Inc.

UCB PHARMACEUTICALS, INC.
1950 Lake Park Drive
Smyrna, GA 30080
770-970-7500
800-477-7877
http://www.ucbpharma.com

62592
UCYCLYD PHARMA, INC.
500 J McCormick Drive
Glen Burnie, MD 21061
410-768-5993
http://www.ucyclyd.com

51079
UDL LABORATORIES, INC.
1718 Northrock Court
Rockford, IL 61103
800-848-0462
http://www.udllabs.com

00127
ULMER PHARMACAL CO.
1614 Industry Ave.
Park Rapids, MN 56470
800-848-5637
http://www.lobanaproducts.com

08222, 08474, 57515
ULTIMED
287 East Sixth Street
St. Paul, MN 55101
651-291-7909
http://www.diabetes-care.com

59640
UNICO HOLDINGS, INC.
1830 2nd Avenue North
Lake Worth, FL 33461
800-367-4477

UNIFIRST CORPORATION
68 Jonspin Rd.
Wilmington, MA 01887
800-225-3364
http://www.unifirst.com

62305
UNIGEN PHARMACEUTICALS, INC.
1221 Tech Court
Westminster, MD 21157
410-751-2108
http://www.unigenpharma.com

UNILEVER HOME AND PERSONAL CARE USA
33 Benedict Place
Greenwich, CT 06830
203-661-2000
800-243-5320
http://www.unilever.com

41785
UNIMED PHARMACEUTICALS
See Solvay Pharmaceuticals

08479
UNIPATH DIAGNOSTICS CO.
See Inverness Medical Innovations

00327
UNITED GUARDIAN LABORATORIES
230 Marcus Blvd.
Hauppauge, NY 11788
631-273-0900
800-645-5566
http://www.u-g.com

00677
UNITED RESEARCH LABORATORIES (URL)
See Mutual Pharmaceutical Co., Inc.

63535
UNITHER PHARMA (UNITED THERAPEUTICS CORP.)
1110 Spring St.
Silver Springs, MD 20910
301-608-9292
888-808-6838
http://www.unitedtherapeutics.com

59730
UNIVAX BIOLOGICS
See Nabi

UPJOHN CO.
See Pfizer US Pharmaceutical Group

00245
UPSHER-SMITH LABS, INC.
6701 Evenstad Dr.
Maple Grove, MN 55369
763-315-2000
800-654-2299
http://www.upsher-smith.com

65580
UPSTATE PHARMA, LLC
1950 Lake Park Drive
Smyrna, GA 30080
770-970-7500
800-477-7877
http://www.ucbpharma.com

92293
UROCARE PRODUCTS, INC.
2735 Melbourne Ave.
Pomona, CA 91767-1931
909-621-6013
800-423-4441
http://www.urocare.com

UROCOR, INC.
See LabCorp

UROLOGIX
14405 21st Ave. North
Minneapolis, MN 55447
763-475-1400
800-475-1403
http://www.urologix.com

US BIOSCIENCE
26111 Miles Rd.
Cleveland, OH 44128
216-765-5000
800-321-9322
http://www.usbio.com

US DENTEK CORP.
307 Excellence Way
Maryville, TN 37801
800-433-6835
http://www.usdentek.com

08463
US DIAGNOSTICS
304 Park Avenue S., Suite 218
New York, NY 10010
866-216-5303

U.S. NEUTRACEUTICALS, LLC
2751 Nutra Lane
Eustis, FL 32726
352-357-2004
http://www.usnutra.com

52747
US PHARMACEUTICAL CORP.
2401-C Mellon Court
Decatur, GA 30035
770-987-4745
http://www.uspco.com

63261
US SURGICAL CORP.
150 Glove Ave.
Norwalk, CT 06856
203-845-1000
800-722-8772
http://www.ussurg.com

00187
VALEANT PHARMACEUTICALS INTERNATIONAL
3300 Hyland Avenue
Costa Mesa, CA 92626
714-545-0100
800-548-5100
http://www.valeant.com

54627
VALMED, INC.
221 Spring Street
Shrewsbury, MA 01545
508-845-3438

VALUE IN PHARMACEUTICALS
3000 Alt Boulevard
Grand Island, NY 14072
800-724-3784
http://www.vipppharm.com

00615
VANGARD LABS, INC.
PO Box 1268
Glasgow, KY 42142-1268
800-825-4123

67537
VARSITY LABORATORIES
PO Box 26708
Birmingham, AL 35260
205-986-1111

VENTANA MEDICAL SYSTEMS, INC.
1910 Innovation Park Dr.
Tucson, AZ 85755
520-887-2155
800-227-2155
http://www.ventanamed.com

11391
VENTLAB CORPORATION
155 Boyce Dr.
Mocksville, NC 27028
336-753-5000
800-593-4654
http://www.ventlab.com

67887
VERACITY PHARMACEUTICALS INC.
3550 Northwest 126th Ave.
Coral Springs, FL 33065
954-426-1919
800-354-8460
http://www.veracitypharma.com

16887
VERNALIS PHARMACEUTICALS
89 Headquarters Plaza
Morristown, NJ 07960
973-993-1855
888-376-2547
http://www.vernalis.com

61748
VERSAPHARM INC.
1775 West Oak Parkway
Marietta, GA 30062-2260
770-499-8100
800-548-0700
http://www.versapharm.com

VERTEX PHARMACEUTICALS, INC.
130 Waverly St.
Cambridge, MA 02139-4211
617-576-3111
http://www.vpharm.com

67000
VERUM PHARMACEUTICALS
See Victory Pharmaceuticals

13436
VERUS PHARMACEUTICALS
12671 High Bluff Dr., Ste. 200
San Diego, CA 92130
858-436-1622
http://www.veruspharm.com/

78112, 75137
VETCO, INC.
90 N. Broadway
Irvington, NY 10553
800-754-8853
http://www.littleremedies.com

78112, 75137
VETCO PHARMACEUTICALS
105 Baylis Rd., Second Floor
Melville, NY 11747-1155
631-755-1155

00702
VHA INC.
220 E. Las Colinas Blvd.
Irving, TX 75039
972-830-0626
800-842-5146
http://www.vha.com

VIASYS HEALTHCARE
227 Washington St., Suite 200
Conshohocken, PA 19428
610-862-0800
866-484-2797
http://www.viasyscriticalcare.com

00149
VICKS HEALTH CARE PRODUCTS
See Procter & Gamble Pharmaceuticals

00149
VICKS PHARMACY PRODUCTS
See Procter & Gamble Pharmaceuticals

67000
VICTORY PHARMACEUTICALS
12707 High Bluff Dr.
San Diego, CA 12797
858-350-4217
866-427-6819

00254
VINTAGE PHARMACEUTICALS, INC.
3241 Woodpark Blvd.
Charlotte, NC 28256
704-596-0516

53459
VIP INTERNATIONAL
1796 Clove Rd.
Staten Island, NY 10304
718-390-0490

00187
VIRATEK
See Valeant Pharmaceuticals International

VIREXX
8223 Roper Road NW
Edmonton, Alberta T6E 6S4
780-433-4411
http://www.virexx.com

66593
VIROPHARMA, INC.
397 Eagleview Blvd.
Exton, PA 19341
610-458-7300
http://www.viropharma.com

54891
VISION PHARMACEUTICALS, INC.
1022 N. Main St.
Mitchell, SD 57301
605-996-3356
800-325-6789
http://www.visionpharm.com

66689, 67043
VISTAPHARM
2224 Cahaba Valley Drive
Birmingham, AL 35242
205-981-1387
877-437-8567
http://www.vistapharm.com

49727
VITA-RX CORP
PO Box 8229
Columbus, GA 31908
706-568-1881

08321
VITAL CARE GROUP
8935 NW 27th St.
Miami, FL 33172
305-620-4007
800-392-4547
http://www.vitalcare.com

08166
VITAL SIGNS INC.
20 Campus Rd.
Totowa, NJ 07512
973-790-1330
800-932-0760
http://www.vital-signs.com

54022
VITALINE CORP. (INTEGRATIVE THERAPEUTICS, INC.)
9755 S.W. Commerce Circle
Wilsonville, OR 97070
800-917-3696

VITALITY INC.
See Vital Care Group

VITAMIN RESEARCH PRODUCT, INC.
4610 Arrowhead Drive
Carson City, NV 89706
775-884-8210
800-877-2447
http://www.vrp.com

62541
VIVUS INC.
1172 Castro Street
Mountain View, CA 94040
650-934-5200
888-345-6873
http://www.vivus.com

WAKEFIELD PHARMACEUTICALS, INC.
See Ivax Pharmaceuticals, Inc.

40805
WAL-MED, INC.
11302 164th Street East
Puyallup, WA 98374-9760
253-845-6633
877-542-3688
http://www.wallace-medical.com

WALLACE-O'FARRELL, INC.
11302 164th Street East
Puyallup, WA 98374-9760
253-845-6633
800-759-7883
http://www.wallace-ofarrell.com

00017
WAMPOLE LABORATORIES
See Inverness Medical Innovations

00047
WARNER CHILCOTT LABORATORIES
100 Enterprise Drive
Rockaway, NJ 07866
973-442-3200
800-521-8813
http://www.warnerchilcott.com

12546
WARNER LAMBERT AMERICAN CHICLE
201 Tabor Road
Morris Plains, NJ 07950
973-540-2000
800-524-2624

59930
WARRICK PHARMACEUTICAL, CORP. (SCHERING PLOUGH CORP.)
12125 Moya Blvd.
Reno, NV 89506
800-547-3869

00591, 52544
WATSON LABORATORIES
311 Bonnie Circle Dr.
Corona, CA 92880
914-767-2000
800-553-4044
http://www.watsonpharm.com

00591, 52544
WATSON PHARMACEUTICALS
311 Bonnie Circle Dr.
Corona, CA 92880
951-493-5300
800-338-9066
http://www.watsonpharma.com

71603
W. E. BASSETT
100 Trap Falls Road Extension
Shelton, CT 06484
203-929-8483
http://www.trim.com

WE PHARMACEUTICALS, INC.
See Airpharma

55946
WELEDA
1 Closter Rd.
Palisades, NY 10964
800-241-1030
http://www.usa.waleda.com

65197
WELLSPRING PHARMACEUTICAL
9040 Town Center Pkwy.
Bradenton, FL 34202
941-552-7880
877-273-1396
http://www.wellspringpharm.com

00917
WESLEY PHARMACAL, INC.
114 Railroad Drive
Ivyland, PA 18974
215-953-1680

00006
WEST POINT PHARMA
See Merck & Co.

00143
WEST-WARD PHARMACEUTICAL CORP.
465 Industrial Way West
Eatontown, NJ 07724
732-542-1191
800-631-2174)

64727
WESTERN RESEARCH LABORATORIES
2404 W. 12th St., Suite 4
Tempe, AZ 85281
623-879-8535
877-797-7997
http://www.wrlonline.com

00072
WESTWOOD SQUIBB PHARMACEUTICALS (BRISTOL-MYERS SQUIBB)
See Bristol-Myers Squibb Company

11444
W. F. YOUNG, INC.
302 Benton Dr.
East Longmeadow, MA 01028-5990
800-628-9653
http://www.absorbine.com

WHITBY PHARMACEUTICALS, INC.
See UCB Pharmaceuticals, Inc.

72695
WHITE LABS, INC.
U7564 Trade St.
San Diego, CA 92121
858-693-3441
888-593-2785
http://www.whitelabs.com

00317
WHORTON PHARMACEUTICALS, INC.
4202 Gary Ave.
Fairfield, AL 35064
205-786-2584

51101
WILLIAM LABORATORIES, INC.
5 Anngina Drive
Enfield, CT 06082
860-749-1350
800-767-7643
http://www.williamlabs.com

52047
WINTEC
1043 East Osage St.
Pacific, MO 63069
636-257-5400

12120
WISCONSIN PHARMACAL CO.
1 Pharmacal Way
Jackson, WI 53037
262-677-4121
800-558-6614
http://www.pharmacalway.com

WM. WRIGLEY JR. CO.
410 N. Michigan Ave.
Chicago, IL 60611
312-644-2121
800-974-4539
http://www.wrigley.com

WOLLFOAM COMPANY
3000 Hempstead Turnpike
Levittown, NY 11756
516-731-5380

64248
WOMEN FIRST HEALTHCARE INC.
See Mutual Pharmaceutical Co., Inc.

64836
WOMENS CAPITAL CORP.
See Barr Laboratories, Inc.

08111, 61168
WOODSIDE BIOMEDICAL INC.
See Hospira

60193
WOODWARD LABORATORIES, INC.
125-B Columbia
Aliso Viejo, CA 92656
949-362-4600
800-780-6999
http://www.woodwardlabs.com

66992
WRASER PHARMACEUTICALS
148 Weisenberger Rd.
Madison, MS 39110
601-605-0664
888-252-3901
http://www.wraser.com

00008
WYETH
5 Giralda Farms
Madison, NJ 07940
800-934-5556
800-999-9384
http://www.wyeth.com

WYETH CONSUMER HEALTH
5 Giralda Farms
Madison, NJ 07940
973-660-5500
800-762-4675
http://www.wyeth.com

39822
X-GEN PHARMACEUTICALS, INC.
PO Box 445
Big Flats, NY 14814
607-732-4411
866-390-4411
http://www.x-gen.us.com

XACTDOSE, INC.
See Actavis Pharma

66479
XANODYNE PHARMACEUTICALS, INC.
1 Riverfront Place
Newport, KY 41071-4563
859-371-6383
877-926-6396
http://www.xanodyne.com

00187
XCEL PHARMACEUTICALS
See Valeant Pharmaceuticals International

XOMA LLC/XOMA LTD.
2910 Seventh Street
Berkeley, CA 94710
510-204-7200
800-544-9662
http://www.xoma.com

00116
XTTRIUM LABORATORIES, INC.
415 West Pershing Road
Chicago, IL 60609
773-268-5800
800-587-3721
http://www.xttrium.com

YOUNG AGAIN PRODUCTS
3608 Oleander Drive
Wilmington, NC 28403-0806
910-371-6775
877-950-4400
http://www.youngagainproducts.com

00273, 60077
YOUNG DENTAL MFG.
13705 Shoreline Court East
Earth City, MO 63045
314-344-0010
800-325-1881
http://www.youngdental.com

90389
ZEE MEDICAL, INC.
22 Corporate Park
Irvine, CA 92606
800-841-8417
http://www.zeemedical.com

ZENITH LABORATORIES
See Ivax Pharmaceuticals, Inc.

18011
ZERXIS
4099 Highway 190
Covington, LA 70433
985-893-4097

51284
ZILA PHARMACEUTICALS, INC.
5227 N. 7th Street
Phoenix, AZ 85014
602-266-6700
866-945-2776
800-922-7887
http://www.zila.com

00053
ZLB BEHRING
1020 First Avenue
King of Prussia, PA 19406 6150
800-683-1288
http://www.hsaexcipient.com

44206
ZLB BIOPLASMA
See ZLB Behring

64909
ZOETICA PHARMACEUTICAL GROUP
See Stada Pharmaceuticals, Inc.

ZONAGEN, INC.
2408 Timberloch Place, B-1
The Woodlands, TX 77380
281-719-3400
http://www.zonagen.com

65224
ZYBER PHARMACEUTICALS, INC.
PO Box 40
Gonzales, LA 70707-0040
225-647-3002
800-793-2145
http://www.zyberphar.com

ZYMETX, INC.
655 Research Pkwy., Suite 554
Oklahoma City, OK 73104
405-809-1314
888-817-1314
http://www.zymetx.com

ZYMOGENETICS, INC.
1201 Eastlake Avenue East
Seattle, WA 98102-3702
206-442-6600
http://www.zymogenetics.com

This **Index** lists all generic names (in bold face), brand names, and group names included in Drug Facts and Comparisons®. Additionally, many synonyms, pharmacological actions, and therapeutic uses for the agents listed are included.

Entries with a prefix preceding the number are found in the ancillary chapters. A prefix of KU indicates the Keeping Up section, a prefix of A indicates placement in the Appendix section.

E

V

This index contains a comprehensive listing of drug trade names unique to Canada. The generic equivalent follows the Canadian trade name in bold. Accessing a *Drug Facts and Comparisons®* (*DFC*) monograph using a Canadian trade name is a two-step process. Use the Canadian Trade Name Index to determine the generic, then use the Quarterly Index to find the page number of the *DFC* drug monograph.

222 (Johnson & Johnson-Merck), *see* **Aspirin/Caffeine Citrate/Codeine Phosphate, Analgesic Combinations**

Accutane Roche (Roche), *see* **Isotretinoin**

Acetoxyl 2.5% and 5% (Valeo Pharma), *see* **Benzoyl Peroxide**

Acetoxyl 10% (Valeo Pharma), *see* **Benzoyl Peroxide**

Aclasta (Novartis Pharmaceuticals), *see* **Zoledronic Acid**

Actifed (Pfizer Consumer Healthcare), *see* **Pseudoephedrine HCl/Triprolidine HCl**

Actifed Plus Extra Strength (Pfizer Consumer Healthcare), *see* **Acetaminophen/ Pseudoephedrine HCl/ Triprolidine HCl**

Activase rt-PA (Roche), *see* **Alteplase**

Adalat XL (Bayer), *see* **Nifedipine**

Adasept Acne Gel (Odan), *see* **Salicylic Acid/Sodium Thiosulfate/Triclosan, Acne Combinations**

Adasept Skin Cleanser (Odan), *see* **Triclosan**

Adrenalin (ERFA Canada), *see* **Epinephrine HCl, Sympathomimetic Bronchodilators**

Advil Cold and Sinus Plus (Wyeth Consumer Healthcare), *see* **Chlorpheniramine Maleate/Ibuprofen/Pseudo-ephedrine HCl, Decongestant, Antihistamine, and Analgesic Combinations**

Aerius (Schering), *see* **Desloratadine**

Aerius Kids (Schering), *see* **Desloratidine**

Airomir (3M Pharmaceuticals), *see* **Albuterol**

Alcomicin (Alcon), *see* **Gentamicin Sulfate**

Aldactazide 25 (Pfizer), *see* **Hydrochlorothiazide/ Spironolactone, Diuretic Combinations**

Aldactazide 50 (Pfizer), *see* **Hydrochlorothiazide/ Spironolactone, Diuretic Combinations**

Alertec (Shire BioChem), *see* **Modafinil**

Alesse 21 (Wyeth Canada), *see* **Ethinyl Estradiol/ Levonorgestrel, Contraceptive Hormones**

Alesse 28 (Wyeth Canada), *see* **Ethinyl Estradiol/ Levonorgestrel, Contraceptive Hormones**

Alka-Seltzer (Bayer Consumer), *see* **Antacid Combinations**

Alka-Seltzer Flavoured (Bayer Consumer), *see* **Aspirin, Salicylates**

Allegra 12 Hour (Aventis Pharma), *see* **Fexofenadine HCl**

Allegra 24 Hour (Aventis Pharma), *see* **Fexofenadine HCl**

Allerdryl (Valeant), *see* **Diphenhydramine HCl**

Allernix (Rougier Pharma), *see* **Diphenhydramine HCl**

Ametop (Smith & Nephew), *see* **Tetracaine HCl**

Amsa PD (ERFA Canada), *see* **Amsacrine**

Anandron (Aventis Pharma), *see* **Nilutamide**

Anbesol Gel Extra Strength (Wyeth Consumer Healthcare), *see* **Benzocaine**

Anexate (Roche), *see* **Flumazenil**

Anugesic-HC (Pfizer Consumer Healthcare), *see* **Hydrocortisone Acetate/Pramoxine HCl/Zinc Sulfate Monohydrate, Steroid-Containing Anorectal Preparations**

Anusol Plus (Pfizer Consumer Healthcare), *see* **Pramoxine HCl/Zinc Sulfate Monohydrate Anesthetic, Anorectal Preparations**

Apo-Acebutolol (Apotex), *see* **Acebutolol HCl**

Apo-Acetaminophen (Apotex), *see* **Acetaminophen**

Apo-Acetazolamide (Apotex), *see* **Acetazolamide**

Apo-Acyclovir (Apotex), *see* **Acyclovir**

Apo-Alendronate (Apotex), *see* **Alendronate Sodium**

Apo-Allopurinol (Apotex), *see* **Allopurinol**

Apo-Alpraz (Apotex), *see* **Alprazolam**

Apo-Alpraz TS (Apotex), *see* **Alprazolam**

Apo-Amiloride (Apotex), *see* **Amiloride HCl**

Apo-Amilzide (Apotex), *see* **Amiloride HCl/ Hydrochlorothiazide, Diuretic Combinations**

Apo-Amiodarone (Apotex), *see* **Amiodarone HCl**

Apo-Amitriptyline (Apotex), *see* **Amitriptyline HCl**

Apo-Amoxi (Apotex), *see* **Amoxicillin Trihydrate**

Apo-Amoxi-Clav (Apotex), *see* **Amoxicillin/Clavulanate Potassium**

Apo-Ampi (Apotex), *see* **Ampicillin Trihydrate**

Apo-Atenidone (Apotex), *see* **Atenolol/Chlorthalidone**

Apo-Atenol (Apotex), *see* **Atenolol**

Apo-Azathioprine (Apotex), *see* **Azathioprine**

Apo-Baclofen (Apotex), *see* **Baclofen**

Apo-Beclomethasone (Apotex), *see* **Beclomethasone Dipropionate, Intranasal Steroids**

Apo-Benztropine (Apotex), *see* **Benztropine Mesylate**

Apo-Bisacodyl (Apotex), *see* **Bisacodyl**

Apo-Bisacodyl DR (Apotex), *see* **Bisacodyl**

Apo-Bisoprolol (Apotex), *see* **Bisoprolol Fumarate**

Apo-Brimonidine (Apotex), *see* **Brimonidine Tartrate**

Apo-Bromocriptine (Apotex), *see* **Bromocriptine Mesylate**

Apo-Buspirone (Apotex), *see* **Buspirone HCl**

Apo-Butorphanol (Apotex), *see* **Butorphanol Tartrate**

Apo-Cal (Apotex), *see* **Calcium Carbonate**

Apo-Calcitonin (Apotex), *see* **Calcitonin Salmon**

Apo-Capto (Apotex), *see* **Captopril**

Apo-Carbamazepine (Apotex), *see* **Carbamazepine**

Apo-Carvedilol (Apotex), *see* **Carvedilol**

Apo-Cefaclor (Apotex), *see* **Cefaclor**

Apo-Cefadroxil (Apotex), *see* **Cefadroxil Monohydrate**

Apo-Cefuroxime (Apotex), *see* **Cefuroxime Axetil**

Apo-Cephalex (Apotex), *see* **Cephalexin**

Apo-Cetirizine (Apotex), *see* **Cetirizine HCl**

Apo-Chlorax (Apotex), *see* **Chlordiazepoxide HCl/Clidinium Bromide, Gastrointestinal Anticholinergic Combinations**

Apo-Chlordiazepoxide (Apotex), *see* **Chlordiazepoxide HCl**

Apo-Chlorhexidine (Apotex), *see* **Chlorhexidine Gluconate**

Apo-Chlorpropamide (Apotex), *see* **Chlorpropamide**

Apo-Chlorthalidone (Apotex), *see* **Chlorthalidone**

Apo-Cimetidine (Apotex), *see* **Cimetidine**

Apo-Ciproflox (Apotex), *see* **Ciprofloxacin**

Apo-Citalopram (Apotex), *see* **Citalopram**

Apo-Clindamycin (Apotex), *see* **Clindamycin**

Apo-Clomipramine (Apotex), *see* **Clomipramine HCl**

Apo-Clonazepam (Apotex), *see* **Clonazepam**

Apo-Clonidine (Apotex), *see* **Clonidine HCl**

Apo-Clorazepate (Apotex), *see* **Clorazepate Dipotassium**

Apo-Cloxi (Apotex), *see* **Cloxacillin Sodium**

Apo-Clozapine (Apotex), *see* **Clozapine**

Apo-Cromolyn Nasal Spray (Apotex), *see* **Cromolyn Sodium**

Apo-Cromolyn Sterules (Apotex), *see* **Cromolyn Sodium**

Apo-Cyclobenzaprine (Apotex), *see* **Cyclobenzaprine HCl**

Apoo-Cyclosporine (Apotex), *see* **Cyclosporine**

Apo-Cyproterone (Apotex), *see* **Cyproterone Acetate**

Apo-Desipramine (Apotex), *see* **Desipramine HCl**

Apo-Desmopressin (Apotex), *see* **Desmopressin Acetate**

Apo-Dexamethasone (Apotex), *see* **Dexamethasone**

Apo-Diazepam (Apotex), *see* **Diazepam**

Apo-Diclo (Apotex), *see* **Diclofenac Sodium**

Apo-Diclo Rapide (Apotex), *see* **Diclofenac Potassium**

Apo-Diclo SR (Apotex), *see* **Diclofenac Sodium**

Apo-Diflunisal (Apotex), *see* **Diflunisal**

Apo-Diltiaz (Apotex), *see* **Diltiazem HCl**

Apo-Diltiaz CD (Apotex), *see* **Diltiazem HCl**

Apo-Diltiaz Injectable (Apotex), *see* **Diltiazem HCl**

Apo-Diltiaz SR (Apotex), *see* **Diltiazem HCl**

Apo-Dimenhydrinate (Apotex), *see* **Dimenhydrinate**

Apo-Dipyridamole (Apotex), *see* **Dipyridamole**

Apo-Divalproex (Apotex), *see* **Divalproex Sodium, Valproic Acid and Derivatives**

Apo-Docusate Calcium (Apotex), *see* **Docusate Calcium**

Apo-Docusate Sodium (Apotex), *see* **Docusate Sodium**

Apo-Doxazosin (Apotex), *see* **Doxazosin Mesylate**

Apo-Doxepin (Apotex), *see* **Doxepin HCl**

Apo-Doxy (Apotex), *see* **Doxycycline Hyclate**

Apo-Doxy-Tabs (Apotex), *see* **Doxycyline Hyclate**

Apo-Erythro Base (Apotex), *see* **Erythromycin**

Apo-Erythro E-C (Apotex), *see* **Erythromycin**

Apo-Tobramycin (Apotex), *see* **Tobramycin**

Apo-Tolbutamide (Apotex), *see* **Tolbutamide**

Apo-Trazodone (Apotex), *see* **Trazodone HCl**

Apo-Trazodone D (Apotex), *see* **Trazodone HCl**

Apo-Triazide (Apotex), *see* **Hydrochlorothiazide/Triamterene, Diuretic Combinations**

Apo-Triazo (Apotex), *see* **Triazolam**

Apo-Trifluoperazine (Apotex), *see* **Trifluoperazine HCl**

Apo-Trihex (Apotex), *see* **Trihexyphenidyl HCl**

Apo-Trimethoprim (Apotex), *see* **Triomethoprim**

Apo-Trimip (Apotex), *see* **Trimipramine Maleate**

Apo-Tryptophan (Apotex), *see* **L-Tryptophan**

Apo-Valproic Acid (Apotex), *see* **Valproic Acid**

Apo-Verap (Apotex), *see* **Verapamil HCl**

Apo-Verap SR (Apotex), *see* **Verapamil HCl**

Apo-Warfarin (Apotex), *see* **Warfarin Sodium**

Aquatain (Wyeth Consumer Healthcare), *see* **Emollients**

Aristospan (Valeo Pharma), *see* **Triamcinolone Hexacetonide**

Asaphen (Pharmascience), *see* **Aspirin**

Asaphen E.C. (Pharmascience), *see* **Aspirin**

Atacand Plus (AstraZeneca), *see* **Candesartan Cilexetil/Hydrochlorothiazide**

Atasol (Church & Dwight), *see* **Acetaminophen**

Atasol-8 (Church & Dwight), *see* **Acetaminophen/Caffeine Citrate/Codeine Phosphate, Narcotic Analgesic Combinations**

Atasol-15 (Church & Dwight), *see* **Acetaminophen/Caffeine Citrate/Codeine Phosphate, Narcotic Analgesic Combinations**

Atasol-30 (Church & Dwight), *see* **Acetaminophen/Caffeine Citrate/Codeine Phosphate, Narcotic Analgesic Combinations**

Auralgan (Wyeth Consumer Healthcare), *see* **Antipyrine/Benzocaine, Otic Preparations**

Avaxim (Sanofi Pasteur), *see* **Hepatitis A Vaccine, Inactivated**

Avaxim-Pediatric (Sanofi Pasteur), *see* **Hepatitis A Vaccine, Inactivated**

Baciguent (Johnson & Johnson-Merck), *see* **Bacitracin**

Baciject (SteriMax), *see* **Bacitracin**

Balminil Codeine + Decongestant + Expectorant (Rougier Pharma), *see* **Codeine Phosphate/Guaifenesin/Pseudoephedrine HCl, Antitussive and Expectorant Combinations**

Balminil Cough & Flu (Rougier Pharma), *see* **Dextromethorphan HBr/Acetaminophen/Guaifenesin/Pseudoephedrine HCl, Antitussive and Expectorant Combinations**

Balminil DM (Rougier Pharma), *see* **Dextromethorphan HBr**

Balminil DM Children (Rougier Pharma), *see* **Dextromethorphan HBr**

Balminil DM + Decongestant (Rougier Pharma), *see* **Dextromethorphan HBr/Pseudoephedrine HCl**

Balminil DM + Decongestant + Expectorant (Rougier Pharma), *see* **Dextromethorphan HBr/Guaifenesin/Pseudoephedrine HCl**

Balminil DM + Expectorant (Rougier Pharma), *see* **Dextromethorphan HBr/Guaifenesin**

Balminil Expectorant (Rougier Pharma), *see* **Guaifenesin**

Balminil Nasal Decongestant (Rougier Pharma), *see* **Xylometazoline HCl**

Benadryl Total/Allergy/Extra Strength (Pfizer Consumer Healthcare), *see* **Acetaminophen/Pseudoephedrine HCl/Diphenhydramine HCl, Decongestant, Antihistamine, and Analgesic Combinations**

Benadryl Total/Allergy/Regular Strength (Pfizer Consumer Healthcare), *see* **Acetaminophen/Pseudoephedrine HCl/Diphenhydramine HCl, Decongestant, Antihistamine, and Analgesic Combinations**

Bengay Arthritis Extra Strength (Pfizer Consumer Healthcare), *see* **Rubs and Liniments**

Bengay Muscle Pain Regular Strength (Original) (Pfizer Consumer Healthcare), *see* **Rubs and Liniments**

Bengay Muscle Pain Ultra Strength (Pfizer Consumer Healthcare), *see* **Rubs and Liniments**

Benoxyl 5% (Stiefel), *see* **Benzoyl Peroxide**

Benoxyl 10% (Stiefel), *see* **Benzoyl Peroxide**

Benoxyl 20% (Stiefel), *see* **Benzoyl Peroxide**

Bentylol (Axcan Pharma), *see* **Dicyclomine HCl**

Benuryl (Valeant), *see* **Probenecid**

Benylin 1 All-in-One Cold and Flu (Pfizer Consumer Healthcare), *see* **Acetaminophen/Dextromethorphan HBR/Guaifenesin/Pseudoephedrine HCl, Antitussive and Expectorant Combinations**

Benylin 2 All-in-One Cold and Flu with Codeine (Non-prescription) (Pfizer Consumer Healthcare), *see* **Codeine Phosphate/Guaifenesin/Pseudoephedrine HCl**

Benylin D for Infants (Pfizer Consumer Healthcare), *see* **Pseudoephedrine HCl**

Benylin DM (Pfizer Consumer Healthcare), *see* **Dextromethorphan HBr**

Benylin DM 12 Hour (Nightime) (Pfizer Consumer Healthcare), *see* **Dextromethorphan HBr**

Benylin DM for Children (Pfizer Consumer Healthcare), *see* **Dextromethorphan HBr**

Benylin DM for Children 12 Hour (Bedtime) (Pfizer Consumer Healthcare), *see* **Dextromethorphan HBr**

Benylin DM-D (Adult) (Pfizer Consumer Healthcare), *see* **Dextromethorphan HBr/Pseudoephedrine HCl**

Benylin DM-D for Children (Pfizer Consumer Healthcare), *see* **Dextromethorphan HBr/Pseudoephedrine HCl**

Benylin DM-D for Infants (Pfizer Consumer Healthcare), *see* **Dextromethorphan HBr/Pseudoephedrine HCl, Pediatric Antitussive Combinations**

Benylin DM-D-E (Pfizer Consumer Healthcare), *see* **Dextromethorphan HBr/Guaifenesin/Pseudoephedrine HCl, Antitussives and Expectorant Combinations**

Benylin DM-D-E Extra Strength (Pfizer Consumer Healthcare), *see* **Dextromethorphan HBr/Guaifenesin/Pseudoephedrine HCl, Antitussive and Expectorant Combinations**

Benylin DM-E (Pfizer Consumer Healthcare), *see* **Dextromethorphan HBr/Guaifenesin, Antitussives with Expectorants**

Benylin DM-E Extra Strength (Pfizer Consumer Healthcare), *see* **Dextromethorphan HBr/Guaifenesin, Antitussives with Expectorants**

Benylin E Extra Strength (Pfizer Consumer Healthcare), *see* **Guaifenesin**

Benztropine Omega (Omega), *see* **Benztropine Mesylate**

Betacaine (Canderm Pharma), *see* **Lidocaine HCl**

Betaderm (Taro), *see* **Betamethasone Valerate**

Betaject (Sandoz), *see* **Betamethasone Sodium Phosphate/Betamethasone Acetate**

Betaloc (AstraZeneca), *see* **Metoprolol Tartrate**

Betaloc Durules (AstraZeneca), *see* **Metoprolol Tartrate**

Betnesol (Shire BioChem), *see* **Betamethasone Sodium Phosphate**

Biaxin BID (Abbott), *see*, **Clarithromycin**

Biobase (Odan), *see* **Ethyl Alcohol, Antiseptics, Miscellaneous**

Biobase-G (Odan), *see* **Ethyl Alcohol/Glycolic Acid, Miscellaneous Antiseptics**

Biquin Durules (AstraZeneca), *see* **Quinidine Sulfate**

Bonamine (Pfizer Consumer Healthcare), *see* **Meclizine HCl**

Brevicon 0.5/35 (Pfizer), *see* **Ethinyl Estradiol/Norethindrone, Contraceptive Hormones**

Brevicon 1/35 (Pfizer), *see* **Ethinyl Estradiol/Norethindrone, Contraceptive Hormones**

Bricanyl Turbuhaler (AstraZeneca), *see* **Terbutaline Sulfate**

Bufferin Extra-Strength (Bristol-Myers Squibb), *see* **Aspirin**

Bugs Bunny and Friends (Bayer Consumer), *see* **Multivitamins with Minerals**

Burinex (LEO), *see* **Bumetanide**

Buscopan (Boehringer Ingelheim), *see* **Hyoscine HBr**

Caelyx (Schering), *see* **Doxorubicin HCl**

Calcite 500 (Riva), *see* **Calcium Carbonate**

Calcite 500 D 400 (Riva), *see* **Calcium/Vitamin D**

Calcite D-500 (Riva), *see* **Calcium Carbonate/Vitamin D**

Calcium 500 (Trianon), *see* **Calcium Carbonate**

Calcium 500 mg with Vitamin D (Novopharm), *see* **Calcium and Vitamin D, Nutritional Combination Products**

Calcium D 500 (Trianon), *see* **Calcium/Vitamin D Combinations**

Calcium Oyster Shell (Novopharm), *see* **Calcium Carbonate, Minerals**

Gen-Buspirone (Genpharm), *see* **Buspirone HCl**

Gen-Captopril (Genpharm), *see* **Captopril**

Gen-Carbamazepine CR (Genpharm), *see* **Carbamazepine**

Gen-Cimetidine (Genpharm), *see* **Cimetidine**

Gen-Ciprofloxacin (Genpharm), *see* **Ciprofloxacin**

Gen-Citalopram (Genpharm), *see* **Citalopram HBr**

Gen-Clindamycin (Genpharm), *see* **Clindamycin HCl**

Gen-Clobetasol (Genpharm), *see* **Clobetasol 17-Propionate**

Gen-Clomipramine (Genpharm), *see* **Clomipramine HCl**

Gen-Clonazepam (Genpharm), *see* **Clonazepam**

Gen-Clozapine (Genpharm), *see* **Clozapine**

Gen-Cyclobenzaprine (Genpharm), *see* **Cyclobenzaprine HCl**

Gen-Cyproterone (Genpharm), *see* **Cyproterone Acetate**

Gen-Diltiazem (Genpharm), *see* **Diltiazem HCl**

Gen-Diltiazem CD (Genpharm), *see* **Diltiazem HCl**

Gen-Doxazosin (Genpharm), *see* **Doxazosin Mesylate**

Gen-Etidronate (Genpharm), *see* **Etidronate Disodium**

Gen-Famotidine (Genpharm), *see* **Famotidine**

Gen-Fenofibrate Micro (Genpharm), *see* **Fenofibrate (Micronized)**

Gen-Fluconazole (Genpharm), *see* **Fluconazole**

Gen-Fluoxetine (Genpharm), *see* **Fluoxetine HCl**

Gen-Fosinopril (Genpharm), *see* **Fosinopril Sodium**

Gen-Gabapentin (Genpharm), *see* **Gabapentin**

Gen-Gemfibrozil (Genpharm), *see* **Gemfibrozil**

Gen-Glybe (Genpharm), *see* **Glyburide**

Gen-Hydroxychloroquine (Genpharm), *see* **Hydroxychloroquine Sulfate**

Gen-Hydroxyurea (Genpharm), *see* **Hydroxyurea**

Gen-Indapamide (Genpharm), *see* **Indapamide Hemihydrate**

Gen-Ipratropium (Genpharm), *see* **Ipratropium Bromide**

Gen-Lamotrigine (Genpharm), *see* **Lamotrigine**

Gen-Lovastatin (Genpharm), *see* **Lovastatin**

Gen-Medroxy (Genpharm), *see* **Medroxyprogesterone Acetate**

Gen-Meloxicam (Genpharm), *see* **Meloxicam**

Gen-Metformin (Genpharm), *see* **Metformin HCl**

Gen-Metoprolol (Type L) (Genpharm), *see* **Metoprolol Tartrate**

Gen-Minocycline (Genpharm), *see* **Minocycline HCl**

Gen-Mirtazapine (Genpharm), *see* **Mirtazapine**

Gen-Nabumetone (Genpharm), *see* **Nabumetone**

Gen-Naproxen EC (Genpharm), *see* **Naproxen**

Gen-Nitro (Genpharm), *see* **Nitroglycerin**

Gen-Nizatidine (Genpharm), *see* **Nizatidine**

Gen-Nortriptyline (Genpharm), *see* **Nortriptyline HCl**

Gen-Oxybutynin (Genpharm), *see* **Oxybutynin Chloride**

Gen-Paroxetine (Genpharm), *see* **Paroxetine**

Gen-Pindolol (Genpharm), *see* **Pindolol**

Gen-Piroxicam (Genpharm), *see* **Piroxicam**

Gen-Propafenone (Genpharm), *see* **Propafenone HCl**

Gen-Ranitidine (Genpharm), *see* **Ranitidine HCl**

Gen-Salbutamol Respirator Solution (Genpharm), *see* **Albuterol Sulfate**

Gen-Salbutamol Sterinebs P.F. (Genpharm), *see* **Albuterol Sulfate**

Gen-Selegiline (Genpharm), *see* **Selegiline HCl**

Gen-Simvastatin (Genpharm), *see* **Simvastatin**

Gen-Sotalol (Genpharm), *see* **Sotalol HCl**

Gen-Tamoxifen (Genpharm), *see* **Tamoxifen Citrate**

Gen-Temazepam (Genpharm), *see* **Temazepam**

Gen-Terbinafine (Genpharm), *see* **Terbinafine HCl**

Gen-Ticlopidine (Genpharm), *see* **Ticlopidine HCl**

Gen-Timolol (Genpharm), *see* **Timolol Maleate**

Gen-Trazodone (Genpharm), *see* **Trazodone HCl**

Gen-Triazolam (Genpharm), *see* **Triazolam**

Gen-Valproic (Genpharm), *see* **Valproic Acid**

Gen-Verapamil (Genpharm), *see* **Verapamil HCl**

Gen-Verapamil SR (Genpharm), *see* **Verapamil HCl**

Gen-Warfarin (Genpharm), *see* **Warfarin Sodium**

Gentlax (Purdue Pharma), *see* **Bisacodyl**

Glaxal Base (WellSpring), *see* **Ointment and Lotion Bases**

GlucoNorm (Novo Nordisk), *see* **Repaglinide**

Glumetza (Bioval Pharmaceuticals), *see* **Metformin HCl**

Gravol (Church & Dwight), *see* **Dimenhydrinate**

Haloperidol LA (Sandoz), *see* **Haloperidol**

Haloperidol-LA Omega (Omega), *see* **Haloperidol**

Hepalean (Organon), *see* **Heparin Sodium**

Hepalean-Lok (Organon), *see* **Heparin Sodium**

Heparin LEO (LEO), *see* **Heparin Sodium**

Heptovir (GlaxoSmithKline), *see* **Lamivudine**

Herplex-D (Allergan), *see* **Idoxuridine**

Hexabrix 200 (tyco Healthcare), *see* **Ioxaglate Meglumine 39.3% and Ioxaglate Sodium 19.6% (32% iodine)**

Hexabrix 320 (tyco Healthcare), *see* **Ioxaglate Meglumine 39.3% and Ioxaglate Sodium 19.6% (32% iodine)**

Hexit (Odan), *see* **Lindane**

Hextend (BioTime), *see* **Hetastarch**

Hip-Rex (3M Pharmaceuticals), *see* **Methenamine Hippurate**

Hp-PAC (TAP Pharmaceuticals), *see* **Amoxicillin Trihydrate/Clarithromycin/ Lansoprazole, *H. pylori* Agents**

Humalog Mix25 (Lilly), *see* **Insulin Analog Injection**

Humulin 20/80 (Lilly), *see* **Insulin Injection (Human)/ Insulin Isophane (Human)**

Hycomine-S (Bristol-Myers Squibb), *see* **Ammonium Chloride/Hydrocodone Bitartrate/Phenylephrine HCl/Pyrilamine Maleate**

Hyderm (Taro), *see* **Hydrocortisone Acetate**

Hydrasense (Schering), *see* **Nasal Products**

Hydromorph Contin (Purdue Pharma), *see* **Hydromorphone HCl**

Hydromorph-IR (Purdue Pharma), *see* **Hydromorphone HCl**

Hydromorphone HP 10 (Sandoz), *see* **Hydromorphone HCl**

Hydromorphone HP 20 (Sandoz), *see* **Hydromorphone HCl**

Hydromorphone HP 50 (Sandoz), *see* **Hydromorphone HCl**

Hydromorphone HP Forte (Sandoz), *see* **Hydromorphone HCl**

Hydrosone (Rougier), *see* **Hydrocortisone**

HydroVal (TaroPharma), *see* **Hydrocortisone Valerate**

HYPERHEP B S/D (Talecris/Bayer), *see* **Hepatitis B Immune Globulin (Human)**

HYPERRAB S/D (Talecris/Bayer), *see* **Rabies Immune Globulin Human**

HYPERRHO S/D (Talecris/Bayer), *see* **Rho(D) Immune Globulin**

HYPERTET S/D (Talecris/Bayer), *see* **Tetanus Immune Globulin (Human)**

Hyzaar DS (Merck Frosst), *see* **Hydrochlorothiazide/ Losartan Potassium, Antihypertensive Combinations**

ICAPS High Potency (Alcon), *see* **Multivitamins with Minerals**

ICAPS Lutein and Zeaxanthin (Alcon), *see* **Multivitamins with Minerals**

Idamycin (Pfizer), *see* **Idarubicin HCl**

Iletin II Pork Lente (Lilly), *see* **Insulin Zinc Suspension (Lente)**

Iletin II Pork NPH (Lilly), *see* **Isophane Insulin Suspension (NPH)**

Iletin II Pork Regular (Lilly), *see* **Insulin Injection**

Imitrex DF (GlaxoSmithKline), *see* **Sumatriptan Succinate**

ImmuCyst (Sanofi Pasteur), *see* **Bacillus Calmette-Guerin, Intravesical**

Imogam Rabies Pasteurized (Sanofi Pasteur), *see* **Rabies Immune Globulin, Human (RIG)**

IMOVAX Rabies (Sanofi Pasteur), *see* **Rabies Vaccine Viral Vaccines, Agents for Active Immunization**

Imunovir (Rivex Pharma), *see* **Inosine Pranobex**

Indocid P.D.A. (Merck Frosst), *see* **Indomethacin Sodium**

Infantol (Church & Dwight), *see* **Multiple Vitamins**

Infufer (Sandoz), *see* **Iron Dextran**

Intralipid 20% (Baxter), *see* **Fat Emulsion, Intravenous**

Intralipid 30% (Baxter), *see* **Fat Emulsion, Intravenous**

Iopidine 0.5% (Alcon), *see* **Apraclonidine HCl**

Iopidine 1% (Alcon), *see* **Apraclonidine HCl**

Isomil STEP 2 (Abbott), *see* **Specialized Infant Foods**

Isotamine (Valeant), *see* **Isoniazid**

K-10 (GlaxoSmithKline), *see* **Potassium Chloride**

K-Dur (Key), *see* **Potassium Chloride**

K-Lyte/Cl (WellSpring), *see* **Potassium Chloride**

Kaopectate (Johnson & Johnson-Merck) *see* **Attapulgite**

Ketoderm (TaroPharma), *see* **Ketoconazole**

Klean-Prep (Rivex Pharma), *see* **Polyethylene Glycol/ Electrolyte, Bowel Evacuants**

Koffex DM (Rougier Pharma), *see* **Dextromethorphan HBr**

Panoxyl 5% Wash (Stiefel), *see* **Benzoyl Peroxide, Anti-infectives, Topical, Antibiotic Agents**

Panoxyl 10% (Stiefel), *see* **Benzoyl Peroxide, Anti-infectives, Topical, Antibiotic Agents**

Panoxyl 15% (Stiefel), *see* **Benzoyl Peroxide, Anti-infectives, Topical, Antibiotic Agents**

Panoxyl 20% (Stiefel), *see* **Benzoyl Peroxide, Anti-infectives, Topical, Antibiotic Agents**

Panoxyl Antibacterial Acne Creamy Wash (Stiefel), *see* **Benzoyl Peroxide, Anti-infectives, Topical, Antibiotic Agents**

Panoxyl Aquagel 2.5% (Stiefel), *see* **Benzoyl Peroxide, Anti-infectives, Topical, Antibiotic Agents**

Panoxyl Aquagel 5% (Stiefel), *see* **Benzoyl Peroxide, Anti-infectives, Topical, Antibiotic Agents**

PANTO IV (ALTANA Pharma), *see* **Pantoprazole Sodium**

Pantoloc (Solvay Pharma), *see* **Pantoprazole Sodium**

Parafon Forte (Johnson & Johnson-Merck), *see* **Acetaminophen/Chlorzoxazone, Skeletal Muscle Relaxant Combinations**

Paraplatin-AQ (Bristol), *see* **Carboplatin**

Pariet (Janssen-Ortho), *see* **Rabeprazole Sodium**

Parvolex (Bioniche), *see* **Acetylcysteine**

Pediatrix (Rougier Pharma), *see* **Acetaminophen**

Pegetron (Schering), *see* **Ribavirin/Interferon Alfa-2b, Recombinant Combination**

PegLyte (Pharmascience), *see* **Polyethylene Glycol/ Electrolyte, Bowel Evacuants**

Penta/3b (Sandoz), *see* **Vitamin B Compound**

Penta/3b + C (Sandoz), *see* **Vitamin Combinations**

Penta/3b Plus (Sandoz), *see* **Multiple Vitamins**

Pentamycetin (Sandoz), *see* **Chloramphenicol**

Pentamycetin/HC (Sandoz), *see* **Chloramphenicol/ Hydrocortisone Acetate, Steroid and Antibiotic Combinations, Ophthalmic**

Percocet-Demi (Bristol-Myers Squibb), *see* **Acetaminophen/Oxycodone HCl, Analgesic Combinations**

Pernox (Westwood-Squibb), *see* **Salicylic Acid/Sulfur, Abrasive Cleansers**

Pharmorubicin PFS (Pfizer), *see* **Epirubicin HCl**

Phenazo (Valeant), *see* **Phenazopyridine HCl**

Phosphates Solution (Pharmascience), *see* **Sodium Phosphates**

PMS-Amiodarone (Pharmascience), *see* **Amiodarone HCl**

PMS-Atenolol (Pharmascience), *see* **Atenolol**

PMS-Baclofen (Pharmascience), *see* **Baclofen**

PMS-Bethanechol (Pharmascience), *see* **Bethanechol Chloride**

PMS-Brimonidine Tartrate (Pharmascience), *see* **Brimonidine Tartrate**

PMS-Bromocriptine (Pharmascience), *see* **Bromocriptine Mesylate**

PMS-Buspirone (Pharmascience), *see* **Buspirone HCl**

PMS-Butorphanol (Pharmascience), *see* **Butorphanol Tartrate**

PMS-Captopril (Pharmascience), *see* **Captopril**

PMS-Carbamazepine (Pharmascience), *see* **Carbamazepine**

PMS-Carvedilol (Pharmascience), *see* **Carvedilol**

PMS-Cholestyramine (Pharmascience), *see* **Cholestyramine Resin**

PMS-Ciprofloxacin (Pharmascience), *see* **Ciprofloxacin HCl**

PMS-Citalopram (Pharmascience), *see* **Citalopram HBr**

PMS-Clonazepam (Pharmascience), *see* **Clonazepam**

PMS-Cyclobenzaprine (Pharmascience), *see* **Cyclobenzaprine HCl**

PMS-Desipramine (Pharmascience), *see* **Desipramine HCl**

PMS-Desonide (Pharmascience), *see* **Desonide**

PMS-Dexamethasone (Pharmascience), *see* **Dexamethasone Acetate, Dexamethasone Sodium Phosphate, Adrenocortical Steroids**

PMS-Diclofenac (Pharmascience), *see* **Diclofenac Sodium**

PMS-Diclofenac SR (Pharmascience), *see* **Diclofenac Sodium**

PMS-Fenofibrate Micro (Pharmascience), *see* **Fenofibrate**

PMS-Fluoxetine (Pharmascience), *see* **Fluoxetine HCl**

PMS-Fluvoxamine (Pharmascience), *see* **Fluvoxamine**

PMS-Gabapentin (Pharmascience), *see* **Gabapentin**

PMS-Gemfibrozil (Pharmascience), *see* **Gemfibrozil**

PMS-Glyburide (Pharmascience), *see* **Glyburide**

PMS-Hydromorphone (Pharmascience), *see* **Hydromorphone HCl**

PMS-Indapamide (Pharmascience), *see* **Indapamide**

PMS-Lactulose (Pharmascience), *see* **Lactulose**

PMS-Lamotrigine (Pharmascience), *see* **Lamotrigine**

PMS-Levobunolol (Pharmascience), *see* **Levobunolol HCl**

PMS-Lindane (Pharmascience), *see* **Lindane**

PMS-Lithium Carbonate (Pharmascience), *see* **Lithium Carbonate**

PMS-Lithium Citrate (Pharmascience), *see* **Lithium Citrate**

PMS-Lorazepam (Pharmascience), *see* **Lorazepam**

PMS-Lovastatin (Pharmascience), *see* **Lovastatin**

PMS-Loxapine (Pharmascience), *see* **Loxapine**

PMS-Meloxicam (Pharmascience), *see* **Meloxicam**

PMS-Metformin (Pharmascience), *see* **Metformin HCl**

PMS-Methylphenidate (Pharmascience), *see* **Methylphenidate HCl**

PMS-Metoprolol-L (Pharmascience), *see* **Metoprolol Tartrate**

PMS-Mirtazapine (Pharmascience), *see* **Mirtazapine**

PMS-Morphine Sulfate SR (Pharmascience), *see* **Morphine Sulfate**

PMS-Nizatidine (Pharmascience), *see* **Nizatidine**

PMS-Oxybutynin (Pharmascience), *see* **Oxybutynin**

PMS-Oxycodone-Acetaminophen (Pharmascience), *see* **Acetaminophen/Oxycodone, Narcotic Analgesic Combinations**

PMS-Paroxetine (Pharmascience), *see* **Paroxetine**

PMS-Phenobarbital (Pharmascience), *see* **Phenobarbital**

PMS-Pravastatin (Pharmascience), *see* **Pravastatin Sodium**

PMS-Ranitidine (Pharmascience), *see* **Ranitidine HCl**

PMS-Simvastatin (Pharmascience), *see* **Simvastatin**

PMS-Sotalol (Pharmascience), *see* **Sotalol HCl**

PMS-Temazepam (Pharmascience), *see* **Temazepam**

PMS-Terazosin (Pharmascience), *see* **Terazosin HCl**

PMS-Terbinafine (Pharmascience), *see* **Terbinafine HCl**

PMS-Timolol (Pharmascience), *see* **Timolol Maleate**

PMS-Trazodone (Pharmascience), *see* **Trazodone HCl**

PMS-Tryptophan (Pharmascience), *see* **L-Tryptophan**

PMS-Valproic Acid (Pharmascience), *see* **Valproic Acid**

PMS-Valproic Acid E.C. (Pharmascience), *see* **Valproic Acid**

Pneumo 23 (Sanofi Pasteur), *see* **Pneumococcal Polysaccharide Vaccine**

Podofilm (Paladin), *see* **Podophyllum Resin**

Polytar AF (Stiefel), *see* **Coal Tar/Menthol/Pyrithione Disulfide/Salicylic Acid, Antiseborrheic Combinations**

Prandase (Bayer), *see* **Acarbose**

PregVit (Duchesnay), *see* **Multivitamins**

Premplus (Wyeth Canada), *see* **Conjugated Estrogens/ Medroxyprogesterone Acetate**

Premplus Cycle (Wyeth Canada), *see* **Conjugated Estrogens/ Medroxyprogesterone Acetate**

Pressyn (Ferring), *see* **Vasopressin**

Pressyn AR (Ferring), *see* **Vasopressin**

Prevex B (TCD), *see* **Betamethasone Valerate**

Prevex Cream (TCD), *see* **Petrolatum**

Prevex HC (TCD), *see* **Hydrocortisone**

Prevex Lotion (TCD), *see* **Petrolatum**

Primene (Baxter), *see* **Amino Acid, Nutritional Therapy, Intravenous**

Priorix (GlaxoSmithKline), *see* **Measles, Mumps and Rubella Virus Vaccine, Live**

Procan SR (ERFA Canada), *see* **Procainamide HCl**

Proctodan-HC (Odan), *see* **Hydrocortisone Acetate/Pramoxine HCl/ Zinc Sulfate Monohydrate, Anorectal Preparations**

Tiamol (TaroPharma), *see* **Fluocinonide**

Tiazac XC (Biovail Pharmaceuticals), *see* **Diltiazem HCl**

Toradol IM (Roche), *see* **Ketorolac Tromethamine**

Trans-Plantar (Westwood-Squibb), *see* **Salicylic Acid**

Transderm-Nitro (Novartis Pharmaceuticals), *see* **Nitroglycerin**

Transderm-V (Novartis Pharmaceuticals), *see* **Scopolamine**

Travasol with Electrolytes (Baxter), *see* **Amino Acids/Dextrose/Electrolytes, Crystalline Amino Acid Infusions with Electrolytes in Dextrose, Nutritional Therapy, Intravenous**

Travasol without Electrolytes (Baxter), *see* **Amino Acids/Dextrose, Crystalline Amino Acid Infusions with Dextrose, Nutritional Therapy, Intravenous**

Triaderm (Taro), *see* **Triamcinolone Acetonide**

Trianal (Trianon), *see* **Aspirin/Butalbital/Caffeine, Analgesic Combinations**

Trianal C1/4 (Trianon), *see* **Aspirin/Butalbital/Caffeine/ Codeine Phosphate, Analgesic Combinations**

Trianal C1/2 (Trianon), *see* **Aspirin/Butalbital/Caffeine/ Codeine Phosphate, Analgesic Combinations**

Triatec-8 (Trianon), *see* **Acetaminophen/Caffeine Citrate/Codeine Phosphate, Analgesic Combinations**

Triatec-8 Strong (Trianon), *see* **Acetaminophen/Caffeine Citrate/Codeine Phosphate, Analgesic Combinations**

Triatec-30 (Trianon), *see* **Acetaminophen/Codeine Phosphate, Analgesic Combinations**

Tri-Cyclen (Janssen-Ortho), *see* **Ethinyl Estradiol/ Norgestimate, Contraceptive Hormones**

Tri-Cyclen LO (Janssen-Ortho), *see* **Ethinyl Estradiol/Norgestimate, Contraceptive Hormones**

Triphasil 21 (Wyeth Canada), *see* **Ethinyl Estradiol/ Levonorgestrel, Triphasic Contraceptive Hormones**

Triphasil 28 (Wyeth Canada), *see* **Ethinyl Estradiol/ Levonorgestrel Triphasic, Contraceptive Hormones**

Triquilar 21 (Berlex Canada), *see* **Ethinyl Estradiol/ Levonorgestrel, Contraceptive Hormones**

Triquilar 28 (Berlex Canada), *see* **Ethinyl Estradiol/ Levonorgestrel, Contraceptive Hormones**

Tri-Vi-Sol with Fluoride (Mead Johnson Nutritionals), *see* **Multivitamins with Fluoride**

Tromboject (Omega), *see* **Sodium Tetradecyl Sulfate**

Tryptan (Valeant), *see* **L-Tryptophan**

Tylenol Aches and Strains (McNeil Consumer Healthcare), *see* **Acetaminophen/ Chlorzoxazone, Skeletal Muscle Relaxant Combinations**

Tylenol Allergy Sinus (Multi-Symptom Relief) (McNeil Consumer Healthcare), *see* **Acetaminophen/ Chlorpheniramine Maleate/ Pseudoephedrine HCl**

Tylenol Allergy Sinus (Nighttime Relief) (McNeil Consumer Healthcare), *see* **Acetaminophen/Pseudo-ephedrine HCl/ Diphenhydramine HCl, Decongestant, Antihistamine, and Analgesic Combinations**

Tylenol Cold Caplets Extra Strength (Daytime) (McNeil Consumer Healthcare), *see* **Acetaminophen/ Dextromethorphan HBr/ Pseudoephedrine HCl**

Tylenol Cold Caplets Extra Strength (Nighttime) (McNeil Consumer Healthcare), *see* **Acetaminophen/ Chlorpheniramine Maleate/ Dextromethorphan HBr/ Pseudoephedrine HCl**

Tylenol Cold Caplets Regular Strength (Daytime) (McNeil Consumer Healthcare), *see* **Acetaminophen/Dextro-methorphan HBr/Pseudo-ephedrine HCl**

Tylenol Cold Caplets Regular Strength (Nighttime) (McNeil Consumer Healthcare), *see* **Acetaminophen/Chlorphen-iramine Maleate/Dextro-methorphan HBr/Pseudo-ephedrine HCl**

Tylenol Cold Suspension Children's (McNeil Consumer Healthcare), *see* **Acetaminophen/Chlorphen-iramine Maleate/ Pseudoephdedrine HCl, Decongestant, Antihistamine and Analgesic**

Tylenol Cold Suspension Children's DM (McNeil Consumer Healthcare), *see* **Acetaminophen/Chlorphen-iramine Maleate/Dextro-methorphan HBr/Pseudo-ephedrine HCl, Antitussive Combinations**

Tylenol Cold Suspension Infant's (McNeil Consumer Healthcare), *see* **Acetaminophen/Chlorphen-iramine Maleate/Pseudo-ephedrine HCl, Decongestant, Antihistamine, and Analgesic Combinations**

Tylenol Cold Tablets Children's Chewable (McNeil Consumer Healthcare), *see* **Acetaminophen/Chlorphen-iramine Maleate/Pseudo-ephedrine HCl, Decongestant, Antihistamine, and Analgesic Combinations**

Tylenol Cold Tablets Children's DM Chewable (McNeil Consumer Healthcare), *see* **Acetaminophen/Chlorphen-iramine Maleate/ Dextromethorphan HBr/Pseudoephedrine HCl, Antitussive Combinations**

Tylenol Cold Tablets Junior Strength DM (McNeil Consumer Healthcare), *see* **Acetaminophen/ Chlorpheniramine Maleate/ Dextromethorphan HBr/ Pseudoephedrine HCl**

Tylenol Cough (McNeil Consumer Healthcare), *see* **Acetaminophen/ Dextromethorphan HBr, Antitussive Combinations**

Tylenol Decongestant (McNeil Consumer Healthcare), *see* **Acetaminophen/ Pseudoephedrine HCl**

Tylenol Flu (Daytime Relief) (McNeil Consumer Healthcare), *see* **Dextromethorphan HBr/ Acetaminophen/Pseudo-ephedrine HCl Antitussive Combinations**

Tylenol Flu (Nighttime Relief) (McNeil Consumer Healthcare), *see* **Acetaminophen/ Pseudoephedrine HCl/ Diphenhydramine HCl, Decongestant, Antihistamine, and Analgesic Combinations**

Tylenol Menstrual (McNeil Consumer Healthcare), *see* **Acetaminophen/Pamabrom/ Pyrilamine Maleate, Nonnarcotic Analgesic Combinations**

Tylenol No. 1 (Janssen-Ortho), *see* **Acetaminophen/ Caffeine/Codeine Phosphate, Narcotic Analgesic Combinations**

Tylenol Sinus Children's (McNeil Consumer Healthcare), *see* **Acetaminophen/Pseudo-ephedrine HCl, Pediatric Decongestant and Analgesic Combinations**

Tylenol Sinus Extra Strength (Daytime Relief) (McNeil Consumer Healthcare), *see* **Acetaminophen/Pseudo-ephedrine HCl, Decongestant and Analgesic Combinations**

Tylenol Sinus Extra Strength (Nighttime Relief) (McNeil Consumer Healthcare), *see* **Acetaminophen/Pseudo-ephedrine HCl/Doxylamine Succinate, Decongestant, Antihistamine, and Analgesic Combinations**

Tylenol Sinus Regular Strength (McNeil Consumer Healthcare), *see* **Acetaminophen/ Pseudoephedrine HCl**

Tylenol Ultra Relief (McNeil Consumer Healthcare), *see* **Acetaminophen/Caffeine, Nonnarcotic Analgesic Combinations**

Typherix (GlaxoSmithKline), *see* **Typhoid Vaccine**

Ultramop (Canderm Pharma), *see* **Methoxsalen**

Ultraquin (Canderm Pharma), *see* **Hydroquinone**

Unisom Extra Strength (Pfizer Consumer Healthcare), *see* **Diphenhydramine HCl**

Unisom Extra Strength Sleepgels (Pfizer Consumer Healthcare), *see* **Diphenhydramine HCl**

Unitron PEG (Schering), *see* **Peginterferon alfa-2b**

Uremol 10 (TCD), *see* **Urea, Topical**

Uremol 20 (TCD), *see* **Urea, Topical**

Uremol HC (TCD), *see* **Hydrocortisone Acetate**

Urisec (Odan), *see* **Urea, Topical**

Uromitexan (Baxter), *see* **Mesna**

URSO DS (Axcan Pharma), *see* **Ursodiol**

Valisone Scalp Lotion (Schering), *see* **Betamethasone Valerate**

Valium Roche Oral (Roche), *see* **Diazepam**

Vaponefrin (Aventis Pharma), *see* **Epinephrine HCl**

Varilrix (GlaxoSmithKline), *see* **Varicella Virus Vaccine**

Varivax III (Merck Frosst), *see* **Varicella Virus Vaccine**

Vaseretic (Merck Frosst), *see* **Enalapril Maleate/ Hydrochlorothiazide, Antihypertensive Combinations**

Vasocon (Novartis Ophthalmics), *see* **Naphazoline HCl**

Vaxigrip (Sanofi Pasteur), *see* **Influenza Virus Vaccine**

Ventodisk (GlaxoSmithKline), *see* **Albuterol**

ISBN-13: 978-1-57439-256-2
ISBN-10: 1-57439-256-5

EAN

9 781574 392562 90000 >